# Stedman's
## MEDICAL
## DICTIONARY

# Stedman's
# MEDICAL
# DICTIONARY

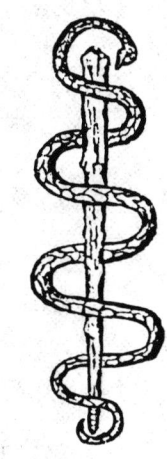

## ILLUSTRATED

*A vocabulary of medicine and
its allied sciences, with pronunciations
and derivations*

### TWENTY-THIRD EDITION

*Completely revised by a staff of 36 editors, covering
46 specialties and subspecialties*

The Williams & Wilkins Company
BALTIMORE

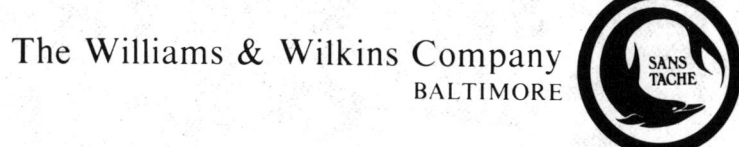

Copyright ©, 1976
The Williams & Wilkins Company
428 E. Preston Street
Baltimore, Md. 21202, U.S.A.

*Made in the United States of America*

Library of Congress Cataloging in Publication Data

Reprinted 1977
Reprinted 1978

Stedman, Thomas Lathrop, 1853–1938.
  Stedman's medical dictionary, illustrated.


  First published in 1911 under title: A practical medical dictionary.
  1. Medicine—Dictionaries. I. Title.
R121.S8 1976     610'.3     75-4993
ISBN 0-683-07924-7


Composed and printed at the
Waverly Press, Inc.
Mt. Royal and Guilford Aves.
Baltimore, Md. 21202, U.S.A

# CONTENTS

# LIST OF COLOR PLATES

*(Between pages 780–781)*

# LIST OF TABLES

*(According to Main Entry Title)*

# EDITORS

sor of Obstetrics and Gynecology, Tulane University School of Medicine, New Orleans, Louisiana

**Immunology and Virology**

THOMAS P. MAGILL, M.D., *Professor Emeritus, Microbiology and Immunology*, College of Medicine, State University of New York, Brooklyn, New York

**Internal Medicine**

DANIEL B. STONE, M.D., *Professor*, Department of Internal Medicine, University of Nebraska Medical Center, Omaha, Nebraska

**Mycology**

HARRY W. MCFADDEN, JR., M.D. (see Clinical Pathology)

**Neurology and Neurosurgery**

A. EARL WALKER, M.D., *Emeritus Professor of Neurological Surgery*, The Johns Hopkins University School of Medicine, Baltimore, Maryland

**Neuropathology**

STANLEY M. ARONSON, M.D., *Dean of Medical Affairs*, Brown University, Providence, Rhode Island

**Nuclear Medicine**

JAMES L. QUINN, III, M.D. (see Radiology)

**Obstetrics**

WOODARD D. BEACHAM, M.D. (see Gynecology)

**Ophthalmology**

JAMES E. LEBENSOHN, M.D., PH.D., *Emeritus Associate Professor of Ophthalmology*, Northwestern University School of Medicine, Chicago, Illinois; *Associate Editor, American Journal of Ophthalmology*

**Otorhinolaryngology**

JOHN P. FRAZER, M.D., *Professor and Chairman*, Division of Otolaryngology, University of Rochester School of Medicine and Dentistry, Rochester, New York

**Parasitology and Tropical Medicine**

DONALD HEYNEMAN, PH.D., *Professor of Parasitology and Assistant Director of the George Williams Hooper Foundation*, University of California, San Francisco, California

**Pathological Anatomy**

COLIN WOOD, M.D., *Professor of Pathology*, University of Maryland School of Medicine, Baltimore, Maryland

**Pharmacology and Toxicology**

DOMINGO M. AVIADO, M.D., *Professor of Phar-*

*macology*, University of Pennsylvania School of Medicine, Philadelphia, Pennsylvania

**Physiology**

RALPH H. KELLOGG, M.D., PH.D., *Professor of Physiology*, University of California School of Medicine, San Francisco, California

**Psychiatry and Psychopharmacology**

RICHARD I. SHADER, M.D., *Associate Professor, Director*, Psychopharmacology Research Laboratory, and *Director of Clinical Psychiatry*, Massachusetts Mental Health Center and Harvard Medical School, Boston, Massachusetts

**Psychology**

JOSEPH D. MATARAZZO, PH.D., *Chairman*, Department of Medical Psychology, University of Oregon Medical School, Portland, Oregon

**Radiology and Nuclear Medicine**

JAMES L. QUINN, III, M.D., *Professor of Radiology*, Northwestern University School of Medicine, and *Director of Nuclear Medicine*, Northwestern Memorial Hospital, Chicago, Illinois

**Respiratory Diseases**

BERNARD J. FREEDMAN, M.B., B.S., F.R.C.P. (London), *Consultant Physician*, King's College Hospital and Medical School, London, England

**Space Medicine**

HOWARD ROBERT UNGER, M.D., *Brigadier General*, United States Air Force, Medical Corps; *Vice Chairman for Aerospace Medicine*, American Board of Preventive Medicine; *Command Surgeon*, United States Air Forces in Europe, Ramstein Air Base, Germany

**Stains and Staining Procedures**

VICTOR M. EMMEL, PH.D., M.D., *Professor of Anatomy*, University of Rochester School of Medicine and Dentistry, Rochester, New York

**Surgery**

DONALD J. FERGUSON, M.D., *Professor of Surgery*, The University of Chicago, Chicago, Illinois

**Toxicology**

DOMINGO M. AVIADO, M.D. (see Pharmacology)

**Tropical Medicine**

DONALD HEYNEMAN, PH.D. (see Parasitology)

**Veterinary Anatomy**

HOWARD E. EVANS, PH.D., *Professor of Veterinary Anatomy*, New York State Veterinary College, Cornell University, Ithaca, New York; *member*, International Committee on Veterinary Anatomical Nomenclature and International Committee on Avian Anatomical Nomenclature of the World Association of Veterinary Anatomists

**Veterinary Medicine**

JOHN B. TASKER, D.V.M., PH.D., *Professor of*

*Clinical Pathology*, New York State Veterinary College, Cornell University, Ithaca, New York

**Virology**

THOMAS P. MAGILL, M.D. (see Immunology)

# ILLUSTRATIONS

**Editor for Art**

JOHN E. PARKER, Medical Illustrator, Washington, D. C.

**Contributing Artists**

RANICE W. CROSBY, *Associate Professor of Art as Applied to Medicine and Director of the Department*, The Johns Hopkins University School of Medicine, Baltimore, Maryland

BIAGIO J. MELLONI, *Chairman*, Department of Medical-Dental Communication, Georgetown University Schools of Medicine and Dentistry, Washington, D. C.

A. HOOKER GOODWIN, *Professor of Medical and Dental Illustration, Director of Curriculum in Medical Art*, and *Head of Illustration Studios*, University of Illinois at the Medical Center, Chicago, Illinois

RAMONA MORGAN, Alexandria, Virginia

# PUBLISHER'S PREFACE TO THE 23RD EDITION

Compilation of a comprehensive vocabulary that will meet the needs of students and professionals in all of the life sciences is indeed a challenge—one that poses innumerable problems.

For example, what are the sources and the criteria for the selection of new entries? Where are the boundaries for definitions that are informative but not encyclopedic in length? In a vocabulary riddled with synonyms, is it possible to search them all out and unequivocally designate preferred nomenclature? When does a medical term become obsolete—and when does an obsolete term lose its value as a dictionary entry?

There are no rule-of-thumb solutions to these problems, but we learned in the 22nd edition that computerized control of the editing process could bring many individual questions into sharp focus, first, by making possible multiple-editor review of subjects in overlapping specialties, and second, by providing an efficient system for correlative cross-checking. In this 23rd edition, we have not only greatly expanded the range of the vocabulary, but we have tried to accomplish a greater degree of integration and coherence, while at the same time allowing the final vocabulary to fulfill the demands made by each of the widely divergent, yet often interrelated, specialties. Some subjects, therefore, have been succinctly treated; others have received necessarily detailed elucidation. Continuous projects have been the quest for elusive synonyms in *Stedman's* massive vocabulary, the correlation of supplementary or related information, and the discrimination between synonyms and "near-synonyms" (as in the case of the "splitters," who classify diseases into small groups according to differences, and the "lumpers," who classify them into large groups because of similarities). Individual editorial preferences were either combined to present definitions broader in scope, or resolved by interchange of ideas. In this way, we have added 15,313 new entries, of which 10,322 are new definitions and 4,991 are new cross-references for synonyms. We have revised 13,094 definitions.

The combined vocabularies for gross anatomy, neuroanatomy, histology, and embryology were subjected to joint editorial review by the editors in these specialties; terminology adheres, as in past editions, to the *Nomina Anatomica* nomenclature, but definitions have been considerably revised and English equivalents (synonyms) for all of the NA terms have been supplied as cross-references. The neuroanatomy terms have been profoundly rewritten to reflect the expanding literature pertaining to the anatomy and physiology of the nervous system; because of the complexity of this subject, many of these definitions are encyclopedic in scope. The accuracy of all chemistry has been confirmed, and in the combined specialties of pharmacology and biochemistry more than a thousand new entries cover drugs, enzymes, pharmacognosy, and toxicology. The vocabularies of the bacteria, viruses, and other parasites have been expanded, and particular attention has been given to the literature of immunology and microbial genetics which during recent years has presented not only many new terms but also applications of old terms that have required relaxation of original restrictive definitions. The several subspecialties of medicine and pathology have received attention from almost all editors, with greater correlation of synonyms, near-synonyms, and the inevitable eponyms; a major concentration of updating is to be found in the dermatological entries. The psychology, psychiatry, and respiratory physiology vocabularies also have been extensively rewritten.

*Stedman's* classical etymology section in the preliminary pages has of course been retained, and in the section, "How to Use This Dictionary," a revised key to simplified phonetic spellings explains related changes made throughout the vocabulary. The gratifying reader response to our experimental "Subentry Index" convinced us of the value of this unique alphabetical master list of cross-references, which is repeated in this edition as Appendix 1.

## ACKNOWLEDGMENTS

Many reference sources have been consulted in our efforts to supply a vocabulary that reflects terminological preferences and specific criteria established by authoritative nomenclature groups. We wish especially to acknowledge the following:

For anatomy, our source and frame of reference is *Nomina Anatomica* (Paris, 1955), as revised by the Seventh and Eighth International Congresses of Anatomists in 1960 and 1965, respectively. For veterinary anatomy, we have consulted *Nomina Anatomica Veterinaria*, Ed. 2, as approved by the General Assembly of the World Association of Veterinary Anatomists in 1971. *Stedman* editorial policy governing anatomical terms is explained on page xvi.

Pharmacological and pharmaceutical sources include *United States Pharmacopeia*, *National Formulary*, *British Pharmacopoeia*, and the *USP Dictionary of Drug Names*, *USAN-10* (with supplements), published for the United States Adopted Names Council. For enzymes, we have devoted special attention to the recommendations of the Enzyme Commission of the International Union of Biochemistry Committee on Nomenclature. *Stedman* treatment of these specialties is described on page xvi.

An important reference source for bacteriology was *Bergey's Manual of Determinative Bacteriology*, Ed. 8, edited by R. E. Buchanan and N. E. Gibbons, published in 1974 by The Williams & Wilkins Company, Baltimore.

*Systematized Nomenclature of Pathology* (*SNOP*), edited by the Committee on Nomenclature and Classification of Disease, College of American Pathologists, was consulted for the vocabulary of pathology and for designations of nomenclatural preferences. *Birth Defects*, *Atlas and Compendium*, edited by Daniel Bergsma and published in 1973 by The Williams & Wilkins Company for the National Foundation—March of Dimes, was also a helpful source.

The *Glossary of Prosthodontic Terms*, Ed. 3, edited by the Nomenclature Commitee of the Academy of Denture Prosthetics, published in 1968 by the *Journal of Prosthetic Dentistry*, C. V. Mosby Company, St. Louis, has supplied many entries, as has the *Glossary of Oral Surgery Terms*, published in 1971 by the American Society of Oral Surgeons' Committee on Hospital Oral Surgery Service, Chicago.

In obstetrics, some of our definitions have been revised to incorporate criteria established by the Committee on Terminology of the American College of Obstetricians and Gynecologists, as set forth in their publication, *Obstetric-Gynecologic Terminology*, published in 1972 by F. A. Davis Company, Philadelphia. Certain recommendations of the Committee on Nomenclature of the International Federation of Gynecology and Obstetrics are also reflected in our definitions.

Through the courtesy of the Congress of Neurological Surgeons and its Committee on the Nomenclature of Neurosurgical Operations, we have included many definitions of operations upon the scalp, skull, cranial contents, spine, and spinal cord.

Special thanks are due to all of the authors, editors, and publishers of the many other texts, journals, and reference sources whose works have been individually cited and duly acknowledged where used throughout the dictionary, and to all of the interested *Stedman* users who write to us.

The monumental editorial accomplishments in this edition of *Stedman's* are entirely attributable to the 36 editors, covering a range of 46 specialties, whose acumen and enthusiasm extended far beyond the limits of their individual concerns and whose spirit of cooperation produced, from a challenge, a hallmark of dictionary compilation.

THE WILLIAMS & WILKINS COMPANY

Anne G. Cutler, *Stedman Managing Editor*

William R. Hensyl, *Stedman Co-managing Editor*

# HOW TO USE THIS DICTIONARY

This section presents the standard explanatory notes pertaining to methods of alphabetization, pronunciation, abbreviation, and derivation; it defines the editorial policies governing the selection and arrangement of special categories of terms such as anatomy, pharmacology, chemistry and biochemistry, eponyms, and synonyms; and it describes in detail the index-type arrangement of main entries with their subentries, and the *Stedman* procedure for cross-referencing, with special emphasis on the unique alphabetical index of subentries (Appendix 1) that is in fact a "master list" of cross-references. A thorough understanding of all of these principles will result not only in time saved through efficient search, but also in increased breadth and depth of information derived.

## PRONUNCIATION

A simplified phonetic spelling, showing pronunciation and syllabification, is given in parentheses immediately following the boldface main entry title and preceding the bracketed derivation. In most words, syllabification determines the vowel sound; *i.e.*, the sound is long if the vowel occurs at the end of a syllable, and short if it is followed by a consonant. Where this general rule is applicable, the diacritical mark is omitted; for exceptions, appropriate diacritical marks (as listed in the "Key to Simplified Phonetic Spellings") are given, and these have been restricted for the most part to only two— the macron (ˉ) for long sounds and the breve (˘) for short sounds. To avoid the introduction of additional, esoteric, diacritical marks, the breve is frequently used arbitrarily to indicate half-long or slurred enunciations. Accent or stress marks *follow* the stressed syllables, and the single accent mark is used for both primary and secondary stress. Where a phonetic spelling is not supplied, the boldface title is accented to show the stressed syllable. Phonetic spellings are not given for subentry titles, and in most of these (except Latin nomenclature) the accent or stress marks are also omitted; however, the significant words comprising a subentry title are listed *per se* in their proper alphabetical location in the vocabulary as main entries with pronunciation and derivation.

### Key to Simplified Phonetic Spellings

**Vowels:**

| | |
|---|---|
| a | at the end of a syllable, long, as in day (phonetically spelled da); before a consonant (except r), short, as in mat. |
| ă | as in mat; usage at the end of a syllable ususally indicates a half-long or slurred enunciation, as in abortion (ă-bor'shun), hep'ă-ti'tis. |
| ā | as in mate (māt). |
| ah | as in father (fah'ther), media (me'dĭ-ah). |
| ar | as in far, artery. |
| ăr | as in care (kăr), fair (făr). |
| ā | as in dairy; because of position of stress mark, is usually avoided (da'rĭ). |
| aw | as in fall (fawl), cause (kawz). |
| e | at the end of a syllable, long, as in bee (phonetically spelled be); before a consonant (except r), short, as in met. |
| ĕ | as in met; usage at the end of a syllable usually indicates a half-long enunciation, as in meridian (mĕ-rid'ĭ-an). |
| ē | as in meet (mēt). |
| er | as in term. |
| ĕr | as in merry (mĕr'ĭ). |
| ēr | as in deer (dēr); because of position of stress mark, sometimes avoided, as in bacteria (bak-tēr'ĭ-ah, or bak-te'rĭ-ah). |
| ë | as the French eu or German oe, nearly as e in her. |
| i | at the end of a syllable, long, as in pie (phonetically spelled pi); before a consonant (except r), short, as in pit. |
| ĭ | as in pit; arbitrarily used to represent the short sound of y, as in pathology (pă-thol'o-jĭ). |
| ī | as in pine (pīn). |
| ir | as in firm. |
| ĭr | as in mirror (mĭr'or). |
| īr | as in fire (fīr). |
| o | at the end of a syllable, long, as in no; before a consonant, short, as in not. |
| ŏ | as in occult (ŏ-kult'). |
| ō | as in note (nōt). |
| oo | as in food. |
| ŏŏ | as in foot, wood. |
| or | as in for. |
| ōr | as in fore, four (fōr). |
| ow | as in cow. |
| oy | as in boy; as the oi in void (voyd), mastoid (mas'toyd). |
| u | at the end of a syllable, as in u'nit; before a consonant, as in bud. |
| ŭ | as in bud. |
| ū | as in dispute (dis-pūt). |
| ü | as the French u or the German ü or ur. |
| ur | as in fur. |
| ūr | as in pūre. |
| y | vowel sound is phonetically represented by long or short i (hi'per-, hip-no'sis, pă-thol'o-jĭ). |

**Consonants:**

| | |
|---|---|
| c | hard, as in cat, represented by k; soft, represented by s. |
| ch | (or kh) a guttural k, as the ch in German bach or Scottish loch. |
| dh | as th in the, this. |
| g | hard, as in get (the soft g is represented |

phonetically by a j).

| | |
|---|---|
| ṅ | as the French nasal n in bon (this sound is also represented by hn). |
| s | hard, as in side, hiss (the soft s is represented by a z). |
| th | as th in think. |
| y | as y in yam, yesterday (but the sound yu is represented by a long u (u'nit), pure (pūr)). |
| zh | as z in azure (azh'ūr). |

**Unusual pronunciations of some initial consonants.** In some words the initial *sound* gives no clue to the initial *letter*, and this may occasion difficulty. Some examples are listed in the table following:

| Initial letters | Pronounced | Examples |
|---|---|---|
| phth- | th-, fth- | phthalein |
| pn- | n- | pneumonia |
| ps- | s- | psoas, psychology |
| pt- | t- | pterygoid, ptosis |
| x- | z- | xanthic, xenon, xiphoid |

## GUIDE TO DERIVATIONS

The section on Medical Etymology, pages xix–xxiv, presents an informative discussion of the origins of our medical vocabulary; a thorough explanation of word formation and syntax, including a series of tables showing the formation of plural, adjectival, and combining forms; a list of Greek and Latin prepositional and adverbial prefixes; and the Root Word List, where specific derivations are discussed in greater detail than is possible in the vocabulary section of the dictionary.

In the vocabulary, etymology is given in square brackets [  ] immediately following the word and its pronunciation. The bracketed material includes (1) the abbreviation indicating the language from which the word is derived, *e.g.*, G. (Greek), L. (Latin), etc. (for other such abbreviations, see "Abbreviations Used in This Dictionary"); (2) in italics, the word from which the term is derived; and (3) in roman type, the English translation. In addition, in many instances references to the Root Word List (pages xxv–xlvii) in the etymological section are given in capital letters, thus: **imperception** [L. *in-*, not, + *per-cipio*, pp. *-ceptus*, to perceive. CAP-].

When a vocabulary entry has the same or approximately the same spelling and/or meaning as that of the language from which it is derived, the information that would be repetitious or that is understood (or given in the definition) is omitted from the bracketed derivation, as in the following examples: **corpus** [L. body]; **linea** [L.].

An effort has been made to reduce the derivation to a simple Greek or Latin word which is easy to remember and which usually occurs in other derivatives. When a verb is hyphenated it indicates that the second part of the word exists as a simple verb with the same or approximately the same meaning, qualified by the addition of the adjectival or adverbial prefix. But if the simple verb

undergoes a change when forming part of a compound it is shown in the derivation, for example, *com-primo*, to press together, fr. *premo*, to press.

In the Root Word List and in vocabulary derivations, the first person singular present of Greek and Latin verbs is used in most instances, rather than the infinitive. Where the English meaning is given in the infinitive it refers to the verb and all its parts.

Combining forms used in the prefix position are listed as separate vocabulary entries with full definitions and with bracketed derivations, often including a reference to the more detailed information in the Root Word List in the etymology section of the dictionary. For the longer lists of compound words containing identical prefixed combining forms, that combining form is given without repeated translation for each, because this information is easily found in a nearby boldface "prefix" entry. For combining forms used within compound words or in the suffix position, derivations are supplied each time used.

## ABBREVIATIONS USED IN THIS DICTIONARY

| | | |
|---|---|---|
| adj | . . . . . . . . . . . . . . . . . . . | adjective. |
| adv | . . . . . . . . . . . . . . . . . . . | adverb. |
| Am. Ind. | . . . . . . . . . . . . . . . | American Indian. |
| Ar | . . . . . . . . . . . . . . . . . . . | Arabic. |
| A.S. | . . . . . . . . . . . . . . . . . | Anglo-Saxon. |
| BP | . . . . . . . . . . . . . . . . . . | British Pharmacopoeia. |
| *cf* | . . . . . . . . . . . . . . . . . . . | L. *confer*, compare. |
| D | . . . . . . . . . . . . . . . . . . . | Dutch. |
| dial | . . . . . . . . . . . . . . . . . | dialect. |
| dim | . . . . . . . . . . . . . . . . . | diminutive. |
| EC | . . . . . . . . . . . . . . . . . . | Enzyme Commission. |
| Eng | . . . . . . . . . . . . . . . . . | English. |
| *e.g.* | . . . . . . . . . . . . . . . . | L. *exempli gratia*, for example. |
| Fr | . . . . . . . . . . . . . . . . . . . | French. |
| fr | . . . . . . . . . . . . . . . . . . . | from. |
| G | . . . . . . . . . . . . . . . . . . . | Greek. |
| Gael | . . . . . . . . . . . . . . . . | Gaelic. |
| gen | . . . . . . . . . . . . . . . . . | genitive. |
| Ger | . . . . . . . . . . . . . . . . . | German. |
| *i.e.* | . . . . . . . . . . . . . . . . | L. *id est*, that is. |
| Ind | . . . . . . . . . . . . . . . . . | Indian. |
| It | . . . . . . . . . . . . . . . . . . . | Italian. |
| Jap | . . . . . . . . . . . . . . . . . | Japanese. |
| L | . . . . . . . . . . . . . . . . . . . | Latin. |
| LL | . . . . . . . . . . . . . . . . . . | Late Latin. |
| M.E | . . . . . . . . . . . . . . . . . | Middle English. |
| Mediev. L | . . . . . . . . . . . . | Medieval Latin |
| Mod. L | . . . . . . . . . . . . . | Modern Latin. |
| NA | . . . . . . . . . . . . . . . . . | Nomina Anatomica. |
| NAV | . . . . . . . . . . . . . . . | Nomina Anatomica Veterinaria. |
| NF | . . . . . . . . . . . . . . . . . | National Formulary. |
| neut. or ntr. | . . . . . . . . . . | neuter |
| obs | . . . . . . . . . . . . . . . . . | obsolete. |
| O.E. | . . . . . . . . . . . . . . . . | Old English. |
| O.Fr | . . . . . . . . . . . . . . . . | Old French. |
| O.H.G. | . . . . . . . . . . . . . . | Old High German. |

Pers ...................Persian.
Pg ....................Portuguese.
p .....................participle.
pl ....................plural
pp ...................perfect participle passive.
priv ..................privative, negative.
*q.v.* ..................*L. quod vide*, which see.
Sansk .................Sanskrit.
sing ..................singular.
Sp ...................Spanish.
thr ...................through.
USAN ...............United States Adopted
                         Names.
USP .................United States Pharmacopeia.
W. Af ...............West African.
* ...................in biographical data, denotes
                         year of birth when year of
                         death is not given.
† ...................in biographical data, denotes
                         year of death when year
                         of birth is not given.

## SPELLING

**Important departures from older spellings.** Some changes in spelling, especially many recommended by the *Nomina Anatomica*, are reflected in this edition of *Stedman's*. For example, annulus is now spelled anulus, chorioid is spelled choroid, calyx has been superseded by calix, mammilla is now mamilla (hence mamillary, for mammillary), the combining forms thyreo- and -physeal now appear as thyro- and -physial, and diphthongs have been omitted from anatomical terms in favor of simpler spellings (though retained for taxonomic classifications of organisms). Cross-referencing has been supplied for these spelling changes.

**Variations in prefixed combining forms.** Combining forms frequently have alternative spellings; for example, hemo- and hemato-, dermo- and dermato-, cine- and kine-, cata- and kata-, phac- and phak-, and sympatho-, sympathico-, sympatheto-. The boldface entries that supply the derivations for these combining forms (see p. xiii, "Guide to Derivations") also serve as guides to their alternative spelling. In addition, strategic cross-referencing for many hundreds of individual terms of this type has been provided.

**Some British and American spellings compared.** Because of differences between British and American spellings, British users may have difficulty in tracking down certain words. When a word can be spelled in two ways—the British way and the American way—look for it in its American form.

The main sources of confusion are *ae* and *oe*, both of which are generally preserved in British use but almost always contracted to *e* in American. Less important differences include the American *-or* for *-our*, *f* for *ph*, and the terminals *-ter* for *-tre*, or *-er* for *-re*, and *-ize* for *-ise*.

British users will experience little or no difficulty when the American equivalent in question occurs toward the end of a word (*e.g.*, diar*rhea* for diar*rhoea*); but when the difference occurs at or near the beginning of a word, the actual entry may be elusive since it is far removed from the alphabetical site at which it is sought. For example, the British reader may be searching for oedema under the letter "o" whereas the American entry will be under "e" (edema).

Most of these occurrences are handled in *Stedman's* by cross-references, for example: "**oe-.** For words so beginning and not found here, see e-." Since such cross-references occur only for prefixes, readers should watch for the same variations within compound words, as these too may change the alphabetical locations of some words.

The following lists are not intended to be complete; rather, they give several examples of British-American equivalents that will serve as guides.

|                  | British       | American       |
|------------------|---------------|----------------|
| **ae for e**     | aegophony     | egophony       |
|                  | aetiology     | etiology       |
|                  | anaemia       | anemia         |
|                  | anaesthetic   | anesthetic     |
|                  | caecum        | cecum          |
|                  | defaecation   | defecation     |
|                  | faeces        | feces          |
|                  | gynaecology   | gynecology     |
|                  | haematuria    | hematuria      |
|                  | haemoglobin   | hemoglobin     |
|                  | haemorrhage   | hemorrhage     |
|                  | paediatric    | pediatric      |
|                  | taenia        | tenia          |
| **ei for i**     | cheiromegaly  | chiromegaly*   |
|                  | cheilitis     | chilitis*      |
|                  | cleidocranial | clidocranial*  |
| **oe for e**     | coeliac       | celiac         |
|                  | foetus        | fetus          |
|                  | oedema        | edema          |
|                  | oesophagus    | esophagus      |
|                  | oestrus       | estrus         |
|                  | -rrhoea       | -rrhea         |
| **-re for -er**  | fibre         | fiber          |
| **-tre for -ter**| goitre        | goiter         |
|                  | litre         | liter          |
|                  | metre         | meter†         |
| **ph for f**     | sulphonamide  | sulfonamide    |
|                  | sulphur       | sulfur         |
| **c for k**      | leucocyte     | leukocyte‡     |
| **miscellaneous**| artefact      | artifact       |
|                  | liquorice     | licorice       |

\* Many American authors apparently prefer the British spellings for some of these terms.

† In linear measures, British usage prefers *-tre* (metre, centimetre); in apparatus for making measurements, both use *-ter* (manometer, micrometer).

‡ British usage prefers leuc- to leuk- except in leukaemia.

## ORGANIZATION OF THE VOCABULARY

**Main entry-subentry arrangement.** In general *Stedman's* adheres to the traditional grouping of multiple-word terms as subentries under governing *noun* main entries. For example, typhoid fever is defined as a subentry under the main entry, fever; crocodile tears syndrome is under syndrome; zona orbicularis, under zona. In a specialty dictionary (as opposed to a language dictionary) the advantages to be gained from such categorization of information are obvious, but this index-like arrangement can create confusion for the reader who either forgets the reiterated injunction, "Look under the noun," or experiences difficulty, and sometimes failure, in locating a given multiple-word term because it has been positioned under some other, synonymous, noun main entry.

**Alphabetical index of subentries.** Appendix 1 is a list of the subentry titles from the vocabulary arranged alphabetically according to the first word of the subentry. It serves as a master cross-referencing system for locating both specific definitions and related information, obviating the need for such cross-references within the vocabulary (see also the introduction to Appendix 1).

In the vocabulary, some deviations from the standard arrangement of noun main entry with adjectival subentries occur for terms that present individual editorial problems; for each of these an appropriate "locating" cross-reference is supplied within the vocabulary. Other deviations occur for categories of terms that have received special handling (*e.g.*, chemical terms), as explained in the following sections.

**Alphabetization of main entries.** For main entries, the letter-for-letter system of alphabetization is used, rather than the word-for-word system. In other words, when a main entry consists of a hyphenated word or of more than one word (as in the case of many chemical terms) such main entry is alphabetized as though all one word. Abbreviations and contractions, too, are alphabetized as written, letter for letter.

With few exceptions, main entries are printed in the singular form. If use of a plural term is mandatory, and if the plural spelling removes it from the alphabetical location it would occupy if singular, a cross-reference has been inserted from the singular to the defined plural form.

**Alphabetization and abbreviation of subentries.** In subentry titles (as well as throughout definitions of both main entries and subentries), the main entry word is represented by its initial letter only. Subentries may be either singular or plural; the plural form is denoted by the addition of an apostrophe-s to the abbreviation, sometimes by the spelled out irregular English plural, or, in the case of Latin nomenclature, by the spelled out Latin plural form. In alphabetizing subentries, the abbreviation for the main entry word, or the pluralized form of that abbreviation, or the spelled out Latin plural, is always completely disregarded. Also disregarded in alphabetizing subentries are prepositions, conjunctions, and arti-

cles, and the apostrophe-s denoting the possessive in eponymic terms. Examples:

**canaliculus**
    auricular c.
    canaliculi dentales
    c. innominatus
    intercellular c.
**law**
    Graham's l.
    l. of gravitation
    l. of the heart
    Mendel's l.'s
    l. of multiple proportion

**Alphabetization and location of compound words.** Compound words that are written closed up (as one word) or that are hyphenated are generally alphabetized as main entries rather than as subentries under the portion of the term that would ordinarily represent a noun main entry. For example, aftercontraction will be found as a main entry in the A's, rather than as a subentry under contraction; counterirritant as a main entry in the C's, rather than under irritant; self-hypnosis is in the S's; end-plate, in the E's. There are many exceptions because spelling usages vary; cheese fly, for example, is usually written as two words, and so will be found as a subentry under fly, whereas horsefly (one word) will be found in the H's as a main entry. Other exceptions have occurred as a result of arbitrary editorial decisions aimed at achieving better correlation of related information. For example, all viruses, including those written as one word (arbovirus, picornavirus, herpesvirus) are listed as subentries under virus. Although extensive cross-referencing has been provided for individual exceptions to the general rule for handling compound terms, it is well to be alert to the possibility that such words may be listed in either of two ways.

**Cross-referencing of synonyms and related terms.** A concerted effort has been made to substitute cross-references for duplicated definitions under synonymous terms. Use of a cross-reference does not denote priority of, or preference for, the defined term over the cross-referenced synonym; however, for the sake of editorial consistency we have routinely endeavored to follow predetermined plans in some classes of terms. These are explained in the section, "Special Categories of Terms."

A cross-reference from a term to its defined synonym consists merely of the name of that synonym, without the word "see." When such a cross-reference leads to a multiple-word term (that is, to a subentry), we have italicized that portion of the term that represents the main entry under which the defined subentry is located, thus:

**disease**
    **Bannister's d.,** angioneurotic *edema.*
**band**
    **iliotibial b.,** *tractus* iliotibialis.

Cross-references to related information rather than to synonyms are identified by the words "see" or "see also." For these cross-references leading to multiple-word subentries, we have similarly italicized the word representing the noun main entry.

Italics have been omitted from cross-references leading from one subentry to another under the same main entry, from cross-references leading to a one-word term (that is, to a main entry *per se*), and from cross-references leading to chemical terms.

The synonyms for a defined term are usually listed at the beginning of the definition, but when the number of synonyms is excessive, or when this procedure would for other reasons be confusing for the reader, the synonyms are listed at the end of the definition, where they are set apart from the definition by such phrases as "also called," "also known as," etc.

## SPECIAL CATEGORIES OF TERMS

**Anatomical terms.** *Nomina Anatomica* (Paris, 1955), as revised by the Seventh and Eighth International Congresses of Anatomists in 1960 and 1965, respectively, is the controlling system for anatomical nomenclature. The terms in the NA list appear in their proper alphabetical order in the *Stedman* vocabulary section and are there defined and identified by the letters NA in brackets [NA]. Alternate names for the same structures, including English equivalents of the NA Latin terms, are listed in the vocabulary as cross-references to the defined NA terms. Anatomical structures that have no NA name are defined under their most commonly used name. Veterinary anatomy terms listed in *Nomina Anatomica Veterinaria* have been selectively added to the vocabulary, and some are identified by the bracketed [NAV].

**Chemical, biochemical, and pharmacological terms.** Multiple-word drug and chemical terms are alphabetized exactly as spelled; this represents a departure from the standard procedure of listing them as subentries under noun main entries. Thus, nicotinic acid is listed in the N's rather than as a subentry under acid, glucose dehydrogenase is in the G's, methyl donors in the M's, vanadium group in the V's. Such multiple-word terms are treated as subentries under the first word of the term when use of the abbreviated first word would cause no confusion. However, compound chemical terms that are written closed up or that are hyphenated are treated as main entries rather than subentries. Examples:

**methyl**
    active m.
    m. alcohol
    m. chloride
    m. donors
    m. red
**methylcellulose**
**methyltransferase**

Greek-letter, numerical, configurational, and most italicized prefixes such as *p-* (*para-*), *o-* (*ortho-*), *m-* (*meta-*), *cis-*, *trans-*, *tert-*, etc., are disregarded in alphabetizing (except for official pharmaceutical spellings in which the prefixes are spelled out and closed up, without italics).

Such components occurring within compound chemical terms are similarly disregarded in alphabetization.

The definitions of drugs, biochemically important compounds (metabolites, hormones), pesticides, etc., accompany the *trivial* (common, short) or *generic* (nonproprietary) names, and these definitions usually include the *systematic* (formal, definitive) names, which are the only fully correct descriptions other than structural formulas. (For further definition of *systematic*, *semisystematic*, *semitrivial*, *trivial*, *generic*, *proprietary*, and *nonproprietary* as applied to the names of chemicals, see these adjectives in the vocabulary.)

In some instances, the definition of a trivial name consists solely of its systematic one, this being considered adequate information (that is, self-defining). Systematic names, generally, are not included as vocabulary entries, though some commonly used ones have been retained; those that are listed usually serve as cross-references to the defined trivial or generic name. The various terms comprising each systematic name are, however, listed and defined. For example, the definition of alanine includes its systematic name, aminopropionic acid, but the latter is not listed as a vocabulary entry, being easily reconstructed from "amino" and "propionic acid," both of which are defined. The definition of cortisone includes its systematic name, 17,21-dihydroxy-4-pregnene-3,11,20-trione, the parts of which are defined by words, formula, or numbered structure, so that the full structure of cortisone may be written.

Special attention has been devoted to the Recommendations of the Enzyme Commission of the International Union of Biochemistry Committee on Nomenclature, and many *Stedman* entries show the EC numbers (rather than the EC Systematic Names) where such exist.

Abbreviations, contractions, or symbols that have earned acceptance by recognized authority or common practice have been made a part of the *Stedman* vocabulary, and are alphabetized letter-for-letter as boldface entries. The terms for which they stand are not always defined, though, if a definition seems unnecessary, as stated above.

Proprietary or trade names for drugs are not listed alphabetically as boldface entries; many commonly used trade names are, however, included as a part of the definition of generic or nonproprietary names. We have tried to identify trade names by the use of small capital letters; our failure to do so in any instance is not to be regarded as indication that the term is not a trade name.

Pharmacological references are identified in parentheses following the boldface vocabulary entry. These include the *United States Pharmacopeia* (USP), *National Formulary* (NF), *British Pharmacopoeia* (BP), and the *USP Dictionary of Drug Names* (USAN), published for the United States Adopted Names Council. The definitions as given in *Stedman's* serve primarily as guides to the information currently available. They do not represent the opinions of the *Stedman* Editorial Committee, nor are the publishers of any of these references responsible for inaccuracies that may occur in our definitions. Our failure to cite an official reference source does not necessarily indicate that the preparation is not official.

**Eponyms.** The names of all persons credited with eponymic nomenclature are listed as main entries in their proper alphabetical location in the vocabulary, usually with additional identifying biographical data. Each biographical entry provides cross-references to all of the eponymic terms attributed to that person.

Whenever feasible, definitions are given under noneponymic rather than under eponymic nomenclature, therefore many eponymic subentries are cross-references to the defined noneponymic synonyms. For example, the biographical entry for Caesar P. M. Boeck contains cross-references to Boeck's disease, Boeck's sarcoid, and Besnier-Boeck-Schaumann syndrome or disease, but each of these subentries is, in turn, a cross-reference to sarcoidosis, where the full definition (including the list of eponyms and other synonyms) is given.

Proper names have been investigated in many sources and contributed by many *Stedman* editors, with additional review by the editor for history and biography. We have followed the spelling most frequently used, and alphabetization is determined precisely by that spelling. Examples to be kept in mind are spellings such as Fränkel *versus* Fraenkel, Löffler *versus* Loeffler, etc. For names beginning with prefixes such as von, Van, de, and others, and which may be used eponymically either with or without the prefix, we have similarly tried to base alphabetical location, for both biographical entries and eponymic subentries, on the most common usage. In many cases we have inserted cross-references, but a double check for such names (with and without the prefix) will be rewarding. When prefixes are considered in determining alphabetization, the name is alphabetized exactly as spelled, letter-for-letter, as though one word. This procedure has also been followed for the prefixes Mac and Mc; if you are not sure which spelling is used, check both.

With the exception of a selected group of Nobel laureates and a few classically historical names, biographical entries are included only for those persons to whom eponymic terms defined in *Stedman's* have been attributed.

**Binomial nomenclature (genera and species).** Definitions for the genera and species of bacteria, protozoan and insect parasites, plants, etc., accompany the proper Latin binominal terms rather than the common or vernacular names; the latter, however, are listed as vocabulary entries, with cross-references to the proper names. Spellings follow official, rather than simplified or Americanized, usages; thus we have *Taenia*, not *Tenia; Haemophilus*, not *Hemophilus; Leucocytozoon*, not *Leukocytozoon*. (See also "Spelling," p. xiv.)

# MEDICAL ETYMOLOGY

As with all modern learning, the vocabularies of the life sciences keep pace with the growth of knowledge. New discoveries, new concepts, new theories—all must have, it seems, new words or new groupings of words to describe and define them in speech and print.

This dictionary—any medical dictionary—any *general* dictionary—contains hundreds of words which are, by philological standards, mis-formed, mis-pronounced, mis-spelled, mis-used; but, by the standards of those who have long used those words, they are familiar, acceptable, and are firmly and irremovably embedded in the language. A dictionary, if it is to be a useful guide to a living language, must spell, pronounce, and define the words as they are used—not, wistfully, as they should have been. *Stedman's* is a working dictionary, a record of a living language.

A dictionary can suggest or set standards—it cannot enforce them. It can point out the right way to go; it cannot bar the writer or speaker from the path which he is accustomed to using, wrong though it may be.

*Stedman's*, however, recognizes its obligation to guide those who would speak more carefully, write more precisely, even coin new words more accurately. To these objectives we dedicate this section on medical etymology.

———————◆———————

Study of the origins of our medical vocabulary can be rewarding fun. Rewarding, because it makes the difficult medical vernacular much easier to learn and retain and at the same time is a hobby that affords much intellectual pleasure and satisfaction. Fun, because many of our commonly used words have intriguing, romantic, or even humorous origins.

The overwhelming majority of our medical terms stem from Greek; another sizable group is derived from Latin. Indeed, it is impossible to appreciate much of the English language itself, let alone the medical vocabulary, without some knowledge of these "dead" languages which are, unfortunately, slipping more and more out of the curricula in both the new and old worlds. Most of the following paragraphs will therefore be devoted to the consideration of terms having a classical origin.

Meanwhile, a few of our words have other sources. From the Arabic we derive a number of terms, especially for our pharmacopeia, such as *alcohol, alkali, camphor, naphtha, senna, syrup, tartar;* others are formed by prefixing the Arabic definite article (*al, el*) to a Greek stem, *e.g., al-*chemy, *el-*ixir.

Most of our simple anatomical terms (*arm, back, bladder, blood, chin, eye, finger, foot, gall, gum, gut, hair, hand, head, heart, hip, knee, liver, lung, mouth,* *neck, thumb, tongue*) are Anglo-Saxon, as are certain other short words of medical flavor, *e.g., ache, fat, hives, sick, swell.* A few other simple monosyllables are of Scandinavian descent: *ill, leg, scab, skin.*

From the French we have adopted a number of medical terms unchanged or slightly modified, *e.g., ballottement, bougie, bruit, chancre, cretin, curette, fontanelle, fourchette, grippe, malaise, pipette, plaque, poison, rale, souffle, tampon, tourniquet, trocar, venom, cul de sac, grand mal, petit mal, mal de mer, tic douloureux.* Others are Anglicized or Americanized forms of French words, *e.g., goiter, gout, malady, malinger, jaundice, ointment, physician, powder.* Still others come from the Greek via a French intermediary: *surgeon, plaster, migraine, quinsy, palsy, frenzy.*

For a few words we are indebted to Italian, *e.g., belladonna, influenza, malaria;* and to Spanish, especially for the names of certain medicaments, *e.g., cascara, guaiacum.* Another small handful of words comes from the Dutch (*cough, litmus, splint, sprue*), German (*anlage, Fahrenheit, magenstrasse*), Persian (*bezoar, borax, talc*), Chinese (*kaolin*), Bengalese (*chaulmoogra*), and Tupian (*curare, ipecacuanha*).

When it comes to a study of the host of words derived from the classical languages, it is interesting to note the number of current words that were used in the same form, though not necessarily with an identical meaning, by the earliest medical writers; much of our present vocabulary has been going strong for 2000 years and more. Hippocrates (460–370 B.C.), for example, used such words as *acromion, adenoma, amblyopia, anthrax, apophysis, borborygmus, bregma, bronchus, cachexia, carcinoma, cholera, chorion, diapedesis, ecchymosis, emphysema, erythema, exanthema, herpes, hippus, ileus, kyphosis, lichen, lochia, lordosis, meninges, nephritis, noma, nystagmus, olecranon, paresis, peritoneum, phagedena, phthisis, polypus, psilosis, symphysis, thorax, typhus, urachus, ureter, urethra.* Galen (131–201 A.D.) had in his medical vocabulary such words as *anthrax, aponeurosis, ascites, chalazion, chemosis, coccyx, diaphoresis, diastole, epididymis, epiphora, gomphosis, hippus, hypophysis, hypospadias, iris, kerion, lysis, mydriasis, pemphigus, peritoneum, phimosis, pityriasis, pterygium, pylorus, sarcoma, skeleton, strabismus, syndrome, systole, tarsus, tenia, thymus, tinea, trichiasis.* Aristotle (384–322 B.C.) used *alopecia, canthus, exophthalmos, glaucoma, leukoma, meconium, nystagmus, pancreas, and podagra.* Others of our present-day terms that first found employment in ancient Greek medical writings include *eczema, kerion, trachoma* (Dioscorides, *fl.* 100 A.D.); *asphyxia, diabetes* (Aretaeus, *fl.* 70 A.D.); *ozena, philtrum, tarsus, zygoma*

(Pollux, *fl.* 180 A.D.); *parenchyma* (Erasistratus, *fl.* 300 B.C.); *amnion* (Empedocles, 504–443 B.C.).

Everyday terms that appeared in ancient medical Latin include *abdomen, anus, cancer, delirium, fistula, hernia, maxilla, omentum, patella, pus, radius, scabies, tibia, valgus, and varsus* (Celsus *fl.* 30 A.D.); and *acetabulum, tinea,* and *verruca* (Pliny, 23–79 A.D.).

Next, it is diverting to group them into miscellaneous categories. There are, for instance, a number of ancient and honorable names, chiefly of important organs, that have come down to us unchanged through the ages; *hepar, gaster, cerebrum,* and *cor* are still what they always were, though each of them by common usage has long since taken second place to *liver, stomach, brain,* and *heart.* On the other hand a number of old anatomical terms have been translated to a nearby part; thus in early medical Greek the original *pleura* was a rib, *bronchus* was the trachea, and *ureter* the urethra. In early Latin, (*h*)*umerus* was the shoulder, *ulna* the elbow, *maxilla* the lower jaw, *femur* the thigh, *anus* the buttocks, and *vulva* the uterus.

Other medical words have deviated from their original meanings: *nausea* (originally *nausia*) must have been reserved for seasickness (G. *naus,* ship) and *hysteria* was clearly a feminine monopoly (G. *hysterikos,* of the womb). *Asphyxia,* which now means suffocation, properly meant a stopping of the pulse (G. *a-* privative + *sphygmos,* pulse).

Another group of words is based on ancient misconceptions. For example, it was formerly thought that the blood vessels carried air; hence *arteries* were named "air-carriers" (G. *aēr* + *tereo,* carry). The *pituitary* was so called because it was believed that the gland was responsible for the secretion of nasal mucus (L. *pituita,* mucus). Again, the state of *melancholia* is no longer believed to be caused by the presence of black bile (G. *melas,* black, + *cholē,* bile). The humoralists are also responsible for the romantic ideas behind such words as *choleric, phlegmatic, sanguine;* and for the "boiling out" of the humors as seen in *eczema* (G. *ekzeō,* boil out).

Then there is a group of terms that started life as adjectives but which now, through usage, have become substantives in their own right. In Greek, *trachea* is the feminine of *trachus,* rough, and it was originally part of the full description, trachea arteria, rough airpipe; then arteria was dropped and trachea alone remained. Similarly all the ancient words ending in -*itis* (*e.g.,* nephritis, arthritis, rhachitis, hepatitis) were originally adjectives indicating whereabouts; thus *hepatitis phleps,* the "in-the-liver vein," was Aristotle's description of the inferior vena cava and affords conclusive evidence that the suffix -*itis* originally contained no inkling of inflammation. Used with *nosos,* disease, such adjectives indicated the site of the lesion—*nephritis nosos,* in-the-kidney disease, and so on. *Nosos* then became taken for granted and the adjectives, *nephritis,* etc., were allowed to stand on their own feet. *Skeleton* was originally *skeleton soma,* a dried-up body.

Among Latin adjectives that have been preserved as anatomical nouns, we have *cecum* (originally *intestinum*

*caecum,* blind intestine), *jejunum* (originally *intestinum jejunum,* hungry intestine—because it was usually found empty at autopsy), and *rectum* (originally *intestinum rectum,* straight intestine). *Decidua* is, of course, the *membrana decidua* (falling-off membrane) and *conjunctiva* is the *tunica conjunctiva* (connecting coat).

By far the largest group of words comprises those that were formed from nonmedical origins, such as *meconium,* poppy-juice; *anthrax,* a hot coal; *pancreas,* all-flesh; *pylorus,* gatekeeper; *scaphoid,* boatlike; *trochlear* (trochlea), pulley, From this largest category it adds interest to separate subgroups that have a common etymological denominator. For example, certain anatomical terms indicate resemblance to letters of the Greek alphabet: *deltoid,* delta-like (Δ); *lambdoid,* lambda-like (Λ); *sigmoid,* sigma-like (s); *hyoid,* upsilon-like (υ); *chiasma,* from *chiazo,* to mark with the letter chi (X).

Then our semantic debt to the grapevine is considerable. *Uva* is Latin for the grape itself and gives us *uvea* and *uvula. Botrys* and *staphyle* are two Greek words meaning a bunch of grapes, and *racemus* is their Latin equivalent; hence our words *staphylococcus, botyroid* and *racemose*—all describing objects that give the appearance of clustering grapes or berries. Finally the vine itself gives us our *pampiniform* plexus (*pampinus,* tendril). Other words with a fruity flavor include *piriform* (pear-shaped), *sycosis* (G. *sykon,* a fig), *morula* (L. *morus,* a mulberry), *nucleus,* a little nut (L. *nux,* nut), *karyo-* (G. *karyon,* nut), *glans* (L. acorn) and *balanitis* (G. *balanos,* acorn), *myrtiformes* (shaped-like-myrtle-berries), *pomum Adami* (Adam's apple), *streptococcus* and other *cocci* (G. *kokkos,* berry).

Vegetables or other crops give us *pisiform* (pea-shaped), *hordeolum* (L. *hordeum,* barley), *pityriasis* (G. *pityra,* bran), *sesamoid* (G. *sēsamon,* sesame seed), *aphakia* (G. *phakos,* lentil), *lens* (L. lentil), *fabella* (a little bean).

Many living creatures lend their descriptive names: *cancer* (L. crab), *carcinoma* (G. *karkinos,* crab), *hippocampus* (sea-horse), *cauda equina* (horse's tail), *lumbrical* (L. *lumbricus,* worm), *vermis* (L. worm), *cochlea* (G. snail), *chemosis* (G. *chēmē,* cockle-shell), *lupus* (L. wolf), *muscle* (L. *musculus,* little mouse), *buphthalmos* (G. ox-eyed), *lagophthalmos* (hare-eyed), *ichthyosis* (G. *ichthys,* fish), *phrynoderma* (G. toadskin), *estrus* (G. *oistros,* gadfly), *formication* (L. *formica,* ant), *coccyx* (G. cuckoo), *coronoid* (G. *korōnē,* crow), *coracoid* (G. *korax,* crow), *chenopodium* (G. *chēnē,* goose), *rostrum* (L. beak). Wings from both Latin (*ala, axilla, pinna*) and Greek (*pterion, pterygium, pterygoid*) are well represented; other parts of avian anatomy are *crista galli* (cox-comb) and *calcar avis* (the spur on a bird's leg). The horse's accouterment is represented by *stapes* (stirrup) and *sella* (saddle).

Weapons and armor are freely borrowed: thus *coryne-* (club), *xiphoid, ensiform* (sword), *vagina* (sheath), *toxic* (bow), *sagittal* (arrow), *galea* (helmet), *thyroid, umbo, umbilicus* (shield), and *thorax* (breastplate) are all featured. Musical instruments are not hard to find: *salpinx* (G. trumpet), *tympanum* (L. drum), *calamus* (L. reed-pipe), *fistula* and *syrinx* (L. and G. pipe or tube, respectively); but the only musician seems to be the trumpeter (*buccinator*).

Household and other utensils make an important contribution. *Pyelos*, a pan or basin, gives us *pyelitis; amnion* and *pellis* (platy*pelloid*) are further Greek words for bowls, while *patella* is a little pan. *Platysma* is a flat plate and *arytenoid* is from *arytaina* (G.), ladle. *Ascites* comes from *askos*, a leather wineskin, and *acetabulum* is a receptacle for vinegar. The *ampulla* was a bottle or pitcher with a narrow neck and relatively bulbous body. The *amphora* was an earthenware storage vessel with two handles from which it got its name (*amphi-*, on both sides, *phoreus*, carrier); we in turn derive *amphoric* breathing from the sound of blowing across the mouth of a hollow vessel. *Calyx* and *cotyle* (*cotyloid*, *cotyledon*) were Grecian drinking vessels, while sieves have given us *cribriform* and *ethmoid*. Finally *infundibulum* is a funnel and *haustrum* a machine for drawing water.

Then one can collect coinages of relatively recent date such as *achalasia* (G. *a-*, privative + *chalasis*, relaxing), *dysdiadochokinesis* (G. *dys-*, prefix expressing difficulty, + *diadoche*, a succession, + *kinesis*, movement) and *hypertension* (G. *hyper*, over, + L. *tensio*, stretch). Such words as the last, composed of both Greek and Latin roots, are often frowned on by the purists and pedants; and it is perhaps true that supertension would be more desirable etymologically than hypertension. However, the medical vocabulary is teeming with such hybrids and the illegitimate admixture of bloods does nothing to lessen the vigor of our jargon. At any rate they are here to stay, they are aften convenient and expressive, and we might as well accept the established ones even if we make an effort to keep our new coinages thoroughbred. Among the common hybrids are *idioventricular* (G.-L.), *sinu-atrial* (L.-G.), *kernicterus* (Ger.-G.), *vagotonia* (L.-G.), *fibroma* (L.-G.), *chancroid* (Fr.-G.), *argentaffinoma* (L.-L.-G.), *autoclave* (G.-L.), *jejunostomy* (L.-G.), *claustrophobia* (L.-G.), *lymphagogue* (L.-G.), and many others (see also "Formation of Compound Words," p. xxii).

Several of our common words remain of doubtful origin. For example, does the *basilic* vein come from the Arabic, *basilik*, inner, or from the Greek, *basilikos*, royal? Is it the inner, medial vein or the royal, hence prominent, vein of the forearm? Then does its antecubital companion, the *cephalic* vein, come the Arabic, *alkifal*, outer, or from the Greek, *kephalē*, head? The Oxford English Dictionary suggests that this vein influences the head and is therefore so named—a conclusion that is hard to justify with current anatomical or physiological knowledge. One school of thought likes to derive *syphilis* from the name of the swineherd in Fracastoro's poem who was supposed to have been the first afflicted with the disease; but others would prefer to derive it from the Greek adjective, *sipholos*, crippled.

Despite a small number of such gray areas, the majority of our medical words have clear-cut, meaningful origins whose study pays handsome dividends in both practical usefulness and academic satisfaction. A by-product of such a study is improvement in our style of writing; for two of the pillars of good style are accurate spelling and the use of words in their proper sense, and a knowledge of word derivation is the best possible insurance against lapses in these two spheres.

# WORD FORMATION AND SYNTAX

The reader whose eye alights for the first time upon such words as hemangioendothelioblastoma, or acrocephalosyndactylism, recoils with something of a shock. But if he knows the individual words that make up these compounds, what appears to be an unintelligible aggregation of letters stands out with stereoscopic clearness as hem-angio-endothelio-blast-oma or acro-cephalo-syn-dactyl-ism.

Not only is a word more easily remembered, spelled, and pronounced when its derivation is understood, but in many cases it contains its own definition, *e.g.*, *poly-chrom-emia*, much-color-blood, an increase in the amount of coloring matter in the blood.

As a preliminary to understanding the formation of compounds from Greek or Latin words, it might be well to review the following terms.

**Root.** A root is that element common to all of a group having kindred meaning that remains after the formative additions (prefixes, suffixes, inflections, etc.) have been removed. For example, the root GEN, GN, is found in Greek, Latin, English, and other Indo-European languages with the sense of "beget"; Greek *gen-os*, birth; Latin *gen-us*, birth; *prae-gn-ans*, before birth, pregnant; English *kin*.

**Root word.** The term "root word" is used loosely in this article to designate a Greek or Latin word that contains the root from which a medical word is derived. A root word, therefore, contains a definite idea which can usually be represented by a single word and which persists through its various derivatives, although it may undergo considerable modification. For example, the Greek verb *kineō* (set in motion, move) is the source of the following Greek and English derivatives: *kinēsis*, movement, hence kinesi-ology, kinesi-meter; *kinēma*, movement, hence cinemat-ics; *kinētos*, movable, kineto-cyte; *kinētikos*, of or for putting in motion, kinet-ic. *Kineō*, thus, contains the idea "movement"; to acquire a working knowledge of a Greek and Latin vocabulary such root words or key words should be learned and remembered.

In the *Stedman* vocabulary bracketed derivations and in the Root Word List, the first person singular present is used for Latin and Greek verbs rather than the true infinitive form of the verb, because the root word is usually more readily recognizable in the former; it refers to the verb and all its parts, although in translation the English infinitive is given.

**Stem.** The stem is the part of an inflected word (see "Inflections," below) that remains after the inflectional additions have been removed. Thus, *vox* (a voice), genitive singular *voc-is* (of a voice), plural *voc-es* (voices). *Voc-* is the stem from which derivatives are formed, *e.g.,* voc-al.

**Inflections.** Inflection is the change in the form of a word to express different grammatical relationships, *i.e.,* the declension of nouns, the conjugation of verbs, and the comparison of adjectives. For example, the English adding of *s* to a noun to form a plural, or *-ed* to a verb to form the past tense, is an inflection. So is the change of the Latin word *os* (a bone) to the genitive singular *ossis* (of a bone).

It is essential that a few of the inflections should be learned. They are as follows:

(a) The genitive singular of some of the Greek and Latin nouns. This is necessary when the nominative case, the form by which the word is known, does not contain the complete stem from which the derivatives are formed, *e.g., sōma* (a body), genitive *sōmat-os;* from this *somat-* is used as a base upon which words are built: somat-o-plasm, psycho-somat-ic. In other nouns, such as *capill-us* (the hair), genitive *capill-i,* the stem or base from which words are built is contained equally in the nominative and genitive cases.

(b) The past participle passive (usually designated by the abbreviation pp.) of Latin verbs, and the future of Greek verbs, when they contain the stem from which derivatives are formed. Examples are L. *solvo* (set free), pp. *solut-us* (having been set free), hence the English derivative, solut-ion; the Greek *klaō* (break), future *klasō,* hence *klasis* (a breaking, a fracture), and the English derivatives arthro-clasis, ana-clasis, etc.

(c) The genitive and the nominative plural of Greek and Latin nouns when these inflections are used in medical terminology, *e.g., caput* (a head), genitive *capitis,* plural *capita.* Many Latin words, and Greek occasionally, are so used. Greek words are often taken into the medical vocabulary and given Latin endings. Words ending in *-os* are given the Latin ending *-us* (*ophthalmos, opthalmus*); those ending in *-on* are given the Latin ending *-um* (*kranion, cranium*).

(d) The changes in the endings of Latin adjectives to denote gender and number. Latin nouns that have become part of the medical vocabulary are occasionally modified by adjectives. These agree with the noun grammatically. The form usually met with is the adjectival ending *-us,* feminine *-a,* neuter *-um* (plurals *-i, -ae, -a);* for example, *deciduus, -a, -um* (falling down); *membrana decidua* (the altered mucous membrane of the pregnant uterus).

Sample plural and adjectival forms are given in the tables on pages xlix–lii.

**Formation of compound words.** A compound word is one that contains more than one stem. A simple word contains one stem. Many compound words have been taken directly from the Greek unchanged, as *ankyloblepharon,* adhesion of the eyelids, but most compounds are formed by taking two or more Greek or Latin words and connecting them by the same technique as the Greeks used. The first part, containing its stem only, is usually joined to the second part by a connecting vowel, especially when the second part begins with a consonant. The vowel is usually *o,* sometimes *i,* and, rarely, *a.* When the first part of a compound ends in a vowel, and the second part begins with one, the vowel-ending of the first part usually disappears, for example, chol-uria, from G. *cholē* + *ouron,* + *-ia.* One exception is that of the compounds of *salpingo-,* as in salpingo-oophorectomy. The forms used for the purpose of creating compound words are called combining forms. Their formation is further illustrated in the tables on pages xlix–lii, and hundreds are listed, with pronunciations, derivations, and definitions, in the *Stedman* vocabulary.

A correctly formed compound word ideally should be composed of words of the same language, whether Latin or Greek. When it contains elements of different languages, it is called a hybrid (see also p. xxi). Chemical compound words are sometimes formed very irregularly. They are often hybrid and greatly abbreviated, *e.g.,* amyl from *am*(ylon) + (h)*yl*(ē), and *formaldehyde* from *form-*(ic acid) + *al*(cohol) + *dehyd* (rogenatum).

**Prefixes.** When a preposition or adverb, prefixed to a Greek or Latin word, ends in a consonant, and the main word begins with a consonant, the final letter of the prefix often undergoes certain changes. Thus final *n* becomes *l* before a following *l,* *e.g.,* sy*l*logism [G. *syn* + *logos*], i*l*lusion [L. *in* + *ludo*]; it becomes *m* before a labial (b, m, p, ph), *e.g.,* emphasis [G. *en* + *phasis*], impel [L. *in* + *pello*]; before *s* it is usually dropped, *e.g.,* systole [G. *syn* + *stellō*].

In Latin, the final consonants of the prepositions *ad* and *ob* are often changed to the same letter as that which follows, *e.g.,* accept [*ad* + *capio*], afferent [*ad* + *fero*], assume [*ad* + *sumo*], occiput [*ob* + *caput*], oppress [*ob* + *premo,* pp. *pressus*]. This change is called assimilation.

In Greek the final vowel of a preposition is dropped before a following vowel, *e.g.,* epencephalon [*epi* + *enkephalos* ], ephemeral [*epi* + *hēmera*], and *cathode* [*kathodos,* from *kata* + *hodos*]. This change is called elision. It does not usually apply, however, to *peri* and *anti.* See also list of Greek and Latin preposition and adverb prefixes, p. xlviii.

## GREEK ALPHABET

A special effort should be made to learn the Greek alphabet. A Greek word seems to have a personality which it loses when transliterated, and it loses at the same time some of the power to impress itself upon the memory.

## THE GREEK ALPHABET

| Letters Capital | Letters Small | Name of Letters | Sound Value |
|---|---|---|---|
| A | α | alpha | a |
| B | β | bēta | b |
| Γ | γ | gamma | g (hard) |
| Δ | δ | delta | d |
| E | ε | epsĭlon | ĕ |
| Z | ζ | zēta | z |
| H | η | ēta | ē |
| Θ | θ | thēta | th |
| I | ι | ĭōta | i |
| K | κ | kappa | k |
| Λ | λ | lambda | l |
| M | μ | mu | m |
| N | ν | nu | n |
| Ξ | ξ | xi | x (= ks) |
| O | ο | ŏmĭkron | ŏ |
| Π | π | pi | p |
| P | ρ | rho | r |
| Σ | σ, s | sigma | s |
| T | τ | tau | t |
| Υ | υ | upsilon | ü |
| Φ | φ | phi | ph |
| X | χ | chi | kh |
| Ψ | ψ | psi | ps |
| Ω | ω | omega | ō |

Of the two signs for sigma, s is used at the end of a word, σ everywhere else.

The letter ρ (rho) at the beginning of a word is almost always represented in Eng. by rh, but has the sound of r; in combinations ρ is doubled after a short vowel and represented by rrh, e.g., dia-rrhea, cata-rrh.

The letter γ (gamma) has the sound of a nasal n (ng) before κ, γ, χ, ξ, for example ἄγγελος, angel, messenger.

In Eng. χ is pronounced like k, ψ like ps.

**Diphthongs.** Pronunciations of Greek diphthongs and their English equivalents are given in the table below:

| Greek diphthong | Greek sound | English equivalents |
|---|---|---|
| αι | ai as in aisle | ae, e |
| ει | ei as in rein | ei, i, e |
| οι | oi as in coin | oe, i, e |
| υι | we | ui |
| αυ | ou as in loud | au |
| ευ | eh-oo | eu |
| ου | ou as in group | u |

In all other combinations each vowel is pronounced separately, as ἀήρ (ah-ēr) air.

**Breathings.** All vowels at the beginning of a word have either the "smooth breathing" (') or the "rough breathing" ('). The former is not pronounced; the latter corresponds to the English h, e.g., ἄρως (erōs, love); ἥρος (heros, hero). Initial ρ or υ always has the rough breathing.

**Accents.** There are the three accents, acute ('), grave (`), and circumflex (^) and every word in Greek has an accent on it. In the pronunciation of Greek, however, we generally follow the Latin accentuation. According to this, words of two syllables are always accented on the first syllable. In words of three or more syllables, the last syllable but one is accented if it is long; if it is short, the syllable before that is accented. A syllable is long if it contains a diphthong or long vowel, or any vowel if followed by two consonants or by x or z.

**Transliteration.** υ is usually represented in English by y; γ before κ, γ, χ, ξ by n; κ by c or k; ρ at the beginning of a word by rh. For diphthongs, see above.

When Greek words are shown in English letters instead of Greek, transliteration is more exact. Diphthongs are changed letter for letter; κ is always k; long ē and ō (eta and omega) are distinguished from short e and o (epsilon and omicron) by the long mark (macron) over the former. Other changes are as above.

## LATIN ALPHABET

The Latin alphabet is the same as the English except that it has no w or j.

**Pronunciation.** The vowels a, e, i, o, u, y, are pronounced as follows: ā as in father, ă as in idea; ē as in they, ĕ as in net; ī as in machine, ĭ as in sit, ō as in tone, ŏ as in obey; ū as in rule, ŭ as in pull; y as in French u.

The diphthongs are pronounced thus: au like ou in house; ae like ai in aisle; oe like oi in spoil; ui like we; eu as eh-oo.

The consonants are pronounced as in English, except for the following: c always as k; g always hard as in get; s as in sin, never as in ease; v like w.

There are other equally acceptable methods of pronouncing Latin, which vary from country to country and from school to school. The "original" or "only correct" pronunciation is not definitely known.

## DIRECTIONS FOR USE OF ROOT WORD LIST

In the following list of the more important Greek and Latin words, from which medical terminology is derived, their meanings are given much more fully than is possible in the dictionary proper. There the root word sometimes recurs frequently in its various derivatives and, in cases where the word has several apparently disconnected meanings, the one most applicable to its derivative has, of necessity, to be given. Although some of the examples given in the Root Word List may no longer be listed in the vocabulary because they are obsolete, they have been retained here because of their illustrative and historic value.

The fundamental meaning is given first (and this is the most important to learn) and its other meanings are given in their chronological order of development. This usually shows the connection between the different meanings.

Where practical, the words from the same root are grouped under a heading which is printed in **CAPITAL** letters. These derivatives may be either Greek or Latin. The heading usually represents the smallest formation of letters common to the derivatives under it and will distinguish such derivatives from other words that are nearly similar in form. It does not correspond to what is known etymologically as a root although it sometimes coincides. In many cases this short combination of letters contains a definite meaning, which is peculiar to itself, and does not occur elsewhere in the medical vocabulary without this meaning, *e.g.*, ANDR-, *man;* CHLOR-, *greenness*; CHROM-, *color*; GAST-, *belly*.

Inflections are given where they are necessary to show the stem from which English words are derived, or when the inflected Greek or Latin word is used in medical terminology. The genitive singular and nominative plural of nouns are then given. Abbreviated forms are used as in dictionaries; for example, *acuo*, pp. *-utus* means *acuo*, perfect participle passive *acutus; helmins, -inthos* means *helmins*, genitive *helminthos; jejunus, -a, -um*, means *jejunus*, masculine, *jejuna*, feminine, *jejunum*, neuter.

All Greek words in the subheadings are followed by the Greek characters, and are so distinguished from the Latin subheadings. Greek or Latin words mentioned under a subheading are of the same language as that subheading unless otherwise indicated by G. or L.

The letters G. or L. in brackets immediately following a derivative indicate that it is a Greek or Latin word taken into the medical vocabulary in its exact form.

Short definitions of medical terms are given where they are necessary to explain the derivation.

The symbol >, the usual sign for *hence* in etymology, separates the classical words from the derivatives: if the Greek or Latin word is used in modern medicine, the classical usage of the word is on the left of this sign, the modern on the right. The words and meanings to the left of it belong to the classical period. If the word is a medieval or modern form it is so stated. (Abbreviations, Mediev. L. and Mod. L.)

Compound derivatives are separated by hyphens to show the part derived from the root word in the subheading. Wherever part of a word with a hyphen is given, the rest is to be supplied from the *last complete derivative preceding it.*

When a Greek or Latin word is used in medicine in its original *form* and *meaning*, the word and meaning are not repeated but are represented by the abbreviation *id.* (*idem*, the same) placed immediately after the symbol >. The initial letter followed by a period is sometimes used to designate the root word in the subheading instead of repeating it in full.

Semicolons are used to separate (1) the different meanings of a word and (2) the different derivatives of the same root word. Commas are used to separate (1) the different shades of the same meaning and (2) words from their definitions.

Special uses of medical words by the ancient writers and physicians are indicated by the following abbreviations: H. (Hippocrates), Arist. (Aristotle), Cels. (Celsus), Aret. (Aretaeus), Gal. (Galenus).

When the derivation given in the dictionary does not require to be enlarged upon, and the root word is not needed for comparison with kindred or similar Greek or Latin words, it is omitted from the following list.

# ROOT WORD LIST

## AC-

AC, a root occurring in many G. and L. words, with sense of *sharpness.*

AKĒ (ἀκή), *a point.* AKAKIA (ἀκακία), *a thorny Egyptian tree.* > Acacia, *a genus of plants of the order Leguminosae;* acacia, *gum arabic.*

AKANTHA (ἄκανθα), *a thorn, prickle; the backbone* of a fish; *one of the spinous processes of the vertebrae.* Gal. > *the spinal column; the spinous process of a vertebra;* acantho-lysis, *a skin disease* characterized by atrophy of the prickle cell layer of the epidermis; -oma, *a cutaneous cancer;* acanth-esthesia; etc. trag-acanth, *a subgenus of leguminous plants.*

AKŌKĒ (ἀκωκή), *a point, edge.* > Acocanthera, *a genus of African plants,* from some species of which the natives obtained an *arrow* poison; antherin.

AKMĒ (ἀκμή), *a point, edge; the culminating point of anything; the crisis* of a disease. H. > acme, *a crisis;* acne (a probable corruption of acme); men-acme [měn, *month*]; an-acmesis, *arrest of development,* [fr. akmēnos, *full-grown.*]; par-acme [G.] *a point at which the prime or crisis is past.*

AKROS (ἄκρος), *highest, topmost;* ntr. as noun AKRON (ἄκρον), *the highest* or *farthest point; peak, extremity.* > In composition usually refers to the extremities of the body; acroataxia; -cephalic; -cyanosis; etc. acrophobia, *fear of heights.* acrot-ic [fr. akrotēs *an extremity*]; acroter-ic [fr. akrōtērion, *any topmost part.*].

ACEO, *to be sour.* ACESCO, pres. p. -ENS -ENTIS, *to turn sour.* > acesc-ent; -ence.

ACETUM, -I, pl. -A, *sour wine; vinegar.* > acet-ous; -ic; -ate, *a salt of acetic acid;* -one; aceton-emia [acetone + G. haima, *blood.*]; -uria; etc. acet-yl, *a univalent radical;* acetylation; -choline; etc.

ACIDUS, -A, -UM, *sour, tart.* > acid; acidum; acid-emia; acidi-fy; -ty; acidopenia; etc.

ACOR, a sour taste, sourness. > *gastric acidity.*

ACER, ACRIS, *sharp, pointed;* of the senses, *keen.* > acrid; -ine; acri-flavina; -monia [L.]

ACERBUS, -A, -UM, *harsh, bitter.* > acerb-ity [acerbitas]; ex-acerb-ation. [fr. exacerbo, pp. -atus, *exasperate.*]

ACERVUS, -I, *a multitude of objects rising in a heap; a multitude.* ACERVULUS, -I, dim. *a little heap.* > brain-sand; acervul-ine; -oma.

ACIES, -EI, *a sharp edge* or *point; keenness.* > margin, edge. ACUO, pp. -UTUS, *to sharpen.* > acu-ity; acu-te; acuminate [fr. acumino, pp. -atus, *to sharpen*].

ACUS, *a needle.* > acu-filopressure; -puncture; -torsion; etc. ACICULA, -AE, dim. *a small pin* for the head-dress. > *a slender needle-like structure.*

## ACOU-

AKOUŌ (ἀκούω), *to hear.* > acou-meter; -lalion; -esthesia; acoustics. bary-ecoia [barys, *heavy*]; oxy-acoia [oxys, *sharp*]. AKOUSMA, -ATOS (ἄκουσμα), *something heard, a rumor.* > *an auditory hallucination;* acousmat-agnosia, *mind-deafness.*

## ACT-, AG-

AGŌ (ἄγω), *to lead, drive, carry.* AGŌGOS (ἀγωγός), *leading.* > -agogue, a suffix with sense of *leading away, drawing forth.* hydr.-agogue; lith-; galact-; etc.

AGŌN (ἀγών), *a gathering, assembly, contest.* > agon-al; -ist; -y [agōnia, *struggle, agony*]; ant-agon-ist.

AGRA (ἄγρα), *a hunting, catching.* > As suffix, *a seizure;* cardi-agra; pod- [G. *a trap for the feet, gout*].

AGO, pp. ACTUS, pres. p. AGENS, *to lead, drive; do, perform.* > act; -or [L.]; re-act.

ACTIO, -ONIS, *a doing, action.* > action; re-; in-.

ACTIVUS, -A, -UM, *active.* > re-active; activ-ate; -ator; etc.

AGITO, pp. -ATUS, *put in motion, drive; excite.* > agito-graphia; -phasia [G. phasis, *speech*].

AGMEN, -INIS, *an army being led; a multitude.* > *an aggregation;* agmin-ate; -ated, *clustered.*

COAGULUM, -I, pl. -A [fr. cogo, contracted fr. co-ago, *to drive together*], *a means of curdling, a coagulator; rennet:* hence COAGULO, pp. -ATUS, *to cause to curdle,* > coagulum, *a clot, a curd* (Mod. L.); coagul-ate; -ase, *a clotting enzyme;* -in.

PURGO, pp. -ATUS, *to cleanse, purify* [fr. purus + ago]. > purg-e; -ation; -ative.

## ACTIN-

AKTIS, -TINOS (ἀκτίς) *a ray, beam.* > actin-ic; -ism; actino-chemistry; -genesis; -gram. Actino-myces, *Ray-fungus,* so called because of its radiating club-shaped roots; -mycosis; -scopy, *examination by x-rays.*

## ADEN-

ADĒN, -ENOS (ἀδήν), *a gland.* H. > adenoid; adeno-cele; etc.

## ADIP-

ADEPS, -IPIS, *the soft fat* of animals. > *lard;* in compounds *fat;* adipo-se, *relating to fat;* -cele; -genous; etc.

## AER-

AĒR, AEROS (ἀήρ), *air.* > aer-endocardia; aero-bion; -pathy, *condition caused by pronounced change in atmospheric pressure.*

AER, AERIS, air. > aeri-al: -ferous; -form.

## AE-, see E-

## AG-, see ACT-

## ALB-

ALBUS, *white.* > alba, *the white substance* of the brain; albo-ferrin; -lene; etc. albino [Pg.].

ALBEDO, -INIS, *whiteness.* > *light reflected from a surface.*

ALBIDUS, -A, -UM, *white.* > *whitish;* albid-uria.

ALBUGO, -INIS, *a white spot* in the eye. > id.; albugin-eous; tunica albugin-ea (Mod. L.); -itis; albugineo-tomy.

ALBUMEN, -INIS, *the white of an egg.* > id.; albumin, *a protein substance;* -ate, *derived albumin;* albumini-meter; albumino-rrhea; etc.

ALBURNUM, -I, *the white layer* between bark and wood of a tree. > id.

## ALG-

ALGOS (ἄλγος), *pain.* > algo-genesis; -lagnia; etc. -algia, a suffix: neuralgia; my-: gastr-; etc.

ALGĒSIS (ἄλγησις) *sense of pain.* > algesi-a; -meter.

## ALI-, ALL-

ALLOS (ἄλλος), *other, another.* > allo-centric; -esthesia; -some; etc. parallax [G.]; allergy; allasso-therapy [allassō, *to alter*].

ALLĒLŌN (ἀλλήλων), gen. pl. with no nom. case in use,

*of one another, mutually, reciprocally.* > allelo-catalytic; -morph; etc.

ALIUS, *other, another;* hence ALIENUS, *belonging to another, strange;* in medic. refers to *strangeness* of the mind, *insane.* > alien; -ist; -ation. ab-alien-ated, *crazy, deranged.*

ALTER, *the other* (of two); ALTERNO, pp. -ATUS, *do by turns.* > alternation.

ALTERO, pp. -ATUS, (Mediev. L.) *to make other, alter.* > alter; -ant; -ation; -ative.

**AMBLY-**

AMBLYS (ἀμβλύς), *blunt, dull;* (metaph.) *dim, weak.* > ambly-opia; -chromatic, *staining faintly;* -acousia; -geustia.

**AMEB-, AMOEB-**

AMOIBĒ (ἀμοιβή), *payment in exchange; change, alteration.* > amoeba or ameba, *a protozoan of non-constant or changing form;* ameb-iasis; -ic; -uria; amebo-cyte; etc.

**AMNI-**

AMNION (ἀμνίον), *a bowl* in which the blood of victims was caught; *the membrane round the fetus.* fr. AMNOS (ἄμνος) *a lamb.* > *the innermost of the fetal membranes;* amnio-rrhea; -rrhexis; ARCH-, -otome, -oma.

**AMYL-,** see MYL-

**ANC-, ANG-, ANK-**

ANKOS (ἄγκος), *a bend* or *hollow.* ANKŌN (ἀγκών) *the bend of the arm; the elbow.* > ancon-eus; -itis; -ad, *toward the elbow;* -agra; etc.

ANKYLOS (ἀγκύλος) *curved, hooked.* > Ancylo-stoma, *a genus of Nematoda, the old-world hook-worm;* ancylostomiasis. ANKYLĒ (ἀγκύλη) 1. *the bend in the arm or wrist;* 2. *a joint bent or stiffened by disease,* or (in compounds) *an abnormal adhesion of parts.* > ankylo-stoma, *lockjaw;* -sis; -chilia, *adhesion of the lips;* -proctia, *a stricture of the anus;* -blepharon, (Cels.).

ANKYRA (ἄγκυρα) *anchor, hook.* > ancyr-oid; etc.

ANGULUS, -I, *angle; corner.* > angle; angular.

**ANDR-**

ANĒR, ANDROS (ἀνήρ), *a man.* > andr-ase; -ecium [oikos, *a house*], *the stamens taken collectively* (bot.); andro-gen; -gyne; etc.

**ANGI-**

ANGEION (ἀγγεῖον), *a vessel for holding liquid or dry substances; a vessel of the body.* > In compounds, usually *a blood vessel;* angi-ectasia; angio-logy; -neurosis; etc. spor-angium, *a sac containing spores.*

**ANISO-,** see ISO-

**ANK-,** see ANC-

**ANTH-**

ANTHOS (ἄνθος), *a flower.* ANTHĒROS (ἀνθηρός) *blooming.* > anther, *pollen bearing part of a stamen;* -idium; -ozoid. acoc-anthera; heli-anth-in; etc.

ANTHEŌ (ἀνθέω), *to bloom;* hence ANTHĒSIS (ἄνθησις), *a flowering;* ANTHĒMA (ἄνθημα), usually in compounds, = anthos. > ex-anthesis [G. *a flowering; eruption*]; en-anthema; ex-anthem, *a skin eruption;* syn-anthem.

**ANTHR-**

ANTHRAX, -AKOS (ἄνθραξ), *charcoal, coal; a precious stone of dark red color, a carbuncle; a malignant pustule or carbuncle.* H. and Gal. > *a carbuncle; an infectious disease of sheep and cattle;* anthrac-emia; -ine, *a hydrocarbon obtained from coal tar;* -osis, *a pulmonary coal-dust disease;* etc.

**ANTR-**

ANTRUM, -I, *a cave;* later *a cavity of the body.* fr. ANTRON (ἄντρον) *a cave.* > *any nearly closed cavity,* esp. one with bony walls; antr-al; -ectomy; antro-cele; -scope; etc.

**AORT-**

AORTĒ (ἀορτή), orig. (in pl.) *the lower extremities of the windpipe.* H.; later, *the artery which proceeds from the left ventricle of the heart.* Arist. > aorta; aort-al; -algia; aortolith; etc.

**AP-,** see HAP-

**AQU-**

AQUA, -AE, *water.* > aqu-eous; aqua-puncture, aqui-ferous; aquo-sity.

**ARACH-**

ARACHNĒ (ἀράχνη), *a spider; a spider's web.* > arachno-

dactyly, *a condition in which the fingers or toes are abnormally long;* -idea, *the middle fibrous membrane covering the brain;* -iditis.

**ARCH-**

ARCHĒ (ἀρχή), *beginning, origin.* > archebiosis, *spontaneous generation;* -genesis.

ARCHAIOS (ἀρχαῖος), *from the beginning, ancient.* > archaeo-cyte; etc.

ARCHI- or ARCHE- (ἀρχι- or ἀρχε-), *inseparable prefix, first, chief.* > archi-plasm; -sperm; etc.

ARCHOS (ἀρχός), *chief, leader; rectum, the anus.* H. > archo-ptosia, *prolapse of the rectum;* -rrhagia; etc.

**ARG-**

ARGOS (ἀργός), *shining, bright.* ARGYROS (ἄργυρος) *silver.* > argyr-ia, *skin discoloration due to administration of silver;* -iasis; argyro-phil, *staining readily with silver dyes.*

ARGENTUM, -I, *silver.* > argent-ine; -ous.

**ARTER-**

ARTĒRIA, -AE (from ἀρτηρία), 1. *the windpipe;* 2. *an artery* as distinct from a vein. If, as some writers stated, Hippocrates made this distinction, no use was made of the knowledge. Long after, the arteries continued to be regarded as airducts. > artery; arteri-agra; arterio-pathy; -le; etc.

**ARTH-**

ARTHRON (ἄρθρον) *a joint; a connecting word.* > arthr-itis [G.]; -oncus; arthro-pathy; -pod; an-arthria [G.]; brady-, *slowness of speech;* dys-; etc.

ARTHROŌ (ἀρθρόω), *fasten by a joint; utter distinctly, articulate;* ARTHROSIS (ἄρθρωσις), *a jointing; articulation* (of speech). > *a joint; degenerative affection of a j.;* cycl-arthrosis; di- [G.]; dys-, 1. *dyslalia,* 2. *malformation of a j.;* en- [G.].

**ARTIC-**

ARTICULUS, -I (dim. of artus, *a joint,* akin to G. arthron), *a small member connecting various parts of the body; a joint.* > *a joint; knuckle;* articul-ation; di-articular.

**ASTER-, ASTRO-**

ASTĒR, ASTEROS (ἀστήρ), *a star.* > *the stellar group surrounding the centrosome;* asteroid; -ion.

ASTRON (ἄστρον), *a star.* > astr-oid; astrosphere, *attraction sphere;* -static; -cyte, *one of the cells forming the neuroglia fibers.*

**ASTH-**

ASTHMA, -ATOS (ἄσθμα), *a short drawn breath, panting.* > asthma; asthmo-lysin; asthmat-ic; etc.

**ASTRAG-**

ASTRAGALOS (ἀστράγαλος), *one of the vertebrae; ball of the ankle joint.* > *the astragalus, the ankle bone;* astragalo-tibial; etc.

**ATM-**

ATMOS (ἀτμός), *steam, vapor.* > In compounds, usually *air, gas,* or *steam;* atmolysis; -meter; -sphere; etc.

ATMIS, -IDOS (ἀτμίς), *steam, vapor.* In compounds, usually *steam;* atmid-albumin, etc.

**AUD-, AUR-, AUS-**

AUDIO, pp. -ITUS, *to hear.* > audi-phone; audio-meter; audito-gnosis; etc.

AURIS, *the ear.* > aur-al; -ist; auri-scope; etc.

AURICULA, -AE (dim. of auris) *the external ear; the ear.* > auricle; auricul-ar; auriculo-cranial; etc.

AUSCULTO, pp. -ATUS, *to listen to.* > auscult; -ate; *to listen to sounds made by thoracic or abdominal viscera.*

**AUX-**

AUXANŌ or AUXŌ (αὐξάνω, αὔξω), *increase in power, strengthen;* AUXĒ or AUXĒSIS (αὔξη) or αὔξησις), *growth, increase.* > auxanography; -logy; auxo-cardia; -hormone; -spore, etc. irid-auxesis; nephr-auxe; aux-etic [auxētikos].

**BAC-**

BACILLUS, gen. and pl. -I (dim. of baculus, *a staff*), *a small staff.* > *a rod-shaped structure; a microorganism;* bacill-ar; bacilli-form; bacillo-phobia; etc.

**BACT-**

BACTERIUM, -I, pl. -A, *a staff* [Mod. L. from BACTĒRION (βακτήριον), *a staff*]. > *a unicellular vegetable microorganism;* bacter-emia; bacterio-genous; etc.

**BALAN-**
BALANOS (βάλανος), an acorn; glans penis; a suppository, pessary. H. > balan-ism, employment of a pessary; balano-rrhagia, inflammation of the glans penis.

**BALL-, BEL-, BOL-**
BALLŌ, fut. BALŌ (βάλλω) to throw. BOLĒ (βολή) a throw. > ball-ismus; ball-istics; belemn-oid [belemnon, βέλεμνον, a dart], dart-shaped; em-bolism, obstruction of a blood vessel [fr. em-ballō, throw or put in]; meta-bolism; ana-; bal-opticon, an instrument for throwing the image of an opaque object on a screen; cata-bolism [kata-bolē]; sym-bol [symbolon, a tally, token, sign, fr. sym-ballō, put together]; amphi-bolia [G.].

**BAS-, BET-**
BASIS (βάσις) a going, a step; foot, base. fr. BAINŌ (βαίνω), to go. > bas-e; basi-lysis; a-basia, inability to walk; ana-basis [G. a going up].
DIABĒTĒS (διαβήτης), a compass (from its outstretched legs); a siphon (literally a passer through); diabetes (Aret); fr. DIABAINŌ (διαβαίνω) to walk or stand with legs well apart; to pass through; diabetes; diabet-ic; diabeto-genic; etc.
BATOS (βατός), passable, accessible, verbal adj. of BAINŌ, to go. > bato-phobia, fear of passing high objects or buildings; hypno-batic.

**BIO-**
BIOS (βίος), life. > bio-gen; -lytic; aero-bion; micro-be; amphi-bia; -bious; sym-bio-sis.

**BLAST-**
BLASTOS (βλαστός), a sprout, shoot; of animals, the germ. > blasto-derm; blast-ema [G. a sprout]; -oma; odonto-blast; osteo-; zoo-; etc.

**BLEN-**
BLENNA (βλέννα), a thick mucous discharge. H. > blenno-rrhea; etc.

**BLEP-**
BLEPŌ, fut. BLEPSŌ (βλέπω), to see. BLEPSIS (βλέψις), sight. > blepso-pathia; a-blepsy.
BLEPHARON (βλέφαρον), an eyelid. > blepharadenitis; blephero-pachynsis, thickening of an eyelid; ankylo-blepharon [G.], adhesion of the eyelids; etc.

**BOL-, see BALL-**

**BRACHI-**
BRACHIŌN (βραχίων), arm; L. BRACHIUM, I, pl -A. > brachi-algia; brachio-cyllosis, curvature of the humerus; etc.

**BRACHY-**
BRACHYS (βραχύς), short. > brachy-odont; -podous; etc.

**BRANCH-**
BRANCHION (βράγχιον), a fin. pl. -IA, gills; L. BRANCHIA, gills. > branchi-al, see dict.; branchiogenic; etc.

**BRONCH-**
BRONCHOS (βρόγχος), the trachea, the windpipe, H. > bronchus [Mod. L.] one of the primary divisions of the trachea; bronchitis; broncho-typhoid; etc.
BRONCHION (βρόγχιον), dim. of bronchos, usually in the pl. BRONCHIA (βρόγχια), the bronchial tubes. > id.; bronchi-al; bronchio-genic; etc. BRONCHIOLUS, Mod. L. dim. of bronchia. > one of the finer subdivisions of the bronchial tubes; bronchiol-itis.

**BUB-**
BOUBŌN (βουβών), the groin; a swelling in the groin, a bubo. H. > bubo, an enlargement of a lymphatic gland; bubon-ic; bubono-cele; etc.

**BUCC-**
BUCCA, the cheek (the part around the mouth; distinguished from GENAE, the cheeks, the side of the face, and from MALA, the upper part of the cheeks under the eyes). > bucca-l, relating to the cheeks or mouth; bucci-lingual; etc.

**BURS-**
BURSA, -AE [mediev. L.], a purse. fr. BYRSA (βύρσα), a skin, hide. > In anat. and zool. a pouch or sac; burso-lith, a calculus formed in a bursa; etc. BURSULA, -AE (Mod. L. dim. of bursa). > a small pouch or sac.

**CAD-, CID**
CADO, pp. CASUS, to fall. > cad-ucous, falling early (bot.); case; casualty; recidivation, relapse; [fr. recidivus, falling

back, fr. re-cido, fall back]; stilli-cidium [L. fr. stilla, a drop]; etc.
INCIDO, to fall into or upon; happen. > incidence; incident-al. semel-incident [semel, once.].
DECIDO, to fall down or off. DECIDUUS, -A, -UM, falling off. > deciduous (of leaves); decidua (fem. adj. sc. membrana) the altered mucous membrane of the pregnant uterus.
CADAVER, -ERIS, corpse. > id.

**CALL-**
CALLUS, -I, hard, thick skin; callousness, insensibility. > callosity; calli-section, vivisection of an anesthetized animal; callositas [L.]; callosal; callous.

**CALX-1, CALCA-**
CALX, CALCIS, the heel. > id.
CALCANEUM, -I, pl. -A, the heel; a rare form of calx, calcis. > the heel bone; the os calcis; calcane-odynia; calcaneo-scaphoid; etc.
CALCAR, a spur. > a spurlike process; calcarine.

**CALX-2, CALCI-, CALCO-**
CALX, CALCIS, limestone, lime. (this word and calx above are from different roots.) > calci-c; -penia; -um; calco-phor-ous; -pherite; etc.
CALCARIUS, pertaining to lime. > calcar-eous; calcari-uria, excretion of lime salts in urine.
CALCULUS, a pebble; a stone in the bladder or kidneys. > a concretion formed in any part of the body; calcul-ous; -ary.

**CAMP-**
KAMPTŌ, fut. KAMPSŌ (κάμπτω, κάμψω), to bend; KAMPTOS (κάμπτος), flexible. > campto-cormia, a condition characterized by flexion of the trunk [kormos, trunk of a tree]; -dactylia; ana-campt-ics, the study of reflection [ana-kamptō, to bend convexly]; etc.
KAMPSIS (κάμψις), a bending. > gony-campsis; osteo-campsia; etc.

**CANC-**
CANCER, -CRI or -CERI, a crab; a malignant tumor, cancer. > cancer; -ation; -ine; -ism; cancero-myces; cancro-logy; etc. canker; chancre [through Fr.].

**CAP-1, CEP-, CIP-**
CAPUT, -ITIS, the head. > id.; the expanded extremity of a structure; capit-ate; -ular; capito-pedal; etc. jani-ceps; multi-.
CAPITELLUM and CAPITULUM (dim). > small head or headlike structure.
ANCEPS, -CIPITIS (an for ambi-) two-headed; two-fold. > ancipit-al; -ate; -ous.
BICEPS, -CIPITIS, two-headed; divided into two parts. > having two heads; the biceps; bicipit-al.
TRICEPS, -CIPITIS, three-headed; threefold. > id., applied to two muscles, t. brachii and t. surae.
PRAECEPS, -CIPITIS, headforemost, headlong, hence PRAECIPITO, pp. -ATUS, to cast down headlong. > precipitat-e; precipit-ant; -atim; -in
SINCIPUT, -PITIS, half a head; the brain; the head (sin- for semi-). > the front part of the head; sincipit-al.
OCCIPUT, -PITIS (obc-), the back of the head. > id.; occipit-al; occipito-mental. centri-ciput (formed on analogy of the two preceding words from centrum and caput), the central portion of the upper surface of the skull).
CAPILLUS, -I (a dim. form akin to caput), the hair of the head; the fibers of plants. > id.
CAPILLARIS, pertaining to the hair. > capillary, as adj. hairlike; as noun, a minute blood vessel. capillar-ectasia; capi-lario-motor; etc.
CAPILLITIUM, the hair collectively. > a network of proto-plasmic threads in a spore capsule.

**CAP-2, CEPT-, CIP-**
CAPIO, pp. CAPTUS, to seize, take. > captation, a seizing, the first stage of hypnotism [fr. capto, pp. -atus, seize, snatch.]; cept-or bi-ceptor; chemo-; contraceptive; cap, abbrev. for capiat, let him take.
RECIPIO, pp. -CEPTUS, take back, receive. > recept-or; recipio-motor; etc.
ACCIPIO, pp. -CEPTUS, accept. > accept-or, a substance that receives or absorbs another. So from CONCIPIO, to take hold of are derived concept; concept-ion; -ive; from INCI-

PIO, *take in hand, begin,* comes incipient; fr. PERCIPIO, *to take wholly, perceive,* are derived perception; imperception; etc.

**CARB-**

CARBO, -ONIS, *coal, charcoal.* > carbon; carb-ide; -olic [oleum, *oil*]; carbo-cyclic; etc.

CARBUNCULUS (dim. of carbo), *a small coal; a kind of tumor.* > carbuncle; carbuncul-ar; -osis.

**CARC-**

KARKINOS (καρκίνος), *a crab; ulcer, cancer.* H. > In compounds, cancer; carcinectomy; -elcosis, carcino-gen; etc.

**CARD-**

KARDIA (καρδία), *heart; mind; the cardiac extremity of the stomach.* H. > cardia, *the heart; the esophageal orifice of the stomach;* cardi-ac; -agra; -ant; cardio-kinetic; peri-cardi-um [G. perikardion]; etc.

**CAROT-**

KAROTIDES, -ŌN (καρωτίδες, -ων), *the great arteries of the neck,* fr. KAROŌ, *to plunge into heavy sleep;* so called from a belief that sleep was caused by increased flow of blood through these arteries. Gal. > the carotids; carot-ic; carotico-tympanic; etc.

**CARP-1**

KARPOS (καρπός), *the joint of the hand and the arm; the wrist.* > carpus, -i, (Mod. L.), *the wrist;* carp-al; -itis; -ectomy; carpo-ptosia; meta-carpus; etc.

**CARP-2**

KARPOS (καρπός), *fruit.* > carp-el, *a simple pistil or one of the members* composing a compound pistil; carpo-gonium; peri-carp.

**CAUS-, CAUT-**

KAIŌ, fut. KAUSŌ (καίω, καύσω), *to set on fire, burn;* of surgeons, *to cauterize.* H. KAUSTIKOS (καυστικός) *capable of burning, corrosive.* > caustic; causticum.

KAUTĒR (καυτήρ), *a branding iron.* > cauter; -y; -ize.

**CELE-**

KĒLĒ (κήλη), *a tumor, a rupture.* H. > celectome, *an instrument for obtaining tumor tissue;* celo-logy. -cele, a suffix denoting *a swelling* or *hernia,* as hydrocele. Compare -cele in the following.

**CELI-, COELI-, CELO**

KOILOS (κοῖλος), *hollow;* KOILIA (κοιλία), *the large hollow of the body, the belly; any hollow or cavity.* > In compounds, *the abdomen;* celi- or coeli-ac; -algia; celio- or coelio-scopy; celo- or coelo-zoic, *inhabiting any of the cavities of the body* (of protozoa). -cele, a suffix denoting *a cavity,* as mesocele. Compare with the preceding CELE-.

**CELL-**

CELLA, -AE, *a storeroom, a chamber, closet.* > a cell, *a minute structure.* CELLULA, -AE (dim. of cella), *a small storeroom.* > a minute cell; cellul-e; -ar; cellulo-neuritis; etc.

**CENT-, CEST-**

KENTEŌ, fut. -ĒSŌ (κεντέω, -ήσω), *prick, stab;* hence, KENTĒSIS (κέντησις), *a pricking.* > centesis, *puncture of a cavity;* cardio-centesis; cerato-, *puncture of the cornea;* entero-; etc.

KENTRON (κέντρον), *any sharp point; the stationary point of a pair of compasses; the center of a circle.* > centro-phose; -cyte; -plasm; ec-centr-ic; etc.

KESTOS (κεστός), *stitched, embroidered;* as noun, *a girdle.* > Cestod-a; -es, *an order of flatworms, the tapeworms;* -iasis; Centro-cestus, *a genus of flukes.*

CENTRUM, -I, *center* [fr. G. kentron]. > center; centr-ad; centri-ciput; -fuge; -petal [fr. peto, *to seek*]; etc.

**CEPH-**

KEPHALĒ (κεφαλή), *head.* > cephal-ad; -emia; -ic; cephalo-cele; -tripsy; etc.

ENKEPHALOS, -ON (ἐγκέφαλος, -ον), *within the head,* as noun, ENKEPHALOS, *the brain.* > encephalon, *brain;* encephal-algia; -atrophy; -itis; encephalo-cele; etc.

**CERAS-, CRAS-**

KERANNYMI, fut. KERASŌ (κεράννυμι, κεράσω), *mix, mingle;* hence, KERASTOS (κεραστός), *mixed, mingled.* > cyto-cerastic; lympho-cerastism.

KRASIS (κρᾶσις), *a mixing, blending; temperament* (of mind or body). > crasis, *constitution, temperament;* dys-crasia; galacto-; ortho-; idiosyn-crasy.

**CERAT-, KERAT-**

KERAS, -ATOS (κέρας), *the horn* of an animal; *horn* (a material). > In compounds, *a horny structure, material,* or *process,* as the cornea or the epidermis; cerato-dermatitis; -centesis; kerat-in; kerato-malacia; etc.

**CERV-**

CERVIX, -ICIS, the neck. > *the neck; any necklike structure;* cervic-al; -ectomy, *amputation of cervix uteri;* cervici-plex; cervico-lingual; etc.

**CES-, CAES-, CID-, CIS-**

CAEDO, pp. CAESUS, *to strike, cut; kill.* > caes-arian section (some derive this word from Julius Caesar, as he is said to have been delivered in this way); caesaro-tomy. amebi-cide; insecti-; etc.

INCIDO, pp. -CISUS, *to cut into.* > incision; -or; -ura [L.].

CIRCUMCIDO, pp. -CISUS, *to cut around.* > circumcision.

**CHEM-**

CHĒMIA or CHĒMEIA (χημία or χημεία), *the Egyptian art,* the art of transmuting the baser metals into gold, fr. Chēmia, *the land of black earth.* The Arabs borrowed the word from the Greek and called the art alchemy [Ar. al, *the +* chēmia; others derive the word fr. Ar. al, *the,* + G. chymeia, *a pouring,* fr. cheō, *to pour,* cf. CHY-] > chem-istry; -ical; chemo-taxis; chemico-cautery; etc.

**CHIR-, CHEIR-**

CHEIR (χείρ), *the hand.* > Chir-acanthus, *a genus of nematoid worms;* chir-algia; -apsia (hapsis, *a touching*): chiro-gnostic; -podist; etc.

CHEIROURGIA (χειρουργία), *a working by hand; a handicraft* or *art; the practice of surgery as opposed to medicine,* fr. ergon (ἔργον) work. H. > chirurgeon; surgeon (abbrev. of preceding).

**CHLOR-**

CHLŌROS (χλωρός), *green, light-green* (like young grass), *yellowish-green.* > chloas-ma [fr. chloazō (χλοάζω), *be* or *become green*]; chlor-al; -ine; chloro-form; -ma; -sis; etc.

**CHOL-**

CHOLĒ (χολή), *gall, bile,* pl. CHOLAI (χολαί), *the gall bladder.* > chol-uria; chole-stasia; -sterol (stereos, στερεός *solid*) with various compounds: cholesterol-emia; -uria; etc. chol-eresis (a word artificially formed on a Greek model).

CHOLERA (χολέρα), "*a disease in which the humors of the body are violently discharged by vomiting and the stool.*" H. > cholera; -ization; choleri-genous; etc.

CHOLĒDOCHOS (χοληδόχος), *containing bile,* as noun, (sc. kystos, *bladder*) the gall bladder, Gal. [fr. dochos, *containing*]. > choledochus, choledoch, *the common bile-duct;* choledocho-plasty; -rraphy; etc.

**CHOND-**

CHONDROS (χόνδρος), *groats of wheat or spelt; a mucilaginous drink made from groats; gristle or cartilage.* H. > chondrus, 1. *cartilage,* 2. *a genus of seaweeds,* 3. *Irish moss;* chondr-al; chondri-gen; chondro-costal; Chondro-myces, *a genus of bacteria,* so called from its gelatinous cysts.

HYPOCHONDRION (ὑποχόνδριον), *the soft part of the body below the cartilage at the breast-bone and above the navel.* H. and Cels. > hypochondria (because imaginary diseases are often seated in this region).

**CHORD-, CORD-**

CHORDĒ (χορδή), *guts, tripe; a string of guts; string* of a lyre or harp. > In compounds any chorda or cord, esp. the notochord; chordo-pexy; chord-itis; -tomy; etc. cephalo-chord; noto- [nōtos, *the back*].

CHORDA, gen. and pl. -AE; Mediev. L. CORDA [fr. G. chordē], *a string or cord made from gut; a rope, cord.* > a *tendon; a stringlike structure;* cord; chord-al; etc.

**CHORI-**

CHORION (χόριον), *the membrane that encloses the fetus, afterbirth,* H.; *any intestinal membrane.* > *the outermost o the fetal envelopes;* in compounds chorion- and chorio- refer also to other membranes, as the *middle coat of the eye, the true skin,* etc. chorion-itis; chorio-retinitis.

CHORIOEIDĒS (χοριοειδής), like the afterbirth; c. chiton, "the coat like an afterbirth," the chorioid coat of the eye. Gal. > chorioidea; chorioid or choroid [the latter form comes fr. choroeidēs, an ancient copyist's error for chorioeidēs].

**CHROM-, CHROS-**

CHRŌMA, -ATOS (χρῶμα), the surface of the body; the complexion; color. fr. CHRŌZŌ (χρώζω) to touch the surface of the body; to tinge, stain. > In many compounds, with sense of color, chrom-affin; chromo-cyte; -lipoid; chromato-genous; -pathy; etc.

CHROIA (χροιά) or CHROA (χρόα), with the same meanings as chrōma. > cyanochroia; allo-chro-ism; etc.

ACHROIA (ἄχροια), absence of color. [a- priv]. > achreo-cythemia.

ACHROOS (ἄχροος), colorless. > achro-ate; -globin.

CHRŌSIS (χρῶσις), a coloring, tinting; fr. CHRŌZŌ. > hema-chrosis; hypo-; meta-, change of color; thermo-.

**CHY-**

CHEŌ (χέω), to pour. > cheo-plasty.

CHYSIS, a pouring. > meta-chysis [G.], transfusion; rhachio-; syn- [G.]; etc.

CHYLOS (χυλός), juice, the juice of plants; the juice produced by digestion. Gal. > chyle; chyl-emia; chyli-ferous; chylo-poiesis; etc. dia-chylon, lead plaster [dia-chylos, juicy].

CHYMOS (χυμός), juice; the juice o' plants; the juices of the body; the taste of a juice, hence the sense of taste. Chymos and chylos were used almost interchangeably by the ancient writers. H. preferred chylos, Arist. chymos. > chyme, the semi-fluid mass of partly digested food passed from the stomach; chymification; chymo-us; etc.

EKCHEŌ (ἐκχέω), to pour out; EKCHYSIS (ἔκχυσις), a pouring out; outflow. > py-ecchysis; ur- [ouron, urine].

ENCHEŌ (ἐγχέω), to pour in; hence, ENCHYMA (ἔγχυμα), a filling; instillation, Gal.; ENCHYSIS (ἔγχυσις), a pouring in. > enchyma; mes-enchyma [mesos, middle]; par- [G. anything poured in beside]: cirs-enchysis [kirsos, varix]; derm-; elaeomy-; etc.

CID-, see CAD- or CES-

**CIL-**

CILIUM, -II, pl. -IA, an eyelid. > 1. eyelash; 2. a hairlike process; Cili-ata, a class of Infusoria; cili-ary (fr. hypothet. L. form ciliarius); ciliaro-tomy; cilio-spinal; etc.

**CIN-, KIN-**

KINEŌ, fut. -ĒSŌ (κινέω), to set in motion. > In compounds the sense of movement. cin-aesthesia, or -esthesia, sense perception of movement; cine-plastics, art of forming a muscular stump capable of movement; etc.

KINĒMA, -ATOS (κίνημα), movement. > cinema; cinemat-ics; cinemato-radiography; etc.

KINĒSIS (κίνησις), movement. > cines-algia; -iatrics; cinesi-meter; lympho-cinesia; etc.

KINĒTOS (κινητός), moveable. > cyneto-cyte; -cytopenia; etc.

**CION-**

KIŌN (κίων), a pillar, column; the uvula. H. > cion, the uvula; ciono-tomy; cion-itis; etc.

CIP-, see CAP-2

**CLAS-**

KLAŌ, fut. klasō (κλάω), to break; in passive, to be broken or deflected (of lines or rays).

KLASMA, -ATOS (κλάσμα), something broken, a fragment. > clasmato-cyte, a connective tissue corpuscle that tends to break up into fragments; -blast.

KLASIS (κλάσις), a breaking, a fracture. > clastic. As suffix, a breaking down: arthroclasis; etc.

ANAKLASIS (ἀνάκλασις), a bending back; reflection of light or sound. > anaclasis, id.

KLASTOS (κλαστός), broken in pieces. > clastic; clasto-thrix; amylo-clast; chondro-; odonto-; osteo-; polio-clastic.

**CLAUS-, CLUS-, CLUD-**

CLAUDO, pp. -CLAUSUS, close, shut; hence CLAUS-TRUM, -I, pl. -A, that by which something is closed, lock, bolt, barrier. > an anatomical structure resembling a barrier; claus-tra-phobia, morbid fear of being enclosed; peri-claustral, sur-rounding the c.

CLAUSURA, gen. and pl. -AE, a lock, bolt. > closure of an opening or passage.

INCLUDO, pp. -CLUSUS, shut in, enclose; include. > in-clude; inclusion.

OCCLUDO, pp. -CLUSUS, to close up. > occlud-e; occlus-ion; -al; -ive.

**CLEID-, CLEIS-, CLID-**

KLEIŌ, fut. KLEISŌ (κλείω), to close, bar, enclose; hence, KLEIS, KLEIDOS (κλείς), that which closes, a key; the collar bone (because it locks the neck and breast together. Cf. L. clavicula fr. clavis, a key. The meaning collar bone was given the word in Mediev. L. but not in classical). > In com-pounds, clavicle; clid-arthritis; -agra; clido-costal; etc.

KLEISIS or KLĒSIS (κλεῖσις or κλῆσις), a closing. > apo-cleisis [G. a shutting off]; arthro-; enteroapo-; hystero-; spleno-; etc.

KLEISTOS (κλειστός), closed. > clistogamy. closed fertile flowers, bot.; a-cleisto-cardia.

**CLIM-, CLIN-, CLIV-**

KLINŌ (κλίνω), to make bend, slope; make recline. > clino-dactyly; -logy; en-clit-ic; syn-clit-ic.

KLIMA, -ATOS (κλίμα), a slope; the supposed slope of the earth from the equator to the pole; a region, zone, climate. > climato-logy; -therapy; climo-graph.

KLIMAX, -AKOS (κλῖμαξ), a ladder or staircase; a climax. > a climax in a disease.

KLIMAKTĒR, -ĒROS (κλιμακτήρ), the rung of a ladder; a dangerous point in a man's life. > climacter; -ic.

KLINĒ (κλίνη), a bed. > clin-ic; -ician; -oid; clino-mania.

KLISIS -EŌS (κλίσις, -εως), a bending, inclination. > cliseo-meter; pelvi-cliseometer.

CLINO = G. klinō (simple verb obsolete in classical L.), to make bend, slope; hence DECLINO, pp. -ATUS, to bend, turn aside. > declin-e; declin-ation; -ator. INCLINO, -ATUS, cause to lean, incline. > inclin-ation; inclinatio pelvis [L.]; inclino-meter. RECLINO, -ATUS, to bend back, recline. > reclin-ation.

CLIVUS, a slope. > a sloping surface, esp. of a bone. DE-CLIVIS, sloping downward. > declive, clivus monticuli.

**COCC-**

KOKKOS (κόκκος), a grain, seed; a berry, specif. the Kerms-berry, that grows upon the Scarlet Oak (Quercus coccifera) from which a scarlet dye was obtained. What was formerly supposed to be a fruit is now known to be the dried bodies of the Kermes insect. > coccus, 1. coch-ineal (thr. Sp. and L.), the dried female insect Pseudococcus cacti. 2. a bacterium of round form. 3. a division of the schizocarp. bot.; cocc-inella; -inellin; cocco-bacillus; -genous. micro-coccus; staphylo-; strepto-; gono-; etc.

**COCCY-**

KOKKYX, -YGOS (κόκκυξ), a cuckoo; the os coccygis (from its resemblance to cuckoo's bill). Gal. > coccyx; coccyg-algia; -eal; -ectomy; -odynia, also coccy-dynia and coccy-odynia; etc.

**COCH-**

COCHLEA, -AE, pl. -AE, a snail; a snail shell; a spiral. > a division of the internal ear; cochle-ate; -ar; cochleo-vestibu-lar.

COCHLEAR or COCHLEARE, a spoon (snail-shell form). > id.; cochlear-iform; cochlear-ia, scurvy-grass, spoon-wort.

COEC-, see CEC-

COEL-, see CEL-

**COLL-1**

KOLLA (κόλλα), glue. > colla-gen; coll-oid; -odium; hemi-collin, a derivative of gelatin.

**COLL-2**

COLLUM, -I, pl. -A, the neck; any necklike part, > id.: colla-pexia; etc.

**COND-**

KONDYLOS (κόνδυλος), a knuckle; the knuckle of any joint, Gal.; any hard bony knob. > condylus; condyle; condyl-ec-tomy; -ar; -oma.

CORD-, see CHORD-

**CORE-**

KORĒ (κορή), a maiden; a puppet, a doll; the pupil of the

eye (because a little image appears in it. *Cf.* L. pupilla fr.
pupa, *a doll*). > In compounds, *the pupil;* cor-ectasia; corelysis; -morphous; coro-meter; -plasty; aniso-coria, etc.

**CORI-**

CORIUM, -I, pl. -A, *hide, skin; leather;* of plants *bark, rind.*
> *the true skin;* cori-aceous.

**CORN-**

CORNU, -US, pl. -UA, *a horn; anything of horny substance;
the horny covering* of the eye. > *a horn; any structure of horny
substance;* corni-fication; cornus, *the dried bark of Cornus
florida.*

CORNEUS, -A, -UM, *of horn, horny.* > cornea (sc. tunica,
*coat*); corneum, *horny layer* of skin.

CORNICULUM, dim. of cornu. > *a small hornlike* or
*horny structure.*

**CORON-**

CORŌNĒ (κορώνη), *a kind of crow; anything shaped or
hooked* like its bill; *a kind of crown; the apophysis of a bone.* H.
> *the coronoid process* of the mandible; coron-ion, *the tip of*
the preceding; coron-oid.

CORONA, gen. and pl. -AE, *a garland, wreath; a crown* [fr.
G. corōnē]. > *any structure suggesting a crown or wreath;*
coron-ad; -ium, a hypothet. *element;* -et, *the upper part of a
horse's hoof.*

CORONARIUS, -A, -UM, *relating to a crown.* > coronaria
(sc. arteria); coronar-y.

**CORP-**

CORPUS, -ORIS, *the body.* > *any body* or *mass; the main
part* of an organ; corpor-al; -eal; corp-se.

CORPUSCULUM, *a little body* (most frequently of atoms).
> corpuscle.

**CRAS-**, see CERAS-

**CRES-, CRET-**

CRESCO, pp. CRETUS, *to grow, arise, increase.* pres. part.
CRESCENS, gen. CRESCENTIS. > crescent (sc. luna, *i.e.
the increasing moon); any crescent-shaped figure; the primitive
sexual form* of the malarial parasite; cresco-graph, *device for
recording growth.*

CONCRESCO, pp. -CRETUS, *to grow together,* > concres-
cence; concre-ment; concret-e; ion.

EXCRESCO, pp. -CRETUS, *to grow out, grow forth.* >
escrescence.

INCRESCO, *grow in* or *upon, increase;* hence INCREMEN-
TUM, -I, *growth, increase.* > id.

**CRET-, CREM-**

CERNO, pp. CRETUS, *to separate; distinguish* by the
senses, *discern;* hence:

CRIMEN, -INIS, (contr. fr. cernimen), *judicial decision,
verdict; crime.* > crime; crinino-logy.

RECREMENTUM, -I, *refuse, dross, filth.* > recrement;
-itious.

DISCERNO, pp. -CRETUS, *separate, divide; discern.* >
discrete, *separate, distinct; made up of separate parts.*

EXCERNO, pp. -CRETUS, *to separate* > excreta (ntr. pl.
of pp. excretus); excret-e; -in; -ion; -ory. EXCREMENTUM,
*feces,* > id.

INCERNO, -CRETUS, *to sift in; add with a sieve.* incretion; -ory; -increto-logy; -pathy; -diagnosis; etc.

SECERNO, pp. -CRETUS, *sever, separate* [fr. se-, *apart*].
> secreta (ntr. pl. of secretus); secret-e; -agogue; -in; -ion;
secreto-motor; -ry; etc.

**CRI-**

KRINŌ (κρίνω), *to separate, distinguish; pick out, choose;
form a judgment, judge;* in medic. *bring to a crisis,* H. and Gal.
[akin to L. cerno]. > dys-crin-ism; hyper-; endo-crin-e;
endo-crin-ism; exo-crine; ec-crino-logy [ek-krino]; etc.

KRISIS (κρίσις), *a separating, distinguishing; decision
judgment; turning point* of a disease, *crisis.* > crisis; eccrisis, *excretion;* paraec-, *a disorder of excretion;* uro-.

KRITĒRION (κριτήριον), *a means of judging, a standard.*
> criterion; uro-.

KRITIKOS (κριτικός), *able to discern critical; decisive.* >
ec-critic; epi-.

**CRY-**

**KRYOS** (κρύος), *icy cold, frost.* > cry-algesia; -esthesia;
cryo-therapy.

**KRYMOS** (κρυμός), *icy cold, frost; a chill.* > crym-odynia;
crymo-philic; etc.

**KRYSTALLOS** (κρυσταλλός), *clear ice; crystal* > crystal;
crystall-ine; -in, *a globulin in the c. lens of the eye;* -itis; -oid;
crystallo-phobia, *morbid fear of glass cbjects* crypto-crystal-
line, *having minute crystals.*

**CUB-**

CUBO, pp. -ITUS, *to recline, lie down; sleep;* hence CU-
BITUS or -UM, *the elbow* (on which one reclines). > cubital; cubito-carpal; etc.

INCUBO, pp. -ITUS, *to lie in a place; to sit upon eggs, to
brood, hatch.* > incubation; -ator.

INCUBUS, *nightmare,* > id.

SUCCUBO (SUBC-), *lie under;* hence SUCCUBA, -AE, *a
strumpet.* > succuba; succubus (Mediev. L.).

**CUSS-, CUT-**

QUATIO, pp. QUASSUS, *to shake, agitate;* hence, CONCU-
TIO, pp. -CUSSUS, *to shake violently, shatter.* > concuss-ion;
-or.

DISCUTIO, pp. -CUSSUS, *strike asunder, shatter, scatter,
disperse.* > discuss, *disperse, cause to disappear;* -ive; discutient (fr. pres. p.).

PERCUTIO, pp. -CUSSUS, *strike through and through.* >
percuss; -ion; -or [L. *one who strikes*]; percusso-punctator.

**CY-, CYT-**

KYŌ (κύω), *to conceive, be pregnant.* > cyasma, *pigmentation
of the skin in pregnancy.*

KYĒSIS (κύησις), *conception.* > cyesis; cyes-edema; cyesiognosis; ec-cyesis, *ectopic gestation;* en- [G. *germination in
plants*], *pregnancy;* encyo-pyelitis [enkyesis].

KYMA (κῦμα), *anything swelling out; a wave; a fetus.* >
dermo-cyma, *fetus in fetu.*

KYOS (κύος), *fetus.* > cyo-phoria [G. fr. phero, *to bear*];
-phoric.

KYTOS (κύτος), *a hollow; any vessel, jar, urn.* > In compounds, *a cell;* cyt-hemolysis; cyto-blast; -zoic; erythro-cyte;
phago-; etc.

**CYAN-**

KYANOS (κύανος), *a dark blue substance* (used to adorn
works in metal). > In compounds, *blue;* cyan-emia; cyano-
pathy; -phil; -gen; -sis [G.]; etc.; antho-cyan-ins.

**CYC-**

KYKLOS (κύκλος), *a ring, circle; any circular body, the
eyeball.* > cycle; in compounds the word has various meanings, *roundness, grouping, rotation,* specif. *the ciliary body;*
cycl-arthrosis, a *rotary joint;* -ectomy, ciliectomy; cyclocephalia; etc.

KYKLŌPS, -ŌPOS (κύκλωψ), Cyclops, *a mythological giant
with one eye* in the middle of his forehead, fr. ōps (ὤψ) an
eye. > cyclop-ia; cyclops, *a monster with fusion of the orbits.*

**CYN-**

KYŌN, KYNOS (κύων), *a dog; unilateral facial paralysis,*
Gal. > cyn-ic spasm; cyn-iatrics; -anthropy; cyno-bex (bēx,
*a cough*); -cephalus.

KYNANCHĒ (κυνάγχη), *dog quinsy; sore throat.* H.; *dog-
collar* [fr. anchō (ἄγχω), to *throttle*]. > cynanche, *sore throat;*
quinsy (a corrupt form of c. through Mediev. L.).

**CYST-**

KYSTIS (κύστις), *the bladder.* > cystis, 1. *bladder.* 2 *cyst;*
cystalgia; cysti-cercosia; cysto-cele; etc.

**CYT-**, see CY-

**DENT-**

DENS, DENTIS, *a tooth.* > 1. id. 2. *the odontoid process;*
dent-al; denti-fication; -labial; etc.

DENTICULUS, (dim.) *a small tooth.* > denticle; denticulate.

DENTATUS, -A, -UM, *toothed.* > dentat-e; dentatum (ntr.)
*nucleus dentatus.*

**DER-**

DERMA, -ATOS (δέρμα), *the skin, hide* of beasts; *the human
skin, bark* of trees; fr. DERŌ (δέρω), *to flay, skin.* > derm,
derma, dermis, *the outer tegument;* derm-ad; -agra and derma-

tagra; Derma-centor *a genus of ticks;* dermato-therapy; etc.
epi-dermis; -dermitis; pachy-derm; -derma-tous; hypodermic.

DEROS (δέρος), poet. form of derma. > ec-deron, *layer of
skin outside the enderon;* en-deron, *the corium.*

**DES-**

DEŌ, fut. DĒSŌ (δέω, δήσω), *to bind, tie; harden, brace up,*
H., hence:

DESIS (δέσις), a *binding together.* > cirso-desis, *ligation of
varicose veins* [kirsos, *varix*]: irido-; etc.

DESMOS or (poet.) DESMA (δεσμός, δέσμα), *a band, bond,
fetter; ligature,* Arist. > desm-itis; desmo-cyte; -id; -pexia;
-some; etc. hemi-desmos; meso-desma.

**DEUT-**

DEUTEROS (δεύτερος), *second.* > deuteranopia, *green-
blindness,* green being the second of the primary colors;
deuteropathic, *relating to a secondary affection;* etc.

**DIDY-**

DIDYMOS (δίδυμος), *twofold, twin;* DIDYMOI (δίδυμοι)
as pl. noun, *the testicles,* Gal. > didym-itis; -odynia; etc.

EPIDIDYMIS, -IDOS (ἐπιδιδυμίς, -ίδος), *the epididymis.*
> epididymis, gen. -idis, pl. -ides (Mod. L.); epididym-al;
-ectomy; -itis; etc.

**DIG-**

DIGITUS, gen. and pl. -I, a *finger* or *toe.* > usually a *finger* as
distinguished from dactylus, a toe; digit-ate; -ation; interdigitation, *the mutual interlocking or processes;* indigitation,
*invagination,* is derived not fr. digitus, but fr. indig-eto or
-ito, pp. -atus, *to call upon, invoke a deity.*

DIGITALIS, *of or belonging to a finger.* > Digitalis purpurea,
*purple foxglove, ladies' fingers;* digitalis, *the drug* derived from
its leaves; digital-in; -ism, *poisoning by d.*

**DIPH-**

DIPHTHERA (διφθέρα), a *prepared hide, leather,* fr.
DEPHŌ (δέφω), *to soften.* > diphther-ia (referring to the
leathery membrane formed in the throat); -ic; -oid; etc.

**DOCH-, DOC-**

DECHOMAI (δέχομαι), *take, receive;* hence, DOCHĒ or
DOCHEION (δοχή or δοχεῖον), a *holder, receptacle.* >
sialo-doch-itis; sialo-docho-plasty; uro-doch-ium.

DOKIMOS (δόκιμος), *acceptable, approved;* hence DOKI-
MAZŌ (δοκιμάζω), *to assay, test.* > dokimasia [G.] *an assay;*
docimas-tic.

DIADECHOMAI (διαδέχομαι), *receive one from another;
succeed;* hence, DIADOCHOS (διάδοχος), *succeeding,
taking over.* > diadocho-cinesis; -cinetic.

**DREP-**

DREPANĒ (δρεπάνη), a *sickle,* fr. DREPŌ (δρέπω), *to
pluck, cull.* > In compounds, *a sickle,* or *crescent-shaped cell;*
drepan-ocyte; -cythemia, *crescent cell anemia.*

**DROM-**

DROMOS (δρόμος), a *running,* a *race.* > drom-ic, *relating
to the flow of nerve impulses;* dromo-graph; -tropic; -mania;
etc.

**DUC-, DUCT-**

DUCO, pp. DUCTUS, *to lead, guide.* DUCTUS, *a leading,
drawing.* > duct; ductulus (dim.) *a minute duct;* caudi-duct,
*to draw toward the tail;* etc. From the following verbs there
are many derivatives similarly formed, mostly from the pp.;
ABDUCO, *lead or draw away;* AD-, *lead to;* CIRCUM-, *draw
around;* CON-, *draw together;* DE-, *lead away;* E-, *lead out;* IN-,
*lead in, admit;* PRO-, *lead forth;* RE-, *lead back;* SE-, *draw
apart.* The pp. of all these verbs is -DUCTUS. Hence ab-
duct-ion; -or. So with the other compounds of duco the words
meaning action and actor, respectively, are formed. Many
words are derived from the pres. p. ending in -ENS, gen.
-ENTIS, as ab-duc-ent; ad-duc-ent. The Eng. verbal derivative has two usual forms, *e.g.,* deduct and deduce; conduct
and conduce.

**EC-, OEC-**

OIKOS (οἶκος), a *house, chamber.* > ec- or oec-oid, *framework
of a red corpuscle:* eco-logy; -mania: aut-ec-ic, *infesting always
the same host* [autos, *self, same*]; di-ec-ious, *having* male and

female flowers *on separate plants* [di-, *two*]; heter-ecious;
met-.

OIKONOMIA (οἰκονομία), *management of a household;
thrift.* > econom-y; -ic.

**ECHIN-**

ECHINOS (ἐχῖνος), *a hedgehog; a sea-urchin.* > In bot. and
zool. compounds the word has the sense of *roughness* or
*prickliness.* echin-ate; -osis, *a condition in which blood corpuscles have lost their smooth outlines;* Echino-coccus, *a genus
of tape worms;* -coccosis.

**ECHO**

ĒCHŌ (ἠχώ), *a sound, an echo.* > *a reverberating sound*
sometimes heard in auscultation of the heart. In compounds,
a sense of *imitation* and *repetition.* echo-lalia; -pathy; -phra-
sia; etc.

**ECT-, EX-, HEX-, SCH-, OCH-**

ECHŌ, fut. HEXŌ or SCHĒSŌ (ἔχω, ἕξω or σχήσω), *to
have, hold;* intrans. *hold one-self, keep in a certain condition,*
etc. > mes-ect-ic; metrap-ectic [mētēr, *mother,* + ap-echō,
*hold off, avoid*]; mion-; pleon-; cat-och-us [katochos, *suffering
from catalepsy.* H.]; syn-och-us [G. -os]; etc.

HEXIS, -EŌS (ἕξις, -εως), *a having; a being in a certain condition, habit of body.* > cac-hexia [G. kakos, *bad*]; cat-hexis
[G.]; mion-exia [meiōn, *less*]; pleon- [pleōn, *more*]; hect-ic
[hectikos, *habitual; consumptive,* Gal.].

SCHESIS, -EŌS (σχέσις, -εως), *a condition; a checking, retention,* H. > galacto-schesis; meno-; sialo-; etc.

ISCHŌ (ἴσχω), a redupl. form of echō, *keep back, restrain.*
> isch-esis, *suppression of a discharge;* -idrosis; -uria; galact-
ischia; hemat-isch-esis.

**EDEM-, OEDEM-**

OIDĒMA, -ATOS (οἴδημα), a *swelling, tumor,* H. fr. OIDEŌ
(οἰδέω) *to swell.* > edema or oedema; edemat-ization; -ous;
etc.

**ELECT-**

ĒLECTRON (ἤλεκτρον), *amber.* > *a separate unit of electricity;* in compounds, *electricity* (so called because the property of developing e. was first observed in amber); electr-ic;
electro-genesis; etc.

**ELYT-**

ELYTRON (ἔλυτρον), a *cover; the sheath* (of a spear); *the
shell* or *husk.* > In compounds, *the vagina;* elytr-itis; elytrocele; -rrhaphy; etc.

**EMB-**

EMBRYON (ἔμβρυον), 1. *a young animal.* 2. *a fetus.* >
embryo, *the offspring of an animal before its birth; the rudimentary plant in the seed;* -cardia, heart sounds resembling
those of the fetus; -geny; -tomy; etc.

**ENTER-**

ENTERON (ἔντερον), a *piece of gut;* in pl. *the intestines*
(formed as a comparative of entos (ἐντός), within, *cf.* Eng.
interior). > *the intestine;* enteron-itis; enteropathy; -pexy;
etc. enter-al; -ic; etc. dys-entery; mes-; li-.

**ER-**

HAIREŌ, fut. -ĒSŌ (αἱρέω, -ήσω), *to take, grasp;* HAIRE-
SIS (αἵρεσις), *a taking.* Hence the foll. verbs each with its
noun derivative; AP-HAIREO, *take away;* noun deriv.
AP-HAIRESIS. > plasm-apheresis; etc. DIAIR-EO, *take
apart, divide;* noun, -ESIS. > dieresis; lipo-; etc. EXAIR-EO,
*take out;* n. -ESIS. > exeresis, *excision;* phrenico-; etc.
KATHAIR-EO, *take down, destroy;* n. -ESIS. > hemocytocatheresis.

SYNAIREO, *grasp together, shorten, contract;* n. -ESIS. >
syneresis.

**ERG-, ORG-**

ERGON (ἔργον), *work.* > erg, *the unit of work* in the metric
system; -in. *a hypothet. substance in the blood;* ergo-esthesio-
graph; -mania; etc. all-erg-y- [allos, *other*]; chir-urg-eon [see
CHIR-)]; hyp-urg-ia (hypourgia, *help*]; etc.

ARGOS, -ON (ἀργός, -όν), *not working, idle* [a- priv.] >
*a gaseous element,* chemically *inert;* arg-amblyopia.

ENERGEIA (ἐνέργεια), *action, energy.* > energ-y; -etic;
-id.

**ERGASIA** (ἐργασία), *work, daily labor.* > id.; ergasio-der-
ma-tosis (of industrial causation); -phobia; cac-ergasia.

**ORGANON** (ὄργανον), *an implement, a tool; an organ of
the body,* Arist.; *a surgical instrument.* H. > an organ;
-acidia; -ic; -ism; organo-genetic; -therapy; etc.

**SYNERGIA** (συνεργία), *co-operation.* > co-ordination;
synerg-ic; -ist; -y; -etic; hemi-a-synergy [a- priv.].

**ERYTH-**

**ERYTHROS** (ἐρυθρός), *red.* > erythr-algia, *painful redness*
of the skin; -emia; -ism, *redness* of hair and complexion;
erythro-blast; etc.

**ERYTHĒMA, -ATOS** (ἐρύθημα), *a redness* or *flush upon
the skin.* H. > id.

**ES-, ET-, HET-**

**HIĒMI,** fut. **HĒSŌ** (ἵημι, ἥσω), *to let go, release; throw.* >
anetic [anetikos, *relaxing,* fr. an-hiĕmi]; aneto-dermia
[anetos, *relaxed*]; apheter [G. *a thrower,* fr. ap-hiĕmi]; catheter [G. *anything let down, catheter; pessary,* fr. kat-hiĕmil];
-ize; -ism; cathetero-stat; paresis [G. *paralysis,* H. fr. par-
iĕmi, *let fall*]; paretic.

**ESOPH-,** see PHAG-

**EST-, OEST-**

**OISTROS** (οἶστρος), *the gadfly; a sting; insane desire.* >
estrus or oestrus, *heat,* the period of sexual excitement in the
female of the lower animals; estru-al; -ation; estro-gen; etc.
an-estrus; pro-.

**ESTH-, AESTH-**

**AISTHĒSIS** (αἴσθησις), *perception* by the senses, *sensation,*
fr. **AISTHANOMAI** (αἰσθάνομαι), *to perceive.* > In compounds *sensation.* esthes-ic; esthesio-gen; -graphy; etc. anesthesia; cin-aesthesia.

**ETH-, AETH-**

**AITHĒR, -EROS** (αἰθήρ), *the upper purer air* (opp. to aēr,
ἀήρ, *the lower air); the sky, heaven.* > ether, aether; ether-eal;
etheri-fication; ethero-bacillin; etc. eth-yl (hylĕ, ὕλη, *substance*); -ylamine; -ylate.

**ETI-, AETI-**

**AITIA** (αἰτία), *a charge, accusation; cause.* > In compounds,
*the cause;* aetio- or etio-logy; -tropic; etc.

**FAC-, FEC-, FIC-**

**FACIO,** pp. **FACTUS,** *to make, build; do, perform.* > fac-tor;
arti-fact; -ficer; -ficial [artificium, *a handicraft*]; cale-facient
[fr. calefacio]; -fier; electri-fy; calcific, *forming a deposit of
lime;* ori-fice; petri-faction; etc. The numerous derivatives of
this verb and its compounds are formed in most cases from
the pp., and less frequently from the present participle. In
prepositional compounds the present becomes -ficio, and the
pp. -fectus, *e.g.* afficio (ad), conficio, deficio, efficio (ex);
inficio; proficio. > affect; -ion; -ive; confect-ion; deficien-cy;
effect, -or; infect; -ion; etc.

**FACILIS,** *easy to do.* > facil-e; -ity; -itation; facult-y [facul-
tas]; -ative.

**FACI-**

**FACIES,** *form, shape, face; appearance.* > countenance; surface; faci-al; facio-brachial; -cervical; fac-et, -ette [thr. Fr.],
*a small smooth area* on a bone.

**FASC-**

**FASCIA,** gen. and pl. -IAE, *a band, fillet; bandage.* > *a sheet
of fibrous tissue* enveloping the body beneath the skin;
*surgical bandage.* fasci-al; -ectomy; fascio-desis [G. desis, *a
binding together*].

**FASCIOLA,** gen. and pl.- -AE (dim. of fascia), *a small
bandage* for the legs. > *a small band of fibers; a genus of flukes;*
Fasciol-opsis.

**FASCIS,** *a bundle of twigs, straw,* or *reeds;* in pl. *a bundle of
rods* and *an ax* carried before the highest magistrates.

**FASCICULUS,** gen. and pl. -I, *a small bundle.* > fascicle,
*a small bundle* of fibers; bot. *a cymose inflorescence;* fascicl-ed;
*growing in a tuft* or *bundle;* fascicul-ar; -ation.

**FEC-1, FAEC-**

**FAEX, FAECIS,** *grounds, dregs, refuse.* > faeces or feces,
*excrement;* fec-al; -ulent; feca-lith.

**DEFAECO,** pp. -atus, *to cleanse from dregs, purify.* > defecate; -ation; -algesiophobia; etc.

**FECULA,** dim. of faex, *burnt tartar,* or *salt of tartar* (deposited in the form of a crust by wine). > starch.

**FEC-2,** see FAC-

**FER-, FERT-**

**FERO,** pp. **LATUS** (irreg. verb), *to bear.* > Chiefly in the
suffix -ferous, *bearing* [fero + Eng. ending -ous]; auri-ferous;
spori-; etc.; and the suffix -fer, the terminal element of nouns
with a corresponding adj. in -ferous, as conifer, *a coniferous
tree.* From compounds of FERO derivatives are formed as
follows: af-fero (adf-) pp. al-latus, *carry to;* au-fero (abf-) pp.
ab-latus, *bear from;* circum-fero, *carry round;* de-, *carry down;*
dif- pp. di-latus, *carry different ways, disperse;* re-fero, *carry
back;* trans-, *carry across.* > afferent; afferentia; ablat-ion;
circumfer-ence; -entia [L.]; defer-ens; -ent; -tial; deferent-
ectomy; -itis; different; -ial; -iation; refer-ence; relative;
transfer; -ence; etc.

**DILATO,** pp. -ATUS, *to spread out, dilate, enlarge* [fr. irreg.
pp. of differo]. > dilatat-ion; dilat-e; -or (short for dilatator).

**FERTILIS,** *fruitful, fertile.* > fertili-zation; -zin.

**FIS-, FID**

**FINDO,** pp. **FISSUS,** perf. **FIDI,** *to cleave, split, divide.* >
fission, *division* of a cell or its nucleus; fission-fungus; fissiparity; Fissi-pedia, *a genus of carnivora with separated toes.*
palmiti-fid; bi-fid [bifidus].

**FISSURA,** gen. and pl. -AE, *a chink, fissure.* > *a cleft, sulcus;*
a fissure; fissur-al; -ed.

**FISTULA,** gen. and pl. -AE, *a tube, a lead water-pipe; a
shepherd's pipe; a kind of ulcer.* Cels. > fistula, *a narrow passage leading from an abscess cavity to the surface,* fistul-ectomy;
etc.

**FLAG-**

**FLAGELLUM,-I,** pl, -A, *a whip; a young branch* or *shoot; the
arm* of a *polypus.* > *a long hairlike process;* Flagell-ata, *a sub
class of Mastigophora;* flagellospore; etc.

**FLAT-**

**FLO,** pp. **FLATUS,** *to blow.* > flatus [L. *a blowing*]; flatulence [Mod. L. flatulentus]; de-flat-e; inflat-e; -ion; insuf-
flat-ion [suf-flo (subf-) pp. -atus, *blow forth, inflate*].

**FLECT-, FLEX-**

**FLECTO,** pp. **FLEXUS,** *to bend.* > flect-ion; flex; -ible; -ion;
-or; re-flex; reflexo-genic; -phile; -therapy; reflect-ion; etc.

**FLEXURA, -AE,** *a bending, flexure.* > id.

**FLU-, FLUX-**

**FLUO,** pp. **FLUXUS** (archaic form **FLUCTUS**), *to flow.* >
con-flu-ence; dif-flu-ence; ef-flu-vium [L.]; in-flu-enza (thr.
Fr. and Sp.); ossi-fluent.

**FLUCTUS, -ŪS,** *a flowing, a wave.* > fluctu-ate; -ation; etc.

**FLUIDUS, -A, -UM,** *flowing, fluid.* > fluid; -ism; fluid-
extractum (Mod. L.); etc.

**FLUOR,** *a flowing, flux.* > fluor-spar; hence, fluor-escein;
-escence; -escin; fluoro-scope; etc.

**FLUXUS, -US.** *a flowing, a flux.* > flux; af-flux; de-; re-;
seri-.

**FOLL-**

**FOLLICULUS,** gen. and pl. -I, *a small bag; shell, skin, follicle.* Dim. of FOLLIS, *a pair of bellows; money-bag.* > a follicle;
follicul-ar; -itis; -oma; etc.

**FOR-**

**FORO,** pp. -ATUS, *to bore, pierce.* > bi-forate; uni-; per-
forat-ion; etc.

**FORAMEN, -INIS,** pl. -INA, *an opening, aperture.* > id;
Foramini-fera, *a subclass of Rhizopoda having anastomosing*
pseudopodia; -ferous, foramin-ulum (Mod. L. dim.).

**FORN-**

**FORNIX, -ICIS,** *an arch* or *vault; a brothel* (situated in
underground vaults). > *a structure of the brain; a vaultlike
space;* forni-column, *the anterior pillar of the cerebral fornix;*
fornic-ate; -ation.

**FRA-**

**FRANGO,** pp. **FRACTUS,** *to break into pieces.* > fract-ure;
-ional; re-fract; re-fract-ion; -ure; -ory; re-frang-ible; *Clos-*

*tridium per-fringens* [per-fringo, *shatter*], *gas bacillus;* saxifrage.

FRAGILIS, *easily broken.* > fragil-e; -ity; fragilo-cyte; -cytosis; etc.

RAGMENTU M, -I, *a piece broken off.* > fragment; fragmentation.

## FUN-, FUS-

FUNDŌ, pp. FUSUS, *to pour; melt;* hence AF-FUNDO (ADF-), *to pour on;* CON-FUNDO, *pour or mix together, confuse;* DIF-FUNDO, *pour forth, diffuse;* EF-FUNDO, *pour out;* IN-; RE-; TRANS-. > fusion; af-fusion; con-; dif-; ef-; in-; infus-ible; -oria; in-fundibulum [L.], *funnel or funnel-like passage* (hence E. funnel); re-fusion; trans-; etc.

## GAL-

GALA, GALAKTOS (γάλα), *milk.* > galactagogue; -idrosis; galacto-blast; -cele; etc. gala-lith; gal-ium, *a plant* (which curdles milk); poly-galact-ia.

## GAM-

GAMOS (γάμος), *marriage* > gam-ont [ōn, ontos, *being*] *a sexual form occurring in the life of some protozoans;* gamo-petalous; -phagia, *disappearance of male or female element in true conjugation;* -phyllous; a-gam-ous; allo-gam-y; crypto-gam.

GAMEŌ (γαμέω), *to marry;* GAMETĒS (γαμέτης), *husband,* GAMETĒ (γαμετή) *wife.* > gamete, *a germ cell;* gameto-blast; -cide; -cinetic; macro-gamete.

## GANGL-

GANGLION (γάγγλιον), *a tumor under the skin.* > *a junction of nerve cells; a cystic swelling* connected with a tendon sheath; *a lymph node;* gangli-al; -ate; gangli-ocyte; ganglion-ectomy; etc.

## GANGR-

GANGRAINA (γάγγραινα), *an eating sore;* fr. GRAŌ (γράω), *to gnaw.* > gangrene, gangren-ous.

## GAST-

GASTĒR, -EROS or -ROS (γαστήρ), 1. *the belly;* 2. *the womb;* 3. *the swelling part* of anything, *the middle or fleshy part* of a muscle. Gal. gaster-hysterotomy; gastr-adenitis; -ic; gastro-cardiac; -cnemius (see meaning 3 above). gastrula (Mod. L. dim. of gastĕr), *the embryo in the stage of development following the blastula.*

## GEN-, GON-

GEN, a root occurring in many G. and L. words with sense of *become, beget, produce.*

GIGNOMAI, fut. GENĒSOMAI (γίγνομαι, γενήσομαι), *to come into being, to be born,* hence, GENESIS (γένεσις), *origin, birth;* GENOS (γένος), *birth, descent.* > gen, gene, *the agent of hereditary transmission of characteristics;* genesi-al; genesio-logy; anthropo-genesis; homo-; etc. Adjs. formed fr. compds. ending in -genesis take the form -genetic.

-GENĒS (-γενής), suffix, actively *producing;* passively *born; produced.* Cf. L. -genus, -gena, fr. root GEN in gigno. > -gen; -gene; -genous; -genic; endo-gen; exo-; hydro-; nitro-; oxy-; phos-gene; homo-genous; crypto-genic; hepato-. The suffix for the corresponding abstract noun is -geny [-GENEIA (-γένεια)] *e.g.,* homogeny; etc.

GONOS (γόνος), *offspring; product* (of plants); *seed; penis.* H. > gon-acratia; gono-cyte; -rrhea; etc. homo-gony; sporo-; sporo-gon-ium, *a sporocarp in mosses.* gon-ad; hence gona-duct (contr. fr. gonad-duct); gonado-gen; -therapy; etc.

GIGNO, pp. GENITUS, *produce, give birth to, beget.* Hence GENUS, -ERIS, *birth, descent, origin;* GENITALIS, *relating to generation or birth.* > genus, *a classification* in natural history between family and species; gener-ic, *relating to a genus;* gener-ate; -ation; -ative; con-gener-ous; de-generate; etc. genital; -alia (ntr. pl.), *the genitals;* con-genital. This root appears also in pre-gn-ant, fr. praegnans, *before birth.*

-GENUS, -GENA, suffix, *producing; produced, born.* See -genĕs above. > -gen; -genous; agglutino-gen; adipo-genous indi-genous [indiginus, *born in*].

## GER-

GĒRAS (γῆρας), *old age.* > geriatrics, gerontology.

## GEST-

GERO, pp. GESTUS, *bear, carry; bring forth, produce.* >

congest-ion; -ine; digest; -ion; -ant; egesta; ingest; -a; -ion; the foregoing fr. the compound verbs con-gero; di-; e-; in-.

## GLAN-

GLANS, GLANDIS, *an acorn; any acorn-shaped fruit; glans penis.* Cels. > *a gland; a goiter;* bot. *a nut.*

GLANDULAE, -ARUM (pl. only; dim. of glans), *the glands of the throat,* called also tonsillae; *enlarged tonsils.* Cels. > glandules, *small glands;* glandul-ar; glanduli-form.

## GLI-

GLIA (γλία), *glue* > *the neuro-glia;* glia-cyte; glio-bacteria, *bacilli in a gluelike mass;* -coccus; -ma, *a tumor formed of neuroglia cells.*

GLISCHROS (γλίσχρος), *glutinous, sticky* > glischr-in, *a mucin-like substance* formed by the Bacillus glischro-genes; glischr-uria.

## GLO-

GLOBUS, *a round body, a ball.* GLOBULUS, dim. *a little ball.* > globule, *a small spherical body,* specif. *a cell of the blood or lymph;* globuli-cide; -ferous; etc. hemo-globin.

GLOMERUS, -ERIS, *a ball* (of thread, yarn, etc.). > *a small rounded swelling,* composed of minute blood vessels.

GLOMERULUS (Mod. L. dim. of glomus). > *a plexus of capillaries;* glomerul-ar; -itis; glomerulo-nephritis; etc.

## GNO-

GIGNŌSKŌ, fut. GNŌSOMAI (γιγνώσκω), *to discern, know;* GNŌSIS (γνῶσις), *knowledge,* > gnosia, *perceptive faculty,* agnosia [G. ignorance]; ana-gnos-asthenia; dia-gnosis [G.]; pro-; physio-.

GNŌMŌN, -ONOS (γνώμων), *a judge, interpreter.* > physio-gnomy; pathognom-ic [pathognōmonikos, *skilled in judging of symptoms or diseases.* Gal.]; etc.

GON-, see GEN-

## GON-, GONY-

GONY, -ATOS (γόνυ), *the knee* [cf. L. genu, knee]. > gon-agra; gonato-cele; gony-oncus; etc.

## GRAM-, GRAPH-

GRAPHŌ (γράφω), *to scratch; write,* GRAMMA, -ATOS (γράμμα), *something written, a document.* > graph; -ite; grapho-logy; -spasm, *writer's cramp.* The suffix -graph originally had the sense of *something written,* as autograph, photograph. In words of more recent formation it has an active sense, *i.e., something that writes,* as helio-graph, cardio-graph.

## GYN-

GYNĒ, GYNAIKOS (γυνή) [Gen *q.v.*], *a woman; the female, mate,* of animals. > In compounds, *woman, female;* in bot. *the female parts of a flower or plant.* gyn-android; -androus; -ase, *a hypothet. substance determining femaleness in heredity;* -atresia; gyneco-gen; -logist; gyne-phobia; gyno-pathy; -phore, *the stalk of the female organ* of a flower. andro-gyne; -gynous; -gyny; poly-gynous, *having many pistils,* bot.

## HAB-, HIB-

HABEO, pp. HABITUS, *to have, hold.* hence, HABITUS (noun), *the condition or state* of a thing; *habit; appearance.* > habit; habitus, *the general characteristic appearance* of the body.

HABITO, pp. -ATUS, *to dwell in a place.* > habitat (lit. *it inhabits) the place where an animal or plant lives in nature.*

COHABITO, pp. -ATUS, *to dwell together,* > cohabit-ation, *a living together; sexual intercourse.*

INHIBEO, pp. -ITUS, *to lay hold of; restrain.* > inhibit; -ion; -or; inhib-in.

HABENA, *that by which a thing is held; a strap.* > *a restricting fibrous band; restraining bandage.*

HABENULA, (dim. of prec.) *a small strip* of diseased flesh cut from the body. Cels. > *a restraining band; peduncle of the pineal body.*

## HAEM-, HEM-, -EM-

HAIMA, -ATOS, (αἷμα, -ατος), *blood.* > haem- or hem-al; haem- or hem-agogue; hema-facient; -therapy; hemo-plastic; hemat-encephalon; hemati-meter; hemato-blast; etc. hydr-em-ia; ur-em-ia; etc.

## HAP-, AP-

HAPTŌ, fut. HAPSŌ (ἅπτω, ἅψω), *to fasten to, lay hold of, grasp.* > hapt-in; hapto-phil; -phore; peri-apt. *an amulet* [periapton, id.]; syn-apsis [G. *a binding together*].

**HAPHĒ** (ἀφή), *a touching, touch.* > haph-algesia; haphe-phobia; di-aphe-metric, *relating to the degree of tactile sensibility;* dys-aphia; -aphic.

**HAPSIS** (ἄψις), *a touching.* > chir-apsia; par-; etc.

**HELIC-**

HELIX, -IKOS, (ἕλιξ, -ικος), *anything which assumes a spiral shape, the convolution* of a shell; *the tendril* of ivy. HELIKĒ (ἑλίκη) *a winding; the convolution* of a shell. fr. HELISSŌ (ἑλίσσω) *to turn round.* > helix, *the margin of the auricle;* helic-ine; helico-pepsin, *a ferment extracted from snails;* -podia, *a gait in which the foot drags and describes a curve.*

**HELM-**

HELMINS, -INTHOS (ἕλμυς, -ινθος), *an intestinal worm,* either flat, plateia, or round, strongylē. H. > helminth; -agogue; -iasis; -ic; helmintho-logy; -phobia. Platy-helmintha, *a class of Vermes;* nema-; an-helminth-ic.

**HEPAT-**

HĒPAR, -ATOS (ἧπαρ, -ατος), *the liver.* > id.; hepat-auxe (auxē, *enlargement);* hepato-cele; etc.

HEPATIKOS (ἡπατικός), *of the liver.* > hepatic; hepatico-tomy, *incision into the hepatic duct;* hepatic-a, *liverwort* (from the shape of its leaves).

**HERM-**

HERMĒS ('Ερμῆς), *the messenger and interpreter of the gods;* the god of the arts and sciences, and later of alchemy when identified with Hermes Trismegistus (thrice greatest), the Egyptian god Thoth. > herm-etic, *airtight (i.e.,* chemically sealed); *pertaining to Hermes, alchemy, chemistry.*

HERMAPHRODITOS ('Ερμαφρόδιτος) *son of Hermes and Aphrodite; a person having characteristics of both sexes.* (Hermaphroditus is said to have become united in one body with the nymph Salmacis while bathing in her fountain). > a hermaphrodit-e, 1. *androgyne;* 2. bot. *a flower with pistil and stamen in the same calyx;* -ism; hermaphrod-ism.

**HERN-**

HERNIA, gen. and pl. -AE, *a rupture, hernia.* Cels. > id.; herni-al; -ation; herniology; etc.

**HET-, see ES-**

**HETER-**

HETEROS (ἕτερος), *other; different;* sometimes with a bad sense = kako-. > heteradelphus; -adenic; hetero-cellular; -lalia; etc.

**HEX-, see ECT-**

**HIPP-**

HIPPOS (ἵππος), *a horse;* in medicine *a complaint of the eyes* such that they are always winking. (H. quoted by Cels.); in compounds often anything *large or coarse, cf.* Eng. horse-chestnut, horseplay. > hippus, *spasmodic movements of the iris* (suggesting galloping of a horse—see above); hipp-iatry; -uric, *relating to urine of horses;* hippo-camp or -campus (hippokampos, *a sea-horse,* fr. h. + kampos, *a sea monster), a raised curved track* on the floor of the lateral ventricle of the brain (so called from its supposed resemblance to the sea-horse); -castanum, *horse-chestnut.*

**HIST-**

HISTOS (ἱστός), *anything set upright; the mast* of a ship; *the beam* of the loom; *the warp* fixed to the loom; *the web; spider's web;* fr. HISTĒMI (ἵστημι), *to set up.* See STA- > In anat. *tissue;* histoblast, *a tissue cell;* -chemistry; -logist; -oma. HISTION (ἱστίον,), *web, cloth; a sail;* dim. of histos. > In compounds also has meaning of *tissue;* histion-ic; histio-cyte; etc.

**HOD-, -OD**

HODOS (ὁδός), *a way, path; a way, manner, method.* > hodo-neuromere; cat-hode [kathodos, *a way down];* cines-od-ic, *pertaining to the path by which motor impulses travel;* met-hod [methodos, fr. meta, *after* + hodos]; peri-od [periodos, *a going round, a cycle, a period];* photoperiod; gastro-periodynia.

HODAIOS (ὁδαῖος), *on the way.* > proct-odaeum; stom-.

**HOM-, -OM-**

HOMOS (ὁμός), *one and the same, common.*

HOMOIOS (ὅμοιος) *like, resembling.* > hom-odont; homo-gony; etc. homeo- or homeo-pathy; -stasis; etc. ANŌMALOS

(ἀνώμαλος), *uneven,* fr. an- priv. + homalos *even,* > anom-al-y; -ous; anomalo-trophy, *abnormality in the nutritive processes.*

**HUM-**

UMERUS (often incorrectly spelled humerus), *the upper arm, shoulder; the bone* of the upper arm. Cels. > the humerus humer-al; humero-ulnar; etc.

**HYDR-**

HYDŌR, -ATOS (ὕδωρ), *water;* combining form HYDR-, HYDRO- (ὑδρ-, ὑδρο-) > hydro- (before a vowel hydr-)—1. *water.* 2. when combined with the name of a part of the body or a disease it denotes an accumulation of *serous fluid* or a *dropsical condition.* 3. prefixed to names of minerals it denotes a *hydrous compound.* 4. in chem. compounds it usually represents *hydrogen.* hydro-therapy; -myelia; -cyanic; hydremia; etc.

HYDATIS, -IDOS (ὑδατίς, -ιδος), *a drop of water; a watery vesicle, a hyatid.* Gal. > a hydatid, *an echinococcus cyst; a vesicular structure;* hydatidi-form; hydatido-cele.

HYDRARGYROS (ὑδράργυρος), *fluid silver, quicksilver.* > hydrargyrum, *quick silver;* hydrargyria, *mercurial poisoning.*

HYDRŌPS, -ŌPOS (ὕδρωψ, -ωπος), *dropsy.* > hydrops-y (of which the word dropsy is a contraction).

**HYGR-**

HYGROS (ὑγρός), *moist, fluid.* > hygro-meter; -phobia; -stomia; etc.

**HYL-, -YL**

HYLĒ (ὕλη), *forest woodland; wood cut down, timber; material.* hylē iatrikē or hylē (alone), *materia medica.* Gal. > In compounds generally in the sense of *matter, material,* and *pulp tissues;* hyl-ic; hyl-oma, *a pulp tumor;* etc. -yl, a common terminal denoting a *monovalent hydrocarbon radical.*

**HYST-1**

HYSTERA (ὑστέρα), *the womb; the ovary* of animals. HYSTERIKOS (ὑστερικός), *suffering in the womb; hysterical,* H.; *relating to the womb.* > In compounds hyster-, hystero- has the sense of 1. *the uterus;* 2. *hysteria.* hyster-algia; -ectomy; -ia; hystero-erotic hysteric-ism; hysterico-neuralgic; etc.

**HYST-2**

HYSTEROS (ὕστερος), *later, following.* > hystero-systole, *delayed contraction* of the heart; hysteresis [G. *a coming later].*

**IATR-, IATRO-**

IATROS (ἰατρός), *physician, surgeon.* > iatro-genic; ped-iatrics; ger-iatrics; psych-iatry.

**ICHOR**

ICHŌR (ἰχώρ), *ichor, the etherial juice* that flows in the veins of the gods instead of blood; *the watery part* of animal juices; *a discharge, matter.* H. > ichor, *the thin watery discharge* from an ulcer; -ous; -rhea; etc.

**ICHTH-**

ICHTHYS (ἰχθύς), *a fish.* > ichth-ermol; ichtho-form; ichthy-ism; ichthyo-toxin.

**IDIO-**

IDIOS (ἴδιος), *one's own, private, peculiar, distinct.* IDIŌTĒS (ἰδιώτης), *a private citizen; one with no special knowledge, a rough, uncouth fellow.* > idio-muscular; -gamist; -crasy; -syncrasy; etc. idiot; idiocy.

**INGUI-**

INGUEN, -INIS, *the front part of the body between the hips and the groin.* > id.; inguin-al; inguino-scrotal; etc.

**INI-, INO-**

IS, INOS (ἴς), *muscle;* (later) *the fibrous vessels in the muscles.* > In compounds, *muscular tissue* or *fiber;* ino-tropic; -lith, *a concretion formed in fibrous tissue;* -ma; inos-itis; etc.

INION (ἰνίον), *the muscle between the occiput and the back.* Arist. (dim. of is, inos). > *the occipital protuberance.* ini-encephalus; ini-ad; inio-pagus.

**INSUL-**

INSULA, gen. and pl. -AE, *an island.* > 1. *island of Reil.* 2. *any circumscribed body,* or *patch* on the skin; insul-ar; -ate; -ator; -in (ref. islands of Langerhans); hence insulino-genic, or insulo-genic, etc.

**IRIS, IRID-**

IRIS, -IDOS ('Ἴρις, -ιδος), *the messenger of the gods, and goddess of the rainbow; any bright colored circle,* as the halo round the moon, *the iris* of the eye. Gal.; *the plant Iris (I. germanica).* > the iris *of the eye; a genus of plants;* ir-itis; ir-itic (iritis + -ic); irid-al; -algia; -escent; -ic; irido-constrictor; etc.

**ISCH-**

ISCHŌ (ἴσχω), *to hold back.* See ECT-. > isch-esis, *suppression of any discharge;* -idrosis; ischo-galactic; etc. an-isch-uria.

**ISCHI-**

ISCHION (ἰσχίον), *the hip joint;* (in later anat.) *the projecting part of the os innominatum* upon which man rests when sitting. Gal. > ischium, -ii. pl. -ia (Mod. L.), *the inferior part of the os innominatum;* ischio-cele; -coccygeal; etc.

ISCHIAS, -ADOS (ἰσχιάς) *pain in the hip.* H. > id.; ischi-ad-ic.

**-ITIS**

-ITIS (ῖτις), fem. ending of adjs. in -ITĒS (-ίτης), *pertaining to; e.g.,* rhach-ites, fem. -itis (ῥαχίτης -ῖτις), *pertaining to the spine;* qualifying the fem. noun nosos (νόσος), *disease* (understood), rhachitis means *spine disease* or *rickets;* so too arthritis (ἀρθρῖτις) *joint disease;* and nephritis (νεφρῖτις) *kidney disease, renal calculus.* > In mod. medicine -itis has come to mean, in most cases, *inflammation of;* appendic-itis; nephr-; etc.

**JAC-, JEC-**

JACIO, pp. JACTUS, *throw, hurl.* JACTO, pp. JACTATUS, *to throw, hurl; to toss about.* > jactat-ion, jact-itation, *a tossing about in bed.* (The last word is formed fr. verb jactito, though its meaning is, *to bring forward in public, to utter.*)

JACULUM, *a dart, javelin.* > jaculiferous, *covered with sharp points.* EJACULO, pp. -ATUS, *hurl out.* > ejaculatio; ejaculat-ion.

DEJICIO, pp. -JECTUS, *to cast down.* > dejection, *depression; feces;* dejecta.

EJICIO, pp. -JECTUS, *cast out.* > ejecta, *egesta,* dejecta. INJICIO, pp. -JECTUS, *to throw in.* > inject; -ion. SUBJICIO, pp. -JECTUS, *to throw* or *lay under* or *near.* > subject; -ive; subjecto-scope.

**JEJ-**

JEJUNUS, -A, -UM, *fasting, hungry; dry, barren.* > jejunum (ntr. of j. so called because it was supposed to be empty after death), *a portion of the small intestine.* jejun-al; jejuno-tomy; etc.

**JUNC-, JUG-**

JUNGO, pp. JUNCTUS, *to join together, unite; harness;* of wounds, *bring together.* JUNCTURA, *a joining; a joint.* > junctura; juncture. CONJUNGO, pp. -JUNCTUS, *bind together; unite.* CONJUNCTIVUS, -A, -UM, *serving to connect, connective.* > conjunctiva (fem. tunica, *a coat* understood) the membrane which lines the inner surface of the eyelids and *conjoins* the lids and the eyeball; conjunctiv-al; -itis; -oma; -iplasty.

JUGUM, -I, pl. -A, *a yoke* for oxen, *a collar* for horses; *a yoke, bond; a ridge of land connecting two points, a height.* > In anat. *a ridge connecting two points.* jug-al; jugo-maxillary; etc.

JUGO, pp. -ATUS, *to join; marry.* hence CONJUGO, *to unite.* > conjugate, *yoked* or *coupled;* conjugat-ion, *sexual union of two cells.*

JUGULUM, -I, p. -A, *the collar bone,* which joins together the shoulders and the breast. Cels.; *the hollow part of the neck above the collar bone, the throat.* > *the neck, throat;* jugul-ar.

JUGULO, -ATUS, *to cut the throat, slay; to confute, silence; drive away.* > jugulation, *the arrest of a disease.*

JUXTA, adv. and prep., *adjoining, near to.* > juxta-position.

**K,** see C

**LAB-, LEPS-, LEPT-**

LAMBANŌ (λαμβάνω), fut. LĒPSOMAI (λήψομαι), infinitive, LABEIN (λαβεῖν), *to take hold of, receive.* LABIS, -IDOS (λαβίς), *a handle, holder; a forceps.* H. > labido-meter; labi-tome, *a forceps with sharp blades.*

LĒPSIS (λῆψις), *a taking, seizing; an attack* of fever or

sickness, *a seizure.* H. > cata-lepsy [katalepsis]; epi-; hypno-; psycho-; syl-lepsis (see under syllambanō).

LĒPTIKOS (ληπτικός), *disposed to accept; assimilative.* > ana-leptic [analeptikos, *restorative*]; anti-; organo-; pro- (proleptikos, *anticipative*]; etc. As a suffix -leptic is the adj. form of -lepsis or -lepsy, *e.g.* cata-leptic; epi-.

SYLLAMBANŌ, fut. -LĒPSOMAI (συλλαμβάνω), *take and bring together, collect; seize.* > syllab-le [syllabē, *a taking together* (of letters)]; a-syllabia; dys- [dys- *difficult*]; syllabus [L. fr Gr.); syllepsis [G. *pregnancy*].

**LABYR-**

LABYRINTHOS (λαβύρινθος), *a labyrinth, a maze; a building with many winding passages, e.g.,* that built in middle Egypt, and later, that built near Gnossus in Crete; *any coiled up body.* > labyrinth, *the internal ear; a labyrinth-like structure;* -ine; -itis; etc.

**LACT-**

LAC, LACTIS, *milk; the milky juice of plants.* > lact-ase; -ation; -escence; lacti-morbus, *milk sickness;* lacto-cele; etc. LACTUCA, *lettuce* (so called fr. its milky juice). > Lactuca, *a genus of plants;* lactucarium, *the dried milk-juice of L. virosa;* lactuc-in, *a bitter principle* derived from the preceding. The Eng. word lettuce is a corrupted form of l.

**LAEV-,** see LEV.

**LAL-**

LALEŌ (λαλέω), *talk, chatter, babble; talk, say.* > lalo-pathy, *speech defect;* -phobia; etc. a-lalia.

LALLO, pp. -ATUS, *to sing a lullaby.* > lall-ing; -ation, *a form of stammering.*

**LARV-**

LARVA, -AE, *a ghost, specter; a mask.* fr. Lares, *tutelary deities, household gods.* > *the wormlike form of an insect* on issuing from the egg; *the early form of any animal, which during its development is unlike its parent,* "because the larval stage of an insect *masks* the true character of the species," Linnaeus; larv-ate; larvi-cide; etc.

**LEC-**

LEKITHOS (λέκιθος,), *the yolk of an egg.* H. > lecith-in; lecitho-protein.

**LEN-**

LENS, LENTIS, *a lentil.* > a lens (so called because shaped like a split lentil); *the crystalline lens of the eye;* lenti-conus; -form.

LENTICULA, -AE (dim. of lens), *a lentil; a lentil shape; freckles.* > *the lenticular nucleus; a freckle.*

LENTICULARIS, *like a lentil; lentil-shaped.* > lenticular, *resembling a lens.*

LENTIGO, -INIS, *a lentil-shaped spot; freckles.* > id.; lentigin-ous.

**LEP-**

LEPŌ, fut. LEPSŌ (λέπω), *to strip off the rind or husks.* LEPIS, -IDOS (λεπίς), *a scale, rind, husk.* > lepid-ic, *relating to a lining membrane of the embryo;* -oma, *rind tumor;* -ine, *scaly;* -osis, *a scaly eruption.*

LEPOS (λέπος), *rind, husk.* > lepo-cyte, *a cell with a distinct envelope;* -thrix; etc.

LEPROS, -A, -ON (λεπρός,), *scaly, rough; leprous,* hence LEPRA (λέπρα), *the leprosy.* H. > lepro-sy; -tic; -phobia; -logy; etc.

LEPTOS (λεπτός), *peeled, husked; thin, fine, slender.* > lepto-dermic; -phonia, *weakness* of voice; etc. kerato-leptynsis [leptynō, *make thin*].

LEMMA (λέμμα), *that which is peeled off, scale, husk.* > lemm-itis; lemmo-cyte; axi-lemma; neuri-, *sheath of Schwann;* neuro- an old term for *the retina.*

**LEPS-,** see LAB-, LEPT-

**LEV-**

LAEVUS, -A, -UM, *left, on the left side.* > levo-duction; etc.

**LIG-**

LIGO, pp. -ATUS, *to tie; bandage; bind together, unite.* > lig-ate; -ation; -ator.

LIGAMENTUM, -I, pl. -A, *a band, tie, bandage.* > ligament, *a band of fibrous tissue* connecting two or more bones; *a band-like structure.*

**LIGATURA**, gen. and pl. -AE, *a band, ligature.* > id.

**LING-, LIG-**

**LINGUA**, gen. and pl. -AE, *the tongue.* > id.; *a tonguelike structure;* lingu-al; linguo-distal; etc.

**LINGULA** or **LIGULA**, gen. and pl. -AE (dim. of lingua) *a little tongue; a tonguelike object.* > lingula, *a tongue-shaped process or structure.* ligula, *a small tongue-shaped structure; the strip of white matter* on the margin of the fourth ventricle (note diff. meanings for two forms of same Latin word).

**LITH-**

**LITHOS** (λίθος), *a stone; a stone in the bladder, calculus.* H. > lith-agogue; litho-logy; lith-ium, *an alkaline metallic element;* -arge (argyros, silver), *lead oxide.*

**LOG-**

**LOGOS** (λόγος), *word, speech, discourse, reason,* fr. LEGŌ (λέγω), *speak, say.* -LOGIA (-λογια), -LOGOS (-λογος), suffixes equiv. to Eng. -logy or -logue (which usu. comes thr. the Fr.) > log-agraphia; -agnosia, *aphasia;* logo-pathy; -plegia; -rrhea; hemato-logy, *science of the blood;* neuro-; oto-; etc.; ana-logue; mono-; etc. Note that carphology (*q.v.* in dict.) is fr. G. verb legō, *pick up*).

**LOPH-**

**LOPHOS** (λόφος), *the back of the neck* of draught-cattle where it is rubbed [lepō *q. v.*]; *crest or tuft* on the head of birds; *tuft of hair.* > lopho-comi, *negroids having tufted hair;* -trichous; ecto-loph.

**LY-, LYS-**

**LYŌ**, fut. LYSŌ (λύω), *to loosen, unfasten; loose, set free, dissolve, break up; destroy.*

**LYSIS** (λύσις), *a setting free; dissolution; remission of a fever.* Gal. > lys-in. *a specific antibody which acts destructively on cells and tissues;* -emia; lyso-zyme. As a suffix, -lysis, *a setting free or a separation;* apo-lysis [G. *a release*]; cata- [G.]; dia- [G. *a separating*]; hydro-; para- [G.]; etc.

**LYTOS** (λυτός), *that may be loosed; soluble.* > actino-lyte; anodo-; electro-; etc.

**LYMPH-**

**LYMPHA**, -AE, *water,* esp. *clear spring water.* > lymph; -aden; -agogue; lympho-cyst; etc.

**MAG-, MANG-**

**MAGNĒSIA** (Μαγνησία), *a region in Thessaly.* MAGNĒS, -ĒTOS (Μάγνης, -ητος), fem. MAGNĒTIS, -IDOS (Μαγνῆτις, -ιδος), *Magnesian.* LITHOS MAGNĒTIS, *the Magnesian stone,* meaning, 1. *a loadstone, magnet.* 2. *a silver-like mineral,* probably *talc.* > magnesia; magnesium [thr. L.]; magnet; -ization; magneto-therapy; etc.

**MANGANESIUM**, a mod. L. corrupted form of magnesium. > manganum; manganese; per-mangan-ate.

**MAL-, MALI-**

**MALUS**, -A, -UM, *bad.* > mal-nutrition; malo-plasty; etc. malaria [thr. Ital. mal'aria fr. L. m. + aer, *air;* formerly believed to be of miasmic origin]; malinger (thr. Fr. L. m. + aeger, *sick*).

**MALIGNUS**, *wicked, malign.* [fr. m. + root GEN, *q.v.*] > malign; -ant; -ancy.

**MALAC-, MALAG-**

**MALAKOS** (μαλακός), *soft, gentle.* MALAKIA (μαλακία), *softness; effeminacy.* > malacia, *a softening* of the tissues; malaco-tomy, *incision of soft parts;* etc.

**MALASSŌ**, fut, -XŌ (μαλάσσω, -ξω), *to soften.* Hence MALAGMA (μάλαγμα) *an emollient, a poultice.* > id.; amalgam (thr. Fr.); amalgam-ate. MALAXIS (μάλαξις), *a softening.* > der-malaxia.

**MALAXO**, *to soften.* > malax-ation.

**MANGA-**, see MAG-

**MANI-1**

**MANIA** (μανία), *madness; enthusiasm.* > id.; mania-c; -cal. As suffix, -mania: clepto-; mono-; etc.

**MANI-2, MANU-**

**MANUS**, gen. and pl. -ŪS, *hand.* > maniphalanx; manu-al; -dynamometer.

**MANIPULUS** [fr. m. + pleo, *to fill, a handful.*] > id.; manipul-ation.

**MANUBRIUM**, -I, pl. -A, *a handle.* > *the upper piece of the sternum; the handle* of the malleus; manubri-ate; -al.

**MARA-, MARC-**

**MARAINŌ**, fut. MARANŌ (μαραίνω), *to put out fire; to make wither.* MARANSIS or MARASMOS (μάρανσις or μαρασμός) Gal. *a dying away; decay.* MARANTIKOS (μαραντικός) *wasting away.* > maransis; marantic; marasmus; -ic; -oid. a-maranth [a- priv. *i.e., never fading*].

**MARCEO**, *wither;* hence MARCESCO, pres. part. MARESCENS, -ENTIS, *to pine away; decay.* MARCIDUS, *withered.* MARCOR, *a withering.* > marcescent, bot. applied to leaves; marcid, *wasting away;* marcor = G. marasmos.

**MAT-, METR-**

**MĒTRA** (μήτρα), *the womb,* H.; *the entrance to the womb,* Arist. > *the womb;* metrypertrophia; metro-scope; etc.

**MATER**, -TRIS (= G. mētōr, *the maker; the mother*), *mother.* MATERNUS, *relating to a mother.* > matern-al; -ity.

**MATRIX**, -ICIS, pl. -ICES, *a breeding animal; the parent stem* of plants; *the womb; source, origin.* > *the womb; formative portion of tooth or nail;* matrix-itis, *inflammation of the nail bed;* matri-caria, *wild chamomile* (so called fr. supposed medicinal value).

**MATERIA**, -AE, or **MATERIES**, -EI, *matter, material of which anything is made; timber; matter, pus.* Cels. > materia medica; materies morbi, *the substance acting as the immediate cause of the disease.*

**MEA-**

**MEO**, pp. MEATUS, *to go, pass.* hence, MEATUS, gen. and pl. -ŪS, *a going, passing; a passage.* > *a passage or canal; an external opening;* meat-al; meato-tome; etc.

**PERMEO**, pp. -ATUS, *to go or pass through, penetrate.* PERMEABILIS, *that can be passed through. passable.* > permeation; permeable; im-.

**MED-**

**MEDIUS**, *middle, mid-,* > medio-tarsal; medi-cornu; etc. medium (ntr. of m.). mediastinum, *a septum between two parts of an organ or cavity* [Mod. L. use; ntr. of mediastinus, lit. *in the middle,* in L. use, *a servant; an assistant.*]

**MEDULLA**, -AE, *the marrow* of bones; *the pith* of plants. > *marrow; any marrow-like substance,* esp. in the center. medullation; medullo-blast; etc.

**MEG-**

**MEGAS**, gen. MEGALOS (μέγας), *great, strong.* > megacardia; megalo-cardia; cardia-megaly (diff. forms with same meaning); mega-cephalic; megalo-gastria; etc.

**MEIO-**, see MIO-

**MEL-1**

**MEL, MELLIS,** honey. MELLITUS, -A, -UM, *of honey; honey-.* > mel, 1. *honey;* 2. *a preparation with honey as the excipient;* mellitum (ntr.), same as mel-2; molasses (formerly melasses fr. mellaceus, *honey-like*).

**MELI**, -ITOS (μέλι), *honey.* MELISSA (μέλισσα), *a bee,* > meli-cera; -lotus; melit-agra; -uria. melisso-phobia; etc., hydro-mel; oxy-.

**MEL-2**

**MĒLON** (μῆλον), *an apple; any tree fruit; the cheeks* (L. malae). > mel-itis, *inflammation of the cheeks;* melono-plasty. camo- or chamo-mile [thr. Mediev. L. fr. chamaimēlon. (χαμαίμηλόν), *the earth-apple,* from the apple-like smell of the flowers]; hama-melis *witch-hazel* [G.].

**MEL-3**

**MELOS** (μέλος), *a limb.* > mel-algia; melo-plasty; etc.

**MEL-4**

**MELOS** (μέλος), *a song.* > melo-mania.

**MELAN-, MELEN-**

**MELAS**, fem. **MELAINA**, ntr. **MELAN** (μέλας, μέλαινα, μέλαν) *black.* > mela-leuca; melan-cholia; melena or melaena. (fem.), *black stool* or *vomit;* melen-emesis; melanocyte; -sis [G.]; calo-mel [kalos, *beautiful*].

**MELASMA** (μέλασμα), *a black or livid spot.* H. > *a patchy pigmentation* of the skin.

**MEN-, MENS-**

**MĒN, MĒNOS** (μήν), *a month.* MĒNĒ (μήνη), *the moon.* > meno-, in most compounds refers to the *menses.* menopause; -rrhagia; etc. cata-menia; em-menia [em-menios, *monthly* fr. en + mĕn]; em-men-agogue; xeno-menia; etc.

**MĒNISKOS** (μηνίσκος dim. of μήνη), *a crescent; any crescent-shaped body.* > meniscus, *a type of lens; a fibro-cartilage of crescent shape.* menisc-itis; menisco-cyte, *a crescent cell;* etc.

**MENSIS, -IS,** pl. -ES, *a month;* (in pl.) *the menses.* MENSTRUO, *to be menstruant.* > the menses; menstru-ate; -ation.

**MENSTRUUS, -A, -UM,** *monthly.* MENSTRUA (ntr. pl. as noun) *the menses.* Cels. > menstruum [Mediev. L.] *a solvent.*

**MENIN-**

MĒNINX, -INGOS (μῆνιγξ), *any membrane,* (of the eye; the drum of the ear; but mostly that enclosing the brain. H.). > *any membrane,* specif. *one of the membranous coverings of the brain and spinal cord.* mening-eal; -itis; meningo-cele; etc.

**METRA-,** see MAT-

**MIO-, MEIO-**

MEIŌN (μείων), *lesser, less* (irreg. comparative of mikros, *small*). > meio- or mio-cardia, *systole;* -pragia; mion-exia [hexis, *habit of body*], *lessened organic resistance;* miosis [G. meiosis, *a lessening*]; mio-tic.

**MIST-, MIX-**

MISCEO, pp. MIXTUS or MISTUS, *to mix, mingle.* MISTURA or MIXTURA, *a mixing,* > mixtura, *a pharmacopeial preparation;* mixture.

MIXIS (μίξις), *a mixing, mingling; sexual intercourse;* fr. MIGNYMI, fut. MIXŌ (μίγνυμι), *to mingle.* > mixo-variation, *transformation in the constitutional germ plasm;* -scopy. pan-mixia.

**MNEM-, MNES-**

MIMNĒSKŌ, fut. MNĒSŌ (μιμνήσκω), *to remind,* in passive *to remember.* MNĒMĒ (μνήμη), *memory,* (in compds. mnēsi-, μνησι-). MNEMON, *mindful.* > mnem-asthenia; -ic; -ism. mnemon-ic; mnemo-technics. a-mnesia [G.]; -mnesic; dys-mnesia; para-; pseudo-; cata-mnesis.

**MOB-,** see MOV-

**MOLAR-**

MOLA, *a mill;* pl. *a jawbone; the teeth;* MOLARIS, *relating to a grinding mill; a grinder, molar* (dens, understood). > molar; molari-form.

**MOLEC-, MOLI-**

MOLES, *a shapeless, huge, heavy mass; a massive structure, a mole; greatness, power.* MOLECULA, -AE, Mod. L. dim. of moles. > a molecul-e; -ar. molimen [L. *a great effort*].

**MOLL-**

MOLLIS, *soft, delicate.* cf. G. malakos. > moll-in; mollities (L. *softness*), *a softening, malacia;* e-mollient.

MOLLUSCUS, -A, -UM, *soft;* MOLLUSCA (f.), *a kind of soft nut with a thin shell;* MOLLUSCUM (ntr.), *a fungus that grows on a maple tree.* > molluscum, *a disease marked by soft round tumors* of the skin; mollusca (ntr. pl.) *one of the leading divisions of invertebrate animals;* mollusc.

**MORB-**

MORBUS, *sickness, disease; grief, distress.* > morbi-fic; -genous.

MORBIDUS, *sickly, diseased.* > morbid; -ity.

MORBILLI, *measles* (Mediev. L. dim. of morbus.) > id.

**MORPH-**

MORPHĒ (μορφή), *form, shape.* > morphea or -aea, *circumscribed scleroderma;* morpho-genesis; -sis (G.); -phyly; etc. a-morphous; anthropo-; di-; hetero-; iso-; etc. meta-morph-osis.

MORPHEUS, *the god of dreams,* so called because of the forms he calls up before the sleeper. First mentioned by Ovid, the word being formed as if from a G. Morpheus (Μορφεύς), from morphē (μορφή). > morph-ina [Mod. L.]; -ine; morphinomania.

**MOV-, MOT-, MOB-**

MOVEO, pp. MOTUS, *move, set in motion.* hence, MOTUS, *a motion.* MOTOR, *a mover;* MOTIO, -ONIS, *a moving.* MOBILIS, *movable.* > move-ment; mov-able; mot-ile; -ility;

moto-facient; motor; -graphic; motor-ium, *the center for motor impulses in the brain;* -ius, *a motor nerve;* -pathy; motion; e-motion; mobil-e; -ity; -ize; im-mob-ile.

**MUSC-**

MUSCA, gen. and pl. -AE, *a fly.* > id.; musca-rine, *an alkaloid found in the fly-agaric* (a poisonous mushroom); muscicide; mosquito (Sp. dim. of mosca fr. musca).

**MUSCU-, MUSCL-, MY-**

MUS, MURIS, *a mouse;* hence, MUSCULUS, gen. and pl. -I (dim. of mus), *a little mouse; a sea-mussel; a muscle of the body.* Cels. > muscle; muscul-ation; -in; musculo-phrenic.

MYS, MYOS (μῦς), *a mouse; a sea-mussel; a muscle of the body.* H. > In compounds, muscle. my-algia; -asthenia; myo-cele; -lysis; etc.

**MY-, MYO-,** see under MUSCU-

**MYC-**

MYKĒS, -ĒTOS (μύκης, -ητος), *a mushroom.* > mycelium [hĕlos, *a nail*]; mycet-hemia; -oma; myco-phylaxin; etc. Actino-myces; blasto-mycet-es; strepto-myc-in; etc.

**MYEL-**

MYELOS (μυελός), *marrow; the pith* of plants. > myel, *the spinal cord;* as a prefix myel-, myelo- refers either 1. to the *spinal cord,* 2. or to *bone marrow.* myel-in; -itis, *inflammation of the spinal cord,* or *the bone marrow;* myelo-plast; -plegia; etc.

**MYI-**

MYIA (μυῖα), *a fly* > myi-asis; -osis; myiocephalon *protrusion of the iris through a wound in the cornea,* so called from its resemblance to the head of a fly; myiodesopsia, *the condition in which muscae volitantes* (dancing flies or spots) *are seen* [myiōdēs, *like flies*].

**MYL-**

MYLĒ (μύλη), *a mill,* in pl. MYLAI (μύλαι), *the grinders, molar teeth.* > myl-abris [G. *a cockroach found in mills*]; mylo-hyoid; litho-myl, *an instrument for crushing a calculus.* AMYLON (ἄμυλον), *fine meal, starch;* ntr. of amylos (ἄμυλος), *especially ground, not at the common mill* [a-priv. + mylĕ]. > In compounds usually *starch;* amyl-oid; amylo-genic; -dyspepsia; -lysis. The hypothet. radical amyl is derived fr. (am)ylon + -yl.

**MYO-**

MYŌ (μύω), *to close the eyes.* MYŌPS, -ŌPOS (μύωψ), *closing* or *contracting the eyes; short sighted;* Arist. (fr. ōps, *the eye*) > myopia [G]; myop-ic.

**NAPH-**

NAPHTHA (νάφθα), *a clear, combustible rock oil,* procured from the Babylonian asphalt. (fr. Persian naft) > naphtha; -lin; -lene; naphtho-formin; etc.

**NEB-, NEPH-**

NEBULA, gen. and pl. -AE, *mist, vapor, fog, smoke.* > 1. *a foglike opacity* of the cornea. 2. *an oily preparation intended for atomization;* nebul-ization; -ium, *a hypothet. element.*

NEPHELĒ (νεφέλη), *a cloud; mass of clouds; clouds in urine,* H. > nephel-opia; nephelometry, *determination of degree of cloudiness in a fluid.*

**NEPHR-**

NEPHROS (νεφρός), in pl. *the kidneys* (rarely in sing.). > nephr-asthenia; nephro-cardiac; -lith; etc. hyperepi-nephria; hypoepi-.

NEPHRITIS (νεφρῖτις), *kidney disease; gravel in the kidneys.* H > *inflammation of the kidneys.*

NEPHRITIKOS (νεφριτικός), *affected with nephritis.* > nephritic.

**NERV-, NEUR-**

NERVUS, gen. and pl. -I, *sinew, nerve, tendon; nerve, force.* > *a long, whitish, cordlike structure that transmits nervous impulses;* nerve; nervi-motion; nervo-cidine; etc. e-nerv-ation [enervo, -atus, *to take out the nerves and sinews; to enervate*]; in-nerv-ation, *nerve distribution.*

NEURON (νεῦρον), *sinew, tendon, the gristly end* of a muscle by which it is attached to the bone; in pl. *nerve, vigor;* neuron enaimon (with blood in it), *a vein.* H. (a nerve, as a transmitter of sensations to the brain, was not known until

Galen's time); *the fiber* of plants. > *the morphological unit of the nervous system; the axis cylinder process of a nerve cell*, neuron-atrophy; -ic; neuro-pathic; -sis; -some; etc. archineuron; tele-.

**NEST-**

NESTIS (νῆστις), *fasting;* as noun, *the jejunum* (from its always being found empty after death. H.). > *the jejunum;* nest-iatria, *hunger cure;* nesti-therapy; nestio-tomy.

**NITR-**

NITRON (νίτρον), *carbonate of soda* (mined in Egypt, combined with oil it was used as soap). > *nitre* or *niter, nitrate of potassium* or *saltpeter;* nitr-ic; -ate; -ous; nitro-gen; nitro- as a prefix = 1. *containing nitrogen.* 2. *combination with the univalent NO₂;* nitroso- as a prefix = *combination with nitrosyl.* The words natrum, natrium, and natron are from Arabic natrūn or nitrūn from G. nitron, whence also L. nitrum.

**NOCT-, NYCT-**

NOX, NOCTIS, *night.* > noct-ambulation; -uria; noctiphobia.

NOCTURNUS, *belonging to the night.* > nocturn-al. (fr. post-classical nocturnalis).

NYX, NYKTOS (νύξ), *night.* > nyct-algia; -aphonia; -uria; nycto-philia;

NYKTERINOS or NYKTEROS (νυκτερινός or νύκτερος), *by night, nightly.* > nycterin-e; nyctero-hemeral, *daily and nightly.*

NYKTALŌPS (νυκτάλωψ), *not seeing at night.* H. and Gal. Though a confusion existed among subsequent ancient writers, many giving it the reverse meaning, *seeing only at night.* [fr. nyx + ōps, *eye.* Some account for otherwise unexplained *l* by deriving it from alaos, *blind*]. > nyctalopia

**NOM-**

NOMOS (νόμος), *custom, usage; law, ordinance.* > nomotopic; -geny, *origin of life by natural causes;* astro-nomy; auto-; bio-; eco- (oikos, *a house)*; gastro-.

**NOMEN-, NOMIN-**

NOMEN, -INIS, *a name.* > nomen-clature [nomenclatura, *a calling by name.* fr. calo, *to call out, proclaim];* in-nominate, *nameless;* os in-nomin-atum; in-nomin-atal.

**NUC-, NUX**

NUX, NUCIS, *a nut,* > nux moschata, *a tincture made from powdered nutmeg;* nux vomica.

NUCELLA (dim. found only once), *a little nut.* > nucellus, *the nucleus of the ovule,* bot.

NUCLEUS, gen. and pl. -I (dim. of nux), *a little nut; a kernel; the inside* of anything > *a kernel; a central mass about which matter is collected or grouped.* nucle-ar; -ated; -ide; nucleo-plasm; etc.

**NYCT-.** see NOCT

**NYMPH-**

NYMPHĒ (νύμφη), *a bride; a married woman; a Nymph, a goddess of lower rank; clear water* (L. lympha); *the chrysalis* or *pupa; the opening rosebud; pudenda muliebria,* Gal. > nympho-lepsy; -leptic (see LAB-); -mania; etc.

NYMPHA, gen. and pl. -AE. *a bride; a young woman; a demi-goddess; the pupa* of an insect. [fr. G. nymphē.] > nympha, -ae (Mod. L. taking its meaning rather fr. G. nymphē), *one* of the labia minora; nymph-itis; nympholabial; etc.

**OCH-,** see ECT-

**OCUL-**

OCULUS, gen. and pl. -I, *the eye; a spot resembling an eye;* of plants, *en eye, bud* > id.; ocul-ar; -ist; -entum, pl. -a [Mod. L.], *eye ointment;* oculo-gyria [G. gyrios, *circular], the limits of motion of the eyeballs;* etc. INOCULO, pp. -ATUS, *to ingraft an eye or bud* of one tree into another. INOCULATIO, -ONIS, *ingrafting.* > inoculation (of virus).

**-OD,** see HOD-

**ODON-**

ODOUS, ODONTOS (ὀδούς), *a tooth, anything pointed* or *sharp.* > odont-agra, *toothache;* odontoschism; etc.

**ODYN-**

ODYNĒ (ὀδύνη), *pain* of body or mind. > odyn-acusis (akouō); odyno-phagia; etc. As suffix; cardi-odynia; odont-, etc.

**OEC-,** see EC-

**-OID, -ODE**

-O-EIDĒS (-ο-ειδής) also contracted to -ŌDĒS (-ώδης), (being EIDOS εἶδος, *form, shape, likeness,* preceded by *o,* which is either the final vowel of the main word, or a combining vowel) a suffix meaning *having the form of, like.* > -oides (three syllables), a Mod. L. form. Hence the Eng. -oid, and -ode, *having the form or resemblance of,* e.g., anthrop-oid; mast-oid; etc. ge-ode. This suffix -ode should be distinguished from -ode in such words as an-ode, cath-ode, etc. from hodos (ὁδός), *a way.*

**OMEN-**

OMENTUM, *adipose membrane, fat; the membrane which encloses the bowels,* Cels.; *any skin that encloses an internal part of the body.* > *a fold of the peritoneum* connecting the abdominal viscera with the stomach; oment-al; -itis; omentoplasty; etc.

**OMM-.** see OPO-

**ONC-1**

ONKOS (ὄγκος), *bulk, mass of a body.* > In compounds onco- often has the sense of *tumor.* The G. word did not have this meaning though the sense of *swelling* is contained in some of its derivatives, as ONKŌMA and ONKŌSIS, words meaning *a swelling,* as in the medical terms oncoma and oncosis. onco-genesis, *origin and growth of a tumor;* -metry, *measurement of the size* of an organ.

**ONC-2**

ONKOS (ὄγκος), *the barb* of an arrow; *a hook,* any *angle.* (fr. root ANC in ankos, ankylos, L. angulus, etc. A different root from that of the preceding.) > Onco-cerca, *a genus of worms of the family Filariidae;* onco-cerosis.

**ONT-**

ON, ONTOS (ὤν, ὄντος), pres. part. of EIMI (εἰμί), *to be.* > onto-genesis, *the history of the evolution of the individual;* -geny; etc. gam-ont; mes-onto-morph; palae-onto-logy; radi-on.

**OO-**

ŌON (ὡόν), *an egg; the seed* of a plant. oo-genesis; -gonium, *the primitive ovum;* or *antenatal egg cell;* oophor- [phoros, *bearing*], a combining form denoting *the ovary;* oophor-itis; oo-theca (Mod. L.) [thēkē, *a chest] an ovary;* ootheco-cele; -pathy; etc.

OARION (ὠάριον), dim. of ōon, *a small egg,* > oarium, *ovary, ootheca;* oar-itis; oario-tomy; mes-oarium.

**OPH-**

OPHTHALMOS (ὀφθαλμός), *the eye.* > ophthalmus; ophthalmia [G.]; ophthalm-odynia; ophthalmo-lith; etc.

**OPIO-, OPO-**

OPOS (ὀπός), *the juice* of plants (as opp. to chylos and chymos). > In compounds opo- is usually of animal extracts as, opo-therapy, etc. hol-opon [holos, *whole*].

OPION (ὄπιον), dim. of opos, *poppy juice; opium.* > opium; opi-ate.

**OPO-, OPS-, OPT-, OMM-**

HORAŌ (ὁράω) irreg. vb. fut. OPSOMAI (ὄψομαι) perf. (pass.) ŌMMAI (ὤμμαι), *to see.*

OPSIS (ὄψις), *the appearance; face; sight.* > opsio-meter; acyan-opsia; micr-; syn-opsis [G. lit. *a seeing all together];* etc.

OPTOS (ὀπτός), *seen; visible.* > opto-gram; -metry; etc.

OPTIKOS (ὀπτικός), *of* or *for sight.* > optic; -ian; optico-ciliary; pan-optic; etc.

DI-OPTRA (διόπτρα), *a levelling instrument.* > diopter, *the unit of refracting power* of lenses; dioptr-ics; dioptro-scopy; etc.

KATOPTRON (κάτοπτρον), *a mirror.* catoptr-ic, *relating to reflected light.*

OMMA, -ATOS (ὄμμα, -ατος), *the eye; sight, vision.* > Ambly-omma, *a genus of ticks;* Hyal- [hyalos, *glass*]; rhin-omm-ectomy, *excision of inner canthus of eye.*

ŌPS, -ŌPOS (ὤψ, ὠπός), the eye, face. > opo-cephalus; -didymus; cycl-ops; -opia; ambyl-opia [G.]; dipl-; hyper-; etc.

METOPON (μέτωπον), the space between the eyes; forehead. > anterior portion of the frontal lobe of the brain; metop-antritis; -odynia; metopo-plasty, etc.

PROSŌPON (πρόσωπον), face. > prosopo-plegia; -schisis; -tocia; a-prosopia; brady-; diprosopus.

**OPSI-**

OPSIOS (ὄψιος), late. > opsi-tocia; -uria; etc.

**OPSO-**

OPSON (ὄψον), cooked meat; a seasoning. > opso-mania; etc.

OPSŌNION (ὀψώνιον), provisions. > opson-in, an element found in serum; -ize; opsono-philia.

**ORA-, see OS**

**ORCH-**

ORCHIS, -IOS or EŌS (ὄρχις), a testicle, H.; the orchid, a plant so called fr. the shape of its root. > id.; orchid (formed as if the stem were orchid-). In compounds both the correct and incorrect forms are used. orchi-ectomy; -lytic; orchid-algia; -ic; orcho-tomy; orch-itis; etc.

**ORG-, see ERG-**

**ORO-**

OROS, or ORRHOS (ὄρος or ὄρρος), the watery part of milk, whey; of blood, serum. > In compounds, blood serum; oro-diagnosis; -immunity; orrho-logy; -meningitis; etc.

**ORTH-**

ORTHOS (ὀρθός), straight; upright, righteous. > In compounds, 1. straight; 2. specific meaning in chem., that a compound is formed by substitutions in the benzene ring arranged consecutively; ortho-acid; -cephalic; -praxy; -sis [G.]; -terion [fr. orthōtēr, one who straightens]; an-orthography.

**OS-, OR-**

OS, ORIS, pl. ORA, the mouth; an opening, entrance. > id.; or-al; -ale; -ad; oralogy. ORIFICIUM, -I, pl. -A (facio), an opening. > id.; orifice.

**OS, OSS-, OST-**

OS, OSSIS, pl. OSSA, a bone. > id.; ossiferous; -fic; etc. OSSEUS, of bone; bony. > osseo-mucoid; etc.
OSSICULUM, -I, pl. -A (dim. of os), a small bone. > id.; ossicle; ossiculotomy; etc.
OSTEON (ὀστέον), a bone. > oste-al; ost-embryon; osteo-genesis; -arthritis; -pathy; etc. crani-ostosis.

**OSM-, OZ-, -OD-**

OSMĒ (ὀσμή), older form ODMĒ (ὀδμή), a smell, odor; a sense of smell. > osmesis [G.]; osm-ics; -idrosis; dys-osmia [G.]; hemian-; par-; an-odmia.
OZŌ (ὄζω), to have a smell, whether sweet or unpleasant. > ozon-e; -ize; -ozono-phore, a red blood corpuscle; ozo-stomia, bad breath; ozaina [G. a fetid polypus].
OSPHRAINOMAI, fut. ŌSPHRĒSOMAI (ὀσφραίνομαι, ὀσφρήσομαι), to catch scent of, smell. OSPHRESIS (ὄσφρησις), sense of smell. > id.; osphresio-lagnia; anosphresia [an- priv.]; hyper-; oxy-; anosphrasia [osphrasia, another form of osphrēsis].
ODOR, a smell, scent. > id.; odori-ferous; -metry; etc.

**OT-**

OUS, ŌTOS (οὖς), an ear; a handle. > ot-acoustic; -helcosis; oto-cranium; cycl-otic; etc.
PARŌTIS, -IDOS (παρωτίς), the gland beside the ear; usually a tumor of the p. gland, Gal. > parotid; parotic.

**OV-**

OVUM, -I, pl. -A, an egg; an egg shape. > an egg or female sexual cell; ov-al; ovi-capsule; -ferous; -form; -parous; -sac, Graafian follicle; ovo-mucoid; -plasm; syn-ovia.
OVARIUM, -I [Mod. L.] ovary. > id.; ovar-aden; ovari-cele; ovario-lytic; mes-ovarium, etc.
OVULUM, -I, pl. -A [Mod. L.], dim. a little egg; an ovule. > ovum contained within the Graafian follicle; ovul-e; ovulogenous; etc.

**OVIN-**

OVIS, a sheep. OVINUS, relating to a sheep. > ovin-ia, sheep pox; -ation, inoculation with sheep pox virus.

**OX-**

OXYS (ὀξύς), sharp, keen; of sight, keen; of taste and smell, pungent; swift. > oxy-gen, so called because at first supposed to be present in all acids. As prefix, oxy- 1. sharp or acid; 2. combined with oxygen. oxy-acouia; -blepsia; -lalia, rapid speech; -iodide; gastr-oxia.
OXALIS (ὀξαλίς), sorrel (from its bitter taste). > oxal-ic acid; -ate.
OXYNŌ (ὀξύνω), to sharpen. > oxyn-tic; acid forming; gastr-oxynsis; para-oxysm [paroxysmos].

**PAED-, see PED-**

**PAG-, PECT-, PEX-**

PĒGNYMI, fut. PĒXŌ, past tense, EPAGĒN (πήγνυμι), to make fast, to fasten; of liquids, to freeze. PĒXIS (πῆξις), a fixing; coagulation. PĒKTOS (πηκτός), fixed, fastened. PAGOS (πάγος), that which is fixed or set; frost. > pegn-in, a preparation containing the milk-curdling enzyme of calf's rennet; -pagus, a suffix denoting a twin monster (fastened together), as cephalo-pagus; etc. pago-plexia, frost-bite; pexis, fixation; cysto-pexy; sym-pexis [G.]; etc. pect-in; -ose; -en; etc.

**PALM-1**

PALMA, gen. and pl. -AE, the palm of the hand; the palm tree (from resemblance of the leaf to outstretched hand). > id.; palm-ar; -ate (bot.); -ature, webbing of the fingers.

**PALM-2, PALMO-**

PALMOS (παλμός), a quivering motion, pulsation; palpitation of the heart. Arist. > palmus, a convulsive tic; palpitation; heart beat; palm-ic; -odic; palmo-scopy; palm-in; -itic acid; etc.

**PALP-**

PALPO, pp. -ATUS, to touch softly, to pat. > palp-able [palpabilis]; -ate; palpation; palpato-metry; etc.
PALPITO, pp. -ATUS, to move quickly and frequently; throb. > palpitation.

**PAN-**

PAS, gen. PANTOS (πᾶς, παντός), all, every; the whole. > panacea (akos, remedy); pano-phobia; pant-amorphic: panto-scopic; etc.
PANKREAS (πάγκρεας), the sweetbread, fr. pas + kreas (κρέας) flesh. > pancreas; pancreat-ic; pancreato-lysis; etc.

**PARI-, PART-**

PARIO, pp. PARTUS, to bring forth, bear; to produce. > pari-ty, the condition of being able to bear children; nulliparity; primi-; multi-. As suffix, ovi-parous; etc.
PARTUS, a bearing, parturition. > id. PARTURIO, to be in travail or labor. > parturi-tion; -ent; -facient.

**PARIE-**

PARIES, -ETIS, pl. -ETES, a wall. > a wall, as of the chest, abdomen, etc.; pariet-al. parieto- as a combining form refers to the wall of a cavity or the parietal bone.

**PAT-**

PATEO, to lie open. > pat-ency; -ent; -ulous; pate-faction [patefacio], a laying open.
PATELLA, gen. and pl. -AE, a small shallow pan; the kneecap; Cels. > the kneecap; patell-ar; patelli-form.

**PATH-**

PATHOS (πάθος), suffering, misfortune; disease. > path-anatomy; patho-gen; -logy; a-pathy; anti-; sym-. As a suffix -pathy usually implies disease or morbid condition, as cardio-pathy. Also a method of treatment, hydro-pathy; homeo-; allo-; etc.

**PECT-, see PAG-**

**PED-, PAED-** (see also PES-, PED-)

PAIS, PAIDOS (παῖς), a child. > paed- or ped-atrophy, marasmus; -iatric; -erasty [eraō, to love]; ortho-pedics; etc.
PAIDION (παιδίον) (dim. of pais), a small child (up to seven years according to H.) > pedio-dontia; pedio-phobia; etc.

**PELV-, PELY-**

PELVIS, a basin. > the pelvis; any basin or cup-shaped

*cavity*, as the pelvis of the kidney; pelvi-cliseometer; -graph; etc.

PELYX, -YKOS (πέλυξ), and PELLIS, -IDOS (πελλίς), *a wooden bowl; a wine-cup.* > In compounds, the pelvis. pelyc-algia; pelyco-graph; dolicho-pellic; platy-; etc.

**PENI-**

PENIS, *a tail; the penis.* > p.; pen-itis; peni-al; -schisis; peno-scrotal; etc.

PENICILLUS, gen. and pl. -I (or PENICILLUM, pl. -A), *a little tail; a painter's brush or pencil;* dim. of peniculus, a dim. of penis. > *one of the tufts* formed by the subdivision of the minute arterial twigs in the spleen; Penicill-ium, *a genus of molds;* penicill-iosis; penicill-in.

**PEP-**

PEPTŌ, fut. PEPSŌ (πέπτω), *to cook; to digest.* PEPSIS (πέψις), *a ripening* of fruit; *cooking; fermentation; digestion; secretion* by the animal organs, Arist. > peps-in; pepsinogen; pepsini-ferous; pept-ic; pepto-crinine, *an extract of the intestinal mucosa;* pepton-e (fr. pres. part.); -emia; -ize; etc. dys-pepsia [G.]; eu- [G.].

**PES-, PED-**

PES, PEDIS, pl. PEDES, *the foot; a footlike part* of anything. > id.; ped-al; pedi-phalanx; pedo-dynamometer; etc. bi-ped; quadru-; im-pede [impedio, *hinder*]; -pedance.
(a) PEDICULUS, -I (dim. of pes), *a little foot; the footstalk* or *pedicle* of a fruit or leaf. > pedicle, 1. *the stemlike process* of a tumor. 2. *the constricted portion* of the arch of a vertebra.
(b) PEDICULUS, -I, or PEDUNCULUS, -I (dim. of pedis, *a louse,* from pes), *a louse.* > pediculus, *a louse;* pediculosis; pedunculus (in Mod. L. regarded as if a dim. of pes), peduncle, *a narrow process* acting as a support, as the brachium of the brain, etc.
PEDICELLUS, -I, a Mod. L. dim. of pediculus (a), *a little foot.* > a pedicel, *a pedicle* or *peduncle;* bot. *the ultimate division of a common peduncle.*
PETIOLUS, -I, dim. of pes, *a little foot* or *leg; the stem* of fruits. > petiole, *the stalk of a leaf; the lower end of the cartilage of the epiglottis;* petiol-ate.

**PEX-, see PAG-**

**PHAG-**

PHAGEIN (φαγεῖν), infinitive with no pres. in use, *to eat,* > phago-cyte; -cytolysis; etc. geo-phag-ist; anthropo-phagous; copro-phagous; eso-phagus (oisō, οἴσω, irreg. fut. of pherō, φέρω, *to bear*); ade-phagia [G. *gluttony*]; brady-; macro-phag; micro-.
PHAGEDAINA (φαγέδαινα), *a canker.* H. > phagedena, a sloughing ulcer.

**PHAN-, PHEN-, PHAS-**

PHAINŌ, fut. PHANŌ (φαίνω), *bring to light; show;* pass. *come to light, appear; shine.* > phaeno- or pheno-gam, *a plant which has true flowers bearing seed;* -logy; -type; phen-ol; -yl; etc. a-phanto-biont; chloro-phane; chromo-phan, *retinal pigment;* chryso-phanic; meno-phania; phos-phene; sa-phenous [saphēnēs, *visible,* sa- intensive prefix].
PHAINOMENON, pl. -A (φαινόμενον), ntr. sing. pres. part. pass. of phainō. > phenomenon, *something seen* or *apparent to the senses.*
PHANEROS (φανερός), *visible.* > phanero-genic, *of obvious origin;* -scope; etc.
PHANTASIA (φαντασία), *an appearance; an imaginary image.* > fantasy; fantastic.
PHANTASMA (φάντασμα), *an imaginary image.* > phantasm, *an illusion;* phantom; phantasmo-logy.
PHASIS (φάσις), *an appearance; phase.* > phase; ana-phase; meta-; em-phasis [G. *a showing clearly*]. Note that a-phasia is derived from phasis (φάσις), *a saying.*
DIAPHANĒS (διαφανής), *transparent.* > diaphane, *a membrane forming the cell wall;* diaphano-scope.

**PHEM-, PHAS-**

PHĒMI, fut. PHĒSŌ, Doric PHASŌ (φημί, φήσω, φασῶ), *to declare, say.* PHĒMĒ (φήμη), *a voice; a saying; speech;*

PHASIS (φάσις), *a saying.* > brady-phemia, *slowness of speech;* para-; a-phasia [G.]; cata-; acata-; dys-; mono-; allophasis, *disordered speech;* etc.

**PHER-, PHOR-**

PHERŌ (φέρω), *to bear, carry; cf.* L. fero > cata-phora [G. fr. katapherō]; epi- [G. *a bringing to,* fr. epipherō]; etc.
PERIPHEREIA (περιφέρεια), *a carrying round; a circumference.* > peripher-y; -ad; -al; periphero-central; etc.
PHOREŌ, fut. PHORĒSŌ (φορέω, φορήσω), *to carry, bear constantly, wear; suffer, bear.* > cyo-phoria [G. fr. kyophoreō]; patho-phor-ic; photo-dys-phoria; etc.
PHORĒSIS (φόρησις), *a wearing; a being borne.* > dia-phoresis [G.]; electro-; ionto-; etc.
PHOROS (φόρος), *bearing.* > phoro-cyte, *a connective tissue cell;* -plast; etc. phos-phorus [Phōsphoros, *Lucifer, the morning star,* fr. phōs, *light*]; phos-phor-escent; phos-phate; hypo-phos-phite; etc. electro-phor-e; phono-phor-e; amphor-ic [amphoreus, *a two-handled jar,* fr. amphi, *on both sides* + phoreus, *a bearer*]. PHORA (φορά), *a carrying; rapid motion, course of movement, range within* which a body moves. > phoro-meter, *an instrument for measuring relative strength of ocular muscles;* -tone, *a prism for exercising eye muscles;* phoria, *position of the eye ball in relation to its visual axis;* hetero-phoria; ortho-; eso-; etc.

**PHIL-**

PHILEŌ (φιλέω), *to love.* > phil-iator; philo-cytase; -neism. As suffix, chromato-phil; -phile; -philous; -philic. hydrophilia, etc.
PHILTRON (φίλτρον), *a love charm; the depression in the center of the upper lip.* > philtrum; philter.

**PHLEG-, PHLOG-**

PHLEGŌ (φλέγω), *to burn; to flame, blaze;* hence, PHLEGMA, -ATOS (φλέγμα), *fire, heat; inflammation,* H.; *a morbid humor* as the result of such heat. > phlegm, 1. *mucus;* 2. *apathy, dullness of character* (supposed to result from excess of mucus in the system); -asia [G.], *severe inflammation;* -atic.
PHLEGMONĒ (φλεγμονή), *fiery heat; inflammation; a boil* (Gal. and H.). > phlegmon; -ous.
PHLOX, PHLOGOS (φλόξ, φλογός) *a flame.* > phlogocyte; -genic; -sis [G. *inflammation*]; etc. PHLOGIZŌ (φλογίζω), *to set on fire.* > phlogis-ton; anti-phlogis-tic; de-phlogis-ticate.

**PHO-**

PHŌS, PHŌTOS (φῶς, φωτός), *light,* esp. *day-light.* contracted fr. phaos (*cf.* phaino) > phose, *subjective sensation of light;* phos-phene, *sensation of light* from pressing on the eyeball; -gene; -phorus; -phate (see PHER-), phot-odynia; photo-genesis; -lysis, *destruction by light.* pheo-chromoblastoma.

**PHRAG-, PHRAX-**

PHRASSŌ, aorist EPHRAXA (φράσσω, ἔφραξα), *to fence in, hedge round.* PHRAGMA, -ATOS (φράγμα, -ατος), *a fence.* > ino-phragma [is, inos, *muscle fiber*]; dia-phragm; etc. EMPHRASSŌ, fut. -XŌ (ἐμφράσσω, -ξω), *to stop up, block;* hence EMPHRAXIS (ἔμφραξις), *a stoppage.* > id; adeno-emphraxis; antio-; gasterangi-; nephr-; pharyng-; pancreat-; etc.

**PHTH-**

PHTHINŌ, fut. PHTHISŌ (φθίνω), *to decline, waste away.* phthin-oid [phthinōdēs].
PHTHISIS (φθίσις), *a wasting away; consumption;* H. > phthisis; phthisio-therapy; etc.

**PHYLL-**

PHYLLON (φύλλον), *a leaf.* > phyll-ode, *a leaflike petiole;* phyllo-porphyrin; -clade; -taxis, *arrangement of leaves* on a stem. chloro-phyll; clado-; etc.

**PHYS-1, PHYM-, PHYT-**

PHYŌ, fut. PHYSŌ (φύω, φύσω), *to beget; produce;* in passive *to grow.* > phy-one; mono-phy-odont; poly-phy-odont.
PHYSIS (φύσις), *the nature* or *form of a person or thing as resulting from growth; nature.* > phys-iatrics; -ic, *pertaining*

to nature, natural philosophy, the science of medicine, hence medicine, esp. a cathartic; -ics; -ician; -ique (thr. Fr.); physiognomy (see GNO-); -logist; physico-chemical; etc. apophysis, an outgrowth, esp. from a bone [G. an offshoot; a bone process, the prominence to which a tendon is attached H.]; dia- [G.], shaft of a long bone; epi- [G. ongrowth, excrescence]; hypo- [G. an undergrowth, a process, Gal.]; sym- [G. a growing together]; osteo-anaphysis [anaphysis, a growing again].

PHYMA, -ATOS (φῦμα), a growth; a tumor, abscess, H. > a localized swelling of the skin; phymat-iasis; -iosis;. -oid; epi-phyma [G. an eruption of pimples, H.]; rhino-.

PHYTON (φυτόν), a plant. > phyto-genesis; -plasm; -phagous; epi-phyte; para-; etc.

**PHYS-2**

PHYSA (φῦσα), a pair of bellows; a breath, blast; hence PHYSAO (φυσάω). to blow, puff up, distend > physo-cele; -metra, distention of uterine cavity with air or gas; -salpinx.

PHYSEMA (φύσημα), something blown or puffed up; a bubble. > emphysema [G.]; -tous; -therapy; emphysemo-dyspnea; etc.

PHYSALLIS, -IDOS (φυσαλλίς), a bladder; bubble. > a brood cell from a cancer; Physalis, a genus of solanaceous herbs; haema-; physali-form; etc.

**PITU-**

PITUITA, phlegm, rheum. > id.; pituit-ary, secreting or containing mucus; pituit-ary body or gland (formerly thought to be source of nasal secretions); -arium (Mod. L.); pituito-trope; etc.

**PLAC-**

PLACENTA, gen. and pl. -AE, a cake. > the organ of attachment of the fetus to the wall of the uterus; placent-al; -ation; -itis; etc. a-placent-al [a- priv.].

PLAKOUS, -OUNTOS (πλακοῦς), a flat cake. > In compounds = placenta; placunt-itis; -oma.

**PLAS-**

PLASSO, fut. PLASO (πλάσσω, πλάσω), to form, mold. > plasson (pres. p.); plasome [soma, body]; Plasso-myxineae. PLASIS (πλάσις), a molding. > cata-plasis [G.]; dia- [G. a putting in order, the setting of a limb. Gal.]; meta- [G. transformation]; a-plasia; cytometa-; dys-; hypo-; etc.

PLASMA, -ATOS (πλάσμα, -ατος), something formed or molded. > plasma; plasmogen; plasmato-gamy; bio-plasm; cata-, a poultice [G. kataplasma]; proto-; etc.

PLASTOS (πλαστός), molded. > plast-id; -idule; -in; plasto-gamy; -some; etc. amylo-plast; peri-; sarco-; chondro-plast-y; neohemo-plast-in.

PLASTIKOS (πλαστικός), fit for molding, plastic. > plastic; -ity; agranulo-plastic; cine-; sym-; etc.

EMPLASTRON (ἔμπλαστρον), a plaster, a salve, Gal. > emplastrum; plaster; plastron [Fr. a breastplate, fr. e.], the sternum with costal cartilages attached.

**PLES-, PLEX-, PLEG-**

PLESSO, fut. PLEXO (πλήσσω), to strike. > pless-esthesia, palpatory percussion; -or, a small hammer; plessi-meter. plex-algia; plexi-meter; apo-plexy; etc.

PLEGE (πληγή), a stroke. > pleg-aphonia; hemi-plegia; irido-; glosso-; para-; di-; lalo-.

PLEKTRON (πλῆκτρον), anything to strike with; an instrument for striking the lyre; a cockspur; an analogous bone on the ankle. > plectrum, the styloid process of the temporal bone; the uvula; the malleus.

**PLEUR-**

PLEURA (πλευρά), a rib; the side. > the serous membrane which envelops the lung; pleur-algia; -isy; pleuro-clyis, a washing out of the pleural cavity; pleurodont, an animal with teeth fixed to the jaw by lateral ankylosis.

**PLIC-, PLEX-**

PLICO, pp. -ATUS or -ITUS, to fold, wind together. > plic-ate; -ation; com-plicate; du-; duplic-itas; -ity; multiple [multiplex]; simplex [L. fr. sim-, same]; simple; etc.

PLICA, gen. and pl. -AE [Mod. L.], a fold or braid. > term applied to various anat. structures, a fold; a matted condition of the hair.

PLECTO, pp. PLEXUS, to plait, braid. > plexus, a network

of nerves, veins, etc. [L. a braid]; amplexus [L.]; complex; -ion.

**PN-**

PNEO (πνέω), to blow; breathe. PNEUMA, -ATOS (πνεῦμα), wind; breath. PNEUMON (πνεύμων), a lung. > pneo-dynamics, mechanics of respiration; -graph. a-pnea; dys-; etc. pneum-arthrosis, presence of air in a joint; -atic; pneumato-cele; etc. pneumon-ectomy; -ia [G.]; etc.

**POD-**

POUS, PODOS (πούς), a foot. (cf. L. pes, pedis, a foot) > pod-agra; -iatrist; podo-gram, an imprint of the sole of the foot. a-pod; -podal. gastro-pod; arthro-.

POLYPOUS, -PODOS (πολύπους), a sea-polypus or octopus; a morbid excrescence in the nose. H. and Gal. > a polypus; polyp.

**POR-1**

POROS (πόρος), a river ford; a passage through; pore of the skin and of plants; any duct or opening of the body. H. > pore; por-encephaly, cavities in the brain substance; Poro-cephalus, a genus of wormlike arthropods; poro-tomy, meatot-omy.

POREIA (πορεία), a going, a journey, a passage. > porio-mania; opistho-poreia, a walking backwards; etc. APORIA (ἀπορία), difficulty of passage; difficulty; discomfort in illness, H.; poverty; fr. aporos, without passage; difficult. > aporio-neur-osis; sial-aporia; etc.

PORUS, gen. and pl. -I [L. fr. G.], a passage, channel in the body. > a pore, meatus, or foramen; por-ous; -osity. Pori-fera, the sponges.

**POR-2**

POROS (πῶρος), a kind of marble; a node on the bones; stone in the bladder, H.; a callus or exudation from fractured bones. > poro-cele, a hernia with indurated coverings; -sis, formation of callus around the ends of fractured bone; -ma.

**PORPH-, PURP-**

PORPHYRA (πορφύρα), the purple-fish; the dye obtained from it; purple. > porphyr-ia; -in; porphyrin-uria; etc. aetio-porphyrin; proto-; oo-; etc.

PURPURA [L. fr. G.], the purple-fish; purple. > a disease characterized by hemorrhage into the skin; purpur-ic; purpuri-ferous, forming a purple pigment; purple.

**PRAG-, PRAC-, PRAX-**

PRASSO, fut. PRAXO (πράσσω), to do; hence PRAGMA, -ATOS, (πρᾶγμα), something done. > praxio-logy, the science of conduct; a-praxia [G.]; dys- [G. ill success.]; chiropractor; mal-praxis; brady-pragia; mio-; practice [thr. Mediev. L.]; pragmat-agnosia; -amnesia.

**PRISM-**

PRISMA, -ATOS [πρίσμα], something sawn; a geometric prism; fr. PRIZO (πρίζω), to saw. > prism; -atic; -oid; prismo-sphere.

**PSEUD-**

PSEUDO (ψεύδω), to cheat, deceive. > pseud-acousma; pseudo-mania; -bacillus; etc.

**PSYCH-**

PSYCHO (ψύχω), to breathe, blow; to make cold; hence, PSYCHE (ψυχή), breath; spirit, soul; mind. > the cerebrospinal nervous system; the mind. psych-algia; -iatry; psychology; -genetic; etc. meta-psyche, the hind-brain; psych-osis [G.]; hypo-psychosis; etc.

PSYCHROS (ψυχρός), cold. > psychro-philic; -phobia; etc.

**PTER-**

PTERON (πτερόν), a feather; a wing. > pter-ion, a craniometric point (see dictionary); ptero-carpous, having winged fruit. a-pteral; Di-ptera, an order of insects having two wings.

PTERYX, -YGOS (πτέρυξ), a wing; anything like a wing. > pteryg-oid, wing-shaped, applied to various anatomical parts near the sphenoid bone; pterygo-palatine; Loxo-pterygium, a genus of trees [loxos, aslant].

PTERYGION (πτερύγιον), dim. of pteryx, anything like a wing; a disease of the eye, when a membrane grows over it from the inner corner. Gal. and Cels. > pterygium, a triangular

*patch of mucous membrane* growing on the conjunctiva; pi-
melo- [pimelē, *fat*].

**PTOM-, PTOS-**

PTŌMA, -ATOS (πτῶμα), *a fall; disaster; a corpse.* PTŌSIS
(πτῶσις), *a falling.* Both fr. PIPTŌ (πίπτω), *to
fall.* > ptom-aine, *an alkaloid derived from decaying animal matter;* ptomaino-toxism; ptomat-opsy, *inspection of a dead body.* sym-ptom (symptōma, -atos, *a falling
together, chance;* in a disease *a symptom*). ptosis, *a falling down*
or *sinking* of any organ; spec. *drooping* of an eyelid; pan-
optosia; pro-ptosis [G.].

**PTY-**

PTYŌ (πτύω), *to spit out.* PTYALON (πτύαλον), *saliva.*
> hemo-ptysis, haemo- [haima, *blood*]; ptyal-agogue; ptyalo-
genic; etc.

**PUNC-**

PUNGO, pp. PUNCTUS, *to prick, puncture; to sting.* >
pung-ent; -ency; punch.
PUNCTUM, -I, pl. -A, *a puncture; a point; a small spot.* >
id.
PUNCTURA, *a pricking; puncture.* > puncture. fili- [filum,
*thread*].

**PUP-**

PUPA, gen. and pl. -AE, *a girl; a doll.* > *a stage in the development of an insect* between larva and imago.
PUPILLA, gen. and pl. -AE, *an orphan girl; the pupil of the
eye* (because a little reflection appears in it; *cf.* G. korē.) >
*the pupil of the eye;* pupillo-scopy; etc.

**PUR-, PUS-**

PUS, PURIS *pus.* > id.; pur-ulent; -uloid; puri-form; puromucous; sup-pur-ate; etc.
PUSTULA, gen. and pl. -AE, *a blister, pustule.* > id.; pustulant; -ation; -osis; pustuli-form; etc.

**PURP-,** see PORPH-

**PYEL-**

PYELOS (πύελος), *a tub; vat.* > In compounds, *the pelvis.*
pyel-itis; pyelo-pathy; etc.

**PYO-,** see PYTH-

**PYR-**

PYR (πῦρ), *fire; violent fever.* > pyr-idine; -ethrum, *the
plant feverfew* [pyrethron, πύρεθρον]; pyro-genic; -mania;
hyper-pyr-emia; etc.
PYRESSŌ, fut. -EXŌ (πυρέσσω, -έξω), *to be feverish.* >
pyrexia; -l.
PYRETOS (πυρετός), *fiery heat; fever.* > pyret-ic; pyretogenesis; -logy; -therapy; etc.
PYRRHOS (πυρρός), *flame colored, reddish-yellow.* >
pyrrh-ol; -oline; bili-pyrrh-in; chole-pyrrh-in; etc.
EMPYREUMA (ἐμπύρευμα), *live coals covered with ashes*
for rekindling later. > *the pungent odor* of organic substances
developed by destructive distillation.

**PYTH-, PYO-**

PYTHŌ (πύθω), *to decay.* > pytho-genic; -genous.
PYON (πύον), *pus. cf.* L. pus > py-aemia or -emia; pyocele; -rrhea; etc. em-py-esis [G. *suppuration*], *a pustular eruption.* em-py-ema [G.].
PYŌSIS (πύωσις), *suppuration.* Gal. > id.; arthro-pyosis;
celio-; dacryo-; encephalo-; nephro-; etc.

**QUAD-, QUAR-**

QUATTUOR, *four.* QUADRI-, QUADRA-, QUADRU-,
QUATRI-, combining forms = *four.* > quadr-angular;
quadri-sect; -valent; quadru-ped; -plet. quarantine (thr. It.
fr. L. quadraginta, *forty;* the original period of detention
being forty days). QUARTUS, *the fourth.* > quart; quart-er;
quarti-para [pario, *to bear*]; -sect; -sternal.

**QUANT-**

QUANTUS, *how much.* > quanti-meter; -valence.

**QUERC-**

QUERCUS, *an oak-tree.* > id.; *the bark of Q. alba;* querc-in;
-ite, *a crystalline substance obtained from acorns;* querci-tan-
nin.

**RAB-**

RABIES, *rage, madness; madness of dogs.*
RABIDUS, *furious, mad.* > rabies; rabid.

**RACE-,** see RHACH-

**RADI-**

RADIUS, gen. and pl. -II, 1. *a staff, rod;* 2. *spoke* of a wheel;
3. *r. of a circle;* 4. *beam or ray;* 5. *the exterior bone of the forearm.*
Cels. > radius, with meanings 3, 4, and 5. radi-able, *capable
of being penetrated by rays;* -al; -ant; -ar; -um; radio-carpal,
*relating to the radius and the bones of the carpus;* -therapy,
*treatment of diseases by radiant energy;* etc.

**RAPH-,** see RHAPH-

**REG-, RECT-, RIG-**

REGO, pp. RECTUS, *to keep straight; guide, direct; rule.*
RECTUS, -A, -UM, as adj. *straight, upright.* > rectum (intestinum understood), "*the straight intestine*"; rect-al; -ec-
tomy; recto-scope; etc. recti-fy. regimen [L. *a guiding*],
*regulation* of mode of living, *diet.*
REGIO, -ONIS, *a boundary line; a district.* > a region; *an
area* of the body.
REGULA, *a straight piece of wood; a ruler; a rule.* > regul-ar;
-ation; regle-men-tation [thr. Fr. from mens, mentis, *mind*],
*regulation* of prostitution.
DIRIGO, pp. -RECTUS, *lay straight, arrange, direct.* > di-
rect-ion; -or; dirigo-motor.
ERIGO, pp. ERECTUS, *to set upright.* > erect; -ion; -ile;
-or.

**RET-**

RETE, *a net.* > reti-form; -al; reto-thelium [G. *thēlē, a nipple*], *the layer of cells covering a reticular tissue.*
RETINA, gen. and pl. -AE (Mediev. L., so called from resemblance to network). > *the inner nervous tunic* of the eyeball; retin-itis; -al; -oid; retino-pathy; etc.
RETICULUM, -I, pl. -A (dim. of rete), *a little net; a network bag.* > 1. *a fine network,* esp. of nerves, etc.; 2. *the second
stomach* of a ruminant. reticul-ation; -ar; reticulo-cyte, *an
erythrocyte containing a network.*

**RHACH-, RACH-**

RHACHIS, -IOS (ῥάχις, -ιος), *the spine, the backbone.* >
id.; rhachi-al; -odynia; rhachio-tomy; -plegia; etc. atelo-
rrhachid-ia; cephalo-rrhachid-ian (this and prec. word
formed on erroneous assumption that stem is rhachid- instead of rhachi-).
RHACHITĒS (ῥαχίτης), *pertaining to the spine,* fem.
RHACHITIS, -IDOS (ῥαχῖτις), *spinal complaint, rickets*
(sc. *nosos, disease*). > rachitis; rachit-ism; rachito-genic-
etc. (the form of these words being influenced by E. rickets).

**RHAG-, RHEG-, RHEX-, -RRHAG-**

RHĒGNYMI, fut. RHĒXŌ (ῥήγνυμι, ῥήξω), *to break
asunder, shatter, burst.* > -rrhagia, as suffix, *a discharge from
a burst vessel;* blenno-rrhagia; metro-; etc. rhagades (G. pl.
of rhagas, *a crack, fissure of the lips.* Gal.) *chaps* or *cracks* in
the skin; cataract [fr. katarrhēgynmi, *break down, rush down*].
RHĒXIS (ῥῆξις), *a bursting* of a vessel. H. > id.; amniorrhexis; etc.
RHĒGMA (ῥῆγμα), *a fracture; fissure.* > id.

**RHAPH-, -RRHA-, RHY-**

RHAPTŌ (ῥάπτω), *to sew, stitch;* hence
RHAPHĒ (ῥάφη), *a seam; suture of the skull,* H.; *a stitching.* > raphe or rhaphe, *the line of union* of two similar structures; entero-rrhaphe, *suture of the intestine;* perineo-; etc.
RHAPHIS, -IDOS (ῥαφίς, -ίδος), *a needle.* > rhaphidio-
spore, *sporozoite.*

**RHE-, -RRHE-**

RHEŌ (ῥέω), *to flow;* hence RHOIA (ῥοία), *a flow, flux.* >
meno-rrhoea or -rrhea; galacto-; dia-; etc. cata-rrh.
RHEOS (ῥέος), *a stream.* > In compounds usually refers
to *electric current* or the *blood stream.* rheo-basic; -meter; -stat,
etc.
RHEUMA, -ATOS (ῥεῦμα), *a flow; stream; a humor* or *discharge* from the body, *a flux.* H. > rheum; rheumat-ic; -ism.
RHYSIS (ῥύσις), *a flowing, flow; issue.* > dysdiemo-rrhysis
[dys- + dia + haima, *blood*], *sluggishness of capillary circulation;* endiemo-; hyperdiemo-; phymato-rrhys-in.

**RHIN-**
RHIS, RHINOS (ῥίς), the nose. > rhin-al; -ism, nasal quality of voice, rhino-plasty; etc.

**RIG-, see REG-**

**RUB-**
RUBER, -BRA, -BRUM, red. > rube-facient; -faction;
rub-edo [L. redness], a flushing; rub-igo [L.], rust; mildew;
rubigin-ous; rub-escent [L. rubesco, to become red]; rub-or
[L.], redness.

**RUPT-**
RUMPO, pp. RUPTUS, to break, burst; hence RUPTURA,
a fracture of a limb or vein. > rupture, hernia, e-rupt-ion;
e-rupt-ive.

**SACC-**
SACCUS, gen. and pl. -I, a sac, bag. > the baglike covering
of a cavity, hernia, cyst, or tumor; a sac; sacc-ate; sacci-form;
etc.
SACCULUS, dim. a little sack. > a small sac; the smaller of
the two sacs in the vestibule of the labyrinth of the ear, a
saccul-e; -ar; -ated; sacculo-cochlear.

**SACCH-**
SAKCHAR, -AROS, or SAKCHARON (σάκχαρ or
σάκχαρον), a sugar made from an Indian cane or palm. >
saccharum, sugar, sucrose; sacchar-in; -ine; -ic; -ide; saccharorrhea; etc.

**SAEPT-, see SEPT-**

**SALP-**
SALPINX, -INGOS (σάλπιγξ), a trumpet. > Anat. a tube,
esp. the fallopian or Eustachian tubes. salping-ectomy;
salpingo-malleus; hemo-salpinx; etc.

**SANG-, SANI-**
SANGUIS, -INIS, blood. > id.; sangui-facient = hematopoietic; Sanguisuga [L. a leech, fr. sugo, to suck]. con-sanguin-
ity.
SANIES, thin bloody matter. > id.

**SARC-**
SARX, SARKOS (σάρξ), flesh; the pulpy substance of fruit.
> sarco-blast, a bud from a germinating cell; -lemma; -logy;
-ma; -carp.

**SCHI-, SCISS-**
SCHIZO, fut. SCHISO (σχίζω), to split, cleave; to separate.
> schiz-axon, a neuraxon divided into two branches; schizo-
cyte; -genesis, multiplication of cells by fission; -mycetes;
-trichia; etc.
SCHINDYLESIS (σχινδύλησις), a cleaving into small
pieces. > a form of synarthrosis.
SCHISIS (σχίσις), a cleaving; division. > cardio-schisis;
gastro-; peni- [penis]; etc.
SCHISTOS (σχιστός), cloven; divided. > schisto-cyte;
-cephalus; Schisto-soma; etc.
SCINDO, pp. SCISSUS, to split, cleave; separate. > scission;
scissi-parity, reproduction by fission; sciss-ura [L.] a fissure;
scissors. ab-scission [abscindo]; di-.

**SCLER-**
SKLEROS (σκληρός), hard. > sclera, the hard outer membrane of the eyeball. In compounds scler-, sclero- denotes
either hardness or the sclera. sclero-derma; -stomy, the operative formation of an opening in the sclera; scler-osis; arteri-
o-scler-osis; splanchno-scler-osis.
SCLEROMA (σκλήρωμα), an induration. H. > id.
SCLEROTICUS, a Mod. L. form fr. G. skleros, hard. >
sclerotica (fem., sc. L. tunica, a coat), sclera (NA); sclerotic,
1. hard, indurated; 2. relating to the sclera; 3. relating to ergot;
etc.
SCLEROTIUM, pl. -IA, Mod. L., a hard mass of mycelia and
reserved food material, the resting stage of certain fungi, as
the ergot.

**SCOP-**
SKOPEO (σκοπέω) to look at, examine. > Usually as suffix,
-scope, -scopy; the adjectival form is -scopic; e.g. micro-scope,
-scopy; -scopic. scopo-meter; -phobia; etc.

**SEB-, SEV-**
SEBUM or SEVUM, the hard fat of animals; tallow, suet. >
In Mod. L. a distinction in meaning is drawn between the
two forms; SEBUM, the secretion of the sebaceous glands; sebaceous; sebi-agogic; sebo-lith, a concretion in a sebaceous follicle; -rrhea; etc. SEVUM, suet or tallow; s. praeparatum, the
prepared suet of the U.S.P.

**SEC-, SEG-**
SECO, pp. SECTUS, to cut. > sect-ile; -io [L.]; -ion; -or [L.];
cuti-sector; bi-sect; dis-; inter-; vivi-; etc. in-sect (cut into,
notched; cf. G. entomon under TOM-).
SEGMENTUM, a cutting; a strip, segment. > segment; -al;
-ation.

**SEP-, SEPS-, SEPT-**
SEPO, fut. SEPSO (σήπω), to make rotten.
SEPSIS (σῆψις), putrification. SEPTOS (σηπτός) and
SEPTIKOS (σηπτικός), putrifying. > sepsis; seps-ine;
sept-emia; septic-emia; -ine; septico-pyremia; etc. a-sepsis;
anti-septic; exo-sepsis.
SEPEDON (σηπεδών), rottenness. > id.; sepedo-genesis.

**SEPT-1, SAEPT-**
SAEPTUM or SEPTUM, -I, pl. -A, a fence, partition; a di-
aphragm. Cels. > a thin wall dividing two cavities or tissues;
septectomy; inter-sept-al, between two septa; inter-saeptum
[L. midriff].
SEPTULUM (Mod. L. dim.), a minute septum.

**SEPT-2**
SEPTEM, seven. > septi-valent; etc.

**SER-**
SERUM, -I, pl. -A, whey (like G. oros), the watery part of
other things. > the watery part of the blood after coagulation;
any clear watery fluid like blood serum; antitoxin; seri-flux;
sero-diagnosis; etc. serosa, a serous membrane (fr. a Mod. L.
form serosus, serous).

**SEV-, see SEB-**

**SINU-**
SINUS, -US, a curve; a hollow; a fold of the toga; the bosom;
a bay. > a hollow or pocket; a channel for the passage of blood;
a cavity within a bone; sinu-itis, -atrial; sinuo-tomy; sinusoid, -itis.

**SIT-**
SITOS (σῖτος), food. > sito-logy; -therapy. para-site; -sitic
SITION (σιτίον), grain; bread; food. > siti-eirgia [eirgo, to
shut out]; sitio-logy; -mania; etc.

**SKEL-**
SKELETOS, -E, -ON (σκελετός), dried up; fr. SKELLO
(σκέλλω), to dry up; SKELETON (ntr.; soma, a body, understood), a mummy; a skeleton. Gal. > skeleton; skelet-al;
-ization; skeleto-logy; exo-skeleton; derma-; endo-.

**SOLU-, SOLV-**
SOLVO, pp. SOLUTUS, release, set free; dissolve. > solv-ent;
-ate; solut-e, the dissolved substance in a solution; solutio [L.];
dissolve; re-solution, arrest of an inflammatory process without suppuration; -solve; -solvent.

**SOM-**
SOMA, -ATOS (σῶμα), the body as opposed to the spirit;
animal body as opposed to plants. > the body without the limbs;
soma-cule, a protoplasmic molecule; som-asthenia, bodily
weakness; somato-pathic; etc. trypano-some; -som-iasis;
schisto-soma; etc.

**SPA-**
SPAO, fut. SPASO (σπάω, σπάσω), to draw a sword; to
draw, stretch; pluck off, snatch, tear; in medic. to cause convulsion or spasm. > spa-giric; hypo-spadias [G. one who has the
orifice of the penis too low, Gal.]; ana-; epi-; para-.
SPASIS (σπάσις), a drawing up or in. > hemo-spasia;
nephro-; etc.
SPASMOS (σπασμός), a drawing tight; a convulsion. >
spasm; -odic; spasmo-lysis; -phemia, stuttering; angio-spasm;
para-; etc.
SPASTIKOS (σπαστικός), drawing in, absorbing; (meanings of mod. derivatives are taken from L. spasticus [fr. the
G.] having cramps or spasms). > spastic; -ity; epi-spastic;
hemo-; etc.

SPADIX (σπάδιξ), *a branch torn off.* > *a thick fleshy spike* of closely set flowers (bot.).

**SPER-, SPOR-**

SPEIRŌ, fut. SPERŌ (σπείρω), *to sow, scatter;* hence

SPERMA, -ATOS, (σπέρμα), *that which is sown, seed; semen.* > sperm, *semen;* -ism, *emission of semen;* spermaturia; -ic; spermato-zoon; -cide; etc. angio-sperm, *a plant that has a seed vessel;* poly-spermia.

SPOROS (σπόρος), *a sowing; seed.* > spore. In compounds a *spore or seed;* spor-angium, *a sac containing spores,* bot.; -ule, *a small spore;* spori-cide; sporo-blast; -zoon; basidiospore; Micro-spor-idia, *an order of Neo-spor-idia,* parasites of invertebrates, *the spores of which are very minute.*

SPORADIKOS (σποραδικός), *scattered;* of diseases, *sporadic.* Gal. > sporadic; sporadoneure, *a nerve cell outside of the nerve centers.*

**SPHIN-**

SPHINKTĒR (σφιγκτήρ), *a band, lace; a muscle closing an aperture,* and remaining naturally in a state of contraction, as the s. ani; fr. SPHINGŌ (σφίγγω), *to bind tight.* > sphincter; -al; -itis; sphinctero-lysis; etc.

**SPHYG-, SPHYX-**

SPHYZŌ (σφύζω), *to throb; to beat* (of the heart). Hence, SPHYGMOS (σφυγμός), or SPHYXIS (σφύξις), *a throbbing* of inflamed parts, H.; *the beating* of the heart. > In compounds sphygm-, sphygmo- relate to *the pulse;* sphygm-ic; sphygmo-logy; -phone; -systole; etc. cardio-sphygmo-graph; hyper-sphyxis; micro-; etc.

ASPHYXIA (ἀσφυξία), *a stopping of the pulse;* fr. a- priv. + sphyzō. > *unconsciousness* due to suffocation; *absence of the pulse beat;* asphyxi-al; -ant; -ate.

**SPIR-1**

SPEIRA (σπεῖρα), *anything wound around, a coil.* > spiradenoma or spir-oma, *adenoma of the sweat glands;* spiro-bacteria; Spiro-chaetaceae [chaetē, *hair*], the single family of *spiral* organisms belonging to the order Spirochaetales; Spiro-chaeta, Sapro-spira, and Cristi-, *genera of this order;* spirochet-e, *an individual of the genus S.;* -al; -osis; -otic; spiro-cheto-lysis. Spiro-nema, *Treponema.*

SPEIRĒMA (σπείρημα), *a coil, a twisted cord or thread.* > spirema, spireme, or spirem, *the mother skein or wreath of chromatin fibrils* appearing in the first stage of mitosis.

SPIRA, gen. and pl. -AE [L. fr. G.], *that which is coiled or twisted; a coil; a fold.* > spir-al; Spirillum [Mod. L. dim. of spiral], *a genus of the tribe Spirilleae;* spirillosis; spirillicidal; etc.

**SPIR-2**

SPIRO, pp. -ATUS, *to breathe* > spiro-graph; -meter; -phore, *a pneumatic cabinet used for artificial respiration;* -scope; etc. expir-e (expiro, *to breathe out);* -ation; -atory; inspir-e; -ation; -ator; per-spir-ation; re-spir-ation; trans-pir-ation; *perspiration;* etc.

SPIRITUS, gen. and pl. -ŪS, *a breathing; the breath of life; life; soul, spirit.* > Pharm. *an alcoholic solution of a gaseous or volatile substance;* spirit; -uous.

**SPLAN-**

SPLANCHNON (σπλάγχνον), usually pl., *the inward parts,* esp. the heart, lungs, liver, and kidneys. > In compounds, *the viscera.* splanchn-ectopia (ektopos, *out of place);* -ic, *visceral;* splanchno-logy; somato-splanchno-pleuric; etc.

**SPLEN-**

SPLĒN (σπλήν), *the spleen,* supposed by the ancients to be the seat of anger and melancholy. > splen-auxe (auxē, *increase);* splen-epatitis, *inflammation of both spleen and liver;* splen-etic 1. *relating to the spleen;* 2. *ill-humored;* splen-unculus, -culus; -ulus, are Mod. L. forms meaning *an accessory spleen.* They are from the L. splen, which comes fr. the G.

**STA-, STEM-**

STA, a root found in many G. and L. words, with sense of *stand or set up.* Cf. Eng. stand.

HISTĒMI, fut. STĒSO (ἵστημι, στήσω), *to make to stand, set upright; to weigh;* intran. *stand.* See also HIST-.

STASIS (στάσις), *a placing, setting; a standing.* > stagnation

of the blood or other fluids; stasi-morphia; -phobia; apostasis [G.]; cata- [G. *an arranging* fr. kathistēmi]; dia- [G. *a standing apart, separation*]; epi- [G.]; *scum;* hypo- [G.]; *sediment;* meta- [G.]; a-stasis [G. *unsteadiness*]; ec-stasy, *a fixed state, a trance, excessive joy;* etc.

STATOS (στατός), verbal adj. of histēmi, *placed, standing.* > stato-liths; -meter; -sphere; hemo-stat, *an agent that arrests flow of blood;* ophthalmo-; thermo-; ana-state; cata-, *a result of catabolism;* meso-, *an intermediate product in metabolism.*

STATIKOS (στατικός), *causing to stand; pertaining to weighing.* > static; static-s; -e [G. *an astringent plant*]; epistatic; clino-, *relating to a recumbent position;* pyo-; aerostatics; bio-; etc.

STADION (στάδιον), *that which stands fast; a fixed standard* of length (about 600 ft.); *a race-course* (because of its length). > stadium [L. fr. G. with Mod. L. meaning], *a stage* in the course of a disease.

STĒMŌN, -ONOS (στήμων, -ονος), *the warp,* which *stood upright* in the ancient loom. > In mod. derivatives *the stamen* of a flower; iso-stemonous; aniso-; etc.

APOSTĒMA, -ATOS (ἀπόστημα, -ατος), *a distance, interval; an abscess.* H. > *an abscess;* aposteme, hemat-apostema.

DIASTĒMA, -ATOS (διάστημα, -ατος), *an interval.* > *a fissure or abnormal opening;* diastemato-pyelia; etc.

SYSTĒMA, -ATOS (σύστημα, -ατος), *an arrangement; an organized whole.* > system; systemat-ization; etc.

PROSTATĒS (προστάτης), *one who stands before.* > prostata [Mediev. L. fr. proistēmi]: prostat-e; -ic; -ectomy; prostato-rrhea; etc.

STO, pp. STATUS, pres. p. STANS, STANTIS, *to stand, stand still; remain, last.* > circum-stant-ial [circumsto]; constant [consto, *stand together*]; contra-st; di-stant; sub-stance [substantia fr. substo].

STABILIS, -E, *firm, stable.* > stabil-e; -ity; stable; metastable [G. meta]; tremo-.

STATUS, -ŪS, *way of standing; condition, state.* > *standing, condition;* state; statu-volence [volo, *wish*], *self-induced hypnotism;* stat-istics; etc.

STATIO, -ONIS, *a standing; position, post.* > station; -ary.

STATURA, -AE, *height of body.* > stature.

STAMEN, -INIS *the warp* (see stēmōn above). > In bot. *the male element of a flower;* stamin-ode [eidos, *form*], *a sterile stamen;* stamina (pl.), *power of endurance.*

STATUO, pp. -UTUS, *cause to stand, set up; establish.* In compds. the *a* is changed to *i, e.g.,* con-stituo; in-; pro-; etc.; the L. noun derivatives are constitutio, -onis, etc. > constitution; in-; pro-; etc.

SISTO, pp. STATUS, *to place, stand* (reduplicated form of sto). > per-sistance; re-; etc.

**STAL-, STOL-**

STELLŌ, fut. STELŌ (στέλλω, στελῶ), *set, place, arrange; despatch, send; check, repress;* hence,

STALSIS (στάλσις), *a compression, restriction,* Gal. > anastalsis [anastellō, *hold back*]; cata- [G. katastellō, *keep down, repress*]; peri- [peristellō].

STALTIKOS (σταλτικός), *contracting; contractile;* also used as terminal element in adjs. from nouns ending in -stalsis or -stolē. > staltic, *styptic;* ana-staltic, *astringent;* cata-; dia-, *reflex;* peri- [peristaltikos, *clasping and compressing,* referring to the p. action of the bowels, Gal.]; etc.

ANASTOLĒ (ἀναστολή), *a drawing back of* flesh from a wound. H. > id., *the gaping of a wound.*

DIASTOLĒ (διαστολή), *a drawing apart, dilation.* > id.; brady-diastole; etc.

SYSTOLĒ (συστολή), *a drawing together, contracting;* fr. systellō (συστέλλω). > id.; a-systole; eury-; hystero- [hysteros, *later*]; etc.

**STAPH-**

STAPHYLĒ (σταφυλή), *a bunch of grapes; the uvula* when swollen so as to resemble a grape. H. > In compounds, *the uvula, or a part or organism suggesting a grape;* staphyl-agra

[G. fr. agra, *a seizing*], *uvula forceps.* H.; -edema; -itis; Staphylococcus, a genus of pathogenic *spherical* organisms.

STAPHYLŌMA (σταφύλωμα), *a blemish* in the eye inside the cornea, *shaped like a grapestone.* > *a bulging of the cornea* due to inflammatory softening.

**STERN-**

STERNON (στερνον), *the chest.* > stern-um -i, pl. -a [Mod. L.]; -al; -ebra, gen. and pl. -ae [Mod. L. formed fr. sternum and vertebra], *a sternal vertebra;* -odynia; sternocostal; etc.

**STHEN-**

STHENOS (σθένος), *strength.* > sthen-ic; -ia; a-sthenia, (a- priv.), *debility;* asthen-ic; -opia, *weak sight;* neur-asthenia; cali-sthenics; hyper-sthenia.

**STIG-**

STIGMA, -ATOS (στίγμα), *the prick* or *mark* of a pointed instrument; *a mark, spot;* fr. STIZŌ (στίζω), *to prick, mark; brand* as a mark of disgrace. > Bot. *the part of the pistil* that receives the pollen; in anat., path., and zool., *a spot, mark,* or *small hole;* stigm-al; stigmat-ic; -ization; -ism; stigmato-dermia; -sis. a-stigmat-ism, *a defect in the eye* or *a lens* such that the rays of light converge, not in *a point,* but in line; physo-stigma [physa, *bellows*] (so called from the shape of the stigma) *calabar bean.*

**STOM-**

STOMA, -ATOS (στόμα), *the mouth; any outlet* or *entrance.* > *an opening* or *pore.* In compounds, 1. *the mouth;* 2. *an artificial opening* between two cavities or canals; stomat-al, *relating to a stoma;* -itis; stomato-cace (kakē, *badness*); -rrhagia; etc. ana-stom-osis [G.], *the interconnection of veins and arteries;* bot. *the interlacing of the veins of leaves.* As a suffix, -stomy denotes an artificial opening, *e.g.,* jejuno-stomy, entero-; etc.

STOMACHOS (στόμαχος), *a mouth, opening; the throat, gullet; the orifice* of the stomach, Gal.; later, *the stomach* itself. > stomach; -ic; -algia; etc.

**STREP-, STRO-**

STREPHŌ (στρέφω), *to turn; twist.* > strepho-symbolia, *perception of objects reversed* as in a mirror; -tome, *a corkscrew shaped surgical instrument;* epistropheus, *a pivot, second cervical vertebra* [G.].

STREPSIS (στρέψις), *a turning round.* > arterio-strepsis; phlebo-; etc.

STREPTOS (στρεπτός), *twisted; curved.* > Strepto-coccus, *a genus of spherical organisms* occurring in large *wavy* chains; strepto-coccemia; -angina, *membranous sore throat* due to streptococci; -cyte; -mycin; Strepto-thrix; -trichal; -trichiasis; etc.

STROBILĒ (στροβίλη), *lint twisted into an oval shape.* H. > strobil-a or -e, *a number of consectuive tapeworm segments;* -oid.

STROPHĒ (στροφή), *a turning; a twist.* > cardia-ana-strophe; syringo-sys-trophe; etc.

STROPHOS (στρόφος), *a twisted band* or *cord; a twisting* of the bowels, *colic.* > stroph-anthus; stropho-cephalus, *a monster with distorted head;* strophulus (Mod. L. dim.), *gum rash.*

**STYP-**

STYPHŌ, fut. STYPSŌ (στύφω), *draw together, contract.* STYPSIS (στύψις), *contraction; astringency.* > stypt-ic; -icin; -ol.

**SUD-**

SUDOR, *sweat;* fr. SUDO, pp. -ATUS, *to sweat,* > id.; sudamen, pl. -amina (Mod. L.), *minute vesicles appearing on the skin* in various fevers; -an, *a name given to several fat-dyes;* sudano-phil; sud-ation; sudor-esis (note G. ending), sudorific; -ferous; etc.

**SULC-**

SULCUS, gen. and pl. -I, *a furrow made by the plough;* fr. SULCO, pp. -ATUS, *to plough.* > *one of the grooves* or *furrows* on the surface of the brain; *any long narrow groove* or *depression;* sulc-al; -ate; sulci-form; sulco-marginal; etc.

SULCULUS, gen. and pl. -I, Mod. L. dim., *a small sulcus.*

**SULF-, SULPH-**

SULFUR or SULPHUR, *brimstone, sulphur.* > id.; as prefix sulf- and sulfo- denote *a content of sulfur or $SO_2$* ; sulf-ate; -ite; -emoglobin; sulfo-hydrate; etc. sulfur-et, *sulfide;* -ous.

**SYRI-**

SYRINX, -INGOS (σῦριγξ), *a pipe, tube.* > *the Eustachian tube; a fistula;* syringadenoma, *a sweat gland tumor;* syringocele; etc.

SYRIGMOS (συριγμός), *a shrill piping sound, a hissing; a ringing* in the ears. > syrigmus, id.; syrigmo-phonia.

**TACH-**

TACHYS (ταχύς), *swift;* superlative, TACHISTOS (τάχιστος); TACHOS (τάχος), *speed.* > tachy-cardia; -phasia; etc. tachography, *recording of the rapidity of the blood current;* tachisto-scope.

**TACT-, TAG-, TIG-**

TANGO, pp. TACTUS, pf. TETIGI, *to touch,* hence, TACTUS, -ŪS, *a touching;* TACTILIS, *tangible.* > tact-ion [tactio]; tacto-meter; tactile; a-tactilia [G. a- priv.].

CONTINGO, pp. -TACTUS, *to touch on all sides, to touch.* > contact; con-tagion [contagio]; contigu-ous; -ity.

**TAL-**

TALUS, -I, *the ankle; ankle-bone; heel.* > *the astragalus;* talo-crural; -fibular; etc. tali-pes-, *clubfoot.*

TALO, -ONIS [Mediev. L.], *the claw of a bird.* > *a low cusp of a tooth.*

**TAR-**

TARSOS (ταρσός), *a wicker-work frame* or *mat; any broad flat surface; the sole* of the foot; *the flat* of an outstretched wing; *the edge of the eyelid and its lashes,* Gal. > tarsus, 1. *the instep;* 2. *the cartilage of the eyelid;* tarsal-e, pl. -ia [Mod. L. form], *any tarsal bone;* tars-al; -algia; -itis, *inflammation of* 1. *the tarsus of the foot;* 2. *the cartilage of the eyelid.* tarso-clasia; etc. meta-tarsus; para-tarsium.

**TAX-, TACT-**

TASSŌ, fut. TAXŌ (τάσσω), *to arrange, put in order;* hence, TAXIS (τάξις), *an arrangement.* > *an arranging; manipulation for reduction of hernia,* etc.; *the reaction of protoplasm to a stimulus;* taxo-logy; -nomy; etc. cyto-taxia; -taxis; -tactic; syn-taxis; hypo-taxia; a-; di-ataxia; psych-.

TAKTIKOS (τακτικός), *pertaining to arranging.* > cyto-tactic; eosino-; etc.

TAGMA, -ATOS (τάγμα, -ατος), *an arrangement; a body of soldiers.* > *a molecular group;* ino-tagma; neuro-.

**TEMP-**

TEMPUS, -ORIS, *time; the right time, opportunity; the right place, the fatal spot; the temple* of the head (usually in the plural, tempora). > temple; tempor-al; temporo-auricular; etc.

TEMPERO, pp. -ATUS, *divide in due proportion; qualify, temper.* > temper-ament [L. -amentum]; -ance [-antia]; -ate; -ature [-atura]; dis-temper [dis- intens.].

**TEN-, TON-, TAS-**

TEINŌ, fut. TENŌ (τείνω), *to stretch, strain;* hence, TATOS (τατός), *that can be stretched.* > ec-tatic; myo-, etc.

TENŌN, -ONTOS (τένων), *a tight stretched band, a sinew, tendon.* > teno-plasty; -tomy tenont-agra; tenonto-plasty; etc.

TONOS (τόνος), *a rope, band* (by which a thing is stretched); *a stretching, straining; a pitching* of the voice; *tension,* > ton-e; -aphasia; -ic; tono-meter; etc. a-ton-y, *lack of tone;* aton-icity; hyper-tonic; iso-; peri-ton-eum, lit. *the membrane stretched around* [peritonaion].

TASIS (τάσις), *a stretching; tension.* > ec-tasis [G.], *dilation* of a tubular structure; en-tasis [G.], or en-tasia, *tonic spasm;* myo-tasis.

TAINIA (ταινία), *a band, head-band; a tapeworm.* Gal. > taenia or tenia, *any anatomical bandlike structure; a tapeworm;* tenia-cide; etc.

TETANOS (τέτανος), *a convulsive tension* of the body. > tetanus; tetan-y; tetano-meter; etc.

TENDO, pp. TENTUS or TENSUS, *to stretch, extend, distend.* > tense; tens-ion; -or; dis-tension; hyper-; hypo- [note

G. preps.]; tent-igo [L. *tension, lust*]; -iginous; -orium [L. *tent*] EXTENDO, *stretch out.* > extend; extens-ion; -or, INTENDO, *stretch forth.* > intens-ity; -ive; intention.

TENDO, -INIS (Mediev. L.), *a tendon.* > id.; tendon; tendino-plasty; -us; etc.

TENTO, pp. -ATUS, *to handle, touch, feel.* > tent, *a probe;* tent-acle; -ative.

TENUIS, *stretched out, fine, thin.* > id.; attenu-ant [at-tenuo, -atus, *make thin*]; -ate; -ation.

TENEO, pp. TENTUS, *to hold, keep, have.* > tenac-ious [tenax]; -ity. CON-TINEO, -TENTUS, *hold together.* > content; contin-ence; -uous; -uity; etc. RETINEO, -TENTUS, *hold back.* > retain; retention; retinaculum [L.].

**TEST-1**

TESTA, *a piece of burned clay; a brick, tile; a shell-fish; a shell.* > *an envelope of certain protozoa;* bot. *a seed covering;* testaceous; Test-aceae, *a group of Amoeba with firm chitinous envelope.*

TESTUM, *a lid of an earthen vessel; an earthen vessel.* In Mediev. L. *an earthen pot for trying or testing metals.* > test; test-tube; -solution; etc.

**TEST-2**

TESTIS, pl. TESTES, *a testicle.* > 1. id. 2. *one of the inferior pair of the corpora quadrigemina;* testi-cond [condo, *to hide*]; -brachial; etc.

TESTICULUS, gen. and pl. -I, dim. *a testicle.* >; id testicul-ar; etc.

**THE-**

TITHĒMI, fut. THĒSŌ, aorist ETHĒKA (τίθημι, θήσω, ἔθηκα), *set, put, place;* hence, THESIS (θέσις), *a setting, placing, arranging.* > *thesis;* cyto-; enthesis [G. *an insertion*]; xen-; meta-thesis [G. *change of position*]; syn- [G. *a putting together*]; electro-synthesis; osteo-; perineo-; etc.

THĒKĒ (θήκη), *a case to put something in, a box.* > theca [L. fr. G.] *a sheath* (esp. of a tendon); thec-al; -itis; apo-thecary [apothēkē, *a storehouse*]; apothec-ium; oo-theca [Mod. L. fr. ōon, egg + thēkē], *ovary.*

THEMA, -ATOS (θέμα, -ατος), *something laid down; a theme.* > apo-theme; epi-; schizo-themia.

THETOS (θετός), verbal adj. of tithēmi, *placed, set.* > athet-osis [athetos, *without place*]; -oid.

**THEL-**

THĒLĒ (θηλή), *the teat, nipple;* fr. THAŌ (θάω), *to suckle.* > thel-oncus; theleplasty; etc.; epi-thelium (originally applied to the thin skin covering the nipples); -theloma; etc.

THĒLYS (θῆλυς), *female.* > thely-tocia, *giving birth to females only;* -blast, *feminonucleus.*

**THER-**

THERAPEUŌ (θεραπεύω), *to be an attendant; to take care of; to treat medically.* H. > therap-y; -eia [G]; therapeu-tics; etc.

**THREP-**, see TREPH-

**THYM-1**

THYMON (θύμον), *thyme.* > thym-e; -ol; -ene, *a volatile oil derived from thyme;* -ic; etc.

THYMOS (θύμος), *a warty excrescence,* so called from its resemblance to a bunch of thyme flowers. Gal.; *the thymus gland* in the chest of young animals; in calves, *the sweetbread.* > *the thymus, a gland* situated in the superior mediastinum and lower part of the neck; thymo-pathy; -ma; etc.

**THYM-2**

THYMOS (θυμός), *the soul; mind.* > a-thymia [G.]; anepi- [an- priv. + epithymia, *desire*]; bary-; cyclo-, *cyclic insanity;* eu-thymia [G.]; lipo- [G. *a swoon,* H. fr. leipō, *leave*]; para-.

**THYR-**

THYREOS (θυρεός), *a door-stone;* later *an oblong shield* (shaped like a door), fr. THYRA (θύρα), *a door;* THYRE-OEIDĒS (θυρεοειδής), *shield-shaped;* chondros th., *the thyreoid cartilage.* Gal. > thyreoid or thyroid; thyr-ine; thyreo-plasty; thyro-hyoid; thyroid-itis; para-thyroid; etc.

**TOM-**

TEMNŌ, fut. TEMŌ (τέμνω, τεμῶ), *to cut;* hence, TOMĒ (τομή), *a cutting;* TOMOS (τομός), *a piece cut off, a slice;* EKTOMĒ (ἐκτομή), *a cutting out.* > tomo-graph; -mania;

-tocia, *cesarean section;* etc. As suffixes, -tomy denotes a *cutting operation,* -tome, *a cutting surgical instrument,* -ectomy, *operative removal of an organ or gland,* e.g., teno-tomy, teno-tome, ten-ectomy. ana-tomy; a-tom (a- priv.) *i.e., something that cannot be cut;* dia-tom-ic; dicho-tomy [dicha, *in two, asunder*]; entomo-logy (entomos, *cut in pieces,* hence entomon *an insect,* from its being nearly *cut in two.* Cf. L. insectum under SEC-; axono-tmesis [tmesis, *a cutting*].

**TON-**, see TEN-

**TONS-**

TONSILLA, gen. and pl. -AE, *a sharp stake* to which vessels were attached; in pl. *the tonsils.* Cels. > tonsils; tonsillitis; tonsillo-tome; etc.

**TORS-, TORT-**

TORQUEO, pp. TORUS, *to turn, twist, wind*

TORSIO, -ONIS, *a wringing, griping.* > torsion; tors-ive; torso-clusion; tort-uous; torti-collis, *wry-neck;* torsio-meter; etc. re-tort, *a vessel used in distilling;* con-torsion; dextro-; levo-; torment [tormentum, *instrument of torture; torture*].

**TOX-**

TOXON (τόξον), *a bow.* > Tox-ascaris, *a genus of Ascaridae;* embryo-toxon; geron-, *arcus senilis.* TOXIKOS (τοξικός), of or for a bow; TOXICON (sc. pharmakon), arrow poison. > tox-emia or -aemia; toxi-cide; toxico-pathic; toxin, *a poisonous substance* produced during the growth of pathogenic organisms. toxin-osis; -emia; etc. toxo- as a combining form often = toxin, e.g., toxo-infection; -lysin, etc. anti-toxin; in-toxication; etc.

**TRACH-1**

TRACHYS, fem. TRACHEIA, ntr. TRACHY (τραχύς), *rough.* > trach-oma, *granular conjunctivitis;* -omatous; trachy-phonia; -chromatic; etc.

TRACHEIA (τραχεῖα), *the windpipe,* properly tracheia arteria, *the rough artery,* so called from the rings of gristle. > trachea, *the windpipe;* trachea-ectasy, *dilation of the trachea;* trache-alis; -algia; etc.

**TRACH-2**

TRACHĒLOS (τράχηλος), *the neck, throat; anything resembling a neck.* > In compounds, *the neck,* or *a necklike part.* trachel-agra; trachelo-cystitis, *inflammation of the neck* of the bladder.

**TREM-, TRES-**

TETRAINŌ, fut. TRĒSŌ (τετραίνω, τρήσω), *to bore through;* TRĒMA, -ATOS (τρῆμα, -ατος), *a perforation, orifice;* TRĒSIS (τρῆσις), *a boring through, a hole;* TRĒTOS (τρητός), verbal adj., *perforated.* > trema, *foramen, vulva;* tremat-ode; -oid; helico-trema; monorcho-; tresis, *perforation;* litho-tresis; spheno-; urethra-; a-tresia; colpo-; a-treto-as prefix *imperforate* [atrētos]; atreto-rrhinia; etc.

**TREP-, TROP-**

TREPŌ, fut. TREPSŌ (τρέπω, τρέψω), *to turn.* > Trepo nema [nema, *a thread*], *a genus of parasites* having rigid or *waving spiral forms.* atropa, *deadly nightshade* [Atropos, *one of the Fates,* fr. atropos, *not to be turned, unchangeable*]; atropine; -ism.

TROPĒ (τροπή), *a turn, turning;* in pl. *the solstices* or *tropics, i.e.,* when the sun appears *to turn* his course and cross the ecliptic. > trop-ism, *the turning of* living cells toward light or darkness, heat or cold, etc. ; tropo-meter; etc. trop ics, -ical; allo-trope; helio-; ectrop-ion [G. *everted eyelid*]; entrop-ion [entropē, *a turning toward*], *inverted eyelid;* irid-ectropium; -entropium; cheil-ectropion; geo-trop-ism; etc.-

**TREPH-**

TREPHŌ, fut. THREPSŌ (τρέφω, θρέψω), *to make grow or increase; rear, support.* > trephocyte, *a cell which supplies nutritious material* to the tissues; trephon-e (fr. pres. part.); threpso-logy; a-threpsia; thremmato-logy [thremma, -atos, *a nursling*]; a-trepsy (badly formed, fr. trephō); thrombus [L. fr. G. thrombos, *a clot*].

TROPHĒ (τροφή), *support, nourishment.* > troph-ism; tropho-logy; -derm; etc. a-trophy; hyper-; dys-; hepato-trophia; etc.

TROPHIKOS (τροφικός), *nursing, tending.* > auto-trophic; histo-; etc.

**TRIB-, TRIP-, TRYP-, TREP-**

TRIBŌ, fut. TRIPSŌ (τρίβω, τρίψω), *to rub, bruise, crush;* TRIPSIS (τρῖψις), *a rubbing.* > trib-ade; -adism; angio-tribe; basio-; tripsis, *massage;* litho-׳ ׳sis; odonto-; clido-tripsy; neuro-; etc.

TRYPAŌ, fut. -ĒSŌ (τρυπάω, -ησω), *to bore, pierce;* TRYPĒSIS, (τρύπησις), *a boring.* > craniotrypesis; etc.

TRYPANON (τρύπανον), *a borer, an auger, a trepan:* H. > Trypano-soma, *a genus of flagellate protozoa;* -somiasis; Trypano-plasma; etc. trepan (thr. old Fr.); -ation; -ize.

**TRICH-**

THRIX, TRICHOS (θρίξ, τριχος), *the hair.* > In compounds, *the hair,* or *a hairlike structure;* trich-atrophia; Trich-ina, *a genus of nematode worms;* -inella; -inosis; trich-osis[G. *a being hairy*], *any disease of the hair;* tricho-bacteria, *flagellated bacteria.* clasto-thrix; mono-trich-ous, *having one flagellum;* etc.

**TYP-**

TYPOS (τύπος), *a blow; mark of a blow; impression* of a seal, etc.; *original form or type.* > typus [L. fr. G.]; typ-ical; arche-type (archetypos, *first-molded, a model*]; homo-; pheno-; stereo-typy; gony-ectyposis [ektypōsis, *modeling in relief*].

**TYPH-**

TYPHOS (τῦφος), *smoke; vapor; stupor* arising from fever. H. > typhus; typh-oid; typho-genic; pyreto-typhosis [typhōsis, *crazy vanity*].

**TYPHL-**

TYPHLOS, -E, -ON, (τυφλός), *blind;* TYPHLON (ntr., enteron understood), *the cecum; cf.* L. caecum (intestinum understood). > typhl-itis; -ectomy; typhlo-ptosis; etc. typhl-osis [G.], *blindness;* typhlo-logy, *science dealing with blindness.*

**UL-1**

OULĒ (οὐλή), *a scar.* > ul-erythema; -oid; -osis; -otic; ulo-dermatitis. See the following.

**UL-2**

OULON (οὖλον), usually pl., *the gums; a gumboil.* H. > ul-emorrhagia, *bleeding from the gums,* -itis; ulo-cace (kakĕ, *badness*); parulis [paroulis, *a gumboil*]; etc. Words such as the following refer either to *a scar,* or to *the gums,* and are derived from OULĒ or OULON acc. to their meaning: ul-ectomy; -etic; ulo-tomy.

**UR-**

OURON (οὖρον), *urine.* > ur-acratia, *incontinence of urine;* -emia; -ic; uric-emia; urico-lysis; uro-logy; urono-phile; glyc-uresis [ourĕsis]; etc.

OURĒTHRA (οὐρήθρα), *urethra.* > urethra; urethr-ism; urethra-l; -scope; urethro-graph; etc.

OURACHOS (οὐραχός), *the urinary canal of a fetus.* H. > urachus, *the portion of the allantois which lies within the body of the fetus.*

OURĒTĒR (οὐρητήρ) = *ourethra* in earlier writers, as H.; later same as mod. anat.; Gal. > ureter; uretero-plasty; etc.

URINA, *urine.* > id.; urin-emia; -al; -ate; urina-lysis; etc.

**UV-**

UVA, *a grape; a bunch of grapes; the soft palate, uvula.* Cels. > uv-ea, *the pigmented layer of the eye;* -eal; uve-itis; uvi-form, *shaped like a grape;* uvae-formis, *the middle layer of the choroid coat.*

UVULA, gen. and pl. -AE, a Mod. L. dim. of uva. > uvula, 1. *pendulum palati;* 2. *a triangular elevation* on the vermis of the cerebellum; uvul-ar; uvula-ptosia; uvolo-tomy; etc.

**VACC-**

VACCA, *a cow;* VACCINUS, -A, -UM, *relating to a cow.* > vaccin-a or -ia, *cowpox;* vaccin-e; -ation; etc.

**VAGI-**

VAGINA, gen. and pl. -AE, *a scabbard, sheath; the covering, sheath* of anything; *the vagina.* > *any sheathlike structure; the female genital canal;* vagin-al; vagino-cele; etc.

**VARI-1**

VARIX, -ICIS, *a dilated vein;* fr. VARUS, *bent, stretched.* > id.; varic-ose; -osis; varici-form; varico-cele; var-isse, *a lump* on the inner side of the hind leg of a horse; VARICULA, gen. and pl. -AE, dim., *a small varix.* Cels. > *conjunctival varix.*

**VARI-2**

VARIUS, *diverse, varying, different; mottled, spotted.* > var-y; vari-ety; -ant; -egate; -ability; -ation, etc.

VARIOLA, Mediev. L., *smallpox.* > id.; variol-ar; -ate; -ous; varioli-form; etc.

VARICELLA, Mod. L. dim. of variola, *chickenpox.* > id.; varicell-ation, *inoculation with chickenpox virus;* -oid; -ous.

**VECT-, VET-, VEX-**

VEHO, pp. VECTUS, pf. VEXI, *to bear, carry, draw.* > vect-ion; vector [L.]; -ial; veh-icle.

VETERIN-US, -A, -UM, *pertaining to beasts of* burden; -ARIUS, noun, *a cattle-doctor.* > veterinar-y; -ian.

CONVEHO, pp. -VECTUS, *carry together,* hence, CON-VEXUS, *vaulted, arched, convex.* > convex, -ity; convect-ion.

**VEL-**

VELUM, -I, pl. -A, *a cover, curtain, veil; a sail.* > *a structure resembling a veil or curtain;* veli-form; vel-ar.

VELAMEN, -INIS, pl. -INA, *a covering, a veil.* > *a membranous envelope or covering.*

VELAMENTUM, -I, pl. -A, same as preceding. > id.; velament-ous.

**VENT-**

VENTER, -TRIS, *the belly; womb; entrails; anything that swells or bellies out.* > *the abdomen; uterus; the swelling part of* a muscle, etc.; ventr-al; -ad; ventri-cornu; ventro-myel, *the anterior portion of the spinal cord;* etc.

VENTRICULUS, gen. and pl. -I, dim., *the belly; the stomach; a ventricle* of the heart. > *the stomach;* a ventricle *of the brain or heart;* ventricul-ar; ventriculo-graphy; etc.

**VERT-, VORT-**

VERTO or VORTO, pp. -SUS, *to turn.* > vert, *to turn, duct;* version, *displacement* of the uterus; *change of position* of fetus in womb; arterio-version; levo-; intro-; etc.

VERTEBRA, gen. and pl. -AE, *a joint; vertebra.* Cels. > *a segment of the spinal column;* vertebr-al; -ate; vertebro-chon-dral; etc. in-vertebr-ate.

VERTIGO, -INIS, *a whirling round; dizziness.* > id.; verti-gin-ous.

VERTEX or VORTEX, -ICIS, *a whirl, eddy, whirlpool; the crown* of the head; *the highest point.* > In mod. medicine the two forms of the word have different meanings, vertex, *the crown or top of the head; the apex of the heart;* vortex, *a whorl-like structure.*

VERTICILLUS, dim., *the whirl* of a spindle. > verticil, *a whorl;* Verticill-ium, *a genus of fungi.*

**VISC-**

VISCUM, *mistletoe; birdlime,* made from its berries. > visc-in, *a glutinous substance from mistletoe;* -ose; visco-meter; etc.

VISCIDUS, *clammy, sticky.* > viscid; -ity.

VISCUS, -ERIS, pl. -ERA, *the soft parts; internal organs.* > id.; viscer-ad; -al; viscero-genic; etc.

**XEN-**

XENOS (ξένος), *guest; host; stranger; foreigner.* > xen-em-bole, *introduction of a foreign substance* into the system; xeno-genesis; -menia; -parasite; -gamy, *cross fertilization,* bot.; etc. Xeno-psylla *a genus of fleas.*

**XER-**

XĒROS (ξηρός), *dry.* > xer-anis [G.], *a gradual loss o₁ moisture in the tissues;* -antic; -aphium (xĕraphion), *a drying powder;* -asia [G. *dryness*], *extreme dryness of the hair;* xero-derma; etc.

**ZE-, ZY-**

ZEŌ (ζέω), *to boil;* hence, ZĒLOS (ζῆλος), *eager rivalry;* ZEMA, -ATOS (ζέμα), *something boiled;* zestos (ζεστός), *boiling hot.* > zeo-scope; zela-typia, *morbid zeal;* zesto-causis, *cauterization by hot steam.*

EKZEŌ (ἐκζέω), *to boil out,* or *over;* of a disease, *to break out;* hence, EKZEMA, -ATOS (ἔκζεμα), *eczema.* Gal. > id.; eczemat-ous; -ization.

ZYMĒ (ζύμη), *leaven.* > zyme, *a ferment;* zym-ad; -ase; -ic; zymo-gen; -logy; -sis [G.]. en-zyme; a-zymia.

**ZO-**

ZAŌ (ζάω), *to live;* hence,

ZŌĒ (ζωή), *a living, life.* > zo-etic, *pertaining to life;* -ic; a-zote (i.e., *not suitable for living beings*) [thr. Fr. fr. a- priv. + zōë] *nitrogen;* a-zoic; meso-; palaeo-; etc.

ZŌON (ζῷον), *a living being, an animal.* > zo-anthropy, *delusion that one is an animal;* zo-iatria, *veterinary medicine;* zoo-biology; -cyst; -phyte; etc. proto-zoon; spermato-; etc.

ZŌDION (ζῴδιον), dim. *a small figure;* in pl. *the signs of the zodiac.* > zodio-philous, bot. *pollinated by animals;* zodiac

# GREEK AND LATIN PREPOSITIONAL AND ADVERBIAL PREFIXES

A knowledge of the following words is very necessary for the proper understanding of the formation of compounds. The rules for assimilation and elision that apply to them are given for reference. (For further discussion pertaining to the prefixes marked with an asterisk, see "Prefixes," p. xxii.

**a-** or **an-** (ἀ- or ἀν-), inseparable particle, a- negative or privative, *un-, in-, not, without;* bef. a vowel usually an-.

**ab, a, abs,** prep., *away from.*

**ad,** prep., *to, toward; at;* unchanged bef. vowels and *b, d, h, m, v;* the d is usually assimilated bef. *c, f, g, l, m, p, r, s, t.**

**ambi-, am-,** insep. prep., *around, on both sides.*

**amphi** (ἀμφί), prep., *about, around, on both sides.**

**ana** (ἀνά), prep., *up to, upwards; back; again.*

**ante,** prep., *before; forwards.*

**anti** (ἀντί), prep., *against; opposite.**

**apo** (ἀπό), prep., *from; asunder; back; again.*

**bis,** in compounds **bi-,** adv., *twice, double, two-.*

**cata,** see kata.

**circum,** adv. and prep., *around, about.*

**contra,** adv. and prep., *opposite; against.*

**cum,** in compounds **com-,** prep., *with, together with;* com- is unchanged bef. *b, p, m;* the m is assimilated bef. *r* as in corrigo and often bef. *l* as in colligo; usually dropped bef. *n;* it is changed to *n* bef. all remaining consonants, con-cutio, etc; usually dropped bef. vowels and *h,* coarguo, cohibeo.

**de,** prep., *from, away from, down from.*

**dia** (διά), prep., *through; in different directions; to the end; completely.*

**dis** (δίς), adv., *twice, doubly;* **di-** in compounds bef. a consonant, except *s, th, t, m, p, ch.*

**dis-,** insep. particle, *asunder, apart; in two;* in compounds sometimes **di-** (bef. *b, d, g, l, m*); it becomes **dif-** bef. *f.*

**dys-** (δυς-), insep. adv., *bad; unlucky; difficult;* like Eng. *mis-, un-.*

**e** or **ex,** prep., *from out of; from;* ex always bef. vowels, and more freq. than e bef. consonants.

**ek** or **ex** (ἐκ or ἐξ), prep., *from out of; from;* ex bef. a vowel.

**ektos** (ἐκτός), adv. and prep., *outside, external;* in Eng. compounds ecto-; opp. to entos.

**en** (ἐν), prep., *in;* in compounds en becomes **em-** bef. *b, m, p, ph, ps;* **el-** bef. *l.*

**endon** (ἔνδον), adv., *in, within;* in compounds **endo-**.

**entos** (ἐντός), adv. and prep., *within;* in Eng. compounds **ento-**.

**epi** (ἐπί), prep., *on, upon; against.**

**eu** (εὖ), adv., *well;* implies *abundance, prosperity, easiness.*

**exō** (ἔξω), adv., *outside, on the outside.*

**extra,** adv. and prep., *outside; beyond; in addition.*

**hemi-** (ἡμί-), insep. prefix, *half-.*

**hyper** (ὑπέρ), prep., *over, above; excessive.*

**hypo** (ὑπό), prep., *under;* in compounds also implies *deficiency.*

**in,** prep., *in, on; into; to;* in compounds in is changed to **im-** bef. a labial; the n is assimilated bef. *l, m, r; cf.* irrigation.

**in-,** insep. negative particle, *un-, in-, not;* **im-** bef. *b* and *p;* the n is assimilated bef. *l, m, r; cf.* irrespirable.

**infra,** adv. and prep., *underneath, below.*

**inter,** adv. and prep., *between; among.*

**intra,** adv. and prep., *on the inside, within; during.*

**intro,** adv., *inwardly, internally; during.*

**kata** (κατά), prep., *down from, down; against; throughout;* in compounds often only strengthens the simple word; in Eng. compounds **cata-**.*

**meta** (μετά), prep., *among; between; along with; after, afterwards;* in compounds often implies *change.**

**ob,** prep., *before; against; on account of;* in compounds the b is unchanged bef. vowels and most consonants; bef. *p, f, c, g,* it is often assimilated.

**para** (παρά), prep., *beside; to the side of, to;* in compounds often means *aside, amiss, wrong;* also *change.*

**per,** prep., *through, throughout;* in compounds may add intensity; *thoroughly, completely.*

**peri** (περί), prep., *round about; above, beyond; exceedingly.**

**post,** adv. and prep., of place *behind;* of time *after.*

**prae,** adv. and prep., *before, in front;* in compounds often enhances meaning, as prae-altus, *very high;* Eng. prefix **pre-**.

**pro** (πρός), prep., *before* (of place and time).

**pro,** adv. and prep., *before, in front of; for* with sense of *protection* or *substitution.*

**pros** (πρός), prep., *motion from* or *to* a place; in compounds motion *toward; besides* (in addition); *beside* (of place).

**re-** or **red-,** insep. particle, *back; again.*

**retro,** adv., *backwards, back.*

**semi-,** insep. particle, *half-, demi-, semi-.*

**sub,** prep., *under, beneath;* of time *during, immediately before* or *after;* in compounds also *rather, slightly;* the b is unchanged bef. vowels and *b, d, j, l, n, s, t, v;* it is assimilated regularly bef. *c, f, g, p,* and often bef. *m* and *r;* sometimes bef. *c, p, t* sub becomes **sus-**.

**super,** adv. and prep., *above, over; in addition.*

**supra,** adv., *on the upper side, above.*

**syn** (σύν), prep., *with, together;* in compounds bef. *b, m, p, ph, ps,* becomes sym- (συμ-); bef. *l* becomes **syl-** (συλ), bef. *s* becomes **sy-** (συ-).*

**trans,** prep., *across, beyond; through;* in compounds unchanged bef. vowels except *i* and bef. consonants *b, c, f, g, p, r, t, v;* either **trans-** or **tra-** bef. *i, j, d, l, m, n;* the *s* of trans is usu. dropped bef. another *s.*

**ultra,** adv. and prep., *beyond; besides; over.*

# PLURAL, ADJECTIVAL, AND COMBINING FORMS OF MEDICAL TERMS

Word formation is discussed on pp. xxi to xxiii of this section on medical etymology. Given below is a series of tables listing examples that will facilitate choice of plural, adjectival, and combining forms for nouns of Greek or Latin derivation. Each table includes (1) the singular nominative-case form of the noun (the form in which the word occurs in the dictionary); (2) its corresponding genitive-case form (with ending underscored, to distinguish this from the word's true stem); (3) its nominative plural form; (4) its corresponding adjective; and (5) its combining form.

Reference numbers (superscribed numbers in the tables) have been provided citing, for words of Greek origin, H. W. Smyth, *Greek Grammar*, Harvard University Press, 1956, and for words of Latin origin, B. L. Gildersleeve and G. Lodge, *Gildersleeve's Latin Grammar*, Macmillan, London, 1960.

Several alternative forms of adjectives are printed in the tables. These multiple forms are not always strictly synonymous. The specific meaning of each is given in the dictionary. Where they occur in the tables these forms have been included merely to call attention to their existence.

In the following tables, stressed syllables are indicated by an accent mark above the vowel. This is a departure from the system of accenting used in the body of the dictionary (see "Key to Simplified Phonetic Spellings," p. xii), but it is the one proper to the Greek language.

TABLE 1. *Greek derivatives*

| Singular, nominative case | | Genitive case | Nominative plural form | Adjectival form | Combining form |
|---|---|---|---|---|---|
| **First declension** | | | | | |
| lennorrhágia | βλεννορραγία | βλεννορραγίας (f.)[216] | blennorrhágiae | blennorrhágic | blennorrhági-o |
| erístole | περιστολή | περιστολῆς (f.)[216] | perístolae | peristólic | perístol-o |
| eróne | περόνη | περόνης (f.)[216] | perónae | peronéal | peroné-o |
| **Second declension** | | | | | |
| sóphagus | οἰσοφάγος | οἰσοφάγου (m.)[231] | esóphagi | esophágeal | esóphag-o |
| ylórus | πυλωρός | πυλωροῦ (m.)[231] | pylóri | pylóric | pylór-o |
| ÿdroperi-cárdium | ὑδροπερικάρδιον | ὑδροπερικαρδίου (n.)[231] | hÿdropericárdia | hÿdropericárdiac, hydroperi-cárdial | hÿdropericárdi-o |
| hállus | φαλλός | φαλλοῦ (m.)[231] | phálli | phállic | pháll-o |
| hórion | χορίον | χορίου (n.)[231] | chória | choriónic | chóri-o |
| eriósteum | περιόστεον | περιοστέου (n.)[235] | perióstea | periósteal | perióste-o |
| **Third declension** | | | | | |
| nasárca | ἀνὰ σάρκα | σάρξ, σαρκός (f.)[256] | anasárcae | anasárcous | anasárc-o |
| lennothórax | βλεννοθώραξ | βλεννοθώρακος (m.)[256] | blennothóraces | blennothorácic | blennothórac-o |
| élix | ἕλιξ | ἕλικος (f.)[256] | hélices | hélicine, hélical | hélic-o |
| ályx | κάλυξ | κάλυκος (f.)[256] | cályces | cálycine | cályc-o |
| álpinx | σάλπιγξ | σάλπιγγος (f.)[256] | salpínges* | salpíngian | salpíng-o |
| ÿdrops | ὕδρωψ | ὕδρωπος (m.)[256] | hýdropes | hydrópic | hýdrop-o |
| hárynx | φάρυγξ | φάρυγγος (f.)[256] | pharýnges* | pharýngeal | pharýng-o |
| tlas | ἄτλας | ἄτλαντος (m.)[257] | atlántes* | atlántic | atlánt-o |
| élminth | ἕλμινς | ἕλμινθος (f.)[257] | helmínthes* | helmínthic | helmínth-o |

TABLE 1. *Greek derivatives—continued*

| Singular, nominative case | Genitive case | Nominative plural form | Adjectival form | Combining form |
|---|---|---|---|---|
| | | Third declension—*continued* | | |
| epidídymis | ἐπιδιδυμίς | ἐπιδιδυμίδος (f.)[257] | epididýmides | epidídymal | epidídym-o |
| schizomýces | σχιζομύκης | σχιζομύκητος (m.)[257] | schizomycétes | schizomycétic | schizomycét-o |
| diaphrágma | διάφραγμα | διαφράγματος (n.)[258] | diaphrágmata | diaphragmátic | diaphrágmat-o |
| kéras | κέρας | κέρατος (n.)[258] | kérata | kerátic, kératose | kérat-o |
| phlégma | φλέγμα | φλέγματος (n.)[258] | phlégmata | phlegmátic | phlégmat-o |
| áxon | ἄξων | ἄξονος (m.)[259] | áxones | axónic, áxonal | áxon-o |
| cremáster | κρεμαστήρ | κρεμαστῆρος (m.)[259] | cremastéres | cremastéric | cremastér-o |
| gáster | γαστήρ | γαστ-έ-ρός (f.)[262] | gastéres | gástric | gástr-o |
| angiostáxis | ἀγγειοστάξις | ἀγγειοστάξεως (f.)[268] | angiostáxes | angiostáctic | angiostáxe-o |
| ecchymósis | ἐκχύμωσις | ἐκχυμώσεως (f.)[268] | ecchymóses | ecchymótic | ecchymóse-o |

\* The accent in asterisked forms (Latinized) follows the Latin rule that, if the second-last syllable long, it receives the accent.

TABLE 2. *Latin derivatives*

| Singular nominative case | Genitive case | Nominative plural form | Adjectival form | Combining form |
|---|---|---|---|---|
| | | First declension | | |
| fístula | fístulae (f.)[29] | fístulae | fístular, fístulate, fístulous | fístul-o |
| lamélla | laméllae (f.)[29] | laméllae | laméllar | laméll-o |
| lámina | láminae (f.)[29] | láminae | láminar, láminated | lámin-o |
| | | Second declension | | |
| acúleus | acúlei (m.)[33] | acúlei | acúleate | acúle-o |
| múcus | múci (m.)[33] | múci | múcous | múc-o |
| músculus | músculi (m.)[33] | músculi | múscular | múscul-o |
| pulvínus | pulvíni (m.)[33] | pulvíni | pulvínar, púlvinate | pulvín-o |
| tóphus | tóphi (m.)[33] | tóphi | topháceous | tóph-o |
| vermículus | vermículi (m.)[33] | vermículi | vermícular, vermícu-lous, vermículose | vermícul-o |
| íleum | ílei (n.)[33] | ílea | íleal | íle-o |
| sérum | séri (n.)[33] | séra | sérous | sér-o |
| divertículum | divertículi (n.)[33] | divertícula | divertícular, diver-tículate | divertícul-o |
| | | Third declension | | |
| sal | sális (m.)[39] | sáles | sáline | sál-o |
| aerúgo | aerúginis (f.)[41.2] | aerúgines | aerúginous | aerúgin-o |
| sudámen | sudáminis (n.)[41.2] | sudámina | sudáminal | sudámin-o |
| téndo | téndinis (f.)[41.2] | téndines | téndinous | téndin-o |
| tussédo | tussédinis (f.)[41.2] | tussédines | tussédinal | tussédin-o |
| cálcar | cálcaris (n.)[44.1] | calcária | cálcarine, cálcarate | cálcar-o |

TABLE 2. *Latin derivatives—continued*

| Singular nominative case | Genitive case | Nominative plural form | Adjectival form | Combining form |
|---|---|---|---|---|
| | | Third declension—*continued* | | |
| cadáver | cadáveris (n.)[44.1] | cadávera | cadáverous, cadáverine | cadáver-o |
| vómer | vómeris (m.)[44.2] | vómeres | vómeral | vómer-o |
| vǎsoconstríctor | vǎsoconstrictóris (m.)[44.3] | vǎsoconstrictóres | vǎsoconstríctoral | vasoconstríctor-o |
| os | óssis (n.)[47.4] | óssa | ósseous | ósse-o; óste-o (Gk.) |
| pus | púris (n.)[47.5] | púra | púrulent | púr-o |
| córpus | córporis (n.)[49] | córpora | córporal, corpóreal | córpor-o |
| ádeps | ádipis (f.)[51.3] | ádipes | adípic, ádipose | ádip-o |
| cicátrix | cicatrícis (f.)[52.3] | cicatríces | cicatrícial | cicátric-o |
| rádix | radícis (f.)[52.3] | radíces | rádical | rádic-o |
| faux | fáucis[52.7] | fáuces | fáucial | fáuc-o |
| nátis | nátis (f.)[53.1] | nátes | nátal | nát-o |
| cávitas | cavitátis (f.)[53.1] | cavitátes | cavit(at)ary: cávitary | cavit(at)-o; cávit-o |
| páries | paríetis (m.)[53.2] | paríetes | paríetal | paríet-o |
| íncus | incúdis (f.)[53.5] | incúdes | íncudal, incúdiform | incúd-o |
| tússis | tússis (f.)[56] | tússes | tússal | túss-i |
| vérmis | vérmis (f.)[56] | vérmes | vermícular, vermículose (from diminutive: vermículus) | vérm-i |
| vérmin | French origin: vermine | vérmin | vérminal, vérminous | vérmin-o |
| cútis | cútis (f.)[56.1] | cútes | cútic | cút-i |
| | | Fourth declension | | |
| spíritus | spíritus (m.)[61] | spíritus | spíritous | spírit-o |
| | | Fifth declension | | |
| cáries | cariéi (f.)[63] | cáries | cárious | cári-o |

TABLE 3. *Compound terms*

| Compound term | Plural form | Adjectival form | Combining form |
|---|---|---|---|
| Latin noun + Latin adjective (the adjective indicates by its ending agreement in grammatical gender, number and case with the noun it modifies) | | | |
| túnica[29] mucósa[73] | túnicae mucósae | mucǒsotúnical, mucǒsotúnicate | mucǒsotúnic-o |
| hílus[33] renális[78] | híli renáles | renihílar, renipórtal | renihíl-o |
| mémbrum[33] viríle[78] | mémbra virília | virimémbral | virimémbr-o |
| cartilágo[41.2] arytenǒídea[73] ἀρυταινοειδής[898a] | cartilágines arytenǒídeae | arytenǒídocartiláginous | arytenǒídocartilágin-o |
| cartilágo[41.2] cuneifórmis[78] | cartilágines cuneifórmes | cǔneocartiláginous | cǔneocartilágin-o |
| articulátio[41.3] selláris[78] | articulatiónes selláres | sěllarticulátional | sěllarticulátion-o |
| jécur[44.4] adipósum[73] | jécura adipósa | ǎdipojécural | ǎdipojécur-o |
| hállux[52.5] fléxus[73] | hálluces fléxi | fléxihállucal | fléxihálluc-o |
| tálipes[53.2] várus[73] | talípedes vári | váritalípedal | váritalíped-o |
| meátus[61] urinárius[73] | meátus urinárii | úrinomeátal | úrinomeát-o |

TABLE 3. *Compound terms—continued*

| Compound term | Plural form | Adjectival form | Combining form |
|---|---|---|---|
| **Latin noun + Latin delimiting genitive** | | | |
| malléolus[33] fíbulae[29] | malléoli fíbulae | fíbulomalléolar | fíbulomalléol-o |
| óstium[33] úteri[33] | óstia úteri | útero-óstial | útero-ósti-o |
| infundíbulum[33] crúris[47.5] | infundíbula crúris | crúro-infundíbular | crúro-infundíbul-o |
| íter[44.5] déntium[53.7] | itínera déntium | dentitíneral | dentitíner-o |
| **Latin noun + Latinized Greek delimiting genitive** | | | |
| cistérna[29] chýli[33] χυλός[231] | cistérnae chýli | chýlocistérnal | chýlocistérn-o |
| **Latinized Greek noun + Latin delimiting genitive** | | | |
| sýmphysis[56.1] púbis[56.2] σύμφυσις, συμφύσεως[268] | sýmphyses púbis | púbosymphýseal | púbosymphýse-o |
| **Anglicized Latin/Greek** | | | |
| bile (bílis)[56.1] | biles | bíliary | bíli-o |
| crícoid cártilage (κρικοειδής: cricoídeus) | crícoid cártilages | crícocartiláginous | crícocartilágin-o |
| hébetude (hebetúdo)[41.2] | hébetudes | hebetúdinal | hebetúdin-o |
| prépuce (praepútium)[33] | prépuces | prepútial | prepúti-o |

# A

α. 1. First letter of the Greek alphabet, alpha, *q.v.* 2. Symbol for Bunsen's solubility *coefficient.*

**A.** 1. Abbreviation for ampere. 2. Symbol for adenosine or adenylic acids in polynucleotides. 3. Symbol (usually capitalized italic) for absorbance. 4. As a subscript, refers to alveolar *gas.*

**°A.** Symbol for degree absolute (an obsolete term replaced by °K, degrees Kelvin).

**Å.** Abbreviation for Ångstrom *unit.*

**a.** 1. Abbreviation for accommodation, anterior, total acidity, area, asymmetric. 2. Symbol (usually italic) for specific absorption *coefficient.* 3. As a subscript, refers to systemic arterial blood.

**aa, āā.** Abbreviation for ana, *q.v.*

**a-, an-** [ G. alpha, privative or negative, inseparable prefix, usually *an-* before a vowel ]. Prefix equivalent to the L. *in-* and E. *un-;* not, without, -less.

**AA.** Abbreviation for amino acids or aminoacyl.

**AAF.** Abbreviation for 2-acetylaminofluorene.

**Aaron,** Charles D., American physician, 1866–1951. See A.'s *sign.*

**ab-** [ L. *ab,* from ]. Prefix signifying from, away from, off.

**abaca** (ah-bah-kah′) [ Native Philippine ]. The plant, *Musa textilis,* and its product, Manila hemp.

**Abadie** (ah-bah-de′), Charles A., French ophthalmologist, 1842–1932. See A.'s *sign* of exophthalmic goiter.

**Abadie** (ah-bah-de′), Joseph L. I. J., French neurosurgeon, 1873–1946. See A.'s *sign* of tabes dorsalis.

**abaissement** (ah-bās-moṅ′) [ Fr. a lowering ]. Couching.

**abalienated** (ab-āl′yen-a-ted) [ L. *ab-alieno,* pp. *-atus,* to separate from. ALI- ]. Mentally deranged.

**abalienation** (ab-āl-yen-a′shun). Mental derangement.

**abam′pere.** The electromagnetic unit of current equal to 10 absolute amperes; a current that exerts on unit magnetic pole at the center of a circle of wire (1 cm. in radius) through which the current passes a force of $2\pi$ dynes.

**abap′ical.** Opposite the apex.

**abarognosis** (ab-ar-og-no′sis) [ G. *a*-priv. + *baros,* weight, + *gnōsis,* knowledge ]. Loss of sense of weight estimation.

**abarthro′sis** [ L. *ab,* from, + G. *arthrōsis,* a joining ]. Dislocation of a joint.

**abartic′ular.** At a distance from, or not involving, a joint.

**abarticula′tion** [ L. *ab,* from, + *articulatio,* joint ]. 1. Dislocation of a joint.

**abasia** (ă-ba′zĭ-ah) [ G. *a-* priv. + *basis,* step. BAS- ]. Inability to walk.
   **a.-asta′sia,** see astasia-abasia.
   **atac′tic a., atax′ic a.,** difficulty in walking by reason of ataxia.
   **choreic a.,** a. related to abnormal movements of the legs.
   **paralytic a.,** a. related to inability to move the leg muscles.
   **paroxysmal trepidant a.,** a. related to spasticity of the legs.
   **spastic a.,** a. due to a spastic contraction of the muscles when an attempt is made to walk.
   **a. trep′idans,** a. due to trembling of the lower limbs.

**abasic, abatic** (ă-ba′sik, ă-bat′ik). Affected by, or associated with, abasia.

**abax′ial, abax′ile.** 1. Lying outside the axis of any body or part. 2. Situated at the opposite extremity of the axis of a part.

**Ab′bau** [ Ger. degradation, deterioration ]. The histologically demonstrable breakdown products noted in many degenerative diseases of the central nervous system.

**Abbé** (ab-a′), Ernst, German physicist, 1840–1905. See A.'s *condenser,* A.-Zeiss *apparatus.*

**Abbé-Estlander operation.** See under operation.

**Abbott,** Alexander C., Philadelphia bacteriologist, 1860–1935. See A.'s *stain* for spores.

**Abbott,** Edville G., American orthopaedic surgeon, 1871–1938. See A.'s *method* of treatment of scoliosis.

**Abbott,** W. Osler, Philadelphia physician, 1902–1943. See A.'s *tube,* Miller-A. *tube.*

**Abderhalden** (ahb′der-hal′den), Emil, Swiss physiologist, 1877–1950. See A.'s *reaction, test.*

**Abderhalden,** F. See A.-Fanconi *syndrome.*

**abdomen** (ab-do′men; ab′do-men) [ L. *abdomen,* etym. uncertain ] [ NA ]. Belly; venter; the part of the trunk that lies between the thorax and the pelvis. The a. does not include the vertebral region posteriorly but is considered by some anatomists to include the pelvis. It contains the greater part of the abdominal cavity, cavum abdominis. The a. is divided by arbitrary planes into nine regions; see also regiones abdominis, under regio.
   **acute a.,** surgical a.; medical jargon for any serious acute intra-abdominal condition (such as appendicitis) attended by pain, tenderness, and muscular rigidity, and requiring an operation.
   **car′inate a.** [ L. *carina,* keel of a ship ], a sinking at the sides with prominence of the central line of the a.
   **navic′ular a.,** scaphoid a.; a condition in which the anterior abdominal wall is sunken and presents a concave rather than a convex contour.
   **a. obsti′pum** [ L. *obstipus,* awry ], deformity of the a. caused by shortness of the recti muscles.
   **pendulous a.,** one with greatly relaxed walls that sag down over the pubic region.
   **scaphoid a.,** navicular a.
   **surgical a.,** acute a.

**abdomin-.** See abdomino-.

**abdom′inal.** Relating to the abdomen.

**abdominalgia** (ab-dom-in-al′je-ah) [ abdomen + G. *algos,* pain ]. Celialgia; celiodynia; abdominal pain.
   **periodic a.,** familial paroxysmal *polyserositis.*

**abdomino-, abdomin-** [ L. *abdomen, q.v.* ]. Combining forms denoting relationship to the abdomen.

**abdom′inocente′sis** [ abdomino- + G. *kentēsis,* puncture ]. Paracentesis of the abdomen.

**abdominocyesis** (ab-dom′ĭ-no-si-e′sis) [ abdomino- + G. *kyēsis,* pregnancy ]. 1. Abdominal *pregnancy.* 2. Secondary abdominal *pregnancy.*

**abdominocystic** (ab-dom-ĭ-no-sis′tik) [ abdomino- + G. *kystis,* bladder ]. Abdominovesical.

**abdom′inogen′ital.** Relating to the abdomen and the genital organs.

**abdom′inohysterec′tomy.** Abdominal *hysterectomy.*

**abdom′inohysterot′omy.** Abdominal *hysterotomy.*

**abdominos′copy** [ abdomino- + G. *skopeō,* to examine ]. Peritoneoscopy.

**abdom′inoscro′tal.** Relating to the abdomen and the scrotum.

**abdom′inothorac′ic.** Relating to both abdomen and thorax.

**abdominouterotomy** (ab-dom′ĭ-no-u-ter-ot′o-mĭ). Abdominal *hysterotomy.*

**abdom′inovag′inal.** Relating to both abdomen and vagina.

**abdom′inoves′ical.** Abdominocystic; relating to the abdomen and urinary bladder, or to the abdomen and gallbladder.

**abduce** (ab-dūs′). Abduct.

**abdu′cens** [ L. ] [ NA ]. Abducent.
   **a. oculi,** *musculus* rectus lateralis oculi.

**abdu′cent** [ L. *abducens* ]. Abducting; drawing away.

**abduct** (ab-dukt′). Abduce; to move away from the axis of the body or of one of its parts.

**abduction** (ab-duk′shun) [ L. *abductio* ]. 1. Movement away from the middle line. 2. Movement (duction) of the eye toward the temple. 3. A position resulting from such movement.

**abduc′tor** [ NA ]. That which abducts or draws something in a direction away from the middle line of the body or of a part, said of various muscles; the opposite of adductor.

**Abegg,** Richard, Danish chemist, 1869–1910. See A.'s *rule.*

**Abel,** John Jacob, "Father of American Pharmacology," 1857–1938. Sometime Professor of Pharmacology of the Johns Hopkins Medical School, and editor of *The Journal of Pharmacology and Experimental Therapeutics.* Inventor of vividiffusion apparatus; see *vividiffusion.*

**Abel,** Rudolf, Jena bacteriologist, 1868–1942. See A.'s *bacillus,*

**ab'embryon'ic** [ L. *ab,* from, + embryonic ]. Opposite the region at which the embryo is formed.

**abenter'ic** [ L. *ab,* from, + G. *enteron,* intestine ]. Apenteric.

**Ab'ercrombie,** John, Scottish physician, 1780–1844. See A.'s *degeneration.*

**Ab'ernethy,** John, London surgeon and anatomist, 1764–1831. See A.'s *fascia, sarcoma.*

**aber'rancy.** Aberration.

**aber'rans** [ L. ] [ NA ]. Aberrant.

**aber'rant** [ L. *aberrans* ]. 1. Wandering off; said of certain ducts, vessels, or nerves taking an unusual course. 2. Differing from the normal, said in botany or zoology of certain atypical individuals in a species. 3. Ectopic.

**aberratio** (ab-er-a'she-o) [ L. ]. Aberration.
  **a. testis,** presence of the testis in a part away from the path followed in a normal descent.

**aberration** (ab-er-a'shun) [ L. *aberratio* ]. Aberrancy. 1. A straying from the normal situation. 2. Deviant development or growth.
  **angle of a.,** see under angle.
  **chromatic a.,** color a.; Newtonian a.; chromatism; a colored fringe on the border of an image produced by the unequal refraction of different wavelengths.
  **chromosome a.,** see under chromosome.
  **diop'tric a.,** spherical a.
  **distan'tial a.,** blurring of the image of a distant object.
  **lateral a.,** the amount of a. expressed as the lateral deviation of a ray from a point reference on the axis ordinarily from an assumed or empiric focal point.
  **longitudinal a.,** displacement of the image, or a series of images, formed by a fixed lens or optical system along the axis.
  **mental a.,** an illogical and unreasonable thought or belief.
  **meridional a.,** an a. produced in the plane of a single meridian of a lens.
  **Newto'nian a.,** chromatic a.
  **optical a.,** failure of rays from a point source to form a perfect image after traversing an optical system.

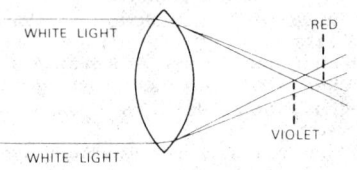

Chromatic Aberration

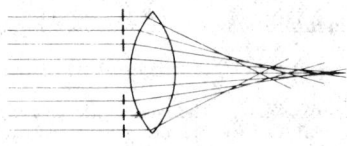

Spherical Aberration

  **spherical a.,** a monochromatic aberration occurring in refraction at a spherical surface in which the paraxial and peripheral rays focus along the axis at different points.
  **ventricular a.,** aberrant ventricular *conduction.*

**aberrom'eter** [ L. *aberratio,* aberration, + G. *metron,* measure ]. An instrument for measuring optical aberration or any error in experimentation.

**abetalipoproteinemia** (a-ba'tah-lip'o-pro'teen-e'mĭ-ah). Bassen-Kornzweig syndrome; a heritable disorder characterized by an absence of plasma lipoproteins having a density less than 1.063, presence of acanthocytes in blood,

retinal pigmentary degeneration, malabsorption, engorgement of upper intestinal absorptive cells with dietary triglycerides, and neuromuscular abnormalities; autosomal recessive inheritance.

**abeyance** (ā-ba'ans) [ fr. O. Fr. ]. A state of temporary abolition of function.

**abfar'ad.** The electromagnetic unit of capacity, equal to $10^9$ farads.

**abhen'ry.** Electromagnetic unit of inductance, equal to $10^{-9}$ henry.

**ab'ient** [ L. *abiens,* pr. p. *ab-eo,* to go from ]. Having a tendency to move away from the source of a stimulus, as opposed to adient.

**Abies** (ab'e-ēz) [ L. the silver fir ]. A genus of evergreen trees, the firs and spruces.
  **A. balsam'ea,** balsam fir, the source of Canada turpentine, or Canada balsam, *Terebinthina canadensis.*
  **A. canaden'sis,** *Tsuga canadensis;* hemlock; the source of Canada pitch.
  **A. excel'sa,** *Picea excelsa;* spruce fir; Norway spruce; the source of Burgundy pitch.

**abietate** (ab-i'ē-tāt). A salt or ester of abietic acid.

**abietic** (ab-e-et'ik). Relating to fir trees or their products.
  **a. acid,** sylvic acid; $C_{20}H_{30}O_2$; a polycyclic acid prepared from rosin and used in the manufacture of varnishes, lacquers, esters; see coniferin.

**abietin** (ab-i'ē-tin). Coniferin.

**abikoviromycin.** Latumicidin; antibiotic produced by *Streptomyces abikoensum* and *S. rubescens;* possesses antiviral activity.

**abil'ity** [ L. *habilitas,* aptitude ]. The physical, mental, or legal competence to function.
  **primary mental a.'s,** a.'s disclosed by factor analysis to be the basic components of intelligence.

**abiogenesis** (ab'ĭ-o-jen'ĕ-sis) [ G. *a-* priv. + *bios,* life, + *genesis,* production ]. The origin of living matter without descent from other living matter; a theory of spontaneous generation.

**ab'iogenet'ic.** Pertaining to spontaneous generation.

**abiol'ogy.** Anorganology; the study of nonliving things.

**abionarce** (ab-i-o-nar'se) [ G. *a-* priv. + *bios,* life, + *narkē,* stupor ]. Lethargy due to infirmity.

**abionergy** (ab-i-on'ur-jĭ) [ G. *a-* priv. + *bios,* life, + *energeia,* action, energy ]. Obsolete term for abiotrophy.

**abiosis** (ab-i-o'sis) [ G. *a-* priv. + *bios,* life ]. 1. Nonviability. 2. Absence of life. 3. Abiotrophy.

**abiot'ic.** Incompatible with life; nonviable.

**abiotrophy** (ab-ĭ-ot'ro-fĭ) [ G. *a-* priv. + *bios,* life, + *trophē,* nourishment ]. Premature loss of vitality or degeneration of certain cells or tissues, usually of genetic etiology; generic term applied to hereditary degenerative diseases.
  **ret'inal a.,** a generic name for several degenerative retinal diseases, *e.g.,* retinitis pigmentosa of genetic etiology.

**abir'ritant.** 1. Abirritative; soothing; relieving irritation. 2. An agent possessing this property.

**abir'ritate.** To soothe, remove irritation, diminish reflex irritability.

**abirrita'tion** [ L. *ab,* from, + *irrito,* pp. *-atus,* to irritate ]. The diminution or abolition of reflex or other irritability in a part.

**abir'ritative.** Abirritant (1).

**ablacta'tion** [ L. *ab,* from, + lactation, *q. v.* ]. Weaning.

**ablastem'ic** [ G. *a-* priv. + *blastēma,* sprout ]. Not germinal or blastemic.

**ablas'tin** [ G. *a-* priv. + *blastos,* germ ]. An antibody that inhibits reproduction of microorganisms; a.'s for bacteria have not been conclusively demonstrated, but they seem to be active in certain protozoal infections.

**ablate** (ab-lāt') [ L. irreg. verb *au-fero,* pp. *ab-latus,* to take away. FER- ]. To remove.

**ablatio** (ab-la'she-o) [ L. see ablate ]. Ablation.
  **a. placen'tae,** *abruptio* placentae.
  **a. ret'inae,** *detachment* of the retina.

**abla'tion** [ L. *ablatio* ]. The removal of a part of the body, as by excision or amputation, or of any growth or noxious substance.

**ablepharia, ablepharon** (ă-blef-a'rī-ah, ah-blef'ah-ron) [ G. *a-* priv. + *blepharon*, eyelid ]. Congenital absence, partial or complete, of the eyelids.

**ableph'arous.** Without eyelids.

**ablephary** (ă-blef'a-rī). Ablepharia.

**ablepsia, ablepsy** (ă-blep'sī-ah, ă-blep'sĭ) [ G. *a-* priv. + *blepō*, to see ]. Blindness.

**ab'luent** [ L. *ab-luo*, pres. p. *-luens* (*luent-*), to wash off ]. 1. Cleansing. 2. Anything with cleansing properties.

**ablu'tion** [ L. *ablutio*, washing off, cleansing ]. Act of washing or bathing.

**ablu'toma'nia** [ L. *ablutio*, washing, + G. *mania*, insanity ]. Morbid preoccupation with thoughts about cleanliness, with frequent washing.

**ab'man** [ L. *ab*, from, + *manus*, hand ]. Anything that transmits human effluvium.

**abner'val.** Abneural (1); away from a nerve; denoting specifically a current of electricity passing through a muscular fiber in a direction away from the point of entrance of the nerve fiber.

**abneural** (ab-nu'ral) [ L. *ab*, away from, + G. *neuron*, nerve ]. 1. Abnerval. 2. Away from the neural axis.

**abnor'mal** [ L. *ab*, from, + *norma*, rule ]. Not normal; differing in any way from the usual state, structure, or condition.

**abnormal'ity.** The state of being abnormal.

    **figure-of-eight a.,** a roentgenographic finding produced by an anomalous drainage of the pulmonary venous return; a large left superior vena cava produces a shadow in the upper mediastinum which is separate from the cardiac silhouette.

**abnor'mity** [ L. *ab*, from, + *norma*, rule ]. Abnormality; deformity.

**ABO blood group.** See appendix 2, Blood Groups.

**ab'oclusion.** Lack of occlusion; a condition in which a tooth or teeth are out of contact with those opposing them.

**abohm** (ab'om). Electromagnetic unit of resistance, equal to $10^{-9}$ ohm.

**aboiement** (ah-bwah-mahn') [ Fr. barking, yelping ]. Involuntary production of abnormal sounds.

**ab'omasi'tis.** Inflammation of the abomasum.

**aboma'sum, aboma'sus** [ L. *ab*, from, + *omasum*, bullock's tripe ]. The fourth compartment and the glandular portion of the stomach of a ruminant; it has a parietal and visceral surface, greater and lesser curvature, fundus, body, and pyloric portion; internally, there are about a dozen longitudinal plicae.

**abo'rad, abo'ral** [ L. *ab*, from, + *os* (*or-*), mouth ]. In a direction away from the mouth.

**abort** [ L. *aborto*, to miscarry ]. 1. To give birth to an embryo or fetus before it is viable. 2. To arrest a disease in its earliest stages. 3. To arrest in growth or development; to cause to remain rudimentary.

**abortient** (ab-or'shent). Abortifacient.

**abortifacient** (ab-or-tĭ-fa'shent) [ L. *abortus*, abortion, + *facio*, to make ]. 1. Abortient; abortigenic; producing abortion. 2. An agent that produces abortion.

**abortigen'ic** [ L. *abortus*, abortion, + *genesis*, production ]. Abortifacient.

**abortion** (ă-bor'shun). 1. Giving birth to an embryo or fetus prior to the stage of viability at about 20 weeks of gestation (fetus weighs less than 500 gm.). A distinction is made between a. and premature birth: premature infants are those born after the stage of viability has been reached but before full term. A. may be either spontaneous (occurs from natural causes) or induced. 2. The product of such nonviable birth. 3. The arrest of any action or process before its normal completion.

    **accidental a.,** a. due to a fall, blow, or other injury.

    **ampullar a.,** a. resulting from pregnancy in tubal ampulla.

    **bovine infectious a.,** bovine *brucellosis.*

    **complete a.,** (1) the complete expulsion or extraction from its mother of a fetus or embryo weighing less than 500 gm. (approximately equal to 22 completed weeks or 154 days of gestation); (2) complete expulsion of any other product of gestation (*e.g.*, hydatidiform mole).

    **contagious a.,** bovine *brucellosis.*

    **criminal a.,** termination of pregnancy without medical or legal justification.

    **enzootic a. of ewes,** a specific infectious a. of sheep caused by *Chlamydia psittaci;* it was formerly thought to be caused by a virus and was designated ovine virus a. or virus a. of ewes.

    **epizootic bovine a.,** a specific infectious a. of cattle first recognized in California in 1956, possibly caused by a chlamydial agent.

    **equine virus a.,** equine rhinopneumonitis; a highly contagious a. of mares, caused by a virus. The same virus causes a mild respiratory infection of young animals shortly after they have been weaned.

    **habitual a.,** a condition in which a woman has had three or more consecutive, spontaneous a.'s.

    **incipient a.,** imminent a.; impending a. in which there is copious vaginal bleeding, uterine contractions and cervical dilation.

    **incomplete a.,** a. in which part of the products of conception have been passed but part (usually the placenta) remains in the uterus.

    **induced a.,** a. brought on purposefully by drugs or mechanical means.

    **inevitable a.,** one signalized by rupture of the membranes in the presence of cervical dilation that has advanced beyond any hope of preventing complete a.

    **infectious a.,** an a. resulting from an infectious disease.

    **justifiable a.,** therapeutic a.

    **missed a.,** one in which the fetus dies *in utero* but the product of conception is retained *in utero* for two months or longer.

    **ovine virus a.,** see enzootic a. of ewes.

    **septic a.,** an infected a. complicated by fever, endometritis, and parametritis.

    **spontaneous a.,** one that has not been artificially induced.

    **therapeutic a.,** a. induced because of the mother's poor health, or to prevent birth of a deformed child or child resulting from rape.

    **threatened a.,** crampy pains and slight show of blood that may or may not be followed by the expulsion of the fetus during the first 20 weeks of pregnancy.

    **tubal a.,** aborted ectopic pregnancy; rupture of an oviduct, the seat of ectopic pregnancy, or extrusion of the product of conception through the fimbriated end of the oviduct.

    **virus a. of ewes,** see enzootic a. of ewes.

**abor'tionist.** One who interrupts a pregnancy before the 20th week of gestation.

**abortive** [ L. *abortivus* ]. 1. Not reaching completion; for example, said of an attack of a disease subsiding before it has fully developed or completed its course. 2. Rudimentary. 3. Ectrotic; cutting short an attack of disease. 4. Abortifacient.

**abortus** [ L. ]. Any product (or all products) of an abortion.

**abouchement** (ah-boosh-mahn') [ Fr. *abouchement*, inosculation, anastomosis ]. Junction of small blood vessel with large.

**aboulia** (ă-boo'lī-ah). Abulia.

**abrachia** (ă-bra'kĭ-ah) [ G *a-* priv. + *brachiōn*, arm ]. The absence of arms.

**abrachiocephalia** (ă-bra'kĭ-o-sĕ-fa'lī-ah). Abrachiocephaly.

**abrachiocephalus** (ă-bra'kĭ-o-sef'al-us). Acephalobrachius; a malformed fetus with abrachiocephaly.

**abrachiocephaly** (ă-bra'kĭ-o-sef'ă-li) [ G. *a-* priv. + *brachiōn*, arm, + *kephalē*, head ]. Abrachiocephalia; acephalobrachia; the absence of arms and head.

**abrachius** (ă-bra'kĭ-us) [ G. *a-* priv. + *brachiōn*, arm ]. An individual without arms.

**abrade** (ă-brād') [ L. *ab-rado*, pp. *-rasus*, to scrape off ]. 1. To wear away by mechanical action. 2. To excoriate; to scrape away the epidermis from a part.

**Abrahams,** Robert, New York physician, 1861–1935. See A.'s *sign.*

**Abrams,** Albert, San Francisco physician, 1863–1924. See A.'s heart *reflex,* lung *reflex.*

**abrasion** (ă-bra'zhun) [ see abrade ]. 1. Abraded wound; an excoriation, or circumscribed removal of the epidermis of skin or mucous membrane. 2. A scraping away of a portion of the surface. 3. Grinding; in dentistry, the grinding or wearing away of tooth substance by mastication, incorrect tooth-brushing methods, or similar causes.

    **brush burn a.,** see brush *burn.*

    **gingival a.,** a circumscribed lesion of the gingiva resulting from mechanical removal of the surface epithelium.

    **mechanical a.,** removal of the epidermis down to the tips of the papillae by rubbing with sand paper, rotating wire brush, or other abrasive material; a method of removing or obliterating cutaneous scars or pits such as those produced by acne vulgaris.

    **tooth a.,** the loss or wearing away of tooth structure caused by the abrasive characteristics of substances other than foods; *cf.* attrition.

**abra'sive.** 1. Causing abrasion. 2. Any material (such as sandpaper or wire brush) used to produce abrasions. 3. A substance used in dentistry for abrading, grinding, or polishing.

**abreact** (ab-re-akt'). 1. To show strong emotion in reliving a previous traumatic experience. 2. To discharge or release repressed emotion.

**abreaction** (ab-re-ak'shun). In Freudian psychoanalysis, an episode of emotional release or catharsis associated with the bringing into conscious recollection previously repressed unpleasant experiences.

    **motor a.,** the release of an unconscious thought, idea, or impulse through motor or muscular expression.

**a'brin.** A toxalbumin obtained from the seed of *Abrus precatorius;* formerly used topically for chronic eye infection.

**abro'sia** [ G. *a-* priv. + *brosis,* food ]. Fasting; starvation or abstaining from food.

**abruptio** (ab-rup'she-o) [ L. fr. *ab-rumpo,* pp. *-ruptus,* to break off. RUPT- ]. Abruption; a tearing away; a rending asunder.

    **a. placen'tae,** ablatio placentae; premature detachment of a normally situated placenta.

**A'brus** [ more correctly *Habrus,* from G. *habros,* graceful ]. A genus of leguminous plants. The root of *A. precatorius,* Indian liquorice, is sometimes used as a substitute for liquorice; the seeds have been used in ophthalmic practice. See abrin.

# ABSCESS

**abscess** (ab'ses) [ L. *abscessus,* a going away ]. 1. A circumscribed collection of pus. 2. A cavity formed by liquefaction necrosis within solid tissue.

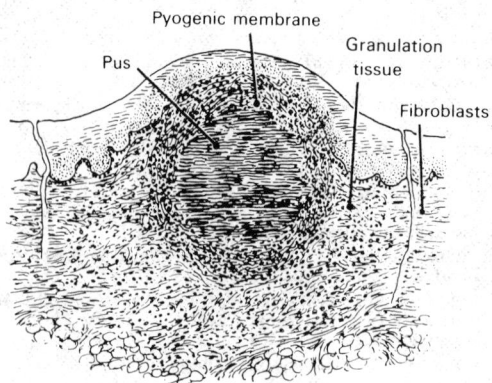

Pyogenic membrane

Pus

Granulation tissue

Fibroblasts

**Abscess of Skin**

**acute a.,** hot a.; a recently found a. with no fibrosis in the wall of the cavity.

**alveolar a.,** an a. in the alveolar process, either pericemental or apical; see also lateral alveolar a.; dental a.

**amebic a.,** an area of liquefaction necrosis of the liver containing amebae, usually following amebic dysentery; the lesion is not a true a., as pus is not present.

**anorectal a.,** perirectal a.

**apical a.,** (1) an a. in the apex of the lung; (2) one in the alveolus at the apex of the root of a tooth.

**appendiceal a.,** an intraperitoneal a., usually in the right iliac fossa, resulting from extension of infection in acute appendicitis, especially with perforation of the appendix.

**appendicular a.,** one in the region of the vermiform appendix.

**Bartholin's a.,** an a. of the vulvovaginal gland.

**Bezold's a.,** an a. deep in the neck associated with suppuration in the mastoid tip cells.

**bicameral a.,** an a. with two separate cavities or chambers.

**bone a.,** suppuration (osteomyelitis) within the medullary cavity of a bone or beneath the periosteum.

**brain a.,** a. within the brain substance.

**branchial cleft cyst a.,** suppuration developing in branchial cleft cyst.

**Brodie's a.,** a chronic, inactive a. of bone marrow, surrounded by dense fibrous tissue and sclerotic bone.

**bursal a.,** suppuration within a bursa.

**canalicular a.,** an a. of the breast discharging into the milk ducts.

**caseous a.,** an a. containing white solid or semisolid material of cheesy consistency; usually tuberculous.

**cerebral a.,** intracerebral a.; an a. of the brain, specifically, of the cerebrum.

**chronic a.,** a long-standing collection of pus surrounded by fibrous tissue; a result of injury or a foreign body.

**cold a.,** (1) an a. without heat or other usual signs of inflammation; (2) tuberculous a.

**collar-button a.,** shirt-stud a.

**crypt a.'s,** a.'s in crypts of Lieberkühn of the large intestinal mucosa; a characteristic feature of ulcerative colitis.

**Delpech's a.,** an a. appearing suddenly with but slight inflammatory symptoms, accompanied by marked adynamia.

**dental a.,** root a.; a walled-off or circumscribed area of inflammation, usually about the apex of a tooth, resulting from extension of dental caries and pulpitis.

**dentoalveolar a.,** an a. confined to the alveolar process investing a tooth root.

**diffuse a.,** a collection of pus not circumscribed by a well defined capsule.

**Douglas' a.,** suppuration in Douglas' pouch.

**dry a.,** the remains of an a. after the pus is absorbed.

**Dubois' a.'s,** thymic a.'s; Dubois' disease; small cysts of the thymus containing polymorphonuclear leukocytes but lined by squamous epithelium; reported in congenital syphilis but also found in the absence of syphilis.

**embolic a.,** an a. arising at the point of arrest of a septic embolus.

**epidural a.,** extradural a.; extradural empyema; an a. lying outside but adjacent to the cerebral or spinal dura mater.

**epiploic a.,** omental a.; a. in or surrounded by omentum majus.

**extradural a.,** epidural a.

**fecal a.,** stercoral a.

**follicular a.,** one in a hair, tonsillar, or other follicle.

**gas a.,** an a. containing gas caused by *Bacillus aerogenes, Escherichia coli,* or other gas-forming microorganisms.

**gingival a.,** gumboil; parulis; a circumscribed, suppurative, inflammatory lesion of the gingiva, usually at the opening of a fistulous tract from an apical a.

**gravitation a.,** hypostatic a.; a wandering a., the pus sinking to dependent parts.

**gummatous a.,** syphilitic a.; one due to the softening and breaking down of a gumma, especially in bone.

**hematogenous a.,** an a. caused by blood-borne organisms.

**hot a.,** acute a.

**hypostatic a.,** gravitation a.

intracerebral a., cerebral a.

intracranial a., an a. within the cranium, *e.g.*, a cerebral, cerebellar, brainstem, epidural, or subdural a.

intradural a., one between the layers of the dura mater.

ischiorectal a., one involving the tissues in the ischiorectal fossa.

lacunar a., one involving the urethral lacunae.

lateral a., lateral alveolar a.

lateral alveolar a., parietal a.; lateral a.; periodontal a.; pericemental a.; a localized suppurative inflammation of the periodontal membrane and the adjacent bone.

lung a., circumscribed area of suppuration in the lung; a complication of uncorrected atelectasis or pneumonia; may extend to involve pleural cavity; see also empyema.

mastoid a., an a. of the mastoid air cells.

metastatic a., a secondary a. formed, at a distance from the primary focus, as a result of the transportation of pyogenic bacteria by the lymph or blood stream.

migrating a., wandering a.

miliary a., one of a number of minute collections of pus, widely disseminated throughout an area or the whole body.

milk a., a mammary a. occurring during lactation.

Munro's a., Munro's *microabscess.*

mycotic a., an a. caused by pathogenic fungi.

omental a., epiploic a.

orbital a., retrobulbar a.; a circumscribed collection of pus within the orbit; frequently an extension of purulent infection of the paranasal sinuses, usually the ethmoids.

otic a., a cerebral a. secondary to suppuration of the middle ear.

Paget's a., obsolete eponym for residual a.

palatal a., a circumscribed collection of pus on the palate; usually caused by a nonvital lateral incisor, double-rooted first bicuspid, second bicuspid, or palatal roots of molars.

pancreatic a., a. originating in or near the pancreas, usually resulting from pancreatic injury or pancreatitis.

parafrenal a., one that occurs on either side of the frenum of the penis.

parametric a., parametritic a.; one in the connective tissue of the broad ligament of the uterus.

parametritic a., parametric a.

paranephric a., one in the region of the kidney, outside the renal fascia.

parietal a., lateral alveolar a.

parotid a., rapidly progressive suppuration in parotid gland; a complication of parotitis.

Pautrier's a., Pautrier's *microabscess.*

pelvic a., an a. in the pelvic peritoneal cavity, developing as a complication of diffuse peritonitis or of localized peritonitis associated with abdominal or pelvic inflammatory disease, such as salpingitis; the pus frequently collects in the rectovesical or rectouterine pouch.

periapical a., apical a.

periappendiceal a., localized collection of purulent exudate around appendix; occurs in association with acute appendicitis with perforation; the exact location varies depending on the position of the appendix.

periarticular a., one surrounding a joint, not usually involving it.

pericemental a., lateral alveolar a.

pericoronal a., infection with collection of pus around the crown of a partially erupted tooth, usually upper or lower third molars. Pus collects in a pocket, either distal, distobuccal and/or distolingual to the tooth crown.

perinephric a., one in the adipose tissue enveloping the kidney, inside the renal fascia.

periodontal a., lateral alveolar a.

perirectal a., anorectal a.; an a. in connective tissue adjacent to the rectum or anus.

peritonsillar a., quinsy; extension of tonsillar infection beyond the capsule with abscess formation usually above and behind the tonsil.

periureteral a., one surrounding the ureter.

periurethral a., one involving the tissues around the urethra.

phlegmonous a., circumscribed suppuration characterized by intense surrounding inflammatory reaction which produces induration and thickening of the affected area.

pilonidal cyst a., suppuration developing in pilonidal cyst.

Pott's a., cold or tuberculous a.

premammary a., one in the subcutaneous tissue covering the mammary gland.

pso'as a., an a., usually tuberculous, originating in vertebral spondylitis (Pott's disease) and extending through the iliopsoas muscle to the inguinal region.

pulp a., an a. of the soft tissue contained in the pulp chamber of a tooth.

pyemic a., septicemic a.; a hematogenous a. resulting from pyemia, septicemia, or bacteremia.

residual a., an a. recurring at the site of a former a. resulting from persistence of microbes and pus.

retrobulbar a., orbital a.

retrocecal a., an a. located posterior to the cecum, usually resulting from perforation of a retrocecal appendix.

retropharyn'geal a., an a. arising, usually, in retropharyngeal lymph nodes, most commonly in infants.

ring a., ring-shaped irregularly bordered leukocytic infiltration of corneal stroma due to infection after trauma with very virulent organisms.

root a., dental a.

satellite a., an a. with intimate relationship to a parent a.

scrofulous a., obsolete term for tuberculous a.

septicemic a., pyemic a.

serous a., periosteal *ganglion.*

shirt-stud a., collar-button a.; two a.'s connected by a narrow channel; usually formed by rupture of an a. through an overlying fascia; originates on palmer (plantar) surface and penetrates to dorsum of hand or foot.

stellate a., a star-shaped necrotic area surrounded by epithelioid cells, seen within swollen inguinal lymph nodes in lymphogranuloma venereum.

stercoral a., fecal a.; a collection of pus and feces.

sterile a., one from which infecting organisms cannot be cultured.

stitch a., an a. in a stitch wound from septic suture material or pyogenic bacteria from the skin.

strumous a., obsolete term for a cold a. of tuberculous origin.

subacute a., an a. of several weeks' duration.

subcranial a., an epidural, intradural, or subdural a.

subdiaphragmatic a., subphrenic a; an a. beneath the diaphragm, most commonly on the right side in one of the peritoneal compartments bounded by the liver and falciform ligament; usually develops after an operation for perforated pelvic ulcer, cholecystitis, or appendicitis.

subdural a., subdural empyema; an a. in the subdural space, *i.e.*, between the dura and arachnoid membranes.

subepidermal a., a microscopic a. located in the dermis just beneath the epidermis.

subgaleal a., a. between the galea aponeurotica and the pericranium.

subhepatic a., collection of pus inferior to the liver.

subphrenic a., subdiaphragmatic a.

subungual a., suppuration beneath a fingernail or toenail.

sudoriparous a., a collection of pus in a sweat gland.

syphilitic a., gummatous a.

thecal a., suppuration in a tendon sheath.

Thornwaldt's a., chronic infection of the pharyngeal bursa; see also Thornwaldt's *syndrome.*

thymic a.'s, Dubois' a.'s.

tropical a., amebic a. of the liver, sometimes but not invariably associated with amebic dysentery.

tuberculous a., an a. caused by the tubercle bacillus; also formerly called cold a.

tubo-ovarian a., a large a. involving a uterine tube and an adherent ovary, resulting from extension of purulent inflammation of the tube.

urinous a., an a. communicating with the bladder or the urethra, and containing urine mixed with pus.

verminous a., worm a.

wandering a., migrating a.; an a. occurring at a distance from the primary focus of disease, pus burrowing along fascial planes or other structures.

worm a., verminous a.; a. due to parasitic worms or in which worms are found.

---

**abscission** (ab-sĭ'shun) [ L. *ab-scindo,* pp. *-scissus,* to cut away from ]. Cutting away.

**corneal a.,** cutting away of the prominence of the cornea in cases of staphyloma.

**absconsio** (ab-skon'she-o) [ Mod. L. fr. *abs-condo,* pp. *-con-ditus* or *-consus,* to hide ]. A recess or cavity.

**absence** (ab'sens). Absentia epileptica; a form of petit mal epilepsy characterized by transient periods of unconsciousness.

**absentia** (ab-sen'she-ah) [ L. ]. Absence.
  **a. epilep'tica,** see absence.

**Absid'ia.** A genus of fungi (family Mucoraceae) belonging to the class Phycomycetes (Zygomycetes). These fungi are commonly found in nature, and may cause phycomycosis.

**absinthe** (ab'sinth, Fr. ab-saṅt'). A liqueur consisting of an alcoholic extract of absinthium and other bitter herbs.

**ab'sinthin.** A bitter principle, $C_{30}H_{40}O_8$; obtained from absinthium.

**ab'sinthism.** Mental and physical deterioration resulting from the habitual overuse of absinthe.

**absin'thium** [ L. fr. G. *apsinthion* ]. Wormwood; the dried leaves and tops of *Artemisia absinthium* (family Compositae). The infusion has been used as a tonic. In large or frequently repeated doses it produces headache, trembling, and epileptiform convulsions.

**absin'thol.** Thujone.

**ab'solute** [ L. *absolutus,* complete, pp. of *ab-solvo,* to loosen from ]. Unconditional; unlimited; complete; entire; fixed; certain.
  **a. cell increase,** see under cell.
  **degrees a.,** see a. *scale.*

**absorb** (ab-sorb') [ L. *ab-sorbeo,* pp. *-sorptus,* to suck in ]. 1. To incorporate or take up gases, liquids, light, or heat. 2. To take any material into the body through the lymphatics or blood vessels. 3. To reduce the intensity of transmitted light.

**absorb'able.** Capable of being absorbed.

**absorb'ance.** Absorbancy; absorbency; optical density; extinction; equal to 2 minus the log of the percentage transmittance; of significance in spectrophotometry. Symbol, *A.*
  **specific a.,** Absorbance per unit of concentration; see specific absorption *coefficient.*

**absorb'ancy.** Absorbance.

**absor'befac'ient** [ L. *ab-sorbeo,* to suck in, + *facio,* to make ]. 1. Causing absorption. 2. Any substance possessing such quality.

**absorb'ency.** Absorbance.

**absorb'ent.** 1. Having the power to absorb, suck up, or take into itself any gas, liquid, light rays, or heat. 2. Any substance possessing such power. 3. Caustic material for removal of carbon dioxide from circuits in which rebreathing occurs, *e.g.,* anesthesia and basal metabolism equipment. Soda lime and barium hydroxide are a.'s.

**absor'ber head.** The portion of a rebreathing anesthesia circuit that contains carbon dioxide absorbent; often referred to as a canister.

**absorptiometer** (ab-sorp'shĭ-om'e-ter) [ L. *absorptio,* absorption, + G. *metron,* measure ]. 1. An instrument for determining the amount of gas absorbed by a given quantity. 2. An appliance for determining the thickness of a layer of liquid between two glass plates in apparent apposition; used in hematoscopy.

**absorp'tion.** 1. The process of absorbing; see absorb; compare adsorb. 2. In dentistry, the taking up of fluids or other substances by the skin, mucous surface, absorbent vessels, or dental materials.
  **cutaneous a.,** the percutaneous a. of drugs, allergens, atopens, toxins, and other substances in contact with the epidermis.
  **disjunctive a.,** a. of living tissue in immediate relation with a necrosed part, producing the line of demarcation.
  **electron resonance a.,** see electron spin *resonance.*
  **external a.,** the a. of substances through skin or other mucous membranes.
  **interstitial a.,** the removal of water or of substances in the interstitial fluid by the lymphatics.
  **paren'teral a.,** a. through the skin or subcutaneous tissues, or by any route other than the alimentary tract.

**pathologic a.,** parenteral a. of any excremental or pathologic material into the blood stream, *e.g.,* pus, urine, bile, etc.

**absorp'tive.** Absorbent.

**absorptiv'ity.** Specific absorption *coefficient.*
  **molar a.,** molar absorption *coefficient.*

**abster'gent** [ L. *abs-tergo,* to wipe off ]. 1. Having cleansing or purgative properties. 2. A cleansing lotion. 3. A purgative.

**abstinence** (ab'stĭ-nens) [ L. *abs-tineo,* to hold back, fr. *teneo,* to hold ]. Specifically, refraining from the use of certain articles of diet or alcoholic beverages, or from sexual intercourse.

**ab'stract** [ L. *ab-straho,* pp. *-tractus,* to draw away ]. 1. A preparation, formerly official in the USP, made by evaporating a fluidextract to a powder and triturating with milk sugar. 2. A condensation or summary of a scientific or literary article or address.

**abstraction** (ab-strak'shun). 1. Bloodletting. 2. Distillation or separation of the volatile constituents of a substance. 3. Exclusive mental concentration; absent-mindedness. 4. The making of an abstract from the crude drug. 5. Teeth or associated structures that are lower than their normal occlusal plane. See odontoptosis.

**abter'minal** [ L. *ab,* from, + *terminus,* end ]. In a direction away from the end and toward the center; denoting the course of an electrical current in a muscle.

**abulia** (ă-bu'lĭ-ah) [ G. *a-* priv. + *boulē,* will ]. Aboulia; loss or impairment of the ability to perform voluntary actions or to make decisions.

**abu'lic.** Relating to, or suffering from, abulia.

**abuse** (ă-būs'). Misuse, wrong use, especially excessive use, of anything.
  **alcohol a.,** alcoholism.
  **analgesic a.,** excessive ingestion of analgesics; reported to cause nephropathy after many years.
  **child a.** physical assault on a child; perpetrated most often by a parent and requiring medical attention.
  **drug a.,** the self-administration of drugs for non-therapeutic purposes; the drug used may or may not be a narcotic.

**abutment** (ah-but'ment). In dentistry, a tooth used for the support or anchorage of a fixed or removable prosthesis.
  **intermediate a.,** a natural tooth, without other natural teeth in proximal contact, which is used as an a., in addition to two primary a.'s.
  **primary a.,** a tooth used for the support or anchorage of a fixed or removable partial denture appliance.

**ab'volt.** Electromagnetic unit of difference of potential, equal to $10^{-8}$ volt.

**AC.** Abbreviation for alternating *current.*

**a.c.** Abbreviation for L. *ante cibum,* before meals.

**Ac.** 1. Chemical symbol for the element actinium. 2. Abbreviation for acetate.

**Acacia** (ă-ka'she-ah) [ G. *akakia* ]. A genus of plants of the family Leguminosae, found especially in tropical and subtropical regions.

**acacia** (USP, BP). Gum arabic; the dried, gummy exudation from *Acacia senegal* and other species of *A.* Molecular weight, about 240,000; contains 15 per cent water. The official preparations are the mucilage and the syrup. Used as an emollient, demulcent and excipient; formerly used as a transfusion fluid; renal and hepatic damage and allergic reactions may follow intravenous use.

**acalcerosis** (a-kal'ser-o'sis). Acalcicosis; calcium deficiency of the diet, or of the body as a result of the loss of the mineral in the excreta.

**acalcicosis** (a-kal'sĭ-ko'sis). Acalcerosis.

**acalculia** (ă-kal-ku'lĭ-ah) [ G. *a-* priv. + L. *calculo,* to reckon ]. A form of aphasia characterized by inability to do simple mathematical problems.

**acal'ypha** [ G. *akalyphēs,* uncovered ]. The herb, dried, or fresh. *Acalypha indica* (family Euphorbiaceae); expectorant and laxative, resembling senega in its action.

**acamp'sia** [ G. *a-* priv. + *kamptō,* to bend ]. Rigidity of a joint; ankylosis.

**acan'tha** [ G. *akantha,* a thorn. AC- ]. A spine or spinous process.

**acanthesthesia** (ă-kan-thes-the′zĭ-ah) [ G. *akantha*, thorn, + *aisthēsis*, sensation ]. A form of paresthesia in which there is a sensation as of a pinprick.

**Acan′thia lectula′ria** [ G. *akantha*, thorn, prickle; L. *lectus*, a bed ]. Early name for *Cimex lectularius*, bedbug.

**acan′thion** [ G. *akantha*, thorn ]. Akanthion; the tip of the anterior nasal spine. See fig. under craniometric *point*.

**acantho-** (ă-kan-tho) [ G. *akantha*, thorn ]. Combining form denoting relationship to a spinous process, or meaning spiny or thorny.

**Acanthoceph′ala** [ acantho- + G. *kephalē*, head ]. The thorny-headed worms; a class (or phylum by some authorities) of nematode-like entozoa without alimentary canal, characterized by a spiny proboscis. In the adult stage they are parasites of vertebrate animals. The larval stage is passed in invertebrates, chiefly crustaceans and insects. Exceptionally, they are parasitic in man; most species are fish parasites.

**acanthocephaliasis** (ă-kan′tho-sef-ă-li′ă-sis) An illness caused by infection with a species of Acanthocephala.

**Acanthocheilonema** (ă-kan′tho-chi-lo-ne′mah). A genus of filarial worm parasitic in man, considered by some to be part of the genus *Dipetalonema*. Adult forms live chiefly in the body cavities, or in skin and subcutaneous tissue. See also *Filaria*, the common name and also the former genus in which *A.* species were classified.

    **A. perstans**, the "persistent filaria," is prevalent in tropical Africa and the northern part of South America; characterized by adult forms that live in the peritoneal, pleural, or pericardial cavities, and by microfilariae that are not sheathed and manifest no periodicity in the circulating blood; transmitted by *Culicoides* species (biting gnats). *A. perstans* is usually regarded as a harmless parasite, but some observers think that it may cause edema and a condition that resembles trypanosomiasis. Formerly termed *Filaria sanguinis hominis*, *F. s. h. perstans*, *F. ozzardi* var. *truncata*. Also called *Dipetalonema perstans*.

    **A. streptocerca**, a species of filarial worm rarely found in natives of tropical Africa; characterized by adult forms that live in the dermis and subcutaneous tissues, and by microfilariae that are not sheathed and manifest no periodicity in the circulating blood; may cause rare examples of chronic edema of the skin. Blood form may be termed *Microfilaria streptocerca*. The worm is also called *Dipetalonema streptocerca*.

**acan′thocheil′onemi′asis.** Infection by the nematode *Acanthocheilonema perstans*, which see.

**acan′thocyte** [ acantho- + G. *kytos*, cell ]. A thorny or peculiarly spiny erythrocyte characterized by multiple spiny cytoplasmic projections; see also acanthocytosis.

**acanthocyto′sis.** A rare condition in which the majority of erythrocytes are acanthocytes; a regular feature of the syndrome of abetalipoproteinemia.

**acanthoid** (ă-kan′thoyd). Spine-shaped; spinous.

**acanthol′ysis** [ acantho- + G. *lysis*, loosening ]. A term used in dermal pathology to denote separation of the prickle cells of the epidermis. It is seen in such conditions as pemphigus vulgaris and keratosis follicularis.

**acantho′ma** [ acantho- + G. suffix -*oma*, tumor ]. A squamous cell tumor that may be malignant, but well differentiated, or benign, or even non-neoplastic; see also adenoacanthoma and keratoacanthoma.

    **a. adenoi′des cys′ticum**, trichoepithelioma.

    **Degos′ a.**, a superficial, scaly, brawny red or brown plaque, usually occurring as a single lesion of an arm or leg.

**acanthopel′vis, acanthopel′yx** [ acantho- + G. *pelvis*, a basin; *pelyx*, a wooden bowl ]. Osteomalacic *pelvis*.

**acantho′sis** [ acantho- + G. suffix -*osis*, condition ]. An increase in the thickness of the prickle cell layer of the epidermis. May be due to an increase in number of individual rete cells or an increase in the size of the cells.

    **a. nig′ricans**, keratosis nigricans; an eruption of velvety, warty growths and hyperpigmentation occurring in the skin of the axillae, neck, anogenital area, and groins. In adults it is indicative of abdominal malignancy. A benign type occurs in children. In the benign or juvenile type the subjects are obese and the skin condition is self-limited.

    **a. verruco′sa**, *keratosis* senilis.

**acanthot′ic.** Pertaining to or characteristic of acanthosis.

**acan′throcyte.** Acanthocyte.

**acan′throcyto′sis.** Acanthocytosis.

**acap′nia** [ G. *a*- priv. + *kapnos*, smoke ]. The absence of carbon dioxide in the blood; sometimes used synonymously with hypocapnia, *q. v.*

**acar′bia** [ G. *a*- priv. + carbon ]. Pronounced reduction in bicarbonate of the blood.

**acar′dia** [ G. *a*- priv. + *kardia*, heart ]. Congenital absence of the heart; a condition sometimes occurring in the smaller parasitic member of conjoined twin when its partner monopolizes the placental blood supply.

**acar′diac.** Without heart.

**acardi′acus** [ G. *a*- priv. + *kardia*, heart ]. A conjoined twin, parasitic on its mate, or utilizing the placental circulation of its mate, and having no heart.

    **a. aceph′alus**, acephalocardius; an acardiac fetus in which the head is absent.

    **a. acormus**, an acardiac fetus with markedly defective trunk.

    **a. amor′phus**, a. anceps.

    **a. an′ceps**, a. amorphus; an acardiac fetus with rudimentary head and extremities.

**acardiotrophia** (ah-kar′de-o-tro′fe-ah) [ G. *a*- priv. + *kardia*, heart, + *trophē*, nourishment ]. Atrophy of the myocardium.

**acar′dius.** Acardiacus.

**acariasis** (ak′ar-i′ah-sis). Acaridiasis; any disease caused by an acarid.

    **demodectic a.**, infestation of hair follicles with *Demodex folliculorum*.

    **psoroptic a.**, infestation of skin with *Psoroptes* mites.

    **pulmonary a.**, infestation of the lungs of monkeys with the mite, *Pneumonyssus simicola*.

    **sarcoptic a.**, scabies; infestation of skin with *Sarcoptes scabiei*.

**acar′icide** [ Mod. L. *acarus*, a mite, fr. G. *akari* + L. *caedo*, to cut, kill ]. 1. Destructive to acarids, or mites. 2. An agent having this property.

**ac′arid.** A member of the order Acarina, a mite.

**Acar′idae.** A family of the order Acarina, including the mites.

**acar′idan.** An acarid.

**acar′idi′asis.** Acariasis.

**Acari′na** [ G. *akari*, a mite ]. An order of Arachnida that includes the mites and ticks.

**acar′ino′sis.** Scabies; mite infestation of the skin.

**ac′aroder′mati′tis** [ G. *akari*, mite, + *derma* (*dermat*-), skin ]. An eruption produced by one of the acarine parasites.

    **a. urticasioides**, infestation with grain itch mite.

**ac′aroid** [ G. *akari*, mite, + *eidos*, resemblance ]. 1. Resembling a mite. 2. An acarus, or mite.

**acarol′ogy** [ G. *akari*, a mite, + *logos*, study ]. Study of acarine parasites, the ticks and mites, and the diseases they transmit.

**ac′aropho′bia** [ G. *akari*, mite, + *phobos*, fear ]. Morbid fear of small parasites, small particles, or of itching.

**Ac′arus** [ G. *akari*, a mite ]. A genus of mites of the family Acaridae.

    **A. balatus**, a tropical variety of mite that causes a particularly severe type of scabies-like irritation.

    **A. folliculo′rum**, *Demodex folliculorum*.

    **A. gallinae**, *Dermanyssus gallinae*.

    **A. hor′de′i**, barley mite that penetrates beneath the skin.

    **A. rhizoglyp′ticus hyacin′thi**, a mite that develops in spoiled onions and may cause dermatitis.

    **A. scabie′i**, *Sarcoptes scabiei*.

    **A. tritici**, *Pediculoides ventricosus*.

**ac′arus.** Any mite or tick; an acarid.

**acar′yote.** Akaryocyte.

**acatalasemia** (a-kat′ah-la-se′mĭ-ah). Acatalasia; anenzymia catalasia; Takahara's disease; the absence of catalase from the blood, a condition that may be associated with extensive ulceration and gangrene of the oral tissues.

**acatalasia** (a-kat-ah-la′zĭ-ah). Acatalasemia.

**acatalep'sia, acat'alepsy** [ G. *a-* priv. + *katalēpsis*, comprehension. LAB- ]. 1. Mental deficiency characterized by a lack of understanding. 2. Uncertainty in diagnosis or prognosis.

**acatalep'tic.** 1. Deficient in comprehension. 2. Uncertain.

**acatamathesia** (ă-kat-ă-mă-the'zĭ-ah) [ G. *a-* priv. + *katamathēsis*, a thorough knowledge or understanding ]. Akatamathesia; loss of the faculty of understanding, *e.g.*, in psychogenic deafness or disease.

**acatapha'sia** [ G. *a-* priv. + *kata-phasis*, affirmation ]. A loss of the power of correctly formulating a statement.

**acatapo'sis** [ G. *a-*priv. + *kata*, down, + *posis*, drinking ]. Difficulty in swallowing liquids; strictly, inability to do so.

**acatastasia** (ă-kat-as-ta'zĭ-ah) [ G. *a-* priv. + *katastasis*, condition ]. Rarely used term meaning deviation from type.

**acatastat'ic** [ G. *a-*priv. + *katastasis*, fixedness ]. Relating to acatastasia.

**acathar'sia, acath'arsy** [ G. *a-* priv. + *katharsis*, a cleansing ]. A failure to obtain a desired purgation.

**acathec'tic.** Relating to acathexia.

**acathex'ia** [ G. *a-* priv. + *kathexis*, a holding in, fr. *kata*, down, + *echō*, fut. *hexō*, to have ]. An abnormal loss of the secretions.

**acathex'is** [ G. *a-* priv. + *kathexis*, retention ]. A mental disorder in which certain objects or ideas fail to arouse an emotional response in the individual.

**acathisia** (ă-kă-thiz'ĭ-ah) [ G. *a-*priv. + *kathisis*, a sitting ]. Akathisia.

**acaudal, acaudate** (ă-kaw'dal, ă-kaw'dāt) [ G. *a-* priv. + L. *cauda*, tail ]. Having no tail.

**acauline** (ă-kaw'lēn) [ G. *a-* priv. + L. *caulis*, stem ] Denoting a group of stemless fungi.

**ACC.** Abbreviation for anodal closure *contraction*.

**accel'erans** [ L. ]. 1. Accelerating; accelerator. 2. The accelerator nerve of the heart.

**Acceleranstoff** [ Ger. ]. The adrenaline-like substance liberated at the terminations of sympathetic fibers in the heart.

**accel'erant.** Accelerator.

**accelera'tion** [ see accelerator ]. 1. The act of accelerating. 2. The rate of increase in velocity per unit of time; commonly expressed in G units; also expressed in centimeters or feet per second squared; in aviation, a. varies directly with the square of the air speed and inversely with the radius of the turn ($a = V^2/r$, where *V* is air speed and *r* is radius of turn).

    **angular a.,** the rate of change of angular velocity; occurs when there is a simultaneous change in velocity and direction, as in an aircraft in a tight spin.

    **linear a.,** the rate of change of velocity without a change in direction; occurs, for example, when the speed of an aircraft increases while flying a straight pathway.

    **radial a.,** the centripetal a. of a particle or vehicle moving along a curved path at a constant velocity; examples include turning a curve in an automobile, pulling out of a dive, or performing a loop maneuver in an aircraft.

**accel'erator** [ L. *accelerans*, pres. part. of *ac-celero*, to hasten, fr. *celer*, swift ]. Accelerant. 1. That which increases rapidity of action or function. 2. In physiology, a nerve, muscle, or substance that quickens movement or response. 3. A catalytic agent used to hasten a chemical reaction (*e.g.*, NaCl or K₂SO₄ added to plaster of Paris and water to hasten setting).

    **linear a.,** a device that produces high energy photons (x-rays) on charged particles for use in radiation therapy.

    **proserum prothrombin conversion a.,** proconvertin.

    **serum a.,** *factor* VII.

    **serum prothrombin conversion a. (SPCA),** *factor* VII.

    **a. uri'nae,** *musculus* bulbospongiosus.

**accelerin** (ak-sel'er-in). Accelerator *globulin*.

**accelerom'eter.** An instrument for measuring the rate of change of velocity per unit of time.

**accentuator** (ak-sent'u-a-tor) [ L. *accentus*, accent, fr. *cano*, to sing ]. A substance, such as aniline, the presence of which allows a combination between a tissue or histologic element and a stain that might otherwise be impossible.

**acceptor** (ak-sep'tor) [ L. *ac-cipio*, pp. *-ceptus*, to accept, fr. *ad*, to, + *capio*, to take. CAP-2 ]. A compound that will take up a chemical group such as an amine group, a methyl group, a carbamyl group, etc., from another compound termed the donor. Thus, under the action of transaminase, glutamic acid is an amine donor while pyruvic acid is an amine a.

**accés pernicieux** [ Fr., pernicious attacks or symptoms ]. A series of phenomena sometimes occurring in apparently mild cases of remittent malarial fever. Pernicious attacks are roughly classified as cerebral and algid.

**accesso'rius** [ L. ] [ NA ]. Acessory.

    **a. willis'ii,** *nervus* accessorius.

**accessory** (ak'ses'o-rĭ) [ L. *accessorius*, fr. *ac-cedo*, pp. *-cessus*, to move toward ]. Supernumerary; adjuvant; denoting certain muscles, nerves, glands, etc.

**accident** (ak'sĭ-dent). A sudden unexpected event or injury occurring without omen or forewarning or developing in the course of a disease.

    **cardiac a.,** sudden cardiac catastrophe, such as may result from coronary occlusion.

    **cerebral vascular a.,** apoplexy.

    **serum a.,** anaphylactic shock resulting from injection of foreign serum for therapeutic purposes; see also serum *disease.*

**accident-prone.** 1. Having a greater number of accidents than would be expected of the average person in similar circumstances. 2. Having personality characteristics predisposing to accidents.

**accipiter** (ak-sip'ĭ-ter) [ L. a hawk ]. A bandage for the nose, so called because its ends branch out like the talons of a hawk grasping the face.

**acclima'tion.** Acclimatization.

**accli'matiza'tion.** Acclimation; physiological adjustment of an individual to a different climate, especially to a change in environmental temperature or altitude.

**accolé forms.** See under form.

**accommodation** (ă-kom'o-da'shun) [ L. *ac-commodo*, pp. *-atus*, to adapt, fr. *modus*, a measure ]. 1. The act or state of adjustment or adaptation. 2. In sensorimotor theory, the alteration of schemata or cognitive expectations to conform with experience. 3. See a. of eye, and related subentries.

    **absolute a.,** a. of an eye independent of its fellow.

    **amplitude of a.,** the total amount of a. between that necessary for distinguishing objects near at hand and for distant vision.

    **a. of eye,** adjustment of the eye for various distances; specifically, alteration of the convexity of the lens of the eye in order to bring light rays from an external object to a focus on the retina.

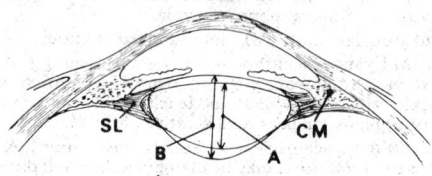

**Accommodation**

Diagram illustrating accommodation of the eye (lens) for near and far vision. *A,* shape of lens for far vision; *B,* shape of lens for near vision; *CM,* ciliary muscle; *SL,* suspensory ligament.

    **histologic a.,** pseudometaplasia; change in shape of cells to meet altered physical conditions, as the flattening of cuboidal cells in cysts as a result of pressure.

    **negative a.,** a. for distant vision by relaxation of the intrinsic muscles.

    **a. of nerve,** the property of nerve by which it adjusts to an electrical stimulus when the rate of change of intensity is not sufficiently rapid to set up an impulse; thus an electrical current of a certain strength excites the nerve if the rate at which the current rises to its maximum strength is sufficiently rapid, but may fail to excite if the rate of change in strength is reduced. The stimulus becomes effective at this slower rate of change in intensity only if the strength of the current is increased. In other words a current in order to excite must rise to its maximum intensity value more abruptly when it is weak than when it is strong.

**positive a.,** a. for near vision.

**relative a.,** quantity of a. required for single binocular vision for any specified distance, or for any particular degree of convergence.

**accom′modative.** Relating to accommodation.

**accouchement** (ă-koosh-moń′) [ Fr.° from *coucher*, to lie down ]. Delivery; childbirth.

**a. forcé** (for-sa′), forced, artificially hastened delivery, by means of forceps, version, etc.; originally applied to rapid dilation of the cervix with the hands, with version and forcible extraction of the fetus.

**accoucheur** (ă-koo-shër′). Obstetrician.

**accoucheuse** (ă-koo-shëz′). Female obstetrician; a skilled midwife with medical education and training.

**accrementition** (ă-kre-men-tish′un) [ L. *accresco*, pp. *-cretus*, to increase ]. 1. Reproduction by budding or germination. 2. Accretion (1).

**accretio cordis.** Adhesion of the pericardium to adjacent extracardiac structures.

**accretion** (ă-kre′shun) [ L. *accretio*, fr. *ad*, to, + *crescere*, to grow ]. 1. Accrementition (2); increase by addition to the periphery of material of the same nature as that already present; *e.g.*, the manner of growth of crystals. 2. In dentistry, foreign material collecting on the surface of a tooth or in a cavity. 3. A growing together.

**accrochage** (ak′ro-shahzh) [ Fr. hooking, hitching ]. Transient synchronization of two inherently independent cardiac rhythms originating in contiguous cardiac elements (*e.g.*, synchronous atrial and ventricular rhythms for a few beats during complete atrioventricular block).

**acebu′tolol** (USAN). (+)-*N*-[ 3-acetyl-4-[ 2-hydroxy-3-[ (1-methylethyl)amino ]propoxy ]phenyl ]butanamide; a β-adrenergic blocking agent.

**acec′lidine** (USAN). GLUCOSTAS; 3-quinuclidinol acetate ester; a cholinergic drug recommended for topical therapy of glaucoma when pilocarpine is not tolerated.

**acedap′sone** (USAN). DADDS; diacetyldiaminodiphenylsulfone; a derivative of dapsone with a longer duration of action. Used to enhance the malaria chemoprophylaxis of quinine or of a combination of chloroquine-primaquine; believed to act by interference with the utilization of folic acid.

**acedia** (ah-se′-de-ah) [ G. *a*-priv. + *kēdos*, care ]. Carelessness, listlessness and apathy; a form of melancholia.

**ace′lius** [ G. *a*-priv. + *celom* ]. An individual with absence of the celom.

**acelom** (a-se′lom) [ G. *a*- priv. + *koilōma*, hollow (celom) ]. Acelomate; lacking a true celom or body cavity lined with mesotholium; condition typically found in Platyhelminthes (flatworms), in which no true body cavity is found, but instead there is a syncytial mass of parenchymal cells.

**acel′omate.** Acelom.

**A.C.E. mixture.** See under mixture.

**acenesthesia** (ă-se-nes-the′zĭ-ah) [ G. *a*- priv. + *koinos*, common, + *aisthēsis*, feeling ]. Absence of the normal sensation of physical existence, or of the consciousness of visceral functioning.

**acenocoumarin** (ă-se′no-koo′mă-rin) (NF). SINTROM; nicoumalone; 3-(α-acetonyl-4-nitrobenzyl)-4-hydroxycoumarin; an orally effective synthetic anticoagulant of the coumarin type, and with similar actions.

**acentric** (ah-sen′trik) [ G. *a*- priv. + *kentron*, center ]. Without a center; in genetics, denoting a chromosome fragment without a centromere.

**acepha′lia, aceph′alism.** Acephaly.

**acephalobrachia** (ă-sef′al-o-bra′kĭ-ah) [ G. *a*- priv. + *kephalē*, head, + *brachiōn*, arm ]. Abrachiocephaly; absence of head and arms.

**acephalobrachius** (ă-sef′al-o-bra′kĭ-us). Abrachiocephalus; a malformed fetus without head or arms.

**aceph′alocar′dia** [ G. *a*- priv. + *kephalē*, head, + *kardia*, heart ]. Absence of head and heart in a parasitic conjoined twin.

**aceph′alocar′dius.** Acardiacus acephalus; a parasitic conjoined twin without head or heart.

**acephalochiria, acephalocheiria** (ă-sef′al-o-ki′rĭ-ah) [ G. *a*- priv. + *kephalē*, head, + *cheir*, hand ]. Absence of head and hands.

**acephalochirus, acephalocheirus** (ă-sef′al-o-ki′rus). A malformed fetus without head or hands.

**acephalocyst** (ă-sef′al-o-sist) [ G. *a*- priv. + *kephalē*, head, + *kystis*, bladder ]. A hydatid cyst with no daughter cyst; a sterile hydatid, so called because it gives origin to no scoleces or tapeworm heads.

**aceph′alogas′ter** [ G. *a*- priv. + *kephalē*, head, + *gastēr*, belly ]. A parasitic conjoined twin consisting only of the lower part of the body. It consists essentially of pelvis and legs.

**aceph′alogaste′ria.** Absence of head, thorax, and abdomen in a parasitic twin with pelvis and legs only.

**aceph′alopo′dia** [ G. *a*- priv. + *kephalē*, head, + *pous*, foot ]. Congenital absence of head and feet.

**aceph′alopo′dius.** A malformed fetus without head or feet.

**acephalorrhachia** (ă-sef′al-o-rak′ī-ah) [ G. *a*- priv. + *kephalē*, head, + *rhachis*, spine ]. Congenital absence of head and spinal column.

**aceph′alosto′mia** [ G. *a*- priv. + *kephalē*, head, + *stoma*, mouth ]. Absence of the greater part of the head with, however, the presence of a mouthlike opening.

**acephalos′tomus.** A malformed fetus having practically no head, but with a mouthlike opening in its uppermost region.

**aceph′alothora′cia** [ G. *a*- priv. + *kephalē*, head, + *thorax*, chest ]. Absence of head and thorax.

**aceph′alotho′rus.** A malformed fetus without head or thorax.

**aceph′alous.** Headless.

**aceph′alus** [ G. *a*- priv. + *kephalē*, head ]. A malformed fetus in which the body lacks a head.

**a. dibrachius,** a fetus lacking a head but having two arms more or less well developed.

**a. dipus,** a fetus lacking a head but showing two recognizably developed feet.

**a. monobrachius,** a fetus lacking a head and showing only one recognizable arm.

**a. monopus,** a fetus lacking a head and with fusion of the lower extremities so extreme that only a single foot is recognizable.

**a. paraceph′alus,** a malformed fetus with only partially developed skull and brain.

**a. sympus,** an a. showing fusion of the lower extremities all the way to the feet.

**aceph′aly** [ G. *a*- priv. + *kephalē*, head ]. Acephalia; acephalism; absence of a head.

**acero′la.** *Malpighia punicifolia* L. (family Malpighiaceae); a fruit of Puerto Rico said to have a higher content of vitamin C (2,000 mg. per 100 gm.) than any other fruit or plant.

**acer′vuline** [ Mod. L. *acervulus*, a little heap ]. Occurring in clusters; aggregated.

**acer′vulus** [ Mod. L. dim. of L. *acervus*, a heap ]. Psammoma *bodies* (1).

**acescence** (ă-ses′ens) [ L. *acesco*, to become sour. AC- ]. 1. A slight degree of acidity. 2. The process of becoming sour.

**acescent** (ă-ses′ent). Slightly acid.

**acestoma** (ă-ses-to′mah) [ G. *akestos*, curable, + *-ōma* ]. Exuberant granulations that are forming a cicatrix.

**acet-.** Combining form denoting the two-carbon fragment of acetic acid (*e.g.*, acetyl, aceto- compounds).

**acetab′ular.** Relating to the acetabulum.

**ac′etab′ulec′tomy** [ L. *acetabulum, q.v.*, *Ā* G. *ektomē*, excision ]. Excision of the acetabulum.

**ac′etab′uloplas′ty** [ L. *acetabulum, q.v.*, + G. *plassō*, to fashion ]. Any operation aimed at restoring the acetabulum to as near a normal state as possible.

**acetab'ulum**, gen. **acetab'uli**, pl. **acetab'ula** [ L. a shallow vinegar vessel or cup ] [ NA ]. Cotyloid cavity; cotyle; a cup-shaped depression on the external surface of the innominate bone, in which the head of the femur fits.

**acetal** (as'et-al). 1. Product of the addition of two moles of alcohol to one of an aldehyde, thus: $RCHO + 2R'OH \rightarrow RCH(OR')_2 + H_2O$. In mixed acetals (e.g., glycosides), two different alcohols are bound to the original aldehyde group. See also hemiacetal. 2. Diethylacetal; 1,1-diethoxyethane; $CH_3CH(OCH_2CH_3)_2$; a synthetic hypnotic, little used today.

    **a. phosphatid(at)e**, alk-1-enylglycerol.

**acetal'dehyde.** Acetic aldehyde; ethaldehyde; ethanal; $CH_3CHO$; an intermediate in yeast fermentation of carbohydrate and in alcohol metabolism; possesses moderate anesthetic activity.

**acetal'dol.** Aldol.

**acetam'ide.** $CH_3CONH_2$; acetic acid amide.

**acetam'idine.** Nitrogen analogue of acetic acid; $CH_3C(NH)NH_2$.

**acetam'inoflu'orene.** $C_6H_4(CH_2)C_6H_3$—$NHCOCH_3$; a carcinogenic compound. For structure, see fluorene.

**acetaminophen** (ă-set-ă-me'no-fen) (USP, NF). TYLENOL; paracetamol; N-acetyl-p-aminophenol; p-acetamidophenol; antipyretic and analgesic.

**acetaminosal'ol.** Phenetsal.

**acetan'ilide.** Antifebrin; $C_6H_5NHCOCH_3$; analgesic and antipyretic; continued use causes cyanosis.

**acetar'sol** (BP). Acetarsone.

**acetar'sone.** STOVARSOL; acetarsol; Fourneau 190; acetylaminohydroxyphenylarsonic acid; N-acetyl-4-hydroxy-m-arsanilic acid; used in amebiasis, and as a local application in Vincent's angina and in trichomonas vaginalis.

    **a. diethylamine**, used as an antisyphilitic.

**ac'etate.** A salt or ester of acetic acid; $CH_3$—$CO$—$O$—.

    **active a.**, acetylcoenzyme A.

    **a. kinase**, acetokinase; a phosphotransferase (EC 2.7.2.1) forming acetylphosphate from ATP and acetate.

    **a. thiokinase**, acetyl-CoA synthetase; see under acetylcoenzyme A.

**ac'etazol'amide** (USP, BP). DIAMOX; the heterocyclic sulfonamide 2-acetylamino-1,3,4-thiadiazole-5-sulfonamide. It inhibits the action of carbonic anhydrase in the kidney, causing an increase in the urinary excretion of sodium, potassium and bicarbonate, reduced excretion of ammonium, a rise in the pH of the urine, and a fall in the pH of the blood. Has been used in respiratory acidosis for diuresis and control of fluid retention, and in epilepsy.

    **a. sodium** (USP), DIAMOX sodium; same actions and uses as a., but more soluble and suitable for parenteral administration.

**acet-dia-mer-sulfon'amides.** A sulfonamide mixture containing equal weights of sulfacetamide, sulfadiazine and sulfamerazine to which there may or may not be added a suitable agent to increase the pH of the urine. Used for its bacteriostatic action.

**ace'tenyl.** Ethynyl.

**ace'tic** [ L. acetum, vinegar ]. Relating to vinegar; sour.

    **a. acid** (USP, BP), ethanoic acid; $CH_3COOH$; a product of the oxidation of ethanol and of the destructive distillation of wood; used locally as a counterirritant and occasionally internally; used also as a reagent.

    **a. acid amide**, acetamide.

    **a. acid, diluted** (NF, BP), contains 6 per cent w/v of a. acid.

    **a. acid, glacial** (USP), contains 99 per cent absolute a. acid; a caustic for removal of corns and warts.

    **a. aldehyde**, acetaldehyde.

**ace'ticocep'tor** [ L. capio, to take. CAP-2 ]. One of the side chains assumed to exist in trypanosomes and other organisms, which have a special affinity for the acetic acid radical.

**acet'ify** [ L. acetum, vinegar, + facio, to make; or fieri, to be made, to become ]. 1. To cause acetic fermentation; to make vinegar. 2. To become vinegar.

**acetim'eter** [ L. acetum, vinegar, + G. metron, measure ]. Acetometer; an apparatus for determining the content of acetic acid in vinegar or other fluid.

**ac'etin.** Glycerol acetate; a condensation product of glycerol and one or more molecules of acetic acid.

**aceto-, acet-.** Prefixes denoting replacement of an H atom by the acetyl radical, as in acetoacetic acid.

**acetoacetate decarboxylase.** A carboxy-lyase (EC 4.1.1.4) cleaving $CO_2$ from acetoacetate to form acetone.

**acetoace'tic acid.** Diacetic acid; $CH_3COCH_2COOH$; one of the ketone bodies, formed in excess and appearing in the urine in starvation or diabetes.

**acetoacetyl-CoA.** Acetoacetylcoenzyme A; intermediate in the oxidation of fatty acids; also formed from two molecules of acetyl-CoA; major role is condensation with acetyl-CoA to form the important β-hydroxy-β-methylglutaryl-CoA.

**acetoacetyl-CoA reductase.** An oxidoreductase (EC 1.1.1.36) catalyzing interconversion of a 3-oxoacyl-CoA and the corresponding 3-hydroxyacyl-CoA, with NADP.

**acetoacetyl-CoA thiolase.** Acetyl-CoA acetyltransferase.

**acetoacetyl-succinic thiophorase.** 3-Ketoacid-CoA transferase.

**acetohexamide** (USP). DYMELOR; 1-[ (p-acetylphenyl)sulfonyl ]-3-cyclohexylurea; an oral hypoglycemic agent that stimulates pancreatic insulin secretion; most useful therapeutically in mild cases of maturity-onset diabetes.

**α-aceto-α-hydroxybutyric acid.** $C_2H_5C(OH)(COCH_3)$-COOH; intermediate in the biosynthesis of isoleucine.

**acetoin** (as-et'-o-in). Acetylmethylcarbinol; $CH_3CH(OH)$-$COCH_3$; a condensation product of two molecules of acetaldehyde.

**acetokinase** (as'e-to-kin-ās'). Acetate kinase.

**ac'etol.** 1-Hydroxy-2-propanone, or hydroxyacetone, $CH_2OH$—$CO$—$CH_3$; also used as a proprietary name for certain commercial items.

**α-acetolac'tic acid.** An intermediate in pyruvic acid catabolism and valine biosynthesis; $CH_3COC(OH)(CH_3)$-COOH.

**ac'etol'ysis.** Decomposition of an organic compound with the addition of the elements of acetic acid at the point of decomposition; a term analogous to hydrolysis and phosphorolysis.

**ac'etomenaph'thone** (BP). Menadiol diacetate.

**ac'etomeroc'tol.** MERBAK; 2-(acetoxymercuri)-4-(1,1,3,3-tetramethylbutyl)phenol; an organic mercurial antibacterial agent.

**acetom'eter.** Acetimeter.

**acetonaph'thone.** Naphthylmethyl ketone.

**acetone** (as'e-tōn). 1. Dimethylketone; a colorless, volatile, inflammable liquid; $CH_3COCH_3$. Extremely small amounts are found in normal urine, but larger quantities occur in urine and blood of diabetic persons; it sometimes imparts an ethereal odor to urine and breath of such patients. 2 (NF). Used as a solvent in some pharmaceutical preparations.

    **a. body**, ketone b.; see under ketone.

    **a. compounds**, β-hydroxybutyric acid, acetoacetic (diacetic) acid, and a.; ketone bodies appearing in the urine in ketosis.

**acetone'mia** [ acetone + G. haima, blood ]. The presence of acetone or acetone bodies in relatively large amounts in the blood, manifested at first by erethism, later by a progressive depression.

**acetone'mic.** Relating to or caused by acetonemia.

**acetoni'trile.** $CH_3CN$; methyl cyanide; a colorless fluid of aromatic odor, soluble in water and alcohol.

**acetonu'ria** [ acetone + G. ouron, urine ]. The excretion in the urine of large amounts of acetone, an indication of incomplete oxidation of large amounts of fat; commonly occurs in diabetic acidosis.

**acetophenazine maleate** (NF). TINDAL maleate; 2-acetyl-10{ 3-[ 4-(2-hydroxyethyl)piperazinyl ]propyl}phenothiazine dimaleate; antipsychotic agent commonly used in the elderly.

**acetophenet'idin.** Phenacetin.

**acetophe′none.** HYPNONE; phenylmethyl ketone; a coal tar derivative, $C_6H_5COCH_3$; hypnotic or mild depressant.

**acetopyr′rothine.** THIOLUTIN; an antibiotic principle obtained from cultures of *Streptomyces albus;* active against Gram-negative and Gram-positive bacteria and many fungi; used to inhibit microbiological growth in beer.

**acetosol′uble.** Soluble in acetic acid.

**acetosul′fone sodium** (NF). PROMACETIN; acetosulphone; sodium 2-*N*-acetylsulfamyl-4,4′-diaminodiphenylsulfone; leprostatic administered orally.

*o*-**acetotoluide.** $CH_3C_6H_4NHCOCH_3$; an isomer of *p*-acetotoluide, having similar properties.

*p*-**acetotoluide.** $CH_3C_6H_4NHCOCH_3$; colorless crystals, slightly soluble in water; antipyretic.

**ac′etous.** Relating to vinegar; sour-tasting.

**ace′tovanil′lon.** Apocynin.

**ace′tozone.** Benzozone; acetyl benzoyl peroxide; germicide.

**acetphenoli′satin.** Oxyphenisatin acetate.

**acetract.** An extract containing acetic acid.

**acetri′zoate sodium** (BP). IODOPAQUE; 3-acetamido-2,4,6-triiodobenzoic acid sodium salt; a radiopaque medium.

**ace′tum,** pl. **ace′ta** [ L. *vinum acetum,* soured wine, vinegar ]. Vinegar.

**acet′urate.** USAN-approved contraction for *N*-acetylglycinate, $CH_3CONHCH_2COO^-$.

**acetyl** (as′et-il). The atom grouping, $CH_3CO-$; an acetic acid molecule from which the hydroxyl group has been removed.

    **a. chloride,** $CH_3COCl$; a colorless liquid; used as a reagent, irritant, and corrosive, causing severe burns.

    **a. transacylase,** ACP acetyltransferase.

    **a. value,** the milligrams of KOH required to neutralize the acetic acid produced by the hydrolysis of 1 gm. of acetylated fat; a measure of the hydroxy acids present in glycerides; notably high in castor oil.

**acetyl-activating enzyme.** Acetyl-CoA synthetase.

**acetyladenylate.** Mixed anhydride between COOH of acetic acid and phosphoric acid residue of adenosine 5′-phosphoric acid, $(Ado)-5′-OP(O_2H)-OCOCH_3$.

**2-acetylaminofluorene.** AAF; *N*-2-fluorenylacetamide; a potent carcinogenic compound. For structure, see fluorene.

**acet′ylase.** Any enzyme catalyzing acetylation or deacetylation, as in the formation of *N*-acetylglutamate from glutamate plus acetyl-CoA or the reverse. A.'s are usually called acetyltransferases, *e.g.,* choline acetyltransferase, phosphate acetyltransferase.

**acetylation** (ă-set-ĭ-la′shun). The formation of an acetyl derivative.

**ace′tylcarbro′mal.** SEDAMYL; *N*-acetyl-*N*-bromodiethylacetylurea; sedative.

**acetylcho′line.** Acetylethanoltrimethylammonium hydroxide; $CH_3CO-OCH_2CH_2N(CH_3)_3OH$; the acetic acid ester of choline isolated from ergot; causes cardiac inhibition, vasodilation, gastrointestinal peristalsis, and other parasympathetic effects. It is liberated from preganglionic and postganglionic endings of parasympathetic fibers and from preganglionic fibers of the sympathetic as a result of nerve injuries, whereupon it acts as a transmitter on the effector organ. It is hydrolyzed into choline and acetic acid by acetylcholinesterase before a second impulse may be transmitted.

    **a. bromide,** available for parasympathomimetic effect.

    **a. chloride** (NF), MIOCHOL; a miotic, administered subcutaneously for parasympathomimetic effect.

**acetylcholinesterase** (as′et-ĭl-ko-lin-es′ter-āz) (EC 3.1.1.7). True cholinesterase; choline esterase I; specific or "e" type cholinesterase; the cholinesterases that hydrolyze acetylcholine within the central nervous system and at peripheral neuroeffector junctions (*e.g.,* motor end-plates and autonomic ganglia).

**acetyl-CoA.** Acetylcoenzyme A; condensation product of coenzyme A and acetic acid; symbolized as $CoAS~COCH_3$; intermediate in transfer of two-carbon fragment, notably in its entrance into the tricarboxylic acid cycle.

**acetyl-CoA acetyltransferase** (EC 2.3.1.9). Acetoacetyl-CoA thiolase; .acetyl-CoA thiolase; thiolase; an acetyl-

transferase forming acetoacetyl-CoA from two molecules of acetyl-CoA, releasing one CoA.

**acetyl-CoA acylase.** Acetyl-CoA hydrolase.

**acetyl-CoA acyltransferase** (EC 2.3.1.16). $\beta$-Ketothiolase; 3-ketoacyl-CoA thiolase; $\beta$-ketothiolase; an enzyme catalyzing the thioclastic cleavage of $\beta$-ketoacyl-CoA, forming an acyl-CoA with a carbon chain shorter by two atoms, the missing two atoms appearing as acetyl-CoA. See also acetyl-CoA acetyltransferase.

**acetyl-CoA carboxylase** (EC 6.4.1.2). A ligase that catalyzes the reaction of acetyl-CoA, $CO_2$, and ATP, with $Mn^{+2}$ as catalyst and covalently bound biotin, to form malonyl-CoA, ADP, and $P_i$, or the reverse (decarboxylase). *N*-Carboxybiotin is an intermediate.

**acetyl-CoA deacylase.** Acetyl-CoA hydrolase.

**acetyl-CoA hydrolase.** Acetyl-CoA acylase; acetyl-CoA deacylase; hydrolase (EC 3.1.2.1) cleaving acetate from acetyl-CoA.

**acetyl-CoA synthetase** (EC 6.2.1.1). Acetyl-activating enzyme; acetate thiokinase; an acid-thiol ligase catalyzing formation of acetyl-CoA from acetate and CoA with splitting of ATP to AMP and $PP_i$. Also acts on propionate and acrylate.

**acetyl-CoA thiolase.** Acetyl-CoA acetyltransferase.

**acetylcys′teine** (NF). MUCOMYST; *N*-acetyl-L-cysteine; a mucolytic agent that reduces the viscosity of mucous secretions.

**acetyldigitox′in** (NF). ACYLANID; the $\alpha$-acetyl ester of digitoxin derived from lanatoside-A. Same actions and uses as digitoxin, but of more rapid onset and shorter duration of action.

**acetyldigox′in.** A digitalis glycoside with properties similar to those of digoxin; derived from digilanide C.

**acet′ylene.** $HC{\equiv}CH$; a colorless explosive gas; anesthetic in concentrations of 40 volumes per cent.

**acet′ylenedicarb′oxamide.** Cellocidin; antibiotic produced by *Streptomyces chibaensis.*

**ac′etylor′nithinase.** Acetylornithine deacetylase.

**acetylornithine deacetylase.** Acetylornithinase; an enzyme (EC 3.5.1.16) catalyzing the hydrolysis of *N*-$\alpha$-acetylornithine to ornithine.

**acetylphos′phate.** $CH_3CO-OPO_3H_2$; a "high energy" phosphate that plays the part of an "active acetate" in the metabolism of various bacteria.

**acetylpro′mazine maleate.** NOTENSIL; 10-[ 3-(dimethylamino)propyl ]phenothiazin-2-yl methyl ketone maleate; used as tranquilizer in veterinary practice.

**3-acetylpyridine** (as′e-til-pir′ĭ-dēn). An antimetabolite of nicotinamide. Produces symptoms of nicotinamide deficiency when fed to mice.

**ac′etylsalicyl′ic acid.** Aspirin.

**acetylstrophan′thidin.** A synthetic ester of strophanthidin; the most rapidly acting digitalis-like preparation available.

*N*1-**acetylsulfanilamide.** Sulfacetamide.

*N*4-**acetylsulfanilamide.** *p*-Sulfamylacetanilide.

**acetyl sulfisoxazole.** See under sulfisoxazole.

**acetyltan′nic acid.** TANNIGEN; diacetyltannic acid; astringent, used for treatment of diarrhea.

**acetyltrans′ferase.** Transacetylase; any enzyme transferring acetyl groups from one compound to another. See also acetyl-CoA, choline, and lipoate acetyltransferases.

**AcG or ac-g.** Abbreviation for accelerator *globulin.*

**achalasia** (ă-kal-a′-zī-ah) [ G. *a-* priv. + *chalasis,* a slackening ]. Failure to relax; referring especially to visceral openings such as the pylorus, cardia or any other sphincter muscles.

    **esophageal a.,** cardiospasm; an obstruction which develops in the terminal esophagus just proximal to the cardioesophageal junction; the upper esophagus becomes dilated and filled with retained food; the defect appears to originate from a loss of motor innervation by fibers originating in the dorsal nucleus of the vagus nerve.

    **pelvirectal a.,** spasm of the pelvic rectum, one cause of constipation.

    **sphincteral a.,** tightness of the sphincters associated with failure of relaxation.

**Achalme** (ash'alm), Pierre J., French etiologist, *1866. See A.'s *bacillus.*

**Achard** (a-shar'), E. Charles, French physician, 1860–1941. See A.-Castaigne *method,* A. *syndrome,* A.-Thiers *syndrome.*

**ache** (āk). A pain of less than severe intensity that persists for a long time.

   **belly-a.,** see bellyache.

   **bone a.** a severe dull pain in the bones, often of syphilitic origin. An extreme variety occurs in dengue (breakbone) fever.

   **stomach a.,** see stomachache.

**acheilia, achilia** (ă-ki'lī-ah) [ G. *a-* priv. + *cheilos,* lip ]. Congenital absence of the lips.

**acheilous, achilous** (ă-ki'lus). Characterized by or relating to acheilia.

**acheiria, achiria** (ă-ki'rī-ah) [ G. *a-* priv. + *cheir,* hand ]. 1. Congenital absence of the hands. 2. Anesthesia in, with loss of the sense of possession of, one or both hands; a condition sometimes noted in hysteria. 3. A form of dyscheiria in which the patient is unable to tell on which side of the body a stimulus has been applied.

**acheiropody, achiropody** (a-ki-rop'o-di) [ G. *a-* priv. + *cheir,* hand, + *podos,* foot ]. Congenital absence of the hands and feet; sutosomal recessive inheritance.

**acheirous, achirous** (ă-ki'rus). Characterized by or relating to acheiria.

**acheirus, achirus** (ă-ki'rus). A malformed individual with acheiria.

**achilia** (ă-ki'lī-ah). Acheilia.

**Achillea** (ă-kil-e'ah). Milfoil; thousand-leaf; oldman's pepper; yarrow. The dried herb of *A. millefolium* (family Compositae), collected when in flower; has been used as an aromatic bitter, diaphoretic and emmenagogue.

**achilleine** (ă-kil'e-ēn). An amorphous bitter substance derived from *Achillea millefolium.* It has been used as an antimalarial, but causes irregular heart action.

**Achilles** (ă-kil'ēz). A mythical Greek warrior who was vulnerable only in the heel. See A. *bursa, reflex, tendon.*

**Achillini** (ak-ĭ-le'nĭ), Alessandro, Bolognese anatomist and physician, 1463–1512. Discovered the malleus, incus, labyrinth, and ileocecal valve.

**achillobursitis** (ă-kil'o-bur-si'tis). Inflammation of a bursa beneath the tendo calcaneus.

**achillodynia** (ă-kil-o-din'ĭ-ah) [ Achilles (tendon) + G. *odynē,* pain ]. Pain due to inflammation of the bursa between the calcaneus and the tendo Achillis (achillobursitis).

**achillorrhaphy** (ă-kil-or'ă-fĭ) [ Achilles (tendon) + G. *rhaphē,* a sewing ]. Suture of the tendo calcaneus.

**achillotenotomy** (ă-kil'o-ten-ot'o-mĭ) [ G. *tenōn,* tendon, + *tomē,* a cutting ]. Achillotomy.

**achillotomy** (ă-kil-ot'o-mĭ) [ Achilles (tendon) + G. *tomē,* incision ]. Achillotenotomy; division of the tendo calcaneus.

**achi'lous.** Acheilous.

**achiria** (ă-ki'rī-ah). Acheiria.

**achiropody** (a-ki-rop'o-dĭ). Acheiropody.

**achi'rous.** Acheirous.

**achi'rus.** Acheirus.

**achlorhydria** (ă-klor-hi'drĭ-ah) [ G. *a-* priv. + chlorhydric (acid) ]. Absence of hydrochloric acid from the gastric juice.

**achlor'ides.** Nonchlorides; salts other than chlorides in the urine.

**achlo'roblep'sia.** Achloropsia.

**achlorop'sia** [ G. *a-* priv. + *chlōros,* green, + *opsis,* vision ]. Green *blindness.*

**Acholeplas'ma.** A genus of bacteria (order Mycoplasmatales) that have characteristics identical to those of the species in the genus *Mycoplasma,* with the exception that the acholeplasmas do not require sterol for growth. Saprophytic and parasitic species occur. The type species is *A. laidlawii.*

   **A. axan'thum,** a species found in a murine leukemia cell line.

**A. granula'rum,** *Mycoplasma granularum;* a species that occurs as a commensal in swine; pathogenicity not determined.

**A. laidlawii,** *Mycoplasma laidlawii;* a species that occurs as a saprophyte in sewage, manure, humus, and soil; type species of the genus *A.*

**acholia** (ă-ko'lī-ah) [ G. *a-* priv. + *cholē,* bile ]. Suppressed secretion of bile.

**achol'ic.** Without bile.

**acholuria** (ă-ko-lu'rīah) [ G. *a-* priv. + *cholē,* bile, + *ouron,* urine ]. Absence of bile pigments from the urine in certain cases of jaundice.

**acholuric** (ă-ko-lu'rik). Without bile in the urine.

**achondrogenesis** (ă-kon'dro-jen'es-is) [ G. *a-* priv., + *chondros,* cartilage, + *genesis,* origin ]. Dwarfism accompanied by various bone aplasias and hypoplasias of all four extremities, with a normal or enlarged skull and a short trunk with delayed ossification of the lower spine; autosomal recessive inheritance.

**achondroplasia** (ă-kon-dro-pla'zī-ah) [ G. *a-* priv. + *chondros,* cartilage, + *plasis,* a molding ]. An abnormality of conversion of cartilage into bone predominantly affecting the epiphyses of long bones; a type of chondrodystrophy. Epiphysial growth is retarded and ceases early, resulting in dwarfism apparent at birth, with short extremities but normal trunk; the head is frequently enlarged, with flattened nose; due to mutation or inherited as an autosomal dominant.

   **homozygous a.,** severe a. affecting an infant whose parents are achondroplastic.

   **mosaic a.,** a. limited to a part of the skeleton, possibly due to delayed mutation occurring after division of the zygote.

**achondroplasty** (ă-kon'dro-plas-tĭ). Achondroplasia.

**achor'date, achor'dal.** Referring to animal forms below the Chordata that do not develop a notochord or chorda.

**achoresis** (ă-ko-re'sis) [ G. *a-* priv. + *chōreō,* to make room, fr. *chōros,* space ]. Permanent contraction of a hollow viscus, such as the stomach or bladder, whereby its capacity is reduced.

**Achorion** (ă-ko'rĭ-on) [ G. *achōr,* dandruff ]. A genus of parasitic fungi. Proper term now *Trichophyton.*

**achreocythemia** (ă-kre-o-si-the'mĭ-ah) [ G. *achroios,* colorless, + *kytos,* receptacle, + *haima,* blood. CHROM- ]. Achroiocythemia; obsolete term for a condition characterized by a lack or deficiency of hemoglobin, and consequent paleness of the red blood cells.

**achroacyte** (ă-kro'ah-sīt) [ G. *a-* priv. + *chroa,* color, + *kytos,* a hollow (cell) ]. A colorless cell; a lymphocyte.

**achroacytosis** (ă-kro-ah-si-to'sis). Obsolete term for lymphocytosis.

**achroglo'bin.** A colorless respiratory protein compound present in certain invertebrates.

**achroiocythemia** (ă-kroy'o-si-the'mĭ-ah). Obsolete term for achreocythemia.

**achromacyte** (ă-kro'mah-sīt). Achromocyte.

**achromasia** (ă-kro-ma'sĭ-ah) [ G. *achrōmos,* colorless ]. 1. Cachectic pallor; pallor associated with the Hippocratic facies of extremely severe and chronic illness, often heralding the moribund state. 2. Achromia.

**achromat** (ak'ro-mat). An achromatic *lens.*

**achromate** (ă-kro'māt) [ G. *a-* priv. + *chrōma,* color ]. An absolutely color-blind person.

**achromatic** (ă-kro-mat'ik) [ G. *a-* priv. + *chrōma,* color ]. 1. Colorless. 2. Not decomposing white light. 3. Not staining readily.

**achro'matin.** The weakly staining components of the nucleus, such as the linin.

**achromatinic** (ă-kro-mă-tin'ik). Relating to or containing achromatin.

**achromatism** (ă-kro'mă-tizm). 1. The quality of being achromatic. 2. The annulment of chromatic aberration by combining glasses of different refractive indexes and different dispersion.

**achromatocyte** (ă-kro-mat'o-sīt). Achromocyte.

**achromatolysis** (ă-kro-mă-tol'ĭ-sis). Plasmolysis; protoplasmolysis; karyoplasmolysis; dissolution of the achromatin of a cell or of its nucleus.

**achromatophil** (ă-kro-mat'o-fil) [ G. *a-* priv. + *chrōma,* color, + *philos,* fond ]. 1. Not being colored by the histologic or bacteriologic stains. 2. A cell or tissue that cannot be stained in the usual way.

**achromatophilia** (ă-kro'mat-o-fil'ĭ-ah). A condition of being refractory to staining processes.

**achromatopsia** (ă-kro-mă-top'sĭ-ah) [ G. *a-* priv. + *chrōma,* color, + *opsis,* vision ]. Monochromatism; complete color blindness; only monochromatic gray in varying luminosity is visible; the totally color-blind person exhibits the characteristics of scotopic vision.

**achro'matopsy.** Achromatopsia.

**achromatosis** (ă-kro-mă-to'sis) [ G. *a-* priv. + *chrōma,* color ]. Achromia.

**achromatous** (ă-kro'mă-tus). Colorless.

**achromaturia** (ă-kro-mă-tu'rĭ-ah) [ G. *a-* priv. + *chrōma,* color, + *ouron,* urine ]. The passage of colorless or very pale urine.

**achro'mia** [ G. *a-*priv. + *chrōma,* color ]. Achromasia (2); achromatosis. 1. Deficiency of natural pigmentation, congenital or acquired. 2. Lack of capacity to accept stains in cells or tissue.

**a. parasit'ica,** a phase of lessening or absence of pigmentation in cutaneous lesions, caused by the fungus *Malassezia furfur;* see also *tinea* versicolor.

**a. unguium,** leukonychia.

**achro'mic.** Colorless.

**achromocyte** (ă-kro'mo-sīt) [ G. *a-*priv. + *chrōma,* color, + *kytos,* hollow (cell) ]. Achromatocyte; achromacyte; a hypochromic, crescent-shaped erythrocyte, probably resulting from artifactual rupture of a red cell with loss of hemoglobin; also called shadow; Ponfick's shadow; or ghost, shadow, Traube's, or phantom corpuscle.

**achromoder'ma.** Leukoderma.

**achro'mophil, achromoph'ilous.** Achromatophil.

**achromotrichia** (ă-kro-mo-trik'ĭ-ah) [ G. *chrōmos,* colorless, + *thrix,* hair ]. 1. Absence or loss of pigment in the hair; see also canities. 2. A graying of the hair of black rats in pantothenic acid deficiency.

**achroodextrin** (ak-ro'o-deks'trin). A dextrin of low molecular weight, formed from starch in a stage of the digestion of the latter by amylase. It gives no color reaction with iodine.

**Achyla.** A genus of aquatic fungi, sometimes saprophytic, sometimes forming molds on animals (fish, insects, etc.).

**achylia** (ă-ki'lĭ-ah) [ G. *a-* priv. + *chylos,* juice. CHY- ]. Achylosis. 1. Absence of gastric juice or other digestive ferment. 2. Absence of chyle.

**a. gas'trica,** diminished or abolished secretion of gastric juice associated with atrophy of the mucous membrane of the stomach.

**a. pancreat'ica,** deficiency or absence of pancreatic secretion causing fatty stools, emaciation and impaired nutrition.

**achylosis** (ă-ki-lo'sis). Achylia.

**achylous** (ă-ki'lus) [ G. *achylos,* without juice ]. 1. Lacking in gastric juice or other digestive secretion. 2. Having no chyle.

**achymia, achymosis** (ă-ki'mĭ-ah, ă-ki-mo'sis) [ G. *a-*priv. + *chymos,* chyme. CHY- ]. Absence or deficiency of chyme.

**acicular** (ă-sik'u-lar) [ L. *acicular,* small pin ]. Needle-shaped, or needle-pointed; applied particularly to leaves and crystals.

**acid** (as'id) [ L. *acidus,* sour ]. 1. A compound of an electronegative element or radical with hydrogen, yielding hydrogen ion in a polar solvent (*e.g.,* in water); it forms salts by replacing all or part of the hydrogen with an electropositive element or radical. An a. containing one displaceable atom of hydrogen in the molecule is called **monobasic;** one containing two such atoms, **dibasic;** and one containing more than two, **polybasic.** 2. In popular language, any chemical compound that has a sour taste (given by the hydrogen ion). 3. Sour; sharp to the taste. 4. Relating to a.; giving an a. reaction. For individual acids, see specific names.

**binary a.,** one containing only two elements.

**fatty a.,** see *fatty acid.*

**inorganic a.,** an a. made up of molecules not containing organic radicals, *e.g.,* HCl, $H_2SO_4$, $H_3PO_4$.

**organic a.,** an a. made up of molecules containing organic radicals; *e.g.,* acetic a., citric a.

**sugar a.'s,** see under sugar.

**ternary a.,** one that contains three elements, such as an inorganic oxacid (*e.g.,* $H_2SO_4$ and $H_3PO_4$).

**vegetable a.,** an acid derived from plants or fruits.

**ac'idam'inu'ria.** Aminoaciduria.

**acide'mia** [ acid + G. *haima,* blood ]. An increase in the H-ion concentration of the blood—a fall below normal in pH, notwithstanding alterations in content of bicarbonate. Individual types of a. are listed by specific name, *e.g.,* isovalericacidemia, aminoacidemia, etc.

**acid-fast.** Acid-proof; a term denoting bacteria that are not decolorized by an acid-alcohol after having been stained with dyes such as basic fuchsin; the mycobacteria and a few nocardiae are the only acid-fast bacteria.

**acid'ify.** 1. To render acid. 2. To become acid.

**acidim'eter.** A device for determining the degree of acidity of a fluid, or the strength of an acid.

**acidim'etry.** The determination of (1) the acidity of a fluid, or (2) the strength of an acid.

**acidis'mus.** Poisoning by acids introduced from without, as contradistinguished from acidosis, or poisoning by acids formed in metabolism.

**acid'ity.** 1. The state of being acid. 2. The acid content of a fluid.

**total a.,** referring to the gastric contents, the a. being determined by titration with sodium hydroxide, using phenolphthalein as indicator. The result is expressed in clinical units.

**acid'ocyte** [ acid + G. *kytos,* cell ]. Eosinophilic *leukocyte.*

**acidocytope'nia** [ acidocyte + G. *penia,* poverty ]. Acidopenia; obsolete term for eosinophilic leukopenia.

**acidocytosis** (ă-sid-o-si-to'sis). Obsolete term for eosinophilic leukocytosis.

**acidope'nia.** Obsolete term for eosinophilic leukocytosis.

**acidophil, acidophile** (ă-sid'o-fil, ă-sid'o-fīl) [ acid + G. *philos,* fond ]. An acidophil *cell.*

**acidophilic** (as'ĭ-do-fil'ik; ă-sid'o-fil'ik). Having an affinity for acid dyes; denoting a cell or tissue element that stains with an acid dye.

**acido'sis** [ acid + G. suffix *-ōsis,* condition ]. A state characterized by actual or relative decrease of alkali in bodily fluids in proportion to the content of acid. Depending on the degree of compensation for the a., the pH of bodily fluids may be normal or decreased. Tissue function is often disturbed in this state, most importantly that of the central nervous system, if compensation is inadequate.

**carbon dioxide a.,** respiratory a.

**compensated a.,** an a. in which the pH of bodily fluids is normal. Compensation may be achieved by enhanced pulmonary excretion of carbon dioxide, utilization of alkaline reserves of bodily fluids, or excretion of a more acidic urine. Commonly, more than one compensatory mechanism is utilized.

**gaseous a.,** respiratory a.

**metabolic a.,** decreased pH and bicarbonate content of the body fluids caused either by the accumulation of excess acids stronger than carbonic acid or by abnormal losses of fixed base from the body, as in diarrhea or renal disease.

**primary renal tubular a.,** see renal tubular a.

**renal tubular a.,** a clinical syndrome characterized by inability to excrete acid urine, and by low plasma bicarbonate and high plasma chloride concentrations, often with hypokalemia; symptoms of chronic acidosis are often complicated by osteomalacia, nephrocalcinosis, or renal stones. **Primary renal tubular a.** is a metabolic defect in the mechanism of urinary acidification, and may be either the transient type, with onset in infancy, or the persistent type, with onset in childhood or adult years; both transient and persistent types are familial, but genetics not clear. **Secondary renal tubular a.** may occur as a complication of hypercalcemic states, hyperglobulinemic disorders, and probably in some other chronic renal conditions; it is a rather regular component of the Fanconi renal syndrome (de Toni-Fanconi syndrome).

**respiratory a.,** carbon dioxide a.; gaseous a.; a. caused by retention of carbon dioxide, owing to inadequate pulmonary ventilation.

**secondary renal tubular a.,** see renal tubular a.

**uncompensated a.,** an a. in which the pH of bodily fluids is subnormal, because restoration of normal acid-base balance is not possible or has not yet been achieved.

**acidosteophyte** (as-ĭ-dos'te-o-fīt) [ G. *akis,* a point, + *osteon,* bone, + *phyton,* growth ]. A sharp-pointed bony outgrowth or osteophyte.

**acidot'ic.** Pertaining to or indicating acidosis.

**acid'ulate.** To render more acid or sour.

**acid'ulous.** Acid or sour.

**acidu'ria** [ acid + G. *ouron,* urine ]. 1. The excretion of an acid urine. 2. Excretion of an abnormal amount of any specified acid. Individual types of a. are listed by specific name, *e.g.,* aminoaciduria, ketoaciduria, etc.

**acidu'ric** [ acid + L. *duro,* to endure ]. Pertaining to bacteria that tolerate an acid environment.

**acidyl** (as'id-il). See acyl.

**acin-.** See also akin-.

**acinar** (as'ĭ-nar). Acinic; pertaining to the acinus.

**Acinetobacter** (a-sī-ne'to-bak'ter). *Lingelsheimia;* a genus of nonmotile, aerobic bacteria (family Neisseriaceae) containing Gram-negative or -variable coccoid or short rods, or cocci, often occurring in pairs. Nonmotile. Spores are not produced. These bacteria grow on ordinary media without the addition of serum. They are oxidase-negative and catalase-positive; carbohydrates are oxidized or not attacked at all, and arginine dihydrolase is not produced. They occur frequently in clinical specimens. The type species is *A. calcoaceticus. (A. stenohalis* is sometimes incorrectly cited as the type species of this genus.)

**A. calcoaceticus,** *Bacterium anitratum; Lingelsheimia anitrata;* a species of bacteria originally found in a quinate enrichment; strains of this organism which were identified as *B. antitratum* were found in the genitourinary tract. It is the type species of the genus *A. (A. stenohalis* is sometimes incorrectly cited as the type species of this genus.)

**acini** (as'ĭ-ne). Plural of acinus.

**acinic** (ah-sin'ik). Acinar.

**acin'iform** [ L. *acinus,* grape, + *forma,* shape ]. Acinous.

**ac'ini'tis.** Inflammation of an acinus.

**ac'inose.** Acinous.

**acinous** (as'ĭ-nus). Resembling an acinus or grape-shaped structure.

**acinus,** gen. and pl. **acini** (as'ĭ-nus) [ L. berry, grape ] [ NA ]. One of the minute grape-shaped secretory portions of an acinous gland. Some authorities use the terms a. and alveolus interchangeably, whereas others differentiate them by the constricted openings of the a. into the excretory duct.

**liver a.,** a somewhat grape-shaped area of liver parenchyma that has as its central axis a terminal branch of the portal vein, hepatic artery, and bile duct; it is composed of segments of several hepatic lobules.

**pulmonary a.,** that part of the airway consisting of a terminal bronchiole and all of its branches.

**acipenserin.** A toxic substance present in the testis of the sturgeon, *Acipenser.*

**Ackee.** A small tree, properly called *Blighia sapida,* commonly found on the island of Jamaica, which bears fruit which is poisonous when unripe or not in good condition (see a. *poisoning*).

**Ackermann,** Conrad T., German physician, 1825–1896. See A.'s *angle.*

**acladio'sis.** A chronic ulcerative skin disease attributed to fungi of the genus *Acladium.* Some believe that the organism is synonymous with *Sporotrichum schenchi.*

**Acla'dium.** An obsolete generic name for a fungus capable of causing acladiosis. Some believe the fungus is identical with *Sporotrichum schencki.*

**ac'lasis** [ G. *a-* priv. + *klasis,* a breaking away, a fragment ]. Failure of modeling during development.

**diaphys'ial a.,** diaphysial juxtaepiphysial exostosis, especially close to the knee; an osteochondrodysplasia characterized by hereditary multiple exostoses.

**aclas'tic** [ G. *a-* priv. + *klastos,* broken in pieces ]. Nonrefractive; not refracting the rays of light.

**acleistocardia** (ā-klīs-to-kar'dī-ah) [ G. *a-* priv. + *kleistos,* closed, + *kardia,* heart ]. Patency of the foramen ovale of the heart.

**aclu'sion** [ G. *a-* priv. + L. *claudo,* pp. *clausus,* to shut. CLAUS- ]. Lack of contact of opposing surfaces of molar and bicuspid teeth when jaws are closed.

**acme** (ak'me) [ G. *akmē,* the highest point ]. The period of greatest intensity of any symptom, sign, or process.

**acmesthesia** (ak-mes-the'zī-ah) [ G. *acmē,* point, + *aisthēsis,* sensation ]. Sensitivity to pinprick. A sensation in the skin of a sharp point.

**acne** (ak'ne) [ probably a corruption (or copyist's error) of G. *akmē,* point of efflorescence. AC- ]. An inflammatory follicular, papular and pustular eruption involving the sebaceous apparatus.

**a. agmina'ta,** Papulonecrotic *tuberculid.*

**a. al'bida,** a. caused by milia.

**a. artificia'lis,** a. venenata; a. produced by external irritants, such as tar (chloracne), or drugs internally administered, such as iodides or bromides.

**asbestos a.,** acneform eruption resulting from occupational exposure to asbestos.

**bromide a.,** follicular eruption on face, trunk, and extremities, due to bromide ingestion.

**a. cachectico'rum,** a. occurring in the subjects who have some debilitating constitutional disease; characterized by large, soft, purulent, ulcerative, cystic, and scarred lesions.

**a. cilia'ris,** follicular papules and pustules on the free edges of the eyelids.

**a. congloba'ta,** severe cystic a., characterized by cystic lesions, abscesses, communicating sinuses, and thickened, nodular scars.

**cystic a.,** a. in which the predominant lesions are cysts and deep-seated scars.

**a. decal'vans,** a rare type of pustular folliculitis of the scalp productive of scarring alopecia.

**a. erythemato'sa,** rosacea.

**a. fronta'lis,** a. of the forehead; possibly synonymous with a. varioliformis.

**a. genera'lis,** a. lesions involving the face, chest and back.

**halogen a.,** an acneform eruption caused by bromides or iodides.

**a. hypertroph'ica,** a. vulgaris in which the lesions, on healing, leave hypertrophic scars.

**a. indura'ta,** deeply seated a., with large papules and pustules, large scars, and hypertrophic scars.

**a. keloid,** see under keloid.

**a. kerato'sa,** an eruption of papules consisting of horny plugs projecting from the hair follicles, accompanied by inflammation.

**a. lupoi'des,** a. varioliformis.

**a. medicamento'sa,** acneform a. caused or exacerbated by several classes of drugs, *e.g.,* antiepileptic, halogens, steroids, tuberculostatic.

**a. necrot'ica,** a. varioliformis.

**a. neonato'rum,** a condition in infants, characterized by papules and comedones on forehead and cheeks; only in rare instances caused by sexual precocity.

**a. papulo'sa,** a. vulgaris in which the papular lesions predominate.

**a. puncta'ta,** a condition that resembles chloracne in that black central comedones are present in all the lesions.

**a. pustulo'sa,** a. vulgaris in which the pustular lesions predominate.

**a. ro'dens,** a. varioliformis.

**a. rosa'cea,** rosacea.

**a. seba'cea,** *seborrhea* oleosa.

**a. simplex, simple a.,** a. vulgaris.

**a. syphilit'ica,** pustular *syphilids.*

**tar a.,** chloracne.

**a. tarsi,** follicular eruptions involving sebaceous glands of the eyelids.

**a. telangiecto'des,** an acneform eruption associated with tuberculosis.

**a. urtica'ta,** an eruption of acne-like lesions, beginning as small urticarial wheals and followed by slight scarring.

**a. variolifor'mis,** a. rodens; a. necrotica; a. lupoides; a pyogenic infection involving follicles occurring chiefly on the forehead and temples; involution of the umbilicated and crusting lesions is followed by scar formation.

**a. venena'ta,** a. artificialis.

**a. vulga'ris,** a. simplex; simple uncomplicated a.; an eruption of papules and pustules on an inflammatory base; condition occurs primarily during puberty and adolescence, due to overactive sebaceous apparatus probably affected by hormonal activity.

**ac'neform.** Acneiform; resembling acne.

**acnegenic** (ak'ne-jen'ik). Pertaining to substances thought to be responsible for causing or exacerbating lesions of acne vulgaris.

**acneiform** (ak-ne'ĭ-form). Acneform.

**acne'mia** [ G. a- priv. + knēmē, leg ]. 1. Congenital absence of legs. 2. Atrophy of the calf muscles.

**acni'tis.** Papulonecrotic *tuberculid.*

**acoasm** (ak'ō-azm). Acousma.

**acocan'thera** [ G. akōkē, a point, + anthēros, blooming ]. Juice from the leaves and stems of *Acocanthera ouabaio* (family Apocynaceae), a South African arrow poison containing ouabain.

**acocan'therin.** Ouabain.

**acognosia, acognosy** (ă-kog-no'sĭ-ah, ă-kog'no-sĭ) [ G. akos, remedy, + gnōsis, knowledge ]. A knowledge of remedies.

**acoin** (ak'o-in). A dianisylphentenyl derivative of quanidine; a local anesthetic characterized by an amidine intermediary linkage; now rarely used, it was one of the first local anesthetics synthesized.

**acola'sia** [ G. akolasia, licentiousness ]. Morbid intemperance or lust.

**acol'ogy** [ G. akos, remedy, + logos, theory ]. Therapeutics.

**acolous** (ak'o-lus) [ G. a- priv. + kōlon, limb ]. Without limbs.

**acoma'nia.** Servile submission to those in authority while being overdomineering at home.

**aco'mia** [ G. a- priv. + komē, hair of head ]. Alopecia.

**acomplemente'mia.** Hypocomplementemia.

**acon'ative** [ G. a- priv. + L. conari, to try ]. Without the desire or wish to act.

**ac'onine.** Hydrolysis product of aconitine; $C_{25}H_{41}NO_9$, in a multicyclic structure.

**acon'itase.** Aconitate hydratase.

**acon'itate hydratase.** Aconitase; an enzyme (EC 4.2.1.3) catalyzing the dehydration of citric acid to cis-aconitic acid, a reaction of significance in the tricarboxylic acid cycle.

**ac'onite.** The dried root of *Aconitum napellus* (family Ranunculaceae), monkshood or wolfsbane. Antipyretic, diuretic, diaphoretic, anodyne, cardiac and respiratory depressant, externally analgesic.

*cis-***aconitic acid.** Dehydration product of citric acid; intermediate in the tricarboxylic acid cycle.

$$HOOCCH_2CCOOH$$
$$\|$$
$$HCCOOH$$

*cis*-Aconitic acid

**acon'itine.** Acetylbenzoylaconine; the active principle (alkaloid) of *Aconitum.* Used as a cardiac sedative. Exceedingly poisonous.

**aconuresis** (ak-on-u-re'sis) [ G. akōn, involuntary, + ourēsis, micturition ]. Enuresis; involuntary urination.

**acopro'sis** [ G. a- priv. + kopros, feces ]. Absence or great scantiness of fecal matter in the intestines.

**aco'prous.** Characterized by the absence of fecal material.

**acorea** (ă-ko-re'ah) [ G. a- priv. + korē, pupil ]. Congenital absence of the ocular pupil.

**aco'ria** [ G. excessive appetite, from a- priv. + koros, satiety ]. 1. Aplesia; absence of the feeling of satiety after eating, from which may arise: 2. Gluttony; to be distinguished from bulimia, in which actual hunger persists.

**acor'mus** [ a- priv. + kormos, trunk of a tree ]. A malformed fetus in which most of the trunk is absent.

**Acosta,** José. See d'Acosta.

**acouasm** (ah-koo'azm). Acousma.

**acousma** (ă-kooz'mah) [ G. akouein, to hear ]. Acouasm; an auditory hallucination in which indefinite sounds, such as ringing or hissing, are heard. See also phoneme.

**acousmatamnesia** (ă-kooz-mă-tam-ne'sĭ-ah) [ G. akousma, something heard, + amnēsia, forgetfulness ]. A loss of memory for sounds.

**acoustic** (ă-koos'tik). Relating to hearing or the perception of sound.

**a. reference level,** the biological reference level for sound measurements. When the term, decibel, is used to indicate the noise level, a reference quantity is implied. This reference value is usually expressed as a sound pressure of 20 micronewtons per square meter. The reference level is referred to as "O decibels," the baseline of the scale of noise levels. This baseline is considered the weakest sound that can be heard by a person with very good hearing in an extremely quiet location. Other equivalent reference levels still being used include 0.0002 microbar and 0.0002 dyne per square centimeter.

**acous'ticopho'bia** [ G. akoustikos, acoustic, + phobos, fear ]. Morbid fear of sounds.

**acoustics** (ă-koos'tiks) [ G. akoustikos, relating to hearing ]. The science that treats of sounds and of their perception.

**ACP.** Abbreviation for acyl carrier protein; see under acyl.

**ACP acetyltransferase.** Acetyl transacylase; enzyme (EC 2.3.1.38) transferring acetyl from acetyl-CoA to ACP to begin fatty acid snythesis.

**acquired** (ă-kwīrd') [ L. ac-quiro (adq-), to obtain, fr. quaero, to seek ]. Denoting a disease, predisposition, habit, etc., that is not congenital but has developed after birth.

**acquisition** (ak'wĭ-zish'un). In psychology, the empirical demonstration of an increase in the strength of the conditioned response in successive trials of pairing the conditioned and unconditioned stimulus.

**acquisitus** (ă-kwiz'ĭ-tus). Acquired.

**acracon'itine.** Pseudoaconitine.

**acral** (ak'ral) [ G. akron, extremity. AC- ]. Relating to or affecting the peripheral parts, e.g., limbs, fingers, ears, etc.

**acramine yellow.** 9- or 5-Aminoacridine hydrochloride; gives a faintly yellow solution with strong bluish violet fluorescence; has been used as a topical antiseptic.

**Acra'nia** [ G. a- priv. + kranion, skull ]. A group of the phylum Chordata whose members possess a notochord, gill slits, and nerve cord but no vertebrae, ribs, or skull; e.g., Amphioxus, tunicates, and acorn worms.

**acra'nia** [ G. a- priv. + kranion, skull ]. Complete or partial absence of a skull; associated with anencephaly.

**acra'nial.** Having no cranium; relating to acrania or an acranius.

**ac'ranil.** 1-(6-Chloro-2-methoxy-9-acridylamino)-3-diethylamino-2-propanol; used for treatment of infections with *Giardia lamblia.*

**acra'nius.** A malformed fetus with acrania. Usually accompanied by markedly defective development of the brain.

**acrasia** (ă-kra'zĭ-ah) [ G. a later form of akrateia. See acratia ]. Incontinence; intemperance.

**Acra'sis.** A species formerly included in the group *Mycetozoa,* but now in the order Acrasiales, consisting of cellular slime molds.

**acratia** (ă-kra'shĭ-ah) [ G. akrateia, incontinence, fr. a- priv. + kratos, strength ]. 1. Incontinence. 2. Loss of strength; weakness. 3. Lack of control.

**acraturesis** (ak-ră-tu-re'sis) [ G. akratēs, powerless, incontinent, + ourēsis, urination ]. 1. Incontinence of urine. 2. Feeble urination due to vesical atony.

**Acree,** Solomon F., American physician, 1875–1957. See A.-Rosenheim test.

**Acrel,** Olof, Swedish surgeon, 1717–1806. See A.'s ganglion.

**acremoniosis** (ak-rĕ-mo-nĭ-o'sis). A condition marked by fever and the occurrence of gumma-like swellings, caused by a fungus *Acremonium potronii*.

**Ac′remo′nium.** A genus of fungi, some members of which are pathogenic for man.

**acribom′eter** [ G. *akribēs*, exact, + *metron*, measure ]. An instrument for measuring very minute objects.

**acrid** (ak′rid) [ L. *acer* (*acr*-), pungent ]. Sharp; pungent; biting; irritating.

**ac′ridine.** Dibenzol[ *b,e* ]pyridine; 10-azaanthracene; derived from coal tar; a dye, dye intermediate, and antiseptic precursor (9-aminoacridine, acriflavine, proflavine). Irritating to skin and mucous membranes.

Acridine

(The inner numbering is that used by *Chemical Abstracts*)

**a. derivatives,** dyes, usually yellow or brown, derived from a. and used in solutions or ointments for their antiseptic properties; *e.g.*, acriflavine, proflavine.

**a. orange,** tetramethyl a.; 3,6-bis(dimethylamino)acridine hydrochloride; a basic fluorescent dye useful as a stain for nucleic acids.

**acrifla′vine.** TRYPAFLAVINE; an acridine dye; a mixture of 2,8-diamino-10-methylacridinium chloride and 2,8-diaminoacridine; a powerful antiseptic used as a local bacteriostatic, especially in gonococcal infections. Also available as a. hydrochloride.

**ac′rimine yellow.** 9-Aminoacridine.

**acrimo′nia** [ L. pungency ]. In ancient humoral pathology, a sharp, pungent, disease-provoking humor.

**acrimony** (ak′rĭ-mo-nĭ) [ L. *acrimonia*, pungency. AC- ]. The quality of being intensely irritant, biting, or pungent.

**ac′rinol.** Ethacridine lactate.

**acrisia** (ă-kris′ĭ-ah) [ G. *a-* priv. + *krisis*, judgment ]. A condition in which diagnosis and especially prognosis are uncertain.

**acrisor′cin** (NF). ARRINOL; 9-aminoacridinium 4-hexylresorcinolate; synthetic antifungal agent.

**acrit′ical** [ G. *a-* priv. + *kritikos*, critical ]. 1. Not critical; marked by no crisis; denoting the diseases terminating by lysis. 2. Indeterminate, especially as regards prognosis.

**acro-** (ak′ro-) [ G. *akron*, extremity, *akros*, extreme ]. A combining form meaning (1) extremity, tip, end, peak, topmost; (2) extreme.

**acroagnosis** (ak′ro-ag-no′sis). [ acro- + G. *agnōsia*, a not knowing ]. Absence of acrognosis or of limb sensibility.

**acroanesthesia** (ak′ro-an-es-the′zĭ-ah) [ acro- + G. *an-* priv. + *aisthēsis* sensation ]. Anesthesia of one or more of the extremities.

**ac′roarthri′tis** [ acro- + G. *arthron*, joint, + *-itis* ]. Inflammation of the joints of the hands or feet.

**acroasphyxia** (ak′ro-as-fik′sĭ-ah) [ acro- + G. *asphyxia*, stoppage of the pulse ]. Dead *fingers.*

**acroataxia** (ak′ro-ah-tak′sĭ-ah) [ acro- + ataxia, *q.v.* ]. Ataxia affecting the distal portion of the extremities: hands and fingers, feet and toes. Opposed to proximoataxia.

**acroblast** (ak′ro-blast) [ acro- + G. *blastos*, germ ]. A component of the developing spermatid. Composed of numerous Golgi elements, it contains the proacrosomal granules.

**acrobrachycephaly** (ak-ro-brak-ĭ-sef′al-e) [ acro- + G. *brachys*, short, + *kephale*, head ]. A type of craniosynostosis in which there is premature closure of the coronal suture, resulting in abnormally short anteroposterior diameter of the skull.

**acrobystiolith** (ak-ro-bis′tĭ-o-lith) [ G. *akrobystia*, prepuce, + *lithos*, stone ]. Obsolete term for preputial calculus.

**acrobysti′tis.** Posthitis.

**ac′rocen′tric.** See acrocentric *chromosome.*

**acrocepha′lia.** Oxycephaly.

**acrocephal′ic.** Oxycephalic.

**acrocephalopolysyndactyly** (ak′ro-sef′al-o-pol′ĭ-sin-dak′tĭ-lĭ). Carpenter's syndrome; congenital malformation in which oxycephaly, brachysyndactyly of hand, and preaxial polydactyly of feet are associated with mental retardation.

**acroceph′alosyndactyl′ia.** Acrocephalosyndactyly.

**acroceph′alosyndac′tylism.** Acrocephalosyndactyly.

**acrocephalosyndactyly** (ak′ro-sef′al-o-sin-dak′tĭ-lĭ) [ acrocephaly + G. *syn,* together, + *daktylos,* finger ]. Acrocephalosyndactylia; acrocephalosyndactylism; acrosphenosyndactyly; acrodysplasia; a congenital syndrome characterized by peaked head, due to premature closure of skull sutures, associated with fusion or webbing of digits. In typical a. (Apert's syndrome), the second, third, and fourth fingers are fused into a mass with a common nail; in atypical a., bony fusion is less and soft tissue webbing of digits predominates.

**acroceph′alous.** Oxycephalic.

**acrocephaly** (ak′ro-sef′ă-lĭ) [ acro- + G. *kephalē,* head ]. Oxycephaly.

**acrochordon** (ak-ro-kor′don) [ acro- + G. *chordē,* cord ]. Skin *tag.*

**acrocinesia** (ak-ro-sin-e′zĭ-ah) [ acro- + G. *kinēsis,* movement ]. Akronkinesia; acrocinesis; excessive movement.

**acrocine′sis.** Acrocinesia.

**ac′rocontrac′ture.** Contracture of the joints of the hands or feet.

**acrocyanosis** (ak′ro-si-an-o′sis) [ acro- + G. *kyanos,* blue, + suffix *-osis,* condition ]. Crocq's disease; a circulatory disorder in which the hands, and less commonly the feet, are persistently cold, blue, and sweaty. Milder forms are closely allied to chilblains.

**ac′rocyanot′ic.** Characterized by acrocyanosis.

**ac′rodermati′tis** [ acro- + G. *derma,* skin, + suffix *-itis,* inflammation ]. Inflammation of the skin of the extremities.

**a. chron′ica atroph′icans,** a gradually progressive dermatitis appearing first on the feet, hands, or elbows and comprised of indurated, erythematous plaques that become atrophic, giving a tissue-paper appearance of the involved sites.

**a. contin′ua,** acrodermatitis perstans; dermatitis repens; Hallopeau's disease (1); a sterile pustular eruption of the fingers and toes, variously attributed to dyshidrosis, pustular psoriasis, and unidentified bacterial infection.

**a. en′teropath′ica,** a disease of young children (3 weeks to 18 months), commencing as a skin eruption on an extremity or around one of the orifices of the body, followed by loss of hair, diarrhea, and other gastrointestinal disturbances; it is intermittently progressive and frequently ends fatally.

**a. hiema′lis,** a. occurring chiefly in winter.

**a. per′stans,** a. continua.

**a. vesiculos′a tropica,** a form occurring in hot climates in which the skin of the extremities is glossy and shows numerous small vesicles.

**ac′rodermato′sis** [ acro- + G. *derma,* skin, + suffix *-osis,* condition ]. Any cutaneous affection involving the more distal portions of the extremities.

**acrodolichomelia** (ak′ro-dol′ĭ-ko-me′lĭ-ă) [ acro- + G. *dolichos,* long, + *melos,* limb ]. Large size and disproportionate growth of the hands and feet.

**ac′rodont** [ acro- + G. *odous,* tooth ]. Applies to tooth attachment in some lower vertebrates (mainly fish) in which the teeth rest on the edge of the jaw bone rather than in sockets or alveoli.

**acrodynia** (ak-ro-din′ĭ-ah) [ acro- + G. *odynē,* pain ]. 1. A disease of infants caused almost exclusively by mercury poisoning and manifested by erythema of the extremities, chest, and nose, polyneuritis, and gastrointestinal symptoms; also known as erythredema; acrodynic erythema; pink disease, Swift's disease; dermatopolyneuritis. 2. A condition caused in rats by a deficiency of pyridoxine (Vitamin B₆), characterized by redness and swelling of the tips of the ears, nose, and paws, leading to necrosis of these parts.

**acrodysesthesia.** (ak'ro-dis-es-the'zĭ-ah) [ acro- + dysesthesia, *q.v.* ]. Abnormal and unpleasant sensation in the peripheral portions of the extremities.

**acrodysplasia** (ak'ro-dis-pla'zĭ-ah) [ acro- + dysplasia, *q.v.* ]. Acrocephalosyndactyly.

**acroedema** (ak'ro-e-de'mah). Edema of hand or foot, often permanent; occurs sometimes after an injury, and in certain nervous diseases.

**acroesthesia** (ak-ro-es-the'zĭ-ah) [ acro- + G. *aisthēsis,* sensation ]. 1. Extreme degree of hyperesthesia. 2 [ G. *akron,* extremity ]. Hyperesthesia of one or more of the extremities.

**acrogeria** (ak'ro-je'rĭ-ah) [ acro- + G. *gerōn,* old ]. A congenital reduction or loss of subcutaneous fat and collagen of the hands and feet, giving the appearance of premature senility.

**acrognosis** (ak-rog-no'sis) [ acro- + G. *gnōsis,* knowledge. GNO- ]. Cenesthesia in relation to the extremities; sensory perception of the limbs and their several parts.

**ac'rohyperhidro'sis.** Hyperhidrosis of the hands and feet.

**acrokerato'sis verruciform'is** [ acro- + keratosis, *q.v.;* L. *verruca,* a wart, + *forma,* form ]. A genodermatosis probably related to Darier's disease and characterized by warty excrescences of the hands and feet.

**acrokinesia** (ak'ro-ki'ne-zĭ-ah). Acrocinesia.

**acroleic acids.** *Acrylic* acids.

**acrolein** (ă-kro'le-in). Acrylic aldehyde; 2-propenal; $CH_2=CHCHO$; a volatile, flammable, oily liquid, giving off irritant vapor, derived from glycerin. Strong irritant of skin and mucous membranes.

**acromega'lia.** Acromegaly.

**ac'romegal'ic.** 1. Pertaining to acromegaly. 2. An individual with acromegaly.

**acromegalogigantism** (ak'ro-meg'al-o-ji'gan-tizm) [ acro- + G. *megas,* great, + *gigas,* giant ]. Gigantism in which the facial features, disproportionate enlargement of the extremities, and other signs of acromegaly are prominent.

**ac'romeg'aloidism.** A condition in which body proportions resemble those of an acromegalic.

**acromegaly** (ak'ro-meg'al-ĭ) [ acro- + G. *megas,* large ]. Acromegalia; Marie's disease (1); a disorder marked by progressive enlargement of the head and face, hands and feet, and thorax, due to excessive secretion of growth hormone by the anterior lobe of the pituitary gland. Diabetes mellitus may eventually develop.

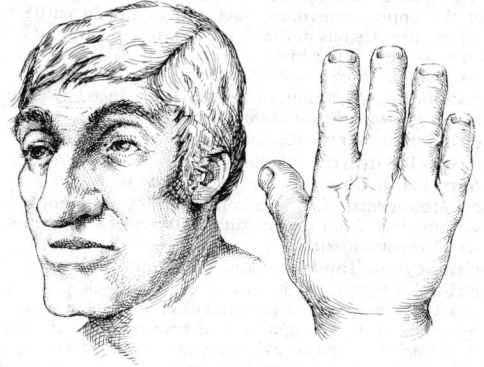

**Acromegaly**
Showing facial features and large, spadelike hand

**acromelalgia** (ak-ro-mel-al'jĭ-ah) [ acro- + G. *melos,* limb, + *algos,* pain ]. A vasomotor neurosis marked by redness, pain, and swelling of the fingers and toes, headache, and vomiting; probably the same as erythromelalgia.

**acromel'ic** [ acro- + G. *melos,* limb ]. Affecting the terminal part of a limb.

**acrometagenesis** (ak'ro-met-ah-jen'e-sis) [ acro- + G. *meta,* beyond, + *genesis,* origin ]. Abnormal development of the extremities resulting in deformity.

**acro'mial.** Relating to the acromion.

**acromic'ria** [ acro- + G. *mikros,* small ]. The antithesis of acromegaly. A condition in which the bones of the face and extremities are small and delicate. Thought by some to be due to a deficiency in the growth hormone of the pituitary gland.

**acro'mioclavic'ular.** Scapuloclavicular; relating to the acromion and the clavicle; denoting the articulation between the clavicle and the scapula and its ligaments.

**acro'miocor'acoid.** Relating to the acromion and the coracoid process; coracoacromial.

**acro'miohu'meral.** Relating to the acromion and the humerus.

**acro'mion** [ G. *akrōmion,* fr. *akron,* tip, + *ōmos,* shoulder ] [ NA ]. Acromial process; the lateral end of the spine of the scapula which projects as a broad flattened process overhanging the glenoid fossa; it articulates with the clavicle and gives attachment to part of the deltoid and of the trapezius muscles.

**acro'mioscap'ular.** Relating to both the acromion and body of the scapula.

**acro'miothora'cic.** Relating to the acromion and the thorax; denoting a branch of the axillary artery, the arteria thoracoacromialis.

**acrom'phalus** [ acro- + G. *omphalos,* umbilicus ]. Abnormal projection of the umbilicus.

**ac'romyco'sis.** Mycosis of a distal part.

**acromyotonia** (ak'ro-mi-o-to'nĭ-ah) [ acro- + G. *mys,* muscle, + *tonos,* tension ]. Acromyotonus; myotonia affecting the extremities only, resulting in spasmodic deformity of the hand or foot.

**acromyot'onus.** Acromyotonia.

**acroneurosis** (ak'ro-nu-ro'sis). Any neurosis, usually vasomotor in nature, manifesting itself in the extremities.

**ac'ronine** (USAN). 3,12-Dihydro-6-methoxy-3,3,12-trimethyl-7$H$-pyrano[ 2,3-$c$ ]acridin-7-one; antineoplastic agent.

**ac'ronyx** [ acro- + G. *onyx,* nail ]. An ingrowing nail.

**acro-osteolysis** (ak'ro-os-te-ol'ĭ-sis). A congenital condition attributed to consanguinity and manifested by palmar and plantar ulcerating lesions with osteolysis.

**acropachy** (ak'ro-pakĭ) [ acro- + G. *pachys,* thick ]. Obsolete term for hypertrophic pulmonary *osteoarthropathy.*

**ac'ropachyder'ma** [ acro- + G. *pachys,* thick, + *derma,* skin ]. Uehlinger's syndrome; idiopathic Bamberger-Marie disease; Brugsch's syndrome; a disorder characterized by thickening of the skin of the face, scalp and extremities together with clubbing of the fingers and deformities of the limb bones.

**ac'roparal'ysis.** Paralysis of the muscles of one or more extremities.

**acroparesthesia** (ak'ro-par'es-the'zĭ-ah) [ acro- + paresthesia, *q.v.* ]. 1. Paresthesia (numbness, tingling, and other abnormal sensations) of one or more of the extremities. 2. An extreme degree of paresthesia.

**ac'ropathol'ogy.** Pathology of the extremities; a study of the morbid changes in orthopaedic affections.

**acrop'athy** [ acro- + G. *pathos,* disease ]. Simple hereditary clubbing of the digits without associated pulmonary or other progressive disease, often more severe in males; autosomal dominant inheritance.

**acrop'etal** [ acro- + L. *peto,* to seek ]. In a direction toward the summit.

**acropho'bia** [ acro- + G. *phobos,* fear ]. Hypsophobia; a morbid dread of heights.

**acropigmentation** (ak'ro-pig-men-ta'shun). Hyperpigmentation of the dorsal surfaces of the fingers and toes beginning in early childhood and usually increasing with age.

**acroposthitis** (ak'ro-pos-thi'tis) [ G. *akroposthia,* prepuce, + suffix -*itis,* inflammation ]. Inflammation of the prepuce.

**acropustulosis** (ak'ro-pus-tu-lo'sis) [ acro- + pustulosis ]. Pustulosis (2); relapsing pustular eruptions of the hands and feet.

**ac'roscler'oder'ma** [ acro- + G. *sklēros*, hard, + *derma*, skin ]. Induration of the skin of the fingers or toes; see also sclerodactyly.

**acrosclerosis** (ak'ro-skle-ro'sis). Stiffness and tightness of the skin of the fingers, with atrophy of the soft tissue and osteoporosis of the distal phalanges of the hands and feet; a form of progressive systemic sclerosis occurring with Raynaud's phenomenon.

**acrose** (ak'rōs). A sugar obtained by the action of a weak alkaline solution on formaldehyde.

**acroso'mal.** Pertaining to the acrosome.

**acrosome** (ak'ro-sōm) [ acro- + G. *soma*, body ]. A membranous caplike covering over the front part of the spermatozoon head; derived from Golgi elements of the spermatid. Associated with the a. are hyaluronidase and a trypsin-like enzyme that are believed to be involved in facilitating the penetration of the ovum by the spermatozoon.

**acroso'min.** A lipoglycoprotein complex present in the acrosome.

**acrosphacelus** (ak'ro-sfas'e-lus) [ acro- + G. *sphakelos*, gangrene ]. Rarely used term for gangrene of the extremities.

**ac'rosphe'nosyndac'tyly** [ acro- + sphenoid + syndactyly ]. Acrocephalosyndactyly.

**acrostealgia** (ak-ros-te-al'ji-ah). Painful inflammation of the bones of the hands and feet.

**acroter'ic** [ G. *akrōtērion*, the topmost point ]. Relating to the extreme periphery, such as the tips of fingers and toes, the end of the nose, etc.

**acrot'ic.** 1 [ G. *akrotēs*, extremity ]. Relating to the surface of the body, especially the cutaneous glands. 2 [ G. *a*- priv. + *krotos*, a striking ]. Marked by great weakness or absence of the pulse; pulseless.

**ac'rotism** [ G. *a*- priv. + *krotos*, a striking ]. Absence or imperceptibility of the pulse; pulselessness.

**acrotrophodynia** (ak'ro-trof'o-din'ĭ-ah) [ acro- + G. *trophē*, nourishment, + *odynē*, pain ]. Neuritis of the extremities occurring as a sequel to trench foot.

**acrotrophoneurosis** (ak'ro-trof'o-nu-ro'sis). A trophoneurosis of one or more of the extremities.

**acryl'ate.** A salt or ester of acrylic acid.

**acryl'ic** (ak-ril'ik). 1. Denoting certain synthetic plastic resins derived from a. acid. 2. For uses in dentistry, see a. *resin*.

   **a. acids,** acroleic acids; a series of unsaturated aliphatic acids of the general formula RH = CH—COOH. The prototype, acrylic acid (R = CH₂) or 2-propenoic acid, is derived from propionic acid by reduction or from glycerol by dehydration.

   **a. aldehyde,** acrolein.

   **a. resin,** see under resin.

**ac'ryloni'trile.** CH₂ = CHCN; vinyl cyanide; used in organic syntheses and in the manufacture of plastics and of synthetic rubber.

**act** (akt). The doing of anything; the performance of any function or the bringing about of any effect.

   **compulsive a.,** an a. that the subject believes he is compelled to do and that he claims he cannot resist.

   **impulsive a.,** (1) an a. performed as a result of an intense urge within the subject's own mind; (2) an act performed without careful deliberation.

**Actae'a** [ fr. G. *actaia*, the elder-tree ]. Baneberry; a genus of plants of the family Ranunculaceae. Has spinal cord-depressing properties similar to those of cimicifuga.

**ACTe.** Abbreviation for anodal closure *tetanus.*

**ACTH.** Abbreviation for adrenocorticotropic *hormone.*

   **big ACTH,** a form of ACTH produced by certain tumors; it is a larger and more acidic molecule than little ACTH, but is not immunochemically distinguishable from little ACTH and does not exert any of the biological effects characteristic of little ACTH; tryptic digestion of big ACTH yields little ACTH.

   **little ACTH,** a term coined to denote conventional ACTH when it is being contrasted with big ACTH.

**actin** (ak'tin). One of the protein components into which actomyosin can be split. Can exist in a fibrous form (F-actin) or a globular form (G-actin).

**F-actin,** the association of G-actin subunits into a fibrous protein (F for fibrous) caused by increase in salt concentration. The conversion of G-actin to F-actin is catalyzed by small concentrations of magnesium ion, is reversible, and is accompanied by the conversion of the bound ATP molecule to ADP and the conversion of one reactive —SH group to an unreactive form.

**G-actin,** the globular (G for globular) subunits of the actin molecule; molecular weight 57,000, containing one molecule of ATP. Soluble in dilute salt, polymerizing to F-actin when ionic strength is increased; see also F-actin.

**acting out.** Overt expression of unconscious emotional feelings.

**actin'ic** [ G. *aktis* (*aktin*-), a ray ]. Relating to the chemically active rays of the electromagnetic spectrum.

**ac'tinism.** The chemical action of rays from a luminous source, residing chiefly though not exclusively in and beyond the violet end of the visible spectrum.

**actin'ium** [ G. *aktis*, a ray ]. An element, symbol Ac, atomic no. 89, discovered by Debierne in pitchblende; it possesses no stable isotopes, and exists in nature only as a disintegration product of uranium and thorium.

   **a. emanation,** radon-219.

**actino-** (ak-tĭ-no-) [ G. *aktis* (*aktin*-), a ray, beam ]. A combining form meaning a ray, as of light; applied to any form of radiation, or to any structure, such as ray fungus or *Actinomyces,* with radiating parts. See also *radio-.*

**ac'tinobacillo'sis.** Wooden tongue; a disease of cattle and swine, occasionally reported in man, caused by *Actinobacillus lignieresi.* It affects the soft tissues often the tongue and cervical lymph nodes, where granulomatous swellings are formed that eventually break down to form abscesses.

**Actinobacillus** (ak'tin-o-bă-sil'lus) [ actino- + L. *bacillus,* a little rod ]. A genus of nonmotile, nonsporeforming, aerobic, facultatively anaerobic bacteria (family Brucellaceae) containing Gram-negative rods interspersed with coccal elements. The metabolism of these bacteria is fermentative; they are pathogenic to animals. The type species is *A. lignieresii.*

   **A. actinoi'des,** a bacterial species of doubtful taxonomic position; it is nonpathogenic for laboratory animals but pathogenic for goats via the intratracheal route. It is isolated from calves with chronic pneumonia.

   **A. actinomycetemcomitans,** a bacterial species of doubtful taxonomic position; it is not pathogenic for laboratory animals, and its pathogenicity in man is questionable; it occurs with actinomycetes in actinomycotic lesions.

   **A. equuli,** a species of bacteria causing suppurative lesions, particularly in the kidneys and joints in foals and piglets, and endocarditis in pigs.

   **A. lignieres'ii,** a species of bacteria producing infections of the upper alimentary tract and mouth in cattle and suppurative lesions in the skin and lungs of sheep; it is the type species of its genus.

   **A. mallei,** *Pseudomonas mallei.*

**actinobolin.** An antibiotic substance produced by *Streptomyces griseoviridis* var. *atrofaciens.*

**ac'tinochem'istry.** Radiochemistry.

**ac'tinoclad'othrix** [ actino- + G. *klados,* branch, + *thrix,* hair ]. Obsolete term for *Actinomyces bovis.*

**actinocongestin** (ak'ti-no-kon-jes'tin). Congestin; a poison obtained from the stinging tentacles of sea anemones; see also actinotoxin.

**ac'tinocymog'raphy.** Actinokymography.

**ac'tinodermati'tis** [ actino- + G. *derma,* skin, + suffix *-itis,* inflammation ]. 1. Inflammation of the skin produced by exposure to sunlight. 2. Adverse reaction of skin to radiation therapy (ultraviolet, x-ray, or radium).

**actin'ogen.** Any radioactive element or, more generally, any substance that produces radiation.

**actinogenesis** (ak'tĭ-no-jen'e-sis) [ actino- + G. *genesis,* production ]. Radiogenesis.

**ac'tinogen'ic.** Radiogenic.

**ac'tinogen'ics.** Radiogenics.

**actin'ogram** Radiogram.

**actin'ograph** [ actino- + G. *graphō,* to write ]. 1. Radiograph. 2. An apparatus for determining the proper exposure of a photographic plate according to the degree of light.

**actinog'raphy.** The making of actinograms; skiagraphy; radiography.

**ac'tinohe'matin.** A red respiratory pigment found in certain forms of *Actinia* (sea anemones).

**actinokymography** (ak'tĭ-no-ki-mog'rah-fĭ) [ actino- + G. *kyma*, wave, + *graphō*, to write ]. Actinocymography; actinography or radiography of organs in motion.

**actin'olite.** 1. Any substance which undergoes a change when exposed to light. 2. A greenish mineral, Ca(MgFe)₃.(SiO₄)₃.

**actinol'ogy.** Radiology.

**actin'olyte** [ actino- + G. *lytos*, soluble, fr. *lyō*, to loose ]. An apparatus used in the application of the actinic rays.

**actinom'eter.** An instrument for determining the intensity and penetrating power of roentgen and other rays.

**actinom'etry** [ actino- + G. *metron*, measure ]. The determination of the photochemical action of light rays.

**ac'tinomyce'lial.** Relating to the mycelium-like filaments of the Actinomycetales.

**Actinomyces** (ak'tĭ-no-mi'sēz) [ actino- + G. *mykēs*, fungus ]. A genus of nonmotile, nonsporeforming, anaerobic to facultatively anaerobic bacteria (family Actinomycetaceae) containing Gram-positive, irregularly staining filaments; diptheroid cells are predominant. Most of the species produce a filamentous microcolony. The metabolism of these chemoheterotrophs is fermentative; the products of glucose fermentation include acetic, formic, lactic and succinic acids but not propionic acid. These organisms are pathogenic for man and/or other animals. The type species is *A. bovis.*

**A. bo'vis,** a species of bacteria causing actinomycosis in cattle; infection in man is not established; it is the type species of its genus.

**A. israe'lii,** a species of bacteria causing human actinomycosis and, occasionally, infections in cattle.

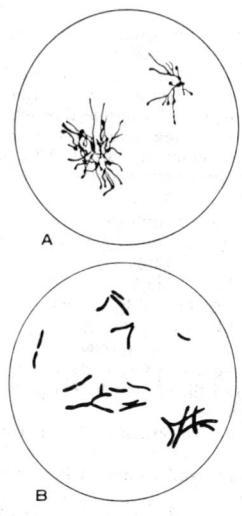

A Microcolony of *Actinomyces israelii*

(Original magnification, *A,* ×400; *B,* ×900)

**Actinomycetaceae** (ak'tĭ-no-mi'se-ta'se-e). A family of nonsporeforming, nonmotile, ordinarily facultatively anaerobic (some species are aerobic and other are anaerobic) bacteria (order Actinomycetales) containing Gram-positive, nonacidfast, predominantly diptheroid cells which tend to form branched filaments in tissue or in some stages of cultural development; the filaments readily fragment, producing diphtheroid or coccoid forms. The metabolism of these chemoheterotrophic bacteria is fermentative. This family contains the genera *Actinomyces* (type genus), *Arachnia, Bacterionema, Bifidobacterium,* and *Rothia.*

**Actinomycetales** (ak'tĭ-no-mi'se-ta'lēz). An order of bacteria consisting of moldlike, rod-shaped, clubbed or filamentous forms with decided tendency to true branching, without endospores, but sometimes developing conidia; it contains four families—Mycobacteriaceae, Actinomycetaceae, Streptomycetaceae and Actinoplanaceae.

**actinomycetes** (ak'tĭ-no-mi-se'tēz). A term used to refer to members of the genus *Actinomyces;* sometimes improperly used to refer to any member of the family Actinomycetaceae or order Actinomycetales.

**ac'tinomyce'tin.** Lytic substance produced by the actinomycete *Streptomyces albus.* Dissolves dead Gram-negative, and, with more difficulty, dead Gram-positive, organisms; also dissolves living organisms in aqueous suspensions.

**actinomy'cins.** Antibiotic agents isolated from a species of *Streptomyces* (*Actinomyces antibioticus*). The a.'s are chromopeptides; most of them contain the chromophore, actinocin. They are derivatives of phenoxazone that differ in the amino acids and their sequence in the peptide chains. They form complexes with DNA and therefore inhibit RNA synthesis, primarily the ribosomal type. A.'s are active against Gram-positive bacteria, fungi, and neoplasms.

**a. A.,** the first of the a.'s isolated in crystalline form.

**a. C,** cactinomycin.

**a. D,** dactinomycin.

**a. F₁,** actinomycin KS4; Ks4; produced by actinomycin C-elaborating strains of *Streptomyces chrysomallus;* used as an antineoplastic agent.

**actinomycoma** (ak'tĭ-no-mi-ko'mah) [ actino- + G. *mykēs*, fungus, + suffix -*oma*, tumor ]. A swelling caused by *Actinomyces.*

**ac'tinomyco'sis** [ actino- + G. *mykēs*, fungus, + suffix -*osis*, condition ]. Actinophytosis; lumpy jaw; a disease primarily of cattle and man caused by *Actinomyces bovis* in cattle and *A. israelii* in man. These actinomycetes are part of the normal bacterial flora of the mouth and pharynx, but when introduced into tissue may produce chronic destructive abscesses or granulomas which eventually discharge a viscid pus containing minute yellowish granules (sulfur granules). In man, the disease commonly affects the cervicofacial area, abdomen, or thorax; in cattle, the lesion is commonly found in the mandible.

**ac'tinomycot'ic.** Relating to actinomycosis.

**Ac'tinomyxid'ia** [ actino- + G. *myxa*, mucus ]. An order of Neosporidia, having a double cellular envelope, three polar capsules, and eight spores.

**ac'tinon.** Radon-219.

**ac'tinoneuri'tis.** Radioneuritis; neuritis caused by prolonged and repeated exposure to x-rays or radium.

**actinophage** (ak-tin'o-fāj) [ actino(myces) + G. *phagein*, to eat ]. A virus specific for actinomycetes.

**actin'ophore** [ actino- + G. *phoros*, bearing ]. A mixture of three parts cerium dioxide and one part thorium dioxide, used in roentgen ray diagnosis.

**ac'tinophyto'sis.** 1. Actinomycosis. 2. Botryomycosis.

**Actinop'oda** [ actino- + G. *pous*, foot ]. A class of Sarcodina having slender pseudopodia with a central axial filament.

**ac'tinoprax'is.** Radiopraxis.

**actin'oqui'nol sodium** (USAN). Sodium tequinol; sodium etoquinol; 8-ethoxy-5-quinolinesulfonic acid sodium salt; ultraviolet screen for topical application to the skin.

**actinorhodine** (ak'tĭ-no-ro'dēn). C₃₂H₂₆O₁₄; an antibiotic pigment produced by *Streptomyces coelicolor.*

**ac'tinos'copy** [ actino- + G. *skopeō*, to view ].    Radioscopy.

**ac'tinostereos'copy.** Radiostereoscopy.

**ac'tinotherapeu'tics.** Radiotherapeutics.

**ac'tinother'apy.** Radiotherapy.

**ac'tinotoxe'mia.** Radiotoxemia.

**actinotoxin** (ak'ti-no-tok'sin) [ fr. Actinozoa, old name for a class of coelenterates that includes the anemones ]. The toxic alcoholic extract from the tentacles of sea anemones.

**action** (ak'shun) [ L. *actio*, from *ago*, pp. *actus*, to do ]. 1. The performance of any of the vital functions, the manner of such performance, or the result of the same. 2. The exertion of any force or power, physical, chemical, or mental. For the actions of some chemical substances (*e.g.,* salt a., nicotinic a., muscarinic a.) see under the name of the substance.

**ball valve a.,** intermittent blockage of a tube or outlet of a cavity by some object or material that permits passage in one direction but not in the other.

**calorigen'ic a.,** thermogenic a.; increasing heat production of the body, as by the thyroid hormone.

**cumulative a.,** cumulative *effect.*

**reflex a.,** see under reflex.

**salt a.,** any physicochemical effect produced by hypertonic concentrations of osmotically active electrolytes.

**sparing a.,** the manner in which a nonessential nutritive component, by its presence in the diet, lowers the requirement for an essential component; thus nonessential cysteine spares essential methionine and nonessential tyrosine spares essential phenylalanine.

**specific a.,** the a. of a drug or a method of treatment which has a direct and especially curative effect upon a disease, *e.g.,* the a. of vitamin $B_{12}$ in pernicious anemia.

**specific dynamic a.,** increase of heat production caused by the ingestion of food, especially of protein.

**thermogen'ic a.,** calorigenic a.

**trigger a.,** the a. of some force, usually slight, that releases a much greater force, bringing about a response that bears little or no relationship to the initiating a., and that otherwise would not occur.

**ac'tithiaz'ic acid.** Mycobacidin.

**ac'tivate.** 1. To render active. 2. To make radioactive.

**activa'tion.** 1. The act of rendering active. 2. An increase in the energy content of an atom or molecule, through the raising of temperature, absorption of light photons, etc., which renders that atom or molecule more reactive. 3. Techniques of altering the physiologic environment of the brain by stimulating it by light, sound, or electricity, in order to produce hidden or latent abnormal activity in the electroencephalogram. 4. Stimulation of cell division in an ovum by fertilization or by artificial means.

**EEG a.,** the low voltage, fast pattern of attentive wakefulness.

**energy of a.,** see under energy.

**ac'tivator.** 1. A substance that renders another substance, or catalyst, active; or that accelerates a process or reaction. 2. The fragment, produced by chemical cleavage of a proactivator (*q.v.*), that induces the enzymic activity of another substance. 3. Cohnheim's term for the internal secretion of the pancreas. 4. An apparatus for making substances radioactive, such as a neutron generator or cyclotron.

**activ'ity.** Quality of being active. 1. In electroencephalography, the presence of neurogenic electrical energy. 2. In physical chemistry, an ideal concentration for which the law of mass action will apply perfectly. The ratio of the a. to the true concentration is the a. coefficient, which becomes 1.00 · · · at infinite dilution.

**blocking a.,** the phenomenon of repression or elimination of electrical activity in the brain because of the arrival of a sensory stimulus.

**insulin-like a.,** see under insulin.

**optical a.,** the ability of a compound in solution (one possessing no plane of symmetry, usually because of the presence of one or more asymmetric carbon atoms) to rotate the plane of polarized light either clockwise or counterclockwise.

**specific a.,** radioactivity per unit mass of the stated element or compound.

**ac'tomy'osin.** A protein complex composed of the globulin myosin and actin in the micellae of the muscle fiber. It is the essential contractile substance of muscle.

**Acto'nia.** A fungus that causes yellowish patches on the pharyngeal mucous membrane which may be mistaken for diphtheria; belongs to order Endomycetales.

**Acuaria spiralis** (ak-u-a'ri-ah spi-ra'lis). A nematode parasite in the proventriculus and esophagus, and sometimes the intestine, of chickens, turkeys, pheasants and other birds.

**acuclosure** (ak'u-klo'zhur) [ L. *acus,* a needle, + *closure* ]. Hemostasis by means of pressure with a needle; similar to acupressure.

**acufilopressure** (ak'u-fi'lo-presh-er) [ L. *acus,* needle, + *filum,* thread, + *pressure* ]. Acupressure fortified by a ligature passed under the needle, increasing the compression of the artery.

**acuity** (ă-ku'ĭ-tĭ) [ thr. Fr. fr. L. *acuo,* pp. *acutus,* sharpen. AC- ]. Sharpness, clearness, distinctness.

**visual a.,** acuteness of vision; it is indicated by a fraction in which the numerator is a number expressing the distance in feet at which the patient sees a line of type on the chart (usually 20 feet), and the denominator a number expressing the distance in feet at which the normal eye would see the smallest letters which the patient sees at the distance at which he is; thus, if at 20 feet he sees only the letters which the normal eye would see at 50 feet, the formula of his vision will be $V = 20/50$.

**acu'leate** [ L. *aculeātus,* pointed, fr. *acus,* needle ]. Pointed; covered with sharp spines.

**acu'minate** [ L. *acumino,* pp. *-atus,* to sharpen ]. Pointed; conical; tapering to a point.

**acuology** (ak'u-ol'o-jĭ) [ L. *acus,* needle, + G. *logos,* study ]. The study of the use of therapeutic needles for injections.

**spinal a.,** a. related to the spine.

**ac'upressure** [ L. *acus,* needle, + pressure ]. A procedure for occluding a wounded artery. A needle is passed in and out of the tissues on either side of the artery, so that its free central portion presses the vessel against the underlying tissues, thereby occluding it.

**ac'upuncture** [ L. *acus,* needle, + *puncture* ]. Puncture with long, fine needles. 1. An ancient Oriental system of therapy. 2. More recently, acupuncture *anesthesia, q.v.*

**acus** (a'kus) [ L. ]. A needle.

**acusection** (ak'u-sek-shun). Section with the electrosurgical needle.

**ac'usector** [ L. *acus,* needle, + *secare,* to cut ]. An electric needle used to cut tissue.

**acu'sis** [ G. *akousis,* hearing ]. Normal hearing; the ability to perceive sound normally.

**acute** (ă-kūt') [ L. *acutus,* sharp ]. 1. Of short and sharp course, not chronic; said of a disease. 2. Sharp; pointed at the end.

**ac'utenac'ulum** [ L. *acus,* needle, + *tenaculum,* holder, fr. *teneo,* to hold ]. Needle-holder.

**acutorsion** (ak'u-tor'shun) [ L. *acus,* needle, + *torsio,* a twisting. TORS- ]. Arrest of hemorrhage from a wounded artery by the passage of a needle through the vessel near the open end, including some of the tissues, and then making a half or a complete turn with the needle, twisting the tissues and the artery, occluding the latter.

**acu'tus** [ L. ] [ NA ]. Acute.

**acyanoblepsia, acyanoblepsy** (ă-si'an-o-blep'sĭ-ah, ă-si'-an-o-blep'sĭ) [ G. *a-* priv. + *kyanos,* a blue substance, + *blepsis,* sight ]. Tritanopia.

**acy'anop'sia.** Tritanopia.

**acyanot'ic.** Characterized by absence of cyanosis.

**acyclic** (ă-si'klik). Not cyclic; denoting especially an a. compound (*q.v.,* under compound).

**acyl** (as'il). An organic radical derived from an organic acid by the removal of the carboxylic hydroxyl group. See, for example, acetyl.

**acyl-ACP dehydrogenase.** Enoyl-ACP reductase (NADPH).

**acyl-ACP reductase.** Enoyl-ACP reductase (NADPH).

**ac'yladenylate.** A compound in which an acyl group is combined with adenosine 5'-phosphate (AMP) by elimination of $H_2O$ between the —COOH of a carboxyl group and the phosphate residue of the AMP, usually initially in the form of ATP and eliminating inorganic pyrophosphate in the condensation.

**acylamidase.** Amidase.

**N-acylamino acid.** RCO—NH—CHR—COOH; an amino acid to the N of which an acyl group is attached, as in hippuric acid (*N*-benzoylglycine) or phenaceturic acid.

**ac'ylase.** Amidase.

**acyla'tion.** The introduction of an acyl radical into an organic compound or the formation of such a radical within an organic compound.

**acyl carrier protein.** ACP; one of the proteins of the complex in cytoplasm that contains all the enzymes required to convert acetyl-CoA and malonyl-CoA to palmitic acid. This complex is tightly bound together in mammalian tissues and in yeast, but that from *Escherichia* *coli* is readily dissociated. The ACP thus isolated is a heat-stable protein with a molecular weight of about 10,000. It contains a free —SH that binds the acyl intermediates in the synthesis of fatty acids as thioesters. This —SH group is part of a 4′-phosphopantetheine, added to the apoprotein by ACP phosphodiesterase (EC 3.1.4.14), which thus plays the same role that it does in coenzyme A. ACP is involved in every step of the fatty acid synthetic process. Some of the individual enzymes involved are acyl-ACP desaturase (EC 1.14.99.6), ACP acetyltransferase (EC 2.3.1.38), ACP malonyltransferase (EC 2.3.1.39), 3-oxoacyl-ACP reductase (EC 1.1.1.100), enoyl-ACP reductase (EC 1.3.19 and .10), and 3-oxoacyl-ACP synthase (EC 2.3.1.41).

**acyl-CoA.** Acylcoenzyme A; $RCH_2CO\sim SCoA$; condensation product of a carboxylic acid and coenzyme A; metabolic intermediates of importance, notably in the oxidation of fat.

**acyl-CoA dehydrogenase (NADP+).** Enoyl-CoA reductase; enzyme (EC 1.3.1.8) catalyzing reduction of enoyl-CoA derivatives of chain length 4 to 16, with NADPH as the hydrogen donor.

**acyl-CoA synthetase** (EC 6.2.1.3). Fatty acid thiokinase (long chain); similar to acetyl-CoA synthetase and butyryl-CoA synthetase, but acts on acids, 3-hydroxy acids, and 2,3- or 3,4-unsaturated acids from $C_6$ to $C_{20}$.

**acyl-malonyl-ACP synthase.** 3-Oxoacyl-ACP synthase.

**acylmercaptan bond.** See under bond.

***N*-acylsphingol.** *N*-Acylsphingosine.

***N*-acylsphingosine.** *N*-Acylsphingol; a condensation product of an organic acid with sphingosine at the amino group of the latter compound.

**ac′yltrans′ferase** (EC Class 2.3). Transacylase; enzymes catalyzing the transfer of an acyl group from an acyl-CoA to various acceptors. The class includes many acetyltransferases.

**acys′tia** [ G. *a-* priv. + *kystis*, bladder ]. Congenital absence of the urinary bladder.

**ad.** A Latin preposition denoting to; it is used in prescription writing to indicate that enough of the ingredient is to be taken to make the entire mixture equal the amount stated.

**ad-** [ L. *ad*, to ]. Prefix denoting increase, adherence, or motion toward, and sometimes with an intensive meaning.

**-ad** [ L. *ad*, to ]. A suffix in anatomical nomenclature having the significance of the English -ward; denoting toward or in the direction of the part indicated by the main portion of the word.

**adactyl′ia, adac′tylism.** Adactyly.

**adac′tylous.** Without fingers or toes.

**adac′tylus.** A congenitally malformed individual with adactyly.

**adactyly** (a-dak′tĭ-lī) [ G. *a-* priv. + *daktylos*, digit ]. A condition characterized by the absence of fingers or toes.

**adaman′tine** [ G. *adamantinos*, very hard, fr. *adamas* (*adamant-*), adamant, a very hard metal, prob. steel, fr. *a-* priv. + *damaō*, to conquer ]. Exceedingly hard; specifically relating to the enamel of the teeth.

**adamantino′ma.** Ameloblastoma.

  **a. of long bones,** a rare tumor of limb bones, usually the tibia, that microscopically resembles an ameloblastoma; the histogenesis is uncertain.

  **pituitary a.,** craniopharyngioma.

**adaman′toblast.** Ameloblast.

**adaman′toblasto′ma.** Ameloblastoma.

**adamanto′ma.** Ameloblastoma.

**Adamkiewicz** (ah-dahm′kya-vits), Albert, Vienna pathologist, 1850–1921. See *arteries* of A., A.'s protein *reaction.*

**Adams,** Robert, Irish physician, 1791–1875. See A.-Stokes or Morgagni-A.-Stokes or Stokes-A. *disease* or *syndrome,* under *syndrome.*

**Adams,** Sir William, English surgeon, 1760–1829. See A.'s *operation* for ectropion.

**Adam's apple.** *Prominentia* laryngea.

**Adanson,** Michel, French naturalist, 1727–1806. Gave his name to *Adansonia.*

**Adanso′nia.** A genus of trees of the family Malvaceae.

  **A. digita′ta,** calabash tree; baobab. The leaves have been used as a febrifuge; the fruit is used as an appetizer.

**adaptation** (ad-ap-ta′shun) [ L. *ad-apto*, pp. *-atus*, to adjust ]. 1. The acquiring of modifications fitting a plant or animal to life in a new environment or under new conditions. 2. An advantageous change in function or constitution of an organ or tissue to meet new conditions. 3. Adjustment of the iris and retina to varying degrees of illumination; see dark a. and light a. 4. A property of certain receptors through which they become less responsive or cease to respond to repeated or continued stimuli the intensity of which is kept constant. 5. The fitting, condensing or contouring of a restorative material, foil, or shell to a tooth or cast so as to be in close contact. 6. Adjustment (2); The dynamic process wherein the thoughts, feelings, behavior, and biophysiologic mechanisms of the individual continually change to adjust to a constantly changing environment.

  **dark a.,** scotopic a.; the adjustment occurring under reduced illumination in which the sensitivity to light is greatly increased; see also dark-adapted *eye.*

  **light a.,** photopic a.; the adjustment occurring under increased illumination in which the sensitivity to light is reduced; see also light-adapted *eye.*

  **photopic a.,** light a.

  **reality a.,** the ability to adjust to the world as it exists.

  **ret′inal a.,** dark or light adjustment to degree of illumination.

  **scotopic a.,** dark a.

  **social a.,** adjustment to living in accordance with interpersonal, social, and cultural restrictions and demands.

**adap′ter.** 1. A connecting part, joining two pieces of apparatus. 2. A converter of electric current to a desired form.

**adaptom′eter.** A device for determining the course of ocular dark adaptation and for measuring the minimum light threshold.

**adaxial** (ad-ak′sī-al). Toward an axis, or on one or other side of an axis.

**adde** (ad′e) [ L. ]. Latin, meaning *add*, used in prescription writing.

**addict.** A person who finds it difficult to stop some habitual practice, especially the taking of drugs or excessive use of alcohol.

**addiction** [ L. *ad-dico*, pp. *-dictus*, consent, fr. *ad-* + *dico*, to say ]. Habituation to some practice considered harmful for the subject.

  **alcohol a.,** alcoholism.

  **drug a.,** pharmacopsychosis; habituation to the use of a drug, the deprivation of which gives rise to symptoms of distress, abstinence or withdrawal symptoms, and an irresistible impulse to take the drug again.

  **opium a.,** o. habit; opiumism; thebaism; opiomania; opiophagism; the habitual use of opium or any of its alkaloids.

**ad′diment** [ L. *additamentum*, an increase, fr. *ad-do*, to add to ]. An obsolete term for complement.

**ad′disin** [ T. *Addison* ]. Factor in gastric tissue and gastric juice that acts upon the extrinsic factor to produce the hematinic principle of liver. Obsolete term now regarded as conceptually inaccurate.

**Addison,** Christopher, English anatomist, 1869–1951. See A.'s clinical *planes.*

**Addison,** Thomas, English physician, 1793–1860. See A.'s *disease, keloid,* Addisonian *anemia, crisis,* A.-Biermer *disease, melasma* addisonii.

**ad′disonism.** A symptom complex resembling in many respects that of Addison's disease, but not due to disease of the suprarenal glands.

**additive** (ad′ĭ-tĭv). A substance not essentially part of a material such as food, fuel, etc., but which is deliberately added to fulfill some specific purpose; for example, solubilizing, flavoring, coloring.

**addu′cens** [ L. pres. p. of *ad-duco*, to bring to. DUC- ]. Adducent.

  **a. oc′uli,** obsolete name for musculus rectus medialis.

**addu′cent** [ L. *adducens, q.v.* ]. Bringing to; adducting; denoting certain adductor muscles, as the adducens oculi.

**adduct** (ă-dukt) [ L. *ad-duco*, pp. -*ductus*, to bring toward ]. 1. To draw toward the median line. 2. An addition product, or complex, or one part of the same.

**adduc'tion.** 1. Movement of a limb toward the central axis of the body, or beyond it. 2. Movement (duction) of the eye toward the nose. 3. A position resulting from such movement.

**adduc'tor.** A muscle drawing a part toward the median line.

**Adelmann** (ah'del-mahn), G. F. B., Russian surgeon, 1811–1888. See A.'s *maneuver*.

**adelomorphous** (ă-del-o-mor'fus) [ G. *adēlos*, uncertain, not clear, + *morphē*, shape ]. Of not clearly defined form. In the past this term was applied to certain cells of the gastric glands.

**adelphotaxis** (ă-del'fo-tak'sis) [ G. *adelphos*, brother; + *taxis*, arrangement ]. A grouping together of cells or organisms in mutual relationship.

**ademo'nia** [ G. *adēmonia*, distress ]. Melancholia.

**aden-.** See adeno-.

**adenal'gia** [ aden- + G. *algos*, pain ]. Adenodynia; pain in a gland.

**ad'enase.** Adenine deaminase; see deaminases.

**ad'enasthe'nia** [ aden- + G. *astheneia*, weakness ]. Abnormally diminished functional activity of a gland.

**aden'dric.** Adendritic.

**adendrit'ic** [ G. *a*- priv. + *dendron*, tree ]. Adendric; without dendrites.

**adenec'tomy** [ aden- + G. *ektomē*, excision ]. Excision of a gland.

**ad'enecto'pia** [ aden- + G. *ek*, out of, + *topos*, place ]. Misposition of a gland; the presence of a gland elsewhere than in its normal anatomical position.

**adenemphraxis** (ad'ĕ-nem-frak'sis) [ aden- + G. *emphraxis*, stoppage ]. Obstruction to the discharge of a glandular secretion.

**ade'nia.** Obsolete term for general enlargement of lymph nodes.

**an'gibro'mic a.,** any diseased condition of the digestive glands.

**aden'iform.** Of glandular appearance; adenoid.

**ad'enine.** 6-Aminopurine; one of the two major purines found in both RNA and DNA; found also in various free nucleotides of importance to the body, *e.g.*, adenylic acid, adenosine triphosphate (ATP), NAD and NADP, flavin-adenine dinucleotide (FAD); in all these compounds, a. is condensed with a sugar molecule at the 9-nitrogen, forming adenosine, *q.v.*

$$NH_2$$

Adenine

a. **arabinoside,** misnomer for arabinosyladenine, *q.v.*
a. **deaminase** (EC 3.5.4.2), see deaminases.
a. **deoxyribonucleotide,** deoxyadenylic acid.
a. **nucleotide,** adenylic acid.
a. **sulfate,** a. conjugated with sulfuric acid; used to stimulate leukocyte production in agranulocytosis.

**adeni'tis** [ aden- + suffix, -*itis*, inflammation ]. Inflammation of a lymph node or of a gland.

**adeniza'tion.** Conversion into glandlike structure.

**adeno-, aden-** [ G. *adēn*, gland ]. Combining forms denoting relation to a gland.

**adenoacanthoma** (ad'ĕ-no-ak-an-tho'mah). A malignant neoplasm consisting chiefly of glandular epithelium (adenocarcinoma), usually well differentiated, with foci of metaplasia to squamous (or epidermoid) neoplastic cells.

**adenoameloblastoma** (ad'ĕ-no-am'el-o-blast-o'mah). Ameloblastic adenomatoid tumor; a benign tumor, usually in the maxilla of young people, composed of ducts lined by cuboidal or columnar cells.

**ad'enoblast** [ adeno- + G. *blastos*, germ ]. A proliferating embryonic cell with the potential to form glandular parenchyma.

**adenocarcinoma** (ad'ĕ-no-kar'sĭ-no'mah) A malignant neoplasm of epithelial cells in glandular or glandlike pattern.

**acinic cell a.,** acinar, acinic cell, acinose, or acinous carcinoma; an a. arising from secreting cells of a racemose gland, particularly the salivary glands.

**a. in situ,** a noninvasive abnormal proliferation of glands believed to precede the appearance of invasive adenocarcinoma; a. in situ has been reported in the endometrium and large intestine.

**Lucké's a.,** Lucké's *carcinoma*.

**mucoid a.,** sometimes applied to mucinous carcinoma, or a. containing mucin secreting neoplastic cells.

**papillary a.,** an a. containing finger-like processes of vascular connective tissue covered by neoplastic epithelium, projecting into cysts or the cavity of glands or follicles; occurs most frequently in the ovary and thyroid gland.

**renal a.,** clear cell carcinoma of the kidney; hypernephroma; Grawitz tumor; a. arising in any part of the renal parenchyma, especially in middle-aged or older people of either sex, although more common in males. Renal a. may form glands resembling renal tubules lined by cells with pale staining cytoplasm; in other cases the cytoplasm is more darkly staining; there may be a papillary or solid alveolar structure, or occasionally the tumor cells may be spindle-shaped. Renal a.'s are frequently of large size before the appearance of symptoms of hematuria due to invasion of the renal vein, flank pain, a palpable mass, or distant metastasis following invasion at renal veins. The tumors commonly have a yellow cut surface and appear well circumscribed grossly, although showing microscopic infiltration of adjacent tissue.

**adenocele** (ad'ĕ-no-sēl) [ adeno- + G. *kēlē*, tumor ]. Obsolete term denoting an adenomatous cystic tumor.

**adenocellulitis** (ad'ĕ-no-sel'u-li'tis). Inflammation of a gland and of the adjacent cellular tissue.

**adenochondroma** ad'ĕ-no-kon-dro'mah) [ adeno- + G. *chondros*, cartilage, + suffix -*oma*, tumor ]. A benign neoplasm or hamartoma with the histologic characteristics of adenoma and chondroma.

**ad'enocyst.** Adenocystoma.

**ad'enocysto'ma.** Adenocyst; adenoma in which the neoplastic glandular epithelium forms cysts.

**ad'enocyte** [ adeno- + G. *kytos*, a hollow (cell) ]. A gland cell.

**adenodiastasis** (ad'ĕ-no-di-as'tah-sis) [ adeno- + G. *diastasis*, a separation ]. Separation or displacement of glands or glandular tissue from their usual anatomical sites, *e.g.*, pancreatic glands in the wall of the small intestine, gastric glands in the wall of the esophagus.

**adenodynia** (ad'ĕ-no-din'ĭ-ah) [ adeno- + G. *odynē*, pain ]. Adenalgia.

**adenoepithelioma** (ad'ĕ-no-ep-ĭ-the-lĭ-o'mah) An epithelioma containing glandular elements. See also epithelioma.

**ad'enofibro'ma.** A benign neoplasm composed of glandular and fibrous tissues, with a relatively large proportion of glands.

**ad'enofi'bromyoma.** Adenomatoid *tumor.*

**ad'enofibro'sis.** Sclerosing *adenosis.*

**adenogenesis** (ad'ĕ-no-jen'e-sis) [ adeno- + G. *genesis*, production ]. The development of a gland.

**adenogenous** (ad-en-oj'en-us) Having an origin in glandular tissue.

**adenog'raphy** [ adeno- + G. *graphō*, to write ]. 1. Anatomy in special relation to the glands. 2. A treatise on the glands.

**adenohypersthenia** (ad'ĕ-no-hi'pers-the'nĭ-ah) [ adeno- + G. *hyper*, in excess, + *sthenos*, strength ]. Excessive functional activity of a gland or set of glands.

**adenohypophysial** (ad'ĕ-no-hi-po-fiz'ĭ-al). Relating to the adenohypophysis.

**adenohypophysis** (ad'ĕ-no-hi-pof'ĭ-sis) [ NA ]. Official alternative name for *lobus* anterior hypophyseos; see also hypophysis.

**ad'enoid** [ adeno- + G. *eidos*, appearance ]. 1. Glandlike; adeniform; lymphoid. 2. See adenoids.

**ad'enoidec'tomy** [ adenoid + G. *ektomē*, excision ]. An operation for the removal of adenoid growths in the nasopharynx.

**ad'enoidism.** Symptoms and signs associated with enlarged adenoids.

**ad'enoidi'tis.** Inflammation of nasopharyngeal lymphoid tissue.

**ad'enoids.** Adenoid disease; Meyer's disease; hypertrophy of the lymphoid nodules in the posterior wall of the nasopharynx, the pharyngeal or Luschka's tonsil, resulting from chronic inflammation.

**adenoleiomyofibroma** (ad'en-o-li'o-mi'o-fi-bro'mah) [ adeno- + G. *leios*, smooth, + *mys*, muscle, + fibroma ]. Adenomatoid *tumor* of the genital tract.

**adenologaditis** (ad'ĕ-no-log'ah-di'tis) [ adeno- + G. *logades*, whites of the eyes, + suffix -*itis*, inflammation ]. Obsolete term for (1) ophthalmia in the newborn, and (2) inflammation of conjunctival glands.

**adenol'ogy** [ adeno- + G. *logos*, treatise, discourse ]. The science that treats of the glands, their development, structure, functions, and diseases.

**adenolymphocele** (ad'ĕ-no-lim'fo-sēl) [ adeno- + L. *lympha*, spring water, + G. *kēlē*, tumor ]. Cystic dilation of a lymph node following obstruction of the efferent lymphatic vessels.

**ad'enolympho'ma.** 1. Benign lymphoepithelial *lesion.* 2. Papillary *cystadenoma* lymphomatosum.

**adenol'ysis** [ adeno- + G. *lysis*, destruction ]. Enzymatic destruction or dissolution of glandular tissue, as in the digestion of a portion or all of the pancreas (by the action of pancreatic enzymes) in acute hemorrhagic necrosis of that organ.

**adeno'ma** [ adeno- + G. suffix -*oma*, tumor ]. An ordinarily benign neoplasm of epithelial tissue in which the tumor cells form glands or glandlike structures in the stroma; usually well circumscribed, tending to compress adjacent tissue rather than infiltrating or invading.

**acidophil a.,** eosinophil a.

**a. adamanti'num,** a term incorrectly used as a synonym of adamantinoma.

**adnexal a.,** an a. arising in, or forming structures resembling, skin appendages.

**adrenal cortical a.,** a benign tumor of adrenal cortical cells; small unencapsulated nodules of adrenal cortex are probably localized areas of hyperplasia rather than a.'s; true a.'s are rare and may be symptomless or associated with Cushing's syndrome or primary aldosteronism.

**apocrine a.,** papillary *hidradenoma.*

**basophil a.,** pituitary basophil a.

**bronchial a.'s,** slowly growing, benign or malignant but slowly progressing, polypoid, epithelial tumors of bronchial mucosa, arising deep to the surface epithelium, possibly from mucous glands or their ducts. There are two histological types, the carcinoid and the cylindromatous.

**chro'mophil a.,** a basophil or an eosinophil a.

**chro'mophobe a.,** a tumor of the chromophobe cells of the anterior pituitary body, sometimes associated with hypopituitarism, hypothalamic disorders, increased intracranial pressure, and visual disturbances; the cell cytoplasm does not stain well with acid or basic dyes.

**colloid a.,** macrofollicular a.; a follicular a. of the thyroid, composed of large follicles containing colloid.

**embryonal a.,** a benign neoplasm in which the glandular epithelial elements are not fully differentiated, resembling immature tissue observed in embryonic development. The concept that such a tumor is derived from a rest of embryonic cells has been generally discarded.

**eosin'ophil a.,** acidophil a.; a tumor of the eosinophilic chromophil cells of the anterior pituitary body, associated with gigantism and acromegaly.

**fetal a.,** an a. occurring in the thyroid or anterior lobe of the pituitary, consisting of tall cylindrical cells arranged in tubular form, and resembling tissue observed in development of the fetus; epithelial elements slightly more mature

than those observed in embryonal a. The concept that such a tumor is derived from a rest of fetal cells has been generally discarded.

**fibroid a.,** fibroadenoma.

**a. fibro'sum,** fibroadenoma.

**follicular a.,** an a. of the thyroid with a simple glandular pattern.

**Fuchs' a.,** a benign epithelial tumor of the ciliary body observed as a small white nodule with a stagnant growth pattern.

**a. gelatino'sa,** colloid *goiter.*

**Getsowa's a.,** an adenocarcinoma of the thyroid gland, formerly thought to originate in a lateral anlage, but probably representing a metastasis from a primary neoplasm in the gland *per se.* Termed also struma postbranchialis.

**a. hidradenoides,** papillary *hidradenoma.*

**Hürthle cell a.,** a follicular a. of the thyroid in which the epithelium has undergone metaplasia into Hürthle cells; see also oxyphil a. and Hürthle cell *tumor.*

**islet cell a.,** a benign neoplasm of the pancreas composed of tissue similar in structure to that of the islets of Langerhans; it may contain functioning beta cells, and may cause hypoglycemia; sometimes termed insuloma, insulinoma, or nesidioblastoma.

**macrofollicular a.,** colloid a.

**malignant a.,** a. malignum; sometimes used for adenocarcinoma, especially when a portion of an a. is thought to be histologically malignant, or metastatic neoplasm of similar type is recognized.

**a. malignum,** malignant a.

**microfollicular a.,** a fetal a. of the thyroid composed of very small follicles and solid alveolar groups of thyroid epithelial cells.

**a. of nipple,** a scaling, crusted or ulcerated tumor of the nipple, resembling Paget's disease but resulting from a benign, localized proliferation of ductal epithelium.

**a. ova'rii testicula're,** arrhenoblastoma.

**ox'yphil a.,** an a. composed of epithelial cells with eosinophilic cytoplasm. The term is a synonym for oncocytoma of salivary glands and has been used for Hürthle cell a. of the thyroid and eosinophil a. of the pituitary. It may also be applied to a parathyroid a. composed of oxyphil cells.

**papillary cystic a.,** an a. in which the lumens of the acini are frequently distended by fluid, and the neoplastic epithelial elements tend to form irregular, fingerlike projections.

**papillary a. of large intestine,** villous a.

**Pick's tubular a.,** androblastoma (1).

**pituitary basophil a.,** basophil a.; a tumor of the basophilic chromophil cells of the anterior pituitary body, associated with Cushing's syndrome.

**pleomorphic a.,** mixed *tumor* of salivary gland.

**polypoid a.,** adenomatous *polyp.*

**renal cortical a.,** one of the usually small a.'s sometimes found in the renal cortex and derived from renal tubular tissue.

**sebaceous a.,** a benign tumor of sebaceous tissue, having a more progressive growth and less mature structure than in sebaceous gland hyperplasia or adenoma sebaceum.

**a. seba'ceum,** pilosebaceous hamartoma; Pringle's disease; a hamartoma occurring on the face, composed of sebaceous glands and fibrovascular tissue and appearing as an aggregation of red or yellow papules which may be associated with tuberous sclerosis. See also sebaceous a.

**sweat duct a.,** a rare tumor of the sweat duct, thought to be a dermal duct tumor (eccrine poroma), except that it originates deeper in the sweat duct and may appear as a verrucous plaque.

**testicular tubular a.,** androblastoma (1).

**tubular a.,** a benign neoplasm composed of epithelial tissue resembling a tubular gland.

**a. tubula're testicula're ova'rii,** arrhenoblastoma.

**villous a.,** papillary a. of the large intestine; usually a solitary and sessile, often large tumor of colonic mucosa composed of mucinous epithelium covering delicate vascular projections; hypersecretion and malignant change occur frequently.

**adeno'matoid.** Having a resemblance to an adenoma.

**adenomato'sis.** The state characterized by multiple glandular overgrowths.

**endocrine a.,** familial polyendocrine a.

**familial polyendocrine a.,** Wermer's syndrome; endocrine a.; pluriglandular a.; the presence of functioning tumors in more than one endocrine gland, commonly the pancreatic islands and parathyroid glands, often associated with peptic ulcers and gastric hypersecretion.

**fibrosing a.,** sclerosing *adenosis.*

**pluriglandular a.,** familial polyendocrine a.

**pulmonary a.,** a neoplastic disease in which the alveoli and distal bronchi are filled with mucus and mucus-secreting columnar epithelial cells. It is characterized by abundant, extremely tenacious sputum, chills, fever, cough, dyspnea, and pleuritic pain.

**pul'monary a. of sheep,** lunger disease; jagziekte (South Africa); Marsh's ovine progressive pneumonia; a chronic pulmonary disease of sheep, probably of viral origin, characterized by adenomatous proliferations in the alveoli and small bronchioles. It occurs in many parts of the world, including the western parts of the United States.

**adeno'matous.** Relating to adenoma, and to some types of glandular hyperplasia.

**adenomere** (ad'ĕ-no-mēr) [ adeno- + G. *meros,* part ]. A structural unit in the parenchyma of a developing gland.

**ad'enomyo'ma.** A benign neoplasm of muscle (usually smooth muscle) with glandular elements; occurs most frequently in uterus and uterine ligaments.

**ad'enomy'ometri'tis** [ adeno- + G. *mys,* muscle, + *metra,* uterus, + suffix *-itis,* inflammation ]. *Adenomyosis* uteri.

**ad'enomy'osarco'ma.** Wilms' *tumor.*

**ad'enomyo'sis.** The ectopic occurrence or diffuse implantation of adenomatous tissue in muscle (usually smooth muscle).

**a. uteri,** adenomyometritis; a benign invasion of myometrium by endometrial tissue.

**ad'enomyxo'ma.** *Cystosarcoma* phyllodes.

**adenonco'sis.** Infrequently used term for a condition in which a gland or glandular organ is grossly enlarged, especially as the result of neoplasm.

**adenoncus** (ad-ĕ-nong'kus) [ adeno- + G. *onkos,* bulk, ONC-1 ]. Enlargement of a gland or glands; a mass composed of enlarged glands.

**ad'enoneu'ral.** Relating to a gland and nervous element.

**adenop'athy** [ adeno- + G. *pathos,* suffering ]. Swelling of or morbid enlargement in the lymph nodes.

**ad'enopharyngi'tis** (ad'ĕ-no-far'in-ji'tis). Inflammation of the adenoids and the pharyngeal lymphoid tissue.

**ad'enophleg'mon** [ adeno- + G. *phlegmonē,* inflammation ]. Acute inflammation of a gland and the adjacent connective tissue.

**ad'enophthal'mia** (ad'en-of-thal'me-ah) [ adeno- + G. *ophthalmos,* eye ]. Obsolete term for inflammation of the Meibomian glands.

**adenophy'ma** [ adeno- + G. *phyma,* tumor ]. Rarely used term for any condition in which a gland or glandular organ is grossly enlarged as the result of an inflammation.

**adenosalpingitis** (ad'e-no-sal-pin-ji'tis). *Salpingitis* isthmica nodosa.

**ad'enosarco'ma.** A malignant neoplasm arising simultaneously or consecutively in mesodermal tissue and glandular epithelium of the same part.

**ad'enose.** Adenous; relating to a gland.

**ad'eno'sinase.** Adenosine nucleosidase.

**aden'osine.** A condensation product of adenine (*q. v.*) and D-ribose; a nucleoside found among the hydrolysis products of all nucleic acids and of the various adenine nucleotides. Symbol, Ado or A. For structure, see adenylic acid.

**a. deaminase** (EC 3.5.4.4), an enzyme found in mammalian tissues, capable of catalyzing the deamination of adenosine, forming inosine in the process.

**a. diphosphate,** see adenosine 5'-diphosphate.

**a. kinase** (EC 2.7.1.20), an enzyme catalyzing the transfer of a phosphate group from ATP to adenosine, forming ADP and adenylic acid.

**a. monophosphate,** adenosine phosphate (USAN); used as a nutrient; see adenylic acid.

**a. nucleosidase** (EC 3.2.2.7), adenosinase; an enzyme cleaving adenosine to adenine and D-ribose.

**a. pyrophosphate,** see adenosine 5'-diphosphate.

**a. tetraphosphate,** A tetra P; a condensation product of adenosine with tetraphosphoric acid at the 5' position. Probably an artifact.

**a. triphosphatase** (EC 3.6.1.3), an enzyme in muscle (myosin) and elsewhere that catalyzes the release of the terminal phosphate group of adenosine triphosphate.

**a. triphosphate,** ATP; adenosine(5')O—$(PO_2H)_2$—$OPO_3H_2$; adenosine with triphosphoric acid at the 5' position. See also entries under ATP.

**adenosine 3':5'-cyclic phosphate.** An activator of phosphorylase kinase; formed in muscle from ATP by adenylate cyclase, and broken down to 5'-AMP by a phosphodiesterase. Sometimes referred to as second messenger; also called cyclic adenylic acid, cyclic phosphate, cyclic AMP (cAMP), although at least one other such compound (2':3') is known.

**adenosine 5'-diphosphate.** ADP; adenosine diphosphate; a condensation product of adenosine with pyrophosphoric acid; formed from ATP by the hydrolysis of the terminal phosphate group of the latter compound. See also entries under ADP.

**adenosine 3'-phosphate.** Yeast adenylic acid (obsolete); see adenylic acid.

**adenosine 5'-phosphate.** Muscle adenylic acid (obsolete); see adenylic acid.

**adenosine 3'-phosphate, 5'-phosphosulfate** PAPS; "active sulfate"; an intermediate in the formation of urinary ethereal sulfates, notable for containing a "high energy" sulfate bond. The 3'-OH of adenosine is replaced by —$OPO_3H_2$, the 5'-OH by $OP(O_2H)$—O—$SO_3H$.

**adeno'sis.** A more or less generalized glandular disease.

**fibrosing a.,** sclerosing a.

**sclerosing a.,** fibrosing a.; adenofibrosis; a nodular, benign breast lesion occurring most frequently in relatively young women and consisting of hyperplastic distorted lobules of acinar tissue with increased collagenous stroma; the changes may be difficult to distinguish microscopically from carcinoma.

**aden'osyl.** The radical of adenosine minus an H or OH from one of the ribosyl OH groups, usually the 5' (see, for example, adenosylmethionine).

**S-aden'osylhomocyst'eine.** The compound formed by the demethylation of S-adenosylmethionine.

**S-aden'osylmethi'onine.** Abbreviated Ado-Met; condensation product of adenosine and methionine; a sulfonium compound bearing a methyl group that is transferred in transmethylation reactions. See also methionine adenosyltransferase.

S-Adenosylmethionine

**adenot'omy** [ adeno- + G. *tomē,* a cutting ]. The cutting or removal of glands.

**ad'enotonsillec'tomy.** Operative removal of tonsils and adenoids.

**ad'enous.** Adenose.

**ad'enovi'rus.** See under virus.

**ad'enyl.** The radical or ion of adenine; sometimes mistakenly used for adenylyl or adenylate (*cf.* a. cyclase).

**a. cyclase,** adenylate cyclase.

**aden'ylate.** Salt or ester of adenylic acid; see also adenylyl.

**a. cyclase** (EC 4.6.1.1), formerly adenyl cyclase or adenylyl cyclase; enzyme acting on ATP to form 3':5'-cyclic AMP.

**a. kinase** (EC 2.7.4.3.), myokinase; a phosphotransferase that catalyzes the phosphorylation of one molecule of ADP at the expense of another, yielding ATP and AMP.

**adenyl'ic acid.** AMP; adenosine monophosphate; adenine ribonucleotide; a condensation product of adenosine and phosphoric acid; a nucleotide found among the hydrolysis products of all nucleic acids. **Yeast adenylic acid** (adenosine 3'-phosphate) and **muscle adenylic acid** (adenosine 5'-phosphate) differ in the place of attachment of the phosphoric acid to the ribose. **Deoxyadenylic acid** differs in having H instead of OH at the 2' position. See also entries under AMP.

Adenylic acid

**cyclic a. acid,** see adenosine 3':5'-cyclic phosphate.

**a. acid deaminase,** AMP deaminase; see under AMP.

**a. acid kinase,** adenylate kinase.

**adenylosuccinase.** Adenylylsuccinate lyase.

**adenylosuccinic acid.** Adenylylsuccinic acid.

**aden'ylyl.** The radical of adenylic acid minus an OH from the phosphoric group.

**a. cyclase,** adenylate cyclase.

**a. pyrophosphate,** adenosine triphosphate.

**adenylylosuccinate lyase.** Adenylosuccinase; an enzyme (EC 4.3.2.2) catalyzing the nonhydrolytic cleavage of adenylylosuccinic acid and also of 5-aminoimidazole-4-N-succinocarboxamide nucleotide to yield fumaric acid.

**adenylylosuccinic acid.** Adenylosuccinic acid; a condensation product of aspartic acid and inosine phosphate; an intermediate in the biosynthesis of adenylic acid.

Adenylylosuccinic acid

**adephagia** (ad-e-fa'jī-ah) [ G. *adēphagia*, gluttony, fr. *adēn*, enough, + *phagein*, to eat ]. Bulimia.

**ad'eps,** gen. **ad'ipis** [ L. lard, fat ]. 1 [ NA ]. Denoting fat or adipose tissue. 2. Lard; axungia porcis; swine fat; purified leaf lard (omental fat of the hog, *Sus scrofa*). Used in the preparation of ointments.

**a. lanae,** wool fat.

**a. lanae hydro'sus,** hydrous or hydrated wool fat; see lanolin.

**a. ovil'lus,** tallow.

**a. renis,** the layer of adipose tissue surrounding the kidney.

**a. suil'lus,** pork lard.

**ader'mia** [ G. *a*- priv. + *derma*, skin ]. Absence of skin.

**ader'mine.** Pyridoxine.

**ader'mogen'esis** [ G. *a*- priv. + *derma*, skin, + *genesis*, production ]. Failure or imperfection in the regeneration of the skin, especially the imperfect repair of a cutaneous defect.

**ad grat. acid.** Abbreviation for the Latin in prescription writing, meaning to a pleasant degree of sourness.

**ADH.** Abbreviation for (1) antidiuretic *hormone,* and (2) *alcohol* dehydrogenase.

**adhat'oda** [ Tamil or Singalese ]. Malabar nut; the leaves of *Adhatoda vasica* (family Acanthaceae); expectorant, antispasmodic, and abortifacient.

**adhe'sio,** pl. **adhesio'nes** [ L. ] [ NA ]. Adhesion.

**a. interthalam'ica** [ NA ], interthalamic adhesion; commissura cinerea or grisea; massa intermedia; columna mollis; the variable connection between the two thalamic masses across the cavity of the third ventricle. It is frequently absent.

**adhesion** (ad-he'zhun) [ L. *adhesio,* fr. *ad-haereo,* pp. *-haesus,* to stock to ]. 1. The process of adhering or uniting of two surfaces or parts, especially the union of the opposing surfaces of a wound. 2. In the plural, bands of more or less organized fibrinous exudate thrown out on the surface of a serous membrane and connecting the opposing surfaces. 3. The physical attraction of unlike molecules for one another. 4. The molecular attraction existing between the surfaces of bodies in contact.

**amniot'ic a.,** amniotic *bands.*

**fi'brinous a.,** consists of fine threads of fibrin resulting from an exudate of plasma or lymph, or an extravasation of blood.

**fibrous a.,** fibrous strands resulting from the organization of fibrinous a.'s.

**interthalamic a.,** *adhesio* interthalamica.

**primary a.,** healing by first intention; see under intention.

**secondary a.,** healing by second intention.

**adhesiot'omy.** Surgical section of adhesions.

**adhe'sive.** 1. Relating to, or having the characteristics of, an adhesion. 2. Any material that is adherent to a surface or causes adherence between surfaces.

**denture a.,** a material to aid in the retention of dentures.

**tissue a.'s,** a.'s utilizing special methacrylates or derivatives of the cyanoacrylate series; they have been used in ophthalmology to seal perforated corneas and scleral incisions, to attach contact lenses to the cornea, and to aid in the removal of an intraocular foreign body or luxated lens.

**adhib.** Abbreviation for L. *adhibendus,* to be administered, fr. *adhibeo,* to apply [ HAB- ].

**a'diactin'ic** [ G. *a*- priv. + *dia,* through, + *aktis,* ray ]. Opaque to photochemically active radiation.

**adiadochocinesia, adiadochocinesis, adiadochokinesia** (ad-e-ad'o-ko-sin-e'sĭ-ah) [ G. *a*-priv. + *diadochos,* successive, + *kinēsis,* movement ]. Inability to perform rapid alternating movements.

**Adian'tum.** A genus of ferns (maidenhair) used in the preparation of demulcents.

**adiaphoresis** (a'dĭ-ah-fo-re'sis, a-di'ah-) [ G. *a*- priv. + *diaphorēsis,* perspiration. PHER- ]. Absence or deficiency of perspiration.

**a'diaphoret'ic.** 1. Suppressing perspiration. 2. A drug that suppresses perspiration.

**adiaphor'ia** [ G. *a*- priv. + *dia,* through, + *phoros,* bearing ]. A failure to respond to stimulation after a series of previously applied stimuli.

**adiapneustia** (ad-i-ap-nu'stĭ-ah) [ G. *a*-priv. + *diapneusis,* an exhaling. PN- ]. Adiaphoresis.

**adiastole** (ă-di-as'to-le) [ G. *a*-priv. + *diastolē,* dilation ]. The absence or imperceptibility of the diastolic movement of the heart.

**adiathermancy** (ă-di'a-ther'man-sī) [ G. *dia-thermainō,* to warm through, fr. *a*- priv. + *dia,* through, + *thermē,* heat ]. Impermeability to heat.

**Adie,** William J., Australian physician, 1886–1935. See A. *syndrome,* Holmes-A. *syndrome.*

**adiemorrhysis** (ad'i-em-or'ĭ-sis) [ G. *a-* priv. + *dia,* through, + *haima,* blood, + *rhysis,* a flowing ]. Arrest of the capillary circulation.

**ad'ient** [ L. *adiens,* pr. p. of *adeo,* to go toward ]. Having a tendency to move toward the source of a stimulus, as opposed to abient.

**Adin'ida** [ G. *a-* priv. + *dien,* a whirling ]. An order of Dinoflagellata, in which the flagella are free and do not lie in furrows.

**ad'iospore** [ G. *a-* priv. + *dia,* through, + *sporos,* seed ]. A fungal spore that increases in size without dividing when inoculated in an animal or cultured at an elevated temperature.

**adip-, adipo-** [ L. *adeps,* fat ]. Combining form relating to fat; for words beginning thus and not found here, see also those beginning with lip-, lipo-.

**adipectomy** (ad'ĭ-pek'to-mĭ) [ L. *adeps,* fat, + G. *ektomē,* excision ]. Lipectomy.

**adiphenine hydrochloride** (ă-dif'ĕ-nēn) (USAN). TRASENTINE; $(C_6H_5)_2CHCOOCH_2CH_2N(C_2H_5)_2$·HCl; antispasmodic with little antimuscarine activity; used to decrease spasm of the biliary tract, gastrointestinal tract, uterus, and ureter.

**adip'ic acid.** Hexanedioic acid; a dicarboxylic acid; $HOOC(CH_2)_4COOH$.

**adipo-.** See adip-.

**adipocele** (ad'ĭ-po-sēl) [ adipo- + G. *kēlē,* tumor ]. Lipocele.

**adipocel'lular.** Relating to both fatty and cellular tissues, or to connective tissue with many fat cells.

**adipoceratous** (ad-ĭ-po-ser'ă-tus). Relating to adipocere.

**adipocere** (ad'ĭ-po-sēr) [ adipo- + G. *cera,* wax ]. A fatty substance of waxy consistency into which dead animal tissues (as those of a corpse) are sometimes converted when kept from the air under certain favoring conditions of temperature; it is thought to be produced by the conversion into fat of the proteins of the tissues.

**ad'ipogen'esis.** Lipogenesis.

**ad'ipogen'ic, adipog'enous.** Lipogenic; lipogenous.

**ad'ipohepat'ic.** Relating to fatty liver.

**ad'ipoid** [ adipo- + G. *eidos,* resemblance ]. Lipoid.

**ad'ipokinet'ic.** Descriptive of an agent that causes mobilization of stored lipid.

**ad'ipoki'nin.** Adipokinetic hormone; an anterior pituitary hormone that brings about mobilization of fat from adipose tissue.

**adipom'eter** [ adipo- + G. *metron,* measure ]. An instrument for determining the thickness of the skin.

**ad'iponecro'sis.** Necrosis of fat, such as may be seen in hemorrhagic pancreatitis.

   **a. neonatorum,** *sclerema* neonatorum.

**ad'ipopec'tic** [ adipo- + G. *pēktos,* fixed ]. Lipopectic.

**ad'ipopex'ia** [ adipo- + G. *pēxis,* fixation ]. Lipopexia.

**ad'iposal'gia** [ adipo- + G. *algos,* pain ]. Painful areas of subcutaneous fat.

**ad'ipose.** Fatty; relating to fat.

**adipo'sis** [ adipo- + G. suffix *-osis,* condition ]. Lipomatosis; liposis (1); an excessive local or general accumulation of fat in the body.

   **a. cardiaca,** *cor* adiposum.

   **a. cerebra'lis,** obesity resulting from intracranial disease, most commonly of the hypothalamus or hypophysis.

   **a. doloro'sa,** Dercum's disease; Anders' disease; lipomatosis neurotica; an affection characterized by a deposit of symmetrical nodular or pendulous masses of fat in various regions of the body, attended with more or less pain.

   **a. or'chica,** *dystrophia* adiposogenitalis.

   **a. tubero'sa simplex,** an affection resembling a. dolorosa, in which the fat occurs in small, more or less circumscribed masses on the abdomen or confined to the extremities; these masses are sensitive to the touch and may be spontaneously painful.

   **a. universa'lis,** excessive deposition of fat throughout all parts of the body, including the viscera.

**adipos'ity.** Obesity.

   **pituitary a.,** obesity resulting from pituitary disease.

**ad'iposu'ria** [ adipo- + G. *ouron,* urine ]. Lipuria.

**adip'sia, adip'sy** [ G. *a-* priv. + *dipsa,* thirst ]. Aposia; absence of thirst or the lack of desire to drink.

**aditus,** pl. **aditus** (ad'ĭ-tus) [ L. access, fr. *ad-eo,* pp. *-itus,* go to ] [ NA ]. An entrance to a cavity or channel.

   **a. ad antrum** [ NA ], the orifice leading from the epitympanic recess to the mastoid antrum.

   **a. ad aqueduc'tum cer'ebri,** *anus* cerebri.

   **a. ad infundib'ulum,** *recessus* infundibuli.

   **a. ad saccum peritonae'i mino'rum,** *foramen* epiploicum.

   **a. glot'tidis inferior,** *cavum* infraglotticum.

   **a. glot'tidis superior,** the lower portion of the ventricle of the larynx.

   **a. laryn'gis** [ NA ], the superior aperture of the larynx, bounded laterally by the aryepiglottic folds.

   **a. or'bitae** [ NA ], the opening of the orbit.

   **a. pelvis,** *apertura* pelvis superior.

**adjust'ment.** 1. In dentistry, a modification made upon a denture, or upon the teeth on a denture after it has been completed and inserted in the mouth. 2. Adaptation (6).

   **occlusal a.,** modification of the occluding surfaces of teeth to develop harmonious relationships between these surfaces.

**ad'juvant** [ L. *ad-juvo,* pres. p. *-juvans,* to give aid to ]. 1. Synergist (1); adminiculum (2); that which aids or assists; denoting a substance that is added to a prescription to assist or increase the action of the main ingredient. 2. In immunology, a vehicle used to enhance antigenicity; *e.g.,* a suspension of minerals (alum, aluminum hydroxide or phosphate) on which antigen is adsorbed; or water-in-oil emulsion in which antigen solution is emulsified in mineral oil (Freund's incomplete a.), sometimes with the inclusion of killed mycobacteria (Freund's complete a.) to further enhance antigenicity.

   **Freund's complete a.,** water-in-oil emulsion of antigen, to which killed mycobacteria are added.

   **Freund's incomplete a.,** water-in-oil emulsion of antigen, without mycobacteria.

**Adler,** Alfred, Austrian psychiatrist, 1870–1937. See Adlerian *psychology, psychoanalysis.*

**Adler,** Oscar, Carlsbad physician, 1879–1932. See A.'s *test.*

**ad lib.** [ Abbreviation for L. *ad libitum,* at pleasure, fr. impers. verb *libet,* it pleases ]. As much as desired; used in directions for taking a remedy when the dose and time of taking are indefinite and unessential.

**admax'illary** [ L. *ad,* to, + *maxilla,* jaw ]. Connected with the jaw.

**adme'dial, adme'dian.** Toward or near the median plane.

**adminic'ulum,** pl. **adminic'ula** [ L. a hand-rest, prop, fr. *ad* + *manus,* hand ]. 1. That which gives support to a part. 2. Adjuvant.

   **a. lin'eae albae** [ NA ], a triangular fibrous expansion, sometimes containing a few muscular fibers, passing from the superior pubic ligament to the posterior surface of the linea alba.

**admov.** Abbreviation in prescription writing for Latin *admove, admoveatur,* let there be added.

**adner'val.** Adneural. 1. Lying near a nerve. 2. In the direction of a nerve; said of an electric current passing through muscular tissue toward the point of entrance of the nerve.

**adneu'ral.** Adnerval.

**adnexa,** sing. **adne'xum** (ad-nek'sah) [ L. connected parts, appendages ]. Annexa; appendages; parts accessory to the main organ or structure.

   **a. oculi,** the eyelids, lacrimal glands, etc., associated with the eyeball.

   **a. uteri,** uterine appendages; the uterine tubes and ovaries.

**adnex'al.** Annexal; relating to the adnexa.

**adnexectomy** (ad-nek-sek'to-mĭ). Annexectomy. 1. Excision of any adnexa. 2. In gynecology, excision of tube and ovary if unilateral and excision of both tubes and ovaries if bilateral. adnexa uteri.

**adnexi'tis** [ L. *annexa,* adnexa, + suffix *-itis,* inflammation ]. Annexitis; inflammation of the adnexa.

**adnex'opexy** [ L. *annexa,* adnexa, + G. *pēxis,* fixation ]. Annexopexy; operation for suspension of tube and ovary; usually, oophoropexy is accomplished without suspension of the tube.

**Ado.** Symbol for adenosine.

**adolescence** (ad'o-les'ens) [ L. *adolescentia* ]. Period of attaining complete growth and maturity.

**adolescent** (ad'o-les'ent). Pertaining to the period or state of adolescence.

**adon'is** [ G. *Adonis*, a mythologic character, the handsome favorite of Aphrodite ]. The herb *Adonis vernalis* (family Ranunculaceae); pheasant's eye; false hellebore. Contains adonitoxin, strophanthidin, aconitic acid, phytosterols, and choline. Used as a cardiac tonic and diuretic in place of digitalis.

**adon'itol.** Ribitol.

**adoral** (ad-o'ral) [ L. *ad*, to, + *os* (*or-*), mouth ]. Near or directed toward the mouth.

**ADP.** Abbreviation for adenosine 5'-diphosphate.

**ADPase.** Apyrase.

**ADP deiminase.** (EC 3.5.4.7); see deiminases.

**adren-, adrenal-, adreno-** [ L. *ad*, toward, + *ren*, kidney ]. Combining forms relating to the adrenal gland.

**adrenal** (ad-re'nal) [ L. *ad*, to, + *ren*, kidney ]. Near or upon the kidney; denoting the glandula suprarenalis.
  **accessory a.,** adrenal rest; an island of cortical tissue separate from the adrenal gland, usually found in the retroperitoneal tissues, kidney, or genital organs.
  **butterfly a.,** *glandula* suprarenalis.
  **Marchand's a.'s,** small collections of accessory a. tissue in the broad ligament of the uterus.

**adrenalectomize** (ad-re-nal-ek'to-mīz). To excise the adrenal glands.

**adrenalectomy** (ad-re-nal-ek'to-mī) [ adrenal + G. *ektomē*, excision ]. Removal of an adrenal gland.

**adrenaline** (ad-ren'al-in, ad-ren'al-ēn) (BP). Epinephrine.
  **a. acid tartrate** (BP), epinephrine bitartrate.
  **a. oxidase,** amine oxidase (flavin-containing).

**adren'aline'mia** [ adrenaline + G. *haima*, blood ]. Adrenemia; the presence of notable or excessive amounts of epinephrine (adrenaline) in the circulation.

**adren'alinu'ria** [ adrenaline + G. *ouron*, urine ]. The presence of epinephrine (adrenaline) in the urine.

**adre'nalism.** A condition resulting from abnormal function of the adrenal glands; obsolete usage.

**adren'alone** (USAN). KEPHRINE; 3'4'-dihydroxy-2-(methylamino)acetophenone; 4-methylaminoacetopyrocatechol; precursor of epinephrine in some manufacturing processes.

**adre'nalop'athy** [ adrenal + G. *pathos*, suffering ]. Any pathologic condition of the adrenal (suprarenal) glands.

**adrenarche** (ad'ren-ar'ke) [ adren- + G. *archē*, beginning ]. 1. Menstruation and other signs of puberty induced by hyperactivity of the adrenal cortex. 2. Physiologic change at puberty caused by adrenocortical secretion of androgenic hormones or precursors of them.

**adrene'mia.** Adrenalinemia.

**adrener'gic** [ adren- + G. *ergon*, work ]. 1. Relating to nerve fibers of the autonomic nervous system that liberate norepinephrine. 2. Relating to drugs that mimic the actions of the sympathetic nervous system; *cf.* cholinergic.

**adre'nic.** Relating to the adrenal gland.

**adreno-.** See adren-.

**adrenoceptive** (ad-re'no-sep'tiv). Referring to chemical sites in effectors with which the adrenergic mediator unites; *cf.* cholinoceptive.

**adrenochrome** (ad-re'no-krōm) [ adreno- + G. *chrōma*, color ]. 3-Hydroxy-1-methyl-5,6-indolinedione; the red oxidation product of epinephrine; was used therapeutically in Germany during the second World War to increase efficiency of diabetic laborers. It is said to produce psychic changes. See also carbazochrome salicylate.

**adre'nocor'tical.** Pertaining to adrenal cortex.

**adre'nocor'ticomimet'ic.** Mimicking adrenocortical function.

**adrenocorticotropic, adrenocorticotrophic** (ad-re'no-kor'tĭ-ko-trop'ik, -trof'ik) [ adrenal cortex + G. *trophē*, nurture; *tropē*, a turning ]. Affecting growth or activity of adrenal cortex.

**adre'nocor'ticotro'pin, adre'nocor'ticotro'phin.** Adrenocorticotropic *hormone*.

**adrenogen'ic.** Adrenogenous; of adrenal origin.

**adrenogenous** (ad-ren-oj'en-us). Adrenogenic.

**adren'olu'tin.** *N*-Methyl-3,5,6-trihydroxyindole; an oxidation product of epinephrine.

**adrenolytic** (ad-ren-o-lit'ik). Denoting antagonism to or inhibition of the action of epinephrine, norepinephrine, and related sympathomimetics; see also adrenergic blocking *agent*.

**adrenomegaly** (ad-re'no-meg'al-ī) [ adreno- + G. *megas*, big ]. Enlargement of the adrenal glands.

**adrenomimetic** (ad-re'no-mī-met'ik). Having an action similar to that of the compounds, epinephrine and norepinephrine, which are liberated from the adrenal medulla and adrenergic nerves. Term coined by W. B. Youmans to replace the less accurate term, sympathomimetic. See also adrenergic and cholinomimetic.

**adrenop'athy.** Adrenalopathy.

**adre'nopause.** The period of life when adrenal function is supposed to be reduced, though such a period has not been specifically delineated.

**adre'nopri'val** [ adreno- + L. *privo*, to deprive ]. Indicating a loss of adrenal function, as a result of either disease or surgical excision.

**adrenoreactive** (ad-re'no-re-ak'tiv). Responding to the catecholamines.

**adre'norecep'tors.** See adrenergic *receptors*.

**adrenos'terone.** Andrenosterone; Reichstein's substance G; 4-androstene-3,11,17-trione (for structure of androstane, see steroids); an androgen isolated from the adrenal cortex.

**adre'notox'in.** A substance toxic for the adrenal glands.

**adre'notroph'ic, adre'notrop'ic.** Adrenocorticotropic.

**adre'notro'phin, adre'notro'pin.** Adrenocorticotropic *hormone*.

**a'driamy'cin.** A cytotoxic antibiotic derived from *Streptomyces peucetius* var. *caesius;* antineoplastic.

**Adrian,** Edgar D., English neurophysiologist, *1889. Nobel laureate, 1932, with Sir Charles S. Sherrington for investigations on the physiology of the nervous system.

**adro'mia** [ G. *a-* priv. + *dromos*, course ]. Failure of muscle innervation.

**ad'rue.** Antiemetic root; cyperus; the root of *Cyperus articulatus*, a West Indian plant; the fluid extract is used as an anthelmintic and antiemetic.

**Adson's test.** See under test.

**adsorb'** [ L. *ad*, to, + *sorbeo*, to suck in ]. To take up by adsorption. Compare absorb.

**adsor'bate.** Any substance adsorbed.

**adsor'bent.** 1. A substance that adsorbs, *e.g.*, carbon, clay, magnesia, etc. 2. In pharmacology, a substance endowed with the property of attaching other substances to its surface without any chemical action; a.'s are used in diarrhea, as an antidote for poisonings, as a protective dusting powder.

**adsorption** (ad-sorp'shun) [ L. *ad*, to, + *sorbeo*, to suck up ]. The property of a substance to attract and hold to its surface a gas, liquid or a substance in solution or in suspension. Compare absorption.
  **chromatographic a., differential a., stratographic a.,** see chromatography.
  **immune a.,** the removal of antibody (agglutinin or precipitin) from antiserum by use of specific antigen; after aggregation has occurred the antigen-antibody complex is separated either by centrifugation or by filtration.

**adster'nal.** Near or upon the sternum.

**ADTe.** Abbreviation for anodal duration *tetanus.*

**adter'minal.** In a direction toward the nerve endings, muscular insertions, or the extremity of any structure.

**ador'sion.** Intorsion.

**adult** (ă-dult'). Fully grown and mature; a fully grown individual.

**adul'terant.** Impurity; additive that is considered to have an undesirable effect.

**adul'tera'tion.** The alteration of any substance by the deliberate addition of a component not ordinarily part of that substance; usually used to imply that the substance is debased as a result.

**adultomor'phism.** Interpretation of children's behavior in adult terms.

**advance** (ad-vans) [ Fr. *avancer*, to set forward ]. To move forward; referring specifically to an operation on the tendinous insertion of a muscle that has become elongated and unable to perform its function properly; the tendon is severed from its attachment (to the globe of the eye, for example) and sutured at a point farther forward.

**advancement** (ad-vans'ment). The moving forward of the tendinous insertion of an elongated muscle.

    **capsular a.,** surgical forward reattachment of the anterior insertion of Tenon's capsule.

    **tendon a.,** excision of the tendon of an eye muscle and fixation of the same farther forward on the globe.

**adventi'cius** [ L. ] [ NA ]. Adventitial.

**adventitia** (ad-ven-tish'yah) [ L. *adventicius*, coming from abroad, foreign, fr. *ad*, to + *venio*, to come ]. The outermost covering of any organ or structure which is properly derived from without and does not form an integral part of such organ or structure. Specifically, the outer coat of an artery, the tunica adventitia.

**adventitial** (ad-ven-tish'al). Relating to the outer coat or adventitia of a blood vessel or other structure.

**adventitious** (ad-ven-tish'us). 1. Coming from without; extrinsic. 2. Accidental. 3. Adventitial.

**ad. 2 vic.** Abbreviation for L. *ad duas vices*, at two times, for two doses.

**adynamia** (ad'ĭ-na'mĭ-ah) [ G. *a-* priv. + *dynamis*, power ]. Weakness; vital debility; asthenia.

    **a. episodica hereditaria,** hyperkalemic periodic *paralysis*.

**adynam'ic.** Relating to adynamia.

**ae-.** For words so beginning and not found here, see under e-.

**Aeby,** Christoph T., Swiss anatomist, 1835–1885. See A.'s *muscle, plane.*

**Aedes** (ah-e'dēz) [ G. *aēdēs*, unpleasant, unfriendly ]. A widespread genus of mosquitos of small size most frequently found in tropical and subtropical regions.

    **A. aegyp'ti,** the yellow fever mosquito, which is also the vector of the pathogen of dengue; it was formerly called *Stegomyia calopus* or *S. Fasciata;* characterized by white lyre-shaped markings on the thorax.

    **A. cabal'lus,** an important vector of Rift Valley fever in South Africa.

    **A. fuscus,** a species found in certain parts of North America.

    **A. leucocelaenus,** transmits yellow fever in South America.

    **A. scapular'is,** a vector of myxomatosis of rabbits.

    **A. sollic'itans,** a common salt-marsh mosquito and vector of eastern equine encephalomyelitis on the Atlantic and Gulf coasts of the United States.

    **A. variegat'us,** an intermediate host of filarial parasites in the Pacific Islands (Gilbert and Ellice group).

**Aeg.** Abbreviation for the Latin *aeger, aegra,* the patient, used in prescription writing.

**aeluropho'bia.** Ailurophobia.

**aeluropsis** (e-loor-op'sis) [ G. *ailouros,* a cat, + *opsis,* vision ]. An obsolete term descriptive of slanting palpebral fissures (similar to those of a cat).

**Aelurostrongylus abstrusus** (e'loor-o-stron'jĭ-lus ab-stru'sus). A common lungworm of cats. The adults live in the terminal bronchioles and alveolar ducts, the eggs hatch in the alveoli, and the larvae ascend the trachea, are swallowed, and pass out of the body in the feces. Land snails and slugs serve as intermediate hosts; snail-eating animals can serve as transport hosts. In heavy infections the affected cat may suffer from cough, diarrhea and emaciation; milder infections usually are not detected during life.

**a'er-, a'ero-** [ G. *aēr*(L. *aer*), air ]. Combining form denoting relationship to air or gas.

**aer** (a'er) [ G. *aēr,* air ]. Atmos.

**aerasthenia** (a-er-as-the'nĭ-ah) [ aer- + G. *asthenia,* weakness ]. Aeroasthenia; aeroneurosis; a psychoneurotic condition marked by worry, lack of self-confidence, and mild depression, occurring in aviators.

**aerated** (a'er-a-ted). Charged with air or other gas.

**aeration** (a-er-a'shun). 1. Airing. 2. Saturating a fluid with air or other gas. 3. The change of venous into arterial blood in the lungs.

**aeremia** (a-er-e'mĭah) [ aer- + G. *haima,* blood ]. Aeroembolism; air *embolism.*

**aerendocardia** (a-er-en-do-kar'dĭ-ah) [ aer- + G. *endon,* within, + *kardia,* heart ]. The presence of undissolved air in the blood within the heart.

**aerenterectasia** (a-er-en-ter-ek-ta'zĭ-ah) [ aer- + G. *enteron,* intestine, + *ektasis,* a stretching out ]. Meteorism; tympanites; pneumatosis cystoides intestinalis; distention of the intestine with gas.

**aeriferous** (a-er-if'er-us). Conducting air.

**aeriform** (a-er'ĭ-form). Gaseous; resembling air.

**aero-.** See aer-.

**aeroasthenia** (a-er-o-as-the'nĭ-ah). Aerasthenia.

**aeroatelectasis** (a'er-o-at-e-lek'tah-sis) [ aero- + atelectasis, *q.v.* ]. A partial, reversible, airless state of lung tissue most likely to occur in pilots exposed to high G forces, breathing 100 per cent oxygen, and wearing an anti-G suit.

**Aerobacter** (a-er-o-bak'tur) [ aero- + *baktērion,* a small staff ]. A rejected generic name of bacteria. The type species is *A. aerogenes.* Organisms previously placed in *A.* belong in *Enterobacter* or *Klebsiella.*

    **A. aerog'enes,** motile organisms formerly placed in this species are now placed in *Enterobacter aerogenes;* the nonmotile organisms have been transferred to *Klebsiella pneumoniae.*

    **A. clo'acae,** *Enterobacter cloacae.*

**a'erobe.** 1. An organism that can live and grow in the presence of oxygen. 2. An organism that can use oxygen as a final electron acceptor in a respiratory chain.

    **ob'ligate a.,** an organism which cannot live or grow in the absence of oxygen.

**aerobic** (a-er-o'bik). Living in air.

**aerobiol'ogy.** The study of atmospheric constituents, living and nonliving, of biological significance, *e.g.,* airborne spores, pathogenic bacteria, allergenic substances, and harmful pollutants.

**aerobioscope** (a-er-o-bi'o-skōp) [ aero- + G. *bios,* life, + *skopeō,* to view ]. An apparatus for determining the bacterial content of the air.

**aerobiosis** (a-er-o-bi-o'sis) [ aero- + G. *biōsis,* mode of living ]. Existence in an atmosphere containing oxygen.

**aerobiotic** (a-er-o-bi-ot'ik). Relating to aerobiosis; living in an oxygen-containing atmosphere; atmosphere.

**aerocele** (a'er-o-sēl) [ aero- + G. *kēlē,* tumor ]. Distention of a small natural cavity with gas.

**Aerococcus** (a-er-o-kok'us) [ aero- + G. *kokkus,* berry ]. A genus of aerobic bacteria containing Gram-positive cocci; they resemble enterococci but do not form chains. They are commonly found in dust in the air of occupied places. These organisms do not produce catalase; they cause greening in blood agar and grow in the presence of 40 per cent bile. The type species is *A. viridans.*

    **A. viridans,** a species originally found in the air of an occupied room; it is the type species of the genus *A.*

**aerocolpos** (a-er-o-kol'pos) [ aero- + G. *kolpos,* womb (vagina) ]. Distention of vagina with gas.

**aerocoly** (a-e-rok'o-li) [ aero- + G. *kolon,* colon ]. Distention of colon with gas.

**aerocystography** (a-er-o-sis-tog'rä-fĭ) [ aero- + G. *kystis,* bladder, + *graphō,* to write ]. Pneumocystography.

**aerocystoscope** (a-er-o-sis'to-skōp) [ aero- + G. *kystis,* bladder, + *skōpeo,* to view ]. An instrument for viewing the interior of the bladder distended with air.

**aerocystoscopy** (a-er-o-sis-tos'ko-pĭ). Inspection of the interior of the bladder, distended with air, by means of a cystoscope.

**aerodermectasia** (a-er-o-der-mek-ta'zĭ-ah) [ aero- + G. *derma,* skin, + *ektasis,* a stretching out ]. Subcutaneous *emphysema.*

**aerodontalgia** (a-er-o-don-tal'jĭ-ah) [ aero- + G. *odous,* tooth, + *algos,* pain ]. Dental pain caused by either increased or reduced atmospheric pressure. It may be experienced during high altitude flying when accompanied by atmospheric decompression.

**primary a.,** dental pain associated with expansion of trapped gases within a tooth, as under a filling, an uncommon condition.

**secondary a.,** pain referred to the dental area from an area of aerosinusitis; more commonly experienced than primary a.

**aerodontia** (ā-er-o-don'she-ah) [ aero- + G. *odous,* tooth ]. The science of the effect of either increased or reduced atmospheric pressure on the teeth.

**aerodynam'ics** [ aero- + G. *dynamis,* force ]. The study of air and other gases in motion, the forces that set them in motion, and the results of such motion.

**aeroembolism** (a'er-o-em'bo-lizm). 1. Air *embolism.* 2. Caisson *disease.*

**aeroemphysema** (a'er-o-em'fi-se-mah). Bubbles of nitrogen in blood and tissue associated with sudden ascent to high altitudes or sudden return to the surface after deep sea diving.

**aerogas'tria.** Distention of the stomach with gas.

**blocked a.,** *aerogastrie* bloquée.

**aerogastrie bloquée** (a-er-o-gas-tre' blo-ka') [ Fr. ]. Blocked aerogastria; spasm of the esophagus which prevents belching.

**aerogel** (a'er-o-jel). A gel in which the liquid (dispersed phase) is replaced by gas.

**aerogen** (a'er-o-jen). A gas-forming microorganism.

**aerogenesis** (a'er-o-jen'ĕ-sis) [ aero- + G. *genesis,* production ]. The production of gas.

**aerogenic** (a'er-o-jen'ik). Gas-forming.

**aerogenous** (a-er-oj'en-us). Gas-forming.

**aerogram** (a'er-o-gram) [ aero- + G. *gramma,* something written ]. Pneumogram.

**aerohydrotherapy** (a-er-o-hi-dro-ther'ă-pĭ) [ aero- + G. *hydōr,* water, + *therapeia,* healing ]. Treatment of disease by means of the application, at different temperatures and in different ways, of both air and water.

**aeroionization** (a-er-o-i'on-i-za'shun). The charging electrically of particles, *e.g.,* fine oil droplets, suspended in air.

**aeroionotherapy** (a-er-o-i'on-o-ther'ă-pĭ). Treatment of respiratory affections by the inhalation of fine electrically charged particles suspended as a mist in the air.

**aeromed'icine.** Aviation *medicine.*

**aerometer** (a-er-om'e-ter) [ aero- + G. *metron,* measure ]. An apparatus for determining the density of, or for weighing, air.

**Aeromo'nas.** A genus of aerobic, facultatively anaerobic bacteria (family Pseudomonaceae) containing Gram-negative, rod-shaped to coccoid cells which occur singly or in pairs or in clumps of chains. Motile cells ordinarily possess a single, polar flagellum; some species are nonmotile. The metabolism of these organisms is both respiratory and fermantative. These bacteria are found in water and sewage; some are pathogenic to fresh water and marine animals. The type species is *A. hydrophila.*

**A. hydrophila,** a species causing red leg disease of frogs; it is the type species of *A.*

**aeroneurosis** (a'er-o-nu-ro'sis). Aerasthenia.

**aero-odontal'gia.** Aerodontalgia.

**aero-odontodynia** (a-er-o-o-don'to-din'ī-ah). Aerodontalgia.

**aeropathy** (a-e-rop'ă-thĭ) [ aero- + G. *pathos,* suffering ]. Any morbid state induced by a pronounced change in the atmospheric pressure, such as mountain sickness, caisson disease, etc.

**aeropause** (a'er-o-pawz). An upper region of the atmosphere, between the stratosphere and outer space, in which gas particles are so sparse as to provide almost no support for man's physiologic requirements or for vehicles that require air for burning fuel.

**aeroperitoneum, aeroperitonia** (a'er-o-pĕr-ĭ-to-ne'um, -to'nĭ-ah). Distention of the peritoneal cavity with gas.

**aerophagia, aerophagy** (a'er-o-fa'jĭ-ah, a-er-of'a-jĭ) [ aero- + G. *phagein,* to eat ]. Pneumophagia; the excessive swallowing of air.

**aerophil** (a'er-o-fil) [ aero- + G. *philos,* fond ]. 1. Air-loving. 2. Aerobic.

**aerophil'ic.** Aerobic.

**aeroph'ilous.** Aerobic.

**aerophobia** (a-er-o-fo'bĭ-ah) [ aero- + G. *phobos,* fear ]. Abnormal and extreme dread of fresh air or of air in motion.

**aerophore** (a'er-o-fŏr) [ aero- + G. *phoros,* bearing ]. 1. Air-conducting. 2. A portable apparatus for purifying air so that it can be breathed over again. 3. An apparatus forcing air into the lungs in the treatment of asphyxia.

**aeropiesotherapy** (a'er-o-pi-e-so-ther'ă-pĭ) [ aero- + G. *piesis,* pressure, + *therapeia,* medical treatment ]. The treatment of disease by means of compressed (or rarified) air.

**aeroplank'ton** [ aero- + G. *planktos,* ntr. *-on,* wandering ]. An organism, *e.g.,* bacterium, pollen grain, etc., carried by air.

**aeroplethysmograph** (a'er-o-plĕ-thiz'mo-graf) [ aero- + G. *plēthysmos,* enlargement, + *graphō,* to write ]. Body *plethysmograph.*

**aeropleura** (a'er-o-plu'ra). Pneumothorax.

**aeroscloscope** (a-er-os'klo-skŏp) [ aero- + G. *sklo,* brachylogy for *sklero,* hard, + *skope,* examination ]. An electronic instrument that counts microscopic airborne germs, dust, and moisture particles, and can distinguish among particles of varying size range, by detecting the light reflection, and the intensity thereof, of each particle.

**aeroscope** (a'er-o-skŏp) [ aero- + G. *skopeō,* to examine ]. An instrument for the examination of air for visible impurities.

**aerosialophagy** (a-er-o-si-al-of'ă-jĭ). Sialoaerophagy.

**aerosinusi'tis.** Inflammation of the paranasal sinuses caused by a difference in pressure within the sinus relative to ambient pressure, secondary to obstruction of the sinus orifice, sometimes brought on by flying at high altitude.

**aero'sis** [ aero- + G. suffix *-osis,* condition ]. The generation of gas in the tissues.

**a'erosol.** 1. A liquid agent or solution dispersed in air in the form of a fine mist for therapeutic, insecticidal, and other purposes. 2. A pharmaceutical a. is a product that is packaged under pressure and contains therapeutically active ingredients, intended for topical application and for introduction into body orifices.

**respirable a.'s,** a.'s with an aerodynamic size under 10 μ.

**aerosoliza'tion.** Dispersion in air of a liquid material or a solution in the form of a fine mist, usually for therapeutic purposes, especially to the respiratory passages.

**aerospace** (a'er-o-spās). The earth's envelope of air and the space beyond it. The two are considered as a single realm for entry of vehicles, satellites, etc.

**aerotaxis** (a'er-o-tak'sis) [ aero- + G. *taxis,* arrangement ]. The movement of living organisms to or away from air; denoting especially the attraction or repulsion by oxygen of aerobic and anaerobic organisms.

**aerotherapeutics, aerotherapy** (a'er-o-ther-ă-pu'tiks, a'er-o-ther'ă-pĭ). 1. Treatment of disease by fresh air. 2. Treatment of disease by air of different degrees of pressure or rarity, or medicated in various ways.

**aerothermotherapy** (a'er-o-ther'mo-ther'ă-pĭ) [ aero- + G. *thermos,* hot, + *therapeia,* healing ]. Treatment of disease by hot air.

**aerothorax** (a'er-o-tho'raks). Pneumothorax.

**aeroti'tis me'dia** [ aero- + G. *ous,* ear, + suffix *-itis,* inflammation ]. An acute or chronic traumatic inflammation of the middle ear caused by a reduction in pressure in the air in the tympanic cavity relative to ambient pressure, secondary to Eustachian tube obstruction. Often occurs on descent in an aircraft from high altitude.

**aerotonom'eter** [ aero- + G. *tonos,* tension, + *metron,* measure ]. 1. An instrument for estimating the tension or pressure of a gas. 2. An instrument for measuring the tension of oxygen and other gases in the blood or other fluids.

**aerotropism** (a-er-ot'ro-pizm) [ aero- + G. *tropos,* a turning ]. The tendency of microorganisms in culture media to group themselves about a bubble of air.

**aerourethroscope** (a'er-o-u-re'thro-skŏp) [ aero- + G. *ourēthra,* urethra, + *skōpeō,* to view ]. An instrument for inspection of the urethra after distending it with air.

**aerugo**, gen. **aeruginis** (e-ru'go) [ L. fr. *aes* (*aer-*), bronze ]. Green *verdigris.*

**aerumna** (e-rum'nah) [ L. contr. from *aegrimonia*, distress ]. Depression associated with a physical ailme ; mental and physical distress combined.

**Aescula'pian** [ L. *Aesculapius*, G. *Asklēpios*, the god of medicine ]. Esculapian. 1. Relating to Aesculapius. 2. Medical. 3. A medical practitioner.

**Aesculapius** (es'ku-la'pī-us). Roman name for the Greek god of medicine, Asclepius, *q. v.*

   staff of A., a rod with only one serpent encircling it and without wings; this is the correct symbol of the medical profession and the emblem of the American Medical Association, the Royal Army Medical Corps, and the Royal Canadian Medical Corps. See also caduceus, and illustrations under caduceus.

**aesculin** (es'ku-lin). Esculin.

**Aes'tival.** Estival.

**afeb'rile.** Nonfebrile; apyretic.

**afetal** (ă-fe'tal). Without relation to a fetus or intrauterine life.

**affect** (af'fekt) [ L. *affectus*, state of mind, fr. *afficio* (*adf-*), pp. - *fectus*, to have influence on. FAC- ]. Emotional feeling tone and mood attached to a thought, including its external manifestations.

   **flat a.**, absence of or diminution in the amount of emotional tone or outward emotional reaction typically shown under similar circumstances.

   **inappropriate a.**, emotional tone or outward emotional reaction out of harmony with the idea, object, or thought accompanying it.

**affec'tion.** 1. Feeling; love. 2. A disease; an abnormal condition of body or mind.

**affec'tive.** Pertaining to emotion, feeling, sensibility, or a mental state.

**affectiv'ity.** Feeling *tone.*

**affectomo'tor.** Pertaining to muscular manifestations associated with emotional or affective tone.

**Affenspalte** (ah'fen-spahl'teh) [ Ger. ]. *Sulcus* lunatus cerebri.

**af'ferens**, pl. **afferen'tia** [ L. ] [ NA ]. Afferent; see also afferentia.

**af'ferent** [ L. *afferens*, fr. *af-fero*, to bring to. FER- ]. Centripeta (1); eisodic; esodic; toward a center, denoting certain arteries, veins, lymphatics, and nerves.

**afferentia** (ă-fer-en'shīah). *Vasa* afferentia (afferent vessels); specifically, the afferent arteries of the kidneys.

**affinity** (ă-fĭn'ĭ-tĭ) [ L. *affinis*, neighboring, fr. *ad*, to, + *finis*, end, boundary ]. Attraction. 1. In chemistry, the force that impels certain atoms to unite with certain others to form compounds. 2. The selective staining of a tissue by a dye or the uptake of a dye, chemical, or other substance selectively by a tissue.

   **residual a.**, the secondary forces that enable apparently saturated atoms, ions, or molecules to attract other atoms or atom groups, giving rise to such phenomena as complex formation, hydration, adsorption, etc.

**affinous** (af'ĭ-nus). Pertaining to a marriage in which the partners are related, not consanguineously, but through another marriage.

**af'firma'tion.** The stage in autosuggestion in which the subject exhibits a positive reactive tendency.

**affix'us** [ L. ] [ NA ]. Attached.

**af'flux, afflux'ion** [ L. *af-fluo*, pp. *-fluxus*, to flow toward ]. A flowing toward; specifically, a flowing of blood toward any part; congestion.

**af'fricate.** A fricative speech sound begun plosively, as the ch in choice and the j in joy.

**affusion** (ă-fu'zhun) [ L. *af-fundo* (*ad-f.*), to pour into ]. The pouring of water upon the body or any of its parts for therapeutic purposes.

**AFH.** Abbreviation for anterior facial *height.*

**afi'brinogene'mia.** The absence of fibrinogen in the plasma. See also hypofibrinogenemia.

   **congenital a.**, a rare, heritable disease in which little or no fibrinogen can be found in plasma.

**af'latoxin.** Toxic metabolites of some strains of *Aspergillus flavus*, which have produced disease in animals eating peanut meal and other feed contaminated by this fungus.

**af'terbirth.** Secundinae; secundines; the placenta and membranes that are extruded from the uterus after birth.

**af'terbrain.** Obsolete term for rhombencephalon.

**af'tercare.** 1. The care and treatment of a patient after operation, or of one convalescing from an acute or serious illness. 2. Following psychiatric hospitalization, the continuing program of rehabilitation designed to reinforce the effects of therapy.

**af'tercat'aract.** Secondary *cataract* (2).

**af'tercontrac'tion.** A muscular contraction persisting a noticeable time after the stimulus has ceased.

**af'tercur'rent.** An electrical current induced in a muscle upon the termination of a constant current that has been passed through it.

**af'terdamp.** Irrespirable gases, chiefly carbon dioxide, left after the explosion of a mixture of fire-damp, or methane, and air in a mine.

**af'terdis'charge.** The prolongation of response of neural elements after cessation of stimulation.

**aftereffect** (af'ter-e-fekt'). A physical, physiologic, psychologic, or emotional phenomenon that continues after removal of the stimulus.

**af'tergild'ing.** The treatment of a histologic specimen of nervous tissue with gold salts.

**af'terhear'ing.** Aftersound.

**afterimage** (af'ter-im'ij). The image of an object of which the subjective sensation persists after the object has disappeared or the eyes are closed. It is called *positive* when its colors are the same as in the original, *negative* when the complementary colors are perceived.

**afterimpression** (af'ter-im-presh'un). Aftersensation.

**af'terload.** 1. The arrangement of a muscle so that, in shortening, it lifts a weight from an adjustable support or otherwise does work against a constant opposing force to which it is not exposed at rest. 2. The load or force thus encountered in shortening.

   **ventricular a.**, the resistance against which a ventricle contracts; contributed to by aortic or pulmonic artery impedance, peripheral vascular resistance, and mass and viscosity of blood.

**aftermovement** (af'ter-moov'ment). See Kohnstamm's *phenomenon.*

**af'terpains.** Painful cramplike contractions of the uterus occurring after childbirth.

**afterperception** (af'ter-per-sep'shun). The appreciation of a stimulus only after it has ceased to act.

**afterpotential** (af'ter-po-ten'shal). The small changes in electrical potential in a stimulated nerve which follow the main, or "spike," potential. They consist of an initial negative deflection followed by a positive deflection in the oscillograph record.

**af'tersensa'tion.** Afterimpression; a sensation persisting after its original cause has ceased to act.

**af'tersound.** Afterhearing; the subjective sensation of a sound after the cause of the sound has ceased.

**af'tertaste.** A taste persisting after contact of the tongue with the sapid substance has ceased.

**af'tertouch.** Persistence of touch sensation after removal of the stimulus.

**aftervision** (af'ter-vizh'un). Afterimage.

**afto'sa** [ Sp. and It. ]. Foot and mouth *disease.*

**Ag.** 1. Chemical symbol for the element silver (argentum). 2. Abbreviation for antigen.

**agalactia** (ă-gal-ak'shĭ-ah) [ G. *a-* priv. + *gala* (*galakt-*), milk ]. Absence of milk in the breasts after childbirth.

   **contagious a.**, a disease of sheep and goats in the Mediterranean region of Europe and Africa, caused by *Mycoplasma agalactiae*; it is a generalized, debilitating disease but one of the most obvious symptoms has been udder infection leading to decrease in milk production.

**agal'acto'sis.** Agalactia.

**agalac'tous.** Relating to agalactia, or to the diminution or absence of breast milk.

**agalorrhea** (ā-gal-ō-re'ah) [ G. *a*- priv. + *gala*, milk, + *rhoia*, a flow ]. Absence of the secretion or flow of milk.

**agamete** (ag'am-ēt) [ G. *a*- priv. + *gametēs*, husband. GAM- ]. A protozoan organism producing spores asexually.

**agam'ic.** Agamous.

**agam'maglob'uline'mia.** Hypogammaglobulinemia; a condition characterized by extremely low levels of γ-globulin in the blood and frequent occurrence of suppurative bacterial infections. Observed in two chief forms, primary (congenital, acquired, and transient forms) and secondary (secondary hypogammaglobulinemia, *q. v.*).

**acquired a.,** a form that becomes evident later in life; may occur in either sex.

**Bruton type a.,** see congenital a.

**congenital a.,** primary a. with congenital deficiency in the rate of production of immunoglobulins. It occurs in two types: (1) sex-linked a. (Bruton type), occurs in males with onset of infections at 4 to 6 months of age, when maternal immunoglobulins disappear from the circulation; plasma cells and pharyngeal lymphoid tissue are absent; sex-linked recessive inheritance; (2) Swiss type, affecting males and females, with onset in the first few weeks of life; there is severe leukopenia, lymphoid tissue is generally deficient, the thymus is small and hypoplastic; autosomal recessive inheritance in most families.

**primary a.,** primary hypogammaglobulinemia; includes transient, congenital, and acquired forms; results from decreased synthesis of γ-globulins, with levels usually less than 100 or 125 mg. per 100 ml.

**secondary a.,** secondary *hypogammaglobulinemia.*

**Swiss type a.,** see congenital a.

**transient a.,** transient hypogammaglobulinemia; a type of primary a.; occurs in infants of both sexes, usually during the second to sixth months of life, probably resulting from immaturity of lymphoid tissue; level of γ-globulin likely to be less than 100 to 150 mg. per 100 ml.

**agamocytogeny** (ă-gam'o-si'toj'ē-nĭ) [ G. *a*-priv. + *kytos*, cell, + *genesis*, becoming ]. Schizogony (2).

**Agamofilaria** (ă-gam'o-fi-la'rĭ-ah) [ G. *agamos*, unmarried, + L. *filum*, thread ]. A name given to immature filarial forms, the genera of the adult forms being undetermined.

**A. streptocerca** [ G. *streptos*, curved, + *kerkos*, tail ], *Dipetalonema streptocerca.*

**agamogenesis** (ag'ă-mo-jen'ē-sis) [ G. *agamos*, unmarried, + *genesis*, production ]. Asexual *reproduction.*

**ag'amogenet'ic.** Indicating asexual reproduction.

**ag'amog'ony** [ G. *a*- priv. + *gamos*, marriage, + *gonos*, offspring ]. Asexual *reproduction.*

**Agamomer'mis cu'licis.** A hairworm or mermithid nematode parasitic in the mosquito. A few cases are recorded of mermithid worms in humans, usually larval worms found emerging from body openings, presumably after injestion of infected insects or application of moist earth bearing free-living larval stages.

**ag'amont** [ G. *a*- priv. + *gamos*, marriage, + *ōn* (*ont-*), being ]. Schizont.

**agamous** (ag'ă-mus) [ G. *agamos*, unmarried ]. Denoting nonsexual reproduction, as by fission, budding, etc.

**aganglion'ic.** Without ganglia.

**agangliono'sis.** The state of being without ganglia; *e.g.,* absence of ganglion cells from Auerbach's plexus (plexus myentericus) is characteristic of congenital megacolon.

**agapism** (ah'gap-ism) [ G. *agapē,* brotherly love ]. The doctrine that exalts nonsexual (brotherly) love.

**agar** (ah'gar, a'gar) [ Bengalese ] (USP). Agar-agar; gelose; polysaccharide (a sulfated galactan) derived from seaweed (various red algae); used as a solidifying agent in culture media.

**ascit'ic a.,** a form of serum a.

**blood a.,** a mixture of blood and nutrient a., used for the cultivation of certain fastidious microorganisms.

**Bordet and Gengou's potato blood a.,** glycerine-potato a. with 25 per cent of blood.

**brilliant green bile salt a.,** a culture medium consisting of a. with peptone, lactose, sodium taurocholate, brilliant green (1:1000 solution), and picric acid solution (1 per cent).

**cholera a.,** an alkaline a. medium for cultures of the cholera vibrio; it is made by dissolving by heat a. 30 in nutrient bouillon 1000, and adding a 10 per cent solution of potassium hydrate 30.

**Conradi-Drigalski a.,** Drigalski-Conradi a.; a selective, nutrient medium for isolation of typhoid and other intestinal pathogens from fecal specimens. It contains the dye crystal violet, which generally inhibits growth of Gram-positive, but not Gram-negative, bacteria (Zeit. Hyg. *39:* 283: 1902).

**Drigalski-Conradi a.,** Conradi-Drigalski a.

**EMB a.,** eosin-methylene blue a.

**Endo a.,** Endo's medium; a medium containing peptone, lactose, dipotassium phosphate, agar, sodium sulfite, basic fuchsin, and distilled water. Originally developed for the isolation of the typhoid bacillus, this medium is now most useful in the bacteriological examination of water. Coliform organisms ferment the lactose, and their colonies become red and color the surrounding medium. Non-lactose-fermenting organisms produce clear, colorless colonies against the faint pink background of the medium.

**Endo's fuchsin a.,** fuchsin a.; nutrient a. containing lactose, alcoholic solution of fuchsin, sodium sulfite, and soda solution. Used as a culture medium to differentiate the typhoid bacillus from the colon bacillus and others of that group.

**eosin-methylene blue a.,** EMB a.; a lactose medium for isolation of coliform organisms.

**fuchsin a.,** Endo's fuchsin a.

**Guarnieri's gelatin a.,** similar to Stoddart's gelatin a. Used for the cultivation of the pneumococcus.

**lactose-litmus a.,** made by adding 2 per cent lactose and litmus to acid-free nutrient a. Used in the differentiation of the typhoid bacillus.

**Novy and MacNeal's blood a.,** a nutrient a. containing 2 volumes of defibrinated rabbit's blood; suitable for the cultivation of a number of trypanosomes.

**nutrient a.,** a simple solid medium containing 3 gm. of beef extract, 5 gm. of peptone, 15 gm. of agar, and 1 liter of water; used for growing many common heterotrophic bacteria.

**Pfeiffer's blood a.,** solid a. with a few drops of human blood smeared on the surface.

**Sabouraud's a.,** French proof a.; contains Chassaing's peptone 1 per cent, agar-agar 1.3 per cent, and maltose or mannite 4 per cent.

**serum a.,** an enriched medium for cultivation of fastidious organisms; prepared by adding sterile serum to melted a.

**Thalmann's a.,** a form of nutrient a., well adapted, it is claimed, to the cultivation of the gonococcus.

**agar-agar** [ Malay ]. Agar.

**agar'ic** [ G. *agarikon,* a kind of fungus ]. White, male, purging, or larch agaric; amadou; the dried fruit body of *Polyporus officinalis,* (family Polyporaceae), occurring in the form of brownish or whitish light masses. Contains agaric acid, which is responsible for the anhidrotic action of the mushroom.

**a. acid,** agaricic acid; agaricinic acid; agaricin; α-hexadecylcitric acid; α-cetylcitric acid; obtained from the white agaric, *Polyporus officinalis;* used in treating the night sweats of phthisis.

**fly a.,** *Amanita muscaria.*

**agar'icin.** Agaric acid.

**Agar'icus** [ L. *agaricum,* fr. G. *agarikon,* a tree fungus ]. A large genus of fungi (mushrooms) of which many are edible, others poisonous.

**A. arvensis,** edible but of coarse fiber.

**A. campestris,** common mushroom of the fields.

**A. hortense,** mushroom of the fields also cultivated commercially.

**A. muscarius,** *Amanita muscaria.*

**ag'arose.** The polysaccharide found in agar preparations, generally comprised of galactose and altered anhydrogalactose residues, with sulfate residues. Used in laboratory work as a chromatographic support.

**agas'tric** [ G. *a*-priv. + *gastēr,* belly ]. Without stomach or digestive tract.

**agastroneuria** (ă-gas-tro-nu'rĭ-ah) [ G. *a*- priv. + *gastēr*, belly, + *neuron*, nerve ]. Lowered nervous control of the stomach.

**Agave** (ā-gah've) [ G. *agauē*, fem. of *agauos*, noble ]. A genus of plants (family Amaryllidaceae) with stiff, spiny, and often succulent leaves; it is found chiefly in Mexico and includes the century plant, *A. americana.*

  **A. atrovi'rens**, a species from which pulque, an alcoholic beverage is made.

  **A. lechuguil'la**, causes lechuguilla poisoning in sheep and goats; see under poisoning.

**age** (āj) [ F. *âge*, L. *aetas* ]. 1. The period that has elapsed since the birth of a living being. 2. One of the periods into which human life is divided, distinguished by physical evolution, equilibrium, and involution. The seven a.'s of man are: infancy, childhood, adolescence, maturity, middle life, senescence, and senility. 3. To grow old; to gradually develop changes in structure which are not due to preventable disease or trauma and which are associated with an increased probability of death. 4. To cause artificially the appearance characteristic of one who has lived long or of a thing that has existed a long time; *e.g.,* to a. wine. 5. In dentistry, to a. an alloy for amalgam by heating it so as to make it set more slowly, increase strength, reduce flow, and have a stable shelf life. Aging occurs by relieving internal strains. Some gold alloys may by aged by heating to cause a phase change.

  **achievement a.**, the relationship between the chronologic age and the age of achievement, as established by standard achievement tests.

  **anatomical a.**, physical a.; a. in terms of structure rather than function.

  **basal a.**, highest mental a. level of the Stanford-Binet intelligence test at which all items are passed.

  **Binet a.**, the a. of the normal child with whose intelligence (as measured by the Binet-Simon tests) the intelligence of the abnormal child corresponds. The Binet a. of the profoundly retarded is 1 to 2 years; of the moderately to severely retarded, 3 to 7 years; of the borderline to mildly retarded; 8 to 12 years.

  **bone a.**, stage of development of bone as adjudged by x-ray, in contrast to chronologic age.

  **childbearing a.**, the period in a woman's life between puberty and the menopause.

  **chronologic a.**, (1) calendar a. or a record of time elapsed since birth; (2) a child's a., expressed in years and months, used as a measurement against which to evaluate the mental a. in computing his Stanford-Binet intelligence quotient.

  **developmental a.**, fetal a.; the period elapsed since implantation.

  **emotional a.**, a measure of emotional maturity by comparison with average emotional development.

  **fetal a.**, developmental a.

  **gestational a.**, the duration of pregnancy as measured from the first day of the last normal menstrual period to the birth; expressed as the number of completed weeks and completed days.

  **mental a.**, a measure, expressed in years and months, of a child's relative intelligence as determined by the Stanford-Binet scale; mental a. antecedes but is related to intelligence quotient.

  **physical a.**, anatomical a.

  **physiologic a.**, a. estimated in terms of function.

**agen'esis** [ G. *a*- priv. + *genesis*, production ]. Absence, failure of formation, or imperfect development of any part.

  **gonadal a.**, gonadal *aplasia.*

  **renal a.**, absence of one or both kidneys, most commonly unilateral with absence of the ipsilateral Müllerian duct and its derivatives; renal function is normal as long as the remaining kidney is intact; bilateral or complete renal a. is associated with Potter's facies and neonatal death.

**agenet'ic.** Pertaining to or characterized by agenesis.

**agenitalism** (a-jen'ĭ-tal-izm). The absence of genitals.

**agen'oso'mia** [ G. *a*- priv. + *genos*, sex, + *soma*, body ]. Markedly defective formation or absence of the genitalia in a fetus. The condition is usually accompanied by protrusion of the abdominal viscera through an incomplete abdominal wall.

**agenoso'mus.** A fetus with agenosomia.

**agent** (a'jent) [ L. *ago*, pres. p. *agens* (*agent*-), to perform ]. An active force or substance capable of producing an effect. For agents not listed here, see the specific name.

  **adrenergic blocking a.**, a compound that selectively blocks or inhibits responses to sympathetic adrenergic nerve activity (sympatholytic a.) and to epinephrine, norepinephrine, and other adrenergic amines (adrenolytic a.). Two distinct classes exist, α- and β-adrenergic receptor blocking a.'s.

  **adrenergic neuronal blocking a.**, a drug (*e.g.,* choline 2,6-xylyl ether bromide and guanethidine sulfate) that prevents the responses evoked by sympathetic nerve impulses; it does not inhibit the responses of the adrenergic receptors to circulating epinephrine, norepinephrine, and other adrenergic amines.

  **adrenolytic a.**, see adrenergic blocking a.

  **adrenomimetic a.**, see adrenergic *amine.*

  **alkylating a.'s**, cytotoxic a.'s such as nitrogen mustards, ethylenimines and alkyl sulfonates, used in the treatment of neoplastic diseases; they alkylate cellular constituents, and their physiological action is thought to arise from such alterations, including cross-linking and cycloalkylation of portions of DNA, of DNA to protein, or of protein to protein—mostly the first.

  **anesthetic a.**, anesthetic (1).

  **antianxiety a.**, minor tranquilizer; a functional category of drugs useful in the treatment of anxiety and able to reduce anxiety at doses which do not cause excessive sedation.

  **antifoaming a.'s**, chemicals, such as ethyl alcohol or 2-ethylhexanol, that lower surface tension (hence production of foam); used in laboratory evaporations; also administered with oxygen to patients in pulmonary edema to relieve the respiratory obstruction aggravated by the foam of edema fluid.

  **antipsychotic a.**, neuroleptic a.; major tranquilizer; a functional category of neuroleptic drugs that are helpful in the treatment of psychosis and have a capacity to ameliorate thought disorder; at present, there are three widely used classes: butyrophenones, phenothiazines, and thioxanthenes.

  **Bittner a.**, mammary cancer *virus* of mice.

  **blocking a.**, a drug that blocks transmission at an autonomic receptor site, autonomic synapse or neuromuscular junction.

  **chela'ting a.**, a compound, such as ethylenediaminetetraacetate, that forms a chelate type of complex with a metal, essentially removing the latter from solution without precipitation. The medicinal use of these a.'s is to render poisonous metal compounds innocuous. The resulting chelate complex is un-ionized, stable, and nonpoisonous, and is excreted in the urine.

  **chimpanzee coryza a.**, abbreviated CCA; respiratory syncytial *virus.*

  **coacervating a.**, see coacervate.

  **Eaton a.**, *Mycoplasma pneumoniae.*

  **embedding a.'s**, materials such as celloidin, paraffin, etc. in which specimens of tissue are set before being cut into sections for microscopic examination.

  **en'terokinet'ic a.**, one used to relieve intestinal atony.

  **F a.**, fertility a.; fertility factor; sex factor; an episome that determines bacterial mating type, conferring capacity to conjugate and to transfer chromosomal elements. $F^+$ (male) strains possess pili (F pili) through which the F a. apparently is transferred to $F^-$ (female) bacteria.

  **F' a.**, F' factor; F genote; originally, any altered F a. (F factor); use now restricted to those that carry chromosomal elements.

  **fertility a.**, F a.

  **foamy a.**, foamy virus; an unclassified agent or virus that commonly contaminates cultures of monkey kidney cells.

  **ganglionic blocking a.**, an a. that impairs the passage of impulses in autonomic ganglia.

  **immunosuppressive a.**, immunosuppressant; immunodepressor; immunodepressant; an a. used to effect immunosuppression.

  **LDH a.**, lactate dehydrogenase *virus.*

  **lissive a.**, a therapeutic or chemical a. that releases spasticity without causing flaccidity.

**luting a.,** a fastening material or cement; *e.g.,* plaster or wax to hold casts to an articulator, or cement to hold teeth on a metal base.

**MS-1 a.,** a strain of hepatitis virus A.

**MS-2 a.,** a strain of hepatitis virus B.

**mutagenic a.,** mutagen.

**neuroleptic a.,** a neurolept or neuroleptic; any of a family of parenterally administered drugs producing analgesia, sedation, and tranquilization; see also antipsychotic a.

**neuromuscular blocking a.,** a compound which, by virtue of its actions on the neuromuscular junction, inhibits the ability of motor nerve stimuli to produce skeletal muscle contraction (*e.g.,* curare, succinylcholine, gallamine, pancuronium).

**nondepolarizing neuromuscular blocking a.,** a compound that paralyzes skeletal muscle primarily by inhibiting transmission of nerve impulses at the meuromuscular junction rather than by affecting the membrane potention of motor end-plate or muscle fibers.

**reducing a.,** any substance that has the power to participate in a reaction involving the transfer of electrons from itself, in the process being oxidized.

**sclero'sing a.,** a compound such as sodium ricinoleate; used in the treatment of varicose veins.

**surface-active a.,** see surfactant.

**sympathetic a.,** see adrenergic *amine.*

**sympatholytic a.,** see adrenergic blocking a.

**sympathomimetic a.,** see adrenergic *amine.*

**therapeutic a.,** see drug.

**transforming a.,** mitogen.

**TRIC a.'s,** abbreviation for trachoma and inclusion conjunctivitis a.'s. See *Chlamydia trachomatis.*

**vagolytic a.,** see vagolytic.

**agerasia** (ă-jer-a'zĭ-ah) [ G. *agērasia,* eternal youth, fr. *a-* priv. + *gēras,* old age ]. An appearance of youth in old age.

**ageusia** (ă-gu'sĭ-ah) [ G. *a-* priv. + *geusis,* taste ]. Loss of the sense of taste.

**ageustia** (ă-gūs'tĭ-ah). Ageusia.

**agger,** pl. **aggares** (aj'er, ag'er, -ēz) [ L. mound ] [ NA ]. An eminence or projection.

    **a. nasi** [ NA ], ridge of the nose; an elevation on the lateral wall of the nasal cavity lying between the atrium of the middle meatus and the olfactory sulcus. It is formed by the mucous membrane covering the base of the ethmoidal crest of the maxilla.

    **a. perpendicula'ris,** *eminentia* fossae triangularis.

    **a. valvae venae,** a slight prominence on the wall of a vein corresponding to the location of a valve.

**agglom'erate, agglom'erated** [ L. *ag-glomero,* to wind into a ball; from *ad,* to, + *glomus,* a ball ]. Crowded together into a mass.

**agglomera'tion.** A crowded mass of independent but similar units; a cluster.

**agglutinant** (ă-glu'tĭ-nant) [ L. *ad,* to + *gluten,* glue ]. 1. Indicating a method of encouraging the healing of a wound by drawing together and holding the edges by adhesion. 2. An adhesive material, *e.g.,* plaster or gluelike material, that holds parts together.

**agglutinate** (ă-glu'tĭ-nāt). To accomplish, or be subjected to, agglutination.

**agglutination** (ă-glu'tĭ-na'shun) [ L. *ad,* to, + *gluten,* glue ]. 1. The process by which suspended bacteria, cells, or other particles of similar size are caused to adhere and form into clumps; agglutination is similar to precipitation, but the particles are larger and are in suspension rather than being in solution. For specific a. reactions in the various blood groups, see appendix 2, Blood Groups. 2. Adhesion of the surfaces of a wound.

    **acid a.,** the clumping together of certain microorganisms at high hydrogen ion concentration.

    **auto-a.,** see autoagglutination.

    **bacte'riogen'ic a.,** the clumpin of erythrocytes as a result of effects of bacteria or their products.

    **cold a.,** a. of red blood cells by their own serum (see autoagglutination), or by any other serum when the blood is cooled below body temperature, but is most pronounced below 25°C. The phenomenon results from cold agglutinins. Although it is seen occasionally in the blood of apparently normal persons, it is more frequent in scarlet fever, staphylococcal infections, pneumonia, certain hemolytic anemias, and trypanosomiasis.

    **cross a.,** group a.

    **group a.,** cross a.; the a., in minor degree, of several varieties of bacteria by a serum specific for another bacterial form.

    **immediate a.,** healing by first intention. See under intention.

    **immune a.,** a. caused by antibody (agglutinin) that is specific for the suspended bacterium, cell, or antigen that has been coated on a particle of suitable size.

    **mediate a.,** healing by second intention. See under intention.

    **mixed a.,** see mixed agglutination *reaction.*

    **nonimmune i.,** (1) a. caused by a lectin, having a degree of specificity the mechanism of which is not understood; (2) a. that results from nonspecific factors, such as in the case of acid a. or spontaneous a.

    **passive a.,** a. of particles that have been coated with soluble antigen, by antiserum specific for the adsorbed antigen.

    **spontaneous a.,** nonspecific clumping of organisms in saline related to lack of polar groups in electrolyte solution.

**agglu'tinative.** Causing, or able to cause, agglutination.

**agglu'tinin.** 1. Immune a.; that causes clumping or agglutination of the bacteria or other cells, which either stimulated the formation of the a., or contain immunologically similar, reactive material; effects of a. may be observed *in vitro* and *in vivo,* under certain conditions. 2. A substance, other than a specific agglutinating antibody, that causes organic particles to agglutinate (for example, a lectin, *q.v.*), commonly with qualifications (for example, plant a.).

    **auto-a.,** see autoagglutinin.

    **bacterio-a.,** see bacterioagglutinin.

    **blood group a.'s,** see appendix 2, Blood Groups.

    **chief a.,** major a.

    **cold a.,** a. that agglutinates human group O erythrocytes at zero to 5°C., but not at 37°C.; found in the serum of less than half of patients with primary atypical pneumonia, and also in certain other diseases, especially trypanosomiasis; titer is usually at a peak relatively early during recovery.

    **cross-reacting a.,** group a.

    **flagel'lar a.,** H a.

    **group a.,** cross-reacting a.; a. (1) specific for a group antigen (*q.v.*).

    **H a.,** (1) flagellar a.; an a. that is formed as the result of stimulation by, and reacts with, the thermolabile antigen(s) in the flagella of motile strains of microorganisms; (2) see ABO blood group, appendix 2.

    **immune a.,** agglutinin (1).

    **major a.,** chief a.; a. (1) present in greatest quantity in an antiserum and that was evoked by the most dominant of a mosaic of antigens.

    **minor a.,** partial a.; a. (1) present in an antiserum in lesser concentration than the major a.

    **O a.,** (1) somatic a.; an a. that is formed as the result of stimulation by, and reacts with, the relatively thermostable antigen(s) in the cell bodies of microorganisms; (2) see ABO blood group, appendix 2.

    **partial a.,** minor a.

    **plant a.,** a lectin.

    **saline a.,** an anti-Rh antibody which causes agglutination of Rh+ erythrocytes when they are suspended either in saline or in a protein medium.

    **serum a.,** an anti-Rh antibody which coats Rh+ erythrocytes; the cells do not agglutinate when suspended in saline, but do agglutinate when suspended in serum or other protein media such as albumin.

    **somatic a.,** O a. (1).

    **warm a.'s,** see autoantibody.

**agglutin'ogen** [ agglutinin + G. suffix *-gen,* production ]. An antigenic substance that stimulates the formation of specific agglutinin, which, under certain conditions, causes agglutination of cells that contain the a.

    **blood group a.'s,** see appendix 2, Blood Groups.

    **T a.,** formed from a latent receptor on human red cells by the action of an enzyme in cultures of certain bacteria.

**agglu'tinogen'ic.** Capable of causing the production of an agglutinin.

**agglu'tinophil'ic** [ agglutination + G. *phileō*, to love ]. Readily undergoing pronounced agglutination.

**agglu'tinophore** [ agglutinin + G. *phoros*, bearing ]. The reactive portion of the antibody molecule, thought to combine with antigen-receptors in such a manner that the cells become physicochemically bound in aggregates (agglutinated).

**agglu'tinoscope** [ agglutination + G. *skopeō*, to view ]. A magnifying glass or simple system of lenses used to observe the phenomenon of agglutination in the test tube.

**agglu'togen.** Agglutinogen.

**agglu'togenic.** Agglutinogenic.

**agglutom'eter** [ agglutination + G. *metron*, measure ]. An apparatus used to observe the results of a microscopic agglutination without resorting to the ordinary microscope.

**aggred. feb.** Abbreviation for during the onset of the fever.

**aggregate** (ag're-gāt) [ L. *ag-grego*, pp. *-atus*, to add to, fr. *grex* (greg-), a flock ]. 1. To unite or come together in a mass or cluster. 2. The total of individual units making up a mass or cluster.

**ag'grega'ted.** Collected together, thereby forming a cluster, clump, or mass of individual units.

**aggres'sin** [ L. *agressor*, an assailant, fr. *ag-gredior*, pp. *-gressus*, to attack, fr. *gradior*, to go, fr. *gradus*, a step ]. A substance postulated to inhibit the resistance mechanisms of the host; also called auxillary pathogenic factor.

**aggression** (ă-gresh'un). A domineering, forceful, or assaultive verbal or physical action toward another person as the motor component of the affects of anger, hostility, or rage.

**aggressiv'ity.** Ability of pathogens to invade.

**aging** (a'jing). The process of growing old, especially by failure of replacement of cells in sufficient number to maintain function; this particularly affects cells like neurons that are incapable of mitotic division.
   **clonal a.,** the deterioration in successive generations of a clone; thus paramecium and other simple forms if allowed to reproduce asexually for a number of generations invariably undergo deterioration, the characters of each group of descendants progressively departing from those of the original sexually produced ancestor.

**agitographia** (aj'ĭ-to-graf'ĭ-ah) [ L. *agito*, to impel, fr. *ago*, to drive, + G. *graphō*, to write ]. A condition in which the patient writes with great rapidity and leaves out words or parts of words.

**agitolalia** (aj'ĭ-to-la'lĭ-ah) Agitophasia.

**agitophasia** (aj'ĭ-to-fa'zĭ-ah) [ L. *agito*, to hurry, + G. *phāsis*, speech ]. Agitolalia; abnormally rapid speech in which words are imperfectly spoken or dropped out of a sentence.

**aglaucopsia** (ă-glaw-kop'sĭ-ah) [ G. *a-* priv. + *glaukos*, bluish green, + *opsis*, vision ]. Green *blindness*.

**aglobu'lia** [ G. *a-* priv. + L. *globulus*, globule. GLO- ]. Obsolete term for anemia.

**a'globulio'sis.** Obsolete term for a condition characterized by anemia.

**aglob'ulism.** Obsolete term for anemia.

**aglomer'ular.** Having no glomeruli; said especially of a kidney in which the glomeruli have been destroyed, or kidneys of certain fish, e.g., toad fish, that possess tubules but no glomeruli.

**aglossia** (ă-glos'ĭ-ah) [ G. *a-* priv. + *glōssa*, tongue ]. Absence of the tongue.

**aglossos'toma** [ G. *a-* priv. + *glōssa*, tongue, + *stoma*, mouth ]. A fetus without a tongue and with a malformed (usually closed) mouth.

**aglucone, aglucon** (a-glu'kōn, -kon). The portion of a glucoside other than the glucose.

**aglutition** (a-gloo-tish'un). Dysphagia.

**aglycone, aglycon** (a-gli'kōn, -kon). The noncarbohydrate portion of a glycoside.

**agly'cosu'ric.** Relating to the absence of glycosuria.

**agmatine.** HN=C(NH₂)NH(CH₂)₄NH₂; 1-amino-4-guanidinobutane; the amine resulting from the decarboxylation of arginine. Found in ergot, sponges, octopus muscle, and the pollen of *Ambrosia artemisifolia*.

**agmatol'ogy** [ G. *agma* (*agmat-*), a fragment + *logos*, study ]. The branch of surgery concerned especially with fractures.

**ag'men,** pl. **agmina** [ L. a multitude ]. A collection; an aggregation.
   **a. peyerian'um,** *folliculi* lymphatici aggregati.

**ag'minate, ag'minated** [ L. *agmen*, a multitude ]. Aggregate; agglomerate; collected together into clusters or masses.

**ag'nail.** Hangnail.

**agnathia** (ag-na'thĭ-ah) [ G. *a-* priv. + *gnathos*, jaw ]. Absence of the lower jaw, usually accompanied by approximation of the ears (see octocephaly).

**agnathous** (ag'na-thus). Relating to agnathia.

**agna'thus.** An individual exhibiting agnathia.

**agnea** (ag-ne'ah) [ G. *agnoia*, want of perception ]. Failure to recognize objects.

**Agnew,** Cornelius R., U. S. ophthalmologist, 1830–1888. See A.-Verhoeff *incision.*

**agnogenic** (ag'no-jen'ik) [ G. *a-* priv. + *gnosis*, knowledge, + *genesis*, origin ]. Idiopathic; of unknown origin or cause.

**agnosia** (ag-no'sĭ-ah) [ G. ignorance; from *a-* priv. + *gnōsis*, knowledge ]. Lack of sensory-perceptual ability to recognize objects.
   **auditory a.,** central auditory imperception of sound; ability to perceive sound at the end organ with inability to interpret it centrally.
   **finger a.,** inability of a patient to recognize his own fingers.
   **ideational a.,** loss of the concept due to damage of association areas.
   **localization a.,** inability to recognize the area where the skin is touched.
   **optic a.,** inability to interpret visual images.
   **position a.,** failure to recognize the posture of an extremity.
   **tactile a.,** inability to recognize objects by the touch.
   **visual-spatial a.,** disturbance in spatial orientation and in understanding of spatial relations.

**agnos'terol.** A sterol differing from lanosterol in having two double bonds at 7,8 and 9,11.

**-agogue, -agog** [ G. *agōgos*, leading forth. ACT- ]. Suffix indicating a promoter or stimulant of; e.g., galactagogue, q. v.

**ago'nad.** A person with absence, congenital or operative, of the sex glands.

**agon'adal.** Relating to the absence of gonads.

**ag'onal.** Relating to the process of dying or the moment of death, so called because of the former erroneous notion that dying is a painful process.

**agoni'adin.** Plumieride.

**ag'onist** [ G. *agōn*, a contest ]. 1. Denoting a muscle in a state of contraction, with reference to its opposing muscle, or antagonist. 2. A drug capable of combining with receptors to initiate drug actions; it possesses affinity and intrinsic activity.

**agony** (ag'o-nĭ) [ G. *agōn*, a struggle, trial ]. 1. Intense pain or anguish of body or mind. 2. The act of dying.

**agoraphobia** (ag'o-rah-fo'bĭ-ah) [ G. *agora*, marketplace, + *phobos*, fear ]. Dread of being in or crossing open spaces.

**agouti** (ah-goo'te) [ Fr. fr. native Indian ]. *Dasyprocta;* a genus of rodents of the guinea pig family. A possible carrier of American cutaneous leishmaniasis.

**-agra** (ag'rah) [ G. *agra*, a seizure. ACT- ]. Suffix meaning sudden onslaught of acute pain.

**agraffe** (ă-graf') [ Fr. *agrafe*, a hook, clasp ]. An appliance for clamping together the edges of a wound, used in lieu of sutures.

**agrammat'ica.** Agrammatism.

**agram'matism** [ G. *agrammatos*, unlearned. GRAPH- ]. Loss, through cerebral disease, of the power to construct a grammatical or intelligible sentence; words are uttered, but not in proper sequence; a form of aphasia.

**agram'matolo'gia.** Agrammatism.

**agran'ulocyte** [ G. *a-* priv. + L. *granulum*, granule, + G. *kytos*, cell ]. A nongranular leukocyte.

**agranulocytopenia** (ah-gran'u-lo-si'to-pe'nĭ-ah) [ agranulocyte + G. *penia*, poverty ]. Agranulocytosis.

**agran'ulocyto'sis.** Acute condition characterized by pronounced leukopenia with great reduction in the number of polymorphonuclear leukocytes (frequently less than 500 granulocytes per cu. mm.); infected ulcers likely to develop in the throat, intestinal tract, and other mucous membranes, as well as in the skin. Termed also agranulocytopenia; agranulocytic angina.

    **feline a.,** panleukopenia.

**agran'uloplas'tic** [ G. *a-* priv. + L. *granulum*, granule, + G. *plastikos*, formative ]. Capable of forming nongranular cells, and incapable of forming granular cells.

**agraph'ia** [ G. *a-* priv. + *graphō*, to write ]. Logographia; loss of the ability to write.

    **absolute a.,** atactic a.; literal a.; a. in which not even unconnected letters can be written.

    **acoustic a.,** acquired inability to write from dictation.

    **amnemonic a.,** a. in which letters and words can be written, but not connected sentences.

    **atactic a.,** absolute a.

    **cerebral a.,** graphic or graphomotor aphasia; mental a.; the inability to express ideas in writing.

    **literal a.,** absolute a.

    **mental a.,** cerebral a.

    **motor a.,** a. due to muscular incoordination.

    **musical a.,** loss of power to write musical notation.

    **optic a.,** inability to copy.

    **verbal a.,** a. in which single letters can be written, but not words.

**agraph'ic.** Relating to or marked by agraphia.

**agrav'ic.** Theoretically, denoting absolute lack of gravity, which does not exist anywhere in the universe but is approached in weightlessness and zerogravity.

**agre'mia** [ G. *agra*, a seizure, + *haima*, blood ]. The state of the blood in gout.

**ag'riothy'mia** [ G. *agriothymos*, wild of temper, fr. *agrios*, wild, + *thymos*, spirit ]. Wild, ferocious mania.

**ag'rius** [ G. *agrios*, wild ]. Rarely used term used to denote a severe, extensive, or rapidly progressive dermatosis.

**agroma'nia** [ G. *agros*, field, + *mania*, frenzy ]. Morbid impulse to live in the open country or in solitude.

**Agropy'ron repens** [ G. *agros*, field, + *pyr*, fire; L. *repens*, creeping ]. Triticum.

**agrypnia** (ă-grip'nĭ-ah) [ G. sleeplessness, fr. *agreō*, to hunt after, + *hypnos*, sleep ]. Insomnia.

**agrypnocoma** (ă-grip'no-ko'mah) [ *agrypnos*, sleepless, + *kōma*, coma ]. A wakeful, apathetic, or lethargic state.

**agryp'node.** Agrypnotic (2).

**agrypnot'ic.** 1. Sleepless: marked by, or suffering from, insomnia. 2. Agrypnode; a drug that prevents sleep.

**ague** (a'gu) [ Fr. *aigu*, acute ]. 1. Archaic term for malarial fever. 2. A chill.

    **brass workers' a.,** a condition in brass workers with clinical manifestations resembling those of malaria.

    **brow a.,** intermittent supraorbital neuralgia.

    **face a.,** trigeminal *neuralgia*.

    **quartan a., quotid'ian a., ter'tian a., malignant tertian a.,** see under malaria.

**ague root** (a'gu). Aletris.

**agyiophobia** (aj'ĭ-o-fo'bĭ-ah) [ G. *agyia*, street, + *phobos*, fear ]. Street phobia; morbid fear of being in a street; a type of agoraphobia.

**agy'ria** [ G. *a-* priv. + *gyros*, circle ]. Lissencephaly; lack of convolutional pattern in the cerebral cortex due to defect of development.

**A.H.** Abbreviation for hyperopic astigmatism.

**AHF.** Abbreviation for antihemophilic factor; see *factor* VIII.

**AHG.** Abbreviation for antihemophilic globulin; see *factor* VIII.

**ahis'tan.** HISTANTIN; 10-(*N*,*N*-dimethylglycyl)phenothiazine; antihistaminic agent.

**ahis'tida'sia.** Histidinemia.

**Ahlfeld,** J.F., German obstetrician, 1843–1929. See A.'s *method, sign.*

**Ahumada,** J. C., Argentinian physician. See A.-Del Castillo *syndrome.*

**a'hylogno'sia** [ G. *a-* priv., + *hyle*, matter, + *gnosis*, recognition ]. Inability to recognize differences of density, weight, and roughness.

**ahyp'nia, ahypno'sis** [ G. *a-* priv. + *hypnos*, sleep ]. Insomnia.

**aichmophobia** (īk'mo-pho'bĭ-ah) [ G. *aichmē*, a point, + *phobos*, fear ]. Morbid fear of being touched by the finger or any slender pointed object.

**AID.** Abbreviation for donor of heterologous (artificial) insemination.

**aid** (ād). Any therapeutic procedure or any device intended to correct or attenuate a handicap.

    **prosthetic speech a.,** an appliance used to close a cleft in the hard or soft palate or both, or to replace lost tissue necessary for the production of good speech.

**aidoi-, aidoio-** [ G. *aidoia*, genitals ]. Archaic combining form relating to the genitals; for some words beginning thus, see ede-, edeo-.

**aidoiomania** (i-doy-o-ma'nĭ-ah). Edeomania;

**AIH.** Abbreviation for homologous (artificial) insemination.

**Ailan'thus** [ of Eastern derivation ]. Tree of heaven; a genus of trees of the Simarubaceae; the bark and leaves of *A. glandulosa* possess anthelmintic and purgative properties.

**aileron** (a'ler-on) [ Fr. *aile*, wing ]. A winglike extension of a fascia or sheath.

**ailurophobia** (i-loo-ro-fo'bĭ-ah) [ G. *ailouros*, cat, + *phobos*, fear ]. Aelurophobia; morbid fear of or aversion to cats.

**ainhum** (ī'yoom) [ from an African (Lagos) word meaning to saw ]. Dactylolysis spontanea; the spontaneous amputation of a toe; a constricting fibrous ring develops in the digitoplantar fold, usually of the little toe, gradually resulting in loss of the toe; it most commonly affects male Negroes in the tropics.

**air** (ār) [ G. *aēr;* L. *aer* ]. The atmosphere; a mixture of gases in the following approximate percentages by volume, after water vapor has been removed: oxygen, 20.94; nitrogen, 78.03; argon and other rare gases, 0.99; carbon dioxide, 0.04. Formerly used to mean any respiratory gas, regardless of its composition. See also related entries under volume and capacity.

    **alkaline a.,** ammonia.

    **alveolar a.,** alveolar *gas*.

    **complemental a.,** inspiratory reserve *volume*.

    **complementary a.,** inspiratory *capacity*.

    **functional residual a.,** functional residual *capacity*.

    **liquid a.,** a. which, by means of intense cold and pressure, has been liquefied.

    **minimal a.,** the volume of a. that remains in the lungs and cannot be expelled after they have been removed from the body, or after the chest has been opened.

    **reserve a.,** expiratory reserve *volume*.

    **residual a.,** residual *volume*.

    **supplemental a.,** expiratory reserve *volume*.

    **tidal a.,** tidal *volume*.

    **vitiated a.,** a. containing a reduced percentage of oxygen.

**airbra'sive.** A device for removal of tooth structure or deposits by means of a stream of $CO_2$ and abrasive directed through a tubular tip.

**Aird,** Robert B., U. S. neurologist, *1903. See Flynn-A. *syndrome.*

**air'way.** 1. Any part of the respiratory tract through which air passes during breathing. 2. In anesthesia or resuscitation, a device for correcting obstruction to breathing, especially oropharyngeal and nasopharyngeal a., endotracheal a., or tracheotomy tube.

    **conducting a.,** the a. from the nasal cavity to a terminal bronchiole.

    **respiratory a.,** that part of the a. where interchange of gases occurs; it includes respiratory bronchioles, alveolar ducts, sacs, and alveoli.

**Ajellomy'ces dermatit'idis.** The perfect state of the fungus *Blastomyces dermatitides;* this sexual state was obtained by pairing compatible strains of this fungus, and is placed in the family Gymnoascaceae.

**ajmaline.** RAUWOLFINE; an alkaloid from roots of *Rauwolfia serpentina;* used for treatment of hypertension.

**aj'owan oil.** Ptychotis oil; a volatile oil distilled from the fruit of *Carum copticum,* one of the sources of thymol; carminative, aromatic, and expectorant.

**akan'thion.** Acanthion.

**akaryocyte** (a-kăr-ĭ-o-sīt) [ G. *a*- priv. + *karyon,* kernel, + *kytos,* a hollow (cell) ]. A cell without a nucleus (karyon), such as the erythrocyte.

**akaryote** (a-kăr'ĭ-ōt) [ G. *a*- priv. + *karyon,* kernel ]. Akaryocyte.

**akatama** (ah-kah-tah'mah) [ a native word ]. An endemic peripheral neuritis affecting the adult natives of West Central Africa. Characterized by burning, prickling, numbness, and erythema.

**akat'amathe'sia.** Acatamathesia.

**akathisia** (a-kă-thiz'ĭ-ah) [ G. *a*- priv. + *kathisis,* a sitting ]. Akatizia; acathisia; a neurosis characterized by an inability to remain in a sitting posture; motor restlessness and a feeling of muscular quivering.

**akatiz'ia.** Akathisia.

**akem'be.** Onyalai.

**akerato'sis.** Deficiency or absence of the horny tissue.

**Akerlund deformity.** See under deformity.

**akinesia** (a-ki-ne'sĭ-ah) [ G. *a*- priv. + *kinēsis,* movement ]. Akinesis. 1. Absence or loss of the power of voluntary motion. 2. Immobility. 3. The postsystolic interval of rest of the heart. 4. A neurosis accompanied by paretic symptoms.
   **a. al'gera** [ G. *algos,* pain ], a condition marked by severe neuralgic pain of indeterminate origin which is excited by any movement.
   **a. amnes'tica** [ G. *amnēsia,* forgetfulness ], loss of muscular power from disuse.
   **reflex a.,** absence of reflex responses.

**akine'sic.** Akinetic.

**akinesis** (a-ki-ne'sis). Akinesia.

**akinesthesia** (a-kin'es-the'zĭ-ah) [ G. *a*- priv. + *kinēsis,* motion, + *aisthēsis,* sensation ]. Absence of the sense of perception of movement; absence of the muscular sense.

**akinet'ic.** Relating to or suffering from akinesia.

**akiyami** (ah-kĭ-yah'mĭ). Hasamiyami.

**ak'lomide** (USAN). NOVASTAT; 2-chloro-4-nitrobenzamide; coccidiostat used in veterinary practice.

**Al.** Chemical symbol of the element aluminum (aluminium).

**Ala.** Symbol for alanine or its mono- or diradical.

**ala,** gen. and pl. **a'lae** (a'lah) [ L. wing ]. 1 [ NA ]. Any winglike or expanded structure. 2. Axilla.
   **a. auris,** auricula.
   **a. cerebel'li,** a. lobuli centralis.
   **a. cine'rea,** *trigonum* nervi vagi.
   **a. cristae galli** [ NA ], wing of the crista galli; a small lateral expansion of the ethmoid bone from the front of the crista galli on each side that articulates with the frontal bone and forms the foramen cecum.
   **alae lin'gulae cerebel'li,** *vincula* lingulae cerebelli.
   **a. lob'uli centralis** [ NA ], a. cerebelli; the lateral winglike projection of the central lobule of the cerebellum.
   **a. major ossis sphenoidalis** [ NA ], a. temporalis; the great wing of the sphenoid bone.
   **a. minor ossis sphenoidalis** [ NA ], Ingrassia's apophysis or wing; the lesser wing of the sphenoid bone.
   **a. nasi** [ NA ], the wing of the nostril; the outer more or less flaring wall of each nostril.
   **a. ossis il'ii** [ NA ], the upper flaring portion of the ilium.
   **a. sacra'lis,** a broad flat projection on either side of the base of the sacrum.
   **a. tempora'lis,** a. major ossis sphenoidalis.
   **a. vespertilio'nis** [ L. bat's wing ], obsolete, but descriptive, term for broad ligament of the uterus.
   **a. vo'meris** [ NA ], wing of the vomer; an everted lip on either side of the upper border of the vomer, between which fits the rostrum of the sphenoid bone.

**al'abam'ine, al'abam'ium.** Astatine.

**alacrima** (a-lak'rĭ-mah) [ G. *a*- priv. + L. *lacrima,* tear ]. A congenital persistent absence of tears.

**Alajouanine,** T. See Foix-A. *myelitis.*

**ala'lia** [ G. *a*- priv. + *lalia,* talking ]. Loss of the power of speech through impairment in the articulatory apparatus; see also aphonia.

**alal'ic.** Relating to alalia.

**al'anine.** 2- or α-Aminopropionic acid; CH₃CH-(NH₂)COOH; one of the amino acids occurring widely in proteins.

**β -alanine.** NH₂CH₂CH₂COOH; a decarboxylation production of aspartic acid.

**alanine aminotransferase.** Alanine transaminase; enzyme (EC 2.6.1.2) transferring amino groups from L-alanine to 2-ketoglutarate, or the reverse (from L-glutamate to pyruvate).

**D-alanine aminotransferase** (EC 2.6.1.21). Effects the same reaction as alanine aminotransferase, but with D-alanine and D-glutamate.

**alanine-oxomalonate aminotransferase** (EC 2.6.1.47). Accomplishes the transfer of the amino groups of L-alanine to oxomalonate, an action similar to that of alanine aminotransferase.

**alanine racemase** (EC 5.1.1.1). An enzyme, requiring pyridoxal phosphate as coenzyme, that catalyzes the racemization of L-alanine to D-alanine. Found in various microorganisms, where it may play a role in the biosynthesis of the D-amino acids present in the capsular proteins.

**alanine transaminase.** Alanine aminotransferase.

**alanosine.** L-2-Amino-3-(*N*-nitroso)hydroxylaminopropionic acid; an antibiotic substance produced by *Streptomyces alanosinicus*; possesses antineoplastic and antiviral activity.

**Alanson,** Edward, British surgeon, 1747–1823. See A.'s *amputation.*

**al'ant camphor.** Alantolactone.

**alan'tin.** Inulin.

**al'antol.** Inulol; a yellowish liquid obtained by distillation from the root of *Inula helenium* or elecampane. Used internally as an irritating tonic. Also used externally as a mild rubefacient.

**alan'tolac'tone.** Alant camphor; helenin; a terpene obtained from elecampane, *Inula helenium;* antiseptic and anthelmintic.

**alant starch.** Inulin.

**al'anyl.** The acyl radical of alanine.

**a'lar.** 1. Relating to a wing; winged. 2. Axillary. 3. Relating to the ala of such structures as the nose, sphenoid, sacrum, etc.

**alas'trim** [ Pg. *alastrar,* to scatter over ]. Cuban itch; amaas; glass-pox; milkpox; variola minor; a mild form of smallpox caused by a less virulent strain of virus.

**alazopep'tin.** An antibiotic, produced by *Streptomyces griseoplanus,* with antitumor activity.

**alba** (al'bah) [ fem. of L. *albus,* white ]. *Substantia* alba.

**Albarran y Dominguez,** Joaquin, Paris urologist, 1860–1912. See A.'s *glands, test, tubules.*

**albas'pidin.** Polystichalbin; a crystalline constituent of aspidium;

**albe'do** [ L. whiteness. ALB- ]. The light reflected from any surface.
   **a. ret'inae,** obsolete term for edema of the retina.

**Albee,** Fred H., New York surgeon, 1876–1945. See A.'s *operation.*

**Albers-Schönberg** (ahl-bärs-shën'bärg), Heinrich E., German radiologist, 1865–1921. See A.-S. *disease.*

**Albert,** Eduard, Vienna surgeon, 1841–1900. See A.'s *operation, suture.*

**Albert,** Henry, U.S. physician, 1878–1930. See A.'s *stair.*

**al'bicans,** pl. **albican'tia** [ L. ]. 1 [ NA ]. 2. *Corpus* albicans.

**albiduria** (al'bĭ-du'rĭ-ah) [ L. *albidus,* whitish, + G. *ouron,* urine ]. Albinuria; the passing of pale or white urine of low specific gravity, as in chyluria.

**al'bidus** [ L. ]. White, whitish.

**Albini,** Giuseppe, Italian physiologist, 1827–1911. See A.'s *nodules.*

**albinism** (al'bĭ-nizm) [ L. *albus,* white ]. Congenital leukoderma; congenital leukopathia; congenital deficiency or absence of pigment in skin, hair, and eyes due to metabolic block in production of melanin; usually autosomal recessive inheritance.

**cutaneous a.,** a heritable condition characterized by patterned loss of skin pigment on extremities and ventral thorax; white forelock often present; no ocular findings.

**ocular a.,** congenital absence of pigment chiefly of the iris and choroid; it may be partial or complete.

**rufous a.,** xanthism.

**total a.,** albinismus totalis; albinismus universalis; congenital total loss of pigment from skin, hair, and choroid.

**universal incomplete a.,** albinoidism.

**albinismus** (al'bĭ-niz'mus) [ L. ]. Albinism.

**a. conscriptus,** piebaldness.

**a. totalis, a. universalis,** total *albinism.*

**albi'no** [ L. *albus,* white ]. An individual with albinism.

**albinoidism** (al'bĭ-noyd-izm) [ albino + G. *eidos,* resemblance ]. Universal incomplete albinism; ocular albinism, nystagmus, myopia, and reduced pigment generally, with some darkening of hair and skin as patient grows older; autosomal recessive inheritance.

**albi'noism.** Albinism.

**albinot'ic.** Pertaining to albinism.

**albinu'ria.** Albiduria.

**Albinus,** Bernhard S., German anatomist and surgeon, 1697–1770. See A.'s *muscle.*

**Albl's ring.** See under ring.

**albocinereous** (al-bo-sin-e're-us) [ L. *albus,* white, + *cinereus,* ashen, fr. *cinis* (*ciner-*), ashes ]. Relating to both the white and the gray matter of the brain or spinal cord.

**Albrecht,** Karl M. P., German anatomist, 1851–1894. See A.'s *bone.*

**Albright,** Fuller, Boston physician, *1900. See A.'s *disease, syndrome,* Forbes-A. *syndrome.*

**Albucas'is** of Cordova. One of the foremost surgeons in Arabian medicine in the 11th century. Wrote a work on medicine called *The Method,* which served as a standard text on surgery in medieval times.

**albuginea** (al-bu-jin'e-ah) [ L. albugineous, *q. v.* ]. 1. Albugeneous. 2. White fibrous tissue layer; see *tunica* albuginea.

**albugineotomy** (al-bu-jin'e-ot'o-mĭ) [ albuginea + G. *tomē,* cutting ]. Incision into any tunica albuginea.

**albugineous** (al-bu-jin'e-us) [ L. *albugineus,* fr. *albugo,* white spot ]. 1. Resembling boiled white of egg. 2. Relating to any tunica albuginea.

**albugin'eus** [ L. ] [ NA ]. Albugineous.

**albu'go** [ L. *albugo* (-*in*-), a white spot. ALB- ]. Leukoma.

**albu'men** [ L. the white of egg ]. 1. Egg *albumin.* 2. Albumin.

**albumim'etry.** Albuminimetry.

**albu'min** [ L. *albumen* (-*min*-), the white of egg. ALB- ]. A type of simple protein widely distributed throughout the tissues and fluids of plants and animals; a.'s are soluble in pure water, precipitable from a solution by mineral acids, and coagulable by heat in acid or neutral solution. Varieties of a. are found in blood, milk, and muscle.

**a. A,** the normal or common type of human serum a.

**acid a.,** syntonin; a derived a. formed by the action of a dilute acid on a native a.; it is not coagulable by heat and is precipitated by neutralization of the solution.

**alkali a.,** a derived a. formed by the action of a weak alkali on native a.; it is not coagulable by heat and is precipitated when the solution is carefully neutralized.

**a. B,** see inherited a. variants.

**Bence Jones a.,** see Bence Jones *protein.*

**blood a.,** serum a.

**derived a.,** an a. formed from native a. by the action of weak acids or alkalies; *e.g.,* albuminate; albumose; metaprotein.

**dried human a.** (BP), normal human serum a.

**egg a.,** ovalbumin; albumen; white of egg; the a. occurring in the white of egg, resembling in many respects serum a.

**a. Gent,** see inherited a. variants.

**inherited a. variants,** several variant types of human serum a. are known, distinguished by characteristic mobility patterns on electrophoresis, either faster or slower than normal a. A; each type is due to a mutation of a gene controlling a. synthesis; the mutant genes are codominant

with the normal gene for a. A, and the group forms a system of genetic polymorphism. The variant types include: a. B (slow), found occasionally in persons of European ancestry; a. Gent (fast), found first at Gent, Belgium; a. Mexico (slow), found in Indians of Mexico and southwestern United States; a. Naskapi (fast), found in the Naskapi and other Indians of northern North America; a. Reading (fast), found first at Reading, England.

**iodinated I 125 serum a.** (USP, BP), ALBUMOTOPE I-125; radioiodinated serum albumin (RISA); a sterile, buffered, isotonic solution prepared to contain not less than 10 mg. of radioiodinated normal human serum albumin per ml., and adjusted to provide not more than 1 millicurie of radioactivity per ml.; used as a diagnostic aid in determining blood volume and cardiac output.

**iodinated I 131 human serum a.** (USP, BP), ALBUMOTOPE I 131; a sterile buffered, isotonic solution prepared to contain not less than 10 mg. of radioiodinated normal human serum albumin per ml., and adjusted to provide not more than 1 millicurie of radioactivity per ml.; used as a diagnostic aid in the measurement of blood volume and cardiac output.

**iodinated I 131 human serum a., aggregated** (USAN), ALBUMOTOPE-LS; prepared with aggregated particles of a.; used for lung scanning.

**a. Mexico,** see inherited a. variants.

**a. Naskapi,** see inherited a. variants.

**native a.,** a protein existing in its natural state in the body; it is soluble in water and not precipitated by diluted acids; the two principal forms are serum a. and egg a.

**normal human serum a.** (USP), dried human a. (BP); a sterile preparation of serum a. obtained by fractionating blood plasma proteins from healthy persons. Used as a transfusion material and to treat edema due to hypoproteinemia.

**Patein's a.,** acetosoluble a.; a substance resembling serum a., but soluble in acetic acid.

**a. Reading,** see inherited a. variants.

**serum a.,** blood a.; a form of a. present in the blood plasma and in serous fluids; the principal protein in plasma.

**a. tannate,** ALBUTANNIN; an astringent powder obtained by the action of tannic acid on a.; contains about 50 per cent tannic acid. Used as an astringent disinfectant in diarrhea and as a dusting powder.

**vegetable a.'s,** a.'s of the plants.

**a. X,** an antithrombin in blood plasma; the normal antithrombin of blood.

**a. X₁,** heparin cofactor, required for the antithrombotic action of heparin.

**albu'minate.** The product of the reaction between native albumin and dilute acids or dilute bases, thereby resulting in acid a.'s or alkali a.'s; both types are characterized by solubility in dilute acid or alkali, and relative insolubility in water, dilute solutions of salts, and alcohol; also termed derived albumin or metaprotein.

**albu'minatu'ria** [ albuminate + G. *ouron,* urine ]. The presence of an abnormally large quantity of albuminates in the urine when voided.

**albuminif'erous** [ albumin + L. *fero,* to bear ]. Producing albumin.

**albuminim'eter.** Albumimeter; an apparatus for determining the quantity of albumin in the urine or other fluids.

**albuminim'etry** [ albumin + G. *metron,* measure ]. Albumimetry; albuminometry; the determination of the amount of albumin present in a fluid.

**albuminip'arous** [ albumin + L. *pario,* to bring forth ]. Forming albumin.

**albuminocholia** (al-bu-min-o-ko'lĭ-ah) [ albumin + G. *cholē,* bile ]. Protein in the bile.

**albuminogenous** (al-bu'mĭ-noj'ĕ-nus). Producing or forming albumin.

**albu'minoid.** Albumoid. 1. Resembling albumin. 2. Any protein. 3. Scleroprotein; glutinoid; a simple type of protein present in horny and cartilaginous tissues and in the lens of the eye; it is insoluble in neutral solvents. Keratin, elastin, and collagen are albuminoids; gelatin, which is formed from collagen, is sometimes called an albuminoid, although it lacks the characteristic a. properties.

**albuminol′ysis** [ albumin + G. *lysis,* dissolution ]. Proteolysis.

**albuminom′etry.** Albuminimetry.

**albu′minone.** Albumone.

**albuminoptysis** (al-bu-mĭ-nop′tĭ-sis) [ albumin + G. *ptysis,* a spitting ]. Albuminous expectoration.

**albu′minoreac′tion.** The presence (positive reaction), or absence (negative reaction) of albumin in the sputum, the positive reaction indicating an inflammatory process in the lungs.

**albuminorrhea** (al-bu-min-o-re′ah) [ albumin + G. *rhoia,* a flow ]. Albuminuria.

**albu′minose.** 1. Albuminous. 2. Albumose.

**albumino′sis.** A condition characterized by an abnormal increase in the albuminous constituents of the blood plasma.

**albu′minous.** Relating in any way to albumin; containing or consisting of albumin.

**albu′minuret′ic** [ albumin + G. *ourētikos,* causing a flow of urine ]. 1. Causing albuminuria. 2. Albuminuric.

**albuminuria** (al-bu′mĭ-nu′rĭ-ah) [ albumin + G. *ouron,* urine ]. The presence of protein in urine, chiefly albumin (but also globulin); usually indicates disease, but sometimes results from a temporary or transient dysfunction (in contrast to a truly pathologic condition).

    **accidental a.,** relatively temporary and incidental a., probably resulting from "accidental" mixing of blood, plasma, or inflammatory exudate with urine as the latter passes downward in the urinary tract, *i.e.,* not from renal disease *per se;* also termed adventitious a., pseudoalbuminuria, or false a.

    **adolescent a.,** functional a. occurring at about the time of puberty; it is usually cyclic or orthostatic a.

    **adventitious a.,** a. resulting from the presence of blood escaping somewhere in the urinary tract, of chyle, or of some other albuminous fluid, not caused by filtration of albumin from the blood through the kidneys; see also accidental a.

    **a. of athletes,** a form of functional a. following excessive muscular exertion.

    **Bamberger's a.,** hematogenous a. that is sometimes observed during the later phases of advanced anemia.

    **benign a.,** orthostatic, dietetic, and similar types of a. that are not the result of pathologic changes in the kidneys.

    **cardiac a.,** a. caused by congestive heart failure.

    **colliquative a.,** an a. that is at first slight in degree, but unexpectedly becomes greatly increased during convalescence from highly febrile disease, *e.g.,* typhoid fever.

    **cyclic a.,** pseudalbuminuria; pseudoalbuminuria; recurrent a.; a functional a. sometimes observed intermittently in cycles of 12 to 36 hours' duration, chiefly in younger persons; the degree of a. is usually slight.

    **dietetic a.,** the excretion of protein in the urine following the ingestion of certain foods; also termed digestive a.

    **essential a.,** a collective term that includes various forms of functional a., *e.g.,* a. of athletes, postural a., etc.; a. not associated with, or the result of, recognizable pathologic conditions.

    **false a.,** adventitious or accidental a.

    **febrile a.,** associated with fever.

    **functional a.,** a collective term designating any a. in which there is no detectable, associated pathologic condition in the kidneys or other tissues; may be observed intermittently during pregnancy or adolescence, in athletes, etc.

    **hematogenous a., hemic a.,** a. occurring in anemia, syphilis, various intoxications, and other conditions characterized by profound changes in the blood.

    **intermittent a.,** functional a., such as cyclic a. or a. of athletes.

    **intrinsic a.,** true a.; serous a.; a. occurring as a result of renal disease in which protein escapes from the plasma and is excreted.

    **lordotic a.,** orthostatic a.; this term was suggested on the theory that the a. is a result of pressure from lordosis in the lumbar spine.

    **neuropathic a.,** a. associated with epilepsy or other convulsive disorders, trauma to the brain, and cerebral hemorrhage.

    **orthostatic a.,** a condition characterized by the appearance of albumin in the urine when the patient is in the erect posture and its disappearance when he is recumbent; also termed postural a.

    **palpatory a.,** a transient a. that sometimes occurs after palpation of the kidneys.

    **paroxysmal a.,** transitory functional a., such as that sometimes observed during pregnancy or adolescence.

    **physiologic a.,** (1) the presence of slight traces of protein in otherwise normal urine; (2) functional a.

    **postrenal a.,** a. caused by disease distal to the kidney.

    **postural a.,** orthostatic a.

    **prerenal a.,** a. caused by disease other than disease of the kidney or genitourinary tract.

    **recurrent a.,** cyclic a.

    **regulatory a.,** transitory a. occurring after unusual physical exertion.

    **serous a.,** intrinsic a.

    **transient a.,** functional or temporary a.

    **true a.,** intrinsic a.

**albuminu′ric.** Relating to, characterized by, or suffering from albuminuria.

**albu′moid.** Albuminoid.

**albu′mone.** A noncoagulable protein contained in blood serum; by some it is regarded as an artifical product formed from the globulins when heat is employed to separate the coagulable proteins.

**albumoscope** (al-bu′mo-skōp) [ albumin + G. *skopeō,* view ]. A specially mounted graduated glass tube, used for determining the presence and the approximate amount of albumin in urine or other fluid; the operation consists of bringing the fluid and nitric acid in contact, without mixing them.

**al′bumose.** A derived albumin, formed during the digestion of a protein, and converted on further digestion into peptone; it is very soluble and is not coagulable by heat.

    **Bence Jones a.,** see Bence Jones *protein.*

**albumosease** (al′bu-mōs-āz). An enzyme that digests albumose by catalyzing its hydrolysis.

**albumose′mia** [ albumose + G. *haima,* blood ]. The presence of albumose in the blood.

**albumosu′ria** [ albumose + G. *ouron,* urine ]. The excretion of an albumose, or proteose, in the urine.

**al′bus** [ L. ] [ NA ]. White.

**albu′terol** (USAN). Salbutamol; VENTOLIN; α1-[ (*tert*-butylamino)methyl ]-4-hydroxy-*m*-xylene-α,α1-diol; a sympathomimetic bronchodilator administered by inhalation.

**Alcaligenes** (al-ka-lij′en-ēz) [ alkali + G. suffix *-gen,* producing ]. A genus of aerobic and facultatively anaerobic bacteria (family Achromobacteraceae) containing Gram-negative rods which are either motile and peritrichous or nonmotile. They do not utilize carbohydrates. They are found mostly in the intestinal canal, decaying materials, dairy products, and soil. These organisms are placed by some authorities in the genus *Brucella.* The type species is *A. faecalis.*

    **A. faeca′lis,** *Bacterium alcaligenes; Bacillus faecalis alcaligenes;* a species of bacteria, generally considered nonpathogenic, found in the intestinal canal.

**alcapton.** Alkapton.

**alcaptonuria.** Alkaptonuria.

**Alcian blue** (al′sĭ-an). A complex phthalocyanin dye used as a stain for acid polysaccharides.

**alclofenac** (al-klo′fē-nak) (USAN). MERVAN; [ 4-(allyloxy)-3-chlorophenyl ]acetic acid; anti-inflammatory agent.

**Alcmaeon** (alk-me′on), Greek philosopher, circa 500 B.C. He placed the seat of intelligence in the brain and was the first to excise the human eye. By tracing the optic nerves to the chiasma he recognized the basis of binocular vision.

**Alcock,** Benjamin, Irish anatomist, *1801. See A.'s *canal.*

**alcogel** (al′ko-jel). Same as a hydrogel, with alcohol instead of water as the dispersion medium.

**alcohol** [ Ar. *al,* the, + *kohl,* fine antimonial powder, the term being applied first to a fine powder, then, to anything impalpable (spirit) ]. 1. One of a series of organic chemical compounds in which a hydrogen (H) attached to carbon is replaced by a hydroxyl (OH), yielding R(OH). Alcohols react with acids to form esters, with alkali metals to form alcoholates. For individual a.'s not listed here, see specific name. 2 (USP, BP). Ethanol; ethyl alcohol; grain alcohol; rectified spirit; $CH_3CH_2OH$; a liquid containing 92.3 per cent by weight, corresponding to 94.9 per cent by volume, at 15.56°, of $C_2H_5OH$. The BP directs it to contain not less than 92 per cent by weight (94.7 per cent by volume) and not more than 92.7 per cent by weight (95.2 per cent by volume) of $C_2H_5OH$. It is made from sugar, starch, and other carbohydrates by fermentation with yeast, and synthetically ethylene or acetyline. Has been used in beverages since antiquity; also used as a solvent, a vehicle, and a preservative; medicinally, it is used externally as a rubefacient, coolant, and disinfectant, and internally as an analgesic, stomachic, sedative, and antipyretic.

**absolute a.,** (1) anhydrous a.; 100 per cent a., water having been removed; (2) dehydrated a.; a. with a minimum admixture of water, at most 1 per cent.

**acid a.,** ethyl a. (70 per cent) containing 1 per cent hydrochloric acid.

**anhy'drous a.,** absolute a. (1).

**dehydrated a.** (BP), absolute a. (2).

**denatured a.,** methylated spirit; industrial methylated spirit (BP); ethyl alcohol (*q. v.,* under ethyl) rendered unfit for consumption as a beverage by the addition of one or several chemicals such as acetone, aldehol, amyl alcohol, aniline dyes, benzene, butyl alcohol, cadmium iodide, camphor, castor oil, chloroform, diethyl ether, diethyl phthalate, gasoline, kerosene, isopropyl alcohol, methyl alcohol, methyl isobutyl ketone, nicotine, pyridine bases, sulfuric acid. Used in industry.

**dihydric a.,** one containing two OH groups in its molecule; *e.g.,* ethylene glycol.

**dilute a.,** eight concentrations are official in the BP: 90, 80, 70, 60, 50, 45, 25 and 20 per cent v/v of $C_2H_5OH$. The USP form contains 41.5 per cent by weight (48.6 per cent by volume) of $C_2H_5OH$.

**fatty a.,** a long chain alcohol (analogous to the fatty acids of which the fatty alcohol may be viewed as a reduction product), *e.g.,* stearyl alcohol.

**monohydric a.,** one containing one OH group.

**primary a.,** an a. characterized by the univalent radical, —$CH_2OH$.

**rubbing a.** (NF), contains not less than 68.5 and not more than 71.5 per cent by volume of absolute alcohol; the remainder consists of water, denaturants (with and without coal tar colors), and perfume oils. It must comply with the requirements of the United States Treasury Department. Used as a rubefacient.

**secondary a.,** an a. characterized by the bivalent atom group, ⟩CHOH.

**sugar a.,** see under sugar.

**tertiary a.,** an a. characterized by the trivalent atom group, ⟩COH.

**trihydric a.,** one containing three OH groups, *e.g.,* glycerol.

**unsaturated a.'s,** those a.'s whose carbon chains contain one or more double or triple bonds.

**alcohol acids.** A group of compounds that contain both the carboxyl and hydroxy radicals, *e.g.,* glycolic acid.

**alcoholate** (al-ko-hol'āt). 1. A tincture or other preparation containing alcohol. 2. A chemical compound in which the hydrogen in the OH group of an alcohol is replaced by an an alkali metal; *e.g.,* sodium methylate, $CH_3ONa$.

**alcohol dehydrogenase.** 1. Aldehyde reductase. 2. Alcohol dehydrogenase (acceptor). 3. Alcohol dehydrogenase (NADP+). 4. Alcohol dehydrogenase (NAD(P)+).

**alcohol dehydrogenase (acceptor).** Alcohol dehydrogenase (2); an oxidoreductase (EC 1.1.99.8) converting primary alcohols to aldehydes with an H acceptor other tahn NAD+.

**alcohol dehydrogenase (NADP+).** Alcohol dehydrogenase (3); an oxidoreductase (EC 1.1.1.2) converting alcohols to aldehydes (or ketones) with NADP+ as H acceptor.

**alcohol dehydrogenase (NAD(P)+).** Alcohol dehydrogenase (4); an oxidoreductase (EC 1.1.1.71) converting alcohols to aldehydes, or the reverse, with NAD+ or NADP+ as H acceptor; also reduces retinal to retinol.

**alcohol'ic.** 1. Relating to, containing, or produced by alcohol. 2. A person addicted to the use of a. beverages in excess.

**alcoholism** (al'ko-hol-izm). Alcohol abuse; alcohol dependence; alcohol addiction; chronic heavy drinking or intoxication resulting in impairment of health, dependency as a coping mechanism, and increased adaptation to the effects of alcohol requiring increasing doses to achieve and sustain a desired effect. Specific signs and symptoms of withdrawal are usually shown upon sudden cessation of such drinking.

**acute a.,** intoxication; drunkenness; a temporary mental disturbance with muscular incoordination and paresis, induced by the ingestion of alcoholic beverages in poisonous amount.

**chronic a.,** a pathologic condition, affecting chiefly the nervous and gastroenteric systems, caused by the habitual use of alcoholic beverages in poisonous amount.

**al'coholiza'tion.** Permeation or saturation with alcohol.

**al'coholize.** 1. To impregnate with alcohol. 2. To convert into alcohol.

**alcoholomania** (al-ko-hol'o-ma'nĭ-ah) [ alcohol + G. *mania,* frenzy ]. 1. A morbid craving for alcoholic beverages. 2. *Delirium* tremens.

**alcoholom'eter** [ alcohol + G. *metron,* measure ]. An apparatus for determining the proportion of alcohol in a fluid.

**alcoholophilia** (al'ko-hol-o-fil'ĭ-ah) [ alcohol + G. *phileō,* to love ]. The craving for alcohol.

**alcoholophobia** (al'ko-hol-o-fo'be-ah) [ alcohol + G. *phobos,* fear ]. A morbid fear of alcohol, or of becoming an alcoholic.

**al'coholu'ria** [ alcohol + G. *ouron,* urine ]. Alcohol in the urine.

**alcoholysis** (al-ko-hol'ĭ-sis) [ alcohol + G. *lysis,* dissolution ]. The splitting of a chemical bond with the addition of the elements of alcohol at the point of splitting.

**al'cosol.** Same as a hydrosol, with alcohol instead of water as the dispersion medium.

**alcuro'nium dichloride** (USAN). ALLOFERIN; *N,N'*-diallylnortoxiferinium dichloride; skeletal muscle relaxant, active as a nondepolarizing neuromuscular blocking agent.

**aldadiene** (al'dah-di'ēn). A metabolite of spironolactone (a steroid lactone, a derivative of androstene) that contains double bonds between C-4 and C-5 and between C-6 and C-7; formed upon removal of the 7α-acetylthiol side chain from spironolactone; as potent a diuretic as the parent compound.

**aldaric acid.** One of a group of sugar acids characterized by the formula HOOC—$(CHOH)_n$—COOH; *e.g.,* saccharic acid.

**al'dehol.** An oxidation product of kerosene; used for denaturing ethyl alcohol.

**aldehyde** (al'de-hīd). A compound containing the radical —CH=O, reducible to an alcohol ($CH_2OH$), oxidizable to an acid (COOH); *e.g.,* acetaldehyde.

**angular a.,** the a. group attached to carbon 10 (between rings A and B) of the steroid nucleus in aldosterone.

**aldehyde base.** A base derived from an ammonia compound of an aldehyde.

**aldehyde dehydrogenase (acylating).** Oxidoreductase (EC 1.2.1.10) converting an aldehyde and CoA to acyl-CoA with NAD+ as H acceptor.

**aldehyde dehydrogenase (NAD+).** Aldehyde → DPN transhydrogenase; an oxidoreductase (EC 1.2.1.3) converting aldehydes to acids with NAD+ as H acceptor.

**aldehyde dehydrogenase (NADP+).** Aldehyde → TPN transhydrogenase; an oxidoreductase (EC 1.2.1.4) converting aldehydes to acids with NADP+ as H acceptor.

**aldehyde dehydrogenase (NAD+ or NADP+).** An oxidoreductase (EC 1.2.1.5) converting aldehydes to acids with NAD+ or NADP+ as H acceptor.

**aldehyde → DPN transhydrogenase.** Aldehyde dehydrogenase (NAD+).

**aldehyde-lyases.** Enzymes (EC sub-subgroup 4.1.2) catalyzing the reversal of an aldol condensation.

**aldehyde reductase.** Alcohol dehydrogenase (1); DPNH → aldehyde transhydrogenase; an oxidoreductase (EC

1.1.1.1) converting alcohols to aldehydes (or ketones) with NAD$^+$ as H acceptor.

**aldehyde → TPN transhydrogenase.** Aldehyde dehydrogenase (NADP$^+$).

**Alder,** A. von. See A.'s *anomaly,* A. *bodies.*

**al'din.** An aldehyde base.

**aldobiuron'ic acid.** The condensation products of an aldose and a uronic acid; such groupings occur among the components of various mucopolysaccharides, notably hyaluronic acid.

**aldohex'ose.** A 6-carbon sugar characterized by the (potential) presence of an aldehyde group in the molecule; *e.g.,* glucose, galactose.

**aldoke'tomu'tase.** Lactoyl-glutathione lyase.

**al'dol.** Acetaldol; $\beta$-hydroxybutyraldehyde; $CH_3$-$CHOHCH_2CHO$; formed by condensation of 2 molecules of $CH_3CHO$ (acetaldehyde). Possesses hypnotic properties. Used in the manufacture of rubber products and perfumes.

**al'dolase.** 1. Generic term for aldehyde-lyase. 2. Name sometimes applied to fructose bisphosphate aldolase.

**aldon'ic acids.** Glyconic acids; monosaccharide derivatives in which the aldehyde group has been oxidized to a carboxyl group.

**aldopen'tose.** A monosaccharide, *e.g.,* ribose, with five carbon atoms, of which one is a (potential) aldehyde group.

**al'dose.** A monosaccharide potentially containing the characteristic group of the aldehydes, —CHO.

   **a. mutarotase,** aldose 1-epimerase.

   **a. reductase** (EC 1.1.1.21), an oxidoreductase (in liver) that converts aldoses to alditols (*e.g.,* glucose to sorbitol) with NADPH as hydrogen donor. See also ketose reductase.

**aldose 1-epimerase** (EC 5.1.3.3), aldose mutarotase; an enzyme catalyzing interconversion of $\alpha$- and $\beta$-D-glucose; also acts on L-arabinose, D-xylose, D-galactose, maltose and lactose.

**al'doside.** A glucoside in which the sugar moiety is an aldose.

**aldos'terone.** A steroid hormone produced by the zona glomerulosa of the adrenal cortex; its major action is to facilitate potassium exchange for sodium in the distal renal tubule, causing sodium reabsorption and potassium and hydrogen loss. For structure, see steroids.

**aldos'teronism.** Hyperaldosteronism; a disorder caused by excessive secretion of aldosterone.

   **primary a.,** Conn's syndrome; an adrenocortical disorder caused by excessive secretion of aldosterone and characterized by headaches (often), nocturia (usually), polyuria (commonly), fatigue, hypertension, hypokalemic alkalosis, potassium depletion, hypervolemia, and decreased plasma renin activity.

   **secondary a.,** pathological a. resulting not from a defect intrinsic to the adrenal cortex but from a stimulation of secretion caused by extra-adrenal disorders; it is associated with increased plasma renin activity and occurs in heart failure, nephrotic syndrome, cirrhosis, and hypoproteinemia.

**al'dotet'rose.** A four-carbon aldose; *e.g.,* threose, erythrose.

**aldox'ime.** A compound derived by the reaction of an aldose with hydroxylamine, thus containing the a. group —HC=NOH.

**Aldrich,** Robert A., American pediatrician, *1917. See A. *syndrome.*

**al'drin.** A hexachlorohexahydrodimethanonaphthalene; a volatile chlorinated hydrocarbon, used as an insecticide. Toxic symptoms (if absorbed through the skin) are irritability followed by depression.

**alecithal** (ă-les'ĭ-thal) [ G. *a*-priv. + *lekithos,* yolk ]. Without yolk; denoting ova with little or no deutoplasm.

**Alectorobius talaje.** An insect commonly found in Mexico and South America. The bites, like those of the bedbug, suppurate.

**alem'bic** [ Ar. *al,* the, + *anbiq,* cup ]. A vessel used in medieval times for distillation, or more properly the cap of this vessel in which the recondensation occurred.

**alem'mal** [ G. *a*-priv. + *lemma,* husk ]. Denoting a nerve fiber lacking a neurolemma.

**alethia** (ă-le'thĭ-ah) [ G. *a*-priv. + *lēthē,* forgetfulness ]. A dwelling upon past events; the incapacity to forget.

**aletocyte** (ă-le'to-sīt) [ G. *alētēs,* a wanderer, + *kytos,* cell ]. A wandering cell of uncertain origin (obsolete or rarely used term).

**al'etris** [ G. a grinder of corn ]. The dried rhizome and roots of *Aletris farinosa* (family Liliaceae); ague root; unicorn root; crow-corn; star-grass; an herb of the eastern United States. A simple bitter, said to be a uterine tonic, diuretic, and antirheumatic.

**aleukemia** (ă-lu-ke'mĭ-ah) [ G. *a*-priv. + *leukos,* white, + *haima,* blood ]. 1. Literally, a lack of leukocytes in the blood. Term is generally used to indicate varieties of leukemic disease in which the white blood cell count in circulating blood is normal or even less than normal (*i.e.,* no leukocytosis), but a few young leukocytes are observed; sometimes used more restrictedly for unusual instances of leukemia with no leukocytosis and no young forms in the blood. 2. Leukopenic myelosis, *i.e.,* leukemic changes in bone marrow, associated with a subnormal number of leukocytes in the blood. See also subleukemia.

**aleuke'mic.** Adjective pertaining to aleukemia, as a. leukemia.

**aleukemoid** (ă-lu-ke'moyd). Resembling aleukemia symptomatically.

**aleukia** (ă-lu'kĭ-ah) [ G. *a*-priv. + *leukos,* white ]. 1. Absence or extremely decreased number of leukocytes in circulating blood; sometimes also termed aleukemic myelosis. 2. Obsolete name for thrombocytopenia.

   **a. hemorrha'gica,** term sometimes used for examples of primary refractory anemia with advanced degrees of granulocytopenia and thrombocytopenia, acellular or extremely hypocellular bone marrow, and extensive purpura. Termed also aplastic anemia, progressive hypocythemia, toxic paralytic anemia, and panmyelophthisis.

**aleukocytic** (ă-lu-ko-sit'ik). Manifesting absence or extremely reduced numbers of leukocytes in blood or lesions.

**aleukocytosis** (ă-lu-ko-si-to'sis) [ G. *a*- priv. + *leukos,* white, + *kytos,* a hollow (cell) ]. Absence or great reduction (relative or absolute) of the number of white blood cells in circulating blood (*i.e.,* an advanced degree of leukopenia), or the lack of leukocytes in an anatomical lesion.

**Aleuris'ma** [ G. *aleuron,* flour ]. A genus of fungi parasitic to man. A number of species have been found in cutaneous lesions.

**aleuron** (al-u'ron) [ G. flour ]. Protein granules in the endosperm of seeds, supposed to contain the vitamins of edible seeds and grains.

**aleuronate** (ă-lu'ro-nāt). Protein from the aleuron layer (endosperm) of cereal grains; used to make bread for diabetics.

**aleu'ronoid.** Resembling flour.

**Alexander** of Tralles, Byzantine eclectic physician, 525–605 A.D. A compiler of the teachings of Galen. Published the *Practica,* a work on medicine containing accounts of gout, cholera, insanity, and many other diseases. First to recommend colchicum for gout.

**Alexander,** W. Stewart, contemporary English pathologist. See A.'s *disease.*

**alexeteric** (ă-lek-se-ter'ik) [ G. *alexētērios,* able to defend, fr. *alexō,* to ward off ]. Protective; defensive; in reference especially to infectious diseases; antidotal.

**alexia** (ă-lek-sĭ-ah) [ G. *a*-priv. + *lexis,* a word or phrase ]. Word blindness or text blindness; loss of the power to grasp the meaning of written or printed words and sentences; called also optical, sensory, or visual a. in distinction to motor a. (aphemia or anarthria), in which there is loss of the power to read aloud although the significance of what is written or printed is understood; musical a., or music blindness, is loss of the power to read musical notation.

   **agnostic a.,** pure word blindness.

**alex'ic.** 1. Possessing the characters of an alexin. 2. Pertaining to alexia.

**alex'idine** (USAN). BISGUADINE; 1,1'-hexamethylenebis[ 5-(2-ethylhexyl)biguanide; antibacterial agent.

**alex'in** [ G. *alexō*, to ward off ]. Buchner's term for the bactericidal substances of cell-free serum, the activity of which is destroyed by heating at 56°C.; applied by Bordet to the heat-labile substance normally present in serum and distinct from the sensitizing substance (antibody) produced by infection or immunization. In this sense it is synonymous with complement.

**alexin'ic.** Resembling, relating to, or having the characteristics of an alexin.

**alexipharmac** (ă-lek'sĭ-far'mak) [ G. *alexipharmakos*, preserving against poison ]. 1. Antidotal. 2. An antidote.

**alexipyretic** (ă-lek'sĭ-pi-ret'ik) [ G. *alexō*, to ward off, + *pyretos*, fever ]. Febrifuge.

**alex'ocyte.** A cell that is thought to secrete alexin or complement. Formerly used as a term for eosinophil.

**alexofix'agen.** Seldom used term for an antigen that stimulates the production of complement-fixing antibodies.

**alexofix'agin** [ alexin + L. *figo*, pp. *fixus*, to fasten ]. Alexofixin; seldom used term for complement-fixing antibody.

**alex'ofixin.** Alexofixagin.

**a-Leydigism** (ah-li'dig-izm). The absence of functioning Leydig cells in the testis.

**algae** (al'je) [ pl. of L. *alga*, seaweed ]. A division of cellular cryptogamous plants, including seaweeds.

**al'gal.** Resembling or pertaining to algae.

**algaroba** (al'gă-ro'bah). Carob flour; locust gum; ground meal of fruit of *Ceratonia siliqua;* used as an adsorbent-demulcent in the treatment of diarrhea.

**al'ge-, alge'si-, al'go-.** Combining forms meaning pain.

**algedonic** (al-je-don'ik) [ G. *algos*, pain, + *hēdonē*, pleasure ]. Relating to a mixed sensation or emotion of pleasure and pain.

**algefacient** (al-je-fa'shent) [ L. *algeo*, to be cold, + *facio*, pr. pl -*iens*, to make ]. An agent that has a cooling action.

**algesia** (al-je'zĭ-ah) [ G. *algēsis*, a sense of pain ]. State of increased sensitivity to pain; sometimes provoked by stimuli not normally painful.

**alge'sic.** Painful; hyperesthetic.

**algesichronometer** (al-je'si-kro-nom'e-tur) [ G. *algēsis*, sense of pain, + *chronos*, time, + *metron*, measure ]. An instrument for recording the time required for the perception of a painful stimulus.

**algesim'eter.** Algesiometer.

**algesiogenic** (al-je'zĭ-o-jen'ik). [ G. *algēsis*, sense of pain, + suffix -*gen*, production ]. Algogenic; pain-producing.

**algesiometer** (al-je-sĭ-om'e-tur) [ G. *algēsis*, sense of pain, + *metron*, measure ]. Algesimeter; algometer; odynometer; an instrument for measuring the degree of sensitivity to a painful stimulus.

**algesthesia** (al-jes-the'ze-ah) [ G. *algos*, pain, + *aisthēsis*, sensation ]. The appreciation of pain, expecially hypersensitivity to painful stimuli; a form of hyperesthesia.

**algesthe'sis.** Algesthesia.

**alges'tone acetophenide** (USAN). DELADROXONE; alphasone acetophenide; 16α,17-dihydroxypregn-4-ene-3,20-dione cyclic acetal with acetophenone; a progestogen used as contraceptive.

**alget'ic.** Painful.

**-algia** [ G. *algos*, pain ]. Suffix meaning pain or painful condition.

**algicide** (al'jĭ-sīd) [ algae, + L. *caedo*, to kill ]. A chemical active against algae.

**algid** (al'jid) [ L. *algidus*, cold ]. Chilly, cold.

**algin** (al'jin). Sodium alginate; a carbohydrate product from a seaweed, *Macrocystis pyrifera;* used as a gel in pharmaceutical preparations.

**alginate** (al'jĭ-nāt). An irreversible hydrocolloid consisting of salts of alginic acid, *q.v.* See also calcium alginate; sodium alginate.

**algin'ic acid** (NF). NORGINE; a colloidal acid polysaccharide obtained from seaweed, composed of mannuronic acid residues; used as sizing material for paper, artificial ivories, and mucilage; alginate dental impression materials are made from it.

**alginuresis** (al'jin-u-re'sis) [ G. *algeinos*, painful, + *ourēsis*, urination ]. Painful micturition.

**algiomo'tor.** Algiomuscular; causing painful muscular contractions.

**algiomuscular** (al'jĭ-o-mus'ku-lar). Algiomotor.

**algiovascular** (al'jĭ-o-vas'ku-lar). Algovascular.

**algo-.** See alge-.

**algogenesis, algogenesia** (al-go-jen'ĕ-sis, al-go-jĕ-ne'zĭ-ah) [ algo- + G. *genesis*, production ]. The production or origin of pain.

**algogen'ic.** Algesiogenic.

**algolag'nia** [ algo- + G. *lagneia*, lust ]. A form of sexual perversion in which the infliction or the experiencing of pain increases the pleasure of the sexual act or causes sexual pleasure independent of the act; a term covering both sadism and masochism.

    **active a.,** sadism.

    **passive a.,** masochism.

**algom'eter** [ algo- + G. *metron*, measure ]. Algesiometer.

**algom'etry.** The process of measuring pain.

**algophilia** (al-go-fil'ĭ-ah) [ algo- + G. *phileō*, to love ]. 1. Pleasure experienced in the thought of pain in others or in oneself. 2. Algolagnia.

**algopho'bia** [ algo- + G. *phobos*, fear ]. Odynophobia; abnormal fear of or sensitiveness to pain.

**algopsychalia** (al-go-si-ka'lĭ-ah) [ algo- + G. *psychē*, mind ]. Psychalgia.

**al'gor** [ L. coldness ]. A chill; cold or the sensation of cold.

    **a. mortis,** the chill of death.

**algos'copy** [ L. *algor*, cold, + G. *skopeō*, to view ]. Cryoscopy.

**al'gospasm** [ G. *algos*, pain, + *spasmos*, convulsion ]. Spasm produced by pain; painful spasm.

**algovas'cular** [ G. *algos*, pain ]. Relating to changes in the lumen of the blood vessels taking place under the influence of pain.

**Alibert,** Jean Louis, French physician; 1768–1838. See A.'s *disease.*

**alible** (al'ĭ-bl) [ L. *alibilis*, nutritive, fr. *alo*, to nourish ]. Nutritive; capable of nourishing.

**alicyclic compounds.** See under compound.

**alienation** (āl'yen-a'shun) [ L. *alieno*, pp. -*atus*, to make strange. ALI- ]. A condition characterized by lack of meaningful relationships to others and sometimes resulting in depersonalization and estrangement from others.

**alienia** (a-li-e'nĭ-ah) [ G. *a*- priv. + L. *lien*, spleen ]. Absence of the spleen.

**alienist** (āl-yen-ist). Obsolete term for one who treats mental diseases.

**al'iform** [ L. *ala*, + *forma*, shape ]. Wing-shaped; resembling a wing; pterygoid.

**al'iment** [ L. *alo*, to nourish ]. 1. Food; nourishment. 2. In sensorimotor theory, that which is assimilated to a schema; analogous to a stimulus.

**alimenta'rius** [ L. ] [ NA ]. Alimentary.

**alimentary** (al'ĭ-men'tar-ĭ) [ L. *alimentarius*, fr. *alimentum*, nourishment ]. Relating to food or nutrition.

**alimenta'tion.** Providing nourishment; see also feeding.

    **forced a.,** forced *feeding.*

    **rectal a.,** feeding by retention enemas.

**alimen'tother'apy.** Dietotherapy.

**alinasal** (al'ĭ-na'sal) [ L. *ala*, + *nasus*, nose ]. Relating to the alae nasi, or flaring portions of the nostrils.

**alinement, alignment** (ă-lin'ment) 1. The act of bringing into line. 2. In dentistry, the line along which the teeth are positioned.

**alinjection** (al'in-jek-shun). The injection of alcohol for hardening and preserving pathologic and histologic specimens.

**aliphat'ic** [ G. *aleiphar* (*aleiphat*-), fat, oil ]. 1. Fatty. 2. Denoting the open chain compounds, most of which belong to the fatty acid series.

    **a. acids,** The acids of nonaromatic hydrocarbons, *i.e.,* acetic, propionic, butyric (and other) acids; the so-called fatty acids, of the formula R-COOH, where R is a nonaromatic hydrocarbon.

**alip'oid** [ G. *a*- priv. + *lipoidēs*, resembling fat ]. Characterized by absence of lipoids.

**alipotrop'ic** [ G. *a*- priv. + *lipos*, fat, + *tropos*, a turning ]. Having no effect upon fat metabolism, or upon the movement of fat to the liver.

**al'iquant.** In chemistry and immunology, pertaining to a portion that results from dividing the whole in a manner that some is left after the a.'s (equal in volume or weight) have been apportioned.

**aliquot** (al'ĭ-kwŏt). In chemistry and immunology, pertaining to (1) a portion that results from dividing the whole into equal parts, leaving no remainder, and (2) loosely, two or more samples of something, of the same volume or weight.

**alisphenoid** (al-ĭ-sfe'noyd) [ L. *ala*, + *sphēn*, wedge ]. Relating to the greater wing of the sphenoid bone.

**aliz'arin.** 1,2-Dihydroxyanthraquinone; a red dye that occurs in the root of madder (*Rubia tinctorum*) in glucose combination (ruberythric acid). Orange needles, slightly soluble in water. Used by the ancients as a dye. Now made synthetically from anthracene, a coal tar product, and used in the manufacture of dyes, *e.g.*, a. blue, a. orange, "Turkey red." Used as an indicator, changing from yellow to red at pH 5.5 to 6.8. Other (modified alizarins have other colors and change color at other pH values.

**a. cyanin,** the disulfonate of hexahydroxyanthraquinone, $C_{14}H_6O_{14}S_2Na_2$; an acid dye used as a nuclear stain and as a fluorochrome in ultraviolet microscopy.

**a. indicator,** a solution consisting of sodium a. sulfonate 1 gm. dissolved in 100 cc. of distilled water. Used as indicator for free acidity in gastric contents.

**a. purpurin,** purpurin.

**a. red S,** sodium a. sulfonate; used as a stain for calcium in bone, and in the determination of fluorine. It changes from yellow to purple between pH 3.7 and 5.2.

**aljodan.** $ICH_2CH_2COO—NHCONH_2$; iodoethyl allophanate; used for iodine effect.

**alkadiene** (al'kah-di'ēn). An acyclic hydrocarbon containing two double bonds.

**alkale'mia** [ alkali + G. *haima*, blood ]. A decrease in H ion concentration of the blood, a rise in pH, irrespective of alterations in the level of bicarbonate ion.

**alkalescence** (al-kal-es'ens). 1. A slight alkalinity. 2. The process of becoming alkaline.

**alkales'cent.** Slightly alkaline; becoming alkaline.

**alkali,** pl. **alkalis** or **alkalies** [ Ar., *al*, the, + *qalīy*, soda ash ]. A strongly basic substance yielding hydroxide ions $(OH^-)$ in solution; *e.g.*, sodium hydroxide, potassium hydroxide.

**caustic a.,** a highly ionized (in solution) alkali (*e.g.*, NaOH).

**fixed a.,** any a. other than ammonia.

**vegetable a.,** (1) alkaloid; (2) a mixture of potassium hydroxide and carbonate.

**volatile a.,** ammonia.

**alkalim'eter.** An instrument for determining the degree of alkalinity of any mixture.

**alkalim'etry** [ alkali + G. *metron*, measure ]. The determination of the degree of alkalinity of a mixture.

**Engel's a.,** a method to determine the alkalinity of the blood; a diluted specimen of blood is titrated with normal tartaric acid solution until the mixture reddens litmus paper, the degree of alkalinity being determined by the amount of tartaric acid solution required to neutralize it.

**al'kaline.** Relating to an alkali; having the reaction of an alkali.

**alkalin'ity.** The condition of being alkaline.

**alkalinization.** Alkalization.

**al'kalinize.** Alkalize.

**alkalinu'ria** [ alkaline + G. *ouron*, urine ]. Alkaluria; the passage of alkaline urine.

**alkalipenia** (al'kă-lĭ-pe'nĭ-ah) [ alkali + G. *penia*, poverty ]. Reduction in alkali, or deprivation.

**al'kalither'apy.** Alkalotherapy.

**alkaliza'tion.** The process of rendering alkaline; alkalinization.

**al'kalize.** Alkalinize; to render alkaline.

**al'kali'zer.** An agent that neutralizes acids, rendering them alkaline.

**al'kaloid.** Any one of hundreds of plant products distinguished by basic reactions (hence the name, given in 1818) arising from heterocyclic nitrogen-containing and often complex structures, and by pharmacological activity. A.'s are synthesized by the plant and are found in the leaf, bark, seed, or other parts usually constituting the active principle of the crude drug. Their trivial names usually end in -ine. They are a loosely defined group and classification is difficult, but they may be classified according to the chemical structure of their main nucleus: phenylalkylamine (ephedrine), pyridine (nicotine), tropine (atropine, cocaine), quinoline (quinine), isoquinoline (papaverine), phenanthrene (morphine), purine (caffeine), imidazole (pilocarpine), and indole (physostigmine, yohimbine). For medicinal purposes the salts of a.'s are usually used.

**fixed a.,** a nonvolatile a.

**alkalom'etry** [ alkaloid + G. *metron*, measure ]. Dosimetry of alkaloids.

**alkalo'sis.** Alkaline intoxication; abnormally high alkali reserve (bicarbonate) of the blood and other body fluids, with a tendency for an increase in pH of the blood, although it may remain normal; a. may result from persistent vomiting, hyperventilation, or excessive ingestion of sodium bicarbonate.

**acapni'al a.,** respiratory a.

**$CO_2$ a.,** respiratory a.

**compensated a.,** a rise in the alkali reserve but, as a result of compensatory readjustments, *e.g.*, retention of $CO_2$ or increased excretion of alkali, no rise in pH occurs. Thus, compensated $CO_2$ a. is usually associated with a subnormal level of bicarbonate ion.

**gaseous a.,** respiratory a.

**metabolic a.,** a condition in which the blood and other body fluids have a pH greater than normal, associated with an increased concentration of bicarbonate, possibly resulting from an excessive intake of alkaline materials or a great loss of chloride (as in persistent vomiting).

**respiratory a.,** acapnial, $CO_2$, or gaseous a.; that resulting from abnormal loss of $CO_2$ produced by hyperventilation, either active or passive; see also compensated and uncompensated a.

**uncompensated a.,** usually related to a rise in the alkali reserve of the blood, possibly resulting from vomiting (loss of HCl) or intake of bicarbonate ion; compensatory mechanisms may fail, thereby leading to alkalemia. Uncompensated $CO_2$ a. may be associated with a normal level of bicarbonate ion.

**al'kalother'apy.** Alkalitherapy; use of alkalis in therapy for local or systemic effect.

**alkalot'ic.** Relating to alkalosis.

**al'kalu'ria.** Alkalinuria.

**al'kamine.** A compound containing both an OH and an $NH_2$ group.

**al'kane.** The general term for a saturated acyclic hydrocarbon as, for example, propane and isobutane.

**al'kanet.** The root of a herb, *Alkanna*, or *Anchusa tinctoria* (family Boraginaceae), that yields a red dye; used as a coloring agent; also used, combined with tannin, as an astringent.

**al'kannin.** Anchusin; 5,8-dihydroxy-2-(1-hydroxy-4-methyl-3-pentenyl)-1,4-naphthoquinone; the red dye from alkanet; used as an astringent; can be used as an indicator: red at pH 6.8, changing to purple at pH 8.8 and blue at pH 10.0.

**alkap'ton** [ Boedeker's coinage fr. alkali, *q.v.*, + G. *kaptein*, to suck up greedily ]. Alcapton; homogentisic acid; resulting from the incomplete oxidation of tyrosine, and the cause of alkaptonuria. See also homogentisic acid.

**alkaptonuria** (al-kap-tŏ-nu'rĭ-ah) [ alkapton + G. *ouron*, urine ]. Alcaptonuria; the excretion of homogentisic acid (alkapton) in the urine due to congenital lack of the enzyme homogentisic acid oxidase, which mediates an essential step in the catabolism of phenylalanine and tyrosine; the urine turns dark if allowed to stand or is alkalinized (a result of formation of polymerization products of homogentisic acid). A. frequently occurs throughout relatively long periods, or may recur and subside at irregular intervals, and arthritis and ochronosis are late complications; autosomal recessive inheritance.

**alkatriene** (al′kah-tri′ēn). An acyclic hydrocarbon containing three double bonds.

**alkaver′vir.** VERILOID; a mixture of alkaloids obtained by the selective extraction of *Veratrum viride* with various organic solvents. Used orally or parenterally as a hypotensive agent. See proveratrines.

**al′kene.** An acyclic hydrocarbon with a molecule containing one double bond, *e.g.,* ethylene.

**alkenyl.** The radical of an alkene.

**alk-1-enyl.** The radical of an alkene in which the double bond indicated by "en(e)" is between carbons 1 and 2 (carbon 1 being the radical carbon), *i.e.,* R—CH=CH—.

**alk-1-enylglycerol (lipid).** A phosphatidate in which at least one of the radicals attached to the glycerol is an alk-1-enyl rather than the usual acyl radical (*i.e.,* is derived from an aldehyde rather than an acid, hence the older trivial names phosphatidal and acetal phosphatidate); also known as plasmalogen (lipid).

**al′kide.** Alkyl (2).

**alkofanone.** ALFONE; 3-phenyl-3-sulfanilylpropiophenone; antidiarrheal agent.

**al′kyl.** 1. A hydrocarbon radical of the general formula $C_nH_{2n+1}$. 2. Alkide; compound, such as tetraethyl lead, in which a metal (Pb, Al, Zn, etc.) is combined with alkyl radicals.

**alkyl′amine.** An alkane containing an —$NH_2$ group in place of one H atom.

**al′kylation.** The substitution of an alkyl radical for a hydrogen atom in a cyclic compound; *e.g.,* the introduction of a side chain into an aromatic compound.

**alkylogen** (al-kil′o-jen). An alkyl ester of a halogen acid, *e.g.,* ethylchloride, methyl bromide.

**allachesthesia** (al-ah-kes-the′sĭ-ah) [ G. *allachē,* elsewhere, + *aisthēsis,* sensation ]. A condition in which a sensation is referred to a point other than that to which the stimulus is applied.

optical a., visual *allesthesia.*

**allantiasis** (al′an-ti′ah-sis) [ G. *allas* (*allant-*), sausage ]. Sausage poisoning, due to botulism in most cases.

**allanto-, allant-** [ G. *allas,* sausage ]. Combining forms for allantois, allantoid.

**allantochorion** (al-lan-to-ko′rī-on). Extraembryonic membrane formed by the fusion of the allantois and chorion.

**allantogenesis** (al-lan-to-jen′ĕ-sis) [ allanto- + G. *genesis,* origin ]. Development of the allantois.

**allanto′ic.** Relating to the allantois.

**allanto′ic acid.** ($NH_2CONH)_2CHCOOH$; produced from allantoin by the hydrolytic action of the enzyme allantoinase.

**allantoicase** (al′lan-to′ĭ-kās) (EC 3.5.3.4). An enzyme (an amididinohydrolase) found in animals other than mammals catalyzing the hydrolysis of allantoic acid to urea and a glyoxylic acid.

**allan′toid** [ allanto- + G. *eidos,* appearance ]. 1. Sausage-shaped. 2. Relating to, or resembling, the allantois.

**allantoidoangiopagus** (al′lan-toyd′o-an-jī-op′ah-gus) [ allantoid + G. *angeion,* vessel, + *pagos,* fastened ]. See allantoidoangiopagous *twins.*

**allantoin** (al-an′to-in). 5-Ureidohydantoin; glyoxyldiureide; cordianine; present in the allantoic fluid, the urine of the fetus, and elsewhere. An oxidation product of uric acid and the end product of purine metabolism in animals other than man and the other primates. Used externally to promote wound healing.

Allantoin

**allanto′inase** (EC 3.5.2.5). An enzyme (an amidohydrolase) that catalyzes the hydrolysis of allantoin to allantoic acid.

**allantoinuria** (al-lan′to-in-u′rĭ-ah) [ allantoin + G. *ouron,* urine ]. The urinary excretion of allantoin. Normal in most mammals, abnormal in man.

**allantois** (al-an′to-is) [ allanto- + G. *eidos,* appearance ]. A fetal membrane developing from the hindgut. In man it is vestigial; externally, in mammals, it contributes to the formation of the umbilical cord and placenta; in birds and reptiles it lies close beneath the porous shell and serves as an organ of respiration.

**allax′is** [ G. *allattein,* to alter ]. Transformation; metamorphosis.

**allele** (ah′lēl) [ G. *allelōn,* reciprocally ]. Any one of a series of two or more different genes that may occupy the same position or locus on a specific chromosome. As autosomal chromosomes are paired, each autosomal locus is represented twice in normal somatic cells. If the same a. occupies both loci, the individual or cell is homozygous for this a. If the a.'s at the two loci are different, the individual or cell is heterozygous for both a.'s. See also dominance of genes, under gene.

**alle′lic.** Relating to one or more of a series of genes that may occupy the same position or locus on a specific chromosome; see also dominance of genes, under gene.

**allelism** (al′e-lizm). State of two or more genes that must occupy the same position or locus on a specific chromosome.

**allelocatalysis** (a-le′lo-kă-tal′ĭ-sis) [ G. *allēlōn,* mutually, reciprocally, + *catalytikos,* able to dissolve. LY- ]. Self-stimulation of growth in a bacterial culture by addition of similar cells.

**alle′locatalyt′ic.** Mutually catalytic; denoting two substances each of which is decomposed in the presence of the other.

**allelomorph** (a-le′lo-morf) [ G. *allēlōn,* reciprocally (ALI-), + *morphē,* shape ]. Allele.

**alle′lomor′phic.** Allelic.

**al′lelomor′phism.** Allelism.

**alle′lotaxis, alle′lotaxy** [ G. *allēlōn,* reciprocally, + *taxis,* an arranging ]. Development of an organ from a number of embryonal structures or tissues.

**Allen,** Edgar, American anatomist, 1892–1943. See A.-Doisy *test, unit.*

**Allen,** Frederick M., American physician, 1879–1964. See A.'s *law, tests, treatment.*

**Allen,** Willard M., American gynecologist, *1904. See Corner-A. *test, unit.*

**Allen's radial compression test.** See radial compression test of A.

**al′lene.** Propadiene; $CH_2CCH_2$; an anesthetic gas (20 to 30 volumes per cent) with considerable cardiorespiratory side effects.

**allenolic acid.** 6-Hydroxy-2-naphthalenepropionic acid; useful in the synthesis of estrogens.

**allen′thesis** [ G. *allos,* other, + *en,* in, + *thesis,* a placing ]. The entrance into the body of any foreign material.

**allergen** (al′er-jen) [ allergy + G. suffix *-gen,* producing ]. Antigen; von Pirquet's term for an incitant of altered reactivity (allergy).

**allergen′ic.** An incitant of allergy.

**allergia** (al-ler′jĭ-ah). Allergy.

**aller′gic.** Relating to any response stimulated by an allergen.

**allergid** (al′er-jid) [ see *-id* (1) ]. A vasculitis manifested by a polymorphous eruption of varying severity ranging from a benign cutaneous allergic disorder to a lethal condition such as polyarteritis nodosa.

**al′lergin.** A seldom used term denoting the reactive substance in the passive transference of anaphylaxis.

**allergiology** (al′er-jĭ-ol′o-ji) [ allergy + G. *logos,* study ]. The science or study of allergy.

**allergization** (al′er-jĭ-za′shun). Active sensitization as a result of allergens being naturally or artificially brought into contact with susceptible tissues.

**allergoder′mia.** An allergic dermatitis.

**allergol'ogy.** Allergiology.

**allergosis** (al'er-go'sis) [ allergy + G. suffix, -osis, condition ]. Any abnormal condition characterized by allergy.

**allergy** (al'er-jī) [ G. allos, other, + ergon, work. ERG- ]. 1. An altered reaction incited by an antigen or allergen, the term having been coined originally by von Pirquet to avoid use of "immune" in processes resulting in induced sensitivity (hypersensitivity), intended to include acquired resistance as well as hypersensitivity; subsequently, for a brief period of time, the term was restricted in usage to reactions resulting from circulating antibodies; sometimes restricted in usage to idiosyncratic sensitivities. The term now is used almost invariably to indicate hypersensitivity of the body cells to a specific substance (antigen, allergen) that results in various types of reaction. Includes anaphylaxis, atopic diseases, serum sickness, and contact dermatitis. 2. That branch of medicine which embraces the study, diagnosis, and treatment of allergic manifestations. 3. An acquired hypersensitivity to certain drugs and biologic preparations.

**bacterial a.,** bacterial hypersensitivity; bacterial sensitivity.

**bronchial a.,** asthma and similar conditions that are allergic in origin.

**cold a.,** physical a. produced by exposure to cold.

**contact a.,** cutaneous reaction caused by direct contact with an allergen to which the person is hypersensitive.

**delayed a.,** delayed type sensitivity (hypersensitivity).

**drug a.,** sensitivity (hypersensitivity) to a drug or other chemical.

**endocrine a.,** sensitivity (hypersensitivity) to an endogenously formed hormone.

**immediate a.,** immediate type sensitivity (hypersensitivity).

**latent a.,** a. that causes no signs or symptoms but can be revealed by means of certain immunologic tests with specific allergens.

**mental a.,** symptoms of a. caused by emotional disturbance.

**physical a.,** erroneous usage of a.; applied to excessive response to factors in the environment such as heat or cold.

**polyvalent a.,** allergic response manifested simultaneously for several or numerous specific allergens.

**Allescheria boy'dii** (al'es-ke'rī-ah boy'di-i). A species of fungi that is parasitic in man and causes maduromycotic mycetoma.

**allesthesia** (al'es-the'zī-ah) [ G. allos, other, + aisthēsis, sensation ]. Allocheiria; alloesthesia; Bamberger's sign (2); a form of allachesthesia in which the sensation of a stimulus in one limb is referred to the opposite limb.

**visual a.,** a disorder characterized by the transposition of images from one half-field to the opposite.

**al'lethrin.** An allylhydroxymethylcyclopentane ester of chrysanthemum-monocarboxylic acid; a viscous liquid, insoluble in water. It is absorbed by lungs, skin, and mucous membranes. It is used as an insecticide, and may cause liver and kidney injury, with lung congestion.

**alli'ance** [ L. alligare, to bind to ]. An association, connection, or union formed for the furtherance of the common interests of its members.

**therapeutic a.,** an implicit agreement between patient and therapist to use insight and control in the resolution of psychic conflict.

**al'licin.** Thio-2-propene-1-sulfinic acid S-allyl ester, $(CH_2=CHCH_2)SO—S(CH_2CH=CH_2)$; an antibacterial agent obtained from Allium saticum (garlic); an irritating liquid with a garlic odor. Active against staphylococci, Bacillus subtilis, and the colon-typhoid-dysentery group of bacteria.

**alliga'tion** [ L. alligatio, fr. al-ligo (adl-), pp. -atus, to bind to ]. A rule of mixtures whereby (a) the cost of a mixture may be determined, given the proportions and prices of the several ingredients; or (b) in pharmacy the relative amounts of solutions of different percentages which must be taken to form a mixture of a given strength.

**alliin.** S-Allylcysteine sulfoxide; $CH_2=CHCH_2(SO)-CH_2CHNH_2COOH$; a sulfur-containing amino acid found in garlic, the odor of which appears upon enzymic conversion to allicin.

**Allis,** Oscar H., Philadelphia surgeon, 1836–1921. See A.'s forceps, sign.

**allit'era'tion** [ Fr. allitération, fr. L. ad, to, + litteram, letter of alphabet ]. In psychiatry, a speech disturbance in which words commencing with the same sounds, usually consonants, are notably frequent.

**allium.** Garlic; Allium sativum (family Liliaceae). The bulb contains up to 0.9 per cent of volatile irritating oil with antiseptic action (see allicin and alliin). It is used as a seasoning, a diaphoretic, diuretic, and expectorant.

**allo-** [ G. allos, other ]. A prefix meaning "other" or differing from the normal or usual.

**al'loalbumine'mia.** The condition of having serum albumin of a variant type that differs in mobility on electrophoresis from the usual type (albumin A); individuals are homozygous for one of the genes for variant albumin types; a genetic polymorphism without known clinical significance. See also inherited albumin variants (under albumin).

**al'loarth'roplasty** [ allo- + G. arthron, joint, + plassō, to form ]. Formation of another or a new joint, using material not from the human body.

**allobar'bital** (USAN). DIAL; 5,5-diallylbarbituric acid; sedative and hypnotic.

**allobiosis** (al-o-bi-o'sis) [ allo- + G. bios, mode of life ]. A change in an organism's responses under altered conditions in the environment.

**allocentric** (al-o-sen'trik). Characterized by or denoting interest centered in other persons rather than in one's self; the antithesis of egocentric.

**allocheiria, allochiria** (al'o-ki'rī-ah) [ allo- + G. cheir, hand ]. Allesthesia.

**allocheiral, allochiral** (al'o-ki'ral). Relating to allocheiria.

**allochezia, allochetia** (al-o-ke'zī-ah, al-o-ke'shī-ah) [ allo- + G. chezō, to defecate ]. The passage of feces through a fistula or other false passage.

**allochiria** (al'-o-ki-rī-ah) Alternative spelling for allocheiria (allesthesia).

**allocholane.** 5α-Cholane.

**allocholesterol** (al-o-ko-les'ter-ōl). Coprostenol; 4-cholesten-3β-ol; an isomer of cholesterol, differing in the position of the one double bond. For structure, see steroids.

**allochro'ic.** Changed or changeable in color; relating to allochroism.

**allochroism** (al-o-kro'izm) [ allo- + G. chrōa, color ]. A change or changeableness in color.

**allochromasia** (al-lo-kro'ma'zī-ah) [ allo- + G. chrōma, color ]. Change of color of the skin or hair.

**alloclamide hydrochloride.** DEGRYP; 2-(allyloxy)-4-chloro-N-[ 2-(diethylamino)ethyl ]benzamide; antitussive with antihistaminic property.

**allocortex** (al'o-kor'teks) [ allo- + L. cortex, bark (cortex) ]. Heterotypic cortex; Vogt's term denoting several regions of the cerebral cortex, in particular the olfactory cortex and the hippocampus, characterized by having fewer cell layers than does the isocortex; see also cortex cerebri.

**α-allocortol.** 5α-Pregnane-3α,11β,17,20α,21-pentaol; differs from cortol in having a 5α H atom (for pregnane structure, see steroids); a metabolite of cortisol found in the urine.

**β-allocortol.** Allo-20β-cortol; 5α-pregnane-3α,11β,17,20β,21-pentaol; 20β isomer of allocortol; 5α enantiomer of β-cortol (for pregnane structure, see steroids); a metabolite of cortisol found in urine.

**α-allocortolone.** 3α,17,20α,21-Tetrahydroxy-5α-pregnane-11-one; 5α enantiomer of cortolone; a metabolite of cortisole found in urine. For structure of pregnane, see steroids.

**β-allocortolone.** 3α,17,20β,21-Tetrahydroxy-5αpregnane-11-one; allo-20β-cortolone; β (at C-20) isomer of allocortolone; a metabolite of cortisol found in urine.

**allocrine** (al'o-krin) [ allo- + G. krinō, to separate ]. Heterocrine.

**allocryp'topine.** $C_{21}H_{23}NO_5$; isomeric with cryptopine; obtained from Chelidonium majus and Sanguinaria canadensis; a mild sedative; locally irritating.

**α-allocryptopine.** α-Fagarine.

**alloeroticism** (al-lo-er-ot'ī-sizm). Alloerotism.

**alloerotism** (al-o-er'o-tizm) [ allo- + G. *erōs*, love ]. Alloeroticism; sexual attraction toward another person, as opposed to autoerotism.

**alloesthe'sia.** Allesthesia.

**allog'amy** [ allo- + G. *gamos*, marriage ]. The fertilization of the ova of one individual by the spermatozoa of another; the opposite of autogamy.

**al'logene'ic, al'logen'ic.** 1. Formerly, pertaining to a different species, or race (heterogeneic). 2. Pertaining to different gene constitutions within the same species, in contradistinction to isogeneic and also to heterogeneic.

**allogotrophia** (al'o-go-tro'fi-ah) [ allo- + G. *trophē*, nourishment ]. Growth or nourishment of one part or tissue at the expense of another part of the body.

**al'lograft.** Allogeneic homograft; a graft from an allogeneic donor of the same species as the recipient, in contradistinction to isograft, on the one hand, and heterograft, on the other.

**allohex'aploid.** See alloploid.

**alloisomer** (al-lo-i'som-er). Geometric *isomer*.

**alloker'atoplasty.** The replacement of opaque corneal tissue with a transparent prosthesis, usually acrylic.

**allokinesis** (al-o-ki-ne'sis) [ allo- + G. *kinēsis*, movement ]. 1. Passive *movement*. 2. Reflex *movement*.

**allola'lia** [ allo- + G. *lalia*, talking ]. Any speech defect, especially one due to disease affecting the speech center.

**allom'erism** [ allo- + G. *meros*, part ]. A characteristic of substances that differ in chemical composition but have the same crystalline form.

**allomet'ron** [ allo- + G. *metron*, measure ]. An evolutionary change in size or proportion of organic beings.

**allometro'pia** [ allo- + G. *metron*, measure, + *ops*, eye ]. Refraction of the eye in indirect vision, as opposed to direct.

**allomorphism** (al-o-mor'fizm) [ allo- + G. *morphē*, form ]. 1. A change of shape in cells due to mechanical causes, such as flattening from pressure, or to progressive metaplasia, such as the change of cells of the bile ducts into liver cells. 2. Similarity of chemical composition, but a difference in crystalline form, especially of crystalline minerals.

**allongement** (al-onzh'-mon) [ Fr. elongation ]. Lengthening of a structure during operation by suitable incisions.

**allon'omous** [ allo- + G. *nomos*, law ]. Governed by external stimuli.

**al'lopath.** 1. One who practices medicine according to the system of allopathy. 2. Erroneously, a physician of the rational or regular school, as distinguished from eclectic or homeopathic practitioners.

**allopath'ic.** Relating to allopathy.

**allop'athist.** Allopath.

**allop'athy** [ allo- + G. *pathos*, suffering ]. Substitutive therapy; auxotherapy; a therapeutic system in which disease is treated by producing a morbid reaction of another kind or in another part—a method of substitution. For example, formerly an injection of a strong solution of silver nitrate might be given early in the course of gonorrhea in order to excite nonspecific inflammation: this procedure employed the principle of a. The gonococcus was unknown at the time.

**allopent'aploid.** See alloploid.

**al'lophanam'ide.** Biuret.

**allophan'ic acid.** *N*-Carboxyurea; carbamoylcarbamic acid; urea carbonic acid; $NH_2CONHCOOH$. The amide is biuret or allophanamide.

**allophasis** (al-of'ă-sis) [ allo- + G. *phasis*, speech ]. Disordered speech.

**al'lophore.** Erythrophore.

**allophthalmia** (al-of-thal'mi-ah). Heterophthalmus.

**alloplasia** (al-o-pla'zi-ah) [ allo- + G. *plasis*, a molding ]. Heteroplasia.

**al'loplast** [ allo- + G. *plastos*, formed ]. 1. A graft of an inert metal or plastic material. 2. An inert foreign body used for implantation into tissues.

**al'loplasty.** The developmental process by which the libido attaches and adapts itself to the environment; the antithesis of autoplasty.

**alloploid** (al'o-ployd) [ allo- + suffix -ploid, *q. v.* ]. Relating to a hybrid individual or cell with two or more sets of chromosomes derived from two different ancestral species. Depending on the number of multiples of haploid sets, alloploids are referred to as alloploids, allotriploids, allotetraploids, allopentaploids, allohexaploids, etc.

**alloploidy** (al-o-ploy'di). The condition of a hybrid individual or cell having two or more sets of chromosomes derived from two different ancestral species.

**allopregnane.** 5α-Pregnane; see pregnane.

**α-allopregnanediol.** 5α-Pregnane-3α,20α-diol; a metabolite of progesterone and adrenocortical hormones, found in urine. For pregnane structure, see steroids.

**β-allopregnanediol.** 5α-Pregnane-3β,20α(and β)-diols; found in urine.

**allopsychic** (al-o-si'kik) [ allo- + G. *psychē*, mind ]. Denoting the mental processes in their relation to the outer world.

**allopurinol** (USP, BP). ZYLOPRIM; 4-hydroxypyrazolo-[ 3,4-*d* ]pyrimidine; HPP; inhibitor of xanthine oxidase, used in the treatment of gout and to retard the rapid metabolic degradation of 6-mercaptopurine.

Allopurinol

**allorhythmia** (al-ō-rith'mi-ah) [ allo- + G. *rhythmos*, rhythm ]. An irregularity in the cardiac rhythm that repeats itself again and again.

**allorhythmic** (al-ō-rith'mik). Relating to or characterized by allorhythmia.

**all or none.** See Bowditch's *law*.

**al'lose.** $C_6H_{12}O_6$; a synthetic sugar isomeric with glucose.

**al'losome** [ allo- + G. *sōma, body* ]. One of the chromosomes differing in appearance or behavior from the ordinary chromosomes, or autosomes, and sometimes unequally distributed among the germ cells; heterochromosome; heterotypical chromosome.

   **paired a.,** diplosome.

   **unpaired a.,** accessory *chromosome*.

**alloster'ic.** Pertaining to or characterized by allosterism.

**allos'terism.** The influencing of an enzyme activity by a change in the conformation of the enzyme, brought about by the noncompetitive binding of a nonsubstrate at a site (the allosteric site) other than the active site of the enzyme.

**allotet'raploid.** See alloploid.

**al'lotherm** [ allo- + G. *thermē*, heat ]. Poikilotherm.

**allothre'onine.** One of four diastereoisomers of threonine, differing from naturally occurring (L) threonine in the configuration of the hydroxyl group in the side chain. Amino acids of the allo series occur whenever the side chain contains an asymmetric carbon, as in alloisoleucine, allohydroxyproline and allohydroxylysine.

**alloto'pia** [ allo- + G. *topos*, place ]. Malposition.

**allotox'in.** Obsolete term for an antitoxin or other substance, formed in the blood or tissues, that checks the injurious action of a toxin.

**al'lotransplanta'tion.** The removal of tissue from one person or animal and grafting it into another of the same species.

**allotrichia circumscripta** (al-o-trik'ĭ-ah sir-kum-skrip'-tah) [ allo- + G. *thrix*, hair, + L. *circumscriptio*, a boundary ]. Woolly-hair *nevus*.

**allotriodontia** (al-ot-rī-o-don'shi-ah) [ G. *allotrios*, foreign, + *odous* (*odont-*), tooth ]. 1. The growth of a tooth in some abnormal location. 2. The transplantation of teeth.

**allotriogeustia** (al-ot'rī-o-gu'sti-ah) [ G. *allotrios*, foreign, + *geusis*, taste ]. Perverted taste for innutritious and unusual objects such as earth.

**allotriophagy** (al-ot-ri-of'ă-ji) [ G. *allotrios*, foreign, + *phagein*, to eat ]. The habit of eating unusual, innutritious, or injurious substances.

**allotriosmia** (al-ot-ri-oz'mĭ-ah) [ G. *allotrios*, foreign, + *osmē*, smell ]. Incorrect recognition of odors.

**allotrip'loid.** See alloploid.

**al'lotrope** [ allo- + G. *tropos*, a turning ]. A substance in one of the allotropic forms that the element may assume.

**allotro'phic** [ allo- + G. *trophē*, nourishment ]. Having an altered nutritive value.

**allotrop'ic.** 1. Relating to allotropy. 2. In psychiatry, denoting a type of personality characterized by a preoccupation with the reactions of others.

**allot'ropism.** Allotropy.

**allot'ropy** [ allo- + G. *tropos*, a turning ]. The existence of certain elements, such as phosphorus and carbon, in several different forms with unlike physical properties.

**allox'an.** An oxidation product of uric acid, 2,4,5,6-pyrimidinetetrone. Its administration to experimental animals causes hypoglycemia due to insulin liberation, followed by hyperglycemia due to destruction of the islets of Langerhans (alloxan diabetes).

**allox'antin.** Uroxin; a condensation product of two molecules of alloxan, formed in the presence of reducing agents; diabetogenic.

**allox'azine.** A heterocyclic compound isomeric to that making up part of the various flavins (isoalloxazine).

**alloxur base.** Obsolete term for purine base.

**alloxure'mia** [ G. *haima*, blood ]. The presence of purine bases in the blood.

**alloxu'ria** [ G. *ouron*, urine ]. The presence of purine bodies in the urine.

**alloy.** A substance composed of a mixture of two or more metals.

**binary a.,** an a. of two metals.

**chrome-cobalt a.'s,** a.'s of cobalt and chromium usually containing nickel plus molybdenum and/or tungsten as well as trace elements; used in dentistry for denture bases, instruments, and other structures.

**Raney a.,** an a. of Ni and Al in equal proportions, used in the preparation of Raney Nickel (*q.v.*, under Raney).

**silver-tin a.,** any a. of silver and tin; Ag 73.15 per cent; Sn 26.83 per cent is Ag₃Sn, the chief intermetallic compound in dental amalgam a.

**ternary a.,** a metal a. having three elements.

**all'spice oil.** Pimenta oil.

**al'lulose.** Psicose.

**allyl** (al'il). The monovalent radical (CH₂=CHCH₂—); included in the molecule of allicin that gives garlic its flavor, also in mustard oil.

**a. alcohol,** 2-propenol; vinyl carbinol; CH₂=CHCH₂OH; a colorless liquid of pungent odor. Used in making resins and plasticizers. Highly irritating to mucous membranes; readily absorbed, causing depression and coma.

**a. cyanide,** 3-butene-nitrile; CH₂=CHCH₂CN; found in some mustard oils.

**a. isothiocyanate,** volatile oil of mustard; allylisosulfocyanate; isothiocyanic acid ester; redskin; CH₂=CH—CH₂—NCS; obtained from *Brassica nigra* or produced synthetically; a vesicant, used in 10 per cent solution in 50 per cent alcohol as a counterirritant in neuralgia; see also mustard oil.

**a. sulfide,** diallyl sulfide; thioallyl ether; "oil garlic"; (CH₂=CHCH₂)S; constituent of garlic oil. Used in the manufacture of flavors.

**al'lylam'ine.** 3-Aminopropylene; CH₂=CH—CH₂—NH₂; a colorless liquid derived from crude oil of mustard. Used in the pharmaceutical industry, *e.g.*, in the manufacture of mercurial diuretics.

**allylbar'bital.** Butalbital.

**allyles'trenol.** GESTANOL; 17-allylestr-4-en-17β-ol; progestational agent.

*N*-**allylnormorphine.** Nalorphine.

**Almeida,** Floriano Paulo de, Brazilian physician. See A.'s *disease*, Lutz-Splendore-A. *disease*.

**Almén,** August T., Swedish physiologist, 1833–1903. See A.'s *test* for blood.

**al'mond oil** (NF, BP). A fixed oil expressed from sweet almonds, the kernels of varieties of *Prunus amygdalus;* used in ointments.

**bitter a. oil,** a volatile oil from the dried ripe kernels of bitter a.'s and from other kernels containing amygdalin; contains between 2 and 4 per cent of hydrocyanic acid and 95 per cent of benzaldehyde.

**al'oe** 1. The dried juice from the leaves of plants of the genus *Aloe* (family Liliaceae), from which are derived aloin, resin, emodin, and volatile oils. 2 (USP, BP). The dried juice from the leaves of *Aloe perryi*, of *A. barbadensis*, or of *A. ferox* and hybrids of this species with *A. africana* and *A. spicata;* it yields not less than 50 per cent of water-soluble extractive; the preparations of the BP are known as aloes and powdered aloes; used as a purgative.

**Barba'dos a.'s,** a variety obtained chiefly from *Aloe chinensis* and *A. vera*.

**Cape a.'s,** Natal a.'s; derived from *Aloe ferox*, used chiefly in veterinary practice.

**Curaçao a.'s,** a variety obtained from the leaves of *Aloe barbadensis*.

**hepatic a.'s,** socotrine a.'s.

**Natal' a.'s,** cape a.'s.

**soc'otrine a.'s,** hepatic a.'s; obtained from *Aloe perryi*.

**aloe-emodin.** 1,8-Dihydroxy-3-(hydroxymethyl)anthraquinone; 3-hydroxymethylchrysazin; rhabarberone; laxative. See aloin and emodin.

**aloetin** (al-o-e'tin). Aloin.

**alogia** (ă-lo'jĭ-ah) [ G. *a*- priv. + *logos*, speech ]. 1. Aphasia. 2. Speechlessness due to mental deficiency or mental confusion.

**alogous** (al'o-gus) [ L. *alogus* fr. G. *alogos*, irrational ]. Unreasonable, irrational.

**aloin** (al'o-in). Barbaloin; aloetin; 1,8-dihydroxy-3-hydroxymethyl-10-(6-hydroxymethyl-3,4,5-trihydroxy-2-pyranyl)anthrone; 10-(1',5'-anhydroglucosyl)-aloe-emodin-9-anthrone; yellow, crystalline principle made up of aloe-emodin and glucose, obtained from aloe. Laxative.

**alope'cia** (al'o-pe'shĭ-ah) [ G. *alōpekia*, a disease like fox mange, fr. *alōpēx*, a fox ]. Acomia; calvities; pelade; baldness; loss of hair.

**a. adna'ta,** a. congenitalis.

**a. area'ta,** a condition of unknown etiology productive of circumscribed, noninflamed areas of baldness on the scalp, eyebrows, and bearded portion of the face. Also called a. circumscripta; Celsus' a. or area; Jonston's a. or area; porrigo decalvans; vitiligo capitis; Cazenave's or Celsus' vitiligo.

**a. cap'itis tota'lis,** total loss of hair from the scalp; see also a. totalis.

**a. celsi, Celsus' a.,** a. areata.

**cicatricial a., a cicatrisa'ta,** a. produced by scar formation as in dermatoses such as folliculitis decalvans, pseudopelade, and lupus erythematosus.

**a. circumscrip'ta,** a. areata.

**congenital sutural a.,** see *dyscephalia* mandibulo-oculofacialis.

**a. congenita'lis,** congenital baldness; a. adnata; absence of all hair at birth.

**a. dissemina'ta,** loss of hair from all parts of the body.

**a. dynam'ica,** hair loss due to some destructive disease process affecting the hair follicles.

**a. follicula'ris,** *folliculitis* decalvans.

**a. hereditaria,** male pattern baldness; sex-influenced dominant inheritance, androgen stimulation required to produce hair loss in heterozygous individuals; homozygous females may have minor hair loss without androgen stimulation.

**Jonston's a.,** a. areata.

**a. leproti'ca,** (1) a rare moth-eaten, patchy type of a. seen in leprosy; (2) the more common lepromatous thinning or total loss of eyebrows and eyelashes.

**a. limina'ris fronta'lis,** hair loss at the hair line; a condition most commonly seen in Negroes; it may be associated with seborrheic dermatitis but the factor of trauma also plays a major role.

**moth-eaten a.,** patchy hair loss of parietal and occipital regions of the scalp, characteristic in secondary syphilis.

**a. mucino'sa,** a relatively unusual condition of unknown origin that may develop as areas of erythema, edema and alopecia in the bearded portion of the face or in the scalp.

**a. neurot'ica,** a. of trophoneurotic origin.

**a. pityro'des** [ G. *pityrōdes*, branny, scurfy ], a falling of the hair, of the body as well as of the scalp, accompanied by an abundant branlike desquamation.

**postoperative pressure a.,** loss of hair over circumscribed area on the posterior scalp from the necessarily continuous pressure on the occiput in a lengthy operative procedure.

**premature a., a. prematu'ra,** ordinary baldness appearing at an unusually early age.

**a. preseni'lis,** ordinary or common baldness occurring in early or middle life without any apparent disease of the scalp.

**a. seni'lis,** the normal falling of the hair of the scalp in old age.

**a. symptomat'ica,** a. occurring in the course of various constitutional or local diseases, or following prolonged febrile illness.

**a. syphilit'ica,** moth-eaten a. (*q. v.*) of secondary syphilis.

**a. tota'lis,** total loss of hair of the scalp (total loss of scalp and body hair is designated a. universalis), not accompanied by any gross inflammatory reaction.

**a. tox'ica,** hair loss attributed to febrile illness.

**a. triangula'ris congenita'lis,** a triangular patch of baldness on the frontal or temporal region; a congenital defect.

**a. universa'lis,** total loss of hair from all parts of the body; *cf.* a. totalis.

**alopecic** (al'-o-pe'-sik). Relating to alopecia.

**Alouette's amputation.** See under amputation.

**alox'idone.** MALIDONE; MALAZOL; 3-allyl-5-methyl-2,4-oxazolidinedione; anticonvulsant (antiepileptic, petit mal) agent.

**alox'iprin.** ALAPRIN; condensation product of aluminum oxide and aspirin; analgesic.

**Alpers,** Bernard J., American neurologist, *1900. See A.'s *disease.*

**alpha** (al'fah). The first letter of the Greek alphabet (α). Used as a classifier in the nomenclature of many sciences. In chemistry denotes the first in a series of isomeric compounds; symbol for specific rotation; denotes a position immediately adjacent to a carboxyl group, as in α-amino acid; the first of a series of closely related compounds, as α-glucose, α-carotene, α-amylase. For most compounds or other terms having this prefix, see under the specific compound or term.

**al'pha am'ylase** (USAN). BUCLAMASE, FORTIZYME; a starch-splitting enzyme obtained from a non pathogenic bacterium of the *Bacillus subtilis* class. Used in the treatment of inflammatory conditions and edema of soft tissues associated with traumatic injury. Its therapeutic usefulness has not been fully established. The mode of action is not known. See also amylase.

**alphaprodine hydrochloride** (NF). PRISILIDENE; NISENTIL; α-1,3-dimethyl-4-phenyl-4-piperidinyl propionate hydrochloride; a narcotic analgesic related to meperidine; physical and psychic dependence may develop.

**alphasone acetophenide.** Algestone acetophenide.

**alphodermia** (al-fo-der'mĭ-ah) [ G. *alphos*, leprosy, + *derma*, skin ]. Absence of cutaneous pigmentation.

**alphon'sin** [ *Alphonse* Ferri ]. A three-pronged bullet forceps.

**alphos** (al'fos) [ G. *alphos*, leprosy ]. Psoriasis.

**al'phyl.** See aralkyl.

**Alport,** A. Cecil, South African physician, 1880–1959. See A.'s *syndrome.*

**alpren'olol hydrochloride** (BP, USAN). APTINE; hydrochloride salt of *dl*-1-(2-allylphenoxy)-3-isopropylaminopropan-2-ol; a β-receptor blocking agent, used for the treatment of cardiac arrhythmias.

**ALS.** Abbreviation for anti-lymphocyte *serum.*

**Alsberg's angle** or **triangle.** See under triangle.

**al'serox'ylon.** RAUWILOID; a fat-soluble alkaloidal fraction extracted from the root of *Rauwolfia serpentina,* containing reserpine and other nonadrenolytic amorphous alkaloids. Used as a sedative in psychoses, in mild

hypertension, and as an adjunct to more potent hypotensive drugs.

**Alston,** Charles, Edinburgh physician, 1683–1760. Gave his name to *Alstonia.*

**alsto'nia** [ C. *Alston* ]. Dita bark; the dried bark of *Alstonia scholaris* and *A. constricta* (family Apocynaceae), tropical trees. It contains about 10 alkaloids, including the strongly alkaline echitenine and ditaine (see echitamine). Formerly used in malaria.

**al'stonine.** Chlorogenin; an alkaloid from alstonia. Antiseptic and antipyretic.

**Alström,** Carl Henry, Swedish geneticist. See A.'s *syndrome.*

**alter** (awl'ter) [ Mediev. L. *altero*, pp. *-atus,* to change, fr. L. *alter,* other ]. 1. To change; to make different; to become different. 2. To remove the gonads from an animal; usually refers to the operation on a male animal.

**alterant** (awl'ter-ant). Alterative. 1. Causing a favorable change in the disordered functions of the body or in metabolism. 2. Obsolete term for drug.

**alteration** (awl-ter-a'shun). 1. A change. 2. A changing; a making different.

**a. cavitaire** [ Fr. ], intracellular edema of the epidermis; it produces a vacuolated appearance of the epithelial cells.

**modal a.,** in electric irritability, a change in the mode of response of degenerated muscle to electric stimulation, the contraction being sluggish instead of quick.

**qualitative a.,** in electric irritability, a change in which the muscle contracts as readily on application of the anode as on that of the cathode.

**quantitative a.,** in electric irritability, a gradual loss of contractility in a muscle in response to static, faradic, and galvanic currents successively.

**alterative** (awl-ter-a'tiv). Alterant.

**alteregoism** (awl-ter-e'go-izm). Identification with people of similar personality to one's own.

**alternans** (awl-ter-nanz') [ L. ]. Alternating; often used substantively for alternation of the heart.

**auditory a.,** auscultatory a.

**auscultatory a.,** auditory a.; alternation in the intensity of heart sounds or murmurs in the presence of a regular cardiac rhythm as a result of alternation of the heart.

**concordant a.,** right ventricular and pulmonary artery a. occur simultaneously with peripheral pulsus a.

**discordant a.,** right ventricular and pulmonary artery a. are present with peripheral pulsus a., but the strong beat of the right ventricle coincides with the weak beat of the left and vice versa.

**electrical a.,** electrical alternation of the heart.

**pulsus a.,** the pulse beats, although regularly spaced, alternate in tension as a result of alternation of the heart.

**visual a.,** alternating excursions of aortic and left ventricular pulsation when observed fluoroscopically.

**Alterna'ria.** A genus of fungi frequently isolated from air and usually considered to be a common laboratory contaminant.

**alternation** (awl-ter-na'shun). The occurrence of two things or phases in succession and recurrently.

**concordant a.,** a. in either the mechanical or electrical activity of the heart, occurring in both systemic and pulmonary circuits.

**discordant a.,** a. in cardiac activities of either the systemic or the pulmonic circuits, but not of both.

**electrical a. of heart,** a disorder in which the ventricular complexes are regular in time but of alternating pattern; a. of P waves occurs rarely.

**a. of generation,** see under generation.

**a. of the heart,** a disorder in which contractions of the heart are regular in time but are alternately stronger and weaker; mechanical a.

**alternocular** (awl-ter-nok'u-lar). Denoting the use of each eye separately instead of binocularly; *e.g.,* one eye for distant vision, the other for near.

**Althe'a** [ L. fr. G. *althaia,* marshmallow ]. Marshmallow root; root of *Althea officinalis* (family Malvaceae). Used in the form of syrup or lozenge as a demulcent in irritation of the mouth and pharynx. Dried leaves have also been used.

**Altherr,** Franz. See Meyenburg-A.-Uehlinger *syndrome*.

**althi′azide** (USAN). Altizide; 3-[ (allythio)methyl ]-6-chloro-3,4-dihydro-2*H*-1,2,4-benzothiadiazine-7-sulfonamide 1,1-dioxide; diuretic also used as antihypertensive agent.

**altizide.** Althiazide.

**Altmann,** Richard, German histologist, 1852–1900. See A.'s *fluid, granule, theory,* A.-Gersh *method.*

**altricious** (al-trish′us) [ L. *altrix* (*altric-*), a nurse, fr. *alo,* to nourish ]. Requiring prolonged nursing care.

**altrigen′drism** [ L. *altri,* fr. *alteri,* other, + Fr. *gendre,* fr. L. *genus,* sort ]. Natural, wholesome, nonerotic activity between the sexes.

**al′trose.** An aldohexose isomeric with glucose, tallose, allose, etc.

**al′um** (NF, BP). A double sulfate of aluminum and of an alkaline earth element or ammonium; chemically an a. is any one of the double salts formed by a combination of a sulfate of aluminum, iron, manganese, chromium, or gallium with a sulfate of lithium, sodium, potassium, ammonium, cesium, or rubidium. The a.'s, markedly astringent, are used locally as styptics.

**burnt a.,** dried a.

**cake a.,** aluminum sulfate octadecahydrate.

**chrome a.,** the sulfate of chromium and potassium; used as a mordant in histologic staining.

**a. curd,** milk coagulated by alum.

**dried a.,** burnt a.; a. deprived of its water of crystallization by heat; an astringent dusting powder.

**ex′siccated a.,** a. heated to complete dryness; a local astringent.

**iron a.,** ferric ammonium sulfate.

**whey a.,** an astringent and styptic preparation made by boiling a. (1 oz.) in milk (10 oz.).

**alum-hematoxylin.** A purple tissue stain used in histology; a mixture of an aqueous solution of ammonium alum and an alcoholic solution of hematoxylin.

**alu′mina.** Aluminum oxide.

**alu′minated.** Containing alum.

**alumino′sis.** A chronic catarrhal affection of the respiratory passages occurring in workers in alum.

**aluminum** [ L. *alumen,* alum ]. A white silvery metal of very light weight. Symbol Al; atomic no. 13, atomic weight 26.98.

**a. acetate,** used as a disinfectant by embalmers; proposed as desiccant and deodorant powder for eczema and chronic skin ulcers.

**a. acetotartrate,** ALSOL; 70 per cent basic aluminum acetate and 30 per cent tartaric acid; antiseptic.

**a. acetylsalicylate,** a. aspirin.

**a. ammonium sulfate,** $AlNH_4(SO_4)_2$; astringent.

**a. aspirin,** a. acetylsalicylate; analgesic and antipyretic.

**a. bismuth oxide,** bismuth aluminate.

**a. bromide,** $AlBr_3$; used in solution as a mouth wash or gargle.

**a. carbonate, basic,** an a. hydroxide-carbonate complex; $Al_2O_3CO_2$; white lumps, insoluble in water. Aqueous suspensions bind phosphorus in the intestine, lower serum inorganic phosphorus resulting in an increase in reabsorption of phosphorus by renal tubules and reduction of urinary excretion of phosphorus. Reduces formation of phosphatic urinary calculi and gastric acidity.

**a. chlorate nonahydrate,** mallebrin; $Al(ClO_3)_3 \cdot 9H_2O$; antiseptic.

**a. chloride hexahydrate** (NF), $AlCl_3 \cdot 6H_2O$; used as an astringent or antiseptic in solution; may be irritating.

**a. diacetate,** a. subacetate.

**a. group,** boron, aluminum, gallium, indium, and thallium.

**a. hydroxide,** hydrated alumina; a. hydrate; $Al(OH)_3$; an astringent dusting powder; also used internally as a mild astringent antacid.

**a. hydroxide gel** (USP, BP), AMPHOJEL; a suspension containing $Al_2O_3$ mainly in the form of a. hydroxide; used as antacid.

**a. hydroxide gel, dried** (USP, BP), obtained by drying the product of interaction in aqueous solution of an a. salt with ammonium or sodium carbonate. Same use as a. hydroxide gel.

**a. hydroxychloride,** CHLORHYDROL; antiperspirant.

**a. magnesium silicate,** magnesium aluminum silicate.

**a. monostearate** (USP), a compound of a. with a mixture of solid organic acids obtained from fats, and consisting chiefly of a. monostearate and a. monopalmitate. Used as a suspending medium in pharmaceutical preparations.

**a. β-naph′tholdisul′fonate,** ALUMNOL; $Al_2[ C_{10}H_5$—OH—$(SO_3)_2 ]_3$; a white powder, soluble in water. Used locally, on mucous membranes, as an astringent antiseptic.

**a. nicotinate,** NICALEX; tris(nicotinato)aluminum; lipopenic agent with peripheral vasodilator action.

**a. o′leate,** $Al(C_{18}H_{33}O_2)_3$; used as an ointment in certain cutaneous affections and in burns.

**a. oxide,** alumina; $Al_2O_3$; used as an abrasive, as a refractory, and in chromatography.

**a. penicil′lin,** see under penicillin.

**a. phe′nolsul′fonate,** $Al(C_6H_4(OH)SO_3)_3$; antiseptic and astringent for local application, usually for cutaneous ulcers.

**a. phosphate,** PHOSPHALJEL; $AlPO_4$; infusible powder, insoluble in water but soluble in alkali hydroxides; used for dental cements with calcium sulfate and sodium silicate.

**a. phosphate gel** (NF), an aqueous suspension of between 4.0 and 5.0 per cent of a. phosphate; antacid.

**a. potassium sulfate,** potassium alum; $AlK(SO_4)_2$; an astringent and styptic; also used in veterinary medicine for ulcerative stomatitis, leukorrhea, and conjunctivitis.

**a. salicylate, basic,** SALUMIN; used in the treatment of ozena and pharyngitis.

**a. salicylate, basic, soluble,** soluble SALUMIN; ammoniated basic a. salicylate; used in solution as a spray for diseases of the upper air passages.

**a. silicate,** kaolin.

**a. subacetate,** a. diacetate; $Al(CH_3CO_2)_2OH$; used in solution as an astringent, as an ingredient in mouth washes, and in embalming fluids.

**a. sulfate octadecahydrate** (USP), cake alum; astringent detergent for skin ulcers.

**Alvegniat's pump.** See under pump.

**alveoalgia** (al′ve-o-al′ji-ah) [ alveolus + G. *algos,* pain ]. Dry socket; alveolalgia; alveolar osteitis; a distressing postoperative sequela to tooth extractions, in which condition the blood clot in the socket disintegrates, leading to an empty socket that becomes secondarily infected. Symptoms start on the second or third day after the extraction and last 10 to 40 days.

**alveobronchiolitis** (al-ve-o-brong′ki-o-li′tis). Bronchopneumonia; inflammation of the bronchioles and pulmonary alveoli; capillary bronchitis with involvement of the alveoli.

**alveolal′gia.** Alveoalgia.

**alve′olar.** Relating to an alveolus.

**alve′olate.** Pitted like a honeycomb.

**alveolec′tomy** [ alveolus + G. *ektomē,* excision ]. 1. Excision of a portion or the whole of the alveolar process. 2. Alveolotomy.

**alveoli** (al-ve′o-li). Plural of alveolus.

**alveolin′gual.** Alveololingual.

**alveoli′tis.** Inflammation of alveoli.

**acute pulmonary a.,** acute inflammation involving the pulmonary alveoli, which may result in necrosis with hemorrhage into the lungs. May be associated with glomerulonephritis, in Goodpasture's syndrome.

**extrinsic allergic a.,** pneumoconiosis resulting from hypersensitivity due to repeated inhalation of organic dust, usually specified according to occupational exposure; in acute form, respiratory symptoms and fever start several hours after exposure to the dust; in chronic form, there is eventual diffuse pulmonary fibrosis after exposure over several years.

**alveolo-** [ L. *alveolus, q.v.* ]. Combining form denoting relation to an alveolus or to the alveolar process.

**alveoloclasia** (al-ve′o-lo-kla′zi-ah) [ alveolo- + G. *klasis,* breaking ]. Destruction of the alveolus.

**alve′oloden′tal.** Relating to the alveoli and the teeth; periodontal.

**alve′olola′bial.** [ alveolo- + Mediev. L. *labialis,* relating to a lip ]. Relating to the labial or outer surface of the alveolar processes.

**alve′ololabia′lis** [ L. ]. Referring to the alveololabial sulcus region.

**alveololingual** (al-ve′o-lo-ling′gwal). Alveolingual; relating to the lingual or inner surface of the alveolar process.

**alve′olomerot′omy** [ alveolo- + G. *meros*, part, + *tomē*, a cutting ]. Surgical removal of a part of the alveolar process.

**alveolopal′atal.** Referring to the palatal surface of the alveolar process.

**alve′oloplas′ty** [ alveolo- + G. *plassō*, to form ]. The surgical preparation of the alveolar ridges for the reception of dentures; also, shaping and smoothing of socket margins after extraction of multiple teeth with subsequent suturing to insure uncomplicated healing.

    **interradicular a.,** intraseptal a.; removal of the interradicular bone and collapsing of the cortical plates to a more desirable alveolar contour.

**alveoloschisis** (al-ve-o-los′kĭ-sis) [ alveolo- + G. *schisis*, cleaving ]. Cleft of the alveolar process.

**alveolot′omy** [ alveolo- + G. *tomē*, incision ]. Alveolectomy (2); the operation of opening into a dental alveolus to give exit to retained pus or other fluid and to gain access to the cavity for treatment.

**alve′olus,** gen. and pl. **alve′oli** [ L. dim. of *alveus*, trough, hollow sac, cavity ] [ NA ]. A small cell or cavity. 1. An air cell; one of the terminal saclike dilations of the alveolar ducts in the lung. 2. One of the terminal secretory portions of an alveolar or racemose gland. 3. One of the honeycomb pits in the wall of the stomach. 4. The a. dentalis.

    **a. dentalis,** pl. **alveoli dentales** [ NA ], alveolus (4); tooth socket; odontobothrion; a socket, of which there are usually 16 in the processus alveolaris of the maxilla or mandible, into which each tooth fits and is attached by means of the periodontal membrane.

    **alveoli pulmo′nis** [ NA ], the air cells of the lungs; bronchic cells; air vesicles; the terminal dilations of the bronchioles where gas exchange is thought to occur.

**alveoplas′ty.** Alveoloplasty.

**al′verine citrate** (USAN). PROFENIL; SPACOLIN; *N*-ethyl-3,3′-diphenyldipropylamine citrate; a smooth muscle relaxant and antispasmodic; may cause hypotension.

**al′veus,** pl. **al′vei** [ L. tray, trough, cavity, fr. *alvus*, belly ] [ NA ]. A channel or trough.

    **a. hippocampi** [ NA ], alveus of the hippocampus; that portion of the fornix covering the ventricular surface of the hippocampus.

    **a. urogenita′lis,** *utriculus* prostaticus.

**alvine** (al′vin, -vīn) [ L. *alvus*, belly ]. Relating to the abdomen or the intestine.

**alvinolith** (al-vin′o-lith, al-vi′no-lith) [ L. *alvus*, belly, + G. *lithus*, stone ]. An enteric calculus.

**alymphia** (ā-lim′fī-ah). Absence or deficiency of lymph.

**alymph′ocyto′sis.** Absence or great reduction of lymphocytes.

**alymphoplasia** (ā-lim′fo-pla′zĭ-ah). Aplasia or hypoplasia of lymphoid tissue.

    **Nezelof type of thymic a.,** Nezelof *syndrome.*

    **thymic a.,** lymphopenic thymic dysplasia; thymic hypoplasia, with absence of Hassell's corpuscles and deficiency of lymphocytes in the thymus and usually in lymph nodes, spleen, and gastrointestinal tract; there is peripheral lymphopenia and often hypogammaglobulinemia and absence of plasma cells; thymic a. presents in early infancy with respiratory infections and leads to death within a few months.

**alymph′opo′tent** [ G. *a*- priv. + lymphocyte + L. *potens*, able ]. Unable to produce lymphocytes or lymphoid cells.

**alysmus** (ā-lis′mus) [ G. *alysmos*, disquiet ]. Restlessness; anguish, especially in a sick person.

**Alzheimer** (altz′hi-mer), Alois, German neurologist, 1864–1915. See A.'s *disease, glia, sclerosis.*

**Am.** 1. Chemical symbol of the element americium. 2. Abbreviation for ametropia, or for mixed astigmatism.

**amaas** (ah′mahs) [ Kaffir, sour milk ]. Alastrim.

**amacrine** (am′ā-krin) [ G. *a*- priv. + *makros*, long, + *is* (*in*-), fiber ]. 1. A cell or structure lacking a long, fibrous

process. 2. Denoting such a cell or structure; see also amacrine *cell.*

**amadou.** Agaric.

**amake′be.** East coast *fever.*

**amal′gable.** Capable of amalgamation.

**amal′gam** [ G. *malagma*, a soft mass. MALAC- ]. A solution of metal in mercury which may set. In dentistry, the metal consists mainly of intermetallic compound Ag₃Sn (approximate formula Ag 67 per cent, Cu 5 per cent, Sn 27 per cent, Zn 1 per cent); zinc and copper are useful but not essential. About one part alloy to two parts mercury are mixed and packed; this hardens to almost full strength in 24 hours. Properties of set a. depend largely on technique, mixing time, packing pressure, etc. Crushing strengths range from 45,000 to 65,000 pounds per square inch for most (A.D.A. specification no. 1).

    **edge-strength of a.,** capability to resist fracture in thin sections; the crushing strength may be used as a measure of strength.

    **flow of a.,** plastic deformation under static load; A.D.A. specification requires less than 4 per cent flow and gives a specific technique for measuring it.

    **pin a.,** an a. restoration held in place largely by small metal rods protruding from holes drilled into tooth structure.

    **spherical a.,** an a. alloy, used in dentistry, composed of spherical particles and claimed to be superior to those composed of filings.

**amal′gamate.** To make an amalgam.

**amal′gama′tion.** The process of combining mercury with a metal or an alloy to form a new alloy.

**amal′gama′tor.** A device for combining mercury with a metal or an alloy to form a new alloy.

**am′andin.** A globulin present in almonds.

**Amanita** (am-ă-ni′tah) [ G. *amanitai*, fungi ]. A genus of fungi, many members of which are highly poisonous.

    **A. muscaria,** fly agaric; fly mushroom; *Agaricus muscarius* (family Agaricaceae); a toxic mushroom with red pileus and white gills. It contains muscarine, and poisoning produces psychosis-like states and other symptoms caused by muscarine, *q. v.*

    **A. phalloides,** deadly agaric; contains a poisonous principle that causes gastroenteritis, hepatic necrosis, and renal necrosis.

**amanozine.** UROFORT; 2-amino-4-anilino-*s*-triazine; diuretic.

**aman′tadine hydrochloride** (NF). SYMMETREL; 1-adamantanamine; an antiviral agent; also used to treat parkinsonism.

**ama′ra** [ neut. pl. of L. *amarus*, bitter ]. Bitters.

**am′arant.** Amaranthum.

**amaran′thum** [ G. *amaranthon*, a never fading flower ] (USP). FD & C Red No. 2; amarant; an azo dye, 1-(4-sulfo-1-naphthylazo)-2-naphthol-3,6-disulfonate (trisodium salt); a soluble reddish brown powder, the color turning to magenta red in solution; a food and cosmetic coloring agent.

**am′aril** [ Sp. *amarillo*, yellow ]. The toxin of Sanarelli's bacillus, *Bacillus icteroides*, at one time asserted to be the specific organism of yellow fever.

**amaril′lic** [ Sp. *amarillo*, yellow ]. Relating to yellow fever.

**amarine** (am′ā-rin) [ L. *amarus*, bitter ]. A name applied to various bitter principles derived from plants. Applied especially to a poisonous substance, 2,4,5-triphenylimidazoline, obtained from oil of bitter almond.

**am′aroid** [ L. *amarus*, bitter, + G. *eidos*, like ]. A bitter extractive that does not belong to the class of glycosides, alkaloids, or any of the known proximate principles of plants.

**amaroi′dal.** Resembling the bitters. Having a slightly bitter taste.

**ama′rum** [ neut. of L. *amarus*, bitter ]. One of a class of vegetable drugs of bitter taste, such as gentian and quassia, used as appetizers and tonics.

**amarylline** (am′ā-ril′ēn). Narcissine.

**amas′tia** [ G. *a*- priv. + *mastos*, breast ]. Absence of the breasts.

**amastigote** (ă-mas'tĭ-gōt) [ G. *a*- priv. + *mastix*, whip ]. Intracellular phase of flagellate protozoan parasites, such as *Leishmania donovani* or *Trypanosoma cruzi;* formerly called Leishman-Donovan (LD) bodies.

**amathophobia** (ă-math-o-fo'bĭ-ah) [ G. *amathos*, dust, + *phobos*, fear ]. Fear of dust or dirt.

**am'ativeness** [ L. *amo*, pp. *amatus*, to love ]. 1. Sexual desire. 2. The propensity to love.

**amaurosis** (am-aw-ro'sis) [ G. *amauros*, dark, obscure, + suffix *-osis*, condition ]. Blindness, especially that occurring without apparent change in the eye itself; *e.g.*, from a cortical lesion.
  **a. centralis,** a. caused by central nervous system disease.
  **a. congenita of Leber,** heredoretinopathia congenita; an autosomal recessive cone-rod abiotrophy causing blindness or amblyopia at birth; frequent in Holland and Sweden.
  **a. fugax,** a temporary blindness; it may result from a transient ischemia due to cerebral arterial disease or to centrifugal force (flight blindness or visual blackout without loss of consciousness in aviators).
  **a. partia'lis fugax,** temporary blindness occurring in attacks, associated with headache, nausea, and scotomas.
  **sabur'ral a.,** a. associated with symptoms of acute gastric disturbance.
  **toxic a.,** blindness due to optic neuritis excited by tobacco, alcohol, wood alcohol, lead, arsenic, quinine, or other poisons.

**amaurotic** (am-aw-rot'ik). Relating to or suffering from amaurosis.

**amaxophobia** (ă-mak-so-fo'bĭ-ah) [ G. *amaxa, hamaxa*, a carriage, + *phobos*, fear ]. Hamaxophobia; morbid fear of meeting or of riding in any sort of vehicle.

**ama'zia.** Amastia.

**Amazo'na aesti'va.** A variety of Amazon parrot, one of the sources of infection in ornithosis.

**ambageusia** (am-bah-gu'sĭ-ah) [ L. *ambo*, both, + *a*- priv. + G. *geusis*, taste ]. Loss of taste from both sides of the tongue.

**Ambard** (ahm-bar'), Léon, Strasbourg pharmacologist, 1876–1962. See A.'s *coefficient, constant, law.*

**ambeno'mium chloride** (NF). MYTELASE; *N,N'*-bis-2-[ (2-chlorobenzyl)diethylammonium chloride ]ethyloxamide; a cholinesterase inhibitor used chiefly in the management of myasthenia gravis and occasionally for intestinal and urinary tract obstruction. It is similar to neostigmine in actions.

**am'ber** [ Mediev. L. *ambra*, amber, fr. Ar. *'anbar*, ambergris ]. Succinite; the pale yellow fossil resin of pine trees found in Northern Europe; contains 5 per cent succinic acid; becomes negatively electrified in friction. It is used for ornaments.
  **a. oil,** a volatile oil distilled from a.

**Amberg,** Emil, American physician, 1868–1948. See A.'s lateral sinus *line.*

**am'bergris** [ Mod. L. *ambra grisea*, gray amber ]. A grayish pathologic secretion from the intestine of the sperm whale; occurs as a flammable, waxy mass, insoluble in water, melting point about 60°C. Contains cholesterol and benzoic acid. Used as a base for perfume.

**ambi-** [ L. *ambo*, both ]. Prefix meaning round; all (both) sides.

**ambidex'ter** [ ambi- + L. *dexter*, right ]. Having equal facility in the use of both hands.

**ambidexter'ity.** The ability to use both hands with equal ease.

**ambidex'trism.** Ambidexterity.

**ambidex'trous.** Ambidexter.

**ambient** (am'bĭ-ent) [ L. *ambiens*, going around ]. Surrounding, environing; pertaining, for example, to the air, noise, temperature, etc., in which an organism or apparatus (such as an electronic pacemaker) functions.

**ambig'uous** [ L. *ambiguus*, fr. *ambigo*, to wander ]. 1. In anatomy, wandering; having more than one direction. 2. Having more than one interpretation.

**ambig'uus** [ L. ] [ NA ]. Ambiguous.

**ambilat'eral** [ ambi- + L. *latus*, side ]. Relating to both sides.

**ambilevous** (am-bĭ-le'vus) [ ambi- + L. *laevus*, left ]. Awkward in the use of both hands.

**ambisex'ual.** Bisexual.

**ambisin'ister** [ ambi- + L. *sinister*, left ]. Ambilevous.

**am'bisinis'trous.** Ambilevous.

**ambiv'alence** [ ambi- + L. *valentia*, strength ]. The coexistence of antithetical attitudes or emotions toward a given person or thing; in psychiatry, often refers to the simultaneous feeling and expression of love and hate toward the same person.

**ambiv'alent.** Relating to or characterized by ambivalence.

**ambiversion** (am-bĭ-ver'zhun) [ ambi- + L. *verto*, pp. *vertus*, to turn ]. A mean between extroversion and introversion.

**am'bivert.** A person who falls between the two extremes of introversion and extroversion, possessing some of the tendencies of each.

**ambly-** [ G. *amblys*, dull ]. Combining form denoting dullness, dimness.

**amblyaphia** (am-blĭ-a'fĭ-ah) [ ambly- + G. *haphē*, touch ]. Diminution in tactile sensibility.

**amblychromasia** (am-blĭ-kro-ma'zĭ-ah) [ ambly- + G. *chrōma*, color ]. A condition in which, chromatin being scanty, a cell nucleus stains faintly.

**amblychromatic** (am-blĭ-kro-mat'ik). Staining faintly; denoting especially a nucleus having but little chromatin.

**amblygeustia** (am-blĭ-gūs'tĭ-ah) [ ambly- + G. *geusis*, taste ]. A blunted sense of taste.

**Amblyomma** (am-ble-om'ah) [ ambly- + G. *omma*, eye, vision ]. A genus of ornate, hard ticks (family Ixodidae) characterized by having eyes, festoons, and deeply imbedded ventral plates near the festoons in males.
  **A. america'num,** Lone-Star tick; it occurs on dogs and many other hosts, including domestic animals, birds, and man; it bites man in larval, nymphal, and adult stages. This tick is an important pest and vector of Rocky Mountain spotted fever, and is found primarily in the southern United States and northern Mexico.
  **A. cajennen'se,** an important pest in Texas, Central and South America, and the West Indies, and the vector of Rocky Mountain spotted fever in Mexico and Central and South America; all stages attack man, domestic animals, and many other hosts.
  **A. hebrae'um,** it occurs on cattle, antelopes, and occasionally man in South Africa and transmits cattle heartwater and African tick typhus to man.
  **A. macula'tum,** the Gulf Coast tick; it occurs in dogs in southeastern United States.
  **A. variega'tum,** vector of cattle heartwater in South Africa and of Nairobi disease.

**amblyopia** (am-blĭ-o'pĭ-ah) [ G. *amblyōpia*, dimness of vision, fr. *amblys* dull, + *ōps*, eye ]. Dimness of vision; partial loss of sight.
  **a. alcohol'ica,** dimness of vision as the result of alcohol poisoning.
  **anisometropic a.,** a functional a. resulting from a marked difference in refractive errors.
  **arsenic a.,** see toxic a.
  **color a.,** see dichromatism.
  **eclipse a.,** solar or eclipse blindness; a macular phototraumatism consequent to watching solar eclipses with inadequate protection; the condition is due to the burning action of thermal rays. See also photoretinopathy.
  **a. ex anop'sia,** dimness of vision from nonuse, occurring in the young as a result of cataract, refractive errors of high degree, etc., which prevent accurate focusing on the retina.
  **hysterical a.,** a manifestation, sometimes, of hysteria.
  **nocturnal a.,** nyctalopia.
  **nutritional a.,** a. resulting from lack of B-complex constituents, thiamin, riboflavin, niacin, or vitamin $B_{12}$; irreversible in prolonged deficiency.
  **quinine a.,** see toxic a.
  **receptor a.,** a result of retinal hemorrhages at birth.
  **strabismic a.,** a cortical suppression of central vision to avoid diplopia and confusion.
  **toxic a.,** chronic retrobulbar optic neuritis caused by tobacco, alcohol liquors, wood alcohol, lead, quinine, arsenic, and certain other poisons.

**uremic a.,** loss of sight, without apparent lesion of the retina, sometimes occurring during an attack of uremia.

**am'blyopiat'rics** [ amblyopia + G. *iatrikos,* relating to medicine ]. Treatment of dimness of vision.

**amblyoscope** (am'blī-o-skōp) [ amblyopia + G. *skopeō,* to view ]. A reflecting stereoscope used for training the fusion sense in strabismus and for stimulation of vision in the amblyopic eye; see also haploscope.

**major a.,** a large, table-supported a.

**Worth's a.,** the original a., a hand-held model consisting of angled tubes which can be swiveled to any degree of convergence or divergence.

**ambo-** [ G. *ambo,* both ]. Prefix meaning round; all (both) sides.

**ambocep'toid.** Obsolete term for an altered amboceptor that has only the complementophil group.

**am'boceptor** [ ambo- + L. *capio,* to take ]. A term originated by Ehrlich expressing his concept, now outmoded, of the structure of complement-fixing antibody; now used chiefly to denote the anti-sheep erythrocyte antibody used in the hemolytic system of complement-fixation tests.

**ambocep'torgen.** Obsolete term for an antigen.

**ambomal'leal.** Relating to the ambos, or incus, and the malleus.

**ambos** [ Ger. ]. Incus.

**ambosexual** (am-bo-seks'u-al). Bisexual.

**ambro'sin.** A principle in ragweed related to absinthin.

**am'bucaine.** SYMPOCAINE; 2-butoxyprocaine; 4-amino-2-butoxybenzoic acid-2-diethylaminoethyl ester; a long-acting, potent, but occasionally irritating local anesthetic.

**ambucet'amide.** DIBUTAMIDE; α-dibutylamino-α-(p-methoxyphenyl)-acetamide; intestinal antispasmodic.

**ambulant** (am'bu-lant) [ L. *ambulans,* walking ]. Ambulatory; walking about or able to walk about; denoting a patient who is not confined to bed with the disease from which he suffers; denoting also the disease in such cases.

**am'bulatory.** Ambulant.

**ambuphylline** (am-bu'fī-lin) (USAN). BUTAPHYLLAMINE; theophylline aminoisobutanol; diuretic and bronchodilator.

**ambustion** (am-bus'chun) [ L. *amb-uro,* pp. *-ustus,* to burn around, scorch ]. A burn or scald.

**ameba** (ă-me'bah). Common name for *Amoeba* and similar naked, lobose, sarcodine protozoa.

**ame'bacide.** Amebicide.

**ame'baism.** 1. Ameboidism (1). 2. Ameboididity.

**amebiasis** (am'e-bi'ah-sis) [ ameba + G. suffix *-iasis,* condition ]. Infection with *Entamoeba histolytica* or other pathogenic amebas.

**a. cu'tis,** a serpiginous, ulcerating eruption with bloody, necrotic crust, appearing usually as an extension of underlying infection (*e.g.,* anus or site of surgical intervention of bowel or liver lesion), but occasionally at site of direct contact.

**hepatic a.,** infection of the liver with *Entamoeba histolytica,* may occur with or without antecedent amebic dysentery.

**ame'bic.** Relating to, resembling, or caused by amebas.

**amebici'dal.** Destructive to amebas.

**amebicide** (ă-me'bī-sid) [ ameba + L. *caedo,* to kill ]. Amebacide; any agent that causes the destruction of amebas.

**ame'biform** [ ameba + L. *forma,* shape ]. Of the shape or appearance of an ameba.

**amebiosis** (ă-me'bi-o'sis) Amebiasis.

**ame'bism.** Amebiasis.

**amebocyte** (ă-me'bo-sit) [ ameba, + *kytos,* cell ]. 1. A wandering cell found in invertebrates. 2. An obsolete term for leukocyte. 3. An *in vitro* tissue culture blood cell.

**ame'boid** [ ameba + G. *eidos,* appearance ]. 1. Resembling an ameba in appearance or characteristics. 2. Of irregular outline with peripheral projections; denoting the outline of a form of colony in plate culture.

**ame'boidid'ity.** Amebaism (2); the power of locomotion after the manner of an ameboid cell.

**ame'boidism.** 1. Amebaism (1); the performance of movements similar to those of an ameba. 2. Denoting a condition sometimes seen in certain nerve cells.

**amebo'ma** [ ameba + G. suffix *-oma,* tumor ]. An amebic granuloma; a nodular, tumor-like focus of proliferative inflammation sometimes developing in chronic amebiasis, especially in the wall of the colon; may occur (1) as a fairly well circumscribed, solitary lesion (from several millimeters to a few centimeters in diameter), or (2) multiple nodular foci of varying sizes, or (3) a relatively large or massive lesion comprised of several smaller foci that become coalescent.

**ame'bule.** A minute ameba.

**ameburia** (am'e-bu'rī-ah) [ ameba + G. *ouron,* urine ]. The presence of amebas in the urine when voided.

**ameiosis** (a'mi-o'sis) [ G. *a-* priv. + *meiōsis,* a lessening ]. A cell division resulting in formation of gametes without reduction in chromosome number.

**a'melanot'ic** [ G. *a-* priv. + *melas,* black ]. Lacking in melanin.

**amel'ia** [ G. *a-* priv. + *melos,* a limb ]. Congenital absence of a limb or limbs.

**complete a.,** tetra-amelia.

**ameliora'tion** [ L. *ad,* to, + *melioro,* to make better, fr. *melior,* compar. of *bonus,* good ]. Improvement; moderation in the intensity of symptoms.

**amel'oblast** [ Early E. *amel,* enamel, + G. *blastos,* germ ]. Adamantoblast; enamel cell; one of the cells of the inner layer of the enamel organ of a develping tooth, concerned with the formation of enamel.

**am'eloblas'todonto'ma.** Ameloblastic *odontoma.*

**am'eloblas'tofibro'ma.** Ameloblastic *fibroma.*

**am'eloblasto'ma.** Adamantinoma; adamantoblastoma; neoplasm originating from epithelial tissue related to the enamel organ; consists of rounded, cordlike, or irregular foci of epithelial cells that frequently surround a stellate reticulum; the basal layers of epithelial cells resemble ameloblasts, but differentiation into keratinizing cells may be observed; enamel is not formed; the stroma is usually loose connective tissue, but is sometimes densely fibrous; the stellate reticulum may degenerate, thereby resulting in one or more cysts. Occurs chiefly in the mandible, especially in the molar region; histologically similar neoplasms rarely occur in the region of the sella turcica (craniopharyngioma) and in the tibia.

**am'eloden'tinal.** Dentinoenamel.

**amelogenesis** (am'el-o-jen'ē-sis). Enamelogenesis; the production and development of enamel.

**a. imperfec'ta,** enamel dysplasia; a group of hereditary defects characterized by faulty metabolism in either of two steps of enamel formation; defective matrix formation leads to enamel hypoplasia, while defective maturation leads to enamel hypocalcification.

**am'elus.** An individual with amelia.

**amenia** (ă-me'nī-ah) [ G. *a-* priv. + *mēn,* month ]. Amenorrhea.

**amenorrhea** (ă-men-o-re'ah) [ G. *a-* priv. + *mēn,* month, + *rhoia,* flow ]. Amenia; absence or abnormal cessation of the menses.

**emotional a.,** a. caused supposedly by some strong emotional disturbance, *e.g.,* fright, grief.

**hypophysial a.,** a. due to inadequate gonadotrophic secretions by the anterior lobe of the hypophysis.

**ovarian a.,** a. due to deficiency of estrogenic hormone.

**pathologic a.,** a. due to organic disease, either uterine or other, such as ovarian or pituitary failure, Simmonds' disease, anemic debility, etc.

**physiologic a.,** a. of pregnancy or the menopause, not associated with an organic disorder.

**postpartum a.,** permanent a. following childbirth, sometimes due to pituitary failure resulting from postpartum hemorrhage and consequent necrosis of the pituitary.

**primary a.,** a. in which the menses have never occurred.

**secondary a.,** any a. in which the menses appeared at puberty but have been suppressed.

**amenorrhe'al, amenorrhe'ic** Relating to, accompanied by, or due to amenorrhea.

**am'ent.** Obsolete term for a mentally retarded person.

**amentia** (ă-men'shĭ-ah) [ L. madness, fr. *ab*, from, + *mens*, mind ]. 1. Mental *retardation*. 2. A form of confusional insanity marked especially by apathy, disorientation, and stupor; the term dementia is more appropriate.

    **a. agita'ta,** a form marked by a high degree of excitement with great motor unrest and incessant hallucinations.

    **a. atton'ita,** a form of passive stupor with semiconsciousness, disorientation, mutism, immobility, and emotional indifference.

    **nevoid a.,** Brushfield-Wyatt *disease*.

    **phen'ylpyru'vic a.,** a. accompanied by the appearance of phenylpyruvate in the urine.

    **Stearns' alcohol'ic a.,** a temporary alcoholic mental disorder resembling delirium tremens but lasting for a longer time and showing a greater degree of amnesia and other mental defects.

**amential** (ă-men'shĭ-al). Pertaining to amentia.

**American Law Institute rule.** See under rule.

**americium** (am'ĕ-ris'ĭ-um). An element obtained by the bombardment of uranium with neutrons; atomic no. 95; symbol Am.

**am'erism** [ G. *a*- priv. + *meros*, part ]. The condition or quality of not dividing into parts, segments, or merozoites.

**ameris'tic.** Endowed with amerism; not dividing into parts or segments.

**ametachromophil, ametachromophile** (ă-met'ah-kro'mo-fil, -fĭl) [ G. *a*- priv. + *meta*, beyond, + *chrōma*, color, + *philos*, fond ]. Orthochromatic; orthochromophil.

**amet'amor'phosis.** Lack of response to stimuli due to undue absorption in thought.

**ametaneutrophil, ametaneutrophile** (ă-met'ah-nu'tro-fil, -fĭl) [ G. *a*- priv. + *meta*, beyond, + L. *neuter* neither, + G. *philos*, fond ]. Orthochromatic; orthoneutrophil.

**amethocaine hydrochloride** (BP). Tetracaine hydrochloride.

**amethop'terin.** Methotrexate.

**ame'tria** [ G. *a*- priv. + *mētra*, uterus ]. Congenital absence of the uterus.

**am'etrom'eter** [ ametropia + G. *metron*, measure ]. An appliance for measuring the degree of ametropia.

**ametropia** (am'ĕ-tro'pĭ-ah) [ G. *ametros*, disproportionate, fr. *a*- priv. + *metron*, measure, + *ōps*, eye ]. A condition in which there is some error of refraction in consequence of which parallel rays, with the eye at rest, are not focused on the retina.

    **axial a.,** that resulting from a shortening or lengthening of the eyeball on the optic axis, causing hyperopia or myopia, respectively.

    **index a.,** that resulting from alteration in the refractive index media of the eye.

**ametro'pic.** Relating to, or suffering from, ametropia.

**amiantaceous** (am'ĭ-an-ta'shus) [ G. *amiantus*, asbestos ]. Asbestos-like; describing a type of crusting of a cutaneous lesion.

**amic** (am'ik). A compound related to or derived from an amide.

**amicetin.** Antibiotic substance produced by *Streptomyces vinaceus-drappus;* possesses antimicrobial activity.

**Amici** (ah-me'che), Giovanni B., Italian physicist, 1784–1863. See A.'s *disk*.

**amicro'bic.** Not microbic; not related to or caused by microorganisms.

**ami'croscop'ic.** Submicroscopic; too small to be seen under the microscope.

**am'idase.** Acylase; acylamidase; enzyme (EC 3.5.1.4) that catalyzes the hydrolysis of monocarboxylic amides to free acid plus NH₃.

**am'idases.** Amidohydrolases.

**amide** (am'id, am'ĭd). A substance that may be derived from ammonia through the substitution of one or more of the hydrogen atoms by acyl groups; R—CO—NH₂; the replacement of one hydrogen atom constitutes a **primary,** that of two hydrogen atoms a **secondary,** and that of three atoms a **tertiary a.**

**amidine** (am'ĭ-din). The monovalent radical —C(NH) —NH₂.

**amidinohydrolases.** Enzymes (EC sub-subgroup 3.5.3) cleaving linear amidines, *e.g.,* arginase, creatinase.

**amidinotransferases.** Transamidinases; enzymes (EC sub-subclass 2.1.4) catalyzing a transamidination reaction (*e.g.,* glycine amidinotransferase).

**amido-.** A prefix denoting the amide radical, R—CO —NH— or R—SO₂—NH—, etc.

**amido black 10B** (am'ĭ-do). An acid disazo dye, $C_{12}H_{14}N_6O_9S_2Na_2$, used as a connective tissue stain and for staining protein in paper chromatography.

**amidogen** (am'ĭ-do-jen'). The amino group —(NH₂).

**amidohydrolases** (am'ĭ-do-hi'dro-la'ses). Deamidases; amidases; deamidating enzymes; enzymes of EC class 3.5.1 and 3.5.2 hydrolyzing C—N bonds of amides; *e.g.,* asparaginase, barbiturase, urease, amidase.

**amidonaphthol red** (am'ĭ -do-naf'thol). An azo dye, $C_{18}H_{13}N_8S_2Na_2$, used in light and fluorescence microscopy.

**amidopy'rine.** Aminopyrine.

**Am'idos'tomum an'seris.** A species of bloodsucking nematodes, similar to those of the genus *Trichostrongylus,* that parasitizes the gizzard and sometimes also the proventriculus and esophagus of domestic and wild ducks and geese; it causes heavy mortality in young birds.

**amidox'imes.** Amide oximes; the oximes of amides with the general formula, R—C(NH₂) = NOH.

**amidoxyl** (am'ĭ-dok'sil). The radical of an amide oxime (amidoxime), the terminal H (of the NOH) having been lost.

**amil'oride hydrochloride** (USAN). COLECTRIL; *N*-amidino-3,5-diamino-6-chloropyrazinecarboxamide mono-hydrochloride dihydrate; a nonsteroidal compound exerting an effect similar to that of an aldosterone inhibitor, *i.e.,* urinary sodium excretion is enhanced and potassium excretion is reduced.

**amim'ia** [ G. *a*- priv. + *mimos,* a mimic ]. Loss of the power to express ideas by gestures or signs.

**aminacrine hydrochloride** (am'ĭ-nak'rin) (BP, USAN). 9-Aminoacridine hydrochloride; bactericidal agent for external use.

**am'inate.** To combine with ammonia.

**am'ine.** A substance that may be derived from ammonia by the replacement of one or more of the hydrogen atoms by hydrocarbon or other radicals. The substitution of one hydrogen atom constitutes a **primary a.,** *e.g.,* NH₂CH₃; that of two atoms a **secondary a.,** *e.g.,* NH(CH₃)₂; that of three, a **tertiary a.,** *e.g.,* N(CH₃)₃; and that of four atoms,

                    +

a **quaternary ammonium ion,** N(CH₃)₄. The a.'s form salts with acids. The quaternary a. is a positively charged ion, which is isolated only in association with a negative ion.

    **adrenergic a.,** sympathomimetic a.

    **adrenomimetic a.,** sympathomimetic a.

    **a. oxidase,** a. oxidase (flavin-containing).

    **a. oxidase (flavin-containing),** monoamine oxidase; tyramine oxidase; tyraminase; amine oxidase; spermine oxidase; adrenaline oxidase; spermidine oxidase; an oxidoreductase (EC 1.4.3.4) containing flavin and oxidizing amines with the aid of 0₂ to aldehydes or ketones with the release of NH₃ and H₂0₂.

    **a. oxidase (pyridoxal-containing),** diamine oxidase; diamino oxyhydrase; histaminase; an oxidoreductase (EC 1.4.3.6) containing pyridoxal phosphate and carrying out the same reaction as a. oxidase (flavin-containing).

    **pressor a.,** pressor *base.*

    **sympathetic a.,** sympathomimetic a.

    **sympathomimetic a.,** adrenergic a.; adrenomimetic a.; sympathetic a.; an agent that evokes responses similar to those produced by adrenergic nerve activity (*e.g.,* epinephrine, ephedrine, and isoproterenol).

**amino-** (ă-me'no-, am'ĭ-no). A prefix denoting a compound containing the radical group, —NH₂.

**amino acid.** An organic acid in which one of the CH hydrogen atoms has been replaced by NH₂. See also α-amino acid.

    **a. acid dehydrogenases,** enzymes catalyzing the oxidative deamination of amino acids to the corresponding keto acids; two relatively nonspecific varieties exist, L- and D- (EC 1.4.1.5 and EC 1.4.99.1), for which L-amino acids and D-amino acids are the respective substrates. The products include NH₃ and a reduced hydrogen acceptor (NADH in the L case). Amino acid dehydrogenases of greater specificity exit, *e.g.*, glycine dehydrogenase. Distinct from amino acid oxidases.

**essential a. acids,** α-amino acids required by animals that must be supplied in the diet (*i.e.*, cannot be synthesized by the animal) either as free a. acids or in proteins.

**nonessential a. acids,** those a. acids that may be synthesized by the organism and are thus not required as such in the diet.

**a. acid oxidases,** distinct from a. acid dehydrogenases; enzymes (EC 1.4.3.2 and 1.4.3.3) oxidizing, with $O_2$, L- and D-amino acids respectively, to the corresponding keto acids, $NH_3$ and $H_2O_2$.

**α-amino acid.** An amino acid of the general formula R—CHNH$_2$—COOH (*i.e.*, the $NH_2$ in the α position). The L forms of these are the hydrolysis products of proteins.

**aminoacidemia** (am'ĭ-no-as'ĭ-de'mĭ-ah) [ amino acid + G. *haima*, blood ]. The presence of excessive amounts of specific amino acids in the blood.

**aminoaciduria** (am'ĭ-no-as'ĭ-du'rĭ-ah) [ amino acid + G. *ouron*, urine ]. Acidaminuria; hyperaminoaciduria; excretion of amino acids in urine, especially in excessive amounts.

**9-aminoac'ridine.** 5-Aminoacridine; acrimine yellow; one of the acridine group of antiseptics (flavins); highly fluorescent in solution. Used topically as an antiseptic; claimed to be less toxic than proflavine.

**9-aminoacridine hydrochloride.** Aminacrine hydrochloride.

**aminoacyl** (am'ĭ-no-as'il). The radical formed from an amino acid by removal of OH from a COOH group.

**aminoacylase** (am'ĭ-no-as'ĭ-las) (EC 3.5.1.14). Enzyme catalyzing hydrolysis of a wide variety of *N*-acyl amino acids to the amino acids. Also known as dehydropeptidase II and hippuricase, from substances on which it acts.

**α-aminoacyl-peptide hydrolases.** Aminopeptidases.

**aminoacyl-tRNA.** See under ribonucleic acid.

**am'inoben'zene.** Aniline.

***p*-am'inobenzo'ic acid** (USP). PABA; a factor (vitamin B$_x$) in the vitamin B complex, being a part of folic acid and required for its formation. It neutralizes the bacteriostatic effects of the sulfonamides since it furnishes an essential growth factor for bacteria, the utilization of which the sulfonamides interfere with.

***p*-aminobenzoic acid diethylamine salt** NEVANIDE; used as hypnotic.

**γ-aminobutyric acid.** $NH_2(CH_2)_3COOH$; a constituent of the central nervous system suggested as a transmitter of inhibitory nerve impulses; abbreviated γAbu or GABA.

**am'inocapro'ic acid** (NF). AMICAR; ε-aminocaproic acid; 6-aminohexanoic acid; an antifibrinolytic agent, used to prevent bleeding in hemophilia, and after heart and prostate surgery when plasminogen or urokinase may be activated.

**aminochlor'thenox'azin hydrochloride.** DEREUMA; 6-amino-2-(2-chloroethyl)-2,3-dihydro-4*H*-1,3-benzoxazin--4-one hydrochloride; antipyretic and analgesic.

**ami'nogluteth'imide.** ELIPTEN; 2-(*p*-aminophenyl)-2-ethylglutarimide. Has been used, in conjunction with other anticonvulsant agents, in the management of mild convulsive disorders. Side effects are frequent. The drug has been withdrawn from the market.

***p*-am'inohippu'ric acid** (USP). *p*-Aminobenzoylglycine; used in determining the renal plasma flow. Abbreviated PAH.

***p*-aminohippuric acid synthetase.** An enzyme in the liver that catalyzes the synthesis of *p*-aminohippuric acid from *p*-aminobenzoic acid and glycine.

**am'inoi'somet'radine.** Amisometradine.

**δ-aminolevulin'ic acid.** $NH_2CH_2COCH_2CH_2COOH$; formed from glycine and succinyl-coenzyme A; a precursor of porphobilinogen, hence an important intermediate in the biosynthesis of hematin.

**δ-aminolevulinic dehydratase.** Porphobilinogen synthase.

**aminolysis** (am'ĭnol'ĭ-sis). Replacement of a halogen in an alkyl or aryl molecule by an amine radical, with elimination of hydrogen halide.

**am'inomet'radine.** Aminometramide.

**am'inomet'ramide.** MINCARD; aminometradine; 1-allyl-6-amino-3-ethyluracil; synthetic uracil derivative; an orally effective diuretic that is believed to act by inhibiting the reabsorption of sodium by the renal tubules; used in the treatment of edema due to congestive heart failure, liver disease, pregnancy, and certain drugs.

**am'inopen'tamide sul'fate.** CENTRINE; 4-dimethylamino-2,2-diphenylvaleramide sulfate; a parasympatholytic agent with atropine-like action; used in the treatment of peptic ulcer, pylorospasm, and certain cases of chronic hypertrophic gastritis.

**aminopeptidase (cytosol).** Leucine aminopeptidase; an enzyme (EC 3.4.11.1) of broad specificity, containing zinc, catalyzing the hydrolysis of the N-terminal amino acid of a peptide.

**aminopeptidase (microsomal).** An aminopeptidase, EC 3.4.11.2 (formerly 3.4.1.2), of broad specificity but preferring alanine and discriminating against proline.

**am'inopep'tidases.** α-Aminoacyl-peptide hydrolases (EC sub-subclass 3.4.11); enzymes catalyzing the breakdown of a peptide, removing the amino acid at the amino end of the chain; found in intestinal juice.

**aminopherase** (am'ĭ-nof'er-ās). Aminotransferase.

**aminophylline** (am'i-no-fil'in, -ēn) (USP, BP). Theophylline ethylenediamine; $(C_7H_8N_4O_2)_2C_2H_4(NH_2)_22H_2O$; diuretic, vasodilator, and cardiac stimulant; also used in asthma that is resistant to epinephrine, and in veterinary medicine.

**aminopro'mazine fumarate.** LISPAMOL; 10-[ 2,3-bis(dimethylamino)propyl ]phenothiazine fumarate; intestinal antispasmodic.

***p*-aminopropiophenone.** PAPP; antidote for cyanide poisoning.

**aminopro'pylon.** AMIPYLO; *N*-(antipyrinyl)-2-(dimethylamino)propionamide; analgesic.

**am'inop'terin.** 4-Aminopteroylglutamic acid; 4-aminofolic acid; a folic acid antagonist; used in treatment of acute leukemia and other neoplastic diseases.

**am'inopy'rine.** PYRAMIDON; amidopyrine; dimethylaminoantipyrine; 4-dimethylamino-2,3-dimethyl-1-phenyl-3-pyrazolin-5-one; used as an antipyretic and analgesic in rheumatism, neuritis, pulmonary tuberculosis, and common colds; may cause leukocytopenia.

**amin'orex** (USAN). APIQUEL; 2-amino-5-phenyl-2-oxazoline; a sympathomimetic appetite suppressant.

***p*-aminosalicylic acid** (am'ĭ-no sal-ĭ-sil'ik as'id). Abbreviated PAS; aminosalicylic acid; 4-amino-2-hydroxybenzoic acid; a bacteriostatic agent against tubercle bacilli, used as an adjunct to streptomycin. The potassium, sodium, and calcium salts have the same use.

**amino-terminal.** The α-$NH_2$ group or the aminoacyl residue containing it at one end of a peptide or protein (usually at left as written); also called NH$_2$-terminal; N-terminal.

**am'inotrans'ferases.** Transaminases; enzymes (EC sub-subclass 2.6.1) transferring amino groups between an α-amino acid to (usually) a 2-keto acid; *e.g.*, alanine and 2-ketoglutarate.

**am'inotri'azole.** Amitrole; 3-amino-1*H*-1,2,4-triazole; an effective weed killer that also possesses some antithyroid activity.

**aminuria** (am'ĭ-nu'rĭ-ah) [ amine + G. *ouron*, urine ]. Excretion of amines in urine.

**amiphen'azole** DAPTAZOLE; 2,4-diamino-5-phenylthiazole; morphine antagonist.

**amisometradine** (am-i'so-met'rah-dēn). ROLICTON; aminoisometradine; 6-amino-3-methyl-1-(2-methylallyl-)uracil; oral diuretic.

**amithi'ozone.** Thiacetazone; TIBIONE; 4'-formylacetanilide thiosemicarbazone; leprostatic agent.

**amito'sis** [ G. *a-* priv. + mitosis ]. Direct division of the nucleus and cell, without the complicated changes in the former that occur in the ordinary process of cell reproduction.

**amitot'ic.** Relating to or marked by amitosis.

**amitriptyline hydrochloride** (USP, BP). ELAVIL; 10,11-dihydro-*N,N*-dimethyl-5*H*-dibenzo[ *a,d* ]cycloheptene-$\Delta^{5,\gamma}$-propylamine hydrochloride; chemically and pharmacologically related to imipramine hydrochloride; an antidepressant agent with mild tranquilizing properties, used in the treatment of mental depression and in the depressive phase of manic-depressive states.

**am'itrole.** Aminotriazole.

**amix'ia** [ G. *a*- priv. + L. *miscere*, pp. *mixtus*, to mix ]. A restriction that prevents general intercrossing in a species, leading to inbreeding.

**am'meter.** An instrument for measuring strength of electric current in amperes.

**Ammon,** Friedrich A. von, German oculist, 1799–1861. See A.'s *operation.*

**ammone'mia.** Ammoniemia.

**ammonia** (ă-mo'nĭ-ah). Alkaline air; a volatile gas, $NH_3$, very soluble in water, forming the base, $NH_4OH$, combining with acids to form ammonium compounds.

    **a. water,** hartshorn.

**ammo'niac.** A gum resin from a plant of western Asia, *Dorema ammoniacum* (family Umbelliferae); used internally as a stimulant and expectorant, and externally as a counterirritant plaster.

**ammoni'acal.** Relating to ammonia or to ammoniac.

**ammonia-lyases.** Enzymes removing nonhydrolytically (hence lyases, EC class 4), by rupture of a C—N bond leaving a double bond (EC subclass 4.3), ammonia (EC sub-subclass 4.3.1); *e.g.,* aspartate ammonia-lyase (aspartase) (EC 4.3.1.1).

**ammo'niated.** Containing or combined with ammonia.

**ammoniemia** (am-mo-nĭ-e'mĭ-ah) [ ammonia + G. *haima,* blood ]. Ammonemia; the presence of ammonia or some of its compounds in the blood, thought to be formed from the decomposition of urea; it usually results in subnormal temperature, weak pulse, gastroenteric symptoms, and coma.

**ammo'nifica'tion.** The production of ammonia from proteins or their cleavage products by the action of bacteria.

**ammonio-.** A prefix meaning ammoniated.

**ammo'nium.** The radical, $NH_4^+$, formed by combination of $NH_3$ and $H^+$; behaves as a univalent metal in forming ammonium compounds.

    **a. benzoate,** $C_6H_5COONH_4$; stimulant diuretic, urinary antiseptic, and antirheumatic.

    **a. bromide,** $NH_4Br$; sedative.

    **a. carbonate** (NF), $(NH_4)_2CO_3$; cardiac and respiratory stimulant and carminative expectorant.

    **a. chloride** (USP), muriate of ammonia; sal ammoniac; $NH_4Cl$; stimulant expectorant, and cholagogue; used to relieve alkalosis and to promote lead excretion.

    **a. ferric sulfate,** ferric ammonium sulfate.

    **a. ichthosulfonate,** ichthammol.

    **a. iodide,** $NH_4I$; expectorant.

    **a. mandelate,** mandelic acid ammonium salt; urinary antiseptic.

    **a. nitrate,** $NH_4NO_3$; used in making nitrous oxide gas, in freezing mixtures, matches, and fertilizers; also used in veterinary medicine.

    **a. phosphate, dibasic,** $(NH_4)_2HPO_4$; used for fire-proofing, in baking powder, and as an antirheumatic.

    **a. phosphate, monobasic,** $NH_4H_2 PO_4$; used in baking powder.

    **quaternary a. base,** any quaternary a. compound.

    **a. salicylate,** used in rheumatism.

    **a. sulfate,** $(NH_4)_2SO_4$; local anesthetic in a 6 per cent solution.

    **a. tartrate,** L-tartaric acid ammonium salt; used for irrigation of alkali burn of the eye.

    **a. val'erate** or **vale'rianate,** $C_{15}H_{33}NO_6$; antispasmodic and sedative.

**ammoniu'ria** [ ammonia + G. *ouron,* urine ]. Ammoniacal urine; excretion of urine that contains an excessive amount of ammonia.

**am'monol'ysis** [ ammonia + G. *lysis,* dissolution ]. The breaking of a chemical bond with the addition of the elements of ammonia ($NH_2$ and H) at the point of breakage.

**ammother'apy** [ G. *ammos,* sand, + *therapeia,* therapy ]. Psammotherapy.

**amnemonic** (am'ne-mon'ik) [ G. *a*- priv. + *mnēmonikos,* pertaining to memory ]. Denoting the ability to write letters and words, but not connected sentences to express an idea; see also agraphia.

**amnesia** (am-ne'zĭ-ah) [ G. *amnēsia,* forgetfulness. MNEM- ]. Disturbance in memory manifested by total or partial inability to recall past experiences.

    **anterograde a.,** a. in reference to events occurring after the trauma or disease that caused the condition.

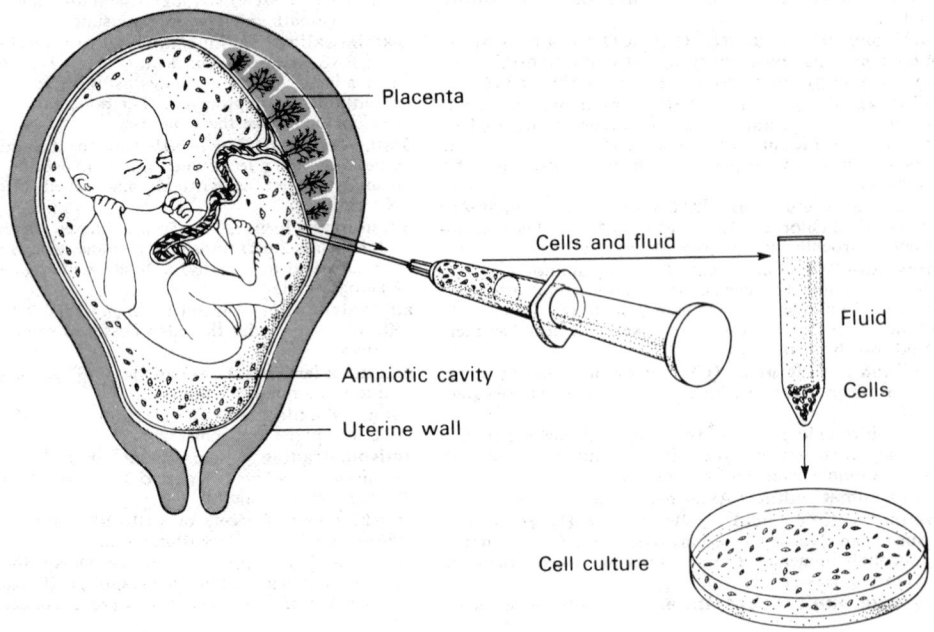

**Amniocentesis**

(From Moment, G. B., and Haberman, H. M.: *Biology: A Full Spectrum,* The Williams & Wilkins Co., Baltimore, 1973.)

**auditory a.,** word *deafness.*

**Broca's a.,** Broca's *aphasia.*

**lacu'nar a.,** localized or patchy a.; a. in reference to isolated events; not a total loss of memory.

**localized a.,** lacunar a.

**patchy a.,** lacunar a.

**posthypnotic a.,** a. following hypnosis.

**retrograde a.,** a. in reference to events that occurred before the trauma or disease that caused the condition.

**tactile a.,** astereognosis.

**traumatic a.,** a. following a sudden, usually accidental, injury.

**verbal a.,** loss of memory for words.

**visual a.,** inability to recall to mind the appearance of objects that have been seen, or to recognize printed words.

**amne'siac.** One suffering from loss of memory.

**amne'sic.** Relating to or affected with amnesia; forgetful.

**amnes'tic.** 1. Amnesic. 2. Agent causing amnesia.

**amnio-** [ G. *amnion, q.v.* ]. Combining form relating to the amnion.

**amniocentesis** (am'nĭ-o-sen-te'sis) [ amnio- + G. *kentēsis,* puncture ]. Transabdominal aspiration of fluid from the amniotic sac.

**amniochorial, amniochorionic** (am'nĭ-o-ko'rĭ-al, -ko-rĭ-on'ik). Relating to both amnion and chorion.

**amnioclepsis** (am'nĭ-o-klep'sis) [ amnio- + G. *kleptō,* fut. *klepsō,* to steal, do secretly ]. The gradual, unperceived escape of the amniotic fluid.

**amniogenesis** (am'nĭ-o-jen'ĕ-sis) [ amnio- + G. *genesis,* production ]. The formation of the amnion.

**amniography** (am'nĭ-og'rȧ-fĭ) [ amnio- + G. *graphō,* to write ]. Roentgenography of the amniotic sac after the injection of an opaque solution into the sac, by which it becomes possible to see the outline of the umbilical cord and the placenta.

**amnioma** (am'nĭ-o'mah) [ amnio- + G. suffix *-oma,* tumor ]. A broad flat tumor of the skin resulting from antenatal adhesion of the amnion.

**amnion** (am'nĭ-on) [ G. the membrane around the fetus, fr. *amnios,* lamb. AMNI- ]. Amniotic sac; the innermost of the membranes enveloping the embryo *in utero.* It consists of a layer of somatopleure with its ectodermal component toward the embryo and its somatic mesodermal component extermal. It is filled with the amniotic fluid in which the embryo is free to move and protected against mechanical injury. In the later stages of pregnancy the amnion

expands to come in contact with and partially fuse to the inner wall of the chorionic vesicle.

**a. nodo'sum,** amniotic caruncles; squamous metaplasia of amnion; nodules in the a. that consist of typical stratified squamous epithelium.

**amnion'ic.** Relating to the amnion.

**amnionitis** (am'nĭ-o-ni'tis) [ amnion + G. suffix *-itis,* inflammation ]. Inflammation resulting from infection of the amniotic sac, usually resulting from premature rupture of the membranes and often associated with neonatal infection.

**amniorrhea** (am-nĭ-o-re'ah) [ amnio- + G. *rhoia,* flow ]. The escape of amniotic fluid, or liquor amnii.

**amniorrhexis** (am-nĭ-ŏ-rek'sis) [ amnio- + G. *rhēxis,* rupture ]. Rupture of the bag of waters.

**am'nioscope.** An endoscope or hollow tube 12 to 20 mm. in diameter by 20 cm. long for studying amniotic fluid through the intact amniotic sac.

**amnioscopy** (am'nĭ-os'ko-pĭ) [ amnio- + G. *skopeō,* to view ]. Examination of the amniotic fluid in the lowest part of the sac by means of an endoscope introduced through the cervical canal.

**Amniota** (am'nĭ-o'tah). A group of vertebrates whose embryos are enclosed in an amnion; it includes all the reptiles, birds, and mammals.

**amniot'ic.** Amnionic.

**amniotome** (am'nĭ-o-tōm) [ amnio- + G. *tomē,* cutting ]. An instrument for puncturing the fetal membranes.

**amniot'omy.** Artificial rupture of the fetal membranes as a means of inducing or expediting labor.

**amobar'bital.** AMYTAL; amylobarbitone; 5-ethyl-5-isoamylbarbituric acid; central nervous system depressant with an intermediate duration of action.

**a. sodium** (USP), amylobarbitone sodium; same action and uses as a.

**amodi'aquine hydrochloride** (NF, BP). CAMOQUINE; 4-(7-chloro-4-quinolylamino)-α-diethylamino-o-cresol dihydrochloride dihydrate; an antimalarial drug, also used in the treatment of amebic hepatitis; but large doses may result in sialorrhea, nausea, vomiting, diarrhea, insomnia, palpitations, spasticity, and possibly convulsions.

**amoeb-.** For several words formed from this stem see ameb-.

**Amoeba,** gen. and pl. **Amoe'bae** (ă-me'bah) [ Mod. L. fr. G. *amoibē,* change. AMEB- ]. A genus of naked, lobose, pseudopod-forming protozoa of the class Sarcodina (or Rhizopoda); common or collective name, ameba (pl. amebae or amebas). Abundant soil-dwellers, especially in rich organic debris; also commonly found as parasites. The typical parasites of man are now placed in the genera *Entamoeba, Endolimax, Iodamoeba,* and *Dientamoeba.*

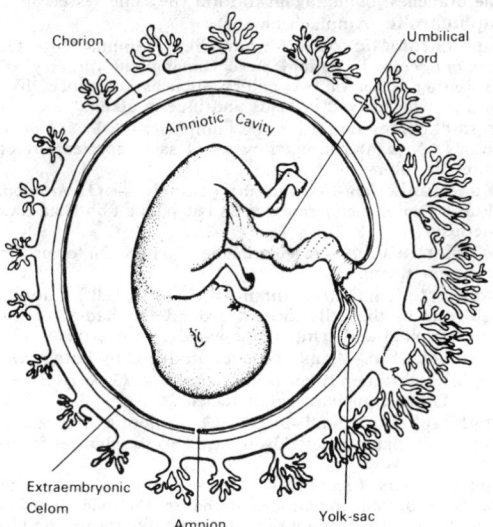

**Amnion**
(From Patten, B. M.: *Human Embryology,* Ed. 3, McGraw-Hill Book Company, New York, 1968. Used with permission.)

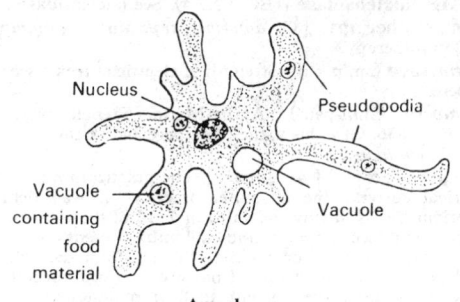

Amoeba

**A. buccalis,** *Entamoeba gingivalis.*

**A. coli,** *Entamoeba coli.*

**A. denta'lis,** *Entamoeba gingivalis.*

**A. dysenter'iae,** *Entamoeba histolytica.*

**A. histolytica,** *Entamoeba histolytica.*

**A. limax,** *Endolimax nana.*

**A. meleag'ridis,** *Histomonas meleagridis.*

**A. proteus,** an abundant, nonparasitic form, remarkable for the number and varied shapes of its pseudopodia.

**Amoebotaenia** (ă-me'bo-te'nĭ-ah). A genus of small (seldom possessing more than 30 segments), intestinal tapeworms of birds.

**A cunea'ta,** *A. sphenoides;* a species common in domestic fowl; the cysticercoid is developed in earthworms.

**A. sphenoi'des,** *A. cuneata.*

**amok** (ă-mok') [ native word ]. 1. A psychic disturbance originally observed in Malaya in which the subject becomes dangerously maniacal ("running amok"). 2. Maniacal, wild or uncontrolled behavior threatening injury to others.

**amolanone hydrochloride.** AMETHONE; 3-(β-diethylaminoethyl)-3-phenyl-2-benzofuranone hydrochloride; anticholinergic and local anesthetic action; used to produce topical anesthesia of the lower urinary tract.

**amor** [ L. ]. Love.

**a. les'bicus,** lesbianism.

**amora'lia** [ G. *a*-priv. + L. *moralis,* moral ]. Moral imbecility; see amoral *imbecile.*

**amora'lis** [ G. *a*- priv. + L. *moralis,* moral ]. Amoral *imbecile.*

**a'morphagno'sia** [ G. *a*-, priv., + *morphē,* shape, + *gnosis,* recognition ]. Inability to recognize the size and shape of objects.

**amor'phia, amor'phism** [ G. *a*- priv. + *morphē,* form ]. The condition of being amorphous or without definite shape.

**amorph'inism.** The condition of an addict deprived of drugs.

**amorphosynthesis** (ă-mor'fo-sin'the-sis) [ G. *a*- priv. + *morphē,* form, + synthesis, *q. v.* ]. A disorder of awareness of space and of body schema.

**amorphous** (ă-mor'fus). 1. Without definite shape or visible differentiation in structure. 2. Not crystallized.

**amorphus** (ă-mor'fus). A malformed fetus with rudimentary head, limbs, and heart.

**Amoss,** Harold L., U. S. physician, 1886–1956. See A.'s *sign.*

**amotio** (ă-mo-shĭ-o) [ L. *a-moveo,* pp. *-motus,* to move from ]. A removal.

**a. placentae,** abruptio placentae.

**a. retinae,** *detachment* of the retina.

**amo'triphene.** MYORDIL; 2,3,3-tris(*p*-methoxyphenyl)-*N,N*-dimethylallylamine; coronary vasodilator.

**amox'ecaine.** LOCASTINE; 2-[ (2-diethylaminoethyl)-ethylamino ]ethyl-*p*-aminobenzoate; local anesthetic.

**AMP.** Abbreviation for adenosine monophosphate (adenylic acid, *q. v.*), specifically the 5'-phosphate.

**AMP deaminase** (EC 3.5.4.6), adenylic acid deaminase; an enzyme converting adenylic acid to inosinic acid and NH₃.

**AMP nucleosidase** (EC 3.2.2.4). See nucleosidases.

**am'pelother'apy** [ G. *ampelos,* grape vine, + therapy ]. Botryotherapy.

**amperage** (am'per-ij). Strength of electric current; see ampere.

**Ampère** (ahm-pair'), André-Marie, French physicist, 1775–1836. Gave his name to ampere and statampere. See A.'s *postulate.*

**ampere** (am-pēr') [ A. *Ampère* ]. The practical unit of electrical current; the absolute, practical a. was defined, originally, as having the value of 1/10 of the electromagnetic unit (see abampere and coulomb). Present definitions are: (1) legal: the current that, flowing for 1 second, will deposit 1.118 mg. of silver from silver nitrate solution; (2) scientific (SI): the current that, if maintained in two straight parallel conductors of infinite length and of negligible circular cross-sections and placed 1 meter apart in a vacuum, produces between them a force of $2 \times 10^{-7}$ newton per meter of length.

**amph-.** See amphi-, and ampho-.

**ampheclexis** (am-fĕ-klek'sĭ-ah) [ G. *amphi,* two-sided, *eklexis,* selection ]. Reciprocal sexual selection, *i.e.,* by both male and female.

**ampheclor'al** (USAN). ACUTRAN; α-methyl-*N*-(2,2,2-trichloroethylidene)-phenethylamine; a sympathomimetic amine used as an anorexigenic.

**amphemerous** (am-fem'er-us) [ G. *amphi,* two-sided, + *hēmera,* day ]. Quotidian.

**amphenone B.** 3,3-bis(*p*-Aminophenyl)-2-butanone; shows antiestrogenic activity in chickens; in man and other animals it suppresses the biosynthesis of adrenal steroids. Derivatives have been tried in the treatment of Cushing's syndrome and primary aldosteronism.

**amphet'amine.** BENZEDRINE; α-methylphenethylamine; 1-phenyl-2-aminopropane; (phenylisopropyl)amine; $C_6H_5CH_2CH(NH_2)CH_3$; closely related in its structure and action to ephedrine and other sympathomimetic amines.

**a. (4-chlorophenoxy)acetate,** SATIETYL; same actions and uses as a. sulfate.

**a. phosphate,** RACEPHAN; same actions and uses as a. sulfate.

**a. sulfate** (BP), BENZEDRINE sulfate; exerts less vasopressor, cardiac and bronchial effect than ephedrine, but has a greater central nervous stimulating effect, decreasing the sensation of fatigue. Used in the treatment of narcolepsy and certain types of paralysis agitans, and to reduce appetite in obesity.

*d*-**amphetamine phosphate.** Dextroamphetamine phosphate.

*d*-**amphetamine sulfate.** Dextroamphetamine sulfate.

**amphi-** [ G. *amphi,* two-sided ]. Combining form meaning on both sides, surrounding, double.

**amphiarthrodial** (am'fĭ-ar-thro'dĭ-al). Relating to amphiarthrosis.

**amphiarthrosis** (am'fĭ-ar-thro'sis) [ amphi- + G. *arthrōsis,* joint ]. Junctura cartilaginea.

**amphias'ter** [ amphi- + G. *astēr,* star ]. The double star, a figure formed by the two asters and the connecting spindle fibers during mitosis.

**amphibar'ic** [ amphi- + G. *baros,* pressure ]. Denoting a pharmacologic material that may lower or elevate arterial blood pressure, depending on the dose.

**amphiblas'tic.** A rarely used term denoting the unequal cleavage of a telolecithal egg.

**amphiblestrodes** (am'fĭ-bles-tro'dēz) [ G. *amphiblēstroeidēs,* netlike. OID- ]. The retina.

**amphibol'ic** [ G. *amphibolos,* doubtful ]. Ambiguous; uncertain; see a. *stage.*

**amphicelous** (am-fĭ-se'lus) [ amphi- + G. *koilos,* hollow ]. Concave at each end, as the body of a vertebra of a fish.

**amphicen'tric** [ amphi- + G. *kentron,* center ]. Centering at both ends, said of a rete mirabile that begins by the vessel breaking up into a number of branches and ends by the branches joining again to form the same vessel.

**amphichro'ic** Amphichromatic.

**amphichromatic** (am'fĭ-kro-mat'ik) [ amphi- + G. *chrōma,* color ]. Amphichroic; having the proerty of exhibiting either of two colors, such as substances like litmus, which is red in acids and blue in alkalis.

**amphichrome** (am'fĭ-krōm) [ amphi- + G. *chrōma,* color ]. A plant bearing flowers of same species but of different colors.

**amphicrania** (am-fĭ-kra'nĭ-ah) [ amphi- + G. *kranion,* skull ]. Double hemicrania; neuralgic pain on both sides of the head.

**am'phicreat'inine.** A leukomaine, $C_8H_{19}N_7O_4$, formed in muscular tissue.

**amphicyte** (am'fĭ-sīt) [ amphi- + G. *kytos,* cell ]. Capsule cell; one of the cells located around the bodies of the cerebrospinal and sympathetic ganglionic neurons.

**am'phigenet'ic.** Amphogenetic; produced by both sexes.

**amphikaryon** (am'fĭ-kăr'ĭ-on) [ amphi- + G. *karyon,* kernel ]. Diploid nucleus; amphinucleus.

**amphileukemic** (am'fĭ-lu-ke'mik). Denoting a leukemic condition that corresponds in degree to the changes in the organ or tissue.

**Amphim'erus** [ amphi- + G. *meros,* segment ]. A genus of opisthorchid trematodes found in the bile ducts of mammals, birds, and reptiles; it is probably transmitted by fish.

**amphimicrobe** (am'fĭ-mi'krōb). A microorganism that is either aerobic or anaerobic according to the environment.

**amphimixis** (am-fĭ-mik'sis) [ amphi- + G. *mixis,* mingling ]. 1. Union of the paternal and maternal chromatin after impregnation of the ovum. 2. In psychoanalysis, a combination of urethral and anal eroticism.

**amphinucleolus** (am'fĭ-nu-kle'o-lus) [ amphi- + L. *nucleolus*, dim. of *nucleus*, kernel ]. A double nucleolus having both basophilic and oxyphilic components.

**Amphiox'us** [ amphi- + G. *oxys*, sharp ]. A genus of small, translucent, fishlike chordates found in warm marine waters. Members are structurally similar to vertebrates in having a notochord, gills, digestive tract, and nerve cord, but they lack paired fins, vertebrae, ribs, or a skull.

**amphistome** (am-fis'tōm) [ amphi- + G. *stoma*, mouth ]. A common name for any trematode of the genus *Paramphistomum*.

**amphitene** (am'fĭ-tēn) [ amphi- + G. *tainia*, band ]. Obsolescent term for zygotene.

**amphithymia** (am'fĭ-thi'mĭ-ah) [ amphi- + G. *thymos*, soul ]. In psychiatry, a mental condition marked by periods of depression and elation.

**amphitrichate, amphitrichous** (am-fĭ-trī'kăt, am-fit'rĭ-kus) [ amphi- + G. *thrix*, hair ]. Having a flagellum or flagella at both extremities of a microbial cell; denoting certain microorganisms.

**amphitypy** (am-fit'ĭ-pĭ). The property of being characteristic of two types.

**ampho-** [ G. *amphō*, both ]. Combining form meaning on both sides, surrounding, double.

**am'phochromat'ophil, am'phochromat'ophile.** Amphophil (2).

**amphochromophil, amphochromophile** (am'fo-kro'-mo-fil, -fil) [ ampho- + G. *chrōma*, color, + *philos*, fond ]. Amphophil.

**amphocyte** (am'fo-sīt). Amphophil (2).

**amphodiplopia** (am'fo-dĭ-plo'pĭ-ah) [ ampho- + G. *diploos*, double, + *ōps*, vision ]. Double vision in each of the two eyes.

**am'phogenet'ic.** Amphigenetic.

**am'pholyte.** Amphoteric *electrolyte*.

**amphomy'cin** (USAN). Antibiotic substance produced by *Streptomyces canus;* used topically for skin infections.

**amphophil, amphophile** (am'fo-fil, -fil) [ ampho- + G. *philos*, fond ]. 1. Amphophilic; having an affinity for both acid and for basic dyes. 2. Amphochromophil; amphocyte; a cell that stains readily with either acid or basic dyes.

**amphophil'ic, amphoph'ilous.** Amphophil (1).

**amphoric** (am-for'ik) [ G. *amphora*, a jar. PHER- ]. Denoting the sound heard in percussion and auscultation resembling the noise made by blowing across the mouth of a bottle.

**amphoricity** (am-fo-ris'ĭ-tĭ). A condition in which amphoric sounds are obtained on auscultation or percussion.

**amphoriloquy** (am-fo-ril'o-kwĭ) [ G. *amphora*, a jar, + *loquor*, to speak ]. The presence of the amphoric voice sound; see under voice.

**amphorophony** (am-fo-rof'o-nĭ) [ G. *amphora*, a jar, + *phōnē*, voice ]. The amphoric voice sound; see under voice.

**amphoter'ic** [ G. *amphoteroi* (pl.), both, fr. *amphō*, both ]. Having two opposite characteristics, especially having the capacity of reacting as either acid or base.

**amphoter'icin B** (USP). FUNGIZONE; amphotericin (BP); $C_{46}H_{73}NO_{20}$; an amphoteric polyene antibiotic prepared from *Streptomyces nodosus;* available as the sodium deoxycholate complex; an antifungal agent, but quite toxic.

**amphot'erism.** Amphotericity; the property of being amphoteric.

**amphothal'ide.** SCHISTOMIDE; *N*-[ 5-(*p*-aminophenoxy)-pentyl ]phthalimide; used for treatment of schistosomiasis.

**amphoto'nia, amphot'ony** [ ampho- + G. *tonos*, tension ]. Increased excitability of both the parasympathetic and sympathetic nervous systems.

**ampicillin** (am'pĭ-sĭ'lin) (USP, BP). α-Aminobenzylpenicillin; acid-stable, semisynthetic penicillin, derived from 6-aminopenicillanic acid; has a broader spectrum of antimicrobial action than penicillin G, inhibiting the growth of Gram-positive and Gram-negative bacteria. It is not resistant to penicillinase. Also available as a. sodium (USP, BP) and a. trihydrate (USP, BP).

**amplexa'tion** [ L. *amplexari*, intens. of *amplecti*, embrace strongly ]. Fixation of fractured clavicle by an apparatus that immobilizes shoulder and neck, with anchor embracing the thorax.

**amplex'us** [ L. an embrace, fr. *amplector*, pp. -*plexus*, to wind around. PLIC- ]. The pairing of male and female at the time that eggs and sperm are discharged simultaneously in those species, such as frogs, in which fertilization occurs externally.

**amplitude** (am'plĭ-tūd) [ L. *amplitudo*, fr. *amplus*, large ]. Largeness; extent.

  **a. of accommodation, a. of convergence,** see the nouns.

  **a. of pulse,** see average pulse *magnitude;* peak *magnitude*.

**am'protro'pine phosphate.** SYNTROPAN; 3-diethylamino-2,2-dimethylpropyl tropate phosphate; antispasmodic, similar in action to atropine.

**ampul, ampule** (am'pūl) [ L. *ampulla*, *q.v.* ]. Ampoule; a hermetically sealed container, usually made of glass, containing a sterile medicinal solution, or powder to be made up in solution, to be used for subcutaneous, intramuscular, or intravenous injection.

**ampulla,** gen. and pl. **ampul'lae** (am-pul'lah) [ L. a two-handled bottle ] [ NA ]. A saccular dilation of a canal or duct.

  **Bryant's a.,** the portion of an artery on the proximal side of a ligature, which contains the clot, its upper boundary being marked by a slight constriction.

  **a. canaliculi lacrimalis** [ NA ], a. ductus lacrimalis; a slight dilation in the lacrimal duct just beyond the punctum lacrimalis.

  **a. chyli,** *cisterna* chyli.

  **a. ductus deferentis** [ NA ], a. of vas deferens; Henle's a.; the dilation of the duct where it approaches its fellow just before it is joined by the duct of the seminal vesicle.

  **a. ductus lacrimalis,** a. canaliculi lacrimalis.

  **duodenal a.,** a. hepatopancreatica.

  **Henle's a.,** a. ductus deferentis.

  **a. hepat'opancreat'ica** [ NA ], duodenal a.; Vater's a.; the dilation within the major duodenal papilla that normally receives both the common bile duct and the main pancreatic duct.

  **a. lactifera,** *sinus* lactiferi.

  **a. membrana'cea,** pl. **ampullae membrana'ceae** [ NA ], membranous a.; a nearly spherical enlargement of one end of each of the three semicircular ducts, anterior, posterior, and lateral, where they connect with the utricle. Each contains a neuroepithelial crista.

  **membranous a.,** a. membranacea.

  **a. of milk duct,** *sinus* lactiferi.

  **a. os'sea,** pl. **ampullae os'seae** [ NA ], osseous a.; a circumscribed dilation of one extremity of each of the three semicircular canals, anterior, posterior, and lateral.

  **osseous a.,** a. ossea.

  **a. recti** [ NA ], a. of rectum; a dilated portion of the rectum just above the anal canal.

  **Thoma's a.,** a dilation of the arterial capillary beyond the sheathed artery of the spleen.

  **a. tu'bae uteri'nae** [ NA ], a. of uterine tube; the wide portion of the uterine (Fallopian) tube near the fimbriated extremity. It has a complexly folded mucosa with a columnar epithelium of mostly ciliated cells between which are secretory cells.

  **a. of uterine tube,** a. tubae uterinae.

  **a. of vas deferens,** a. ductus deferentis.

  **Vater's a.,** a. hepatopancreatica.

**ampul'lar.** Relating in any sense to an ampulla.

**ampullitis** (am-pul-li'tis). Inflammation of any ampulla, especially of the dilated extremity of the vas deferens.

**ampullula** (am-pul'u-lah) [ Mod. L. dim. of L. *ampulla* ]. A circumscribed dilation of any minute lymphatic or blood vessel or duct.

# AMPUTATION

**amputation** (am-pu-ta'shun) [ L. *amputatio,* fr. *am-puto,*
pp. *-atus,* to cut around, prune ]. 1. The cutting off of a limb
or part of a limb, the breast, or other projecting part. 2. In
dentistry, a. may be of the root of a tooth, or of the pulp,
or even of a nerve root or ganglion, *e.g.,* the Gasserian
ganglion. A modifying adjective must therefore be used
(pulp a.; root a.).

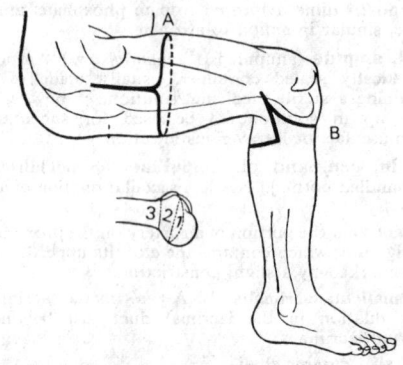

**Amputation**

*A,* racket incision for amputation of the hip; *B,* incision
for Carden's, Gritti's, and Stokes' amputations. The inset
shows the lines of section of the femur for (*1*) Carden's, (*2*)
Gritti's, and (*3*) Stokes' amputations.

**Alanson's a.,** circular a., the stump shaped like a cone.
**Alouette's a.,** a. of the hip.
**aperiosteal a.,** one with removal of periosteum from bone
at site of a.
**Bier's a.,** osteoplastic a. of tibia and fibula.
**bloodless a.,** dry a.; one in which, by means of an
Esmarch bandage or some other appliance, the escape of
blood from the cut surfaces is slight.
**Callander's a.,** tenontoplastic a. through the femur at the
knee.
**Carden's a.,** transcondylar a. of the leg, the femur being
sawn through the condyles just above the articular surface.
**central a.,** one in which the flaps are so united that the
cicatrix runs across the end of the stump.
**cervical a.,** a. of the uterine cervix.
**chop a.,** a. by a circular cut through soft parts and bone
without flaps.
**Chopart's a.,** disarticulation at the midtarsal joint,
leaving only the astragalus and calcaneum, with the soft
parts of the sole of the foot to cover the stump.
**cinematic a.,** cineplastic a.
**cineplas'tic a.,** cinematic a.; cineplastics; kineplastics;
cinematization; a method of a. of an extremity whereby the
muscles and tendons are so arranged in the stump that they
are able to execute independent movements and to communicate motion to a specially constructed prosthetic apparatus.
**circular a.,** one performed by a circular incision through
the skin, the muscles being similarly divided higher up, and
the bone higher still.
**coat-sleeve a.,** one in which there is one long skin flap
folded over the stump.
**congenital a.,** intrauterine a.; spontaneous a.; one
produced *in utero,* formerly attributed to the pressure of
adventitious constricting bands; more recently regarded as
the result of an intrinsic deficiency of embryonic tissue.
**consecutive a.,** an a. performed during or following
suppuration.
**a. in contiguity,** disarticulation.

**a. in continuity,** a. through a segment of a limb, not at
a joint.
**cutaneous a.,** one leaving only flaps of skin.
**diclas'tic a.,** one performed without the knife or saw, the
bone being broken and the soft tissues bitten off with an
écraseur.
**Dieffenbach's a.,** circular a. at the hip joint with
temporary elastic ligature.
**double flap a.,** a. in which a flap is cut from the soft parts
on either side of the limb.
**dry a.,** bloodless a.
**Dupuytren's a.,** a. of arm at shoulder joint.
**eccentric a.,** one with scar of stump off-center.
**elliptical a.,** circular a. in which the sweep of the knife
is not exactly vertical to the axis of the limb, the outline
of the cut surface being therefore elliptical.
**excentric a.,** one in which the line of union of the flaps
does not run across the end of the stump.
**Farabeuf's a.,** (1) a. of the leg, the flap being large and
on the outer side; (2) a. of the foot; subastragaloid
disarticulation.
**flap a.,** one in which flaps of the muscular and cutaneous
tissues are made to cover the end of the bone; see also flap
operation.
**flapless a.,** an a. without any tissue to cover stump.
**forequarter a.,** interscapulothoracic a.
**Gritti's a.,** Gritti's operation; supracondylar a. of the
femur, the patella being preserved and applied to the end
of the bone, its articular cartilage being removed so as to
obtain union.
**guillotine a.,** linear a.; a direct, sweeping section of all
tissues of a limb, without dissection or flaps.
**Guyon's a.,** a. above the malleoli, a modification of
Syme's operation.
**Hancock's a.,** a. of foot through astragalus.
**Hey's a.,** Hey's operation; a. of the foot in front of the
tarsometatarsal joint.
**immediate a.,** one necessitated by irreparable injury to
the limb, which is performed within twelve hours after the
injury.
**interilioabdominal a.,** a. of entire leg and a part of the
pelvis.
**intermediate a.,** one performed during the period of
reaction from shock, and in older days before the period
of inevitable suppuration.
**interpel'viabdom'inal a.,** Jaboulay's operation; a. of the
thigh with removal of the corresponding lateral half of the
pelvis.
**interscap'ulothorac'ic a.,** forequarter a.; a. of the arm
with removal of the scapula and a portion of the clavicle
on the same side.
**intrapyretic a.,** intermediate a.; one performed at a stage
between trauma or incipient gangrene and suppuration.
**intrauterine a.,** congenital a.
**Jaboulay's a.,** interpelviabdominal a.
**kineplastic a.,** cineplastic a.
**Kirk's a.,** a. at lower end of femur, using tendon of
quadraceps extensor to cover end of bone.
**Langenbeck's a.,** a. of foot.
**Larrey's a.,** a. at shoulder joint.
**Le Fort's a.,** a modification of Pirogoff's a.; the calcaneus
is sawed through horizontally instead of vertically so that
the patient steps on the same part of the heel as before.
**linear a.,** guillotine a.
**Lisfranc's a.,** Lisfranc's operation; a. of the foot at the
tarsometatarsal joint, the sole being preserved to make the
flap.
**Mackenzie's a.,** a modification of Syme's a. at the ankle
joint, the flap being taken from the inner side.
**major a.,** a. of the lower or upper extremity above the
ankle or the wrist, respectively.
**Malgaigne's a.,** subastragalar a.
**mediotar'sal a.,** a. of the forepart of the foot through the
tarsal region; Chopart's a.
**Mikulicz-Vladimiroff a.,** Mikulicz-Vladimiroff operation; an osteoplastic resection of the foot in which the talus
and calcaneus are exsected, the anterior row of tarsal bones
being united to the lower end of the tibia, the articular
surfaces of both being removed; the lower end of the stump
is therefore the anterior portion of the foot, the patient
walking thereafter on tiptoe.

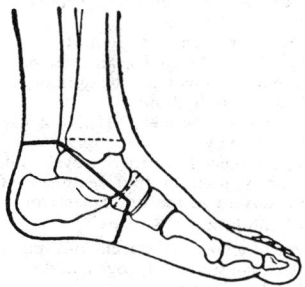

**Mikulicz-Vladimiroff Amputation**
Osteoplastic resection of the ankle. *Heavy line*, line of incision; *dotted line*, line of section through the bones.

**minor a.,** a. of a hand or foot or any of its parts.
**multiple a.,** a. of two or more limbs or parts of limbs performed at the same operation.
**musculocutaneous a.,** one with a flap of muscle and skin.

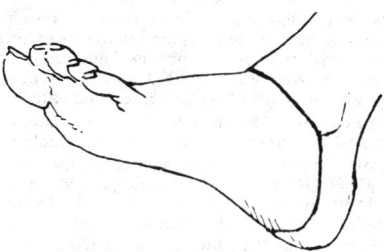

**Skin Incision in Syme's Amputation**

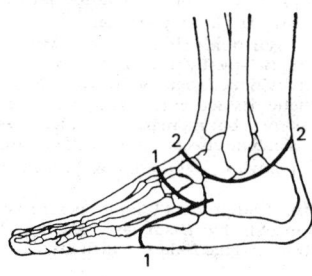

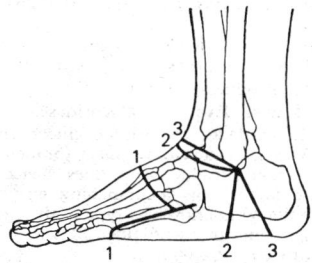

**Tarsal Amputations**
*Above: 1,* Chopart's; *2,* Mackenzie's. *Below:* Lines of incision for amputations: *1-1,* Lisfranc's; *2-2,* Pirogoff's; *3-3,* Syme's.

**oblique a.,** one in which the line of section through an extremity is at other than a right angle; this yields an oval appearance to the cut surface (hence sometimes, though rarely, referred to as an oval a.).
**osteoplastic a.,** an a., such as several through the tarsus, in which the cut surface of another bone is brought in apposition with the one primarily divided so that the two unite, thus giving a better stump.
**oval a.,** (1) one in which the flaps are obained by oval incisions through the skin and muscle; (2) rarely used synonym for oblique a.
**pathologic a.,** one necessitated by cancer or other disease of the limb and not by an injury.
**periosteoplastic a.,** subperiosteal a.
**Pirogoff's a.,** a. of the foot, the lower articular surfaces of the tibia and fibula being sawn through and the ends covered with a portion of the os calcis which has also been sawn through from above posteriorly downward and forward.
**primary a.,** intermediate a.
**pulp a.,** pulpotomy.
**quadruple a.,** a. of both arms and both legs.
**racket a.,** a circular or slightly oval a., in which a long incision is made in the axis of the limb.
**rectangular a.,** one in which the flaps are fashioned in this shape.
**Ricard's a.,** a. of foot, using calcaneus in stump as weight-bearer.
**root a.,** apicoectomy.
**secondary a.,** one performed some time after an injury; *not* intermediate a.
**spontaneous a.,** congenital a.
**Stokes' a.,** a modification of Gritti's a. in that the line of section of the femur is slightly higher.
**subastrag'alar a.,** Malgaigne's a.; a. of the foot in which only the astragalus is retained.
**subperios'teal a.,** periosteoplastic a.; one in which the periosteum is stripped back from the bone and replaced afterward, forming a periosteal flap over the cut end.
**Syme's a.,** Syme's operation (1); a. of the foot at the ankle joint, the malleoli being sawed off, and a flap being made with the soft parts of the heel.
**tarsotibial a.,** a. through the ankle joint.
**Teale's a.,** (1) a. of the forearm in its lower half, or of the thigh, with a long posterior rectangular flap and a short anterior one; (2) a. of the leg, with a long anterior rectangular flap and a short posterior one.

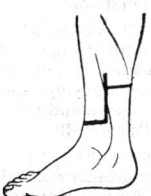

**Teale's Leg Amputation**
Showing lines of incision. The bone section is made at the upper extremity of the vertical line.

**tertiary a.,** a. after infection has been controlled.
**a. by transfixion,** one performed by transfixing the soft parts with a long knife and cutting the flap or flaps from within outward.
**transverse a.,** one in which the line of section through the extremity is at right angles to the long axis.
**traumatic a.,** a. resulting from accidental or nonsurgical injury; may be complete, subtotal, or incomplete.
**Tripier's a.,** a modification of Chopart's a., in that a part of the calcaneus is also removed.
**Vladimiroff-Mikulicz a.,** Mikulicz-Vladimiroff a.

**am'putee.** A person with an amputated limb.
**ampyrone.** 4-Amino-2,3-dimethyl-1-phenyl-3-pyrazolin-5-one; antipyretic and analgesic.

**amquin'ate** (USAN). Amquinolate; methyl-7-(diethyl-amino)-4-hydroxy-6-propyl-3-quinolinecarboxylate; antimalarial agent.

**Amsler,** Marc, Swiss ophthalmologist, *1891. See A.'s *chart, marker.*

**amuck** (ă-muk'). Amok.

**amu'sia** [ G. *a-* priv. + *mousa,* music ]. A form of aphasia characterized by loss of the faculty of musical expression or of the recognition of simple musical tones.

    **sensory a.,** failure to interpret or appreciate musical sounds.

    **vocal a.,** the inability to sing, although the individual is capable of other motor and speech performance.

**Amussat** (am-ü-să'), Jean Z., French surgeon, 1796–1856. See A.'s *valves, valvula.*

**amychophobia** (am-i-ko-fo'bĭ-ah) [ G. *amychē,* a scratch, + *phobos,* fear ]. Morbid fear of being scratched.

**amyctic** (ă-mik'tik) [ G. *amyssein,* to scratch, scarify ]. Pruritic; irritating.

**amydricaine hydrochloride.** ALYPINE; 1-(dimethyl-amino)-2-[ (dimethylamino)-methyl ]-2-butanol hydrochloride; topical anesthetic.

**amyelencephalia** (a-mi'el-en-sĕ-fa'lĭ-ah) [ G. *a-* priv. + *myelos,* marrow, + *enkephalos,* brain ]. Absence of both brain and spinal cord.

**amy'elencephal'ic, amy'elenceph'alous.** Without brain or spinal cord.

**amy'elenceph'alus.** An individual without brain or spinal cord.

**amyelia** (ă-mi-e'lĭ-ah) [ G. *a-* priv. + *myelos,* marrow ]. Absence of the spinal cord, found only in association with anencephaly.

**amyelic** (ă-mi-el'ik). Amyelous.

**amyelinated** (ă-mi'ĕ-lĭ-na'ted). Unmyelinated.

**amyelination** (ă-mi'ĕ-lĭ-na'shun). Loss of the myelin sheath of a nerve.

**amyelinic** (ă-mi'ĕ-lin'ik). Unmyelinated.

**amyeloic, amyelonic** (ă-mi'ĕ-lo'ik, ă-mi-ĕ-ion'ik) [ G. *a-* priv. + *myelos,* marrow ]. 1. Amyelous. 2. Terms sometimes used in hematology to indicate the absence of bone marrow, or the lack of functional participation of bone marrow, in hemopoiesis.

**amyelous** (ă-mi'e-lus). Amyelic; amyeloic (1); amyelonic (1); without spinal cord.

**amyelus** (ă-mi'e-lus) [ G. *a-* priv. + *myelos,* marrow ]. An individual without spinal cord.

**amygdala,** gen. and pl. **amyg'dalae** (ă-mig'dah-lah) [ L. fr. G. *amygdalē,* almond; in Mediev. & Mod. L. a tonsil ]. 1. *Corpus* amygdaloideum. 2. Tonsilla; denoting the cerebellar tonsil, as well as the lymphatic tonsils (pharyngeal, palatine, lingual, laryngeal, and tubal).

    **a. cerebel'li,** *tonsilla* cerebelli.

**amyg'dalase.** β-Glucosidase.

**amyg'dalin.** Amygdaloside; mandelonitrile-β-gentiobioside; a glucoside present in almonds and seeds of other plants of the family Rosaceae. The addition of emulsin splits a. into oil of bitter almond and hydrocyanic acid.

**amyg'daline.** 1. Relating to an almond. 2. Relating to a tonsil, or to the brain structure called amygdala or amygdaloid nucleus.

**amyg'daloid** [ amygdala + G. *eidos,* appearance ]. Resembling an almond or a tonsil.

**amyg'dalose.** Gentiobiose.

**amyg'daloside.** Amygdalin.

**amyl-.** See amylo-.

**a'myl.** Pentyl; the radical formed from a pentane, $C_5H_{12}$, by removal of one H. Several isomeric forms exist, the more important being $CH_3CH_2CH_2CH_2CH_2$— (amyl or pentyl); $(CH_3)_2CHCH_2CH_2$— isoamyl or isopentyl); $CH_3CH_2CH_2CH(CH)_3$— and $(CH_3CH_2)_2CH$— secondary amyls); and $CH_3CH_2C(CH_3)_2$— tertiary amyl or pentyl).

    **a. acetate,** $CH_3CO$—$C_5H_{11}$; an ester naturally occurring in, and lending flavor to, fruits such as strawberry.

    **a. alcohol,** (1) commercial amyl alcohol: fusel oil; a mixture of various isomers of amyl alcohol, mostly isoamyl alcohol; (2) normal amyl alcohol: 1-pentanol; used as a

solvent for varnishes and oils. The vapors are irritating; highly toxic.

    **a. alcohol, tertiary,** amylene hydrate.

    **a. butyrate,** $C_3H_7CO$—$C_5H_{11}$; an ester occurring naturally in, and lending flavor to, the apricot.

    **a. hydrate,** amylene hydrate.

    **a. nitrite** (NF), VAPOROLE; $C_5H_{11}NO_2$; vasodilator, in angina pectoris and cyanide poisoning.

    **a. val'erate,** apple oil; isoamyl isovalerate; used as a sedative; formerly used in the treatment of gallstones because of its solvent action on cholesterol.

**amylaceous** (am'i-la'shus). Starchy.

**am'ylase.** One of a group of starch-splitting or amylolytic enzymes that cleave starch, glycogen, and related polysaccharides, all α-1,4-glucans.

    **pancreatic a.,** amylopsin; an α-amylase (*q.v.*) in pancreatic juice.

    **salivary a.,** ptyalin; the α-amylase (*q.v.*) of saliva.

**α-amylase.** Diastase; ptyalin; glycogenase; a glucanohydrolase (EC 3.2.1.1) yielding α-glucose and maltose in a random manner from starch, glycogen, etc. (1,4-α-glucans).

**β-amylase.** Diastase; saccharogen amylase; glycogenase; a glucanohydrolase (EC 3.2.1.2) yielding β-maltose units from the nonreducing ends of 1,4-α-glucans.

**γ-amylase.** Exo-1,4-α-glucosidase.

**amylasu'ria.** Diastasuria; the excretion of starch-splitting enzyme (amylase, sometimes termed diastase) in the urine, especially with reference to increased amounts; the normal level ranges from 200 to 1000 units, but considerably greater amounts are likely in acute pancreatitis.

**amylemia** (am-i-le'mĭ-ah) [ amylo- + G. *haima,* blood ]. The hypothetic presence of starch in the circulating blood.

**am'ylene.** Trimethylethylene; pentene; 2-methyl-2-butene; $(CH_3)_2C$=$CHCH_3$; a flammable liquid hydrocarbon formed by the decomposition of amyl alcohol. It has anesthetic properties but undesirable side actions.

    **a. chloral,** DORMIOL; dimethylethylcarbinolchloral; hypnotic.

    **a. hydrate** (NF), dimethylethylcarbinol; tertiary amyl alcohol; amyl hydrate; *tert*-pentanol; hypnotic; used as a solvent for tribromethanol for rectal anesthesia.

**am'ylin.** The cellulose of starch; the insoluble envelope of starch grains.

**amylo-, amyl-** [ G. *amylon,* starch. AMYL- ]. Combining forms indicating starch or polysaccharide nature or origin.

**amylobar'bitone** (BP). Amobarbital.

**am'ylocaine hydrochloride.** STOVAINE; 1-(dimethylaminomethyl)-1-methylpropyl benzoate hydrochloride; benzoylethyldimethylaminopropanol hydrochloride; a local anesthetic. Its action is slightly stronger than that of cocaine, less toxic but more irritant. It has been used for spinal anesthesia. Side effects and aftereffects are frequent.

**am'yloclast** [ amylo- + G. *klastos,* broken in pieces ]. Amylase.

**amylodex'trin.** End product ("limit" dextrin) of hydrolysis of amylopectin by β-amylase. Further hydrolysis requires dextrin-1,6-glucosidase, which attacks the branch points.

**amylodyspepsia** (am'i-lo-dis-pep'sĭ-ah) [ amylo- + G. *dys-,* difficult, + *pepsis,* digestion ]. Inability to digest starchy food.

**amylogenesis** (am'i-lo-jen'ĕ-sis) [ amylo- + G. *genesis,* production ]. Amylosynthesis; the biosynthesis of starch.

**am'ylogen'ic.** Producing starch.

**amyloglucosidase.** Exo-1,4-α-glucosidase.

**amylo-1,6-glucosidase.** Dextrin 6-α-glucosidase; enzyme (EC 3.2.1.33) hydrolyzing α-1,6 links (branch points) in chains of 1,4-linked α-glucose residues, hence the terms "debranching factor" or "debranching enzyme." Deficiency (Hereditary) is known as type 3 glycogenosis. See also dextranase, and oligo-1,6-glucosidase.

**am'ylohydrol'ysis.** Amylolysis.

**am'yloid** [ amylo- + G. *eidos,* resemblance ]. A protein (probably combined with chondroitin sulfuric acid) that is microscopically homogeneous, but that is composed of fine fibrils when seen under the electron microscope, staining dark brown with iodine and becoming birefringent when

stained with Congo red; occurs characteristically as pathologic extracellular deposits beneath the endothelium of
capillaries or sinusoids, in the walls of arterioles, and
especially in association with reticuloendothelial tissue. See
also amyloidosis.

**amyloido′sis** [ amyloid + G. suffix -*osis*, condition ]. A
disease of unknown cause characterized by the extracellular accumulation of amyloid in various organs and tissues
of the body.

**a. cu′tis,** infiltration of skin by amyloid, an abnormal
protein substance. The eruption consists of itching papules, small nodules, and plaques. There is no evidence of
infiltrate in other organs.

**familial a. with febrile urticaria and deafness,** Muckle-Wells *syndrome.*

**focal a.,** nodular a.

**a. of multiple myeloma,** foci of a. in mesenchymal tissues
of some persons (5 to 10 per cent) with multiple myeloma;
no direct relation between amyloid and Bence Jones
protein is conclusively known.

**nodular a.,** focal a.; a form of a. in which the protein
occurs as small masses or nodules beneath the skin or
mucous membranes, *e.g.,* in the larynx.

**primary a.,** a form of a. not associated with other
recognized disease (see also secondary a.); sometimes
familial; tends to involve diffusely the arterial walls and
mesenchymal tissues in the tongue, lungs, intestinal tract,
skin, skeletal muscle, and myocardium; the amyloid in this
condition frequently does not manifest the usual affinity
for Congo red, and sometimes provokes a foreign-body
type of inflammatory reaction in the adjacent tissue.

**renal a.,** amyloid nephrosis (1); renal deposits of amyloid,
especially in glomerular capillary walls, which may cause
albuminuria and the nephrotic syndrome.

**secondary a.,** the most frequent form of a., occurs in
association with another chronic disease, *e.g.,* tuberculosis,
osteomyelitis, rheumatoid arthritis, and so on; organs
chiefly involved are the liver, spleen, and kidneys, and the
adrenal glands less frequently.

**senile a.,** a common form of a. in very old people, usually
mild and limited to the heart.

**urticaria, deafness, and a.,** Muckle-Wells *syndrome.*

**amylol′ysis** [ amylo- + G. *lysis,* dissolution ]. Amylohy-
drolysis; hydrolysis of starch into sugar.

**amylomal′tase.** 4-α -Glucanotransferase.

**amylopec′tin.** A branched chain polyglucose (glucan) in
starch.

**amylopectin 6-glucanohydrolase.** Debranching enzyme
(*q. v.*); an enzyme (EC 3.2.1.69) with action similar to that
of isoamylase and pullulanase, but limited to amylopectin
as substrate; cleaves 1,6-α -glucosidic linkages.

**amylopectin 1,6-glucosidase.** Formerly R enzyme, EC
3.2.1.9; now known to be at least three enzymes, pullulanase, isoamylase, amylopectin 6-glucanohydrolase, enzymes hydrolyzing 1,6-α-glucosidic links. See also
oligo-1,6-glucosidase, amylo-1,6-glucosidase.

**am′ylopectino′sis** [ amylopectin + G. suffix -*osis*, condition ]. Glycogenosis due to deficiency of brancher enzyme.

**brancher deficiency a.,** type 4 *glycogenosis.*

**amylophagia** (am′ĭ-lo-fa′jĭ-ah) [ amylo- + G. *phagein*, to
eat ]. A craving for starchy foods.

**am′ylophosphor′ylase.** Glycogen phosphorylase; see under glycogen.

**am′yloplast** [ amylo- + G. *plastos,* formed ]. Amylogenic
body; a granule in the protoplasm of a vegetable cell that
is the center of a starch-forming process.

**am′yloplas′tic.** Amylogenic.

**amylop′sin.** A pancreatic α-amylase.

**amylorrhea** (am-ĭ-lor-re′ah) [ amylo- + G. *rhoia*, flow ].
Passage of undigested starch in the stools.

**am′ylose.** Unbranched polyglucose (glucan) in starch.

**am′ylosu′ria.** Amyluria; excretion of starch in the urine.

**am′ylosyn′thesis.** Amylogenesis.

**amylo-1-4,1-6-transglucosidase.** 1,4-α -Glucan 6-α -
glucosyltransferase.

**amylo-(1,4 → 1,6)-transglucosylase.** 1,4-α -Glucan 6-α-
glucosyltransferase.

**amylpenicillin sodium.** Flavacidin; flavicin; sodium
*n*-amylpenicillinate; penicillin dihydro F sodium; an antibi-

otic derived from cultures of *Aspergillus flavus;* a naturally
occurring F type penicillin, active against Gram-positive
microorganisms.

**amylphosphorylase.** Phosphorylase (2).

**am′ylum.** Starch.

**amylu′ria.** Amylosuria.

**amy′ocar′dia** [ G. a- priv. + *mys*, muscle, + *kardia,*
heart ]. Myasthenia cordis; weakness of the heart muscle.

**amyoesthesia, amyoesthesis** (ă-mi′o-es-the′zĭ-ah, -the′-
sis) [ G. a- priv. + *mys*, muscle, + *aisthēsis*, perception ].
Loss of muscle sensation.

**amy′opla′sia** [ G. a- priv. + *mys*, muscle, + *plasis*, a
molding ]. Deficient formation of muscle tissue.

**a. congenita,** *arthrogryposis* multiplex congenita.

**amyostasia** (ă-mi′o-pla′zĭ-ah) [ G. a- priv. + *mys*, muscle,
+ *stasis,* standing ]. Difficulty in standing, due to muscular
tremor or incoordination.

**amy′ostat′ic.** Showing muscular tremors.

**amyosthenia** (ă-mi′os-the′nĭ-ah) [ G. a- priv. + *mys*, muscle, + *sthenos,* strength ]. Muscular weakness.

**amyosthen′ic.** Relating to or causing muscular weakness.

**amy′otaxy, amyotax′ia** [ G. a- priv. + *mys*, muscle, +
*taxis,* order ]. Muscular ataxia.

**amyoto′nia** [ G. a- priv. + *mys*, muscle, + *tonos*, tone ].
Myatonia.

**a. congenita,** Oppenheim's syndrome; myatonia congenita; an absence of muscular tone, observed especially in
infants and affecting only the muscles innervated by the
spinal nerves; atonic pseudoparalysis of congenital origin,
but neither familial nor hereditary.

**amy′otro′phia.** Amyotrophy.

**amyotro′phic.** Relating to muscular atrophy.

**amyotrophy** (ă-mi-ot′ro-fĭ) [ G. a- priv. + *mys*, muscle, +
*trophē*, nourishment ]. Muscular wasting or atrophy.

**diabet′ic a.,** a. in patients with diabetes.

**neuralgic a.,** atrophy of muscle due to neuralgia or
neuritis.

**progressive spinal a.,** progressive muscular *atrophy.*

**amyous** (am′i-us) [ G. a- priv. + *mys*, muscle ]. Lacking in
muscular tissue, or in muscular strength.

**amyxia** (ă-mik′sĭ-ah) [ G. a- priv. + *myxa*, mucus ]. Absence of mucus.

**amyxorrhea** (ă-mik-sor-re′ah) [ G. a- priv. + *myxa*, mucus, + *rhoia,* flow ]. Absence of the normal secretion of
mucus.

**an-.** See a-.

**An.** Chemical symbol of the element actinium.

**ana-** (an′ah) [ G. *ana,* up ]. Prefix meaning up, toward,
apart. Distinguish from *an-*, which is *a-* privative with *n*
before a vowel.

**ana** (an′ah). A distributive Greek preposition, meaning of
each; used in prescription writing in the abbreviated form
āā, or more correctly āā, to denote that the stated amount
of each of the indicated substances is to be taken.

**Anabaena.** A genus of Cyanobacteria causing odors in
water supplies.

**anab′asine.** Neonicotine; 2-(3-pyridyl)piperidine; a tobacco alkaloid with a piperidine ring in the place of the
pyrrol ring present in nicotine.

**anab′asis** [ G. a going up. BAS- ]. A stage of progression
or worsening in a disease.

**anabat′ic.** Relating to the anabasis of a disease; increasing
in severity.

**anabiosis** (an-ah-bi-o′sis) [ G. a reviving, fr. *ana*, again, +
*biōsis*, life ]. Resuscitation after apparent death.

**anabiot′ic.** 1. Resuscitating; restorative. 2. A revivifying
remedy; a powerful stimulant.

**anabolergy** (an′ah-bol′er-jĭ) [ G. *anabolē*, a building up, +
*ergon*, work ]. Energy consumed in the process of
anabolism.

**anabol′ic.** Relating to or promoting anabolism.

**anab′olin.** Anabolite.

**anab′olism** [ G. *anabolē*, a raising up ]. The process of
assimilation of nutritive matter and its conversion into
living substance. This includes synthetic processes and
requires energy.

**anab'olite.** Anabolin; any substance formed as a result of anabolic processes.

**anabro'sis** [ G. fr. *ana*, up, + *bibrōskō*, to eat up ]. Superficial erosion or ulceration.

**an'abrot'ic.** A substance that produces ulceration or erosion of the skin surface.

**anacamp'tic.** In optics or acoustics, rarely used term meaning reflecting or reflected.

**anacamp'tics** [ G. *anakamptō*, to bend back ]. Rarely used term meaning the study of reflection of sound or light.

**anacamptom'eter** [ G. *anakampsis*, a bending back, reflection, + *metron*, measure ]. Instrument for measuring the intensity of the deep reflexes.

**anacardiol.** 3-Ethoxy-*N,N*-diethyl-4-hydroxybenzamide; analeptic.

**anacatadidymus** (an'ah-kat-ah-did'ĭ-mus) [ G. *ana*, up, + *kata*, down, + *didymos*, twin ]. Conjoined twins united in the middle but separated above and below.

**anacatesthesia** (an'ah-kat'es-the'zĭ-ah) [ G. *ana*, up, + *kata*, down, + *aisthēsis*, sensation ]. A hovering sensation.

**anacatharsis** (an'ah-kă-thar'sis) [ G. *ana*, up, + *katharsis*, cleansing ]. Severe and long-continued vomiting.

**anacathar'tic.** Emetic; causing anacatharsis.

**anacholia** (an'ah-ko'lĭ-ah) [ G. *ana*, backward, + *cholē*, bile ]. Retention or lessened secretion of bile.

**anachoresis** (an'ah-ko-re'sis) [ G. a retiring, a refuge, fr. *ana*, *Ā chĭreī*, to give room, retire ]. 1. The accumulation of particulate material (from the circulating blood) in certain sites in the tissues. 2. The aggregation of various microorganisms in the region of syphilitic, tuberculous, or other inflammations, a phenomenon usually associated with induced sensitivity to the specific infection.

**an'achoret'ic, an'achor'ic.** Relating to anachoresis.

**anacidity** (an'ă-sid'ĭ-tĭ). Absence of acidity; denoting especially absence of hydrochloric acid in the gastric juice.

**anac'idogen'esis.** Failure to form acid.

    **renal a.,** failure of the renal tubules to acidify the urine, which leads to acidosis, decalcification of the skeleton, and spontaneous fractures.

**anaclasis** (ă-nak'lă-sis) [ G. a bending back, reflection. CLAS- ]. 1. Reflection of light or sound. 2. Refraction of the ocular media. 3. Forcible flexion of a joint to break up the adhesion in fibrous ankylosis.

**anaclit'ic** [ G. *ana*, toward, + *klinein*, to lean ]. Leaning or depending upon; in psychoanalysis, relating to the dependence of the infant on the mother or mother substitute.

**anac'mesis.** Obsolete spelling for anakmesis.

**anacrot'ic** [ G. *ana*, up, + *krotos*, a beat ]. Referring to the upstroke or ascending limb of the arterial pulse tracing; abbreviation for anadicrotic, twice beating on the upstroke; see pulse.

**anacrotism** (ă-nak'ro-tizm). Peculiarity of the pulse wave as described under anacrotic pulse.

**an'acul'ture** Obsolete term for a formalinized whole culture used as a vaccine.

**anacusis** (an'ă-ku'sis) [ G. *an-* priv. + *akousis*, hearing ]. Total loss or absence of the ability to perceive sound as such.

**anade'nia** [ G. *an-* priv. + *adēn*, gland ]. Absence of glands or abeyance of glandular function.

    **a. ventriculi,** the absence of glands from the stomach.

**anadicrot'ic** [ G. *ana*, up, + *di-krotos*, double beating ]. Anacrotic.

**anadicrotism** (an-ah-dik'ro-tizm). Anacrotism.

**anadidymus** (an-ah-did'ĭ-mus) [ G. *ana*, up, + *didymos*, twin ]. Conjoined twins, united below but separated above; duplicitas anterior.

**anadip'sia** [ G. *ana*, intensive, + *dipsa*, thirst ]. Extreme thirst; see polydipsia.

**anadre'nalism.** Complete lack of adrenal function.

**anaerobe** (an'a-er-ōb, an-a'er-ōb) [ G. *an-* priv. + *aēr*, air, + *bios*, life ]. A microorganism that thrives best, or only, in the absence of oxygen.

    **facultative a.,** one able to grow in the presence or absence of free oxygen.

    **obligate (obligatory) a.,** one that will grow only in the absence of free oxygen.

**anaerobic** (an-a-er-o'bik). Relating to an anaerobe; living without oxygen.

**anaerobiosis** (an-a-er-o-bi-o'sis) [ G. *an-* priv. + *aēr*, air, + *biōsis*, way of living ]. Existence in an oxygen-free atmosphere.

**anaerogen'ic** [ G. *an-* priv. + *aēr*, air, + suffix *-gen*, producing ]. Not producing gas.

**anaerophyte** (an-a'er-o-fīt) [ G. *an-* priv. + *aēr*, air, + *phyton*, plant ]. 1. A plant that grows without air. 2. An anaerobic bacterium.

**anaeroplasty** (an-a'er-o-plas-tĭ) [ G. *an-* priv. + *aēr*, air, + *plassō*, to form ]. Treatment of wounds by exclusion of air.

**anagen** (an'ah-jen) [ G. *ana*, up, + suffix *-gen*, producing ]. Growth phase of hair cycle.

**anagenesis** (an'ah-jen'ĕ-sis) [ G. *ana*, up, + *genesis*, production ]. Repair of tissue; regeneration of lost parts.

**an'agenet'ic.** Pertaining to anagenesis.

**anages'tone acetate** (USAN). ANATROPIN; 17-hydroxy-6α-methylpregn-4-en-20-one acetate; progestational agent.

**anagnosasthenia** (an'ag-nōs-as-the'nĭ-ah) [ G. *anagnōsis*, reading, + *astheneia*, weakness ]. A form of neurasthenia in which the attempt to read causes distressing symptoms.

**Anagnostakis,** Andrei, Cretan ophthalmologist, 1826–1897. See A.'s operation.

**anagogy** (an-ă-go'jĭ) [ G. *anagōgē*, fr. *an-ago*, to lead up. ACT-, AG- ]. Psychic content of an idealistic or spiritual nature.

**an'agraph** [ G. *anagraphē*, a writing out ]. Prescription.

**anagyrine** (an-aj'ĭ-rēn) [ G. *anagyros*, the stinking bean trefoil, fr. *ana*, up, + *gyros*, circle ]. Monolupine; rhombinin; an alkaloid, related to sparteine, from *Anagyris foetida*, a leguminous shrub of the Mediterranean region, having properties somewhat similar to scoparius (Irish broom). Has been used as a circulatory stimulant (edema).

**anákhré** (an-ah-kra') [ native term on the French Ivory Coast in Africa, meaning "big nose" ]. Goundou.

**anakmesis** (an-ak'me-sis) [ G. *an-* priv. + *akmēnos*, full grown, fr. *akmē*, highest point ]. Arrest of maturation of leukocytes in their production centers, thereby resulting in greater numbers of young forms and progressively smaller proportions of mature granular cells in the bone marrow, as observed in agranulocytosis.

**anaku'sis.** Anacusis.

**a'nal.** Relating to the anus.

**analbumine'mia** [ G. *an-* priv. + albumin, *q.v.*, + G. *haima*, blood ]. Absence of albumin from the serum.

**analep'tic** [ G. *analēptikos*, restorative. LAB- ]. 1. Strengthening; stimulating; invigorating. 2. A restorative remedy. 3. A central nervous system stimulant.

**analgesia** (an-al-je'zĭ-ah) [ G. insensibility, fr. *an-* priv. + *algēsis*, sensation of pain ]. A condition in which nociceptive stimuli are perceived but are not interpreted as pain; usually accompanied by sedation without loss of consciousness.

    **a. al'gera,** spontaneous pain in a part, associated with loss of sensibility.

    **conduction a.,** sensory denervation in a portion of the body (regional anesthesia), produced by pharmacological means.

    **a. doloro'sa,** a. algera.

    **spinal a.,** sensory denervation produced by injection of local anesthetic into the subarachnoid space; a euphemism for spinal *anesthesia, q.v.*

    **surface a.,** topical *anesthesia.*

**analgesic** (an-al-je'zik). 1. Analgetic (1); a compound capable of producing analgesia, *i.e.,* one that relieves pain by altering perception of nociceptive stimuli without producing anesthesia or loss of consciousness. 2. Characterized by altered response to painful stimuli.

**analgesimeter** (an'al-je-zim'ĭ-ter) [ analgesia + G. *metron*, measure ]. A device for measuring experimental pain.

**analget'ic.** 1. Analgesic (1). 2. Associated with altered pain perception.

**anal'ity.** Referring to the psychic organization derived from, and characteristic of, the anal period of psychosexual development.

**anallergic** (an-al-lur'jik). Not allergic.

**analogous** (ă-nal'o-gus). Resembling functionally, but having a different origin or structure.

**analogue** (an'ă-log) [ G. *ana-logos,* analogous ]. 1. One of two organs or parts in different species of animals or plants, which differ in structure or devlopment but are similar in function. 2. Chemistry: a compound that resembles another in structure; may be an isomer, but not necessarily (*e.g.,* fluorouracil is an analogue of uracil). Often used to block enzymatic reactions by combining with enzymes (*e.g.,* isopropylthiogalactoside *versus* lactose).

**analphalipoproteinemia** (an'al'fah-lip'o-pro'te-in-e'-mĭ-ah). Tangier *disease.*

**anal'ysand.** In psychoanalysis, the person being analyzed.

**analysis,** pl. **analyses** (ă-nal'ĭ-sis) [ G. a breaking up, fr. *ana,* up, + *lysis,* a loosening. LY- ]. 1. The breaking up of a chemical compound into simpler elements; a process by which the composition of a substance is determined. 2. The separation of any compound substance or concept into the parts composing it. 3. See psychoanalysis. 4. Applied in electroencephalography to the estimation or recording of the components of a complex wave form in terms of their frequency and amplitude.

  **activation a.,** the identification and quantification of unknown elements from their characteristic electromagnetic spectra and decay constants after they have been made radioactive by exposure to high levels of particulate radiation.

  **adsorption a.,** chromatographic a.; see chromatography.

  **bite a.,** occlusal a.

  **brad'ykinet'ic a.,** the a. of a movement by means of slow cinematography.

  **character a.,** a. of the defenses and personality traits that characterize an individual.

  **chromat'ograph'ic a.,** chromatography.

  **cluster a.,** a statistical procedure, using correlation, by which the dynamic interaction of a number of factors can be studied simultaneously.

  **colorimet'ric a.,** determination of structure or quantity by means of color, *i.e.,* light absorption, at specific wavelengths (usually in the visible range) of a compound or its derivatives.

  **content a.,** any of a variety of techniques for classification and study of the verbal products of normal or of psychologically disabled individuals.

  **densimetric a.,** estimation of the amount of solids in a solution by the specific gravity.

  **didactic a.,** training a.

  **distributive a.,** in psychobiology, term used to describe the a. of information gained about the patient and its distribution by the physician along the lines that are indicated by the patient's complaint and symptoms.

  **ego a.,** psychoanalytic study of the ways in which the ego deals with intrapsychic conflicts.

  **existential a.,** existential *therapy.*

  **factor a.,** a statistical procedure, involving the further a. of a table of intercorrelations, to discover the constituent irreducible traits in such a complex mass of data, as in a statistical search for the core factors of intelligence or personality.

  **fractional gastric a.,** see gastric a.

  **gasometric a.,** the determination of structure or quantity of a substance by means of gaseous derivatives.

  **gastric a.,** a. of the contents of the stomach after the ingestion of a test meal. The gastric contents are aspirated through a specially designed stomach tube (Rehfuss', Ryle's, etc.), and the free and total acidities, the pH, and the peptic activity are determined; they may also be examined for food residue, bile, blood, mucus, etc. In the fractional method of gastric a., which is now generally used, a sample is aspirated 15 minutes after the ingestion of the test meal, and every 15 minutes thereafter until the stomach is empty. The free acidity with or without the previous administration of histamine can be determined by means of quinine: this is the so-called tubeless method of gastric a. See also quinine test.

  **gravimet'ric a.,** quantitative a. by weighing separately each constituent as such or in a form of known constitution.

  **interaction process a.,** in psychology, a. of small group behavior in terms of 12 specific categories, *e.g.,* solidarity, tension release, agreement, and others.

  **occlusal a.,** bite a.; a study of the relations of the occlusal surfaces of opposing teeth and their effect upon related structures.

  **percept a.,** psychologic survey of an individual's personality using Rorschach's series of inkblots.

  **qualitative a.,** the determination of the nature, as opposed to the quantity, of the elements entering into the composition of any substance.

  **quantitative a.,** the determination of the amount, as well as the nature, of each of the elements composing a substance.

  **spectrophotometric a.,** determination of structure and/or quantity by means of light absorption, *i.e.,* spectrophotometry; colorimetric a. at any wavelength, visible or not.

  **spectroscopic a.,** determination of the components of a substance by means of its emission spectrum.

  **stratographic a.,** chromatography.

  **thermal a.,** in binary alloys, a method to determine the per cent composition where the elements are known by plotting a cooling curve and referring to the constitution diagram.

  **training a.,** didactic a.; the psychoanalytic treatment of an analytic candidate (usually a physician), carried out under the official auspices of a psychoanalytic training institute.

  **transactional a.,** a psychotherapy system, used in both individual and group treatment, involving a systematic understanding of the qualities of interpersonal interactions in the treatment sessions. The system includes four components: structural analysis of intrapsychic phenomena; transactional a. proper, the determination of the currently dominant ego state (parent, child, or adult) of each participant; game analysis, the identification of the games played in their interactions and of the gratifications provided; and script analysis, the uncovering of the causes of the patient's emotional problems.

  **a. of variance,** a statistical technique by which sets of measurements are investigated to determine to what extent the individual measures obtained are determined by experimental influences or by chance influences.

  **volumetric a.,** Quantitative a. by the addition of graduated amounts of a standard test solution to a solution of a known amount of the substance analyzed, until the reaction is just at an end. Depends upon stoichiometric nature of the reaction between test solution and unknown.

**an'alyst.** 1. One who makes analytical determinations. 2. Short term for psychoanalyst.

**analyt'ical.** 1. Relating to analysis. 2. Relating to psychoanalysis.

**an'alyzer, an'alyzor.** 1. The prism in a polariscope by means of which the polarized light is examined. 2. The neural basis of the conditioned reflex (Pavlov). It includes all the sensory side of the reflex arc and its central connections. 3. An instrument attached as a separate unit to the electroencephalographic apparatus to determine the frequency and amplitude components of a particular channel of the record. 4. Any instrument that performs an analysis.

  **wave a.,** an apparatus that can take a complex mixture of wave forms, separate out their component frequencies, and indicate their distribution on a record.

**anamne'sis** [ G. *anamnēsis,* recollection. MNEN- ]. 1. The act of remembering. 2. The medical history of a patient.

**anamnes'tic.** 1. Relating to the anamnesis or previous medical history of a patient. 2. Mnemonic; assisting the memory.

**anamnion'ic, anamniot'ic.** Without an amnion.

**Anamniota** (an-am-nĭ-o'tah). A group of vertebrates whose embryos are not enclosed in an amnion; it includes the Cyclostomata, fish, and amphibians.

**an'amorpho'sis** [ G. *ana,* up, + *morphē,* form ]. 1. In phylogeny, a progressive series of changes in the evolution of a group of animals or plants. 2. In optics, the process of correcting a distorted image by the use of a curved mirror.

**ananaphylaxis** (an-an-ah-fi-lak'sis). Antianaphylaxis.

**ananastasia** (an-an-ah-sta'zī-ah) [ G. *a-* priv. + *anastasis,* stand up ]. Inability to stand up.

**anancasm** (an'an-kazm) [ G. *anagkasma,* compulsion ]. Any form of repetitious stereotyped behavior which, if prevented, results in anxiety.

**anancas'tia** [ G. *anankastos,* compelled ]. An obsession in which a person feels himself forced to act or think against his will.

**an'ancas'tic.** Pertaining to anancasm or anancastia.

**anan'dria** [ G. want of manhood, fr. *an-* priv. + *anēr-* (*andr-*), man ]. Absence of masculinity.

**anangioid** (an-an'jī-oyd) [ G. *an-* priv. + *angeion,* vessel, + *eidos,* resemblance ]. Seemingly avascular.

**anangioplasia** (an-an'jī-o-pla'zī-ah) [ G. *an-* priv. + *angeion,* vessel, + *plassō,* to form ]. Imperfect vascularization of a part due to nonformation of vessels, or vessels with inadequate caliber.

**anan'gioplas'tic.** Relating to, characterized by, or due to defective development of the vascular system.

**anapeiratic** (an'ah-pi-rat'ik) [ G. *ana-peiraomai,* to try again, fr. *peiraō,* to try ]. Resulting from overuse; denoting certain occupational neuroses.

**anaphase** (an'ah-fāz) [ G. *ana,* up, + *phasis,* appearance ]. The stage of mitosis or meiosis in which the chromosomes move from the equatorial plate toward the poles of the cell. In mitosis a full set of daughter chromosomes (46 in man) moves toward each pole. In the first division of meiosis one member of each homologous pair (23 in man), now consisting of two chromatids united at the centromere, moves toward each pole. In the second division of meiosis the centromere has divided and the two chromatids separate, one moving to each pole.

**anaphia** (an-a'fī-ah, an-af'ī-ah) [ G. *an-* priv. + *haphē,* touch ]. Anhaphia; absence of the sense of touch.

**anaphoresis** (an'ă-fo-re'sis) [ G. *ana,* up, + *phorēsis,* a being borne ]. 1 [ G. *ana,* up + *phorēsis,* a being borne ]. The movement of electrically charged particles (anions) in a solution or suspension toward the anode; see electrophoresis. 2 [ G. *an-* priv. + (dia) phoresis ]. Reduction or absence of sweat secretion.

**anaphoria** (an'ă-fo'rī-ah) [ G. *ana,* up, + *phoros,* bearing. PHER- ]. Anatropia; a tendency of the eyes, when in a state of rest, to turn upward.

**anaphrodisia** (an-af'ro-diz'ī-ah) [ G. insensibility to love, from *an-* priv. + *Aphroditē,* the goddess of love, fr. *aphros,* sea foam ]. Sexual anesthesia; frigidity; sexual coldness; absence of sexual feeling.

**anaph'rodis'iac.** Antaphrodisiac; antaphroditic (1). 1. Relating to anaphrodisia (absence of sexual feeling). 2. Repressing or destroying sexual desire. 3. An agent that lessens or abolishes sexual desire.

**anaphylactic** (an'ah-fi'lak'tik). Relating to anaphylaxis; manifesting extremely great sensitivity to foreign protein or other material.

**an'aphylac'tin.** Seldom-used term for specific antibody thought to react with shocking antigen, thereby resulting in anaphylactic shock. See also toxogenin.

**an'aphylac'togen.** Any substance (antigen) capable of rendering a person or animal susceptible to anaphylaxis; a substance (antigen) that will cause an anaphylactic reaction in such a sensitized person or animal.

**an'aphylac'togen'esis.** The production of anaphylaxis.

**an'aphylac'togen'ic.** Producing anaphylaxis; pertaining to substances that result in an animal becoming susceptible to anaphylaxis.

**an'aphylac'toid** [ anaphylaxis + G. *eidos,* resemblance ]. Resembling anaphylaxis; pseudoanaphylactic. A. shock does not require the incubation period characteristic of induced sensitivity (anaphylaxis) and may result from intravenous injection of serum that is pretreated with kaolin or starch, trypsin, organic colloids, peptone, or other materials.

**anaphylatoxin** (an-ă-fil'ă-tok'sin) [ anaphylaxis + toxin ]. Anaphylotoxin. 1. A substance postulated to be the immediate cause of anaphylactic shock and which is assumed to result from the *in vivo* combination of specific antibody and the specific sensitizing material, when the latter is injected as a shock dose in a sensitized animal. 2. The small fragment (C3a) split from the third component (C3) of complement by C3 convertase (*q. v.*) and that releases histamine from rat peritoneal mast cells, causes pig ileum to contract, and produces a local wheal following intracutaneous injection in man. Also used with reference to a small fragment (C5a) split from the fifth component (C5) of complement by the EAC1243 complex (*q. v.* under complement) that has chemotactic properties, as well.

**anaphylaxis** (an-ah-fi-lak'sis) [ G. *ana,* away from, back from, + *phylaxis,* protection ]. A term coined by Portier and Richet to indicate a lessened resistance to a toxin which results from a previous inoculation of the same material, and in this sense was synonymous with hypersensitivity in its original usage of a postulated increased sensitivity to a toxin; shortly thereafter, a. was used by Arthus to indicate an induced sensitivity; at times a. is used for anaphylactic *shock, q.v.* The term is commonly used to denote the immediate, transient kind of immunological (allergic) reaction characterized by contraction of smooth muscle and dilation of capillaries due to release of pharmacologically active substances (histamine, bradykinin, serotonin, and slow-reacting substance), classically initiated by the combination of antigen (allergen) with cell-fixed, cytophilic antibody; the reaction can be initiated, also, by relatively large quantities of serum aggregates (antigen-antibody complexes, and other) that seemingly activate complement leading to production of anaphylatoxin (*q.v.*)—a reaction sometimes termed "aggregate a."

**active a.,** reaction following inoculation of antigen in a subject previously sensitized to the specific antigen, in contrast to passive a.

**aggregate a.,** see a.

**antiserum a.,** passive a.

**chronic a.,** *enteritis* anaphylactica.

**generalized a.,** systemic a.; the immediate response involving smooth muscles and capillaries throughout the body of a sensitized person or animal, that follows intravenous (and occasionally intracutaneous) injection of antigen (allergen); see also anaphylactic *shock.*

**inverse a.,** anaphylactic shock in an animal (*e.g.,* guinea pig) whose tissues contain Forssman antigen, resulting from an intravenous injection of serum that contains Forssman's antibody.

**local a.,** the immediate, transient kind of response that follows the injection of antigen (allergen) into the skin of a sensitized person or animal and is limited to the area surrounding the site of inoculation; see also skin *test.*

**passive a.,** reaction resulting from inoculation of antigen in an animal previously inoculated intravenously with specific antiserum from another animal, a latent period being required between the two inoculations.

**passive cutaneous a.,** a reaction that occurs in the guinea pig when antiserum is injected into the skin and, 6 to 24 hours later, specific antigen and a dye such as Pontamine blue or Evans blue are inoculated intravenously; the size of the blue areas at the sites of the antibody injections is a measure of the degree of altered permeability to dye-bound albumin.

**reversed a.,** reversed passive a.

**reversed passive a.,** reversed a.; an anaphylactic reaction induced in an animal that is injected (1) with a specific antigen, which will bind to reactive tissue, and then after a latent period (2) with serum from another animal previously sensitized to the identical antigen; a form of passive a.

**slow-reacting substance of a.,** see slow-reacting *substance.*

**systemic a.,** generalized a.

**anaphylotox'in.** Anaphylatoxin.

**anaplasia** (an-ah-pla'sī-ah) [ G. *ana,* again, + *plasis,* a molding ]. 1. Loss of structural differentiation, especially as seen in most, but not all, malignant neoplasms. 2. A supposed reversion, in the case of a cell, to a more primitive, embryonic type in which reproductive activity is marked.

**Anaplas'ma** [ G. *an-* priv. + *plasma,* something formed or molded ]. A genus of microorganisms (family Anaplasmataceae) which parasitize red blood cells. There is no demonstrable multiplication of these organisms in other tissues. In erythrocytes the organisms appear as spherical, chromatic granules. These organisms are natural parasites of ruminants (families Bovidae and Camelidae) and are transmitted by arthropods. Initially regarded as protozoa, they are now placed in the order Rickettsiales. The type species is *A. marginale*.

**A. centra′le**, a species that causes benign anaplasmosis of cattle.

**A. margina′le**, a species that causes malignant anaplasmosis of cattle; it is the type species of the genus *A.*

**A. o′vis**, a species that is the agent of anaplasmosis in sheep and goats; cattle are refractory.

**an′aplasmo′sis.** Gallsickness; galsiekte (1); an infectious disease of ruminants varying from peracute to chronic, caused by *Anaplasma marginale* in its various forms, characterized by anemia, icterus, and fever; blood-feeding arthropods, chiefly ticks, may serve as vectors, though mechanical transmission by tabanid flies may occur.

**anaplas′tic.** 1. Relating to anaplasty. 2. Characterized by or pertaining to anaplasia.

**an′aplasty** [ G. *ana*, again, + *plassō*, to form ]. Plastic surgery.

**anaplero′sis** [ G. a filling up ]. The form of plastic surgery that consists in the transplantation of tissue to fill a defect resulting from injury or disease.

**anaplerot′ic.** Relating to anaplerosis.

**anapne′a** [ G. *anapnoia.* PN- ]. 1. Respiration. 2. Recovery of breath.

**anapne′ic.** Relating to anapnea.

**anap′nograph** [ G. *anapnoē*, respiration, + *graphō*, to record ]. Spirograph.

**anapnom′eter** [ G. *anapnoē*, respiration, + *metron*, measure ]. Spirometer.

**anap′nother′apy.** Any form of inhalation therapy, including resuscitation and inhalation anesthesia.

**anapophysis** (an′ă-pof′ĭ-sis) [ G. *ana*, back, + *apophysis*, offshoot. PHYS- ]. An accessory spinal process of a vertebra, found especially in the thoracic or lumbar vertebrae.

**anap′tic.** Relating to anaphia.

**anarith′mia** [ G. *an-* priv. + *arithmos*, number ]. Aphasia marked by inability to count or use numbers.

**anarrhexis** (an-ă-rek′sis) [ G. *ana*, back, again, + *rhēxis*, rupture ]. Refracturing of a bone by operation.

**anar′thria** [ G. fr. *an-arthos*, without joints; (of sound) inarticulate. ARTH- ]. The loss of power of articulate speech. See also aphasia, aphemia, and alexia.

**anasarca** (an′ah-sar′kah) [ G. *ana*, through, + *sarx* (*sark*-), flesh ]. Hydrosarca; a generalized infiltration of edema fluid into subcutaneous connective tissue.

**fetoplacental a.**, edema of fetus and placenta as found in fetal hydrops.

**anasar′cous.** Dropsical; marked by anasarca.

**anascitic** (an′ah-sit′ik). Characterized by the absence of ascites.

**anastal′sis** [ G. *ana*, throughout, up, + *stalsis*, constriction. STAL- ]. 1. Astriction; styptic action. 2. Antiperistalsis.

**anastal′tic.** 1. Astringent. 2. An astringent or styptic remedy. 3. Antiperistaltic.

**anastate** (an′ah-stāt) [ G. *anastatos*, made to rise ]. Any product of anabolism.

**anastigmatic** (an′as-tig-mat′ik). Not astigmatic.

**anastole** (an-as′to-le) [ G. *anastolē*, the laying bare of a wound. STAL- ]. Gaping of a wound.

**anas′tomose.** 1. To open one into the other directly or by connecting channels, said of blood vessels and lymphatics, and also of nerves. 2. To unite by means of an anastomosis.

**anastomo′sis,** pl. **anastomo′ses** [ G. *anastomōsis*, from *anastomoō*, to furnish with a mouth ]. 1 [ NA ]. A natural communication, direct or indirect, between two blood vessels or other tubular structures; also, by extension, a passage of nerve fibers from one nerve to another. 2. An operative union of two hollow or tubular structures, as divided ends of intestine or blood vessels.

**antiperistaltic a.**, one against the normal flow of contents.

**arteriolovenular a.**, a. arteriovenosa.

**a. arterioveno′sa** [ NA ], arteriovenous or arteriolovenular a.; vessels through which blood is shunted from arterioles to venules without passing through the capillaries.

**arteriovenous a.**, a. arteriovenosa.

**Braun′s a.**, after gastroenterostomy, prevention of reverse peristalsis by a. between loops of jejunum on either side of stomach a.

**Clado′s a.**, a. in the broad ligament between the appendicular and ovarian arteries.

**crucial a.**, an a. between branches of the perforating, gluteal and circumflex femoral arteries located behind the upper part of the femur.

**Galen′s a.**, a nerve at the posterior surface of the larynx connecting the superior and inferior laryngeal nerves, supplying sensory fibers to the latter.

**heterocladic a.**, a. between branches of different arteries.

**Hofmeister-Pólya a.**, see Hofmeister′s *operation*, and Pólya′s *operation*.

**homocladic a.**, a. between branches of same artery.

**Hyrtl′s a.**, Hyrtl′s *loop.*

**intestinal a.**, enteroenterostomy.

**isoperistaltic a.**, one to allow flow of contents in the same and natural direction.

**Jacobson′s a.**, a portion of the tympanic plexus.

**postcostal a.**, longitudinal a. of intersegmental arteries giving rise to vertebral artery.

**Potts′ a.**, Potts′ *operation.*

**precapillary a.**, an a. between minute arteries just before they become capillaries.

**precostal a.**, longitudinal a. of intersegmental arteries giving rise to thyrocervical and costocervical trunks.

**Riolan′s a.**, a. of the superior and inferior mesenteric arteries.

**Schmidel′s anastomoses**, abnormal channels of communication between the caval and portal venous systems, as for example, a communication between the right and left gastric veins and the azygos vein.

**termino-terminal a.**, an operation by which the central end of an artery is connected with the peripheral end of the corresponding vein, and the peripheral end of the artery with the central end of the vein.

**transureteroureteral a.**, an a. from one ureter to the opposite ureter.

**ureterotubal a.**, an a. between ureter and Fallopian tube.

**ureteroureteral a.**, a. from one part of a ureter to another part of the same ureter.

**anas′tomot′ic.** Pertaining to any anastomosis.

**anastomot′ica magna.** 1. *Arteria* collateralis ulnaris inferior. 2. *Arteria* genus descendens.

**anas′tral.** Lacking an aster.

**anatherapeusis** (an′ah-ther′ah-pu′sis). Therapeusis by steadily increasing doses.

**anatomical** (an′ă-tom′ĭ-kal). 1. Relating to anatomy. 2. Structural.

**a. snuffbox**, tabatière anatomique; a hollow seen on the radial aspect of the wrist when the thumb is extended fully; it is bounded by the prominences of the tendon of the musculus extensor pollicis longus posteriorly and of the tendons of the musculus extensor pollicis brevis and musculus abductor pollicis longus anteriorly; the radial artery crosses the floor which is formed by the scaphoid and the trapezium bone.

**anatom′icomed′ical.** Referring to both medicine and anatomy.

**anatom′icopatholog′ic.** Relating to pathologic anatomy.

**anatom′icosur′gical.** Relating to surgical anatomy.

**anat′omist.** A specialist in the science of anatomy.

**anatomy** (ă-nat′o-mĭ) [ G. *anatomē*, dissection, from *ana*, up, + *tomē*, a cutting ]. 1. The structure of an organism; morphology. 2. The science of the morphology or structure of organisms. 3. Dissection. 4. A work describing the form and structure of an organism and its various parts.

**applied a.**, the practical application of anatomical knowledge to diagnosis and treatment.

**artificial a.**, the manufacture of models of anatomic structures, or the study of a. from such models.

**artistic a.,** the study of a. for artistic purposes, as applied to painting, drawing, or sculpture.

**clastic a.,** plastic a.; the construction or study of models in layers which can be removed one after the other to show the structure of the organism and/or organ.

**comparative a.,** the comparative study of animal structure in regard to homologous organs or parts.

**dental a.,** that branch of gross a. that deals with the morphology of teeth (structure and form), their location, position, and relationships.

**descriptive a.,** systematic a.; a description of, especially a treatise describing, physical structure, more particularly that of man.

**developmental a.,** a. of the structural changes of an individual from fertilization to adulthood; includes embryology, fetology, and postnatal development.

**general a.,** the study of gross and microscopic structures as well as of the composition of the body, its tissues and fluids.

**gross a.,** macroscopic a.; general a., so far as it can be studied without the use of the microscope.

**living a.,** the study of a. in the living individual by inspection.

**medical a.,** a. in its bearing upon the diagnosis and treatment of internal disorders.

**macroscopic a.,** gross a.

**microscopic a.,** the branch of a. in which the structure of cells, tissues, and organs is studied with the light microscope; see histology.

**morbid a.,** rarely used term for pathological anatomy.

**pathological a.,** the study of diseased, altered, or injured organs and tissues.

**physiologic a.,** a. studied in its relation to function.

**plastic a.,** clastic a.

**practical a.,** a. studied by means of dissection.

**radiological a.,** the study of the body through radiograms.

**regional a.,** topographic a.; a. of certain related parts or divisions of the body.

**special a.,** the a. of certain definite organs or groups of organs concerned in the performance of special functions; descriptive a. dealing with the separate systems.

**surface a.,** the study of the configuration of the surface of the body, especially in its relation to deeper parts.

**surgical a.,** applied a. in reference to surgical diagnosis and treatment.

**systematic a.,** descriptive a.

**systemic a.,** a. of the systems of the body.

**topographic a.,** regional a.

**transcendental a.,** the theories and deductions based upon the morphology of the organs and individual parts of the body.

**ultrastructural a.,** the ultramicroscopic study of structures too small to be seen with a light microscope.

**veterinary a.,** the anatomy of animals, with emphasis on domestic species.

**visceral a.,** viscerotomy; splanchnotomy; dissection of viscera.

**anatopism** (ă-nat′o-pizm) [ G. *ana,* backward, + *topos,* place ]. Failure to conform to the cultural pattern.

**anatox′ic.** Pertaining to the characteristic properties of anatoxin (toxoid).

**anatox′in.** Toxoid.

**anatricrotic** (an′ah-tri-krot′ik). Characterized by anatricrotism; denoting a sphygmographic tracing with three waves on the ascending limb.

**anatricrotism** (an′ah-trik′ro-tizm) [ G. *ana,* up, + *tri-*, thrice, *krotos,* beating ]. The condition of the pulse manifesting itself by a triple beat on the ascending limb of the sphygmographic tracing.

**anatrip′sis** [ G. a rubbing, fr. *tribō,* fut. *tripsō,* to rub ]. Therapeutic use of friction with or without simultaneous application of a medicament.

**anatrip′tic.** 1. Pertaining to anatripsis. 2. A remedy to be applied by friction or inunction.

**anatrophic** (an′ah-trof′ik). 1 [ G. *ana,* up, + *trophē,* nourishment ]. Nourishing. 2 [ G. *an-* priv. + *atrophia* ]. Preventing or curing atrophy.

**anatro′pia** [ G. *ana,* up, + *trope,* a turning ]. Anaphoria.

**anaudia** (an-aw′dī-ah) [ G. *an-* priv. + *audān,* to speak ]. Aphonia.

**Anaxag′oras** of Clazomenae, Greek philosopher, 500–428 B.C. Taught that all matter was made of four primordial elements, *earth, air, fire* and *water.*

**Anaximan′der** of Miletus, Greek philosopher, 611–547 B.C. He conceived of a primary substance between water and air, and through the separation of this primordial material into opposites, heat and cold, wet and dry, etc., all matter was formed.

**anax′on, anax′one** [ G. *an-* priv. + *axōn,* axis ]. Having no axon; denoting certain nerve cells first described by Ramón y Cajal as amacrine cells in the retina, and later discovered in several brain regions.

**anaz′olene sodium** (USAN). 4′-Anilino-8-hydroxy-1,1′-azonaphthalene-3,5′,6-trisulfonic acid trisodium salt; plasma volume indicator.

**anazoturia** (an′az-o-tu′rī-ah) [ G. *an-* priv. + azoturia ]. A deficiency or lack of nitrogenous metabolic products excreted in urine; pertains especially to unusually small quantities of urea in urine.

**AnCC.** Abbreviation for anodal or positive pole closure *contraction.*

**anchone** (ang-ko′ne) [ G. *agchonē,* a strangling ]. Spasm of the throat muscles, often a conversion reaction.

**anchorage** (ang′kor-ij) [ L. *ancora,* fr. G. *ankyra,* anchor ]. 1. The operative fixation of loose or prolapsed abdominal or pelvic organs. 2. The part to which anything is fastened; specifically, in dentistry, a tooth to which a bridge or a fixed partial denture is fastened, the root to which a crown is fastened, or one of the points serving to retain a filling.

**compound a.,** in orthodontics, a. involving more than one tooth.

**anchusin** (an′ku-sin). Alkannin.

**ancillary** (an′sī-lēr-ī) [ L. *ancillaris,* relating to a maid servant ]. Auxiliary, accessory, or secondary.

**ancip′ital, ancip′itate, ancip′itous** [ L. *anceps,* two-headed. CAP- ]. Two-headed; two-edged.

**an′con** [ G. *ankon,* elbow ] [ NA ]. Elbow.

**anconad** (an′ko-nad) [ G. *ankōn,* elbow, + L. *ad,* to ]. Toward the elbow.

**anconag′ra** [ G. *ankōn,* elbow, + *agra,* a seizure ]. Obslete term for gout in the elbow.

**an′conal, anco′neal.** Relating to the elbow (ancon); to the anconeus muscle.

**anco′neus** [ L. ]. 1. Anconal. 2. *Musculus* anconeus.

**anconitis** (an′ko-ni′tis) [ G. *ankōn,* elbow, + suffix *-itis,* inflammation ]. Inflammation of the elbow joint.

**anconoid** (an′ko-noyd). Resembling the elbow.

**ancylo-.** For words beginning thus and not found here, see ankylo-.

**Ancylostoma** (an′sī-los′to-mah) [ G. *ankylos,* curved, hooked, + *stoma,* mouth ]. A genus of Nematoda, the Old World hookworm, the members of which are parasitic in the duodenum. They attach themselves to clusters of villi in the mucous membrane, sucking blood and causing a state of anemia, especially in cases of malnutrition. The eggs are passed with the feces and the larvae develop in moist soil; infectious third-stage larvae enter the body of man through the skin of the feet and ankles, possibly also in drinking water, and reach maturity in the intestine.

**A. brazilien′se,** a species with only one pair of ventral teeth, normally an intestinal parasite of dogs and cats but also found in man; a cause of human cutaneous larva migrans.

**A. cani′num,** a species, with three pairs of ventral teeth in the oral cavity, that infects dogs; it occurs in man, but is usually restricted to the skin; see cutaneous *larva migrans.*

**A. ceylanicum,** found in the civet cat of Ceylon. Rarely reported from man.

**A. duodena′le,** the Old World hookworm of man, widespread in temperate areas, in contrast to the more tropical distribution of *Necator americanus,* the New World hookworm.

**an′cylostomat′ic.** Referring to hookworm.

**ancylostomiasis** (an-sī-los-to-mi′ah-sis). Hookworm disease; Egyptian or tropical chlorosis; tunnel disease or anemia; miner's anemia; brickmaker's anemia; pronounced anemia, emaciation, dyspepsia, and swelling of the abdomen with mental and physical inertia due to the presence of a species of *Ancylostoma* or *Necator* in the intestine.

    **cutaneous a.,** small vesicles and pustules on the skin at the sites of penetration of the larvae of *Ancylostoma* or other hookworms. These itching lesions, which begin most commonly on the feet and between the toes, frequently precede the onset of intestinal symptoms, particularly after sensitizing exposures. Also called a. cutis; ancylostomiasis dermatitis; coolie, ground, swimmer's, toe, water, or swamp itch; water sore.

    **a. cutis,** cutaneous a.

**ancyroid** (an'sĭ-royd) [ G. *ankyra*, anchor, + *eidos*, resemblance ]. Ankyroid; shaped like the fluke of an anchor; denoting the cornua of the lateral ventricles of the brain and the coracoid process of the scapula.

**Andernach** (ahn'der-nahkh), Johann W. (Jean Guinter of Andernach), German physician, 1505–1574. He was one of Vesalius' teachers in Paris. See A.'s *ossicle.*

**Anders,** James M., Philadelphia physician, 1854–1936. See A.'s *disease.*

**Andersch,** Carl D., German anatomist, 1732–1777. See A.'s *ganglion, nerve.*

**Andersen,** Dorothy H., American pediatrician, *1901. See A.'s *disease.*

**Anderson,** Roger, Seattle surgeon, *1891. See A. *splint.*

**Anderson-Collip test.** See under test.

**andi'ra** [ West Indian native name ]. Worm bark; cabbage tree; the bark of *Andira inermis,* a leguminous tree of tropical America. Emetic, purgative, and anthelmintic.

**andirine** (an-di'rin). *N*-Methyltyrosine; an alkaloid from *Andira;* has negligible stimulating action.

**Andral,** Gabriel, French physician, 1797–1876. See A.'s *decubitus.*

**andrenos'terone.** Adrenosterone.

**Andrews,** C. J., U. S. surgeon. See Brandt-A. *maneuver.*

**andriatrics, andriatry** (an-drĭ-at'riks, an-dri'ă-trĭ) [ G. *anēr*, a man, + *iatreia*, medical treatment ]. Medical science relating to diseases of male genital organs and diseases of men in general.

**andro-** [ G. *anēr* (gen. andros), male ]. Combining form meaning masculine; pertaining to the male of the species.

**an'droblasto'ma.** 1. Pick's tubular adenoma; testicular tubular adenoma; Sertoli cell tumor; a testicular tumor microscopically resembling fetal testis, with varying proportions of tubular and stromal elements; the tubules contain Sertoli cells, which may cause feminization. 2. *Arrhenoblastoma* of the ovary.

**androcyte** (an'dro-sĭt) [ andro- + G. *kytos,* cell ]. Spermatid.

**androgamones** (an'dro-gam'ōnz) [ andro- + G. *gamos,* marriage ]. Gamones believed to be present in sperm; a. I appears to play a part in holding spermatozoa inactive

Mouth and buccal cavity of *Ancylostoma duodenale* (left) and *Necator americanus* (right).

until after ejaculation; a. II seems to play a part in helping the sperm cell to penetrate the ovum.

**an'drogen.** A generic term for an agent, usually a hormone, *e.g.,* testosterone or androsterone, that stimulates the activity of the accessory sex organs of the male, encourages the development of the male sex characteristics, or prevents the changes in the latter, *e.g.,* the comb and wattles of the cockerel, which follow castration. The natural a.'s are steroids, derivatives of androstane (for structure of androstane, see steroids).

    **adrenal a.,** any androgenic hormone of andrenocortical origin; the known adrenal a.'s are dehydroepiandrosterone (and its sulfate), androstenedione, 11β-hydroxyandrostenedione, and possibly testosterone.

**androgenesis** (an-dro-jen'e-sis) [ andro- + G. *genesis,* production ]. Egg development in the presence only of paternal chromosomes.

**androgen'ic.** Andromimetic; relating to an androgen; having a masculinizing effect.

**androg'enous** (an-droj'en-us). Giving birth to males.

**androgyne** (an'dro-jin). Androgynus.

**androgynism** (an-droj'ĭ-nizm). Androgyny.

**androgynoid** (an-droj'ĭ-noyd) [ andro- + G. *gynē,* woman, + *eidos,* resemblance ]. A male resembling a female, or possessing hermaphroditic features.

**androgynos** (an-droj'ĭ-nos). Androgynus.

**androgynous** (an-droj'ĭ-nus). Pertaining to androgyny.

**androgynus** (an-droj'ĭ-nus). Female *pseudohermaphrodite.*

**androgyny** (an-droj'ĭ-nĭ) [ andro- + G. *gynē,* woman ]. Female *pseudohermaphroditism.*

**an'droid** [ andro- + G. *eidos,* resemblance ]. Resembling a man in form and structure.

**androisox'azole.** NEO-PONDEN; 17α-methylandrostan [ 3,2-c ]isoxazol-17β-ol; anabolic agent.

**androl'ogy** [ andro- + G. *logos,* treatise ]. The branch of medicine that treats of the man and of the diseases peculiar to the male sex.

**an'droma'nia** [ andro- + G. *mania,* frenzy ]. Nymphomania.

**Androm'eda.** A genus of plants of the family Ericaceae, several species of which contain andromedotoxin.

**androm'edotox'in.** The active principle obtained from several species of the genera *Andromeda* and *Rhododendron.*It is a heart poison, first stimulating and then paralyzing the vagus, and it also paralyzes the motor nerve ends in striped muscle. It is strongly emetic.

**andromimetic** (an-dro-mĭ-met'ik). Androgenic.

**andromorphous** (an'dro-mor'fus) [ andro- + G. *morphē,* form ]. Having a man's form or build; male conformation.

**androp'athy** [ andro- + G. *pathos,* suffering ]. Any disease, such as prostatitis, peculiar to the male sex.

**andropho'bia** [ andro- + G. *phobos,* fear ]. Morbid fear of men, or of the male sex.

**an'drostane.** The parent hydrocarbon of the androgenic steroids. The 5α isomer has also been called etioallocholane; the 5β isomer, testane, etiane, and etiocholane. For structure, see steroids.

**androstanediol** (an-dro-stăn'di-ol). 5α-Androstane-3β,17β-diol; the 3α isomer is also called dihydroandrosterone; the 5β isomers are also known; steroid metabolites. For structure of androstane, see steroids.

**androstanedione** (an-dro-stăn'di-ōn). 5α-Androstane-3,17-dione; the 5β isomer is also known; steroid metabolites. For structure, see steroids.

**androstene** (an'dro-stēn). Androstane with an unsaturated (*i.e.,* —CH=CH—) bond in the molecule. For androstane structure, see steroids.

**androstenediol** (an-dro-stēn'di-ol). 5-Androsten-3β,17β-diol; a steroid metabolite differing from androstanediol in the possession of a double bond between C-5 and C-6. For structure, see steroids.

**5-androstene-3β,16α-diol.** CETADIOL; differs from androstenediol in location of one OH group (for structure, see steroids); tranquilizer.

**androstenedione** (an-dro-stēn'di-ōn). 4-Androstene-3,17-dione (androstanedione with a double bond between C-4 and C-5; for structure, see steroids). An androgenic steroid of weaker biological potency than testosterone; secreted by the testis, ovary, and adrenal cortex.

**androstenolone** (an-dro-stēn-o-lōn). 3β-Hydroxy-5-androsten-17-one (for structure, see steroids).

**andros'terone.** *cis*-Androsterone (see also epiandrosterone); 3α-hydroxy-5α-androstan-17-one; (3α-hydroxyetioallocholan-17-one; 3-epihydroxyetioallocholan-17-one); for structure, see steroids. A steroid metabolite, found in male urine, having weak androgenic potency.

**AnDTe.** Abbreviation for anodal duration *tetanus.*

**anectasis** (an-ek'tah-sis) [ G. *an-* priv. + *ektasis,* dilation ]. Primary *atelectasis.*

**Anel,** Dominique, French surgeon, 1679–1725. See A.'s *method, probe.*

**anelec'trode.** Anode.

**anelectroton'ic.** Relating to anelectrotonus.

**anelectrotonus** (an'e-lek-trot'o-nus) [ anelectrode + G. *tonos,* tension ]. The changes in excitability and conductivity in a nerve or muscle cell in the neighborhood of the anode during the passage of a constant electric current.

---

# ANEMIA

---

**anemia** (ă-ne'mĭ-ah) [ G. *anaimia,* fr. *an-* priv. + *haima,* blood ]. Any condition in which the number of red blood cells per cu. mm., the amount of hemoglobin in 100 ml. of blood, and the volume of packed red blood cells per 100 ml. of blood are less than normal. Thus, clinically, the term generally pertains to the concentration of oxygen-transporting material in a designated volume of blood, in contrast to total quantities (see also oligocythemia, oligochromemia, and oligemia). A. is frequently manifested by pallor of the skin and mucous membranes, shortness of breath, palpitations of the heart, soft systolic murmurs, lack of the usual energy, fatigability, and so on.

**achlorhy'dric a.,** Faber's a. or syndrome; a form of chronic hypochromic microcytic a. associated with achlorhydria or achylia gastrica; observed most frequently in women in the 3rd to 5th decades.

**achres'tic a.** [ G. *a-* priv. + *chrēsis,* a using ], a form of chronic, progressive macrocytic a. in which the changes in bone marrow and circulating blood closely resemble those of pernicious a.; on the other hand, there is only transient or no response to therapy with liver extract. The condition is frequently fatal; glossitis, gastrointestinal disturbances, disease in the central nervous system, and pyrexia are not observed, and there is only little bleeding or hemolysis.

**acquired hemolyt'ic a.,** nonhereditary acute or chronic a. associated with or caused by extracorpuscular factors, *e.g.,* certain infectious agents, chemicals (including therapeutic agents), burns, toxic materials from higher plant and animal forms (including snake venoms), autoantibodies, and so on; see also idiopathic a. h. a. and symptomatic a. in this section.

**acute a.,** any anemic condition that develops rather rapidly and persists for a relatively short time, *e.g.,* a. resulting from profuse hemorrhage.

**acute hemolyt'ic a.,** characterized by destruction of erythrocytes, with symptoms developing rapidly within a few days or progressively increasing during a 3- to 5-week period; condition frequently associated with aching pain in the back, abdomen, or extremities, as well as headache, malaise, chill, and fever. See also hemolytic a.

**Addisonian a.,** pernicious a.

**African a.,** sickle cell a.

**agastric a.,** a. following removal of the stomach.

**alimentary a.,** nutritional or deficiency a.

**an'cylostome a.,** a. resulting from infection with hookworms, *Ancylostoma duodenale* or *Necator americanus,* a greater degree of a. usually occurs in the former type.

**anhem'atopoiet'ic a., anhemopoietic a.,** a. resulting from faulty production of erythrocytes.

**aplas'tic a.,** aleukia hemorrhagica; Ehrlich's a.; a. gravis; characterized by a greatly decreased formation of erythrocytes and hemoglobin, and usually associated with pro-

nounced granulocytopenia and thrombocytopenia, as a result of hypoplastic or aplastic bone marrow.

**asiderotic a.,** chlorosis.

**autoallergic hemolytic a. of the cold-antibody type,** cold hemagglutinin *disease.*

**autoimmune hemolytic a.,** acquired hemolytic a. due to serum autoantibodies that react with the patient's red blood cells; the Coombs test is positive.

**Belgian Congo a.,** kasai.

**Biermer's a.,** pernicious a.

**a. of Blackfan and Diamond,** congenital hypoplastic a.

**brickmaker's a.,** a. associated wih ancylostomiasis.

**cam'eloid a.,** elliptocytic a.

**chlorot'ic a.,** chlorosis.

**congenital a.,** a. neonatorum (*q. v.*), a form of erythroblastosis fetalis.

**congenital aplastic a.,** Fanconi's a.

**congenital aregen'erative a.,** congenital hypoplastic a.

**congenital dyserythropoietic a.,** a group of a.'s characterized by ineffective erythropoiesis, bone marrow erythroblastic multinuclearity, and secondary hemochromatosis; probably autosomal recessive inheritance. Three types are described: type I, macrocytic, megaloblastic a. with erythroblastic internuclear chromatin bridges; type II, normoblastic a. with multinucleated erythroblasts; type III, macrocytic a. with erythroblastic multinuclearity and gigantoblasts.

**congenital hemolyt'ic a.,** hereditary *spherocytosis.*

**congenital hypoplastic a.,** congenital aregenerative a.; familial hypoplastic a.; erythrogenesis imperfecta; a. of Blackfan and Diamond; a normocytic, normochromic a. resulting from congenital hypoplasia of the bone marrow; the marrow is grossly deficient in erythroid precursors but other elements are normal; a. is progressive and severe, but leukocyte and platelet counts are normal or slightly reduced; survival of transfused erythrocytes is normal; minor congenital anomalies are found in some patients.

**Cooley's a.,** *thalassemia* major.

**cow's milk a.,** a. occurring in some children fed on formula containing cow's milk.

**crescent cell a.,** sickle cell a.

**cytogen'ic a.,** primary progressive pernicious a.

**deficiency a.,** any a. resulting from a deficit or lack of an essential substance in the diet, as in pernicious a. or idiopathic hypochromic a.; also termed nutritional a., alimentary a.

**Diamond-Blackfan a.,** congenital hypoplastic a.

**dilution a.,** hydremia.

**dimorphic a.,** an a. caused by a dual deficiency.

**diphyl'loboth'rium a.,** tapeworm or fish tapeworm a.; sometimes associated with diphyllobothriasis, and thought to be caused by differential absorption of vitamin $B_{12}$ by the tapeworm.

**drepan'ocyt'ic a.,** sickle cell a.

**dyshe'mopoiet'ic a.,** any a. resulting from defective function of the bone marrow.

**Ehrlich's a.,** aplastic a.

**elliptocyt'ic a.,** cameloid a., characterized by elliptical erythrocytes (ovalocytes) resembling those observed normally in camels; 1 to 15 per cent of erythrocytes in nonanemic persons may be oval, but greater proportions are observed in certain patients with microcytic anemia; latter conditions frequently termed "symptomatic ovalocytosis." See also elliptocytosis.

**equine infectious a.,** swamp fever (1); a disease of horses marked by general debility, remittent fever, staggering gait, progressive anemia, and loss of flesh; the causative agent is a virus that is transmitted by bloodsucking insects.

**erythroblas'tic a.,** thalassemia or Cooley's a.

**erythroblast'ic a. of childhood,** thalassemia or Cooley's a., occurring classically in infants and young children.

**erythronor'moblastic a.,** hypochromic a.

**essential a.,** primary a.

**Faber's a.,** achlorhydric a.

**false a.,** pseudoanemia.

**familial erythroblastic a.,** thalassemia.

**familial hypoplas'tic a.,** congenital hypoplastic a.

**familial microcytic a.,** 1. target cell a.; see also *thalassemia* minor. 2. A rare type of hypochromic microcytic a. associated with a defect of iron metabolism characterized by high serum iron, hepatic iron deposits, and absence of stainable bone marrow iron stores.

**familial splenic a.,** cerebroside *lipidosis.*

**Fanconi's a.,** Fanconi's pancytopenia; congenital pancytopenia; congenital aplastic a.; a type of idiopathic refractory a. characterized by pancytopenia, hypoplasia of the bone marrow, and congenital anomalies, occurring in members of the same family. The a. is normocytic or slightly macrocytic (but not megaloblastic), and macrocytes and target cells may be found in the circulating blood; the leukopenia usually represents a neutropenia, but all types of leukocytes may be affected. Congenital anomalies include dwarfism, microcephaly, hypogenitalism, strabismus, anomalies of the thumbs and kidneys, mental retardation, and microphthalmia. The condition is thought to be hereditary, probably resulting from a recessive gene, and is usually detected between the ages of 4 and 12 years.

**fish tapeworm a.,** diphyllobothrium a.

**general a.,** a. affecting the total volume of blood and all of the organs and tissues, *i.e.,* the complete person.

**genetic a.,** any a. associated with an inherited defect in the structure or function of the erythrocytes and erythropoietic tissue.

**globe cell a.,** hereditary *spherocytosis.*

**globular a.,** oligocythemia.

**goat's milk a.,** nutritional a. in infants who are maintained chiefly with goat's milk, which is relatively poor in content of iron.

**a. gravis,** aplastic a.

**ground itch a.,** a. associated with ancylostomiasis.

**Hayem-Widal a.,** a chronic and acquired type of hemolytic a. of unknown origin.

**hemolyt′ic a.,** any a. resulting from abnormal destruction of erythrocytes in the body.

**hemorrhag′ic a.,** resulting directly from loss of blood, *i.e.,* actual bleeding or hemorrhage.

**hemotox′ic a.,** toxic a.

**hookworm a.,** occurring as a part of disease (ancylostomiasis) caused by *Ancylostoma duodenale,* or by *Necator americanus.*

**hy′perchromat′ic a.,** hyperchromic a.

**hyperchromic a.,** characterized by an increase in the ratio of the weight of hemoglobin to the volume of the erythrocyte, *i.e.,* the mean corpuscular hemoglobin concentration (MCHC) is greater than normal; with the exception of some instances of hereditary spherocytosis, such "supersaturation" does not occur. Although the weight of hemoglobin per cell may be greater in the macrocytes of pernicious a., the increase is proportional to the larger volume, and such cells are not truly hyperchromic.

**hypochro′mic a.,** erythronormoblastic a.; characterized by a decrease in the ratio of the weight of hemoglobin to the volume of the erythrocyte, *i.e.,* the mean corpuscular hemoglobin concentration (MCHC) is less than normal; the individual cells contain less hemoglobin than they could have under optimal conditions.

**hypochro′mic microcyt′ic a.,** hypoferric a.; a type of a. caused by a deficiency of iron; the amount of hemoglobin is reduced to a greater degree than the red blood cell count, as a result of (1) less than normal percentage of hemoglobin per cell, and (2) the smaller than normal size of most of the erythrocytes. The mean corpuscular volume (MCV), mean corpuscular hemoglobin (MCH), and mean corpuscular hemoglobin concentration (MCHC) are less than normal.

**hypoferric a.,** hypochromic microcytic or iron deficiency a.

**hypoplas′tic a.,** progressive nonregenerative a. resulting from greatly depressed, inadequately functioning bone marrow; as the process persists, aplastic a. may occur.

**ic′terohemolyt′ic a.,** hereditary *spherocytosis.*

**idiopath′ic a.,** so-called primary or essential a. See primary a.

**idiopathic hypochromic a.,** chronic a. affecting chiefly 30- to 50-year-old women, but frequently observed in other decades. Only few examples (4 to 6 per cent) are found in men. It is characterized by hypochromic microcytic erythrocytes, pallor, weakness, and fatigue; frequently associated with hypo- or achlorhydria and gastrointestinal disorders and "neuroses." Cause not known, but deficiency

of iron and loss of blood (menses) are probably significant factors.

**a. infan′tum pseudoleuke′mica,** Jaksch's a. or disease; infantile pseudoleukemia; syndrome observed in infants and young children, characterized by a deficiency of hemoglobin, anisocytosis and poikilocytosis, numerous erythroblasts, conspicuous leukocytosis with relative lymphocytosis, splenomegaly, hepatomegaly, and enlarged lymph nodes; now known to be associated with a variety of conditions, *e.g.,* malnutrition, gastrointestinal disorders, thalassemia, iron deficiency, or tuberculosis or other infections.

**infectious a.,** developing as a complication of various infections, especially in persistent suppurative disease and septicemia; probably results from depressed formation and short survival of erythrocytes.

**intertrop′ical a.,** a. occurring in ancylostomiasis.

**iron deficiency a.,** hypoferric a.; any hypochromic microcytic a., with the exception of that occurring in thalassemia, and a. produced in certain experimental animals that are deficient in vitamin $B_6$ or copper.

**isochro′mic a.,** any a. in which the concentration of hemoglobin in the cells (MCHC) is normal, but there is a reduction in the amount of hemoglobin, in proportion to the lesser number of erythrocytes.

**Jaksch's a.,** a. infantum pseudoleukemica.

**lead a.,** a. associated with poisoning from lead; thought to result from a defect in synthesis of hemoglobin based on the failure of iron being combined in the porphyrin ring.

**Lederer's a.,** a form of acute acquired hemolytic a. associated with abnormal hemolysins, and sometimes with hemoglobinuria; successfully treated by means of a blood transfusion.

**leukoerythroblastic a.,** myelophthisic a.

**local a.,** resulting from a decreased supply of blood to a part, as in the occlusion of a vessel.

**a. lymphatica,** Hodgkin's *disease.*

**macrocyt′ic a.,** megalocytic a.; any a. in which the average size of circulating erythrocytes is greater than normal, *i.e.,* the mean corpuscular volume (MCV) is 94 cu. $\mu$ or more (normal range, 82 to 92 cu. $\mu$); includes such syndromes as pernicious a., sprue, celiac disease, macrocytic a. of pregnancy, a. of diphyllobothriasis, and others.

**macrocyt′ic achy′lic a.,** pernicious a.

**macrocytic a. of pregnancy,** a relatively rare condition, except for instances of macrocytic a. in tropical regions, many of which are associated with pregnancy; characterized by a low level of hemoglobin and a reduced number of erythrocytes, which are larger than normal (macrocytes); clinical syndrome (including pallor, asthenia, dyspepsia, diarrhea, and so on) persists, and may be progressive, during pregnancy; usually recedes after pregnancy is terminated. Formerly incorrectly termed pernicious a. of pregnancy.

**malignant a.,** pernicious a.

**Marchiafava-Micheli a.,** paroxysmal nocturnal *hemoglobinuria.*

**Mediterranean a.,** thalassemia.

**megaloblastic a.,** any a. in which there is a predominant number of megaloblasts, and relatively few normoblasts, among the hyperplastic erythroid cells in the bone marrow (as in pernicious a.).

**meg′alocytic a.,** macrocytic a.

**metaplastic a.,** pernicious a. in which the various formed elements in the blood are changed, *e.g.,* multisegmented, unusually large neutrophiles (macropolycytes), immature myeloid cells, bizarre platelets, and so on.

**microcytic a.,** any a. in which the average size of circulating erythrocytes is smaller than normal, *i.e.,* the mean corpuscular volume (MCV) is 80 cu. $\mu$ or less (normal range, 82 to 92 cu. $\mu$); includes such syndromes as nutritional hypochromic a., chlorosis, hypochromic a. of pregnancy, and so on.

**mi′crodrepanocyt′ic a.,** sickle cell-thalassemia disease; patients are heterozygous for both the sickle cell and a thalassemia gene; about 60 to 80 per cent of hemoglobin is Hb S, up to 20 per cent, Hb F, and the remainder Hb A; clinically resembles sickle cell a.

**milk a.,** sometimes occurring in infants who are fed a milk diet (excluding other foods) for too long a time; a type of hypochromic microcytic a., resulting from deficiency of iron.

**miner's a.,** miner's disease (1); occupational disease in miners exposed to infection by hookworms; see ancylostomiasis.

**molecular a.,** a. due to the presence in the blood of an abnormal hemoglobin; *e.g.*, sickle cell a., thalassemia.

**mountain a.,** a condition resulting from inadequate adjustment to the lower partial pressures of oxygen at high altitudes; occurs more frequently at elevations greater than 10,000 or 12,000 feet; usually termed mountain sickness, especially when the condition is chronic.

**myelophthi′sic a., myelopath′ic a.,** resulting from space-occupying pathologic processes that replace hemopoietic tissue; characterized by immature myeloid cells as well as nucleated erythroid cells in the circulating blood, the latter frequently out of proportion to the a. See also leukoerythroblastosis.

**negative a.,** term used infrequently to designate a. characterized by erythroblasts in circulating blood, but with no decrease in the red blood cell count.

**neona′tal a.,** *erythroblastosis* fetalis.

**a. neonator′um,** term sometimes used for less advanced examples of erythroblastosis fetalis in which a. is chief feature.

**normochro′mic a.,** any a. in which the concentration of hemoglobin in the erythrocytes is within the normal range, *i.e.*, the mean corpuscular hemoglobin concentration (MCHC) is from 32 to 36 per cent.

**normocyt′ic a.,** any a. in which the erythrocytes are normal in size, *i.e.*, the mean corpuscular volume (MCV) ranges from 82 to 92 cu. $\mu$.

**nutritional a.,** alimentary a.; any a. resulting from a deficiency of certain essential materials in the diet, *e.g.*, iron, vitamins, protein.

**os′teosclerot′ic a.,** a form of myelophthisic a., resulting from pathologic formation of bone and dense fibrous tissue that destroys and replaces bone marrow, as in osteopetrosis.

**ovalocyt′ic a.,** elliptocytic a.

**pernicious a.,** Addisonian a.; Biermer's a.; macrocytic achylic a.; malignant a.; a chronic, progressive a. of older adults, occurring more frequently during the fifth and later decades, but rarely in persons less than 30 years old; thought to result from a defect of the stomach, with atrophy and associated lack of an "intrinsic" factor; characterized by numbness and tingling, weakness, and a sore smooth tongue, as well as shortness of breath after slight exertion, faintness, pallor of the skin and mucous membranes, anorexia, diarrhea, loss of weight, and fever; laboratory studies usually reveal greatly decreased red blood cell counts, low levels of hemoglobin, numerous macrocytic erythrocytes (color index greater than normal, but not truly hyperchromic), and hypo- or achlorhydria, in association with a predominant number of megaloblasts and relatively few normoblasts in the bone marrow; the leukocyte count in peripheral blood may be less than normal, with relative lymphocytosis and multisegmented neutrophils; administration of vitamin $B_{12}$ results in a characteristic reticulocyte response, relief from symptoms, and an increase in erythrocytes, provided that pernicious a. is not complicated by another disease; when properly treated, the condition is not actually "pernicious," as it was prior to the use of liver and vitamin $B_{12}$.

**physiologic a.,** apparent a. caused by increased fluid volume of the blood.

**polar a.,** a form of a. sometimes observed in natives of temperate climates when they migrate to the Arctic or Antarctic regions.

**posthemorrhag′ic a.,** an acute a. caused by fairly sudden and rapid loss of blood, *e.g.*, the traumatic laceration of a relatively large vessel, erosion of an artery in a duodenal ulcer, hemorrhage in an ectopic pregnancy, or the result of such diseases as hemophilia and acute leukemia.

**postoperative cerebral a.,** a form of local a. following surgery that may result in cerebral malfunction.

**primary a.,** a. occurring as the result of disease originating in the hemopoietic tissues; also termed essential or cytogenic a. None of these terms is entirely suitable, inasmuch as any a. is now regarded as a symptom of a basic disorder, and is actually "secondary" to that condition; for

example, even pernicious a. results from a defect in the gastrointestinal tract.

**primary erythroblas′tic a.,** *thalassemia* major.

**primary refractory a.,** any of a group of anemic conditions in which there is persistent, frequently advanced a. that is not successfully treated by any means except blood transfusions, and that is not associated with another primary disease, such as a malignant neoplasm, chronic disease of the liver or kidneys, various infections, and so on. Includes acquired and idiopathic aplastic a.'s (pancytopenia), acute transitory erythroblastopenia, congenital hypoplastic a., and acquired erythrocytic hypoplasia.

**progressive pernicious a.,** a term sometimes used to emphasize the advancing course of pernicious a.

**pure red cell a.,** congenital hypoplastic a.

**radiation a.,** hypoplastic a. sometimes occurring after high level acute or low level chronic exposure to ionizing radiation.

**Runeberg's a.,** a clinical type of progressive pernicious a. in which brief periods of apparent improvement occur from time to time.

**secondary a.,** a. occurring as a complication or sequela in another condition (*e.g.*, bleeding peptic ulcer, chronic poisoning, inanition, and so on), as distinguished from disease originating in hemopoietic tissues. See also primary a.

**secondary refractory a.,** any persistent a. that is successfully treated only by blood transfusions, and that is associated with another condition, *e.g.*, malignant neoplasms, chronic infections, various diseases of the liver or kidneys, and so on.

**sickle cell a.,** crescent cell a.; African a.; drepanocytic a.; meniscocytosis; an a. characterized by the presence of crescent-shaped or sickle-shaped erythrocytes in peripheral blood, excessive hemolysis, and active hemopoiesis; symptoms include those of a., leg ulcers, arthritic manifestations, and acute attacks of pain; the hemoglobin is abnormal, up to 85 per cent or more being sickle cell hemoglobin (Hb S) and the remainder fetal hemoglobin (Hb F); patients are homozygous for the sickle cell gene; individuals heterozygous for this gene have sickle cell trait.

**slaty a.,** pertaining to an ash-gray pallor in poisoning from acetanelid or silver (argyria).

**spastic a.,** local a. resulting from nontransitory contraction of the arterial vessels in the affected region.

**spherocytic a.,** hereditary *spherocytosis*.

**splenic a.,** Banti's *syndrome*.

**splenic a. of infants,** a. infantum pseudoleukemica.

**symptomatic a.,** so-called "secondary" a. See also primary a.

**tapeworm a.,** diphyllobothrium a.

**target cell a.,** any a. with a conspicuous number of target cells in the peripheral blood; characteristic of thalassemia minor, also found in several hemoglobinopathies; target cells also appear after splenectomy.

**toxic a.,** hemotoxic a.; any a. resulting from the destructive effects of a chemical, metabolic poison, bacterial toxin, venom, and similar materials.

**traumatic a.,** hemorrhagic a.

**trophoneurotic a.,** a. presumably resulting from a profound nervous shock.

**tropical a.,** various syndromes frequently observed in persons in tropical climates, usually resulting from nutritional deficiencies or disease caused by hookworms.

**tunnel a.,** a. associated with ancylostomiasis.

---

**ane′mic.** Pertaining to or manifesting the various features of anemia.

**anemom′eter** [ G. *anemos*, wind, + *metron*, measure ]. An instrument for measurement of velocity of air flow.

**anem′onol.** A volatile oil, possessing markedly toxic properties, obtained from plants of the genus *Anemone*.

**anemop′athy** [ G. *anemos*, wind, + *pathos*, suffering ]. A disease caused by winds, especially high winds.

**anemophobia** (an′e-mo-fo′bī-ah) [ G. *anemos*, wind, + *phobos*, fear ]. Morbid fear of wind.

**anemotrophy** (an′e-mot′ro-fī) [ G. *an-* priv. + *haima*, blood, + *trophē*, nourishment ]. Lack of substances essential to the formation of blood, thereby resulting in hypoplastic anemia.

**anencephalia** (an'en-sef-a'lĭ-ah). Anencephaly.

**anencephal'ic.** Relating to anencephaly; without brain.

**anenceph'alous.** Anencephalic.

**anenceph'alus.** An individual without a brain.

**anencephaly** (an'en-sef'al-e) [ G. *an-* priv. + *enkephalos*, brain ]. Anencephalia; markedly defective development of the brain, together with absence of the bones of the cranial vault. The cerebral and cerebellar hemispheres are usually wanting, with only a rudimentary brain stem and some traces of basal ganglia present. Colloquially, individuals with this malformation are sometimes called "frog-babies." The condition is incompatible with life.

**anen'terous** [ G. *an-* priv. + *entera*, intestines ]. Having no intestine; denoting certain parasites, such as tapeworms.

**anenzymia** (an-en-zi'mĭ-ah). Congenital absence of a specific enzyme.

   **a. catala'sia,** acatalasemia.

**anephric** (ă-nef'rik). Lacking kidneys.

**anep'ia** [ G. *an-* priv. + *epos*, word ]. Aphasia.

**anep'iplo'ic.** Lacking an omentum (epiploon).

**anerga'sia** [ G. *an-* priv. + *ergasia*, work ]. Absence of psychic activity as the result of organic brain disease.

**an'ergas'tic.** Pertaining to or characterized by anergasia.

**anergia** (an-er'jĭ-ah). Anergy (2).

**anergic** (an-er'jik). Relating to, or marked by, anergy.

**anergy** (an'er-jĭ) [ G. *an-* priv. + *energeia*, energy, from *ergon*, work ]. 1. Absence of sensitivity reactions in a subject previously inoculated with substances that would be antigenic (immunogenic) in most other subjects; often used to indicate relative or reduced sensitivity either specifically (*i.e.*, as a type of reaction to an allergen) or nonspecifically (*i.e.*, as a result of the alteration of the immunologic responses by fever, cachexia, or other crises. 2. Anergia; lack of energy.

   **negative a.,** nonspecific a.; a reduction of the normal or usual immunologic responses because of unrelated intervening disease.

   **nonspecific a.,** negative a.

   **positive a.,** specific a.; a reduction of the normal or usual immunologic response resulting from a reaction to a specific allergen.

   **specific a.,** positive a.

**an'eroid** [ G. *a-* priv. + *nēros*, wet, + *eidos*, form ]. Without fluid; denoting a form of barometer and sphygomomanometer, without mercury, in which the varying air pressure is indicated by a pointer governed by the movement of a metallic disk occluding a chamber exhausted of air.

**an'eryth'roblep'sia.** Obsolete term for anerythropsia.

**anerythrocyte** (an'e-rith'ro-sīt) [ G. *an-* priv. + *erythros*, red, + *kytos*, cell ]. Mature, anuclear red blood cell that contains no hemoglobin; termed also lympherythrocyte.

**anerythroplasia** (an-e-rith'ro-pla'zĭ-ah) [ G. *an-* priv. + erytho(cyte) + G. *plasis*, a molding ]. A condition in which there is no formation of red blood cells.

**anerythroplastic** (an-e-rith'ro-plas'tik). Anerythroregenerative; characterized by anerythroplasia.

**anerythropsia** (an-er-ĭ-throp'sĭ-ah) [ G. *an-* priv. + *erythros*, red, + *opsis*, vision ]. Protanopia.

**anerythroregenerative** (an-e-rith'-thro-re-jen'er-a-tiv). Anerythroplastic; pertaining to or characterized by lack of regeneration of red blood cells.

**anesthecinesia** (an-es'the-sĭ-ne'ze-ah). Anesthekinesia.

**anesthekinesia** (an-es'the-kĭ-ne'ze-ah) [ G. *an-* priv. + *aesthēsis*, sensation, + *kinēsis*, movement ]. Combined sensory and motor paralysis.

**anesthesia** (an'es-the'zĭ-ah) [ G. *anaisthēsia*, fr. *an-* priv. + *aisthēsis*, sensation ]. A state characterized by loss of sensation, the result of pharmacological depression of nerve function or of neurological disease.

   **acupuncture a.,** acupuncture (2); percutaneous insertion of, and stimulation by, needles placed in critical areas of the body in order to produce loss of sensation in another area.

   **axillary a.,** loss of sensation in the distal two-thirds of the upper extremity following injection of a local anesthetic solution about the nerve trunks in the axilla.

   **balanced a.,** a technique of general a. based on the concept that administration of a mixture of small amounts of several neuronal depressants summates the advantages but not the disadvantages of the individual components of the mixture.

   **basal a.,** parenteral administration of one or more sedatives to produce a state of depressed consciousness short of a general a.

   **block a.,** conduction a.

   **brachial a.,** anesthetization of an upper extremity by injection of local anesthetic solution about the brachial plexus.

   **caudal a.,** regional a. by injection of local anesthetic into the epidural space *via* the caudal canal.

   **cerebral a.,** loss of sensation due to a lesion of the cerebral cortex or other parts of the cerebrum.

   **cervical a.,** regional a. of the neck by injection of a local anesthetic about the cervical nerves.

   **circle absorption a.,** inhalation a. in which a circuit with carbon dioxide absorbent is used for complete (closed) or partial (semiclosed) rebreathing of exhaled gases.

   **compression a.,** pressure a. (2).

   **conduction a.,** block a.; regional a. in which local anesthetic solution is injected about nerves to inhibit nerve transmission; includes spinal, epidural, nerve block, and field block a., but not infiltration or topical a.

   **continuous epidural a.,** fractional epidural a.; insertion of a catheter into the lumbar or caudal epidural space for the repeated injection of local anesthetic solutions as a means of prolonging duration of anesthesia.

   **continuous spinal a.,** fractional spinal a.; a malleable spinal needle or catheter is inserted into the spinal subarachnoid space and left *in situ* to permit serial intermittent injection of the local anesthetic drug for prolonged spinal a.

   **crossed a.,** a. of one side of the body due to a lesion on the other side of the brain.

   **dental a.,** general or conduction a. for operations upon the teeth, gingivae, or associated structures.

   **diagnostic a.,** conduction a. administered for evaluation of etiology of painful conditions.

   **differential spinal a.,** blockade of different types of nerves in the subarachnoid space, based upon their differences in sensitivity to local anesthetics; a form of diagnostic spinal a.; also observed during surgical spinal a.

   **dissociated a.,** loss of sensation for pain and temperature without loss of tactile sense.

   **dissociative a.,** a form of general a. characterized by catalepsy, catatonia, and amnesia, especially that produced by phenylcyclohexylamine compounds, including ketamine.

   **a. doloro'sa,** painful a.; severe spontaneous pain occurring in an anesthetic zone.

   **electric a.,** a., usually general a., produced by application of an electrical current.

   **endotracheal a.,** an inhalation anesthetic technique in which anesthetic and respiratory gases pass through a tube placed in the trachia *via* the mouth or nose.

   **epidural a.,** peridural a.; regional a. produced by injection of local anesthetic solution into the peridural space.

   **extradural a.,** anesthetization, by local anesthetics, of nerves near the spinal canal external to the dura mater; often refers to epidural a., but may include paravertebral a.

   **field block a.,** conduction a. in which small nerves are not anesthetized individually, as in nerve block a., but instead are blocked *en masse* by local anesthetic solution injected to form a barrier proximal to the operative site.

   **fractional a.,** continuous spinal or continuous epidural a.

   **fractional epidural a.,** continuous epidural a.

   **fractional spinal a.,** continuous spinal a.

   **general a.,** loss of ability to perceive pain associated with loss of consciousness; produced by intravenous or inhalation anesthetic agents. General a. is differentiated from regional a., in which consciousness is retained. Signs of general a. and the physiological responses to it vary with individual anesthetic agents and the concentrations in which they are administered.

**girdle a.,** a. distributed as a band encircling the abdomen.

**glove a.,** loss of sensation in the hand, from the tips of the fingers to the wrist.

**gus'tatory a.,** loss of the sense of taste.

**high spinal a.,** spinal a. in which the level of sensory denervation extends to the second or third thoracic dermatome.

**hyperbaric a.,** inhalation of depressant gases or vapors at pressures greater than 1 atmosphere, especially as a means of producing general a. with agents too weak to produce a. at 1 atmosphere.

**hyperbaric spinal a.,** spinal a. in which spread of local anesthetic in the subarachnoid space is controlled by adjusting the position of the patient after the specific gravity of the local anesthetic solution has been made greater than that of cerebrospinal fluid by addition of glucose.

**hypobaric spinal a.,** spinal a. in which spread of local anesthetic in the subarachnoid space is controlled by adjusting the position of the patient after the specific gravity of the local anesthetic solution has been made lower than that of cerebrospinal fluid by addition of distilled water.

**hypotensive a.,** a. in which arterial hypotension is deliberately induced as a means of decreasing operative blood loss.

**hypothermic a.,** general a. administered in conjunction with artificial lowering of body temperature.

**hysterical a.,** a. as a manifestation of hysteria, usually involving half the body or isolated patches that cannot be explained on an organic basis.

**infiltration a.,** local a.

**inhalation a.,** general a. resulting from breathing of anesthetic gases or vapors.

**insufflation a.,** maintenance of inhalation a. by delivery of anesthetic gases or vapors directly to the airway of a patient spontaneously breathing room air.

**intercostal a.,** regional a. produced by injection of local anesthetic solution about intercostal nerves.

**intramedullary a.,** intraosseous a.; general a. by injection of intravenous anesthetic agent(s) into the medullary canal of long bones; now rarely used.

**intranasal a.,** (1) insufflation a. in which an inhalation anesthetic is added to inhaled air passing through the nose or nasopharynx; (2) a. of nasal passages by infiltration and topical application of local anesthetic solution to nasal mucosa.

**intraoral a.,** (1) insufflation a. in which an inhalation anesthetic is added to inhaled air passing through the mouth; (2) regional a. of the mouth and associated structures when local anesthetic solutions are used by topical application to oral mucosa, by local infiltration, or as nerve blocks.

**intraosseous a.,** intramedullary a.

**intraspinal a.,** injection of local anesthetic solution directly into the spinal cord; inaccurately used as a synonym for spinal a.

**intratracheal a.,** endotracheal a.

**intravenous a.,** general a. in which venipuncture is used as a means of injecting central nervous system depressants into the circulation.

**intravenous regional a.,** Bier's method (1); regional a. by intravenous injection of local anesthetic solution distal to an occlusive tourniquet in an extremity previously exsanguinated by pressure or gravity.

**isobaric spinal a.,** spinal a. in which spread of local anesthetic solution within the subarachnoid space is limited by making the specific gravity of the solution equal to that of cerebrospinal fluid.

**local a.,** infiltration a.; regional a. produced by direct infiltration of local anesthetic solution into the operative site or, rarely, by freezing.

**low spinal a.,** spinal a. in which the level of sensory denervation is caudad to the umbilicus.

**muscular a.,** loss of the muscle sense, of the power to determine the position of a limb or to recognize a difference in weights.

**nerve block a.,** conduction a. in which local anesthetic solution is injected about peripheral nerves.

**nonrebreathing a.,** a technique for inhalation a. in which carbon dioxide accumulation is prevented by valves that exhaust exhaled air from the circuit.

**olfactory a.,** anosmia.

**open drop a.,** inhalation a. by vaporization of a liquid anesthetic placed drop by drop on a gauze mask covering the mouth and nose.

**optic a.,** temporary amaurosis.

**paracervical block a.,** regional a. of the cervix uteri by injection of local anesthetic solution into tissues adjacent to the cervix.

**paravert'ebral a.,** (1) a. by injection of local anesthetic solution about nerves as they exit from the vertebral canal; (2) combined presynaptic, postsynaptic, and ganglionic sympathetic block by injection of local anesthetic solution about paravertebral sympathetic chains.

**peridural a.,** epidural a.

**periodontal a.,** a. of the periodontal ligament, produced by injection of a local anesthetic drug.

**pharyngeal a.,** a. of the pharynx occasionally complicating nervous disorders; most common in hysterical patients.

**presacral a.,** injection of local anesthetic solution anterior to the sacrum, to block nerves as they exit from the sacral foramina.

**pressure a.,** compression a.; loss of sensation produced by pressure applied to a peripheral nerve.

**pudendal a.,** local a. produced by blocking the pudendal nerves near the spinal processes of the ischium; used in obstetrics.

**rebreathing a.,** a technique for inhalation a. in which a portion or all of the gases that are exhaled pass back into the a. circuit, with carbon dioxide being absorbed prior to subsequent inhalation.

**rectal a.,** general a. following instillation into the rectum of liquid inhalation anesthetics or intravenous anesthetics.

**refrigeration a.,** cryoanesthesia.

**regional a.,** use of local anesthetic solution(s) to produce circumscribed areas of loss of sensation; a generic term, regional a. includes conduction, nerve block, spinal, epidural, field block, infiltration, and topical a.

**sacral a.,** regional a. limited to those areas innervated by sacral sensory nerves.

**saddle block a.,** a form of spinal a. limited in area to the buttocks, perineum, and inner surfaces of the thighs.

**segmental a.,** loss of sensation limited to an area supplied by one or more spinal nerve roots.

**semi-closed a.,** inhalation a. using a circuit in which a portion of the exhaled air is exhausted from the circuit and a portion is rebreathed following absorption of carbon dioxide.

**semi-open a.,** inhalation a. in which a portion of inhaled gases is derived from an anesthesia circuit while the remainder consists of room air.

**sexual a.,** anaphrodisia.

**spinal a.,** (1) subarachnoid a.; sensory denervation produced by injection of local anesthetic solution(s) into the spinal subarachnoid space; (2) loss of sensation produced by disease of the spinal cord.

**splanchnic a.,** visceral a.; loss of sensation in those areas of the visceral peritoneum innervated by the splanchnic nerves.

**stocking a.,** loss of sensation in the area covered by a stocking.

**subarachnoid a.,** spinal a. (1).

**surgical a.,** (1) any a. administered for the purpose of permitting performance of an operative procedure, as differentiated from obstetrical a., diagnostic a., therapeutic a.; (2) loss of sensation with muscle relaxation adequate for operation.

**tactile a.,** loss or impairment of the sense of touch.

**therapeutic a.,** administration of an anesthetic as a means of treatment, (e.g., for asthma, causalgia).

**thermal a., thermic a.,** loss of heat sense.

**to-and-fro a.,** a. by means of a valveless closed a. circuit in which respired gases pass back and forth through a carbon dioxide absorbent interposed between patient and respiratory reservoir bag.

**topical a.,** surface analgesia; superficial loss of sensation in mucous membranes or skin, produced by direct application of local anesthetic solutions, ointments, or jellies.

**total spinal a.,** spinal a. extensive enough to produce loss of sensation in all extracranial sensory roots.

**traumatic a.,** loss of sensation resulting from nerve injury.

**unilateral a.,** hemianesthesia.

**visceral a.,** splanchnic a.

**an'esthe'siol'ogist.** A physician specializing solely in anesthesiology and related areas (to be differentiated from anesthetist, *q. v.*).

**anesthesiology** (an'es-the'zĭ-ol-o-jĭ) [ anesthesia + G. *logos*, treatise ]. The science concerned with the pharmacological, physiological, and clinical basis of anesthesia and related fields, including resuscitation, intensive respiratory care, pain.

**anesthesiophore** (an'es-the'zĭ-o-fōr) [ anesthesia + G. *phoros*, bearing ]. The active group of a molecule that confers anesthetic or hypnotic effect.

**anesthet'ic.** 1. An anesthetic agent; a compound (*e.g.*, ether) that reversibly depresses neuronal function, producing loss of ability to perceive pain and/or other sensations. 2. Collective designation for anesthetizing agents administered to an individual subject at a particular time (she had an anesthetic for her operation; he gave four anesthetics today). 3. Characterized by loss of sensation (the hand was anesthetic). 4. Capable of producing loss of sensation (an anesthetic gas). 5. Associated with or due to the state of anesthesia (anesthetic complication).

**flammable a.,** an a. agent that supports combustion and forms explosive mixtures with air or oxygen.

**general a.,** a compound that produces loss of sensation and loss of consciousness.

**inhalation a.,** a gas or a liquid with a vapor pressure great enough to produce general anesthesia when breathed.

**intravenous a.,** a compound that produces anesthesia when injected into the circulation *via* venipuncture.

**local a.,** a compound that, when applied directly to mucous membranes or when injected about nerves, produces loss of sensation by inhibiting nerve excitation or conduction.

**primary a.,** the compound that contributes most to loss of sensation when a mixture of anesthetics is administered.

**secondary a.,** a compound that contributes to, but is not primarily responsible for, loss of sensation when two or more anesthetics are simultaneously administered.

**spinal a.,** (1) a local anesthetic agent capable of producing loss of sensation when injected into the subarachnoid space; (2) the provision of anesthesia by the subarachnoid injection of a local anesthetic (he had a spinal anesthetic for his operation).

**volatile a.,** a liquid a. drug that volatilizes to a vapor; when the vapor is inhaled, general anesthesia is produced; see also anesthetic *vapor.*

**anes'thetist.** The person who administers an anesthetic, whether an anesthesiologist, a physician who is not an anesthesiologist, a nurse anesthetist, etc.

**anes'thetiza'tion.** The act of producing loss of sensation.

**anes'thetize.** To produce loss of sensation.

**anestrous** (an-es'trus). Relating to the anestrus.

**ane'strum.** Anestrus.

**anestrus** (an-es'trus) [ G. *a-* priv. + *oistros*, a gadfly, mad desire (estrus). EST- ]. Anestrum; the period of sexual quiescence between the estrus cycles of mammals. This may be (a) a prolonged period in monestrous animals (dogs) or seasonally polyestrous animals (sheep), or (b) a prolonged period of failure of estrus in mature nonpregnant, polyestrous animals.

**anethole** (an'e-thōl) (USP). 1-Methoxy-4-propenylbenzene; *p*-propenylanisole; anise camphor; a derivative of fennel and anise oils; a flavoring substance.

**ane'thopath** [ G. *an-* priv. + *ethos*, custom, + *pathos*, suffering ]. A morally uninhibited person.

**anet'ic** [ G. *anetikos*, relaxing. ES- ]. Soothing; relaxing.

**anetiologic** (an-e'tĭ-o-loj'ik). Not etiologic; not in accordance with the laws of etiology.

**anetoderma** (an-e'to-der'mah) [ G. *anetos*, relaxed (ES-), + *derma*, skin ]. Primary idiopathic macular atrophy; atrophia maculosa cutis; an unusual form of atrophoderma characterized by circumscribed translucent lesions in which the skin becomes baglike and wrinkled.

**Jadassohn-Pellizari a.,** atrophy preceded by erythema or urticaria.

**Schweninger-Buzzi a.,** atrophy with no preceding inflammation.

**an'etus.** Intermittent *fever.*

**aneuploid** (an'u-ployd) [ G. *an-* priv. + euploid ]. Having an abnormal number of chromosomes not an exact multiple of the haploid number.

**an'euploid'y.** State of having an abnormal number of chromosomes not an exact multiple of the haploid number.

**partial a.,** a type of mosaicism in which some cells have a normal number of chromosomes and some have an abnormal number.

**aneuria** (ă-nu'rĭ-ah) [ G. *a-* priv. + *neuron*, nerve ]. Lack of nervous energy; see also neurasthenia.

**aneu'ric.** Relating to or affected by aneuria.

**aneurine** (an'u-rēn). Thiamin.

**aneurolemmic** (ă-nu'ro-lem'ik). Without a neurolemma.

**aneurysm** (an'u-rizm) [ G. *aneurysma* (*-mat-*), an aneurysm, fr. *eurys*, wide ]. Circumscribed dilation of an artery, or a blood-containing tumor connecting directly with the lumen of an artery.

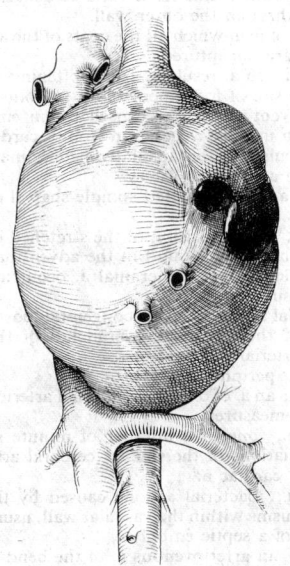

Abdominal Aortic Aneurysm

**ampul'lary a.,** saccular a.

**a. by anastomo'sis,** a mass of dilated anastomosing vessels that produce a pulsating tumor usually in a superficial position.

**arteriosclerotic a.,** atherosclerotic a.; the commonest type of a., occurring in the abdominal aorta and other large arteries in the elderly; due to weakening of the media by severe atherosclerosis.

**arteriovenous a.,** a dilated arteriovenous shunt.

**atherosclerotic a.,** arteriosclerotic a.

**axial a.,** one involving the entire circumference of a blood vessel.

**bacte'rial a.,** mycotic a.

**benign bone a.,** aneurysmal bone *cyst.*

**Bérard's a.,** an arteriovenous a. in the tissues outside of the injured vein.

**berry a.,** a small a. of a cerebral artery that communicates by a narrow channel with the lumen of the vessel.

**cardiac a.,** mural a.; ventricular a.; thinning, stretching and bulging of a weakened ventricular wall, usually as a result of myocardial infarction.

**cavernous-carotid a.,** a fistulous communication, usually of traumatic origin, between the cavernous sinus and the traversing internal carotid artery; a pulsating unilateral exophthalmos and a detectable cranial bruit are common accompaniments.

**a. of Charcot,** a. of Charcot and Bouchard; a small round nodular a. of a small artery or arteriole of the cerebral cortex or basal ganglia; thought by some to be the cause of massive cerebral hemorrhage. Frequency of a.'s of Charcot is greatly increased in hypertensive persons.

**a. of Charcot and Bouchard,** a. of Charcot.

**cir'soid a.,** racemose a. or hemangioma; dilation of a group of blood vessels due to congenital malformation with arteriovenous shunting.

**compound a.,** an a. in which some of the coats of the artery are ruptured, others intact.

**congenital cerebral a.,** localized dilation of a primitive vessel; often a berry a.

**consecutive a.,** diffuse a.

**cylin'droid a.,** tubular a.

**diffuse a.,** one that has enlarged and spread to the surrounding tissues in consequence of rupture of its walls.

**dissecting a.,** splitting or dissection of an arterial wall by blood entering through an intimal tear or by interstitial hemorrhage; dissecting a.'s are most common in the aorta, with an intimal tear near the aortic valve and distal dissection of the media for a variable distance, frequently rupturing through the outer wall.

**ectatic a.,** one in which all the coats of the artery, though stretched, are unruptured.

**embolic a.,** an a. resulting from softening of the arterial wall at the site of lodgement of an embolus.

**em'bolomycot'ic a.,** one caused by an embolism composed of an infected vegetation from a cardiac valve.

**false a.,** pulsating, encapsulated hematoma in communication with a ruptured artery.

**fu'siform a.,** an elongated spindle-shaped dilation of an artery.

**hernial a.,** the protrusion of the stretched inner coats of an artery through a wound in the adventitia.

**infraclinoid a.,** an intracranial a. occurring within the cavernous sinus or below.

**intracranial a.,** an a., either congenital, posttraumatic, or mycotic, of the intracranial branches of the carotid or vertebral arterial systems.

**lateral a.,** peripheral a. (1).

**medical a.,** an a. of one of the internal arteries inaccessible to surgical measures.

**mil'iary a.,** one of a number of minute sacculated or fusiform dilations of the smaller cerebral arteries.

**mural a.,** cardiac a.

**mycotic a.,** bacterial a.; one caused by the growth of microorganisms within the vascular wall, usually following impaction of a septic embolus.

**Park's a.,** an arteriovenous a. of the bend of the elbow, in which the brachial artery communicates with the brachial and median basilic veins.

**peripheral a.,** (1) lateral a.; a a saclike a. springing from one side of an artery; (2) an a. of one of the smaller branches of an artery.

**phantom a.,** student's a.; aortismus abdominalis; a palpable throbbing aorta, mistaken by novices for an a.

**Pott's a.,** aneurysmal *varix.*

**rac'emose a.,** cirsoid a.

**Rasmussen's a.,** aneurysmal dilation of a branch of a pulmonary artery in a tuberculous cavity, rupture of which may cause serious hemoptysis.

**saccular a., sacculated a.,** a saclike bulging on one side of an artery.

**serpentine a.,** dilation and tortuosity of an artery, sometimes affecting the temporal artery in the aged.

**student's a.,** phantom a.

**supraclinoid a.,** an intracranial a. of the internal carotid artery, occurring above the clinoid bone.

**surgical a.,** an a. of one of the external arteries, amenable to surgical treatment.

**syphilitic a.,** an a. affecting mainly the aortic arch, resulting from tertiary syphilitic aortitis, usually involving the thoracic aorta.

**traction a.,** an aortic a. assumed to be due to the pull of a persistent ductus arteriosus.

**traumatic a.,** an a. resulting from physical damage to the wall of an artery in a wound or by a fragment of fractured bone; usually a false a. or arteriovenous a.

**true a.,** localized dilation of an artery with an expanded lumen lined by stretched remnants of the arterial wall.

**tubular a.,** the uniform dilation of an artery along a considerable distance.

**varicose a.,** a blood-containing sac, communicating with both an artery and a vein.

**ventricular a.,** cardiac a.

**verminous a.,** worm a.; a. in horses caused by the migrations of larvae of *Strongylus vulgaris,* usually involving the mesenteric arteries.

**worm a.,** verminous a.

**aneurysmal** (an-u-riz'mal). Aneurysmatic; relating to an aneurysm.

**aneurysmatic** (an-u-riz-mat'ik). Aneurysmal.

**aneurysmectomy** (an-u-riz-mek'to-mĭ) [ aneurysm + G. *ektomē,* excision ]. Excision of the sac of an aneurysm.

**aneurysmograph** (an'u-riz'mo-graf). X-ray of an aneurysm.

**aneurysmoplasty** (an-u-riz'mo-plas'tĭ) [ aneurysm + G. *plassō,* to form ]. Matas' operation; endoaneurysmorrhaphy; endoaneurysmoplasty; treatment of an aneurysm by opening the sac and suturing its walls together so as to obliterate it and restore the lumen of the artery. See also aneurysmorrhaphy.

**aneurysmorrhaphy** (an'u-riz-mor'ă-fĭ) [ aneurysm + G. *raphē,* suture ]. Closure by suture of the sac of an aneurysm.

**cerebral a.,** repair of an intracranial aneurysm; various techniques may be used, including clipping, ligature, trapping, reinforcement by various methods, and induced thrombosis by piloinjection.

**aneurysmotomy** (an'u-riz-mot'o-mĭ) [ aneurysm + G. *tomē,* incision ]. Incision into the sac of an aneurysm.

**angei-.** For words so beginning, see those beginning angi-.

**angelica root** (an-jel'ĭ-kah). The root of *Angelica archangelica* (family Umbelliferae); a tonic and stimulant, and may cause nausea; used as a carminative, diuretic, and externally as a counterirritant.

**Angelucci** (ahn-jĕ-loot'che), Arnaldo, Italian ophthalmologist, 1854–1934. See A.'s *syndrome.*

**Anghelescu** (ahn-jĕ-les'koo), Constantin, Roumanian surgeon, 1869–1948. See A.'s *sign.*

**angi-.** See angio-.

**angialgia** (an'jĭ-al'jĭ-ah) [ angio- + G. *algos,* pain ]. Pain in blood vessel.

**an'giasthe'nia** [ angio- + G. *astheneia,* weakness ]. Vascular instability.

**angiectasia, angiectasis** (an-jĭ-ek-ta'sĭ-ah, an-jĭ-ek'ta-sis) [ angio- + G. *ektasis,* a stretching ]. Dilation of a lymphatic or blood vessel.

**congenital dysplastic a.,** Klippel-Trenaunay-Weber *syndrome.*

**angiectat'ic** [ angio- + G. *ektatos,* capable of extension ]. Marked by the presence of dilated blood vessels.

**angiectomy** (an-jĭ-ek'to-mĭ) [ angio- + G. *ektomē,* excision ]. Excision of a section of a blood vessel.

**angiecto'pia** [ angio- + G. *ektopos,* out of place ]. Abnormal location of a blood vessel.

**angiitis, angitis** an-jĭ-i'tis, an-ji'tis) [ angio- + G. suffix *-itis,* inflammation ]. Vasculitis; inflammation of a blood vessel (arteritis, phlebitis) or of a lymphatic vessel (lymphangitis).

**consecutive a.,** a. caused by extension of the inflammatory process from the surrounding tissues.

**hypersensitivity a.,** an inflammatory reaction in a blood vessel, the result of a specific reaction to an antigenic (allergic) substance or other agents to which the individual expresses unusual vascular sensitization.

**necrotizing a.,** inflammatory reaction of blood vessels resulting in fibrinoid necrosis of tissue.

**angileucitis** an-jĭ-lu-si'tis) [ angio- + G. *leukos,* white, + suffix *-itis,* inflammation ]. Lymphangitis.

**angina** (an'jĭ-nah, an-ji'nah) [ L. quinsy ]. 1. Sore throat from any cause. 2. A severe constricting pain; commonly used in the term a. pectoris.

**abdominal a.,** a. abdominis; intestinal a.; angor abdominis; intermittent abdominal pain, frequently occurring at a fixed time after eating, caused by inadequacy of the mesenteric circulation from arteriosclerosis or spasm.

**a. abdom′inis,** abdominal a.

**agranulocyt′ic a.,** agranulocytosis.

**a. cruris,** intermittent *claudication.*

**a. decubitus,** a. pectoris decubitus.

**a. diphtheritica,** pharyngeal or laryngeal diphtheria.

**a. dyspep′tica,** a. associated with gastroenteric upset.

**a. of effort,** a. pectoris precipitated by physical exertion.

**a. epiglottid′ea,** inflammation of epiglottis.

**false a.,** a. pectoris vasomotoria.

**Henoch's a.,** necrotic a.

**hypercyanotic a.,** anginal pain in cyanotic patients with congenital heart disease or chronic pulmonary disease, the pain developing with intensification of the cyanosis during activity.

**intestinal a.,** a. abdominis.

**lymphatic a.,** monocytic a.; an affection resembling Vincent's a. marked by an increase in the number of lymphocytes in the blood.

**a. lymphomato′sa,** agranulocytosis.

**a. membrana′cea,** membraneous *croup.*

**monocyt′ic a.,** lymphatic a.

**necrotic a.,** Henoch's a.; a form, occurring usually as a complication of scarlet fever and more rarely of diphtheria, in which gangrenous patches are found in the mucous membrane of the air passages.

**neutropenic a.,** agranulocytosis.

**a. notha,** a. vasomotoria.

**a. pec′toris,** breast pang; heart stroke; stenocardia; coronarism; Elsner's asthma; Heberden's asthma; cardiagra; severe constricting pain in the chest, often radiating from the precordium to the left shoulder and down the arm, due to ischemia of the heart muscle, usually caused by coronary disease.

**a. pec′toris decu′bitus,** a decubitus; anginal pain developing while the subject is recumbent.

**a. pec′toris si′ne do′lore,** Gairdner's *disease.*

**a. pec′toris vasomoto′ria,** reflex a.; a. spuria; a. pseudangina; pseudoangina; a. vasomotoria; a. pectoris in which the breast pain is comparatively slight, but pallor, followed by cyanosis, and coldness and numbness of the extremities are marked.

**Plaut's a.,** Vincent's *disease.*

**reflex a.,** a. pectoris vasomotoria.

**a. scarlatino′sa,** sore throat of scarlet fever.

**a. sine dolore,** symptoms of coronary insufficiency occurring without pain.

**a. spuria,** a. pectoris vasomotoria.

**ulceromembranous a.,** Vincent's *disease.*

**a. vasomotor′ia,** a. pectoris vasomotoria.

**Vincent's a.,** Vincent's *disease.*

**anginal** (an′jĭ-nal). Relating to angina in any sense.

**anginiform** (an-jin′ĭ-form). Resembling angina.

**anginoid** (an′jin-oid). Resembling an angina, especially angina pectoris.

**an′ginopho′bia** [ angina + G. *phobos,* fear ]. Extreme fear of an attack of angina pectoris.

**an′ginose, an′ginous.** Relating to any angina.

**angio-, angi-** [ G. *angeion,* vessel ]. Combining forms relating to blood or lymph vessels.

**angioarchitecture** (an′jĭ-o-ar′kĭ-tek-tūr). 1. The arrangement and distribution of the blood vessels of any organ. 2. The vascular framework of an organ or tissue.

**angioatax′ia** (an′jĭ-o-ă-tak′sĭ-ah) [ angio- + G. *ataxia,* confusion ]. A condition of irregular spasmodic variability in arterial tonus.

**an′gioblast** [ angio- + G. *blastos,* germ ]. 1. A cell taking part in blood vessel formation. 2. The primordial mesenchymal tissue from which embryonic blood cells and vascular endothelium are differentiated.

**an′gioblasto′ma.** Hemangioblastoma.

**angiocardiography** (an′jĭ-o-kar-dĭ-og-rah-fe) [ angio- + G. *kardia,* heart, + *graphō,* to write ]. X-ray study of the heart and great vessels made visible by the intravenous injection of a radiopaque solution.

**rapid biplane a.,** synchronous a. in two planes at right angles to each other at a speed of 10 to 12 exposures a second.

**selective a.,** a method designed to improve visualization by concentrating the contrast medium in the region to be studied; with the aid of a pressure apparatus the medium is injected through a catheter into the area for study. Selective arteriography can be accomplished by injecting contrast material through a small catheter into any small artery, *e.g.,* the pancreaticoduodenal artery.

**an′giocar′diokinet′ic, an′giocar′diocinet′ic** [ angio- + G. *kardia,* heart, + *kinēsis,* movement ]. Causing dilation or contraction in the heart and blood vessels.

**an′giocardiop′athy** [ angio- + G. *kardia,* heart, + *pathos,* disease ]. Disease affecting both heart and blood vessels.

**an′giocardi′tis** [ angio- + G. *kardia,* heart, + suffix *-itis,* inflammation ]. Inflammation of the heart and blood vessels.

**angiocavernoma** (an′jĭ-o-kav-er-no′mah). *Angioma* cavernosum.

**angiocav′ernous.** Relating to the condition present in angioma cavernosum.

**angiochiloscope** (an′jĭ-o-ki′lo-skōp) [ angio- + G. *cheilos,* lip, + *skopeō,* to examine ]. Angiocheiloscope; an instrument used to study blood circulation of the lips.

**angiocholecystitis** (an-jĭ-o-ko-le-sis-ti′tis) [ angio- + G. *cholē,* bile, + *kystis,* bladder, + suffix *-itis,* inflammation ]. Inflammation of the bile vessels and gallbladder.

**angiocholitis** (an-jĭ-o-ko-li′tis). Cholangitis.

**an′gioclast** [ angio- + G. *klastos,* broken ]. A forceps for controlling bleeding from an artery.

**angiocyst** (an′jĭ-o-sist). A small vesicular aggregation of embryonic mesodermal cells that may give rise to vascular endothelium and blood cells.

**an′giodermati′tis** [ angio- + G. *derma,* skin, + suffix *-itis,* inflammation ]. Inflammation of the cutaneous vessels.

**an′giodias′copy** (an′jĭ-o-di-as′ko-pī) [ angio- + G. *dia,* through, + *skopeō,* to view ]. Examination of the vessels in a part by transillumination.

**angiodiathermy** (an′jĭ-o-di′ah-ther-mĭ) [ angio- + G. *dia,* through, + *thermē,* heat ]. Treatment of glaucoma by coagulation, using diathermy applied to the long posterior ciliary arteries.

**angiodynia** (an-jĭ-o-din′ĭ-ah) [ angio- + G. *odynē,* pain ]. Angialgia.

**an′giodystro′phia.** Angiodystrophy.

**angiodystrophy** (an′jĭ-o-dis′tro-fī) [ angio- + G. *dys-,* bad, + *trophē,* nourishment ]. A nutritional disorder associated with marked vascular changes.

**angioedema** an-jĭ-o-e-de′mah). Angioneurotic *edema.*

**angioelephantiasis** (an′jĭ-o-el′e-fan-ti′ah-sis). Extensive increase in vascularity of the subcutaneous tissue, producing great thickening simulating large, diffuse angioma formation.

**an′giofi′brolipo′ma.** A neoplasm composed of fibrocytes, capillaries, and adipose tissue.

**angiofibro′ma.** Telangiectatic *fibroma.*

**juvenile a.,** juvenile hemangiofibroma; a markedly vascular fibrous tumor occurring in the nasopharynx of males, usually in the second decade of life; epistaxis and local invasion may result, but spontaneous regression is usual after sexual maturity.

**an′giofibro′sis.** Fibrosis of the walls of blood vessels.

**angiogenesis** (an′jĭ-o-jen′e-sis) [ angio- + G. *genesis,* production ]. Development of blood vessels.

**angiogen′ic.** 1. Relating to angiogenesis. 2. Of vascular origin.

**angioglioma** (an′jĭ-o-gli-o′mah). A mixed glioma and angioma.

**angiogliomatosis** (an′jĭ-o-gli′o-mah-to′sis). The occurrence of multiple areas of proliferating capillaries and neuroglia.

**angiogliosis** (an′jĭ-o-gli-o′sis). The occurrence of an angioglioma.

**angiogram** (an′jĭ-o-gram) [ angio- + G. *gramma,* a writing ]. Radiogram obtained in angiography.

**angiography** (an-jĭ-og′ră-fī) [ angio- + G. *graphō,* to write ]. 1. Radiography of vessels after the injection of a radiopaque material. 2. Description of the blood vessels or lymphatics.

**cerebral a.,** cerebral arteriography; radiographic visualization of the blood vessels supplying the brain, including their extracranial portions. The injection may be made by percutaneous puncture (closed a.) or after exposure (open a.) of: aortic arch; brachial artery, by catheterization or retrograde injection; carotid artery; femoral artery with catheterization and serial selective visualization of carotid and vertebral systems; subclavian artery; and vertebral artery.

**radionuclide a.,** the display, by means of a stationary scintillation camera device, of the passage of a bolus of a rapidly injected radiopharmaceutical.

**spinal a.,** spinal arteriography; radiographic visualization of the spinal cord vessels by controlled injection of contrast media into the appropriate vessels, performed by artery catheterization.

**an′giohe′mophil′ia.** von Willebrand's *disease*.

**angiohyalinosis** (an′jĭ-o-hi′al-ĭ-no′sis) [ angio- + G. *hyalos*, glass, + suffix *-osis*, condition ]. Hyaline degeneration of the walls of the blood vessels.

**an′giohyperto′nia** [ angio- + G. *hyper*, over, + *tonos*, tension ]. Vasospasm.

**an′giohy′poto′nia, an′giohy′poto′nus** [ angio- + G. *hypo*, under, + *tonos*, tension ]. Vasoparesis or vasoparalysis.

**angioid** (an′jĭ-oyd) [ angio- + G. *eidos*, resemblance ]. Resembling blood vessels.

**angioinvasive** (an′jĭ-o-in-va′siv). Denoting a neoplasm or other pathologic condition capable of entering the vascular bed.

**an′giokerato′ma** [ angio- + G. keras, horn, + suffix *-ōma*, tumor ]. Telangiectatic wart; telangiectasia verrucosa; keratoangioma; an intradermal cavernous hemangioma, over which there is a wartlike thickening of the horny layer of the epidermis.

**a. corpo′ris diffu′sum** Fabry's *disease*.

**Fordyce's a.,** asymptomatic vascular papules of the scrotum, appearing in late adolescence; much less common in the vulva.

**Mibelli's a.'s,** telangiectatic small papules of the dorsa of the hands and feet, as well as on the elbows and knees, that enlarge to over 0.05 cm.; familial incidence.

**an′giokerato′sis.** The occurrence of multiple angiokeratomas.

**angiokinesis** (an′jĭ-o-kin-e′sis) [ angio- + G. *kinēsis*, movement ]. Vasomotion.

**an′giokinet′ic.** Vasomotor.

**angioleiomyoma** (an′jĭ-o-li′o-mi-o′mah). Vascular *leiomyoma*.

**an′giolip′ofibro′ma.** Angiofibrolipoma.

**an′giolipo′ma.** A lipoma that contains an unusually large number, or foci of proliferated, neoplastic-like, frequently dilated vascular channels.

**an′giolith** [ angio- + G. *lithos*, stone ]. 1. A venous calculus; phlebolith. 2. A calcareous deposit in the wall of an artery.

**an′giolith′ic.** Relating to an angiolith.

**an′giolo′gia** [ NA ]. Angiology.

**angiol′ogy** [ angio- + G. *logos*, treatise, discourse ]. The science that treats of the blood vessels and lymphatics in all their relations.

**an′giolu′poid** [ angio- + L. *lupus*, wolf, + G. *eidos*, resemblance ]. A tuberculous lesion of the skin. The lesions are telangiectatic papules distributed over the nose and cheeks.

**angiolysis** (an-jĭ-ol′ĭ-sis) [ angio- + G. *lysis*, destruction ]. Obliteration of a blood vessel, such as occurs in the newborn infant after tying of the umbilical cord.

**angioma** (an-jĭ-o′mah) [ angio- + G. suffix *-ōma*, tumor ]. A swelling or tumor due to proliferation with or without dilation of the blood vessels (hemangioma) or lymphatics (lymphangioma).

**capillary a.,** *nevus* vascularis.

**cavernous a.,** cavernous *hemangioma*.

**cherry a.'s,** senile *hemangioma*.

**encephal′ic a.,** a collection of dilated arteries in the brain.

**a. lymphat′icum,** lymphangioma.

**petechial a.'s,** multiple lesions resembling petechiae but due to dilation of capillary walls; they are obliterated by pressure.

**a. pigmento′sum et atroph′icum,** *xeroderma* pigmentosum.

**a. serpigino′sum,** essential telangiectasia (2); Hutchinson's disease (2); nevus lupus; the presence of rings of red dots on the skin, which tend to widen peripherally, due to proliferation, with subsequent atrophy, of the superficial capillaries.

**spider a.,** arterial *spider*.

**superficial a.,** *nevus* vascularis.

**telangiectatic a.,** a. composed of dilated vessels.

**a. venosum racemo′sum,** the appearance (tortuous swelling) caused by varicosities of superficial veins.

**angiomatoid** (an-jĭ-o′mah-toid). Resembling a tumor of vascular origin.

**an′giomato′sis.** A condition characterized by multiple angiomas.

**ceph′alotrigem′inal a.,** Sturge-Weber *syndrome*.

**congenital dysplastic a.,** congenital dysplastic angiopathy; a. in which there is dysplasia of the underlying tissues, sometimes with overgrowth of bone as in the Klippel-Trenaunay syndrome; or the cephalotrigeminal a. (the Sturge-Weber syndrome), in which there is an angioma in the distribution of one or more branches of the trigeminal nerve with calcification of the cortex, underlying vascular anomalies, amentia, epilepsy, sometimes glaucoma.

**encephalofacial a.,** Sturge-Weber *syndrome*.

**encephalotrigeminal a.,** Sturge-Weber *syndrome*.

**oculoencephalic a.,** an incomplete form of Sturge-Weber syndrome consisting of angiomas of choroid and meninges only.

**retinocerebral a.,** Lindau's *disease*.

**telangiectatic a.,** disseminated capillary and venous vascular malformations of the cerebral hemispheres and leptomeninges, occurring in Sturge-Weber syndrome.

**angio′matous.** Relating to or resembling an angioma.

**an′giomeg′aly** [ angio- + G. *megas*, large ]. Enlargement of blood vessels or lymphatics.

**angiom′eter** [ angio- + G. *metron*, measure ]. An instrument for measuring the diameter of a blood vessel.

**an′giomy′ocar′diac** [ angio- + G. *mys*, muscle, + *kardia*, heart ]. Relating to the blood vessels and the cardiac muscle.

**angiomyofibroma** (an′jĭ-mi′o-fi-bro′mah). Vascular *leiomyoma*.

**an′giomy′olipo′ma** [ angio- + G. *mys*, muscle, + *lipos*, fat, + suffix *-oma*, tumor ]. A benign neoplasm of adipose tissue (lipoma) in which muscle cells and vascular structures are fairly conspicuous. The most common form is a renal tumor containing smooth muscle.

**an′giomyo′ma** [ angio- + G. *mys*, muscle, + suffix *-ōma*, tumor ]. Vascular *leiomyoma*.

**angiomyoneuroma** (an′jĭ-o-mi′o-nu-ro′sis). Glomus *tumor*.

**angiomyopathy** (an′jĭ-o-mi′op′ă-thĭ) [ angio- + G. *mys*, muscle, + *pathos*, suffering ]. Disease of blood vessels involving muscular layer.

**an′giomy′osarco′ma.** A myosarcoma that has an unusually large number of proliferated, frequently dilated vascular channels.

**angiomyxoma** (an′jĭ-o-mik-so′mah). An infiltrative neoplasm of primitive mesenchyme (*i.e.*, myxoma) in which there is an unusually large number of vascular structures.

**angioneuralgia** (an′jĭ-o-nu-ral′jĭ-ah). An affection, marked by a burning pain in an extremity, accompanied by redness and edema of the affected area, thought to be an early stage of Raynaud's disease.

**angioneurectomy** (an′jĭ-o-nu-rek′to-mĭ) [ angio- + G. *neuron*, nerve, + *ektomē*, excision ]. 1. Exection of the vessels and nerves of a part. 2 [ G. *neuron*, cord ]. Exection of a segment of the spermatic cord for the relief of an enlarged prostate or to produce sterility.

**an′gioneurede′ma** [ angio- + G. *neuron*, + *oidēma*, a swelling ]. Edema due to an angioneurosis, or vasomotor disorder.

**an′gioneu′romyo′ma.** Glomus *tumor*.

**an'gioneuro'sis.** Vasoneurosis; a disorder due to disease or injury of the vasomotor nerves or center.

**an'gioneurot'ic.** Relating to an angioneurosis.

**an'gioneurot'omy** [ angio- + G. *neuron*, nerve, + *tomē*, a cutting ]. Division of both nerves and vessels of a part.

**angioparalysis** (an'jī-o-pă-ral'ī-sis). Vasoparalysis.

**an'giopar'esis.** Vasoparesis.

**an'giopathol'ogy.** The morbid changes in diseases of the blood vessels.

**angiop'athy** [ angio- + G. *pathos*, suffering ]. Angiosis; any disease of the blood vessels or lymphatics.
   **congenital dysplastic a.,** congenital dysplastic *angiomatosis.*

**angiophacomatosis** (an'jī-o-fak'o-mah-to'sis). Angiophakomatosis; the angiomatous phacomatoses: Lindau's disease and the Sturge-Weber syndrome.

**an'gioplan'y** [ angio- + G. *planē*, a wandering ]. Angiectopia.

**an'gioplas'ty** [ angio- + G. *plassō*, to form ]. Reconstruction of an injured blood vessel.

**angiopneumography** (an'jī-o-nu-mog'rah-fī). Roentgenologic visualization of the pulmonary vessels.

**angiopoiesis** (an'jī-o-poy-e'sis) [ angio- + G. *poiesis*, making ]. Vasifaction; vasoformation; the formation of blood or lymphatic vessels.

**angiopoietic** (an'jī-o-poy-et'ik). Relating to angiopoiesis.

**an'giopressure.** Pressure on a vessel for the arrest of bleeding.

**angiorrhaphy** (an-jī-or'ă-fī) [ angio- + G. *rhaphē*, a seam ]. Suture of any vessel, especially of a blood vessel.

**angiorrhexis** (an'jī-o-rek'sis) [ angio- + G. *rhēxis*, rupture ]. Rupture of a blood vessel or lymphatic.

**an'giosarco'ma.** A rare malignant neoplasm believed to originate from blood lymphatic vessels; grossly soft and poorly circumscribed; microscopically composed of closely packed round or spindle-shaped cells, some of which line small spaces resembling vascular clefts. See also hemangioendothelioma; hemangiosarcoma; lymphangiosarcoma; and Kaposi's *sarcoma.*

**angiosclerosis** (an'jī-o-skle-ro'sis) [ angio- + G. *sklērōsis*, hardening ] Fibrous disease involving the entire vascular system.

**an'giosclerot'ic.** Marked by angiosclerosis.

**an'gioscope** [ angio- + G. *skopeō*, to view ]. A modified microscope for studying the capillary vessels.

**angioscotoma** (an'jī-o-sko-to'mah) [ angio- + G. *skotōma*, dizziness, vertigo ]. Ribbon-shaped defect of the visual fields caused by the retinal vessels, perivascular spaces, and lymphatics.

**an'gioscotom'etry.** The measurement or projection of the angioscotoma tree.

**an'giosi'ali'tis** [ angio- + G. *sialon*, saliva, + suffix *-itis*, inflammation ]. Inflammation of a salivary duct.

**angiosis** (an-jī-o'sis). Angiopathy.

**angiospasm** (an'jī-o-spazm). Vasospasm.
   **labyrin'thine a.,** Lermoyez' *syndrome.*

**an'giospas'tic.** Vasospastic.

**angiosperms** (an'jī-o-spermz) [ angio- + G. *sperma*, seed ]. A subdivision of the Spermatophyta, or seed-bearing plants, comprising over 140,000 species. The ovules or future seeds are in a closed ovary and fertilization takes place through the stigma.

**angiostaxis** (an'jī-o-stak'sis) [ angio- + G. *staxis*, a trickling, fr. *stazō*, to drip ]. 1. Oozing of blood. 2. Hemophilia.

**an'giosteno'sis** [ angio- + G. *stenōsis*, a narrowing ]. Narrowing of one or more blood vessels.

**angios'tomy** [ angio- + G. *stoma*, mouth ]. Artificial opening into an artery in the operation preliminary to an implantation.

**Angiostrongylus** (an'jī-o-stron'jī-lus). A genus of strongyle nematodes that are lungworms of rodents and Canidae, and are transmitted by slugs or land snails.
   **A. cantonen'sis,** metastrongylid nematode lungworm of rodents, transmitted by infected molluscs ingested by rodents. They develop in the brain and migrate to lungs, where the adult worms are found. These organisms are thought to cause eosinophilic encephalomeningitis in man

in the Pacific basin; larvae have been removed from the anterior chamber of the eye from men in Thailand who had eaten raw snails.
   **A. vaso'rum,** a species occurring in the pulmonary artery and, rarely, in the right ventricle of the dog and fox. Thrombi may occur in the lungs; hypertrophy of the heart and liver may result in ascites. Affected animals suffer from dyspnea and occasionally may die from cardiac insufficiency.

**angios'trophy** [ angio- + G. *strophē*, a twist. STREP- ]. Twisting the cut end of an artery to arrest bleeding.

**an'giotelec'tasis, an'giotel'ecta'sia** [ angio- + G. *telos*, end, + *ektasis*, a stretching out ]. Dilation of the terminal arterioles.

**angioten'sin.** Formerly called angiotonin; a vasoconstrictive principle produced by enzymatic action of renin upon a serum $\alpha_2$-globulin (angiotensinogen) formed by the liver. See a. I and a. II.
   **a. I,** a decapeptide of slightly variable sequence, depending on the animal source, formed from the tetradecapeptide angiotensinogen by the removal of four amino acid residues, a reaction catalyzed by renin; a peptidase cleaves two more residues to yield a. II, the physiologically active form.
   **a. II,** an octapeptide formed by the removal of two amino acid residues from a. I; a potent vasopressor agent and the most powerful stimulus for production and release of aldosterone.
   **a. amide** (NF), HYPERTENSIN; a synthetic substance closely related to the naturally occurring a. II; a potent vasopressor agent useful in the management of certain types of shock and circulatory collapse.
   **a. precursor,** angiotensinogen.

**angioten'sinase.** Angiotonase; hypertensinase; former name for the enzyme responsible for converting angiotensin I to II; it is now applied to the enzyme that degrades angiotensin II.

**angiotensin'ogen.** Hypertensinogen; a tetradecapeptide (formerly considered to be a circulating $\alpha_2$-globulin) that is converted by the enzyme renin to angiotensin II.

**angiot'omy** [ angio- + G. *tomē*, cutting ]. Section of an artery or vein.

**angiot'onase.** Angiotensinase.

**an'gioto'nia.** Vasotonia.

**an'gioton'ic.** Increasing vascular tension, particularly arteriolar.

**angiotonin** (an'jī-o-to'nin). Former name for angiotensin.

**an'giotribe** [ angio- + G. *tribō*, to bruise ]. A crushing instrument, in the shape of strong forceps with screw attachment, used to crush the end of an artery together with the tissue in which it is embedded, to arrest hemorrhage.

**an'giotrip'sy** [ angio- + G. *tripsis*, friction, bruising ]. The use of the angiotribe to arrest hemorrhage.

**angiotrophic** (an'jī-o-trof'ik) [ angio- + G. *trophē*, nourishment ]. Vasotrophic; relating to the nutrition of the blood vessels or lymphatics.

**angitis** (an-ji'tis). Angiitis.

**Angle,** Edward H., American dentist, 1855–1930. See A.'s *classification.*

# ANGLE

**angle** (ang'gl) [ L. *angulus* ]. The meeting point of two lines or planes; the figure formed by the junction of two lines or planes; the space bounded on two sides by lines or planes that meet. See also angulus.
   **a. of aberration,** obsolete synonym for a. of refraction.
   **Ackermann's a.'s,** a.'s at base of skull with hydrocephalus and encephalocele.
   **acromial a.,** *angulus* acromialis.
   **acute a.,** any a. less than 90°.
   **adjacent a.,** one with a line in common with another a.

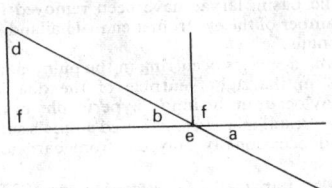

**Geometric Angles**

*a*, Acute angle; *b*, adjacent angle; *d*, oblique angle; *e*, obtuse angle; *f*, *f*, right angles.

**alpha a.,** the a. between the axis of vision and the corneal axis.

**Alsberg's a.,** a. of direction; a. of elevation; the a. within Alsberg's triangle, formed by lines passing through the long axis of the neck and the long axis of the shaft of the femur. Usually about 41°, it is supplementary to the a. of inclination. See fig. under Alsberg's *triangle*.

**alve'olar a.,** the a. between the horizontal plane and a line connecting the base of the nasal spine and the middle point of the projection of the alveolus of the maxilla.

**ANS a.,** SNA a.; in cephalometrics, an a. measurement of the anteroposterior positioning of the maxilla relative to the cranial base.

**a. of aperture,** a. formed by lines drawn from the ends of the diameter of a lens to its point of focus.

**axial a.,** an a. formed by two surfaces of a body, the line of union of which is parallel with its axis; the axial a.'s of a tooth are the distobuccal, distolabial, distolingual, mesiobuccal, mesiolabial, and mesiolingual.

**axioincisal, axiolabial, axiolabiolingual, axiolingual, axiolinguocervical, axiolinguoclusal, axiolinguogingival, axiomesial, axiomesiocervical, axiomesiogingival, axiomesioincisal,** and **axioclusal a.'s,** see these terms.

**bas'ilar a.,** one formed by the intersection at the basion of lines coming from the nasal spine and the nasal point.

**Bennett a.,** the a. formed by the sagittal plane and the path of the advancing condyle during lateral mandibular movement as viewed in the horizontal plane.

**beta a.,** the a. formed by a line connecting the bregma and hormion meeting the radius fixus.

**bior'bital a.,** that formed by the meeting of the axes of the orbits.

**Broca's a.'s,** (1) Broca's basilar a.; (2) Broca's facial a.; (3) *angulus* occipitalis.

**Broca's basilar a.,** the a. formed at the basion of lines drawn from the nasion and the alveolar point.

**Broca's facial a.,** the a. formed by the intersection at the biauricular axis of lines drawn from the supraorbital point and the alveolar point.

**buccal a.'s,** those formed by the buccal surface of a tooth joining the other surfaces.

**bucco-occlu'sal a.,** line of junction of the buccal and occlusal surfaces of a tooth.

**Camper's facial a.,** the a. formed by the intersection of a line drawn from the glabella through the anterior surface of the incisors and a line drawn from the inferior nares point through the porion.

**cardiohepatic a.,** a. formed by upper border of liver and right border of heart, especially as defined by percussion.

**carrying a.,** the a. made between the median plane of arm and median plane of extended forearm.

**cavity line a.,** the a. formed by two walls of a cavity meeting along a line.

**cavosurface a.,** see cavosurface.

**cephal'ic a.,** one of several a.'s formed by the intersection of two lines passing through certain points of the face or cranium.

**cephalomedullary a.,** the a. made by the junction of the cerebrum and the brain stem.

**cerebel'lopon'tile a.,** cerebellopontine a.

**cerebel'lopon'tine a.,** cerebellopontile a.; pontine a.; the recess at the junction of the cerebellum and pons.

**a. of convergence,** the a. that the visual axis makes with the median line when a near object is looked at.

**costal a.,** *angulus* costae.

**craniofacial a.,** the a. formed by the basifacial and basicranial axes at the midpoint of the sphenoethmoidal suture.

**critical a.,** the a. of incidence of a ray of light which results in the refractive ray being on the surface between the two media; a greater angle results in total reflection.

**cusp a.,** (1) the a. made by the slopes of a cusp with the plane which passes through the tip of the cusp and which is perpendicular to a line bisecting the cusp, measured mesiodistally or buccolingually; (2) the a. made by the slopes of a cusp with a perpendicular line bisecting the the cusp, measured mesiodistally or buccolingually; (3) one-half of the included a. between the buccal and lingual or mesial and distal cusp inclines.

**Daubenton's a.,** occipital a. (2); an a. formed by the junction, at the opisthion, of lines coming from the basion and from the projection in the median plane of the lower border of the orbits.

**a. of declination,** the a. formed by a line drawn through the center of the long axis of the neck of the femur meeting a line drawn in the transverse axis of the condyles, when the bone is viewed from above, looking, as it were, straight down through the head of the femur. Used as an index of deviation of the head of the femur posteriorly as occurs in coxa vara. Normally the a. is about 12°, but may be 45° in coxa vara.

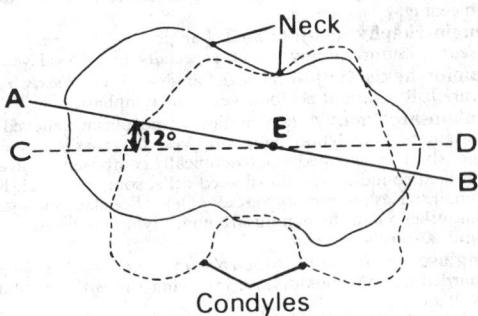

**Angle of Declination of Femur**

Superior view of right femur, showing angle of declination (*AEC*), with proximal end (*continuous line*) projected over distal end (*interrupted line*); *AB*, long axis of neck; *CD*, transverse axis of condyles.

**a. of depression,** a. of inclination.

**a. of deviation,** a. of refraction.

**a. of deviation of the electrical axis of the heart,** the a. between the manifest vector in the frontal plane and the horizontal plane.

**a. of direction,** Alsberg's *angle.*

**distobuccal, distobucco-occlusal, distobuccopulpal, distocervical, distoclusal, distogingival, distoincisal, distolabial, distolabiopulpal, distolingual, distolinguo-occlusal, disto-occlusal, distopulpal a.'s,** see these terms.

**duode'nojeju'nal a.,** *flexura* duodenojejunalis.

**a. of elevation,** Alsberg's *angle.*

**epigastric a.,** the a. formed by the xiphoid process with the body of the sternum.

**ethmoid a.,** the a. made by the plane of the cribriform plate of the ethmoid bone extended to meet the basicranial axis.

**facial a.,** any of several variously named (Broca's, Camper's, Jacquart's, ophryospinal, Topinard's) and variously defined anatomical a.'s that have been used to quantify facial protrusion.

**filtration a.,** *angulus* iridocornealis.

**Frankfort mandibular plane a.,** cant of the mandible; the a. formed by the intersection of the mandibular plane (gonion-gnathion) with the sella-nasion or Frankfort plane.

**frontal a.,** *angulus* frontalis.

**gamma a.,** the a. between the axis of the eyeball and line of vision.

**hypsiloid a.,** y-a.

**impedance a.,** a term expressing the ratio of electric resistance to electric capacity (ohms to microfarads) in the tissues of the body or any other substance.

**a. of incidence,** (1) the a. that a ray entering a refracting medium makes with a line drawn perpendicular to the surface of this medium; (2) the a. that a ray striking a reflecting surface makes with a line perpendicular to this surface.

**incident a.,** a. of incidence.

**inci'sal a.,** the a. formed by the junction of either the mesial or distal surfaces with the cutting edge of an incisor or cuspid tooth.

**incisal guide a.,** the a. formed with the horizontal plane by drawing a line in the sagittal plane between incisal edges of the maxillary and mandibular central incisors when the teeth are in centric occlusion.

**a. of inclination,** a. of depression; the a. formed by the meeting of a line drawn through the shaft of the femur with one passing through the long axis of the femoral neck; normally it is about 127°. See fig. under Alsberg's *triangle.*

**inferior a. of scapula,** *angulus* inferior.

**iridocor'neal a.,** *angulus* iridocornealis.

**a. of the iris,** *angulus* iridocornealis.

**Jacquart's facial a.,** similar to Camper's facial a., but intersection is always at nasal spine point; additional variation uses supraorbital point instead of glabella, and this latter version is also known as ophryospinal facial a. or Topinard's facial a.

**a. of the jaw,** *angulus* mandibulae.

**kappa a.,** the a. between the pupillary axis and the visual axis, measured at the nodal point.

**labiogingival a.,** see labiogingival.

**lambda a.,** the a. between the pupillary axis and the line of sight, measured from the pupil of the eye.

**lateral a. of eye,** *angulus* oculi lateralis.

**lateral a. of scapula,** *angulus* lateralis.

**lateral a. of the uterus,** the upper part of the side of the uterus at the point of its junction with the uterine tube.

**limiting a.,** critical a.

**line a.,** see cavity line a.

**linguogingival, linguo-occlusal a.'s,** see these terms.

**Louis' a.,** *angulus* sterni.

**Ludwig's a.,** *angulus* sterni.

**lumbosacral a.,** the angle between the long axis of the lumbar part of the vertebral column and that of the sacrum.

**a. of the mandible,** *angulus* mandibulae.

**mastoid a.,** *angulus* mastoideus.

**maxillary a.,** the a. formed by a line drawn from the ophryon and another from the point of the mandible and meeting at the contact between the upper and lower incisor teeth.

**medial a. of eye,** *angulus* oculi medialis.

**mesial a.,** the a. formed by the meeting of the mesial with the labial (or buccal) or lingual surface of a tooth.

**mesiobuccal, mesiobucco-occlusal, mesiobuccopulpal, mesiocervical, mesiogingival, mesioincisal, mesiolabial, mesiolingual, mesiolinguo-occlusal, mesiolinguopulpal, mesio-occlusal a.'s,** see these terms.

**metafacial a.,** a. between the pterygoid processes and the base of the skull; Serres' a.

**meter a.,** the unit of convergence; the a. that the visual line makes with the median line when looking at an object one meter distant.

**a. of mouth,** *angulus* oris.

**Mulder's a.,** the a. formed by the intersection of Camper's horizontal line and a line drawn from the sphenoccipital suture to the root of the nose.

**occipital a.,** (1) *angulus* occipitalis; (2) Daubenton's a.

**olfactory a.,** the a. formed by the plane of the lamina cribrosa and the basicranial axis.

**ophryospi'nal a.,** see Jacquart's facial a.

**optic a.,** the a. formed by the meeting of the visual axes.

**parietal a.,** one formed by the meeting of the prolongation of two lines tangential to the most prominent part of the zygomatic arch and to the parietofrontal suture on each

side; when the lines remain parallel the a. is zero, when they diverge it is negative; also called Quatrefages's a.

**pelviver'tebral a.,** the a. made by the pelvis with the general axis of the trunk or spine.

**phren'opericar'dial a.,** the a. made by the pericardium with the upper surface of the diaphragm.

**Pirogoff's a.,** venous a. (1).

**point a.'s,** a.'s formed by the junction of three walls of a cavity. It is usually desirable that no two walls meet at an a. of more than 90° except in the inlay preparation, where a slight divergence of lateral walls is necessary.

**a. of polarization,** the a. of incidence at which the reflected light is all polarized.

**pontine a.,** cerebellopontine a.

**proximobuccal, proximolabial, proximolingual a.'s,** see these terms.

**pubic a.,** *angulus* subpubicus.

**Quatrefages' a.,** parietal a.

**Ranke's a.,** the a. formed by the horizontal plane of the head and a line passing from the center of the margin of the alveolar arch of the maxilla, below the nasal spine to the center of the frontonasal suture.

**a. of reflection,** the a. that a ray reflected from a surface makes with a line drawn perpendicular to this surface; it is equal to the a. of incidence (2).

**a. of refraction,** a. of deviation; the a. that a ray leaving a refracting medium makes with a line drawn perpendicular to the surface of this medium.

**Rolando's a.,** the a. which the fissure of Rolando makes with the midplane.

**Serres' a.,** metafacial a.

**SNA a.,** ANS a.

**solid a.,** point (trihedral) a.

**sphe'noid a., sphenoi'dal a.,** (1) one formed by the intersection of the top of the sella turcica (dorsum sellae), of lines coming from the nasal point and from the tip of the rostrum of the sphenoid; (2) *angulus* sphenoidalis.

**squint a.,** the a. formed by the line of vision of the strabismic eye and a line drawn to the object which should be fixed.

**sternal a.,** *angulus* sterni.

**ster'noclavic'ular a.,** the a. formed by the junction of the clavicle with the sternum.

**subpubic a.,** *angulus* subpubicus.

**superior a. of scapula,** *angulus* superior.

**Sylvian a.,** the a. formed by the Sylvian line and a line perpendicular to the horizontal plane tangential to the highest point of the hemisphere.

**tentor'ial a.,** the a. made by the plane of the tentorium and the basicranial axis.

**Topinard's facial a.,** see Jacquart's facial a.

**a. of torsion,** the a. formed by the axes of two portions of a long bone; denotes the amount of rotation either along one axis or between two axes.

**venous a.,** (1) Pirogoff's a.; the junction of the internal jugular and subclavian veins, toward which converge the external and the anterior jugular and the vertebral veins, the thoracic duct in the left a. and the right lymphatic duct in the right a.; (2) in neuroradiology, the a. of unison of the thalamostriate vein (vena terminalis) with the internal cerebral vein, usually closely behind the interventricular foramen of Monro.

**Virchow's a.,** Virchow-Holder a.; an a. formed by the meeting of a line drawn from the middle of the nasofrontal suture to the base of the anterior nasal spine with a line drawn from this last point to the center of the external auditory meatus.

**Virchow-Holder a.,** Virchow's a.

**visual a.,** the a. formed at the retina by the meeting of lines drawn from the periphery of the object seen.

**Vogt's a.,** a craniometric a. formed by the nasobasilar and alveolonasal lines.

**Weisbach's a.,** a craniometric a. formed by the junction, at the alveolar point, of lines passing from the basion and from the middle of the frontonasal suture.

**Welcker's a.,** *angulus* sphenoidalis.

**y-a.,** in craniometry, the a. at the inion formed by lines drawn from the hormion and the lambda.

**ang'licus su'dor** [ Mediev. L. + L. *sudor*, sweat ]. English sweating fever or sickness; infectious fever, characterized by profuse sweating which occurred in epidemic form during the Middle Ages.

**angor** (ang'gor) [ L. quinsy, anguish ]. Extreme distress or mental anguish.

    **a. abdom'inis,** *angina* abdominis.

    **a. animi,** a. pectoris (2); the sense of being in the act of dying, differing from the fear of death or the desire for death; a symptom that may occur with angina pectoris and occasionally in diseases of the medulla.

    **a. pectoris,** (1) Gairdner's *disease;* (2) a. animi.

**angostu'ra bark.** Cusparia bark; the bark of *Galipea offic-inalis;* formerly used as bitter tonic and antipyretic.

**Ångström** (awng'strem), Anders J., Swedish physicist, 1814–1874. See Å.'s *law, scale, unit.*

**Anguil'lula** [ Mod. L. dim. of L. *anguilla,* eel ]. A name no longer considered valid for a genus of free-living nematodes; see *Turbatrix.*

**ang'ula'tion.** Formation of an angle; an abnormal angle or bend in an organ.

**an'gulus,** gen. and pl. **an'guli** [ L. ] [ NA ]. An angle or corner; see angle.

    **a. acromia'lis** [ NA ], acromial angle; the prominent angle at the junction of the posterior and lateral borders of the acromion.

    **a. cos'tae** [ NA ], costal angle; the rather abrupt change in curvature of the body of a rib posteriorly, such that the neck and head of the rib are directed upward.

    **a. frontalis** [ NA ], frontal angle; the anterior superior angle of the parietal bone.

    **a. infectio'sus,** angular stomatitis.

    **a. infe'rior** [ NA ], inferior angle of the scapula; the acute angle formed by junction of the medial and lateral borders of the scapula.

    **a. infrasterna'lis** [ NA ], the angle between the lower borders of the costal cartilages of the two sides as they approach the sternum.

    **a. ir'idis,** a. iridocornealis.

    **a. iridocornea'lis** [ NA ], a. iridis; angle of the iris; iridocorneal a.; the acute a. between the iris and the cornea at the periphery of the anterior chamber of the eye.

    **a. latera'lis** [ NA ], lateral angle of the scapula; the blunt, concave head of the scapula forming the glenoid cavity at the junction of the superior and lateral borders of the bone.

    **a. mandib'ulae** [ NA ], angle of the mandible; angle of the jaw; the angle formed by the lower margin of the body and the posterior margin of the ramus of the mandible.

    **a. mastoid'eus** [ NA ], mastoid angle; the posteroinferior point of the parietal bone.

    **a. occipitalis** [ NA ], occipital angle; the posterior superior angle of the parietal bone.

    **a. oculi latera'lis** [ NA ], canthus; lateral angle of the eye; a. oculi temporalis; lateral canthus; external canthus; the angle formed by the junction of the lateral parts of the upper and lower eyelids.

    **a. oculi media'lis** [ NA ], canthus; medial angle of the eye; a. oculi nasalis; medial canthus; internal canthus; the angle formed by the union of the upper and lower eyelids medially.

    **a. oculi nasa'lis,** a. oculi medialis.

    **a. oculi temporalis,** a. oculi lateralis.

    **a. oris** [ NA ], angle of the mouth; the lateral limit of the oral fissure.

    **a. sphenoidalis** [ NA ], sphenoid angle (2); Welcker's angle; the anterior inferior angle of the parietal bone.

    **a. sterni** [ NA ], sternal angle; angle of Louis; angle of Ludwig; the angle between the manubrium and the body of the sternum.

    **a. subpu'bicus** [ NA ], subpubic or pubic a.; the a. formed by the inferior rami of the pubic bones.

    **a. supe'rior** [ NA ], superior angle of the scapula; formerly named the medial angle, it lies at the junction of the superior and medial borders of the bone.

**anhalon'idine.** 1,2,3,4-Tetrahydro-6,7-dimethoxy-1-methyl-8-isoquinolinol; an alkaloid from *Lophophora williamsii* (peyote).

**anhal'onine.** $C_{12}H_{15}NO_3$; an alkaloid from *Lophophora williamsii;* has been used in asthma and angina pectoris.

**Anhalon'ium lewin'ii.** *Lophophora williamsii.*

**anhaph'ia.** Anaphia.

**anhedonia** (an-he-do'nĭ-ah) [ G. *an-* priv. + *hedonē,* pleasure ]. Absence of pleasure from the performance of acts that would ordinarily be pleasurable.

**anhelation** (an-hĕ-la'shun) [ L. *anhelatio* ]. Panting; shortness of breath.

**anhe'lous.** Dyspneic.

**anhematopoietic** (an-he-mă-to-poy-et'ik) [ G. *an-* priv. + *haima,* blood, + *poieō,* to make ]. Pertaining to a deficiency or lack of formation of blood, or anhematosis.

**anhematosis** (an-he-mă-to'sis) [ G. *an-* priv. + *haimatōsis,* a changing into blood ]. A condition in which there is inadequate formation of blood, as a result of defective function of bone marrow.

**anhemolytic** (an-he-mo-lit'ik) [ G. *an-* priv. + *haima,* blood, + *lytikos,* capable of loosing or dissolving ]. Not hemolytic, *i.e.,* not capable of destroying red blood cells by means of lysis.

**anhepatogenic** (an-hep'ă-to-jen'ik) [ G. *an-* priv. + *hepar,* liver, + suffix *-gen,* to produce ]. Not produced in or by the liver.

**anhidrosis, anidrosis** (an-hi-dro'sis, an-ĭ-dro'sis) [ G. *an-* priv. + *hidrōs,* sweat ]. Absence of sweating.

**anhidrotic, anidrotic** (an-hi-drot'ik, an-ĭ-drot'ik). 1. Relating to, or characterized by, anhidrosis. 2. An agent that reduces, prevents, or stops sweating. 3. Denoting a reduction or absence of sweat glands, characteristic of congenital ectodermal defect.

**anhis'tic, anhis'tous** [ G. *an-* priv. + *histos,* web ]. Without apparent structure.

**an'hormo'nia.** State of hormone deficiency.

**anhy'drase.** An enzyme that catalyzes the removal of water from a compound. Most such enzymes are known as hydrases, hydro-lyases, or dehydratases.

    **carbonic a.,** carbonate dehydratase; see under carbonate.

**anhydration** (an'hi-dra'shun). Dehydration.

**anhydremia** (an-hi-dre'mĭ-ah) [ G. *an-* priv. + *hydōr,* water, + *haima,* blood ]. A decreased volume of the fluid portion (plasma) of blood.

**anhy'dride.** An oxide that can combine with water to form an acid or that is derived from an acid by the abstraction of water. For individual anhydrides, see specific name.

**anhydro-** (an-hi'dro-) [ G. *an-*priv., + *hydōr,* water ]. Chemical prefix denoting the removal of water.

**anhydrohemoglobin** (an-hi'dro-he'mo-glo'bin). The hemoglobin obtained upon drying, with the water molecule, ordinarily bound to the ferrous ion of heme, removed.

**anhy'droleucovor'in.** 5,10-Methenyltetrahydrofolic acid; an intermediate formed in the folic acid-catalyzed glycine-serine interconversion.

**anhy'drosug'ars.** Sugars from which one or more molecules of water have been eliminated.

**anhydrous** (an-hi'drus). Containing no water, especially water of crystallization.

**anhypno'sis** [ G. *an-* priv. + *hypnos,* sleep ]. Insomnia.

**aniacinamidosis** (ă-ni'ă-sin-am'ĭ-do'sis). Aniacinosis; deficiency of niacinamide, which if severe and protracted may lead to pellagra.

**ani'acino'sis.** Aniacinamidosis.

**anianthinopsy** (an-ĭ-an'thĭ-nop'sĭ) [ G. *an-* priv. + *ianthinos,* violet colored, + *opsis,* vision ]. Violet blindness; inability to recognize violet or purple.

**anicteric** (an-ik-ter'ik). Not icteritious.

**anidean** (an-id'e-an) [ see anideus ]. Shapeless; amorphous; denoting a formless mass of tissue.

**anideus** (an-id'e-us) [ G. *an-* priv. + *eidos,* shape ]. Fetu anideus; a parasitic fetus consisting of a poorly different ated mass of tissue with slight indications of parts.

    **embryonic a.,** a blastoderm without axial organization

**ani'dous.** Anidean.

**anidro'sis.** Anhidrosis.

**anile** (an'il) [ L. *anilis,* fr. *anus,* an old woman ]. In one dotage; imbecile.

**anileridine** (an'ĭ-lĕr'ĭ-dēn) (NF). LERITINE; ethyl 1-(4 aminophenethyl)-4-phenylisonipecotate; related chem cally and pharmacologically to meperidine hydrochlorid Used for the relief of moderate to severe pain; also mildl antihistaminic and spasmolytic. Its addiction liability is equivalent to that of morphine.

**anilide** (an'ĭ-lid). An *N*-acyl aniline, *e.g.*, acetanilide, $CH_3CONHC_6H_5$.

**an'ilinc'tion, an'ilinc'tus** [ L. *anus* + *linctio* (*lingere*), licking ]. Sexual stimulation by licking or kissing.

**aniline** (an'ĭ-lin, -lēn) [ Ar. *an-nil*, indigo ]. Phenylamine; aminobenzene; $C_6H_5(NH_2)$; an oily, colorless or brownish fluid, of aromatic odor and acrid taste, that is the parent substance of many synthetic dyes. It is derived from benzene by the substitution of the group —$NH_2$ for one of the hydrogen atoms.

**a. blue**, a mixture of sulfonated triphenylmethane dyes used widely as a connective tissue stain.

**an'ilinism.** Anilism.

**anilinophil, anilinophile** (an-ĭ-lin'o-fil, -fil) [ aniline + G. *philos*, fond ]. Anilinophilous; denoting a cell or histologic structure that takes readily an aniline stain.

**anilinoph'ilous.** Anilinophil.

**an'ilism.** Anilinism; chronic aniline poisoning characterized by gastric and cardiac weakness, vertigo, muscular depression, intermittent pulse, and cyanosis.

**anil'ity** [ L. *anilitas*, fr. *anus*, an old woman ]. Dotage; imbecility.

**an'il-quin'oline.** Quinoline prepared synthetically from aniline.

**anima** (an'ĭ-mah) [ L. air, breath, soul ]. 1. The soul or spirit; see animus (4). 2. In Jungian psychology, the inner self, in contrast with the outer aspect of the personality (persona); a female archtype in a man.

**animal** [ L. ]. 1. A living, sentient organism that has membranous cell walls, requires oxygen and organic foods, and is capable of voluntary movement as distinguished from a plant or mineral. 2. One of the lower a. organisms as distinguished from man.

**cold-blooded a.,** poikilotherm.

**control a.,** in laboratory or clinical experimentation, the rabbit, guinea pig, or other a. submitted to the same conditions as the others used for the experiment, with the crucial factor (such as the injection of antitoxin, the administration of a drug, etc.) omitted. See also control, and control *experiment*.

**Houssay a.,** one that has been pancreatectomized and hypophysectomized. Named after the discoverer of the principle that a.'s are more sensitive to insulin after removal of the pituitary, and that after this operation the intensity of diabetes in depancreatized a.'s is diminished.

**normal a.,** in bacteriology, an experimental a. that has neither suffered an attack of a particular disease nor received an injection of the specific microorganism or its toxin.

**thalamic a.,** an experimental a. whose brain anterior to the optic thalami has been removed.

**warm-blooded a.,** hematherm.

**animalcule** (an-ĭ-mal'kūl) [ Mod. L. *animalculum*, dim. of L. *animal*, a living being ]. 1. Obsolete term for a microscopic animal organism or protozoan. 2. Term used by believers in the defunct preformation theory to designate the supposed miniature body contained in one of the sex cells.

**animal'ity.** The sum of characteristics distinguishing an animal from a vegetable organism.

**animation** (an'ĭ-ma'shun) [ L. *animo*, pp. *-atus*, to make alive; *anima*, breath, soul ]. 1. The state of being alive. 2. Liveliness; high spirits.

**suspended a.,** a temporary state resembling death, with cessation of respiration; may also refer to certain forms of hibernation in animals or to endospore formation by some bacteria.

**an'imatism.** The attribution of mental or spiritual qualities to both living beings and nonliving things; see also animism.

**an'imism.** The view that all things in nature, both animate and inanimate, contain a spirit or soul; held by primitive peoples and small children. See also animatism.

**an'imus** [ L. *animus*, breath, rational soul in man, intellect, conscious power, will, disposition ]. 1. An animating or energizing spirit. 2. Intention to do something; disposition. 3. In psychiatry, a spirit of active hostility or grudge. 4. The

soul; anima; the ideal image toward which a person strives. 5. In Jungian psychology, a male archetype in a woman.

**anincretinosis** (an'ĭn-kre-tĭ-no'sis) [ G. *an-* priv. + incretion, + suffix *-osis*, condition ]. A disorder arising from failure of one or more of the organs of internal secretion.

**anion** (an'i-on). An ion that carries a negative charge, going therefore to the positively charged anode. In salts the acid radicals are a.'s.

**anion exchange.** The process by which an anion in a mobile (liquid) phase exchanges with another anion previously bound to a solid, positively charged phase, the latter being an anion exchanger. An anion-exchange process takes place when $Cl^-$ is exchanged for $OH^-$ in desalting. The reaction is $Cl^-$ (in solution) + ($OH^-$ on anion exchanger$^+$) → ($Cl^-$ on anion exchanger) + $OH^-$ (in solution). Combined with cation exchange, *q.v.*, NaCl is removed from solution. Anion exchange may also be used chromatographically, to separate anions, and medicinally, to remove an anion (*e.g.* $Cl^-$) from gastric contents or bile acids in the intestine.

**anion exchanger.** An insoluble solid, usually a polystyrene or a polysaccharide, that has attached to it cation groups such as —$NR_3^+$ or —$NHR_2^+$, which can attract and hold anions that pass by in a moving solution in exchange for anions in the solution.

**anionic** (an'i-on'ĭk). Referring to a negatively charged ion.

**an'ionot'ropy.** The migration of a negative ion in tautomeric changes.

**aniridia** (an'ĭ-rid'ĭ-ah). Almost complete absence of the iris; see also irideremia.

**an'isate.** 1. A salt of anisic acid, usually possessing antiseptic properties. 2. To flavor with anise.

**anischuria** (an-is-ku'rĭ-ah) [ G. *an-* priv. + *ischouria*, retention of urine ]. Incontinence of urine.

**anise** (an'is). The fruit of *Pimpinelĺla anisum* (family Umbelliferae); aromatic and carminative.

**a. camphor,** anethole.

**a. oil** (USP, BP), the volatile oil distilled with steam from the dried ripe fruit of *Pimpinella anisum* or *Illicium verum;* a flavoring agent.

**aniseiko'nia** (an'ĭ-si-ko'nĭ-ah) [ G. *anisos*, unequal, + *eikōn*, an image ]. A relative difference in size or shape of the ocular images, correctable by iseikonic lenses when clinically significant.

**anis'ic.** Relating to anise.

**a. acid,** umbellic acid; *p*-methoxybenzoic acid; a crystalline volatile acid obtained from aniseed; it forms the antiseptic anisates.

**anisindione** (an'ĭ-sin-di'ōn). MIRADON; 2-*p*-anisylindan-1,3-dione; an anticoagulant with pharmacologic actions similar to those of phenindione and bishydroxycoumarin.

**aniso-** (an-i'so-, an'ĭ-so-) [ G. *anisos*, unequal ]. Combining form meaning unequal or dissimilar.

**anisoaccommodation** (an-i'so-ă-kom-o-da'shun) [ aniso- + L. *accommodare*, to adapt ]. Variation between the two eyes in accommodation capacity.

**anisochromasia** (an-i'so-kro-ma'zĭ-ah) [ aniso- + G. *chroma*, color ]. The unequal distribution of hemoglobin in the red blood cells, such that the periphery is pigmented and the central region is virtually colorless, as observed in films of blood from persons with certain forms of anemia caused by deficiency of iron. Normal red blood cells show mild a. because of their biconcave shape.

**anisochromatic** (an-i'so-kro-mat'ĭk). 1. Not uniformly of one color. 2. Term frequently used in referring to mixtures of two colors in which characters may be recognized differently by persons with dichromatic perception (partial color blindness) than by those with normal perception.

**anisocoria** (an-i'so-ko'rĭ-ah) [ aniso- + G. *korē*, pupil ]. A condition in which the two pupils are not of equal size.

**anisocytosis** (an-i'so-si-to'sis) [ aniso- + G. *kytos*, cell, + suffix *-osis*, condition ]. Considerable variation in the size of cells that are normally uniform, especially with reference to red blood cells.

**anisodactylous** (an-i'so-dak'tĭ-lus). Having corresponding digits of unequal length.

**anisodactyly** (an-i'so-dak'tĭ-lĭ) [ aniso- + G. *daktylon*, finger ]. Unequal length in corresponding fingers.

**anisogamy** (an'ĭ-sog-ă-mĭ) [ aniso- + G. *gamos*, marriage ]. Fusion of two gametes unequal in size or form; fertilization as distinguished from isogamy or conjugation.

**anisognathous** (an'ĭ-sog'nă-thus) [ aniso- + G. *gnathos*, jaw ]. Having jaws of abnormal relative size, the upper being wider than the lower.

**an'isohy'percyto'sis** [ aniso- + G. *hyper*, above, + *kytos*, a hollow (cell) ]. An abnormally high white blood cell count, with changes in the normal percentages of the various types, especially with reference to cells of the granulocytic series.

**an'isohy'pocyto'sis** [ aniso- + G. *hypo*, beneath, + *kytos*, a hollow (cell) ]. An abnormally low white blood cell count, with changes in the normal percentages of the various types, especially with reference to cells of the granulocytic series.

**anisoiconia** (an-i'so-i-ko'nĭ-ah). Rarely used term for aniseikonia.

**anisokaryosis** (an-i'so-kar-ĭ-o'sis) [ aniso- + G. *karyon*, nut (nucleus), + suffix *-osis*, condition ]. Variation in size of nuclei, greater than the normal range for a tissue.

**an'isole.** Methoxybenzene; $C_6H_5OCH_3$; obtained from anisic acid; used in perfumery.

**anisoleukocytosis** (an-i'so-lu'ko-si-to'sis) [ aniso- + G. *leukos*, white, + *kytos*, cell ]. Anisonormocytosis.

**anisomastia** (an-i'so-mas'tĭ-ah) [ aniso- + G. *mastos*, breast ]. Asymmetrical breasts.

**anisomelia** (an-i'so-me'lĭah) [ aniso- + G. *melos*, limb ]. A condition of inequality between two paired limbs.

**ani'sometro'pia** [ aniso- + G. *metron*, measure, + *ōps*, sight ]. A difference in the power of refraction of the two eyes.

**ani'sometrop'ic.** 1. Relating to anisometropia. 2. Having eyes of unequal refractive power.

**anisomy'cin.** Flagecidin; 2-*p*-methoxyphenylmethyl-3-acetoxy-4-hydroxypyrrolidine; antibiotic trichomonacide.

**anisomyopia** (an-i'so-mi-o'pĭ-ah). Unequal myopia in the two eyes.

**an'isonor'mocyto'sis** [ aniso- + L. *norma*, rule, + G. *kytos*, a hollow (cell) ]. A white blood cell count within the normal range, although there are abnormal percentages of the various types, especially cells of the granulocytic series.

**anisophoria** (an-i-so-fo'rĭ-ah) [ aniso- + G. *phora*, a carrying ]. Heterophoria in which the degree of phoria varies with the direction of gaze.

**aniso'pia** [ aniso- + G. *ōps*, eye ]. A condition of inequality in visual power between the two eyes.

**anisopiesis** (an-i'so-pi-e'sis) [ aniso- + G. *piesis*, pressure ]. Unequal arterial blood pressure on the two sides of the body.

**anisorrhythmia** (an-i-so-rith'mĭ-ah) [ aniso- + G. *rhythmos*, rhythm ]. Irregular action of the heart, or absence of synchronism in the rate of auricles and ventricles.

**anisosphygmia** (an-i-so-sfig'me-ah) [ aniso- + G. *sphygmos*, pulse ]. Difference in volume, force, or time of the pulse in the corresponding arteries on two sides of the body, *e.g.*, the two radials, or femorals.

**anisospore** (an-i'so-spōr) [ aniso- + G. *sporos*, seed ]. A sexual cell capable of uniting with one of the opposite sex to form a new organism, as distinguished from the nonsexual cell, or isospore.

**anisosthenic** (an-i-sos-then'ik) [ aniso- + G. *sthenos*, strength ]. Of unequal strength; denoting two muscles or groups of muscles either paired or antagonists.

**anisoton'ic** [ aniso- + G. *tonus*, tension ]. Not having equal tension; having unequal osmotic pressure.

**anisotropic** (an'i-so-trop'ik) [ aniso- + G. *tropos*, a turning ]. 1. Not equal in all directions. 2. Doubly refractive; birefringent. See refraction.

**anisotro'pine methylbromide** (USAN). VALPIN; 8-methyltropinium bromide 2-propylvalerate; anticholinergic, intestinal antispasmodic.

**anisu'ria** [ aniso- + G. *ouron*, urine, + suffix *-ia*, condition ]. Excretion of urine at varying rates, as measured from hour to hour.

**anisylbu'tamide.** 1-Butyl-3-(*p*-methoxyphenylsulfonyl)-urea; hypoglycemic agent.

**anitrogenous** (ă-ni-troj'e-nus). Non-nitrogenous.

**Anitschkow,** Nikolai, Russian pathologist, *1885. See A. *cell, myocyte.*

**ankle** (ang'kl). 1. The joint between the leg and foot in which the tibia and fibula above articulate with the talus below. 2. The region of the a. joint. 3. Talus.

**ankylo-** (ang'kĭ-lo-) [ G. *ankylos*, bent, crooked; *ankylōsis*, stiffness or fixation of a joint ]. Combining form meaning bent, crooked, stiff, or fixed. See also words beginning with ancylo-.

**ankyloblepharon** (ang'kĭ-lo-blef'ar-on) [ ankylo- + G. *blepharon*, eyelid ]. Blepharosynechia.

**ankylocolpos** (ang'kĭ-lo-kol'pos) [ ankylo- + G. *kolpos*, womb (vagina) ]. Adhesion of the walls of the vagina; atresia or imperforation of vagina.

**ankylodactyly, ankylodactylia** (ang'kĭ-lo-dak'tĭ-lĭ, -dak-til'ĭ-ah) [ ankylo- + G. *daktylos*, finger ]. Adhesion between two or more fingers or toes. See also syndactyly.

**ankyloglossia** (ang'kĭ-lo-glos'ĭ-ah) [ ankylo- + G. *glōssa*, tongue ]. Tongue-tie.

**ankylomele** (ang'kĭ-lo-me'le) [ ankylo- + G. *mēlē*, probe ]. A curved or bent probe.

**ankylopoietic** (ang'kĭ-lo-poi-et'ik). Forming ankylosis.

**ankyloproctia** (ang'kĭ-lo-prok'shĭ-ah) [ ankylo- + G. *prōktos*, anus ]. Imperforation or stricture of the anus.

**an'kylosed.** Stiffened; bound by adhesions; denoting a joint in a state of ankylosis.

**ankylosis** (ang'kĭ-lo'sis) [ G. *ankylōsis*, stiffening of a joint ]. Stiffening or fixation of a joint.

    **artificial a.,** arthrodesis.

    **bony a.,** synostosis.

    **dental a.,** rigid fixation of tooth to the surrounding bony alveolus as a result of periodontal membrane ossification.

    **extracapsular a.,** spurious a.; stiffness of a joint due to induration of the surrounding tissues.

    **false a.,** fibrous a.

    **fibrous a.,** false a.; ligamentous a.; stiffening of a joint due to the presence of fibrous bands between the bones forming the joint.

    **intracapsular a.,** stiffness of a joint due to the presence of bony or fibrous adhesions between the bones forming the joint.

    **ligamen'tous a.,** fibrous a.

    **spurious a.,** extracapsular a.

    **true a.,** synostosis.

**Ankylos'toma.** *Ancylostoma.*

**ankylos'toma** [ ankylo- + G. *stoma*, mouth ]. Trismus.

**ankylostomi'asis.** Ancylostomiasis.

**an'kylot'ic.** Characterized by or pertaining to ankylosis.

**ankylot'omy.** The surgical procedure for relieving ankyloglossia.

**ankylurethria** (ang-kil-u-re'thrĭ-ah) [ ankylo- + G. *ourēthra*, urethra, + suffix *-ia*, condition ]. Imperforation or stricture of the urethra.

**an'kyroid.** Ancyroid.

**anlage,** pl. **anla'gen** (ahn'lah-gheh) [ Ger. hereditary factor ]. 1. Primordium; a term frequently appearing in embryological literature. 2. In psychoanalysis, genetic predisposition to a given trait or personality characteristic.

**Annandale,** Thomas, Scottish surgeon, 1838–1907. See A.'s *operation.*

**anneal** (an-nēl') [ A.S. *anaelan*, to burn ]. 1. To soften or temper a metal by controlled heating and cooling; the process makes a metal more easily adapted, bent, or swaged, and less brittle. 2. In dentistry, to heat gold leaf preparatory to its insertion into a cavity, in order to drive off adsorbed gases and other contaminants. See also annealing *lamp,* annealing *tray.*

**annec'tent** [ L. *an-necto,* pres. p. *-nectnes,* pp. *-nexus,* to join to ]. Connected with; joined.

**annex'a.** Adnexa.

**annex'al.** Adnexal.

**annexec'tomy.** Adnexectomy.

**annexi'tis** Adnexitis.

**annex'opexy** Adnexopexy.

**annotto** (ah-not′o). Also spelled arnotta, annotta, annatto. Coloring matter extracted from the seeds of *Bixa orellana*. Contains bixin and several other yellow to orange-red pigments. Used for coloring butter, margarine, cheese, and oils.

**an′nular** [ L. *annulus*, ring ]. Ring-shaped.

**an′nuloplasty** [ L. *annulus*, ring, + G. *plassō*, to form ]. Plastic reconstruction of an incompetent (usually mitral) cardiac valve.

**annulorrhaphy** (an-u-lor′a-fī) [ L. *annulus*, ring, + G. *raphē*, seam ]. Closure of a hernial ring by suture.

**an′nulus.** See anulus. (In *Nomina Anatomica* the spelling has been changed from annulus to anulus.)

**AnOC.** Abbreviation for anodal opening *contraction*.

**anochlesia** (an′o-kle′zī-ah) [ G. *an*- priv. + *ochlēsis*, disturbance ]. 1. Catalepsy. 2. Quietude.

**anochromasia** (an′o-kro-ma′zī-ah) [ G. *anō*, upward, + *chrōma*, color ]. 1. Failure of cells or other elements of tissue to be colored in the usual manner when treated with a stain (or stains). 2. Accumulation of hemoglobin in the peripheral zone of erythrocytes, thereby resulting in a pale, virtually colorless central portion.

**anociassociation** (ă-no′sī-ă-so′sī-a′shun) [ G. *a*- priv. + L. *noceo*, to injure, + association ]. The theory that afferent stimuli, especially pain, contribute to the development of surgical shock, and, as a corollary, that nerve blocks protect against shock.

**anococcygeal** (a-no-kok-sij′e-al). Relating to both anus and coccyx.

**ano′dal.** Anodic; of, pertaining to, or emanating from an anode.

**anode** (an′ōd) [ G. *anodos*, a way up, fr. *ana*, up, + *hodos*, a way ]. Anelectrode; the positive pole of a galvanic battery or the electrode connected with it; an electrode toward which negatively charged ions (anions) migrate; *cf.* cathode.

**ano′dic.** Anodal.

**anod′mia** [ G. *an*- priv. + *odmē*, stench ]. Anosmia.

**an′odont.** A person without teeth.

**anodontia** (an-o-don′shī-ah) [ G. *an*- priv. + *odous*, tooth ]. Absence of teeth.

  **partial a.,** hypodontia.

**anodont′ism.** The state in which all tooth germs have failed to develop.

**anodyne** (an′o-dīn) [ G. *an*- priv. + *odynē*, pain ]. A compound less potent than an anesthetic or a narcotic but capable of relieving pain.

**anoesia** (an-o-e′sī-ah) [ G. *anoēsia*, from *a*- priv. + *noos*, perception ]. Anoia; lack of the power of comprehension, as in severe and profound levels of mental retardation.

**anoetic** (an-o-et′ic). 1. Relating to or suffering from anoesia. 2. Incomprehensible.

**a′nogen′ital.** Relating in any way to both the anal and the genital regions.

**anoia** (an-oy′ah). Anoesia.

**anomalopia** (ă-nom′ă-lo′pī-ah) [ G. *anōmalos*, irregular, + *ōps*, eye ]. Partial color blindness in which the appreciation of red or of green is less than normal. A person whose perception of red is defective (protanomaly), to match a yellow light with a mixture of red and green light, requires the addition of more red than does a normal person; one who is defective in green perception (deuteranomaly) requires the addition of more green light to make a match.

**anom′aloscope** [ G. *anōmalos*, irregular, + *skopeō*, to examine ]. An instrument used for the detection of color blindness; *i.e.*, of dichromatism and of anomalous trichromatism.

**anomalot′rophy** [ G. *anōmalos*, irregular, + *trophē*, nourishment ]. Abnormality in the nutritive processes.

**anomaly** (ă-nom′ă-lī) [ G. *anōmalia*, irregularity ]. Deviation from the average or norm; anything unusual or irregular or contrary to a general rule.

  **Alder's a.,** coarse azurophilic granulation of leukocytes, especially granulocytes, which may be associated with gargoylism and Morquio's disease.

  **Aristotle's a.,** when a small object is held between the first and second fingers crossed in such a way that it touches or presses upon skin surfaces which ordinarily are not pressed upon simultaneously by a single object, it is perceived falsely as two.

  **Chediak-Steinbrinck-Higashi a.,** Chediak-Steinbrinck-Higashi *syndrome*.

  **developmental a.,** an a. established during intrauterine life; a congenital a.

  **Ebstein's a.,** Ebstein's disease; congenital downward displacement of the tricuspid valve into the right ventricle.

  **eugnathic a.,** eugnathia.

  **Freund's a.,** a narrowing of the upper aperture of the thorax by shortening of the first rib and its cartilage, resulting in defective expansion of the apex of the lung and consequent predisposition to tuberculosis.

  **Hegglin's a. of constitutional changes in neutrophils and platelets,** May-Hegglin a.; a disorder in which neutrophils and eosinophils contain basophilic structures known as Döhle or Amato bodies and in which there is faulty maturation of platelets, with thrombocytopenia.

  **May-Hegglin a.,** Hegglin's a. of constitutional changes in neutrophils and platelets.

  **morning glory a.,** an unusual congenital a. of the optic disk in which the nerve head is funnel-shaped, with a dot of white tissue at the end of the excavation, and is surrounded by an elevated pigmented anulus; the retinal vessels seen are multiple narrow bands at the edge of the disk.

  **Pelger-Huët nuclear a.,** an inherited congenital inhibition of lobulation of nuclei of neutrophilic leukocytes; most cells present band or bilobulate appearance, only an occasional cell has trilobed structure; not associated with disease, but may be confused with leukocyte "shift to left."

  **Peters' a.,** anterior chamber cleavage *syndrome*.

  **Rieger's a.,** iridocorneal mesodermal *dysgenesis*.

  **Shone's a.,** coarctation of the aorta, subaortic stenosis and stenosing ring of the left atrium found in association with a parachute mitral valve.

**an′omer.** One of two sugar molecules that are epimeric (see epimer) at the hemiacetal carbon atom (carbon-1 in aldoses, carbon-2 in ketoses); example, α-D-glucose and β-D-glucose are anomers.

**ano′mia** [ G. *a*- priv. + *ōnoma*, name ]. Visual aphasia; inability to name objects, although they are subjectively perceived.

**anomie** (an′o-me) [ Fr., fr. G. *anomia*, lawlessness ]. 1. Lawlessness; absence or weakening of social norms or values, with corresponding erosion of social cohesion. 2. In psychiatry, absence or weakening of individual norms or values, characterized by anxiety, isolation, and personal disorientation.

**anonychia, anonychosis** (an-o-nik′ī-ah, an-o-ni-ko′sis) [ G. *an*- priv. + *onyx* (*onych*-), nail ]. Absence of the nails.

**anon′yma** [ G. *an*- priv. + *onyma*, name ]. Innominate; unnamed; term formerly applied to the large vessels in the thorax, now called the truncus brachiocephalicus and the venae brachiocephalicae.

**anoopsia** (an-o-op′sī-ah) [ G. *anō*, upward, + *opsis*, vision ]. Obsolete term for hyperphoria.

**Anopheles** (an-of′e-lēz) [ G. *anōphelēs*, useless, harmful, fr. *an*- priv. + *ōpheleō*, to be of use ]. A genus of mosquitoes of the family *Culicidae*, subfamily *Anophelinae*. The sporogenous cycle of the malarial parasite is passed in the body cavity of female mosquitoes of certain species of this genus. A few selected important vectors for major malarious areas are listed below.

  **A. albima′nus** [ L. *albus*, white, + *manus*, hand ], a species having white hind feet, a common carrier of the malaria parasite in the West Indies and Central America.

  **A. albitar′sus,** a South American species that transmits malaria.

  **A. balabacensis,** vector in southeast Asia, Burma, and India.

  **A. culicifacies,** common malaria vector in India and Ceylon, China and the Oriental region.

  **A. darlingi,** a South American species, an important carrier of the malarial parasite.

  **A. fluviatilis,** important vector in India and Pakistan.

  **A. freeborni,** vector in western United States (although endemic cases are no longer present).

  **A. funestus,** an important African species that transmits malaria.

**A. gambiae,** an African species, important vector of malaria.

**A. labranchiae,** important vector in southern Europe and the Mediterranean basin.

**A. maculatus,** vector in Malaya and Indonesia.

**A. maculipen'nis,** the type species of this genus; the wings are marked by spots formed of collections of scales; one of the most widely spread species and active in the dissemination of malaria; formerly an important vector in continental Europe.

**A. minimus,** important vector throughout Oriental region.

**A. pseudopunctipennis,** a South American vector.

**A. quadrimaculatus,** formerly an important carrier of malaria in the southern United States.

**A. stephensi,** widespread important vector of malaria in Asia.

**A. sundaicus,** important vector in the Orient and southeast Asia.

**A. superpictus,** important vector in the Mediterranean region, Middle East, and southern Asia.

**anophelicide** (an-of'el-ĭ-sīd). An agent that destroys the *Anopheles* mosquito.

**anophelifuge** (an-of'el-ĭ-fūj). An agent that drives away or prevents the bite of *Anopheles* mosquitoes.

**Anopheli'nae.** A subfamily of the mosquitoes (Culicidae) consisting of several genera, including the carriers of the malarial parasite, all of which are included in the genus *Anopheles.*

**anoph'eline.** Referring to the *Anopheles* mosquito.

**anoph'elism.** The habitual presence in any region of *Anopheles* mosquitoes.

**anophoria** (an'o-fo'rī-ah) [ G. *anō*, upward, + *phora*, a carrying ]. Hyperphoria.

**anophthalmia** (an-of-thal'mĭ-ah) [ G. *an*- priv. + *ophthalmos*, eye ]. Congenital absence of one or both eyes.

**anophthal'mos.** Anophthalmus (1).

**anophthal'mus** [ G. *an*- priv. + *ophthalmos*, eye ]. 1. Congenital absence of one or both eyes, their place being taken by small solid or cystic bodies. 2. A person born without eyes.

**ano'pia** [ G. *an*- priv. + *ōps* (*ōp-*), eye ]. Obsolete term for (1) anophthalmia, (2) anopsia, and (3) hyperphoria.

**a'noplasty.** Plastic operation on the anus.

**Anoplocephala** (an-op'lo-sef'ă-lah) [ G. *anoplos*, unarmed, + *kephalē*, head ]. A genus of large tapeworms with strong linear segmentation that are found in mammals.

**A. perfolia'ta,** *Taenia equina;* a cosmopolitan tapeworm of the horse, donkey, mule, and zebra; cysticercoid larvae are found in arthropods.

**anop'sia** [ G. *an*- priv. + *opsis*, sight ]. Nonuse of the faculty of vision, such as results from congenital cataract, or high degrees of refractive errors, or from the disuse of one eye in marked strabismus with consequent amblyopia.

**anorchid** (an-or'kid). Anorchis; a male without testes.

**anorchidism** (an-or'kĭ-dizm) [ G. *an*- priv. + *orchis*, testis ]. Anorchism; absence of the testes.

**anorchis** (an-or'kis). Anorchid.

**anorchism** (an-or'kizm). Anorchidism.

**anorectal** (a'no-rek'tal). Relating to both anus and rectum.

**anorectic** (an-o-rek'tik). Anoretic. 1. Causing, or characterized by, anorexia. 2. An agent that causes anorexia.

**anoret'ic.** Anorectic.

**anorexia** an'o-rek'sī-ah) [ G. fr. *an*- priv. + *orexis*, appetite ]. Asitia; diminished appetite; aversion to food.

**a. nervo'sa,** a personality disorder manifested by extreme aversion to food, resulting in life-threatening weight loss and usually occurring in young women; considered a hysterical illness, but sometimes resembling or preceding a psychosis.

**anorex'iant.** A drug, process, or event that leads to anorexia.

**anorexigenic** (an'o-rek-sī-jen'ik). Promoting or causing anorexia.

**anorgan'ic.** Inorganic.

**anorganology** (an'or-gan-ol'o-jī) [ G. *an*- priv., + *organon*, tool, + *logos*, study ]. Abiology.

**anorgasmy** (an-or-gaz'mĭ). Failure to experience an orgasm.

**anorthog'raphy** [ G. *an*- priv. + *orthos*, straight, + *graphō*, to write ]. Agraphia.

**anortho'pia** [ G. *an*-priv. + *orthos*, straight, + *ōps*, eye ]. Obsolete term for heterophoria.

**anortho'sis** [ G. *an*- priv. + *orthos*, straight ]. Inability to experience penile erection, as in impotence.

**a'noscope.** A short speculum for examining the anal canal and lower rectum.

**Bacon's a.,** an instrument resembling a rectal speculum, with a long slit on one side and an electric light opposite.

**a'nosig'moidos'copy.** Endoscopy of the anus, rectum and sigmoid.

**anosmia** (an-oz'mĭ-ah) [ G. *an*- priv. + *osmē*, sense of smell ]. Olfactory anesthesia; loss of the sense of smell. It may be essential or true, due to lesion of the olfactory nerve; mechanical or respiratory, due to obstruction of the nasal fossae; reflex, due to disease in some other part or organ; functional, without any apparent causal lesion.

**anosmic** (an-oz'mik). Relating to anosmia.

**ano'sodiaphor'ia** [ G. *a*- priv. + *nosos*, disease, + *diaphoria*, difference ]. Indifference, real or assumed, regarding the presence of disease, specifically of paralysis.

**anosognosia** (ă-no'sog-no'sī-ah) [ G. *a*-priv. + *nosos*, disease, + *gnōsis*, knowledge ]. Ignorance, real or feigned, of the presence of disease, specifically of paralysis.

**anosogno'sic.** Relating to anosognosia.

**a'nospi'nal.** Relating to the anus and the spinal cord.

**anos'teopla'sia.** [ G. *an*- priv. + *osteon*, bone, + *plassō*, to form ]. Failure of bone formation.

**anostosis** (an'os-to'sis) [ G. *an*- priv. + *osteon*, bone ]. Failure of ossification.

**anotia** (an-o'shī-ah) [ G. *an*- priv. + *ous*, ear ]. Congenital absence of one or both ears.

**anotropia** (an'o-tro'pī-ah) [ G. *anō*, up, + *tropē*, a turning ]. Rarely used term meaning upward squint, hyperphoria.

**ano'tus** [ G. *an*- priv. + *ous* (*ōt-*), ear ]. An individual without ears.

**a'noves'ical.** Relating in any way to both anus and urinary bladder.

**anov'ular.** Anovulatory; not related to or coincident with ovulation.

**anovula'tion.** Suspension or cessation of ovulation.

**anov'ulatory.** Anovular.

**anoxemia** (an'ok-se'mĭ-ah) [ G. *an*- priv. + oxygen + G. *haima*, blood ]. Absence of oxygen in arterial blood; often erroneously used in place of hypoxemia.

**anoxia** (an-ok'sĭ-ah) [ G. *an*- priv. + oxygen + suffix -*ia*, condition ]. Absence of oxygen in inspired gases, arterial blood, or tissues; to be differentiated from hypoxia.

**altitude a.,** hypobaropathy.

**anemic a.,** a. resulting from a decreased concentration of functional hemoglobin or a reduced number of erythrocytes; it is caused by hemorrhage or anemia of various types, or by poisoning with CO, nitrites, or chlorates.

**anoxic a.,** a. resulting from a defective mechanism of oxygenation in the lungs; may be caused by: (1) a low tension of oxygen, *e.g.*, high altitudes, foreign gases; (2) abnormalities in pulmonary tissues, as in pneumonia, asthma, emphysema, drowning, paralysis of respiratory muscles, and so on; and (3) a right-to-left shunt in the heart.

**diffusion a.,** abrupt, transient decrease in alveolar oxygen tension when room air is inhaled at the conclusion of a nitrous oxide anesthesia.

**fulminant a.,** stuporous or comatose condition resulting from an unusually rapid decrease in the content of oxygen in arterial blood and tissues, especially the brain.

**histotox'ic a.,** poisoning of the respiratory enzyme systems of the tissues, as in the inhibition of cytochrome oxidase by cyanides or the depression of dehydrogenases by barbiturates and morphine; owing to the inability of tissue cells to utilize oxygen, its tension in arterial and capillary blood is usually greater than normal.

**a. neonator'um,** any a. observed in newborn infants.

**stagnant a.,** as a result of slower peripheral circulation through the tissues, the oxygen tension in capillary blood is less than normal; on the other hand, the saturation, total load, and tension in arterial blood is normal; the condition is associated with congestive cardiac failure, postoperative shock, and impaired venous return.

**anoxiate** (an-ok′sĭ-āt). To cause anoxia; to deprive of an adequate supply of oxygen, either locally or in the blood and tissues generally, as a result of interference with respiratory or circulatory functions.

**ansa,** gen. and pl. **an′sae** (an′sah) [ L. loop, handle ] [ NA ]. Any anatomical structure in the form of a loop or an arc.

**a. cervica′lis** [ NA ], a loop in the cervical plexus formerly known as the a. hypoglossi. It consists of fibers from the first three cervical nerves, some of which accompany the hypoglossal nerve for a short distance.

**Haller′s a.,** a communicating branch between the facial nerve and the glossopharyngeal nerve below the stylomastoid foramen.

**Henle′s a.,** nephronic *loop.*

**a. hypoglos′si,** a. cervicalis.

**lenticular a.,** a. lenticularis.

**a. lenticula′ris** [ NA ], lenticular a. or loop; the tortuous efferent pathway of the globus pallidus, after Monakow′s description consisting of three parts: (1) a *ventral division* composed of thick, heavily myelinated fibers originating from the medial segment of the globus pallidus, forming a thick fiber plate beneath the latter′s ventral border, then curving dorsally around the medial margin of the internal capsule to join with (2) the *dorsal division,* formed by fibers likewise arising in the medial pallidal segment but perforating rather than circumventing the internal capsule; the fusion of both divisions forms the fasciculus lenticularis which courses caudomedialward through the subthalamic region, forming a fiber sheet, field H₂ of Forel, over the dorsal surface of the subthalamic nucleus and entering field H from the lateral side, most of its fibers then sharply curving dorsally and laterally into field H₁ with which they enter the thalamus to end in the nuclei centromedianus, ventralis lateralis, and ventralis anterior; fewer fibers of the fasciculus lenticularis continue their caudal course to terminate in the midbrain tegmentum. (3) An *intermediate division* of the ansa lenticularis is composed of fibers which arise from the lateral segment, perforate the cerebral peduncle, and terminate in the subthalamic nucleus.

**ansae nervo′rum spina′lium,** loops of the spinal nerves, connecting branches between the anterior spinal nerves.

**peduncular a.,** a. peduncularis.

**a. peduncula′ris** [ NA ], peduncular a. or loop; Reil′s a.; a complex fiber bundle curving around the medial edge of the internal capsule and connecting the anterior part of the temporal lobe—temporal cortex, amygdala, and olfactory cortex—with the mediodorsal nucleus of the thalamus; it enters the thalamus as a component of the inferior thalamic peduncle which also contains a major part of the fibers connecting the mediodorsal nucleus to the orbitofrontal cortex.

**Reil′s a.,** a. peduncularis.

**a. sacra′lis,** a nerve cord connecting the sympathetic nerve trunk and ganglion impar.

**a. subcla′via** [ NA ], subclavian loop; Vieussens′ loop or a.; the cord connecting the middle and inferior cervical sympathetic ganglia, forming a loop around the anterior and inferior aspects of the subclavian artery.

**Vieussens′ a.,** a. subclavia.

**a. vitellina,** term, used rarely, denoting a loop of vitelline blood vessels on the embryonic yolk sac.

**an′sate.** Ansiform.

**an′serine** [ L. *anserinus,* fr. *anser,* goose ]. 1. Relating to or resembling a goose or any part of one; see cutis anserina and pes anserinus. 2. Methylcarnosine; *N-β*-alanyl-1-methyl-L-histidine; present in muscle.

**anseri′nus** [ L. ] [ NA ]. Anserine (1).

**an′siform** [ L. *ansa,* handle, + *forma,* shape ]. Ansate; in the shape of a loop or arc.

**ansot′omy** [ L. *ansa,* handle + G. *tomē,* cutting ]. 1. Surgical division of a loop, usually a constricting loop. 2. Section of the ansa lenticularis for treatment of striatal syndromes.

**ant-.** See anti-.

**ant.** One of the most numerous insects (order Hymenoptera), characterized by an extraordinary development of colonial dwelling and caste specialization.

**harvester a.,** *Pogonomyrmex.*

**velvet a.,** a wingless mutilid wasp (family Mutilidae, order Hymenoptera) known for its venomous sting.

**antac′id.** 1. Neutralizing an acid. 2. Any agent that reduces or neutralizes acidity, as of the gastric juice or any other secretion.

**antag′onism** [ G. *antagōnisma,* from *anti,* against, + *agōnizomai,* to fight, fr. *agōn,* a contest ]. Opposition; mutual resistance; denoting mutual opposition in action between muscles, drugs, diseases, or physiologic processes or between drugs and diseases or drugs and physiologic processes.

**bacterial a.,** the killing, injury or inhibition of one bacterium by products of another.

**antag′onist.** Something opposing or resisting the action of another; denoting certain muscles, drugs, etc., that tend to neutralize or impede the action or effect of other muscles, etc. Reverse of synergist.

**associated a.,** one of two muscles or groups of muscles which pull in nearly opposite directions, but which, when acting together, move the part in a path between their diverging lines of action.

**competitive a.,** antimetabolite.

**enzyme a.,** antimetabolite, or inhibitor of enzyme action.

**antal′kaline.** Reducing or neutralizing alkalinity.

**antanalgesia** (ant′an-al-je′zĭ-ah) [ anti- + analgesia, *q.v.* ]. The ability of certain drugs to lower pain thresholds.

**antaphrodisiac** (ant′af-ro-diz′ĭ-ak). Anaphrodisiac.

**antaphrodit′ic.** 1. Anaphrodisiac. 2. Antivenereal.

**antapoplectic** (ant′ap-o-plek′tik). Having a supposed power to prevent apoplexy or relieve its effects.

**ant′arthrit′ic.** Antiarthritic. 1. Relieving arthritis. 2. A remedy for arthritis.

**antasthen′ic** [ anti- + G. *astheneia,* weakness ]. 1. Strengthening; invigorating. 2. An agent possessing such qualities.

**antasthmatic** (ant′az-mat′ik). 1. Tending to relieve or prevent asthma. 2. An agent that prevents or arrests an asthmatic attack.

**antatrophic** (ant′ă-trof′ik). 1. Preventing or curing atrophy. 2. An agent that promotes the restoration of atrophied structures.

**antaz′oline hydrochloride** (BP). ANTISTINE hydrochloride; phenazoline hydrochloride; 2-(*N*-benzylanilinomethyl)-2-imidazoline hydrochloride; a histamine-antagonizing agent used in treating allergy. Also available as a. phosphate (NF).

**ante-** [ L. *ante,* before ]. Prefix meaning before.

**antebrachial** (an′te-bra′kĭ-al). Antibrachial; relating to the forearm.

**antebrachium** (an-te-bra′kĭ-um) [ ante- + L. *brachium,* arm ]. [ NA ]. Forearm; also written antibrachium.

**antecar′dium.** Precordia.

**ante cibum** (an′te si′bum) [ L. ]. Before a meal.

**antecu′bital** [ ante- + L. *cubitum,* elbow ]. In front of the elbow.

**an′tecur′vature.** Anterior *curvature,* anteflexion.

**antefebrile** (an′te-feb′ril) [ ante- + L. *febris,* fever ]. Antepyretic.

**anteflex** [ ante- + L. *flecto,* pp. *flexus,* to bend ]. Anteflect; to bend forward, or cause to bend forward.

**anteflexed.** Anteflected; in a state of anteflexion.

**anteflexion** (an′te-flek′shun). Anteflection; a bending forward; a sharp forward curve or angulation; denoting especially a foward bend in the uterus at the junction of corpus and cervix. See fig. on p. 86.

**antemet′ic.** Antiemetic.

**an′te mor′tem** [ L. acc. case of *mors* (*mort*-), death ]. Before death. As an adjective, usually written as one word (antemortem examination).

**antena′tal** [ ante- + L. *natus,* birth ]. Occurring or existing before the birth of the individual.

**ante par′tum** [ ante- + L. *pario,* pp. *partus,* to bring forth. PARI- ]. Before labor or childbirth; as an adjective usually

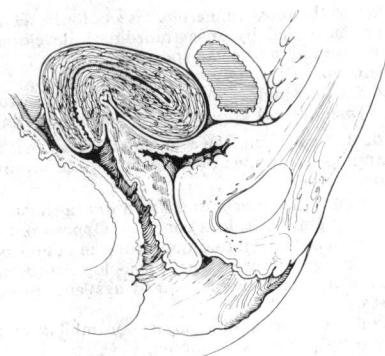

**Acute Anteflexion of the Uterus**

written as one word, antepartum; contrasted with intrapartum, during labor or delivery, and postpartum, after delivery.

**antephialtic** (ant'ef-ī-al'tik) [ anti- + G. *ephialtēs*, nightmare ]. Tending to prevent nightmares or distressing dreams.

**an'teposi'tion.** Forward or anterior position.

**an'te pran'dium** [ L. ]. Before a meal; in prescription writing (abbreviated a.p.), usually means before dinner.

**antepros'tate.** *Glandula* urethralis.

**antepyret'ic** [ ante- + G. *pyretos*, fever ]. Antefebrile; before the occurrence of fever; before the period of reaction following shock.

**ante'rior** [ L. ]. 1. Before, in relation to time or space; in front of or in the front part of; ventral; hemal; as contrasted with dorsal, neural. This is the NA general term applied to the front part of the body or any structure. 2. Sometimes used to designate a cranial and rostral position in quadrupeds or certain embryos. 3. A veterinary anatomy term restricted to parts of the eye and inner ear.

**antero-.** A prefix denoting anterior.

**an'teroexter'nal.** In front and to the outer side.

**an'terograde** [ L. *gradior*, pp. *gressus*, to step, go ]. Moving forward.

**an'teroinfer'ior.** In front and below.

**an'terointer'nal.** In front and to the inner side.

**an'terolat'eral.** In front and to the side, especially the outer side.

**an'terome'dial.** In front and toward the inner side or middle line.

**an'terome'dian.** In front and in the central line.

**an'teroposte'rior.** 1. Relating to both front and rear. 2. In x-ray describing the path of the beam from anterior to posterior through the patient to expose the film, *e.g.*, an A-P view of the abdomen.

**an'terosupe'rior.** In front and above.

**ant'erot'ic** [ anti- + G. *erōtikos*, pertaining to love ]. Pertaining to an effort to avoid erotic feelings.

**antever'sion** [ ante- + Mediev. L. *versio*, a turning ]. Turning forward, inclining forward as a whole without bending.

**antevert'ed.** Tilted forward; in a position of anteversion.

**antexion** (an-tek'-shun). Flexion of the spine.

**anthelix** (ant'he-liks, an'the-liks) [ anti- + G. *helix*, coil ] [ NA ]. Antihelix; an elevated ridge of cartilage anterior and roughly parallel to the posterior portion of the auricle helix.

**anthelmin'thic.** Anthelmintic.

**anthelmintic** (ant'hel-min'tik, an'thel-) [ anti- + G. *helmins*, worm ]. 1. Anthelminthic; helminthagogue; helminthic; vermifuge; an agent that destroys or expels intestinal worms. 2. Vermifugal; having the power to destroy or expel intestinal worms.

**an'thelone.** Urogastrone.

**a. E,** enterogastrone.

**a. U,** urogastrone.

**anthelotic** (ant'he-lot'ik) [ anti- + G. *hēlos*, nail, callus ]. A remedy for corns.

**anthema** (an-the'mah, an'the-mah) [ G. *anthein*, to blossom ]. Generalized eruption with sudden onset.

**antheridiol** (an'ther-id'ī-ōl). A sterol, with a molecular weight of 470, that serves as an ectohormone for several species of the genus *Achyla*, an aquatic fungus. Secreted by female strains, it promotes selective male somatic development and initiates a male hormonal secretion that induces formation of female sexual organs.

**anthiolimine.** ANTHIOMALINE; lithium antimony thiomalate; used in the treatment of filariasis and schistosomiasis.

**an'thocy'anins** [ G. *anthos*, flower, + *kyanos*, a blue substance ]. A group of floral pigments ranging from red to blue. They are soluble in water and alcohol but not in ether.

**Anthomyia** (an-tho-mi'ya) [ G. *anthos*, flower, + *myia*, fly ]. A genus of muscoid flies similar in appearance to the common housefly.

**A. canicula'ris,** a small black horsefly, the larvae of which have been reported as accidental parasites in the intestine of man, being hatched there from the ingested eggs; symptoms of gastroenteric irritation may be caused by it; adults may transport eggs of the tropical warble fly of man, *Dermatobia hominis*, a cause of myiasis.

**anthormone** (an-thor'mōn). Obsolete synonym for chalone.

**anthoxanthins** (an'tho-zan'thinz). Compounds responsible for the yellow and ivory shades of flowers; usually divided into flavones and flavonols.

**anthrace'mia.** Anthrax septicemia; the presence of *Bacillus anthracis* in the circulating blood, usually resulting from previously developed anthrax of the skin or lungs.

**an'thracene** [ G. *anthrax*, coal ]. A hydrocarbon obtained from coal tar; occurs as colorless crystals with violet fluorescence. The alizarin dyes are manufactured from it.

**Anthracene**

**anthra'cia** [ G. *anthrax*, carbuncle ]. The occurrence of carbuncles.

**anthracic** (an-thras'ik). Relating to anthrax.

**an'thracin.** 1. Anthracene. 2. A toxin of the anthrax bacillus.

**anthraco-** (an'thrā-ko-) [ G. *anthrax*, coal, charcoal, carbuncle. ANTHR- ]. Combining form relating to coal or to carbuncle.

**an'thracoid** [ G. *anthrax*, carbuncle, + *eidos*, resemblance ]. 1. Resembling a carbuncle or a malignant pustule. 2. Resembling anthrax or its bacillus.

**anthracom'eter** [ G. *anthrax*, coal (carbon), + *metron*, measure ]. An instrument for determining the amount of carbon dioxide in the air or other gaseous mixture.

**anthracosilicosis.** (an'thrā-ko-sil'ī-ko'sis) [ anthraco- + silicosis, *q.v.* ]. Accumulation of carbon and silica in the lungs from inhaled coal dust. The silica content produces fibrous nodules.

**anthraco'sis** [ anthraco- + G. suffix -osis, condition ]. Accumulation of carbon from inhaled smoke or coal dust in the lungs. Also called collier's lung; miner's lung; melanedema; pneumomelanosis.

**an'thracot'ic.** Characterized by anthracosis.

**an'thragal'lol.** 1,2,3-Trihydroxyanthraquinone; used as a brown dye and for the treatment of chronic dermatoses.

**an'thralin** (USP). Dithranol; 1,8,9-anthracenetriol; 1,8,9-dihydroxyanthranol; used as a substitute for chrysarobin in ointment for treatment of psoriasis and ringworm infestation.

**anthramu'cin.** A neutralizing material from the capsule of *Bacillus anthracis* that neutralizes serum and tissue antimicrobial action.

**anthramy′cin** (USAN). Antibiotic produced by *Streptomyces refuineus;* possesses antineoplastic activity.

**anthranil′ic acid.** *o*-Aminobenzoic acid; one of the products of tryptophan catabolism.

**anthraniloyl** (an-thrǎ-nil′o-il). The radical of anthranilic acid (R—CO—).

**anthrapurpurin** (an′thrǎ-pur′pu-rin). Trihydroxyanthraquinone; $C_{14}H_8O_5$; a purple dye used in histology as a reagent for calcium.

**9,10-anthraquinone** (an′thrǎ-kwǐ′nōn). 9,10-Dioxoanthracene; the basis of natural cathartic principles in plants; see quinone. 2. A yellow substance used in the manufacture of alizarin and as a reagent.

9,10-Anthraquinone

**anthraro′bin.** 1,2,10-Anthracenetriol; parasiticide.

**anthrax** [ G. *anthrax* (*anthrak*-), charcoal, coal, a carbuncle. ANTHR- ]. 1. Carbuncle. (2); occurs in man from infection of subcutaneous tissues with *Bacillus anthracis,* the disease is marked by hemmorrhage and serous effusions in the organs and cavities in the body, and symptoms of extreme prostration. 2. Splenic fever; charbon; an infectious disease of animals, especially the herbivora, due to the presence in the blood of *Bacillus anthracis.*

　**cerebral a.,** a form of internal a., associated with pulmonary or intestinal a., in which the specific bacilli invade the capillaries of the brain; in addition to the symptoms of pulmonary or intestinal a. there is violent delirium; cerebral a. is frequently associated with a hemorrhagic meningitis.

　**cutaneous a.,** malignant *pustule.*

　**emphysem′atous a.,** blackleg.

　**intestinal a.,** a form of internal a. marked by chill, high fever, pain in the head, back, and extremities, vomiting, bloody diarrhea, great prostration, and frequently hemorrhages from the mucous membranes and in the skin (petechiae); the disease is usually fatal; see also *mycosis intestinalis.*

　**pul′monary a.,** wool sorters′ disease; a form of internal a. acquired by inhalation of dust containing *Bacillus anthracis,* there is an initial chill followed by pain in the back and legs, rapid respiration, dyspnea, cough, fever, rapid pulse, and extreme prostration.

　**symptomatic a.,** blackleg.

**an′throne.** 9,10-Dihydro-9-oxoanthracene; a reagent used in the detection of carbohydrates.

**an′thropo-** [ G. *anthrōpos,* man ]. A combining form meaning human, or denoting some relationship to man.

**anthropobiology** (an′thro-po-bi-ol′o-jĭ). The study of the biologic relationships of the human race.

**anthropocentrism** (an′thro-po-sen′trizm). The assumption that man is the central fact of the universe.

**anthropogenesis** (an′thro-po-jen′ĕ-sis). Anthropogeny.

**anthropogen′ic, anthropogenet′ic.** Relating to anthropogeny.

**anthropogeny** (an-thro-poj′en-ĭ) [ anthropo- + G. *genesis,* origin ]. Anthropogenesis; the origin and development of man, both individual and racial.

**anthropog′ony.** Anthropogeny.

**anthropography** (an′thro-pog′rǎ-fĭ) [ anthropo- + G. *graphō,* to write ]. The geography of man; the distribution of the varieties of mankind.

**anthropoid** (an′thro-poyd) [ G. *anthrōpo-eidēs,* man-like ]. 1. Resembling man in structure and form. 2. One of the monkeys resembling man; an ape.

**Anthropoidea** (an-thro-po-id′e-ah). A suborder of Primates, including man and the monkeys.

**anthropol′ogy** [ anthropo- + G. *logos,* treatise ]. The branch of science that treats of man in all his relations.

　**applied a.,** a fusion of modern cultural a. and some aspects of sociology in the study of literate peoples in their cultures and deriving applications therefrom.

　**criminal a.,** a. in its relation to the criminal, his physical and mental characteristics, heredity, social relations, etc. See also criminology.

　**cultural a.,** study of the culture of nonliterate peoples and the application of the findings to more civilized groups.

　**physical a.,** the study of the physical attributes of man.

**anthropom′eter.** An instrument for measuring various dimensions of the human body.

**anthropomet′ric.** Relating to anthropometry.

**anthropom′etry** [ anthropo- + G. *metron,* measure ]. The branch of anthropology that deals with the comparative measurements of the human body and its several parts.

**anthropomorphism** (an′thro-po-mor′fizm) [ anthropo- + G. *morphē,* form ]. Humanization; the ascription of human shape or qualities to nonhuman creatures or inanimate objects, as contrasted with theriomorphism; an interpretation of what is not human or personal in human or personal terms or characteristics.

**an′thropon′omy** [ anthropo- + G. *nomos,* law ]. The study of the laws governing the development of the human race and the relation of man to his environment.

**anthroponosis** (an′thro-po-no′sis) [ anthropo- + G. *nosis,* disease ]. An infectious disease restricted to man, originally derived from animals (zoonosis, either an anthropozoonosis or zooanthroponosis) for example, the urban form of Old World cutaneous leishmaniasis in the USSR, caused by *Leishmania tropica* var. *minor.*

**anthropopathy** (an′thro-pop′ǎ-thĭ) [ anthropo- + G. *pathos,* suffering ]. The possession or experiencing of human feelings.

**anthropophagy** (an′thro-pof′ǎ-jĭ) [ anthropo- + G. *phagein,* to eat ]. Cannibalism.

**anthropophilic** (an′thro-po-fil′ik) [ anthropo- + G. *phileō,* to love ]. Man-seeking or man-preferring, generally with reference to bloodsucking arthropods; designates preference of a parasite for the human host as a source of blood or tissues over an animal host.

**anthropophobia** (an′thro-po-fo′bǐ-ah) [ anthropo- + G. *phobos,* fear ]. A morbid aversion to or dread of human companionship; phobanthropy.

**an′thropos′copy.** [ anthropo- + G. *skopeō,* to view ]. Judging the type of body build by inspection.

**anthroposomatology** (an′thro-po′so-mǎ-tol′o-jĭ) [ anthropo- + G. *sōma,* body, + *logos,* study ]. That part of anthropology which has to do with the human body, such as anatomy, physiology, pathology, etc.

**anthroposophy** (an′thro-pos′o-fĭ) [ anthropo- + G. *sophia,* wisdom ]. Knowledge conncerning human attributes.

**an′thropotox′in.** An alleged poison exhaled in the breath.

**anthropozoonosis** (an′thro-po-zo′o-no′sis) [ anthropo- + G. *zōon,* animal, + *nosis,* disease ]. A zoonosis maintained in nature by animals and transmissible to man; *e.g.,* rabies, brucellosis.

**anti-** [ G. *anti,* against ]. A prefix signifying against, opposing, or, in relation to symptoms and diseases, curative.

**antiac′id.** Antacid.

**antiagglu′tinin.** A specific antibody that inhibits or destroys the action of an agglutinin.

**antialex′in.** Anticomplement.

**antialler′gic.** Relating to any agent or measure that prevents, inhibits, or alleviates an allergic reaction.

**an′tiam′ylase.** A substance that neutralizes the action of amylase.

**antianaphylaxis** (an′tǐ-an′ǎ-fi-lak′sis). A condition in which an anaphylactic reaction in the tissues is avoided (*i.e.,* anaphylaxis is "neutralized") by means of a series of injections of extremely small, but progressively increased doses of the antigen to which there is hypersensitivity. Termed also desensitization or anergy, in relation to the specific antigen.

**antiandrogen** (an′ti-an′dro-jen). Any substance capable of preventing full expression of the biological effects of androgenic hormones on responsive tissues, either by producing antagonistic effects on the target tissue, as estrogens do, or by merely inhibiting androgenic effects, as do agents like cyproterone.

**an'tiane'mic.** Pertaining to factors or substances that prevent or correct anemic conditions.

**an'tian'tibody.** Antibody specific for another antibody contained in whole or fractionated immune serum with which a person or animal has been inoculated.

**an'tiantitox'in.** An antibody that inhibits or counteracts the effects of an antitoxin. See also antiantibody.

**antiarachnolysin** (an-tĭ-ar-ak-nol'ĭ-sin) [ anti- + G. *arachnē*, spider, + lysin ]. An antivenin counteracting the poison (lysin) of the spider.

**antiarrhythmic** (an'tĭ-ă-rith'mik). Andidysrhythmic; combating an arrhythmia.

**antiarthritic** (an'tĭ-ar-thrit'ik). Antarthritic.

**antiasthmatic** (an'tĭ-az-mat'ik). 1. Relieving or preventing asthma. 2. A remedy that may prevent or shorten an asthmatic paroxysm.

**antiautolysin** (an'ti-aw-tol'ĭ-sin). An antibody that inhibits or neutralizes the activity of an autolysin.

**antibacterial** (an'tĭ-bak'te'rĭ-al). Destructive to or preventing the growth of bacteria.

**antibechic** (an-tĭ-bek'ik) [ anti- + G. *bēx* (*bēch*-), cough ]. Antitussive.

**antibi'ogram.** A record of the resistance of microbes to various antibiotics.

**antibi'ont.** A microorganism producing antimicrobial substance.

**antibio'sis** [ anti- + G. *biōsis*, life ]. An association of two organisms which is detrimental to one of them.

**antibiot'ic.** 1. Relating to antibiosis. 2. Prejudicial to life. 3. A soluble substance derived from a mold or bacteria that inhibits the growth of other microorganisms; relating to such an action.

   **broad spectrum a.,** one having a wide range of activity against both Gram-positive and Gram-negative organisms.

**antibiotic-resistant.** Indicating microorganisms that continue to multiply although exposed to antibiotic agents.

**antibi'otin.** Avidin.

**antiblennorrhagic** (an-tĭ-blen-o-raj'ik). 1. Preventive or curative of mucous discharge (blennorrhagia). 2. A remedy possessing such properties.

**antibody** (an'tĭ-bod'ĭ). Originally, a body or substance evoked in man or other animal by an antigen, and characterized by reacting specifically with the antigen in some demonstrable way—antibody and antigen each being defined in terms of the other, but it is now supposed that antibodies may also exist naturally without being present as a result of the stimulus provided by the introduction of an antigen: (1) in the broad sense any body or substance, soluble or cellular, which is evoked by the stimulus provided by the introduction of antigen and which reacts specifically with antigen in some demonstrable way; (2) one or other of the classes of globulins (immunoglobulins, *q.v.*) present in the blood serum or body fluids of an animal as a result of antigenic stimulus or "naturally." Different genetically inheritant determinants, Gm and Inv, control the antigenicity of the antibody molecule; the various classes differ widely in abilities to react in different kinds of serologic tests. For a discussion of the various blood group reactions, see appendix 2, Blood Groups. Cross-references to the specific blood groups are also listed under antigen.

   **agglutinating a.,** agglutinin; a. that causes clumping or aggregation of particulate forms with specific antigen, as in bacterial cells and erythrocytes.

   **anaphylac'tic a.,** a special form of a. in certain tissues of various animals sensitized in such a manner that anaphylaxis occurs when a subsequent dose of the same antigen is administered; also formerly termed sensibilisin.

   **anti-kidney a.'s,** a.'s produced in an animal, usually of another species, by the injection of kidney substance.

   **antinuclear a.,** an a. showing an affinity for cell nuclei demonstrated by exposing a cell substrate to the serum to be tested followed by exposure to an antihuman-globulin serum conjugated with fluorescein; development of specific nuclear fluorescence is a positive reaction. This a. is found in the serum of a high proportion of patients with systemic lupus erythematosus rheumatoid arthritis and certain collagen diseases, in some of their healthy relatives, and in about 1 per cent of normal controls.

   **auto-a.,** see autoantibody.

   **bivalent a.,** a. that causes a visible reaction with specific antigen as in agglutination, precipitation, and so on; so-called because according to the "lattice theory" aggregation occurs when the antibody molecule has two or more receptors which link across from one particle of antigen to another; probably a characteristic of the class of immunoglobulin.

   **blocking a.,** (1) univalent a.; (2) noncytophilic a., in general of the IgG class, that is free to combine with circulating antigen (allergen) and thus prevent the antigen (allergen) from combining with cell-fixed cytophilic a.

   **blood group a.'s,** see appendix 2, Blood Groups.

   **cell-bound a.,** a term sometimes used for supposed a. on the surface of cells that effects cell-mediated (delayed type) sensitivity, a supposition still unsupported by definite evidence. Not to be confused with cytophilic a.

   **CF a.,** complement-fixing a.

   **complement-fixing a.,** CF a.; a. that combines with and sensitizes antigen to the action of complement, sometimes, but not always, resulting in lysis.

   **complete a.,** bivalent a.; term frequently used as a distinctive designation, especially with reference to blood groups and types; for example, a. that causes visible agglutination of Rh-positive erythrocytes in 0.85 per cent solution of NaCl.

   **cross-reacting a.,** (1) a. specific for group antigens, *i.e.,* those with identical functional groups; (2) a. for antigens that have functional groups of closely similar, but not identical, chemical structure.

   **cytophilic a.,** a. that in addition to, and unrelated to, its specific affinity for the antigen that induced it, has, because of the properties of the Fc portion of the heavy chain, an affinity for certain kinds of cells; frequently applied to cytophilic a.'s other than the Prausnitz-Küstner kind and especially to those that can be determined by tests *in vitro*. See also cytophilic antibody *test*.

   **Forssman a.,** heterophil a.; a heterogenetic a. specific for the Forssman group of heterogenetic antigens.

   **heterocytotropic a.,** a kind of cytophilic a. similar in activity to homocytotropic a. (*q.v.*), but seemingly of a different immunoglobulin class and having an affinity for cells of a different species rather than for cells of the same or a closely related species.

   **het'erogenet'ic a.,** one that not only causes a visible reaction with the antigen that stimulated its formation, but also cross-reacts with certain antigens that are not phylogenetically related to the specific antigen. See also heterogenetic antigen.

   **het'erophil a., heterophile a.,** Forssman a.

   **homocytotropic a.,** a kind of cytophilic a. that has an affinity for tissues (notably mast cells) of the same, or closely related, species, and that upon combining with specific antigen triggers the release of pharmacological mediators of anaphylaxis from the cells to which it is attached; the tropism seems to be dependent upon the Fc portion of the antibody molecule.

   **immobilizing a.,** treponema-immobilizing a.

   **incomplete a.,** univalent a.

   **inhibiting a.,** univalent a.

   **lymphocytotoxic a.'s,** a.'s specific for histocompatibility antigens of lymphocytes and which, upon combining with the antigens, induce cellular damage or death.

   **natural a.,** normal a.

   **neutralizing a.,** a form of a. that reacts with an infectious agent (usually a virus) and destroys or inhibits its infectivity and virulence; may be demonstrated by means of mixing serum with the suspension of infectious agent, and then injecting the mixture into animals that are susceptible to the agent in question.

   **nonprecipitable a.,** nonprecipitating a.

   **nonprecipitating a.,** nonprecipitable a.; a. that, under conditions normally employed in precipitin tests, is refractory to precipitation by specific a., demonstrable when antigen is added serially in small amounts; nonprecipitating a. will precipitate under special conditions such as addition of complement.

**normal a.,** that demonstrable in the serum or plasma of various persons or animals not known to have been stimulated by specific antigen, either artificially or as the result of naturally occurring contact.

**Prausnitz-Küstner a.,** reaginic a.; one of the IgE class of a.'s first demonstrated by Prausnitz and Küstner by passive transfer to the skin.

**precipitating a.,** precipitin.

**reaginic a.,** Prausnitz-Küstner a.

**treponema-immobilizing a.,** immobilizing a.; treponemal a.; a., evoked during syphilitic infections, possessing specific affinity for *Treponema pallidum,* and which in the presence of complement immobilizes the organism.

**treponemal a.,** treponema-immobilizing a.

**univalent a.,** blocking a. (1); an "incomplete" form of a. that may coat antigen, but which according to the "lattice theory" does not have a second receptor for attachment to another molecule of antigen. In the case of Rh+ erythrocytes such an anti-Rh antibody may coat the cells but not cause them to agglutinate in saline; however, agglutination does occur when such coated cells are suspended in serum or other protein media, such as albumin, therefore called serum agglutinin.

**Vi a.,** a form of a. that agglutinates highly virulent strains of *Salmonella typhosa, i.e.,* cells with Vi antigen; such bacteria are not agglutinable with O antiserum until the Vi antigen is destroyed. See Vi antigen.

**Wassermann a.,** a., evoked during syphilitic infections, that combines with cardiolipin in the presence of lecithin and cholesterol; it is distinct from the treponema-immobilizing a.

**antibrachial** (an-tĭ-bra′kĭ-al). Antebrachial.

**antibrachium** (an-tĭ-bra′kĭ-um). Antebrachium.

**antibro′mic** [ anti- + G. *brōmos,* smell ]. 1. Deodorizing. 2. A deodorizer.

**anticachectic** (an′tĭ-kă-kek′tik). Counteracting cachexia.

**antical′culous.** Antilithic.

**antican′crin.** A postulated antibody (or a principle resembling antibody) that is thought to react with malignant neoplastic cells and lead to degeneration or necrosis.

**anticarious** (an′tĭ-ka′rĭ-us). Preventing or inhibiting caries.

**anticataphylaxis** (an′tĭ-kat′ă-fi-lak′sis). Interference with or inhibition of cataphylaxis.

**anticathexis** (an′tĭ-kă-thek′sis). Counterinvestment; in psychoanalysis, the shifting of an emotional charge to an impulse or action of an opposite character; for example, unconscious hatred expressed as conscious love. See also cathexis.

**anticath′ode.** Target; a metal plate in an x-ray tube on which the cathode rays impinge, giving origin to the x-rays.

**anticephalalgic** (an′tĭ-sef′al-al′jik). Headache-relieving.

**antichlorotic** (an′ti-klo-rot′ik). Helpful in the treatment of chlorosis.

**anticholagogue** (an-tĭ-kol′ă-gog). An agent or process reducing or suspending the flow of bile.

**anticholinergic** (an′tĭ-kol-in-er′jik). Antagonistic to the action of parasympathetic or other cholinergic nerve fibers.

**anticholinesterase** (an′tĭ-kol-in-es′ter-ās). One of the drugs that inhibit or inactivate acetylcholinesterase, either reversibly, *e.g.,* physostigmine, or irreversibly, *e.g.,* the organophosphates (tetraethyl pyrophosphate).

**antic′ipate** [ L. *anticipo,* pp. *-cipatus,* to anticipate, fr. *anti* (old form of *ante*), before, + *capio,* to take. CAP-2 ]. To come before the appointed time; said of a periodic symptom or disease, such as a malarial paroxysm, when it recurs at progressively shorter intervals.

**anticipa′tion.** 1. Appearance before the appointed time of a periodic symptom or sign, such as a malarial paroxysm. 2. Progressively earlier age of onset of a hereditary disease in successive generations.

**anticli′nal** [ anti- + G. *klinō,* to incline ]. Inclined in opposite directions, as two sides of a pyramid.

**anticne′mion** (an-tik-ne′mĭ-on) [ G. *antiknēmion* ]. The shin.

**anticoagulant** (an′tĭ-ko-ag′u-lant). 1. Preventing coagulation. 2. An agent that prevents coagulation.

**an′ticoag′ulin.** A substance that inhibits or destroys the effects of coagulin.

**antico′don.** The trinucleotide sequence complementary to a codon. Thus, if a codon is A-G-C, its anticodon is U (or T)-C-G. The complementarity principle arises from Watson-Crick base-pairing, in which A is complementary to U (or T), G is complementary to C. Anticodon is sometimes called "nodoc." See fig. under anticodon.

**anticom′plement.** Antialexin; a substance that combines with a complement and so neutralizes its action by preventing its union with the antibody.

**an′ticomplemen′tary.** Denoting a substance possessing the power of diminishing or abolishing the action of a complement.

**anticontagious** (an′tĭ-kon-ta′jus). Preventing contagion.

**an′ticonvul′sant.** Anticonvulsive. 1. Preventing or arresting convulsions. 2. An agent that prevents or arrests convulsions.

**an′ticonvul′sive.** Anticonvulsant.

**anticorrosive** (an′tĭ-kŏ-ro′siv). Preventing corrosion.

**anti′cus** [ L. in the very front, fr. *ante,* before ]. A term in anatomical nomenclature to designate a muscle or other structure which of all similar structures is nearest the front or ventral surface; the NA uses "anterior" in place of a.

**anticy′totox′in.** A specific antibody that inhibits or destroys the activity of a cytotoxin.

**antidepres′sant.** 1. Counteracting depression. 2. An agent or drug used in treating depression; the most common types are tricyclic antidepressants and monoamine oxidase inhibitors.

**antidiabetic** (an′tĭ-di-ă-bet′ik). Counteracting diabetes.

**antidiarrheal, antidiarrhetic** (antĭ-di-ă-re′al, -di-ă-ret′-ik). Having the property of opposing or correcting diarrhea.

**antidiastase** (an′tĭ-di′as-tās). An antibody or similar material formed in the blood as a result of injections of diastase; a. inhibits or destroys the activity of diastase.

**antidin′ic** [ anti- + G. *dinos,* dizziness ]. 1. Relieving vertigo. 2. An agent that prevents or relieves vertigo.

**antidiuresis** (an′tĭ-di-u-re′sis). Reduction of urinary volume.

**antidiuret′ic.** An agent that reduces the output of urine.

**an′tido′tal.** Relating to or acting as an antidote.

**an′tidote** [ G. *antidotos,* from *anti,* against, + *dotos,* what is given, fr. *didōmi,* to give ]. An agent that neutralizes a poison or counteracts its effects.

**chemical a.,** a substance that unites with a poison to form an innocuous chemical compound.

**mechanical a.,** a substance that prevents the absorption of a poison.

**physiologic a.,** an agent that produces systemic effects contrary to those of a given poison.

**antidrom′ic** [ anti- + G. *dromos,* a running ]. Relating to propagation of an impulse along an axon in a direction the reverse of the normal; *cf.* dromic.

**antidysenteric** (an′tĭ-dis-en-ter′ik). Relieving or preventing dysentery.

**antidysrhythmic** (an′tĭ-dis-rith′mik). Antiarrhythmic.

**antidysuric** (an′tĭ-dis-u′rik). Preventing or relieving strangury or distress in urination.

**antiemetic** (an′tĭ-e-met′ik) [ anti- + G. *emetikos,* emetic ]. Antemetic. 1. Preventing or arresting vomiting. 2. A remedy that tends to control nausea and vomiting.

**an′tiendotox′in.** An antibody to endotoxins, especially one which neutralizes their injurious effects.

**antienergic** (an′tĭ-en-er′jik) [ anti- + G. *energos,* active ]. Acting against or in opposition.

**antienzyme** (an′tĭ-en′zīm). An agent or principle that retards, inhibits, or destroys the activity of an enzyme; may be an inhibitory enzyme or an antibody to an enzyme.

**ant′iepilep′tic.** Indicating a drug or any measure that tends to prevent an epileptic seizure.

**antiestrogen** (an′tĭ-es′tro-jen). Any substance capable of preventing full expression of the biological effects of estrogenic hormones on responsive tissues, either by producing antagonistic effects on the target tissue, as androgens do, or by merely inhibiting estrogenic effects, as do agents like ethamoxytriphetol.

**antieurodontic** (an'tĭ-u-ro-don'tik) [ anti- + G. *euros*, mold, + *odous*, tooth ]. An agent or process designed to prevent tooth decay.

**antifebrile** (an'tĭ-fe'brĭl, -feb'rĭl) [ anti- + L. *febris*, fever ]. Antipyretic.

**antife'brin.** Acetanilide.

**antifer'ment.** Antienzyme.

**an'tifermen'tative.** Preventing or arresting fermentation.

**ant'ifibrinol'ysin.** Antiplasmin.

**an'tiflux.** A material, such as graphite or iron rouge or whiting in alcohol, used to limit the flow of solder.

**antifo'lic.** 1. Antagonistic to the action of folic acid. 2. Any agent with this effect. See also folic acid antagonist.

**antifung'al.** Antagonistic to fungi (fungistatic or fungicidal).

**anti-G.** A term in the strict sense that means "antigravity" but, as commonly used, the adjectival term implies protection against the effects of gravity (*e.g.*, anti-G *suit*).

**antigalactagogue** (an'tĭ-gă-lak'tă-gog). Antigalactic.

**antigalac'tic** [ anti- + G. *gala*, milk ]. Antigalactagogue. 1. Diminishing or arresting the secretion of milk. 2. An agent so acting.

**antigen** (an'tĭ-jen) [ anti(body) + G. suffix -*gen*, producing ] (abbreviated Ag). Allergen; immunogen; any of various sorts of material (*e.g.*, microorganisms, toxoids, exotoxins, foreign proteins, foreign cells or tissues and others) that, as a result of coming in contact with appropriate tissues of an animal body, after a latent period, usually of from 8 to 14 days, induces a state of sensitivity and/or resistance to infection or toxic substances, and which will react in a demonstrable way with tissues and/or antibody of the sensitized subject, *in vivo* or *in vitro*. Modern usage tends to retain the broad meaning of a., employing the terms determinant group and antigenic determinant for the particular chemical group of a molecule that confers antigenic specificity. See also hapten.

**ABO a.'s.** see ABO blood group, appendix 2.

**acetone-insoluble a.,** cardiolipin.

**Au a.,** (1) see Auberger blood group, appendix 2; (2) see hepatitis-associated a.

**Au(1) a.,** hepatitis-associated a.

**Australia a.,** hepatitis-associated a.

**Beᵃ a., Becker a.,** see low frequency blood groups, appendix 2.

**Bi a., Bile's a.,** see low frequency blood groups, appendix 2.

**blood group a.,** generic term for any inherited antigen found on the surface of erythrocytes that determines a blood grouping reaction with specific antiserum. A.'s of the ABO and Lewis blood groups may be found also in saliva and other body fluids. The genes controlling development of blood group a.'s vary in frequencies in different population and ethnic groups. See also appendix 2, Blood Groups.

**By a.,** see low frequency blood groups, appendix 2.

**capsular a.,** that found only in the capsules of certain microorganisms; *e.g.*, the specific polysaccharides of various types of pneumococci.

**carcinoembryonic a.** (abbreviated CEA), oncofetal a.; a glycoprotein constituent of the glycocalyx of embryonic entodermal epithelium, generally absent from adult cells with the exception of some carcinomas in which it may also be detected in the patient's serum.

**CDE a.'s,** see Rh blood group, appendix 2.

**choles'terinized a.,** cardiolipin to which cholesterol has been added.

**Chrᵃ a.,** see low frequency blood groups, appendix 2.

**complete a.,** any a. capable of stimulating the formation of antibody with which it reacts *in vivo* or *in vitro*, as distinguished from incomplete a. (hapten).

**Di a.,** see Diego blood group, appendix 2.

**Duffy a.'s.,** see Duffy blood group, appendix 2.

**flagellar a.,** the heat-a labile a.'s associated with bacterial flagella which with specific antibody are agglutinated into loose, fluffy masses which are easily disintegrated by shaking, in contrast to somatic a.; *cf.* H a.

**Forssman a.,** a type of heterogenetic a. found in dogs, horses, sheep, cats, turtles, and eggs of some fish, and also in certain bacteria (*e.g.*, some strains of enteric organisms and pneumococci) and varieties of corn; usually found in the tissues and organs (not in blood), but is present in sheep erythrocytes and not in this animal's tissues. With the exception of guinea pigs and hamsters, Forssman a. is not found in rodents, or in frogs, hogs, and most of the primate group. The antibody that develops in infectious mononucleosis of man reacts specifically with the Forssman a.

**Fy a.'s.,** see Duffy blood group, appendix 2.

**G a.** [ Ger. *gebundenes*, bound ], internal a.; an antigenic viral nucleoprotein.

**Ge a.,** see high frequency blood groups, appendix 2.

**Good a.,** see low frequency blood groups, appendix 2.

**Gr a.,** Vw a.; see MNSs blood group, appendix 2.

**group a.'s,** a.'s that are shared by related genera of microorganisms.

**H a.,** (1) the a. in the flagella of motile bacteria; so named because they were first identified in motile bacteria from a film (German, *Hauch*) of spreading growth on agar medium; see also O a.; (2) see ABO blood group, appendix 2.

**He, Hu a.'s,** see MNSs blood group, appendix 2.

**heart a.,** cardiolipin.

**hepatitis-associated a.,** abbreviated HAA; also known as Australia a., Au a., Au(1) a., Aus a.; hepatitis B a.; a serum a. associated with serum hepatitis, electron microscopically shown to be composed of spherical particles about 20 nm in diameter, lamellated spheres about 40 nm in diameter, or larger tubular forms. It is recommended that the term hepatitis-associated a. be replaced by the name hepatitis B surface a. (HBₛAg) in order to avoid ambiguity, there being another a.: hepatitis B core a. (HBᶜAg).

**hepatitis B a.,** hepatitis-associated a.

**hepatitis B core a.** (abbreviated HBᶜAg), the a. found in the core of the Dane particle (seemingly the hepatitis B virus) and also in hepatocyte nuclei in hepatic B infections.

**hepatitis B surface a.** (abbreviated HBₛAg), hepatitis-associated a.; a. of the small (20 nm) spherical and filamentous forms of hepatitis B a., and a surface a. of the larger (42 nm) Dane particle (seemingly the hepatitis B virus).

**het'erogenet'ic a.,** heterophil a.; an a. which is possessed by a variety of different phylogenetically unrelated species; examples are the various organ or tissue specific a.'s, the alpha- and beta-crystalline protein of the lens of the eye, and Forssman a.

**het'erophil a.,** heterogenetic a.

**HL-A a.'s,** any of the tissue transplantation compatibility a.'s controlled by genes at the HL-A chromosome locus; there are many alleles for this locus and most individuals are heterozygotes.

**Ho a.,** see low frequency blood groups, appendix 2.

**I and i a.'s,** see I blood group, appendix 2.

**incomplete a.,** hapten.

**internal a.,** G a.

**Jk a.'s,** see Kidd blood group, appendix 2.

**Jobbins a.,** see low frequency blood groups, appendix 2.

**Js a.,** see Sutter blood group, appendix 2.

**K and k a.'s,** see Kell blood group, appendix 2.

**Lan a.,** see high frequency blood groups, appendix 2.

**Le a.'s,** see Lewis blood group, appendix 2.

**Levay a.,** see low frequency blood groups, appendix 2.

**Lu a.'s,** see Lutheran blood group, appendix 2.

**lymphogranuloma venereum a.** (USP), a sterile suspension of the inactivated agent of *Miyagawanella lymphogranulomatis* (*Chlamydia trachomatis*), prepared by growing the organism in the embryonic tissues of the domestic fowl (*Gallus domesticus*); used for diagnosis. See also Frei *test*.

**M₁, M₂, Mᶜ, Mᴳ a.'s,** see MNSs blood group, appendix 2.

**Miᶻ, Mu a.'s,** see MNSs blood group, appendix 2.

**MNSs a.'s,** see MNSs blood group, appendix 2.

**mumps skin test a.,** a sterile suspension of killed mumps virus in isotonic sodium chloride solution. Used to determine susceptibility to mumps or to confirm a tentative diagnosis.

O a., (1) somatic a., which is situated in the bodies of microorganisms, in contrast to that in the flagella or capsules; so termed because such a. was first identified in nonmotile bacterial cells that colonized without forming a film (German, *ohne Hauch*); see also H a.; (2) see ABO blood group, appendix 2.

oncofetal a., carcinoembryonic a.

organ-specific a., a heterogenetic antigen with organ specificity; for example, in addition to species specific a., kidney of one species contains a. that is identical to that in kidney of other species.

Ot a., see low frequency blood groups, appendix 2.

P a.'s, see P blood group, appendix 2.

partial a., hapten.

pollen a., an extract of the antigenic protein from the pollen of plants; *i.e.*, pollen allergen, used in the diagnosis and treatment of hay fever.

private a.'s, see low frequency blood groups, appendix 2.

public a.'s, see high frequency blood groups, appendix 2.

Rh a.'s, see Rh blood group, appendix 2.

Rhus toxicodendron a., a solution of an extract from the fresh leaves of poison ivy, with 0.4 per cent of procaine hydrochloride. Used by intradermal injection to determine sensitiveness to the poison of *Rhus toxicodendron,* and intramuscularly injected to relieve poison ivy dermatitis.

Rhus venenata a., a solution from an extract of the fresh leaves of poison sumach. Used to determine sensitiveness to the plant or to relieve the dermatitis caused by contact with the leaves.

S a., viral a. that remains in solution after the particles of virus have been removed by means of centrifugation; in the case of the influenza viruses, it is the internal helical structure, free of the external envelope.

sensitized a., the complex formed when a. combines with specific antibody; so called because the a., by the mediation of antibody, is rendered sensitive to the action of complement.

shock a., an a. capable of producing anaphylactic shock in an animal that has been sensitized to it.

Sm a., see high frequency blood groups, appendix 2.

somatic a., O a. (1).

species-specific a., antigenic components in the tissues and fluids of members of a species of animal, by means of which various species may be immunologically distinguished; for example, serum albumin of horses is immunologically different from that of man, dogs, sheep, and so on.

specific a.'s, a.'s that characterize a single genus of microorganisms.

Stobo a., see low frequency blood groups, appendix 2.

Streptococcus M a., M protein; the somatic a. associated with virulence and type specificity of group A streptococci; removed from cell surface by trypsin digestion.

Swᵃ a., see low frequency blood groups, appendix 2.

Swann a.'s, see low frequency blood groups, appendix 2.

T a., see neoantigen.

tissue-specific a., organ-specific a.

Tj a., see P blood group, appendix 2.

Trᵃ a., see low frequency blood groups, appendix 2.

V a., viral a. that is intimately associated with the virus particle, is protein in nature, has multiple antigenicities, and is strain-specific. Antibody to such a. is demonstrable as protective or neutralizing antibody.

Vel a., see high frequency blood groups, appendix 2.

Ven a., see low frequency blood groups, appendix 2.

Vi a., "virulence a.," an external nonflagellar a. of enterobacteria formerly thought to be related to increased virulence.

Vw a., see MNSs blood group, appendix 2.

Webb a., see low frequency blood groups, appendix 2.

Wrᵃ a., see low frequency blood groups, appendix 2.

Wright a.'s, see low frequency blood groups, appendix 2.

Xg a., see Xg blood group, appendix 2.

Ytᵃ a., see high frequency blood groups, appendix 2.

antigenemia (an'tĭ-jĕ-ne'mĭ-ah) [ antigen + G. *haima,* blood ]. Persistence of antigen in circulating blood; *e.g.,* Au-antigenemia (presence of Australia antigen in blood serum).

an'tigen'ic. Immunogenic; having the properties of an antigen.

antigenicity (an'tĭ-jĕ-nis'ĭ-tĭ). Immunogenicity; the state or property of being antigenic.

antigen'other'apy. The use of an antigen as a means of stimulating active immunity (formation of antibody) in the treatment of disease, either preventing its development or modifying its course.

antigonorrheic (an'ti-gon-o-re'ik). Curative of gonorrhea.

antigrav'ity. See anti-G.

antihe'lix. Anthelix.

an'tihemagglu'tinin. A substance (including antibody) that inhibits or prevents the effects of hemagglutinin.

an'tihemol'ysin. A substance (including antibody) that inhibits or prevents the effects of hemolysin.

an'tihemolyt'ic. Preventing hemolysis.

antihemorrhagic (an-tĭ-hem-or-raj'ik). Hemostatic; arresting hemorrhage.

antihidrotic (an'tĭ-hi-drot'ik, -hĭ-drot'ik). Antiperspirant.

antihis'tamines. Drugs having an action antagonistic to that of histamine. Used in the treatment of allergy symptoms.

an'tihistamin'ic. 1. Tending to neutralize or antagonize the action of histamine or to inhibit its production in the body. 2. An agent having such an effect, used to relieve the symptoms of allergy.

antihor'mones. Substances demonstrable in serum that inhibit or prevent the usual effects of certain hormones, and which, in certain instances at least, are specific antibodies.

antihyaluron'idase. A hyaluronidase inhibitor.

antihydriotic (an'tĭ-hi-drī-ot'ik). Antiperspirant.

antihydropic (an'tĭ-hi-drop'ik). 1. Relieving dropsy. 2. An agent that causes dropsical effusions to disappear.

an'tihyperten'sive. Indicating a drug or mode of treatment that reduces the blood pressure of hypertensive subjects.

antihypnotic (an'ti-hip-not'ik). 1. Preventing or tending to prevent hypnosis. 2. An arousing agent, or one that antagonizes sleep.

anti-icteric (an'tĭ-ik-ter'ik). Preventing or curing icterus (jaundice).

anti-immune (an'tĭ-im-mūn'). Interfering with the production of immunity.

anti-inflam'matory. Reducing inflammation by acting on body mechanisms, without directly antagonizing the causative agent; examples of anti-inflammatory agents are antihistamines and glucocorticoids.

anti-isol'ysin. A substance, probably antibody, that inhibits or prevents the effects of isolysin.

antiketogenesis (an'tĭ-ke'to-jen'ĕ-sis). 1. The prevention or reduction of ketosis through the formation of oxaloacetic acid and allied substances in the body, thus stimulating the action of the tricarboxylic acid cycle and oxidizing the ketone bodies that would otherwise accumulate. 2. Inhibition of the formation of ketone bodies by depression of fat utilization.

antike'togen'ic. Inhibiting the formation of ketone bodies, or accelerating their utilization.

antike'toplas'tic. Reducing the amount of ketone bodies excreted in urine or breath.

antiki'nase. A substance, probably antibody, that inhibits or prevents the effects of a kinase.

antilac'tase. An antienzyme that inhibits or prevents the activity of lactase.

antilem'ic [ anti- + G. *loimos,* plague ]. Preventive or curative of the plague.

antilep'sis [ G. *antilēpsis,* laying hold of in turn, reciprocation ]. Revulsive treatment; lessening of disease in a part by drawing blood away from it by counterirritation.

antilep'tic. Pertaining to or characterized by antilepsis.

an'tileuko'cidin. 1. A substance that inhibits or prevents the effects of leukocidin. 2. A leukocidin-specific antibody.

antileukotoxin (an'tĭ-lu-ko-tok'sin). A substance (including antibody) that inhibits or prevents the effects of leukocytoxin; frequently regarded as synonymous with antileukocidin.

antilewisite (an'tĭ-lu'ĭ-sit). Dimercaprol.

an'tilipotrop'ic. Pertaining to substances depressing choline synthesis (*e.g.,* by competing for methyl groups) and thus enhancing dietary fatty liver.

**antilith'ic** [ anti- + G. *lithos*, stone ]. 1. Anticalculous; preventing the formation of calculi or promoting their dissolution. 2. An agent so acting.

**antilo'bium** [ L., fr. G. *antilobion* ]. Tragus.

**antiluetic** (an-tī-lu-et'ik). Antisyphilitic.

**antiluteogenic** (an'tī-lu-te-o-jen'ik). Inhibiting the growth or hastening involution of the corpus luteum.

**antily'sin.** An antibody that inhibits or prevents the effects of lysin.

**antily'sis.** [ anti- + G. *lysis*, loosening ]. The effect of an antilysin, whereby destruction of cells (as a result of complement-fixing) is inhibited or prevented.

**antilyt'ic.** Inhibiting or preventing lysis; pertaining to antilysis.

**antimala'rial.** Preventing or curing malaria.

**an'timer.** Enantiomer.

**antimere** (an'tī-mēr). [ anti- + G. *meros*, a part ]. 1. A segment of an animal body formed by planes cutting the axis of the body at right angles. 2. One of the symmetrical parts of a bilateral organism. 3. The right or left half of the body.

**an'times.enter'ic.** Pertaining to the part of the intestine that lies opposite the mesenteric attachment.

**an'timetab'olite.** A substance that competes with, replaces, or antagonizes a particular metabolite; *e.g.*, ethionine is an a. of methionine.

**an'timetro'pia** [ anti- + G. *metron*, measure, + *ōps*, eye ]. A form of anisometropia in which the refractive errors in the two eyes are of different kinds, as when one eye is myopic and the other hypermetropic.

**antimicrobial** (an'tī-mi-kro'bī-al). Tending to destroy microbes, to prevent their development, or to prevent their pathogenic action.

**an'timitot'ic.** 1. Having an arresting action upon mitosis. 2. A drug having such an effect (*e.g.*, a folic acid antagonist that is used in leukemia to inhibit the multiplication of white cells).

**antimon'goloid.** Denoting an obliquity of the palpebral fissures laterally downward, in contrast to the laterally upward slant seen in Mongolian races.

**antimo'nial.** Containing or relating to antimony.

**antimonic** (an-tī-mo'nik, -mon'ik). 1. Antimonial. 2. Denoting antimony in its quinquivalent state, Sb5+.
  **a. acid,** one of three acids: *ortho*-antimonic acid, $H_3SbO_4$; *meta*-, $HSbO_3$; and *pyro*-, $H_4Sb_2O_7$.
  **a. oxide,** antimony pentoxide.

**antimo'nid.** A chemical compound containing antimony in union with a more positive element, *e.g.*, sodium a., $Na_3Sb$.

**antimo'nous.** 1. Antimonial. 2. Denoting antimony in its trivalent state, Sb3+.
  **a. oxide,** antimony trioxide.
  **a. sulfide,** black *antimony.*

**an'timony.** Antimonium; stibium; symbol Sb (*stibium*); a metallic element, atomic no. 51, atomic weight 121.77, valences +3, +5. Used in alloys. Toxic and irritating to the skin and mucous membranes.
  **black a.,** the native sulfide of a.; antimonous sulfide; stibmite; $Sb_2S_3$; freed from impurities. Used in glass-making.
  **a. chloride,** see a. trichloride.
  **a. dimercaptosuccinate,** ASTIBAN; stibocaptate; 2,3-dimercaptosuccinic acid cyclic thioantimonate; an antiparasitic effective against *Schistosoma mansoni* and *Schistosoma haematobium.*
  **a. oxide,** a. trioxide.
  **a. potassium tartrate** (USP), tartar emetic; tartrated a.; potassium antimonyl tartrate; expectorant; also the drug of choice for schistosomiasis japonicum, though it is extremely toxic and must be administered very slowly intravenously. Common toxic manifestations are phlebitis, tachycardia, and hypotension; sudden deaths have been reported, chiefly from circulatory collapse.
  **a. sodium gluconate** stibogluconate sodium.
  **a. sodium tartrate** (BP), sodium antimonyl tartrate; $Na(SbO)C_4H_4O_6$; used in the treatment of schistosomiasis, and as an emetic.

**a. sodium thioglycollate,** a compound of a trioxide and thioglycolic acid; used for tropical parasites.
  **tartrated a.,** a. potassium tartrate.
  **a. thioglycollamide,** the triamide of a. thioglycolic acid; $Sb(SCH_2CONH_2)_3$. Used in the treatment of trypanosomiasis, kala azar, and filariasis.
  **a. trichloride** $SbCl_3$; butter of a.; with vitamin A to form a blue compound, with β-carotene to form a green one, thus affording a widely employed method for assay of these substances. Used externally as a caustic for the removal of warts and other small growths.
  **a. trioxide,** a. oxide; antimonous oxide; flowers of antimony; $Sb_2O_3$. Used technically in paints and flame-proofing; also used as an expectorant and emetic.

**antim'onyl.** The univalent radical SbO—.

**antimuscarinic** (an'tī-mus'kă-rin'ik). Inhibiting or preventing the actions of muscarine and muscarine-like agents, or the effects of parasympathetic stimulation at the neuroeffector junction (*e.g.*, atropine).

**antimyasthenic** (an'tī-mi'as-then'ik). Tending toward the correction of the symptoms of myasthenia gravis, *e.g.*, the action of neostigmine.

**antimy'cin.** Citrinin.

**antimy'cin A.** An antibiotic isolated from cultures of an unidentified species of *Streptomyces*; $C_{28}H_{40}O_9N_2$; an active fungicide, insecticide, and miticide.

**an'timycot'ic** [ anti- + G. *mykēs*, fungus ]. Destructive to fungi.

**antinauseant** (an'tī-naw'se-ant). Having an action to prevent nausea, *e.g.*, motion sickness.

**antineoplastic** (an'tī-ne-o-plas'tik). Preventing the development, maturation, or spread of neoplastic cells.

**antinephritic** (an'tī-nĕ-frit'ik). Preventing or relieving inflammation of the kidneys.

**antineuralgic** (an'tī-nu-ral'jik). Relieving the pain of neuralgia.

**antineuritic** (an'tī-nu-rit'ik). Relieving neuritis.

**an'tineurotox'in.** An antibody to a neurotoxin.

**antin'iad.** Toward the antinion.

**antin'ial.** Relating to the antinion.

**antin'ion** [ anti- + G. *inion*, nape of the neck ]. The space between the eyebrows; the point on the skull opposite the inion.

**antin'omy** [ anti- + G. *nomos*, law ]. A contradiction between two principles, each of which is considered true.

**antinuclear** (antī-nu'kle-ar). Having an affinity for or reacting with the cell nucleus.

**antioc'ular.** Directed against the tissues of the eye; *e.g.*, a. antibodies.

**an'tiodontal'gic** [ anti- + G. *odous*, tooth, + *algos*, pain ]. 1. Relieving toothache. 2. A toothache remedy.

**an'tiorgas'tic.** Pertaining to an effort to avoid orgasm.

**an'tiox'idant.** An agent that inhibits oxidation and thus prevents rancidity of oils or fats or the deterioration of other materials through oxidative processes.

**an'tioxida'tion.** The retardation of oxidation of one substance by the addition of another.

**an'tiparasit'ic.** Destructive to parasites.

**antiparastata** (an'tī-pă-ras'tă-tak) [ anti- + G. *parastatēs*, a testicle. STA- ]. *Glandula* bulbourethralis.

**antip'athy** [ anti- + G. *pathos*, suffering ]. Enantiopathy.

**an'tipedic'ular.** Destructive to lice.

**antipep'tone.** A peptic digest resistant to trypsin; trypsin limit digest. Undefined and obsolete.

**antiperiodic** (an'tī-pe-rī-od'ik). Preventing the regular recurrence of a disease (*e.g.*, malaria) or a symptom.

**an'tiperistal'sis.** Reversed peristalsis; intestinal contractions forcing the contents upward.

**an'tiperistal'tic.** 1. Relating to antiperistalsis. 2. Impeding or arresting peristalsis.

**an'tiper'spirant.** Antihidrotic; antihydriotic; antisudorific. 1. Having an inhibitory action upon the secretion of sweat. 2. An agent having such an action.

**antiphagocytic** (an'tī-fag'o-sit'-ik). Impeding or preventing the action of the phagocytes.

**antiphlogistic** (an'tĭ-flo-jis'tik) [ anti- + G. *phogistos*, burnt up ]. 1. Preventing or relieving inflammation. 2. An agent that subdues inflammation.

**antipho'bic.** A mechanism or drug designed to control phobias.

**antiplasmin** (an-tĭ-plaz'min). Antifibrinolysin; a substance that inhibits or prevents the effects of plasmin; found in plasma and some tissues, especially the spleen and liver.

**antiplas'tic.** Preventing cicatrization.

**antiplate'let.** A substance that manifests a lytic or agglutinative action on the blood platelets, thereby inhibiting or destroying the effects of the latter.

**antipneumococcic** (an'tĭ-nu'mo-kok'sik). Destructive to, or repressing the growth of, the pneumococcus.

**antip'odal.** Opposite; occupying the opposite side of a cell or other body.

**an'tipode** [ G. *antipous*, with the feet opposite ]. A thing diametrically opposite.

   **optical a.,** enantiomer.

**antipo'sic.** 1. Inhibitory to the drinking of water and other beverages. 2. An agent that has this effect.

**an'tiprecip'itin.** A specific antibody that inhibits or prevents the effects of a precipitin.

**antiproges'tin.** A substance that inhibits progesterone formation, that interferes with its carriage or stability in the blood, or that reduces its uptake by, or effects on, target organs. Many such substances have been identified; each commonly exerts only one of the possible antagonistic actions mentioned.

**an'tipros'tate.** *Glandula* bulbourethralis.

**antiprotease** (an'tĭ-pro'te-ās). A substance inhibiting proteinase activity.

**an'tiprothrom'bin.** An anticoagulant that inhibits or prevents the conversion of prothrombin into thrombin; examples are heparin, which is present in various tissues (especially in liver), and dicoumarin, which is isolated from partially decomposed sweet clover.

**an'tiprurit'ic.** 1. Preventing or relieving itching. 2. An agent that relieves itching.

**antipsoric** an-tĭ-so'rik) [ anti- + G. *psōra*, itch ]. Curative of scabies, or the itch.

**antipsychotic** (an'tĭ-si-kot'ik). 1. An antipsychotic *agent*, *q.v.* 2. Denoting the actions of such an agent.

**an'tiputrefac'tive.** Preventing putrefaction.

**antipyogenic** (an'tĭ-pi-o-jen'ik) [ anti- + G. *pyon*, pus, + suffix *-gen*, production ]. Preventing suppuration.

**antipyre'sis.** Symptomatic treatment of fever rather than of the underlying disease.

**an'tipyret'ic** [ anti- + G. *pyretos*, fever. PYR- ]. 1. Antithermic; reducing fever. 2. Febrifuge; an agent tending to reduce fever.

**antipy'rine.**          PHENAZONE;          2,3-dimethyl-1-phenyl-3-pyrazoline-5-one; analgesic and antipyretic.

   **a. acetylsal'icylate,** ACETOPYRINE; ACOPYRINE; a compound of a. and aspirin; antirheumatic and analgesic.

   **a. sal'icylac'etate,** PYROSAL; analgesic, antirheumatic, antipyretic.

   **a. sal'icylate,** SALIPYRINE; analgesic and antipyretic, used in dysmenorrhea, influenza, and all acute catarrhs in the early stages.

**antipyrot'ic** [ anti- + G. *pyrōtikos*, burning, inflaming ]. 1. Antiphlogistic. 2. Relieving the pain and promoting the healing of superficial burns. 3. An application for burns.

**antirachitic** (an'tĭ-rä-kit'ik). Promoting the cure of rickets or preventing its development.

**antiren'net, antiren'nin.** An antienzyme found in the serum of animals injected with the enzyme rennin (or rennet); inhibits or prevents the milk-coagulating action of the enzyme.

**antirheumatic** (an'tĭ-ru-mat'ik). Preventive or curative of rheumatism.

**antiri'cin.** An antibody or antitoxin that inhibits or prevents the effects of ricin.

**antiru'minant.** Denoting a method to (1) control regurgitation of food or (2) break a compulsive trend of thought.

**anti-S.** An agglutinin for certain types of human erythrocytes; it causes rare instances of hemolytic transfusion reactions.

**an'tiscorbu'tic** 1. Preventive or curative of scorbutus or scurvy. 2. A remedy for scurvy.

**antiseborrheic** (an'tĭ-seb-or-re'ik). 1. Preventing or relieving excessive flow of sebum; preventing or relieving seborrheic dermatitis. 2. An agent having such actions.

**antisecretory** (an'tĭ-se-kre'to-rĭ). Inhibitory to secretion, *e.g.*, as said of certain drugs that reduce or suppress gastric secretion.

**antisep'sis** [ anti- + G. *sēpsis*, putrefaction ]. Prevention of infection by inhibiting the growth of infectious agents; see also disinfection.

**antisep'tic.** 1. Relating to antisepsis. 2. An agent or substance capable of effecting antisepsis.

**an'tise'rum.** Immune serum; serum that contains demonstrable antibody or antibodies specific for one (monovalent or specific a.) or more (polyvalent a.) antigens; may be prepared from the blood of animals inoculated parenterally (under certain conditions) with an antigenic material or from the blood of animals and persons that have been stimulated by natural contact with an antigen (as in those who recover from an attack of disease). For a discussion of the various blood group reactions, see appendix 2, Blood Groups. Cross-references to the specific blood groups are also listed under antigen.

   **blood group a.'s,** see appendix 2, Blood Groups.

   **Félix's a.,** an a. against enteric fever produced from horses.

   **heterol'ogous a.,** one that reacts with (*e.g.*, agglutinates) certain microorganisms or other complexes of antigens, even though the a. was produced by means of stimulation with a different microorganism or antigenic material; see also homologous a.

   **homol'ogous a.,** one in which there is complete correspondence between the content of antibodies and the antigenic material used for producing the a.; thus, if Bacterium I (with antigens *a, b, c,* and *d*) is used to produce an a., the latter would contain antibodies *A, B, C,* and *D*. Such an a. is homologous for Bacterium I, but it is also *heterologous* for various bacteria that might contain any 1, 2, or 3 (but not all 4) of the same antigens.

   **monovalent a.,** see a.

   **nerve growth factor a.,** NGF a.; an a. containing antibodies against nerve growth *factor (q.v.)*. When injected into newborn animals the majority of sympathetic ganglion cells are permanently destroyed, resulting in hypoinnervation of peripheral tissues.

   **polyvalent a.,** see a.

   **specific a.,** see a.

**antishock.** An agent used to relieve shock or hypotension.

**antisialagogue** (antĭ-si-al'ă-gog) [ anti- + G. *sialon*, saliva, + *agōgos*, drawing forth ]. An agent that diminishes or arrests the flow of saliva.

**antisialic** (an-tĭ-si-al'ik). Reducing the flow of saliva.

**antisid'eric** [ anti- + G. *sideros*, iron ]. Counteracting the physiological action of iron, probably by complexing or precipitation; *e.g.*, tannin is a.

**antiso'cial.** Behaving in violation of the social or legal norms of society; for example, the psychopathic personality; *cf.* asocial.

**an'tispasmod'ic.** 1. Preventive or curative of convulsions or spasmodic affections. 2. An agent that quiets spasm.

**antispermatox'in.** An antibody that inhibits or prevents the effects of a spermatoxin.

**antistaphylococci** (an'tĭ-staf'ĭ-lo-kok-sĭ). Antagonistic to staphylocci or their toxins.

**an'tistaph'ylol'ysin.** A substance that antagonizes or neutralizes the action of staphylolysin.

**antisteapsin** (an-tĭ-ste-ap'sin). An antibody counteracting the action of pancreatic lipase (steapsin).

**antistreptococcic** (an'tĭ-strep-to-kok'sik). Destructive to streptococci or antagonistic to their toxins.

**antistrep'toki'nase.** An antibody that inhibits the dissolution of fibrin by streptokinase; orig. antifibrinolysin.

**an'tistreptol'ysin.** An antibody that inhibits or prevents the effects of fibrinolytic antigen elaborated by certain group A streptococci; the amount of a. in the serum is frequently increased during and after streptococcal disease, and comparative titers may be a diagnostic and prognostic aid.

**antisub'stance.** Antibody.

**antisudorific** (an'tĭ-su'dor-if'if). Antiperspirant.

**antisyphilitic** (an'tĭ-sif'ĭ-lit'ik). Antiluetic. 1. Curative of syphilis. 2. A specific remedy for syphilis.

**an'titetan'ic.** Denoting an agent that tends to relax tetanic muscular contraction.

**antithe'nar.** Hypothenar.

**antither'mic** [ anti- + G. *thermē*, heat ]. Antipyretic.

**antithrom'bin.** Any substance that inhibits or prevents the effects of thrombin in such a manner that blood does not coagulate.

　　**normal a.,** an a. naturally occurring in blood and certain tissues under normal conditions in contrast to abnormal states or a. from other sources.

**antithy'roid.** Relating to an agent such as thiouracil that suppresses thyroid function.

**antithyroi'din.** A serum prepared from the blood of sheep from which the thyroid gland has been removed. Has been used in the treatment of Graves' disease and other conditions supposed to be due to hypersecretion of the thyroid gland.

**antiton'ic.** Diminishing muscular or vascular tonus.

**antitox'ic.** Antidotal; neutralizing the action of a poison; specifically, relating to an antitoxin.

**antitox'igen.** Antitoxinogen.

**antitoxin** (an'tĭ-tok'sin) [ anti- + G. *toxicon,* poison ]. Antibody formed in response to antigenic poisonous substances of biologic origin, such as bacterial exotoxins (*e.g.,* those elaborated by *Clostridium tetani* or *Corynebacterium diphtheriae*), phytotoxins, and zootoxins; a. neutralizes the pharmacologic effects of its specific toxin *in vitro,* and also *in vivo* if the toxin is not already fixed in the tissue cells. The combination of a. with toxin does not necessarily result in destruction of either substance, and the union may frequently be dissociated by means of appropriate procedures. In general usage, the term antitoxin refers to whole, or globulin fraction, of serum from animals (usually horses) immunized by injections of the specific toxoid. *Clostridium perfringens* and *C. septicum.*

　　**bothropic a., Bothrops a.,** a. specific for the venom of pit vipers of the genus *Bothrops* (*Bothrophora*) of the family Crotalidae.

　　**botulinum a.,** botulism a.

　　**botulism a.,** a specific for a toxin of one or another strain of *Clostridium botulinum* (*q.v.*).

　　**bovine a.,** one prepared from cattle instead of horses, used in the treatment of persons who are sensitive to horse serum; the cattle are immunized against the toxin for which specific a. is desired.

　　**Cro'talus a.,** a. specific for venom of rattlesnakes (*Crotalus* species).

　　**despe'ciated a.,** an antitoxic serum treated in an appropriate manner to alter the species-specific protein, such that a person who is sensitized to the animal protein is not likely to have a serious reaction when the a. is administered.

　　**diphtheria a.** (BP), a. specific for the toxin of *Corynebacterium diphtheriae.*

　　**dysentery a.,** a. specific for the neurotoxin of the Shiga dysentery bacillus (*Shigella dysenteriae*).

　　**fatigue a.,** see fatigue *toxin.*

　　**gas gangrene a.** (BP), pentavalent gas gangrene a. (NF); a. specific for the toxin of one or more species of *Clostridium* that cause gaseous gangrene and associated toxemia, especially *C. perfringens* (*C. welchii*), *C. novyi, C. septicum, C. histolyticum,* and *C. oedematiens.* Commercially available preparations are usually polyvalent, *i.e.,* contain a. for two or more species. The BP also lists monovalent a. for *C. welchii* or *C. septicum.*

　　**normal a.,** serum that is capable of neutralizing an equivalent quantity of a normal toxin solution.

　　**plant a.,** a. specific for a phytotoxin.

**scarlet fever a.,** a. specific for the erythrogenic toxin of strains of group A β-hemolytic streptococci.

　　**staphylococcus a.** (BP), a preparation from native serum containing antitoxic globulins or their derivatives that specifically neutralize the lethal, skin-necrosing, and hemolytic properties of the α-toxin of *Staphylococcus aureus.*

　　**tetanus a.** (USP, BP), a. specific for the toxin of *Clostridium tetani.*

　　**tetanus and gas gangrene a.'s** (NF), a solution of antitoxic substances obtained from animals immunized against the toxins of *Clostridium tetani, C. perfringens,* and *C. septicum.*

　　**tetanus-perfrin'gens a.,** an a. prepared from animals immunized against the toxins of *Clostridium tetani* and *C. perfringens* (*C. welchii*).

**an'titoxin'ogen** [ antitoxin + suffix *-gen,* producing ]. Any antigen that stimulates the formation of antitoxin in an animal or person, *i.e.,* a toxin or a toxoid.

**antitragicus** (an'tĭ-traj'ĭkus). See *musculus* antitragicus.

**an'titra'gohel'icine.** See *fissura* antitragicohelicina.

**antitra'gus** [ G. *anti-tragos,* the eminence of the external ear, fr. *anti,* opposite, + *tragos,* a goat, the tragus ] [ NA ]. A projection of the cartilage of the auricle, in front of the cauda helicis, just above the lobule, and posterior to the tragus from which it is separated by the intertragic notch.

**antitreponemal** (an'tĭ-trep-o-ne'mal). Treponemicidal.

**antitrismus** (an'tĭ-triz'mus). A condition of tonic muscular spasm preventing closure of the mouth.

**an'titrope** [ anti- + G. *tropē,* a turn ]. An organ or appendage that forms a symmetrically reversed pair with another of the same type, *e.g.,* the right and left legs of a vertebrate.

**antitro'pic** Similar, bilaterally symmetrical, but in an opposite location (as in a mirror image), *e.g.,* the right thumb in relation to the left thumb.

**antytryp'sic.** Antitryptic.

**antitryp'sin.** A substance that inhibits or prevents the action of trypsin.

**antitryp'tic.** Antitrypsic; possessing properties of antitrypsin.

**ant'itu'morigen'esis.** Inhibition of the growth of a neoplasm.

**antitus'sive** [ anti- + L. *tussis,* cough ]. Antibechic. 1. Relieving cough. 2. A cough remedy.

**antity'phoid.** Preventive or curative of typhoid fever.

**antiuratic** (an'tĭ-u-rat'ik). Restricting the formation or preventing the precipitation of urates.

**antiurease** (an-tĭ-u're-āz). A substance that inhibits or prevents the hydrolysis of urea by urease.

**antiven'ene** [ anti- + L. *venenum,* poison ]. Antivenin.

**antivenereal** (an-tĭ-vĕ-ne're-al). Preventive or curative of venereal diseases.

**antiven'in.** Antivenene; an antitoxin specific for an animal or insect venom.

**antivi'ral.** Opposing a virus, weakening or abolishing its action.

**antivi'tamin.** A substance that prevents a vitamin from exerting its typical biological effects. Most a.'s have chemical structures similar to vitamins (*e.g.,* pyridoxine and its a., deoxypyridoxine) and appear to function as competitive antagonists. Some a.'s produce effects, in addition, that are unrelated to vitamin antagonism.

**an'tivivisec'tion.** Opposition to the use of living animals for experimentation; see vivisection.

**an'tivivisec'tionist.** One who is opposed to experimentation on living animals.

**antixerophthalmic** an'tĭ-ze'rof-thal'mik) [ anti- + G. *xēros,* dry, + *ophthalmos,* eye ]. Applied to vitamin A, a deficiency of which results in drying of the conjunctiva.

**antixerotic** (an-tĭ-ze-rot'ik). Preventing xerosis.

**Anton,** Gabriel, German neuropsychiatrist, 1858–1933. See A.'s *syndrome.*

**Antoni types A and B neurilemoma.** See under neurilemoma.

**antra** (an'trah). Plural of antrum.

**an'tral.** Relating to an antrum.

**antrec'tomy** [ antrum + G. *ektomē,* excision ]. 1. Removal of the walls of an antrum. 2. Removal of the antrum (distal half) of the stomach; often combined with bilateral excision of vagus nerve trunks (vagectomy) in treatment of peptic ulcer.

**antro-** [ L. *antrum,* from G. *antron,* a cave ]. Combining form denoting relationship to any antrum.

**an'troduodenec'tomy.** Surgical removal of the antrum of the stomach and the ulcer-bearing part of the duodenum.

**antronalgia** (an'tro-nal'jĭ-ah) [ antro- + G. *algos,* pain ]. Pain in an antrum.

**antrona'sal.** Relating to a maxillary sinus and the corresponding nasal fossa.

**antroneurolysis** (an'tro-nu-rol'ĭ-sis) [ antro- + G. *neuron,* nerve, + *lysis,* loosening ]. Antrum dissection, interrupting all the nerve elements present in the submucosa.

**an'trophore** [ antro- + G. *phoros,* bearing ]. A medicated bougie for the local treatment of disease in any accessible cavity or canal, especially the urethra.

**antrophose** (an'tro-fōz) [ antro- + G. *phos,* light ]. A subjective sensation of light or color originating in the visual centers of the brain.

**antropyloric** (an'tro-pi-lor'ik). Related to or affecting the antrum pyloricum.

**an'troscope** [ antro- + G. *skopeō,* to view ]. An instrument to aid in the ocular examination of any cavity; specifically, an electric light bulb for transillumination of the antrum of Highmore to determine the presence or absence of an accumulation of fluid or a tumor in that cavity.

**antros'copy.** Examination of any cavity, especially of the antrum of Highmore, by means of an antroscope.

**antros'tomy** [ antro- + G. *stoma,* mouth ]. The formation of a more or less permanent opening into any antrum.

**antrot'omy** [ antro- + G. *tomē,* incision ]. Incision through the wall of any antrum.

**an'troto'nia.** Tonus of an antrum.

**an'trotympan'ic.** Relating to the mastoid antrum and the tympanic cavity.

**antrum,** gen. **antri,** pl. **antra** [ L. fr. G. *antron,* a cave ]. 1 [ NA ]. Any nearly closed cavity, particularly one with bony walls. 2. The pyloric end of the stomach, partially shut off, during digestion, from the cardiac end, or fundus, by the prepyloric sphincter.

**a. cardi'acum,** forestomach; a dilation that occasionally occurs in the aboral end of the esophagus near the stomach.

**a. ethmoida'le,** *sinus* ethmoidalis.

**a. of Highmore,** *sinus* maxillaris.

**mastoid a.,** a. mastoideum.

**a. mastoid'eum** [ NA ], tympanic a.; mastoid a.; a cavity in the petrous portion of the temporal bone, communicating posteriorly with the mastoid cells and anteriorly with the epitympanic recess of the middle ear.

**max'illary a.,** *sinus* maxillaris.

**a. pylor'icum** [ NA ], a bulging of the pyloric end of the stomach wall along the greater curvature when the organ is distended; see antrum (2).

**tympan'ic a.,** a. mastoideum.

**antu'itarism** [ ant(erior lobe) + (pit)uitar(y) ]. A condition resulting from hyperactivity of the anterior lobe of the pituitary body, gigantism or acromegalia.

**Antyllus** (an-til'us), Greek physician, *circa* 150 A.D., greatest surgeon of his era. See A.'s *method.*

**an'ulus,** pl. **an'uli** [ L. ] [ NA ]. A ring; a circular or ring-shaped structure. See also ring.

**a. abdomina'lis,** a. inguinalis profundus.

**a. cilia'ris,** *orbiculus* ciliaris.

**a. conjuncti'vae** [ NA ], conjunctival ring; a narrow ring at the junction of the periphery of the cornea with the conjunctiva.

**a. femora'lis** [ NA ], femoral ring; the superior opening of the femoral canal, bounded anteriorly by the inguinal ligament, posteriorly by the pectineus muscle, medially by the lacunar ligament, and laterally by the femoral vein.

**a. fibrocartilagin'eus** [ NA ], the thickened portion of the circumference of the tympanic membrane that is fixed in the tympanic sulcus.

**a. fibro'sus** [ NA ], (1) coronary tendon; Lower's ring; one of four fibrous rings that surround atrioventricular and arterial orifices of the heart; (2) the fibrous ring forming the circumference of the intervertebral disk.

**a. of fibrous sheath,** *pars* anularis vaginae fibrosae.

**Haller's a.,** Haller's *insula.*

**a. hemorrhoida'lis,** *zona* hemorrhoidalis.

**a. inguina'lis profun'dus** [ NA ], a. abdominalis; deep inguinal ring; abdominal ring; the opening in the transversalis fascia through which the ductus deferens (or round ligament in the female) enters the inguinal canal.

**a. inguina'lis superficia'lis** [ NA ], subcutaneous ring; superficial inguinal ring; external inguinal ring; the slit-like opening in the aponeurosis of the external oblique muscle of the abdominal wall through which the spermatic cord (round ligament in the female) emerges from the inguinal canal.

**a. ir'idis,** ring of the iris; one of two zones on the anterior surface of the iris, separated by a circular line concentric with the pupillary border; the **a. iridis minor** [ NA ] is the inner of the two zones and is much narrower than the other, **a. iridis major** [ NA ].

**a. ova'lis,** *limbus* fossae ovalis.

**a. preputia'lis,** the circular line of junction between the outer and the inner leaf at the anterior extremity of the prepuce.

**a. tendin'eus communis** [ NA ], ligament of Zinn; a fibrous ring that surrounds the optic foramen and the medial part of the superior orbital fissure. It gives origin to the four rectus muscles of the eye and is partially fused with the sheath of the optic nerve.

**a. tympanicus** [ NA ], tympanic ring; tympanic bone; a more or less complete bony ring at the inner end of the external auditory meatus, giving attachment to the tympanic membrane.

**a. umbilica'lis** [ NA ], umbilical ring; canalis umbilicus; an opening in the linea alba through which pass the umbilical vessels in the fetus. In young embryos it is relatively nearer to the pubis, but gradually ascends to the center of the abdomen. It is closed in the adult, its site being indicated by the umbilicus or navel.

**a. urethra'lis,** *musculus* sphincter vesicae.

**Vieussens' a.,** *limbus* fossae ovalis.

**anuresis** (an-u-re'sis) [ G. *an-* priv. + *ourēsis,* urination ]. Absence of the act of urination, in contradistinction to anuria, the state characterized by the failure to urinate (the words are not true synonyms).

**anuret'ic, anu'ric.** Relating to anuresis, or anuria.

**anu'ria.** Total suppression of urine formation.

**a'nus,** gen. **a'ni,** pl. **a'nus** [ L. ] [ NA ]. Anal orifice; the lower opening of the digestive tract, lying in the fold between the nates, through which fecal matter is extruded.

**artificial a.,** an opening into the bowel, usually in the right or left flank, made by the operation of colostomy.

**Bartholin's a.,** a. cerebri.

**a. cer'ebri,** Bartholin's a.; aditus ad aqueductum cerebri; entrance to the cerebral aqueduct (of Sylvius) immediately caudal to the third ventricle.

**imperforate a.,** anal *atresia.*

**preternatural a.,** artificial a.

**a. vesica'lis,** rectal emptying into the urinary bladder.

**vestib'ular a., vulvovag'inal a.,** a congenital malformation in a female in whom the a. is imperforate, but the rectum opens into the vagina just above the vulva.

**an'vil.** Incus.

**anxi'etas** [ L. fr. *anxius,* distressed, fr. *ango,* pp. *anxus,* to cause pain ]. Anxiety.

**a. preseni'lis,** anxiety caused by approaching senility.

**a. tibia'rum,** restless legs *syndrome.*

**anxiety** (ang'zi'ĕ-tĭ) [ L. *anxietas, q. v.* ]. 1. In psychoanalysis, apprehension of danger and dread accompanied by restlessness, tension, tachycardia, and dyspnea unattached to a clearly identifiable stimulus. 2. In experimental psychology, a drive or motivational state learned from previously neutral cues.

**castration a.,** castration *complex.*

**free-floating a.,** term used in psychoanalysis to describe a pervasive, unrealistic expectation unattached to a clearly formulated concept or object of fear; observed particularly in a. neurosis and may be seen in some cases of latent schizophrenia.

**noetic a.,** in existential psychotherapy, a. caused by confusion or loss of meaning in life.

**separation a.,** in psychiatry, a child's apprehension or fear associated with his removal from or loss of a parent.

**situation a.,** a. related to current life problems.

**AOC.** Abbreviation of anodal opening *contraction*, also written AnOC.

**aorta,** pl. and gen. **aortae** (a-or'tah) [ Mod. L. fr. G. *aortē*, from *aeirō*, to lift up. AORT- ] [ NA ]. A large artery of the elastic type which is the main trunk of the systemic arterial system, arising from the base of the left ventricle; the **thoracic a.** is divided into the *ascending* portion, the *arch*, and the *descending* portion; at the diaphragm it becomes the **abdominal a.** and bifurcates at the left side of the body of the fourth lumbar vertebra into the right and left common iliac arteries.

**a. abdomina'lis** [ NA ], abdominal a.; the a. from the diaphragm to the bifurcation into right and left common iliac arteries.

**a. angus'ta,** congenital narrowness of a.

**a. ascen'dens** [ NA ], ascending a.; the first part of the a. between its origin from the heart and the arch of the a.

**buckled a.,** pseudocoarctation.

**a. descendens** [ NA ], descending a.; the part of the a. between the arch and the bifurcation into the common iliac arteries, it includes the thoracic and abdominal aortae.

**dynamic a.,** abnormally marked pulsations of abdominal a.

**kinked a.,** pseudocoarctation.

**overriding a.,** a congenitally malpositioned a. whose origin straddles the ventricular septum and so receives ejected blood from the right ventricle as well as from the left; it is found especially in tetralogy of Fallot.

**primitive a.,** the paired aortic primordia in young embryos.

**a. thoracica** [ NA ], thoracic a.; the a. from its origin to the diaphragm; its branches are the coronary, innominate or brachiocephalic, left subclavian and common carotid, intercostal, subcostal, diaphragmatic, vas aberrans, bronchial, esophageal, pericardial, and mediastinal arteries.

**ventral a.'s,** the paired vessels ventral to the pharynx, which give rise to the aortic arches.

**aor'tal.** Aortic.

**aortal'gia** [ aorta + G. *algos*, pain ]. Pain assumed to be due to aneurysm or other pathologic condition of the aorta.

**aortarctia** (a-or-tark'shĭ-ah) [ aorta + L. *arcto*, properly *arto*, to narrow ]. Aortostenosis.

**aortar'tia.** Aortostenosis.

**aortectasis, aortectasia** (a-or-tek'tă-sis, -tek-ta'zĭ-ah) [ aorta + G. *ektasis*, a stretching ]. Dilation of aorta.

**aortectomy** (a-or-tek'to-mĭ) [ aorta + G. *ektomē*, excision ]. Excision of a portion of the aorta.

**aor'tic.** Relating to the aorta or the a. orifice of the left ventricle of the heart.

**aor'ticore'nal.** Related to the aorta and kidney, specifically the ganglion aorticorenale.

**aortis'mus abdomina'lis** [ L. ]. Phantom *aneurysm*.

**aorti'tis.** Inflammation of the aorta.

**giant cell a.,** giant cell arteritis involving the aorta, sometimes with dissecting aneurysm.

**syphilitic a.,** the commonest manifestation of tertiary syphilis; involves the thoracic aorta; replacement of elastic tissue in the media by vascular scars results in dilation that may lead to aneurysm formation.

**aor'tocor'onary.** Relating to the aorta and the coronary arteries.

**aor'togram.** X-ray picture of aorta after the injection of contrast medium (may be direct puncture or intravenous).

**aortography** (a-or-tog'ră-fĭ) [ aorta + G. *graphō*, to write ]. Radiographic visualization of the aorta and its branches by injection of contrast media using percutaneous puncture or catheterization technique.

**ret'rograde a.,** a. by the injection of the contrast medium into the aorta through one of its branches, *e.g.*, the brachial; that is, in a direction against the blood stream.

**translum'bar a.,** injection into the abdominal aorta through a needle just below the 12th rib and 4 fingerbreadths to the left of the spinal processes of the vertebrae.

**aor'toil'iac.** Relating to the aorta and the iliac arteries.

**aortopathy** (a-or-top-ă-thĭ) [ aorta + G. *pathos*, suffering ]. Disease affecting the aorta.

**aortoptosia, aortoptosis** (a-or-top-to'zĭ-ah, -top-to'sis) [ aorta + G. *ptōsis*, a failing ]. A sinking down of the abdominal aorta in splanchnoptosia.

**aortorrhaphy** (a-or-tor'af-e) [ aorta + G. *rhaphē*, seam ]. Suture of the aorta.

**aortosclerosis** (a-or'to-skle-ro'sis). Arteriosclerosis of the aorta.

**aor'tosteno'sis** [ aorta + G. *stenōsis*, a narrowing ]. Aortarctia; aortartia; narrowing of the aorta.

**aortot'omy** [ aorta + G. *tomē*, a cutting ]. Incision into the aorta.

**a. p.** Abbreviation for L. *ante prandium*, before dinner.

**APA.** Abbreviation for antipernicious anemia *factor*.

**apallesthesia** (ă-pal-es-the'zĭ-ah) [ G. *a-* priv. + *pallo*, to tremble, quiver, + *aisthēsis*, feeling ]. Pallanesthesia.

**apancreatic** (ă-pan'kre-at'ik). Without pancreas.

**apan'dria** [ G. *apo*, from, + *anēr* (*andr-*), man ]. Aversion to men, *i.e.*, members of the male sex.

**apanthropia, apanthropy** (ap'an-thro'pĭ-ah, ă-pan'thro-pĭ) [ G. *apo*, from, + *anthrōpos*, man ]. Aversion to man, to human society.

**aparalytic** (a-par'ă-lit'ik). Not paralyzed; without paralysis.

**apar'athy'roidism.** Lack of parathyroid glands.

**aparathyrosis** (ă-par-ă-thi-ro'sis). An extreme degree of hypoparathyroidism where no parathyroid function is detectable.

**apareunia** (ă-par-u'nĭ-ah) [ G. *a-* priv. + *para*, alongside, + *eunē*, bed ]. Absence or impossibility of coitus.

**ap'arthro'sis** [ G. fr. *apo*, from, + *arthron*, joint ]. Disarticulation.

**apas'tia** [ G. *apastia*, fasting ]. Failure to eat.

**ap'athet'ic.** Exhibiting apathy; indifferent.

**ap'athism.** A sluggishness of reaction, the opposite of erethism.

**ap'athy** [ G. *apatheia*, fr. *a-* priv. + *pathos*, suffering ]. Absence of emotion; indifference; insensibility.

**apatite** (ap'ah-tīt). Name given to a group of minerals of the general formula $Ca_{10}F_2(PO_4)_6$ (fluorapatite). It is thought to be closely similar to the mineral salt of bones and teeth.

**ap'azone** (USAN). 5-(Dimethylamino)-9-methyl-2-propyl-1$H$-pyrazolo[ 1,2-$\alpha$ ][ 1,2,4 ]benzotriazine-1,3(2$H$)-dione; anti-inflammatory agent.

**apeidosis** (ap'i-do'sis) [ G. *apo*, away, + *eidos*, form ]. Departure from the normal histologic picture or the characteristic manifestations of a disease.

**apel'lous** [ G. *a-* priv. + L. *pellis*, skin ]. 1. Without skin. 2. Without foreskin; circumcised.

**apenteric** (ap'en-ter'ik) [ G. *apo*, from, + *enteron*, intestine ]. Abenteric; away from the intestine, said of a morbid process which would normally occur in the intestine.

**apep'sia** [ G. *a-* priv. + *pepsis*, a digesting ]. Extreme dyspepsia; complete cessation of digestion.

**apepsin'ia.** Lack of pepsin in the gastric juice.

**aperient** (ă-pe'rĭ-ant) [ L. *aperio*, pres. p. *aperiens*, to open ]. 1. Slightly cathartic. 2. A laxative or mild cathartic.

**aperiodic** (a-pe'rĭ-od'ik). Not occurring periodically.

**aperistal'sis.** Absence of peristalsis.

**aper'itive** [ Fr. *apéritif*, from L. *aperio*, to open ]. 1. Aperient. 2. Stimulating the appetite.

**Apert,** Eugène, Paris pediatrician, 1868–1940. See A.'s *hirsutism, syndrome.* Cooke-A.-Gallais *syndrome.*

**apertognathia** (ă-per'to-nath'ĭ-ah) [ L. *apertus*, open, + G. *gnathos*, jaw ]. Open *bite*.

**ap'ertom'eter.** Instrument for measuring the angular aperture of a microscope objective.

**apertu'ra,** pl. **apertu'rae** [ L. fr. *aperio*, pp. *apertus*, to open ] [ NA ]. An opening or aperture.

**a. exter'na aqueduc'tus vestib'uli** [ NA ], the external opening of the vestibular aqueduct on the posterior surface of the petrous part of the temporal bone.

**a. externa canalic'uli cochleae** [ NA ], the external opening of the cochlear aqueduct on the temporal bone medial to the jugular fossa.

**a. latera'lis ventric'uli quar'ti** [ NA ], lateral aperture of the 4th ventricle; foramen lateralis ventriculi quarti; foramen of Luschka, of Retzius, or of Key-Retzius; one of the two lateral openings of the fourth ventricle into the subarachnoid space.

**a. media'na ventric'uli quar'ti** [ NA ], median aperture of the 4th ventricle; arachnoid foramen; foramen of Magendie; the large midline opening in the posterior inferior part of the roof of the 4th ventricle, connecting the ventricle with the cerebellomedullary cistern of the subarachnoid space.

**a. pelvis inferior** [ NA ], a. pelvis minoris; pelvic plane of outlet; fourth parallel pelvic plane; inferior strait; plane of outlet; the lower opening of the true pelvis, bounded anteriorly by the pubic arch, laterally by the rami of the ischium and the sacrotuberous ligament on either side, and posteriorly by these ligaments and the tip of the coccyx.

**a. pelvis minoris,** a. pelvis inferior.

**a. pelvis superior** [ NA ], pelvic plane of inlet; aditus pelvis; first parallel pelvic plane; superior strait; pelvic brim; plane of inlet; the upper opening of the true pelvis, bounded anteriorly by the symphysis pubica and the pubic crest on either side, laterally by the iliopectineal lines, and posteriorly by the promontory of the sacrum.

**a. pirifor'mis** [ NA ], piriform opening; the anterior nasal openings in the skull.

**a. sinus frontalis** [ NA ], the opening of the frontal sinus on the nasal part of the frontal bone.

**a. sinus sphenoidal'is** [ NA ], one of the pair of openings in the body of the sphenoid bone through which the sphenoid sinuses communicate with the sphenoethmoidal recess of the nasal cavity.

**a. thoracis inferior** [ NA ], the inferior boundary of the bony thorax composed of the twelfth thoracic vertebra and the lower margins of the rib cage and sternum.

**a. thoracis superior** [ NA ], the upper boundary of the bony thorax composed of the first thoracic vertebra and the upper margins of the first ribs and manubrium of the sternum.

**a. tympan'ica canalic'uli chordae tympani** [ NA ], tympanic opening of the canal for the chorda tympani; the opening of the canal for the chorda tympani into the middle ear.

**aperture** (ap'er-tūr) [ L. *apertura,* an opening ]. 1. Apertura; an opening; orifice. 2. The diameter of the objective of a microscope.

**angle of a.,** see under angle.

**angular a.,** the diameter of the object glass of a microscope measured by the angle made by lines from periphery of objective to focus.

**lateral a. of the fourth ventricle,** *apertura* lateralis ventriculi quarti.

**median a. of the fourth ventricle,** *apertura* mediana ventriculi quarti.

**numerical a.** (abbr. N.A.), defined by the formula *n* sine *a,* where *n* is the refractive index of the medium between the object and objective lens and *a* is the angle between the central and the marginal ray entering the objective.

**apetinil.** ADIPARTHROL; *N*-ethyl-α-methylphenethylamine; sympathomimetic with anorexigenic effect.

**a'pex,** gen. **ap'icis,** pl. **ap'ices** [ L. summit or tip ] [ NA ]. The extremity of a conical or pyramidal structure, such as the heart or the lung.

**a. of arytenoid cartilage,** a. cartilaginis arytenoideae.

**a. auric'ulae** [ NA ], a. satyri; tip of the auricle; a point projecting upward and posteriorly from the free outcurved margin of the helix a little posterior to its upper end.

**a. capit'is fib'ulae** [ NA ], a. of the head of the fibula; also called styloid process of the fibula.

**a. cartila'ginis arytenoi'deae** [ NA ], a. of the arytenoid cartilage; the pointed upper end of the cartilage which supports the corniculate cartilage and the aryepiglottic fold.

**a. cor'dis** [ NA ], vertex cordis; the blunt extremity of the heart formed by the left ventricle; see a. *beat.*

**a. cornus posterioris** [ NA ], tip of the horn; caput cornus; the pointed extremity of each posterior gray column or cornu of the spinal cord.

**a. cuspidis** [ NA ], a. of a cusp of a tooth.

**a. of head of fibula,** a. capitis fibulae.

**a. linguae** [ NA ], tip of the tongue.

**a. na'si** [ NA ], tip of the nose.

**or'bital a.,** the posterior part of the orbit into which the optic foramen opens.

**a. ossis sacri** [ NA ], a. of the sacrum; the tapering lower end of the sacrum that articulates with the coccyx.

**a. par'tis petro'sae** [ NA ], apex of the petrous part of the temporal bone; the blunt medial extremity of the petrous part that forms the posterior wall of the foramen lacerum. The carotid canal opens at the apex.

**a. of patella,** a. patellae.

**a. patel'lae** [ NA ], apex of the patella; the pointed lower end of the patella from which the ligamentum patellae passes to insert on the tibial tuberosity.

**a. prosta'tae** [ NA ], apex of the prostate; the lowermost part of the prostate, situated above the urogenital diaphragm.

**a. of prostate,** a. prostatae.

**a. pulmonis** [ NA ], the rounded, upper extremity of each lung that extends into the cupula of the pleura.

**a. radicis dentis** [ NA ], the terminal end of a dental root.

**root a.,** extreme tip of r. of a tooth; the part farthest from the incisal or occlusal side.

**a. of sacrum,** a. ossis sacri.

**a. sat'yri,** a. auriculae.

**a. of urinary bladder,** a. vesicae.

**a. vesicae** [ NA ], a. of the urinary bladder; the junction of the superior and anteroinferior surfaces of the bladder, continuous above with the median umbilical ligament.

**apexcar'diogram.** Graphic recording of the movements of the chest wall produced by the apex beat of the heart.

**apex'igraph** [ apex + G. *graphō,* to write ]. A device for determining the size and position of the apex of a tooth root.

**APF.** Abbreviation for animal protein *factor.*

**Apgar,** Virginia, U. S. anesthesiologist, 1909–1974. See A. *score.*

**apha'cia.** Obsolete spelling for aphakia.

**aphagia** (ă-fa'jĭ-ah) [ G. *a*- priv. + *phagein,* to eat ]. Dysphagia.

**a. al'gera,** failure to eat or swallow because it causes pain.

**aphagopraxia** (ă-fag'o-prak'sĭ-ah) [ G. *a*- priv. + *phagein,* to eat, + *praxis,* doing ]. Dysphagia.

**aphakia** (ă-fa'kĭ-ah) [ G. *a*- priv. + *phakos,* lentil, anything shaped like a lentil. LEN- ]. Absence of the crystalline lens.

**apha'kial, apha'kic.** Devoid of crystalline lens.

**aphalangia** (a-fă-lan'gĭ-ah) [ G. *a*- priv. + phalanx, *q.v.* ]. Absence of fingers or toes.

**aphanisis** (ă-fan'ĭ-sis) [ G. *aphaneia,* disappearance ]. Fear of losing sexual power.

**aphantobi'ont** [ G. *aphantos,* invisible, + *bion,* pres. p. ntr. of *bioō,* to live, a living thing ]. Virus; obsolete term for one of a number of ultramicroscopic, filtrable particles, some the pathogens of certain diseases, and others assumed to be back of vital processes.

**aphasia** (ă-fa'zĭ-ah) [ G. speechlessness, fr. *a*- priv. + *phasis,* speech ]. Logagnosia; logamnesia; logasthenia; impaired or absent communication by speech, writing, or signs, due to dysfunction of brain centers in the dominant hemisphere.

**acoustic a.,** auditory a.

**amnestic a., amnesic a.,** inability to find or remember words.

**anom'ic a.,** nominal a.

**associative a.,** conduction a.

**ataxic a.,** motor a.

**auditory a.,** word deafness; acoustic a.; disability in comprehending speech or sounds.

**Broca's a.,** motor a.

**conduction a.,** associative a.; a form of a. in which the subject can speak and write in a way, but skips or repeats words or substitutes one word for another, the lesion being in the association tracts connecting the various language centers.

**expressive a.,** motor a.

**functional a.,** a. related to conversion hysteria.

**global a.,** loss of all forms of communication.

**graphic a., graphomotor a.,** cerebral or mental agraphia; the inability to express ideas in writing.

**impressive a.,** sensory a.

**jargon a.,** a. in which the patient talks in nonsense syllables or in which several words are run together as one.

**Kussmaul's a.,** mutism in psychosis.

**mixed a.,** a mixture of motor and sensory a.

**motor a.,** any of the varieties of a. in which the power of expression by writing, speaking, or signs is lost. Also called ataxic, expressive, or Broca's a.

**nominal a.,** optic a.; anomic a.; a. in which the patient has difficulty in recalling or is unable to recall the names of persons and things.

**optic a.,** nominal a.

**pathematic a.,** mutism related to anger or strong emotions.

**psychosensory a.,** inability to comprehend written or spoken words.

**receptive a.,** sensory a.

**semantic a.,** a. in which objects are correctly named, there is little disturbance in articulation or words and individual words are understood, but the broader meaning of what is heard cannot be grasped.

**sensory a.,** impressive or receptive a.; loss of the power to comprehend written (or printed) or spoken words.

**syntactial a.,** a. in which the words are fairly well pronounced but short phrases or poorly constructed sentences without articles, prepositions or conjunctions are spoken.

**total a.,** global a.

**transcortical a.,** a. caused by damage to association pathways.

**visual a.,** (1) word *blindness;* (2) anomia.

**Wernicke's a.,** word deafness and anomia.

**apha'siac, apha'sic.** Relating to or suffering from aphasia.

**Aphasmid'ia.** Subclass of class Nematoda lacking phasmids (caudal sensory organs). Includes *Trichuris* and *Trichinella,* important human parasites.

**apheliotropism** (ap-he-lī-ot'ro-pizm) [ G. *apo,* away, + *helios,* sun, + *tropein,* to turn ]. Negative heliotaxis.

**aphemesthesia** (af'e-mes-the'zīah) [ G. *a-* priv. + *phēmē,* speech, + *aisthēsis,* sensation ]. Loss of the sense of articulate speech; inability to recognize what oneself is saying.

**aphe'mia** [ G. *a-* priv. + *phēmē,* speech ]. 1. A form of motor aphasia in which the power of expressing one's ideas in spoken words is lost. 2. Anarthria. 3. Obsolete term for aphasia.

**aphe'mic.** Relating to or suffering from aphemia.

**aphepho'bia.** Haphephobia.

**aphilopony** (a'fil-op'o-nī) [ G. *a-* priv. + *philō,* to like, + *ponos,* work ]. Fear of or lack of desire to work.

**aphonia** (ā-fo'nī-ah) [ G. *a-* priv. + *phōne,* voice ]. Loss of the voice in consequence of disease or injury of the organ of speech.

**hysterical a.,** loss of voice for psychogenic reasons; common in some varieties of hysteria.

**a. paralyt'ica,** a. due to paralysis of the vocal cords.

**a. parano'ica,** loss of voice due to anger.

**spastic a.,** a spasmodic contraction of the adductor muscles excited by an attempt at phonation.

**aphon'ic.** Aphonous; voiceless; relating to or suffering from aphonia.

**aphon'oge'lia** [ G. *a-* priv. + *phonē,* sound, + *gelān,* to laugh ]. Lack of ability to laugh out loud.

**aph'onous.** Aphonic.

**aphorisms of Hippocrates.** See under Hippocrates.

**aphose** (af'ōz) [ G. *a-* priv. + *phōs,* light ]. A subjective sensation of a dark spot or patch in the line of vision.

**aphotesthesia** (ā-fo-tes-the'zī-ah) [ G. *a-* priv. + *phōs,* light, + *aisthēsis,* perception ]. A condition, caused by overexposure to the sun's rays, in which there is decreased sensitivity of the retina to light.

**aphrasia** (ă-fra'zī-ah) [ G. *a-* priv. + *phrasis,* speaking ]. Speechlessness; dumbness; inability to speak, from any cause.

**a. parano'ica,** stubborn mutism (silence) of the insane (paranoiac).

**aphrenia** (ă-fre'nī-ah) [ G. *a-* priv. + *phrēn,* mind ]. 1. Dementia. 2. Unconsciousness. 3. Apoplexy.

**aphrodisia** (af-ro-diz'ī-ah) [ G. *aphrodisios,* relating to Aphrodite or Venus ]. 1. Sexual desire, especially when excessive. 2. Sexual congress.

**aphrodis'iac.** 1. Increasing sexual desire. 2. Anything that arouses or increases sexual desire.

**aphrodisiomania** (af-ro-diz'ī-o-ma'nī-ah) [ G. *aphrodisia,* sexual pleasures, + *mania,* insanity ]. Abnormal and excessive erotic interest.

**aphrone'sia** [ G. *a-* priv. + *phronēsis,* common sense, fr. *phroneō,* to think, fr. *phrēn,* mind ]. 1. Silliness. 2. Dementia.

**aphronia** (ă-fro'nī-ah) [ G. *aphrōn,* witless ]. Defect in thinking.

**aphtha,** pl. **aph'thae** (af'thah) [ G. ulceration ]. A minute ulcer on a mucous membrane, often covered by a gray or white exudate. See also aphthae and aphthosis.

**aph'thae** [ G. *aphthai,* pl. of *aphtha,* ulceration ]. Small white spots often associated with small ulcerations on the mucous membrane of the mouth seen in thrush, sprue, or with Vincent's infection; though usually caused by a virus or fungus, they may occur after enteric use of the broad spectrum antibiotics. See also aphthosis.

**Bednar's a.,** a traumatic affection of the newborn consisting of two yellow, flattened, slightly elevated patches, one on either side of the median raphe of the palate; they are often ulcerated.

**contagious a.,** foot and mouth *disease.*

**a. epizooticae,** foot and mouth *disease.*

**Mikulicz' a.,** *periadenitis* mucosa necrotica recurrens.

**a. orienta'les, a. trop'icae,** tropical *sprue.*

**aph'thoid.** Resembling aphthae.

**aphthoi'des chronica.** Sprue (1).

**aphthongia** (af-thon'jī-ah) [ G. *a-* priv. + *phthongos,* voice ]. A form of lingual spasm sometimes affecting public speakers; a variety of occupational neurosis analogous to writer's cramp.

**aphthosa** (af-tho'sah). Foot and mouth *disease.*

**aph'tho'sis.** Any condition characterized by the presence of aphthae (*q. v.*).

**habitual a.,** recurrent ulcerative *stomatitis.*

**aph'thous.** Characterized by or relating to aphthae or aphthosis.

**aphylaxis** (a-fi-lak'sis) [ G. *a-* priv. + *phylaxis,* a guarding ]. Nonimmunity; lack of protection against disease.

**ap'ical.** Relating to or situated at or near the apex of any structure.

**apicectomy** (ap'ī-sek'to-mī) [ L. *apex,* summit or tip, + G. *ektomē,* excision ]. 1. Opening and exenteration of air cells in the apex of the petrous pyramid of the temporal bone. 2. In dental surgery, an obsolete synonym for apicoectomy.

**apiceotomy** (ā-pis'e-ot'o-mī). Apicotomy.

**ap'ices.** Plural of apex.

**apicitis** (ap'ī-si'tis). Inflammation of the apex of any structure, particularly the apex of the lung.

**apico-** (ap'ī-ko-) [ L. *apex,* summit or tip ]. Combining form relating to any apex.

**apicoectomy** (ap'ik-o-ek'tom-e) [ apico- + G. *ektomē,* excision ]. Root amputation or resection; excision of the apex of a dental root.

**ap'icolo'cator.** A device for locating the root apex of a tooth.

**apicolysis** (ap-ī-kol'ī-sis) [ apico- + G. *lysis,* destruction ]. Artificial collapse of the upper portion of the lung by the operative detachment of the parietal pleura allowing a mesial displacement of the pulmonary apex.

**Apicomplex'a.** A subphylum of the phylum Protozoa, which includes the Sporozoa and Piroplasma and is characterized by the presence of an apical *complex, q. v.*

**apicostome** (ap'ī-ko-stōm). The trocar and cannula used in apicostomy.

**apicos'tomy** [ apico- + G. *stoma*, mouth ]. An operation in which the labial or buccal alveolar plate is perforated with a trocar and cannula; done to reach the root apex, and to take cultures from this area.

**apicot'omy** [ apico- + G. *tome*, a cutting ]. Apiceotomy; incision into an apical structure.

**apicurettage** (ap'ĭ-ku'rē-tahzh). Apical curettage after removal of an infected tooth.

**apigen'in.** 4',5,7-Trihydroxyflavone; a plant pigment; the aglucone of apiin, a glycoside present in parsley, and of apigenin-7-glucoside.

**apinealism** (ă-pin'e-al-izm). Absence of the pineal gland.

**apiol.** Parsley camphor; 1-allyl-2,5-dimethoxy-3,4-methylenedioxybenzene; antipyretic.

**apiphobia** (a'pĭ-fo'bĭ-ah) [ L. *apis*, bee, + G. *phobos*, fear ]. Melissophobia; morbid fear of bees.

**apitu'itarism.** Total lack of functional pituitary tissue; may be iatrogenic (*e.g.*, as a consequence of hypophysectomy) or the result of a spontaneous disease process.

**A'pium.** See celery seed.

**aplacen'tal.** Without a placenta; denoting the monotremes (which lay eggs and have no placenta) and the marsupials (which have a transitory simple yolk-sac placenta).

**aplanatic** (ă-plă-nat'ik). Pertaining to aplanatism, or to an aplanatic lens.

**aplan'atism** [ G. *a-* priv. + *planetos*, wandering ]. Freedom from chromatic or spherical aberration; said of a lens.

**aplasia** (ă-pla'zĭ-ah) [ G. *a-* priv. + *plasis*, a molding ]. 1. Defective development or congenital absence of an organ or tissue. 2. In hematology, incomplete or retarded or defective development. or a cessation of the usual regenerative process.

   **a. axia'lis extracortica'lis,** Merzbacher-Pelizaeus *disease*.

   **a. cu'tis congen'ita,** congenital absence or deficiency of a localized area of skin, with the base of the defect covered by a thin translucent membrane; most often a single area near the vertex of the scalp, but may involve other areas.

   **germinal a.,** seminiferous tubule *dysgenesis*.

   **gonadal a.,** gonadal agenesis; the congenital absence of essentially all gonadal tissue; in this state, the external genitalia and genital ducts are female; if Leydig cells are present, however, the external genitalia are commonly ambiguous and the genital ducts are female.

   **a. pilorum propia,** monilethrix.

**aplas'tic.** Pertaining to aplasia, or conditions characterized by defective regeneration, as in a. anemia.

**aplesia** (ă-ple'zĭ-ah) [ G. *aplesotos*, insatiate, fr. *a-* priv. + *pletho*, to become full ]. Acoria (1).

**apleuria** (a-plu'rĭ-ah). Congenital absence of one or more ribs; usually associated with absent transverse process or processes.

**aplo'na.** A preserved apple powder, made in Switzerland. Used in the treatment of chronic bacillary dysentery.

**aplysin.** A neurotoxin obtained from the marine nudibranch *Aplasia* (the sea hare).

**apnea** (ap'ne-ah) [ G. *apnoia*, want of breath. PN- ]. The absence of breathing.

   **chemoreceptor a.,** administration of oxygen to a patient whose respiratory drive consists of a hypoxemic stimulus to the carotid body when the respiratory center is depressed by general anesthesia or hypercarbia.

   **deglutition a.,** inhibition of breathing during swallowing.

   **ether a.,** ether anesthesia administered to the point of a. and then maintained with controlled respiration.

   **induced a.,** intentional respiratory arrest during general anesthesia produced by hypocarbia, a muscle relaxant drug, chemoreceptor a., or sudden cessation of rhythmic intermittent pressure during controlled respiration.

   **vagal a.,** cessation of respiration during general anesthesia following stimulation of the vagus nerve in the chest above the heart level or in the cervical and higher regions.

   **a. vera,** true a.; absence of respiratory movements, owing to acapnia and the consequent lack of stimulus by carbon dioxide to the respiratory centers; sometimes induced by oxygen therapy in chronic emphysema.

**apneic** (ap'ne-ik). Related to or suffering from apnea.

**apneumatic** (ap-nu-mat'ik) [ G. *a-* priv. + *pneuma*, breath ]. Containing no air, denoting a lung in the state of collapse.

**apneumatosis** (ap-nu-mă-to'sis) [ G. *a-* priv. + *pneumatoō*, to inflate, + suffix *-osis*, condition ]. Congenital atelectasis.

**apneumia** (ap-nu'mĭ-ah) [ G. *a-* priv. + *pneumōn*, lung ]. Congenital absence of the lungs.

**apneusis** (ap-nu'sis) [ G. *a-* priv. + *pneusis*, a breathing, fr. *pneō*, to breathe ]. An abnormal form of respiration following experimental section of the pons just behind its anterior border and consisting of prolonged inspirations alternating with short expiratory movements.

**apneus'tic.** Pertaining to apneusis.

**apo-** [ G. *apo*, away from, off ]. Combining form meaning, usually, separated from or derived from.

**apobio'sis** [ G. death, fr. *apo*, from, + *biōsis*, life ]. Death; especially local death of a part of the organism.

**apocamno'sis** [ G. *apokamnō*, to grow very weary, fr. *kamnō*, to toil ]. Rapidly induced fatigue.

**ap'ocartere'sis** [ G. *apocarterein*, to starve oneself to death ]. Suicide by starvation.

**apocleisis** (ap'o-kli'sis) [ G. *apo*, away, + *kleisis*, closure ]. Aversion to food.

**apocodeine** (ap-o-ko'dēn). $C_{18}H_{19}NO_2$; monomethyl ether of apomorphine. Has been used as an expectorant, mild emetic and hypnotic, and cathartic.

**apocope** (ă-pok'o-pe) [ G. *apokopē*, a cutting off ]. Amputation.

**apocop'tic** [ G. *apo-koptō*, to cut off ]. Relating to, or occurring as a result of an amputation; see *plethora apocoptica*.

**apocrine** (ap'o-krin) [ G. *apo-krinō*, to separate ]. See apocrine *gland*.

**apocrus'tic** [ G. *apokroustikos*, able to beat off, fr. *apo*, off, + *krouō*, to strike ]. 1. Astringent and repellent. 2. A drug so acting.

**apocupreine** (ap'o-ku'pre-in). Apoquinine.

**apocynein** (ap-o-si'ne-in). An active principle of *Apocynum cannabinum*, acting upon the heart like digitalis.

**apocynin** (ă-pos'ĭ-nin). 4-Hydroxy-3-methoxyacetophenone; acetovanillon; an active principle of *Apocynum cannabinum;* has been used for its digitalis-like effect.

**Apocynum** (ă-pos'i-num) [ G. *apokynon*, dogbane; fr. *apo*, from, + *kyōn*, dog ]. A genus of herbs of the family Apocynaceae.

   **A. androsaemifo'lium,** dogbane; wild ipecac; bitter-root; rheumatism weed; the rhizome is diuretic, cathartic, and diaphoretic.

   **A. cannab'inum,** Canadian hemp; Indian physic; formerly used for its digitalis-like effect.

**apodal** (a-po'dal) [ G. *a-* priv. + *pous*, foot ]. Without feet.

**apodemialgia** (ap'o-de'mĭ-al'jĭ-ah) [ G. *apodēmia*, being away from home, + *algos*, pain ]. A longing to get away from home or to travel; wanderlust; the opposite of nostalgia.

**apo'dia** [ G. *a-* priv. + *pous*, foot ]. Apody; congenital absence of feet.

**ap'odous.** Apodal.

**ap'ody.** Apodia.

**apoenzyme** (ap'o-en-zīm). The protein portion of an enzyme as contrasted with the nonprotein portion, or coenzyme, or prosthetic portion (if present).

**apofer'ment.** Apoenzyme.

**apofer'ritin.** A protein in the intestinal wall. It combines with a ferric hydroxide-phosphate compound to form ferritin, which is thought to be the first stage in the absorption of iron.

**apogam'ia, apog'amy** [ G. *apo*, away, + *gamein*, to wed ]. Parthenogenesis.

**apo'lar.** Having no poles; denoting specifically embryonic nerve cells (neuroblasts) that have not yet begun to sprout processes.

**apomix'ia** [ G. *apo*, from, + *mixis*, a mingling ]. Parthenogenesis.

**apomor'phine hydrochloride** (NF, BP). $C_{17}H_{17}NO_2$·HCl; a derivative of morphine; expectorant, emetic, and hypnotic.

**apone'a** [ G. *aponoia, q.v.* ]. Amentia

**aponeurectomy** (ap'o-nu-rek'to-mī). Excision of an aponeurosis.

**aponeurology** (ap'o-nu-rol'o-jī). The branch of anatomy that treats of aponeuroses and their relations.

**aponeurorrhaphy** (ap'o-nu-ror'ă-fī) [ aponeurosis + G. *rhaphē,* suture ]. Fasciorrhaphy.

**aponeurosis,** pl. **aponeuroses** (ap'o-nu-ro'sis) [ G. the end of the muscle where it becomes tendon, fr. *apo,* from, + *neuron,* sinew ] [ NA ]. A fibrous sheet or expanded tendon, giving attachment to muscular fibers and serving as the means of origin or insertion of a flat muscle; it sometimes also performs the office of a fascia for other muscles.

    **Denonvilliers' a.,** *septum* rectovesicale.

    **epicra'nial a., a. epicrania'lis** [ NA ], *galea* aponeurotica.

    **extensor a.,** a triangular tendinous expansion including the tendon of the extensor digitorum centrally, interosseus tendons on each side, and a lumbrical tendon laterally. It covers the dorsal aspect of the metacarpophalangeal joint and the proximal phalanx.

    **a. of insertion,** a tendinous sheet serving for the insertion of a broad muscle.

    **a. of investment,** a fibrous membrane covering and keeping in place a muscle or group of muscles.

    **a. linguae** [ NA ], lingual a.; the thickened lamina propria of the tongue to which the lingual muscles attach.

    **lingual a.,** a. linguae.

    **a. musculi bicipitis brachii** [ NA ], lacertus fibrosus, or semilunar fascia; bicipital fascia; radiating fibers from the tendon of insertion of the biceps passing obliquely over the hollow of the elbow to the ulnar side and becoming merged into the deep fascia of the forearm.

    **a. of origin,** a tendinous expansion serving as the attachment of origin of a broad muscle.

    **palatine a.,** the tendinous lamina in the anterior two-thirds of the soft palate into which all of the palatal muscles insert. It is attached to the posterior border of the hard palate.

    **a. palmaris** [ NA ], palmar fascia; Dupuytren's fascia; the tough fascia investing the muscles of the palm.

    **Petit's a.,** the posterior layer of the broad ligament of the uterus.

    **a. pharynge'a,** *fascia* pharyngobasilaris.

    **a. plantaris** [ NA ], plantar fascia; the tough fascia investing the muscles of the sole.

    **Sibson's a.,** *membrana* suprapleuralis.

    **temporal a.,** *fascia* temporalis.

    **thoracolumbar a.,** *fascia* thoracolumbalis.

**ap'oneurosi'tis.** Inflammation of an aponeurosis.

**ap'oneurot'ic.** Relating to an aponeurosis.

**aponeurotome** (ap'o-nu'ro-tōm). An instrument for dividing an aponeurosis.

**aponeurotomy** (ap'o-nu-rot'o-mī). Incision of an aponeurosis.

**apon'ia** [ G. *a-* priv. + *ponos,* toil, pain ]. 1. Nonexertion, abstention from labor. 2. Absence of pain.

**apon'ic.** Relating to aponia; analgesic; relieving fatigue.

**aponoia** (ă-pon-oy'ah) [ G. *aponoia;* fr. *apo,* away, + *nous,* mind ]. Amentia.

**apopathet'ic** Describing a form of behavior in which a person conspicuously alters his conduct in the presence of other people.

**apophylaxis** (ap'o-fi-lak'sis). A diminution of the phylactic power of the body fluids, as sometimes observed in the negative phase of therapy with immunizing agents.

**apophysary** (ă-pof'ī-sa-rī). Apophysial.

**apophysial, apophyseal** (ă-po-fiz'e-al). Apophysary; relating to or resembling an apophysis.

**apophysis,** pl. **apoph'yses** (ă-pof'ī-sis) [ G. an offshoot. PHYS- ] [ NA ]. An outgrowth or projection, especially one from a bone. A bony process or outgrowth that lacks an independent center of ossification.

    **bas'ilar a.,** the basilar process of the occipital bone.

    **a. conchae,** *eminentia* conchae.

    **a. hel'icis,** *spina* helicis.

    **Ingras'sia's a.,** *ala* minor.

    **lentic'ular a.,** *processus* lenticularis.

    **temporal a.,** *processus* mastoideus.

**apophysitis** (ă-pof-ī-si'tis). 1. Inflammation of any apophysis. 2. Appendicitis.

    **a. tibia'lis adolescen'tium,** Osgood-Schlatter *disease.*

**apoplasmia** (ap'o-plaz'mī-ah). A decrease in the amount of blood plasma.

**apoplec'tic.** Relating to, suffering from, or predisposed to apoplexy.

**apoplec'tiform.** Apoplectoid.

**apoplec'toid.** Resembling apoplexy; apoplectiform.

**apoplexy** (ap'o-plek-sī) [ G. *apoplēxia.* PLES- ]. 1. A classical term for cerebral hemorrhage, thrombosis, embolism, or vasospasm usually characterized by some degree of paralysis; also called stroke, cerebrovascular accident, cerebral crisis, ictus. 2. An effusion of blood into a tissue or organ.

    **abdominal a.,** mesenteric hemorrhage, thrombosis or embolus involving mesenteric or abdominal blood vessels.

    **adrenal a.,** hemorrhage into the adrenal, or thrombosis of the adrenal veins followed by acute adrenal insufficiency; induced in animals by pantothenic acid deficiency, and in man occurring in the Waterhouse-Friderichsen syndrome.

    **bulbar a.,** a. due to vascular lesion in the brain stem.

    **capillary a.,** a. due to damage of capillaries.

    **congestive a.,** a. caused by temporary disturbance of circulation.

    **cutaneous a.,** sudden rush of blood to skin and subcutaneous tissue.

    **embol'ic a.,** a. caused by the plugging of an artery of the brain by an embolus.

    **functional a.,** a condition simulating a. without any cerebral lesion; a form of conversion hysteria.

    **heat a.,** (1) heat *stroke;* (2) ardent *fever.*

    **ingraves'cent a.,** the slowly progressive onset of stroke.

    **neonatal a.,** a. of the newborn; intracranial hemorrhage in newborn children.

    **pontile a.,** bulbar a.

    **pulmonary a.,** hemorrhagic infarct of the lung; a circumscribed infiltration of the lung with blood in consequence of embolism or thrombosis of a branch of the pulmonary artery.

    **Raymond type of a.,** a form of ingravescent a. in which there is paresthesia of the hand on the side to become paralyzed.

    **serous a.,** a. due to edema or local exudation of serum.

    **spasmodic a.,** the occurrence of apoplectic symptoms caused by a temporary spasm of a cerebral artery.

    **spinal a.,** hematorrhachis.

    **splenic a.,** peracute anthrax often seen in ruminants, in which death occurs very quickly after the appearance of the first signs of the disease. Grossly enlarged spleen and capillary hemorrhages are often the only lesions.

    **thrombot'ic a.,** a. caused by thrombosis.

    **ure'thral a.,** hemorrhage from the urethra which occasionally occurs in severe (malignant) hypertension.

    **uterine a.,** hemorrhagic necrosis of the endometrium, seen especially in old women with cardiac failure; sometimes associated with superficial hemorrhagic necrosis of the bowel.

**apoprotein** (ap'o-pro'te-in, -tēn). See apoenzyme.

**apoptosis** (ă-pop-to'sis, ă-po-to'sis) [ G. a falling or dropping off, fr. *apo,* off, + *ptosis,* a falling ]. Cell deletion by fragmentation into membrane-bound particles which are phagocytosed by other cells.

**ap'oqui'nine.** Homoquinine; apocupreine; demethylated quinine; a crystalline alkaloid from cinchona bark with some actions similar to those of quinine.

**ap'orepres'sor.** Inactive *repressor.*

**apor'ia** [ G. *aporia,* difficulty, doubt ]. Doubt, especially deriving from incompatible views on the same subject.

**aporioneurosis** (ă-po'rī-o-nu-ro'sis) [ G. *aporia,* difficulty, doubt, + *neurosis* ]. 1. Embarrassment or hesitation. 2. Anxiety *neurosis.*

**aposia** (a-po'zĭ-ah) [ G. *a-* priv. + *posis,* drink ]. Adipsia.

**apositia** (ap'o-sish'ī-ah) [ G. *apo,* away, + *sitos,* food ]. Distaste for food.

**aposit'ic.** Decreasing the appetite for food; relating to apositia.

**ap'osome** [ G. *apo*, from, + *sōma*, body ]. A cytoplasmic inclusion produced by the cell itself.

**apos'tasis** [ G. a departure from, an abscess. STA- ]. The termination of a disease.

**apostax'is** [ G. a trickling down ]. A slight hemorrhage, or bleeding by drops.

**ap'ostem, aposte'ma, ap'osteme** [ G. *apostēma*, abscess. STA- ]. An abscess.

**apos'thia** [ G. *a-* priv. + *posthē*, foreskin ]. Congenital absence of the prepuce.

**apostilb** (apo-stilb) [ G. *apo*, from + *stilbe*, lamp ]. A unit of brightness equal to 0.1 millilambert.

**ap'othana'sia** [ G. *apo*, away, + *thanatos*, death ]. Postponement of death; prolongation of life; see also orthothanasia (2).

**apothecary** (ā-poth'e-kĕr-ī) [ G. *apothēkē*, a barn, storehouse, fr. *apo*, from, + *thēkē*, a box ]. 1. Obsolescent term for pharmacist or druggist. 2. In England, a medical practitioner licensed by the Society of Apothecaries of London to practice medicine and dispense drugs; in Ireland one similarly licensed by the Apothecaries' Hall of Ireland.

**surgeon-a.,** see *surgeon-apothecary.*

**ap'othem, ap'otheme** [ G. *apo*, from, + *thema*, something set down, fr. *tithēmi*, to place. THE- ]. A precipitate caused by long boiling of a vegetable infusion or by its exposure to air.

**apotox'in.** Richet's term for the anaphylactic substance resulting from the union of the special antibody (toxogenin) with the subsequently injected antigen; the a. was thought to cause the signs and symptoms of anaphylaxis.

**apoxesis** (apok-se'sis) [ G. *apo*, away, + *xeein*, to scrape ]. Subgingival *curettage.*

**ap'ozem, apoz'ema** [ G. See ZE- ]. A decoction.

**ap'ozy'mase.** The protein portion of zymase.

**apparatother'apy.** Mechanicotherapy.

**apparatus,** pl. **apparatus** (ap-ă-ra'tus, -rat'us) [ L. equipment. fr. *ap-paro*, pp. *-atus*, to prepare ]. 1. A collection of instruments adapted for a special purpose. 2. An instrument made up of several parts. 3 [ NA ]. A system; the group of glands, ducts, blood vessels, muscles, or other anatomical structures concerned in the performance of some function; see also system, systema.

**Abbé-Zeiss a.,** an a. for counting the blood corpuscles, consisting of a mixer for diluting the blood and a cell $1/10$ mm. deep, marked off into divisions of $1/400$ sq. mm. so that each division contains $1/4000$ cu. mm.; also called Thoma-Zeiss hemocytometer.

**Abel's vividiffusion a.,** see under vividiffusion.

**achromatic a.,** the nonstaining asters and spindle fibers in a dividing cell.

**attachment a.,** the tissues that attach the tooth to the alveolar process: cementum, periodontal membrane, and alveolar bone.

**Barcroft-Warburg a.,** Warburg's a.

**Beckmann's a.,** a. for the accurate measurement of melting points and boiling points in connection with molecular weight determinations.

**Benedict-Roth a.,** a device employed to measure the amount of oxygen utilized in quiet breathing in the basal state for the estimation of the basal metabolic rate.

**branchial a.,** the aggregate of the pharyngeal arches, pouches, clefts, and membranes seen in the developing embryo or lower vertebrates.

**central a.,** the centrosome and centrosphere.

**chromatic a.,** the deeply staining mass of chromosomes in a dividing cell.

**chromidial a.,** the aggregate of extranuclear network, irregular strands, and masses of basophilic staining material permeating the protoplasm of the cell. See also ribosome and cytoplasmic *reticulum.*

**dental a.,** the masticatory *system.*

**a. digesto'rius** [ NA ], systema digestorium [ NA ]; alimentary or digestive apparatus or system; the digestive tract from the mouth to the anus with all its associated glands and organs.

**Golgi a.,** Golgi complex; Golgi internal reticulum; Holmgren-Golgi canals; with the electron microscope it is seen to consist of a complex of parallel, flattened saccules, vesicles, and vacuoles; it lies adjacent to the nucleus of a cell. Concerned with intracellular formation of secretory products.

**Haldane's a.,** a device used for the analysis of respiratory gases.

**hyoid a.,** a. hyoideus.

**a. hyoi'deus,** hyoid a.; veterinary anatomy term for hyoid bones, a modified portion of the ancestral brachial skeleton consisting of an articulated chain of bones extending from the mastoid region of the skull on each side to the base of the tongue; in man, it is reduced to a single bone, os hyoideum; in a typical mammal (dog), it consists of a tympanohyoid cartilage attached to the skull, followed by the stylohyoid, epihyoid, keratohyoid, basihyoid, and thyrohyoid bones.

**juxtaglomerular a.,** juxtaglomerular complex; the juxtaglomerular body together with the macula densa of the distal tubule and the granular mesangial cells.

**Kirschner's a.,** Kirschner's *wire.*

**Kjeldahl a.,** an a. for distilling ammonia arising from acid decomposition of an organic compound; used in nitrogen analysis.

**a. lacrima'lis** [ NA ], lacrimal a., consisting of the lacrimal gland, the lacrimal lake, the lacrimal canaliculi, the lacrimal sac, and the nasolacrimal duct.

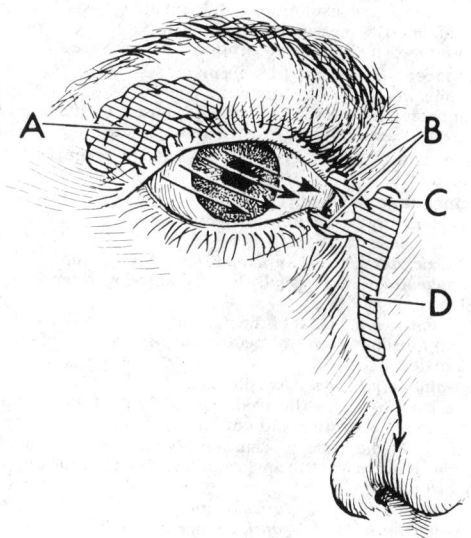

**Lacrimal Apparatus**
*A*, lacrimal gland; *B*, lacrimal canaliculi; *C*, lacrimal sac; *D*; nasolacrimal duct; *arrows* indicate the direction of flow of tears secreted by the lacrimal gland (*A*).

**a. ligamento'sus colli,** *ligamentum* nuchae.

**a. ligamento'sus Weitbrecht'i,** *membrana* tectoria.

**a. major, a. minor,** old terms for median and lateral *lithotomy,* respectively.

**Malgaigne's a.,** a double-inclined plane for fracture of the thigh.

**masticatory a.,** (1) masticatory *system;* (2) stomatognathic *system.*

**mental a.,** mental structure; a term used in psychoanalysis to describe the structure of topography of the mind.

**a. respirato'rius** [ NA ], systema respiratorium [ NA ]; respiratory apparatus or system; all the air passages from the nose to the pulmonary alveoli.

**Roughton-Scholander a.,** Roughton-Scholander syringe; a syringe-like device for analyzing the respiratory gases in a small sample of blood.

**Sayre's suspension a.,** a tripod derrick with rope and pulley for head traction during the application of a plaster of Paris jacket.

**Scholander a.,** a device used for determining the oxygen and carbon dioxide percentage in 0.5 ml. of a respiratory gas.

**subneural a.,** modified sarcoplasm in a motor end-plate.

**a. suspenso'rius lentis,** *zonula* ciliaris.

**Tallerman a.,** an a. in which one extremity or the trunk can be enclosed and submitted to dry air of a high temperature; used in the treatment of chronic rheumatism and other affections.

**Taylor's a.,** Taylor's splint; a steel spinal support for the treatment of Pott's disease.

**Tiselius a.,** an a. for separating proteins in solution by electrophoresis and thus for determining the isoelectric point, molecular weight, and related physical properties; the direction and rate of migration of the protein and the characteristics of the boundary phase between the protein solution and the supernatant salt solution are recorded by photography of the changes in refractive index at the boundary.

**urinary a.,** urinary *system.*

**a. urogenita'lis** [ NA ], systema urogenitale [ NA ]; urogenital or genitourinary apparatus or system; includes all the organs concerned in reproduction and in the formation and voidance of the urine.

**Van Slyke a.,** an a. for determining amounts of respiratory gases in blood.

**Warburg's a.,** Barcroft-Warburg a.; an a. for measuring the oxygen consumption of incubated tissue slices by manometric measurement of changes in gas pressure produced by oxygen absorption in an enclosed flask.

**apparent** (ă-păr'ent) [ L. *apparens,* visible, fr. *appareo,* to come in sight ]. 1. Manifest; obvious; *e.g.,* a clinically apparent infection. 2. Frequently used (confusingly) to mean "seeming to be," ostensible, pseudo-.

**appearance** (ă-pēr'ans) [ L. *appareo,* to come in sight ]. Aspect.

**appendage** (ă-pen'dij) [ L. *appendix, q.v.* ]. Appendix; annexum; any part, subordinate in function or size, attached to a main structure.

**auric'ular a.'s,** (1) auricula (2); a. of the atrium; (2) small congenital tumors usually located anterior to the auricle of the ear.

**drumstick a.,** an a. of the nucleus that represents the XX chromosome seen in neutrophil leukocytes of human females.

**epiploic a.,** *appendix* epiploica.

**a.'s of the eye,** the eyelids with their lashes, eyebrows, lacrimal apparatus, and conjunctiva.

**a.'s of the fetus,** amnion, yolk-sac, and the fetal (chorionic) part of the placenta together with the umbilical cord.

**left auricular a.,** *auricula* sinistra.

**right auricular a.,** *auricula* dextra.

**a.'s of the skin,** the hairs, nails, and sweat, sebaceous, and mammary glands.

**uterine a.'s,** the ovaries, uterine (Fallopian) tubes, and ligaments.

**vermiform a.,** *appendix* vermiformis.

**appendal'gia** [ appendix + G. *algos,* pain ]. Pain in the right iliac fossa in the region of the vermiform appendix.

**appendectomy** (ap'pen-dek'to-mĭ) [ appendix + G. *ek-tomē,* excision ]. Appendicectomy; scolecoidectomy; scolectomy; removal of any appendix, specifically, the vermiform appendix.

**auricular a.,** excision of the heart's auricular appendix.

**appen'dical.** Appendiceal.

**appendiceal** (ap-pen-dis'ĭ-al). Relating to an appendix.

**appen'dicec'tasis.** Ectasia of the appendix.

**appendicectomy** (ap-pen'dĭ-sek'to-mĭ). Appendectomy.

**appen'dicism.** Appendicosis; any chronic disease of the vermiform appendix, or a symptomatic uneasiness in the region of this structure.

**appendicitis** (ap-pen'dĭ-si'tis) [ appendix + G. suffix *-itis,* inflammation ]. Apophysitis; scolecoiditis; inflammation of the vermiform appendix.

**actinomycotic a.,** chronic suppurative a. due to infection by *Actinomyces israelii,* sometimes resulting in a fecal fistula following appendectomy.

**acute a.,** aute inflammation of the appendix, usually due to bacterial infection, which may be precipitated by obstruction of the lumen by a fecalith. Symptoms of periumbilical colicky pain and vomiting are followed by fever, leukocytosis, and signs of peritoneal inflammation in the right lower quadrant of the abdomen. Perforation is a frequent complication.

**bilharzial a.,** caused by the deposition of the eggs of the blood fluke, *Schistosoma mansoni,* in the vermiform appendix.

**catarrhal a.,** mild acute a. without suppuration.

**chronic a.,** fibrous adhesions, scarring, or deformity of the appendix following subsidence of acute a.; other than fibrous obliteration of the distal lumen which is not abnormal in older persons.

**focal a.,** acute a. involving only part of the appendix, sometimes at the site of, or distal to, an obstruction of the lumen.

**gangrenous a.,** acute a. with necrosis of the wall of the appendix, most commonly developing in obstructive a. and frequently causing perforation and acute peritonitis.

**lumbar a.,** a retrodisplaced appendix in the lumbar region.

**obstructive a.,** acute a. due to infection of retained secretion behind an obstruction of the lumen by a fecalith or some other cause, including carcinoma of the cecum.

**stercoral a.,** a. following a lodgment of fecal material in the appendix.

**subperitoneal a.,** a. of a subperitoneally placed appendix.

**suppurative a.,** acute a. with purulent exudate in the lumen and wall of the appendix.

**verminous a.,** a. caused by obstruction or response to the presence of parasitic worms such as *Ascaris lumbricoides, Strongyloides stercoralis,* or the pinworm *Enterobius vermicularis.*

**appendiclausis** (ap-pen'dĭ-klaw'sis) [ appendix + L. *clausus,* closed ]. Atrophy or obstruction of the appendix.

**appendico-** (ă-pen'dĭ-ko-) [ L. *appendix,* appendage ]. Combining form relating, usually, to the vermiform appendix.

**appendicocele** (ă-pen'dĭ-ko-sēl) [ appendico- + G. *kēlē,* hernia ]. The vermiform appendix in a hernial sac.

**appen'dicoenteros'tomy** [ appendico- + G. *enteron,* intestine, + *stoma,* mouth ]. 1. The establishment of an artificial opening between the appendix and the small intestine. 2. Appendicostomy.

**appen'dicolithi'asis** [ appendico- + G. *lithos,* stone ]. A state characterized by stones in the vermiform appendix.

**appendicolysis** (ă-pen-dĭ-kol'ĭ-sis) [ appendico- + G. *lysis,* a loosening ]. An operation for freeing the appendix from adhesions.

**appen'dicopath'ia** [ appendico- + G. *pathos,* disease ]. Any disease of the vermiform appendix.

**a. oxyu'rica,** lesion of the mucosa of the appendix, supposed to be caused by the presence of pinworms, *Enterobius vermicularis.*

**appendico'sis.** Appendicism.

**appendicos'tomy** [ appendico- + G. *stoma,* mouth ]. Appendicoenterostomy (2); Weir's operation; operation for opening into the intestine through the tip of the appendix vermiformis, previously attached to the anterior abdominal wall, for the purpose of flushing out the cecum and colon.

**appendicular** (ap'pen-dik'u-lar). 1. Relating to an appendix or appendage. 2. Relating to the limbs, as opposed to axial, which refers to the trunk and head.

**ap'pendic'uloradiog'raphy.** X-ray of the vermiform appendix.

**appen'dix,** gen. **appen'dicis,** pl. **appen'dices** [ L. appendage, fr. *ap-pendo (adp-),* to hang something on ]. [ NA ]. An appendage. Specifically the appendix vermiformis.

**auricular a.,** auricula (2).

**a. ceci,** a. vermiformis.

**a. epididym'idis** [ NA ], a small pedunculated body attached to the head of the epididymis.

**a. epiplo'ica,** pl. **appendices epiploicae** [ NA ], epiploic appendage; one of a number of little processes or sacs of peritoneum projecting from the serous coat of the large intestine, except the rectum; they are generally distended with fat.

**a. fasci'olae,** sternal prolongation of the "neck band" lesion of pellagra.

**a. fibro'sa hep'atis** [ NA ], a fibrous process, into which the tip of the left lobe of the liver may taper out, that passes with the left triangular ligament to be attached to the diaphragm.

**Morgagni's a.,** *lobus* pyramidalis.

**a. tes'tis** [ NA ], ovarium masculinum; a vesicular nonpedunculated structure attached to the cephalic pole of the testis, which is a vestige of the cephalic end of the Paramesonephric (Müllerian) duct.

**a. ventric'uli laryn'gis,** *sacculus* laryngis.

**a. vermifor'mis** [ NA ], vermiform process; vermiform appendage; a. ceci; a wormlike intestinal diverticulum extending from the blind end of the cecum. It varies from 3 to 6 inches in length and ends in a blind extremity.

**a. vesiculo'sa,** pl. **appendices vesiculosae** [ NA ], vesicular appendage; hydatid of Morgagni; a small fluid-filled cyst attached by a slender stalk to the fimbriated end of the uterine tube; a vestigial remnant of the embryonic mesonephric duct.

**appercep'tion** [ L. *ad,* to, + *per-cipio,* pp. *-ceptus,* to take wholly, perceive, fr. *capio,* to take ]. 1. Comprehension; conscious perception; the full apprehension of any psychic content. 2. The process of referring the perception of ideas to one's own personality.

**appercep'tive.** Relating to, involved in, or capable of apperception.

**appersona'tion, ap'person'ifica'tion.** A delusion in which the person assumes the character of another person.

**ap'pestat** [ appetite + G. *statos,* standing ]. The mechanism in the brain (possibly in the hypothalamus) concerned with the appetite and controlling the amount of food intake.

**appetite** (ap'ĕ-tīt) [ L. *ad-peto,* pp. *-petitus,* to seek after, desire ]. A desire or longing to satisfy any conscious physical or mental need.

**excessive a.,** bulimia.

**perverted a.,** pica.

**appetition** (ap-ĕ-tish'un) [ L. *appetitio,* strong desire; see appetite ]. Desire directed toward a definite goal or object.

**applanation** (ap'lan-a'shun) [ L. *ad,* toward, + *planum,* plane ]. In tonometry, the flattening of the cornea by pressure. Intraocular pressure is directly proportional to external pressure, inversely proportional to area flattened. See also applanation *tonometer.*

**applanom'etry.** Use of an applanation tonometer.

**apple** (ap'l). The fruit of *Pyrus malus* (family Rosaceae).

**Adam's a.,** *prominentia* laryngea.

**bitter a.,** colocynth.

**May a.,** podophyllum.

**a. oil,** amyl valerate.

**thorn a.,** *Datura stramonium.*

**appliance** (ă-pli'ans). A device used to provide function or for therapeutic purposes (*e.g.,* dental prosthesis, fixation splint, removable occlusal overlay, obturator). See also restoration.

**craniofacial a.,** a device used to immobilize and/or reduce mandibular or midfacial fractures; see also subentries under fixation.

**edgewise a.,** an orthodontic a. employing a rectangular labial arch wire attached to bands fitted to individual teeth; sometimes called Tweed edgewise treatment.

**Hawley a.,** a removable orthodontic a. used to retain the position of teeth after active treatment.

**light wire a.,** an orthodontic a. utilizing small gauge labial wires with expansion and contraction loops formed into it and attached to bands fitted to individual teeth; sometimes called Begg light wire differential force technique.

**Roger-Anderson pin fixation a.,** an a. used in extraoral fixation of mandibular fractures and prognathisms; see also external pin *fixation.*

**ap'plicator** [ L. *ap-plico,* to attach to. PLIC- ]. A slender rod of wood or flexible metal, at one end of which is attached a pledget of cotton or other substance for making local applications to the nose or any other accessible surface.

**apposition** (ap'o-zish'un) [ L. *ap-pono,* pp. *-positus,* to place at or to ]. 1. The putting in contact of two substances. 2. The condition of being placed or fitted together.

**approach** (ă-prōch). A term used in psychiatry to describe how interpersonal relationships are negotiated.

**idiographic a.,** the comprehensive study of an individual as a basis for understanding human behavior in general.

**nomothetic a.,** this frame of psychologic reference attempts to provide norms and general principles of behavior by the study of groups.

**regressive-reconstructive a.,** a form of psychotherapy in which regression, in order to resurrect some original psychic trauma, is an integral part of the treatment.

**approx'imate** [ L. *ad,* to, + *proximus,* nearest ]. To bring close together. In dentistry: 1. Proximate, denoting the contact surfaces, either mesial (proximal) or distal, of two adjacent teeth. 2. Close together; denoting the teeth in the human jaw, as distinguished from the separated teeth in certain of the lower animals.

**approxima'tion.** In surgery, bringing tissue edges into apposition for suturing in the desired position.

**APR.** Abbreviation for anterior pituitary *reaction.*

**apractognosia** (a-prak'tog-no'zī-ah) [ G. *a-*priv. + *practa,* things to be done, + *gnosis,* recognition ]. Failure to perform tasks involving spatial analysis; disorganization of construction and drawing.

**aprag'matism** [ G. *a-*priv. + pragmatism, *q.v.* ]. An interest in theory or dogmatism rather than practical results.

**apraxia** (ă-prak'sī-ah) [ G. *a-*priv. + *prattō,* to do ]. 1. A disorder of voluntary movement, consisting in a more or less complete incapacity to execute purposeful movements, notwithstanding the preservation of muscular power, sensibility, and coordination in general. 2. A psychomotor defect in which one is unable to apply to its proper use an object which he is nevertheless able to name and the uses of which he can describe.

**a. al'gera,** a hysterical condition in which speaking, reading, writing, or consecutive thinking is impossible owing to the severe headache it causes.

**cortical a.,** motor a.

**ideational** or **ideatory a.,** a misuse of objects due to a disturbance of identification (agnosia).

**ideokinet'ic** or **ideomo'tor a.,** transcortical a.; a form in which there is a break between the limb center and the ideational center: thus, simple movements, for which memories in the limb center suffice, are well executed, but unusual or complicated ones fail as the command cannot be carried to the limb center.

**innervation a.,** motor a.

**limb-kinet'ic a.,** motor a.

**motor a.,** cortical a.; innervation a.; limb-kinetic a.; an inability to make movements or to use objects for the purpose intended by the will.

**transcortical a.,** ideokinetic a.

**aprax'ic, aprac'tic.** Marked by or pertaining to apraxia.

**apricot kernel oil** (a'prĭ-kot). See persic oil.

**aprobar'bital.** ALURATE; 5-allyl-5-isopropylbarbituric acid; allylisopropylmalonylurea; hypnotic and sedative (intermediate action). Also available as a. sodium, with the same uses.

**aproctia** (ă-prok'shyah) [ G. *a-*priv. + *prōktos,* anus ]. Absence or imperforation of the anus.

**aprofen.** Aprophen.

**a'pron** [ O. Fr. *naperon,* a cloth ]. 1. An outer garment, covering the front of the body, to protect the clothing during surgical operations and other maneuvers. 2. A structure resembling an a.

**Hottentot a.,** *velamen* vulvae.

**aprophen.** Aprofen; 2,2-diphenylpropionic acid 2-diethylaminoethyl ester; analgesic and antispasmodic.

**aprophoria** (ap'ro-fo'rī-ah) [ G. *a-*priv. + *prophora,* utterance ]. Aphasia, including agraphia.

**aprosex'ia** [ G. *a-*priv. + *prosexis,* attention, fr. *pros-echō,* to hold to ]. Inattention, due to ocular, aural, or nasal defects or to mental weakness.

**aprosody** (ă-pros'o-dĭ) [ G. a- priv. + prosōdia, voice modulation ]. Absence, in speech, of the normal pitch, rhythm, and variations in stress.

**aproso'pia** [ G. a- priv. + prosōpon, face ]. Congenital absence of the greater part or all of the face, usually associated with other malformations.

**aproti'nin** (USAN). TRASYLOL; a protease and kallikrein inhibitor obtained from animal organs; a polypeptide with a molecular weight of about 6000. May be useful in the treatment of pancreatitis.

**apsithyria** (ap'sĭ-thi'rĭ-ah) [ G. a- priv. + psithyrizō, to whisper ]. Loss of the ability to whisper.

**aptyalia** (ap-ti-a'le-ah). Asialism.

**aptyalism** (ap-ti'al-ism) [ G. a- priv. + ptyalon, saliva ]. Asialism.

**APUD** (from amine precursor uptake, decarboxylase). Proposed designation for a group of cells in different organs secreting polypeptide hormones; cells in this group have certain biochemical characteristics in common, the first letters of which form the name. They contain amines, such as catecholamine and 5-hydroxytryptamine, take up precursors of these amines *in vivo*, and contain amino-acid decarboxylase. Recognition of these characteristics helped to identify the cell-type secreting calcitonin.

**apurin'ic acid.** DNA from which the purine bases have been removed by mild acid treatment.

**a'pus** [ G. a- priv. + pous, foot ]. An individual without feet or with entire absence of the lower extremities.

**apyetous** (ă-pi'ĕ-tus) [ G. a- priv. + pyēsis, suppuration ]. Apyous; nonsuppurative; not purulent.

**apyknomorphous** (ă-pik'no-mor'fus) [ G. a- priv. + pyknos, thick, + morphē, shape, form ]. Denoting a cell or other structure that does not stain deeply owing to the fact that the stainable or chromophil material is not closely aggregated.

**apyous** (ă-pi'us) [ G. a- priv. + pyon, pus ]. Apyetous.

**apy'rase.** An enzyme (EC 3.6.1.5) catalyzing hydrolytic removal of one orthophosphate residue from adenosine triphosphate to yield adenosine diphosphate; *i.e.,* ATP + $H_2O \rightarrow$ ADP + $P_i$. Also known as ADPase; ATP-diphosphatase.

**apyret'ic.** Nonfebrile; without fever.

**apyrexia** (a-pi-rek'sĭ-ah) [ G. a- priv. + pyrexis, fever ]. Absence of fever.

**apyrex'ial.** Apyretic.

**apyrimidin'ic acid.** DNA from which the pyrimidine bases have been removed by chemical treatment.

**aq.** Abbreviation for L. *aqua,* water.

**aqua,** gen. and pl. **aquae** (ak'wah, ah'kwah) [ L. ]. Water; $H_2O$; hydrogen monoxide. The pharmaceutical waters, aquae, are aqueous solutions of volatile substances (see water). The pharmaceutical solutions, liquors, are aqueous solutions of nonvolatile substances (see solution).
   **a. aera'ta,** aerated or carbonated water.
   **a. fortis,** weak nitric acid.
   **a. frig'ida,** pl. **aquae frigidae,** cold water.
   **a. pluvia'lis,** rain water.
   **a. re'gia, a. rega'lis** [ L. royal water, so called from its power to dissolve gold ], nitrohydrochloric acid.
   **a. vinae,** brandy or alcohol.

**aquacobalamin** (ak'wah-ko-bal'ă-min). Aquocobalamin; vitamin $B_{12a}$ (tautomeric with $B_{12b}$); a cobalamin derivative in which the sixth coordinate bond of the cobaltic ion is attached to a water molecule. See also vitamin $B_{12}$.

**aq'uacul'ture.** The systematic cultivation of aquatic plants and animals to serve as sources of food.

**aquaphobia** (ak'wah-fo'bĭ-ah) [ L. *aqua,* water, + G. *phobos,* fear ]. Morbid fear of water.

**aquapunc'ture** [ L. *aqua,* water, + *punctura,* puncture ]. Hypodermic injection of water to produce counterirritation or for any other purpose.

**Aquaspirillum** (ah-kwah-spi-ril'um) [ L. *aqua,* water, + *spirillum,* coil ]. A genus of motile, nonsporeforming, aerobic bacteria (family Spirillaceae) containing Gram-negative, rigid, helical or helically curved cells which are 0.2 to 1.5 μm in diameter. Motile cells contain fascicles of flagella at one or both poles. Some species can grow anaerobically with nitrate instead of oxygen as the terminal electron acceptor. These organisms are chemoorganotrophic, possessing a strictly respiratory metabolism. They do not ferment carbohydrates; a few species can oxidize a limited variety of carbohydrates. The habitat of these organisms is fresh water. Thirteen species are presently included in this genus, and the type species is *A. serpens.*

**aquatic** (ah-kwat'ik). 1. Of or pertaining to water. 2. Denoting an organism that lives in water.

**aqueduct** (ak'we-dukt) [ L. *aqueductus, q. v.* ]. Aqueductus.
   **a. of cerebrum,** *aqueductus* cerebri.
   **cochlear a.,** *ductus* perilymphaticus.
   **Cotunnius' a.,** *aqueductus* vestibuli.
   **Fallopian a.,** *canalis* facialis.
   **Sylvian a.,** *aqueductus* cerebri.
   **a. of vestibule,** *aqueductus* vestibuli.

**aqueduc'tus,** pl. **aqueduc'tus** [ L. fr. *aqua,* water, + *ductus,* a leading, fr. *duco,* pp. *ductus,* to lead ] [ NA ]. Aqueduct; a conduit or canal.
   **a. cer'ebri** [ NA ], aqueduct of the cerebrum; a. sylvii; Sylvian aqueduct; a canal about 3/4 inch long, lined with ependymal cells, leading downward through the mesencephalon from the third to the fourth ventricle.
   **a. cochleae** [ NA ], *ductus* perilymphaticus.
   **a. cotun'nii,** a. vestibuli.
   **a. fallo'pii,** *canalis* facialis.
   **a. syl'vii,** a. cerebri.
   **a. vestib'uli** [ NA ], aqueduct of the vestibule; a. cotunnii; Cotunnius' aqueduct or canal; a canal running from the vestibule and opening on the posterior surface of the petrous portion of the temporal bone, giving passage to the endolymphatic duct and a small vein.

**aqueous** (ak'we-us, a'kwe-us). Watery; of, like, or containing water.
   **a. humor,** *humor* aquosus.

**aquiparous** (ă-kwip'er-us) [ L. *aqua,* water, + *pario,* to bring forth ]. Secreting or excreting a watery fluid.

**aquocobalamin** (ak'wo-ko-bal'ă-min). Aquacobalamin.

**aquo-ion** (ak'wo-i'on). A hydrated ion; an ion containing one or more water molecules, *e.g.,* $Cu(H_2O)_4^{++}$.

**aquosity** (ă-kwos'ĭ-tĭ). 1. The state of being watery. 2. Moisture.

**aquo'sus** [ L. ] [ NA ]. Aqueous.

**aquula** (ak'woo-lah) [ L. a small stream ]. Obsolete term for the endolymph (**a. interna**) and perilymph (**a. externa**) in the membranous labyrinth.

**Ar.** Chemical symbol of argon.

**ara.** 1. Prefix for arabinose or arabinosyl (see araC). 2. Symbol for arabinose or its mono- or diradical.

**ar'aban.** A polysaccharide that yields arabinose on hydrolysis; a constituent of some pectins.

**ar'abic.** Relating to or derived from various species of acacia giving a gummy or resinous exudate.
   **a. acid,** arabin.

**ar'abin.** Arabic acid; a carbohydrate gum, hydrolyzing to arabinose and hexoses, found naturally in union with calcium, potassium, and magnesium, when it is called gum arabic.

**ar'abinoaden'osine.** Arabinosyladenine.

**arabinose** (ă-rab'ĭ-nōs, ar'ă-bin-ōs). Pectin sugar; a pentose widely distributed in plants, usually in complex polysaccharides (for structure, see sugars). Used in culture media.

**arab'ino'sis.** Disordered metabolism of the pentose arabinose.

**arab'inosu'ria.** Excretion of arabinose in the urine.

**ar'abinosyla'denine.** Arabinoadenosine; 9-β-D-arabinofuranosyladenine; used for herpes simplex corneae and vaccinial keratitis.

**ar'abinosylcy'tosine.** Symbol araC or aC (sometimes CA); arabinofuranosylcytosine; arabinocytidine; cytarabine; sometimes mistakenly called cytosine arabinoside. The compound of arabinose and cytosine, analogous to ribosylcytosine (cytidine). A chemotherapeutic agent with antiviral and tumor-growth inhibiting properties. It inhibits the biosynthesis of DNA.

**arab'itol.** A sugar alcohol, $C_5H_{12}O_5$, 1,2,3,4,5-pentanepentol, obtained from the reduction of arabinose.

**2-araboke'tose.** Ribulose (*erythro*pentulose).

**araC.** Symbol for arabinosylcytosine.

**arachic acid** (ă-rak'ik). Arachidic acid.

**arachidic acid** (ăr'ă-kid'ik). Arachic acid; *n*-eicosanoic acid; $CH_3(CH_2)_{18}COOH$; a fatty acid contained in peanut oil, butter, and other fats.

**arachidon'ic acid.** 5,8,11,14-Eicosatetraenoic acid; $CH_3(CH_2)_4CH=(CHCH_2CH=)_3CH(CH_2)_3COOH$; a liquid, unsaturated fatty acid essential in nutrition and used in infantile eczema, usually administered as soybean extract. It is a precursor of prostaglandins, rapidly converted by the lung into prostaglandin E or F.

**arachis oil** (ar'ă-kis) (BP). Peanut oil.

**arachnephobia** (ă-rak'ne-fo-be-ah) [ G. *arachne*, spider, + *phobos*, fear ]. Morbid fear of spiders.

**Arachnia** (ă-rak'nĭ-ah). A genus of nonmotile, non-sporeforming, facultatively anaerobic bacteria (family Actinomycetaceae) containing Gram-positive, non-acid fast branched, diphtheroid rods (0.2 to 0.3 by 3.0 to 5.0 $\mu$m and longer). These organisms produce filamentous microcolonies. Their metabolism is fermentative. Primarily propionic and acetic acids are produced from glucose. Catalase is not produced. The cell wall contains diaminopimelic acid but not arabinose. These organisms are pathogenic for man, causing lacrimal canaliculitis and typical actinomycosis. The type species is *A. propionica*.

  **A. propionica,** a species causing lacrimal canaliculitis and typical actinomycosis. It is the type species of the genus *A*.

**Arachnida** (ă-rak'nĭ-dah) [ G. *arachne*, spider ]. A class of arthropods in the subphylum Chelicerata, consisting of spiders, scorpions, harvestmen, mites, ticks, and allies.

**arachnidism** (ă-rak'nĭ-dizm). Arachnoidism; araneism; systemic poisoning following the bite of a spider (especially of the black widow spider).

**arachnitis** (ar-ak-ni'tis). Arachnoiditis.

**arachnodactyly** (ă-rak-no-dak'tĭ-lĭ) [ G. *arachnē*, spider, + *daktylos*, finger ]. Dolichostenomelia; spider fingers; a condition in which the hands and fingers, and often the feet and toes, are abnormally long and slender; a regular feature of Marfan's syndrome and Achard syndrome.

**arachnoid** (ar-ak'noyd) [ G. *arachnē*, spider, cobweb, + *eidos*, resemblance ]. Resembling a cobweb; denoting specifically the arachnoidea covering the brain and spinal cord.

**arachnoidal** (ar-ak-noy'dal). Relating to the arachnoid membrane, or arachnoidea.

**arachnoidea, arachnoi'des** (ar-ak-noyd'ĭ-ah) [ Mod. L. *arachnoideus*, fem. -*ea* (sc. *tela*, web), fr. G. *arachnē*, spider, + *eidos*, resemblance ] [ NA ]. Arachnoid membrane; meninx serosa; a delicate fibrous membrane forming the middle of the three coverings of the brain (**a. enceph'ali**) and spinal cord (**a. spina'lis**); it is closely applied to the outer membrane, the dura mater, from which it is separated only by the subdural cleft, but between it and the inner layer, the pia mater, lies the subarachnoid space.

**arach'noidism.** Arachnidism.

**arachnoiditis** (ă-rak'noy-di'tis). Arachnitis; leptomeningitis (*q.v.*); inflammation of the arachnoid membrane and subjacent subarachnoid space.

  **adhesive a.,** obliterative a.; thickening of the leptomeninges, sometimes with obliteration of the subarachnoid space; probably related to acute or chronic leptomeningitis of bacterial or chemical origin; see also leptomeningeal *fibrosis.*

  **neoplastic a.,** neoplastic *meningitis.*

  **obliterative a.,** adhesive a.

**arachnolysin** (ar-ak-nol'ĭ-sin). A hemolytic substance in the venom of certain spiders.

**arachnopho'bia** [ G. *arachne*, spider + *phobos*, fear ]. Fear of spiders.

**ar'ack** [ Hindoo word ]. A strong alcoholic liquor distilled from dates, rice, sap of the coconut palm, and other substances.

**Ara'lia.** A genus of plants (family Araliaceae), several species of which have been used in domestic medicine for their aromatic properties. The rhizome and roots of *A. nudicaulis* (wild sarsaparilla, wild licorice, small spikenard) and *A. racemosa* (American spikenard), plants growing in eastern and central North America, are stimulant, diaphoretic, and alterative.

**aral'kyl.** Arylated alkyl; a radical in which an aryl group is substituted for a hydrogen atom of an alkyl group; *e.g.*, $C_6H_5CH_2$—.

**Aran** (ar-on') Francçois A., Paris physician, 1817–1861. See A.'s *cancer,* A.-Duchenne *disease,* Duchenne-A. *disease.*

**araneism** (ă-ra'ne-izm). Arachnidism.

**Arantius** (Aranzi), Giulio C., Italian anatomist and physician, 1530–1589. See A.'s *canal,* venous *canal* of A., *corpora* Arantii, *duct* of A., A.'s *ligament, nodule, ventricle.*

**araphia** (ă-ra'fĭ-ah) [ G. *a*- priv. + *rhaphe*, a seam ]. Holorachischisis.

**ar'aro'ba** [ Brazil Indian, bark ]. Goa powder; crude chrysarobin; the dried and powdered concretion found in the wood of *Vouacapoua (Andira) araroba* (family Leguminosae), a forest tree of Brazil; it contains about 50 per cent of chrysarobin.

**ar'bor,** pl. **arbo'res** [ L. tree ] [ NA ]. In anatomy, one of the treelike or branching structures.

  **a. vitae cerebel'li** [ NA ], the arborescent appearance presented in sagittal sections of the cerebellum, formed by the contrasting outlines of the white and gray matter.

  **a. vi'tae u'teri,** *plicae* palmatae.

**arborescent** (ar-bo-res'ent). Treelike; branching; dendritic.

**arboriza'tion.** Ramification; denoting especially (1) the terminal branching of nerve fibers or blood vessels; (2) the leaflike pattern formed under certain conditions by a dried smear of cervical mucus.

**ar'borize.** To ramify.

**ar'boroid** [ L. *arbor,* tree, + G. *eidos,* resemblance ]. Denoting a colony of protozoa, each of which remains attached to another cell or to the main stem at one point, forming a branching or dendritic figure.

**ar'borvi'rus.** Arbovirus (see under virus).

**arborvitae** (ar'bor-vi'te) [ L. tree of life ]. Any of the trees of the genus *Thuja.*

  **a. oil,** cedar leaf oil.

**ar'bovi'rus.** See under virus.

**ar'butin.** Ursin; hydroxyquinone-$\beta$-D-glucopyranoside; a glucoside from uva ursi; diuretic and urinary antiseptic.

**Ar'butus** [ L. wild strawberry tree ]. A genus of evergreen shrubs (family Ericaceae).

  **A. uva ursi,** *Arctostaphylos uva ursi.*

**arc** [ L. *arcus,* a bow ]. 1. A curved line or segment of a circle. 2. Continuous luminous passage of an electric current in a gas or vacuum between two or more separated carbon or other electrodes.

  **auric'ular a., binauric'ular a.,** a line carried over the cranium from the center of one external auditory meatus to that of the other.

  **breg'matolamb'doid a.,** the line running along the sagittal suture from the bregma to the apex of the lambdoid suture.

  **crater a.,** an a. of a direct current that forms a pitlike excavation at the positive pole.

  **a. de cercle** [ Fr. ], a pathological and exaggerated arching backward of the body, as in opisthotonos; was a common symptom of hysteria and hysteroepilepsy; now rarely seen.

  **flame a.,** an a. between two impregnated electrodes that causes volatilization of the core with resultant flame.

  **longitudinal a. of the skull,** the line carried over the skull from the nasion to the opisthion.

  **mercury a.,** an a. between quartz tubes containing mercury as the cathode and mercury or tungsten as the anode; it produces ultraviolet rays.

  **na'sobregmat'ic a.,** a line running through the midline of the forehead from the nasion to the bregma.

  **na'sooccip'ital a.,** the a. from the root of the nose to inferior limit of the external occipital protuberance.

  **pulmonary a.,** pulmonary *salient.*

  **reflex a.,** the route followed by nerve impulses in the production of a reflex act, from the periphery through the afferent nerve to the nervous system and thence through the efferent nerve to the effector organ. See fig. under gamma *loop.*

**arcade** (ar-kād) [ L. *arcus,* arc, bow ]. An anatomical structure resembling a series of arches.

**anomalous mitral a.,** short cordae tendineae extending from both papillary muscles to the central portion of the anterior leaflet of the mitral valve and resulting in stenosis or incompetence of the valve.

**Flint's a.,** a series of vascular arches at the bases of the pyramids of the kidney.

**Riolan's a.,** the anastomoses of the intestinal vessels in the mesentery.

**ar'cate.** Arched; bow-shaped.

**arch-, arche-, archi-, archo-** [ G. *archē*, origin, beginning. ARCH- ]. Combining forms meaning primitive, or ancestral; also first, or chief.

---

# ARCH

---

**arch** [ thru O. Fr. fr. L. *arcus*, bow ]. In anatomy, any vaulted or archlike structure. See arcus.

**abdom'inothorac'ic a.,** the line of the false ribs on either side with the lower end of the sternum, marking roughly the boundary line between the abdomen and thorax.

**alveolar a.,** *arcus* alveolaris.

**anterior a. of atlas,** *arcus* anterior atlantis.

**anterior palatine a.,** *arcus* palatoglossus.

**aortic a., a. of the aorta,** *arcus* aortae.

**aortic a.'s,** a series of arterial channels encircling the embryonic pharynx in the mesenchyme of the branchial a.'s. There are potentially 6 pairs, but in mammals pair 5 is poorly developed or wanting. Pairs 1 and 2 are functional only in very young embryos; pair 3 is involved in the formation of the carotids; a. 4 on the left is incorporated in the a. of the aorta; the 6th a.'s form the proximal part of the pulmonary arteries.

**arterial a.'s of colon,** branches of the colic arteries that form a.'s in the mesocolon from which the walls of the colon are supplied.

**arterial a.'s of ileum,** those formed by branches of the superior mesenteric artery from which vessels pass between the layers of the mesentery to the wall of the ileum.

**arterial a.'s of jejunum,** those formed by branches of the superior mesenteric artery which supply the walls of the jejunum.

**arterial a. of lower eyelid,** *arcus* palpebralis inferior.

**arterial a. of upper eyelid,** *arcus* palpebralis superior.

**axillary a.,** Langer's a.; Langer's muscle; an anomalous muscle or tendinous slip that passes across the axilla from the pectoralis major to insert with the latissimus dorsi onto the humerus.

**branchial a.'s,** visceral a.'s; pharyngeal a.'s; typically, six a.'s in vertebrates; in the lower vertebrates they bear gills; they transiently appear in the higher vertebrates and give rise to specialized structures in the head and neck.

**carpal a.'s,** two anastomotic arterial twigs running transversely across the wrist: the anterior lies in front of the carpus, being formed by anterior carpal branches of the radial and ulnar arteries; it is distributed to the structures of the wrist and carpal joints; the posterior or dorsal lies on the posterior surface of the carpus, being formed by the dorsal carpal branches of the radial and ulnar arteries; it is distributed to the structures of the carpal and wrist joints and gives off two dorsal interosseous branches.

**Corti's a.,** the a. formed by the junction of the heads of Corti's inner and outer pillar cells.

**cortical a.'s of kidney,** the portions of renal substance (cortex) intervening between the bases of the pyramids and the capsule of the kidney.

**costal a.,** *arcus* costalis.

**a. of cricoid cartilage,** *arcus* cartilaginis cricoideae.

**crural a.,** *ligamentum* inguinale.

**deep palmar a.,** *arcus* palmaris profundus.

**deep palmar venous a.,** *arcus* venosus palmaris profundus.

**dental a.,** *arcus* dentalis.

**dorsal venous a. of foot,** *arcus* venosus dorsalis pedis.

**expansion a.,** an orthodontic appliance that moves the dental structures distally, bucally, or labially, creating increased molar to molar width and arch length.

**fallen a.'s,** a breaking down of the bony a.'s—either longitudinal or transverse or both—of the foot; the resulting deformity is flat foot or spread foot or both.

**Fallopian a.,** *ligamentum* inguinale.

**fem'oral a.,** *ligamentum* inguinale.

**a.'s of the foot,** (1) longitudinal a.; (2) plantar a.; (3) transverse a.

**glossopal'atine a.,** *arcus* palatoglossus.

**Gothic a.,** needle point *tracing*.

**Haller's a.'s,** (1) *ligamentum* arcuatum laterale; (2) *ligamentum* arcuatum mediale.

**hemal a.'s,** three or four V-shaped bones located ventral to the bodies of the third to sixth coccygeal vertebrae; they represent intercentra and usually enclose the ventral caudal artery and vein.

**hyoid a.,** the second visceral, or branchial, a.

**iliopectineal a.,** *arcus* iliopectineus.

**jugular a.,** *arcus* venosus juguli.

**labial a.,** an orthodontic a. wire that approximates the labial surfaces of the teeth.

**Langer's a.,** axillary a.

**lateral longitudinal a.,** *arcus* pedis longitudinalis, pars lateralis.

**lingual a.,** an orthodontic a. wire that approximates the lingual surfaces of the teeth.

**longitudinal a.,** *arcus* pedis longitudinalis.

**medial longitu'dinal a.,** *arcus* pedis longitudinalis, pars medialis.

**malar a.,** *arcus* zygomaticus.

**mandib'ular a.,** mandibular process; the first postoral a. in the branchial a. series.

**nasal venous a.,** formed at the root of the nose by the two supratrochlear veins connected by a transverse vein.

**neural a.,** *arcus* vertebrae.

**a. of the palate,** the vaulted roof of the mouth.

**pal'atoglos'sal a.,** *arcus* palatoglossus.

**pal'atopharynge'al a.,** *arcus* palatopharyngeus.

**pharyngeal a.'s,** branchial a.'s.

**pharyn'gopal'atine a.,** *arcus* palatopharyngeus.

**plantar a.,** (1) *arcus* plantaris; (2) either of two bony a.'s of the foot, longitudinal a. or transverse a.

**plantar venous a.,** *arcus* venosus plantaris.

**posterior palatine a.,** *arcus* palatopharyngeus.

**postoral a.,** the series of branchial a.'s caudal to the mouth. The first is the mandibular, the second is the hyoid. Caudal to the hyoid the a.'s are unnamed, and designated only by their postoral number.

**primitive costal a.'s,** formed in the thoracic region of the vertebral column in the embryo from the costal processes or costal elements which give rise to the ribs.

**pubic a.,** *arcus* pubis.

**ribbon a.,** a thin, ribbon-shaped, rectangular orthodontic a. wire applied to the dental a.'s so that its widest dimension is parallel to the labial or buccal surfaces of the teeth.

**Shenton's a.,** Shenton's *line*.

**superciliary a.,** *arcus* superciliaris.

**superficial palmar a.,** *arcus* palmaris superficialis.

**superficial palmar venous a.,** *arcus* venosus palmaris superficialis.

**supraor'bital a.,** *margo* supraorbitalis.

**tarsal a.,** see *arcus* palpebralis inferior and *arcus* palpebralis superior.

**tendinous a.,** *arcus* tendineus.

**transverse a.'s,** *arcus* pedis transversalis.

**Treitz' a.,** a vascular a. formed by the left superior colic artery and the inferior mesenteric vein, between the left border of the ascending portion of the duodenum and the medial border of the left kidney.

**vascular a.'s,** old term for aortic a.'s.

**vertebral a.,** *arcus* vertebrae; see also hemal a.

**visceral a.'s,** branchial a.'s.

**wire a.,** a wire conforming to the dental a.; used to restore the normal curve to the denture.

**zygomat'ic a.,** *arcus* zygomaticus.

---

**archae'us,** pl. **archaei** (ar-ke'us) [ L. fr. G. *archaios*, chief, leader ]. Term first used by Valentine and later by Paracelsus and van Helmont to denote a spirit that presided over and governed bodily processes.

**archaic** (ar-ka′ik) [ G. *archaikos,* ancient ]. Ancient; old; in psychiatry, denoting the ancestral past of mental processes.

**Archambault,** LaSalle, U. S. neurologist, 1879–1940. See Meyer-A. *loop.*

**arche-.** See arch-.

**archenteron** (ark-en′ter-on) [ G. *archē,* beginning, + *enteron,* intestine ]. Celenteron; gastrocele (1); the primitive gut cavity formed by the invagination of the blastula.

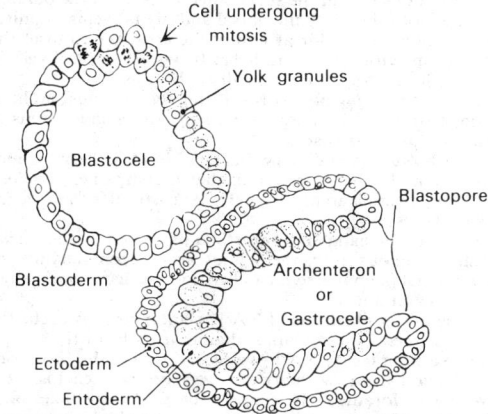

**Formation of the Archenteron**
(From Patten, B. M.: *Foundations of Embryology,* McGraw-Hill Book Co., Inc., New York, 1958. Used with permission.)

**archeocyte** (ar′ke-o-sīt) [ G. *archaios,* ancient, + *kytos,* cell ]. Obsolete term for a wandering cell.

**archeokinetic** (ar-ke-o-kin-et′ik) [ G. *archaios,* ancient, + *kinētikos,* relating to movement ]. Denoting a low, and primitive, type of motor nerve mechanism such as is found in the peripheral and the ganglionic nervous systems; differentiated from the neokinetic and the paleokinetic systems.

**archetype** (ar′ke-tīp) [ G. *archetypos,* first molded, fr. *arche,* first, + *typiō,* to beat, stamp ]. 1. A primitive structural plan from which various modifications have evolved. 2. Imago (2); in Jungian psychology, structural manifestation of the collective unconscious.

**archi-.** See arch-.

**archiater** (ar-kī-a′ter) [ archi- + G. *iatros,* physician ]. 1. A chief physician of any institution. 2. A physician to royalty.

**Archibald's fever.** See under fever.

**archicortex** (ar′ki-kor′teks) [ archi- + L. *cortex, q. v.* ]. Archipallium. 1. Typically, the phylogenetically older parts of the cerebral cortex. 2. More specifically, the cortex forming the hippocampus. See also allocortex, and *cortex* cerebri.

**archil** (ar′kil). Roccellin; a violet dye from the lichens *Rocella tinctoria* and *R. fuciformis.*

**archin** (ar′kin). Emodin.

**archinephron** (ar-kī-nef′ron) [ archi- + G. *nephron,* kidney ]. The pronephros.

**archipallium** (ar-kī-pal′ī-um) [ archi- + L. *pallium, q. v.* ]. Archicortex.

**archiplasm** (ar′kī-plazm). Archoplasm; the protoplasm which Boveri believed formed the centrosomes, asters, and spindles.

**architectonics** (ar-kī-tek-ton′iks). Cytoarchitectonics.

**architecture** (ar′kī-tek′chur). The character or style of any structure.

    **bone a.,** in dentistry, the pattern of trabeculae and associated structures; see also Wolff's *law.*

    **gingival a.,** in dentistry, the shape or contour of the gingiva around the teeth.

**architis** (ar-ki′tis) [ arch- + G. suffix *-itis,* inflammation ]. Proctitis.

**archo-.** See arch-.

**archocele** (ar′ko-sēl) [ archo- + G. *kēlē,* tumor ]. Prolapse of the rectum; hernia of the rectum.

**archocystosyrinx** (ar′ko-sis′to-sir′inks) [ archo- + G. *kystis,* bladder, + *syrinx,* fistula ]. A rectovesical fistula.

**archoplasm** (ar′ko-plazm). Archiplasm.

**archoptoma** (ar-kop-to′mah) [ archo- + G. *ptōma,* a fall ]. Archoptosia.

**archoptosia, archoptosis** (ar-kop-to′zī-ah, ar-kop-to′sis) [ archo- + G. *ptōsis,* a falling ]. Prolapse of the rectum.

**archorrhagia** (ar-ko-ra′jī-ah) [ archo- + G. *rhēgnymi,* to burst forth ]. A discharge of blood from the anus.

**archorrhea** (ar-ko-re′ah) [ archo- + G. *rhoia,* flow ]. A discharge of pus from the anus.

**archostenosis** (ar′ko-stě-no′sis) [ archo- + G. *stenōsis,* narrowing ]. Stricture of the rectum or anus.

**archosyrinx** (ar-ko-sir′inks) [ archo- + G. *syrinx,* tube, fistula ]. Fistula in the anus.

**arch′wire.** A device consisting of a wire conforming to the alveolar or dental arch, used as an anchorage in correcting irregularities in the position of the teeth.

**ar′ciform.** Arcuate.

**arcta′tion** [ L. *arto* (improp. *arcto*), pp. *-atus,* to tighten ]. Narrowing; contraction; stricture; coarctation.

**Arctostaph′ylos** [ G. *arktos,* a bear, + *staphylē,* bunch of grapes ]. A genus of evergreen shrubs of the family Ericaceae.

    **A. uva ursi,** *Arbutus uva ursi;* bearberry; the source of the drug uva ursi. The ground leaves contain the glucoside, arbutin. Formerly used as a mild antiseptic diuretic.

**ar′cual.** Relating to an arch.

**arcuate** (ar′ku-āt) [ L. *arcuatus,* bowed ]. Arciform; arched; having the shape of a bow (arcus).

**arcuation** (ar-ku-a′shun). 1. A bending. 2. A curvature.

**arcua′tus** [ L. ] [ NA ]. Arcuate.

---

# ARCUS

---

**arcus,** gen. and pl. **arcus** (ar′kus) [ L. a bow ] [ NA ]. Any structure resembling a bent bow or an arch; an arc.

    **a. adipo′sus,** a. senilis.

    **a. alveolaris mandibulae** [ NA ], alveolar arch of the mandible; the free margin of the alveolar process of the mandible.

    **a. alveola′ris maxillae** [ NA ], alveolar arch of the maxilla; the free border of the alveolar process of the maxilla.

    **a. anterior atlan′tis** [ NA ], the anterior arch of the atlas that connects the lateral masses of the atlas anteriorly and articulates with the dens of the axis.

    **a. aor′tae** [ NA ], aortic arch; arch of the aorta; the curve between the ascending and descending portions of the aorta; it lies behind the manubrium sterni; it gives off the brachiocephalic trunk, the left common carotid, and the left subclavian arteries.

    **a. cartila′ginis cricoi′deae** [ NA ], arch of the cricoid cartilage; the narrow part of the cartilage that encircles the air passage anterior to the lamina.

    **a. costalis** [ NA ], costal arch; a. costarum; consisting of the lateral borders of the inferior aperture of the thorax that meet at the infrasternal angle.

    **a. costa′rum,** a. costalis.

    **a. dentalis,** dental arch; (1) the curved contour of the natural dentition or of the residual ridge; (2) the composite structure of the natural dentition and the residual ridge, or the remains thereof after the loss of some or all of the natural teeth.

    **a. dentalis inferior** [ NA ], the mandibular dentition.

    **a. dentalis superior** [ NA ], the maxillary dentition.

    **a. glossopalati′nus,** a. palatoglossus.

    **a. iliopectin′eus** [ NA ], iliopectineal arch; iliopectineal ligament; ligamentum iliopectineale; the fascial partition that separates the vascular and muscular lacunae deep to the inguinal ligament.

**a. juveni'lis,** anterior embryotoxon; a grayish ring at the corneal margin resembling the a. senilis, but occurring in a young person; it may be associated with hyperlipoproteinemia type II.

**a. lipoi'des,** a. senilis.

**a. lumbocosta'lis latera'lis,** *ligamentum* arcuatum laterale.

**a. lumbocosta'lis media'lis** *ligamentum* arcuatum mediale.

**a. palati'ni,** pillars of the fauces; see a. palatoglossus and a. palatopharyngeus.

**a. palatoglos'sus** [ NA ], palatoglossal arch; glossopalatine arch; anterior palatine arch; anterior pillar of the fauces; one of a pair of ridges or folds of mucous membrane passing from the soft palate to the side of the tongue. It encloses the palatoglossus muscle.

**a. palatopharyngeus** [ NA ], palatopharyngeal arch; pharyngopalatine arch; posterior palatine arch; posterior pillar of the fauces; one of a pair of ridges or folds of mucous membrane which passes downward from the posterior margin of the soft palate to the lateral wall of the pharynx. It encloses the palatopharyngeus muscle.

**a. palmaris profundus** [ NA ], deep palmar arch; a. volaris profundus; the arterial arch located deep to the long flexor tendons in the hand. It is formed by the radial artery in conjunction with the deep palmar branch of the ulnar artery.

**a. palmaris superficia'lis** [ NA ], superficial palmar arch; a. volaris superficialis; the arterial arch in the hand located superficial to the long flexor tendons. It is formed principally by the ulnar artery and is usually completed by a communication with the superficial palmar branch of the radial artery.

**a. palpebralis inferior** [ NA ], the arterial arch of the lower eyelid, formed by the medial palpebral artery which communicates with a branch of the lacrimal artery along the tarsal margin.

**a. palpebralis superior** [ NA ], the arterial arch of the upper eyelid, formed by communicating branches of the medial and lateral palpebral arteries. Often two arches are present, one located near the free border of the tarsal plate, the other along the upper border of the tarsus.

**a. pedis longitudinalis** [ NA ], longitudinal arch of the foot; it consists of a *pars medialis* including the calcaneus, talus, navicular, three cuneiform bones, and the three medial metatarsals, and a *pars lateralis* formed by calcaneus, cuboid and two lateral metatarsals. The arch is supported normally by ligaments, intrinsic muscles, and the tendons of extrinsic muscles of the foot.

**a. pe'dis transversa'lis** [ NA ], transverse arch of the foot; the arch formed by the proximal parts of the metatarsal bones, the three cuneiform bones, and the cuboid.

**a. planta'ris** [ NA ], plantar arch; the arterial arch formed by the lateral plantar artery running across the bases of the metatarsal bones and anastomosing with the dorsal pedal artery.

**a. posterior atlan'tis** [ NA ], the posterior arch of the atlas that connects the lateral masses of the atlas posteriorly.

**a. pubis** [ NA ], pubic arch; the arch formed by the inferior rami of the pubic bones.

**a. seni'lis,** an opaque, grayish ring at the periphery of the cornea just within the sclerocorneal junction, of frequent occurrence in the aged; it results from a deposit of fatty granules in, or hyaline degeneration of, the lamellae and cells of the cornea. Also called a. adiposus; a. lipoides; gerontoxon; lipoidosis corneae.

**a. supercilia'ris** [ NA ], superciliary arch; a fullness extending laterally from the glabella on either side, above the orbital margin of the frontal bone.

**a. tar'seus,** a. palpebralis.

**a. tendin'eus** [ NA ], tendinous arch; a fibrous band arching over a vessel or nerve as it passes through a muscle, and protecting it from injurious compression.

**a. tendin'eus fas'ciae pelvis** [ NA ], tendinous arch of the pelvic fascia; a linear thickening of the superior fascia of the pelvic diaphragm extending posteriorly from the body of the pubis alongside the bladder (and vagina in the female) and giving attachment to the supporting ligaments of the pelvic viscera.

**a. tendin'eus mus'culi levato'ris ani** [ NA ], tendinous arch of the levator ani muscle; a thickened portion of the obturator fascia that extends in an arching line from the pubis posteriorly to the ischial spine and gives origin to part of the levator ani muscle.

**a. tendin'eus musculi solei** [ NA ], a tendinous arch stretching over the popliteal vessels between the tibia and fibula, that gives origin to the central portion of the soleus muscle.

**a. unguium,** whitish area near the root of the nail.

**a. veno'sus dorsa'lis pedis** [ NA ], dorsal venous arch of the foot; the arch in the subcutaneous tissue of the dorsum of the foot formed by the dorsal and digital veins; it unites medially with the dorsal vein of the great toe to form the great saphenous vein, and laterally with the dorsal vein of the little toe to form the small saphenous.

**a. veno'sus jug'uli** [ NA ], jugular venous arch; a connecting vein between the two anterior jugular veins in the suprasternal space.

**a. veno'sus palma'ris profun'dus** [ NA ], deep palmar venous arch; the venous arch that accompanies the deep palmar arterial arch; it usually consists of paired venae comitantes.

**a. veno'sus palma'ris superficia'lis** [ NA ], superficial palmar venous arch; the venous arch accompanying the superficial palmar arterial arch; it consists usually of paired venae comitantes.

**a. veno'sus planta'ris** [ NA ], plantar venous arch; the arch formed by the plantar digital veins from the toes.

**a. ver'tebrae** [ NA ], vertebral arch; the posterior projection from the body of a vertebra that encloses the vertebral foramen. It consists of paired pedicles and laminae. The spinous, transverse, and articular processes arise from the arch.

**a. vola'ris profun'dus,** a. palmaris profundus.

**a. vola'ris superficia'lis,** a. palmaris superficialis.

**a. zygomat'icus** [ NA ], zygomatic arch; malar arch; zygoma (2); the arch formed by the temporal process of the zygomatic bone that joins the zygomatic process of the temporal bone.

---

**ARD.** Abbreviation for acute respiratory *disease.*

**ardanesthe'sia** [ L. *ardor,* heat, + G. *an-* priv. + *aisthēsis,* sensation ]. Thermoanesthesia.

**ar'dor** [ L. fire, heat ]. A hot or burning sensation.

**a. urinae,** a scalding sensation on urinating.

**a. ventric'uli,** pyrosis.

---

# AREA

**area** (a're-ah) [ L. a courtyard ] 1 [ NA ]. Any circumscribed surface or space. 2. All of the part supplied by a given artery or nerve. 3. A part of an organ having a special function, as the motor a. of the brain. See also regio, region, space, zone.

**acoustic a.,** a. acustica.

**a. acu'stica,** acoustic a.; the floor of the lateral recess of the fourth ventricle, extending medially to the sulcus limitans and overlying the cochlear and vestibular nuclei of the rhombencephalon.

**anterior intercondylar a.,** a. intercondylaris anterior.

**aortic a.,** the region of the chest wall over the second right costal cartilage, where sounds produced at the aortic orifice are often best heard.

**apical a.,** the a. about the root end of a tooth.

**association a.'s,** association *cortex.*

**auditory a.,** auditory *cortex.*

**bare a. of liver,** a. nuda hepatis.

**bare a. of stomach,** the part of posterior surface of the fundus of the stomach between the two diverging layers of the gastrophrenic ligament, that is not covered by peritoneum.

**basal seat a.,** that portion of the oral structures which is available to support a denture.

**Broca's a.,** Broca's *center.*

Broca's parolfactory a., a. parolfactoria.

Brodmann's a.'s, a.'s of the cerebral cortex mapped out on the basis of the cortical cytoarchitectural patterns; see *cortex* cerebri.

**a. of cardiac dullness,** a triangular a. determined by percussion of the front of the chest; it corresponds to the part of the heart that is not covered by lung tissue.

**catchment a.,** the a. delineated on a map, representing the community served by a mental health center.

Celsus' a., *alopecia* areata.

**a. centra'lis,** *macula* retinae.

**a. coch'leae** [ NA ], cochlear a.; the a. inferior to the transverse crest of the fundus of the internal acoustic meatus through which the filaments of the cochlear nerve pass to enter the cochlea.

**cochlear a.,** a. cochleae.

Cohnheim's a.'s, Cohnheim's field; a polygonal mosaic-like figure formed by a group of myofibrils as seen in the cross-section of a skeletal muscle fiber examined under the microscope.

**cribriform a.,** a. cribrosa.

**a. cribrosa** [ NA ], cribriform a.; the apex of a renal papilla pierced by 10 to 22 openings of the papillary ducts, the foramina papillaria. See also *macula* cribrosa.

**denture-bearing a.,** denture foundation a.

**denture foundation a.,** denture-bearing a.; that portion of the basal seat that supports the complete or partial denture base under occlusal load.

**denture-supporting a.,** denture *foundation.*

**dermatomic a.,** dermatome (3).

**embryonal a., embryonic a.,** the a. of the blastoderm on either side of, and immediately cephalic to the primitive streak where the component cell layers have become thickened.

**entorhinal a.,** Brodmann's a. 28; a cytoarchitecturally well defined a. of multilaminate cerebral cortex on the medial aspect of the parahippocampal gyrus, immediately behind the olfactory cortex of the uncus; the a. is the origin of the major fiber system afferent to the hippocampus, the so-called perforant pathway.

**excitable a.,** motor *cortex.*

**a. of facial nerve,** a. nervi facialis.

Flechsig's a.'s, three divisions of each lateral half of the medulla as seen on transverse section, marked off by the root fibers of the hypoglossal and vagus nerves; the a.'s are called anterior, lateral, and posterior.

**frontal a.,** frontal *cortex.*

**fronto-orbital a.,** orbitofrontal *cortex.*

**fusion a.,** Panum's a.

**a. gas'trica** [ NA ], one of a number of small polygonal a.'s, separated by linear depressions, on the surface of the mucous membrane of the stomach; they contain the gastric foveolae.

**germinal a.,** a. germinativa; the place in the blastoderm where the embryo begins to be formed.

**a. germinati'va,** germinal a.

Head's a.'s, a.'s of skin innervated by the spinal cord segments, *i.e.,* a.'s corresponding to the distribution of the fibers in single spinal nerves.

**hysterogenic a.'s** hysterogenic *zones.*

**impression a.,** in dentistry, that surface which is recorded in an impression.

**inferior vestibular a.,** a. vestibularis inferior.

**insular a.,** insula (1).

**a. intercondyla'ris ante'rior** [ NA ], anterior intercondylar a.; the broad depressed a. between the tibial condyles anteriorly.

**a. intercondyla'ris poste'rior** [ NA ], posterior intercondylar a.; popliteal notch; the deep notch between the tibial condyles posteriorly.

Jonston's a., *alopecia* areata.

Kiesselbach's a., Little's a.; an a. on the anterior portion of the nasal septum rich in capillaries and often the seat of epistaxis.

Krönig's a., a resonant field over the apex of the lung anteriorly and posteriorly.

Little's a., Kiesselbach's a.

**macular a.,** the portion of the retina used for central vision; the center area of the fovea centralis retinae appears free of vessels and is much reduced in thickness.

Martegiani's a., Martegiani's *funnel.*

**mitral a.,** the region of the chest over the apex of the heart, where the sounds, normal or pathologic, produced at the mitral valve are usually heard most distinctly.

**motor a.,** motor *cortex.*

**a. nervi facialis** [ NA ], a. of the facial nerve; the a. in the fundus of the internal acoustic meatus superior to the transverse crest through which the facial nerve passes to enter the facial canal.

**a. nuda hepatis** [ NA ], bare area of the liver; the a. on the posterior surface of the liver which is fused with the diaphragm and therefore not covered by peritoneum.

**obeliar a.,** the rhomboid region limited by lines uniting the parietal foramen of each side to the extremities of the straight portion of the sutura sagittalis.

**olfactory a.,** *substantia* perforata anterior.

**a. opa'ca,** the peripheral a. of the blastoderm of birds and reptiles which is opaque because of adherent yolk.

**oval a. of Flechsig,** see *fasciculus* semilunaris.

Panum's a., fusion a.; the a. in and about the macula in which stimulation of corresponding retinal points results in stereoscopic vision.

**parastriate a.,** see visual *cortex.*

**a. parolfacto'ria (Brocae)** [ NA ], parolfactory a.; Broca's parolfactory a.; a small region of cerebral cortex on the medial surface of the frontal lobe, formed by the junction of the gyrus rectus with the gyrus cinguli, demarcated from the gyrus subcallosus by the sulcus parolfactorius posterior.

**parolfactory a.,** a. parolfactoria.

**pear-shaped a.,** retromolar *pad.*

**a. pellu'cida,** the translucent central part of the blastoderm of birds and reptiles.

**peristriate a.,** see visual *cortex.*

**piriform a., pyriform a.,** piriform *cortex.*

Pitres' a., prefrontal cortex of the cerebral hemisphere; see frontal *cortex.*

**postcentral a.,** the cortex of the postcentral gyrus; see somatic sensory *cortex.*

**post dam a.,** posterior palatal seal a.

**posterior intercondylar a.,** a. intercondylaris posterior.

**posterior palatal seal a.,** post dam a.; postpalatal seal a.; the soft tissues along the junction of the hard and soft palates on which pressure within the physiologic limits of the tissues can be applied by a denture to aid in the retention of the denture.

**postpalatal seal a.,** posterior palatal seal a.

**a. postre'ma,** a small, elevated a. in the lateral wall of the inferior recess of the fourth ventricle; one of the few loci in the brain where the blood-brain barrier is lacking.

**precentral a.,** the cortex of the precentral gyrus; see motor *cortex.*

**precommissural septal a.,** a. subcallosa.

**prefrontal a.,** prefrontal cortex; see frontal *cortex.*

**premotor a.,** premotor *cortex.*

**preoptic a.,** preoptic *region.*

**pressoreceptive a.'s,** vascular zones containing pressoreceptors. They are located principally in the carotid sinus and the cardioaortic regions.

**pressure a.,** an a. of excessive displacement of tissue.

**prestriate a.,** secondary visual cortex; see visual *cortex.*

**pretectal a.,** pretectal region; pretectum; a narrow, transversally oriented rostral zone of the mesencephalic tectum, bounded caudally by the superior colliculus, rostrally by the trigonum habenulae, and laterally by the pulvinar thalami; the a. contains several nuclei that receive fibers from the optic tract; it has efferent connections with the nucleus of Edinger-Westphal of both sides, by way of which it mediates the pupillary light reflex.

**primary visual a.,** see visual *cortex.*

**pulmonary a.,** the region of the chest at the second left intercostal space, where sounds produced at the pulmonary orifice of the right ventricle are heard most distinctly.

**relief a.,** in dentistry, the portion of the surface of the mouth upon which pressures are reduced or eliminated.

**rest a.,** rest seat; (1) the portion of the tooth selected and prepared to receive an occlusal, incisal, or lingual rest; (2) the portion of tooth structure or of a restoration in a tooth prepared so that it is spoon-shaped on some posterior teeth and V-shaped or hook-shaped on some anterior teeth, into which seats the metallic occlusal or incisal rest of a partial denture.

**retention a.,** retention groove; retention point; a provision made within a cavity preparation of a tooth to hold in place the first pieces of gold when placing a direct gold restoration.

**Rolando's a.,** motor *cortex.*

**secondary visual a.,** see visual *cortex.*

**sensorial or sensory a.'s,** see *cortex* cerebri.

**sensorimotor a.,** the precentral and postcentral gyri of the cerebral cortex.

**septal a.,** the region of the cerebral hemisphere that stretches as a thin sheet of brain tissue between the fornix bundle and the ventral surface of the corpus callosum, forming the medial wall of the lateral ventricle's frontal horn; it extends ventrally through the narrow interval between the anterior commissure and the rostrum corporis callosi as the precommissural septum or gyrus subcallosus, which is continuous caudally with the preoptic a. and hypothalamus, as well as more laterally with the substantia innominata. The septal a.'s major functional connections are with the hippocampus and hypothalamus.

**silent a.,** any a. of the cerebral or cerebellar surface, lesion of which occasions no definite sensory or motor symptoms.

**skip a.'s,** subsidiary segments of diseased intestine in regional enteritis, separated from the region of major involvement.

**somesthetic a.,** somatic sensory *cortex.*

**stress-bearing a.,** (1) the portion of the mouth capable of providing support for a denture; (2) surfaces of oral structures that resist forces, strains, or pressures brought upon them during function; see also denture *foundation,* supporting a., tissue-bearing a.

**striate a.,** see visual *cortex.*

**strip a. of Hines,** a narrow band of the cerebral cortex lying in front of the motor cortex and fusing with it; injury in this a. causes spasticity, increased tendon jerks and forced grasping.

**Stroud's pectinated a.,** a. of anal canal lying just below the columnae rectales.

**a. subcallo'sa** [ NA ], gyrus subcallosus.

**subcallosal a.,** *gyrus* subcallosus.

**superior vestibular a.,** a. vestibularis superior.

**supporting a.,** (1) the surface of the mouth available for the support of a denture; see also denture *foundation;* (2) those areas of the maxillary and mandibular edentulous ridges which are considered best suited to carry the forces of mastication when the dentures are in function.

**tissue-bearing a.,** denture *foundation.*

**tricuspid a.,** the region of the chest wall over the lower part of the body of the sternum, where the sounds produced at the right atrioventricular orifice are heard most distinctly.

**trigger a.,** any point or circumscribed a., irritation of which will give rise to functional action or disturbance elsewhere.

**vagus a.,** a portion of the floor of the fourth ventricle overlying the vagoglossopharyngeal nuclei.

**a. vasculo'sa,** the part of the a. opaca of the embryonic blastoderm of the chick, where the first blood vessels appear.

**vestibular a.,** a. vestibularis inferior and a. vestibularis superior.

**a. vestibula'ris inferior** [ NA ], inferior vestibular a.; the a. of the fundus of the internal acoustic meatus inferior to the transverse crest through which the saccular nerve passes.

**a. vestibula'ris superior** [ NA ], superior vestibular a.; the a. in the fundus of the internal acoustic meatus superior to the transverse crest through which the superior part of the vestibular nerve passes to reach the utriculus and the ampullae of the anterior and lateral semicircular ducts.

**visual a.,** visual *cortex.*

**Wernicke's a.,** Wernicke's *center.*

---

**area'tus, area'ta** [ L. ]. Occurring in patches or circumscribed areas.

**Ar'eca** [ Malay ]. A genus of palms of India and the Malay Archipelago. The a. nuts, or betel nuts, contain arecoline and 15 per cent red tannin. They are chewed in the East Indies, and have an anthelmintic action. See also betel nut.

**A. cat'echu,** a large handsome tree of the East Indies that furnishes the betel nut or areca nut. Astrigent and anthelmintic.

**arecaidine.** Arecaine; 1,2,5,6-tetrahydro-1-methylnicotinic acid; crystalline alkaloid resembling betaine, derived from the betel nut.

**arec'aine.** Arecaidine.

**arec'oline.** $C_8H_{13}NO_2$; a colorless oily alkaloid from the betel nut.

**a. hydrobromide,** methyl-1,2,5,6-tetrahydro-1-methylnicotinate hydrobromide; anthelmintic for veterinary use.

**areflexia** (a-re-flek'sĭ-ah). Absence of reflexes.

**arenaceous** (ar'ĕ-na'shus) [ L. *arena,* sand ]. Sandy.

**arena'tion** [ L. *arena,* sand ]. Psammotherapy.

**areola,** pl. **areolae** (ă-re'o-lah, ă-re'o-le) [ L. dim. of *area* ]. 1 [ NA ]. Any small area. 2. One of the spaces or interstices in areolar tissue. 3. a. mammae. 4. A pigmented, depigmented, or erythematous zone surrounding a papule, pustule, wheal, or cutaneous neoplasm.

**Chaussier's a.,** a ring of indurated tissue surrounding the lesion of malignant pustule.

**a. mammae** [ NA ], a. papillaris; areola (3); a circular pigmented area surrounding the nipple or papilla mammae; its surface is dotted with little projections due to the presence of the areolar, or Montgomery's glands beneath.

**a. papilla'ris,** a. mammae.

**a. umbilica'lis, a. umbilica'ris,** a pigmented ring around the umbilicus in the pregnant woman.

**are'olar.** Relating to an areola in any sense.

**areom'eter** [ G. *araios,* thin, + G. *metron,* measure ]. Hydrometer.

**Aretaeus of Cappadocia** (ar-et-e'us). A Greek physician practicing in Rome *circa* 120–200 A.D.; the most outstanding physician of the Pneumatic School. Gave excellent descriptions of pneumonia, pleurisy, empyema, epilepsy and diabetes, and described several types of insanity.

**Arg.** Symbol for arginine or its mono- or diradical.

**argamblyopia** (ar'gam-blĭ-o'pĭ-ah) [ G. *argos,* not working, fr. *a-* priv. + *ergon,* work ]. Obsolete term for amblyopia from disuse of the eye.

**Ar'gas.** A genus of soft ticks of the family Argasidae, some species of which, usually infesting birds, may attack man.

**A. american'us,** *A. persicus.*

**A. minia'tus,** *A. persicus.*

**A. per'sicus,** fowl tick; adobe tick; Persian tick; blue bug; a bloodsucking parasite of poultry; in Australia it may transmit fowl spirochetosis.

**A. reflex'us,** pigeon tick; may cause a cutaneous inflammatory lesion in man.

**argas'id.** Common name for members of the family Argasidae.

**Argasidae** (ar-gas'ĭ-de). Family of ticks (superfamily Ixodoidea, order Acarina), the soft ticks, so called because of their wrinkled, leathery, tuberculated appearance that fills out when the tick is engorged with blood. A dorsal shield (scutum) is not present; the mouthparts (capitulum) are subterminal or ventral in a depression (camerostome) that extends above the capitulum to form the anterior margin of the cephalothorax (hood). A. contains about 85 species in 4 genera: *Argas, Ornithodoros, Otobius,* and *Antricola;* argasid ticks, chiefly species of the genus *Ornithodoros,* harbor and transmit spirochetes of the genus *Borrelia* that cause relapsing fever in birds and mammals.

**argentaffin, argentaffine** (ar-jen'tă-fin, -fēn) [ L. *argentum,* silver, + *affinitas,* affinity, *q.v.* ]. Pertaining to cells or tissue elements that reduce silver ions in solution, thereby becoming stained brown or black.

**ar'gentaffino'ma.** Carcinoid.

**argentation** (ar'jen-ta'shun). Impregnation with a silver salt; when tissues or organs are involved during life, the condition is termed argyria.

**argentic** (ar-jen'tik). 1. Argyric (1); relating to silver. 2. Denoting a chemical compound containing silver as the rare, doubly charged ($Ag^{++}$) ion.

**ar'gentine.** Relating to, resembling, or containing silver.

**argentophil, argentophile** (ar-jen'to-fil, -fil). Argyrophil.

**argen'tous.** Denoting a chemical compound containing silver as a singly charged (Ag) ion. The vast majority of silver compounds contain the a. ion; where the ionic state of silver is not specifically stated, as in silver nitrate, the a. state is assumed.

**argentum,** gen. **argen'ti** (ar-jen'tum) [ L. ]. Silver; symbol Ag.

**ar'ginase.** An enzyme (EC 3.5.3.1) of the liver that catalyzes the hydrolysis of arginine to ornithine and urea; a key enzyme of the urea cycle.

**ar'ginine.** 2-Amino-5-guanidinovaleric acid; one of the amino acids occurring among the hydrolysis products of protein; particularly abundant in the basic proteins such as histones and protamines. Forms, along with lysine and histidine, the group of basic amino acids, otherwise called hexone bases or 6-carbon amino acids.

**a. deiminase** (EC 3.5.3.6), a. dihydrolase; a. iminohydrolase; an enzyme catalyzing the hydrolytic deamination of arginine to citrulline.

**a. dihydrolase,** a. deiminase.

**a. glutamate** (USAN), MODUMATE; composed of arginine and glutamic acid; given intravenously to detoxify ammonia; used in the treatment of ammoniemia resulting from liver dysfunction.

**a. hydrochloride** (NF), ARGIVENE; used for intravenous administration as an adjunct in the treatment of encephalopathies associated with liver diseases and ammoniacal azotemia.

**a. iminohydrolase,** a. deiminase.

**a. oxytocin,** oxytocin with arginine at position 8 (identical with a. vasotocin); see also a. vasopressin.

**a. phosphate,** phosphoarginine.

**a. vasopressin,** [ Arg[8] ]vasopressin; vasopressin containing arginine in position 8 (as in most mammals and in the chicken).

$$Cys-Tyr-Phe-Gln-Asn-Cys-Pro-\overset{8}{Arg}-Gly-NH_2$$

[8-Arginine]vasopressin

**a. vasotocin,** vasotocin with arginine at position 8 (identical with a. oxytocin); see also a. vasopressin.

**argininosuccinase.** Argininosuccinate lyase.

**argininosuccinate lyase** (EC 4.3.2.1). Argininosuccinase; enzyme cleaving L-argininosuccinate nonhydrolytically to L-arginine and fumarate.

**argininosuccinic acid.** HOOC—CH₂—CH(COOH)— NH—C(NH)—NH(CH₂)₃—CHNH₂—COOH; formed as an intermediate in the conversion of citrulline to arginine in the urea cycle, in a reaction involving aspartic acid and adenosine triphosphate.

**arginosuccinicaciduria** (ar'jin-o-suk-sin'ik-as-id-ūr-ĭ-ah). A possibly heritable disorder characterized by excessive urinary excretion of arginosuccinic acid, epilepsy, ataxia, mental retardation, liver disease, and friable, tufted hair. Presumed to be the consequence of the deficiency of an enzyme responsible for splitting arginosuccinic acid to arginine and fumaric acid.

**arginyl** (ar'jin-il). The aminoacyl radical of arginine.

**ar'gon** [ G. ntr. of *argos,* lazy, inactive, fr. *a-* priv. + *ergon,* work ]. A gaseous element, symbol Ar, atomic no. 18, atomic weight 39.9, present in the atmosphere in the proportion of about 1 per cent. It is one of the inert or noble gases.

**Argonz,** J., Argentinian physician. See A.-Del Castillo *syndrome.*

**Argyll Robertson.** See Robertson, Douglas Argyll.

**argyria** (ar-jir'ĭ-ah, ar-ji'rĭ-ah) [ G. *argyros,* silver ]. Argyriasis; argyrosis; argyrism; a slate-gray or bluish discoloration of the skin and deep tissues, due to the deposit of insoluble albuminate of silver, occurring after the medicinal administration for a long period of a soluble silver salt; formerly fairly common after the use of installations of silver-containing materials into the nose and sinuses.

**argyriasis** (ar'jĭ-ri'ah-sis). Argyria.

**argyr'ic.** 1. Argentic (1). 2. Relating to argyria.

**argyrism** (ar'jir-izm). Argyria.

**argyritis** (ar'jĭ-ri'tis) [ G. *argyros,* silver, + suffix *-itis,* inflammation ]. Silver or yellow litharge; lead oxide when of a decidedly yellow color.

**argyrophil, argyrophile** (ar-ji'ro-fil, -fil) [ G. *argyros,* silver, + *philos,* fond ]. Argentophil, argentophile; pertaining to tissue elements that are capable of impregnation with silver and being made visible after a reducing agent is used.

**argyrosis** (ar'jĭ-ro'sis). Argyria.

**arhinencephalia** (ā-rin'en-sĕ-fa'lĭ-ah). Arrhinencephaly.

**arhinia** (ă-rin'ĭ-ah). Arrhinia.

**Arias-Stella,** Javier M. D., Peruvian pathologist, *1924. See A.-S. *effect, phenomenon.*

**ariboflavinosis** (a-ri'bo-fla-vĭ-no'sis). Properly hyporiboflavinosis; a state produced by a deficiency of riboflavin in the diet, in which chilosis or angular stomatitis and magenta tongue may be found.

**aris'togen'ics** [ G. *aristos,* best, + *genikos,* pertaining to race ]. Eugenics.

**aristolochic acid.** 8-Methoxy-6-nitrophenanthro[ 3,4-d ]-1,3-dioxole-5-carboxylic acid; aromatic bitter.

**Aristotle** (ar'ĭ-stot-l) of Stagira, 384–322 B.C., one of the greatest of the world's philosophers and scientists. His writings dominated scientific thought for many centuries and included books on botany, zoology, embryology, comparative anatomy, and physiology. See A.'s *anomaly,* Aristotelian *method.*

**arith'moma'nia.** The morbid impulse to count.

**Arizona** (ār'ĭ-zo'nah). A genus of motile, peritrichous, nonsporeforming, aerobic to facultatively anaerobic bacteria (family Enterobacteriaceae) containing Gram-negative rods. These organisms do not produce urease and do not grow in media containing potassium cyanide. They decarboxylate lysine, arginine, and ornithine. Lactose is generally fermented. These organisms have been isolated from a wide variety of animals, including man; they may cause gastroenteritis in man, and frequently are involved in localized lesions in man and lower animals. There is a single species, *A. hinshawii,* the type species.

**Arlt,** Carl F. R. von, Vienna oculist, 1812–1887. See A.'s *operation, sinus, trachoma.*

**arm** [ L. *armus,* fore-quarter of an animal; G. *harmos,* a shoulder joint ]. The segment of the superior limb between the shoulder and the elbow; inaptly used by the general population to mean the whole superior limb.

**bar clasp a.,** a clasp a. which has its origin in the denture base or major connector; it consists of the a. which traverses but does not contact the gingival structures, and a terminal end which approaches its contact with the tooth in a gingivo-occlusal direction.

**bird a.,** nonmedical term for atrophy of a. muscles.

**brawny a.,** a swollen arm of lymphedema, particularly after homolateral radical mastectomy.

**circumferential clasp a.,** a clasp a. which has its origin in a minor connector and which follows the contour of the tooth approximately in a plane perpendicular to the path of insertion of the partial denture.

**circumferential clasp a., retentive,** one that is flexible and engages the infrabulge at the terminal end of the a.

**circumferential clasp a., stabilizing,** one that is relatively rigid and embraces the height of contour of the tooth.

**reciprocal a.,** a clasp a. or other extension used on a removable partial denture to oppose the action of some other part or parts of the appliance.

**retention a.,** retentive a.

**retentive a.,** retention a.; a flexible segment of a removable partial denture that engages an undercut on an abutment and is designed to retain the denture.

**armamenta'rium** [ L. an arsenal, fr. *armamenta* (pl. only), implements, tackle, fr. *arma* (pl. only), armor, arms ]. In medicine, all the means (drugs, instruments, etc.) at the disposal of the physician or of the surgeon to fit him for the practice of his profession or the treatment of a specific disease.

**Armanni-Ebstein kidney.** See under kidney.

**arma'rium** [ L. a closet, chest, fr. *arma* (pl. only), armor ]. Armamentarium, especially the literary part, or the physician's library.

**Armil'lifer.** A genus of Pentastomida (tongue worms) of the order Porocephalida, family Porocephalidae; adults are found in the lungs of reptiles, young in many mammals, including man.

**A. armillatus,** a species occurring in the python, the larva or nymph being occasionally found in man; also known as *Porocephalus armillatus* and *Netterhynchus armillatus.*

**armoracia** (ar-mo-ra'sĭ-ah) [ L. and G. ]. Horseradish; obtained from the roots of *Radicula armoracia* (Cruciferae); a condiment.

**arm'pit.** *Fossa* axillaris; axilla.

**Armstrong,** A. R. See King-A. *unit.*

**Armstrong,** Henry E., English physician. See King-A. *unit.*

**Arndt,** G., German physician. See A.-Gottron *syndrome.*

**Arndt** (arnt), Rudolph, German psychiatrist, 1835–1900. See A.'s *law.*

**Arneth** (ar'nāt), Joseph, German physician, 1873–1955. See A. *classification, count, formula, index, stages.*

**arnica** (ar'nĭ-kah) [ Mod. L. ]. The dried flower heads of *Arnica montana* (family Compositae); leopard's bane; mountain tobacco; a cardiac sedative, but seldom given internally; used externally for sprains and bruises.

**Arnold,** Friedrich, German anatomist, 1803–1890. See A.'s *bundle, canal, ganglion, nerve, tract.*

**Arnold,** Julius, German pathologist, 1835–1915. See A.'s *bodies,* A.-Chiari *deformity, malformation, syndrome.*

**Arnold,** V., Austrian physician, 19th century. See A.'s *test.*

**aromatic** (ar-o-mat'ik) [ G. *arōmatikos,* fr. *arōma,* spice, sweet herb ]. 1. Having an agreeable, somewhat pungent, spicy odor. 2. One of a group of vegetable drugs having a fragrant odor and slightly stimulant properties.

**aromatic L-amino-acid decarboxylase** (EC 4.1.1.26). Dopa decarboxylase; tryptophan decarboxylase; hydroxytryptophan decarboxylase; catalyzes the decarboxylation of dopa to dopamine and of tryptophan to tryptamine. It also decarboxylates hydroxytryptophan. This enzyme is important in the biosynthetic pathway of catecholamines and melanin.

**aro'matize.** To render aromatic; to treat with aromatics in order to disguise the taste or smell.

**aroyl** (ā'o-il). The radical of an aromatic acid, *e.g.,* benzoyl; analogous to acyl.

**arrachement** (ä-rash-moñ') [ Fr. tearing out ]. Pulling out the capsule, in membranous cataract, by means of a capsule forceps inserted through a corneal incision.

**arrec'tor,** pl. **arrecto'res** [ L. that which raises, fr. *ar-rigo,* pp. *-rectus,* to raise up ] [ NA ]. Erector.

    **arrecto'res pilo'rum,** A bundle of smooth muscle inserted between the connective sheath of the hair follicle and the papillary layer of the dermis. Contraction of the muscle erects the hair and causes cutis anserina (goose flesh).

**arrest** [ O.Fr. *arester,* fr. LL. *adresto,* to stop behind ]. 1. To stop; check; restrain. 2. A stoppage; an interference with or a checking of the regular course of a disease or symptom or the performance of a function. 3. Inhibition of a developmental process; usually the ultimate stage of development; premature a. may lead to a congenital abnormality.

    **cardiac a.,** a loss of effective cardiac function, which results in cessation of circulation; may be due to asystole in which there is no observable myocardial activity or to ventricular fibrillation.

    **circulatory a.,** cessation of the circulation of blood as a result of ventricular standstill or fibrillation.

    **epiphysial a.,** early and premature fusion between epiphysis and diaphysis.

    **maturation a.,** cessation of complete differentiation of cells at an immature stage: in spermatogenic maturation a. the seminiferous tubules contain spermatocytes but no spermatozoa develop.

    **sinus a.,** cessation of sinus activity; the ventricles may continue to beat under A-V nodal or idioventricular control; sinus standstill; atrial standstill; complete S-A block.

**arrhenic** (ā-rĕn'ic). Relating to arsenic.

**Arrhenius** (ah-ra'ne-us), Svante A., Swedish chemist, 1859–1927. See A.'s *doctrine, equation, law,* A.-Madsen *theory.*

**arrhenoblastoma** (ă-re-no-blas-to'mah) [ G. *arrhēn,* male, + *blastos,* germ, + suffix *-ōma,* tumor ]. Adenoma ovarii testiculare; adenoma tubulare testiculare ovarii; gynandroblastoma (1); a rare ovarian tumor that produces masculinization and often contains tubules and luteinized cells.

**arrhenogenic** (ă-re-no-jen'ik). Productive of males only.

**arrhenoplasm** (ă-re'no-plazm) [ G. *arrhēn,* male, + *plasma,* something formed ]. The male element of idioplasm.

**arrhenotocia** (ă-re-no-to'sĭ-ah) [ G. *arrhēn,* male, + *tokos,* birth ]. A form of parthenogenesis in which the virgin female gives birth to males only, as in the case of the queen bee.

**arrhigosis** (ă-rĭ-go'sis) [ G. *a-* priv. + *rigoun,* to shiver ]. Lack of perception of cold.

**arrhinencephaly, arrhinencephalia** (ă-rin-en-sef'al-ĭ, -sĕ-fa'lĭ-ah) [ G. *a-*priv. + *rhis(rhin-),* nose, + *enkephalos,* brain ]. An absence or rudimentary state of the rhinencephalon, or olfactory lobe of the brain, on one or both sides, with a corresponding lack of development of the external olfactory organs.

**arrhinia** (ă-rin'ĭ-ah) [ G. *a-* priv. + *rhis* (*rhin-*), nose ]. Absence of the nose.

**arrhythmia** (ă-rith'mĭ-ah) [ G. *a-* priv. + *rhythmos,* rhythm ]. Irregularity; loss of rhythm; denoting especially an irregularity of the heart beat. See also entries under rhythm.

    **juvenile a.,** sinus a.

    **nonphasic sinus a.,** sinus a. in which variations in rhythm are not related to the phases of respiration.

    **phasic sinus a.,** respiratory a.; sinus a. in which the irregularity is related to the phases of respiration, the rate being faster in inspiration and slower in expiration.

    **respiratory a.,** phasic sinus a.

    **sinus a.,** juvenile a.; irregularity of the heart beat, the heart being under the control of its normal pacemaker, the sinus (S-A) node.

**arrhyth'mic.** Marked by loss of rhythm; pertaining to arrhythmia.

**arrhythmogenic** (ă-rith-mo-jen'ik) [ G. *a-* priv. + *rhythmos,* rhythm, + suffix *-gen,* production ]. Capable of inducing arrhythmias.

**arrhythmokinesis** (ă-rith'mo-kĭ-ne'sis) [ G. *a-* priv. + *rhythmos,* rhythm, + *kinēsis,* movement ]. Inability to preserve the rhythm of voluntary alternating movements.

**ar'row.** An arrow-shaped instrument; a slender, sharp-pointed rod of silver nitrate or other caustic adapted for insertion into a tumor.

**ar'rowroot.** The rhizome of *Maranta arundinacea,* a plant of tropical America; the source of a form of starch formerly much used in the diet of children and invalids.

**Arroy'o,** Carlos F., American physician, 1892–1928. See A.'s *sign.*

**Arruga,** Hermenegilde, Spanish ophthalmologist, *1886. See A.'s *forceps.*

**arsacetin.** *p*-Acetamidobenzenearsonic acid; formerly used as an antisyphilitic agent.

**arsan'ilate.** A salt or ester of arsanilic acid.

**arsanil'ic acid.** $H_2N—C_6H_4—AsO(OH)_2.$

**arsen'amide.** CARPASIDE; *p*-[ bis(carboxymethylmercapto)arsino ]benzamide; used in treatment of filariasis.

**ar'senate.** A salt of arsenic acid, $H_3AsO_4.$

**arseni'asis.** Chronic arsenical poisoning.

**arsenic** (ar'sĕ-nik) [ Mod. L. fr. G. *arsenikon,* fr. *arsēn,* strong ]. Arsenium; ratsbane. 1. An element, a steel-gray metal, symbol As, atomic no. 33, atomic weight 74.9; forms a number of poisonous compounds, some of which are used in medicine. 2. Relating to the element arsenic, or one of its compounds; denoting especially arsenic acid, $H_3AsO_4 \cdot 1/2 H_2O,$ which forms arsenates with certain bases; not to be confused with what is sometimes called arsenic, which is arsenic trioxide, $As_2O_3.$

    **a. acid,** $H_3AsO_4;$ hydrate of arsenic oxide or arsenic trioxide, $As_2O_3.$

    **a. trihydride,** arsine.

    **a. trioxide,** arsenous oxide; so-called "arsenous acid"; white arsenic; $As_2O_3;$ dissolves in water to give arsenous acid, $H_3AsO_3$. Used in the treatment of skin diseases and malaria, and as a tonic; also used externally as a caustic. **white a.,** a. trioxide.

**arsen'ical, arsen'ic.** Relating to or containing arsenic.

**arsen'icalism.** Arseniasis.

**arsenic-fast.** Resistant to the poisonous action of arsenic; denoting especially spirochetes and other protozoan parasites, which acquire resistance after repeated administration of the drug.

**ar'senide.** Arseniuret; a compound of arsenic with a metal or other positively charged atoms or groups in which the arsenic is not bound to any atoms of oxygen, *e.g.,* $Ba_3As_2$, barium arsenide.

**arse'nious.** Arsenous.

**ar'senite.** A salt of arsenous acid.

**arse'nium.** Arsenic.

**arseniuret** (ar-se'nyu-ret). Arsenide.

**arseniureted** (ar-se'nyu-ret-ed). Combined with arsenic so as to form an arsenide.

**ar'seniza'tion.** Permeation with arsenic.

**ar'senoblast** [ G. *arsēn*, male, + *blastos*, germ ]. Masculonucleus; male pronucleus; the male element of the zygote or fertilized ovum.

**ar'senorelap'sing.** Obsolete term denoting a case of syphilis in which the symptoms recur after an apparent cure by arsphenamine or other arsenical.

**ar'senother'apy.** Treatment with arsenic, usually by intravenous injection, for syphilis.

**ar'senous.** Arsenious; relating to the metal arsenic or one of its compounds, denoting especially a compound of arsenic with a valence of +3, *e.g.,* $H_3AsO_3$.
 **a. acid,** arsenic trioxide.
 **a. hydride,** arsine.
 **a. oxide,** arsenic trioxide.

**arsenox'ides.** Oxidation products in the body of arsphenamines; believed to be the agents active against the spirochetes.

**ar'sine.** Arsenic trihydride; arseniureted hydrogen; arsenous hydride; $AsH_3$; a cell and blood poison. Many of its organic derivatives have been used in chemical warfare.

**arson'ic acid.** A derivative of arsenic acid by replacement of a hydroxyl group by an organic radical.

**arso'nium.** The positively charged ion, $AsH_4^+$; analogous to the ammonium ion $(NH_4^+)$.

**arsphenamine** (ars-fen'ămin). SALVARSAN; Ehrlich 606; phenarsenamine; 3,3'-diamino-4,4'-dihydroxyarsenobenzene dihydrochloride; formerly used in the treatment of syphilis, yaws, and some other diseases of protozoan origin, after neutralization with NaOH. The synthesis of a. in 1907 and the demonstration of its usefulness as a therapeutic agent by Paul Ehrlich and co-workers (1909) marked the beginning of chemotherapy.

**arsthinol.** BALARSEN; 3-acetamido-4-hydroxydithiobenzenearsonous acid, cyclic (hydroxymethyl)ethylene ester; amebicide.

**ar'tarine.** An alkaloid, $C_{21}H_{23}NO_4$, from artar root, *Xanthoxylum senegalense* (family Rutaceae); said to be similar to veratrine in its action as a cardiac stimulant.

**ar'tefact.** Artifact.

**artegraft** (USAN). Graft composed of a section of bovine artery that has been treated with ficin and tanned with dialdehyde starc; used as a prosthetic for arterial grafting.

**Artemis'ia.** A genus of plants of the family Compositae, found chiefly in Europe, Asia, and North America.

*l*-**arter'enol.** *l*-Norepinephrine.

**arteri-.** See arterio-.

# ARTERIA

**arteria,** gen. and pl. **arteriae** (ar-te'rī-ah, ar-te'rī-e) [ L. from G. *artēria*, the windpipe, later an artery as distinct from a vein. ARTER-] [ NA ]. Artery; a blood vessel conveying blood in a direction away from the heart. With the exception of the pulmonary and umbilical arteries, the arteries convey red or aerated blood. Arterial branches are given in the definition of the major artery; many are also listed and defined under ramus, which see. See color plates 10 to 13.

 **a. acetab'uli,** *ramus* acetabularis arteriae obturatoriae.

 **a. alveola'ris inferior** [ NA ]. inferior alveolar artery; inferior dental artery; *origin,* maxillary artery; *distribution,* through mandibular canal to lower teeth; *branches,* mylohyoid, mental, dental.

 **a. alveola'ris superior anterior** [ NA ]. anterior superior alveolar artery; anterior superior dental artery; *origin,* infraorbital artery; *distribution,* upper incisors and canine teeth, maxillary sinus.

 **a. alveola'ris superior posterior** [ NA ], posterior superior alveolar artery; posterior dental artery; *origin,* maxillary artery; *distribution,* molar and premolar teeth, gingiva.

 **a. anastomot'ica magna,** (1) a. collateralis ulnaris inferior; (2) a. genus descendens.

 **a. angula'ris** [ NA ], angular artery; the terminal branch of the facial; *distribution,* muscles and skin of side of nose; *anastomoses,* lateral nasal, and dorsal artery of nose and palpebrals from the ophthalmic.

 **a. anon'yma,** *truncus* brachiocephalicus.

 **a. appendicula'ris** [ NA ], appendicular artery; the branch of the ileocolic artery that supplies the vermiform appendix.

 **a. arcua'ta** [ NA ], arcuate artery; a. metatarsalis; metatarsal artery; *origin,* dorsalis pedis; *branches,* deep plantar, dorsal metatarsals and dorsal digitals.

 **arteriae arcua'tae renis** [ NA ], arcuate arteries of the kidney; arciform arteries; branches of the interlobar arteries of the kidney which at the junction of the cortex and medulla turn and run at right angles to the parent stem and approximately parallel to surface of the kidney.

 **a. articula'ris az'ygos,** a. genus media.

 **a. ascen'dens** [ NA ], ascending artery; the branch of the ileocolic artery that communicates with a branch of the right colic artery and supplies the ascending colon.

 **a. auditi'va interna,** a. labyrinthi.

 **a. auricula'ris posterior** [ NA ], posterior auricular artery; *origin,* external carotid; *branches,* muscular, posterior tympanic, auricular, occipital, and stylomastoid.

 **a. auricula'ris profun'da** [ NA ], deep auricular artery; *origin,* maxillary; *distribution,* articulation of jaw, parotid gland, and external acoustic meatus; *anastomoses,* branches of superficial temporal and posterior auricular.

 **a. axilla'ris** [ NA ], axillary artery; the continuation of the subclavian in the axilla, becoming the brachial in the arm; *branches,* superior thoracic, thoracoacromial, lateral thoracic, subscapular, circumflex humeral, posterior and anterior.

 **a. basila'ris** [ NA ], basilar artery; formed by union of the two vertebral arteries; runs from the lower to the upper border of the pons, where it bifurcates into the two posterior cerebral arteries; *branches,* anterior spinal artery, two inferior cerebellar arteries, labyrinthine, pontine, and superior cerebellar artery.

 **a. brachia'lis** [ NA ], brachial artery; humeral artery; *origin,* is a continuation of the axillary; *branches,* profunda brachii, superior ulnar collateral, inferior ulnar collateral, muscular, and nutrient branches; bifurcates at the elbow into radial and ulnar.

 **a. brachia'lis superficia'lis** [ NA ], superficial brachial artery; an occasional variation in which the brachial artery lies superficial to the median nerve in the arm.

 **a. bucca'lis** [ NA ], buccal artery; buccinator artery; *origin,* maxillary; *distribution,* buccinator muscle, skin, and mucous membrane of cheek; *anastomoses,* buccal branch of facial.

 **a. bulbi pe'nis** [ NA ], artery of the bulb of the penis; a. bulbi urethrae; a branch of the internal pudendal artery which supplies the bulb of the penis.

 **a. bulbi ure'thrae** a. bulbi penis.

 **a. bulbi vestib'uli** [ NA ], artery of the bulb of the vestibule; the branch of the internal pudendal artery in the female that supplies the bulb of the vestibule.

 **a. calcari'na,** calcarine artery; a continuation of the posterior cerebral artery along the calcarine fissure.

 **a. cana'lis pterygoid'ei** [ NA ], artery of the pterygoid canal; Vidian artery; *origin,* maxillary or descending palatine; *distribution*, upper part of pharynx, auditory tube, levator and tensor palati muscles; *anastomoses*, through tympanic branch with other tympanic arteries.

**a. carot'is commu'nis** [ NA ], common carotid artery; *origin*, right from brachiocephalic, left from arch of aorta; runs upward in the neck and divides opposite upper border of thyroid cartilage into *terminal branches*, external and internal carotid.

**a. carot'is externa** [ NA ], external carotid artery; *origin*, common carotid; *branches*, superior thyroid, lingual, facial, occipital, posterior auricular, ascending pharyngeal, and *terminal branches*, maxillary and superficial temporal.

**a. carot'is interna** [ NA ], internal carotid artery; arises from the common carotid opposite upper border of thyroid cartilage, and terminates in the middle fossa of the skull, dividing into the middle and anterior cerebral arteries; *branches*, caroticotympanic, artery of semilunar ganglion, inferior and superior hypophysial, ophthalmic, posterior communicating, choroid, anterior and middle cerebral.

**a. cau'dae pancrea'tis** [ NA ], caudal pancreatic artery; *origin*, splenic artery near the left gastroepiploic; *distribution*, the tail of the pancreas; *anastomoses*, with other pancreatic arteries.

**a. ceca'lis ante'rior** [ NA ], anterior cecal artery; *origin*, ileocolic artery; *distribution*, anterior region of cecum.

**a. ceca'lis poste'rior** [ NA ], posterior cecal artery; *origin*, ileocolic artery; *distribution*, posterior region of cecum.

**a. celia'ca**, *truncus* celiacus.

**a. centra'lis ret'inae** [ NA ], central artery of the retina; a. retinae centralis; Zinn's artery; a branch of the ophthalmic artery which penetrates the optic nerve 1 cm. behind the eye to enter the eye at the optic papilla in the retina; it divides into superior and inferior temporal and nasal branches.

**a. cerebel'li infe'rior ante'rior** [ NA ], anterior inferior cerebellar a.; *origin*, basilar; *distribution*, lower surface of lateral lobes of cerebellum; *anastomoses*, posterior inferior cerebellar.

**a. cerebel'li inferior posterior** [ NA ], posterior inferior cerebellar a.; *origin*, vertebral; *distribution*, medulla, choroid plexus, and cerebellum; *anastomoses*, superior cerebellar and anterior inferior cerebellar.

**a. cerebel'li superior** [ NA ], superior cerebellar a.; *origin*, basilar; *distribution*, upper surface of cerebellum and colliculi; *anastomoses*, posterior inferior cerebellar.

**a. cer'ebri anterior** [ NA ], anterior cerebral artery; one of the two terminal branches of the internal carotid; it passes posteriorly in the interhemispheric fissure along with its fellow of the opposite side, the two being joined by the anterior communicating artery. Branches supply anterobasal parts of the caudate nucleus and putamen, medial parts of the frontal and parietal lobes, and the corpus callosum.

**a. cer'ebri me'dia** [ NA ], middle cerebral artery; one of the two large terminal branches of the internal carotid artery. It passes laterally around the pole of the temporal lobe, then posteriorly, lying in the depth of the lateral cerebral fissure. It supplies blood to a very large central part of the cortical convexity including, on the left side, both Broca's and Wernicke's speech centers. Perforating branches supply the putamen, caudate nucleus, and anterior part of the internal capsule.

**a. cer'ebri posterior** [ NA ], posterior cerebral artery, formed by the bifurcation of the basilar artery; it passes around the cerebral peduncle to reach the medial aspect of the hemisphere. It supplies blood to the ventral surface of the temporal lobe, all of the occipital lobe, and the largest part of the thalamus. It is usually joined to the middle cerebral artery by the posterior communicating artery.

**a. cervica'lis ascendens** [ NA ], ascending cervical artery; cervicalis ascendens; *origin*, inferior thyroid, sometimes independently from the thyrocervical trunk; *distribution*, muscles of neck and spinal cord; *anastomoses*, branches of vertebral, occipital, ascending pharyngeal, and deep cervical.

**a. cervica'lis profunda** [ NA ], deep cervical artery; *origin*, costocervical trunk; *distribution*, posterior deep muscles of neck; *anastomoses*, branches of occipital, ascending cervical, and vertebral.

**a. cervica'lis superficia'lis** [ NA ], superficial cervical artery; a variation in which the superficial branch of the transverse cervical artery arises independently.

**a. cervicovagina'lis**, cervicovaginal *artery*.

**a. choroi'dea ante'rior** [ NA ], anterior choroidal artery; *origin*, internal carotid or middle cerebral artery; *distribution*, optic tract, crus cerebri, uncus, hippocampus, globus pallidus, posterior part of internal capsule, geniculate bodies of the thalamus, and choroid plexus in the inferior horn of the lateral ventricle.

**a. choroi'dea posterior**, posterior choroidal artery; one of several branches (*rami choroidei posteriores* [ NA ]) of the posterior cerebral artery that supply the choroid plexus of the body of the lateral ventricle and of the 3rd ventricle.

**a. cilia'ris anterior** [ NA ], anterior ciliary artery; one of several arteries derived from muscular branches of the ophthalmic which perforate the anterior part of the sclera and anastomose with posterior ciliary arteries.

**a. cilia'ris posterior brevis** [ NA ], short posterior ciliary artery; one of several ciliary branches of the ophthalmic distributed to the choroid coat of the eye.

**a. cilia'ris posterior longa** [ NA ], long posterior ciliary artery; one of two branches of the ophthalmic running forward between the sclerotic and choroid coats to the iris, at the outer and inner margins of which they form by anastomosis two circles.

**a. circumflex'a fem'oris latera'lis** [ NA ], lateral circumflex a. of the thigh; *origin*, profunda femoris; *distribution*, hip joint, thigh muscles; *anastomoses*, medial circumflex femoral, inferior gluteal, superior gluteal, popliteal.

**a. circumflex'a fem'oris media'lis** [ NA ], medial circumflex artery of the thigh; *origin*, profunda femoris; *distribution*, hip joint, muscles of thigh; *anastomoses*, inferior gluteal, superior gluteal, lateral circumflex femoral.

**a. circumflex'a hu'meri anterior** [ NA ], anterior circumflex humeral artery; *origin*, axillary; *distribution*, shoulder joint and biceps muscle; *anastomoses*, posterior circumflex humeral.

**a. circumflex'a hu'meri posterior** [ NA ], posterior circumflex humeral artery; *origin*, axillary; *distribution*, muscles and structures of shoulder joint; *anastomoses*, anterior circumflex humeral, suprascapular, thoracoacromial, and profunda brachii.

**a. circumflex'a il'ium profun'da** [ NA ], deep circumflex iliac artery; *origin*, external iliac; *distribution*, muscles and skin of lower abdomen, sartorius and tensor fasciae latae; *anastomoses*, lumbar, epigastric, gluteal, iliolumbar, and superficial circumflex iliac.

**a. circumflex'a il'ium superficia'lis** [ NA ], superficial circumflex iliac artery; *origin*, femoral; *distribution*, inguinal lymph nodes and integument of that region; sartorius, and tensor fasciae latae muscles; *anastomoses*, deep circumflex iliac.

**a. circumflex'a scap'ulae** [ NA ], circumflex scapular artery; *origin*, subscapular; *distribution*, muscles of shoulder and scapular region; *anastomoses*, branches of suprascapular and transverse cervical.

**a. col'ica dextra** [ NA ], right colic artery; *origin*, superior mesenteric, sometimes by a common trunk with the ileocolic; *distribution*, ascending colon; *anastomoses*, middle colic, ileocolic.

**a. col'ica media** [ NA ], *origin*, superior mesenteric; *distribution*, transverse colon; *anastomoses*, right and left colic.

**a. col'ica sin'istra** [ NA ], left colic artery; *origin*, inferior mesenteric; *distribution*, descending colon and splenic flexure; *anastomoses*, middle colic, sigmoid.

**a. collatera'lis media** [ NA ], middle collateral artery; the posterior terminal branch of the profunda brachii, anastomosing with the arteries which form the rete articulare cubiti.

**a. collatera'lis radia'lis** [ NA ], radial collateral artery; the anterior terminal branch of the profunda brachii, anastomosing with the radial recurrent.

**a. collatera'lis ulna'ris inferior** [ NA ], inferior ulnar collateral artery; *origin*, brachial; *distribution*, arm muscles at back of elbow; *anastomoses*, ulnar recurrent, anterior and posterior, superior ulnar collateral, profunda brachii, and recurrent interosseous.

**a. collatera'lis ulna'ris superior** [ NA ], superior ulnar collateral artery; *origin*, brachial; *distribution*, elbow joint;

*anastomoses,* posterior ulnar recurrent and inferior ulnar collateral.

**a. co'mes nervi phren'ici,** a. pericardiacophrenica.

**a. com'itans nervi ischiad'ici** [ NA ], companion artery to the sciatic nerve; *origin,* inferior gluteal; *distribution,* sciatic nerve; *anastomoses,* branches of profunda femoris.

**a. commu'nicans anterior** [ NA ], anterior communicating artery; a short vessel joining the two anterior cerebral arteries and completing the *circulus* arteriosus cerebri (circle of Willis) anteriorly.

**a. commu'nicans posterior** [ NA ], posterior communicating artery; *origin,* internal carotid; *distribution,* optic tract, crus cerebri, interpeduncular region, and hippocampal gyrus; *anastomoses,* with posterior cerebral to form the cerebral arterial circle (circle of Willis).

**a. conjunctiva'lis,** conjunctival artery; one of a number of minute arteries derived from muscular branches of the ophthalmic.

**a. conjunctiva'lis anterior** [ NA ], anterior conjunctival artery; one of a number of small branches of the anterior ciliary arteries that supplies the conjunctiva.

**a. conjunctiva'lis posterior** [ NA ], posterior conjunctival artery; one of a series of branches from the tarsal arterial arches that supplies the conjunctiva.

**a. corona'ria dextra** [ NA ], right coronary artery; *origin,* right aortic sinus; *distribution,* it passes around the right side of the heart in the coronary sulcus, giving branches to the right atrium and ventricle, including the atrioventricular branches and the posterior interventricular branch.

**a. corona'ria sin'istra** [ NA ], left coronary artery; *origin,* left aortic sinus; *distribution,* it divides into two major branches, an anterior interventricular which descends in the anterior interventricular sulcus, and a circumflex branch which passes to the diaphragmatic surface of the left ventricle; gives atrial, ventricular, and atrioventricular branches.

**a. cremaster'ica** [ NA ], cremasteric artery; external spermatic artery; *origin,* inferior epigastric; *distribution,* coverings of spermatic cord; *anastomoses,* external pudendal, spermatic, and perineal a.

**a. cystica** [ NA ], cystic artery; *origin,* right branch of hepatic; *distribution,* gall bladder and visceral surface of the liver.

**a. deferentia'lis,** a. ductus deferentis.

**a. digita'lis dorsa'lis** [ NA ], dorsal digital artery; one of the collateral digital branches of the dorsal metatarsal arteries in the foot, and of the dorsal metacarpal arteries in the hand.

**a. digita'lis palma'ris commu'nis** [ NA ], common palmar digital artery; one of three arteries arising from the superficial palmar arch and running to the interdigital clefts where each divides into two proper palmar digital arteries.

**a. digita'lis palma'ris pro'pria** [ NA ], palmar digital artery proper; collateral digital artery; the artery that passes along the side of each finger.

**a. digita'lis planta'ris commu'nis** [ NA ], common plantar digital artery; one of four arteries arising from a superficial plantar arch, when present as a variation. They unite with the plantar metatarsal arteries.

**a. digita'lis planta'ris pro'pria** [ NA ], plantar digital artery proper; one of the digital branches of the plantar metatarsal arteries.

**a. dorsalis clitori'dis** [ NA ], dorsal artery of the clitoris; one of the two terminal branches of the internal pudendal artery in the female, the other being the a. profunda clitoridis.

**a. dorsa'lis na'si** [ NA ], dorsal artery of the nose; *origin,* ophthalmic; *distribution,* skin of side of nose; *anastomoses,* angular.

**a. dorsa'lis pe'dis** [ NA ], dorsal artery of the foot; a continuation of the anterior tibial; *branches,* lateral tarsal, arcuate, dorsal metatarsal; *anastomoses,* with the lateral plantar to form the plantar arch.

**a. dorsa'lis pe'nis** [ NA ], dorsal artery of the penis; the dorsal terminal branch of the internal pudendal artery in the male.

**a. duc'tus deferen'tis** [ NA ], artery of the ductus deferens; a. deferentialis; *origin,* anterior division of internal iliac, or sometimes superior vesical; *distribution,* ductus deferens, seminal vesicles, testicle, ureter; *anastomoses,* testicular, cremasteric branch of inferior epigastric.

**a. epigas'trica inferior** [ NA ], inferior epigastric artery; deep epigastric a.;*origin,* external iliac; *branches,* cremasteric, muscular and pubic; *anastomoses,* superior epigastric, obturator.

**a. epigas'trica superficia'lis** [ NA ], superficial epigastric artery; *origin,* femoral; *distribution,* inguinal glands and integument of lower abdomen; *anastomoses,* inferior epigastric, superficial circumflex iliac and external pudendal.

**a. epigas'trica superior** [ NA ], superior epigastric artery; *origin,* the medial terminal branch of internal thoracic; *distribution,* abdominal muscles and integument, falciform ligament; *anastomoses,* inferior epigastric.

**a. episclera'lis** [ NA ], episcleral artery; one of many small branches of the anterior ciliary arteries that perforate the sclera behind the cornea to supply the iris and ciliary body.

**a. ethmoida'lis anterior** [ NA ], anterior ethmoidal artery; *origin,* ophthalmic; *distribution,* cerebral membranes in anterior cranial fossa, anterior ethmoidal cells, frontal sinus, anterior upper part of nasal mucous membrane, skin of dorsum of nose.

**a. ethmoida'lis posterior** [ NA ], posterior ethmoidal artery; *origin,* ophthalmic; *distribution,* posterior ethmoidal cells and upper posterior part of lateral wall of nasal cavity.

**a. facia'lis** [ NA ], facial artery; a. maxillaris externa; external maxillary artery; *origin,* external carotid; *branches,* ascending palatine, tonsillar and glandular branches, submental, inferior labial, superior labial, masseteric, buccal, and lateral nasal branches, and angular.

**a. femora'lis** [ NA ], femoral artery; crural artery; *origin,*continuation of external iliac, beginning at inguinal ligament; *branches,* external pudendal, superficial epigastric, superficial circumflex iliac, profunda femoris, descending genicular, terminating in the popliteal at the upper part of the popliteal space.

**a. fibula'ris** [ NA ], a. peronea.

**a. fronta'lis,** a. supratrochlearis.

**arteriae gas'tricae bre'ves** [ NA ], short gastric arteries; vasa brevia; four or five small arteries given off from the splenic, passing to the greater curvature of the stomach, and anastomosing with the other arteries in that region.

**a. gas'trica dextra** [ NA ], right gastric artery; pyloric artery; *origin,* hepatic; *distribution,* pyloric portion of stomach on the lesser curvature; *anastomoses,* left gastric.

**a. gas'trica sin'istra** [ NA ], left gastric artery; coronary artery; *origin,* celiac; *distribution,* lesser curvature of stomach, abdominal part of the esophagus, and, frequently, a portion of the left lobe of the liver; *anastomoses,* esophageal, right gastric.

**a. gastroduodena'lis** [ NA ], gastroduodenal artery; *origin,* hepatic; terminal *branches,* right gastroepiploic, superior pancreaticoduodenal.

**a. gastroepiplo'ica dextra** [ NA ], right gastroepiploic artery; *origin,* gastroduodenal; *distribution,* greater curvature and walls of stomach and greater omentum; *anastomoses,* frequently unites with left gastroepiploic and branches from this arch anastomose with branches of right and left gastric.

**a. gastroepiplo'ica sin'istra** [ NA ], left gastroepiploic artery; *origin,* splenic; *distribution,* greater curvature of stomach and greater omentum; frequently joining right gastroepiploic, which see for anastomoses.

**a. ge'nus descen'dens** [ NA ], descending artery of the knee; *origin,* femoral; *distribution,* knee joint and adjacent parts; *anastomoses,* medial superior genicular, medial inferior genicular, lateral superior genicular, lateral circumflex femoral, and anterior tibial recurrent.

**a. ge'nus inferior latera'lis** [ NA ], lateral inferior artery of the knee; *origin,* popliteal; *distribution,* knee joint; *anastomoses,* lateral superior genicular and anterior tibial recurrent (and posterior).

**a. ge'nus inferior media'lis** [ NA ], medial inferior artery of the knee; *origin,* popliteal; *distribution,* knee joint; *anastomoses,* anterior and posterior tibial recurrent and medial superior genicular.

**a. ge'nus media** [ NA ], middle artery of the knee; a. articularis azygos; *origin,* popliteal; *distribution,* synovial membrane and cruciate ligaments of knee joint.

**a. ge'nus superior latera'lis** [ NA ], lateral superior artery of the knee; *origin,* popliteal; *distribution,* knee joint; *anastomoses,* lateral circumflex femoral, third perforating, anterior tibial recurrent, lateral inferior genicular.

**a. ge'nus superior media'lis** [ NA ], medial superior artery of the knee; *origin,* popliteal; *distribution,* knee joint; *anastomoses,* descending genicular, lateral superior genicular.

**a. glu'tea inferior** [ NA ], inferior gluteal artery; a. ischiadica (ischiatica); *origin,* internal iliac; *distribution,* hip joint and gluteal region; *anastomoses,* branches of internal pudendal, lateral sacral, superior gluteal, obrurator, medial and lateral circumflex femoral.

**a. glu'tea superior** [ NA ], superior gluteal artery; *origin,* internal iliac; *distribution,* gluteal region; *anastomoses,* lateral sacral, inferior gluteal, internal pudendal, deep circumflex iliac, lateral circumflex femoral.

**a. helici'na** [ NA ], helicine artery; one of the coiled arteries in the erectile tissue of the penis.

**a. hepat'ica commu'nis** [ NA ], common hepatic artery; *origin,* celiac; *branches,* right gastric, gastroduodenal, and proper hepatic.

**a. hepat'ica pro'pria** [ NA ], proper hepatic artery; *origin,* common hepatic; *branches,* right and left hepatic.

**a. hyaloi'dea** [ NA ], hyaloid artery; the terminal branch of the primitive ophthalmic artery which forms in the embryo an extensive ramification in the primary vitreous and a vascular tunic around the lens; by $8^1/_2$ months, these vessels have atrophied almost completely, but a few persistent remnants are evident entopically as muscae volitantes.

**a. hypogas'trica,** a. iliaca interna.

**arteriae il'ei** [ NA ], ileal arteries; intestinal arteries; *origin,*superior mesenteric; *distribution,* ileum; *anastomoses,* other branches of superior mesenteric.

**a. ileocol'ica** [ NA ], ileocolic artery; *origin,* superior mesenteric, often by a common trunk with the right colic; *distribution,* terminal part of ileum, cecum, vermiform appendix, and ascending colon; *anastomoses,* right colic and ileal.

**a. ili'aca commu'nis** [ NA ], common iliac artery; one of the two terminal branches of the abdominal aorta; opposite the lumbosacral articulation, it becomes the internal iliac and also gives off the external iliac.

**a. ili'aca externa** [ NA ], external iliac artery; *origin,* common iliac; *branches,* inferior epigastric, deep circumflex iliac; becomes the femoral at the inguinal ligament.

**a. ili'aca interna** [ NA ], internal iliac artery; hypogastric artery; *origin,* common iliac; *branches,* iliolumbar, lateral sacral, obturator, superior gluteal, inferior gluteal, umbilical, superior vesical, inferior vesical, middle rectal; the artery itself usually divides into an anterior and a posterior division, the anterior terminating in the internal pudendal, the posterior in the superior gluteal.

**a. iliolumba'lis** [ NA ], iliolumbar artery; *origin,* internal iliac; *distribution,* pelvic muscles and bones; *anastomoses,* deep circumflex iliac, obturator, lumbar.

**a. infraorbita'lis** [ NA ], infraorbital artery; *origin,* maxillary; *distribution,* upper canine and incisor teeth, inferior rectus and inferior oblique muscles, lower eyelid, lacrimal sac, and upper lip; *anastomoses,* branches of ophthalmic, facial, superior labial, transverse facial, and buccinator.

**a. intercosta'lis posterior** [ NA ], posterior intercostal artery; one of nine pairs of arteries arising from the thoracic aorta and distributed to the nine lower intercostal spaces, spinal column, spinal cord, and muscles and integument of the back; they anastomose with branches of the musculophrenic, internal thoracic, superior epigastric, subcostal and lumbar.

**a. intercosta'lis supre'ma** [ NA ], highest intercostal artery; a. intercostalis superior; *origin,* costocervical trunk; *distribution,* structures of first and second intercostal spaces; *anastomoses,* anterior intercostal branches of internal thoracic.

**arteriae interlobula'res** [ NA ], interlobular arteries; (1) arteries which pass between lobules of an organ; (2) the many terminal branches of the hepatic artery passing between hepatic lobules; (3) branches of the interlobar arteries of the kidney passing outward through the cortex and supplying the glomeruli.

**a. interos'sea anterior** [ NA ], anterior interosseous artery; a. interossea volaris; volar interosseous artery; *origin,* common interosseous; *distribution,* deep parts of the forearm anteriorly; *anastomoses,* posterior interosseous.

**a. interos'sea communis** [ NA ], common interosseous artery; *origin,* ulnar; *branches,* anterior and posterior interosseous.

**a. interos'sea posterior** [ NA ], posterior interosseous artery; dorsal interosseous artery; *origin,* common interosseous; *distribution,* deep parts of forearm posteriorly.

**a. interos'sea recur'rens** [ NA ], recurrent interosseous artery *origin,* posterior interosseous; *distribution,* elbow joint; *anastomoses,* branches of profunda brachii and inferior ulnar collateral.

**a. interos'sea vola'ris,** a. interossea anterior.

**arteria intestina'les,** arteriae ilei and arteriae jejunales.

**a. ischiad'ica, a. ischiat'ica,** a. glutea inferior.

**arteriae jejuna'les** [ NA ], jejunal arteries; intestinal arteries; *origin,* superior mesenteric; *distribution,* jejunum; *anastomoses,* by a series of arches with each other and with ileal arteries.

**arteriae labiales anteriores,** *rami* labiales anteriores.

**a. labia'lis inferior** [ NA ], inferior labial artery; *origin,* facial; *distribution,* structures of lower lip; *anastomoses,* the artery from the opposite side, mental and sublabial.

**a. labia'lis superior** [ NA ], superior labial artery; superior coronary artery; *origin,* facial; *distribution,* structures of upper lip and, by a septal branch, the anterior and lower part of the nasal septum; *anastomoses,* the artery of the opposite side and the sphenopalatine.

**a. labyrin'thi** [ NA ], artery of the labyrinth; a. auditiva interna; internal auditory artery; a branch of the basilar artery that enters the labyrinth through the internal acoustic meatus.

**a. lacrima'lis** [ NA ], lacrimal artery; *origin,* ophthalmic; *distribution,* lacrimal gland, lateral and superior rectus muscles, superior eyelid, forehead, and temporal fossa.

**a. laryn'gea inferior** [ NA ], inferior laryngeal artery; *origin,* inferior thyroid; *distribution,* muscles and mucous membrane of larynx; *anastomoses,* superior laryngeal.

**a. laryn'gea superior** [ NA ], superior laryngeal artery; *origin,* superior thyroid; *distribution,* muscles and mucous membrane of larynx; *anastomoses,* cricothyroid branch of superior thyroid and terminal branches of inferior laryngeal.

**a. liena'lis** [ NA ], splenic artery; *origin,* celiac trunk; *branches,* pancreatic, left gastroepiploic, short gastric, and splenic.

**a. ligamen'ti'tere'tis'u'teri** [ NA ], artery of the round ligament of the uterus; *origin,* inferior epigastric; *distribution,* round ligament.

**a. lingua'lis** [ NA ], lingual artery; *origin,* external carotid; *distribution,* runs along under surface of tongue, terminates as ranine artery, a. profunda linguae; *branches,* suprahyoid and dorsal lingual branches and sublingual artery.

**a. lo'bi cauda'ti** [ NA ], artery of the caudate lobe; *origin,* left branch of proper hepatic; *distribution,* caudate lobe of the liver.

**a. lumba'lis** [ NA ], lumbar artery; one of four or five pairs; *origin,* abdominal aorta; *distribution,* lumbar vertebrae, muscles of back, abdominal wall; *anastomoses,* intercostal, subcostal, superior and inferior epigastric, deep circumflex iliac, and iliolumbar.

**a. lumba'lis i'ma** [ NA ], lowest lumbar artery; *origin,* middle sacral; *distribution,* sacrum and iliac muscle; *anastomosis,* circumflex iliac artery.

**a. luso'ria,** an abnormally placed artery or vascular ring producing dysphagia by pressure on the esophagus.

**a. malleola'ris anterior latera'lis** [ NA ], anterior lateral malleolar artery; *origin,* anterior tibial; *distribution,* ankle joint; *anastomoses,* peroneal, lateral tarsal.

**a. malleola'ris anterior media'lis** [ NA ], anterior medial malleolar artery; *origin,* anterior tibial; *distribution,* ankle joint and neighboring integument; *anastomoses,* branches of posterior tibial.

**arteriae malleola'res posterio'res latera'les,** *rami* malleolares laterales.

**arteriae malleola'res posterio'res media'les,** *rami* malleolares mediales.

**a. mamma'ria interna,** a. thoracica interna.

**a. masseter'ica** [ NA ], masseteric artery; *origin,* maxillary; *distribution,* deep surface of masseter muscle; *anastomoses,* branches of transverse facial and masseteric branches of facial.

**a. maxilla'ris** [ NA ], maxillary artery; internal maxillary artery; *origin,* external carotid; *branches,* deep auricular, anterior tympanic, middle meningeal, inferior alveolar, masseteric, deep temporal, buccal, superior posterior alveolar, infraorbital, descending palatine, artery of pterygoid canal, sphenopalatine.

**a. maxilla'ris externa,** a. facialis.

**a. media'na** [ NA ], median artery; a. comes nervi mediani; *origin,* anterior interosseous; *distribution,* accompanies median nerve to palm; *anastomoses,* branches of superficial palmar arch.

**a. mediastina'lis anterior,** *rami* mediastinales arteriae thoracicae internae.

**a. menin'gea anterior** [ NA ], anterior meningeal artery; *origin,* ophthalmic; *distribution,* meninges in middle cranial fossa; *anastomoses,* branches of middle meningeal and meningeal branches of internal carotid and lacrimal.

**a. menin'gea media** [ NA ], middle meningeal artery; *origin,* maxillary; *branches,* petrosal, ganglionic, superior tympanic, frontal and parietal; *distribution,* to parts mentioned and through terminal branches to anterior and middle cranial fossae; *anastomoses,* meningeal branches of occipital, ascending pharyngeal, ophthalmic and lacrimal, stylomastoid, accessory meningeal branch of maxillary, and deep temporal.

**a. menin'gea posterior** [ NA ], posterior meningeal artery; *origin,* ascending pharyngeal; *distribution,* dura mater of posterior cranial fossa; *anastomoses,* branches of middle meningeal and vertebral.

**a. menta'lis** [ NA ], mental artery; terminal branch of inferior alveolar; *distribution,* chin; *anastomosis,* inferior labial artery.

**a. mesenter'ica inferior** [ NA ], inferior mesenteric artery; *origin,* aorta; *branches,* left colic, sigmoid, superior rectal; *anastomoses,* middle colic and middle rectal.

**a. mesenter'ica superior** [ NA ], superior mesenteric artery; *origin,* aorta; *branches,* inferior pancreaticoduodenal, jejunal, ileal, ileocolic, appendicular, right colic, middle colic; *anastomoses,* superior pancreaticoduodenal and left colic.

**a. metacar'pea dorsa'lis** [ NA ], dorsal metacarpal artery; dorsal interosseous artery; one of three branches of the posterior carpal arch, running in the back of the 2d, 3d, and 4th interosseous muscles.

**a. metacar'pea palma'ris** [ NA ], palmar metacarpal artery; palmar interosseous artery; one of the three arteries springing from the deep palmar arch and running in the three medial interosseous spaces; they anastomose with the dorsal metacarpal arteries.

**a. metatarsa'lis,** a. arcuata.

**a. metatar'sea dorsa'lis** [ NA ], dorsal metatarsal artery; one of the three branches of the arcuate supplying the three lateral toes and the lateral side of the second toe through the collateral branches, the dorsal digital.

**a. metatar'sea planta'ris** [ NA ], plantar metatarsal artery; one of four branches of the plantar arch that divide into plantar digital arteries to supply the toes.

**a. musculophren'ica** [ NA ], musculophrenic artery; *origin,* the lateral terminal branch of internal thoracic; *distribution,* diaphragm and intercostal muscles; *anastomoses,* branches of pericardiacophrenic, inferior phrenic, and posterior intercostal arteries.

**arteriae nasa'les posterio'res latera'les** [ NA ], posterior lateral nasal arteries; branches of the sphenopalatine artery that supply the posterior parts of the conchae and lateral nasal wall.

**a. nasa'lis poste'rior sep'ti** [ NA ], posterior septal artery of the nose; a branch of the sphenopalatine artery that supplies the nasal septum and accompanies the nasopalatine nerve.

**a. nutri'cia** [ NA ], nutrient artery; nutrient vessel; an artery of variable origin that supplies the medullary cavity of a long bone.

**arteriae nutri'ciae hu'meri** [ NA ], nutrient arteries of the humerus; *origin,* deep brachial; *distribution,* the medullary cavity of the humerus.

**a. obturato'ria** [ NA ], obturator artery; *origin,* anterior division of the internal iliac; *distribution,* ilium, pubis, obturator and adductor muscles; *anastomoses,* iliolumbar, inferior epigastric, medial circumflex femoral; *branches,* pubic, acetabular, anterior, and posterior.

**a. obturato'ria accesso'ria** [ NA ], accessory obturator artery; the term applied to the pubic branch of the inferior epigastric artery when it contributes a significant supply through the obturator canal.

**a. occipita'lis** [ NA ], occipital artery; *origin,* external carotid; *branches,* sternocleidomastoid, and muscular, meningeal, auricular, occipital mastoid, and descending.

**a. ophthal'mica** [ NA ], ophthalmic artery; *origin,* internal carotid; *branches,* ciliary, central artery of retina, anterior meningeal, lacrimal, conjunctival, episcleral, supraorbital, ethmoidal, palpebral, dorsal nasal, and supratrochlear.

**a. ova'rica** [ NA ], ovarian artery; *origin,* aorta; *distribution,* ureter, ovary, ovarian ligament and uterine tube; *anastomoses,* uterine.

**a. palati'na ascen'dens** [ NA ], ascending palatine artery; *origin,* facial; *distribution,* lateral walls of pharynx, tonsils, auditory tubes, and soft palate; *anastomoses,* tonsillar branch of facial, dorsal lingual, and descending palatine.

**a. palati'na descen'dens** [ NA ], descending palatine artery; *origin,* maxillary; *distribution,* soft palate, gums, and bones and mucous membrane of hard palate; *anastomoses,* sphenopalatine, ascending palatine, ascending pharyngeal, and tonsillar branches of facial.

**a. palati'na major** [ NA ], greater palatine artery; anterior branch of descending palatine artery, supplying the gums and mucous membrane of the hard palate.

**a. palati'na minor** [ NA ], lesser palatine artery; one of several posterior branches of the descending palatine in the greater palatine canal, distributed to the soft palate and tonsil.

**arteriae palpebra'les** [ NA ], palpebral arteries; branches of the ophthalmic supplying the upper and lower eyelids, consisting of two sets, *lateral* and *medial.*

**a. pancreat'ica dorsa'lis** [ NA ], dorsal pancreatic artery; great superior pancreatic artery; *origin,* splenic; *distribution,* head and body of pancreas; *anastomoses,* superior pancreaticoduodenal.

**a. pancreat'ica infe'rior** [ NA ], inferior pancreatic artery; transverse pancreatic artery; *origin,* dorsal pancreatic; *distribution,* body and tail of pancreas; *anastomoses,* pancreatica magna.

**a. pancreat'ica mag'na** [ NA ], great pancreatic artery; *origin,* splenic; *distribution,* tail of pancreas; *anastomoses,* inferior and caudal pancreatic arteries.

**a. pancreat'icoduodena'lis inferior** [ NA ], inferior pancreaticoduodenal artery; one of two arteries, *origin,* superior mesenteric; *distribution,* head of pancreas, duodenum; *anastomoses,* superior pancreaticoduodenal.

**a. pancreat'icoduodena'lis superior** [ NA ], superior pancreaticoduodenal artery; one of two arteries, *origin,* gastroduodenal; *distribution,* head of pancreas, duodenum, common bile duct; *anastomoses,* inferior pancreaticoduodenal, splenic.

**arteriae perforan'tes** [ NA ], perforating arteries; *origin,* a. profunda femoris; *distribution,* as three or four vessels that pass through the adductor magnus to the posterior and lateral parts of the thigh.

**a. pericardiacophren'ica** [ NA ], pericardiacophrenic artery; comes nervi phrenici; *origin,* internal thoracic; *distribution,* pericardium, diaphragm, and pleura; *anastomoses,* musculophrenic, inferior phrenic, mediastinal and pericardial branches of the internal thoracic.

**a. perinea'lis** [ NA ], perineal artery; *origin,* internal pudendal; *distribution,* superficial structures of the perineum; *anastomoses,* external pudendal arteries.

**a. pero'nea** [ NA ], peroneal artery; fibular artery; arteria fibularis; *origin,* posterior tibial; *distribution,* soleus, tibialis posterior, flexor longus hallucis, peroneal muscles, inferior tibiofibular articulation, and ankle joint; *anastomoses,* anterior lateral malleolar, lateral tarsal, lateral plantar, dorsalis pedis.

**a. pharyn'gea ascen'dens** [ NA ], ascending pharyngeal artery; *origin,* external carotid; *distribution,* wall of pharynx and soft palate.

**a. phren'ica inferior** [ NA ], inferior phrenic artery; *origin*, the first paired branch from the abdominal aorta inferior to the diaphragm; *distribution*, diaphragm; *anastomoses*, superior phrenic, internal thoracic, and musculophrenic.

**a. phren'ica superior** [ NA ], superior phrenic artery; one of a pair of small arteries given off from the thoracic aorta just superior to the diaphragm; *distribution*, diaphragm; *anastomoses*, musculophrenic, pericardiacophrenic, and inferior phrenic.

**a. planta'ris latera'lis** [ NA ], lateral plantar artery; larger of the two terminal branches of the posterior tibial; *distribution*, forms the plantar arch and through it supplies the sole of the foot and plantar surfaces of the toes; *anastomoses*, medial plantar, dorsalis pedis.

**a. planta'ris media'lis** [ NA ], medial plantar artery; one of the terminal branches of the posterior tibial; *distribution*, medial side of the sole of the foot; *anastomoses*, dorsalis pedis, lateral plantar.

**a. poplit'ea** [ NA ], popliteal artery; continuation of femoral in the popliteal space, bifurcating at the lower border of the popliteus muscle into the anterior and posterior tibial; *branches*, lateral and medial superior genicular, middle genicular, lateral and medial inferior genicular, and sural arteries.

**a. prin'ceps pol'licis** [ NA ], chief artery of thumb; principal artery of thumb; *origin*, radial; *distribution*, palmar surface and sides of thumb; *anastomoses*, arteries on dorsum of thumb.

**a. profun'da bra'chii** [ NA ], deep brachial artery; *origin*, brachial; *distribution*, humerus and muscles and integument of arm; *anastomoses*, radial recurrent, recurrent interosseous, ulnar collateral, posterior circumflex humeral.

**a. profun'da clitori'dis** [ NA ], deep artery of the clitoris; the deep terminal branch of the pudendal artery in the female; it supplies the crus of the clitoris.

**a. profun'da fem'oris** [ NA ], deep artery of the thigh; *origin*, femoral; *branches*, lateral circumflex femoral, medial circumflex femoral, perforating (3 or 4).

**a. profun'da lin'guae** [ NA ], deep artery of the tongue; a. ranina; ranine artery; termination of lingual; *distribution*, muscles and mucous membrane of under surface of tongue.

**a. profun'da pe'nis** [ NA ], deep artery of the penis; *origin*, terminal branch of the internal pudendal artery; *distribution*, corpus cavernosum of the penis.

**a. puden'da inter'na** [ NA ], internal pudendal artery; *origin*, internal iliac; *branches*, inferior rectal, perineal, posterior scrotal (or labial), urethral, artery of bulb of penis (or of vestibule), deep artery of penis (or clitoris), dorsal artery of penis (or clitoris).

**arteriae puden'dae externae** [ NA ], external pudendal arteries; *origin*, femoral; *distribution*, skin over pubis, skin over penis, scrotum, or labium majus; *anastomoses*, dorsal artery of penis or clitoris, posterior scrotal or labial arteries.

**a. pulmona'lis,** *truncus* pulmonalis.

**a. pulmona'lis dextra** [ NA ], right pulmonary artery; one of two branches of the pulmonary trunk, it passes transversely across the mediastinum to enter the hilus of the right lung. Branches are distributed with the bronchi and there are frequent variations in which subsegmental bronchi receive independent branches. The NA lists the following branches; ramus apicalis, r. posterior descendens, r. anterior descendens, r. anterior ascendens, r. posterior ascendens, r. lobi medii (r. lateralis, r. medialis), r. apicalis [ superior ] lobi inferioris, pars basalis, from which arise r. subapicalis [ subsuperior ], r. basalis medialis [ cardiacus ], r. basalis anterior, r. basalis lateralis, and r. basalis posterior.

**a. pulmona'lis sin'istra** [ NA ], left pulmonary artery; it enters the hilus of the left lung. Its branches accompany the segmental and subsegmental bronchi and are listed as follows in the NA: ramus apicalis, r. anterior descendens, r. posterior, r. anterior ascendens, r. lingularis (r. lingularis superior, r. lingularis inferior), r. apicalis [ superior ] lobi inferioris, pars basalis, from which arise r. subapicalis [ subsuperior ], r. basalis medialis, r. basalis anterior, r. basalis lateralis and r. basalis posterior.

**a. radia'lis** [ NA ], radial artery; *origin*, brachial; *branches*, radial recurrent, dorsal metacarpal, dorsal digital, princeps pollicis, palmar metacarpal, and muscular, carpal, and perforating.

**a. radia'lis in'dicis** [ NA ], radial index artery; a. volaris indicis radialis; *origin*, radial; *distribution*, radial side of index finger.

**a. ranina,** a. profunda linguae.

**a. recta'lis inferior** [ NA ], inferior rectal artery; inferior hemorrhoidal artery; *origin*, internal pudendal; *distribution*, anal canal, muscles and skin of the anal region, and skin of the buttock; *anastomoses*, middle rectal, perineal, and gluteal.

**a. recta'lis media** [ NA ], middle rectal artery; middle hemorrhoidal artery; *origin*, internal iliac; *distribution*, middle portion of rectum; *anastomoses*, superior and inferior rectal.

**a. recta'lis superior** [ NA ], superior rectal artery; superior hemorrhoidal artery; *origin*, inferior mesenteric; *distribution*, upper part of rectum; *anastomoses*, middle and inferior rectal.

**a. recur'rens radia'lis** [ NA ], radial recurrent artery; *origin*, radial; *distribution*, ascends around lateral side of elbow joint; *anastomoses*, radial collateral, interosseous recurrent.

**a. recur'rens tibia'lis anterior** [ NA ], anterior tibial recurrent artery; a branch of the anterior tibial artery which ascends to supply the front and sides of the knee joint.

**a. recur'rens tibia'lis posterior** [ NA ], posterior tibial recurrent artery; an inconstant branch of the posterior tibial artery which ascends anterior to the popliteus muscle, anastomoses with branches of the popliteal artery and sends a twig to the tibiofibular joint.

**a. recur'rens ulnaris** [ NA ], recurrent ulnar artery; *origin*, ulnar artery; *distribution*, two branches, anterior and posterior, pass medially in front of and behind the elbow joint; *anastomoses*, superior and inferior ulnar collateral.

**a. rena'lis** [ NA ], renal artery; *origin*, aorta; *branches*, ureteral, perirenal, and glandular, and inferior suprarenal; *distribution*, kidney.

**arteriae re'nis** [ NA ], arteries of the kidney; the branches of the renal artery that supply the kidney tissue. Usually five in number, they give off interlobar, arcuate and interlobular arteries in sequence. The latter send afferent arterioles to the glomeruli as well as branches to the kidney capsule.

**a. ret'inae centra'lis,** a. centralis retinae.

**a. retroduodena'lis** [ NA ], retroduodenal artery; *origin*, one of several small branches from the gastroduodenal artery posterior to the duodenum; *distribution*, first part of duodenum.

**a. sacra'lis latera'lis** [ NA ], lateral sacral artery; one of two arteries which arise from the internal iliac artery; they supply muscles and skin in the neighborhood and send branches into the sacral canal.

**a. sacra'lis media'na** [ NA ], median sacral artery; middle sacral artery; *origin*, back of abdominal aorta just above the bifurcation; *distribution*, lower lumbar vertebrae, sacrum, and coccyx; *anastomoses*, lateral sacral, superior and middle rectal.

**a. scapula'ris descen'dens** [ NA ], a. scapularis dorsalis [ NA ]; descending scapular artery; dorsal scapular artery; *origin*, subclavian or transverse cervical; *distribution*, muscles and skin along the medial border of the scapula; *anastomoses*, suprascapular and circumflex scapular.

**a. scapula'ris dorsa'lis** [ NA ], alternate term for a. scapularis descendens.

**a. segmen'ti anterio'ris inferio'ris re'nis** [ NA ], artery to the anterior inferior segment of the kidney; *origin*, anterior branch of renal; *distribution*, anterior inferior renal segment.

**a. segmen'ti anterio'ris superio'ris re'nis** [ NA ], artery to the anterior superior segment of the kidney; *origin*, anterior branch of renal; *distribution*, anterior superior renal segment.

**a. segmen'ti inferio'ris re'nis** [ NA ], artery to the inferior segment of the kidney; *origin*, anterior branch of renal; *distribution*, inferior renal segment.

**a. segmen'ti posterio'ris re'nis** [ NA ], artery to the posterior segment of the kidney; *origin*, continuation of the posterior branch of renal; *distribution*, posterior renal segment.

**a. segmen'ti superio'ris re'nis** [ NA ], artery to the superior segment of the kidney; *origin,* anterior branch of renal; *distribution,* superior renal segment.

**arteriae sigmoi'deae** [ NA ], sigmoid arteries; *origin,* inferior mesenteric; *distribution,* descending colon and sigmoid flexure; *anastomoses,* left colic, superior rectal.

**a. spermat'ica interna,** a. testicularis.

**a. sphe'nopalati'na** [ NA ], sphenopalatine artery; *origin,* maxillary; *distribution,* posterior portion of lateral nasal wall and septum; *anastomoses,* branches of descending palatine, superior labial, and infraorbital.

**a. spina'lis anterior** [ NA ], anterior spinal artery; *origin,* vertebral; *distribution,* spinal cord and pia mater; *anastomoses,* branches of intercostal and lumbar arteries.

**a. spina'lis posterior** [ NA ], posterior spinal artery; *origin,* vertebral; *distribution,* medulla, spinal cord, and pia mater; *anastomoses,* spinal branches of intercostal arteries.

**a. stylomastoi'dea** [ NA ], stylomastoid artery; *origin,* posterior auricular; *distribution,* external acoustic meatus, mastoid cells, semicircular canals, stapedius muscle, and vestibule; *anastomoses,* tympanic branches of internal carotid and ascending pharyngeal, and auditory branch of basilar.

**a. subcla'via** [ NA ], subclavian artery; *origin,* right from brachiocephalic, left from arch of aorta; *branches,* vertebral, thyrocervical trunk, internal thoracic; costocervical trunk, descending scapular; it is directly continuous with the axillary.

**a. subcosta'lis** [ NA ], subcostal artery; *origin,* thoracic aorta; *distribution,* inferior to twelfth rib in a manner similar to posterior intercostal arteries.

**a. sublingua'lis** [ NA ], sublingual artery; *origin,* lingual; *distribution,* extrinsic muscles of tongue, sublingual gland, mucosa of region; *anastomoses,* the artery of opposite side and submental.

**a. submenta'lis** [ NA ], submental artery; *origin,* facial; *distribution,* mylohyoid muscle, submandibular and sublingual glands, and structures of lower lip; *anastomoses,* inferior labial, mental branch of inferior dental and sublingual.

**a. subscapula'ris** [ NA ], subscapular artery; *origin,* axillary; *branches,* circumflex scapular, thoracodorsal; *distribution,* muscles of shoulder and scapular region; *anastomoses,* branches of transverse cervical, suprascapular, lateral thoracic, and intercostals.

**a. supraduodena'lis** [ NA ], supraduodenal artery; *origin,* gastroduodenal; *distribution,* first part of duodenum.

**a. supraorbita'lis** [ NA ], supraorbital artery; *origin,* ophthalmic; *distribution,* frontalis muscle and scalp; *anastomoses,* branches of the superficial temporal and supratrochlear.

**a. suprarena'lis inferior** [ NA ], inferior suprarenal artery; *origin,* renal; *distribution,* suprarenal gland.

**a. suprarena'lis media** [ NA ], middle suprarenal artery; *origin,* aorta; *distribution,* suprarenal gland; *anastomoses,* superior and inferior suprarenal.

**a. suprarena'lis superior** [ NA ], superior suprarenal artery; *origin,* inferior phrenic artery; *distribution,* suprarenal gland.

**a. suprascapula'ris** [ NA ], suprascapular artery; transverse scapular artery; *origin,* thyrocervical trunk; *distribution,* clavicle, scapula, muscles of shoulder, and shoulder joint; *anastomoses,* transverse cervical circumflex scapular.

**a. supratrochlea'ris** [ NA ], supratrochlear artery; a. frontalis; frontal artery; *origin,* ophthalmic; *distribution,* anterior portion of scalp; *anastomoses,* branches of supraorbital.

**a. sura'lis** [ NA ], sural artery; artery of the calf; one of four or five arteries arising (sometimes by a common trunk) from the popliteal; *distribution,* muscles and integument of the calf; *anastomoses,* posterior tibial, medial and lateral inferior genicular.

**a. tar'sea latera'lis** [ NA ], lateral tarsal artery; *origin,* dorsalis pedis; *distribution,* tarsal joints and extensor digitorum brevis muscle; *anastomoses,* arcuate, peroneal, lateral plantar, anterior lateral malleolar.

**a. tar'sea media'lis** [ NA ], medial tarsal artery; one of two small branches of the dorsalis pedis; *distribution,* medial malleolar rete.

**a. tempora'lis media** [ NA ], middle temporal artery; *origin,* superficial temporal; *distribution,* temporal fascia and muscle; *anastomoses,* branches of maxillary.

**a. tempora'lis profun'da** [ NA ], deep temporal artery, two in number, anterior and posterior; *origin,* maxillary; *distribution,* temporal muscle; *anastomoses,* branches of superficial temporal, lacrimal, and middle meningeal.

**a. tempora'lis superficia'lis** [ NA ], superficial temporal artery; *origin,* a terminal branch of the external carotid; *branches,* transverse facial, middle temporal, orbital, parotid, anterior auricular, frontal, and parietal.

**a. testicula'ris** [ NA ], testicular artery; a. spermatica interna; internal spermatic artery; *origin,* aorta; *branches,* ureteral, cremasteric, epididymal; *distribution,* testicle and parts designated by names of branches; *anastomoses,* branches of renal, inferior epigastric, deferential.

**a. thora'cica interna** [ NA ], internal thoracic artery; a. mammaria interna; internal mammary artery; *origin,* subclavian; *branches,* pericardiacophrenic, anterior mediastinal, thymic, bronchial, muscular, and perforating branches, and bifurcates into the musculophrenic and superior epigastric.

**a. thora'cica latera'lis** [ NA ], lateral thoracic artery; external mammary artery; long thoracic artery; *origin,* axillary; *distribution,* muscles of chest or breast (in females).

**a. thora'cica supre'ma** [ NA ], highest thoracic artery; superior thoracic artery; *origin,* axillary; *distribution,* muscles of chest; *anastomoses,* branches of suprascapular, internal thoracic, and thoracoacromial.

**a. thoracoacromia'lis** [ NA ], thoracoacromial artery; acromiothoracic artery; thoracic axis; *origin,* axillary; *distribution,* muscles and skin of shoulder and upper chest; *anastomoses,* branches of superior thoracic, internal thoracic, lateral thoracic, posterior and anterior circumflex humeral, and suprascapular.

**a. thoracodorsa'lis** [ NA ], thoracodorsal artery; dorsal thoracic artery; *origin,* subscapular; *distribution,* muscles of upper part of back; *anastomoses,* branches of lateral thoracic.

**a. thy'mica,** rami thymici arteriae thoracicae internae.

**a. thyroi'dea i'ma** [ NA ], lowest thyroid, an inconstant artery; Neubauer's artery; *origin,* arch of aorta or brachiocephalic artery; *distribution,* thyroid gland.

**a. thyroi'dea inferior** [ NA ], inferior thyroid artery; *origin,* thyrocervical trunk; *branches,* ascending cervical, inferior laryngeal, and muscular, esophageal, and tracheal.

**a. thyroi'dea superior** [ NA ], superior thyroid artery; *origin,* external carotid; *branches,* infrahyoid, superior laryngeal, sternocleidomastoid, cricothyroid and two terminal branches.

**a. tibia'lis anterior** [ NA ], anterior tibial artery; *origin,* popliteal; *branches,* posterior and anterior tibial recurrent, lateral and medial anterior malleolar, dorsalis pedis, lateral tarsal, medial tarsal, arcuate, dorsal metatarsal, and dorsal digital.

**a. tibia'lis posterior** [ NA ], posterior tibial artery; the larger and more directly continuous of the two terminal branches of the popliteal; *branches,* peroneal, nutrient of fibula, lateral and medial posterior malleolar, nutrient of tibia, medial and lateral plantar.

**a. transver'sa col'li** [ NA ], transverse cervical artery; transverse artery of the neck; *origin,* thyrocervical trunk; *branches,* superficial and deep (descending scapular).

**a. transver'sa facie'i** [ NA ], transverse facial artery; *origin,* superficial temporal; *distribution,* parotid gland, parotid duct, masseter muscle, and overlying skin; *anastomoses,* infraorbital and buccal branches of maxillary, and buccal and masseteric branches of facial.

**a. tympan'ica anterior** [ NA ], anterior tympanic artery; Glaserian artery; *origin,* maxillary; *distribution,* middle ear; *anastomoses,* tympanic branches of internal carotid and ascending pharyngeal and stylomastoid.

**a. tympan'ica inferior** [ NA ], inferior tympanic artery; *origin,* ascending pharyngeal; *distribution,* middle ear; *anastomoses,* tympanic branches of other arteries.

**a. tympan'ica posterior** [ NA ], posterior tympanic artery; *origin,* stylomastoid; *distribution,* tympanic cavity; *anastomoses,* other tympanic arteries.

**a. tympan'ica superior** [ NA ], superior tympanic artery; *origin*, middle meningeal; *distribution*, middle ear; *anastomoses*, other tympanic arteries.

**a. ulna'ris** [ NA ], ulnar artery; *origin*, brachial; *branches*, ulnar recurrent, interosseous, dorsal and palmar carpal, deep palmar, and superficial palmar arch with its digital branches.

**a. umbilica'lis** [ NA ], umbilical artery; before birth is continuation of common iliac; after birth it is obliterated between bladder and umbilicus, forming the medial umbilical ligament, the remaining portion, between internal iliac artery and bladder, being reduced in size and giving off the superior vesical arteries.

**a. urethra'lis** [ NA ], urethral artery; *origin*, perineal artery; *distribution*, membranous urethra.

**a. uteri'na** [ NA ], uterine artery; *origin*, internal iliac; *distribution*, uterus, upper part of vagina, round ligament, and inner part of uterine (Fallopian) tube; *anastomoses*, ovarian, vaginal, inferior epigastric.

**a. vagina'lis** [ NA ], vaginal artery; *origin*, internal iliac; *distribution*, vagina, base of bladder, rectum; *anastomoses*, uterine, internal pudendal.

**a. vertebra'lis** [ NA ], vertebral artery; *origin*, subclavian; *branches*, posterior spinal, anterior spinal, posterior inferior cerebellar, and various muscular, meningeal, and spinal branches; the two vertebrals unite to form the basilar; *anastomoses*, descending branch of occipital and deep cervical.

**a. vesica'lis inferior** [ NA ], inferior vesical artery; *origin*, internal iliac; *distribution*, base of bladder, ureter, and (in the male) seminal vesicles, ductus deferens, and prostate; *anastomoses*, middle rectal, and other vesical branches.

**a. vesica'lis superior** [ NA ], *origin*, umbilical; *distribution*, bladder, urachus, ureter; *anastomoses*, other vesical branches.

**a. zygomat'icoorbita'lis** [ NA ], zygomaticoorbital artery; *origin*, superficial temporal, sometimes middle temporal; *distribution*, orbicularis oculi muscle and portions of the orbit; *anastomoses*, lacrimal and palpebral branches of ophthalmic.

---

**arte'rial.** Relating to one or more arteries or to the entire system of arteries.

**arte'rializa'tion.** 1. Making or becoming arterial. 2. Aeration of the blood whereby it is changed in character from venous to arterial. 3. Vascularization. 4. Conversion of venous structure to resemble the artery.

**arteriarctia** (ar-te-rī-ark'shǐ-ah) [ L. *arteria*, artery, + *arcto*, to constrict ]. Narrowing of the arteries; vasconstriction.

**arteri'asis.** Generalized arteriosclerosis.

**arteriectasis, arteriectasia** (ar-te-rī-ek'tă-sis, -ek-ta'zĭ-ah) [ L. *arteria*, artery, + G. *ektasis*, distention ]. Dilation of the arteries; vasodilation.

**arteriectomy** (ar-te-rī-ek'to-mĭ) [ L. *arteria*, artery, + G. *ektomē*, excision ]. Excision of part of an artery.

**arterio-, arteri-** [ L. *arteria*, fr. G. *artēria*, artery ]. Combining forms meaning artery.

**arterioatony** (ar-te-rī-o-at'o-nĭ) [ arterio- + G. *atonia*, atony ]. A relaxed state of the arterial walls.

**arteriocap'illary.** Relating to both arteries and capillaries.

**arte'riogram** [ arterio- + G. *gramma*, something written ]. X-ray picture of artery after injection of contrast medium into it.

**arteriog'raphy** [ arterio- + G. *graphō*, to write ]. 1. Sphygmography. 2. Description of the arteries. 3. Visualization of an artery or arteries by x-rays after injection of a radiopaque contrast medium.

**cerebral a.,** cerebral *angiography*.

**selective a.,** see selective *angiocardiography*.

**spinal a.,** spinal *angiography*.

**arteriola,** pl. **arteriolae** (ar-te-rī-o'lah, ar-te-rī-o'le) [ Mod. L. dim. of *arteria*, artery ] [ NA ]. Arteriole; a minute artery with a muscular wall; a terminal artery continuous with the capillary network.

**a. macula'ris inferior** [ NA ], inferior macular arteriole; *origin*, central artery of retina; *distribution*, inferior part of macula.

**a. macula'ris superior** [ NA ], superior macular arteriole; *origin*, central artery of retina; *distribution*, upper part of macula.

**a. media'lis ret'inae** [ NA ], medial arteriole of the retina; an arteriole supplying the medial part of the retina between the areas supplied by the inferior nasal and superior nasal arterioles.

**a. nasa'lis ret'inae inferior** [ NA ], inferior nasal arteriole of the retina; the branch of the central artery of the retina that supplies the lower medial, or nasal, part of the retina.

**a. nasa'lis ret'inae superior** [ NA ], superior nasal arteriole of the retina; the branch of the central artery of the retina that passes to the upper medial, or nasal, part of the retina.

**arteriolae rec'tae** [ NA ], straight vessels into which the efferent arteriole of the juxtamedullary glomeruli breaks up; they form a leash of vessels which, arising at the bases of the pyramids, run through the renal medulla toward the apex of each pyramid, then reverse direction in a hairpin turn, and run straight back again toward the base of the pyramid.

**a. tempora'lis ret'inae inferior** [ NA ], inferior temporal arteriole of the retina; the branch of the central artery of the retina that passes laterally below the macula to supply the lower lateral or temporal part of the retina.

**a. tempora'lis ret'inae superior** [ NA ], superior temporal arteriole of the retina; the branch of the central artery of the retina that passes laterally above the macula to supply the upper lateral or temporal part of the retina.

**arterio'lar.** Of or pertaining to an arteriole or the arterioles collectively.

**arteriole** (ar-te'rī-ōl). Arteriola.

**afferent glomerular a.,** a branch of an interlobular artery of the kidney that conveys blood to the glomerulus.

**capillary a.,** a minute artery that terminates in a capillary.

**efferent glomerular a.,** the vessel that carries blood from the glomerular capillary network to the capillary bed of the proximal convoluted tubule.

**inferior macular a.,** *arteriola* macularis inferior.

**inferior nasal a. of retina,** *arteriola* nasalis retinae inferior.

**inferior temporal a. of retina,** *arteriola* temporalis retinae inferior.

**medial a. of retina,** *arteriola* medialis retinae.

**superior macular a.,** *arteriola* macularis superior.

**superior nasal a. of retina,** *arteriola* nasalis retinae superior.

**superior temporal a. of retina,** *arteriola* temporalis retinae superior.

**arte'riolith** [ L. *arteria*, artery, + G. *lithos*, a stone ]. A calcareous deposit in the wall of an artery or in a thrombus.

**arte'rioli'tis.** [ L. *arteriola*, arteriole, + G. suffix -*itis*, inflammation ]. A degenerative or inflammatory condition of the arterioles.

**necrotizing a.,** arteriolonecrosis; necrosis in the media of arterioles, characteristic of malignant hypertension.

**arteriolo-** [ L. *arteriola*, arteriole ]. Combining from relating to arterioles.

**arteriol'ogy** [ L. *arteria*, artery, + G. *logos*, study ]. The anatomy of the arteries: usually associated with the study of the other vessels under the name angiology.

**arterio'lonecro'sis** [ L. *arteriola*, arteriole, + G. *nekrōsis*, a killing ]. Necrotizing *arteriolitis*.

**arteriolosclerosis** (ar-te-rī-o'lo-skle-ro'sis). Arteriolar sclerosis; arteriosclerosis affecting mainly the arterioles.

**arteriolovenous** (ar-te-rī-o'lo-ve'nus). Involving both the arterioles and veins.

**arterio'love'nular.** Arteriolovenous.

**arteriomalacia** (ar-te'rī-o-mă-la'shǐ-ah) [ arterio- + G. *malakia*, softness ]. Softening of the arteries.

**arteriom'eter** [ arterio- + G. *metron*, measure ]. An instrument for measuring the diameter of an artery, or its change in size during pulsation.

**arteriomo'tor.** Causing changes in the caliber of an artery; vasomotor with special reference to the arteries.

**arteriomy'omato'sis** [ arterio- + G. *mys*, muscle, + suffix -*oma*, tumor, + suffix -*osis*, condition ]. Thickening of the walls of an artery by an overgrowth of muscular fibers arranged irregularly, intersecting each other without any definite relation to the axis of the vessel.

**arte'rionecro'sis.** Necrosis of an artery or arteries.

**arterionephrosclerosis** (ar-te'rĭ-o-nef'ro-skle-ro'sis). Arterial *nephrosclerosis.*

**arte'riopal'mus** [ arterio- + G. *palmos,* throbbing ]. Subjective sensation of throbbing of an artery.

**arteriop'athy** [ arterio- + G. *pathos,* suffering ]. Any disease of the arteries.

**hypertensive a.,** arterial degeneration resulting from arterial hypertension.

**arteriophlebotomy** (ar-te'rĭ-o-flĕ-bot'o-mĭ) [ arterio- + G. *phleps* (*phleb-*), vein, + *tomē,* a cutting ]. Bloodletting from the minute arterioles and venules by scarification.

**arte'riopla'nia** [ arterio- + G. *planē,* a straying ]. The presence of an anomaly in the course of an artery.

**arte'rioplas'ty** [ arterio- + G. *plassō,* to form ]. Matas' operation for aneurysm; any operation for the reconstruction of the wall of an artery.

**arte'riopres'sor.** Causing increased arterial blood pressure.

**arteriorrhaphy** (ar-te'rĭ-or'ă-fĭ) [ arterio- + G. *rhaphē,* seam ]. Suture of an artery.

**arteriorrhexis** (ar-te'rĭ-o-rek'sis) [ arterio- + G. *rhēxis,* rupture ]. Rupture of an artery.

**arte'risclero'sis** [ arterio- + G. *sklērōsis,* hardness ]. Arterial sclerosis; sclerosis or hardening of the arteries; the types generally recognized are: atherosclerosis (intimal sclerosis), medial calcification (Mönckeberg's a.), hypertensive a., and arteriolar sclerosis.

**hyperplastic a.,** hyperplasia of the intima and internal elastic layer and hypertrophy of the media independent of atheromatous lesions.

**hypertensive a.,** progressive increase in muscle and elastic tissue of arterial walls, resulting from hypertension. In longstanding hypertension elastic tissue forms numerous concentric layes in the intima and there is replacement of muscle by collagen fibers and hyaline thickening of the intima of arterioles. Such changes can develop with increasing age in the absence of hypertension and may then be referred to as senile a.

**medial a.,** Mönckeberg's a.

**Mönckeberg's a.,** medial a.; Mönckeberg's degeneration, sclerosis, or calcification; arterial sclerosis involving the peripheral arteries, especially of the legs of older people, with deposition of calcium in the medial coat (pipe-stem arteries) but with little or no encroachment on the lumen.

**nodular a.,** atheromas occurring in the arterial intima as more or less discrete tumors.

**a. oblit'erans,** a. producing narrowing and occlusion of the arterial lumen.

**senile a.,** see hypertensive a.

**arte'riosclerot'ic.** Relating to or affected by arteriosclerosis.

**arterios'ity.** A state of being arterial; denoting the aeration of the blood.

**arteriospasm** (ar-te'-rĭ-o-spazm). Spasm of an artery or arteries.

**arte'riosteno'sis** [ arterio- + G. *stenōsis,* a narrowing ]. Narrowing of the caliber of an artery, either temporary, through vasoconstriction, or permanent, through arteriosclerosis.

**arte'riostrep'sis** [ arterio- + G. *strepsis,* a twisting ]. Twisting of the divided end of an artery for the arrest of bleeding.

**arte'riotome.** A lancet for performing arteriotomy.

**arteriot'omy** [ arterio- + G. *tomē,* incision ]. Bloodletting from an artery, or any surgical incision into the lumen of an artery, as to remove a lodged embolus.

**arteriot'ony** [ arterio- + G. *tonos,* tension ]. Blood *pressure.*

**arteriovenous** (ar-te'rĭ-o-ve'nus). Relating to both an artery and a vein or to both arteries and veins in general; both arterial and venous.

**arte'riover'sion** [ arterio- + L. *versio,* a turning ]. The arrest of hemorrhage from the open end of an artery by everting the wall of the vessel.

**arte'riover'ter.** An instrument for facilitating arterioversion.

**arteri'tis** [ L. *arteria,* artery, + G. suffix *-itis,* inflammation ]. Inflammation involving an artery or arteries.

**cranial a.,** temporal a.

**equine viral a.,** "pinkeye"; epizootic cellulitis; an acute epizootic disease of horses, formerly misdiagnosed as equine influenza; a highly contagious viral disease characterized by a high fever and respiratory and digestive tract signs; abortion is a common result.

**giant cell a.,** temporal a.

**granulomatous a.,** temporal a.

**a. nodo'sa,** *polyarteritis* nodosa.

**a. oblit'erans,** obliterating a.; *endarteritis* obliterans.

**rheumatic a.,** a. due to rheumatic fever; Aschoff bodies are frequently found in the adventitia of small arteries, especially in the myocardium, and may lead to fibrosis and constriction of the lumens.

**rheumatoid a.,** a. associated with rheumatoid arthritis, especially aortitis with aortic valve incompetence reported with ankylosing spondylitis.

**temporal a.,** cranial a.; giant cell a.; granulomatous a.; panarteritis with medial necrosis and multinucleated giant cells in temporal, retinal, or intracerebral arteries. The patients are elderly and may present with constitutional symptoms, severe bitemporal headache, and ocular symptoms including sudden loss of vision in one eye.

---

# ARTERY

---

**ar'tery** [ L. *arteria,* fr. G. *artēria.* ARTER- ]. Arteria.

**ab'errant a.,** one having an unusual origin or course.

**accessory obturator a.,** *arteria* obturatoria accessoria.

**acetab'ular a.,** *ramus* acetabularis arteriae obturatoris.

**acro'mial a.,** *ramus* acromialis arteriae thoracoacromialis.

**acromiothora'cic a.,** *arteria* thoracoacromialis.

**a.'s of Adamkiewicz,** *rami* spinales (1c).

**a'lar a. of nose,** a branch of the angular a. that supplies the ala of the nose.

**angular a.,** *arteria* angularis.

**anonymous a.,** *truncus* brachiocephalicus.

**anterior cecal a.,** *arteria* cecalis anterior.

**anterior cerebral a.,** *arteria* cerebri anterior.

**anterior choroidal a.,** *arteria* choroidea anterior.

**anterior ciliary a.,** *arteria* ciliaris anterior.

**anterior circumflex humeral a.,** *arteria* circumflexa humeri anterior.

**anterior communicating a.,** *arteria* communicans anterior.

**anterior conjunctival a.,** *arteria* conjunctivalis anterior.

**anterior descending a.,** *ramus* interventricularis anterior.

**anterior ethmoidal a.,** *arteria* ethmoidalis anterior.

**anterior inferior cerebellar a.;** *arteria* cerebelli inferior anterior.

**a. of anterior inferior segment of kidney,** *arteria* segmenti anterioris inferioris renis.

**anterior intercostal a.'s,** *rami* intercostales anteriores.

**anterior interosseous a.,** *arteria* interossea anterior.

**anterior interventricular a.,** *ramus* interventricularis anterior.

**anterior labial a.'s,** *rami* labiales anteriores.

**anterior lateral malleolar a.,** *arteria* malleolaris anterior lateralis.

**anterior medial malleolar a.,** *arteria* malleolaris anterior medialis.

**anterior meningeal a.,** *arteria* meningea anterior.

**anterior peroneal a.,** *ramus* perforans arteriae peroneae.

**anterior spinal a.,** *arteria* spinalis anterior.

**anterior superior alveolar a.,** *arteria* alveolaris superior anterior.

**anterior superior dental a.,** *arteria* alveolaris superior anterior.

**a. of anterior superior segment of kidney,** *arteria* segmenti anterioris superioris renis.

**anterior tibial a.,** *arteria* tibialis anterior.

**anterior tibial recurrent a.,** *arteria* recurrens tibialis anterior.

**anterior tympanic a.,** *arteria* tympanica anterior.

**appendicular a.,** *arteria* appendicularis.

**arciform a.'s,** *arteriae* arcuatae renis.

**arcuate a.,** *arteria* arcuata.

**arcuate a.'s of kidney,** *arteriae* arcuatae renis.

**ascending a.,** *arteria* ascendens.

**ascending cervical a.,** *arteria* cervicalis ascendens.

**ascending palatine a.,** *arteria* palatina ascendens.

**ascending pharyngeal a.,** *arteria* pharyngea ascendens.

**axillary a.,** *arteria* axillaris.

**azygos a. of vagina,** one of two a.'s that run longitudinally in the midline on the anterior and posterior aspects of the vagina. They take *origin* from the uterine a.

**basilar a.,** *arteria* basilaris.

**brachial a.,** *arteria* brachialis.

**bronchial a.'s,** *rami* bronchiales aortae thoracicae.

**buccal a., buccinator a.,** *arteria* buccalis.

**a. of bulb of penis,** *arteria* bulbi penis.

**a. of bulb of vestibule,** *arteria* bulbi vestibuli.

**calca'neal a.'s,** *rami* calcanei.

**cal'carine a.,** *arteria* calcarina.

**a. of calf,** *arteria* suralis.

**carot'icotympan'ic a.,** *rami* caroticotympanici arteriae carotis internae.

**carotid a.,** *arteria* carotis.

**carpal a.,** see under *ramus* carpeus.

**caudal pancreatic a.,** 12 *arteria* caudae pancreatis.

**a. of caudate lobe,** *arteria* lobi caudati.

**cavernous a.'s,** a number of small branches of the internal carotid a. which supply the trigeminal ganglion and the walls of the cavernous and petrosal sinuses.

**cecal a.'s,** *arteria* cecalis anterior; *arteria* cecalis posterior.

**ce'liac a.,** *truncus* celiacus.

**central a. of retina,** *arteria* centralis retinae.

**cerebellar a.'s,** see subentries under *arteria* cerebelli.

**cerebral a.'s,** see subentries under *arteria* cerebri.

**a. of cerebral hemorrhage,** lenticulostriate a.

**cervicovaginal a.,** arteria cervicovaginalis; an anastomotic communication between the uterine a. and the vaginal a.; it courses along the lateral aspect of the cervix and vagina.

**Charcot's a.,** lenticulostriate a.

**chief a. of thumb,** *arteria* princeps pollicis.

**circumflex fibular a.,** *ramus* circumflexus fibulae arteriae tibialis posterioris.

**circumflex scapular a.,** *arteria* circumflexa scapulae.

**coiled a. of uterus,** see spiral a.

**collateral a.,** one through which a collateral circulation is established.

**collateral digital a.,** *arteria* digitalis palmaris propria.

**common carotid a.,** *arteria* carotis communis.

**common hepatic a.,** *arteria* hepatica communis.

**common iliac a.,** *arteria* iliaca communis.

**common interosseous a.,** *arteria* interossea communis.

**common palmar digital a.,** *arteria* digitalis palmaris communis.

**common plantar digital a.,** *arteria* digitalis plantaris communis.

**communicating a.,** one that connects two larger a.'s.

**conjunctival a.,** *arteria* conjunctivalis.

**coronary a.,** (1) *arteria* gastrica sinistra; (2) *arteria* coronaria.

**cortical a.'s,** branches of the anterior, middle and posterior cerebral a.'s that supply the cerebral cortex.

**costocer'vical a.,** *truncus* costocervicalis.

**cremasteric a.,** *arteria* cremasterica.

**cricothyroid a.,** *ramus* cricothyroideus arteriae thyroideae superioris.

**crural a.,** *arteria* femoralis.

**cystic a.,** *arteria* cystica.

**deep auricular a.,** *arteria* auricularis profunda.

**deep brachial a.,** *arteria* profunda brachii.

**deep cervical a.,** *arteria* cervicalis profunda.

**deep circumflex iliac a.,** *arteria* circumflexa ilium profunda.

**deep a. of clitoris,** *arteria* profunda clitoridis.

**deep epigastric a.,** *arteria* epigastrica inferior.

**deep a. of penis,** *arteria* profunda penis.

**deep temporal a.,** *arteria* temporalis profunda.

**deep a. of thigh,** *arteria* profunda femoris.

**deep a. of tongue,** *arteria* profunda linguae.

**descending a. of knee,** *arteria* genus descendens.

**descending palatine a.,** *arteria* palatina descendens.

**descending scapular a.,** *arteria* scapularis descendens.

**digital collateral a.,** *arteria* digitalis palmaris propria.

**distributing a.,** see muscular a.

**dorsal a. of the clitoris,** *arteria* dorsalis clitoridis.

**dorsal digital a.,** *arteria* digitalis dorsalis.

**dorsal a. of foot,** *arteria* dorsalis pedis.

**dorsal interos'seous a.,** (1) *arteria* interossea posterior; (2) *arteria* metacarpea dorsalis.

**dorsal metacarpal a.,** *arteria* metacarpea dorsalis.

**dorsal metatarsal a.,** *arteria* metatarsea dorsalis.

**dorsal a. of nose,** *arteria* dorsalis nasi.

**dorsal pancreatic a.,** *arteria* pancreatica dorsalis.

**dorsal a. of the penis,** *arteria* dorsalis penis.

**dorsal scapular a.,** *arteria* scapularis descendens.

**dorsal thoracic a.,** *arteria* thoracodorsalis.

**a. of ductus deferens,** *arteria* ductus deferentis.

**elastic a.,** a large a., such as the aorta or pulmonary a., which has many elastic membranes in its tunica media.

**end a.,** an a. with insufficient anastomoses to maintain viability of the tissue supplied if occlusion of the a. occurs. circulation.

**episcleral a.,** *arteria* episcleralis.

**esophageal a.,** *ramus* esophageus aortae thoracicae.

**external carotid a.,** *arteria* carotis externa.

**external iliac a.,** *arteria* iliaca externa.

**external mammary a.,** *arteria* thoracica lateralis.

**external maxillary a.,** *arteria* facialis.

**external pudendal a.'s,** *arteriae* pudendae externae.

**external spermatic a.,** *arteria* cremasterica.

**facial a.,** *arteria* facialis.

**femoral a.,** *arteria* femoralis.

**fibular a.,** *arteria* peronea.

**frontal a.,** *arteria* supratrochlearis.

**gastroduodenal a.,** *arteria* gastroduodenalis.

**Glaserian a.,** *arteria* tympanica anterior.

**great anastomotic a.,** (1) *arteria* collateralis ulnaris inferior; (2) *arteria* genus descendens.

**great pancreatic a.,** *arteria* pancreatica magna.

**great superior pancreatic a.,** *arteria* pancreatica dorsalis.

**greater palatine a.,** *arteria* palatina major.

**helicine a.,** *arteria* helicina.

**highest intercostal a.,** *arteria* intercostalis suprema.

**highest thoracic a.,** *arteria* thoracica suprema.

**humeral a.,** *arteria* brachialis.

**hyaloid a.,** *arteria* hyaloidea.

**hypogas'tric a.,** *arteria* iliaca interna.

**ileal a.'s,** *arteriae* ilei.

**ileocolic a.,** *arteria* ileocolica.

**iliolumbar a.,** *arteria* iliolumbalis.

**inferior alveolar a.,** *arteria* alveolaris inferior.

**inferior dental a.,** *arteria* alveolaris inferior.

**inferior epigastric a.,** *arteria* epigastrica inferior.

**inferior gluteal a.,** *arteria* glutea inferior.

**inferior hemorrhoidal a.,** *arteria* rectalis inferior.

**inferior labial a.,** *arteria* labialis inferior.

**inferior laryngeal a.,** *arteria* laryngea inferior.

**inferior mesenteric a.,** *arteria* mesenterica inferior.

**inferior pancreatic a.,** *arteria* pancreatica inferior.

**inferior pancreaticoduodenal a.,** *arteria* pancreaticoduodenalis inferior.

**inferior phrenic a.,** *arteria* phrenica inferior.

**inferior rectal a.,** *arteria* rectalis inferior.

**a. of inferior segment of kidney,** *arteria* segmenti inferioris renis.

**inferior suprarenal a.,** *arteria* suprarenalis inferior.

**inferior thyroid a.,** *arteria* thyroidea inferior.

**inferior tympanic a.,** *arteria* tympanica inferior.

**inferior ulnar collateral a.,** *arteria* collateralis ulnaris inferior.

**inferior vesical a.,** *arteria* vesicalis inferior.

**infraorbital a.,** *arteria* infraorbitalis.

**infrascapular a.,** a small branch of the arteria circumflexa scapulae.

**innominate a.,** *truncus* brachiocephalicus.

**interlobular a.'s,** *arteriae* interlobulares.

**internal auditory a.,** *arteria* labyrinthi.

internal carotid a., *arteria* carotis interna.
internal iliac a., *arteria* iliaca interna.
internal mammary a., *arteria* thoracica interna.
internal maxillary a., *arteria* maxillaris.
internal pudendal a., *arteria* pudenda interna.
internal spermatic a., *arteria* testicularis.
internal thoracic a., *arteria* thoracica interna.
intestinal a.'s, *arteriae* ilei; *arteriae* jejunales.
jejunal a.'s, *arteriae* jejunales.
a.'s of the kidney, *arteriae* renis.
a. of labyrinth, *arteria* labyrinthi.
lacrimal a., *arteria* lacrimalis.
large a., see elastic a.
lateral circumflex a. of thigh, *arteria* circumflexa femoris lateralis.
lateral inferior a. of knee, *arteria* genus inferior lateralis.
lateral nasal a., a branch of the facial a. which supplies the dorsum and ala of the nose.
lateral plantar a., *arteria* plantaris lateralis.
lateral sacral a., *arteria* sacralis lateralis.
lateral splanchnic a.'s, a rise in the embryo from the dorsal aorta to supply the mesonephros, testis (or ovary), and the adrenal gland.
lateral stri'ate a.'s, *rami* striati arteriae cerebri mediae.
lateral superior a. of knee, *arteria* genus superior lateralis.
lateral tarsal a., *arteria* tarsea lateralis.
lateral thoracic a., *arteria* thoracica lateralis.
left colic a., *arteria* colica sinistra.
left coronary a., *arteria* coronaria sinistra.
left gastric a., *arteria* gastrica sinistra.
left gastroepiploic a., *arteria* gastroepiploica sinistra.
left pulmonary a., *arteria* pulmonalis sinistra.
lentic'ulostri'ate a., Charcot's a.; a. of cerebral hemorrhage; any one of a variety of small a.'s entering the base of the brain through the substantia perforata anterior and supplying the striatum, globus pallidus, and internal capsule; most of these perforating a.'s are branches of the middle cerebral and anterior choroidal a.'s.
lesser palatine a., *arteria* palatina minor.
lingual a., *arteria* lingualis.
long posterior ciliary a., *arteria* ciliaris posterior longa.
long thoracic a., *arteria* thoracica lateralis.
lowest lumbar a., *arteria* lumbalis ima.
lowest thyroid a., *arteria* thyroidea ima.
lumbar a., *arteria* lumbalis.
mac'ular a.'s, *arteriolae* maculares.
marginal a. of colon, formed by anastomoses between the right and left colic a.'s. It passes downward from the left colic flexure to the aboral end of the pelvic colon.
masseteric a., *arteria* masseterica.
mastoid a., *ramus* mastoideus arteriae occipitalis.
maxillary a., *arteria* maxillaris.
medial circumflex a. of thigh, *arteria* circumflexa femoris medialis.
medial inferior a. of knee, *arteria* genus inferior medialis.
medial plantar a., *arteria* plantaris medialis.
medial striate a.'s, *rami* striati arteriae cerebri mediae.
medial superior a. of knee, *arteria* genus superior medialis.
medial tarsal a., *arteria* tarsea medialis.
median a., *arteria* mediana.
median sacral a., *arteria* sacralis mediana.
medium a., see muscular a.
medullary a.'s of brain, branches of the cortical a.'s which penetrate to and supply the white matter of the cerebrum.
mental a., *arteria* mentalis.
metatarsal a., *arteria* arcuata.
middle cerebral a., *arteria* cerebri media.
middle collateral a., *arteria* collateralis media.
middle hemorrhoidal a., *arteria* rectalis media.
middle a. of knee, *arteria* genus media.
middle meningeal a., *arteria* meningea media.
middle rectal a., *arteria* rectalis media.
middle sacral a., *arteria* sacralis mediana.
middle suprarenal a., *arteria* suprarenalis media.
middle temporal a., *arteria* temporalis media.
muscular a., medium a.; distributing a.; an a. with a tunica media composed principally of circularly arranged smooth muscle.

musculophrenic a., *arteria* musculophrenica.
myometrial arcuate a.'s, branches of the uterine and ovarian a.'s.
myometrial radial a.'s, continuations of the myometrial arcuate a.'s.
Neubauer's a., *arteria* thyroidea ima.
nutrient a., *arteria* nutricia.
nutrient a. of the femur, one of two a.'s, superior and inferior, arising from the first and third perforating respectively (sometimes second and fourth).
nutrient a. of the fibula, *origin,* peroneal (fibular); *distribution,* fibula.
nutrient a.'s of the humerus, *arteriae* nutriciae humeri.
nutrient a. of the tibia, derived from the upper part of the posterior tibial and enters through the nutrient foramen on the posterior surface of the tibia.
obturator a., *arteria* obturatoria.
occipital a., *arteria* occipitalis.
om'phalomes'enter'ic a., an occasional branch of the superior mesenteric a. which passes to the region of the umbilicus, its terminals connecting with capillaries in the falciform ligament of the liver.
ophthalmic a., *arteria* ophthalmica.
ovarian a., *arteria* ovarica.
palmar digital a. proper, *arteria* digitalis palmaris propria.
palmar interosseous a., *arteria* metacarpea palmaris.
palmar metacarpal a., *arteria* metacarpea palmaris.
palpebral a.'s, *arteriae* palpebrales.
a.'s of the penis, *arteria* dorsalis penis; *arteria* profunda penis.
perforating a.'s, *arteriae* perforantes.
perforating a.'s of foot, *rami* perforantes arteriae metatarsearum plantares.
perforating a.'s of hand, *rami* perforantes arteriae metacarpalium palmares.
perforating a.'s of internal mammary, *rami* perforantes arteriae thoracicae internae.
perforating a. of peroneal, *ramus* perforans arteriae peroneae.
pericardiacophrenic a., *arteria* pericardiacophrenica.
perineal a., *arteria* perinealis.
peroneal a., *arteria* peronea.
pipe-stem a.'s, a.'s hardened by calcification as seen in Mönckeberg's arteriosclerosis. The term describes the characteristic feeling which they give to the finger of an examiner.
plantar metatarsal a., *arteria* metatarsea plantaris.
popliteal a., *arteria* poplitea.
posterior alveolar a., *arteria* alveolaris superior posterior.
posterior auricular a., *arteria* auricularis posterior.
posterior cecal a., *arteria* cecalis posterior.
posterior cerebral a., *arteria* cerebri posterior.
posterior choroidal a., *arteria* choroidea posterior.
posterior circumflex humeral a., *arteria* circumflexa humeri posterior.
posterior communicating a., *arteria* communicans posterior.
posterior conjunctival a., *arteria* conjunctivalis posterior.
posterior dental a., *arteria* alveolaris superior posterior.
posterior descending a., *ramus* interventricularis posterior.
posterior ethmoidal a., *arteria* ethmoidalis posterior.
posterior inferior cerebellar a., *arteria* cerebelli inferior posterior.
posterior intercostal a., *arteria* intercostalis posterior.
posterior interosseous a., *arteria* interossea posterior.
posterior interventricular a., *ramus* interventricularis posterior.
posterior labial a.'s, *rami* labiales posteriores arteriae pudendae internae.
posterior lateral nasal a.'s, *arteriae* nasales posteriores laterales.
posterior meningeal a., *arteria* meningea posterior.
posterior pancreat'icoduode'nal a., a branch of the gastroduodenal a. that descends behind the head of the pancreas.
posterior peroneal a., *ramus* malleolaris lateralis arteriae peroneae.
a. of posterior segment of kidney, *arteria* segmenti posterioris renis.

**posterior septal a. of nose,** *arteria* nasalis posterior septi.

**posterior spinal a.,** *arteria* spinalis posterior.

**posterior superior alveolar a.,** *arteria* alveolaris superior posterior.

**posterior tibial a.,** *arteria* tibialis posterior.

**posterior tibial recurrent a.,** *arteria* recurrens tibialis posterior.

**posterior tympanic a.,** *arteria* tympanica posterior.

**princeps cervi'cis a.,** *ramus* descendens (2).

**principal a. of thumb,** *arteria* princeps pollicis.

**proper hepatic a.,** *arteria* hepatica propria.

**proper plantar digital a.,** *arteria* digitalis plantaris propria.

**a. of pterygoid canal,** *arteria* canalis pterygoidei.

**pubic a.,** (1) *ramus* pubicus arteriae epigastricae inferioris; (2) *ramus* pubicus arteriae obturatoriae.

**pulmonary a.,** *truncus* pulmonalis; see also *arteria* pulmonalis dextra and *arteria* pulmonalis sinistra.

**a. of the pulp,** the first section of a penicillus of the spleen.

**pylor'ic a.,** *arteria* gastrica dextra.

**quadriceps a. of the femur,** *ramus* descendens arteriae circumflexae femoris lateralis.

**radial a.,** *arteria* radialis.

**radial collateral a.,** *arteria* collateralis radialis.

**radial index a.,** *arteria* radialis indicis.

**radial recurrent a.,** *arteria* recurrens radialis.

**radic'ular a.,** one of those that accompany the anterior or posterior spinal nerve roots into the vertebral canal.

**ra'nine a.,** *arteria* profunda linguae.

**recurrent interosseous a.,** *arteria* interossea recurrens.

**recurrent ulnar a.,** *arteria* recurrens ulnaris.

**renal a.,** *arteria* renalis.

**retroduodenal a.,** *arteria* retroduodenalis.

**right colic a.,** *arteria* colica dextra.

**right coronary a.,** *arteria* coronaria dextra.

**right gastric a.,** *arteria* gastrica dextra.

**right gastroepiploic a.,** *arteria* gastroepiploica dextra.

**right pulmonary a.,** *arteria* pulmonalis dextra.

**a. of round ligament of uterus,** *arteria* ligamenti teretis uteri.

**a. to sciatic nerve,** *arteria* comitans nervi ischiadici.

**screw a.'s,** coiled a.'s into the uterine mucosa or in the macular region of the retina.

**scrotal a.'s,** *rami* scrotales.

**septal a.,** a branch of the superior labial a. that supplies the lower part of the nasal septum.

**sheathed a.,** a subdivision of the penicillus of the spleen surrounded by reticular cells.

**short gastric a.'s,** *arteriae* gastricae breves.

**short posterior ciliary a.,** *arteria* ciliaris posterior brevis.

**sigmoid a.'s,** *arteriae* sigmoideae.

**small a.'s,** unnamed muscular a.'s, usually with fewer than six or seven layers of muscle.

**somatic a.'s,** arise in the embryo from the dorsal aorta and supply the body wall. They persist almost unchanged as the posterior intercostal, subcostal and lumbar a.'s.

**sphenopalatine a.,** *arteria* sphenopalatina.

**spiral a.,** a coiled a. of the uterus; one of the corkscrew-like a.'s in premenstrual or progestational endometrium.

**splenic a.,** *arteria* lienalis.

**stape'dial a.,** a small a. in the embryo that passes through the ring of the stapes; it is later obliterated. It is a second aortic arch derivative.

**sternal a.'s,** small branches of the internal thoracic that are distributed to the transverse thoracic muscle and posterior surface of the sternum.

**sternomas'toid a.,** *ramus* sternocleidomastoideus arteriae occipitalis.

**stylomastoid a.,** *arteria* stylomastoidea.

**subclavian a.,** *arteria* subclavia.

**subcostal a.,** *arteria* subcostalis.

**sublingual a.,** *arteria* sublingualis.

**submental a.,** *arteria* submentalis.

**subscapular a.,** *arteria* subscapularis.

**sulcal a.,** a small branch of the anterior spinal a. running in the anterior median fissure of the spinal cord.

**superficial brachial a.,** *arteria* brachialis superficialis.

**superficial cervical a.,** *arteria* cervicalis superficialis.

**superficial circumflex iliac a.,** *arteria* circumflexa ilium superficialis.

**superficial epigastric a.,** *arteria* epigastrica superficialis.

**superficial palmar a.,** *ramus* palmaris superficialis arteriae radialis.

**superficial temporal a.,** *arteria* temporalis superficialis.

**superficial volar a.,** *ramus* palmaris superficialis arteriae radialis.

**superior cerebellar a.,** *arteria* cerebelli superior.

**superior coronary a.,** *arteria* labialis superior.

**superior epigastric a.,** *arteria* epigastrica superior.

**superior gluteal a.,** *arteria* glutea superior.

**superior hemorrhoidal a.,** *arteria* rectalis superior.

**superior labial a.,** *arteria* labialis superior.

**superior laryngeal a.,** *arteria* laryngea superior.

**superior mesenteric a.,** *arteria* mesenterica superior.

**superior pancreaticoduodenal a.,** *arteria* pancreaticoduodenalis superior.

**superior phrenic a.,** *arteria* phrenica superior.

**superior rectal a.,** *arteria* rectalis superior.

**a. of superior segment of kidney,** *arteria* segmenti superioris renis.

**superior suprarenal a.,** *arteria* suprarenalis superior.

**superior thoracic a.,** *arteria* thoracica suprema.

**superior thyroid a.,** *arteria* thyroidea superior.

**superior tympanic a.,** *arteria* tympanica superior.

**superior ulnar collateral a.,** *arteria* collateralis ulnaris superior.

**supraduodenal a.,** *arteria* supraduodenalis.

**supraorbital a.,** *arteria* supraorbitalis.

**suprascapular a.,** *arteria* suprascapularis.

**supratrochlear a.,** *arteria* supratrochlearis.

**sural a.,** *arteria* suralis.

**terminal a.,** end a.

**testicular a.,** *arteria* testicularis.

**thoracoacromial a.,** *arteria* thoracoacromialis.

**thoracodorsal a.,** *arteria* thoracodorsalis.

**transverse cervical a.,** *arteria* transversa colli.

**transverse facial a.,** *arteria* transversa faciei.

**transverse a. of neck,** *arteria* transversa colli.

**transverse pancreatic a.,** *arteria* pancreatica inferior.

**transverse scapular a.,** *arteria* suprascapularis.

**ulnar a.,** *arteria* ulnaris.

**umbilical a.,** *arteria* umbilicalis.

**urethral a.,** *arteria* urethralis.

**uterine a.,** *arteria* uterina.

**vaginal a.,** *arteria* vaginalis.

**venous a.,** *truncus* pulmonalis.

**ventral splanchnic a.'s,** a.'s that arise on the embryo from the dorsal aorta and are distributed to the digestive tube.

**vertebral a.,** *arteria* vertebralis.

**Vid'ian a.,** *arteria* canalis pterygoidei.

**volar interosseous a.,** *arteria* interossea anterior.

**Wilkie's a.,** the right colic a. when it occasionally crosses the duodenum.

**Zinn's a.,** *arteria* centralis retinae.

**zygomat'ico-or'bital a.,** *arteria* zygomaticoorbitalis.

---

**arthr-.** See arthro-.

**arthrag'ra** [ G. *arthron*, joint, + *agra*, seizure ]. Articular gout.

**ar'thral.** Relating to a joint; articular.

**arthralgia** (ar-thral'jĭ-ah) [ G. *arthron*, joint, + *algos*, pain ]. Arthrodynia; severe pain in a joint, especially one not inflammatory in character.

    **intermittent a.,** periodic a.

    **periodic a.,** a condition in which pain and swelling of one or more joints, most commonly the knee, occurs at regular intervals; there is sometimes abdominal pain, purpura, or edema; the disease may show a familial tendency.

    **a. saturni'na,** severe pain, chiefly on flexion of the joints of the lower extremities, in lead poisoning.

**arthral'gic.** Arthrodynic; relating to or affected with arthralgia.

**arthrec'tomy** [ G. *arthron*, joint, + *ektomē*, excision ]. Exsection of a joint.

**arthrempyesis** (ar-threm-pi-e'sis) [ G. *arthron*, joint, + *empyēsis*, suppuration. PYO- ]. Arthroempyesis; the presence of pus in a joint.

**arthresthe'sia** [ G. *arthron*, joint, + *aisthesis*, sensation ]. Articular *sensibility*.

**arthrifuge** (ar'thrĭ-fūj) [ arthritis + L. *fugo*, to chase away ]. A gout remedy.

**arthrit'ic.** Relating to arthritis.

**arthritide** (ar'thrĭ-tēd) [ Fr. ]. A skin eruption of assumed gouty or rheumatic origin.

**arthritides** (ar-thrit'ĭ-dēz). Plural of arthritis.

**arthritis,** pl. **arthrit'ides** (ar-thri'tis) [ G. fr. *arthron,* joint, + suffix -*itis,* inflammation ]. Inflammation of a joint; state characterized by inflammation of joints.

**acute rheumatic a.,** rheumatic *fever.*

**atroph'ic a.,** neuropathic *arthropathy.*

**chronic absorptive a.,** a. accompanied by pronounced resorption of bone with shortening and deformity, especially of the hands; when the deformity is extreme the condition has also been termed a. mutilans.

**chronic proliferative a.,** rheumatoid a.

**chronic rheumatic a.,** rheumatoid a.

**chylous a.,** filarial a.

**colitic a.** a form of a. sometimes resembling rheumatoid a. which may complicate the course of ulcerative colitis; the etiology is unknown.

**a. defor'mans,** rheumatoid a.

**degenerative a.,** degenerative joint *disease.*

**dysenteric a.,** an effusion into the cavity and ligaments surrounding the joints, which may come on during the acute stage of bacillary dysentery.

**filarial a.,** chylous a.; a. occurring in filariasis, probably due to extravasation of lipid-rich lymph resembling chyle into the joint space.

**a. fungo'sa,** white swelling; chronic inflammation, usually tuberculous, of a joint, commonly the knee or the vertebrae, with proliferation of the synovial fringes producing a boggy swelling.

**gouty a.,** inflammation of the joints (especially of the great toe) in gout.

**hemophilic a.,** joint disease resulting from hemophilic bleeding into a joint.

**hypertroph'ic a.,** degenerative joint *disease.*

**juvenile rheumatoid a.,** Still's disease; polyarticular joint disease, associated with lymph node and splenic enlargement, occurring in infants and young children; it is accompanied by profuse sweating, mild fever of intermittent type, and anemia.

**a. mu'tilans,** a form of rheumatoid a. in which osteoporosis occurs with destruction of the joint cartilages and pronounced deformities of chiefly the hands and feet. May be associated with psoriasis. It has been suggested that the joint and skin diseases may have a common etiology.

**a. nodo'sa,** (1) rheumatoid a.; (2) gout.

**ochronot'ic a.,** a complication of ochronosis; an inborn error of metabolism characterized by brownish discoloration of the sclera, gunmetal staining of cartilages, especially of the nose and ears, and urine that turns black on standing or when rendered alkaline.

**proliferative a.,** rheumatoid a.

**psoriat'ic a.,** the concurrence of psoriasis and a., sometimes thought to be a specific disease entity; see a. mutilans.

**rheu'matoid a.,** chronic rheumatoid a.; a. deformans; a. nodosa (1); chronic proliferative a.; osseous or nodose rheumatism; a systemic disease, especially common in women, affecting connective tissue. A. is the dominant clinical manifestation. There is thickening of articular soft tissue, with extension of synovial tissue over articular cartilages, which become eroded. The course is variable but tends to be chronic and progressive, leading to deformities and disability.

**suppurative a.,** pyarthrosis; empyema articuli; suppurative synovitis; purulent synovitis; acute inflammation of synovial membranes, with purulent effusion into a joint, due to bacterial infection. The usual route of infection is hematogenous, to the synovial tissue. Suppurative a. causes lysis of the articular cartilage, and may become chronic, with sinus formation and ankylosis.

**a. urat'ica,** gout.

**arthro-, arth-** [ G. *arthron,* joint ]. Combining forms denoting a joint, or articulation, of the skeleton.

**arthrocace** (ar-throk'a-se) [ arthro- + G. *kakē,* badness ]. Caries of a joint.

**arthrocele** (ar'thro-sēl) [ arthro- + G. *kēlē,* hernia, tumor ]. 1. Hernia of the synovial membrane through the capsule of a joint. 2. Any swelling of a joint.

**arthrocentesis** (ar'thro-sen-te'sis) [ arthro- + G. *kentēsis,* puncture ]. Incision into a joint; arthrotomy; withdrawal of fluid through a puncture needle.

**arthrochondritis** (ar'thro-kon-dri'tis) [ arthro- + G. *chondros,* cartilage, + suffix -*itis,* inflammation ]. Inflammation of an articular cartilage.

**arthrocla'sia** [ arthro- + G. *klasis,* a breaking ]. The forcible breaking up of the adhesions in ankylosis.

**arthrod'esis** [ arthro- + G. *desis,* a binding together ]. Syndesis; the stiffening of a joint by operative means.

**arthro'dia** [ G. *arthrōdia,* a gliding joint, fr. *arthron,* joint, + *eidos,* form ]. *Articulatio* plana.

**arthro'dial.** Relating to arthrodia.

**arthrodynia** (ar-thro-din'ĭ-ah) [ arthro- + G. *odynē,* pain ]. Arthralgia.

**arthrodyn'ic.** Arthralgic.

**arthrodysplasia** (ar'thro-dis-pla'zĭ-ah) [ arthro- + G. *dys,* bad, + *plasis,* a molding ]. Abnormal joint development.

**hereditary a.,** nail-patella *syndrome.*

**arthroempyesis** (ar'thro-em-pi-e'sis). Arthrempyesis.

**ar'throendos'copy.** Endoscopic examination of the interior of a joint.

**arthroereisis** (ar-thro-er-i'sis). Arthrorisis.

**arthrogenous** (ar-throj'en-us). 1. Of articular origin; starting from a joint. 2. Forming an articulation.

**ar'throgram.** An x-ray of a joint.

**arthrography** (ar-throg'rā-fī) [ arthro- + G. *graphō,* to describe ]. 1. Roentgenography of a joint. 2. A treatise on the joints.

**arthrogryposis** (ar'thro-grĭ-po'sis) [ arthro- + G. *gryphōsis,* a crooking ]. Retention of a joint in a flexed position, caused by developmental failure of differentiation of intraarticular structure.

**a. mul'tiplex congen'ita,** amyoplasia congenita; myodystrophia fetalis; limitation of range of joint motion and contractures present at birth, usually involving multiple joints; a syndrome probably of diverse etiology that may result from changes in spinal cord, muscle, or connective tissue.

**arthrokatadysis** (ar'thro-kă-tad'ĭ-sis) [ arthro- + G. *katadysis* a dipping under, a setting, fr. *dyō,* to make sink ]. Otto's *disease.*

**ar'throlith** [ arthro- + G. *lithos,* stone ]. A gouty deposit in a joint.

**arthrolithi'asis.** Articular *gout.*

**arthrol'ogy** [ arthro- + G. *logos,* study ]. The branch of science that has to do with the joints.

**arthrol'ysis** [ arthro- + G. *lysis,* a loosening ]. The restoration of mobility in stiff and ankylosed joints.

**arthromeningitis** (ar'thro-men-in-ji'tis) [ arthro- + G. *mēninx,* membrane, + suffix -*itis,* inflammation ]. Synovitis.

**arthrom'eter.** An instrument for measuring the degree of motion in a joint, the range of mobility being registered on a dial.

**arthrom'etry** [ arthro- + G. *metron,* measure ]. Measurement of the range of movement in a joint.

**arthroncus** (ar-throng'kus) [ arthro- + G. *onkos,* bulk, ONC-1 ]. 1. Swelling of a joint. 2. A joint tumor.

**ar'throno'sos** [ arthro- + G. *nosos,* disease ]. Joint disease.

**ar'thro-on'ychodyspla'sia.** Nail-patella *syndrome.*

**arthro-ophthalmopathy** (ar'thro-of'thal-mop'ă-thī). Disease affecting joints and eyes.

**hereditary progressive a.,** Stickler syndrome; progressive myopia and abnormal epiphysial development in the vertebrae and long bones, inherited as an autosomal dominant trait.

**ar'thropath'ia** [ L. ]. Arthropathy.

**a. psoriat'ica,** inflammatory involvement of small joints in persons suffering from psoriasis.

**ar'thropathol'ogy.** The study of diseases of joints.

**arthrop'athy** [ arthro- + G. *pathos,* suffering ]. Arthropathia; any disease affecting a joint.

**diabetic a.,** a neuropathic a. occurring in diabetes.

**neuropath'ic a.**, atrophic arthritis; a. with a nervous basis, *e.g.*, Charcot's joint, diabetic a., in which the joint undergoes a gradual, usually painless, destruction. Such a.'s are now thought to be due to minor accidental injuries that, as a result of the lack of sensation in the part, are disregarded and not shielded from further damage and given rest and appropriate attention.

**static a.**, secondary involvement of a joint following disease in a joint of the same extremity, as knee or ankle with hip disease.

**tabetic a.**, charcot's disease (2); an enlargement of a joint, due to rarefying osteitis, often associated with spontaneous fractures, occurring in tabes dorsalis.

**arthrophlysis** (ar-throf'li-sis) [ arthro- + G. *phlysis*, eruption, fr. *phlyō*, to boil over ]. An eczematous eruption in gouty or rheumatic subjects.

**arthrophyma** (ar-thro-fi'mah) [ arthro- + G. *phyma*, swelling, tumor, PHYS- ]. An articular tumor or swelling.

**ar'throplasty** [ arthro- + G. *plassō*, to form ]. 1. The making of an artificial joint in case of ankylosis. 2. An operation to restore as far as possible the integrity and functional power of a joint.

    **gap a.**, the surgical correction of ankylosis by creating a space between the ankylosed part and the portion for which movement is desired.

    **interposition a.**, surgical correction of ankylosis by separation of the immobile fragment from the mobilized fragment and interposition of a substance (*e.g.*, fascia, cartilage, metal, or plastic) between them.

    **intracapsular temperomandibular joint a.**, operative recontouring of the articular surface of the mandibular condyle without the removal of the articular disk.

**arthropneumoroentgenography** (ar'thro-nu'mo-rent'-gen-og'raf-e). X-ray examination of a joint after it has been injected with air.

**ar'thropod** [ arthro- + G. *pous*, foot ]. A member of the phylum Arthropoda.

**Arthrop'oda** [ see arthropod ]. Joint-footed animals; a phylum of the Metazoa that includes the classes Crustacea (crabs, shrimps, crayfish, lobsters), Insecta, Arachnida (spiders, scorpions, mites, ticks), Chilopoda (centipedes), Diplopoda (millipedes), Merostomata (horseshoe crabs), and various other extinct or lesser known groups. A. forms the largest assemblage of living organisms, 75 per cent insects, of which over a million species are known.

**ar'thropo'dic, arthrop'odous.** Pertaining to arthropods.

**arthropyosis** (ar'thro-pi-o'sis) [ arthro- + G. *pyōsis*, suppuration ]. Suppuration in a joint.

**arthrorisis** (ar'thro-ri'sis) [ arthro- + G. *ereisis*, a propping up ]. Arthroerisis; an operation for limiting motion in a joint in cases of undue mobility from paralysis.

**arthrosclerosis** (ar'thro-skle-ro'sis) [ arthro- + G. *sklērō-sis*, hardening ]. Stiffness of the joints, especially in the aged.

**ar'throscope.** An instrument for examining joint interiors.

**arthros'copy** [ arthro- + G. *skopeō*, to view ]. Examination of the interior of a joint.

**arthro'sis** [ (1) G. *arthrōsis*, a jointing; (2) arthro- + G. suffix -*ōsis*, condition ]. 1. A joint. 2. A trophic degenerative affection of a joint.

    **temporomandibular a.**, a degenerative, noninfectious condition of the temporomandibular joint, characterized by pain, cracking, and limited mandibular opening.

**ar'throspore** [ arthro- + G. *sporos*, seed ]. A form of thallospore; a spore formed by septation of a hypha with subsequent separation of the a.'s at the septa.

**arthrosteitis** (ar-thros-te-i'tis) [ arthro- + G. *osteon*, bone, + suffix -*itis*, inflammation ]. Inflammation of the osseous structures of a joint.

**arthros'tomy** [ arthro- + G. *stoma*, mouth ]. The establishment of a temporary opening into a joint cavity.

**arthrosynovitis** (ar'thro-sin-o-vi'tis). Inflammation of the synovial membrane of a joint.

**ar'throtome.** A large, strong scalpel used in cutting cartilaginous and other tough joint structures.

**arthrot'omy** [ arthro- + G. *tomē*, a cutting ]. Cutting into a joint.

**ar'throtrop'ic** [ arthro- + G. *tropos*, a turning ]. Tending to affect joints.

**ar'throty'phoid.** Typhoid fever with joint symptoms simulating rheumatism.

**arthroxesis** (ar-throk'se-sis) [ arthro- + G. *xesis*, a scraping ]. Removal of diseased tissue from a joint by means of the sharp spoon or other scraping instrument.

**Arthus** (ar-tüs'), N. Maurice, French bacteriologist, 1862–1945. See A. *reaction, phenomenon*.

**artiad** (ar'ti-ad) [ G. *artios*, exact, (of numbers) even ]. Obsolete term for an element of even valence.

**artic'ular.** Relating to a joint.

**articula're.** In cephalometrics, the point of intersection of a line drawn along the posterior border of the ramus where it crosses a line drawn along the base of the cranium.

**artic'ulate** [ L. *articulo*, pp. -*atus*, to articulate. ARTIC- ]. 1. Articulated; jointed; to join or connect together loosely to allow motion between the parts. 2. To speak distinctly and connectedly.

**artic'ulated.** Jointed.

---

# ARTICULATIO

**articulatio**, pl. **articulatio'nes** (ar-tik'u-la-shi'-o) [ L. a forming of vines. ARTIC- ] [ NA, NAV ]. In anatomy, articulation (1); junctura ossium [ NA, NAV ]; joint; articulus; the place of union, usually more or less movable, between two or more bones. Joints between skeletal elements exhibit a great variety of form and function, and are classified into three general morphological types: *juncturae* fibrosae; *juncturae* cartilagineae; and *juncturae* synoviales.

    **a. acromioclavicula'ris** [ NA ], acromioclavicular joint; a plane joint between the acromial end of the clavicle and the medial margin of the acromion.

    **a. antebrachiocar'pea** [ NAV ], antebrachiocarpal joint; in domestic animals, the joint where the radius and ulna articulate with the carpal bones.

    **a. atlantoaxia'lis** [ NAV ], atlantoaxial articulation; in domestic animals, a joint formed by the joining of the lateral and median atlantoaxial joints.

    **a. atlantoaxia'lis latera'lis** [ NA ], lateral atlantoaxial joint; lateral atlantoepistrophic joint; a condylar joint between the inferior articular pits of the atlas and the superior articular surfaces of the axis.

    **a. atlantoaxia'lis media'na** [ NA ], median atlantoaxial joint; middle atlantoepistrophic joint; a pivot joint between the dens of the axis and the ring formed by the anterior arch and the transverse ligament of the atlas.

    **a. atlan'tooccipita'lis** [ NA ], atlantooccipital joint; a condylar joint between the superior articular pits of the atlas and the condyles of the occipital bone.

    **a. calca'neocuboi'dea** [ NA ], calcaneocuboid joint; a somewhat saddle-shaped joint between the anterior surface of the calcaneus and the posterior surface of the cuboid.

    **a. calcaneoquarta'lis** [ NAV ], in domestic mammals, the joint between the calcaneus and fourth tarsal bone; it corresponds to the a. calcaneocuboidea in man.

    **a. capitis costae** [ NA ], joint of the head of a rib; the joint between a rib and bodies of two adjacent vertebrae; the joint cavity is divided by an intraarticular ligament which attaches to the intervertebral disk. The first, tenth, eleventh, and twelfth ribs articulate with only one vertebra.

    **articulationes carpometacar'peae** [ NA ], carpometacarpal joints; the joints between the carpal and metacarpal bones; these are all plane joints except that of the thumb, which is saddle-shaped.

    **a. carpometacar'pea pol'licis** [ NA ], carpometacarpal joint of the thumb; the saddle-shaped articulation between the trapezium and the base of the first metacarpal bone.

    **a. centrodista'lis** [ NAV ], centrodistal joint in domestic animals; it corresponds to the a. cuneonavicularis in man.

    **a. compos'ita** [ NA ], compound joint; a joint in which more than two skeletal elements participate.

**a. condyla'ris** [ NA ], condylar joint; condyloid joint; a joint in which two, more or less distinct, rounded surfaces of one bone articulate with shallow depressions on another bone.

**a. costochondra'lis** [ NA ], costochondral joint; the cartilaginous joint between the sternal end of a rib and the lateral end of a costal cartilage.

**a. cos'totransversa'ria** [ NA ], costotransverse joint; the articulation between the neck and tubercle of a rib and the transverse process of a vertebra.

**articulationes costovertebra'les** [ NA ], costovertebral joints; the joints uniting ribs and vertebrae; they consist of the a. capitis costae and the a. costotransversaria.

**a. cotylica** [ NA ], a. spheroidea.

**a. coxae** [ NA ], hip joint; the ball-and-socket joint between the head of the femur and the acetabulum.

**a. cricoarytenoid'ea** [ NA ], cricoarytenoid articulation; the joint between the base of each arytenoid cartilage and the upper border of the lamina of the cricoid cartilage.

**a. cricothyroid'ea** [ NA ], cricothyroid articulation; the articulation between the inferior horn of the thyroid cartilage and the side of the cricoid cartilage.

**a. cu'biti** [ NA ], elbow joint; a compound hinge joint between the humerus and the bones of the forearm. It consists of the a. humeroradialis and the a. humeroulnaris.

**a. cuneonavicula'ris** [ NA ], cuneonavicular articulation; the joint between the anterior surface of the navicular and the posterior surfaces of the three cuneiform bones.

**a. ellipsoi'dea** [ NA ], ellipsoidal joint; a modified ball-and-socket joint in which the joint surfaces are elongated or ellipsoidal. It is a biaxial joint, *i.e.*, two axes of motion at right angles to each other, the radiocarpal being an example.

**a. femoropatella'ris** [ NAV ], femoropatellar joint (2); in domestic animals, a part of the a. genus between the patella and the trochlea of the femur.

**a. femorotibia'lis** [ NAV ], femorotibial joint; knee (4); in domestic animals, the condyloid part of the a. genus between the femur and tibia.

**a. genus** [ NA ], knee joint; a compound condylar joint consisting of the joint between the condyles of the femur and the condyles of the tibia, the semilunar cartilages being interposed, and the articulation between femur and patella.

**a. hu'meri** [ NA ], humeral articulation; shoulder joint; a ball-and-socket joint between the head of the humerus and the glenoid cavity of the scapula.

**a. humeroradia'lis** [ NA ], humeroradial articulation; the portion of the elbow joint between the capitulum of the humerus and the head of the radius.

**a. humeroulna'ris** [ NA ], humeroulnar joint; the portion of the elbow joint between the trochlea of the humerus and the trochlear notch of the ulna.

**a. incudom llea'ris** [ NA ], incudomalleolar joint; the saddle joint between the incus and the malleus.

**a. incudostape'dia** [ NA ], incudostapedial articulation; the joint between the lenticular process on the long crus of the incus and the head of the stapes.

**articulationes intercarpeae** [ NA ], intercarpal joints; the articulations between the carpal bones.

**articulationes interchondra'les** [ NA ], interchondral articulations; the joints between the contiguous surfaces of the fifth, sixth, seventh, eighth, ninth, and tenth costal cartilages.

**articulationes intermetacarpeae** [ NA ], intermetacarpal joints; the articulations between the bases of the second, third, fourth, and fifth metacarpal bones.

**articulationes intermetatarseae** [ NA ], intermetatarsal articulations; the joints between the bases of the five metatarsal bones.

**articulationes interphalangeae** [ NA ], interphalangeal articulations; digital joints; the hinge joints between the phalanges of the fingers (articulationes interphalangeae manus) or toes (articulationes interphalangeae pedis).

**articulationes intertarseae** [ NA ], intertarsal articulations; the joints which unite the tarsal bones.

**a. intrachondra'lis** [ NAV ], intrachondral joint; a synovial joint within some of the rib cartilages in artiodactyls.

**a. mandibula'ris,** a. temporomandibularis.

**articulationes ma'nus** [ NA ], articulations of the hand; these joints include the radiocarpal or wrist joint; intercar-

pal, carpometacarpal, intermetacarpal; metacarpophalangeal and interphalangeal joints.

**a. mediocarpea** [ NA ], middle carpal joint; the joint between the proximal and distal rows of carpal bones.

**articulationes metacar'pophalangeae** [ NA ], metacarpophalangeal articulations; the spheroid joints between the heads of the metacarpals and the bases of the proximal phalanges.

**articulationes metatar'sophalangeae** [ NA ], metatarsophalangeal articulations; the spheroid joints between the heads of the metatarsals and the bases of the proximal phalanges of the toes.

**articulationes ossiculo'rum audi'tus** [ NA ], joints of the ear bones; the joints of the ossicular chain consisting of a. incudomallearis, a. incudostapedia, and syndesmosis tympanostapedia.

**a. os'sis car'pi accesso'rii** [ NAV ], articulation of the accessory carpal bone in domestic mammals, corresponding to the a. ossis pisiformis in man; the flexor carpi ulnaris inserts upon it.

**a. ossis pisifor'mis** [ NA ], articulation of the pisiform bone; the joint between the pisiform and triquetrum; it is separate from the other intercarpal joints.

**articulationes pe'dis** [ NA ], articulations of the foot, including the talocrural, intertarsal, tarsometatarsal, intermetatarsal, metatarsophalangeal and interphalangeal joints.

**a. plana** [ NA ], plane joint; arthrodia; gliding joint; a synovial joint in which the opposing surfaces are nearly planes and in which there is only a slight, gliding motion as in the intermetacarpal joints.

**a. radiocarpea** [ NA ], radiocarpal articulation; carpal articulation; wrist joint; the joint between the distal end of the radius and its articular disk and the proximal row of carpal bones with the exception of the pisiform bone.

**a. radioulna'ris distalis** [ NA ], distal radioulnar articulation; the pivot joint between the head of the ulna and the ulnar notch on the radius; an articular disc passes across the distal part of the joint.

**a. radioulna'ris proxima'lis** [ NA ], proximal radioulnar articulation; the pivot joint between the head of the radius and the ring formed by the radial notch of the ulna and the anular ligament.

**a. sacroiliaca** [ NA ], sacroiliac articulation; the synovial joint on either side between the auricular surface of the sacrum and that of the ilium.

**a. sellar'is** [ NA ], saddle joint; a biaxial joint in which the double motion is effected by the opposition of two surfaces each of which is concave in one direction and convex in the other; as in the carpometacarpal articulation of the thumb.

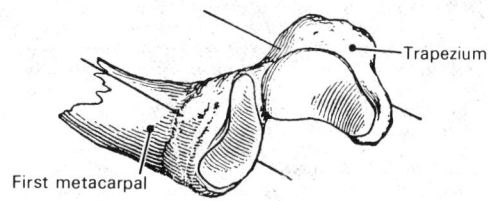

Trapezium

First metacarpal

**Articulatio Sellaris (Saddle Joint)**

**a. simplex** [ NA ], simple joint; one composed of two bones only.

**a. spheroi'dea** [ NA ], spheroid articulation; a. cotylica; cotyloid joint; enarthrosis; ball-and-socket joint; a multiaxial joint in which a more or less extensive sphere on the head of one bone fits into a rounded cavity in the other bone, as in the hip joint.

**a. sternoclavicula'ris** [ NA ], sternoclavicular joint; the articulation between the medial end of the clavicle and the manubrium of the sternum and cartilage of the first rib; an articular disc subdivides the joint into two cavities.

**articulationes sternocosta'les** [ NA ], sternocostal articulations; the joints between the cartilages of the first seven ribs and the sternum; synovial cavities are variable in occurrence in these joints.

**a. subtala'ris** [ NA ], subtalar joint; a plane joint between the inferior surface of the talus and the posterior articular surface of the calcaneus.

**a. synovia'lis manubriosterna'lis** [ NAV ], manubriosternal synovial joint; the synovial joint between the first sternebra or manubrium and the rest of the sternum in the goat, ox, pig, and sheep.

**a. talocalca'nea** [ NAV ], talocalcaneal joint; in domestic animals, the joint cavity between the talus and the central tarsal; it also extends between the talus and the calcaneus.

**a. talocalcaneocentra'lis** [ NAV ], the talocalcaneocentral joint in domestic animals; it corresponds to a talocalcaneonavicularis in man.

**a. tal'ocalca'neonavicula'ris** [ NA ], talocalcaneonavicular joint; a ball-and-socket joint, part of the transverse tarsal joint, formed by the head of the talus articulating with the navicular bone and the anterior part of the calcaneus.

**a. talocrural'is** [ NA ], talocrural articulation; ankle joint; mortise joint; a hinge joint between the tibia and fibula above and the talus below.

**a. tarsi transversa** [ NA ], transverse tarsal articulation; Chopart's joint; midtarsal joint; the joint between the talus and calcaneus posteriorly and the navicular and cuboid bones anteriorly.

**a. tarsocrura'lis** [ NAV ], tarsocrural joint; the most proximal joint of the foot in domestic animals; both the talus and the calcaneus articulate with the bones of the crus, except in the horse.

**articulationes tarsometatar'seae** [ NA ], tarsometatarsal joints; cuneometatarsal joints; the three joints between the tarsal and metatarsal bones, consisting of a medial joint between the first cuneiform and first metatarsal, an intermediate joint between the second and third cuneiforms and corresponding metatarsals, and a lateral joint between the cuboid and fourth and fifth metatarsals.

**a. tem'poromandibula'ris** [ NA ], temporomandibular articulation or joint; a. mandibularis; mandibular joint; the articulation between the head of the mandible and the mandibular fossa and articular tubercle of the temporal bone; an articular disc divides the joint into two cavities.

**a. tibiofibula'ris**, tibiofibular articulation; superior tibial articulation; (1) [ NA ], the plane joint between the lateral condyle of the tibia and the head of the fibula; (2) [ NAV ], in domestic animals there is a proximal and a distal articulation.

**a. trochoid'ea** [ NA ], helicoid or lateral ginglymus; trochoid, rotary, or pivot joint, in which a section of a cylinder of one bone fits into a corresponding cavity on the other, as in the proximal radioulnar articulation.

---

**articula'tion** [ L. *articulatio, q.v.* ]. 1. Articulatio. 2. A joining or connecting together loosely so as to allow motion between the parts. 3. Distinct connected speech or enunciation. 4. In dentistry, *tooth* arrangement.

**atlantoaxial a.**, see entries under *articulatio* atlantoaxialis.

**atlantooccipital a.**, *articulatio* atlantooccipitalis.

**balanced a.**, balanced *occlusion.*

**carpal a.**, *articulatio* radiocarpea.

**condylar a.**, *articulatio* condylaris.

**confluent a.**, a tendency to run the syllables together in speech.

**cricoarytenoid a.**, *articulatio* cricoarytenoidea.

**cricothyroid a.**, *articulatio* cricothyroidea.

**cuneonavicular a.**, *articulatio* cuneonavicularis.

**dental a.**, gliding occlusion; the contact relationship of the upper and lower teeth when moving into and away from centric occlusion.

**distal radioulnar a.**, *articulatio* radioulnaris distalis.

**a.'s of foot**, *articulationes* pedis.

**a.'s of hand**, *articulationes* manus.

**humeral a.**, *articulatio* humeri.

**humeroradial a.**, *articulatio* humeroradialis.

**incudostapedial a.**, *articulatio* incudostapedia.

**inferior tibial a.**, *syndesmosis* tibiofibularis.

**interchondral a.'s**, *articulationes* interchondrales.

**intermetatarsal a.'s**, *articulationes* intermetatarseae.

**interphalangeal a.'s**, *articulationes* interphalangeae.

**intertarsal a.'s**, *articulationes* intertarseae.

**metacarpophalangeal a.'s**, *articulationes* metacarpophalangeae.

**metatarsophalangeal a.'s**, *articulationes* metatarsophalangeae.

**a. of pisiform bone**, *articulatio* ossis pisiformis.

**proximal radioulnar a.**, *articulatio* radioulnaris proximalis.

**radiocarpal a.**, *articulatio* radiocarpea.

**sacroiliac a.**, *articulatio* sacroiliaca.

**spheroid a.**, *articulatio* spheroidea.

**sternocostal a.'s**, *articulationes* sternocostales.

**superior tibial a.**, *articulatio* tibiofibularis.

**talocrural a.**, *articulatio* talocruralis.

**temporomandibular a.**, *articulatio* temporomandibularis.

**tibiofibular a.**, *articulatio* tibiofibularis.

**transverse tarsal a.**, *articulatio* tarsi transversa.

**trochoid a.**, *articulatio* trochoidea.

**artic'ulator.** A mechanical device which represents the temporomandibular joints and jaw members to which maxillary and mandibular casts may be attached.

**adjustable a.**, (1) an a. which may be adjusted to permit movement of the casts into recorded eccentric relationships; (2) an a. capable of adjustment to more than one eccentric position.

**artic'ulatory.** Relating to articulate speech.

**artic'ulo mortis** [ ART- ]. At the point or instant of death; in the jaws of death.

**artic'ulostat.** A research instrument that will position dentures and the head of an x-ray machine in such a manner that films made at separate times may be accurately superimposed.

**artic'ulus** [ L. joint ]. Articulatio.

**ar'tifact** [ L. *ars*, art, + *facio*, pp. *factus*, to make ]. Anything, especially in a histologic specimen or a graphic record, that is caused by the technique used and is not a natural occurrence, but is merely incidental.

**artifactitious** (ar'tĭ-fak-tish'us). Produced by an artifact; unnatural.

**artifistula'tion.** Fenestration (3).

**ar'tiodac'tyl.** Common name for a member of the order Artiodactyla.

**Artiodactyla** (ar'tĭ-o-dak'tĭlah) [ G. *artios*, even in number, + *daktylos*, finger ]. An order of even-toed ungulates having either two or four digits, with the axis between the third and fourth; *e.g.*, pig and hippopotamus with four; camel, deer, giraffe, antelope, and cow with two.

**aryepiglottic** (ăr'ĭ-ep-ĭ-glot'ik). Arytenoepiglottidean; relating to the arytenoid cartilage and the epiglottis; denoting a fold of mucous membrane (plica aryepiglottica) and a muscle contained in it (musculus aryepiglotticus).

**aryl** (ăr'il). An organic radical derived from an aromatic compound by removing a hydrogen atom.

**a. acylamidase**, arylamidase; an amidohydrolase (EC 3.5.1.13) cleaving the acyl group from an anilide by hydrolysis.

**arylam'idase.** Aryl acylamidase.

**arylarson'ic acid.** An arsonic acid containing an aryl radical.

**arylsul'fatase.** An enzyme (EC 3.1.6.1) that cleaves phenol sulfates, including cerebroside sulfates. A deficit of arylsulfatase-A has been demonstrated in the tissues of patients with metachromatic leukodystrophy. See also sulfatase.

**arytena** (ăr'ĭ-te'nah) [ G. *arytaina*, a ladle ] [ NA ]. Any ladle-shaped structure.

**arytenoepiglottidean** (ar-it'e-no-ep'ĭ-glŏ-tid'e-an). Aryepiglottic.

**arytenoid** (ăr-ĭ-te'noyd) [ see arytenoideus ]. Denoting a cartilage (cartilago arytenoidea) and a muscle (musculus arytenoideus) of the larynx.

**arytenoidectomy** (ăr'ĭ-te-noy-dek'to-mĭ) [ arytenoid + G. *ektomē*, excision ]. Excision of an arytenoid cartilage.

**arytenoi'deus** [ G. *arytainoeides*, ladle-shaped, applied to cartilage of the larynx, fr. *arytaina*, a ladle, + *eidos*, resemblance ]. *Musculus* arytenoideus.

**arytenoiditis** (ă-rit'ĕ-noy-di'tis). Inflammation of an arytenoid cartilage.

**ar'ytenoi'dopex'y** [ arytenoid + G. *pēxis,* fixation ]. Fixation by surgery of cartilages or muscles of arytenoids.

**As.** 1. Abbreviation for astigmatism or astigmatic. 2. Chemical symbol of the element of arsenic.

**asafet'ida** [ Pers. *aza,* mastic, + L. *fetidus,* fetid ] (BP). A gum resin, the inspissated exudate from the root of *Ferula foetida* (family Umbelliferae). Used as a repellant against dogs, cats, and rabbits, and formerly used as an antispasmodic. In Asia, it is used as a condiment and flavoring agent.

**asaphia** (ă-saf'ĭ-ah, ă-sa'fĭ-ah) [ G. *asapheia,* obscurity, fr. *a-* priv. + *saphēs,* clear ]. Indistinctness in speech.

**As'arum** [ L. fr. G. *asaron,* hazelwort ]. A genus of plants of the family Aristolochiaceae.

**A. canaden'se,** wild ginger; Indian ginger; Canada snakeroot; an aromatic stimulant and diaphoretic.

**A. europae'um,** hazelwort; European snakeroot; emetic and cathartic.

**asbes'tos** [ G. unquenchable ]. A fibrous material made of a calcium and magnesium silicate, and used for thermal insulation and fireproofing; inhalation of a. particles can cause asbestosis.

**asbesto'sis.** Pneumoconiosis due to inhalation of asbestos particles; sometimes complicated by pleural endothelioma or bronchial carcinoma.

**ascariasis** (as'kă-ri'ah-sis). Disease caused by infection with *Ascaris* or related ascarid nematodes.

**ascaricide** (as-kăr'ĭ-sīd) [ ascarid + L. *caedo,* to kill ]. 1. Causing the death of ascarid nematodes. 2. An agent that destroys ascarid nematodes.

**as'carid.** 1. A general name for any nematode of the superfamily Ascaroidea. 2. Pertaining to such nematodes.

**Ascaridia** (as'kă-rid'ĭ-ah). A genus of relatively large nematodes (family Heterakidae) that inhabit the intestine of birds and cause ascaridiasis. Their life cycle is direct, without an intermediate host; their appearance and habits are much like those of members of the family Ascaroidea.

**A. colum'bae,** a common species that occurs in domestic and wild pigeons.

**A. gal'li,** a species abundant in the small intestine of chickens, turkeys, geese, guinea fowl, and many wild birds in most parts of the world.

**ascaridiasis** (as-kă'rĭ-di'ă-sis). Disease caused by infection with a species of the genus *Ascaridia,* commonly occurring in the intestine of fowl.

**Ascarid'icae.** Ascaroidea.

**Ascaridid'ea.** Ascaroidea.

**ascar'idole.** Ascarisin; 1,4-peroxido-*p*-menthene-2; a major constituent of oil of chenopodium; anthelmintic.

**Ascaris** (as'kă-ris) [ G. *askaris,* an intestinal worm ]. A genus of large, heavy-bodied roundworms parasitic in the small intestine; abundant in man and many other vertebrates.

**A. equo'rum,** *Parascaris equorum.*

**A. lumbricoi'des,** large roundworm of man; one of the commonest human parasites (8 to 12 inches in length). Various symptoms such as restlessness, fever, and some-

times diarrhea, are attributed to its presence, but usually it causes no definite symptoms. The similar species, *A. suis* (or *A. lumbricoides suis*) is very common in swine. The swine type is not readily transmitted to man, and *vice versa.* The types are morphologically and immunologically indistinguishable but apparently are host-adapted types, considered distinct species or races.

**A. vitulorum,** occurs in the small intestine of cattle, zebu, and water buffalo.

**ascar'isin.** Ascaridole.

**Ascaroi'dea.** Ascaridicae; Ascarididea; a superfamily of parasitic worms of the subphylum Nematoda, including the important ascarids of man and domestic animals and heterakids of birds.

**Ascarops strongylina.** A small, bloodsucking worm found in the stomach of pigs and wild boars in many parts of the world. Larvae develop in coprophagous beetles; worms adhere to the gastric mucosa of the pig, and may cause inflammation and ulceration in heavy infections.

**ascen'dens** [ L. ] [ NA ]. Ascending.

**ascen'sus** [ L. ascent ]. A moving upward; having an abnormally high position.

**ascertain'ment.** In genetic research, the method by which patients with hereditary disease are located or selected for study.

**complete a.,** method by which essentially all affected individuals in a population are located by survey or an appropriate random sampling technique.

**incomplete a.,** method of locating affected individuals in which probability of locating any specific patient has a known value between zero and 1.

**single a.,** method of locating affected individuals by hospital or clinic admission or other way in which probability of encountering same family twice approaches zero.

**truncate a.,** incomplete a.

**Aschelminthes** (ask-hel-min'thēz). Nemathelminthes; a phylum of the Metazoa, including the class Nematoda and a disparate assortment of other roundworms; they are nonsegmented, bilaterally symmetric, and cylindric or filiform, with a pseudocele body cavity and rounded or pointed ends; they vary considerably in size, and the male is usually smaller than the female.

**Ascher,** Karl W., Cincinnati ophthalmologist, *1887. See A.'s aqueous influx *phenomenon,* A.'s *syndrome.*

**Aschheim** (ahsh'hīm), Selmar, German obstetrician and gynecologist, *1878. See A.-Zondek *test.*

**aschistodactyly, aschistodactyl'ia** (ah-skis'to-dak'tī-lĭ), [ G. *a-* priv. + *schistos,* cleft, + *daktylos,* finger ]. Syndactyly.

**Aschner** (ahsh'ner), Bernhard, Austrian gynecologist, 1883–1960. See A.'s *phenomenon, reflex,* A.-Dagnini *reflex.*

**Aschoff** (ahsh'off), K. A. Ludwig, Berlin pathologist, 1866–1942. See A.'s *bodies, node, nodules;* Rokitansky-A. *sinus.*

**ascites** (ă-si'tēz) [ L. fr. G. *askos,* a bag, + suffix -*ites, q. v.* ]. Hydroperitoneum; abdominal dropsy; an accumulation of serous fluid in the peritoneal cavity.

**a. adipo'sus,** chylous a.

**chyliform a.,** chylous a.

**chylous a.,** a. chylosus; chyliform a.; a. adiposus; fatty or milky a.; chyloperitoneum; the presence in the peritoneal cavity of a milky fluid containing suspended fat, ordinarily caused by an obstruction of the thoracic duct from neoplasm or other lesion, causing rupture of distended lacteals.

**fatty a.,** chylous a.

**gelatinous a.,** pseudomyxoma peritonei; the presence of pseudomucinous a., usually resulting from rupture of a pseudomucinous ovarian cyst with generalized implantations upon the peritoneum and omentum; also found occasionally in myxedema.

**hemorrhagic a.,** bloody or blood-stained serous fluid, frequently resulting from metastatic carcinoma in the peritoneal cavity.

**milky a.,** chylous a.

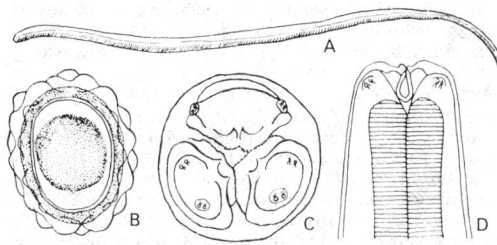

A

B C D

*Ascaris lumbricoides*

A, female; B, fertilized egg; C, head-on view of worm, showing lips and papillas; D, ventral view, showing anterior extremity of mature worm. Reduced from original magnifications of × ⅓ (A), ×500 (B), ×10 (C), ×5 (D). (From Blacklock and Southwell: *Guide to Human Parasitology,* edited by T. H. Davey, H. K. Lewis & Co., Ltd., 1958.)

**preag'onal a.,** an outpour of serum in the peritoneal cavity consequent upon an intense congestion of the viscera, sometimes immediately preceding death.

**a. precox,** a. appearing earlier than peripheral edema in cases of constrictive pericarditis.

**pseu'dochy'lous a.,** the presence in the peritoneum of an opalescent or cloudy fluid which does not contain fat.

**ascitic** (ă-sit'ik). Relating to ascites.

**ascitogenous** (as'ĭ-toj'ĕ-nus). Producing ascites.

**Asclepiadae** (as'kle-pi'ă-de). Asclepiads.

**Asclepi'ades** of Bithynia (born circa 124 B.C.). Established Greek medicine in Rome, 91 B.C. He taught a theory of disease based on the atomic theories of Democritus and rejected the humoral theory of Hippocrates.

**Asclepiads** (as-klēp'e-adz) [ G. *Asklēpiadēs,* a descendant of *Asklēpios* (L. *Aesculapius*) pl. *Asclēpiadai,* used as a name for physicians ]. An order of Greek physicians, priests of Asclepius, (*q. v.*), whose descendants they claimed and were supposed to be.

**Ascle'pias** [ G. *Asklēpios,* Aesculapius ]. A genus of plants (family Asclepiadaceae), commonly called milkweeds; some species, *e.g., A. eriocarpa* and *A. galioides,* are toxic to herbivorous animals and fowl.

**A. syri'aca,** wild cotton; silkweed. The root is used in amenorrhea, dropsy, rheumatism, and asthma.

**A. tubero'sa,** butterfly weed; yellow milkweed; pleurisy root. Formerly used as a diuretic and cathartic and in pleurisy.

**Asclepi'eia.** A temple of Aesculapius in ancient Greece, as at Cos, Cnidus, Pergamos or Epidaurus.

**Asclepius** (as-kle'pĭ-us) [ G. *Asklēpios* ]. In Greek mythology, son of Apollo and god of medicine. Daughters attributed to him are Hygeia, the goddess of health, and Panakeia (Panacea), "the all healing." See also Aesculapius.

**ascocarp (as'ko-karp)** [ G. *askos,* bag, + *karpos,* fruit ]. Fruiting body of the Ascomycetes, bearing asci and ascospores.

**Ascoli** (ahs-ko'le), Alberto, Italian serologist, 1877–1957. See A. *reaction.*

**Ascomycetes** (as'ko-mi-se'tēz) [ G. *askos,* a bag, + *mykēs,* mushroom ]. A class of fungi characterized by the presence of a sac-like structure (ascus) containing ascospores. Such fungi have generally two distinct reproductive phases, the sexual or perfect stage and the asexual or imperfect stage. Ergot, truffles, molds, and yeasts belong to the class.

**ascor'bate.** A salt or ester of ascorbic acid.

**a. oxidase** (EC 1.10.3.3), a copper-containing enzyme that catalyzes the oxidation of ascorbic acid to dehydroascorbic acid.

**ascor'bic acid** (as-kor'bik) (USP, BP). Vitamin C; cevitamic acid; 2,3-didehydro-L-*threo*-hexono-1,4-lactone; the antiscorbutic vitamin, specifically preventing scurvy. It is a strong reducing agent and is also used as an antioxidant in foodstuffs.

CH₂OH

H—C₅—OH

C'⁴

HO
C³        O

C²   C¹

HO        O

Ascorbic acid

**ascor'byl pal'mitate** (NF). L-Ascorbic acid-6-palmitate; used as a preservative in pharmaceutical preparations.

**asco'sin.** An antibiotic produced by *Streptomyces canescus;* an antifungal active against yeasts and some filamentous fungi.

**ascospore** (as'ko-spor) [ G. *askos,* bag, + *sporos,* seed ]. A spore formed within an ascus; the sexual spore of Ascomycetes.

**as'cus,** pl. **as'ci** (as'kus) [ G. *askos,* bag ]. The saclike cell of Ascomycetes in which ascospores are formed; the spore mother cell from which ascospores develop following nuclear fusion and meiosis.

**-ase.** A termination denoting an enzyme; it is suffixed to the name of the substance (substrate) upon which the enzyme acts. Thus, starch-splitting enzymes are amylases, fat-splitting enzymes are lipases, etc. Coagulating enzymes may be called thrombases, oxidizing enzymes, oxidases, etc. Enzymes named before the convention was established generally have an -*in* ending; *e.g.,* pepsin, trypsin, ptyalin, steapsin, etc.

**asecretory** (a-se-kre'to-rī). Without secretion.

**Aselli** (or **Asello** or **Aselius**), Gaspar, Italian anatomist at Cremona, 1581–1626. He rediscovered the lacteal vessels, and his *De lactibus* (1628) contained the earliest anatomical color plate. See A.'s *glands, pancreas.*

**asema'sia** [ G. *a-* priv. + *sēmasia,* the giving of a signal, fr. *sēma,* sign ]. Asymbolia (2).

**ase'mia** [ G. *a-* priv. + *sēma,* sign ]. Asymbolia (2).

**asepsis** (ā-sep'sis) [ G. *a-* priv. + *sēpsis,* putrefaction ]. A condition in which living pathogenic organisms are absent.

**asep'tic.** Marked by or relating to asepsis.

**asep'ticism.** The practice of aseptic surgery.

**asep'ticize.** To render aseptic or sterile.

**asequence** (ā-se'kwens). Lack of normal sequence, specifically, between atrial and ventricular contractions.

**asex'ual.** 1. Without sex, as in a. reproduction. 2. Having no sexual desire or interest.

**asexualization** (a-seks'u-al-ĭ-za'shun). Sterilization, as by castration.

**ash** [ O.E. *asce* ]. What remains after any substance has been burned; the nonvolatile (mineral) constituents of any substance.

**bone a.,** the mineral matter obtained by burning or calcining bones.

**Ashley's phenomenon.** See under phenomenon.

**Ashman's phenomenon.** See under phenomenon.

**asialad'enism** [ G. *a-* priv. + *sialon,* saliva, + *adēn,* gland ]. A postulated state in which parotin secretion is deficient. The possible consequences of such a deficiency are said to be fetal chondrodystrophia, arthritis deformans, spondylitis deformans, and alveolar pyorrhea. It is claimed that such disorders respond favorably to parotin therapy.

**asialia** (a-si-a'lĭ-ah). Asialism.

**asi'alism** [ G. *a-* priv. + *sialon,* saliva ]. Aptyalism; aptyalia; asialia; diminished or arrested secretion of saliva.

**asitia** (a-sish'ĭ-ah) [ G. *a-* priv. + *sitos,* food ]. Anorexia.

**Askanazy cell.** See under cell.

**askiatic** (a-ski-at'ik) [ G. *a-* priv. + *skia,* shadow ]. Absence of shadow.

**asleep.** 1. In a state of sleep. 2. Paresthetic; denoting numbness and tingling in an extremity which usually occurs on the resumption of the blood flow to a nerve following temporary pressure or mild injury.

**Asn.** Symbol for asparagine or its mono- or diradical.

**asocial** (a-so'shul). Not social; indifferent to social rules or customs; withdrawn from society, *e.g.,* a recluse or a regressed schizophrenic person.

**aso'mus,** pl. **asoma'ta** [ G. *a-* priv. + *sōma,* body ]. A fetus with only a rudimentary body.

**Asp.** Symbol for aspartic acid or its radical forms.

**aspalasomus** (as'pal-ă-so'mus) [ G. *aspalax,* a mole, + *sōma,* body ]. A malformed fetus with eventration at the lower part of the abdomen, presenting separate openings for intestine, bladder, and sexual organs.

**aspar'aginase.** L-Asparaginase. 1. An enzyme (EC 3.5.1.1) catalyzing the hydrolysis of asparagine to aspartic acid and ammonia. (The term asparaginase II was formerly used for glycine aminotransferase.) 2 (USP). CRASNITIN; the enzyme from *Escherichia coli,* used in the treatment of acute leukemia and other neoplastic diseases.

**L-asparaginase.** Asparaginase.

**asparagine** (as-par'ă-jin). Symbol, Asn or Asp (NH₂); the β-amide of aspartic acid; α-amino-β-succinamic acid; NH₂COCH₂CH(NH₂)COOH; a nonessential amino acid occurring in proteins. Diuretic.

**a. synthetase** (EC 6.3.1.1), an acid-ammonia ligase (amide synthetase) forming asparagine from aspartate and NH₃ with cleavage of ATP to AMP.

**aspar'aginyl.** The aminoacyl radical of asparagine.

**aspar'agosin.** A fructosan occurring in asparagus roots.

**Aspar'agus** [ L. fr. G. *asparagos* ]. A genus of plants of the family Liliaceae.

    **A. officinalis,** an edible vegetable, the rhizome and roots of which, together with the young edible shoots, are used as a diuretic.

**aspar'tase.** Aspartate ammonia-lyase.

**aspar'tate.** A salt or ester of aspartic acid.

    **a. aminotransferase** (EC 2.6.1.1), a. transaminase; glutamic oxaloacetic transaminase (GOT, sometimes SGOT for serum aspartate aminotransferase); an enzyme catalyzing the transfer of an amine group from glutamic acid to oxaloacetic acid, forming α-ketoglutaric acid and aspartic acid, or *vice versa.* The serum level of this enzyme is increased in myocardial infarction and in diseases involving destruction of liver cells.

    **a. ammonia-lyase** (EC 4.3.1.1), an enzyme catalyzing the conversion of aspartic acid to fumaric acid, splitting out ammonia. Also called aspartase.

    **a. carbamoyltransferase** (EC 2.1.3.2), enzyme catalyzing formation of ureidosuccinate (*N*-carbamoylaspartate) by the transfer of carbamoyl from carbamoylphosphate to the α-NH₂ of aspartate.

    **a. decarboxylases,** enzymes removing one or the other CO₂ from aspartate, denoted as aspartate 1-decarboxylase (formerly EC 4.1.1.11, now included with glutamate decarboxylase, EC 4.1.1.15) and aspartate 4-decarboxylase (EC 4.1.1.12), respectively.

    **a. kinase** (EC 2.7.2.4), an enzyme catalyzing the phosphorylation by ATP of aspartate to 4-phosphoaspartate (β-aspartyl phosphate.

    **a. transaminase,** a. aminotransferase.

**aspartate 4-decarboxylase.** Aspartate β-decarboxylase; a carboxy-lyase (EC 4.1.1.12) converting aspartate to alanine, releasing CO₂, also decarboxylating aminomalonate and (in bacteria) removing SO₂ from cysteinesulfinate (see desulfinase).

**aspar'tic acid.** α-Aminosuccinic acid; asparaginic acid; HOOCCHNH₂CH₂COOH; one of the amino acids occurring in proteins.

    **a. acid decarboxylase,** see aspartate decarboxylase.

**aspar'tyl.** The aminoacyl radical of aspartic acid.

**β-aspartyl(acetylglucosamine).** Misnomer for *N*β-asparagino-*N*-acetylglucosamine or *N*β-aspartamido-*N*-acetylglucosamine, or, formally, L-β-aspartamido-2-acetamido-1,2-dideoxy-β-D-glucose; a compound of *N*-acetylglucosamine and asparagine, linked via the amide nitrogen of the latter and carbon-1 of the former.

**aspar'tylgly'cosamine.** Generic term for compounds of asparagine and a 2-amino sugar; see β-aspartyl(acetylglucosamine), the chief representative.

**aspartylglycosaminuria** (as-par'til-gli-ko'să-mī-nu'rī-ah). A disorder of glycoprotein catabolism characterized by the presence of an aspartylglycosamine in the urine and a gargoyle-like syndrome: progressive mental retardation, coarse face, impaired speech and motor function, connective tissue and skeletal changes; autosomal recessive inheritance.

**β-aspartyl phosphate.** H₂O₃PCOCH₂CHNH₂COOH; 4-phosphoaspartate.

**aspecific** (a'spe-sif'ik). Not specific.

**as'pect** [ L. *aspectus*, fr. *a-spicio*, pp. *-spectus*, to look at ]. 1. Appearance; looks. 2. The side of an object that is directed in any designated direction.

**as'per** [ L. ] [ NA ]. Rough.

**Aspergillales** (as'pur-jil'a-lez). An order of the Ascomycetes that includes the molds *Aspergillus* and *Penicillium.*

**aspergillic acid** (as-per-jil'ik). 2-Hydroxy-3-isobutyl-6-(1-methylpropyl)pyrazine-1-oxide; produced by *Aspergillus flavus;* an antibiotic agent moderately active against Gram-positive and Gram-negative bacteria; toxic to animal tissues.

**aspergil'lin.** A black pigment obtained from various species of *Aspergillus;* improperly used to designate various antibiotics obtained from *Aspergillus.*

**aspergilloma** (as'pur-jil-o'mah). An infectious granuloma caused by *Aspergillus.*

**aspergillomycosis** (as'pur-jil'o-mi-ko'sis). Mycotic infection with *Aspergillus* organisms.

**aspergillosis** (as-pur-jil-o'sis). 1. The presence of any species of *Aspergillus* in the tissues or on a mucous surface of man and animals, and the symptoms produced thereby. 2. Infection of the lungs and air sacs of birds, especially chickens and turkeys, with a common mold, *Aspergillus fumigatus.* Frequently introduced in spoiled, moldy feed, the disease often destroys whole flocks.

    **aural a.,** otomycosis due to an *Aspergillus* organism.

    **bronchopulmonary a.,** pulmonary a.

    **pulmonary a.,** bronchopulmonary a.; an inflammatory and destructive disease of the bronchi and lungs due to the pressure and growth of *Aspergillus fumigatus,* associated with recurrent pulmonary segmental consolidation, obstruction of segmental bronchi by mucous plugs, and bronchiectasis.

**Aspergillus,** pl. **aspergil'li** (as-pur-jil'us) [ Mediev L. a sprinkler, fr. L. *aspergo,* to sprinkle ]. A genus of fungi of the class Ascomycetes. It contains many species of molds, several with black, brown, or green spores.

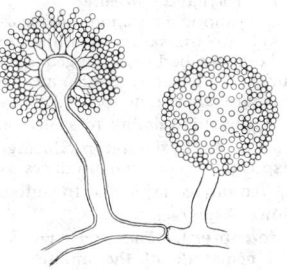

*Aspergillus*
Showing cross section (*left*)

    **A. auricular'is,** a. *niger,* a species found in the external auditory meatus; see otomycosis. It is used commercially in place of malt for the conversion of starch to fermentable sugars.

    **A. bouffardi,** a fungus seen in Bouffardi's black grain mycetoma.

    **A. clavatus,** yields an antibiotic substance known as clavacin; isolated from soil and feces.

    **A. flaves'cens,** a pathogenic form with yellowish spores.

    **A. flavus,** a form with yellow spores. It produces the antibiotic aspergillic acid. It has been isolated from the human external ear.

    **A. fumigatus,** yields the antibiotics fumigacin and fumigatin. This fungus is the common cause of aspergillosis in man and birds.

    **A. glaucus,** a blue-green mold on fruit; a common saprophyte.

    **A. mucuroid'es,** a form found in the lungs.

    **A. nid'ulans,** a species that causes one form of white mycetoma.

    **A. niger,** a pathogenic form, with black spores, often present in the external auditory meatus. Citric and gluconic acids are manufactured commercially by the use of *A. niger.*

    **A. terreus,** produces the antibiotic citrinin; has been isolated from otomycosis.

**aspermatism** (a-sper'mă-tizm) [ G. *a-* priv. + *sperma,* seed ]. Aspermia; lack of secretion or of expulsion of semen.

**aspermatogen'ic** [ G. *a-* priv. + *sperma,* seed, + suffix -*gen,* production ]. Failing in the production of spermatozoa.

**asper'mia.** Aspermatism.

**asper'sion** [ L. *aspersio*, a sprinkling ]. A form of hydrotherapy in which water of a given temperature is sprinkled on the body.

**aspheric** (a-sfer'ik) [ G. *a*-priv. + *sphaira*, sphere ]. Denoting a lens or mirror with paraboloidal surface that eliminates spherical aberration.

**asphyctic** (as-fik'tik). 1. Relating to or suffering from asphyxia. 2. Pulseless.

**asphyg'mia** (as-fig'mī-ah) [ G. *a*- priv. + *sphygmos*, pulse ]. Temporary absence of pulse.

**asphyxia** (as-fik'sī-ah) [ G. *a*- priv. + *sphyzō*, to throb. SPHYG- ]. Asphyxiation; impaired exchange of oxygen and carbon dioxide, usually on a ventilatory, not circulatory, basis; combined hypercarbia and hypoxia or anoxia.
  **blue a.,** a. livida.
  **cyanotic a.,** traumatic a.
  **a. liv'ida,** blue a.; a form of a. neonatorum in which the skin is cyanotic, but the heart is strong and the reflexes are preserved. Prognosis is usually good.
  **local a.,** stagnation of the circulation, sometimes resulting in local gangrene especially of the fingers; one of the symptoms usually associated with the local syncope of Raynaud's disease.
  **a. neonato'rum,** a. occurring in the newborn.
  **a. pal'lida,** a form of a. of the newborn, in which the skin is pale, the pulse weak and slow, and the reflexes abolished. Prognosis is usually poor.
  **symmetric a.,** Raynaud's *disease.*
  **traumatic a.,** cyanotic a.; ecchymotic mask; the extravasation of blood into the skin and conjunctivae, formerly common in those who had been hanged; seen occasionally in crush injuries; produced by sudden mechanical increase in venous pressure, analogous to the Rumpel-Leede sign.

**asphyx'ial.** Asphyctic; relating to asphyxia.

**asphyx'iant.** 1. Asphyxiating; producing asphyxia. 2. Anything, especially a gas, that produces asphyxia.

**asphyx'iate.** To induce asphyxia; to suffocate.

**asphyx'ia'tion.** Asphyxia.

**Aspiculuris tetraptera.** The mouse pinworm; an abundant oxyurid nematode of the mouse cecum or large intestine, along with another common oxyurid pinworm of mice, *Syphacia obvelata;* it is also found in other rodents, including *Rattus.*

**aspidin.** A toxic active principle, $C_{25}H_{32}O_8$, contained in aspidium.

**aspid'inol.** An alcohol, $C_{12}H_{16}O_4$, occurring in aspidium.

**aspid'ium** [ G. *aspidion*, a little shield, dim. of *aspis*, shield ]. Male fern (BP); filix mas; the rhizomes and stipes of *Dryopteris filix-mas* (European a. or male fern), or of *Dryopteris marginalis* (American a. or marginal fern) (family Polypodiaceae). The BP recognizes the rhizome, frond-bases and apical bud of *D. filix-mas* only. Used in the treatment of tapeworm infestation, usually in the form of the oleoresin or extract.
  **a. oleoresin,** male fern oleoresin; extract of male fern; used as a tapeworm anthelmintic; because of its potential toxicity, its use is restricted to patients who do not respond to treatment with safer drugs such as dichlorophen, niclosamide, or quinacrine.

**as'pidosam'ine.** A strong base, $C_{22}H_{28}N_2O_2$, derived from aspidosperma, or quebracho; a toxic irritant.

**Aspidosperma** (as'pĭ-do-sper'mah). A genus of trees of the family Apocynaceae. The dried bark of *A. quebrachoblanco* is the drug quebracho, which has been used as a respiratory stimulant.

**as'pidosper'mine.** A base, vallesine, $C_{22}H_{30}N_2O_2$, obtained from aspidosperma, or quebracho; an irritant.

**aspirate** (as'pĭ-rāt) [ L. *a-spiro*, pp. *-atus*, to breathe on, give the H sound ]. 1. A sound having the breathing character of the letter *h.* 2. To remove by negative pressure, suction, or aspiration.

**aspira'tion.** 1. Removal, by suction, of air or fluid from a body cavity, from a region where unusual collections have accumulated, or from a container. 2. The inspiratory sucking into the airways of fluid or foreign body, as the a. of vomitus. 3. A surgical technique for congenital cataracts, requiring only a small corneal incision, severance lens capsule, lens material well stirred, and aspiration with

an 18-gauge blunt needle. 4. A strong desire, longing, or ambition to obtain or achieve.

**as'pirator.** An apparatus for removing fluid by aspiration from any of the body cavities; it consists usually of a hollow needle or trocar and cannula, connected by rubber tubing with a bottle or metal cylinder from which the air is exhausted by means of a syringe or reversed air pump.
  **water a.,** a jet ejector pump operated by water and commonly used as a laboratory suction pump.

**as'pirin** (USP, BP). Acetylsalicylic acid; $C_6H_4(OCOCH_3)$-COOH; readily absorbed from mucous membranes, and excreted in urine within 6 hours; widely used as an analgesic and antipyretic, and in the treatment of rheumatism.

**asple'nia.** Absence of the spleen.

**asplen'ic.** Having no spleen.

**Asple'nium.** A genus of ferns (family Polypodiaceae), sometimes thought to have vermicidal actions.
  **A. adian'tum,** black maidenhair; the extracts are mildly stimulant and astringent.

**asporogen'ic.** Asporogenous.

**asporogenous** (as-po-roj'en-us) [ G. *a*- priv. + *sporos*, seed, + suffix *-gen*, production ]. Asporogenic; not producing spores.

**aspor'ous** [ G. *a*-priv. + *sporos*, seed ]. Having no spores.

**aspor'ulate.** Nonsporeforming.

**assassin bug.** Insect of the family Reduviidae, order Hemiptera, which inflicts irritating, painful bites in animals and man.

**assay** (as'sā, ă-sā'). 1. Analysis; test of purity; trial. 2. To examine; to subject to analysis.
  **biologic a.,** bioassay.
  **immunochemical a.,** immunoassay.

**assem'bly** [ O.Fr. *assembler*, to assemble ]. The act or process of bringing together parts to form a complete unit.
  **cell a.,** in psychology, a hypothetical unit of interacting neural pathways within the brain.

**Assézat** (ah-sa-zā'), Jules, French anthropologist, 1832–1876. See A.'s *triangle.*

**assim'ilable.** Capable of being assimilated.

**assimila'tion** [ L. *as-similo*, pp. *-atus*, to make alike ]. 1. The incorporation of digested materials from food, into the tissues of the organism. 2. The amalgamation and modification of newly perceived information and experiences into the existing cognitive structure.
  **primary a.,** chylopoiesis.
  **reproductive a.,** in sensorimotor theory, an active cognitive process by which past experience is applied to novel situations.

**Assmann,** Herbert, German internist, 1882–1950. See A.'s tuberculous *infiltrate.*

**asso'ciate.** 1. Any item or individual grouped with others by some common factor. 2. To accomplish association.
  **paired a.'s,** words, syllables, digits, or other items learned in pairs, so that when one is given, its a. is to be recalled.

**association** (ă-so'sī-a'shun) [ L. *as-socio*, pp. *-sociatus*, to join to; *ad Ā socius*, companion ]. Union; connection of persons, things, or ideas by some common factor. 2. A functional two ideas, events, or psychological phenomena that is established through learning or experience. See conditioning.
  **clang a.,** psychic a.'s that are the result of sounds or clangs; often encountered in the manic phase of manic-depressive psychosis.
  **dream a.'s,** the memories and emotions which arise when a patient tries to understand a dream.
  **free a.,** An investigative psychoanalytic technique in which the patient verbalizes, with reservation or censor, the passing contents of his mind; the verbalized conflicts that emerge constitute resistances tht are the basis of the psychoanalyst's interpretations.

**associationism** (ă-so'sī-a'shun-izm). In psychology, the theory that man's understanding of the world occurs through ideas associated with sensory experience rather than through innate ideas.

**asso'cius** [ L. ] [ NA ]. Associated with.

**as'sonance.** Similarity in vowel sounds.

**astasia** (ă-sta'zĭ-ah) [ G. unsteadiness, from *a*- priv. + *stasis*, standing. STA- ]. Inability, through muscular incoordination, to stand.

**asta'sia-aba'sia.** Blocq's disease; the inability to either stand or walk in the normal manner; the person affected seems to collapse when attempting to walk, as if to prove that he cannot do so; a symptom of conversion hysteria.

**astat'ic.** Pertaining to astasia.

**as'tatine** [ G. *astatos*, unstable ]. An artificial radioactive element of the halogen series; symbol At, atomic number 85.

**asteatodes** (ă'ste-ă-to'dēz). Asteatosis.

**asteatosis** (ă-ste-ă-to'sis) [ G. *a*- priv. + *stear* (*steat*-), fat ]. Diminished or arrested action of the sebaceous glands.

 **a. cutis,** dry, scaly integument with decrease in sebaceous secretion.

**as'ter** [ Mod. L. fr. G. *astēr*, a star ]. Astrosphere.

 **sperm a.,** see sperm-aster.

**astereognosis** (ă-ster'e-og-no'sis) [ G. *a*- priv. + *stereos*, solid, + *gnōsis*, knowledge ]. Stereoagnosis; stereoanesthesia; loss of the power of judging the form of an object by touch.

**aste'rion** [ G. *asterios*, starry ]. A craniometric point in the region of the posterolateral, or mastoid, fontanel, at the junction of the lambdoid, occipitomastoid and parietomastoid sutures. See fig. under craniometric *point*.

**asterixis** (ă-ster-ik'sis) [ G. *a*- priv. + *stērixis*, fixed position ]. An abnormal flapping tremor consisting of involuntary jerking movements, especially in the hands, best elicited by having the patient extend his arms, dorsiflex his wrists, and spread his fingers. Commonly called a "liver flap" because of its frequent occurrence in patients with impending hepatic coma, although it also may be seen in other forms of metabolic encephalopathy.

**aster'nal** [ G. *a*- priv. + *sternon*, chest ]. Not related to or connected with the sternum, *e.g.*, a. rib. 2. Without a sternum.

**aster'nia.** The condition of being without a sternum.

**Asterococcus** (as-ter-o-kok'kus) [ Mod. L. fr. G. *astēr*, a star, + *kokkos*, a berry ]. *Mycoplasma*.

**as'teroid** [ G. *astēr*, star, + *eidos*, resemblance ]. Resembling a star.

**as'terotoxin.** A poison obtained from the starfishes, Asteroidea.

**asthenia** (as-the'nĭ-ah) [ G. *astheneia*, weakness, fr. *a*- priv. + *sthenos*, strength. STHEN- ]. Weakness; debility.

 **a. gra'vis hypophy'seogen'ea,** severe weakness from loss of pituitary function.

 **neu'rocir'culatory a.,** effort syndrome; irritable heart; soldier's heart; anxiety; a syndrome of functional nervous and circulatory irregularities characterized by increased susceptibility to fatigue, palpitation, dyspnaea, rapid pulse, precordial pain, and anxiety; observed especially in soldiers on active duty but also in civil life.

 **a. pigmento'sa,** Addison's *disease*.

**asthen'ic.** Relating to asthenia; weak.

**asthenocoria** (as-the'no-ko'rĭ-ah) [ G. *astheneia*, weakness, + *korē*, pupil of the eye ]. Slow reaction of the pupil to the light stimulus.

**asthenom'eter** [ G. *astheneia*, weakness, + *metron*, measure ]. 1. An instrument for measuring the degree of asthenopia. 2. An instrument for measuring the degree of muscular weakness or strength; dynamometer.

**as'thenope.** An individual with asthenopia.

**astheno'pia** [ G. *astheneia*, weakness, + *ōps*, eye ]. Subjective symptoms arising from use of the eyes; see also eyestrain.

 **accom'modative a.,** a. due to errors of refraction and the consequent strain on the ciliary muscle.

 **muscular a.,** a. due to imbalance of the extrinsic ocular muscles.

 **nervous a.,** a. due to functional or organic nervous disease.

 **neurasthenic a.,** a. due to neurasthenia, frequently after a debilitating disease.

 **retinal a.,** neurasthenic a.

 **tarsal a.,** a. due to abnormal pressure of the eyelids on the globe of the eye.

**asthenop'ic.** Relating to or suffering from asthenopia.

**asthenopyra** (as-the'no-pi'rah) [ G. *astheneia*, weakness, + *pyr*, fire ]. A weak or low grade fever.

**asthe'nosper'mia** [ G. *astheneia*, weakness, + *sperma*, seed, semen ]. Loss or reduction of motility of the spermatozoa, frequently associated with infertility.

**asthma** (az'mah) [ G. ]. Originally, a term used to mean "difficult breathing"; the present trend is to use this term to denote bronchial a. (*q.v.*) and to discard all other usages, such as cardiac a., renal a., and the like.

 **atop'ic a.,** dyspnea not due to cardiac, renal, or thymic disease, chronic bronchitis, emphysema, or external allergens.

 **bronchial a.,** a condition of the lungs in which there is widespread narrowing of airways, varying over short periods of time either spontaneously or as a result of treatment; the narrowing is due in varying degrees to contraction (spasm) of smooth muscle, edema of the mucosa, and mucus in the lumen of the bronchi and bronchioles; these changes ae caused by the local release of spasmogens and vasoactive substances (*e.g.*, histamine, or the slow-reacting substance of anaphylaxis) in the course of an allergic process.

 **bronchit'ic a.,** catarrhal a.

 **cardiac a.,** cardiasthma; an asthmatic attack, the bronchoconstriction being secondary to the pulmonary congestion and edema of left ventricular failure.

 **catar'rhal a.,** bronchitic a.; spasmodic dyspnea accompanying bronchitis.

 **Cheyne-Stokes a.,** the dyspnea of advanced myocardial degeneration.

 **Elsner's a.,** *angina* pectoris.

 **essential a.,** nervous a.; a. occurring without any perceptible changes in the bronchial mucous membrane.

 **extrinsic a.,** bronchial a. resulting from an allergic reaction to foreign substances, such as inhaled particles, vapors, or gases, or ingested foods, beverages, or drugs.

 **grinder's a.,** the dyspnea of siderosis or silicosis.

 **hay a.,** the asthmatic stage of hay fever.

 **Heberden's a.,** *angina* pectoris.

 **horse a.,** a. caused by sensitivity to the hair, dander, or other emanations from horses.

 **hyperthyroid a.,** asthmatic attacks occurring in toxic goiter, sometimes probably caused by congestive failure and sometimes related to thyroid crises.

 **intrinsic a.,** bronchial a. in which no extrinsic causes can be identified, and which is assumed to be due to an endogenous process, possibly allergic.

 **miller's a.,** a. caused by flour or grain allergens.

 **miner's a.,** the dyspnea of anthracosis.

 **nervous a.,** essential a.

 **potter's a.,** the dyspnea of pneumoconiosis.

 **printer's a.,** a. occurring in printers exposed to certain allergens used in color printing. At the present time this is extremely rare.

 **reflex a.,** symptomatic a.

 **renal a.,** the dyspnea accompanying disease of the kidneys.

 **spasmodic a.,** a. due to spasm of the bronchioles.

 **steam-fitter's a.,** a. associated with asbestosis.

 **stone a.,** a feeling of pressure and burning pain in the chest, caused by the presence of a bronchial calculus, relieved at once when the concretion is dislodged by a violent paroxysm of coughing.

 **stripper's a.,** a. associated with byssinosis.

 **summer a.,** a. associated with rose cold or hay fever.

 **symptomatic a.,** reflex a.; a. occurring as a reflex in disease of the viscera, the nose, or other parts.

**asthmatic** (az-mat'ik). Relating to or suffering from asthma.

**asthma-weed.** 1. Lobelia. 2. *Euphorbia pilulifera*.

**asthmogenic** (az'mo-jen'ik). Causing asthma.

**astig'magraph.** An instrument for demonstrating the presence of astigmatism.

**astigmatic** (as'tig-mat'ik). Relating to or suffering from astigmatism.

**astigmatism** (ă-stig'mă-tizm) [ G. *a*- priv. + *stigma* (*stigmat*-), a point. STIG- ]. A condition of unequal curvatures along the different meridians in one or more of the refractive surfaces (cornea, anterior or posterior surface of the lens) of the eye, in consequence of which the rays from a luminous point are not focused at a single point on the retina, but are spread out as a line in one or another direction.

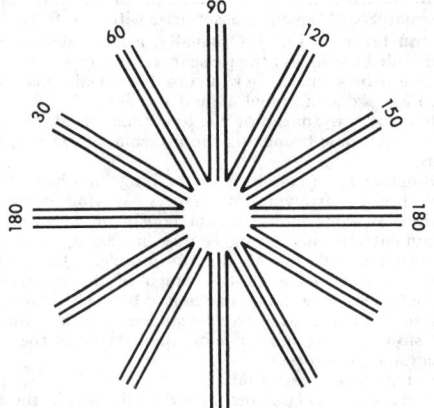

The Clock Dial for Testing Astigmatism

**a. against the rule,** reversed a.; a. when the greater curvature or refractive power is in the horizontal meridian.

**a. with the rule,** direct a.; a. when the greater curvature or refractive power is in the vertical meridian.

**compound hyperop'ic a.,** a. in which both vertical and horizontal meridians are hyperopic.

**compound myop'ic a.,** a. in which both vertical and horizontal meridians are myopic.

**cor'neal a.,** a. due to defect in the curvature of the corneal surface.

**direct a.,** a. with the rule.

**irregular a.,** a. in which different parts of the same meridian have different degrees of curvature.

**lentic'ular a.,** a. due to defect in the curvature or position of the lens.

**mixed a.,** a. in which the vertical or horizontal meridian is hyperopic while the other is myopic.

**myopic a.,** that form of a. in which the abnormality in curvature or in the refractive power of the media brings the focus in front of the retina.

**regular a.,** a. in which the curvature in each meridian is equal throughout its course, and the meridians of greatest and least curvature are practically at right angles to each other.

**reversed a.,** a. against the rule.

**simple hyperop'ic a.,** a. in which the curvature in one meridian is hyperopic while that of the meridian at right angles to it is normal, or emmetropic.

**simple myop'ic a.,** a. in which the curvature of either the vertical or the horizontal meridian is myopic while that of the other is normal.

**astigmatom'eter, astigmom'eter.** An instrument for measuring the degree and determining the variety of astigmatism.

**astigmatom'etry, astigmom'etry.** Determination of the form and measurement of the degree of astigmatism.

**astigmat'oscope.** Astigmoscope; an instrument for detecting and measuring the degree of astigmatism.

**astigmatos'copy.** Astigmoscopy; the use of the astigmatoscope.

**astig'mia.** Astigmatism.

**astig'mic.** Astigmatic.

**astig'moscope.** Astigmatoscope.

**astigmos'copy.** Astigmatoscopy.

**asto'matous.** Without a mouth.

**astomia** (ă-sto'mǐ-ah) [ G. *a*- priv. + *stoma*, mouth ]. The condition of having no mouth.

**as'tomous.** Astomatous.

**astrag'alar.** Relating to the astragalus or talus.

**astrag'alec'tomy** [ astragalus, + G. *ektomē*, excision ]. Removal of the astragalus, or talus.

**astrag'alocalca'nean.** Relating to both the astragalus, or talus, and the calcaneus, or os calcis.

**astrag'alofib'ular.** Relating to both the astragalus, or talus, and the fibula.

**astrag'aloscaph'oid.** Talonavicular; relating to both the astragalus, or talus, and the scaphoid or navicular bone.

**astrag'alotib'ial.** Relating to both the astragalus, or talus, and the tibia.

**astrag'alus** [ G. *astragalos*, ball of the ankle joint. ASTRAG- ]. Talus.

**Astrag'alus.** A genus of plants (family Leguminosae), notably *A. mollissimus* (locoweed), on the range lands of western North America; capable of taking selenium from the soil, causing poisoning in sheep, cattle, and horses. *A. gummate* is a source of tragacanth. The common species of North America are called milk vetch. The genus is among the largest, containing approximately 1600 species.

**as'tral.** Relating to an astrosphere.

**astrapophobia** (as'trah-po-fo'bǐ-ah) [ G. *astrapē*, lightning, + *phobos*, fear ]. Morbid fear of lightning.

**astriction** (as-trik'shun). 1. Constipation. 2. Astringent action. 3. Compression for the arrest of hemorrhage.

**astringent** (as-trin'jent) [ L. *astringens* ]. 1. Causing contraction of the tissues. 2. Arresting secretion. 3. Styptic; arresting hemorrhage. 4. An agent that causes contraction of the tissues, arrest of the secretion, or the control of bleeding.

**as'trobiol'ogy.** The branch of biology concerned with study of life on planets or satellite bodies.

**as'troblast** [ G. *astron*, star, + *blastos*, germ ]. A primitive cell developing into an astrocyte.

**as'troblasto'ma.** Grade II astrocytoma; grade III astrocytoma; a relatively poorly differentiated glioma composed of young, immature, neoplastic cells of the astrocytic series in a somewhat scanty stroma of delicate fibrillary material; the cells frequently manifest a radial arrangement about small blood vessels, being attached to the walls of the vessels by means of short fibrils that terminate in so-called "sucker feet." A.'s usually grow more rapidly and invade more irregularly that astrocytomas, and the average survival (after symptoms develop) is approximately 24 to 28 mo., *i.e.*, from one-half to one-third that observed with astrocytomas; approximately two-thirds occur in the cerebrum, and the cerebellum is the second most frequent site.

**astrocele** (as'tro-sēl) [ G. *astron*, star, + *koilia*, hollow ]. Centrosphere.

**as'trocyte** [ G. *astron*, star, + *kytos*, hollow (cell) ]. Astroglia; macroglia; spider cell (1); Cajal's cell (2); Deiter's cell (2); one of the large neuroglia cells of nervous tissue. See also neuroglia.

**ameboid a.,** protoplasmic a. (1).

**fibrous a.,** stellate cell with long processes found in the white substance of the brain and spinal cord and characterized by having bundles of fine filaments in its cytoplasm.

**protoplasmic a.,** (1) gemistocyte; gemästete cell; ameboid a. or cell; reactive a. or cell; gemistocytic a. or cell; a swollen neural cell possessing a well defined acidophilic cytoplasm; (2) one form of a., found in gray substance, having few fibrils and numerous branching processes.

**reactive a.,** protoplasmic a. (1).

**astrocyto'ma** [ G. *astron*, star, + *kytos*, cell, + suffix *-oma*, tumor ]. A relatively well differentiated glioma composed of neoplastic cells that resemble one of the types of astrocytes, with varying amounts of fibrillary stroma; a.'s in children and persons less than 20 years of age usually arise in a cerebellar hemisphere, and there is a reasonably good prognosis if the neoplasm is resected; a's in adults usually occur in the cerebrum, are frequently only moderately or poorly differentiated, and the prognosis is not as good as in the a.'s in children; in adults, the neoplasms sometimes grow rapidly and invade extensively.

**chiasmatic a.,** a. of the optic chiasm; it is often of piloid type and slow-growing.

**gemistocytic a.,** protoplasmic a.

**grade I a.,** solid or cystic a. of high differentiation.

**grade II a.,** astroblastoma.

**grade III a.,** astroblastoma.

**grade IV a.,** glioblastoma multiforme.

**piloid a.,** a slowing growing a. composed histologically of elongated fibrous astrocytes; often located in the optic chiasm or hypothalamus.

**protoplasmic a.,** gemistocytoma; gemistocytic a.; a neoplasm composed of large, plump, swollen, acidophilic astrocytes.

**as'trocyto'sis.** An increase in the number of astrocytes, frequently observed in an irregular, poorly or moderately well defined zone adjacent to degenerative lesions (*e.g.,* encephalomalacia), focal inflammations (*e.g.,* abscesses), or certain neoplasms in the brain; in some instances, a. may be diffuse in a relatively large region; a. represents a reparative defense mechanism.

**a. cer'ebri,** *glioblastosis* cerebri.

**astroependymoma** (as'tro-e-pen'dī-mo'mah). Mixed glioma; a glial neoplasm composed of a mixed population of astrocytic and ependymal cells.

**astrog'lia** [ G. *astron,* star, + neuroglia ]. Astrocyte.

**as'troid** [ G. *astroeidēs,* fr. *astron,* star, + *eidos,* resemblance ]. Star-shaped.

**as'trokinet'ic.** Relating to movement of the centrosome and astrosphere of a dividing cell.

**astrosphere** (as'tro-sfēr) [ G. *astron,* star, + *sphaira,* ball ]. Aster; an attraction sphere; Lavdovsky's nucleoid; set of radiating fibrils extending outward from the cytocentrum and centrosphere of a dividing cell.

**Astwood,** Edwin B., American endocrinologist, *1909. See A.'s *test.*

**astyclinic** (as'tī-klin'ik) [ G. *asty,* city, + *klinē,* bed ]. Polyclinic.

**astysia** (a-stī'zī-ah) [ G. *a-* priv. + *stuein,* to erect, stiffen ]. Sexual impotence.

**asurre'nalism, asu'prarenalism.** State of adrenal absence or adrenocortical insufficiency.

**asverin.** 1-Methyl-3-piperidylidenedi(2-thienyl)methane; antitussive.

**Asx.** Symbol meaning "Asp or Asn."

**asyllabia** (a-sil-la'bī-ah) [ G. *a-* priv. + *syllablē,* syllable ]. A form of alexia in which one recognizes the individual letters, but cannot comprehend them when arranged collectively in syllables or words.

**asylum** (ă-si'lum) [ L. fr. G. *asylon,* a sanctuary, fr. *a-* priv. + *sylē,* right of seizure ]. An institution for the housing and care of those who by reason of age or mental or bodily infirmities are unable to care for themselves; colloquialism for insane asylum, which is an obsolete term for mental hospital or state mental hospital.

**asymbolia** (a'sim-bo'lī-ah) [ G. *a-* priv. + *symbolon,* an outward sign. BAL- ]. 1. A loss of the power of appreciation by touch of the form and nature of an object. 2. Sign blindness; asemasia; asemia; a form of aphasia in which the significance of signs is not appreciated.

**asymmet'rical.** Not symmetrical; denoting a lack of symmetry between two or more like parts.

**asym'metry.** 1. Want of symmetry; disproportion between two or more like parts. 2. Significant difference in amplitude or frequency of two brain wave tracings taken simultaneously from the two sides of the brain under identical conditions of recording.

**asymptomat'ic.** Without symptoms, or producing no symptoms.

**asynclitism** (ă-sin'klī-tizm) [ G. *a-* priv. + *syn-klino,* to incline together ]. Obliquity; absence of synclitism or parallelism between the axis of the presenting part of the child and the pelvic planes in childbirth.

**anterior a.,** Nägele *obliquity.*

**posterior a.,** Litzmann *obliquity.*

**asyndesis** (ă-sin'de-sis) [ G. *a-* priv. + *syn,* together, + *desis,* binding ]. 1. A mental defect in which separate ideas or thoughts cannot be joined into a coherent concept. 2. A breaking up of the connecting links in language, said to be characteristic of language disturbance of schizophrenics.

**asynechia** (a-sī-nek'ī-ah) [ G. *a-* priv. + *synecheia,* continuity ]. Discontinuity of structure.

**asynergia, asynergy** (ă-sin-ur'jī-ah, ă-sin'ur-je) [ G. *a-* priv. + *syn,* with, + *ergon,* work ]. Lack of cooperation or working together of parts that normally act in unison.

**a'syner'gic.** Characterized by asynergia.

**asynesia, asynesis** (ă-sī-ne'zī-ah, a-sī-ne'sis) [ G. *a-* priv. + *synesis,* union, understanding ]. Lack of quick comprehension or mother wit.

**asynodia** (ă-sī-no'dī-ah) [ G. *a-* priv. + *synodia,* a journey together, fr. *syn,* with, + *odos,* road, way ]. Sexual impotence; lack of coincidence in the orgasms in sexual intercourse.

**asyntaxia** (a-sin-tak'sī-ah) [ G. *a-* priv. + *syntaxis,* orderly arrangement ]. Failure of proper embryonic development.

**a. dorsa'lis,** failure of the neural groove to close.

**asystemat'ic.** Not systematic; not relating to one system or set of organs.

**asystole** (ă-sis'to-le) [ G. *a-* priv. + *systolē,* a contracting. STAL- ]. Cardiac standstill; absence of contractions of the heart.

**asysto'lia.** Asystole.

**asystol'ic.** 1. Relating to asystole. 2. Not systolic.

**AT-10.** Dihydrotachysterol.

**atac'tic.** Ataxic.

**atactil'ia** [ G. *a-* priv. + L. *tactilis,* relating to touch, fr. *tango,* pp. *tactus,* to touch ]. Loss of the sense of touch.

**ataractic** (at'ă-rak'tik) [ G. *ataraktos,* calm ]. 1. Ataraxic; having a quietening or tranquilizing effect. 2. A tranquilizer.

**ataraxia** (at'ă-rak'sī-ah) [ G. *a-* priv. + *taraktos,* disturbed, + *-ia* ]. Calmness and peace of mind; imperturbability; tranquility.

**atarax'ic.** Ataractic.

**atav'ic.** Atavistic.

**at'avism** [ L. *atavus,* a remote ancestor ]. The appearance in an individual of characteristics presumed to have been present in some remote ancestor; reversion to an earlier biological type.

**atavis'tic.** Atavic; relating to atavism.

**at'avus** [ L. remote grandfather ] [ NA ]. Throwback; a structure not commonly found in man that resembles a structure known to have existed in remote ancestral forms.

**ataxia** (ă-tak'sī-ah) [ G. *a-* priv. + *taxis,* order. TAX- ]. Dyssynergia; a loss of the power of muscular coordination.

**acute a.,** progressive a. of cerebellar type developing after severe infections.

**Briquet's a.,** weakening of the muscle sense and increased sensibility of the skin, in hysteria.

**Bruns' a.,** difficulty in initiation of movements of the feet when they are in contact with the ground; a condition related to a frontal lobe lesion.

**cerebel'lar a.,** loss of muscular coordination as a result of disease in the cerebellum.

**a. cordis,** atrial *fibrillation.*

**equine spinal a.,** see wobblers.

**Friedreich's a.,** hereditary spinal a.

**hereditary cerebel'lar a.,** Marie's disease (3); Marie's a.; a disease of later childhood and early adult life, marked by ataxic gait, hesitating and explosive speech, nystagmus, and sometimes optic neuritis.

**hereditary spinal a.,** Friedreich's a., heredoataxia; tabes hereditaria; sclerosis of the posterior and lateral columns of the spinal cord, occurring in children; it is marked by a. in the lower extremities, extending to the upper, followed by paralysis and contractures.

**kinetic a.,** motor a.

**Leyden's a.,** pseudotabes.

**locomotor a.** (1) motor a.; (2) *tabes* dorsalis.

**Marie's a.,** hereditary cerebellar a.

**moral a.,** inconstancy of ideas and the will; a manifestation of hysteria.

**motor a.,** kinetic a.; locomotor a.; inability to perform coordinated muscular movements.

**ocular a.,** nystagmus.

**pseudoataxia,** pseudotabes.

**Sanger-Brown a.,** a familial spinocerebellar degeneration.

**spinal a.,** a. due to spinal cord disease, as in tabes dorsalis.

**static a.,** inability to preserve the equilibrium in standing through loss of the deep sensibility.

**a. telangiecta'sia,** Louis-Bar syndrome; a familial syndrome of progressive cerebellar a., with oculocutaneous telangiectases and proneness to pulmonary infections; coarse nystagmoid oscillations appear.

**vasomo'tor a.,** a form of autonomic a. causing irregularity in the peripheral circulation, marked by alternations of pallor and suffusion, due to spasm of the smaller blood vessels.

**atax'iadynam'ia.** Muscular weakness combined with incoordination.

**atax'iagram.** The tracing made by means of an ataxiagraph.

**atax'iagraph.** An instrument for measuring the degree and direction of the swaying of the head in static ataxia; a stylus attached to the top of the head records the movements on a disk supported just above it.

**ataxiaphasia** (ă-tak'sĭ-ă-fa'zĭ-ah) [ G. *a-* priv. + *taxis,* order, + *phasis,* an affirmation, speech ]. Inability to form connected sentences, although single words may perhaps be used intelligibly.

**atax'ic.** Atactic; relating to, marked by, or suffering from ataxia.

**atax'iophe'mia** [ G. *a-* priv. + *taxis,* order, + *phēmē,* voice, speech ]. Incoordination of the muscles concerned in speech production.

**atax'y.** Ataxia.

**atelectasis** (at'e-lek'tă-sis) [ G. *atelēs,* incomplete, + *ektasis,* extension. TEN- ]. Airlessness of the lungs, due to failure of expansion or resorbtion of air from the alveoli. See also pulmonary *collapse.*

**primary a.,** anectasis; nonexpansion of the lungs after birth, found in all stillborn infants and in liveborn infants who die before respiration is established.

**secondary a.,** pulmonary collapse (*q.v.*), particularly of infants, due to hyaline membrane disease or elastic recoil of the lungs while dying from other causes.

**atelectat'ic.** Relating to atelectasis.

**atel'encepha'lia.** Ateloencephalia.

**ate'lia.** Ateliosis.

**ateliosis** (ă-te'lĭ-o'sis) [ G. *atelēs,* incomplete, + suffix *-osis,* condition ]. Atelia; incomplete development of the body or any of its parts, as in infantilism and dwarfism.

**a. cordis,** atelocardia.

**ateliot'ic.** Marked by ateliosis.

**atelo-** (at'e-lo-) [ G. *atelēs,* incomplete, fr. *a-* priv. + *telos,* end, fulfillment ]. Combining form meaning incomplete or imperfect.

**at'elocar'dia** [ atelo- + G. *kardia,* heart ]. Ateliosis cordis; incomplete development of the heart.

**at'eloceph'aly, at'elocepha'lia** [ atelo- + G. *kephalē,* head ]. Incomplete development of the head.

**atelocheilia, atelochilia** (at'e-lo-ki'lĭ-ah) [ atelo- + G. *cheilos,* lip ]. Defective development of the lip; *e.g.,* cleft lip.

**atelocheiria, atelochiria** (at'e-lo-ki'rĭ-ah) [ atelo- + G. *cheir,* hand ]. Imperfect development of the hands.

**at'eloenceph'aly, at'eloencepha'lia** [ atelo- + G. *enkephalos,* brain ]. Imperfect formation of the brain structures.

**at'eloglos'sia** [ atelo- + G. *glōssa,* tongue ]. Imperfect development of the tongue.

**atelognathia** (at'e-log-nath'ĭ-ah) [ atelo- + G. *gnathos,* jaw ]. Defective formation of a jaw, especially of the lower jaw.

**atelomyelia** (at'e-lo-mi-e'lĭ-ah) [ atelo- + G. *myelon,* marrow ]. Imperfect development of the spinal cord.

**atelopidtoxin.** A potent dialyzable poison from the skin of the golden arrow frog (*Atelopus zeteki*) of Central and South America; it differs chemically and pharmacologically from other dendrobatid frog toxins that have been used as arrow-tip poisons.

**atelopodia** (at'e-lo-po'dĭ-ah) [ atelo- + G. *pous,* foot ]. Imperfect formation of the feet.

**at'eloproso'pia** [ atelo- + G. *prosōpon,* face ]. Imperfect development of the face.

**atelorrhachidia** (at'el-o-ră-kid'ĭ-ah) [ atelo- + G. *rhachis,* spinal column ]. Defective formation of the vertebral column.

**At'elosac'charomy'ces.** A genus of yeastlike fungi associated with blastomycotic lesions of man but apparently not the causative agent.

**atelostomia** (at'e-lo-sto'mĭ-ah) [ atelo- + G. *stoma,* mouth ]. Imperfect development of the mouth or its contained parts.

**Atetra P.** Abbreviation for adenosine tetraphosphate.

**athe'lia** [ G. *a-* priv. + *thēlē,* nipple ]. Absence of the nipples.

**ather'mancy** [ G. *athermantos,* not heated, fr. *a-* priv. + *thermaino,* to heat, fr. *thermē,* heat ]. Impermeability to heat.

**ather'manous.** Absorbing radiant heat; not permeable to heat rays.

**ather'mic.** Apyretic.

**ather'mosystal'tic** [ G. *a-* priv. + *thermos,* hot, + *systaltikos,* constringent. STAL- ]. Not contracted or constricted by ordinary variations of temperature; said of certain tissues.

**athero-** [ G. *athere,* gruel ]. Combining form relating to the deposit of gruel-like, soft, pasty materials, for example, in arteries.

**atheroembolism** (ath'er-o-em'bo-lizm). Cholesterol *embolism.*

**ath'erogen'esis.** Formation of atheroma, important in the pathogenesis of arteriosclerosis.

**atherogen'ic.** Having the capacity to initiate, increase, or accelerate the process of atherogenesis.

**athero'ma** [ G. *athērē,* gruel, + suffix *-ōma,* tumor ]. Atherosis. 1. Lipid deposits in the intima of arteries producing a yellow swelling on the endothelial surface. 2. The lesions of atherosclerosis.

**athero'matous.** Relating to or affected by atheroma.

**atheronecrosis** (ath'er-o-ne-kro'sis). The regressive alteration accompanying arteriosclerosis.

**atherosclero'sis** (ath'er-o-skle-ro'sis). Nodular sclerosis; arteriosclerosis characterized by lipid deposits in the intima, irregularly distributed in large and medium-sized arteries. The lipid deposits are associated with fibrosis and calcification, and are almost always present to some degree in the middle-aged and elderly. Severe a. leads to reduction of the arterial lumen and predisposes to thrombosis. The resulting ischemic manifestations include angina pectoris and myocardial infarction, strokes, intermittent claudication and gangrene of the lower extremities, and some cases of renal hypertension.

**athero'sis.** Atheroma.

**ath'erothrombo'sis.** Clot formation in an atheromatous vessel.

**ath'etoid.** Resembling athetosis.

**ath'eto'sic, ath'etot'ic.** Pertaining to, or marked by, athetosis.

**atheto'sis** [ G. *athetos,* without position or place. THE- ]. A condition in which there is a constant succession of slow, writhing, involuntary movements of flexion, extension, pronation, and supination of the fingers and hands, and sometimes of the toes and feet.

**double a.,** Vogt *syndrome.*

**double congenital a.,** congenital bilateral a., often associated with spastic paraplegia.

**posthemiplegic a.,** posthemiplegic chorea; abnormal jerking or athetotic movements associated with hemiplegia.

**pupillary a.,** rarely used term meaning hippus.

**athrepsia** (ă-threp'sĭ-ah) [ G. *a-* priv. + *threpsis,* nourishment. TREPH- ]. 1. Marasmus. 2. Term suggested by Ehrlich for the presumed immunity of a host when neoplastic cells failed to grow after injection into the host; thought to result from a deficiency or lack of an essential nutritive substance (or substances) required for development of the neoplastic cells.

**ath'repsy.** Athrepsia.

**athrep'tic.** Relating to athrepsia.

**ath'rocyto'sis.** The capacity of cells to absorb and retain electronegative colloids, as shown by macrophages and at the apical surface of proximal convoluted tubule cells of the kidney.

**athrombia** (ă-throm-bĭ-ah) [ G. *a-* priv. + thrombin, *q.v.* ]. A defect of blood clotting characterized by deficiency in formation of thrombin.

**athymia** (ă-thi'mĭ-ah) [ G. *a-* priv. + *thymos,* mind, also thymus. THYM-1 and THYM-2 ]. 1. Absence of affect or emotivity; morbid impassivity. 2. Athymism; absence of the thymus gland or its secretion.

**athy'mism.** Athymia (2).

**athy'rea.** Athyroidism.

**athy'ria.** Athyroidism.

**athyroidemia** (ă-thi'roy-de'mĭ-ah). Absence of the thyroid secretion and the effect of its loss upon the condition of the blood.

**athy'roidism.** Athyria; athyrea; athyrosis; absence of the thyroid gland or suppression of its secretion.

**athyro'sis.** Athyroidism.

**athyrot'ic.** Relating to athyrosis, or athyroidism.

**atictia** (ă-tik'shĭ-ah) [ G. *a-* priv. + *ticto,* to beget ]. Rarely used term for male sterility.

**atlan'tad.** In a direction toward the atlas.

**atlan'tal.** Atloid; relating to the atlas.

**atlanto-, atlo-** [ G. *atlas, q.v.* ]. Combining forms relating to the atlas.

**atlan'toax'ial.** Atloaxoid; atlantoepistrophic; pertaining to the atlas and the axis; denoting the joint between the two vertebrae.

**atlantodidymus** (at-lan'to-did'ĭ-mus) [ atlanto- + G. *didymos,* twin ]. Atlodidymus; conjoined twins with two heads on one neck and a single body.

**atlantoepistrophic** (at-lan'to-ep'ĭ-strof'ik). Atlantoaxial.

**atlantooccipital** (at-lan'to-ok-sip'ĭ-tal). Atlooccipital; relating to the atlas and the occipital bone.

**atlantoodontoid** (at-lan'to-o-don'toyd). Relating to the atlas and the dens of the axis.

**at'las** [ G. *Atlas,* in Greek mythology a Titan who supported the earth on his shoulders ] [ NA ]. First cervical vertebra, articulating with the occipital bone and rotating around the dens of the axis.

**atlo-.** See atlanto-.

**atloax'oid.** Atlantoaxial.

**atlodid'ymus.** Atlantodidymus.

**at'loid.** Atlantal.

**atlooccipital** (at'lo-ok-sip'ĭ-tal). Atlantooccipital.

**atmiat'rics** [ G. *atmos,* vapor, + *iatrikē,* practice of medicine ]. Atmotherapy; the use of sprays in the treatment of diseases of the respiratory passages.

**atmo-** [ G. *atmos,* vapor. ATM- ]. Prefix denoting steam or vapor, or derived by action of same.

**at'mograph** [ atmo- + G. *graphō,* to write ]. Pneumograph.

**atmol'ysis** [ atmo- + G. *lysis,* dissolution ]. The separation of mixed gases by passing them through a porous diaphragm, the lighter gases diffusing through at a faster rate.

**atmom'eter** [ atmo- + G. *metron,* measure ]. An instrument for measuring the rate of evaporation.

**atmos** [ abbreviation of atmosphere ]. Aer; a unit of air pressure, being the pressure of one dyne per square centimeter.

**at'mosphere** [ atmo- + G. *sphaira,* sphere ]. 1. The air; its composition is: 20.94 per cent oxygen, 0.04 per cent carbon dioxide, 78.03 per cent nitrogen, and 0.99 per cent inert gases. 2. Any gas surrounding a given body; a gaseous medium. 3. A unit of air pressure (see atmos).

**atmos'pheriza'tion.** Conversion of venous into arterial blood.

**at'mother'apy.** Atmiatrics.

**Atmungsferment** [ Ger. ]. Warburg's respiratory enzyme; a system of oxidases that participate in respiratory processes; probably identical with the cytochrome system.

**ato'cia** [ G. *atokia,* fr. *a-* priv. + *tokos,* childbirth ]. 1. Nulliparity. 2. Sterility in the female.

**a'tolide** (USAN). 2-Amino-4'-(diethylamino)-*o*-benzotoluidide; anticonvulsant agent.

**at'om** [ G. *atomos,* indivisible, uncut. TOM- ]. The ultimate particle of an element, believed, prior to the 1890's, to be as indivisible as its name indicates The discovery of radioactivity demonstrated the existence of subatomic particles. The a. is now known to be composed of smaller particles, notably protons, neutrons and electrons, the first two being most of the atomic nucleus.

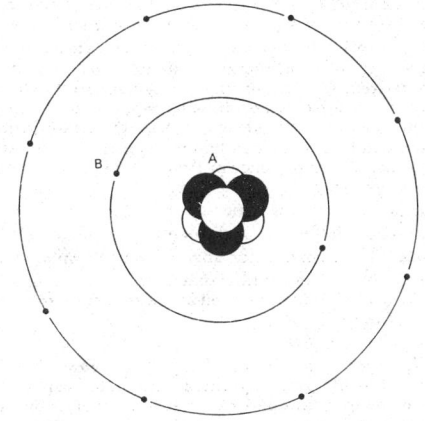

**Structure of the Atom**

*A,* nucleus, containing protons (*open circles*) and neutrons (*black circles*); *B,* electrons, traveling in orbit around nucleus.

**activated a.,** excited a.; an a. possessing more than normal energy as a result of input of energy.

**Bohr's a.,** a concept or model of the a. in which the negatively charged electrons move in circular or elliptical orbits around the positively charged nucleus, energy being emitted or absorbed when electrons change from one orbit to another.

**ionized a.,** an a. that possesses an electrostatic charge as a result of loss or gain of electrons; a monoatomic ion, *e.g.,* H+.

**nuclear a.,** a concept or model of the a. characterized by the presence of a small, massive nucleus at its center (this concept was first advanced by Rutherford).

**radioactive a.,** an a. with an unstable nucleus, which emits particulate or electromagnetic radiation (radiactive emission) to achieve greater stability.

**recoil a.,** the remainder of a. from which a nuclear particle has been emitted or ejected; since this occurs with high velocity, the remainder recoils with a velocity inversely proportional to its mass.

**stripped a.,** an a. minus all its electrons; the nucleus.

**tagged a.,** a radioactive a., or a stable but rare one, which by its presence in a molecule helps identify that molecule; a labeled a.; see also radioactive a.

**atom'ic.** Relating to an atom.

**atomicity** (at-om-is'ĭ-tĭ). 1. The valence or replaceable atoms in a molecule. 2. The number of atoms in a molecule of an element.

**at'omism.** In psychology, the approach to the study of a psychological phenomenon through the analysis of the elementary parts of which it is assumed to be composed; the opposite of holism.

**atomis'tic.** Pertaining to the characteristic of atomism, as opposed to holism; for example, psychoanalysis as opposed to Gestalt psychology.

**atomiza'tion.** Spray production; the reducing of a fluid to small droplets.

**at'omi'zer.** A device for making vapor or spray; see also nebulizer; vaporizer.

**ato'nia** [ G. languor. TEN- ]. Atony.

**aton'ic.** Relaxed; without normal tone or tension.

**atonicity** (at-o-nis'ĭ-tĭ). Atony.

**at'ony** [ *atonia,* languor ]. Atonia; atonicity; relaxation; flaccidity; lack of tone or tension.

**at'open.** The exciting cause of any form of atopy.

**atopic** (ă-top'ik) [ G. *atopos,* out of place ]. Displaced; misplaced; relating to or marked by atopy.

**atopognosia, atopognosis** (ă-top-og-no′zĭ-ah, -og-no′sis) [ G. *a-* priv. + *topos*, place, + *gnōsis*, knowledge ]. Inability to locate a sensation properly.

**atopomenorrhea** (at′o-po-men-or-re′ah) [ G. *atopos*, out of place, + menorrhea ]. Vicarious *menstruation.*

**atopy** (at′o-pĭ) [ G. *atopia*, strangeness, fr. *a-* priv. + *topos*, a place ]. A form of allergy occurring only in man and characterized by: (1) immediate vascular, exudative reaction of the sensitive tissue following exposure to the specific exciting agent; (2) a tendency to acquire certain forms of familial conditions such as hay fever, asthma, and atopic dermatitis; (3) the presence of Prausnitz-Küstner antibodies or atopic reagins.

**atoxic** (a-tok′sik). Not toxic.

**ATP.** Abbreviation for adenosine triphosphate.

**ATPase.** Abbreviation for adenosine triphosphatase.

**ATPD.** Symbol indicating that a gas volume has been expressed as if it had been dried at the ambient temperature and pressure.

**ATP-diphosphatase.** Apyrase.

**ATPS.** Symbol indicating that a gas volume has been expressed as if it were saturated with water vapor at the ambient temperature and barometric pressure; this is the condition of an expired gas equilibrated in a spirometer.

**atrabil′iary** [ L. *atra bilis*, black bile (*cf.* melancholy) ]. Depressed in mind; melancholic.

**atrachelocephalus** (ă-trak′e-lo-sef′a-lus) [ G. *a-* priv. + *trachēlos*, neck, + *kephalē*, head ]. A fetus with its head and neck absent or very poorly developed.

**atractylic acid.** See atractyloside.

**atractyligenin.** See atractyloside.

**atractyloside.** Atractylic acid; potassium atractylate; atractylin; atractosylidic acid; a highly poisonous steroid from *Atractylis gummifera* L. (*Compositae*). with a strychnine-like action, producing convulsions of a hypoglycemic nature. The aglycon, atractyligenin, is combined with glucose and isovaleric acid and is the toxic principle. A. interferes with oxidative reactions, the citric acid cycle, and nerve conduction.

**atranorin.** Parmelin; $C_{19}H_{18}O_8$; isolated from lichens; antimicrobial agent.

**atre′mia** [ G. a keeping still, fr. *a-* priv. + *tremō*, to tremble ]. Absence of tremor.

**atrep′sy** [ G. *a-* priv. + *trephō*, to nourish ]. A condition in which a living virus perishes after inoculation into the tissues because of the absence of adaptable nourishment there; an old hypothesis offered in explanation of certain cases of immunity.

**atrep′tic.** Relating to atrepsy.

**atresia** (ă-tre′zĭ-ah) [ G. *a-* priv. + *trēsis*, a hole ]. Absence of a normal opening or normally patent lumen.

    **anal a.,** a. ani; imperforate anus; congenital absence of an anal opening due to the presence of a membranous septum (persitence of the cloacal membrane), or to complete absence of the anal canal.

    **aortic a.,** congenital absence of the normal valvular orifice into the aorta.

    **biliary a.,** a. of the major bile ducts, causing cholestasis and jaundice; it does not become apparent until several days after birth. Periportal fibrosis develops and leads to cirrhosis, with proliferation of small bile ducts unless these are also atretic. Giant cell transformation of liver cells occurs. See also neonatal *hepatitis.*

    **choanal a.,** congenital failure to open of one or both choanae.

    **esophageal a.,** congenital failure of the full esophageal lumen to develop.

    **a. follic′uli,** a normal process affecting the ovarian primordial follicles in which death of the ovum results in cystic degeneration followed by cicatricial closure.

    **intestinal a.,** an obliteration of the lumen of the small intestine; ileum is involved in 50 per cent of cases, with the jejunum and duodenum following in frequency; most frequent cause of intestinal obstruction in the newborn; etiology may be related to a failure of recanalization during early development or to some impairment of blood supply during intrauterine life.

    **a. iridis,** atretopsia; congenital absence of pupillary opening.

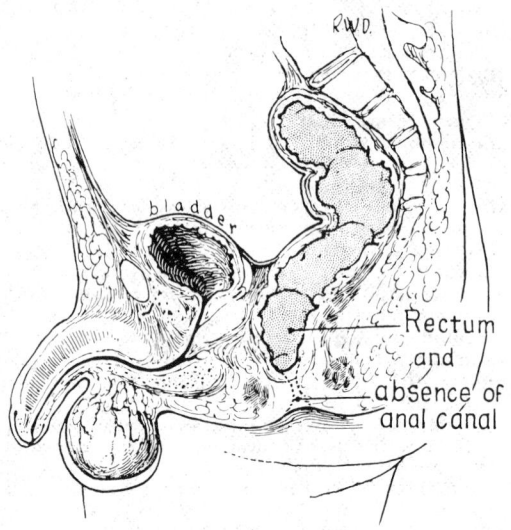

**Anal Atresia**

    **laryngeal a.,** congenital failure of the laryngeal opening to develop, resulting in partial or total obstruction at or just above or below the glottis.

    **mitral a.,** congenital absence of the normal mitral valve orifice.

    **pulmonary a.,** congenital absence of the normal valvular orifice into the pulmonary artery.

    **tricus′pid a.,** congenital lack of the tricuspid orifice.

    **vaginal a.,** colpatresia; imperforation or occlusion of the vagina.

**atre′sic.** Atretic.

**atret′ic.** Atresic; imperforate; lacking a normal opening or a normally patent lumen; relating to atresia.

**atreto-** (ă-tre′to-) [ G. *atrētos*, imperforate ]. A prefix denoting lack of opening of the part named.

**atretoblepharia** (ă-tre′to-blĕ-fa′rĭ-ah) [ atreto- + G. *blepharon*, eyelid ]. Symblepharon.

**atretocystia** (ă-tre′to-sis′tĭ-ah) [ atreto- + G. *kystis*, bladder ]. Lack of opening of a bladder.

**atre′togas′tria** [ atreto- + G. *gastēr*, stomach ]. Lack of opening of the stomach.

**atretop′sia** [ atreto- + G. *ōps*, eye ]. *Atresia* iridis.

**atreturethria** (ă-tre′tu-re′thrĭ-ah). Lack of opening of the urethra.

**atria** (a′trĭ-ah). Plural of atrium.

**atrial** (a′trĭ-al). Relating to an atrium.

**at′rialized.** Incorporated into the atrium, as of part of the right ventricle in Ebstein's anomaly.

**atrican.** MONIFLAGON; *N*-(5-nitro-2-thiazolyl)-2-thiophenecarboxamide; antiprotozoal and antimycotic agent.

**atrichia** (ă-trik′ĭ-ah) [ G. *a-* priv. + *thrix* (*trich-*), hair ]. Atrichosis; absence of hair, congenital or acquired.

**atrichosis** (ă-trik-o′sis). Atrichia.

**atrich′ous.** Without hair.

**atrio-** (a′trĭ-o-) [ L. *atrium, q.v.* ]. Combining form relating to the atrium.

**a′triomeg′aly** [ atrio- + G. *megas*, great ]. Enlargement of the atrium.

**a′trionec′tor** [ atrio- + L. *necto*, to join ]. *Nodus* sinuatrialis.

**atrioseptopexy** (a′trĭ-o-sep′to-pek′sĭ) [ atrio- + L. *septum*, partition, + G. *pexis*, fixation ]. A closed surgical technique for repairing atrial septal defects, in which a portion of the free wall of the right atrium is sutured down to occlude the defect.

**atrioseptoplasty** (a'trī-o-sep'to-plas-tĭ) [ atrio- + L. *septum*, partition, + G. *plassō*, to form ]. Surgical repair of an atrial septal defect.

**atrioseptostomy** (a'trī-o-sep-tos'to-mĭ) [ atrio- + L. *septum*, partition, + G. *stoma*, mouth ]. The establishment of a communication between the two atria of the heart.

   **balloon a.**, a. produced by pulling a balloon-bearing catheter across the interatrial septum for the purpose of establishing an interatrial mixing of blood in the treatment of congenital heart disease.

**a'triotome.** An instrument for opening an atrium.

**atriotomy** (a'trī-ot'o-mĭ) [ atrio- + G. *tomē*, incision ]. Surgical opening of an atrium.

**atrioventricular** (a'trī-o-ven'trik'u-lar). Relating to both the atria and the ventricles of the heart; auriculoventricular.

**atrip'licism** [ L. *atriplex* (-*plic*-), the orach, a vegetable ]. An intoxication caused by the ingestion of certain species of *Atriplex*, eaten as greens in China; it is marked by pain and swelling of the fingers, spreading to the forearm; bullae and ulcers form and the fingers may become gangrenous.

**atrium,** pl. **a'tria** (a'trī-um) [ L. entrance hall ]. 1 [ NA ]. A chamber or cavity to which are connected several chambers or passageways. 2. A. cordis. 3. The tympanum proper, that part of the tympanic cavity that lies immediately to the inner aspect of the drum membrane. 4. A. meatus medii. 5. In the lung, a subdivision of the alveolar duct from which alveolar sacs open.

   **accessory a.**, *cor* triatriatum.

   **a. cordis** [ NA ], a. of the heart; the upper chamber of each half of the heart.

   **a. dextrum** [ NA ], the a. of the right side of the heart which receives the blood from the venae cavae and coronary sinus.

   **a. glot'tidis,** *vestibulum* laryngis.

   **a. of heart,** a. cordis.

   **infection a.,** an obsolete term for the portal of entry of pathogenic microorganisms.

   **a. mea'tus medii** [ NA ], the anterior expanded portion of the middle meatus of the nose, just above the vestibule.

   **a. pulmona'le,** a. sinistrum.

   **a. sinis'trum** [ NA ], a. pulmonale; a. of the left side of the heart which receives the blood from the pulmonary veins.

**atrolact'amide.** THEMISONE; α-hydroxy-α-phenylpropionamide; anticonvulsant.

**At'ropa** [ named for G. *Atropos*, one of the Fates cutting the thread of life, because of the lethal effects of the plant. TREP- ]. A genus of plants (family Solanaceae) of which *A. belladonna* is typical.

   **A. belladon'na,** the source of the drug belladonna; contains atropine and related alkaloids.

   **A. mandrag'ora,** *Mandragora officinarum;* contains atropine alkaloids.

**atroph'ede'ma.** Angioneurotic *edema*.

**atro'phia** [ G. fr. *a*- priv. + *trophē*, nourishment ]. Atrophy.

   **a. bulborum hereditaria,** Norrie's *disease*.

   **a. cutis,** atrophoderma.

   **a. infan'tum,** *tabes* mesenterica.

   **a. maculo'sa cu'tis.** anetoderma.

   **a. musculo'rum lipomato'sa,** pseudohypertrophic muscular *paralysis.*

   **a. pilo'rum pro'pria,** a general term that includes fragilitas crinium, trichorrhexis nodosa, monilethrix, and atrophy of the hair.

**atrophic** (ă-trof'ik). Relating to atrophy; atrophied; characterized by atrophy.

**at'rophied.** Marked by atrophy; wasted.

**atrophoderma** (at'ro-fo-der'mah). Atrophy of the skin; may be discrete localized areas or widespread areas; see also anetoderma.

   **a. al'bidum** [ L. *albidus*, whitish ], a stocking-like type of atrophy affecting the extremities. It is probably congenital and begins in early childhood on the lower limbs. It is a symmetric thinning that renders the parts sensitive.

   **a. biotripticum,** senile cutaneous atrophy.

   **a. diffu'sum,** diffuse idiopathic cutaneous atrophy.

   **a. macula'tum,** primary macular atrophy of the skin; a rare condition in which a macular lesion involutes, leaving a depressed spot.

   **a. neurit'icum,** glossy *skin.*

   **a. pigmento'sum,** *xeroderma* pigmentosum.

   **a. reticula'tum symmet'ricum fa'ciei,** a rarely used term for *folliculitis* ulerythematosa reticulata.

   **senile a., a. seni'lis,** the loss of fat, increased pigmentation and other involuntary changes of the skin in old age.

   **a. stria'tum,** the condition marked by the presence of lineae albicantes.

   **a. vermiculatum,** *folliculitis* ulerythematosa reticulata.

**at'rophodermato'sis.** Any cutaneous affection in which a prominent symptom is skin atrophy.

**atrophy** (at'ro-fī) [ G. *atrophia*, fr. *a*- priv. + *trophē*, nourishment ]. A wasting of tissues, organs or the entire body; it may result from death and reabsorption of cells, diminished cellular proliferation, pressure, ischemia, malnutrition, decreased work, hormone changes.

   **acute yellow a. of the liver,** Rokitansky's disease (1); acute parenchymatous hepatitis; a lesion in which there is extensive and rapid death of parenchymal cells of the liver, sometimes with fatty degeneration, a., softening and shrinkage of the liver, characterized by jaundice, hemorrhage, gastric dysfunction, and mental disorders, usually terminating in coma and death. The necrosis may result from fulminant viral infection or chemical poisoning.

   **alveolar a.,** diminution in size of the supportive tissues of the teeth due to age.

   **arthrit'ic a.,** a. of muscles rendered inactive by a chronically inflamed or fixed joint.

   **blue a.,** depressed blue atrophic scars due to injections in the skin of impure substances; seen in narcotics addicts.

   **brown a.,** a. of the heart wall, probably due to malnutrition especially in the elderly, in which the muscle is dark reddish brown and reduced in volume; the muscle fibers become pigmented especially about the nuclei, by lipochrome granules.

   **Buchwald's a.,** a progressive form of cutaneous a.

   **cerebellar a.,** degeneration of the cerebellum during the course of certain abiotrophic disorders.

   **cerebellar a., nutritional type,** a moderately circumscribed cortical a. restricted largely to the anterior vermis and noted in cachectic patients, particularly those with chronic alcoholism.

   **compensatory a.,** a. especially of an endocrine organ as a result of its function being assumed by a new source of hormone, *e.g.,* the parathyroid glands undergo a. and fail to produce their normal amount of hormone in the presence of an adenoma of parathyroid tissue; testicular, ovarian, or adrenal cortical atrophy may follow prolonged treatment with androgens, estrogens, or adrenal cortical steroids.

   **cyanot'ic a.,** a. due to destruction of the parenchymatous cells of an organ in consequence of chronic venous congestion.

   **cyanotic a. of the liver,** cardiac *cirrhosis.*

   **disuse a.,** a. of a part from long disuse, as that of the muscles or bone, or both, of a fractured limb.

   **Erb's a.,** progressive muscular *dystrophy.*

   **essential progressive a. of iris,** progressive a. of the iris without inflammatory signs, characterized by loss of the epithelium with hole formation, progressive displacement of the pupil, ectropion of the pupillary margin and eventually glaucoma; typically unilateral.

   **exhaustion a.,** a. especially of glandular cells, *e.g.,* islet cells of pancreas or parenchyma of thyroid, from excessive functional activity or overstimulation.

   **facioscapulohumeral a.,** Landouzy and Dejerine *dystrophy.*

   **familial spinal muscular a.,** infantile muscular a.

   **fatty a.,** fatty infiltration secondary to an a. of the essential elements of an organ or tissue.

   **gingival a.,** decrease in size and/or cellular elements of the gingiva; often termed gingival recession.

   **gray a.,** a degeneration of the optic disk in which it assumes a grayish or bluish gray color.

   **gyrate a. of choroid and retina,** a slowly progressive a. of the choroid, pigmentary epithelium, and retina, with irregular confluent atrophic areas having a ring-shaped contour; autosomal recessive inheritance.

**Hoffmann's muscular a.,** infantile muscular a.

**horizontal a.,** horizontal resorption; a progressive loss of alveolar and supporting bone surrounding the teeth, beginning at the most coronal level of the bone.

**Hunt's a.,** neural a. of the small muscles of the hand without sensory disturbances; two types are recognized: *thenar,* from compression neuritis of the thenar branch of the median nerve; *hypothenar,* from compression neuritis of the deep palmar branch of the ulnar nerve.

**idiopathic muscular a.,** progressive muscular *dystrophy.*

**infantile muscular a.,** Hoffmann's a.; Werdnig-Hoffmann disease; familial spinal muscular a.; infantile progressive spinal muscular a.; progressive muscular wasting due to degeneration of motor neurons in anterior horns of the spinal cord; onset is usually in the first year, with 80 per cent mortality by the age of 4 years; autosomal recessive inheritance.

**infantile progressive spinal muscular a.,** infantile muscular a.

**interstitial a.,** decalcification of a living bone.

**ischemic muscular a.,** see Volkmann's *contracture.*

**juvenile muscular a.,** Kugelberg-Welander disease; Wohlfart-Kugelberg-Welander disease; slowly progressive proximal muscular weakness with fasciculation and wasting, electromyographic and muscle biopsy findings of lower motor neuron disease; onset usually at age 2 to 17 years; autosomal recessive inheritance is usual.

**Kienböck's a.,** acute a. of bone of extremity following inflammation.

**Leber's hereditary optic a., Leber's optic a.;** Leber's disease; degeneration of the optic nerve and papillomacular bundle with resulting rapid loss of central vision, progressive for several weeks, then usually stationary for years with permanent central scotoma; age of onset is variable, most often in the third decade. The mechanism of inheritance is complex and not well understood; males are predominantly affected, transmission by normal females, but X-linkage is unlikely because affected males do not transmit the condition to descendants.

**linear a.,** *striae* cutis distensae.

**a. of the liver,** a condition in which one or more essential structures of the liver become atrophic from wasting, inanition, ischemia, or toxic effect.

**macular a.,** rare condition characterized by discrete, sharply defined areas of atrophy. The surface protrudes as small bladder-like tumors. The cause is unknown.

**marantic a.,** marasmus.

**muscular a.,** a wasting of muscular tissue, especially due to lack of use; see also myopathic a.

**myopathic a.,** muscular a. due to disease of the muscle itself and not of paralytic or central nervous origin.

**neuritic a.,** neurotrophic a.

**neurogenic a.,** fascicular *degeneration.*

**neurotrophic a.,** neuritic a.; trophic change; a. of a muscle resulting from neuritis or degeneration of the motor nerves, usually beginning in the lower extremities, reaching the greatest extent in the legs, less in the upper extremities.

**olivopontocerebellar a.,** olivopontocerebellar degeneration; a progressive neurologic disease characterized by loss of neurons in the cerebellar cortex, basis pontis, and inferior olivary nuclei; it results in ataxia, tremor, involuntary movement, and dysarthria; five clinical types (four dominant in inheritance, one recessive) have been described, depending on additional findings, such as sensory loss, retinal degeneration, ophthalmoplegia, and extrapyramidal signs.

**periodontal a.,** decrease in size and/or cellular elements of the periodontium after it has reached normal maturity.

**peroneal muscular a.,** Charcot-Marie-Tooth disease; neurogenic a. characterized by slowly progressive wasting of distal muscles of the extremities, usually involving the legs before the arms; pes cavus is often the first sign. autosomal dominant, autosomal recessive, and X-linked recessive types exist, with severity related to genetic type.

**Pick's a.,** circumscribed a. of the cerebral cortex.

**postmenopausal a.,** a. following the menopause, for example, a. of the genital organs, or of the oral mucosa.

**pressure a.,** the wasting of hard or soft tissue resulting from excessive pressure applied to tissue by a denture base.

**primary macular a. of the skin,** *atrophia* maculatum.

**progressive choroidal a.,** choroideremia (2).

**progressive muscular a.,** Duchenne-Aran or Aran-Duchenne disease; Cruveilier's disease; muscular trophoneurosis; creeping palsy; wasting paralysis or palsy; a. of the cells of the anterior cornua of the spinal cord, resulting in a slow progressive wasting and paralysis of the muscles of the extremities and of the trunk.

**pseudohypertrophic muscular a.,** see pseudohypertrophic muscular *dystrophy.*

**red a.,** a. of an organ associated with chronic passive congestion, seen sometimes in the liver in connection with disease of the heart.

**remitting spinal a.,** chronic anterior *poliomyelitis.*

**scapulohumeral a.,** Vulpian's a.

**senile a.,** wasting of tissues and organs with advancing age, probably from decreased anabolic processes, due to endocrine changes and vascular obstruction.

**serous a.,** a degenerative change occurring in fat cells, the fat being absorbed and its place being taken by a serous fluid.

**a. of the skin,** atrophoderma.

**spinal a.,** *tabes* dorsalis.

**striate a. of the skin,** linear pink striations occurring in the skin of debilitated, usually bedfast patients.

**traction a.,** *striae* cutis distensae.

**transneuronal a.,** a transsynaptic deafferentation change, noted especially in the lateral geniculate body of the central nervous system.

**trophoneurotic a.,** a. related to loss of innervation.

**Vulpian's a.,** scapulohumeral a.; progressive spinal muscular a. beginning in the shoulder.

**yellow a. of the liver,** acute yellow a. of the liver.

**Zimmerlin's a.,** a variety of hereditary progressive muscular a. in which the a. begins in the upper half of the body.

**at′ropine** (NF, BP). *dl*-Hyoscyamine; *dl*-tropyl tropate; tropine tropate; $C_{17}H_{23}NO_3$; alkaloid obtained from *Atropa belladonna;* antispasmodic, antisudorific, anticholinergic, and mydriatic.

**a. methonitrate** (BP), the methylnitrate of a.; same actions and uses as a.

**a. methylbromide,** methylatropine bromide.

**a. sulfate** (USP, BP), anticholinergic.

**at′ropinism.** The symptoms of poisoning by atropine or belladonna.

**atro′piniza′tion.** The administration of atropine or belladonna to the point of achieving the pharmacologic effect.

**at′roscine.** Scopolamine.

**attach′ment.** 1. A connection of one part with another. 2. In dentistry, a mechanical device for the fixation and stabilization of a dental prosthesis.

**epithelial a.,** a collar of epithelial cells, continuous with the crevicular epithelium, adherent to the tooth at the base of the gingival sulcus.

**frictional a.,** precision a.

**internal a.,** precision a.

**key a.,** precision a.

**keyway a.,** precision a.

**muscle-tendon a.,** muscle-tendon junction; the union of a muscle and tendon fiber in which sarcolemma intervenes between the two; the end of the muscle fiber may be rounded, conical, or tapered.

**parallel a.,** precision a.

**pericemen′tal a.,** the tissues surrounding the cementum of the tooth, *i.e.,* the periodontal ligament and alveolar bone.

**precision a.,** internal a.; frictional a.; slotted a.; key a.; keyway a.; parallel a.; (1) a frictional retainer used in fixed and removable denture construction; consists of closely fitting male and female parts, the latter of which is contained usually within the normal or expanded contours of the crown of the abutment tooth; (2) a frictional retainer used in fixed and removable partial denture construction that consists of closely fitting male and female parts; (3) one that depends upon resistance between parallel walls of male and female parts.

**slotted a.,** precision a.

**snap a.,** a type of precision a. in which the male portion replaces the entire crown and is attached to a post embedded within the root portion of the tooth; the female portion is included within the denture base.

**attack.** The occurrence of some disease or episode, ordinarily with a dramatic onset, such as an a. of shingles or heart a.

**drop a.,** attacks characterized by falling without warning, often upon movement of the head.

**transient ischemic a.,** brief episodes of neurological dysfunction due to transient cerebral ischemia; abbreviated TIA.

**uncinate a.,** the aura or hallucination of taste or smell preceding an epileptic seizure.

**vagal a.,** vasovagal a., syncope, or syndrome; a paroxysmal condition marked by a slow pulse, fall in blood pressure, and sometimes convulsions; it is thought to be due to sudden stimulation of the vagus nerve mediated through receptors in the carotid sinus, the aortic arch, or the heart.

**vasovagal a.,** vagal a.

**at'tar of rose** [ Pers. *attara,* to smell sweet ]. Rose oil.

**attend'ing** [ L. *attendo,* to bend to, notice ]. In psychology, readiness to perceive, as in listening or looking; focusing of sense organs is sometimes involved.

**atten'uant.** 1. Diluting; making thin or less, as of a fluid. 2. A diluent. 3. Any agent, means or method used to reduce the virulence of a pathogenic microorganism or virus, or the action of a drug.

**attenuate** (ă-ten'u-āt) [ L. *at-tenuo,* pp. *-tenuatus,* to make thin or weak, fr. *tenuis,* thin. TEN- ]. 1. To dilute; to make thinner. 2. To reduce the virulence of a pathogenic microorganism. 3. To reduce or weaken.

**attenua'tion.** 1. Dilution; thinning. 2. Diminution of virulence in a strain of an organism, obtained through selection of variants which occur naturally or through experimental means. 3. Reduction or weakening.

**attic,** or **tympanic attic.** *Recessus* epitympanicus.

**at'ticomas'toid.** Relating to the attic of the tympanum, and the mastoid antrum or cells.

**atticot'omy** [ attic + G. *tomē,* incision ]. Operative opening into the tympanic attic.

**at'titude** [ Mediev. L. *aptitudo,* fr. L. *aptus,* fit ]. 1. Posture; position of the body and limbs. 2. Manner of acting. 3. In social or clinical psychology, a relatively stable and enduring predisposition or set to behave or react in a certain way toward persons, objects, institutions, or issues.

**emotional a.'s,** passional a.'s.

**passional a.'s,** a.'s expressive of any of the great passions, *e.g.,* anger, lust, etc.

**attitu'dinal.** Relating to a posture of the body, *e.g.,* attitudinal (statotonic) reflex.

**atto-** [ Danish *atten,* eighteen ]. A prefix denoting one quintillionth (10-18).

**attol'lens** [ L. *at-tollo* (*adt-*), pres. p. *-tollens,* to lift up ]. Lifting up; raising.

**a. aurem, a. auric'ulam,** *musculus* auricularis superior.

**a. oc'uli,** *musculus* rectus superior.

**attraction** (ă-trak'shun) [ L. *at-traho,* pp. *-tractus,* to draw toward ]. The tendency of two bodies to approach each other.

**cap'illary a.,** the force that causes fluids to rise up very fine tubes or through the pores of a loose material.

**chemical a.,** the force impelling atoms of different elements or molecules to unite to form new substances or compounds.

**magnetic a.,** the force that draws iron or steel toward a magnet.

**neurotropic a.,** the pull of a regenerating axon toward the motor end-plate.

**at'trahens** [ see attraction ]. Drawing toward, denoting a muscle (attrahens aurem or auriculam) rudimentary in man, that tends to draw the pinna of the ear forward; see musculus auricularis anterior.

**attrition** (ă-trish'un) [ L. *at-tero,* pp. *-tritus,* to rub against, rub away ]. 1. Wearing away by friction or rubbing. 2. In dentistry, the loss of tooth structure caused by the abrasive character of food or from bruxism (night grinding); *cf.* abrasion.

**atypia** (a-tip'ī-ah). Atypism; state of being not typical.

**atypical** (a-tip'ī-kal) [ G. *a-* priv. + *typikos,* conformed to a type. TYP- ]. Not typical; not corresponding to the normal form or type.

**atypism.** Atypia.

**Au** [ L. *aurum,* gold ]. Chemical symbol of the element gold.

**Aub,** Joseph C., Boston physician, *1890. See A.-Dubois *table.*

**Auberger (Au) blood group.** See appendix 2, Blood Groups.

**Aubert** (o-bair'), Hermann, German physiologist, 1826–1892. See A.'s *phenomenon.*

**au'cubin.** $C_{15}H_{24}O_9$; a glycoside contained in the seeds of *Acuba japonica* (family Cornaceae) and *Plantago ovata* (family Plantaginaceae). The seeds are used in the treatment of chronic dysentery in India.

**audile** (aw'dil). 1. Relating to audition. 2. Denoting the type of mental imagery in which a person recalls most readily that which he has heard, as contrasted with visile and motile. 3. Auditive.

**audio-** [ L. *audio,* to hear ]. Combining form relating to hearing.

**au'dioanalge'sia.** Analgesia produced by sound or sounds.

**aud'iogen'ic** [ audio- + G. *genesis,* production ]. 1. Caused by sound, especially a loud noise; convulsive seizures, for example, or a rise in blood pressure can be produced in rats by sudden loud sounds. 2. Sound-producing.

**au'diogram** [ audio- + G. *gramma,* a drawing ]. The graphic record drawn from the results of hearing tests with the audiometer which charts threshold of hearing at various frequencies against sound intensity in decibels.

**pure tone a.,** a chart of the threshold for hearing acuity at various frequencies usually expressed in decibels above normal threshold and usually covering frequencies from 128 to 8000 cps.

**speech a.,** the record of thresholds for spondaic word lists and scores for phonetically balanced word lists.

**audiol'ogist.** A specialist in evaluation, habitation, and rehabilitation of those whose communication disorders center in whole or in part in the hearing function.

**audiol'ogy.** The study of hearing disorders through the identification and measurement of hearing function loss as well as the rehabilitation of persons with hearing impairments.

**audiom'eter** [ audio- + G. *metron,* measure ]. An electrical instrument for measuring the threshold of hearing for pure tones of frequencies generally varying from 200 to 8000 cps (recorded in terms of decibels). It also records thresholds for lists of spoken words and discrimination percentage for phonetically balanced word lists.

**audiom'etrist.** A person trained in the use of the audiometer in testing hearing acuity.

**audiom'etry.** Use of the audiometer.

**Békésy a.,** semiautomatic a. in which the tone sweeps the audiometric scale while the patient controls intensity by pressing a signal when the tone is not heard.

**PGSR a.,** psychogalvanic skin resistance test for the measurement of hearing acuity without conscious cooperation of the patient.

**audiovisual** (aw'dī-o-vizh'u-al). Pertaining to a communication or teaching technique that combines both audible and visible symbols.

**audition** (aw-dish'un). Hearing.

**chromatic a.,** the subjective perception of color caused by the hearing of certain sounds.

**gustatory a.,** a form of synesthesia in which a sensation of taste is noted when certain sounds are heard.

**au'ditive.** Audile (3); a person who learns and remembers more readily through hearing than through sight.

**au'ditory** [ L. *audio,* pp. *auditus,* to hear ]. Pertaining to the sense of hearing or to the organs of hearing.

**auditus** [ L. ] [ NA ]. The sense of hearing.

**Auenbrugger,** Leopold J., Austrian physician, 1722–1809. See A.'s *sign.*

**Auer** (ow'er), John, American physician, 1875–1948. See A. *bodies,* Meltzer and A. *test.*

**Auerbach,** Leopold, German anatomist, 1828–1897. See A.'s *ganglion, plexus.*

**Aufrecht** (owf'rekht), Emanuel, German physician, 1844–1933. See A.'s *sign.*

**augnathus** (awg-na'thus) [ G. *au,* again, + *gnathos,* jaw ]. An individual with a double mandible.

**Aujeszky** (aw-jes'ke), Aládár, Budapest pathologist, 1869–1933. See A.'s *disease.*

**aura,** pl. **au'rae** (aw'rah) [ L. breeze, odor, gleam of light ]. The beginning of a seizure as recognized by the patient; a peculiar sensation felt by the patient immediately preceding an epileptic attack; it may be a paresthesia in the epigastric region or in the hand or leg ascending to the head, noises in the ears, flashes of light, vertigo, etc.; it is called auditory, epigastric, vertiginous, etc., according to its seat or nature.

    **intellectual a.,** a dreamy, detached, or reminiscent mental state preceding the epileptic seizure; also called reminiscent a.

    **kinesthetic a.,** a feeling of movement of a part of the body when no movement occurs.

**au'ral.** 1. Relating to the ear (auris). 2. Relating to an aura.

**au'ramine O.** A yellow fluorescent dye, $C_{17}H_{22}N_3Cl$, used as a stain for the tubercle bacillus.

**auranti'asis cutis** [ L. *aurantium,* orange, + suffix *-iasis,* condition; *cutis,* skin ]. Carotinosis cutis; carotenosis cutis; yellow coloration of the skin caused by increase in carotene content.

**auran'tiogliocla'din.** 2,3-Dimethoxy-5,6-dimethyl-*p*-benzoquinone; an antibiotic obtained from *Gliocladium roseum.*

**auriasis** (aw-ri'ah-sis). Chrysiasis.

**au'ric.** Relating to gold (aurum).

**auricle** (aw'rĭ-kl). Auricula.

    **accessory a.'s,** small, fleshy nodules or folds, sometimes with supporting cartilage, occasionally found along the margins of the embryonic branchial clefts.

    **cervical a.,** accessory a. on the neck.

    **left a.,** *auricula* sinistra.

    **right a.,** *auricula* dextra.

**auricula,** pl. **auric'ulae** (aw-rik'u-lah) [ L. the external ear. dim. of *auris,* ear ]. Auricle. 1 [ NA ]. Pinna; ala auris; the projecting shell-like structure on the side of the head, constituting, with the external acoustic meatus, the external ear. 2. The appendage of the atrium.

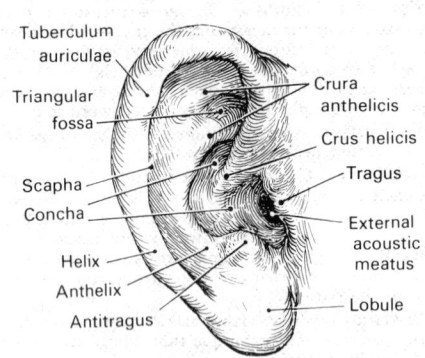

**The Auricle of the Ear**
(From Spalteholz, W.: *Hand Atlas of Human Anatomy,* J. B. Lippincott Co., Philadelphia, 1959. Used with permission.)

    **a. atrii** [ NA ], atrial auricula (auricle) or appendage of the atrium; a small conical pouch projecting from the upper anterior portion of each atrium of the heart.

    **a. dextra** [ NA ], right auricle; right auricular appendage; the small conical projection from the right atrium.

    **a. sinistra** [ NA ], left auricle; left auricular appendage; the small conical projection from the left atrium.

**auric'ular.** Relating to the ear, or to an auricle in any sense.

**auriculare,** pl. **auricula'ria** (aw-rik-u-la're) [ L. *auricularis,* pertaining to the ear ]. Auricular point; a craniometric point at the center of the opening of the external auditory

canal; or, in certain cases, the middle of the upper edge of this opening.

**auric'ulocra'nial.** Relating to the auricle or pinna of the ear and the cranium.

**auric'ulotem'poral.** Relating to the auricle or pinna of the ear and the temporal region.

**auric'uloventric'ular.** Obsolete synonym for atrioventricular.

**aurid,** pl. **aurides** (aw'rid, aw'rī-dēz) [ L. *aurum,* gold, + *-id* (1), *q.v.* ]. A skin lesion due to injection of gold salts.

**au'riform.** Ear-shaped.

**au'rin.** Corallin; *p*-rosolic acid; a triphenylmethane derivative, $C_{19}H_{14}O_3$, used as an indicator; it changes from yellow to red at pH 6.8 to 8.2.

**au'rintricarboxyl'ic acid.** A chelating agent that has a special affinity for beryllium and may therefore be of use in combating beryllium poisoning. The ammonium salt is known as ALUMINON.

**auris,** pl. **au'res** (aw'ris) [ L. ] [ NA ]. Ear.

    **antrum a.,** *meatus* acusticus externus.

    **a. externa** [ NA ], the external ear constituted by the auricula and the external acoustic meatus; see also auricula, pinna.

    **a. interna** [ NA ], internal ear; see ear; labyrinth, and labyrinthus.

    **a. media** [ NA ], the middle ear; see also *cavum* tympani.

**auriscope** (aw'rĭ-skōp) [ L. *auris,* ear, + *skopeō,* to view ]. Otoscope.

**aurochromoderma** (aw'ro-kro'mo-der-mah) [ L. *aurum,* gold, + *chrōma,* color, + *derma,* skin ]. Chrysiasis.

**au'romercap'toacetan'ilid.** LAURON; aurothiglycamide; (1-D-glucosylthio)gold; $AuSCH_2CONH—C_6H_5$; an organic gold compound, insoluble in water; used in the treatment of rheumatoid arthritis, administered by intramuscular injection. It is more slowly absorbed than the water-soluble gold salts.

**au'rone.** 2-Benzylidene-3(2*H*)-benzofuranone; the parent compound of a series of plant pigments; a.'s may be formed from chalcones; they are substituted coumaranones.

$$\text{Aurone}$$

**Aurone**

**aurother'apy.** Chrysotherapy.

**au'rothi'oglu'cose** (USP). SOLGANAL; gold thioglucose; organic gold preparation with —SAu group in place of 1-OH group of glucose; used in rheumatoid arthritis and nondisseminated lupus erythematosus.

**aur'othiogly'canide.** α-Auromercaptoacetanilid.

**aurum** (aw'rum) [ L. ]. Gold.

**auscult** (aws-kult'). To auscultate.

**auscultate** (aws'kul-tāt) [ L. *ausculto,* pp. *-atus,* to listen to ]. To listen to the sounds made by the thoracic or abdominal viscera as a means of diagnosis.

**ausculta'tion.** Listening to the sounds made by the thoracic or abdominal viscera, by the contracting muscles, by the blood in the vessels, by the fetus *in utero,* or to sounds in any of the other internal parts of the body; used as a diagnostic method.

    **direct a.,** immediate a.

    **immediate a.,** direct a.; a. by application of the ear to the surface of the body.

    **mediate a.,** a. using a stethoscope.

**auscul'tatory.** Relating to auscultation.

**auscul'toscope.** Stethoscope.

**austenit'ic** [ W. C. *Roberts-Austen* ]. In stainless steels, denoting those that are not ferromagnetic and contain chromium and nickel. They are high in resistance to corrosion.

**Austin Flint.** See Flint.

**aut-.** See auto-.

**au′tacoid** [ G. *autos*, self, + *akos*, a remedy ]. Obsolete term for hormone.

**duodenal a.,** secretin.

**excitatory a.,** obsolete term for hormone.

**inhibitory a., restraining a.,** obsolete terms for chalone.

**autarcesis** (awt′ar-se′sis) [ G. *autos*, self, + *arkesis*, a warding off ]. Innate *immunity.*

**autechoscope** (aw-tek′o-skōp) [ G. *autos*, self, + *ēchō*, sound, + *skopeō*, to examine ]. Autostethoscope.

**aute′cic, aute′cious** [ G. *autos*, same, + *oikion*, house ]. Denoting a parasite that infects, throughout its entire existence, the same host.

**autemesia** (awt′ē-me′zī-ah) [ G. *autos*, self, + *emesis*, vomiting ]. Idiopathic or functional vomiting; also, vomiting induced by provoking the gag reflex.

**authenticity** (aw′then-tis′ī-tī) [ G. *authentikōs*, original, primary ]. 1. The quality of being authentic, genuine, and valid. 2. In psychological functioning and personality, applied to the conscious feelings, perceptions, and thoughts that a person expresses and communicates.

**autism** (aw′tizm) [ G. *autos*, self ]. A tendency to morbid self-absorption at the expense of regulation by outward reality.

**infantile a.,** Kanner's syndrome; severe emotional disturbance of childhood characterized by inability to form meaningful interpersonal relationships; believed by some to be a form of childhood schizophrenia.

**autis′tic.** 1. Pertaining to autism. 2. A person suffering from autism.

**auto-, aut-** [ G. *autos*, self ]. A prefix meaning self, same.

**au′toactiva′tion.** Autocatalysis.

**au′toagglutina′tion.** 1. Nonspecific agglutination or clumping together of cells (*e.g.*, bacteria, erythrocytes, and the like) due to physical-chemical factors. 2. The a. of a person's red blood cells in his own serum, as a consequence of specific autoantibody.

**au′toagglu′tinin.** A type of "cold" agglutinin, occasionally found in serum of persons with hepatic diseases, trypanosomiasis, and certain other conditions, and even in persons who have no evidence of disease; at room and refrigerator temperatures, a.'s react with red blood cells of all groups, including the person's own cells; usually do not react at 37°C.

**au′toal′lergy.** Autoimmunity.

**au′toanal′ysis.** Self-analysis; the attempted analysis, or psychoanalysis, of one's own self.

**autoanaphylaxis** (aw′to-an′ă-fi-lak′sis). Reaction induced by the injection of one's own blood or secretions, as in autoserotherapy.

**au′toan′tibody.** An antibody that has affinity for one or other of subject's own tissues.

**cold a.,** one that reacts at zero to 5°C., but not at 37°C.

**Donath-Landsteiner cold a.,** a. responsible for paroxysmal cold hemoglobinuria; it is of the IgG class and is adsorbed to red cells only at temperatures of 20° or lower, causing the red cells to lyse in the presence of complement at higher temperatures; it has only slight agglutinating properties in spite of its marked lytic activity; has a specificity within the blood group P (that is, it is an anti-P autoantibody). It formerly was frequently associated with syphilis, also occasionally present for short periods of time following measles and other infections.

**hemagglutinating cold a.,** an a. of the IgM class with marked capacity to agglutinate erythrocytes but with somewhat less affinity for complement than the Donath-Landsteiner type; the cause of cold-hemagglutinin disease (autoallergic hemolytic anemia of the cold-antibody type).

**warm a.,** one that reacts optimally at 37°C.

**au′toanticom′plement.** An anticomplement that is formed in the body of an animal and inhibits or destroys the complement of the same animal.

**au′toassay.** Detection or estimation of the amount of a substance produced in an organism by means of a test object in that organism, as, for example, use of the denervated heart *in situ* of a cat to assay for epinephrine or sympathin liberated into its blood stream.

**au′toblast** [ auto- + G. *blastos*, germ ]. 1. An independent cell. 2. Protozoon.

**autocatalysis** (aw′to-kă-tal′ī-sis). A reaction in which one or more of the products formed acts to catalyze the reaction; beginning slowly, the rate of such a reaction rapidly increases.

**au′tocatalyt′ic.** Relating to autocatalysis.

**autocath′eterism.** Passage of a catheter upon oneself.

**autochthonous** (aw-tok′thon-us) [ auto- + G. *chthon*, land, ground, country ]. 1. Native to the place inhabited; aboriginal. 2. Originating in the place where found; said of a disease originating in the part of the body where found, or of a disease acquired in the place where the patient is.

**autoclasia** (aw′to-kla′sī-ah) [ auto- + G. *klasis*, breaking ]. Especially in opthalmology, term used to denote progressive destruction of a tissue or organ as a result of immunologically induced damage; *cf.* autoclasis.

**autoclasis** (aw-tok′lah-sis) [ auto- + G. *klasis*, breaking ]. A breaking up or rupturing from intrinsic or internal causes; *cf.* autoclasia.

**au′toclave** [ auto- + L. *clavis*, a key, in the sense of self-locking ]. 1. An apparatus for sterilization by steam under pressure; it consists of a strong closed boiler containing a small quantity of water and, in a wire basket, the articles to be sterilized. 2. To sterilize in an autoclave.

**au′toconduc′tion.** Therapeutic induction of a high frequency current in tissues by means of a solenoid.

**autocys′toplasty.** Autoplasty of the bladder.

**autocytol′ysin.** Antibody formed in a person or animal and, in the presence of complement, destructive to various cells of the same individual.

**autocytolysis** (aw′to-si-tol′ī-sis). Autolysis.

**autocytotox′in.** A toxic substance that destroys cells of the person's or animal's body in which the toxin is formed.

**autoder′mic** [ auto- + G. *derma*, skin ]. Relating to one's own skin; denoting the method of skin grafting (autodermic graft; dermatoautoplasty) in which the grafts are taken from the patient's own skin.

**au′todestruc′tion.** Autolysis.

**au′todiges′tion.** Autolysis.

**au′todip′loid.** Relating to autodiploidy.

**au′todip′loidy.** The condition of an individual or cell with two sets of chromosomes derived from duplication of a single haploid set.

**au′todrain′age.** Drainage into contiguous tissues.

**autoecholalia** (aw′to-ek-o-la′lī-ah) [ auto- + echolalia, *q. v.* ]. The repetition of some or all the words in one's own statements.

**aut′oeczematiza′tion.** A generalized reaction, called an absorption reaction, which is usually attributed to overzealous therapy of a localized stasis dermatitis, or chronic eczematous eruption.

**au′toepila′tion.** Spontaneous hair loss.

**autoerotic** (aw-to-er-ot′ik). Pertaining to autoerotism.

**autoeroticism** (aw-to-er-ot′ī-sizm). Autoerotism.

**autoerotism** (aw-to-er′o-tizm) [ auto- + G. *erōtikos*, relating to love ]. Autoeroticism. 1. Sexual arousal or gratification using one's own body, as in masturbation. 2. Sexual self love, in contrast with alloerotism. See also narcissism.

**autofluorescence** (aw′to-flu-or-es′ens). The emission of visible light from a substance when irradiated.

**autofluoroscope** (aw′to-flu′or-o-skōp). A type of scintillation camera consisting of a matrix of individual sodium iodide crystals, each with their separate light pipe and photomultiplier tube; used for radioisotope scanning procedures.

**au′tofun′doscope.** An instrument with which an observer can visualize the vessels of his own eye.

**autog′amous.** Relating to or characterized by autogamy.

**autogamy** (aw-tog′ă-mī) [ auto- + G. *gamos*, marriage ]. Automixis; a form of self-fertilization, in which fission of the cell nucleus occurs without division of the cell, the two pronuclei so formed reuniting to form the synkaryon. In other cases the cell body also divides, but the two daughter cells immediately conjugate.

**autogenesis** (aw′to-jen′ē-sis) [ auto- + G. *genesis*, production ]. Self-production; abiogenesis.

**autogenet′ic, autogen′ic.** Relating to autogenesis. Self-producing; self-produced.

**autogenous** (aw-toj'en-us) [ G. *autogenēs*, self-produced ]. 1. Autogenetic. 2. Endogenous; originating within the body, applied to vaccines prepared from bacteria obtained from the infected person.

**autognosis** (aw'tog-no'sis) [ auto- + G. *gnōsis*, knowledge ]. Self-knowledge; recognition of one's own character, tendencies, and peculiarities.

**au'tograft.** Autotransplant; autologous graft; autoplastic graft; tissue or an organ transferred by grafting into a new position in the body of the same individual; not taken from another member of the same species (allograft or homograft; isograft) or from a member of another species (heterograft).

**autograft'ing.** Autotransplantation.

**au'togram** [ auto- + G. *gramma*, something written ]. A wheal-like lesion on the skin following pressure by a blunt instrument or by stroking.

**autog'raphism.** Dermatographism.

**au'tohemagglutina'tion.** Autoagglutination of erythrocytes.

**autohemol'ysin.** An antibody that (with complement) causes lysis of erythrocytes in the same person or animal in whose body the lysin is formed.

**autohemol'ysis.** Hemolysis occurring in certain diseases as a result of a hemolysin, an autoantibody, induced within the afflicted individual.

**au'tohemother'apy.** Treatment of disease by the withdrawal and reinjection of the patient's own blood.

**au'tohemotransfu'sion.** Autotransfusion.

**autohypnosis** (aw'to-hip-no'sis). Autohypnotism; statuvolence; idiohypnotism; self-induced hypnosis (as opposed to heterohypnosis), accomplished by concentrating on self-absorbing thought or on the idea of being hypnotized.

**autohypnot'ic.** Relating to autohypnosis.

**autohypnotism** (aw'to-hip'no-tizm). Autohypnosis.

**autoimmunity** (aw'to-im-mu'nĭ-tĭ). The condition in which antibodies are produced against the subject's own tissues.

**au'toimmuniza'tion.** Induction of autoallergy. Some diseases may result from a., either by the action of serum antibodies, as in acquired hemolytic anemia, or by the action of sensitized lymphocytes. In some other diseases, a. may be a secondary process resulting from the liberation of antigens from damaged tissues. The liability to a. appears to have a genetic basis.

**autoinfec'tion.** Autoreinfection. 1. Reinfection by microbes or parasitic organisms on or within the body that have already passed through an infective cycle, such as a succession of boils, or a new infective cycle with production of a new generation of larvae and adults by the nematode *Strongyloides stercoralis* or the cestode *Hymenolepsis nana.* 2. Self-infection by direct contagion as with parasite eggs passed in the infectious state transmitted by fingernails (anal-oral route), as with the pinworm, *Enterobius vermicularis.*

**autoinfu'sion.** Forcing the blood from the extremities by the application of an Esmarch bandage, in order to raise the blood pressure and fill the vessels in the vital centers; resorted to after excessive loss of blood or other body fluids.

**autoinoculable** (aw-to-in-ok'u-lă-bl). Susceptible of autoinoculation.

**au'toinoc'ula'tion.** A secondary infection originating from a focus of disease already present in the body; it may be local, as when an ulcerated surface produces another sore in a part in contact with it, or systemic, by the setting free of bacteria or their products from a local infective focus.

**autointox'icant.** A toxic agent produced within an animal which causes autointoxication.

**au'tointoxica'tion.** Self-poisoning; autotoxicosis; enterointoxication; enterotoxism; intestinal intoxication; the result of absorption of the waste products of metabolism, decomposed matter from the intestine, or the products of dead and infected tissue as in gangrene.

**autoisolysin** (aw-to-i-sol'ĭ-sin). An antibody that (with complement) causes lysis of blood cells in the person or animal in whose body the lysin is formed, as well as in others of the same species.

**autoker'atoplas'ty** [ auto- + G. *keras*, horn, + *plassō*, to fashion ]. Grafting of corneal tissue from one eye of the patient to his other eye.

**autokinesia, autokinesis** (aw-to-kin-e'sĭ-ah, aw-to-kin-e'-sis) [ auto- + G. *kinēsis*, movement ]. Voluntary movement.

**autokinet'ic.** Relating to autokinesis.

**autolesion** (aw'to-le'zhun). Self-inflicted injury.

**autol'ogous** [ auto- + G. *logos*, relation ]. 1. Occurring naturally and normally in a certain type of tissue or a specific structure of the body; sometimes used to indicate a neoplasm derived from cells that occur normally in that site, *e.g.,* a squamous cell carcinoma in the esophagus. 2. In transplantation, referring to a graft in which the donor and recipient areas are in the same individual.

**autol'ysate.** The complex of substances resulting from autolysis.

**autol'ysin.** An antibody that (with complement) causes lysis of the cells and tissues in the body of the person (or animal) in whom the lysin is formed.

**autol'ysis** [ auto- + G. *lysis*, dissolution ]. 1. The enzymatic digestion of cells (especially when dead or degenerate) by enzymes present within them (autogenous). 2. Destruction of cells as a result of a lysin formed in those cells or others in the same organism.

**autolysosome** (aw'to-li'so-sōm). A lysosome to which hydrolases have been fused.

**autolyt'ic.** Pertaining to or causing autolysis.

**au'tolyze.** To undergo autolysis.

**au'tomal'let.** Obsolete term for automatic *plugger.*

**autom'atism.** Telergy. 1. The state of being independent of the will or of central innervation, applicable, for example, to the heart's action. 2. An act performed without intent or conscious exercise of the will, often without realization of its occurrence. 3. A condition in which an individual is consciously or unconsciously, but involuntarily, compelled to the performance of certain motor or verbal acts, often purposeless and sometimes foolish or harmful.

 **ambulatory a.,** a person's automatic performance of an action or series of actions without being consciously aware of the processes involved in the performance.

 **immediate posttraumatic a.,** a posttraumatic state in which the patient performs automatically without immediate or late memory of his behavior.

**automat'ograph.** An instrument for recording automatic movements.

**automix'is** [ auto- + G. *mixis,* intercourse ]. Autogamy.

**automnesia** (aw-tom-ne'zĭ-ah) [ auto- + G. *mnēsis,* a remembering ]. Spontaneous revival of memories of an earlier condition of life.

**automysophobia** (aw'to-mis'o-fo'bĭ-ah) [ auto- + G. *mysos,* dirt, + *phobos,* fear ]. A morbid dread of personal uncleanliness.

**autonom'ic** [ G. *autonomos,* fr. *autos,* self, + *nomos,* law ]. 1. Autonomous; relating to or characterized by autonomy. 2. Relating to the autonomic nervous system.

**autonom'icus** [ L. ] [ NA ]. Autonomic.

**autonomotropic** (aw'to-nom-o-trop'ik) [ autonomic + *trepein,* to turn. ]. Acting on the autonomic nervous system.

**auton'omous.** Autonomic.

**auton'omy** [ auto- + G. *nomos,* law ]. Independence of outside control, or of control by the cerebrospinal nerve centers.

 **functional a.,** in social psychology, the tendency of a developed motive system (*e.g.,* motive of acquisition) to become independent of the primary or innate drive from which it originated (*e.g.,* need for food).

**au'to-ophthal'moscope.** An ophthalmoscope for the examination of the fundus of one's own eyes.

**au'to-oxida'tion.** Autoxidation; the direct combination of a substance with molecular oxygen at ordinary temperatures.

**au'to-oxidi'zable.** Referring to compounds and certain components of enzyme systems in the tissues that react directly with oxygen, *e.g.*, *b* hemochromogen in cytochrome, which do not require the action of dehydrogenases.

**autopath'ic.** Rarely used synonym for idiopathic.

**autopathog'raphy** [ auto- + G. *pathos*, suffering, + *graphō*, to write ]. The writing of one's own medical history.

**autopep'sia** [ auto- + G. *pepsis*, digestion ]. Self-digestion, said of ulceration of the gastric mucous membrane by its own secretion, or the digestion of the skin surrounding a gastrostomy or colostomy opening.

**autophagia** (aw-to-fa'jǐ-ah) [ auto- + G. *phagein*, to eat ]. Self-eating. 1. Biting one's own flesh. 2. Segregation and disposal of damaged organelles within a cell. 3. Maintenance of the nutrition of the whole body by metabolic consumption of some of the body tissues.

**autopha'gic.** Relating to or characterized by autophagia.

**autophil'ia** [ auto- + G. *phileō*, to love ]. Narcissism.

**autophobia** (aw-to-fo'bǐ-ah) [ auto- + G. *phobos*, fear ]. Pathologic self-hatred; fear of solitude.

**autophony** (aw-tof'o-nǐ) [ auto- + G. *phōnē*, sound ]. Tympanophonia; increased resonance of one's own voice, breath sounds, arterial murmurs, etc., noted especially in disease of the middle ear or of the nasal fossae.

**autopho'tograph.** Autoradiogram.

**au'toplast** [ auto- + G. *plassō*, to form ]. Autograft.

**autoplas'tic.** Relating to autoplasty; autologous.

**autoplas'ty.** The repair of defects by transplanting or grafting tissues from the patient's own body. See autograft.

**autoploid** (aw'to-ployd) [ auto- + suffix -ploid, *q.v.* ]. Relating to an individual or cell with two or more sets of chromosomes derived from duplication of a single haploid set. Depending on the number of multiples of the haploid set, autoploids are referred to as autodiploids, autotriploids, autotetraploids, autopentaploids, autohexaploids, etc.

**au'toploi'dy.** The condition of an individual or cell with two or more sets of chromosomes derived from duplication of a single haploid set.

**au'toplug'ger.** Obsolete term for automatic *plugger*.

**au'topod.** Autopodium.

**autopodium,** pl. **autopodia** (aw'to-po'dǐ-um, -ah) [ auto- + G. *pous (pod-)*, foot ]. Autopod; the distal major subdivision of a limb (the hand or foot).

**au'topoi'sonous.** Autotoxic.

**autopol'ymer.** See autopolymer *resin*.

**autopol'ymeriza'tion.** Polymerization without the use of external heat, as a result of the addition of an activator and a catalyst.

**au'topol'yploid.** See autoploid.

**au'topolyploi'dy.** See autoploidy.

**autop'sia** [ G. ]. Autopsy.

    **a. in vivo,** examination of the organs, especially the abdominal organs, during life by means of an exploratory incision.

**au'topsy** [ G. *autopsia*, seeing with one's own eyes ]. 1. Postmortem examination; an examination of the internal organs of a dead body for the purpose of determining the cause of death or of studying the pathologic changes present. 2. In the terminology of the ancient Greek school of empirics, the intentional reproduction of an effect, event or circumstance that occurred in the course of a disease and observation of its influence in ameliorating or aggravating the patient's symptoms.

**au'topy'other'apy** [ auto- + G. *pyon*, pus, + *therapeia*, treatment ]. Autotherapy (4); treatment in which a person is injected with pus obtained from himself; a modification of this is autogenous vaccine therapy.

**autora'diogram.** Radioautogram.

**au'toradiog'raphy.** Radioautography.

**au'toregula'tion.** 1. The tendency of the blood flow to an organ or part to remain at or return to the same level despite changes in the pressure in the artery which conveys blood to it. 2. In general, any biologic system equipped with inhibitory feedback systems such that a given change tends to be largely or completely counteracted. For example, baroreceptor reflexes form a basis for autoregulation of the systemic arterial blood pressure.

    **heterometric a.,** the a. of the strength of contraction of the ventricle that occurs in direct relation to the end-diastolic fiber length in accordance with Starling's law of the heart.

    **homeometric a.,** the a. of strength of contraction of the ventricle by mechanisms or agents (*e.g.*, the staircase phenomenon or treppe, sympathetic nerves, norepinephrine) that do not depend upon change in the end-diastolic fiber length.

**autoreinfection** (aw'to-re-in-fek'shun). Autoinfection.

**au'toreproduc'tion.** Replication (2); the ability of a gene or virus, or nucleoprotein molecule generally, to bring about the synthesis of another molecule like itself from smaller molecules within the cell.

**autorrhaphy** (aw-tor'ă-fǐ) [ auto- + G. *raphē*, sewing ]. Wound closure by using tissues from area of wound.

**au'toscope** [ auto- + G. *skopeō*, to inspect ]. Any instrument used in the visual examination of one's own organs or cavities.

**autosen'sitize.** To sensitize against one's own body cells.

**autosepticemia** (au'to-sep-ti-se'mǐ-ah) [ auto- + G. *sēpsis*, decay, + *haima*, blood ]. Endosepsis; septicemia apparently originating from microorganisms existing within the animal and not introduced from without.

**au'toserother'apy.** The treatment of certain conditions, such as dermatoses, by hypodermic injection of the patient's own blood serum obtained at an earlier time.

**au'tose'rum.** A serum obtained from the patient's own blood and used in autoserotherapy.

**au'tosex'ualism.** 1. Autoeroticism. 2. Narcissism.

**au'tosite** [ auto- + G. *sitos*, food ]. See conjoined unequal *twins*.

**autosmia** (awt-oz'mǐ-ah) [ auto- + G. *osmē*, smell ]. Smelling one's own body odor.

**au'toso'mal.** Pertaining to an autosome.

**autosomatognosis** (aw'to-so'mă-tog-no'sis) [ auto- + G. *sōma*, body, + *gnōsis*, recognition ]. The feeling that a portion of the body which has been removed is still present, *e.g.*, phantom limb.

**autoso'matognos'tic.** Pertaining to autosomatognosis.

**au'tosome** [ auto- + G. *sōma*, body ]. Any chromosome other than a sex chromosome; a.'s normally occur in pairs in somatic cells and singly in gametes.

**autosuggestibility** (aw'to-sug-jes-tǐ-bil'ǐ-tǐ). A mental state in which autosuggestion readily occurs.

**autosuggestion** (aw'to-sug-jes'chun). 1. The constant dwelling upon an idea or concept, thereby inducing some change in the mental or bodily functions. 2. The reproduction in the brain of impressions previously received which become then the starting point of new acts or ideas.

**autosynnoia** (aw-to-sin-noy'ah) [ auto- + G. *synnoia*, deep thought, fr. *syn*, with + *noeō*, to think ]. Self-centeredness; a mental disorder in which one never has a thought unconnected with himself.

**autosynthesis** (aw'to-sin'the-sis). Self-reproduction.

**autotel'ic** [ auto- + G. *telos*, end, completeness, purpose ]. Denoting those traits closely bound up with the central purposes of an individual.

**autotemnous** (aw'to-tem'nus) [ auto- + G. *temnō*, to cut. TOM- ]. Denoting a cell that propagates itself by fission without previous conjugation.

**autother'apy.** 1. Self-treatment. 2. Spontaneous cure. 3. autoserotherapy. 4. A now outmoded method of treating disease by the administration of the patient's own pathologic excretions, as, for example, the swallowing of the discharge from a wound, or the subcutaneous injection of the filtered sputum in the case of tuberculosis.

**autot'omy** [ auto- + G. *tomē*, a cutting ]. 1. The act of casting off a body part as a means of escape; *e.g.*, the limb of a crab or the tail of a lizard. 2. Fission; spontaneous division.

**autotopagnosia** (aw'to-top-ag-no'zǐ-ah) [ auto- + G. *topos*, place, + agnosia, *q.v.* ]. Inability to recognize any part of the body; a condition resulting from a lesion of the major hemisphere.

**autotoxemia** (aw'to-tok-se'mĭ-ah). Autointoxicants within the blood usually resulting in autointoxication.

**autotox'ic.** Autopoisonous; relating to autointoxication.

**au'totoxico'sis.** Autointoxication.

**autotox'in.** Any poison originating within the body upon which it acts.

**au'totransfu'sion.** Transfusing back into the body of blood removed; see also autoinfusion.

**autotrans'plant.** Autograft.

**au'totransplanta'tion.** Autografting; the performance of an autograft.

**autotroph** (aw'to-trōf) [ auto- + G. *trophē*, nourishment ]. A microorganism which uses only inorganic materials as its source of nutrients; carbon dioxide serves as the sole carbon source.

**autotroph'ic.** Pertaining to an autotroph.

**au'totuber'culin.** Tuberculin prepared from cultures made from the patient's own sputum.

**autotyphization** (aw'to-ti'fĭ-za'shun). The production of symptoms resembling those of typhoid fever occurring as a result of autointoxication.

**autourotherapy** (aw'to-u'ro-ther'ă-pĭ) [ auto- + G. *ouron,* urine, + *therapeia,* treatment ]. Treatment (now outmoded) of various allergic diseases, laryngospasm, urticaria, angioneurotic edema, etc., by subcutaneous or intramuscular injection of the patient's own sterilized urine.

**au'tovac'cina'tion.** A second vaccination with virus from a vaccine sore on the same individual.

**autoxidation** (aw-tok'sĭ-da'shun). Auto-oxidation.

**autox'idator.** A substance that hastens the process of autoxidation.

**autozygous** (aw'to-zi'gus) [ auto- + G. *zygōtos,* yoked ]. Relating to genes in different individuals that are identical because of descent from ancestors common to both.

**auxano-, aux-, auxo-** [ G. *auxanō,* to increase ]. Prefix denoting relation to increase, *e.g.,* in size, intensity, speed.

**auxanogram** (awk-san'o-gram) [ auxano- + G. *gramma,* something written ]. A plate culture of bacteria in which variable conditions are provided in order to determine the effect of these conditions on the growth of the bacteria.

**auxanograph'ic.** Pertaining to auxanogram or auxanography.

**auxanog'raphy.** The study, using auxanograms, of the effects of different conditions on the growth of bacteria.

**auxanol'ogy** [ auxano- 'G. *logos,* study ]. The study of growth.

**auxenolonic acid** (awk'sen-o-lon-ik). Auxin b.

**aux'entriol'ic acid.** Auxin a.

**auxesis** (awk-se'sis) [ G. increase ]. 1. Increase in size. 2. Hypertrophy.

**auxetic** (awk-set'ik) [ G. *auxētikos,* promoting growth ]. A hypothetical chemical substance, the supposed specific action of which is to excite proliferation in leukocytes and other cells.

**auxiliomotor** (awg-zil'ĭ-o-mo'tor). Aiding motion.

**auxilytic** (awk'sĭ-lit'ik) [ G. *auxō,* to increase, + *lysis,* dissolution ]. Increasing the destructive power of a lysin, or favoring lysis.

**auxins** (awk'sinz). Plant hormones; chemical substances, in plants, that control plant growth. They are formed in one part of the plant and transferred to other parts where their action is exerted.

   **auxin a,** auxin in the tips of oats, corn and in fungi.

   **auxin b,** auxin in malt and maize germ. It is the β-keto acid of auxin a.

**auxo-** (awk'so-). See auxano-.

**auxocar'dia** [ auxo- + G. *kardia,* heart ]. 1. Enlargement of the heart, either hypertrophy or dilation. 2. the cardiac *diastole.*

**auxochrome** (awk'so-krōm) [ auxo- + G. *chrōma,* color ]. The atomic group within a dye molecule by which the dye is bound to reactive groups in tissues.

**aux'ocyte** [ auxo- + G. *kytos,* cell ]. An early stage of oocyte, spermatocyte, or sporocyte.

**auxodrome** (awk'so-drōm) [ auxo- + G. *dromos,* course ]. A course of growth as plotted on a Wetzel grid.

**aux'oflore.** An atom or group of atoms that, by its presence in a molecule, shifts its fluorescent radiation in the direction of the shorter wavelength, or increases the fluorescence. Opposite of bathoflore.

**auxogluc** (awk'so-glook). An atomic grouping that, when present in a molecule, intensifies its sweetness.

**auxol'ogy.** Obsolete term for embryology.

**auxom'eter** [ auxo- + G. *metron,* measure ]. An instrument for measuring the magnifying power of a lens.

**aux'other'apy.** Allopathy.

**aux'oton'ic.** In botany, induced by growth.

**aux'otox.** An atomic grouping that, when present in a molecule, intensifies its poisonous characteristics.

**auxotroph** (awk'so-trōf) [ auxo- + G. *trophē,* nourishment ]. A mutant microorganism that requires some nutrient that is not required by the organism (prototroph) from which the mutant was derived.

**auxotrophic** (awk'so-trof'ik, -tro'fik). Pertaining to an auxotroph.

**A-V.** Abbreviation for (1) arteriovenous, and (2) atrioventricular.

**aval'vular.** Nonvalvular; without valves.

**avas'cular.** Nonvascular; without blood or lymphatic vessels. May be a normal state as in certain forms of cartilage, or the result of disease.

**avas'culariza'tion.** The expulsion of blood from a part by means of an Esmarch bandage.

**Avel'lis,** Georg, German laryngologist, 1864–1916. See A.'s *syndrome.*

**Ave'na sati'va.** The common oat (family Gramineae) of cultivation; yields the albuminoid, avenin.

**av'enin.** A protein (prolamin) in oats (*Avena*), about 25 per cent glutamic acid; considered highly nutritious.

**Avenzo'ar** (Ibn Zuhr), Arabian physician of Cordova, 1113–1162. Wrote the *Theisir* or "Rectification of Health." He did not hesitate to question the *Canon* of Avicenna and strongly opposed astrology and mysticism in medicine.

**a'vian** [ L. *avis,* bird ]. Pertaining to birds.

**Avicenna** (av-is-en'ah), or **Ibn Sina,** Persian physician, 980–1037. Was renowned as physician, poet, scientist, and philosopher. Osler spoke of his book, the *Canon,* as "the most famous medical textbook ever written." See A.'s *gland.*

**av'idin.** Antibiotin; protein in nondenatured egg white that binds biotin and prevents its absorption, thus leading to biotin deficiency.

**avir'ulent.** Not virulent.

**avi'tamino'sis.** Properly hypovitaminosis, a deficiency disease state resulting from an inadequate supply of one or more vitamins in the diet; scurvy and beriberi are examples.

   **conditioned a.,** a. caused by any number of pathologic states or dysfunctions in which the supply of a vitamin absorbed by the body is inadequate for the needs under particular circumstances; an example is the reduced bacterial synthesis of the vitamins in the alimentary canal produced by antibiotic agents.

**avivement** (ah-vēv-moñ') [ Fr. *aviver,* to quicken, revive ]. Excision of the edges of a wound to revive the healing process.

**Avogad'ro,** Amadeo, Italian physicist, 1766–1856. See A.'s *constant, hypothesis, law, number, postulate.*

**avoirdupois** (av'er-dĕ-poyz') [ Fr. to have weight, corrupted fr. O. Fr. *avoir,* property, + *de,* of, + *pois,* weight ]. A system of weights in which 16 ounces make a pound; the pound is the equivalent of 453.6 gm. See appendix 5.

**avulsion** (ă-vul-zhun) [ L. *a-vello,* pp. *-vulsus,* to tear away ]. A tearing away or forcible separation; *cf.* evulsion.

   **complete scalp a.,** an extensive laceration separating all or almost all of the scalp from underlying tissues and the skin of the face and neck.

   **incomplete scalp a.,** laceration in which only a portion of the scalp is separated from underlying tissues.

   **phrenic a.,** the pulling out of a portion of the phrenic nerve, producing an elevation of that side of the diaphragm and partial collapse of the corresponding lung.

   **tooth a.,** the traumatic separation of a tooth from its alveolus.

**aware'ness.** The state of being conscious, cognizant, or alert.

 **reality a.,** the ability to distinguish external objects as being different from oneself.

**Ax.** Abbreviation for axis.

**axanthopsia** (ak'san-thop'sĭ-ah) [ G. *a-* priv. + *xanthos,* yellow, + *opsis,* vision ]. Yellow blindness; inability to see yellow tints.

**Axelrod,** Julius, U. S. pharmacologist, \*1912. Nobel laureate, 1970, with Ulf von Euler and Bernard Katz for their work on humoral transmitter substances and mechanisms at nerve terminals.

**Axenfeld,** Karl T. P. P., German ophthalmologist, 1867–1930. See A.'s *syndrome,* Morax-A. *conjunctivitis, diplobacillus.*

**axenic** (a-zen'ik) [ G. *a-* priv. + *xenos,* foreign ]. 1. Sterile; used especially of a living organism devoid of other living organisms; denoting a pure culture. 2. Also used to denote "germ-free" animals, *e.g.,* animals born and raised in sterile environment (housing, air, food).

**axerol.** Obsolete term for retinol.

**axeroph'thol.** Obsolete term for retinol.

**axes** (ak'sēz). Plural of axis.

**ax'ial.** 1. Axile; relating to an axis. 2. Relating to or situated in the central part of the body, in the head and trunk as distinguished from the extremities. 3. In dentistry, relating to or parallel with the long axis of a tooth.

**axif'ugal** [ L. *axis* + *fugio,* to flee from ]. Axofugal; extending away from an axis or axon.

**ax'il.** Axilla.

**ax'ile.** Axial.

**axilla,** gen. and pl. **axillae** (ak'sil'ah, ak-sil'e) [ L. ] [ NA ]. Armpit; maschale; axillary space or cavity; axil; the cavity beneath the shoulder joint, bounded roughly by the pectoralis major anteriorly, the latissimus dorsi posteriorly, the chest wall medially, the humerus laterally, the shoulder joint above, and the axillary fascia and hairy integument below; it contains the axillary artery and vein, the brachial plexus, lymphatic nodes, and areolar tissue.

**ax'illary.** Relating to the axilla.

**axio-** (ak'sĭ-o-) [ L. *axis* ]. Combining form relating to an axis. See also axo-.

**axiobuc'cal.** Referring to the junction of the axial and buccal planes, usually a line.

**ax'iobuccogin'gival.** Referring to the junction of the axial, the buccal and the gingival planes; usually a point.

**axioincisal** (ak'sĭ-o-in-si'sal). Referring to the line angle formed by the junction of the incisal edge and axial walls of a tooth.

**axiola'bial.** Pertaining to the line angle of a cavity formed by the junction of the axial and the labial walls of a tooth.

**ax'iola'biolin'gual.** Referring to a section from labial to lingual along the longitudinal axis of a tooth.

**ax'iolin'gual.** Refers to the line angle of a cavity formed by the junction of an axial and a lingual wall; see cavity line *angle.*

**ax'iolin'guocer'vical.** Refers to the point (trihedral) angle formed by the junction of an axial, lingual and cervical (gingival) wall of a cavity; see point *angle.*

**ax'iolin'guoclu'sal.** Refers to the point (trihedral) angle formed by the junction of an axial, lingual, and occlusal wall of a cavity; see point *angle.*

**ax'iolin'guogin'gival.** Refers to the point (trihedral) angle formed by the junction of an axial, lingual, and gingival (cervical) wall of a cavity; see point *angle.*

**ax'iome'sial.** Refers to the line angle of a cavity formed by the junction of an axial and a mesial wall; see cavity line *angle.*

**ax'iome'siocer'vical.** Refers to the point (trihedral) angle formed by the junction of an axial, mesial, and cervical (gingival) wall of a cavity; see point *angle.*

**ax'iome'siodis'tal.** See under plane.

**ax'iome'siogin'gival.** Refers to the point (trihedral) angle formed by an axial, mesial, and gingival (cervical) wall of a cavity; see point *angle.*

**ax'iome'sioinci'sal.** Refers to the point (trihedral) angle formed by the junction of an axial, mesial, and incisal wall of a cavity; see point *angle.*

**axion** (ak'sĭ-on). The brain and spinal cord (cerebrospinal axis).

**ax'io-occlu'sal.** Pertaining to the line angle formed by the junction of the axial and occlusal walls of a tooth.

**ax'ioplasm.** Axoplasm.

**axiopo'dium,** pl. **axiopo'dia** [ Mod. L. fr. L. *axis* + G. *podion,* dim. of *pous* (*pod-*), foot ]. A permanent pseudopodium containing a stiff axial filament of differentiated protoplasm.

**ax'iopul'pal.** Refers to the line angle formed by the junction of an axial and pulpal wall of a cavity; see cavity line *angle.*

**ax'iover'sion.** Abnormal inclination of the long axis of a tooth.

**axip'etal** [ L. *axis* + *peto,* to seek ]. Centripetal.

**ax'iramif'icate.** Denoting a nerve cell whose axon, usually short, breaks up into many branches, *e.g.,* Golgi's type II cells.

**axis,** pl. **axes** (ak'sis, ak'sēz) [ L. axle, axis ]. 1. A straight line passing through a spherical body between its two poles, and about which the body may revolve. 2. The central line of the body or any of its parts. 3. The spinal column. 4. The central nervous system. 5 [ NA ]. Epistropheus; toothed or odontoid vertebra; vertebra dentata; the second cervical vertebra. 6. An artery that divides, immediately upon its origin, into a number of branches.

 **basibregmat'ic a.,** a line extending from the basion to the bregma.

 **basicra'nial a.,** a line drawn from the basion to the midpoint of the sphenoethmoidal suture.

 **basifa'cial a.,** facial a.; a line drawn from the subnasal point to the midpoint of the sphenoethmoidal suture.

 **biauric'ular a.,** a straight line joining the two auricularia (*cf.* auriculare).

 **a. bulbi externus** [ NA ], external a. of the eye; that part of the optic a. from the anterior surface of the cornea to the posterior surface of the sclera.

 **a. bulbi internus** [ NA ], internal a. of the eye; that part of the optic a. from the posterior surface of the cornea to the anterior surface of the retina.

 **ce'liac a.,** *truncus* celiacus.

 **cephalocaudal a.,** the long a. of the body.

 **cerebrospi'nal a.,** encephalomyelonic a.; neural a.; axion; the central nervous system; the brain and spinal cord.

 **condylar a.,** a line through the two mandibular condyles around which the mandible may rotate during a part of the opening movement.

 **conjugate a.,** conjugata.

 **craniofa'cial a.,** a straight line passing through the mesethmoid, presphenoid, basisphenoid, and basioccipital bones.

 **a. deviation,** see under deviation.

 **electrical a.,** the general direction of the electromotive force developed in the heart during its activation, usually represented in the frontal plane; see triaxial reference *system.*

 **embryonic a.,** the cephalocaudal a. established in the embryo by the primitive streak.

 **enceph'alomyelon'ic a.,** cerebrospinal a.

 **external a. of eye,** a. bulbi externus.

 **facial a.,** basifacial a.

 **frontal a.,** the transverse a. of the eyeball, a line running transversely through the center of the globe of the eye.

 **hinge a.,** mandibular a.; an imaginary line between the mandibular condyles around which the mandible can rotate without translatory movement.

 **instantaneous electrical a.,** the resultant of the electromotive forces developing in the heart at any given moment.

 **internal a. of eye,** a. bulbi internus.

 **a. len'tis** [ NA ], axis of the lens; a line connecting the anterior and posterior poles of the crystalline lens.

 **long a.,** a line parallel to an object lengthwise; in dentistry, the line extending inciso- (occluso-) cervically parallel to axial surfaces of a tooth.

 **long a. of body,** cephalocaudal a.

 **mandibular a.,** hinge a.

mean electrical a., the average magnitude and direction of all the electromotive forces developed during the cardiac event under consideration (*e.g.*, atrial depolarization, ventricular depolarization, or ventricular repolarization. See also axis *deviation.*

neural a., cerebrospinal a.

normal a., a mean electrical a. of the heart situated between −30° and +90°; see hexaxial reference *system.*

opening a., an imaginary line around which the condyles may rotate during opening and closing movements of the mandible; *cf.* fulcrum *line.*

optic a., a. opticus.

a. op'ticus [ NA ], optic a.; the a. of the eye connecting the anterior and posterior poles; it usually diverges from the visual a. by 5 degrees or more.

orbital a., the line from the middle of the orbital opening to the center of the optic foramen.

a. pelvis [ NA ], pelvic a., plane of pelvic canal; a hypothetical curved line joining the center point of each of the four planes of the pelvis.

principal optic a., a line passing through the center of a lens of refracting system at right angles to its surface.

pupillary a., a line perpendicular to the surface of the cornea, and passing through the center of the pupil.

rotational a., fulcrum *line.*

sag'ittal a., the anteroposterior a. of the eyeball.

secondary a., any ray passing through the optical center of a lens.

a. of symmetry, an a. through a particle (*e.g.*, a virus) on such a plane that, if the particle is rotated on the a., there are two or more positions at which the particle appears identical.

thora'cic a., (1) *arteria* thoracoacromialis; (2) *vena* thoracoacromialis.

thyroid a., *truncus* thyrocervicalis.

transporionic a., an imaginary line connecting the upper central points of the external auditory meatuses; used in roentgenographic cephalometry (see porion).

vertical a., the vertical line passing through the center of the eyeball.

visual a., line of vision; the straight line extending from the object seen, through the center of the pupil, to the macula lutea of the retina.

**axo-** (ak'so) [ G. *axōn,* axis ]. Combining form meaning axis; usually relating to axon, *q.v.*

**axoaxonic** (ak'so-ak-son'ik). Refers to the synaptic contact between the axon of one nerve cell and that of another; see synapse.

**axodendrit'ic.** Referring to the synaptic relationship of an axon with a dendrite; see synapse.

**axof'ugal** [ axo- + L. *fugio,* to flee ]. Axifugal.

**ax'ograph** [ axo- + G. *graphō,* to write ]. A device for recording scales or axes of predetermined magnitude on kymographic records.

**ax'olem'ma** [ axo- + G. *lemma,* husk. LEP- ]. Mauthner's sheath; the delicate plasma membrane of the axon.

**axol'ysis** [ axo- + G. *lysis,* dissolution ]. Destruction of the axon of a nerve.

**axom'eter.** Axonometer; an instrument for determining the axis of a spectacle lens.

**axon** (ak'son) [ G. *axōn,* axis ]. Formerly also known as axis cylinder, cylindraxile, neuraxon, neurite, axonal process, Deiters' process. The single one among a nerve cell's processes that under normal conditions conducts nervous impulses away from the cell body and its remaining cell processes (dendrites). The a. is a relatively even filamentous process varying in thickness from about 0.25 to more than 10 μ. In contrast to dendrites, which rarely exceed 1.5 mm. in length, a.'s can extend far away from the parent cell body (some a.'s of the pyramidal tract are 40 to 50 cm. long). A.'s 0.5 μ thick or over are generally enveloped by a segmented myelin sheath provided by oligodendroglia cells (in brain and spinal cord) or Schwann cells (in peripheral nerves); the accompanying fig. shows a node of Ranvier between two adjacent myelin-sheath segments. Like dendrites and nerve cell bodies, a.'s contain a large number of longitudinal threadlike filaments, the neurofibrils. With some exceptions, nerve cells can synaptically transmit impulses to other nerve cells or to effector cells (muscle cells, gland cells) exclusively by way of the

synaptic terminals of their a. See also axon *terminal;* synapse; neurofibril; myelin *sheath.*

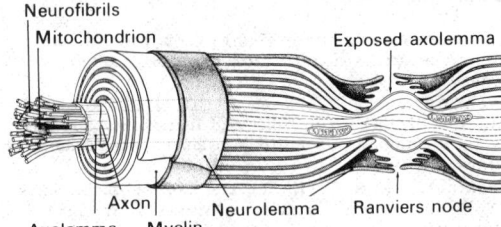

Neurofibrils
Mitochondrion
Exposed axolemma
Axon
Axolemma Myelin
Neurolemma Ranviers node

**Detail of an Axon, Myelin Sheath, and Neurolemma**

**ax'onal.** Pertaining to an axon.

**axoneme** (ak'so-nēm) [ axo- + G. *nēma,* a thread ]. 1. The central thread running in the axis of the chromosome. 2. A central cylinder common to all cilia and flagella, consisting of nine double microtubules and an inner core of two individual fibrils.

**axonog'raphy.** Electroaxonography; the recording of electrical changes in axons.

**axonom'eter.** Axometer.

**axonotme'sis** [ axo- + G. *tmēsis,* a cutting. TOM- ]. Interruption of the axons of a nerve followed by complete degeneration of the peripheral segment, without severance of the supporting structure of the nerve. Such a lesion may result from pinching, crushing, or prolonged pressure.

**axop'etal** [ axo- + L. *peto,* to seek ]. Extending in a direction toward an axon.

**axoph'theral.** Obsolete term for retinal(dehyde).

**ax'oplasm.** Neuroplasm of the axon.

**axosomat'ic** [ axo- + G. *sōma,* body ]. Referring to the synaptic relationship of an axon with a nerve cell body; see synapse.

**axostyle** (ak'so-stil) [ axo- + G. *stylos,* pillar ]. An elongate supporting rod or tubule that runs the length of certain flagellate protozoans, frequently projecting out of the posterior end. Single or multiple, filamentous or rigid, they vary with the species but serve as an endoskeletal framework and may function in locomotion as well.

**axotomy** (ak-sot'o-mī) [ axo- + G. *tomē,* to cut ]. The incision or cutting of an axon.

**Ayala's index** or **quotient.** See under index.

**Ayerza** (ah-yer'thah or ah-yer'sah), Abel, Argentinian physician, 1861–1918. See A.'s disease.

**Ayre,** J. Ernest, American gynecologist, *1910. See A. brush.

**azocarmine B, azocarmine G** (az-o-kar'min). Red acid dyes, the former more soluble in water, used in differential staining of pituitary acidophil cells.

**azacos'terol hydrochloride** (USAN). Diazasterol hydrochloride;  17β-[ 3-(dimethylamino)propyl ]methylamino ]androst-5-en-3β -ol hydrochloride; hypocholesteremic agent.

**a'zacrine.** 2-Methoxy-6-chloro-9-(5'-diethylamino-2'-pentyl)amino-3-azoacridine hydrochloride; an antimalarial; an effective schizontocide in acute falciparum infection.

**azacyclonol hydrochloride** (a'zah-si'klo-nol). FRENQUEL hydrochloride; γ-pipradol hydrochloride; α,α-diphenyl-4-piperidine-methanol hydrochloride; a structural isomer of pipradol hydrochloride and partially antagonistic to the actions of the latter agent; used with varying results in the treatment of hallucinations and confusion.

**8-azaguanine** (a'zah-gwah'nēn). Guanazolo; triazologuanine; a guanine antagonist that retards the growth of some cancers in mice.

**azalein** (ă-za'-le-in). Fuchsin.

**azametho'nium bromide.** PENIOMID; [ (methylimino)-diethylene ]bis-[ ethyldimethylammonium bromide ]; ganglionic blocking agent.

**a'zaperone** (USAN). 4'-Fluoro-4-[ 4-(2-pyridyl)-1-piperazinyl ]butyrophenone; tranquilizing agent.

**azapetine phosphate** (a-zap'ĕ-tēn) (NF). ILIDAR; 6-al-lyl-6,7-dihydro-5*H*-dibenz[ *c.e* ]azepine phosphate. A potent adrenergic (α-receptor) blocking agent similar in action and uses to those of tolazoline. Used in the treatment of peripheral vascular diseases.

**azar'ibine** (USAN). TRIAZURE; 2-β-D-ribofuranosyl-*as*-triazine-3,5(2*H*,4*H*)-dione 2',3',5'-triacetate; antipsoriatic agent.

**azarin** (a'ză-rin). A yellow dye from coal tar.

**azaserine** (a'ză-sēr'ēn) (USAN). *O*-Diazoacetyl-L-serine; $N_2CH$—CO—O—$CH_2CH(NH_2)COOH$; an antibiotic inhibitor of purine synthesis.

**azathi'oprine** (USP, BP). IMURAN; 6-(1-methyl-4-nitro-5-imidazolyl)thiopurine; a derivative of 6-mercaptopurine, used as a cytotoxic and immunosuppressive agent in organ transplantation and in the treatment of autoimmune hemolytic anemias, systemic lupus erythematosus, leukemias, and rheumatoid arthritis.

**azathy'mine.** 6-Azathymine; an antimetabolite of thymine.

Azathymine

**6-azauridine** (az-aw'rĭ-dēn). AzUR; a triazine analogue of uridine; antimetabolite with selectivity for human neoplastic leukocytes; produces partial remissions in certain acute leukemias of adults.

**azela'ic acid.** Nonanedioic acid; $HOOC(CH_2)_7COOH$; one of the products of the oxidative cleavage of oleic acid at the double bond.

**aze'otrope** [ G. *a*- priv. + *zeein*, to boil, + *tropos*, a turning ]. A mixture of two liquids that boils without change in proportion of the two liquids, either in the liquid or the vapor phase; 95 per cent ethanol and 6 N HCl are both azeotropes or azeotropic mixtures.

**halothane-ether a.,** an azeotropic mixture in the proportions halothane 68 to diethyl ether 32, by volume.

**azide** (az-id). A compound that contains the monovalent —$N_3$ group.

**azo-** (a'zo-, az-o-). A prefix denoting the presence in a molecule of the group —N=N—; the prefix *diazo-* is also used.

**azoamyly** (az-o-am'i-lĭ) [ G. *a*- priv. + *zōon*, animal, + *amylon*, starch ]. Absence or diminution in the amount of glycogen in the liver, presumed to result from defective metabolism of hepatic cells. Obsolete usage.

**azobiliru'bin.** The red-violet pigment formed by the condensation of diazotized sulfanilic acid with bilirubin in the van den Bergh reaction.

**azocarmine.** A dye giving a dark purplish red color as a histological stain.

**azo compound.** An organic compound containing the diazo (—N=N—) group linked to two carbon atoms; if linked to other than a carbon atom (or to -CN) on one side, the term "diazo" is used.

**azo dyes.** Dyes in which the azo group is the chromophore and joins benzene or naphthalene rings; they are used as

8-Azaguanine

biological stains, clinically to promote epithelial growth in the treatment of sluggish ulcers, burns, and other wounds, and in histology as fat stains; many have anticoagulant action. See *scarlet* red; *scarlet* red sulfonate; dimazon.

**azo'ic.** Containing no living things; without organic life.

**azolit'min.** A purplish red coloring matter obtained from litmus. Used as an indicator of pH; red at 4.5, blue at 8.3.

**azomy'cin.** 2-Nitroimidazole; antibiotic substance produced by an unidentified *Streptomyces* species; antimicrobial agent.

**azoospermia** (a-zo-o-sper'mĭ-ah) [ G. *a*- priv. + *zōon*, animal, + *sperma*, seed ]. Absence of living spermatozoa in the semen; failure of spermatogenesis.

**azopro'teins.** Modified proteins produced by treatment with diazonium derivatives of various aromatic amines. Used to elicit antibody formation and demonstrate antibody specificity.

**azoru'bin S.** A dark red mono-azo dye that may be used as a means of detecting hepatic dysfunction; after intravenous injection in a normal person, most of the dye is excreted in bile, but approximately 5 per cent is found in urine; larger amounts are excreted by the kidneys when the liver is diseased.

**azosul'famide.** NEOPRONTOSIL; PRONTOSIL-soluble; 2-(4'-sulfamylphenylazo) -7- acetamido-1- hydroxynaphthalene-3,6-disulfonate; a reddish derivative, soluble in water, less toxic but less effective than sulfanilamide. It owes its antibacterial activity to the sulfanilamide released.

**azote** (a'zōt, az'ōt). Nitrogen; a name proposed originally by Lavoisier and not used outside France; nevertheless, the origin of the stem azo (*q.v.*).

**azote'mia** [ azote + G. *haima*, blood ]. Uremia.

**nonrenal a.,** nitrogen retention from something other than primary renal disease, also called prerenal a.

**azother'mia** [ azote + G. *therme*, heat ]. Fever from nitrogen retention.

**az'otize.** To combine with nitrogen.

**az'otized.** Nitrogenized; containing nitrogen.

**azotom'eter.** A device for determining the amount of urea and uric acid in the urine.

**azotorrhea** (a-zo-to-re'ah) [ azote, *q.v.*, + G. *rheō*, to flow ]. Excessive discharge of nitrogenous material in the urine or feces, indicating impaired digestion or utilization of protein of albumin. Obsolete usage.

**azoturia** (az'o-tu'rĭ-ah) [ azote + G. *ouron*, urine ]. An increased elimination of urea in the urine.

**a. of horses,** paralytic myoglobinuria; Monday morning sickness; hemoglobinemia paralytica; black water (colloquialism); usually occurring in the heavier work type of horse, it appears suddenly, shortly after the horse has returned to work after a few days' rest. The disease is afebrile; it presents a rapidly developing paralysis of the hind legs due to massive muscle degeneration, especially of the muscles of the loin and croup, the urine becomes dark brown in color because of the presence of myoglobin derived from the degenerating muscles.

**azotu'ric.** Relating to the urinary excretion of nitrogen.

**azovan blue** (B.P.). *Evans* blue.

**az'ul.** Pinta.

**az'ulin.** A blue aniline dye.

**AzUR.** 6-Azauridine.

**azure** (azh'ūr). A term for a group of basic, blue methylthionine or phenothiazine dyes; the a.'s are used as biological stains.

**a. A,** a blue dye; asymmetrical dimethylthionine chloride, $(CH_3)N \cdot C_6H_3(SN)C_6H_3NH \cdot HCl$.

**a. B,** trimethylthionine chloride, $(CH_3)_2N \cdot C_6H_3(SN)C_6H_3 \cdot NCH_3 \cdot HCl$.

**a. C,** monomethylthionine chloride, $(CH_3)NH \cdot C_6H_3(SN)C_6H_3 \cdot NH \cdot HCl$.

**a. I,** trade name for a mixture containing a. A and a. B; methylene azure.

**a. II,** a mixture of a. I and methylene blue.

**az'ures'in** (NF). DIAGNEX blue; a complex of azure A and carbacrylic resin; used as an indicator for the detection of gastric achlorhydria without intubation.

**azurophil, azurophile** (azh-u-ro-fil, -fīl) [ azure + G. *philos*, fond ]. Staining readily with an azure dye, denoting especially the hyperchromatin.

**az'ygogram.** X-ray picture of the azygos venous system after injection of contrast medium.

**azygography** (az'i-gog'ră-fī). Radiography of the azygos venous system after injection of contrast medium.

**azygos** (az'i-gos) [ G. *a*- priv. + *zygon*, a yoke ] [ NA ]. An unpaired (azygous) anatomical structure.

**azygous** (az'i-gus, ă-zi'gus) [ L. *azygos* ]. Unpaired; single.

**azy'mia** [ G. *a*- priv. + *zymē*, ferment. ZE- ]. Absence of an enzyme.

**azy'mic, az'ymous.** 1. Without an enzyme. 2. Unfermented; unleavened.

# B

$\beta$. The Greek letter, beta, *q.v.*

**B.** 1. Abbreviation for base. 2. Chemical symbol of the element boron. 3. As a subscript, refers to barometric *pressure.*

**b.** As a subscript, refers to blood.

**Ba.** Chemical symbol of the element barium.

**Babbitt,** Isaac, American inventor, 1799–1862. See B. *metal.*

**Babcock,** S. M., American chemist, 1843–1931. See B's *test, B. tube.*

**Babcock,** William Wayne, American surgeon, 1872–1963. See B.'s *forceps, operation.*

**Babès,** Victor, Roumanian bacteriologist, 1854–1926. Gave his name to *Babesia.* See B.-Ernst *bodies,* B.'s *node, stain.*

**Babesia** (bă-be'zĭ-ah) [ V. *Babès* ]. *Piroplasma;* the most economically important genus of the family Babesiidae. These parasites multiply in the red blood cells to form pairs or tetrads. An extremely important pathogen in many parts of the world, it causes babesiosis (piroplasmosis) in most types of domestic animals; known vectors are ixodid or argasid ticks.

**B. argenti'na,** a species morphologically similar to *B. bovis,* but occurring in cattle in Central and South America and Australia; the disease caused by this parasite in Australia is particularly severe. It is transovarially transmitted by *Boophilus microplus* in South America and by *B. australis* in Australia.

**B. ber'bera,** a species described from cattle in North Africa, U.S.S.R. and southern Europe; may prove to be a synonym of *B. bovis.*

**B. bigem'ina,** the etiologic agent of bovine babesiosis, also known as cattle tick fever.

**B. bo'vis,** the most important cause of bovine babesiosis in Europe, occurring also in the U.S.S.R. and Africa; this parasite is smaller than *B. bigemina* and the disease caused by it generally less severe; it is transmitted by ticks of the genera *Boophilus, Rhipicephalus* and *Ixodes.*

**B. cabal'li,** a cause of equine babesiosis in many parts of the world, including the southeastern United States; vector ticks are species of *Dermacentor, Hyalomma,* and *Rhipicephalus.*

**B. ca'nis,** found in dogs, wolves and jackals in many tropical and subtropical areas of the Americas, Europe, Asia, and Africa; it is most pathogenic in dogs, causing mild to severe canine babesiosis, the severest disease occurring in dogs imported into areas where the disease is enzootic; the most important vector is *Rhipicephalus sanguineus.*

**B. diver'gens,** the commonest species of *Babesia* in western and central Europe, causing a disease of cattle similar to that produced by *B. bovis,* the vector tick is *Ixodes ricinus.*

**B. e'qui,** occurs in horses, mules, donkeys and zebras and has geographic distribution similar to that of *B. caballi,* but is smaller and more pathogenic.

**B. fe'lis,** found in domestic and wild members of the cat family, chiefly in Africa and India, causing babesiosis less severe than that caused by *B. canis.*

**B. gibsoni,** *Nuttallia gibsoni;* infects dogs, wolves and jackals, chiefly in India, Ceylon and China, and is smaller than *B. canis;* it is only slightly pathogenic for the natural host, the jackal, but highly pathogenic in the dog.

**B. motasi,** causes acute or chronic disease of sheep and goats in southern Europe, Africa, the Middle East, the U.S.S.R., and other areas; transmitted by ticks of the genera *Rhipicephalus, Haemaphysalis* and *Dermacentor.*

**B. ovis,** described from sheep and goats in many tropical and subtropical areas of the eastern hemisphere; it is smaller and less pathogenic than *B. motasi,* and immunologically distinct.

**B. trautmanni,** causes mild or fatal babesiosis in pigs in southern Europe, the U.S.S.R., and Africa; the vector is *Rhipicephalus sanguineus.*

**babesiasis** (bă-be-zi'ă-sis). Babesiosis.

**Babesiidae** (bab'e-zi'e-de, -ze'e-de) A family of protozoan parasites of the order Piroplasmida (Haemosporidia) occurring in the red blood cells of various mammals. The organisms are piriform, round, or oval in shape and reproduce by schizogony to form tetrads or by binary fission to form pairs in the red blood cells; transmission is effected by ticks. The family includes the genera *Babesia* and *Echinozoon; Aegyptianella,* formerly included, is now thought to be a rickettsia.

**babesiosis** (bă-be'zĭ-o'sis). Babesiasis; piroplasmosis; any disease caused by infection with a species of *Babesia,* the infection being transmitted by ticks.

**bovine b.,** bovine hemoglobinuria; redwater fever (1); Texas cattle fever; tick fever (3); an infectious disease of cattle caused by *Babesia bigemina* and transmitted by *Boophilus annulatus;* the disease was once prevalent in the southern United States but has now been eradicated; a similar disease occurs in many other countries, but the intermediate tick host varies in different areas.

**canine b.,** malignant fever in dogs caused by *Babesia canis* and transmitted by a tick.

**equine b.,** equine biliary fever; a disease of horses caused by species of *Babesia* and characterized by high fever, icterus, and enlargement of the spleen and lymph nodes.

**Babinski,** Joseph F., Paris neurologist, 1857–1932. See B.'s *phenomenon, reflex, sign.*

**baby.** An infant; a newborn child; a child yet unable to walk.

**blue b.,** a child born cyanotic because of a congenital cardiac or pulmonary defect causing incomplete oxygenation of the blood.

**collodion b.,** a newborn in whom the skin, at birth, is bright red, shiny, translucent, and drawn tight, giving a distorted appearance (as if having been painted with collodion) of immobilization of the face; the contraction of the skin causes ectropion, a pressed down appearance of the nose, and a gaping of the mouth and the labia; the condition is also called lamellar exfoliation of the newborn.

**baccate** (bak'āt) [ L. *bacca,* berry ]. Berry-like.

**Baccelli,** Guido, Italian physician, 1832–1916. See B.'s *sign.*

**bacciform** (bak'se-form) [ L. *bacca,* berry ]. Berry-shaped.

**Bachman,** George W., American parasitologist, *1890. See B. and Pettit *test.*

**Bachmann.** See Rivinus.

**Bachmann's bundle.** See under bundle.

**Bacillaceae** (bă-sil-la'se-e). A family of aerobic or facultatively anaerobic, sporeforming, ordinarily motile bacteria (order Eubacteriales) containing Gram-positive rods. These organisms are chemoheterotrophic. Some species are pathogenic. Ordinarily two genera, *Bacillus* and *Clostridium,* are included. The type genus is *Bacillus.*

**bacillar, bacillary** (bas'il-ar, bas'il-a-rĭ). Shaped like a rod; consisting of rods or rodlike elements.

**Bacille bilié de Calmette-Guérin** [ Fr. ]. Calmette-Guérin bacillus; BCG, a strain of *Mycobacterium bovis* used in the preparation of a vaccine against tuberculosis.

**bacille'mia** [ bacillus + G. *haima,* blood ]. The presence of rod-shaped bacteria in the circulating blood.

**bacilli** (bă-sil'i). Plural of bacillus.

**bacil'liform** [ L. *bacillus,* a rod, + *forma,* form ]. Rod-shaped.

**bacil'lin.** An antibiotic substance produced by *Bacillus subtilis.*

**bacillomyx'in.** An antibiotic active against certain pathogenic fungi obtained from cultures of *Bacillus subtilis.*

**bacillosis** (bas'ĭ-lo'sis). A general infection with bacilli.

**bacilluria** (bas'ĭ-lu'rĭ-ah) [ bacillus + G. *ouron,* urine ]. The passage of urine containing bacilli.

**Bacil'lus** [ L. dim. of *baculus,* rod, staff ]. A genus of aerobic or facultatively anaerobic, sporeforming, ordinarily motile bacteria (family Bacillaceae) containing Gram-positive rods. Motile cells are peritrichous. These organisms are chemoheterotrophic. They are found primarily in soil. A few species are animal pathogens; some species produce antibodies. The type species is *B. subtilis.*

**B. al'vei,** a species found in foulbrood in bees.

**B. amyloliquefa'ciens,** a highly amylolytic species of soil bacteria that produces subtilism.

**B. an'thracis,** Davaine's bacillus; a species which causes anthrax in man, cattle, swine, sheep, rabbits, guinea pigs, and mice.

**B. brevis,** a species found in soil, air, dust, milk, and cheese; some strains produce the antibiotic gramicidin or tyrocidin.

**B. hemoly'ticus,** *Clostridium haemolyticum.*

**B. histoly'ticus,** *Clostridium histolyticum.*

**B. ili'acus,** *Escherichia iliacus; Proteus iliacus,* a Gram--negative, nonsporing, motile, rod-shaped organism found in the intestinal canal. Its taxonomic relationships are not clear.

**B. in'dicus,** *Chromobacterium indicum; Serratia indica.*

**B. influen'zae,** *Haemophilus influenzae.*

**B. larvae,** a species that causes American foulbrood of honeybees.

**B. lentimor'bus,** a species that causes type B milky disease of the Japanese beetle, *Popillia japonica.*

**B. megate'rium,** a saprophytic species much studied experimentally, strains of which produce bacteriocins (megacins).

**B. polymyxa,** a species found in soil, water, milk, feces, and decaying vegetables; some strains produce the antibiotic polymyxin.

**B. popil'liae,** a species that causes type A milky disease of the Japanese beetle, *Popillia japonica.*

**B. pseudodiphtheriae,** *Corynebacterium bovis.*

**B. pulvifa'ciens,** a species that possibly causes the death of honeybee larvae.

**B. subtilis,** grass bacillus; hay bacillus; a species found in soil and decomposing organic matter; some strains produce the antibiotic subtilin, subtenolin, or bacillomycin. It is the type species of the genus *B.*

**B. thuringien'sis,** a species that causes the death of the larvae of certain insects.

**bacil'lus,** pl. **bacil'li** [ L. dim. of *baculus,* a rod, staff ]. 1. A rod-shaped bacterium. 2. The vernacular form of the generic name *Bacillus;* used to refer to a member of the genus *Bacillus.*

**Abel's b.,** *Klebsiella ozaenae.*

**abortus b.,** *Brucella abortus.*

**acne b.,** *Propionibacterium acnes.*

**Bang's b.,** *Brucella abortus.*

**Battey b.,** *Mycobacterium intracellulare.*

**blue pus b.,** *Pseudomonas aeruginosa.*

**Bordet-Gengou b.,** *Bordetella pertussis.*

**Calmette-Guérin b.,** *Bacille* bilié de Calmette-Guérin.

**cholera b.,** *Vibrio cholerae.*

**colon b.,** see *Escherichia coli.*

**comma b.,** *Vibrio cholerae.*

**Davaine's b.,** *Bacillus anthracis.*

**Döderlein's b.,** a large, Gram-positive bacterium occurring in normal vaginal secretions; although thought by some to be identical with *Lactobacillus acidophilus,* the identity of Döderlein's b. is still doubtful.

**Ducrey's b.,** *Haemophilus ducreyi.*

**dysentery b.,** an organism of the genus *Shigella* which causes dysentery.

**Eberth's b.,** *Salmonella typhi.*

**Flexner's b.,** *Shigella flexneri.*

**Friedländer's b.,** *Klebsiella pneumoniae.*

**fusiform b.,** *Fusobacterium fusiforme.*

**Gärtner's b.,** *Salmonella enteritidis.*

**gas b.,** *Clostridium perfringens.*

**Ghon and Sachs b.,** *Clostridium septicum.*

**glanders b.,** *Pseudomonas mallei.*

**grass b.,** *Bacillus subtilis.*

**Hansen's b.,** *Mycobacterium leprae.*

**hay b.,** *Bacillus subtilis.*

**Hoffmann's b.,** *Corynebacterium pseudodiphtheriticum.*

**hog cholera b.,** *Salmonella choleraesuis.*

**influenza b.,** *Haemophilus influenzae.*

**Johne's b.,** *Mycobacterium paratuberculosis.*

**Kitasato's b.,** *Yersinia pestis.*

**Klebs-Loeffler b.,** *Corynebacterium diphtheriae.*

**Koch's b.,** (1) *Mycobacterium tuberculosis,* (2) *Vibrio cholerae.*

**Koch-Weeks b.,** *Haemophilus influenzae.*

**lactic acid b.,** a member of the genus *Lactobacillus.*

**leprosy b.,** *Mycobacterium leprae.*

**Loeffler's b.,** *Corynebacterium diphtheriae.*

**mist b.,** *Mycobacterium smegmatis,* formerly *M. lacticola.*

**Moeller's grass b.,** *Mycobacterium phlei.*

**Morgan's b.,** *Proteus morganii.*

**Much's b.,** an alleged non-acid fast granular form of the tubercle b.; not demonstrable by the Ziehl stain, but takes a modified Gram stain; it is said to be the form present in the tuberculous skin lesion.

**necrosis b.,** *Sphaerophorus necrophorus.*

**Nicolaier's b.,** *Clostridium tetani.*

**paraco'lon b.,** any one of a number of diverse enteric bacteria which fail to ferment lactose promptly.

**paradysentery b.,** *Shigella flexneri.*

**paratyphoid b.,** one of the three organisms causing the three forms, A, B, and C, of paratyphoid fever; see under *Salmonella.*

**Park-Williams b.,** a special strain of *Corynebacterium diphtheriae* used for toxin production.

**Pfeiffer's b.,** *Haemophilus influenzae.*

**plague b.,** *Pasteurella pestis.*

**Plaut's b.,** *Fusobacterium fusiforme,* differentiated by some from Vincent's b.; the former is motile and nonpathogenic, the latter is nonmotile and pathogenic.

**Plotz b.,** a small, Gram-positive bacterium suggested as the pathogenic agent of typhus fever.

**Preisz-Nocard b.,** *Corynebacterium pseudotuberculosis.*

**rest b.,** Behring's term for the tubercle b. after the removal of the constituents soluble, respectively, in pure water, in a 10 per cent salt solution, and in alcohol and ether. It is from this that TC, or tuberculase, is prepared.

**Sachs' b.,** *Clostridium septicum.*

**Schimmelbusch's b.,** an alleged organism causing cancrum oris.

**Schmorl's b.,** *Sphaerophorus necrophorus.*

**Schottmüller's b.,** *Salmonella schottmuelleri.*

**Shiga b.,** *Shigella dysenteriae.*

**Shiga-Kruse b.,** *Shigella dysenteriae.*

**Sonne b.,** *Shigella sonnei.*

**tubercle b.,** (1) *Mycobacterium tuberculosis* (human); (2) *M. bovis* (bovine); (3) *M. avium* (avian).

**typhoid b.,** *Salmonella typhi.*

**Vincent's b.,** *Fusobacterium fusiforme.*

**vole b.,** an acid-fast b. isolated from voles by Wells and used in the production of a vaccine against human and bovine tuberculosis.

**Weeks' b.,** *Haemophilus influenzae.*

**Welch's b.,** *Clostridium perfringens.*

**Whitmore's b.,** *Pseudomonas pseudomallei.*

**bacitra'cin** (USP, BP). An antibacterial polypeptide of known chemical structure isolated from cultures of an aerobic, Gram-positive, spore-bearing bacillus (member of the *Bacillus subtilis* group). It is active against hemolytic streptococci, staphylococci, and several types of Gram-positive, aerobic, rod-shaped organisms. Usually applied locally. Zinc bacitracin (USP) is also available.

**back.** Dorsum.

**hollow b.,** lordosis.

**poker b.,** spondylitis deformans.

**saddle b.,** lordosis.

**backache** (bak'āk). Nonspecific term used to describe back pain; generally refers to pain below cervical level.

**back'bone.** Columna vertebralis.

**back'cross.** Mating of an individual heterozygous for one or more gene pairs to an individual homozygous for the same gene pairs.

**back'ing.** In dentistry, a metal support which serves to attach a facing to a prosthesis.

**back-knee.** Genu recurvatum.

**bac'lofen** (USAN). LIORESAL; β-{ aminomethyl)-*p*-chlorohydrocinnamic acid; muscle relaxant.

**Bacon,** Harry E., American physician, *1900. See B.'s *anoscope.*

**bacteremia** (bak'tēr-e'mĭ-ah) [ bacteria + G. *haima,* blood ]. Bacteriemia; the presence of viable bacteria in the circulating blood.

**bacteria** (bak-tēr'ĭ-ah). Plural of bacterium.

**bacte'rial.** Relating to bacteria.

**bactericholia** (bak'tēr-ĭ-ko'lĭ-ah). Bacteria in bile.

**bacterici'dal.** Bacteriocidal; causing the death of bacteria.

**bactericide** (bak'tēr'ĭ-sīd) [ bacteria + L. *caedo*, to kill ]. An agent that destroys bacteria.

   **specific b.,** a bacteriolytic immune serum destructive to one bacterial species or genus only.

**bacterid** (bak'ter-id) [ bacteria + suffix -*id* (1), *q.v.* ]. 1. A recurrent or persistent eruption of discrete, sterile pustules of the palms and soles, thought to be an allergic response to infection at a remote site. 2. A dissemination of a previously localized bacterial skin infection.

**bacteriemia** (bak-tēr-ĭ-e'mĭ-ah). Bacteremia.

**bac'terin.** A bacterial vaccine a suspension of bacteria, killed generally by heat or chemical means, used to enhance immunity.

**bacterina'tion.** Vaccination (2).

**bacterin'ia.** The systemic reaction sometimes following an injection of bacterins.

**bacterio-** [ see bacterium ]. Combining form relating to bacteria.

**bacte'rioagglu'tinin.** An antibody that agglutinates bacteria.

**bacte'rioci'dal.** Bactericidal.

**bacte'rioci'din.** Antibody having bactericidal activity.

**bacte'riocin'ogens.** Bacteriocin factors; bacterial episomes responsible for the elaboration of bacteriocins; in certain respects they resemble defective prophages.

**bacte'riocins.** Proteins which are produced by certain bacteria possessing bacteriocinogens, and which exert a lethal effect on closely related bacteria; in general, b.'s have a narrower range of activity than antibiotics and are more potent.

**bacterioclasis** (bak-tēr-ĭ-ok'lă-sis) [ bacterio- + G. *klasis*, a breaking ]. Fragmentation of bacteria, as in the Twort phenomenon.

**bacte'riofluores'cin.** A fluorescent material produced by bacteria.

**bacteriogenic** (bak-tēr'ĭ-o-jen'ik). Caused by bacteria.

**bacteriogenous** (bak-tēr-ĭ-oj'en-us). 1. Producing bacteria. 2. Of bacterial origin or causation.

**bacte'riohemagglu'tinin.** A hemagglutinin formed in the body as a result of stimulation by bacteria or their component antigens.

**bacte'riohemol'ysin.** A hemolysin formed in the body as a result of stimulation by bacteria or their component antigens.

**bacterioid** (bak-tēr'ĭ-oyd) [ bacterio- + G. *eidos*, resemblance ]. Resembling bacteria.

**bacteriolog'ical.** Relating to bacteriology.

**bacteriol'ogist.** One who primarily studies or works with bacteria.

**bacteriology** (bak-tēr-ĭ-ol'o-jĭ) [ bacterio- + G. *logos*, study ]. The branch of science which deals with the study of bacteria.

   **systematic b.,** that branch of b. dealing with nomenclature and classification.

**bacteriol'ysin.** Specific antibody that combines with bacterial cells (*i.e.*, antigen) and, when adequate complement is available, causes lysis or dissolution of the cells.

**bacteriolysis** (bak-tēr'ĭ-ol'ĭ-sis) [ bacterio- + G. *lysis*, dissolution ]. The dissolution of bacteria, *e.g.*, by means of hypotonic solutions or by specific antibody and complement.

**bacteriolyt'ic.** Pertaining to lytic destruction of bacteria; manifesting the ability to cause dissolution of bacterial cells.

**bacte'riolyze.** To cause the digestion or solution of bacterial cells.

**Bacterionema.** A genus of nonmotile, nonsporeforming, aerobic to facultatively anaerobic (some are strictly anaerobic) bacteria (family Actinomycetaceae) containing Gram-positive, non-acid fast, septate and nonseptate filaments (1.0 to 2.5 by 3 to μm). They may or may not produce catalase. Filamentous microcolonies are produced. The metabolism of these organisms is fermentative.

The products of glucose fermentation include carbon dioxide and formic, acetic, propionic, and lactic acids. The cell wall contains both diaminopimelic acid and arabinose. Catalase may or may not be produced. These organisms are found in the oral cavity of man and other primates. The type species is *B. matruchotii*.

   **B. matruchotii,** a species found in the oral cavities of man and other primates. It is the type species of the genus *B*.

**bacte'riopathol'ogy.** The study of disease in relation to bacteria or their products (*e.g.*, toxins), or both, as causal agents.

**bacte'riopex'y** [ bacterio- + G. *pēxis*, fixation ]. The immobilization of bacteria by phagocytic cells.

**bacteriophage** (bak-tēr'ĭ-o-fāj) [ bacterio- + G. *phagein*, to eat ]. A virus with specific affinity for bacteria and the active agent in d'Herelle's phenomenon. B.'s have been found in association with essentially all groups of bacteria, including the blue-green "algae"; like other viruses they contain either (but never both) ribonucleic acid (RNA b.) or deoxyribonucleic acid (DNA b.); they vary in structure from seemingly simple filamentous (fibrous) virus (*q.v.*) to relatively complex forms with contractile "tails"; their relationships to the host bacteria are rather specific and, as in the case of temperate b., may be genetically intimate; they are named after the bacterial species, group, or strain for which they are specific, *e.g.*, corynebacteriophage, coliphage, etc.; see also coliphage.

   **defective b.,** defective phage; a temperate b. mutant whose genome does not contain all of the normal components and cannot become fully infectious virus, yet can replicate indefinitely in the bacterial genome as defective probacteriophage; many defective b.'s are mediators of transduction.

   **mature b.,** the complete, infective form of b.

   **temperate b.,** b. whose genome incorporates with, and replicates with, that of the host bacterium; dissociation (and resultant development of vegetative b.) occurs at a slow rate resulting occasionally in lysis of a bacterium and release of mature b., thus rendering the bacterial culture capable of inducing general lysis if transferred to a culture of a susceptible bacterial strain.

   **typhoid b.,** b. specific for *Salmonella typhosa*.

   **vegetative b.,** the form of b. that multiplies freely within the host bacterium, independently of bacterial multiplication.

   **virulent b.,** a b. that regularly causes lysis of the bacteria that it infects; it may exist in one or the other of only two forms, vegetative or mature. It does not have a probacteriophage form (*i.e.*, its genome does not incorporate with that of the host bacterium), therefore it does not effect lysogenization.

**bacteriophagia** (bak-tēr'ĭ-o-fa'jĭ-ah). Twort-d'Herelle phenomenon.

**bacteriophagology** (bak-tēr'ĭ-o-fā-gol'o-jĭ). The study of bacteriophages.

**Bacterioph'agum intestinale.** An early name for bacteriophage.

**bacteriophobia** (bak-tēr-ĭ-o-fo'bĭ-ah) [ bacterio- + G. *phobos*, fear ]. A morbid fear of bacteria and other microbes.

**bacteriophytoma** (bak-tēr'ĭ-o-fi-to'mah) [ bacterio- + G. *phytos*, plant, + suffix -*oma*, growth ]. A growth in plant tissues produced by bacteria.

**bacte'rioplas'min.** A plasmin found in bacteria.

**bacterioprotein** (bak-tēr'ĭ-o-pro'tēn). One of the albuminous substances, or proteins, within the cells of bacteria; these substances vary in character and properties.

**bacteriop'sonin.** An opsonin acting upon bacteria, as distinguished from a hemopsonin which affects red blood corpuscles.

**bacterio'sis.** A morbid state caused by a bacterial microparasite; a localized or generalized bacterial infection.

**bacteriostasis** (bak-tēr'ĭ-os'tă-sis) [ bacterio- + G. *stasis*, a standing still ]. An arrest or retardation of growth of bacteria.

**bacte'riostat.** Any agent that inhibits or retards bacterial growth.

**bacte'riostat'ic.** Inhibiting or retarding the growth of bacteria.

**bacte′riother′apy.** Treatment of disease by means of bacteria or their products.

**bacte′riotox′ic.** 1. Poisonous or toxic to bacteria. 2. Caused by or pertaining to a bacteriotoxin.

**bacte′riotox′in.** A specific substance injurious to bacteria, usually a bacteriolysin.

**bacte′riotrop′ic** [ bacterio- + G. *tropē*, a turning ]. Turning toward or moving in the direction of bacteria; having an affinity for bacteria.

**bacte′riot′ropin.** A constituent of the blood, usually a specific antibody, *i.e.*, opsonin, that combines with bacterial cells and causes them to be more susceptible to phagocytes.

**bacte′riotryp′sin.** Enzyme produced by bacteria, particularly *Vibrio cholerae.*

**Bacterium** (bak-tēr′ĭ-um) [ Mod. L. fr. G. *baktērion*, dim. of *baktron*, a staff or club ]. A bacterial generic name placed in the list of rejected names by the Judicial Commission and the International Committee on Systematic Bacteriology of the International Association of Microbiological Societies. As a consequence, *B.* is no longer used in bacteriology. Identifiable organisms formerly placed in the genus *B.* have all been transferred to other genera.

    **B. anitratum,** *Acinetobacter calcoaceticus.*
    **B. coli** *Escherichia coli.*

**bacterium,** pl. **bacte′ria** (bak-tēr′ĭ-um) [ Mod. L. fr. G. *baktērion*, dim. of *baktron*, a staff ]. A prokaryotic microorganism that differs from blue-green algae primarily in that the blue-green algae perform photosynthesis accompanied by oxygen evolution and have a photosynthetic pigment system that includes chlorophyll *a* and β-carotene.

    **Binn′s b.,** a type of the typhoid-paratyphoid subgroups of the nonlactose fermenting bacteria.
    **Chauveau′s b.** *Bacillus anthracis symptomatici; Clostridium chauvei.*
    **endoter′ic b.,** one that forms an endotoxin.
    **exoter′ic b.,** a b. that secretes an exotoxin.
    **lysogenic b.,** (1) a b. in the symbiotic condition in which its genome includes the genome (probacteriophage) of a temperate bacteriophage; in occasional instances the probacteriophage dissociates from the bacterial genome, develops into vegetative bacteriophage causing lysis of the respective host b. and release, into the culture medium, of mature, infective temperate bacteriophage. The majority of bacteria in the culture retain bacteriophage genomes within their own and are "immune" to reinfection; accordingly, obvious bacteriolysis does not occur and the lysogenic bacterial culture may be maintained indefinitely; however, because of the contained free mature bacteriophage, general lysis may be induced in cultures of other, susceptible, bacterial strains; (2) formerly, a pseudolysogenic bacterial strain (*i.e.*, a "carrier" strain of bacteriophage of low infectivity).

**bacteriuria** (bak-tēr′ĭ-u′rĭ-ah). The passage of bacteria in the urine.

**bac′teroid.** Resembling bacteria.

**Bacteroidaceae** (bak′te-roy-da′se-e). A family of obligately anaerobic (microaerophilic species may occur), nonsporeforming bacteria (order Eubacteriales) containing Gram-negative rods which vary in size from minute, filterable forms to long, filamentous, branching forms; pronounced pleomorphism may occur. Motile and nonmotile species occur; motile cells are peritrichous. Body fluids are frequently required for growth. Carbohydrates are usually fermented with the production of acid; gas may be produced in glucose or peptone media. These organisms occur primarily in the intestinal tracts and mucous membranes of warm-blooded animals. They may be pathogenic. The type genus is *Bacteroides.*

**Bacteroides** (bak′ter-oy′dēz) [ G. *bacterion* + *eidos*, form ]. A genus of obligately anaerobic, nonsporeforming bacteria (family Bacteroidaceae) containing Gram-negative rods. Motile species and nonmotile species occur; motile cells are peritrichous. Some species ferment carbohydrates and produce combinations of succinic, lactic, acetic, formic, or propionic acids, sometimes with short-chained alcohols; butyric acid is not a major product. Those species which do not ferment carbohydrates produce from peptone either trace to moderate amounts of

succinic, formic, acetic, and lactic acids or major amounts of acetic and butyric acids with moderate amounts of alcohols and isovaleric, propionic, and isobutyric acids. Some species are pathogenic to man and other animals. The type species is *B. fragilis.*

    **B. biacutus,** a species isolated from a case of appendicitis.
    **B. coagulans,** a species isolated from human feces and lung.
    **B. constella′tus,** a species isolated from an inflamed lacrimal sac.
    **B. corrodens,** a species isolated from infections of the respiratory tract, buccal cavity, intestinal tract, and blood after a dental extraction; probably occurs normally in man and other animals.
    **B. frag′ilis,** a species which is one of the predominant organisms in the lower intestinal tracts of man and other animals; also found in specimens from appendicitis, peritonitis, rectal abscesses, pilonidal cysts, surgical wounds, and lesions of the urogenital tract. It is the type species of the genus *B.*
    **B. furco′sus,** a species found in an infected appendix, in lung abscesses, and in feces.
    **B. melaninogen′icus,** a species found in the mouth, feces, infections of the mouth, soft tissue, respiratory tract, urogenital tract, and the intestinal tract. Pathogenic, but ordinarily in association with other organisms.
    **B. nodo′sus,** a species causing foot rot in sheep and possibly in goats.
    **B. ora′lis,** a species found in the gingival crevice area of man and in infections of the oral cavity and upper respiratory and genital tracts.
    **B. pneumosintes,** *Dialister pneumosintes;* a species found in nasopharyngeal washings from normal individuals; it may be involved in secondary infections of the upper respiratory tract.
    **B. pneumosin′tes** subsp. **septice′miae** a subspecies found in blood and brain abscesses.
    **B. pneumosin′tes** subsp. **sep′ticus,** a subspecies found in blood from a patient with chronic polyarthritis and endocarditis.
    **B. praeacu′tus,** a species found in the intestinal tracts of infants and in a gangrenous lesion.
    **B. putredi′nis,** a species found in feces and cases of acute appendicitis.
    **B. serpens,** a species found in infections of the intestinal tract, middle ear, and blood; also found in contaminated sea water.
    **B. trichoi′des,** a species found in blood, abdominal abscesses, intestinal tract infections, prostatic aspirate, wounds, and in a burn infection.

**bacteroidosis** (bak′ter-oy-do′sis). Infection with *Bacteroides.*

**baculiform** (bă-ku′lĭ-form) [ L. *baculum*, a rod, + *forma*, form ]. Rod-shaped.

**baculum** (bak′yu-lum) [ L. a rod ]. *Os penis.*

**Badal,** Antoine J., Bordeaux ophthalmologist, 1840–1929. See B.'s *operation.*

**Baehr-Lohlein lesion.** See under lesion.

**Baelz** (bālts), Erwin B., German physician in Tokyo, 1849–1913. See B.'s *disease.*

**Baer,** Karl E. von, Russian embryologist, 1793–1876. Founder of modern descriptive and comparative embryology.

**Baer,** William S., American orthopedic surgeon, 1872–1931. See B.'s *method.*

**Baeyer,** Johann F. W. A. von, German chemist, 1835–1917. See B.'s *theory.*

**bag** [ A.S. *baelg* ]. 1. A pouch; sac; receptacle. 2. The mammary glands or udder of a cow.

    **Ambu b.,** a self-reinflating bag to produce positive-pressure respiration during resuscitation, foam rubber being built into the walls of the b. so that its shape is automatically restored after compression and air is drawn in from the atmosphere.
    **Barnes′ b.,** Barnes' dilator; a dilatable, hourglass-shaped, rubber b., made in various sizes; formerly used for dilating the cervix uteri.
    **breathing b.,** a collapsible reservoir from which gases are inhaled and into which gases are sometimes exhaled during general anesthesia or artificial ventilation.

**Champetier de Ribes b.,** an elongated conical silk and rubber b. filled with water; formerly used to dilate the cervix and to provoke uterine contractions, in order to induce premature labor or in cases of placenta previa.

**Douglas b.,** a large b. (60 to 80 liters), made of airtight fabric, for the collection of expired air to determine oxygen consumption in man under many conditions of actual work.

**ice b.,** a rubber b. into which crushed ice is put to produce local cooling.

**nuclear b.,** the aggregation of nuclei occurring in the nonstriated center of an intrafusal muscle fiber of a neuromuscular spindle.

**Petersen's b.,** a rubber b. introduced into the rectum and inflated, in order to push up the bladder so as to facilitate the operation of suprapubic cystotomy.

**Plummer b.,** Plummer's *dilator.*

**Politzer b.,** a pear-shaped rubber b. used for forcing air through the Eustachian tube by the Politzer method.

**reservoir b.,** a collapsible container from which gases are inhaled and into which they may be exhaled during general anesthesia or artificial ventilation.

**Voorhees b.,** a hydrostatic b. formerly used for dilating the cervix in *accouchement forcé.*

**b. of waters,** the amniotic sac and contained amniotic fluid.

**bagasse** (bă-gas') [ Fr. fr. Sp. *bagazo,* husks or refuse ]. The crushed fibers or refuse from sugar cane.

**bagassosis** (bag'ă-so'sis). Extrinsic allergic alveolitis due to the inhalation of the spores of *Thermoactinomyces vulgaris* contaminating sugar cane fiber (bagasse).

**Baggenstoss change.** See under change.

**Bah'nung** [ Ger. ]. The increased ease of transmission of a nerve impulse in a nerve tract as a result of prior stimulation.

**baicalein.** Noroxylin; 5,6,7-trihydroxyflavone; astringent.

**Bail's hypothesis.** See under hypothesis.

**Baillarger** (bi-yar-zha'), Jules G. F., French neurologist, 1809–1890. See B.'s *band, lines.*

**Bailliart,** (bi-yar'), Paul, French ophthalmologist, 1877–1969. See B.'s *ophthalmodynamometer.*

**Bainbridge reflex.** See under reflex.

**bakand'jia.** Murine *typhus.*

**Baker,** James P. See Charcot-Weiss-B. *syndrome.*

**Baker,** William M., English surgeon, 1839–1896. See B.'s *cyst.*

**bak'kola.** A fungus growth on birch trees in Finland, a decoction of which is popularly used in cancer; it contains a principle resembling chrysarobin.

**BAL.** Abbreviation for British anti-Lewisite; see dimercaprol.

**balan-.** See balano-.

**bal'ance** [ L. *bi-,* twice, + *lanx,* dish, scale ]. 1. Scales; an apparatus for weighing. 2. The normal state of action and reaction between two or more parts or organs of the body. 3. Quantities, concentrations, and proportionate amounts of bodily constituents, *e.g.,* water and electrolyte b. 4. The difference between intake and outgo, as of nitrogen or other metabolite. See also equilibrium.

**acid-base b.,** acid-base equilibrium; the normal b. between acid and base in the blood plasma, expressed in the hydrogen ion concentration, pH.

**cholesterol b.,** see under cholesterol.

**electrolyte b.,** usually designates the bodily content of sodium and potassium and the concentrations of these ions in extracellular and intracellular fluids.

**fluid b.,** water b.; b. in the intake and loss of water.

**genic b.,** see balance theory of sex, under theory.

**nitrogen b.,** see under nitrogen.

**occlusal b.,** a condition in which there are simultaneous contacts of the occluding units of the opposing dental arches in centric and eccentric positions within the functional range.

**b. theory of sex,** see under theory.

**water b.,** fluid b.

**Wilhelmy b.,** a device for measuring surface tension in terms of the pull exerted on a thin plate of platinum or other material suspended vertically through the surface; used in a Langmuir trough to study pulmonary surfactant.

**balaneutics** (bal'ă-nu'tiks) [ G. *balaneutica,* things pertaining to bathing ]. Balneology.

**balan'ic** [ G. *balanos,* acorn, glans ]. Relating to the glans penis or glans clitoridis.

**bal'anism** [ G. *balanos,* acorn, glans, pessary ]. Obsolete term for the use of a pessary or suppository.

**Balani'tes aegypti'aca** [ L. *balanos,* acorn ]. A genus of trees growing in the Near East, whose berries contain an active principle deadly to mollusks, miracidia, cercariae, tadpoles, and fish. Added to drinking water it is used as a prophylactic against bilharziasis.

**balani'tis** [ G. *balanos,* acorn, glans, + suffix *-itis,* inflammation ]. Inflammation of the glans penis or glans clitoridis.

**b. circina'ta,** a form thought to be due to the presence of *Spirochaeta balanitidis.*

**b. diabet'ica,** a form in diabetics resulting from irritation by the saccharine urine or urine contaminated with bacteria.

**b. xerot'ica oblit'erans,** atrophy and shrinking of the skin of the glans penis, which may result in urethral stenosis. The cause is unknown, but the condition is believed to be lichen sclerosus et atrophicus of the glans penis.

**balano-, balan-** [ G. *balanos,* acorn, glans ]. Combining forms relating to the glans penis.

**balanoblennorrhea** (bal'an-o-blen-or-e'ah) [ balano- + G. *blennos,* mucus, + *rhoia,* flow ]. Gonorrheal inflammation of the external surface of the glans penis.

**balanocele** (bal'an-o-sēl) [ balano- + G. *kēlē,* hernia ]. Protrusion of the glans penis through a gangrenous opening in the prepuce.

**balanochlamyditis** (bal'an-o-klam-ĭ-di'tis) [ balano- + G. *chlamys* (*chlamyd-*), a short mantle, + suffix *-itis,* inflammation ]. An inflammatory condition of the glans and prepuce of the clitoris.

**bal'anoplasty.** Any plastic operation upon the glans penis.

**balanoposthitis** (bal'an-o-pos-thi'tis) [ balano- + G. *posthē,* prepuce, + suffix *-itis,* inflammation ]. Inflammation of the glans penis and overlying prepuce.

**balanopreputial** (bal'an-o-pre-pu'shĭ-al). Relating to the glans penis and the prepuce.

**balanorrhagia** (bal'an-ō-ra'jĭ-ah) [ balano- + G. *rhēgnymi,* to burst forth ]. A running discharge from the glans penis.

**balanorrhea** (bal-an-ō-re'ah) [ balano- + G. *rhoia,* flow ]. Purulent balanitis.

**bal'antidi'asis.** Balantidosis; a disease caused by the presence of *Balantidium coli* in the large intestine; characterized by diarrhea, dysentery, and occasionally ulceration.

**Balantid'ium** [ G. *balantidion,* dim of *ballantion,* a bag ]. A genus of Ciliata, a class of Protozoa consisting largely of free-living aquatic ciliated forms.

**B. coli,** a parasitic ciliate, a cause of colitis resembling amebic dysentery. Normally, a parasite of pigs, transmitted by ingestion of infective cysts.

**B. suis,** originally considered distinct from the ciliate parasite of man, *B. coli,* but now considered synonymous with *B. coli.*

**balantido'sis.** Balantidiasis.

**bal'anus** [ G. *balanos,* acorn, glans penis. BALAN- ]. Glans penis.

**balbuties** (bal-bu'shĭ-ēz) [ L. *balbutio,* to stammer, fr. *balbus,* stammering ]. Stammering; stuttering.

**bald** [ M.E. *balled* ]. With no hair, or with a decrease in the amount of hair.

**bald'ness.** Alopecia.

**congenital b.,** *alopecia* congenitalis.

**male pattern b.,** *alopecia* hereditaria.

**Balduzzi's reflex.** See under reflex.

**Baldy,** John M., Philadelphia gynecologist, 1860–1934. See B.'s *operation.*

**baleri** (bal-a-re') [ a Peuhl (African) term meaning south ]. A name applied to *Trypanosoma brucei* infections of animals in the upper Niger valley region of West Africa; nagana.

**Balfour,** George W., English physician, 1823–1903. See B.'s *disease.*

**Balint,** Rudolph. See B.'s syndrome.

**Ball,** Sir Charles B., Dublin surgeon, 1851–1916. See B.'s *operation.*

**ball.** 1. A round mass; see bezoar. 2. In veterinary medicine, a large pill or bolus, about the size of a man's thumb. It contains medicinal agents held together by inert excipients.

    **chondrin b.,** one of the globular masses formed by a group of cells inclosed in a capsule, in hyaline cartilage.

    **dust b.,** a mass sometimes found in the stomach or intestine of an animal fed on mill cleanings.

    **food b.,** phytobezoar.

    **b. of the foot,** the padded portion of the sole at the anterior extremity of the metatarsus, upon which the weight rests when the heel is raised.

    **hair b.,** trichobezoar.

    **wool b.,** a trichophytobezoar formed chiefly of wool and vegetable matter in the stomach of sheep.

**Ballance,** Sir Charles A., English surgeon, 1856–1936. See B.'s *sign,* Koerte-B. *operation.*

**Ballet,** Gilbert, French neurologist, 1853–1916. See B.'s *disease, sign.*

**balling gun, balling iron.** An instrument used for administering boluses or capsules to animals.

**ballism** (bal'izm) [ G. *ballismos,* a jumping about. BALL- ]. Ballismus. 1. The occurrence of lively jerking or shaking movements, especially as observed in chorea. 2. Obsolete term for paralysis agitans.

**ballismus** (bal-iz'mus). Ballism.

**ballis'tocar'diogram** [ G. *ballō,* to throw, + *kardia,* heart, + *gramma,* something written ]. A record of the body's recoil caused by cardiac contraction and the ejection of blood into the aorta; may be used as a basis for calculating the cardiac output in man.

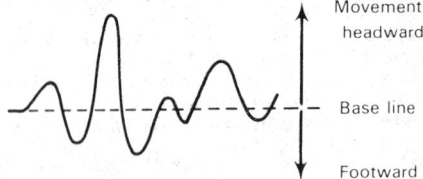

Movement headward

Base line

Footward

A Ballistocardiogram

**ballis'tocar'diograph.** Instrument for taking a ballistocardiogram, consisting either of a moving table suspended from the ceiling, or of an apparatus that rests upon the patient's body, usually on the shins, together with an optically recording system.

**ballis'tocardiog'raphy.** 1. The graphic recording of movements of the body imparted by ballistic forces (cardiac contraction and ejection of blood, deceleration of blood flow through the great vessels). These minute movements are amplified and recorded on moving chart paper after being translated into an electrical potential by a pickup device. 2. The study and interpretation of ballistocardiograms.

**ballistophobia** (bal-is-to-fo'bī-ah) [ G. *ballo,* to throw, + *phobos,* fear ]. A morbid fear of missiles.

**balloon.** To distend a cavity with air to facilitate its examination.

    **Shea-Anthony antral b.,** sinus b.

    **sinus b.,** Shea-Anthony antral b.; a hollow rubber structure, expandable with either liquid or air, used to support depressed fractures of the walls of the maxillary sinus; the b. of a Foley catheter is frequently used for this purpose.

**ballot'table.** Capable of exhibiting the phenomenon of ballottement.

**ballottement** (bal-ot-moń') [ Fr. *balloter,* to toss up ]. 1. A maneuver in physical examination to estimate the size of an organ not near the surface, particularly when there is ascites, by a flicking motion of the hand or fingers similar to that of dribbling a basketball. 2. An infrequently used method of diagnosis of pregnancy: with the tip of the forefinger in the vagina, a sharp tap is made against the lower segment of the uterus; the fetus, if present, is tossed upward, and if the finger is retained in place will be felt to strike against the wall of the uterus as it falls back.

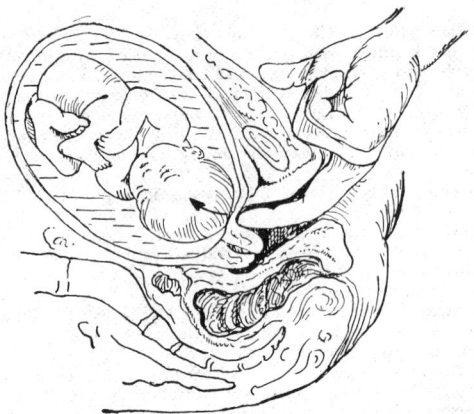

Ballottement

    **renal b.,** a maneuver in which the kidney is tossed between the fingertips of the two hands to identify it and determine its mobility.

**balm** [ L. *balsanum,* fr. G. *balsamon,* the balsam tree ]. 1. Balsam. 2. An ointment, especially a fragrant one. 3. A soothing application.

    **b. of Gil'ead,** Mecca balsam; opobalsamum; an oleoresin from *Commiphora opobalsamum* (family Burseraceae), probably the myrrh of the Bible; used in perfumery.

    **mountain b.,** eriodictyon.

    **sweet b.,** melissa.

**Bal'me,** Paul J., French physician, *1857. See B. *disease.*

**bal'nea.** Plural of balneum.

**balneary** (bal'ne-a-rī). An institution for the administration of balneotherapy.

**balneation** (bal'ne-a'shun). Balneotherapy.

**balneog'raphy** [ L. *balneum,* bath, + G. *graphō,* to write ]. A treatise on mineral springs and baths.

**balneol'ogy** [ L. *balneum,* bath, + G. *logos,* study ]. Balaneutics; the branch of medical science that treats of the constitution of natural mineral waters and their therapeutic use, especially in the form of baths.

**bal'neotherapeu'tics, bal'neother'apy** [ L. *balneum,* bath ]. The therapeutic application of baths.

**bal'neum,** pl. **bal'nea** [ L. ]. A bath; see also bath.

    **b. are'nae,** a sand bath.

    **b. cal'idum,** a hot bath.

    **b. frig'idum,** a cold bath.

    **b. mari'ae,** a salt water bath.

    **b. maris,** a salt water bath.

    **b. tep'idum,** a warm bath.

**Baló,** Jozsef, Hungarian physician, *1896. See B.'s *disease.*

**balsam** (bawl'sam) [ G. *balsamon;* L. *balsamum* ]. 1. A fragrant, resinous or thick, oily exudate from various trees and plants. 2. Balm.

    **Canada b.,** Canada turpentine; a yellowish liquid resin from the b. fir, *Abies balsamea* (family Pinaceae); contains kinene and bornyl acetate; used for mounting histologic specimens and as a cement for lenses.

    **b. of copai'ba,** copaiba.

    **gurjun b.,** wood oil; an oleoresin from *Dipterocarpus alatus* (family Dipterocarpaceae), a tree of India and other regions of southern Asia; formerly used in leprosy and in catarrhal conditions.

    **Mecca b.,** *balm* of Gilead.

    **b. of Peru,** a thick, dark brown liquid b. obtained from *Toluifera pereirae* (family Leguminosae); contains 60 per cent cinnamein. Used as a healing application to wounds.

    **Tolu b.** (USP, NF, BP), a yellowish brown soft mass obtained from *Toluifera balsamum* (family Leguminoseae); contains cinnamic and benzoic acids and esters. Used as a stimulant expectorant.

**balsam'ic.** 1. Relating to balsam. 2. Fragrant.

**Balser** (bahl'zer), W. August, German physician, 19th century. See B.'s *necrosis.*

**Bamberger,** Heinrich von, Vienna physician, 1822–1888. See B.'s *albuminuria, disease,* B.-Marie *disease,* B.'s *sign.*

**bamethan sulfate** (USAN). VASCULAT; α-[ (butylamino)-methyl ]-*p*-hydroxybenzyl alcohol sulfate; sympathomimetic amine used as peripheral vasodilator.

**bamifylline hydrochloride** (ba-mif'ĭ-lin) (USAN). TRENTADIL; 8-benzyl-7-{2-[ ethyl(2-hydroxyethyl)amino ] ethyl}theophylline hydrochloride; vasodilator and smooth muscle relaxant.

**bamipine.** SOVENTOL; 4-N-benzylanilino-1-methylpiperidine; antihistaminic.

**bancrofti'asis, bancrofto'sis.** Infection with *Wuchereria bancrofti.*

**band.** 1. Any appliance or part of an apparatus that encircles or binds the body or a limb. 2. Any ribbon-shaped or cordlike anatomical structure that encircles or binds another structure or that connects two or more parts; see fascia, line, stripe, stria, tenia.

**A b.'s,** Q b.'s; Q disks; A disks; anisotropic disks; the dark-staining anisotropic cross striations occurring in the myofibrils of muscle fibers.

**absorption b.,** that part of a broad spectrum of incident light that is absorbed by passage through a gaseous, liquid, or dissolved substance; the absorption b. is exploited for analytical purposes in colorimetry or spectrophotometry, and is usually described in terms of the wavelength where maximum absorbance occurs (*i.e.,* $\lambda_{max}$).

**amniotic b.'s,** strands of amniotic tissue adherent to the embryo or fetus; they may cause constriction of embryonic limbs; also called amniotic adhesions, Streeter's b.'s, and Simonart's b.'s, threads, or ligaments.

**anchor b.,** a b. that serves as a source of resistance when orthodontic forces are applied.

**anogen'ital b.,** the first indication of the perineum in the embryo.

**at'rioventric'ular b.,** *fasciculus* atrioventricularis.

**Baillarger's b.'s,** Baillarger's *lines.*

**Bechterew's b.,** *line* of Bechterew.

**belly b.,** a strip of flannel or other material encircling the abdomen.

**Broca's diagonal b.,** a white fiber bundle descending in the precommissural septum toward the base of the forebrain, immediately rostral to the lamina terminalis; at the base, the bundle turns in the caudolateral direction; traveling through a ventral stratum of the substantia innominata alongside the optic tract, it fades before reaching the amygdala.

**Clado's b.,** the suspensory ligament of the ovary covered with peritoneum.

**clamp b.,** an anchor b. secured to the tooth by means of a clamping device.

**b.'s of colon,** *teniae* coli.

**coronary b.,** corium coronae; a region of the pododerm; a prominent ridge of corium and underlying tela subcutanea at the top of the hoof from which most of the wall of the hoof grows.

**Gennari's b.,** *line* of Gennari.

**b of Giacomini,** uncus b. of Giacomini.

**H b.,** Hensen's line; Hensen's disk; H disk; the paler area in the center of the A band of a striated muscle fiber.

**His' b.,** *fasciculus* atrioventricularis.

**I b.,** I disk; isotropic disk; a light b. on each side of the Z line of striated muscle fibers.

**iliotibial b.,** *tractus* iliotibialis.

**Lane's b.,** Lane's kink; congenital b. on distal ileum causing stasis.

**M b.,** see M *line.*

**Mach's b.,** a relatively bright or dark b. perceived in a zone where the brightness increases or decreases rapidly.

**Maissiat's b.,** *tractus* iliotibialis.

**Meckel's b.,** a portion of the anterior ligament binding the malleus to the wall of the tympanum.

**moderator b.,** *trabecula* septomarginalis.

**pecten b.,** a fibrous induration of the anal pecten resulting from passive congestion or a low form of inflammation in this region.

**perioplic b.,** a narrow b. of corium and underlying tela subcutanea proximal to the coronary b. at the top of the hoof; the periople develops from it.

**Q b.'s,** see A b.'s.

**Reil's b.,** (1) *trabecula* septomarginalis; (2) *lemniscus* medialis.

**Simonart's b.'s,** amniotic b.'s.

**Soret's b.,** a dark b. in the violet end of the spectrum for hemoglobin.

**Streeter's b.'s,** amniotic b.'s.

**tooth b.,** the metal b. placed around the crown of a tooth for attaching an orthodontic appliance.

**uncus b. of Giacomini,** frenulum or b. of Giacomini; tail of the dentate gyrus; cauda fasciae dentatae; a slender whitish b., the attenuated anterior continuation of the dentate gyrus (fascia dentata), crossing transversally the surface of the recurved part of the uncus gyri parahippocampalis.

**ventricular b. of the larynx,** *plica* vestibularis.

**Weltmann's coagulation b.,** a b. of coagulation in a test tube that contains blood serum of the patient mixed in varying proportions with a solution of calcium chloride in distilled water; the presence of the b. is regarded as a nonspecific laboratory result suggesting the presence of exudative, fibrotic, or septic states.

**Z b.,** see Z *line.*

**zon'ular b.,** *zona* orbicularis.

**bandage** (ban'dij). A piece of cloth or other material, of varying shape and size, applied to a limb or other part of the body, to make compression, prevent motion, retain surgical dressings, etc.

**adhesive b.,** a sterile individual dressing consisting of a plain absorbent gauze affixed to a film or fabric coated with a pressure-sensitive, adhesive composition.

**Barton's b.,** a figure-of-8 b. supporting the lower jaw below and anteriorly; used in fracture.

**Baynton's b.,** adhesive plaster spiral b. for ulcer of the leg.

**cap'eline b.,** [ L. *capella,* a cap ]. a b. covering the head or an amputation stump like a cap.

**circular b.,** one encircling a limb or the trunk.

**crucial b.,** a b. in the shape of a T; T-b.

**demigauntlet b.,** one that covers only the hand, leaving the fingers exposed.

**Desault's b.,** a b. for fracture of the clavicle; the elbow is bound to the side, a pad being previously placed in the axilla.

**elastic b.,** one containing rubber or webbing; used to make pressure on a limb or other part.

**Esmarch's b.,** a rubber b. wound tightly about limb from the periphery toward the center in order to exsanguinate the member and offer a bloodless field for operation.

**figure-of-8 b.,** a b. applied alternately to two parts, usually two segments of a limb above and below the joint, in such a way that the turns describe the figure 8.

**Fricke's b.,** enveloping the scrotum with adhesive plaster strips in inflammation of the testicles and epididymis.

**Galen's b.,** a head b. consisting of a broad piece of cloth split into three tails at each of the two ends; these strips or tails are tied together over the forehead, under the chin, and at the nucha.

**gauntlet b.,** a b. for hand and fingers; see fig.

**gauze b.** see gauze, and subentries.

**Gibney's fixation b.,** herring-bone strapping of the foot and leg for sprain of the ankle.

**Gibson's b.,** a b., resembling Barton's b., for retaining the bone in fracture of the lower jaw.

**hammock b.,** a b. for retaining dressings on the head; the dressings are covered by a wide gauze strip the ends of which are brought down over the ears and held while a narrow circular b. is passed around the head, the ends are then turned up over the b. and other turns are made securing them firmly.

**Hippocrates' b.,** Hippocrates' *cap.*

**immovable b.,** a b. of cloth impregnated with plaster of Paris, liquid glass, or the like, which hardens soon after its application.

**many-tailed b.,** a large oblong cloth, the ends of which are cut into narrow strips, which is applied to the abdomen, the strips being tied or overlapped and safety pinned.

**Martin's b.,** a roller b. of soft rubber used to make compression on a limb in the treatment of varicose veins or ulcers.

**oblique b.,** one in which the successive turns proceed obliquely up or down the limb.

**plaster b.,** a roller b. impregnated with plaster of Paris, and applied moist, in order to make a permanent dressing for a fracture or diseased joint.

**recurrent b.,** (1) a spiral b. in which a second layer is formed by turns made in a direction the reverse of the first; (2) a b. applied to the end of an amputation stump, the head, etc., overlapping strips being carried forward and backward, retained by a circular b. at each equatorial turn.

**reverse b.,** a spiral b. in which with each turn the strip of cloth is turned back on itself, so as to facilitate adjustment to the swelling portion of a limb.

**roller b.,** a strip of cheese cloth or other material, of variable width, rolled into a compact cylinder so as to facilitate its application.

**scarf b.,** triangular b.

**Scultetus' b.,** one with several overlapping tails, usually applied on the thorax or abdomen.

**spica b.,** [ L. *spica*, ear of grain ]. a figure-of-8 b. applied to the body and the first part of a limb, or to the hand and a finger, in which the successive strips overlap slightly, giving a fancied resemblance to an ear of wheat.

**spiral b.,** an oblique b. encircling a limb, the successive turns overlapping those preceding by one-half or one-third.

**spiral reverse b.,** one with alternate obverse and reverse turns, to conform to a cone-shaped extremity.

**suspen'sory b.,** a bag of silk or cotton for supporting the scrotum and testes.

**T-b.,** a b. of two strips of cloth attached at right angles, used for retaining dressings on the perineum, etc.

**triangular b.,** a piece of cloth cut in the shape of a right-angled triangle, used as a sling for the arm and for other purposes.

**Tuffnell's b.,** a permanent b., consisting of a cheese-cloth roller impregnated with a mixture of flour and white of egg.

**Velpeau's b.,** a b. which serves to immobilize arm to chest wall; the forearm goes obliquely across and upward on front of chest.

**Bandi,** Ivo, 1867–1926. See B.'s *method* for identifying bacillus.

**Bandl,** Ludwig, German obstetrician, 1842–1892. See B.'s *ring*.

**bandy-leg.** *Genu* varum.

**bane.** A poison or blight.

**bane'berry.** Actaea.

**Bang,** Bernhard L. F., Copenhagen physician, 1848–1932. See B.'s *bacillus, disease, method* (for eliminating tuberculosis from dairy herds), abortus-B.-ring *test*.

**Bang,** Ivar, Swedish physiologic chemist, 1869–1918. See B.'s *method* (for microestimation of blood constituents).

**Bangerter,** Alfred P. D., Swiss ophthalmologist. See B.'s *method*.

**banis'terine.** Harmine.

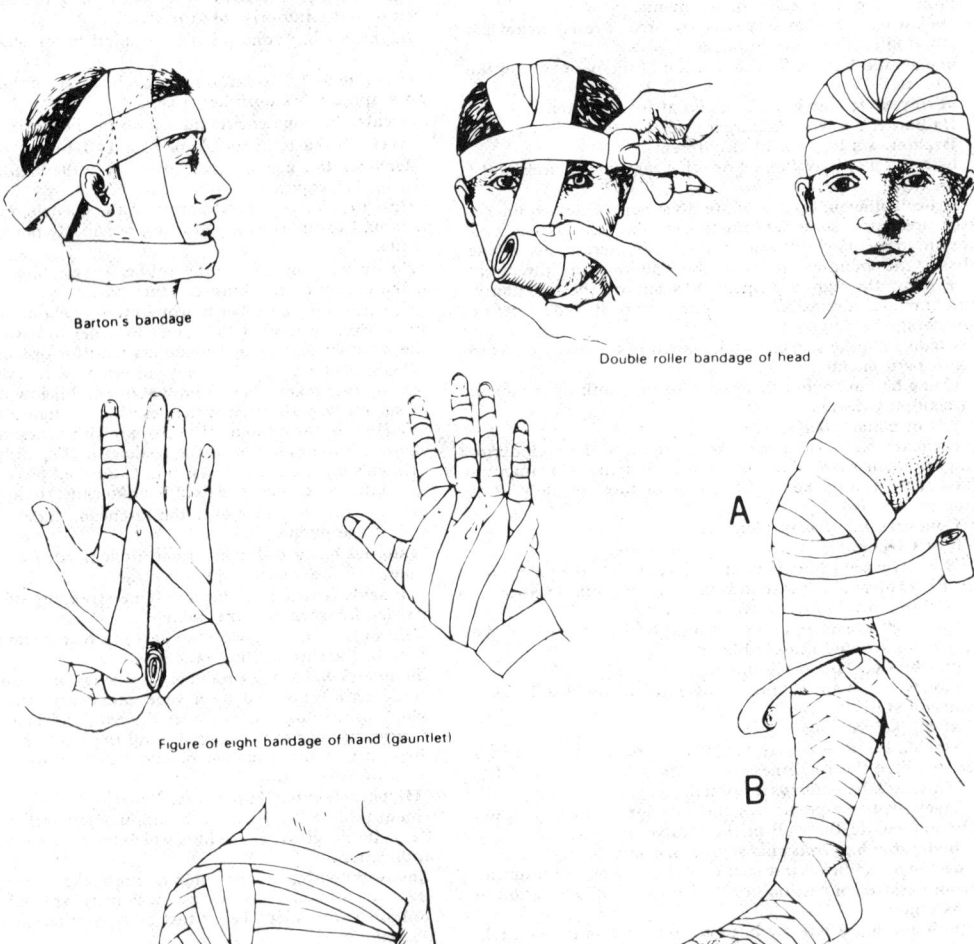

Barton's bandage

Double roller bandage of head

Figure of eight bandage of hand (gauntlet)

A Figure of eight of knee

B Spiral reverse

Spica of shoulder

**Bandaging**
(From Ellison, E. L.: *Practical Bandaging*, J. B. Lippincott Co., Philadelphia, 1914)

**Bannister,** Henry M., U. S. physician, 1844–1920. See B.'s *disease.*

**Banti,** Guido, Italian physician, 1852–1925. See B.'s *disease, syndrome.*

**Banting,** Sir Frederick G., Canadian physician, 1891 –1941. Nobel laureate, 1923, with John J. R. Macleod, for the discovery of insulin.

**Banting,** William, London physician, 1797–1878. Gave his name to bantingism.

**ban'tingism** [ W. *Banting* ]. A method of reducing obesity by a diet consisting chiefly of lean meat, avoiding fats other than those found in lean meat and carbohydrates.

**baptitox'ine.** Ulexine.

**Bar,** Paul, French obstetrician, 1853–1945. See B.'s *incision.*

**bar.** 1. The international unit of pressure; it is equal to 1 megadyne (10$^6$ dyne) per sq. cm. or 0.987 atmosphere. 2. One of the two convergent ridges on the ground surface of the hoof of a horse, united by the frog, and fused with the sole in front. 3. A metal segment of greater length than width which serves to connect two or more parts of a removable partial denture; see also major *connector;* 4. a segment of tissue or bone which unites two or more similar structures.

**arch b.,** (1) a connector used in the retention and stabilization of prosthetic appliances; it extends from one side of the a. to the other; may be palatal or lingual; (2) any one of several types of wires, b.'s, or splints conforming to the arch of the teeth and used for the treatment of fractures of the jaws and/or stabilization of injured teeth.

**b. of bladder,** *plica interureterica.*

**clasp b.,** see clasp.

**connector b.,** (1) b. (2); (2) see major or minor *connector.*

**Kennedy b.,** see continuous bar *retainer.*

**labial b.,** a major connector located labial to the dental arch joining two or more bilateral parts of a mandibular removable partial denture.

**lingual b.,** a major connector located lingual to the dental arch joining two or more bilateral parts of a mandibular removable partial denture.

**median b.,** Mercier's barrier; valvula prostatica; enlarged central or median portion of prostate.

**Mercier's b.,** *plica interureterica.*

**occlusal rest b.,** a minor connector used to attach an occlusal rest to a major part of a removable partial denture.

**palatal b.,** a major connector which crosses the palate and unites two or more parts of a maxillary removable partial denture.

**Passavant's b.,** Passavant's *cushion.*

**sternal b.,** one of the transverse units of the developing sternum formed by the union of paired primordia.

**terminal b.,** the attachment between epithelial cells consisting of the zonula occludens and zonula adherens.

**baragnosis** (băr-ag-no'sis) [ G. *baros,* weight + *a*- priv., + *gnōsis,* a knowing ]. Failure to appreciate the weight of objects held in the hand.

**Bárány** (băr'a-nē), Robert, Vienna otologist, 1876–1936. Nobel laureate, 1914, for his work on the physiology and pathology of the vestibular apparatus. See B.'s *sign, test.*

**barba** (bar'bah) [ L. ] 1 [ NA ]. The beard. 2. A hair of the beard.

**bar'bak.** *N,N'*-Mercuridicarbanilonitrile; fungicide.

**barbaloin** (bar-bal'o-in). Aloin.

**bar'barala'lia** [ G. *barbará*(fem. of adj. *barbaros*), foreign, + *lalia,* prattle ]. Dyslalia in attempting to speak a foreign language.

**barber-chair.** An adjustable type seat, quickly movable from upright to supine or semisupine positions; used to increase tolerance to high accelerations.

**bar'berry.** Berberis.

**barbiero** (bar-bī-a'ro). Brazilian term for the bloodsucking hemipteran triatomid bug, *Panstrongylus megistus,* an important vector of Chagas' disease, caused by *Trypanosoma* (or *Schizotrypanum*) *cruzi.*

**barbiers.** Beriberi.

**bar'bital.** VERONAL; barbitone; 5,5-diethylbarbituric acid; diethylmalonylurea; hypnotic and sedative.

**b. sodium,** barbitone sodium (BP); soluble b.; soluble barbitone; sodium salt of b., with same action as b.

**bar'bitone** (BP). Barbital.

**barbit'urate.** A salt of barbituric acid.

**barbitu'ric acid.** Malonylurea; 2,4,6-trioxohexahydropyrimidine; 2,4,6-(1*H*,3*H*,5*H*) pyrimidinetrione; a crystalline dibasic acid from which barbital and other barbiturates are derived; has no sedative action.

Barbituric acid

**bar'biturism.** Chronic poisoning by any of the derivatives of barbituric acid. The symptoms, which are not very distinctive, are a cutaneous eruption accompanied by chills, fever, and headache.

**barbone** (bar-bo'na) [ It. bearded ]. An old name for hemorrhagic septicemia.

**barbotage** (bar-bo-tahzh') [ Fr. *barboter,* to dabble ]. A method of spinal anesthesia in which a portion of the anesthetic solution is injected into the cerebral spinal fluid; cerebral spinal fluid is then aspirated into the syringe and a second portion of the contents of the syringe is injected; this process is repeated until the entire contents of the syringe are injected.

**bar'bula hirci** [ L. dim. of *barba,* beard, + gen. sing. of *hircus,* goat ]. The hairs growing from the tragus, antitragus, and incisura intertragica at the opening of the external acoustic meatus.

**Barclay,** Alfred E., English physician, 1877–1949. See B.-Baron *disease.*

**Barcroft,** Joseph F., English physiologist, 1872–1947. See B.-Warburg *apparatus, technique.*

**Bard,** Louis, Swiss physician, 1857–1930. See B.'s *sign.*

**Bard,** Philip, U. S. physiologist, *1898. See Cannon-B. *theory.*

**Bardet,** Georges, French physician, *1885. See B.-Biedl *syndrome;* Laurence-Moon-B.-Biedl *syndrome.*

**Bardinet** (bar-de-na'), Barthélemy A., French physician, 1809–1874. See B.'s *ligament.*

**bare'foot.** An unshod horse.

**baresthesia** (bar-es-the'zĭ-ah) [ G. *baros,* weight, + *aisthēsis,* sensation ]. Pressure *sense.*

**baresthesiometer** (bar'es-the'zĭ-om'e-tur) [ G. *baros,* weight, + *aisthēsis,* sensation, + *metron,* measure ]. An instrument for measuring the pressure sense.

**Baréty,** Jean P., French surgeon, 1887–1912. See B.'s *method.*

**bariatric** (băr-ĭ-at'rik). Relating to bariatrics.

**bariatrician** (băr'ĭ-ă-trish'un). A physician or surgeon skilled in bariatrics.

**bariatrics** (băr-ĭ-at'riks) [ G. *baros,* weight, + *iatreia,* medical treatment ]. That branch of medicine or surgery that deals with the management (prevention or control) of obesity and allied diseases.

**baric** (băr'ik). Relating to barium, or to barometric pressure (as in isobar), or to weight generally.

**baric'ity** [ G. *baros,* weight ]. The weight of one substance compared to the weight of an equal volume of another substance at the same temperature.

**baril'la.** Commercial, usually impure, sodium carbonate and sulfate.

**barito'sis.** A form of pneumoconiosis caused by barite or barium dust.

**barium** (băr'ĭ-um, ba'rĭ-um) [ G. *barys,* heavy ]. A metallic divalent element, symbol Ba, atomic weight 137.36, atomic no. 56; an alkaline earth element.

**b. chloride,** formerly used as a heart tonic and for varicose veins; extremely toxic.

**b. hydroxide,** Ba(OH)$_2$; a caustic compound combined with calcium hydroxide in a carbon dioxide absorbent; used in anesthetic circuits. See also absorbent (3).

**b. oxide,** barium monoxide; baryta; calcined baryta; BaO; it is caustic, forming the strong base, Ba(OH)$_2$, in water. Used as a dehydrating agent.

**b. sulfate** (USP, BP), terra alba; terra ponderosa; BaSO$_4$; given orally or rectally as a suspension for x-ray visualization of the gastrointestinal tract.

**b. sulfide,** a grayish yellow powder, poisonous. Used as a depilatory.

**bark.** 1. The envelope or covering of the roots, trunk, and branches of plants. B.'s of pharmacological significance not listed below are alphabetized under specific names. 2. Cinchona.

**crown b.,** pale b.

**druggists' b.,** cinchona b., removed from the trunk and dried in quills.

**manufacturers' b.,** cinchona b., broken and pressed flat to facilitate transportation.

**mossed b.,** light colored cinchona b., the result of binding the trunk with paper, cloth, leaves, etc.

**pale b.,** crown b.; the dried b. of *Cinchona officinalis*.

**red b.,** cinchona rubra.

**renewed b.,** cinchona b. that has been formed to cover portions of the tree previously denuded.

**yellow b.,** yellow *cinchona.*

**Barkman's reflex.** See under reflex.

**Barkow,** Hans K. L., German anatomist, 1798–1873. See B.'s *ligament.*

**bar'ley.** The seeds of *Hordeum distichon* (family Gramineae).

**Barlow,** Sir Thomas, London physician, 1845–1945. See B.'s *disease.*

**barn** [ fr. "big as the side of a barn" by humorous comparison with much smaller areas ]. A unit of area for nuclear cross-section equal to 10⁻²⁴ cm.² 

**Barnes,** Robert, London obstetrician, 1817–1907. See B.'s *bag, curve, dilator, speculum, zone.*

**Barnes' dystrophy.** See under dystrophy.

**baro-** [ G. *baros,* weight ]. Combining form relating to weight or pressure.

**baroceptor** (băr'o-sep-tor). Baroreceptor.

**bar'ograph.** Barometrograph; a device that gives a continuous record of barometric pressure.

**bar'omet'rograph.** Barograph.

**barophilic** (băr-o-fil'ik) [ G. *baros,* weight, + *phileō,* to love ]. Thriving under high environmental pressure; applied to microorganisms.

**baroreceptor** (băr'o-re-sep'tor). Baroceptor; pressoreceptor; sensory nerve endings in the wall of the auricles of the heart, vena cava, aortic arch, and carotid sinus, sensitive to stretching of the wall resulting from increased pressure from within, and functioning as the elicitation points of central reflex mechanisms that tend to reduce that pressure.

**baroscope** (băr'o-skōp). An instrument measuring changes in atmospheric pressure.

**bar'osinusi'tis** [ G. *baros,* weight, pressure, + sinusitis ]. Aerosinusitis.

**Baros'ma** [ G. *barys,* heavy, + *osmē,* odor ]. A genus of shrubs of the family Rutaceae.

**B. betuli'na,** a South African shrub, the leaves of which furnish buchu.

**bar'ospirator** [ G. *baros,* weight, + *spiro,* pp. -*atus,* to breathe ]. An instrument used in artificial respiration; produces variations in the air pressure within a closed chamber, *e.g.,* Drinker respirator.

**bar'ostat.** A pressure-regulating device or structure, such as the baroreceptors of the carotid sinus and aortic arch.

**barotax'is** [ G. *baros,* weight, + *taxis,* order ]. Reaction of living tissue to changes in pressure.

**bar'otitis me'dia.** Aerotitis media.

**barotrauma** (băr'o-traw'mah) [ G. *baros,* weight, + trauma ]. Injury, generally to the middle ear or paranasal sinuses, resulting from imbalance between ambient pressure and that within the affected cavity.

**otic b.,** injury caused to the ear by imbalance in pressure between ambient air and the air in the middle ear.

**sinus b.,** aerosinusitis, injury to air sinuses, resulting from imbalance in pressure between ambient air and air in the paranasal sinuses.

**barot'ropism** [ G. *baros,* weight, + *tropē,* a turning ]. Barotaxis.

**Barr,** Murray L., Canadian microanatomist, *1908. See B. chromatin *body.*

**Barraquer** (bah-rah-kair'), Ignacio, Barcelona ophthalmologist, 1884–1965. See B.'s *method.*

**Barraquer Roviralta,** (bah-rah-kair') J. A., Spanish physician, *1852. See B.'s *disease.*

**Barré** (bar-a'), Jean A., French neurologist, *1880. See Guillain-B. *reflex,* B.'s *sign,* Guillain-B. *syndrome.*

**barren** (băr'en) [ M.E. *bareyne* ]. Unable to produce a pregnancy.

**Barrett,** N. R. See B.'s *syndrome.*

**Barrier** (băr-re-a'), François M., French physician, 1813–1870. See B.'s *vacuoles.*

**barrier** (băr'rĭ-er). 1. Obstacle; impediment. 2. In psychiatry and social psychiatry, a conflictual agent that blocks resolving behavior.

**blood-air b.,** the material intervening between alveolar air and the blood; it consists of a nonstructural film or surfactant, alveolar epithelium, basement lamina, and endothelium.

**blood-aqueous b.,** a membrane of the capillary bed of the ciliary body that permits two-way transfer of fluids between the aqueous chamber and the blood stream.

**blood-brain b.,** blood-cerebrospinal fluid b.; blood-CSF b.; a selective mechanism opposing the passage of most large-molecular compounds from the blood to the cerebrospinal fluid and brain tissue. Traditionally thought to be a property of the pial-glial membrane surrounding the intracerebral blood vessels, it now appears likely that the b. largely is a function of the cerebral blood vessels proper.

**blood-cerebrospinal fluid b.,** blood-brain b.

**incest b.,** in psychoanalysis, the learning or internalization of parental and social prohibitions against incest.

**Mercier's b.,** median *bar.*

**placental b.,** the tissue intervening between fetal and maternal blood in the placenta. It differs widely in composition in different mammals and at different stages of pregnancy in the human placenta. It acts as a selective membrane regulating the passage of substances from the maternal to the fetal blood. See placenta.

**barrow** (băr'o) [ O.E. *barowe* ]. A castrated male hog.

**Barth,** Jean B., Strasburg physician, 1806–1877. See B.'s *hernia.*

**Bartholin** (bar'to-lin), Caspar, Copenhagen anatomist, 1655–1738. See B.'s *abscess, cyst, cystectomy, duct, gland.*

**Bartholin** (bar'to-lin), Thomas, Danish anatomist, 1616–1680. See B.'s *anus.*

**bartholinitis** (bar-to-lin-i'tis). Inflammation of a vulvovaginal (Bartholin's) gland.

**Bartholomew,** Rudolph A., U. S. obstetrician-gynecologist, *1886. See B.'s *rule.*

**Barton,** John R., Philadelphia surgeon, 1794–1871. See B.'s *bandage, forceps, fracture.*

**Bartonel'la** [ A. L. *Barton* ]. A genus of microorganisms (family Bartonellaceae) placed in the order Rickettsiales; they multiply in fixed-tissue cells and in erythrocytes, and reproduce by binary fission; they are found in man and in arthropod vectors.

**B. bacilliformis,** a species of microorganisms found in the blood and epithelial cells of lymph nodes, spleen, and liver of human cases of oroya fever; also found in blood and in eruptive elements in verruga peruana. Probably also found in sand flies (*Phlebotomus verrucarum*). Known to be established only on the South American continent and perhaps in Central America. It is the type species of the genus *Bartonella.*

**bartonello'sis.** A disease that is endemic in certain valleys of the Andes in Peru, Chile, Ecuador, Bolivia, and Colombia; caused by *Bartonella bacilliformis* and transmitted by the bite of the nocturnally biting sandfly, *Phlebotomus verrucarum.* It occurs in three forms: (1) Oroya fever (Carrion's disease), a generalized, acute, febrile, systemic infection, frequently fatal; (2) verruga peruana, a chronic form of the disease followed by nodular eruptions; and (3) a combination (or sequence) of these.

**Bartter,** F. C., U. S. physician, *1914. See B.'s *syndrome*.

**Baruch,** Simon, New York physician, 1840–1921. See B.'s *law*.

**baruria** (bar-u'ri-ah) [ G. *barys*, heavy, + *ouron*, urine ]. Excretion of urine that has an unusually high specific gravity, *e.g.*, greater than 1.025 to 1.030.

**Barwell,** Richard, English surgeon, 1826–1916. See B.'s *operation*.

**bary-** [ G. *barys*, heavy ]. Combining form meaning heavy.

**barye** bar'e) [ G. *barys*, heavy ]. The centimeter-gram-second unit of pressure, equal to a pressure of 1 dyne per sq. cm.

**baryglossia** (bar-i-glos'i-ah) [ bary- + G. *glōssa*, tongue ]. Barylalia.

**baryla'lia** [ bary- + G. *lalia*, speech ]. Baryphonia.

**baryma'zia** [ bary- + G. *mazos*, breast ]. Hypertrophy of the breast.

**barypho'nia** [ bary- + G. *phōnē*, voice ]. Baryglossia; barylalia; a deep voice.

**bary'ta** [ G. *barytēs*, weight ]. See barium oxide.
    **calcined b.,** barium oxide.

**barythy'mia** [ G. *barythymos*, heavy in spirit, fr. *barys*, heavy, + *thymos*, mind, disposition ]. Depression of spirits.

**baryto-.** A prefix indicating the presence of barium in a mineral.

**ba'sad.** In a direction toward the base of any object or structure.

**ba'sal.** 1. Relating to a base. 2. In dentistry, denoting the floor of a cavity in the grinding surface of a tooth.

**basalio'ma.** Basal cell *carcinoma*.

**ba'saloid.** Resembling that which is basal, but not necessarily basal in origin or position.

**basalo'ma.** Basal cell *carcinoma*.

**basculation** (bas-ku-la'shun) [ Fr. *basculer*, to swing ]. 1. The replacement of a retroverted uterus by a sort of seesaw movement. 2. Systolic recoil of the heart.

**base** [ L. and G. *basis*. BAS- ]. 1. The lower part or bottom; the part opposite the apex; the foundation; see basis. 2. In pharmacy, the chief ingredient of a mixture. 3. In chemistry, an electropositive element (cation) that unites with an anion to form a salt; a compound ionizing to yield hydroxyl ion. 4. A Brønsted b. is any molecule or ion that combines with hydrogen ion; *e.g.*, OH⁻, CN⁻, NH₃. This more general definition is gradually replacing the older and more limited definitions given in (3). 5. Nitrogen-containing organic compounds (*e.g.*, purines, pyrimidines, amines, alkaloids, ptomaines) that act as Brønsted b.'s. 6. Cations, or substances forming cations. 7. Element or radical containing an unshared pair of electrons (Lewis concept), *e.g.,*

$$ \begin{matrix} \text{H} \\ \ddot{} \\ :\text{N}:\text{H} \\ \ddot{} \\ \text{H} \end{matrix} \; + \; \text{H}^+ \; \rightarrow \; \begin{bmatrix} \text{H} \\ \ddot{} \\ \text{H}:\text{N}:\text{H} \\ \ddot{} \\ \text{H} \end{bmatrix}^+ $$

    **acrylic resin b.,** a form made of acrylic resin molded to conform to the tissues of the alveolar process and used to support the teeth of a prothesis.
    **al'dehyde b.,** see under aldehyde.
    **b. of arytenoid cartilage,** *basis* cartilaginis arytenoideae.
    **b. of bladder,** *fundus* vesicae urinariae.
    **b. of brain,** *facies* inferior cerebri.
    **Brønsted b.,** see b. (4).
    **cement b.,** for dental usage, see cement (2).
    **b. of cochlea,** *basis* cochleae.
    **denture b.,** saddle (2); (1) that part of a denture which rests on the oral mucosa and to which teeth are attached; (2) that part of a complete or partial denture which rests upon the basal seat and to which teeth are attached.
    **b. of heart,** *basis* cordis.
    **hexone b.'s,** the basic α-amino acids found among the hydrolysis products of proteins, namely, arginine, histi-

dine, and lysine, which are basic by virtue of the presence in the side chains of a guanidine, imidazole, and amine group, respectively; called "hexone" because each is a six-carbon compound.
    **histone b.,** hexone b.
    **b. of lung,** *basis* pulmonis.
    **b. of mandible,** *basis* mandibulae.
    **b. material,** see under material.
    **b. of metacarpal bone,** *basis* ossis metacarpalis.
    **metal b.,** a metallic portion of a denture base forming a part of wall of the basal surface of the denture; it serves as a base for the attachment of the plastic (resin) part of the denture and the teeth.
    **b. of metatarsal bone,** *basis* ossis metatarsalis.
    **b. of modiolus,** *basis* modioli.
    **nucleinic (nucleic acid) b.,** purine b.
    **b. pair,** see under pair.
    **b. of patella,** *basis* patellae.
    **b. of phalanx,** *basis* phalangis.
    **plastic b.,** a denture or record b. made of a plastic material.
    **pressor b.,** pressor amine; (1) one of several products of intestinal putrefaction believed to cause functional hyperpiesis, or high blood pressure, when absorbed; (2) any alkaline substance that raises blood pressure.
    **b. of prostate,** *basis* prostatae.
    **purine b.,** any purine.
    **b. of pyramid,** *basis* pyramidis.
    **pyrim'idine b.,** any pyrimidine.
    **quaternary ammo'nium b.'s,** see under ammonium.
    **record b.,** baseplate.
    **b. of sacrum,** *basis* ossis sacri.
    **Schiff b.,** a condensation (dehydration) product of a primary amine and an aldehyde with production of an N = C link; intermediates formed by pyridoxal phosphate in transaminations and amino acid decarboxylations are Schiff b.'s.
    **Schreiner's b.,** spermine.
    **shellac b.,** a resinous wafer adapted to maxillary or mandibular casts to form baseplates.
    **b. of skull,** *basis* cranii.
    **b. of stapes,** *basis* stapedis.
    **temporary b.,** baseplate.
    **tinted denture b.,** a denture b. that simulates the coloring and shading of natural oral tissues.
    **b. of tongue,** *radix* linguae.
    **tooth-borne b.,** the denture b. restoring an edentulous area which has abutment teeth at each end for support; the tissue which it covers is not used for support.
    **trial b.,** baseplate.
    **vegetable b.,** alkaloid.
    **xanthine b.,** purine b.

**basedoid** (baz'e-doyd). Denoting a condition resembling Basedow's disease, but without toxic symptoms.

**Basedow** (bah'zeh-do). Karl A. von, German physician, 1799–1854. See B.'s *disease*, Basedowian *insanity*, B.'s *pseudoparaplegia*.

**basedowian** (bah-ze-do'vi-an) [ K. *Basedow* ]. A sufferer from Basedow's or Graves' disease.

**base'ment.** 1. Base (1). 2. A cavity or space partly or completely separated from a larger space above it.

**baseplate** (bas'plat). Record base; temporary base; trial base; a temporary form representing the base of a denture; used for making maxillomandibular (jaw) relation records and for the arrangement of teeth.
    **stabilized b.,** a b. lined with plastic material to improve its fit and stability.

**bas-fond** (bah-fawn'). Fundus.

**basi-, basio-, baso-** [ G. and L. *basis*, base. BAS- ]. Combining forms meaning base, or basis.

**basia'lis.** Basal; relating to a basis or the basion.

**basialveolar** (ba-si-al-ve'o-lar). Relating to both basion and alveolar point; denoting especially the b. length, or the shortest distance between these two points.

**basiarachnitis,** **basiarachnoiditis** (ba-si-ar-ak-ni'tis, ba-se-ar-ak-noy-di'tis). Rarely used terms for basilar *leptomeningitis*.

**ba'sic.** Basilar; basal; relating to a base of any kind.

**basicity** (ba-sis'ĭ-tĭ). 1. The valence or combining power of an acid, or the number of replaceable atoms of hydrogen in its molecule. 2. The quality of being basic.

**ba'sicra'nial.** Relating to the base of the skull.

**Basidiobolus** (bă-sĭd'e-o-bo'lus) [ Mod. L. *basidium*, dim. of G. *basis*, base, + L. *bolus*, fr. G. *bolos*, lump or clod ]. A genus of fungi belonging to the class Phycomycetes (Zygomycetes); several strains of this fungus have been isolated from cases of subcutaneous phycomycosis in man.

**Basidiomycetes** (bă-sĭd' e-o-mi-sēt'es) [ Mod. L. *basid-ium*, dim. of G. *basis*, base, + *mykēs* (*mykēt*), fungus ]. A class of the fungi. The basidium which is a characteristic of this class is a peculiar type of reproductive organ; it is a swollen terminal cell situated on a slender stalk; it gives rise to slender filaments (sterigmata), usually four in number, from the ends of which the spores are developed. The class comprises the smuts, rusts, mushrooms, and puffballs.

**basid'iospore** [ G. *basidon*, small base, + *sporos*, seed ]. A spore (fungus) borne on a basidium, resulting from karyogamy and meiosis; such spores are found on mushrooms and related forms.

**basid'ium,** pl. **basid'ia** [ L. fr. G. *basis*, base ]. A spore-bearing organ or conidiophore, the spore mother cell of Basidiomycetes, that bears a fixed number of asexual spores (basidiospores or conidia) externally after karyogamy and meiosis.

**ba'sifa'cial.** Relating to the lower portion of the face.

**ba'sihy'al, basihy'oid.** The base or body of the hyoid bone.

**bas'ilar.** Relating to a base.

**ba'silat'eral.** Relating to the base and one or more sides of any part.

**ba'silem'ma** [ basi- + G. *lemma*, rind. LEP- ]. Basement *membrane*.

**basil'icus** [ L. fr. G. *basilikos*, royal ] [ NA ]. Denoting a prominent or important part or structure.

**basil'ysis** [ basi- + G. *lysis*, a loosening ]. Crushing the base of the skull of a fetus when delivery of a living child is impossible.

**bas'ilyst.** An instrument for crushing and extracting the head after craniotomy.

**ba'sin.** A receptacle or container for fluids, as for water used in washing.

**pus b.,** a receptacle curved so as to fit closely the surface to which it is applied, used to receive the pus from a wound during its cleansing and redressing.

**ba'sina'sal.** Relating to the basion and the nasion; denoting especially the b. length, or the shortest distance between the two points.

**ba'sio-.** See basi-.

**basioccipital** (ba'sĭ-ok-sip'ĭ-tal). Relating to the basilar process of the occipital bone.

**basioglos'sus.** The portion of the hyoglossus muscle that originates from the body of the hyoid bone.

**ba'sion** [ G. *basis*, a base ]. The middle point on the anterior margin of the foramen magnum, opposite the opisthion.

**basiotrip'sy** [ G. *basis*, base, + *tripsis*, a rubbing ]. Basilysis.

**basip'etal** [ basi- + L. *peto*, to seek ]. In a direction toward the base.

**basipho'bia** [ G. *basis*, a stepping, + *phobos*, fear ]. A morbid fear of walking.

**basis** [ L. and G. BAS- ]. [ NA ]. Base; foundation.

**b. cartilaginis arytenoideae** [ NA ], base of the arytenoid cartilage. It articulates with the cricoid cartilage and from it the muscular process extends laterally and the vocal process projects anteriorly.

**b. cerebri,** *facies* inferior cerebri.

**b. cochleae** [ NA ], base of the cochlea. It is directed posteriorly and medially and lies close to the internal acoustic meatus.

**b. cordis** [ NA ], base of the heart. It is formed mainly by the left atrium but to a small extent by the posterior part of the right atrium. It is directed backward and to the right and is separated from the vertebral column by the esophagus and aorta.

**b. cra'nii** [ NA ], the base of the skull. The inferior aspect is termed the **b. cranii externa** [ NA ], or norma basilaris. The interior aspect on which the brain rests is the **b. cranii interna** [ NA ].

**b. mandib'ulae** [ NA ], base of the mandible; the rounded inferior border of the body of the mandible.

**b. modi'oli** [ NA ], base of the modiolus; the part of the modiolus enclosed by the basal turn of the cochlea; it faces the lateral end of the internal acoustic meatus.

**b. os'sis metacarpa'lis** [ NA ], base of metacarpal bone; the expanded proximal extremity of each metacarpal that articulates with one or more of the distal row of carpal bones.

**b. os'sis metatarsa'lis** [ NA ], base of metatarsal bone; the expanded proximal extremity of each metatarsal bone; it articulates with one or more of the distal row of tarsal bones.

**b. os'sis sa'cri** [ NA ], base of the sacrum; the central part of the upper end of the sacrum that articulates with the body of the fifth lumbar vertebra. Most frequently the median ventral point of its anterior border forms the promontory and posteriorly it supports the superior articular processes.

**b. patel'lae** [ NA ], base of the patella; the superior border of the patella to which the tendon of the rectus femoris attaches.

**b. pedun'culi,** *crus* cerebri.

**b. phalan'gis** [ NA ], base of the phalanx; the expanded proximal end of each phalanx in the hand or foot that articulates with the head of the next proximal bone in the digit.

**b. prosta'tae** [ NA ], base of the prostate; the broad upper surface of the prostate contiguous with the bladder wall.

**b. pulmonis** [ NA ], base of the lung; the lower concave part of the lung that rests upon the convexity of the diaphragm.

**b. pyram'idis** [ NA ], base of the pyramid; the outer broad part of a renal pyramid that lies next to the cortex.

**b. stape'dis** [ NA ], base of the stapes; footplate (1); the flat portion of the stapes that fits in the oval window.

**basisphenoid** (ba'sĭ-sfe'noyd). Relating to the base or body of the sphenoid bone; denoting the independent center of ossification in the embryo that forms the posterior portion of the body of the sphenoid bone.

**ba'sitem'poral.** Relating to the lower part of the temporal region.

**ba'siver'tebral.** Relating to the body of a vertebra.

**bas'ket.** A basket-like arborization of the axon of cells in the cerebellar cortex, surrounding the cell body of Purkinje cells.

**fibrillar b.'s,** the scleral end of neuroglia fibers of Müller which as fine, tapering, needlelike fibrillae ascend the proximal parts of rods and cones, giving them a fibrillar appearance.

**Basle Nomina Anatomica.** Basel anatomical nomenclature; a list of Latin terms in anatomy adopted by the German Anatomical Society at its meeting in Basle in 1895. This system is commonly known as the BNA. A moderate revision of the BNA terminology was adopted at the meeting of the International Congress of Anatomists in Paris in 1955 and was modified in New York (1960), Wiesbaden (1965), and Leningrad (1970). See also *Nomina Anatomica*.

**ba'so-.** See basi-.

**basocyte** (ba'so-sit) [ G. *basis*, base, + *kytos*, cell ]. Basophilic *leukocyte*.

**ba'socytope'nia.** Basophilic *leukopenia*.

**ba'socyto'sis.** Basophilic *leukocytosis*.

**basoerythrocyte** (ba'so-e-rith'ro-sit). A red blood cell that manifests changes of basophilic degeneration, such as basophilic stippling, punctate basophilia or basophilic granules.

**basoerythrocytosis** (ba'so-e-rith'ro-si-to'sis). An increase of red blood cells with basophilic degenerative changes, frequently observed in diseases characterized by prolonged hypochromic anemia.

**ba'sograph** [ baso- + G. *graphō*, to write ]. An instrument that makes graphic records of abnormalities of gait.

**basolat'eral.** Basal and lateral; term used with reference to one of the two major subdivisions of the corpus amygdaloideum, the other subdivision being the corticomedial group of nuclei.

**basometachromophil, basometachromophile** (ba'so-met'ah-krō'mo-fil, -fil). Staining metachromatically with a basic dye. See metachromasia.

**ba'sope'nia** [ baso- + G. *penia*, poverty ]. Basophilic *leukopenia*.

**basophil, basophile** (ba'so-fil, -fil) [ baso- + G. *phileō*, to love ]. 1. A leukocyte of the granulocytic series, characterized by a relatively pale, lobate nucleus and conspicuous, large or coarse, densely basophilic granules; Ordinarily comprise only 0.5 to 1 per cent of the leukocytes in circulating blood. See color plate 14. 2. A parenchymatous cell with distinctive basophilic granules, as the b. of the pituitary gland. 3. Basophilic.

   **tissue b.,** mast *cell.*

**ba'sophil'ia.** Basophilism. 1. A condition in which there is more than the usual number of basophilic leukocytes in the circulating blood (basophilic leukocytosis) or an increase in the proportion of parenchymatous basophilic cells in an organ (in the bone marrow, basophilic hyperplasia). 2. A condition in which basophilic erythrocytes are found in circulating blood, as in certain instances of leukemia, advanced anemia, malaria, plumbism, and so on.

   **Grawitz' b.,** see b. (2).

   **pituitary b.,** obsolete name for pituitary basophil *adenoma.*

   **punctate b.,** stippling.

**ba'sophil'ic.** Basophil (3); having an affinity for basic dyes.

**basophilism** (ba-sof'ĭ-lizm). Basophilia.

   **Cushing's b.,** obsolete name for pituitary basophil *adenoma.*

   **pituitary b.,** obsolete name for pituitary basophil *adenoma.*

**ba'soplasm.** That part of the cytoplasm which stains readily with basic dyes.

**Bassen,** F. A. See B.-Kornzweig *syndrome.*

**Bassini,** Edoardo, Italian surgeon, 1844–1924. See B.'s *operation.*

**Bassler,** Anthony New York physician, 1874–1959. See B.'s *sign.*

**bas'sorin.** The insoluble portion, 60 to 70 per cent, of tragacanth that swells to form a gel; contains complex methoxylated acids, particularly bassoric acid.

**bast** [ A.S. *baest*]. The fibrous inner portion of the bark of linden and other trees.

**Baste'do,** Walter A., New York physician, 1873–1952. See B.'s *sign.*

**bat** [ M.E. *bakke* ]. A member of the mammalian order Chiroptera.

   **vampire b.,** a member of the genus *Desmodus.*

**bath** [ A.S. *baeth* ]. 1. The immersion of the body or any of its parts in water or any other yielding or fluid medium; or the application of such medium in any form (spray, vapor, affusion, jets, etc.) to a part or the whole of the body. 2. The apparatus employed in giving a b. of any form. The term is qualified according to the medium used: water b. air b., sand b., mud b., hot, warm, tepid, etc.; according to the temperature of the medium: temperate, cool, and cold (see below); according to the form in which the medium is applied: spray b., vapor b., douche b., etc.; according to the medicament added to the medium: acid b., alkaline b., alum b., astringent b., mustard b., sulfur b., etc.; and according to the part bathed: full b., foot b., sitz b., etc. B.'s are given in therapeutics for their local effect upon the skin in cutaneous disorders or for their effect upon the nervous or circulatory system, either relaxing or stimulating. The science which treats of bathing, especially bathing in the sea or in the waters of mineral springs, is called balneology. Hydrotherapy is the branch of therapeutics which deals with the local or general application of water in various forms and at various temperatures, chiefly for its systemic effects.

   **air b.,** the exposure of the naked body to the air, either cold or warm.

   **blood b.,** a b. in the warm, freshly drawn blood of an animal.

   **cold b.,** one in water at a temperature of 45°F. or lower.

   **contrast b.,** one in which a part is immersed in hot water (110°F. to 60°F.) for a period of a few minutes and then in cold (43°F. to 15.6°F.). The hot and cold periods are alternated regularly at half-hour intervals. Used to increase the blood flow to the part.

   **cool b.,** one in water at a temperature of about 68°F. (20°C.)

   **douche b.,** the local application of water in the form of a large jet or stream.

   **dousing b.,** a luminous electric hot air b. given at a very high temperature.

   **electric b., electrotherapeu'tic b.,** (1) hydroelectric b.; one in which the medium is charged with electricity; (2) the application of static electricity, the patient standing on an insulated platform.

   **Finnish b.,** sauna.

   **full b.,** one in which the entire body is immersed.

   **graduated b.,** one in which the temperature of the water is gradually lowered.

   **Greville b.,** a nonluminous electric hot air b. given at a very high temperature.

   **gymnoco'lon b.,** an intestinal b. by means of a special apparatus allowing of the injection of 8 to 16 ounces of an isotonic salt solution and the immediate evacuation of water and fecal masses, this being repeated until several quarts of water have been used.

   **hafus'si b.** [ Ger. *hand*, hand, + *fuss*, foot ], a modification of the Nauheim b., the hands and feet only of the patient being immersed in hot water through which carbon dioxide gas is made to pass.

   **half b.,** one in which only the hips and lower extremities are immersed.

   **hot b.,** one in water at a temperature of about 106°F. or over.

   **hydroelectric b.,** electric b. (1).

   **light b.,** exposure of the uncovered skin of the patient to light rays from the sun, a battery of electric light bulbs, or other source.

   **moor b.,** immersion of the body in thin mud taken from a swamp or other uncultivated tract.

   **Nauheim b.,** Nauheim *treatment.*

   **needle b.,** one in which water is thrown forcibly against the body in the shape of many very fine jets.

   **rain b.,** (1) one taken by standing naked in the rain; (2) a very gentle form of shower b.

   **Russian b.,** a steam b. followed by rubbing and a cold plunge; also called Finnish b.

   **sand b.,** (1) covering the body with warm dry sand; see also psammotherapy; (2) an arrangement whereby a substance to be treated (in chemical operations) is in a vessel which is protected from the direct action of the fire by a layer of sand.

   **sitz b.** [ Ger. *sitzen*, to sit ], a hip b., the patient sitting in the tub, the legs being outside.

   **sun b.,** exposure of the more or less naked person to the sun.

   **temperate b.,** one at a temperature of about 78°F.

   **tepid b.,** one in water at a temperature of about 86°F.

   **transcu'tan b.,** a b. in water containing in solution or suspension various remedial agents, which exerts a curative action by the heat of the water and the absorption of the chemical constituents of the added substances.

   **Turkish b.,** a hot air b. followed by rubbing and hot and cold dousing.

   **warm b.,** one at a temperature of about 98°F.

   **water b.** in chemistry, a vessel containing water, in which a container holding a substance to be heated or evaporated can be immersed.

**bathmotro'pic** [ G. *bathmos*, threshold (BAS-), + *tropē*, a turning ]. Influencing nervous and muscular excitability in response to stimuli.

   **negatively b.,** lessening nervous or muscular irritability.

   **positively b.,** increasing nervous or muscular irritability.

**batho-, bathy-** [ G. *bathos*, depth; *bathys*, deep ]. Combining forms relating to depth.

**bathochrom'ic** (bath'o-kro'mik). Denoting the shift of an absorption spectrum maximum to a longer wavelength.

**bath'oflore.** An atom or group of atoms that, by its presence in a molecule, shifts its fluorescent radiation in the direction of longer wavelength, or reduces the fluorescence. Opposite of auxoflore.

**bathopho'bia** [ G. *bathos*, depth, + *phobos*, fear ]. Morbid fear of deep places, or of looking into deep places.

**bath'yanesthe'sia** [ G. *bathys*, deep, + *an-* priv. + *aisthēsis*, sensation ]. Loss of deep or mesoblastic sensibility.

**bathycar'dia** [ G. *bathys*, deep, + *kardia*, heart ]. A condition in which the heart occupies a lower position than normal, but is fixed there, being thereby distinguished from cardioptosis.

**bathyesthesia** (bath'ĭ-es-the'zĭ-ah) [ G. *bathys*, deep, + *aisthēsis*, sensation ]. Sensation in the parts below the surface of the body; the muscle sense; deep or mesoblastic sensibility.

**bathygas'try** [ G. *bathys*, deep, + *gastēr*, stomach ]. Low lying stomach; gastroptosis.

**bathyhyperesthesia** (bath-ĭ-hi'per-es-the'zĭ-ah) [ G. *bathys*, deep, + *hyper*, above, + *aisthēsis*, sensation ]. Exaggerated sensitiveness of the muscular tissues and other deep structures.

**bathyhypesthesia** (bath-ĭ-hip'es-the'zĭ-ah) [ G. *bathys*, deep, + *hypo*, under, + *aisthēsis*, sensation ]. Impairment of sensation in the deeper parts; partial loss of the muscle sense.

**batrachophobia** (bat-rak-o-fo'be-ah) [ G. *batrachos*, frog, + *phobos*, fear ]. Morbid fear of frogs.

**Batten,** Frederick Eustace, London ophthalmologist, 1865–1918. See B.-Mayou *disease*.

**Battle,** William H., English surgeon, 1855–1936. See B.'s *incision, sign*.

**batyl alcohol.** $CH_2OHCHOHCH_2$—O—$(CH_2)_{17}CH_3$; a compound formed by the condensation of stearyl alcohol with one of the hydroxyl groups of glycerol, producing an ether (C—O—C) linkage; found in shark oil.

**Baudelocque** (bōd-lok'), Jean L., Paris obstetrician, 1746–1810. See B.'s *diameter*, uterine *circle*.

**Baudelocque** (bōd-lok'), Louis A., Paris obstetrician, 1800–1864. See B.'s *operation*.

**Bauhin** (bo-an'), Kaspar, Swiss anatomist, 1560–1624. See B.'s *gland, valve*.

**Baumé** (bo-ma'), Antoine, French chemist and pharmacist, 1728–1805. See B.'s *scale*.

**Baumès** (bo-mes'), Jean B. T., French physician, 1777–1828. See B.'s *symptom*.

**Baumès** (bo-mes'), Pierre P. F., French physician, 1791–1871. See B.'s *law*, Colles-B. *law*.

**Baumgarten,** P. Clemens von, German pathologist, 1848–1928. See B.'s *stain*, Cruveilhier-B. *disease, murmur, syndrome*.

**Baunscheidt,** Carl, German mechanic, 19th century. Gave his name to baunscheidtism.

**baunscheidtism** (bown'shid-tizm) [ C. *Baunscheidt* ]. A method of producing counterirritation in the treatment of various diseases, by puncturing the skin with an instrument set with numerous needles, and then rubbing in croton oil or other irritant.

**bay.** In anatomy, a recess containing fluid. Especially, the lacrimal b.

**celomic b.'s,** medial and lateral recesses at either side of the urogenital mesentery of the embryo.

**lacrimal b.,** a slight recess at the medial angle of the eye in which are the puncta lacrimalia, or openings into the lacrimal ducts.

**Bayard,** Henri L., French physician, 1812–1852. See B.'s *ecchymoses*.

**bay'berry.** 1. The fruit of *Myrica cerifera*; see myrica. 2. The fruit of *Laurusnobilis*, the baytree.

**b. bark,** myrica.

**Bayle,** Antoine L. J., French physician, 1799–1858. See B.'s *disease*.

**Bayle,** Gaspard L., French physician, 1774–1816. See B.'s *granulations*.

**Baynton,** Thomas, English surgeon, 1761–1820. See B.'s *bandage*.

**bay rum.** A toilet preparation distilled from a maceration of bay leaves from *Myrica* (*Pimenta*) *acris* in Santa Cruz rum.

**Bazett's formula.** See under formula.

**Bazin,** Antoine P.E., Paris dermatologist, 1807–1878. See B.'s *disease*.

**BBOT.** Abbreviation for 2,5-bis-2-(5-*t*-butylbenzoxazolyl)-thiophene; see under butylbenzoxazolyl.

**BCG.** Abbreviation for (1) Bacille bilié de Calmette-Guérin; (2) ballistocardiograph.

**b.d.** Abbreviation for L. *bis die*, twice a day.

**bdella** (del'ah) [ G. leech ]. A leech; hirudo.

**bdellepithecium** (del-ep-ĭ-the'sĭ-um) [ G. *bdella*, leech, + *epi*, upon, + *thēkē*, a box ]. A cylinder for holding a leech until it has fastened itself to the skin.

**bdellium** (del'ĭ-um) [ G. *bdellion*, a plant that exudes a fragrant gum ]. A gum from *Balsamodendron africanum*, a common adulterant of myrrh. Also a gum from *B. mukul* of India, and another from *Hyphoene thebaica* of Egypt.

**bdellometer** (del-om'e-tur). An artificial leech.

**bdellotomy** (del-ot'o-mĭ) [ G. *bdella*, leech, + *tomē*, incision ]. Incision into or cutting off the end of a sucking leech so that the blood may escape from its body allowing it to continue sucking.

**bdelyg'mia** [ G. *bdelygmia*, nausea ]. Nausea; loathing for food.

**B.D.S.** Abbreviation for Bachelor of Dental Surgery.

**B.D.Sc.** Abbreviation for Bachelor of Dental Science.

**Be.** Chemical symbol of the element beryllium.

**beaded** (be'ded). 1. Marked by numerous small rounded projections, often arranged in a row like a string of beads. 2. Applied to a series of noncontinuous bacterial colonies along the line of inoculation in a stab culture. 3. Denoting stained bacteria in which more deeply stained granules occur at regular intervals in the organism.

**beading of the ribs.** Rachitic *rosary*.

**Beadle** (be'del), George W., U. S. geneticist, *1903. Nobel laureate, 1958, with Edward L. Tatum and Joshua Lederberg for the discovery that genes act by regulating definite chemical events.

**beak** (bēk) [ L. *beccus* ]. 1. Nose of pliers used in dentistry for contouring and adjusting wrought or cast metal dental appliances. 2. Sometimes used to describe a beak-shaped anatomical structure; see rostrum.

**beak'er.** A thin glass vessel, with a lip (beak) for pouring, used by chemists as containers for liquids.

**Beale,** Lionel S., English physician, 1828–1906. See B.'s *cell, stain*.

**beam** (bēm) [ O.H.G. *boum* ]. Any bar whose curvature changes under load.

**cantilever b.,** a b. that is supported by only one fixed support at only one of its ends.

**continuous b.,** one that continues over three or more supports, those supports not at the b. ends being equally free supports.

**neutral axis of straight b.,** at stresses within the proportional limit, the axis is perpendicular to the plane of loading and lies at the gravity axis of the cross-section of the b.

**restrained b.,** one that has two or more supports, at least one of which permits some freedom of rotation to the point of support but not as much as if the support were a free support.

**simple b.,** a straight b. that has two, and only two, supports, one at either end.

**bean** (bēn). The flattened seed, contained in a pod, of various leguminous plants. B.'s of pharmacological significance are alphabetized by specific name.

**bear'berry.** *Arctostaphylos uva ursi*.

**bearing** (bār'ing). A supporting point or surface.

**central b.,** in dentistry, application of forces between the maxillae and mandible at a single point located as near as possible to the center of the supporting areas of the upper and lower jaws. This procedure is used for the purpose of distributing closing forces evenly throughout the areas of the supporting structures during the recording of maxillomandibular (jaw) relations and during the correction of occlusal errors.

**bearing down.** The expulsive effort of a parturient woman in the second stage of labor.

**beat** [ A.S. *beatan* ]. 1. To strike; to throb or pulsate. 2. A stroke, impulse, or pulsation, as of the heart or pulse.

**apex b.,** the visible and/or palpable pulsation made by the apex of the left ventricle as it strikes the chest wall in systole; normally in the fifth intercostal space, about 10 cm. to the left of the median line.

**automatic b.,** automatic contraction; in contrast to forced b.; an ectopic b. that arises *de novo* and is not precipitated by the preceding b.; thus escaped and parasystolic b.'s are automatic.

**capture b.,** ventricular capture; the cardiac cycle resulting when, after a period of atrioventricular (A-V) dissociation, the atria regain control of the ventricles.

**combination b.,** fusion b.

**coupled b.'s,** see bigeminal *pulse.*

**dependent b.,** forced b.

**dropped b.,** a heart b. that fails to appear owing to A-V block.

**echo b.,** see reciprocal *rhythm.*

**ectop'ic b.,** a cardiac b. originating elsewhere than at the sinoatrial node.

**escape b., escaped b.,** escaped contraction; an automatic b., usually arising from the A-V node or ventricle, occurring *after* the next expected normal b. has defaulted; it is therefore always a *late* b., terminating a longer cycle than the normal.

**forced b.,** dependent b.; (1) an extrasystole; a premature b. supposedly precipitated in some way by the preceding normal b. to which it is coupled; (2) an extrasystole caused by artificial stimulation of the heart.

**fusion b.,** combination b.; mixed b.; summation b.; the atrial or ventricular complex in the electrocardiogram when either atria or ventricles are activated by two simultaneously invading impulses; in an atrial fusion b. the atria are activated in part by the sinus impulse and in part by a retrograde impulse from A-V node or ventricle; in a ventricular fusion b. the ventricles are activated partly by the descending sinus or A-V nodal impulse and partly by an ectopic ventricular impulse.

**heart b.,** ictus cordis; a complete cardiac cycle, including spread of the electrical impulse and the consequent mechaniical contraction. See also cardiac *contraction*, cardiac *systole.*

**interference b.,** ventricular capture in A-V dissociation.

**mixed b.,** fusion b.

**paired b.'s,** see bigeminy.

**premature b.,** extrasystole.

**reciprocal b.,** see reciprocal *rhythm.*

**summation b.,** fusion b.

**Beau** (bo), Joseph H. S., Paris physician, 1806–1865. See B.'s *lines.*

**Beaumont,** William, American army surgeon and pioneer physiologist, 1785–1853. Famous for his observations and experiments upon the stomach of Alexis St. Martin, whose stomach wall was partly destroyed by a gun-shot wound leaving a fistula through which Beaumont could observe the gastric interior.

**Beauperthuy** (bo-per-tü-e'), Louis D., West Indian physician, 1803–1871. See B.'s *treatment.*

**bebee'rine.** Curine; an alkaloid closely related to *d*-tubocurarine, present in several species of *Chondodendron.* Methylation of b. results in the formation of an isomer of *d*-tubocurarine.

**becan'thone hydrochloride** (USAN). LORANIL; 1-{[2-[ ethyl (2-hydroxy-2-methylpropyl) amino ]ethyl ]amino}-4-methylthioxanthen-9-one; schistosomicide.

**Beccaria** (bek-kah'-rah), Augusto, Italian physician, 20th century. See B.'s *sign.*

**Bechterew** (bekh-ter'yef), Vladimir M. von, Russian neurologist, 1857–1927. See B.'s *band, disease, line, nucleus,* B.-Mendel *reflexes,* Mendel-B. *reflex,* B.'s *sign.*

**Beck,** Claude S., American surgeon, *1894. See B.'s *operation, triad.*

**Beck,** Emil G., American surgeon, 1866–1932. See B.'s *method.*

**Beck,** E. V. See Bek, E. V.

**Becker's disease.** See under disease.

**Becker,** Otto H. E., German oculist, 1828–1890. See B.'s *phenomenon, test.*

**Beckmann's apparatus.** See under apparatus.

**Beckwith,** John Bruce, U. S. pathologist, *1933. See B.-Wiedemann *syndrome.*

**Béclard** (ba-klar'), Pierre A., French anatomist, 1785–1825. See B.'s *hernia, triangle.*

**beclometh'asone dipropionate** (BP). PROPADERM; dipropionate salt of 9-chloro-11$\beta$,17,21-trihydroxy-16$\beta$-methylpregna-1,4-diene-3,20-dione; topical anti-inflammatory agent.

**Becquerel** (bek-rel'), Antoine H., French physicist, 1852–1908. See B. *rays.*

**bed.** In anatomy, a base or structure giving support to another.

**capillary b.,** the capillaries considered collectively and their volume capacity.

**fracture b.,** a narrow b. with supports under the mattress to prevent sagging, for a patient under treatment for fracture.

**Gatch b.,** one with cranks and screws for elevating patient's head and knees.

**water b.,** a mattress in the form of a closed rubber bag filled with water.

**bed'bug.** *Cimex lectularius.*

**bed'lam** [ corruption or contraction of St. Mary of *Bethlehem* Hospital in London ]. 1. An insane asylum or mental hospital. 2. A place or scene of wild or riotous behavior. 3. A disturbing uproar.

**Bednar,** Alois, Vienna physician, 1816–1888. See B.'s *aphthae.*

**Bedso'nia.** The former genus name for *Chlamydia;* now used as a common term denoting species of *Chlamydia, e.g.,* bedsonias, bedsonia organisms, bedsonial agents.

**bed'sore.** Decubitus *ulcer.*

**bed-wetting.** Enuresis.

**bee** [ A.S. *beó, bi* ]. An insect of the genus *Apis;* the honeybee, *A. mellifica,* is the source of honey and wax.

**b. glue,** propolis.

**beech oil.** Beechwood tar.

**beech'wood tar.** Beech oil; a thick, oily liquid of dark brown color and the odor of creosote; largely used as a source of creosote.

**beef.** Meat or skeletal muscle from mature cattle.

**baby b.,** very young b.; it is redder and less watery than veal.

**Beer,** Georg J., Austrian ophthalmologist, 1763–1821. See B.'s *knife, operation.*

**Beer's law.** See under law.

**Beers,** W. George, Canadian dentist, 19th century. See B.'s *crown.*

**bees'wax.** Wax (1).

**white b.** (BP), white *wax.*

**Beevor's sign.** See under sign.

**Begbie,** James, Edinburgh physician, 1798–1869. See B.'s *disease.*

**Begg,** P. R. See B. *light wire differential force* technique.

**Béguez César,** Antonio, Cuban pediatrician. See B. C. *disease.*

**beha'vior.** 1. Any response emitted by or elicited from an organism. 2. Any mental or motor act or activity. 3. Specifically, parts of a total response pattern.

**adaptive b.,** any b. that enables an organism to adjust to a particular situation or environment.

**adient b.,** appetitive b.

**ambient b.** aversive b.

**appetitive b.,** adient b.; movement of an organism toward a certain type of stimulation, such as food; *cf.* aversive b.

**aversive b.,** ambient b.; movement of an organism away from a certain type of stimulation, such as electric shock; *cf.* appetitive b.

**Hookean b.,** the b. of a perfectly elastic body; *i.e.,* the strain is directly proportional to the stress; see also Hooke's *law.*

**molar b.,** in psychology, b. described in large response units rather than smaller ones; *cf.* molecular b.

**molecular b.,** in psychology, b. described in small response units rather than larger ones; a specific response; *cf.* molar b.

**obsessive b.,** the repetitive, stylized b. of an obsessive-compulsive personality.

**operant b.,** response (2).

**passive-aggressive b.,** apparently compliant b., with intrinsic obstructive or stubborn qualities, to cover deeply felt aggressive feelings.

**respondent b.,** b. in response to a specific stimulus; usually associated with classical conditioning.

**ritualistic b.,** automatic b. of psychogenic or cultural origin.

**target b.,** operant.

**beha′vioral.** Pertaining to behavior.

**beha′viorism.** Behavioral psychology; a branch of psychology that attempts to formulate, through systematic observation and experimentation, the laws and principles which underlie the behavior of man and animals. Its major contributions have been made in the areas of conditioning and learning.

**beha′viorist.** An adherent of behaviorism.

**Behçet** (ba′chet), Hulusi, Turkish dermatologist, 1889–1948. See B.'s *disease, syndrome.*

**behen′ic acid.** *N*-Docosanoic acid.

**Behr's disease.** See under disease.

**Behring** (ba′ring), Emil A. von, German bacteriologist, 1854–1917. First Nobel laureate, 1901, for his work on serum therapy, especially its application against diphtheria. See B.'s *law.*

**BEI.** Abbreviation for butanol-extractable iodine.

**Beierinck** (bi′er-ink), W. M., Dutch physician. See B.'s *reaction.*

**Beigel,** Hermann, Austrian physician, 1830–1879. See B.'s *disease.*

**bej′el.** Nonvenereal endemic syphilis found chiefly among Arab children; apparently due to *Treponema pallidum.*

**Bek** (or Beck), E. V. See Kashin-B. *disease.*

**Békésy,** Georg von. See von Békésy.

**bel** [ A. G. *Bell*]. Unit expressing the relative intensity of a sound. The intensity in bels is the logarithm (to the base 10) of the ratio of the power of the sound to that of a reference sound. Ordinarily, the reference sound is assumed to be one with a power of $10^{-16}$ watts per sq. cm., approximately the threshold of a normal human ear at 1000 cycles per second.

**belam′erine.** Narcissine.

**belch** [ A.S. *baelcian* ]. To eructate.

**Belcher gastrectomy.** See under gastrectomy.

**belch′ing.** Eructation.

**belem′noid** [ G. *belemnon,* a dart, + *eidos,* resemblance. BALL- ]. Dart-shaped; styloid.

**Belfield,** William T., Chicago surgeon, 1856–1929. See B.'s *operation.*

**Bell,** Sir Charles, Scottish surgeon, anatomist, and physiologist, 1774–1842. See B.'s *law,* respiratory *nerve, palsy, phenomenon, spasm.*

**Bell,** John, Scottish surgeon and anatomist, 1763–1820. See B.'s *muscle.*

**Bell,** Luther V., American physician, 1806–1862. See B.'s *delirium.*

**Bell,** William Blair, Liverpool physician, 1871–1936. See B.'s *calcimeter.*

**belladon′na** [ It. *bella,* beautiful, + *donna,* lady ]. Deadly nightshade; *Atropa belladonna* (family Solanaceae); a perennial herb with dark purple flowers and shining purplish black berries. The leaves and root (0.5 per cent b. alkaloids) contain atropine and related alkaloids which are anticholinergic. Used as powder and tincture in asthma, colic, and hyperacidity.

**b. leaf** (USP), the dried leaf of *Atropa belladonna,* containing 0.3 per cent of b. alkaloids.

**powdered b. herb** (BP), the herb reduced to a fine powder; contains 0.3 per cent of alkaloids, calculated as hyoscyamine.

**belladon′nine.** An artificial alkaloid derived from atropine by warming with hydrochloric acid.

**bell-crowned.** Denoting a tooth the crown of which has a cross-sectional diameter much greater than that of the neck.

**Bellini** (bel-e′ne), Lorenzo, Italian physician and anatomist, 1643–1704. See B.'s *ducts, ligament.*

**Belloc (Belloq)** (bel-ok′), Jean J., French surgeon, 1732–1807. See B.'s *cannula, sound.*

**belly** (bel′i) [ O.E. *belig,* bag ]. 1. The abdomen. 2. Venter (2); the prominent thick central part of a muscle. 3. Popularly, the stomach or womb.

**b.'s of digastric muscle,** see under *venter.*

**drum b.,** tympanites.

**frog b.,** the slightly distended b. in rickets.

**frontal b.,** *venter* frontalis.

**occipital b.,** *venter* occipitalis.

**b.'s of omohyoid muscle,** see under *venter.*

**bellyache** (bel′i-āk). Colic.

**belly-bound.** Constipated.

**belly-button.** Umbilicus.

**belonephobia** (bel′o-ne-fo′bi-ah) [ G. *belonē,* needle, + *phobos,* fear ]. Morbid fear of needles, pins, and other sharp-pointed objects.

**belo′noskias′copy** [ G. *belonē,* needle, + *skia,* shadow, + *skopeō,* to examine ]. A subjective form of retinoscopy, using the shadow phenomena of needle movements in front of eye to determine the refractive condition of the eye.

**bem′egride** (BP). MEGIMIDE; 3-ethyl-3-methylglutarimide; a central nervous system stimulant. Used as an analeptic in intoxications due to barbiturates and other central nervous system depressant drugs.

**bem′idone.** Oxypetidin; 4-(*m*-hydroxyphenyl)-1-methylisonipecotic acid ethyl ester; narcotic analgesic.

**benac′tyzine hydrochloride.** SUAVITIL; 2-diethylaminoethyl benzilate hydrochloride. An anticholinergic drug with the same actions but with approximately only one-fifth the activity of atropine. It is thought to raise the threshold of emotional reaction to external stimuli. It is used as a psychotherapeutic and tranquilizing agent.

**Bence Jones,** Henry, London physician, 1814–1873. See B. J. *albumin, albumose, cylinders, protein, reaction.*

**ben′dazac** (USAN). [ (1-Benzyl-1 *H*-indazol-3-yl)oxy ]-acetic acid; anti-inflammatory agent.

**Bender,** Lauretta, New York psychiatrist, *1897. See B. gestalt *test.*

**ben′droflu′azide** (BP). Bendroflumethiazide.

**ben′droflu′methi′azide** (NF). NATURETIN; bendrofluazide; 3-benzyl-3,4-dihydro-6-(trifluoromethyl)-2 *H*-1,2,4-benzothiadiazine-7-sulfonamide-1,1-dioxide. An orally effective diuretic and antihypertensive drug that produces an increase in the urinary excretion of sodium, chloride and water, and a moderate increase in the excretion of potassium and bicarbonate. It enhances the action of other antihypertensive agents, *e.g.,* methyldopa or rauwolfia alkaloids.

**bends.** One of the manifestations of caisson disease or high altitude flight, characterized by pain in the arms, legs, and joints and weakness caused by the liberation in the tissues of bubbles composed largely of nitrogen.

**beneceptor** (ben′e-sep′tor) [ L. *bene,* well, + *capio,* to take ]. A nerve organ or mechanism (ceptor) for the appreciation and transmission of stimuli of a beneficial character; *cf.* nociceptor.

**Benedek's reflex.** See under reflex.

**Benedict,** F. G., U. S. metabolist, 1870–1957. See B.-Roth *apparatus, calorimeter.*

**Benedict,** Stanley R., American chemist, 1884–1936. See B.-Hopkins-Cole *reagent,* B.'s *solution, test.*

**Benedikt,** Moritz, Vienna physician, 1835–1920. See B.'s *syndrome.*

**Benian's stain.** See under stain.

**benign** (be-nin) [ thru O. Fr. fr. L. *benignus,* kind ]. The mild character of an illness or the nonmalignant character of a neoplasm.

**Béniqué** (ba-ne-ka′), Pierre Jules, Paris physician, 1806–1851. See B.'s *sound.*

**benne oil** (ben′nĕ). Sesame oil.

**Bennet,** James H., English obstetrician, 1816–1891. See B.'s *corpuscles.*

**Bennett,** Edward H., Dublin surgeon, 1837–1907. See B.'s *fracture.*

**Bennett,** John H., English physician, 1812–1875. See B.'s *disease.*

**Bennett,** Norman G., British dentist, 1870–1947. See B. *movement, angle.*

**Benois** (bĕ-nwahz'), Louis, French physicist, *1856. See B.'s *scale.*

**benox'inate hydrochloride.** DORSACAINE; 2-diethylaminoethyl-4-amino-3-*n*-butoxybenzoate hydrochloride; a soluble benzoic acid ester related to procaine; a surface anesthetic that also has bacteriostatic action; used especially in ophthalmology.

**benper'idol** (USAN). Benzperidol; FRENACTYL; 1-{1-[ 3-(*p*-fluorobenzoyl) propyl ]-4-piperidyl}-2-benzimidazolinone; tranquilizer.

**ben'salan** (USAN). 3,5-Dibromo-*N*-(*p*-bromobenzyl)-salicylamide; disinfectant.

**Bensley,** Robert R., American-Canadian anatomist, 1867–1956. See B.'s specific *granules.*

**Benson,** Arthur H., English ophthalmologist, 1860–1912. See B.'s *disease.*

**ben'tonite** (USP, BP). Native colloidal, hydrated aluminum silicate; an absorbent clay found in the western United States; it is sometimes used in the treatment of diarrhea and skin disorders.

**benz-.** Combining form denoting association with benzene.

**ben'zalac'etophe'none.** Chalcone.

**benzalcoumaram-3-one.** Aurone.

**benzal'dehyde** (USP). $C_6H_5CHO$; benzoic aldehyde; essential oil of bitter almond; an aldehyde produced artificially or obtained from oil of bitter almond, containing not less than 80 per cent of b.; a flavoring agent.

**benzalko'nium chloride** (USP, BP). ZEPHIRAN chloride; a mixture of alkylbenzyldimethylammonium chlorides in which the alkyls are long-chain compounds ($C_8$ to $C_{18}$); a surface-active germicide for many pathogenic nonsporulating bacteria and fungi. Aqueous solutions of this agent have a low surface tension, and possess detergent, keratolytic, and emulsifying properties that aid the penetration and wetting of tissue surfaces.

**benzan'idin.** Bethanidine sulfate.

**benzan'threne.** Benz[ α ]anthracene; 1,2-benzanthracene; naphthanthracene; a carcinogenic hydrocarbon.

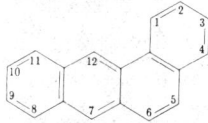

**Benz[α]anthracene**

**ben'zathine penicillin G.** See under penicillin.

**ben'zene.** Benzol; coal tar naphtha; $(CH)_6$ (not to be confused with benzin, petroleum ether); a hydrocarbon from light coal tar oil. The basic structure in the aromatic compounds of dentistry. Used as a solvent; has been used in the treatment of leukemia, Hodgkin's disease, and polycythemia and locally for the destruction of pediculi.

**Benzene**

**b. bromide,** a lacrimator or tear gas.

**b. nucleus,** the six carbon atoms of the b. ring.

**b. ring,** the closed chain arrangement of the carbon and hydrogen atoms in the b. molecule, as shown in the graphic formula of that substance; see closed chain *compound.*

**(γ)-benzene hexachloride** (USP, BP). Incorrect name for 1,2,3,4,5,6-hexachlorocyclohexane, or lindane.

**benzes'trol** (NF). CHEMESTROGEN; 3-ethyl-2,4-bis(*p*-hydroxyphenyl)acetate; synthetic estrogenic substance for oral use.

**benzetho'nium chloride** (NF). PHEMEROL chloride; a synthetic quaternary ammonium compound; one of the cationic class of detergents. Germicidal and bacteriostatic.

**benzet'imide hydrochloride** (USAN). 2-(1-Benzyl-4-piperidyl)-2-phenylglutarimide monohydrochloride; anticholinergic agent for gastrointestinal use.

**benzhexol hydrochloride** (BP). Trihexyphenidyl hydrochloride.

**ben'zidine.** *p*-Diaminodiphenyl; $NH_2C_6H_4C_6H_4NH_2$; used to detect sulfates in water analysis, or for the identification of blood.

**benzilo'nium bromide** (USAN). PORTYN; 1,1-diethyl-3-hydroxypyrrolidinium bromide benzilate; anticholinergic drug for treatment of peptic ulcer.

**benzimidazole.** A ring system made up of a benzene ring fused with an imidazole ring. Occurs in nature as part of the vitamin $B_{12}$ molecule.

**Benzimidazole**

**benzin, benzine.** Petroleum benzin.

**benzin'damine hydrochloride.** Benzydamine hydrochloride.

**benziodarone.** AMPLIVIX; 2-ethyl-3-benzofuranyl 4-hydroxy-3,5-diiodophenyl ketone; coronary vasodilator.

**benzoate** (ben'zo-āt). A salt or ester of benzoic acid.

**ben'zoated.** Containing benzoic acid or a benzoate, usually sodium benzoate.

**benzobu'tamine.** β-(Dimethylaminomethyl)-β-ethylphenethyl alcohol benzoate; antitussive.

**ben'zocaine** (NF, BP). ANESTHESIN; ethyl aminobenzoate; $NH_2C_6H_4—COO(C_2H_5)$; the ethyl ester of *p*-aminobenzoic acid; surface anesthetic in cream (NF) and aerosol (NF).

**benzoc'tamine hydrochloride** (USAN). TACITIN; *N*-methyl-9,10-ethanoanthracene-9(10*H*)-methylamine hydrochloride; a sedative, also with muscle-relaxing agent.

**ben'zodep'a** (USAN). DUALAR; [ bis(1-acridinyl)phosphinyl ]carbamic acid, benzyl ester; antineoplastic agent.

**benzodiazepine** (ben'zo-di-az'ĕ-pēn). Parent compound for the synthesis of a number of psychoactive compounds (*e.g.*, diazepam, chlordiazepoxide), with a common molecular configuration:

**Benzodiazepine**

**benzo'ic.** Relating to or derived from benzoin.

**b. acid** (USP, BP), benzoyl hydrate; flowers of benzoin; $C_6H_5COOH$; occurs naturally in gum benzoin; used as a food preservative, locally as a fungistatic, and orally as an antiseptic, diuretic, and expectorant. It is excreted rapidly as hippuric acid.

**b. aldehyde,** benzaldehyde.

**benzoin** (ben'zo-in, ben'zoyn). 1 (USP). Gum benzoin; gum benjamin; a balsamic resin, obtained from *Styrax benzoin* (family Styraceae); stimulant expectorant, but usually used by inhalation in laryngitis and bronchitis; retards rancidification of fats and is used for this purpose in the official benzoinated lard. 2. Benzoylphenylcarbinol; $C_6H_5CHOHCOC_6H_5$.

**ben'zol.** Benzene.

**benzo'natate** (NF). TESSALON; nonaethyleneglycol monomethyl ether *p-n*-butylaminobenzoate; an antitussive agent related chemically to tetracaine. It suppresses cough due to acute and chronic bronchitis, bronchial asthma and other conditions.

**benzopurpurin** (ben-zo-pur'pu-rin). A red acid dye, $C_{34}H_{26}N_6O_6S_2Na_2$, used as a plasma stain and as an indicator; it changes from violet to red in the pH range 1.2 to 4.0.

**1,4-benzoquinone.** Quinone (2); essential part of coenzyme Q and vitamin E; reducible to hydroquinone.

1,4-Benzoquinone

**benzoquinonium chloride** (ben'zo-kwĭ-no'nĭ-um). MYTOLON; a doubly substituted diaminobenzoquinone.

**benzores'inol.** A resinous constituent of benzoin (1).

**benzosul'fimide.** Saccharin.

**benzothi'adi'azides.** A class of diuretics that increase the excretion of sodium and chloride and an accompanying volume of water, independent of alterations in acid-base balance; most of the compounds in this group are analogues of 1,2,4-benzothiadiazine-1,1-dioxide. See also benzthiazide.

**benzox'iquine** (USAN). DIOXYLINE; 8-quinolinol benzoate ester; disinfectant.

**benzoyl** (ben'zo-il). The benzoic acid radical, $C_6H_5CO$—, forming benzoyl compounds (see b. chloride).
  **b. chloride,** $C_6H_5COCl$; a colorless liquid of pungent odor; a reagent.
  **b. cholinesterase,** cholinesterase.
  **b. peroxide** (USP), $C_6H_5CO$—O—O—$COC_6H_5$; made by the interaction of sodium peroxide and b. chloride. Used in oil as an application to ulcers and to burns and scalds. Also used in promoting the polymerization of denture base resins.
  **b. sal'icin,** populin.

**benzoylpas calcium.** THEREPAS; 4-benzamidosalicylic acid calcium salt; antituberculous agent.

**ben'zozone.** Acetozone.

**benzper'idol.** Benperidol.

**benzphet'amine hydrochloride.** DIDREX; *N*-benzyl-*N,α*-dimethylphenethylamine hydrochloride; a sympathomimetic agent used as an anorexiant.

**benzpyrin'ium bromide.** STIGMONENE; 1-benzyl-3-hydroxypyridinium bromide diethylcarbamate; a cholinergic drug with action and uses similar to those of neostigmine.

**benzquin'amide** (USAN). QUANTRIL; a benzoquinoline amide used in the treatment of anxiety in psychoneurotic and psychotic disorders.

**benzthi'azide** (NF). AQUATAG; EXNA; PROAQUA; 3-[ (benzylthio)methyl ]-6-chloro-2*H*-1,2,4-benzothiadiazine-7-sulfonamide 1,1-dioxide; a diuretic and antihypertensive agent.

**benztro'pine mesylate** (USP, BP). COGENTIN methansulfonate; 3-diphenylmethoxytropane methanesulfonate; a parasympatholytic agent with atropine-like action, antihistaminic and local anesthetic properties; used in paralysis agitans and drug-induced parkinsonism.

**benzydamine hydrochloride** (ben-zid'ă-mēn) (USAN). Benzindamine hydrochloride; DORINAMIN; 1-benzyl-3-[ 3-dimethylamino)propoxy ]-1*H*-indazole; analgesic and antipyretic.

**benzyl** (ben'zil). The hydrocarbon radical, $C_6H_5CH_2$—.
  **b. alcohol** (NF, BP), phenmethylol; phenylcarbinol; $C_6H_5CH_2OH$; possesses local anesthetic and bacteriostatic properties.

**b. benzoate** (USP, BP), $C_6H_5CO$—$OCH_2C_6H_5$; reduces the contractility of unstriated muscular tissue, possessing marked antispasmodic properties. Formerly used in biliary and renal colic, spastic constipation, vesical spasm, asthma, high blood pressure, uterine colic, etc. Used now as a pediculicide and scabicide.
  **b. benzoate-chlorophenothane-ethyl aminobenzoate,** a mixture of three components used in emulsions or ointments.
  **b. carbinol,** phenylethyl alcohol.
  **b. cin'namate,** cinnamein; *trans*-cinnamic benzyl ester; a constituent of balsams of Peru, tolu, and styrax.
  **b. fu'marate,** dibenzyl fumarate; $C_6H_5CH_2OOCCHCH$-$COOCH_2C_6H_5$; used for the same purposes as b. benzoate.
  **b. man'delate,** the b. ester of mandelic acid, having an antispasmodic action similar to that of b. benzoate.
  **b. suc'cinate,** dibenzyl succinate; $(C_6H_5CH_2)_2(CH_2CO_2)_2$; action and dosage are the same as those of b. benzoate.

**benzyl'ic.** Relating to or containing benzyl.

**benzyl'idene.** The hydrocarbon radical, $C_6H_5$—CH=.

**ben'zylox'ycar'bonyl.** Amino-protecting radical, used (as the chloride) in peptide synthesis, yielding $PhCH_2OCO$—NHR. Preferred term for carbobenzoxy, but still symbolized Z or Cbz.

**ben'zylpenicill'in** (BP). Penicillin G.

**bephenium hydroxynaphthoate** (USP). ALCOPAR; benzyldimethyl- (2-phenoxyethyl) ammonium-3-hydroxy-2-naphthoate; effective against *Ancylostoma duodenale* and *Necator americanus* (hookworms of man), though somewhat less effective against the latter; drug of choice for hookworms, but much less effective against other human helminths. Poorly absorbed from the alimentary tract and relatively nontoxic.

**Bérard** (ba-rar'), Auguste, French surgeon, 1802–1846. See B.'s *aneurysm*.

**Béraud** (ba-ro'), Bruno J., French surgeon, 1825–1865. See B.'s *valve*.

**ber'bamine.** An alkaloid from berberis, $C_{37}H_{40}N_2O_6$, isomeric with oxyacanthine.

**ber'berine.** Umbellatine; $C_{20}H_{19}NO_5$; an alkaloid from *Hydrastis canadensis* (family Berberidaceae); has been used as antimalarial, antipyretic, and carminative, and externally for indolent ulcers.

**ber'beris.** Barberry; Oregon grape root; root bark of *Berberis vulgaris* (family Berberidaceae); formerly used as a bitter tonic.

**ber'bine.** Oxyacanthine.

**berdache** (ber-dash') [ Fr. ]. A person who adopts the dress and manner of the opposite sex.

**Berengario da Carpi,** Jacopo, Italian anatomist, *c.* 1460–1530. He made several anatomical discoveries and was the author, among other books, of *Isagogae Breves,* one of the first anatomical textbooks with illustrations taken from dissections.

**ber'gamot** [ *Bergamo,* a town in Italy ]. The fruit of *Citrus aurantium* var. *bergamia* (family Rutaceae); Wild b. is known as monarda, or American horsemint, a source of thymol.
  **b. oil,** a volatile oil distilled from the fresh rind of b.; used chiefly as a perfume.

**bergap'ten.** A camphor-like substance obtained from the bergamot oil.

**Bergenhem,** Bengt, Swedish surgeon, *1898. See B.'s *operation*.

**Berger,** Hans, Jena neurologist, 1873–1941. See B. *rhythm*.

**Berger** (bair-zha'), Oskar, Breslau physician, 1844–1885. See B.'s *paresthesia*.

**Berger cells.** See under cell.

**Bergmann,** Ernst von, German surgeon, 1836–1907. See B.'s *incision*.

**Bergmann,** Gottlieb H., German neurologist and anatomist, 1781–1861. See B.'s *cords, fibers*.

**Bergmeister's papilla.** See under papilla.

**Bergonié** (bair-gŭ-ne-a'), Jean A., Bordeaux physician, 1857–1925. See B. *method*.

**beriberi** (ber'ĭ-ber'ĭ) [ Singhalese, extreme weakness ]. Kakké; endemic neuritis; barbiers; panneuritis endemica; a specific polyneuritis, occurring in endemic form in eastern and southern Asia, and sporadically in other parts of the world without reference to climate. It is a disease resulting mainly from a deficiency of thiamin in the diet, and prevails where there is starvation or famine. Sensory nerves are likely to be affected more than motor nerves, symptoms beginning in the feet and working upward, with the hands affected later. In this country it is now very rare, even in alcoholics.

**dry b.,** paraplegic b.; affects chiefly the peripheral nerves. Its clinical pattern is predominantly that of a neuropathy without congestive failure.

**wet b.,** edematous b., in which congestive heart failure occurs in addition to peripheral neuropathy.

**Berkefeld,** Wilhelm, German manufacturer, 1836–1897. See B. *filter.*

**berkelium** (berk'li-um) [ *Berkeley,* Calif., city where first prepared ]. An artificial transuranium radioactive element; symbol Bk, atomic no. 97.

**Berlin,** Rudolf, German ophthalmologist, 1833–1897. See B.'s *disease, edema.*

**Berlin blue.** Prussian blue; used as a dye in histology.

**Berman-Moorhead locator.** See under locator.

**Bernard** (ber-nar'), Claude, French physiologist, 1813–1878. See B.'s *canal, duct puncture,* B.-Horner *syndrome,* B.-Sergent *syndrome.*

**Bernays** (ber'naz), Augustus C., St. Louis surgeon, 1854–1907. See B.'s *sponge.*

**Bernhardt,** Martin, Berlin neurologist, 1844–1915. See B.'s *disease,* Roth-B. *disease,* B.-Roth *syndrome.*

**Bernhardt's formula.** See under formula.

**Bernheim's syndrome.** See under syndrome.

**Bernoulli,** Daniel, Swiss mathematician, 1700–1782. See B. *effect;* B.'s *law, principle, theorem.*

**Berry,** Sir James, Canadian surgeon, 1860–1946. See B.'s *ligament.*

**berserk'** [ Old Norse *berserkr* ]. Mad; term used to describe a condition in which the emotions are completely out of hand.

**Berson,** Solomon A., U. S. internist, *1918. See B. *test.*

**Berthollet** (ber-to-la'), Claude L., French chemist, 1748–1822. See B.'s *fluid, law.*

**Bertin** (bair-tan'), E. J., French anatomist, 1712–1781. See B.'s *bone, column, ligament, ossicle.*

**beryl'lio'sis.** Beryllium poisoning characterized by the occurrence of sarcoid-like granulomas in the skin by accidental implantation and a granulomatous fibrosis of the lungs occurring particularly when a person inhales beryllium over a period of time.

**beryl'lium.** One of the elements; symbol Be, atomic weight 9.013, atomic no. 4; a white metal belonging to the alkaline earths; formerly called glucinum.

**berythromycin** (be-rith'ro-mi'sin) (USAN). Erythromycin B; 12-deoxyerythromycin; antiamebic and antibacterial agent.

**Besnier,** Ernest, French dermatologist, 1931–1909. See B.'s *prurigo,* B.-Boeck-Schauman *disease, syndrome.*

**Besnoi'tia.** A genus of protozoan parasites (family Besnoitiidae, class Sporozoa) that localize in subcutaneous, connective, serous, and other tissues and are surrounded by a heavy, nucleated wall of host tissue, forming a pseudocyst. The genus, related to *Toxoplasma,* has been erroneously called *Globidium* and has often been confused with *Eimera* and *Sarcocystis.* Hosts include domestic ruminants, reindeer, caribou, rodents, opossums, and reptiles.

**B. bennet'ti,** occurs in horses and asses in North America and Africa, causing a chronic disease with scabbing, scarring, and thickening of the skin.

**B. besno'iti,** the cause of besnoitiosis of cattle, goats, and larger antelopes in Europe, Africa, the Middle East, South America, and Asia; mechanical transmission is by blood-sucking flies; it primarily causes a chronic low grade infection.

**B. gilru'thi,** found in the walls of the abomasum and intestines of sheep, where it is suspected of causing diarrhea.

**B. jelliso'ni,** a species causing acute or chronic disease in mice.

**B. leuckar'ti,** occurs in the intestine of the horse.

**B. taran'di,** a species occurring in reindeer and caribou, giving rise to a condition called "corn-meal disease" because of the granular nature of the lesions on the skin.

**Besnoitiidae.** A family of protozoan parasites, similar to those of the family Toxoplasmatidae, to which the genus Besnoitia belong.

**bes'noitio'sis.** A disease of cattle primarily caused by *Besnoitia besnoiti.* Pseudocysts occur chiefly in the connective tissue of the skin, nasal mucous membranes, and serous membranes. Following a febrile stage, depilatory and seborrheic changes occur in the skin.

**Best,** Franz, Dresden pathologist, 1878–1920. See B.'s *disease,* carmine *stain.*

**bestiality** (bes'ti-al'i-ti). Sexual relations with an animal.

**bes'ylate.** USAN-approved contraction for benzesulfonate, $C_6H_5SO_3^-$.

**beta** (ba'tah) [ G. ]. The second letter of the Greek alphabet, $\beta$. 1. Used in chemical nomenclature to indicate substitution of a hydrogen atom at the 2nd carbon atom from a functional group. 2. The second in a series of isomeric compounds. For compounds having this prefix, and not listed below, see the specific name.

**betacism** (ba'tah-sizm) [ G. *beta,* the second letter of the alphabet ]. A defect in speech in which the sound of *b* is given to other consonants.

**betahis'tine hydrochloride** (USAN). SERC; 2-[ 2-(methylamino)ethyl ]pyridine dihydrochloride; used as a histamine-like agent for treatment of Ménière's disease.

**betaine** (be'tah-in). Trimethylglycocoll anhydride; oxyneurine; $(CH_3)_3N^+—CH_2COO^-$; an oxidation product of choline and a transmethylating intermediate in metabolism.

**b. aldehyde,** $(CH_3)_3N^+CH_2CHO$; an intermediate in the interconversion of betaine and choline.

**b. aldehyde oxidase (hydrogenase)** (EC 1.2.1.8), an oxidizing enzyme that catalyzes the oxidation of betaine aldehyde to betaine; part of the choline oxidase system.

**betameth'asone** (NF, BP). CELESTONE; betadexamethasone; 9-fluoro-11$\beta$,17,21-trihydroxy-16$\beta$-methyl-1,4-pregnadiene-3,20-dione (for structure of pregnadione, see steroids); 9$\alpha$-fluoro-16$\beta$-methylprednisolone. A semisynthetic glucocorticoid with anti-inflammatory effects and toxicity similar to those of cortisol; not useful in the treatment of adrenal insufficiency because it causes little sodium retention. For systemic and topical therapy, its actions are similar to those of prednisone, but more potent. Also available as b. sodium phosphate (BP, NF), b. acetate (NF), and b. valerate (NF, BP).

**betanaph'thol.** See $\beta$-naphthol.

**betatron** (ba'tah-tron). A circular electron accelerator that is a source of either high energy electrons or x-rays.

**betazole hydrochloride** (USP). HISTALOG; an analogue of histamine that stimulates gastric secretion with less tendency to produce the side effects seen with histamine; used in place of histamine, to measure the gastric secretory response.

**betel** (be'tl) [ Pg. *betel, betle,* fr. Malayalam or Tamil *vetila* ]. The dried leaves of *Piper betle* (family Piperaceae), a climbing East Indian plant; stimulant and narcotic. The fresh leaves are wrapped around the b. nut and lime, and chewed. Used topically as a counterirritant, internally as an antitussive.

**b. nut,** areca nut; the nut of the areca palm, *Areca catechu* (family Palmae), of the East Indies, chewed by the natives. An alkaloid, arecoline, obtained from it is used in veterinary practice in the treatment of gastrointestinal disorders.

**bethanechol chloride** (be-than'e-kol). URECHOLINE chloride; carbamoylmethylcholine chloride; (2-hydroxypropyl)trimethylammonium chloride carbamate; a parasympathomimetic agent, used to relieve constipation, paralytic ileus, and urinary retention.

**bethan'idine sulfate** (USAN). Bethanidine sulphate (BP); benzanidin; ESBATAL; 1-benzyl-2,3-dimethylguanidine; adrenergic blocking agent used for palliative treatment of hypertension.

**Bethea** (beth-a'), Oscar W., New Orleans physician, *1878. See B.'s *method.*

**Bethes'da-Bal'lerup Group.** A group of citrate-utilizing, slow lactose-fermenting bacteria (family Enterobacteriaceae) which share a similar series of antigens with the lactose-fermenting citrobacters; these organisms are now included in the genus *Citrobacter* without a distinction between prompt and slow lactose fermentation.

**bethox'ycaine hydrochloride.** MILLICAINE; 3-amino-4-butoxybenzoic acid 2-(diethylamino)ethyl hydrochloride; local anesthetic.

**Bettendorff,** Anton J., German chemist, 1839–1902. See B.'s *test.*

**Betula** (bet'u-lah) [ L. the birch tree ]. A genus of trees or shrubs of the family Betulaceae, birch, yielding an oil containing methyl salicylate. Used internally and externally to meet the same indications as wintergreen oil.
  **B. alba,** white birch; the source of rectified birch tar oil.
  **B. lenta,** sweet birch; yields the official methyl salicylate; formerly called oil of sweet birch, or oil of teaberry.

**betula oil.** Oil of sweet birch; a volatile oil obtained by distillation from the bark of *Betula lenta;* see also *methyl* salicylate.

**bet'ulin.** An alcohol obtained from the white birch, *Betula* alba.

**between-brain.** Obsolete term for diencephalon.

**Betz,** Vladimir A., Russian anatomist, 1834–1894. See B. cells.

**Beurmann** (bowr'man), C. Lucien de, French physician, 1851–1923. See B.'s *disease.*

**Beuttner** (boyt'ner), Oskar, Swiss gynecologist, 1866–1929. See B.'s *method.*

**Bevan,** Arthur D., American surgeon, 1861–1943. See B.'s *incision.*

**Bevan-Lewis,** William, English physician and physiologist, 1847–1929. See B.-L. *cells.*

**bev'el.** 1. A surface having a sloped edge that usually forms an obtuse angle. 2. The edge of a cutting instrument.

**bezoar** (be'zōr) [ Pers. *padzahr,* antidote ]. A concretion formed in the alimentary canal of animals, especially ruminants, and occasionally man; formerly considered to be a useful medicine with magical properties, and apparently still used for this purpose in the Far East. According to the substance forming the ball, it may be termed trichobezoar (hairball), trichophytobezoar (hair and vegetable fiber mixed), and phytobezoar (foodball).

**Bezold** (bets'ölt), Albert von, German physiologist, 1836–1868. See B.'s *ganglion.*

**Bezold** (bets'ölt), Friedrich, Munich otologist, 1842–1908. See B.'s *abscess, mastoiditis, perforation, sign, symptom,* triad.

**Bezold-Jarisch reflex.** See under reflex.

**bhang** (bang) [ Hind. ]. The name given in the East to powdered preparation of *Cannabis sativa* (family Moraceae), which is chewed or smoked by the local residents.

**BHN.** Abbreviation for Brinell hardness *number.*

**Bi.** Chemical symbol of the element bismuth.

**bi-** [ L. ]. Prefix meaning twice or double; used in referring to double structures, dual actions, etc.; see also di- and bis-.

**Bial** (be'ahl), Manfred, Berlin physician, 1869–1908. See B.'s *test.*

**bialamicol hydrochloride** (bi'ă-lam'ĭ-kol) (USAN). CAMOFORM; 6,6'-diallyl-α,α'-bis(diethylamino)-4,4'-bi-o-cresol hydrochloride; amebicide.

**Bianchi** (be-ahn'ke), Giovanni B., Italian anatomist, 1681–1761. See B.'s *nodule, valve.*

**bi'artic'ular.** Diarthric.

**biasterionic** (bi-as-ter-ĭ-on'ik). Relating to both asterions, especially the b. diameter, or b. width, the shortest distance from one asterion to the other.

**biauricular** (bi-aw-rik'u-lar). Relating to both auricles, in any sense.

**bi'ba'sic.** Dibasic.

**bibenzo'nium bromide.** SEDOBEX; [ 2-(1,2-diphenylethoxy)ethyl ]trimethylammonium bromide; antitussive.

**bi-bi.** See bi-bi *reaction.*

**bib'lioclast** [ G. *biblion,* book, + *klastos,* broken ]. One who mutilates or destroys books.

**bib'lioklept** [ G. *biblion,* book, + *kleptō,* to steal ]. One who steals books.

**bib'liokleptoma'nia.** Morbid tendency to steal books.

**bib'lioma'nia.** Morbidly intense desire to collect and possess books, especially rare books.

**bib'liopho'bia** [ G. *biblion,* book, + *phobos,* fear ]. Morbid dread or hatred of books.

**bibrocathol.** BIBROCATHIN; 4,5,6,7-tetrabromo-2-hydroxy-1,3,2-benzodioxabismole; topical anesthetic.

**bib'ulous** [ L. *bibulus,* drinking freely, absorbent ]. Absorbent.

**bicam'eral** [ bi- + L. *camera,* chamber ]. Having two cavities or hollows, denoting especially an abscess divided by a more or less complete septum.

**bicap'sular.** Having a double capsule.

**bicar'bonate.** $HCO_3^-$; the ion remaining after the first dissociation of carbonic acid.

**bicar'diogram.** The composite curve of an electrocardiogram representing the combined effects of the right and left ventricles.

**bicel'lular.** 1. Composed of two cells. 2. Having two compartments or chambers.

**bicephalus** (bi-sef'al-us). Dicephalus.

**biceps** (bi'seps) [ bi- + L. *caput,* head, CAP-1 ] [ NA ]. Bicipital.

**biceptor** [ bi- + L. *capio,* to take, CAP-2 ]. A receptor having two complementophil groups.

**Bichat** (be-shă'), Marie F. X., French anatomist, physician, and biologist, 1771–1802. See B.'s *canal, fat-pad, fissure, foramen, fossa, ligament, membrane, protuberance, tunic.*

**bichloride** (bi-klo'rīd). A compound with a molecule containing two atoms of chlorine to one of another element, *e.g.,* $CaCl_2$.

**bicho** (be'cho). Epidemic gangrenous *proctitis.*

**bichro'mate.** Dichromate.

**bicil'liate.** Having two cilia.

**bicip'ital** [ bi- + L. *caput,* head. CAP-1 ]. 1. Two-headed. 2. Relating to a biceps muscle.

**Bickel,** Gustav, German physician, 19th century. See B.'s *ring.*

**bicon'cave.** Concave on two sides; denoting especially a form of lens.

**bicon'vex.** Convex on two sides; denoting especially a form of lens.

**bicor'nis** [ L. ] [ NA ]. Bicornous.

**bicor'nous, bicor'nuate, bicor'nate** [ bi- + L. *cornu,* horn ]. Two-horned; having two processes or projections.

**bicro-.** Pico-.

**bicron.** Picometer.

**bicuspid** (bi-kus'pid) [ bi- + L. *cuspis,* point ]. Having two points, prongs, or cusps.

**bicus'pidiza'tion.** Change of a normally tricuspid aortic valve into a functioning bicuspid valve; performed in correction of aortic insufficiency.

**b.i.d.** Abbreviation for L. *bis in die,* twice a day.

**bidactyly** (bi-dak'tĭ-lĭ) [ bi- + G. *daktylos,* finger ]. An abnormality in which the medial digits are lacking with only the 1st and 5th represented; see also lobster-claw *deformity.*

**Bidder,** Friedrich H., German anatomist in Dorpat, 1810–1894. See B.'s *organ.*

**bidet'** [ Fr. a small horse ]. A tub for a sitz bath, having also an attachment for giving vaginal or rectal injections.

**bidiscoidal** (bi'dis-koy'dal). Resembling, or consisting of, two disks.

**biduous** (bid'u-us) [ L. *biduus,* lasting two days, fr. *bi-* + *dies,* day ]. Of two days' duration.

**Biebl,** M. See B. *loop.*

**Biebrich scarlet red** (be'brik). Scarlet red; see under scarlet.

**Biederman** (be'dur-man), J. B., Cincinnati physician *1907. See B.'s *sign.*

**Biedl** (be'dl), Artur, Austrian physician, 1869–1933. See Laurence-B. *syndrome* or Laurence-Moon-B. *syndrome.*

**Bielschowsky,** Alfred, German ophthalmologist, 1871–1940. See B.'s *method, sign.*

**Bielschowsky** (be-al-show'skī), Max, German neuropathologist, 1869–1940. See B.'s *disease,* Jansky-B. *disease.*

**Bier** (bēr), August K. G., Berlin surgeon, 1861–1949. See B.'s *amputation, hyperemia, method.*

**Biermer** (bēr'mer), Anton, German physician, 1827–1892. Gave his name to biermerin. See B.'s *anemia,* B.'s *disease,* Addison-B. *disease,* B.'s *sign.*

**Biernacki** (byer-naht'ske), Edmund A., Polish pathologist, 1866–1912. See B.'s *sign.*

**Biesiadecki** (bya-syah-det'ske), Alfred von, Polish physician, 1839–1888. See B.'s *fossa.*

**Biett** (be-et'), Laurent Théodore, Paris physician, 1781–1840. See B.'s *disease.*

**bifascicular** (bi'fā-sik'u-lar). Involving two of the three fascicles of the ventricular conduction system of the heart.

**bi'fid** [ L. *bifidus,* cleft in two parts. FIS- ]. Split or cleft; separated into two parts.

**Bi'fidobacte'rium** [ L. *bifidus,* cleft in two parts, + bacterium, *q.v.* ]. A genus of anaerobic bacteria containing Gram-positive rods of highly variable appearance; freshly isolated strains characteristically show bifurcated V and Y forms, uniform or branched, and club or spatulate forms. They frequently stain irregularly; two or more granules may stain with methylene blue, while the remainder of the cell is unstained. They are not acid-fast, are nonmotile, and do not produce spores; acetic and lactic acids are produced from glucose. Pathogenicity for man or other animals has not been reported, though they have been found in the feces and alimentary tracts of infants, older people, and other animals. The type species is *B. bifidum.*
    **B. bifidum,** *Lactobacillus bifidus;* type species of the genus *Bifidobacterium;* found in the feces and alimentary tracts of breast- and bottle-fed infants, and of older persons, rats, turkeys, and chickens; also found in the rumen of cattle; pathogenicity for man or other animals has not been reported; see also *Lactobacillus bifidus* subsp. *pennsylvanicus.*

**bi'fidus** [ L. ] [ NA ]. Bifid.

**bifocal** (bi-fo'kal). Having two foci.

**bifo'rate** [ bi- + L. *foro,* pp. -*atus,* to bore, pierce ]. Having two openings.

**bifur'cate, bifur'cated** [ bi- + L. *furca,* fork ]. Forked; two-pronged; having two branches.

**bifurcatio** (bi'fur-ka'she-oh). [ NA ]. Bifurcation.
    **b. tra'cheae** [ NA ], bifurcation of the trachea; the division of the trachea into the right and left main bronchi; it occurs at the level of the 5th or 6th thoracic vertebral body and is marked internally by the presence of a carina or keel-like ridge between the diverging bronchi.

**bifurca'tion.** A forking; a division into two branches. See bifurcatio.

**bifur'cus** [ L. ] [ NA ]. Bifurcate.

**Bigelow,** Henry J., Boston surgeon, 1818–1890. See B.'s *ligament, septum.*

**bigemina** (bi-jem'ī-mah). Bigeminal *pulse.*

**bigeminal** (bi-jem'ī-nal) [ bi- + L. *geminus,* twin ]. Paired; double; twin.

**bigem'ini.** Bigeminy.

**bigem'inum** [ L. ntr. of *bigeminus,* doubled ]. One of the bigeminal bodies.

**bigeminy** (bi-jem'ī-nī). Bigemini; twinning; pairing; especially, the occurrence of heart beats in pairs.
    **atrial b.,** pairing of atrial beats, as when an atrial extrasystole is coupled to each sinus beat.
    **atrioventricular nodal b.,** A-V nodal b.; nodal b.; paired beats, each pair consisting of an A-V nodal extrasystole coupled to a beat of the dominant, usually sinus, rhythm.
    **escape-capture b.,** paired beats, each couplet consisting of an escape beat followed by a conducted sinus beat.
    **nodal b.,** atrioventricular nodal b.
    **reciprocal b.,** paired beats, each pair consisting of an A-V nodal beat followed by a reciprocal beat.
    **ventricular b.,** paired ventricular beats, the common form consisting of ventricular extrasystoles coupled to sinus beats.

**biger'minal.** Relating to two germs or ova.

**big-head.** 1. In horses, usually denotes osteodystrophia fibrosa. 2. Gas gangrene infection of tissues of the head, caused by *Clostridium novyi* in sheep, usually young rams with head wounds. 3. Photosensitization in sheep.

**bigitalin** (bi-jit'ā-lin) Gitoxin.

**big-knee.** In cattle, a bursitis over the carpus.

**Bignami,** Amico, Italian physician, 1862–1929. See Marchiafava-B. *disease.*

**bilabe** (bi'lāb) [ bi- + L. *labium,* lip ]. A slender forceps for seizing and removing urethral or small vesical calculi.

**bilat'eral** [ bi- + L. *latus,* side ]. Relating to, or having, two sides.

**bilat'eralism.** A condition in which the two sides are symmetrical.

**bile** [ L. *bilis* ]. Gall; fel; the yellowish brown or green fluid secreted by the liver. It contains sodium glycocholate and sodium taurocholate, cholesterol, biliverdin and bilirubin, mucus, fat, lecithin and cells and cellular debris. It is discharged into the duodenum where it aids in the emulsification of fats, increases peristalsis, and retards putrefaction.
    **A b.,** b. from the common duct.
    **b. acids,** taurocholic and glycocholic acids; used when biliary secretion is inadequate and for prevention of gallstone colic.
    **B b.,** b. from the gallbladder.
    **C b.,** b. from the hepatic duct.
    **b. pigments,** coloring matter in the b., derived from porphyrins by rupture of a methene bridge (*e.g.,* bilirubin, biliverdin).
    **b. salts,** the salt forms of bile acid conjugates (*e.g.,* taurocholate, glycocholate).
    **white b.,** the contents of the gallbladder when the cystic duct is obstructed; it is a pigment-free fluid consisting largely of mucus.

**Bilharz,** Theodor, German helminthologist, 1825–1862. Gave his name to *Bilharzia.*

**Bilhar'zia** [ T. *Bilharz* ]. An early name for *Schistosoma,* the genus of trematode worms causing animal and human blood fluke disease.

**bilharzi'asis, bilharzio'sis.** Schistosomiasis.

**bilharzioma** (bil-har-zī-o'mah). A tumor-like swelling of the skin, due to schistosomiasis.

**bili-** [ L. *bilis,* bile ]. Combining form relating to bile.

**bil'iary.** Relating to bile.

**bil'icy'anin.** Obsolete term denoting a pigment, resulting from the oxidation of biliverdin, that is blue in an alkaline medium, purple in an acid one.

**bilifac'tion, bilifica'tion** [ bili- + L. *facio,* pp. *factus,* to make ]. Rarely used terms meaning bile formation.

**bilif'erous.** Containing or carrying bile.

**bilifla'vin.** Obsolete term denoting a yellow bile pigment derived from biliverdin.

**biliful'vin** [ bili- + L. *fulvis,* tawny ]. Bilirubin plus other biliary substances, thereby resulting in a tawny mixture; also, a tawny component of bile from oxen, not found in normal human bile; obsolete.

**bilifuscin** (bil-ī-fus'in). A dark green-brown pigment found in bile and gallstones. See also bilirubinoids.

**biligen'esis.** Bile production.

**biligen'ic.** Bile-producing.

**bilihu'min** [ bili- + L. *humus,* earth ]. An obsolete term denoting an insoluble black (or almost black) residue that may remain after bile and pigmented gallstones are treated with various organic solvents.

**bi'lin, bi'line.** The chain of four pyrrole residues resulting from the cleavage of one bond of one of the four methylidene residues of the porphin part of a porphyrin; specifically, the unsubstituted tetrapyrrole. Sometimes called porphobilin. Biliribun and biliverdin are bilins.

**bilineur'ine.** Choline.

**bilious** (bil'yus). 1. Biliary; relating to bile. 2. Relating to or suffering from biliousness.

**bil'iousness.** An imprecisely delineated congestive disturbance with anorexia, coated tongue, constipation, headache, dizziness, pasty complexion, and, rarely, slight jaundice; assumed to result from hepatic dysfunction.

**biliphein** (bil'ĭ-fe'in). Bilifulvin or cholophein, or a complex of bilirubin and other components of bile, resulting in a red-brown or dusky orange-red mixture of unidentified compounds; obsolete.

**bilipra'sin.** A green pigment in bile, closely similar and possibly identical to biliverdin; obsolete.

**bilip'tysis** [ bili- + G. *pytalon*, saliva ]. The occurrence of bile in the sputum.

**bilipur'pin, bilipur'purin.** A purple bile pigment of ruminants, presumably derived from chlorophyl; obsolete.

**bilirachia** (bil-ĭ-ra'kĭ-ah) [ bili- + G. *rachis*, spine ]. Bile in the spinal fluid.

**bilirubin** (bil-ĭ-roo'bin) [ bili- + L. *ruber*, red ]. A red bile pigment found as sodium bilirubinate (soluble), or as an insoluble calcium salt in gallstones; formed from hemoglobin during normal and abnormal destruction of erythrocytes by the reticuloendothelial system.

**bilirubinemia** (bil-ĭ-roo-bin-e'mĭ-ah) [ bilirubin + G. *haima*, blood ]. The presence of bilirubin in the blood, where it is normally present in relatively small amounts; the term is usually used in relation to increased concentrations observed in various pathologic conditions where there is excessive destruction of erythrocytes or interference with the mechanism of excretion in the bile. Determination of the quantity of bilirubin in the blood serum reveals two fractions, namely direct reacting (conjugated) and indirect reacting (nonconjugated) bilirubin. Determination of conjugated and total bilirubin in serum is an important and frequently clinical laboratory test.

**biliru'binglob'ulin.** A bilirubin-globulin complex; a transport form of bilirubin to the liver, where bilirubin is converted to a diglucuronic acid derivative and passes into the bile.

**biliru'binoids.** A generic term denoting intermediates in the conversion of bilirubin to stercobilin by reductive enzymes in intestinal bacteria. Included are mesobilirubin, mesobilane (mesobilirubinogen, urobilinogen IX-α), mesobilene-b (urobilin IX-α), urobilinogen, urobilin, reduction products of mesobilane (stercobilinogen) and mesobilene (stercobilin), and mesobiliviolin. Most are found in normal urine and feces. Products related to these intermediates and found in pathological conditions (jaundice, liver disease), are the probilifuscins, bilifuscins, and propentdyopents, structurally indefinite, found in gallstones.

**biliru'binu'ria** [ bilirubin + G. *ouron*, urine ]. The presence of bilirubin in the urine.

**bilither'apy.** Treatment with bile, or with bile salts.

**biliuria** (bil'ĭ-u'rĭ-ah) [ bili- + G. *ouron*, urine ]. Choluria; choleuria; the presence of various bile salts, or bile, in the urine.

**bilivaccine** (bil'ĭ-vak-sēn). An oral bacterial vaccine given along with ox-bile.

**biliver'dine, biliver'din.** Uteroverdine; verdine; dehydrobilirubin; a green bile pigment formed from the oxidation of bilirubin.

**biliverdinglobin** (bil-ĭ-ver'din-glo'bin). Verdoglobin; choleglobin; a first product in the destruction of hemoglobin, caused by rupture of the α-methene bridge in heme to yield a biliverdin-globin compound; further degraded to bilirubin, with destruction of the globin.

**bilixanthin** (bil-ĭ-zan'thin). A yellow oxidation product of biliverdin; obsolete.

**Bill,** Arthur H. See B.'s *maneuver.*

**Billings,** John S., U. S. army surgeon, 1838–1913. He founded the Surgeon General's Library and in 1880 began issuing the *Index Medicus,* an alphabetical index of medical publications.

**Billroth** (bil'rōt), C. A. Theodor, Zurich and Vienna surgeon, 1829–1894. See B.'s *cords, operations, venae cavernosae.*

**bilo'bate.** Having two lobes.

**bilob'ular.** Having two lobules.

**biloc'ular** [ bi- + L. *loculus*, dim. of *locus*, a place ]. Bicellular; bicameral.

**biloc'ulate.** Bilocular.

**biloph'odont** [ bi- + G. *lophos*, ridge, + *odous*, tooth ]. Having two longitudinal ridges on the premolar and molar teeth; designating certain animals, such as the kangaroo.

**biman'ual** [ bi- + L. *manus*, hand ]. Relating to, or performed by, both hands.

**bimas'toid.** Relating to both mastoid processes.

**bimeth'adol.** Dimepheptanol.

**bimo'dal.** Denoting a frequency curve characterized by two peaks.

**bimolec'ular.** Involving two molecules; for example, a b. reaction.

**binangle** (bin-ang'-ul) [ L. *bini*, pair, + *angulus*, angle ]. 1. The second angle given the shank of an angled instrument to bring its working end close to the axis of the handle in order to prevent it from turning about the axis. 2. A dental instrument possessing the above characteristics.

**bi'nary** [ L. *binarius*, consisting of two, fr. *bini*, double ]. Denoting two.

**binau'ral** [ L. *bini*, a pair, + *auris*, ear ]. Relating to both ears; binotic.

**bind** [ A.S. *bindan* ]. 1. To bandage; confine; encircle with a band. 2. To join together with a band or ligature. 3. To combine or unite molecules by means of reactive groups, either in the molecules *per se* or in a chemical added for that purpose; frequently used especially in relation to chemical bonds that may be fairly easily broken (*i.e.*, noncovalent), as in the binding of a toxin with antitoxin, or a heavy metal with a chelating agent, and so on. 4. A close interpersonal relationship in which one person feels compelled to act in a certain way to obtain the approval of the other person.

**double b.,** a type of personal interaction in which one receives two mutually conflicting verbal or nonverbal instructions or demands from the same person or different individuals, resulting in a situation in which either compliance or noncompliance with either alternative threatens a needed relationship.

**bind'er.** 1. A broad bandage; especially one encircling the abdomen. 2. Anything that binds; see bind (3).

**obstetrical b.,** a supporting garment covering the abdomen from the ribs to the trochanters, tightly pinned at the back, affording support after childbirth or, rarely, during childbirth.

**bineg'ative.** Carrying a double negative charge, *e.g.*, sulfate ion, $SO_4^=$.

**Binet** (be-na'), Alfred, French psychologist, 1857–1911. See B. *age, scale, test,* B.-Simon *scale, test,* Stanford-B. intelligence *scale.*

**Bing,** Richard J., American physician, \*1909. See Taussig-B. *disease, syndrome.*

**Bing's reflex.** See under reflex.

**Bingham,** E. C., U. S. chemist, 1878–1945. See B. *flow, model, plastic.*

**bini'odide.** Diiodide.

**Binn's bacterium.** See under bacterium.

**binocular** (bin-ok'u-lar) [ L. *bini*, paired, + *oculus*, eye ]. Adapted to the use of both eyes; said of an optical instrument.

**binomial** (bi-no'mĭ-al) [ bi- + G. *nomos*, name ]. Consisting of two terms or names. See also binary *combination.*

**binotic** (bin-o'tik) [ L. *bini*, a pair, + G. *ous* (*ōt-*), ear ]. Binaural.

**binov'ular** [ L. *bini*, pair, + Mod. L. *ovulum*, dim. of L. *ovum*, egg ]. Relating to two ova.

**binox'ide.** Dioxide.

**Binswanger,** Otto Ludwig, German neurologist, 1852–1929. See B.'s *disease, encephalopathy.*

**binuclear, binucleate** (bi-nu'kle-ar, bi-nu'kle-āt). Having two nuclei.

**binu'cleolate.** Having two nucleoli.

**Binz** (bints), Carl, German pharmacologist, 1832–1913. See B.'s *test.*

**bio-** [ G. *bios*, life ]. Combining form denoting life.

**bioacoustics** (bi'o-ă-koos'tiks). The science dealing with the effects of sound fields or mechanical vibrations in living organisms.

**bioassay** (bi-o-as-a'). The determination of the potency or concentration of a compound by its effect upon animals, isolated tissues, or microorganisms, as compared with a standard preparation.

**bioastronautics** (bi'o-as'tro-naw'tiks). The study of the effects of space travel and space habitation on living organisms.

**bioavailability** (bi'o-ă-văl'ă-bil'ĭ-tĭ). The physiological availability of a given amount of a drug, as distinct from its chemical potency.

**biocat'alyst.** Enzyme.

**biocat'alyzer.** Enzyme.

**biocenosis** (bi-o-se-no'sis) [ bio- + G. *koinos*, common ]. The relationships between different organisms living in association and under similar conditions.

**biochem'ical.** Relating to biochemistry, or physiological chemistry.

**biochemistry** (bi-o-kem'is-trĭ). Physiological chemistry; biological chemistry; the chemistry of living organisms and of the changes occurring therein.

**biochemorphic** (bi'o-kem-or'fik). Denoting the relation between the biologic action of foods and drugs and their chemical structure.

**biochemorphology** (bi'o-kem-or-fol'o-je) [ bio- + chemistry + G. *morphē*, shape, + *logos*, study ]. 1. The study of the relationship between chemical structure and biological action. 2. Macroscopic or gross morphology, as revealed by biochemical techniques such as selective staining of enzymes, antibodies, and other materials.

**biocidal** (bi-o-si'dal) [ bio- + L. *caedo*, to kill ]. Active against life; particularly pertaining to microorganisms.

**bioclimatology** (bi-o-kli-mă-tol'o-jĭ). The science of the relation of climate to life.

**biocol'loid.** A colloid existing in a plant or animal.

**biocytin.** ε-N-Biotinyl-L-lysine; biotin condensed through its carboxyl group with the ε-amino group of a lysine in the apoenzymes to which biotin is the coenzyme; the predominant form in which biotin occurs.

**biocytinase.** An enzyme in human blood, catalyzing the hydrolysis of biocytin to biotin and lysine.

**biodynam'ic.** Relating to biodynamics.

**biodynamics** (bi'o-di-nam'iks) [ bio- + G. *dynamis*, force ]. The science dealing with the force or energy of living matter.

**bioecology** (bi-o-e-kol'o-jĭ). Ecology.

**bioelectri'city.** Electrical phenomena occurring in living tissues.

**bioel'ement.** An element essential to the functioning of living tissue.

**bioenergetics** (bi'o-en-er-jet'iks). The study of energy changes involved in the chemical reactions within living tissue.

**bioengineer'ing.** See biomedical *engineering.*

**biofeed'back.** A training technique being developed by experimental and clinical psychologists to enable an individual to gain some element of voluntary control over autonomic body functions. The technique is based on the learning principle that a desired response is learned when one received information (feedback) that a specific thought complex or action produced the desired response.

**bioflav'onoids.** Naturally occurring flavone or coumarin derivatives showing so-called vitamin P activity, notably rutin and esculin.

**bi'ogen.** 1. Archaic word for protoplasm. 2. One of a number of unstable molecules in protoplasm that are assumed to be continually undergoing assimilation and disassimilation.

**biogenesis** (bi'o-jen'e-sis) [ bio- + G. *genesis*, origin ]. The term given by Huxley to the now generally accepted view that life originates only from preexisting life and never from nonliving material; see also spontaneous *generation,* and recapitulation *theory.*

**biogenet'ic.** Relating to biogenesis.

**biogeochemistry** (bi'o-je'o-kem'is-trĭ). The study of the influence of living organisms and life processes on the chemical structure and history of the earth.

**biograv'ics** [ bio- + L. *gravis,* weight ]. That field of study dealing with the effect on living organisms (particularly man) of abnormal gravitational effects produced, *e.g.,* by acceleration or by free fall; in the former case, heavier than normal weight is induced, and in the latter weightlessness.

**bi'oinstrument.** A sensor or device usually attached to or embedded in the human body or other living animal to record and to transmit physiologic data to a receiving or monitoring station.

**biokinet'ics** [ bio- + G. *kinēsis,* motion ]. The study of the growth changes and movements that developing organisms undergo.

**biologic, biological** (bi'o-loj'ik, -loj'ĭ-kal). Relating to biology.

**biologist** (bi-ol'o-jist). A student of biology.

**biology** (bi-ol'o-jĭ) [ bio- + G. *logos,* study ]. The branch of science that deals with living organisms. It consists of several branches: morphology, physiology, pathology, ecology, paleontology, etc.

  **molecular b.,** that aspect of b. that seeks to understand, explain, or rationalize biological phenomena in terms of molecular (or chemical) interactions. It differs from biochemistry in that the latter is concerned primarily with the chemical behavior of biologically important substances and analogues thereof, and differs from general biology or parts thereof in its emphasis on chemical interactions, especially those involved in the replication of hereditary material (DNA), its "transcription" into RNA, and its "translation" into or expression in protein—in other words, in the chemical reactions connecting genotype and phenotype.

  **radiation b.,** that field of science which studies the biological effects of ionizing radiation on living systems.

**bi'olumines'cence** [ bio- + L. *lumen* (-*inis*), light ]. Light produced by certain forms of life, including crustacea, bacteria, and fungi, from the oxidation of substances termed luciferins through the action of enzymes called luciferases; "cold" light, as opposed to light generated by heating materials to high temperature (incandescent light).

**biolysis** (bi-ol'ĭ-sis) [ bio- + G. *lysis,* dissolution ]. The disintegration of organic matter through the chemical action of living organisms, *e.g.,* bacteria.

**biolytic** (bi-o-lit'ik). Capable of destroying life.

**bi'omass.** The total weight of all living things in a given area, biotic community, species population, or habitat; a measure of total biotic productivity.

**biomathemat'ics.** Mathematics applied to processes occurring in living organisms.

**bi'ome.** The total complex of biotic communities occupying and characterizing a particular area or zone; *e.g.,* desert, grassland, deciduous forest.

**biomechan'ics.** The science of the action of forces, internal or external, on the living body.

  **dental b.,** dental *biophysics.*

**biomed'ical.** 1. Pertaining to those aspects of the natural sciences, especially the biological and physiologic sciences, that relate to or underlie medicine. 2. Biological and medical; *i.e.,* encompassing both the science(s) and the art.

**biom'eter** [ bio- + G. *metron,* measure ]. A device for measuring carbon dioxide given off by small organisms and, hence, for determining the quantity of living matter present.

**biometrician** (bi-o-mē-trish'an). One who specializes in the science of biometry.

**biomet'rics.** Biometry.

**biom'etry.** The statistical analysis of biological data.

**biomi'croscope.** Slitlamp microscope; corneal microscope; a binocular microscope used with a slitlamp for viewing the segments of the living eye.

**biomicroscopy** (bi-o-mi-kros'ko-pĭ). 1. Microscopic examination of living tissue in the body. 2. Examination of the cornea, lens, vitreous, retina by use of a slitlamp combined with a binocular corneal microscope.

**bi'on** [ G. pres. p. ntr. of *bioō,* to live ]. A living thing.

**Biondi** (byon'de), D., †1914. See B.-Heidenhain *stain.*

**bionecrosis** (bi-o-ne-kro'sis). Necrobiosis.

**bion'ics** [ bio- + G. *electronika,* things electronic ]. The science of biologic functions and mechanisms as applied to electronic devices, such as computers, employing various aspects of physics, mathematics, and chemistry. A specific example is that of improving cybernetic engineering by reference to the organization of the vertebrate nervous system.

**bionom'ics.** 1. Bionomy. 2. Ecology.

**bion'omy** [ bio- + G. *nomos,* law ]. Bionomics (1); the laws of life; the science that treats of the laws regulating the vital functions.

**biono'sis** [ bio- + G. *nosos,* disease ]. Any disease resulting from the effects of living agents (*e.g.,* bacteria, viruses, helminths, etc.,) in the tissues.

**biophage** (bi'o-fāj). An organism that derives the nourishment for its existence from another living organism; a parasite.

**biophagism** (bi-of'ă-jizm) [ bio- + G. *phagein,* to eat ]. Biophagy; the deriving of nourishment from living organisms.

**biophagous** (bi-of'ă-gus). Feeding on living organisms; denoting certain parasites.

**biophagy** (bi-of'ă-jĭ). Biophagism.

**biopharmaceutics** (bi'o-far-mă-su'tiks). The study of the physical and chemical properties of a drug, and its dosage form, as related to the onset, duration, and intensity of drug action.

**biophil'ia** [ bio- + G. *philia,* love, fondness for ]. Instinct of self-preservation.

**bi'ophore** [ bio- + G. *phoreō,* to carry ]. The ultimate unit, according to Weissmann, an aggregation of which composes the determinant, which in turn is one of the units forming the id; it is so named on the supposition that in it resides the vitality of the cell.

**biophotometer** (bi-o-fo'tom'e-ter). An instrument used for measuring the rate and degree of dark adaptation.

**bi'ophylac'tic.** Relating to biophylaxis.

**biophylaxis** (bi-o-fi-lak'sis) [ bio- + G. *phylaxis,* protection ]. Nonspecific defense reactions of the body, *e.g.,* phagocytosis, vascular and other reactions of inflammatory processes.

**biophys'ics.** 1. The study of biological processes and materials by means of the theories and tools of physics. 2. The study of physical processes (*e.g.,* electricity, luminescence) occurring in organisms.

   **dental b.,** dental biomechanics; the relationship between the biologic behavior of oral structures and the physical influence of a dental restoration.

**biophysiog'raphy** [ bio- + G. *physis,* nature, + *graphō,* to write ]. The branch of biology that deals with the natural history of living organisms; descriptive biology.

**bi'oplasm** [ bio- + G. *plasma,* thing formed ]. Protoplasm, especially in its relation to living processes and development.

**bioplas'mic.** Relating to bioplasm.

**bioplas'min.** The hypothetical constituent of the cytoplasm upon which the life and functional activity of the cell depend.

**bi'opsy** [ bio- + G. *opsis,* vision ]. 1. The process of removing tissue from living patients for diagnostic examination. 2. A specimen obtained by b.

   **aspiration b.,** needle b.

   **biochemical b.,** a combined procedure in which tissue is removed for diagnostic gross and histologic observation, and also for biochemical study; for example, a neoplasm may be identified histologically, and the diagnosis confirmed by means of chemical analysis or assay of a distinctive constituent or product.

   **endoscopic b.,** b. obtained by long instruments through an endoscope or obtained by a needle from the outside under endoscopic guidance.

   **needle b.,** aspiration b.; any method in which the specimen for b. is removed by means of aspirating it through a hypodermic needle or trocar that is pierced through the skin, or the external surface of an organ, and into the underlying tissue to be examined.

   **open b.,** surgical incision, exposure, and inspection of the region from which the b. is taken.

   **punch b.,** trephine b.; any method in which a small cylindroid piece of tissue for b. is removed by means of a special instrument that may be pierced directly into an organ, or through the skin or a small incision in the skin.

   **sponge b.,** abrasion of a lesion with cellulose sponge.

   **total b.,** total *excision.*

   **trephine b.,** punch b.

   **wedge b.,** excision of a pie-shaped portion.

**biopsychology** (bi'o-si-kol'o-je). An area of study at the interface of psychology, biology, physiology, biochemistry, the neural sciences, and related areas.

**biopterin.** A pterin found in yeast, the fruit fly, and in normal human urine.

**biopy'oculture** [ bio- + G. *pyon,* pus, + culture ]. A culture made from purulent exudate in which various cells, including the phagocytes, are still viable.

**biorbital** (bi-or'bĭ-tal) [ bi- + G. *orbita,* orbit ]. Relating to both orbits.

**biorheology** (bi'o-re-ol'o-jĭ) [ bio- + G. *rheō,* to flow, + *logos,* study ]. The science of deformation and flow in biological systems.

**biorhythm** (bi'o-rith'm) [ bio- + G. *rhythmos,* rhythm ]. A biologically inherent cyclic variation or recurrence of an event or state, such as the sleep cycle, circadian rhythms, periodic diseases.

**bioroentgenography** (bi'o-rent'gen-og'raf-e). The making of x-ray pictures of subjects in motion.

**bi'os** [ G. *bios,* life ]. The name given to an extract of beerwort made by Wildiers in 1901; this extract was required for the initial growth of certain types of yeast. It is a mixture of many substances, including growth factors, coenzymes, and vitamins, these being responsible for the effect.

**biosat'ellite.** An artificial satellite capable of transporting living animals or man through space.

**bi'ose.** Glycol aldehyde; a 2-carbon sugar, CHO—CH₂OH.

**bi'oside.** Disaccharide (biose).

**bio'sis** [ G. *biōsis,* way of living ]. Life in general.

**bioso'cial.** Involving the interplay of biological and social influences.

**bi'ospectrom'etry** [ bio- + L. *spectrum,* an image, + G. *metron,* measure ]. Clinical spectrometry; the spectroscopic determination of the types and amounts of various substances in living tissue or fluid from a living body.

**bi'ospectros'copy** [ bio- + L. *spectrum,* image, + G. *skopeō,* to examine ]. Clinical spectroscopy; the spectroscopic examination of specimens of living tissue, including fluids removed therefrom.

**biospeleology** (bi'o-spe'le-ol'o-je) [ bio- + G. *spēliaion,* cave ]. The study of organisms whose natural habitat is wholly or partly subterranean.

**biosphere** (bi'o-sfēr) [ bio- + G. *sphaira,* sphere ]. All the regions in the world where living organisms are found.

**biostatics** (bi-o-stat'iks) [ bio- + G. *statikos,* causing to stand ]. The science of metabolism; of the relation between structure and function.

**biostatis'tics.** The science of statistics applied to biological or medical data.

**bios'terin.** An early term applied to vitamin A.

**biosynthesis** (bi-o-sin'the-sis). The formation of a chemical compound by enzymes, either in the organism (*in vivo*) or by fragments or extracts of cells (*in vitro*).

**biosystem** (bi'o-sis'tem). A living organism or any complete system of living things that can, directly or indirectly, interact with others.

**Biot** (be-o'), Camille, French physician, 19th century. See B.'s *breathing.*

**biota** (bi-o'tah) [ Mod. L. fr. G. *bios,* life ]. The collective flora and fauna of a region.

**biotax'is** [ bio- + G. *taxis,* arrangement ]. 1. The classification of living beings according to their anatomical characteristics. 2. Cytoclesis.

**biotelemetry** (bi-o-tel-em'e-trĭ). Technique of monitoring vital processes and transmitting data without wires to a point remote from the subject.

**biot'ic.** Pertaining to life.

**biot'ics** [ G. *biōtikos,* relating to life ]. The science that deals with the functions of life, or vital activity and force.

**bi'otin.** Coenzyme R; W factor; formerly designated vitamin H or factor H of the B₂ complex. The methyl ester has been crystallized from raw egg white. It is a growth factor for most yeast organisms, especially *Saccharomyces cerivisiae.* Deficiency in animals (possible only on sterilized diets because of bacterial synthesis of b. in the intestine) produces a dermatitis called "egg white injury"; excess may be carcinogenic in rats. B. is inactivated by avidin with which it combines. Chemical name: *cis*-tetrahydro-2-oxothieno[ 3,4-*d* ]imidazoline-4-valeric acid.

Biotin

**b. oxidase,** an enzyme catalyzing the beta-oxidation of the biotin side chain.

**b. sulfoxide,** an oxidation product of b. found in, *inter alia,* cow's milk residues.

**biotinidase.** (EC 3.5.1.12). An enzyme catalyzing the hydrolysis of biotin amide, biocytin, and other biotinides to biotin.

**biotinyllysine** (bi'o-tin'il-li'sin). Biocytin.

**biot'omy** [ bio- + G. *tome,* a cutting ]. Vivisection.

**biotope** (bi'o-tōp) [ G. *bios,* life, + *topos,* place ]. A distinctive habitat or biological niche.

**biotoxicol'ogy.** The study of poisons produced by living organisms.

**biotox'in.** Any toxic substance formed in an animal body, and demonstrable in its tissues or body fluids, or both.

**biotransforma'tion.** The conversion of drugs and other substances to their metabolites in the living organism.

**biotussal.** PECTIPRONT; 1-[ 2-hexahydro-1*H*-azepin-1-yl)-ethyl ]-2-oxocyclohexanecarboxylic acid benzoyl ester; antitussive.

**bi'otype.** 1. A population or group of individuals composed of the same genotype. 2. A group (infrasubspecific) of bacterial strains distinguishable from other strains of the same species on the basis of physiological characters.

**bipal'atinoid.** A capsule with two compartments, used for making remedies in nascent form; the reaction between the two substances takes place as the capsule dissolves in the stomach, and so sets free the remedy.

**bipara** (bip'ā-rah) [ bi- + L. *pario,* to give birth ]. Secundipara.

**biparasitism** (bi-păr'ā-sit-izm). Hyperparasitism.

**bi'paren'tal.** Having two parents, male and female.

**biparietal** (bi-pā-ri'e-tal) [ bi- + L. *paries,* wall ]. Relating to both parietal bones of the skull.

**bip'arous** [ bi- + L. *pario,* to give birth ]. Bearing two young.

**bi'ped** [ bi- + L. *pes,* foot ]. 1. Two-footed. 2. Any animal with only two feet.

**bi'pedal.** 1. Relating to a biped. 2. Capable of locomotion on two feet; *e.g.,* an iguana and some other lizards have this capability.

**bipen'nate, bipen'niform** [ bi- + L. *penna,* feather ]. Having a double feather arrangement.

**bipep'tide.** Dipeptide.

**biper'forate.** Having two foramina or perforations.

**biper'iden** (NF). AKINETON; α-5-norbornen-2-yl-α-phenyl-1-piperidinepropanol; an anticholinergic agent with sedative and central effects on the basal ganglia; used in the symptomatic treatment of parkinsonism and drug-induced parkinsonism. Also official (NF) as the hydrochloride.

**biphen'amine hydrochloride** (USAN). ALVININE; MELSAPHINE; β-diethylaminoethyl 2-hydroxy-3-phenylbenzoate hydrochloride; antiseborrheic agent.

**biphenyl.** The aromatic hydrocarbon,

Biphenyl

**bipo'lar.** 1. Having two poles; denoting those nerve cells in which the branches project from two, usually opposite, points. 2. Relating to both ends or poles of a bacterial or other cell.

**bi'pos'itive.** Carrying a double positive charge, *e.g.,* the calcium ion, $Ca^{++}$.

**bi'potential'ity.** The capability of differentiating along two developmental pathways.

**bipubiotomy** (bi-pu-bī-ot'o-mī). Double pubiotomy; division of the pubis on both sides.

**biramous** (bi-ra'mus) [ bi- + L. *ramus,* branch ]. Having two branches.

**Birbeck,** M. S. See B.'s *granule.*

**birch.** *Betula.*

**rectified b. tar oil,** b. tar; pyroligneous oil obtained by the dry distillation of the wood of *Betula alba,* white birch, and rectified by steam distillation; used externally in the treatment of skin diseases.

**sweet b.,** *Betula lenta.*

**sweet b. oil,** see betula oil, and methyl salicylate.

**b. tar,** rectified b. tar oil.

**white b.,** *Betula alba.*

**Birch-Hirschfeld** (berkh-hersh'felt), Felix V., German pathologist, 1842–1899. See B.-H.'s *stain.*

**Bird,** Golding, English physician, 1814–1854. See B.'s *formula.*

**Bird,** Samuel D., Australian physician, 1833–1904. See B.'s *sign.*

**bi'rect'ifica'tion.** A method of analysis for fermented liquors by fractional distillation.

**birefractive** (bi-re-frak'tiv). Birefringent; refracting twice; splitting a ray of light in two.

**birefringent** (bi-re-frin'-jent). Birefractive.

**bi'rota'tion.** Mutarotation.

**birth.** 1. The passage of the offspring from the uterus to the outside world; the act of being born. 2. Specifically, in the human, the complete expulsion or extraction from its mother of a fetus weighing 500 gm. or more (equivalent to approximately 22 completed weeks or 154 days of gestation), irrespective of gestational age, and regardless of whether or not the umbilical cord has been cut or whether or not the placenta is attached.

**cross b.,** parodynia perversa; an abnormal presentation, neither of head nor of breech, the fetus lying transversely in the uterus, across the axis of the parturient canal.

**premature b.,** the b. of an infant after the period of viability (20-week gestation or 500-gm. birth weight) but before full term.

**birth'mark.** Nevus (1).

**strawberry b.,** strawberry *nevus.*

**bis-** [ L. ]. Prefix signifying two or twice. In chemical terminology, used to denote the presence of two complex groups in one molecule. Thus, bis(4-aminophenyl)sulfone contains two 4-aminophenyl groups; see also bi-.

**bisacodyl** (bis-ak'o-dil) (USP, BP). DULCOLAX; 4,4'-(2-pyridylmethylene)diphenol diacetate; bis(*p*-acetoxyphenyl)-2-pyridylmethane. A relatively nontoxic laxative used orally or rectally for constipation.

**bis'acro'mial.** Relating to both acromion processes.

**bis'albu'mine'mia.** The condition of having two kinds of serum albumin that differ in mobility on electrophoresis: normal albumin (albumin A), and any one of several variant types that migrate slower or faster than albumin A. Individuals are heterozygous for the gene for albumin A and the gene for a variant albumin type; a genetic polymorphism without known clinical significance. See also inherited *albumin* variants.

**bi'salt.** An acid salt, for example, $NaHSO_4$.

**bisaxillary** (bis-ak'sī-lēr-ī). Relating to both axillae.

**Bischof,** W., German neurosurgeon. See B.'s *myelotomy.*

**Bischoff,** Johann J., German gynecologist, *1841. See B.'s *operation.*

**biscuit** (bis'kit). A term associated with the firing of porcelain, and applied to the fired article before glazing. May be any stage after the fluxes have flowed enough to provide rigidity to the structure up to the stage where shrinkage is complete. Referred to as low, medium or high b., depending on the completeness of vitrification, also as hard or soft b.

**biscuit-bake.** Biscuit-firing; the initial bake(s) given fusing procelain at lower than glazing temperature to control shrinkage during the process of building up the dental restoration.

**biscuit-firing.** Biscuit-bake.

**bisdehydrodoisynolic acid.** Tetradehydro-doisynolic acid.

**bis'dequalin'ium chloride.** SALVIZOL; 1,1'-decamethyl-ene-4,4'-(1,10-decamethylenediimino)bis[ quinaldinium c-hloride ]; antiseptic.

**bisethylxanthogen.** LENISARIN; dithiobis[ thioformic acid ]-*O,O*-diethyl ester; topical parasiticide.

**bisex'ual.** Ambisexual; having gonads of both sexes. See also hermaphroditism and subentries.

**bisferious** (bis-fe'rĭ-us) [ L. *bis*, twice, + *ferio*, to strike ]. Striking twice, said of the pulse; see *pulsus* bisferiens.

**Bishop's sphygmoscope.** See under sphygmoscope.

**bishydrox'ycoum'arin.** Dicumarol.

**bisiliac** (bis-il'ĭ-ak). Relating to any two corresponding iliac parts or structures, as the iliac bones or iliac fossae.

**Bismarck brown Y.** A diazo dye used for staining histologic sections and in the Papanicolaou technique for vaginal smears.

**bismuth** (biz'muth) [ Ger. *Wismut* ]. A reddish, crystalline, brittle, trivalent metal, chemical symbol Bi, atomic no. 83, atomic weight 209. Several of its salts are used in medicine. Some of these are salts containing $BiO^+$ rather than $Bi^{+++}$, hence carry the prefix sub- (*e.g.*, b. subgallate, b. subsalicylate, b. subnitrate).

**b. aluminate,** aluminum b. oxide; BISMANAT; gastric antacid.

**b. ammonium citrate,** ammoniocitrate of b.; intestinal astringent.

**b. carbonate,** b. subcarbonate.

**b. chloride oxide,** b. oxychloride.

**b. citrate,** used in the making of b. and ammonium citrate.

**b. eth'ylcam'phorate,** an antisyphilitic compound for intramuscular injection.

**milk of b.** (NF), a suspension of b. hydroxide and b. subcarbonate in water. Used in gastric and intestinal disorders.

**b. oxide,** $Bi_2O_3$; used for the same purposes as the subnitrate.

**b. oxycarbonate,** b. subcarbonate.

**b. oxychloride,** BiOCl; basic b. chloride; bismuthyl chloride; b. chloride oxide; used for the same purposes as the subnitrate.

**b. oxyni'trate,** b. subnitrate.

**b. potassium tartrate,** $BiK(C_4H_4O_6)_2$; potassium bismuthyl tartrate; formerly used in the treatment of syphilis.

**b. salic'ylate,** see b. subsalicylate.

**b. sodium tartrate,** a basic sodium b. tartrate; antisyphilitic agent.

**b. sodium tri'glycol'lamate,** BISTRIMATE; sodium b. complex of nitrilotriacetic acid; a double salt useful in certain diseases of the skin.

**b. subcar'bonate,** b. oxycarbonate; b. carbonate; bismuthyl carbonate; $(BiO)_2CO_3$; used for the same purposes as b. subnitrate, but has lower toxicity.

**b. subgal'late,** DERMATOL; used internally in diarrhea and externally as an astringent and protective dusting powder.

**b. subni'trate,** b. oxynitrate; a basic salt, the composition of which varies with the conditions of preparation; used internally as an intestinal astringent and in gastric ulcer; used externally as a mild astringent and antiseptic. External and internal use have resulted in serious methemoglobinemia.

**b. subsalic'ylate,** used as an intestinal antiseptic, or as an antisyphilitic by intramuscular injection.

**b. tribromophenate,** XEROFORM; b. tribromphenol; used as an intestinal antiseptic, and externally as a substitute for iodoform.

**b. trichloride,** $BiCl_3$; butter of bismuth; addition of water results in formation of b. oxychloride.

**bismutho'sis.** Chronic bismuth *poisoning*.

**bis'muthyl.** The group, BiO, that behaves chemically as an atom of a univalent metal; its salts are the oxysalts or subsalts of bismuth.

**b. carbonate,** *bismuth* subcarbonate.

**bis'obrin lactate** (USAN). *meso*-1,1'-Tetramethylenebis[1,2,3,4-tetrahydro-6,7-dimethoxyisoquinoline]-dilactate; a fibrinolytic agent.

**bisox'atin acetate** (USAN). LAXONALIN; 2,2-bis(*p*-hydroxyphenyl)-2*H*-1,4-benzoxazin-3(4*H*)-one diacetate; a laxative.

**bi'stephan'ic.** Relating to both stephanions; denoting particularly the b. width of the cranium, or b. diameter, the shortest distance from one stephanion to the other.

**bisteroid** (bi-stĕr'oid). A molecule composed of two molecules of a given steroid joined together by a carbon-to-carbon bond.

**bistoury** (bis'too-rĭ) [ Fr. *bistouri*, fr. *bisorit*, dagger ]. A long, narrow-bladed knife, straight or curved on the edge, sharp or blunt pointed (probe-pointed); used for opening abscesses, slitting up sinuses and fistulas, etc.

**bi'stra'tal.** Having two strata or layers.

**bisul'fate.** Acid sulfate; disulfate; a salt containing $HSO_4^-$.

**bisul'fide.** 1. Disulfide (1). 2. A compound of the anion $HS^-$; an acid sulfide.

**bisul'fite.** A salt or ion of $HSO_3^-$, for example, $NaHSO_3$.

**bitar'trate.** A salt or anion resulting from the neutralization of one of tartaric acid's two acid groups.

**bitch** [ O.E. *bicche* ]. A female dog of breeding age.

**bite** [ A.S. *bītan* ]. 1. To incise or seize with the teeth. 2. The act of incision or seizure with the teeth. 3. A morsel of food held between the teeth. 4. Term used to denote the amount of pressure developed in closing the jaws. 5. Undesirable jargon for terms such as interocclusal record, checkbite, maxillomandibular registration, denture space, and interarch distance. 6. A wound or puncture of the skin made by animal or insect; see bites.

**balanced b.,** balanced *occlusion.*

**biscuit b.,** see maxillomandibular *record.*

**close b.,** small interarch *distance.*

**closed b.,** reduced interarch *distance.*

**cross b.,** an arrangement whereby the mandibular teeth are labial or buccal to the maxillary teeth in a horizontal plane.

**deep b.,** an abnormally large overlap of anterior teeth in centric occlusion.

**edge-to-edge b.,** edge-to-edge *occlusion.*

**end-to-end b.,** edge-to-edge *occlusion.*

**jumping the b.,** an orthodontic technique for correcting a crossbite, usually anterior.

**locked b.,** an occlusion in which the cusp arrangement restricts lateral excursions.

**normal b.,** normal occlusion.

**open b.,** (1) see large interarch *distance;* (2) a condition in which the anterior, or posterior, mandibular teeth cannot be brought into the proper occlusal relation to the maxillary dentition because of a dislocation of the temporomandibular articulation, a mandibular fracture, malunion of an old fracture, a deformity of either the alveolar processes of the maxillae or mandible, or abnormal tongue habits.

**rest b.,** a contradictory term that should not be used; see physiologic rest *position.*

**working b.,** working *contacts.*

**bitem'poral.** Relating to both temples or temporal bones.

**bites** [ see bite ]. The pentration of the skin (puncture or laceration) by a great variety of phylla and species of the animal kingdom (including *Homo sapiens*), with reactions as the result of (1) mechanical injury; (2) injection of toxic material such as snake or scorpion venom; (3) injection of antigenic substance capable of inducing and eliciting allergic sensitization; (4) introduction of otherwise saprophytic flora such as *Staphylococcus pyogenes* in the instance of human bites; (5) invasion of the tissue as in myiasis; and (6) transmission of disease such as typhus and rabies. Depending on the nature of the material propelled into the puncture of the skin, and, in the case of antigenic material, on the previous exposure and immunity of the host, the local reaction will be immediate or delayed, accompanied by varying degrees of pain, itching and burning, and systemic manifestations specific for the offending agent.

**bithi'onol.** ACTAMER; BITHIN; 2,2'-thiobis[ 4,6-dichlorophenol ]; an effective drug against the human lungworm, *Paragonimus westermani;* less effective against the Oriental liver fluke, *Clonorchis sinensis;* also used as a bacteriostat in soaps and detergents, and sodium bithionate is used as a topical bactericide and fungicide. Photosensitivity reactions may occur.

**b. sulfoxide,** BTS; same systemic uses as b.; greater intestinal absorption permits the administration of lower doses.

**Bitot** (be-to'), Pierre A., Bordeaux physician, 1822–1888. See B.'s *spots.*

**bitrochanteric** (bi-tro-kan-ter'ik). Relating to two trochanters, either to the two trochanters of one femur or to both great trochanters.

**bitrop'ic** [ bi- + G. *tropē,* a turning ]. Having a dual affinity, as in tissues or organisms.

**bit'ters.** 1. An alcoholic liquor in which bitter vegetable substances, quinine, gentian, or the like, have been steeped. 2. Bitter vegetable drugs, usually used as tonics; such are quassia, gentian, cinchona, etc.

**aromat'ic b.,** b. with a pleasant aromatic flavor.

**bittersweet.** Dulcamara.

**Bittner agent.** See under agent.

**Bittner's milk factor.** See under factor.

**Bittorf,** Alexander, German physician, 1876–1949. See B.'s *reaction.*

**biuret** (bi'u-ret'). Allophanamide; $H_2NCO$—$NH$—$CONH_2$; derived from urea by heating, eliminating $NH_3$ between two ureas.

**bivalence, bivalency** (bi-va'lens, biv'ă-lens, bi-va'len-sī). Divalence, divalency; a combining force, or valence, double that of the hydrogen atom.

**bivalent** (bi-va'lent, biv'ă-lent) [ bi- + L. *valere,* to have power ]. 1. Divalent; having a combining power equal to two atoms of hydrogen, for example, $Ca^{++}$. 2. In cytology, a structure consisting of two paired homologous chromosomes, each split into two sister chromatids, as seen during the pachytene stage of prophase in meiosis.

**biven'ter** [ bi- + L. *venter,* belly ]. Two-bellied; digastric; denoting several muscles.

**b. cervi'cis,** *musculus* spinalis capitis.

**b. mandib'ulae,** *musculus* digastricus.

**biven'tral.** Digastric.

**bix'in.** A carotenoid (a carotene-dioic acid); the orange-red coloring matter from seeds of *Bixa orellana.* The ester is used as a food and colorant. See annotto.

**bi'zygomat'ic.** Relating to both zygomas.

**Bizzozero** (bit-sot'ser-o), Giulio, Italian physician, 1846–1901. See B.'s red *cells,* B.'s *corpuscles.*

**Bjerrum** (byer'oom), J., Danish ophthalmologist, 1827–1892. See B.'s *scotoma, sign.*

**Bk.** Chemical symbol of the element berkelium.

**Black,** J. A., British army surgeon. See B.'s *formula.*

**Black,** Joseph, Scottish chemist and physicist, 1728–1799. Noted for his discovery that carbon dioxide was a constituent of the atmosphere. He enunciated the principles of specific heat, heat capacity, and latent heat.

**Blackfan,** Kenneth D., American physician, 1883–1941. See Diamond-B. *anemia.*

**black'head.** 1. Comedo. 2. Histomoniasis.

**black'leg.** Quarter ill; black quarter; quarter evil; emphysematous or symptomatic anthrax; a specific infectious disease of cattle and sheep caused by *Clostridium chauvei (feseri).* It is essentially a gas gangrene usually affecting the upper parts (heavily muscled) of the legs of young animals, and is highly fatal.

**black'out.** Temporary loss of consciousness due to decreased blood flow to the brain as a result of centrifugal acceleration when an aviator makes a turn with his head toward the center of the curve, as when he pulls out of a power dive. See also red-out.

**visual b.,** see *amaurosis* fugax.

**blad'der** [ A.S. *blaedre* ]. Vesica.

**air b.,** swim b.; a two-chambered gas-filled sac that is present in most fish and functions as a hydrostatic organ; it is located beneath the vertebral column, and is connected with the esophagus in some fish.

**allantoic b.,** a type of b. formed as an outgrowth of the cloaca.

**atonic b.,** a large, dilated, and nonemptying b.; usually due to disturbance of innervation.

**autonomic b.,** involuntary spontaneous or induced periodic reflex emptying of the urinary b.

**cord b.,** neurogenic dysfunction of the b.; a condition resulting from paresis of the nervous supply of the b., marked by weakness of the detrusor muscle and sphincters, and generally by residual urine.

**fascic'ulate b.,** one with hypertrophied walls, the muscular bundles standing out like interlacing cords on the inner surface of the viscus.

**gall b.,** see gallbladder, and *vesica* fellea.

**ileal b.,** a surgically produced b. for adsorption disorders.

**nervous b.,** a b. condition in which there is a neurotic wish to urinate frequently but with failure to empty the b. completely.

**neurogenic b.,** defective functioning of bladder due to impaired innervation.

**stammering of the b.,** irregular halting or interruption of the stream in micturition.

**swim b.,** air b.

**u'rinary b.,** *vesica* urinaria.

**blad'derworm.** See *Cysticercus.*

**bladevent** (blăd'vent). A thin wedge-shaped ventplant.

**Blagden's law.** See under law.

**blain** [ A.S. *blegen* ]. A lesion on the skin.

**Blainville** (blan-vēl'), Henri M. D. de, French zoologist and anthropologist, 1777–1850. See B.'s *ears.*

**Blair,** V. P., American surgeon, 1871–1955. See B.-Brown *graft.*

**Blair Bell.** See Bell, William Blair.

**Blalock,** Alfred, American surgeon, 1899–1965. See B.-Hanlon *operation,* B.-Taussig *operation.*

**Blandin** (blahn-dan'). Philippe F., Paris surgeon, 1798–1849. See B.'s *gland.*

**blas** [ a Middle E. variant of *blast* ]. Term invented by van Helmont to denote a mystical spirit or vital force which presided over and governed the various processes of the body. Each bodily function was supposed to have its own special b.; b. appears to be the counterpart of the archaeus of Paracelsus.

**Blasius** (blah'se-oos), Gerardus, Dutch anatomist, 17th century. See B.'s *duct.*

**Blaskovics,** Laszlo, Hungarian ophthalmologist, 1869–1938. See B.'s *operation.*

**-blast** [ G. *blastos,* germ ]. A combining form (suffix) indicating an immature precursor cell of the type indicated by the preceding word, *e.g.,* lymphoblast, an immature cell in the lymphocyte series.

**blaste'ma** [ G. a sprout ]. 1. The primordial cellular mass from which an organ or part is formed. 2. A cluster of cells competent to initiate the regeneration of a damaged or ablated structure.

**blastem'ic.** Relating to the blastema.

**blastici'din S.** Antibiotic substance produced by *Streptomyces griseochromogenes.*

**blas'tin** [ G. *blastanō,* to cause to grow ]. A substance that stimulates cell growth, such as allantoin.

**blasto-** [ G. *blastos,* germ ]. A combining form used in terms pertaining to the process of budding (and the formation of buds) by cells or tissue, as in *Blastomyces,* a genus of fungi that reproduce by means of budding.

**blastocele** (blas'to-sēl) [ blasto- + G. *koilos,* hollow ]. Blastocoele; cleavage cavity; segmentation cavity; the cavity in the blastula of a developing embryo.

**blastoce'lic.** Relating to the blastocele.

**blastocoele** (blas'to-sēl). Blastocele.

**blastocoelic** (blas'to-se'lik). Blastocelic.

**blastocyst** (blas'to-sist) [ blasto- + G. *kystis,* bladder ]. Blastodermic vesicle; the modified blastula stage of mammalian embryos. It consists of the inner cell mass, and a thin trophoblast layer enclosing the blastocele.

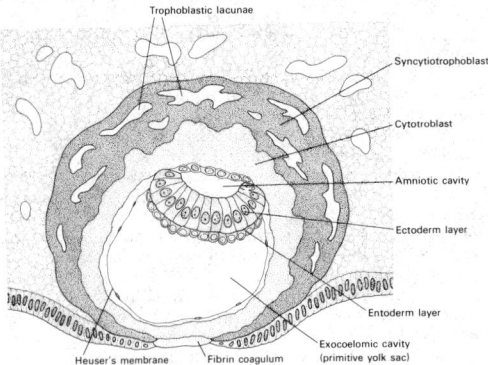

**Human Blastocyst, Ninth Day**
(After Hertig and Rock, from Langman, J.: *Medical Embryology*, Ed. 2, The Williams & Wilkins Co., Baltimore, 1969.

**blastocyte** (blas'to-sīt) [ blasto- + G. *kytos*, cell ]. An undifferentiated cell of the morula or blastula stage of an embryo. A blastomere.

**blastocyto'ma.** Blastoma.

**blas'toderm, blastoder'ma** [ blasto- + G. *derma*, skin ]. The thin disk-shaped cell mass of a young embryo and its extraembryonic extensions over the surface of the yolk. When it is fully formed all three of the primary germ layers (ectoderm, entoderm, and mesoderm) are present.

**bilaminar b.,** the b. of a young embryo when it consists of only two of the three primary germ layers it will ultimately have.

**embryonic b.,** that part of the b. that takes part in the formation of the embryonic body.

**extraembryonic b.,** that part of the b. which is not incorporated in the embryo but forms membranes concerned in its nourishment and protection.

**trilaminar b.,** the b. after all three of the primary germ layers have been established.

**blastoder'mal, blastoder'mic.** Relating to the blastoderm.

**blas'todisk.** 1. The disk of active cytoplasm at the animal pole of a telolecithal egg. 2. The blastoderm, especially in very young stages when its extent is small.

**blastogenesis** (blas'to-jen'ĕ-sis) [ blasto- + G. *genesis*, origin ]. 1. Reproduction of unicellular organisms by budding. 2. Development of an embryo during cleavage and germ layer formation. 3. The transformation of small lymphocytes of human peripheral blood in tissue culture into large, morphologically primitive blastlike cells capable of undergoing mitosis; this phenomenon can be induced by a variety of agents including phytohemagglutinin, certain antigens to which the cell donor has been previously immunized, and leukocytes from an unrelated individual.

**blastogen'ic, blastogenet'ic.** Relating to blastogenesis.

**blastolysis** (blas-tol'ĭ-sis) [ blasto- + G. *lysis*, loosening ]. Dissolution of the blastocyst and subsequent death.

**blastolytic** (blas-to-lit'ik). Relating to blastolysis.

**blasto'ma** [ blasto- + G. suffix, *-oma*, tumor ]. Blastocytoma; a neoplasm composed chiefly or entirely of immature, undifferentiated cells (*i.e.*, blast forms), with only little or virtually no stroma.

**blas'tomere** [ blasto- + G. *meros*, part ]. Cleavage cell; one of the cells into which the egg divides after its fertilization.

**blastomerot'omy.** Blastotomy.

**Blastomyces, pl. blastomyce'tes** (blas-to-mi'sēz) [ blasto- + G. *mykēs*, fungus ]. A genus of yeastlike budding fungi usually including *B. dermatitidis*, the cause of North American blastomycocis, and *Paracoccidioides braziliensis*, the cause of South American blastomycosis.

**B. brazilien'sis,** the cause of South American blastomycosis. The preferred scientific name is *Paracoccidioides braziliensis*.

**B. coccidioi'des,** *Coccidioides immitis.*

**B. dermatit'idis,** the pathogen of North American blastomycosis.

**blastomycetes** (blas-to-mi-se'tēz). Plural of *Blastomyces.*

**blastomyce'tic.** Relating to or caused by blastomycetes.

**blastomy'cin.** A sterile liquid concentrate of the soluble growth products of *Blastomyces dermatitidis* when grown in the mycelial phase on a synthetic medium; used as a dermal reactivity indicator.

**blastomycosis** (blas'to-mi-ko'sis). Term used to describe several distinctive infections: (1) North American b.; (2) South American b.; (3) cryptococcosis.

**Brazilian b.,** South American b.

**European b.,** cryptococcosis.

**keloidean b.,** lobomycosis.

**North American b.,** Gilchrist's disease or mycosis; a suppurative, granulomatous chronic disease caused by *Blastomyces dermatitidis;* it starts as a respiratory infection and disseminates, usually with cutaneous, osseous, and pulmonary manifestations.

**South American b.,** paracoccidioidal granuloma; Brazilian b.; Lutz-Splendore-Almeida disease; infection with *Paracoccidioides brasiliensis* that produces a chronic, fatal mycosis with ulcerative granulomas of the buccal and nasal mucosa; regional and generalized lymphadenopathy occurs, with involvement of the skin and spread to lungs, spleen, and other viscera.

**blas'toneu'ropore** [ blasto- + neuropore, *q. v.* ]. A temporary opening formed in some embryos by the union of the blastopore and neuropore.

**blas'tophore** [ blasto- + G. *phorōs*, bearing ]. An early stage of division of a coccidial schizont in which spheroid or ellipsoid structures are formed, each with a single peripheral layer of nuclei; merozoites form at the surface of the b. over each nucleus, grow out radially, and separate from the residual body (remnant of the b.); in a first-generation schizont such as *Eimeria bovis*, about 120,000 merozoites are produced.

**blastophthoria** (blas'tof-tho'rĭ-ah) [ blasto- + G. *phthora*, ruin, corruption ]. Degeneration of the germ cells as a result of poisoning by syphilis, lead, alcohol, opium, etc.

**blastophthoric** (blas'tof-thor'ik). Relating to blastophthoria.

**blastopore** (blas'to-pōr) [ blasto- + G. *poros*, opening, POR-1 ]. The opening into the archenteron formed by the invagination of the blastula to form a gastrula; the gastropore; protostoma.

**blastospore** (blas'to-spōr) [ blasto- + G. *sporos*, seed ]. A thallospore of round or ovoid shape developed by budding from a hypha.

**blastot'omy** [ blasto- + G. *tomē*, incision ]. Blastomerotomy; the experimental destruction of one or more blastomeres.

**blas'tula** [ G. *blastos*, germ ]. An early stage of an embryo formed by the rearrangement of the blastomeres of the morula to form a hollow sphere.

**blas'tular.** Pertaining to the blastula.

**blastula'tion.** The formation of the blastula or blastocyst.

**Blatin** (blă-tan'), Marc, French physician, *1878. See B.'s *syndrome.*

**Blatta.** A genus of insect that includes the common cockroach; family Blattidae. The cockroach yields a diuretic principle: antihydropin. The genus is composed of several species; the common cockroach is *B. orientalis.*

**blaze** [ Old Ger. *blase* ]. A wide white marking on a horse's face, running from the nose to the forehead.

**bleb.** A collection of fluid beneath the skin; usually the lesions are smaller than bullae or blisters.

**bleed'er.** A sufferer from hemophilia, Christmas disease, Osler's disease, or other bleeding disorders. 2. A phlebotomist.

**bleed'ing.** Losing blood as a result of rupture or severance of blood vessels.

**dysfunctional uterine b.,** uterine b. due to an endocrine imbalance rather than to any organic disease.

occult b., see occult *blood*.

**blem'ish.** 1. A small, circumscribed alteration of the skin considered to be unesthetic but insignificant. 2. To alter the skin, rendering an unesthetic appearance. 3. In a horse, any abnormality that detracts from a horse's appearance but does not interfere with his usefulness.

**blennadeni'tis** [ G. *blennos,* mucus, + *adēn,* gland, + suffix *-itis,* inflammation ]. Inflammation of the mucous glands.

**blennem'esis** [ G. *blennos,* mucus, + *emesis,* vomiting ]. Vomiting of mucus.

**blenno-, blenn-** [ G. *blennos,* mucus ]. Combining form relating to mucus.

**blennogen'ic** [ blenno- + G. suffix *-gen,* to produce ]. Muciparous; forming mucus.

**blennogenous** (blen-oj'en-us). Blennogenic.

**blennoid** (blen'oyd) [ blenno- + G. *eidos,* resemblance ]. Mucoid; resembling mucus.

**blennometri'tis** [ blenno- + G. suffix *-itis,* inflammation ]. Obsolete designation for inflammation of the uterine mucous membrane, especially when accompanied by a discharge.

**blennophthalmia** (blen-of-thal'mī-ah). 1. Conjunctivitis. 2. Gonorrheal *ophthalmia.*

**blennorrhagia** (blen'o-ra'jī-ah) [ blenno- + G. *rhēgnymi,* to burst forth ]. Discharge from mucous surfaces.

**blennorrhagic** (blen-o-raj'ik). Relating to blennorrhagia.

**blennorrhea** (blen'o-re'ah) [ blenno- + G. *rhoia,* a flow ]. 1. Any mucous discharge, especially from the urethra or vagina. 2. An obsolete term for gonorrhea.

   **b. adulto'rum,** an obsolete term for gonorrhea.

   **b. conjunctiva'lis,** gonorrheal *ophthalmia.*

   **inclusion b.,** inclusion conjunctivitis of the newborn caused by *Chlamydia oculogenitale* and acquired during birth from the genital tract of the mother.

   **b. neonato'rum,** *ophthalmia* neonatorum; usually gonorrheal.

   **Stoerk's b.,** chronic, first purulent then dry, catarrh of the upper air passages with hypertrophy of the mucous membrane and submucosa, in many cases the same as scleroma.

**blennorrhe'al.** Relating to blennorrhea.

**blennostasis** (blen-os'tā-sis) [ blenno- + G. *stasis,* standing ]. Diminution or suppression of secretion from the mucous membranes.

**blennostat'ic.** Diminishing mucous secretion.

**blennotho'rax.** An accumulation of mucous secretion in the bronchi.

**blennu'ria** [ blenno- + G. *ouron,* urine ]. The excretion of an excess of mucus in the urine.

**blephar-.** See blepharo-.

**bleph'aradeni'tis** (blef'ar-ad-ē-ni'tis) [ blephar- + G. *adēn,* gland, + suffix *-itis,* inflammation ]. Blepharoadenitis; inflammation of the Meibomian glands or the marginal glands of Moll or Zeiss.

**bleph'aral.** Referring to the eyelids.

**blepharectomy** (blef'ar-ek'to-me) [ blepharo- + G. *ektomē,* excision ]. Excision of all or part of an eyelid.

**blepharedema** (blef'ar-ě-de'mah). Edema of the eyelids, causing swelling and often a baggy appearance.

**blepharitis** (blef'ă-ri'tis) [ blepharo- + G. suffix *-itis,* inflammation ]. Inflammation of the eyelids.

   **b. angula'ris,** inflammation of the lid margins at the angles of the commissure.

   **ciliary b.,** b. marginalis.

   **b. marginalis,** psorophthalmia; ciliary or marginal b.; inflammation of the margins of the eyelids.

   **b. parasit'ica, b. phthiriat'ica,** pediculous b.; marginal b. due to the presence of lice.

   **b. squamo'sa,** a chronic inflammation of the margins of the lids with the formation of branny scales.

   **b. ulcero'sa,** marginal b. with ulceration.

**blepharo-, blephar-** [ G. *blepharon,* eyelid ]. Combining forms meaning eyelid.

**bleph'aroadeni'tis.** Blepharadenitis.

**bleph'aroadeno'ma** [ blepharo- + G. *adēn,* gland, + suffix *-oma,* tumor ]. A glandular tumor, or adenoma, of the eyelid.

**blepharochalasis** (blef'ar-o-kal'as-is) [ blepharo- + G. *chalasis,* a slackening ]. Ptosis adiposa; dermatolysis palpebrarum; a condition in which there is a redundancy of the upper eyelids so that a fold of skin hangs down, often concealing the tarsal margin when the eye is open.

**blepharochromidrosis** (blef'ar-o-kro-mī-dro'sis) [ blepharo- + G. *chrōma,* color, + *hidrōsis,* sweat ]. Chromidrosis of the eyelids.

**blepharoclonus** (blef'ar-ok'lo-nus) [ blepharo- + G. *klonos,* a tumult ]. Clonic spasm of the eyelids.

**bleph'arocolobo'ma** [ blepharo- + coloboma, *q.v.* ]. A defect, as a fissure, of the eyelid. It may be congenital, pathologic, or artificial.

**bleph'aroconjunctivi'tis.** Inflammation of the palpebral conjunctiva.

**bleph'arodias'tasis** [ blepharo- + G. *diastasis,* separation ]. Abnormal separation or inability to close completely the eyelids.

**blepharokeratoconjunctivitis** (blef'ar-o-ker'ă-to-konjunk'tī-vi'tis). An inflammation of infective, allergic, or irritative origin involving the margins of the lids, cornea, and conjunctiva.

**blepharomelasma** (blef'ar-o-mě-laz'mah) [ blepharo- + melasma, *q.v.* ]. A dark discoloration of the skin of the eyelid.

**bleph'aron** [ G. *blepharon,* eyelid ]. Palpebra.

**blepharon'cus** (blef'ar-ong'kus) [ blepharo- + G. *onkos,* a mass ]. A tumor of the eyelid.

**blepharopachynsis** (blef'ar-o-pā-kin'sis) [ blepharo- + G. *pachynsis,* a thickening ]. A pathological thickening of an eyelid.

**bleph'arophimo'sis** [ blepharo- + G. *phimōsis,* an obstruction ]. Blepharostenosis; inability to open the eye to the normal extent.

**bleph'arophy'ma** [ blepharo- + G. *phyma,* a tumor ]. Tumor of the skin of the eyelid.

**bleph'aroplast** [ blepharo- + G. *plastos,* formed ]. Basal *body.*

**bleph'aroplas'tic.** Relating to blepharoplasty.

**bleph'aroplasty** [ blepharo- + G. *plassō,* to form ]. Any operation for the restoration of a defect in the eyelid.

**blepharoplegia** (blef'ar-o-ple'jī-ah) [ blepharo- + G. *plēgē,* stroke ]. Paralysis of an eyelid.

**blepharoptosis** (blef'ar-o-to'sis, blef'ar-op'to-sis) [ blepharo- + G. *ptōsis,* a falling ]. Blepharoptosia; drooping of the upper eyelid.

**blepharorrhaphy** (blef-ar-or'af-e) [ blepharo- + G. *rhaphē,* seam ]. Tarsorrhaphy.

**bleph'arospasm, bleph'arospas'mus.** Spasmodic winking, or contraction of the orbicularis palpebrarum muscle.

**bleph'arostat** [ blepharo- + G. *statos,* fixed ]. Eye *speculum.*

**bleph'arosteno'sis** [ blepharo- + G. *stenōsis,* a narrowing ]. Blepharophimosis.

**blepharosynechia** (blef'ar-o-sin-ek'ī-ah) [ blepharo- + G. *synecheia,* continuity, fr, *syn-echō,* to hold together ]. Ankyloblepharon; temporary or permanent adhesion of eyelid edges to each other.

**blepharot'omy** [ blepharo- + G. *tomē,* incision ]. A cutting operation on an eyelid.

**Blessig,** Robert, German physician, 1830–1878. See B.'s cysts, groove, lacuna.

**blind.** Unable to see; without useful sight; see blindness.

**blind'ness.** Loss of useful sight; legal b. in the United States is corrected vision of the better eye to 20/200 or less, or visual field contraction to 20 degrees or less; with 4/200 vision, help is required in traveling; absolute b. connotes no light perception. See also amaurosis.

   **blue b.,** tritanopia.

   **blue-yellow b.,** see tritanopia and tetartanopsia.

   **color b.,** an inability to recognize one or more of the seven primary colors. See also anomalopia.

   **complete color b.,** achromatopsia.

   **cortical b.,** psychic b.; cortical psychic b.; loss of sight due to a lesion in the cortical representation of vision; the fundus and pupillary reflexes are normal.

   **cortical psychic b.,** cortical b.

   **day b.,** hemeralopia.

**eclipse b.,** eclipse *amblyopia.*

**flash b.,** see flashblindness.

**flight b.,** visual blackout in aviators; see also *amaurosis fugax.*

**functional b.,** loss of vision related to conversion hysteria.

**green b.,** deuteranopia.

**letter b.,** a form of aphasia in which one is unable to recognize the significance of letters.

**mind b.,** psychanopsia; a division of aphasia in which the person no longer understands what he sees.

**moon b.,** periodic *ophthalmia.*

**music b.,** musical *alexia.*

**night b.,** nyctalopia.

**note b.,** musical *alexia.*

**object b.,** apraxia (2).

**partial color b.,** dichromatism.

**psychic b.,** cortical b.

**red b.,** protanopia.

**red-green b.,** a general term for protanopia, deuteranopia, protanomaly, and deuteranomaly, since these are not sharply differentiated by pseudoisochromatic charts or yarn tests; also called xanthocyanopsia, *q. v.*

**sign b.,** asymbolia (2).

**snow b.,** actinic conjunctivitis with obscuration of vision caused by sunlight reflected from snow.

**solar b.,** eclipse *amblyopia.*

**taste b.,** the lack of ability to appreciate a substance by taste.

**text b.,** alexia.

**twilight b.,** a defect of vision greater in bright light than in dull light; may be due to posterior subcapsular cataract.

**word b.,** alexia.

**yellow b.,** axanthopsia.

**blis'ter.** 1. A collection of fluid under the epidermis or within the epidermis (subepidermal or intradermal). 2. To form a b. with heat or other blistering agent.

**blood b.,** one containing blood; resulting from a minor pinch or crushing injury.

**fever b.,** *herpes* simplex of the lips.

**fly b.,** a cantharidal b. caused by discharge of a vesicating body fluid by certain beetles, particularly members of the family Meloidae which produce cantharidin, for example, *Lytta* (*Cantharis*) *vesicatoria,* the notorious "Spanish fly." Non-cantharidin vesicating fluid is produced by other beetles, such as rove beetles (family Staphylinidae), especially the genus *Paederus,* whose fluid, on contact with the skin, produces an intensely painful blister.

**flying b.,** a misnomer for a vesicator agent applied successively to different skin areas and kept in one place just long enough to cause redness but not long enough to cause a b.

**blis'tering.** 1. Vesicating; causing a blister to form. 2. Vesication; the formation of a blister, bleb, or vesicle.

**bloat, bloating** (blōt). 1. Abdominal distention from swallowed air or intestinal gas from fermentation. 2. Hoven; tympany of the rumen; a distention of the rumen of cattle, caused by the accumulation of gases of fermentation. Particularly likely to occur when the animals are pastured on rich legume grasses. If unrelieved the condition may quickly lead to death.

**Bloch,** Bruno, Swiss dermatologist, 1878–1933. See B.-Sulzberger *disease.*

**Bloch** (blokh), Konrad, U. S. biochemist, *1912. Nobel laureate, 1964, with Feodor Lynen, for contributions to the knowledge of reactions involved in biosynthesis of cholesterol and fatty acids.

**Bloch** (blokh), Marcel, Paris physician, 1885–1925. See B.'s *reaction, scale.*

**block** [ Fr. *bloquer*]. 1. To obstruct; to arrest passage through. 2. A condition in which the passage of a nervous impulse is arrested, wholly or in part, temporarily or permanently. 3. Heart b. 4. See anesthesia.

**anterograde b.,** atrioventricular b.

**arboriza'tion b.,** intraventricular b. supposedly due to widespread blockage in the Purkinje ramifications and manifested in the electrocardiogram by a pattern similar to bundle-branch b. but with complexes of low amplitude.

**atrioventricular b.,** A-V b.; anterograde b.; heart b.; impairment of the normal conduction between atria and ventricles; in **first degree A-V b.** there is prolongation of A-V conduction time (P-R interval); in **second degree A-V b.** some but not all atrial impulses fail to reach the ventricles, thus some ventricular beats are dropped; in **complete A-V b.** no impulses can reach the ventricles despite a slow ventricular rate (under 45 per minute); atria and ventricles beat independently.

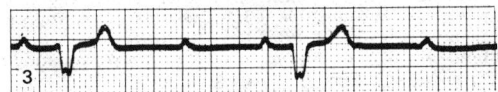

**Complete Atrioventricular Block**

**biochemical b.,** (1) the halting of a portion of the metabolic pathway, through the absence of an enzyme necessary for the catalysis of one of the chemical reactions involved in that pathway. Thus, phenylketonuria is a biochemical b. caused by the absence of phenylalanine hydroxylase, which converts phenylalanine to tyrosine; (2) the production of such a b. by the use of chemical inhibitors, such as an antimetabolite or a metabolic "poison."

**bite b.,** occlusion *rim.*

**bundle-branch b.,** intraventricular b. due to interruption of conduction in one of the two main branches of the bundle of His and manifested in the electrocardiogram by marked prolongation of the QRS complex.

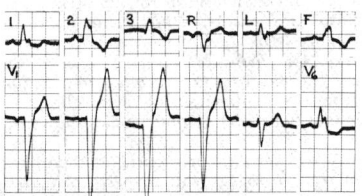

**Left Bundle-Branch Block**

(From Marriott, H. J. L.: *Practical Electrocardiography,* Ed. 4, The Williams & Wilkins Co., Baltimore, 1968.)

**entrance b.,** protective b.

**exit b.,** inability of an impulse to leave its point of origin, the mechanism for which is conceived as an encircling zone of refractory tissue denying passage to the emerging impulse.

**fascicular b.,** a condition based on the concept that two fascicles in the left branch of the bundle of His provide three fascicles of a system of conduction, of which the right bundle branch constitutes the third, for the transmission of the cardiac impulse from atrium above to ventricle below the A-V node; block may occur in any or all fascicles, all three together producing complete A-V block; see also hemiblock.

**heart b.,** atrioventricular b.

**intra-atrial b.,** impaired conduction through the atria, manifested by widened and often notched P waves in the electrocardiogram.

**intraventricular b.,** I-V b.; delayed conduction within the ventricular conducting system or myocardium, including bundle-branch and peri-infarction b.'s, and the hemiblocks.

**Mobitz types atrioventricular b.,** type I, the dropped beat of the Wenckebach phenomenon, *q.v.;* type II, a dropped cardiac cycle that occurs without alteration in the conduction of the preceding intervals.

**peri-infarction b.,** an electrocardiographic abnormality associated with an old myocardial infarct and caused by delayed activation of the myocardium in the region of the infarct; characterized by an initial vector directed away from the infarcted region with the terminal vector directed toward it.

**protective b.,** protection; an unexplained mechanism whereby a pacemaker is protected from being discharged by the impulse from another center; the mechanism, usually conceived as an encircling zone of unidirectionally refractory tissue permitting egress of impulses from the center but preventing access to the center, is seen in operation in ventricular parasystole where the parasystolic center is protected from discharge by the sinus pacemaker and so is able to maintain its intrinsic rhythm undisturbed.

**retrograde b.,** impaired conduction backward from the ventricles or A-V node into the atria.

**sinus, sinoatrial,** or **sinoauricular (S-A) b.,** failure of the impulse to leave the sinus node so that a complete cardiac cycle is dropped.

**stellate b.,** anesthesia produced by injection of local anesthetic solution in the vicinity of the stellate ganglion.

**unidirectional,** b. that prevents passage of an impulse when it approaches from one direction but not from the other, as when b. in the A-V node prevents anterograde conduction to the ventricles while retrograde conduction to the atria remains intact.

**Wilson b.,** the commonest form of right bundle-branch b. characterized in lead I by a tall slender R wave followed by a wider S wave of lower voltage.

**block'ade.** 1. The intravenous injection of large amounts of colloidal dyes or other substances whereby the reaction of the reticuloendothelial cells to other influences (by phagocytosis for example) is temporarily prevented. 2. Arrest of transmission at autonomic synaptic junctions, autonomic receptor sites, or myoneural junctions by a drug. See also anesthesia; block; and blocking.

**adrenergic b.,** selective inhibition by a drug of the responses of effector cells to adrenergic sympathetic nerve impulses (sympatholytic) and to epinephrine and related amines (adrenolytic).

**cholinergic b.,** inhibition by a drug of nerve impulse transmission at autonomic ganglionic synapses (ganglionic b.), at postganglionic parasympathetic effector cells (*e.g.,* by atropine); and at myoneural junctions (myoneural b.) or the inhibition of a cholinergic agent.

**ganglionic b.,** inhibition of nerve impulse transmission at autonomic ganglionic synapses by drugs such as nicotine, hexamethonium, etc.

**myoneural b.,** inhibition of nerve impulse transmission at myoneural junctions by a drug such as curare.

**narcotic b.,** the use of drugs to inhibit the effects of narcotic substances; commonly adjunctive to treatment of opiate addiction.

**sympathetic b.,** b. between a preganglionic sympathetic fiber and the ganglion cell.

**virus b.,** the interference of one virus by another either attenuated or unrelated.

**block'er.** An instrument used to block a passage.

**Macintosh b.'s,** a series of tubes used during thoracic surgery for the blocking of one lung, or lobe, from the other.

**block'ing.** 1. Obstructing; the arrest of passage through; 2. In psychoanalysis, a sudden break in free association occurring when a painful subject or repressed complex is touched.

**alpha b.,** the desynchronization of the brain waves produced by opening the eyes or by intense thought or emotion.

**field b.,** regional anesthesia produced by infiltration of local anesthetic solution into the tissues surrounding operative field.

**nerve b.,** interruption of the passage of impulses through a nerve by the injection of alcohol or local anesthetic solutions.

**block out.** The elimination of undercuts by filling such areas with a medium such as wax or wet pumice.

**Blocq,** Paul O., Paris physician, 1860–1896. See B.'s *disease.*

**blood** (blud) [ A.S. blōd ]. Sanguis; the "circulating tissue" of the body; the fluid and its suspended formed elements that are circulated through the heart, arteries, capillaries, and veins; b. is the means by which (1) oxygen and nutritive materials are transported to the tissues, and (2) carbon dioxide and various metabolic products are removed for excretion. The b. consists of a pale yellow or gray-yellow fluid, plasma, in which are suspended red b. cells (erythrocytes), white b. cells (leukocytes), and platelets. See also arterial b. and venous b.

*Blood of domestic animals*

| Species | Erythrocytes* | Diameter | Hemoglobin* |
|---|---|---|---|
| | *millions* | *microns* | *gm. per cent* |
| Horse | 6.9–12.5 (8.5) | 5.6 | 9–18 (12) |
| Cow | 6.3–10.5 (7) | 5.6 | 8.5–14 (11) |
| Sheep | 8.0–15.0 (12) | 4.8 | 8–15 (12) |
| Goat | 8.0–18.0 (13) | 4.0 | 8–14.5 (11) |
| Swine | 5.0–8.0 (7) | 6.0 | 10–16 (13) |
| Dog | 6.0–8.0 (6.8) | 7.0 | 11–18 (15) |
| Cat | 5.0–10.0 (7.8) | 5.9 | 8–15 (12) |

\* Averages are shown in parentheses.

**arterial b.,** b. that is oxygenated in the lungs, found in the left chambers of the heart and in the arteries, and relatively bright red.

**b. count,** see *blood count.*

**b. dust,** hemoconia.

**b. factor,** according to one school of thought, b. group antigens or agglutinogens are subdivided into b. factors, each with a specific reaction with an antibody. A single antigen, produced by a single gene, may consist of a set of b. factors and react with a corresponding set of antisera. Another school of thought considers agglutinogens and b. factors to be essentially synonymous, each controlled by a single gene.

**b. group,** a system of genetically determined antigens or agglutinogens located on the surface of the erythrocyte. Each blood group is determined by a series of two or more genes that are allelic or at least very closely linked on a single chromosome. Because of the antigen differences existing between individuals, b. groups are important with respect to b. transfusions, maternal-fetal b. group incompatibilities (erythroblastosis fetalis), and tissue and organ transplantation. B. groups have medicolegal uses, particularly in disputed paternity cases, and are useful in genetic and anthropologic studies. Certain b. groups have been supposed to be related to susceptibility or resistance to certain diseases. The term "blood group" is often used as synonymous with "blood type," *q.v.* See appendix 2, Blood Groups, for individual b. groups: ABO, Auberger, Diego, Duffy, I, Kell, Kidd, Lewis, Lutheran, MNSs, P, Rh, Sutter, Xg, and the low frequency and high frequency b. groups.

**b. grouping,** the classification of b. samples by means of appropriate laboratory tests according to their agglutination reactions with respect to one or more b. groups. In general, a suspension of erythrocytes to be tested is exposed to a known specific antiserum; agglutination of the erythrocytes indicates that they possess the antigen for which the antiserum is specific, while absence of agglutination indicates absence of the antigen. Certain antiserums require special testing conditions.

**b. group specific substances A and B** (NF), solution of complexes of polysaccharides and amino acids that reduces the titer of anti-A and anti-B isoagglutinins in serum from group O persons. Used to render group O b. reasonably safe for transfusion into persons of group A, B, or AB, but does not affect any incompatibility that results from various other factors, such as Rh.

**laky b.,** b. that is undergoing or has undergone laking; see lake (2) and laky.

**occult b.,** occult bleeding; b. in the feces in amounts too small to be seen but detectable by chemical tests.

**packed human b. cells** (USP), whole b. from which plasma has been removed; may be prepared any time during the dating period of the whole b. from which it is derived, but not later than 6 days after the b. has been drawn if separation of plasma and cells is achieved by centrifugation.

**b. puzzles,** foreign bodies or deformed b. cells that may be misinterpreted as infectious agents (*e.g.,* bacteria, fungi, etc.) in stained films, as a result of similarities in morphology and staining properties.

**sludged b.,** b. in which the corpuscles, as a result of some general abnormal state, *e.g.,* burns, traumatic shock, and similar stresses, become massed together in the capillaries, and thereby block the vessels or move slowly through them.

**strawberry-cream b.,** the appearance of the b. in advanced degrees of lipemia.

**b. substitute,** human plasma, serum albumin, or a solution of such substances as dextran, gum acacia, gelatin, isinglass, etc., used for transfusion in hemorrhage and shock.

**b. type,** the specific reaction pattern of erythrocytes of an individual to the antisera of one blood group; *e.g.,* the ABO b. group consists of four major b. types, O, A, B, and AB, depending on agglutination of erythrocytes by neither, one, the other or both anti-A and anti-B testing sera. The b. type is the genetic phenotype of the individual for one b. group system and may vary in detail with the number of different antisera available for testing. See also appendix 2, Blood Groups.

**b. typing,** b. grouping.

**venous b.,** b. which has passed through the capillaries of various tissues, except the lungs, and is found in the veins, the right chambers of the heart, and the pulmonary arteries; it is usually dark red as a result of a lower content of oxygen.

**b. vessel,** see *blood vessel.*

**whole b.** (USP), b. drawn from a selected donor under rigid aseptic precautions; contains citrate ion or heparin as an anticoagulant; used as a b. replenisher.

**whole human b.** (BP), b. mixed with a suitable anticoagulant obtained from a human subject who is free from disease transmissible by b. transfusion. Not more than 420 ml. are drawn from one subject on one occasion.

**blood count.** Calculation of the number of red or white blood cells in a cubic millimeter of blood, by means of counting the cells in an accurate volume of diluted blood; also, the determination of the percentages of various types of leukocytes, *i.e.,* a differential count, as observed in a stained film of blood.

**differential b. c.,** an enumeration of the number of white blood cells in a given amount (cubic millimeter) of blood, including a determination of the approximate percentage of each variety of leukocyte present.

**Schilling's b. c.,** Schilling's index; a method of counting blood in which the polymorphonuclear neutrophils are separated into four groups according to the number and arrangement of the nuclear masses in these cells.

**blood'less.** Without blood; anemic; exsanguinated.

**blood'letting.** Abstraction (1); removing blood, usually from a vein as remedial measure; used now in congestive heart failure and polycythemia.

**general b.,** removing blood by an incision into an artery (arteriotomy) or a vein (venesection, phlebotomy).

**local b.,** removing blood from the smaller vessels by wet cupping or leeching.

**blood'root.** Sanguinaria.

**blood'shot.** Locally congested, the smaller blood vessels of the part, *e.g.,* the conjunctiva, being dilated and visible.

**blood stream, bloodstream.** The flowing blood as it is encountered in the organism, as distinguished from blood which has been removed from the organism or sequestered in a part; thus, something added to the blood stream may be expected to become distributed to all parts of the body through which blood is flowing.

**blood vessel.** A tube (artery, capillary, vein, or sinus) conveying blood.

**blood'worm.** 1. The filarial parasite of sheep, *Elaeophora schneideri.* 2. Red aquatic larvae of certain dipterous gnats and midges. 3. Marine annelids in the family Terobellidae with soft bodies and red blood. 4. Blood-inhabiting worms, such as the *Schistosoma* of man.

**Bloom,** David, U. S. dermatologist, *1892. See B.'s *syndrome.*

**blotch.** Commonly used term to denote a pigmented or erythematous lesion.

**Blount,** Walter P., U. S. orthopaedist, *1900. See B.'s *disease,* B.-Barber *disease.*

**blow'fly.** See *Calliphora, Lucilia, Phormia.*

**blue.** Of the color of the clear sky, between green and violet on the spectrum. For individual blue dyes not listed below, see the specific name.

**sky b.,** a pigment mixture of cobaltous stannate and calcium sulfate used biologically as an injection mass.

**blue'bag.** Ovine *mastitis.*

**blue'comb.** Bluecomb *disease.*

**blues.** Mental depression or despondency.

**blue'tongue.** Soremuzzle; an infectious disease of sheep, possibly of cattle, caused by a virus. It has long been known in South Africa, in recent years it has been recognized in the United States. It is manifested by catarrhal inflammation of the mucosae of the mouth, nose, and intestinal tract, accompanied frequently by foot involvement and lameness. Bloodsucking midges of the genus *Culicoides* have been implicated in transmission of b. in South Africa and the United States.

**Blum,** Paul, French physician, 1878–1933. See Gougerot and B. *disease.*

**Blumenau** (bloo'men-ow), Leonid, Russian neurologist, 1862–1932. See B.'s *nucleus.*

**Blumenbach,** Johann F., German physiologist, 1752–1840. See B.'s *clivus.*

**Blumer,** George, American physician, 1858–1940. See B.'s *shelf.*

**blunt'hook.** See under hook.

**blush.** A sudden and brief redness of the face and neck due to emotion.

**BMR.** Abbreviation for basal metabolic *rate.*

**BNA.** Abbreviation for *Basle Nomina Anatomica.*

**boar** (bōr). A male hog.

**bobbing.** An up-and-down movement.

**ocular b.,** a movement disorder of the eye observed in comatose patients with lesions of the lower pons; the eyeballs intermittently dip briskly downward and more slowly return to the primary position in a bobbing action.

**Bobroff,** V. F., Moscow surgeon, *1858. See B.'s *method.*

**Boc.** Abbreviation for *t*-butoxycarbonyl.

**BOC, t-BOC.** Abbreviations formerly used for *t*-butoxycarbonyl; current usage is Boc.

**Bochdalek** (bokh-dal'ek), Vincent A., Prague anatomist, 1801–1883. See B.'s *flower basket, foramen, ganglion, gap, hernia, muscle, valve.*

**Bock,** August C., German anatomist, 1782–1833. See B.'s *ganglion, nerve.*

**Bockhart,** Max, German physician, 1883–1921. See B.'s *impetigo.*

**Bodansky,** Aaron, American biochemist, 1896–1941. See B. *unit.*

**Bodecker index.** See under index.

**Bo'do.** A genus of free-living, ovoid or slightly pyriform protozoa with two flagella, one projecting anteriorly and the other posteriorly; may be ingested as encysted forms in food or drink, or possibly deposited in feces or urine after excretion; in either instance, cysts frequently develop into trophozoites if the specimen is permitted to remain at room temperature for a few hours prior to examination; the organisms are not pathogenic in man.

**B. cauda'tus,** a species that is found in specimens of human feces (especially in tropical regions); the organisms are frequently termed coprozoic flagellates.

**B. saltans,** a protozoan flagellate of intestinal tract sometimes observed in ulcers.

**B. urina'rius,** a species found occasionally in the urine.

# BODY

**body** (bod'ĭ) [ A.S. *bodig* ]. Corpus; soma (see both). 1. The head, neck, trunk, and extremities. 2. The material part of man, as distinguished from the mind and spirit. 3. The principal mass of any structure. 4. A thing; a substance.

**acetone b.,** ketone b.; see under ketone.

**adrenal b.,** *glandula* suprarenalis.

**alcoholic hyaline b.'s,** Mallory b.'s.

**Alder b.'s,** granular inclusions in polymorphonuclear leukocytes; they take on a dark color with Giemsa-Wright stain and react metachromatically with toluidine blue. See also Alder's *anomaly.*

**amylogenic b.,** amyloplast.

**am'yloid b.'s of the prostate,** small masses of colloid material often present in the tubules of the gland. See also *corpus* amylaceum.

**anococcygeal b.,** *ligamentum* anococcygeum.

**aortic b.,** *glomus* aorticum.

**Arnold's b.'s,** small portions or minute fragments of erythrocytes (sometimes mistaken for blood platelets), or small "ghosts" of erythrocytes.

**Aschoff b.'s,** Aschoff nodules; a form of granulomatous inflammation characteristically observed in acute rheumatic carditis. Fully developed Aschoff b.'s (100 μ to 900 μ in diameter) consist of fibrinoid change in connective tissue, lymphocytes, occasional plasma cells, and peculiar histiocytes. The latter are ovoid, rounded, or irregular, with an abundant, granular, basophilic or amphophilic cytoplasm; the nuclei are irregularly ovoid and relatively large, with a conspicuous, hyperchromatic, sometimes bar-shaped central mass of chromatin from which fine strands radiate toward the nuclear membrane, in some instances larger and multinucleated. During healing of Aschoff nodules, the characteristic cells and fibroblasts appear, collagen is formed, and the foci gradually become small scars.

**asteroid b.,** (1) an eosinophilic inclusion resembling a star with delicate radiating lines, occurring in a vacuolated area of cytoplasm of a multinucleated giant cell; asteroid b.'s are especially frequent in sarcoidosis, but occur also in other granulomas; (2) a rounded fungal spore, seen in tissue sections, with radiating peripheral eosinophilic projections produced by the host's tissue reaction; seen occasionally in sporotrichosis.

**Auer b.'s.** rod-shaped structures of uncertain nature in the cytoplasm of immature myeloid cells, especially myeloblasts, in acute myelocytic leukemia; stained red by azure-eosin stains; contain peroxisomes and may be an abnormal form of lysosomes.

**Babès-Ernst b.'s,** intracellular granules, present in many species of bacteria, which posses a strong affinity for nuclear stains; also referred to as volutin or metachromatic granules.

**Barr chromatin b.,** sex *chromatin.*

**basal b.,** basal corpuscle or granule; blepharoplast; a minute body at the origin of each cilium or flagellum; it is not part of the kinetoplast, as formerly believed, but the origin of the outer fibrils of the flagellar axoneme; it lies alongside the flagellar vacuole as a small cylinder from which the nine peripheral double fibrils of the flagellar axoneme emerge.

**bigeminal b.'s,** *corpora* bigemina.

**Bollinger b.'s,** relatively large, spheroid or ovoid, usually somewhat granular, acidophilic, intracytoplasmic inclusion b.'s observed in the infected tissues of birds with fowlpox; when b.'s are ruptured large numbers of fowlpox virus particles are released.

**Borrel b.'s,** particles of fowlpox virus; aggregates of Borrel b.'s in infected cells result in the formation of Bollinger b.'s.

**brassy b.,** a dark-colored, usually shrunken erythrocyte in which there is a malarial parasite.

**Buchner's b.'s,** obsolete term for defensive *proteins.*

**Cabot's ring b.'s,** ring-shaped or figure-of-eight structures staining red with Wright's stain found in red blood cells in severe anemias, probably a remnant of the nuclear membrane; a form of basophilic degenerative process.

**Call-Exner b.'s,** small fluid-filled spaces between granulosal cells in ovarian follicles and in ovarian tumors of granulosal origin; they may form a rosette-like structure.

**cancer b.'s,** discrete, acidophilic or amphophilic, hyaline b.'s of various shapes and sizes, occurring in the cytoplasm of some of the neoplastic cells and also extracellularly in the stroma of various carcinomas and sarcomas; formerly regarded by some observers as parasitic causal agents, but now generally thought to be simple inclusions or the products of degenerative changes.

**carotid b.,** *glomus* caroticum.

**cavernous b.,** see *corpus* cavernosum.

**central b.,** cytocentrum.

**chromaffin b.'s,** paraganglia.

**chromatin b.,** the genetic apparatus of bacteria; see nucleus (2).

**cil'iary b.,** *corpus* ciliare.

**Civatte b.'s,** colloid b.'s.

**b. of clitoris,** *corpus* clitoridis.

**coccyge'al b.,** *corpus* coccygeum.

**colloid b.'s,** Civatte b.'s; eosinophilic hyaline b.'s seen in or just beneath the epidermis, particularly in lichen planus.

**compressible cavernous b.'s,** submucous venous plexuses found at the level of the pharyngoesophageal junction and anal canal, which assist in reducing or obliterating the lumen.

**Councilman (hyaline) b.,** Councilman's lesion; an eosinophilic globule, seen in the liver in yellow fever, derived from necrosis of a single hepatic cell.

**Cowdry's type A inclusion b.'s,** dropletlike masses of acidophilic material surrounded by clear halos within nuclei, with margination of chromatin on the nuclear membrane, and cellular changes believed to result from infection by a virus.

**Cowdry's type B inclusion b.'s,** dropletlike masses of acidophilic material surrounded by clear halos within nuclei, without other changes indicative of virus infection.

**cytoid b.'s,** swollen retinal nerve fibers which, cut transversely, look like cells; found in cotton-wool spots.

**cytoplasmic inclusion b.'s,** see inclusion b.'s.

**Deetjen's b.'s,** blood *platelets.*

**demilune b.,** a circular b. of extreme transparency except for a crescentic punctate substance on one side which contains hemoglobin. The b. is much larger than a red blood cell, but is thought possibly to be a degenerated red blood cell swollen by imbibition; it has been found in malaria and in convalescence from typhoid fever; the transparent portion is called the glass b.

**Döhle b.'s,** Döhle's inclusions; discrete, round or oval b.'s ranging in diameter from just visible to 2 μ which stain sky blue to gray blue with Romanowsky stains, found in neutrophils of patients with infections or burns.

**Donovan b.'s,** Leishman-Donovan b.'s.

**Ehrlich's inner b.,** Heinz-Ehrlich b., a round oxyphil b. found in the red blood cell in case of hemocytolysis due to a specific blood poison.

**elementary b.'s,** (1) old term for virions, especially the largest virus particles, seen by light microscopy when stained; (2) blood *platelets.*

**end b.,** old term for complement.

**endoglobular b.,** nucleoid.

**b. of epididymis,** *corpus* epididymidis.

**epithe'lial b.,** *glandula* parathyroidea.

**fat b. of the cheek,** *corpus* adiposum buccae.

**fat b. of ischiorectal fossa,** *corpus* adiposum fossae ischiorectalis.

**fat b. of the orbit,** *corpus* adiposum orbitae.

**foreign b.,** anything in the tissues or cavities of the b. that has been introduced there from without, and that is not rapidly absorbable.

**b. of fornix,** *corpus* fornicis.

**fuchsin b.'s,** (1) Russell b.'s; (2) hyaline b.'s.

**b. of gallbladder,** *corpus* vesicae felleae.

**Gamna-Favre b.'s,** characteristic, relatively large, intracytoplasmic, basophilic inclusion b.'s observed in endothelial cells in lymphopathia venereum, probably composed of degenerated nuclear material; see also Miyagawa b.'s.

**Gamna-Gandy b.'s,** Gandy-Gamna b.'s; siderotic nodules; small, firm, spheroidal or irregular foci that are yellow-brown, brown, or rustlike in color, occurring chiefly in the spleen in such conditions as fibrocongestive splenomegaly, sickle cell disease, and some examples of hemochromatosis. The b.'s consist of relatively dense fibrous tissue or collagenous fibers impregnated with iron pigment, probably resulting from organization and scarring of sites where small perivascular hemorrhages occurred.

**Gandy-Gamna b.'s,** Gamna-Gandy b.'s.

**glass b.,** see demilune b.

**globoid b.,** a minute ultramicroscopic filtrable form observed during early work with poliomyelitis, and thought to be etiologically related to the disease.

**Guarnieri b.'s,** intracytoplasmic acidophilic inclusion b.'s observed in epithelial cells in variola (smallpox) and vaccinia infections, and which include aggregations of Paschen b.'s or virus particles.

**Halberstaedter-Prowazek b.'s,** trachoma b.'s.

**Hassall's b.'s,** Hassall's concentric *corpuscles.*

**Hassall-Henle b.'s,** Henle's warts; hyaline b.'s on the posterior surface of Descemet's membrane at the periphery of the cornea.

**Heinz b.'s,** minute b.'s sometimes seen in erythrocytes by the dark ground illumination method, after staining with azur I, regarded by Heinz as particles of dead cytoplasm, by others as composed of cholesterinolein; called also beta-substance and substantia metachromaticogranularis.

**Heinz-Ehrlich b.,** Ehrlich's inner b.

**hematoxylin b.'s,** hematoxyphil b.'s; poorly defined, homogeneous basophilic remnants of whole nuclei, an occasional finding in the fixed tissues of patients with systemic lupus erythematosus; the b.'s are so named on the basis of their affinity for hematoxylin stain; they are observed more frequently in the renal glomeruli and the walls of blood vessels, and probably are related to the L.E. phenomenon.

**hematoxyphil b.'s,** hematoxylin b.'s.

**Herring b.'s,** neurosecretory *substance.*

**Highmore's b.,** *mediastinum* testis.

**Howell-Jolly b.'s,** spherical or ovoid, eccentrically located granules, approximately 1 micron in diameter, occasionally observed in the stroma of circulating erythrocytes, especially in stained preparations (as compared with wet unstained films); probably represent nuclear remnants, inasmuch as they can be stained with dyes that are rather specific for chromatin, *e.g.,* methyl green. The significance of the b.'s is not exactly known, but they occur more frequently, and in greater numbers, after splenectomy.

**hyaline b.'s,** homogeneous eosinophilic inclusions in the cytoplasm of epithelial cells; in renal tubules hyaline b.'s represent droplets of protein reabsorbed from the lumen; see also Mallory b.'s.

**hyaline b.'s of the pituitary,** herring's b.'s; cells filled with hyaline material seen in the posterior lobe of the hypophysis, thought by some to represent an internal secretion; others believe them to be artifacts.

**hyaloid b.,** *corpus* vitreum.

**b. of hyoid bone,** *corpus* ossis hyoidei.

**b. of ilium,** *corpus* ossis ilii.

**immune b.,** an early term for antibody.

**inclusion b.'s,** distinctive structures frequently formed in the nucleus or cytoplasm (occasionally in both locations) in cells infected with certain filtrable viruses, observed especially in nerve, epithelial, or endothelial cells; may be demonstrated by means of various stains, especially Mann's eosin methylene blue or Giemsa's techniques. **Nuclear inclusion b.'s** are usually acidophilic and are of two morphologic types: (1) granular, hyaline, or amorphous, and of various sizes, *i.e.,* the Cowdry type A b.'s, occurring in such diseases as herpes simplex infection or yellow fever; (2) more circumscribed, frequently with several in the same nucleus (and no reaction in adjacent tissue), *i.e.,* the type B b.'s, occurring in such diseases as Rift Valley fever and poliomyelitis. **Cytoplasmic inclusion b.'s** may be: (1) acidophilic, relatively large, spherical or ovoid, and somewhat granular, as in variola or vaccinia, rabies, and molluscum contagiosum; basophilic, relatively large, complex combinations of viral and cellular material, as in trachoma, psittacosis, and lymphopathia venereum. In some instances, inclusion b.'s are known to be infective and probably represent aggregates of virus particles in combination with cellular material, whereas others are apparently not infective and may represent only abnormal products formed by the cell in response to the virus. Inclusion b.'s that resemble some of those known to be related to viral infections are occasionally observed in degenerative diseases and in lead poisoning.

**b. of incus,** *corpus* incudis.

**infrapatellar fat b.,** *corpus* adiposum infrapatellare.

**intercarotid b.,** *glomus* caroticum.

**intermediary b.,** Ehrlich's early noncommittal term for antibody.

**intermediate b. of Flemming,** residual interzonal spindle fibers between daughter cells following mitosis.

**interre′nal b.'s,** distinct paired or unpaired structures in all fishes, which lie in close proximity to the kidney. They are homologous to the cortical tissue of the mammalian adrenal gland.

**b. of ischium,** *corpus* ossis ischii.

**Jaworski's b.'s,** mucous shreds in the gastric contents in hyperchlorhydria.

**Joest b.'s,** intranuclear inclusion b.'s produced in certain nerve cells by the virus of Borna disease.

**Jolly b.'s,** Howell-Jolly b.'s.

**juxtaglomerular b.,** a collection of cells around the renal glomerular arterioles which contain cytoplasmic granules, probably composed of renin.

**juxtarestiform b.,** a medial subdivision of the inferior cerebellar peduncle (corpus restiforme) composed of fibers reciprocally connecting the vestibular nuclei with the cerebellum, in particular the latter's nodulus, flocculus, and nucleus fastigii. It also carries primary sensory fibers from the vestibular ganglia to the cerebellum, as well as cerebellar projections to the rhombencephalic reticular formation.

**ketone b.,** see under ketone.

**Koch's blue b.'s,** schizonts of *Theileria parva,* the causative agent of east coast fever of cattle. They are found principally within endothelial cells of the spleen and lymph nodes.

**Kurloff's b.'s,** palely basophilic, granular inclusions sometimes observed in the cytoplasm of the large mononuclear leukocytes (probably lymphocytes) of guinea pigs and certain other animals; thought by some observers to be an intracellular phase in the life cycle of the protozoan parasite *Leukocytozoon cobayae,* whereas others regard the b.'s as a stage in the development of leukocytic granules.

**Lafora b.,** an intraneuronal inclusion b. composed of acid mucopolysaccharides, seen in familial myoclonus epilepsy.

**Lallemand's b.'s,** old term for small, gelatinoid concretions sometimes observed in seminal fluid; also an old term for Bence Jones cylinders.

**Landolt's b.'s,** bipolar nerve cells lying between the retinal rods and cones in amphibia, reptiles, and birds.

**lateral geniculate b.,** *corpus* geniculatum laterale.

**LCL b.'s,** Levinthal-Cole-Lillie b.'s.

**L-D b.,** Leishman-Donovan b.

**L.E. b.,** the amorphous round b. in the cytoplasm of an L.E. cell.

**Leishman-Donovan b.,** L-D b.; the intracytoplasmic, nonflagellated (amastigote) form of the protozoan parasite, *Leishmania donovani,* the causal agent of kala azar (visceral leishmaniasis). See also amastigote.

**Levinthal-Cole-Lillie b.'s,** LCL b.'s; psittacosis inclusion b.'s named for three workers who discovered these b.'s independently and almost simultaneously.

**Lewy b.'s,** intracytoplasmic inclusion b.'s especially noted in pigmented brainstem neurons and seen in Parkinson's disease.

**Lieutaud's b.,** *trigonum* vesicae.

**Lindner b.'s,** initial b.'s resembling inclusion b.'s found in epithelial cells in scrapings in trachoma.

**loose b.,** a solid tissue fragment lying free in a body cavity, especially a joint or the peritoneal cavity; see also melon-seed b. and joint mice.

**Luys' b.,** *nucleus* subthalamicus.

**Mallory b.'s,** alcoholic hyalin; alcoholic hyaline b.'s; large, poorly defined accumulations of eosinophilic material in the cytoplasm of damaged hepatic cells in certain forms of cirrhosis and marked fatty change especially due to alcoholism.

**Malpighian b.'s,** *folliculi* lymphatici lienales.

**mamillary b.,** *corpus* mamillare.

**b. of mammary gland,** *corpus* mammae.

**b. of mandible,** *corpus* mandibulae.

**b. of maxilla,** *corpus* maxillae.

**medial geniculate b.,** *corpus* geniculatum mediale.

**melon-seed b.,** a small fibrous b. lying loose in the joints or tendon sheaths. See also loose b.

**metachromatic b.'s,** concentrated deposits, primarily of polymetaphosphate, which occur in many bacteria as well as in algae, fungi, and protozoa; these granules differ in staining properties from the surrounding protoplasm.

**Michaelis-Gutmann b.**, a rounded homogenous b., 1 to 10 $\mu$ in diameter, containing calcium and iron; found within macrophages in the bladder wall in malakoplakia.

**Miyagawa b.'s**, *Chlamydia trachomatis* (*Miyagawanella lymphogranulomatosis*); the elementary b.'s which develop in the intracytoplasmic microcolonies of lymphogranuloma venereum.

**molluscum b.**, the central caseous mass contained in the lesions of molluscum contagiosum. It consists of degenerated cells and the inclusion b.'s (virus).

**Mooser b.'s**, a term used to refer to the rickettsiae found in the exudate (and in tissue) from the tunica vaginalis in endemic typhus fever (caused by *Rickettsia typhi*); first described by Mooser during experimental studies of Mexican typhus fever.

**multilamellar b.**, cytosome (2).

**multivesicular b.'s**, membrane-bound b.'s 0.2 to 0.3 $\mu$ wide containing a number of small vesicles; hydrolases (especially acid phosphatase) occur in the matrix.

**myelin b.**, myelin *figure*.

**b. of nail**, *corpus* unguis.

**Negri b.'s**, Negri corpuscles; inclusion b.'s found in the cytoplasm of certain nerve cells containing the virus of rabies, especially in Ammon's horn of the hippocampus.

**nerve cell b.**, the part of the neuron that includes the nucleus but excludes the processes.

**Nissl b.'s**, chromophil *substance*.

**nuclear inclusion b.'s**, see inclusion b.'s.

**olivary b.**, oliva.

**onion b.'s**, epithelial *nests*.

**Pacchionian b.'s**, *granulationes* arachnoideales.

**pampin'iform b.**, epoophoron.

**b. of pancreas**, *corpus* pancreatis.

**paraaortic b.'s**, *corpora* paraaortica.

**parabasal b.**, a term formerly equivalent to the DNA kinetoplast, part of the giant mitochondrion of certain parasitic flagellates (see also kinetoplast). The parabasal b. plus the blepharoplast were previously thought to comprise a kinetoplast, or locomotory apparatus, but kinetoplast is now restricted to part of the DNA giant mitochondrion, blepharoplast is the flagellar basal body, and parabasal b. is a distinct structure near the nucleus, probably equivalent to the metazoan Golgi apparatus.

**paraneph'ric b.**, a mass of fat lying behind the renal fascia.

**paranu'clear b.**, attraction *sphere*.

**parater'minal b.**, *gyrus* subcallosus.

**Paschen b.'s**, particles of virus observed in relatively large numbers in squamous cells of the skin (or the cornea of experimental animals) in variola (smallpox) or vaccinia.

**b. of penis**, *corpus* penis.

**perin'eal b.**, *centrum* tendineum perinei.

**b. of phalanx**, *corpus* phalangis.

**Pick's b.'s**, intracytoplasmic argentophilic inclusion b.'s seen in neurons in Pick's disease.

**pineal b.**, *corpus* pineale.

**Plimmer's b.'s**, small, rounded or ovoid, hyaline, possibly encapsulated b.'s sometimes observed in the cytoplasm of malignant neoplastic cells, and formerly thought by Plimmer to be causal parasite; see also cancer b.'s.

**polar b.**, one of the two small cells formed by the ovum during its maturation. The first polar b. is usually released just prior to ovulation, and the second not until after the ovum has been discharged from the ovary. In mammals the second polar b. may fail to form unless the ovum has been penetrated by a sperm cell. See fig. under oocyte.

**Prowazek b.'s**, historic term for either of two types of inclusion b.'s associated with diseases caused by filtrable viruses: (1) trachoma b.'s, also termed Halberstaedter-Prowazek b.'s; (2) tiny, ovoid, granular forms, frequently in pairs, observed in the cytoplasm and in Guarnieri b.'s in the cutaneous squamous cells of man and animals infected with variola (smallpox) or vaccinia virus; probably the same as Paschen b.'s.

**Prowazek-Greeff b.'s**, trachoma b.'s.

**psammoma b.'s**, (1) acervulus; brain sand; corpora arenacea; sabulum; sand b.'s; mineralized b.'s occurring in the meninges, choroid plexus, and in certain meningiomas, composed usually of a central capillary surrounded by concentric whorls of meningocytes in various stages of hyaline change and mineralization; (2) calcospherite.

**psittacosis inclusion b.'s**, intracytoplasmic microcolonies of *Chlamydia* observed in the bronchial epithelial cells infected with *C. psittaci*.

**pubic b.**, *corpus* ossis pubis.

**purine b.'s**, any purine.

**quadrigeminal b.'s**, *corpora* quadrigemina.

**residual b.**, a cytoplasmic vacuole containing accumulated particulate products of metabolism, *e.g.*, lipofuscin.

**rest b.**, a small mass of cytoplasm remaining after the nucleus and cytoplasm of the schizont of certain sporozoan protozoa have divided into asexual spores or merozoites.

**res'tiform b.**, *pedunculus* cerebellaris inferior.

**b. of rib**, *corpus* costae.

**rice b.**, one of the ricelike b.'s found in hygromas, tendon sheaths, and joints.

**Russell b.'s**, small, discrete, variably sized, spherical, intracytoplasmic, acidophilic, hyaline b.'s that stain deeply with fuchsin; first observed in neoplastic cells and formerly thought (by some workers) to be the causal agent of carcinoma, presumably a blastomycete, but now known to be secretory or degenerative products of the cell. They occur frequently in plasma cells in chronic inflammation, where they are believed to consist of $\gamma$-globulin.

**sand b.'s**, psammoma b.'s (1).

**Sandström's b.'s**, *glandula* parathyroidea.

**Savage's perineal b.**, *centrum* tendineum perinei.

**Schaumann b.'s**, conchoidal calcified b.'s found in granulomas, particularly in sarcoidosis.

**seg'menting b.**, schizont.

**b. of sphenoid bone**, *corpus* ossis sphenoidalis.

**spongy b. of penis**, *corpus* spongiosum penis.

**b. of sternum**, *corpus* sterni.

**b. of stomach**, *corpus* ventriculi.

**striate b.**, *corpus* striatum.

**suprarenal b.**, *glandula* suprarenalis.

**b. of sweat gland**, *corpus* glandulae sudoriferae.

**Symington's anococcyg'eal b.**, *ligamentum* anococcygeum.

**b. of talus**, *corpus* tali.

**threshold b.**, threshold substance; any material in the blood plasma that is excreted in the urine only when the level exceeds a certain physiologic value, *e.g.*, glucose.

**thyroid b.**, *glandula* thyroidea.

**b. of tibia**, *corpus* tibiae.

**tigroid b.'s**, chromophil *substance*.

**b. of tongue**, *corpus* linguae.

**trachoma b.'s.**, Prowazek-Greeff b.'s; Halberstaedter-Prowazek b.'s; Prowazek b.'s (1); distinctive, complex, intracytoplasmic forms found in the conjunctival epithelial cells of persons in the acute phase of trachoma, and less frequently in later stages; vary from (1) discrete acidophilic granules (approximately 250 millimicrons in diameter), to (2) irregular clumps of such material embedded in a basophilic matrix, to (3) relatively large basophilic b.'s (approximately 700 to 1000 millimicrons in diameter), to (4) large basophilic b.'s that include discrete, tiny, acidophilic granules (as described above).

**trapezoid b.**, *corpus* trapezoideum.

**Trousseau-Lallemand b.'s**, Lallemand's b.'s.

**turbinated b.**, (1) turbinal; the turbinated bone or concha with its covering of mucous membrane and other soft parts; (2) *concha* nasalis (inferior, media, superior, and suprema).

**tympanic b.**, tympanic *gland*.

**b. of ulna**, *corpus* ulnae.

**ul'timobranch'ial b.**, a diverticulum from the 4th pharyngeal pouch of an embryo; by some regarded as a rudimentary 5th pharyngeal pouch; by others as a lateral thyroid primordium. The ultimobranchial b.'s of lower vertebrates contain large amounts of calcitonin. In mammals the b.'s fuse with the thyroid gland and are thought to develop into the parafollicular cells.

**b. of urinary bladder**, *corpus* vesicae urinariae.

**b. of uterus**, *corpus* uteri.

**vaccine b.'s**, old term pertaining to intracellular b.'s that were erroneously thought to be forms in the life cycle of a protozoan organism, *Cytorrhyctes vaccinae*, postulated to be the causal agent of vaccinia.

**Verocay b.'s,** "clear" spaces outlined by opposing rows of parallel nuclei seen microscopically in neurilemomas.

**b. of vertebra,** *corpus* vertebrae.

**Virchow-Hassall b.'s,** Hassall's concentric *corpuscles.*

**vitreous b.,** *corpus* vitreum.

**Wolf-Orton b.'s,** intranuclear inclusion b.'s of nonviral origin that are noted in cells of malignant neoplasms, especially those of glial cell origin.

**Wolffian b.,** mesonephros.

**x-b.'s,** (1) certain granules and flecks noted in specimens of blood in malaria and other febrile conditions, and in specimens of apparently normal ox blood and rabbit blood; their nature and significance are not known, and it has been claimed that they are artifacts occurring in old slides, especially after long use in the tropics; (2) Plimmer's b.'s.

**yellow b.,** *corpus* luteum.

**Zuckerkandl's b.'s,** *corpora* paraaortica.

---

**Boeck** (bĕkh), Caesar P. M., Norwegian dermatologist, 1845–1917. See B.'s *disease, sarcoid,* Besnier-B.-Schaumann *disease, syndrome.*

**Boeck,** Carl Wilhelm, Norwegian physician, 1808–1875, noted for his work in leprosy. See Danielssen-B. *disease.*

**Boedeker** (bĕ'da-ker), Carl H. D., German chemist, 1815–1895. See B.'s *test.*

**Boehmer's hematoxylin.** See under hematoxylin.

**Boerhaave** (boor'hah-veh), Hermann, Dutch physician, 1668–1738. See B.'s *glands.*

**Bogaert,** Ludo van. See van Bogaert, Ludo.

**bog'bean.** Buckbean.

**Bogorad,** F. A., 20th century. See B.'s *syndrome.*

**Bogros** (bog-ro'), Annet J., French anatomist, 1786–1823. See B.'.s *space.*

**Bogros** (bog-ro'), Antoine, French anatomist, 1786–1823. See B.'s serous *membrane.*

**bohe'mium.** Rhenium.

**Bohn's nodule.** See Epstein's *pearls.*

**Bohr,** Christian, Scandinavian physiologist, 1855–1911. See B. *effect.*

**Bohr,** Neils H. D., Danish physicist, 1885–1962. See B.'s *atom, magneton, theory.*

**boil** [ A.S. *byl,* a swelling ]. Furuncle.

**Aleppo b.** [ *Aleppo,* a vilayet and its capital in Asiatic Turkey ], see cutaneous *leishmaniasis.*

**Bagdad b.,** see cutaneous *leishmaniasis.*

**blind b.,** a furuncle that does not have a fluctuant central point; appears as a dull red painful papule.

**date b.,** see cutaneous *leishmaniasis.*

**Delhi b.,** see cutaneous *leishmaniasis.*

**Jericho b.,** see cutaneous *leishmaniasis.*

**Madura b.,** maduromycosis.

**oriental b.,** tropical b.; oriental or tropical sore or ulcer; the tropical sore of Old World cutaneous *leishmaniasis* ( *q. v.* ).

**salt water b.'s,** furuncles on hands and forearms of fishermen.

**shoe b.,** olecranoid bursitis in the horse; so called because it may be caused by trauma from the shoe in the recumbent animal.

**tropical b.,** oriental b.; see cutaneous *leishmaniasis.*

**bolandi'ol dipropionate** (USAN). Norpropandrolate; ANABIOL; 3β,17β-dipropionyloxy-4-estrene; anabolic agent.

**bolas'terone** (USAN). MYAGEN; 7α,17-dimethyltestosterone; anabolic agent.

**boldenone undecylenate** (USAN). PARENABOL; 17β-hydroxyandrosta-1,4-dien-3-one; an anabolic steroid.

**bol'din.** Boldoglucin; a glycoside from boldus. Cholagogue and diuretic.

**bol'dine.** A bitter alkaloid obtained from boldus.

**bol'do.** Boldus.

**bol'dus** [ Chilean ]. Boldo; the leaves of *Boldu boldus* or *Peumus boldus* (family Monimiaceae), an evergreen shrub of Chile; used in various disturbances of liver function.

**bole** (bōl) [ G. *bōlos,* a lump of clay ]. An argillaceous earth or clay; chiefly a hydrated aluminum silicate with ferric

hydrate. Used as a pigment and as adsorbent and protective in gastrointestinal inflammation.

**white b.,** kaolin.

**bo'lenol** (USAN). 19-Nor-17α-pregn-5-en-17-ol; an anabolic steroid.

**Boley gauge.** See under gauge.

**Boll,** Franz C., German histologist and physiologist, 1849–1879. See B.'s *cells.*

**Bollinger,** Otto, German pathologist, 1843–1909. See B. *bodies, granules.*

**Bollman,** Jesse L., American physiologist, *1896. See Mann-B. *fistula.*

**Bolognini's symptom.** See under symptom.

**bolom'eter** [ G. *bolē,* a throw, a sunbeam, + *metron,* measure ]. 1. An instrument for measuring the force of the heart beat as distinguished from the blood pressure. 2. An instrument for determining minute degrees of radiant heat.

**boloscope** [ G. *bolē,* a throw, a sunbeam, + *skopeō,* to veiw ]. An instrument for the location of metal foreign bodies in the body by which two pencils of x-rays are focused to intersect at the foreign object. Visible rays from two lamps are coupled with the x-rays and converge in the same way upon the object; the surgeon is thus able to cut down upon it in natural light.

**Bolton plane, Bolton point.** See the nouns.

**bo'lus** [ L. fr. G. *bōlos,* lump, clod ]. 1. A very large pill, usually of soft consistency, made extemporaneously and to be taken at once. 2. A masticated morsel of food ready to be swallowed. 3. Bole.

**bombard'.** To expose a substance to particulate or electromagnetic radiations for the purpose of making it radioactive.

**bond.** In chemistry, the force holding two neighboring atoms in place and resisting their separation; a bond is electrovalent if it consists of the attraction between oppositely charged groups, or covalent if it results from the sharing of one, two, or three pairs of electrons by the bonded atoms; see also hydrogen b. and hydrophobic b.

**acylmercaptan b.,** —CO—S—; a "high energy" b. formed by the condensation of a carboxyl group (—COOH) and a mercaptan (or thiol) group (—SH); widely formed in the course of intermediary metabolism, notably in the oxidation of fats, where the —SH is part of coenzyme A and the —COOH is part of the fatty acid being oxidized.

**conjugated double b.'s,** two double b.'s separated by one single b.

**disulfide b.,** the —S—S— link binding two peptide chains (or different parts of one peptide chain). It occurs as part of the molecule of the amino acid, cystine, and is important as a structural determinant in many protein molecules, notably keratin, insulin, and oxytocin.

**double b.,** a covalent b. resulting from the sharing of two pairs of electrons; commonly represented as, *e.g.,* $CH_2=CH_2$ (ethylene).

**high energy phosphate b.,** see high energy *phosphate.*

**hydrogen b.,** a b. arising from the sharing of a hydrogen atom, covalently bound to N or O, with another N or O. In substances of biological importance the most common hydrogen b.'s are those in which H links N to O or N. Such

**Hydrogen bonding between purines and pyrimidines**

In these structures, hydrogen bonds are indicated by dotted lines; *R* = deoxyribose in chains.

b.'s link purines on one strand to pyrimidines in the other strand of nucleic acids, thus maintaining double-stranded structures. See also Watson-Crick *helix.*

**peptide b.,**  the common link (—CO—NH—) between amino acids in proteins, actually a form of amide linkage.

**semipolar b.,**  coordinate b.; one in which the two electrons shared by a pair of atoms belonged originally to only one of the atoms; often represented by a small arrow pointing toward the electron receiver as in nitric acid, O(OH)N→O, or phosphoric acid. (OH)$_3$P→O.

**single b.,**  a covalent b. resulting from the sharing of one pair of electrons; *e.g.,* CH$_3$—CH$_3$ (ethane).

**triple b.,**  a covalent b. resulting from the sharing of three pairs of electrons; *e.g.,* CH≡CH (acetylene).

# BONE

**bone**  [ A.S. *bān* ]. 1. A hard tissue consisting of cells in a matrix of ground substance and collagen fibers. The fibers are impregnated with mineral substance, chiefly calcium phosphate and carbonate; this inorganic matter comprises about 67 per cent by weight of adult bone. 2. For definitions of bones as part of the animal skeleton, see os, and color plates 17 and 18.

**aitch b.,**  H b.; term used by butchers for the cut edge of the ossa coxarum on the ventral midline, when the hindquarters are divided.

**Albrecht's b.,**  a small b. between the basioccipital and basisphenoid.

**alveolar b.,**  (1) *processus* alveolaris; (2) in dentistry, denotes the specialized b. structure which supports the teeth, and is also called alveolar supporting bone.

**alve'olar supporting b.,**  *processus* alveolaris; see also alveolar b. (2).

**ankle b.,**  talus.

**basal b.,**  the osseous tissue of the mandible and maxillae except the alveolar processes.

**bas'ilar b.,**  os basilare; basioccipital b.; the basilar process of the occipital b. which unites with the condylic portions in about the fourth or fifth year.

**basioccip'ital b.,**  basilar b.

**Bertin's b.'s,**  *conchae* sphenoidales.

**blade b.,**  scapula.

**breast b.,**  sternum.

**Breschet's b.'s,**  *os* suprasternale.

**brittle b.'s,**  *osteogenesis* imperfecta.

**bundle b.,**  the part of alveolar b. containing perforating fibers of Sharpey.

**calca'neal b.,**  calcaneus.

**calf b.,**  fibula.

**cancellous b.,**  *substantia* spongiosa.

**cannon b., canon-b.,**  shank b. (1).

**capitate b.,**  *os* capitatum.

**carpal b.'s,**  ossa carpi; see carpus.

**cartilage b.,**  endochondral b.

**cavalry b.,**  rider's b.

**central b.,**  *os* centrale.

**central b. (of ankle),**  *os* naviculare.

**b.'s of cerebral cranium,**  *ossa* cranii.

**cheek b.,**  *os* zygomaticum.

**coccygeal b.,**  *os* coccygis.

**coffin b.,**  *os* ungulare.

**collar b.,**  clavicula.

**compact b.,**  *substantia* compacta.

**convoluted b.,**  see entries under *concha* nasalis.

**cortical b.,**  *substantia* corticalis.

**coxal b.,**  *os* coxae.

**cranial b.'s,**  *ossa* cranii.

**cubital b.,**  *os* triquetrum.

**cuboid b.,**  *os* cuboideum.

**cuneiform b.,**  *os* triquetrum.

**dermal b.,**  a b. formed by ossification of the cutis.

**b.'s of digits of foot,**  *ossa* digitorum pedis.

**b.'s of digits of hand,**  *ossa* digitorum manus.

**dorsal talonavicular b.,**  Pirie's b.

**ear b.,**  *ossiculum* auditus.

**elbow b.,**  ulna.

**endochondral b.,**  replacement b.; cartilage b.; a b. that develops in a cartilage after the latter is partially or entirely destroyed; b. preformed in cartilage.

**epac'tal b.'s,**  *ossa* suturarum.

**epihyal b.,**  an ossified stylomastoid ligament.

**epipter'ic b.,**  Flower's b.; a Wormian b. occasionally present at the pterion or junction of the parietal, frontal, great wing of the sphenoid, and squamous portion of the temporal b.'s.

**episternal b.,**  *os* suprasternale.

**ethmoid b.,**  *os* ethmoidale.

**exercise b.,**  rider's b.

**exoccipital b.** (eks-ok-sip'ĭ-tal), *pars* lateralis ossis occipitalis.

**facial b.'s,**  *ossa* faciei.

**first cuneiform b.,**  *os* cuneiforme mediale.

**flank b.,**  *os* ilium.

**flat b.,**  *os* planum.

**Flower's b.,**  a sutural b. at the pterion; epipteric b.

**frontal b.,**  *os* frontale.

**Goethe's b.,**  (1) large sutural b. at the lambda; (2) *os* incisivum.

**greater multangular b.,**  *os* trapezium.

**H b.,**  aitch b.

**hamate b.,**  *os* hamatum.

**haunch b.,**  huckle b. (1).

**heel b.,**  calcaneus.

**heterotopic b.'s,**  b.'s that do not belong to the main skeleton but that regularly develop in certain organs: heart, penis, clitoris, and snout of some animals.

**hip b.,**  *os* coxae.

**hollow b.,**  *os* pneumaticum.

**hooked b.,**  *os* hamatum.

**huckle b.,**  (1) haunch b.; the os coxae in the pelvis of the horse; (2) the astragalus in the tarsus of the horse.

**hyoid b.,**  (1) *os* hyoideum; (2) see *apparatus* hyoideus.

**iliac b.,**  *os* ilium.

**inca'rial b.,**  *os* interparietale.

**incisive b.,**  *os* incisivum.

**b.'s of the inferior limb,**  *ossa* membri inferioris.

**innom'inate b.,**  *os* coxae.

**intermaxillary b.,**  *os* incisivum.

**intermediate cuneiform b.,**  *os* cuneiforme intermedium.

**interparietal b.,**  *os* interparietale.

**ischial b.,**  *os* ischii.

**jaw b.,**  mandibula.

**jugal b.,**  *os* zygomaticum.

**Krause's b.,**  small b. (secondary ossification center) between the ilium and the pubic b. in the growing acetabulum.

**lacrimal b.,**  *os* lacrimale.

**lamellar b.,**  b. in which the tubular lamellae are formed that are characterized by having collagen fibers arranged in a parallel, spiral manner.

**lateral cuneiform b.,**  *os* cuneiforme laterale.

**lentic'ular b.,**  *processus* lenticularis incudis.

**len'tiform b.,**  *os* pisiforme.

**lesser multangular b.,**  *os* trapezoideum.

**lin'gual b.,**  *os* hyoideum.

**long b.,**  *os* longum.

**lunate b.,**  *os* lunatum.

**malar b.,**  *os* zygomaticum.

**marble b.'s,**  osteopetrosis.

**b. marrow,**  *medulla* ossium.

**mastoid b.,**  *processus* mastoideus.

**medial cuneiform b. of foot,**  *os* cuneiforme mediale.

**medullary b.,**  areas of b. formation present in the marrow spaces of the long b.'s of birds, which serve as a readily mobilized source of calcium for shell formation.

**membrane b.,**  a b. developed within a connective tissue membrane, as contrasted with endochondral b.

**middle cuneiform b.,**  *os* cuneiforme intermedium.

**multangular b.,**  see *os* trapezium; *os* trapezoideum.

**nasal b.,**  *os* nasale.

**navicular b.,**  *os* naviculare.

**navicular b. of hand,**  *os* scaphoideum.

**nonlamellar b.,**  woven b.

**occipital b.,**  *os* occipitale.

**orbic'ular b.,**  *processus* lenticularis incudis.

**palatine b.,**  *os* palatinum.

**parietal b.,** *os* parietale.

**pastern b.,** one of three b.'s in the foot of the horse; see *os* coronale, *os* compedale, *os* ungulare.

**pedal b.,** *os* ungulare.

**penis b.,** *os* penis.

**perichondral b.,** periosteal b.; in the development of a long b. a collar or cuff of osseous tissue forms in the perichondrium of the cartilage model; the connective tissue membrane of this perichondral b. then becomes periosteum.

**periosteal b.,** perichondral b.

**periotic b.,** the petrous and mastoid portions of the temporal b.

**petrosal b.,** the petrous portion of the temporal b. In antenatal life it appears as a separate ossification center.

**petrous b.,** *pars* petrosa ossis temporalis.

**pin b.,** butchers' and livestock judges' term for the tuber ischii.

**ping-pong b.,** the thin shell of osseous tissue at the periphery of a giant cell tumor in a b.

**pipe b.,** *os* longum.

**Pirie's b.,** the dorsal talonavicular b.; an anomalous b. of the foot located near the head of the talus.

**pisiform b.,** *os* pisiforme.

**pneumatic b.,** *os* pneumaticum.

**postsphe′noid b.,** the posterior portion of the body of the sphenoid b.

**preinterpari′etal b.,** a large sutural b. occasionally found detached from the anterior portion of the interparietal b.

**premax′illary b.,** *os* incisivum.

**presphe′noid b.,** the anterior portion of the body of the sphenoid b.

**pubic b.,** *os* pubis.

**pyramidal b.,** *os* triquetrum.

**replacement b.,** endochondral b.

**reticulated b.,** woven b.

**rider's b.,** cavalry b.; exercise b.; ossification of the tendon of the adductor longus from strain in horseback riding.

**ring-b.,** see ringbone.

**Riolan's b.'s,** several small sutural b.'s sometimes present in the petrooccipital suture.

**sacred b.,** *os* sacrum.

**scaphoid b.,** *os* scaphoideum.

**scroll b.,** *concha* nasalis.

**second cuneiform b. of tarsus,** *os* cuneiforme intermedium.

**semilunar b.,** *os* lunatum.

**septal b.,** alveolar bone between tooth roots.

**sesamoid b.,** *os* sesamoideum.

**sesamoid b.'s of the fingers,** *ossa* digitorum manus.

**sesamoid b.'s of the toes,** *ossa* digitorum pedis.

**shank b.,** (1) cannon b.; the middle metacarpal (or metatarsal) b. in the horse; (2) the tibia.

**shin b.,** tibia.

**short b.,** *os* breve.

**sieve b.,** the cribrose plate of the ethmoid bone.

**sphenoid b.,** *os* sphenoidale.

**sphenoid′al turbinated b.'s,** *conchae* sphenoidales.

**splint b.,** (1) the second or fourth, or internal or external small metacarpal b.'s in the horse; these are splinter-like in shape, and lie on either side of the metacarpal, or cannon b.; (2) fibula.

**spongy b.,** (1) *substantia* spongiosa; (2) one of the turbinated b.'s.

**stifle b.,** the patella of the stifle joint of a horse.

**b.'s of the superior limb,** *ossa* membri superioris.

**su′prainterpari′etal b.,** a sutural b. at the posterior portion of the sagittal suture.

**suprasternal b.,** *os* suprasternale.

**su′tural b.'s,** *ossa* suturarum.

**tail b.,** *os* coccygis.

**tarsal b.'s,** see tarsus.

**temporal b.,** *os* temporale.

**thigh b.,** femur.

**third cuneiform b.,** *os* cuneiforme laterale.

**three-cornered b.,** *os* triquetrum.

**tongue b.,** *os* hyoideum.

**trabecular b.,** *substantia* spongiosa.

**trapezium b.,** *os* trapezium.

**trapezoid b.,** *os* trapezoideum.

**triangular b.,** *os* trigonum.

**triquetral b.,** *os* triquetrum.

**turbinated b.'s,** see entries under *concha* nasalis.

**tympanic b.,** *anulus* tympanicus.

**tympanohy′al b.,** a small nodule of b. forming the base of the cartilaginous styloid process of the petrosal b. at birth.

**unciform b.,** *os* hamatum.

**Vesalius' b.'s,** *os* vesaleanum.

**b.'s of the visceral cranium,** *ossa* faciei.

**wedge b.,** *os* cuneiforme mediale.

**wedge b. of foot,** *os* cuneiforme laterale.

**Wormian b.'s,** *ossa* suturarum.

**woven b.,** reticulated b.; nonlamellar b.; bony tissue characteristic of the embryonal skeleton in which the collagen fibers of the matrix are arranged irregularly in the form of interlacing networks.

**yoke b.,** *os* zygomaticum.

**zygomatic b.,** *os* zygomaticum.

---

**bone black.** Animal *charcoal.*

**bonelet** (bōn′let). Ossicle.

**bone-salt.** The main chemical compound in bone, deposited as minute crystals in a netlike matrix of collagenous fibers containing the protein collagen (ossein). It closely resembles the naturally occurring fluorapatite $3Ca_3(PO_4)_2$.$CaF_2$, but is probably a hydroxyapatite in which F is replaced by OH.

**Bonhoeffer,** Karl, Berlin psychiatrist, 1868–1948. See B.'s *sign.*

**Bonner's position.** See under position.

**Bonnet** (bon-na′), Amédée, French surgeon, 1809–1858. See B.'s *capsule, operation.*

**Bonnevie,** Kristine, German physician, 1872–1950. See B.-Ullrich *syndrome.*

**Bonnier** (bon-e-a′), Pierre, French clinician, 1861–1918. See B.'s *syndrome.*

**Bonwill,** W. G. A., American dentist, 1833–1899. See B. *triangle.*

**boo′hoo.** Name formerly given to a fever with malaise, indigestion, and pain in various parts of the body, from which newcomers to the Hawaiian Islands sometimes suffered.

**Böök,** Jan Avid. See B. *syndrome.*

**Boophilus** (bo-of′ĭ-lus) [ G. *bous,* ox, + *philos,* fond ]. A genus of hard ticks (family Ixodidae) infesting cattle; members are important vectors of bovine babesiosis and anaplasmosis in various parts of the world. Previously considered to be synonymous with *Margaropus,* but now considered distinct, *B.* is distinguished by presence of eyes, palpi and hypostome characteristics, and lack of festoons.

**B. annula′tus,** the cattle tick; formerly the vector of bovine babesiosis in the southern United States; it was eliminated after a long tick-eradication program but is still an important tick in Mexico and certain other countries; it is a one-host tick, which makes control easier than with the two- and three-host ticks.

**B. decolora′tus,** a vector of bovine babesiosis and anaplasmosis in certain parts of Africa.

**B. microplus,** the tropical cattle tick; an important vector of bovine babesiosis and anaplasmosis in Mexico, Central and South America, Africa, Australia, and oriental countries; it was eliminated from the United States along with *B. annulatus* after a tick-eradication program.

**boos′ter.** See under dose.

**boot.** A boot-shaped appliance.

**Junod's b.,** an airtight case into which the arm or leg is inserted and the air is then exhausted; used to divert a portion of the blood temporarily from the general circulation.

**bo′rate.** A salt of boric acid.

**bo′rated.** Mixed or impregnated with borax or boric acid.

**bo′rax** (BP). Sodium borate.

**borboryg′mus,** pl. **borboryg′mi** (bor′bo-rig′mus) [ G. *borborygmos,* rumbling in the bowels ]. Rumbling or gurgling noises, produced by movement of gas in the alimentary canal, audible at a distance.

**Bordeau,** or **Bordeu,** Théophile de. See *de Bordeau.*

**bor'der.** 1. Edge; margin. 2. See margo.

**alveolar b.,** (1) the most occlusal edge of the alveolar bone; (2) alveolar ridge.

**anterior b.,** *margo* anterior.

**brush b.,** limbus penicillatus; the epithelial surface consisting of microvilli about 2 $\mu$ long, such as occur on the cells of the proximal tubule of the nephron.

**denture b.,** denture edge; periphery; (1) the limit or boundary or circumferential margin of a denture base; (2) the margin of the denture base at the junction of the polished surface with the impression (tissue) surface; (3) the extreme edges of a denture base at the buccolabial, lingual, and posterior limits; (4) the extreme margins of a denture base.

**inferior b.,** *margo* inferior.

**posterior b. of petrous part of temporal bone,** *margo* posterior partis petrosae ossis temporalis.

**radial b.,** *margo* lateralis (2).

**sagittal b.,** *margo* sagittalis.

**sphenoidal b.,** *margo* sphenoidalis.

**striated b.,** limbus striatus; the free surface of the columnar absorptive cells of the intestine formed by microvilli about 1 $\mu$ long, giving the appearance of parallel striations with the light microscope.

**superior b. of petrous part of temporal bone,** *margo* superior partis petrosae ossis temporalis.

**tibial b.,** *margo* medialis (3).

**vermilion b.,** vermilion zone; vermilion transitional zone; the red margin of the upper and lower lip that commences at the exterior edge of the intraoral labial mucosa ("moist line") and extends outward, terminating at the extraoral labial cutaneous junction; a thinly keratinized intergrade type of stratified squamous epithelium with a well developed stratum lucidum.

**Bordet** (bor-da'), Jules, Belgian bacteriologist, 1870–1961. Nobel laureate, 1919, for his discoveries relating to immunity. Gave his name to *Bordetella*. See B. and Gengou's potato blood *agar,* B.-Gengou *bacillus,* B.'s *phenomenon,* B.-Gengou *phenomenon,* B.'s *test* (for precipitin), B.'s serologic *test.*

**Bordetella** [J. *Bordet*]. A genus of strictly aerobic bacteria (family Brucellaceae) containing minute, Gram-negative coccobacilli. Motile and nonmotile species occur; motile cells are peritrichous. The metabolism of these organisms is respiratory. These organisms require nicotinic acid, cysteine, and methionine. Hemin (X factor) and coenzyme I (V factor) are not required. They are parasites and pathogens of the mammary respiratory tract. The type species is *B. pertussis.*

**B. bronchiseptica,** a species which frequently is the cause of bronchopneumonia in rodents and of bronchopneumonia complicating distemper in dogs.

**B. parapertus'sis,** a species that causes a whooping cough-like disease.

**B. pertussis,** *Haemophilus pertussis;* a species which causes whooping cough. It is the type species of the genus *B.*

**Borel'li,** Giovanni A., Italian mathematician and physicist, 1608–1679. Professor of mathematics at Messina and later at Pisa. Applied mechanical principles to explain physiologic processes, especially of the muscular, digestive, and circulatory systems. His ideas and experiments were recorded in a work entitled *De Motu Animalium* (1680).

**bo'ric acid** (BP). Boracic acid; $H_3BO_3$; a very weak acid, used as an antiseptic dusting powder, in saturated solution as a collyrium, and with glycerin in aphthae and stomatitis.

**bo'rism.** Symptoms caused by the ingestion of borax or any compound of boron.

**Börjeson,** Mats, Swedish physician. See B.-Forssman-Lehmann *syndrome.*

**Born,** Gustav Jacob, German embryologist, 1851–1900. See B. *method* (of wax plate reconstruction).

**bornane** (bor'nān). Camphane; 1,7,7-trimethylnorbornane; parent of borneols, camphene, and similar essential oils (terpenes).

**bor'neol.** Borneo camphor; bornyl alcohol; camphyl alcohol; 2-camphanol; 2-hydroxycamphane; occurs in deposits in the wood of *Dryobalanops aromatica* (family Dipterocarpaceae), a tree of Borneo and Sumatra; used in the manufacture of perfume and incense.

**Bornane**

**bor'nyl alcohol.** Borneol.

**boroglycerin** (bo-ro-glis'er-in). Glyceryl borate; boroglycerol; a soft mass obtained by heating glycerin and boric acid; antiseptic, usually used mixed with equal parts of glycerin, constituting glycerite.

**boroglycerol** (bo-ro-glis'er-ol). Boroglycerin.

**bo'ron.** A nonmetallic trivalent element, symbol B, atomic weight 10.82, atomic no. 5. Occurs as a hard crystalline mass or as a brown powder.

**bo'rosalicyl'ic acid.** A mixture of 1 part boric acid and 2 parts salicylic acid; used in antiseptic washes and ointments, chiefly in veterinary medicine.

**Borrel,** Amédée, French bacteriologist, 1867–1936. See B. *bodies,* B. blue *stain.*

**Borrelia** (bor-re'li-ah, bor-rel'i-ah) [A. *Borrell*]. A genus of bacteria (family Treponemataceae) containing cells 8 to 16 micrometers in length, with coarse, shallow, irregular spirals. The cells generally taper at the ends into fine filaments. These organisms are parasitic on many forms of animal life. They are generally hematophytic or are found on mucous membranes. Some borreliae are transmitted by the bites of arthropods. The type species is *B. anserina.*

**B. anseri'na,** a species which causes a spirochaetosis of fowls; found in the blood of infected geese, ducks, other fowls, and vector ticks. It is the type species of the genus *B.*

**B. babylonen'sis,** a species isolated from a tick (*Ornithodoros tholozani* var. *babylonensis*) from a rodent burrow in the ruins of Kish near Babylon.

**B. ber'bera,** a species causing relapsing fever in the Arab countries of Northern Africa; probably transmitted by lice.

**B. brasilien'sis,** a species isolated from a tick (*Ornithodoros brasiliensis*) from Rio Grande do Sul, Brazil.

**B. buccalis,** a species found in normal mouths; it invades lesions formed on the respiratory mucous membrane.

**B. car'teri,** a species causing relapsing fever in India and probably other southern Asian countries; it is transmitted by a bedbug, *Cimex rotundatus.*

**B. cauca'sica,** a species found as a cause of relapsing fever in the Caucasus; transmitted by *Ornithodoros verrucosus.*

**B. crocidu'rae,** a species isolated from the shrew-mouse (*Crocidura stampflii*) in Senegal.

**B. dipodil'la,** a species isolated from the pigmy gerbille (*Dipodillus* sp.) from Crescent Island on the east shore of Lake Naivasha, Kenya.

**B. duge'sii,** a species isolated from a tick (*Ornithodoros dugesi*) in Mexico.

**B. dut'tonii,** a species causing Central and South African relapsing fever, transmitted by a tick, *Ornithodoros moubata.*

**B. glossi'nae,** a species found in the stomach contents of the tsetse fly, *Glossina palpalis.*

**B. grain'geri,** a species isolated from a tick (*Ornithodoros graingeri*) from caves near Tiwi, south of Mombasa, Kenya.

**B. har'veyi,** a species found in the blood of a grivet monkey (*Cercopithecus aethiops centralis*) captured in the forest of Southern Mau, Kenya Colony.

**B. herm'sii,** a species found as a cause of relapsing fever in British Columbia, Canada, California, Colorado, Idaho, Nevada, Oregon, and Washington; transmitted by a tick, *Ornithodoros hermsi.*

**B. hispan'ica,** a species causing relapsing fever in Spain, Portugal, and northwest Africa.

**B. hyos,** a species found in the blood and in intestinal ulcers and other lesions of hogs suffering from hog cholera.

**B. koch'ii** a species causing African relapsing fever and transmitted by *Ornithodoros savigni*.

**B. latysche'wii,** a species isolated from the gerbilles *Rhombombys opimus* and *Gerbillus eversmanni* in Fergana, Usbekistan; also found in Iran.

**B. novyi,** a species found as a cause of American relapsing fever; arthropod vectors are unknown.

**B. par'keri,** a species found as a cause of relapsing fever in the western United States; transmitted by a tick, *Ornithodoros parkeri*.

**B. per'sica,** a species found as a cause of Persian relapsing fever; the vector, *Ornithodoros tholozani*, is known from the Egyptian western desert, Cyprus, Israel, Iraq, and the USSR to the western border of China, Afghanistan, and Kashmir.

**B. recurren'tis,** *Spirochaeta obermeieri;* Obermeier's spirillum; a species causing European relapsing fever; transmitted by the bedbug, *Cimex lectularius, and the louse, Pediculus humanus* subsp. *humanus.*

**B. refrin'gens,** a species found in genital mucous membranes and in unclean states or in necrotic lesions of the genitalia of man; apparently nonpathogenic.

**B. thei'leri,** a species found in the blood of cattle and other mammals in South Africa.

**B. turica'tae,** a species found as a cause of relapsing fever in Mexico, New Mexico, Texas, Oklahoma, and Kansas; transmitted by *Ornithodoros turicata*.

**B. venezuelen'sis,** a species causing spirochetal relapsing fever in Central and South America; transmitted by *Ornithodoros rudis* and *O. venezuelensis*.

**B. vincent'ii,** a species found on normal respiratory mucous membranes; also found in association with *Fusobacterium fusiforme* in cases of Vincent's angina.

**Borst,** Maximilian, German pathologist, 1869–1946. See B.-Jadassohn type intraepidermal *epithelioma*.

**Borthen** (bor'ten), Johan, Norwegian ophthalmologist. See B.'s *operation*.

**boss.** 1. A protuberance; a circumscribed rounded swelling. 2. The prominence of a kyphosis, or humpback.

**bos'selated** [ Fr. *bosseler*, to emboss ]. Marked by numerous bosses or rounded protuberances.

**bossela'tion.** 1. A boss. 2. A condition in which one or more bosses, or rounded protuberances are present.

**Bossi,** Luigi M., Italian obstetrician, 1859–1919. See B.'s *dilator*.

**Boston,** Leonard N., U. S. physician, 1871–1931. See B.'s *sign*.

**Bostroem** (bos'trem), Eugen W., Jena physician, 1850 –1928. See B.'s *stain*.

**bot.** See (1) botfly; (2) bots.

**Botallo (Botallus),** Leonardus, Italian physician in Paris, *1530. See B.'s *duct, foramen, ligament.*

**bot'fly.** Robust, hairy fly, often strikingly marked in black and yellow or gray, whose larvae produce a variety of myiasis conditions in man and various domestic animals, especially the herbivorous groups of animals; also known as warble flies, heel flies, skin bots, head bots, and stomach or horse bots for various groups of these economically important parasites.

**head b.'s,** members of the dipterous families Oestridae and Cuterebridae; robust, hairy, black, yellow, or gray flies that deposit newly hatched larvae on, in some cases, eggs, on or near the nostrils of sheep, goats, deer, horses, camels, and, rarely, man. These swift flies deposit their larvae on the wing, their hosts often showing great alarm and distress at the presence of these insects.

**human b.,** *Dermatobia hominis*.

**skin b.'s,** hairy, robust flies of the family Cuterebridae, whose larvae develop in the skin of man and domestic animals (*Dermatobia hominis*), or of rodents, rabbits, cats, and, rarely, dogs (*Cuterebra* species).

**warble b.,** warble fly, heel fly, or gadfly of the genus *Dermatobia* or *Hypoderma, q.v.*

**both'ria.** Plural of bothrium.

**Bothriocephalus** (both'rĭ-o-sef'al-us) [ G. *bothrion*, dim. of *bothros*, pit or trench, + *kephalē*, head ]. A genus of pseudophyllid tapeworms with both plerocercoid and adult stages in fishes; sometimes historically confused with *Diphyllobothrium*.

**B. corda'tus,** a species common in dogs and man in Greenland.

**B. la'tus,** incorrect name for *Diphyllobothrium latum*.

**B. mansoni,** incorrect name for *Spirometra mansoni*.

**B. mansonoides,** incorrect name for *Spirometra mansonoides*.

**both'rium,** pl. **both'ria** [ G. *bothros*, pit or trench ]. One of the slitlike sucking grooves found on the scolex of pseudophyllidean tapeworms, such as the broad fish tapeworm of man, *Diphyllobothrium latum*.

**Botkin,** Sergei P., Russian physician, 1832–1889. See B.'s *disease*.

**botryoid** (bot'rĭ-oyd) [ G. *botryoeidēs*, like a bunch of grapes (*botrys*) ]. Having numerous rounded protuberances resembling a bunch of grapes.

**Botryomyces** (bot'rĭ-o-mi'sēz) [ G. *botrys*, a bunch of grapes, + *mykēs*, fungus ]. A generic name applied to a supposed fungus causing botryomycosis. Since this disease is now known to be caused by several kinds of bacteria, staphylococci most commonly, the name is invalid and rarely used. The name of the disease has been retained, nevertheless, to indicate a peculiar type of tissue reaction.

**bot'ryomyco'sis.** A chronic granulomatous condition of horses, cattle, swine, and man caused by bacteria. It is characterized by granules in the pus, these consisting of masses of bacteria, generally staphylococci but sometimes other types, surrounded by a hyaline capsule which sometimes exhibits clublike bodies around its periphery. The anatomical structure of the lesion resembles actinomycosis and mycetoma. The lesions usually involve the skin but occasionally also the viscera.

**botryomycot'ic.** Relating to or affected by botryomycosis.

**bot'ryother'apy** [ G. *botrys*, a cluster of grapes ]. Grape cure; a method of treatment of chronic constipation, abdominal plethora, etc., by an exclusive or nearly exclusive diet of grapes—a fad now extinct.

**bots** [ Gael. *boiteag*, maggot ]. The larvae of several species of flies (botflies, *q.v.*).

**horse b.,** *Gastrophilus* larvae.

**ox b.,** cattle grub; the larvae of the warble flies, *Hypoderma bovis* and *H. lineatum*.

**sheep b.,** *Oestrus ovis* larvae.

**Böttcher** (bet'kher), Arthur, German anatomist, 1831– 1889. See B.'s *canal, cells, crystals, ganglion, space*, Charcot-B. *crystalloids*.

**bottle.** A container for liquids.

**wash-b.,** (1) a bottle containing water, with a tube passing to the bottom, through which gases are forced to purify them; (2) a stoppered bottle containing fluid, provided with two tubes, one ending above the other below the fluid, so that by blowing through the short tube the liquid is forced in a small stream from the free end of the long one; used for washing chemical apparatus.

**Woulfe's b.,** a b. with two or three necks, used in a series, connected with tubes, for working with gases (washing, drying, absorbing, etc.).

**bot'uline.** Botulinus *toxin*.

**bot'ulinogen'ic.** Botulogenic.

**botulism** (bot'u-lizm) [ L. *botulus,* sausage ]. Lamziekte; sal-lamziekte; loin disease; midland disease; allantiasis; duck sickness; limber neck; a food poisoning, really an intoxication, due to the ingestion of *Clostridium botulinum* toxin in "spoiled" food. Problem in man, chickens, and water fowl; occurs in cattle, sheep, and horses; swine, dogs, and cats are somewhat resistant. When phosphorus-starved cattle eat the toxin-containing bones of animals which have died on the range, the disease is called lamziekte (S. Africa), loin disease (southwest United States), and midland disease (Australia). Characterized by paralysis in all species, hence the name limber neck in fowl. See also *Clostridium botulinum*.

**botulismotoxin** (bot'u-liz-mo-tok'sin). Botulinus *toxin*.

**botulogenic** (bot'u-lo-jen'ik). Botulinogenic; botulism-producing.

**boubas** (bo-oo'bahs) [ native Brazilian word ]. Yaws.

**Bouchard,** Charles Jacques, French physician, 1837–1915. See B.'s *disease*.

**bouche de tapir** [ Fr. ]. Tapir *mouth*.

**Boucheron speculum.** See under speculum.

**Bouchut** (boo-shü'), Jean A. E., Paris physician, 1818–1891. See B.'s *method, respiration, tube.*

**Bouffardi's mycetomas.** See under mycetoma.

**bougie** (boo-zhē') [ Fr. candle ]. A cylindrical instrument, resembling a sound, usually more or less flexible and yielding, used in the diagnosis and treatment of strictures of tubular passages, such as the urethra or rectum. It is sometimes made of a soluble material, containing a medicament, and is used for making local applications to the urethra, etc.

**b. à boule** (boo-zhe'ä-bool'), one with a bulbous extremity; also called acorn tipped, bulbous, olive pointed, etc.

**filiform b.,** a very slender b. of firm but yielding structure.

**wax b.,** one used to locate sharp-edged calculi.

**whip b.,** a b. that decreases in size, to end in a threadlike tip.

**bougienage** (boo-zhe-nazh'). Examination or treatment of the interior of any canal by the passage of a bougie or cannula.

**Bouillaud** (boo-yo'), Jean B., French physician, 1796–1881. See B.'s *disease.*

**bouillon** (boo-yawn') [ Fr. broth, fr. *bouillir*, to boil ]. A clear beef tea.

**Bouilly** (boo-ye'), Vincent G., French gynecologist, 1848–1903. See B.'s *operation.*

**Bouin** (bwan), Paul, French histologist, 1870–1962. See B.'s *fluid, solution.*

**boulim'ia.** Bulimia.

**bound.** 1. To limit; circumscribe; enclose. 2. Indicating a substance such as iodine, phosphorus, calcium, morphine, etc., that is not in readily soluble form but exists in combination with a colloid, especially protein.

**bouquet** (boo-ka') [ Fr. ]. 1. A cluster or bunch of structures, especially of blood vessels, suggesting a b.

**Riolan's b.,** the muscles and ligaments, "les fleurs rouges et les fleurs blanches" (the red and white flowers), arising from the styloid process.

**Bourgery** (boor'jer-e), Marc Jean, French anatomist and surgeon, *1797. See B.'s *ligament.*

**Bourneville,** Désiré-Magloire, French physician, 1840–1909. See B.'s *disease*, B.-Pringle *disease.*

**Bourquin,** Anne, American chemist, *1897. See Sherman-B. *unit.*

**bouton** (boo-ton') [ Fr. button ]. 1. Button, pustule, knoblike swelling. 2. Boil.

**axonal terminal b.'s,** axon *terminals.*

**b. de Bagdad, b. de Biskra,** or **d'Orient,** the tropical sore of cutaneous *leishmaniasis, q.v.*

**b. en chemise,** small abscess of the intestinal mucosa, occurring in amebic dysentery.

**b.'s en passage,** consecutive synapses along the course of an axon.

**terminal b.'s,** axon *terminals.*

**b.'s terminaux,** axon *terminals.*

**boutonnière** (boo-ton-yair') [ Fr. buttonhole ]. An artificially produced slit or buttonhole-like opening in a membrane.

**Bouveret** (boo-ve-ra'), Leon, French physician, 1850–1929. See B.'s *sign.*

**Bovet** (bo-va'), Daniel, Swiss pharmacologist in Italy, *1907. Nobel laureate, 1957, for his discoveries relating to synthetic compounds that inhibit the action of certain body substances.

**Bovic'ola.** A genus of biting lice that is considered by some to be a subgenus of *Damalinia;* see also *Trichodectes.*

**B. bo'vis,** *Trichodectes scalaris;* the common red or biting ox louse of cattle.

**B. ca'prae,** *Trichodectes climax;* found on sheep and goats, as are *B. crassipes* and *B. limbatus.*

**B. e'qui,** *Trichodectes parumpilosus;* the common biting louse of horses.

**B. o'vis,** *Trichodectes sphaerocephalus;* the common biting louse of sheep.

**bovine** (bo'vin, -vin) [ L. *bos* (*bov-*), ox ]. Relating to cattle.

**bovovaccine** (bo-vo-vak'sēn). A vaccine against bovine tuberculosis, elaborated by v. Behring. It was widely used in the latter part of the 19th century but is now obsolete.

**bow, Logan's.** A lip traction bow; used to prevent tension on sutures used for closing cleft lip.

**Bowditch,** Henry P., Boston physiologist, 1840–1911. See B.'s *law.*

**bow'el** [ through the Fr. from L. *botulus*, sausage ]. The intestine.

**Bowen,** John T., American dermatologist, 1857–1941. See B.'s *disease*, B.'s *disease* of cornea.

**bowleg** (bo'leg). *Genu varum.*

**Bowles type stethoscope.** See under stethoscope.

**Bowman,** Sir William, English ophthalmologist, anatomist, and physiologist, 1816–1892. See B.'s *capsule, disks, gland, membrane, muscle, operation, probe, theory.*

**box.** Container; receptacle.

**fracture b.,** a long container of bottom and sides only, to support a fractured leg.

**Skinner b.,** an experimental apparatus in which an animal presses a lever to obtain a reward.

**box'idine** (USAN). 1-[ 2-[ [ 4'-(Trifluoromethyl)-4-biphenylyl ]oxy ]ethyl ]pyrrolidine; an anticholesteremic agent.

**box'ing.** In dentistry, pertains to b. an impression: the building up of vertical walls, usually in wax, around the impression to produce the desired size and form of the base of the cast, and to preserve certain landmarks of the impression.

**box-note.** A hollow reverberating sound, like that produced by tapping an empty box, heard on percussion of the chest in emphysema.

**Boyden,** Edward A., American anatomist, *1886. See B.'s *meal, sphincter.*

**Boyer** (bwa-ya'), Baron Alexis, Paris surgeon, 1757–1833. See B.'s *bursa, cyst.*

**Boyle,** Hon. Robert, British physicist and chemist, 1627–1691. See B.'s *law.*

**Bozeman,** Nathan, American surgeon, 1825–1905. See B.-Fritsch *catheter*, B.'s *operation, position, speculum.*

**Bozzi's foramen.** See under foramen.

**Bozzolo** (bot'tso-lo) Camillo, Italian physician, 1845–1920. See B.'s *sign.*

**BP.** Abbreviation for *British Pharmacopoeia.* See Pharmacopeia.

**Br.** Chemical symbol of the element bromine.

**bracelet** (brās'let). An appliance for the wrist.

**Nussbaum's b.,** an appliance designed for the use of one with writer's cramp.

**braces** (bra'sez). Colloquialism for orthodontic appliances.

**bra'chia.** Plural of brachium.

**bra'chial.** Relating to the arm.

**brachialgia** (bra'kī-al'jī-ah) [ L. *brachium*, arm, + *algos*, pain ]. Pain in the arm.

**b. statica paresthetica,** pain in the arm and transient paresthesia occurring only at night.

**brachio-** (bra'kī-o-, brak'ī-o-) [ L. *brachium* (*q.v.*), arm ]. Combining form meaning (1) arm, (2) radial.

**brachiocephalic** (bra'kī-o-sē-fal'ik). Relating to both arm and head.

**bra'chiocru'ral.** Relating to both arm and thigh.

**bra'chiocu'bital.** Relating to both arm and forearm.

**bra'chiogram.** Tracing of the brachial artery pulse.

**brachiotomy** (bra'kī-ot'o-mī) [ brachio- + G. *tomē*, incision ]. Incision into or amputation of an arm; especially removal of the arm of the fetus to allow for delivery.

**brachium,** pl. **bra'chia** (bra'kī-um, brak'ī-um) [ L. arm, prob. akin to G. *brachiōn* ] [ NA ]. 1. The arm, specifically the segment of the upper limb between the shoulder and the elbow. 2. An anatomical structure resembling an arm.

**b. collic'uli inferio'ris** [ NA ], b. of the inferior colliculus; b. quadrigeminum inferius; inferior quadrigeminal b.; a fiber bundle passing from the inferior colliculus on either side of the brain stem along the lateral border of the superior colliculus to the posterior part of the thalamus where it enters the medial geniculate body. It forms part of the major ascending auditory pathway.

**b. collic'uli superio'ris** [ NA ], radix medialis tractus optici [ NA ]; b. of the superior colliculus; medial root of the optic tract; superior quadrigeminal b.; b. quadrigeminum superius; a band of fibers of the optic tract extending past the lateral geniculate body to terminate in the superior colliculus and pretectal region.

**b. conjuncti'vum cerebel'li,** *pedunculus* cerebellaris superior.

**b. of the inferior colliculus,** b. colliculi superioris. **inferior quadrigeminal b.,** b. colliculi inferioris.

**b. pontis,** *pedunculus* cerebellaris medius.

**b. quadrigem'inum inferius,** b. colliculi inferioris.

**b. quadrigem'inum superius,** b. colliculi superioris. **superior quadrigeminal b.,** b. colliculi superioris.

**Bracht,** Erich Franz, German obstetrician and gynecologist, *1882. See B. *maneuver.*

**Bracht-Wachter lesion.** See under lesion.

**brachy-** (brak'ĭ-) [ G. *brachys,* short ]. Combining form meaning short.

**brachybasia** (brak'ĭ-ba-sĭ'ah) [ brachy- + G. *basis,* a stepping ]. The shuffling gait characteristic of partial paraplegia.

**brachycardia** (brak-ĭ-kar'dĭ-ah). Bradycardia.

**brachycephalia** (brak'ĭ-sĕ-fa'lĭ-ah). Brachycephaly.

**brachycephalic** (brak-ĭ-sef-al'ik). 1. Relating to or characterized by brachycephaly. 2. A b. individual.

**brachycephalism** (brak-ĭ-sef'al-izm) [ brachy- + G. *kephalē,* head ]. Brachycephaly.

**brachyceph'alous.** Brachycephalic.

**brachycephaly** (brak-ĭ-sef'al-ĭ) [ brachy- + G. *kephalē,* head ]. Brachycephalia; brachycephalism; disproportionate shortness of head, the skull having a cephalic index of over 80; among the brachycephalic races are the American Indians, Malayans, and Burmese.

**brachycheilia** (brak'ĭ-ki'lĭ-ah). Brachychilia.

**brachychilia** (brak'ĭ-ki'lĭ-ah) [ brachy- + G. *cheilos,* lip ]. Brachycheilia; brachychily; abnormally short lips.

**brachycnemic** (brak-ĭ-ne'mik) [ brachy- + G. *knēmē,* leg ]. Having short legs; specifically, relating to a tibiofemoral index of less than 82 with a shank disproportionately shorter than the thigh.

**brachycranic** (brak'ĭ-kra'nik) [ brachy- + G. *kranion,* skull ]. Brachycephalic with a cephalic index of 80.0 to 84.9.

**brachydactyl'ic.** Having short fingers; relating to brachydactyly.

**brachydactyly, brachydactylia** (brak-ĭ-dak'tĭ-lĭ, -dak-til'ĭ-ah) [ brachy- + G. *daktylos,* finger ]. Shortness of the fingers.

**brachyesophagus** (brak'ĭ-e-sof'ă-gus) [ brachy- + esophagus ]. An abnormally short esophagus.

**brachyfacial** (brak-ĭ-fa'shal). Brachyprosopic.

**brachyglossal** (brak'ĭ-glos'al) [ brachy- + G. *glōssa,* tongue ]. Denoting an abnormally short tongue.

**brachygnathia** (brak-ig-na'thĭ-ah) [ brachy- + G. *gnathos,* jaw ]. Bird face; abnormal shortness or recession of the mandible.

**brachygnathous** (brak-ig'na-thus). Having a receding underjaw.

**brachykerkic** (brak'ĭ-ker'kik) [ brachy- + G. *kerkis,* radius ]. Relating to a radiohumeral index of less than 75, with a forearm relatively shorter than the upper arm.

**brachymet'acar'pia.** Brachymetacarpalism; brachymetacarpalia; abnormal shortening of the metacarpals, especially the 4th and 5th.

**brachymetapody** (brak'ĭ-met-ap'od-ĭ) [ brachy- + G. *meta-* (tarsal) + *pous* (*pod-*), foot ]. Apparent shortness of toes or fingers resulting from shortness or hypoplasia of the metacarpals or metatarsals.

**brachymetatarsia** (brak'ĭ-met-ă-tar'sĭ-ah). Shortness of the metatarsals.

**brachymetropia** (brak-ĭ-me-tro'pĭ-ah) [ brachy- + G. *metron,* measure, + *ōps,* eye ]. Obsolete synonym for myopia.

**brachymorphic** (brak'ĭ-mor'fik) [ brachy- + G. *morphē,* form ]. Having, or denoting, a shorter form than that of the usually accepted norm.

**brachyodont** (brak'ĭ-o-dont) [ brachy- + G. *odous,* tooth ]. Having short teeth.

**brachypellic** (brak'ĭ-pel'ik) [ brachy- + pelvis ]. Brachypelvic; denoting a transverse oval pelvis; see brachypellic *pelvis.*

**brachypelvic.** (brak'ĭ-pel'vik). Brachypellic.

**brachyphalangia** (brak'ĭ-fă-lan'jĭ-ah) [ brachy- + phalanx, *q.v.* ]. Excessive shortness of the phalanges.

**brachypodous** (brak-ip'o-dus) [ brachy- + G. *pous,* foot ]. Having short feet.

**brachyprosopic** (brak-ĭ-pro-sop'ik) [ brachy- + G. *prosōpikos,* facial ]. Having a short face.

**brachyrhinia** (brak'ĭ-ri'nĭ-ah) [ brachy- + G. *rhis,* nose ]. Abnormal shortness of the nose.

**brachyrhynchus** (brak'ĭ-ring'kus) [ brachy- + G. *rhynchos,* snout ]. Abnormal shortness of the nose and maxilla, often associated with cyclopia.

**brachyskelic** (brak'ĭ-skel'ik) [ brachy- + G. *skelos,* leg ]. Relating to abnormally short legs.

**brachystaphyline** (brak-ĭ-staf'ĭ-lin) [ brachy- + G. *staphylē,* uvula ]. Having a short palate; having a palatomaxillary index above 85.

**brachytype** (brak'ĭ-tip). Endomorph.

**brachyuranic** (brak-ĭ-u-ran'ik) [ brachy- + G. *ouranos,* the sky, roof of the mouth ]. Having a palatomaxillary index above 115.

**bracing.** In dentistry, denotes resistance to horizontal components of masticatory force; see *component* of force.

**Bradford,** Edward H., Boston orthopedist, 1848–1926. See B. *frame.*

**bradsot.** Braxy.

**brady-** (brad'ĭ-) [ G. *bradys,* slow ]. Combining form meaning slow.

**bradyarrhythmia** (brad'ĭ-ă-rith'mĭ-ah) [ brady- + G. *a-* priv. + *rhythmos,* rhythm ]. Any disturbance of the heart's rhythm resulting in a rate under 60 beats per minute.

**bradyarth'ria** [ brady- + G. *arthroō,* to utter distinctly, fr. *arthron,* a joint, ARTH- ]. A form of dysarthria characterized by an abnormal slowness or deliberation in speech; also called bradyglossia; bradylalia; bradylogia.

**bradycardia** (brad-ĭ-kar'dĭ-ah) [ brady- + G. *kardia,* heart ]. Brachycardia; bradyrhythmia; oligocardia; slowness of the heart beat, usually defined as a rate under 60 beats per minute.

**cardiomuscular b.,** b. due to disease of the cardiac musculature.

**central b.,** b. due to disease of the central nervous system, usually with increased intracranial pressure.

**essential b.,** idiopathic b.; a slow pulse for which no cause can be discovered.

**fetal b.,** a fetal heart rate of less than 100 beats per minute.

**idiopathic b.,** essential b.

**nodal b.,** b. when the A-V node is pacemaker of the heart; see A-V nodal *rhythm.*

**postinfectious b.,** a toxic b. occurring during convalescence from various infectious diseases, such as influenza.

**sinus b.,** S-A b.; b. originating in the normal sinus pacemaker.

**ventric'ular b.,** slowness of ventricular rate, usually implying the presence of atrioventricular block.

**bradycar'dic.** Relating to or characterized by bradycardia.

**bradycine'sia.** Bradykinesia.

**bradycrotic** (brad-ĭ-krot'ik) [ brady- + G. *krotos,* a striking ]. Relating to or characterized by a slow pulse.

**bradydiastole** (brad-ĭ-di-as'to-le). Prolongation of the diastole of the heart.

**bradyesthesia** (brad-ĭ-es-the'zĭ-ah) [ brady- + G. *aisthēsis,* sensation ]. A retardation in the rate of transmission of sensory impressions.

**bradyglos'sia** [ brady- + G. *glōssa,* tongue ]. 1. Slow or difficult tongue movement. 2. Bradyarthria.

**bradykinesia** (brad-ĭ-kin-e'zĭ-ah) [ brady- + G. *kinēsis,* movement ]. Bradycinesia; extreme slowness in movement.

**bradykinet'ic.** Characterized by or pertaining to slow movement.

**brad′yki′nin.** Kallidin I; kallidin 9; the nonapeptide Arg-Pro-Pro-Gly-Phe-Ser-Pro-Phe-Arg, produced from a decapeptide (kallidin II or kallidin 10; bradykinin with an α-terminal lysine; bradykininogen) that is produced from $\alpha_2$-globulin by a proteolytic enzyme termed kallikrein, normally present in blood in an inactive form, and similar to trypsin in action. Bradykinin is one of a number of so-called kinins, polypeptides formed in blood by proteolysis (also found in wasp stings and damaged skin, and in sweat, saliva, and pancreatic juice) but not normally present in blood, that stimulate visceral smooth muscle but relax vascular smooth muscle, thus producing vasodilation, and that increase capillary permeability. Bradykinin is the most potent vasodilator for man yet discovered.

**brad′ykinin′ogen.** A decapeptide present in blood. Through the action of trypsin, proteolytic enzymes of certain snake venoms or kallikreins, lysine is split off from b. to yield bradykinin.

**bradyla′lia** [ brady- + G. *lalia*, speech ]. Bradyarthria.

**bradylex′ia** [ brady- + G. *lexis*, word ]. Abnormal slowness in reading.

**bradylo′gia** [ brady- + G. *logos*, word ]. Bradyarthria.

**brad′ymenorrhe′a** [ brady- + G. *mēn*, month, + *rhoia*, flow ]. A slow menstrual flow or prolonged menstrual bleeding.

**bradypep′sia** [ brady- + G. *pepsis*, digestion ]. Slowness of digestion.

**bradypha′gia** [ brady- + G. *phagein*, to eat ]. Extreme slowness in eating.

**bradypha′sia** [ brady- + G. *phasis*, speaking ]. Bradyphemia; a form of aphasia characterized by slowness of speech.

**bradyphe′mia** [ brady- + G. *phēmē*, speech ]. Bradyphasia.

**bradypnea** (brad-ip-ne′ah) [ brady- + G. *pnoē*, breathing ]. Abnormal slowness of respiration, specifically a low respiratory frequency.

**bradypragia** (bra′de-pra′je-ah) [ brady- + G. *prassō*, to do, act. PHRAG- ]. Sluggish action; slow movement.

**bradypsychia** (brad-ĭ-si′ke-ah) [ brady- + G. *psychē*, soul ]. Slow cerebration; slowness of mental reactions.

**bradyrhythmia** (brad-ĭ-rith′mĭ-ah). Bradycardia.

**bradysper′matism.** Absence of ejaculatory force, so that the semen trickles away slowly.

**bradysphygmia** (brad-ĭ-sfig′mĭ-ah) [ brady- + G. *sphygmos*, pulse. SPHYG- ]. Slowness of the pulse; bradycardia. (Note: b. can occur without bradycardia, as in ventricular bigemi ny when every alternate beat may fail to produce a peripheral pulse.)

**bradystal′sis** [ G. *bradys*, slow, + (*peri*)*stalsis*, contracting around ]. Slow bowel motion.

**bradyteleocinesia** (brad′ĭ-tel-e-o-sin-e′sĭ-ah) [ brady- + G. *teleos*, complete, + *kinēsis*, movement ]. Bradyteleokinesis; sudden arrest of a movement just before its intended termination, then after a pause it is completed slowly or by jerks; a symptom of cerebellar disease.

**bradyteleokinesis** (brad′ĭ-tel-e-o-kin-e′sis). Bradyteleocinesia.

**bradyto′cia** [ brady- + G. *tokos*, childbirth ]. Tedious labor; slow delivery.

**bradyuria** (brad-ĭ-u′rĭ-ah) [ brady- + G. *ouron*, urine ]. Slow micturition.

**bradyzoite** (brad-ĭ-zo′īt) [ brady- + G. *zōē*, life ]. A slowly multiplying encysted form of sporozoan parasite typical of chronic infection with *Toxoplasma gondii*. It has also been called a merozoite or zoite; the complex of b.'s within an enclosing membrane has also been called pseudocyst or cyst.

**Bragard′s test.** See under test.

**Brahn reaction.** See under reaction.

**Braid,** James, English surgeon, 1795–1860. Gave his name to braidism.

**braid′ism.** Obsolete term for hypnotism.

**Brailey,** William A., London ophthalmologist, 1845–1915. See B.'s operation.

**Braille,** Louis, French teacher of blind, 1809–1852. Invented braille.

**braille** (brāl) [ Louis *Braille* ]. A system of writing and printing by means of raised points representing letters, to enable the blind to read by touch.

**Brailsford,** James Frederick, English radiologist, †1961. See B.-Morquio *disease.*

**Brain,** W. Russell, British physician, 1895–1966. See B.'s *reflex.*

**brain** [ A.S. *braegen* ]. Encephalon; the mass of nervous matter within the cranium; the cerebral hemispheres, basal ganglia, brain stem, and cerebellum.

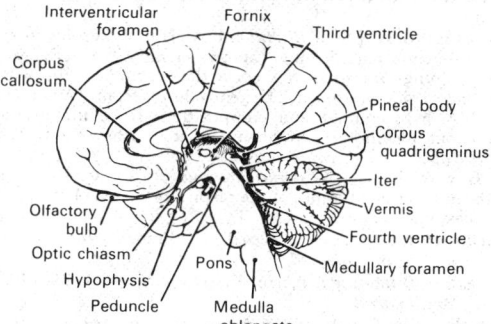

**Parts of the Brain**

Diagram of a brain which has been divided by a sagittal section between the hemispheres.

**abdominal b.,** *plexus* celiacus.
**olfactory b.,** rhinencephalon.
**smell b.,** rhinencephalon.
**thalamic b.,** obsolete term for diencephalon.
**visceral b.,** limbic *system.*

**brain′case.** The cranium in its restricted sense, the part of the skull that encloses the brain.

**brain′stem, brain stem.** The midbrain, pons and medulla oblongata.

**brain′washing.** Inducing a person to modify his attitudes and behavior in certain directions through various forms of pressure or torture.

**brallobar′bital.** VESPERONE; 5-allyl-5-(2-bromoallyl)barbituric acid; hypnotic.

**bran.** A by-product of the milling of wheat, containing approximately 20 per cent of indigestible cellulose; a bulk cathartic, usually taken in the form of cereal or special bran products.

**branch.** An offshoot; in anatomy, one of the primary divisions of a nerve or blood vessel. See branch.

**branchia,** pl. **bran′chiae** (brang′kĭ-ah) [ G. gills. BRANCH- ] [ NA ]. The gills, or organs of respiration in water-living animals. In embryological terminology, used usually adjectively to denote the branchial *apparatus* (*q. v.*).

**branchial** (brang′kĭ-al). 1. Relating to branchiae or gills. 2. In embryology, denoting the various structures constituting the branchial *apparatus, q. v.*

**branch′ing** [ Fr. *branche*, related to L. *branchium*, arm ]. Dividing into parts; sending out offshoots; bifurcating.
 **false b.,** in bacteriology, the appearance of b. produced when a cell is pushed out of the general line of growth and develops a new line of growth while the remaining cells continue to develop along the original line of growth.

**branchiogenic, branchiogenous** (brang′kĭ-o-jen′ik, brang′kĭ-oj′en-us) [ G. *branchia*, gill, + suffix -*gen*, to produce ]. Originating from the branchial arches.

**branchioma** (brang-kĭ-o′mah). A rare form of carcinoma that originates in remnants of epithelium in the branchial structures. Most of the carcinomas occurring in this site are likely to be metastases from a primary neoplasm in another location.

**branchiomere** (brang-kĭ-o-mēr) [ G. *branchia*, gill, + *meros*, part ]. An embryonic segment corresponding to one of the branchial arches.

**branchiomerism** (brang-kī-om′er-izm). An arrangement into branchiomeres.

**branchiomotor** (brang′kī-o-mo′tor). Relating to or controlling the movement of muscles derived from the branchial arches.

**Brandt,** M. L., U. S. obstetrician. See B.-Andrews *maneuver.*

**bran′dy.** Spiritus vini vitis; an alcoholic liquid obtained by the distillation of the fermented juice of sound ripe grapes and usually containing 48 to 54 per cent ethyl alcohol.

**Branham,** H. H., American surgeon, 19th century. See B.'s *sign.*

**Branhamel′la** [ Sara *Branham* ]. A genus of aerobic, nonmotile, nonsporeforming bacteria (family Neisseriaceae) containing Gram-negative cocci that occur in pairs with adjacent sides flattened. The genus differs from *Neisseria* in DNA base content and composition. It occurs in the mucous membranes of the upper respiratory tract. The type species is *B. catarrhalis.*

**B. catarrha′lis,** *Neisseria catarrhalis;* a species found in the mucous membranes of the respiratory tract of humans; occasionally causes disease. Type species of the genus *B.*

**Braquehaye** (brak-a′e), Jules P. L., French gynecologist, *1865. See B.'s *method.*

**Brasdor** (brah-dor′), Pierre, French surgeon, 1721–1798. See B.'s *method.*

**brash.** Any disorder of the digestive system accompanied by a burning sensation.

**water b.,** pyrosis.

**weaning b.,** diarrhea from which the infant may suffer at the time of being weaned.

**Bras′sica.** A genus of plans (family Cruciferae) that includes the mustards, *q. v.*

**Brauer,** Ludolph, German physician, 1865–1951. See B.'s *operation.*

**Braun,** Gustav von, Vienna gynecologist, 1829–1911. See B.'s *hook.*

**Braun's anastomosis.** See under anastomosis.

**Braun graft, Braun-Wangensteen graft.** See both under graft.

**Braune,** Christian W., German anatomist, 1831–1892. See B.'s *canal, muscle, valve.*

**Braun von Fernwald,** Carl R., Vienna obstetrician, 1822–1891. See B.'s *sign.*

**Braxton Hicks,** John. See Hicks, John Braxton.

**braxy** (brak′sĭ) [ Nor. *brad sot,* quick plague ]. A fatal disease of sheep, marked by inflammation of the abomasum and duodenum; the symptoms preceding death in the less acute form are weakness, coma, dyspnea; the pathogenic organism is *Clostridium septicum.*

**German b.,** black *disease.*

**Bray,** Charles William, U. S. otologist, *1904. See Wever-B. *phenomenon.*

**braye′ra.** Cusso; kousso; the dried panicles of the pistillate flowers of *Hagenia abyssinica* (*Brayera anthelmintica*) (family Rosaceae), a tree of the elevated region of Abyssinia. Has been used as a vermifuge. See also kosin.

**brazil′in.** A red natural dye, $C_{16}H_{14}O_5$, obtained from several species of tropical trees; it is used as a nuclear stain and as an indicator; red in alkalies, yellow in acids.

**bra′zing.** Soldering.

**break′down.** A failure, collapse, or sudden loss of health or the ability to function efficiently.

**nervous b.,** a nonmedical term for emotional or mental illness; often, a euphemism for psychiatric illness.

**break′off.** A feeling of physical separation from the earth when piloting an aircraft at high altitude.

**break′through.** A sudden manifestation of new and more constructive attitudes following a period of resistance during psychotherapy.

**breast** [ A.S. *breōst* ]. 1. The anterior surface of the thorax. 2. The mamma.

**caked b.,** stagnation *mastitis.*

**chicken b.,** *pectus carinatum.*

**funnel b.,** *pectus* excavatum.

**irritable b.,** swelling and induration of the b., not due to a neoplasm, and usually of comparatively brief duration.

**pigeon b.,** *pectus* carinatum.

**breath** [ A.S. *braeth* ]. 1. The respired air. 2. An inspiration.

**bad b.,** halitosis; fetor ex ore.

**out of b.,** dyspneic.

**shortness of b.,** dyspnea.

**breath-holding.** Cessation of breathing, usually in the inspiratory position; seen during the induction of inhalation anesthesia.

**breath′ing.** Respiration (2); the inhalation and exhalation of air.

**apneustic b.,** a series of slow, deep inspirations in very deep general anesthesia, each one held for 30 to 90 seconds, after which the air is suddenly expelled by the elastic recoil of the lung.

**Biot's b.,** Biot's respiration; completely irregular b. such as may occur in meningitis.

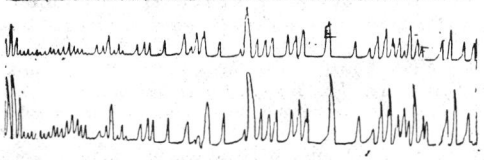

Biot's Breathing

**bronchial b.,** breath sounds of an abnormal quality, heard, on auscultation, over consolidated lung, over a pulmonary cavity, and (rarely) over a pleural effusion with underlying collapsed lung.

**goose b.,** a peculiar hissing type of respiration.

**intermittent positive pressure b.,** abbreviated IPPB; artificial respiration produced by the intermittent inflation of the lungs with air or oxygen under pressure; exhalation usually is passive.

**luxus b.,** unnecessarily deep and forcible inspiration.

**mouth b.,** habitual respiration through the mouth instead of the nose.

**positive-negative pressure b.,** abbreviated PNPB; inflation of the lungs with positive pressure and deflation with negative pressure by an automatic ventilator.

**positive pressure b.,** the inhalation and exhalation of air or oxygen that is under a small constant positive pressure relative to the ambient pressure.

**shallow b.,** a type of b. that occurs in acute pulmonary disease, *e.g.,* bronchopneumonia, in which parts of the lung are overventilated and other parts underventilated.

**Breda** (bra′dah), Achille, Italian dermatologist, 1850–1933. See B.'s *disease.*

**bredouillement** (bra-dwe-maw′) [ Fr. ]. Omission of parts of words related to extremely rapid speech.

**breech** [ A.S. *brēc* ]. The nates.

**breed′ing.** Selected mating of individuals to produce a desired strain. See also crossbreeding; linebreeding; inbreeding.

**bregma** (breg′mah) [ G. the forepart of the head ]. The point on the skull corresponding to the junction of the coronal and sagittal sutures. See fig. under craniometric *point.*

**bregmat′ic.** Relating to the bregma.

**brei** (bri). A fine mince or mush of tissue in which the cells are for the most part intact, used in biochemical research; *cf.* homogenate.

**Breisky** (bri′ske), August, German gynecologist, 1832–1889. See B.'s *disease.*

**Brenner,** Fritz, German pathologist, *1877. See B. *tumor.*

**brephic** (bref′ik) [ G. *brephos,* embryo ]. Relating to a very primitive stage of development.

**brephoplastic** (bref′o-plas′tik) [ G. *brephos,* embryo, + *plastos,* formed ]. Developed from embryonic tissue; formed during embryonic life.

**brephopolysarcia** (bref′o-pol-ĭ-sar′kī-ah) [ G. *brephos,* embryo, + *polys,* much, + *sarx,* flesh ]. A condition characterized by excessive flesh in embryo or newborn.

**brephotrophic** (bref'o-trof'ik) [ G. *brephos*, embryo, + *trophē*, nourishment ]. Relating to the nutrition of embryo or newborn.

**Breschet** (brĕ-sha'), Gilbert, French anatomist, 1784–1845. See B.'s *bones, canals, hiatus, sinus, veins*.

**bretylium tosylate.** DARENTHIN; (*o*-bromobenzyl)ethyl-dimethylammonium *p*-toluenesulfonate. A sympatholytic agent that prevents the release of norepinephrine from the nerve ending; used in the treatment of essential hypertension.

**Breuer,** Josef, German physician, 1842–1925. See Hering-B. *reflex.*

**Breus** (broys), Carl, Austrian obstetrician, 1852–1914. See B. *mole.*

**brevicol'lis** [ L. *brevis*, short, + *collum*, neck ]. Short neck.

**brevis** [ L. ] [ NA ]. Short.

**Bricker operation.** See under operation.

**Brickner's position.** See under position.

**bridge.** 1. The upper part of the ridge of the nose formed by the nasal bones. 2. One of the threads of protoplasm that appears to pass from one cell to another. 3. Fixed partial *denture.*

**arteriolovenular b.,** the largest capillary connecting arteriole to venule.

**cell b.'s,** intercellular b.'s.

**cytoplasmic b.'s,** intercellular b.'s.

**Gaskell's b.,** *fasciculus* atrioventricularis.

**intercellular b.'s,** cell b.'s; cytoplasmic b.'s; slender cytoplasmic strands connecting adjacent cells. In the epidermis and other stratified squamous epithelia the b.'s are processes separated by a desmosome. True b.'s exist between incompletely divided germ cells.

**removable b.,** removable partial *denture.*

**Wheatstone's b.,** an apparatus for measuring electrical resistance. Four resistors are connected to form the four sides or "arms" of a square. A voltage is applied to one diagonal pair of connections, while the voltage between the other diagonal pair is measured, *e.g.,* by a galvanometer. The bridge is "balanced" when the measured voltage is zero. Then, the ratios of the two pairs of adjoining resistances must be identical.

**bridge'work.** See partial *denture.*

**bri'dle.** 1. Frenum. 2. A band of fibrous material stretching across the surface of an ulcer or other lesion or forming adhesions between opposing serous or mucous surfaces.

**Brieger** (bre'ger), Ludwig, Berlin physician, 1849–1919. See B.'s *reaction.*

**Bright,** Richard, English internist and pathologist, 1789–1858. See B.'s *disease.*

**Brill,** Nathan E., New York physician, 1860–1925. See B.'s *disease,* B.-Symmers *disease,* B.-Zinsser disease.

**brilliant cresyl blue.** A basic oxazin dye, $C_{17}H_{20}N_3OCl$, used as a supravital stain for reticulocytes in blood.

**brilliant green.** See under green.

**brim.** The upper edge or rim of a hollow structure.

**pelvic b.,** *apertura* pelvis superior.

**brim'stone** [ A.S. *brinnan*, to burn ]. Sulfur; specifically, sublimed sulfur remelted and cast in cylindrical molds.

**brin'dle** [ diminutive of O.E. *brinded* ]. A hair coat color in which there is a uniform mixture of gray or tawny hairs with others of white or black; a composite color.

**Brinell,** J. A., Swiss engineer, *1849. See B. hardness *number.*

**Brinkerhoff,** William C., American physician, 19th century. See B.'s *speculum.*

**brinotab.** 4,4'-(Decamethylenedithio)bis[ 1-methyl-pyridinium-*p*-toluenesulfonate ]; topical antiseptic.

**Brinton,** William, London physician, 1823–1867. See B.'s *disease.*

**Briquet** (bre-ka'), Paul, Paris physician, 1796–1881. See B.'s *ataxia, syndrome.*

**brisement forcé** (brĕz-moń' for-sa') [ Fr. forcible breaking ]. The breaking by forcible means of the adhesions in ankylosis.

**bris'ket** [ O.E. *brusket* ]. The part of a beef animal (sometimes used of other species) that constitutes the caudoventral part of the neck and lies cranially to and between the forelimbs of the animal.

**Brissaud** (bre-so'), Edouard, French physician, 1852–1909. See B.'s *disease, infantilism, reflex,* B.-Marie *syndrome.*

**British anti-Lewisite.** Dimercaprol.

**British Pharmacopoeia.** See Pharmacopeia.

**broach.** A dental instrument for removing the pulp of a tooth or exploring the canal.

**barbed b.,** a root canal instrument set with barbs; used for removing a dental pulp, pulp tissue remnants or dentinal debris.

**smooth b.,** an exploring instrument used in endodontic practice; a root canal tine.

**Broadbent,** Sir William H., London physician, 1835–1907. See B.'s *law,* Bolton-B. *plane,* B.'s *sign.*

**broad-spectrum.** See under spectrum.

**Broca,** Pierre P., French surgeon, neurologist, and anthropologist, 1824–1880. See B.'s *amnesia, angle, aphasia, area, parolfactory area,* diagonal *band, center, field, fissure, formula,* visual *plane, pouch.*

**Brock's knife.** See under knife.

**Brock operation.** See under operation.

**Brock's syndrome.** See under syndrome.

**Brocq** (brok), Anne J. L., French dermatologist, 1856–1928. See B.'s *disease.*

**brocre'sine** (USAN). α-(Aminooxy)-6-bromo-*m*-cresol; a histidine decarboxylase inhibitor.

**Brödel,** Max, German medical artist in the U. S., 1870–1941. See B.'s bloodless *line.*

**Brodie,** Sir Benjamin C., English surgeon, 1783–1862. See B.'s *abscess, bursa, disease, knee.*

**Brodie,** Charles Gordon, Scottish anatomist, 1786–1818. See B.'s *ligament.*

**Brodie fluid.** See under fluid.

**Brodmann,** Korbinian, German neurologist, 1868–1918. See B.'s *areas.*

**Broesike** (brë'ze-keh), Gustav, German anatomist, *1853. See B.'s *fossa.*

**broken-wind.** Heaves in horses; pulmonary emphysema in horses.

**brom-, bromo-** [ G. *brōmos*, a stench ]. A prefix most commonly indicating the presence of bromine in a compound.

**bro'manylpro'mide.** 3-(*p*-Bromoanilino)-*N,N*-dimethylpropionamide; analgesic.

**bro'mate.** Salt or anion of bromic acid.

**bro'mated.** Brominated; combined or saturated with bromine or any of its compounds.

**broma'zepam** (USAN). 7-Bromo-1,3-dihydro-t-(2-pyridyl)-2*H*-1,4-benzodiazepin-2-one; an antianxiety agent.

**bromchlor'enone** (USAN). VINYZENE; 6-bromo-5-chloro-2-benzoxazolinone; fungicide.

**bromcre'sol green.** A substituted triphenylmethyl; minute, slightly yellow crystals, sparingly soluble in water, readily soluble in alcohol, ether, and ethyl acetate. Used as an indicator of pH, yellow at pH 3.8, blue-green at pH 5.4.

**bromcre'sol purple.** A substituted triphenylmethyl; minute, slightly yellow crystals, practically insoluble in water, but soluble in alcohol and dilute alkalies. Used as an indicator of pH, yellow at pH 5.2, purple at pH 6.8.

**Bromel,** Olaf, Swedish botanist. Gave his name to bromelain.

**bromelain** (bro'mĕ-lān) (USAN). Bromelin; one of a number of SH-proteinases (peptide hydrolases class) from plant latexes; obtained from pineapple; classified with papain, ficin, and asclepain as EC 3.4.17.2; orally administered in the treatment of inflammation and edema of soft tissues associated with traumatic injury.

**bro'melin.** Bromelain.

**bromhex'ine hydrochloride** (USAN). BISOLVON; 3,5-dibromo-*N*ᵃ-cyclohexyl-*N*ᵃ-methyltoluene-α,2-diamine hydrochloride; expectorant with mucolytic, antitussive and bronchodilator properties.

**brom'hidro'sis.** Bromidrosis.

**bro'mic.** Relating to bromine; denoting especially bromic acid, $HBrO_3$.

**bro'mide.** The anion Br⁻; salt of HBr.

**bromidrosiphobia** (brom'ĭ-dro'sĭ-fo'bĭ-ah) [ bromidrosis + G. *phobos*, fear ]. A morbid fear of giving forth a bad odor from the body, with sometimes the belief that such odor is present.

**bromidrosis** (brom'ĭ-dro'sis) [ G. *brōmos*, a stench, + *hidrōs*, perspiration ]. Bromhidrosis; osmidrosis; ozochrotia; fetid or foul smelling perspiration.

**bro'mindi'one** (USAN). FLUIDANE; 2-(*p*-bromophenyl)-1,3-indandione; oral anticoagulant.

**bromine** (bro'mēn, -min). Bromum; a nonmetallic, reddish, volatile, liquid element, symbol Br, atomic no. 35, atomic weight, 79.9. It unites with hydrogen to form hydrobromic acid, and this reacts with many metals to form bromides, some of which are used in medicine.

**bro'minism.** Bromism.

**bro'mism.** Brominism; chronic bromide intoxication. The main symptoms are headache, mental inertia, occasionally violent delirium, muscular weakness, cardiac depression, an acneform eruption, a foul breath, anorexia, and gastric distress. Treatment: removal of all sources of bromide ingestion and administration of ammonium chloride and sodium chloride to hasten the elimination of bromide.

**bromo-.** See brom-.

*p*-**bromoacetan'ilide.** Bromoanilide; ANTISEPSIN; analgesic and antipyretic.

**bro'moac'etone.** $CH_2BrCOCH_3$; a lacrimatory gas.

**bromoan'ilide.** *p*-Bromoacetanilide.

**bro'moben'zyl cy'anide.** $C_6H_5CHBrCN$; a lacrimator.

**bro'moder'ma** [ bromide + G. *derma*, skin ]. An acneform or granulomatous eruption due to allergic hypersensitivy to bromide, unrelated to blood bromide levels.

**bro'modi'phenhy'dramine hydrochloride.** AMBODRYL; 2- (*p*-bromo-α-phenylbenzyloxy) -*N*,*N*-dimethylethylamine hydrochloride; an antihistamine; may cause drowsiness and xerostomia.

**bro'moform.** Tribromomethane; $CHBr_3$; formerly used as an antitussive, antispasmodic, and sedative. It is more toxic than most other cough preparations.

**bro'mofor'mism.** Chronic bromoform poisoning; bromoform addiction.

**bromoguanide** (bro'mo-gwah'nid). Bromine analogue of chloroguanide; antimalarial agent.

**bro'mohy'perhidro'sis** (bro'mohy'peridro'sis [ G. *brōmos*, a stench, + *hyper*, over, + *hidrōsis*, sweating ]. Excessive secretion of sweat of a fetid odor.

**bro'moma'nia.** Delirium caused by poisoning with bromine or any of its salts.

**bromomenorrhea** (bro-mo-men-or-e'ah) [ G. *brōmos*, stench, + *mēn*, month, + *rhoia*, flow ]. The discharge of menses characterized by an offensive odor.

**bromomethyl ethyl ketone.** $BrCH_2COC_2H_5$; a lacrimating gas.

**bromophe'nol blue** (USP). Bromphenol blue.

**bromopnea** (bro-mop-ne'ah) [ G. *brōmos*, a stench, + *pnoē*, breath ]. Obsolete term meaning offensive breath.

**bromosaligenin.** BROMSALIZOL; 5-bromo-2-hydroxybenzyl alcohol; used for treatment of arthritis.

**bromosulfophthalein** (bro'mo-sul'fo-thal'e-in, -fthal'e-in). Sulfobromophthalein.

**5-bromouracil** (bro'mo-u'rä-sil). Synthetic analogue (antimetabolite) of thymine, in which a bromine atom takes the place of the methyl group in thymine.

**brom'phenir'amine maleate** (NF). DIMETANE; parabromdylamine maleate; 2-[ *p*-bromo-α-(2-dimethylaminoethyl)benzyl ]pyridine maleate; a potent antihistaminic agent with low incidence of side effects.

**bromphe'nol blue.** Bromophenol blue; a substituted triphenylmethyl; an acid-base indicator with a pK at 4.0; yellow at pH less than 3.1, blue at pH more than 4.7; used as a reagent for measuring the pH of urine.

**bromsulfophthalein** (brom-sul'fo-thal'e-in, -fthal'e-in). Sulfobromophthalein.

**bromthy'mol blue.** A substituted triphenylmethyl; a dye used primarily as a hydrogen ion indicator with pK at 7.0; yellow at pH 6.0, blue at pH 7.6; a weak but toxic vital stain.

**bro'mural.** BROMISOVALUM; α-bromisovaleryl urea; sedative and hypnotic.

**broncatar.** Camphoric acid compound with 2-amino-2-thiazoline (1:2); antitussive and respiratory stimulant.

**bronch-, bronchi-.** See broncho-.

**bronch'adeni'tis** [ bronch- + G. *adēn*, gland, + suffix -*itis*, inflammation ]. Inflammation of the bronchial glands.

**bronchi** (brong'kī). Plural of bronchus.

**bronchia** (brong'kĭ-ah) [ G. pl. of *bronchion*, dim. of *bronchos*, trachea. BRONCH- ]. The bronchial tubes.

**bronchial** (brong'kĭ-al). Relating to the bronchi and the bronchial tubes.

**bronchiarctia** (brong-kĭ-ark'shĭ-ah) [ bronchi- + L. *arcto* (improp. form of *arto*), to compress ]. Bronchiostenosis.

**bron'chiecta'sia.** Bronchiectasis.

**bronchiectasic** (brong-kĭ-ek-ta'zik). Relating to bronchiectasis.

**bronchiectasis** (brong-kĭ-ek'tă-sis) [ bronchi- + G. *ektasis*, a stretching ]. Bronchiectasia; bronchodilation (1); dilation of a bronchus or of the bronchial tubes.

  **capillary b.,** bronchiolectasis.

  **cylindrical b.,** a general symmetrical dilation of a bronchus or bronchial tube.

  **dry b.,** bronchiectasia sicca; characterized by lack of productive cough and occasional hemoptysis.

  **sacculated b.,** an irregular dilation occurring in pockets of varying size and shape.

**bronchiloquy** (brong-kil'o-kwī) [ bronchi- + L. *loquor*, to speak ]. Bronchophony.

**bronchiocele** (brong'kĭ-o-sēl). Bronchocele.

**bronchiocrisis** (brong-kĭ-o-kri'sis). Bronchial *crisis.*

**bronchiogenic** (brong-kĭ-o-jen'ik). Bronchogenic; of bronchial origin; emanating from the bronchi.

**bronchiole** (brong'kĭ-ōl). Bronchiolus.

  **respiratory b.'s,** *bronchioli* respiratorii.

  **terminal b.,** the final part of the purely conducting portion of the pulmonary airway.

**bron'chiolecta'sia.** Bronchiolectasis.

**bronchiolectasis** (brong'kĭ-o-lek'tă-sis) [ bronchiole + G. *ektasis*, a stretching ]. Bronchiolectasia; capillary bronchiectasia; dilation of the minute bronchial tubules, or bronchioles.

**bronchiolitis** (brong-kĭ-o-li'tis) [ bronchiole + suffix -*itis*, inflammation ]. Inflammation of the smallest bronchial tubes.

  **ex'udative b.,** inflammation of the bronchioles, with fibrinous exudation.

  **b. fibro'sa oblit'erans,** obstruction of bronchioles, especially terminal bronchioles, by fibrous granulation arising from ulcerated mucosa; the condition may follow inhalation of irrant gases, or complicate pneumonia.

  **vesic'ular b.,** bronchopneumonia.

**bronchiolo-** [ L. *bronchiolus, q.v.* ]. Combining form relating to the bronchiolus.

**bron'chiolopul'monary.** Relating to the bronchioles and the lungs.

**bronchiolus,** pl. **bronchioli** (brong-ki'o-lus, brong-ki'o-lī) [ Mod. L. dim. of *bronchus* ]. [ NA ]. Bronchiole; one of the finer subdivisions of the bronchial tubes, less than 1 mm. in diameter, and having no cartilage in its wall, but relatively abundant smooth muscle and elastic fibers.

  **bronchioli respiratorii** [ NA ], respiratory bronchioles; the smallest bronchioles (0.5 mm. in diameter) that connect the terminal bronchioles to alveolar ducts. Alveoli rise from part of the wall.

**bronchiosteno'sis.** Narrowing of the lumen of a bronchial tube.

**bronchit'ic.** Relating to bronchitis.

**bronchitis** (brong-ki'tis). Inflammation of the mucous membrane of the bronchial tubes.

  **asthmat'ic b.,** b. which aggravates an existing asthma.

  **cap'illary b.,** bronchopneumonia.

  **Castellani's b.,** hemorrhagic b.

  **croupous b.,** fibrinous b.

  **dry b.,** a form with scanty secretion.

  **epidem'ic b.,** bronchial influenza.

  **fi'brinous b.,** pseudomembranous, croupous, or plastic b.; Championniére's disease; Lucas-Championniére disease; inflammation of the bronchial mucous membrane, accompanied by a fibrinous exudation which often forms a cast of the bronchial tree.

**hemorrhagic b.,** Castellani's b.; bronchopulmonary spirochetosis; bronchospirochetosis; a chronic b. due to infection with spirochetes (though other bacteria are usually present and contribute to the infection); the chief symptoms are cough and bloody sputum.

**infectious avian b.,** a specific infectious disease of young birds, caused by a virus. It is highly transmissible and often causes heavy losses of young chicks, and heavy production losses among older, laying birds.

**b. kettle,** *croup* kettle.

**oblit'erative b., b. obliterans,** a fibrinous b. in which the exudate is not expectorated but becomes organized, obliterating the affected portion of the bronchial tubes.

**plastic b.,** fibrinous b.

**pseudomembranous b.,** fibrinous b.

**putrid b.,** b. accompanied by an expectoration of foul smelling material.

**summer b.,** rose *cold;* hay *fever.*

**verminous b.,** hoose; b. and bronchopneumonia caused by invasion of the bronchi by lungworms. Occurs commonly in cattle, swine, and sheep; rarely in other species.

**vesic'ular b.,** capillary b. with extension of the inflammation to the pulmonary alveoli.

**bronchium,** pl. **bronchia** (brong'kĭ-um, brong'kĭ-ah) [ Mod. L. fr. G. *bronchion* ]. A bronchial tube.

**broncho-** (brong-ko-) [ G. *bronchos,* windpipe. BRONCH- ]. Combining form denoting bronchus, and, in ancient usage, the trachea.

**bronchoalveolar** (brong-ko-al-ve'o-lar). Bronchovesicular.

**bronchocavernous** (brong-ko-kav'er-nus). Relating to a bronchus or bronchial tube and a pulmonary pathologic cavity.

**bronchocele** (brong'ko-sēl) [ broncho- + G. *kēlē,* hernia ]. Bronchiocele; a circumscribed dilation of a bronchus.

**bronchocephalitis** (brong-ko-sef-al-i'tis) [ broncho- + G. + *kephalē,* head, + suffix *-itis,* inflammation ]. Whooping cough.

**bronchoconstric'tion.** Bronchostenosis.

**bronchoconstrictor** (brong-ko-kon-strik'tor). 1. Causing a reduction in caliber of a bronchus or bronchial tube. 2. An agent that possesses this action.

**bronchodilatation** (brong'ko-dil-ă-ta'shun). Bronchodilation (2); increase in caliber of the bronchi and bronchioles in response to pharmacologically active substances or autonomic nerve activity.

**bronchodilation** (brong'ko-di-la'shun). 1. Rarely used synonym for bronchiectasis. 2. Sometimes used as an alternative spelling for bronchodilatation.

**bronchodilator** (brong-ko-di-la'tor). 1. Causing an increase in caliber of a bronchus or bronchial tube. 2. An agent that possesses this power.

**bronchoedema** (brong'ko-ē-de'mah). Swelling of the mucosa of the bronchial tubes.

**bronchoegophony** (brong-ko-e-gof'o-nĭ). An accentuated or exaggerated egophony.

**bron'choesophagol'ogy** [ broncho- + G. *oisophagos,* esophagus, + *logos,* study ]. The specialty that deals with peroral endoscopic examination of the esophagus and tracheobronchial tree.

**bron'choesophagos'copy.** Examination of the tracheobronchial tree or esophagus through appropriate endoscopes.

**bronchofiberscope** (brong-ko-fi'ber-skōp). A fiberscope particularly adapted for visualization of the trachea and bronchi.

**bronchogenic** (brong-ko-jen'ik). Bronchiogenic.

**bron'chogram.** The radiogram obtained at bronchography.

**bronchography** (brong-kog'ră-fĭ) [ broncho- + G. *graphē,* a drawing ]. Radiographic examination of the tracheobronchial tree by the injection of one of several radiopaque materials.

**broncholith** (brong'ko-lith) [ broncho- + G. *lithos,* stone ]. Bronchial calculus; a hard concretion in a bronchus or bronchial tube.

**bron'cholithi'asis.** Bronchial inflammation or obstruction caused by broncholiths.

**bronchomalacia** (brong'ko-mă-la'shĭ-ah) [ broncho- + G. *malakia,* a softening ]. Degeneration of elastic and connective tissue of bronchi and trachea.

**bronchomoniliasis** (brong'ko-mo-nĭ-li'ah-sis). Infection of the bronchial mucous membrane with a species of *Candida,* formerly called *Monilia.*

**bronchomo'tor.** 1. Causing a change in caliber, dilation or contraction, of a bronchus or bronchial tube. 2. An agent that possesses this action.

**bronchomycosis** (brong-ko-mi-ko'sis) [ broncho- + G. *mykēs,* fungus ]. Any fungus disease of the bronchial tubes or bronchi.

**broncho-oidiosis** (brong'ko-o-id-ĭ-o'sis). A bronchitis, prevalent in Ceylon, simulating tuberculosis, caused by the presence of *Candida tropicalis.*

**bronchopathy** (brong-kop'ă-thĭ). Any bronchial disease.

**bronchophony** (brong-kof'o-nĭ) [ broncho- + G. *phōnē,* voice ]. Exaggerated vocal resonance heard over a bronchus surrounded by consolidated lung tissue; see also tracheophony.

**whispered b.,** a hollow reverberating whisper heard in auscultating over a bronchus through solid or compressed lung tissue.

**bronchoplasty** (brong'ko-plas-tĭ) [ broncho- + G. *plassō,* to form ]. The surgical repair of any defect in the bronchi.

**bronchopneumonia** (brong'ko-nu-mo'nĭ-ah). Acute inflammation of the walls of the smaller bronchial tubes, with irregular areas of consolidation due to spread of the inflammation into peribronchiolar alveoli and the alveolar ducts; may become confluent or may be hemorrhagic; complications may include necrosis and abscess formation. Also called catarrhal pneumonia; lobular pneumonia; capillary bronchitis; vesicular bronchiolitis.

**tuberculous b.,** usually an acute form of tuberculosis.

**bronchopneumonitis** (brong'ko-nu-mo-ni'tis). Bronchopneumonia.

**bronchopulmonary** (brong-ko-pul'mo-nĕ-rĭ). Relating to the bronchial tubes and the lungs.

**bronchorrhagia** (brong-ko-ra'jĭ-ah) [ broncho- + G. *rhēgnymi,* to burst forth ]. Hemoptysis.

**bronchorrhaphy** (brong-kor'ă-fĭ) [ broncho- + G. *raphē,* a seam ]. Suture of a wound of the bronchus.

**bronchorrhea** (brong-ko-re'ah) [ broncho- + G. *rhoia,* a flow ]. Excessive secretion from the bronchial mucous membrane.

**bronchoscope** (brong'ko-skōp) [ broncho- + G. *skopeō,* to view ]. An instrument for use in inspecting the interior of the tracheobronchial tree for diagnostic purposes or for the removal of foreign bodies.

**bronchoscopy** (brong-kos'ko-pĭ). Inspection of the interior of the tracheobronchial tree by means of an electrically lighted endoscope.

**bronchospasm** (brong'ko-spazm). Spasmodic narrowing of the lumen of a bronchus.

**bronchospirochetosis** (brong'ko-spi'ro-ke-to'sis). Hemorrhagic *bronchitis.*

**bron'chospirog'raphy.** A method for studying the functioning of one lung or a portion of a lung. A catheter equipped with inflatable cuff is placed in the bronchus and thus the same studies which ordinarily are made for both lungs simultaneously can be made for one lung.

**bronchospirom'eter** [ broncho- + L. *spiro,* to breathe, + G. *metron,* measure ]. An appliance for measuring the air capacity of each individual lung separately with a double bronchoscope.

**bron'chospirom'etry.** Use of a double lumen catheter to determine respiratory function of the two separate lungs.

**bronchostaxis** (brong'ko-stak'sis) [ broncho- + G. *staxis,* a dripping ]. Hemorrhage from the bronchi.

**bronchostenosis** (brong-ko-sten-o'sis). Stenosis or narrowing of the caliber of a bronchus.

**bronchostomy** (brong-kos'to-mĭ) [ broncho- + G. *stoma*, mouth ]. Formation of an opening from without into a bronchus.

**bronchotome** (brong'ko-tōm) [ broncho- + G. *tomē*, a cutting ]. An instrument for incising a bronchus.

**bronchotomy** (brong-kot'o-mĭ). Incision of a bronchus.

**bronchotracheal** (brong-ko-tra'kĭ-al). Relating to the trachea and bronchi.

**bronchovesicular** (brong-ko-ves-ik'u-lar). Bronchoalveolar; relating to the bronchial tubes and alveoli in the lungs.

**bronchus,** pl. **bronchi** (brong'kus, brong'kĭ) [ Mod. L. fr. G. *bronchos*, windpipe. BRONCH- ] [ NA ]. One of the subdivisions of the trachea serving to convey air to and from the lungs. The trachea divides into right and left main bronchi which in turn form lobar, segmental and subsegmental bronchi. In structure the intrapulmonary bronchi have a lining of pseudostratified ciliated columnar epithelium, and a lamina propria with abundant longitudinal networks of elastic fibers. There are spirally arranged bundles of smooth muscle, abundant mucoserous glands, and in the outer part of the wall irregular plates of hyaline cartilage.

   **eparte'rial b.,** obsolete term for the right superior lobe b. which passes above the right pulmonary artery.

   **hyparte'rial bronchi,** obsolete term for those bronchi which pass below the pulmonary arteries, *i.e.,* right middle and inferior lobar bronchi and left superior and inferior lobar bronchi.

   **bronchi lobares** [ NA ], lobar bronchi; the divisions of the main bronchi that supply the lobes of the lungs. On the right there are three lobar bronchi (*b. lobaris superior, b. lobaris medius* and *b. lobaris inferior*) and on the left there are two (*b. lobaris superior* and *b. lobaris inferior*). The lobar bronchi divide into segmental bronchi.

   **primary b.,** the main b. arising at the tracheal bifurcation and extending into the developing lung of the embryo.

   **b. principalis dexter** [ NA ], right main b.; it arises at the bifurcation of the trachea and enters the hilus of the right lung giving off the superior lobe b. and continuing downward to give off the middle and inferior lobe bronchi.

   **b. principalis sinister** [ NA ], left main b.; it arises at the bifurcation of the trachea, passes in front of the esophagus and enters the hilus of the left lung where it divides into a superior lobe b. and an inferior lobe b.

   **b. segmenta'lis** [ NA ], segmental b.; one of the divisions of a lobar b. that supplies a bronchopulmonary segment. In the right lung there are commonly ten: *in the superior lobe,* b. segmentalis apicalis, b. segmentalis posterior, b. segmentalis anterior; *in the middle lobe,* b. segmentalis lateralis, b. segmentalis medialis; *in the inferior lobe,* b. segmentalis apicalis or superior, b. segmentalis basalis medialis or cardiacus, b. segmentalis basalis anterior, b. segmentalis basalis lateralis, b. segmentalis basalis posterior. In the left lung there are commonly nine: *in the*

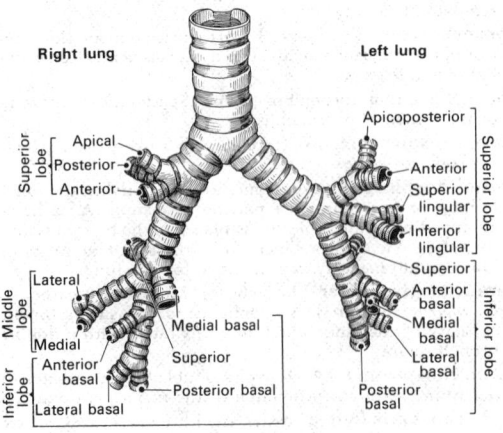

Right lung     Left lung

Superior lobe — Apical, Posterior, Anterior

Apicoposterior

Superior lobe — Anterior, Superior lingular, Inferior lingular

Middle lobe — Lateral, Medial

Medial basal, Superior

Inferior lobe — Anterior basal, Lateral basal, Posterior basal

Inferior lobe — Superior, Anterior basal, Medial basal, Lateral basal, Posterior basal

**Segmental Bronchi**

*superior lobe,* b. segmentalis apicoposterior, b. segmentalis anterior, b. lingularis superior, b. linqularis inferior; *in the inferior lobe,* b. segmentalis apicalis or superior, b. segmentalis basalis medialis or cardiacus, b. segmentalis basalis anterior, b. segmentalis basalis lateralis, b. segmentalis basalis posterior.

   **stem b.,** the main b. from which the branches of the bronchial tree arise.

**Brønsted,** J. N., Danish physical chemist. See B. *base, theory.*

**brontophobia** (bront-o-fōb'ĭ-ah) [ G. *brontē*, thunder, + *phobos*, fear ]. Morbid fear of thunder.

**brood.** 1. Litter (2). 2. To sit on and hatch eggs. 3. To ponder anxiously; to meditate morbidly.

**Brooke,** Henry A. G., English dermatologist, 1854–*1919.* See B.'s *disease,* B.'s *tumor.*

**broom.** Scoparius.

**broparoes'trol.**     LONGESTROL;   1-bromo-2-(*p*-ethylphenyl)-1,2-diphenylethylene; estrogenic substance.

**brossage** (bro-sazh') [ Fr. brushing ]. 1. Scraping with a stiff brush to remove granulations, as in trachoma. 2. To excite adhesive inflammation, as in omentopexy.

**Broussais** (broo-sa'), Francis J. V., Paris physician, 1772–1838. Gave his name to broussaisism.

**broussaisism** (broo-sa'izm) [ F. *Broussais* ]. The doctrine that living matter has but one property, that of contractility, which is excited into action by irritation and becomes quiescent when no irritation is present. The notion that irritation, proceeding from inflammation of the gut, was the cause of all disease led to much futile treatment misdirected at the alimentary canal.

**brow** [ A.S. *brū* ]. 1. The eyebrow. 2. The forehead.

**Brown,** James B., U. S. plastic surgeon, 1899–1971. See Blair-B. *graft.*

**Brown,** John, Scottish physician, 1735–1788. See *brunonianism,* Brunonian *system.*

**Brown,** Robert, English botanist, 1773–1858. See Brownian *movement,* Brownian-Zsigmondy *movement.*

**Brown,** Wade H., U. S. pathologist, *1878. See B.-Pearce *tumor.*

**Browning,** William, Brooklyn anatomist and neurologist, 1855–1941. See B.'s *vein.*

**Browning's phenomenon.** See under phenomenon.

**brown'ism.** Brunonianism.

**Brown-Séquard** (sa-kar'), Charles E., French physiologist and neurologist, 1817–1894. See B.-S.'s *paralysis, syndrome.*

**Bruce,** J., African traveler, 1730–1794. Gave his name to brucine.

**Brucella** (bru-sel'lah) [ Sir David Bruce ]. A genus of encapsulated, nonmotile bacteria (family Brucellaceae) containing short, rod-shaped to coccoid, Gram-negative cells. These organisms do not produce gas from carbohydrates. They are parasitic, invading all animal tissues and causing infection of the genital organs, the mammary gland, and the respiratory and intestinal tracts, and are pathogenic for man and various species of domestic animals. The type species is *B. melitensis.*

   **B. abor'tus,** Bang's bacillus; a species which causes abortion in cows, mares, and sheep, undulant fever in man, and a wasting disease in chickens; probably identical with or closely allied to *B. melitensis.*

   **B. meliten'sis,** a species which causes undulant fever (brucellosis, Malta fever) in man, abortion in goats, and a wasting disease in chickens. It may infect cows and hogs and be excreted in their milk. It is the type species of the genus *B.*

   **B. su'is,** a species causing abortion in swine, undulant fever (brucellosis) in man, and a wasting disease in chickens. It may also infect horses, dogs, cows, monkeys, goats, and laboratory animals.

**Brucellaceae** (bru-sel-a'se-e). A family of bacteria (order Eubacteriales) containing small, coccoid to rod-shaped, Gram-negative cells which occur singly, in pairs, in short chains, or in groups. The cells may or may not show bipolar staining. Motile and nonmotile species occur; motile cells are peritrichous. V (phosphopyridine nucleotide) and/or X (hemin) factors are sometimes cold-blooded for growth. Blood serum may be required or may enhance growth. Increased carbon dioxide tension may also favor growth, especially on primary isolation. These organisms are parasites and pathogens which affect warm-blooded animals, including man, rarely cold-blooded animals. The type genus is *Brucella*.

**brucellemia** (bru-sel-e'mĭ-ah). Brucellosis.

**brucellergin** (bru-sel'er-jin). A fat-free nucleoprotein antigen derived from brucella. Used in skin testing for brucellosis.

**brucelliasis** (bru-sel-li'ah-sis). Infection with any of the *Brucella* (*Acaligenes*) group of organisms.

**brucel'lin.** A vaccine prepared from several species of *Brucella*, formerly thought to prevent or cure brucellosis.

**brucellosis** (bru-sel-o'sis). Undulant fever; Rio Grande fever; rock fever; Mediterranean fever (1); abortus fever; Cyprus fever; gastric remittent fever; melitensis; melitococcosis; an infectious disease characterized by fever, sweating, weakness, pains, and aches, sometimes becoming chronic and producing long-lasting disability, caused by *Brucella abortus, B. melitensis*, or *B. suis*. It is ordinarily transmitted from animals, and is thus a hazard particularly to farmers, veterinarians, and slaughter-house workers. Characteristically, *B. melitensis* affects goats, *B. abortus*, cattle, and *B. suis*, swine; a certain amount of crossing over may occur. There is considerable variation in the strain causing human disease, depending chiefly upon the prevalent species of animal. The organism may be spread from milk or cheese, or from direct contact with diseased animals.

**bovine b.**, bovine infectious abortion; contagious abortion; Bang's disease; a disease in cattle caused by *Brucella abortus*. In pregnant cows, it is characterized by abortion late in pregnancy, followed by retained placenta and metritis; in bulls, orchitis and epididymitis may occur. The organism may localize in the udder and thus appear in milk from infected cows.

**Bruch** (brookh), Carl W. L., German anatomist, 1819–1884. See B.'s *glands, membrane*.

**brucine** (bru-sēn, -in) [ J. *Bruce* ]. Dimethoxystrychnine; an alkaloid from *Strychnos nuxvomica* and *S. ignatia* (family Loganiaceae). Produces paralysis of sensory nerves and peripheral motor nerves; the convulsive action which is characteristic of strychnine is almost entirely absent. Used as local anodyne and tonic.

**Bruck**, Alfred, German physician, *1865. See B.'s *disease*.

**Brücke** (brük'eh), Ernst v., Vienna physiologist, 1819–1892. See B.'s *muscle, tunic*.

**Brudzinski**, Josef von, Polish physician, 1874–1917. See B.'s *reflex, sign*.

**Brugia** (bru'jĭ-ah). A genus of filarial worms transmitted by mosquitoes to man, primates, carnivores, and a number of other mammals.

**B. malayi**, the Malayan filaria, formerly called *Wuchereria malayi;* an important agent of human filariasis and elephantiasis in Malaya, Borneo, Java, Sumatra, Ceylon, India, southern China, and South Korea. Two nuclei are present in the tip of the tail of the microfilariae. The nuclei-free area of the head is longer than broad, and the body assumes kinky rather than sinuous curves; otherwise, these microfilariae are similar to those of *Wuchereria bancrofti*. Transmitted to man by species of *Mansonia* and of *Anopheles* mosquitoes; adult parasites cause lymphangitis and lymphadenitis (similar to *W. bancrofti*), but, in contrast, there is less involvement of the genital region and lower extremities, and a relatively greater incidence of disease in the upper extremities. Recently, zoonotic subperiodic forest forms have been discovered in cats and other animals in Malaya.

**Brugsch** (broogsh), Theodor, German internist, *1878. See B.'s *syndrome*.

**bruise** (brooz). Contusion usually producing a hematoma without rupture of the skin. See also contusion.

**bruissement** (brwēs'moñ) [ Fr. ]. A purring auscultatory sound.

**bruit** (brwe) [ Fr. ]. An auscultatory sound, especially an abnormal one.

**aneurysmal b.**, blowing murmur heard over an aneurysm.

**carotid b.**, a systolic murmur heard at the root of the neck but not at the aortic area; any b. produced by blood flow in a carotid artery.

**b. de canon**, cannon sound; the loud first heart sound heard intermittently in complete atrioventricular block when the ventricles, happening to contract shortly after the atria, find the atrioventricular valves widely opened by atrial contraction and loudly slam them shut.

**b. de diable** [ Fr. humming-top ], venous *hum*.

**b. de galop** [ Fr. ]. gallop *rhythm*.

**b. de lime** [ Fr. file ], introduced by Laënnec to describe a rough rasping murmur.

**b. de moulin**, gurgling or splashing mill-wheel sounds heard when both fluid and air are present in the pericardial sac.

**b. de rappel** [ Fr. drum-beat ], double-shock sound; applied by Bouilland to describe the cadence of a split second heart sound, or of the second sound followed by an opening snap.

**b. de Roger**, Roger's *murmur*.

**b. de scie ou de rape** [ Fr. saw, rasp ], introduced by Laënnec to describe harsh, rasping murmurs.

**b. de soufflet** [ Fr. bellows ], introduced by Laënnec to describe a blowing murmur.

**b. de tabourka**, a loud tambour-like or bell-like second heart sound heard at the aortic area in syphilitic aortitis.

**b. de triolet** [ Fr. a little trio ], introduced by Gallavardin to describe the triple cadence produced by a systolic click.

**thyroid b.**, vascular murmur heard over hyperactive thyroid gland.

**Traube's b.**, gallop (2).

**Brumpt**, Emile, *1877. See B.'s *mycetoma*.

**Brunn** (broon), Albert von, German anatomist, 1849–1895. See B.'s *membrane, nest*.

**Brunner** (broo'ner), Johann C., Swiss anatomist, 1653–1727. See B.'s *gland*.

**brunnero'ma**. An adenoma of Brunner's glands; a rare solitary tumor.

**brunnero'sis**. Benign nodular hyperplasia of Brunner's glands.

**brunonianism** (bru-no'nĭ-an-izm) [ J. *Brown* ]. Brownism; a hypothesis resembling that of Broussais—that all disease resulted from excessive or deficient stimulation. Those with excessive stimulation were bled excessively and sometimes fatally, and those with deficient stimulation were stimulated with excessive brandy, sometimes fatally. See also Brunonian *system*.

**Bruns**, Ludwig, German neurologist, 1858–1916. See B.'s *ataxia*.

**Brunschwig**, Alexander, Chicago surgeon, *1901. See B.'s *operation*.

**brush** [ A.S. *byrst*, bristle ]. An instrument made of some flexible material, such as bristles, attached to a handle.

**Ayre b.**, a device for collecting gastric mucosal cells in cancer detection studies. It consists of a long flexible tube with a b. at the distal end. After positioning in the stomach the b. is rotated and "sweeps" cells from the mucosa.

**bronchoscopic b.**, a small b. for insertion through a bronchoscope for the purpose of wiping off cells for microscopic identification in suspected bronchial carcinoma.

**denture b.**, a b. used to clean removable dentures.

**Haidinger's b.'s**, an appearance produced when polarized light from an evenly illuminated surface falls upon the eye; it consists of a dark yellowish b. or tuft, narrowest in its center, which separates from each other two lighter bluish tufts, placed vertically to the first.

**Kruse's b.**, a bunch of fine platinum wires attached to a holder; used in bacteriological work to spread material over the surface of a culture medium.

**polishing b.**, a b. usually mounted in a rotating instrument, used to polish teeth or artificial replacements.

**Brushfield**, Thomas, British physician, 1858–1937. See B.'s *spots*, B.-Wyatt *disease*.

**brush'ite.** $CaHPO_4 \cdot 2H_2O$; a naturally occurring acid calcium phosphate.

**Bruton**, Ogden C., U. S. pediatrician, *1908. See Bruton type *agammaglobulinemia*.

**bruxism** (bruk'sizm) [ G. *brucho*, to grind the teeth ]. a clenching of the teeth, associated with forceful lateral or protrusive jaw movements, resulting in rubbing, gritting, or grinding together of the teeth, usually during sleep (sometimes a pathologic condition).

**Bryant,** Sir Thomas, English surgeon, 1828–1914. See B.'s *ampulla, line, sign, traction, triangle.*

**bryo'nia.** The dried root of *Bryonia alba* or *B. dioica* (family Cucurbitaceae). An active irritant hydragogue cathartic that has caused serious poisoning, hence is no longer used.

**bryon'idin.** A glycoside from bryonia that exercises a paralytic effect upon the central nervous system.

**bry'onin.** Mixture of a glycoside and an alkaloid from bryonia, neither of which is physiologically active.

**bryoresin** (bri-o-rez'in). Dark brown resin obtained from bryonia to which its purgative properties are probably due.

**BSP.** Abbreviation for BROMSULPHALEIN, bromosulfophthalein, or sulfobromophthalein sodium; see the latter.

**BTPS.** Symbol indicating that a gas volume has been expressed as if it were saturated with water vapor at body temperature (37°C) and at the ambient barometric pressure; used for measurements of lung volumes.

**BTU.** Abbreviation for British thermal *unit.*

**buaki.** A nutritional (protein deficiency) disease observed in natives of the Congo and characterized by edema, skin lesions, and anemia. Perhaps related to kwashiorkor.

**bubas** (boo'bahs). Yaws.
   **b. brazilia'na,** espundia.

**bu'bo** [ G. *boubōn*, the groin, a swelling in the groin ]. Inflammatory swelling of one or more lymph nodes in the groin; the confluent mass of nodes suppurates.
   **bullet b.,** a hard, painless swelling of a gland in the groin, accompanying a chancre.
   **chancroid'al b.,** an ulcerating b., due to *Haemophilus ducreyi.*
   **climatic b.,** *lymphogranuloma* venereum.
   **Frei's b.,** *lymphogranuloma* venereum.
   **indolent b.,** an indurated enlargement of an inguinal node.
   **malignant b.,** the b. associated with bubonic plague.
   **parot'id b.,** a swelling of the parotid gland due to secondary septic infection.
   **primary b.,** one occurring as the first sign of venereal infection.
   **venereal b.,** an enlarged gland in the groin associated with any venereal disease, especially chancroid.
   **virulent b.,** a chancroidal b.

**bubonal'gia** [ G. *boubōn*, groin, + *algos*, pain ]. Pain in the groin.

**bubon'ic.** Relating in any way to a bubo.

**bubonocele** (bu-bon'o-sēl) [ G. *boubōn*, groin, + *kēlē*, tumor ]. Inguinal hernia; especially one in which the knuckle of intestine has not yet emerged from the external abdominal ring.

**bubon'ulus** [ Mod. L. dim. of *bubo* ]. 1. An abscess occurring along the course of a lymphatic vessel. 2. One of a number of hard nodules, often breaking down into ulcers, which form along the course of acutely inflamed lymphatic vessels of the dorsum of the penis; also called Nisbet's chancre.

**bucar'dia** [ G. *bous,* ox, + *kardia,* heart ]. Cor bovinum; extreme hypertrophy of the heart.

**bucca,** gen. and pl. **buccae** (buk'ah, buk'e) [ L. BUCC- ]. [ NA ]. The cheek.

**buc'cal.** Pertaining to or adjacent to the cheek.

**buc'cally.** In the direction of the cheek.

**buccina** [ L. ] [ NA ]. The cheek.

**buccinator** (buk'sĭ-na'tor) [ L. *buccinator,* trumpeter ]. See *musculus* buccinator.

**bucco-** (buk'o-) [ L. *bucca,* cheek ]. Combining form relating to the cheek.

**buc'coax'ial.** Refers to the line angle formed by the buccal and axial walls of a cavity; see line *angle.*

**buc'coax'iocer'vical.** Refers to the point (trihedral) angle formed by the junction of the buccal, axial, and cervical (gingival) walls of a cavity; see point *angle.*

**buc'coax'iogin'gival.** Refers to the point (trihedral) angle formed by the junction of a buccal, axial, and gingival (cervical) wall; see point *angle.*

**buccocervical** (buk'o-ser'vĭ-kal). 1. Relating to the cheek and the neck. 2. In dental anatomy, referring to that portion of the buccal surface of a bicuspid or molar tooth adjacent to its cemento-enamel junction.

**buccoclusal** (buk'o-klu'sal). An incorrect term; refers to the line angle formed by the junction of a buccal and pulpal wall; see buccopulpal; see line *angle.*

**buc'codis'tal.** Refers to the line angle formed by the junction of a buccal and distal wall of a cavity; see line *angle.*

**buccogingival** (buk'o-jin'jĭ-val). Relating to the cheek and the gum.

**buc'cola'bial.** 1. Relating to both cheek and lip. 2. In dentistry, referring to that aspect of the dental arch or those surfaces of the teeth in contact with the mucosa of lip and cheek, the surfaces opposite the lingual surfaces.

**buccolingual** (buk'o-ling'wal). Pertaining to the cheek and the tongue.

**buccomesial** (buk'o-me'zĭ-al). Refers to the line angle formed by the junction of a buccal and mesial wall of a cavity; see line *angle.*

**buccopharyngeal** (buk'o-fā-rin'jĭ-al). Relating to both cheek or mouth and pharynx.

**buc'copul'pal.** Refers to the line angle formed by the junction of a buccal and pulpal wall of a cavity; see line *angle.*

**buc'cover'sion.** Malposition of a posterior tooth axially inclined in a direction toward the cheek.

**buccula** (buk'u-lah) [ L. dim. of *bucca,* cheek ]. A fatty puffing under the chin; double chin.

**Buchner** (bookh'ner), Eduard, German chemist, 1860–1917. See B. *funnel.*

**Buchner** (bookh'ner), Hans, German bacteriologist, 1850–1902. See B.'s *body, stain.*

**buchu** (bu'ku) [ native ]. Hottentot tea; the dried leaves of *Barosma betulina, B. crenulata* or *B. serratifolia* (family Rutaceae), a shrub growing in South Africa. Carminative, diuretic, and urinary antiseptic. It seems unlikely that it exerts any antibacterial action in the bladder.

**Buchwald,** Hermann Edmund. German physician, *1903. See B.'s *atrophy.*

**Buck,** Gurdon, New York surgeon, 1807–1877. See B.'s *extension, fascia.*

**buck.** A male antelope, deer, pronghorn, rabbit, or sheep.

**buck'bean.** Bogbean; water shamrock; marsh trefoil; menyanthes; the leaves of *Menyanthes trifoliata* (family Gentianaceae); credited with emmenagogue, antiscorbutic, and simple bitter properties.

**buck'thorn.** *Rhamnus.*
   **alder b.,** *Rhamnus frangula.*

**Bucky,** Gustav, American radiologist, 1880–1963. See B. *diaphragm,* B.'s *rays.*

**bu'clizine hydrochloride** (USAN). SOFTRAN; 1-(*p*-*tert-* butylbenzyl) -4- (*p*-phenylbenzl)piperazine dihydrochloride; a mild sedative used for motion sickness, vertigo, and anxiety accompanying psychosomatic disorders; should not be used for nausea of pregnancy.

**buclosamide.** *N*-Butyl-4-chlorosalicylamide; topical antifungal agent.

**bu'crylate** (USAN). Isobutyl 2-cyanoacrylate; a tissue adhesive used in surgery.

**Bucy,** Paul C., U. S. neurosurgeon, *1904. See Klüver-B. *syndrome.*

**bud.** A structure that resembles the b. of a plant.
   **bronchial b.,** one of the outgrowths from the primordial entodermal bronchus, giving rise to pulmonary epithelium.
   **end b.,** tail b.
   **gustatory b.,** *caliculus gustatorius.*
   **limb b.,** an ectodermally covered mesenchymal outgrowth on the embryonic flank giving rise to either the forelimb or hindlimb.
   **liver b.,** the primordial cellular diverticulum from foregut entoderm of the embryo that gives rise to the parenchyma of the liver.

**lung b.,** the endodermal lung primordium which will give rise to the epithelial lining of the respiratory tract.

**metanephric b.,** ureteric b.; the primordial cellular outgrowth from the mesonephric duct that gives rise to the epithelial lining of the ureter, pelvis and calyces of the kidney, and the straight collecting tubules.

**syncytial b.,** syncytial *knot.*

**tail b.,** end b.; the rapidly proliferating mass of cells at the caudal extremity of the embryo.

**taste b.,** *caliculus* gustatorius.

**tooth b.,** the primordial structures from which a tooth is formed; the enamel organ, dental papilla, and the dental sac enclosing them.

**ureteric b.,** metanephric b.

**vascular b.,** an endothelial sprout arising from a blood vessel.

**Budd,** George, London physician, 1808–1882. See B.'s *cirrhosis, jaundice, syndrome.*

**Budde** (bood'deh), E., Danish sanitary engineer, *1871. See B. *process.*

**buddeize** (bood'de-īz). To treat by the Budde process.

**bud'ding.** Gemmation.

**Budge** (bood'ga), Julius L., German physiologist, 1811–1888. See B.'s *center.*

**Budin** (bü-dän'), Pierre C., French gynecologist, 1846–1907. See B.'s obstetrical *joint,* B.'s *pelvimeter.*

**Buerger,** Leo, New York physician, 1879–1943. See B.'s *disease,* Winiwarter-B. *disease,* B.'s *stain.*

**bufa-, bufo-.** Combining forms that denote origin from toads. They are used in the systematic and trivial names of a great number of toxic substances (genins) isolated from plants and animals containing the bufanolide structure (see bufanolide). Prefixes denoting species origin are often attached, *e.g.,* marinobufagin, marinobufotoxin.

**bufagenins** (bu'fä-jen-inz). Bufagins.

**bufagins** (bu'fä-jinz). Bufagenins; a group of steroids (bufanolides) in the venom of a family of toads, the Bufonidae, having a digitalis-like action upon the heart (*e.g.,* bufotalin); *cf.* bufotoxins. For structure of bufanolides, see steroids.

**bu'falin.** A specific type of bufanolide, containing 3β,14-dihydroxy-5β,14β-bufa-20,22-dienolide. For structure of bufanolide, see steroids.

**bufanolide** (bu-fan'o-līd). Fundamental steroid lactone of several squill-toad (Bufonidae) venoms or toxins; also found in the form of glycosides in plants (*cf.* digitalis). The steroid is essentially that of 5β-androstane, with a 14β-H. The lactone at C-17 is structurally related to the —CH(CH$_3$)CH$_2$CH$_2$CH$_3$ radical attached to C-17 in the cholanes, and is in the same configuration as that of cholesterol (*i.e.,* 20R); in some species, b. is formed from cholesterol. Various b. derivatives having unsaturation in the lactone ring (20,22) or elsewhere (4) are known as bufenolides (one double bond), bufadienolides (*e.g.,* bufalin, telecinobufagin, marinobufagin, bufogenin B, bufotalin, bufotoxin), bufatrienolides (*e.g.,* scillarenin), etc. They have varying numbers of hydroxyl groups at positions 3, 5, 14, and 16, and these may be further substituted (*e.g.,* bufatalin, bufotoxin, gitoxigenin). For structure, see steroids.

**buf'fer.** 1. A mixture of an acid and its conjugate base (salt), such as $H_2CO_3/HCO_3^-$; $H_2PO_4^-/HPO_4^=$, which when present in a solution reduces any changes in pH that would otherwise occur in the solution when acid or alkali is added to it. Thus the pH of the blood and body fluids is maintained virtually constant (pH 7.45) although acid metabolites are continually being formed in the tissues and $CO_2$ ($H_2CO_3$) is lost in the lungs. See also conjugate acid-base pair, under conjugate. 2. To add a b. to a solution and thus give it the property of resisting a change in pH when it receives a limited amount of acid or alkali.

**b. capacity,** the amount of hydrogen ion (or hydroxyl ion) required to bring about a specific pH change in a specified volume of a b. (see b. value).

**b. pair,** an acid and its conjugate base (anion).

**secondary b.,** see Hamburger's *law.*

**b. value,** the power of a substance in solution to absorb acid or alkali without change in pH; this is highest at a pH equal to the pK of the acid of the b. pair (see b. capacity).

**b. value of the blood,** the ability of the blood to compensate for acid-alkali fluctuations without disturbance of the pH.

**Buffon** (boo'-fon), Compt de (Georges Louis Leclerc), French naturalist, 1707–1788. Published *Histoire Naturelle.* Some of his views on evolution and the origin of species anticipated Darwin by more than a hundred years.

**bufo-.** See bufa-.

**bufogenin B** (bu'fo-jen-in). A steroid toxin from Chinese toads; a 3β,14,16-trihydroxy-bufa-20,22-dienolide; *cf.* bufalin.

**Bufonidae** (bu-fon'ī-de) [ L. *bufo,* toad ]. A family of toads whose dermal glands secrete several kinds of pharmacologically active substances having a cardiac action similar to that of digitalis.

**bufor'min** (USAN). 1-Butylbiguanide; oral hypoglycemic agent.

**bufotalin** (bu'fo-tal'in). The steroid of a bufotoxin (bufogenin). It is bufogenin B acetylated at the C-16 OH.

**bufoten'ine.** Mappine; 3-(2-dimethylaminoethyl)indol-5-ol; N,N-dimethylserotonin; a psychotomimetic agent isolated from the venom of certain toads. It raises the blood pressure by a vasoconstrictor action and produces psychic effects including hallucinations. It is also present in several plants and is one of the active principles of cohoba.

**bufotox'in.** Vulgarobufotoxin; a toxic substance in venom of *Bufa vulgaris,* the common European toad; bufotalin esterified with suberylarginine at C-14 OH group.

**bufotox'ins.** A group of steroid lactones (conjugates of bufogenins and suberylarginine at C-14) of digitalis present in the venoms of the Bufonidae. Their effects are similar to but weaker than those of the bufagins.

**bug'gery** [ O.F. *bougre,* heretic, fr. Med. L. *Bulgaris,* a Bulgar (hence a heretic) ]. Bestiality; sodomy.

**bu'gleweed.** Lycopus.

**Buhl** (bool), Ludwig von, German pathologist, 1816–1880. See B.'s *disease.*

**Buist,** Robert C., Scottish obstetrician, 1860–1939. See B.'s *method.*

**bulb** [ L. *bulbus,* a bulbous root ]. 1. Bulbus; any globular or fusiform structure. 2. *Medulla* oblongata. 3. A short, vertical underground stem of plants such as scilla and allium.

**aortic b.,** *bulbus* aortae.

**arterial b.,** *bulbus* aortae.

**carotid b.,** *sinus* caroticus.

**b. of corpus spongiosum,** *bulbus* penis.

**dental b.,** the papilla, derived from mesoderm, that forms the part of the primordium of a tooth which is situated within the cup-shaped enamel organ.

**duode'nal b.,** duodenal *cap.*

**end b.,** one of the oval or rounded bodies in which the sensory nerve fibers terminate in mucous membrane.

**b. of eye,** *bulbus* oculi.

**hair b.,** *bulbus* pili.

**ju'gular b.,** *bulbus* venae jugularis.

**Krause's end b.'s,** *corpuscula* bulboidea.

**b. of lateral ventricle,** a rounded elevation in the dorsal part of the medial wall of the posterior horn of the lateral ventricle, produced by the forceps major.

**olfac'tory b.,** *bulbus* olfactorius.

**b. of penis,** *bulbus* penis.

**Rouget's b.,** a venous plexus on the surface of the ovary.

**taste b.,** *caliculus* gustatorius.

**b. of ure'thra,** *bulbus* penis.

**b. of vestibule,** *bulbus* vestibuli.

**bul'bar.** 1. Relating to a bulb. 2. Relating to the rhombencephalon (hindbrain). 3. Bulb-shaped; resembling a bulb.

**bulbi'tis.** Inflammation of the bulbous portion of the urethra.

**bulbo-** [ L. *bulbus,* bulb ]. Combining form relating to a bulb, or bulbus.

**bulbocap'nine** [ G. *bolbos,* bulb, + *kapnoeidēs,* smoke-colored ]. An alkaloid from *Corydalis cava* or *Capnoides cavum* (family Fumariaceae). Produces a state of catalepsy in lower animals; recommended in the treatment of vestibular nystagmus, Ménière's disease, paralysis agitans, and other tremors.

**bul'bocaverno'sus.** See under musculus.

**bulboid** (bul'boyd) [ bulbo- + G. *eidos*, resemblance ]. Bulb-shaped.

**bulbonuclear** (bul-bo-nu'kle-ar). Relating to the nuclei in the medulla oblongata.

**bulbopon'tine.** Relating to the rostral part of the rhombencephalon composed of the pons and overlying tegmentum.

**bulbosacral** (bul'bo-sa'kral). See bulbosacral *system*.

**bulbospi'nal.** Relating to the medulla oblongata and spinal cord, particularly to nerve fibers interconnecting the two.

**bulbourethral** (bul'bo-u-re'thral). Urethrobulbar; relating to the bulbus penis and the urethra.

**bul'bus,** gen. and pl. **bul'bi** [ L. a plant bulb ] [ NA ]. Bulb, *q. v.*

   **b. aor'tae** [ NA ], aortic bulb; arterial bulb; the dilated first part of the aorta containing the aortic semilunar valves and the aortic sinuses.

   **b. cor'dis,** a transitory dilation in the embryonic heart where the arterial trunk joins the ventral roots of the aortic arches.

   **b. cornus posterior'is** [ NA ], bulb of the posterior horn of the lateral ventricle of the brain; a curved elevation on the inner wall of the posterior horn produced by the fibers of the forceps major of the corpus callosum as they bend backward into the occipital lobe.

   **b. oc'uli** [ NA ], bulb of the eye; eyeball; globe of the eye; the eye proper without the appendages.

   **b. olfacto'rius** [ NA ], olfactory bulb; the grayish expanded anterior extremity of the olfactory tract, lying on the cribriform plate of the ethmoid and receiving the olfactory filaments.

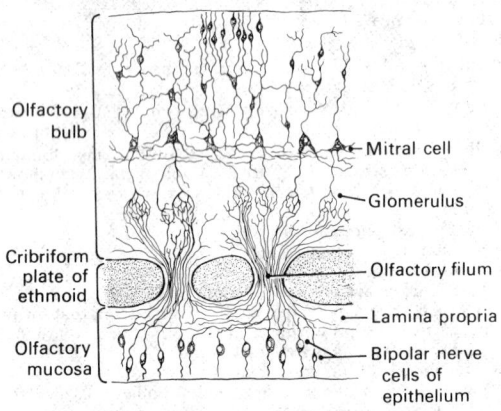

**Bulbus Olfactorius**

Diagram of olfactory mucosa and olfactory bulb (Ramón y Cajal), showing neuronal relations. (Slightly modified from Copenhaver, W. F.: *Bailey's Textbook of Histology*, Ed. 15, The Williams & Wilkins Co., Baltimore, 1964.)

   **b. penis** [ NA ], bulb of corpus spongiosum, penis, or urethra; b. urethrae; the expanded posterior part of the corpus spongiosum penis lying in the interval between the crura of the penis.

   **b. pili** [ NA ], hair bulb; the lower expanded extremity of the hair that fits like a cap over the papilla pili at the bottom of the hair follicle.

   **b. ure'thrae,** b. penis.

   **b. venae jugula'ris** [ NA ], bulb of the jugular vein; one of two dilated parts of the internal jugular vein; the superior is a dilation at the beginning of the internal jugular vein in the jugular fossa of the temporal bone; the inferior bulb is a dilated portion of the vein just before it reaches the anonyma.

   **b. vestib'uli** [ NA ], bulb of vestibule; a mass of erectile tissue on either side of the vagina united in front by a slender portion, the pars intermedia.

**bule'sis** [ G. *boulēsis*, a willing ]. The will; a willing.

**bulimia** (bu-lim'ī-ah) [ G. *bous*, ox, + *limos*, hunger ]. Morbidly increased appetite, often alternating with periods of anorexia.

**bulim'ic.** Relating to bulimia.

**bulk'age.** Anything, such as agar, that increases the bulk of material in the intestine, thereby stimulating peristalsis.

**bulla,** gen. and pl. **bul'lae** (bul'ah, bŏŏ'lah) [ L. bubble ]. 1. A bleb; blister; a circumscribed area of separation of the epidermis, due to the presence of clear serum. 2 [ NA ]. A bubble-like structure.

   **b. ethmoida'lis** [ NA ], ethmoidal b.; a bulging of the inner wall of the ethmoidal labyrinth in the middle meatus of the nose, just below the middle nasal concha; it is regarded as a rudimentary turbinal.

   **pulmonary b.,** (1) an air-filled blister on the surface of the lung; (2) a similar abnormality within the lung presenting as a thin-walled cavity.

   **b. tympan'ica,** the bony capsule enclosing the middle ear of the cat and dog.

**Buller,** Frank, Canadian ophthalmic surgeon, 1844–1905. See B.'s *shield.*

**bull'nose.** Necrotic *rhinitis* of pigs.

**bullock** (bŏŏ'ok). A steer; particularly one that is used for work.

**bullous** (bul'us). Relating to, of the nature of, or marked by, bullae.

**Bumke** (boom'ke), O. C. E., German neurologist, 1877–1950. See B.'s *pupil.*

**BUN.** Abbreviation for blood urea *nitrogen.*

**bunam'idine hydrochloride** (USAN). *N,N*-Dibutyl-4-hexyloxynaphthamidine monohydrochloride; anthelmintic.

**bundle.** A structure composed of a group of fibers, muscular or nervous; a fasciculus.

   **aberrant b.'s,** a group, or groups, of fibers from the corticobulbar or corticonuclear tract, directed to each of the motor nuclei of cranial nerves.

   **anterior ground b.,** fasciculus anterior proprius; see *fasciculi* proprii.

   **Arnold's b.,** *tractus* temporopontinus.

   **atrioventricular b.,** *fasciculus* atrioventricularis.

   **A-V b.,** *fasciculus* atrioventricularis.

   **Bachmann's b.,** division of the anterior internodal tract which continues into the left atrium providing a specialized path for interatrial conduction.

   **comma b. of Schultze,** *fasciculus* semilunaris.

   **Flechsig's ground b.'s,** the fasciculus anterior proprius and fasciculus lateralis proprius; see *fasciculi* proprii.

   **Gantzner's accessory b.,** see Gantzner's *muscle.*

   **Gierke's respiratory b.,** *tractus* solitarius.

   **ground b.'s,** *fasciculi* proprii.

   **Held's b.,** a vertically arched b. of fibers in the superficial layer of the myometrium.

   **Helweg's b.,** olivospinal tract.

   **His' b.,** *fasciculus* atrioventricularis.

   **Hoche's b.,** see *fasciculus* semilunaris.

   **hook b. of Russell,** uncinate b. of Russell.

   **Keith's b.,** *fasciculus* atrioventricularis.

   **Kent's b.,** *fasciculus* atrioventricularis.

   **Kent-His b.,** *fasciculus* atrioventricularis.

   **Killian's b.,** the lowest fibers of the inferior constrictor of the pharynx.

   **Krause's respiratory b.,** *tractus* solitarius.

   **lateral ground b.,** fasciculus lateralis proprius; see *fasciculi* proprii.

   **Lissauer's b.,** *fasciculus* dorsolateralis.

   **Loewenthal's b.,** *tractus* tectospinalis.

   **medial forebrain b.,** a fiber system coursing longitudinally through the lateral zone of the hypothalamus, connecting the latter reciprocally with the midbrain tegmentum and with various components of the limbic system; it also carries fibers from norepinephrin- and serotonin-containing cell groups in the brainstem to the hypothalamus and cerebral cortex, as well as dopamine-carrying fibers from the substantia nigra to the caudate nucleus and putamen.

   **medial longitudinal b.,** *fasciculus* longitudinalis medialis.

   **Meynert's retroflex b.,** *fasciculus* retroflexus.

   **Monakow's b.,** *tractus* rubrospinalis.

**muscle b.,** a group of muscle fibers held together by connective tissue.

**oblique b. of pons,** *fasciculus* obliquus pontis.

**olfactory b.,** a fiber system, described by Zuckerkandl as "Reichbundel," descending from the septum pellucidum in front of the anterior commissure toward the base of the forebrain. It contains precommissural fibers of the fornix, fibers from the septum to the hypothalamus and substantia innominata, as well as fibers ascending to the septum and hippocampus from the hypothalamus and midbrain. It bears no special relation to the sense of smell.

**olivocochlear b.,** a group of fibers originating from small cell groups surrounding the superior olive (nucleus dorsalis corporis trapezoidei), passing out with the contralateral vestibular nerve, then bridging over into the cochlear nerve, and terminating synaptically on the hair cells of Corti's organ. This efferent system in the cochlear nerve modulates the responsiveness of the auditory receptor cells.

**Pick's b.,** a b. of nerve fibers recurving rostralward from the pyramidal tract in the medulla oblongata, and believed to consist of corticonuclear fibers.

**posterior longitudinal b.,** *fasciculus* longitudinalis medialis.

**precommissural b.,** see olfactory b.

**predorsal b.,** *tractus* tectospinalis.

**Schütz' b.,** *fasciculus* longitudinalis dorsalis.

**solitary b.,** *tractus* solitarius.

**tendon b.,** a group of tendon fibers surrounded by a sheath of irregular connective tissue, the peritendineum.

**Türck's b.,** *tractus* frontopontinus.

**uncinate b. of Russell,** hook b. of Russell; that component of the fastigiobulbar tract that loops over the dorsal surface of the brachium conjunctivum (superior cerebellar peduncle) before turning ventrally and caudally in the restiform body.

**Vicq d'Azyr's b.,** *fasciculus* mamillothalamicus.

**Weismann's b.,** muscle fibers within the muscle spindle; intrafusal fibers.

**Bunge** (boong'eh), Gustav von, German physiologist, 1844–1920. See B.-Trantenroth *stain*.

**bungpag'ga.** *Myositis* purulenta tropica.

**bunion** (bun'yun) [ O.F. *buigne*, bump on the head ]. A localized swelling at either the medial or dorsal aspect of the first metatarsophalangeal joint; can be related to an underlying inflammatory bursa; the medial b. is usually associated with hallux valgus.

**tailor's b.,** a b. on the lateral side of the fifth toe.

**Bunnell,** Sterling, U. S. surgeon, *1882. See B.'s *suture*.

**bu'nodont** [ G. *bounos*, mound, + *odous* (*odont*-), tooth ]. Having molar teeth with rounded or conical cusps; opposed to lophodont.

**bu'nolol hydrochloride** (USAN). DL-5-[ 3-*tert*-Butylamino)-2-hydroxypropoxy ]-3,4-dihydro-1(2*H*)-naphthalenone hydrochloride; a β-adrenergic blocking agent for treatment of cardiac arrhythmias.

**Bunosto'mum.** A genus of hookworms (family Ancylostomatidae, subfamily Necatorinae) found in cattle and other herbivores; similar to *Necator*.

**B. phlebot'omum,** a species that occurs in cattle, sheep, and some wild ruminants in many parts of the world.

**B. trigonoceph'alum,** a cosmopolitan parasite in the small intestines of sheep and goats.

**Bunsen,** Robert W., German chemist and physicist, 1811–1899. See B. *burner*, B.'s solubility *coefficient*, B.-Roscoe *law*.

**buphthalmia** (buf-thal'mi-ah). Buphthalmos.

**buphthalmos, buphthalmus** (buf-thal'mus) [ G. *bous*, ox, + *ophthalmos*, eye ]. Congenital glaucoma; hydrophthalmos; an affection of infancy, marked by an increase of intraocular fluid with enlargement of the eyeball.

**bupiv'acaine** (BP, USAN). MARCAINE; *dl*-1-butyl-pipecoloxylidide; a potent, long-acting local anesthetic used in epidural anesthesia and nerve blocks.

**bur.** 1. A small shaft of steel or other hard metal with fluting or cutting planes on one end. It is inserted into a dental handpiece. Designed in various end shapes, it may be used at various rotational velocities for excavating decay, shaping cavity forms, and in general for any reduction of tooth structure. 2. See burr.

**fissure b.,** a cylindrical or tapered rotary cutting tool intended for extending or widening fissures in a tooth, as for general surface reduction of tooth substance.

**inverted cone b.,** a dental drill in the shape of a truncated cone with the smaller end attached to the shaft; generally used for entering carious pits or creating undercuts in cavity preparations.

**round b.,** a dental b. with the cutting blades spherically arranged.

**bu'ramate** (USAN). Benzylcarbamic acid 2-hydroxyethyl ester; anticonvulsant.

**bur'bot liver oil.** Oil extracted from the liver of the burbot, *Lota maculosa;* used for the same purposes as cod liver oil.

**Burchard-Liebermann reaction,** and **Liebermann-Burchard test.** See the nouns.

**Burdach** (boor'dakh), Karl F., German anatomist and physiologist, 1776–1847. See B.'s *column, fasciculus,* nucleus, tract.

**bur'dock.** Lappa.

**buret', burette'** [ Fr. ]. A graduated glass tube with a tap as its lower end, used for measuring liquids in volumetric chemical analyses. See fig. under titration.

**Bürger,** Max. See B.-Grütz *syndrome*.

**Burk,** D. See Lineweaver-B. *equation*.

**Burkitt,** Denis. See B.'s *lymphoma*.

**Burlew disk.** See under disk.

**Burn,** J. H. See B. and Rand *theory*.

**burn** [ A.S. *baernan* ]. 1. To consume with fire. 2. To cause a lesion of the skin by heat. 3. To cause a lesion by acid or any other agent, similar to that caused by heat; to cauterize. 4. To suffer pain caused by excessive heat, or

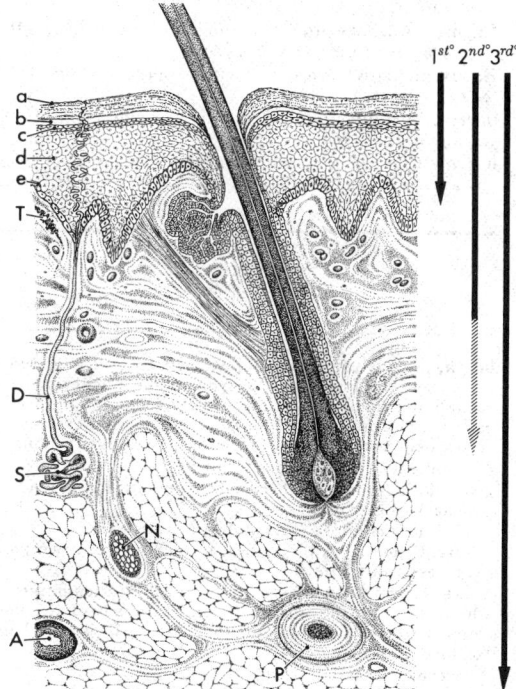

**Burns**

The five layers of epidermis, showing (*vertical arrows*) 1st, 2nd, and 3rd degree burns. *a,* Stratum corneum; *b,* stratum lucidum; *c,* stratum granulosum; *d,* stratum spinosum; *e,* stratum basale; *A,* artery; *D,* duct of sudoriferous gland; *G,* sebaceous gland; *H,* hair follicle; *N,* nerve; *P,* Pacinian corpuscle; *S,* sudoriferous gland; *T,* tactile corpuscle.

similar pain from any cause. 5. A lesion caused by heat or any chemical cauterizing agent, including friction, electricity (lighting), electromagnetic energy (ultraviolet, x-ray, laser, atomic explosion); types of burns resulting from different agents are relatively specific and diagnostic. The division of burns into three degrees is recognized for geographical designation: first, involving only the epidermis and causing erythema and edema without vesiculation; second, involving the epidermis and dermis and usually forming blisters that may be superficial or deep dermal necrosis, but epithelial regeneration may extend from the skin appendages; third, destruction of the entire skin; deep third-degree b.'s extend into subcutaneous fat, muscle, or bone and often cause much scarring.

**brush b.,** mat b.; rope b.; a b. caused by friction of a rapidly moving object against the skin or ground into the skin.

**chemical b.,** one due to a caustic chemical.

**flash b.,** one due to very brief exposure to intense radiant heat; the typical b. produced by atomic explosion.

**radiation b.,** one caused by overexposure to radium, x-rays, atomic energy in any form, ultraviolet rays, etc.

**thermal b.,** one caused by heat.

**burn′er.** The part of a lamp that holds the wick or where the fuel is burned.

**Bunsen b.,** a gas b. supplied with lateral openings admitting so much air that the carbon is completely burned, giving a very hot but only slightly luminous flame.

**Burnet** (bur-net′), Sir F. Macfarlane, Australian virologist, *1899. Nobel laureate, 1960, with Peter B. Medawar for the discovery of acquired immunological tolerance.

**Burnett,** Charles H., American physician, *1901. See B.'s *syndrome.*

**burning-bush.** Euonymus.

**bur′nisher** [ O. F. *burnir,* to polish ]. An instrument for smoothing and polishing the surface or edge of a dental restoration.

**Burns,** Allan, Scottish anatomist, 1781–1813. See B.'s *ligament,* falciform *process, space.*

**Burow** (boo′rov), Karl A., German surgeon, 1809–1874. See B.'s *operation, vein.*

**burr.** 1. A drilling tool for enlarging a trephine hole in the cranium. 2. See bur.

**burrow** (bur′ro). 1. A subcutaneous tunnel or tract made by a parasite such as the itch mite. 2. A sinus or fistula.

# BURSA

**bursa,** pl. **bur′sae** (bur′sah) [ Mediev. L. a purse ] [ NA ]. A closed sac lined with a synovia-like membrane and containing fluid. Bursae are usually found or formed in areas subject to friction, for example, over an exposed or prominent part or where a tendon passes over a bone.

**Achil′les b.,** b. tendinis calcanei.

**b. achil′lis** [ NA ], official alternate term for b. tendinis calcanei.

**b. of acro′mion,** b. subcutanea acromialis.

**adventitious b.,** a b.-like cyst formed between two parts as a result of friction.

**b. anserina** [ NA ], anserine b.; tibial intertendinous b.; the b. between the tibial collateral ligament of the knee joint and the tendons of the sartorius, gracilis and semitendinosus muscles.

**anserine b.,** b. anserina.

**bicipitoradial b.,** b. bicipitoradialis.

**b. bicip′itoradia′lis** [ NA ], bicipitoradial b.; the b. between the tendon of the biceps brachii muscle and the anterior part of the tuberosity of the radius.

**Boyer's b.,** b. retrohyoidea.

**Brodie's b.,** b. subtendinea musculi gastrocnemii medialis.

**Calori's b.,** a b. between the arch of the aorta and the trachea.

**b. cubita′lis interos′sea** [ NA ], interosseous b. of the elbow; an inconstant b. located between the tendon of the biceps and the ulna.

**deep in′frapatel′lar b.,** b. infrapatellaris profunda.

**b. fabricii,** the b. of Fabricius in poultry, a blind saclike structure located on the posterodorsal wall of the cloaca.

**Fleischmann's b.,** b. sublingualis; an inconstant serous b. at the level of the frenulum linguae, between the surface of the genioglossus muscle and the mucous membrane of the floor of the mouth.

**b. of gastrocne′mius,** b. subtendinea musculi gastrocnemii.

**glu′teofem′oral b.,** between the tendon of the gluteus maximus muscle and the tendon of the vastus lateralis muscle.

**b. of great toe,** between the lateral side of the base of the first metatarsal bone and the medial side of the shaft of the second metatarsal.

**b. of hyoid,** b. retrohyoidea.

**iliac b.,** b. subtendinea iliaca.

**b. iliopectinea** [ NA ], iliopectineal b.; a large b. between the iliopsoas tendon and the iliopubic eminence.

**iliopectineal b.,** b. iliopectinea.

**infracardiac b.,** a small serous sac sometimes present on the medial side of the base of the right lung in the embryo. See also pneumatoenteric *recess.*

**infrahyoid b.,** b. infrahyoidea.

**b. infrahyoi′dea** [ NA ], infrahyoid b.; a b. sometimes found between the inferior margin of the body of the hyoid bone and the median thyrohyoid ligament.

**b. infrapatella′ris profunda** [ NA ], deep infrapatellar b.; between the upper part of the tibia and the patellar ligament.

**b. intermuscula′res musculi gluteorum** [ NA ], intermuscular gluteal bursae.

**interosseous b. of elbow,** b. cubitalis interossea.

**b. intratendin′ea olec′rani** [ NA ], b. of Monro; a b. sometimes present within the tendon of insertion of the triceps brachii.

**b. ischiad′ica musculi glutei maximi** [ NA ], ischial b.; between the gluteus maximus muscle and the tuberosity of the ischium.

**b. ischiad′ica musculi obturato′rii interni** [ NA ], the large, constant b. between the obturator internus tendon and the lesser sciatic notch.

**is′chial b.,** b. ischiadica musculi glutei maximi.

**b. of latiss′imus dorsi,** b. subtendinea musculi latissimus dorsi.

**Luschka's b.,** b. pharyngea.

**b. of Monro,** b. intratendinea olecrani.

**b. mucosa,** b. synovialis.

**b. musculi bicipitis femoris superior** [ NA ], a b. frequently found between the tendon of origin of the long head of the biceps femoris and the ischial tuberosity and origin of the semimembranosus.

**b. musculi coracobrachia′lis** [ NA ], a b. frequently present between the tendon of origin of the coracobrachialis and the subscapularis muscle.

**b. musculi extenso′ris carpi radia′lis brevis** [ NA ], the b. between the tendon of insertion of the extensor carpi radialis brevis and the base of the third metacarpal.

**b. musculi pirifor′mis** [ NA ], a small b. located between the tendons of the piriformis and superior gemellus and the femur.

**b. musculi semimembrano′si** [ NA ], b. of the semimembranosus; it lies between the muscle, the head of the gastrocnemius, and the knee joint.

**b. musculi tenso′ris veli palati′ni** [ NA ], b. of the tensor veli palatini muscle; a small b. located where the tendon of the tensor passes around the pterygoid hamulus.

**b. of ob′turator internus,** b. subtendinea musculi obturatoris interni.

**b. of olec′ranon,** b. subcutanea olecrani.

**omental b.,** b. omentalis.

**b. omenta′lis** [ NA ], omental b.; omental sac; the lesser peritoneal sac or cavity; an isolated portion of the peritoneal cavity lying dorsal to the stomach and extending craniad to the liver and diaphragm and caudad into the greater omentum. It opens into the general peritoneal cavity at the epiploic foramen.

**b. ovar'ica,** the peritoneal recess between the medial aspect of the ovary and the mesosalpinx.

**b. pharynge'a** [ NA ], pharyngeal b.; Luschka's b.; Thornwaldt's cyst; a cystic notochordal remnant found inconstantly in the posterior wall of the nasopharynx at the lower end of the pharyngeal tonsil.

**pharyngeal b.,** b. pharyngea.

**b. of poplite'us,** recessus subpopliteus.

**prepatel'lar b.,** b. subcutanea prepatellaris.

**b. quadra'tus fem'oris,** between the front of the quadratus femoris muscle and the lesser trochanter of the femur.

**radial b.,** *vagina* tendinis musculi flexoris pollicis longi.

**retrohyoid b.,** b. retrohyoidea.

**b. retrohyoi'dea** [ NA ], retrohyoid b.; Boyer's b.; b. of hyoid; subhyoid b.; a b. between the posterior surface of the body of the hyoid bone and the thyrohyoid membrane.

**rider's b.,** an adventitious b. on the inner side of the knee caused by horseback riding.

**b. of sem'imembrano'sus,** b. musculi semimembranosi.

**subacromial b.,** b. subacromialis.

**b. subacromia'lis** [ NA ], subacromial b.; between the acromion and the capsule of the shoulder joint.

**b. subcuta'nea acromia'lis** [ NA ], the b. between the acromion and the skin.

**b. subcuta'nea calca'nea** [ NA ], a b. in the sole of the foot superficial to the calcaneus.

**b. subcuta'nea infrapatella'ris** [ NA ], subcutaneous infrapatellar b.; between the patellar ligament and the skin.

**b. subcuta'nea malle'oli latera'lis** [ NA ], the b. overlying the lateral malleolus.

**b. subcuta'nea malle'oli media'lis** [ NA ], the b. overlying the medial malleolus.

**b. subcuta'nea olecrani** [ NA ], b. of olecranon; subcutaneous b. over olecranon process of the ulna.

**b. subcuta'nea prepatella'ris** [ NA ], prepatellar b.; between the skin and the lower part of the patella.

**b. subcuta'nea prominen'tiae laryn'geae** [ NA ], the subcutaneous b. located in front of the junction of the laminae of the thyroid cartilage.

**b. subcuta'nea trochanter'ica** [ NA ], the b. overlying the greater trochanter of the femur.

**b. subcuta'nea tuberos'itas tib'iae** [ NA ], the b. located superficial to the tibial tuberosity, either subcutaneous or subfascial.

**subcutaneous infrapatellar b.,** b. subcutanea infrapatellaris.

**subdeltoid b.,** b. subdeltoidea.

**b. subdeltoid'ea** [ NA ], subdeltoid b.; the b. between the deltoid muscle and the capsule of the shoulder joint. It may be combined with the subacromial b.

**b. subfascia'lis prepatella'ris** [ NA ], a b. between the fascia lata and the quadriceps tendon anterior to the patella.

**subhy'oid b.,** b. retrohyoidea.

**b. sublingua'lis,** Fleischmann's b.

**subscap'ular b.,** b. subtendinea musculi subscapularis.

**b. subtendinea iliaca** [ NA ], subtendinous iliac b.; iliac b.; the b. at the insertion of the iliopsoas muscle into the lesser trochanter.

**b. subtendinea musculi bicipitis femoris inferior** [ NA ], the b. between the tendon of insertion of the biceps femoris and the fibular collateral ligament of the knee joint.

**b. subtendineae musculi gastrocnemii** [ NA ], b. of gastrocnemius; subtendinous b. of the gastrocnemius, consisting of lateral and medial b. between the heads of the gastrocnemius and capsule of the knee joint.

**b. subtendin'ea musculi infraspinat'i** [ NA ], the b. located between the tendon of the infraspinatus and the capsule of the shoulder joint.

**b. subtendinea musculi latissimus dorsi** [ NA ], b. of latissimus dorsi; a constant b. between the tendons of the teres major and the latissimus dorsi near their intersections.

**b. subtendinea musculi obturato'rii interni** [ NA ], b. between the tendon of the obturator internus muscle and the femur.

**bursae subtendin'eae musculi sarto'rii** [ NA ], bursae, sometimes separate from the b. anserina, located between the tendons of the sartorius, semitendinosus, and gracilis muscles.

**b. subtendinea musculi subscapularis** [ NA ], subscapular b.; between the tendon of the subscapularis muscle and the neck of the scapula; it communicates with the shoulder joint.

**b. subtendinea musculi teretis majoris** [ NA ], b. of teres major; b. under the tendon of the teres major near its insertion.

**b. subtendin'ea musculi tibia'lis anterio'ris** [ NA ], the small b. between the medial surface of the first cuneiform bone and the tendon of the tibialis anterior.

**b. subtendinea musculi trapezii** [ NA ], b. of trapezius; a b. between the tendon of the trapezius muscle and the medial end of the scapular spine.

**b. subtendin'ea musculi tricip'itus brachii** [ NA ], the b. located deep to the tendon of the triceps brachii near its insertion on the olecranon.

**b. subtendin'ea prepatella'ris** [ NA ], a b. between the tendon of the quadriceps and the patella.

**suprapatellar b.,** b. suprapatellaris.

**b. suprapatella'ris** [ NA ], suprapatellar b.; a large b. between the lower part of the femur and the tendon of the quadriceps femoris muscle. It usually communicates with the cavity of the knee joint.

**synovial b.,** b. synovialis.

**synovial trochlear b.,** *vagina* synovialis musculorum obliqui superioris.

**b. synovia'lis** [ NA ], synovial b.; b. mucosa; a sac containing synovial fluid which occurs at sites of friction, as between a tendon and a bone over which it plays, or subcutaneously over a bony prominence. The NA lists the following types: b. synovialis subcutanea, b. synovialis submuscularis, b. synovialis subfascialis, and b. synovialis subtendinea.

**b. tendinis calcanei** [ NA ], bursa achillis [ NA ]; b. of tendo calcaneus; Achilles b.; b. between the tendo calcaneus and the upper part of the posterior surface of the calcaneum.

**b. of tendo calca'neus,** b. tendinis calcanei (achillis).

**b. of tensor veli palatini muscle,** b. musculi tensoris veli palatini.

**b. of te'res major,** b. subtendinea musculi teretis majoris.

**tib'ial interten'dinous b.,** b. anserina.

**b. of trape'zius,** b. subtendinea musculi trapezii.

**trochanter'ic b.,** b. trochanterica musculi glutei maximi.

**b. trochanter'ica musculi glutei maximi** [ NA ], trochanteric b.; a multilocular b. between the gluteus maximus muscle and the great trochanter of the femur.

**bursae trochanter'icae musculi glutei medii** [ NA ], the b. between the tendon of the gluteus medius and the greater trochanter and the b. between the piriformis and gluteus medius.

**b. trochanter'ica musculi glutei minimi** [ NA ], a fairly large b. usually located between the gluteus minimus and the greater trochanter.

**trochlear synovial b.,** *vagina* synovialis musculorum obliqui superioris.

**ulnar b.,** *vagina* synovialis communis musculorum flexorum.

**bur'sal.** Relating to a bursa.

**bursautee** (bur-saw'te) [ E. Indian ]. An old term for chronic, granulomatous skin diseases of horses, now known more specifically as cutaneous habronemiasis and phycomycosis. Also spelled bursatti and bursattee.

**bursec'tomy** [ bursa + G. *ektomē,* excision ]. Surgical removal of a bursa.

**bur'sicon.** A substance secreted by various elements of the insect nervous system after molting; it promotes hardening and tanning of the new cuticle.

**bur'sine.** Choline.

**bursi'tis.** Inflammation of a bursa.

　**bicipital b.,** intertubercular b.

　**calcaneal b.,** capped hock; inflammation of one of the bursae related to the tuber calcanei, usually a result of trauma to the subcutaneous bursa; occurs most frequently in the horse.

　**intertubercular b.,** shoulder b.; bicipital b.; inflammation of the intertubercular bursa of the biceps brachii muscle of the shoulder of the horse, usually the result of trauma.

　**prepatellar b.,** housemaid's *knee.*

**shoulder b.,** intertubercular b.

**subacromial b.,** scapulohumeral *periarthritis.*

**subdeltoid b.,** scapulohumeral *periarthritis.*

**trochanteric b.,** inflammation of one of the trochanteric bursae of the horse, and a common cause of hip lameness.

**bur'solith** [ bursa + G. *lithos,* stone ]. A calculus formed in a bursa.

**bursop'athy.** Any disease of a bursa.

**bursot'omy** [ bursa + G. *tomē,* a cutting ]. Incision through the wall of a bursa.

**bur'sula** [ Mod. L. dim. of Mediev. L. *bursa,* purse ]. A small pouch or bag.

**b. tes'tium,** scrotum.

**Burton,** Henry, English physician, 1799–1849. See B.'s *line.*

**Bury,** Judson S., English dermatologist, 1852–1944. See B.'s *disease.*

**Buschke,** Abraham, German dermatologist, 1868–1943. See B.'s *disease,* Busse-B. *disease, B.-.Löwenstein tumor.*

**Busquet** (büs-ka'), G. Paul, French physician, *1866. See B.'s *disease.*

**Busse-Buschke disease.** See under disease.

**busulfan** (USP). MYLERAN; busulphan (BP); 1,4-butanediol dimethanesulfonate; tetramethylene *bis*(methanesulfonate); $CH_3O_2SO(CH_2)_4OSO_2CH_3$. It is absorbed from the mucous membranes, and selectively depresses proliferation of granulocytic elements. Used in the treatment of chronic myelocytic leukemia; known to be teratogenic in humans.

**bu'tabar'bital.** BUTISOL; butabarbitone; 5-*sec*-butyl-5-ethylbarbituric acid; sedative and hypnotic with intermediate duration of action.

**b. sodium** (NF), BUTISOL sodium; same uses as b.

**bu'tabar'bitone** (BP). Butabarbital.

**bu'tacaine sulfate** (BP). BUTYN sulfate; 3-(dibutylamino)-1-propanol *p*-aminobenzoate sulfate; a local anesthetic, recommended especially for the eye.

**butalbital** (bu-tal'bĭ-tal) (USAN). SANDOPTAL; allylbarbital; 5-allyl-5-isobutylbarbituric acid; a barbiturate of intermediate duration of action; sedative and hypnotic.

**butallylonal** (bu'tä-lil-o-nal). PERNOSTON; 5-(2-bromoallyl)-5-*sec*-butylbarbituric acid; barbiturate with intermediate duration of action; a hypnotic once widely used, especially in Europe.

**butam'ben.** Butyl aminobenzoate.

**bu'tane.** $C_4H_{10}$; a gaseous hydrocarbon present in natural gas. Various isomers are known, many of which are anesthetically active, as is butane itself.

**butanedioic acid** (bu'tän-di-o'ik). Succinic acid.

**butanilicaine phosphate.** HOSTACAINE; 2-(butylamino)-6'-chloro-*o*-acetotoluidide; an aminoacyl anilide local anesthetic used for regional nerve blocks.

**butano'ic acid.** Butyric acid.

**bu'tanol.** Butyl alcohol.

**butaper'azine** (USAN). REPOISE; 1-{ 10-[ 3-(4-methyl-1-piperazinyl)propyl ]-phenothiazin-2-yl}-1-butanone; antipsychotic.

**butav'erine hydrochloride.** GEMORA; β-phenyl-1-piperidinepropionic acid butyl ester; intestinal antispasmodic.

**butazol'amide.** BUTAMIDE; *N*-(5-sulfamoyl-1,3,4-thiadiazol-2-yl)butyramide; carbonic anhydrase inhibitor, used for induction of diuresis.

**butethal** (bu'te-thal). BUTOBARBITAL; NEONAL; butobarbitone; 5-butyl-5-ethylbarbituric acid; sedative and hypnotic.

**buteth'amate.** PHENESIN; 2-phenylbutyric acid 2-(diethylamino)ethyl ester; intestinal antispasmodic agent.

**buteth'amine hydrochloride.** MONOCAINE hydrochloride; local anesthetic.

**buthal'ital sodium.** TRANSITHAL; thialbutone sodium; 5-allyl-5-isobutyl-2-thiobarbituric acid sodium salt; used for intravenous anesthesia.

**buthi'azide** (USAN). 6-Chloro-3, 4-dihydro-3-isobutyl-2*H*-1,2,4-benzothiadiazine-7-sulfonamide 1,1-dioxide; a diuretic, also with antihypertensive action.

**bu'tobar'bitone.** Butethal.

**bu'topyr'onox'yl.** INDALONE; butyl mesityl oxide oxalate; an insect repellent, effective against the biting stable fly (*Stomoxys calcitrans*).

**butox'amine hydrochloride** (USAN). α-{ 1-(*tert*-Butylamino)ethyl ]-2,5-dimethoxybenzyl alcohol hydrochloride; experimental agent that inhibits mobilization of fatty acid.

**t-butoxycarbonyl.** Abbreviated Boc (formerly BOC or *t*-BOC); *tert*-butyloxycarbonyl; $(CH_3)_3$ C—O—CO—; an amino-protecting group used in peptide synthesis.

**2-butox'ypro'caine.** Ambucaine.

**butrip'tyline hydrochloride** (USAN). *dl*-10,11-Dihydro-*N,N,β* -trimethyl-5*H*-dibenzo [*a,d*]cycloheptene-5- pro pylamine; antidepressant.

**butt.** 1. To bring any two square-ended surfaces in contact so as to form a joint. 2. In dentistry, to place a restoration directly against the tissues covering the alveolar ridge.

**butter** [ L. *butyrum,* G. *boutyron,* prob. fr. *bous,* cow, + *tyron,* cheese ]. 1. A coherent mass of milk fat, obtained by churning or shaking cream until the separate fat globules run together, leaving a liquid residue, buttermilk. 2. A soft solid having more or less the consistency of butter.

**b. of an'timony,** antimony trichloride.

**b. of bismuth,** bismuth trichloride.

**caca'o b., co'coa b.,** theobroma oil; see also cacao.

**b. of tin,** stannic chloride pentahydrate, $SnCl_4 \cdot 5H_2O$.

**b. yellow,** methyl y.; dimethylaminoazobenzene; *p*-dimethylaminoazobenzene, $C_6H_5N:NC_6H_4N(CH_2)_2$, occurs as yellow leaflets or as a yellow crystalline powder. It is a fat-soluble yellow dye which has a carcinogenic action in experimental animals. Used as an indicator pH: red, 2.9; yellow, 4.0.

**b. of zinc,** zinc chloride.

**Butter's cancer.** See under cancer.

**but'terfly.** 1. Any structure or apparatus resembling in shape a butterfly with outstretched wings. 2. Butterfly eruption, patch, or rash; a scaling lesion on each cheek, joined by a narrow band across the nose; seen in lupus erythematosus and seborrheic dermatitis.

**but'termilk.** The fluid containing casein and lactic acid, left after the process of making butter.

**but'ternut.** Juglans.

**but'tock.** Nates.

**but'ton** [ Middle Fr. *boton,* a bud, probably fr. L. *bottere,* to thrust ]. 1. A structure or lesion of knob shape. 2. An apparatus or part of an apparatus of the shape of a small ball or knob.

**Amboy'na b.** [ *Amboyna,* one of the Spice Islands in the Malay Archipelago ], yaws.

**Biskra b.,** the tropical sore of cutaneous leishmaniasis.

**Murphy's b.,** an appliance for intestinal anastomosis; it consists of two hollow cylinders, one of which is sutured into each open end of the intestine; the two are then joined and fasten automatically, maintaining the two ends of intestine in apposition by their serous surfaces; after firm union has occurred the cylinders slough away and are passed in the stools.

**Oriental b.,** the tropical sore of cutaneous leishmaniasis.

**peritoneal b.,** a device used to drain ascitic fluid to subcutaneous space.

**Villard's b.,** a modified Murphy's b.

**but'tonhole.** 1. A short straight cut made through the wall of a cavity or canal. 2. The contraction of an orifice down to a narrow slit; *i.e.,* the so-called mitral b. in extreme mitral stenosis.

**bu'tyl.** A radical of butane; $C_4H_9$—.

**b. alcohol,** $C_4H_9OH$; several isomeric forms are known: primary normal butyl alcohol, the butyl alcohol of fermentation, $CH_3CH_2CH_2CH_2OH$; isobutyl alcohol, $(CH_3)_2CHCH_2OH$; secondary butyl alcohol, $CH_3CH_2CH(CH_3)OH$; and tertiary butyl alcohol, $(CH_3)_3COH$; or propylcarbinol, isopropylcarbinol, ethylmethylcarbinol, and trimethylcarbinol, respectively.

**b. aminobenzoate** (NF). BUTESIN; butamben; *n*-butyl *p*-aminobenzoate; local anesthetic, very insoluble and only slightly absorbed; applied directly to wounds or burns as a dusting powder, or in the form of troches, ointment, suppositories, or oil solution.

**b. chloral hydrate,** trichlorobutyl aldehyde; 1,1,2-tri-chloro-*n*-butylaldehyde hydrate; $CH_3CHCl—CCl_2—CH(OH)_2$; formerly called, incorrectly, croton-chloral hydrate; formerly used for the temporary relief of trigeminal neuralgia.

**butyl'amine.** A colorless, transparent liquid, $C_4H_{11}NH_2$, miscible with water. Intermediate for pharmaceuticals, dyestuffs, etc.

**butylated hydroxyanisole** (BP). 2-*t*-Butyl-4-methoxy-phenol; an antioxidant.

**butylated hydroxytoluene** (NF, BP). 2,6-Di-*t*-butyl-*p*-cresol; an antioxidant.

**2,5-*bis*-2-(5-*t*-butylbenzoxazolyl)-thiophene.** BBOT; a scintillator used in radioactivity measurements by scintillation counting.

*tert*-**butyloxycarbonyl.** See *t*-butoxycarbonyl.

**butylpar'aben** (USP). BUTEBEN; butyl *p*-hydroxybenzoate; antifungal preservative.

**butylvi'nal.** SPEDA; 5-(1-methylbutyl)-5-vinylbarbituric acid; hypnotic with intermediate duration of action.

**butyraceous** (bu'tir-a'shĭ-us). Buttery in consistence.

**bu'tyrate.** A salt or ester of butyric acid.

**butyr'ic.** Relating to butter.

**b. acid,** butanoic acid; an acid of unpleasant odor, occurring in butter, cod liver oil, sweat, and many other substances. It exists in two forms: **normal butyric acid,** butanoic acid; ethylacetic acid, propylformic acid; $(CH_3CH_2CH_2COOH)$; occurs as a glyceride in cow's butter; **isobutyric acid,** dimethylacetic acid, $(CH_3)_2CHCOOH)$; one of the intermediates in valine catabolism, found as a glyceride in croton oil and elsewhere.

**bu'tyrocho'lines'terase.** Cholinesterase.

**bu'tyroid.** 1. Buttery. 2. Resembling butter.

**butyrom'eter** [ G. *boutyron*, butter, + *metron*, measure ]. An instrument for determining the amount of butterfat in milk.

**butyrophe'none.** One of a group of derivatives of 4-phenylbutylamine that have neuroleptic activity; *e.g.*, haloperidol.

**bu'tyrous.** Denoting a tissue or bacterial growth of butter-like consistency.

**bu'tyryl.** The radical of butyric acid, $C_3H_7COO—$.

**butyrylcholine esterase.** Cholinesterase.

**butyryl-CoA synthetase** (EC 6.2.1.2). Fatty acid thiokinase (medium chain); similar to acyl-CoA synthetase, but acts on acids from $C_4$ to $C_{11}$.

**bu'tystat.** 5-Butyl-6-methyl-2-thiouracil; antithyroid agent.

**Buzzard,** Thomas, London physician, 1831–1919. See B.'s *maneuver.*

**Buzzi,** S. See Schweninger-B. *anetoderma.*

**by'pass.** Shunt.

**aortocoronary b.,** coronary b.

**aortoiliac b.,** an operation in which a vascular prosthesis is used between the aorta and femoral artery to relieve obstruction of the lower abdominal aorta, its bifurcation, and the proximal iliac branches.

**cardiopulmonary b.,** a method of maintaining extracorporeal circulation by diversion of the blood flow away from the heart; blood is passed through a pump oxygenator (heart-lung machine) and then returned to the arterial side of the circulation; used in operations upon the heart.

**coronary b.,** aortocoronary b.; an operation to shunt blood through vein grafts or other conduits from the aorta to branches of the coronary arteries, in order to increase the flow beyond the local obstruction.

**femoropopliteal b.,** an operation in which a vascular prosthesis is used to bypass an obstruction in the femoral artery; graft may be synthetic material (Dacron), autologous tissue (saphenous vein), or heterologous tissue (bovine carotid artery).

**jejunoileal b.,** jejunoileal shunt; anastomosis of the upper jejunum to the terminal ileum, retaining the excluded intestine, which is closed proximally and anastomosed to the colon distally; for treatment of morbid obesity.

**byssinosis** (bis'ĭ-no'sis) [ G. *byssos*, flax, + suffix -*osis*, condition ]. Cotton-mill fever; an occupational respiratory disease of cotton, flax, and hemp workers. It is characterized by symptoms (especially wheezing) most severe at the beginning of each work week.

**byssocausis** (bis'o-kaw'sis) [ G. *byssos*, flax, + *kausis*, burning ]. Use of the moxa.

# C

**C.** 1. Abbreviation for cylinder, cylindrical lens, cathode, cathodal, centigrade, Celsius, contraction, closure (of an electrical circuit), congius (gallon), large calorie (Calorie). 2. Chemical symbol for the element carbon. 3. Symbol for cytidine (ribosylcytosine). 4. When followed by a subscript, indicates renal clearance of a substance (*e.g.*, $C_{In}$, clearance of inulin), compliance (*e.g.*, $C_L$, compliance of the lungs), or concentration (3).

**c.** 1. Abbreviation for L. *centum* (one hundred), *cum* (with), and small calorie. 2. As a subscript, refers to blood *capillary*.

**CA.** Abbreviation for (1) carcinoma; (2) cancer; (3) cytosine arabinoside; (4) *Chemical Abstracts* Service.

**Ca.** 1. Abbreviation for cathode. 2. Chemical symbol of the element calcium.

**ca.** Abbreviation for Latin *circa* (about, approximately).

**caapi.** Aya huasca; wild rue; a hallucinogenic preparation obtained from *Banisteria caapi* (family Malpighaceae), a South American jungle vine; contains harmine and other psychotomimetic principles.

**cab'bage tree.** Andira.

**cab'inet.** A box or small chamber.

    **pneumatic c.,** an airtight box of steel with plate glass front, large enough to hold a person sitting, in which the air may be condensed or rarified at will.

    **Sauerbruch's c.,** an airtight chamber permitting operation on the thorax under negative air pressure, the patient lying within the c. with his head outside.

**Cabot,** Arthur T., American surgeon, 1852–1912. See C.'s *splint*.

**Cabot,** Richard C., Boston physician, 1868–1939. See C.'s ring *bodies*.

**Cabot-Locke murmur.** See under murmur.

**cac-, caci-.** See caco-.

**cacao** (kă-ka'o) [ native Mexican origin ] (USP). Prepared c.; cocoa; a powder prepared from the roasted cured kernels of the ripe seed of *Theobroma cacao Linné* (family Sterculiaceae). The tree is a handsome evergreen cultivated in the tropics. It yields chocolate and "cocoa," used as beverages, and a fat, theobroma oil. The latter is used in the making of suppositories and for other pharmaceutical purposes.

    **c. oil,** theobroma oil.

**cacation** (kă-ka'shun) [ L. *caco*, pp. *-atus*, to go to stool ]. Defecation.

**cacatory** (kak'ă-to-rĭ). Relating to bowel movements, especially excessive discharges or diarrhea.

**CaCC,** or **CCC.** Abbreviation for cathodal closure *contraction*.

**Cacchione,** Aldo. See De Sanctis-C. *syndrome*.

**cacergasia** (kak-er-gas'ĭ-ah) [ G. *kakergasia*, fr. *kakos*, bad, + *ergasia*, work. ERG- ]. Kakergasia; poor functioning of mind or body.

**cacesthesia** (kak-es-the'zĭ-ah) [ G. *kakos*, bad, + *aisthēsis*, sensation ]. Kakesthesia. 1. Malaise. 2. Any disorder of sensibility.

**caché** (kă-sha') [ Fr. hidden, covered ]. A lead cone covered with several layers of paper, having a mica window at the bottom. Used as an applicator in radiotherapy, the radium or other radioactive substance being at the apex of the cone and filters being placed below as required.

**cachectic** (kă-kek'tik). Relating to or suffering from cachexia.

**cachet** (kă-sha') [ Fr. a seal ]. A seal-shaped capsule or wafer for enclosing powders of disagreeable taste.

**cachexia** (kă-kek'sĭ-ah) [ G. *kakos*, bad, + *hexis*, a habit of body ]. A general lack of nutrition and wasting occurring in the course of a chronic disease or emotional disturbance.

    **African c.,** geophagia.

    **c. aphtho'sa,** sprue (2).

    **c. aquo'sa,** an edematous form of ancylostomiasis.

    **Grawitz' c.,** a fatal c., resembling pernicious anemia but with no degenerative changes in the red blood cells, occurring especially in the aged.

    **c. hypophysea,** Simmonds' *disease*.

    **c. hypophys'eopri'va,** a condition following total removal of the hypophysis cerebri, marked by a fall of body temperature, electrolyte imbalance, and hypoglycemia, followed by coma and death.

    **hypophysial c.,** Simmonds' *disease*.

    **lymphatic c.,** obsolete term for lymphoma.

    **malarial c.,** chronic *malaria*.

    **mercurial c.,** chronic mercurial *poisoning*.

    **c. ovariopri'va,** ill health resulting from removal or destruction of ovaries.

    **pituitary c.,** Simmonds' *disease*.

    **sat'urnine c.,** chronic lead *poisoning*.

    **c. suprarenalis,** obsolete term for Addison's *disease*.

    **c. strumipri'va,** c. thyropriva, resulting from removal of a goiter.

    **c. thyroid'ea,** c. thyropriva.

    **c. thyropri'va,** c. thyroidea; signs and symptoms of myxedema resulting from the loss of thyroid tissue, either at surgery or by radiotherapy.

    **c. urina'ria, urinary c.,** (1) toxic symptoms occurring with renal infection caused by back pressure from an overdistended bladder, *e.g.*, in prostatic hypertrophy; (2) the constitutional disturbance accompanying suppuration anywhere in the urinary tract.

**cachinnation** (kak-ĭ-na'shun) [ L. *cachinnare*, to laugh immoderately and loudly ]. Laughter without apparent cause often found in schizophrenia.

**caco-, caci-, cac-** (kak-o-) [ G. *kakos*, bad ]. Combining forms meaning bad or ill.

**cacocholia** (kak'o'ko'lĭ-ah) [ caco- + G. *cholē*, bile ]. An abnormal state of the bile.

**cacochylia** (kak-o-ki'lĭ-ah) [ caco- + G. *chylos*, juice, CHY- ]. 1. An abnormal state of the gastric juice. 2. Indigestion.

**cacochymia** (kak-o-ki'mĭ-ah) [ caco- + G. *chymos*, juice, CHY- ]. 1. Cacochylia. 2. Disordered metabolism.

**cacodemonomania** (kak-o-de'mon-o-ma'nĭ-ah) [ caco- + G. *daimōn*, spirit, + *mania*, frenzy ]. A mental condition in which the patient believes himself to be inhabited by or possessed by an evil spirit.

**cacodyl** (kak'o-dil). Tetramethyldiarsine; dicacodyl; $(CH_3)_2As$—$As(CH_3)_2$; an evil smelling oil resulting from the distillation together of arsenous acid and potassium acetate.

**cacodylate** (kak'o-dil-āt). A salt or ester of cacodylic acid.

**cacodyl'ic.** Relating to cacodyl; denoting especially c. acid.

    **c. acid,** dimethylarsinic acid; $(CH_3)_2AsOOH$; prepared by treating cacodyl and cacodyl oxide with mercuric oxide; forms cacodylates with various bases which were used in skin diseases, tuberculosis, malaria, and other affections in which arsenic was considered of value.

**cacoethic** (kak-o-e'thik). Ingravescent, ill-conditioned, or malignant.

**cacogenesis** (kak-o-jen'ĕ-sis) [ caco- + G. *genesis*, origin ]. Abnormal growth or development.

**cacogenic** (kak-o-jen'ik). 1. Relating to cacogenesis. 2. Tending toward racial deterioration through bad sexual selection.

**cacogenics** (kak-o-jen'iks). The opposite of eugenics; the aggregation of factors tending, through adverse sexual selection, to the deterioration of the race.

**cacogeusia** (kak-o-ju'sĭ-ah) [ caco- + G. *geusis*, taste ]. A bad taste.

**cacomelia** (kak-o-me'lĭ-ah) [ caco- + G. *melos*, limb ]. A congenital deformity of one or more of the limbs.

**cacoplas'tic** [ caco- + G. *plastikos*, formed ]. 1. Relating to or causing morbid growth. 2. Incapable of normal or perfect formation.

**cacorhythmic** (kak-o-rith'mik). Marked by disturbance of cardiac rhythm.

**cacos′mia** [ G. *kakosmia,* a bad smell, fr. *kakos,* bad, + *osmē,* the sense of smell ]. Kakosmia; a subjective perception of disagreeable odors that do not exist; a variety of parosmia.

**cacostomia** (kak-o-sto′mĭ-ah) [ caco- + G. *stoma,* mouth ]. Kakostomia; obsolete term for noma, severe stomatitis.

**cac′othen′ic.** Cacogenic.

**cac′othen′ics.** Cacogenics.

**cacotrophy** (kă-kot′ro-fĭ) [ caco- + G. *trophē,* nourishment ]. Obsolete term for malnutrition.

**cactinomycin** (kak′tĭ-no-mi′sin) (USAN). Actinomycin C; SANAMYCIN; produced by *Streptomyces chrysomallus.* It is a mixture of actinomycins C₁ (dactinomycin), C₂, and C₃. Used as an antineoplastic, immunosuppressive agent. See also actinomycin.

**cacumen,** pl. **cacu′mina** (kak-u′men) [ L. summit ]. 1. The top or apex of anything, of a plant or an anatomical structure. 2. The anterior portion of the superior vermis of the cerebellum; culmen.

**cacu′minal.** Relating to the top or apex of anything.

**cadaver** (kă-dav′er) [ L. fr. *cado,* to fall. CAD- ]. A dead body; corpse.

**cadav′eric.** Relating to a dead body.

**cadav′erine.** H₂N(CH₂)₅NH₂; a foul-smelling diamine formed by bacterial decarboxylation of lysine.

**cadav′erous.** Having the pallor and appearance of a corpse.

**cade oil.** Juniper tar.

**cad′mium** [ L. *cadmia,* G. *kadmeia* or *kadmia,* an ore of zinc, calamine ]. A metallic element, symbol Cd, atomic no. 48, atomic weight 112.40, resembling tin in appearance and zinc in its chemical relations. Its salts are poisonous and little used in medicine. Various compounds of c. (acetate, chloride, hydroxide, selenide, sulfate, etc.) are used in metallurgy, photography, electrochemistry, and other industries; a few (oxide, salicylate, succinate, sulfide, sulfate) have been used as toxic agents (ascaricide, antiseptic, fungicide).

**c. sulfide,** CAPSEBON; used in seborrheic dermatitis of the scalp. Appears to be as effective as selenium sulfide but less irritating and essentially nontoxic.

**CaDTe.** Abbreviation for cathodal duration *tetanus.*

**caduca** (kă-du′kah) [ L. fem. of *caducus,* fallen, falling, fr. *cado,* to fall ]. *Membrana* decidua.

**caduceus** (kă-du′se-us) [ L. the staff of Mercury ]. A staff with two oppositely twined serpents and surmounted by two wings. The emblem of the Medical Corps, U.S. Army. The staff of Aesculapius (see under Aesculapius) is the

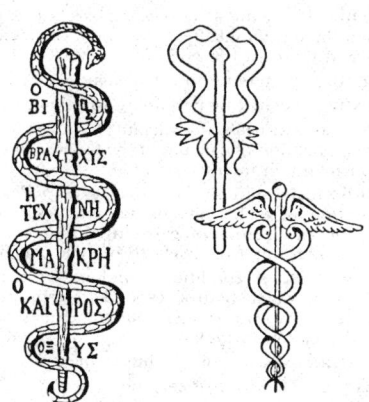

**Caduceus**

*Upper right,* caduceus carried by Mercury; *left,* wand of of Aesculapius; *lower right,* insignia of the United States Army Medical Corps. (From Skinner, H. A.: *The Origin of Medical Terms,* The Williams & Wilkins Co., Baltimore, 1961.)

correct symbol of the medical profession. For veterinary medicine the double serpent was changed in 1972 to its present form with a single serpent.

**cae-.** For words so beginning, see under ce-.

**Caelius Aurelianus** (se′lĭ-us aw-re-lĭ-a′nus), *ca.* 5th century A.D. The outstanding physician and medical writer (*De morbis acutis et chronicis*) following Galen.

**Caesalpinus,** Andrea. See Cesalpino.

**caffeic** (kă-fe′ik). Relating to coffee.

**caffeine** (kaf′ēn) (USP, BP). Guaranine; thein; 1,3,7-trimethylxanthine; an alkaloid obtained from the dried leaves of *Thea sinensis,* tea, or the dried seeds of *Coffea arabica,* coffee; used as a diuretic and circulatory and respiratory stimulant, and in the treatment of headaches.

**c. citrate,** citrated c., a mixture of equal parts of c. and citric acid.

**c. hydrate** (BP), monohydrate of c.; central nervous system stimulant.

**c. and sodium ben′zoate** (USP), a mixture of equal parts of sodium benzoate and c. Used to meet the indication of c.

**c. and sodium salic′ylate,** a mixture of sodium salicylate and c. Used for the relief of headache and neuralgia.

**caffeinism** (kaf′ēn-izm). Chronic coffee poisoning, characterized by palpitation, dyspepsia, irritability, and insomnia.

**caf′feol.** Caffeone; caffeon; an aromatic oil obtained by roasting coffee; consists of 50 per cent of furfurol alcohol, and small quantities of valerianic acid, phenol, pyridine, and a nitrogenous aromatic substance. The coffee aroma is believed to be due to this substance.

**caf′feon, caf′feone.** Caffeol.

**Caffey,** John, U. S. pediatrician, *1895. See C.'s *disease,* *syndrome,* C.-Silverman *syndrome.*

**cage** (kāj). An enclosure made partly or completely of open work and commonly used to house animals; a structure resembling such an enclosure.

**Faraday c.,** an enclosure screened from external electrical waves, used in electroencephalography.

**thoracic c.,** the skeletal thorax consisting of the thoracic vertebrae, the ribs with their costal cartilages, and the sternum; it supports and protects the thoracic organs and is important in respiration.

**cahinca root** (ka-hing′kah). David's root; snowberry; cainca; the root of *Chiococca racemosa* and other species of *Chiococca* (family Rubiaceae), plants of tropical America; diuretic and purgative.

**cainca.** Cahinca root.

**cainogen′esis.** Cenogenesis.

**cainopho′bia.** Cenotophobia.

**Cajal** (ka-hal′) (Ramon y Cajal), Santiago, Spanish histologist, 1852–1934. Nobel laureate, 1906, with Camillo Golgi, in recognition of their work on the structure of the nervous system. See C.'s *cells,* interstitial *nucleus* of C., C.'s astrocyte *stain.*

**caj′eputene.** Limonene.

**cajeput oil** (kaj′e-put). Cajuput oil; a volatile oil distilled from the fresh leaves of *Cajuputi viridiflora,* a tree of tropical Asia and Australia; stimulant, counterirritant, and expectorant.

**caj′eputol, caj′uputol.** Cineole.

**Cal′abar bean.** Physostigma.

**calabarine** (kal′ă-bar-ēn). A liquid alkaloid believed to be a mixture of physostigmine decomposition products.

**cal′abash tree.** *Adansonia digitata.*

**calage** (kal-azh′) [ Fr. wedging ]. Wedging the body in the berth by means of pillows, in order to prevent rolling in case of seasickness.

**cal′amine.** 1. Zinc oxide with a small amount of ferric oxide (USP) or basic zinc carbonate suitably colored with ferric oxide (BP); used in dusting powders, lotions, and ointments, as a mild astringent and protective agent for skin disorders. 2. Hydrous zinc silicate; Zn₂SiO₄H₂O. 3. Native form of zinc carbonate. 4. An alkaloid. 5. An alloy.

**cal′amus** [ L. reed, a pen ]. 1. Sweet flag; the dried, unpeeled rhizome of *Acorus calamus* (family Araceae); aromatic and stomachic. 2. A reed-shaped structure.

c. scripto′rius [ L. writing pen ], Arantius' ventricle; inferior part of the rhomboid fossa; the narrow lower end of the fourth ventricle between the two clavae.

calcaneal, calcanean (kal-ka′ne-al, kal-ka′ne′an). Relating to the calcaneus or heel bone.

calcaneo- (kal-ka′ne-o-) [ L. calcaneum, heel. CALX-1 ]. Combining form relating to the calcaneus.

calca′neoapoph′ysi′tis. Inflammation at posterior part of os calcis, at insertion of Achilles tendon.

calca′neoastrag′aloid. Relating to the calcaneus, or os calcis, and the astragalus, or talus.

calca′neocu′boid. Relating to the calcaneus and the cuboid bone.

calcaneodynia (kal-ka′ne-o-din′ĭ-ah) [ calcaneo- + G. odynē, pain ]. Painful heel.

calca′neonavic′ular. Calcaneoscaphoid; relating to the calcaneus and the navicular bone.

calca′neoscaph′oid. Calcaneonavicular.

calca′neotib′ial. Relating to the calcaneus and the tibia.

calcaneovalgus (kal-ka′ne-o-val′gus). See talipes calcaneovalgus.

calcaneovarus (kal-ka′ne-o-va′rus). See talipes calcaneovarus.

calca′neum [ L. the heel. CALX-1 ]. Calcaneus.

calca′neus, gen. and pl. calca′nei (kal-ka′ne-us) [ L. the heel (another form of calcaneum) ]. 1 [ NA ]. Calcaneum; calcaneous bone; heel bone; os calcis; the largest of the tarsal bones; it forms the heel and articulates with the cuboid anteriorly and the talus above. 2. Talipes calcaneus.

calcar (kal′kar) [ L. spur, cock's spur. CALX-1 ]. Spur or spurlike process. 1 [ NA ]. A small projection from any structure; internal spurs (septa) at the level of division of arteries and confluence of veins when branches or roots form an acute angle. 2. A dull spine or projection from a bone. 3. A horny outgrowth from the skin. See also subentries under spur.

c. a′vis [ NA ], hippocampus minor; Morand's spur; Haller's unguis; unguis avis; the lower of two elevations on the medial wall of the posterior horn of the lateral ventricle of the brain, caused by the proximity of the bottom of the calcarine fissure.

c. femora′le, Bigelow's septum; a bony spur springing from the under side of the neck of the femur above and anterior to the lesser trochanter, adding to the strength of this part of the bone.

c. pedis, heel; calx.

calca′reous [ L. calcarius, pertaining to lime, fr. calx, lime. CALX-2 ]. Chalky; relating to or containing lime or calcium, or calcific material.

cal′carine. 1. Relating to a calcar. 2. Spur-shaped.

calcariuria (kal-kar-ĭ-u′rĭ-ah) [ L. calcarius, of lime, + G. ouron, urine ]. Excretion of calcium (lime) salts in the urine.

calcergen (kal′ser-jen). Any substance that produces calcergy at the site of its injection.

calcergy (kal′ser-jĭ) [ L. calx, chalk, calcium, + G. ergon, work, production ]. Local calcification of soft tissue occurring at the site of injection of certain chemical compounds such as lead acetate or cerium chloride. Hydroxylapatite deposits are found in the calcified areas.

calcic (kal′sik). Relating to lime.

calcicosis (kal-sĭ-ko′sis). Pneumoconiosis from the inhalation of limestone dust; sometimes called marble cutter's phthisis.

calcif′erol (BP). Ergocalciferol.

calcif′erous. Containing lime; producing any of the salts of calcium.

calcifica′tion [ L. calx, lime, + facio, to make ]. 1. Deposition of lime or other insoluble calcium salts. 2. A process in which tissue or noncellular material in the body becomes hardened as the result of precipitates or larger deposits of insoluble salts of calcium (and also magnesium), especially calcium carbonate and phosphate.

dystrophic c., that occurring in degenerated or necrotic tissue, as in hyalinized scars, degenerated foci in leiomyomas, caseous nodules and so on.

c. inhibitor, see under inhibitor.

metastat′ic c., that occurring in nonosseous, viable tissue (i.e., tissue that is not degenerated or necrotic), as in the

stomach, lungs, and kidneys (and rarely in other sites); the cells of the organs mentioned secrete acid materials, and, under certain conditions in instances of hypercalcemia, the alteration in pH seems to cause precipitation of calcium salts in these sites.

Mönckeberg's c., Mönckeberg's arteriosclerosis.

pulp c., calcified nodules or amorphous deposits in the pulp of a tooth.

cal′cify. To deposit or lay down calcium salts, as in the formation of bone.

calcimeter (kal-sim′ĭ-ter) [ calcium + G. metron, measure ]. A device for estimating the amount of calcium in the blood or other materials.

Bell's c., a graduated pipet in which a mixture is made for determining the calcium index (see Bell's method).

calcina′tion. The process of calcining.

cal′cine. To expel water and volatile matter by heat; to roast metals, bone, etc.

calcino′sis [ calcium + suffix -osis, condition ]. A condition characterized by the deposition of calcium salts in nodular foci in various tissues other than the parenchymatous viscera; two well known forms of the condition are recognized, i.e., c. circumscripta and c. universalis, as well as a third form that is reversible and is described under several names.

c. circumscrip′ta, Profichet's disease; localized deposits of calcium salts in the skin and subcutaneous tissues; the deposits are usually surrounded by a zone of granulomatous inflammation; clinically, the lesions resemble the tophi of gout.

c. cutis, a deposit of calcium in the skin; it usually occurs secondary to a preexisting inflammatory, degenerative, or neoplastic dermatosis.

c. intervertebralis, calcium deposit in vertebral disk.

reversible c., a form of c. sometimes observed in patients who constantly ingest large quantities of milk and alkaline medicines, as in the treatment of peptic ulcer.

c. universa′lis, diffuse deposits of calcium salts in the skin and subcutaneous tissues, connective tissue, and other sites; this form of c. may be associated with dermatomyositis, occurs more frequently in young persons, and is usually fatal. The serum levels of calcium and phosphorus are generally within normal limits.

cal′ciostat [ calcium + G. statos, standing ]. Rarely used term denoting a postulated mechanism by which the parathyroid hormone production is increased when serum calcium is low and decreased when it is high.

cal′ciotraumat′ic. Relating to the c. line of disturbed calcification that appears in the dentin of the incisor teeth of young rats placed on a rachitogenic diet: high in calcium and low in phosphorus and with no vitamin D.

calcipe′nia [ calcium + G. penia, poverty ]. A condition in which there is an insufficient amount of calcium in the tissues and fluids of the body.

cal′cipe′nic. Pertaining to calcipenia.

calcipex′ic. Related or pertaining to calcipexis.

calcipexis (kal′sĭ-pek′sis) [ calcium + G. pēxis, a fixing ]. Calcipexy; fixation of calcium in the tissues, an occasional cause of tetany in infants.

calciphilia (cal-sĭ-fil′ĭ-ah) [ calcium + G. phileō, to love ]. A condition in which the tissues manifest an unusual affinity for, and fixation of, calcium salts circulating in the blood; manifesting a tendency to become calcified.

cal′ciphylax′is. A condition of induced systemic hypersensitivity in which tissues respond to appropriate challenging agents with a sudden, but sometimes evanescent, local calcification (Selye).

calcipriv′ia. Absence of calcium in diet.

calcipriv′ic. Deprived of calcium.

cal′cite. Calcium carbonate; CaCO₃; calcspar; a naturally occurring mineral found in several forms, e.g., chalk, Iceland spar, limestone, marble. See also calcium carbonate.

calcito′nin (USAN). See thyrocalcitonin. (Calcitonin is a word that was devised to designate a hypocalcemic hormone thought to be secreted by the parathyroid glands, but now known to be of thyroidal origin.)

# CALCIUM

**calcium,** gen. **cal'cii** (kal'sĭ-um) [ Mod. L. fr. L. *calx,* lime. CALX-2 ]. A metallic dyad element, of a lustrous yellow color, symbol Ca, atomic no. 20, atomic weight 40.09, density 1.54, melting point 810°. The oxide of c. is an alkaline earth, CaO, quicklime, which on the addition of water becomes c. hydrate, Ca(OH)$_2$, slaked lime. Several of the salts of c. are used in medicine. For some organic c. salts not listed below, see the name of the organic acid portion. 2. *Factor* IV.

**c. alginate,** a topical hemostatic.

**c. aminosalic'ylate** (NF, BP), the c. salt of *p*-aminosalicylic acid, with the same uses.

**c. ben'zoate,** soluble in 20 parts of water; used as an internal antiseptic and in albuminuria.

**c. benzoylpas** (NF), BENZAPAS; calcium 4-benzamidosalicylate. An effective antituberculous agent for concomitant use with other antituberculous drugs. It is more palatable and produces fewer gastrointestinal disturbances than most of the other aminosalicylates.

**c. bromide,** used to meet the same indications as potassium bromide.

**c. carbas'pirin** (USAN), CALURIN; salicylic acid acetate calcium salt, compound with urea (1:1) complex; analgesic.

**c. carbide,** CaC$_2$; c. acetylide; occurs in blackish crystalline lumps; when in contact with water it yields acetylene gas.

**c. carbimide,** c. cyanamide; Ca = N—C≡N; a fertilizer and weed seed killer that also exhibits antithyroid activity. Like disulfiram, it impairs ethanol metabolism; workers in cyanamide-producing plants exhibit systemic symptoms ("Monday-morning illness") after ingestion of alcohol.

**c. carbimide, citrated,** TEMPOSIL; ABSTEM; a mixture of 2 parts citric acid to 1 part c. carbimide; in the metabolism of ethanol, it slows the conversion of acetaldehyde to acetate; used in the treatment of alcoholism.

**c. car'bonate** (NF, BP), chalk; CaCO$_3$; astringent and antacid; see also calcite.

**c. carbonate, precipitated** (USP), CaCO$_3$; used as an antacid in the management of peptic ulcers and other conditions of gastric hyperacidity.

**c. ca'seinate,** the form of casein present in cow's milk; used in dietetic preparations; has been used for diarrhea in infants.

**c. chloride** (USP, BP), used to correct increased capillary permeability as in urticaria and dermatitis herpetiformis, also in alkalosis and to acidify the urine. It is not well tolerated. Intravenous use requires great caution. The hexahydrate is official in the BP.

**c. cyanamide,** c. carbimide.

**c. cyclamate** (BP), salt of c. and cyclamic acid; noncaloric sweetening agent.

**c. disodium edetate** (USP), edetate calcium disodium.

**c. disodium ethylenediaminetetraacetate,** edetate calcium disodium.

**c. folinate,** leucovorin calcium.

**c. glubi'onate** (USAN), CALGLUCON; calcium D-gluconate lactobionate monohydrate; a calcium replenisher.

**c. gluceptate** (USP), c. glucoheptonate; used as a nutrient.

**c. glucoheptonate,** c. gluceptate.

**c. glu'conate** (USP, BP), a salt of c. more palatable than the chloride.

**c. glycerophos'phate,** a c. and phosphorus dietary supplement.

**c. group,** the metals of the alkaline earths, beryllium, magnesium, calcium, strontium, barium, and radium.

**c. hip'purate,** said to be a solvent of uratic gravel and calculi.

**c. hydroxide** (USP, BP), used to make lime water.

**c. hypophos'phite,** has been used for rickets and impaired nutrition.

**c. index,** see Bell's *method.*

**c. i'odate,** used as a dusting powder and, in lotion and ointment, as an antiseptic and deodorant.

**c. iodobehenate,** c. monoiodobehenate.

**c. ipodate** (USP), calcium 3-[ (dimethylaminomethylene)amino ]-2,4,6-triiodohydrocinnamate; a radiopaque medium used in cholangiography and cholecystography.

**c. lactate** (USP, BP), used for rickets.

**c. lactophos'phate,** a mixture of c. lactate, c. acid lactate, and c. acid phosphate; used as a c. and phosphorus dietary supplement.

**c. leucovorin,** see under leucovorin.

**c. levulinate** (USP), a hydrated c. salt of levulinic acid; it has the usual effects of c. administered orally or intravenously.

**c. man'delate,** urinary anti-infective agent; excreted unchanged in the urine, where it exerts a bacteriostatic and bacteriocidal action against *Escherichia coli, Streptococcus faecalis,* and organisms of the *Proteus, Alcaligenes, Salmonella,* and *Shigella* groups.

**c. mon'ohy'drogen phosphate,** c. phosphate, dibasic.

**c. monoiodobehenate,** CALIOBEN; c. iodobehenate; (C$_{21}$H$_{42}$ICOO)$_2$Ca; used to meet the indications of the ordinary iodides.

**c. ox'alate,** CaC$_2$O$_4$; found as sediment in the urine and in urinary calculi.

**c. oxide,** lime (2).

**c. pantothenate** (USP), the c. salt of pantothenic acid; vitamin B filtrate factor.

**c. pantothenate, racemic** (USP), a mixture of the c. salts of the dextrorotatory and levorotatory isomers of pantothenic acid; same uses as c. pantothenate.

**c. paracaseinate,** the insoluble curd formed by the reaction of Ca$^{++}$ with paracasein.

**c. perman'ganate,** an intestinal antiseptic.

**c. peroxide,** used in acid dyspepsia and as in intestinal antiseptic.

**c. phosphate, dibasic** (NF), c. monohydrogen phosphate; secondary c. phosphate; CaHPO$_4$·2H$_2$O; used as a c. and phosphorus dietary supplement.

**c. phosphate, tribasic** (NF), tricalcium phosphate; tertiary c. phosphate; bone phosphate; bone ash; Ca$_3$-(PO$_4$)$_2$; used as an antacid.

**c. propionate,** the c. salt of propionic acid; antifungal agent.

**c. saccharate,** c. D-saccharate; used as an antacid in dyspepsia and flatulence, as an antidote in carbolic acid poisoning, and as a stabilizer for c. gluconate solution for parenteral administration.

**c. stearate** (NF), used in the preparation of tablets.

**c. sulfate** (NF), dried gypsum; plaster of Paris; used for making plaster splints and other fixed dressings.

**c. sulfide, crude,** sulfurated lime; used in the treatment of boils and acne, and externally as an application to scabies and ringworm.

**c. sulfite,** used as an intestinal antiseptic, and locally in the treatment of parasitic skin diseases.

**c. trisodium pentetate,** Pentetate trisodium calcium.

---

**calcium-45** ($^{45}$Ca). Most easily available of the radioactive c. isotopes; beta-emitter with a half-life of 164 days; used as a tracer.

**calciuria** (kal'sĭ-u're-ah). The urinary excretion of calcium; sometimes used as a synonym for hypercalciuria.

**calcodynia** (kal-ko-din'ĭ-ah) [ L. *calx,* heel, + G. *odynē,* pain ]. Painful *heel.*

**calcoid** (kal'koyd) [ L. *calx,* lime, + G. *eidos,* resemblance ]. Obsolete term for a neoplasm of the tooth pulp.

**calcoph'orous** [ L. *calx,* lime, + G. *phoros,* bearing ]. Calciferous.

**calcospherite** (kal-ko-sfe'rĭt) [ L. *calx,* lime, + G. *sphaira,* sphere ]. Psammoma body (2) a tiny, spheroidal, concentrically laminated body containing accretive deposits of calcium salts; found most frequently in papillary carcinomas of the thyroid and ovary, probably as the result of degenerative changes in the fibrovascular stroma.

**calc'spar.** Calcite.

**cal'culary.** Relating to a calculus or calculi.

**cal'culi.** Plural of calculus.

**calculif'ragous** [ L. *calculus,* stone, + *frango,* pp. *fractus,* to break, FRA- ]. Relating to the crushing of a stone in the bladder.

**calculosis** (kal-ku-lo'sis) [ L. *calculus,* small stone, + suffix *-osis,* condition ]. The tendency or disposition to form calculi or stones.

**cal'culous.** Relating to calculi.

**calculus,** gen. and pl. **cal'culi** (kal'ku-lus) [ L. a pebble, a calculus. CALX-2 ]. A concretion formed in any portion of the body, usually composed of salts of inorganic or organic acids, or of other material, such as cholesterol.

**alvine c.,** intestinal "stone," from hardening of feces.

**arthritic c.,** gouty *tophus.*

**bil'iary c.,** gallstone.

**blood c.,** hemic c.; a phlebolith, or concretion of coagulated blood, or a c. formed in a thrombus.

**cardiac c.,** cardiolith.

**coral c.,** dendritic c.; a large kidney stone molded to the pelvis with branches filling the calices.

**dendritic c.,** coral c.

**dental c.,** (1) calcified deposits formed around the teeth; (2) tartar; (3) salivary c.; (4) serumal c.

**fu'sible c.,** one composed of ammoniomagnesium phosphate and calcium phosphate.

**gastric c.,** gastrolith.

**hematogenet'ic c.,** serumal c.

**hemic c.,** blood c.

**hempseed c.,** a small urinary c. of calcium oxalate, when multiple, forming gravel.

**intestinal c.,** a concretion in the bowel, either a coprolith or an enterolith.

**lacrimal c.,** dacryolith.

**mammary c.,** a concretion in one of the ducts of the breast.

**mulberry c.,** a hard, dark brown or gray, usually nodulated concretion in the bladder, composed chiefly of calcium oxalate.

**nasal c.,** rhinolith.

**pancreat'ic c.,** a concretion, usually multiple, in the pancreatic duct, associated with chronic pancreatitis.

**preputial c.,** a c. in the space between the prepuce and the glans penis; phimosis is the most important predisposing cause.

**prostat'ic c.,** prostatolith; a c. formed in the prostate, usually from corpora amylacea.

**pulp c.,** pulp *stone.*

**renal c.,** stone in the kidney, renal pelvis, or calices.

**sal'ivary c.,** (1) a c. in a salivary duct or gland; (2) tartar of the teeth; (3) calcified deposits formed around the teeth, supragingivally or subgingivally.

**se'rumal c.,** (1) hematogenetic c.; a greenish or dark brown deposit on the roots of the teeth in periodontal disease; (2) subgingival c.

**stag-horn c.,** a c. with several branches, usually within an obstructed renal pelvis.

**subgingival c.,** calcareous deposit found on the tooth apical to the gingival margins.

**supragingival c.,** (1) calcified plaques adherent to tooth surface above free gum margin; (2) tartar; (3) salivary c.; (4) dental c.

**ton'sillar c.,** tonsillolith.

**urinary c.,** a c. in the kidney, ureter, bladder, or urethra.

**u'terine c.,** womb stone; uterolith; hysterolith; a calcareous concretion in the uterus.

**venous c.,** phlebolith.

**vesical c.,** cystolith; stone in the bladder; a urinary c. formed or lodged in the bladder.

**Caldani,** Leopoldo M. A., Italian anatomist, 1725–1813. See C.'s *ligament.*

**Caldwell,** George W., American physician, 1834–1918. See C.-Luc *operation.*

**Caldwell,** William E., American obstetrician, 1880–1943. See C.-Moloy *classification.*

**calef.** Abbreviation for L. *calefacio,* to make warm, or *calefiat,* let (it) be warmed.

**calefa'cient** [ L. *calefacio,* fr. *caleo,* to be warm, + *facio,* to make ]. 1. Making warm or hot. 2. An agent causing a sense of warmth in the part to which it is applied.

**calen'din.** Calendulin.

**calen'dula** [ L. *Calendae,* the first day of the month, the plant flowering nearly every month ]. Marigold; the dried florets of *Calendula officinalis* (family Compositae); used chiefly externally as an application to sprains and bruises.

**calen'dulin.** Calendin; physiologically active substance isolated from *Calendula officinalis.*

**calf,** pl. **calves** (kaf, kavz) [ Gael. *kalpa* ]. 1. Sura. 2. A young bovine animal, male or female.

**bull-dog c.,** a c. with a short muzzle and brachycephalic skull, usually resulting from chondrodystrophy; associated with this condition are shortened limbs and anomalies of the vertebral centra; it often results in respiratory and feeding difficulties, and is sometimes fatal.

**football c.,** term used to describe the doughy sensation elicited on palpation of the c. when muscle necrosis has developed as a consequence of acute ischemia produced by acute arterial embolism.

**gnome's c.,** the very full rounded c. occurring in pseudohypertrophic muscular dystrophy affecting the gastrocnemius muscles.

**calf-bone.** Fibula.

**cal'iber** [ Fr. *calibre,* of uncert. etym. ]. The diameter of a tube or canal.

**cal'ibrate.** 1. To graduate or standardize any measuring instrument. 2. To measure the diameter of a tube.

**caliceal** (kal'ĭ-se'al). Calyceal; relating to the calix.

**calicectasis** (kal-ĭ-sek'tă-sis) [ calix, *q.v.,* + G. *ektasis,* dilation ]. Caliectasis; calycectasis; pyelocaliectasis; dilation of the pelvis and calices of the kidney.

**calicectomy** (kal'ĭ-sek'to-mĭ) [ calix, *q.v.* + G. *ektomē,* excision ]. Caliectomy; calycectomy; excision of a calix.

**calices** (kal'ĭ-sēz). Plural of calix.

**caliciform** (kă-lis-ĭ-form) [ L. *calix, q.v.,* + *forma,* form ]. Calyciform; shaped like a calix.

**cal'icine.** Calycine; of the nature of, or resembling a calix.

**caliculus,** pl. **calic'uli** (kă-lik'u-lus) [ L. dim. from G. *kalyx,* the cup of a flower ]. Calycle; calyculus; a bud-shaped or cup-shaped structure, resembling the closed calyx of a flower.

**c. gustato'rius** [ NA ], taste or gustatory bud, bulb, or corpuscle; Schwalbe's corpuscle; one of a number of flask-shaped cell nests located in the epithelium of vallate, fungiform, and foliate papillae of the tongue and also in the soft palate, epiglottis, and posterior wall of the pharynx. The c. consists of sustentacular, gustatory, and basal cells between which the intragemmal sensory nerve fibers terminate. See fig. under *papilla* vallata.

**c. ophthal'micus** [ NA ], optic cup; ocular cup; the double-walled cup formed by the invagination of the embryonic vesicle; its inner component becomes the sensory layer of the retina, its outer layer, the pigment layer.

**caliec'tasis.** Calicectasis.

**caliec'tomy.** Calicectomy.

**califor'nium** [ *California,* state and university where first prepared ]. An artificial transuranium element, symbol Cf, atomic no. 98. Half-life of the most stable known isotope ($^{251}$Cf) is 700 years.

**caliga'tion.** Caligo.

**caligo** (kă-li'go) [ L. fog, darkness ]. Caligation; dimness of vision.

**cal'ipers** [ a corruption of *caliber* ]. An instrument consisting of two legs hinged at one extremity, used for measuring diameters (in obstetrics, the pelvic diameters).

**calirrhaphy** (kal-ir'raf-ĭ) [ L. *kalix, q.v.,* + G. *raphē,* suture ]. Plastic surgery on a calyx of the kidney.

**calisa'ya bark** [ S. Am. ]. Yellow *cinchona.*

**calisthen'ics** [ G. *kalos,* beautiful, + *sthenos,* strength ]. The practice of various exercises ("setting-up exercises," the use of dumb-bells, Indian clubs, etc.) with the object of preserving health and increasing physical strength.

**calix,** pl. **cal'ices** (ka'liks) [ L. fr. G. *kalyx,* the cup of a flower ] [ NA ]. Calyx; infundibulum; one of the branches or recesses of the pelvis of the kidney into which the orifices of the Malpighian renal pyramids project.

**calices rena'les majo'res** [ NA ], the primary subdivisions of the renal pelvis, usually two or three in number

**calices rena'les mino'res** [ NA ], the subdivisions of the major calices, varying in number from 7 to 13, which receive the renal papillae.

**Calkins,** Leroy Adelbert, U. S. obstetrician-gynecologist, 1894–1960. See C.'s *sign.*

**calks, calkins** (kawlks, kawl'kinz). Projections of varying shapes and sizes attached to the lower surface of a horse's shoe. Usually there is a single toe c. and two heel c.'s, one at the end of each prong. They are usually attached to prevent the animal slipping on hard surfaces. Sometimes they are used to level the bearing surface of the foot.

**Call-Exner bodies.** See under body.

**Callahan,** J. R. See C.'s *method.*

**Callander,** C. Latimer, San Francisco surgeon, 1892–1947. See C.'s *amputation.*

**Calleja** (cahl-ya'ha), Camilo, Madrid anatomist, †1913. See *islands* of C.

**Calliphora** (kă-lif'o-rah). A genus of blowfies, the bluebottle flies, the larvae of which feed on dead flesh. *C. vomitoria* and *C. vicina* are common species in the United States.

**Callison,** James S., New York physician, *1873. See C.'s *fluid.*

**Callitro'ga.** A genus of flesh flies of the family Calliphoridae, whose larvae develop in decaying flesh or carrion or in wounds or sores (myiasis). The "secondary invaders" are flies attracted to decaying flesh, and their larvae may develop in neglected wounds (they were formerly used as "surgical maggots"). "Primary invaders," such as the American screw worm fly, *C. hominivorax,* are attracted by fresh blood and deposit eggs in or near small sores such as tick bites; larvae of these flies feed on living flesh and produce many serious cases of myiasis in man and domestic animals from the U. S. Gulf states to Argentina.

    *C. hominivorax,* the American screw worm fly; a serious pest of livestock from the Gulf Coast states to Argentina. The fly deposits eggs on wounds, tick bites, or intact moist areas of the body, and the larvae invade living tissues, causing severe myiasis and often death. It is known to attack man, especially in the nose, though wounds, eyes, body openings have also been attacked. It is a primary cause of myiasis in the New World.

**callo'sal.** Relating to the corpus callosum.

**callose** (kal'ōs). A β-1,3-glucan formed by appropriate enzymes from UDP-glucose, differing from cellulose, a β-1,4-glucan formed from GDP-glucose, and starch amylose, an α-1,4-glucan formed from ADP-glucose.

**callos'itas.** Callosity.

**callos'ity** [ L. fr. *callosus,* thick skinned ]. Callus; callositas; tyloma; keratoma; poroma; a circumscribed thickening of the keratin layer of the epidermis as a result of friction or intermittent pressure.

**callo'somar'ginal.** Relating to the corpus callosum and the gyrus cinguli; denoting the sulcus between them.

**callo'sus** [ L. ] [ NA ]. Callosal.

**callous** (kal'us). Relating to a callus or callosity.

**callus** (kal'us) [ L. hard skin ]. 1. Callosity. 2. The hard bonelike substance thrown out between and around the ends of a fractured bone.

    **central c.,** the provisional c. within the medullary cavity.

    **definitive c.,** the c. between the two ends of the fractured bone which becomes converted into osseous tissue.

    **ensheathing c.,** the mass of provisional c. around the outside of the bone.

    **provisional c.,** temporary c.; the c. thrown out as nature's splint to keep the ends of the bone in apposition; it is absorbed after union is complete.

    **temporary c.,** provisional c.

**cal'mative.** 1. Calming; quieting; sedative. 2. An agent that quiets excitement; a sedative.

**Calmette,** L. C. A., French bacteriologist, 1863–1933. See *bacille* bilié de C.-Guérin, C. *test,* C.-Guérin *vaccine.*

**cal'omel.** Mercurous chloride.

    **vegetable c.,** podophyllum.

**calor** (ka'lor) [ L. ]. Heat; one of the four signs of inflammation (c., rubor, tumor, dolor) enunciated by Celsius.

**caloradiance** (kal'o-ra'dī-ans). The emission of heat rays.

**calorescence** (kal'o-res'ens). The heating to incandescence of a body by infrared radiation.

**Calori** (kah-law're), Luigi, Italian anatomist, 1807–1896. See C.'s *bursa.*

**calor'ic** [ L. *calor,* heat ]. 1. Relating to a calorie. 2. Relating to heat.

    **c. value,** the heat evolved by a food when burnt or metabolized.

**calorie, calory** (kal'o-rī) [ L. *calor,* heat ]. A unit of heat content or energy. The **large calorie** (usually written with a capital C or abbreviated Cal. or kcal.) is used in measurements of the heat production of chemical reactions, including those involved in biology, *e.g.,* caloric content of foodstuffs; it is defined as the quantity of energy required to raise the temperature of 1 kg. of water 1°C., or more precisely from 15° to 16°C.; it is 1000 times the value of the **small calorie** (written with a lower case c or abbreviated cal.), the quantity of energy required to raise the temperature of 1 gm. of water 1°C. (from 15° to 16°C. in case of normal or standard c.), therefore often referred to as the gram c. See also British thermal *unit. The c. is being replaced by the SI unit, the joule* (=0.24 cal.).

    **gram c.,** small c.

    **kilogram c., kilocalorie,** large c. (Calorie).

    **mean c.,** $1/100$ of the heat required to raise 1 gm. of water from 0°C. to 100°C.

**calorifa'cient** [ L. *calor,* heat, + *facio,* to make ]. Calorific; producing heat.

**calorif'ic.** Calorifacient.

**calor'igenic.** Capable of generating heat.

**calorim'eter** [ L. *calor,* heat, + G. *metron,* measure ]. An apparatus for measuring the amount of heat liberated in a chemical reaction.

    **Benedict-Roth c.,** see Benedict-Roth *apparatus.*

    **bomb c.,** an instrument for determining the potential energy of organic substances, including those in foods; consists of a hollow, steel container lined with platinum and filled with pure oxygen. A weighed quantity of food is placed therein and ignited with an electric fuse. The heat produced is absorbed by water surrounding the bomb; from the rise in temperature, the calories liberated are calculated.

**cal'orimet'ric.** Relating to calorimetry.

**calorim'etry.** The measurement of the amount of heat given off by a reaction or group of reactions (as by an organism).

    **direct c.,** measurement of the heat produced by a reaction, as distinguished from indirect methods, which involve measurement of something other than heat production itself.

    **indirect c.,** determination of heat production of an oxidation reaction by measuring uptake of oxygen and/or liberation of $CO_2$ and nitrogen excretion and then calculating the amount of heat produced.

**cal'oripunc'ture.** Ignipuncture.

**calor'itrop'ic.** Relating to thermotropism.

**cal'ory.** Calorie.

**calum'ba.** Columbo; colomba; the dried root of *Jateorrhiza palmata* (family Menispermaceae), a tall climbing vine of East Africa. Used as a bitter tonic.

**cal'umbin.** Columbin; $C_{21}H_{24}O_7$; an amaroid from calumba that accounts for the bitterness of the crude drug.

**calu'sterone** (USAN). METHOSARB; 17β-hydroxy-7β,17-dimethylandrost-4-en-3-one; antineoplastic agent.

**calvaria,** pl. **calvariae** (kal-va'rī-ah) [ L. a skull ] [ NA ]. Skullcap; cranium cerebrale; the upper, domelike portion of the skull.

**calva'rial.** Relating to the skullcap.

**calva'rium.** Incorrectly used for calvaria.

**calve** (kav) In cows, to give birth to one or more calves.

**Calvé,** Jacques, French orthopedic surgeon, 1875–1954. See C.-Perthes *disease,* Legg-C.-Perthes *disease.*

**calves.** Plural of calf.

**calvities** (kal-vish'e-ēz) [ L. fr. *calvus,* bald ]. Alopecia.

**calx,** gen. **calcis,** pl. **calces.** 1 [ L. limestone. CALX-2 ]. Lime. 2 [ CALX-1 ] [ NA ]. The heel.

**calyceal** (kal'ĭ-se'al). Caliceal.

**calycec'tasis.** Calicectasis.

**calycec'tomy.** Calicectomy.

**calyciform** (kă-lis'ĭ-form). Caliciform.

cal'ycine. Calicine.

cal'ycle, calyc'ulus. Caliculus.

calyec'tasis. Calicectasis.

Calym'matobacte'rium [ G. *kalymma*, hood, veil, + *bakterion*, rod ]. A genus of nonmotile bacteria (family Brucellaceae) containing Gram-negative, pleomorphic rods with single or bipolar condensations of chromatin. The cells occur singly and in clusters. Outside of the human body growth occurs only in the yolk sac or amniotic fluid of a developing chick embryo or in a medium containing embryonic yolk. These organisms are pathogenic for man. The type species is *C. granulomatis*.

C. granulo'matis, a species of bacteria causing granulomatous lesions in man, particularly in the inguinal region. It is the type species of the genus *C*.

calyx (ka'liks) [ G. cup of a flower ]. Calix.

camben'dazole (USAN). Isopropyl 2-(4-triazolyl)-5-benzimidazolecarbamate; anthelmintic.

cam'bium [ L. exchange ]. 1. The inner layer of the periosteum. 2. A layer between the wood and bark in plants.

cambo'gia [ *Camboja* or *Cambodia* ] (NF, BP). Gamboge; a gum resin obtained from *Garcinia hanburii* (family Guttiferae); purgative and anthelmintic.

c. in'dica, Indian gamboge; the gum resin from *Garcinia morella*; cathartic.

cam'elpox. Photo-shootur; a disease of camels that may produce local lesions in man from contact; little information is available with respect to etiological agent.

camera, pl. camerae, cameras (kam'er-ah) [ L. a vault ]. 1. A closed box; especially one used to contain the lens and the plates in photography. 2 [ NA ]. In anatomy, any chamber or cavity, such as one of the chambers of the heart, or eye.

c. anterior bulbi [ NA ], c. oculi anterior; c. oculi major; anterior chamber of the eye; the space between the cornea and the iris, filled with a watery fluid (aqueous humor) and communicating through the pupil with the posterior chamber.

c. cordis, pericardium; pericardial sac.

c. lucida, an optical instrument which by means of prisms or mirrors projects the image of an object, drawing, etc., to a paper upon which a facsimile can be readily traced.

c. obscura, (1) photographic c.; (2) the eye.

c. oculi major, c. oculi anterior, c. anterior bulbi.

c. oculi minor, c. oculi posterior, c. posterior bulbi.

c. posterior bulbi [ NA ], c. oculi posterior; c. oculi minor; posterior chamber of the eye; the ringlike space between the iris, the crystalline lens, and the ciliary body; it is filled with aqueous humor.

retinal c.'s, floor-standing and hand-held models available for ocular fundus photography; for fluorescein angiography, accessory equipment provides appropriate exciter and barrier filters, a high power, rapid charge flash generator, and automatic picture intervals of 0.2 to 2 seconds.

c. vitrea bulbi [ NA ], vitreous c.; vitreous chamber of the eye; the large space between the lens and the retina; it is filled with the vitreous body.

vitreous c., c. vitrea bulbi.

camerostome (kam'er-o-stōm) [ L. *camera*, a vault, + G. *stoma*, mouth ]. Ventral depression of the anterior cephalothorax of soft ticks (family Argasidae) in which the mouthparts (capitulum) lie.

cam'isole. Straitjacket.

camomile (kam'o-mil). Chamomile.

cAMP. Abbreviation for adenosine 3':5'-cyclic phosphate (cyclic AMP).

Campbell, William F., Brooklyn surgeon, 1867–1926. See C.'s *ligament*.

Camper, Pieter, Dutch physician and anatomist, 1722–1789. See C.'s *angle, chiasm, fascia, ligament, line*.

camphamed'rine. CARDENYL; *N*-β-hydroxy-α-methylphenyl)-*N*-methyl-10-camphorsulfonamide; analeptic.

cam'phane. Bornane.

cam'phene. 2,2-Dimethyl-3-methylene-norbornane; a terpenoid occurring in many essential oils, *e.g.*, turpentine, camphor, citronella.

cam'phor [ mediev. L. fr. Ar. *kāfure* ] (USP, BP). 2-Bornanone. 1. A solid, tough, crystalline, translucent substance; a ketone distilled from the bark and wood of *Cinnamomum camphora*, an evergreen tree of Southeastern Asia and the adjoining islands; also prepared synthetically from oil of turpentine. 2. Any stearoptene resembling this. Stimulant, carminative, expectorant, and diaphoretic.

Borneo c., borneol.

cantharis c., cantharidin.

c. liniment (BP), camphorated oil; a mixture of camphor and cottonseed oil, or camphor and arachis oil; a mild counterirritant.

monobromated c., antispasmodic, soporific, and sedative.

tar c., naphthalene.

thyme c., thymol.

camphora'ceous. Resembling camphor in appearance or odor.

cam'phorated. Containing camphor.

c. oil, camphor liniment.

camphor'ic acid. 1,2,2-Trimethyl-1,3-cyclopentanedicarboxylic acid; respiratory stimulant.

cam'phorism. Camphor poisoning, marked by gastroenteritis, coma or convulsions, and other cerebral symptoms.

camphotamide. TONICORINE; 3-diethylcarbamoyl-1-methylpyridinium camphorsulfonate; analeptic agent.

cam'phyl alcohol. Borneol.

cam'pi foreli [ L. pl. of *campus*, field ]. *Fields* of Forel.

campim'eter [ L. *campus*, field, + G. *metron*, measure ]. A portable, hand-held type of tangent screen.

campim'etry. Investigation of the visual field by means of a campimeter.

camptocormia (kamp'to-kor'mi-ah) [ G. *kamptos*, bent, + *kormos*, trunk of a tree ]. Prosternation; posture characterized by flexion at hips and trunk when individual is erect, but it is not fixed deformity.

camptodactyly, camptodactylia (kamp-to-dak'ti-li, -dak-til'i-ah) [ G. *kamptos*, bent, + *daktylos*, finger ]. Campylodactyly.

camptome'lia [ G. *kamptos*, bent, + *melos*, limb ]. A bending of the limbs, producing a fixed deformity.

camptospasm (kamp'to-spazm). A nervous or hysterical forward bending of the trunk.

campylodactyly (kam'pi-lo-dak'ti-li) [ G. *campylos*, curved, + *daktylos*, finger ]. Camptodactyly; streblodactyly; permanent flexion of one or both interphalangeal joints of one or more fingers, usually the little finger.

camsylate. USAN-approved contraction for camphorsulfonate.

camylofine. SPASMOCAN; *N*-[ 2-(diethylamino)ethyl ]-2-phenylglycine isopentyl ester; anticholinergic agent.

Canada, Wilma J., U. S. radiologist. See Cronkhite-C. *syndrome*.

can'adine. Tetrahydroberberine; xanthopuccine; $C_{20}H_{21}NO_4$; an alkaloid present in *Hydrastis canadensis* (family Ranunculaceae) and in *Corydalis cava* (family Fumaraceae).

# CANAL

canal (kă-nal') [ L. *canalis* ]. A duct or channel; a tubular structure. See also canalis and duct.

abdom'inal c., canalis inguinalis.

accessory c., a branch of the canalis radicis dentis extending laterally in the apical half or furcation area of the root of a tooth.

adductor c., canalis adductorius.

Alcock's c., canalis pudendalis.

alimen'tary c., canalis alimentarius.

alve'olar c.'s, canales alveolares.

alveolar anterior c.'s, canales alveolares.

alveoloden'tal c.'s, canales alveolares.

a'nal c., canalis analis.

anterior condyloid c. of occipital bone, canalis hypoglossi.

**anterior dental c.'s,** *canales* alveolares.

**Arantius' c.,** *ductus* venosus.

**archenteric c.,** notochordal c.; the invagination of the blastopore into the notochordal process to form a cavity.

**Arnold's c.,** a bony c. in the petrous portion of the temporal bone through which passes the lesser petrosal nerve.

**arterial c.,** *ductus* arteriosus.

**atrioventricular c.,** the c. in the embryonic heart leading from the common sinuatrial chamber to the ventricle.

**auditory c.,** *meatus* acusticus externus.

**basipharyn'geal c.,** *canalis* vomerovaginalis.

**Bernard's c.,** *ductus* pancreaticus accessorius.

**Bichat's c.,** *cisterna* venae magnae cerebri.

**blastopor'ic c.,** an opening marking the remains of the neurenteric c.

**bony semicircular c.'s,** *canales* semicirculares ossei.

**Böttcher's c.,** c. between the saccule and the utricle.

**Braune's c.,** the parturient c. formed by the uterine cavity, dilated cervix, vagina, and vulva.

**Breschet's c.'s,** see *canalis* diploicus.

**carot'id c.,** *canalis* caroticus.

**carpal c.,** *canalis* carpi; *sulcus* carpi.

**caudal c.,** in anesthesiology, the space occupied by the sacral extension of the epidural space.

**central c.,** *canalis* centralis.

**central c.'s of cochlea,** *canales* longitudinales modioli.

**cervical c.,** *canalis* cervicis uteri.

**cil'iary c.'s,** *spatia* anguli iridocornealis.

**Civinini's c.,** *iter* chordae anterius.

**Cloquet's c.,** *canalis* hyaloideus.

**coch'lear c.,** *canalis* spiralis cochleae.

**con'dylar c., con'dyloid c.,** *canalis* condylaris.

**Corti's c.,** corti's *tunnel.*

**Cotunnius' c.,** *aqueductus* vestibuli.

**cra'niopharyn'geal c.,** pituitary *diverticulum.*

**crural c.,** *canalis* femoralis.

**deferent c.,** *ductus* deferens.

**dental c.'s,** *canales* alveolares.

**dentinal c.'s,** *canaliculi* dentales.

**diploic c.'s,** *canales* diploici.

**Dorello's c.,** a bony c. sometimes found at the tip of the temporal bone enclosing the abducens nerve and inferior petrosal sinus as these two structures enter the cavernous sinus.

**Dupuytren's c.,** *vena* diploica.

**entodermal c.,** the gut tube of young embryos.

**facial c.,** *canalis* facialis.

**Fallopian c.,** *canalis* facialis.

**fem'oral c.,** *canalis* femoralis.

**Ferrein's c.,** *rivus* lacrimalis.

**Fontana's c.,** *sinus* venosus sclerae.

**galactoph'orous c.'s,** *ductus* lactiferi.

**Gartner's c.,** *ductus* epoophori longitudinalis.

**gastric c.,** *canalis* ventriculi.

**greater palatine c.,** *canalis* palatinus major.

**gynecophoric c.,** a ventral groove running the length of male schistosome flukes, into which the threadlike female worm fits.

**Hannover's c.,** the space between the ciliary zonule and the vitreous body.

**Haversian c.'s,** Leeuwenhoek's c.'s; vascular c.'s in osseous tissue.

**Hensen's c.,** *ductus* reuniens.

**c. of Hering,** cholangiole.

**Hirschfeld's c.'s,** interdental c.'s.

**His' c.,** *ductus* thyroglossus.

**Holmgrén-Golgi c.'s,** Golgi *apparatus.*

**c. of Hovius,** an anastomotic circle between the anterior twigs of the venae vorticosae in the eyes of some animals, but not in normal human eyes.

**Hoyer's c.'s,** arteriovenous (arteriolovenular) anastomoses.

**Huguier's c.,** *iter* chordae anterius.

**Hunter's c.,** *canalis* adductorius.

**hyaloid c.,** *canalis* hyaloideus.

**hypoglossal c.,** *canalis* hypoglossi.

**incisive c., incisor c.,** *canalis* incisivus.

**inferior dental c.,** *canalis* mandibulae.

**infraor'bital c.,** *canalis* infraorbitalis.

**inguinal c.,** *canalis* inguinalis.

**interdental c.'s,** Hirschfeld's c.'s; c.'s that extend vertically through alveolar bone between roots of mandibular and maxillary incisor and maxillary bicuspid teeth.

**interfacial c.'s,** intercellular spaces occurring in relation to intercellular bridges in stratified squamous epithelium.

**irruption c.,** the channel along which the periosteal vascular bud invades the cartilaginous matrix of growing bone.

**Jacobson's c.,** *canaliculus* tympanicus.

**Kürsteiner's c.'s,** small embryonic epithelial tubules connecting the cervical part of the developing thymus and the inferior parathyroid.

**Laurer's c.,** a slender tube that forms part of the ovarian complex of trematodes; the c. connects the sperm duct (between seminal receptacle and ootype) to the dorsal surface of the worm, though it frequently ends blindly without reaching the surface. Laurer's c. is thought to have served as a vagina (and may still do so in some instances) or an exit drain for surplus seminal material from the seminal receptacle.

**Lauth's c.,** *sinus* venous sclerae.

**Leeuwenhoek's c.'s,** Haversian c.'s.

**c.'s for lesser palatine nerves,** *canales* palatini minores.

**longitudinal c.'s of modiolus,** *canales* longitudinales modioli.

**Löwenberg's c.,** *ductus* cochlearis.

**Malpighian c.,** *ductus* epoophori longitudinalis.

**mandibular c.,** *canalis* mandibulae.

**marrow c.,** *canalis* radicis dentis.

**mental c.,** *foramen* mentale.

**Müller's c.,** *ductus* paramesonephricus.

**musculotu'bal c.,** *canalis* musculotubarius.

**nasolacrimal c.,** *canalis* nasolacrimalis.

**neural c.,** the c. within the embryonic neural tube; the primordium of the canalis centralis.

**neurenter'ic c.,** a transitory communication between the neural tube and the gut which appears in the embryos of some lower forms.

**notochordal c.,** archenteric c.

**Nuck's c.,** see *processus* vaginalis peritonei.

**nutrient c.,** *canalis* nutricius.

**obturator c.,** *canalis* obturatorius.

**optic c.,** *canalis* opticus.

**palatovagi'nal c.,** *canalis* palatovaginalis.

**partu'rient c.,** the cavity of the uterus and the vagina through which the fetus passes.

**pelvic c.,** the passage from the superior to the inferior strait of the pelvis.

**pericardioperitoneal c.,** the constricted portion of the embryonic celom that joins the pericardial cavity to the peritoneal cavity, developing into the pleural cavities.

**persistent atrioventric'ular c.,** endocardial cushion defect; persistent A-V communis; developmentally atrial and ventricular septa fail to meet, resulting in a low atrial and high ventricular septal defect or common atrioventricular c.

**Petit's c.,** *spatia* zonularia.

**pharyn'geal c.,** *canalis* palatovaginalis.

**pleur'opericard'ial c.'s,** in the embryo, spaces or channels, one on each side, connecting the pericardial and pleural cavities.

**pleuroperitoneal c.,** the communication between the embryonic pleural and peritoneal cavities.

**portal c.'s,** the spaces in the substance of the liver which are occupied by connective tissue and the ramifications of the bile ducts, portal vein, hepatic artery, nerves, and lymphatics.

**posterior dental c.'s,** *canales* alveolares.

**pter'ygoid c.,** *canalis* pterygoideus.

**pter'ygopal'atine c.,** *canalis* palatinus major.

**pudend'al c.,** *canalis* pudendalis.

**pulp c.,** *canalis* radicis dentis.

**pyloric c.,** *canalis* pyloricus.

**Rivinus' c.'s,** see entries under *ductus* sublinguales.

**root c.,** *canalis* radicis dentis.

**Rosenthal's c.,** *canalis* spiralis cochleae.

**sacral c.,** *canalis* sacralis.

**Santorini's c.,** *ductus* pancreaticus accessorius.

**Schlemm's c.,** *sinus* venosus sclerae.

**semicircular c.'s,** *canales* semicirculares ossei.

**small c. of chorda tympani,** *canaliculus* chordae tympani.

**spinal c.,** *canalis* vertebralis.

**spiral c. of the cochlea,** *canalis* spiralis cochleae.

**spiral c. of modiolus,** *canalis* spiralis modioli.

**Stilling's c.,** *canalis* hyaloideus.

**subsartor'ial c.,** *canalis* adductorius.

**Sucquet's c.'s,** communications between venules and small arteries; arteriovenous (arteriolovenular) anastomoses.

**tarsal c.,** *sinus* tarsi.

**temporal c.,** a c. in the zygomatic bone transmitting the zygomaticofacial and zygomaticotemporal nerves and vessels.

**Theile's c.,** the serous space formed by the reflexion of the pericardium on the aorta and pulmonary artery.

**tubotympanic c.,** the first pharyngeal pouch of the embryo during its modification to form the auditory (Eustachian) tube and the tympanic cavity.

**tympan'ic c.,** *canaliculus* tympanicus.

**uniting c.,** *ductus* reuniens.

**urogenital c.,** urethra.

**u'terovagi'nal c.,** a median tubular structure produced in the embryo from the fusion of the caudal parts of the Müllerian (paramesonephric) ducts.

**van Hoorne's c.,** *ductus* thoracicus.

**Velpeau's c.,** *canalis* inguinalis.

**venous c. of Arantius,** *ductus* venosus.

**ver'tebral c.,** *canalis* vertebralis.

**vesicourethral c.,** the cranial portion of the primitive urogenital sinus; it gives rise to the bladder and part of the urethra.

**Vidian c.,** *canalis* pterygoideus.

**Volkmann's c.'s,** vascular c.'s in bone which, unlike those of the Haversian system, are not surrounded by concentric lamellae of bone; they run for the most part transversely, perforating the lamellae of the Haversian system, and communicate with the c.'s of that system.

**vo'merine c.,** *canalis* vomerovaginalis.

**vomerobasilar c.,** a passage at the union of the vomer and the sphenoid bone.

**vom'erovagi'nal c.,** *canalis* vomerovaginalis.

**Walther's c.'s,** *ductus* sublinguales minores.

**Wirsung's c.,** *ductus* pancreaticus.

---

**cana'les.** Plural of canalis.

**canalic'ular.** Relating to a canaliculus.

**canalic'uli.** Plural of canaliculus.

**canalic'uliza'tion.** The formation of canaliculi, or small canals, in any tissue.

**canaliculus,** pl. **canalic'uli** (kan-ă-lik'u-lus) [ L. dim. fr. *canalis,* canal ] [ NA ]. A small canal or channel.

**auric'ular c.,** c. mastoideus.

**biliary c.,** bile capillary; one of the intercellular channels, about 1 $\mu$ or less in diameter, that occurs between liver cells.

**bone c.,** the c. interconnecting bone lacunae with one another or with a Haversian canal.

**canaculi caroticotympanici** [ NA ], small openings within the carotid canal that afford passage to the tympanic cavity of branches of the internal carotid artery and carotid sympathetic plexus.

**c. chordae tym'pani** [ NA ], small canal of the chorda tympani; iter chordae posterius; a canal leading from the facial canal to the tympanic cavity through which the chorda tympani nerve enters this cavity.

**c. cochleae** [ NA ], cochlear canaliculus; a minute canal in the temporal bone that passes from the cochlea inferiorly to open in front of the medial side of the jugular fossa. It contains the perilymphatic duct.

**cochlear c.,** c. cochleae.

**canaliculi denta'les** [ NA ], dentinal tubules; dentinal canals; minute, wavy, branching tubes or canals in the dentin; they contain the dentinal fibers and extend radially from the pulp to the dentoenamel junction.

**c. innomina'tus,** an occasional opening in the great wing of the sphenoid bone, between the foramen spinosum and foramen ovale, which transmits the lesser petrosal nerve.

**intercellular c.,** secretory c.; one of the fine channels between adjoining secretory cells, such as those between serous cells in salivary glands.

**intracellular c.,** a fine c. extending deeply into the cytoplasm of a cell such as the gastric parietal cell.

**c. lacrima'lis** [ NA ], lacrimal canaliculus; lacrimal duct; a curved canal beginning at the punctum lacrimale in the margin of each eyelid near the medial commissure and running transversely medially to empty with its fellow into the lacrimal sac. See fig. under apparatus.

**c. mastoid'eus** [ NA ], mastoid c.; auricular c.; the canal that extends from the jugular fossa laterally through the mastoid process. It transmits the auricular branch of the vagus.

**c. reu'niens,** *ductus* reuniens.

**secretory c.,** intercellular c.

**Thiersch's canaliculi,** minute channels in newly formed reparative tissue, permitting the circulation of nutritive fluids, precursors of new vascularization.

**c. tympan'icus** [ NA ], tympanic c.; Jacobson's canal; a minute canal passing from the inferior surface of the petrous portion of the temporal bone between the jugular fossa and carotid canal to the floor of the tympanic cavity. It transmits the tympanic branch of the glossopharyngeal nerve.

**canaline.** $NH_2$—O—$CH_2CH_2CH(NH_2)COOH$; precursor of canavanine, into which it can be converted by an enzyme (transamidinase), found in kidney and in the jack-bean, which transfers the amidine group of arginine to canaline; notable for the presence of an N—O—C link.

**canalis,** pl. **cana'les** (kan-a'lis) [ L. ] [ NA ]. A canal or channel.

**c. adductor'ius** [ NA ], adductor canal; Hunter's canal; subsartorial canal; the space in the thigh between the vastus medialis and adductor muscles, converted into a canal by the overlying sartorius muscle. It gives passage to the femoral vessels.

**c. alimenta'rius** [ NA ], alimentary canal; digestive tube; digestive tract; the mouth, pharynx, esophagus, stomach, and intestine.

**canales alveola'res** [ NA ], alveolar (anterior) canals; alveolodental canals; posterior dental canals; canals in the body of the maxilla that transmit nerves and vessels to the molar teeth.

**c. ana'lis** [ NA ], anal canal; the terminal portion of the alimentary canal; it extends from the upper level of the pelvic diaphragm to the anal orifice.

**c. caroticus** [ NA ], carotid canal; a passage through the petrous part of the temporal bone from its inferior surface upward, medially, and forward to the apex where it opens into the foramen lacerum. It transmits the internal carotid artery and plexuses of veins and autonomic nerves.

**c. carpi** [ NA ], carpal canal; the space deep to the flexor retinaculum of the wrist through which the median nerve and the flexor tendons of the fingers and thumb pass.

**c. centra'lis** [ NA ], central canal; syringocele (1); tubus medullaris; (1) in the adult, the minute and usually obliterated canal that extends from the fourth ventricle down throughout the length of the spinal cord; (2) in the embryo, the ependyma-lined lumen (cavity) of the neural tube, the cerebral part of which remains patent to form the ventricles of the brain, while the spinal part dwindles and is often reduced to a solid strand of modified ependyma cells.

**c. cervicis uteri** [ NA ], cervical canal; a fusiform canal extending from the isthmus of the uterus to the opening of the uterus into the vagina.

**c. condyla'ris** [ NA ], condylar canal; condyloid canal; the opening through the occipital bone posterior to the condyle on each side that transmits the occipital emissary vein.

**canales diplo'ici** [ NA ], diploic canals; channels in the diploë that accommodate the diploic veins.

**c. facia'lis** [ NA ], facial canal; Fallopian aqueduct; aqueductus fallopii; Fallopian canal; the bony passage in the temporal bone through which the facial nerve passes. It commences in the internal auditory meatus, passes at first anteriorly, then turns posteriorly to pass medial to the tympanic cavity. Finally, it turns downward to reach the stylomastoid foramen.

**c. femora'lis** [ NA ], femoral canal; crural canal; the medial compartment of the femoral sheath.

**c. hyaloid'eus** [ NA ], hyaloid canal; canal of Stilling; Cloquet's canal; a minute canal running through the vitreous from the discus nervi optici to the lens, containing in fetal life a prolongation of the central artery of the retina, the hyaloid artery.

**c. hypoglos'si** [ NA ], hypoglossal canal; anterior condyloid canal of the occipital bone; the canal through which the hypoglossal nerve emerges from the skull.

**c. incisi'vus** [ NA ], incisive canal; one of several bony canals leading from the floor of the nasal cavity into the incisive fossa on the palatal surface of the maxilla. They convey the nasopalatine nerves and branches of the greater palatine arteries which anastomose with the septal branch of the sphenopalatine artery.

**c. infraorbita'lis** [ NA ], infraorbital canal; a canal running beneath the orbital margin of the maxilla from the infraorbital groove, in the floor of the orbit, to the infraorbital foramen; it transmits the infraorbital artery and nerve.

**c. inguina'lis** [ NA ], inguinal canal; abdominal canal; Velpeau's canal; the obliquely directed passage through the layers of the lower abdominal wall that transmits the spermatic cord in the male and the round ligament in the female.

**canales longitudina'les modioli** [ NA ], longitudinal canals of the modiolus; centrally placed channels that convey vessels and nerves to the apical turns of the cochlea.

**c. mandib'ulae** [ NA ], mandibular canal; inferior dental canal; the canal within the mandible that transmits the inferior alveolar nerve and vessels. Its posterior opening is the mandibular foramen.

**c. musculotuba'rius** [ NA ], musculotubal canal; a canal beginning at the anterior border of the petrous portion of the temporal bone near its junction with the squamous portion, and passing to the tympanic cavity; it is divided by the cochleariform process into two canals: one for the auditory (Eustachian) tube, the other for the tensor tympani muscle.

**c. nasolacrima'lis** [ NA ], nasolacrimal canal; the bony canal formed by the maxilla, lacrimal bone, and inferior concha that transmits the nasolacrimal duct from the orbit to the inferior meatus of the nose.

**c. nervi petro'si superficial'is minoris,** *hiatus* canalis nervi petrosi minoris.

**c. nutri'cius** [ NA ], nutrient canal; a canal in the shaft of a long bone or in other locations in irregular bones through which the nutrient artery enters a bone.

**c. obturato'rius** [ NA ], obturator canal; the opening in the superior part of the obturator membrane through which the obturator nerve and vessels pass from the pelvic cavity into the thigh.

**c. opticus** [ NA ], optic canal; optic foramen; foramen opticum; the short canal through the lesser wing of the sphenoid bone at the apex of the orbit that gives passage to the optic nerve and the ophthalmic artery.

**c. palati'nus major** [ NA ], greater palatine canal; pterygopalatine canal; the c. formed between the maxilla and palate bones. It transmits the descending palatine artery and the greater palatine nerve.

**canales palati'ni minores** [ NA ], canals for the lesser palatine nerves located in the posterior part of the palatine bone.

**c. palatovagina'lis** [ NA ], palatovaginal c.; pharyngeal canal; on the under surface of the vaginal process of the sphenoid bone a furrow is converted into a canal by the sphenoidal process of the palatine bone; it transmits the pharyngeal branch of the maxillary artery and the pharyngeal nerve from the sphenopalatine ganglion.

**c. pterygoi'deus** [ NA ], pterygoid canal; Vidian canal; an opening through the pterygoid process of the sphenoid bone through which pass the artery, vein, and nerve of the pterygoid canal.

**c. pudenda'lis** [ NA ], pudendal canal; Alcock's canal; the space within the obturator fascia lining the lateral wall of the ischiorectal fossa that transmits the pudendal vessels and nerves.

**c. pyloricus** [ NA ], pyloric canal; the aboral segment (about 2 to 3 cm. long) of the stomach; it succeeds the antrum and ends at the gastroduodenal junction.

**c. radicis dentis** [ NA ], marrow canal; (1) the root canal of a tooth; (2) the chamber of the dental pulp lying within the root portion of a tooth.

**c. reuniens,** *ductus* reuniens.

**c. sacralis** [ NA ], sacral canal; the continuation of the vertebral canal in the sacrum.

**canales semicircula'res ossei** [ NA ], bony semicircular canals; the three bony tubes in the labyrinth of the ear within which the membranous semicircular ducts are located. They lie in planes at right angles to each other and are known as **canales semicirculares anterior, posterior,** and **lateralis.**

**c. spiralis cochleae** [ NA ], spiral canal of the cochlea; cochlear canal; Rosenthal's canal; the winding tube of the bony labyrinth which makes two and a half turns about the modiolus of the cochlea; it is divided incompletely into two compartments by a winding shelf of bone, the lamina spiralis ossea.

**c. spira'lis modio'li** [ NA ], spiral canal of the modiolus; the space in the modiolus in which the spiral ganglion of the cochlear nerve lies.

**c. umbilica'lis,** *anulus* umbilicalis.

**c. ventric'uli** [ NA ], gastric canal; the part of the body of the stomach that follows the lesser curvature; it is characterized by longitudinal mucosal folds.

**c. vertebra'lis** [ NA ], vertebral canal; spinal canal; tubus vertebralis; the canal that contains the spinal cord, spinal meninges, and related structures. It is formed by the vertebral foramina of successive vertebrae of the articulated vertebral column.

**c. vomerovagina'lis** [ NA ], vomerovaginal canal; basipharyngeal canal; vomerine canal; an opening between the vaginal process of the sphenoid and the ala of the vomer on either side. It conveys a branch of the sphenopalatine artery.

**canaliza'tion.** The formation of canals or channels in any tissue.

**canav'alin.** A bactericidal mixture consisting of an enzyme obtained from jack bean, *Canavalia ensiformis* (family Leguminosae) and a coenzyme associated with the vitamin B complex; it attacks the polysaccharide component of certain pathogenic bacteria.

**Canavan,** M. M. See C.'s *disease, sclerosis.*

**canav'anine.** 2-Amino-4-(guanidinooxy)butyric acid; obtained from the jack bean, *Canavalia ensiformis* (family Leguminosae). It inhibits the growth of many microorganisms.

**can'cellated** [ L. *cancello,* to make a lattice work ]. Having a lattice work structure; reticular.

**cancellous** (kan'se-lus). Cancellated; denoting the reticular or spongy tissue of bone. See also *substantia* spongiosa.

**cancel'lus,** pl. **cancel'li** [ L. a grating, lattice ] [ NA ]. A lattice-like structure such as spongy bone.

**cancer** (kan'ser) [ L. a crab, a cancer. CANC- ]. A general term frequently used to indicate any of various types of malignant neoplasms, most of which invade surrounding tissues, may metastasize to several sites, and are likely to recur after attempted removal and to cause death of the patient unless adequately treated; any carcinoma or sarcoma (or other malignant neoplasm), but, in ordinary usage, especially the former.

**c. à deux** [ Fr. *deux,* two ], carcinomas occurring at approximately the same time, or in fairly close succession, in two persons who live together.

**Aran's c.,** chloroma.

**c. atroph'icans,** a scirrhous carcinoma in which there are relatively few neoplastic cells in a conspicuously dense, sclerotic, collagenous matrix.

**betel c.,** buyo cheek c.; carcinoma of the mucous membrane of the cheek, observed in certain East Indian natives, probably as a result of irritation from chewing a preparation of betel nut and lime rolled within a betel leaf.

**Butter's c.,** carcinoma of the hepatic flexure of the colon.

**buyo cheek c.** [ Phillipine *buyo,* betel ], betel c.

**chimney sweep's c.,** a carcinoma of the skin of the scrotum, occurring as an occupational disease in chimney sweeps and thought to result from chronic irritation by soot.

**colloid c.,** mucinous *carcinoma.*

**con'jugal c.,** c. à deux occurring in man and wife.

**contact c.,** one that develops in a portion of the body where there is direct contact with a carcinoma already present in another site in the same person.

**cystic c.,** cystic *carcinoma.*

duct c., duct *carcinoma.*

enceph'aloid c., medullary *carcinoma.*

c. en cuirasse (on-kwe-rahs') [ Fr. breastplate ], a carcinoma that involves a considerable portion of the skin of one or both sides of the thorax.

epidermoid c., squamous cell *carcinoma.*

epithe'lial c., any malignant neoplasm originating from epithelium, *i.e.,* a carcinoma.

glandular c., adenocarcinoma.

green c., chloroma.

he'matoid c., a soft, highly vascularized, malignant neoplasm, with numerous thin-walled vascular channels that bleed easily; sometimes termed fungus haematodes.

kang c., kangri c., a carcinoma of the skin of the thigh or abdomen in certain Indian or Chinese workers; thought to result from irritation by heat from a hot brick oven (kang) or fire basket (kangri).

med'ullary c., medullary *carcinoma.*

melanot'ic c., malignant *melanoma.*

mouse c., any of various types of malignant neoplasms that occur naturally in mice, especially in certain inbred "c. strains" used for research studies.

mule-spinner's c., carcinoma of the scrotum or adjacent skin exposed to oil, observed in some workers in cotton-spinning mills.

paraffin c., carcinoma of the skin occurring as an occupational disease in paraffin workers.

pipe-smoker's c., squamous cell carcinoma of the lip or tongue, formerly thought to result from long-continued irritation by hot tobacco smoke or by the stem of a clay pipe.

pitch-worker's c., carcinoma of the skin of the face or neck, arms and hands, or the scrotum, resulting from irritation by chemical compounds in pitch, which occurs naturally as asphalt, or as a residue in the distillation of tar.

rodent c., rodent *ulcer.*

scirrhous c., scirrhous *carcinoma.*

spider c., an infrequently used term for a malignant neoplasm with a rhizoid or filamentous edge of thin, threadlike, red lines that represent dilated vascular channels associated with the neoplasm; a form of telangiectatic c.

telangiectat'ic c., a c. with numerous dilated capillaries and "lakes" of blood within relatively large endothelium-lined channels.

water c., obsolete term for noma.

cancera'tion. A change that results in properties and features usually associated with malignant neoplasms, *e.g.,* as in the development of a carcinoma in a site previously involved by a benign condition.

cancericidal (kan'ser-ĭ-si'dal) [ cancer + L. *caedo,* to kill ]. Cancerocidal; capable of destroying the neoplastic cells of carcinomas or sarcomas.

can'cerigen'ic. Carcinogenic.

canceroci'dal. Cancericidal.

cancerol'ogy. Cancrology; the science pertaining to, or the study of, the causation, pathogenesis, biologic features, prevention, diagnosis, and treatment of cancers. See also oncology (a more commonly used term).

canceromyces (kan'ser-o-mi'sēz) [ cancer + *mykēs,* fungus ]. An obsolete term for an organism apparently intermediate between a mycete and a mold, regarded by Niessen as pathogenic for cancer.

cancerophobia (kan-sur-o-fo'bĭ-ah) [ cancer + G. *phobos,* fear ]. Carcinophobia; a morbid fear of acquiring a malignant growth.

cancerous (kan'ser-us). Relating to or pertaining to a malignant neoplasm, or being afflicted with such a process.

cancra (kang'krah). Plural of cancrum.

Cancriamoe'ba macroglos'sa [ L. *cancer* (*cancr-* or *cancer-*), cancer, + amoeba; G. *makros,* large, + *glossa,* tongue ]. Tumor cells mistakenly identified at one time as amebae with long pseudopodia, postulated as a cause of the cancer.

cancriform (kang'krĭ-form). Resembling cancer.

cancroid (kang'kroyd) [ cancer + G. *eidos,* resemblance ]. 1. Cancriform. 2. A malignant neoplasm (*e.g.,* basal cell carcinoma, and also certain others) that manifests a lesser degree of malignancy than that frequently observed with other types of carcinoma or sarcoma.

cancrology (kang-krol'o-jĭ) [ cancer + G. *logos,* study ]. Cancerology.

cancrum, pl. can'cra (kang'krum) [ Mod. L. fr. L. *cancer* (*cancr-*), cancer ]. A gangrenous, ulcerative, inflammatory lesion.

c. nasi, gangrenous, necrotizing, and ulcerative rhinitis (inflammation of the nasal mucous membrane), especially in children.

c. oris, noma.

can'dela [ L. ]. Candle; the unit of luminous intensity; the luminous flux emitted per unit of solid angle (steradian) by a full radiator having a temperature of the freezing point of platinum and an area of $1/60$ sq. cm. The c. is a basic unit in the SI system.

can'dicans [ L. *candico,* pres. p. -*ans,* to be whitish ]. One of the corpora albicantia.

can'dici'din (NF). Candeptin; a fungistatic and fungicidal polyene antibiotic agent derived from a soil actinomycete similar to *Streptomyces griseus;* used in the treatment of vaginal candidiasis.

Can'dida [ L. *candidus,* dazzling white ]. A large genus of yeastlike fungi commonly found in nature; some are frequently isolated from the skin, feces, vaginal vault, or pharynx of man. Some species cause candidiasis (moniliasis); others produce primary or secondary diseases in man.

c. al'bicans, *Monilia albicans;* the usual cause of candidiasis (moniliasis). Infection of the oropharynx, vagina, and gastrointestinal tract is common; pneumonia, meningitis, and similar lesions are less common. It is ordinarily saprophytic but may become pathogenic after the administration of certain antibiotics, probably from disturbance in the balance of the bacterial flora of the body.

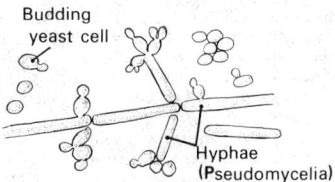

*Candida albicans*
(Original magnification, ×1000)

candide'mia [ *Candida* + G. *haima,* blood ]. The presence of cells of the yeastlike fungus, *Candida albicans,* in the peripheral blood.

candidiasis (kan'dĭ-di'ă-sis). Candidosis; moniliasis; infection with, or disease caused by, *Candida* or *Monilia albicans.*

candido'sis. Candidiasis.

candid'ulin. A crystalline antibacterial agent obtained from cultures of *Aspergillus candidus,* $C_{11}H_{15}O_3N$. It is active against many mycobacteria (but not *Mycobacterium tuberculosis*) and a variety of other bacteria.

candle (kan'dl). Candela.

candle-meter. Lux.

candle-power. Luminous *intensity.*

Can'idae [ L. *canis,* dog ]. A family of the *Carnivora* including the dogs, wolves, and foxes.

canine (ka'nin) [ L. *caninus* ]. 1. Relating to a dog. 2. Relating to the c. teeth. 3. A c. tooth. 4. Referring to the cuspid tooth.

canin'iform. Resembling a canine tooth.

Ca'nis familia'ris. The domestic dog.

can'ister. A box or container; in anesthesiology, the container for carbon dioxide absorbent; see also *absorber* head.

canities (kan-ish'e-ēz) [ L. fr. *canus,* hoary, gray ]. Poliosis; trichopoliosis; grayness of the hair.

c. unguium, leukonychia.

canker (kang'ker) [ L. *cancer* ]. 1. In cats and dogs, acute inflammation of the external ear and auditory canal. 2. In the horse, a process similar to but more advanced than thrush. The horny frog is generally under-run with a whitish, cheeselike exudate, and the entire sole and even the wall of the hoof may be undermined. 3. Obsolete term for aphthous stomatitis.

**water c.,** noma.

**cannabidiol.** $C_{21}H_{30}O_2$; a constituent of *Cannabis*, related to cannabinol.

**can'nabin.** A resinoid obtained from *Cannabis sativa* var. *indica* (family Moraceae); has been used in hysteria, neuralgia, delirium tremens, and insomnia.

**cannab'inol.** 6,6,9-Trimethyl-3-pentyl-6*H*-dibenzo[ *b,d* ]-pyran-1-ol; a constituent of the resinous exudate of the pistillate flowers of *Cannabis sativa;* it has no psychotomimetic action, but the tetrahydro derivatives isolated from marijuana do.

**can'nabis** [ L. fr. G. *kannabis,* hemp ]. *Cannabis indica;* American hemp; Indian hemp; Indian cannabis; marijuana; marihuana; bhang, charas; ganja; hashish; and many slang terms; the dried flowering tops of the pistillate plants of *Cannabis sativa* var. *indica* (family Moraceae) containing isomeric tetrahydrocannabinols, cannabinol, and cannabidiol. Preparations of c. are smoked or ingested by members of various cultures and subcultures to induce psychotomimetic effects such as euphoria, hallucinations, drowsiness, and other mental changes. C. was formerly used as a sedative and analgesic.

**can'nabism.** Poisoning by Indian hemp or hashish (related to marijuana). Associated with hallucinations and other subjective manifestations.

**Cannizzaro's reaction.** See under reaction.

**Cannon,** Walter B., Boston physiologist, 1871–1945. See C.'s *ring,* C.'s *test,* C. and La Paz *test,* Rosenblueth and C. *test,* C.'s *theory,* C-Band *theory.*

**cannula** (kan'u-lah) [ L. dim. of *canna,* reed ]. A tube that is inserted into a cavity by means of a trocar filling its lumen; after insertion the trocar is withdrawn leaving the c. as a channel for the escape of fluid in the cavity. See fig. under trocar.

**Belloc's c.,** Belloc's sound; a hollow sound containing a curved spring, used for passing a thread through the nostril and mouth in order to draw in a plug in case of profuse epistaxis.

**Lindeman's c.,** a c. used in blood transfusion.

**perfusion c.,** a double-barreled c. used for irrigation of a cavity, the wash fluid passing into the cavity through one tube and out through the other.

**washout c.,** one that can be irrigated without removal from the artery.

**cannula'tion, cannuliza'tion.** Insertion of a cannula.

**Canomyces** (ka'no-mi'sēz). Pleuropneumonia organism from canine distemper.

**canren'one** (USAN). 17-Hydroxy-3-oxo-17α-pregna-4,9-diene-21-carboxylic acid γ-*l* lactone; an aldosterone antagonist.

**cant.** A sloping, slanted, or angled surface.

**c. of the mandible,** Frankfort mandibular plane *angle.*

**Cantelli's sign.** See under sign.

**can'thal.** Relating to a canthus.

**canthar'idal.** Relating to or containing cantharides.

**canthar'idate.** A salt of cantharidic acid.

**cantharides** (kan-thăr'ĭ-dēz). Plural of cantharis.

**canthar'idic acid.** $C_{10}H_{14}O_5$; an acid, derived from cantharis, that forms salts (cantharidates) with alkalis.

**canthar'idin.** Cantharis camphor; $C_{10}H_{12}O_4$; hexahydro-3α,7α-dimethyl-4,7-epoxyisobenzofuran-1,3-dione; the active principle of cantharis; the anhydride of cantharic acid.

**can'tharis,** gen. **canthar'idis,** pl. **canthar'ides** [ L. fr. G. *kantharis,* a beetle ]. Spanish fly; Russian fly; a dried beetle, *Cantharis vesicatoria.* Counterirritant and vesicant.

**canthec'tomy** [ G. *kanthos,* canthus, + *ektomē,* excision ]. Excision of a canthus.

**canthi'tis.** Inflammation of a canthus.

**canthol'ysis** [ G. *kanthos,* canthus, + *lysis,* loosening ]. Incision of the canthus to widen the slit between the lids; canthoplasty (1).

**can'thoplasty** [ G. *kanthos,* canthus, + *plassō,* to form ]. 1. An operation for lengthening the palpebral fissure by cutting through the external canthus. 2. An operation for restoration of the canthus in case of pathologic or traumatic defect.

**canthorrhaphy** (kan-thor'ă-fī) [ G. *kanthos,* canthus, + *rhaphē,* suture ]. Suture of the eyelids at either canthus.

**canthot'omy** [ G. *kanthos,* canthus, + *tomē,* incision ]. Slitting of the canthus; cantholysis; canthoplasty (1).

**canthus,** pl. **can'thi** (kan'thus) [ G. *kanthos,* corner of the eye ]. See *angulus* oculi lateralis and *angulus* oculi medialis.

**Cantor,** Meyer O., Detroit physician, *1907. See C. *tube.*

**CaOC.** Abbreviation for cathodal opening *contraction.*

**caoutchin** (kow'chin). Limonene.

**caoutchouc** (kow'chook) [ S. A. Indian, *cahuchu* ]. Rubber; India rubber; the prepared inspissated milky juice of *Hevea brasiliensis* and other species of *Hevea* (family Euphorbiaceae), known in commerce as pure Para rubber. Used in the manufacture of various plasters, tissues, bandages, etc.

**cap.** 1. Abbreviation for L. *capiat,* let (him or her) take, *capiatur,* let it be taken, or *capiendus, a, um,* to be taken, fr. *capio,* to take. 2. Any anatomical structure that resembles a c. or cover. 3. A protective covering for an incomplete tooth. 4. Colloquial reference to the restoration of the coronal part of a natural tooth by means of an artificial crown.

**acrosomal c.,** a thin covering over the anterior part of the nucleus of the spermatozoon; derived from the acrosomal granule.

**chin c.,** a device designed to put force upon the chin to restrain forward growth.

**cradle c.,** Colloquialism for seborrheic dermatitis of the scalp of the newborn.

**dental c.'s,** deciduous cheek teeth in the horse which remain attached to erupting permanent teeth.

**duode'nal c.,** the first portion of the duodenum, pileus ventriculi, as seen in the x-ray picture.

**Dutch c.,** a contraceptive vaginal diaphragm.

**enamel c.,** the enamel covering the crown of a tooth.

**Hippocrates' c.,** a roller bandage for the head.

**ice c.,** an ice bag shaped to fit the head.

**metanephric c.,** the concentrated mass of mesodermal cells about the ureteral (metanephric) bud in a young embryo. The cells of the cap form the uriniferous tubules of the permanent kidney.

**phrygian c.,** on x-ray, a fold in the fundus of the gallbladder.

**pyloric c.,** duodenal c.

**skull c.,** calvaria.

**x-ray c. of Zinn,** prominence of the pulmonary arc in the cardiac silhouette in cases of patent ductus arteriosus.

**capac'itance.** The quantity of electric charge that may be stored upon a body per unit electric potential; expressed in farads, abfarads, or statfarads.

**capacitation** (kă-pas'ĭ-ta'shun) [ L. *capacitas,* fr. *capax,* capable of ]. The process whereby spermatozoa acquire the ability to fertilize ova. This process occurs in the female genital tract and, depending on species, requires 1 to 6 hours for completion. It is characterized by loss of the acrosome cap by spermatozoa and an increase in their respiratory metabolism and content of DNA.

**capac'itor.** Condenser (4); a device for holding a charge of electricity.

**capacity** (kă-pas'ĭ-tī) [ L. *capax,* able to contain; fr. *capio,* to take ]. 1. The potential cubic contents of a cavity or receptacle. 2. Ability; power to do. 3. See also fig. and subentries under volume.

**buffer c.,** see under buffer.

**cranial c.,** the cubic content of the skull obtained by determining the cubage of small shot, seeds, or beads required to fill the skull.

**diffusing c.** (symbol, D, followed by subscripts indicating location and chemical species), the amount of oxygen taken up by pulmonary capillary blood per minute per unit average oxygen pressure gradient between alveolar gas and pulmonary capillary blood; units are: ml/min/mm Hg; also applied to other gases such as carbon monoxide.

**functional residual c.,** functional residual air; the volume of gas remaining in the lungs at the end of a normal expiration; it is the sum of expiratory reserve volume and residual volume.

**heat c.,** thermal c.; the quantity of heat required to raise the temperature of a system 1°C.

**inspiratory c.,** complemental air; complementary air; the volume of air that can be inspired after a normal expiration; it is the sum of the tidal volume and the inspiratory reserve volume.

**maximum breathing c.** (MBC), maximum voluntary ventilation (MVV); the volume of air breathed when a subject breathes as deeply and as quickly as possible for 15 seconds, as measured by a spirometer without a carbon dioxide absorber. The difference between the maximum breathing capacity and the pulmonary ventilation is called the breathing reserve.

**oxygen c.,** the maximum quantity of oxygen that will combine chemically with the hemoglobin in a unit volume of blood; normally it amounts to 1.34 ml. of $O_2$ per gm. of Hb or 20 ml. of $O_2$ per 100 ml. of blood.

**resid'ual c.,** residual *volume.*

**respiratory c.,** vital c.

**thermal c.,** heat c.

**total lung c.,** abbreviated TLC; the inspiratory c. plus the functional residual c.; *i.e.,* the volume of air contained in the lungs at the end of a maximal inspiration. Also equals vital c. plus residual volume.

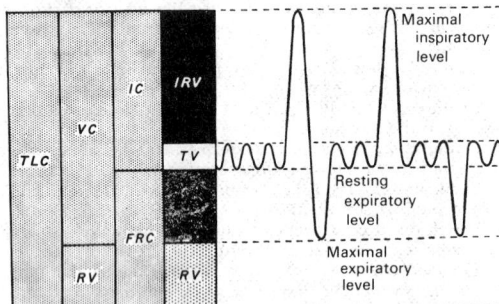

**Subdivisions of the Total Lung Capacity**

*TLC,* total lung capacity; *VC,* vital capacity; *RV,* residual volume; *IC,* inspiratory capacity; *FRC,* functional residual capacity; *IRV,* inspiratory reserve volume; *TV,* tidal volume; *ERV,* expiratory reserve volume. (From Comroe, J. H., Jr., et al.: *The Lung: Clinical Physiology and Pulmonary Function Tests,* Ed. 2, © 1962, Year Book Medical Publishers, Inc. Used by permission of Year Book Medical Publishers.)

**vital c.,** respiratory c.; the greatest volume of air that can be exhaled from the lungs after a maximum inspiration.

**Capdepont,** C., French physician. See C.'s *disease.*

**capeline** (kap'e-lin). See under bandage.

**Capgras,** Jean Marie Joseph, French psychiatrist, 1873–1950. See C.'s *syndrome.*

**cap'illarecta'sia** [ capillary + G. *ektasis,* extension ]. Dilation of the capillary blood vessels.

**Capillaria** (kap-ĭ-la'rĭ-ah). A genus of aphasmid nematode worms, characized by threadlike appearance; related to *Trichuris,* the whipworm.

  **C. aeroph'ila,** a small nematode occurring in the bronchi, bronchioles, and nasal sinuses of dogs, cats, and foxes; it causes rhinotracheitis, bronchitis, and nasal discharge in young animals.

  **C. bo'vis,** occurs in the small intestine of cattle, sheep and goats.

  **C. brev'ipes,** found in the small intestine of cattle, sheep and goats.

  **C. hepat'ica,** threadworm of rodents infecting the liver; rarely reported from man.

  **C. philippinen'sis,** a species of threadworm that has been implicated as a cause of intestinal capillariasis among northern Philippine fishermen.

  **C. pli'ca,** a fine threadworm occurring in the urinary bladder and sometimes the kidney pelvis of the dog and cat; it apparently causes little damage in many instances.

**capillariasis** (kap-ĭ-lār-i'ah-sis). A parasitic disease caused by an infection with the threadworm (nematode) belonging to the genus *Capillaria,* generally *C. philippinensis.*

  **intestinal c.,** a malabsorption syndrome caused by infection with *Capillaria philippinensis;* characterized by abdominal pain, edema, diarrhea, cachexia, hypoproteinemia, hypotension, cardiac failure, and hyporeflexia; severe infection is often manifested as a fulminating disorder that leads to death; thiabendazole is usually an effective therapeutic agent.

**capillar'iomo'tor.** Vasomotor, with special reference to the capillaries.

**capillarios'copy.** Microangioscopy; capillaroscopy; viewing the cutaneous capillaries at the base of the fingernail through the low power of the microscope.

**capillaritis** (kap'ĭ-lār-i'tis). Inflammation of a capillary or capillaries.

**capillar'ity.** The rise of liquids in narrow tubes.

**cap'illarop'athy.** Microangiopathy; any disease of the capillaries.

**capillaros'copy.** Capillarioscopy.

**cap'illary** [ L. *capillaris,* relating to hair. CAP-1 ]. 1. Resembling a hair; fine; minute. 2. A capillary vessel; *e.g.,* blood c. and lymph c. 3. Relating to a blood or lymphatic c. vessel.

  **arterial c.,** a c. opening from an arteriole or metarteriole.

  **bile c.,** biliary *canaliculus.*

  **blood c.** (symbol c, as a subscript), a vessel whose wall consists of endothelium and its basement membrane. Its diameter when the c. is open is about 8 $\mu$. With the electron microscope, fenestrated c.'s and continuous c.'s are distinguished. The former occur in renal glomeruli, intestinal villi, and some glands; the latter, in muscle.

  **continuous c.,** one in which pinocytotic vesicles are numerous and pores are absent.

  **fenestrated c.,** one in which ultramicroscopic pores of variable size occur; usually these are closed by a delicate diaphragm, although diaphragms are not seen in the renal glomerular c.'s.

  **lymph c.,** the beginning of the lymphatic system of vessels; the lymph c., which is lined with flattened endothelium, has a lumen of variable caliber; see lacteal.

  **sinusoidal c.,** a c. with caliber of from 10 $\mu$ to 20 $\mu$ or more; it is lined with a nonphagocytic, fenestrated type of endothelium and occurs in such organs as the anterior lobe of the hypophysis and adrenal cortex.

  **venous c.,** one opening into a venule.

**capil'lus,** gen. and pl. **capil'li** [ L. hair ] [ NA ]. A hair of the head.

**capistra'tion** [ L. *capistrum,* muzzle: phimosis ]. Paraphimosis.

**capita** (kap'ĭ-tah). Plural of caput.

**capita'lis** [ L. *caput,* head ] [ NA ]. Relating to the head.

**cap'itate** [ L. *caput* (*capit*-), head ]. 1. Head-shaped; having a rounded extremity. 2. *Os* capitatum.

**capita'tus** [ L. ] [ NA ]. Capitate (1).

**capitel'lum** [ L. dim. of *caput,* head. CAP-1 ]. 1. Capitulum; 2. *Capitulum* humeri.

**capit'ium** [ L. *caput,* head ]. A bandage for the head.

**capitoped'al** [ L. *caput,* head, + *pes* (*ped*-), foot ]. Relating to the head and the feet.

**capitonnage** (kap'i-to-nahzh') [ Fr. *capitonnage,* upholstering ]. Surgical closure of a cyst cavity by use of sutures.

**capitula** (kă-pit'u-lah). Plural of capitulum.

**capit'ular.** Relating to a capitulum.

**capitulum,** pl. **capit'ula** (kă-pit'u-lum) [ L. dim. of *caput,* head. CAP-1 ]. 1 [ NA ]. A small head or rounded articular extremity of a bone; see also caput. 2. The bloodsucking, probing, sensing, and holdfast mouthparts of a tick, including the basal supporting structure (basis capituli); relative size and shape of mouthparts forming the c. are characteristic for the genera of hard ticks.

  **c. hu'meri** [ NA ], small or radial head, capitellum, of the humerus.

**Caplan,** Anthony, British physician, 20th century. See C.'s *nodule, syndrome.*

**cap'nogram** [ G. *kapnos*, smoke, + *gramma*, something written ]. A continuous record of the carbon dioxide content of expired air.

**cap'nograph.** Instrument by which a continuous graph of the carbon dioxide content of expired air is obtained.

**ca'pon.** A castrated male bird, generally a chicken.

**ca'ponize.** To castrate a male bird, making a capon.

**cap'ping.** Covering.

    **direct pulp c.,** a procedure for covering and protecting an exposed vital pulp under favorable conditions.

    **indirect pulp c.,** the application of a suspension of calcium hydroxide to a thin layer of dentin overlying the pulp (near exposure) in order to stimulate secondary dentin formation and protect the pulp.

**Capps,** Joseph A., U. S. physician, \*1872. See C.'s *reflex.*

**cap'rate.** A salt or ester of capric acid.

**capreomy'cin sulfate** (USP). CAPASTAT; sulfate salt of the cyclic peptide antibiotic obtained from *Streptomyces capreolus.* In combination with *p*-aminosalicylic acid, used in the treatment of tuberculosis; cochlear nerve damage may develop.

*n*-**cap'ric acid.** Decanoic acid, $CH_3(CH_2)_8COOH$, found among the hydrolysis products of fat in goat's milk, cow's milk, and other substances; it has a more or less pronounced goatlike odor.

**capriloquism** (kă-pril'o-kwizm) [ L. *caper*, goat, + *loquor*, to speak ]. Egophony.

**cap'rin.** Decanoin; tridecanoylglycerol (glyceryl caprate is a misnomer); found in butter, and one of the substances upon which the flavor of that substance depends.

**caprine** (că'prin) [ L. *caprinus*, of goats ]. Relating to goats; goatlike.

**cap'rizant.** Bounding; leaping; denoting a form of pulse beat.

**cap'roate.** 1. A salt or ester of caproic acid. 2. USAN-approved contraction for hexanoate, $CH_3$-$(CH_2)_4COO^-$.

**caprochlor'one.** 4-(*o*-Chlorobenzyl)-5-oxo-4-phenylhexanoic acid; antiviral agent.

*n*-**capro'ic acid.** Hexanoic acid; $CH_3(CH_2)_4COOH$; found among the hydrolysis products of fat in butter and some other substances.

**caproin** (kap'ro-in). Octanoin; trioctanoylglycerol (glyceryl caproate is a misnomer); found with caprin and butyrin in butter.

**caproyl** (kap'ro-il). Hexanoyl; the radical of caproic acid, $CH_3(CH_2)_4CO—$.

**caproylamine** (kap-ro-il'am-in). Hexanoyl amide; caproamide; $CH_3(CH_2)_4CONH_2$; a ptomaine from cod liver oil.

**caproylate** (kap'ro-ĭ-lāt). Hexanoylate; a salt or ester of caproic acid.

**cap'rylate.** Octanoylate; a salt or ester of caprylic acid.

*n*-**capryl'ic acid.** Octanoic acid; $CH_3(CH_2)_6COOH$, found among the hydrolysis products of fat in butter and other substances.

**capsaicin** (cap-sa'ĭ-sin). STYPTYSAT; *trans*-8-methyl-*N*-vanillyl-6-nonenamide; alkaloidal principle in the fruits of various species of *Capsicum*, with same uses as capsicum.

**cap'sicin.** A yellowish red oleoresin containing the active principle of capsicum.

**cap'sicum** [ Mod. L. fr. L. *capsa*, a box (from the shape of the fruit) ]. The dried ripe fruit of *Capsicum frutescens* (family Solanaceae); cayenne, African, or red pepper. Carminative, gastrointestinal stimulant, and externally rubefacient.

    **c. oleoresin,** gastrointestinal stimulant and carminative; also used externally as a counterirritant.

**capsid** (kap'sid). See virion.

**capsomer** (kap'so-mĕr). See virion.

**capsula,** gen. and pl. **cap'sulae** (kap'su-lah) [ L. dim. of *capsa*, a chest or box ] [ NA ]. Capsule. 1. A membranous structure enveloping an organ or any other part, or a joint. 2. An anatomical structure resembling a capsule or envelope.

    **c. adipo'sa re'nis** [ NA ], adipose capsule; the perirenal fat.

    **c. articula'ris** [ NA ], articular capsule; joint capsule; a fibrous sac, enclosing a joint, formed by an outer fibrous membrane and an inner synovial membrane.

    **c. articula'ris cricoarytenoi'dea** [ NA ], cricoarytenoid articular capsule; the capsule enclosing the joint between the arytenoid and cricoid cartilages.

    **c. articula'ris cricothyroi'dea** [ NA ], cricothyroid articular capsule; the capsule enclosing the cricothyroid joint.

    **c. bulbi,** *vagina* bulbi.

    **c. cordis,** the pericardium.

    **c. externa** [ NA ], external capsule; periclaustral lamina; a thin lamina of white substance separating the claustrum from the putamen or lateral portion of the lenticular nucleus. It joins the internal capsule at either extremity of the putamen, forming a capsule of white matter over the lateral side of the lenticular nucleus.

    **c. extre'ma,** extreme capsule; the layer of white matter separating the claustrum from the cortex of the insula, probably representing largely the white matter (incoming and outgoing fibers) of the insular cortex.

    **c. fibrosa glan'dulae thyroid'eae** [ NA ], the fibrous sheath of the thyroid gland.

    **c. fibro'sa perivascularis hep'atis** [ NA ], Glisson's capsule; a layer of connective tissue ensheathing the hepatic artery, portal vein, and bile ducts as these ramify within the liver.

    **c. fibrosa renis** [ NA ], fibrous capsule of the kidney; a fibrous membrane that encases the kidney; normally it is easily stripped away from the underlying renal tissue.

    **c. glomer'uli** [ NA ], Bowman's capsule; Malpighian capsule; Müller's capsule; the expanded beginning of a renal tubule. The visceral layer consists of podocytes which surround a tuft of capillaries, the glomerulus. The parietal c. is a flat epithelium which becomes cuboidal at the tubular pole.

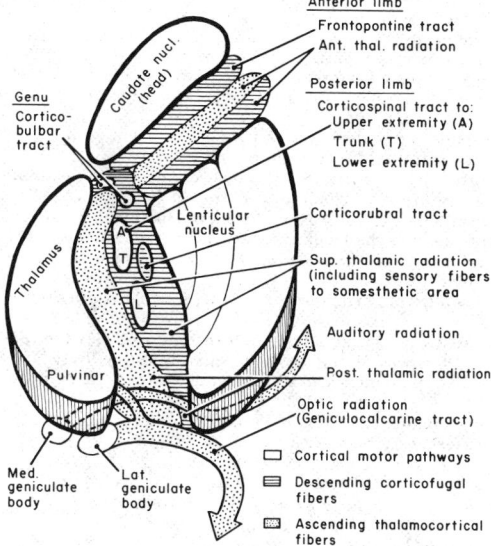

**Capsula Interna**
Right internal capsule and neighboring structures. (From Truex, R. C., and Carpenter, M. B.: *Human Neuroanatomy,* Ed. 6, The Williams & Wilkins Co., Baltimore, 1969.)

    **c. interna** [ NA ], internal capsule; a massive layer (8 to 10 mm. thick) of white matter separating the caudate nucleus and thalamus on the medial side from the more laterally situated lentiform nucleus (globus pallidus and putamen). It is made up of (a) fibers ascending from the thalamus to the cerebral cortex that compose, among others, the visual, auditory, and somatic sensory radiations, and (b) fibers descending from the cerebral cortex to the thalamus, subthalamic region, midbrain, hindbrain, and spinal cord. The internal capsule is the major route by which the cerebral cortex is connected with the brainstem and spinal cord. Laterally it is directly continuous with the corona radiata which forms a major part of the cerebral hemisphere's white matter; caudally and medially it continues, much reduced in size, as the crus cerebri which contains, among others, the pyramidal tract. On horizontal section it appears in the form of a V opening out laterally; the V's obtuse angle is called genu (knee); its anterior and posterior limbs, respectively, the crus anterior and crus posterior.

   **c. lentis** [ NA ], lenticular capsule; crystalline capsule; capsule enclosing the crystalline lens.

   **c. li'enis,** *tunica* fibrosa lienis.

   **c. vasculosa lentis,** in the embryo, the vascular mesenchymal capsule which invests the crystalline lens; the vessels of the dorsal part of the capsule are branches of the hyaloid artery, those of the ventral part are derived from the anterior ciliary arteries. Normally all the vessels are atrophied by the end of the eighth month of intrauterine life.

**cap'sular.** Relating to any capsule.

**capsula'tion.** Enclosure in a capsule.

**capsule** (kap'sūl) [ L. *capsula* ]. 1. Capsula. 2. A membranous structure, consisting usually of dense collagenous connective tissue, which envelopes an organ or part. 3. A fibrous tissue layer enveloping a tumor. 4. A solid dosage form in which the drug is enclosed in either a hard or soft soluble container or "shell" of a suitable form of gelatin. 5. In space medicine, a small sealed pressurized cabin with a satisfactory artificial environment for containing man or animals for orbital space, for very high altitude space, or as an emergency escape device.

   **adipose c.,** *capsula* adiposa renis.

   **adrenal c.,** *glandula* suprarenalis.

   **articular c.,** *capsula* articularis.

   **atrabil'iary c.,** *glandula* suprarenalis.

   **auditory c.,** the cartilage that, in the embryo, surrounds the developing auditory vesicle.

   **bacterial c.,** a layer of slime of variable composition which covers the surface of some bacteria. Capsulated cells of pathogenic bacteria are usually more virulent than cells without capsules for the former are more resistant to phagocytic action.

   **Bonnet's c.,** the anterior part of the vagina bulbi.

   **Bowman's c.,** *capsula* glomeruli.

   **brood c.'s,** small hollow projections from the lining membrane of a hydatid cyst from which arise the scolices.

   **cartilage c.,** the basophilic matrix in hyaline cartilage surrounding the lacunae in which lie the cartilage cells.

   **cricoarytenoid articular c.,** *capsula* articularis cricoarytenoidea.

   **cricothyroid articular c.,** *capsula* articularis cricothyroidea.

   **Crosby c.,** an attachment to the end of a flexible tube, used for peroral biopsy of the small intestine, by which a piece of mucosa is sucked into an opening in the c. and cut off.

   **crys'talline c.,** *capsula* lentis.

   **external c.,** *capsula* externa.

   **extreme c.,** *capsula* extrema.

   **eye c.,** *vagina* bulbi.

   **fibrous articular c.,** *membrana* fibrosa.

   **fibrous c. of kidney,** *capsula* fibrosa renis.

   **Gerota's c.,** the renal *fascia.*

   **Glisson's c.,** *capsula* fibrosa perivascularis hepatis.

   **internal c.,** *capsula* interna.

   **joint c.,** *capsula* articularis.

   **lentic'ular c.,** *capsula* lentis.

   **Malpighian c.,** (1) *capsula* glomeruli; (2) a thin fibrous membrane enveloping the spleen and continued over the vessels entering at the hilus.

   **Müller's c.,** *capsula* glomeruli.

   **nasal c.,** the cartilage around the developing nasal cavity of the embryo.

   **optic c.,** the concentrated zone of mesenchyme around the developing optic cup; the primordium of the sclera of the eye.

   **otic c.,** the cartilage c. surrounding the inner ear mechanism. In elasmobranchs, it remains cartilaginous in

the adult. In the embryos of higher vertebrates, it is cartilaginous at first but later becomes bony.

   **radiotelemetering c.,** radiopill; an instrument that transmits measurements by radio impulses, from within the body; for example, measurements of pressure from within the small bowel.

   **seminal c.,** *vesicula* seminalis.

   **space c.,** c. (4).

   **suprare'nal c.,** *glandula* suprarenalis.

   **Tenon's c.,** *vagina* bulbi.

**capsulitis** (kap'su-li'tis). Inflammation of the capsule of an organ or part, as of the liver or crystalline lens.

   **hepat'ic c.,** perihepatitis.

   **c. of the lab'yrinth,** otosclerosis.

**cap'sulolentic'ular.** Referring to the crystalline lens and its capsule.

**cap'suloplas'ty** [ L. *capsula,* capsule, + G. *plassō,* to fashion ]. Plastic surgery of a capsule, more particularly the capsule of a joint.

**capsulorrhaphy** (kap-su-lor'ă-fī) [ L. *capsula,* capsule, + *raphē,* suture ]. Suture of a tear in any capsule; specifically, suture of a joint capsule to prevent recurring dislocation of the articulation.

**cap'sulotome.** Cystitome.

**capsulot'omy** [ L. *capsula,* capsule, + G. *tomē,* a cutting ]. 1. Incision through a capsule, specifically, the capsule of the lens in the extracapsular cataract operation. 2. Cystotomy.

**captation** (kap-ta'shun) [ L. *captatio,* seizure ]. Early stages of hypnotism.

**captodi'amine.** SUVREN; 2[ *p*-(butylthio)-α-phenylbenzylthio ]-*N,N*-dimethylethylamine; sedative and antianxiety agent.

**cap'ture.** A taking; a catch.

   **atrial c.,** control of the atria after a period of independent beating, as in complete A-V block, by the retrograde impulse.

   **ventricular c.,** c. *beat.*

**cap'uride** (USAN). PACINOX; (2-ethyl-3-methylvaleryl)-urea; used as hypnotic.

**Capuron,** Joseph, French physician, 1767–1850. See C.'s *points.*

**caput,** gen. **cap'itis,** pl. **cap'ita** (kap'ut, ka'put) [ L. See CAP-1 ]. 1[ NA ]. The head. 2[ NA ]. Any head, or expanded or rounded extremity of an organ or other anatomical structure.

   **c. breve** [ NA ], short head; in biceps brachii and biceps femoris, the head that has the more distal origin.

   **c. cornus,** *apex* cornus posterioris.

   **c. costae** [ NA ], the head of a rib articulating by two facets with the bodies of two contiguous vertebrae.

   **c. epididymid'is** [ NA ], head of epididymis; globus major; the upper and larger extremity of the epididymis.

   **c. fem'oris** [ NA ], head of the femur; hemispheric articular surface at the upper extremity of the femur, which fits into the acetabulum to form the hip joint.

   **c. fib'ulae** [ NA ], head of the fibula; the superior extremity of the fibula, which articulates by a facet with the under surface of the lateral condyle of the tibia.

   **c. gallinaginis** (gal-lin-aj'in-is) [ Mod. L. snipe's head ], *colliculus* seminalis.

   **c. humera'le** [ NA ], humeral head; the name applied to the heads of some of the muscles of the forearm that attach to the humerus.

   **c. hu'meri** [ NA ], head of the humerus; the upper rounded extremity fitting into the glenoid cavity of the scapula.

   **c. humeroulna're** [ NA ], humeroulnar head; the head of the superficial flexor of the digits that attaches to both the humerus and the ulna.

   **c. latera'le** [ NA ], lateral head; one of the heads of origin of the triceps brachii and of the gastrocnemius.

   **c. long'um** [ NA ], long head; the head that has the more proximal origin in the biceps and triceps brachii and the biceps femoris.

   **c. mallei** [ NA ], the head of the malleus articulating with the body of the incus.

   **c. mandib'ulae** [ NA ], head of the mandible; the expanded articular portion of the condylar process of the mandible.

**c. media'le** [ NA ], medial head; one of the heads of origin of the triceps brachii and of the gastrocnemius.

**c. medu'sae** [ *Medusa,* a mythologic character whose scalp consisted of a mass of serpents ] Cruveilhier's sign; varicose veins radiating from the umbilicus, seen in the Cruveilhier-Baumgarten *syndrome.*

**c. mor'tuum,** impure ferrous oxide left after the ignition of iron pyrites.

**c. nu'clei cauda'ti** [ NA ], the head or anterior extremity of the caudate nucleus projecting into the anterior horn of the lateral ventricle.

**c. obli'quum** [ NA ], oblique head; one of the heads of origin of the adductor of the thumb and of the adductor of the great toe.

**c. os'sis metacarpa'lis** [ NA ], head of a metacarpal bone; the expanded distal end of a metacarpal that articulates with the proximal phalanx of the same digit.

**c. pancre'atis** [ NA ], head of the pancreas; that portion of the pancreas lying in the concavity of the duodenum.

**c. phalangis** [ NA ], head of the phalanx; trochlea phalangis; the rounded articular surface at the distal end of the proximal and middle phalanx of each finger and toe.

**c. profun'dum** [ NA ], deep head; the head of short flexor of the thumb that arises from the trapezoid and capitate bones.

**c. quadra'tum,** a head of large size and square shape, owing to thickened parietal and frontal eminences, seen in rachitic children.

**c. radia'le** [ NA ], radial head; the name applied to one of the heads of origin of several forearm muscles that arise from the ulna.

**c. radii** [ NA ], head of the radius; the disk-shaped upper extremity articulating with the capitulum of the humerus.

**c. sta'pedis** [ NA ], the head of the stapes that articulates with the lenticular process of the incus.

**c. superficia'le** [ NA ], superficial head; the head of the short flexor of the thumb that arises from the flexor retinaculum and the trapezium.

**c. succeda'neum** [ L. *succedaneus,* following, substituting ], an edematous swelling formed on the presenting portion of the scalp of an infant during birth. The effusion overlies the periosteum and consists of serum. Contrasted with cephalhematoma, in which condition the effusion lies under the periosteum and consists of blood.

**c. tali** [ NA ], the head, or anterior portion, of the talus.

**c. transver'sum** [ NA ], transverse head; one of the heads of origin of the adductor of the thumb and of the great toe.

**c. ulnae** [ NA ], head or distal extremity of the ulna.

**c. ulna're** [ NA ], ulnar head; the name applied to one of the heads of several muscles of the forearm that arise from the ulna.

**Carabelli,** Georg C., Vienna dentist, 1787–1842. See C. *tubercle.*

**caramel** (kar'ah-mel) (USP). Burnt sugar; a concentrated solution of the substance obtained by heating sugar with an alkali; a thick, dark brown liquid. Used as a coloring and flavoring agent in pharmaceutical preparations.

**caram'iphen ethanedisulfonate.** TAORYL; TORYN; diethylaminoethyl 1-phenylcyclopentane-1-carboxylate ethanedisulfonate; antitussive.

**caramiphen hydrochloride** (kă-ram'ĭ-fen) (BP). PANPARNIT; diethylaminoethyl-1-phenylcyclopentane-1-carboxylate hydrochloride; a synthetic spasmolytic drug; used in the treatment of diseases of the basal ganglia, *e.g.,* parkinsonism and hepatolenticular degeneration.

**carat** (kăr'at) [ Ar. *girat,* bean ]. In precious metals, the amount of the main metal present expressed in twenty-fourths; *e.g.,* 24-c. gold is 100 per cent gold. See also fineness.

**cara'te.** Pinta.

**car'away** (NF, BP). Caraway seed; carum; the dried ripe fruit of *Carum carvi* (family Umbelliferae); a biennial plant cultivated in northern Europe, Siberia and the United States. Used as a flavoring agent.

**c. oil** (NF), a volatile oil distilled from the fruit of *Carum carvi;* a flavoring agent.

**powdered c.** (BP), similar uses as for c.

**carb-, carba-, carbo-.** Prefixes indicating the attachment of a group containing a carbon atom.

**car'bachol** (USP, BP). CHARCHOLIN; carbamoylcholine chloride; choline chloride carbamate; parasympathetic stimulant.

**car'bacryl'amine res'ins.** See under resin.

**car'badox** (USAN). Methyl 3-(2-quinoxalvinylmethylene)carbazate $N^1,N^4$-dioxide; antibacterial agent.

**car'bamate.** A salt or ester of carbamic acid; it forms the basis of urethane hypnotics.

**c. kinase,** a phosphotransferase (EC 2.7.2.2) catalyzing the reaction of carbamoyl phosphate and ADP to form ATP, $NH_3$, and $CO_2$ (the reverse of the reaction catalyzed by carbamoylphosphate synthase).

**carbamaz'epine** (USP, BP). TEGRETAL; TEGRETOL; 5-*H*-dibenz[ *b,f* ]azepine; anticonvulsant; also analgesic, especially useful in trigeminal neuralgia.

**carbam'ic.** Relating to the amide of carbonic acid.

**c. acid,** a hypothetical acid, $NH_2$—COOH, forming carbamates.

**car'bamide.** Urea or one of its derivatives.

**carbamino compound.** Any carbamic acid derivative formed by the combination of carbon dioxide with a free amino group to form an *N*-carboxy group, —NH—COOH, as in the hemoglobin molecule, where it accounts for the carriage in the blood of about 20 per cent of the $CO_2$ produced in the tissues.

**car'baminohemoglo'bin.** Carbon dioxide bound to hemoglobin by means of a reactive amino group on the latter, *i.e.,* HbNHCOOH. Approximately 20 per cent of the total content of carbon dioxide in blood is combined with hemoglobin in this manner.

**carbamoyl** (kar-bam'o-il). The radical, $NH_2$—CO—, the transfer of which plays an important role in some biochemical reactions, *e.g.,* the urea cycle, carbamoyl phosphate.

**carbamoylaspartate dehydrase.** Dihydro-orotase.

***N*-carbamoylaspartic acid.** *Ureidosuccinic* acid.

**carbamoylation** (kar-bam'o-il-a'shun). Carbamylation; transfer of the carbamoyl of carbamoyl phosphate to an amino group with elimination of inorganic phosphate.

**carbamoylglutamic acid.** $HOOC(CH_2)_2CH(NH-CONH_2)COOH$; an intermediate in the carbamoylation of ornithine to citrulline in the urea cycle.

**carbamoylphosphate.** $H_2NCO$—$OPO_3H_2$; a reactive intermediate capable of transferring its carbamoyl group $(H_2NCO—)$ to an acceptor molecule, forming citrulline from ornithine in the urea cycle, and ureidosuccinic acid from aspartic acid in pyrimidine ring formation.

**c. synthase,** a phosphotransferase (EC 2.7.2.5) catalyzing condensation of 2 ATP, $NH_3$, $CO_2$, and $H_2O$ to yield 2 ADP + $P_i$ + carbamoylphosphate (the reverse of carbamate kinase).

***O*-carbamoylserine.** $H_2NCO$—$OCH_2CH(NH_2)COOH$; the L form is an antibiotic isolated from *Streptomyces;* the D form (synthetic) is inactive.

**carbamoyltransferase** (EC group 2.1.3). Transcarbamoylase; any enzyme transferring carbamoyl groups from one compound to another (*e.g.,* aspartate carbamoyltransferase, ornithine carbamoyltransferase).

**carbamoylurea.** Biuret.

**car'bamyl.** Carbamoyl.

**carbamyla'tion.** Carbamoylation.

**carbar'sone** (NF, BP). 4-Ureidobenzenearsonic acid; *N*-carbamoylarsanilic acid; recommended in the treatment of amebiasis and other protozoal infections.

**car'basus** [ L. fr. G. *karpasos,* flax, cotton ]. Gauze; lint.

**car'batrine hydrochloride.** PAVATRINE hydrochloride; ROBITRIN; 2-diethylaminoethyl-9-fluorenecarboxylate hydrochloride; a smooth muscle relaxant, used in the treatment of gastrointestinal, ureteral, and uterine spasms.

**car'bazides.** Carbohydrazides; 1,3-diaminoureas; RNH—NHCONH—NHR .

**carbazochrome salicylate** (kar-ba'zo-krōm). ADRENOSEM salicylate; adrenochrome monosemicarbazone sodium salicylate complex; an oxidation product of epinephrine used for the systemic control of capillary bleeding associated with increased capillary permeability.

**car'bazole.** Diphenyleneimine; 9-azafluorene; reacts with carbohydrates (including uronates and deoxypentoses) giving colors characteristic of the sugar type; used for assay and analysis of carbohydrates and formaldehyde.

**carbenicil'lin disodium** (USAN). Carbenicillin sodium (BP); PYOPEN; disodium salt of 6-($\alpha$-carboxyphenylacetamido)penicillamic acid; a semisynthetic form of penicillin administered parenterally.

**carbenox'alone disodium.** BIOGASTRONE; SANODIN; $3\beta$-hydroxy-11-oxoolean-12-en-30-oic acid hydrogen succinate disodium salt; used as anti-inflammatory agent for treatment of peptic ulcer.

**car'betapen'tane citrate.** TOCLASE; 2-(diethylaminoethoxy)ethyl 1-phenylcyclopentyl-1-carboxylate citrate; it has atropine-like and local anesthetic actions and effectively suppresses acute cough due to common upper respiratory infections.

**carbet'idine** ATENOS; 1-[ 2-(2-hydroxyethoxy ethyl ]-4-phenylisonipecotic acid ethyl ester; analgesic.

**carb'hemoglo'bin.** Carbaminohemoglobin.

**car'bide.** A compound of carbon with an element more electropositive than itself, e.g., CaC$_2$, calcium carbide.

**carbido'pa** (USAN). (−)-L-$\alpha$-Hydrazino-3,4-dihydroxy-$\alpha$-methylhydrocinnamic acid monohydrate; a decarboxylation inhibitor.

**carbimazole** (BP). 1-Methyl-2-imidazolethiol ethyl carbonate; used in the treatment of hyperthyroidism; it is less toxic than thiouracil.

**car'binol.** Methyl alcohol.

**carbinox'amine mal'eate** (NF). CLISTIN; 2-[ $p$-chloro-$\alpha$-(2-dimethylaminoethoxy)benzyl ]pyridine maleate; an antihistaminic agent.

**car'biphene hydrochloride** (USAN). BANDOL; etymide; 2-ethoxy-$N$-methyl-$N$-[ 2-(methylphenethylamino)ethyl ]-2,2-diphenylacetamide; analgesic.

**carbo-.** See carb-.

**carbo** [ L. coal. CARB- ]. Charcoal.

**carboangiocardiography** (kar'bo-an-jĭ-og'rǎ-fĭ). A form of angiocardiography in which carbon dioxide is injected as a negative contrast medium.

**carbobenzoxy.** Abbreviated Cbz; see benzyloxycarbonyl.

**carboclor'al** (USAN). URAL; chloral-urethane; (2,2,2-trichloro-1-hydroxyethyl)carbamic acid ethyl ester; used as hypnotic.

**carbocyclic compound** (kar'bo-si'klik). See under compound.

**carbohe'mia.** Carbonemia; a greater than normal amount of carbon dioxide in the blood, as the result of abnormal retention or a defect in the mechanism of elimination. Rarely used term.

**car'bohemoglo'bin.** Carbaminohemoglobin.

**carbohy'drases.** A generic term for enzymes that hydrolyze carbohydrates, e.g., maltase, lactase, sucrase, amylase, etc.

**carbohy'drate.** Sugar; saccharide; aldehydic or ketonic derivative of polyhydric alcohols. The name is derived from the fact that the most common examples of such compounds have formulas that may be written $C_x(H_2O)_y$; thus glucose may be written $C_6(H_2O)_6$ and sucrose $C_{12}(H_2O)_{11}$. They are nevertheless not true hydrates and the name is in that sense a misnomer. The group includes compounds with relatively small molecules, such as those mentioned above (i.e., the simple sugars or saccharides) as well as macromolecular substances such as starch, glycogen, and cellulose (the polysaccharides). The c.'s most typical of the class contain carbon, hydrogen, and oxygen only, but c. intermediates in tissue contain phosphorus, and mucopolysaccharides contain nitrogen and often sulfur.

**carbohydratu'ria.** The excretion of one or more carbohydrates in the urine, e.g., glucose, galactose, lactose, a pentose, and so on; thus, c. is a general term that includes such conditions as glycosuria (melituria), galactosuria, lactosuria, pentosuria, etc.

**car'bolate.** 1. A salt or ester of carbolic acid (phenol). 2. To carbolize.

**carbol-fuchsin** (kar'bol-fook'sin). 1. See Ziehl's solution. 2. See carbol-fuchsin paint.

**carbol'ic acid.** Phenol.

**car'bolize.** To mix with or add carbolic acid (phenol).

**carbolu'ria** [ carbolic acid + G. ouron, urine ]. The presence of phenol (carbolic acid) in the urine.

**car'bomer** (USAN). A polymer of acrylic acid crosslinked with a polyfunctional compound; a suspending agent for pharmaceuticals.

**carbom'etry.** Carbonometry.

**carbomy'cin.** MAGNAMYCIN; a basic antibiotic obtained from cultures of Streptomyces halstedii; active against Gram-positive bacteria, rickettsia, and certain large viruses.

**car'bon** [ L. carbo, coal ]. A nonmetallic tetravalent element, symbol C, atomic no. 6, atomic weight 12.011. Two natural isotopes ($^{12}$C, $^{13}$C); two artificial, radioactive isotopes of interest ($^{11}$C, $^{14}$C). The element occurs in two pure forms, diamond and graphite, in impure form in charcoal, coke, and soot, and in the atmosphere as CO$_2$. Its compounds are found in all living tissues, and the study of its vast number of compounds constitutes most of organic chemistry.

**anomeric c.,** the reducing c. of a sugar; C-1 of an aldose, C-2 of a 2-ketose.

**c. bisulfide,** c. disulfide.

**c. cycle,** or **c. dioxide cycle,** see under cycle.

**c. dioxide,** (1) carbonic acid gas; CO$_2$; the product of the combustion of c. with a free supply of air; (2) (USP, BP), contains not less than 99.0 per cent by volume of CO$_2$; used as a respiratory stimulant.

**c. dioxide, active,** the form in which c. dioxide is added to methylcrotonyl-CoA to form $\beta$-methylglutaconyl-CoA in the catabolism of leucine and to acetyl-CoA to form malonyl-CoA. It is a complex of $N$-carboxybiotin (biotin + CO$_2$) and an enzyme. See acetyl-CoA carboxylase, under acetyl.

**c. dioxide snow,** DRY ICE; solid c. dioxide (USP); used in the treatment of warts, lupus, nevi, and other skin affections, and as a refrigerant.

**c. disulfide,** CS$_2$; a colorless liquid of a characteristic ethereal odor, fetid when impure. It is a parasiticide, but is seldom used other than as a solvent. It is extremely flammable.

**c. monox'ide,** CO; formed by the incomplete combustion of c. A colorless, odorless, and poisonous gas. Its toxic action is due to its strong affinity for hemoglobin and cytochrome, reducing oxygen transport and blocking oxygen utilization.

**quaternary c. atom,** an atom of c. to which four other c. atoms are attached.

**c. tetrachloride** (NF), tetrachloromethane; CCl$_4$; a colorless, mobile liquid having a characteristic ethereal odor resembling that of chloroform; used as a cleansing fluid, a fire extinguisher, and an anthelmintic, especially against hookworm.

**therapeutic c.'s,** therapeutic electrodes.

**carbon-11.** $^{11}$C; a cyclotron-produced, positron-emitting radioisotope of carbon with a half-life of 20 minutes.

**carbon-12.** $^{12}$C; 98.89 per cent of natural carbon; the standard of atomic mass.

**carbon-13.** $^{13}$C; 1.11 per cent of natural carbon.

**carbon-14.** $^{14}$C; a beta-emitter with a half-life of 5600 years; widely used as a tracer in studying various aspects of metabolism, notably photosynthesis; naturally occurring $^{14}$C, arising from cosmic rays, is used to date relics containing natural carbonaceous materials.

**car'bonate.** A salt of carbonic acid; CO$_3$=.

**c. dehydratase** (EC 4.2.1.1), c. hydro-lyase; carbonic anhydrase; a zinc-containing enzyme in red blood cells that catalyzes the conversion of carbon dioxide (CO$_2$) entering the blood from the tissues into carbonic acid (H$_2$CO$_3$). The reverse reaction occurs when the blood reaches the lungs and carbon dioxide is liberated.

**c. dehydratase inhibitor,** carbonic anhydrase inhibitor; an agent, usually chemically related to the sulfonamides, that inhibits the activity of carbonate dehydratase (carbonic anhydrase), producing a general decrease in the formation of H$_2$CO$_3$ in the tissues. This results in a transient diuresis, a metabolic acidosis, a decreased rate of formation of aqueous humor (and a reduction in intraocular pressure), and, with large doses, a reduced formation of gastric hydrochloric acid. See also acetazolamide and dichlorphenamide.

**c. hydro-lyase,** c. dehydratase.

**carbone′mia.** Carbohemia.

**carbon′ic.** Relating to carbon.

  **c. acid,** $H_2CO_3$, formed from $H_2O$ and $CO_2$.

  **c. anhydrase,** carbonate dehydratase.

  **c. anhydrase inhibitor,** carbonate dehydratase inhibitor.

  **c. anhydride,** carbon dioxide; $CO_2$.

**car′bonize.** To char.

**carbonom′eter** [ L. *carbo* (*carbon-*), coal, + G. *metron*, measure ]. A device for determining the proportion of carbon dioxide in the air or expired breath by the precipitation of calcium carbonate from lime water.

**carbonom′etry.** Carbometry; the determination of the presence and the proportion of carbon dioxide by means of the carbonometer.

**carbonu′ria.** Term used but rarely to denote the excretion of carbon dioxide or other carbon compounds in the urine.

**car′bonyl.** The characteristic group, —CO—, of the ketones, aldehydes, and organic acids.

**carborun′dum.** Carbide of silicon; SiC; a substance of extreme hardness used for polishing in place of emery.

**carbox′amide.** Aminocarbonyl; a molecular configuration (—CONH₂) that, together with the related carboximides (iminocarbonyls) (—CONH—) is a constituent of many hypnotics, including barbiturates, hydantoins, thiazines.

**carboxy-.** Combining form indicating addition of CO or $CO_2$.

*N*-**carboxyaminoacid anhydrides.** See *N*-carboxyanhydrides.

*N*-**carbox′yanhy′drides.** Heterocyclic derivatives of amino acids from which polypeptides may be synthetized.

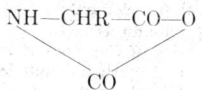

NH—CHR—CO—O

CO

*N*-Carboxyanhydride

**carbox′ydis′mutase.** Ribulosebisphosphate carboxylase.

**carbox′yhemoglo′bin.** Carbon monoxide hemoglobin; abbreviated HbCO; a fairly stable union of carbon monoxide with hemoglobin. The formation of c. prevents the normal transfer of carbon dioxide and oxygen during the circulation of blood; thus, increasing levels of c. result in various degrees of asphyxiation, including death.

**carbox′yhemoglobine′mia.** The presence of carboxyhemoglobin in the blood.

**carbox′yl.** The characterizing group (—COOH) of certain organic acids; *e.g.*, HCOOH (formic acid), $CH_3COOH$ (acetic acid), etc.

**carbox′ylase.** One of several carboxy-lyases, trivially named carboxylases or decarboxylases (EC group 4.1.1), catalyzing the addition of $CO_2$ to all or part of another molecule to create an additional —COOH group (*e.g.*, ribulosebisphosphate carboxylase, EC 4.1.1.39).

**carboxyla′tion.** Addition of $CO_2$ to an organic acceptor, as in photosynthesis, to yield a —COOH group; catalyzed by carboxylases.

**carbox′yltrans′ferase** (EC group 2.1.3). Transcarboxylase; any enzyme transferring carboxyl groups from one compound to another.

**carboxymeth′yl cel′lulose.** See under cellulose.

**carbox′ypep′tidase.** One of several hydrolases removing the amino acid at the free carboxyl end of a polypeptide chain.

**carboxypeptidase A** (EC 3.4.12.2). Carboxypolypeptidase; releases C-terminal amino acids, with exception of arginine, lysine, and proline.

**carboxypeptidase B** (EC 3.4.12.3). Protaminase; releases C-terminal lysine or arginine preferentially.

**carboxypeptidase C** (EC 3.4.12.1). A carboxypeptidase that has broad specificity for all C-terminal α-amino acids, including proline.

**carboxypeptidase G.** Glutamate γ-carboxypeptidase.

**carboxypolypeptidase.** Carboxypeptidase A.

**carbro′mal** (BP). ADALIN; Bromdiethylacetylurea; bromdiethylacetyl carbamide; formerly widely used as a sedative.

**carbubar′bital.** NOGEXAN; carbamic acid ester with 5-butyl-5-(2-hydroxyethyl)barbituric acid; sedative with intermediate duration of action.

**carbuncle** (kar′bung′kl) [ L. *carbunculus*, dim. of *carbo*, a live coal, a carbuncle. CARB- ]. 1. Deep-seated pyogenic infection of several contiguous hair follicles, with formation of connecting sinuses and underlying necrosis and ulceration; often preceded or accompanied by fever, malaise, and prostration. 2. Anthrax (1).

  **renal c.,** abscess within the kidney which may open into the renal pelvis or may extend outward and give rise to perinephric abscess.

**carbun′cular.** Relating to a carbuncle.

**carbunculo′sis.** A condition marked by the occurrence of several carbuncles in rapid succession.

**car′buret.** 1. Archaic for carbide. 2. To combine with carbon. 3. To enrich a gas with volatile hydrocarbons, as in a carburetor.

**carbu′tamide.** NADISAN; 1-butyl-3-sulfanilylurea; oral hypoglycemic agent.

**carbu′terol hydrochloride** (USAN). [ 5-[ 2-(*tert*-Butylamino)-1-hydroxyethyl ]-2-hydroxyphenyl ]urea monohydrochloride; a sympathomimetic drug with bronchodilatory activity.

**carcass** (kar′kas) [ F. *carcasse*, fr. It. *carcassa* ]. 1. The body of a dead animal. 2. In butcher's terminology, refers to animals used for human food; the body after the hide, head, tail, extremities, and viscera have been removed.

**carceag** (kar′se-ag). Carciag; a disease of sheep in the Balkan States caused by *Babesia* (*Piroplasma*) *motasi* and transmitted chiefly by ticks of the genus *Rhipicephalus.*

**car′ciag.** Carceag.

**carcin-.** See carcino-.

**carcinec′tomy** (kar′sin-ek′to-mī) [ G. *karkinos*, cancer, + *ektomē*, excision ]. Carcinosectomy; carcinomectomy; excision of a cancerous tumor.

**car′cinelco′sis** [ G. *karkinos*, cancer, + *helkōsis*, ulceration ]. A chronic, progressive ulcer caused by a malignant neoplasm, such as a rodent ulcer (basal cell carcinoma).

**carcino-, carcin-** (kar′sĭ-no-) [ G. *karkinos*, crab, cancer. CARC- ]. Combining form relating to cancer.

**carcinogen** (kar′sĭ-no-jen). Any cancer-producing substance. The most potent c.'s, including those isolated from coal tar, are polycyclic aromatic hydrocarbons.

**car′cinogen′esis** [ carcino- + G. *genesis*, generation ]. The origin or production of cancer, including carcinomas and other malignant neoplasms.

**car′cinogen′ic.** Cancerigenic; causing cancer.

**car′cinoid** [ G. *karkimōdēs*, cancerous, + *eidos*, form ]. Carcinoid tumor; argentaffinoma; a neoplasm composed of islands of rounded cells of medium size, with moderately small vesicular nuclei, thought to be derived from Kulchitsky cells in the crypts of Lieberkühn; the neoplastic cells are frequently palisaded at the periphery of the small groups, and the latter have a tendency to extend into the muscularis. Cytoplasmic granules are demonstrable by impregnation with silver, and the granules are known to contain 5-hydroxytryptamine (see carcinoid *syndrome*). C. neoplasms occur anywhere in the gastrointestinal tract (and in the lungs and other sites), but approximately 90 per cent are in the appendix; the remainder are found chiefly in the ileum, but also in the stomach, other parts of the small intestine, the colon, and the rectum. The neoplasms are usually small and covered by intact mucosa, with a yellow cut surface. C.'s of the appendix hardly ever metastasize, but reported incidences of metastases from other primary sites vary from 25 to 75 per cent; lymph nodes in the abdomen and the liver may be conspicuously involved, but metastases above the diaphragm are rare.

**car′cinolyt′ic** [ carcino- + G. *lytikos*, causing a solution ]. Destructive to the cells of carcinoma.

# CARCINOMA

**carcinoma** (kar-sĭ-no'mah) [ G. *karkinōma*, fr. *karkinos*, cancer, + suffix *-oma*, tumor ]. Any of the various types of malignant neoplasm derived from epithelial tissue in several sites, occurring more frequently in the skin and large intestine in both sexes, the bronchi, stomach, and prostate gland in men, and the breast and cervix in women. C.'s are identified histologically on the basis of invasiveness and the changes that indicate anaplasia, *i.e.*, loss of polarity of nuclei, loss of orderly maturation of cells (especially in squamous cell type), variation in the size and shape of cells, hyperchromatism of nuclei (with clumping of chromatin), and increase in the nuclear-cytoplasmic ratio. C.'s may be undifferentiated, or the neoplastic tissue may resemble (to varying degree) one of the types of normal epithelium.

**acinar c.,** acinic cell *adenocarcinoma.*

**acinic cell c.,** acinic cell *adenocarcinoma.*

**acinose c., acinous c.,** acinic cell *adenocarcinoma.*

**adenoid cystic c.,** cylindromatous c.; a histologic type of c. characterized by large epithelial masses containing round, glandlike spaces or cysts; the cysts frequently contain mucus and are bordered by a few or many layers of epithelial cells without intervening stroma, forming a cribriform pattern like a slice of Swiss cheese. Adenoid cystic c.'s occur most commonly in salivary glands; the stroma is often hyalinized, and these c.'s may also be called cylindromas.

**adnexal c.,** a c. arising in, or forming structures resembling, skin appendages.

**adrenal cortical c.'s,** large invasive and metastasizing tumors which may cause virilism or Cushing's syndrome.

**alveolar cell c.,** bronchiolar c.

**basal cell c.,** basal cell epithelioma; basaloma; basalioma; a slow-growing, locally invasive, but rarely metastasizing neoplasm derived from basal cells of the epidermis or hair follicles; see also rodent *ulcer.*

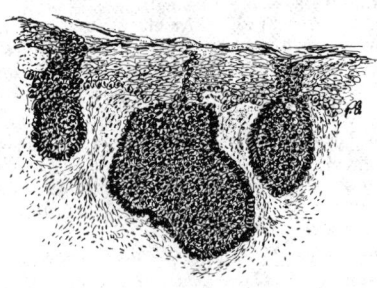

**Basal Cell Carcinoma of the Skin**

**basal squamous cell c.,** basosquamous c.

**basaloid c.,** a poorly differentiated squamous cell c. of the anus that has some microscopic resemblance to basal cell c. of the skin, but which frequently metastasizes.

**basisquamous c.,** basosquamous c.

**basosquamous c.,** basisquamous c.; basal squamous cell c.; a c. of the skin which structurally and in behavior is considered transitional between basal cell and squamous cell c. The term should not be used for the much more common keratotic variety of basal cell c., in which the tumor cells are of basal type but which contains small foci or abrupt keratinization. The behavior of such tumors does differ from that of other types of basal cell c.

**bronchiolar c.,** an unusual c. that is thought to be derived from epithelium of terminal bronchioles; the neoplastic tissue extends along the alveolar walls and grows in small masses within the alveoli, involving the lung (1) in a fairly uniformly diffuse, frequently massive manner (resembling the stage of "hepatization" in pneumococcal lobar pneu-

monia), or (2) in a nodular or lobular manner, with the lesion (or lesions) being more prominent in the peripheral portion; there is only little tendency to invasion, and the architectural pattern of the lung is usually preserved, or altered only slightly in relatively small foci. Microscopically, the neoplastic cells are cuboidal or columnar, and some of the latter may be ciliated; mucin may be demonstrated in some of the cells and in the material in the alveoli, which also includes denuded cells and cellular debris; fibrosis of pulmonary septums is frequently conspicuous. Although metastases in regional lymph nodes, and even in more distant sites, are known to occur, this is not a frequent feature. Termed also terminal bronchiolar c., alveolar cell c., diffuse pulmonary c., cancerous pulmonary adenomatosis, c. bronchiolorum, and carcinomatoides alveogenica multicentrica.

**bronchogenic c.,** c. of the lung, arising from a bronchus.

**cervical c.,** c. of the uterine cervix.

**clear cell c. of kidney,** renal *adenocarcinoma.*

**colloid c.,** mucinous c.

**c. cuta'neum,** squamous or basal cell c. of the skin.

**cylindromatous c.,** adenoid cystic c.

**cystic c.,** cystic cancer; a c. in which (1) true, epithelium-lined cysts are formed, or (2) degenerative changes may result in cystlike spaces.

**duct c.,** ductal c., duct cancer; a c. derived from epithelium of ducts, *e.g.,* in the breast or pancreas.

**ductal c.,** duct c.

**embryonal c.,** a malignant neoplasm of the testis, composed of large anaplastic cells with indistinct cellular borders, amphophilic cytoplasm, and ovoid, round, or bean-shaped nuclei that may have multiple large nucleoli; in some instances, the neoplastic cells may form tubular structures. Embryonal c.'s may be malignant teratomas without differentiated elements.

**epidermoid c.,** squamous cell c.

**follicular c.'s,** c.'s of the thyroid composed of well or poorly differentiated epithelial follicles without papillary formation. It is difficult to distinguish them from adenomas; the criteria include blood vessel invasion and the finding of metastases of follicular thyroid tissue in other structures such as cervical lymph nodes and bone. Follicular c.'s may take up radioactive iodine.

**giant cell c.,** a malignant epithelial neoplasm characterized by unusually large anaplastic cells.

**giant cell c. of thyroid gland,** an apparently rapidly progressive undifferentiated c. observed in the thyroid gland, and characterized by numerous, unusually large, anaplastic cells derived from glandular epithelium of the thyroid gland. Termed also spindle cell c. or carcinosarcoma of thyroid gland.

**glandular c., c. glandula're,** adenocarcinoma.

**hair-matrix c.,** a form of basal cell c. forming partially differentiated hair follicles.

**hepatocellular c.,** malignant *hepatoma.*

**Hürthle cell c.,** see Hürthle cell *tumor.*

**c. in situ,** intraepithelial c.; a lesion observed chiefly in stratified squamous epithelium, and characterized by cytologic changes of the type associated with invasive c.; on the other hand, the pathologic process is limited to the lining epithelium, without conclusive histologic evidence of extension to adjacent structures. The distinctive changes are more apparent in the nucleus, *i.e.,* variation in size and shape, loss of orderly maturation, increase in chromatin, and numerous mitoses (including several that are atypical) in all layers of the epithelium. The lesion is presumed to be the histologically recognizable precursor of invasive epidermoid c., or, in other words, a localized and curable phase of c. A similar process is also observed in glandular epithelium, but intraepithelial c. in such sites is more difficult to identify.

**intraductal c.,** a form of c. derived from the epithelial lining of ducts, especially in the breast, where most c.'s arise from ductal epithelium; the neoplastic cells proliferate in irregular papillary projections or masses, filling the lumens, that are solid, cribriform, or centrally necrotic. Intraductal c. frequently invades surrounding stroma and may then metastasize.

**intraepidermal c.,** Bowen's *disease.*

**intraepithelial c.,** c. in situ.

**invasive c.,** a neoplasm in which collections of epithelial cells infiltrate or destroy the underlying stroma.

**kangri burn c.,** kangri *cancer.*

**latent c.,** an epithelial neoplasm showing microscopic features of malignancy believed to have remained localized and asymptomatic for a long period; for example, small c.'s of the prostate in old men, found incidentally at autopsy.

**c. lenticula're,** a form of c. tuberosum, or scirrhous cancer of the skin, characterized by multiple, small, relatively flat nodules that frequently become coalescent, thereby resulting in larger, irregular, patchy foci that manifest some resemblance to fungus disease in the skin.

**liver cell c.,** malignant *hepatoma.*

**lobular c.,** a form of acinous c., especially of the breast, where lobular c. is much less common than ductal c.

**lobular c. in situ,** noninfiltrating lobular c.

**Lucké c.,** L.'s adenocarcinoma; a virus-associated adenocarcinoma of the kidney in adult frogs.

**medullary c., c. medulla're,** medullary or encephaloid cancer; a malignant neoplasm that consists chiefly of neoplastic epithelial cells, with only a scant amount of fibrous stroma; medullary c.'s are comparatively soft and brainlike in consistency.

**melanotic c., c. melano'des, c. melanot'icum,** malignant *melanoma.*

**mesometanephric c.,** mesonephroma.

**metastatic c.,** secondary c.; a c. that has appeared in a region remote from its site of origin; for example, in axillary lymph nodes, from the breast.

**microinvasive c.,** a variety of c. seen most frequently in the uterine cervix, in which c. in situ of squamous epithelium, on the surface or replacing the lining of glands, is accompanied by small collections of abnormal epithelial cells that infiltrate a very short distance into the stroma. It is believed that this may represent the earliest stage of invasion, in which the neoplastic cells are capable of intrusion but not of sustained growth in connective tissue.

**mucinous c.,** colloid c. or cancer; a variety of adenocarcinoma in which the neoplastic cells secrete conspicuous quantities of mucin, and, as a result, the neoplasms are likely to be glistening, sticky, and gelatinoid in consistency.

**mucoepidermoid c.,** a malignant tumor of glandular tissues, arising especially from the ducts of salivary gland, composed of a mixture of mucus-secreting and epidermoid squamous cells.

**c. myxomato'des,** a form of colloid cancer in which there is myxomatous metaplasia of the cellular fibrous stroma.

**noninfiltrating lobular c.,** lobular c. in situ; c. of the breast in which tumor cells fill preexisting acini within lobules, without invading the surrounding stroma.

**oat cell c.,** an anaplastic, small-celled c., usually bronchogenic.

**occult c.,** a small c., either asymptomatic or giving rise to metastases without symptoms due to the primary c.

**papillary c.,** a malignant neoplasm characterized by the formation of numerous, irregular, finger-like projections of fibrous stroma that is covered with a surface layer of neoplastic epithelial cells.

**primary c.,** c. at the site of origin, with local invasion in that organ.

**renal cell c.,** renal *adenocarcinoma.*

**sarcomatoid c.,** spindle cell c.

**scirrhous c.,** scirrhous cancer; fibrocarcinoma; a hard c., fibrous in nature, resulting from a desmoplastic reaction by the host tissue to the presence of the neoplasm.

**secondary c.,** metastatic c.

**signet ring cell c.,** a poorly differentiated adenocarcinoma composed of cells with a cytoplasmic droplet of mucus that compresses the nucleus to one side along the cell membrane; arises most frequently in the stomach.

**c. simplex,** (1) any form of c. in which the relative proportions of stroma and neoplastic epithelial cells are not unusual, *i.e.,* stromal elements are not comparatively abundant, nor are they reduced in amount or lacking; (2) a c. lacking any identifiable microscopic pattern, such as glandular structure.

**spindle cell c.,** sarcomatoid c.; a c. composed of elongated cells, generally a poorly differentiated squamous cell c. which may be difficult to distinguish from a sarcoma.

**squamous cell c.,** epidermoid cancer or c.; a malignant neoplasm that is derived from stratified squamous epithelium, but that may also occur in sites where glandular or columnar epithelium is normally present; variable amounts of keratin are formed, in relation to the degree of differentiation, and, if the keratin is not on the surface, it accumulates in the neoplasm as a "keratin pearl"; in instances in which the cells are well differentiated, intercellular bridges may be observed between adjacent cells.

**transitional cell c.,** a malignant neoplasm derived from transitional epithelium, occurring chiefly in the urinary bladder, ureters, or renal pelves, especially if well differentiated. Transitional cell c.'s are frequently papillary. They are graded 1 to 3 according to the degree of anaplasia, grade 1 appearing histologically benign but being liable to recurrence. So-called transitional cell c. of the upper respiratory tract is more properly classified as squamous cell c.

**c. of uterine cervix,** observed especially in middle-aged women, usually a squamous cell c., but adenocarcinoma sometimes occurs. In addition to intraepithelial c., four clinical stages are defined, as follows: stage I, c. involving only the cervix; stage II, c. extends beyond the cervix, but not to the lower third of the vagina or the wall of the pelvis; stage III, c. involving the lower third of the vagina or extending to the wall of the pelvis, or both; stage IV, c. extending into the rectum or urinary bladder (or both), or to other sites beyond those previously indicated.

**V-2 c.,** a transplantable, highly malignant c. of experimental animals, that developed as a result of malignant change in a virus-induced papilloma of a domestic rabbit.

**verrucous c.,** a well differentiated papillary squamous cell c., especially of the oral cavity, that may invade locally but rarely metastasizes.

**villous c., c. villo'sum,** a form of c. in which there are numerous, closely packed, papillary projections of neoplastic epithelial tissue.

**Walker c.,** Walker *carcinosarcoma.*

**Wolffian duct c.,** mesonephroma.

---

**carcinomato'sis.** Carcinosis; a condition resulting from widespread dissemination of carcinoma in multiple sites in various organs or tissues of the body; sometimes also used in relation to involvement of a relatively large region of the body.

**carcino'matous.** Pertaining to or manifesting the characteristic properties of carcinoma.

**carcinomec'tomy.** Carcinectomy.

**carcinosarcoma** (kar'sī-no-sar-ko'mah). A malignant neoplasm that contains elements of carcinoma and sarcoma so extensively intermixed as to indicate neoplasia of epithelial and mesenchymal tissue; see also collision *tumor.*

**renal c.,** Wilms' *tumor.*

**Walker c.,** Walker carcinoma; a transplantable c. of the rat that originally appeared spontaneously in the mammary gland of a pregnant albino rat, and which now resembles a carcinoma in young transplants and a sarcoma in older transplants.

**carcinosec'tomy.** Carcinectomy.

**carcino'sis.** Carcinomatosis.

**carcinostat'ic.** 1. Pertaining to an arresting or inhibitory effect on the development or progression of a carcinoma. 2. An agent that manifests such an effect.

**carcoma** (kar-ko'mah) [ Sp. wood dust under the bark of a tree, caused by the wood louse ]. Dark red-brown or mahogany-colored granular material that occurs in human feces in tropical regions. It yields a chemical reaction similar to that of urobilinogen and is composed of calcium oxide, iron, phosphoric and carbonic acids, urobilinogen, cholerythrogen, and other organic matter in varying proportions.

**car'damon** [ L. *cardamonum,* fr. G. *kardamōmon,* the spice of cardamum ]. *Elletaria cardamomum* (family Zingiberaceae), a plant of India and Ceylon.

**c. fruit** (BP) the dried, nearly ripe fruit of *Elettaria cardamomum* var. *minuscula.*

**c. oil** (NF), a volatile oil distilled from the seeds of *Elletaria cardamomum;* a flavoring agent.

**c. seed** (NF), the dried ripe seed of *Elletaria cardamomum;* flavoring agent and aromatic carminative.

**Cardarel'li,** Antonio, Italian physician, 1831–1926. See C.'s *sign,* Oliver-C. *sign.*

**Carden,** Henry D., British surgeon, *1872. See C.'s *amputation.*

**cardi-.** See cardio-.

**car'dia** [ G. *kardia,* heart ] [ NA ]. That part of the stomach immediately adjacent to the esophageal opening.

**car'diac** [ L. *cardiacus* ]. 1. Pertaining to the heart or to the esophageal opening of the stomach. 2. A sufferer from heart disease. 3. A remedy for heart disease.

**cardi'acus** [ L. ] [ NA ]. Cardiac (1).

**cardiagra** (kar-dī-ag'rah) [ cardi- + G. *agra,* seizure ]. Obsolete term for (1) a gouty affection of the heart; (2) *angina pectoris.*

**cardial'gia** [ cardi- + G. *algos,* pain ]. 1. Heartburn; peratodynia; an uncomfortable burning sensation in the stomach. 2. Cardiodynia.

**cardianastrophe** (kar-de-an-as'tro-fe) [ G. *kardia,* heart, + *anastrophē,* a turning back. STREP- ]. Dextrocardia.

**cardiasthenia** (kar-dī-as-the'nī-ah) [ cardi- + G. *astheneia,* weakness ]. Weakness in the action of the heart.

**cardiasthma** (kar-dī-az'mah). Cardiac *asthma.*

**car'diatax'ia** [ cardi- + G. *ataxia,* disorder ]. Extreme irregularity in the action of the heart.

**cardiatelia** (kar'dī-ā-te'lī-ah) [ cardi- + G. *atelēs,* incomplete ]. Incomplete development of the heart.

**car'dicente'sis.** Cardiocentesis.

**car'dicin.** An antibiotic obtained from a species of *Nocardia.* Active against fungi, bacteria, and viruses, but toxic for animals and man.

**cardiectasia** (car'dī-ek-ta'zī-ah) [ cardi- + G. *ektasis,* a stretching ]. Dilation of the heart.

**cardiectomy** [ cardi- + G. *ektomē,* excision ]. Excision of the cardiac extremity of the stomach.

**cardiectopia** (kar-dī-ek-to'pī-ah) [ cardi- + G. *ektopos,* out of place ]. Abnormal placement of the heart.

**cardinal** (kar'dī-nal) [ L. *cardinalis,* principal ]. Chief or principal; in embryology, relating to the main venous drainage.

**card'ing.** The procedure of placing individual sets of anterior or posterior teeth in trays lined with a wax strip.

**cardio-, cardi-** [ G. *kardia,* heart ]. Combining forms relating (1) to the heart, and (2) to the cardia (ostium cardiacum).

**car'dioaccel'erator.** Accelerating the heart beat.

**car'dioac'tive.** Influencing the heart.

**car'dioangiog'raphy.** Angiocardiography.

**cardioangiology** (kar'de-o-an'jī-ol-o-je) [ cardio- + G. *angeion,* vessel, + *logos,* study ]. Cardiovasology; science dealing in general with the heart and blood vessels.

**car'dioaor'tic.** Relating to the heart and the aorta.

**car'dioarte'rial.** Relating to the heart and the arteries.

**cardiocairograph** (kar-dī-o-ki'ro-graf) [ cardio- + G. *kairos,* the right point of time, + *graphō,* to write ]. An instrument that synchronizes roentgen exposures of the thorax with selected phases of the cardiac cycle.

**cardiocele** (kar'dī-o-sēl) [ cardio- + G. *kēlē,* hernia ]. A herniation or protrusion of the heart through an opening in the diaphragm, or through a wound.

**car'diocente'sis** [ cardio- + G. *kentēsis,* puncture ]. Cardicentesis; paracentesis cordis; operative puncture of the heart.

**cardiochalasia** (kar'dī-o-kā-la'zī-ah). Achalasia of the cardia.

**cardiocirrhosis** (kar'dī-o-sī-ro'sis). Cardiac *cirrhosis.*

**car'diocla'sia.** Cardiorrhexis.

**car'diodio'sis** [ cardio- (2) + G. *diōsis,* a spreading open ]. Maneuver of dilating the gastric cardia.

**car'diodynam'ics.** The mechanics of the heart's action, including its movement and the forces generated thereby.

**car'diodyn'ia** [ cardio- + G. *odynē,* pain ]. Cardialgia; pain in the heart.

**car'diogen'esis.** The formation of the heart in the embryo.

**car'diogen'ic.** Of cardiac origin.

**cardioglo'bin.** A complex system of interacting proteins that increases myocardial contractility.

**car'diogram** [ cardio- + G. *gramma,* a diagram ]. 1. The graphic curve made by the stylet of a cardiograph. 2. Used colloquially as an abbreviation for electrocardiogram. 3. Generally used for any tracing derived from the heart, such prefixes as apex-, electro-, phono-, or vector- being understood.

**esophageal c.,** tracing of left atrial contractions made by recording displacements of column of air in an esophageal tube.

**car'diograph** [ cardio- + G. *graphō,* to write ]. An instrument for recording graphically the movements of the heart, constructed on the principle of the sphygmograph.

**cardiog'raphy.** The use of the cardiograph.

**ultrasound c.,** echocardiography.

**vector c.,** see vectorcardiography.

**car'diohe'mothrom'bus.** Cardiothrombus.

**car'diohepat'ic.** Relating to the heart and the liver.

**car'diohep'atomeg'aly.** Enlargement of both heart and liver.

**cardioid** (kar'dī-oyd) [ cardi- + G. *eidos,* resemblance ]. Resembling a heart.

**car'dioinhib'itory.** Arresting or slowing the action of the heart.

**car'diokinet'ic** [ cardio- + G. *kinēsis,* movement ]. Influencing the action of the heart.

**car'diolip'in.** Acetone-insoluble antigen; heart antigen; a 1,3-diphosphatidyl glycerol with immunological properties; used in serological diagnosis of syphilis. When mixed with lecithin and cholesterol c. will combine with the Wassermann antibody but not with the treponema-immobilizing antibody.

**car'diolith** [ cardio- + G. *lithos,* stone ]. Cardiac calculus; a concretion in the heart, or an area of calcareous degeneration in its walls or valves.

**cardiol'ogist.** One having special knowledge and experience in the diagnosis and treatment of heart disease.

**cardiol'ogy** [ cardio- + G. *logos,* study ]. The science of the heart and its diseases.

**cardiolysis** (kar-dī-ol'ĭ-sis) [ cardio- + G. *lysis,* loosening ]. Brauer's operation; an operation for breaking up the adhesions in chronic mediastinopericarditis. Access is gained by resection of a portion of the sternum and the corresponding costal cartilages.

**car'diomala'cia** [ cardio- + G. *malakia,* softness ]. Softening of the walls of the heart.

**car'diomeg'aly** [ cardio- + G. *megas,* large ]. Macrocardia; megacardia; enlargement of the heart.

**glycogen c.,** c. due to abnormal storage of glycogen within the heart muscle cells; glycogen storage disease of the heart.

**cardiom'etry** [ cardio- + G. *metron,* measure ]. Measuring the dimensions of the heart or the force of its action.

**car'diomotil'ity.** Movements of the heart.

**cardiomuscular** (kar'dī-o-mus'ku-lar). Pertaining to the cardiac musculature.

**car'diomy'olipo'sis** [ cardio- + G. *mys,* muscle, + *lipos,* fat, + suffix -*osis,* condition ]. Fatty degeneration of the myocardium.

**car'diomyop'athy** [ cardio- + G. *mys,* muscle, + *pathos,* disease ]. Myocardiopathy; disease of the myocardium.

**alcoholic c.,** myocardial disease occurring in some chronic alcoholic persons; it may either result from thiamin deficiency or be of unknown pathogenesis.

**beer-drinker's c.,** beer heart; myocardial degeneration with pericardial effusion, reported in heavy beer-drinkers in Quebec and Omaha, probably due to the use of cobalt sulfate in the beer as a foam stabilizer.

**idiopathic c.,** primary c.

**postpartum c.,** cardiomegaly and congestive heart failure developing in the puerperium in the absence of any of the known causes of heart disease.

**primary c.,** idiopathic c.; disease that affects primarily the heart muscle, sparing other cardiac structures and usually resulting in fibrosis or hypertrophy. Primary c. may be divided into four groups: (1) hypertrophic (left or biventricular hypertrophy); (2) obstructive hypertrophic (idiopathic hypertrophic subaortic *stenosis, q.v.*); (3) congestive biventricular dilatation; and (4) restrictive stiffening of the wall by amyloid deposits or fibrosis.

**secondary c.,** disease that affects the myocardium secondarily to systemic disease, infection, or metabolic disease.

**cardiomyot'omy** [ cardio- (2) + G. *mys,* muscle, + *tomē,* cutting ]. Esophagomyotomy.

**cardionecrosis** (kar'dĭ-o-nĕ-kro'sis). Necrosis of the myocardium.

**car'dionec'tor** [ cardio- + L. *necto,* to join ]. Rarely used synonym for conducting system of the heart; see under system.

**car'dioneph'ric.** Cardiorenal.

**cardioneural** (kar'dĭ-o-nu'ral) [ cardio- + G. *neuron,* nerve ]. Relating to the nervous control of the heart.

**cardioneurosis** (kar'dĭ-o-nu-ro'sis). Cardiac *neurosis.*

**car'dio-omen'topexy** [ cardio- + omentum, + G. *pēxis,* fixation ]. Operation for the attachment of omentum to the heart with the object of improving its blood supply.

**car'diopal'mus** [ cardio- + G. *palmos,* palpitation ]. Palpitation of the heart.

**car'diopal'udism** [ cardio- + paludism (malaria) ]. Irregularity in the heart's action due to malaria.

**car'diopath.** A sufferer from heart disease.

**cardiop'athy** [ cardio- + G. *pathos,* disease ]. Any disease of the heart.

**car'diopericar'diopexy** [ cardio- + pericardium, *q.v.,* + G. *pēxis,* fixation ]. An operation to increase the blood supply to the myocardium; it consists in spreading sterile magnesium silicate (a form of talc) within the pericardial sac, which causes an adhesive pericarditis and an increase in blood supply through the stimulation of the development of interarterial coronary anastomoses.

**car'dioper'icardi'tis.** Inflammation of both myocardium and pericardium.

**car'diopho'bia.** Fear of heart disease.

**car'diophone** [ cardio- + G. *phōnē,* sound ]. A stethoscope specially designed to aid in listening to the sounds of the heart.

**cardiophony** (kar'dĭ-of'o-nĭ). Auscultation of the heart, or reproducing the heart sounds by means of a microphone and amplifier.

**car'diophre'nia.** Phrenocardia.

**car'dioplas'ty** [ cardio- + G. *plassō,* to fashion ]. Esophagogastroplasty; plastic surgery on the cardiac sphincter of the stomach.

**cardioplegia** (kar'dĭ-o-ple'jĭ-ah) [ cardio- + G. *plēgē,* stroke. PLES- ]. 1. Paralysis of the heart. 2. An elective procedure for stopping cardiac activity temporarily by means of the injection of chemicals, the use of selective hypothermia, or electrical stimuli.

**cardiople'gic.** Relating to cardioplegia.

**cardiopneumatic** (kar'dĭ-o-nu-mat'ik) [ cardio- + G. *pneuma,* breath ]. Relating to the heart's action and the respiration.

**cardiopneumograph** (kar'dĭ-o-nu'mo-graf) [ cardio- + G. *pneuma,* breath, + *graphō,* to write ]. An instrument for recording graphically the cardiac and respiratory movements.

**cardioptosia** (kar'dĭ-op-to'sĭ-ah) [ cardio- + G. *ptōsis,* a falling ]. Cor mobile; cor pendulum; drop heart; a condition in which the heart is unduly movable and displaced downward; to be distinguished from bathycardia, in which the heart is fixed in a lower position.

**car'diopul'monary.** Relating to the heart and lungs.

**car'diopunc'ture.** Cardiocentesis.

**cardiopyloric** (kar'dĭ-o-pi-lor'ik, -pĭ-lor'ik). Relating to the cardiac and pyloric extremities of the stomach.

**car'diore'nal.** Cardionephric; nephrocardiac; renicardiac; relating to the heart and the kidney.

**cardiorrhaphy** (kar-dĭ-or'ă-fĭ) [ cardio- + G. *rhaphē,* suture ]. Suture of the heart wall.

**cardiorrhexis** (kar-dĭ-o-rek'sis) [ cardio- + G. *rhēxis,* rupture, RHAG- ]. Cardioclasia; rupture of the heart wall.

**cardioschisis** (kar-dĭ-os'kĭ-sis) [ cardio- + G. *schisis,* a division ]. The division of adhesions between the pericardium and the chest wall.

**cardiosclerosis** (kar-dĭ-o-skle-ro'sis) [ cardio- + G. *sklērōsis,* hardening ]. Ethmocarditis; a condition of fibrous, or connective tissue, overgrowth in the heart wall, usually associated with coronary arterial obstruction.

**car'dioscope** [ cardio- + G. *skopeō,* to view ]. An instrument for inspecting the interior of the living heart.

**car'diospasm.** esophageal *achalasia.*

**cardiosphygmograph** (kar'dĭ-o-sfig'mo-graf) [ cardio- + G. *sphygmos,* pulse, + *graphō,* to write ]. An instrument for recording graphically the movements of the heart and the radial pulse.

**cardiotachometer** (kar'dĭ-o-tă-kom'e-tur) [ cardio- + G. *tachos,* rapidity, + *metron,* measure ]. An instrument for measuring the rapidity of the heart beat.

**car'diother'apy.** Treatment directed at heart diseases.

**car'diothrom'bus.** Cardiohemothrombus; a clot of blood within one of the heart's chambers.

**car'diothy'rotoxico'sis.** Hyperthyroidism with cardiac complications.

**cardiot'omy** [ cardio- + G. *tomē,* incision ]. 1. Incision into the heart wall. 2. Incision into the cardiac end of the stomach.

**car'dioton'ic** [ cardio- + G. *tonos,* tension ]. Exerting a favorable, so-called tonic, effect upon the action of the heart.

**cardiotopometry** (kar'dĭ-o-to-pom'ĕ-trĭ) [ cardio- + G. *topos,* place, + *metron,* measure ]. Determination of the area of cardiac dullness.

**car'diotox'ic** [ cardio- + G. *toxikon,* poison ]. Having a deleterious effect upon the action of the heart, due to poisoning of the cardiac muscle or of its conducting system.

**car'diovalvuli'tis.** Inflammation of the heart valves.

**car'diovalvulot'omy** [ cardio- + Mod. L. *valvula,* a little value, + G. *tomē,* a cutting ]. An operation for the correction of mitral stenosis consisting of cutting or excising a part of the mitral valve.

**car'diovas'cular** [ cardio- + L. *vasculum,* vessel ]. Relating to the heart and the blood vessels or the circulation.

**car'diovas'culore'nal.** Relating to the heart, arteries, and kidneys, especially as to function or disease.

**car'diovasol'ogy.** Cardioangiology.

**car'diover'sion.** Restoring the heart's rhythm to normal by means of electrical countershock.

**car'dioverter.** Machine for administering electrical countershock for the purpose of restoring the heart's rhythm to normal.

**cardi'tis.** Inflammation of the heart.

**rheumatic c.,** pancarditis occurring in rheumatic fever, characterized by formation of Aschoff bodies in the cardiac interstitial tissue; may be associated with acute cardiac failure, endocarditis with small fibrin vegetations on the margins of closure of valve cusps (especially the mitral), and fibrinous pericarditis; it is frequently followed by scarring of the valves with stenosis.

**care.** In medicine and public health, a general term for the application of knowledge to the benefit of a community or individual.

**comprehensive medical c.,** a concept that includes not only the traditional c. of the acutely or chronically ill patient, but also the prevention and early detection of disease and the rehabilitation of the disabled.

**health c.,** c. that encompasses the social, economic, and environmental influences, in addition to medical c.

**intensive c.,** management and c. of critically ill patients; see also intensive c. *unit.*

**medical c.,** the portion of c. under a physician's direction.

**primary medical c.,** medical c. by a physician who is the first contact with the patient and who provides entry for the patient into the health c. system.

**secondary medical c.,** medical c. by a physician who acts as a consultant at the request of the primary physician.

**tertiary medical c.,** specialized consultative c. by specialists working in a center that has a wide catchment area and has personnel and facilities that encourage special investigation and treatment.

**careba'ria** [ G. *kara,* head, + *barutēs,* heaviness ]. Pressure or heaviness in the head.

**caribi** (kă-re′be). Epidemic gangrenous *proctitis.*

**car′ica.** Papaya.

**car′icin.** Papain.

**car′icous** [ L. *carica,* a dried fig, fr. province of *Caria* in Asia Minor ]. Relating to or having the semblance of a fig.

**caries** (ka′rĭ-ēz, kăr-ēz) [ L. dry rot ]. Destruction or necrosis of teeth or bone (the latter usage, however, is obsolete).

    **active c.,** presence of lesions in teeth that prolapse toward pulp.

    **arrested dental c.,** lesions that have healed spontaneously.

    **backward c.,** retrograde or secondary enamel c.; spread of decay back toward enamel surface after primary penetration toward pulp.

    **dental c.,** a localized, progressively destructive disease of the teeth that starts at the external surface (usually the enamel) with the apparent dissolution of the inorganic components by organic acids. These acids are produced in immediate proximity to the tooth by the enzymatic action of masses of microorganisms (in the bacterial plaque) on carbohydrates. The initial demineralization is followed by an enzymatic destruction of the protein matrix. Cavitation and direct bacterial invasion follow. In the dentin, demineralization of the walls of the tubules is followed by bacterial invasion and destruction of the organic matrix. Untreated dental c. progresses to the pulp, resulting in infection and its sequelae.

    **c. fungo′sa,** an obsolete term for a form of c. of tuberculous origin accompanied with a fungus proliferation of the tissues.

    **interdental c.,** c. between the teeth.

    **Pott's c.,** tuberculous *spondylitis.*

    **primary c.,** initial lesions produced by direct extension from an external surface.

    **secondary c.,** backward c.

    **senile dental c.,** lesions occurring in old age, usually interproximally and in cementum.

    **spinal c.,** tuberculous *spondylitis.*

**carina,** pl. **cari′nae** (kă-ri′nah) [ L. the keel of a boat ]. 1. In man, a term applied or applicable to several anatomical structures forming a projecting central ridge. 2. That portion of the sternum in a bird, bat, or mole that serves as the origin of the pectoral muscles; it is not found in flightless birds and most mammals.

    **c. for′nicis,** a ridge running along the undersurface of the fornix of the brain.

    **c. tracheae** [ NA ], the ridge separating the openings of the right and left main bronchi at their junction with the trachea.

    **c. urethra′lis vagi′nae** [ NA ], c. vaginae; the lower part of the anterior column of the vagina, in relation with the urethra.

    **c. vagi′nae,** c. urethralis vaginae.

**car′inate** [ see carina ]. Keel-shaped, relating to or resembling a carina.

**cario-** (kăr-ĭ-o-). Combining form relating to caries.

**cariogen′esis.** The process of producing caries; the mechanism of caries production.

**cariogen′ic.** Producing caries; usually said of diets.

**cariogenic′ity.** Potential for caries production.

**carios′ity.** Cariousness; state of being carious.

**cariostat′ic.** Exerting an inhibitory action upon the progress of dental caries.

**carious** (kăr′ĭ-us). Relating to or affected with caries.

**cariso′prodol.** RELA; SOMA; *N*-isopropyl-2-methyl-2-propyl-1,2-propanediol dicarbamate; a skeletal muscle relaxant, chemically related to meprobamate. It appears to give relief in muscular disorders involving pain and spasm, *e.g.,* strains and sprains.

**caris′sin.** A glucoside obtained from *Carissa ovata stolonifera* of Australia. A powerful heart poison.

**Carlen's catheter.** See under catheter.

**carmal′um.** A 1 per cent solution of carmine in 10 per cent alum water. Used as a stain in histology.

**Carmichael,** J. P., American dentist, 1856–1946. See C. *crown.*

**car′minate.** A red salt of carminic acid with an alkali.

**carmin′ative** [ L. *carmino,* pp. *-atus,* to card wool; special Mod. L. use of the word, to expel wind ]. 1. Preventing the formation or causing the expulsion of flatus. 2. An agent that relieves flatulence.

**carmine** (kar′min, kar′mēn) [ Mediev. L. *carminus,* contr. fr. *carmisinus,* fr. Ar. *qirmizē,* the cochineal insect ]. Red coloring matter extracted from the cochineal insect, *Coccus cacti,* by treatment with a solution of alum. See also Best's c. *stain,* Orth's *stain.*

    **Schneider's c.,** a stain consisting of a saturated solution of c. in concentrated acetic acid.

**carmin′ic acid.** $C_{22}H_{20}O_{13}$; the essential constituent of carmine.

**carmin′ophil, carmin′ophile, carminoph′ilous** [ G. *phileō,* to love ]. Staining readily with carmine dyes.

**carneous** (kar′ne-us) [ L. *carneus* ]. Fleshy.

**car′nes** (kar′nēz) [ L. ]. Plural of caro.

**carneus** [ L. ] [ NA ]. Carneous.

**Carnett's sign.** See under sign.

**carnifica′tion** [ L. *caro* (*carn*-), flesh, + *facio,* to make ]. A change in tissues, whereby they become fleshy, resembling muscular tissue.

**car′nine.** Obsolete term for a nondescript mixture of purines, probably hypoxanthine and inosine, extracted from sugar beets and meats.

**car′nitine.** γ-Amino-β-hydroxybutyric acid trimethylbetaine; vitamin $B_T$; $B_T$ factor; a betaine isolated from muscle and liver.

**Carniv′ora** [ L. *carnivorus,* fr. *caro* (*carn*-), flesh, + *voro,* to devour ]. An order of chiefly flesh-eating mammals that includes the cats, dogs, bears, civets, minks, and hyenas, as well as the raccoon and panda; some species are omnivorous or herbiverous.

**carnivore** (kar′nĭ-vōr). One of the *Carnivora.*

**carniv′orous.** Flesh-eating.

**car′nosine.** β-Alanylhistidine; inhibitine; ignotine; found in muscle, sometimes *N*-methylated (anserine).

**carnos′ity.** 1. Fleshiness. 2. A fleshy protuberance.

**caro,** gen. **car′nis,** pl. **car′nes** (ka′ro) [ L. ]. Flesh; muscle.

    **c. quadra′ta Syl′vii** [ J. *Sylvius* ], *musculus* quadratus plantae.

**car′ob flour.** Algaroba.

**car′otenase.** β-Carotene 15,15′-dioxygenase.

**car′otene.** A class of carotenoid (*q. v.*); name for a group of yellow-red pigments (lipochromes) widely distributed in plants and animals, notably in carrots, of particular interest in that they include precursors of the vitamins A (provitamin A carotenoids). Chemically, they consist of 8 isoprene units in a symmetrical chain with the 2 isoprenes at each end cyclized in α-carotene and β-carotene (γ-carotene has only one end cyclized). The cyclic ends of β-carotene are identical β-ionine-like structures; thus, on oxidative fission (see β-carotene-15,15′-dioxygenase), β-carotene yields 2 molecules of vitamin A. The cyclic ends of α-carotene differ; one is an α-ionone, the other a β-ionone; on fission, α-carotene, like γ-carotene, yields 1 molecule of vitamin A (β-ionone derivative). The carotenes are closely related in structure to the xanthophylls and lycopenes and to the open chain squalene, a $C_{30}$ compound.

*β-Carotene*

    **c. oxidase,** lipoxygenase.

**β-carotene cleavage enzyme.** β-Carotene-15,15′-dioxygenase.

**$\beta$-carotene-15,15'-dioxygenase** (EC 1.13.11.21). $\beta$-Carotene cleavage enzyme; carotenase; enzyme converting $\beta$-carotene to vitamina A aldehyde (retinal), adding $O_2$.

**carotene'mia.** Carotinemia; carotene in the blood, especially pertaining to increased quantities, which sometimes cause a pale yellow-red pigmentation of skin that may resemble icterus; pseudojaundice.

**carot'enoid.** Carotinoid. 1. Resembling carotene, having a yellow color. 2. See carotenoids.

**carot'enoids.** Generic term for a class of hydrocarbons (carotenes) and their oxygenated derivates (xanthophylls) consisting of 8 isoprenoid units joined so that the orientation of these units is reversed at the center, placing the two central methyl groups in a 1,6 relationship in contrast to the 1,5 of the others. All carotenoids may be formally derived from the acyclic $C_{40}H_{56}$ structure (part *IA* of the accompanying group of structures) with its long central chain of conjugated double bonds by (1) hydrogenation, (2) dehydrogenation, (3) oxidation, or (4) cyclization, or combinations of these. Included as carotenoids are some compounds arising from certain rearrangements or degradations of the carbon skeleton (structure *IB*), but not retinol (vitamin A) and related $C_{20}$ compounds. The $C_9$ end groups may be acyclic with 1,2 and 5,6 double bonds (as in structure *IA*) or cyclohexanes with a single double bond at 5,6 or 5,4, or cyclopentanes or aryl groups; these are now designated by Greek letter prefixes (illustrated in part II of the accompanying group of structures) preceding "carotene" ($\alpha$ and $\gamma$, which are used in the trivial names $\alpha$-carotene and $\gamma$-carotene, are not used for that reason).

Suffixes (-oic acid, -oate, -al, -one, -ol) indicate certain oxygen-containing groups (acid, ester, aldehyde, ketone, alcohol). All other substitutes appear as prefixes (alkoxy-, epoxy-, hydro-, etc.). The configuration about all double bonds is *trans* unless *cis* and locant numbers appear. The term *retro-* (prefix) is used to indicate a shift of one position of all single and double bonds. *Apo* indicates shortening of the molecule. The trivial names of some natural carotenoids are: capsorubin (a $\kappa$,$\kappa$-carotenedione); bixin (a 9'-*cis*-diapo-carotenedioate); phytoene (a 15-*cis*-octahydro-$\psi$,$\psi$-carotene); $\beta$-carotene ($\beta$,$\beta$-carotene); $\alpha$-carotene ($\beta$,$\epsilon$-carotene); $\gamma$-carotene ($\beta$,$\psi$-carotene); lycopene ($\psi$,$\psi$-carotene); provitamin A; zeaxanthin ($\beta$,$\beta$-carotene-3,3'diol); $\zeta$-carotene (7,8,7',8'-tetrahydro-$\psi$,$\psi$-carotene).

**caroteno'sis cutis.** *Aurantiasis* cutis.

**carot'ic** [ G. *karōtikos*, stupefying. CAROT- ]. 1. Carotid. 2. Stuporous.

**carot'icotympan'ic.** Relating to the carotid canal and the tympanum.

**carot'id** [ G. *karōtides*, the carotid arteries, fr. *karoō*, to put to sleep (because compression of the c. artery results in unconsciousness). CAROT- ]. Pertaining to any c. structure.

**carot'idyn'ia.** Carotodynia.

**carot'igram.** Tracing of the carotid pulse.

**car'otin.** Carotene.

**car'otinase.** Carotenase.

**carotine'mia.** Carotenemia.

**car'otinoid.** Carotenoid.

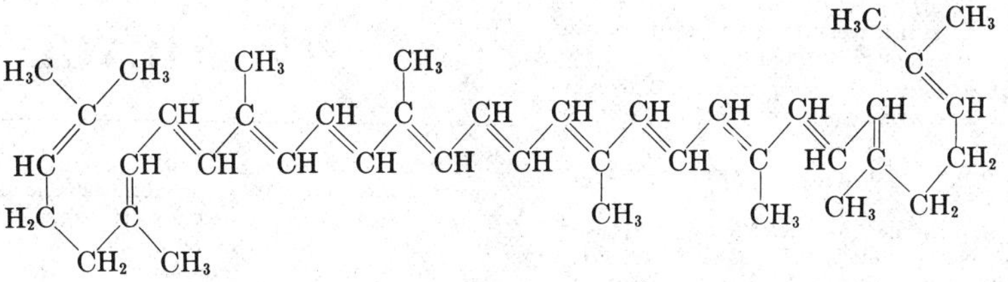

*IA*. Acyclic structures from which carotenoids are derived

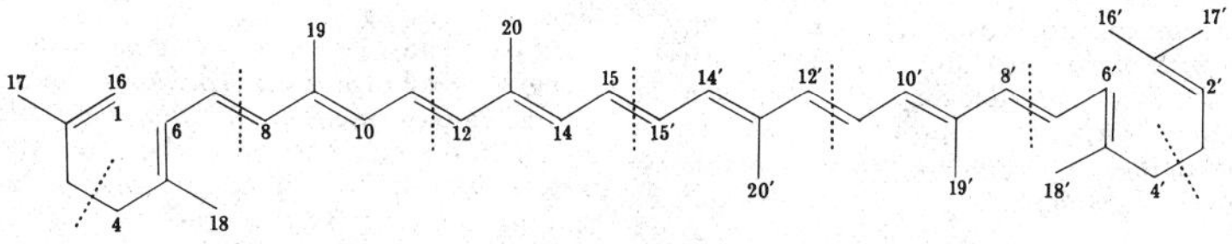

*IB*. General formula. For convenience, carotenoid formulas are often written in shorthand form as shown here; broken lines indicate formal division into isoprenoid units; numbering system is shown.

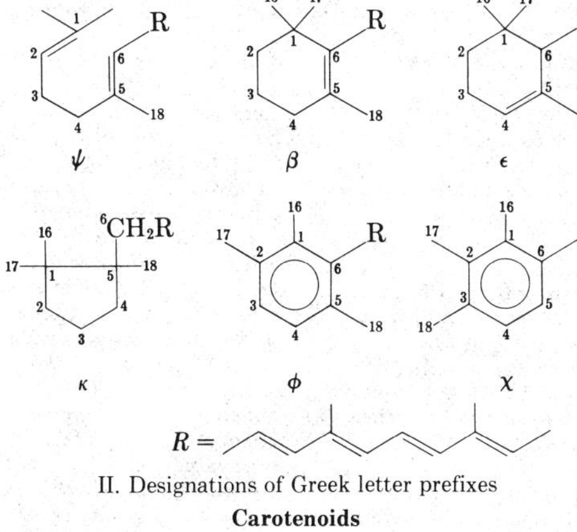

II. Designations of Greek letter prefixes

**Carotenoids**

**carotino'sis cutis.** *Aurantiasis* cutis.

**carot'odyn'ia** [ G. *odynē*, pain ]. Carotidynia; pain caused by pressure on the carotid artery.

**carpaine** (kar'pa-in). $C_{14}H_{25}NO_2$; an alkaloid from the leaves of *Carica papaya* (family Caricaceae). Diuretic and cardiac tonic, resembling digitalis.

**car'pal.** Relating to the carpus.

**carpec'tomy** [ G. *karpos*, wrist, + *ektomē*, excision ]. Ex-section of a portion or all of the carpus.

**Carpenter,** Charles C. J., U. S. immunologist, *1931. See C.'s *syndrome*.

**Carpenter,** George, British physician, 1859–1910. See C.'s *syndrome*.

**carphen'azine maleate** (NF). PROKETAZINE maleate; 1-{10-(3-[ 4-(2-hydroxyethyl)-1-piperazinyl ]propyl)pheno-thiazine-2-yl{-1-propanone bis(hydrogen maleate); a phe-nothiazine tranquilizer of the piperazine group. Functionally classified as an antipsychotic agent, it is used in the treatment of chronic and acute schizophrenia. It also possesses antiemetic, adrenolytic, anticholinergic, and dopamine-blocking actions.

**carpholo'gia, carphol'ogy** [ G. *karphologia*, a gathering of twigs, fr. *karphos*, bits of wood, straw, wool, etc., + *legō*, to pick up ]. Floccillation.

**carpi'tis.** Carpal arthritis in the horse and other animals.

**carpocar'pal.** Midcarpal; referring to the articulation be-tween the two rows of carpal bones.

**Carpoglyp'tus** [ G. *karpos*, fruit, + *glyphō*, to carve ]. A genus of mites including *C. passularum*, the fruit mite, which causes a dermatitis among handlers of dried fruit.

**car'pometacar'pal.** Relating to both carpus and metacar-pus.

**carpopedal** (kar'po-ped'al) [ G. *karpos*, wrist, + L. *pes* (*ped*-), foot ]. Relating to the wrist and the foot, or the hands and feet; denoting especially c. spasm.

**carpoptosis, carpoptosia** (kar-pop-to'sis, kar-pop-to'zī-ah) [ G. *karpos*, wrist, + *ptōsis*, a falling ]. Wrist-drop.

**Carpue,** Joseph C., English surgeon, 1764–1846. See C.'s *method*.

**carpus,** gen. and pl. **car'pi** (kar'pus) [ Mod. L. fr. Gr. *karpos* ] [ NA ]. The wrist. 1. The proximal segment of the hand consisting of the carpal bones and the associated soft parts. 2. The ossa carpi, *viz.*, the os scaphoideum, os lunatum, os triquetrum, os pisiforme, os trapezium, os trapezoideum, os capitatum, and os hamatum, which articulate proximally with the radius and indirectly with the ulna, and distally with the five metacarpal bones. 3. In domestic mammals, the bones of the proximal row are called radial, intermediate, ulnar and accessory, while those of the distal row are termed first, second, third and fourth carpal bones.

　**c. curvus,** Madelung's *deformity*.

**Carr,** Francis H., British chemist, *1874. See C.-Price *test*.

**car'rageen, car'ragheen.** Chondrus (2).

**carrageenan.** Carrageenin; a polysaccharide obtained from Irish moss; a galactosan sulfate resembling agar in molecular structure.

**Carré,** M. H. See C. 's *disease*.

**carre-four sensitif** (kar-foor'son-se-tēf') [ Fr. sensory crossroads ]. A term given by Charcot to the posterior portion of the posterior limb of the internal capsule.

**Carrel** (kä-rel'), Alexis, French-American surgeon in the U. S., 1873–1944. Nobel laureate, 1912, for his work on vascular suture and the transplantation of blood vessels and organs. See C.'s *mixture*, C.-Lindbergh *pump*, C.'s *treatment*, Dakin-C. *treatment*.

**car'rier.** 1. Vector (1); bacilli or bacteria c. 2. A person in apparent health who is infected with some pathogenic organism which in him evokes no manifestations of disease, but which, when accidentally transferred to another, may produce an attack of the specific disease. 3. Any chemical capable of accepting an atom, radical, or subatomic particle from one compound, then passing it to another; thus, the cytochromes may be viewed as electron c.'s, homocysteine as a methyl c., and so on.

　**amalgam c.,** an instrument used to transport triturated amalgam to a cavity preparation and to deposit it therein.

**convalescent c.,** an excreter of pathogenic organisms who has had a clinically recognizable attack of the disease.

　**genetic c.,** a person in apparent health whose chromo-somes contain a pathologic mutant gene which may be transmitted to his children. In some conditions a c. may be detected by an appropriate laboratory test or physical sign.

　**translocation c.,** a person with balanced translocation; see under translocation.

**Carrión** (kahr-rī-ōn'), Daniel A., Peruvian student, 1850–1886, who inoculated himself with the disease later designated as C.'s disease, and lost his life thereby. See C.'s *disease*.

**Carron oil** [ *Carron* iron works in Scotland, where the mixture was first used ]. Lime liniment; a mixture of equal parts of lime water and olive or linseed oil, applied for the relief of burns and scalds.

**car'rot** [ L. *carota*, G. *karōton* ]. The fruit or seed of *Daucus carota* (family Umbelliferae), a herb yielding a common vegetable.

**car'salam.** BEAPRINE; $2H$-1,3-benzoxazine-2,4($3H$)-dione; analgesic.

**Carswell,** Sir Robert, English physician, 1793–1857. See C.'s *grapes*.

**Carter,** Henry V., Anglo-Indian physician, 1831–1907. See C.'s *fever, mycetoma*.

**Carte'sian.** Relating to Descartes (Latinized, Cartesius), to his philosophy or to his mathematical methods.

**car'thamus** [ Ar. *qurtum*, fr. *qartama*, paint; the plant yields a dye ]. Safflower; parrot-seed; false or bastard saffron; the dried florets of *Carthamus tinctorius* (family Compositae); see also safflower oil.

# CARTILAGE

**cartilage** (kar'tĭ-lij) [ L. *cartilago* (*cartilagin*-), gristle ]. Cartilago; a connective tissue characterized by its nonvas-cularity and firm consistency. It consists of cells (chon-drocytes) and interstitial substance (matrix) of fibers and a ground substance (chondromucoid). There are three kinds of c.: hyaline c., elastic c. (see below), and fibrocarti-lage (*q.v.*).

　**accessory c.,** a sesamoid c.

　**accessory nasal c.'s,** *cartilagines* nasales accessoriae.

　**accessory quadrate c.,** *cartilagines* alares minores.

　**c. of acoustic meatus,** *cartilago* meatus acustici.

　**alisphenoid c.,** the c. in the embryo from which the greater wing of the sphenoid bone is developed.

　**annular c.,** *cartilago* cricoidea.

　**arthrodial c.,** *cartilago* articularis.

　**articular c.,** *cartilago* articularis.

　**aryten'oid c.,** *cartilago* arytenoidea.

　**auditory c.,** *auditory capsule*.

　**c. of auditory tube,** *cartilago* tubae auditivae.

　**auric'ular c.,** *cartilago* auriculae.

　**bas'ilar c.,** the c. filling the foramen lacerum; fibrocarti-lago basalis.

　**branchial c.'s,** c.'s developing within the vertebrate or embryonic branchial arches; they form the viscerocranium.

　**calcified c.,** c. in which calcium salts are deposited in the matrix; it occurs prior to replacement by osseous tissue and sometimes in aging c.

　**cariniform c.,** the keel-shaped, laterally compressed cartilaginous prolongation at the cranial end of the sternum of the horse.

　**cellular c.,** an embryonic or immature stage of c. in which it consists chiefly of cells with very little ground substance.

　**ciliary c.,** incorrect term sometimes applied to the tarsus inferior and tarsus superior; see tarsus (2).

　**circumferen'tial c.,** *labrum* acetabulare; *labrum* glenoid-ale.

　**conchal c.,** *cartilago* auriculae.

　**connecting c.,** interosseous c.; uniting c.; the c. in an immovable joint such as the symphysis pubis.

　**corniculate c.,** *cartilago* corniculata.

　**costal c.,** *cartilago* costalis.

**cricoid c.,** *cartilago* cricoidea.

**cuneiform c.,** *cartilago* cuneiformis.

**diarthro'dial c.,** *cartilago* articularis.

**elastic c.,** yellow c.; a variety in which the cells are surrounded by a territorial capsular matrix outside of which is an interterritorial matrix containing elastic fiber networks in addition to the collagen fibers and ground substance.

**en'siform c.,** *processus* xiphoideus.

**ensisternum c.,** *processus* xiphoideus.

**epiglottic c.,** *cartilago* epiglottica.

**epiphysial c.,** *cartilago epiphysialis.*

**fal'ciform c.,** *meniscus* medialis.

**floating c.,** a loose piece of c. within a joint cavity, detached from the articular c. or from a meniscus.

**greater alar c.,** *cartilago* alaris major.

**Huschke's c.'s,** two horizontal cartilaginous rods at the edge of the cartilaginous septum of the nose.

**hyaline c.,** c. having a frosted glass appearance. In adult c. the cells are present in isogenous groups. The interstitial substance contains fine collagenous fibers obscured by the ground substance (chondromucoid).

**hypsiloid c.,** Y c.

**innom'inate c.,** *cartilago* cricoidea.

**interos'seous c.,** connecting c.

**interver'tebral c.,** *discus* intervertebralis.

**intraartic'ular c.,** *discus* articularis.

**intrathyroid c.,** a narrow slip of c. sometimes found joining the laminae of the thyroid c. of the larynx in infancy.

**investing c.,** *cartilago* articularis.

**Jacobson's c.,** *cartilago* vomeronasalis.

**c.'s of larynx,** *cartilagines* laryngis.

**lateral c.,** cartilaginous plates that extend above the hoof from the caudal angles of the distal phalanx of the horse. They are readily palpated under the skin of the sides of the hoof. They assist in distributing the animal's weight during locomotion.

**lateral c. of nose,** *cartilago* nasi lateralis.

**lesser alar c.'s,** *cartilagines* alares minores.

**loose c.,** floating c.

**Luschka's c.,** a small cartilaginous nodule sometimes found in the anterior portion of the vocal cord.

**mandib'ular c.,** Meckel's c.; a c. bar in the mandibular arch. It forms a temporary supporting structure in the embryonic mandible. Its proximal end gives rise to the cartilaginous primordium of the malleus.

**me'atal c.,** *cartilago* meatus acustici.

**Meckel's c.,** mandibular c.

**Meyer's c.'s,** the anterior sesamoid c.'s at the anterior attachments of the inferior thyroarytenoid ligaments.

**Morgagni's c.,** *cartilago* cuneiformis.

**c. of the nasal septum,** *cartilago* septi nasi.

**orbitosphenoid c.,** the embryonic c. that develops on the side of the cartilaginous neurocranium into the lesser wing of the sphenoid bone.

**parachor'dal c.,** c. primordia adjacent on either side to the cephalic portion of the notochord in young embryos; they represent an initial step in the formation of the chondrocranium.

**parasep'tal c.,** *cartilago* vomeronasalis.

**perio'tic c.,** a cartilaginous mass on either side of the chondrocranium surrounding the developing auditory vesicle in the fetus; the otic capsule in its early cartilaginous stage.

**permanent c.,** c. that remains as such and does not become converted into bone.

**c. of the pharyng'otympan'ic tube,** *cartilago* tubae auditivae.

**precur'sory c.,** temporary c.

**primor'dial c.,** c. in an early stage in its development.

**quadrangular c.,** *cartilago* septi nasi.

**Reichert's c.,** a c. in the mesenchyme of the second branchial arch in the embryo, from which are developed the styloid processes, the stylohyoid ligaments, and the lesser cornua of the hyoid bone.

**retic'ular c., ret'iform c.,** rarely used terms for fibrocartilage.

**Santorini's c.,** *cartilago* corniculata.

**secondary c.,** c., such as that in certain joints, which undergoes a direct transformation into bone.

**Seiler's c.,** a small rod of c. attached to the vocal process of the arytenoid c.

**semilu'nar c.,** one of the articular menisci of the knee joint; see meniscus lateralis and meniscus medialis.

**septal c.,** *cartilago* septi nasi.

**sesamoid c. of larynx,** *cartilago* sesamoidea laryngis.

**sesamoid c.'s of the nose,** *cartilagines* nasales accessoriae.

**slipping rib c.,** subluxation of rib c., usually at junction with sternum, causing pain and audible click.

**sternal c.,** a costal c. of one of the true ribs.

**supra-arytenoid c.,** *cartilago* corniculata.

**tarsal c.,** incorrect term sometimes applied to the tarsus inferior and tarsus superior; see tarsus (2).

**temporary c.,** precursory c.; a c. that normally becomes replaced by bone, to form a part of the skeleton.

**thyroid c.,** *cartilago* thyroidea.

**tracheal c.'s,** *cartilagines* tracheales.

**triangular c.,** *discus* articularis radioulnaris.

**triquet'rous c.,** (1) *discus* articularis radioulnaris; (2) *cartilago* arytenoidea.

**tubal c.,** *cartilago* tubae auditivae.

**uniting c.,** connecting c.

**vo'merine c., vomerona'sal c.,** *cartilago* vomeronasalis.

**Weitbrecht's c.,** the articular disc of the acromioclavicular joint.

**Wrisberg's c.,** *cartilago* cuneiformis.

**xiphoid c.,** *processus* xiphoideus.

**Y c.,** hypsiloid c.; Y-shaped c.; the connecting c. for the ilium, ischium, and pubis, it extends through the acetabulum.

**yellow c.,** elastic c.

---

**cartila'gines.** Plural of cartilago.

**cartilaginoid** (kar'tĭ-laj'ĭ-noyd). Resembling cartilage; chondroid.

**cartilaginous** (kar'tĭ-laj'ĭ-nus). Relating to or consisting of cartilage.

**cartila'go,** pl. **cartila'gines** [ L. gristle ] [ NA ]. Cartilage.

**c. ala'ris major** [ NA ]. greater alar cartilage; one of a pair of cartilages that form the tip of the nose. It consists of a medial crus that extends into the nasal septum with its fellow of the opposite side, and a lateral crus that forms the anterior part of the wing of the nose.

**cartila'gines ala'res mino'res** [ NA ], lesser alar cartilages; accessory quadrate cartilage; the two to four cartilaginous plates of the ala nasi posterior to the greater alar cartilage.

**c. articula'ris** [ NA ]; articular cartilage; arthrodial, diarthrodial, or investing cartilage; the cartilage covering the articular surfaces of the bones forming a synovial joint.

**c. arytenoi'dea** [ NA ], arytenoid cartilage; triquetrous cartilage (2); one of a pair of small pyramidal laryngeal cartilages that articulate with the lamina of the cricoid cartilage. It gives attachment to the posterior part of the corresponding vocal ligament and to several muscles. The base of the cartilage is hyaline but the apex is elastic.

**c. auric'ulae** [ NA ], the cartilage of the concha or auricle.

**c. cornicula'ta** [ NA ], corniculate cartilage; supra-arytenoid cartilage; corniculum laryngis; Santorini's c.; a conical nodule of elastic cartilage surmounting the apex of each arytenoid cartilage.

**c. costa'lis** [ NA ], costal cartilage; the cartilage forming the anterior continuation of a rib.

**c. cricoi'dea** [ NA ], cricoid cartilage; annular cartilage; innominate cartilage; the lowermost of the laryngeal cartilages; it is shaped like a seal-ring, being expanded into a nearly quadrilateral plate (lamina) posteriorly; the anterior portion is called the arch (arcus).

**c. cuneifor'mis** [ NA ], cuneiform cartilage; Morgagni's cartilage or tubercle; Wrisberg's c.; a small rod of elastic cartilage in the aryepiglottic fold above the corniculate cartilage.

**c. epiglot'tica** [ NA ], epiglottic cartilage; a thin lamina of elastic cartilage forming the central portion of the epiglottis.

**c. epiphysia'lis** [ NA ], epiphysial cartilage; the disk of cartilage between the shaft and the epiphysis of a long bone during its growth.

**cartila'gines laryn'gis** [ NA ], the cartilages of the larynx, including the thyroid, cricoid, arytenoid, corniculate, and cuneiform cartilages and the epiglottis.

**c. mea'tus acus'tici** [ NA ], cartilage of the acoustic meatus; meatal cartilage; the cartilage that forms the wall of the lateral part of the external acoustic meatus. It is incomplete above and is firmly attached to the margins of the bony part of the external meatus.

**cartila'gines nasa'les accessor'iae** [ NA ], accessory nasal cartilages; sesamoid cartilages of the nose; variable small plates of cartilage located in the interval between the greater alar and lateral nasal cartilages.

**cartilagines na'si** [ NA ], the cartilages of the nose, including the lateral, greater alar, lesser alar, accessory, vomeronasal, and septal cartilages.

**c. nasi latera'lis** [ NA ], lateral cartilage of the nose; the cartilage located in the lateral wall of the nose above the alar cartilage.

**c. septi nasi** [ NA ], cartilage of the nasal septum; quadrangular cartilage; septal cartilage; pars cartilaginea septi nasi; a thin cartilaginous plate located between vomer, perpendicular plate of the ethmoid, and nasal bones, and completing the nasal septum anteriorly.

**c. sesamoi'dea laryngis** [ NA ], sesamoid cartilage of the larynx; a small nodule of elastic cartilage sometimes present on the lateral border of the arytenoid cartilage.

**c. thyroid'ea** [ NA ], thyroid cartilage; the largest of the cartilages of the larynx; it is formed of two approximately quadrilateral plates (*laminae*) joined anteriorly at an angle of from 90° to 120°, the prominence so formed constituting the laryngeal prominence (Adam's apple).

**cartilagines trachea'les** [ NA ], tracheal cartilages; the 16 to 20 incomplete rings of hyaline cartilage forming the skeleton of the trachea; the rings are deficient posteriorly for from one-fifth to one-third of their circumference.

**c. tritic'ea** [ L. *triticum*, wheat ] [ NA ], corpus triticeum; a rounded nodule of cartilage, the size of a grain of wheat, occasionally present in the posterior margin of the lateral hyothyroid ligament.

**c. tubae auditi'vae** [ NA ], cartilage of the auditory tube; tubal cartilage; the trough-shaped cartilage that forms the medial wall, roof, and part of the lateral wall of the auditory tube.

**c. vomeronasa'lis** [ NA ], vomeronasal, vomerine, para-septal, or Jacobson's cartilage; vomer cartilagineus; a narrow strip of cartilage located between the lower edge of the cartilage of the nasal septum and the vomer.

**ca'rum** [ Mod L. fr. L. *careum*, G. *karon*, caraway ]. Caraway.

**caruncle** (kăr'ung-kl). Caruncula.

**amniotic c.'s,** *amnion* nodosum.

**Morgagni's c.,** *lobus medius* prostatae.

**Santorini's major c.,** *papilla* duodeni major.

**Santorini's minor c.,** *papilla* duodeni minor.

**ure'thral c.,** a small, fleshy, sometimes painful growth from the mucous membrane, usually occurring at the meatus of the female urethra. It may be angiomatous, papillomatous, or granulomatous.

**caruncula,** pl. **carun'culae** (kă-rung'ku-lah) [ L. a small fleshy mass, fr. *caro*, flesh ]. Caruncle. 1 [ NA ]. A small, fleshy protuberance, or any structure suggesting such a shape. 2. In ungulates, one of about 200 specific disklike areas of the uterine endometrium that, in conjunction with the fetal cotyledon, forms a placentome of the placenta; as a site of fetal-maternal contact, the c. remains constant in position but enlarges greatly in size during pregnancy.

**c. hymena'lis,** pl. **carunculae hymenales** [ NA ], c. myrtiformis; one of the numerous tabs or projections surrounding the orifice of the vagina after rupture of the hymen.

**c. lacrima'lis** [ NA ], a small reddish body at the medial canthus of the eye, containing modified sebaceous and sweat glands.

**c. myrtifor'mis,** pl. **carunculae myrtiformes,** c. hymenalis.

**c. saliva'ris,** c. sublingualis.

**c. sublingua'lis** [ NA ], c. salivaris; a papilla on each side of the frenulum linguae marking the opening of the submandibular (Wharton's) duct.

**Carus** (kah'roos), Karl G., German obstetrician, 1789–1869. See C.'s *circle, curve*.

**car'vacrol.** 2-*p*-Cymenol; an isomer of thymol; occurs in several volatile oils (majoram, origanum, savory and thyme). Its properties and activity closely resemble those of thymol. It has antiseptic properties, but it is used chiefly as a perfume.

**Carvallo's sign.** See under sign.

**car'ver.** A dental hand instrument appearing in a wide variety of end shapes, used for forming and contouring wax, filling materials, etc., in many procedures.

**caryo-** [ G. *karyon*, nut, kernel ]. For most words so beginning, and not listed here, see karyo-.

**caryophyl'lus, caryophyl'lum** [ G. *karyophyllon*, clove tree, fr. *karyon*, nut, + *phyllon*, leaf ]. Clove.

**caryotheca** (kār'ĭ-o-the'kah) [ caryo- + G. *thēkē*, sheath, box ]. Nuclear *envelope*.

**Casal,** Gasper, Spanish physician, 1691–1759. See C.'s *necklace*.

**casamino acids.** Trivial term for the mixture of amino acids derived by hydrolysis of casein; used in bacterial and similar growth media.

**cascara** (kas-kār'ah) (BP). C. sagrada.

**c. amara,** Honduras bark; the dried bark of a species of *Picramnia* (family Simarubaceae); used as a bitter tonic and alterative.

**c. sagrada** (USP), cascara (BP); the dried bark of *Rhamnus purshiana* (family Rhamnaceae); used as a laxative.

**cascaril'la.** [ Sp. dim of *cascara*, bark ] Sweetwood bark; the dried bark of *Croton eluteria* (family Euphorbiaceae), a shrub of the Bahama Islands. Aromatic stimulant.

**case** [ L. *casus,* an occurrence. CAD- ]. 1. An instance of disease with its attendant circumstances. The patient is not the c.: the patient dies or recovers, the c. terminates fatally or ends in recovery; the surgeon operates *in* a c., but operates *on* the patient. 2. A box or container.

**trial c.,** in opthalmology, a box containing a set of trial lenses.

**casease** (ka'se-ās). An albumin-digesting enzyme of bacterial origin; used to hasten ripening of cheese; see also cathepsin.

**caseation** (ka-se-a'shun) [ L. *caseus,* cheese ]. A form of coagulation necrosis in which the necrotic tissue resembles cheese and contains a mixture of protein and fat that is absorbed very slowly; it occurs particularly in tuberculosis.

**casein** (ca'se-in, ka'sēn). The principal protein of cow's milk; the chief constituent of cheese; rather insoluble in water but soluble in dilute alkaline and salt solutions; forms a hard insoluble plastic with formaldehyde. It is a constituent of some glues. Various components are designated α-, β-, and κ-caseins.

**c. iodine,** caseo-iodine; iodinated c.; a compound of c. with iodine formed by incubating the protein with the element, which becomes attached to tyrosine groups in the protein.

**caseinase** (ka'se-in-ās). See cathepsin.

**caseinate** (ka'se-in-āt). A salt of casein.

**caseinogen** (ka'se-in'o-jen). "Soluble" casein; κ-casein; when acted upon by rennin, c. is converted into paracasein.

**caseose** (ka'se-ōs). A product resulting from the hydrolysis or digestion of casein (a nondescript term).

**caseous** (ka'se-us). Pertaining to or manifesting the gross and microscopic features of tissue affected by caseation; see also caseous *necrosis*.

**cashé** (kă-sha'). Caché.

**ca'sings.** The membranous coverings of sausages; they may consist of intestines, stomachs, esophagi, and urinary bladders of animals, or of synthetic materials.

**Caslick's operation.** See under operation.

**cassava starch** (kă-sah'vah). Tapioca.

**Casselberry,** William E., American laryngologist, 1858–1916. See C. *position*.

**Casser (Casserio),** Giulio, Italian anatomist, 1556–1616. See C.'s *fontanelle,* perforated *muscle*.

**Casse'rian.** Relating to or described by Casser.

**cassette** (kă-set') [ Fr., dim. of *casse,* box ]. A plate holder for use in photography and roentgenography, especially for rapid sequence filming—such as is necessary in the rapid changes of angiography.

**Cassia** (kash'yah) [ L. fr. G. *kasia* ]. A genus of herbs and trees of the family Leguminosae.

**C. acutifo'lia,** the source of Alexandrine senna.

**C. angustifo'lia,** the source of Indian or Tinnevelly senna.

**c. bark,** cinnamon.

**c. buds,** the immature fruits of various species of cinnamon.

**c. caryophylla'ta,** clove bark; a cinnamon-like bark.

**c. fistula,** cassiae pulpa, purging c.; C. pods; C. sticktree; the dried ripe fruit of *Cassia fistula*, pudding-stick; used as a laxative.

**C. marilan'dica,** the source of American senna; a drug of the same properties as the official senna, but much weaker.

**C. occidenta'lis,** furnishes ovate seeds used as a substitute for coffee, called Mogdad or Negro coffee.

**c. oil,** cinnamon oil.

**Saigon c.,** cinnamon.

**C. zeylan'icum,** *Cinnamomum zeylanicum*; see cinnamon.

**cassiopeium** (kas-ī-o'pe-um) [ L. *Cassiopeia*, mother of Andromeda; a constellation ]. Lutetium.

**cast.** 1. An object formed by the solidification of a liquid poured into a mold. 2. The rigid encasement of a part, usually with plaster of Paris, for purposes of immobilization. 3. An elongated or cylindroid mold formed in a tubular structure (*e.g.,* renal tubule, bronchiole) that may be observed in histologic sections or in material such as urine or sputum; results from inspissation of fluid material secreted or excreted in the tubular structures. 4. The act of restraining a large animal, usually a horse, with ropes and harnesses in a recumbent position. 5. In dentistry, a positive reproduction of the form of the tissues of the upper or lower jaw, which is made by the solidification of plaster, metal, etc., poured into an impression, and over which denture bases or other dental restorations may be fabricated.

**blood c.,** a c. usually formed in renal tubules, but may occur in bronchioles; consists of inspissated material that includes various elements of blood (*i.e.*, erythrocytes, leukocytes, fibrin, and so on), resulting from bleeding into the glomerulus or tubule, or into the alveolus or bronchiole.

**coma c.,** Külz's cylinder; a renal c. of strongly refracting granules said to be indicative of imminent coma in diabetes.

**decid'ual c.,** a mold of the interior of the uterus formed of the exfoliated mucous membrane in cases of extrauterine gestation.

**dental c.,** a positive likeness of a part or parts of the oral cavity.

**diagnostic c.,** study c.; study model; a positive likeness of dental structures used for the purposes of study and treatment planning. When it is retained for use after the initial study and treatment to serve as a pattern for reproducing esthetics of the natural dentition in dentures, it is sometimes referred to as a pre-extraction c. or record.

**epithe'lial c.,** one that contains epithelial cells and their remnants; occurs most frequently in renal tubules and urine.

**false c.,** pseudocast.

**fatty c.,** a renal or urinary c. consisting largely of fat globules. Fatty c.'s containing doubly refractile bodies (composed of cholesterol) are found in the nephrotic syndrome.

**fi'brinous c.,** a yellow c. that somewhat resembles a waxy c.; more likely to occur in urine of certain patients with acute nephritis.

**granular c.,** a relatively dark, dense c. of coarsely or finely particulate cellular debris and other proteinaceous material. See also waxy c.

**hair c.,** trichobezoar.

**hy'aline c.,** a relatively transparent renal c. composed of proteinaceous material derived from disintegration of cells. See also waxy c.

**investment c.,** refractory c.

**master c.,** a replica of the prepared tooth surfaces, residual ridge areas, and/or other parts of the dental arch as reproduced from an impression.

**mucous c.,** one type of pseudocast.

**pre-extraction c.,** see diagnostic c.

**preoperative c.,** see diagnostic c.

**refractory c.,** investment c.; a c. made of material that will withstand the high temperatures of casting or soldering without disintegrating.

**renal c.,** tube c.; any type of c. formed in a renal tubule, and found in urine, consisting of various materials, *e.g.*, albumin, cells, blood, and so on.

**spurious c.,** pseudocast.

**study c.,** diagnostic c.

**tube c.,** renal c.

**urinary c.'s,** c.'s discharged in the urine.

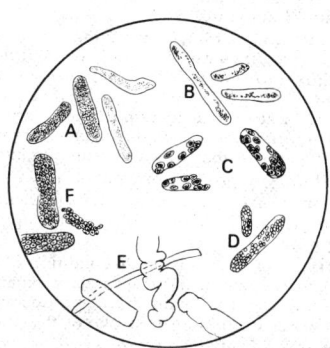

**Urinary Casts**

*A,* coarsely and finely granular casts; *B,* hyaline casts; *C,* leukocyte casts; *D,* erythrocyte casts; *E,* waxy casts; *F,* epithelial casts.

**vacuum c.,** the c. of a metal in the presence of a vacuum.

**waxy c.,** a form of renal c. consisting of homogeneous proteinaceous material that has a high refractive index, in contrast to the low refractive index of hyaline c.'s; waxy c.'s probably represent an advanced stage of the disintegrative process that results in coarsely and finely granular c.'s, and are usually indicative of oliguria or anuria.

**Castaigne,** Joseph, French physician, *1871. See Achard-C. *method.*

**casta'nea** [ L. the chestnut tree ]. The dried leaves, collected late in the season, of *Castanea dentata* (family Fagaceae), the American chestnut. Formerly used in the treatment of whooping cough in the form of a tea or infusion.

**Castellani,** Sir Aldo, Italian physician, 1878–1971. See C.'s *bronchitis, paint,* C.-Low *sign,* C.'s absorption *test.*

**cast'ing.** 1. A metallic object formed in a mold. 2. The act of forming a c. in a mold.

**centrifugal c.,** c. molten metal into a mold by spinning the metal from a crucible at the end of a revolving arm.

**Castle,** William B., Boston physician, *1897. See C.'s extrinsic and intrinsic *factors.*

**castor bean** *Ricinus.*

**cas'tor oil** (USP, BP). A fixed oil expressed from the seeds of *Ricinus communis* (family Euphorbiaceae); purgative.

**aromatic c. oil** (NF), contains cinnamon oil 3, clove oil 1, vanillin 1, saccharin 0.5, alcohol 30, in c. oil to make 1000; a cathartic.

**castrate** (kas'trāt) [ L. *castro,* pp. *-atus,* to deprive of generative power (male or female) ]. 1. To remove the testicles or the ovaries. 2. One from whom the testicles or ovaries have been removed.

**cas'trated.** Deprived of the testicles or of the ovaries.

**castra'tion** [ see castrate ]. 1. Removal of the testicles or ovaries. 2. In psychiatry, usually the fantasied actual loss of the penis by the female or fear of its potential loss by the male.

**functional c.,** gonadal atrophy produced by prolonged treatment with sex hormones.

**casualty** (kaz'u-al-tī). An injury, or the victim of an accident.

**casuistry** (kaz'u-is-trī) [ Fr. *casuiste,* fr. L. *casus,* case ]. Examination of how the general principles of ethics apply to a particular case.

**cata-** [ G. *kata*, down ]. Combining form meaning down. For words so beginning and not found here, see also kata-.

**cataba'sial** [ cata- + Mod. L. *basion* ]. Denoting a skull in which the basion is lower than the opisthion.

**cat'abiot'ic** [ cata- + G. *biotikos*, relating to life ]. 1. Used up in the carrying on of the vital processes other than growth, or in the performance of function, referring to the energy derived from food. 2. Functional; denoting an activity of the cell; opposed to bioplastic or vegetative. Conceptually obscure and rarely used term.

**catabol'ic.** Relating to catabolism.

**catab'olin.** Catabolite.

**catab'olism** [ G. *katabolē*, a casting down. BALL- ]. 1. The breaking down in the body of complex chemical compounds into simpler ones, often accompanied by the liberation of energy, as opposed to anabolism, the reverse process. 2. Retrograde metamorphosis; retromorphosis; the tendency to degeneration during development, as in the case of the eyes of many cave-dwelling animal species.

**catab'olite.** Any product of catabolism.

**catacrot'ic** [ cata- + G. *krotos*, beat ]. Denoting a pulse tracing in which the down stroke is interrupted by one or more upward waves.

**catacrotism** (kă-tak'ro-tizm). A condition of the pulse in which there are one or more secondary expansions of the artery following the main beat, producing secondary upward waves on the down stroke of the pulse tracing.

**cat'adicrot'ic** [ cata- + G. *di-*, two, + *krotos*, beat ]. Denoting a pulse tracing in which there are two minor elevations interrupting the descending limb.

**catadicrotism** (kat'ah-di'kro-tizm). A condition of the pulse marked by two minor expansions of the artery following the main beat producing two secondary upward waves on the downstroke of the pulse tracing.

**catadidymus** (kat'ah-did'ĭ-mus) [ cata- + G. *didymus*, twin ]. A twin fetus joined above but double below; duplicitas posterior.

**catadiop'tric.** Employing both reflecting and refractive optical systems.

**catagen** (kat'ah-jen). An intermediate phase of the hair cycle during which proliferation ceases and regression of the hair follicle occurs.

**catagenesis** (kat'ah-jen'ĕ-sis) [ cata- + G. *genesis*, production ]. Involution.

**cat'alase.** An enzyme (EC 1.11.1.6; a hemoprotein) catalyzing the decomposition of hydrogen peroxide to water and oxygen.

**cat'alepsy** [ G. *katalēpsis*, a seizing, catalepsy, fr. *kata*, down, + *lēpsis*, a seizure. LAB- ]. A morbid state, allied to autohypnosis or hysteria, in which there is a waxy rigidity of the limbs that may be placed in various positions which they will maintain for a time. The subject is irresponsive to stimuli; the pulse and respiration are slow, and the skin is pale.

**catalept'ic.** Relating to, or suffering from, catalepsy.

**catalep'toid.** Simulating or resembling catalepsy.

**catalogia** (kat'ah-lo'jĭ-ah) [ cata- + G. *logion*, declaration ]. Verbigeration.

**catalysis** (kă-tal'ĭ-sis) [ G. *katalysis*, dissolution ]. The effect that a catalyst exerts upon a chemical reaction.

   **contact c.,** a process wherein the catalyst is a solid and the catalyzed reaction is produced in gases making contact with the solid.

   **surface c.,** c. at the surface of a solid particle or a macromolecule.

**cat'alyst.** A substance that accelerates a chemical reaction but is not consumed or changed permanently thereby. Enzymes are c.'s. Inorganic c.'s include finely divided metals (Pt, Rh), carbon, etc.

   **negative c.,** one that retards a reaction.

   **organic c.,** enzyme.

   **positive c.,** one that accelerates a reaction.

   **Raney c.,** Raney Nickel; see under Raney.

**catalyt'ic.** Relating to or effecting catalysis.

**cat'alyze.** To act as a catalyst.

**cat'alyzer.** Catalyst.

**catame'nia** [ G. the menses, ntr. pl. of *katamēnios*, monthly, fr. *mēn*, month ]. Menses.

**catame'nial.** Relating to the catamenia.

**catamen'ogen'ic.** Causing menstruation.

**catamnesis** (kat-am-ne'sis) [ cata- + G. *mnēmē*, memory, MN- ]. The medical history of a patient after an illness; the follow-up history.

**catamnes'tic.** Related to catamnesis.

**cat'apasm** [ G. *katapasma*, a powder; *katapassō*, to sprinkle over ]. A dusting powder applied to raw surfaces or ulcers.

**catapha'sia** [ cata- + G. *phasis*, a saying ]. A disorder of speech in which there is an involuntary repetition several times of the same word.

**cataph'ora** [ G. a falling down. PHER- ]. Semicoma, or somnolence interrupted by intervals of partial consciousness.

**cataphoresis** (kat'ah-fo-re'sis) [ cata- + G. *phorēsis*, a being carried ]. Movement toward the cathode in electrophoresis; opposite of anaphoresis.

**cataphoret'ic.** Relating to cataphoresis.

**catapho'ria** [ cata- + G. *phora*, movement ]. Catatropia; a downward deviation of either eye while the other fixes.

**cataphor'ic.** Relating to cataphora or cataphoria.

**cataphylaxis** (kat-ă-fi-laks'is) [ cata- + G. *phylaxis*, protection ]. A seldom used term to designate a deterioration in the natural defense mechanisms by which the body resists infectious disease.

**catapla'sia, catapla'sis** [ cata- + G. *plasis*, a molding ]. Reversionary metamorphosis; a degenerative change in cells or tissues that is the reverse of the constructive or developmental change; a return to an earlier or embryonic stage.

**cat'aplasm** [ G. *kataplasma*, poultice, from *kataplassō*, to spread over. PLAS- ]. Poultice.

**cataplec'tic.** 1. Developing suddenly. 2. Pertaining to cataplexy.

**cataplexy** (kat'ah-plek'sī) [ cata- + G. *plēxis*, a blow, stroke. PLES- ]. A transient attack of extreme muscular weakness, resembling apoplexy, related to an emotional state such as laughing heartily.

**cataract** (kat'ă-rakt) [ L. *cataracta*, fr. G. *katarrhakiēs*, a downrushing, a waterfall, fr. *kata-rrhēgnymi*, to break down, rush down. RHAG- ]. A loss of transparency of the lens of the eye, or of its capsule.

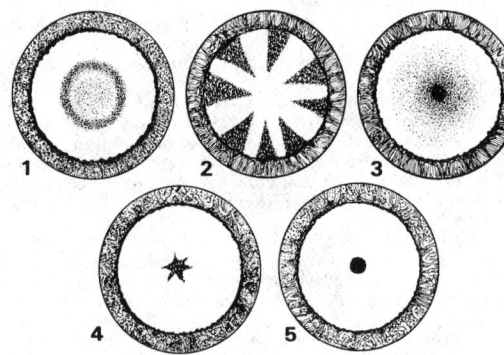

**Cataracts**

Appearance as observed by indirect ophthalmoscopic examination. *1*, Lamellar; *2*, senile cortical; *3*, senile nuclear; *4*, posterior polar; *5*, anterior polar.

   **after-c.,** secondary c. (2).

   **arborescent c.,** one in which the opacity has an appearance of branching lines.

   **atopic c.,** a c. associated with atopic dermatitis.

   **axial c.,** a lenticular opacity in the sagittal axis of the lens.

   **axillary c.,** a type of congenital (hereditary) c. with opacities deep and central.

   **black c.,** cataracta brunescens; cataracta nigra; one in which the lens is hardened and of a dark brown color.

**blue c.,** coronary c. of bluish color.

**capsular c.,** one in which the opacity affects the capsule only.

**capsulolenticular c.,** one in which both the lens and its capsule are involved; see also membranous c.

**central c.,** nuclear c.

**choroidal c.,** slowly developing c. due to choroidal disease, high myopia, and retinitis pigmentosa.

**complete c.,** one involving the entire lens.

**complicated c.,** secondary c. (1).

**congenital c.,** embryonal c.; c. present at birth.

**copper c.,** *chalcosis* lentis.

**coralliform c.,** opacities resembling coral, associated with atopic dermatitis.

**coronary c.,** c. characterized by club-shaped opacities in the periphery of the cortex near the equator of the lens.

**cortical c.,** one in which the opacity affects the cortex of the lens.

**cuneiform c.,** cortical c. in which the opacities radiate from the periphery like spokes of a wheel.

**diabetic c.,** c. in diabetes, rapidly developing and bilateral.

**electric c.,** cataracta electrica; a c. that follows contact with a high power electric current, or a lightning flash.

**embryonal c.,** congenital c.

**fibroid c., fibrinous c.,** a sclerotic hardening of the capsule of the lens, following exudative iridocyclitis.

**floriform c.,** a congenital c. with opacities arranged like the petals of a flower.

**fusiform c.,** spindle c.

**galactose c.,** a neonatal c. associated with galactosemia, *q. v.*

**glassworker's c.,** one occurring in glassmakers and due to the heat from the molten glass.

**gray c.,** a cataract of gray color, usually senile, mature, cortical.

**green c.,** glaucoma.

**hard c.,** a c. in which the lens nucleus has become hard.

**hypermature c.,** overripe c.; one in which the lens becomes either dehydrated and flattened (phacosclerosis) or liquid and soft, with the nucleus at the bottom of the capsule (Morgagnian c.).

**immature c.,** intumescent incipient stage of lens opacification.

**infantile c.,** juvenile c. affecting a very young child.

**intumescent c.,** immature c., swollen because of water absorption.

**juvenile c.,** a soft c. occurring in a child or young adult.

**lamellar c.,** zonular c.; one in which the opacity is limited to certain of the layers of the lens external to the nucleus.

**lenticular c.,** one in which the opacity is confined to the substance of the lens.

**mature c.,** one in which the entire lens substance has become opaque to directly beneath the capsule so that there is no longer any iris shadow present.

**membranous c.,** a secondary c. composed of the remains of the thickened capsule with more or less degenerated lens substance.

**Morgagni's c.,** sedimentary c.; a hypermature c. in which the cortex becomes soft and of a milky opacity while the hard dark nucleus sinks.

**nuclear c.,** central c.; one involving the nucleus only.

**peripheral c.,** peripheral coronal type distribution of small cortical opacities.

**perinuclear c.,** one in which the nucleus is clear but is surrounded by a ring or sphere of opacity.

**polar c.,** a capsular c. limited to a certain area over the anterior or posterior pole of the lens.

**primary c.,** one occurring independently of any other disease of the eye.

**progressive c.,** one in which clouding process advances and finally involves the entire lens.

**punctate c.,** an incomplete c. in which there are opaque dots scattered through the lens.

**pyramidal c.,** a cone-shaped, anterior polar c.

**radiation c.,** c. due to excessive or prolonged exposure to x-rays, radium, beta rays, heat, or radioactive isotopes.

**reduplicated c.,** a type of congenital c. with opacities situated at various levels in the lens.

**ripe c.,** mature c.

**secondary c.,** (1) complicated c.; one that accompanies or follows some other eye disease such as glaucoma; (2) aftercataract; one that occurs in the remains of the lens or capsule after a cataract operation.

**sedimentary c.,** Morgagni's c.

**senile c.,** c. occurring spontaneously in old age.

**siliculose c., siliquose c.,** calcareous degeneration of the capsule of the lens.

**soft c.,** a c. of soft consistency throughout and white in color.

**spindle c.,** fusiform c.; one in which the opacity is fusiform, extending from one pole to the other.

**stationary c.,** one that does not progress beyond a certain stage, *e.g.,* a polar c.

**stellate c.,** central lens opacities radiating toward the periphery with subcapsular and cortical changes.

**subcapsular c.,** opacities concentrated beneath the capsule.

**sutural c.,** congenital type of c. with opacities along the sutures of the lens.

**tetany c.,** one that develops in presenile patients as a result of postoperative tetany.

**total c.,** one involving the entire lens.

**toxic c.,** c. due to drugs or chemicals.

**traumatic c.,** one due to contusion, rupture, or foreign body.

**zonular c.,** lamellar c.

**catarac'ta** [ L. ]. Cataract.

**c. brunescens,** black *cataract.*

**c. dermatogenes,** cataract with skin disease.

**c. membrana'cea accre'ta,** adhesions between the lens capsule and the iris.

**c. neurodermat'ica,** cataract associated with atopic dermatitis.

**c. nigra,** black *cataract.*

**cataractogenesis** (kat'ă-rak-to-jen'ĕ-sis) [ cataract + G. *genesis,* production ]. The state of cataract formation.

**cat'aractogen'ic.** Cataract-producing.

**catarac'tous.** Relating to a cataract.

**cata'ria** [ L. *cattus,* male cat (post-class) ]. Catnep; catnip; catmint; the dried flowering tops of *Nepeta cataria* (family Labiatae). Emmenagogue and antispasmodic; reported to produce psychic effects.

**catarrh** (kă-tahr') [ G. *katarrheō,* to flow down. RHE- ]. Simple inflammation of a mucous membrane; popularly, chronic rhinitis.

**autumnal c.,** hay *fever.*

**malignant c. of cattle,** malignant catarrhal *fever.*

**nasal c.,** rhinitis.

**catarrhal** (kă-tah'ral). Relating to or affected with catarrh.

**Catarrhi'na** [ G. *kata,* down, + *rhis* (*rhin-*), nose ]. A genus of old world monkeys in the superfamily Cercopithecoidea.

**cat'arrhine.** Relating to a genus of monkeys, the *Catarrhina.*

**catastalsis** (kat'ah-stal'sis) [ G. *kata-stellō,* to put in order, check. STAL- ]. A contraction wave resembling ordinary peristalsis but not preceded by a zone of inhibition.

**catastal'tic.** 1. Inhibitory; restricting; restraining. 2. An inhibitory or checking agent, such as an astringent or antispasmodic.

**catastasis** (kă-tas'tă-sis) [ G. ]. 1. A condition or state. 2. Restoration to a normal condition or a normal place.

**cat'astate** [ G. *katastatos,* settled down ]. Catabolite.

**catastat'ic** Relating to a catastate.

**catatasis** (kă-tat'ă-sis) [ cata- + G. *teinein,* to stretch ]. Obsolete term for traction.

**cat'athermom'eter.** Psychrometer.

**catato'nia** [ G. *katatonos,* stretching down, depressed, fr. *kata,* down, + *tonos,* tone ]. 1. Stupor. 2. A type of schizophrenia characterized by periods of physical rigidity, negativism, excitement, and stupor.

**cataton'ic, catato'niac.** Relating to, or characterized by, catatonia; stuporous.

**catatricrotic** (kat'ah-tri-krot'ik). Denoting a pulse curve with three minor elevations interrupting the down stroke.

**catatricrotism** (kat'ah-tri'kro-tizm). The condition in which the pulse curve is catatricrotic.

**catatro'pia** [ cata- + G. *trope*, a turn ]. Cataphoria.

**catax'ia** [ G. *kataxis*, a breaking, fr. *katagnymi*, fut. *kataxo*, to break in pieces ]. The breaking of a pathogenic symbiosis of microorganisms.

**catechase** (kat'e-kās). Catechol 1,2-dioxygenase.

**catechin** (kat'e-kin). Catechuic acid; catechinic acid; 3,3',4',5,7-flavanpentol (for structure, see flavone and note chemical relationship to pyrocatechol and chalcone); derived from catechu; used as an astringent in diarrhea and as a stain.

**catechol** (kat'e-kol). 1. Pyrocatechol. 2. Term loosely used for catechin, which contains a pyrocatechol moiety, and as the root of catecholamines, which are pyrocatechol derivatives.

   **c. oxidase,** Monophenol monooxygenase.

**cat'echolam'ines.** Pyrocatechols with an alkylamine side chain; examples of biochemical interest are epinephrine, norepinephrine, and dopa.

**catechol 1,2-dioxygenase** (EC 1.13.11.1). Catechase; pyrocatechase; an oxidoreductase catalyzing oxidation of pyrocatechol with $O_2$ to *cis-cis*-muconate.

**catechol 2,3-dioxygenase** (EC 1.13.11.2). An oxidoreductase oxidizing catechol, with $O_2$, to 2-hydroxymuconate semialdehyde.

**catechu** (kat'e-choo, kat'e-ku) [ East Indian name ]. Gambir.

   **c. nigrum,** black c.; cutch; an extract of the heart wood of *Acacia catechu* (family Leguminosae). Used as an astringent in diarrhea.

**catechu'ic acid.** Catechin.

**catelectrotonus** (kat'e-lek-trot'o-nus) [ cathode + electrotonus ]. The changes in excitability and conductivity in a nerve or muscle in the neighborhood of the cathode during the passage of a constant electric current.

**Catenabacterium** (kat'e-nah-bak-tēr-ī-um) [ L. *catena*, chain, + bacterium ]. An obsolete genus of nonmotile, anaerobic bacteria containing Gram-positive, straight or curved rods which ordinarily occur in long chains or filaments. These organisms may be pathogenic. The type species is *C. helminthoides*. This genus is no longer recognized, and most of its species have been transferred to *Eubacterium* or *Lactobacillus*.

   **C. catenafor'me,** *Lactobacillus catenaforme*.

   **C. contor'tum,** *Eubacterium contortum*.

   **C. filamento'sum,** *Eubacterium filamentosum*.

   **C. helminthoi'des,** type species of the genus; this organism may be slightly pathogenic; it causes minor abscesses in rabbits.

**cat'enating.** Occurring in a chain or series.

**cat'enoid** [ L. *catena*, chain, + G. *eidos*, resemblance ]. Catenulate; like a chain; denoting a colony of protozoa in which the individuals are joined end to end.

**caten'ulate.** Catenoid.

**caten'ulin.** An antibiotic of the neomycin group produced by an unidentified streptomycete.

**catgut** [ probably from *kit*, a small violin, through confusion with kit, a small cat ]. Sheep's intestine twisted into cords of varying thickness, used in surgery as an absorbable suture and ligature material. See also suture (3).

   **IKI c.,** c. sterilized in a solution of 1 part of iodine in 100 parts of a solution of potassium iodide.

   **silverized c.,** prepared by immersion in a 2 per cent solution of colloidal silver for 1 week and then in 95 per cent alcohol for a quarter to half an hour.

   **sterilized surgical c.** (BP), consists of a strand prepared from the collagen derived from healthy mammals purified and sterilized; it is official in 13 gauges ranging from a diameter of 0.025 to 1.105 mm.

**Catha** (kath'ah) [ Arab. *khat* ]. A genus of African plants of the family Celastraceae.

   **C. ed'ulis,** "flower of paradise"; a plant of Abyssinia and Arabia, cultivated for use as a stimulant; khat (the fresh leaves and twigs) is chewed or used in the preparation of a beverage. The active principle is pharmacologically related to the amphetamines, probably *d*- norisoephedrine.

**catharom'eter.** An instrument for measuring thermal conductivity of air.

**catharsis** (kā-thar'sis) [ G. purification, fr. *katharos*, pure ]. 1. Purgation; excessive action of the bowels. 2. The release or discharge of emotional tension or anxiety by psychoanalytically guided emotional reliving of past, especially repressed, events.

**cathar'tic.** 1. Purging; relating to catharsis. 2. An agent causing active movement of the bowels.

**cathectic** (kā-thek'tik). Pertaining to cathexis.

**cathec'ting.** See investing (2).

**cathemoglo'bin.** An artificial derivative of hemoglobin in which the globin is denatured and the iron oxidized.

**cathep'sins.** Proteinases and peptidases (peptide hydrolases) of animal tissues of varying specificities.

   **c. B,** c. $B_1$.

   **c. $B_1$** (EC 3.4.17.1), c. B; intracellular proteinase in vertebrates.

   **c. C,** dipeptidyl peptidase.

   **c. D** (EC 3.4.23.5), c. E; a proteinase active at acid pH, somewhat similar to pepsin A.

   **c. E,** c. D.

**cathepsis** (kā-thep'sis) [ G. *kathepsis*, a boiling down, fr. *hepso*, to boil ]. Protein hydrolysis or synthesis in living cells or hydrolysis in dead animal tissues (autolysis) due to cathepsins.

**cathep'tic.** Relating to the action of cathepsins, *i.e.*, to cathepsis.

**cath'eter** [ G. *katheter*, fr. *kathiemi*, to send down. ES- ]. 1. A hollow cylinder of silver, India rubber, or other material, designed to be passed through the urethra into the bladder to drain this viscus of urine in case of retention from cause. 2. A similar instrument used for passage through other canals.

   **c. à demeure** (ă-dem-ēr') [ Fr. *demeurer*, to dwell ], one which is retained permanently or for a considerable period in the urethra.

   **bicoudate c.,** one with a double bend.

   **Bozeman-Fritsch c.,** a slightly curved double-current uterine c. with several openings at the tip.

   **cardiac c.,** intracardiac c.

   **Carlen's c.,** a double lumen, flexible c. for separate intubation of the two main bronchi.

   **c. coudé** (koo-da'), elbowed c.

   **elbowed c.,** c. coudé; prostatic c.; one with an angular bend near the beak, of use when there is obstruction by the prostate.

   **c. en chemise,** used to control hemorrhage following external (perineal) urethrotomy. It consists of a piece of gauze fastened to a c.; the c. is passed through the perineal wound onto the bladder until the open end of the gauze lies flush with the perineum. The space between the c. and the "chemise" of gauze is then packed with absorbent cotton.

   **Eusta'chian c.,** one used for catheterization of the middle ear through the Eustachian tube.

   **female c.,** a short, nearly straight c. for passage into the female bladder.

   **Fogarty c.,** a c. with an inflatable balloon near its tip, used to remove thrombi from major veins, *e.g.*, iliofemoral; also used to remove stones from the biliary ducts.

   **Foley c.,** a retention c. with a device for inflating a retaining balloon.

   **indwelling c.,** one left in place in the bladder.

   **intracardiac c.,** cardiac c.; a c. that can be passed into the heart via a vein or artery; by means of it samples of blood may be withdrawn (to determine oxygen saturation, etc.), pressures may be measured within the heart's chambers or great vessels and contrast media injected; used mainly in the diagnosis and evaluation of congenital, rheumatic, and coronary artery lesions.

   **Nélaton's c.,** a flexible c. of red rubber.

   **pacing c.,** a cardiac c. with one or two electrodes at its tip, which when connected to a pulse generator and advanced pervenously into the right atrium or ventricle is used for artificial pacing of the heart.

   **Pezzer c.,** a self-retaining c. with a bulbous extremity.

   **Phillips' c.,** one with filiform guide, for urethra.

   **prostat'ic c.,** elbowed c.

   **self-retaining c.,** one so constructed that it remains in urethra and bladder until removed.

   **two-way c.,** a c. used for irrigation.

**vertebrated c.,** one made of several segments moving on each other like the links of a chain.

**whistle-tip c.,** one with opening at end as well as on side.

**winged c.,** a soft rubber c. with little flaps at each side of the beak in order to retain it in the bladder.

**catheteriza'tion, cath'eterism.** The passage of a catheter.

**cath'eterize.** To subject a person to the passage of a catheter.

**cath'eterostat** [ catheter + G. *statos,* standing ]. A stand for holding catheters.

**cathexis** (kă-thek'sis) [ G. *kathexis,* a holding in, retention ]. Attachment of libido to a specific idea or object.

**cath'odal.** Abbreviated C or Ca; relating to the cathode.

**cath'ode** [ G. *kathodos,* a way down, fr. *kata,* down, + *hodos,* a way ]. Abbreviated C, or Ca; the negative pole of a galvanic battery or the electrode connected with it; an electrode toward which positively charged ions (cations) migrate; *cf.* anode.

**cathod'ic.** Relating to the cathode; electropositive.

**cathod'olyte.** Cation.

**cathol'ysis.** Electrolysis with a cathode needle.

**cation** (kat'i-on) [ G. *kation,* going down ]. An ion carrying a charge of positive electricity, therefore going to the negatively charged cathode.

**cation exchange.** The process by which a cation in a liquid phase exchanges with another cation present as the counter-ion of a negatively charged polymer, the latter being a cation exchanger. A cation-exchange reaction in removal of the $Na^+$ of a sodium chloride solution is $RSO_3^-H^+ + Na^+ \rightarrow RSO_3^-Na^+ + H^+$ (R is the polymer, $RSO_3^-$ the cation exchanger). If this is combined with the anion-exchange reaction given under anion exchange, NaCl is removed from the solution. Cation exchange may also be used chromatographically, to separate cations, and medicinally, to remove a cation, *e.g.,* $H^+$, from gastric contents, or $Na^+$ and $K^+$ in the intestine.

**cation exchanger.** An insoluble solid (usually a polystyrene or a polysaccharide) that has negatively charged radicals attached to it (*e.g.,* $—COO^-$, $—SO_3^-$), which can attract and hold cations that pass by in a moving solution.

**cation'ic.** With reference to positively charged ions and their properties.

**cationogen** (kat-i-on'o-jen). A substance that gives rise to positively charged ions.

**cat'lin, cat'ling.** A long, sharp-pointed, double-edged knife used in amputations.

**cat'nep, cat'nip.** Cataria.

**cat'ochus** [ G. *katochē,* epilepsy (Galen), fr. *katechō,* to hold fast ]. The trancelike phase of catalepsy in which the patient is conscious but cannot move or speak.

**catop'tric** [ G. *katoptron,* mirror. OPO- ]. Relating to reflected light.

**catop'troscope** [ G. *katoptron,* mirror, + *skopeō,* to view ]. An instrument fitted with mirrors to reflect reflected light.

**cauda,** pl. **caudae** (kaw'dah) [ L. a tail ]. Tail. 1 [ NA ]. Any tail, or tail-like structure, or tapering or elongated extremity of an organ or other part. 2 [ NAV ]. In veterinary anatomy, a free appendage representing the caudal end of the vertebral column; it is covered by skin and hair, feathers, or scales.

**c. epididym'idis** [ NA ], tail of the epididymis; globus minor of the epididymis; the inferior part of the epididymis that leads into the ductus deferens; part of the reservoir of spermatozoa.

**c. equi'na** [ L. horse's tail ] [ NA ], the bundle of spinal nerve roots arising from the lumbar enlargement and conus medullaris and running through the lower part of the subarachnoid space within the vertebral canal below the first lumbar vertebra; it comprises the roots of all the spinal nerves below the first lumbar.

**c. fas'ciae denta'tae,** uncus *band* of Giacomini.

**c. hel'icis** [ NA ], a flattened process terminating the cartilage of the helix posteriorly and inferiorly.

**c. nu'clei cauda'ti** [ NA ], cauda striati; tail of the caudate nucleus; the elongated posterior extension of the caudate nucleus that parallels the body and inferior horn of the lateral ventricle.

**c. pancre'atis** [ NA ], tail of the pancreas; the left extremity of the pancreas within the lienorenal ligament.

**c. stria'ti,** c. nuclei caudati.

**caudad** (kaw'dad). In a direction toward the tail.

**caudal** (kaw'dal) [ Mod. L. *caudalis* ]. 1. Relating to any cauda, or anatomical structure resembling a tail. 2. Toward the tail end of the organism; depending on context, the term can be synonymous with inferior or posterior; antonyms are rostral, oral, cephalad.

**cauda'lis** [ NA ]. Caudal; toward the tail.

**caudate** (kaw'dāt). 1. Tailed; possessing a tail. 2. *Nucleus* caudatus.

**cauda'tolentic'ular.** Caudolenticular; relating to the nuclei caudatus and lenticularis.

**cauda'tum.** *Nucleus* caudatus.

**caudocephalad** (kaw-do-sef'al-ad). In a direction from the tail toward the head.

**cau'dolentic'ular.** Caudatolenticular.

**caul** (kawl) [ Gaelic, *call,* a veil ]. 1. Galea (4); velum (2); veil (2); the amnion forming the bag of waters, sometimes delivered unruptured with the baby; a piece of amnion capping the baby's head when born. 2. *Omentum* majus.

**caumesthesia** (kaw-mes-the'zī-ah) [ G. *kauma,* heat (CAU-), + *aisthēsis,* sensation ]. A sense of heat irrespective of the temperature of the air.

**causalgia** (kaw-zal'jī-ah) [ G. *kausis,* burning (CAU-), + *algos,* pain ]. Persistent severe burning sensation of the skin, usually following direct or indirect (vascular) injury of sensory fibers of a peripheral nerve, and accompanied by cutaneous changes (temperature and sweating).

**cause** (kawz) [ L. *causa* ]. That which produces an effect or condition; that by which a morbid change or disease is brought about.

**constitutional c.,** a c. acting from within or through some systemic process or inborn error.

**exciting c.,** the direct provoking c. of a disease.

**predisposing c.,** anything that produces a susceptibility or disposition to a disease without itself causing the disease.

**proximate c.,** the immediate actual c.

**specific c.,** one the action of which produces only one definite disease; *e.g.,* the specific micro-organism causing diphtheria, tuberculosis, or tetanus.

**caustic** (kaws'tik) [ G. *kaustikos,* fr. *kaiō,* to burn. CAU- ]. Corrosive; escharotic. 1. Exerting an effect resembling a burn. 2. An agent producing this effect.

**lunar c.,** toughened silver nitrate.

**cauter** (kaw'ter) [ G. *kautēr,* a branding iron. CAU- ]. A cautery iron.

**cauterant** (kaw'ter-ant). 1. Cauterizing. 2. A cauterizing agent.

**cauteriza'tion.** The act of cauterizing.

**gas c.,** c. by means of a lighted gas jet.

**solar c.,** sun c.

**sun c.,** c. by means of the sun's rays focused by a lens or a mirror.

**cauterize** (kaw'ter-iz). To apply a cautery; to burn with the actual or potential cautery.

**cautery** (kaw'ter-ī) [ G. *kautērion,* a branding iron. CAU- ]. 1. An agent used for scarring or burning the skin or tissues by means of heat or of caustic chemicals. 2. The destructive effect produced by a cauterizing agent.

**actual c.,** technocausis; a c., such as electrocautery or a hot iron, acting directly through heat and not by chemical means.

**bipolar c.,** surgical c. by high frequency electrical current passed through tissue between tips of forceps; used for hemostasis.

**button c.,** Corrigan's c.; an actual c. in which the heated part is a knob on the end of a nonconducting handle.

**chemical c.,** chemocautery.

**cold c.,** cryocautery.

**Corrigan's c.,** button c.

**electric c.,** galvanocautery.

**galvanic c.,** galvanocautery.

**monopolar c.,** surgical c. by high frequency electrical current passed from a locally applied instrument, where the action takes place, through tissues to a distant grounded metal plate.

**Paquelin's c.,** a cauterizing apparatus consisting of a hollow platinum body, in the shape of a knife, needle, ball, etc., which is heated by the forcing into it of a mixture of the vapor of benzin and air.

**potential c.,** virtual caustic; an agent such as potassium hydroxide that forms an eschar without the agency of actual fire.

**virtual c.,** potential c.

**cava** (ka'vah). *Vena cava.*

**cav'agram.** Cavogram.

**ca'val.** Relating to a vena cava.

**cav'ascope** [ L. *cavum*, hole, + G. *skopeō*, to view ]. An instrument for examining the interior of any cavity.

**cave.** A hollow or enclosed space or cavity; see cavum, cavitas, caverna.

**caveo'la,** pl. **caveo'lae** [ L. ]. A small pocket, vesicle, cave or recess communicating with the outside of a cell and extending inward, indenting the cytoplasm and the cell membrane. Such caveolae may be pinched off to form free vesicles within the cytoplasm. They are considered to be sites of uptake of materials into the cell, expulsion of materials from the cell, or sites of addition or removal of cell (unit) membrane to or from the cell surface.

**cavern** (kav'ern) [ L. *caverna*, a grotto, fr. *cavus*, hollow ]. 1. Caverna. 2. A pathologic cavity or excavation from loss of pulmonary tissue in tuberculosis.

**caverna,** pl. **caver'nae** (kă-ver'nah) [ L. ] [ NA ]. Cavern; an anatomical cavity.

**cavernae corpo'ris spongio'si** [ NA ], cavities of the corpus spongiosum; the vascular spaces forming the erectile tissue of the corpus spongiosum penis in the male and the bulb of the vestibule in the female.

**cavernae corpo'rum cavernoso'rum** [ NA ], cavities of the corpora cavernosa; the endothelium-lined blood-filled spaces of the corpora cavernosa that, together with the intervening fibrous trabeculae, form the erectile tissue of the penis or clitoris.

**cavernicole** (kav'er-nĭ-kōl) [ Fr. ]. A plant or animal that lives in naturally occurring subterranean spaces such as caves.

**caverniloquy** (kav'er-nil'o-kwĭ) [ L. *caverna*, cavern, + *loqui*, to talk ]. Low pitched pectoriloquy heard over a lung cavity.

**caverni'tis.** Cavernositis; inflammation of the corpus cavernosum penis.

**fibrous c.,** Peyronie's *disease.*

**caverno'ma.** Cavernous *hemangioma.*

**c. lymphat'icum,** *lymphangioma* cavernosum.

**cav'ernoscope.** An instrument for inspecting a cavity.

**cavernoscopy** (kav'er-nos'ko-pĭ) [ L. *caverna*, cavern, + G. *skopeō*, to view ]. Inspection of a cavity by means of a cavernoscope.

**cavernosi'tis.** Cavernitis.

**cavernos'tomy** [ L. *caverna*, cavern, + G. *stoma*, mouth ]. The opening of any cavity to establish drainage; speleostomy.

**cav'ernous.** Relating to a cavern or a cavity; containing many cavities.

**Ca'via** [ Mod. L. from native Indian ]. A genus of the family Caviidae that includes the guinea pigs.

**C. porcel'lus,** guinea pig; a 1- to 2-pound rodent with a very short tail that is not visible externally; native to South America, where it is raised for food; used widely as a laboratory animal in bacteriologic, pathologic, and pharmacologic research.

**Caviidae.** The family of rodents that includes the genus *Cavia* (guinea pigs).

**cav'itary.** 1. Relating to a cavity or having a cavity or cavities. 2. Denoting any animal parasite that has an enteric canal or body cavity and that lives within the host's body.

**cav'itas,** pl. **cavita'tes** [ Mod. L. ]. A cavity.

**c. glenoida'lis** [ NA ], glenoid cavity; the hollow in the head of the scapula that receives the head of the humerus to make the shoulder joint.

**cavita'tion.** The formation of a cavity, as in the lung in tuberculosis.

**cavitis** (ka-vi'tis). Celophlebitis.

**cavity** (kav'ĭ-tĭ) [ L. *cavus*, hollow ]. 1. A hollow space; see cavum. 2. Defect or loss of tooth structure produced by dental caries.

**abdominal c.,** *cavum* abdominis.

**allantoic c.,** the lumen of the allantois.

**amniot'ic c.,** the fluid-filled c. surrounding the developing embryo.

**axillary c.,** axilla.

**body c.,** the celom (2).

**buccal c.,** (1) *vestibulum* oris; (2) in dentistry, a c. beginning by decay on the buccal surface of a tooth.

**cleavage c.,** the blastocele.

**complex c.,** compound c.

**compound c.,** a c. involving more than one surface of a tooth; two or more c.'s joined to form one c.

**c. of the concha,** *cavum* conchae.

**cot'yloid c.,** acetabulum.

**cranial c.,** the space contained within the skull.

**crown c.,** *cavum* coronale.

**distal c.,** loss of tooth structure on the surface of an anterior tooth away from the midline; on posterior teeth, on the posterior surface.

**ectoplacental c.,** epamniotic c.

**ectotrophoblastic c.,** a developmental c. appearing between the trophoblast and the embryonic disk ectoderm in some mammals.

**epamniotic c.,** ectoplacental c.; a developmental c. derived by division of the proamniotic space; it is further removed from the embryo than the amniotic c.

**epidur'al c.,** *cavum* epidurale.

**fissure c.,** in dentistry, a c. beginning in a fissure on the occlusal surfaces of posterior teeth.

**glenoid c.,** *cavitas* glenoidalis.

**head c.,** the cephalic region in the embryos of vertebrates containing the modified somites that give rise to the eye muscles.

**c. of larynx,** *cavum* laryngis.

**Meckel's c.,** *cavum* trigeminale.

**medullary c.,** *cavum* medullare.

**nasal c.,** *cavum* nasi.

**nephrotomic c.,** nephrocele (2).

**occlu'sal c.,** a carious c. starting from the occlusal surface of a tooth.

**oral c.,** *cavum* oris.

**pelvic c.,** *cavum* pelvis.

**pericardial c.,** (1) in the adult, the *cavum* pericardii; (2) in the embryo, that part of the primary celom containing the heart; originally it is in open communication with the pleural c.'s and indirectly, through them, with the peritoneal part of the celom.

**peritone'al c.,** *cavum* peritonei.

**perivisceral c., primitive perivisceral c.,** the space between the ectoderm and entoderm in the gastrula.

**pharyngonasal c.,** *pars* nasalis pharyngis.

**c. of pharynx,** *cavum* pharyngis.

**pit c.,** in dentistry, a c., usually small, beginning in a pit on the labial, buccal, lingual, or occlusal tooth surface.

**pleural c.,** *cavum* pleurae.

**pleuroperitoneal c.,** that part of the embryonic celom later partitioned to give rise to the pleural and peritoneal c.'s.

**proximal c.,** a c. occurring in the proximal surface, either distal or mesial, of a tooth.

**pulp c.,** *cavum* dentis.

**Retzius' c.,** *spatium* retropubicum.

**segmentation c.,** the blastocele.

**c. of the septum pellucidum,** *cavum* septi pellucidi.

**somite c.,** myocele (2).

**splanchnic c.,** visceral c.; the celom or one of the body c.'s derived from it.

**subarach'noid c.,** *cavum* subarachnoideale.

**subdu'ral c.,** subdural *space.*

**subgerminal c.,** the c. beneath the embryonic area; the archenteron.

**tension c.,** tension *pneumothorax.*

**thorac'ic c.,** *cavum* thoracis.

**trigeminal c.,** *cavum* trigeminale.

**tympan'ic c.,** *cavum* tympani.

**c. of uterus,** *cavum* uteri.

**vis'ceral c.,** splanchnic c.

**cav'ogram.** An angiogram of a vena cava.

**cavog'raphy.** Angiography of vena cava.

**ca'vosur'face.** Relating to a cavity and the surface of a tooth; denoting especially the c. angle formed by the junction of the cavity wall and the surface of the tooth.

**cavum,** pl. **ca'va** (ka'vum) [ L. ntr. of adj. *cavus,* hollow ] [ NA ]. A hollow, hole, or cavity.

**c. abdominis** [ NA ], abdominal cavity; enterocele; the space bounded by the abdominal walls, the diaphragm, and the pelvis. It may be arbitrarily separated from the pelvic cavity by a plane across the superior aperture of the lesser pelvis. However, it may include the pelvis with the abdomen. Within the c. lie the greater part of the organs of digestion, the spleen, the kidneys, and the suprarenal glands. Most of these organs are partially invested by a serous membrane, the peritoneum, which also lines the interior of the abdominal wall and the pelvic cavity.

**c. articula're** [ NA ], a joint cavity.

**c. conchae** [ NA ], cavity of the concha; the lower, larger portion of the concha below the crus helicis; it forms the vestibule to the external acoustic meatus.

**c. corona'le** [ NA ], crown cavity; the space within the crown of a tooth continuous with the root canal.

**c. den'tis** [ NA ], cavity of the tooth; pulp cavity; the central hollow of a tooth consisting of the crown cavity and the root canal. It is lined throughout with odontoblasts.

**c. doug'lasi,** *excavatio* rectouterina.

**c. epidurale** [ NA ], epidural space or cavity; the space between the walls of the vertebral canal and the dura mater of the spinal cord.

**c. infraglotticum** [ NA ], aditus glottidis inferior; the part of the cavity of the larynx immediately below the glottis.

**c. laryn'gis** [ NA ], cavity of the larynx; it is continuous above with the pharynx at the level of the aryepiglottic folds and extends downward through the rima vestibuli and rima glottidis to the trachea.

**c. mediastina'le,** an inappropriate name sometimes applied to the mediastinum.

**c. medulla're** [ NA ], medullary cavity; the marrow cavity in the shaft of a long bone.

**c. na'si** [ NA ], nasal cavity; the cavity on either side of the nasal septum, lined with ciliated respiratory mucosa,

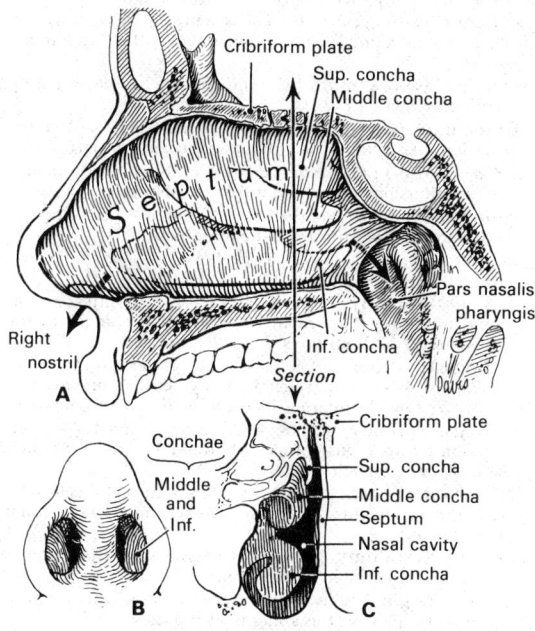

**Cavum Nasi**

*A,* sagittal section showing right nasal cavity as seen through septum; *B,* nares viewed from below; *C,* coronal section at level indicated showing relationship between air passages and mucosal surfaces.

extending from the naris anteriorly to the choana posteriorly, and communicating with the paranasal sinuses through their orifices in the lateral wall, from which also project the three choanae. The cribriform plate, through which the olfactory nerves are transmitted, forms the roof; the floor is formed by the hard palate.

**c. oris** [ NA ], oral cavity; mouth; the region consisting of the *vestibulum oris* [ NA ], the narrow cleft between the lips and cheeks, and the teeth and gums, and the *cavum oris proprium* [ NA ], the oral cavity proper, the space between the dental arches, limited posteriorly by the isthmus of the fauces.

**c. pelvis** [ NA ], pelvic cavity; the space bounded at the sides by the bones of the pelvis, above by a plane passing through the arcuate lines, and below by the pelvic diaphragm. It contains the pelvic viscera.

**c. pericar'dii** [ NA ], pericardial cavity; the potential space between the parietal and the visceral layers of the serous pericardium.

**c. peritonei** [ NA ], peritoneal cavity; greater peritoneal sac; the interior of the peritoneal sac, normally only a potential space between the parietal and visceral layers of the peritoneum.

**c. pharyn'gis** [ NA ], cavity of the pharynx; it consists of a nasal part continuous anteriorly with the nasal cavity and receiving the openings of the auditory tubes, an oral part opening through the fauces into the oral cavity, and a laryngeal part leading into the vestibule of the larynx and to the esophagus.

**c. pleurae** [ NA ], pleural cavity; the potential space between the parietal and visceral layers of the pleura.

**c. psalte'rii,** Verga's *ventricle.*

**c. ret'zii,** *spatium* retropubicum.

**c. sep'ti pellu'cidi** [ NA ], cavity of the septum pellucidum; fifth ventricle; Duncan's, Sylvian, Vieussens', or Wenzel's ventricle; ventriculus quintus; a slitlike, fluid-filled space of variable width enclosed between the left and right septum pellucidum of the human brain. Usually isolated, the space in some cases communicates with the third ventricle through an opening between the two fornix columns and can then appear on a ventriculogram. Present in less than 10 per cent of humans, the c. is probably the result of a developmental anomaly that is usually asymptomatic.

**c. subarachnoidea'le** [ NA ], subarachnoid space or cavity; the space between the arachnoidea and pia mater, traversed by delicate fibrous trabeculae and filled with cerebrospinal fluid. Since the pia mater immediately adheres to the surface of the brain and spinal cord, the space is greatly widened whereever the brain surface exhibits a deep depression (for example, the deep grooves of the cerebral cortex); such widenings are called cisternae. All of the large blood vessels supplying the brain and spinal cord lie suspended in the subarachnoid space.

**c. subdura'le,** subdural *space.*

**c. thoracis** [ NA ], thoracic cavity; the space within the thoracic walls, bounded below by the diaphragm and above by the neck.

**c. trigemina'le** [ NA ], trigeminal cavity; Meckel's cave or cavity; the evagination of the meningeal layer of dura from the posterior cranial fossa near the tip of the petrous part of the temporal bone downward and medially beneath the dura of the middle cranial fossa. It encloses the roots of the trigeminal nerve and the trigeminal ganglion.

**c. tympani** [ NA ], tympanic cavity; cavity of the middle ear; an air chamber in the temporal bone containing the ossicles. It is lined with mucous membrane and is continuous anteriorly with the auditory tube and posteriorly with the tympanic antrum and mastoid air cells. See fig., p. 242.

**c. u'teri** [ NA ], cavity of the uterus.

**c. ves'icouteri'num,** excavatio vesicouterina.

**c. ver'gae,** Verga's *ventricle.*

**cavy.** Common name for a member of the genus *Cavia* (the guinea pig).

**Cazenave** (kahz-nav'), P. L. Alphée, Paris dermatologist, 1795–1877. See C.'s *disease, vitiligo.*

**Cb.** Chemical symbol of the element columbium, now niobium (Nb).

**CBG.** Abbreviation for corticosteroid-binding *globulin.*

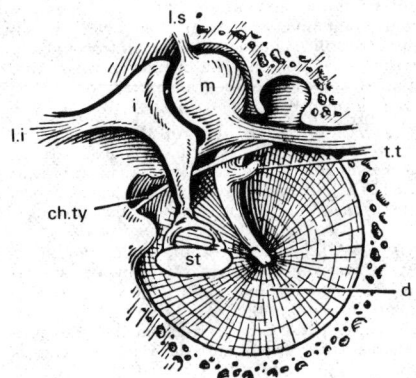

**Cavum Tympani Viewed from Within Outward**

*d,* Drum membrane; *i,* incus; *m,* malleus; *st,* stapes; *ch.ty,* chorda tympani nerve; *l.s,* ligament of malleus; *l.i,* ligament of incus; *t.t,* tendon of tensor tympani muscle.

**Cbz.** Abbreviation for carbobenzoxy (benzyloxycarbonyl) radical.

**cc.** or **c.c.** Abbreviation for cubic centimeter; see milliliter.

**CCC.** Abbreviation of cathodal closing, or closure, *contraction.*

**CCTe.** Abbreviation for cathodal closing, or closure, *tetanus.*

**Cd.** Chemical symbol of the element cadmium.

**CDE blood group.** See Rh blood group, appendix 2.

**CDP.** Abbreviation for *cytidine* diphosphate.

**Ce.** Chemical symbol of the element cerium.

**CEA.** Abbreviation for carcinoembryonic *antigen.*

**cebocephalus** (se'bo-sef'ā-lus). [ G. *kebos,* monkey, + *kephalē,* head ]. An individual with cebocephaly.

**cebocephaly** (se'bo-sef'ā-lī) [ G. *kebos,* monkey, + *kephalē,* head ]. A malformation in which the features are suggestive of those of a monkey; there is usually a tendency toward cyclopia, with defective or absent nose and closely set eyes.

**cec-.** See ceco-.

**cecal** (se'kal). 1. Relating to the cecum. 2. Ending blindly or in a cul-de-sac.

**cecectomy** (se-sek'to-mī) [ ceco- + G. *ektomē,* excision ]. Typhlectomy; excision of the cecum.

**cecitis** (se-si'tis). Typhlitis; inflammation of the cecum.

**ceco-, cec-** [ L. *caecum,* cecum ]. Combining forms relating to the cecum.

**cecocele** (se'ko-sēl) [ ceco- + G. *kele,* tumor, rupture ]. Typhlocele; cecum in a hernia sac.

**cecocolostomy** (se'ko-ko-los'to-mī). Formation of an anastomosis between cecum and colon.

**ce'cofixa'tion.** Cecopexy.

**cecoileostomy** (se-ko-il'e-os'to-mī). Ileocecostomy.

**cecopexy** (se'ko-pek'sī) [ ceco- + G. *pexis,* fixation ]. Typhlopexy; cecofixation; operation for anchoring a movable cecum.

**cecoplication** (se'ko-pli-ka'shun) [ ceco- + L. *plico,* pp. *-atus,* to fold ]. Operative reduction in size of a dilated cecum by the formation of folds or tucks in its wall.

**cecoptosis** (se'kop-to'sis) [ ceco- + G. *ptōsis,* a falling ]. Typhloptosis; downward displacement of the cecum.

**cecorrhaphy** (se-kor'ā-fī) [ ceco- + G. *rhaphē,* suture ]. Typlorrhaphy; suture of the cecum.

**cecosigmoidostomy** (se'ko-sig-moy-dos'to-mī). The formation of a communication between the cecum and the sigmoid colon.

**cecostomy** (se-kos'to-mī) [ ceco- + G. *stoma,* mouth ]. Typhlostomy; the operative formation of a cecal fistula.

**cecotomy** (se-kot'o-mī) [ ceco- + G. *tome,* incision ]. Typhlotomy; incision into the cecum.

**cecum,** pl. **ce'ca** (se'kum) [ L. ntr. of *caecus,* blind ] [ NA ]. Caecum. 1. Typhlon; blind gut, the cul-de-sac, about 2½ inches in depth, lying below the terminal ileum forming the first part of the large intestine. 2. Any similar structure ending in a cul-de-sac.

   **c. cupula're** [ NA ], cupular blind sac; the upper blind extremity of the cochlear duct.

   **c. vestibula're** [ NA ], vestibular blind sac; the lower extremity of the cochlear duct, occupying the cochlear recess in the vestibule.

**cecutient** (se'ku-shunt) [ L. *caecus,* blind ]. A person with partial sight.

**ce'dar leaf oil.** Thuja oil; arbor vitae oil; obtained by steam distillation from the fresh leaves of *Thuja occidentalis;* used as an insect repellent and counterirritant, and in perfumery.

**ce'dar wood oil.** Volatile oil obtained from the wood of *Juniperus virginiana* (family Pinaceae); used as an insect repellent, in perfumery, and as a clearing agent in microscopy.

**cel** [ L. *celer,* swift ]. A unit of velocity; 1 cm. per second.

**cela'tion** [ L. *celo,* pp. *-atus,* to conceal ]. Concealment of pregnancy or of the birth of a child.

**-cele** (-sēl) [ G. *kēlē,* tumor, hernia ]. A suffix denoting a swelling or hernia of the part signified by the main word.

**celectome** (se'lek-tōm) [ G. *kēlē,* tumor, + *ektomē,* excision ]. An instrument, such as the harpoon, for obtaining a bit of tissue from the interior of a tumor for examination.

**celenteron** (se-len'ter-on) [ G. *koilos,* hollow, + *enteron,* intestine ]. Archenteron.

**cel'ery seed.** The dried ripe fruit of *Apium graveolens* (family Umbelliferae); has been used in dysmenorrhea and as a sedative.

**celestice'tin.** Antibiotic produced by *Streptomyces caelestis;* possesses antimicrobial activity.

**ce'liac** [ G. *koilia,* belly. CELI- ]. Relating to the abdominal cavity.

**celi'acus** [ L. ] [ NA ]. Celiac.

**celiadelphus** (se-lī-ā-del'fus) [ G. *koilia,* belly, + *adelphos,* brother ]. Conjoined twins with fused abdomens.

**celiagra** (se-lī-ag'rah) [ G. *koilia,* belly, + *agra,* seizure ]. A gouty affection of the stomach or other abdominal organs.

**celialgia** (se-lī-al'jī-ah) [ G. *koilia,* belly, + *algos,* pain ]. Abdominalgia.

**celiectomy** (se-lī-ek'to-mī) [ G. *koilia,* belly, + *ektomē,* excision ]. Excision of any abdominal organ, or part of one.

**celio-** (se'lī-o-) [ G. *koilia,* belly. Combining form denoting relationship to the abdomen; see also celo-.

**celiocentesis** (se'lī-o-sen-tē'sis) [ celio- + G. *kentēsis,* puncture ]. Paracentesis of the abdomen.

**celiodynia** (se-lī-o-din'-ī-ah) [ celio- + G. *odynē,* pain ]. Abdominalgia.

**ce'lioenterot'omy** [ celio- + G. *enteron,* intestine, + *tomē,* incision ]. Laparoenterotomy (2); opening into the intestine through an incision in the abdominal wall.

**ce'liogastros'tomy** [ celio- + G. *gastēr,* stomach, + *stoma,* mouth ]. Laparogastrostomy; establishment of a gastric fistula through an incision in the abdominal wall.

**ce'liogastrot'omy** [ celio- + G. *gastēr,* stomach, + *tomē,* incision ]. Laparogastrotomy; abdominal section with incision of the stomach.

**ce'liohysterec'tomy** (se'lī-o-his-ter-ek'to-mī) [ celio- + G. *hystera,* womb, + *ektomē,* excision ]. Abdominal *hysterectomy.*

**ce'liohysterot'omy** [ celio- + G. *hystera,* womb, + *tomē,* incision ]. Abdominal *hysterotomy.*

**ce'liomyal'gia** [ celio- + G. *mys,* muscle, + *algos,* pain ]. Rheumatic pain in the abdominal muscles.

**ce'liomy'omec'tomy** [ celio- + myoma, *q.v.,* + G. *ektomē,* excision ]. Abdominal *myomectomy.*

**ce'liomy'omot'omy** [ celio- + myoma, *q.v.,* + G. *tomē,* incision ]. Laparomyomotomy; incision into a myoma after abdominal incision.

**ce'liomy'osi'tis** [ celio- + G. *mys,* muscle, + suffix *-itis,* inflammation ]. Inflammation of the abdominal muscles.

**ce′liopar′acente′sis** [ celio- + G. *parakentēsis*, a puncture for dropsy (Galen). CENT- ]. Paracentesis of the abdomen.

**celiop′athy** [ celio- + G. *pathos*, disease ]. Any abdominal disease.

**celiorrhaphy** (se-lī-or′ă-fī) [ celio- + G. *rhaphē*, seam ]. Laparorrhaphy; suture of a wound in the abdominal wall.

**celiosalpingectomy** (se′lī-o-sal-pin-jek′to-mī) [ celio- + G. *salpinx*, trumpet + *ektomē*, excision ]. Abdominal *salpingectomy*.

**celiosalpingotomy** (se′lī-o-sal-pin-got′o-mī) [ celio- + G. *salpinx*, trumpet, + *tomē*, incision ]. Abdominal *salpingotomy*.

**celios′copy** [ celio- + G. *skopeō*, to view ]. Peritoneoscopy.

**celiot′omy** [ celio- + G. *tomē*, incision ]. Laparotomy (2); abdominal section; ventrotomy; incision through the abdominal wall.

　**vaginal c.,** opening the peritoneal cavity through the vagina.

**celi′tis** [ G. *koilia*, belly, + suffix -*itis*, inflammation ]. Any inflammation of the abdomen.

---

# CELL

---

**cell** [ L. *cella*, a storeroom, a chamber ]. 1. A minute structure, the living, active basis of all plant and animal organization, composed of a mass of protoplasm, enclosed in a delicate membrane and containing a nucleus. C.'s are of the most varied form and structure according to the function which they have to perform. 2. A small closed or partly closed cavity.

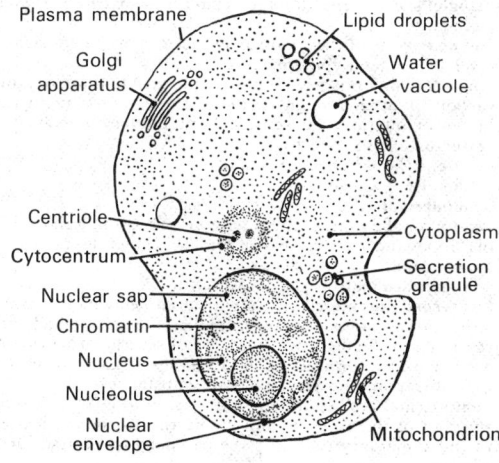

Plasma membrane — Lipid droplets — Golgi apparatus — Water vacuole — Centriole — Cytoplasm — Cytocentrum — Secretion granule — Nuclear sap — Chromatin — Nucleus — Nucleolus — Nuclear envelope — Mitochondrion

**Schematic Diagram of a Cell**

**A c.'s,** see alpha c.'s of pancreas and of hypophysis.

　**absolute c. increase,** refers to an actual or real increase of one of the types of leukocytes. The absolute number of any variety of leukocyte in 1 cu. mm. of blood is obtained by multiplying the total leukocyte count by the percentage of the cell types in question.

　**absorption c.,** a small glass chamber with parallel sides, in which absorption spectra of solutions can be obtained.

　**absorptive c.'s of intestine,** c.'s on the surface of villi of the small intestine and the luminal surface of the large intestine which are characterized by having microvilli on their free surface.

　**acid c.,** parietal c.

　**acid′ophil c.,** acidophil; a c. whose cytoplasm or its granules stain with acid dyes.

**ac′inar c.,** acinous c.; any secreting c. lining an acinus, especially applied to the c.'s of the pancreas which furnish pancreatic juice, to distinguish them from the c.'s of the islets of Langerhans.

　**ac′inous c.,** acinar c.

　**acoustic c.,** a hair c. of the organ of Corti.

　**ad′ipose c.,** fat c.

　**adventi′tial c.,** pericyte.

　**air c.'s,** (1) *alveoli* pulmonis; (2) air-containing spaces in the skull.

　**albu′minous c.,** (1) serous c.; (2) zymogen c.

　**algoid c.,** one appearing like c.'s of algae sometimes found in chronic diarrhea.

　**alpha c. of anterior lobe of hypophysis,** acidophil c.

　**alpha c. of pancreas,** a c. of the islets of Langerhans believed to secrete glucagon; also called A c.'s.

　**alveolar c.'s,** (1) thin epithelial c.'s lining alveoli of lung; (2) c.'s lining a secretory alveolus.

　**am′acrine c.,** a nerve c. with short branching dendrites but believed to lack an axon; Cajal described and named such cells in the retina.

　**ame′boid c.,** wandering c.; a c. such as a leukocyte, having ameboid movements, with a power of locomotion; (2) protoplasmic *astrocyte* (1).

　**amniogenic c.'s,** c.'s that give rise to the amnion.

　**anabiotic c.'s,** c.'s that are capable of resuscitation after apparent death; the existence of anabiotic tumor c.'s is postulated to explain the recurrence of a cancer after a very long symptomless period following operation.

　**anaplastic c.,** (1) a c. that has reverted to an embryonal state; (2) an undifferentiated c., characteristic of malignant neoplasms.

　**angioblastic c.'s,** those c.'s that, in the early embryo, give rise to primitive blood c.'s and endothelium.

　**Anitschkow c.,** cardiac *histiocyte*.

　**anterior c.'s,** *cellulae* anteriores.

　**antigen-responsive c.,** antigen-sensitive c.

　**antigen-sensitive c.,** antigen-responsive c.; a small lymphocyte that, although not itself an immunologically activated c., responds to antigenic (immunogenic) stimulus by a process of division and differentiation that results in the production of immunologically activated cells.

　**apo′lar c.,** a neuron without processes.

　**APUD c.'s,** see APUD.

　**argen′taffin c.'s,** enterochromaffin c.'s; Kulchitsky c.'s; pheochrome c.'s; c.'s located in the glands of the gastrointestinal tract; their basally located granules show silver and chromate reactions, fluoresce after formalin fixation, and couple with kiazonium salts. They are believed to contain 5-hydroxytryptamine and to be of endocrine nature.

　**argyrophilic c.'s,** c.'s whose granules react with silver salts after the use of a reducing agent; in the gastric mucosa, especially the pylorus, they are believed to produce gastrin.

　**Askanazy c.,** Hürthle c.

　**astroglia c.,** astrocyte.

　**auditory receptor c.'s,** columnar c.'s in the epithelium of the organ of Corti, having hairs; see Corti's c.'s.

　**autosynthetic c.,** an artificial c., such as one made by mixing together brain lipoids, the protein of any organ, and brain ash (electrolyte) solution (Crile).

　**B c.'s,** (1) beta c.'s of pancreas or hypophysis; (2) B *lymphocyte*.

　**balloon c.,** an unusually large degenerated tissue c. with pale-staining vacuolated or reticulated cytoplasm, as in viral hepatitis or in degenerated epidermal c.'s in herpes zoster.

　**band c.,** band neutrophil; rod nuclear c.; Schilling's band c.; stab c.; staff c.; any c. of the granulocytic (leukocytic) series that has a nucleus which could be described as a curved or coiled band, no matter how marked the indentation, if it does not completely segment the nucleus into lobes connected by a filament.

　**basal c.,** basilar c.; a c. of the deepest layer of an epithelium.

　**basaloid c.,** a c., usually of the epidermis, resembling a basal c.

　**basilar c.,** basal c.

　**basket c.,** (1) a neuron enmeshing the cell body of another neuron with its terminal axon ramifications; (2) smudge c.; (3) myoepithelial c.'s with branching processes which occur basal to the secretory c.'s of certain salivary gland and lacrimal gland alveoli.

**ba'sophil c. of anterior lobe of the hypophysis,** beta c. of anterior lobe of hypophysis.

**beaker c.,** goblet c.

**Beale's c.,** a bipolar ganglion c. of the heart with one spiral and one straight prolongation.

**Berger c.'s,** hilus c.'s.

**beta c. of anterior lobe of hypophysis,** basophil c. of anterior lobe of hypophysis; one that contains basophil granules and is believed to furnish the gonadotrophic hormones.

**beta c.'s of the pancreas,** B c.'s (1); the predominant c.'s of the islets of Langerhans; they furnish insulin.

**Betz c.'s,** Bevan-Lewis c.'s; large pyramidal c.'s in the motor area of the precentral gyrus of the cerebral cortex.

**Bevan-Lewis c.'s,** Betz c.'s.

**bipo'lar c.,** a neuron having two processes, as those of the retina or the spiral and vestibular ganglia of the eighth nerve.

**Bizzozero's red c.'s,** nucleated red blood c.'s in human blood.

**blast c.,** an immature precursor c. (*e.g.*, erythroblast, lymphoblast, neuroblast); see also -blast.

**blood c.,** one of the formed elements of the blood, a leukocyte or erythrocyte. See color plates 14 to 16.

**Boll's c.'s,** basal c.'s in the lacrimal gland.

**bone c.,** osteocyte.

**border c.'s,** c.'s forming the inner boundary of the organ of Corti.

**Böttcher's c.'s,** c.'s of the basilar membrane of the cochlea.

**branchial c.'s,** cartilage c.'s forming the branchial apparatus; possibly derived from the neural crest.

**bristle c.,** hair c. of the internal ear.

**bronchic c.'s,** *alveoli* pulmonis.

**brood c.,** mother c.

**burr c.,** a crenated red blood c.

**C c.,** (1) gamma c.; a c. of the pancreatic islets of the guinea pig; (2) parafollicular c.

**Cajal's c.,** (1) horizontal c. of Cajal; (2) astrocyte.

**calic'iform c.,** goblet c.

**cam'eloid c.,** elliptocyte.

**capsule c.,** amphicyte.

**carrier c.,** phagocyte.

**cartilage c.,** chondrocyte.

**castrate c.'s,** castration c.'s.

**castration c.'s,** castrate c.'s; signet ring c.'s (1); altered basophilic c.'s of the anterior lobe of the pituitary that develop following castration; the body of the c. is occupied by a large vacuole that displaces the nucleus to the periphery, giving the c. a resemblance to a signet ring.

**caterpillar c.,** cardiac *histiocyte*.

**centroac'inar c.,** Langerhans' c. (2); a nonsecretory c. of a pancreatic ductule that occupies the lumen of an acinus.

**chalice c.,** goblet c.

**chief c. of corpus pineale,** pinealocyte.

**chief c. of parathyroid gland,** a dark, water-clear or transitional c.; the clear c. has abundant glycogen, the others a varying content of fine granules.

**chief c. of stomach,** zymogenic c.

**chro'maffin c.,** a c. that stains with chromic salts, in adrenal medulla and paraganglia of sympathetic nervous system.

**chromophobe c.'s of anterior lobe of hypophysis,** c.'s without specific granules, so that the cytoplasm is essentially unstained after the usual histological procedures.

**Claudius' c.'s,** columnar c.'s on the floor of the ductus cochlearis external to the organ of Corti.

**clear c.,** present in the deepest layer of the epidermis or between it and the dermis; thought to be derived from neuroectoderm and to give rise to melanocytes of the skin.

**clear c. of the parathyroid gland,** chief c. of parathyroid gland.

**cleavage c.,** blastomere.

**cochlear hair c.'s,** sensory c.'s in the organ of Corti in synaptic contact with sensory as well as efferent fibers of the cochlear (auditory) nerve; from the apical end of each c. about 100 stereocilia extend from the surface and make contact with the tectorial membrane.

**column c.'s,** neurons in the gray matter of the spinal cord, the axons of which pass into the fasciculi proprii, or ground bundles, of the spinal cord's white matter.

**colum'nar c.,** cylindric c.; a c. taller than it is broad, usually epithelial; it may be tall columnar or low columnar.

**commissural c.,** heteromeric c.; a spinal neuron whose axon passes to the opposite side.

**compound granule c.,** gitter c.; gitterzelle; a microglial c. distended with phagocytosed debris.

**cone c. of retina,** one of the two types of visual receptor c.'s, particularly essential for visual acuity and color vision; the second type is the rod c.

**connective tissue c.,** any of the c.'s of varied form occurring in connective tissue.

**Corti's c.'s,** hair c.'s of the organ of Corti; the receptor c.'s for hearing; the peripheral processes of the cochlear nerve are applied to their base and their short hairs are in contact with the tectorial membrane.

**counting c.,** see under chamber; see also hemocytometer.

**crescent c.,** sickle c.

**cylindric c.,** columnar c.

**cytomegalic c.'s,** large intranuclear and intracytoplasmic c.'s containing cytomegalic inclusion bodies.

**daughter c.,** one of the c.'s resulting from the division of a parent c.

**Davidoff's c.'s,** Paneth's granular c.'s.

**decidual c.,** an enlarged, ovoid connective tissue c. appearing in the endometrium of pregnancy.

**deep c.,** mesangial c.

**Deiters' c.'s,** (1) the outer phalangeal c.'s of the organ of Corti; (2) astrocytes or spider c.'s of the neuroglia.

**delta c. of anterior lobe of hypophysis,** a variety of c. having basophilic granules.

**delta c. of pancreas,** a c. of the islets with fine granules stainable with aniline blue.

**dem'ilune c.'s,** serous c.'s that form a crescent.

**dendritic c.'s,** in embryonic ectoderm, c.'s of neural crest origin with extensive processes; they early develop melanin.

**Dogiel's c.'s,** the different cell types in cerebrospinal ganglia.

**dome c.,** one of the rounded surface c.'s of the epitrichial layer of the fetal epidermis.

**dust c.,** coniophage; an alveolar phagocyte that contains carbon or other foreign particles; these c.'s occur in the lumen or interalveolar septum of pulmonary alveoli.

**effector c.,** see effector.

**egg c.,** the unfertilized ovum.

**enamel c.,** ameloblast.

**endodermal c.'s,** entodermal c.'s.

**endothelial c.,** one of the squamous c.'s forming the lining of blood and lymph vessels and the inner layer of the endocardium.

**en'terochro'maffin c.'s,** argentaffin c.'s.

**en'teroen'docrine c.'s,** c.'s with granules which may be either argentaffinic or argyrophilic; the c.'s, which are scattered in the digestive tract, are of several varieties and are believed to produce such hormones as gastrin, serotonin, glucagon, and perhaps other substances.

**entodermal c.'s,** endodermal c.'s; embryonic c.'s forming the roof of the yolk sac and giving rise to the epithelium of the alimentary tract and the parenchyma of associated glands.

**epen'dymal c.,** a c. lining the central canal of the spinal cord (those of pyramidal shape) or one of the brain ventricles (those of cuboidal shape).

**epidermic c.,** one of the c.'s of the epidermis.

**epithelial c.,** one of the many varieties of c.'s that form epithelium.

**epithe'lioid c.,** large mononuclear histiocytes having certain epithelial characteristics, particularly in tubercles where they are polygonal and have eosinophilic cytoplasm.

**er'ythroid c.,** a c. of the erythrocytic series.

**ethmoidal c.'s,** *cellulae* ethmoidales.

**exudation c.,** exudation *corpuscle*.

**Fañanas c.,** a specialized astrocyte found in the cerebellar cortex.

**fat c.,** adipose c.; a connective tissue c. distended with one or more fat globules, the cytoplasm usually being compressed into a thin envelope, with the nucleus at one point in the periphery.

**floor c.,** an obsolete term for the cell body of pillar c.'s in the floor of the arch of Corti.

**foam c.'s,** c.'s with abundant, pale-staining, finely vacuolated cytoplasm, usually histiocytes which have ingested or accumulated material that dissolves during tissue preparation, especially lipids; see also lipophage.

**follic′ular epithe′lial c.,** a c. lining a follicle such as that of the thyroid gland.

**follicular ovarian c.'s,** c.'s of an ovarian follicle that surround the developing ovum; they form the stratum granulosum ovarii and cumulus oophorus.

**foreign body giant c.,** a multinucleate "cell" or syncytium formed around particulate mater in chronic inflammatory reactions.

**formative c.'s,** inner cell mass c.'s of the blastocyst.

**foveolar c.'s of stomach,** theca c.'s of the foveolae of the stomach.

**fuchsin′ophil c.,** a c. with a special affinity for fuchsin dye.

**fusiform c.'s of cerebral cortex,** spindle-shaped c.'s in the sixth layer of the cortex cerebri.

**gamma c. of pancreas,** C c. (1).

**ganglion c.,** originally, any nerve c. (neuron); in current usage, a neuron the c. body of which is located outside the limits of the brain and spinal cord, hence forms part of the peripheral nervous system. Ganglion c.'s are either (a) the pseudounipolar c.'s or origin of the sensory spinal and cranial nerves (sensory ganglia), or (b) the peripheral multipolar motor neurons innervating the viscera (visceral or autonomic ganglia).

**ganglion c.'s of dorsal spinal root,** pseudounipolar nerve c. bodies in the ganglia of the dorsal spinal nerve roots; the sensory spinal nerves are composed of the peripheral axon branches of these sensory ganglion c.'s, whereas the central axon branch of each such c. enters the spinal cord as a component of the dorsal root.

**ganglion c.'s of retina,** the nerve c.'s of the retina whose central processes (fibers) form the optic nerve. Their peripheral processes connect with the bipolar c.'s and through them with the rod and cone c.'s. These c. bodies are round or flask-shaped and vary considerably in size. See fig. under retina.

**Gaucher c.'s,** large c.'s derived from the reticuloendothelial system, and found especially in the spleen, lymph nodes, liver, and bone marrow of patients with Gaucher's disease, a form of reticuloendotheliosis or lipid histiocytosis; Gaucher c.'s are finely, uniformly vacuolated and contain kerasin (a cerebroside), which accumulates as a result of a genetically determined metabolic abnormality.

**gemästete c.,** protoplasmic *astrocyte* (1).

**gemistocytic c.,** protoplasmic *astrocyte* (1).

**germ c.,** the ovum or spermatozoon.

**germinal c.,** a c. from which other c.'s are proliferated.

**ghost c.,** (1) a dead c. in which the outline remains visible, but without other cytoplasmic structures or stainable nucleus; (2) an erythrocyte after loss of its hemoglobin.

**Giannuzzi's c.'s,** c.'s of serous demilunes.

**giant c.,** a c. of large size, often with many nuclei; see Betz c.

**gitter c.** [ Ger. *gitterzelle,* fr. *gitter,* lattice, wire-net ], compound granule c.

**Gley's c.'s,** interstitial c.'s of the testis.

**glia c.'s,** neuroglia c.'s; see neuroglia.

**globoid c.,** a large c. of mesodermal origin that is found clustered in the intracranial tissues in globoid cell leukodystrophy.

**goblet c.,** beaker c.; caliciform c.; chalice c.; an epithelial c. that has been distended with mucin, and when this is discharged as mucus a crateriform or goblet-shaped shell remains. See fig. under epithelium.

**Golgi's c.'s,** type I: nerve c.'s whose long axons leave the gray matter of which they form part; type II: c.'s with short axons which ramify in the gray matter.

**Goormaghtigh's c.'s,** juxtaglomerular c.'s.

**granule c.'s,** (1) small nerve cell bodies in the external and internal granular layers of the cerebral cortex; (2) nerve cell bodies, of which only the nuclei are usually seen, in the granular layer of the cerebellar cortex.

**granule c. of connective tissue,** mast c.

**granulosa c.,** a c. of the membrana granulosa lining the vesicular ovarian follicle which becomes a luteal c. after ovulation.

**granulosa lutein c.'s,** c.'s derived from the membrana granulosa of a mature ovarian follicle which forms the major component of the corpus luteum.

**Grawitz' slumbering c.'s,** an obsolete eponym referring to c.'s in the body tissue that are normally inconspicuous but which, in certain inflammatory states, suddenly increase in size and become easily visible.

**great alveolar c.'s,** cuboidal c.'s connected with the flattened pulmonary alveolar c.'s and having in their cytoplasm lamellated bodies (cytosomes) which perhaps represent the source of the surfactant that coats the alveoli.

**guan′ine c.,** one whose cytoplasm contains glistening crystals of guanine.

**gustatory c.'s,** taste c.'s.

**gyrochrome c.,** see gyrochrome.

**hair c.'s,** sensory epithelial c.'s present in the organ of Corti, in the maculae and cristae of the membranous labyrinth of the ear, and in taste buds; they are characterized by having long stereocilia or kinocilia (or both) which, with the light microscope, appear as fine hairs. See also vestibular hair c.'s, cochlear hair c.'s, and taste c.'s.

**heart failure c.'s,** large extravasated mononuclear phagocytes containing the granules of hemosiderin found in the sputum or in the lungs of patients with longstanding pulmonary congestion from left-sided heart failure.

**HeLa c.'s,** the first continuously cultured human malignant c.'s, derived from a carcinoma of the cervix; used in the cultivation of viruses.

**HEMPAS c.'s,** (abbreviation for hereditary erythroblastic multinuclearity associated with positive acidified serum); the abnormal erythrocytes of type II congenital dyserythropoietic *anemia, q.v.*

**Hensen's c.,** one of the supporting c.'s in the organ of Corti, immediately to the outer side of the c.'s of Deiters.

**heteromer′ic c.,** commissural c.

**hilus c.'s,** Berger c.'s; c.'s in the hilus of the ovary which produce androgens; they are thought to be the ovarian counterpart of the interstitial c.'s of the testis.

**Hofbauer c.,** a large c. in the connective tissue of the chorionic villi; it appears to be a type of phagocyte.

**horizontal c. of Cajal,** a small fusiform c. found in the superficial layer of the cerebral cortex with its long axis placed horizontally.

**horizontal c.'s of retina,** c.'s in the outer part of the inner nuclear layer of the retina which lie with their axes more or less parallel with the surface. They are thought to connect the rods of one part of the retina with cones of another part.

**Hortega c.'s,** see microglia.

**Hürthle c.,** Askanazy c.; a large, granular eosinophilic c. derived from thyroid follicular epithelium by accumulation of mitochondria, *e.g.,* in Hashimoto's disease.

**I c.,** inclusion c.; a cultured skin fibroblast containing membrane-bound inclusions; see I cell *disease.*

**immunologically activated c.,** an immunocyte that carries out an immune response, in contradistinction to an immunologically competent c.

**immunologically competent c.,** a small lymphocyte that is able to be immunologically activated by exposure to a substance that is antigenic (immunogenic) for the respective c., activation involving either the capacity to produce antibody or the capacity to participate in the delayed type of sensitivity.

**inclusion c.,** I c.

**indifferent c.,** an undifferentiated, nonspecialized c.

**intercapillary c.,** mesangial c.

**interstitial c.'s,** (1) Leydig's c.'s; c.'s between the seminiferous tubules of the testis, believed to furnish the male sex hormone; (2) c.'s derived from the theca interna of atretic follicles of the ovary; they are prominent in animals, but not in man, and are believed to be secretory; (3) pineal c.'s similar to glial c.'s with long processes.

**irritation c.,** Türk's c.

**islet c.,** one of the c.'s of the pancreatic islets.

**juvenile c.,** term used by Schilling to designate young forms of granulocytic leukocytes in which the nucleus (1) is not segmented (*i.e.,* not polymorphonuclear) and (2) contains a nucleolus; see metamyelocyte.

**juxtaglomerular c.'s,** Goormaghtigh's c.'s; polkissen of Zimmermann; specialized myoepithelial c.'s cuffing the afferent arterioles; they produce and release renin.

**karyochrome c.,** see karyochrome.

**Kulchitsky c.'s,** argentaffin c.'s.

**Kupffer c.'s,** stellate c.'s of liver; reticuloendothelial c.'s lining the hepatic sinusoids.

**lacis c.** (lah-see) [ Fr. *lacis,* meshwork ], one of the c.'s of the juxtaglomerular apparatus found at the vascular pole of the renal corpuscle.

**Langerhans' c.'s,** (1) dendritic c.'s in the epidermis and dermis, having a clear cytoplasm with characteristic platelike granules and occasional melanosomes but lacking desmosomes. (2) centroacinar c.'s.

**Langhans' c.'s,** (1) Langhans'-type giant c.'s; multinucleated giant c.'s seen in tuberculosis and other granulomas; the nuclei are arranged in an arciform manner at the periphery of the c.'s; (2) cytotrophoblast c.'s.

**Langhans'-type giant c.'s,** Langhans' c.'s (1).

**L.E. c.,** abbreviation for lupus erythematosus c.; a leukocyte containing an amorphous round body which is a phagocytosed nucleus from another cell and exposed to serum antinuclear globulin. L.E. c.'s are formed *in vitro* in the blood of patients with systemic lupus erythematosus, or by the action of the patient's serum on normal leukocytes.

**Leishman's chrome c.'s,** basophilic granular leukocytes (basophils) observed in the circulating blood of some persons with blackwater fever.

**lepra c.'s,** distinctive, large, mononuclear phagocytes (macrophages) with a foamlike cytoplasm, and also poorly staining saclike structures resulting from degeneration of such c.'s, observed characteristically in leprous inflammatory reactions. In either instance, the indistinct staining results from the fact that the c.'s and saclike structures contain numerous, fairly closely packed leprosy bacilli, which are acid-fast and resistant to staining by ordinary methods; the organisms may be vividly demonstrated by means of acid-fast staining procedures.

**Leydig's c.,** interstitial c. of the testis.

**light c.'s of thyroid,** parafollicular c.'s.

**lining c.,** littoral c.

**Lipschütz c.'s,** centrocytes.

**littoral c.,** [ L. *littoralis,* the seashore ] the reticuloendothelial lining c.'s of lymphatic sinuses of lymph nodes and the blood sinuses of bone marrow.

**Loevit's c.'s,** erythroblasts.

**lupus erythematosus c.,** L.E. c.

**luteal c., lutein c.,** a c. of the corpus luteum of the ovary.

**lymph c.,** lymphocyte.

**lymphoid c.,** lymphocyte.

**macroglia c.,** astrocyte.

**Marchand's wandering c.,** a c. of the reticuloendothelial system; see under system.

**marrow c.,** any c. of bone marrow, especially hemopoietic c.'s. See color plates 14 to 16.

**Martinotti's c.,** a small multipolar nerve c. with short branching dendrites scattered through various layers of the cerebral cortex; its axon extends toward the surface of the cortex.

**mast c.,** labrocyte; granule c. of connective tissue; tissue basophil; a connective tissue c. that contains coarse, basophilic, metachromatic granules; the c. is believed to contain heparin and histamine.

**mastoid c.'s,** *cellulae* mastoideae.

**Mauthner's c.,** a large neuron of the spinal cord with its c. body located in the metencephalon of fish and amphibia.

**Merkel's tactile c.,** *meniscus* tactus.

**mesame'boid c.,** (1) an unattached embryonic c. of mesodermal origin; (2) Minot's term for a primordial wandering hemocytoblast.

**mesangial c.,** deep c.; intercapillary c.; a phagocytic c. in the capillary tuft of the renal glomerulus, interposed between endothelial c.'s and the basement membrane in the central regions of the tuft.

**mesenchymal c.'s,** fusiform or stellate c.'s found between the ectoderm and entoderm of young embryos. The shape of the c.'s in fixed material is indicative of the fact that in life they were on the move from their place of origin to areas where they will become reaggregated and specialized. Most mesenchymal c.'s are derived from already established mesodermal layers, but in the cephalic region they arise also from neural crest or neural tube ectoderm. They are the most strikingly pluripotential c.'s in the embryonic

body, giving rise in different locations to any of the types of connective or supporting tissues, to smooth muscle, or to vascular endothelium, or to blood cells (see mesenchyme).

**mesoglia c.'s,** mesoglia.

**mesothe'lial c.,** one of the flat c.'s of mesothelium lining serous membranes.

**Mexican hat c.,** target c.

**Meynert's c.'s,** solitary pyramidal c.'s found in the cortex in the region of the calcarine fissure.

**microglia c.'s,** see microglia.

**middle c.'s,** *cellulae* mediae.

**midget bipolar c.'s,** bipolar c.'s in the inner nuclear layer of the retina that synapse with individual cone c.'s in the outer plexiform layer. Other larger bipolar c.'s in the inner nuclear layer synapse with both rod and cone c.'s. The axons of both types synapse in the inner plexiform layer with the dendrites of the ganglion c.'s.

**Mikulicz' c.'s,** foamy macrophages containing *Klebsiella rhinoscleromatis;* found in the mucosal nodules in rhinoscleroma.

**mirror-image c.,** (1) a cell whose nuclei have identical features and are placed in the cytoplasm in similar fashion; (2) a binucleate form of Reed-Sternberg c. often found in Hodgkin's disease; the twin nuclei are disposed in relation to an imaginary plane between them like a single nucleus together with its image in a mirror.

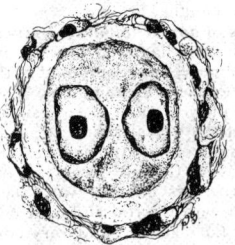

**Mirror-Image Cell**

**mitral c.'s,** large nerve c.'s in the olfactory lobe of the brain whose dendrites synapse (in glomeruli) with axons of the olfactory receptor c.'s of the nasal mucous membrane, and whose axons pass centrally in the olfactory tract to the olfactory cortex.

**monocytoid c.,** one having morphological characteristics of a monocyte but which is nonphagocytic.

**mossy c.,** one of the two types of neuroglia c.'s, consisting of a rather large body with numerous short branching processes.

**mother c.,** metrocyte; a c. which, by division, gives rise to two or more daughter c.'s.

**motor c.,** a neuron whose axon innervates peripheral effector c.'s such as muscle fibers or gland c.'s.

**mucoalbuminous c.'s,** mucoserous c.'s.

**mucoserous c.'s,** mucoalbuminous c.'s; glandular c.'s intermediate in histologic characteristics between serous and mucous c.'s.

**mucous c.,** a c. secreting mucus; goblet c.

**mucous neck c.,** one of the mucin-secreting c.'s in the neck of a gastric gland.

**Müller's radial c.'s,** Müller's *fibers* (2).

**multipolar c.,** a nerve c. with a number of dendrites arising from the c. body.

**mural c.,** a nonendothelial c. enclosed within the basement membrane of retinal capillaries.

**my'eloid c.,** specifically, any young c. that develops into a mature granulocyte, but frequently used as a synonym for marrow c.

**myoepithe'lial c.,** a smooth muscle c. of ectodermal origin, found in a number of organs such as mammary, sweat, and lacrimal glands.

**myoid c.,** one resembling a muscle c.

**Nageotte c.'s,** c.'s found in the cerebrospinal fluid, one or two per cubic millimeter in health, but in greater numbers in various diseases.

**nerve c.,** neuron.

**Neumann's c.'s,** nucleated c.'s in the bone marrow developing into red blood c.'s.

**neurilemma c.'s,** Schwann c.'s.

**neuroendocrine c.'s,** see neuroendocrine.

**neuroepithelial c.'s,** see neuroepithelium.

**neuroglia c.'s,** see neuroglia.

**neurolemma c.'s,** Schwann c.'s.

**neuromuscular c.,** a c. of a lower metazoan organism that is both sensitive and contractile.

**neurosecre'tory c.'s,** nerve c.'s, such as those of the hypothalamus, that elaborate a chemical substance (such as a releasing factor or, more rarely, a true hormone) that influences the activity of another structure (*e.g.*, anterior lobe of the hypophysis). See also neurosecretion.

**Niemann-Pick c.,** Pick c.

**noble c.'s,** the c.'s of the organs, nerves, and muscles; the differentiated c.'s of the body as distinguished from the fixed or connective tissue and wandering c.'s having phagocytic properties. An obsolete usage.

**nurse c.,** Sertoli c.

**oat c.,** a short, bluntly spindle-shaped c. that contains a relatively large, hyperchromatic nucleus, frequently observed in some forms of undifferentiated bronchogenic carcinoma.

**olfactory receptor c.'s,** Schultze's c.'s; very slender nerve c.'s, with large nuclei and surmounted by long, sensitive cilia in the olfactory epithelium at the roof of the nose; they are the receptors for smell.

**oligodendroglia c.'s,** see oligodendroglia.

**Opalski c.,** a characteristically altered glial c. in the basal ganglia and thalamus in hepatolenticular degeneration.

**osseous c.,** osteocyte.

**os'teochondrogen'ic c.,** one of the undifferentiated c.'s in the inner layer of the periosteum of a bone developing endochondrally which is capable of developing into an osteoblast or a chondroblast.

**osteogen'ic c.,** one of the c.'s in the inner layer of the periosteum which forms osseous tissue.

**oxyntic c.,** parietal c.

**oxyphil c.'s,** c.'s of the parathyroid gland which increase in number with age. The cytoplasm contains numerous mitochondria and stains with eosin.

**P c.,** a characteristic specialized c., with probable pacemaker function, found in the S-A node and A-V junction.

**Paget's c.'s,** relatively large, neoplastic epithelial c.'s (carcinoma c.'s) with hyperchromatic nuclei and palely staining cytoplasm; in Paget's disease of the breast, such c.'s occur in neoplastic epithelium in the ducts and in the epidermis of the nipple, areola, and adjacent skin.

**Paneth's granular c.'s,** Davidoff's c.'s; granular c.'s located in the fundus of intestinal glands of the small intestine and appendix.

**parafollicular c.'s,** "C" c.'s (2); light c.'s of thyroid; c.'s present between follicles or interspersed among follicular c.'s; they are rich in mitochondria and are believed to be the source of thyrocalcitonin.

**paraganglionic c.'s,** c.'s of the embryonic sympathetic nervous system that become chromaffin c.'s.

**par'alu'teal c.,** one of the c.'s derived from the theca interna that enter into the formation of the corpus luteum.

**parenchymatous c. of corpus pineale,** pinealocyte.

**parent c.,** mother c.

**pari'etal c.,** oxyntic c.; acid c.; one of the c.'s of the gastric glands; it lies upon the basement membrane covered by the chief c.'s. It secretes hydrochloric acid which reaches the lumen of the gland through fine canals (canaliculi).

**peptic c.,** zymogenic c.

**pericapillary c.,** pericyte.

**perithe'lial c.,** pericyte.

**pes'sary c.,** a red blood c. in which the hemoglobin has disappeared from the center, leaving only the periphery visible.

**phalangeal c.'s,** Deiter's c.'s (1); the supporting c.'s of the organ of Corti, attached to the basement membrane and receiving between their free extremities the hair c.'s. See also phalanx (2).

**pheochrome c.,** see chromaffin c. and argentaffin c.

**physaliphorous c.,** c.'s containing a bubbly or vacuolated cytoplasm, *e.g.*, as characteristically seen in chordoma.

**Pick c.,** Niemann-Pick c.; a relatively large, rounded or polygonal, mononuclear c., with indistinctly or palely staining, foamlike cytoplasm that contains numerous droplets of a phosphatide, sphingomyelin; such c.'s are widely distributed in the spleen and other tissues, especially those rich in reticuloendothelial components, in patients with Niemann-Pick disease.

**pigment c.,** a c. containing pigment granules.

**pigment c.'s of iris,** c.'s of the stromal layer of the iris; in dark eyes (but not in blue) they contain granules of pigment.

**pigment c.'s of retina,** c.'s in the outermost layer of the retina that contain pigment granules.

**pigment c. of skin,** melanocyte.

**pillar c.'s,** pillar c.'s of Corti; Corti's pillars or rods; external and internal pillar c.'s; tunnel c.'s; c.'s forming the center and inner walls of the tunnel in the organ of Corti.

**pin'eal c.,** c.'s of the corpus pineale or epiphysis.

**plasma c.,** plasmocyte; plasmacyte; an ovoid c. with an eccentric nucleus having chromatin arranged like a clock face or spokes of a wheel. The cytoplasm is strongly basophilic because of the abundant ribonucleic acid (RNA) in its cytoplasmic reticulum. Plasma c.'s are active in the formation of antibodies. See color plate 15.

**pluripotent c.'s,** primordial c.'s which may still differentiate into various specialized types of tissue elements, *e.g.*, mesenchymal c.'s.

**polar c.,** polar *body*.

**pol'ychromat'ic c.,** polychromatophil c.; a primitive erythrocyte in bone marrow, with basophilic material as well as hemoglobin (acidophilic) in the cytoplasm.

**polychromatophil c.,** polychromatic c.

**posterior c.'s,** *cellulae* posteriores.

**pregnancy c.'s,** hypophysial chromophobe c.'s that increase in number and accumulate eosinophil granules during pregnancy.

**pregranulosa c.'s,** capsular c.'s surrounding the primordial ova in the embryonic ovary; they are derived from celomic epithelium.

**prickle c.,** spine c.; one of the c.'s of the stratum spinosum of the epidermis; so called because of the intercellular bridges; see fig. under epidermis.

**primary embryonic c.,** in a very young embryo, a c. still capable of differentiating in different directions.

**primitive reticular c.,** a c. with processes making contact with those of other similar c.'s to form a cellular network; along with the network of reticular fibers, the reticular c.'s form the stroma of bone marrow and lymphatic tissues.

**primordial c.,** a c. from a group that constitutes the primordium (anlage) of an organ or part of the embryo.

**primordial germ c.,** gonocyte; the most primitive undifferentiated sex cell, found initially outside the gonad.

**principal c.,** chief c.

**procaryotic c.,** prokaryotic c.; a c. with a procaryotic characteristics; sometimes applied to bacteria and blue-green algae, although neither is, in the strict sense, a c.

**prokaryotic c.,** prokaryotic c.

**pseudounipolar c.** unipolar *neuron*.

**pseu'doxantho'ma c.,** relatively large phagocytic c.'s (macrophages) that contain numerous small lipid vacuoles or hemosiderin (or both), in organizing hemorrhagic or inflammatory lesions.

**pulpal c.,** the specific macrophagic c. of the spleen substance.

**Purkinje's c.'s,** Purkinje's corpuscles; large nerve c.'s of the cerebellar cortex with a piriform cell body and dendrites arranged in a plane transverse to the folium. See fig. under neuron.

**pus c.,** pyocyte; pus corpuscle; a neutrophilic leukocyte.

**pyram'idal c.'s,** neurons of the cerebral cortex which, in sections perpendicular to the cortical surface, exhibit a triangular shape with a long apical dendrite directed toward the surface of the cortex; there are also lateral dendrites, and a basal axon which descends to deeper layers. See fig. 7 under neuron.

**pyrrol c., pyrrhol c.,** (1) a reticuloendothelial element that has a special affinity for pyrrol blue, taking up the dye by a process of ultraphagocytosis; (2) a leukocyte that gives a reaction with *p*-aminobenzaldehyde and hydrochloric acid.

**reactive c.,** protoplasmic *astrocyte* (1).

**red blood c.,** erythrocyte.

**Reed-Sternberg c.'s,** Reed c.'s; Sternberg c.'s; Sternberg-Reed c.'s; large reticulum c.'s generally regarded as pathognomonic of Hodgkin's disease; a typical Reed-Sternberg c. has a pale-staining, acidophilic cytoplasm and one or two large nuclei showing marginal clumping of chromatin and unusually conspicuous, deeply acidophilic nucleoli. Binucleate Reed-Sternberg c.'s frequently show a mirror-image form (see mirror-image c.).

**Renshaw c.'s,** inhibitory interneurons that are innervated by collaterals from motoneurons and in turn form synapses with the same and adjacent motoneurons to exert inhibition.

**resting c.,** a quiescent c.; one not undergoing mitosis.

**resting wandering c.,** a reticuloendothelial c.

**reticular c.,** see primitive reticular c.

**retic'uloendothe'lial c.,** a c. of the reticuloendothelial system; see under system.

**rhag'iocrine c.,** reticuloendothelial c.

**Rieder c.'s,** abnormal myeloblasts (12 to 20 microns in diameter) in which the nucleus may be widely and deeply indented (*i.e.,* suggestive of lobulation), or may actually be a bi- or multi-lobate structure; such c.'s are frequently observed in acute leukemia, and probably represent a more rapid maturation of the nucleus than that of the cytoplasm.

**Rindfleisch's c.'s,** eosinophilic granular leukocytes (eosinophils).

**rod nuclear c.,** band c.

**rod c. of retina,** rod (2); see also retina.

**Rolando's c.'s,** the nerve c.'s in Rolando's gelatinous substance of the spinal cord.

**rosette-forming c.'s,** T-lymphocytes (*q.v.*) with an affinity for sheep erythrocytes and which, when suspended in serum, bind the uncoated, nonsensitized erythrocytes in a rosette formation.

**Rouget c.,** spider c. (2); capillary pericyte; a c. with several slender processes that embraces the capillary wall in amphibia.

**sarcogenic c.,** myoblast.

**satellite c.'s,** c.'s surrounding the c. body of a ganglion c. and continuous with the neurolemma of the processes.

**satellite c.'s of skeletal muscle,** elongated c.'s occupying depressions in the sarcolemma and between it and the endomysium.

**scavenger c.,** phagocyte.

**Schilling's band c.,** band c.

**Schultze's c.'s,** olfactory receptor c.'s.

**Schwann c.'s,** neurolemma c.'s; neurilemma c.'s; c.'s of ectodermal (neural crest) origin that compose a continuous envelope around each nerve fiber of peripheral nerves. Schwann c.'s are comparable to the oligodendroglia c.'s of brain and spinal cord; like the latter, they may form membranous expansions that wind around axons and thus form the axon's myelin sheath.

**segmented c.,** a polymorphonuclear leukocyte matured beyond the band c. so that two or more lobes of the nucleus occur.

**sensitized c.,** (1) a c., or bacterium, that has combined with specific antibody to form a complex capable of reacting with complement components; (2) a small, "committed," c. derived, by division and differentiation, from a transformed lymphocyte (see lymphocyte *transformation*).

**septal c.,** a round pale c. of the lungs in the septa between the pulmonary alveoli.

**seromucous c.'s,** c.'s that are morphologically and histochemically intermediate between serous and mucous c.'s.

**serous c.,** a c. especially of the salivary gland that secretes a watery or thin albuminous fluid, as opposed to a mucous c.

**Sertoli c.'s,** nurse c.'s; elongated c.'s in the seminiferous tubules to which spermatids are attached during spermiogenesis.

**sex c.,** a spermatozoon or an ovum.

**Sézary c.,** an atypical mononuclear c. seen in the peripheral blood in the Sézary syndrome; it has a large, convoluted nucleus and scanty cytoplasm containing PAS (periodic acid-Schiff)-positive vacuoles.

**shadow c.,** smudge c.

**sickle c.,** crescent c.; drepanocyte; meniscocyte; an abnormal, crescentic erythrocyte that is characteristic of sickle c. anemia, resulting from an inherited abnormality of hemoglobin (hemoglobin S) causing decreased solubility at low oxygen tension.

**signet ring c.'s,** (1) castration c.'s; (2) c.'s containing a cytoplasmic droplet of mucus that compresses the nucleus to one side of the c.; found in certain adenocarcinomas.

**silver c.,** one of a number of c.'s seen in plaques of multiple sclerosis, having round or oval nuclei, the body of the c. containing many yellow or light brown particles. The c.'s are characteristic of multiple sclerosis, but are found in other conditions, including syphilis.

**skein c.,** reticulocyte.

**smudge c.'s,** basket c.'s (2); shadow c.'s; Gumprecht's shadows; immature leukocytes of any type that have undergone partial breakdown during preparation of a stained smear or tissue section, because of their greater fragility; smudge c.'s are seen in largest numbers in acute leukemia.

**somatic c.'s,** the c.'s of an organism, other than the germ c.'s.

**sperm c.,** a spermatozoon.

**spider c.,** (1) astrocyte; (2) Rouget c.; (3) a c. in a rhabdomyoma of the heart, with central nucleus and cytoplasmic mass connected to the cell wall by strands of cytoplasm separated by clear, glycogen-filled areas.

**spindle c.,** a fusiform c., such as those in the deeper layers of the cerebral cortex.

**spine c.,** prickle c.

**splenic c.'s,** large round ameboid c.'s (macrophages) in the splenic pulp.

**squamous c.,** a flat scalelike epithelial c.

**stab c.,** band c.

**staff c.,** band c.

**standard c.,** an electrical c. having a definite known voltage.

**stellate c.'s of cerebral cortex,** small star-shaped c.'s in the second and fourth layers of the cortex, and large stellate c.'s in the deeper part of the third layer in the visual cortex. See also Golgi c.'s (type II).

**stellate c.'s of liver,** Kupffer c.'s.

**stem c.,** hemocytoblast.

**Sternberg c.'s,** Reed-Sternberg c.'s.

**stichochrome c.,** see stichochrome.

**strap c.,** an elongated tumor c. of uniform width which may show cross-striations; found in rhabdomyosarcoma.

**summer c.,** a spherical or elliptical c. densely populated with acidophilic granules, seasonally prevalent in amphibian interrenal (adrenocortical) tissue during the spring and summer months.

**supporting c.,** sustentacular c.

**surface c.'s of stomach,** theca c.'s of stomach.

**sustentac'ular c.,** supporting c.; one of the ordinary elongated c.'s resting on the basement membrane, that surround and serve as a support to the shorter specialized c.'s in certain organs, such as the labyrinth of the inner ear or olfactory epithelium.

**sympathetic formative c.,** a neuroblast of the embryonic autonomic nervous system.

**sympathicotropic c.'s,** c.'s in the hilus of the ovary associated with unmyelinated nerve fibers.

**sym'pathochro'maffin c.,** one of the c.'s in the embryo from which both sympathetic ganglion c.'s and chromaffin c.'s are developed.

**syno'vial c.,** a c. in the synovial membrane of joints lying between the collagenous fibers.

**T c.,** T *lymphocyte.*

**tactile c.,** touch c.; one of the epithelioid c.'s of a corpusculum tactus.

**tanned red c.'s,** erythrocytes subjected to mild treatment with tannic acid so that they adsorb onto their surface soluble antigens; used in hemagglutination tests; chemicals other than tannic acid have also been used.

**target c.,** Mexican hat c.; an erythrocyte in target c. anemia with a dark center, surrounding by a light band which again is encircled by a darker ring; it thus resembles a shooting target.

**tart c.,** a monocyte with an engulfed nucleus in which the structure is still well preserved.

**taste c.'s,** gustatory c.'s; darkly staining c.'s in a taste bud (caliculus gustatorius) that appear to have fine hairs extending into the gustatory pore; the hairs are long microvilli containing a number of closely packed microtubules. The taste c.'s stand in synaptic contact with sensory nerve fibers of the facial, glossopharyngeal, or vagus nerves.

**tendon c.'s,** elongated fibroblastic c.'s arranged in rows between the collagenous tendon fibers.

**theca c.'s of stomach,** surface c.'s of stomach; the c.'s lining the surface and foveolae; after mucin is released the apical part of the c. has the appearance of an empty sac or theca.

**theca-lutein c.,** a c. of the corpus luteum that comes from the theca interna of the ovarian follicle after ovulation.

**Tiselius electrophoresis c.,** the special container in a Tiselius apparatus containing the solution to be electrophoretically analyzed.

**totipo'tent c.,** an undifferentiated c. capable of developing into any type of c., *e.g.*, the fertilized ovum.

**touch c.,** tactile c.

**Touton giant c.,** a xanthoma c. in which the multiple nuclei are grouped around a small island of nonfoamy cytoplasm.

**transitional c.,** any c. thought to represent a phase of development from one form to another.

**tubal air c.'s,** *cellulae* pneumaticae tubae auditivae.

**tunnel c.'s,** pillar c.'s.

**Türk's c.,** irritation c.; a relatively large, immature c. with certain morphologic features resembling those of a plasma c., although the nuclear pattern is similar to that of a myeloblast; found in circulating blood only in pathologic conditions.

**tympanic c.'s,** small depressions in the walls of the middle ear.

**Tzank c.'s,** acantholytic c.'s seen in the Tzank *test, q.v.*

**undifferentiated c.,** a primitive c. that has not assumed the morphologic and functional characteristics which it will later acquire.

**unipo'lar c.,** unipolar *neuron.*

**vasoformative c.,** angioblast.

**vestibular hair c.'s,** c.'s in the sensory epithelium of the maculae and cristae of the membranous labyrinth of the inner ear; afferent and efferent nerve fibers of the vestibular nerve end synaptically upon them; from the apical end of each c. a bundle of stereocilia and a kinocilium extend into the membrana statoconiorum of the maculae and the cupula of the cristae.

**Virchow's c.'s,** (1) the lacunae in osseous tissue containing the bone c.'s; also the bone c.'s themselves; (2) corneal *corpuscles.*

**visual receptor c.'s,** the rod and cone c.'s of the retina.

**wandering c.,** ameboid c.

**Warthin-Finkeldey c.'s,** giant c.'s with multiple overlapping nuclei, found in lymphoid tissue in measles, especially during the prodromal stage.

**wasserhelle c.'s,** the water-clear c.'s (chief c.'s) of the parathyroid glands.

**water-clear c. of parathyroid,** a variety of chief c.

**white blood c.,** leukocyte.

**wing c.,** one of the polyhedral c.'s in the corneal epithelium beneath the surface layer.

**yolk c.'s,** primitive embryonic c.'s lying between the entoderm and mesoderm; they probably give rise to the endothelium of vitelline vessels.

**zymogen'ic c.,** a c. that secretes an enzyme; specifically a chief c. of a gastric gland or an acinar c. of the pancreas.

---

**cel'la,** gen. and pl. **cel'lae** (sel'ah) [ L. storeroom, or compartment ]. [ NA ]. A room or cell.

**c. media,** *pars* centralis ventriculi lateralis.

**cellaburate** (sel'ä-bu'rat) (USAN). Cellulose acetate butyrate; a plastic filming agent for pharmaceuticals.

**cellicolous** (sel-lik'o-lus) [ L. *cella*, cells, + *colere*, to abide in ]. Living within cells.

**cellobi'ase.** β-Glucosidase.

**cellobi'ose.** A disaccharide obtained from cellulose; a glucose-β-1,4-glucoside, differing only in the nature of the glycoside bond from maltose, which is a glucose-α-glucoside.

**celloci'din.** Acetylenedicarboxamide.

**cellohex'ose.** Glucose.

**celloi'din.** A solution of pyroxylin in ether and alcohol. Used for embedding histologic specimens.

**cello'na.** A cellulose bandage impregnated with plaster of Paris.

**cel'lose.** Cellobiose.

**cellula,** gen. and pl. **cel'lulae** (sel'u-lah) [ L. a small chamber, dim. of *cella* ]. 1 [ NA ]. In gross anatomy, a cellule; a small but macroscopic compartment. 2. In histology, a cell.

**cellulae anterio'res,** anterior cells; the anterior group of air cells in the ethmoidal labyrinth; each cell communicates with the middle meatus of the nasal cavity.

**c. coli,** haustrum.

**cellulae ethmoida'les** [ NA ], ethmoidal cells; the numerous small air-filled cells in the ethmoidal labyrinth; see also cellulae anteriores, cellulae mediae, and cellulae posteriores.

**cellulae mastoid'eae** [ NA ], mastoid cells; numerous small intercommunicating cavities in the mastoid process of the temporal bone that empty into the mastoid or tympanic antrum.

**cellulae me'diae,** middle cells; the middle group of air cells in the ethmoidal labyrinth; each cell communicates with the middle meatus of the nasal cavity.

**cellulae pneumat'icae tubae auditivae** [ NA ], tubal air cells; occasional small air cells in the inferior wall of the auditory tube, near the tympanic orifice, communicating with the cavity of the tympanum.

**cellulae posterio'res,** posterior cells; the posterior group of air cells in the ethmoidal labyrinth; each cell communicates with the superior meatus of the nasal cavity.

**cellulae tympan'icae** [ NA ], tympanic cells; numerous groovelike depressions in the walls of the tympanic cavity, communicating with the tubal air cells.

**cel'lular** [ L. *cellula*, dim. of *cella*, storeroom ]. 1. Relating to, derived from, or composed of cells. 2. Areolar; having numerous compartments or interstices.

**cellula'rity.** The degree, quality, or condition of cells which are present.

**cel'lulase** (EC 3.2.1.4). An enzyme catalyzing the hydrolysis of cellulose to cellobiose; found in a variety of microorganisms in soil and in the digestive tracts of herbivores.

**cellule** (sel'ul). In gross anatomy, a cellula.

**cel'lulici'dal** [ cellula + L. *caedo*, to kill ]. Destructive to cells.

**cellulif'ugal** [ cellula + L. *fugio*, to flee ]. Moving from, or extending in a direction away from, a cell or cell body; denoting certain cells repelled by other cells, or processes extending from the body of a cell.

**cel'lulin.** Cellulose.

**cellulip'etal** [ cellula + L. *peto*, to seek ]. Moving toward, or extending in a direction toward, a cell or cell body.

**celluli'tis.** Inflammation of cellular or connective tissue.

**acute scalp c.,** nonlocalized inflammation of the scalp without suppuration.

**dissecting c.,** *perifolliculitis* abscedens et suffodiens.

**epizootic c.** equine viral *arteritis.*

**ligneous pelvic c.,** marked chronic, painful induration of pelvic tissues.

**pelvic c.,** parametritis.

**phlegmonous c.,** diffuse *phlegmon.*

**cel'lulosan.** Hemicellulose.

**cel'lulose.** A polysaccharide made up of cellobiose residues, differing in this respect from starch, which is made up of maltose residues. Forms the basis of vegetable fiber (cotton is 90 per cent cellulose). It is the most abundant organic compound in the world.

**c. acetate phthalate** (USP), a reaction product of phthalic anhydride and a partial acetate ester of c.; used as a tablet-coating agent.

**carboxymethyl c.,** CM-cellulose.

**CM-cellulose,** carboxymethyl c.; c. in which some of the OH groups are modified to contain $-CH_2-COOH$ groups; used for column chromatography.

**CM-cellulose sodium,** see sodium carboxymethyl cellulose.

**DEAE-cellulose,** diethylaminoethyl c.; c. to which diethylaminoethyl groups have been attached; used in anion-exchange chromatography.

**ECTEOLA-cellulose,** c. treated with epichlorhydrin and triethanolamine, to add tertiary amine groups to the c. and convert it to an anion-exchange material, for which use it is manufactured and sold.

**microcrystalline c.** (NF), purified, partially depolymerized c., prepared by treating α-cellulose, obtained as a pulp from fibrous plant material, with mineral acids. Used as a tablet diluent.

**oxidized c.,** (1) (USP), OXYCEL; cellulosic acid in the form of gauze; it is absorbable. Used as a hemostatic in operations where ligation is not feasible (capillary or venous bleeding from small vessels). The cellulosic acid has a pronounced affinity for hemoglobin and produces an artificial clot; (2) (BP), a sterile, absorbable substance prepared by the oxidation of cotton; it contains not less than 16 and not more than 22 per cent of carboxyl. See also oxycellulose.

**TEAE-cellulose,** triethylaminoethyl-substituted c.; used in ion-exchange chromatography.

**cellulos'ic acid.** Oxidized *cellulose.*

**celo-.** 1 [ G. *koilōma,* hollow (celom) ]. Combining form relating to the celom. 2 [ G. *kēlē,* hernia ]. Combining form meaning hernia. 3 [ G. *koilia,* belly ]. Combining form relating to abdomen; see also celio-.

**celol'ogy** [ G. *kēlē,* hernia, + *logos,* study ]. The branch of surgery that has to do with hernia.

**ce'lom, celo'ma** (se'lom, se-lo'mah) [ G. *koilōma,* a hollow ]. 1. The cavity between splanchnic and somatic mesoderm. 2. The general body cavity in the adult.

**extraembryonic c.,** that portion of the c. that extends beyond the confines of the embryonic body.

**celom'ic.** Relating to the celom, or body cavity.

**celonychia** (se-lo-nik'ī-ah) [ G. *koilos,* hollowed, + *onyx* (*onych-*), nail ]. Koilonychia.

**celophlebitis** (se-lo-fle-bi'tis) [ G. *koilos,* hollow, + *phlebitis, q.v.* ]. Cavitis; inflammation of a vena cava.

**celoschisis** (se-los'kī-sis) [ G. *koilia,* belly, + *schisis,* a fissure ]. Gastroschisis.

**ce'loscope** [ G. *koilos,* hollow, + *skopeō,* to view ]. A device for examining the interior of a cavity of the body.

**celos'copy.** Examination of any cavity of the body.

**celosomia** (se'lo-so'mī-ah) [ G. *kēlē,* hernia, + *sōma,* body ]. Congenital protrusion of the abdominal or thoracic viscera, usually with defect of the sternum and ribs as well as of the abdominal walls.

**ce'loso'mus.** A malformed individual with celosomia.

**ce'lothe'lium.** Obsolete term for mesothelium.

**celot'omy** [ G. *kēlē,* hernia, + *tomē,* incision ]. Herniotomy.

**celozo'ic** [ G. *koilos,* hollow, + *zoikos,* pertaining to animals. ZO- ]. Inhabiting any of the cavities of the body (therefore extracellular). Applied to certain parasitic protozoa, chiefly gregarines.

**Cel'sius,** Anders, Swedish astronomer, 1701–1744. See C.'s *scale.*

**Cel'sus,** Aulus (Aurelius) Cornelius, Roman physician and medical writer, 1st century. See C.'s *area, chancre, kerion, operation, papules, vitiligo.*

**cement** (se-ment') [ L. *cementum, q.v.* ]. 1. Cementum. 2. In dentistry, any oxyphosphate or other material used in filling a tooth cavity or as an adherent sealer in attaching various dental restorations in or on the tooth. 3. Any ground substance holding together cells or other structures.

**dental c.,** tooth c.

**intercellular c.,** a presumably adhesive substance that occurs between some epithelial cells.

**oxyphosphate of copper c.,** a dental preparation, the combination of a solution of orthophosphoric acid with a c. powder (usually zinc oxide, pretreated) modified with varying proportions of copper oxide.

**oxyphosphate of zinc c.,** see zinc phosphate c.

**polycarboxylate c.,** a powder containing primarily zinc oxide mixed with a liquid containing polyacrylic acid which reacts to form a hard crystalline mass upon standing. When used to lute metal castings to teeth, it has

the potential of bonding to the calcium contained in tooth structure as well as to any base metals contained in the casting.

**silicate c.,** a dental filling material prepared by mixing a modified phosphoric acid solution with a powdered silica alumina fluoride glass. It has about eight times the crushing strength of construction c. It is translucent and resembles porcelain on hardening. Various shades matching tooth opacity are available.

**tooth c.,** (1) cementum; (2) dental c.; a filling material; *e.g.,* zinc c., copper c., silicate c., and zinc oxide-eugenol c.

**zinc-eugenol c.** (USP), 10 parts of the powder are mixed with 1 part of the liquid to a thick paste immediately before use. The powder contains zinc acetate, zinc stearate, zinc oxide, and rosin. The liquid contains eugenol and cottonseed oil. Used as a dental protective.

**zinc phosphate c.,** a powder containing primarily zinc oxide, mixed with a liquid containing orthophosphoric acid; they react to form a hard crystalline mass on standing. Used in dentistry as a luting agent for cast metal restorations and orthodontic bands, and as a temporary restorative material, or as a base under restorations, particularly in deep cavities.

**cementa'tion.** 1. The process of attaching parts by means of a cement. 2. In dentistry, attaching a restoration to natural teeth by means of a cement.

**cemen'ticle.** A calcified spherical body, composed of cementum lying free within the periodontal membrane, attached to the cementum or imbedded within it.

**cemen'tifica'tion.** The metaplastic production of cementum or cementoid within a less differentiated connective tissue, *e.g.,* c. of a fibroma.

**cemen'tite.** Iron carbide; an intermetallic compound which by its hard brittle nature hardens steel.

**cement'oblast** [ L. *cementum,* cement, + G. *blastos,* germ ]. One of the cells concerned with the formation of the layer of cementum on the roots of teeth.

**cement'oblasto'ma.** Cementifying *fibroma.*

**cementoclasia** (se-men'to-kla'zī-ah) [ L. *cementum,* cement, + G. *klasis,* fracture ]. The destruction of cementum by cementoclasts.

**cement'oclast** [ L. *cementum,* cement, + G. *klastos,* broken ]. One of the multinucleated giant cells, identical with osteoclasts, that are associated with the destruction of cementum.

**cement'ocyte** [ L. *cementum,* cement, + G. *kytos,* cell ]. A cell with numerous processes, present in the secondary cementum of the tooth.

**cement'oden'tinal.** Dentinocemental.

**cementoma** (se'men-to'mah) [ L. *cementum,* cement, + G. suffix, -*ōma,* tumor ]. 1. A painless nodular accumulation of cementum attached to the apex of a tooth. 2. Cementifying *fibroma.*

**cementum** (se-men'tum) [ L. *caementum,* rough quarry stone, fr. *caedo,* to cut. CES- ] [ NA ]. Cement; substantia ossea dentis; a layer of modified bone covering the dentin of the root and neck of a tooth.

**primary c.,** noncellular c.

**secondary c.,** c. that forms on the root surface after eruption; it contains cementocytes.

**cenadelphus** (se'nă-del'fus) [ G. *koinos,* common, + *adelphos,* brother ]. Diplopagus.

**cenesthesia** (se'nes-the'zī-ah) [ G. *koinos,* common, + *aisthēsis,* sensation ]. Sixth sense; the general sense of bodily existence; the sensation caused by the functioning of the internal organs.

**cenesthe'sic, cenesthet'ic.** Relating to cenesthesia.

**cenesthopathy** (se-nes-thop'ă-thī) [ G. *koinos,* common, + *aisthēsis,* sensation, + *pathos,* suffering ]. A feeling or sense of general ill-being not related to any particular organ or part of the body.

**ceno-** (se'no-). 1 [ G. *koinos,* common ]. Combining form meaning shared in common. 2 [ G. *kainos,* new ]. Combining form meaning new or fresh. 3 [ G. *kenos,* empty ]. Rarely used combining form denoting emptiness. See also alternative spellings under coeno- and keno-.

**cenocyte** (se'no-sit). Coenocyte.

**cenocytic** (se'no-sit-ik). Coenocytic.

**cenogenesis** (se-no-jen′es-is) [ G. *kainos*, new, + *genesis*, a producing ]. The production in an individual of characters differing from those of its ancestors, as opposed to palingenesis.

**ce′nosite** [ G. *koinos*, common, + *sitos*, food ]. A facultative commensal organism; one that can sustain itself apart from its usual host.

**cenotoxin** (se′no-tok′sin). Kenotoxin.

**cenotrope** (sē′nō-trōp) [ G. *koinos*, common, + *tropē*, a turning ]. The behavior pattern shown by all members of a large group having the same biologic equipment and same experience.

**censor** (sen′sor) [ L. a judge, critic, fr. *censeo*, to value, judge ]. The psychic barrier which, according to psychoanalytic theory, prevents certain unconscious thoughts and wishes from coming to consciousness unless they are so cloaked or disguised as to be unrecognizable.

**cen′talum.** 2-Methyl-1-phenyl-3-butyne-1,2-diol; hypnotic and sedative.

**cen′ter** [ L. *centrum;* G. *kentron*. CENT- ]. 1. The middle point of a body; loosely, the interior of a body. 2. A group of nerve cells governing a specific function. 3. A community-oriented or community-based agency or facility.

**anospinal c.,** the c. in the spinal cord that controls the contraction of the anal sphincter.

**Broca's c.,** Broca's field or area; motor speech c.; a small posterior part of the inferior frontal gyrus of the left hemisphere, corresponding approximately to Brodmann's area 44 (see fig. under *cortex* cerebri); Broca identified this region as an essential component of the motor mechanisms governing articulated speech.

**Budge's c.** ciliospinal c.

**cell c.,** cytocentrum.

**ciliospinal c.,** Budge's c.; the preganglionic motor neurons in the first thoracic segment of the spinal cord which give rise to the sympathetic innervation of the dilator muscle of the eye's pupil.

**community mental health c.,** a psychiatric facility, based in the community, for the prevention and treatment of mental disorder.

**diaphysial c.,** primary c. of ossification in the shaft of a long bone.

**epio′tic c.,** the c. of ossification of the petrous part of the temporal bone that appears posterior to the posterior semicircular canal.

**expiratory c.,** the region of the medulla oblongata that is electrically active during expiration and where electrical stimulation produces sustained expiration.

**feeding c.,** colloquial and somewhat provisional term indicating a region of the lateral zone of the hypothalamus, electrical stimulation of which in the rat elicits uninterrupted eating; destruction of the region causes long-lasting anorexia (aversion to food).

**germinal c. of Flemming,** a secondary nodule of lymphatic tissue in which numerous medium and large lymphocytes are in mitotic division.

**inspiratory c.,** the region of the medulla oblongata that is electrically active during inspiration and where electrical stimulation produces sustained inspiration.

**Kerckring's c.,** Kerckring's ossicle; an occasional independent ossification c. in the occipital bone; it appears in the posterior margin of the foramen magnum at about the 16th week of gestation.

**medullary c.,** *centrum* semiovale.

**motor speech c.,** Broca's c.

**optic c.,** the point in the crystalline lens where the rays cross each other in proceeding from the cornea to the retina.

**ossific c.,** the area of earliest destruction of cartilage prior to onset of ossification.

**ossification c.,** the area in a developing bone where osteogenesis occurs; the primary c. is in the shaft and the secondary in the epiphysis of a long bone.

**reaction c.,** the lightly staining center in a lymphatic nodule in which the predominant cells are macrophages.

**respiratory c.,** the region in the medulla oblongata concerned with integrating afferent information to determine the signals to the respiratory muscles; the inspiratory and expiratory c.'s considered together.

**rotation c.,** a point or line around which all other points in a body move. See axis.

**satiety c.,** colloquial term referring to the region of the ventromedial nucleus in the hypothalamus; destruction of this small region in the rat leads to continuous eating and extreme obesity.

**semioval c.,** *centrum* semiovale.

**sensory speech c.,** Wernicke's c.

**speech c.'s,** areas of the cerebral cortex centrally involved in speech function; one is in the left inferior frontal gyrus, a second one in the supramarginal, angular, and first and second temporal gyri; see also Broca's c. and Wernicke's c.

**sphenotic c.,** one of the paired c.'s of ossification of the sphenoid bone.

**suicide prevention c.,** a mental health facility devoted especially to the prevention of suicide by the treatment of suicidally prone persons and by maintaining a telephone answering service operating 24 hours a day to receive calls from suicidal persons.

**vital c.,** c. essential to life, usually refers to the centers located in the medulla oblongata which are necessary for the maintenance of respiration and circulation.

**Wernicke's c.,** Wernicke's area, field, region, or zone; sensory speech c.; the region of the cerebral cortex thought to be essential for understanding and formulating coherent, propositional speech; it encompasses a large region of the parietal and temporal lobes of the left cerebral hemisphere, corresponding approximately to Brodmann's areas 40, 39, and 22 (see fig. under *cortex* cerebri).

**centesis** (sen-te′sis) [ G. *kentēsis*, puncture, fr. *kenteō*, to prick, pierce. CENT- ]. Puncture; when used as a suffix, usually denotes paracentesis (*q.v.*) of a given organ or site.

**centi-** [ L. *centum*, one hundred ]. A prefix used in the metric system to signify one one-hundredth ($10^{-2}$).

**cen′tibar** A unit of atmospheric pressure, the hundredth part of a bar.

**cen′tigrade** [ L. *centum*, one hundred, + *gradus*, step, degree ]. 1. Consisting of 100 degrees. 2. One hundredth part of a circle, equal to 3.6° of the astronomical circle. 3. See centigrade *scale*.

**cen′tigram.** The hundredth part of a gram; 0.1543 grain.

**centiliter** (sen′ti-le-ter). The hundredth part of a liter; ten milliliters; 162.3 minims.

**cen′timeter.** The hundredth part of a meter; 0.3937 inch.

**centinor′mal.** One hundredth normal (0.01 N); denoting the concentration of a solution.

**centipede** (sen′ti-pēd). A venomous predaceous arthropod of the order Chilopoda, characterized by one pair of legs per leg-bearing segment. The venom is injected through the first pair of leg-like appendages, modified into piercing poison claws. The bites may be painful and locally necrotic, but seldom are dangerous, except to very young children. Genera found in the United States include *Scutigera, Lithobius, Scolopendra,* and *Geophilus,* which see.

**centipoise** (sen′ti-poyz). One one-hundredth of a poise.

**cen′tistoke.** A unit of kinematic viscosity equal to $1/100$ of a stoke.

**centra** (sen′trah). Plural of centrum.

**cen′trad.** 1. Toward the center. 2. A unit of measurement of the refracting strength of a prism; it corresponds to the deviation of a ray of light, the arc of which is $1/100$ of the radius of the circle, or 0.57°; it is expressed by the symbol $\nabla$ .

**centrage** (sen′trāj). The condition in which the center of curvature of all the relecting and refracting surfaces of an optical system are on a single straight line.

**centra′lis** [ L. ] [ NA ]. Central; in the center.

**cen′traphose** [ G. *kentron*, center, + *a-* priv. + *phōs*, light ]. Centrophose.

**centre** [ Fr. ]. Center.

**c. médian of Luys,** *nucleus* centromedianus.

**cen′trencephal′ic.** Relating to the center of the encephalon.

**centric** (sen′trik). Pertaining to a center.

**centriciput** (sen-tris′ĭ-put) [ L. *centrum*, center, + *caput*, head. CAP- ]. The central portion of the upper surface of the skull, between the occiput and the sinciput.

**centrif'ugal** [ L. *centrum*, center, + *fugio*, to flee ]. 1. Efferent. 2. Denoting the direction of the force pulling an object outward (away) from an axis of rotation.

**centrif'ugaliza'tion.** Centrifugation.

**centrif'ugalize.** To submit to rapid rotary action, as in a centrifuge.

**centrifuga'tion.** Subjection to sedimentation, by means of the centrifuge, of solids suspended in a fluid.

**density gradient c.,** ultracentrifugation of substances in concentrated solution of cesium salts; at equilibrium, the medium exhibits a concentration (hence density) gradient increasing in the direction of centrifugal force and the substances of interest collect in layers at the levels of their densities.

**centrifuge** (sen'trĭ-fūj). 1. An apparatus by means of which particles in suspension in a fluid may be separated; this is done by whirling the vessel containing the fluid about in a circle, the centrifugal force throwing the particles to the peripheral part of the rotated vessel. 2. To centrifugalize.

**human c.,** a machine used to expose men or animals to high degrees of centripetal acceleration.

**cent'rilob'ular.** At or near the center of a lobule, *e.g.*, of the liver.

**centriole** (sen'trĭ-ōl) [ G. *kentron*, a point, center ]. Usually paired organelles lying in the cytocentrum; they are tubular structures 150 mμ by 300 to 500 mμ, with a wall having nine triple microtubules. The c.'s may be multiple and numerous in some cells such as the giant cells of bone marrow. See schematic diagram under cell.

**distal c.,** the c., in the developing spermatozoon, that gives rise to the flagellum.

**proximal c.,** the c. that lies next to the head of the developing spermatozoon.

**centrip'etal** [ L. *centrum*, center, + *peto*, to seek ]. 1. Afferent. 2. Denoting the direction of the force pulling an object toward an axis of rotation.

**centro-** [ G. *kentron*, center ]. Combining form relating to a center.

**Centroces'tus** [ G. *kentron*, point, center, + *kestos*, belt, both words fr. *kenteo*, to pierce ]. A genus of extremely small flukes of the family Heterophyidae.

**C. cuspida'tus,** a species reported from man in Formosa, probably identical with *Stamnosoma formosanum.*

**cen'trocyte** [ centro- + G. *kytos*, cell ]. Lipschütz cell; a cell whose protoplasm contains single and double granules of varying size stainable with hematoxylin; seen in lesions of lichen planus.

**centrokinesia** (sen'tro-kin-e'sĭ-ah) [ centro- + G. *kinēsis*, movement ]. Movement excited by a stimulus of central origin.

**centrokinet'ic.** 1. Relating to centrokinesia. 2. Excitomotor.

**centrolecithal** (sen-tro-les'ith-al) [ centro- + G. *lekithos*, yolk ]. Denoting an ovum in which the deutoplasm accumulates centrally.

**centromere** (sen'tro-mēr) [ centro- + G. *meros*, part ]. 1. Kinetochore; the nonstaining primary constriction of a chromosome which is the point of attachment of the

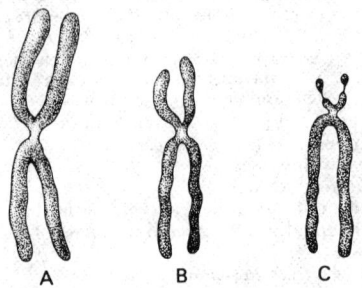

**Normal Positions of the Centromere**
*A*, metacentric; *B*, submetacentric; *C*, acrocentric, with satellites.

spindle fiber and is concerned with chromosome movement during cell division. The c. divides the chromosome into two arms, and its position is constant for a specific chromosome. The position of the c. may be near one end of the chromosome (acrocentric), near the center (metacentric), or between (submetacentric). 2. Obsolete term for the neck of the spermatozoon.

**centrophose** (sen'tro-fōz) [ centro- + G. *phōs*, light ]. Centraphose; a subjective sensation of a dark or light spot originating in the central visual system.

**cen'troplasm** [ centro- + G. *plasma*, thing formed ]. The substance of the cytocentrum.

**centrosclerosis** (sen'tro-skle-ro'sis). Myelofibrosis.

**cen'troscope.** An instrument for producing successive vertical and horizontal afterimages.

**cen'trosome** [ centro- + G. *sōma*, body ]. Cytocentrum.

**centrosphere** (sen'tro-sfēr) [ centro- + G. *sphaira*, a ball, sphere ]. The specialized, often gelated cytoplasm of the cytocentrum from which the astral fibers (microtubules) extend during mitosis.

**centrostal'tic** [ centro- + G. *stallein*, set forth, fetch ]. Relating to the center of motion.

**centrum,** pl. **cen'tra** (sen'trum) [ L. fr. G. *kentron*. CENT- ] [ NA ]. A center of any kind, especially an anatomical center.

**c. media'num,** *nucleus* centromedianus.

**c. medulla're,** c. semiovale.

**c. ova'le,** c. semiovale.

**c. semiova'le,,** semioval center, medullary center; c. medullare; c. ovale; Vicq d'Azyr's c. semiovale; Vieussen's c.; the great mass of white matter composing the interior of the cerebral hemisphere; the name refers to the general shape of this white core in horizontal sections of the hemisphere.

**c. tendin'eum** [ NA ], central tendon; trefoil tendon; a three-lobed fibrous sheet occupying the center of the diaphragm.

**c. tendineum perinei** [ NA ], central tendon of the perineum; perineal body; the fibromuscular mass between the anal canal and the urogenital diaphragm in the median plane.

**c. of a vertebra,** (1) the ossification center of the central mass of the body of a vertebra; (2) the body of a vertebra as distinct from the arches.

**Vicq d'Azyr's c. semiova'le,** c. semiovale.

**Vieussens' c.,** c. semiovale.

**Willis' c. nervo'sum,** *ganglia* celiaca.

**Centruroides** (sen'troo-roy'dēz). A genus of North American scorpions, the commonest of which are *C. gracilis*, the margarite scorpion; *C. vittatus*, the stripe-back scorpion; and *C. sculpturatus*, the deadly sculptured scorpion. See also Scorpionida.

**cephaeline** (sef-a'e-lēn). Desmethylemetine; dihydropsychotrine; $C_{28}H_{38}N_2O_2$; an alkaloid of ipecac; emetic and amebicide.

**Cephaelis** (sef-ah-el'is) [ G. *kephalē*, head, + *eilō*, to roll up, pack close ]. *Uragoga.*

**cephal-.** See cephalo-.

**cephalad** (sef'al-ad). Oral; rostral; situated or oriented toward the head end of an organism.

**cephalalgia** (sef'al-al'jĭ-ah) [ cephal- + G. *algos*, pain ]. Headache.

**histamin'ic c.,** cluster *headache.*

**Horton's c.,** cluster *headache.*

**cephalan'thin.** An amorphous bitter, toxic glucoside from cephalanthus.

**cephalan'thus** [ cephal- + G. *anthos*, flower ]. The bark, especially the bark of the root, of *Cephalanthus occidentalis* (family Rubiaceae), buttonwood, buttonbush, a North American tree; antipyretic and laxative.

**cephalea** (sef-al-e'ah). Headache.

**c. agita'ta, c. atton'ita,** violent headache sometimes occurring in influenza and in the early stages of other infectious diseases.

**cephaledema** (sef'al-ĕ-de'mah). Edema of the head.

**cephale'mia** [ cephal- + G. *haima*, blood ]. Congestion, active or passive, of the brain.

**cephalex'in** (USP). KEFLEX; a broad spectrum antibiotic derived from cephalosporin C; it is rapidly absorbed from the gastrointestinal tract, is minimally bound to serum protein, and appears to be useful for the same infections that respond to cephalothin.

**cephalhematocele** (sef'al-he-mat'o-sēl) [cephal- + G. *haima*, blood, + *kēlē*, tumor]. Cephalohematocele; a cephalhematoma communicating with the cerebral sinuses.

**cephalhematoma** (sef'al-he-mă-to'mah) [cephal- + G. *haima*, blood, + suffix -*ōma*, tumor]. Cephalohematoma; a blood cyst of the scalp in a newborn infant, due to an effusion of blood beneath the pericranium; contrasted with caput succedaneum, in which the effusion overlies the periosteum and consists of serum.

**cephalhydrocele** (sef'al-hi'dro-sēl) [cephal- + G. *hydōr*, water, + *kēlē*, tumor]. An extracranial serous cyst.

**cephal'ic.** Cranial; relating to the head.

**ceph'alin.** Kephalin; a term formerly applied to a group of phosphatidic acids resembling lecithin but containing ethanolamine or serine in the place of choline; these are now known as phosphatidylethanolamine and phosphatidylserine Widely distributed in the body, especially in the brain and spinal cord. Used as a local hemostatic and as a reagent in liver function test.

**cephali'tis.** Encephalitis.

**cephaliza'tion.** 1. The evolutionary tendency for important functions of the nervous system to move forward in the brain. 2. The initiation and concentration of the growth tendency at the anterior end of the embryo.

**ceph'alo-, cephal-** [G. *kephalē*, head]. Combining forms denoting the head.

**cephalocaudal** (sef-al-o-kaw'dal) [cephalo- + L. *cauda*, tail]. Cephalocercal; relating to both head and tail, *i.e.*, to the long axis of the body.

**ceph'alocele.** Encephalocele.

**cephalocentesis** (sef'al-o-sen-te'sis) [cephalo- + G. *kentēsis*, puncture]. Paracentesis capitis; passage of a hollow needle or trocar and cannula into the brain to drain an abscess or the fluid of a hydrocephalus.

**ceph'alocer'cal** [cephalo- + G. *kerkos*, tail]. Cephalocaudal.

**cephalochord** (sef'al-o-kord). The intracranial portion of the notochord in the embryo.

**cephalodidymus** (sef'al-o-did'ĭ-mus) [cephalo- + G. *didymos*, twin]. Conjoined twins fused except in the cephalic region, which has remained paired; a variety of duplicitas anterior

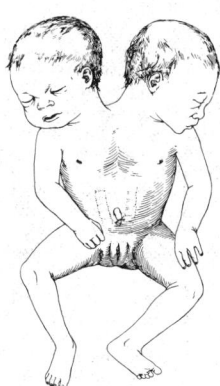

**Cephalodidymus**

**cephalodiprosopus** (sef'al-o-di-pros'o-pus) [cephalo- + G. *di-*, two, + *prosōpon*, face]. Asymmetrical conjoined twins with the head of the autosite carrying a more or less reduced parasitic head; see also *diprosopus* parasiticus.

**cephalodynia** (sef'al-o-din-ĭ-ah) [cephalo- + G. *odynē*, pain]. Cephalalgia; headache; specifically, rheumatism of the fibrous structure of the scalp muscle.

**cephalogenesis** (sef'al-o-jen'e-sis) [cephalo- + G. *genesis*, production]. The formation of the head in the embryonic period.

**cephalogly'cin** (NF). KAFOCIN; a semisynthetic broad spectrum antibiotic produced from cephalosporin C. It appears to be less potent than cephalothin but is well absorbed from the gastrointestinal tract.

**ceph'alogram.** cephalometric *roentgenogram.*

**cephalography** (sef-al-og'ră-fĭ) [cephalo- + G. *graphō*, to write]. Cephalology; description of or treatise on the head.

**cephalogyric** (sef-ă-lo-ji'rik) [cephalo- + G. *gyros*, a circle]. Relating to circular movements of the head.

**cephalohemat'ocele,** Cephalhematocele.

**cephalohemato'ma.** Cephalhematoma.

**ceph'alohemom'eter** [cephalo- + G. *haima*, blood, + *metron*, measure]. An instrument showing the degree of intracranial blood pressure.

**cephalol'ogy.** Cephalography.

**cephalomeg'aly** [cephalo- + G. *megas*, great]. Enlargement of the head.

**cephalomelus** (sef'ă-lom'e-lus) [cephalo- + G. *melos*, a limb]. A malformed individual with an excrescence resembling a leg or arm, growing from the head.

**cephalome'nia** [cephalo- + G. *mēn*, month]. Vicarious menstruation from the nose or other part of the head.

**ceph'alomeningi'tis** [cephalo- + G. *mēninx* [*mening-*], membrane]. Inflammation of the membranes of the brain.

**cephalom'eter.** Craniometer.

**cephalomet'rics** [cephalo- + G. *metron*, measure]. In oral surgery: 1. The scientific measurement of the bones of the cranium by utilizing a fixed, reproducible position for the exposure of lateral skull measurements. 2. A scientific study of the measurements of the head with relation to specific reference points.

**cephalom'etry.** Measurements on the living head, or head without removal of the soft parts. See also cephalometrics.
  **ultrasonic c.,** mensuration of the fetal head by ultrasound waves.

**cephalomo'tor.** Relating to movements of the head.

**Cephalomyia** (sef'ă-lo-mi'yah). Former name for *Oestrus*, a genus of sheep botflies.

**ceph'alont** [cephalo- + G. *ōn* (*ont-*), being]. Adult stage of a cephaline gregarine, a sporozoan parasite commonly found in arthropods and other invertebrate hosts. The body is usually divided by a septum into an anterior epimerite and protomerite and a posterior deutomerite. (The acephaline gregarines lack a dividing septum.)

**cephalopagus** (sef-ă-lop'ă-gus) [cephalo- + G. *pagos*, something fixed]. Conjoined twins with heads fused but the remainder of the bodies separate; see also craniopagus; *duplicitas* posterior.

**cephalop'athy** [cephalo- + G. *pathos*, suffering]. Any disease affecting the head or brain.

**ceph'alopel'vic.** Pertaining to the size of the fetal head in relation to the maternal pelvis.

**ceph'alopelvim'etry.** Roentgenographic measurement of the dimensions of the pelvis and the fetal head.

**cephalopharyngeus** (sef'al-o-fă-rin'je-us). See *musculus* constrictor pharyngis superior.

**cephaloridine** (sef'ă-lor'ĭ-dēn) (NF). LORIDINE; a chemically modified cephalosporin C.; a broad spectrum antimicrobial for persons allergic to penicillin; it is poorly absorbed from the gastrointestinal tract.

**cephalorrhachidian** (sef'al-o-ra-kid'ĭ-an) [cephalo- + G. *rhachis*, spine. RHACH- ]. Relating to the head and the spine.

**cephalospor'in.** One of several antibiotic substances obtained from *Cephalosporium acremonium, C. salmosynnematum,* and other fungi.
  **c. C,** its antibiotic activity is due to the 7-aminocephalosporinic acid portion of the molecule; it is effective against Gram-positive and Gram-negative bacteria, but is less potent than c. N. Addition of side chains produced semisynthetic broad spectrum antibiotics with greater antibacterial activity than that of c. C. They are stable in dilute acid and resistant to penicillinase. The antibiotic activity is due to interference with bacterial cell-wall synthesis.

**c. N,** synnematin B; penicillin N; D-4-amino-4-carboxy-butyl penicillinic acid; an antibiotic substance active against Gram-positive and Gram-negative bacteria; it is inactivated by penicillinase; on hydrolysis it yields penicillamine.

**c. P,** a steroid antibiotic produced by *Cephalosporium;* it is chemically related to fusidic and helvolic acids; active only against Gram-positive bacteria.

**ceph'alosporin'ic acid.** The basic structure of cephaloridine, cephalosporin C, cephalothin.

Cephalosporinic acid

**Ceph'alospo'rium.** A genus of spore-bearing fungi.

**C. granulo'matis,** causes granulomatous lesions; the form has been isolated from mycetoma.

**ceph'alothin.** KEFLIN; 7-(thiophene-2-acetamido)cephalosporanic acid; chemically modified cephalosporin C; a broad spectrum antibiotic substance effective against penicillin-resistant staphylococci, and recommended for treating respiratory, urinary and gastrointestinal infections; side effects are few and mild. *Pseudomonas* is resistant to this antibiotic. C. is poorly absorbed from the gastrointestinal tract. Cephalothin sodium is official in the USP and BP.

**cephalothoracic** (sef'al-o-tho-ras'ik). Relating to the head and the chest.

**cephalothoracoiliopagus** (sef'ă-lo-tho-ră-ko-il-ĭ-op'ă-gus). Synadelphus.

**cephalothoracopagus** (sef'al-o-tho-ră-kop'ă-gus) [ cephalo- + G. *thorax,* chest, + *pagos,* something fixed ]. Conjoined twins with the bodies fused in the cephalic and thoracic regions.

**c. asym'metros,** c. monosymmetros.

**c. disym'metros,** a form of c. with the fused head showing equally developed faces directed laterally.

**c. monosym'metros,** c. asymmetros; a form of c. in which only one of the faces is well developed.

**ceph'alotome** [ cephalo- + G. *tomē,* a cutting ]. An instrument for cutting into the fetal head to permit its compression in cases of dystocia.

**cephalot'omy.** The operation of cutting into the head of the fetus.

**cephalotoxin** (sef'ă-lo-tok'sin). A poison, believed to be a protein, found in the salivary glands of cephalopods (octopus); see also eledoisin.

**cephalotribe** (sef'al-o-trib) [ G. *tribō,* to rub, bruise ]. A forceps-like instrument, with strong blades and a screw handle, by means of which the fetal head can be crushed.

**ceph'alotrip'sy** [ cephalo- + G. *tripsis,* a bruising ]. Crushing of the fetal head in cases of dystocia.

**ceptor** (sep'tor) [ L. *capio,* to take ]. 1. In Ehrlich's theory of immunity, a receptor which has been thrown off as a result of overproduction; intermediary body; immune body; haptin; it may be an amboceptor (cytolysin or bacteriolysin) or a uniceptor (the antitoxin molecule). 2. A nervous mechanism adapted to the appreciation and transmission of stimuli from the periphery to nerve centers.

**chemical c.,** c. that initiates chemical reactions in response to the appropriate stimuli.

**contact c.,** a nerve c. in the surface layer of skin or mucous membrane by means of which impulses contributed by direct physical impact are received.

**distance c.,** a nerve mechanism of one of the organs of special sense whereby the being is brought into relation with his distant environment.

**nerve c.,** ceptor (2).

**cera** (se'rah) [ L. ]. Wax.

**ceraceous** (se-ra'shus) [ L. *cera,* wax ]. Waxen.

**cer'amide.** Generic term for a class of sphingolipid, N-acyl (fatty acid) derivatives of a long chain base (*e.g.,* sphinga-

nine or sphingosine) of the general formula $CH_3$-$(CH_2)_{12}CH=CH—CHOH—CH(CH_2OH) NH—CO—R$, where R is the fatty acid residue, attached in this case to 4-sphingenine (sphingosine) in amide linkage. Formerly termed N-acylsphingol.

**c. dihexoside,** the accumulated glycolipid noted in glycolipid lipidosis.

**c. saccharide,** glycosphingolipid.

**cer'asin.** Kerasin.

**cer'asinose.** A carbohydrate in the gummy exudation from the bark of the cherry tree (cerasin from gum).

**cer'asus** [ L. ]. Cherry.

**cerat-.** For words beginning thus, and not given here, see kerat-.

**cerate** (se'rāt) [ L. *cera,* wax ]. An unctuous solid preparation, harder than an ointment, containing sufficient wax to prevent it from melting when applied to the skin. Use has practically ceased.

**cer'atin.** Keratin.

**ceratocricoid** (sĕr'a-to-kri'koyd). Keratocricoid; relating to the inferior cornua of the thyroid cartilage and to the cricoid cartilage, or the cricothyroid articulation.

**cer'atoglos'sus** [ L. ]. *Musculus* chondroglossus.

**ceratohyal** (sĕr'a-to-hi'al). Keratohyal; relating to one of the cornua of the hyoid bone.

**Ceratophyllus** (sĕr'a-tof'ĭ-lus). The rat flea of temperate climates which transmits plague bacillus.

**cer'beroside.** Thevetin B.

**cercaria,** pl. **cerca'riae** (ser-ka'rĭ-ah) [ G. *kerkos,* tail ]. The free-swimming trematode larva that emerges from its host snail. It may penetrate the skin of a final host (as in *Schistosoma* of man), encyst on vegetation (as in *Fasciola*) or on fish (as in *Clonorchis*), or penetrate and encyst in various arthropod hosts. Body and tail are greatly varied in form, and specialized function is adapted to the particular life cycle demands of each species. See also sporocyst (1).

**cerci** (ser'se). Plural of cercus.

**cerclage** (sair-klazh') [ Fr. an encircling, hooping, banding ]. 1. Binding together the ends of an obliquely fractured bone or the fragments of a broken patella, brought into close apposition, by an encircling wire loop or bandage, tightly drawn, or a ring. 2. Operation for retinal detachment in which the choroid is brought in contact with the detached retina by a taut encircling silicone band around the sclera. 3. The placing of a nonabsorbable suture around an incompetent cervical os.

**cercocystis** (ser-ko-sis'tis) [ G. *kerkos,* tail, + *kystis,* bladder ]. A specialized form of the tapeworm cysticercoid larva that develops within the vertebrate host villus rather than in an invertebrate host; *e.g.,* the c. of *Hymenolepis nana* in its direct or egg-borne cycle in man.

**cercomer** (ser'ko-mer) [ G. *kerkos,* tail ]. The caudal appendage of a larval cestode, the procercoid stage of pseudophyllid cestodes; it may also be found on the cysticercoid larvae of taenioid cestodes, as well as in many of the hymenolepidids (*e.g., Hymenolepis nana*). This appendage frequently bears the hooks originally used by the hexacanth in clawing its way into the intermediate host in which the procercoid or other larval stage develops.

**cercomo'nad.** A general name for members of the genus *Cercomonas.*

**Cercomo'nas** [ G. *kerkos,* tail + *monas* (*monad*-), unit, monad ]. A genus of freshwater and coprophilic protozoan flagellates in which members have one anterior and one posterior flagellum. Species have been described from the intestine or feces of man and several types of domestic livestock, but have usually proved to be other genera such as *Trichomonas* or *Chilomastix.*

**C. longicau'da,** a fecal protozoan flagellate.

**Cercopithecoidea** (ser'ko-pith-e-koy'dĭ-ah) [ G. *kerkos,* tail, + *pithēkos,* monkey ]. One of the three superfamilies of the suborder Anthropoidea; includes apes, old world monkeys, and man.

**Cercopithe'cus.** A genus of the family Cercopithecidae, represented by guenons and common African monkeys.

**cercus,** gen. and pl. **cer'ci** (ser'kus) [ Mod. L. fr. G. *kerkos,* tail ]. A stiff hairlike structure.

**ce'rea flexibil'itas** [ L. ]. "Waxy flexibility," in which the limb remains where placed; often seen in catatonic schizophrenia.

**cereal** (se're'al) [ L. *Cerealis*, pertaining to *Ceres*, the goddess of agriculture ]. Relating to any edible grain or the plant producing it.

**cerebellar** (sĕr'e-bel'ar). Relating to the cerebellum.

**cerebelli'tis.** Inflammation of the cerebellum.

**cerebello-** (sĕr-e-bel'o-) [ L. *cerebellum, q.v.* ]. Combining form relating to the cerebellum.

**cerebel'lolen'tal.** Relating to the cerebellum and the lens of the eye.

**cerebel'lomed'ullary.** Relating to the cerebellum and the medulla oblongata.

**cerebel'lo-ol'ivary.** Relating to the connection of the cerebellum with the inferior olive.

**cerebel'lopon'tine.** Relating to the cerebellum and the pons; denoting especially the c. recess or angle between these two structures.

**cerebel'loru'bral** [ cerebello- + L. *ruber*, red ]. Relating to the connection of the cerebellum with the red nucleus.

**cerebellum,** pl. **cerebel'la** (sĕr'e-bel'um) [ L. dim. of *cerebrum*, brain ] [ NA ]. The large posterior brain mass lying above the pons and medulla and beneath the posterior portion of the cerebrum; it consists of two lateral hemispheres united by a narrow middle portion, the vermis.

**cerebr-.** See cerebro-.

**cerebral** (sĕr'ē-bral, sĕ-re'bral). Relating to the cerebrum.

**cer'ebral'gia** [ cerebrum + G. *algos*, pain ]. Cephalalgia; headache.

**cer'ebrasthe'nia.** Psychasthenia.

**cerebration** (sĕr-e-bra' shun). Activity of the mental processes, conscious or unconscious.

**cer'ebrin.** 1. A nondescript derivative of phrenosin, probably sphingosine. 2. Phrenosin.

**cerebritis** (sĕr'e-bri'tis). Nonlocalized inflammation of the brain without suppuration.

   **suppurative c.,** nonlocalized inflammation (phlegmon) of the brain with suppuration.

**cerebro-, cerebr-, cerebri-** (sĕr'e-bro-, sĕ-re'bro-) [ L. *cerebrum*, brain ]. Combining form relating to the cerebrum.

**cerebrocuprein** (sĕr'e-bro-ku'pre-in). A copper-containing protein isolated from brain.

**cer'ebrogalac'tose.** D-Galactose.

**cer'ebrogalac'toside.** Cerebroside.

**cer'ebro'ma.** Encephaloma.

**cer'ebromala'cia.** Encephalomalacia.

**cerebromeningitis** (sĕr'e-bro-men-in-ji'tis). Meningoencephalitis.

**cer'ebron.** Phrenosin.

   **c. sulfuric acid,** a glycolipid sulfate isolated from brain.

**cerebron'ic acid.** Phrenosinic acid; 2-hydroxylignoceric acid, $CH_3$—$(CH_2)_{21}$—CHOH—COOH. A constituent of phrenosin (cerebron).

**cer'ebropath'ia.** Encephalopathy.

   **c. psychica toxemica,** Korsakoff's *syndrome.*

**cerebropathy** (sĕr'e-brop'ă-thī). Encephalopathy.

**cer'ebrophysiol'ogy.** The physiology of the cerebrum.

**cerebropsychosis** (sĕr'e-bro-si-ko'sis) Organic mental illness; a mental disorder asso·iated with or dependent upon a lesion of the cerebrum.

**cerebrosclerosis** (sĕr'e-bro-skle-ro'sis) [ cerebro- + G. *sklērōsis*, hardening ]. Encephalosclerosis, specifically of the cerebral hemispheres.

**cerebroscope** (sĕ-re'bro-skōp). 1. Encephaloscope. 2. The ophthalmoscope applied to diagnosis of brain disease.

**cerebroscopy** (sĕr'e-bros'ko-pī). Encephaloscopy.

**cer'ebrose.** D-Galactose.

**cer'ebroside.** Galactolipid; a class of glycosphingolipid; specifically a monoglycosylceramide (ceramide monosaccharide). C.'s are found in the myelin sheath of nerve tissue. Examples are kerasin, phrenosin, nervon, oxynervon, these names also being used for the fatty acid involved. C. is sometimes prefixed by gluco-, galacto-, etc., in place of the

correct glucosylceramide, etc. The sulfate esters of c.'s are known as sulfatides.

   **c. sulfatase,** c. sulfatidase; an enzyme (EC 3.1.6.8.) that cleaves sulfate from a cerebroside 3-sulfate; it is deficient in metachromatic leukodystrophy.

   **c. sulfatidase,** c. sulfatase.

**cer'ebrosido'sis.** Gaucher's *disease.*

**cer'ebro'sis.** Encephalosis.

**cerebrospinal** (sĕr'e-bro-spi-nal, sĕ-re'bro-). Encephalorrhachidian; encephalospinal; relating to the brain and the spinal cord.

**cer'ebrospi'nant.** 1. Acting upon the cerebral nervous system, the brain and spinal cord. 2. An agent affecting the cerebrospinal system.

**cerebrosterol.** 24β-Hydroxycholesterol; a hydroxylated cholesterol found in brain and spinal cord.

**cer'ebrosu'ria** [ cerebrose + G. *ouron*, urine ]. The excretion of cerebrose in the urine.

**cer'ebrot'omy** [ cerebro- + G. *tomē*, incision ]. The incision of the brain substance to evacuate an abscess.

**cer'ebroto'nia** [ cerebro- + G. *tonos*, tone ]. A personality pattern associated with ectomorphic bodily type and with predominance of intellective processes; characterized by traits of inhibition, restraint, and concealment.

**cer'ebrovas'cular.** Relating to the blood supply to the brain, particularly with reference to pathologic changes.

**cerebrum,** pl. **cerebrums, cerebra** (sĕr'e-brum, sĕ-re'-brum) [ L. *brain* ] [ NA ]. Originally referred to the largest portion of the brain, including practically all parts within the skull except the medulla, pons, and cerebellum; it now usually refers only to the parts derived from the telencephalon and includes mainly the cerebral hemispheres (cerebral cortex and basal ganglia).

   **c. abdomina'le,** *plexus* celiacus.

   **c. exsicca'tum** [ L. dried brain ], cerebrinin; the brain of the calf, dried and pulverized.

**cerecloth** (sĕr'kloth) [ L. *cera*, wax ]. Gauze or cheese cloth impregnated with wax containing an antiseptic, used in surgical dressings.

**Cerenkov radiation.** See under radiation.

**cer'esin.** Purified ozokerite; cerin; earth wax; mineral wax; a mixture of hydrocarbons of high molecular weight; a substitute for beeswax, and used in dentistry for impressions.

**Ce'reus** [ L. *cereus*, of wax, as noun, a wax taper ]. A genus of cacti.

**cerin** (se'rin). Ceresin.

**cerium** (se'rī-um) [ named after the planetoid *Ceres* ]. A metallic element, symbol Ce, atomic no. 58, atomic weight 140.13.

   **c. oxalate,** cerous oxalate; a mixture of the oxalates of c., neodymium, praseodymium, lanthanum, and other earths; has been used in the treatment of vomiting.

**cero-** (se'ro-, sĕr-o-) [ L. *cera*, wax ]. Combining form relating to wax.

**ceroid** (se'royd). A waxlike, golden or yellow-brown pigment first found in fibrotic livers of choline-deficient rats, and also known to be present in some of the cirrhotic livers (and certain other tissues) of human beings. C. is acid-fast, insoluble in fat solvents, and probably a type of lipofuscin.

**ceroplasty** (se'ro-plas-tī) [ G. *kēros*, wax, + *plassō*, to mold ]. The manufacture of wax models of anatomical and pathologic specimens or of skin lesions.

**certifi'able.** 1. That which can or must be certified; said of infectious, industrial, and other diseases that are required by law to be reported to health authorities. 2. Denoting a person showing psychotic behavior of sufficient gravity to justify involuntary mental hospitalization.

**certifica'tion.** 1. The reporting to health authorities of notifiable disease. 2. The attainment of board certification in a specialty. 3. The court procedure by which a patient is committed to a mental institution. 4. Involuntary mental hospitalization.

**cer'tify** [ L. *certus*, certain, + *facio*, to make ]. 1. To give information regarding; to notify; specifically, to report to the health authorities the occurrence of a contagious or other reportable disease. 2. To commit a patient to a mental hospital in accordance with the laws of the state.

**ceru'lean** [ L. *caeruleus*, blue, fr. *caelum*, sky ]. Blue.

**ceru'leus** [ L. ] [ NA ]. Cerulean.

**ceruloplasmin** (sĕ-roo'lo-plaz'min) [ L. *caeruleus*, dark blue ]. A blue, copper-containing α-globulin of blood plasma, with a molecular weight of 150,000 and 8 atoms of copper per molecule; believed to play a part in erythropoiesis; it is reduced in amount in hepatolenticular degeneration.

**cerumen** (sĕ-roo'men) [ L. *cera*, wax ]. Earwax; the soft, brownish yellow, waxy secretion (a modified sebum) of the ceruminous glands of the external auditory meatus.

**c. inspissa'tum**, inspissated c.; dried earwax plugging the external auditory canal.

**ceru'minal.** Relating to cerumen.

**ceruminolytic** (sĕ-roo'mĭ-no-lit'ik) [ cerumen, *q.v.*, + G. *lysis*, a loosening ]. One of several substances instilled into the external auditory canal to soften wax.

**ceruminoma** (sĕ-roo-mĭ-no'mah). Tumor of ceruminous glands of the external auditory canal; usually benign.

**ceru'mino'sis.** Excessive formation of cerumen.

**ceru'minous.** Relating to cerumen.

**ce'ruse** [ L. *cerussa* ]. 1. Basic lead carbonate. 2. Native lead carbonate.

**cerveau isolé** (ser-vo' ē-so-la') [ Fr. detached brain ]. A cat with its brain transected at the level of the mesencephalon.

**cervical** (ser'vĭ-kal) [ L. *cervix* (*cervic*-), neck ]. Relating to a neck, or cervix, in any sense.

**cervica'lis.** Cervical.

**c. ascen'dens**, (1) *musculus* iliocostalis cervicis; (2) *arteria* cervicalis ascendens.

**cervicectomy** (ser-vĭ-sek'to-mĭ) [ cervix + G. *ektomē*, excision ]. Trachelectomy; excision of the cervix uteri.

**cervices** (ser'vĭ-sēz). Plural of cervix.

**cervicitis** (ser-vĭ-si'tis). Trachelitis; inflammation of the mucous membrane, frequently involving also the deeper structures, of the cervix uteri.

**cervico-** (ser'vĭ-ko-) [ L. *cervix*, neck ]. Combining form relating to a cervix, or neck, in any sense.

**cervicobrachial** (ser-vĭ-ko-bra'kĭ-al). Relating to the neck and the arm.

**cervicobuccal** (ser'vĭ-ko-buk'al). Relating to the buccal region of the neck of a premolar or molar tooth.

**cervicodyn'ia** [ cervico- + G. *odynē*, pain ]. Trachelodynia; neck pain.

**cer'vicofa'cial.** Relating to the neck and the face.

**cer'vicola'bial.** Relating to the labial region of the neck of an incisor or canine tooth.

**cervicolingual** (ser'vĭ-ko-ling'gwal). Relating to the lingual region of the cervix of a tooth.

**cervicolinguoaxial** (ser'vĭ-ko-ling'gwo-ak'sĭ-al). Refers to the point (trihedral) angle formed by the junction of the cervical (gingival), lingual, and axial walls of a cavity; see axiolinguocervical; see point *angle*.

**cervico-occipital** (ser'vĭ-ko-ok-sip'ĭ-tal). Relating to the neck and the occiput.

**cer'vicoplasty.** Plastic surgery on the cervix uteri or on the neck.

**cervicothoracic** (ser'vĭ-ko-tho-ras'ik). Relating (1) to the neck and thorax, (2) to their transition, (3) to the disk between the 7th cervical vertebra and 1st thoracic vertebra, and (4) to the fusion of these vertebrae.

**cervicotomy** (ser'vĭ-kot'o-mĭ) [ cervico- + G. *tomē*, incision ]. Trachelotomy; incision into the cervix uteri.

**cer'vicoves'ical.** Relating to the cervix of the uterus and the bladder.

**cervix**, gen. **cervi'cis**, pl. **cervi'ces** (ser'viks) [ L. neck ]. 1 [ NA ]. Collum. 2 [ NA ]. Any necklike structure.

**c. of the axon**, the constricted portion of the axon just before the myelin sheath begins.

**c. colum'nae posterio'ris**, a slight constriction of the posterior gray column of the spinal cord, seen on cross-section a little behind the gray commissure.

**c. dentis**, *collum* dentis.

**c. uteri** [ NA ], neck of the uterus; the lower part of the uterus extending from the isthmus of the uterus into the vagina. It is divided into supravaginal and vaginal parts by its passage through the vaginal wall.

**c. vesicae urina'riae** [ NA ], neck of the urinary bladder; the lowest part of the bladder formed by the junction of the fundus and the inferolateral surfaces.

**ce'ryl.** 1-Hexacosanol; the hydrocarbon radical, $C_{26}H_{53}$—, of ceryl alcohol.

**Cesalpino** (se-sal-pe'no), Andrea, Italian physician and anatomist, 1519–1603. In his *Peripatetic Questions* he foreshadowed the discovery of the circulation of the blood and on this account some would give him priority over Harvey. But he offered very little experimental evidence, his views were obscured by a disputatious exposition, and he left little impression upon his contemporaries.

**cesarean section** and **hysterectomy.** See the nouns.

**cesium** (se'zĭ-um) [ L. *caesius*, bluish gray ]. Caesium, a metallic element, symbol Cs, atomic no. 55, atomic weight 132.91. A member of the alkali metal group.

**Cestan**, Raymond, French neurologist, 1872–1934. See C.-Chenais *syndrome*.

**Cestoda** (ses-to'dah). Eucestoda; a subclass of tapeworms of the class Cestoidea, containing the typical members of this group, including the tapeworms that parasitize man and domestic animals.

**ces'tode, ces'toid.** Common name for tapeworm of the class Cestoidea (*q.v.*) or its subclass, Cestoda (or Eucestoda).

**cestodiasis** (ses'to-di'ă-sis). Disease caused by infection with a cestode.

**Cestoidea** (ses-toy'de-ah) [ G. *kestos*, girdle, + *eidos*, form ]. The tapeworms; a class of platyhelminth flatworms characterized by lack of an alimentary canal and, in typical forms, by a strobilate or segmented body with a scolex or holdfast organ at one end. Adult worms are vertebrate parasites, usually found in the small intestine.

**cetaceum** (sĕ-ta'she-um) [ G. *kētos*, a whale ]. Spermaceti.

**cetalkonium chloride** (set'al-ko'nĭ-um) (USAN). BANICOL; benzylhexadecyldimethylammonium chloride; antibacterial agent.

**cethox'ium bromide.** BIOCIDAN; hexadecyl(2-hydroxycyclohexyl)-dimethylammonium bromide; antiseptic.

**cetiprin.** Ethyldimethyl(1-methyl-3,3-diphenylpropyl)ammonium bromide; intestinal antispasmodic agent.

**ce'tophen'icol** (USAN). D-*threo*-N-[ *p*-Acetyl-β-hydroxy-α-(hydroxymethyl)phenethyl ]-2,3-dichloroacetamide; antibacterial agent.

**cetostearyl alcohol** (BP). A component of the hydrophilic ointment ingredient known as emulsifying wax. It is a mixture of solid aliphatic alcohols consisting chiefly of stearyl and cetyl alcohols.

**cetox'ine.** 2-(*N*-Benzylanilano)acetamidoxine; antihistaminic agent.

**cetraria** (se-tra'rĭ-ah) [ L. *caetra*, a short Spanish shield (from shape of the apothecia) ]. Iceland moss; the dried plant, *Cetraria islandica* (family Parmeliaceae). Used as a demulcent, and as a folk-remedy for bronchitis. It is not a moss but a lichen.

**cetra'rin.** A bitter acid principle from *Cetraria islandica*, a mixture of three distinct substances: cetraric acid, lichen-stearic acid, and the green pigment thallochlor.

**cet'rimide** (BP). Cetyltrimethylamine bromide.

**cetrimo'nium bromide.** CETAVLON; hexadecyltrimethylammonium bromide; antiseptic.

**ce'tyl.** The univalent alcohol radical $C_{16}H_{33}$— of cetyl alcohol (hexadecanol).

**c. alchohol** (NF), 1-hexadecanol; palmityl alcohol; used as an emulsifying aid and in the preparation of "washable" ointment bases. It is the 16-carbon alcohol corresponding to palmitic acid; so called because it is isolated from among the hydrolysis products of spermaceti.

**c. palmitate**, $C_{15}H_{31}CO$—$OC_{16}H_{31}$; the chief constituent of spermaceti.

**ce'tylpyridin'ium chloride** (NF, BP). CEEPRYN chloride; the monohydrate of the quaternary salt of pyridine and cetyl chloride; a cationic detergent with antiseptic action against nonsporulating bacteria.

**ce'tyltrimethyl'amine bromide.** Cetrimide; a mixture of dodecyl-, tetradecyl-, and hexadecyltrimethylammonium bromides; an odorless surface-active agent, readily soluble in water. It is a disinfectant with a strong bacteriostatic action, used for the sterilization of instruments and utensils.

**cevadil'la** [ Sp. dim. of *cebada*, barley ]. Sabadilla.

**cev'adine.** $C_{32}H_{49}NO_9$; an alkaloid occurring in the seeds of *Schoenocaulon officinale (Sabadilla officinarum)*, family Liliaceae; highly irritating to skin and mucous membranes. See also veratrine.

**cevitam'ic acid.** Ascorbic acid.

**ceyssatite** (sēs'at-it) [ *Ceyssat*, a French village ]. A white earth consisting of nearly pure silica. Used as a dusting powder in eczema.

**CF.** Abbreviation for citrovorum *factor*.

**Cf.** Chemical symbol of the artificial element, californium.

**CGS, cgs.** Abbreviation for centimeter-gram-second *system* or *unit*.

**Chaber'tia ovi'na.** The bowel worm; a strongyle nematode parasitic in the digestive tracts of sheep, goats, cattle, and some wild animals; it is not a bloodsucker ordinarily, but feeds on the mucosa of the gut, where it produces considerable damage.

**Chaddock,** Charles G., St. Louis neurologist, 1861–1936. See C.'s *reflex, sign*.

**Chadwick,** James R., American gynecologist, 1844–1905. See C.'s *sign*.

**chaeta** [ Mod. L. fr. G. *chaite*, stiff hair ]. Seta.

**chafe** (chāf) [ Fr. *chauffer*, to heat, fr. L. *calefacio*, to make warm ]. To cause irritation of the skin by friction.

**Chagas** (chah'gahs), Carlos, Brazilian physician, 1879–1934. See C.'s *disease*, C.-Cruz *disease*.

**chago'ma.** The skin lesion in Chagas' disease.

**Chain** (chān), Ernst B., German biochemist in England, *1906. Nobel laureate, 1945, with Sir Alexander Fleming and Sir Howard Florey for the discovery of penicillin and its curative effect in various infectious diseases.

**chain** (chān) [ L. *catena* ]. 1. In chemistry, a series of atoms held together by one or more covalent bonds. 2. In bacteriology, a linear arrangement of living cells which have divided in one plane and which have remained attached to each other.

**A c.,** glycyl c.; a polypeptide component of insulin containing 21 amino acids; insulin is formed by the linkage of an A c. to a B c. by two disulfide bonds. The amino acid composition of the A c. is a function of species.

**B c.,** phenylalanyl c.; a polypeptide component of insulin containing 30 amino acids. Insulin is formed by the linkage of a B c. to an A c. by two disulfide bonds. The amino acid composition of the B c. is a function of species.

**behavior c.,** related behaviors in a series in which each response serves as a stimulus for the next response.

**closed c. compound,** cyclic *compound*.

**glycyl c.,** see A c.

**hemolyt'ic c.,** the hemolysis that occurs when complement fixes with the previously formed union of erythrocytes and specific antibody.

**lateral c.,** side c.

**long c.,** in bacteriology, a continuous line of more than 8 cells.

**open c. compound,** see under compound.

**ossicular c.,** the bridge of three ossicles, the malleus, incus, and stapes, between the tympanic membrane and the oval window.

**phenylalanyl c.,** see B c.

**short c.,** in bacteriology, a string of 2 to 8 cells.

**side c.,** lateral c.; a c. of atoms linked to a benzene ring, or any closed c. compound, by replacement of H atoms.

**chain'ing.** Learning related behaviors in a series in which each response serves as a stimulus for the next response.

**chalasia, chalasis** (kā-la'zī-ah, kā-la'sis) [ G. *chalaō*, to loosen ]. The inhibition and relaxation of any previously sustained contraction of muscle, usually of a synergic group of muscles.

**chalaza** (kā-la'zah) [ G. hail; a small tubercle, a sty (Galen) ]. 1. Chalazion. 2. The suspensory ligament of the yolk in a bird's egg.

**chalazion,** pl. **chala'zia** (kal-a'zī-on) [ G. dim. of *chalaza*, a sty ]. Meibomian cyst; tarsal cyst; a chronic inflammatory granuloma in the tarsus of the eyelid, due to infammation of a Meibomian gland.

**collar-stud c.,** a c. that extends through the tarsal plate anteriorly (c. externum) and toward the conjunctiva.

**chalcomycin** (kal'ko-mi'sin). $C_{35}H_{56}O_{14}$; a macrolide antibiotic, isolated from *Streptomyces bikiniensis* NRRL 2737; contains two carbohydrate moieties, chalcose and mycinose, each attached by glycoside linkage to a 15-membered lactone; active against Gram-positive cocci, particularly *Staphylococcus aureus*.

**chalcone** (kal'kōn). 3-Phenylacrylphenone; benzylidene acetophenone; $C_6H_5CH = CH—CO—C_6H_5$; the parent compound of a series of plant pigments.

**chalcosis** (kal-ko'sis) [ G. *chalkos*, copper, brass ]. 1. Chronic copper poisoning. 2. A deposit of fine particles of copper in the lungs or other parts.

**c. lentis,** cataract due to copper foreign body.

**chalicosis** (kal-e-ko'sis) [ G. *chalix*, gravel ]. Flint disease; pneumonoconiosis caused by the inhalation of dust incident to the occupation of stone cutting.

**chalinoplasty** (kal'in-o-plas'tī) [ G. *chalinos*, bridle, corner of the mouth, + *plassō*, to form ]. The correction of defects of the mouth and lips, especially of the corners of the mouth.

**chalk** (chawk) [ L. *calx* ]. Creta. 1. Calcium carbonate. 2 (BP). See prepared c.

**French c.,** talc.

**prepared c.** purified native calcium carbonate, usually molded into cones. Used as a mild astringent and antacid.

**chalkitis** (kal-ki'tis) [ G. *chalkos*, copper, brass ]. Chalcosis.

**chalk'stone.** Gouty *tophus*.

**chalone** (ka'lōn). Originally, a hormone (*e.g.*, enterogastrone) that inhibits rather than stimulates. Now, any one of a number of mitotic inhibitors elaborated by a tissue and active within that tissue rather than, like hormones, on another tissue; a reversible tissue-specific mitotic inhibitor.

**chalybeate** (kal-ib'e-āt) [ G. *chalyps* (*chalyb-*), steel ]. 1. Ferruginous; martial; relating to or containing iron. 2. A therapeutic agent containing iron.

**chamazulene.** 1,4-Dimethyl-7-ethylazulene; anti-inflammatory agent.

**chamber** (chăm'ber) [ L. *camera* ]. A compartment or enclosed space. See also camera.

**altitude c.,** high altitude c.; a decompression c. for simulating a high altitude environment, particularly its low barometric pressure.

**anechoic c.,** a room designed to absorb all sound so as to eliminate all echoes; used for isolation and sound research on human subjects.

**anterior c. of the eye,** *camera* anterior bulbi.

**aqueous c.'s,** the anterior and posterior c.'s of the eye containing the aqueous humor; see *camera* anterior bulbi and *camera* posterior bulbi.

**decompression c.,** a c. for exposing organisms to pressures below that of the atmosphere.

**Haldane c.,** a c. for metabolic studies on animals.

**high altitude c.,** altitude c.

**hyperbaric c.,** one employing high pressure oxygenation; useful in conditions such as heart abnormalities, gas gangrene, circulatory inadequacies, and decompression sickness.

**ionization c.,** a c. for detecting ionization of the enclosed gas. Used for determining intensity of ionizing radiation.

**posterior c. of the eye,** *camera* posterior bulbi.

**pulp c.,** that portion of the pulp cavity which is contained in the crown or body of the tooth.

**relief c.,** a recess in the impression surface of a denture to reduce or eliminate pressure from that specific area of the mouth.

**Sandison-Clark c.,** a c. which can be fitted over a hole punched in a rabbit's ear, so that tissue will grow to fill the defect between two transparent plates. If the distance between the plates is small the living tissue can be studied microscopically.

**sinuatrial c.,** the common c. formed by the single embryonic atrium and the right and left horns of the sinus venosus.

**Thoma's counting c.,** see Thoma-Zeiss *hemocytometer*.

**vitreous c.,** *camera* vitrea bulbi.

**Zappert counting c.,** a special, standardized glass slide used for counting cells (especially erythrocytes and leukocytes) and other particulate material in a measured volume of fluid; the central portion is precisely ground in such a manner that the uniformly flat surface is exactly 0.1 mm. lower than that of two parallel ridges on which a special, uniformly flat coverslip may be placed; accurately etched lines on the flat central portion form the boundaries of groups of squares of known areas, thereby providing the basis for determining the volume of fluid in which the cells are counted. Glass slides of this type are frequently known as hemocytometers.

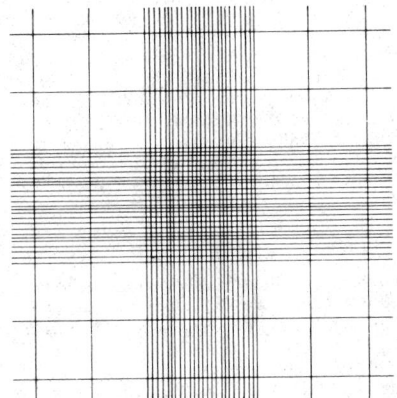

Diagram of Ruled Portion of Zappert
Counting Chamber

**Chamberlain,** W. E., U. S. radiologist, 1891–1947. See C.'s *line.*

**Chamberland,** Charles E., French bacteriologist, 1851–1908. See C. *filter,* Pasteur-C. *filter.*

**Chamberlen,** Peter, English obstetrician, 1560–1631. See C. *forceps.*

**chamecephalic** (kam-e-sef-al'ik) [ G. *chamai,* on the ground (low, stunted), + *kephalē,* head ]. Having a flat head; denoting a skull with a vertical index of 70 or less; similar to tapinocephalic.

**chamecephalous** (kam-e-sef'al-us). Chamecephalic.

**chameprosopic** (kam'e-pro-sop'ik) [ G. *chamai* (adv.), on the ground (low, spread out), + *prosōpikos,* facial. OPO- ]. Having a broad face.

**chamomile** (kam'o-mil) [ G. *chamaimēlon,* chamomile, fr. *chamai,* on the ground, + *mēlon,* apple ]. Camomile; Roman or English chamomile; the flowering heads of *Anthemis nobilis* (family Compositae); stomachic.

**Champetier de Ribes,** Camille Louis Antoine, French obstetrician, 1848–1935. See C. de R. *bag.*

**Championnière,** J. M. L. See Lucas Championnière.

**chancre** (shang'ker) [ Fr. indirectly from L. *cancer* ]. Hard sore; syphilitic, autochthonous, or hard ulcer; primary lesion; the site of infection of syphilis or chancroid (soft chancre); it begins as a papule or area of infiltration, of dull red color, hard, and insensitive; the center usually becomes eroded or breaks down into an ulcer.
　　**Celsus' c.,** obsolete eponym for chancroid.
　　**eating c.,** obsolete term for chancroid.
　　**hard c.,** a syphilitic c.
　　**Hunter's c.,** obsolete eponym for a syphilitic c.
　　**mixed c.,** a sore resulting from simultaneous inoculation with syphilis and chancroid.
　　**monorecidive c.,** a c. that recurs at the site of a previously healed lesion.
　　**Nisbet's c.,** obsolete eponym for bubonulus (2).
　　**c. redux,** a second c. occurring in a syphilitic subject, possibly an allergic reaction without the presence of the specific spirochete.
　　**soft c.,** chancroid.
　　**sporotrichositic c.,** the initial lesion at the site of infection in sporotrichosis.
　　**sulcus c.,** obsolete term for a syphilitic c.

　　**syphilitic c.,** see c.
　　**true c.,** syphilitic c.
　　**tularemic c.,** primary lesion, usually of finger, thumb, or hand, in tularemia.

**chan'criform.** Resembling chancre.

**chancroid** (shang'kroyd) [ chancre + G. *eidos,* resemblance ]. Soft chancre; an infectious venereal ulcer at the site of infection by *Haemophilus ducreyi.*

**chancroid'al.** Relating to or of the nature of chancroid.

**chancrous** (shang'krus). Characterized by having a chancre.

**change.** Alteration; in pathology, structural alteration of which the cause and significance is uncertain.
　　**Armanni-Ebstein c.,** Armanni-Ebstein *kidney.*
　　**Baggenstoss c.,** distention of pancreatic acini by proteinaceous secretion, seen in dehydration.
　　**Crooke's hyaline c.,** Crooke's hyaline degeneration; replacement of cytoplasmic granules of basophil cells of the anterior pituitary by homogenous hyaline material; a characteristic finding in Cushing's syndrome, but usually not present in the cells of a basophil adenoma.
　　**fatty c.,** fatty *metamorphosis.*
　　**c. of life,** menopause; climacteric.
　　**trophic c.,** neurotrophic *atrophy.*

**chan'nel** [ L. *canalis* ]. Canal; canalis.

**Chantemesse** (shahnt-mes'), André, French bacteriologist, 1851–1919. See C. *reaction.*

**chaparro amargoso** (chah-pahr'ro ah-mar-go'so) [ Sp. *chaparro,* live oak or bramble, + *amargoso,* bitter ]. Mexican name of a plant, *Castela nicholsoni,* family Simarubaceae, used in the treatment of intestinal protozoal infections.

**chappa** (chap'pah) [ W. Af. ]. A disease marked by subcutaneous nodules, the size of a pigeon's egg, which break down, giving exit to a fatty looking material, and form ulcers; the eruption is preceded by severe muscular and articular pains.

**chapped** (chapt) [ M.E. *chap,* to chop, split ]. Having or pertaining to skin that is dry, scaly, and fissured, owing to the action of cold or to the excess rate of evaporation of moisture from the skin surface.

**character** (kăr'ak-ter). Characteristic (1); an attribute, trait, or definite and distinct structural feature of an animal or plant.
　　**acquired c.,** a c. developed in a plant or animal as a result of environmental influences during the individual's life.
　　**c. armor,** a habitual pattern of organized defenses against anxiety.
　　**compound c.,** an inherited c. dependent upon two or more distinct genes.
　　**dominant c.,** an inherited c. determined by a dominant gene; see gene.
　　**inherited c.,** Mendelian c.; unit c.; a single attribute of an animal or plant that is transmitted from generation to generation in accordance with genetic principles; see gene.
　　**Mendelian c.,** inherited c.
　　**primary sex c.'s** the sex glands, testes or ovaries, and the accessory sex organs.
　　**recessive c.,** an inherited c. determined by a recessive gene; see dominance of genes, under gene.
　　**secondary sex c.'s,** those c.'s peculiar to the male or female, *e.g.,* the beard of men and the breasts of women, which develop at puberty.
　　**sex-linked c.,** an inherited c. determined by sex-linked gene; see gene.
　　**unit c.,** inherited c.

**characteristic** (kăr'ak-ter-is'tik). 1. Character. 2. Pertaining to a character.
　　**time c.,** chronaxie.

**characterization** (kăr'ak-ter-ī-za'shun) The description or attributing of distinguishing traits.
　　**denture c.,** modification of the form and color of the denture base and/or teeth to produce a more lifelike appearance.

**char'acterol'ogy.** Study of character.

**charas.** A resin obtained from *Cannabis sativa.*

**charbon** (shar-boṅ') [ Fr. coal ]. Anthrax (2).

**char'coal.** Carbo; carbon obtained by heating or burning wood with restricted access of air.

**activated c.** (USP), medicinal c.; the residue from the destructive distillation of various organic materials, treated to increase its adsorptive. power. Used in diarrhea, as antidote in various forms of poisoning, and in purification processes in industry and research.

**animal c.,** bone black; ivory black; bone c.; produced by incomplete combustion of animal tissues, especially bone.

**vegetable c.,** wood c.; c. obtained by charring vegetable tissues, especially the wood of willow, beech, birch, or oak.

**wood c.,** vegetable c.

**Charcot** (shar-ko'), Jean M., French neurologist, 1825–1893. See *aneurysm* of C., *aneurysm* of C. and Bouchard, C.'s *artery,* C.-Böttcher *crystalloids,* C.-Leyden *crystals,* C.-Neumann and C.-Robin *crystals,* C.'s *disease,* C.-Marie-Tooth *disease,* Erb-C. *disease,* C.'s *intermittent fever,* C.'s *gait,* C.'s *joint,* C.'s *syndrome.* C.-Weiss-Barber *syndrome;* C.'s *triad,* C.'s *vertigo,* C.'s *zone.*

**charge.** A quantity of electricity.

**electronic c.,** a quantity of electricity that is equal numerically to the c. on an electron.

**charlatan** (shar'lä-tan). Quack; a medical fraud claiming to cure disease by useless procedures, secret remedies, and worthless diagnostic and therapeutic machines.

**charlatanism** (shar'lä-tan-izm). Quackery; a fraudulent claim to medical knowledge; treating the sick without knowledge of medicine or authority to practice medicine.

**Charles,** Jacques C., French physicist, 1746–1823. See C.'s *law.*

**char'ley horse** [ slang ]. Localized pain or muscle stiffness following sudden or excessive muscular activity; distinguished from an athletic cramp by its persistence; probably caused by fluid distention in muscle sheath.

**Charlouis' disease.** See under disease.

**Charlton,** Willy, German physician, *1889. See Schultz-C. *phenomenon,* Schultz-C. *reaction.*

**Charrière** (shä-re-air'), Joseph F. B., Paris instrument maker, 1803–1876. See C. *scale.*

**chart.** 1. A sheet of paper on which various data relating to the disease, pulse, respiration, temperature, urinary analysis, etc., are recorded in tabular form. 2. Curve (2). 3. In ophthalmology, test-types for examining far or near vision; see *test-type.*

**alignment c.,** d'Ocagne *nomogram.*

**Amsler's c.'s,** finely squared c.'s held at 30 cm. for the rapid detection of central and paracentral irregularities in the visual field.

**Walker's c.,** a system of plotting the relative fetal and placental sizes.

**charta,** gen. and pl. **chartae** (kar'tah) [ L. a sheet of paper (Egyptian papyrus) ]. Paper.

**Charters,** W. J. See C.'s *method.*

**chart'ing.** Clinical recording; making a record in tabular or graph form of the progress of the disease.

**chartreusin.** Antibiotic produced by *Streptomyces chartreusis;* tuberculostatic agent.

**chasma** (kaz'mah) [ G. fr. *chainō,* to yawn ]. Pandiculation; yawning; an expanse; an opening.

**Chassaignac** (shas-a-nyak'), Edouard P. M., French surgeon, 1804–1879. See C.'s *écraseur, space, tubercle.*

**Chastek paralysis.** See under paralysis.

**Chaudhry,** Amand P. See Gorlin-C.-Moss *syndrome.*

**Chauffard** (sho-far'), Anatole M. E., French physician, 1855–1932. See C.'s *syndrome,* Still-C. *syndrome.*

**Chauliac** (sho'lĭ-ak), Guy de, French surgeon, 1300–1368. Considered by some to be the most eminent authority on surgery during the 14th century.

**chaulmoogra, chaulmugra, chaulmaugra** (chawl-moo'-grah, chawl-maw'grah) [ E. Ind. ]. The ripe seed of *Hydnocarpus wightiana* (family Flacourtiaciae) or *Taraktogenos kurzi* (family Bixaceae).

**c. oil,** hydnocarpus oil; gynocardia oil; the fixed oil expressed from seeds of *Taraktogenos kurzii* and *Hydnocarpus wightiana;* formerly used in the treatment of leprosy.

**chaulmoo'gric acid.** A cyclic fatty acid found among the hydrolysis products of the glycerides of chaulmoogra oil.

**Chaussier** (sho-se-a'), François, French physician, 1746–1828. See C.'s *areola, line, sign.*

**Chauveau** (sho-vo'), Auguste, Paris veterinary surgeon, 1827–1917. See C.'s *bacterium.*

**Chayes,** Herman. See C.'s *method.*

**Ch.B.** Abbreviation for Chirurgiae Baccalaureus, Bachelor of Surgery.

**Ch.D.** Abbreviation for Chirurgiae Doctor; Doctor of Surgery.

**Cheadle,** Walter B., English pediatrician, 1835–1910. See C.'s *disease.*

**check'bite.** Interocclusal *record.*

**centric c.,** see maxillomandibular *record;* interocclusal *record.*

**eccentric c.,** interocclusal *record.*

**lateral c.,** interocclusal *record.*

**protrusive c.,** protrusive *record.*

**check'erberry oil.** Gaultheria oil.

**Chédiak,** Moisés. See C.-Higashi *disease,* C.-Steinbrinck-Higashi *anomaly* or *syndrome.*

**cheek** [ A. S. *ceáce* ]. Bucca; mala; gena; the side of the face forming the lateral wall of the mouth.

**cheil-.** See cheilo-.

**cheilalgia, chilalgia** (ki-lal'jĭ-ah) [ cheil- + G. *algos,* pain ]. Pain in the lip.

**cheilectomy, chilectomy** (ki-lek'to-mĭ) [ cheil- + G. *ektomē,* excision ]. 1. Excision of a portion of the lip. 2. Chiseling away bony irregularities on the lips of a joint cavity that interfere with movements of the joint.

**cheilectropion, chilectropion** (ki-lek-tro'pĭ-on) [ cheil- + G. *ektropos,* a turning out ]. Eversion of the lips or a lip.

**cheilitis, chilitis** (ki-li'tis) [ cheil- + G. suffix -*itis,* inflammation ]. Inflammation of the lips or of a lip, with redness and the production of fissures radiating from the angles of the mouth. A form of c. has been induced by riboflavin deficiency and cured with riboflavin and other B-complex vitamins or a good diet, see also cheilosis.

**actinic c.,** dry lips, with or without keratoses, due to excessive exposure to sunlight.

**commissural c.** (1) perlèche; fissures at angles of the mouth, possibly due to *Candida albicans* and attributed by some to riboflavin deficiency; (2) fissures at the angles of the mouth caused by inadequately constructed or improperly worn dentures, sagging cheeks, atopic dermatitis of the perioral area, excessive licking of the lips, hypersalivation and drooling, and nutritional deficiencies.

**c. exfoliati'va,** an exfoliative dermatitis; it may be related to atopic dermatitis or to contact sensitivity.

**c. glandula'ris,** myxadenitis labialis; Volkmann's c.; Baelz' disease; a congenital condition characterized by hypertrophy of the mucous glands of the lips.

**impetiginous c.,** pyoderma of the lips.

**c. venena'ta,** allergic contact dermatitis of the lips.

**Volkmann's c.,** c. glandularis.

**cheilo-, cheil-** [ G. cheilos, lip ]. Combining forms denoting relationship to the lips; for some words beginning thus and not found here, see also chilo- and chil-.

**cheiloalveoloschisis, chiloalveoloschisis** (ki'lo-al've-o-los'kĭ-sis) [ cheilo- + L. *alveolus, q.v.,* + G. *schisis,* cleft ]. Cleft of the prepalate.

**cheilognathoglossoschisis, chilognathoglossoschis** (ki'lo-nath'o-glos-os'kĭ-sis, ki-log'nă-tho-) [ cheilo- + G. *gnathos,* jaw, + *glōssa,* tongue, + *schisis,* cleft ]. An associated condition of cleft mandible and lower lip, and bifid tongue.

**cheilognathopalatoschisis, chilognathopalatoschisis** (ki'lo-nath-o-pal-ă-tos'kĭ-sis, ki-log'nă-tho-). Cheilognathouranoschisis.

**cheilognathoprosoposchisis, chilognathoprosoposchisis** (ki'lo-nath-o-pros-o-pos'kĭ-sis, ki-log'nă-tho-) [ cheilo- + G. *gnathos,* jaw, + *prosōpon,* face, + *schisis,* cleft ]. Oblique facial cleft, with cleft of lip and jaw.

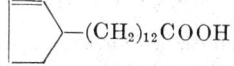

$$\rangle\!-\!(CH_2)_{12}COOH$$

**Chaulmoogric acid**

**cheilognathoschisis, chilognathoschisis** (ki′lo-nă-thos′kī-sis, ki-log′nă-thos′kī-sis) [ cheilo- + G. *gnathos*, jaw, + *schisis*, cleft ]. Cleft lip with a cleft in the jaw.

**cheilognathouranoschisis, chilognathouranoschisis** (ki′lo-nath′o-u-ra-nos′kī-sis, ki-log′nă-tho-) [ cheilo- + G. *gnathos*, jaw, + *ouranos*, sky (roof of mouth), + *schisis*, cleft ]. Cheilognathopalatoschisis; cleft lip with cleft jaw and palate.

**cheilophagia, chilophagia** (ki′lo-fa′jī-ah) [ cheilo- + G. *phagein*, to eat ]. Biting the lips.

**cheiloplasty, chiloplasty** (ki′lo-plas-tī) [ cheilo- + G. *plassō*, to form ]. Plastic surgery of the lips.

**cheilorrhaphy, chilorrhaphy** (ki-lor′ă-fī) [ cheilo- + G. *raphē*, suture ]. Suturing of the lip.

**cheiloschisis, chiloschisis** (ki-los′kī-sis) [ cheilo- + G. *schisis*, cleft ]. Cleft *lip.*

**cheilosis, chilosis** (ki-lo′sis) [ cheil- + G. suffix *-osis*, condition ]. Angular stomatitis seen in riboflavin deficiency and other B-complex deficiencies; it begins with a small fissure, without much inflammation, and accumulation of dried serum; it may eventuate in deep fissures, see also cheilitis.

**cheilostomatoplasty, chilostomatoplasty** (ki-lo-sto′mă-to-plas-tī) [ cheilo- + G. *stoma*, mouth, + *plassō*, to form ]. Plastic surgery of the lips and mouth.

**cheilotomy, chilotomy** (ki-lot′o-mī) [ cheilo- + G. *tomē*, incision ]. 1. Incision into the lip.

**cheir-.** See cheiro-.

**cheirarthritis, chirarthritis** (ki′rahr-thri′tis) [ cheir- + arthritis ]. Obsolete term for inflammation of the joints of the hand.

**cheiro-, cheir-** [ G. *cheir*, hand ]. Combining forms meaning hand. For words beginning thus and not found here, see also chiro-.

**cheirobrachialgia, chirobrachialgia** (ki′ro-bra′kī-al′jī-ah) [ cheiro- + G. *brachiōn*, arm, + algos, pain ]. Obsolete term for pain and paresthesia in the hand and arm.

**cheirocinesthesia** (ki′ro-sin-es-the′zī-ah). Cheirokinesthesia.

**cheirognostic, chirognostic** (ki′rog-nos′tik) [ cheiro- + G. *gnostikos*, perceptive ]. Able to recognize the hand, or to distinguish between right and left.

**cheirokinesthesia, chirokinesthesia** (ki′ro-kin-es-the′zī-ah) [ cheiro- + G. *kinēsis*, movement, + *aisthēsis*, sensation ]. Cheirocinesthesia; chirocinesthesia; the subjective sensation of movement of the hands.

**cheirokinesthetic** (ki′ro-kin-es-thet′ik). Relating to cheirokinesthesia.

**cheirology, chirology** (ki-rol′o-jī) [ cheiro- + G. *logos*, word ]. Dactylology.

**cheiromegaly, chiromegaly** (ki′ro-meg′ă-lī) [ cheiro- + G. *megas*, large ]. Macrocheiria.

**cheiroplasty, chiroplasty** (ki′ro-plas-ti) [ cheiro- + G. *plassō*, to form ]. A plastic operation upon the hand.

**cheiropodalgia, chiropodalgia** (ki′ro-po-dal′jī-ah) [ cheiro- + G. *pous*, foot, + *algos*, pain ]. Pain in the hands and in the feet.

**cheiropompholyx, chiropompholyx** (ki′ro-pom′fo-liks) [ cheiro- + G. *pompholyx*, a bubble, fr. *pomphos*, a blister ]. Dyshidrosis.

**cheirospasm, chirospasm** (ki′ro-spazm) [ cheiro- + G. *spasmos*, spasm ]. Spasm of the muscles of the hand, as in writers' cramp.

**chelate** (ke′lāt). 1. To effect chelation. 2. Pertaining to chelation. 3. A complex formed through chelation.

**chelation** (ke-la′shun) [ G. *chēlē*, claw ]. Bond formation between a metal ion and two or more polar groupings of a single molecule; thus, in heme, the $Fe^{++}$ ion is chelated by the porphyrin ring. Chelation can be used to remove an ion from participation in biological reactions, as in the chelation of $Ca^{++}$ of blood by EDTA, which thus acts as an anticoagulant.

**chelicera**, pl. **cheli′cerae** (kĕ-lis′ĕ-rah) [ G. *chēlē*, claw, + *keras*, horn ]. One of the two anterior appendages of arachnids. In ticks and parasitic mites the chelicerae are protrusible and constitute important organs of attachment.

**chelidon** (kel′e-don) [ G. *chelidōn*, a swallow, because of fancied resemblance to the shape of a swallow's tail ]. Fossa cubitalis.

**chelidonium** (kel-e-do′nī-um) [ G. *chelidonion*, swallow-wort, celandine, fr. *chelidōn*, a swallow ]. The dried plant, *Chelidonium majus* (family Papaveraceae), or garden celandine; purgative.

**cheliped** (kel′ī-ped, ke′lī-ped) [ G. *chēlē*, claw, + L. *pes, pedis*, foot ]. The first thoracic appendage (pincer) of crustaceans, such as the crayfish, etc.

**che′loid.** Keloid.

**Chelonia** (ke-lo′nī-ah) [ G. *chelōnē*, a tortoise ]. An order of reptiles, embracing the turtles, tortoises, and terrapins. The body is enclosed in a bony shell covered with epidermal scutes and formed dorsally by expanded ribs, the carapace, and ventrally by a sternal plastron.

    **C. imbrica′ta,** the hawksbill sea turtle; the source of commercial tortoise shell.

    **C. my′das,** the green sea turtle of commerce.

**chelo′nian.** Resembling or relating to a turtle or tortoise.

**chem-.** See chemo-.

**chem′exfolia′tion.** A chemosurgical technique designed to remove acne scars or treat chronic skin defects caused by exposure to sunlight. Buffered phenol solution is used, among other substances.

**chemi′atry.** Iatrochemistry.

**chem′ical.** Relating to chemistry, to the mutual relations and interaction of the elements, and to the phenomena resulting therefrom.

**chem′icocau′tery.** Chemocautery.

**chemiotax′is.** Chemotaxis.

**chemise** (shem-ez′) [ Fr. shirt ]. A square of linen tied to a catheter passed through its center; used to retain a tampon packed around the catheter inserted into a wound, such as that resulting from a perineal section.

**chem′ist.** One educated in and practicing the science of chemistry.

**chemistry** (kem′is-trī) [ G. *chēmeia*, alchemy. CHEM- ]. The science dealing with the atomic composition of substances, with the elements and their reactions, and with the formation, decomposition and properties of molecules.

    **analytic c.,** the application of c. to the determination of composition.

    **applied c.,** the employment of the theory and principles of chemistry to practical processes in home and factory.

    **biological c.,** biochemistry.

    **clinical c.,** (1) the c. of human health and disease; (2) c. in connection with the management of patients, as in a hospital laboratory.

    **epithermal c.,** hot atom c.; the science dealing with the chemical reactions of recoil atoms and free radicals produced in low energy nuclear processes.

    **hot atom c.,** epithermal c.

    **inorganic c.,** the c. of compounds not involving covalent bonds.

    **macromolecular c.,** the c. of macromolecules (*e.g.,* proteins, nucleic acids) and polymers (nylon, polyethylene, etc.).

    **medical c.,** c. in its relation to pharmacy, physiology, or any science connected with medicine.

    **medicinal c.,** pharmaceutical c.

    **nuclear c.,** the science dealing with the c. of nuclear reactions and processes.

    **organic c.,** that branch of c. dealing with covalently linked atoms, centering around carbon compounds of this type; originally, and still including, the c. of natural products, whence the name "organic."

    **pharmaceutical c.,** medicinal c.; pharmacochemistry; c. in its application to the analysis and the manufacture of drugs.

    **physiological c.,** biochemistry.

    **radiation c.,** the science dealing with the effects of ionizing or nuclear radiation on chemical reactions or materials.

    **synthetic c.,** the formation or building up of complex compounds by uniting the more simple ones.

**chemo-, chem-** (kem′o-, ke′mo-) [ G. *chēmeia*, alchemy. CHEM- ]. Combining forms relating to chemistry.

**chemoautotroph** (kem'o-aw'to-trōf) [ chemo- + G. *autos,* self, + *trophikos,* nourishing ]. An organism which depends on chemicals for its energy and principally on carbon dioxide for its carbon.

**chemoautotrophic** (kem'o-aw'to-trof'ik). Pertaining to a chemoautotroph.

**chemobiodynamics** (kem'o-bi'o-di-nam'iks) [ chemo- + G. *bios,* life, + *dynamis,* power ]. Study devoted to elucidation of correlations between the chemical constitution of various materials and their ability to modify the function and morphology of biological systems.

**chemobiot'ic.** A combination of an antibiotic with a chemotherapeutic agent; *e.g.,* penicillin plus sulfanilamide.

**chem'ocar'cinogen'esis.** The production of cancer by chemical agents.

**chem'ocau'tery.** Any substance (*e.g.,* potassium hydroxide) by the application of which tissue is destroyed.

**chemoceptor** (kem'o-sep-tor). Chemoreceptor.

**chem'odecto'ma.** Nonchromaffin paraganglioma; relatively rare, usually benign neoplasm originating in the chemoreceptor tissue of the carotid body, glomus jugulare, and aortic bodies; c.'s resemble paragangliomas, except that the latter contain chromaffin cells, whereas the former do not; histologically, c.'s consist of numerous, rounded or ovoid, hyperchromatic cells that tend to be grouped in an alveolus-like pattern within a scant to moderate amount of fibrous stroma; several relatively large thin-walled vascular channels are usually present; depending on the site, it is also termed aortic body tumor, carotid body tumor, or glomus jugulare tumor.

**chem'odectomato'sis.** Multiple tumors of perivascular tissue of carotid body or presumed chemoreceptor type, which have been reported in the lungs as minute neoplasms.

**chem'odifferentiation.** Differentiation of the cellular chemical constituents in the embryo prior to cytodifferentiation; sometimes recognizable histochemically.

**chemoheterotroph** (kem'o-het'er-o-trōf) [ chem- + G. *heteros,* other, + *trophē,* nourishment ]. Chemoorganotroph.

**chem'oheterotroph'ic.** Chemoorganotrophic; pertaining to a chemoheterotroph.

**chemoimmunology** (kem'o-im'u-nol'o-jī). Immunochemistry.

**chem'okine'sis** [ chemo- + G. *kinēsis,* movement ]. Stimulation of an organism by presence of a chemical.

**chem'okinet'ic.** Referring to chemokinesis.

**chemoluminescence** (kem'o-lu-min-es'ens). 1. Light produced by chemical action. 2. Radiation causing chemical action.

**chemol'ysis** [ chemo- + G. *lysis,* dissolution ]. Chemical decomposition.

**chemonucleolysis** (kem'o-nu-kle-ol'ī-sis). The enzymatic dissolution of the nucleus pulposus by injection of chymopapain; the procedure is used in the treatment of intervertebral disk lesions.

**chemoorganotroph** (kem'o-or'gā-no-trof) [ chemo- + G. *organon,* organ, + *trophē,* nourishment ]. Chemoheterotroph; an organism that depends on organic chemicals for its energy and carbon.

**chemoorganotrophic** (kem'o-or-gan-o-trof'ik). Chemoheterotrophic; pertaining to a chemoorganotroph.

**chem'opallidec'tomy** [ chemo- + globus pallidus + G. *ektomē,* excision ]. Destruction of the globus pallidus by injection of a chemical agent.

**chem'opal'lidothalamec'tomy** [ chemo- + L. *pallidus,* pale, + G. *thalamos,* bed, + *ektomē,* excision ]. Destruction of portions of the globus pallidus and thalamus by injection of a chemical substance.

**chem'opallidot'omy** [ chemo- + pallidum, + G. *tomē,* incision ]. The injection of a chemical (usually necrotizing) into the globus pallidus.

**chemoprophylaxis** (kem'o-pro-fi-lak'sis) [ chemo- + prophylaxis, *q.v.* ]. The prevention of disease by the use of chemicals or drugs.

**chem'orecep'tor.** Chemoceptor; any cell that is activated by a change in its chemical milieu and thereby originates a flow of nervous impulses. Such cells can be either (1) "transducer" cells innervated by sensory nerve fibers (*e.g.,* the gustatory receptor cells of the taste buds; cells in the carotid body that are sensitive to changes in the oxygen and carbon dioxide content of the blood); or (2) nerve cells proper, such as the olfactory receptor cells of the olfactory mucosa, and certain cells in the brainstem that are sensitive to changes in the composition of the blood or cerebrospinal fluid.

**medullary c.,** the c.'s in or near the ventrolateral surface of the medulla that are stimulated by local acidity.

**peripheral c.,** the c.'s in the carotid and aortic bodies that are stimulated by chemical changes in the composition of the blood such as hypoxia.

**chemoreflex** (kem'o-re'fleks). A reflex initiated by the stimulation of chemoreceptors, *e.g.,* of a carotid body.

**chem'oresis'tance.** Indicating the resistance of bacteria or malignant cells to the inhibiting action of certain chemical substances used in treatment.

**chem'osen'sitive.** Capable of perceiving changes in the chemical composition of the environment, *e.g.,* changes in the oxygen and carbon dioxide content of the blood.

**chem'ose'rotherapy.** Combination of treatment with serum and drugs.

**chemosis** (ke-mo'sis) [ G. *chēmē,* a yawning, the cockle (from its gaping shell) ]. Edema of the ocular conjunctiva, forming a swelling around the cornea.

**chemosmosis** (kem'os-mo'sis). Chemical action transmitted through a membrane.

**chem'osurgery.** Removal of diseased tissue by repeated application of cauterizing chemicals such as zinc chloride.

**chemosyn'thesis.** The formation of definite compounds by chemical action.

**chemotac'tic.** Relating to chemotaxis.

**chemotax'is** [ chemo- + G. *taxis,* orderly arrangement ]. Chemotropism; attraction of living protoplasm to chemical stimuli, whereby the cells are attracted (positive c.) or repelled (negative c.) by acids, alkalies, or other bodies exhibiting chemical properties; see also phagocytosis.

**chem'othalamec'tomy** [ chemo- + thalamus, + G. *ektomē,* excision ]. Chemothalamotomy; chemical destruction of a part of the thalamus, usually for relief of pain or dyskinesia.

**chem'othalamot'omy.** Chemothalamectomy.

**chem'otherapeu'tic.** Relating to chemotherapy.

**chem'otherapeu'tics.** The branch of therapeutics that deals with chemotherapy.

**chem'other'apy.** Treatment of disease by means of chemical substances or drugs; see also pharmacotherapy.

**chemotic** (ke-mot'ic). Relating to chemosis.

**chem'otrans'mitter.** A chemical substance produced to diffuse and cause responses of neurons or effector cells.

**chemotropism** (kĕ-mot'ro-fĭ) [ chemo- + G. *tropos,* direction, turn ]. Chemotaxis.

**Chenais** (shē-na'), Louis J., French physician, 1872–1950. See Cestan-C. *syndrome.*

**chenodeoxychol(an)ic acid.** See *cholic* acid.

**chenopodium** (ke-no-po'dī-um) [ G. *chēn,* goose, + *pous* (*pod-*), foot ]. American wormseed; Mexican tea; Jesuit tea; the dried ripe fruit of *Chenopodium ambrosoides* (family Chenopodiaceae).

**c. oil,** oil of American wormseed; a volatile oil distilled from c.; anthelmintic.

**cher'ry.** Cerasus; the edible fruit of *Prunus cerasus* (family Rosaceae).

**c. juice,** the juice expressed from the fresh ripe fruit of *Prunus cerasus*; it contains not less than 1.0 per cent of malic acid; used as a flavoring agent, and as a vehicle for cough syrups and other preparations for oral administrations.

**cher'ubism** [ Hebr. *kerubh,* cherub ]. Familial fibrous dysplasia of the jaws; a familial multilocular fibro-osseous disease, with enlargement of the jaw bones in young children (producing the characteristic facies) that tends to regress in adult life; in c., bone formation is by osteoblasts (unlike fibrous dysplasia of bone).

**Chervin** (sher-vaṅ'), Claudius, French pedagogue, 1824 –1896. See C.'s *method.*

**chest** [ A.S. *cest,* a box ]. The thorax.

**a'lar c.,** phthinoid c.

**barrel c.,** a c. permanently the shape of a c. during full inspiration, seen in cases of emphysema.

**blast c.,** trauma to c. and lungs by shock wave.

**cobbler's c.,** characterized by a depression of the lower half of the sternum; seen in shoemakers and others whose occupation causes pressure to be made in this locality.

**flail c.,** flapping chest wall; loss of stability of thoracic cage following fracture of sternum and/or ribs.

**flat c.,** one in which the anteroposterior diameter is shorter than the average.

**fo'veated c.,** *pectus* excavatum.

**funnel c.,** *pectus* excavatum.

**keeled c.,** *pectus* carinatum.

**phthinoid c.,** (tin'oyd) alar c.; pterygoid c.; a long narrow c., the lower ribs being more oblique than usual and sometimes reaching almost to the crest of the ilium; the scapulae project backward, the manubrium sterni is depressed, and Louis' angle is sharper than normal.

**pter'ygoid c.,** phthinoid c.

**chest'nut.** 1. Castanea. 2. A small oval or round horny structure in the skin on the inner side of the legs of the horse. Since the architecture of c.'s varies in every individual, they may be used, like fingerprints of man, for positive identification of individuals.

**Cheyne** (chān), John, Scottish physician, 1777–1836. See C.-Stokes *asthma,* C.'s *nystagmus,* C.-Stokes *psychosis,* C.-Stokes *respiration.*

**Chiari** (ke-ah're), Hans, German pathologist, 1851–1916. See Arnold-C. *deformity, malformation, syndrome,* C.'s *disease,* C.'s *net,* C.'s *syndrome,* C.-Frommel *syndrome.*

**chiasm** (ki'azm) [ G. *chiasma, q.v.* ]. 1. Chiasma. 2. The crossing of intertwined chromosomes during prophase.

**Camper's c.,** *chiasma* tendinum.

**optic c.,** *chiasma* opticum.

**chiasma,** pl. **chias'mata** (ki-az'mah) [ G. *chiasma,* two crossing lines, fr. the letter *chi, X* ] [ NA ]. Chiasm (1); a decussation or crossing of two tracts, such as tendons or nerves.

**c. op'ticum** [ NA ], optic chiasm; optic decussation; a flattened quadrangular body in front of the tuber cinereum and infundibulum, the point of crossing or decussation of the fibers of the optic nerves; most of the fibers cross to the opposite side, some run directly forward on each side without crossing, some pass transversely on the posterior surface between the two optic tracts and others pass transversely on the anterior surface between the two optic nerves.

**c. ten'dinum** [ NA ], crossing of the tendons; Camper's chiasm; the passage of the tendons of the flexor digitorum profundus (flexor digitorum longus in the foot) through the interval left by the decussation of the fibers of the tendons of the flexor digitorum superficialis (flexor digitorum brevis in the foot).

**chiasmatic** (ki-az-mat'ik). Relating to a chiasm.

**chiasmometer** (ki'az-mom'e-ter) [ G. *chiasma,* decussation, + *metron,* measure ]. Chiastometer; an instrument to measure the distance between the centers of rotation of the eyes.

**chi'astom'eter.** Chiasmometer.

**chick'enpox.** Varicella.

**Chick-Martin test.** See under test.

**Chievitz** (che'wits), Johan H., Copenhagen anatomist, 1850–1901. See C.'s *layer, organ.*

**chig'ger.** The larva of *Trombicula* species; a bloodsucking stage of mites of the family Trombiculidae, which includes the vectors of scrub typhus.

**chignon** (she-nyon') [ Fr. nape of the neck ]. Beigel's *disease.*

**chigoe** (chig'o). Common name for *Tunga penetrans.*

**chil-.** See cheilo- and chilo-.

**Chilaiditi,** Demetrius. See C.'s *syndrome.*

**chilalgia.** Cheilalgia.

**chilblain** [ chill + A.S. *blegen,* a blain, *q.v.* ]. Erythema pernio; perniosis; erythema, itching, and burning, especially of the dorsa of the fingers and toes, and of the heels, nose, and ears on exposure to extreme cold (usually associated with high humidity); lesions can be single or multiple, and can become blistered and ulcerated.

**child'bearing.** Pregnancy and parturition.

**child'birth.** Parturition; labor; delivery.

**childhood.** The period of life between infancy and puberty.

**chilectomy.** Cheilectomy.

**chilectropion.** Cheilectropion.

**chilitis.** Cheilitis.

**chill** [ A.S. *cele,* cold ]. 1. A sensation of cold. 2. Rigor; a feeling of cold with shivering and pallor, accompanied by an elevation of temperature in the interior of the body. Usually it is a prodromal symptom of an infectious disease due to the invasion of the blood by the toxins.

**congestive c.,** historical term for a form of pernicious malaria in which the paroxysm is accompanied by congestion of the gastroenteric tract and profuse diarrhea preceded by a c., vomiting, and prostration.

**chilo-, chil-** [ G. *cheilos,* lip ]. Combining form denoting relationship to the lips; for some words beginning thus, and not found here, see also cheilo- and cheil-.

**chiloalveoloschisis** (ki'lo-al-ve-o-los'kĭ-sis). Cheiloalveoloschisis.

**chi'lognathos'chisis.** Cheilognathoschisis.

**chilomastigiasis** (ki'lo-mas'tĭ-gi'ah-sis). Chilomastosis; infection with *Chilomastix* organisms.

**Chilomastix** (ki-lo-mas'tiks) [ chilo- + G. *mastix,* whip ]. A genus of flagellated protozoa parasitic in the intestine of man and other primates, and in many other mammals, birds, amphibia and reptiles. It is ordinarily nonpathogenic, but one species, *C. mesnili,* is thought to be an occasional cause of diarrhea in children.

**chilomastosis** (ki'lo-mas-to'sis). Chilomastigiasis.

**chilopa.** Onyalai.

**chi'lopha'gia.** Cheilophagia.

**chi'loplas'ty.** Cheiloplasty.

**Chilopoda** (ki-lop'o-dah) [ chilo- + G. *pous,* foot ]. A class of Arthropoda, the centipedes.

**chilopodiasis** (ki-lo-po-di'ā-sis). Invasion of one of the cavities, especially the nasal cavity, by a species of Chilopoda, or centipede.

**chilor'rhaphy.** Cheilorrhaphy.

**chiloschisis** (ki-los'kĭ-sis) [ chilo- + G. *schisis,* fissure ]. Cleft *lip.*

**chilosis** (ki-lo'sis). Cheilosis.

**chilot'omy.** Cheilotomy.

**chimaphilin.** 2,7-Dimethyl-1,4-naphthoquinone; from *Chimaphila carymbosa;* urinary antiseptic.

**chimera** (ki-mēr-ah, kī-mēr'ah) [ L. *chimoera,* fr. G. *chimaira* (lit. a she-goat), a fabulous monster: the front a lion, the rear a dragon ]. 1. In experimental embryology, the individual produced by grafting an embryonic part of one animal on to the embryo of another, either of the same or of another species. 2. An individual who has received a transplant of genetically and immunologically different tissue, such as bone marrow. 3. Twins with two immunologically different types of erythrocytes. 4. Sometimes used as a synonym for mosaic. 5. The rat-fish; a cartilaginous, mollusc-eating fish of the group Holocephali in the class Chondrichthys (*q.v.*), believed to be related to the ancient placoderms.

**radiation c.,** an individual with mosaicism induced by exposure to ionizing radiation; see mosaic.

**chimeric** (ki-mer'ik). Relating to a chimera.

**chimerism** (ki-mer'izm). The state of being a chimera.

**chimpanzee** (chim-pan'ze, chim'pan-ze') [ Native Guinea ]. *Anthropopithecus troglodytes;* anthropoid apes; used in biologic experiments.

**chimyl alcohol.** $CH_2OHCHOHCH_2$—O—$(CH_2)_{15}CH_3$; an ether formed by the condensation of cetyl alcohol with one of the terminal hydroxyl groups of glycerol; found in shark oil.

**chin** [ A.S. *cin* ]. Mentum; the prominence formed by the anterior projection of the mandible, or lower jaw.

**double c.,** buccula.

**galoche c.** (ga-lōsh), an abnormally narrow, protruding c.

**chiniofon** (kin'-ī-o-fon). ANAYODIN; YATREN; a mixture of 7-iodo-8-hydroxyquinoline-5-sulfonic acid and sodium bicarbonate. Used in the treatment of amebic dysentery.

**chinkum'bi.** Chiufa.

**chionablepsia** (ki-ōn-a-blep'sī-ah) [ G. *chiōn*, snow, + *ablepsia*, blindness, fr. *a*- priv. + *blepō*, to see ]. An obsolete word meaning snow blindness.

**chip.** A small fragment resulting from breakage or cutting.
   **bone c.'s,** small pieces of cancellous bone generally used to fill in bony defects and to precipitate recalcification.

**chip-blower.** An instrument for blowing the debris out of, or drying, a tooth cavity that is being excavated for a filling; it consists of a rubber bulb with a metal nozzle.

**chiro-, chir-** [ G. *cheir*, hand ]. Combining forms denoting the hand. For words beginning thus and not found here, see also cheiro- and cheir-.

**chirocinesthesia** (ki-ro-sin-es-the'zī-ah). Cheirokinesthesia.

**chi'rognos'tic.** Cheirognostic.

**chirokinesthesia** (ki-ro-kin-es-the'-zī-ah). Cheirokinesthesia.

**chirology** (ki-rol'o-jī). Dactylology.

**chiromegaly** (ki-ro-meg'al-ī). Macrocheiria.

**chiroplasty** (ki'ro-plas-tī). Cheiroplasty.

**chi'ropodal'gia.** Cheiropodalgia.

**chiropodist** (ki-rop'o-dist) [ chiro- + G. *pous*, foot ]. Podiatrist.

**chiropody** (ki-rop'o-dī). Podiatry.

**chiropompholyx** (ki'ro-pom'fo-liks). Dyshidrosis.

**chiropractic** (ki-ro-prak'tik) [ chiro- + G. *praktikos*, efficient ]. A philosophic system of mechanical therapeutics that attributes disease to vertebral subluxations; it treats disease with manipulation of the vertebra in order to relieve pressure on the nerves at the intervertebral foramina, "so that nerve force may flow freely from the brain to the rest of the body." Many of its devotees also use orthodox methods of medical management.

**chiropractor** (ki-ro-prak'tor). One who employs the doctrine and dogma of chiropractic.

**Chiroptera** (ki-rop'ter-ah) [ chiro- + G. *pteron*, wing ]. Bats; an order of placental mammals (of worldwide distribution) characterized by a modification of the forelimbs that enables them to fly, and they are capable of emitting ultrasonic sounds that enable them to echolocate and avoid objects in the dark; they are mostly insectivorous, but some species feed on nectar, fruit, fish, and blood; the blood-feeding species are important vectors of rabies.

**chiroscope** (ki'ro-skōp) [ chiro- + G. *skopeō*, to view ]. A haploscopic instrument used for training ocular muscles in strabismus; it coordinates hand and eye as the patient draws while looking through it.

**chi'rospasm.** Cheirospasm.

**chirurgeon** (ki-rur'jon) [ G. *cheirourgus*, fr. *cheir*, hand, + *ergon*, work. ERG- ]. Surgeon.

**chirurgery** (ki-rur'jer-ī) [ G. *cheirourgia* ]. Surgery.

**chirurgical** (ki-rur'jī-kal). Surgical.

**chisel** (chiz'l). A single beveled end-cutting blade with a straight or angled shank used with a thrust along the axis of the handle for cutting or splitting dentin and enamel. When angled for access a second angle is added to bring the cutting edge nearly in line with the axis of the handle so as to restore balance. This is known as binangling and the c. is called a binangled c.

**chi-square.** A statistical technique whereby variables are categorized to determine whether a distribution of scores is due to chance or experimental factors.

**chitin** (ki'tin). The horny substance in the exoskeleton of beetles, crabs, certain microorganisms; a polymer of *N*-acetyl-D-glucosamine, similar in structure to cellulose. Second most abundant polysaccharide in nature.

**chitinase** (ki'tī-nās). Chitodextrinase; poly-$\beta$-glucosaminidase; an enzyme (EC 3.2.1.14) catalyzing the hydrolysis of chitin to *N*-acetylglucosamine. Some enzymes of this type display lysozyme activity.

**chitinous** (ki'tin-us). Of or relating to chitin.

**chitobiose** (ki'to-bi'ōs). The disaccharide repeating unit in chitin; differs from cellobiose only in the presence of an *N*-acetylamino group on carbon-2 in place of the hydroxyl group.

**chitodextrinase** (ki'to-deks'trī-nās). Chitinase.

**chitoneure** (ki'to-nūr) [ G. *chiton*, tunic, + *neuron*, sinew, nerve ]. A rarely used collective term for the sheaths of nerves, nerve bundles, and nerve fibrils.

**Chittenden,** Russell H., American physiologic chemist, 1856–1943. See C.'s standard *diet.*

**chiu'fa.** Chinkumbi; kanyemba; disease seen in North Rhodesia and South America; it is an acute gangrenous proctitis and colitis with high fever; in women the vulva and vagina may be affected. It occurs at high altitudes (2000 to 2500 ft.).

**Chlamydia** (klā-mid'ī-ah) [ G. *chlamys*, cloak ]. *Bedsonia; Chlamydozoon; Miyagawanella;* the single genus of the family Chlamydiaceae, including all the agents of the psittacosis-lymphogranuloma-trachoma disease groups. Two species are recognized, *C. psittaci* and *C. trachomatis;* the latter is differentiated from the former by its intracytoplasmic production of glycogen and its susceptibility to sulfadiazine. The type species is *C. trachomatis.*
   **C. oculogenita'lis,** Former name for *C. trachomatis.*
   **C. psitta'ci,** *Rickettsia psittaci;* organisms that resemble *C. trachomatis,* but which form loosely bound intracytoplasmic microcolonies up to 12 μm in diameter, do not produce glycogen in sufficient quantity to be detected by iodine stains, and are not susceptible to sulfadiazine. Various strains of this species cause psittacosis in man and ornithosis in nonpsittacine birds; pneumonitis in cattle, sheep, swine, cats, goats, and horses; epizootic bovine abortion and enzootic abortion of ewes; bovine sporadic encephalomyelitis; enteritis of calves; epizootic chlamydiosis of muskrats and hares; encephalitis of opossum; and conjunctivitis of cattle, sheep, and guinea pigs. A number of agents previously described on clinical grounds as separate species of *C.* or as species of the invalid genus *Miyagawanella* are now recognized as belonging to *C. psittaci;* also formerly called ornithosis virus and psittacosis virus.
   **C. tracho'matis,** spherical, nonmotile organisms that form compact intracytoplasmic microcolonies up to 10 μm in diameter which (by division) give rise to infectious spherules 0.3 μm or more in diameter, accumulate glycogen for a limited period in sufficient quantity to be detected by iodine stain, and are sensitive to sulfadiazine; various strains of this species cause trachoma, inclusion conjunctivitis, lymphogranuloma venereum, mouse pneumonitis, nonspecific urethritis, and proctitis; it is the type species of the genus *C.;* formerly known as inclusion conjunctivitis virus, lymphogranuloma venereum virus, and trachoma virus.

**Chlamydiaceae** (klā-mid'ī-a'se-e). Chlamydozoaceae; a family of the order Chlamydiales (formerly included in the order Rickettsiales) that includes the agents of the psittacosis-lymphogranuloma-trachoma-group. The family contains small, coccoid, Gram-negative microorganisms that resemble rickettsiae but which differ from them significantly by possessing a unique, obligately intracellular developmental cycle; intracytoplasmic microcolonies give rise to infectious forms by division. The classification of these organisms previously was in a state of flux, but they are now placed in a single genus, *Chlamydia,* the type genus of the family.

**Chlamydophrys** (klā-mid'o-fris) [ G. *chlamys*, cloak, + *ophrys*, brow ]. A shelled ameba, commonly found as a fecal protozoan.

**chlamydospore** (klam'ī-do-spōr) [ G. *chlamys*, cloak, + *sporos*, seed ]. A form of thallospore; a thick-walled, terminal or intercalary, vegetative cell of certain fungi that is modified into a resting spore.

**Chlamydozoaceae** (kla-mid'o-zo-a'se-e). Chlamydiaceae.

**Chlam'ydozo'on.** Chlamydia.

**chloasma** (klo-az'mah) [ G. *chloazō*, to become green ]. Moth patch; melanoderma or melasma characterized by the occurrence of extensive brown patches of irregular shape and size on the skin of the face and elsewhere; the pigmented patches are also called the mask of pregnancy, and are associated with pregnancy, menopause, and use of oral contraceptives.
   **c. bronzi'num,** tropical mask; a bronze-colored pigmentation, probably produced by hormone imbalance, occurring in gradually increasing areas on the face, neck, and chest in persons exposed continuously to the tropical sun;

similar to c. of the temperate zone, but intensified because of intense sunlight.

**c. uteri'num,** c. of the face occurring in pregnancy and in disorders of the uterus or ovaries.

**chlophedianol hydrochloride** (klo'fē-di'ä-nol) (USAN). ULO; 2-chloro-α-(2-dimethylaminoethyl)benzhydrol hydrochloride; an antitussive agent related chemically to the antihistamines.

**chlor-** [ G. *chloros*, green ]. Combining form denoting (1) green; (2) association with chlorine. See also chloro-.

**chlor'ace'tic acid.** Chloroacetic acid.

**chloracne** (klor-ak'ne). Tar acne; an acne-like eruption due to prolonged contact with certain chlorinated compounds (naphthalenes and diphenyls). Keratinous plugs (comedones) form in the pilosebaceous orifices. Variously sized, small papules (2 to 4 mm.) develop.

**chlo'ral.** Trichloroacetic aldehyde; $CCl_3$—CHO; anhydrous chloral; a thin oily liquid of a pungent odor, formed by the action of chlorine gas on alcohol.

**c. betaine** (NF), BETA-CHLOR; the adduct formed by chloral hydrate and betaine; it is slowly hydrolyzed in the alimentary tract to chloral hydrate. Used as a hypnotic and sedative.

**c. hydrate** (USP, BP), $CCl_3CH(OH)_2$; hypnotic, sedative, and anticonvulsant, and externally as a rubefacient, anesthetic, and antiseptic.

*m*-**chloral.** *p*-Chloral; metachloral; trichloral; trichloracetaldehyde; obtained from chloral by prolonged contact with sulfuric acid; a polymer of chloral with properties similar to those of chloral hydrate.

*p*-**chloral.** *m*-Chloral.

**chlo'ralism.** The habitual use of chloral as an intoxicant, and the symptoms caused thereby.

**chlo'ralose.** α-Chloralose; glucochloral; hypnotic but not reliable for human use. It is principally used to produce general anesthesia in laboratory animals.

**chloral-urethane.** Carbochloral.

**chlorambucil** (klor-am'bu-sil) (USP, BP). LEUKERAN; |*p*-[ bis(2-chloroethyl)amino ]phenyl|butyric acid; a nitrogen mustard derivative that depresses lymphocytic proliferation and maturation. Used in chronic lymphocytic leukemia, lymphosarcoma, and Hodgkin's disease.

**chlo'ramine B.** Sodium *N*-chlorobenzenesulfonamide; a nontoxic antiseptic substance used in wound irrigation as a substitute for chloramine T.

**chlo'ramine T.** Chloramine; sodium *N*-chloro-*p*-toluenesulfonamide; $CH_3C_6H_4SO_2N(Cl)Na3H_2O$; a nontoxic but strong antiseptic used in the irrigation of wounds and infected cavities.

**chloraminophen'amide.** SALAMID; 4-amino-6-chloro-*m*-benzenedisulfonamide; diuretic.

**chloramphen'icol** (USP, BP). CHLOROMYCETIN; D-(−)-*threo*-2,2-dichloro-*N*-[ β-hydroxy-α-(hydroxymethyl)-*p*-nitrophenethyl ]acetamide; an antibiotic obtained from a streptomyces found in a sample of soil from Caracas, Venezuela. Effective against a number of pathogenic microorganisms including *Staphylococcus aureus*, *Brucella abortus*, Friedländer's bacillus, and the organisms of typhoid, typhus, and Rocky Mountain spotted fever; active by mouth. A serious reaction resulting in marrow damage with agranulocytosis or aplastic anemia may occur.

$O_2N$—⬡—$CHOH$—$CH$—$CH_2OH$
                       |
                      $NH$—$CO$—$CHCl_2$

Chloramphenicol

**c. pal'mitate** (USP), same action and use as c.

**c. sodium succinate** (USP), CHLOROMYCETIN succinate; chloramphenicol-α-(sodium succinate); the water-soluble sodium succinate derivative of c., suitable for parenteral administration. Antibacterial activity, uses, and side effects are similar to those of the parent compound.

**chlorane'mia.** Chlorosis.

**chlo'rate.** A salt of chloric acid.

**chloraz'anil.** DIURAZINE; 2-amino-4-(*p*-chloroanilino)-*s*-triazine; diuretic.

**chlor'azol black E.** An acid dye, $C_{34}H_{25}N_9O_7S_2Na_2$, used as a fat and general tissue stain.

**chlorbenzox'amine.** LIBRATAR; chlorbenzoxyethamine; 1-[ 2-(*o*-chloro-α-phenylbenzyloxy)ethyl ]-4-*o*-methylbenzylpiperazine; anticholinergic agent.

**chlorbenzox'yeth'amine.** Chlorbenzoxamine.

**chlorbet'amine.** MONTAMIDE; 2,2-dichloro-*N*-(2,4-dichlorobenzyl)-*N*-(2-hydroxyethyl)acetamide; amebicide.

**chlorbu'tol** (BP). Chlorobutanol.

**chlorcyc'lizine hydrochloride** (NF, BP). DI-PARALENE hydrochloride; 1-(*p*-chlorobenzhydryl)-4-methylpiperazine hydrochloride. An antihistaminic agent.

**chlor'dane.** A chlorinated hydrocarbon used as an insecticide. It may be absorbed through the skin with resultant severe toxic effects: hyperexcitability of central nervous system, tremors, lack of muscular coordination, convulsions, and death. It also causes damage to the liver, kidneys, and spleen. It is only mildly toxic to animals.

**chlordantoin** (klor-dan'to-in) (NF). SPOROSTACIN; 5-(1-ethylpentyl)-3-(trichloromethylthio)-hydantoin; topical antifungal agent.

**chlordiazepoxide hydrochloride** (klor-di-a'ze-pok'sīd) (USP, BP). LIBRIUM; the hydrochloride of 7-chloro-2-methylamin ·5-phenyl-3*H*-1, 4-benzodiazepine-4-oxide; antianxiety agent.

**chlorel'lin.** An antibiotic obtained from algae (*Chlorella vulgaris*); active against *Escherichia coli*, staphylococci, and hemolytic streptococci.

**chlore'mia.** 1. Chlorosis. 2. Abnormally large amounts of chloride in the blood.

**chloreth'yl.** Ethyl chloride.

**chlorguanide hydrochloride** (klor-gwah'nid). Chloroguanide hydrochloride.

**chlorhex'adol.** LORA; 2-methyl-4-(2,2,2-trichloro-1-hydroxy-ethoxy)-2-pentanol; hypnotic.

**chlorhex'idine hydrochloride** (BP, USAN). HIBITANE; 1,1'-hexamethylenebis[ 5-(*p*-chlorophenyl)biguanide ] dihydrochloride; topical antiseptic.

**chlorhy'dria.** Presence of excessive hydrochloric acid in the stomach.

**chlo'ric.** Relating to chlorine.

**c. acid,** $HClO_3$.

**chlo'ride.** A compound containing chlorine, especially salts of hydrochloric acid.

**c. shift,** Hamburger's phenomenon; when $CO_2$ enters the blood from the tissues, it passes into the red cell and is converted by the enzyme, carbonic anhydrase, to carbonic acid ($H_2CO_3$). $HCO_3^-$ ion passes into the plasma while $Cl^-$ migrates into the red cell. Reverse changes occur in the lungs when $CO_2$ is eliminated from the blood.

**chloridimetry** (klor-ĭ-dim'e-trĭ). The process of determining the amount of chlorides in the blood or urine, or in other fluids.

**chloridom'eter.** An apparatus for turbidimetric analysis of chlorides.

**chlor'idu'ria.** Chloruresis.

**chlo'rin, chlo'rine.** Dihydroporphine, the two additional hydrogens being at positions 7 and 8 of the chlorophyll type of porphine.

**chlo'rinated.** Containing chlorine.

**chlorin'danol** (USAN). LANESTA; 7-chloro-4-indanol; spermicide.

**chlorine.** A greenish toxic, gaseous element; symbol Cl, atomic no. 17, atomic weight 35.46; a halogen. Used as a disinfectant and bleaching agent in the form of hypochlorite or of c. water, because of its oxidizing power.

**c. group,** see halogen.

**chloriodized** (klor-i'o-dīzd). Containing both chlorine and iodine.

**c. oil,** iodochlorol; chlorinated and iodized peanut oil formed by the chemical addition of iodine monochloride; contains chlorine 7.5 and iodine 27 per cent; used for roentgenography of sinus and bronchial tract.

**chlor'ison'damine chlo'ride.** ECOLID chloride; 4,5,6,7-tetrachloro- (22- -dimethylaminoethyl) -2 -methylisoindolinium chloride; a quaternary ammonium compound with ganglionic blocking action similar to, but more potent than, hexamethonium and pentolinium. Used in the management of severe hypertension including the malignant phase.

**chlo'rite.** A salt of chlorous acid; it contains the radical $ClO_2{}^-$.

**chlormad'inone acetate** (BP, USAN). GESTAFORTIN; LORMIN; LUTERAN; LUTESTRAL; LUTORAL; 6-chloro-17-hydroxy-4,6-pregnadiene-3,20-dione acetate (for pregnadiene structure, see steroids); 6-chloro-6-dehydro-17$\alpha$-acetoxyprogesterone; a progesterone derivative. Used in conjunction with estrogen as an oral contraceptive.

**chlormer'odrin** (USP). NEOHYDRIN; 1-[ 3-(chloromercuri)-2-methoxypropyl ]urea; a mercurial diuretic chemically related to meralluride.

**chlormez'anone.** TRANCOPAL; 2-(4-chlorophenyl)-3-methyl-4-metathiazanone-1,1-dioxide; a muscle relaxant and tranquilizing agent with pharmacologic actions and uses similar to those of meprobamate.

**chloro-** [ G. *chlōros*, green ]. Combining form denoting (1) green; (2) association with chlorine. See also chlor-.

**chlo'roace'tic acid.** Chloracetic acid; an acetic acid in which one or more of the hydrogen atoms are replaced by chlorine. According to the number of atoms so displaced the acid is called monochloroacetic (chloroacetic), dichloroacetic, or trichloroacetic.

**chlo'roace'tophenone.** A lacrimatory gas; $C_6H_5$-$COCH_2Cl$.

**chloroane'mia.** Chloranemia.

**chloroaz'odin.** AZOCHLORAMIDE; $\alpha,\alpha'$-azo-bis(chloroformamidine); a bactericidal agent used as a surgical antiseptic.

**chlo'roblast** [ chloro- + G. *blastos*, germ ]. Erythroblast.

**chlorobu'tanol** (USP). CHLORETONE; chlorbutol; trichloro-*tert*-butyl alcohol; $Cl_3CC(CH_3)_2OH$; acetone chloroform; hypnotic sedative and local anesthetic; used chiefly as a preservative in multiple-dose vials for parenteral use.

**chlorocre'sol** (BP). *p*-Chloro-*m*-cresol; used as an antiseptic and disinfectant; is more active in acid than in alkaline solutions.

**chlorocruorin** (klo-ro-kru'or-in). A hemoglobin like pigment greenish in color, found in certain worms. It contains a porphyrin differing from protoporphyrin by a formyl group in place of the 2-vinyl group.

**chloroeth'ane.** Ethyl chloride.

**chlo'roform** [ chlor(ine) + form(yl) ] (NF, BP). Trichloromethane; methylene trichloride; $CHCl_3$; used by inhalation to produce general anesthesia, and internally as an anodyne, sedative, and antispasmodic; also used as a solvent.

   **ac'etone c.,** chlorobutanol.

**chlorofor'min.** An old term for a substance extracted from tubercle bacilli by means of chloroform.

**chlo'roformism.** The habit of chloroform inhalation and the symptoms caused thereby.

**chlor'ogenin.** Alstonine.

**chloroguanide hydrochloride** (klor'o-gwah'nid) (NF). PALUDRINE; proguanil hydrochloride; chlorguanide hydrochloride; 1-(*p*-chlorophenyl)-5-isopropylbiguanide monohydrochloride; an antimalarial drug.

**chlorohe'min.** Hemin.

**chlo'rolabe.** Term proposed for one of two pigments presumed to reside in the cones of the eye, absorbing in the green portion of the spectrum (opposed to erytrolabe).

**chloroleukemia** (klo'ro-lu-ke'mī-ah) [ chloro- + G. *leukos*, white, + *haima*, blood ]. Chloroma.

**chlorolymphosarcoma** (klo'ro-lim'fo-sar-ko'mah). An obsolete term, formerly used to designate a form of chloroma in which the characteristic abnormal cells were thought to be lymphoblastic in origin; it is now doubted that lymphocytic leukemia and lymphosarcoma ever result in chloroma.

**chloro'ma** [ chloro- + G. suffix -*ōma*, tumor ]. Chloroleukemia; chloromyeloma; Aran's cancer; green cancer; Balfour's disease; a condition characterized by the development of multiple, localized green masses of abnormal cells, especially in relation to the periosteum of the skull, spine, and ribs. In most instances, the abnormal cells are myeloblasts. The clinical course of c. is similar to that of acute leukemia, and the findings in blood and bone marrow are not distinguishable; the condition is observed more frequently in children and young adults.

*p*-**chlo'romercuriben'zoate.** Organic mercury compound; $ClHgC_6H_4COO^-$; reacts with —SH groups of proteins, etc.; inhibitor of action of those proteins (enzymes) that depend on —SH reactivity. Abbreviated ClHgBzOH, or PCMB, or *p*CMB.

**chlorometh'ane.** Methyl chloride; a refrigerant; also an inhalation anesthetic. It hydrolyzes to methanol.

**chlorom'etry.** The measurement of chlorine content, or the use of analytical techniques involving the release or titration of chlorine.

**chloromyeloma** (klo'ro-mi-ē-lo'mah) [ chloro- + G. *myelos*, marrow, + suffix -*ōma*, tumor ]. Chloroma.

**chlorope'nia** [ chloro- + G. *penia*, poverty ]. Hypochloremia; abnormally low content of chlorides in the blood.

**chloroper'cha.** A solution of base-plate gutta-percha in chloroform, used in dentistry for coating the root canal wall prior to the insertion of a gutta-percha cone or cones, to effect a better seal of the root canal.

**chlo'rophane** [ chloro- + G. *phainō*, to show ]. A greenish yellow pigment in the retina.

**chlorophe'nol.** One of several substitution products obtained by the action of chlorine on phenol. Used as antiseptics.

*o*-**chlorophe'nol.** An antiseptic liquid, used in the treatment of lupus.

*p*-**chlorophe'nol.** Parachlorophenol.

**chlorophen'othane.** Dichlorodiphenyltrichloroethane.

**chlo'rophyll.** The green pigment of plants; the porphyrin (phorbin) pigment found in photosynthetic organisms; the light-absorbing plant pigments that, in living plants, convert light energy into oxidizing and reducing power, thus fixing $CO_2$ and evolving $O_2$. The naturally occurring forms are chlorophyll *a, b, c,* and *d.* See structure and subentries.

**Chlorophyll**

   **c. a,** the phytylester of 1,3,5,8-tetramethyl-4-ethyl-2-vinyl-9-oxo-10-carbomethoxyphorbin-7-propionic acid (see structure); the major pigment found in all oxygen-evolving photosynthetic organisms (higher plants and red and green algae).

   **c. b,** generally characteristic of the higher plants, including the *Chlorophyta, Euglenophyta,* and green algae; has a formyl (—CHO) group in place of a methyl at position 3.

   **c. c,** present in *Phaeophyta* (brown algae), *Bacillariophyta* (diatoms), and *Pyrrophyta* (dinoflagellates).

   **c. d,** present in the *Rhodophyta* (red algae), along with chlorophyll *a;* and has the chlorophyll *a* structure with formyl in place of the 2-vinyl.

   **c. esterase,** chlorophyllase.

   **water-soluble c. derivatives,** CHLORESIUM; the copper complex of sodium and/or potassium salts of saponified c.

Used topically for deodorization of chronic lesions and to promote wound repair.

**chlorophyllase** (klo'ro-fil-ās). A hydrolyzing enzyme (EC 3.1.1.14) catalyzing the removal of the phytyl group from chlorophyll, leaving chlorophyllide.

**chlo'rophyllide, chlo'rophyllid.** What is left of the chlorophyll molecule when the phytyl group is removed.

**chloro'pia.** Chloropsia.

**chloropic'rin.** $CCl_3NO_2$; trichloronitromethane; nitrochloroform; toxic lung irritant and lacrimatory gas; also causes vomiting, colic, and diarrhea, and therefore called vomiting gas.

**chlo'roplast** [ chloro- + G. *plastos*, formed ]. A plant cell inclusion body containing chlorophyll; occurs in cells of leaves and young stems.

**chloropred'nisone.** $6\alpha$-Chloro-17,21-dihydroxypregna-1,4-diene-3,11,20-trione; topical anti-inflammatory agent.

**chloropriv'ic.** Deprived of the chlorides or hydrochloric acid.

**chloroprocaine hydrochloride** (klo'ro-pro'kān) (NF). NESACAINE hydrochloride; $\beta$-diethylaminoethyl-2-chloro-4-aminobenzoate hydrochloride. Local anesthetic similar in action and use to procaine hydrochloride.

**chloropsia** (klo-rop'sĭ-ah) [ chloro- + G. *opsis*, eyesight ]. Green vision; chloropia; a condition in which all objects appear to be colored green, as may occur in digitalis intoxication.

**chloropyr'amine.** SYNOPEN; 2-[ *p*-chlorobenzyl-(2-dimethylaminoethyl)amino ]pyridine; antihistaminic agent.

**chlo'roquine phosphate** (USP, BP). SN7618; ARALEN; 7-chloro-4-(4-diethylamino-1-methylbutylamino)quinoline phosphate; an antimalarial agent used for the treatment and suppression of *Plasmodium vivax, P. malariae,* and *P. falciparum*; it does not produce a radical cure because it has no effect on the exoerythrocytic stages; resistant strains have developed in Southeast Asia and South America. Also used for hepatic amebiasis and for certain skin diseases, *e.g.,* lupus erythematosus and lichen planus.

**chlo'roquine sulfate** (BP). Sames uses as chloroquine phosphate.

**chloro'sis** [ chloro- + suffix *-osis*, condition ]. A form of chronic hypochromic microcytic (iron deficiency) anemia, characterized by a great reduction in hemoglobin that is out of proportion to the decreased number of red blood cells. The condition is observed chiefly in girls, from puberty to the third decade, rarely occurring in women more than 25 years of age. C. is usually associated with diets deficient in iron and protein. A similar condition is observed extremely rarely in boys and young men. Also called chlorotic or asiderotic anemia; chloranemia; green sickness.

**Egyptian c.,** ancylostomiasis.

**late c.,** a form of chronic hypochromic anemia (iron-deficient), affecting chiefly women in the third to fifth decades; the condition is frequently associated with poor diets, multiple pregnancies, or chronic wasing diseases.

**tropical c.,** ancylostomiasis.

**chlo'rothen citrate.** TAGATHEN; chloromethapyrilene citrate; *N,N*-dimethyl-*N'*-(2-pyridyl)-*N'*-(5-chloro-2-thenyl ) ethylenediamine citrate. An antihistaminic agent.

**chlorothi'azide** (USP, BP). DIURIL; 6-chloro-7-sulfamyl-1,2,4-benzothiadiazine-1,1-dioxide. An orally effective diuretic inhibiting renal tubular reabsorption of sodium; used in the treatment of edema due to congestive heart failure, liver disease, pregnancy, premenstrual tension, and drugs; also used as an adjunct in the management of hypertension.

**c. sodium** (USAN), suitable for parenteral administration.

**chlorothy'mol.** Monochlorothymol; chlorthymol; $C_{10}H_{13}OCl$; antibacterial for topical use.

**chlorot'ic.** Pertaining to or having the characteristic features of chlorosis.

**chlo'rotrian'isene** (NF, BP). TACE; chlorotris-(*p*-methoxyphenyl)ethylene; tri-*p*-anisylchloroethylene; a synthetic estrogen derived from stilbene. Active by mouth.

**chlo'rous.** Relating to chlorine; denoting compounds of chlorine containing a larger proportion of the element than the chloric compounds.

**c. acid,** $HClO_2$; an acid forming chlorites with bases.

**chlo'rovinyldichloroar'sine.** Lewisite.

**chlorphen'esin** (BP). MYCIL; 3-(*p*-chlorophenoxy)-1,2-propenediol; topical antifungal agent.

**c. carbamate** (USAN), MAOLATE; carbamic acid 3-(*p*-chlorophenoxy)-2-hydroxypropyl ester; skeletal muscle relaxant.

**chlorphenindione.** INDALITON; an anticoagulant related chemically to phenindione.

**chlor'phenir'amine mal'eate** (USP, BP). CHLOR-TRIMETON; ($\pm$)-2-[ *p*-chloro-$\alpha$-[ -2-(dimethylamino)ethyl ]-benzyl ]pyridine maleate; an antihistamine.

**chlorphe'nol red.** An acid-base indicator with a pK value of 6.0; yellow at pH values below 5.1, red above 6.7.

**chlorphenox'amide.** MEBINOL; N-($\beta$-hydroxyethyl)-*N*-[ *p*-(4-nitrophenoxy)benzyl ]dichloroacetamide; amebicide.

**chlor'phenox'amine hydrochloride** (NF). PHENOXENE; SYSTRAL; 2-(*p*-chloro-$\alpha$-methyl-$\alpha$-phenylbenzyloxy)-*N,N*-dimethylethylamine hydrochloride. Used in the management of idiopathic, arteriosclerotic, and postencephalitic parkinsonism, usually with concomitant administration of other anti-Parkinsonian agents.

**chlorphen'termine hydrochloride** (USAN). PRE-SATE; 4-chloro-$\alpha,\alpha$-dimethylphenethylamine hydrochloride; a sympathomimetic amine used as an anorexiant.

**chlorproeth'azine hydrochloride.** NEURIPLEGE; 2-chloro-10-(3-diethylaminopropyl)phenothiazine; skeletal muscle relaxant.

**chlorproguanil hydrochloride** (klor-pro'gwah-nil) (BP). LAPUDRINE; the 3,4-dichloro homologue of chloroguanide; used for causal prophylaxis and suppression of falciparum malaria.

**chlorpro'mazine** (USP). THORAZINE; 10-(3-dimethylaminopropyl)-2-chlorophenothiazine; an antiemetic, antiadrenergic, anticholinergic drug with little ganglion-blocking action. Though chemically related to promethazine, it has no antihistamine action. It depresses conditioned reflexes and the hypothalamic centers, and has a hypotensive action of central origin. Used in psychoses.

**c. hydrochloride** (USP, BP), suitable for oral, intramuscular, and intravenous administration.

**chlorpro'pamide** (USP, BP). DIABINESE; 1-(*p*-chlorophenylsulfonyl)-3-propylurea; an orally effective hypoglycemic agent related chemically and pharmacologically to tolbutamide; used in controlling hyperglycemia in selected patients with diabetes mellitus.

**chlorprothixene** (klor-pro-thik'sēn) (NF, USAN). TARACTAN; 2-chloro-9-(3-dimethylaminopropylidene)thiaxanthene; antipsychotic of the thioxanthene group; it also possesses antiemetic, adrenolytic, spasmolytic, and antihistaminic actions. It must be used with caution in patients with epilepsy and kidney disease.

**chlorquin'aldol.** STEROSAN; 5,7-dichloro-8-hydroxyquinaldine. Keratoplastic, antibacterial, and antifungal agent. Used in the treatment of cutaneous bacterial and mycotic infections.

**chlor'tetracy'cline.** AUREOMYCIN; an antibiotic agent; a naphthacene derivative, obtained from *Streptomyces aureofaciens*. It is active against a wide range of pathogenic microorganisms including hemolytic streptococci, staphylococci, typhoid bacilli, and brucellae, as well as certain viruses. Also available as c. calcium and c. hydrochloride (NF, BP).

**chlorthal'idone** (USP, BP). HYGROTON; 2-chloro-5-(1-hydroxy-3-oxo-1-isoindolinyl)benzenesulfonamide; an orally effective diuretic and antihypertensive agent, used in steroid therapy and the treatment of edema associated with congestive heart failure, renal disease, hepatic cirrhosis, pregnancy, obesity and premenstrual tension. It produces an increase in the excretion of sodium, chloride, potassium, and water.

**chlorthenox'azin.** APIRAZIN; 2-(2-chloroethyl)-2,3-dihydro-4*H*-1,3-benzoxazin-4-one; antipyretic and analgesic.

**chlorthy'mol.** Chlorothymol.

**chloruresis** (klor-u-re'sis). Chloruria; chloriduria; the excretion of chloride in the urine.

**chloruretic** (klor'u-ret'ik). Relating to an agent that increases the excretion of chloride in the urine, or to such an effect.

**chloru'ria.** Chloruresis.

**chlorzox'azone.** PARAFLEX; 5-chloro-2-benzoxazolol; a skeletal muscle relaxant used in the treatment of painful muscle spasm due to musculoskeletal disorder of non-neurologic origin.

**choana,** pl. **choa'nae** (ko'an-ah) [ Mod. L. fr. G. *choanē*, a funnel ] [ NA ]. Posterior naris; postnaris; the opening into the nasopharynx of the nasal cavity on either side.

　　**primary c.,** the initial opening of the nasal pits of the embryo into rostral part of the primordial oronasal cavity, before the formation of the secondary palate.

　　**secondary c.,** the definitive c. opening into the nasopharynx, after the nasal chambers have been lengthened by the formation of the secondary palate.

**cho'anal.** Pertaining to a choana.

**choanate** (ko'an-āt). Having a funnel, *i.e.*, with a ring or collar.

**choanoid** (ko'an-oyd) [ G. *choanē*, funnel, + *eidos*, resemblance ]. Funnel-shaped; infundibuliform.

**choanomastigote** (ko'an-o-mas'ti-gōt) [ G. *choanē*, a funnel, + *mastix*, whip ]. A term in the series used to describe developmental stages of the parasitic flagellates (see amastigote, epimastigote, promastigote, trypomastigote). Denotes the "barleycorn" form of the flagellate in the genus *Crithidia*, found parasitic in insects (stages are often confused with developmental forms of human or other vertebrate parasitic flagellates). The flagellum arises anterior to the nucleus and emerges through a wide funnel-shaped reservoir.

**Choanotae'nia infundib'ulum.** An important cosmopolitan tapeworm of fowls, occurring in the small intestine and transmitted by houseflies and stableflies; it is related to *Dipylidium*, the double-pored dog tapeworm.

**choc** (shok) [ Fr. ]. A poorly coordinated response elicited by stimuli for which the body has no ready prepared adaptation.

　　**c. en dôme,** the accentuated apical impulse of left ventricular hypertrophy, originally regarded as characteristic of aortic insufficiency.

**Chodzko's reflex.** See under reflex.

**choice.** 1. That which is selected. 2. The act of selecting.

　　**object c.,** in psychoanalysis, the object (usually a person) upon which psychic energy is centered.

**choke.** 1. To prevent respiration by compression or obstruction of the larynx or trachea. 2. Any obstruction of the esophagus in herbivorous animals by a partly swallowed foreign body, *e.g.*, an apple, a turnip, or a portion of an ear of corn.

　　**ophthalmovascular c.,** a condition in which the blood supply of the retina is interfered with by mutual pressure of retinal vessels ramifying in such a way as to lie across each other.

　　**thorac'ic c.,** obstruction by a foreign body in the thoracic portion of the esophagus of an animal.

**chokes.** A manifestation of caisson disease or altitude sickness characterized by dyspnea, coughing, and choking.

**chol-.** [ G. *cholē*, bile ]. Combining form denoting relationship to bile.

**cholagogic** (kol-ă-goj'ik). Cholagogue (2).

**cholagogue** (kol'ă-gog) [ chol- + G. *agōgos*, drawing forth ]. 1. An agent that promotes the flow of bile into the intestine, especially as a result of contraction of the gallbladder. 2. Relating to such an agent or effect.

**chola'ic acid.** Taurocholic acid.

**cholalic** (ko-lal'ik). Relating to bile.

　　**c. acid,** cholic acid.

**cho'lane.** Parent hydrocarbon of the cholanic acids (found in cholic acids); androstane with a —CH(CH₃)-CH₂CH₂CH₃ group in the 17 position. 5α-Cholane is sometimes called allocholane. For structures, see steroids.

**cho'laner'esis.** Increase in output of cholic acid or its conjugates.

**cholangeitis** (ko-lan-je-i'tis). [ chol- + G. *angeion*, vessel, + suffix -*itis*, inflammation ]. Cholangitis.

**cholangiectasis** (ko-lan'ji-ek'tā-sis) [ chol- + G. *angeion*, vessel, + *ektasis*, a stretching ]. Dilation of the bile ducts, usually a sequel to obstruction.

**cholangiocarcinoma** (ko-lan'ji-o-kar-sĭ-no'mah). An adenocarcinoma, primary in intrahepatic bile ducts.

**cholangioenterostomy** (ko-lan'ji-o-en'ter-os'to-mĭ). Surgical anastomosis of bile duct to intestine.

**cholangiogastrostomy** (ko-lan'ji-o-gas-tros'to-mĭ) [ chol- + G. *angeion*, vessel, + *gastēr*, belly, + *stoma*, mouth ]. The formation of a communication between a bile duct and the stomach.

**cholangiography** (ko-lan-ji-og'ră-fĭ) [ chol- + G. *angeion*, vessel, + *graphō*, to write ]. Roentgenographic examination of the bile ducts.

　　**cystic duct c.,** introduction of contrast medium through the cystic duct into the biliary system.

　　**percutaneous c.,** visualization of biliary ducts by inserting a needle into the substance of the liver. The needle is introduced through the skin inferior to the right costal margin.

**cholangiole** (ko-lan'ji-ōl) [ chol- + G. *angeion*, vessel, + -*ole*, dim. suffix ]. Canal of Hering; a ductule occurring between a bile canaliculus and an interlobular bile duct.

**cholangiolitis** (ko-lan'ji-o-li'tis). An inflammation of the small bile radicles or cholangioles sometimes leading to cholangiolitic cirrhosis.

**cholangioma** (ko-lan'ji-o'mah) [ chol- + G. *angeion*, vessel, + suffix -*oma*, tumor ]. A neoplasm of bile duct origin, especially within the liver; may be either benign or malignant (the latter is termed a cholangiocarcinoma).

**cholangios'copy** (ko-lan'ji-os'ko-pĭ) [ chol- + G. *angeion*, vessel, + *skopeō*, to examine ]. Visual examination of bile ducts by aid of cystoscope.

**cholangios'tomy** (ko-lan-ji-os'to-mĭ) [ chol- + G. *angeion*, vessel, + *stoma*, mouth ]. The surgical formation of a fistula into a bile duct.

**cholangiotomy** (ko-lan-ji-ot'o-mĭ) [ chol- + G. *angeion*, vessel, + *tomē*, incision ]. Incision into a bile duct.

**cholangitis** (ko-lan-ji'tis) [ chol- + G. *angeion*, vessel, + suffix -*itis*, inflammation ]. Cholangeitis; angiocholitis; inflammation of a bile duct.

**cholanic acids** (ko-lan'ik). 1. Cholic acids; cholan-24-oic acids. 2. Ursocholanic acid; see also cholic acid.

**cholan-24-oic acids.** Cholanic acids; see *cholic* acids.

**cholanopoiesis** (ko'lă-no-poy-e'sis) [ chol- + G. *anō*, upward, + *poiēsis*, making ]. The synthesis by the liver of cholic acid or its conjugates, or of natural bile salts.

**cho'lanopoiet'ic.** Pertaining to or promoting cholanopoiesis.

**cholan'threne.** A polycyclic, somewhat carcinogenic hydrocarbon, structural parent of the highly carcinogenic 3 (or 20)-methylcholanthrene, *q.v.*

**cholascos** (ko-las'kos) [ chol- + G. *askos*, bag ]. The escape of bile into the free peritoneal cavity.

**cho'late.** A salt or ester of a cholic acid.

　　**c. synthetase or thiokinase,** choloyl-CoA synthetase; see under choloyl.

**chole-** (ko'le-, kol'e) [ G. *cholē*, bile ]. Combining form relating to bile.

**cho'lecalcif'erol.** 1. Vitamin D₃; 9,10-secocholesta-5,7,10(19)-trien-3β-ol; formed by breakage of 9,10 bond in 7-dehydrocholesterol by ultraviolet irradiation, yielding a double bond between C-10 and C-19. Probably the vitamin D of animal origin; found in skin, fur, feathers of animals and birds exposed to sunlight, also in butter, brain, fish oils, and egg yolk. 2 (USP). Activated 5,7-cholestadien-3β-ol; an antirachitic, oil-soluble vitamin; one unit is defined as the activity of 0.025 μg. of vitamin D₃ present in the USP vitamin D reference standard.

**cholechrome** (ko'le-krōm). Bile pigment.

**cholechromopoiesis** (ko'le-kro-mo-poy-e'sis) [ chole- + G. *chrōma*, color, + *poiesis*, making ]. The synthesis of bile pigments by the liver.

**cholecyanin** (ko-le-si'an-in). Bilicyanin.

**cholecyst** (ko'le-sist). *Vesica fellea*.

**cholecystagogic** (ko-le-sis'tăgoj'ik). Stimulating activity of the gallbladder.

**cholecystagogue** (ko'le-sis'tă-gog) [ chole- + G. *kystis,* bladder, + *agōgos,* leader ]. A substance that stimulates activity of the gallbladder.

**cho'lecystat'ony.** [ chole- + G. *kystis,* bladder, + *atonia,* atony ]. Atonia, weakness, or failure of function of the gallbladder.

**cholecystectasia** (ko-le-sis-tek-ta'zī-ah) [ chole- + G. *kystis,* bladder, + *ektasis,* extension ]. Dilation of the gallbladder.

**cholecystectomy** (ko-le-sis-tek'to-mī) [ chole- + G. *kystis,* bladder, + *ektomē,* excision ]. Surgical removal of the gallbladder.

**cholecystendysis** (ko-le-sis-ten'dī-sis) [ chole- + G. *kystis,* bladder, + *endysis,* an entering in ]. Cholecystotomy.

**cho'lecysten'teroanas'tomo'sis.** Cholecystenterostomy.

**cholecystenterorrhaphy** (ko-le-sist-en-ter-or'ă-fī) [ chole- + G. *kystis,* bladder, + *enteron,* intestine + *rhaphē,* suture ]. Suture of the gallbladder to the intestinal wall.

**cholecystenterostomy** (ko-le-sist-en-ter-os'to-mī) [ chole- + G. *kystis,* bladder, + *enteron,* intestine, + *stoma,* mouth ]. Cholecysteroanastomosis; enterocholecystostomy; surgical formation of a direct communication between the gallbladder and the intestine.

**cholecystic** (ko-le-sis'tik). Relating to the cholecyst, or gallbladder.

**cholecystis** (ko-le-sis'tis) [ chole- + G. *kystis,* bladder ]. *Vesica fellea.*

**cholecystitis** (ko-le-sis-ti'tis) [ chole- + G. *kystis,* bladder, + suffix *-itis,* inflammation ]. Inflammation of the gallbladder.

    **acute c.,** acute inflammation with congestion and edema or hemorrhagic necrosis of the gallbladder wall, usually due to impaction of a stone in the cystic duct; infrequently due to infection.

    **chronic c.,** chronic inflammation of the gallbladder, usually secondary to lithiasis.

    **emphysematous c.,** c. with a gas-producing organism, giving rise to gas in the gallbladder.

    **c. glandularis proliferans,** Rokitansky-Aschoff sinuses; possibly a misnomer, as the sinuses may be diverticula which do not result from inflammation.

    **xanthogranulomatous c.,** chronic c. with sometimes conspicuous nodular infiltration by lipid macrophages; may be associated with biliary obstruction by calculi.

**cholecys'tocele.** A swelling or hernia of the gallbladder.

**cholecystocolostomy** (ko-le-sis-to-ko-los'to-mī) [ chole- + G. *kystis,* bladder, + *kolon,* colon, + *stoma,* mouth ]. Cystocolostomy; operative establishment of a communication between the gallbladder and the colon.

**cholecystoduodenostomy** (ko-le-sis'to-du-o-de-nos'to-mī) [ chole- + G. *kystis,* bladder, + L. *duodenum* + G. *stoma,* mouth ]. Operative establishment of a direct communication between the gallbladder and the duodenum.

**cholecystogastrostomy** (ko-le-sis'to-gas-tros'to-mī) [ chole- + G. *kystis,* bladder, + *gastēr,* stomach, + *stoma,* mouth ]. The operative establishment of a communication between the gallbladder and the stomach.

**cholecystog'raphy** [ chole- + G. *kystis,* bladder, + *grapho,* to write ]. Visualization of the gallbladder by roentgen rays after the administration of a radiopaque substance such as sodium tetraiodophenolphthalein which is excreted by the liver and concentrated by the normal gallbladder.

**cholecystoileostomy** (ko-le-sis'to-il-e-os'to-mī) [ chole- + G. *kystis,* bladder, + *ileum* + G. *stoma,* mouth ]. The operative establishment of a communication between the gallbladder and the ileum.

**cholecystojejunostomy** (ko-le-sis'to-je-ju-nos'-to-mī) [ chole- + G. *kystis,* bladder, + *jejunum* (see JEJ-), + G. *stoma,* mouth ]. The surgical establishment of a communication between the gallbladder and the jejunum.

**cho'lecys'tokin'ase.** An enzyme catalyzing the hydrolysis of cholecystokinin.

**cho'lecys'tokinet'ic.** Promoting emptying of the gallbladder.

**cholecystoki'nin.** A hormone liberated by the upper intestinal mucosa on contact with gastric contents; stimulates the contraction of the gallbladder.

**cholecystolithiasis** (ko-le-sis'to-lith-i'ă-sis) [ chole- + G. *kystis,* bladder, + *lithos,* stone ]. The presence of one or more gallstones in the gallbladder.

**cholecystolithotripsy** (ko-le-sis'to-lith'o-trip-sī) [ chole- + G. *kystis,* bladder, + *lithos,* stone, + *tripsis,* a rubbing ]. The crushing of a gallstone by manipulation of the unopened gallbladder.

**cholecystomy** (ko-le-sis'to-mī). Cholecystotomy.

**cholecyston'cus.** An undesirable term formerly used for a neoplasm of the gallbladder.

**cho'lecystop'athy.** Disease of the gallbladder.

**cholecystopexy** (ko-le-sis'to-pek-sī) [ chole- + G. *kystis,* bladder, + *pēxis,* fixation ]. Suture of the gallbladder to the abdominal wall.

**cholecystorrhaphy** (ko-le-sis-tor'ă-fī) [ chole- + G. *kystis,* bladder, + *rhaphē,* sewing ]. Suture of the incised or ruptured gallbladder.

**cholecystostomy** (ko-le-sis-tos'to-mī) [ chole- + G. *kystis,* bladder, + *stoma,* mouth ]. The surgical establishment of a fistula into the gallbladder.

**cholecystotomy** (ko-le-sis-tot'o-mī) [ chole- + G. *kystis,* bladder, + *tomē,* incision ]. Cholecystendysis; incision into the gallbladder.

**choledoch-.** See choledocho-.

**choledoch** (ko'le-dok) [ G. *cholēdochos,* containing bile, fr. *cholē,* bile, + *dechomai,* to receive ]. *Ductus choledochus.*

**choledochal** (ko-le-dok'al, ko-led'o-kal). Relating to the common bile duct.

**choledochectomy** (ko-led-o-kek'to-mī) [ choledoch- + G. *ektomē,* excision ]. Surgical removal of a portion of the common bile duct.

**choledochendysis** (ko-le-dok-en'di-sis) [ choledoch- + G. *endysis,* an entering in ]. Choledochotomy.

**choledochiarctia** (k0-le-dok-e-ark'te-ah) [ choledoch- + L. *artus* (improperly *arctus*), narrow ]. Stenosis of the gall duct.

**choledochitis** (ko-led-o-ki'tis) [ choledoch- + G. suffix *-itis,* inflammation ]. Inflammation of the common bile duct.

**choledocho-, cholodoch-** [ G. *cholēdochos,* containing bile, fr. *cholē,* bile, + *dechomai,* to receive ]. Combining forms relating to the ductus choledochus (the common bile duct).

**choledochocholedocostomy** (ko-led'o-ko-ko-led'o-kos'-to-mī). Operative joining of divided portions of common bile duct.

**choledochoduodenostomy** (ko-led'o-ko-du-o-de-nos'to-mī) [ choledocho- + duodenum + G. *stoma,* mouth ]. Surgical formation of a communication, other than the natural one, between the common bile duct and the duodenum.

**choledochoenterostomy** (ko-led'o-ko-en-ter-os'to-mī) [ choledocho- + G. *enteron,* intestine, + *stoma,* mouth ]. Surgical establishment of a communication, other than the natural one, between the common bile duct and any part of the intestine.

**choledochography** (ko-led'o-kog'rā-fī). Roentgenographic examination of the bile duct after the administration of a radiopaque substance.

**choledochojejunostomy** (ko-led'o-ko-jĕ-ju-nos'to-mī). Surgical anastomosis between common bile duct and jejunum.

**choledocholith** (ko-led'o-ko-lith) [ choledocho- + G. *lithos,* stone ]. Stone in the common bile duct.

**choledocholithiasis** (ko-led'o-ko-lith-i'ă-sis). The presence of a gallstone in the common bile duct.

**choledocholithotomy** (ko-led'o-ko-lī-thot'o-mī) [ choledocho- + G. *lithos,* stone, + *tomē,* incision ]. Incision of the common bile duct for the extraction of an impacted gallstone.

**choledocholithotripsy** (ko-led'o-ko-lith'o-trip-sī) [ choledocho- + G. *lithos,* stone, + *tripsis,* rubbing ]. Choledocholithotrity; crushing of a gallstone in the common duct by manipulation without opening of the duct.

**choledocholithot'rity.** Choledocholithotripsy.

**choledochoplasty** (ko-led'o-ko-plas'tī). A plastic operation on the common bile duct.

**choledochorrhaphy** (ko-led-o-kor′ră-fĭ) [ choledocho- + G. *rhaphē*, suture ]. Suturing together the divided ends of the common bile duct.

**choledochostomy** (ko-led-o-kos′to-mĭ) [ choledocho- + G. *stoma*, mouth ]. The surgical establishment of a fistula into the common bile duct.

**choledochotomy** (ko-led-o-kot′o-mĭ) [ choledocho- + G. *tomē*, incision ]. Choledochendysis; incision into the common bile duct.

**choledochous** (ko-led′o-kus). Containing or conveying bile.

**choledochus** (ko-led′o-kus) [ see choledoch ]. *Ductus* choledochus.

**choleglobin** (ko′le-glo′bin). A pigmented compound of globin and iron porphyrin (with an open ring due to cleavage of the α-methene bridge by α-methyl oxygenase). The first intermediate in the degradation of hemoglobin; Further degraded to verdohemochrome, biliverdin, and bilirubin. Also termed bile pigment hemoglobin; verdohemoglobin.

**cholehematin** (ko′le-he′mah-tin). A red pigment in the bile of herbivorous animals, derived from chlorophyll. A product of hematin oxidation.

**cholehemia** (ko-le-he′mĭ-ah) [ chole- + G. *haima*, blood ]. Cholemia.

**cholehemochro′mogen.** A substance derived from choleglobin or hemoglobin by chemical treatment; obsolete.

**choleic** (ko-le′ik). Cholic.

**c. acids,** complexes of bile acids with sterols.

**cholelith** (ko′le-lith) [ chole- + G. *lithos*, stone ]. Gallstone.

**cholelithiasis** (ko′le-lĭ-thi′ă-sis). A condition in which concretions are present in the gallbladder or bile ducts.

**cholelithotomy** (ko′le-lĭ-thot′o-mĭ) [ chole- + G. *lithos*, stone, + *tomē*, incision ]. Operative removal of a gallstone.

**cholelithotripsy** (ko-le-lith′o-trip-sĭ) [ chole- + G. *lithos*, stone, + *tripsis*, a rubbing ]. Cholelithotrity; the crushing of a gallstone.

**cholelithotrity** (ko-le-lĭ-thot′rĭ-tĭ) [ chole- + G. *lithos*, stone, + L. *tero*, pp. *tritus*, to rub ]. Cholelithotripsy.

**cholemesis** (ko-lem′e-sis) [ chole- + G. *emesis*, vomiting ]. Vomiting of bile.

**cholemia** (ko-le′mĭ-ah). [ chole- + G. *haima*, blood ]. The presence of bile salts in the circulating blood.

**chole′mic.** Relating to cholemia.

**cholepathia** (ko-le-path′ĭ-ah). 1. Disease of bile ducts. 2. Irregularity in contractions of the bile ducts.

**c. spas′tica,** spastic contraction of the bile ducts.

**cho′leper′itone′um.** Bile in the peritoneum, which may lead to bile peritonitis.

**cho′leperitoni′tis.** Inflammation resulting from bile in the peritoneal cavity.

**cholepoiesis** (ko′le-poi-e′sis) [ chole- + G. *poiēsis*, a making ]. Cholopoiesis; formation of bile.

**cholepoietic** (ko′le-poi-et′ik). Relating to the formation of bile.

**cholepyrrhin** (ko-le-pir′in). Impure bilirubin.

**cholera** (kol′er-ah) [ L. a bilious disease, fr. G. *cholē*, bile. CHOL- ]. 1. Formerly, a nonspecific term for a variety of gastrointestinal disturbances. 2. Asiatic c.; an acute epidemic infectious disease of man caused by *Vibrio cholerae* and occurring chiefly in Asia. A soluble toxin elaborated in the intestinal tract by the vibrio alters the permeability of the mucosa, causing a profuse watery diarrhea, extreme loss of fluid and electrolytes, and a state of collapse. The toxin does not cause any morphologic change in the intestinal mucosa. Dramatic recovery follows intravenous replacement of electrolytes and fluid.

**Asiatic c.,** c. (2); so called because it occurs chiefly in Asia (especially India and Pakistan), also to distinguish it from c. morbus, formerly very common in the western world.

**chicken c.,** fowl c.

**fowl c.,** a destructive disease of domestic fowls caused by *Pasteurella multocida;* chicken c.

**hog c.,** swine fever; swine c.; swine pest; an acute, highly infectious, highly fatal virus disease of swine characterized by a sudden onset and high fever; the United States has an eradication program.

**c. infan′tum,** an old term for a disease of infants, characterized by vomiting, profuse watery diarrhea, fever, great prostration, and collapse.

**c. morbus,** an old term for acute severe gastroenteritis of unknown etiology, marked by severe colic, vomiting, and watery stools, formerly common during hot weather.

**c. sicca** [ L. dry ], an old term for a malignant form of disease seen during epidemics of Asiatic c. in which death occurs without diarrhea.

**swine c.,** hog c.

**typhoid c.,** an old term for Asiatic c. with predominantly cerebral manifestations.

**choleragen** (kol′er-ah-jen) [ cholera + G. suffix -*gen*, producing ]. A term suggested for a factor (or factors) that is produced during growth *in vitro* of the cholera vibrio and that causes diarrhea.

**choleraic** (kol′er-a′ik). Relating to cholera.

**choleraphage** (kol′er-ă-fāj) [ cholera + G. *phagein*, to eat ]. Bacteriophage of the cholera bacillus.

**choleresis** (kol-er-e′sis). The secretion of bile as opposed to the expulsion of bile by the gallbladder.

**choleretic** (ko-ler-et′ik). Relating to choleresis.

**choleriform** (kol′er-ĭ-form). Resembling cholera.

**cholerigenic** (kol′er-ĭ-jen′ik). Cholerigenous; causing or engendering cholera.

**cholerigenous** (kol-er-ij′en-us). Cholerigenic.

**cholerine** (kol′er-ēn). A mild form of diarrhea seen during epidemics of Asiatic cholera.

**cholerization** (kol′er-ĭ-za′shun). Inoculation with cholera as a prophylactic measure.

**choleroid** (kol′er-oyd). Resembling cholera; choleriform.

**cholerrhagia** (kol′er-ra′jĭ-ah) [ chole- + G. *rhegnymi*, to burst forth ]. Extensive flow of bile.

**cholerrhagic** (kol-e-raj′ik). Referring to the flow of bile.

**cholestane** (ko′les-tān). The parent hydrocarbon of cholesterol; androstane with a —CH(CH₃)CH₂CH₂CH₂CH-(CH₃)₂ group in position 17(β). The 5β form is sometimes known as coprostane; for structure, see steroids.

**choles′tanol.** Dihydrocholesterol; 3(β)-hydroxycholestane; differing from cholesterol in the absence of the double bond. For structure of cholestane, see steroids.

**choles′tanone.** An oxidation product of dihydrocholesterol, differing from it in the presence of a ketone oxygen in place of the 3-hyroxyl group; an isomer of coprostanone.

**cholestasia, cholestasis** (ko-les-ta′sĭ-ah, ko-les′ta-sis) [ chole- + G. *stasis*, a standing still ]. An arrest in the flow of bile.

**cholestat′ic.** Tending to diminish or stop the flow of bile.

**cholesteatoma** (ko-les-te-ă-to′mah) [ chole- + steatoma ]. A tumor-like mass of keratinizing squamous epithelium and cholesterol in the middle ear, usually resulting from chronic otitis media, with squamous metaplasia or extension of squamous epithelium inward to line an expanding cystic cavity that may involve the mastoid and erode surrounding bone. 2. An epidermoid cyst arising in the central nervous system in man or animals, commonly in the lateral ventricle of old horses.

**choles′tenone.** A dehydrocholestanone, differing from cholestanone in the presence of a double bond between carbons 4 and 5.

**cholesteremia** (ko-les-ter-e′mĭ-ah) [ cholesterol + G. *haima*, blood ]. Cholesterinemia; cholesterolemia; the presence of enhanced quantities of cholesterol in the blood.

**choles′teride.** A cholesteryl ester of a fatty acid, *e.g.*, cholesteryl palmitate.

**cholesterin** (ko-les′ter-in) Cholesterol.

**cholesterinemia** (ko-les-ter-in-e′mĭ-ah) Cholesteremia.

**cholesterino′sis.** Cholesterolosis.

**cerebrotendinous c.,** cerebrotendinous *xanthomatosis*.

**cholesterinuria** (ko-les-ter-in-u′rĭ-ah) [ cholesterin + G. *ouron*, urine ]. Cholesteroluria.

**choles′teroder′ma.** Xanthochromia.

**choles′terohy′drotho′rax.** Hydrothorax in which the fluid contains cholesterol.

**cholesterol** (ko-les′ter-ol). Cholesterin; 5-cholesten-3β-ol (cholestane with a 5,6 double bond and a 3β hydroxyl group). For structure of cholestane, see steroids. The most abundant steroid in animal tissues, especially in bile and gallstones. It is official in the USP; used in the preparation of hydrophilic petrolatum.

**c. balance,** the relationship between the intake of c. and its manufacture by the body to its utilization, sequestration, or excretion from the body. When the input equals output, a state of balance exists; when c. accumulates, the balance is positive; when it declines, the balance is negative.

**c. es′tersturz,** decrease in the ratio of ester to total c. of blood, a phenomenon noted in parenchymatous hepatic disease.

**cholesterolemia** (ko-les-ter-ol-e′mi-ah) [ cholesterol + G. *haima,* blood ]. Cholesteremia.

**choles′terologen′esis.** The biosynthesis of cholesterol.

**cholesterolosis** (ko-les′ter-ol-o′sis). Cholesterinosis; cholesterosis. 1. A condition resulting from a disturbance in metabolism of lipids, characterized by deposits of cholesterol in tissue, as, for example, in Tangier disease. 2. Cholesterol crystals in the anterior chamber of the eye; it occurs occasionally in blindness following severe trauma and may be followed by hyphema and secondary glaucoma.

**cholesteroluria** (ko-les′ter-ol-u′rī-ah). The excretion of cholesterol in urine.

**cholestero′sis.** Cholesterolosis.

**c. cu′tis,** xanthomatosis.

**choletelin** (ko-let′el-in). Bilixanthin.

**choletherapy** (ko-le-ther′ă-pī). Treatment of disease by the use of oxgall.

**choleuria** (ko-le-u′rī-ah). Biliuria.

**cho′lever′din.** Biliverdin.

**Cholewa** (kho-la′vah), Erasmus R., German physician, *1845. See Itard-C. *sign.*

**cholic** (kol′ik). Relating to the bile.

**c. acid,** accepted trivial name (replacing cholalic and cholanic acids) for a family of steroids comprising the bile acids (or salts), generally in conjugated form (*e.g.,* glycocholic and taurocholic acids). Chemically, cholic acids are cholan-24-oic (cholanic) acids (the terminal $C_{24}$ of cholane becoming a —COOH group; for structure of cholane, see steroids). Biologically, cholic acids are derived from cholesterol (a cholestane derivative) and display varying degrees of oxidation (OH groups) and orientation at positions 3, 6, 7, and 12. It is these oxidations and orientations that distinguish the several cholic acids. Thus, cholic acid is 3α,7α,12α-trihydroxy-5β-cholan-24-oic acid; ursocholic acid is 3α,7β,12α-tri-. . .; deoxycholic acid is 3α,12α-di-. . .; chenodeoxycholic acid is 3α,7α-di- . . .; hyodeoxycholic acid is 3α,6α-di-. . .; ursodeoxycholic acid is 3α,7β-di-. . .; and lithocholic acid is 3α-. . . (ellipses stand for hydroxy-5β-cholan-24-oic acid or hydroxy-5β-cholanic acid).

**cholicele** (ko′lē-sēl) [ G. *cholē,* bile, + *kēlē,* tumor ]. Enlargement of the gallbladder due to retained fluids.

**choline** (ko′lēn). (2-Hydroxyethyl)trimethylammonium ion; $HOCH_2$—$CH_2$—$N(CH_3)_3^+$; lipotropic factor; transmethylation factor; found in most animal tissues either free or in combination with lecithin (phosphatidyl choline) or acetate (acetylcholine) or cytidine diphosphate. It is included in the vitamin B complex; in experimental animals, a lack of this factor causes fatty liver or hepatic cirrhosis; it prevents the fatty degenerative changes that frequently occur in pancreatectomized animals. As acetylcholine, it is essential for synaptic transmission. Several salts of choline are used in medicine. Amanitine, bilineurine, bursine, fagine, gossypine, luridine, sincaline, and vidine are all more or less archaic terms for choline.

**c. acetylase,** c. acetyltransferase.

**c. acetyltransferase** (EC 2.3.1.6), c. acetylase; an enzyme catalyzing the condensation of choline and acetyl-coenzyme A, forming acetylcholine.

**c. chloride,** HEPACHOLINE; lipotropic agent.

**c. dihydrogen citrate,** (2-hydroxyethyl)trimethylammonium citrate; lipotropic agent.

**c. esterase I,** acetylcholinesterase.

**c. esterase II,** cholinesterase.

**c. gluconate,** (2-hydroxyethyl)trimethylammonium D-gluconate; same use as c. dihydrogen citrate.

**c. kinase** (EC 2.7.1.32), c. phosphokinase; an enzyme which, in the presence of ATP, catalyzes the formation of phosphorylcholine from choline.

**c. phosphatase,** phospholipase D.

**c. phosphokinase,** c. kinase.

**c. salicylate,** ACTASAL; salicyclic acid choline salt; (2-hydroxyethyl)trimethylammonium salicylate; analgesic and antipyretic.

**c. theophyllinate** (BP), CHOLEDYL; theophylline cholinate; choline salt of theophylline; a bronchodilator administered orally.

**cho′linephosphotrans′ferase** (EC 2.7.8.2), enzyme catalyzing the reaction between CDP-choline and 1,2-diacylglycerol to form phosphatidylcholine.

**cholinergic** (kol-in-er′jik) [ choline + G. *ergon,* work ]. Relating to nerve fibers that cause effects similar to those induced by acetylcholine; introduced by H. H. Dale; *cf.* adrenergic.

**chol′inester.** An ester of choline, *e.g.,* acetylcholine.

**cholinesterase** (ko′lin-es′ter-as). (EC 3.1.1.8). Pseudocholinesterase; benzoyl cholinesterase; butyrylcholine esterase; butyrocholinesterase; choline esterase II; nonspecific or "s"-type cholinesterase; one of a family of enzymes capable of catalyzing the hydrolysis of acylcholines and a few other compounds. See also acetylcholinesterase.

**"e"-type c.** [ "e" in erythrocyte ], acetylcholinesterase.

**nonspecific c.,** cholinesterase.

**c. reactivator,** a drug that reacts directly with the alkylphosphorylated enzyme to free the active unit; the drugs used therapeutically to reactivate phosphorylated forms of acetylcholinesterase are oximes, *e.g.,* diacetylmonoxime and monoisonitrosoacetone.

**"s"-type c.** [ "s" in serum ], cholinesterase.

**specific c.,** acetylcholinesterase.

**true c.,** acetylcholinesterase.

**chol′inocep′tive.** Refers to chemical sites in effector cells with which acetylcholine unites to exert its actions; *cf.* adrenoceptive.

**chol′inolyt′ic.** Preventing the action of acetylcholine.

**chol′inomimet′ic.** Having an action similar to that of acetylcholine, the substance liberated by cholinergic nerves. Term coined by W. B. Youmans and proposed by him to replace the less accurate term, parasympathomimetic; *cf.* adrenomimetic.

**cholinoreactive** (kol′in-o-re-ak′tiv). Responding to acetylcholine and related compounds.

**chol′inorecep′tors.** See cholinergic *receptors.*

**cholis′tine sulphometh′ate sodium** 56 (BP). Colistimethate sodium.

**cholo-** (kol-o-, ko-lo-) [ G. *cholē,* bile ]. Combining form denoting relationship to bile.

**chol′ogen′ic.** Bile-producing.

**chololith** (kol′o-lith). Cholelith.

**chololithiasis** (kol′o-lith-i′ă-sis). Cholelithiasis.

**chololithic** (kol′o-lith′ik). Relating in any way to gallstones.

**choloplania** (kol-o-pla′nī-ah) [ cholo- + G. *planē,* a wandering ]. The presence of bile salts in the blood or tissues.

**cholopoiesis** (kol′o-poy-e′sis). Cholepoiesis.

**cholorrhea** (kol-or-re′ah) [ cholo- + G. *rhoia,* a flow ]. An excessive secretion of bile.

**cholos′copy.** [ cholo- + G. *skopeō,* to view ]. Examination of the interior of the bile ducts through an endoscope.

**cholotho′rax.** Bile in the pleural cavity.

**choloyl** (ko′lo-il). The radical of cholic acid (or cholate), as in choloyl-CoA, etc.

**choloyl-CoA synthetase.** Cholate thiokinase (EC 6.2.1.7); converts cholate to choloyl-CoA with cleavage of ATP to AMP.

**choluria** (ko-lu′rī-ah) [ G. *cholē,* bile, + *ouron,* urine ]. Biliuria.

**cholylcoenzyme A** (ko′lil-ko-en′zim). A condensation product of cholic acid and coenzyme A, an intermediate in the formation of bile salts from bile acids, as taurocholic acid from cholic acid.

**cholysteramine resin.** See under resin.

**Chondodendron** (kon'do-den'dron). A small genus of woody vines or high-climbing shrubs with large leaves, indigenous to Brazil, Peru, and Ecuador; certain species, particulary *C. tomentosum*, yield curare and are the source of *d*-tubocurarine. The root of *C. tomentosum* yields pareira brava, a crude drug formerly used in the treatment of disorders of the urinary bladder.

**chondral** (kon'dral) [ G. *chondros*, cartilage ]. Relating to cartilage.

**chondralgia** (kon-dral'jī-ah) [ G. *chondros*, cartilage, + *algos*, pain ]. Chondrodynia.

**chondralloplasia** (kon'dral-o-pla'zī-ah) [ G. *chondros*, cartilage, + *allos*, other, + *plasia*, a molding ]. The occurrence of cartilage in abnormal situations in the bony skeleton.

**chondrectomy** (kon-drek'to-me) [ G. *chondros*, cartilage, + *ektomē*, excision ]. Excision of a cartilage.

**Chondrich'thyes** [ G. *chondros*, cartilage, + *ichthys*, a fish ]. The cartilaginous fishes; a class comprising the sharks, rays, and chimeras.

**chondrification** (kon-drī-fī-ka'shun) [ G. *chondros*, cartilage, + L. *facio*, to make ]. Conversion into cartilage.

**chondrify** (kon-drī-fi). To become cartilaginous.

**chondrin** (kon'drin). A gelatin-like substance obtained from cartilage by boiling.

**chondrio-.** For words beginning thus, see chondro-.

**chondritis** (kon-dri'tis) [ G. *chondros*, cartilage, + suffix -*itis*, inflammation ]. Inflammation of cartilage.

   **costal c.,** inflammation with pain and sometimes with swelling of the costal cartilages. May be mistaken for angina or heart trouble; it is sometimes associated with respiratory infection.

**chondro-, chondrio-** [ G. *chondrion*, dim. of *chondros*, groats (coarsely ground grain), grit, gristle, cartilage. CHOND- ]. Combining forms meaning, or relating to, (1) cartilage or cartilaginous, and (2) granular or gritty substance.

**chon'droalbumoid.** One of the proteins of cartilage.

**chondroblast** (kon'dro-blast) [ chondro- + G. *blastos*, germ ]. Chondroplast; a cell of growing cartilage tissue.

**chon'droblasto'ma.** A highly cellular but benign tumor arising in the epiphyses of long bones in young people; it consists of tissue resembling fetal cartilage; also called benign epiphysial c.; Codman's tumor.

**chondrocalcinosis** (kon'dro-kal-sī-no-sis) [ chondro- + calcium + G. suffix -*osis*, condition ]. Calcification of cartilage.

   **articular c.,** pseudogout; a disease characterized by calcified deposits, free from urate and consisting of calcium pyrophosphate crystals, in articular cartilage and adjacent soft tissue; it leads to goutlike attacks of pain and swelling of the involved joints, and to eventual osteoarthrosis. It seems to be inherited in some families, and associated with hyperparathyroidism in others.

**chondroclast** (kon'dro-klast) [ chondro- + G. *klastos*, broken in pieces ]. A multinucleated cell concerned with reabsorption of cartilage.

**chondrocostal** (kon-dro-kos'tal) [ chondro- + L. *costa*, rib ]. Relating to the costal cartilages.

**chondrocranium** (kon-dro-kra'nī-um) [ chondro- + G. *kranion*, skull ]. A cartilaginous skull; the cartilaginous parts of the developing skull.

**chondrocyte** (kon'dro-sit) [ chondro- + G. *kytos*, a hollow (cell) ]. Cartilage cell; a connective tissue cell that occupies a lacuna within the cartilage matrix.

   **isogenous c.'s,** a group derived from one cell by division.

**chondrodermati'tis nodular'is chron'ica hel'icis.** Winkler's disease; a benign, chronic, small, painful nodule (or nodules) on the helix of the ear; may occasionally ulcerate.

**chondrodynia** (kon-dro-din'ī-ah) [ chondro- + G. *odyne*, pain ]. Chondralgia; pain in cartilage.

**chondrodysplasia** (kon'dro-dis-pla'zī-ah) [ chondro- + G. *dys*, bad, + *plasis*, a molding ]. Chondrodystrophy.

   **hereditary deforming c.,** obsolete term for hereditary multiple *exostoses*.

**chondrodystro'phia.** Chondrodystrophy.

   **c. calcif'icans congen'ita,** *dysplasia* epiphysialis punctata.

   **c. congen'ita puncta'ta,** Conradi's *disease*.

**chondrodystrophy** (kon-dro-dis'tro-fī) [ chondro- + G. *dys*, bad, + *trophe*, nourishment ]. Chondrodysplasia; a disturbance in the development of the cartilage primordia of the long bones involving especially the region of the epiphysial plates, and resulting in arrested growth of the long bones and a condition of stocky dwarfism. The head and trunk are of essentially normal proportions but the extremities are abnormally short.

   **asymmetrical c.,** Ollier's *disease*.

   **hereditary deforming c.,** hereditary multiple *exostoses*.

**chondroectodermal** (kon'dro-ek'to-der'mal). Relating to ectodermally derived cartilage, e.g., branchial cartilages that may have developed from the neural crest.

**chondrofibroma** (kon-dro-fi-bro'mah). Chondromyxoid *fibroma*.

**chondrogenesis** (kon-dro-jen'e-sis) [ chondro- + G. *genesis*, origin ]. The formation of cartilage.

**chondroglossus** (kon-dro-glos'us) [ chondro- + G. *glossa*, tongue ]. See *musculus* chondroglossus.

**chon'drohypopla'sia.** A mild form of achondroplasia; affected individuals survive into adult life.

**chondroid** (kon'droyd) [ chondro- + G. *eidos*, resemblance ]. 1. Cartilaginoid; resembling cartilage. 2. Cartilaginous; relating to or consisting of cartilage. 3. Cartilage not characteristically developed which is primarily cellular with capsules thin or lacking and with a basophilic matrix.

**chondroitin** (kon-dro'ī-tin). A mucopolysaccharide which upon hydrolysis yields acetic acid, glucuronic acid, and galactosamine. Present in chondrin, generally as the c. sulfate.

   **c. sulfate,** a combination of sulfuric acid with glycuronic acid, galactosamine, and acetic acid; found in connective tissue.

   **c. sulfate B,** dermatan sulfate.

**chondrology** (kon-drol'o-jī) [ chondro- + G. *logos*, treatise ]. Science in relation to cartilage and the cartilages.

**chondroma** (kon-dro'mah) [ chondro- + G. suffix -*ōma*, tumor ]. A benign neoplasm derived from mesodermal cells that form cartilage; c.'s that develop within a bone are termed enchondromas; c.'s that develop from periosteum or parosteal connective tissue are termed juxtacortical or periosteal c.'s.

   **c. sarcomato'sum,** obsolete term for chondrosarcoma.

**chondromalacia** (kon-dro-mal-a'shī-ah) [ chondro- + G. *malakia*, softness ]. Softening of any cartilage.

   **c. feta'lis,** an intrauterine form of c. in which the fetus is born dead with soft pliable limbs.

   **generalized c.,** relapsing *perichondritis*.

   **c. of larynx,** laryngomalacia; the presence of soft laryngeal cartilage, most often seen in chronic atrophic polychondritis.

**chondromatosis** (kon-dro-mā-to'sis). The presence of multiple tumor-like foci of cartilage.

   **synovial c.,** c. occurring in the synovial membrane of a joint.

**chondromatous** (kon-dro'mā-tus). Pertaining to or manifesting the features of a chondroma.

**chon'dromere** [ chondro- + G. *meros*, part ]. A cartilage unit of the axial skeleton developing within a single metamere of the body; a primordial cartilaginous vertebra together with its costal component.

**chon'dromu'cin.** Chondromucoid.

**chondromucoid** (kon'dro-mu'koyd). A mucoprotein found in cartilage; it contains chondroitin sulfate.

**chondromyxoma** (kon'dro-mik-so'mah). Chondromyxoid *fibroma*.

**chondro-osseous** (kon'dro-os'e-us). Relating to cartilage and bone either as a mixture of the two tissues or as a junction between the two such as the union of a rib and its costal cartilage.

**chon'dro-os'teodys'trophy.** Osteochondrodystrophy.

**chondropathy** (kon-drop'ā-the) [ chondro- + G. *pathos*, suffering ]. Any disease of cartilage.

**chondropharyngeus** (kon'dro-făr-in-je'us). See *musculus* constrictor pharyngis medius.

**chondrophyte** (kon'dro-fit) [ chondro- + G. *phytos*, a growth ]. An abnormal cartilaginous mass that develops at the articular surface of a bone.

**chondroplast** (kon'dro-plast) [ chondro- + G. *plastos*, formed ]. Chondroblast.

**chondroplasty** (kon'dro-plas-tī) [ chondro- + G. *plassō*, to form ]. Reparative or plastic surgery of cartilage.

**chondroporosis** (kon'dro-po-ro'sis) [ chondro- + L. *porosus*, porous ]. A condition of cartilage in which spaces appear, either normal (in the process of ossification) or pathologic.

**chon'dropro'tein.** A protein occurring normally in cartilage, such as chondromucoid, chondrogen, etc.

**chondro'samine.** Galactosamine.

**chondrosarcoma** (kon'dro-sar-ko'mah). A malignant neoplasm derived from cartilage cells, occurring most frequently near the ends of long bones, in middle-aged and old people. C.'s are composed of cartilage cells that may have multiple nuclei. Histological evidence of malignancy may be slight.

**chon'drosin.** The repeating disaccharide in chondroitin sulfate, containing acetylgalactosamine and glucuronic acid.

**chondrosis** (kon-dro'sis). 1. The formation of cartilage 2. A cartilaginous tumor.

**chon'droskel'eton.** A skeleton formed of hyaline cartilage; for example, that of the human embryo or of certain adult fishes such as the shark or ray.

**chondrosome** (kon'dro-sōm) [ chondro- + G. + *sōma*, body ]. Obsolete term for mitochondrion.

**chondrosternal** (kon-dro-ster'nal). Relating to a sternal cartilage; chondroxiphoid; relating to the costal cartilages and the sternum.

**chon'droster'noplas'ty.** Correction of malformations of sternum.

**chondrotome** (kon'dro-tōm) [ chondro- + G. *tomē*, cutting ]. Cartilage knife; a very strong scalpel-shaped knife used in cutting cartilage.

**chondrotomy** (kon-drot'o-mī) [ chondro- + G. *tomē*, a cutting ]. Division of a cartilage.

**chondrotrophic** (kon-dro-trof'ik) [ chondro- + G. *trophē*, nourishment ]. Influencing the nutrition and thereby the development and growth of cartilage.

**chondroxiphoid** (kon'dro-sif'oyd) [ chondro- + G. *xiphos*, sword, + *eidos*, appearance ]. Relating to the xiphoid or ensiform cartilage.

**chondrus** (kon'drus) [ G. *chondros*, gristle. CHOND- ]. 1. Cartilage. 2. Irish moss; carrageen; pig wrack; pearl moss; the plant *Chondrus crispus*, *Fucus crispus*, or *Gigartina mamillosa* (family Gigartinaceae). Demulcent in chronic and intestinal disorders.

**chonechondrosternon** (ko'ne-kon'dro-ster-non) [ G. *choanē* (chōnə̄), funnel, + *chondros*, cartilage, + *sternon*, sternum ]. *Pectus excavatum.*

**Chopart** (sho-par'), François, Paris surgeon, 1743–1795. See C.'s *amputation, joint.*

**chord-** [ G. *chordē*, cord ]. Combining form meaning cord. For words beginning thus not found here, see cord-.

**chorda,** pl. **chor'dae** (kor'da) [ L., cord ]. 1. A tendon. 2 [ NA ]. A tendinous or a cordlike structure.
  **c. chirurgica'lis,** see suture (3).
  **c. dorsa'lis,** notochord.
  **c. magna,** *tendo* calcaneus.
  **c. obli'qua** [ NA ], oblique cord; Weitbrecht's cord; oblique or round ligament of the elbow joint; a slender band extending from the lateral part of the coronoid process of the ulna distad and laterad to the radius immediately distal to the bicipital tuberosity.
  **c. ser'ica chirurgica'lis,** surgical *silk.*
  **c. spermat'ica,** *funiculus* spermaticus.
  **chordae tendineae** [ NA ], tendinous cords; the tendinous strands running from the papillary muscles to the atrioventricular valves (mitral and tricuspid).
  **c. tympani** [ NA ]. cord of the tympanum, a nerve given off from the facial nerve in the facial canal. It passes through the canaliculus of the chorda tympani into the tympanic cavity, crosses over the tympanic membrane and handle of the malleus, and passes out through the

petrotympanic fissure to join the lingual branch of the mandibular nerve. It conveys taste sensation from the anterior two-thirds of the tongue and carries parasympathetic preganglionic fibers to the submandibular and sublingual salivary glands.
  **c. umbilica'lis,** *funiculus* umbilicus.
  **c. vertebra'lis,** notochord.
  **c. voca'lis,** pl. **chordae voca'les,** *plica* vocalis.
  **chordae willis'ii,** Willis' *cords.*

**chordal** (kor'dal). Relating to any chorda or cord, especially to the notochord.

**chor'da-mes'oderm.** That part of the protoderm of a young embryo which has the potentiality of forming notochord and mesoderm.

**Chorda'ta** [ L. *chorda*, fr. G. *chordē*, a string ]. The phylum of animals with a notochord, transient or persistent, *i.e.*, in the adult or at a stage in their development; includes the subphyla Hemicaudata, Urochordata, Cephalocaudata, and Vertebrata.

**chor'date.** An animal of the phylum *Chordata.*

**chordee** (kor-de') [ Fr. corded ]. Penis lunatus; painful erection of the penis in gonorrhea or Peyronie's disease, with curvature resulting from lack of distensibility of the corpus cavernosum urethrae.

**chorditis** (kor-di'tis) [ G. *chordē*, cord, + suffix -*itis*, inflammation ]. Inflammation of a cord; usually a vocal cord.
  **c. fibrino'sa,** inflammation of the vocal cords with fibrinous exudation.
  **c. nodo'sa,** singer's *nodes.*
  **c. tubero'sa,** singer's *nodes.*
  **c. voca'lis,** inflammation of the vocal cords.
  **c. vocalis inferior,** chronic subglottic laryngitis; an inflammation limited mainly to the undersurface of the vocal cords and adjacent parts.

**chordo'ma** [ (noto)chord + G. suffix -*oma*, tumor ]. A rare neoplasm of skeletal tissue, thought to be derived from persistent portions of the notochord; such remnants are found in the intervertebral disks (as the nuclei pulposi), on the clivus between the sella turcica and foramen magnum, and sometimes in the sacrum. More than half of c.'s occur in the sacrococcygeal region, one fourth at the base of the skull, and others chiefly in the cervical segment of the vertebral column. The neoplasms are composed of microscopic lobules, with abundant quantities of extracellular mucus; some of the cells contain vacuoles of mucus, whereas others do not; the vacuoles may be situated among thin strands of cytoplasm, thereby manifesting a structure that resembles that of soap bubbles, and such cells are termed physaliphorous cells. Metastases occur in less than 10 per cent of instances, but the neoplasms impinge on nerves and ganglia, and frequently cause death as a result of being in surgically inaccessible sites.

**chordoskeleton** (kor-do-skel'e-ton). The part of the skeleton in the embryo that develops in relation with the notochord.

**chordot'omy.** Cordotomy.

**chorea** (ko-re'ah) [ L. fr. G. *choreia*, a choral dance, fr. *choros*, a dance ]. Saint Anthony's, Saint John's, or Saint With's dance, a disorder usually of childhood, characterized by irregular, spasmodic, involuntary movements of the limbs or facial muscles.
  **automatic c.,** uncontrollable abnormal movements.
  **buttonmaker's c.,** ataxic movements of the hand and arm, a professional neurosis in buttonmakers.
  **chronic progressive c.,** hereditary c.
  **c. cordis,** heart irregularity related to c.
  **dancing c.,** procursive c.;
  **degenerative c.,** hereditary c.
  **c. dimidia'ta,** hemichorea.
  **electric c.,** (1) Dubini's disease; progressively fatal spasmodic disorder, possibly of malarial origin, occurring chiefly in Italy; (2) a severe form of Sydenham's c., in which the spasms are rapid and of a specially jerky character.
  **c. festi'nans** [ L. *festinare*, to hasten ]. procursive c.
  **fibrillary c.,** Morvan's c.; fasciculations of the muscles of the legs and trunk.
  **c. gravida'rum,** c. in pregnancy.
  **habit c.,** tic.
  **hemilateral c.,** hemichorea.
  **Henoch's c.,** spasmodic *tic.*

**hereditary c.,** Huntington's c.; chronic progressive c.; degenerative c.; a chronic disorder, beginning usually between the ages of 30 and 50 years, characterized by choreic movements in the face and extremities accompanied by a gradual loss of the mental faculties ending in dementia. Autosomal dominant inheritance.

**Huntington's c.,** hereditary c.

**hysterical c.,** conversion hysteria in which choreiform movements constitute the chief feature.

**c. insa′niens,** maniacal c.; a severe form of c. marked by the occurrence of delirium, chiefly found in association with pregnancy.

**juvenile c.,** Sydenham's c.

**laryn′geal c.,** a spasmodic tic involving the muscles, resulting in an explosive manner of talking.

**local c.,** occupation or professional *neurosis.*

**c. major,** a spasmodic attack occurring in patients with conversion hysteria.

**mani′acal c.,** c. insaniens.

**methodical c.,** c. in which the movements recur at definite intervals.

**mimet′ic c.,** imitation of the c. movements of another person.

**c. minor,** Sydenham's c.

**Morvan's c.,** fibrillary c.

**c. nu′tans,** a functional manifestation characterized by rhythmic nodding.

**paralytic c.,** a form in which there is weakness or paresis of an extremeity or portion of the body, with slight jerking movements.

**posthemiple′gic c.,** posthemiplegic *athetosis.*

**procursive c.,** c. festinans; dancing c.; a form in which the child whirls around, runs forward, or exercises a sort of rhythmic dancing movement.

**rheumatic c.,** Sydenham's c.

**rhythmic c.,** patterned movement in conversion hysteria.

**c. rotato′ria,** a form in which the head is rotated or oscillates rapidly.

**saltatory c.,** rhythmic dancing movements.

**senile c.,** a disorder resembling Sydenham's c., not associated with rheumatism or cardiac disease, occurring in the aged.

**Sydenham's c.,** c. minor; juvenile c.; rheumatic c.; Sydenham's disease St. Vitus' dance; an acute toxic or infective disorder of the nervous system, usually associated with acute rheumatism occurring in young persons and characterized by involuntary, semipurposeful but ineffective movements; they involve the facial muscles and muscles of the neck and limbs; they are intensified by voluntary effort but disappear in sleep.

**tetanoid c.,** c. due to lenticular degeneration.

**choreal** (ko-re′al). Relating to chorea.

**choreic** (ko-re′ik). Relating to or of the nature of chorea.

**choreiform** (ko-re′ĭ-form). Resembling chorea.

**choreo-** [ see chorea ]. Combining form relating to chorea.

**choreoathetoid** (ko′re-o-ath′e-toyd). Pertaining to or characterized by choreoathetosis.

**choreoathetosis** (ko′re-o-ath-e-to′sis) [ choreo- + G. *athētos,* unfixed, + suffix -*ōsis,* condition ]. Abnormal movements of body of combined choreic and athetoid pattern.

**choreoid** (ko′re-oyd). Choreiform; resembling chorea.

**choreophrasia** (ko′re-o-fra′zi-ah) [ choreo- + G. *phrasis,* speaking ]. The continual repetition of meaningless phrases.

**chorio-** [ G. *chorion,* membrane. CHORI- ]. Combining form relating to any membrane, but especially that which encloses the fetus.

**chorioadenoma** (ko′rĭ-o-ad-e-no′mah). A benign neoplasm of chorion, especially with hydatidiform mole formation.

**c. destruens,** invasive mole; hydatidiform mole in which there is an unusual degree of invasion of the myometrium or its blood vessels. C. destruens is clinically benign.

**chorioallantoic** (ko′rĭ-o-al′an-to′ik). Pertaining to the chorioallantois.

**chorioallantois** (ko′rĭ-o-ă-lan′to-is). The extraembryonic membrane formed by the fusion of the allantois with the serosa or false chorion, especially in avian embryos.

**chorioamnionitis** (ko′rĭ-o-am′nĭ-o-ni′tis). See amnionitis.

**chorioangioma** (ko′rĭ-o-an-jĭ-o′mah) [ chorion + angioma ]. A benign tumor of placental blood vessels (hemangioma), usually of no clinical significance; large tumors may be associated with placental insufficiency or hydramnios. In some instances, the stroma is edematous and may resemble myxomatous tissue.

**choriocapillaris** (ko′rĭ-o-kap-ĭ-la′ris). *Lamina* choroidocapillaris.

**choriocarcinoma** (ko′rĭ-o-kar-sĭ-no′mah). Chorionic epithelioma; chorioepithelioma; syncytioma malignum; trophoblastoma; a highly malignant neoplasm derived from syncytial trophoblasts and cytotrophoblasts that form irregular sheets and cords, which are surrounded by irregular "lakes" of blood; villi are not formed. The neoplastic cells invade the myometrium and blood vessels; metastases develop relatively early in the course of the illness, and are frequently found in the lungs, liver, brain, vagina and various other pelvic organs. Rarely, metastases have disappeared spontaneously. The proportion of c.'s which originate from hydatidiform moles is disputed. C.'s occasionally originate in teratoid neoplasms of the ovaries or testes, and are then poorly responsive to chemotherapy.

**choriocele** (ko′rĭ-o-sēl) [ chorio- + G. *kēlē,* hernia ]. A hernia of the choroid coat of the eye through a defect in the sclera.

**chorioepithelioma** (ko′rĭ-o-ep-ĭ-the-lĭ-o′mah). Choriocarcinoma.

**chorioid-, chorioido-.** For words beginning thus, see those beginning with choroid-, choroido-.

**chorioma** (ko-rĭ-o′mah). 1. Rarely used term for a benign or malignant tumor of chorionic tissue. 2. Choriocarcinoma.

**c. benig′num,** obsolete term for hydatidiform mole.

**c. malig′num,** obsolete term for choriocarcinoma.

**choriomeningitis** (ko-rĭ-o-men-in-ji′tis). A cerebral meningitis in which there is a more or less marked cellular infiltration of the meninges, often with a lymphocytic infiltration of the choroid plexuses particularly of the third and fourth ventricles.

**lymphocytic c.,** virus infection of mice and other animals including man. This disease often appears in animals used for experimental work, as a result of provocation by the injection of foreign materials into the nervous system.

**chorion** (ko′rĭ-on) [ G. *chorion,* membrane enclosing the fetus. CHORI- ]. Chorionic sac; the outermost fetal membrane; it is multilayered, consisting of extraembryonic somatic mesoderm and trophoblast; on the maternal surface it possesses villi that are bathed by maternal blood; as pregnancy progresses part of the c. becomes the definitive placenta.

**c. frondo′sum** [ leafy ], the part of the c. where the villi persist, forming the fetal part of the placenta.

**c. laeve** [ smooth ], the portion of the c. from which the villi disappear in the later stages of pregnancy.

**primitive c.,** previllous c.; the c. before its villi are well formed.

**shaggy c.,** old term for c. frondosum.

**smooth c.,** old term for c. laeve.

**yolk-sac c.,** omphalochorion.

**chorionepithelioma** (ko′rĭ-on-ep-ĭ-the-lĭ-o′mah). Choriocarcinoma.

**chorionic** (ko-rĭ-on′ik). Relating to the chorion.

**chorionitis** (ko-rĭ-on-i′tis). Inflammation of the chorion.

**Chorioptes** (ko-rĭ-op′tez) [ G. *chorion,* membrane, + *optos,* visible. OPO- ]. A genus of cosmopolitan and very common mange mites (family Psoroptidae) that cause chorioptic or symbiotic mange, characterized by restriction of the mange to certain parts of the animal's body. Various species described, *i.e.* C. *equi* of horses, C. *caprae* of goats, C. *ovis* of sheep, C. *cunniculi* of rabbits, are now thought to be strains of one species, C. *bovis* of cattle.

**chorioretinal** (ko-rĭ-o-ret′in-al). Relating to the choroid coat of the eye and the retina.

**chorioretinitis** (ko-rĭ-o-ret-in-i′tis). Choroidoretinitis; inflammation of the choroid and retina; see also retinochoroiditis.

**chorista** (ko-ris′tah) [ G. *chōristos,* separated ]. A focus of tissue that is histologically normal *per se,* but not in the organ or structure in which it is located; tissues displaced, during development, from their normal position; see also choristoma.

**choris'toblasto'ma** [ choristoma + blastoma ]. An autonomous neoplasm composed of relatively undifferentiated cells of a choristoma.

**choristoma** (ko-ris-to'mah) [ G. *chōristos*, separated, + *-ōma* ]. A mass formed by maldevelopment of tissue of a type not normally found at that site.

**choroid** (ko'royd) [ G. *choroeidēs*, a false reading for *chorioeidēs*, like a membrane. CHORI- ]. 1. Resembling the chorion, the corium, or any membrane. 2. The middle coat of the eyeball; choroidea, *q.v.*

**choroidal** (ko-roy'dal). Choroid; relating to the choroid coat of the eye.

**choroidea** (ko-royd'e-ah) [ see choroid ] [ NA ]. Choroid; the middle, vascular tunic of the eye lying between the retina and the sclera. Although formerly spelled chorioidea, omission of the first *i* is the current *Nomina Anatomica* spelling.

**choroideremia** (ko-roy-der-e'mĭ-ah) [ choroid + G. *erēmia*, absence ]. 1. Congenital absence of the choroid of the eye. 2. Progressive tapetochoroidal dystrophy; progressive choroidal atrophy; progressive degeneration of the choroid in males, beginning with peripheral pigmentary retinopathy, followed by atrophy of the pigmentary epithelium and sclerosis of the choroidal vessels; night blindness, progressive constriction of visual fields, and finally complete blindness. X-linked inheritance; heterozygous females show atypical pigmentary retinopathy but no visual defect and no progression.

**choroiditis** (ko-roy-di'tis). Posterior uveitis; inflammation of the choroid. This term is now restricted to inflammatory conditions; *cf.* choroidopathy.

**anterior c.,** c. characterized by round spots about the size of $1/2$ to $1/3$ optic disk diameter in front of and in the region of the equator.

**diffuse c.,** disseminated c.

**disseminated c.,** diffuse c.; inflammation of the choroid in which there are numerous spots of exudation scattered over the fundus.

**Tay's central guttate c.,** senile guttate *choroidopathy.*

**choroido-.** Combining form relating to the choroid, *q.v.*

**choroidocyclitis** (ko-roy'do-si-kli'tis) [ choroido- + G. *kyklos*, circle ]. Inflammation of the choroid coat and the ciliary body.

**choroidoiritis** (ko-roy'do-i-ri'tis). Inflammation of the choroid coat and the iris.

**choroidopathy** (ko'roy-dop'ă-thī). Choroidosis; noninflammatory degeneration of the choroid.

**acute serous c.,** bullous retinal detachment induced by fluid from the choriocapillary layer underlying the retinal pigment cells; may either regress spontaneously or require restricted photocoagulation.

**areolar c.,** central areolar choroidal sclerosis; a slowly progressive pigmentary degeneration of young persons; characterized by black foci closely set together and coalescent at the posterior pole and macular region.

**Doyne's honeycomb c.,** a slowly progressive degeneration of the macular area of the retina characterized by the appearance of small, round, white spots that form a mosaic resembling a honeycomb; deterioration of central vision late in life; irregular autosomal dominant inheritance.

**guttate c.,** a degenerative disorder marked by widespread distribution of colloid excrescences.

**myopic c.,** chronic degeneration of the sclerotic and choroid with posterior staphyloma, accompanying high myopia.

**senile guttate c.,** Hutchinson's disease; Tay's disease; Tay's central guttate choroiditis; a condition characterized by the presence of colloid bodies in the macular region.

**choroidoretinitis** (ko-roy'do-ret-in-i'tis). Chorioretinitis.

**choroidosis** (ko-roy-do'sis). Choroidopathy.

**Christ,** J., German dermatologist. See C.-Siemens *syndrome.*

**Christensen,** Erna, Danish neurologist. See C.-Krabbe *disease.*

**Christian,** Henry A., Boston internist, 1876–1951. See C.'s *disease,* Hand-Schüller-C. *disease, Weber–C. disease,* C.'s *syndrome.*

**Christison,** Sir Robert, Scottish physician, 1797–1882. See C.'s *formula.*

**Christmas disease, factor.** See the nouns.

**Chrobak** (khro'bak), Rudolf, Austrian gynecologist, 1843–1910. See C. *pelvis.*

**chrom-, chromat-, chromato-, chromo-** [ G. *chroma,* color ]. Combining forms meaning color. For words beginning with chrom- or chromo- and not listed thus, see chromat- and chromato-.

**chro'maffin** [ chrom- + L. *affinis,* affinity ]. Chromophil (3); chromaphil; giving a brownish yellow reaction with chromic salts; denoting certain cells in the medulla of the adrenal glands.

**chromaffinoma** (kro-maf-in-o'mah). A neoplasm composed of chromaffin cells derived from primitive sympathogonia, and occurring in the medullae of adrenal glands, the organs of Zuckerkandl, or the paraganglia of the thoracolumbar sympathetic chain. See also pheochromocytoma.

**chromaffinopathy** (kro'maf-in-op'ă-thī) [ chromaffin, *q.v.,* + G. *pathos,* suffering ]. Any pathologic condition of chromaffin tissue in the medulla of adrenal glands, the organs of Zuckerkandl, and so on.

**chro'man, chro'mane.** 3,4-Dihydro-2$H$-1-benzypyran; fundamental unit of the tocopherols (vitamin E). See also chromanol, chromenol.

**Chroman (Chromane)**

**chro'manol.** Hydroxychroman; 6-hydroxychroman (6-chromanol) is the fundamental unit of the tocopherols (vitamin E), tocols, and tocotrienols, as well as of ubiquinone-, toco-, and phyllochromanol. See also chromenol.

**chro'maphil.** Chromophil.

**chromat-.** See chrom-.

**chro'mate.** A salt of chromic acid.

**chromat'ic.** Of or pertaining to color or colors; produced by, or made in, a color or colors.

**chro'matid** [ G. *chrōma,* color, + *-id*(2), *q.v.* ]. Each of the two strands formed by longitudinal duplication of a chromosome that becomes visible during prophase of mitosis or meiosis; the two c.'s are joined by the still undivided centromere. After the centromere has divided at metaphase and the two c.'s have separated, each c. becomes a chromosome.

**chro'matin** [ G. *chrōma,* color ]. The portion of the nucleus of a cell that is readily stained by dyes; distinguished from the nonstainable portion, or achromatin. It may form a fibrillar network or granules of various sizes and shapes, composed of deoxyribonucleic acid combined with a basic protein, and is the carrier of the genes. See schematic diagram under cell.

**sex c.,** Barr c. body; a small, condensed mass of c. representing an inactivated X-chromosome usually located at the periphery of the interphase nucleus just inside the nuclear membrane; the number of sex c. bodies per nucleus is one less than the number of X-chromosomes, hence normal males and females with Turner's syndrome (XO) have none (sex c. negative), normal females and males with Klinefelter's syndrome (XXY) have one, and (XXX) females have two c. masses. For technical reasons only about half the cells in a preparation show typical masses. See also Lyon *hypothesis.*

**chro'matinol'ysis.** Chromatolysis (1).

**chromatinorrhexis** (kro-mat'ĭ-no-rek'sis) [ chromatin + G. *rhēxis,* rupture ]. Fragmentation of the chromatin.

**chro'matism** [ G. *chrōma*, color ]. 1. Abnormal pigmentation. 2. Chromatic *aberration*.

**chromato-.** See chrom-.

**chro'matodermato'sis** [ chromato- + G. *derma*, skin, + suffix -*osis*, condition ]. Chromatosis; chromatopathy; chromopathy; a disease of the skin accompanied by pigmentation.

**chromatogenous** (kro-mă-toj'en-us) [ chromato- + suffix -*gen*, producing ]. Producing color; causing pigmentation.

**chromat'ogram.** The record produced by chromatography.

**chromat'ograph.** To perform chromatography.

**chromatography** (kro-mă-tog'ră-fī) [ chromato- + G. *graphō*, to write ]. Absorption analysis; chromatographic analysis; absorption c.; the separation of chemical substances and particles (originally pigments and other highly colored compounds) by differential movement through a two-phase system. The mixture of materials to be separated is percolated through a column or sheet of some suitable chosen absorbent (*e.g.*, an ion-exchange material). The substances least absorbed are least retarded and emerge the soonest; those more strongly absorbed emerge later. The name derives from the first uses of c., to separate plant pigments.

    **gas c.,** a chromatographic procedure in which the moving phase is a mixture of gases or vapors, which are separated in the process by their differential adsorption on a stationary phase.

    **gas-liquid c.,** abbreviated GLC; the same as gas c., with the stationary phase being liquid rather than solid.

    **paper c.,** c. in which the moving phase is a liquid and the stationary phase is paper; see also partition c.

    **partition c.,** the separation of similar substances by repeated divisions between two immiscible liquids, so that the substances, in effect, cross the partition between the liquids in opposite directions. Where one of the liquids is bound as a film on filter paper, the process is termed paper partition c. or paper c.

    **thin-layer c.,** abbreviated TLC; c. through a thin layer of cellulose or similar inert material supported on a glass or plastic plate.

    **two-dimensional c.,** paper c. in which a spot, located originally in one corner of the sheet, is developed in one direction, after which the sheet is rotated 90 degrees and developed, with another solvent, in the new direction. The resultant spots are thus spread over the entire paper, giving a "map" or "fingerprint." Generalized to include c. followed by electrophoresis (or *vice versa*), column c. followed by paper c., etc.

**chro'matoid** [ chromato- + G. *eidos*, form ]. A refractile substance composed of chromatin and contained within the cytoplasm of the mature cyst of *Entamoeba histolytica*.

**chro'matokine'sis** [ chromato- + G. *kinēsis*, movement ]. Rearrangement of the chromatin into various forms.

**chromatolysis** (kro-mă-tol'ĭ-sis) [ chromato- + G. *lysis*, dissolution ]. Chromatinolysis; chromolysis; the disintegration of the granules of chromophil substance (Nissl bodies) in a nerve cell body which may occur after exhaustion of the cell or damage to its peripheral process.

    **central c.,** retrograde c.; c. associated with significant axonal injury.

    **retrograde c.,** central c.

    **transsynaptic c.,** transsynaptic *degeneration*.

**chromatolyt'ic.** Relating to chromatolysis.

**chromatom'eter** [ chromato- + G. *metron*, measure ]. Colorimeter; a scale of various shades of color, used for determining the color or depth of color of a liquid.

**chromatopathy** (kro'mă-top'ă-thī). Chromatodermatosis.

**chro'matopec'tic.** Chromopectic; relating to or causing chromatopexis.

**chromatopexis** (kro'mă-to-pek'sis) [ chromato- + G. *pēxis*, fixation ]. Chromopexis; the fixation of color or staining fluid.

**chromatophagous** (kro-mă-tof'a-gus) [ chromato- + G. *phagein*, to eat ]. Removing pigment; denoting certain microorganisms that cause a loss of pigment; see chromophage.

**chromat'ophil, chromat'ophile, chromatophil'ic, chromatoph'ilous.** See chromophil, etc.

**chro'matophil'ia.** Chromophilia.

**chromatopho'bia.** Chromophobia.

**chromatophore** (kro-măt'o-fōr) [ chromato- + G. *phoros*, bearing ]. 1. A colored plastid, due to the presence of chlorophyll, found in certain forms of protozoa. 2. A pigment-bearing cell found chiefly in the skin, mucous membrane, and choroid coat of the eye, and also in melanomas. 3. Chromophore.

**chro'matophor'otro'phin.** See melanocyte-stimulating *hormone*.

**chro'matophor'otrop'ic** [ chromatophore + G. *tropos*, a turning ]. Denoting the attraction of chromophores to the skin or other organs.

**chro'matoplasm.** The part of the cytoplasm containing pigment.

**chromatop'sia** [ chromato- + G. *opsis*, vision ]. Colored vision; a condition in which all objects appear abnormally colored. C.'s are designated according to color as: *xanthopsia*, yellow vision; *erythropsia*, red vision; *chloropsia*, green vision, and *cyanopsia*, blue vision.

**chromatoptometry** (kro'mă-top-tom'e-trī) [ chromato- + G. *optikos*, referring to vision, + *metron*, measure ]. Chromoptometry; measurement of the degree of color perception.

**chromatosis** (kro-mă-to'sis) [ chromato- + G. suffix -*osis*, condition ]. 1. Chromatodermatosis. 2. Pigmentation.

**chromatotropism** (kro'mă-tot'ro-pizm) [ chromato- + G. *tropē*, turn ]. 1. A change of color. 2. The phenomenon of orientation in response to color.

**chro'matrope 2R.** A red acid dye, $C_{16}H_{10}N_2O_8S_2Na_2$, used as a counterstain and for staining red blood cells in sections.

**chromatu'ria** [ chromato- + G. *ouron*, urine ]. Abnormal coloration of the urine.

**chrome** (krōm). Chromium, especially as a source of pigment.

    **c. red,** basic lead chromate, $PbCrO_4PbO$.

    **c. yellow,** Leipzig yellow; lemon yellow; Paris yellow; basic lead chromate; a fine yellow powder used in paints and dyes.

**chro'mene.** 2*H*-1-Benzopyran; fundamental unit of the tocopherolquinones. See also chroman, chromenol.

Chromene

**chro'menol.** Hydroxychromene; 6-hydroxychromene (6-chromenol) is the fundamental unit of the tocopherolquinones (oxidized vitamin E) and plastochromenol. See also chromanol.

**chromesthesia** (kro-mes-the'zĭ-ah) [ G. *chrōma*, color, + *aisthēsis*, sensation ]. 1. The color sense. 2. A condition in which another sensation, such as taste or smell, is excited by the perception of color.

**chromhidro'sis.** Chromidrosis.

**chro'mic acid.** $H_2CrO_4$ or $H_2Cr_4O_7$, formed by dissolving chromium trioxide ($CrO_3$) in water.

**chro'micize.** To mix with a chromium salt.

**chromidia** (kro-mid'ĭ-ah). Plural of chromidium.

**chromidiation** (kro-mid-ĭ-a'shun). Chromidiosis.

**chromidiosis** (kro-mid-ĭ-o'sis). Chromidiation; an outpouring of nuclear substance and chromatin into the cell protoplasm.

**chromidium, pl. chromid'ia** (kro-mid'ĭ-um) [ G. *chrōma*, color, + -*idion*, a diminutive termination ]. A basophilic particle or structure in the cell cytoplasm, rich in ribonucleic acid, often found in specialized cells.

**chromidro'sis** [ G. *chrōma*, color, + *hidros*, sweat ]. Chromhidrosis; the excretion of sweat containing pigment.

**chro'mium.** A metallic element, symbol Cr, atomic no. 24, atomic weight 52.01.

**c. trioxide,** chromic acid, $CrO_3$; used as a caustic in the removal of warts and other small growths from the skin and genitals. The hydrated acid, $H_2CrO_4$, forms variously colored salts with potassium, lead, and other bases.

**chromo-.** See chrom-.

**Chromobacte'rium** (kro-mo-bak-te'rĭ-um). A genus of bacteria (family Rhizobiaceae) containing Gram-negative, motile rods. These microorganisms produce a violet pigment (violacein) and are occasionally pathogenic to man and other animals. The type species is *C. violaceum.*

**C. janthi'num,** a species believed to cause a fatal septicemia in man and other animals.

**C. viola'ceum,** type species of the genus *C.;* it is found in soil and water.

**chro'moblast.** [ chromo- + G. *blastos,* germ ]. An embryonic cell with the potentiality of developing into a pigment cell.

**chro'moblas'tomyco'sis** [ chromo- + G. *blastos,* germ, + *mykēs,* fungus, + suffix - *osis,* condition ]. Chromomycosis; dermatitis verrucosa; a pigmented, verrucous fungus infection of the skin and subcutaneous tissues caused by dematiaceous fungi belonging to the genera *Cladosporium* ( *Hormodendrum* ) or *Phialophora.*

**chro'mocenter.** Karyosome.

**chromocystoscopy** (kro'mo-sis-tos'ko-pī) [ chromo- + G. *kystis,* bladder, + *skopeō,* to view ]. Inspection of the ureteral orifices in the bladder after the giving of methylene blue or other aniline dye by mouth, in order to determine the functional activity of the kidneys.

**chromocyte** (kro'mo-sit) [ chromo- + G. *kytos,* cell ]. Any pigmented cell, such as a red blood corpuscle.

**chro'mocytom'eter** [ chromo- + G. *kytos,* cell, + *metron,* measure ]. A form of hemoglobinometer.

**chromogen** (kro'mo-jen). 1. A substance, itself without definite color, that may be transformed into a pigment; denoting especially benzene and its homologues toluene, xylene, quinone, naphthalene, and anthracene, from which the aniline dyes are manufactured. 2. A microorganism that produces pigment.

**Porter-Silber c.'s,** yellow phenylhydrazones formed by the reaction of 17,21-dihydroxy-20-oxosteroids with a phenylhydrazine-ethanol-sulfuric acid reagent. Used chiefly to determine plasma cortisol concentrations and the urinary output of 17-hydroxycorticoids.

**chromogenesis** (kro-mo-jen'ĕ-sis) [ chromo- + G. *genesis,* production ]. The production of coloring matter or pigment.

**chromogen'ic.** Chromoparic. 1. Relating to chromogen. 2. Producing pigment; denoting certain bacteria that produce pigment.

**chromoisomerism** (kro'mo-i-som'er-izm). Isomerism in which the isomers display different colors.

**chromolipoid** (kro'mo-lip'oyd). Lipochrome; any pigmented lipid, such as carotene.

**chromolune** (kro'mo-lūn) [ chromo- + L. *lumen,* light ]. An apparatus for producing colored light rays.

**chromol'ysis.** Chromatolysis.

**chromomere** (kro'mo-mēr) [ chromo- + G. *meros,* a part ]. A condensed segment of a chromonema.

**chromom'eter.** Chromatometer.

**chro'momy'cin.** TOYOMYCIN; antibiotic produced by *Streptomyces griseus;* possesses antineoplastic and antimicrobial activity.

**chro'momyco'sis.** Chromoblastomycosis.

**chro'monar hydrochloride** (USAN). INTENSAIN; [ { 3-[ 2-(diethylamino)ethyl ]-4-methyl-2-oxo-2 *H*-1-benzo-pyran-7-yl|oxy ] acetic acid ethyl ester hydrochloride; used as coronary vasodilator for treatment of angina pectoris.

**chromone** (kro'mōn). 4 *H*-1-Benzopyran-4-one; fundamental unit of various plant pigments and other substances. See flavone, chromene, chromane.

**chromone'ma,** pl. **chromone'mata** [ chromo- + G. *nema,* thread ]. Chromatic fiber; the coiled filament which extends the entire length of a chromosome and exhibits an

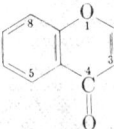

Chromone

intensely positive Feulgen test for deoxyribonucleic acid; the genes are located on the c.

**chro'monucle'ic acid.** Deoxyribonucleic acid.

**chromopar'ic** [ chromo- + L. *pario,* to bring forth ]. Chromogenic.

**chromop'athy.** Chromatodermatosis.

**chromopec'tic.** Chromatopectic.

**chromopex'is.** Chromatopexis.

**chromophage** (kro'mo-fāj) [ chromo- + G. *phagein,* to eat. PHAG- ]. A phagocyte that destroys pigment; term applied by Metchnikoff to the cells believed by him to be active in the blanching of the hair.

**chro'mophanes** [ chromo- + G. *phaino,* to show ]. The colored oil globules in the retinal cones of some animals; believed to be concerned with the mechanism of color vision.

**chro'mophil, chro'mophile** (kro'mo-fil, kro'mo-fil) [ chromo- + G. *phileō,* to love ]. 1. Chromophilic. 2. A cell or any histologic element that stains readily. 3. Chromaffin.

**chro'mophil'ia** [ chromo- + G. *phileō,* to love ]. Chromatophilia; the property possessed by most cells of staining readily with appropriate dyes.

**chromophil'ic, chromoph'ilous.** Staining readily; denoting certain cells and histologic structures.

**chro'mophobe, chromopho'bic** [ chromo- + G. *phobos,* fear ]. Resistant to stains, staining with difficulty or not at all; denoting certain cells or tissues.

**chro'mopho'bia** [ chromo- + G. *phobos,* fear ]. Chromatophobia. 1. Resistance to stains on the part of cells and tissues. 2. A morbid dislike of colors.

**chromophore** (kro'mo-fōr) [ chromo- + G. *phoros,* bearing ]. Chromatophore (3); color radical; the atomic grouping upon which the color of a substance depends.

**chromophor'ic, chromoph'orous.** 1. Relating to a chromophore. 2. Producing or carrying color; denoting certain microorganisms.

**chro'mophose** [ chromo- + G. *phōs,* light ]. A subjective sensation of a spot or patch of color in the eye.

**chro'mopho'tother'apy.** Chromotherapy.

**chro'mophyto'sis.** An obsolete synonym for tinea versicolor.

**chromoplas'tid.** A pigmented plastid, containing chlorophyll, formed in certain protozoans.

**chromopro'tein.** One of a group of conjugated proteins, consisting of a combination of pigment with a protein; *e.g.,* hemoglobin.

**chromop'sia.** Chromatopsia.

**chromoptometry** (kro'mop-tom'e-trī). Chromatoptometry.

**chro'moretinog'raphy.** Color photography of the retina.

**chro'moscope** [ chromo- + G. *skopeō,* to view ]. An apparatus for testing the color sense.

**chromos'copy.** The operation of testing the color sense.

**chro'mosin.** Obsolete term for an acid tryptophan-containing protein found in chromosomes.

**chro'moso'mal.** Pertaining to chromosomes.

**chromosome** (kro'mo-sōm) [ chromo- + G. *sōma,* body ]. One of the bodies (normally 46 in man) in the cell nucleus that is the bearer of genes; it has the form of a delicate chromatin filament during interphase, contracts to form a compact cylinder segmented into two arms by the centromere during metaphase and anaphase stages of cell division, and is capable of reproducing its physical and chemical structure through successive cell divisions. In the case of microbes, the c. is prokaryotic, not being enclosed within a nuclear membrane and not being subject to a mitotic mechanism.

**c. aberration,** any deviation from the normal number or morphology of c.'s.

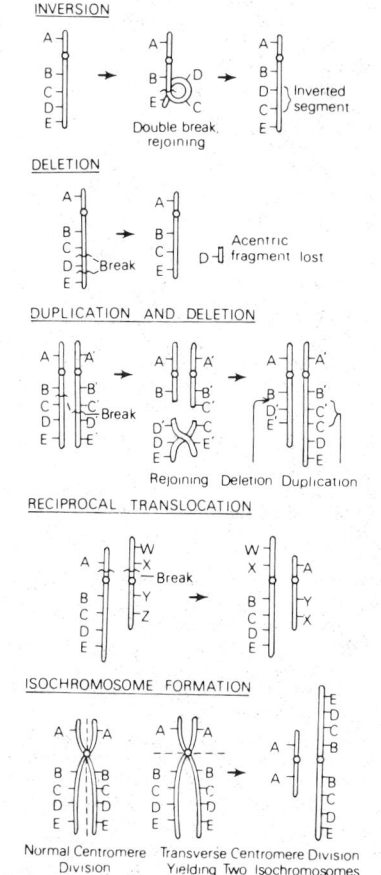

INVERSION

A B C D E → Double break, rejoining → Inverted segment

DELETION

A B C D E → Break → Acentric fragment lost

DUPLICATION AND DELETION

A B C D E → Break → → Rejoining Deletion Duplication

RECIPROCAL TRANSLOCATION

A W X Y Z → Break → W X A B C D E Y X

ISOCHROMOSOME FORMATION

Normal Centromere Division      Transverse Centromere Division Yielding Two Isochromosomes

**Chromosome Aberrations**

(From Herndon, C. N., in Morehead, R. P.: *Human Pathology*, McGraw-Hill Book Co., Inc., New York, 1965.)

**accessory c.,** monosome; heterotropic c.; unpaired allosome or c.; a c. existing without its normal homologous c.; at the reduction division of gametogenesis an accessory c. is likely to be included in one daughter cell and not in the other, but may be lost completely by lagging behind on the equatorial plate.

**acrocentric c.,** a c. with the centromere placed very close to one end so that the shorter arm is very small, often with a satellite. See fig. under centromere.

**bivalent c.,** a pair of c.'s temporarily united.

**Christchurch (Ch¹) c.,** an abnormal small acrocentric c. (no. 21 or 22) with complete or almost complete deletion of the short arm, resulting in horseshoe or dumbbell shape; found in cultured leukocytes in some cases of chronic lymphocytic leukemia, also in some normal relatives of patients.

**deletion of c.'s,** a c. aberration resulting from breakage of a c., failure of refusion of the segments, and loss of a fragment. A single break that fails to reunite results in loss of the part of the c. arm that does not contain the centromere. Two breaks may result in refusion of the end fragments with exclusion of the segment between the fracture lines; the segment that does not contain the centromere is lost. Deletion of a small fragment may occur as a result of unequal crossing over or exchange of segments between two homologous c.'s.

**dicentric c.,** a c. with two centromeres, an abnormality that may result from reciprocal translocation. See translocation.

**duplication of c.'s,** a c. aberration resulting from unequal crossing over or exchange of segments between two homologous c.'s; one c. of the pair loses a small segment while the other gains this segment. The c. gaining the segment has undergone duplication while its homologue has undergone deletion.

**endoreduplication of c.'s,** see endoreduplication.

**giant c.,** (1) polytene c.; (2) lampbrush c.

**heterotrop'ic c.,** accessory c.

**heterotypical c.,** allosome.

**homologous c.'s,** members of a single pair of c.'s.

**inversion of c.'s,** a c. aberration resulting from a double break, turning end for end of the fragment between the fracture lines and refusion of the fragments. This results in reversal of the order of genes in a segment of the c.

**lampbrush c.,** a large c. found in oocytes of certain animals characterized by many fine lateral projections giving the appearance of a test tube brush or lampbrush.

**metacentric c.,** a c. with a centrally placed centromere that divides the c. into two arms of approximately equal length. See fig. under centromere.

**mosaicism of the c.'s,** see mosaic (2).

**nonhomologous c.'s,** c.'s that are not members of the same pair.

**nucleolar c.,** one regularly associated with a nucleolus.

**odd c.,** accessory c.

**Philadelphia (Ph¹) c.,** an abnormal minute c. probably derived from a small acrocentric (No. 21 or 22) by loss of a large part of the long arm; found in cultured leukocytes of many patients with chronic myelocytic leukemia.

**polytene c.,** stage of c. division; forms the giant c. found in the salivary gland of dipterous insects; the great width is the result of repeated divisions of the chromonema without subsequent separation of the filaments.

**reduction of c.'s,** the process occurring during the meiotic cell division in gametogenesis whereby one member of each homologous pair of c.'s is distributed to each sperm or ovum; the somatic number of c.'s (46 in man) is thus reduced to the haploid number (23 in man) in each gamete. Union of the sperm and ovum then restores the diploid or somatic number in the one-cell zygote.

**ring c.,** a c. with ends joined to form a circular structure; the normal form of the c. in certain bacteria.

**c. satellite,** a small chromosomal segment separated from the main body of the c. by a secondary constriction; in man, usually associated with the short arm of an acrocentric c.

**sex c.'s,** the pair of c.'s responsible for sex determination; in one sex the members of the sex c. pair are alike (homologous), while in the opposite sex they are different. In man and most animals the sex c.'s are designated X and Y; females have two X c.'s, whereas males have one X c. and one Y c. In certain birds, insects and fishes the sex c.'s are designated Z and W; males have two Z c.'s, whereas females may have one Z c. and one W c., or may have one Z c. and no W c. Genes located on sex c.'s are sex-linked.

**sex c. imbalance,** an abnormal pattern of sex c.'s; such patterns may be associated with developmental disorders; thus, the pattern in men with seminiferous tubule dysgenesis is XXY, and in women with Turner's syndrome it is XO; rarer patterns of sex c. imbalance are XXX, XXXY, XXYY, and XYY.

**submetacentric c.,** a c. with the centromere so placed that it divides the c. into two arms of unequal length. See fig. under centromere.

**telocentric c.,** a c. with a terminal centromere; such c.'s are unstable and arise by misdivision or breakage within the centromere region; they are usually eliminated in a few cell divisions or transformed into isochromosomes.

**translocation of c.'s,** see translocation.

**W, X, Y,** and **Z c.'s,** see sex c.'s.

**chromother'apy.** Treatment of disease by colored light.

**chromotox'ic.** Caused by a toxic action on the hemoglobin, as in chromotoxic hyperchromemia, or resulting from the destruction of hemoglobin.

**chromotrichia** (kro-mo-trik'ĭ-ah) [chromo- + G. *thrix* (*trich-*), hair]. Colored or pigmented hair.

**chro'motrich'ial.** Pertaining to colored hair.

**chronax'ia, chronax'is, chronaxy.** Chronaxie.

**chronaxie** (kro'nak-sī) [ G. *chronos*, time, + *axia*, value ]. Chronaxia; chronaxis; chronaxy; a time characteristic; a measurement of excitability of nervous or muscular tissue. It is the shortest duration of an effective electrical stimulus having a strength equal to twice the minimum strength required for excitation.

**chro'naxim'eter.** An instrument for measuring chronaxie.

**chronaximetry** (kron'ak-sim'e-tre) [ G. *chronos*, time, + *axia*, value, + *metrein*, to measure ]. The measurement of chronaxie.

**chronic** (kron'ik) [ G. *chronos*, time ]. Of long duration; denoting a disease of slow progress and long continuance.

**chronicity** (kron-is'ĭ-tĭ). The state of being chronic.

**chrono-** (kron-o-) [ G. *chronos*, time ]. Combining form relating to time.

**chron'obiol'ogy** [ chrono- + G. *bios*, life, + *logos*, study ]. The science that deals with the duration of life and the means of prolonging it; see geriatrics and gerontology.

**chronognosis** (kron-og-no'sis) [ chrono- + G. *gnōsis*, knowledge ]. Perception of the passage of time.

**chronograph** (kron'o-graf) [ chrono- + G. *graphō*, to record ]. An instrument for measuring and recording brief periods of time.

**chronom'etry** [ chrono- + G. *metron*, measure ]. Measurement of intervals of time.

   **mental c.,** study of the duration of mental and behavorial processes.

**chron'opho'tograph.** A photograph taken as one of a series for the purpose of showing successive phases of a motion.

**chronotaraxis** (kron'o-tă-rak'sis) [ chrono- + G. *taraxis*, confusion ]. Confusion of the time sense.

**chronotropic** (kron'ŏ-trop'ik). Affecting the rate of rhythmic movements such as the heart beat.

**chronotropism** (kron-ot'ro-pizm) [ chrono- + G. *trope*, turn, change ]. Modification of the rate of a periodic movement, *e.g.*, the heart beat, through some external influence.

   **negative c.,** retardation of movement, especially of the heart rate.

   **positive c.,** acceleration of movement; especially of the heart rate.

**chrys-, chryso-** [ G. *chrysos*, gold ]. Combining forms meaning gold. See also auro-.

**chrysarobin** (kris-ă-ro'bin) [ G. *chrysos*, gold, + Brazil Ind. *araroba*, bark ]. An extract of Goa powder; a complex mixture of reduction products of chrysophanic acid, emodin, and emodin monomethyl ether. Used locally in ringworm, psoriasis, and eczema.

**chrys'azin.** Danthron.

**chrysiasis** (krī-si'ă-sis) [ G. *chrysos*, gold ]. Chrysoderma; auriasis; aurochromoderma; a permanent slate-gray discoloration of the skin and sclerae resulting from deposition of gold in the connective tissue of the skin after administration of excessive amounts of gold.

**chrysocyanosis** (kris'o-si-ă-no'sis). Pigmentation of skin due to reaction to therapeutic use of gold salts.

**chrysoderma** (kris'o-der'mah) [ G. *chrysos*, gold, + *derma*, skin ]. Chrysiasis.

**chrysoidine** (kris-oy-dēn). 2,4-Diaminoazobenzene hydrochloride; chrysoidine orange; a dye made from aniline; c. citrate and c. thiocyanate are used as antiseptics.

**Chrysomyia** (kris-o-mi'yah) [ G. *chrysos*, gold, + *myia*, fly ]. A genus of myiasis-producing fleshflies with medium-sized metallic-colored adults; includes Old World screw worm, *C. bezziana* (sometimes called *Cochliomyia bezziana*).

**Chrysops** (kris'ops). Deer fly; a genus of biting flies characterized by a splotched wing pattern; intermediate hosts for *Pasteurella tularensis* in the United States and for *Loa loa* in Africa.

   **C. dimidiata,** vector of *Loa loa.*

   **C. discalis,** vector of *Pasteurella tularensis,* cause of deer fly fever (tularemia).

   **C. distinctipennis,** vector of *Loa loa.*

   **C. silacea,** vector of *Loa loa.*

**chrysotherapy** (kris-o-ther'ă-pī) [ G. *chrysos*, gold ]. Aurotherapy; treatment of disease by the administration of gold salts.

**chthonophagia, chthonophagy** (thon-o-fa'jī-ah; thon-of'a-jī) [ G. *chthōn*, earth, + *phagein*, to eat ]. Geophagia.

**chut'ta.** Cancer of the roof of the mouth developing in Asians who smoke cigars with the lighted end inside the mouth. A similar association has been reported from South America and Sardinia.

**Chvostek** (khvosh'tek), Franz, Austrian surgeon, 1834–1884. See C.'s *habitus, sign.*

**chyl-.** See chylo-.

**chylangioma** (ki-lan-jī-o'mah) [ chyl- + G. *angeion*, vessel, + suffix *-oma*, tumor ]. A mass of prominent, dilated lacteals and larger intestinal lymphatic vessels.

**chylaqueous** (ki-la'kwe-us) [ chyl- + L. *aqua*, water ]. Referring to watery chyle.

**chyle** (kĭl) [ G. *chylos*, juice. CHY- ]. A turbid, white or pale yellow fluid taken up by the lacteals from the intestine during digestion. It consists of lymph and finely emulsified fat, is alkaline in reaction and coagulates, outside the body, into fibrin and serum. It is conveyed by the thoracic duct to the left subclavian vein, where it becomes mixed with the blood.

**chylemia** (ki-le'mĭ-ah) [ chyl- + G. *haima*, blood ]. The presence of chyle in the circulating blood.

**chylidrosis** (ki-lī-dro'sis) [ chyl- + G. *hidrōs*, sweat ]. Sweating of a milky fluid like chyle.

**chylifaction** (ki-lī-fak'shun) [ chyl- + L. *facio*, to make ]. Chylopoiesis.

**chylifactive** (ki-lī-fak'tiv). Chylopoietic.

**chyliferous** (ki-lif'er-us) [ chyl- + L. *fero*, to carry ]. Chylophoric; conveying chyle.

**chylification** (ki-lī-fi-ka'shun). Chylopoiesis.

**chyliform** (ki'-lī-form). Resembling chyle.

**chylo-, -chyl** (ki'lo) [ G. *chylos*, juice, chyle. CHY- ]. Combining form relating to chyle.

**chylocele** (ki'lo-sēl) [ chylo- + G. *kēlē*, tumor ]. A cystlike lesion resulting from the effusion of chyle into the tunica vaginalis propria and cavity of the tunica vaginalis testis.

**chylocyst** (ki'lo-sist) [ chylo- + G. *kystis*, bladder ]. *Cisterna* chyli.

**chyloderma** (ki-lo-der'ma) [ chylo- + G. *derma*, skin ]. Lymph *scrotum.*

**chylomediastinum** (ki'-lo-me'de-as-ti'num). The abnormal presence of chyle in the mediastinum.

**chylomicron,** pl. **chylomicrons** (ki'lo-mi-kron) [ chylo- + G. *micros*, small ]. A microscopic particle of fat, about 1 μ in diameter, occurring in lymph (chyle); especially numerous after a meal of fat; C.'s also occur in blood.

**chylomicronemia** (ki-lo-mi-kro-ne'me-ah). Chylomicrons in the circulating blood, especially with reference to an increased number.

**chylopericarditis** (ki'lo-per-ĭ-kar-di'tis). Chylopericardium.

**chylopericardium** (ki'lo-per-ĭ-kar'dī-um). A milky pericardial effusion resulting from obstruction of the thoracic duct or from trauma.

**chyloperitoneum** (ki'lo-per-ĭ-to-ne'um). Chylous *ascites.*

**chylophoric** (ki-lo-for'ik) [ chylo- + G. *phoros*, bearing ]. Chyliferous.

**chylopleura** (ki-lo-plu'rah). An accumulation of a milky fluid in the pleural cavity; see also chylothorax.

**chylopneumothorax** (ki'-lo-nu'mo-tho'raks). The presence of free chyle and air in the chest.

**chylopoiesis** (ki-lo-poy-e'sis) [ chylo- + G. *poiesis*, a making ]. Chylifaction; chylification; the formation of chyle in the intestine and its absorption by the lacteals.

**chylopoietic** (ki-lo-poy-et'ik). Chylifactive; relating to chylopoiesis.

**chylorrhea** (ki'lo-re'ah) [ chylo- + G. *rhoia*, flow ]. The flow or discharge of chyle.

**chylosis** (ki-lo'sis). The formation of chyle from the food in the intestine, its absorption by the lacteals, and its mixture with the blood and conveyance to the tissues.

**chylothorax** (ki-lo-tho′raks). Chylopleura; an accumulation of milky chylous fluid in the pleural space, usually on the left.

**chylous** (ki′lus). Relating to chyle.

**chyluria** (ki-lu′rī-ah) [ chyl- + G. *ouron*, urine ]. The passage of chyle, or a turbid, white fluid containing suspended fat globules, in the urine; one form of albiduria.

**chymase** (ki′mās). Rennin.

**chyme** (kīm) [ G. *chymos*, juice. CHY- ]. The semifluid mass of partly digested food passed from the stomach into the duodenum.

**chymification** (ki-mī-fī-ka′shun) [ G. *chymos*, juice, + L. *facio*, to make ]. Chymopoiesis.

**chymopapain** (ki-mo-pā′pain). A sulfhydryl enzyme, related to papain, that acts partly on chondromucoprotein.

**chymopoiesis** (ki′mo-poy-e′sis) [ G. *chymos*, juice, chyme, + *poiesis*, a making ]. Chymification; the production of chyme; the physical state of the food (semifluid) brought about by digestion in the stomach.

**chymorrhea** (ki′mo-re′ah) [ G. *chymos*, juice, + *rhoia*, flow ]. The flow of chyme.

**chymosin** (ki′mo-sin). Rennin.

**chymosinogen** (ki-mo-sin′o-jen). The zymogen of rennin.

**chy′motryp′sin** (USP). CHYMAR; ENZEON; QUIMOTRASE; chymotrypsin A; chymotrypsin B; proteinase (EC 3.4.21.1) of gastrointestinal tract, preferentially cleaving carboxyl links of hydrophobic amino acids; synthesized in the pancreas as chymotrypsinogen, and subsequently converted to $\pi$-, $\delta$-, and finally $\alpha$-chymotrypsin by successive trypsin cleavages. Has been proposed for use in the treatment of inflammation and edema associated with trauma and to facilitate intracapsular cataract extraction. It may be administered by the buccal, oral, intraocular, or intramuscular routes. Sterile chymotrypsin is official in the NF.

**c. A,** chymotrypsin.

**c. B,** chymotrypsin.

**c. C** (EC 3.4.21.2), similar to chymotrypsin, but with broader specificity.

**c. with trypsin,** CHYMOLASE oral; CHYMORAL; HAUGASE; ORENZYME; same uses as c.

**chy′motrypsin′ogen.** Precursor of chymotrypsin.

**chymous** (ki′mus). Relating to chyme.

**Ci.** Abbreviation for curie.

**C.I.** Abbreviation for Colour *Index* (q.v.).

**Ciaccio** (chah′cho), Carmelo, Italian pathologist, *1877. See C.'s *method*.

**Ciaccio** (chah′cho), Giuseppe V., Italian anatomist, 1824–1901. See C.'s *glands*.

**cibophobia** (si′bo-fo′bī-ah) [ L. *cibus*, food, + G. *phobos*, fear ]. Fear of eating, or loathing for, food.

**cicatrectomy** (sik′ă-trek′to-mī) [ L. *cicatrix*, scar, + G. *ektomē*, excision ]. Excision of a scar.

**cicatrice** (sik′ă-tris). Cicatrix.

**cicatricial** (sik-ă-trish′al). Relating to a cicatrix.

**cicatrisot′omy, cicatrisot′omy** (sik′ă-trī-kot′o-mī, -sot′-o-mī) [ L. *cicatrix*, scar, + G. *tomē*, cutting ]. Uletomy.

**cicatrix,** pl. **cicatri′ces** (sik′ă-triks, sī-ka′triks) [ L. ]. Scar; the fibrous tissue replacing the normal tissues destroyed by injury or disease.

**brain c.,** a lesion, resulting from repair of brain injury (reactive gliosis), characterized by proliferation of mesodermal and ectodermal (glial) elements; clinical manifestations (*e.g.*, posttraumatic epilepsy) are due to associated neural involvement rather than to the cicatrix itself. See also isomorphous *gliosis*.

**filtering c.,** a c. through which fluid may seep, although no visible openings are present; denoting especially a form of c. sometimes obtained after operation for glaucoma, through which there is a slight constant drainage of aqueous humor.

**meningocerebral c.,** scarring and adhesions involving contiguous brain and meninges; typically caused by head injury.

**u′loid c.,** see uloid (2).

**vicious c.,** one that by its contraction causes a deformity.

**cicat′rizant.** Causing or favoring cicatrization.

**cicatrization** (sik′ă-trī-za′shun). 1. The process of scar formation. 2. The healing of a wound otherwise than by first intention.

**cic′atrize.** To heal, to be closed by scar tissue; said of a wound or tissue defect.

**cichor′igenin.** Esculetin.

**cic′utine.** Coniine.

**cicutox′in.** (−)-Heptadeca-*trans*-8,10,12-triene-4,6-diyne-1,4-diol; a toxic principle present in water hemlock, *Cicuta virosa* (family Umbelliferae); pharmacologic action is similar to that of picrotoxin.

**cidoxepin hydrochloride** (si-dok′sĕ-pin) (USAN). *cis*-N, N-Dimethyldibenz [ *b, e* ] oxepin-$\Delta^{11(6H)}$,$\alpha$-propylamine hydrochloride; antipsychotic agent.

**ciguatera** (sēg′wah-tēr′ah) [ Sp., prob. *cigua*, sea snail ]. Poisoning due to the ingestion of the flesh or viscera of various marine fishes; the symptoms are gastrointestinal upset, muscular weakness, and other neurological disturbances; see also ciguatoxin.

**ciguatoxin** (sēg′wah-tok′sin). A marine saponin of unknown structure but with the empirical formula $C_{35}H_{65}NO_8$; the toxic substance causing ciguatera.

**cilia** (sil′ī-ah). Plural of cilium.

**ciliarotomy** (sil′ī-ăr-ot′o-mī). Surgical division of the zona ciliaris.

**ciliary** (sil′ī-ă-rī) [ Mod. L. *ciliaris*, relating to or resembling an eyelid, or eyelash, fr. L. *cilium*, eyelid ]. Relating to (1) any cilia or hairlike processes, (2) the eyelashes, (3) certain of the structures of the eyeball.

**ciliastatic** (sil-ī-ah-stat′ik). Denoting a drug or condition that slows or stops the beating of cilia (generally used with reference to respiratory mucosal cilia).

**Ciliata** (sil-ī-a′tah). Ciliates; a class of Protozoa whose members bear cilia or structures derived from them, such as cirri or membranelles. Typical members, such as *Paramecium* or *Balantidium coli* (a parasite of man) possess two distinctive nuclei, a macronucleus and a micronucleus; only the latter bears the hereditary material exchanged in conjugation (a form of sexual reproduction found only in the C.).

**cil′iated.** Having cilia.

**ciliectomy** (sil-ī-ek′to-me). Cyclectomy.

**cilio-, cili-** (sil′ī-o, sil′ī) [ L. *cilium*, q.v. ]. Combining forms relating to cilia or meaning ciliary, in any sense.

**ciliogenesis** (sil′ī-o-jen′ē-sis). The formation of cilia.

**Ciliophora** (sil′ī-of′o-rah) [ cilio- + G. *phoros*, bearing ]. A subphylum of protozoa that includes the abundant free-living ciliates (the parasite *Balantidium* among others) and the sessile suctorians.

**cil′ioret′inal.** Pertaining to the ciliary body and the retina.

**ciliosscleral** (sil′ī-o-skle′ral). Relating to the ciliary body and the sclera.

**cil′iospi′nal.** Relating to the ciliary body and the spinal cord; denoting in particular the c. *center*.

**ciliotomy** (sil′ī-ot′o-mī) [ cilio- + G. *tomē*, incision ]. Surgical section of the ciliary nerves.

**ciliotoxicity** (sil′ī-o-tok-sis′ī-tī). The characteristic of a drug or condition which impairs ciliary activity (generally refers to respiratory mucosal cilia).

**cilium,** pl. **cil′ia** (sil′ī-um) [ L. an eyelid ]. 1 [ NA ]. Eyelash. 2. A motile extension of a cell surface, for example, of certain epithelial cells, containing nine longitudinal double filaments or microtubules arranged in a peripheral ring, together with a central pair.

**cil′lo.** Cillosis.

**Cillobacterium** (sil′lo-bak-tēr-ī-um). An obsolete genus of motile, anaerobic bacteria containing Gram-positive, straight or curved rods. Motile cells are peritrichous. These organisms may be pathogenic. The type species is *C. moniliforme*. This genus is no longer recognized, and most of its species have been transferred to *Eubacterium*.

**C. combesi,** *Eubacterium combesi*.

**C. moniliforme,** *Eubacterium moniliforme*.

**C. multiforme,** *Eubacterium multiforme*.

**C. tenue,** *Eubacterium tenue*.

**cillo′sis** [ Mod. L., spelling influenced by Fr. *ciller*, to wink ]. Cillo; spasmodic twitching of an eyelid.

**Cimex lectularius.** Bedbug; member of the family Cimicidae, with a flat, reddish-brown wingless body, prominent lateral eyes, and a three-jointed beak. These insects have a characteristic pungent odor from thoracic stink glands and are abundant pests in human abodes, especially in the tropics under poor sanitary conditions. Though the bedbug's bite produces an urticarial wheal, no important human disease has been proved to be routinely transmitted by this common household pest.

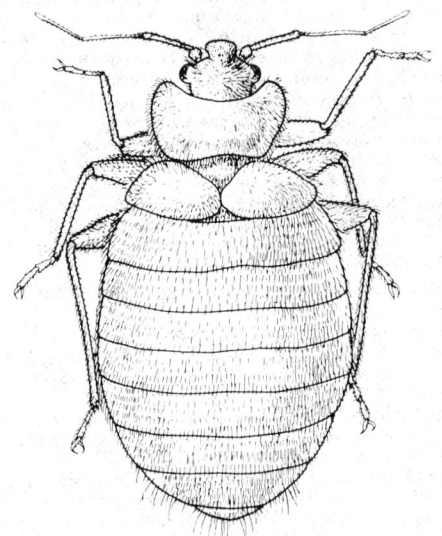

*Cimex lectularius*
(From Najarian, H. H.: *Textbook of Medical Parasitology*, The Williams & Wilkins Co., Baltimore, 1967.)

**cimicifuga** (sim-ĭ-sif′u-gah) [ L. *cimex* (*cimic*-), bedbug, + *fugo*, to chase ]. Macrotys; black snakeroot; black cohosh; rhizome and roots of *Cimicifuga racemosa* (*Actaea racemosa*) (family Ranunculaceae); a herb of eastern and central United States and Canada. Formerly used as alterative, emenagogue, antispasmodic, and antirheumatic.

**cimicosis** (sim-ĭ-ko′sis). Lesions produced by bedbug (*Cimex*) bites.

**cin-.** See cine-.

**cinanesthesia** (sin-an-es-the′zī-ah). Kinanesthesia.

**cinan′serin hydrochloride** (USAN). 2′-[ [ 3-(Dimethylamino)propyl ]thio ]cinnamanilide monohydrochloride; a serotonin inhibitor.

**cincham′idine.** Hydrocinchonidine.

**cinchol** (sin′kol). β-Sitosterol.

**cinchona** (sin-ko′nah). Cinchona bark; Peruvian bark; quina; quinaquina; quinquina; Jesuits' bark; the dried bark of root and stem of various species of *Cinchona*, a genus of evergreen trees (family Rubiaceae), native of South America but cultivated in various tropical regions. The cultivated bark contains 7 to 10 per cent of total alkaloids; about 70 per cent is quinine. C. contains more than 20 alkaloids, of which two pairs of isomers are most important: quinine and quinidine, and cinchonidine and cinchonine. See also subentries under bark.

   **c. rubra**, red bark; the dried bark of *C. succirubra* (more often probably *C. robusta*).

   **yellow c.**, yellow bark; calisaya bark; the dried bark of *Cinchona calisaya*.

**cinchonamine** (sin-ko′nă-mēn). An indole alkaloid derived from cuprea bark, *Remijia purdieana* (family Rubiaceae), related to cinchona.

**cinchonic** (sin-kon′ik). Relating to cinchona.

**cinchonicine** (sin-kon′ĭ-sēn). Cinchotoxine.

**cinchonidine** (sin-kon′ĭ-dēn). An isomer of cinchonine; an alkaloid obtained from the bark of several species of

cinchona. Indications the same as those of quinine, but it must be given in larger doses. Several c. salts are available.

**cinchonine** (sin′-ko-nēn). A quinoline alkaloid prepared from the bark of several species of cinchona; tonic and antimalarial. Several c. salts are available.

**cinchoninic acid** (sin-ko-nin′ik). Quinoline-4-carboxylic acid; fundamental structure of cinchonidine, cinchonine, cincophen, cinchotoxin.

$$\text{COOH}$$

Cinchoninic acid

**cinchonism** (sin′ko-nizm). Quininism; poisoning by cinchona, quinine, or quinidine; characterized by tinnitus aurium, headache, deafness, and occasionally anaphylactoid shock.

**cin′chophen.** ATOPHAN; 2-phenylquinoline-4-carboxylic acid; 2-phenylcinchoninic acid; $C_6H_5$—($C_9H_5N$)—COOH; analgesic, antipyretic, and uricosuric agent. May produce liver damage and gastric lesions and is considered a dangerous drug. Used in experimental animals to produce gastric ulcer.

**cinchotine** (sin′ko-tēn). Hydrocinchonine.

**cinchotoxine** (sin-ko-tok′sin). Cinchonicine; an isomer of cinchonine; a rearrangement product of cinchonine or cinchonidine. It is more toxic than the former and has no febrifugal activity.

**cinclisis** (sing′-klī-sis) [ G. *kinglizein*, to wag the tail, change constantly ]. Rapid repetition of a movement, *e.g.*, rapidly repeated winking.

**cincon′ifine.** Hydrocinchonine.

**cine-** (sin′e-) [ G. *kineō*, fut. *kinēsō*, to move. CIN- ]. Combining forms denoting movement (and when spelled this way, usually relating to motion pictures); for words beginning thus and not found here, see kin- and kine-.

**cinean′giocardiog′raphy.** Motion pictures of the passage of a contrast medium through chambers of the heart and great vessels.

**cineangiography** (sin′e-an-jī-og-ră-fī). Motion pictures of the passage of a contrast medium through blood vessels.

**cinedensigraphy** (sin′e-den-sig′ră-fī). Recording of movements of parts of the body or organs by means of x-rays and radiosensitive cells.

**cinefluorography** (sin′e-flu-or-og′ră-fī). The taking of motion pictures of fluoroscopic views, especially of the heart and great vessels or gastrointestinal tract after the administration of a contrast medium.

**cinefluoroscopy** (sin′e-flu-or-os′ko-pī). Motion pictures of fluoroscopic study.

**cinegastroscopy** (sin′e-gas-tros′ko-pī). Motion pictures of gastroscopic observations.

**cinemat′ics.** Kinematics.

**cinematization** (sin-e-mat-ĭ-za′shun). Cineplastic *amputation.*

**cinemat′ofluorog′raphy.** Cinefluorography.

**cinematography** (sin′e-mă-tog′ră-fī). The taking of motion pictures to record actions and reactions of a subject and of surgical procedures.

**cinemat′oradiog′raphy.** Radiography of an organ in motion, *e.g.*, the heart.

**cin′ene.** Limonene.

**cin′eole, cin′eol.** Eucalyptol; cajeputol; 1,8-epoxy-*p*-menthane; obtained from the volatile oil of *Eucalyptus globulus* and other species of *Eucalyptus*; a stimulant expectorant.

**cinephotomicrography** (sin′e-fo′to-mi-krog′ră-fī). The making of a motion picture of microscopic objects. Often time lapse photography is used whereby pictures are taken at intervals so that the motion appears to be speeded up.

**cineplas′tics** (sin-e-plas′tiks). See cineplastic *amputation.*

**cineradiography** (sin'e-ra-dī-og'ră-fī). Cinematoradiography.

**cinerea** (sin-e're-ah) [ L. fem. of *cinereus*, ashy, fr. *cinis*, ashes ]. 1. The gray matter of the brain and other parts of the nervous system. 2. Old term for the mantle layer of the embryonic neural tube; see under layer.

**cinereal** (sin-e're-al). Relating to the gray matter of the nervous system.

**cineritious** (sin-er-ish'us). Ashen; denoting the gray matter of the brain, spinal cord, and ganglia.

**cineroentgenography** (sin'e-rent-gen-og'ră-fī). The production of moving x-ray pictures.

**cinetoplasm, cinetoplasma** (sin-et'o-plazm, sin-et-o-plaz'mah). Kinetoplasm.

**cineurography** (sin'e-u-rog'ră-fī). Motion picture urography.

**cingulate** (sin'gu-lāt). Relating to a cingulum.

**cingulectomy** (sin'gu-lek'to-mī) [ cingulum + G. *ektomē*, excision ]. Cingulotomy; bilateral surgical excision of the anterior half of the cingular gyrus; performed for certain psychoses.

**cingulot'omy.** Cingulectomy.

**cin'gulum,** gen. **cin'guli,** pl. **cin'gula** (sin'gu-lum) [ L. girdle, fr. *cingo*, to surround ] [ NA ]. 1. A structure that has the form of a belt or girdle. 2. A well marked fiber bundle passing longitudinally in the white matter of the gyrus cinguli (collateral gyrus); the bundle extends from the region of the anterior perforated substance back over the dorsal surface of the corpus callosum; behind the latter's splenium it curves down and then forward in the white matter of the parahippocampal gyrus. It is composed largely of fibers from the anterior thalamic nucleus to the cingulate and parahippocampal gyri, but also contains association fibers connecting these gyri with the frontal cortex, and their various subdivisions with each other. 3. Lingual lobe; basal r. (2); a U- or W-shaped ridge at the base of the lingual surface of the crown of the upper incisors and cuspid teeth, the lateral limbs running for a short distance along the linguoproximal line angles, the central portion just above the gingiva.

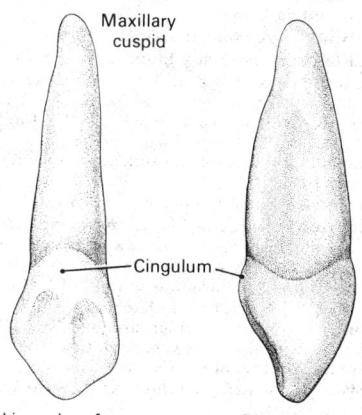

Maxillary cuspid

Cingulum

Lingual surface    Distal surface

**Cingulum of a Tooth**

**c. athlet'icum,** a zone of dilated venules in the skin outlining the insertion of the diaphragm; it is said to be common in athletes and those subject to severe physical strain, and occurs in asthmatics, especially those with the gouty diathesis; emphysematous girdle.

**c. membri inferior'is** [ NA ], pelvic girdle; the bony ring formed by the hip bones and the sacrum, to which the inferior limbs are attached.

**c. membri superior'is** [ NA ], shoulder girdle; thoracic girdle; the bony ring, incomplete posteriorly, that serves for the attachment and support of the superior limbs. It is formed by the manubrium sterni, the clavicles, and the scapulae.

**cin'nabar** [ G. *kinnabari* ]. Mercuric sulfide, red.

**cinnamal'dehyde.** Cinnamic aldehyde; chief constituent of cinnamon oil.

**cin'namate.** A salt or ester of cinnamic acid.

**cin'namein.** Benzyl cinnamate.

**cin'namene.** Styrene.

**cinnam'ic.** Relating to cinnamon.
  **c. acid,** phenylacrylic acid; 3-phenylpropenoic acid; cinnamylic acid; $C_6H_5CH=CHCOOH$; obtained from cinnamon oil, Peruvian and tolu balsams, or storax. Has been used in lupus as paint and in infectious diseases to promote leukocytosis.
  **c. alcohol,** styrone.
  **c. aldehyde,** cinnamaldehyde.

**cinnamon** (sin'ă-mon) [ L. fr. G. *kinnamōmon*, cinnamon ]. 1 (NF). Saigon c.; Saigon cassia; the dried bark of *Cinnamomum loureirii* Nees (family Lauraceae), an aromatic bark used as a spice, and in medicine as an adjuvant, carminative, and aromatic stomachic. 2 (BP). The dried inner bark of the shoots of coppiced trees of *Cinnamomum zeylanicum*, known as Ceylon c.
  **cassia c.,** Chinese c.; *Cinnamomum cassia* Nees (family Lauraceae); the unofficial source of most of the cinnamon in the shops; the source of c. oil (USP).
  **c. oil** (USP), cassia o.; the vollatile oil distilled with steam from the leaves and twigs of *Cinnamomum cassia*, contains not less than 80 per cent by volume of the total aldehydes of c. oil.

**cinnamyl'ic acid.** Cinnamic acid.

**cinnarizine** (si-năr'ī-zēn) (USAN). DIMITRON; 1-cinnamyl-4-diphenylmethylpiperazine; antihistaminic agent.

**cinobu'fagin.** A cardiac poison (a bufadienolide; for structure, see steroids) secreted in the venoms of certain toads.

**cinocentrum** (sin-o-sen'trum). Kinocentrum.

**cinox'ate** (USAN). 2-Ethoxyethyl-*p*-methoxycinnamate; an ultraviolet screen for topical application on the skin.

**cin'perene** (USAN). 2-(1-Cinnamyl-4-piperidyl)-2-phenylglutarimide; a tranquilizer.

**cin'tazone** (USAN). 2-Pentyl-6-phenyl-1*H*-pyrazolo[ 1,2-*a* ]cinnoline-1,3(2*H*)-dione; an anti-inflammatory agent.

**cion** (si'on) [ G. *kiōn*, pillar, the uvula ]. Archaic term for uvula.

**circadian** (ser'kă-de'an, ser-ka'de-an) [ L. *circa*, about, + *dies*, day ]. Relating to biologic variations or rhythms with a cycle of about 24 hours.

**circel'lus** [ L. ]. Circle.
  **c. veno'sus hypoglos'si,** *plexus venosus canalis hypoglossi.*

**circinate** (sur'sĭ-nāt) [ L. *circinatus*, made round, pp. of *circino*, to make round, fr. *circinus*, a pair of compasses ]. Circular; ring-shaped.

**circle** (sur'kl) [ L. *circulus* ]. 1. A ring-shaped structure or group of structures. 2. A line or process with every point equidistant from the center.
  **arterial c. of cerebrum,** *circulus arteriosus cerebri.*
  **articular vascular c.,** *circulus articularis vasculosus.*
  **Baudelocque's uterine c.,** pathologic retraction *ring.*
  **Carus' c.,** Carus' *curve.*
  **closed c.,** a circuit for administration of an inhalation anesthetic in which there is complete rebreathing with carbon dioxide absorption.
  **defensive c.,** the addition of a secondary disease limiting or arresting the progress of the primary affection, as when pneumothorax supervenes on pulmonary tuberculosis, the two affections exerting a reciprocally antagonistic action.
  **diffusion c.,** diffusion spot; one of a number of c.'s formed on the plane of projection of an image when it is not in the focus of the lens.
  **greater arterial c. of iris,** *circulus* arteriosus iridis major.
  **Haller's c.,** (1) *circulus* vasculosus nervi optici; (2) *plexus* venosus areolaris; (3) *circulus* callosus or fibrosus halleri.
  **Huguier's c.,** anastomosis around the isthmus of the uterus (junction of the cervix with the body) between the right and left uterine arteries.
  **lesser arterial c. of iris,** *circulus* arteriosus iridis minor.
  **Pagenstecher's c.,** in the case of a freely movable abdominal tumor, the mass is moved throughout its entire range, its position at intervals being marked on the abdominal wall; when these points are joined a c. is

formed, the center of which marks the point of attachment of the tumor.

**Ridley's c.,** *sinus* circularis (1).

**semi-closed c.,** a circuit for administration of an inhalation anesthetic in which partial rebreathing with carbon dioxide absorption is combined with loss from the circuit of a portion of respired gases through valves.

**vascular c.,** (1) the c. around the mouth formed by the inferior and superior labial arteries; (2) *circulus* vasculosus nervi optici; (3) *plexus* venosus areolaris.

**vascular c. of optic nerve,** *circulus* vasculosus nervi optici.

**venous c. of mammary gland,** *plexus* venosus areolaris.

**vicious c.,** (1) the mutually accelerating action of two independent diseases, or of a primary and secondary affection; (2) the passage of food, after a gastroenterostomy, from the artificial opening through the intestinal loop by antiperistaltic action, into the stomach again by the pyloric orifice, or the reverse.

**c. of Willis,** *circulus* arteriosus cerebri.

**Zinn's vascular c.,** *circulus* vasculosus nervi optici.

**cir'clecuf.** An inflatable sleeve-like device used in place of the usual bandage-type cuff employed for the clinical measurement of the blood pressure. It is drawn into place by passing the hand and forearm through it. This device is particularly suitable for the self-measurement of the blood pressure.

**circuit** (sur'kit) [ L. *circuitus,* a going round, fr. *circum,* around, + *eo,* pp. *itus,* to go ]. The path or course of an electric or other current.

**anesthetic c.,** equipment used during inhalation anesthesia to control concentration of inhaled gases; includes breathing tubes, directional valves, a reservoir bag, and a mechanism for prevention of carbon dioxide accumulation.

**reverberating c.,** a theory of periodic conduction through the cerebral cortex of trains of impulses traveling in c.'s of neurons.

**circulation** (sur-ku-la'shun) [ L. *circulatio* ]. Movements in a circle, or through a circular course, or through a course which leads back to the same point.

**blood c.,** the course of the blood from the heart through the arteries, capillaries, and veins back again to the heart. See plate 23.

**capillary c.,** course of the blood through the capillaries.

**collateral c.,** c. maintained in small anastomosing vessels when the main artery is obstructed.

**compensatory c.,** c. established in dilated collateral vessels when the main artery of the part is obstructed.

**cross c.,** c. to an animal or one of its parts from the c. of another animal.

**derivative c.,** arteriovenous *shunt.*

**embryonic c.,** the basic plan of the c. of a young mammalian embryo is at first similar to that in water-living forms, with an unpartitioned heart and conspicuous aortic arches in the branchial region. As gestation progresses the arrangement of the major blood vessels gradually approaches more and more closely that of the adult, but the routing of blood through the heart that is characteristic of the adult cannot be attained until lung breathing begins at the time of birth. See plate 23.

**enterohepatic c.,** refers to c. of substances such as bile salts which are absorbed from the intestine and carried to the liver, where they are secreted into the bile and again enter the intestine.

**extracorporeal c.,** the c. of blood outside of the body through a heart-lung machine, artificial kidney, etc.

**fetal c.,** the c. which serves the fetus *in utero,* with the placental conduit responsible for supplying oxygen and nutritive material and for eliminating $CO_2$ and nitrogenous wastes. See also embryonic c. and plate 23.

**greater c.,** systemic c.

**lesser c.,** pulmonary c.

**lymph c.,** the slow passage of lymph through the lymphatic vessels and glands.

**placental c.,** the c. of blood through the placenta during intrauterine life, serving the needs of the fetus for aeration, absorption, and excretion.

**portal c.,** the c. of blood to the liver from the small intestine via the portal vein.

**postnatal c.,** see color plate 23.

**primitive c.,** see embryonic c.

**pulmonary c.,** lesser c.; the passage of blood from the right ventricle through the pulmonary artery to the lungs and back through the pulmonary veins to the left atrium.

**Servetus' c.,** obsolete term for the pulmonary c.

**systemic c.,** greater c.; the c. of blood through the arteries, capillaries, and veins of the general system, from the left ventricle to the right atrium.

**cir'culatory.** Relating to the circulation.

**circulus,** gen. and pl. **cir'culi** (sur'ku-lus) [ L. dim. of *circus,* circle ]. 1 [ NA ]. Any ringlike structure. 2. A circle formed by connecting arteries, veins, or nerves.

**c. arterio'sus cerebri** [ NA ], arterial circle of the cerebrum; circle of Willis; an anastomotic "circle" (roughly pentagonal in outline) at the base of the brain, formed, in order from before backward, by the anterior communicating artery, the two anterior cerebral, the two internal carotid, the two posterior communicating, and the two posterior cerebral arteries.

**c. arterio'sus hal'leri,** c. vasculosus nervi optici.

**c. arterio'sus ir'idis major** [ NA ], greater arterial circle of the iris; an arterial circle at the ciliary border of the iris.

**c. arterio'sus ir'idis minor** [ NA ], lesser arterial circle of the iris; an arterial circle near the pupillary margin of the eye.

**c. articula'ris vasculo'sus** [ NA ], articular vascular circle; an anastomosis of vessels encircling a joint.

**c. callo'sus hal'leri,** circulus fibrosus halleri; Haller's circle (3); one of the fibrous rings surrounding the opening of the mitral and tricuspid valves in the heart.

**c. fibrosus halleri,** c. callosus halleri.

**c. vasculo'sus nervi op'tici** [ NA ], vascular circle of the optic nerve; Zinn's vascular circle; Zinn's corona; Haller's circle (1); circulus arteriosus halleri; a network of branches of the short ciliary arteries on the sclera around the point of entrance of the optic nerve.

**c. veno'sus hal'leri,** *plexus* venosus areolaris.

**c. veno'sus rid'leyi,** *sinus* circularis (1).

**c. zin'nii,** c. vasculosus nervi optici.

**circum-** (sur-kum-) [ L. around ]. A prefix denoting a circular movement, or a position surrounding the part indicated by the word to which it is joined.

**circuma'nal.** Perianal; periproctic; surrounding the anus.

**cir'cumartic'ular** [ circum- + L. *articulus,* joint ]. Periarthric; surrounding a joint.

**circumax'illary.** Around the axilla.

**circumbul'bar.** Around any bulb, especially the eyeball.

**circumcision** (sur-kum-sizh'un) [ L. *circumcido,* to cut around, fr. *circum,* around, + *caedo,* to cut ]. The operation of removing part or all of the foreskin, or prepuce.

**pharaonic c.,** infibulation; causing scar tissue to join the labia to prevent coitus.

**circumcor'neal.** Surrounding the cornea.

**circumduc'tion** [ circum- + L. *duco,* pp. *ductus,* to draw ]. Cycloduction; movement of a part, as the eye or an extremity, in a circular direction.

**circumferentia** (sur-kum-fe-ren'shi-ah) [ L. a bearing around. FER- ] [ NA ]. Circumference.

**c. articula'ris** [ NA ], articular circumference. There are two structures with this title: **c. articularis ul'nae,** articular circumference of the ulna, (at its distal end), and **c. articularis ra'dii,** articular circumference of the radius, (at its proximal end).

**cir'cumflex** [ circum- + L. *flexus,* to bend ]. Describing an arc of a circle; denoting several anatomical structures: arteries, veins, nerves, and muscles.

**circumflex'us** [ L. ] [ NA ]. Circumflex.

**circumgemmal** (sur-kum-jem'al) [ circum- + L. *gemma,* a bud ]. Surrounding a budlike or bulblike body; denoting a mode of nerve termination by fibrils surrounding an end bulb.

**cir'cuminites'tinal.** Surrounding the intestine.

**circumlen'tal.** Surrounding the crystalline lens.

**circumnuclear** (sur-kum-nu'kle-ar). Surrounding any nucleus.

**circumocular** (sur-kum-ok'u-lar) [ circum- + L. *oculus,* eye ]. Around the eye.

**circumo'ral** [ circum- + L. *os* (*oris*), mouth ]. Encircling the mouth.

**circumor'bital.** Around the orbit.

**circumre'nal** [ circum- + L. *ren,* kidney ]. Perinephric.

**circumscribed** (sur'kum-skrībd) [ circum- + L. *scribo,* to write ]. Bounded by a line; limited or confined.

**circumscrip'tus** [ L. ]. Circumscribed.

**circumstantiality** (sur'kum-stan-shī-al'ī-tī) [ L. *circumsto,* pr. p. -*stans,* to stand around. STA- ]. A term for a type of conversation in which a patient voluntarily or involuntarily avoids any direct statement or answer to a question by digression into tangential, elaborate and irrelevant details. It is observed in the schizophrenias and in obsessional disorders.

**circumval'late** [ circum- + L. *vallum,* wall ]. Denoting a structure surrounded by a wall, as the c. papillae of the tongue.

**circumvas'cular** [ circum- + L. *vasculum,* vessel ]. Surrounding any vessel, especially a blood vessel.

**circumvol'ute** [ L. *circum-volvo,* pp. -*volutus,* to roll around ]. Twisted around; rolled about.

**cirolemy'cin** (USAN). A substance produced by *Streptomyces bellus;* antibacterial, also with antineoplastic action.

**cirrhogenic** (sīr-o-jen'ik). Cirrhogenous.

**cirrhogenous** (sīr-roj'e-nus) [ G. *kirrhos,* yellow, with reference to the liver, + suffix -*gen,* producing ]. Cirrhogenic; tending to the development of cirrhosis.

**cirrhonosus** (sīr-ron'o-sus) [ G. *kirrhos,* tawny, + *nosos,* disease ]. A disease of the fetus marked anatomically by a yellow staining of the peritoneum and pleura.

**cirrhosis** (sīr-ro'sis) [ G. *kirrhos,* tawny, + suffix -*osis,* condition ]. Fibroid or granular induration; progressive disease of the liver characterized by diffuse damage to hepatic parenchymal cells, with nodular regeneration, fibrosis, and disturbance of normal architecture. C. is associated with failure in the function of hepatic cells and interference with blood flow in the liver, frequently resulting in jaundice, portal hypertension and ascites.

**alcoholic c.,** c. that frequently develops in chronic alcoholism, characterized in an early stage by enlargement of the liver due to fatty change, and later by Laënnec's c. with contraction of the liver. It is uncertain whether alcoholism leads to c. by a direct effect of alcohol on the liver cells, or because of an associated nutritional deficiency (the latter hypothesis being supported by experiments with rats).

**bil'iary c.,** c. due to biliary obstruction, which may be a primary intrahepatic disease or secondary to obstruction of extrahepatic bile ducts. The latter may lead to inflammatory changes and proliferation in small bile ducts with fibrosis, but marked disturbance of the lobular pattern is infrequent. See also primary biliary c.

**Budd's c.,** chronic enlargement of the liver without jaundice, formerly thought to be of intestinal origin.

**capsular c. of the liver,** glisson's c.

**cardiac c.,** cardiac liver; cyanotic atrophy of the liver; pseudocirrhosis; cardiocirrhosis; stasis c.; an extensive fibrotic reaction within the liver as a result of prolonged congestive heart failure.

**cholangiolitic c.,** a form of c. in which there is diffuse inflammation of the cholangioles, with inflammation, fibrosis, and regeneration; characterized by chronicity, relapses, and febrile episodes.

**cryptogenic c.,** c. of unknown etiology, with no history of alcoholism or previous acute hepatitis.

**fatty c.,** early nutritional c., especially in alcoholics, in which the liver is enlarged by fatty change, with mild fibrosis.

**Glisson's c.,** capsular c. of the liver; chronic perihepatitis with thickening and subsequent contraction, resulting in atrophy and deformity of the liver.

**Hanot's c.,** primary biliary c.

**juvenile c.,** active chronic *hepatitis.*

**Laënnec's c.,** portal c.; hobnail liver (*q. v.*); c.; c. in which normal liver lobules are replaced by small regeneration nodules, sometimes containing fat, separated by a fairly regular framework of fine and fibrous tissue strands.

**necrotic c.,** postnecrotic c.

**nutritional c.,** c. occurring in persons or animals with general or specific dietary deficiencies; methionine and cystine deficiency may produce changes of c. in animals,

but the relationship of human malnutrition to c. is uncertain.

**pigmentary c.,** see hemochromatosis.

**portal c.,** Laënnec's c.,

**posthepatitic c.,** active chronic *hepatitis.*

**postnecrotic c.,** necrotic c.; c. characterized by necrosis involving whole lobules, with collapse of the reticular framework to form large scars. Regeneration nodules are also large. Postnecrotic c. may follow viral or toxic necrosis or develop as a result of ischemic necrosis in the course of nutritional c.

**primary biliary c.,** Hanot's c.; a rare condition occurring mainly in women, characterized by obstructive jaundice with hyperlemia; no obstruction of large bile ducts is found. The liver shows c. with marked portal infiltration by lymphocytes and plasma cells and frequently by epithelioid cell granulomas. Proliferation of small bile ducts is not seen.

**stasis c.,** cardiac c.

**toxic c.,** c. of the liver resulting from chronic poisoning by lead, carbon tetrachloride, etc.

**cirrhotic** (sīr-rot'ik). Relating to or affected with cirrhosis.

**cirrose, cirrous** (sīr'ōs, sīr'us). Relating to or having cirri.

**cirrus,** pl. **cirri** (sīr'rus) [ L. a curl ]. A structure formed from a cluster or tuft of fused cilia constituting one of the sensory or locomotor organs of certain ciliate protozoa.

**cirsectomy** (sur-sek'to-me) [ G. *kirsos,* varix, + *ektomē,* excision ]. Excision of a section of a varicose vein.

**cirsocele** (sur'so-sēl) [ G. *kirsos,* varix, + *kēlē,* tumor ]. Varicocele.

**cirsodesis** (sur-sod'e-sis) [ G. *kirsos,* varix, + *desis,* a binding, fr. *deō,* to bind ]. Ligation of varicose veins.

**cirsoid** (sur'soyd) [ G. *kirsos,* varix, + *eidos,* appearance ]. Varicose; resembling a varix.

**cirsomphalos** (sur-som'fā-los) [ G. *kirsos,* varix, + *omphalos,* umbilicus ]. The presence of varicose veins around the umbilicus; caput medusae.

**cirsophthalmia** (ser-sof-thal'mi-ah) [ G. *kirsos,* varix, + *ophthalmos,* eye ]. Varicose dilation of the conjunctival blood vessels.

**cirsotome** (sur'-so-tōm). A cutting instrument used in removing varicose veins.

**cirsotomy** (sur-sot'o-mī) [ G. *kirsos,* varix, + *tomē,* incision ]. Treatment of varicose veins by multiple incisions.

**cis-** [ L. ]. 1. A prefix meaning on this side, on the near side. Opposite of trans-. 2. In genetics, a prefix denoting the location of two or more genes on the same chromosome of a homologous pair. 3. In organic chemistry, a form of isomerism in which similar functional groups are attached on the same side of the plane that includes two adjacent, fixed carbon atoms (*e.g.,* the 2- and 3-OH groups of ribofuranose); see also trans-.

**cissa** (sis'ah) [ G. *kissa* ]. Citta; cittosis; craving for unusual or unwholesome articles of food; the unnatural longings of pregnancy. See also pica.

**cistern** (sis'tern) [ L. *cisterna* ]. Cisterna.

**cerebellomedullary c.,** *cisterna* cerebellomedullaris.

**c. of chiasm,** *cisterna* chiasmatis.

**chyle c.,** *cisterna* chyli.

**c. of cytoplasmic reticulum,** see cisterna (2).

**c. of great vein of cerebrum,** *cisterna* venae magnae cerebri.

**interpeduncular c.,** *cisterna* interpeduncularis.

**c. of lateral fossa of cerebrum,** *cisterna* fossae lateralis cerebri.

**c. of nuclear envelope,** *cisterna* caryothecae.

**Pecquet's c.,** *cisterna* chyli.

**pontine c.,** *cisterna* pontis.

**subarachnoidal c.'s,** *cisternae* subarachnoideales.

**cisterna,** gen. and pl. **cister'nae** (sis-ter'nah) [ L. an underground cistern for water, fr. *cista,* a box ]. Cistern. 1 [ NA ]. Any cavity or enclosed space serving as a reservoir, especially for chyle, lymph, or cerebrospinal fluid. 2. An ultramicroscopic space occurring between the membranes of the flattened sacs of the cytoplasmic reticulum, the Golgi complex, or the two membranes of the nuclear envelope.

**c. ambiens, ambient c.,** c. venae magnae cerebri.

**c. basa'lis,** c. interpeduncularis.

**c. caryothe′cae,** cistern of the nuclear envelope; the space between the internal and external membranes of the envelope; may be continuous in places with cisterns of the cytoplasmic reticulum.

**c. cerebellomedulla′ris** [ NA ], cerebellomedullary cistern; c. magna; the largest of the subarachnoid cisterns between the undersurface of the cerebellum and the dorsal surface of the medulla oblongata.

**c. chias′matis** [ NA ], cistern of the chiasm; a dilation of the subarachnoid space below and anterior to the optic chiasm.

**c. chy′li** [ NA ], chyle cistern; receptaculum chyli; ampulla chyli; Pecquet′s cistern; chylocyst; a dilated sac at the lower end of the thoracic duct into which the intestinal trunk and two lumbar lymphatic trunks open. It occurs inconstantly and when present is located behind the aorta opposite the 1st and 2nd lumbar vertebrae.

**c. crura′lis,** c. interpeduncularis.

**c. fossae latera′lis cer′ebri** [ NA ], cistern of the lateral fossa of the cerebrum; an elongated expansion of the subarachnoid space where the arachnoid bridges over the opening of the Sylvian fissure.

**c. interpeduncula′ris** [ NA ], interpeduncular cistern; c. basalis; c. cruralis; a dilation of the subarachnoid space in front of the pons, where the arachnoid membrane stretches across between the two temporal lobes over the base of the diencephalon.

**c. magna,** c. cerebellomedullaris.

**c. perilymphat′ica,** *spatium* perilymphaticum.

**c. pontis,** pontine cistern; an upward continuation of the subarachnoid space of the spinal cord, continuous about the medulla with the c. cerebellomedullaris.

**cisternae subarachnoidea′les** [ NA ], subarachnoidal cisterns; widening portions of the subarachnoid space within the cranium where the arachnoid bridges over a depression on the surface of the brain.

**subsurface c.,** a cistern of the cytoplasmic reticulum that lies close to the plasma membrane; such cisternae occur especially in the cell bodies of neurons.

**terminal cisternae,** pairs of transversely oriented tubules occurring at regular intervals in skeletal muscle fibers; together with an intermediate tubule they make up a triad.

**c. ve′nae mag′nae cer′ebri,** cistern of the great vein of the cerebrum; c. ambiens; ambient c.; Bichat′s canal or foramen; an expansion of the subarachnoid space extending forward between the corpus callosum and the thalamus; it encloses the internal cerebral veins which caudally join to form the vena magna cerebri (Galen′s vein).

**cister′nal.** Relating to a cisterna.

**cisternography** (sis′tern-og′rä-fī). The roentgenographic study of the basal cisterns of the brain after the subarachnoid introduction of an opaque contrast medium.

**pontocerebellar c.,** the roentgenographic study of the cerebellar pontine angle and contiguous structures after the introduction of a radiopaque contrast medium into the subarachnoid space.

**cistron** (sis′tron). The smallest functional unit of heredity; a length of chromosomal deoxyribonucleic acid (DNA) associated with a single biochemical function. Under classical concepts a gene might consist of more than one cistron; in modern molecular biology the cistron is essentially equivalent to the gene; see also gene.

**cisvestism** (sis-ves′tizm) [ L. *cis*, on the near side of, + *vestio*, to dress ]. Cisvestitism; the practice of dressing in clothes that are not appropriate to one′s position or status; *cf.* transvestism.

**cisvest′itism** (sis-ves′tī-tizm). Cisvestism.

**Citel′lus** [ Mod. L. ]. A genus of ground squirrel. *C. beecheyi, C. grammurus, C. pygmaeus, C. townsendi,* and several other species act as an important resevoir of *Yersina pestis.*

**citen′amide** (USAN). 5*H*-Dibenzo[ *a,d* ]cycloheptene-5-carboxamide; an anticonvulsant drug.

**cit′ral.** An aldehyde from oils of lemon, orange, verbena, and lemon grass.

**cit′ramalic acid.** 2-Methylmalic acid.

**cit′rase.** Citrate lyase.

**cit′ratase.** Citrate lyase.

**citrate** (sit′rāt, si′trāt). A salt or ester of citric acid.

**c. aldolase,** c. lyase.

**c. lyase** (EC 4.1.3.6), citratase; citrase; citridesmolase; citrate aldolase; an enzyme that catalyzes the cleavage of citric acid to oxaloacetic acid and acetic acid, in the absence of coenzyme A.

**c. synthase** (EC 4.1.3.7), citrogenase; condensing enzyme; oxaloacetate transacetase; an enzyme catalyzing the condensation of oxaloacetic acid and acetyl-CoA, forming citric acid and coenzyme A.

**cit′rated.** Containing a citrate; specifically denoting blood serum or milk to which has been added a solution of potassium or sodium citrate, or both.

**cit′ric acid** 1. 2-Hydroxy-1,2,3-propanetricarboxylic acid; the acid of citrus fruits, widely distributed in nature; a key intermediate in intermediary metabolism. 2 (USP, BP). Available for use as a scurvy preventive.

**c. acid cycle,** tricarboxylic acid cycle; see under cycle.

**cit′rides′molase.** Citrate lyase.

**cit′rin.** Vitamin P.

**cit′rinin.** Antimycin; a substituted benzpyran carboxylic acid, with antibiotic properties; isolated from *Aspergillus niveus,* also from *Penicillium citrinum;* active against Gram-positive bacteria only.

**Citrobacter** (sit′ro-bak-ter). A genus of motile bacteria (tribe Salmonelleae) containing Gram-negative rods which utilize citrate as a sole source of carbon; the motile cells are peritrichous. The fermentation of lactose by these organisms is delayed or absent. They produce trimethylene glycol from glycerol. The pathogenicity of these organisms is problematical. The type species is *C. freundii.*

**C. freundii,** *Escherichia freundii;* a species found in water, feces, and urine. It appears to be an inhabitant of the normal intestine but it may occur in alimentary infections and in infections of the urinary tract, gallbladder, middle ear, and meninges. It is the type species of the genus *Citrobacter.*

**C. interme′dius,** *Escherichia intermedia;* a species of bacteria found in soil, water, and the intestinal tracts of man and other animals.

**citrogenase.** Citrate synthase.

**citronel′la.** *Cymbopogon (Andropogon) nardis* (family Gramineae); a fragrant grass of Ceylon, from which is distilled a volatile oil used as a perfume and insect repellent.

**c. oil,** a volatile oil distilled from *Cymbopogon (Andropogon) nardus,* used as an insectifuge and in perfume.

**citronel′lal.** 3,7-Dimethyl-6-octenal; $(CH_3)_2C=CH(CH_2)_2CH(CH_3)CH_2CHO$; a terpene aldehyde found in the essential oils of eucalyptus, orange peel, lemon peel, and citronella.

**citrovorum factor** (si-trov′o-rum). Folinic acid.

**citrul′line.** $\alpha$-Amino-$\delta$-ureidovaleric acid; 5-ureidonorvaline; an amino acid formed from ornithine in the course of the urea cycle. It is found in watermelon (*Citrullus vulgaris*) and in casein.

**citrulline′mia.** Citrullinuria; a disease of amino acid metabolism (usually classed as a type of aminoaciduria) in which citrulline concentrations in blood, urine, and cerebrospinal fluid are elevated; vomiting, ammonia intoxication, and mental retardation beginning in infancy; autosomal recessive inheritance.

**cit′rullinu′ria.** Enhanced urinary excretion of citrulline; one manifestation of citrullinemia, *q.v.*

**citta** (kit′ah, sit′-ah) [ G. *kitta, kissa,* longing for strange food by pregnant women ]. Cissa.

**citto′sis.** Cissa.

**Civatte** (siv-ät′), French dermatologist, 1877-1956. See C. bodies, disease, poikiloderma.

**civet** (siv′et). The secretion from the anal glands of *Viverra civetta* and *V. zibetha,* animals of Africa and southern Asia, respectively. Used, like musk, in perfumery.

**civetone** (siv′ĕ-tōn). A cyclic ketone, 9-cycloheptadecen-1-one, the glandular secretion of the civet cat; notable for the size of the ring, which contains 17 carbon atoms; used in perfumes.

**Civinini** (che-ve-ne′ne), Filippo, Italian anatomist, 1805–1844. See C.′s *canal, ligament, process.*

**Cl.** Chemical symbol for the element chlorine.

**clad'inose.** 3-*O*-Methylmycarose; a methylated hexose derived from erythromycins by mild hydrolysis.

**clad'io'sis** [ G. *klados*, branch or root, + suffix *-osis*, condition ]. Verrucous lesions and ascending lymphangitis due to *Scopulariopsis blochii;* a dermatomycosis.

**Clado,** Spiro, French gynecologist, 1856–1905. See C.'s. *anastomosis, band, ligament, point.*

**Clador'chis watsoni.** Incorrect term for *Watsonius watsoni.*

**cladosporiosis** (klad'o-spo-rī-o'sis). Infection with a fungus belonging to the genus *Cladosporium.*

**Cladospor'ium** [ G. *klados*, a branch, + *sporos*, seed ]. A genus of fungi having dark-colored conidiophores with oval or round spores and commonly isolated in soil or plant residues. The genus is often called *Hormodendrum.* Found in chromoblastomycosis in man.

  **C. bantianum,** a species which has been isolated from several cases of brain abscess in humans; the species appears to be neurotropic.

  **C. werneckii,** a species commonly designated as the causitive agent of tinea nigra in tropical areas.

**clad'othrico'sis.** An obsolete term for infection with *Cladothrix* (*Actinomyces*) *asteroides.*

**clairvoyance** (klăr-voy'ans) [ Fr. ]. The ability to perceive or see that which is not discernible by ordinary means; a type of extrasensory perception.

**clamox'yquin hydrochloride** (USAN). 5-Chloro-7-{ [ (3-diethylaminopropyl) amino ]-methyl} -8-quinolinol dihydrochloride; amebicide.

**clamp.** An instrument for making compression of an artery, the pedicle of a tumor, or other structures.

  **Cope's c.,** one used in excision of colon and rectum.

  **Crafoord c.,** one used in heart and lung surgery.

  **Crile's c.,** a rubber-covered c. for temporary stoppage of blood flow.

  **Gant's c.,** a right-angled c. used in hemorrhoidectomy.

  **Gaskell's c.,** an instrument for crushing the atrioventricular bundle in experimental animals and thus producing heart block.

  **gingival c.,** a springlike metal piece encircling or grasping the cervix of a tooth and shaped so as to retract the gingival tissue.

  **Goldblatt's c.,** a c. applied experimentally to the renal artery to produce chronic hypertension by renal ischemia.

  **Mikulicz' c.,** one used to crush walls between proximal and distal colon in two-stage colectomy.

  **mogen c.** [ Hebrew star ], a circumcision instrument.

  **Payr's c.,** one used in gastrectomy or enterectomy.

  **Rankin's c.,** a three-bladed c. used in resection of colon.

  **rubber dam c.,** a springlike metal piece encircling or grasping the cervix of a tooth and so shaped as to prevent a rubber dam from riding off the tooth.

  **Willet's c.,** Willet's *forceps.*

**clap.** Colloquialism for gonorrhea.

**clapotage, clapotement** (klă-pŭ-tazh', klă-put-moń') [ Fr. ]. The splashing sound heard on succussion of a dilated stomach.

**Clapton's line.** See under line.

**clarif'icant** [ L. *clarus*, clear, + *facio*, to make ]. 1. Making a turbid liquid clear. 2. Any agent having this property.

**clarifica'tion.** The process of making a turbid liquid clear.

**Clark,** Leland C., Jr., U.S. biochemist, \*1918. See C. *electrode.*

**Clark's weight rule.** See under rule.

**Clarke,** Cecil. See C.-Hadfield *syndrome.*

**Clarke,** Sir Charles M., English physician, 1782–1857. See C.'s *ulcer.*

**Clarke,** Jacob A. L., English anatomist, 1817–1880. See C.'s *column, nucleus.*

**clasmatocyte** (klaz-mat'o-sīt) [ G. *klasma*, a fragment, + *kytos*, a hollow (cell) ]. Macrophage.

**clasmatosis** (klaz-mă-to'sis) [ G. *klasma*, a fragment, + suffix *-osis*, condition ]. The extension of pseudopodia-like processes in unicellular organisms and blood cells by plasmolysis rather than by a true pseudopodia formation.

**clasp.** 1. A part of a removable partial denture which acts as a direct retainer and/or stabilizer for the denture by partially surrounding or contacting an abutment tooth. 2.

A direct retainer of a removable partial denture, usually consisting of two arms joined by a body which connects with an occlusal rest. At least one arm of a clasp usually terminates in the infrabulge (gingival convergence) area of the tooth enclosed.

  **bar c.,** Roach c.; (1) a c. whose arms are bar type extensions from major connectors or from within the denture base; the arms pass adjacent to the soft tissues and approach the point of contact on the tooth in a gingivo-occlusal direction; (2) a c. which consists of two or more separate and distinct arms located opposite to each other on the tooth. The bar arms arise from the framework or a connector and may traverse the soft tissue. One arm (bar) usually terminates in the infrabulge (gingival convergence) area of the tooth and is retentive, and the other usually on the suprabulge (occlusal convergence) area, and acts as a reciprocal arm.

  **circumferential c.,** (1) a c. that encircles more than 180 degrees of a tooth, including opposite angles, and which usually contacts the tooth throughout the extent of the c., at least one terminal being in the infrabulge (gingival convergence) area; (2) a c. consisting of two circumferential c. arms, both of which originate from the same minor connector and are located on opposite surfaces of the abutment tooth.

  **continuous c.,** continuous bar *retainer.*

  **Roach c.,** bar c.

**class** [ L. *classis*, a class, division ]. In biologic classification, the division next below the phylum (or subphylum) and above the order.

**classifica'tion.** A systematic arrangement into classes or groups.

  **Angle's c.,** a list of the several forms of malocclusion.

  **Arneth's c.,** a c. of the polymorphonuclear neutrophils according to the number of their nuclear lobes; see Arneth's *stages.*

  **Caldwell-Moloy c.,** a c. of the variations in the female pelvis; namely gynecoid, android, anthropoid, and platypelloid pelvis, based on the type of the posterior and anterior segments of the inlet.

  **Cummer's c.,** a listing of several types of removable partial dentures in accordance with the distribution of direct retainers.

  **Denver's c.,** a system of nomenclature for human mitotic chromosomes, classifying them on the basis of length and position of the centromere.

  **Duke's c.,** a c. of the extent of spread of operable carcinoma of the large intestine in surgical specimens.

  **Galton's system of c. of fingerprints,** see under fingerprint.

  **Jansky's c.,** the c. of the blood groups of the human race into I, II, III, and IV, now designated, respectively, as O, A, B, and AB.

  **Kennedy c.,** a listing of several forms of partially edentulous jaws in accordance with the distribution of the missing teeth.

  **Lancefield c.,** a serologic c. dividing hemolytic streptococci into groups which bear a definite relationship to their sources; the classification is based upon precipitation tests depending upon group-specific substances which are probably carbohydrate in nature. *Group A* contains strains pathogenic for man; *B*, strains from mastitis in cows and from normal milk, including a few strains from the human throat and vagina: *C*, strains from various lower animals, including a number from cattle; *D*, strains from cheese; *E*, strains from certified milk; *F*, strains mainly from the human throat, associated with tonsillitis; *G*, strains from man, a few from monkeys and dogs; and *H* and *K*, nonpathogenic strains from normal human nose and throat.

**clastic** (klas'tik) [ G. *klastos*, broken ]. Breaking up into pieces, or exhibiting a tendency so to break or divide.

**clastothrix** (klas'to-thriks) [ G. *klastos*, broken, + *thrix*, hair ]. *Trichorrhexis* nodosa.

**cla'thrates.** A type of inclusion compound in which small molecules are trapped in the cage-like lattice of macromolecules.

**Clau'berg,** Karl W., German bacteriologist, \*1893. See C.'s *test, unit.*

**Claude,** Albert, Belgian electron microscopist, *1899. Nobel laureate, 1974, with Christian deDuve and George Palade, for their discoveries concerning the structural and functional organization of the cell.

**Claude,** Henri, French psychiatrist, 1869–1945. See C.'s *syndrome.*

**claudication** (klaw-dĭ-ka'shun) [ L. *claudicatio,* fr. *claudico,* to limp ]. Limping, usually referring to intermittent c.

   **cerebral c.,** insufficient blood supply to the brain related to narrowing of the arteries.

   **intermittent c.,** Charcot's syndrome; myasthenia angiosclerotica; a condition caused by ischemia of the leg muscles due to sclerosis with narrowing of the arteries of the legs; it is characterized by attacks of lameness and pain, brought on by walking, chiefly in the calf muscles.

**claudicatory** (klaw'dĭ-ka-to-rī). Relating to claudication, especially intermittent claudication.

**Claudius,** Friedrich M., Austrian anatomist, 1822–1869. See C.'s *cells, fossa.*

**clause, Delaney.** A clause of the Food Additives Amendment of the U. S. Federal law specifying that no substance that has been found to induce cancer in any animal species may be incorporated into food.

**claus'tral.** Relating to the claustrum.

**claustrophobia** (klaw-stro-fo'bĭ-ah) [ L. *claustrum,* an enclosed space, + G. *phobos,* fear ]. A morbid fear of being in a closed place.

**claustrum,** pl. **claus'tra** (klaw'strum) [ L. barrier ]. One of several anatomical structures bearing a fancied resemblance to a barrier. Specifically [ NA ], a thin vertically placed lamina of gray matter lying close to the outer portion (putamen) of the lenticular nucleus, from which it is separated by the external capsule.

   **c. gut'turis, c. o'ris,** *palatum* molle.

   **c. virgina'le,** a rare term for hymen.

**clausura** (klaw-su'rah) [ L. a lock, bolt, fr. *claudo,* to close ]. Atresia.

**clava** (kla'vah) [ L. a club ]. *Tuberculum* nuclei gracilis.

**clav'acin.** Patulin.

**cla'val.** Relating to the clava.

**clavate** (kla'vāt) [ L. *clava,* a club ]. Club-shaped.

**clav'atin.** Patulin.

**clavicle** (klav'ĭ-kl). Clavicula.

**clavicotomy** (klav'ĭ-kot'o-mĭ) [ clavicle + G. *tomē,* incision ]. Surgical division of the clavicle.

**clavicula,** pl. **clavic'ulae** (klă-vik'u-lah) [ L. *clavicula,* a small key, fr. *clavis,* key. CLEID- ] [ NA ]. Clavicle; collar bone; a doubly curved long bone that forms part of the shoulder girdle. Its medial end articulates with the manubrium sterni, its lateral end with the acromion of the scapula.

**clavic'ular.** Relating to the clavicle.

**claviculus,** pl. **klavic'uli** (klă-vik'u-lus) [ Mod. L. dim. of L. *clavus,* a nail ]. One of Sharpey's fibers.

**clav'iformin.** Patulin.

**clavus** (kla'vus) [ L. a nail, wart, corn ]. 1. Corn; a small conical callosity caused by pressure over a bony prominence, usually on a toe. 2. A severe pain in the head, sharply limited in area, as if caused by the driving of a nail. 3. A condition resulting from healing of a granuloma of the foot in yaws. A core falls out, leaving an erosion.

   **c. hyster'icus,** a lancinating pain felt in the sagittal suture.

**claw** [ L. *clavus,* a nail ]. A sharp, slender, usually curved nail on the paw of an animal.

   **dew c.,** a rudimentary digit, not reaching the ground, on the feet of many quadrupeds.

**claw'hand.** A deformity resulting from atrophy of the interosseous muscles, with hyperextension at the metacarpophalangeal joints and flexion at the interphalangeal joints.

**Claybrook,** Edwin B., Maryland surgeon, *1871. See C.'s *sign.*

**Clayton gas.** See under gas.

**cleaning.** In dentistry, a procedure whereby accretions are removed from the teeth or from a dental prosthesis. See also prophylaxis.

   **ultrasonic c.,** in dentistry, the use of a high frequency vibrating point to remove deposits from tooth structure; also the process of cleaning dentures by placing them in a special liquid in a container that generates high frequency vibrations.

**clear'ance.** 1. Removal of a substance from the blood, *e.g.,* by the kidney, expressed in terms of the volume flow of arterial blood or plasma that would contain the amount of substance removed per unit time. Abbreviated C with a subscript indicating the substance removed. Units: ml/min. 2. A condition in which bodies may pass each other without hindrance. 3. The distance between bodies.

   **interocclusal c.,** interocclusal *distance.*

   **inulin c.,** a fairly accurate method for determining the rate of filtration in the renal glomeruli, since inulin is completely filterable through them and is neither excreted nor reabsorbed by the renal tubules; after the intravenous administration of inulin, the amount excreted in the urine is divided by the plasma concentration; the average c. in an adult person is 120 ml. of plasma per minute (normal range is from 100 to 150 ml. per minute), the figures being corrected to a standard body surface of 1.73 sq. m.

   **maximum urea c.,** the urea c. when the urine flow exceeds 2 ml. per minute; normal value is about 75 ml. of blood per minute in an adult.

   **occlusal c.,** a condition in which the opposing occlusal surfaces may glide over one another without any interfering projection.

   **standard urea c.,** the value obtained when the square root of the urine flow (when below 2 ml. per minute) is multiplied by the ratio of urinary urea to whole blood urea concentrations; the normal value is about 54 ml. per minute in an adult.

   **urea c.,** the volume of plasma or blood that would be completely cleared of urea by one minute's excretion of urine, *i.e.,* the urinary urea excretion rate divided by the plasma or blood concentration.

**clearer** (klēr'er). An agent, used in histological preparations, which is miscible in both the dehydrating or fixing fluid and the embedding substance.

**cleavage** (klēv'ij). 1. Segmentation; the series of cell divisions occurring in the ovum immediately following its fertilization; see also cleavage *division.* 2. The splitting of a complex molecule into two or more simpler molecules. 3. The linear clefts in the skin indicating the direction of the fibers in the dermis. See illustration of cleavage lines, under line.

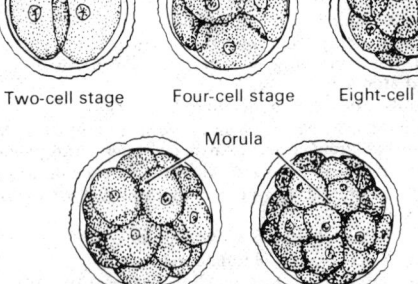

Polar bodies

Two-cell stage     Four-cell stage     Eight-cell stage

Morula

**Cleavage (Segmentation) of Ovum and Formation of Morula**

   **abnormal c. of cardiac valve,** congenital malformation of a valve leaflet with a defect extending from the free margin.

   **adequal c.,** c. resulting in the formation of blastomeres of approximately equal size.

   **complete c.,** holoblastic c.

   **determinate c.,** c. resulting in blastomeres each destined to give rise to some particular part of the embryo.

**discoidal c.,** meroblastic c. limited to the small cap of protoplasm of large-yolked eggs, such as the telolecithal eggs of birds.

**enamel c.,** the splitting of enamel in a plane parallel to the direction of the enamel rods.

**equal c.,** producing blastomeres of like size.

**equatorial c.,** c. in which the plane of cytoplasmic division is at right angles to the axis of the ovum.

**holoblastic c.,** c. in which the blastomeres are completely separated.

**hydrolytic c.,** hydrolysis; c. accompanied by taking up the constituents of water.

**incomplete c.,** meroblastic c.

**indeterminate c.,** c. resulting in blastomeres of similar developmental potencies, each capable, when isolated, of producing an entire embryonic body.

**meridional c.,** c. in a plane through the axis of the zygote.

**meroblastic c.,** incomplete separation of the blastomeres, with the divisions being limited to the nonyolked portion of the egg.

**phosphoroclastic c.,** phosphorolysis.

**progressive c.,** a type of sporulation in a fungal sporangium; the c. planes in the cytoplasm first produce multicellular spores (protospores) and subsequently sporangiospores.

**puden'dal c.,** *rima* pudendi.

**superficial c.,** meroblastic c. with the divisions limited to the peripheral cytoplasm of a centrolecithal egg.

**thioclastic c.,** the splitting of a bond in fashion analogous to hydrolysis or phosphorolysis except that the elements of a substituted hydrogen sulfide (usually coenzyme A) are added across the break.

**unequal c.,** that producing blastomeres of different sizes.

**yolk c.,** segmentation of the vitellus.

**cleaver** (kle'ver). A heavy knife for cutting or chopping.

**enamel c.,** an instrument with a heavy shank and a very short blade at about 90° to the axis of the handle; used with a hoeing motion to strip enamel from the axial surfaces of a tooth in preparation for a crown.

**Cleemann's sign.** See under sign.

**cleft.** A fissure.

**anal c.,** *crena* ani.

**branchial c.'s,** gill c.'s; a bilateral series of slitlike openings into the pharynx through which water is drawn by aquatic animals. In the walls of the c.'s are the vascular gill filaments that take up oxygen from the water passing through the c.'s. Sometimes loosely applied to the branchial ectodermal grooves of mammalian embryos which are their imperforate, rudimentary homologues.

**cholesterol c.,** a space caused by the dissolving out of cholesterol crystals in sections of tissue embedded in paraffin.

**facial c.,** a c. resulting from incomplete merging or fusion of embryonic processes normally uniting in the formation of the face and jaws, as c. lip, or oblique facial c.

**first visceral c.,** hyomandibular c.

**gill c.'s,** branchial c.'s.

**gingival c.,** a fissure associated with pocket formation and lined by mixed gingival and pocket epithelium.

**gluteal c.,** *crena* ani.

**hyobranchial c.,** the c. caudal to the hyoid arch of the embryo.

**hy'omandib'ular c.,** first visceral c.; the external auditory meatus is developed from its dorsal portion.

**interneuromeric c.'s,** c.'s between the neuromeric or segmental elevations in the primitive rhombencephalon.

**Larrey's c.,** *trigonum* sternocostale.

**Maurer's c.'s,** Maurer's *dots.*

**natal c.,** *crena* ani.

**oblique facial c.,** prosoposchisis.

**residual c.,** residual lumen; the remnants of the pituitary lumen (Rathke's pouch) which occurs between the pars distalis and pars intermedia; a distinct lumen is present in some animals but in man one is present only during prenatal development and sometimes in young children.

**Schmidt-Lantermann c.'s,** Schmidt-Lantermann *incisures.*

**synaptic c.,** the space about 200 Å wide between the axolemma and the postsynaptic surface; see also synapse.

**vis'ceral c.,** any c. between two branchial (visceral) arches in the embryo.

**cleid-.** See cleido-.

**cleidagra, clidagra** (kli-dag'rah) [ cleid- + G. *agra,* seizure ]. Rarely used term meaning gouty pain in the clavicle.

**cleidal, clidal** (kli'dal). Relating to the clavicle.

**cleidarthritis, clidarthritis** (kli'dar-thri'tis) [ cleid- + G. *arthron,* joint, + suffix *-itis,* inflammation ]. Rarely used term meaning inflammation of either of the articular ends of the clavicle.

**cleido-, cleid-** (kli'do-) [ G. *kleis,* clavicle. CLEID- ]. Combining forms relating to the clavicle; also spelled clido-, clid-.

**cleidocostal, clidocostal** (kli-do-kos'tal) [ cleido- + L. *costa,* rib ]. Relating to the clavicle and a rib.

**cleidocranial, clidocranial** (kli'do-kra'nĭ-al) [ G. *kleis,* clavicle, + *kranion,* cranium ]. Relating to the clavicle and the cranium.

**cleidoic, clidoic** (kli-do'ik) [ G. *kleidoun,* to lock up ]. Shut in from the external environment, as the embryo within the uterus.

**cleidorrhexis, clidorrhexis** (kli-do-rek'sis) [ cleido- + G. *rhēxis,* rupture ]. Reduction of the diameter of the shoulder girdle of the fetus by fracture or bending of the clavicles.

**cleidotomy, clidotomy** (kli-dot'o-mĭ) [ cleido- + G. *tomē,* a cutting ]. Division of the clavicles to reduce the width of the shoulders of the fetus in certain cases of dystocia.

**cleidotripsy, clidotripsy** (kli'do-trip'sĭ) [ cleido- + G. *tripsis,* a rubbing ]. Crushing of the clavicle of the fetus in order to reduce the width of the shoulder girdle in cases of dystocia.

**-cleisis** [ G. *kleisis,* a closing ]. Suffix meaning closure.

**Cleland,** W. Wallace. See C.'s *reagent.*

**clem'astine** (USAN). TAVIST; D-2-[ 2-[ (*p*-chloro-α-methyl-α-phenylbenzyl)oxy ]ethyl ]-1-methylpyrrolidine; antihistaminic.

**clemizole hydrochloride** (klem'ĭ-zōl). ALLERCUR; 1-chlorobenzyl-2-(1-pyrrolidinylmethyl)benzimidazole hydrochloride; an antihistaminic agent. It has little anticholinergic activity and apparently no effect on gastric secretion.

**clench'ing.** The intermittent forceful contacting of the upper and lower teeth usually associated with emotional tensions.

**cleoid** (kle'oyd) [ A. S. *cle,* claw + G. *eidos,* resemblance ]. A dental instrument with a pointed elliptical cutting end, used in excavating cavities or carving fillings and waxes.

**Cléret,** M., French physician. See Launois-C. *syndrome.*

**Clevenger** (klev'en-jer), Shobal V., American neurologist, 1843–1920. See C.'s *fissure.*

**click.** A slight sharp sound.

**ejection c.,** a clicking ejection sound; see under sound.

**mitral c.,** the opening snap of the mitral valve.

**systolic c.,** a sharp, clicking sound heard during cardiac systole; when heard in early systole it is usually an ejection sound; in late systole usually signifies mitral insufficiency but may be due to pleuropericardial adhesions or other extracardiac mechanisms.

**clicking.** A snapping, crepitant noise noted on excursions of the temperomandibular articulation; due to an asynchronous movement of the disk and condyle.

**clidag'ra.** Cleidagra.

**cli'dal.** Cleidal.

**clidarthritis** (kli-dar-thri'tis). Cleidarthritis.

**clidin'ium bro'mide** (USAN). 3-Hydroxy-1-methyl-quinuclidinium bromide benzilate; an anticholinergic agent.

**clido-, clid-** (kli'do-) [ G. *kleis,* clavicle. CLEID- ]. Combining forms relating to the clavicle; see also cleido-.

**cli'docos'tal.** Cleidocostal.

**cli'docra'nial.** Cleidocranial.

**clido'ic.** Cleidoic.

**cli'dorrhex'is.** Cleidorrhexis.

**clidot'omy.** Cleidotomy.

**cli'dotripsy.** Cleidotripsy.

**climacophobia** (kli'mă-ko-fo'bĭ-ah) [ G. *klimax,* ladder, + *phobos,* fear ]. Fear of stairs or of climbing.

**climac'ter** [ G. *klimaktēr*, the round of a ladder. CLIM- ]. Climacteric (1).

**climacteric** (kli-mak'ter-ik, kli-mak-ter'ik). 1. Climacter; climacterium; a period of life, occurring in women preceding termination of the reproductive period, and characterized by endocrine, somatic, and psychic changes, and ultimately menopause; no corresponding period occurs in men. 2. Relating to a climacter, or critical period of life.

**grand c.,** the sixty-third year, the ninth of the seven-year periods, each of which from the third (twenty-first year) on used to be regarded as a critical time.

**climacte'rium.** The climacteric.

**c. precox,** premature climacteric.

**c. virile,** the supposed period in males when procreative power ceases; physiologically untrue.

**climatol'ogy.** The branch of meteorology that has to do with a study of climate and its relation to disease.

**cli'matother'apy.** The treatment of disease by removal to a region having a different climate from the one at home.

**climax** (kli'maks) [ G. *klimax,* staircase. CLIM- ]. 1. The height of a disease; the stage of greatest severity. 2. Orgasm.

**cli'mograph** [ G. *klima,* climate, + *graphō,* to record ]. A diagram showing the effect of climate on health.

**clindamy'cin hydrochloride** (USP). CLEOCIN; clinimycin hydrochloride; hydrochloride salt of 7(*S*)-chloro-7-deoxylincomycin; antibacterial agent.

**clinic** (klin'ik) [ G. *klinē,* bed ]. 1. An institution, building, or part of a building where ambulatory patients are cared for. 2. An institution, building, or part of a building in which medical instruction is given to students by means of demonstrations in the presence of the sick. 3. A clinical lecture.

**clinical** (klin'ĭ-kl). 1. Relating to the bedside of a patient or to the course of his disease. 2. Denoting the symptoms and course of a disease as distinquished from the laboratory findings of anatomical changes. 3. Relating to a clinic.

**clinician** (klin-ish'un). A physician, investigator, or teacher engaged in clinical practice, as distinguished from an investigator or teacher working in preclinical fields.

**clinicopathologic** (klin'ĭ-ko-path-o-loj'ik). Pertaining to the signs and symptoms manifested by a patient, and also the results of laboratory studies, as they relate to the findings in the gross and histologic examination of tissue by means of biopsy or autopsy, or both.

**clinimycin hydrochloride.** Clindamycin hydrochloride.

**clino-** (kli'no-) [ G. *klinō,* to slope, incline, or bend. CLIM- ]. Combining form denoting a slope (inclination or declination) or bend.

**clinocephal'ic, clinoceph'alous.** Relating to clinocephaly.

**clinocephaly** (kli'no-sef'ă-lī) [ clino- + G. *kephalē,* head ]. Saddle head; a condition in which the upper surface of the skull is more or less concave, presenting a saddle-shaped appearance in profile.

**clinodactyly** (kli'no-dak'tĭ-lī) [ clino- + G. *daktylos,* finger ]. Permanent deflection of one or more fingers.

**clinog'raphy** [ G. *klinē,* bed, + *graphō,* to write ]. Graphic representation of signs and symptoms exhibited by a patient.

**clinoid** (kli'noyd) [ G. *klinē,* bed, + *eidos,* resemblance ]. 1. Resembling a bed. 2. *Processus* clinoideus.

**clinoi'deus** [ L. ] [ NA ]. Clinoid.

**clinometer** (kli-nom'e-ter) [ clino- + G. *metron,* measure ]. Clinoscope.

**clinoscope** (kli'no-skōp) [ clino- + G. *skopeō,* to view ]. Clinometer; an instrument for measuring cyclophoria.

**clioquinol** (BP). Iodochlorhydroxyquin.

**cliox'amide** (USAN). TREMERAD; 4'-chloro-3,5-diiodosalicylanilide acetate; anthelmintic.

**cliseometer** (klis'e-om'e-ter) [ G. *klisis,* inclination (CLIM-), + *metron,* measure ]. An instrument for measuring the angle which the axis of the pelvis makes with that of the body.

**clithrophobia** (klith-ro-fo'bĭ-ah) [ G. *kleithron,* a bolt, + *phobos,* fear ]. Morbid dread of being locked in.

**clition** (klit'ĭ-on) [ G. *klitos,* a declivity ]. A craniometric point in the middle of the highest part of the clivus on the sphenoid bone.

**clitoridauxe** (klit'o-rī-dawk'se) [ clitoris + G. *auxē,* increase ]. Obsolete term for hypertrophy of the clitoris.

**clitoridean** (klit'o-rī-de'an). Relating to the clitoris.

**clit'oridec'tomy** [ clitoris + G. *ektomē,* excision ]. Removal of the clitoris.

**clitoriditis** (klit'o-rī-di'tis) [ clitoris + G. suffix -*itis,* inflammation ]. Clitoritis; inflammation of the clitoris.

**clitoris,** pl. **clitor'ides** (klit'o-ris, kli'to-ris) [ G. *kleitoris* ] [ NA ]. A small cylindric, erectile body, rarely exceeding 2 cm. in length, situated at the most anterior portion of the vulva and projecting between the branched extremities of the labia minora, which form its prepuce and frenulum. It consists of a glans, a corpus, and two crura, and is the homologue of the penis in the male except that it is not perforated by the urethra and does not possess a corpus spongiosum.

**clit'orism.** 1. Prolonged and usually painful erection of the clitoris; the analogue of priapism. 2. Clitoridauxe.

**clitori'tis.** Clitoriditis.

**clit'oromeg'aly** [ clitoris + G. *megas,* great ]. Enlarged clitoris.

**clival** (kli'val). Pertaining to the clivus.

**clivus,** pl. **cli'vi** (kli'vus) [ L. slope. CLIM- ] [ NA ]. 1. A downward sloping surface. 2. Blumenbach's c.; the sloping surface from the dorsum sellae to the foramen magnum composed of part of the body of the sphenoid and part of the pars basilaris of the occipital bone.

**Blumenbach's c.,** clivus (2).

**cloaca** (klo-a'kah) [ L. sewer ]. 1. In early embryos, the entodermally lined chamber into which hindgut and allantois empty. 2. In birds and monotremes, the common chamber into which open hindgut, bladder, and genital ducts.

**ectodermal c.,** the proctodeum of the embryo.

**entodermal c.,** the terminal portion of the hindgut internal to the cloacal membrane of the embryo.

**persistent c.,** sinus urogenitalis (2); a condition in which the urorectal fold has failed to divide the c. of the embryo into rectal and urogenital portions.

**cloacal** (klo-a'kal). Pertaining to the cloaca.

**cloacitis** (klo-ă-si'tis). An inflammation of the cloacal mucosa of fowls, with ulceration and chronic discharge.

**clobenz'tropine.** TEPRIN; 3-(*p*-chloro-α-phenylbenzyloxy)tropane; antihistaminic drug.

**clo'dazon hydrochloride** (USAN). 5-Chloro-1-[ 3-(dimethylamino)propyl ]-3-phenyl-2-benzimidazoline monochloride monohydrate; antidepressant.

**clofazimine** (klo-fa'zĭ-mēn) (USAN). 3-(*p*-Chloroanilino)-10-(*p*-chlorophenyl)-2,10-dihydro-2-(isopropylimino)-phenazine; tuberculostatic and leprostatic agent.

**clofenet'amine.** KEITHON; 2-(*p*-chloro-α-methyl-α-phenylbenzyloxy)-triethylamine; used as anticholinergic agent for treatment of parkinsonism.

**clofibrate** (klo-fī'brāt) (USP, BP). Ethyl chlorophenoxyisobutyrate; it reduces plasma levels of cholesterol, triglycerides, and uric acid; used in the treatment of hypercholesterolemia and atherosclerosis.

**clo'forex.** FRENAPYL; (*p*-chloro-α,α-dimethylphenethyl)-carabamic acid ethyl ester; anorexic agent.

**cloges'tone acetate** (USAN). 6-Chloro-3β,17-dihydroxypregna-4,6-dien-20-one diacetate; a progestational agent.

**clo'macran phosphate** (USAN). 2-Chloro-9-[ 3-(dimethylamino)propyl ]acridan phosphate; a tranquilizer.

**clo'meges'tone acetate** (USAN). 6-Chloro-17-hydroxy-16α-methylpregna-4,6-diene-3,20-dione acetate; a progestational drug.

**clomiphene citrate** (klo'mĭ-fēn) (USP). CLOMID; 2-[ *p*-(2-chloro-1,2-diphenylvinyl)phenoxy ]triethylamine dihydrogen citrate; an analogue of the nonsteroid estrogen, chlorotrianisene. It has antifecundity properties and inhibits the production of gonadotropins in rats. In anovulatory women it stimulates fertility by promoting the secretion of gonadotropins, probably by competing (as an antiestrogen) with endogenous circulating estrogen arising from excessive immature ovarian follicles. It is also possible that clomiphene acts on the hypothalamic neuroendocrine apparatus. Many questions remain unanswered in regard to the precise mechanism of its action.

**clomipramine hydrochloride** (klo-mip'ră-mēn) (USAN). 3-Chloro-5-[3-(dimethylamino)propyl]-10,11-dihydro-5*H*-dibenz[*b,f*]azepine monohydrochloride; antidepressant.

**clo'nal.** Pertaining to a clone.

**clona'zepam** (USAN). 5-(*o*-Chlorophenyl)-1,3-dihydro-7-nitro-2*H*-1,4-benzodiazepin-2-one; anticonvulsant drug.

**clone, clon** [ G. *klōn*, slip, cutting used for propagation ]. A colony or group of organisms which have arisen from a single individual as a result of asexual reproduction (*e.g.*, a group of plants, identical in characters, which have been propagated from cuttings or by budding from a single individual).

**clon'ic.** Of the nature of clonus, marked by alternate contraction and relaxation of muscle.

**clonicity** (klon-is'ĭ-tĭ). The state of being clonic.

**clon'icoton'ic.** Both clonic and tonic; said of certain forms of muscular spasm.

**clo'nidine hydrochloride** (USAN). CATAPRES; 2-(2,6-dichloroanilino)-2-imidazoline hydrochloride; an antihypertensive agent with central and peripheral actions.

**clon'ism.** A long continued state of clonic spasms.

**cloni'trate** (USAN). DYLATE; 3-chloro-1,2-propanediol dinitrate; used as coronary vasodilator for treatment of angina pectoris.

**clonix'eril** (USAN). 2,3-Dihydroxypropyl 2-(3-chloro-*o*-toluidino)nicotinate; analgesic.

**clonix'in** (USAN). 2-(3-Chloro-*o*-toluidino)nicotinic acid; analgesic.

**clonogen'ic.** Arising from or consisting of a clone.

**clon'ograph** [ G. *klonos*, tumult, + *graphō*, to write ]. An instrument for registering the movements in clonic spasm.

**clonorchiasis** (klo-nor-ki'ă-sis). Clonorchiosis; a disease caused by the presence of *Clonorchis sinensis* in the distal bile ducts; repeated infection induces an intense proliterative and granulomatous condition with considerable tissue pathology; infection may be benign, but chronic infection may last for many years.

**clonorchiosis** (klo-nor-kĭ-o'sis). Chlonorchiasis.

**Clonor'chis sinen'sis.** Chinese fluke; Oriental fluke; a trematode of the family Opisthorchiidae, sometimes called *Opisthorchis sinensis*, which in the Far East infects the bile passages of man and many animals, *e.g.*, cat, dog, and other fish-eating animals. Infection is caused by eating raw, smoked, or undercooked fish, and has been reported from eating raw crayfish. Cyprinoid fish serve as chief second intermediate hosts; various operculate snails serve as the first intermediate hosts.

**clon'ospasm.** Clonus.

**clonus** (klo'nus) [ G. *klonos*, a tumult ]. Clonospasm; a form of movement marked by contractions and relaxations of a muscle, occurring in rapid succession; see also contraction.

 **ankle c.,** foot phenomenon; a rhythmical contraction of the calf muscles following a sudden passive dorsal flexion of the foot, the leg being semiflexed.

 **cathodal opening c.,** abbreviated COCL; c. produced near a cathode when the flow of current is stopped.

 **toe c.,** toe reflex (2); alternating movements of flexion and extension of the great toe following forcible extension at the metatarsophalangeal joint.

 **wrist c.,** rhythmic contractions and relaxations of the muscles of the forearm excited by a forcible passive extension of the hand.

**clopam'ide** (USAN). BRINALDIX; 1-(4-chloro-3-sulfamoylbenzamido)-2,6-dimethylpiperidine; diuretic.

**clo'pidol** (USAN). COYDEN; clopindol; 2,5-dichloro-2,6-dimethyl-4-pyridinol; a coccidiostat for poultry.

**Cloquet** (klo-ka'), Hippolyte, French anatomist, 1787–1840. See C.'s *ganglion, space.*

**Cloquet** (klo-ka'), Jules G., French anatomist, 1790–1883. See C.'s *canal, hernia, node, septum, sign.*

**clorpren'aline hydrochloride** (USAN). VORTEL; isoprophenamine hydrochloride; *o*-chloro-α-(isopropylaminomethyl)benzyl alcohol hydrochloride; bronchodilator.

**closir'amine aceturate** (USAN). 8-Chloro-11-[ 2-(dimethylamino)ethyl ]-6,11-dihydro-5*H*-benzo[ 5,6 ]cyclohepta-[ 1,2,-*b* ]pyridine compound with *N*-acetylglycine; antihistaminic.

**clostrid'ial.** Relating to any bacterium of the genus *Clostridium.*

**clostrid'iopep'tidase A.** Collagenase.

**clostrid'iopep'tidase B.** *Clostridium histolyticum* proteinase B.

---

# CLOSTRIDIUM

---

**Clostridium,** pl. **clostrid'ia** (klos-trid'ĭ-um) [ G. *klōstēr*, a spindle ]. A genus of anaerobic (or anaerobic, aerotolerant), sporeforming, motile (occasionally nonmotile) bacteria (family Bacillaceae) containing Gram-positive rods; motile cells are peritrichous. Many of the species are saccharolytic and fermentative, producing various acids and gases and variable amounts of neutral products; other species are proteolytic, some attacking proteins with putrefaction or more complete proteolysis. Some species fix free nitrogen. Exotoxins are sometimes produced by these organisms. They may cause disease in man and other animals. They are generally found in soil and in the intestinal tracts of man and other animals. The type species is *C. butyricum.*

 **C. aerofoetidum,** a species found in a case of gaseous gangrene and in feces.

 **C. bifermentans,** a species found in putrid meat and gaseous gangrene; also commonly found in soil, feces, and sewage. Its pathogenicity varies from strain to strain.

 **C. botuli'num,** a species which occurs widely in nature and which is a frequent cause of food poisoning (botulism) from preserved meats, fruits, or vegetables which have not been properly sterilized before canning. Including *C. parabotulinum* strains, there are six main types, A to F, characterized by antigenically distinct but pharmacologically similar, very potent neurotoxins, each of which can be neutralized only by the specific antitoxin; group C toxin contains at least two components; the recorded cases of human botulism have been due mainly to types A, B, E, and F; type C*α* causes botulism in domestic and wild water fowl; C*β* and D are associated with intoxications in cattle.

 **C. butyr'icum,** a species which occurs in naturally soured milk, in naturally fermented starchy plant substances, and in soil; it is not pathogenic. It is the type species of the genus *C.*

 **C. cadaveris,** a species found in a human cadaver and in the peritoneum of a rabbit; it is not pathogenic for guinea pigs or rabbits.

 **C. capitova'le,** a species found in the pleural fluid of a sheep dead of gas gangrene, in cases of septicemia in humans, and in the feces of normal infants.

 **C. carnis,** a species found in a rabbit inoculated with soil; it is pathogenic for laboratory animals, in which an exotoxin produces edema, necrosis, and death.

 **C. chauvoei,** *C. feseri;* a species which causes black leg, black quarter, or symptomatic anthrax in cattle and other animals; it produces an exotoxin.

 **c. chromog'enes,** a species found in pus from a perinephritic abscess in a human; weakly pathogenic for laboratory animals.

 **C. cochlearium,** a species found in human war wounds and septic infections; it is not pathogenic for guinea pigs.

 **C. difficile,** a species found in the feces of newborn infants; pathogenic for guinea pigs and rabbits.

 **C. fallax,** a species found in war wounds, appendicitis, and black leg of sheep; it produces a weak exotoxin.

 **C. feseri,** *C. chauvoei.*

 **C. gummosum,** a species found in gaseous gangrene and in normal human (adult and infant) feces.

 **C. haemoly'ticum,** a species found in cattle dying of icterohemoglobinuria; it is pathogenic and toxic for guinea pigs and rabbits and produces an unstable, hemolytic toxin.

**C. histoly′ticum,** a species found in war wounds, where it induces necrosis of tissue; it produces a cytolytic exotoxin which causes local necrosis and sloughing on injection; it is not toxic on feeding; it is pathogenic for small laboratory animals.

**C. innomina′tum,** a species found in septic and gangrenous war wounds.

**C. microspo′rum,** a species found in the abdominal contents of a fatal case of peritonitis.

**C. multifermentans,** a species found in a human muscle infected with gas gangrene; also found in fermented olives and spoiled chocolate candy.

**C. nigri′ficans,** a species found in canned corn showing "sulfur stinker spoilage." It is not pathogenic.

**C. no′vyi,** a species consisting of three types, A, B, and C. Type A, from a case of gaseous gangrene and from human necrotic hepatitis, produces γ-toxin (a hemolytic lecithinase); B, from black disease (infectious necrotic hepatitis) of sheep, produces β-toxin (a hemolytic lecithinase); and C, found in bacillary osteomyelitis of water buffaloes, does not produce toxin.

**C. oedema′tiens,** *C. novyi.*

**C. parabotuli′num,** a species containing organisms formerly referred to as *C. botulinum* types A and B. The types are identified by protection tests with known type antitoxin. Pathogenic for man and animals. Produces a powerful exotoxin.

**C. paraputri′ficum,** a species found in feces, especially those of infants, gaseous gangrene, and postmortem fluid and tissue cultures; it is not pathogenic for rabbits or guinea pigs.

**C. perfrin′gens,** a species which is the chief causative agent of gas gangrene in man. It may also be involved in causing enteritis, appendicitis, food poisoning, and puerperal fever. It causes gas gangrene in other animals, especially sheep. This organism is found in soil, water, milk, dust, sewage, and intestinal tract of man and other animals.

**C. ramo′sum,** *Ramibacterium ramosum;* a species found in the natural cavities of man and other animals as well as in sea water; it is also found in association with mastoiditis, otitis, pulmonary gangrene, putrid pleurisy, appendicitis, intestinal infections, balanitis, liver abscess, osteomyelitis, septicemia, urinary infections, in the vagina and in feces. It is the type species of the genus *Ramibacterium.*

**C. sep′ticum,** Ghon and Sach's bacillus; a species found in malignant edema of animals, in human war wounds, and in cases of appendicitis. It is pathogenic for guinea pigs, rabbits, mice, and pigeons and produces an exotoxin which is lethal and hemolytic.

**C. sphenoi′des,** a species found in gangrenous war wounds; it is not pathogenic for guinea pigs or rabbits.

**C. sporo′genes,** a species found in intestinal contents, gaseous gangrene, and soil; it is not pathogenic for guinea pigs or rabbits, but does produce a slight, temporary, local tumefaction.

**C. tale,** a species found in a case of acute appendicitis and in canned fish; pathogenicity for laboratory animals is variable.

**C. ter′tium,** a species found in wounds, but nonpathogenic for laboratory animals.

**C. te′tani,** a species that causes tetanus; it produces a potent exotoxin (neurotoxin) which is intensely toxic for

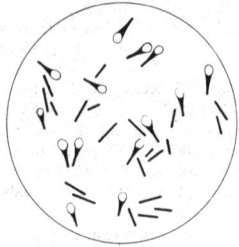

*Clostridium tetani*

Cells stained to show spores (original magnification, ×3200).

man and animals when formed in tissues or injected, but not when ingested.

**C. tetanoi′des,** a species found in war wounds, post-morten blood cultures, and garden soil.

**C. tetanomor′phum,** a species found in war wounds and soil; it is not pathogenic for rabbits or guinea pigs.

**C. thermosaccharoly′ticum,** a species of thermophilic bacteria found in "hard swell" of canned goods; it is not pathogenic to laboratory animals.

**C. welch′ii,** *C. perfringens.*

---

**Clostridium histolyticum proteinase B** (EC 3.4.22.8). Clostridiopeptidase B; clostripain; a proteinase cleaving preferentially at arginine CO— bonds.

**clostripain.** *Clostridium histolyticum* proteinase B.

**closure** (klo′zhur). 1. The completion of a reflex pathway. 2. The place of coupling between stimuli in the establishment of conditioned learning. 3. To achieve or experience a sense of completion in a mental task.

**flask c.,** in dentistry, the procedure of bringing the two halves or parts of a flask together.

**flask c., final,** the last c. of a flask before curing after trial packing the mold with a denture-base material.

**flask c., trial,** preliminary c.'s made for the purpose of eliminating excess denture-base material, and to ensure that the mold is completely filled.

**velopharyngeal c.** the apposition of the palate to the upper posterior pharyngeal wall as in deglutition and in some speech sounds.

**clo′sylate.** USAN-approved contraction for *p*-chlorobenzenesulfonate.

**clot.** 1. To coagulate. 2. A coagulation; a thrombus.

**agony c.,** a c. formed in the heart during the act of dying.

**antemortem c.,** a blood c. found at autopsy, which was formed in any of the heart cavities or the great vessels before death.

**blood c.,** crassamentum; the coagulated phase of b.; the soft, coherent, jelly-like red mass resulting from the conversion of fibrinogen to fibrin, thereby entrapping the red b. cells (and other formed elements) within the coagulated plasma.

**chicken fat c.,** c. formed *in vitro* or postmortem from leukocytes and plasma of sedimented blood.

**currant jelly c.,** a jelly-like mass of red blood cells and fibrin formed by the *in vitro* or postmortem clotting of whole or sedimented blood.

**lam′inated c.,** a c. formed in a succession of layers such as occurs in the natural cure of an aneurysm.

**passive c.,** a c. formed in an aneurysmal sac in consequence of the circulation through the aneurysm having ceased.

**postmortem c.,** a c. formed in the heart or great vessels after death.

**Schede's c.,** see Schede's *method.*

**clot′tage.** The blocking of any canal or duct by a blood clot.

**Cloudman,** Arthur M. See C. *melanoma.*

**clove.** Caryophyllus; the dried flower bud of *Eugenia caryophyllata* (family Myrtaceae), containing eugenol and caryophillin. Used as a flavor, and is the source of clove oil.

**c. bark,** *Cassia caryophyllata.*

**c. oil** (USP, BP), the volatile oil distilled with steam from cloves; it contains not less than 85 per cent by volume of total phenolic substances, chiefly eugenol; used as a dental analgesic.

**clown′ism.** A stage in hysteroepilepsy in which the patient assumes grotesque attitudes.

**clox′acil′lin sodium** (USP, BP). [ 5-Methyl-3-(*o*-chlorophenyl)-4-isoxazolyl ]penicillin sodium; a penicillinase-resistant penicillin.

**clo′zapine** (USAN). 8-Chloro-11-(4-methyl-1-piperazinyl)-5*H*-dibenzo[ *b,e*][ 1,4 ]diazepine; sedative.

**club′bing.** Broadening and thickening of ends of fingers, seen in chronic pulmonary disease.

**club′foot.** Talipes.

**club′hand.** Talipomanus.

**clump** [ A.S. *clympre*, a lump ]. To form into clusters, small aggregations, or groups.

**clump'ing.** Agglutinating; the massing together of bacteria or other cells suspended in a fluid.

**cluneal** (klu'ne-al). Pertaining to the clunes.

**clunes** (klu'nēz) [ pl. of L. *clunis*, buttock ] [ NA ]. Nates; buttocks.

**clupan'odon'ic acid.** 4,8,12,15,19-Docosapentaenoic acid ($C_{22}H_{34}O_2$).

**clupeine** (klu'pe-ēn). A protamine in the sperm of the herring.

**clut'tering.** The dropping of letters or syllables by a hurried or nervous speaker.

**Clutton,** Henry H., English surgeon, 1850–1909. See C.'s *joints*.

**clysis** (kli'sis) [ G. *klysis*, a drenching by a clyster ]. An infusion of fluid for therapeutic purposes. Formerly the word meant an enema, and then the washing out of material from any body space or cavity by fluids. Also used as combining form, in suffix position, to denote injection.

**clysma** (kliz'mah) [ G. *klysma*, a drenching ]. An enema or clyster.

**clyster** (klis'ter) [ G. *klystēr*, fr. *klyzō*, fut. *klysō*, to wash out ]. Enema; clysma; a rectal injection of water, gas, or other fluid.

**clys'terize.** To administer a rectal injection.

**cm.** Abbreviation for centimeter.

**Cm.** Chemical symbol of the element curium.

**C.M.** Abbreviation for the degree *chirurgiae magister*, master in surgery.

**CM-.** Symbol for carboxymethyl radical.

**CM-cellulose.** See under cellulose.

**CMP.** Symbol for cytidine 5'-phosphate (or for any cytidine monophosphate).

**CN.** The cyanide radical, $CN^-$ or —CN.

**cnemial** (ne'mĭ-al) [ G. *knēmē*, leg ]. Relating to the leg, especially to the shin.

**cnemis** (ne'mis) [ G. *knēmis* (*knēmid-*), a legging ]. The shin.

**cnemitis** (ne-mi'tis). Inflammation of the tibia, especially periostitis of the anterior edge of the tibia.

**cnemoscoliosis** (ne-mo-sko-lĭ-o'sis) [ G. *knēmē*, leg, + *skoliōsis*, crookedness, fr. *skolios*, curved ]. Curvature of the bones of the leg as in bowleg.

**cnida,** pl. **cnidae** (ni'dah, ni'de) [ G. *knidē*, nettle ]. Nematocyst.

**Cnidian** (ni'dĭ-an). Relating to the city of Cnidus or to the teachings of its physicians.

**cnidocyst** (ni'do-sist). Nematocyst.

**cnidosis** (ni-do'sis) [ G. *knidōsis*, nettle-rash, fr. *knidē*, a nettle ]. Urticaria.

**Cnidosporidia** (ni'do-spo-rid'ĭ-ah). A subphylum of Protozoa that includes parasitic organisms (formerly classified with the Sporozoa) possessing spores bearing one or more polar filaments.

**Cnidus** (ni-dus). An ancient Greek city of Caria in Asia Minor, the seat of a famous school of medicine (5th and 4th centuries B.C.) and site of a temple to Aesculapius.

**CNS.** 1. Abbreviation for central nervous system; see *systema nervosum centrale*. 2. The thiocyanate radical, $CNS^-$ or —CNS.

**Co.** Chemical symbol for the element cobalt.

**CoA.** Abbreviation for coenzyme A.

**coacervate** (ko-as'er-vāt). Cohesil; cluster of molecules; generic term indicating an aggregate of colloidal particles, aggregates separated out of an emulsion (coacervation) by the addition of some third component (coacervating agent).

**coac'erva'tion.** Formation of a coacervate from an emulsion.

**coagglutinin** (ko-ă-glu'tĭ-nin). A substance that *per se* does not agglutinate an antigen, but does result in agglutination of antigen that is appropriately coated with univalent antibody. See also conglutination.

**coag'ula.** Plural of coagulum.

**coag'ulable.** Capable of being coagulated or clotted.

**coagulant** (ko-ag'u-lant). 1. An agent that causes, stimulates, or accelerates coagulation, especially with reference to blood. 2. Coagulative; causing coagulation.

**coag'ulate** [ L. *coagulo*, pp. *-atus*, to curdle ]. 1. To convert a fluid or a substance in solution into a solid or gel. 2. To clot; to curdle; to change from the liquid state to a solid or gel.

**coagulation** (ko-ag-u-la'shun). 1. Clotting; the process of changing from liquid to solid, especially of blood 2. A clot or coagulum. 3. The transforming of a sol into a gel or semisolid mass, *e.g.*, the c. of the white of an egg by means of boiling. In any colloidal suspension, the dispersion of the disperse phase from the continuous phase is greatly reduced, thereby leading to a complete or partial separation of the latter. C. is usually an irreversible phenomenon.

**coag'ulative.** Coagulant; causing coagulation.

**coag'ulin.** An antibody causing coagulation of the antigen.

**coag'ulinoid.** A coagulin in which the function group has been destroyed by heating to 65° to 70°C.

**coagulometer** (ko-ag-u-lom'e-ter) [ L. *coagulum*, a means of curdling, + G. *metron*, measure ]. An apparatus for measuring the time required for a drop of blood to coagulate. One form (that of Russell and Brodie) consists of a truncated glass cone, on which is placed a drop of blood that projects in a moist chamber; through a fine tube passing into the moist chamber a current of air is blown; the apparatus is placed under a microscope and the movements of the corpuscles observed. The time elapsing from the moment that the blood was shed to that when the motion of the individual corpuscles ceases is taken as the coagulation time.

**coagulop'athy.** A disease affecting the coagulability of the blood.

  **consumption c.,** a disorder in which marked reductions develop in blood concentrations of platelets and of certain circulating coagulation factors; may be accompanied by widespread intravascular coagulation.

**coagulum,** pl. **coag'ula** (ko-ag'u-lum) [ L. a means of coagulating, rennet. ACT- ]. Crassamentum; a clot; a curd; a soft, nonrigid, insoluble mass formed when a sol is coagulated. The process is usually not reversible, and a c. cannot be converted to a colloidal suspension, unless its basic nature is chemically altered.

**coal oil.** Petroleum.

**coal tar** (USP, BP). A by-product obtained during the destructive distillation of bituminous coal; a very dark semisolid of characteristic naphthalene-like odor and a sharp, burning taste; used in the treatment of skin diseases.

  **c. tar naphtha,** benzene.

  **prepared c. tar** (BP), obtained by heating commercial c. tar in a shallow vessel for 1 hour at 50°C. Used in the preparation of c. tar solution.

**Coan.** Relating to the island of Cos or to the teachings of its physicians.

**coapt** (ko'apt). To join together. See coaptation.

**coaptation** (ko-ap-ta'shun) [ L. *co-apto*, pp. *-aptatus*, to fit together ]. The joining together or fitting of two surfaces, as the lips of a wound or the ends of a broken bone.

**coarct** (ko-arkt') [ L. *co-arcto*, pp. *-arctatus*, to press together ]. To press together.

**coarc'tate.** 1. Coarct. 2. Pressed together.

**coarctation** (ko-ark-ta'shun). 1. A narrowing. 2. A compression.

  **reversed c.,** aortic arch syndrome in which blood pressure in the arms is lower than in the legs.

**coarctotomy** (ko-ark-tot'o-mĭ) [ L. *coarctatus*, pressed together (see coarct), + G. *tomē*, cutting ]. Division of a stricture.

**CoAS-, CoASH.** Symbol for coenzyme A radical or reduced coenzyme A.

**coat.** 1. The outer covering or envelope of an organ or part. 2. One of the layers of membranous or other tissues forming the wall of a canal or hollow organ; see tunica.

  **buffy c.,** crusta inflammatoria; crusta phlogistica; leukocyte cream; the upper, lighter portion of the blood clot (coagulated plasma and white blood cells), occurring when coagulation is delayed so that the red blood cells have had time to settle; the portion of centrifuged, anticoagulated blood which contains leukocytes and platelets.

**sclerotic c.,** sclera.

**coat'ing.** A covering; a layer of some substance spread over a surface.

**antireflection c.,** a film of magnesium fluoride spread on lens to minimize reflections.

**CoA transferases.** See under coenzyme A.

**Coats,** George, English ophthalmologist, 1876–1915. See C.'s *disease.*

**cobal'amin.** A general term for compounds containing the dimethylbenzimidazolylcobamide nucleus of vitamin $B_{12}$ (*q. v.*).

**c. concentrate** (NF), the dried, partially purified product resulting from the growth of selected *Streptomyces* cultures or other cobalamin-producing microorganisms; contains at least 500 $\mu$g. of c. in each gram.

**cobalt** (ko'bawlt) [ Ger. *kobalt* ]. A steel-gray metallic element, symbol Co, atomic no. 27, atomic weight 58.94. It is a constituent of vitamin $B_{12}$. Its compounds afford pigments, the protoxide being the beautiful c. blue.

**co'balt-58.** $^{58}$Co; positron emitter with half-life of 72 days.

**co'balt-60.** $^{60}$Co; half-life, 5.3 years; emits beta particles and energetic gamma rays and is used in radiation therapy and diagnosis, in place of radium (radon) and x-rays.

**cobaltous chloride** (ko-bawl'tus). $CoCl_2 \cdot 6H_2O$; used in the treatment of various types of refractory anemia, to improve the hematocrit, hemoglobin, and erythrocyte count.

**cobamic acid.** Cobinic acid with a ribofuranose phosphate attached to the aminopropanol unit. It is a part of the vitamin $B_{12}$ structure.

**cobamide.** The hexa-amide of cobamic acid.

**cobaya** (ko-ba'yah) [ Native Ind. ]. Guinea pig; *Cavia cobaya.*

**cobinamide.** The hexa-amide of cobinic acid; part of the vitamins $B_{12}$ (the cobalamins).

**cobinic acid.** Cobyrinic acid with a 1-aminopropan-2-ol side chain attached to the —$CH_2CH_2COOH$ group on carbon-17 (side chain *f*). It is a part of the vitamin $B_{12}$ structure.

**cobra** (ko'brah) [ Port. snake, from L. *coluber,* snake ]. Dangerous venomous snakes of India, Africa and Asia in the family Elapidae; the genus *Naja* includes the common cobra of India and Africa and the Egyptian asp; typical behavior includes spreading of the neck (hood), rearing one-third of the body off of the ground, and, in some species, the spitting of venom which is primarily neurotoxic.

**c. venom cofactor,** see under cofactor.

**c. venom factor,** see under factor.

**cobra-lecithid** (ko'brah-les'ĭ-thid). A mixture of phospholipase A and lysolecithin.

**cobral'ysin.** Phospholipase A and direct lytic factor, acting in concert to produce hemolysis of erythrocytes.

**cobyric acid.** Cobyrinamide; the hexa-amide of cobyrinic acid; factor $V_{1a}$; part of the vitamins $B_{12}$ (the cobalamins).

**cobyrinamide.** Cobyric acid.

**cobyrinic acid.** Corrin with methyl groups at positions 1, 2, 5, 7, 12 (2), 15, 17; —$CH_2COOH$ groups at positions 2, 7, 18; —$CH_2CH_2COOH$ groups at positions 3, 8, 13, 17; and divalent cobalt centered among the four nitrogens. The acid side chains are designated, in numerical order, *a, b, c, d, e, f, g.* It is a part of vitamin $B_{12}$.

**c. acid hexa-amide,** cobyric acid.

**COC.** Abbreviation for cathodal opening *contraction.*

**coca** (ko'kah) [ S. Am. ]. The dried leaves of *Erythroxylon coca,* yielding not less than 0.5 per cent of ether-soluble alkaloids; the source of cocaine and several other alkaloids.

**cocaine** (ko-kān) (NF, BP). Benzoylmethylecgonine; an alkaloid obtained from the leaves of *Erythroxylon coca* (family Erythroxylaceae), and other species of *Erythroxylon,* or by synthesis from ecgonine or its derivatives. Has moderate vasoconstrictor activity. The salts are used as a topical anesthesia. C. hydrochloride is official in the USP and BP.

**cocainidine** (ko-kān'ĭ-dēn). An alkaloid from coca leaves, similar to cocaine but much weaker, and perhaps isomeric with it.

**cocainism** (ko'kān-izm). The habitual use of cocaine as an intoxicant.

**co'cainist.** One suffering from cocaine addiction.

**cocainization** (ko'kān-ĭ-za'shun). The production of local anesthesia by the topical application or injection of cocaine.

**co'carbox'ylase.** Thiamin pyrophosphate.

**cocar'cinogen.** The material that works symbiotically with a carcinogen in the production of cancer.

**Coccaceae** (kok-ka'se-e) [ G. *kokkos,* a berry, COCC- ]. An obsolete term for a family of Eubacteriales which included all the spherical cells dividing in one (*Streptococcus*), two (*Micrococcus*), or three (*Sarcina*) planes, then forming cells, pairs, tetrads, cubes or larger packets, or chains.

**coccal** (kok'al). Relating to cocci.

**cocci** (kok'si). Plural of coccus.

**Coccidia.** (kok-sid'ĭ-ah). Coccidiasina; a subclass of important protozoa in the class (or subphylum) Sporozoa, in which schizogony and sporogony can occur in the same host, in contrast to the gregarines, which do not reproduce by schizogony, and the haemosporines, in which schizogony takes place in a vertebrate and sporogony in an invertebrate host.

**coccidia** (kok-sid'ĭ-ah). Plural of coccidium.

**coccidial** (kok-sid'ĭ-al). Relating to coccidia.

**Coccidiasi'na.** Coccidia.

**coccidioidal** (kok-sid-ĭ-oy'dal). Referring to the disease coccidioidomycosis or the infecting organism.

**Coccidioides** (kok-sid-ĭ-oy'dēz) [ coccidium + G. *eidos,* resemblance ]. A genus of fungi, some of which are parasitic in man.

**C. im'mitis** [ L. rough ], a species of fungi causing coccidioidomycosis.

**coccidioidin** (kok-sid-ĭ-oy'din) (USP). A sterile solution containing the by-products of growth of *Coccidioides immitis;* used as a dermal reactivity indicator.

**coccidioidoma** (kok-sid-ĭ-oy-do'mah). Infectious granuloma caused by *Coccidioides immitis.*

**coccidioidomeningitis** (kok-sid-ĭ-oy'do-men-in-ji'tis). Meningitis associated with coccidioidomycosis.

**coccidioidomycosis** (kok-sid-ĭ-oy'do-mi-ko'sis) [ coccidioides + G. *mykēs,* fungus, + suffix -*osis,* condition ]. California disease; desert rheumatism; a disease caused by infection with *Coccidioides immitis.*

**latent or asymptomatic c.,** a form of the disease not recognized clinically; detected by skin test or by measuring antibodies in the blood serum.

**primary c.,** valley fever; desert fever; a disease common in the San Joaquin Valley of California and certain additional areas in the Southwest United States as well as the Chaco region of Argentina caused by inhalation of the arthrospores of the fungus *Coccidioides immitis,* with acute onset of symptoms resembling pneumonia or pulmonary tuberculosis, productive of sputum containing the fungus followed by the development of erythematous nodules in skin. The coccidioidin test is positive.

**secondary c.,** coccidioidal granuloma; may occur late as a secondary manifestation.

**coccidiosis** (kok-sid-ĭ-ō'sis). Group name for diseases due to any species of coccidia; c. is a common and serious disease of many species of domestic animals and birds (not often serious in dogs and cats) and many wild animals kept in captivity; man and horses do not often suffer from c.

**coccidiostat** (kok-sid'ĭ-o-stat). A chemical agent that generally is added to animal feed to partially inhibit or delay the development of animal coccidiosis; *e.g.,* nicarbazin.

**coccidium, pl. coccidia** (kok-sid'ĭ-um) [ Mod. L. dim. of G. *kokkos,* berry ]. Common name given to protozoan parasites of the family Eimeriidae (order Coccidia) in which schizogony occurs within epithelial cells, generally in the intestine, but in some species in the bile ducts and kidney; the final product of sexual fusion and differentiation within the host, the oocyst, generally passes to the soil in the feces, undergoes sporulation, and then acts as the infective form for another host. The c. are parasitic in most domestic and wild birds and mammals, and occasionally in man; they are highly host-specific. The majority are nonpathogenic, but certain species rank among the most serious and economically important pathogens of diseases, such as coccidiosis, in birds and mammals.

**coccinella** (kok-sin-el'ah). Cochineal.

**coccinellin** (kok-sin'el-in). The coloring matter derived from cochineal.

**coc'cobac'illary.** Relating to a coccobacillus.

**coccobacillus** (kok'o-bă-sil'us) [ G. *kokkos*, berry ]. A short, thick bacterial rod of the shape of an oval or slightly elongated coccus.

**coc'coid** [ G. *kokkos*, berry, + *eidos*, resemblance ]. Resembling a coccus.

**cocculin** (kok'u-lin). Picrotoxin.

**cocculus** (kok'u-lus) [ Mod. L. dim. of G. *kokkos*, berry ]. Fish berry, Indian berry; the dried fruit of *Anamirta cocculus* (family Menispermaceae), a climbing shrub of India. The source of picrotoxin.

**coccus,** pl. **coc'ci** (kok'us) [ G. *kokkos*, berry ]. 1. A bacterium of round, spheroidal, or ovoid form. 2. See cochineal.
  **Neisser's c.** *Neisseria gonorrhoeae.*
  **Weichselbaum's c.,** *Neisseria meningitidis.*

**Coc'cus cac'ti.** See cochineal.

**coccyalgia** (kok-sī-al'jī-ah) [ coccyx + G. *algos*, pain ]. Coccygodynia.

**coccycephalus** (kok'sī-sef'al-us) [ G. *kokkyx*, cuckoo, + kephalē, head ]. A malformed individual in whom the cephalic profile suggests a beak.

**coccydyn'ia.** Coccygodynia.

**coccygalgia** (kok-sī-gal'jī-ah) [ coccyx + G. *algos*, pain ]. Coccygodynia.

**coccygeal** (kok-sij'e-al). Relating to the coccyx.

**coccygectomy** (kok-sī-jek'to-mī) [ coccyx + G. *ektomē*, excision ]. Removal of the coccyx.

**coccygeus** (kok-sī-je'us). See under musculus.

**coccygodynia** (kok'sī-go-din'ī-ah) [ coccyx + G. *odynē*, pain ]. Coccyalgia; pain in the coccygeal region.

**coccygotomy** (kok'sī-got'o-mī) [ coccyx + G. *tomē*, a cutting ]. Operation for freeing the coccyx from its attachments.

**coccyodynia** (kok'sī-o-din'ī-ah). Coccygodynia.

**coccyx,** gen. **coc'cygis,** pl. **coc'cyges** (kok'siks) [ G. *kokkyx*, a cuckoo, the coccyx. COCCY- ]. *Os* coccygis.

**cochineal** (kotch'ī-nēl) [ L. *coccineus*, scarlet ]. Coccus (2); the dried female insects, *Coccus cacti*, enclosing the young larvae, or (BP), the dried female insect, *Dactylopius coccus*, containing eggs and larvae; used as a coloring agent and a stain. See carmine.

**cochlea,** pl. **coch'leae** (kok'le-ah) [ L. snail shell. COCH- ] [ NA ]. A cone-shaped cavity in the petrous portion of the temporal bone, forming one of the divisions of the labyrinth or internal ear. It consists of a spiral canal making two and a half turns around a central core of spongy bone, the *modiolus*, this spiral canal of the cochlea contains the membranous cochlea, or *ductus cochlearis*, in which is the spiral organ Corti).
  **membranous c.,** *ductus* cochlearis.

**cochlear** (kok'le-ar). Relating to the cochlea.

**cochleare** (kok-le-a're) [ L. ]. A spoon.

**cochleariform** (kok-le-ar'ī-form) [ L. *cochleare*, spoon (COCH-), + *forma*, form ]. Spoon-shaped.

**cochleate** (kok'le-āt) [ L. *cochlea*, a snail shell ]. Resembling more or less a snail shell; denoting the appearance of a form of plate culture.

**cochleitis** (kok-le-i'tis). Cochlitis.

**cochleovestibular** (kok'le-o-ves-tib'u-lar). Relating to the cochlea and the vestibule of the ear.

**Cochliomyia americana** (kok-le-o-mi'yah). Incorrect name often used for *Callitroga hominivorax.*

**cochlitis** (kok-li'tis). Cochleitis; inflammation of the cochlea.

**cocillana** (ko'se-yah'nah). The dried bark of *Guarea rusbyi,* a Bolivia tree. Used as an expectorant in bronchitis.

**Cock,** Edward, English surgeon, 1805–1892. See C.'s peculiar *tumor.*

**Cockayne,** Edward A., English physician, 1880–1956. See C.'s *disease, syndrome.*

**cock'tail.** Mixed drink.
  **lytic c.,** local term for a quick-acting depressant solution to be taken by mouth.
  **Philadelphia c.,** Rivers' c.
  **Rivers' c.,** Philadelphia c.; an intravenous slow injection of from 1000 to 2000 cc. of 10 per cent dextrose in isotonic saline to which thiamine hydrochloride and 25 units of insulin are added. Used in acute alcoholism.

**COCl.** Abbreviation for cathodal opening *clonus*, written also CaOCl.

**cocoa** (ko'ko) (USP). A powder prepared from the roasted kernels of ripe seed of *Theobroma cacao* (family Sterculiaceae); used in the preparation of c. syrup, a flavoring agent. See also cacao.

**coconsciousness** (ko-kon'shus-nes). A splitting of consciousness into two streams.

**cocto-** (kok'to-) [ L. *coctus*, boiled ]. Prefix indicating boiled or modified by heat.

**coctolabile** (kok'to-la'bil). Subject to alteration or destruction when exposed to the temperature of boiling water.

**coctostabile, coctostable** (kok'to-sta'bil, -sta'bl). Resisting the temperature of boiling water without alteration or destruction.

**cod.** 1. The fat-filled scrotum of a castrated bovine animal. 2. A common marine fish (family Gadidae) related to the haddock and pollack.

**co'damine.** A benzylisoquinoline alkaloid derived from the mother liquor of morphine, isomeric with laudanine.

**code.** 1. A set of rules, principles, or ethics. 2. Any system devised to convey information or facilitate communication.
  **genetic c.,** the genetic information carried by the specific DNA molecules of the chromosomes; specifically, the system whereby particular combinations of three adjacent nucleotides in a DNA molecule control the insertion of particular amino acids in equivalent places in a protein molecule.

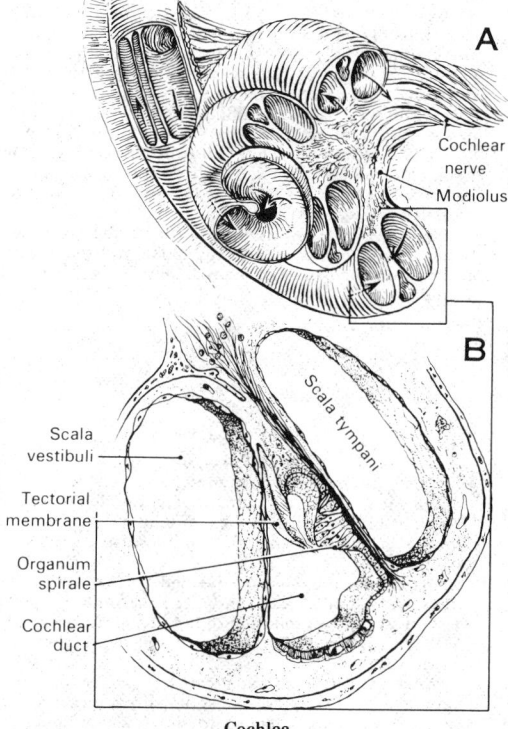

**Cochlea**

*A*, frontal view of right cochlea, with sections of spiral canal removed to show internal structure; *B*, section across spiral canal.

**codecarboxylase** (ko'de-kar-bok'sĭ-lās). Pyridoxal 5'-phosphate.

**codehydrogenase I** (ko'de-hi-droj'ĕ-nās). Nicotinamide adenine dinucleotide.

**codehydrogenase II.** Nicotinamide adenine dinucleotide phosphate.

**codeine** (ko'dēn) [ G. *kōdeia*, head, poppy head ] (NF). Methylmorphine; morphine monomethyl ether; morphine 3-methyl ether; obtained from opium, which contains 0.7 to 2.5 per cent, but usually made from morphine. Used as an analgesic and antitussive; drug dependence (physical and psychic) may develop, but c. is less liable to produce addiction than is morphine. Codeine sulfate is official in the NF; codeine phosphate, in the USP and BP.

**Co'dex medicamenta'rius** [ L. a book pertaining to drugs ]. The official title of the French Pharmacopeia.

**Codivilla,** Alessandro, Italian surgeon, 1851–1913. See C.'s *extension, operation.*

**cod liver oil** (NF, BP). The partially destearinated fixed oil extracted from the fresh livers of *Gadus morrhuae* and other species of the family Gadidae; it contains in each gram at least 850 USP units of vitamin A and at least 85 USP units of vitamin D; the preparation official in the BP contains not less than 600 units of vitamin A and not less than 85 units of vitamin D per gram. Used as a supplementary source of vitamins A and D.

**Codman,** Ernest Amory, Boston surgeon, 1869–1940. See C.'s *sign, tumor.*

**codominant** (ko-dom'ĭ-nant). In genetics, denoting an equal degree of dominance of two genes, both being expressed in the phenotype of the individual; *e.g.*, genes A and B of the ABO blood group are codominant; individuals with both are type AB.

**co'don.** Triplet (3); a sequence of three bases in a strand of DNA that provides genetic code information for a specific amino acid. See also fig. under protein.

**codox'ime** (USAN). Dihydrocodeinone O-(carboxymethyl)oxime; antitussive drug.

**coe-.** For words so beginning, and not found here, see ce-.

**coefficient** (ko-ē-fish'ent) [ L. *co-* + *efficio* (*exfacio*), to accomplish ]. The expression of the amount or degree of any quality possessed by a substance, or of the degree of physical or chemical change normally occurring in that substance under stated conditions.

**absorption c.,** (1) the milliliters of a gas at standard temperature and pressure that will saturate 100 ml. of liquid; (2) the amount of light absorbed in passing through 1 cm. of a 1 molar solution of a given substance, expressed as a constant in Beer's law. See also specific absorption c.

**activity c.,** see activity (2).

**Ambard's c.,** ureosecretory constant; the relation between the amount of urea in the blood and that excreted in the urine, a measure of renal activity; it is given by the formula:

$$K = \frac{Ur}{\sqrt{D \times \dfrac{70}{P} \times \dfrac{\sqrt{C}}{25}}}$$

in which *Ur* means gm. of urea per L. of blood; *C*, gm. of urea per L. of urine; *D*, gm. of urea excreted in 24 hours; *P*, weight of the patient in kg., *K*, urea index. The normal figure is from 0.06 to 0.08; an increase denotes renal insufficiency.

**biological c.,** the energy expended by the body at rest.

**Bunsen's solubility c.,** symbol $\alpha$; the milliliters of gas STPD dissolved per milliliter of liquid and per atmosphere (760 mm Hg) partial pressure of the gas at any given temperature.

**correlation c.'s,** a statistical term referring to the relationship between two sets of paired measurements. Correlation c.'s are intended to show degree of relationship, but do not mean that one variable causes the other. Correlation c.'s may be positive, negative, or curvilinear, depending on whether the variations are in the same, opposite, or both directions.

**creatinine c.,** see under creatinine.

**c. of demineralization,** see under demineralization.

**distribution c.,** sometimes called the partition c.; the ratio of concentrations of a substance in two immiscible phases at equilibrium; the basis of many chromatographic separation procedures.

**extinction c.,** specific absorption c.

**hygienic laboratory c.,** Rideal-Walker c.

**c. of inbreeding,** a figure expressing the degree of inbreeding of an individual as the probability that he may possess identical genes at any pair of loci because of inheritance of these genes through both father and mother from an ancestor common to both; in general the c. of inbreeding of a child is one-half the c. of relationship of its parents.

**isoton'ic c.,** the amount of salts in the blood plasma, or the amount that should be added to distilled water in order to prepare an isotonic solution.

**Lancet c.,** a figure expressing the disinfecting power of any substance; it is obtained by dividing the figure representing the percentage strength of the weakest killing dilution of phenol by that representing the percentage strength of the weakest killing dilution of the disinfectant, both at $2\frac{1}{2}$ and at 30 minutes.

**lethal c.,** that concentration of disinfectant that kills bacteria at 20–25°C. in the shortest period of time.

**Long's c.,** Long's *formula.*

**molar absorption c.,** molar absorbancy index; molar extinction c.; molar absorptivity; absorbance (of light) per unit path length (usually the centimeter) and per unit of concentration (moles per liter); a fundamental unit in spectrophotometry. Symbol, $\epsilon$.

**molar extinction c.,** molar absorption c.

**Ostwald's solubility c.,** symbol, $\lambda$; the milliliters of gas dissolved per milliliter of liquid and per atmosphere (760 mm. of Hg) partial pressure of the gas at any given temperature. This differs from $\alpha$, Bunsen's solubility c. in that the amount of dissolved gas is expressed in terms of its volume at the temperature of the experiment, instead of STPD. Thus, $\lambda = \alpha (1 + 0.00367t)$, where $t$ = temperature in degrees centigrade.

**oxygen utilization c.,** the quotient obtained by dividing the figure for the volumes of oxygen in 100 ml. of venous blood by that for the volumes per cent of oxygen in arterial blood. Thus, if the venous blood contains 14 volumes per cent and the arterial blood 19 volumes per cent, then the coefficient is $^{14}/_{19} = 0.74$.

**partition c.,** distribution c.

**phenol c.,** Rideal-Walker c.

**Poiseuille's viscosity c.,** an expression of the viscosity as determined by the capillary tube method; the coefficient $\eta = (\pi P r t / 8 \, vl)$, where $P$ is the pressure difference between the inlet and outlet of the tube, $r$ the radius of the tube, $l$ its length, and $v$ the quantity of liquid delivered in the time $t$.

**reflection c.** (symbol $\sigma$), a measure of the relative permeability of a particular membrane to a particular solute; calculated as the ratio of observed osmotic pressure to that calculated from van't Hoff's law; also equal to 1 minus the ratio of the effective pore areas available to solute and to solvent.

**c. of relationship,** a figure expressing the degree of genetic relationship between two individuals in terms of the proportion of genes identical because of inheritance from ancestors common to both; it is obtained by raising $\frac{1}{2}$ to the power equal to the number of pedigree links (parent-child or sib-sib) separating the individuals, and summing all paths of relationship. The c. also expresses the probability that a rare gene found in one person will be present in any relative.

**reliability c.,** an index of the consistency of measurement often based on the correlation between scores obtained on the initial test and a retest (test-retest reliability) or between scores on two similar forms of the same test (equivalent-form reliability).

**respiratory c.,** respiratory *quotient.*

**Rideal-Walker c.,** phenol c.; hygienic laboratory c.; a figure expressing the disinfecting power of any substance; it is obtained by dividing the figure indicating the degree of dilution of the disinfectant that kills a microorganism in a given time by that indicating the degree of dilution of phenol which kills the organism in the same space of time under similar conditions.

**selection c.**, see under selection.

**specific absorption c.**, absorptivity; absorbancy index; specific extinction; extinction coefficient; abosrbance (of light) per unit path length (usually the centimeter) and per unit of mass concentration; symbol, *a* (not *k*); *cf.* molar absorption c.

**temperature c.**, the fractional change in any physical property per degree rise in temperature.

**velocity c.**, the rate of transformation of a unit mass of substance in a chemical reaction.

**c. of viscosity**, the value of the force per unit area required to maintain a unit relative velocity between two parallel planes a unit distance apart.

**Coelenterates** (se-len'ter-āts). One of the major phyla of invertebrates, to which such forms as jellyfish belong.

**coelom.** Celom.

**coenesthesia** (sē'nes-thē'zhe-ah). Cenesthesia.

**coeno-** (se'no-) [ G. *koinos*, common ]. Combining form meaning shared in common; for words beginning thus and not found here, see ceno-.

**coenocyte** (se'no-sīt) [ G. *koinos, common, + kytos*, cell ]. Cenocyte; a multinucleate cell or hypha without cross walls, characteristic of the hyphae of Phycomycetes; see also nonseptate *mycelium*.

**coenocytic** (se'no-sit-ik). Cenocytic; pertaining to or having the characteristics of a coenocyte.

**coenurosis** (se-nu-ro'sis). Infection of sheep, goats, cattle and other species with *Coenurus cerebralis*, the encysted larvae of the tapeworm, *Multiceps multiceps*.

**Coenurus** (se-nu'rus) [ G. *koinos*, common, + *oura*, tail ]. Larval form of taenioid cestodes in which a bladder is formed with a number of invaginated scoleces developing within. Distinguished from hydatid by the absence of free-floating daughter cyst colonies budded off within the bladder. C. larvae are found in members of the genus *Multiceps*.

**C. cerebra'lis**, the coenurus larvae of the tapeworm *Multiceps multiceps*, found in the brain and spinal cord of sheep, goats, and other ruminants (a few have been recorded in man); adults are found in the intestine of dogs, foxes, coyotes, and jackals.

**C. seria'lis**, the coenurus larvae of the tapeworm *Multiceps serialis*, found in subcutaneous and intramuscular tissues of rabbits and hares (a few have been recorded in man); adult worms are found in the intestine of dogs, foxes, and jackals.

**coenzyme.** (ko-en'zīm). A substance that enhances or is necessary for the action of enzymes; c.'s are of smaller molecular size than the enzymes themselves, are dialyzable and relatively heat-stable, and are usually easily dissociable from the protein portion of the enzyme. Several vitamins are c.'s, *e.g.* thiamin, pyridoxal, nicotinamide, riboflavin.

**coenzyme I.** Nicotinamide adenine dinucleotide.

**coenzyme II.** Nicotinamide adenine dinucleotide phosphate.

**coenzyme A.** CoA; CoASH; a coenzyme containing pantothenic acid, adenosine 3'-phosphate, 5'-pyrophosphate, and 2-aminoethanethiol ("2-mercaptoethylamine," cysteamine); involved in the transfer of acyl groups, notably in transacetylations.

**CoA transferases** (EC Class 2.8.3), thiaphorases; enzymes transferring CoA from acetyl-CoA or succinyl-CoA to other acyl radicals.

**coenzyme Q.** Quinones with isoprenoid side chains (specifically, ubiquinones) that mediate electron transfer between cytochrome *b* and cytochrome *c*. Chemically similar to vitamins E and K, and to other tocopherols, quinones, and tocols.

**coenzyme R.** Biotin.

**coeur** [ Fr. ]. Heart.

**c. en sabot**, sabot heart; wooden-shoe heart; descriptive term for the roentgenographic configuration of the heart in the tetralogy of Fallot; the elevated apex combined with a transverse rectangular enlargement is likened to a wooden shoe.

**co'factor.** A prosthetic group such as heme, coenzymes, and inorganic ions such as magnesium ion, essential for enzyme action.

**cobra venom c.**, properdin factor B; glycine-rich β-glycoprotein; $\beta_2$-glycoprotein II; the normal serum component, designated C3 proactivator, that participates with a component of cobra venom (and perhaps another serum factor) in the activation of C3 (the third component of complement; see also *properdin* factor B; *properdin* system; and component of *complement*.

**platelet c.**, see *factor* VIII.

**platelet c. II**, see *factor* IX.

**c. of thromboplastin**, see *factor* V.

**c. V**, see *factor* VII.

**cofer'ment.** Coenzyme.

**Coffey**, Robert C., American surgeon, 1869–1933. See C. *suspension.*

**Cogan**, David G., American ophthalmologist, *1908. See C.'s *syndrome.*

**cognition** (kog-nī'shun) [ L. *cognitio* ]. A generic term embracing the quality of knowing, which includes perceiving, recognizing, conceiving, judging, sensing, reasoning, and imagining.

**cognitive** (kog'nī-tiv). Pertaining to cognition.

**Cohen's test.** See under test.

**cohe'sil.** Coacervate.

**cohesion** (ko-he'zhun) [ L. *co-haereo*, pp. *-haesus*, to stick together ]. The attraction between molecules or masses that holds them together.

**Cohn**, Hermann L., German ophthalmologist, 1838–1906. See C.'s *test.*

**Cohnheim**, Julius F., German histologist, pathologist, and physiologist, 1839–1884. See C.'s *areas, fields, theory.*

**Cohnistreptothrix** (ko-nī-strep'to-thriks). An obsolete generic name applied to a bacterium which is probably not identifiable. The organism, *C. foersteri* (*Streptothrix foersteri*), was originally found in an inflamed tear duct, and it may have been the first streptomycete described. The type species is *C. foersteri*.

**cohoba** (ko-ho'bah). A psychotomimetic hallucinogenic substance obtained from *Acacia niopo* (family Leguminosae), a Central American plant, *Piptadenia peregrina*, and other plants. Among its constituents are bufotenine and dimethyltryptamine. Used in native localities as snuff or enema.

**cohoba'tion** [ Mediev. L. *cohobo*, to redistill ]. Redistillation of a liquid, to obtain it in still greater purity.

**cohor'mone.** A chemical substance that enhances or prolongs the action of a hormone; thus certain heavy metals enhance the action of gonadotrophins and zinc prolongs the action of insulin. Rarely used term.

**coin-counting.** A sliding movement of the tips of the thumb and index finger, occurring in paralysis agitans.

**coin'osite.** Cenosite.

**coital** (ko'ī-tal). Pertaining to coitus.

**Coiter**, Volcher, Dutch surgeon and anatomist, 1534–1600. See C.'s *muscle.*

**coition** (ko-ish'un) [ L. *co-eo*, pp. *-itus*, to come together ]. Coitus.

**coitophobia** (ko-ī-to-fo'bī-ah) [ L. *coitus*, sexual intercourse, + G. *phobos*, fear ]. A morbid fear of the sexual act.

**coitus** (ko'ī-tus) [ L. ]. Copulation; coition; sexual union.

**c. interrup'tus**, onanism (1); withdrawal of the penis before ejaculation.

**oral c.**, fellatio.

**c. reservatus**, c. in which ejaculation is postponed or suppressed.

**col.** A crater-like area of the interproximal oral mucosa joining the lingual and buccal interdental papillae.

**co'la.** Kola.

**colchiceine** (kol'chī-se-in). Demethylated colchicine; $C_{21}H_{23}NO_6$; a derivative of colchicum, obtained by hydrolysis; used for gout.

**colchicine** (kol'chī-sin) (USP, BP). $C_{22}H_{25}NO_6$; an alkaloid obtained from colchicum; used for gout.

**colchicum** (kol'chī-kum) [ L. fr. G. *kolchikon*, meadow-saffron ]. Meadow saffron; autumn crocus; the plant

*Colchicum autumnale* (family Liliaceae); the source of colchicine, which is used for gout.

**c. corm** (BP), the corm of *C. autumnale* collected in the early summer, deprived of its coats, sliced and dried.

**c. corm, powdered** (BP), used to prepare a liquid extract and a tincture.

**c. seed,** the dried ripe seed of *Colchicum autumnale;* it contains the alkaloids desacetylmethylcolchicine and colchiceine.

**cold.** A virus infection involving the upper respiratory tract; characterized by lack of fever, watery nasal discharge, and sneezing, with a duration of 3 to 5 days. See also common cold *virus.*

**c. in the head,** coryza; rhinitis.

**c. on the chest,** bronchitis.

**rose c.,** allergic rhinitis occurring in the spring and early summer.

**cold-blooded.** Poikilothermal.

**cold work.** In metals, the shaping of a structure by plastic deformation without melting and casting. This atomic rearrangement increases hardness and other properties.

**Cole,** Laurent, French pathologist, \*1903. See Benedict-Hopkins-C. *reagent,* Hopkins-C. *test.*

**Cole,** Lewis Gregory, U. S. radiologist, 1874–1954. See C.'s *sign.*

**Cole-Cecil murmur.** See under murmur.

**colectasia** (ko-lek-ta′zī-ah) [ G. *kolon,* colon, + *ektasis,* a stretching ]. Distention of the colon.

**colectomy** (ko-lek′to-mī) [ G. *kolon,* colon, + *ektomē,* excision ]. Excision of a segment or all of the colon.

**coleitis** (kol-e-i′tis) [ G. *koleos,* sheath, + suffix *-itis,* inflammation ]. Vaginitis.

**Coleman,** Warren U. S. physician, 1869–1948. See C.-Shaffer *diet.*

**coleo-** (kol′e-o-, ko′le-o-) [ G. *koleos,* sheath ]. Combining form meaning sheath or, specifically, the vagina.

**coleocele** (kol′e-o-sēl) [ G. *koleos,* sheath, + *kēlē,* tumor ]. Colpocele (1).

**coleocystitis** (kol′e-o-sis-ti′tis) [ G. *koleos,* sheath, + *kystis,* bladder, + suffix *-itis,* inflammation ]. Colpocystitis.

**Coleoptera** (ko′le-op′ter-ah) [ G. *koleos,* sheath + *pteron,* wing ]. An order of insects, the beetles, characterized by having a pair of hard, horny elytra (wing covers) overlying a pair of delicate, membranous flying wings; it is the largest of the insect orders and the largest order of any group.

**coleoptosis** (ko′le-op′to-sis). Coloptosis.

**col′eospas′tia** [ G. *koleos,* sheath, + *spastikos,* drawing in ]. Rarely used term meaning vaginismus.

**coleotomy** (kol-e-ot′o-mī) [ G. *koleos,* sheath, + *tomē,* incision ]. 1. Incision into the pericardium. 2. Vaginotomy.

**coles′tipol** (USAN). Tetraethylenepentamine polymer with 1-chloro-2,3-epoxypropane; an antilipemic drug.

**colibacillemia** (ko′li-bas-il-le′mī-ah) [ colibacillus + G. *haima,* blood ]. The presence of *Escherichia coli* in the circulating blood.

**colibacilluria** (ko′li-bas-il-u′rī-ah) [ colibacillus + G. *ouron,* urine ]. Coliuria; the presence of *Escherichia coli* in aseptically or "cleanly" voided urine.

**colibacillus,** pl. **colibacilli** (ko′li-ba-sil′us). Colon bacillus; *Escherichia coli.*

**colic** (kol′ik) [ G. *kōlikos,* relating to the colon ]. 1. Relating to the colon. 2. Enteralgia; spasmodic pains in the abdomen.

**appendic′ular c.,** colicky pain in the vermiform appendix.

**bil′iary c.,** colica hepatica; intense pain felt in the right upper quadrant of the abdomen from impaction of a gallstone in the cystic or hepatic duct or the ampulla of Vater.

**bil′ious c.,** more or less severe pain accompanying acute indigestion, diarrhea, and the presence of bile in the stools and vomitus.

**copper c.,** an affection similar to lead c. occurring in chronic poisoning by copper.

**Devonshire c.,** lead c.

**flatulent c.,** tympanites.

**gallstone c.,** biliary c.

**gastric c.,** bellyache; stomachache.

**hepatic c.,** hepatalgia; biliary c.

**lead c.,** Devonshire c.; painter's c.; saturnine c.; severe abdominal pain, with constipation, symptomatic of lead poisoning.

**meco′nial c.,** abdominal pain of newborn infants.

**menstrual c.,** intermittent crampy abdominal pains associated with menstruation.

**milk c.,** enterotoxemia.

**mucous c.,** abdominal pain in mucous colitis or enteritis.

**nephrit′ic c.,** (1) pain occasionally present in cases of acute renal inflammation; (2) renal c.

**ovarian c.,** ovarian neuralgia or pain due to any disease of the ovaries.

**painter's c.,** lead c.

**pancreat′ic c.,** severe abdominal pain, resembling that of biliary colic, caused by the passage of a pancreatic calculus.

**pseudomem′branous c.,** mucous c.

**renal c.,** severe pain caused by the impaction or passage of a calculus in the ureter or renal pelvis.

**sal′ivary c.,** periodical attacks of pain in the region of a salivary duct or gland, accompanied by an acute swelling of the gland, occurring in cases of salivary calculus.

**sat′urnine c.,** lead c.

**tubal c.,** pain due to spasmodic contraction of the oviduct excited by a blood clot, other irritant, or the injection of gas or oil.

**u′terine c.,** painful cramps of the uterine muscle sometimes occurring at the menstrual period, or in association with uterine disease.

**vermic′ular c.,** appendicular c.

**zinc c.,** c. resulting from chronic zinc poisoning.

**col′ica.** 1. A colic artery; see under arteria. 2. Colic; abdominal pain.

**c. hepat′ica,** biliary *colic.*

**c. muco′sa,** mucomembranous *enteritis.*

**c. picto′num, c. picto′rum,** lead *colic.*

**c. scorto′rum,** prostitutes' colic; abdominal pain occurring in prostitutes, attributed variously to neuralgia of the hypogastric plexus, to salpingitis, or to other inflammatory conditions of the internal genital organs.

**col′icin.** Bacteriocin produced by strains of *Escherichia coli* and by other enterobacteria (*Shigella* and *Salmonella*).

**colicinogeny** (kol′ī-sī-noj-ĕ-nī). The bacterial property of producing a colicin.

**colicoplegia** (kol′ī-ko-ple′jī-ah) [ G. *kolikos,* suffering from colic, + *plēgē,* stroke ]. Lead poisoning marked by both colic and palsy.

**coliform** (ko′lī-form, kol′ī-form). Denoting enterobacteria other than *Salmonella, Shigella,* and *Proteus.*

**colimy′cin.** Colistin.

**col′ione.** Obsolete synonym for chalone.

**coliphage** (ko′lī-fāj, kol′ī-fāj). A bacteriophage with an affinity for one or another strain of *Escherichia coli.* Because of the ready availability of strains of *E. coli,* the c.'s have played a dominant role in the bacteriophage studies from which were derived many concepts of modern microbial genetics. In general, the c.'s, like other bacteriophages, are known by symbols that have significance only as a means of laboratory identification. Additional notations, however, specifically identify variant characteristics; for instance, λdg denotes the deficient prophage (coliphage) λ carrying the bacterial gene *gal* (galactose).

**c. f-1,** the first filamentous virus (bacteriophage) recognized, and one of a group of seven c.'s (numbered f-1 through f-7) that were the first recognized bacteriophages with an affinity for only male (Hfr, $F^+$, and F′) bacterial strains, and all but c. f-1 being spherical RNA bacteriophages.

**c. f-2,** a spherical RNA c. with affinity only for male (Hfr, $F^+$, and F′) bacterial strains; see also c. f-1.

**c. λ,** coliphage lambda; phage lambda; a c. for which the *Escherichia coli* strain K12 is lysogenic; used extensively in studies of lysogeny and the source of the discovery of specialized transduction.

**c. X174,** a bacteriophage with single-stranded DNA and, therefore, of great experimental interest.

**T c.** [ T fr. *type* ], any one of a group of seven c.'s that have the same bacterial host strain (strain "B" of *Escherichia coli*); selection was by chance and numbering (T-1 through T-7) was arbitrary, but the so-called T-even phages (T-2, T-4, and T-6) are related antigenically and morphologically, as are, also, T-3 and T-7.

**co'liplica'tion.** An operation for reducing the lumen of a dilated colon by making folds or tucks in its walls.

**co'lipuncture.** Colocentesis.

**colis'timeth'ate sodium** (USP, USAN). Colistin (or cholistin) sulphomethate sodium (BP); pentasodium colistinmethanesulfonate; contains the pentasodium salt of the penta(methanesulfonic acid) derivative of colistin A as the major component, with a small proportion of the pentasodium salt of the same derivative of colistin B. An effective antibiotic against most Gram-negative bacilli (except *Proteus*); given intramuscularly. See also colistin sulfate and polymyxin.

**colis'tin.** Colimycin; a mixture of cyclic polypeptide antibiotics from *Bacillus colistinus;* separable into polymyxins.

**c. sulfate** (USP, BP), COLY-MYCIN; the sulfate salt of an antibacterial substance produced by the growth of *Bacillus polymyxa* var. *colistinus,* and consisting primarily of colistin A with small amounts of colistin B. It is effective against most Gram-negative bacteria (except *Proteus*); given orally for intestinal antibacterial action. See also colistimethate sodium and polymyxin.

**c. sulphomethate sodium** (BP), colistimethate sodium.

**colitis** (ko-li'tis) [ G. *kolon,* colon, + suffix - *itis,* inflammation ]. Inflammation of the colon.

**amebic c.,** inflammation of the colon in amebiasis.

**c. cys'tica superficia'lis,** a form of c. in which there is superficial cyst formation in the colon.

**granulomatous c.,** changes, identical to those of regional enteritis, involving the colon.

**c. gravis,** ulcerative c.

**mucous c.,** myxomembranous c.; colic myxoneurosis; an affection of the mucous membrane of the colon, characterized by more or less colicky pain, constipation or diarrhea, sometimes alternating, and the passage of mucous or slimy pseudomembranous shreds and patches.

**myxomembranous c.,** mucous c.

**pseudomem'branous c.,** pseudomembranous *enterocolitis.*

**ulcerative c.,** a chronic disease of unknown cause, characterized by ulceration of the colon and rectum, with bleeding, mucosal crypt abscesses, and inflammatory pseudopolyps. Ulcerative c. frequently causes anemia, hypoproteinemia, and electrolyte imbalance, and is less frequently complicated by perforation or carcinoma of the colon.

**uremic c.,** c. characterized by hemorrhages in the mucosa, occurring in renal failure, possibly owing to the irritant effect of ammonia formed by breakdown of increased urea in the intestinal secretions.

**co'litoxe'mia.** A condition resulting from the toxic effects of *Escherichia coli* or its products (or both) in the circulating blood.

**coliuria** (ko-lī-u'rī-ah). Colibacilluria.

**col'lacin.** Collastin; degenerated collagen.

**collagen** (kol'lă-jen) [ G. *koila,* glue, + suffix *-gen,* producing ]. 1. The major protein of the white fibers of connective tissue, cartilage, and bone, insoluble in water, altered to easily digestible, soluble gelatins by boiling in water, dilute acids, or alkalies. Comprises over half the protein of the mammal. High in glycine, alanine, proline, hydroxyproline; poor in sulfur; no tryptophan. Prepared from bone by dissolving the mineral part of bone with acid. 2. See c. *fiber.*

**collagenase** (kol'lă-jĕ-nās). Clostridiopeptidase A; an enzyme (EC 3.4.24.3) that catalyzes the hydrolysis of collagen.

**collagenation** (kol'ă-jĕ-na'shun). Collagenization.

**collagen'ic.** Collagenous.

**collagenization** (kol-laj'ĕ-nĭ-za'shun). Collagenation. 1. Replacement of tissues or fibrin by collagen. 2. Synthesis of collagen by fibroblasts.

**collagenolytic** (kol-laj'ĕ-no-lit'ik). Causing the lysis of collagen, gelatin, and other proteins containing proline.

**collagenosis** (kol-laj-ĕ-no'sis). Collagen *disease.*

**collagenous** (kol-laj'ĕ-nus). Collagenic; producing or containing collagen.

**collapse** (ko-laps') [ L. *col-labor,* pp. *-lapsus,* to fall together ]. 1. A condition of extreme prostration, similar to shock and due to the same causes, often with the added

hazard of a great loss of fluid, as in cholera. 2. To fall into a state of profound physical depression. 3. A falling together of the walls of a structure.

**circulatory c.,** failure of the circulation, either cardiac or peripheral.

**massive c.,** relatively sudden atelectasis of entire lung, or lobe.

**pulmonary c.,** secondary atelectasis (*q.v.*) due to bronchial obstruction, pleural effusion or pneumothorax, cardiac hypertrophy, or enlargement of other structures adjacent to the lungs.

**collap'sother'apy.** See collapse *therapy.*

**col'lar.** A band, usually denoting one encircling the neck.

**renal c.,** in the embryo, a ring of veins around the aorta below the origin of the superior mesenteric artery.

**c. of Venus,** syphilitic *leukoderma.*

**collarette** (kol'er-et'). The line of junction of the ciliary and pupillary zones of the iris, visible as a sinuous, scalloped, circular line in the iris.

**collas'tin.** Collacin.

**collas'tromin.** An insoluble material in connective tissue, to which procollagen is attached.

**collat'eral.** 1. Indirect, subsidiary or accessory to the main thing; side by side. 2. A side branch of a nerve axon or blood vessel.

**Colles,** Abraham, Irish surgeon, 1773–1843. See C.'s *fascia, fracture, law, C.-Baumès law, C.'s ligament, space.*

**collic'ulec'tomy.** Excision of the colliculus seminalis.

**colliculi'tis.** Inflammation of the urethra in the region of the colliculus seminalis.

**collic'ulus,** pl. **collic'uli** (kol-lik'u-lus) [ L. mound, dim. of *collis,* hill ] [ NA ]. A small elevation above the surrounding parts.

**c. cartila'ginis arytenoi'deae** [ NA ], the elevation on the anterolateral surface of the arytenoid cartilage above the triangular fovea.

**facial c.,** c. facialis.

**c. facia'lis,** [ NA ], facial c. eminence, or hillock; eminentia abducentis or facialis; a prominent portion of the eminentia medialis, just above the striae medullares in the rhomboidal fossa; it is caused by the curve of the genu of the facial nerve around the nucleus of the abducens nerve.

**inferior c.,** c. inferior.

**c. infe'rior** [ NA ], inferior c.; corpus quadrigeminum posterius; the ovoid, paired, inferior eminence of the lamina tecti mesencephali or lamina quadrigemina; it receives the lateral lemniscus and projects by way of the brachium colliculi inferioris to the medial geniculate body of the thalamus. It is thus an essential way-station in the central auditory pathway.

**seminal c.,** c. seminalis.

**c. semina'lis** [ NA ], seminal c.; c. urethralis; verumontanum; caput gallinaginis; an elevated portion of the urethral crest upon which open the two ejaculatory ducts and the prostatic utricle.

**superior c.,** c. superior.

**c. supe'rior** [ NA ], superior c.; corpus quadrigeminum anterius; the paired, larger, rounded anterior eminence of the lamina tecti mesencephali or lamina quadrigemina. Its major afferent connection is with the retina, but it receives additional fibers from the cerebral cortex, in particular from the visual cortex. Its efferent connections are with the lower brainstem and spinal cord—tractus tectobulbaris and tectospinalis—and with the pulvinar and other cell groups in the caudal part of the thalamus.

**c. urethra'lis,** c. seminalis.

**Collier,** James S., English physician, 1870–1935. See C.'s *tract.*

**col'liga'tion** [ L. *cum,* together, + *ligāre,* to bind ]. 1. A combination in which the units are distinguishable one from the other (vs. fusion). 2. The bringing of isolated events into a unified experience.

**col'liga'tive.** Referring to properties of solutions that depend only on the concentration of dissolved substances and not on their nature (*e.g.,* osmotic pressure, elevation of boiling point).

**collima'tion** [ L. *collineare,* to direct in a straight line ]. The process of restricting the detection from a given area of interest.

**col'limator.** A device of high absorption coefficient material used in x-ray to restrict and confine the x-ray beam to a given area and in nuclear medicine to restrict the detection of emitted radiations from a given area of interest.

**Collins,** Edward Treacher, English ophthalmologist, 1862–1919. See Treacher Collins *syndrome.*

**colliot'omy** [ G. *kolla,* glue, + G. *tomē,* incision ]. The cutting of adhesions.

**Collip,** James B., Canadian biochemist, 1892–1965. See Noble-C. *procedure,* Anderson-C. *test.*

**colliquation** (kol'lĭ-kwa'shun) [ L. *col-,* together, + *liquo,* pp. *liquatus,* to cause to melt ]. 1. Excessive discharge of fluid. 2. Softening. 3. Wasting away.

　　**ballooning c.,** ballooning *degeneration.*

　　**retic'ulating c.,** reticular *degeneration.*

**colliquative** (kol-lik'wă-tiv). Denoting a discharge, liquid in character and excessive in amount, as a c. diarrhea or a c. sweat.

**collo'dion** (USP, BP). Collodium; made by dissolving pyroxylin or gun cotton in ether and alcohol. On evaporation it leaves a glossy contractile film. Used as a protective for cuts or as a vehicle for the local application of medicinal substances.

　　**canthar'idal c.,** c. vesicans; blistering c.; composed of a powdered chloroform extract of cantharides in flexible c.; vesicant.

　　**flexible c.** (USP), a mixture of camphor, castor oil, and collodion; (BP), a mixture of castor oil, Canada turpentine, and collodion; used for the same purposes as collodion, but its film possesses the advantage, for certain conditions, of not contracting.

　　**hemostat'ic c.,** styptic c.

　　**iodized c.,** a 5 per cent solution of iodine in flexible c.; a counterirritant.

　　**salicylic acid c.** (USP), salicylic acid and flexible c.; a keratolytic agent used in the treatment of corns and verrucae.

　　**styptic c.,** styptic colloid; hemostatic c.; xylostyptic ether; made of tannic acid in flexible c.; astringent and local hemostatic.

　　**c. vesicans,** cantharidal c.

**collo'dium** [ G. *kolla,* glue, + *eidos,* appearance ]. Collodion.

**colloid** (kol'loyd) [ G. *kolla,* glue, + *eidos,* appearance ]. 1. Aggregates of atoms or molecules in a finely divided state (submicroscopic), dispersed in a gaseous, liquid, or solid medium, and resisting sedimentation, diffusion, and filtration, thus differing from precipitates ( *e.g.,* fog-liquid in gas; smoke-solid in gas; emulsions; gels; suspensions). 2. Glue-like. 3. Colloidin; a translucent, yellowish, homogeneous material of the consistency of glue, less fluid than mucoid or mucinoid, found in the cells and tissues in a state of c. degeneration. 4. The stored secretion within follicles of the thyroid gland. 5. For dentistry, see hydrocolloid.

　　**bovine c.,** conglutinin.

　　**dispersion c.,** dispersoid.

　　**emulsion c.,** emulsoid.

　　**hy'drophil** or **hydrophil'ic c.,** emulsoid.

　　**hydropho'bic c.,** suspensoid.

　　**irreversible c.,** one, *e.g.,* egg white, that is not again soluble in water after having been dried at ordinary temperature.

　　**lyophil'ic c.,** emulsoid.

　　**lyopho'bic c.,** suspensoid.

　　**protective c.,** a c. that has the power of preventing the precipitation of suspensoids under the influence of an electrolyte.

　　**reversible c.,** one that is again soluble in water after having been dried at ordinary temperature.

　　**stable c.,** reversible c.

　　**styptic c.,** styptic *collodion.*

　　**suspension c.,** suspensoid.

　　**thyroid c.,** the semifluid material that occupies the lumen of thyroid follicles; it contains thyroglobulin mainly.

　　**unstable c.,** irreversible c.

**colloid'al.** Relating to colloid.

**colloi'din.** Colloid (3).

**colloidocla'sia, colloidocla'sis** [ colloid + G. *klasis,* fracture ]. A rupture of the colloid equilibrium in the body.

**colloidoclas'tic.** Relating to colloidoclasia.

**colloidogen** (kol-loy'do-jen). A substance capable of giving rise to a colloidal solution or suspension.

**col'lotox'ism** [ perhaps fr. L. *collum,* neck (of clam), + G. *toxikon,* poison ]. Food poisoning from eating clams, occasionally associated with a thiaminase in clams.

**collox'ylin** [ G. *kolla,* glue, + *xylinos,* woody, fr. *xylon,* wood ]. Pyroxylin.

**collum,** pl. **col'la** (kol'um) [ L. ]. 1 [ NA ]. The neck; cervix; the part between the shoulders or thorax and the head. 2. A constricted or necklike portion of any organ or other anatomical structure.

　　**c. anatom'icum hu'meri** [ NA ], anatomical neck of the humerus; a groove separating the head from the tuberosities, giving attachment to the capsular ligament.

　　**c. chirur'gicum hu'meri** [ NA ], surgical neck of the humerus; the narrowing portion below the head and tuberosities.

　　**c. costae** [ NA ], neck of the rib; the flattened portion of a rib between the head and the tuberosity.

　　**c. den'tis** [ NA ], neck of a tooth; cervical zone of a tooth; the slightly constricted part of a tooth, between the crown and the root.

　　**c. distortum,** torticollis.

　　**c. fem'oris** [ NA ], neck of the femur; a short constricted strong bar projecting at a more or less obtuse angle (about 125°) from the upper end of the shaft of the femur, and supporting the head.

　　**c. folli'culi pili,** the narrowed part of the hair follicle between the hair bulb and the surface of the skin.

　　**c. glandis penis** [ NA ], of the glans penis; a constriction behind the corona glandis penis.

　　**c. hu'meri,** neck of the humerus; see c. anatomicum and c. chirurgicum.

　　**c. mallei** [ NA ], neck of the malleus.

　　**c. mandib'ulae** [ NA ], neck of the condylar process of the mandible.

　　**c. ra'dii** [ NA ], neck of the radius; the narrow part of the shaft just below the head.

　　**c. scap'ulae** [ NA ], neck of the scapula; a slight constriction marking the separation of that portion bearing the glenoid cavity and coracoid process from the remainder of the scapula.

　　**c. tali** [ NA ], neck of the talus; a constriction separating the head, or anterior portion, from the body.

　　**c. vesicae felleae** [ NA ], neck of the gallbladder; the narrow portion between the body of the gallbladder and beginning of the cystic duct.

**collunarium** (kol'u-na'rĭ-um) [ L. *col-luo* (*conl-*), to wash thoroughly, + *nares,* nostrils ]. A nose wash; nasal douche.

**collutorium** (kol'u-to'rĭ-um) [ Mod. L. fr. *col-luo,* pp. *-lutus,* to wash thoroughly ]. Collutory; mouthwash; gargle; a medicated liquid used for cleansing the mouth and treating diseased states of the mucous membrane.

**col'lutory** [ L. *colluere,* to rinse ]. Collutorium.

**Collyric'ulum fa'ba.** A fluke that causes the formation of subcutaneous cysts (cutaneous monostomidosis) in chickens, turkeys and other birds.

**collyrium** (kol-līr'ĭ-um) [ G. *kollyrion,* poultice, eye salve ]. 1. A soothing eye water. 2. Originally, any preparation for the eye.

**colo-** (ko'lo-, kol'o-) [ G. *kolon,* colon ]. Combining form relating to the colon.

**colobo'ma** [ G. *kolobōma,* lit., the part taken away in mutilation, fr. *koloboō,* to dock, mutilate ]. Any defect, congenital, pathologic, or artificial, especially of the eye.

　　**c. of the choroid,** a congenital defect of the choroid and retina, seen as a white patch (the exposed sclera) usually situated below the optic disk, causing a scotoma in that region.

　　**Fuchs' c.,** congenital conus; a congenital crescentic defect in the choroid at the lower edge of the optic disk.

　　**c. iridis,** c. of the iris; a congenital cleft of the iris, often associated with c. of the choroid, or the defect resulting from iridectomy.

　　**c. lentis,** a segment of the lens which is shorter and thicker than normal, giving the appearance of a notch.

　　**c. lobuli,** congenital fissure of the lobule of the ear.

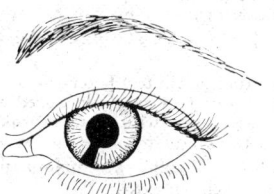

**Coloboma Iridis**
(From Langman, J.: *Medical Embryology*, Ed. 2, The Williams & Wilkins Co., Baltimore, 1969.)

**c. of optic nerve,** a congenital notch in the formation of the optic nerve, appearing as a craterlike excavation at the optic disk.

**c. palpebra'le,** a congenital notch in the lid margin.

**c. retinae,** a condition in which a portion of the retina is lacking.

**c. of vitreous,** a congenital indentation of the vitreous body by mesoderm; severe cases involve a high degree of myopia.

**colocentesis** (ko'lo-sen-te'sis) [ colo- + G. *kentēsis,* a puncture ]. Colipuncture; colopuncture; puncture of the colon with a trochar or scalpel to relieve distention.

**colocholecystostomy** (ko'lo-ko-le-sis-tos'to-mĭ). Cholecystocolostomy.

**colocolic** (ko'lo-kol'ik). From colon to colon; said of a spontaneous or induced anastomosis between two parts of the colon.

**co'locolos'tomy** [ colon + colon + G. *stoma,* mouth ]. The establishment of a communication between two noncontinuous segments of the colon.

**col'ocynth** [ G. *kolokynthē,* the round gourd or pumpkin ]. Colocynthis; colocynthidis pulpa; bitter apple; the peeled dried fruit of *Citrullus colcynthis* (family Cucurbitaceae), a herb of the sandy shores of the Mediterranean, resembling somewhat the watermelon plant. A hydrogogue cathartic.

**colocyn'thin.** A glucoside, $C_{56}H_{54}O_{23}$, from colocynth; occurs in the form of an amorphous yellow powder. Has been used hypodermically as a purgative.

**co'lodyspep'sia.** Pain from disorder of the colon.

**co'loenteri'tis.** Enterocolitis.

**co'lohep'atopex'y** [ colo- + G. *hēpar (hēpat-),* liver, + *pēxis,* fixation ]. Attachment of the colon to the liver to form protective adhesions after gall bladder operations.

**cololysis** (ko-lol'ĭ-sis) [ colo- + G. *lysis,* loosening ]. Procedure of freeing the colon from adhesions.

**colom'ba.** Calumba.

**colominic acid.** Polymer of *N*-acetylneuraminic acid.

**colon** (ko'lon) [ G. *kolon* ] [ NA ]. The division of the large intestine extending from the cecum to the rectum.

**c. ascen'dens** [ NA ], ascending c.; the portion of the c. between the ileocecal orifice and the right colic flexure.

**ascending c.,** c. ascendens.

**c. descen'dens** [ NA ], descending c.; the part of the c. extending from the left colic flexure to the pelvic brim.

**descending c.,** c. descendens.

**giant c.,** megacolon.

**iliac c.,** that portion of the descending c. which lies in the left iliac fossa, between the crest of the left ilium and the pelvic brim.

**irritable c.,** tendency to colonic hyperperistalsis, sometimes with colicky pains and diarrhea.

**lead-pipe c.,** scarred, rigid colon of advanced ulcerative colitis.

**c. pelvinum,** c. sigmoideum.

**sigmoid c.,** c. sigmoideum.

**c. sigmoideum** [ NA ], sigmoid c.; c. pelvinum; the part of the c. describing an S-shaped curve between the pelvic brim and the third sacral segment. It is continuous with the rectum.

**transverse c.,** c. transversum.

**c. transver'sum** [ NA ], transverse c.; the part of the c. between the right and left colic flexures. It extends more or less transversely across the abdomen.

**colonalgia** (ko-lon-al'jĭ-ah) [ colon + G. *algos,* pain ]. Colic; pain in the colon.

**colon'ic.** Relating to the colon.

**colonization** (kol'on-ĭ-za'shun). 1. Innidiation.2. The formation of compact population groups of the same type of microorganism, as the colonies that develop when a bacterial cell begins reproducing. 3. The care of certain persons, *e.g.* lepers, mental patients, and so on, in community groups.

**colon'ogram.** Graphic recording of movements of the colon.

**co'lonom'eter.** A device for counting bacterial colonies.

**co'lonop'athy.** Colopathy; any disordered condition of the colon.

**colonorrhagia** (ko-lon-or-ra'jĭ-ah). Colorrhagia.

**colonorrhea** (ko'lon-or-re'ah). Colorrhea.

**colon'oscope.** An elongated rectal speculum.

**colonos'copy** [ colon + G. *skopeō,* to view ]. Inspection of the upper portion of the rectum by means of a colonoscope.

**col'ony** [ L. *colonia,* a colony ]. 1. A group of cells growing on a solid nutrient surface, each arising from the multiplication of an individual cell; a clone. 2. A group of people with similar interests, living in a particular location or area.

**daughter c.,** a secondary c. growing on the surface of an older c.; it is smaller and may have characteristics different from those of the mother c.

**filamentous c.,** in bacteriology, a c. composed of long, interwoven, irregularly disposed threads.

**Gheel c.,** a c. in Gheel, Belgium, originating in the 13th century, for the informal communal care, in private homes, of severely mentally disordered persons.

**H. c.,** a c. of motile organisms forming a thin film (*Hauch*) of growth; see Hauch.

**lenticular c.,** (1) a bacterial c., shaped like a lentil, within the subject of the medium; (2) a bacterial colony, of the shape of a planoconvex lens, on the surface of the medium.

**mother c.,** a c. which gives rise to a secondary c. (a daughter c.), the latter growing on the surface of the former; the daughter c. is smaller than the mother c., and the characteristics of the c.'s may differ.

**mucoid c.,** a c. showing viscous or sticky growth typical of an organism producing large quantities of a carbohydrate capsule.

**O. c.** [ Ger. *ohne Hauch,* without film ], growth of a nonmotile bacterium in discrete, compact c.'s in contrast to a film (*Hauch*) of growth produced by some motile bacteria.

**rough c.,** a bacterial c. with a granular, flattened surface; this type of c. is usually associated with loss of virulence with respect to that of smooth c.'s.

**smooth c.,** a bacterial c. with a glistening, rounded surface; this type of c. is usually associated with increased virulence with respect to that of rough c.'s.

**spheroid c.,** a c. of protozoa in which the individual cells are held together in a coherent spherical mass by a gelatinous material.

**colop'athy.** Colonopathy.

**colopexy, colopexia** (kol'o-pek'sĭ, ko'lo-pek'sĭ-ah) [ colo- + G. *pēxis,* fixation ]. Attachment of a portion of the colon to the abdominal wall.

**colopexos'tomy** [ colo- + G. *pēxis,* fixation, + *stoma,* mouth ]. The establishment of an artificial anus by opening into the colon after its fixation to the abdominal wall.

**colopexot'omy** [ colo- + G. *pēxis,* fixation, + *tomē,* incision ]. Incision into the colon after its fixation to the abdominal wall.

**colophony** (ko-lof'o-nĭ) [ *Colophōn,* Summit, a town in Ionia ] (BP). 1. Rosin. 2. Resin.

**coloplication** (ko'lo-plĭ-ka'shun) [ colo- + Mod. L. *plica,* fold ]. Taking a tuck in a dilated colon.

**co'loproc'tia.** Colostomy.

**coloproctitis** (ko-lo-prok-ti'tis) [ colo- + G. *prōktos,* anus (rectum), + suffix -*itis,* inflammation ]. Colorectitis; proctocolitis; inflammation of both colon and rectum.

**co'loproctos'tomy** [ colo- + G. *prōktos,* anus (rectum), + *stoma,* mouth ]. Colorectostomy; establishment of a communication between the rectum and a segment of the colon not continuous with it.

**coloptosis, coloptosia** (ko-lop-to'sis, -to'sī-ah) [ colo- + G. *ptōsis,* a falling ]. Coleoptosis; downward displacement, or prolapse, of the colon, especially of the transverse portion.

**co'lopunc'ture.** Colocentesis.

**color** (kul'or) [ L. ]. Hue; the quality other than shape and texture that an object presents to the eye.

　**complementary c.'s,** two primary c.'s which, when combined, produce white light.

　**confusion c.'s,** a set of c.'s (usually of colored wools), cream, buff, pale blue, gray, brown, green, violet, etc., used in tests for c. blindness.

　**incidental c.,** a c. the impression of which remains fixed on the retina after the object causing it is no longer present; afterimage.

　**primary c.,** one of the seven c.'s composing the solar spectrum; violet, indigo, blue, green, yellow, orange, red.

　**pure c.,** visual sensations produced by light of specific wave length.

　**saturated c.,** a simple c. of the spectrum which cannot be further decomposed; the smaller the admixture of white light with the simple c., the greater the degree of saturation.

　**simple c.,** primary c.

　**tone c.,** timbre.

**colorectitis** (ko'lo-rek-ti'tis). Coloproctitis.

**colorectostomy** (ko'lo-rek-tos'to-mī). Coloproctostomy.

**colorim'eter.** Chromatometer.

　**Duboscq's c.,** an apparatus for measuring the depth of tint in a fluid by comparing it with a standard fluid; glass cylinders are immersed in each of two cups containing, one the standard fluid, the other the fluid to be tested; on looking through the cylinders the tints are equalized by raising or lowering the cylinder in one cup, and the extent of this raising or lowering is indicated on a scale and gives the exact difference in tint.

**colorim'etry.** A procedure for quantitative chemical analysis, based on comparison of the color developed in a solution of the test material with that in a standard solution. The two solutions are observed simultaneously in a colorimeter, and quantitated on the basis of the absorption of light.

**colorrhagia** (ko-lo-ra'je-ah) [ colo- + G. *rhēgnymi,* to burst forth ]. Colonorrhagia; an abnormal discharge from the colon.

**color'raphy** [ colo- + G. *raphē,* suture ]. Suture of the colon.

**colorrhea** (ko-lo-re'ah) [ colo- + G. *rhoia,* a flow ]. Colonorrhea; diarrhea thought to originate from the process confined to or affecting chiefly the colon.

**colos'copy** [ colo- + G. *skopeō,* to view ]. Visual examination of the colon by use of a sterilized sigmoidoscope during laparotomy.

**colosigmoidostomy** (ko'lo-sig-moy-dos'ko-pī). Formation of an anastomosis between any part of the colon and the sigmoid colon.

**colostomy** (ko-los'to-mī) [ colo- + G. *stoma,* mouth ]. Establishment of an artificial anus by an opening into the colon.

**colostra'tion.** Infantile diarrhea attributed to the action of the colostrum.

**colos'tric.** Relating to the colostrum.

**colostrorrhea** (ko-los-tror-re'ah) [ colostrum, *q.v.,* + G. *rhoia,* flow ]. An abnormally profuse secretion of colostrum.

**colos'trous.** Relating to colostrum.

**colostrum** (ko-los'trum) [ L. ]. Foremilk (1); a thin, white, opalescent fluid, the first milk secreted at the termination of pregnancy; it differs from the milk secreted later in containing more lactalbumin and lactoprotein.

**colot'omy** [ colo- + G. *tomē,* incision ]. Incision into the colon.

**colp-.** See colpo-.

**colpal'gia** [ colp- + G. *algos,* pain ]. Vaginodynia.

**colpatresia** (kol-pā-tre'zī-ah) [ colp- + G. *atrētos,* imperforate ]. Vaginal *atresia.*

**colpec'tasis, colpecta'sia** [ colp- + G. *aktasis,* stretching ]. Distention of the vagina.

**colpec'tomy** [ colp- + G. *ektomē,* excision ]. Vaginectomy (1).

**colpeurynter** (kol'pu-rin'ter) [ colp- + G. *eurynō,* to dilate, fr. *eurys,* wide ]. A bag introduced empty into the vagina and then filled with water, formerly used as a tampon or in the uterus to dilate the cervix.

**colpi'tis** [ colp- + G. suffix *-itis,* inflammation ]. Vaginitis.

　**c. mycotica,** vaginomycosis.

**colpo-, colp-** [ G. *kolpos,* any fold or hollow; specifically, bosom (vagina) ]. Combining forms denoting the vagina. For words beginning thus and not found here, see vagino-, vagin-.

**colpocele** (kol'po-sēl) [ colpo- + G. *kēlē,* hernia ]. 1. Vaginocele; coleocele; elytrocele; a hernia projecting into the vagina. 2. Colpoptosis.

**colpocleisis** (kol-po-kli'sis) [ colpo- + G. *kleisis,* closure ]. Simon's operation (1); operation for obliterating the lumen of the vagina.

**col'pocysti'tis** [ colpo- + G. *kystis,* bladder, + suffix *-itis,* inflammation ]. Coleocystitis; inflammation of both vagina and bladder.

**col'pocys'tocele** [ colpo- + G. *kystis,* bladder, + *kēlē,* hernia ]. Cystocele.

**colpocys'toplasty** [ colpo- + G. *kystis,* bladder, + *plassō,* to mold ]. A surgical plastic procedure to repair the vesicovaginal wall.

**colpocystot'omy** [ colpo- + G. *kystis,* bladder, + *tomē,* incision ]. Incision into the bladder through the vagina.

**colpocystoureterotomy** (kol'po-sis'to-u-re-ter-ot'o-me) [ colpo- + G. *kystis,* bladder, + *ourēter,* ureter, + *tomē,* incision ]. Colpoureterocystotomy; incision into the ureter by way of the vagina and the bladder.

**colpodynia** (kol-po-din'ī-ah) [ colpo- + G. *odynē,* pain ]. Vaginodynia.

**col'pohy'perpla'sia** [ colpo- + hyperplasia, *q.v.* ]. A condition marked by thickening of the vaginal mucous membrane.

　**c. cys'tica,** pachyvaginitis cystica; an infectious form, occurring usually in pregnancy, in which the thickened mucous membrane is studded with retention cysts.

　**c. emphysemato'sa,** c. cystica in which the fluid in the cysts is partly or wholly replaced by a gas.

**colpohysterectomy** (kol'po-his'ter-ek'to-mī) [ colpo- + G. *hystera,* uterus, + *ektomē,* excision ]. Vaginal *hysterectomy.*

**col'pohys'teropexy** [ colpo- + G. *hystera,* uterus, + *pēxis,* fixation ]. An operation for fixation of the uterus performed through the vagina.

**col'pohysterot'omy** [ colpo- + G. *hystera,* uterus, + *tomē,* incision ]. Vaginal *hysterotomy.*

**col'pomi'croscope.** A special microscope for direct visual examination of the cervix.

**col'pomicros'copy.** Direct observation and study of cells in the vagina and cervix magnified *in vivo,* in the undisturbed tissue, by means of a special instrument.

**colpomycosis** (kol'po-mi-ko'sis). Vaginomycosis.

**colpomyomectomy** (kol'po-mi-o-mek'to-mī) [ colpo- + myoma + G. *ektomē,* excision ]. Vaginal *myomectomy.*

**colpop'athy.** [ colpo- + G. *pathos,* suffering ]. Vaginopathy.

**colpoperineoplasty** (kol'po-pĕr'ĭ-ne'o-plas-tī) [ colpo- + perineum, + G. *plassō,* to form ]. Vaginoperineoplasty.

**colpoperineorrhaphy** (kol'po-per-ĭ-ne-or'ă-fī) [ colpo- + perineum, + G. *rhaphē,* sewing ]. Vaginoperineorrhaphy.

**colpopexy** (kol'po-pek-sī) [ colpo- + G. *pēxis,* fixation ]. Vaginofixation.

**col'poplasty** [ colpo- + G. *plassō,* to form ]. Vaginoplasty.

**colpopoiesis** (kol'po-poy-e'sis) [ colpo- + G. *poiēsis,* a making ]. McIndoe's operation; Williams' operation; surgical construction of an artificial vagina.

**colpoptosis, colpoptosia** (kol-pop-to'sis, kol-po-to'sis, -to'sī-ah) [ colpo- + G. *ptōsis,* a falling ]. Colpocele (2); elytroptosis; prolapse of the vaginal walls.

**col´porec´topex´y** [ colpo- + rectum + G. *pēxis*, fixation ]. Repairing a prolapsed rectum by suturing it to the wall of the vagina.

**colporrhagia** (kol-pŏ-ra´jĭ-ah) colpo- + G. *rhēgnymi*, to burst forth ]. Vaginal hemorrhage.

**colporrhaphy** (kol-por´ă-fĭ) [ colpo- + G. *rhaphē*, suture ]. Elytrorrhaphy; repair of a rupture of the vagina by freshening and suturing the edges of the tear.

**colporrhexis** (kol-po-rek´sis) [ colpo- + G. *rhēxis*, rupture ]. A tearing of the vaginal wall; vaginal laceration.

**col´poscope.** An endoscopic instrument that magnifies cells of the vagina and cervix *in vivo* to allow direct observation and study of these tissues.

**colpos´copy** [ colpo- + G. *skopeō*, to view ]. Examination of vagina and cervix by means of an endoscope.

**colpospasm** (kol´po-spazm). Spasmodic contraction of the vagina.

**col´postat** [ colpo- + G. *statos*, standing ]. An appliance for use in the vagina, such as a radium applicator for treatment of cancer of the cervix.

**colposteno´sis** [ colpo- + G. *stenōsis*, narrowing ]. Elytrostenosis; narrowing of the lumen of the vagina.

**colpostenot´omy** [ colpo- + G. *stenōsis*, narrowing, + *tomē*, incision ]. Division of a colpostenosis.

**colpot´omy** [ colpo- + G. *tomē*, incision ]. Vaginotomy.

**colpoureterocystotomy** (kol´po-u-re´ter-o-sis-tot´o-me). Colpocystoureterotomy.

**colpoureterotomy** (kol´po-u-re-ter-ot´o-me) [ colpo- + G. *tomē*, incision ]. Incision into a ureter through the vagina.

**colpoxerosis** (kol-po-ze-ro´sis) [ colpo- + G. *xērōsis*, dryness ]. Abnormal dryness of the vaginal mucous membrane.

**Colubridae** (kol-u´brĭ-de) [ L. *coluber*, serpent ]. A family of serpents. This family contains two-thirds of all species of snakes. The majority are harmless, but it includes a few rear-fanged poisonous species.

**Colubrinae** (kol-u´brĭ-ne). A subfamily of the *Colubridae*. These are the typical harmless snakes of the world. The teeth vary in size, but no poison glands are present.

**colum´bin.** Calumbin.

**colum´bium** [ *Columbia* ]. Former name for the element, symbol Cb, atomic no. 41, atomic weight 92.91. The internationally accepted name is now niobium, symbol Nb.

**colum´bo.** Calumba.

**columella,** pl. **columel´lae** (kol´u-mel´lah) [ L. dim. of *columna*, column ]. 1. Columnella; a column, or a small column. 2. In fungi, especially the Phycomycetes, a sterile invagination or inflated end of a sporangiophore that extends into the sporangium.

    **c. au´ris.** the middle ear ossicle of amphibians, reptiles, and birds; it is homologous with the stapes of mammals.

    **c. coch´leae,** modiolus.

    **c. nasi,** the lower margin of the septum nasi.

**column** (kol´um) [ L. *columna* ]. An anatomical part or structure in the form of a pillar or cylindric funiculus; see also fasciculus.

    **anal c.'s,** *columnae* anales.

    **anterior c. of medulla oblongata,** *pyramis* medullae oblongatae.

    **anterior c. of spinal cord,** *columna* anterior.

    **anterolateral c. of spinal cord,** *funiculus* lateralis.

    **Bertin's c.'s,** *columnae* renales.

    **branchial efferent c.,** special visceral or splanchnic efferent c.; a c. of gray matter in the brainstem of the embryo which is represented in the adult by the nucleus ambiguus and the motor nuclei of the trigeminal and facial nerves.

    **Burdach's c.,** *fasciculus* cuneatus.

    **Clarke's c.,** *nucleus* thoracicus.

    **dorsal c. of spinal cord,** *columna* posterior.

    **c. of fornix,** *columna* fornicis.

    **general somatic afferent c.,** in the embryo, a c. of gray matter in the hindbrain and upper segments of the spinal cord which is represented in the adult by the sensory nuclei of the trigeminal nerve.

    **general somatic efferent c.,** a c. of gray matter in the embryo which is represented in the adult by the nuclei of

the oculomotor, trochlear, abducens, and hypoglossal nerves.

    **general visceral** or **splanchnic afferent c.,** a column of gray matter in the hindbrain of the embryo, in further development giving rise to the nucleus of the solitary tract.

    **general visceral** or **splanchnic efferent c.,** a c. of gray matter in the hindbrain of the embryo which is represented in the adult by the dorsal nucleus of the vagus, the superior and inferior salivatory nuclei, and the nucleus of Edinger-Westphal.

    **Goll's c.,** *fasciculus* gracilis.

    **Gowers' c.,** *tractus* spinocerebellaris anterior.

    **gray c.'s,** *columnae* griseae.

    **intermediolateral cell c. of spinal cord,** *nucleus* intermediolateralis.

    **lateral c. of spinal cord,** *columna* lateralis.

    **Morgagni's c.'s,** *columnae* anales.

    **muscle c.,** sarcostyle; a term formerly applied to a single myofibril or sometimes to a group of them.

    **positive c.,** a luminous stream, usually pinkish in color, seen in passing a current of high potential through a tube from which the air has been partly exhausted.

    **posterior c. of spinal cord,** (1) *columna* posterior; (2) in clinical parlance, the term often refers to the funiculus posterior of the spinal cord's white matter.

    **renal c.'s,** *columnae* renales.

    **Rolando's c.,** a slight ridge on either side of the medulla oblongata related to the descending trigeminal tract and nucleus.

    **Sertoli's c.'s,** see Sertoli's *cells.*

    **special somatic afferent c.,** a c. of gray matter in the hindbrain of the embryo, represented in the adult by the nuclei of the auditory and vestibular nerves.

    **special visceral** or **splanchnic efferent c.,** branchial efferent c.

    **spinal c.,** *columna* vertebralis.

    **Stilling's c.,** *nucleus* thoracicus.

    **Türck's c.,** *tractus* pyramidalis anterior.

    **vaginal c.'s,** *columnae* rugarum.

    **ventral c. of spinal cord,** *columna* anterior.

    **vertebral c.,** *columna* vertebralis.

**columna,** gen. and pl. **colum´nae** (kol-um´nah) [ L. ] [ NA ]. Column.

    **columnae ana´les** [ NA ], anal columns; Morgagni's columns; a number of vertical ridges in the mucous membrane of the upper half of the anal canal.

    **c. ante´rior** [ NA ], anterior or ventral column of the spinal cord; the pronounced, ventrally oriented ridge of gray matter in each half of the spinal cord; it corresponds to the anterior or ventral horn appearing in transverse sections of the cord, and contains the motor neurons innervating the skeletal musculature of the trunk, neck, and extremities; see also columnae griseae.

    **colum´nae car´neae,** *trabeculae* carneae.

    **c. for´nicis** [ NA ], column of the fornix; anterior pillar of the fornix; that part of the fornix that curves down in front of the thalamus and the interventricular foramen of Monro, then continues through the gray matter of the hypothalamus to the mamillary body. Consisting primarily of fibers originating in the hippocampus, the c. fornicis is the direct continuation of the crus fornicis (that stretch of the fornix passing forward and medialward closely below the corpus callosum).

    **columnae gris´eae** [ NA ], gray columns; the three somewhat ridge-shaped masses of gray matter (columna posterior or dorsalis, columna anterior or ventralis, and columna lateralis) that extend longitudinally through the center of each lateral half of the spinal cord; in transverse sections these columns appear as gray horns and are therefore commonly called ventral or anterior horn (cornu anterius), dorsal or posterior horn (cornu posterius), and lateral horn (cornu laterale).

    **c. latera´lis** [ NA ], lateral column of spinal cord; a slight protrusion of the gray matter of the spinal cord into the lateral funiculus of either side, especially marked in the thoracic region where it encloses preganglionic motor neurons of the sympathetic division of the autonomic nervous system; it corresponds to the lateral horn (cornu laterale) appearing in transverse sections of the spinal cord; see also columnae griseae.

**c. mol'lis,** *adhesio* interthalamicus.

**c. nasi,** the fleshy termination of the septum nasi.

**c. poste'rior** [ NA ], posterior or dorsal column of the spinal cord; the pronounced, dorsolaterally oriented ridge of gray matter in each lateral half of the spinal cord, corresponding to the cornu posterius (posterior or dorsal horn) appearing in transverse sections of the cord; see also *columnae griseae*.

**columnae rena'les** [ NA ], renal columns; Bertin's columns; the prolongations of cortical substance separating the pyramids of the kidney.

**columnae ruga'rum** [ NA ], vaginal columns; two slight longitudinal ridges, anterior and posterior, in the vaginal mucous membrane, each marked by a number of transverse mucosal folds.

**c. vertebra'lis** [ NA ], vertebral or spinal column; spine; backbone; the series of vertebrae that extend from the cranium to the coccyx, providing support and forming a flexible bony case for the spinal cord.

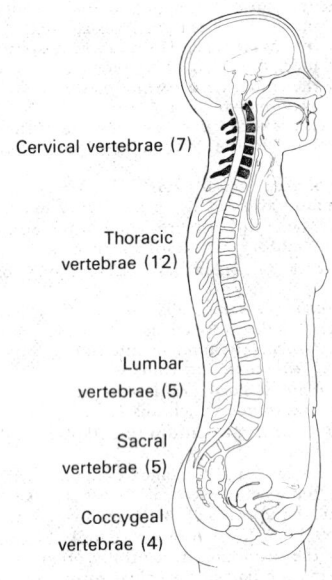

Cervical vertebrae (7)

Thoracic vertebrae (12)

Lumbar vertebrae (5)

Sacral vertebrae (5)

Coccygeal vertebrae (4)

**Columna Vertebralis**

Adult vertebral column, shown in relation to the body

**columnel'la** [ L. dim. of *columna*, a column; another form of *columella* ]. Columella.

**columniza'tion** [ L. *columna*, column ]. Filling the vagina with a tampon in order to prevent prolapse of the uterus.

**colyone** (ko'li-ōn). Obsolete synonym for chalone.

**colypeptic** (ko-li-pep'tik) [ G. *kōlyō*, to hinder, + *pepsis*, digestion. PEP- ]. Retarding digestion.

**coma** (ko'mah) [ G. *kōma*, deep sleep ]. A state of profound unconsciousness from which one cannot be roused; it may be due to the action of an ingested poison, such as alcohol or opium, or of one formed in the body, as in uremic or diabetic c., to injury or disease of the brain, as in apoplexy, or to hysteria. See also consciousness.

**c. carcinomato'sum,** c. occurring in the final stage of cancerous cachexia.

**diabetic c.,** Kussmaul's c.; c. that developes in severe and inadequately treated cases of diabetes mellitus; results from reduced oxidative metabolism of the central nervous system that, in turn, stems from severe ketoacidosis and possibly also from the histotoxic action of the ketone bodies and disturbances in water and electrolyte balance. Commonly fatal, unless appropriate therapy is instituted promptly.

**hepat'ic c.,** c. occurring in advanced cirrhosis, hepatitis, poisoning, or other severe liver disease. Mental confusion or delirium may precede, as may flapping tremor. The patient may or may not be deeply jaundiced and may have acute disorders of ammonia, nitrogen, and amino acid metabolism.

**hyperosmolar hyperglycemic nonketonic c.,** c. in which blood glucose concentration is increased but without the presence of ketone bodies in plasma.

**Kussmaul's c.,** diabetic c.

**thyrotox'ic c.,** c. preceding death in thyroid storm or thyrotoxic crisis.

**co'matose.** In a state of coma.

**combina'tion.** 1. The act of combining (*i.e.*, by joining, uniting, or otherwise bringing into close association) separate entities. 2. The state of being so combined.

**binary c.,** the name of a species of bacteria consisting of two parts: a generic name and a specific epithet.

**combus'tible.** Capable of rapid combination with oxygen, or of burning.

**combus'tion** [ L. *comburo*, pp. -*bustus*, to burn up, fr. *com-*, intensive, + hypothet. *buro* = *uro*, to burn ]. Burning; the rapid oxidation of any substance accompanied by the production of heat and light.

**c. equivalent,** see under equivalent.

**heat of c.,** see under heat.

**nuclear c.,** a nuclear reaction yielding energy; nuclear fusion or fission.

**slow c.,** decay.

**sponta'neous c.,** the ignition of a mass of material by heat developed within it by the oxidation of the substances composing it without external ignition.

**Comby,** Jules, Paris pediatrician, 1853–1947. See C.'s *sign.*

**comedo,** pl. **comedo'nes** (kom'e-do, ko-me'do) [ L. a glutton, fr. *com-edo*, to eat up ]. Blackhead; a plug of sebaceous matter, capped with a blackened mass of dust and epithelial debris, filling the pilosebaceous orifice.

**come'docarcino'ma.** A form of carcinoma in which plugs of necrotic malignant cells may be expressed from the ducts.

**comes,** pl. **com'ites** (ko'mēz) [ L. a companion, fr. *com-*, together, + *eo*, pp. *itus*, to go ] [ NA ]. A blood vessel accompanying another vessel or a nerve; the veins accompanying an artery, often two in number, are called venae comitantes or venae comites.

**c. nervi phrenici,** *arteria* pericardiacophrenica.

**Comessatti test.** See under test.

**commen'sal** [ L. *con-*, with, together + *mensa*, table ]. Denoting two organisms which live together, neither bearing a parasitic relation to the other, without harm or prejudice to either but with one or both members deriving benefit.

**commen'salism.** The state of being commensal.

**epizoic c.,** phoresis (2).

**comminuted** (kom'i-nu-ted) [ L. *com-minuo*, pp. -*minutus*, to make smaller, break into pieces, fr. *minor*, less ]. Broken into a number of fragments; denoting especially a fractured bone.

**comminution** (kom-i-nu'shun). A breaking into a number of small fragments.

**commissu'ra,** gen. and pl. **commissu'rae** [ L. a joining together, seam, fr. *com-mitto*, to send or bring together, combine ] [ NA ]. Commissure. 1. Angle or corner of the eye, lips, or labia. 2. A bundle of nerve fibers passing from one side to the other in the brain or spinal cord.

**c. al'ba** [ NA ], white commissure; anterior white commissure; commissura ventralis alba; a narrow band of white substance bordering on the anterior median fissure of the spinal cord in front of the anterior gray commissure, and consisting of nerve fibers crossing over from one half of the spinal cord to the other.

**c. ante'rior** [ NA ], anterior commissure; a round bundle of nerve fibers that crosses the midline of the brain near the anterior limit of the third ventricle. It consists of a smaller pars anterior, the fibers of which pass in part to the olfactory bulbs, and a larger pars posterior, which interconnects the left and right temporal lobes.

**c. anterior gris'ea,** see *substantia* intermedia centralis et lateralis.

**c. bulbor'um,** pars intermedia (2); a narrow median band that connects the two masses of erectile tissue (the bulb of the vestibule) on either side of the vaginal orifice.

**c. cine'rea,** *adhesio* interthalamica.

**c. for'nicis** [ NA ], commissure of the fornix; hippocampal commissure; commissura hippocampi; transverse fornix; delta fornicis; lyra davidis; psalterium (1); it consists of fibers that interconnect the hippocampi by way of the fimbriae fornicis.

**c. gris'ea,** (1) *adhesio* interthalamica; (2) see *substantia* intermedia centralis et lateralis.

**c. habenula'rum** [ NA ], commissure of the habenulae; habenular commissure; the connection between the right and left habenular nuclei; the decussation of fibers of the two striae medullares, forming the dorsal portion of the peduncle of the pineal body.

**c. hippocam'pi,** c. fornicis.

**c. labio'rum** [ NA ], commissure of the lips; the junction of the lips lateral to the angle of the mouth.

**c. labio'rum anterior** [ NA ], the junction of the labia majora anteriorly at the mons pubis.

**c. labio'rum posterior** [ NA ], a slight fold uniting the labia majora posteriorly in front of the anus.

**c. palpebra'rum latera'lis** [ NA ], lateral palpebral commissure; the union of the upper and lower eyelids adjacent to the lateral angle.

**c. palpebra'rum media'lis** [ NA ], medial palpebral commissure; the union of the upper and lower eyelids adjacent to the medial angle and lacus lacrimalis.

**c. poste'rior cer'ebri** [ NA ], posterior cerebral commissure; a thin band of white matter, crossing from side to side beneath the habenula of the pineal body and over the aditus ad aqueductum cerebri; it is largely composed of fibers interconnecting the left and right pretectal region and related cell groups of the midbrain.

**c. posterior gris'ea,** see *substantia* intermedia centralis et lateralis.

**commissurae supraop'ticae** [ NA ], supraoptic commissures; commissures of Ganser, Gudden, and Meynert; the commissural fibers that lie above and behind the optic chiasm.

**c. ventra'lis alba,** c. alba.

**commissu'ral.** Relating to a commissure.

**com'missure.** Commissura.

**anterior c.,** *commissura* anterior.

**anterior white c.,** *commissura* alba.

**c. of the cerebral hemispheres,** *corpus* callosum.

**c. of fornix,** *commissura* fornicis.

**Ganser's c.'s,** *commissurae* supraopticae.

**Gudden's c.'s,** *commissurae* supraopticae.

**c. of habenulae,** *commissura* habenularum.

**habenular c.,** *commissura* habenularum.

**hippocampal c.,** *commissura* fornicis.

**lateral palpebral c.,** *commissura* palpebrarum lateralis.

**c. of lips,** *commissura* labiorum.

**medial palpebral c.,** *commissura* palpebrarum medialis.

**Meynert's c.'s,** *commissurae* supraopticae.

**posterior cerebral c.,** *commissura* posterior cerebri.

**supraoptic c.'s,** *commissurae commissura* supraopticae.

**Wernekinck's c.,** the decussation of the brachia conjunctiva before their entrance into the red nucleus of the tegmentum.

**white c.,** *commissura* alba.

**commissurot'omy.** 1. The surgical division of any commissure, fibrous band, or ring. 2. Midline *myelotomy.*

**mitral c.,** sectioning of the fibrous ring surrounding the mitral orifice in the heart for the relief of mitral stenosis.

**commit'ment.** Certification for mental illness; involuntary mental hospitalization.

**commotio** (kŏ-mo'shyo) [ L. a moving, commotion, fr. *com-moveo*, pp. - *motus*, to set in motion, agitate ]. Concussion.

**c. cer'ebri,** brain *concussion.*

**c. ret'inae,** *concussion* of retina.

**c. spinalis,** concussion of the spinal cord.

**commun'icable.** Capable of being communicated or transmitted.

**commu'nicans,** pl. **communicantes** [ L. pres. p. of *communico*, pp. - *atus*, to share with someone, make common ]. Communicating; connecting or joining.

**commu'nica'tion** [ L. *communicatio* ]. In anatomy, a joining or connecting, *e.g.,* anastomosis.

**arteriovenous c.,** an abnormal opening, permitting blood to pass directly from an artery to a vein.

**nonverbal c.,** c. without words, *e.g.,* by pictures, symbols, facial expressions, gestures, posture.

**commu'nis** [ L. common ] [ NA ]. Common; relating to more than one.

**commu'nity.** A given segment of a society or a population.

**biotic c.,** the complex of all biological elements comprising a given biotype; see also ecosystem.

**therapeutic c.,** a specially structured mental hospital or community health center milieu that provides an effective environment for behavioral changes in patients through resocialization and rehabilitation.

**Comol'li,** Antonio, Italian pathologist, *1879. See C.'s *sign.*

**comp.** Abbreviation for L. *compositus, -a, -um,* compound.

**compacta** (kom-pak'tah). *Stratum* compactum.

**compar'ascope** [ L. *comparo,* to compare, + G. *skopeō,* to view ]. A microscope accessory by means of which an observer may directly compare simultaneously the findings in two microscopic preparations.

**compatibil'ity.** The condition of being compatible.

**compat'ible** [ L. *con-,* with, + *patior,* to suffer ]. 1. Capable of being mixed without undergoing destructive chemical change or exhibiting mutual antagonism; said of the elements in a properly constructed pharmaceutical mixture. 2. Relating to two samples of blood the serum of either of which does not agglutinate the red blood cells from the other; blood that causes no reaction when transfused; tissues or organs that are not rejected when transplanted from one person or animal to another 3. Denoting satisfactory relationships in marriage or in sexual activities.

**com'pensated.** Designating that compensation has occurred. See, for example, c. *acidosis.*

**compensa'tion** [ L. *com-penso,* pp. *-atus,* to weigh together, counterbalance ]. 1. Term used to describe a process in which a tendency for a change in a given direction is counteracted by another change so that the original change is not evident. 2. An unconscious mechanism by which the individual tries to make up for fancied or real deficiencies.

**compen'satory.** Providing compensation; making up for loss.

**com'petence.** 1. The quality of being competent or capable of performing an allotted function. 2. Integrity; especially the normal tight closure of a cardiac valve. 3. The ability of a group of embryonic cells to respond to an organizer. 4. The ability of a (bacterial) cell to take up free DNA, which may or may not be transforming DNA and lead to transformation. 5. Immunological c.; the capacity of a lymphocyte to respond to an antigen (immunogen) and exhibit specific immunological activity. 6. In psychiatry, the mental ability to distinguish right from wrong and to manage one's own affairs.

**cardiac c.,** ability of the ventricles to pump the blood returning to the atria, so that atrial pressure does not rise abnormally.

**immunological c.,** c. (5).

**competition** (kom'pe-tish'un). The process by which the activity or presence of one substance interferes with, or suppresses, the activity of another substance with similar affinities.

**antigenic c.,** c. that occurs when two different antigens, each of which can evoke an immunological response when inoculated alone, are mixed in equal quantities and inoculated together; the response may be to only one, that to the other being largely or entirely suppressed.

**complaint** (kom-plānt'). A malady, disease, or symptom, or the description of it.

**summer c.,** summer *diarrhea.*

**com'plement** [ L. *complementum,* that which completes, fr. *com-pleo,* to fill up ]. Ehrlich's term for the thermolabile substance, normally present in serum, that is destructive to certain bacteria and other cells which have been senstitized by specific complement-fixing antibody; it is a complex of not less than nine components which combine with the antigen-antibody complex in a definite sequence, and which are named C1 through C9. All nine components seem to be required for immune lysis; the first seven are involved in chemotaxis, but only the first four are involved in immune adherence or phagocytosis or are fixed by conglutinins. See also alexin, and component of c.

**c. chemotactic factor,** the activated complex of the fifth, sixth, and seventh components of complement (C567) which induces chemotaxis in the case of polymorphonuclear leukocytes.

**component of c.,** any one of the nine distinct protein units (designated C1 through C9 and distributed in the $\alpha$, $\beta$, and $\gamma$ electrophoretic partitions of normal serum) that effect the immunological activities long associated with complement (*q.v.*). C1 (a complex of three subunits, C1q, C1r, and C1s), after activation by erythrocyte-antibody complex (EA) or other sensitized antigen, is enzymic (as C1 esterase) for C4 and (owing to the reaction with C4) for C2. The C42 moiety (C3 convertase) of the EAC142 complex then cleaves C3, the active fragment of which enters the EAC1423 complex that cleaves C5. The complex EAC14235 then combines sequentially with C6, C7, C8, and C9 to form lytic complement. C1 may be activated, also, by aggregated antibody. C3 may also be activated by bacterial endotoxin seemingly in conjunction with "normal" IgM antibody with only minimal use of C1, C4, and C2; by the properdin system (*q.v.*, under properdin); and by a component of cobra venom in association with the normal serum cofactor, C3 proactivator (properdin factor B), and perhaps one other.

**c. fixation,** fixation of c. in a serum by an antigen-antibody combination whereby it is rendered unavailable to complete a reaction in a second antigen-antibody combination for which c. is necessary; the second system usually serves as an indicator (red blood cells plus specific hemolysin); if c. is fixed with the first antigen-antibody union, hemolysis does not occur, but, if c. is not so removed, it causes hemolysis in the second system; see also Bordet-Gengou *phenomenon,* and Wassermann *test.*

**complementa′tion.** Functional interaction between two defective viruses permitting replication under conditions inhibitory to the single virus.

**complex** (kom′pleks [ L. *complexus,* woven together. PLIC- ]. 1. An organized constellation of feelings, thoughts, perceptions, and memories which may be in part unconscious and may strongly influence associations and attitudes. 2. In chemistry, the relatively stable combination of two or more compounds into a larger molecule; *e.g.,* hemoglobin is a c. of globin and heme. 3. A composite of chemical or immunological structures. 4. A structural anatomical entity made up of three or more interrelated parts. 5. An informal term used to denote a group of individual structures known or believed to be anatomically, embryologically, or functionally related.

**aberrant c.,** an anomalous c., more specifically an abnormal ventricular c. caused by abnormal intraventricular conduction of a supraventricular impulse.

**amygdaloid c.,** *corpus* amygdaloideum.

**anom′alous c.,** a c. in the electrocardiogram differing significantly from the physiologic type in the same heart and lead.

**antigenic c.,** a composite of different antigenic structures, such as a cell or a bacterium, or, by extension, a molecule containing two or more determinant groups of different antigenic specificities.

**apical c.,** a structural c. found among sporozoans and piroplasms constituting the subphylum Sporozoa; components of this system, visible under the electron microscope, include a polar ring, conoid, micronemes, rhoptries, and subpellicular tubules.

**atrial c.,** auricular c.; P wave in the electrocardiogram.

**auricular c.,** atrial c.

**avian leukosis-sarcoma c.,** a term applied to avian sarcoma, myeloblastosis, erythroblastosis, leukosis, osteopetrosis, and lymphomatosis in the belief that these may all be different expressions of infection by the avian leukosis-sarcoma virus.

**brain wave c.,** a specific combination of fast and slow activity that recurs enough times to be identified as a discrete phenomenon.

**Cain c.,** brother c.; extreme envy or jealousy of a brother, leading to hatred.

**castration c.,** (1) a child's fear of injury to the genitals by the parent of the same sex as punishment for unconcious guilt over oedipal feelings; (2) unconscious fear of injury from those in authority.

**caudal pharyngeal c.,** the ultimobranchial body associated with the embryonic fourth and transitory fifth pharyngeal pouches.

**charge transfer c.,** a c. between two organic molecules in which an electron from one (the donor) is transferred to the other (the acceptor), becoming generally distributed throughout the latter. These c.'s are generally highly colored and may be so observed. Subsequent transfer of a hydrogen atom completes the reduction of the acceptor.

**Diana c.,** ideas leading to the adoption of masculine traits and behavior in a female.

**diphasic c.,** a c. consisting of both positive and negative deflections.

**Eisenmenger's c.,** Eisenmenger's tetralogy; Eisenmenger's disease; the combination of ventricular septal defect with pulmonary hypertension and consequent right-to-left shunt through the defect, with or without an associated overriding aorta.

**Electra c.,** father c.; female counterpart of the Oedipus c., *q.v.*

**electrocardiographic c.,** a deflection or group of deflections in the electrocardiogram.

**equiphasic c.,** isodiphasic c.

**feminin′ity c.,** in psychoanalysis, the unconscious fear, in boys and men, of castration at the hands of the mother with resultant identification with the aggressor and envious desire for breasts and vagina.

**Golgi c.,** Golgi *apparatus.*

**immune c.,** antigen combined with specific antibody, to which complement may also be fixed, and which may precipitate or remain in solution.

**inferiority c.,** a sense of inadequacy which is expressed in extreme shyness, diffidence, or timidity, or as a compensatory reaction in exhibitionism or aggressiveness.

**isodiphasic c.,** equiphasic c.; a diphasic c. whose positive and negative deflections are approximately equal.

**Jocasta c.,** a mother's libidinous fixation on a son.

**jumped process c.,** see dislocation of articular processes (vertebral, cervical), under dislocation.

**junctional c.,** the attachment zone between epithelial cells; typically, the complex consists of the zonula occludens, the zonula adherens, and the macula adherens (desmosome).

**juxtaglomerular c.,** juxtaglomerular *apparatus.*

**K c.,** slow waves in the electroencephalogram related to arousal from sleep by a sound.

**Lear c.,** a father's libidinous fixation on a daughter.

**Meyenburg's c.,** clusters of small bile ducts occurring in polycystic livers, separate from the portal areas.

**monophasic c.,** a c. in the electrocardiogram that is entirely negative or entirely positive.

**mother superior c.,** the tendency of a psychotherapist to play a mother's role to the detriment of the therapeutic process.

**Oedipus c.,** a developmentally distinct group of associated ideas, aims, instinctual drives, and fears generally observed in male children 3 to 6 years old; in female children, it is referred to as the Electra c. During this period, coinciding with the peak of the phallic phase of psychosexual development, the child's sexual interest is attached primarily to the parent of the opposite sex and is accompanied by aggressive feelings toward the parent of the same sex. The passing of the Oedipus c. is, in psychoanalytic theory, the dissolution of the Oedipus c. at about the age of 5 or 6 and its replacement by the castration c., *q.v.*

**persecution c.,** a feeling that others have evil designs against one's well-being.

**primary c.,** the typical lesions of primary pulmonary tuberculosis, consisting of a small peripheral focus of infection, with hilar or paratracheal lymph node involvement.

**QRS c.,** the principal deflection in the electrocardiogram, representing ventricular depolarization.

**spike and wave c.,** a c. of a slow wave and a fast one usually seen in the electroencephalogram in petit mal seizures.

**Steidele's c.,** congenital absence of the aortic arch.

**superiority c.,** term sometimes given to the compensatory behavior, *e.g.*, aggressiveness, self-assertion, associated with inferiority c.

**symptom c.,** (1) syndrome; (2) complex (1).

**ternary c.,** term used to describe the tripartite combination of, for example, enzyme-cofactor-substrate, the active form involved in many enzyme reactions.

**triple symptom c.,** Behçet's *syndrome.*

**ventricular c.,** the QRST wave in the electrocardiogram.

**complexion** (kom-plek'shun) [ L. *complexio,* a combination, (later) physical condition. PLIC- ]. The color, texture, and general condition of the skin of the face.

**complex'us** [ L. an embracing, encircling ]. Obsolete term for *musculus* semispinalis capitis.

**compliance** (kom-pli'ans). Abbreviated C; a measure of the ease with which a structure or substance may be deformed. In medicine and physiology, usually a measure of the ease with which a hollow viscus (*e.g.* lung, urinary bladder, gallbladder) may be distended; the volume change resulting from the application of a unit pressure differential between the inside and outside of the viscus. The reciprocal of elastance, *q.v.*

**dynamic c. of lung,** the value obtained when lung c. is estimated during breathing by dividing the tidal volume by the difference in instantaneous transpulmonary pressures at the ends of the respiratory excursions, when flow in the airway is momentarily zero. This value deviates markedly from static c. in patients in whom resistances and compliances are not uniform throughout the lung (*i.e.,* uneven time constants).

**specific c.,** (1) the c. of a structure divided by its initial volume; (2) more specifically for the lungs, the c. divided by the functional residual capacity.

**static c.,** the value obtained when c. is measured at true equilibrium, *i.e.,* in the absence of any motion.

**complicated** (kom'pli-ka-ted) [ L. *com-plico,* pp. *-atus,* to fold together ]. Made complex; denoting a disease upon which another disease or episode has been superimposed, altering symptoms and modifying its course for the worse.

**complica'tion.** A morbid process or event occurring during a disease which is not an essential part of the disease, although it may result from it or from independent causes.

**compo'nent** [ L. *com-pono,* pp. *-positus,* to place together ]. An element forming a part of the whole.

**anterior c. of force,** a force operating to move teeth anteriorly.

**c. of complement,** see under complement.

**c. of force,** (1) one of the factors from which a resultant force may be compounded or into which it may be resolved; (2) one of the vectors into which a force may be resolved.

**c.'s of mastication,** the various jaw movements that are made during the act of mastication, as determined by the neuromuscular system, the temporomandibular articulations, the teeth, and the food being chewed. The c.'s of mastication may be separated (for purposes of analysis or description) into opening, closing, left lateral, right lateral, and anteroposterior c.'s.

**c.'s of occlusion,** the various factors involved in occlusion, such as the temporamandibular joint, the associated neuromusculature, the teeth, and the denture-supporting structures.

**composition** (kom-po-zish'un) [ L. *compono,* to arrange ]. In chemistry, the kind and number of atoms constituting a molecule.

**modeling c.,** modeling *plastic.*

**compos mentis** [ L. possessed of one's mind; *compos,* having control, fr. *potis,* able ]. Of sound mind; sane.

**com'pound** [ thru O. Fr., fr. L. *compono* ]. 1. In chemistry, a substance formed by the covalent or electrostatic union of two or more elements, generally differing entirely in physical characteristics from any of its components. 2. In pharmacy, denoting a preparation containing several ingredients. For c.'s not listed here, see the specific chemical or pharmaceutical names.

**c. 20,** laudexium methyl sulfate.

**c. A, Kendall's,** 11-dehydrocortiscosterone.

**acy'clic c.,** open chain c.

**addition c.,** strictly, an association of two or more complete molecules in which each preserves its fundamental structure and no covalent bonds are made or broken (hydrates of salts, coordination c.'s, adducts); more loosely, association of acids with basic organic c.'s (as of amines with HCl); still more loosely, addition of two molecules without loss of any atom but forming new covalent bonds (*e.g.*, $CH_2 = CH_2 + Br_2 \rightarrow BrCH_2 - CH_2Br$).

**alicyclic c.'s,** c.'s with molecules containing saturated rings (*e.g.*, cyclohexane), and possessing properties more similar to those of acyclic compounds (*e.g.*, hexane) than to those of aromatic c.'s containing rings with conjugated double bonds (*e.g.*, benzene).

**aliphat'ic c.,** open chain c.

**aromat'ic c.,** a cyclic c. characterized by the prescence of conjugated double bonds within the ring; benzene and its derivatives are the most common examples.

**c. B, Kendall's,** corticosterone. (Kendall's desoxy compound B is 11-deoxycorticosterone; see deoxycorticosterone.)

**c. B, Wintersteiner's,** $3\beta,17,21$-trihydroxy-$5\alpha$-pregnane-11,20-dione ($5\alpha$-pregnane = allopregnane; see steroids for structure).

**bi'nary c.,** a c. whose molecules contain only two elements or two atoms of different kinds, such as HCl.

**carbocyclic c.,** a closed chain c. in which the atoms of the closed chain (or ring) are all carbon, *e.g.*, benzene, $(CH)_6$. See also cyclic c.

**closed chain c.,** cyclic c.

**condensation c.,** a complex c. resulting from the combination of two more simple substances, with the splitting off of some other substance, such as alcohol or water.

**conjugated c.,** one formed by the union of two c.'s (as by the elimination of water between an alcohol and an organic acid to form an ester) and easily converted to the original c.'s (hydrolysis).

**cyclic c.,** any c. in which the constituent atoms, or any part of them, form a ring; this is used mainly in organic chemistry where numerous c.'s contain rings of carbon atoms (isocyclic or carbocyclic) or carbon atoms plus one or more atoms of other types, usually nitrogen, oxygen, or sulfur (heterocyclic); where the ring is saturated or contains nonconjugated double bonds (alicyclic), the c. is similar in properties to the corresponding open chain c. (*e.g.*, cyclohexane resembles hexane); where the ring contains conjugated double bonds (aromatic, with benzene and pyridine the prime examples), it is more stable than the corresponding saturated ring and exhibits unusual chemical properties, characteristic of itself and not of other types of rings or of open chain c.'s.

**c. E, Kendall's,** cortisone.

**endothermic c.,** a c. that involves the absorption of heat when formed from its elements.

**exothermic c.,** a c. that involves the emission of heat when formed from its elements.

**c. F, Kendall's,** hydrocortisone.

**c. F, Wintersteiner's,** cortisone.

**fatty c.,** open chain c.

**heterocyclic c.,** a closed chain c. in which the ring contains atoms of more than one element. Applied to organic cyclic compounds in which the ring is made up of carbon atoms plus at least one other type of atom (*e.g.*, pyridine). See also cyclic c.

**high energy c.'s,** classically, a group of phosphoric acid esters whose hydrolysis takes place with a free energy change of $-5,000$ to $-11,000$ calories per mole (in contrast to $-1,000$ to $-4,000$ for simple phosphoric acid esters like glucose 6-phosphate or $\alpha$-glycerophosphates), thus being capable of driving energy-consuming reactions in living cells or reconstituted cell-free systems. Adenosine 5'-triphosphate, with respect to the $\beta$ and $\gamma$ phosphates, is the best known and is regarded as the immediate energy source for most metabolic syntheses. Others are acetyl phosphate, creatine phosphate, phosphoenolpyruvate. The general types are acid anhydrides, phosphoric esters of enols, phosphamic acid ($R-NH-PO_3H_2$) derivatives, acyl thioesters (*e.g.*, of coenzyme A), sulfonium c.'s ($R_3-S^+$) and aminoacyl esters of ribosyl moieties. See also high energy *phosphate.*

**homocyclic c.,** isocyclic c.

**impression c.,** modeling *plastic.*

**inclusion c.,** the mechanical trapping of small molecules within spaces between other molecules; *e.g.,* the inclusion of iodine molecules by starch molecules to form the well known red-to-black "addition c."

**inorganic c.,** a c. in which the atoms or radicals are held together by electrostatic forces rather than covalent bonds; capable of dissociation into ions in polar solvents (*e.g.,* $H_2O$); *cf.* organic c.

**isocyclic c.,** a closed chain c. in which the atoms are all of the same element (*e.g.,* benzene). See also cyclic c.

**Kendall's c.'s,** see c. A, B, E, and F.

**meso c.'s,** c.'s containing more than one asymmetric carbon atom, with configurations about them so balanced that the molecule as a whole possesses a plane of symmetry, although the individual carbon atoms do not; such compounds are not optically active; *e.g.,* ribitol, mucic acid, and meso-inositol.

**modeling c.,** modeling *plastic.*

**nonpolar c.,** one made up of molecules that possess a symmetrical distribution of charge so that no positive or negative poles exist; they are not ionizable in solution. Hydrocarbons are the most notable examples. See also organic c.

**onium c.'s,** (o'ne-um), a generic term for c.'s such as those of the ammonium, phosphonium, or sulfonium type, all being complex cations.

**open chain c.,** acyclic c.; aliphatic c.; fatty c.; an organic c. in which the chain does not form a ring.

**organic c.,** a c. composed of atoms held together by covalent (shared electron) bonds; not dissociable into ions by polar solvents; *cf.* inorganic c.

**polar c.,** one that ionizes in solution, or one in the molecule of which electric charge is not symmetrically distributed so that there is a separation of charge, *i.e.,* the formation of a definite positive and negative pole; water is the most familiar example of this latter case. See inorganic c.

**quaternary c.,** one that contains four different components.

**Reichstein's c.'s,** see *substance* Fa, G, H, M, Q, and S.

**ring c.,** cyclic c.

**saturated c.,** one in which all the atoms of the molecule are connected by single bonds.

**substitution c.,** one formed by the substitution of a new element or radical for one previously present (as in substitution of Cl for H in $CH_4$ to yield $CH_3Cl$ or $CCl_4$).

**ter'nary** or **ter'tiary c.,** one that contains three components.

**unsaturated c.,** organic c.'s containing double or triple bonds, thus capable of adding other atoms to become saturated without loss of any atom. See addition c.

**Wintersteiner's c.'s,** see c. B and F.

**com'press** [ L. *com-primo,* pp. *-pressus,* to press together ]. A pad of gauze or other material bandaged over a part where it is desired to make compression.

**graduated c.,** one made of layers of cloth in such a way that it is thickest in the center, becoming thinner toward the periphery.

**wet c.,** one moistened with saline or antiseptic solution.

**compression** (kom-presh'un). A squeezing together; the exertion of pressure on a body in such a way as to tend to increase its density; the decrease in a dimension of a body under the action of two external forces directed toward one another in the same straight line.

**cer'ebral c., c. of the brain,** pressure upon the intracranial tissues by an effusion of blood or cerebrospinal fluid, an abscess, a neoplasm, a depressed fracture of the skull, or an edema of the brain.

**c. of tissue,** tissue *displaceability.*

**compres'sor.** 1. A muscle contraction of which causes compression of any structure. 2. An instrument for making pressure on a part, especially on an artery to prevent loss of blood.

**c. venae dorsalis penis,** Houston's muscle; a part of the musculus ischiocavernosus which passes to the dorsum of the penis.

**compresso'rium.** Compressor (2).

**Compton,** Arthur H., U. S. physicist *1892. See C. *effect.*

**compto'nia.** Sweet fern; the leaves of *Comptonia asplenifolia* (family Myricaceae); used in colic and diarrhea and externally as a poultice.

**compulsion** (kom-pul'shun) [ L. *com-pello* pp. *-pulsus,* to drive together, compel ]. Uncontrollable thoughts or impulses to perform an act, often repetitively, as an unconscious mechanism to avoid unacceptable ideas and desires which, by themselves, arouse anxiety. The anxiety becomes fully manifest if performance of the compulsive act is prevented.

**compul'sive.** Influenced by compulsion.

**con-.** Prefix fr. L. preposition meaning with; appears as com- before p, b, or m, and as co- before a vowel.

**con'albu'min.** A glycoprotein containing mannose and galactose, constituting about 14 per cent of egg white.

**cona'men** [ L. *conamen,* an attempt ]. A suicidal attempt.

**conanine.** A steroid alkaloid; pregnane with a methylimino group bridging C-18 and C-20 (in α-configuration). For pregnane structure, see steroids.

**con'arach'in.** A protein in peanuts.

**conarium** (ko-na'rĭ-um) [ G. *kōnarion* (dim. of *kōnos,* cone), the pineal body ]. *Corpus* pineale.

**cona'tion** [ L. *conātio,* an undertaking, effort ]. The conscious tendency to act; willing active effort; in human context usually an aspect of mental process; historically aligned with cognition and affection, more recently used in the wider sense of impulse, desire, purposive striving.

**con'ative.** Pertaining to conation, *i.e.,* the act of striving or making an effort: by natural active force in plants or animals; in analogous human effort usually conscious and willed.

**conatus** (ko-nah'tus, ko-na'tus) [ L. attempt ]. Striving toward self-preservation and self-affirmation.

**concamera'tion** [ L. *concameratio,* a vault; fr. *concamero,* pp. *-atus,* to vault over, fr. *camera,* a vault ]. A system of interconnecting cavities.

**con'canav'alin.** Either of two crystalline globulins, occurring with canavalin in the jack bean, that will agglutinate the blood of mammals and that react with polyglucosans.

**concat'enate** [ L. *con-cateno,* pp. *-atus,* to link together, fr. *catena,* a chain ]. Denoting the arrangement of a number of structures, enlarged lymph glands for example, in a row like the links of a chain.

**Concato,** Luigi M., Italian physician, 1825–1882. See C.'s *disease.*

**concave** (kon'kāv) [ L. *concavus,* arched or vaulted ]. Having a depressed or hollowed surface.

**concav'ity.** A hollow or depression, with more or less evenly curved sides, on any surface.

**conca'vocon'cave.** Concave on two opposing surfaces.

**conca'vocon'vex.** Concave on one surface and convex on the opposite surface.

**concentration** (kon'sen-tra'shun) [ L. *con-,* together, + *centrum,* center ]. 1. A preparation made by extracting a crude drug, precipitating from the solution, and drying; resinoid. 2. Increasing the strength of a fluid by evaporation. 3. The quantity of a substance per unit volume or weight. In renal physiology, symbol U for urinary c., P for plasma c.; in respiratory physiology, symbol C for amount per unit volume in blood, F for fractional c. (mole fraction or volume per volume) in dried gas. Subscripts indicate location and chemical species.

**minimal alveolar (anesthetic) c.,** abbreviated MAC; the end-alveolar c. of an inhalation anesthetic which prevents somatic response to a painful stimulus in 50 per cent of individuals treated; proposed as an index of relative potency of inhalation anesthetics.

**molar c.,** see molar (4).

**normal c.,** see normal (3).

**urea c.,** see Ambard's *coefficient* and Ambard's *law.*

**concentric** (kon-sen'trik). Having a common center, such that more spheres, circles, or segments of circles are within one another.

**concept** [ L. *conceptum,* something understood, pp. ntr. of *concipio,* to receive, apprehend, fr. *con-,* together, + *capio,* to take. CAP-2 ]. 1. An abstract idea or notion. 2. An explanatory variable or principle in a scientific system.

**no-threshold c.,** that the biologic effect of radiation is proportional to dose, even for minutely small doses.

**conception** [ L. *conceptio;* see concept ]. 1. Concept. 2. The act of forming a general idea or notion. 3. Implantation of the blastocyst; see implantation.

**colony c.,** an aggregation of individually distinct organs possessing specific functions.

**imper'ative c.,** a concept that does not arise from association but appears spontaneously and refuses to be banished; obsession.

**concept'ual.** Relating to the formation of ideas, to mental conceptions.

**concep'tus.** The products of conception, *i.e.,* embryo and membranes.

**concha,** pl. **con'chae** (kon'kah) [ L. a shell ] [ NA ]. In anatomy, a structure comparable to a shell in shape, as the auricle or pinna of the ear or a turbinated bone in the nose.

**c. auric'ulae** [ NA ], the large hollow, or floor of the auricle, between the anterior portion of the helix and the antihelix; it is divided by the crus of the helix into the cymba above and the cavum below.

**Morgagni's c.,** c. nasalis superior.

**c. nasa'lis inferior** [ NA ], inferior turbinated bone; a thin spongy bony plate with curved margins, on the lateral wall of the lower part of the nasal fossa, separating the middle from the inferior meatus; it articulates with the ethmoid, lacrimal, maxilla, and palate bones.

**c. nasa'lis me'dia** [ NA ], middle turbinated bone; the lower and larger of two bony plates with up-curved margins, projecting from the inner wall of the ethmoidal labyrinth; it separates the superior from the middle meatus of the nose.

**c. nasa'lis superior** [ NA ], superior turbinated bone; Morgagni's c. the upper of the bony plates with up-curved margins, projecting from the inner wall of the ethmoidal labyrinth; it forms the upper boundary of the superior meatus of the nose.

**c. nasa'lis suprema** [ NA ], supreme or highest or fourth turbinated bone; c. santorini; a small c. frequently present on the posterosuperior part of the lateral nasal wall. It overlies the supreme nasal meatus.

**Santorini's c.,** c. nasalis suprema.

**c. sphenoida'lis** [ NA ], sphenoidal c.; Bertin's bones; sphenoidal turbinals; sphenoidal turbinated bones; paired ossicles of pyramidal shape, the spines of which are in contact with the medial pterygoid lamina, the bases forming the roof of the nasal cavity.

**conchitis** (kon-ki'tis). Inflammation of any concha.

**conchoidal** (kon-koy'dal). Shaped like a shell; having alternate convexities and concavities on the surface.

**conchoscope** (kon'ko-skōp) [ concha + G. *skopeō,* to view ]. A form of nasal speculum.

**con'clina'tion.** Intorsion.

**con'crement** [ L. *con-cresco,* to grow together. CRES- ]. A concretion; a deposit of calcareous material in a part.

**concres'cence** [ see concrement ]. 1. Coalescence; the growing together of originally separate parts. 2. In dentistry, the union of the roots of a tooth, or of two adjacent teeth, by an outgrowth of cementum.

**concre'tio** [ L. ]. Concretion.

**c. cor'dis,** internal adhesive pericarditis; synechia pericardii; extensive adhesion between parietal and visceral layers of the pericardium with partial or complete obliteration of the pericardial cavity.

**concre'tion** [ L. *cum,* together, + *crescere,* to grow ]. The aggregation or formation of solid material.

**alvine c.,** fecalith; coprolith.

**prostatic c.,** *corpus* amylaceum.

**concus'sion** [ L. *concussio,* fr. *con-cutio,* pp. *-cussus,* to shake violently, fr. *con-* (intens.) + *quatio,* to shake ]. 1. A violent shaking or jarring. 2. An injury of a soft structure, as the brain, resulting from a blow or violent shaking; commotio.

**brain c.,** commotio cerebri; a clinical syndrome, due to mechanical forces, characterized by immediate and transient impairment of neural function, such as alteration of consciousness, disturbance of vision and equilibrium, etc.

**c. of the retina,** an edematous condition of the macular area, due to trauma terminating in some degree of macular degeneration; also called commotio retinae, concussion edema, Berlin's edema.

**spinal c.,** a sudden, transient loss of function of the spinal cord, caused by injury but without permanent gross damage.

**concus'sor.** A hammer-like instrument for tapping the parts as a form of massage.

**condensa'tion** [ L. *con-denso,* pp. *-atus,* to make thick, condense, fr. *densus,* thick ]. 1. Compression; making more solid or dense. 2. The change of a gas to a liquid, or of a liquid to a solid. 3. In psychoanalysis, an unconscious mental process in which one symbol stands for a number of others. 4. In dentistry, the process of packing a filling material, particularly amalgam, into a cavity, using such force and direction that excess mercury is expressed from the filling mass and no voids result.

**condense.** To pack; to increase the density of; applied particularly to insertion of gold foil or silver amalgam in a cavity prepared in a tooth.

**condenser.** 1. An apparatus for cooling a gas to a liquid, or a liquid to a solid. 2. In dentistry, a manual or powered instrument used for packing a plastic or unset material into a cavity of a tooth. Variation in sizes and shapes allows conformation of the mass to the cavity outline. 3. Microscopic c.; see Abbé's c. and dark-field c. 4. Capacitor.

**Abbé's c.,** a system of two or three wide angle, achromatic, convex and planoconvex lenses that may be moved upward or downward beneath the stage of a microscope, thereby regulating the concentration of light (directly from a bulb or reflected from a mirror) that passes through the material to be examined on the stage.

**cardioid c.,** a type of dark-field c.

**dark-field c.,** an apparatus for throwing reflected light through the microscope field, so that only the object to be examined is illuminated, the field itself being dark.

**paraboloid c.,** a type of dark-field c.

**condition.** 1. To train. 2. A certain response that is elicited by a specifiable stimulus or emitted in the presence of certain stimuli with reward of the response during prior occurrence. 3. Referring to several classes of learning in the behavioristic branch of psychology.

**conditioning.** The process of acquiring, developing, educating, establishing, learning, or training new responses in animal or man. The term is used to describe both respondent and operant behavior. In both usages it refers to a change in the frequency or form of behavior as a result of the influence of the environment.

**avoidance c.,** the technique whereby an organism learns to avoid unpleasant or punishing stimuli by learning the appropriate anticipatory response to protect it from further such stimuli; *cf.* escape c.

**classical c.,** stimulus substitution; a form of learning, as in Pavlov's experiments, in which a previously neutral stimulus becomes a conditioned stimulus when presented together with an unconditioned stimulus; called stimulus substitution because the new stimulus evokes the response in question; see also respondent c.

**escape c.,** the technique whereby an organism learns to terminate unpleasant or punishing stimuli by making the appropriate new response which ceases the delivery of such stimuli.

**higher order c.,** the use of a previously conditioned stimulus to condition further responses, in much the same way unconditioned stimuli are used.

**instrumental c.,** that in which the response is a prerequisite to achieving some goal; often used as a synonym for operant c., but some psychologists make distinctions in the usages of these two terms.

**operant c.,** Skinnerian c.; a type of c. developed by Skinner in which an experimenter waits for the response to be conditioned to occur spontaneously, immediately after which the organism is given a reinforcer (reward). After this procedure is repeated many times, the frequency of target response emission will have significantly increased over its pre-experiment base rate.

**Pavlovian c.,** respondent c.

**respondent c.,** Pavlovian c.; a type of c., first studied by I. P. Pavlov, in which a neutral stimulus (bell sound) elicits a response (salivation) as a result of pairing it (associating it contiguously in time) a number of times with an unconditioned or natural stimulus for that response (food shown to a hungry dog).

**second-order c.,** the use of a previously successfully used stimulus as the unconditioned stimulus for further c.

**Skinnerian c.,** operant c.

**trace c.,** c. when there is no temporal overlap between c. stimulus and the unconditioned stimulus.

**condom.** A sheath or cover for the penis, for use in the prevention of conception or of infection during coitus.

**conduc'tance.** 1. A measure of conductivity; the ratio of the current flowing through a conductor to the difference in potential between the ends of the conductor; the c. of a circuit is the reciprocal of its resistance. 2. The ease with which a fluid or gas enters and flows through a conduit, air passage, or respiratory tract.

**conduction** [ L. *con-duco,* pp. *ductus,* to lead, conduct. DUC- ]. 1. The act of transmitting or conveying certain forms of energy, such as heat, sound, or electricity from one point to another, without evident movement in the conducting body. 2. The transmission of stimuli of various sorts by living protoplasm.

**aberrant ventricular c.,** ventricular aberration; abnormal intraventricular c. of a supraventricular beat, especially where surrounding beats are normally conducted;

**accelerated c.,** the defect in the Wolff-Parkinson-White and Lown-Ganong-Levine syndromes, according to one theory, whereby the impulse travels abnormally rapidly from atrium to ventricle, gaining early access to the ventricular myocardium.

**air c.,** in relation to hearing, the transmission of sound to the inner ear through the external auditory canal and the structures of the middle ear.

**anterograde c.,** forward c. from sinus node to ventricular myocardium.

**antidromic c.,** see antidromic.

**atrial c.,** intra-atrial c.

**atrioventricular c.,** A-V c.; forward c. of the cardiac impulse from atria to ventricles via the A-V node, represented in the electrocardiogram by the P-R interval.

**avalanche c.,** the discharge of an impulse from a neuron into a large number of neurons of the same physiologic system thus producing the liberation of a very large amount of nervous energy by a given stimulus.

**bone c.,** osteophony; in relation to hearing, the transmission of sound to the inner ear through vibrations applied to the bones of the skull.

**concealed c.,** c. of an impulse through a part of the heart without direct evidence of its presence in the electrocardiogram; c. is inferred only because of its influence on the subsequent cardiac cycle.

**decremental c.,** impaired c. in a portion of a fiber because of progressively lessening response of the unexcited portion of the fiber to the action potential coming toward it; it is manifested by decreasing speed of c., amplitude of action potential, and extent of spread of the impulse.

**delayed c.,** first degree atrioventricular (A-V) heart block; see under block.

**forward c.,** anterograde c.

**intra-atrial c.,** atrial c.; c. of the cardiac impulse through the atrial myocardium, represented by the P wave in the electrocardiogram.

**intraventricular c.,** ventricular c.; c. of the cardiac impulse through the ventricular myocardium, represented by the QRS complex in the electrocardiogram.

**nerve c.,** the transmission of an impulse along a nerve fiber.

**orthodromic c.,** see orthodromic.

**Purkinje c.,** c. of the cardiac impulse through the Purkinje system.

**retrograde c.,** retroconduction; ventriculoatrial c.; conduction backward from ventricles or from A-V node into and through the atria.

**saltatory c.,** the conduction in which the nerve impulse 'jumps' from one node of Ranvier to the next.

**synaptic c.,** the c. of a nerve impulse across a synapse.

**ventricular c.,** intraventricular c.

**ventriculoatrial c.,** V-A c.; retrograde c.

**conductiv'ity.** 1. The power of transmission or conveyance of certain forms of motion, as heat, sound, and electricity, without perceptible motion in the conducting

body. 2. The property, inherent in living protoplasm, of transmitting a state of excitation, *e.g.,* in muscle or nerve.

**conductor** 1. A probe or sound with a groove through which a knife is passed in slitting open a sinus or fistula; a grooved director. 2. Any substance possessing conductivity.

**conduit.** A channel.

**ileal c.,** use of a segment of ileum to serve as a replacement for another tubular organ, *i.e.,* used to form an artificial bladder into which ureters can be implanted following total cystectomy; proximal end of ileal segment is closed, while the distal opening is brought to skin level as a stoma; urine is collected in an ileostomy bag.

**condu'plicate** [ L. *con-,* with, + *duplico,* pp. *-atus.* PLIC- ]. Folded upon itself lengthwise.

**conduplicato corpore.** *Uterus* didelphys.

**conduran'go** [ Peruv. ]. The bark of *Gonolobus condurango, Marsdenia condurango* (family Asclepiadaceae), a shrub of Ecuador and Peru. Aromatic bitter and astringent.

**con'dylar.** Relating to a condyle.

**con'dylarthro'sis** [ G. *kondylos,* condyle, + *arthrōsis,* a jointing ]. A joint, like that of the knee, formed by condylar surfaces.

**condyle** (kon'dil). Condylus.

**c. of humerus,** *condylus* humeri.

**lateral c.,** *condylus* lateralis.

**lateral c. of femur,** *condylus* lateralis femoris.

**lateral c. of tibia,** *condylus* lateralis tibiae.

**mandibular c.,** *processus* condylaris.

**medial c.,** *condylus* medialis.

**medial c. of femur,** *condylus* medialis femoris.

**medial c. of tibia,** *condylus* medialis tibiae.

**condylec'tomy** [ G. *kondylos,* condyle, + *ektomē,* excision ]. The cutting away of a condyle.

**condyl'ion** [ G. *kondylion,* dim. of *kondylos,* condyle ]. A point on the outer (lateral) or inner (medial) surface of the condyle of the mandible.

**con'dyloid** [ G. *kondylōdēs,* like a knuckle, fr. *kondylos,* condyle, + *eidos,* resemblance ]. Relating to or resembling a condyle.

**condylo'ma** [ G. *kondylōma,* a knob ]. Verruca mollusciformis; a wartlike excrescence at the anus or vulva, or on the glans penis.

**c. acumina'tum,** a projecting warty growth on the external genitals or at the anus, consisting of fibrous overgrowths covered by thickened epithelium, possibly due to viral infection. It is almost always benign, although malignant change has been reported. Also called pointed c.; papilloma acuminatum; papilloma venereum; verruca acuminata; cauliflower excrescence; and fig, moist, pointed, or venereal wart.

**flat c.,** c. latum.

**giant c.,** Buschke-Löwenstein tumor; a large type of c. acuminatum found in the preputial sac of the penis of middle-aged, uncircumcized men; it tends to extend deeply and recur.

**c. la'tum,** flat c.; a secondary syphilitic eruption of flat-topped papules, occurring in groups covered by a necrotic layer of epithelial detritus, and secreting a seropurulent fluid; they are found at the anus and wherever contiguous folds of skin produce heat and moisture.

**pointed c.,** c. acuminatum.

**c. subcuta'neum,** *molluscum* contagiosum.

**condylo'matous.** Relating to a condyloma.

**condylot'omy** [ G. *kondylos,* condyle, + *tomē,* incision ]. Division through, without removal of, a condyle.

**con'dylus** [ L. fr. G. *kondylos,* knuckle, the knuckle of any joint ] [ NA ]. Condyle; a rounded articular surface at the extremity of a bone.

**c. humeri** [ NA ], condyle of the humerus; the distal end of the humerus, including the trochlea, capitulum and the fossae olecranae, coronoidea and radialis.

**c. latera'lis** [ NA ], lateral condyle; (1) **c. l. femoris,** lateral condyle of the femur; (2) **c. l. tibiae,** lateral condyle of the tibia.

**c. media'lis** [ NA ], medial condyle; (1) **c. m. femoris,** medial condyle of the femur; (2) **c. m. tibiae,** medial condyle of the tibia.

**c. occipita'lis** [ NA ], occipital condyle; one of two elongated oval facets on the under surface of the occipital bone, one on each side of the foramen magnum, which articulate with the atlas.

**-cone.** Suffix denoting the cusp of a tooth in the upper jaw, e.g., paracone.

**cone** [ G. *kōnos*, cone ]. 1. A figure having a circular base with sides inclined so as to meet at a point above; see conus. 2. One of the visual receptors in the retina; see retinal c.'s. 3. *Corpus* pineale.

**antipodal c.,** the set of astral rays of a dividing cell extending from the centriole in a direction opposite to the equatorial plate.

**arterial c.,** *conus* arteriosus.

**ether c.,** apparatus employed in the administration of ether by the open-drop technique.

**fertilization c.,** a protuberance of the cytoplasm of the ovum at the point where the effective spermatozoon is attached.

**Haller's c.'s,** *lobuli* epididymidis.

**implantation c.,** axon *hillock.*

**keratosic c.'s,** horny pointed or rounded elevations on the hands and feet, occasionally observed in cases of gonorrheal rheumatism.

**c. of light,** Politzer's luminous c.; light reflex; Woelde's triangle; Wilde's triangle; a bright area seen on inspection of the tympanic membrane; it is triangular in shape, extending downward from the umbo.

**med'ullary c.,** *conus* medullaris

**ocular c.,** the c. of light in the interior of the eyeball formed by the rays entering through the pupil and focused on the retina.

**Politzer's luminous c.,** c. of light.

**pulmonary c.,** *conus* arteriosus.

**retinal c.'s,** the photosensitive, outward-directed, cone-shaped process of a cone cell, one of the two types of photoreceptor cell of the retina (the other being the rod cell). Cones are essential for sharp vision and for color vision. The only type of photoreceptor present in the macula lutea of the retina's fovea centralis, they become interspersed with increasing numbers of rods toward the periphery of the retina. See fig. under retina.

**theca interna c.,** the conical thickening of thecal cells with its apex pointed toward the ovarian surface.

**twin c.,** two retinal c.'s fused together.

**vascular c.'s,** lobuli epididymidis; see under lobulus.

**conenine.** Con-5-enine; conanine with a 5-6 double bond.

**cones'si** [ E. Ind. ]. Kurchi bark; the bark of *Holarrhena antidysenterica* (family Apocynaceae), an Indian tree; used as an astringent and in the treatment of dysentery and amebiasis.

**con'essine.** Wrightine; neriine; 3β-(dimethylamino)-con-5-enine; 3β-dimethylamino-18α:20α-methylimino-5-pregnene (for structure of pregnene, see steroids); an alcohol derived from *Holarrhena antidysenterica* (conessi, kurchi bark); a yellow astringent, used in the treatment of amebic dysentery and vaginal trichomoniasis.

**conex'us,** pl. **conex'us** [ L. ] [ NA ]. Connexus; a connecting structure.

**c. intertendin'eus** [ NA ], intertendinous connections; juncturae tendinum; fibrous bands passing obliquely between the diverging tendons of the extensor digitorum on the dorsum of the hand.

**confabula'tion** [ L. *con-fabular,* pp. *-fabulatus,* to talk together, fr. *fabula,* narrative ]. The making up of tales and recitals and a readiness to give a fluent answer, with no regard whatever to facts, to any question put; a symptom of presbyophrenia.

**confectio,** gen. **confectio'nis,** pl. **confectio'nes** (kon-fek'shyo) [ L. fr. *conficio,* pp. *-fectus,* to make ready, prepare. FAC- ]. Confection.

**confection** [ L. *confectio, q.v.* ]. Confectio; conserve; electuary; a pharmaceutical preparation consisting of a drug mixed with honey or syrup; a soft solid, sometimes used as an excipient for pill masses.

**confer'tus** [ L. *confercio,* pp. *-fertus,* to cram together, fr. *farcio,* to fill full, cram ]. Arranged closely together; confluent; coalescing.

**configura'tion.** 1. The general form of the body and its parts. 2. In chemistry, the spatial arrangement of atoms in a molecule. The c. of a compound (e.g., a sugar) is the unique spatial arrangement of its atoms such that no other arrangement of these atoms is superimposable thereon with complete correspondence, regardless of changes in conformation (i.e., twisting or rotation about single bonds). Change of c. requires breaking and rejoining of bonds, as in going from D to L c.'s of sugars (see also conformation). 3. See gestalt.

**confinement** [ L. *confine* (ntr.), a boundary, confine, fr. *con-* + *finis,* boundary ]. Lying-in; giving birth to a child.

**conflict.** The tension or stress experienced by an organism when satisfaction of a need, drive, or motive is thwarted by the presence of other attractive or unattractive needs, drives, or motives.

**approach-approach c.,** a situation of indecision and vacillation in which an individual is confronted with two equally attractive alternatives.

**approach-avoidance c.,** a situation of indecision and vacillation in which the individual is confronted with a single object or event which has both attractive and unattractive qualities.

**avoidance-avoidance c.,** a situation of indecision and vacillation in which the individual is confronted with two equally unattractive alternatives.

**role c.,** the need of an individual to play two different parts that cannot be harmonized; see also *role-playing.*

**con'fluence** [ L. *confluens* ]. A flowing together; a joining of two or more streams.

**c. of the sinuses,** *confluens* sinuum.

**conflu'ens** [ L. ] [ NA ]. Confluence.

**c. sinuum** [ NA ], confluence of the sinuses; torcular herophili; a meeting place, at the internal occipital protuberance, of the superior sagittal, straight, occipital, and two transverse sinuses of the dura mater.

**con'fluent** [ L. *con-fluo,* to flow together ]. 1. Joining; running together; denoting certain skin lesions which become merged, forming a patch; denoting a disease characterized by lesions which are not discrete, or distinct one from the other. 2. Denoting a bone formed by the blending together of two originally distinct bones.

**conformation.** Arrangement of a molecule in space achieved by rotation of groups about single, covalent bonds, without breaking any covalent bonds. The latter restriction differentiates conformation from configuration (as in anomers and related stereoisomers) where a bond or bonds must be broken in going from one form (configuration) to another. Conformation is one of the most important aspects of sugar chemistry and is basic to an understanding of the chemical properties of sugars (see Haworth formulas, under sugars).

**envelope c.,** see Haworth conformational formulas, under sugars.

**conformer** [ L. *conformo,* to fashion ]. A mold, usually of plastic material, cartilage, or bone. Used in plastic surgical repair; to maintain space in a cavity; to prevent closing by healing of an artificial or natural opening affected by neighboring surgical repair.

**confrontation** (kon-fron-ta'shun). The act of informing a person what one's position is in relationship to him, what one is experiencing, and how one perceives him.

**confusion.** A mental state in which reactions to environmental stimuli are inappropriate; a state in which the person is bewildered or perplexed or unable to orientate himself, occurring often in amentia.

**confusional.** Characterized by or pertaining to confusion.

**cong.** Abbreviation for congius, a gallon.

**congela'tion** [ L. *con-gelo,* pp. *-atus,* to freeze ]. 1. Freezing. 2. Frostbite.

**congener** (kon'je-ner) [ L. *con-,* with, + *genus,* race ]. 1. One of two or more things of the same kind, as of animal or plant with respect to classification. 2. One of two or more muscles with the same function.

**congen'erous** [ see congener ]. 1. Having the same function; denoting certain muscles that are synergistic. 2. Derived from the same source, or of a similar nature.

**congen'ital** [ L. *congenitus,* born with, fr. *con-,* with, + *gigno,* pp. *genitus,* to beget. GEN- ]. Existing at birth, referring to certain mental or physical traits or pecularities, malformations, diseases, etc.; may be either hereditary or due to some influence occurring during gestation, even up to the moment of birth.

**congen'itus** [ L. ] [ NA ]. Congenital.

**congested.** Containing an abnormal amount of blood; in a state of congestion.

**congestin** (kon-jes'tin). Actinocongestin.

**congestion** [ L. *congestio*, a bringing together, a heap, fr. *con-gero*, pp. *-gestus*, to bring together. GEST- ]. The presence of an abnormal amount of blood in the vessels of a part, due either to increased afflux or to an obstruction to the return flow. See also hyperemia.

    **active c.,** an increased flow of arterial blood to a part.

    **brain c.,** encephalemia; increased volume of the intravascular compartment; usually results in brain *swelling, q. v.*

    **functional c.,** physiologic c.; hyperemia occurring during functional activity of an organ.

    **hypostatic c.,** hypostasis; c. due to pooling of venous blood in a dependent part.

    **passive c.,** c. due to partial stagnation of blood in the capillaries and venules in consequence of obstruction or slowing of the venous drainage.

    **physiologic c.,** functional c.

    **venous c.,** overfilling and distention of the veins with blood as a result of mechanical obstruction or right ventricular failure.

**congestive.** Relating to congestion.

**congius,** pl. **con'gii** [ L. ]. A gallon.

**conglo'bate** [ L. *con-globo*, pp. *-atus*, to gather into a *globus*, ball ]. Formed in a single, rounded mass.

**congloba'tion.** An aggregation of numerous particles into one rounded mass.

**conglom'erate** [ L. *con-glomero*, pp. *-atus*, to roll together, fr. *glomus*, a ball. GLO- ]. Composed of several parts aggregated into one mass.

**conglu'tin.** A protein, contained in almonds and various seeds, resembling casein.

**conglu'tinant** [ L. *con-glutino*, pp. *-atus*, to glue together, fr. *gluten*, glue ]. Adhesive; promoting the union of the lips of a wound.

**conglutina'tion.** 1. Adhesion; coalescence. 2. Agglutination of antigen(erythrocyte)-antibody-complement complex by normal bovine serum (and certain other colloidal materials). The procedure provides a means of detecting the presence of nonagglutinating antibody.

**conglu'tinin.** Bovine serum protein that when absorbed by erythrocyte-antibody-complement complexes, causes them to agglutinate. It is comparatively thermostable; it apparently dissociates when diluted with physiologic saline solution. Certain colloids, *e.g.*, acacia, gelatin, and dextran, may be substituted for c.

**Congo red** (NF). An acid dye, sodium diphenyl-diazo-bis-α-naphthylaminesulfonate; used as an indicator (pH 3.0, blue-violet, to pH 5.0, red) in testing for free hydrochloric acid in gastric contents; the dye is frequently absorbed by amyloid, and special preparations may be administered intravenously as a laboratory aid in the diagnosis of secondary amyloidosis.

**conhy'drine.** Oxyconine; 2-(α-hydroxypropyl)piperidine; α-ethyl-2-piperidinemethanol; an alkaloid obtained from conium.

**coni.** Plural of conus.

**con'ic, con'ical.** Resembling a cone.

**-conid.** Suffix denoting the cusp of a tooth in the lower jaw, *e.g.*, paraconid.

**conid'ia.** Plural of conidium.

**conid'ial.** Relating to a conidium.

**conidiophore** (kon-id'ĭ-o-fōr) [ conidium + G. *phoros*, bearing ]. The mycelial stalk of a fungus which bears conidia.

**Conidiosporales** (ko-nid'ĭ-o-spo-ra lēs) An order of fungi which includes the genera *Acladium, Glenospora,* and *Trichothecium.*

**conidiospore** (kon-id'i-o-spōr) [ conidium + G. *sporos,* seed ]. Conidium.

**conid'ium,** pl. **conid'ia** [ Mod. L. dim. fr. G. *konis,* dust ]. Conidiospore; a nonsexual unenclosed or walled spore, or exospore, of certain fungi, produced asexually.

**conif'erin.** Abietin; laricin; 4-hydroxy-3-methoxy-1-(γ-hydroxypropenyl)benzene-4-D-glucoside; the principal glucoside of the conifers.

**coniine** (ko'ne-ēn). Cicutine; conicine; conine; 2-propyl-piperidine; the active alkaloid of conium; the hydrobromide and hydrochloride salts have been used as an antispasmodic.

**co'niofibro'sis** [ G. *konis,* dust, + fibrosis ]. Fibrosis produced by dust.

**coniol'ogy** [ G. *konis,* dust, + *-logia* ]. The science that treats of dust and of its effects.

**co'niolymph'stasis.** Stasis of lymph caused by dust, presumably through the intervention of fibrosis.

**coniom'eter** [ G. *konis,* dust, + *metron,* measure ]. A device for estimating the amount of dust in the air.

**co'niophage.** Dust *cell.*

**conio'sis** [ G. *konis,* dust ]. Any disease or morbid condition caused by dust.

**co'niot'omy.** Cricothyrotomy.

**coni'um** [ L. fr. G. *kōneion,* hemlock ]. Conii fructus; the dried unripe fruit of *Conium maculatum* (family Umbelliferae); poison hemlock; spotted cowbane poison; spotted parsley. Has been used as a sedative, antispasmodic, and anodyne.

**coniza'tion.** Excision of a cone of tissue, *e.g.,* mucosa of the cervix.

    **cold c.,** obtaining a cone of endocervical tissue with a cold knife blade so as to preserve histological characteristics and avoid charring.

**con'jugant** [ L. *con-jugo,* to join ]. A member of a mating pair of organisms or gametes undergoing conjugation, *q. v.*

**con'jugase.** Glutamate γ-carboxypeptidase.

    **vitamin B$_c$ c.,** see under vitamin.

**conjuga'ta** [ L. fem. of *conjugatus,* pp. of *con-jugo,* to join together ] [ NA ]. Conjugate, or anteroposterior, diameter of the pelvic inlet; conjugate axis; internal conjugate; true conjugate; diameter medianus; the distance from the promontory of the sacrum to the upper edge of the pubic symphysis.

    **c. diagonal'is,** diagonal *conjugate.*

**con'jugate** [ L. *conjugatus,* joined together. See conjugata ]. 1. Conjugated; joined or paired. 2. Conjugating.

    **diag'onal c.,** false c. (1); conjugata diagonalis; the anteroposterior dimension of the inlet that measures the clinical distance from the promontory of the sacrum to the lower margin of the symphysis pubis.

    **effective c.,** false c. (2); the internal c. measured from the nearest lumbar vertebra to the symphysis, in spondylolisthesis.

    **external c.,** Baudelocque's diameter; the distance in a straight line between the depression under the last spinous process of the lumbar vertebrae and the upper edge of the symphysis pubis.

    **false c.,** (1) diagonal c.; (2) effective c.

    **folic acid c.,** see under folic acid.

    **c. of the inlet,** conjugata.

    **internal c.,** conjugata.

    **obstetric c.,** the diameter that represents the shortest diameter through which the head must pass in descending into the superior strait and measures, by means of x-ray, the distance from the promontory of the sacrum to a point on the inner surface of the symphysis a few millimeters below its upper margin.

    **obstetric c. of the outlet,** the c. of the outlet lengthened by the backward displacement of the coccyx.

    **c. of the outlet,** the distance from the tip of the coccyx to the lower edge of the symphysis pubis; see obstetric c. of the outlet.

    **true c.,** conjugata.

**conjuga'tio** [ L. ] [ NA ]. A combining, mixing, or connection.

**conjuga'tion** [ L. *con-jugo,* pp. *-jugatus,* to join together. JUG- ]. 1. The union of two unicellular organisms or of the male and female gametes of multicellular forms followed by partition of the chromatin and the production of two new cells. 2. In bacterial c., "mating" is by simple contact, the sex factor (F agent) seemingly being transferred by means of F pili. 3. Sexual reproduction among protozoan ciliates, during which two individuals of appropriate mating types fuse along part of their lengths. Their macronuclei degenerate, and the micronuclei in each macronucleus divide several times (including a meiotic division); one of the resulting haploid pronuclei passes from each conjugant into the other and fuses with the remaining haploid nucleus in each conjugant. The organisms then separate (becoming exconjugants), undergo nuclear reorganization, and subsequently divide by asexual mitosis. 4. The combination, especially in the liver, of certain toxic substances formed in the intestine, drugs or steroid hormones with glucuronic or sulfuric acid. A means by which the biological activity of certain chemical substances can be terminated.

**conjuncti′va,** pl. **conjuncti′vae** [ L. fem. of *conjunctivus,* from *conjungo,* pp. -*junctus,* to bind together. JUG- ]. The mucous membrane covering the anterior surface of the eyeball (tunica conjunctiva bulbi, bulbar c.) and lining the lids (tunica conjunctiva palpebrarum, palpebral c.).

**conjuncti′val.** Relating to the conjunctiva.

**conjunctive.** Joining; connecting; connective.

**conjunctiviplasty** (kon′jungk-ti′vĭ-plas′tĭ). Conjunctivoplasty.

**conjunctivi′tis.** Inflammation of conjunctiva.

**actinic c.,** arc-flash c., Klieg c., snow c.; welder's c.; a c. resulting from exposure to ultraviolet rays, as from acetylene torches, therapeutic lamps, Klieg lights, or glare from snow.

**acute contagious c., acute epidemic c.,** pinkeye; Koch-Weeks c.; an acute c. marked by intense hyperemia and profuse mucopurulent discharge; caused by *Haemophilus aegypticus* (Koch-Weeks bacillus).

**allergic c.,** atopic c.; a conjuctival reaction to a substance producing an allergic response, either immediate or delayed.

**angular c.,** Morax-Axenfeld c.; diplobacillary c.; a subacute bilateral conjunctival inflammation caused by the Morax-Axenfeld diplobacillus, marked by redness of the lateral canthi and scanty, stringy discharge that adheres to the lashes.

**arc-flash c.,** actinic c.

**c. arida,** xerophthalmia.

**atopic c.,** allergic c.

**blenorrheal c.,** gonococcal c.

**calcareous c.,** c. petrificans; lithiasis c.; a common condition in which the palpebral conjunctiva displays minute yellow concretions due to products of cellular degeneration in Henle's glands.

**catarrhal c., chronic,** a chronic conjunctival hyperemia with slight mucoid discharge, due to irritation from dust, glare, insomnia, or depressed sympathetic tone.

**chemical c.,** conjunctival inflammation due to chemical irritants.

**cicatricial c.,** a chronic, progressive ocular affection that produces scarring of the conjunctiva primarily and of the cornea sequentially, transient small vesicles, a viscid ropy discharge, symblepheron, xerosis, and trichiasis; eventually bilateral. Sometimes (erroneously) called ocular pemphigus.

**croupous c.,** acute c. with membranous exudation without infiltration of the underlying conjunctiva.

**diphtherit′ic c.,** membranous c.; a severe conjunctival inflammation caused by the Klebs-Loeffler bacillus (*Corynebacterium diphtheriae),* characterized by an infiltrating membrane which cannot be removed without leaving a raw surface; the eyelids are swollen, painful, and of boardlike hardness.

**diplobacillary c.,** angular c.

**follic′ular c.,** c. associated with the presence of granules of lymphoid tissue on inner surface of lower lid.

**follicular c., acute,** an epidemic mucopurulent inflammation of the conjunctiva marked by follicles, especially in the lower fornix; may be caused by *Chlamydia,* adenoviruses, herpes virus, and Newcastle disease virus.

**gonococcal c.,** blenorrheal c.; a severe c. caused by gonococci and marked by intensely swollen, congested conjunctiva, swollen eyelids, and profuse purulent discharge.

**granular c.,** trachomatous c.

**inclusion c.,** inclusion blenorrhea; a follicular c. caused by *Chlamydia trachomatis* and characterized by slight discharge and a benign course.

**infantile pu′rulent c.,** *ophthalmia* neonatorum.

**Klieg c.,** actinic c.

**Koch-Weeks c.,** acute contagious c.

**larval c.,** c. due to imbedding of larvae in the eye.

**ligneous c.,** characterized typically by ligneous induration of upper tarsal conjunctiva, whitish pseudomembrane, and, in severe cases, corneal opacity; usually bilateral.

**lithiasis c.,** calcareous c.

**c. medicamentosa,** a c. caused by medicine instilled into the conjunctival sac.

**Meibomian c.,** a c. accompaning chronic inflammation of the Meibomian glands, presenting swollen tarsal plates and frothy seborrheic secretion.

**mem′branous c.,** diphtheritic c.

**molluscum c.,** c. associated with lesions of molluscum contagiosum of the eyelid.

**Morax-Axenfeld c.,** angular c.

**necrotic infectious c.,** Pascheff's c.; a unilateral, suppurative, necrotic inflammation of the conjunctiva characterized by scattered, elevated white spots in the fornices and palpebral conjunctiva, and ipsilateral swelling of preauricular, parotid, and submaxillary lymph glands.

**Parinaud's c.,** leptothricosis conjunctivae; a subacute inflammation of the conjunctiva due to infection with *Leptothrix;* it is characterized by the presence of large irregular reddish granulations in the connective tissue of the lids and fornix with simultaneous swelling of the preauricular, submaxillary, and cervical lymph glands, presumably contracted by contagion from animals. The syndrome described by Parinaud is now believed to be oculogranular tularemia caused by *Francisella* (*Pasteurella*) *tularensis.*

**Pascheff's c.,** necrotic infectious c.

**c. petrif′icans,** calcareous c.

**phlycten′ular c.,** a circumscribed c. accompanied by the formation of small red nodules of lymphoid tissue (phlyctenulae) on the conjunctiva.

**prairie c.,** a chronic c., characterized by the presence of small white spots on the palpebral conjunctiva, especially of the lower lid.

**pseudomembranous c.,** a rare, nonspecific inflammatory reaction characterized by the appearance upon, but not within, the conjunctiva of a coagulated fibrinous network which may be peeled off from intact epithelium.

**snow c.,** actinic c.

**spring c.,** vernal c.

**squirrel plague c.,** tularemic c.

**swimming pool c.,** an inclusion c. caused by adenovirus contamination of swimming pools.

**toxicogenic c.,** c. produced by topical application of a microbial toxin.

**trachomatous c.,** granular c.; a chronic infection of the conjunctiva characterized by conjunctival follicles and subsequent cicatrization; see also trachoma.

**tularemic c.,** squirrel plague c.; c. tularensis; a c. due to *Pasteurella tularensis* (*Francisella tularensis*), transmitted to man from rabbits and other rodents; characterized by chemosis, small necrotic ulcers, and enlargement of preauricular, parotid, cervical, and submaxillary lymph glands.

**vernal c.,** spring c.; spring ophthalmia; a chronic, bilateral conjunctival inflammation with photophobia and intense itching that recurs seasonally during warm weather; characterized in the palpebral form by cobblestone papillae in the upper palpebral conjunctiva; in the bulbar form, by gelatinous nodules adjacent to the limbus.

**welder's c.,** actinic c.

**conjunctivodacryocystorhinostomy** (kon-jungk′tĭ-vo-dak′rĭ-o-sis′to-ri-nos′to-mĭ) [ conjunctiva + G. *dakryon,* tear, + *kystis,* cyst, + *ris* (*rhin-*), nose, + *stoma,* mouth ]. A procedure for providing lacrimal drainage when the canaliculi are closed; silicon tubes are inserted that extend from the conjunctival sac to the nose, and allowed to remain there for a year or two.

**conjunc′tivodac′ryocystos′tomy** [ conjunctiva + G. *dakryon,* tear, + *kystis,* sac, + *stoma,* mouth ]. 1. A surgical procedure through the conjunctiva, resulting in an opening into the lacrimal sac. 2. The opening so produced.

**conjunctivo'ma.** A homeoplastic tumor of the conjunctiva.

**conjunctivoplasty** (kon'jungk-ti'vo-plas'tī, konjungk'tī-vo-). Conjunctiviplasty; plastic surgery of the conjunctiva.

**conjunctivorhinos'tomy** [ conjunctiva + G. *ris* (*rhin*), nose, + *stoma*, mouth ]. 1. A surgical procedure resulting in a passageway through the conjunctiva into the nasal cavity. 2. The opening so produced.

**conjuncti'vus** [ L. ] [ NA ]. Conjunctiva.

**Conn,** J., American physician, 20th century. See C.'s *syndrome*.

**connector.** In dentistry, a part of a partial denture which unites its components.

   **major c.,** a plate or bar (lingual bar, palatal bar) used for the purpose of uniting partial denture bases.

   **minor c.,** the connecting link (tang) between the major c. or base of a partial denture and other units of the prosthesis, such as clasps, indirect retainers, and occlusal rests.

**Connell,** F. G., American surgeon, *1875. See C.'s *suture*.

**connex'us.** Conexus.

**co'noid** [ G. *kōnoeidēs*, cone-shaped ]. 1. A cone-shaped structure. 2. An organelle at the anterior end of sporozoites and merozoites in the developmental stages of *Sarcocystis*, *Besnoitia*, and *Frankelia*, all closely related coccidian sporozoans (family Sarcocystidae); the structure is absent from the haemosporidians and piroplasms, which are more distantly related sporozoans. The function of the c. is unknown, but it is thought to be an organelle of penetration into the host cell, possibly aided by a protrusible form of the c.

   **Sturm's c.,** term used in ophthalmic optics to refer to rays, emerging from an astigmatic system, that are enveloped by a surface that is a type of c.

**conomyoidin** (ko-no-mi'oy-din) [ G. *kōnos*, cone, + *mys*, muscle, + *eidos*, resemblance ]. Contractile protoplasm at inner end of inner segment of visual cells; activity is most evident in fishes and amphibians, slight in mammals.

**con'quinine.** Quinidine.

**Conradi,** A. C., Norwegian physician, 1809–1869. See C.'s *line*.

**Conradi,** E., German physician. See C.'s *disease*.

**Conradi,** Heinrich German bacteriologist, *1876. See C.-Drigalski *agar*, Drigalski-C. *agar*.

**consanguineous** (kon'sang-gwīn'ē-us) [ L. *cum*, with, + *sanguis*, blood: *consanguineus* ]. Related by blood.

**consanguinity** (kon'sang-gwīn'ī-tī) [ L. *consanguinitas*, blood relationship ]. Blood relationship; kinship because of common ancestry.

**conscious** (con'shus) [ L. *conscius*, knowing ]. 1. Aware; having present knowledge or perception of oneself, one's acts and surroundings. 2. Denoting something occurring with the perceptive attention of the individual, as a c. act or idea, distinguished from automatic or instinctive.

**consciousness** (con'shus-nes) [ L. *con-scio*, to know, to be aware of ]. Awareness; perception of physical facts or mental concepts; a state of general wakefulness and responsiveness to environment. Impairment of consciousness may be of any degree of severity. Terms such as elation, lethargy, drowsiness, stupor, semicoma, and coma are commonly used with varying connotations to describe levels of consciousness. There is no unanimity of opinion on the precise meanings of these terms.

   **clouding of c.,** a state in which the patient is not in contact with the environment.

   **double c.,** a condition in which one lives in two seemingly unrelated mental states, being, while in one, unaware of the other or of the acts performed in the other. See also *dual personality*.

   **field of c.,** the material of awareness at any given moment.

**consensual** [ L. *con-*, with, + *sensus*, sensation ]. Reflex; denoting what is done in response to a stimulus without the cooperation of the will.

**conservation** (kon-ser-va'shun) [ L. *conservatio*, a preserving, keeping ]. In sensorimotor theory, the mental operation by which an individual retains the idea of an object after its removal in time or space.

**conserv'ative.** 1. Preservative. 2. Opposed to radical or heroic measures of treatment.

**conserve.** Confection.

**consol'idant.** A substance that promotes healing or union.

**consolidation** [ L. *consolido*, to make thick, condense, fr. *solidus*, solid ]. Solidification into a firm, dense mass; applied especially to the inflammatory solidification of the lung in pneumonia.

**con'solute.** Completely miscible.

**con'sonant.** Speech sound chiefly characterized by a non-musical friction noise generated by driving expired air through a narrow orifice.

**conspecific.** Of the same species.

**con'stancy.** The quality of being constant.

   **object c.,** the tendency for objects to be perceived as unchanging despite variations in the positions in and conditions under which the objects are observed.

**constant.** A quantity which, under stated conditions, does not vary with changes in the environment.

   **Ambard's c.,** see Ambard's *coefficient*, and Ambard's *law*.

   **association c.,** in experimental immunology, a mathematical expression of hapten-antibody interaction: average association c., $K = $ [ hapten-bound antibody ]/[ free antibody ][ free hapten ].

   **Avogadro's c.,** Avogadro's *number*.

   **decay c.,** the mathematical expression for the number of atoms of a radionuclide decaying in a unit of time.

   **dissociation c.,** the equilibrium c. involved in the dissociation of a compound into two or more ions.

   **dissociation c. of an acid,** symbol, $K_a$; expressed by general equation $(H^+)(A^-)/(HA) = K_a$, where HA is the acid.

   **dissociation c. of a base,** symbol, $K_b$; expressed by the general equation $(B^+)(OH^-)/(BOH) = K_b$, where BOH is the base.

   **dissociation c. of water,** symbol $K_w$; $(H^+) (OH^-) = K_w = 10^{-14}$ at 25°C.

   **equilibrium c.,** in the reaction $A + B \rightleftarrows C + D$ at equilibrium (*i.e.*, no net change in *A*, *B*, *C*, or *D*), the concentrations of the four components are related by the

equation $K = \dfrac{[\,C\,][\,D\,]}{[\,A\,][\,B\,]}$ ; $K$ is the equilibrium con-

stant. If any component in the reaction has a multiplier (*e.g.*, $H_2 \rightleftarrows 2H$), that multiplier appears as an exponent in the calculation of $K = ([\,H\,]^2/[\,H_2\,])$. When this equation is applied to the ionization of a substance in solution, $K$ is called the dissociation constant and its negative logarithm (base 10) is the pK. See also Henderson-Hasselbalch *equation*.

   **Faraday's c.,** the faraday (96,500 coulombs).

   **flotation c.,** symbol $S_f$; characteristic sedimentation behavior of a lipoprotein fraction of plasma in a centrifugal field in a medium of appropriate density, achieved by adding a salt or $D_2O$ to the plasma. Also called Svedberg of flotation; negative S.

   **gas c.,** $R$ (symbol for the constant) $= 8.314 \times 10^7$ ergs per degree centigrade per mole.

   **Michaelis** or **Michaelis-Menten c.,** symbol $K_m$; equal to the concentration of the substrate at which half the maximum velocity of a reaction is achieved; the ratio of the rate c.'s $(k_2 + k_3)/k_1$ in the reaction Enzyme + Substrate $\underset{k_2}{\overset{k_1}{\rightleftarrows}}$ ES complex $\overset{k_3}{\rightarrow}$ Products + Enzyme; equal to substrate concentration $\times$ [ $(V_{max} - V_{obs})/V_{obs}$ ]. The latter is the Michaelis-Menten equation. See also Lineweaver-Burk *equation*.

   **Newtonian c. of gravitation,** G (symbol for the constant) $= (6.73 \pm 0.03) \times 10^{-8}$ dyne cm.²; used in centrifugation and aviation physiology to express the force developed by centrifugal motion; plus or minus notation is used according to the direction of the force in relation to the body. When the body is accelerated or decelerated, it is subjected to a change in G. At rest, 1 G, i.e., the pull of gravity, is being exerted on the body. See also G *force*.

**Planck's c.,** a c., $6.6256 \times 10^{-34}$ J s (Joule-seconds) or $6.6256 \times 10^{-27}$ erg-seconds. Symbol, $h$.

**radioactive c.,** the fraction of a radioactive substance disintegrating in a given unit of time; symbol $\lambda$.

**rate c.,** velocity c.

**sedimentation c.,** see under sedimentation.

**time c.,** that part of the rate meter circuit that determines the time interval over which the rate of incoming events will be averaged.

**velocity c.'s,** rate c.'s; in enzymic reactions, $k_1$, $k_2$, and $k_3$ in the Michaelis-Menten c. ($q. v.$).

**Constantine the African,** Constantinus Africanus, c. 1020–1087. A monk at Salerno and Monte Cassino who translated Arabic medical works into Latin which had great influence on European medicine.

**con'stella'tion.** In psychiatry, all the factors that determine a particular action.

**constipate** [ L. *con-stipo,* pp. *-atus,* to press together ]. To cause a sluggishness in the action of the bowels.

**constipated.** Costive; suffering from constipation.

**constipation.** A condition in which bowel movements are infrequent or incomplete.

**constitution** [ L. *constitutio,* constitution, disposition, fr. *constituo,* pp. *-stitutus,* to establish, fr. *statuo,* to set up. STA- ]. 1. The physical makeup of the body, including the mode of performance of its functions, the activity of its metabolic processes, the manner and degree of its reactions to stimuli, and its power of resistance to the attack of pathogenic organisms. 2. In chemistry, the number and kind of atoms in the molecule and the relation they bear to each other.

**constitutional.** 1. Relating to the constitution. 2. General; relating to the system as a whole; not local.

**constriction** (kon-strik'shun) [ L. *con-stringo,* pp. *-strictus,* to draw together ]. 1. Binding or contraction of a part. 2. Stricture; stenosis. 3. A subjective sensation as if the body or any part were tightly bound or squeezed.

**constrictor** (kon-strik'tor) [ L. fr. *constringo,* to draw together ]. 1. Anything that binds or squeezes a part. 2 [ NA ]. A muscle the action of which is to narrow a canal; a sphincter.

**constructive** [ L. *con-struo,* pp. *-structus,* to build up ]. 1. Building up. 2. Anabolic.

**consultant** [ L. *consulto,* pp. *-atus,* to deliberate, ask advice ]. 1. A physician or surgeon who does not take actual charge of a patient, but acts in an advisory capacity, deliberating with and counseling the personal attendant. 2. A member of a hospital staff who has no active service but stands ready to advise in any case, at the request of the attending physician or surgeon.

**consultation.** Meeting of two or more physicians to evaluate the nature and progress of disease in a particular patient and to establish diagnosis, prognosis, and therapy.

**consumption** [ L. *con-sumo,* pp. *-sumptus,* to take up wholly, use up, waste ]. 1. The using up of something, especially the rate at which it is used. 2. An obsolete term for a wasting of the tissues of the body, usually tuberculous.

**oxygen c.,** (1) symbol QO or $QO_2$, the rate at which oxygen is used by a tissue; units: microliters of oxygen STPD used per milligram of tissue per hour; (2) symbol V $O_2$, the rate at which oxygen enters the blood from alveolar gas, equal in the steady state to the consumption of oxygen by tissue metabolism throughout the body; units: ml/min STPD.

**consumptive.** Relating to, or a sufferer from, consumption.

**contact** [ *con-tingo,* pp. *-tactus,* to touch, seize, fr. *tango,* to touch ]. 1. The touching or apposition of two bodies. 2. A person who has been exposed to contagion.

**balancing c.,** balancing occlusal surface; (1) the c.'s between upper and lower dentures on the balancing side for the purpose of stabilitizing the dentures; (2) the c.'s between upper and lower dentures at the opposite side from the working side (anteroposteriorly or laterally) for the purpose of stabilizing the dentures; (3) the c.'s between upper and lower natural or artificial teeth at the opposite side from the working side.

**centric c.,** centric *occlusion.*

**deflective occlusal c.,** cuspal interference; a condition of tooth c.'s which diverts the mandible from a normal path of closure to centric jaw relation.

**initial c.,** (1) the first meeting of opposing teeth upon elevation of the mandible toward the maxillae; (2) the initial occlusal c. of opposing teeth when the jaw is closed.

**interceptive occlusal c.,** see deflective occlusal c.

**premature c.,** see deflective occlusal c.

**proximal c., proximate c.,** the point or area of touching of the surfaces of two adjacent teeth in the same arch.

**c. with reality,** correctly interpreting external phenomena in relation to the norms of one's social or cultural milieu; this ability is impaired in some psychoses.

**working c.'s,** working bite; working occlusion; c.'s of teeth made on the side of the occlusion toward which the mandible has been moved.

**contactant.** Any of a heterogeneous group of allergens that elicit manifestations of induced sensitivity (hypersensitivity) by direct contact with skin or mucosa.

**contagion** (kon-ta'jun) [ L. *contagio;* fr. *contingo,* to touch closely ]. 1. Contagium. 2. Transmission of disease by contact. with the sick. The term originated long before development of modern ideas of infectious disease and has since lost much of its significance, being included under the more inclusive term "communicable disease." 3. The production of a neurosis or psychosis through imitation or autosuggestion.

**immediate c.,** direct c. occurring as the result of actual contact with the sick.

**mediate c.,** indirect c. effected through the medium of persons or objects that have been in contact with the sick.

**psychic c.,** communication of a nervous disorder by imitation.

**contagious.** Communicable; relating to contagion; transmissible by contact with the sick.

**contagiousness.** Communicableness; the quality of being contagious or transmissible by contact.

**conta'gium** [ L. a touching, another form of *contagio* ]. The virus or essential causative substance of any infectious (not merely contagious) disease.

**contam'inant.** That which contaminates; an impurity; any material of an extraneous nature associated with a chemical, a pharmaceutical preparation or a physiologic principle.

**contam'inate.** To soil with infectious material.

**contamina'tion** [ L. *contamino,* pp. *-atus,* to stain, defile ]. 1. Pollution; soiling with infectious material. 2. In chemistry or pharmacy, the presence of any extraneous material that renders a substance or preparation impure. 3. The Freudian term for a fusion and condensation of words.

**content** [ L. *contentus,* fr. *con-tineo,* pp. *-tentus,* to hold together, contain, fr. *teneo,* to hold ]. 1. That which is contained within something else, usually in this sense in the plural form, contents. 2. In psychology, the form of a dream as presented to consciousness. 3. Sometimes used to mean concentration (3), but this is ambiguous; *e.g.,* blood hemoglobin c. could mean either its concentration or the product of its concentration and the blood volume.

**latent c.,** the hidden, unconscious meaning of thoughts or actions, especially in dreams or fantasies.

**manifest c.,** those elements of fantasy and dreams which are consciously available and reportable.

**contiguity** (kon-tĭ-gu'ĭ-tĭ) [ L. *contiguus,* touching, fr. *contingo,* to touch ]. 1. Contact without actual continuity; see also continuity. 2. The occurrence of two or more objects, events, or mental impressions together in space (spatial c.) or time (temporal c.).

**contig'uous.** Adjacent or in actual contact.

**con'tinence** [ L. *continentia,* fr. *con-tineo,* to hold back, fr. *teneo,* to hold ]. Moderation, temperance, or self-restraint, in respect to the appetites, especially to the sexual act.

**con'tinent.** Temperate or abstinent as regards sexual indulgence.

**continued** [ L. *continuo,* to join together, make continuous ]. Continuous; without intermission; said especially of protracted fever without apyretic intervals, such as typhoid fever, compared with the paroxysms of fever in malaria.

**continu'ity** [ L. *continuus,* continued ]. Absence of interruption, a succession of parts intimately united. A single bone of the skull has the quality of *continuity* in all its parts; a cranial suture is marked by *contiguity* of the bones entering into its formation.

**contour** (kon'toor) [ L. *con-* (intens.), + *torno,* to turn (in a lathe), fr. *tornus,* a lathe ]. 1. The outline of a part; the surface configuration. 2. In dentistry, to restore the normal outlines of a broken or otherwise misshapen tooth, or to create the external shape or form of a prosthesis.

**flange c.,** the design of the flange of a denture.

**gingival c.,** gingival architecture; gum c.; the shape or form of the gingiva, either natural or artificial, around the necks of the teeth.

**gum c.,** gingival c.

**height of c.,** see under height.

**contra-** [ L. ]. A prefix signifying opposed, against. For some words so beginning and not listed here, see counter-.

**contra-angle.** 1. One of the double or triple angles in the shank of an instrument by means of which the cutting edge or point is brought into the axis of the handle. 2. An extension piece added to the end of a dental handpiece which, through a set of bevel gears, changes the angle of the drill.

**contra-aperture.** Counteropening.

**contracep'tion.** The prevention of conception or impregnation.

**contracep'tive** [ L. *contra,* against, + conceptive ]. An agent for the prevention of conception or relating to any measure or agent designed to prevent conception.

**"combination" oral c.,** a mixture of a steroid having progestational activity and an estrogen; one such pill is taken daily for approximately 19 days of each menstrual cycle.

**intrauterine c. device,** see under device.

**oral c.,** any orally effective preparation designed to prevent conception.

**"sequential" oral c.,** a preparation providing two types of medication; the first type, containing only an estrogen, is taken daily from the 5th to approximately the 19th day of the menstrual cycle; the second, containing an estrogen and a semisynthetic progestational steroid, is taken daily from the 20th to the 24th days of the cycle.

**contract** [ L. *con-traho,* pp. *-tractus,* to draw together ]. 1 (kon-trakt'). To shorten; to become reduced in size; in the case of muscle, either to shorten or to undergo an increase in tension. 2. To acquire by contagion or infection. 3. (kon'trakt). An explicit, bilateral commitment by psychotherapist and patient to a defined course of action to attain the goal of the psychotherapy.

**contrac'tile.** Having the property of contracting.

**contractil'ity.** The ability or property of a substance, especially of muscle, of shortening, or becoming reduced in size, or developing increased tension.

**contractin.** A protein extracted from contracted muscle.

**contractio** (kon-trak'shyo) [ L. ]. Contraction.

**contrac'tion** [ L. *contractio,* fr. *kon-traho,* pp. *-tractus,* to draw together ]. 1. A shortening or increase in tension; denoting the normal function of muscular tissue. 2. A shrinkage or reduction in size. 3. Heart beat, as in premature c.; see also subentries under beat.

**after-c.,** see aftercontraction.

**ano'dal closure c.,** ACC or AnCC; the momentary c. of a muscle under the influence of the positive pole when the electrical circuit is established.

**ano'dal opening c.,** AOC or AnOC; the momentary c. of a muscle under the influence of the positive pole when the circuit is broken.

**automatic c.,** automatic *beat.*

**carpoped'al c.,** carpopedal *spasm.*

**catho'dal closure c.,** CCC or CaCC; the momentary c. of a muscle under the influence of the negative pole when an electrical circuit is established.

**catho'dal opening c.,** COC or CaOC; the momentary c. of a muscle under the influence of the negative pole when the circuit is broken.

**closing c.,** c. produced at the time of closing of the circuit when using direct current to stimulate the muscle.

**escaped c.,** escaped *beat.*

**escaped ventricular c.,** an escaped beat arising in the ventricle.

**fibrillary c.'s,** c.'s occurring spontaneously in individual muscle fibers; they are seen commonly a few days after damage to the motor nerves supplying the muscle, and this type of activity is distinguished from fasciculation, which is related to activation of motor units.

**front-tap c.,** Gowers' c.; c. of the calf muscles when the anterior surface of the leg is struck.

**Gowers' c.,** front-tap c.

**hourglass c.,** constriction of the middle portion of a hollow organ, such as the stomach or the gravid uterus.

**hunger c.'s,** strong c.'s of the pylorus associated with hunger pains.

**idiomuscular c.,** myoedema.

**isometric c.,** see isometric (2).

**isotonic c.,** see isotonic (3).

**myotat'ic c.,** (1) reflex c. of a muscle induced by its passive stretching; (2) tendon *reflex.*

**opening c.,** a c. produced at the time of opening the circuit when using direct current to stimulate the muscle or a motor nerve.

**paradoxical c.,** a tonic c. of the anterior tibial muscles when a sudden passive dorsal flexion of the foot is made.

**postural c.,** maintenance of muscular tension (usually isometric) sufficient to maintain posture.

**premature c.,** premature *beat.*

**tetanic c.,** see tetanus (2).

**tonic c.,** sustained contraction of a muscle, as employed in the maintenance of posture.

**contrac'ture** [ L. *contractura,* fr. *con-traho,* to draw together ]. A permanent muscular contraction due to tonic spasm or to loss of muscular equilibrium, the antagonists being paralyzed.

**Dupuytren's c.,** Nodular proliferation of fibrous tissue of the palmar fascia, leading to c. with permanent flexion of the fingers, especially the fourth and fifth, of one or both hands. May be associated with similar deformity in feet as well as with Peyronie's disease.

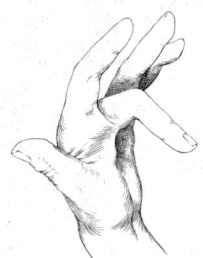

**Dupuytren's Contracture**

**functional c.,** a muscular shortening that ceases during sleep or general anesthesia.

**organic c.,** c., usually due to fibrosis within the muscle, that persists whether the subject is conscious or unconscious.

**Volkmann's c.,** tissue degeneration produced by ischemia leading to a late c. involving muscles, tendons, fascia, and other soft tissues; caused by interference with blood flow, thus by direct vessel compression or prolonged spasm.

**contrafissura** (kon'trah-fi-shu'rah) [ L. *contra,* against, counter, + *fissura,* fissure ]. Fracture by contrecoup; fracture of a bone, as in the skull, at a point opposite that where the blow was received.

**contraindicant** (kon-trah-in'di-kant). Indicating the contrary; that is to say, showing that a method of treatment which would otherwise be proper is forbidden by special circumstances in the individual case.

**contraindication** (kon-trah-in-di-ka'shun). Any special symptom or circumstance that renders the use of a remedy or the carrying out of a procedure inadvisable.

**contralat'eral** [ L. *contra,* opposite, + *latus,* side ]. Relating to the opposite side, as when pain is felt or paralysis occurs on the side opposite to that of the lesion.

**contrast** [ L. *contra*, against, + *sto*, pp. *status*, to stand ]. A comparison in which the differences between two objects are shown.

**simultaneous c.,** the enhancement of the visual sensation of white when a white object is placed beside a black one; the black object also appears blacker as a result of the contiguity of white. Complementary colors also appear brighter when placed in juxtaposition; thus green appears a brighter green and red a brighter red if these two colors are placed beside one another.

**successive c.,** the visual effect caused by staring at a brightly colored object and then at a gray surface; the latter appears tinged with the color which is the complementary of the color of the object. Or if instead of directing the eyes to a gray surface they are turned to a surface colored in the complementary of the object, the color intensity of the surface is enhanced; for example, after looking first at red a green surface appears a brighter green.

**contrastim'ulant.** 1. Annulling the effect of a stimulant. 2. An agent whose action opposes that of a stimulant.

**contrecoup** (kawn-tr-koo') [ Fr. counter-blow ]. Denoting the manner of a contrafissura, or fracture of a bone, as in the skull, at a point opposite that at which the blow was received. See also contrecoup injury of the brain, under injury.

**contracta'tion** [ L. *con-trecto*, pp. -*trectatus*, to handle, fr. *tracto*, to drag, take hold of, fr. *traho*, to draw ]. 1. Sexual dalliance. 2. The impulse to embrace one of the opposite sex.

**control** [ Mediev. L. *contrarotulum*, a counterroll for checking accounts, fr. L. *rotula*, dim. of *rota*, a wheel ]. 1. To verify an experiment by means of another with the crucial variable omitted, as when a given amount of toxin is injected into two rabbits of equal weight, one receiving antitoxin, the other not; if the animal not receiving antitoxin (the c.) dies, the assumption is that the other would also have succumbed without the protective injection of antitoxin. 2. A control organism or experiment. 3. The regulation of maintenance of a function, action, reflex, etc.

**associative automatic c.,** nerve impulses from the corpus striatum acting finally upon the muscles.

**birth c.,** oligogenics; (1) restriction of the number of offspring by means of contraceptive measures; (2) projects, programs, or methods to control reproduction, by either improving or diminishing fertility.

**idiodynam'ic c.,** nervous impulses from the medulla that preserve the normal trophic condition of the muscles.

**own c.'s,** a method of experimental c. in which the same subjects are used in both experimental and c. conditions.

**reflex c.,** nerve impulses transmitted to the muscles to maintain normal reflex action.

**Schick c.,** (BP), Schick test toxin (see Schick test) that has been heated at a temperature not lower than 70° and not higher than 85° for not less than 5 minutes; it is used in conjunction with Schick test toxin in order to exclude reactions due to nonspecific substances.

**social c.,** the influence on the behavior of a person exerted by other persons or by society as a whole; for example, through social ostracism or the criminal law.

**stimulus c.,** the use of conditioning techniques to bring the target behavior of an individual under environmental c.

**syner'gic c.,** impulses transmitted from the cerebellum regulating the muscular activity of the synergic units of the body.

**tonic c.,** nerve impulses that maintain a normal tonus or level of activity in muscle or other effector organs.

**vestib'ulo-equilib'ratory c.,** nerve impulses transmitted from the semicircular canals, saccule, and utricle that serve to maintain the equilibrium of the body.

**contuse'** [ L. *con-tundo*, pp. -*tusus*, to beat, bruise ]. To bruise.

**contu'sion** [ L. *contusio*, a bruising ]. A bruise.

**brain c.,** a bruising, usually of the surface, of the brain with extravasation of blood but without rupture of the pia-arachnoid; healing results in a superficial depressed siderotic area, possibly with incorporated meninges; see also brain *cicatrix*.

**scalp c.,** intracutaneous or subcutaneous extravasation of blood without gross disruption of skin.

**wind c.,** windage.

**con'ular.** Cone-shaped.

**Conus.** A genus of shellfish that inhabits the shores of some South Pacific islands. Several species, *C. geographus, C. textilis, C. aulicus, C. tulipa,* and *C. marmoreus* are poisonous, their sting or spine causing acute pain, edema, numbness, spreading paralysis, and sometimes coma and death.

**conus,** pl. **co'ni** [ L. fr. G. *kōnos*, cone ]. 1 [ NA ]. Cone. 2. Posterior staphyloma in myopic choroiditis.

**c. arterio'sus** [ NA ], infundibulum (4) [ NA ]; arterial cone; pulmonary cone; the left or anterior portion of the cavity of the right ventricle of the heart, which terminates in the pulmonary artery.

**congenital c.,** Fuch's *coloboma*.

**distraction c.,** a c. where the optic nerve proceeds through the scleral canal in a strongly oblique direction.

**c. elas'ticus** [ NA ], the thicker lower portion of the elastic membrane of the larynx.

**co'ni epididym'idis** [ NA ], *lobuli* epididymidis.

**c. medulla'ris** [ NA ], medullary cone; the tapering lower extremity of the spinal cord.

**myopic c.,** myopic *crescent*.

**pulmonary c.,** c. arteriosus.

**supertraction c.,** a reddish yellow c. or ring at the nasal margin of the optic disk, produced by displacement of the pigment layer and lamina vitrea of the choroid; occurs in high myopia.

**co'ni vasculo'si,** *lobuli* epididymidis.

**convalescence** [ L. *con-valesco*, to grow strong, fr. *valeo*, to be strong ]. A period between the end of a disease and the patient's restoration to complete health.

**convalescent.** 1. Getting well or one who is getting well. 2. Denoting the period of convalescence.

**convallam'arin.** The genin of the glycoside convallamarogenin, present in the root of *Convallaria;* diuretic and cardiac stimulant.

**convallamarogenin.** $C_{27}H_{42}O_4$; the major glycoside present in the roots of *Convallaria.*

**convallaria** [ L. *convallis,* an enclosed valley ]. The flower, rhizome, and roots of *Convallaria majalis* (family Liliaceae), lily of the valley. They contain glycosides with digitalis-like action.

**conval'larin.** An acrid glycoside obtained from convallaria.

**convallatoxin.** $C_{29}H_{42}O_{10}$; a glycoside from the blossoms of *Convallaria ornithogalum* (family Liliaceae) and Antiaris (family Moraceae).

**convection** [ L. *con-veho*, pp. -*vectus*, to carry or bring together ]. The conveyance of heat in liquids or gases movement of the heated particles, as when the layer of water at the bottom of a heated pot rises or the warm air of a room ascends to the ceiling.

**convergence** [ L. *con-vergo*, to incline together ]. 1. The tending of two or more objects toward a common point. 2. The direction of the visual lines to a near point.

**amplitude of c.,** range of c.; the distance between the near point and far point of c.

**angle of c.,** see under angle.

**far point of c.,** the point to which the visual lines are directed when c. is at rest.

**near point of c.,** the point to which the visual lines are directed when c. is at its maximum.

**negative c.,** the slight divergence of the visual axes when c. is at rest, as when looking at the far point of normal vision or during sleep.

**positive c.,** inward deviation of the visual axes even when c. is at rest, as in cases of convergent squint.

**range of c.,** amplitude of c.

**unit of c.,** see meter *angle*.

**convergent.** Tending toward a common point.

**conversion** (kon-ver'zuhn) [ L. *con-verto,* pp. -*versus,* to turn around, to change ]. 1. Change; transmutation. 2. Transformation of an emotion into a physical manifestation, as in hysteria. 3. In virology, lysogenic c.; the acquisition, by bacteria, of a new property associated with presence of a prophage.

lysogenic c., c. (3).

**convertase.** A term of limited usage applied to an enzyme that "converts" a substance to an active state.

C3 c., the complexed and activated fourth and second (C42a) components of complement that activates the third component (C3); see component of *complement*.

C3 proactivator c., C3PA convertase; *properdin* factor D (*q.v.*); a seeming enzyme that converts C3 proactivator (properdin factor B) to the activator state.

**convertin.** *Factor VII.*

**convex** [ L. *convexus*, vaulted, arched, convex, fr. *con-veho*, to bring together ]. Applied to a surface that is evenly curved or bulging outward, the segment of a sphere.

high c., the segment of a sphere of short radius.

low c., the segment of a sphere of long radius.

**convexity.** 1. The state of being convex. 2. A convex structure.

cortical c., *facies* superolateralis cerebri.

**convexoba'sia** [ L. *convexus*, outwardly curved, + *basis*, foundation ]. Forward bending of the occipital bone.

**convex'ocon'cave.** Convex on one surface and concave on the opposite surface.

**convex'us** [ L. ] [ NA ]. Convex.

**convex'ocon'vex.** Biconvex; convex on two opposite surfaces.

**con'volute** [ L. *con-volvo*, pp. *-volutus*, to roll together ]. Rolled together with one part over the other; in the shape of a roll or scroll.

**con'voluted.** Convolute.

**convolutio** (kon-vŏ-lu'shyo). Convolution.

**convolution** [ L. *convolutio* ]. 1. A coiling or rolling of an organ. 2. Specifically, a gyrus of the cerebral or cerebellar cortex.

angular c., *gyrus* angularis.

anterior central c., *gyrus* precentralis.

ascending frontal c., *gyrus* precentralis.

ascending parietal c., *gyrus* postcentralis.

callosal c., *gyrus* cinguli.

cingulate c., *gyrus* cinguli.

first temporal c., *gyrus* temporalis superior.

hippocampal c., *gyrus* parahippocampalis.

inferior frontal c., *gyrus* frontalis inferior.

inferior temporal c., *gyrus* temporalis inferior.

middle frontal c., *gyrus* frontalis medius.

middle temporal c., *gyrus* temporalis medius.

posterior central c., *gyrus* postcentralis.

second temporal c., *gyrus* temporalis medius.

superior frontal c., *gyrus* frontalis superior.

superior temporal c., *gyrus* temporalis superior.

supramarginal c., *gyrus* supramarginalis.

third temporal c., *gyrus* temporalis inferior.

transitional c., transitional *gyrus.*

transverse temporal c.'s, *gyri* temporales transversi.

Zuckerkandl's c., *gyrus* subcallosus.

**convolu'tus** [ L. ] [ NA ]. Convolute.

**convol'vulin.** A high molecular, amorphous principle obtained from jalap, *Exogonium purga.*

**Convol'vulus** [ L. a plant, bindweed, fr. *con-volvo*, to roll together ]. A genus of twining plants of the *Convolvulaceae*, e.g., jalap.

**convul'sant.** Causing convulsions; convulsive; eclamptogenic; eclamptogenous.

**convulsion** [ L. *convulsio*, fr. *con-vello*, pp. *-vulsus*, to tear up ]. A violent spasm.

clonic c., one in which the contractions are intermittent, the muscles alternately contracting and relaxing.

coordinate c., a clonic c. in which the movements are seemingly purposeful, being exaggerations of those that may occur naturally.

ether c., c. associated with the triad of deep ether anesthesia, hyperthermia, and hypercapnia.

hysterical c., see hysteria.

hysteroid c., see hysteria.

immediate posttraumatic c., c. beginning within minutes after injury.

infantile c., c. in infancy that may be associated with fever, teething (tooth spasm), etc.

mimic c., facial *tic.*

puerperal c.'s, puerperal *eclampsia.*

salaam c.'s, nodding *spasm.*

static c., saltatory *spasm.*

tetanic c., tonic c.

tonic c., tetanic c.; one in which muscle contraction is sustained.

**convulsive.** Relating to convulsions; marked by or producing convulsions.

**Cooke,** A. Bennett, American physician, *1869. See C.'s *speculum.*

**Cooke-Apert-Gallais syndrome.** See under syndrome.

**Cooley,** Thomas B., American pediatrician, 1871–1945. See C.'s *anemia.*

**Coolidge,** William D., American physicist, *1873. See C. *tube.*

**Coombs,** Carey F., British physician, 1879–1932. See C. *murmur.*

**Coombs,** R. R. A., British immunologist, *1921. See Gell and C. *reactions*, C.'s *test*, direct C.'s *test*, indirect C.'s *test.*

**Cooper,** Sir Astley P., English anatomist and surgeon, 1768–1841. See C.'s *disease, fascia, hernia, herniotome, ligaments.*

**Coope'ria.** A genus of small, slender nematodes (family Trichostrongylidae) inhabiting the small intestine, rarely the abomasum, of ruminants. They are of a bright reddish color when fresh. They suck blood and produce serious effects when present in large numbers. In partly immune animals, these worms become enclosed in nodules in the wall of the intestine.

C. biso'nis, occurs in cattle, sheep, bison, and pronghorn antelopes.

C. curti'cei, occurs in sheep, goats, and wild deer in Europe, although cosmopolitan in distribution.

C. oncoph'ora, occurs in cattle and domestic and wild sheep, but rarely in the horse; although worldwide in distribution, it is most common in the northern United States and Canada.

C. pectina'ta, occurs in cattle, sheep, water buffalo, dromedary camels, and various wild ruminants; it is common in the southern United States.

C. puncta'ta, *Strongyloides bovis;* occurs mainly in cattle, less commonly in sheep, water buffalo, and several wild ruminants; although worldwide in distribution, it is especially widespread in North America and common in Hawaii.

C. spatula'ta, occurs in cattle and sheep in the southern United States, Kenya, Australia, and Malaysia.

**Coopernail,** George P., American surgeon, *1876. See C.'s *sign.*

**coordinate** (ko-or'dĭ-nāt) [ see coordination ]. 1. Any of the scales or magnitudes that serve to define the position of a point. 2. To perform the act of coordination.

Cartesian c.'s, rectangular c.'s in which the position of a point is determined in terms of $x$, $y$, and $z$, representing scales for the three dimensions of space.

polar c.'s, a system of c.'s in which the position of a point is specified in terms of the distance and the angle or direction from a reference point.

**coordination** (ko-or'dĭ-na'shun) [ L. *co-*, together, + *ordino*, pp. *-atus*, to arrange, fr. *ordo* (*ordin-*), arrangement, order ]. The harmonious working together; especially of several muscles or muscle groups in the execution of complicated movements.

**Coors filter.** See under filter.

**co-os'sifica'tion.** State of being joined by bone formation.

**co-os'sify** [ L. *co-*, together, + *os*, bone, + *facio*, to make ]. To unite into one bone.

**copaiba** (ko-pi'bah) [ Sp. ]. Copaiva; balsam of c. or copaiva; the oleoresin of *Copaifera officinalis* and other species of *Copaifera* (family Leguminosae), a South American plant; expectorant, diuretic, and stimulant.

c. oil, a volatile oil obtained by distillation from c.; used for the same purposes as c.

**copar'affinate.** A mixture of water-insoluble isoparaffinic acids partially neutralized with isooctyl hydroxybenzyldialkyl amines. Used as an antifungal agent for external application.

**cope.** 1. The upper half of a flask in the casting art; hence applicable to the upper or cavity side of a denture flask. 2.

In psychiatry and psychology, to confront a challenge, conflict, or anxiety with intent to resolve.

**Cope's clamp.** See under clamp.

**co'pepod.** Any member of the order Copepoda.

**Copep'oda** [ G. *kōpē*, an oar, + *pous* (*pod-*), a foot ]. An order of fresh water and marine crustacea, some species of which are commonly called water fleas; abundant free-living crustaceans of basic importance in the aquatic food chain in both the marine and fresh water environments. Some are ectoparasites of both cold-blooded and warm-blooded aquatic vertebrates; the parasitic copepods of fish and whales are often highly modified for deep penetration of the skin or for adherence by suckers and hooks (*e.g.*, the fish lice, *Argulus*). Certain copepods (*Cyclops, Diaptomus*) are important as intermediate hosts of the broad fish tapeworm of man (*Diphyllobothrium latum*) and of the guinea worm of man (*Dracunculus madinensis*).

**coping.** A thin metal covering or cap.

transfer c., in dentistry, a metallic, acrylic resin or other covering or cap used to position a die in an impression.

**copiopia** (kop-e-o'pe-ah) [ G. *kopos*, fatigue, + *ōps*, eye ]. Obsolete term for asthenopia.

**copodyskinesia** (kop-o-dis-kin-e'sī-ah) [ G. *kopos*, fatigue, + *dys-*, bad, + *kinēsis*, movement ]. Occupation *neurosis*.

**copolymer.** A polymer in which two or more monomers or base units are combined.

c. resin, see under resin.

**copper** [ L. *cuprum*, orig. *Cyprium*, after the island of *Cyprus*, where it was mined ]. A metallic element, symbol Cu, atomic no. 29, atomic weight 63.54. Several of its salts (see under cupric) are used in medicine.

aluminated c., lapis divinus; made by fusing together potassium alum, c. sulfate, and potassium nitrate and camphor; has been used as a mild caustic and as a collyrium.

**copper-64.** $^{64}$Cu; beta and positron emitter with a half-life of 12.82 hours.

**copper-67.** $^{67}$Cu; beta and gamma emitter with a half-life of 59 hours.

**cop'peras.** Impure commercial variety of ferrous sulfate, *q.v.*

**copperhead.** A poisonous snake of the genus *Denisonia* in Australia and *Agkistrodon* in the United States.

**Coppet** (kŏ-pa'), Louis C. de, French physicist, 1841–1911. See C.'s *law*.

**coprem'esis** [ G. *kopros*, dung, + emesis ]. Fecal *vomiting*.

**copro-** [ G. *kopros*, dung ]. Combining form meaning filth or dung, usually used in referring to feces.

**cop'roan'tibodies.** Antibodies occurring in the intestinal content; they probably are formed by plasma cells in the intestinal mucosa and consist chiefly of the IgA class.

**coprolag'nia** [ copro- + G. *lagneia*, lust ]. A form of sexual perversion in which the thought or sight of excrement causes pleasurable sensation.

**coprola'lia** [ copro- + G. *lalia*, talk ]. The involuntary utterance of vulgar or obscene words.

**cop'rolith** [ copro- + G. *lithos*, stone ]. A hard mass consisting of inspissated feces.

**coprol'ogy** [ copro- + G. *logos*, study ]. Scatology.

**copro'ma** [ copro- + G. suffix, -*ōma*, tumor ]. Scatoma; fecaloma; stercoroma; a fecal mass; an accumulation of inspissated feces in the colon or rectum giving the appearance of an abdominal tumor.

**Cop'romas'tix prowazek'i.** A fecal protozoan flagellate.

**Coprom'onas subti'lis.** A fecal protozoan flagellate.

**coprophagous** (ko-prof'a-gus). Feeding on excrement.

**coprophagy** (kop-rof'a-jī) [ copro- + G. *phagein*, to eat ]. The eating of human or animal excrement.

**cop'rophil, coprophil'ic.** 1. Denoting bacteria, protozoa, etc. occurring in fecal matter. 2. Relating to coprophilia.

**coprophil'ia** [ copro- + G. *philos*, fond ]. 1. Attraction of microorganisms for fecal matter. 2. In psychiatry, a morbid attraction to, and love for (with a sexual element) fecal matter.

**cop'ropho'bia** [ copro- + G. *phobos*, fear ]. Morbid fear of defecation and feces.

**cop'rophra'sia.** Coprolalia.

**coproplanesia** (kop-ro-plan-e'sī-ah) [ copro- + G. *planesis*, a wandering ]. The passage of feces through a fistula or artificial anus.

**coproporphyrin** (kop'ro-por'fi-rin). One of two porphyrin compounds found normally in feces as a decomposition product of bilirubin (hence, from hemoglobin); excreted in urine in a metabolic disorder known as coproporphyrinuria.

**coprostane.** $5\beta$-Cholestane, the parent hydrocarbon of coprosterol. For structure, see steroids.

**$3\beta$-copros'tanol.** Coprosterol.

***epi*-coprostanol.** $5\beta$-Cholestan-3α-ol. (For structure of cholestane, see steroids.)

**coprosta'sia** [ copro- + G. *stasis*, a standing ]. Constipation; costiveness; fecal impaction.

**coprostenol.** Allocholesterol.

**copros'terin.** Coprosterol.

**copros'terol.** $3\beta$-Coprostanol; $5\beta$-cholestan-5$\beta$-cholastan-3$\beta$-ol; a sterol of the feces produced by the reduction of cholesterol. For structure, see steroids.

***epi*-coprosterol.** *epi*-Coprostanol.

**coprostigmastane.** $5\beta$-Stigmastane.

**coprozoa** (kop-ro-zo'ah) [ copro- + G. *zōon*, animal ]. Protozoa that can be cultivated in fecal matter, although not necessarily living in feces within the intestine.

**coprozoic** (kop-ro-zo'ik). Relating to coprozoa; coprophil.

**coptosis** [ G. *kopto*, to tire, + suffix *osis*, condition ]. The state of perpetual fatigue.

**cop'ula** [ L. a bond, tie ]. 1. Zygote. 2. An infrequently used term for complement-fixing antibody. 3. In anatomy, a narrow part connecting two structures, *e.g.*, the body of the hyoid bone; the hypobranchial eminence.

His' c., hypobranchial *eminence*.

c. linguae, hypobranchial *eminence*.

**copula'tion** [ L. *copulatio*, a joining, fr. prec. ]. 1. Coitus; sexual intercourse; sexual union between two individuals, male and female. 2. In protozoology, conjugation between two cells that do not fuse but separate after mutual fertilization; observed in the infusoria.

**coq.** Abbreviation for L. *coque*, imperative of *coquo*, to cook, boil.

**coquille** (ko-kēl) [ Fr. ]. A spherical curved lens of uniform thickness.

**cor,** gen. **cordis** [ L. ] [ NA ]. Heart.

c. adipo'sum, adiposis cardiaca; fatty heart (2); accumulation of adipose tissue beneath the visceral pericardium, associated with obesity.

c. bilocula're, a heart in which the interatrial and interventricular septa are absent or incomplete.

c. bovi'num, bucardia.

c. hirsu'tum, fibrinous *pericarditis*.

c. mobile, movable heart; a heart that moves unduly on change of bodily position.

c. pendulum, pendulous heart; an extreme form of c. mobile in which the heart appears to be suspended by the great vessels.

c. pulmona'le, (1) chronic cor pulmonale: hypertrophy of the right ventricle resulting from disease of the lungs, except for lung changes in diseases that primarily affect the left side of the heart and excluding congenital heart diease; (2) acute cor pulmonale: dilation and failure of the right side of the heart due to pulmonary embolism.

c. tomento'sum, fibrinous *pericarditis*.

c. triatria'tum, accessory atrium; a heart with three atrial chambers, the left atrium being subdivided by a transverse septum with a single small opening which separates the openings of the pulmonary veins from the mitral valve.

c. trilocula're, three-chambered heart due to absence of the interatrial or of the interventricular septum.

c. trilocula're biatria'tum, absence of the interventricular septum.

c. trilocula're biventricula're, absence of the interatrial septum.

c. villo'sum, fibrinous *pericarditis*.

**coracidium** (ko-rā-sid'ī-um). The ciliated first-stage aquatic embryo of pseudophyllid and other cestodes with aquatic cycles. Within the ciliated embryophore is a hooked larva, the hexacanth, that develops in the intermediate host, usually an aquatic crustacean, into the next larval stage, the procercoid.

**coracoacromial** (kor'ă-ko-ă-kro'mĭ-al). Acromiocoracoid; relating to the coracoid and acromial processes.

**coracobrachialis** (kor'ă-ko-bra-kĭ-a'lis). Relating to the coracoid process of the scapula and the arm. See also *musculus* coracobrachialis.

**cor'acoclavic'ular.** Relating to the coracoid process and the clavicle.

**cor'acohu'meral.** Relating to the coracoid process and the humerus.

**cor'acoid** [ G. *korakōdēs*, like a crow's beak, fr. *korax*, raven, + *eidos*, appearance ]. Shaped like a crow's beak; denoting a process of the scapula.

**cor'acoidi'tis.** Inflammation of the coracoid process.

**cor'allin.** Aurin.
    **red c.,** peony red; peonin; produced from c. by the action of ammonia.

**cord-.** For words beginning thus, not found here, see chord-.

**cord** [ L. *chorda*, a string ]. 1. In anatomy, any long, rope-like structure. 2. To become corded or stringlike, or having the appearance of a cord.
    **Bergmann's c.'s,** *striae* medullares ventriculi quarti.
    **Billroth's c.'s.,** splenic c.'s.
    **condyle c.,** condylar *axis.*
    **dental c.,** an aggregation of epithelial cells forming the rudimentary enamel organ.
    **false vocal c.,** *plica* vestibularis.
    **Ferrein's c.'s,** *plica* vocalis.
    **gan'gliated c.,** *truncus* sympathicus.
    **genital c.,** one of a pair of mesenchymal ridges bulging into the caudal part of the celom of a young embryo and containing the mesonephric (Wolffian) and Müllerian duct.
    **germinal c.'s,** the ovigerous c.'s of the embryonic ovary or the primordial seminiferous tubules of the embryonic testis.
    **hepatic c.'s,** liver laminae as seen in sections.
    **lateral c. of brachial plexus,** *fasciculus* lateralis plexus brachialis.
    **medial c. of brachial plexus,** *fasciculus* medialis plexus brachialis.
    **medullary c.'s,** (1) the c.'s of dense lymphoid tissue between the sinuses in the medulla of a lymph node; (2) the primordial cell c.'s in the medulla of the embryonic gonad from which the rete testis is formed in the male and the rete ovarii in the female.
    **nephrogenic c.,** the definitive connecting stalk between the embryo or fetus and the placenta; at birth it consists of loose mesenchyme (Wharton's jelly) in which are embedded the umbilical vessels.
    **oblique c.,** *chorda* obliqua.
    **ovigerous c.'s,** columns of cells growing into the ovarian stroma from the germinal epithelium and giving rise to ova and ovarian (Graafian) follicles.
    **posterior c. of brachial plexus,** *fasciculus* posterior plexus brachialis.
    **psalte'rial c.,** *stria* vascularis ductus cochlearis.
    **red pulp c.'s,** splenic c.'s.
    **rete c.'s,** primordial cell c.'s in the embryonic gonads that become the rete testes of the male and the rete ovarii of the female.
    **sex c.'s,** germinal c.'s.
    **spermatic c.,** *funiculus* spermaticus.
    **spinal c.,** *medulla* spinalis.
    **splenic c.'s,** red pulp c.'s; Billroth's c.'s; the tissue occurring between the venous sinuses in the spleen.
    **tendinous c.'s,** *chordae* tendineae.
    **testicular c.,** *funiculus* spermaticus.
    **testis c.'s,** the germinal c.'s of the embryonic testis.
    **umbil'ical c.,** *funiculus* umbilicalis.
    **vocal c.,** *plica* vocalis.
    **Weitbrecht's c.,** *chorda* obliqua.
    **Wilde's c.'s,** transverse markings on the corpus callosum.
    **Willis' c.'s,** chordae willisii; several fibrous c.'s crossing the superior sagittal sinus.

**cord'abrasion.** Abrasion of vocal cords to remove lesions.

**cordate.** Heart-shaped.

**cordec'tomy** [ G. *chordē*, cord, + *ektomē*, excision ]. Excision of a cord.

**cordial** (kor'dĭ-al, kor'jul). A sweet aromatic liquor.

**cordi'anine.** Allantoin.

**cor'diform** [ L. *cor* (*cord-*), heart, + *forma*, shape ]. Heart-shaped.

**cor'dis** [ gen. of L. *cor*, heart ]. Of the heart.

**cord'opexy** [ G. *chordē*, cord, + *pēxis*, fixation ]. The operative fixation of any displaced anatomical cord; specifically the fixation to one side of one or both vocal cords for the relief of laryngeal stenosis.

**cordot'omy** [ G. *chordē*, cord, + *tomē*, a cutting ]. Chordotomy; anterolateral, spinal, or spinothalamic tractotomy; division of tracts of the spinal cord, usually of the anterolateral quadrant; may be performed percutaneously (stereotactic c.) or after laminectomy (open c.) by various techniques such as incision or radiofrequency coagulation.

**cordy'cepin.** 3'-Deoxyadenosine; 9-cordyceposidoadenine; a crystalline antibiotic obtained from *Cordyceps militaris.* Active against strains of *Bacillus subtilis* and certain mycobacteria.

**core-, coreo-, coro-** [ G. *korē*, pupil ]. Combining forms relating to the pupil.

**core** [ L. *cor*, heart ]. 1. The central mass of necrotic tissue in a boil. 2. A metal casting, usually with a post in the canal of a root, designed to retain an artificial crown. 3. A sectional record, usually of plaster of Paris or one of its derivatives, of the relationships of parts, such as teeth, metallic restorations, or copings.
    **atomic c.,** the nucleus plus the nonvalence electrons.
    **central transactional c.,** the reticular activating system of the brain.

**corecleisis, coreclisis** (kor-e-kli'sis) [ G. *korē*, pupil, + *kleisis*, a closing ]. Occlusion of the pupil.

**corecta'sia, corec'tasis** [ G. *korē*, pupil, + *ektasis*, a stretching out ]. Pathologic dilation of the pupil.

**corec'tomedial'ysis** [ G. *korē*, pupil, + *ektomē*, excision, + *dialysis*, a loosening ]. A peripheral iridectomy to form an artificial pupil.

**corecto'pia** [ G. *korē*, pupil, + *ektopos*, out of place ]. Presence of the pupil to one side of the center of the iris.

**coredias'tasis** [ G. *kore*, pupil, + *diastasis*, a separation ]. A dilated state of the pupil.

**corelysis** (ko-re-li'sis) [ G. *korē*, pupil, + *lysis*, a loosening ]. The loosening of adhesions between the capsule of the lens and the iris.

**coremor'phosis** [ G. *korē*, pupil, + *morphōsis*, formation ]. The formation of an artificial pupil.

**coreom'eter** [ G. *korē*, pupil, + *metron*, measure ]. Obsolete term for pupillometer.

**coreom'etry.** Obsolete term for pupillometry.

**cor'eoplasty** [ G. *korē*, pupil, + *plassō*, to form ]. Coroplasty; the reestablishment of an occluded, or correction of a deformed, pupil.

**corepex'y** [ G. *korē*, pupil, + *pēxis*, a fixing in place ]. Corepraxy.

**coreprax'y** [ G. *korē*, pupil, + *praxis*, action ]. Corepexy; an operation to centralize an eccentric pupil.

**co'repres'sor.** A molecule, usually a product of a specific enzyme pathway, that combines with inactive repressor (produced by a regulator gene) to form active repressor, which then attaches to an operator gene site and inhibits activity of the structure genes controlled by the operator; a homeostatic mechanism for regulating enzyme production in repressible enzyme systems.

**corestenoma** (kor-e-stě-no'mah) [ G. *korē*, pupil, + *stenōma*, a narrow pass ]. A narrowing of the pupil.
    **c. congen'itum,** a partial occlusion of the pupil by congenital outgrowths from the sphincter margin.

**Corey,** R. B., U. S. chemist, *1897. See Pauling-C. *helix.*

**Cori** (kor'e), Carl F., U. S. biochemist, *1896. Nobel laureate, 1947, with Gerty T. Cori, for their discovery of the course of the catalytic conversion of glycogen. See C. *cycle, ester.*

**Cori,** Gerty Theresa, U. S. biochemist, 1896–1957. Nobel laureate, 1947, with Carl F. Cori. See C.'s *disease.*

**coriamyrtin** (ko-re-am'ur-tin). A bitter principle, $C_{15}H_{18}O_5$, from *Coriaria myrtifolin* and *C. japonica* (family Coriaraceae); a convulsant resembling picrotoxin. Has been used as a central nervous system stimulant.

**co'rian'der** (BP). The dried ripe fruit of *Coriandrum sativum* (family Umbelliferae). A mild stimulant aromatic; used as a flavoring agent.

  **c. oil** (USP, BP), a volatile oil distilled from c.; a flavor.

  **powdered c.** (BP), used for flavor.

**coring.** A metallurgical phenomenon occurring during the formation of alloys; a similar event takes place during the setting of certain gels. It is of interest in dentistry because so many different alloys are used and silicate cements are believed to set by means of the formation of a gel structure. It also occurs during the formation of certain gels such as the setting of silicate cements used in dentistry.

**co'rium,** pl. **co'ria** [ L. skin, hide, leather ] [ NA ]. Dermis; cutis vera; enderon; it is composed of a superficial, thin layer that interdigitates with the epidermis, the stratum papillare, and a deeper thick layer of dense, irregular connective tissue, the stratum reticulare. The c. contains blood and lymphatic vessels, nerves and nerve endings, glands, and, except for glabrous skin, hair follicles.

**Corium**

Section of thin skin, with portion of tela subcutanea

  **c. coro'nae** [ NAV ], coronary *band*.

  **c. lim'bi** [ NAV ], periople.

  **c. pari'etis** [ NAV ], the wall of the pododerm, *q.v.*

  **c. so'lae** [ NAV ], the sole of the pododerm, *q.v.*

**Corlett,** William T., American dermatologist, 1854–1948. See C.'s *pyosis.*

**corm** [ G. *kormos,* tree trunk without boughs ]. A solid, thick, erect underground stem of plants, *e.g.,* colchicum.

**corn** [ L. *cornu,* horn, hoof ]. 1. Clavus (1). 2. A small inflammatory focus under the sole of the hoof of the horse usually between the bar and the wall. The forefeet are most often affected. It is sometimes seen in other hoofed animals.

  **asbestos c.,** asbestos wart; a granulomatous or hyperkeratotic lesion of the skin at the site of deposit of asbestos particles.

  **hard c.,** heloma durum; the usual form of c. over a toe joint.

  **seed c.,** a papilloma or wart on the sole of the foot.

  **soft c.,** heloma molle; a c. formed by pressure between two toes, the surface being macerated and yellowish in color.

**cor'nea** [ L. fem. of *corneus,* horny, sc. *tunica, coat* ] [ NA ]. A transparent membrane, forming the anterior sixth of the outer coat of the eyeball; it is more curved (*i.e.,* is a segment of a smaller sphere. It consists of thin, stratified, squamous epithelium, substantia propria mainly of collagen, and an inner endothelium.

  **conical c.,** keratoconus.

  **c. farina'ta,** a bilateral type of degenerative change in the deep stroma of the c. of the elderly; marked by fine, dustlike opacities.

  **c. gutta'ta,** *dystrophia* endothelialis corneae.

  **c. pla'na congen'ita familia'res,** a form of c. flatter than normal.

  **c. verticilla'ta,** congenital whorl-like opacities in the c.

**cor'neal.** Relating to the cornea.

**cor'neobleph'aron** [ cornea + G. *blepharon,* eyelid ]. Attachment of the lid margin to the cornea.

**corneosclera** (kor'ne-o-skle'rah). The combined cornea and sclera when considered as forming the external coat of the eyeball.

**cor'neoscle'ral.** Pertaining to, or denoting simultaneous involvement of, the cornea and sclera.

**cor'neous** [ L. corneus, fr. *cornu,* horn ]. Horny.

**Corner,** Edred M., English surgeon, 1873–1950. See C.'s *tampon.*

**Corner,** George W., American anatomist, *1889. See C.-Allen *test, unit.*

**corners** (kor'nerz). The deciduous incisors of the horse external to the intermediates; the outermost of the three incisors.

**cor'neum** [ L., ntr. of *corneus,* horny, fr. *cornu,* horn ]. *Stratum* corneum.

**cornic'ulate** [ L. *corniculatus,* horned ]. 1. Resembling a horn. 2. Having horns or horn-shaped appendages.

**cornicula'tus** [ L. ] [ NA ]. Corniculate.

**cornic'ulum** [ L. dim. of *cornu,* horn ]. A cornu of small size.

  **c. laryn'gis,** *cartilago* corniculata.

**cornifica'tion** [ L. *cornu,* horn, + *facio,* to make ]. Keratinization.

**cornified.** Keratinized.

**corn oil** (USP). Maise oil (BP); maize oil; the refined fixed oil expressed from the embryo of *Zea mays* (family Gramineae); a solvent.

**cor'nu,** gen. **cor'nus,** pl. **cor'nua** [ L. horn ]. A horn. 1 [ NA ]. Any structure resembling a horn in shape. 2. Any structure composed of horny substance. 3. One of the coronal extensions of the dental pulp underlying a cusp or lobe. 4. The major subdivisions of the lateral ventricle in the cerebral hemisphere (the frontal horn, occipital horn, and temporal horn); see also *ventriculus* lateralis.

  **c. ammo'nis,** see hippocampus.

  **c. ante'rius** [ NA ], anterior horn; ventral horn; (1) the anterior or frontal division of the lateral ventricle of the brain, extending forward from Monro's interventricular foramen (see *ventriculus* lateralis); (2) the anterior or ventral gray column of the spinal cord as appearing in cross section (see also *columna* anterior; *columnae* griseae).

  **c. coccy'geum** [ NA ], coccygeal c.; one of two processes that project upward from the dorsum of the base of the coccyx.

  **c. cuta'neum,** cutaneous *horn.*

  **c. huma'num,** cutaneous *horn.*

  **c. infe'rius** [ NA ], inferior horn; underhorn; (1) c. inferius cartilaginis thyroideae [ NA ], inferior horn of the thyroid cartilage; one of the pair of downward prolongations at the back of the thyroid cartilage; it articulates on each side with the cricoid cartilage; (2) c. inferius marginis falciformis [ NA ], inferior horn of the saphenous opening; the lower part of the falciform margin of the opening in the fascia lata through which the greater saphenous vein passes; (3) c. inferius ventriculi lateralis [ NA ], the inferior division of the lateral ventricle of the brain extending downward and forward into the medial part of the temporal lobe (see *ventriculus* lateralis).

  **cornua of lateral ventricle,** see c. anterius (1), c. inferius (3), c. posterius (1).

**c. latera'le** [ NA ], lateral horn; the small lateral gray column of the spinal cord as appearing in transverse section; see also *columna* lateralis; *columnae* griseae.

**c. ma'jus** [ NA ], greater horn; the larger and more lateral of of the two processes on either side of the hyoid bone.

**c. mi'nus** [ NA ], lesser horn; styloid c.; the shorter and more medial of the two processes on either side of the hyoid bone.

**c. poste'rius** [ NA ], posterior horn; dorsal horn; (1) the posterior or occipital division of the lateral ventricle of the brain, extending backward into the occipital lobe (see *ventriculus* lateralis); (2) the posterior gray column of the spinal cord as appearing in cross section (see also *columna* posterior; *columnae* griseae).

**c. sacra'le** [ NA ], sacral horn; the most caudal part of the intermediate sacral crest. On each side it forms the lateral margin of the sacral hiatus and articulates with the coccygeal c.

**cornua of saphenous opening,** c. inferius (2); c. superius (2).

**cornua of spinal cord,** see c. anterius (2), c. laterale, c. posterius (2).

**styloid c.,** c. minus.

**c. supe'rius** [ NA ], (1) c. superius cartilaginis thyroideae [ NA ], superior horn of the thyroid cartilage; one of the pair of upward prolongations from the thyroid cartilage to which the lateral hyothyroid ligament attaches; (2) c. superius marginis falciformis [ NA ], superior horn of the saphenous opening; the upper part of the falciform margin of the opening in the fascia lata through which the greater saphenous vein passes.

**cornua of thyroid cartilage,** c. inferius (1); c. superius (1).

**cor'nua.** Plural of cornu.

**cor'nual.** Relating to a cornu.

**cornus** [ L. *cornus*, the cornel cherry-tree ]. The dried bark of the root of *Cornus florida* (family Cornaceae), dogwood. A feeble, astringent bitter.

**coro-** [ G. *korē*, pupil ]. Combining form relating to the pupil. For words beginning thus and not found here, see also those beginning core- and coreo-.

**corom'eter.** Obsolete synonym for pupillometer.

**coro'na,** pl. **coro'nae** [ L. garland, crown, fr. G. *korōnē*. CORON- ] [ NA ]. Any structure, normal or pathologic, resembling or suggesting a crown or a wreath.

**c. cap'itis,** crown of the head; the topmost part of the head.

**c. cilia'ris** [ NA ], ciliary crown or wreath; the circular figure on the inner surface of the ciliary body, formed by the processes and folds (plicae) taken together.

**c. clin'ica** [ NA ], clinical crown; that part of the crown of a tooth visible in the oral cavity.

**c. dentis** [ NA ], crown of a tooth; anatomical crown; the portion of a tooth covered with enamel.

**c. glandis** [ NA ], the prominent posterior border of the glans penis.

**c. radia'ta,** radiate crown; (1) [ NA ], a fan-shaped fiber mass on the white matter of the cerebral cortex, composed of the widely radiating fibers of the internal capsule; (2) an investment of the oocyte, composed of several layers of epithelial cells derived from the cumulus oophorus of the ovarian (Graafian) follicle.

**c. seborrhe'ica,** a red band at the hair line along the upper border of the forehead and temples occasionally observed in seborrheic dermatitis involving the scalp.

**c. vene'ris,** papular syphilitic lesions (secondary eruption) along the anterior margin of the scalp or on the back of the neck.

**Zinn's c.,** *circulus* vasculosus nervi optici.

**cor'onad.** In a direction toward any corona.

**cor'onal.** Relating to a corona.

**coronale** (kor-o-na'le) [ L. neuter of *coronalis*, pertaining to a *corona*, crown ]. 1. *Os* frontale. 2. One of the two most widely separated points on the coronal suture at the poles of the greatest frontal diameter.

**corona'lis** [ NA ]. Coronal; referring to the coronal plane.

**corona'ria.** A coronary artery, of the heart.

**cor'onarism** [ coronary (artery) + -*ism* ]. Coronary insufficiency; *angina* pectoris.

**cor'onari'tis.** Inflammation of coronary artery or arteries.

**cor'onary** [ L. *coronarius;* fr. *corona*, a crown ]. 1. Relating to or resembling a crown. 2. Encircling; denoting various anatomical structures.

**coro'navi'rus.** See under virus.

**cor'oner** [ L. *corona*, a crown ]. An official whose duty it is to investigate sudden, suspicious, or violent death to determine the cause. In some communities in the United States the office has been replaced by that of medical examiner.

**coronet** [ Fr. *coronette;* L. *corona*, crown ]. The line of junction between the skin and the hoof or claw.

**coro'nion** [ G. *korōnē*, crow ]. The tip of the coronoid process of the mandible; a craniometric point.

**coroni'tis.** Inflammation of the coronary band of the horse's hoof, resulting in imperfect horn formation.

**cor'onoid** [ G. *korōnē*, a crow, + *eidos*, resembling ]. Shaped like a crow's beak; denoting certain processes and other parts of bones.

**cor'onoidec'tomy** [ coronoid, *q.v.*, + G. *ektomē*, excision ]. The surgical removal of the coronoid process of the mandible.

**cor'oparel'cysis** (ko'ro-par-el'si-sis) [ G. *korē*, pupil, + *parelkō*, to draw aside ]. An operation for displacing the pupil to one side in cases of central corneal opacity.

**cor'oplasty.** Coreoplasty.

**coros'copy** [ G. *korē*, pupil, + *skopeō*, to view ]. Obsolete synonym for retinoscopy.

**corot'omy.** Iridotomy.

**cor'pora.** Plural of corpus.

**corpo'real.** Pertaining to the body, or to a corpus.

**cor'porin.** Obsolete term for corpus luteum hormone.

**corpse** [ L. *corpus*, body ]. A dead body; cadaver.

**corps ronds** (kor-roń') [ Fr. round bodies ]. Dyskeratotic cells occurring in the prickle cell layer. These are characteristically found in keratosis follicularis.

**cor'pulence, cor'pulency** [ L. *corpulentia*, magnification of *corpus*, body ]. Obesity; fatness.

# CORPUS

**corpus,** gen. **cor'poris,** pl. **cor'pora** [ L. body ] [ NA ]. 1. The human body, consisting of head (caput), neck (collum), trunk (truncus), and limbs (membra). 2. Any body or mass. 3. The main part of an organ or other anatomical structure, as distinguished from the caput (head) or cauda (tail). See also body and soma.

**c. adipo'sum buccae** [ NA ], sucking pad or cushion; Bichat's fat-pad; fat body of the cheek; an encapsuled mass of fat in the cheek on the outer side of the buccinator muscle, especially marked in the infant; supposed to strengthen and support the cheek during the act of sucking.

**c. adipo'sum fossae ischiorecta'lis** [ NA ], fat body of the ischiorectal fossa; the fat within the ischiorectal fossa. It is traversed by the inferior rectal vessels and nerves.

**c. adipo'sum infrapatella're** [ NA ], infrapatellar fat body; the fatty mass that occupies the area between the patellar ligament and the patellar synovial fold of the knee joint.

**c. adipo'sum or'bitae** [ NA ], fat body of the orbit; a mass of fat contained in the orbit.

**c. albicans** [ NA ], atretic c. luteum; c. candicans; a retrogressed c. luteum characterized by increasing cicatrization and shrinkage of the cicatricial core with an amorphous, convoluted, completely hyalinized lutein zone surrounding the central plug of scar tissue.

**corpora alla'ta,** a pair of endocrine glands which are located near the brain in insects and which produce juvenile hormone; when there is a high concentration at the time of molting another larval stage will result; removal at an early larval stage causes pupation and the formation of a midget adult; implantation at late larval stages can result in very large adults. The action of the juvenile hormone is interrelated with that of brain hormone and ecdysone.

c. amygdaloi'deum [ NA ], amygdala (1); amygdaloid nucleus; nucleus amygdalae; almond nucleus; amygdaloid complex; a rounded mass of gray matter in the anterior portion of the temporal lobe of the cerebrum, underneath the olfactory cortex of the uncus, immediately anterior to the inferior horn of the lateral ventricle; its major efferent fiber connections are with the hypothalamus and mediodorsal nucleus of the thalamus; it is also reciprocally associated with the cortex of the temporal lobe.

c. amyla'ceum, pl. cor'pora amyla'cea, one of a number of small, ovoid or rounded bodies, sometimes laminated, resembling a grain of starch, found in nervous tissue, in the prostate, and in pulmonary alveoli; of little pathological significance; apparently derived from degenerated cells or proteinaceous secretions. Also called amniotic, amylaceous, amyloid, or colloid corpuscle.

c. aorticum, aortic *body*.

corpora arantii, *nodulus* valvulae semilunaris.

corpora arena'cea, psammoma *bodies* (1).

atret'ic c. lu'teum, c. albicans.

c. atret'icum, atretic ovarian *follicle*.

corpora bigem'ina, bigeminal bodies; a bilateral single swelling of the roofplate of the embryonic midbrain that later in development becomes subdivided into a superior and an inferior colliculus.

c. callo'sum [ NA ], commissure of the cerebral hemispheres; the great commissural plate of nerve fibers interconnecting the cortical hemispheres (with the exception of most of the temporal lobes which are interconnected by the anterior commissure). Lying at the bottom of the longitudinal fissure, and covered on each side by the gyrus cinguli, it is arched from behind forward and is thick at each extremity (splenium and genu) but thinner in its long central portion (truncus); it curves back underneath itself at the genu to form the rostrum of the corpus callosum.

c. can'dicans, c. albicans.

c. caverno'sum clitor'idis [ NA ], cavernous body of the clitoris; one of the two parallel columns of erectile tissue forming the body of the clitoris; they diverge at the root to form the crura of the clitoris.

c. caverno'sum conchae, *plexus* cavernosi concharum.

c. caverno'sum penis [ NA ], cavernous body of the penis one of two parallel columns of erectile tissue forming the dorsal part of the body of the penis; they are separated posteriorly, forming the crura of the penis.

c. caverno'sum ure'thrae, c. spongiosum penis.

c. cepifor'me, pl. corpora cepiformia [ L. *cepa*, onion, + *forma*, form ], a multilayered, encapsulated body seen with the electron microscope.

c. cilia're [ NA ], ciliary body; a thickened portion of the tunica vasculosa of the eye between the choroid and the iris; it consists of three parts or zones; orbiculus ciliaris, corona ciliaris, and musculus ciliaris.

c. clitoridis [ NA ], the body of the clitoris.

c. coccy'geum [ NA ], coccygeal body; glomus coccygeum; arteriococcygeal gland; an arteriovenous (arteriolovenular) anastomosis supplied by the middle sacral artery and located on the pelvic surface of the coccyx. It was formerly called a gland (of Luschka) or a glomus and included with the paraganglia.

c. costae [ NA ], the body of a rib.

c. denta'tum, *nucleus* dentatus cerebelli.

c. epididym'idis [ NA ], body of the epididymis; the middle part that extends downward from the head to the tail of the epididymis on the posterior surface of the testis.

c. fem'oris [ NA ], the shaft of the femur.

c. fibro'sum, the small, fibrous mass (scar) in the ovary which is formed following the atresia of an ovarian follicle; it is similar to a corpus albicans but smaller.

c. fibulae [ NA ], the shaft of the fibula.

c. fimbria'tum [ L. *fimbriatus*, fringed ], (1) *fimbria* hippocampi; (2) the outer, ovarian, extremity of the oviduct.

c. fornicis [ NA ], body of the fornix; the middle part of the fornix situated beneath the corpus callosum.

c. genicula'tum externum, c. geniculatum laterale.

c. genicula'tum internum, c. geniculatum mediale.

c. genicula'tum latera'le [ NA ], lateral geniculate body; c. geniculatum externum; the lateral one of a pair of small oval masses that protrude slightly from the posteroinferior

aspects of the thalamus. The main (dorsal) subdivision of the lateral geniculate body serves as a processing ("relay") station in the major pathway from the retina to the cerebral cortex, receiving fibers from the optic tract and giving rise to the geniculocalcarine radiation to the visual cortex in the occipital lobe.

c. genicula'tum media'le [ NA ], c. geniculatum internum; medial geniculate body; the medial one of a pair of prominent cell groups in the posteroinferior parts of the thalamus; it functions as the last of a series of processing stations along the auditory conduction pathway to the cerebral cortex, receiving the brachium of the inferior colliculus and giving rise to the auditory radiation to the auditory cortex in the superior temporal gyrus.

c. glan'dulae sudorif'erae [ NA ], body of a sweat gland; the coiled tubular portion of a sweat gland located in the subcutaneous tissue or deep in the corium and connected to the surface of the skin by a long duct.

c. hemorrhag'icum, c. luteum hematoma; the lining of such hematomas is formed by the thinned-out bright yellow lutein zone. The gradual resorption of the blood elements may take many weeks, leaving a cavity filled with a clear fluid, *i.e.*, a. c. luteum cyst.

c. high'mori, c. highmoria'num, *mediastinum* testis.

c. hu'meri [ NA ], shaft of the humerus.

c. in'cudis [ NA ], body of the incus; the main part of the incus that articulates with the malleus and from which the short and long limbs arise.

c. lin'guae [ NA ], body of the tongue; the oral part of the tongue anterior to the terminal sulcus.

c. lu'teum [ NA ], the yellow endocrine body formed in the ovary in the site of a ruptured ovarian follicle. The life history of the c. luteum begins immediately after ovulation. There is an early stage of proliferation or hyperemia and of vascularization before full maturity. There is a festooned and bright yellowish lutein zone, traversed by trabeculae of theca interna containing numerous blood vessels. The structure measures 1 to 1.5 cm. in diameter. If pregnancy does not occur, it is called a c. luteum spurium, which undergoes progressive retrogression to a c. albicans. Although the c. luteum secretes an estrogenic hormone, it elaborates a second hormone known as progesterone which is much more characteristic of it. In the event of pregnancy, the c. luteum verum becomes even larger and persists to the 5th or 6th month of pregnancy before beginning to retrogress.

c. luysi, *nucleus* subthalamicus.

c. mamilla're [ NA ], mamillary body; mamillary tubercle of hypothalamus; a small, round, paired cell group that protrudes into the interpeduncular fossa from the inferior aspect of the hypothalamus. It receives a major bundle of hippocampal fibers from the fornix and projects fibers to the anterior thalamic nuclei and into the tegmentum of the brainstem.

c. mam'mae [ NA ], body of the mammary gland; the principal part of the breast, consisting of glandular tissue and its supporting fibrous tissue. It forms a conical mass converging toward the nipple and is surrounded by adipose tissue.

c. mandib'ulae [ NA ], body of the mandible; the heavy, U-shaped, horizontal portion of the mandible extending posteriorly to the angle where it is continuous with the ramus; it supports the lower teeth.

c. maxil'lae [ NA ], body of the maxilla; the central portion of the maxilla hollowed out by the maxillary sinus; it presents orbital, nasal, anterior, and infratemporal surfaces and supports four process, frontal, zygomatic, palatine, and alveolar.

c. medulla're cerebel'li [ NA ], the interior white substance of the cerebellum.

c. nu'clei cauda'ti [ NA ], that part of the caudate nucleus lying in the floor of the central part of the lateral ventricle.

c. oliva're, oliva.

c. oryzoid'eum, rice *body*.

c. ossis hyoi'dei [ NA ], the body of the hyoid bone.

c. ossis ilii [ NA ], body of the ilium; it forms the upper two-fifths of the acetabulum and joins the pubis and ischium in the acetabulum. It continues above into the ala or wing of the ilium.

c. ossis ischii [ NA ], body of the ischium; the entire ischium with the exception of the ramus.

**c. ossis metacarpa'lis** [ NA ], the shaft of one of the metacarpal bones.

**c. ossis pubis** [ NA ], body of the pubic bone; pubic body; the flattened medial portion of the pubic bone entering into the pubic symphysis. From it extend the superior and inferior rami.

**c. ossis sphenoida'lis** [ NA ], body of the sphenoid bone; the central portion of the sphenoid bone from which the greater and lesser wings and the pterygoid processes arise. The sphenoidal sinuses lie within it.

**c. pampinifor'me,** paroophoron.

**c. pancre'atis** [ NA ], body of the pancreas; the part of the pancreas from the point where it crosses the portal vein to the point where it enters the lienorenal ligament.

**c. papilla're** *stratum* papillare corii.

**cor'pora paraaor'tica** [ NA ], paraaortic bodies; organs of Zuckerkandl; Zuckerkandl's bodies; small masses of chromaffin tissue found near the sympathetic ganglia along the abdominal aorta; they are more prominent during fetal life.

**c. paratermina'le,** *gyrus* subcallosus.

**c. pe'nis** [ NA ], body of the penis; scapus penis; the free pendulous portion of the penis.

**c. phalangis** [ NA ], body of the phalanx; the shaft of each phalanx of the hand or foot.

**c. pinea'le** [ NA ], pineal body; pineal gland; conarium; epiphysis cerebri; a small, unpaired, flattened body, shaped somewhat like a pine cone (whence two of its names), attached at its anterior pole to the region of the posterior and habenular commissures, and lying in the depression between the two superior colliculi below the splenium of the corpus callosum. It is a glandular structure, composed of follicles containing epithelioid cells and lime concretions called brain sand. Despite its attachment to the brain, it appears to receive nerve fibers exclusively from the peripheral autonomic nervous system.

**c. pon'tobulba're,** a collection of nerve cells in the lower part of the medulla oblongata forming a ridge which crosses the restiform body obliquely.

**corpora quadrigemina,** quadrigeminal bodies; the *colliculus* inferior and *colliculus* superior, *q.v.;* four hemispherical elevations (a pair of superior and a pair of inferior colliculi) forming the roof of the mesencephalon.

**c. quadrigem'inum ante'rius,** *colliculus* superior.

**c. quadrigem'inum poste'rius,** *colliculus* inferior.

**c. radii** [ NA ], shaft of the radius; the triangular body of the radius located between the expanded proximal and distal extremities of the bone.

**c. restifor'me,** *pedunculus* cerebellaris inferior.

**c. spongio'sum penis** [ NA ], spongy body of the penis; the median column of erectile tissue located between and ventral to the two corpora cavernosa penis. Posteriorly it expands into the bulbus penis and anteriorly it terminates as the enlarged glans penis. It is traversed by the urethra.

**c. spongio'sum urethrae muliebris,** the submucous coat of the female urethra, containing a venous network that insinuates itself between the muscular layers, giving to them an erectile nature.

**c. sterni** [ NA ], body of the sternum; mesosternum; midsternum; gladiolus; the middle and largest portion of the sternum.

**c. stria'tum** [ NA ], striate body; the caudate and lentiform (lenticular) nuclei considered as one structure, a striate appearance on section being caused by slender fascicles of myelinated fibers. Histologically, the c. striatum can be subdivided into the generally small-celled striatum, consisting of the nucleus caudatus and the large outer segment of the lentiform nucleus (the putamen), and a large-celled pallidum composed of the two inner segments of the lentiform nucleus.

**c. ta'li** [ NA ], body of the talus; the large posterior part of the talus forming the trochlea above for articulation with the tibia and fibula and articulating below with the calcaneus.

**c. tib'iae** [ NA ], body of the tibia; the shaft of the tibia.

**c. trapezoid'eum** [ NA ], trapezoid (4); trapezoid body; a plate of transverse fibers running over the dorsal (deep) border of the pontine nuclei; it is formed by those fibers of the ascending auditory pathway that cross over to the opposite side of the brainstem.

**c. triti'ceum,** *cartilago* triticea.

**c. ul'nae** [ NA ], body of the ulna; the shaft of the ulna between the proximal extremity and the head.

**c. un'guis** [ NA ], body of the nail; the exposed portion of the nail distal to its root.

**c. u'teri** [ NA ], body of the uterus; the part of the uterus above the isthmus, comprising about two thirds of the non-pregnant organ.

**c. ventric'uli** [ NA ], body of the stomach; the part of the stomach that lies between the fundus above and the pyloric antrum below; its boundaries are poorly defined.

**c. ver'tebrae** [ NA ], body of a vertebra.

**c. ves'icae fel'leae** [ NA ], body of the gallbladder; the main part of the gallbladder terminating in the rounded fundus below and continuing into the neck of the gallbladder above.

**c. ves'icae urina'riae** [ NA ], body of the urinary bladder; the portion of the bladder between the apex and fundus.

**c. vit'reum** [ NA ], vitreous (2); vitreum; vitreous or hyaloid body; a transparent jelly-like substance filling the interior of the eyeball behind the lens of the eye; it is composed of a delicate network (vitreous stroma) enclosing in its meshes a watery fluid (vitreous humor), and surrounded by a membranous condensation of the stroma, the vitreous membrane. See also subentries under vitreous.

---

**corpuscle** (kor'pus-l) [ L. *corpusculum,* dim. of *corpus,* body. CORP- ]. 1. Corpusculum; any small mass or body. 2. A blood cell.

**amniot'ic c., amyla'ceous c., am'yloid c.,** *corpus* amylaceum.

**articular c.'s,** *corpuscula* articularia.

**axis c., axile c.,** the central portion of a tactile c.

**basal c.,** basal *body.*

**Bennet's c.'s,** large and small types, respectively identical to Nunn's gorged c.'s and Drysdale's c.'s; an obsolete eponym.

**Bizzozero's c.'s,** blood *platelets.*

**blood c.** blood *cell,* leukocyte or erythrocyte.

**bone c.,** bone *cell.*

**bridge c.,** desmosome.

**bulboid c.'s,** *corpuscula* bulboidea.

**cartilage c.,** chondrocyte.

**cement c.,** a cementocyte contained within a lacuna or crypt of the cementum of a tooth; an entrapped cementoblast.

**chyle c.,** a cell of the same appearance as a leukocyte, present in chyle.

**colloid c.,** *corpus* amylaceum.

**colostrum c.,** one of numerous bodies present in the colostrum; they are supposed to be modified leukocytes containing fat droplets; galactoblast.

**concentrated human red blood c.** (BP), prepared from one or more preparations of whole human blood which are not more than 14 days old and each of which has already been directly matched with the blood of the intended recipient.

**corneal c.'s,** Toynbee's c.'s; Virchow's c.'s; connective tissue cells found between the laminae of fibrous tissue in the cornea.

**Dogiel's c.,** an encapsulated sensory nerve ending.

**Donné's c.'s,** leukocytes containing fat droplets, found in colostrum.

**Drysdale's c.'s,** degenerated cells with a pyknotic nucleus and a large vacuole (frequently lipid) that occupies all or most of the cytoplasmic portion, observed in fluid from certain examples of ovarian cysts; an obsolete term.

**dust c.'s** hemoconia.

**Eichhorst's c.'s,** the globular forms sometimes occurring in the poikilocytosis of pernicious anemia.

**exudation c.,** inflammatory c.; plastic c.; exudation cell; a cell present in an exudate which assists in the organization of new tissue.

**genital c.'s,** *corpuscula* genitalia.

**ghost c.,** achromocyte.

**Gluge's c.'s,** large pus cells containing fat droplets.

**Golgi-Mazzoni c.,** an encapsulated sensory nerve ending similar to a Pacinian c. but simpler in structure.

**Grandry's c.'s,** general sensory endings in the beak, mouth, and tongue of birds; similar to Merkel's c.'s.

**Hassall's concentric c.'s,** Hassall's bodies; Virchow-Hassall bodies; thymus c.'s; small bodies of flattened epithelial cells arranged around a granular nucleated c., found in the medulla of the lobules of the thymus.

**Herbst's c.'s,** tactile c.'s, resembling Pacinian c.'s, but much smaller, found in birds.

**inflammatory c.,** exudation c.

**Key-Retzius c.'s,** tactile c.'s, resembling those of Pacini, found in the beak of certain aquatic birds.

**lam'ellated c.'s,** *corpuscula* lamellosa.

**lymph c., lymphat'ic c., lymphoid c.,** a mononuclear type of leukocyte formed in lymph nodes and other lymphoid tissue, and also in the blood.

**Malpighian c.,** (1) *corpusculum* renis; (2) *folliculus* lymphaticus lienalis.

**Mazzoni's c.,** a tactile c. apparently identical with Krause's end-bulb.

**Meissner's c.,** *corpusculum* tactus.

**Merkel's c.,** *meniscus* tactus.

**Mexican hat c.,** see target cell *anemia.*

**milk c.,** one of the fat droplets in milk.

**mollus'cum c.'s,** Paterson's c.'s; the degenerated cells containing the inclusion bodies (virus) causative of molluscum contagiosum.

**Negri c.'s,** Negri *bodies.*

**Norris' c.'s,** decolorized red blood cells that are invisible or almost invisible in the blood plasma, unless they are appropriately stained.

**Nunn's gorged c.'s,** an obsolete term designating epithelial cells observed in ovarian cysts, showing marked degeneration.

**oval c.,** *corpusculum* tactus.

**Pacinian c.'s,** *corpuscula* lamellosa.

**Paterson's c.'s,** molluscum c.'s.

**pessary c.,** an elongated red blood cell with hemoglobin concentrated in the peripheral portion.

**phantom c.,** achromocyte.

**plastic c.,** exudation c.

**Purkinje's c.'s,** Purkinje's *cells.*

**pus c.,** pyocyte; one of the polymorphonuclear leukocytes that comprise the chief portion of the formed elements in pus.

**Rainey's c.'s,** rounded, ovoidal, or sickle-shaped spores, 12 to 16 by 4 to 9 $\mu$, found within the elongated cysts (Meischer's tubes) of the protozoan *Sarcocystis.*

**red c.,** erythrocyte.

**renal c.,** *corpusculum* renis.

**reticulated c.,** reticulocyte.

**Ruffini's c.'s,** sensory end-structures in the subcutaneous connective tissues of the fingers, consisting of an ovoid capsule within which the sensory fiber ends with numerous collateral knobs.

**salivary c.,** one of the leukocytes present in saliva.

**Schwalbe's c.,** *caliculus* gustatorius.

**shadow c.,** achromocyte.

**splenic c.,** *folliculus* lymphaticus lienalis.

**tactile c.,** *corpusculum* tactus.

**taste c.,** *caliculus* gustatorius.

**terminal nerve c.'s,** *corpuscula* nervosa terminalia.

**third c.,** platelet.

**thymus c.,** Hassall's concentric c.

**touch c.,** *corpusculum* tactus.

**Toynbee's c.'s,** corneal c.'s.

**Traube's c.'s,** achromocyte.

**Tröltsch's c.'s,** minute spaces, resembling c.'s, between the radial fibers of the drum membrane of the ear.

**Valentin's c.'s,** small bodies, probably amyloid, found occasionally in nerve tissue.

**Vater's c.'s,** *corpuscula* lamellosa.

**Vater-Pacini c.'s,** *corpuscula* lamellosa.

**Virchow's c.'s,** corneal c.'s.

**white c.,** any type of leukocyte.

**Zimmermann's c.,** platelet.

**corpus'cula.** Plural of corpusculum.

**corpus'cular.** Relating to a corpuscle.

**corpus'culum,** pl. **corpus'cula** [ NA ]. Corpuscle; a small mass or body.

**corpuscula articula'ria** [ NA ], articular corpuscles; encapsulated nerve terminations within joint capsules.

**corpuscula bulboi'dea** [ NA ], end bulbs of Krause; bulboid corpuscles; nerve terminals in skin, mouth, conjunctiva, and other parts; they consist of a laminated capsule of connective tissue enclosing the terminal, branched, convoluted ending of an afferent nerve fiber. They are generally believed to be sensitive to cold.

**corpuscula genita'lia** [ NA ], genital corpuscles; special encapsulated nerve endings found in the skin of the genitalia and nipple.

**corpuscula lamello'sa** [ NA ], lamellated corpuscles (of Vater, of Herbst, or of Pacini); small oval bodies in the skin of the fingers, in the mesentery, tendons, and elsewhere, formed of concentric layers of connective tissue with a soft core in which the axon of a nerve fiber runs, splitting up into a number of fibrils that terminate in bulbous enlargements; they are sensitive to pressure.

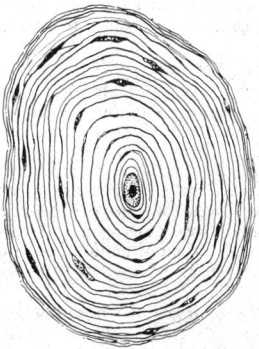

**Cross Section of a Corpusculum Lamellosum (Pacinian Corpuscle)**

**corpuscula nervo'sa termina'lia** [ NA ], terminal nerve corpuscles; generic term denoting specialized encapsulated nerve endings such as corpuscula bulboidea, corpuscula lamellosa, corpuscula tactus, corpuscula genitalia, corpuscula articularia, and menisci tactus.

**c. renis,** pl. **corpuscula renis** [ NA ], renal corpuscle; Malpighian corpuscle; the tuft of glomerular capillaries and the capsula glomeruli that encloses it.

**c. tactus,** pl. **corpuscula tactus** [ NA ], tactile corpuscle; oval corpuscle; touch corpuscle; Meissner's corpuscle; one of numerous oval bodies found in the papillae of the corium, especially that of the fingers and toes; they consist of a connective tissue capsule in which the axon fibrils terminate around and between a pile of wedge-shaped epithelioid cells.

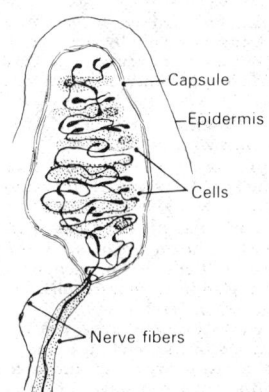

Capsule
Epidermis
Cells
Nerve fibers

**Corpusculum Tactus (Meissner's Corpuscle)**

**correc'tion.** The act of reducing a fault; the elimination of an unfavorable quality.

**occlusal c.,** (1) the c. of malocclusion, by whatever means is employed; (2) the elimination of disharmony of occlusal contacts.

**corrective** [ L. *cor-rigo* (*conr-*), pp. -*rectus,* to set right, fr. *rego,* to keep straight ]. 1. Counteracting, modifying, or changing what is injurious. 2. A drug that modifies or corrects an undesirable or injurious effect of another drug.

**correlation** (kor-re-la'shun). 1. The mutual or reciprocal relation of two or more items or parts. 2. The act of bringing into mutual or reciprocal relation.

**product-moment c.,** a statistical procedure which yields the correlation coefficient referred to as r. and involves the actual values, rather than the ranks (rank order) of the measurements.

**rank-difference c.,** the relationship between paired series of measurements, each ranked according to magnitude, which yields a coefficient known as *rho;* the value of *rho* varies from zero (no relationship) to 1.00 (perfect relationship).

**Correra's line.** See under line.

**correspondence.** In ophthalmology, the condition in which corresponding points on the retina have the same directional value, that is, they see things in the same direction.

**anomalous c.,** a condition, frequent in strabismus, in which the foveas do not give rise to the same visual direction, the fovea of one eye functioning with an extrafoveal area of the other eye.

**harmonious c.,** a type of anomalous retinal c. in which the angle of anomaly is equal to the objective angle of strabismus.

**Corrigan,** Sir Dominic J., Irish pathologist and clinician, 1802–1880. See C.'s *cautery, disease, pulse.*

**cor'rigent** [ L. see corrective ]. Corrective.

**corrin.** The cyclic system of four pyrrole rings forming corrinoids, which are the central structure of the vitamins $B_{12}$ and related compounds, differing from porphyrin in that two of the pyrrole rings are directly linked.

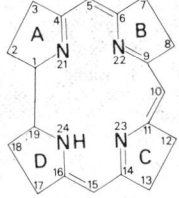

Corrin

**corrode.** To cause, or to be affected by, corrosion.

**corro'sion** [ L. *cor-rodo* (*conr-*), pp. -*rosus,* to gnaw ]. 1. The wearing away gradually by pressure, as in the case of the tissues by a tumor or aneurysm. 2. Disintegration of a metal by oxidation or other chemical reaction. See also erosion.

**corrosive.** 1. Causing corrosion. 2. An agent that produces corrosion, such as an acid.

**corrugator** [ L. *cor-rugo* (*conr-*), pp. -*atus,* to wrinkle, fr. *ruga,* a wrinkle ] [ NA ]. A muscle that draws together the skin, causing it to wrinkle.

**cortex,** gen. **cor'ticis,** pl. **cor'tices** [ L. bark ] [ NA ]. The outer portion of an organ such as the kidney, as distinguished from the inner, or medullary, portion.

**adrenal c.,** c. glandulae suprarenalis.

**agranular c.,** see c. cerebri.

**association c.,** association areas; generic term denoting the large expanses of the cerebral c. that are not sensory or motor in the customary sense, and instead are thought to be involved in advanced stages of sensory information processing, multisensory integration, or sensorimotor integration; see also c. cerebri.

**auditory c.,** auditory area; the region of the cerebral c. that receives the auditory radiation from the medial geniculate body, a cell group of the thalamus in turn receiving the auditory pathway ascending from the coch-

lear nuclei in the rhombencephalon; the auditory c. corresponds approximately to Brodmann's areas 41 and 42 (see fig. under c. cerebri).

**cerebellar c.,** c. cerebelli.

**c. cerebel'li** [ NA ], cerebellar c.; the thin gray surface layer of the cerebellum, consisting of an outer molecular layer or stratum moleculare (including a single layer of Purkinje cells, the ganglionic layer), and an inner granular layer or stratum granulosum.

**cerebral c.,** c. cerebri.

**c. cer'ebri** [ NA ], cerebral c.; the layer of gray matter (1 to 4 mm. thick) covering the entire surface of the cerebral hemisphere of mammals. It is characterized by a laminar organization of its cellular and fibrous components such that its nerve cells are stacked in more or less sharply defined layers varying in number from one, as in the archicortex of the hippocampus, to five or six in the larger neocortex; the outermost (molecular or plexiform) layer contains very few cell bodies and is composed largely of the distal ramifications of the long apical dendrites issued perpendicularly to the surface by pyramidal and fusiform

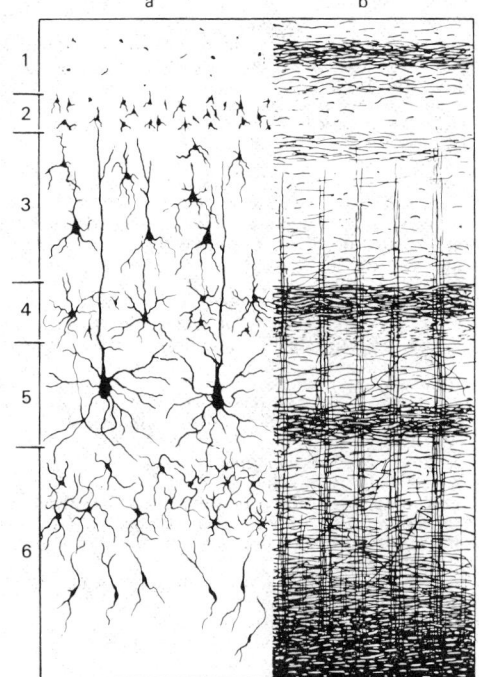

**Layers of the Homotypic Cerebral Cortex**

*a,* Cells; *b,* fibers; *1,* molecular layer; *2,* outer granular layer; *3,* pyramidal cell layer; *4,* inner granular layer; *5,* ganglionic layer; *6,* multiform cell layer. (After Brodmann.)

cells in deeper layers. From the surface inward, the layers (see fig.) in Brodmann's classification, are: (1) molecular or plexiform layer; (2) layer of outer granule cells; (3) pyramidal cell layer; (4) inner granular layer; (5) layer of large pyramidal cells (ganglionic layer); and (6) layer of multiform cells, many of which are fusiform. This multilaminate organization is typical of the neocortex (homotypic c.; isocortex in Vogt's terminology), which in man covers the largest part by far of the cerebral hemisphere. The more primordial heterotypic c. or allocortex (Vogt) has fewer cell layers, *e.g.,* a single pyramidal cell layer in the c. of the hippocampus (archicortex), a pyramidal and a multiform layer in the olfactory c. (piriform c.) of the uncus (paleocortex). A form of c. intermediate between isocortex and allocortex, called juxtallocortex (Vogt) covers the ventral part of the cingulate gyrus and the entorhinal area of the parahippocampal gyrus.

On the basis of local differences in the arrangement of

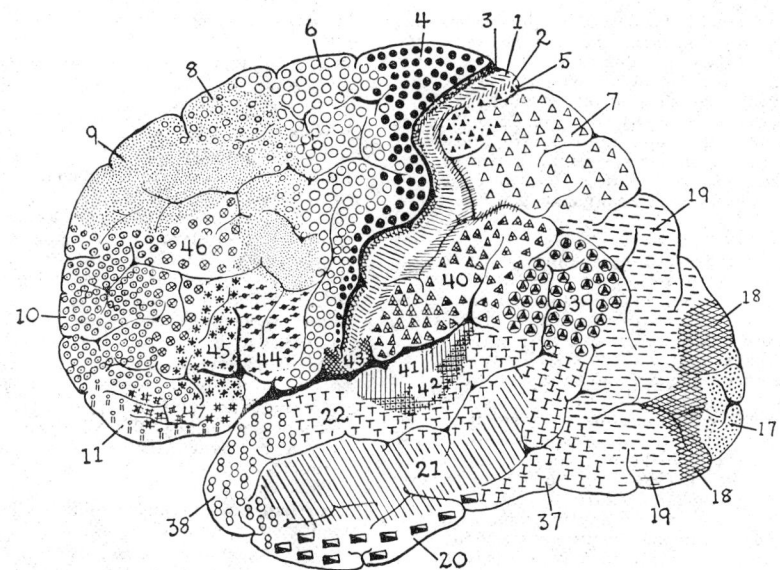

**Brodmann's Areas**

Cytoarchitectural map of convex surface of the human cortex. The numbered patterns (47) are distinctive areas that differ from each other in total thickness, in the thickness and density of individual layers, and in the arrangement and number of cells and fibers. Investigators since Brodmann (1909) have parceled the cerebral cortex into more than 200 areas; Brodmann's map, however, is still widely used as a reference. (After Brodmann, from Truex, R. C., and Carpenter, M. B.: *Human Neuroanatomy*, Ed. 6, The Williams & Wilkins Co., Baltimore, 1969.)

nerve cells (cytoarchitecture), Brodmann outlined 47 areas in the cerebral c. (see fig.). In functional terms these can be classified in three categories; (1) motor c. (areas 4 and 6), having a poorly developed inner granular layer (agranular c.) and prominent pyramidal cell layers; (2) sensory c., characterized by a prominent inner granular layer (granular c. or koniocortex) and comprising the somatic sensory c. (areas 1 to 3), the auditory c. (areas 41 and 42), and the visual c. (areas 17 to 19); and (3) association c., the vast remaining expanses of the cerebral c. See also association c., auditory c., frontal c., koniocortex, motor c., premotor c., piriform c., somatic sensory c., visual c., and speech *center*.

**deep c.,** paracortex.

**dysgranular c.,** the region of the cerebral c. that is transitional between the agranular c. of the precentral gyrus and the granular frontal cortex: area 8 of Brodmann (see fig. under c. cerebri).

**fetal c.,** provisional c.; an extensive area of the adrenal gland present in primates during fetal life and for a short period after birth; located between the definitive cortex and the medulla, it contains large cells arranged in a reticular pattern. Involution of this zone in man is largely completed by 3 months after birth. See also androgenic *zone*.

**frontal c.,** frontal area; c. of the frontal lobe of the cerebral hemisphere; (1) originally, the entire cortical expanse anterior to the sulcus centralis, including the agranular motor cortex (Brodmann's areas 4 and 6), the dysgranular c. (area 8), and the granular frontal (prefrontal) c. anterior to the latter; (2) now more often refers to the granular frontal (prefrontal) c. See fig. under c. cerebri.

**c. glandulae suprarena'lis** [ NA ], adrenal c.; suprarenal c.; the outer part of the adrenal gland, consisting of three zones: zona glomerulosa, zona fasciculata, and zona reticularis, from without inward. This part of the adrenal c. yields several steroid hormones: corticosterone, deoxycorticosterone, estrone, etc.

**granular c.,** see c. cerebri.

**c. of hair shaft,** the outer portion of the hair, composed of flat, nucleated, epithelial cells.

**heterotypic c.,** allocortex.

**homotypic c.,** Isocortex.

**insular c.,** insula (1).

**lam'inated c.,** neocortex and allocortex.

**c. of lens,** c. lentis.

**c. len'tis** [ NA ], c. of lens; the softer more superficial part of the crystalline lens which encloses the central part or nucleus. Its refractive power is less than that of the nucleus.

**c. of lymph node,** c. nodi lymphatici.

**motor c.,** motor area; excitable area; Rolando's area; the region of the cerebral c. most nearly immediately influencing movements of the face, neck and trunk, and arm and leg; it corresponds approximately to Brodmann's areas 4 and 6 of the precentral gyrus (see fig. under c. cerebri). Its effects upon the motor neurons innervating the skeletal musculature are mediated by the pyramidal tract and are particularly essential for man's capacity to perform finely graded movements of arm and leg.

**c. nodi lymphat'ici** [ NA ], c. of a lymph node; the outer portion of the lymph node underneath its capsule, consisting of fibrous trabeculae separating densely packed masses of lymphocytes arranged in nodules and separated from the trabeculae and capsule by lymph sinuses. See fig. under nodus lymphaticus.

**olfactory c.,** piriform c.

**orbitofrontal c.,** fronto-orbital area; the cerebral c. covering the basal surface of the frontal lobes.

**c. of ovary,** the layer of the ovarian stroma lying immediately beneath the tunica albuginea. This layer is composed of connective tissue cells and fibers, among which are scattered primary and vesicular (Graafian) follicles in various stages of development. The c. varies in thickness according to the age of the individual, becoming thinner with advancing years.

**parastriate c.,** see visual c.

**peristriate c.,** see visual c.

**piriform c.,** piriform area; the olfactory c., corresponding to the rostral half of the uncus. Receiving its major afferent connection from the olfactory bulb, the piriform c. is to be classified as allocortex; see also c. cerebri.

**prefrontal c.,** see frontal c.

**premotor c.,** premotor area; a somewhat ill-defined term usually referring to areas 6 and 8 of Brodmann (see fig. under c. cerebri).

**primary visual c.,** see visual c.

**provisional c.,** fetal c.

**renal c.,** c. renis.

**c. renis** [ NA ], renal c.; the part of the kidney consisting of renal lobules in the outer zone beneath the capsule and also the lobules of the renal columns which are extensions inward between the pyramids; it contains the glomeruli and the proximal and distal convoluted tubules.

**secondary sensory c.,** a cortical region occupying the parietal operculum (upper lip of the Sylvian fissure) closely posterior to the foot of the postcentral gyrus; like the primary somatic-sensory c. of the postcentral gyrus, this region receives sensory impulses originating in face, trunk, and limbs.

**secondary visual c.,** see visual c.

**sensory c.,** formerly denoting specifically the somatic sensory c., this term now refers collectively to the somatic sensory, auditory, visual, and olfactory regions of the cerebral c.; see also c. cerebri and related subentries.

**somatic sensory c., somatosensory c.,** somesthetic area; sensory c. (obsolete); the region of the cerebral c. receiving the somatic sensory radiation from the ventrobasal nucleus of the thalamus; it represents the primary cortical processing mechanism for sensory information originating at the body surfaces (touch) and in deeper tissues such as muscle, tendons, and joint capsules (position sense); it corresponds approximately to Brodmann's areas 1 to 3 on the postcentral gyrus (see fig. under c. cerebri).

**supplementary motor c.,** a region from which, by electrical stimulation, the musculature of all bodily parts (face, trunk, arm, and leg) can be activated, as it also can by stimulation of the motor c. of the precentral gyrus; the region corresponds approximately to the expansion of area 6 (Brodmann) over the radial surface of the cerebral hemisphere.

**suprarenal c.,** c. glandulae suprarenalis.

**tertiary c.,** paracortex.

**c. of thymus,** the outer part of a lobule of the thymus; it surrounds the medulla and is composed of masses of closely packed lymphocytes.

**visual c.,** visual area; the region of the cerebral c. occupying the entire surface of the occipital lobe, and composed of Brodmann's area 17 to 19 (see fig. under c. cerebri). Area 17 (also called striate c. or area because of Gennari's line, a thin white fiber band running parallel to the surface about the middle thickness of the cross section of the c.) is the primary visual c., receiving the optic or visual radiation from the lateral geniculate body of the thalamus. The surrounding areas 18 (parastriate c.) and 19 (peristriate c.) are probably involved in subsequent steps of visual information processing; together they are also referred to as the secondary visual c.

**cortexolone.** 11-Deoxycortisol.

**Corti,** Alfonso, Italian anatomist, 1822–1888. See C.'s auditory *teeth* (under tooth), *arch, canal, cells, ganglion, membrane, organ, pillars, rods, tunnel.*

**cor'tical.** Relating to a cortex.

**corticalization.** Encephalization; telencephalization; in phylogenesis, the migration of function from subcortical centers to the cortex.

**cor'ticalosteot'omy.** An osteotomy through the cortex at the base of the dentoalveolar segment, which serves to weaken the resistance of the bone to the application of orthodontic forces.

**cor'tices.** Plural of cortex.

**corticifugal** (kor-tĭ-sif'u-gal) [ L. *cortex,* rind, bark, + *fugio,* to flee ]. Corticoefferent; passing in a direction away from the outer surface; denoting especially nerve fibers conveying impulses away from the cerebral cortex.

**corticipetal** (kor-tĭ-sip'e-tal) [ L. *cortex,* rind, bark, + *peto,* to seek ]. Corticoafferent; passing in a direction toward the outer surface; denoting especially nerve fibers conveying impulses toward the cerebral cortex.

**cor'ticoaf'ferent.** Corticipetal.

**cor'ticobul'bar.** Connecting cortex and motor cranial nuclei in the medulla.

**cor'ticoef'ferent.** Corticifugal.

**cor'ticoid.** 1. Having an action similar to that of a steroid hormone of the adrenal cortex. 2. Any principle exhibiting this action.

**formaldehydogenic c.'s,** those c.'s that yield formaldehyde upon oxidation with periodic acid; included are those

with α-ketol(—COCH$_2$OH) and α-glycol(—CHOHC-H$_2$OH) side chains on carbon-17. See also glucocorticoid, mineralocorticoid.

**cor'ticonu'clear.** See *fibrae* corticonucleares.

**cor'ticopon'tine.** See *tractus* corticopontini.

**cor'ticoretic'ular.** See *fibrae* corticoreticulares.

**corticospi'nal.** See *tractus* corticospinalis.

**corticosteroid.** (kor'tĭ-ko-stĕr'oid). A steroid produced by the adrenal cortex; a corticoid containing a steroid.

**corticos'terone.** 11β,21-Dihydroxy-4-pregnene-3,20-dione (for structure, see steroids); Kendall's compound B; Reichstein's substance H; a steroid obtained from the adrenal cortex. It induces some deposition of glycogen in the liver, sodium conservation, and potassium excretion.

**cor'ticothal'amic.** Pertaining to cortex and thalamus; the term is applied to fibers leading from the cerebral cortex to the thalamus.

**corticotroph** (kor'tĭ-ko-trof). A cell of the adenohypophysis that produces adrenocorticotropic hormone (ACTH).

**corticotro'pin, corticotro'phin** [ G. *tropē,* a turning; *trophē,* nourishment ] (BP). Adrenocorticotropic *hormone* (ACTH).

**c.-zinc hydroxide** (BP), purified c. absorbed on zinc hydroxide; same uses as c. but with a prolonged duration of action.

**β-corticotropin,** A polypeptide fraction of ACTH, containing 40 amino acids in a known sequence.

**cortin.** An acetone extract of the cortical cells of the adrenal glands containing several steroid principles, *e.g.,* corticosterone, deoxycorticosterone, etc., adrenocortin.

**cortisol.** Hydrocortisone.

**c. acetate,** Hydrocortisone acetate.

**cortisone.** 17,21-Dihydroxy-4-pregnene-3,11,20-trione (for pregnene structure, see steroids; the double bond at C4-C5 is sometimes expressed as Δ4); Kendall's compound E; Reichstein's substance Fa; Wintersteiner's compound F. A steroid isolated from the adrenal cortex; not normally secreted in significant quantities by the human adrenal cortex. Endogenously, it is probably a metabolite of hydrocortisone. When exogenous c. is given, it exhibits no biological activity until it is converted to hydrocortisone (cortisol). It acts upon carbohydrate metabolism (glucocorticoid), and influences the nutrition and growth of the connective (collagenous) tissues. It is used in rheumatoid arthritis, adrenal insufficiency, certain allergic states, diseases of the collagenous tissues, inflammatory conditions, pemphigus, and some neoplastic diseases of the lymphatic system. C. is contraindicated in psychosis, peptic ulcer, herpes simplex of the eye, and infections that cannot be controlled by antibiotics.

**c. acetate** (USP, BP), CORTOGEN acetate; CORTONE acetate; 11-dehydro-17-hydroxycorticosterone-21-acetate. Same action and uses as c.

**cortol.** α-Cortol; 5β-pregnane-3α,11β,17,20α,21-pentaol; 5β enantiomer of allocortol. A reduction product of cortisone, present in the urine; it differs from cortisone in that the three keto groups are reduced to hydroxyls.

**β-cortol.** Same as cortol, but with 20β—OH group; 5β enantiomer of β-allocortol; found in urine.

**cortolone.** α-Cortolone; 5β-pregnane-3α,17,20α,21-tetraol-11-one; 5β enantiomer of allocortolone (for structure, see steroids). A reduction product of cortisone, present in the urine; it differs from cortisone in that two of the keto groups (at positions 3 and 20) are reduced to hydroxyls.

**β-cortolone.** Same as cortolone, but with the OH at C-20 in β configuration; 5β enantiomer of β-allocortolone; found in urine.

**corun'dum** [ Hind. *kurand* ]. Native crystalline aluminum oxide.

**corusca'tion** [ L. *corusco,* to flash ]. A psychiatric term for a subjective sensation as of a flash of light before the eyes.

**Corvisart des Marets** (kor-ve-sar' da mah-ret'), Jean N., French clinician, 1755–1821. See C.'s *disease, facies.*

**coryban'tism** [ G. *korybas* (*-bant-*), a priest of Cybele ]. Wild delirium with hallucinations.

**coryd'alis** [ G. *korydallis,* the crested lark, fr. *korys,* helmet; referring to the shape of the flower ]. The tuber of *Dicentra* (*Bicuculla*) *cucullaria* and *D. canadensis* (family Fumariaceae); turkey pea; wild hyacinth; turkey corn;

squirrel corn. Contains a number of physiologically active alkaloids of which bulbocapnine is the only one showing possible therapeutic value.

**corymbiform** (kor-im′bĭ-form) [ L. *corymbus,* cluster, garland ]. Denoting the flower-like clustering of skin lesions in granulomatous diseases, *e.g.,* syphilis, tuberculosis.

**corynebacteriophage** (kŏ-ri′ne-bak-te′rĭ-o-fāj). Any one of the bacteriophages specific for corynebacteria.

β **c.,** β phage; a DNA-containing bacteriophage that induces toxigenicity in strains of *Corynebacterium diphtheriae* that are lysogenic for its prophage.

**Corynebacterium** (kŏ-ri′ne-bak-te′rĭ-um) [ G. *coryne,* a club, + *bacterium,* a small rod; M. L. *Corynebacterium,* club bacterium ]. A genus of nonmotile (except for some plant pathogens), aerobic to anaerobic bacteria (family Corynebacteriaceae) containing irregularly staining, Gram-positive, straight to slightly curved, often club-shaped rods which, as a result of snapping division, show a picket fence arrangement. These organisms are widely distributed in nature. The best known species are parasites and pathogens on humans and domestic animals. The type species is *C. diphtheriae.*

**C. acnes,** *Propionibacterium acnes.*

**C. bovis,** *Bacillus pseudodiphtheria;* a nonpathogenic species of bacteria found in freshly drawn cow's milk.

**C. diphthe′riae,** *C. ulcerans;* Kleb-Loeffler bacillus; a species which causes diphtheria and produces a powerful exotoxin causing degeneration of various tissues, notably myocardium, in man and experimental animals. Virulent strains of this organism are lysogenic. This organism is commonly found in membranes in the pharynx, larynx, trachea, and nose in cases of diphtheria. It is also found in apparently healthy pharynx and nose in carriers, and is occasionally found in the conjunctiva and in superficial wounds. It also occasionally infects the nasal passages and wounds of horses. It is the type species of the genus *C.*

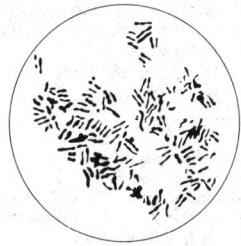

*Corynebacterium diphtheriae*
(Original magnification, × 2250)

**C. enzy′micum,** a species found in human lungs, blood, and joints; pathogenic for laboratory animals.

**C. e′qui,** a species found in spontaneous pneumonia of foals and in other infections of horses; also found in swine, cattle, and buffaloes.

**C. hof′manii,** *C. pseudodiphtheriticum.*

**C. murisep′ticum,** a species which causes septicemia in mice.

**C. o′vis,** *C. pseudotuberculosis.*

**C. parvum,** a species found in female urogenital organs; pathogenic to white mice.

**C. phocae,** a species found in an erysipelas occurring in the transition between the corium and the blubber of seals.

**C. pseudodiphtheriticum,** *C. hofmanii;* Hofmann's bacillus; a nonpathogenic species found in normal throats.

**C. pseudotuberculosis,** *C. ovis;* a species found in necrotic areas in sheep kidney, in caseous lymphadenitis in sheep, and in ulcerative lesions in horses, cattle, and other warm-blooded animals.

**C. pyog′enes,** a species which is probably the most frequently occurring pyogenic organism in cattle, swine, and sheep. It is frequently found alone, or with other bacteria, in a great variety of suppurative processes. It is not pathogenic for man. It produces a toxin and a heat-labile hemolysin.

**C. renale,** a species of bacteria which occurs in purulent infections of the urinary tract in cattle, sheep, horses, and dogs; pathogenic to laboratory animals.

**C. striatum,** a species found in nasal mucus and in the throat; also found in udders of cows with mastitis. Pathogenic to laboratory animals.

**C. xerosis,** a species found in normal and diseased conjunctiva. There is no evidence that this organism is pathogenic.

**coryza** (kŏ-ri′zah) [ G. ]. Acute rhinitis; cold in the head.

**allergic c.,** a rhinitis in an allergic individual due to the presence of an agent to which he is hypersensitive.

**pollen c.,** allergic *rhinitis.*

**c. spasmod′ica,** hay *fever.*

**cory′zavi′rus.** See rhinovirus, under virus.

**Cos.** An island in the Aegean Sea, birthplace of Hippocrates and origin of the Dogmatic School of ancient Greek medicine.

**cosme′sis** [ G. *kosmēsis,* an adorning, fr. *kosmeō,* to order, arrange, adorn, fr. *kosmos,* order ]. A concern in therapeutics, especially in surgical operations, for the appearance of the patient; a resort to an operation which will improve the appearance, or avoidance of an operation which will mutilate or disfigure in any way; see also cosmetic.

**cosmet′ic.** 1. Relating to cosmesis. 2. Relating to the use of cosmetics.

**cosmet′ics.** Composite term for a variety of camouflages applied to the skin, hair, and nails for purposes of beautifying in accordance with cultural dictates.

**cosmo′bion,** pl. **cosmo′bia.** Term used by H. H. Wilder to designate monovular twins as a biological entity, whether separate or conjoined.

**cosmopol′itan** [ G. *kosmos,* universe, + *polis,* city-state ]. In the biological sciences, a term denoting worldwide distribution.

**costa,** gen. and pl. **costae** [ L. ]. 1 [ NA ]. Rib; one of the twenty-four elongated curved bones forming the main portion of the bony wall of the chest. 2. Basal rod; a rodlike internal supporting organelle that runs along the base of the undulating membrane of certain flagellate parasites such as Trichomonas.

**c. fluc′tuans,** floating *rib.*

**costae spu′riae** [ NA ], false ribs; vertebrochondral ribs; five lower ribs on either side that do not articulate with the sternum directly.

**costae verae** [ NA ], true ribs; vertebrosternal ribs; seven upper ribs on either side whose cartilages articulate directly with the sternum.

**costal.** Relating to a rib.

**costal′gia** [ L. *costa,* rib, + G. *algos,* pain ]. Pleurodynia.

**costec′tomy** [ L. *costa,* rib, + G. *ektomē,* excision ]. Exsection of a rib.

**Costen,** James B., American physician, *1895. See C.'s *syndrome.*

**costicar′tilage.** *Cartilago* costalis.

**cos′tiform** [ L. *costa,* rib, + *forma,* form ]. Rib-shaped.

**costive** [ contraction from L. *constipo,* to press together ]. Constipated; especially by reason of dryness of the feces rather than as a consequence of muscular atony.

**cos′tiveness.** Constipation; a condition in which the stools are infrequent, scanty, and dry.

**costo-** [ G. *costa,* rib ]. Combining form relating to the ribs.

**costocen′tral.** Costovertebral.

**costochondral** (kos-to-kon′dral). Relating to the costal cartilages.

**costoclavic′ular.** Relating to the ribs and the clavicle.

**costocor′acoid.** Relating to the ribs and the coracoid process of the scapula.

**costogen′ic.** Arising from a rib; pleurogenic (2).

**costoinferior.** Relating to the lower ribs.

**costoscap′ular.** Relating to the ribs and the scapula.

**costoscapula′ris.** *Musculus* serratus anterior.

**costoster′nal.** Pertaining to the ribs and the sternum.

**cos′toster′noplasty** [ costo- + G. *sternon,* chest, + *plassō,* to fashion ]. An operation to correct a malformation of the anterior chest wall.

**costosuperior.** Relating to the upper ribs.

**cos′totome.** An instrument, knife or shears, designed for cutting through a rib.

**costot′omy** [ costo- + G. *tomē*, a cutting ]. Division or exsection of a rib.

**costotransverse** (kos-to-trans-vurs′). Relating to the ribs and the transverse processes of the vertebrae articulating with them.

**cos′totransvesec′tomy.** Excision of a proximal portion of a rib and the articulating transverse process.

**costover′tebral.** Costocentral; relating to the ribs and the bodies of the thoracic vertebrae with which they articulate.

**costoxiphoid** (kos-to-zi′foyd). Relating to the ribs and the xiphoid cartilage of the sternum.

**cosyntropin** (ko-sin-tro′pin) (USAN). CORTROSYN; synthetic form of adrenocorticotropin.

**Cotard** (kŭ-tar′), Jules, French neurologist, 1840–1887. See C.'s *syndrome.*

**cotar′nine.** An alkaloidal principle, $C_{12}H_{15}NO_4$, derived from narcotine by oxidation. Astringent.

**COTe.** Abbreviation of cathodal opening *tetanus.*

**cothromb′oplas′tin.** *Factor VII.*

**co′tinine.** 1-Methyl-5-(3-pyridyl)-2-pyrrolidinone; one of the major detoxication products of nicotine. It is eliminated rapidly and completely by the kidneys.
  **c. fumarate** (USAN), SCOTINE; a psychomotor stimulant.

**cotransport** (ko-trans′port). The transport of one substance across a membrane, coupled with the simultaneous transport of another substance across the same membrane in the same direction.

**Cotte** (cot), Gaston, French surgeon, 1879–1951. See C.'s *operation.*

**Cotting,** Benjamin E., American surgeon, 1812–1898. See C.'s *operation.*

**Cotton,** A., physical chemist, See C. *effect.*

**cotton** [ Ar. *qútun* ]. The white, fluffy, fibrous covering of the seeds of a plant of the genus *Gossypium* (family Malvaceae). It is used extensively in surgical dressings.
  **absorbent c.,** c. from which all fatty matter has been extracted, so that it readily takes up fluids.
  **purified c.** (USP), absorbent c.; the hairs of the seed of varieties of *Gossypium* and other allied species, freed from adhering impurities, deprived of fatty matter, bleached, and sterilized. Used for tampons, etc.
  **soluble gun c.,** pyroxylin.
  **styptic c.,** absorbent c. wet with a dilute solution of ferric chloride, and then dried. Applied locally as a hemostatic.

**cottonseed oil** (USP, BP). The refined fixed oil obtained from the seed of cultivated plants of various varieties of *Gossypium hirsutum* or of other species of *Gossypium* (family Malvaceae); a solvent.

**Cotugno** (ko-toon′yo). See Cotunnius.

**Cotunnius (Cotugno),** Domenico, Neapolitan anatomist, 1736–1822. See C.'s *aqueduct, canal, disease, liquid, liquor* cotunnii, C.'s *space.*

**cotyla** (kot′ĭ-lah) [ L. ] [ NA ]. Cotyle.

**cotyle** (kot′ĭ-le) [ G. *kotylē,* anything hollow, the cup or socket of a joint ]. 1. Any cup-shaped structure. 2. Specifically, the acetabulum.

**cotyle′don** [ G. *kotylēdon,* any cup-shaped hollow ]. A unit of the placenta visible grossly on the maternal surface as an irregularly shaped lobe circumscribed by depressed areas. It is made up of trophoblastic cells, fibrous tissue, and abundant blood vessels. The fetal vessels traverse the villous structures and are in close contact with the maternal blood of the intervillous space where gaseous and metabolic exchange occurs.

**Cotylogon′imus** [ G. *kotylē,* cup, + *gonimos,* productive, fr. root GEN- ]. A group of heterophyid flukes, now properly included in the genus *Heterophyes.*

**cot′yloid** [ G. *kotylē,* a small cup, + *eidos,* appearance ]. 1. Cup-shaped; cuplike. 2. Acetabular; relating to the cotyloid cavity or acetabulum.

**couching** [ Fr. *coucher,* to lay down, to put to bed ]. Abaissement; an outmoded operation for cataract, consisting in displacing the lens downward out of the line of vision by means of a needle-shaped instrument, the couching needle.

**cough.** 1. A sudden explosive forcing of air through the glottis, excited by an effort to expel mucus or other matter from the bronchial tubes or larynx. 2. To force air through the glottis by a series of expiratory efforts.
  **brassy c.,** loud metallic clanging c. caused by pressure on the trachea or laryngeal nerves, as by an aneurysm of the aortic arch.
  **compression c.,** c. excited by a growth compressing one of the larger bronchial tubes.
  **ear c.,** a reflex c., through the auricular branch of the vagus, excited by irritation in the external auditory canal.
  **gander c.,** the characteristic clanging, brassy c. of tracheal obstruction.
  **hebet′ic c.,** nervous c. occurring frequently at puberty, and sometimes simulating tuberculosis.
  **kennel c.,** a highly contagious form of laryngitis, tracheitis, and bronchitis in dogs, probably caused by a virus.
  **privet c.,** an allergic c., occurring in China during May and June, supposed to be caused by inhalation of the pollen of a species of privet (*Lingustrum*); it is analogous to the laurel fever seen in New England.
  **reflex c.,** a c. excited reflexly by irritation in some distant part, as the ear or the stomach.
  **stomach c.,** a reflex c. excited at times by irritation of the gastric mucous membrane.
  **tooth c.,** c. of reflex origin, due to caries or other disease or malformation of the teeth.
  **trigeminal c.,** a reflex c. due to irritation of the terminals of the trigeminus nerve in the upper respiratory passages.
  **weaver's c.,** c., dyspnea, and sense of constriction of the chest, caused in persons working with mildewed yarns.
  **whooping c.,** pertussis.
  **winter c.,** chronic bronchitis, of the aged especially, coming on with the advent of cold weather and continuing until late spring.

**Coulomb,** Charles A. de, French physicist, 1736–1806. Gave his name to coulomb and statcoulomb.

**coulomb** (koo-lom′) [ C. *Coulomb* ]. Symbol Q; the amount of electricity delivered by a current of 1 ampere in 1 second; equal to 1/96,500 faraday.

**coumaran.** 2,3-Dihydrobenzofuran; contrast coumarin.

**coumaranone.** 3(2*H*)-Benzofuranone; basis of many plant products. See aurone.

**cou′marin** [ *coumarou,* native name of Tonka bean ]. Cumarin; coumaric anhydride; *ortho*-oxycinnamic anhydride; 2*H*-1-benzopyran-2-one; a fragrant neutral principle obtained from Tonka bean, *Dypterix* (*Coumarouma*) *odorata,* and made synthetically from salicylic aldehyde. It is used to disguise unpleasant odors.

**coumestrol.** δ-Lactone of 2-(2,4-dihydroxyphenyl)-6-hydroxy-3-benzofurancarboxylic acid; an estrogenic hormone isolated from clover.

**Councilman,** William T., American pathologist, 1854–1933. Gave his name to *Councilmania.* See C. *body,* C.'s *lesions.*

**Councilman′ia** [ W. *Councilman* ]. Obsolete generic term for a group of amebas now recognized as *Entamoeba.*

**counseling** (kown′sel-ing) [ L. *consilium,* deliberation ]. The giving of advice, opinion, and instruction to direct the judgment or conduct of another.
  **marital c.,** the process whereby a trained counselor assists married couples to resolve problems that arise and trouble them in their relationship; husband and wife are seen by the same counselor in separate and joint c. sessions focusing on immediate family problems.
  **pastoral c.,** the use of psychotherapeutic methods by clergymen for parishioners seeking help with personal problems.

**count.** 1. A reckoning, enumeration, or accounting. 2. To enumerate or score.
  **Arneth c.,** the percentage distribution of polymorphonuclear neutrophils, based on the number of lobes in the nuclei (from 1 to 5). See also Arneth *index.*
  **blood c.,** see *blood count.*
  **Feulgen c.,** see Feulgen *test.*
  **filament-nonfilament c.,** a differential c. of the number of neutrophils showing nuclear division and those showing no such division.

**counter.** A device that counts.

**Geiger-Müller c.,** an instrument for measuring radioactivity by counting the emission of radioactive particles. It consists of a metallic cylinder, negatively charged, in a vacuum tube containing a fine, positively charged wire at its center. Radiations produce negative ions by ionization of the residual gas molecules; the ions bombard the wire and are detected by electrical amplification.

**proportional c.,** a Geiger-Müller c. operating in the voltage range and under conditions in which pulse height is proportional to the energy of the particles being counted, thus making discrimination between particles of different energies possible.

**scintillation c.,** used for the detection of radioactivity; the radiation is absorbed by a crystal resulting in minute flashes of light, which are detected by a photomultiplier and an amplifier. Also called scintillascope; scintillator; scintillometer; spinthariscope.

**counter-** [ L. *contra,* against ]. Combining form meaning opposite, opposed, against. For some words so beginning and not found here, see also those beginning with contra-.

**counterbal'ancing.** A procedure in behavorial research for distributing unwanted but unavoidable influences equally among the different experimental conditions or subjects.

**counterconditioning** (kown'ter-kon-dish'un-ing). Any of a group of specific behavior therapy techniques in which a second conditioned response is instituted for the express purpose of counteracting or nullifying a previously conditioned or learned response.

**countercurrent.** 1. Flowing in an opposite direction. 2. A current flowing in a direction opposite to another current.

**countercurrent exchanger.** A system in which heat or chemicals passively diffuse across a membrane separating two c. streams so that at each end the fluid leaving along one side of the membrane nearly resembles, in temperature or composition, the fluid entering the other; *e.g.,* the venae comites in the arms serve as a c. exchanger, the arterial blood serving to rewarm the cooler venous blood.

**countercurrent multiplier.** A system in which energy is used to transport material across a membrane separating two c. tubes connected at one end to form a hairpin shape; by this means a concentration can be achieved in the fluid in the hairpin bend, relative to the inflow and outflow fluids, that is much greater than the transport mechanism could produce between the two sides of the membrane at any point; *e.g.,* the nephronic loops in the renal medulla act as c. multipliers.

**counterdepressant.** 1. A drug or agent that prevents or antagonizes the depressing action of another drug or agent. 2. Having a counterdepressing effect.

**counterdie.** The reverse image of a die, usually made of a softer and lower fusing metal than the die. See also die.

**coun'terexten'sion.** Countertraction.

**counterimmunoelectrophoresis** (cown'ter-im'u-no-e-lek'tro-fo-re'sis). A modification of immunoelectrophoresis in which antigen (*e.g.,* serum containing hepatitis B virus) is placed in wells cut in the sheet of agar gel toward the cathode, and antiserum is placed in wells toward the anode; antigen and antibody, moving in opposite directions, form precipitates in the area between the cells where they meet in concentrations of optimal proportions.

**coun'terincis'ion.** A second incision opposite to a first incision; see also counteropening.

**coun'terinvest'ment.** Anticathexis.

**counterir'ritant.** 1. An agent that causes irritation or a mild inflammation of the skin with the object of relieving a deep seated inflammatory process; a derivative. 2. Relating to or producing counterirritation.

**counterirrita'tion.** Derivation; irritation or mild inflammation (redness, vesication, or pustulation) of the skin excited for the purpose of relieving an inflammation of the deeper structures.

**counteropening.** Contra-aperture; counterpuncture; a second opening made at the dependent part of an abscess or other cavity containing fluid, which is not draining satisfactorily through an opening previously made.

**coun'terpho'bic.** 1. Denoting a state of actual preference, on the part of a phobic person, for the very situation of which he is afraid. 2. Opposed to the phobic impulse, as in

c. mastery of a feared action by repeated engagement in the action.

**coun'terpoi'son.** 1. Antidote. 2. Antitoxin.

**coun'terpulsa'tion.** A means of assisting the failing heart by automatically removing arterial blood just before and during ventricular ejection and returning it to the circulation during diastole.

**counterpuncture.** Counteropening.

**countershock.** An electric (A.C. or D.C.) shock applied to the heart to terminate a disturbance of its rhythm.

**counterstain.** A second stain of different color, having affinity for other tissues, cells, or parts of cells than those taking the primary stain, used to render more distinct the parts taking the first stain.

**countertraction.** Counterextension; the resistance, or back-pull, made to extension on a limb; in the case of extension made on the leg, for example, c. may be effected by raising the foot of the bed so that the weight of the body pulls against the weight attached to the limb.

**coun'tertransfer'ence.** In psychoanalysis, the analyst's transference (often unconscious) of his emotional needs and feelings toward the patient; personal involvement to the detriment of the desired objective analyst-patient relationship.

**coun'tertrans'port.** The transport of one substance across a membrane, coupled with the simultaneous transport of another substance across the same membrane in the opposite direction.

**coup** (koo) [ Fr. ]. Stroke (1).

**c. de sabre,** linear scleroderma usually found over the scalp or forehead.

**couple.** To copulate; denoting especially the performance of the act by the lower animals.

**coupling.** Bigeminal rhythm; usually the result of the repeated pairing of a normal sinus beat with a ventricular extrasystole.

**constant c.,** fixed c.

**fixed c.,** constant c.; where several premature beats are seen, the interval between each of them and the preceding normal beat is constant.

**c. interval,** see under interval.

**variable c.,** where several extrasystoles are seen, the interval between each of them and the preceding sinus beat varies.

**Cournand** (koor'nand), André F., French physiologist in U. S. *1895. Nobel laureate, 1956, with Werner T. O. Forssmann and Dickinson W. Richards, for their discoveries concerning heart catheterization and pathological changes in the circulatory system.

**courses** [ Fr. *course;* L. *curses,* a running, flowing ]. Menses.

**Courvoisier** (koor-vwah-ze-a'), Ludwig G., French surgeon, 1843–1918. See C.'s *law, sign.*

**Coutard** (koo-tar'), Henri, French radiologist in the U.S., 1876–1950. See C.'s *technique.*

**couvade** (koo-vahd') [ Fr. hatch, cover ]. A custom among primitive peoples in accordance with which, when a child is born, the father takes to his bed as if he also had delivered a child; he usually also submits to various rituals pertaining to childbirth.

**Couvelaire** (koo-vel-air'), Alexandre, Paris obstetrician, 1873–1948. See *uterus.*

**couvercle** (koo-ver'kl) [ Fr. cover, lid ]. An external coagulum, especially a blood clot formed extravascularly.

**co'valent.** An interatomic bond characterized by the sharing of 2, 4, or 6 electrons.

**coverslip.** Cover *glass.*

**Cowdria ruminan'tium.** The rickettsial agent causing heartwater in cattle, sheep and goats in South Africa, transmitted by ticks of the genus *Amblyomma.*

**Cowdry's type A and B inclusion bodies.** See under body.

**Cowling's rule.** See under rule.

**Cowper,** William, London anatomist, 1666–1709. See C.'s *cyst, gland.*

**Cowpe'rian.** Relating to Cowper.

**cowperi'tis.** Inflammation of Cowper's gland.

**cowpox.** Vaccinia (1).

**coxa,** gen. and pl. **coxae** [ L ]. 1. *Os* coxae. 2 [ NA ]. Hip or hip joint.

**c. adduc'ta,** c. vara.

**c. flexa,** c. vara.

**c. magna,** enlargement and deformation of femoral head; usually a sequela of avascular necrosis.

**c. plana,** epiphysial aseptic *necrosis* (of the upper end of the femur).

**c. valga** [ L. *valgus,* bowlegged ], alteration of the angle made by the axis of the femoral neck to the axis of the femoral shaft; in c. valga the angle tends to approach 180 degrees; the femoral neck is in more of a straight line relationship to the shaft of the femur.

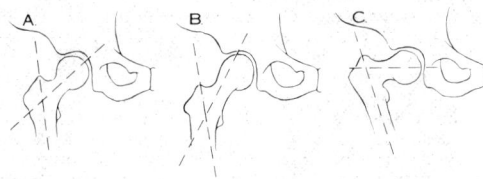

**Coxa Valga and Coxa Vara**
*A,* normal femoral neck; *B,* coxa valga; *C,* coxa vara

**c. vara,** c. adducta; c. flexa; alteration in angulation of neck to shaft of femur so that it approaches 90 degrees or less; the neck becomes more horizontal.

**c. vara, false,** approximation of the head of the femur to the shaft, due not to deformity of the neck of the femur, but to curvature of the shaft.

**c. vara lux'ans,** c. vara with dislocation of the head.

**coxag'ra** [ L. *coxa,* hip, + G. *agra,* seizure ]. Obsolete term meaning gout in the hip joint.

**coxal'gia** [ L. *coxa,* hip, + G. *algos,* pain ]. 1. Coxodynia. 2. Coxitis.

**c. fugax,** transient pain in the hip.

**Coxiel'la** [ H. R. Cox ]. A genus of filterable bacteria (order Rickettsiales) containing small, pleomorphic, rod-shaped or coccoid, Gram-negative cells which occur intracellularly in the cytoplasm of infected cells and possibly extracellularly in infected ticks. These organisms have not been cultivated in cell-free media; they are parasitic on man and other animals. The type species is *C. burnetii.*

**C. burnetii,** *Rickettsia burnetii;* a species (order Rickettsiales) which causes Q fever in man. It is the type species of the genus *C.*

**coxi'tis.** Rarely used term for inflammation of the hip joint.

**c. fugax,** recurrent inflammation of hip joint without known cause. No concurrent abnormal laboratory findings; may follow 3 to 4 weeks after upper respiratory infection; to be distinguished from pain of neuropathy of one or more nerves about the hip.

**coxodyn'ia** [ L. *coxa,* hip, + G. *odynē,* pain ]. Coxalgia; pain in the hip joint.

**coxofem'oral.** Relating to the hip bone and the femur.

**coxot'omy** [ L. *coxa,* hip, + G. *tomē,* cutting ]. Incision into the hip joint.

**cox'otuber'culo'sis.** Tuberculous hip-joint disease.

**coyotillo** (ko'yo-tēl'yo). *Karwinskia humboldtiana.*

**cozy'mase.** Nicotinamide adenine dinucleotide.

**c.p.** Abbreviation for chemically *pure.*

**c.p.s.** Abbreviation for cycles or counts per second.

**CR.** Abbreviation for (1) conditioned *reflex;* (2) crown-rump *length* (which is also abbreviated CRL).

**Cr.** 1. Chemical symbol of the element chromium. 2. Abbreviation for creatinine.

**crab.** 1. A crustacean, many varieties of which are edible. 2. An insect, the crab louse, *Phthirius pubis.*

**Crabtree,** Herbert G. See C. *effect.*

**cradle** (kra'dl). A frame used to keep the bedclothes from pressing on a fractured or wounded part.

**Crafoord,** Clarence, Stockholm surgeon, *1899. See C. *clamp.*

**Craigia** (kra'gī-ah) [ C. *Craig* ]. Obsolete generic term for a group of amebas now recognized as *Entamoeba.*

**Cramer,** Friedrich, German surgeon, 1847–1903. See C.'s *splint.*

**cramp.** 1. A painful spasm. 2. Colic; gripping pain in the intestine colic. 3. A professional neurosis, qualified according to the occupation of the sufferer; *e.g.,* seamstress's c.; writer's c.

**accessory c.,** torticollis.

**dactylographer's c.,** typist's c.; an occupation neurosis; see also writer's c.

**heat c.'s,** muscle spasm induced by hard work in intense heat, accompanied by severe pain; sometimes related to salt deficiency, hyperventilation, and overindulgence in alcohol.

**intermittent c.,** tetany.

**miner's c.'s,** stoker's c.'s; c.'s caused by excessive salt loss through perspiration.

**musician's c.,** an occupation neurosis, affecting those who play on musical instruments, and named usually according to the instrument played upon.

**pianist's c., piano-player's c.,** a professional neurosis affecting the muscles of the fingers and forearms in piano players.

**seamstress's c.,** sewing spasm; an occupation neurosis occurring in the fingers of needle-women.

**shaving c.,** keirospasm; xyrospasm; an occupation neurosis affecting barbers.

**stoker's c.'s,** miner's c.'s.

**tailor's c.,** tailor's spasm; a spasmodic neurosis of the muscles of the forearm and hand.

**telegrapher's c.,** Morse finger; an occupation neurosis characterized by spasm of the extensor muscles of the fingers of the right hand, on grasping the telegraphic key.

**violinist's c.,** a professional neurosis affecting the fingers of the left hand, or sometimes the right arm, in violin players.

**waiter's c.,** a professional neurosis characterized by spasm of the muscles of the back and right arm in waiters.

**watchmaker's c.,** a professional neurosis consisting in (1) spasm of the orbicularis palpebrarum muscle, from holding the lens to the eye; (2) spasm of the muscles of the hand in attempting the delicate movements of watch repairing.

**writer's c.,** mogigraphia; graphospasm; scrivener's palsy; an occupation neurosis affecting chiefly the muscles of the thumb and two adjoining fingers of the right hand, induced by excessive use of the pen; it occurs in one of four main forms; spastic, paralytic, neuralgic, and tremulous.

**cramp bark.** *Viburnum opulus.*

**Crampton,** C. Ward, American physician, *1877. See C. *test.*

**Crampton,** Sir Philip, Irish surgeon, 1777–1858. See C.'s *line, muscle.*

**crani-.** See cranio-.

**cra'nial.** 1. Relating to the cranium. 2. Toward the head; in human anatomy, synonymous with superior.

**crania'lis** [ NA ]. Cranial.

**craniamphitomy** (kra-nĭ-am-fit'o-mĭ) [ G. *kranion,* skull, + *amphi,* around, + *tomē,* cutting ]. A decompression operation of wide extent, the entire circumference of the calvarium being divided.

**Crania'ta** [ Mediev. L. *cranium,* fr. G. *kranion,* skull ]. Vertebrata.

**craniectomy** (kra'nĭ-ek'to-mĭ) [ G. *kranion,* skull, + *ektomē,* excision ]. Excision of a portion of the skull, *e.g.,* subtemporal and suboccipital.

**linear c.,** production of an artificial cranial suture.

**cranio-, crani-** (kra'nĭ-o-) [ G. *kranion,* skull ]. Combining forms denoting relation to the cranium.

**cranio-aural** (kra'nĭ-o-aw'ral). Relating to the skull and the ear.

**craniocele** (kra'nĭ-o-sēl) [ cranio- + G. *kēleō,* hernia ]. Encephalocele.

**craniocerebral** (kra'nĭ-o-sĕr'e-bral). Relating to the skull and the brain.

**cranioclasia, cranioclasis** (kra-nĭ-o-kla'sĭ-ah, kra-nĭ-ok'la-sis) [ cranio- + G. *klasis,* a breaking ]. Crushing of the fetal skull in cases of dystocia.

**cra'nioclast** [ cranio- + G. *klaō*, to break in pieces ]. An instrument like a strong forceps used for crushing and extracting the fetal head after perforation.

**craniocleidodysostosis** (kra′nĭ-o-kli′do-dis-os-to′sis) [ cranio- + G. *kleis*, clavicle, + dysostosis, *q.v.* ]. Cleidocranial *dysostosis.*

**craniodidymus** (kra′nĭ-o-did′ĭ-mus) [ cranio- + G. *didymos*, twin ]. Conjoined twins with fused bodies but two heads.

**craniofacial** (kra′nĭ-o-fa′shal). Relating to both the face and the cranium.

**cra'niofenes'tria** [ cranio- + L. *fenestra*, window ]. Craniolacunia; incomplete formation of the bones of the vault of the fetal skull so that there are nonossified areas in the calvarium.

**craniognomy** (kra′nĭ-og′no-mĭ) [ cranio- + G. *gnōme*, judgment ]. Phrenology.

**cra'niograph.** An instrument for making drawings to scale of the diameters and general configuration of the skull.

**craniography** (kra-nĭ-og′ră-fĭ) [ cranio- + G. *graphō*, to write ]. The art of representing, by drawings made from measurements, the configuration of the skull and the relations of its angles and craniometric points.

**craniolacunia** (kra′nĭ-o-lă-ku′nĭ-ah) [ cranio- + L. *lacuna*, cleft, + suffix *-ia*, condition ]. Craniofenestria.

**craniology** (kra-nĭ-ol′o-jĭ) [ cranio- + G. *logos*, study ]. The science dealing with variations in size, shape, and proportion of the cranium, especially with the variations characterizing the different races of men.

   **Gall's c.,** phrenology.

**craniomalacia** (kra′nĭ-o-mal-a′shĭ-ah) [ cranio- + G. *malakia*, softness ]. Softening of the bones of the skull.

**craniomeningocele** (kra′nĭ-o-men-in′go-sēl) [ cranio- + G. *mēninx*, membrane, + *kēlē*, hernia ]. Protrusion of the meninges through a defect in the skull.

**craniom'eter.** An instrument for measuring the diameters of the skull.

**craniomet'ric.** Relating to craniometry.

**craniom'etry** [ cranio- + G. *metron*, measure ]. Measurement of the dry skull after removal of the soft parts, and study of its topography.

**craniopagus** (kra-nĭ-op′ă-gus) [ cranio- + G. *pagos*, something fixed ]. Conjoined twins with fused skulls: see also janiceps, and syncephalus.

   **c. occipita'lis,** iniopagus; conjoined twins united at the occipital region of the skull.

   **c. parasit'icus,** a variety of c. in which one fetus is rudimentary in form and parasitic on the other. See also epicomus.

**craniopathy** (kra-nĭ-op′ă-thĭ) [ cranio- + G. *pathos*, suffering ]. Any pathological condition of the cranial bones.

   **metabolic c.,** Morgagni's *syndrome.*

**craniopharyngeal** (kra′nĭ-o-fă-rin′je-al). Relating to the cavity of the skull and to the pharynx.

**craniopharyngioma** (kra′nĭ-o-fă-rin-jĭ-o′mah). A neoplasm that develops between the brain and the pituitary gland, frequently in the sella turcica presumably from the nests of epithelium (derived from Rathke's pouch) that have been observed along the hypophysial stalk. The histologic pattern is similar to that observed in ameloblastomas of the primitive enamel organ (adamantinomas), with intersecting bands of epithelium bordered by radially arranged cells; the epithelial cells are frequently stellate and loosely arranged, or of squamous type and compactly grouped. Termed also pituitary adamantinoma, Rathke's pouch tumor, Erdheim tumor, and suprasellar cyst.

   **cystic papillomatous c.,** a form characterized by large cysts within which are fungating, irregular outgrowths of stratified squamous epithelium.

**craniophore** (kra′nĭ-o-fōr) [ cranio- + G. *phoros*, bearing ]. An apparatus for holding a skull while its angles and diameters are measured.

**cra'nioplasty** [ cranio- + G. *plassō*, to form ]. The operative repair of a defect of the skull.

**cra'niopunc'ture.** Puncture of the skull.

**craniorrhachidian** (kra′nĭ-o-ră-kid′ĭ-an) [ cranio- + G. *rhachis*, spine ]. Craniospinal.

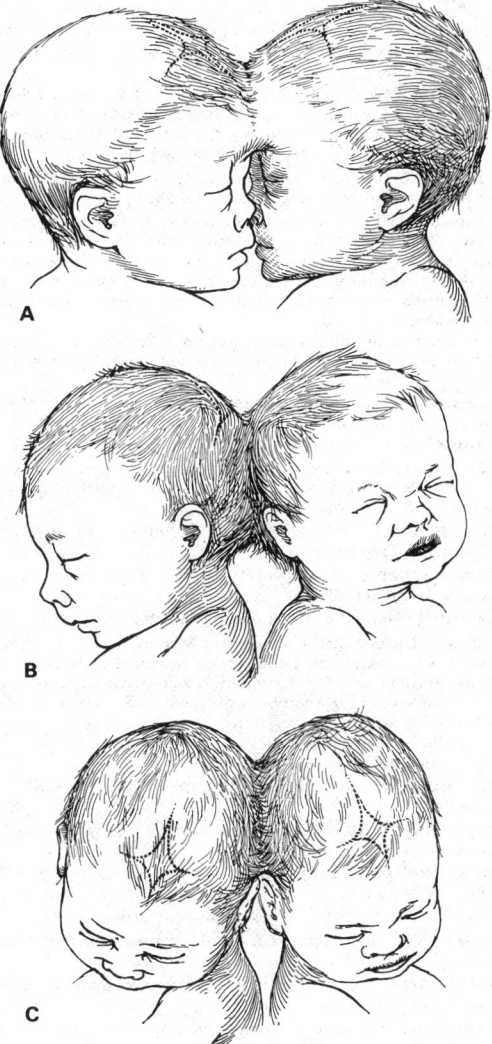

**Craniopagus**
*A*, frontal; *B*, occipital; *C*, parietal

**craniorrhachischisis** (kra′nĭ-o-ră-kis′kĭ-sis) [ cranio- + G. *rhachis*, spine, + *schisis*, a cleaving ]. Congenitally unclosed skull and spinal column.

**cra'niosa'cral.** A term that indicates the cranial and sacral origins of the parasympathetic division of the autonomic nervous system.

**cranioschisis** (kra′nĭ-os′kĭ-sis) [ cranio- + G. *schisis*, a cleavage ]. Congenital failure of the skull to close mid-dorsally, usually accompanied by grossly defective development of the brain.

**craniosclerosis** (kra′nĭ-o-skle-ro′sis) [ cranio- + G. *skleros*, hard, + suffix *-osis*, condition ]. Thickening of the skull.

**cranioscopy** (kra-nĭ-os′ko-pĭ) [ cranio- + G. *skopeō*, to view ]. Examination of the skull in the living subject for craniometric or diagnostic purposes.

**cra'niospi'nal.** Craniorrhachidian; relating to the cranium and spinal column.

**cra'niosteno'sis** [ cranio- + G. *stenōsis*, a narrowing ]. Premature closure of cranial sutures resulting in malformation of the skull.

**craniostosis** (kra'nĭ-os-to'sis) [ cranio- + G. *osteon*, a bone, + suffix *-osis*, condition ]. Craniosynostosis.

**craniosynostosis** (kra'nĭ-o-sin'os-to'sis). Craniostosis; premature ossification of the skull and obliteration of the sutures; see also oxycephaly.

**craniotabes** (kra'nĭ-o-ta'bēz) [ cranio- + L. *tabes*, a wasting ]. Circumscribed craniomalacia; a disease marked by the presence of areas of thinning and softening in the bones of the skull, usually of syphilitic or rachitic origin.

**craniotome** (kra'nĭ-o-tōm). An instrument designed for perforation and crushing of the fetal skull.

**craniotomy** (kra'nĭ-ot'o-mĭ) [ cranio- + G. *tomē*, incision ]. 1. Opening into the skull, either by attached or detached c. or by trephination. 2. Perforation of the head of the fetus, removal of the contents, and compression of the empty skull, when delivery by natural means is impossible.

    **attached c.,** attached cranial section; osteoplastic c.; bone flap; c. with section of the skull attached to muscles and / or other structures as a hinge.

    **detached c.,** detached cranial section; free bone flap; c. with section of cranium separated from its attachments.

    **osteoplastic c.,** attached c.

**craniotonoscopy** (kra'nĭ-o-to-nos'ko-pĭ) [ cranio- + G. *tonos*, tone, + *skopeō*, to examine ]. Auscultatory percussion of the cranium.

**craniotrypesis** (kra'nĭ-o-trĭ-pe'sis) [ cranio- + G. *trypēsis*, a boring ]. Trephining of the skull.

**craniotympanic** (kra'nĭ-o-tim-pan'ik). Relating to the skull and the middle ear.

**cranitis** (kra-ni'tis). Inflammation of the bones of the skull.

**cranium,** pl. **cra'nia** (kra'nĭ-um) [ Mediev. L. fr. G. *kranion* ] [ NA ]. Skull; the bones of the head collectively; in a more limited sense, the brain pan, the bony case containing the brain, excluding the bones of the face. See color plates 19 and 20, and fig. under skull.

    **c. bif'idum,** encephalocele.

    **c. cerebra'le,** calvaria.

    **c. viscera'le,** visceral c.; those parts of the skull of branchial arch origin.

**crap'ulent, crap'ulous** [ L. *crapula*, drunkenness ]. Drunken; suffering from alcoholic intoxication.

**crassamen'tum** [ L. thickness, fr. *crassus*, thick ]. 1. Blood clot. 2. Coagulum.

**cras'sus** [ L. ] [ NA ]. Thick, dense, or gross.

**cra'ter.** The most depressed, usually central portion of an ulcer.

**crater'iform** [ L. *crater*, bowl, + *forma*, shape ]. Hollowed like a bowl or a saucer.

**craw-craw.** Kra-kra; a term applied in West Africa to a vesiculopustular skin eruption, attended with itching, which may lead to ulceration. Some cases are caused by *Onchocerca*. The name has also been given to papular and pustular eruptions in the French Congo and on the Cameroon Coast.

**Crawford,** B. H., British physiologist. See Stiles-C. *effect*.

**cra'zing.** In dentistry, denotes the appearance of minute cracks on the surface of plastic restorations such as filling materials, denture teeth, or denture bases.

**CRD.** Abbreviation for chronic respiratory *disease*.

**cream** (krēm) [ L. *cremor*, thick juice, broth ]. 1. The upper fatty layer which forms in milk on standing or which is separated from it by centrifugalization. It contains about the same amount of sugar and protein as milk, but from 12 to 40 per cent more fat. 2. Any whitish viscid fluid resembling c. 3. A semisolid emulsion of either the oil-in-water or the water-in-oil type, ordinarily intended for topical use.

    **cleansing c.,** a form of cold c. used to remove grime and cosmetics from the skin.

    **cold c.,** a water-in-oil emulsion of various oils, waxes, and water; the standard formula, rose water ointment, contains expressed almond oil, rose water, spermaceti, white paraffin wax, and sodium borate; used as a cleansing or lubricating c.

    **greaseless c.,** vanishing c.

    **leukocyte c.,** buffy *coat*.

    **lubricating c.,** a form of cold c. used as a massage c. or night c.; it contains lanolin or its derivatives.

    **vanishing c.,** greaseless c.; an oil-in-water emulsion containing potassium, ammonium, or sodium stearate with water and holding in emulsified form more or less free stearic acid; it also contains a hygroscopic ingredient such as glycerol, and a small amount of a fatty ingredient; it leaves a protective, invisible film of stearic acid on the skin.

**crease** (krēs). See fold.

**creatinase** (kre'ă-tĭ-nās). 1. An enzyme catalyzing the cyclic condensation of creatine phosphate into creatinine. 2. A bacterial enzyme degrading creatine to smaller products.

**creatine** (kre'ă-tēn, -tin). ($N$-Methylguanidine)acetic acid; $H_2N—C(NH)—N(CH_3)—CH_2—COOH$; occurs in urine, sometimes as such, but generally as creatinine, and in muscle, generally as phosphocreatine.

    **c. kinase** (EC 2.7.3.2), an enzyme catalyzing the transfer of phosphate from phosphocreatine to ADP, forming creatine and ATP; of importance in muscle contraction.

    **c. phosphate,** a compound of creatine (through its $NH_2$ group) with phosphoric acid. A source of energy in the contraction of muscle, its breakdown furnishing energy phosphate for the resynthesis of ATP from ADP by creatine kinase.

**creatinemia** (kre'ă-tĭ-ne'mĭ-ah) [ creatine + G. *haima*, blood ]. The presence of abnormal concentrations of creatine in peripheral blood.

**creatinine** (kre-at'ĭ-nēn, -nin). A component of urine and the final product of creatine catabolism; formed by the dephosphorylative cyclization of phosphocreatine.

$$HN—C(NH)—N(CH_3)—CH_2—CO$$

    **c. coefficient,** the number of milligrams of c. excreted daily per kilogram of body weight.

**creatinuria** (kre-ă-tĭ-nu'rĭ-ah) [ creatine + G. *ouron*, urine ]. The urinary excretion of increased amounts of creatine.

**Credé** (kreh-da'), Karl S. F., German obstetrician and gynecologist, 1819–1892. See C.'s *methods*.

**creep.** Time-dependent strain due to stress.

    **c. recovery,** the time-dependent portion of the decrease in strain following unloading of the specimen.

**cremas'ter** [ G. *kremastēr*, a suspender, in pl. the muscles by which the testicles are suspended, fr. *kremannymi*, to hang ]. See *fascia* cremasterica; *musculus* cremaster.

**cremasteric** (kre-mas-tĕr'ik). Relating to the cremaster.

**cremnocele** (krem'no-sēl) [ G. *krēmnos*, overhanging cliff, labium pudendi, + *kēlē*, hernia ]. Labial hernia; a protrusion of intestine into a labium majus.

**cremnophobia** (krem-no-fo'bĭ-ah) [ G. *krēmnos*, precipice, + *phobos*, fear ]. Morbid fear of precipices or steep places.

**cremor** (kre'mor) [ L. thick juice or broth ]. Cream.

**crena,** pl. **cre'nae** (kre'nah) [ L. a notch ] [ NA ]. A notch; a cleft; one of the notches into which the opposing projections fit in the cranial sutures.

    **c. ani** [ NA ], anal, natal, or gluteal cleft, c. clunium; the sulcus between the nates.

    **c. clu'nium** [ L. *clunis*, buttock ], c. ani.

    **c. cordis,** sulcus interventricularis anterior; sulcus interventricularis posterior.

**cre'nate, cre'nated** [ L. *crena*, a notch ]. Notched; indented; denoting the outline of a shriveled red blood cell, as observed in a hypertonic solution.

**crena'tion.** The process of becoming, or state of being, crenated.

**crenocyte** (kre'no-sit) [ L. *crena*, a notch, + G. *kytos*, a hollow (cell) ]. A red blood cell with serrated, notched edges.

**cre'nocyto'sis** [ crenocyte + G. suffix *-osis*, condition ]. The presence of crenocytes in the blood.

**Cre'nosoma vul'pis.** A metastrongyle lungworm of the fox, wolf, dog, raccoon, and other small carnivores in Europe, Asia, and North America; it occurs in the bronchi, where it causes bronchitis.

**cren'other'apy** [ G. *krēnē*, spring, + *therapeia*, treatment ]. Crounotherapy.

**creophagy, creophagism** (kre-of'ah-jī, kre-of'ah-jizm) [ G. kreas, meat, + phagein, to eat ]. Carnivorousness; flesh-eating.

**cre'osol.** 2-Methoxy-*p*-cresol; a slightly yellowish aromatic liquid distilled from guaiac or from beechwood tar. Constituent of creosote (*cf.* cresol).

**cre'osote** [ G. *kreas*, flesh, + *sōtēr*, to preserve ]. A mixture of phenols (chiefly methyl guaiacol, guaiacol, and creosol) obtained during the distillation of wood-tar, preferably that derived from beechwood. Used as a disinfectant.

**crep'itant.** 1. Relating to or characterized by crepitation. 2. Denoting a fine rale heard in pneumonia and in certain other conditions. 3. The sensation imparted to the palpating finger by gas or air in the subcutaneous tissues.

**crepita'tion** [ L. *crepitus, q.v.* ]. 1. Crackling; the quality or sound of a rale which resembles noise heard on rubbing hair between the fingers. 2. The sensation felt on placing the hand over the seat of a fracture when the broken ends of the bone are moved, or over tissue, in which gas gangrene is present. 3. Noise or vibration produced by rubbing bone or irregular cartilage surfaces together as by movement of patella against femoral condyles in arthritis and other conditions.

**crepitus** (krep'ĭ-tus) [ L. fr. *crepo*, to rattle ]. 1. Crepitation. 2. A noisy discharge of gas from the intestine.

   **artic'ular c.,** the grating of a joint.

   **bony c.,** crepitation (2).

   **c. index, c. redux,** see rale.

**crepus'cular** [ L. *crepusculum*, twilight ]. Pertaining to a twilight state of consciousness.

**crescent** (kres'ent) [ L. *cresco*, pp. *cretus*, to grow. CRES- ]. 1. Any figure of the shape of the moon in its first quarter. 2. The figure made by the gray columns or cornua on cross-section of the spinal cord. 3. Malarial c.

   **artic'ular c.,** *meniscus* articularis.

   **Giannuzzi's c.'s,** serous *demilunes*.

   **glomerular c.,** proliferated epithelial cells partly encircling a renal glomerulus; it occurs in glomerulonephritis.

   **Heidenhain's c.'s,** serous *demilunes*.

   **malarial c.,** sickle form; the primitive sexual form of *Plasmodium falciparum*, developing into the male or female gametocyte.

   **myop'ic c.,** myopic conus; a white or grayish white crescentic patch in the fundus of the eye to the outer side of the optic disk, due to atrophy of the choroid, allowing the sclera to become visible.

   **sublingual c.,** the crescent-shaped area on the floor of the mouth formed by the lingual wall of the mandible and the adjacent part of the floor of the mouth.

**crescentic** (kres-sen'tik). Shaped like a crescent.

**crescograph** (kres'ko-graf) [ L. *cresco*, to grow, + G. *graphō*, to draw or write ]. A device for recording the degree and rate of growth.

**cre'sol** (BP). Hydroxytoluene; methylphenol; HO—$C_6H_4$—$CH_3$; a mixture of the three isomeric cresols, *o*-, *m*-, and *p*-cresol, obtained from coal tar. Its properties are similar to those of phenol, but it is less poisonous. Used as a disinfectant.

   **c. red,** an acid-base indicator with a pK value of 8.3; yellow at pH values below 7.4, red above 9.0.

***m*-cresol.** See metacresol.

**cre'solase.** Monophenol monooxygenase.

---

# CREST

---

**crest** [ L. *crista* ]. 1. A ridge, especially a bony ridge; see crista. 2. The ridge of the neck of a male animal, especially of a stallion or bull. 3. Feathers on the top of a bird's head, or finrays on the top of a fish's head.

   **acous'tic c.,** *crista* ampullaris.

   **acousticofacial c.,** the part of the neural crest from which the ganglia of the 7th and 8th cranial nerves develop.

   **alve'olar c.,** (1) the portion of the alveolar bone extending beyond the periphery of the socket, lying interproximally; (2) the top of the residual alveolar bone.

   **ampul'lary c.,** *crista* ampullaris.

   **anterior lacrimal c.,** *crista* lacrimalis anterior.

   **arched c.,** *crista* arcuata.

   **ar'cuate c.,** *crista* arcuata.

   **articular c.'s,** *cristae* sacrales intermediae.

   **basilar c. of cochlear duct,** *crista* basilaris ductus cochlearis.

   **buc'cinator c.,** crista buccinatoria; a ridge passing from the base of the coronoid process of the mandible to the region of the last molar tooth; it gives attachment to the buccinator muscle.

   **c. of cochlear opening,** *crista* fenestrae cochleae.

   **conchal c.,** *crista* conchalis.

   **deltoid c.,** *tuberositas* deltoidea.

   **dental c.,** crista dentalis; a ridge on the alveolar processes of the jaw bones in the fetus.

   **ethmoidal c.,** *crista* ethmoidalis.

   **external occipital c.,** *crista* occipitalis externa.

   **falciform c.,** *crista* transversa.

   **frontal c.,** *crista* frontalis.

   **ganglionic c.,** neural c.

   **gingival c.,** the edge or ridge of the free gingiva that separates the gingival sulcus from the external gingiva.

   **gluteal c.,** *tuberositas* glutea.

   **c. of greater tubercle,** *crista* tuberculi majoris.

   **iliac c.,** *crista* iliaca.

   **inci'sor c.,** the front part of the nasal c. of the palatine process of the maxilla.

   **infratem'poral c.,** *crista* infratemporalis.

   **infundib'uloventric'ular c.,** *crista* supraventricularis.

   **inguinal c.,** an elevation in the body wall of the embryo at the internal opening of the inguinal canal. Part of the gubernaculum develops within it.

   **intermediate sacral c.'s,** *cristae* sacrales intermediae.

   **internal occipital c.,** *crista* occipitalis interna.

   **interos'seous c.,** *margo* interosseus.

   **intertrochanter'ic c.,** *crista* intertrochanterica.

   **Kölliker's dental c.,** *os* incisivum.

   **c. of lesser tubercle,** *crista* tuberculi minoris.

   **marginal c.,** *crista* marginalis.

   **medial c.,** *crista* medialis.

   **c.'s of nailbed,** *cristae* matricis unguis.

   **nasal c.,** *crista* nasalis.

   **c. of neck of rib,** *crista* colli costae.

   **neural c.,** ganglionic c.; ganglion ridge; a band of neuroectodermal cells along either side of the line of closure of the embryonic neural groove. With the closure of the neural groove to form the neural tube, these bands come to lie dorsolateral to the developing spinal cord, where they separate into clusters of cells that develop into dorsal-root ganglion cells, autonomic ganglion cells, the chromaffin cells of the adrenal medulla, or neurolemmal cells (Schwann cells).

   **ob'turator c.,** *crista* obturatoria.

   **c. of palatine bone, palatine c.,** *crista* palatina.

   **posterior lacrimal c.,** *crista* lacrimalis posterior.

   **pubic c.,** *crista* pubica.

   **c. of ridge,** see under ridge.

   **sacral c.,** *crista* sacralis.

   **sagittal c.,** a prominent ridge along the sagittal suture of the skull, present in some animals as a result of temporal muscle development.

   **c. of scapular spine,** the posterior subcutaneous border of the spine of the scapula that expands in its medial part into a smooth triangular area.

   **sphenoid c.,** *crista* sphenoidalis.

   **spiral c.,** *labium* limbi vestibulare.

   **su'pinator c.,** *crista* musculi supinatorius.

   **supramas'toid c.,** crista supramastoidea; the posterior root of the zygomatic process of the temporal bone.

   **supraventric'ular c.,** *crista* supraventricularis.

   **terminal c.,** *crista* terminalis.

   **tibial c.,** *margo* anterior tibiae.

   **transverse c.,** (1) *crista* transversa; (2) *crista* transversalis.

   **triangular c.,** *crista* triangularis.

trigeminal c., that part of the cranial neural c. from which the ganglion of the 5th cranial nerve develops.

**trochanter'ic c.,** *crista* intertrochanterica.

**tur'binated c.,** *crista* conchalis.

**tympan'ic c.,** crista tympanica; a ridge on the tympanic ring.

**ure'thral c.,** *crista* urethralis.

**vestibular c., c. of vestibule,** *crista* vestibuli.

**cresta** (kres'tah) [ L. *crispus,* trembling ]. A small membrane organelle characteristic of certain flagellate protozoa. The c. is located near the pelta and frequently can be seen in the living organism as an independently moving structure.

**cres'ylate.** A salt of cresylic acid, or cresol.

**cres'yl blue (brilliant).** Aminodimethylaminoethyldiphenazonium chloride; a dye used for staining the reticulum in young erythrocytes (reticulocytes).

**cres'yl violet acetate.** A basic oxazin dye, $C_{18}H_{15}N_3O_3$, used as a stain for nuclei and Nissl bodies.

**creta** (kre'tah) [ L. orig. adj. fr. *Creta,* Crete, *i.e.* Cretan earth, chalk ]. Chalk.

**cre'tin** [ Fr. *crétin* ]. An individual exhibiting cretinism.

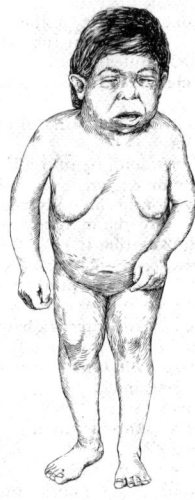

Cretin

**cre'tinism.** Infantile hypothyroidism; may arise from thyroid agenesis or inadequate maternal intake of iodine during gestation. It appears during the first years of life and results in stunting of bodily growth and of mental development.

**cre'tinis'tic.** Cretinous.

**cre'tinoid.** Resembling a cretin; presenting symptoms similar to those of cretinism.

**cre'tinous.** Relating to cretinism or a cretin.

**Creutzfeld,** Hans Gerhard, German neuropsychiatrist, 1885–1964. See C.-Jakob *disease.*

**crevice** (krev'is) [ Fr. *crevasse* ]. A crack or small fissure, especially in a solid substance.

**gingival c.,** gingival *sulcus.*

**crevicular** (krĕ-vik'u-lar). Relating to any crevice; especially, in dentistry, to the gingival crevice or subgingival space.

**CRF.** Abbreviation for corticotropin-releasing *factor.*

**crib'ber.** Windsucker; a horse that has the habit of cribbing.

**crib'bing.** Crib-biting; windsucking; a habit, formed by a horse when young, of biting at the manger or other objects; air is often sucked in at this time, and the horse may become chronically bloated.

**crib-biting.** Cribbing.

**crib'rate.** Cribriform.

**cribra'tion.** 1. Sifting; passing through a sieve. 2. The condition of being cribrate or numerously pitted or punctured.

**crib'riform** [ L. *cribrum,* a sieve, + *forma,* form ]. Cribrate; sievelike; containing many perforations.

**cribrifor'mis** [ L. ] [ NA ]. Cribriform.

**cribro'sus** [ L. ] [ NA ]. Cribriform.

**cribrum,** pl. **cri'bra** (kri'brum, krib'rum) [ L. a sieve ]. *Lamina* cribrosa ossa ethmoidalis.

**Cricetinae** (kri-se'tĭ-ne). A subfamily of rodents (family Muridae) that includes the hamsters and the native American rats.

**Cricetulus griseus.** The striped hamster; a small rodent native to Europe and Asia; reservoir for kala azar infection.

**Crice'tus.** See hamster.

**Crichton-Browne** (kri'ton), Sir James, English physician, 1840–1938. See C.-B.'s *sign.*

**Crick** (krik), Francis H. C., English biochemist, *1916. Nobel laureate, 1962, with James D. Watson and Maurice H. F. Wilkins, for their discoveries concerning the molecular structure of nucleic acids and its significance for information transfer in living materials. See Watson-C. *helix.*

**cricoarytenoid** (kri'ko-ăr-ĭ-te'noyd). Relating to the cricoid and arytenoid cartilages.

**cricoarytenoideus** (kri-ko-ă-rit'e-no-id'e-us). See under musculus.

**cricoid** (kri'koyd) [ L. *cricoideus,* fr. G. *krikos,* a ring, + *eidos,* form ]. Ring-shaped; denoting the cricoid cartilage.

**cricoidectomy** (kri'koy-dek'to-mĭ) [ cricoid + G. *excision* ]. Excision of the cricoid cartilage.

**cricoideus** [ L. ] [ NA ]. Cricoid.

**cricoidynia** (kri'koy-din'ĭ-ah) [ cricoid + G. *odynē,* pain ]. Pain in the cricoid.

**cricopharyngeal** (kri'ko-fă-rin'je-al). Relating to the cricoid cartilage and the pharynx; a part of the inferior constrictor muscle of the pharynx. See *musculus* constrictor pharyngis inferior.

**cricothyroid** (kri-ko-thi'royd). Relating to the cricoid and thyroid cartilages.

**cricothyroideus** (kri'ko-thi-roy'de-us). See under musculus.

**cri'cothyroidot'omy.** An incision between the cricoid and thyroid cartilages for the purpose of maintaining a patent airway.

**cricothyrotomy** (kri'ko-thi-rot'o-mĭ) [ cricoid + thyroid + G. *tomē,* incision ]. Intercricothyrotomy; inferior laryngotomy; incision through the skin and cricothyroid membrane for relief of respiratory obstruction. Used prior to tracheotomy in certain emergency respiratory obstructions.

**cricotomy** (kri-kot'o-mĭ) [ cricoid + G. *tomē,* incision ]. Division of the cricoid cartilage.

**Crigler,** John F., U. S. physician, *1919. See C.-Najjar disease, syndrome.

**Crile's clamp.** See under clamp.

**criminology** (krī-mĭ-nol'o-jĭ) [ L. *crimen,* crime (CRET-), + G. *logos,* study ]. The branch of science that deals with the physical and mental characteristics and behavior of criminals.

**crinin** (krin'in). A substance that will stimulate the production of secretions by specific glands.

**crinis,** pl. **cri'nes** (kri'nis) [ L. ]. Hair.

**crinogenic** (krin'o-jen'ik) [ G. *krinō,* to separate, + suffix *-gen,* to produce ]. Causing secretion; stimulating a gland to increased function.

**cripple** (krip'l) [ A.S. *creopan,* to creep ]. A lame person or one who owing to a physical defect or injury is partially or completely disabled.

**crisis,** pl. **cri'ses** (kri'sis) [ G. *krisis,* a separation, crisis. CRI- ]. 1. A sudden change in the course of an acute disease. A disease that terminates by c. is one in which a change for the better occurs suddenly (as in pneumonia), as distinguished from one that terminates by lysis. 2. A paroxysmal pain in an organ or circumscribed region of the body occurring in the course of tabes dorsalis. 3. A convulsive attack.

**Addisonian c.,** acute adrenocortical *insufficiency.*

**adolescent c.,** the emotional turmoil often accompanying adolescence.

**adrenal c.,** acute adrenocortical *insufficiency.*

**anaphylac'toid c.,** colloidoclastic shock; symptoms resembling those of anaphylaxis arising from colloidoclasis; see also anaphylactoid.

**blood c.,** (1) appearance of a large number of nucleated red blood cells in the peripheral blood, accompanied by reticulocytosis and occurring in "exhausted" bone marrow in pernicious anemia and in hemolytic icterus; (2) a suddenly appearing leukocytosis, indicating a change for the better in the course of a grave blood disease.

**cerebral c.,** apoplexy.

**Dietl's c.,** paroxysmal attacks of lumbar and abdominal pain with nausea and vomiting resulting from kinking of the ureter in persons with wandering kidney.

**febrile c.,** the stage in a febrile disease when spontaneous defervescence occurs.

**gastric c.,** an attack, usually of several days' duration, of severe pain in the abdomen or around the waist, accompanied by nausea and vomiting and occasionally diarrhea, occurring in the course of, or preceding, tabes dorsalis.

**glaucomatocyclitic c.,** a form of secondary open angle glaucoma, due to recurring mild cyclitis in one eye; the elevated ocular tension lasts 4 to 8 weeks.

**identity c.,** a disorientation concerning one's sense of self and role in society, often of acute onset and related to a particular and significant event in one's life.

**laryn'geal c.,** an attack of paralysis of the abductor, or spasm of the adductor, muscles of the larynx with dyspnea and noisy respiration, occurring in tabes dorsalis.

**myelocyt'ic c.,** a temporary but conspicuous and sudden increase in cells of the myelocytic series in the circulating blood.

**ocular c.,** sudden and intense pain in the eyes.

**oculogyric crises,** attacks of forced eye movement, usually upward rotation, seen in encephalitis lethargica.

**Pel's crises,** ocular crises occurring in tabes dorsalis.

**sickle cell c.,** protean acute symptoms developing recurrently in patients with sickle cell anemia; it is caused by vascular occlusion or hemolysis and may follow infection, dehydration, or hypoxia from blood loss or high altitudes.

**tabet'ic c.,** c. (2).

**therapeutic c.,** a turning point leading to positive or negative change in psychiatric treatment.

**thyroid c.,** thyrotoxic c.

**thyrotox'ic c.,** thyroid c.; thyroid storm; the exacerbation of symptoms which occurs in thyrotoxicosis following some shock or injury or after thyroidectomy; it is marked by rapid pulse (140 to 170 per minute), nausea, diarrhea, fever, loss of weight, extreme nervousness, and a sudden rise in the basal metabolic rate; coma is usual and death is common. occasionally the entire clinical picture is that of profound prostration, weakness, and collapse, without the phase of muscular overactivity and tachycardia.

**crispa'tion** [ L. *crispo,* pp. *-atus,* to curl ]. 1. A "creepy" sensation due to slight, fibrillary muscular contractions. 2. Retraction of a divided artery or of muscular fibers or other tissues when cut across.

# CRISTA

**crista,** pl. **cris'tae** (kris'tah) [ L. crest ] [ NA ]. A ridge, crest, or elevated line projecting from a level or evenly rounded surface. See also crest.

**c. ampulla'ris** [ NA ], ampullary crest; acoustic crest; transverse septum (1); an elevation on the inner surface of the ampulla of each semicircular duct. Filaments of the vestibular nerve pass through the c. to reach hair cells on its surface. The hair cells are capped by the cupula, a gelatinous protein-polysaccharide mass.

**c. arcua'ta** [ NA ], arcuate or arched crest; the ridge on the anterior surface of the arytenoid cartilage that separates the triangular from the oblong fovea.

**c. basila'ris ductus cochlea'ris** [ NA ], basilar crest of cochlear duct; an inward projection of the spiral ligament of the cochlea to which is attached the basilar membrane forming the floor of the cochlear duct.

**c. buccinator'ia,** buccinator *crest.*

**c. cap'itis cos'tae** [ NA ], the ridge that separates the superior and inferior articular surfaces of the head of a rib.

**c. colli costae** [ NA ], crest of neck of rib; the sharp upper margin of the neck of a rib.

**c. concha'lis** [ NA ], conchal crest; turbinated crest; (1) the ridge of the nasal surface of the body of the maxilla that articulates with the inferior nasal concha; (2) the ridge on the nasal surface of the perpendicular part of the palate bone to which the inferior nasal concha attaches.

**cristae cu'tis** [ NA ], skin ridges; ridges of the epidermis of the palms and soles, where the sweat pores open.

**c. denta'lis,** dental *crest.*

**c. dividens,** the lower free edge of the septum secundum, forming the upper margin of the fetal foramen ovale.

**c. ethmoida'lis** [ NA ], nasal concha; ethmoidal crest; (1) a ridge on the upper part of the nasal surface of the frontal process of the maxilla that gives attachment to the anterior portion of the middle nasal concha; (2) a ridge located high on the medial surface of the perpendicular part of the palate bone to which the middle nasal concha attaches posteriorly.

**c. fenes'trae coch'leae** [ NA ], crest of the cochlear opening; the edge of the opening of the cochlear window to which the secondary tympanic membrane is attached.

**c. fronta'lis** [ NA ], frontal crest; a ridge arising at the termination of the sagittal sulcus on the cerebral surface of the frontal bone and ending at the foramen caecum.

**c. gal'li** [ NA ], cock's comb; the superior triangular portion of the perpendicular plate of the ethmoid bone, projecting above the level of the cribriform plate; it gives attachment to the falx cerebri.

**c. glutea,** *tuberositas* glutea.

**c. hel'icis,** *crus* helicis.

**c. ilia'ca** [ NA ], iliac crest; the long, curbed upper border of the ilium.

**c. infratempora'lis** [ NA ], infratemporal crest; pterygoid ridge of the sphenoid bone; a rough ridge making the angle of union of the temporal and infratemporal surfaces of the greater wing of the sphenoid bone.

**c. intertrochanter'ica** [ NA ], intertrochanteric crest; trochanteric crest; the rounded ridge that connects the greater and lesser trochanters of the femur posteriorly and marks the junction of the neck and shaft of the bone.

**c. lacrima'lis anterior** [ NA ], anterior lacrimal crest; a vertical ridge on the lateral surface of the frontal process of the maxilla that forms part of the medial margin of the orbit.

**c. lacrima'lis posterior** [ NA ], posterior lacrimal crest; a vertical ridge on the orbital surface of the lacrimal bone which, together with the anterior lacrimal crest, bounds the fossa for the lacrimal sac.

**c. margina'lis** [ NA ], marginal crest, marginal ridge; the rounded borders which form the mesial and distal margins of the occlusal surface of a tooth.

**cristae ma'tricis un'guis** [ NA ], crests of the nailbed; the numerous longitudinal ridges of the nailbed distal to the lunula.

**c. media'lis** [ NA ], medial crest; a ridge of bone, on the posterior surface of the fibula, separating the attachment of the posterior tibial muscle from that of the flexor hallucis longus and soleus muscles.

**cristae of mitochondria,** cristae mitochondriales; shelf-like infoldings of the inner membrane of a mitochondrion.

**c. musculi supinator'ius** [ NA ], supinator crest; crest of the supinator muscle; the proximal part of the interosseous border of the ulna.

**c. nasa'lis** [ NA ], nasal crest; the midline ridge in the floor of the nasal cavity, formed by the union of the paired maxillae and palatine bones. The vomer attaches to the crest.

**c. obturato'ria** [ NA ], obturator crest; a ridge that extends from the pubic tubercle to the acetabular notch, giving attachment to the pubofemoral ligament of the hip joint.

**c. occipita'lis externa** [ NA ], external occipital crest; linea nuchae mediana; a ridge extending from the external occipital protuberance to the border of the foramen magnum.

**c. occipita'lis interna** [ NA ], internal occipital crest; a ridge running from the internal occipital protuberance to the posterior margin of the foramen magnum, giving attachment to the falx cerebelli.

**c. palatina** [ NA ], palatine crest; crest of the palatine bone; a transverse ridge near the posterior border of the bony palate, located on the inferior surface of the horizontal lamina of the palatine bone.

**c. phal'lica,** *crista* urethralis (1).

**c. pu'bica** [ NA ], pubic crest; the rough anterior border of the body of the pubis, continuous laterally with the pubic tubercle.

**c. quar'ta,** a ridge that projects into the posterior end of the lateral semicircular duct of the labyrinth.

**c. sacralis** [ NA ], sacral crest; one of five rough irregular ridges on the posterior surface of the sacrum. The unpaired **c. sacralis mediana** is formed by the fused spinous processes of the upper four sacral vertebrae, the **cristae sacrales intermediae,** intermediate or articular crests, are formed by the fusion of articular processes of all the sacral vertebrae, and the **cristae sacrales laterales,** which are rough lips lying lateral to the sacral foramina, represent the fused transverse processes of sacral vertebrae.

**c. sphenoida'lis** [ NA ], sphenoid crest; a vertical ridge in the midline of the anterior surface of the sphenoid bone. It articulates with the perpendicular plate of the ethmoid bone.

**c. spiralis,** *labium* limbi vestibulare.

**c. supramastoidea,** supramastoid *crest.*

**c. supraventricula'ris** [ NA ], supraventricular crest; infundibuloventricular crest; the internal muscular ridge that separates the conus arteriosus from the remaining part of the cavity of the right ventricle of the heart.

**c. termina'lis** [ NA ], terminal crest; tenia terminalis; a vertical crest on the interior wall of the right atrium that lies to the right of the sinus venarum cavarum and separates this from the remainder of the right atrium.

**c. transver'sa** [ NA ], transverse crest (1); falciform crest; a horizontal ridge that divides the fundus of the internal acoustic meatus into a superior and an inferior area. In the former are the internal opening of the facial canal and openings for the branches of the vestibular nerve to the utricle and to the ampullae of the anterior and lateral semicircular canals. In the latter are openings for the cochlear nerve, and for branches of the vestibular nerve to the saccule and to the ampulla of the posterior semicircular canal.

**c. transversa'lis** [ NA ], transverse crest (2); transverse ridge; a crest or ridge on the occlusal surface of a tooth formed by the union of two triangular crests.

**c. triangula'ris** [ NA ], triangular crest; triangular ridge; a crest or ridge which extends from the apex of a cusp of a premolar or molar tooth toward the central part of the occlusal surface.

**c. tuber'culi major'is** [ NA ], crest of greater tubercle; the ridge below the greater tubercle of the humerus into which the pectoralis major muscle inserts.

**c. tuber'culi minor'is** [ NA ], crest of lesser tubercle; the ridge below the lesser tubercle of the humerus into which the teres major muscle inserts.

**c. urethra'lis** [ NA ], urethral crest; (1) in the male, c. phallica; a longitudinal fold on the posterior wall of the urethra extending from the uvula of the bladder through the prostatic urethra; prominent in its midportion is the seminal colliculus; (2) in the female a conspicuous longitudinal fold of mucosa on the posterior wall of the urethra.

**c. vestib'uli** [ NA ], crest of the vestibule; vestibular crest; an oblique ridge on the inner wall of the vestibule of the labyrinth, bounding the spherical recess above and posteriorly.

---

**cristobalite.** A form of silica used in dental casting investment.

**Critchett,** George, English ophthalmoligist, 1817–1882. See C.'s *operation.*

**crite'ria.** Plural of criterion.

**criterion,** pl. **criteria** (kri-tēr'ĭ-on, -ĭ-ah) [ G. *kritērion,* a standard ]. 1. A standard or rule for judging; usually plural (criteria) denoting a set of standards or rules. 2. In psychology, a standard against which test scores on intelligence tests or other measured behaviors are validated.

**Spiegelberg's criteria** (for diagnosis of ovariocyesis), (1) the oviduct on the affected side must be intact; (2) the gestation sac must occupy the position of the ovary; (3) the gestation sac must be connected to the uterus by the ovarian ligament; and (4) ovarian tissue must be present in the wall of the gestation sac.

**crith** [ G. *krithē,* barley corn ]. The weight of 1000 cc. of hydrogen gas at 0°C. and 760 mm. Hg pressure; taken as the unit of weight of gases.

**Crithid'ia.** A genus of asexual, monogenetic, insect-parasitizing flagellates in the family Trypanosomatidae.

**crithid'ia.** Epimastigote (*q.v.*); stage of development of certain flagellate parasites of vertebrates in the insect host, such as the multiplying form of the agent of African sleeping sickness in the salivary glands of the tsetse fly host, or that of the agent of Chagas' disease in the triatomine bug; also the form developed in culture in these organisms.

**critical** (krit-ĭ-kal). Referring to a crisis.

**crocidismus** (kro-si-diz'mus) [ G. *krokydismos,* the plucking of the nap of a woolen blanket or garment, fr. *krokys,* the nap ]. Floccillation.

**Crocq,** Jean, Belgian physician, 1868–1925. See C.'s *disease.*

**crocus** (kro'kus) [ L. fr. G. *krokos,* the crocus, saffron (made from its stigmas) ]. Saffron; the dried stigmas of *Crocus sativus* (*C. officinalis*) (family Iridaceae). Used occasionally in flatulent dyspepsia and as an antispasmodic in asthma and dysmenorrhea and as a coloring and flavoring agent.

**autumn c.,** colchicum.

**Crohn,** Burrill, B., New York physician, *1884. See C.'s *disease.*

**cromolyn sodium** (kro'mo-lin) (USAN). INTAL; sodium cromoglycate; disodium 5,5'-[ (2-hydroxytrimethylene)-dioxy ]bis[ 4-oxo-4*H*-1-benzopyran-2-carboxylate ]; a bronchodilator drug used for the prevention of asthmatic attack.

**Cronkhite,** L. W., Jr., U. S. physician *1919. See C.-Canada *syndrome.*

**Crooke,** Arthur C., English pathologist, *1905. See C.'s hyaline *change,* C.'s hyaline *degeneration,* C.'s *granules.*

**Crosby,** William Holmes, Jr., American physician, *1914. See C. *capsule.*

**Cross,** Howard B., U. S. bacteriologist, 1873–1921. See C. *stain.*

**cross** [ F. *croix,* L. *crux* ]. 1. Any figure in the shape of a c. formed by two intersecting lines, + or ×. 2. *Crux* of the heart.

**hair c.'s,** *cruces* pilorum.

**Ranvier's c.'s,** black or brown figures in the shape of a c., marking Ranvier's nodes in the longitudinal section of a nerve stained with silver nitrate.

**cross'breed.** 1. A hybrid. 2. To breed a hybrid.

**cross'breeding.** Hybridization.

**cross-eye.** See crossed *eyes.*

**cross-firing.** A defect in the gait of a horse, generally a pacer, as a result of which the inner quarter or ground surface (or shoe) of a front foot is struck by the toe (or shoe) of the hind foot of the opposite side.

**crossing-over.** See under gene.

**cross matching.** In testing for compatibility of bloods before choosing a donor, the red blood cells of the donor are mixed with serum of the recipient, and the red blood cells of the recipient with the serum of the donor. The former is frequently termed the *major cross match,* and the latter the *minor cross match.*

**cross'way.** The crossing of two nerve paths.

**sensory c.,** the postlenticular portion of the posterior limb of the internal capsule of the brain.

**Crosti,** A. See Gianotti-C. *syndrome.*

**Crotalidae** (kro-tal'ĭ-de). Family of New World pit vipers; see viper.

**crot'alin** [ *Crotalus,* a genus of rattlesnakes ]. A protein in rattlesnake venom.

**crot'aline.** Monocrotaline.

**cro'talism.** Crotalaria *poisoning.*

**Crot'alus** [ G. *krotalon,* a rattle, fr. *krotos,* a rattling noise ]. A genus of rattlesnakes native to North America; these live-bearing pit vipers (family Crotalidae) are found from coast to coast and from Canada to Mexico; they have large fangs that are replaced periodically throughout life and a venom that is both neurotoxic and hemolytic. The largest species are the diamondbacks of the southern states (*C. adamanteus*) and western states (*C. atrox*); the smallest are the pigmy rattlers, *Sistrurus,* of New York and several other localities.

**crotamiton** (kro-tam'ĭ-ton) (BP). EURAX; *N*-ethyl-*o*-crotonotoluide. Sarcopticide for topical use in scabies.

**crotaphion** (kro-taf'ĭ-on) [ G. *krotaphos,* the temple of the head ]. The tip of the greater wing of the sphenoid bone; a point in craniometry.

**cro'tin.** A toxic mixture of albuminoids from the seeds of *Croton tiglium* (family Euphorbiaceae).

**cro'tonase.** Enoyl-CoA hydratase.

**croton'ic acid.** $CH_3CH=CHCOOH$; an unsaturated fatty acid present in croton oil; also found in clay soil in Texas and formed during the dry distillation of wood.

**cro'ton oil.** A fixed oil expressed from the seeds of *Croton tiglium* (family Euphoriaceae), an East Indian shrub; used as an irrigant purgative, and externally as a counterirritant and vesicant.

**cro'tonyl-ACP reductase.** Enoyl-ACP reductase.

**crounotherapy** (kroo'no-ther'ă-pĭ) [ G. *krounos,* a spring ]. Treatment of disease by the internal administration of mineral waters, as distinguished from balneotherapy, or the external use of the same.

**croup** (kroop) [ Scots, probably from A.S. *kropan,* to cry aloud ]. 1. Laryngotracheobronchitis in infants and young children caused by parainfluenza virus types 1 and 2. 2. Any affection of the larynx in children, characterized by difficult and noisy respiration and a hoarse cough. 3. The part of the top line of a horse that lies back of the pin or hip bones and in front of the tailhead; the rump.

**croupous** (kroo'pus). Relating to croup; marked by a fibrinous exudation.

**croupy** (kroo'pĭ). Having the characteristics of croup, as a c. cough.

**Crouzon,** Octave, French physician, 1874–1938. See C.'s *disease.*

**crown** [ L. *corona* ]. 1. Corona. 2. In dentistry, that part of a tooth that is covered with enamel or an artificial substitute for that part.

**anatomical c.,** *corona* dentis.

**artificial c.,** a fixed restoration of the major part of the entire coronal part of a natural tooth; usually of gold, porcelain, or acrylic resin.

**Beers' c.,** a gold shell c. described in 1880 by Beers. The type of c. was described as early as 1746 by Mouton.

**bell-shaped c.,** a c. of a tooth with an exaggerated occlusogingival contour; human deciduous molars typify the bell-shaped c.

**Carmichael c.,** a three-quarter c. for anterior teeth made by reducing the proximal and lingual surfaces with disks and stones and cutting longitudinal grooves on the proximal surfaces for retention. As it preceded the casting technique, the early Carmichael c. was made by burnishing a thin plate of pure gold over the preparation, flowing a lower carat gold or gold solder over the matrix, and obtaining the desired contour with stones and disks.

**cast gold c.,** casting of gold in a mold made by the investment of a wax pattern carved to represent a replacement of coronal tooth structure.

**ceramo-metal c.,** a c. of metal with porcelain fused to exposed surfaces for esthetic reasons.

**ciliary c.,** *corona* ciliaris.

**clinical c.,** *corona* clinica.

**collar c.,** Richmond c.; a c. consisting of a porcelain facing and a coping united and held together by means of solder or by an intermediary casting. The coping consists of a metal cap fitted to the root face and a dowel extending into the root canal.

**extra-alveolar c.,** that portion of a tooth extending occlusally or incisally from the junction of the tooth root and the supporting bone.

**c. of the head,** *corona* capitis.

**jacket c.,** a hollow c. of acrylic resin, fused porcelain or cast gold, combinations of gold and acrylic or gold and porcelain; it fits over the prepared stump of the natural c.

**post-c.,** see postcrown.

**radiate c.,** *corona* radiata.

**Richmond c.,** collar c.

**c. of a tooth,** *corona* dentis.

**crown'ing.** 1. The capping of a tooth. 2. That stage of childbirth when the fetal head has negotiated the pelvic outlet and the largest diameter of the head is encircled by the vulvar ring.

**cru'ces.** Plural of crux.

**cruciate** (kru'shi-at) [ L. *cruciatus* ]. Shaped like, or resembling, a cross.

**crucia'tus** [ L. ] [ NA ]. Cruciate.

**crucible** (kroo'sĭ-bl) [ Mediev. L. *crucibulum,* a night lamp, later, a melting pot ]. A pot of clay, graphite, platinum, or other material used as a container or reactions or meltings at high temperature.

**cru'fomate** (USAN). 4-*tert*-Butyl-2-chlorophenyl methyl methylphosphoramide; a veterinary anthelmintic.

**cru'or** (kroo'or) [ L. blood (that flows from a wound) ]. Coagulated blood.

**crura** (kroo'rah). Plural of crus.

**crureus** (kroo-re'us) [ Mod. L. ]. *Musculus* vastus intermedius.

**crural** (kroo'ral). Relating to the leg or thigh, or any crus; femoral.

**crus,** gen. **cru'ris,** pl. **cru'ra** [ L. ] [ NA ]. 1. The leg, the segment of the inferior limb between the knee and the ankle. 2. Any anatomical structure resembling a leg; usually (in the plural) a pair of diverging bands or elongated masses.

**c. ante'rius cap'sulae inter'nae** [ NA ], anterior limb of the internal capsule; the portion of the internal capsule that passes between the head of the caudate nucleus and the putamen; it lies anterior to the genu of the internal capsule.

**c. ante'rius stape'dis** [ NA ], anterior limb of the stapes; the anterior of the two delicate curving limbs of the stapes that pass from the head of the bone to the base or foot-plate.

**c. anthel'icis** [ NA ], leg of the antihelix; one of two ridges, inferior and superior, bounding the fossa triangularis, by which the antihelix begins at the upper part of the auricle.

**c. breve incu'dis** [ NA ], the short process of the incus, fitting into a depression (fossa incudis) in the epitympanic recess.

**c. cer'ebri** [ NA ], cerebral peduncle; basis pedunculi; pes pedunculi; specifically, the massive bundle of corticofugal nerve fibers passing longitudinally over the dorsal surface of the midbrain on each side of the midline. It consists of fibers descending from the cortex to the tegmentum of the brainstem, pontine gray matter, and spinal cord. See also *pedunculus* cerebri.

**c. clitor'idis** [ NA ], c. of the clitoris; the continuation on each side of the corpus cavernosum of the clitoris which diverges from the body posteriorly and is attached to the pubic arch.

**c. of clitoris,** c. clitoridis.

**c. cor'poris caverno'si penis,** c. penis.

**c. dex'trum diaphrag'matis** [ NA ], right c. of the diaphragm; the muscular origin of the diaphragm from the bodies of the upper three or four lumbar vertebrae that passes upward to the right of the aorta toward the central tendon.

**c. for'nicis** [ NA ], c. of the fornix; posterior pillar of the fornix; that part of the fornix that rises in a forward curve behind the thalamus to continue forward as the corpus fornicis below the corpus callosum; see also fornix.

**c. of fornix,** c. fornicis.

**c. hel'icis** [ NA ], limb of the helix; crista helicis; a transverse ridge continuing backward the helix of the auricle, dividing the concha into an upper portion, cymba, and a lower portion, cavum conchae.

**c. latera'le** [ NA ], lateral limb; (1) lateral limb of the superficial inguinal ring; (2) lateral limb of the greater alar cartilage of the nose.

**left c. of diaphragm,** c. sinistrum diaphragmatis.

**c. longum incu'dis** [ NA ], the long process of the incus terminating in the processus lenticularis or os orbiculare.

**c. media'le** [ NA ], medial limb; (1) medial limb of the superficial inguinal ring; (2) medial limb of the greater alar cartilage of the nose.

**crura membrana'cea ampulla'ria** [ NA ], ampullary limbs of the semicircular ducts; the dilated ends of the three semicircular ducts, each of which contains a specialized thickening of the epithelium known as the crista ampullaris.

**c. membrana'ceum commu'ne duc'tus semicircula'ris** [ NA ], common limb of the membranous semicircular ducts; the united, nonampullary ends of the superior and posterior semicircular ducts.

**c. membrana'ceum sim'plex duc'tus semicircula'ris** [ NA ], simple membranous limb of the semicircular duct; the end of the lateral semicircular duct that opens into the utricle.

**crura os'sea cana'les semicircula'res** [ NA ], limbs of the bony semicircular canals; the extremities of the bony semicircular canals in which the corresponding membranous limbs of the semicircular ducts are located; they are the c. osseum commune, c. osseum simplex, and crura ossea ampullaria.

**c. penis** [ NA ], c. corporis cavernosi penis; the posterior portion of the corpus cavernosum penis attached to the ischiopubic ramus.

**c. poste'rius cap'sulae inter'nae** [ NA ], posterior limb of the internal capsule; that subdivision of the internal capsule that lies behind the genu of the internal capsule between the thalamus and lentiform nucleus.

**c. poste'rius stape'dis** [ NA ], posterior limb of the stapes; the posterior of the two delicate limbs of the stapes that connect the head and base or foot-plate of the bone.

**right c. of diaphragm,** c. dextrum diaphragmatis.

**c. sinis'trum diaphrag'matis** [ NA ], left crus of the diaphragm; the muscular origin of the diaphragm from the upper two or three lumbar vertebrae that ascends to the left of the aorta to reach the central tendon.

**crush** [ O. Fr. *cruisir* ]. 1. To squeeze injuriously between two hard bodies. 2. A bruise or contusion from pressure between two solid bodies.

**crusot'omy** (krus-ot'o-mĭ) [ L. *crus, q.v.,* + G. *tomē,* incision ]. A mesencephalic pyramidal *tractotomy.*

**crust** [ L. *crusta* ]. 1. An outer layer or covering. 2. A scab; a coagulation product of blood, serum, pus, or a combination of two or more of these.

**milk c.,** *crusta* lactea.

**crusta,** pl. **crus'tae** (krus'tah) [ L. ]. Crust.

**c. inflammato'ria,** buffy *coat.*

**c. lac'tea,** milk crust, scall, or tetter; seborrhea of the scalp in an infant.

**c. phlogis'tica,** buffy *coat.*

**Crustacea** (krus-ta'she-ah) [ L. *crusta,* a crust ]. A class of aquatic animals (phylum Arthropoda) with a chitinous exoskeleton and jointed appendages, *e.g.,* the crab, lobster, crayfish, shrimp. isopods, ostracods, and amphipods. Some, such as certain copepods, are parasitic, others serve as intermediate hosts for parasitic worms which cause disease in man and various vertebrates. See also Copepoda.

**crutch** [ A. S. *cryce* ]. A device used to assist in walking when the act is impaired by a lower extremity (or trunk) disability. It transfers all or part of weight-bearing to the upper extremity; may be used singly or in pairs.

**Cruveilhier** (krü-vāl-ya'), Jean, French pathologist and anatomist, 1791–1874. See C.'s *disease, fascia, fossa, joint, ligaments, plexus, sign,* C.-Baumgarten *disease, murmur, syndrome,* and *fossa* navicularis C.

**crux,** pl. **cru'ces** (kruks) [ L. ]. Cross.

**c. of the heart,** the area of junction of the walls of the four chambers of the heart.

**cruces pilo'rum** [ NA ], hair crosses; the growth of hair in crosslike figures.

**Cruz,** Oswaldo, Brazilian physician, 1872–1917. See Chagas-C. *disease,* C. *trypanosomiasis.*

**cry.** A loud inarticulate vocal utterance. 2. To make a loud vocal sound. 3. To weep.

**c. of anger,** a passionate crying accompanied by kicking.

**arthrit'ic c.,** joint c.

**epileptic c.,** a c. that may occur at the onset of a convulsion.

**c.'s for help,** telephone calls, notes suggesting suicide and left in conspicuous places, and other behaviors which communicate extreme distress and potential suicide.

**c. of illness,** a feeble c., better described as a moan.

**joint c.,** arthritic c.; a night c. uttered by a sufferer from chronic tuberculous arthritis.

**night c.,** a loud scream uttered by a child during sleep; it is sometimes without apparent significance; at one time it was thought to be indicative of tuberculous arthritis.

**c. of pain,** a continuous, or, if due to colic, intermittent c., quite characteristic and hardly to be mistaken.

**cry-.** See cryo-.

**cryalgesia** (kri-al-je'zĭ-ah) [ G. *kryos,* cold, + *algos,* pain. CRY- ]. Crymodynia; pain caused by cold.

**cryanesthesia** (kri-an-es-the'zĭ-ah) [ G. *kryos,* cold, + *an-priv.* + *aisthēsis,* sensation ]. A loss of sensation or perception of cold.

**cryesthesia** (kri-es-the'zĭ-ah) [ G. *kryos,* cold, + *aisthēsis,* sensation ]. 1. A subjective sensation of cold. 2. Sensitiveness to cold.

**crymo-** (kri'mo-) [ G. *krymos,* cold ]. Combining form relating to cold; see also cryo-, psychro-.

**crymoanesthesia** (kri'mo-an-es-the'zĭ-ah) [ crymo- + anesthesia ]. Refrigeration *anesthesia.*

**crymodynia** (kri-mo-din'ĭ-ah) [ crymo- + G. *odynē,* pain ]. Cryalgesia.

**crymophilic** (kri-mo-fil'ik) [ crymo- + G. *philos,* fond ]. Cryophilic; preferring cold; denoting microorganisms which grow best at low temperatures.

**crymophylactic** (kri-mo-fĭ-lak'tik) [ crymo- + G. *phylaxis,* a guarding against ]. Cryophylactic; resistant to cold; said of certain microorganisms which are not destroyed even by freezing temperatures.

**crymother'apy.** Cryotherapy.

**cryo-** (kri'o-) [ G. *kryos,* cold ]. Combining form relating to cold; see also crymo-, psychro-.

**cryoaerotherapy** (kri'o-a'er-o-ther'ah-pĭ). The use of cold air in treatment.

**cryoanesthesia** (kri'o-an-es-the'zĭ-ah). Refrigeration anesthesia; localized application of cold as a means of producing regional anesthesia.

**cry'obiol'ogy.** The study of the effects of low temperatures on living organisms.

**cryocautery** (kri'o-kaw'ter-ĭ). Any substance, such as liquid air or carbon dioxide snow, the application of which causes destruction of tissue by freezing.

**cryoconization** (kri'o-kon-ĭ-za'shun). Freezing of a cone of endocervical tissue with a cryoprobe.

**cryode** (kri'ōd). Cryoextractor.

**cry'oextrac'tion.** Removal of cataract by means of an applicator that has been artifically cooled to make frozen contact with the lens.

**cry'oextrac'tor.** Cryode; cryostylet; an instrument, artifically cooled, for extraction of the lens by freezing contact.

**cryofibrinogen** (kri'o-fi-brin'o-jen). An abnormal type of fibrinogen very rarely found in human plasma; it is precipitated upon cooling, but redissolves when warmed to room temperature.

**cry'ofibrin'ogene'mia.** The presence in the blood of cryofibrinogens.

**cryoflu'orane.** Dichlorotetrafluoroethane.

**cryogen** (kri'o-jen). Refrigerant; freezing mixture.

**cryogenic** (kri-o-jen'ik) [ cryo- + G. suffix *-gen,* producing ]. Producing, or relating to the production of, low temperatures.

**cryogen'ics.** The science of producing and maintaining very low temperatures, particularly temperatures in the range of liquid helium ( < 4.2°K.).

**cryoglob'ulin.** Abnormal plasma proteins (paraproteins) characterized by precipitating, gelling, or crystallizing when serum or solutions of them are cooled. They may appear in patients with multiple myeloma. They are distinguished from Bence Jones proteins by their larger molecular weight (180,000 compared with 35,000 to 50,000).

**cry'oglobuline'mia.** The presence of abnormal quantities of cryoglobulin in the blood plasma.

    **crystal c.,** a syndrome of repeated episodes of widespread purpura and cutaneous ulcerations in a patient whose serum contains a homogenous cryoglobulin that spontaneously forms crystals.

**cry'ohy'drate.** A eutectic system of a salt and water.

**cryohypophysectomy** (kri'o-hi-pof'ĭ-sek'to-mĭ) [ cryo- + hypophysis, + G. *ektomē*, excision ]. Destruction of hypophysis by cold.

**cryolysis** (kri-ol'ĭ-sis) [ cryo- + G. *lysis*, dissolution ]. Destruction by cold.

**cryom'eter** [ cryo- + G. *metron*, measure ]. A device for measuring very low temperatures.

**cryopallidectomy** (kri'o-pal-id-ek'to-me) [ cryo- + globus pallidus, *q.v.*, + G. *ektomē*, excision ]. Destruction of the globus pallidus by cold.

**cryopathy** (kri-op'ă-thĭ) [ cryo- + G. *pathos*, suffering ]. A condition (*e.g.*, disease or injury) in which exposure to cold is an important factor.

**cryopexy** (kri'o-pek-sĭ) [ cryo- + G. *pēxis*, a fixing in place ]. In retinal detachment surgery, sealing retina to choroid by probe cooled with liquid nitrogen applied to sclera.

**cryophilic** (kri-o-fil'ik) [ cryo- + G. *philos*, fond ]. Crymophilic.

**cry'ophylac'tic.** Crymophylactic.

**cry'opill.** A solid cylinder of compressed carbon dioxide, for use in a cryosurgical instrument.

**cry'oprecip'itate.** Precipitate which forms when soluble material is cooled, especially with reference to the precipitate that forms in normal blood plasma which has been subjected to cold precipitation and which is rich in antihemophilic globulin (factor VIII).

**cry'oprecipita'tion.** The process of forming a cryoprecipitate from solution.

**cry'oprobe.** The instrument used in cryosurgery.

**cryoprostatectomy** (kri'o-pros-tă-tek'to-mĭ) [ cryo- + L. *prostata*, prostate, + G. *ektomē*, excision ]. Destruction of the prostate gland by cold.

**cryopro'tein.** A protein that precipitates from solution when cooled and redissolves upon warming.

**cryopulvinectomy** (kri'o-pul-vĭ-nek'to-mĭ) [ cryo- + L. *pulvinar*, *q.v.*, + G. *ektomē*, excision ]. Destruction of the pulvinar by cold.

**cry'oscope.** An instrument for measuring the freezing point.

**cryoscopy** (kri-os'ko-pĭ) [ cryo- + G. *skopeō*, to examine ]. Algoscopy; the determination of the freezing point of a fluid, usually blood or urine, compared with that of distilled water.

**cry'ospasm** [ cryo- + G. *spasmos*, convulsion ]. Spasm produced by cold.

**cry'ostat** [ cryo- + G. *statos*, standing ]. A freezing chamber.

**cryostylet, cryostylette** (kri'o-sti-let). Cryoextractor.

**cry'osur'gery.** Surgery with use of decreased temperature, either locally or generally.

**cryothalamectomy** (kri'o-thal-ă-mek'to-mĭ) [ cryo- + thalamus, + G. *ektomē*, excision ]. Destruction of the thalamus by cold.

**cry'otherapy.** 1. Crymotherapy; frigotherapy; the use of cold in the treatment of disease. 2. Refrigeration *anesthesia*.

**cry'otol'erant.** Tolerant to very low temperatures.

**crypt-.** See crypto-.

**crypt.** Crypta.

    **dental c.,** the space filled by the dental follicle.

    **enamel c.,** enamel niche; the narrow, mesenchymally filled space between the dental ledge and an enamel organ.

    **c.'s of the iris,** pits near the pupillary margin of the anterior surface of the iris.

    **Lieberkühn's c.'s,** *glandulae* intestinales.

    **lingual c.,** a pit lined with epithelium in the lingual tonsil.

    **Morgagni's c.'s,** *sinus* anales.

    **sebaceous c.,** *glandula* sebacea.

    **syno'vial c.,** a diverticulum of the synovial membrane of a joint.

    **tonsillar c.,** *crypta* tonsillaris.

**crypta,** pl. **cryp'tae** (krip'tah) [ L. fr. G. *kryptos*, hidden ] [ NA ]. Crypt; a pitlike depression or tubular recess.

    **c. tonsilla'ris,** pl. **cryptae tonsilla'res** [ NA ], tonsillar crypt; one of the variable number of deep recesses that extend into the palatine and pharyngeal tonsils from the free surface where they open at the fossulae tonsillares.

**cryptanamnesia** (krip-tan-am-ne'sĭ-ah) [ G. *kryptos*, concealed, + *anamnēsis*, memory. MN- ]. Subconscious *memory*.

**cryptectomy** (krip-tek'to-mĭ) [ crypt, + G. *ektomē*, excision ]. Excision of a tonsillar or other crypt.

**crypten'amine acetates** or **tannates.** UNITENSIN acetates or tannates; acetate or tannate salts of alkaloids from a nonaqueous extract of *Veratrum viride*, containing the hypotensive alkaloids protoveratrines A and B, germitrine, neogermetrine, germerine, germidine, jervine, rubijervine, isorubijervine, and germubide. Used as an antihypertensive agent. See also protoveratrines.

**cryptesthesia** (krip-tes-the'zĭ-ah) [ G. *kryptos*, concealed, + *aisthesis*, sensation, perception ]. Subconscious perception; awareness of facts or occurrences not ordinarily perceptible to the senses; intuition.

**cryptic** (krip'tik) [ G. *kryptikos* ]. Hidden; occult; larvate.

**crypti'tis.** Inflammation of a follicle or glandular tubule, particularly in the rectum.

**crypto-, crypt-** [ G. *kryptos*, hidden, concealed ]. Combining form relating to a crypt, or meaning hidden, obscure, without apparent cause.

**cryptocavine.** Cryptopine.

**cryp'toceph'alus** [ crypto- + G. *kephalē*, head ]. A malformed fetus with an underdeveloped and very small head.

**cryptococcoma** (krip'to-kok-o'mah). Toruloma; an infectious granuloma, typically in the brain, caused by *Cryptococcus neoformans*.

**cryptococcosis** (krip'to-kok-o'sis). European blastomycosis; torulosis; Buschke's disease (2); Busse-Buschke disease; an acute, subacute, or chronic infection by *Cryptococcus neoformans*, causing a pulmonary, systematic, or meningeal mycosis.

**Cryptococcus** (krip'to-kok'us) [ crypto- + G. *kokkos*, berry ]. A genus of fungi that reproduce by budding; no spores are developed. The old term is *Torula*.

    **C. capsula'tus,** *Histoplasma capsulatum*. This organism is not a member of the genus *Cryptococcus*.

    **C. dermatit'idis,** obsolete name for *Blastomyces dermatitidis*.

    **C. farcimino'sus,** the cause of epizootic lymphangitis or pseudofarcy in members of the horse family. It is now known as *Zymonema farciminosum*, a yeastlike organism that causes a purulent inflammation of the lymphatic channels of the legs, leading to ulcerations.

    **C. gilchris'ti,** obsolete name for *Blastomyces dermatitidis*.

    **C. hom'inis,** *C. neoformans*.

    **C. hystolyt'icus,** *C. neoformans*.

    **C. linguae pilosae,** a form that infects the tongue and causes hypertrophy of the filiform papillae (lingua nigra).

    **C. meningit'idis,** *C. neoformans*.

    **C. neofor'mans,** *C. hominis; C. hystolyticus; C. meningitidis;* a form that attacks the skin, lungs, and especially the brain and its membranes; cause of cryptococcosis or European blastomycosis.

**cryp'tocrys'talline.** Having very minute crystals.

**Cryptocys'tis trichodec'tis.** A term no longer used for the larval form of dog tapeworm, *Dipylidium caninum*.

**cryptodidymus** (krip'to-did'ĭ-mus) [ crypto- + G. *didymos*, twin ]. Conjoined twins, one of which (the "parasite") small, poorly developed, and more or less concealed within the larger ("host") twin.

**Cryptogamia** (krip-to-gam'ĭ-ah) [ crypto- + G. *gamos*, marriage ]. A division of the plant kingdom containing all forms of plant life which do not reproduce by means of seeds. Included are three phyla: the Thallophyta (algae, bacteria, fungi and lichens), the Bryophyta (mosses and liverworts), and the Pteridophyta or (ferns, horsetails, and club mosses).

**cryptogenet'ic, cryptogen'ic** [ crypto- + G. *genesis*, origin ]. Of obscure, indeterminate origin; opposed to phanerogenic.

**cryp'tolith** [ crypto- + G. *lithos*, stone ]. A concretion in a gland follicle.

**cryptomenorrhea** (krip-to-men-or-e'ah) [ crypto- + G. *men*, month, + *rhoia*, flow ]. The occurrence each month of the general symptoms of the menses without any flow of blood, as in cases of imperforate hymen.

**cryptomerorachischisis** (krip'to-me'ro-rā-kis'-kī-sis) [ crypto- + G. *meros*, part, + *rachis*, spine, + *schisis*, cleavage ]. *Spina* bifida occulta.

**cryptomnesia** (krip-tom-ne'zī-ah). Cryptanamnesia.

**cryptophthalmia** (krip-tof-thal'me-ah). Cryptophthalmus.

**cryptophthalmus** (krip-tof-thal'mus) [ crypto- + G. *ophthalmos*, eye ]. Cryptophthalmia; congenital absence of eyelids with skin passing continuously from forehead onto cheek over a rudimentary eye.

**cryp'topine.** Cryptocavine; an alkaloid derived from opium; $C_{21}H_{22}NO_5$; resembles papaverine in its action.

**cryptopo'dia** [ crypto- + G. *pous*, foot ]. A condition of swelling of the lower part of the leg and the foot, in such a manner that there is great distortion and the sole seems to be a flattened pad.

**cryptopy'ic** [ crypto- + G. *pyon*, pus ]. Pertaining to a condition characterized by concealed suppuration; denoting a pyemia without apparent cause.

**cryptopyr'role.** 3-Ethyl-2,4-dimethylpyrrole; one of the pyrrole derivatives obtained by the drastic reduction of heme.

**cryp'tora'diom'eter** [ crypto- + L. *radius*, ray, + G. *metron*, measure ]. A device for estimating the degree of penetrative power of x-rays.

**cryptorchid** (krip-tor'kid) [ crypto- + G. *orchis*, testis ]. Cryptorchis; one whose testes have not descended into the scrotum.

**cryptorchidectomy** (krip'tor-kī-dek'o-mī) [ crypto- + G. *orchis*, testis, + *ektome*, excision ]. Surgical removal of an undescended testis.

**cryptorchidism** (krip-tor'kī-dizm). Cryptorchism.

**cryptorchidopexy** (krip-tor'kī-do-pek'sī) [ crypto- + G. *orchis*, testis, + *pexis*, fixation ]. Orchiorrhaphy.

**cryptorchis** (krip-tor'kis). Cryptorchid.

**cryptorchism** (krip-tor'kizm). Cryptorchidism; the failure of descent of a testis.

**Cryptosporid'ium** [ crypto- + G. *sporos*, seed ]. A genus of coccidia in which the oocyst is said to have four naked sporozoites, although this is unsubstantiated because oocysts have not been found in feces and the normal mode of transmission is unknown; there are two species in domestic fowl, three in laboratory rodents.

C. **meleag'ridis,** occurs in the lower small intestine of turkeys and is an occasional cause of illness and low mortality in young poults, as described from Scotland.

C. **tyzze'ri,** a relatively rare, nonpthogenic species occurring in the ceca of chickens, as described from Massachusetts.

**Cryptotermes** (krip-to-ter'mēz) [ crypto- + late L. *termes*, woodworm ]. A genus of termites, considered by some as responsible for sprue through ingestion of their fecal pellets.

**cryptoxanthin** (krip'to-zan'thin). Carotenoid yielding 1 mole of vitamin A per mole.

**cryp'tozo'ite** [ crypto- + G. *zoe*, life ]. The exoerythrocyte stage that develops directly from the sporozoite inoculated by the infected mosquito; development of the first generation of merozoites in the vertebrate host tissues, usually the liver parenchyma.

**cryptozygous** (krip-toz'ī-gus) [ crypto- + G. *zygon*, yoke ]. Having a narrow face as compared with the width of the cranium, so that, when the skull is viewed from above, the zygomatic arches are not visible.

**crystal** (kris'tal) [ G. *krystallos*, clear ice, crystal. CRYS- ]. A solid of regular shape and, for a given compound, characteristic angles, formed when an element or compound solidifies slowly enough, as a result either of freezing from the liquid form or of precipitating out of solution, to allow the individual molecules to take up regular positions with respect to one another.

**asthma c.,** Charcot-Leyden c.

**blood c.'s,** hematoidin c.'s; see hematoidin.

**Böttcher's c.'s,** small c.'s observed microscopically in prostatic fluid that is treated with a drop or two of 1 per cent solution of ammonium phosphate.

**Charcot-Leyden c.'s,** Charcot-Neumann c.'s; Leyden's c.'s; Charcot-Robin c.'s; c.'s of the shape of elongated double pyramids, formed from eosinophils, found in the sputum in bronchial asthma and in other exudates or transudates containing eosinophils.

**Charcot-Neumann c.'s,** Charcot-Leyden c.'s.

**Charcot-Robin c.'s,** Charcot-Leyden c.'s.

**chiral c.,** an enantiomorphic, dissymmetric, optically active c.

**clathrate c.,** lattice-like arrangement of molecules of one substance surrounding molecules of another substance; proposed as a basis for mode of action of inhalation anesthetics.

**ear c.'s,** statoconia.

**Florence's c.'s,** brown rhombic c.'s formed at the interface between a drop of Lugol's solution and a drop of fluid that contains semen; not a specific test for the latter.

**hydrate c.,** one of several possible microstructural arrangements of water molecules based on intermolecular forces; suggested as being involved in the mode of action of inhalation anesthetics.

**knife-rest c.,** a c. of ammoniomagnesium phosphate found in alkaline urine.

**Leyden's c.'s,** Charcot-Leyden c.'s.

**Lubarsch's c.'s,** intracellular c.'s in the testis resembling sperm c.'s.

**sperm c., spermin c.,** a c. of spermin phosphate found in the semen; possibly identical to Böttcher's c.'s.

**Teichmann's c.'s,** c.'s of hemin, the chloride of heme.

**thorn apple c.'s,** ammonium urate c.'s in the shape of rounded bodies with many projecting points.

**twin c.,** two c.'s that have grown together along a common face.

**Virchow's c.'s,** yellow-brown, amber, or burnt orange c.'s of hematoidin, frequently observed in extravasated blood in tissues.

**whetstone c.'s,** xanthine c.'s occasionally observed in urine.

**crys'tallin.** A globulin in the crystalline lens of the eye.

**crys'talline.** 1. Clear; transparent. 2. Relating to a crystal or crystals.

**crystalli'tis.** Obsolete term for phacitis.

**crys'talliza'tion.** The assumption of a crystalline form when a vapor or liquid becomes solidified, or a solute precipitates from solution.

**heat of c.,** see under heat.

**cryst'allogram** [ G. *crystallos*, crystal, + *gramma*, something written ]. A photograph produced when x-rays are diffracted by a crystal.

**crystallography** (kris'tal-log'rā-fī). The study of the shape and atomic structure of crystals.

**crys'talloid.** 1. Resembling a crystal, or being such. 2. A body which in solution can pass through a semipermeable membrane, as distinguished from a colloid, which cannot do so.

**Charcot-Böttcher c.'s,** spindle-shaped c.'s 10 to 25 μ long, found in human Sertoli cells.

**Reinke c.'s,** rod-shaped crystal-like structures with pointed or rounded ends present in the interstitial cells of the testis (Leydig cells) and ovary.

**crystallophobia** (kris'tal-lo-fo'bī-ah) [ G. *krystallon*, crystal, + *phobos*, fear ]. Morbid fear of glass objects.

**crystalluria** (kris'tal-lu'rī-ah). The excretion of crystalline materials in the urine.

**crystal violet.** Gentian violet (USP); methylrosanilin chloride (USP); methyl violet; hexamethyl-pararosanilin chloride ($C_{25}H_{30}N_3Cl$), a dark green powder or greenish, glistening, small particles with metallic luster; soluble in water, alcohol, glycerine, and chloroform. Under the several names, these products are variable mixtures of tetra-, penta-, and hexamethyl-pararosanilin of which the latter appears to be the most important. It has been used in the treatment of burns, wounds, infections of skin and mucous membranes, and (internally) for pinworm and certain fluke infections. It is also used as a stain in histology and bacteriology; see Gram *stain*.

**Cs.** Chemical symbol of the element cesium.

**CSF.** Abbreviation for cerebrospinal fluid (*liquor* cerebrospinalis, *q.v.*).

**Csillag,** J. See C.'s disease.

**Ctenocephalides** (te′no-sef-al′ĭ-dēz) [ G. *ktenodēs,* like a cockle, + *kephalē,* head ]. A genus of fleas. *C. canis* (dog flea) and *C. felis* (cat flea) are nearly universal ectoparasites of household pets; will attack man when starving owing to absence of pets.

**CTP.** Abbreviation of cytidine triphosphate.

**Cu.** Chemical symbol of the element copper (cuprum).

**cu′beb** [ Ar. and Hindu, *kababa* ]. Cubebs; the dried unripe, nearly full-grown fruit of *Piper cubeba* (family Piperaceae), a climbing plant of the West Indies. Used as stimulant, carminative, and local irritant; has been used as a mild urinary antiseptic.

  **c. oil,** a volatile oil distilled from the fruit of *Piper cubeba;* for uses, see c.

**cubital** (ku′bĭ-tal). Relating to the elbow or to the ulna.

**cu′bitocar′pal.** Radiocarpal.

**cu′bitum** [ L. ] [ NA ]. Cubital.

**cubitus,** gen. and pl. **cu′biti** (ku′bĭ-tus) [ L. elbow. CUB- ] [ NA ]. Elbow; ulna.

  **c. valgus,** deviation of the extended forearm to the outer (radial) side of the axis of the limb.

  **c. varus,** deviation of the extended forearm inward (toward ulnar) side of forearm.

**cuboid, cuboidal** (ku′boyd, ku-boy′dal) [ G. *kybos,* cube, + *eidos,* resemblance ]. 1. Resembling a cube in shape. 2. Relating to the os cuboideum.

**Cuboni test.** See under test.

**cucur′bocit′rin.** A saponin from watermelon seeds. Causes dilation of capillaries and a consequent fall in blood pressure. See citrin.

**cud** (kud). Material regurgitated from the rumen for rechewing. All ruminants chew the c.

**cud′bear** [ coined fr. *Cuthbert* by Dr. *Cuthbert* Gordon, who patented the powder ]. Persio; a red-brown powder obtained from certain lichens, especially *Lecanora tartarea, Roccella montagnei,* and *Dendrographa leucophoea,* by macerating for several days with diluted ammonia. It is used in the arts as a dye and in pharmacy as a coloring agent.

**cue** (kū). A term used in conditioning and learning theory to describe a pattern of stimuli to which a person or animal has learned to respond.

  **response-produced c.'s,** successive stimulus c.'s in a behavior chain; each response serves as a reinforcer for the previous response and as a stimulus, or cue, for the next response.

**cuff.** Any structure shaped like a c.

  **rotator c. of the shoulder,** musculotendinous c.; the upper half of the capsule of the shoulder joint reinforced by the tendons of insertion of the supraspinatus, infraspinatus, teres minor, and subscapularis muscles.

**Cuignet** (kū-e-nya′), Ferdinand L. J., French ophthalmologist, *1823. See C.'s *method.*

**cuirass** (kwe-ras′) [ Fr. *cuirasse,* a breastplate ]. A term in symptomatology and pathology having reference to the thorax.

  **tabet′ic c.,** an anesthetic area on the chest sometimes noted in cases of tabes dorsalis.

**cul-de-sac,** pl. **culs-de-sac** (kul-de-sak′) [ Fr. bottom of a sack ]. A blind pouch or tubular cavity closed at one end; *e.g.,* diverticulum; cecum.

  **conjuncti′val c.,** *fornix* conjunctivae.

  **Douglas′ c.,** *excavatio* rectouterina.

  **greater c.,** *fundus* ventriculi.

**Gruber's c.,** a lateral diverticulum in the suprasternal space beside the medial extremity of the clavicle behind the sternal fasciculus of the sternocleidomastoid muscle.

**lesser c.,** *antrum* pyloricum.

**culdocentesis** (kul′do-sen-te′sis) [ cul-de-sac + G. *kentesis,* puncture ]. Aspiration of fluid from the cul-de-sac (rectouterine excavation) by puncture of the vaginal vault near the midline between the uterosacral ligaments.

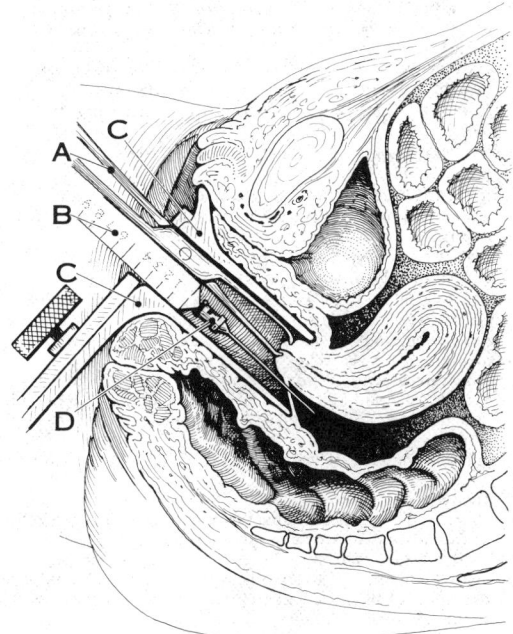

**Culdocentesis**
The instruments are: *A,* Allis forceps; *B,* syringe; *C,* speculum; *D,* 18-gauge spinal needle.

**culdoplasty** (kul′do-plas′tĭ) [ cul-de-sac + G. *plasso,* to fashion ]. A plastic procedure to remedy relaxation of the posterior fornix of the vagina.

**culdoscope** (kul′do-skōp). An endoscopic instrument used in culdoscopy.

**culdoscopy** (kul-dos′ko-pĭ) [ cul-de-sac + G. *skopeō,* to view ]. Introduction of an endoscope through the posterior vaginal wall and viewing the rectovaginal pouch and pelvic viscera.

**culdotomy** (kul-dot′o-mĭ) [ cul-de-sac + G. *tomē,* incision ]. Cutting into the cul-de-sac of Douglas.

**Culex** (ku′leks) [ L. gnat ]. A genus of mosquitoes including over 2,000 species, largely tropical but worldwide in distribution; they are vectors for a number of diseases of man and of domestic and wild animals and birds.

  **C. pi′piens,** the common, nocturnal brown house mosquito of temperate climates; breeds commonly in standing water, especially in artificial containers, and has a 5- to 6-day cycle under optimal conditions; closely related forms are found in tropical areas.

  **C. tarsa′lis,** an important vector of St. Louis and western equine encephalomyelitis viruses and other viruses in horses, birds and man.

**Culicidae** (ku-lis′ĭ-de). A family of insects (order Diptera) that includes the true mosquitoes, which are all included in the subfamily Culicinae.

**culicidal** (ku-lĭ-si′dal) [ L. *culex,* gnat, + *caedo,* to kill ]. Destructive to mosquitoes.

**cu′licide.** An agent that destroys mosquitoes.

**culicifuge** (ku-lis′ĭ-fūj) [ L. *culex,* gnat + *fugo,* to drive away ]. 1. Driving away gnats and mosquitoes. 2. An agent that keeps mosquitoes from biting.

**Culicoides** (ku-lĭ-koy′dēz) [ L. *culex*, gnat ]. A genus of minute biting gnats or midges, vectors of several nonpathogenic human filariae, *Anchocerca* of horses and cattle, and several viral agents of domestic sheep and fowl.

**C. aus′teni,** an intermediate host of the filarial worm, *Acanthocheilonema* (or *Dipetalonema*) *perstans*, chiefly in equatorial Africa.

**C. fu′rens,** vector of the human nonpathogenic filarial worm, *Mansonella ozzardi*, in the West Indies.

**C. milne′i,** one of the vectors of the human nonpathogenic filarial worm, *Acanthocheilonema perstans*, in West Africa.

**C. variipen′nis,** believed to be a vector of bluetongue disease of sheep in southwest United States.

**culicosis** (ku′lĭ-ko′sis). Dermatitis caused by mosquitoes ( *Culex*).

**Cullen,** Thomas S., American gynecologist, 1868–1953. See C.'s *sign*.

**culmen,** pl. **cul′mina** (kul′men) [ L. summit ] [ NA ]. Lobulus culminis; the anterior prominent portion of the monticulus of the vermis of the cerebellum.

**cultiva′tion** [ Mediev. L. *cultivo*, pp. -*atus*, fr. L. *colo*, pp. *cultus*, to till ]. Culture.

**culture** (kul′tūr) [ L. *cultura*, tillage, fr. *colo*, pp. *cultus*, to till ]. 1. The propagation of microorganisms on or in media of various kinds. 2. A mass of microorganisms on or in a medium.

**hanging-block c.,** the propagation of microorganisms on a cube of solidified agar medium which is inoculated, attached to a cover glass, and inverted over a moist chamber or hollowed slide.

**mixed lymphocyte c.,** see mixed lymphocyte culture *test*.

**needle c.,** stab c.

**neotype c.,** neotype *strain*.

**pure c.,** in the ordinary bacteriologic sense, a c. consisting of the descendants of a single cell.

**roll-tube c.,** a c. in a tube of medium which has been melted and allowed to solidify while the tube is being spun; the inside of the tube is thereby coated with a thin layer of solidified medium.

**sensitized c.,** a live c. of an organism to which a specific antiserum is added; after the mixture is incubated for several minutes (during which antibody in the serum combines with the organisms), the excess serum is removed by means of centrifugation, washing in physiologic saline solution, and recentrifugation; the sensitized organisms may then be resuspended in physiologic saline solution.

**shake c.,** a c. made by inoculating a liquefied gelatin or agar medium, distributing the inoculum thoroughly by agitation, and then allowing the medium to solidify in the tube in an upright position.

**slant c.,** slope c.; a c. made on the slanting surface of a medium which has been solidified in a test tube inclined from the perpendicular so as to give a greater area than that of the lumen of the tube.

**slope c.,** slant c.

**smear c.,** a c. obtained by spreading material presumed to be infected on the surface of a solidified medium.

**stab c.,** needle c.; a c. produced by inserting an inoculating needle with inoculum down the center of a solid medium contained in a test tube.

**stock c.,** a c. of a microorganism maintained solely for the purpose of keeping the microorganism in a viable condition by subculture, as necessary, into fresh medium.

**streak c.,** a c. produced by lightly stroking an inoculating needle or loop with inoculum over the surface of a solid medium.

**tissue c.,** the maintenance of live tissue after removal from the body, by placing in a vessel with a sterile nutritive medium.

**type c.,** type *strain*.

**Culver's physic** or **root.** Leptandra.

**cu′marin.** Coumarin.

**cumeth′arol.** DICUMOXANE; cumethoxaethane; 3,3′-(2-methoxyethylidene)bis[ 4-hydroxycoumarin ]; oral anticoagulant.

**cumethoxaethane.** Cumetharol.

**cu′minal′dehyde thiosemicarbazone.** CUTHIZONE; *p*-isopropylbenzaldehyde thiosemicarbazone; antiviral agent.

**Cummer,** W. E. See C.'s *classification*, C.'s *guideline*.

**cumulative** (ku′mu-la-tiv). Tending to accumulate or pile up; as certain drugs may have a cumulative effect; see also cumulative *effect*.

**cumulus,** pl. **cu′muli** (ku′mu-lus) [ L. a heap ] [ NA ]. A collection or heap of cells.

**c. ooph′orus** [ NA ], discus proligerus; proligerous disk; c. ovaricus; proligerous membrane; a mass of epithelial cells surrounding the ovum in the ovarian follicle.

**c. ova′ricus,** c. oophorus.

**cuneate** (ku′ne-āt) [ L. *cuneus*, wedge ]. Wedge-shaped.

**cuneiform** (ku′ne-ĭ-form). Wedge-shaped.

**cuneocuboid** (ku′ne-o-ku′boyd). Relating to the lateral cuneiform and the cuboid bones.

**cuneonavic′ular.** Relating to the cuneiform and the navicular bones.

**cuneoscaph′oid.** Cuneonavicular.

**cuneus,** pl. **cu′nei** (ku′ne-us) [ L. wedge ] [ NA ]. That region of the medial aspect of the occipital lobe of each cerebral hemisphere that is bounded by the parietooccipital fissure and the calcarine fissure.

**cuniculus,** pl. **cunic′uli** (ku-nik′u-lus) [ L. a rabbit; an underground passage ]. The burrow of the itch mite in the epidermis.

**Cunisset's test.** See under test.

**cunnilinction, cunnilinctus** (kun-ĭ-lingk′shun, -lingk′-tus). Cunnilingus.

**cunnilinguist** (kun′ĭ-ling′gwist) [ L. *cunnus*, pudendum, + *lingua*, tongue ]. One who practices cunnilinction.

**cunnilingus** (kun-ĭ-ling′gus) [ L. *cunnus*, pendulum, + *lingo*, to lick ]. Cunnilinction; cunnilinctus; sexual stimulation by licking or kissing the vulva or clitoris; a type of oral genital sexual activity.

**cunnus** (kun′us) [ L. ]. Vulva.

**cup** [ A. S. *cuppe* ]. 1. An excavated or cup-shaped structure, either anatomical or pathologic. 2. A cupping *glass*.

**Diogenes c.,** poculum diogenis; the palm of the hand when contracted and deepened by the action of the muscles on either side.

**dry c.,** a cupping glass applied to the unbroken surface for the purpose of drawing blood to the part without abstracting any; see also wet c.

**eye c.,** (1) a small oblong cuplike receptacle, fitting over the eye, intended to facilitate the application of a liquid medicament to the conjunctiva; (2) the optic c.

**glauco′matous c.,** glaucomatous excavation; a deep depression of the optic disk characterized by overhanging walls over which the central retinal vessels bend sharply.

**Klapp's suction c.'s,** cupping glasses of special shapes to fit various portions of the body, used to induce hyperemia in Bier's method.

**ocular c.,** *caliculus* ophthalmicus.

**optic c.,** *caliculus* ophthalmicus.

**perilimbal suction c.,** an aid in diagnosis of open-angle glaucoma; after application of negative pressure, the subsequent rise of ocular tension is less in glaucoma than in normal eyes.

**physiolog′ic c.,** a funnel-shaped excavation of the optic disk, an exaggeration of the normal depression.

**suction c.,** (1) one of the cupping glasses of various shapes, used to produce local hyperemia according to Bier's method; (2) an obsolete method which utilized rubber cups to retain dentures through attachment to the oral mucosa by suction.

**wet c.,** a cupping glass applied to a part previously scarified or incised, in order to draw away blood.

**cu′pola.** Cupula.

**cupped.** Hollowed; made cup-shaped.

**cup′ping.** 1. Formation of a hollow, or cup-shaped excavation. 2. Application of a c. glass; formerly used as one of the methods to produce slow bleeding.

**cu′pralylna′trium.** CUPRELON; cupralylsodium; *m*-[ (*N*-allyl-1-mercaptoformimidoyl)-amino ]benzoic acid copper derivative sodium salt; antiarthritic agent.

**cupreine** (ku′pre-ēn). Ultraquinine; an alkaloid, $C_{19}H_{22}N_2O_2 2H_2O$, from cuprea bark; used in the synthesis of ethylhydrocupreine.

**cu′pric.** Pertaining to copper, particularly to copper in the form of a doubly charged positive ion.

**c. acetate, normal,** $Cu(CH_3COOH)_2 \cdot H_2O$; crystallized verdigris; a stimulating local caustic to ulcers.

**c. arsenite,** copper arsenite; Scheele's green; $CuHAsO_3$; a green crystalline powder. Obsolete as medicinal agent; used as insecticide and pigment.

**c. chloride,** copper chloride; copper bichloride; copper dichloride; $CuCl_2 \cdot 2H_2O$. Has been used as an antiseptic in the treatment of water supplies, ponds, and pools.

**c. citrate,** copper citrate; used for the same indications as the other salts of copper, as astringent and antiseptic.

**c. sulfate** (NF), copper sulfate; copper sulphate (BP); blue vitriol; blue stone; $CuSO_4 \cdot 5H_2O$; it is highly poisonous to algae, is a prompt and active emetic, and is used as an irritant, astringent, and fungicide. It was formerly used, in a wooden holder, to treat trachoma.

**cupriuresis** (ku-prī-u-re'sis) [ L. *cuprum*, copper, + G. *ourēsis*, a urinating ]. The urinary excretion of copper.

**cuprohe'mol.** Hemol with 2 per cent copper in organic combination.

**cuprox'oline.** DICUPRENE; 8-hydroxy-5,7-quinolinedisulfonic acid copper derivative compound with diethylamine; antiarthritic agent.

**cupula,** pl. **cu'pulae** (ku'pu-lah) [ L. dim. of *cupa*, a tub ] [ NA ]. Cupola; a cup-shaped or domelike structure.

**c. cochleae** [ NA ], the domelike apex of the cochlea.

**c. cristae ampulla'ris** [ NA ], cap of the ampullary crest; a gelatinous mass that overlies the hair cells of the cristae ampullares of the semicircular ducts.

**c. pleurae** [ NA ], cervical pleura; the dome-shaped roof of the pleural cavity extending up through the superior aperture of the thorax.

**cu'pular.** 1. Relating to a cupula. 2. Cupulate; dome-shaped.

**cu'pulate.** Cupular (2); dome-shaped.

**cu'pulogram.** A graphic representation of vestibular function relative to normal performance.

**curaçao** (ku-rä-so') [ Curaçao, island in the Netherlands West Indies ]. A liqueur or cordial made of alcohol, sugar, and bitter-orange peel.

**curage** (ku'rij, ku-rahzh') [ Fr. a cleansing ]. Curettage by means of the finger rather than the curet.

**curare** (ku'rah-re, koo'rah-re) [ S. Am. ]. Curara; curari; ourari; urari; wourara; wourali; woorari, etc.; Indian arrow poison; an extract of various plants, especially *Strychnos toxifera, S. Castelnaei, S. crevauxii,* and *Chondodendron tomentosum.* Orally it is practically inert. Used intravenously or intramuscularly, it produces muscular paralysis by preventing motor nerve impulses from causing normal contraction of skeletal muscles. Death results from paralysis of the respiratory muscles. The antidote to excessive curarization is neostigmine methylsulfate.

**curar'iform.** Denoting a drug having an action like curare.

**curar'imimet'ic.** Having a curare-like action.

**curarine** (ku'rah-rēn). C-Curarine I; $C_{40}H_{44}N_4O^{++}$; the alkaloid principle of calabash curare.

**curariza'tion.** The induction of a condition of muscular relaxation or paralysis by the administration of curare or related compounds that have the ability to block nerve impulse transmission at the myoneural junction.

**cu'rarize.** To induce motor, but not sensory paralysis by the administration of curare.

**curative** (kūr'ă-tiv). 1. That which heals or cures. 2. Tending to heal or cure.

**curb.** A hard, painful, inflammatory swelling on the back part of the hock of the horse. It occurs in the plantar ligament near its insertion. It is characterized by swelling and heat in the part, and generally by lameness. It is believed to be caused by straining the ligament in falling, jumping, or pulling.

**cur'cuma** [ Ar. *kurkum,* saffron ]. Turmeric; the rhizome of *Curcuma longa* (family Zingiberaceae) or *C. rotunda* (*Amomum curcuma*), an Indian plant of the ginger family. Formerly used as a stimulant and in the treatment of functional disorders of the liver and biliary tract; now used only as a condiment and dyestuff.

**curd.** The coagulum of milk.

**alum c.,** milk coagulated by alum.

**cure** (kūr) [ L. *curo,* to care for ]. 1. To heal; to make well. 2. A restoration to health. 3 [ Ger. *kur.* ]. A special method or course of treatment. 4. See dental *curing.*

**diet c.,** a system of treatment by regulation of the diet.

**faith c.,** a psychotherapeutic treatment based upon prayer and a profound belief in divine intervention in human affairs.

**gold c.,** Keeley c.

**grape c.,** botryotherapy.

**hunger c.,** hunger *therapy.*

**Keeley c.,** a secret method of treatment of alcoholism, said to be by the administration of strychnine and of gold chloride.

**radical c.,** a c. that completely and permanently corrects the condition.

**rest c.,** in psychiatry, the treatment of mental illness by rest and change of environment.

**terrain c.,** system of treatment by means of diet and of walking exercises taken in accurate dosage, along paths of measured ascent and measured length.

**thirst c.,** dipsotherapy.

**water c.,** hydrotherapy.

**curet** (ku-ret'). Curette.

**curetment** (ku-ret'ment). Curettage.

**curettage** (ku'rĕ-tahzh'). Curettement; curetment; a scraping of the interior of a cavity for the removal of new growths or other abnormal tissues, or to obtain material for tissue diagnosis.

**periapical c.,** (1) removal of a cyst or granuloma from its pathologic bony crypt, utilizing a curette; (2) the removal of tooth fragments and debris from sockets at the time of extraction or of bone sequestra subsequently.

**subgingival c.,** removal of subgingival calculus, ulcerated epithelial and granulomatous tissues found in periodontal pockets.

**curette** (ku-ret') [ Fr. ]. Curet. 1. An instrument in the form of a loop, ring, or scoop, with sharpened edges, attached to a rod-shaped handle, used to scrape the interior of a cavity for the removal of new growths or altered tissues. 2. To use a c.

**Hartmann's c.,** a. c., cutting on the side, for the removal of adenoids.

**curettement** (ku-ret'ment). Curettage.

**Curie** (koo're), Marie S., French chemist and physicist of Polish birth, 1867–1934. Celebrated as the codiscoverer, with her husband, of radioactivity and of the elements radium and polonium.

**Curie,** Pierre C., French chemist and physicist (husband of Marie S.), 1859–1906.

**curie** (ku'rī) [ Pierre and Marie S. *Curie* ]. Abbreviated Ci (formerly c); a unit of measurement of radioactivity, 3.70 × 10¹⁰ disintegrations per second. One gram of ²²⁶Ra emits 1 Ci of radioactivity.

**cu'riegram** [ M. *Curie* ]. Autoradiogram.

**cu'rine.** Bebeerine.

**curing** (ku'ring). The act of accomplishing a cure.

**dental c.,** the procedure by which the denture-base materials are hardened to the form of a denture in a denture mold; see also process (4).

**curium** (ku're-um) [ P. and M. *Curie* ]. Element of atomic no. 96, symbol Cm; not occurring naturally on earth, but first formed artificially in 1944 by bombarding plutonium-239 with alpha particles; the most stable of the c. isotopes is c.-247, with a half-life of approximately 90 million years.

**Curling,** Thomas B., English surgeon, 1811–1888. See C.'s *ulcer.*

**current** (kur'rent) [ L. *currens,* pres. p. of *curro,* to run ]. A stream or flow of fluid, air or electricity.

**action c.,** an electrical c. induced in muscle fibers when they are effectively stimulated. Normally it is followed by contraction.

**after-c.,** see aftercurrent.

**alternating c.,** AC; c. which flows first in one direction then in the other, *e.g.,* 60-cycle c.

**anodal c.,** a c. produced in tissues under the anode when the circuit is closed.

**ascending c.,** the direction of c. flow in a nerve when the anode is placed peripheral to the cathode. The convention used is that c. flows from positive to negative.

**axial c.,** the central, rapidly moving portion of the blood stream in an artery.

**centrif'ugal c.,** descending c.

**centrip'etal c.,** ascending c.

**constant c., continuous c.,** a nonalternating and unbroken electrical c.

**d'Arsonval c.,** high frequency c.

**demarcation c.,** c. of injury.

**descending c.,** centrifugal c.; direction of c. flow in a nerve when cathode is placed peripheral to anode; opposite of ascending c.

**direct c.,** DC; a c. of the type derived from a battery; sometimes referred to as galvanic c.

**electrotonic c.,** see electrotonus.

**high frequency c.,** d'Arsonval c.; Tesla c.; an alternating electric c. having a frequency of 10,000 or more per second; it produces no muscular contractions and does not affect the sensory nerves.

**high tension c.,** one produced by a high electromotive force.

**inducing c.,** the primary c. that gives rise to a secondary c. in the induction coil.

**c. of injury,** the c. set up when an injured part of a nerve, muscle, or other excitable tissue is connected through a conductor with the uninjured region; the injured tissue is negative to the uninjured.

**labile c.,** an electrical c. applied to the body by means of electrodes that are constantly shifted about.

**Leduc c.,** a direct electric c., which is interrupted approximately 110 times a second by means of the Leduc interrupter, used to produce electric anesthesia or electric narcosis.

**Morton's c.,** electrical discharges from a Leyden jar passed through the patient, the jar being continuously recharged by means of a static machine.

**Ouidin c.,** a monopolar desiccating c. used in electrosurgery.

**primary c.,** inducing c.

**reversed c.,** a c. of changed direction.

**secondary c.,** see inducing c.

**Curschmann** (koorsh'mahn), Heinrich, German physician, 1846–1910. See C.'s *disease, spirals.*

**Curtis,** A. H. See Fitz-Hugh and C. *syndrome.*

**curvatura,** pl. **curvatu'rae** (kur'vă-tu'rah) [ L. ] [ NA ]. Curvature.

**c. ventric'uli major** [ NA ], greater curvature of the stomach; the border of the stomach to which the greater omentum is attached.

**c. ventric'uli minor** [ NA ], lesser curvature of the stomach; the right border of the stomach to which the lesser omentum is attached.

**curvature** (kur'vă-tūr) [ L. *curvatura,* fr. *curvo,* pp. *-atus,* to bend, curve ]. Curvatura (*q. v.*); a bending or flexure.

**angular c.,** the sharp bend in the spine in Pott's disease.

**anterior c.,** kyphosis.

**backward c.,** lordosis.

**gingival c.,** the rounding of the gum along its line of attachment to the neck of a tooth.

**hyperopia of c.,** see under hyperopia.

**lateral c.,** scoliosis.

**occlusal c.,** *curve* of occlusion.

**Pott's c.,** the kyphosis of Pott's disease.

**spinal c.,** see kyphosis, lordosis, and scoliosis.

**curve** (kurv) [ L. *curvo,* to bend ]. 1. Curvature; a nonangular continuous bend. 2. Chart; a graphic representation, by means of a continuous line of shifting direction, of the course of the temperature or pulse, of the numbers of cases of a disease in a given period, or of any other group of parts which might be otherwise presented by a table of figures; a sphygmogram or any other tracing made by a recording instrument.

**alinement c.,** the line passing through the center of the teeth laterally in the direction of the c. of the dental arch.

**anti-Monson c.,** reverse c.

**Barnes' c.,** a c. corresponding in general with Carus' c., being the segment of a circle whose center is the promontory of the sacrum.

**buccal c.,** the line of the dental arch from the canine, or cuspid tooth to the third molar.

**Carus' c.,** an imaginary curved line obtained from a mathematical formula, supposed to indicate the outlet of the pelvic canal.

**compensating c.,** the anteroposterior and lateral curvature in the alignment of the occluding surfaces and incisal edges of artificial teeth; used to develop balanced occlusion.

**distribution c.,** a graph of a frequency distribution.

**"dromedary" c.,** a c. with two humps (like those of a camel); usually a fever c.

**dye-dilution c.,** indicator-dilution c.; graph of the serial concentrations (dilutions) of a dye, *e.g.,* Evans blue, following its intravascular or intracardiac injection; useful in the diagnosis of congenital cardiac shunts, measurement of cardiac output, and detection of cardiovalvular incompetence.

**frequency c.,** a graph of a frequency distribution.

**Friedman c.,** a graph on which hours of labor are plotted against cervical dilation in centimeters.

**Gaussian c.,** Gaussian *distribution.*

**indicator-dilution c.,** dye-dilution c.

**intracardiac pressure c.,** c. of pressure recorded within the atrium or ventricle (intraatrial and intraventricular pressure c.'s).

**isovolume pressure-flow c.,** the relationship between transpulmonary pressure and respiratory air flow, expressed as a function of lung volume.

**logistic c.,** an S-shaped c. which depicts the growth of a population in an area of fixed limits.

**milled-in c.'s,** milled-in *paths.*

**Monson c.,** the c. of occlusion in which each cusp and incisal edge touches or conforms to a segment of the surface of a sphere 8 inches in diameter with its center in the region of the glabella.

**muscle c.,** myogram.

**c. of occlusion,** occlusal curvature; (1) a curved surface which makes simultaneous contact with the major portion of the incisal and occlusal prominences of the existing teeth; (2) the c. of a dentition on which the occlusal surfaces lie.

**Pleasure c.,** an occlusal c. described by Pleasure; see reverse c.

**Price-Jones c.,** a distribution c. of the measured diameters of red blood cells; it is to the right of the normal c. (*i.e.,* indicating larger diameters) in instances of pernicious anemia and other forms in which macrocytes are present, and to the left (*i.e.,* indicating smaller diameters) in iron deficiency and other forms of microcytic anemia.

**probability c.,** a graph of the normal distribution representing relative probabilities.

**pulse c.,** sphygmogram.

**reverse c.,** anti-Monson c.; in dentistry, a c. of occlusion which is convex upward.

**c. of Spee,** von Spee's c.; anatomic curvature of the occlusal alignment of teeth beginning at the tip of the lower cuspid and following the buccal cusps of the natural bicuspids and molars, continuing to the anterior border of the ramus.

**Starling's c.,** a graph in which cardiac output is plotted against atrial pressure; with increasing venous return and atrial pressure the output proportionately increases until further increments overload the heart and the output falls.

**strength-duration c.,** a graph relating the intensity of an electrical stimulus to the length of time it must flow to be effective; see chronaxie and rheobase.

**stress-strain c.,** a c. showing the ratio of deformation to load during the testing of a material in tension.

**tension c.,** the direction of the trabeculae in cancellous bone tissue adapted to resist stress.

**Traube-Hering c.'s,** Traube-Hering waves; slow oscillations in blood pressure usually extending over several respiratory cycles; related to variations in vasomotor tone; rhythmical variations in blood pressure.

**von Spee's c.,** c. of Spee.

**Cusco** (küs-ko'), Edouard G., Paris surgeon, 1819–1894. See C.'s *speculum.*

**cusco bark** (ku'sko). The bark of *Cinchona pubescens* and *C. pelletieriana;* see cinchona.

**Cushing,** Harvey W., American neurosurgeon, 1869–1939. See C.'s *basophilism, disease, law, phenomenon, syndrome.*

**Cushing,** Hayward W., Massachusetts surgeon, 1854–1934. See C.'s *suture.*

**cushion** (koosh'un). In anatomy, any structure resembling a pad or c.

**a'trioventric'ular canal c.'s,** endocardial c.'s; a pair of mounds of embryonic connective tissue covered by endothelium, bulging into the embryonic atrioventricular canal. Located one dorsally and one ventrally, they grow together and fuse, dividing the originally single canal into right and left atrioventricular orifices.

**endocardial c.'s,** atrioventricular canal c.'s.

**c. of epiglottis,** *tuberculum* epiglotticum.

**Eusta'chian c.,** *torus* tubarius.

**levator c.,** *torus* levatorius.

**Passavant's c.,** Passavant's bar, pad, or ridge; a prominence on the posterior wall of the nasal pharynx formed by contraction of the superior constrictor of the pharynx during swallowing.

**pharyngoesophageal c.'s,** pharyngoesophageal pads; venous plexuses on the anterior and posterior walls of the pharyngoesophageal junction.

**plantar c.,** a dense mass of fibrofatty tissue overlying the frog in the foot of the horse. It serves an important shock-absorbing function.

**sucking c.,** *corpus* adiposum buccae.

**cusp** (kusp) [ L. *cuspis,* point ]. Cuspis. 1. In dentistry, a conical elevation arising on the surface of a tooth from an independent calcification center; see also tuberculum dentis. 2. A leaflet of one of the heart's valves.

**anterior c.,** *cuspis* anterior.

**posterior c.,** *cuspis* posterior.

**septal c.,** *cuspis* septalis.

**c. of tooth,** *cuspis* dentis.

**cuspad** (kus'pad) [ L. *ad,* to ]. In a direction toward the cusp of a tooth.

**cuspal** (kus'pal). Pertaining to a cusp.

**cusparia bark.** Angostura bark.

**cuspid** (kus'pid) [ L. *cuspis,* point ]. 1. Cuspidate; having but one cusp. 2. *Dens* caninus.

**cus'pidate.** Cuspid (1).

**cuspis,** pl. **cus'pides** (kus'pis) [ L. a point ] [ NA ]. Cusp.

**c. anterior** [ NA ], anterior cusp; the anterior leaflet of either the right or left atrioventricular valve.

**c. coro'nae** [ NA ], an alternate term for c. dentis.

**c. den'tis** [ NA ], cusp of a tooth; c. coronae; an elevation or mound on the crown of a tooth making up a part of the occlusal surface.

**c. posterior** [ NA ], posterior cusp; the posterior leaflet of either the right or left atrioventricular valve.

**c. septa'lis** [ NA ], septal cusp; the leaflet of the right atrioventricular valve located adjacent to the interventricular septum.

**cusso** (ku'so). Brayera.

**cutaneous** (ku-ta'ne-us) [ L. *cutis,* skin ]. Relating to the skin.

**cutch.** Catechu nigrum.

**cut'down.** Venostomy; dissection of a vein for insertion of a cannula or needle for the administration of intravenous fluids or medication.

**Cuterebra cuniculi.** A fly belonging to the botfly group, which deposits its larvae on rabbits. The larvae develop into large grubs, usually in the subcutaneous connective tissue of the neck. Similar grubs, probably of other species, are not uncommon in cats and are sometimes found in dogs and in man.

**cuticle** (ku'ti-kl) [ L. *cuticula,* dim. of *cutis,* skin ]. 1. Cuticula. 2. The layer, sometimes chitinous in invertebrates, which occurs on the surface of epithelial cells.

**dental c.,** *cuticula* dentis.

**enamel c.,** *cuticula* dentis.

**ker'atose c.,** the outer layer of the choroid coat of the eye, next to the cornea.

**Nasmyth's c.,** *cuticula* dentis.

**c. of the root sheath,** a thin layer of cells lining the hair follicle.

**cuticula,** pl. **cutic'ulae** (ku-tik'u-lah) [ L. cuticle ]. 1 [ NA ]. Cuticle; an outer thin layer, usually horny in nature. 2. Epidermis.

**c. dentis** [ NA ], dental or enamel cuticle; Nasmyth's membrane or cuticle; skin of the teeth; it consists of two extremely thin layers (the inner one clear and structureless, the outer one cellular) covering the enamel of recently erupted teeth. It is soon abraded.

**c. pili,** cuticle of the hair.

**c. vaginae folliculi pili,** cuticle of the sheath of the follicle of the hair.

**cutic'ulariza'tion.** Covering an abraded area with epidermis.

**cu'tin** [ L. *cutis,* skin ]. A specially prepared, thin, animal membrane used as a protective covering for wounded surfaces.

**cu'tireac'tion** [ L. *cutis,* skin, + reaction ]. The inflammatory reaction in the case of a skin test in a sensitive (allergic) subject.

**cutis** ku'tis) [ L. ] [ NA ]. Pellis [ NA ]; skin; the membranous, protective covering of the body; it consists of epidermis and corium (dermis). See figs. under epidermis and corium.

**c. anseri'na,** gooseflesh; contraction of the arrectores pilorum produced by cold, fear, or other stimulus, causing the follicular orifices to become prominent.

**c. hyperelas'tica,** elastic skin; a congenital condition in which the skin is abnormally elastic and can be pulled out sometimes to an extraordinary distance, returning to its normal shape when released.

**c. laxa,** loose skin; dermatochalasis; pachydermatocele (1); a congenital condition in which there appears to be an excessive amount of skin hanging in folds.

**c. marmora'ta,** a pink, marble like mottling of the skin on exposure to cold, common in children and some adults; also associated with debilitating diseases.

**c. rhomboida'lis nu'chae,** geometric configurations of the skin of the back of the neck as a result of aging or prolonged exposure to sunlight.

**c. unctuo'sa,** *seborrhea* oleosa.

**c. vera,** corium.

**c. ver'ticis gyra'ta,** a congenital condition in which the skin of the scalp is hypertrophied and thrown into folds forming anterior to posterior furrows.

**cu'tisec'tor** [ L. *cutis,* skin, + *sector,* a cutter ]. 1. An instrument for cutting small pieces of skin for grafting. 2. An instrument used to remove a section of skin for microscopic examination.

**cutiza'tion.** The transition from mucous membrane to skin at the mucocutaneous margins.

**Cutler-Powell-Wilder test.** See under test.

**cut'ting.** In dentistry, the penetration, division, or removal of tooth structure with a sharp-edged or rotary instrument.

**ultrasonic c.,** the use of a high frequency vibrating cutting point and an abrasive slurry to remove tooth structure.

**cut'weed.** *Fucus vesiculosus.*

**cuvet, cuvette** (ku-vet'). A small container or cup in which solutions are placed for photometric analysis.

**Cuvier** (ku-ve-a), Georges L., French scientist, 1769–1832. See C.'s *ducts, veins.*

**cyamepro'mazine.** CIANATIL; 10-(3-dimethylamino-2-methylpropyl)-phenothiazine-2-carbonitrile; sedative with antihistaminic and antispasmodic properties.

**cyan-.** See cyano-.

**cyanal'cohol.** Cyanohydrin.

**cyan'amide.** Toxic, water-soluble substance, $H_2NCN$ or $NH=C=NH$; sometimes used in referring to calcium cyanamide, $CaCN_2$.

**cy'anate.** A compound containing the radical $-O-C\equiv N$ or ion (OCN)·.

**cyanemia** (si-an-e'mi-ah) [ cyan- + G. *haima,* blood ]. Imperfect aeration of the blood, that in the arteries resembling venous blood.

**cyanephidrosis** (si-an-ef-i-dro'sis) [ cyan- + G. *ephidrosis,* sweating ]. Cyanhidrosis; the excretion of sweat with a bluish tint.

**cyanhidrosis** (si-an-hi-dro'sis). Cyanephidrosis.

**cyanhy'dric acid.** Hydrocyanic acid.

**cy'anide.** A compound containing the radical —CN or ion (CN)⁻.

   **c. methemoglobin,** cyanmethemoglobin.

**cyan'idin.** (3')-Oxidation product of pelargonidin component of anthocyanins.

**cyanmethemoglobin** (si'an-met'he-mo-glo'bin). Cyanide methemoglobin; compound of cyanide with methemoglobin, which is formed when methylene blue is administered in cases of cyanide poisoning, the compound being relatively nontoxic.

**cy'anmetmy'oglo'bin.** Compound in which a cyanide group is bound to the iron atom $Fe^{3+}$) of metmyoglobin.

**cyano-, cyan-** [ G. *kyanos,* a dark blue mineral ]. 1. Combining form meaning blue. 2. A chemical prefix frequently used in naming compounds that contain the cyanide group, CN, as part of the molecule.

**cy'anoace'tic acid.** Nitrilomalonic acid; malonic mononitrile; $CNCH_2COOH$.

**cy'anoac'rylate adhesives.** Synthetic products possessing good host acceptance, relative permanency, and tissue barrier action. In strabismus surgery, isobutyl-2-cyanoacrylate monomer after polymerization prevents postoperative fibrotic adhesions.

**Cyanobacteria** (si'ā-no-bak-tēr'ĭ-ah). Cyanophyceae; a division of the kingdom Procaryotae. These organisms are unicellular or filamentous and are either nonmotile or possess a gliding motility. They reproduce by binary fission and perform photosynthesis with the production of oxygen. These blue-green bacteria were formerly referred to as blue-green algae.

**cyanochroic, cyanochrous** (si-an-o-kro'ik, si-an-ok'rus) [ cyano- + G. *chroia,* color ]. Cyanotic.

**cy'anocobal'amin** (USP, BP). Vitamin$B_{12}$, *q.v.;* hematopoietic agent apparently identical with the antianemia factor of liver; used in the treatment of pernicious anemia, tropical and nontropical sprue, and certain cases of nutritional macrocytic and megaloblastic anemias.

   **radioactive c.,** cyano[ ⁵⁷Co ]cobalamin or cyano[ ⁵⁸Co ]-cobalamin, produced by the growth of certain microorganisms on a medium containing cobalt-57 or cobalt-58; used in the investigation of the absorption and metabolism of cyanocobalamin.

**cy'anoder'ma** [ cyano- + G. *derma,* skin ]. Cyanosis.

**cyan'ogen.** A compound of two atoms each of carbon and nitrogen $(CN)_2$.

   **c. chloride,** CNCl; a highly volatile liquid; a systemic poison used as a warning agent in fumigation with hydrogen cyanide.

**cyanogen'ic.** Capable of producing hydrocyanic acid; said of plants such as sorghum, Johnson grass, arrowgrass and wild cherry which may cause cyanide poisoning in herbivorous animals.

**cy'anohy'drin.** RCHOHCN; cyanalcohol; an addition compound of HCN and an aldehyde.

**cyanophil, cyanophile** (si'an-o-fil, -fĭl) [ cyano- + G. *philos,* fond ]. A cell or element which is differentially colored blue by a staining procedure.

**cyanophilous** (si'ā-nof'ĭ-lus). Readily stainable with a blue dye.

**cyanophose** (si'an-o-fōz). A phose of a bluish color.

**Cyanophyceae** (si'ā-no-fi'se-e) [ cyano- + G. *phykos,* seaweed ]. Cyanobacteria.

**cyano'pia.** Cyanopsia.

**cyanop'sia** (si-ā-nop'sĭ-ah) [ cyano- + G. *opsis,* vision ]. Cyanopia; blue vision; a condition in which all objects appear blue; may temporarily follow cataract extraction.

**cyanop'sin.** A photochemical pigment present in the cones of the retina of some species; formed by the combination of opsin and vitamin $A_2$ instead of $A_1$, as with rhodopsin.

**cyanose tardive.** Cyanosis that is slow to appear; applied to the potentially cyanotic group of congenital heart diseases with an abnormal communication between systemic and pulmonary circulations; cyanosis is absent while the shunt is from left to right, but if the shunt reverses, as after exercise or late in the course of the disease, cyanosis appears.

**cyanosed** (si'ā-nozd). Cyanotic.

**cyanosis** (si-ā-no'sis) [ G. dark blue color, fr. *kyanos,* blue substance ]. Cyanoderma; a dark bluish or purplish coloration of the skin and mucous membrane due to deficient oxygenation of the blood. It becomes evident when reduced hemoglobin in the blood exceeds 5 gm. per 100 ml.

   **compression c.,** c. due to severe compression of the thorax or abdomen, resulting in a venous reflex that causes c., edema, and petechial hemorrhages over the head, neck, and upper part of the chest; the conjunctiva and retinas are similarly affected.

   **enterogenous c.,** apparent c. caused by the absorption of nitrites or other toxic materials from the intestine with the formation of methemoglobin or sulfhemoglobin. The skin color change is due to the chocolate color of methemoglobin.

   **false c.,** c. due to the presence of an abnormal pigment, such as methemoglobin, in the blood, and not resulting from a deficiency of oxygen.

   **hereditary methemoglobinemic c.,** congenital *methemoglobinemia.*

   **tardive c.,** *cyanose* tardive.

   **toxic c.,** c. due to methemoglobin formation resulting from the action of certain drugs, *e.g.,* nitrites.

**cyanot'ic.** Relating to or marked by cyanosis.

**cyanuria** (si'ā-nu'rĭ-ah) [ cyano- + G. *ouron,* urine ]. Dark blue urine.

**cyanu'ric acid.** 2,4,6-Trihydroxy-1,3,5-triazine, a cyclic product formed by heating urea.

**Cyathos'toma.** One of two genera of gapeworms of poultry, the other being *Syngamus,* in the nematode family Strongylidae.

   **C. bronchia'lis,** gapeworm of wild geese and domestic ducks, geese, and swans; occurs in the larynx, trachea, and bronchi and causes distress and symptoms similar to those produced by the chicken gapeworm, *Syngamus trachea;* its life cycle is thought to be similar to that of *Syngamus trachea.*

**Cyathos'tomum.** A genus of strongyle nematodes (family Strongylidae, subfamily Cyathostominae); it includes many of the small strongyles of horses formerly placed in the genus *Trichonema,* which some American scientists have divided into several similar genera, *e.g., C., Cylicocercus, Cylicocyclus, Cylicodontophorus, Cylicostephanus, Cylicotetrapedon, Cylicobrachytus,* and *Poterostomum.*

**cybernetics** (si'ber-net'iks) [ G. *kybernētica,* things pertaining to control or piloting ]. 1. The comparative study of electronic calculators and the human nervous system, with intent to explain the functioning of the brain. 2. The science of control and communication in both living and nonliving systems; characteristically, control is governed by feedback, that is, by communication within the system concerning the difference between the actual and the desired result, action then being modified so as to minimize this difference. See also feedback.

**cycl-** [ G. *kyklos,* circle ]. See cyclo-.

**cyclamate sodium** (si'klā-māt). See under sodium.

**cyclam'ic acid.** Cyclohexanesulfamic acid; cyclohexylsulfamic acid; *N*-cyclohexylsulfamic acid; a sweetening agent.

**cyc'lamin.** 3-β-Glucoside of malvidin chloride; a saponin-like body, $C_{13}H_{25}ClO_{12}.4H_2O$, obtained from the tuber of the herb *Cyclamen europaeum* (family Primulaceae); hemolytic agent, emetic, and purgative.

**cyclan'delate.** CYCLOSPASMOL; 3,3,5-trimethylcyclohexyl mandelate; an antispasmodic similar in action to papaverine; used for obliterative vascular diseases and vasospastic conditions.

**cyclar'bamate.** CALMALONE; 1,1-cyclopentanedimethanol dicarbanilate; tranquilizer with antispasmodic properties.

**cyclarthrodial** (si-klar-thro'di-al). Relating to a cyclarthrosis.

**cyclarthrosis** (si-klar-thro'sis) [ cyclo- + G. *arthrōsis,* articulation ]. A rotary, or trochoid, joint.

**cy'clase.** Descriptive name applied to an enzyme that forms a cyclic phosphodiester, *e.g.,* adenylate cyclase.

**cycla'zocine** (USAN). A potent analgesic of the benzomorphan series; an antagonist of morphine, precipitating withdrawal symptoms in man.

# CYCLE

**cycle** (si'kl) [ G. *kyklos*, circle ]. 1. A recurrent series of events. 2. A recurring period of time.

**anovulatory c.,** a sexual c. in which no ovum is discharged.

**brain wave c.,** the complete upward and downward excursion of a single wave, complex, or impulse.

**carbon dioxide c., carbon c.,** the circulation of carbon as $CO_2$ from the expired air of animals and decaying organic matter to plant life where it is synthesized (through photosynthesis) to carbohydrate material, from which, as a result of catabolic processes in all life, it is again ultimately released to the atmosphere as $CO_2$.

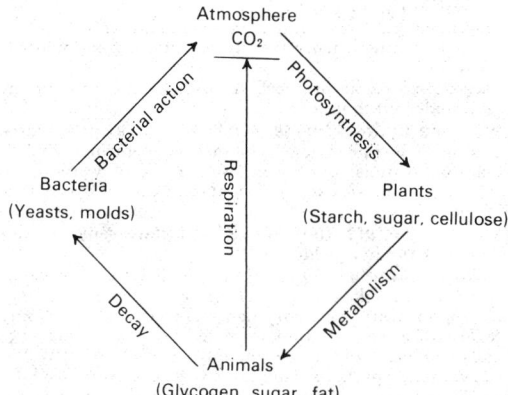

**Carbon Dioxide Cycle**
(After Haekle)

**cardiac c.,** the complete round of cardiac systole and diastole with the intervals between, or commencing with any event in the heart's action to the moment when that same event is repeated.

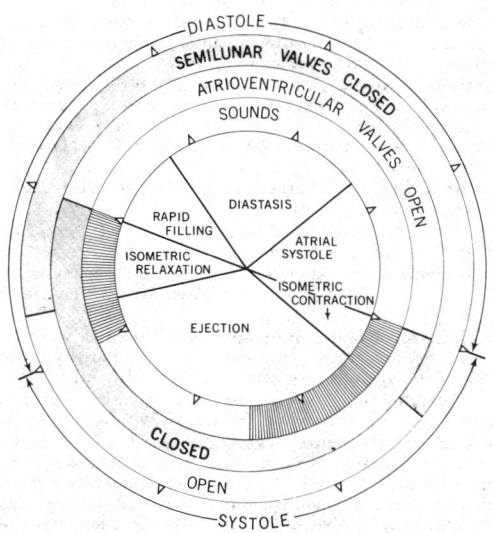

**Cardiac Cycle**
Divisions marked by △ indicate tenths of a second

**chewing c.,** a complete course of movement of the mandible during a single masticatory stroke.

**citric acid c.,** tricarboxylic acid c.

**Cori c.,** term given to the phases in the metabolism of carbohydrate: glycogenolysis in the liver; passage of glucose into the circulation; deposition of glucose in the muscles as glycogen; glycogenolysis during muscular activity and conversion to lactate, which is converted to glycogen in the liver.

**dicarboxylic acid c.,** that portion of the tricarboxylic acid c. involving the dicarboxylic acids; succinic, fumaric, malic, and oxaloacetic acids.

**dies'trous c.,** the estrous c. of diestrous animals.

**endog'enous c.,** the growth and reproduction of a parasite, such as the malarial organism, within the body of the vertebrate host.

**estrous c.,** the series of physiologic uterine, ovarian, and other changes that occur in higher animals, consisting of proestrus, estrus, postestrus, and anestrus or diestrus.

*Estrous cycles of the common domesticated animals*

| Species | Length | | Estrus | |
|---|---|---|---|---|
| | Days | Average | Days | Average |
| Horse | 19–23 | 21 | 4.5–5.5 | 5.3 days |
| Cow | 18–24 | 21 | 0.5–1.0 | 18 hr. |
| Sheep | 14–20 | 17 | 0.5–2.0 | 20 hr. |
| Goat | 15–24 | 20 | 2–5 | 40 hr. |
| Swine | 18–24 | 21 | 1–5 | 2 days |
| Dog | Usually 2 cycles per year | | 4–13 | 7–8 days |
| Cat | 2 or 3 cycles per year | | 15–21 | 8 days |

**exog'enous c.,** the development of a parasite, such as the malarial parasite, in the body of the invertebrate host.

**fatty acid oxidation c.,** a series of reactions involving acyl-coenzyme A compounds, whereby these undergo beta oxidation and thioclastic cleavage, with the formation of acetylcoenzyme A; the major pathway of fatty acid catabolism in living tissue.

**forced c.,** a cardiac c. (atrial or ventricular) that is cut short by a forced beat.

**genesial c.,** the reproductive period of a woman's life.

**glycine succinate c.,** a series of metabolic steps in which glycine, probably as pyruvate, is condensed with succinic acid and is then oxidized to $CO_2$ and $H_2O$ with regeneration of the succinic acid.

**glyoxylic acid c.,** a catabolic c. in plants and microorganisms replacing the tricarboxylic acid c. of animals. Its key reaction is the condensation of acetate with glyoxylic acid to malic acid (analogous to the condensation of acetate and oxaloacetic acid to form citric acid in the tricarboxylic acid c.).

**hair c.,** the phases of growth (anagen), regression (catagen), and quiescence (telogen) in the life of a hair.

**Krebs c.,** tricarboxylic acid c.

**Krebs-Henseleit c.,** urea c.

**Krebs' ornithine c.,** urea c.

**Krebs' urea c.,** urea c.

**life c.,** the entire life history of a living organism.

**masticating c.'s,** the patterns of mandibular movements formed during the chewing of food.

**menstrual c.,** the period in which an ovum matures, is ovulated, and enters the uterine lumen via the Fallopian tubes. Ovarian hormonal secretions effect endometrial changes such that, if fertilization occurs, nidation will be possible. In the absence of fertilization, ovarian secretions wane, the endometrium sloughs, and menstruation begins. This c. is commonly said to last, on the average, for 28 days, with day 1 of the c. designated as that day on which menstrual flow begins.

**mitotic c.,** the cyclic events of cells undergoing growth and division; the c. is subdivided into the following phases or periods: mitosis (M); gap 1 ($G_1$); synthesis of DNA (S); and gap 2 ($G_2$).

**nitrogen c.,** the series of events in which the nitrogen of the atmosphere is fixed and made available for plant and animal life and then returned to the atmosphere. Nitrifying bacteria convert $N_2$ and $O_2$ to $NO_2^-$ and $NO_3^-$; the latter is absorbed by plants and converted to protein. If the plants decay, the nitrogen is, in part, given up to the atmosphere, and the remainder is converted by microorganisms to ammonia, nitrites, and nitrates; if the plants are eaten by animals, their excreta or bacterial decay return the nitrogen to the soil and air.

**ornithine c.,** urea c.

**ovarian c.,** the normal sex c. which includes development of an ovarian (Graafian) follicle, rupture of the follicle and discharge of the ovum, formation and regression of a corpus luteum. See fig. under ovary.

**reproductive c.,** the c. which begins with conception and extends through gestation and parturition.

**restored c.,** an atrial or ventricular cardiac c. that follows the returning c. and resumes the normal rhythm.

**returning c.,** an atrial or ventricular cardiac c. that begins with an extrasystole or a forced beat.

**succinic acid c.,** a series of oxidation reduction reactions in which succinic acid and other 4-carbon atoms acids (fumaric, malic, oxaloacetic) take part in the oxidation of pyruvic acid as part of the tricarboxylic acid c. See also dicarboxylic acid c.

**tricarboxylic acid c.,** Krebs c.; citric acid c.; a series of reactions, beginning and ending with oxaloacetic acid, during the course of which a two-carbon fragment is completely oxidized to carbon dioxide and water with the production of twelve high energy phosphate bonds; the main source of energy in the mammalian body; the end toward which carbohydrate, fat, and protein metabolism all point; so called because the first four substances involved, *e.g.,* citric acid, *cis*-aconitic acid, isocitric acid, and oxalosuccinic acid are all tricarboxylic acids. From oxalosuccinate, the others are, in order, α-ketoglutarate, succinate, fumarate, L-malate and oxaloacetate, which condenses with acetyl-CoA (from fatty acid degradation) to form citrate (citric acid) again.

**urea c.,** the sequence of chemical reactions, taking place in the liver, that results in the production of urea; the key reaction is the hydrolysis of arginine, by arginase, to ornithine and urea; ornithine is then converted to citrulline by a carbamoylation reaction involving glutamic acid and then to arginine again by an amination reaction involving aspartic acid. Also known as Krebs' urea c., Krebs-Hanseleit c., ornithine c.

**visual c.,** the transformation of carotenoids involved in the bleaching and regeneration of the visual pigment:

$$\text{rhodopsin} \xrightarrow{\text{(light)}} trans\text{-retinene} (+ \text{ opsin}) \rightarrow$$

$$trans\text{-vitamin A}_1 \xrightarrow{\text{(liver)}} cis\text{-vitamin A}_1 \rightarrow cis\text{-retinene}$$
$$(+ \text{ opsin}) \rightarrow \text{rhodopsin.}$$

**cyclectomy** (si-klek'to-mī, sik-lek'to-mī) [ cyclo- + G. *ektomē,* excision ]. Excision of a portion of the ciliary muscle or body.

**cyclencephalia** (si-klen-se-fa'lī-ah). Cyclencephaly.

**cyclencephaly** (si-klen-sef'ă-lī) [ cyclo- + G. *enkephalos,* brain ]. Cyclencephalia; cyclocephaly; a condition, in a malformed fetus, characterized by poor development and more or less fusion of the two cerebral hemispheres.

**cyclex'edrine.** EVENTIN; ethylhexedrine; *N,β*-dimethylcyclohexaneethylamine; sympathomimetic drug with anorexigenic properties.

**cyclic** (si'klik, sik'lik). 1. Occurring periodically; denoting especially the course of the symptoms in certain mental affections. 2. In chemistry, continuous, without end; see cyclo-.

**c. adenylic acid,** or **c. AMP,** adenosine 3':5'-cyclic phosphate.

**c. compound,** see under compound.

**c. phosphoric acid,** see under phosphoric acid.

**cyclic AMP.** Adenosine 3':5'-cyclic phosphate.

**3':5'-cyclic AMP synthetase.** Trivial name for an enzyme that catalyzes formation of adenosine 3':5'-cyclic phosphate from ATP, with liberation of $PP_i$; stimulated by epinephrine. Sometimes also called adenylate cyclase or (erroneously) adenyl cyclase.

**cyclicot'omy.** Cyclotomy.

**cyclitis** (si-kli'tis) [ G. *kyklos,* circle (ciliary body), + suffix *-itis,* inflammation ]. Inflammation of the ciliary body.

**heterochromic c.,** a mild inflammatory form of c. in which the irises become different in color.

**plastic c.,** inflammation of the ciliary body, and usually of the entire uveal tract, with a fibrinous exudation into the anterior chamber and vitreous.

**pure c.,** uncomplicated c., the iris not being involved in the inflammatory process.

**pu'rulent c.,** suppurative inflammation of the ciliary body, including usually the iris, constituting endophthalmitis.

**serous c.,** serous iridocyclitis with keratic precipitates (*q. v.* under precipitate).

**cy'clizine hydrochloride** (USP, BP). MAREZINE hydrochloride; 1-diphenylmethyl-4-methylpiperazine hydrochloride. Antihistamine agent useful in the prevention and relief of motion sickness and symptoms caused by vestibular disorders.

**cy'clizine lactate** (NF). MAREZINE lactate; same use and action as the hydrochloride.

**cyclo-** (si'klo-, sik'lo-) [ G. *kyklos,* circle. CYC- ]. 1. Combining form relating to a circle or cycle, or denoting association with the ciliary body. 2. Chemical combining form indicating a continuous molecule, without end (*e.g.,* cyclopentane), or the formation of such a structure between two parts of a molecule (*e.g.,* cyclonucleoside).

**cyclobar'bital.** Cyclobarbitone; PHANODORN; 5-(1-cyclohexen-1-yl)-5-ethylbarbituric acid; used as a mild hypnotic and for pre- and postoperative sedation.

**c. calcium,** cyclobarbitone calcium (BP); calcium salt used as intravenous hypnotic.

**cyclobar'bitone** (BP). Cyclobarbital.

**cyclobu'tane.** Tetramethylene; $(CH_2)_4$; a potent inhalation anesthetic; predisposes to arrhythmias.

**cyclocephaly, cyclocephalia** (si-klo-sef'ă-lī, -sĕ-fa'lī-ah) [ cyclo- + G. *kephalē,* head ]. Cyclencephaly.

**cyclochoroiditis** (si-klo-ko-royd-i'tis). Inflammation of the ciliary body and the choroid coat of the eye.

**cyclocu'marol.** CUMOPYRAN; 4-hydroxycoumarin anticoagulant No. 63; a synthetic anticoagulant compound, related to bishydroxycoumarin.

**cyclodialysis** (si-klo-di-al'ĭ-sis) [ cyclo- + G. *dialysis,* separation ]. Heine's operation; establishment of a communication between the anterior chamber and the suprachoroidal space in order to relieve intraocular pressure in glaucoma.

**cy'clodiather'my.** Diathermy applied to the ciliary region in treatment of glaucoma.

**cycloduction** (si-klo-duk'shun) [ cyclo- + L. *duco,* pp. *ductus,* to draw ]. Circumduction.

**cycloelectrolysis** (si'klo-e-lek-trol'ĭ-sis). Electrolysis applied to the ciliary body to lessen ocular tension in glaucoma.

**cy'cloform.** Isobutyl-*p*-aminobenzoate; used as a dusting powder for its local anesthetic effect, in burns, painful ulcers, tuberculous laryngitis, hemorrhoids, and itching.

**cy'clogram** [ cyclo- + G. *gramma,* a drawing ]. A graphic representation of the visual field made with a cycloscope.

**cycloguanil pamoate** (si'klo-gwahn'il) (USAN). CAMOLAR; chloroguanide triazine pamoate; CI-501; 4,6-diamino-1-(*p*-chlorophenyl)-1,2-dihydro-2,2-dimethyl-*s*-triazine pamoate; a long-acting antimalarial agent that prevents the growth or survival of the pre-erythrocytic and erythrocytic parasites.

**cyclohex'amine.** *n*-Ethyl-1-phenylcyclohexylamine hydrochloride; a dissociative anesthetic.

**cyclohexanesulfamic acid** (USP). Cyclamic acid.

**cyclohex'imide.** An antibiotic principle, $C_{15}H_{23}NO_4$, obtained from certain strains of *Streptomyces griseus;* it is also an effective repellent for rats, which will die of thirst or starvation rather than ingest water or food containing as little as 1 mg. per liter.

**cyclohex'itol.** Inositol.

**cyclohexylsulfamic acid** (BP). Cyclamic acid.

**cycloid** (si'kloyd) [ cyclo- + G. *eidos*, resembling ]. Suggesting cyclothymia; a term applied to a physical type including rubicund, round-faced, jovial, happy-go-lucky individuals who, however, tend to have periods of mild depression; see schizoid.

**cyclokerati'tis.** Dalrymple's disease; inflammation of both the ciliary body and the cornea.

**cy'clol.** A cyclic peptide structure, postulated at one time (but never confirmed) as occurring in proteins. Occurs in some of the ergot alkaloids. A diketopiperazine.

Cyclol

**cyclomastopathy** (si'klo-mas-top'ă-thī) [ cyclo- + G. *mastos*, breast, + *pathos*, suffering ]. Chronic cystic *mastitis.*

**cyclometh'ycaine sulfate** (BP). SURFACAINE; 3-(2-methylpiperidino)propyl-*p*-cyclohexyloxybenzoate sulfate; effective topical anesthetic for abrasions and certain skin lesions.

**cyclopent'amine hydrochloride** (NF). CLOPANE hydrochloride; *N*,α-dimethylcyclopentaneethylamine hydrochloride; 1-cyclopentyl-2-methylaminopropane hydrochloride. A sympathomimetic amine, similar in action to ephedrine, except that it causes only slight central excitation.

**cyclopen'tane.** Pentamethylene; $(CH_2)_5$; a closed ring hydrocarbon containing 5 carbon atoms, isomeric with pentene.

**cy'clopenta'noperhy'drophenan'threne.** Incorrect name for cyclopenta[ *a* ]phenanthrene, the tetracyclic steroid nucleus (*q.v.* under steroid).

**cyclopenthi'azide** (BP, USAN). NAVIDREX; $C_{13}H_{18}$-$ClN_3O_4S_2$; a benzothiadiazide diuretic.

**cy'clopen'tolate hydrochloride** (USP, BP). CYCLOGYL hydrochloride; 2-(dimethylamino)ethyl-1-hydroxy-α-phenylcyclopentaneacetate hydrochloride; an anticholinergic, spasmolytic drug, used in refraction determinations; causes cycloplegia and mydriasis.

**cyclopep'tide.** Polypeptide lacking terminal —NH and —COOH groups by virtue of their combination to form another peptide link (*e.g.*, gramicidin).

**cyclophen'azine hydrochloride** (USAN). 10-[ 3-(4-Cyclopropyl-1-piperazinyl) propyl-2-(trifluoromethyl)phenothiazine dihydrochloride; a tranquilizing drug.

**cy'clophor'ases.** The group of enzymes in mitochondria, catalyzing the complete oxidation of pyruvic acid to carbon dioxide and water; essentially those enzymes and coenzymes involved in the tricarboxylic acid cycle.

**cyclophoria** (si'klo-fo'rĭ-ah) [ cyclo- + G. *phora*, movement ]. Heterophoria caused by lack of equilibrium of the oblique muscles of the eye; it results in deviation of corresponding retinal meridians from parallelism.

    **accommodative c.,** a cyclical or rotative deviation of the eye due to oblique astigmatism.

    **essential c.,** a type of c. attributable to anatomical anomalies.

**cy'clophorom'eter.** An instrument designed to measure cyclophoria.

**cyclophos'phamide** (USP, BP). CYTOXAN; *N*,*N*-bis-(2-chloroethyl)-*N*'-(3-hydroxypropyl)phosphordiamidic acid cyclic ester monohydrate; an alkylating agent with the same antitumor activity and uses as the parent compound, nitrogen mustard (mechlorethamine hydrochloride). It is not a vesicant or tissue irritant and is less toxic than nitrogen mustard.

**cyclophotocoagulation** (si'klo-fo'to-ko-ag-u-la'shun) [ cyclo- + photocoagulation, *q.v.* ]. Photocoagulation with the argon laser through the pupil to selectively destroy individual ciliary processes; a procedure useful in stubborn glaucoma; the approach is effective and safe for depression of aqueous humor formation.

**cy'clophre'nia** [ cyclo- + G. *phrēn*, the mind ]. Manic-depressive *psychosis.*

**Cyclophyllidae** (si'klo-fil'ĭ-de) [ cyclo- + G. *phyllon*, leaf ]. An order of tapeworms that includes most of the common parasites of man and domestic animals.

**cyclo'pia** [ G. *Kyklōps*, fr. *kyklos*, circle, + *ōps*, eye ]. Synophthalmia; a congenital defect in which the two orbits merge to form a single cavity containing one eye, which is likely to show more or less evidence of its origin by fusion of the right and left optic primordia. It is usually combined with cyclencephaly.

**cycloplegia** (si-klo-ple'jī-ah) [ cyclo- + G. *plēgē*, stroke ]. Paralysis of accommodation; loss of power in the ciliary muscle of the eye; pathologic or induced.

**cyclople'gic.** 1. Relating to cycloplegia. 2. A drug that paralyzes the ciliary muscle and thus the power of accommodation.

**cyclopro'pane** (USP, BP). Trimethylene; $(CH_2)_3$; a colorless gas of characteristic odor resembling petroleum benzin, and having a pungent taste. It is usually supplied in compressed form in metallic cylinders, and is used for producing general anesthesia. It is flammable.

**cyclopro'pene.** An unsaturated 3-carbon cyclic hydrocarbon; very unstable and prone to polymerize. The c. ring occurs in nature in sterculic acid.

Cyclopropene

**cyclopro'pyl ethyl ether.** CYPRETH ether; $CH_3CH_2$-$OCH(CH_2)_2$; a volatile liquid used for inhalation anesthesia.

**cyclopro'pyl methyl ether.** CYPROME ether; $CH_3$-$OCH(CH_2)_2$; a liquid inhalation anesthetic.

**cyclopro'pyl vinyl ether.** CYPRETHYLENE ether; $CH_2$-$CHOCH(CH_2)_2$; a liquid inhalation anesthetic.

**cyclops** (si'klops) [ see cyclopia ]. An individual with cyclopia; also called monoculus, monops, monophthalmus.

**cycloser'ine** (USP, BP). SEROMYCIN; orientomycin; D-4-amino-3-isoxazolidinone; cyclic anhydride of serine amide. An antibiotic produced by strains of *Streptomyces orchidaceus* or *S. garyphalus* with a wide spectrum of antibacterial activity. Used in tuberculosis and in certain upper and lower urinary tract infections.

**cyclo'sis** [ G. fr. *kykloō*, to move around ]. The movement of the protoplasm and contained plastids within the protozoan cell.

**Cyclostoma'ta** [ cyclo- + G. *stoma*, mouth ]. An order of fishes possessing a cartilaginous skeleton, a circular mouth without true jaws (agnatha), and no paired fins; because of their eel-like form they are often mistaken for eels, which are bony fish with paired fins. The cyclostomes include the parasitic hagfishes (Myxinoidea) and sea lamprey (*Petromyzon marinus*), as well as some nonparasitic freshwater forms.

**cy'clotate.** USAN-approved contraction for 4-methylbicyclo[ 2.2.2 ]oct-2-ene-1-carboxylate.

**cyclothi'azide** (NF). ANHYDRON; 6-chloro-3,4-dihydro-3-(2-norbornen-5-yl)-2*H*-1,2,4-benzothiadiazine-7-sulfonamide-1,1-dioxide; a diuretic and antihypertensive.

**cy'clothy'mia** [ cyclo- + G. *thymos*, rage. THYM-2 ]. Manic-depressive *psychosis.*

**cyclothy'miac, cyclothy'mic.** Relating to cyclothymia.

**cy'clotome.** A delicate knife for use in cyclotomy.

**cyclotomy** (si-klot'o-mī) [ cyclo- + G. *tomē*, incision ]. Operation of cutting the ciliary muscle.

**cy'clotron.** An accelerator that produces high speed ions (*e.g.*, protons and deuterons) under the influence of an alternating magnetic field, for the bombardment of atomic nuclei.

**cyclotropia** (si-klo-tro'pī-ah) [ cyclo- + G. *trope*, a turn, turning ]. A meridional deviation around the anterior-posterior axis of one eye with respect to the other.

**cyclotus** (si-klo'tus) [ cyclo- + G. *ous*, ear ]. Synotus.

**cyclozoonosis** (si'klo-zo-o-no'sis) [ cyclo- + G. *zōon*, animal, + *nosos*, disease ]. A zoonosis that requires more than one vertebrate host (but no invertebrate) for completion of the life cycle; *e.g.*, various taenioid cestodes such as *Taenia saginata* and *T. solium* in which man is an obligatory host; hydatid disease, a c. in which man is not an obligatory host.

**cy'crimine hydrochloride** (NF). PAGITANE hydrochloride; 1-phenyl-1-cyclopentyl-3-piperidino-1-propanol hydrochloride. An anticholinergic drug used in the treatment of parkinsonism.

**Cyd.** Symbol for cytidine.

**Cydonia oblongata** (si-do'nī-ah). Quince.

**cyema,** pl. **cyemata** (si-e'mah) [ G. *kyēma*, embryo ]. The conceptus at any stage in its development, whether normal or abnormal.

**cyesedema** (si'e-sē-de'mah) [ G. *kyēsis*, pregnancy, + *oidēma*, a swelling (edema) ]. Gestational *edema*.

**cyesiognosis** (si-e-sī-og-no'sis) [ G. *kyēsis*, pregnancy, + *gnōsis*, knowledge ]. The diagnosis of pregnancy.

**cyesis** (si-e'sis) [ G. *kyēsis* ]. Pregnancy.

**cyestein, cyesthein** (si-es'te-in, si-es'the-in) [ G. *kyēsis*, pregnancy, + *esthēs*, garment ]. A scum or pellicle occasionally seen on the surface of the standing urine from a pregnant woman; formerly regarded as one of the signs of pregnancy.

**cyhep'tamide**  (USAN).  10,11-Dihydro-5*H*-dibenzo-[*a,d*]- cycloheptene-5-carboxamide; anticonvulsant.

**cyl.** Abbreviation for cylinder, or cylindrical *lens*.

**cyl'inder** [ G. *kylindros*, a roll ]. 1. A cylindrical *lens*. 2. A cylindrical or rodlike renal cast. 3. A cylindrical metal container for gases stored under high pressure.

**axis c.,** obsolete term for axon.

**Bence Jones c.'s,** slightly irregular, relatively smooth, rod-shaped or cylindroid bodies of fairly tenacious, viscid proteinaceous material in the fluid of the seminal vesicles.

**crossed c.'s,** a combination of two cylindrical lenses the axes of which are at right angles to each other.

**Külz's c.,** coma *cast*.

**cylindraxis** (sil'in-drak'sis). Historical precursor of the term axon, based on an interpretation of the myelinated nerve fiber as a cylinder of which the axon formed the axis.

**cylin'drical.** Cylinder-shaped; referring to a cylinder.

**cylindroadenoma** (sil'in-dro-ad-e-no'mah). Cylindroma.

**cyl'indroid** [ G. *kylindrōdēs*, fr. *kylindros*, roll, cylinder, + *eidos*, appearance ]. A mucous cast; false cast; an elongated mass of mucus or nucleoprotein in the urine. C.'s resemble hyaline casts, but usually have a tapered end that is slightly curved, hooked, or twisted, in contrast to the rounded or blunt ends of the latter.

**cylindroma** (sil-in-dro'mah) [ G. *kylindros*, cylinder, suffix *-oma*, tumor ]. Cylindroadenoma; a histologic type of epithelial neoplasm characterized by islands of neoplastic cells embedded in a hyalinized stroma which may represent a thickened basement membrane. They may form from ducts of glands, especially in salivary glands, skin, and bronchi. C.'s are frequently malignant; those in the salivary glands are also termed adenoid cystic carcinomas.

**cylindrosarcoma** (sil'in-dro-sar-ko'mah). A sarcoma that manifests several foci of hyaline degenerative changes such as those observed in cylindromas.

**cylindruria** (sil-in-dru'rī-ah). The presence of renal cylinders or casts in the urine.

**cyllosis** (sil-lo'sis) [ G. *kyllōsis*, a crippling ]. Deformity of the foot, particularly clubfoot (talipes).

**cyl'loso'ma** [ G. *kyllos*, deformed, esp. clubfooted or bandylegged, + *sōma*, body ]. Congenital defect of the lower abdominal wall on one side with defective development of the leg on that side.

**cyl'loso'mus.** A malformed individual with cyllosoma.

**cymarin.** K-Strophanthin-2; a glycoside of cymarose, present in the seeds of *Strophanthus kombé;* the aglycone is strophanthidin.

**cym'arose.** 3-Methyldigitose; an isomer of diginose; a constituent of some cardiac glycosides.

**cymba conchae** [ G. *kymbē*, the hollow of a vessel, a cup, bowl, a boat ] [ NA ]. The upper, smaller part of the external ear lying above the crus helicis.

**cymbocephalic, cymbocephalous** (sim-bo-sē-fal'ik, sim-bo-sef'ā-lus). Relating to cymbocephaly.

**cymboceph'aly** [ G. *kymbē*, the hollow of a vessel, a boat-shaped structure, + *kephalē*, head ]. The condition characterized by a boat-shaped skull, one with a depression of the upper surface.

**cynanche** (sin-ang'ke) [ L. fr. G. *kynanchē*, dog quinsy, sore throat, fr. *kyon* (*kym*-), dog, + *anchō*, to throttle. CYN- ]. Sore *throat*.

**cynan'thropy** [ G. *kyon*, dog, + *anthrōpos*, man ]. A delusion in which the patient barks and growls, imagining himself to be a dog.

**cynic** (sin'ik) [ G. *kynikos*, doglike ]. Doglike; denoting a spasm of the muscles of the face; see *risus* caninus.

**cynocephalus** (si-no-sef'ā-lus) [ G. *kyon*, dog, + *kephalē*, head ]. A malformed individual with a head sloping back from the orbits, so that it resembles the head of a dog.

**cy'nopho'bia** [ G. *kyon*, dog, + *phobos*, fear ]. Morbid fear of dogs.

**cynorex'ia** [ G. *kyon*, dog, + *orexis*, appetite ]. Bulimia.

**Cyon,** Elie de, Russian physiologist, 1843–1912. See C.'s *nerve.*

**cyophoria** (si-o-for'ī-ah) [ *kyos*, fetus, + *phoros*, bearing ]. Pregnancy.

**cyophor'ic** [ G. *kyophoros*, pregnant ]. Relating to pregnancy.

**Cyperus.** See adrue.

**cypionate** (sip'ī-o-nāt). USAN-approved contraction for cyclopentanepropionate.

**cyprenor'phine hydrochloride.** *N*-(Cyclopropylmethyl)-tetrahydro-7α-(1-hydroxy-1-methyl)-6,14-endoethenonororipovine hydrochloride; narcotic antagonist.

**cypridology** (si-prī-dol'o-jī) [ G. *Kypris*, Cyprian name for Aphrodite or Venus, goddess of love, + *logos*, study ]. Venereology.

**cypridopathy** (si-prī-dop'ā-thī) [ G. *Kypris*, Aphrodite, + *pathos*, disease ]. Any venereal disease.

**cypridophobia** (si'prī-do-fo'bī-ah) [ G. *Kypris*, Aphrodite, + *phobos*, fear ]. Morbid fear of veneral disease or of sexual intercourse.

**Cyprin'idae** [ G. *kyprinos*, a carp ]. A family of bony freshwater fishes including the goldfishes, carp, chubs, and minnows.

**cyprohep'tadine hydrochloride** (NF, BP). PERIACTIN; 1-methyl-4-(5-dibenzo-[ a,e ]-cycloheptatrienylidine)-piperidine; a potent antagonist of histamine and serotonin.

**cyproquinate** (si'pro-kwin'āt) (USAN). COXYTROL; 6,7-bis(cyclopropylmethoxy)-4-hydroxy-3-quinolinecarboxylate; a coccidiostat for poultry.

**cypro'terone acetate** (USAN). 6-Chloro-17-hydroxy-1α,2α-methylene-4,6-pregnadiene-3,20-dione acetate (for structure of pregnadiene, see steroids); a synthetic steroid capable of inhibiting the biological effects exerted by endogenous or exogenous androgenic hormones; an antiandrogen.

**cyprox'imide** (USAN). 1-(*p*-Chlorophenyl)-1,2-cyclopropanedicarboximide; a tranquilizer with antidepressant action.

**cyrtometer** (sur-tom'e-ter) [ G. *kyrtos*, bent, + *metron*, measure ]. An instrument for determining the size and shape of the chest.

**cyrtosis** (sur-to'sis) [ G. fr. *kyrtos*, bent ]. Obsolete term denoting any abnormal curvature of the spine or extremities.

**Cys (Cys-).** Symbol for cysteine (half-cystine) or its mono- or diradical.

# CYST

**cyst** (sist) [ G. *kystis,* bladder ]. 1. A bladder. 2. An abnormal sac containing gas, fluid, or a semisolid material.

**adventitious c.,** false c.; a c. resulting from the formation of an enclosing wall around a blood effusion or other foreign body.

**allanto'ic c.,** urachal c.; a circumscribed dilation of the urachus.

**alveolar hydatid c.,** multilocular hydatid c.; a hydatid c. of a multiloculate type, usually in the liver of man; an uncommon infection in central and eastern Europe and northern temperate boreal regions. It is caused by the minute tapeworm, *Echinococcus multilocularis,* adults of which are in foxes, larvae (alveolar hydatid), chiefly in microtine rodents, rarely in man. Growth is by exogenous budding and is not limited by an outer laminated membrane; necrosis, cavitation, contiguous spread, and death usually ensue.

**alveoloden'tal c.,** odontocele; a c. in relation to an unerupted tooth either in the tissues over it (extracapsular) or originating from the aplastic tooth structures (intracapsular).

**aneurysmal bone c.,** benign bone aneurysm; a benign osteolytic lesion expanding a long bone or within a vertebra, consisting of blood-filled spaces.

**apoplec'tic c.,** an adventitious c. formed of the effused blood in apoplexy.

**arachnoid c.,** a fluid-filled c. lined with arachnoid membrane and usually congenital in origin; it is frequently situated near the lateral aspect of the fissure of Sylvius.

**atheromatous c.,** sebaceous c.

**Baker's c.,** a collection of synovial fluid which has escaped from a bursa and formed a new sac in the muscles or other tissues outside of the joint; seen in severe osteoarthritis.

**Bartholin's c.,** a c. arising from the major vestibular gland or its ducts.

**bile c.,** *vesica* fellea.

**Blessig's c.'s,** Iwanoff's c.'s; peripheral cystoid degeneration of the retina found in some children and almost universal after the age of 20.

**blood c.,** hemorrhagic c.

**blue dome c.,** (1) one of a number of small dark blue nodules or c.'s in the vaginal fornix due to retained menstrual blood in endometriosis affecting this region; (2) a benign retention c. of the mammary gland in fibrocystic disease, containing a pale slightly yellow fluid which gives a blue color to the c. when viewed from a certain angle.

**bone c.,** see solitary bone c.

**Boyer's c.,** a subhyoid c.

**branchial c.,** branchial cleft c.

**branchial cleft c.,** branchial c.; a cervical c. arising from persistence of ectodermal branchial cleft (groove) or entodermal pharyngeal pouches.

**bursal c.,** a retention c. in a bursa.

**butter c.,** soap c.; a focus of saponified or partly saponified necrotic tissue in a lipoma.

**cerebellar c.,** a c. usually occurring in the lateral cerebellar white matter; it is often a part of cerebellar astrocytoma.

**chocolate c.,** Sampson's c.; c. of the ovary with intracavitary hemorrhage and hematoma formation; often seen with endometriosis of the ovary but occasionally with other types of c.'s.

**choledochal c.,** c. originating from common bile duct; usually becomes apparent early in life as a right upper abdominal mass in association with jaundice.

**chyle c.,** a circumscribed dilation of a lymphatic channel of the mesentery, containing chyle.

**colloid c.,** one with gelatinous contents.

**compound c.,** multilocular c.

**cor'pora lu'tea c.'s,** persistent corpora lutea with c. formation.

**Cowper's c.,** a retention c. of one of Cowper's glands.

**cuta'neous c., cutic'ular c.,** any c. of the skin.

**daughter c.,** a secondary c.; a c. usually multiple, derived from a primary c.

**degeneration c.,** involution c.

**dental c.,** radicular c.

**dentig'erous c.,** a c. arising from tooth germ after formation of the hard tissues.

**dermoid c.,** a tumor consisting of displaced epiblastic structures, the wall being formed of epithelium-lined connective tissue and containing epithelium, hair, and other appendages of the skin.

**dermoid c. of ovary,** a common benign cystic teratoma of the ovary, lined for the most part by skin, and containing hair and sebum, but also usually containing a variety of other well differentiated structures within a small inwardly projecting mass of solid tissue.

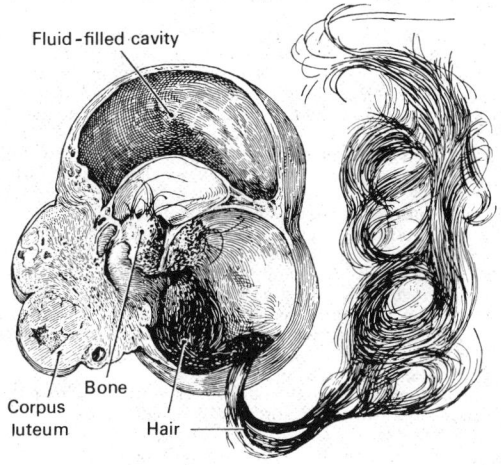

Fluid-filled cavity

Corpus luteum

Bone

Hair

**Dermoid Cyst of Ovary**
Contains bone and hair

**dila'tion c.,** retention c.

**distention c.,** retention c.

**duplication c.,** a congenital malformation, usually cystic in nature, attached to or originating from any part of the alimentary canal, from the base of the tongue to the anus. Duplication may be spherical when there is no direct connection with the parent lumen; in other instances, the duplication assumes a tubular appearance, especially when there is an enteric communication.

**echinococ'cus c.,** hydatid c.

**endometrial c.,** a c. resulting from endometrial implantation outside the uterus.

**endothe'lial c.,** a serous c. whose sac is lined with endothelium.

**epen'dymal c.,** neural c.; a circumscribed distention of some portion of the central canal of the spinal cord or of the cerebral ventricles.

**epider'mal c.,** implantation or inclusion c.; implantation or sequestration dermoid; a c. formed of a mass of epidermal cells which, as a result of trauma, has been pushed beneath the epidermis; the c. is lined with stratified squamous epithelium and contains concentric layers of keratin.

**epidermoid c.,** a spherical, firm, unilocular c. of the dermis, comprised of encysted, lamellated, birefringent keratin and a variable amount of sebum; the c. is lined by a keratinizing epithelium resembling the epidermis, and may be derived by metaplasia from a sebaceous cyst.

**epithe'lial c.,** a c. lined with epithelium.

**Epstein's c.'s,** Epstein's *pearls.*

**extravasa'tion c.,** hemorrhagic c.

**exuda'tion c.,** a c. resulting from distention of a closed cavity, such as a bursa, by an excessive secretion of its normal fluid contents.

**false c.,** adventitious c.

**follic'ular c.,** tubulocyst.

**Gartner's c.,** a c. of the chief duct in the vestigial structures of the parovarium corresponding to the sexual portion of the Wolffian body.

**gas c.,** one with gaseous instead of the ordinary liquid or pultaceous contents.

**glomerular c.'s,** c.'s some of which contain glomerular tufts, found in occasional cases of congenital polycystic kidneys.

**granddaughter c.,** a tertiary c. sometimes developed within a daughter c., as in the hydatid cyst of *Echinococcus.*

**hemorrhag'ic c.,** sanguineous or extravasation c.; hematocyst; a c. containing blood or resulting from the encapsulation of a hematoma.

**hepatic c.'s,** congenital c.'s thought to originate from an obstruction of biliary ductules; they may be solitary and range in size from small to enormous. Polycystic disease may also occur.

**hydat'id c.,** echinococcus c.; a c. formed in the liver, or, less frequently, elsewhere, by the larval stage of the taenioid tapeworm, *Echinococcus,* chiefly in ruminants. Two morphological forms caused by *Echinococcus granulosus* are found in man: the unilocular hydatid c. and the osseous hydatid c. A third form in man is the alveolar hydatid c., caused by *Echinococcus multilocularis.* Final host is the dog or wild canid, in the small intestine of which the very small adult tapeworm matures and produces infectious eggs that pass out in the feces.

**implantation c.,** epidermal c.

**inclusion c.,** epidermal c.

**involution c.,** degeneration c.; a mammary c. occurring at the menopause, due to cystic degeneration of the gland.

**iodine c.'s,** a term used to indicate the c.'s of *Iodamoeba butschlii,* characterized by a large iodine-positive glycogen vacuole.

**Iwanoff's c.'s,** Blessig's c.'s.

**junctional c.,** a c. of the testis arising from the structures connecting the rete testis with the epididymis.

**Kobelt's c.,** *appendix* vesiculosa.

**lac'teal c.,** milk c.; a retention c. in the mammary gland resulting from closure of a lactiferous duct.

**Meibo'mian c.,** chalazion.

**milk c.,** lacteal c.

**Morgagn'ian c.,** *appendix* vesiculosa.

**mother c.,** the echinococcus c., from the inner, or germinal layer of which secondary c.'s containing scoleces (daughter c.'s) are developed; sometimes tertiary c.'s (granddaughter c.'s) are developed within the daughter c.'s. It occurs most frequently in the liver, but may be found in other organs and tissues. The symptoms are those of a tumor of the part affected.

**mucous c.,** a retention c. resulting from obstruction in the duct of a mucous gland. See also mucocele; ranula.

**multiloc'ular c.,** compound c.; one containing several compartments formed by membranous septa.

**multilocular (or multiloculate) hydatid c.,** alveolar hydatid c.

**Nabothian c.,** Nabothian gland or follicle; a retention c. that develops when a mucous gland of the cervix uteri is obstructed, often as the result of its duct becoming plugged with squamous epithelium; the latter is formed from metaplasia of the normal epithelium during chronic inflammation of the cervix.

**necrot'ic c.,** one due to a circumscribed encapsulated area of necrosis with subsequent liquefaction of the dead tissue.

**neural c.,** ependymal c.

**nevoid c.,** one with a very vascular sac.

**odontogenic c.,** a c. of tooth germ origin.

**oil c.,** a c. resulting from fatty degeneration of the epithelial lining of a sebaceous, dermoid, or lacteal c., or from the injection of oil or fat material subcutaneously.

**oophorit'ic c.,** an ovarian c. arising from the ovary proper rather than from the parovarium.

**osseous hydatid c.,** a morphological form caused by *Echinococcus granulosus,* and found in the long bones or the pelvic arch of man if the embryo is filtered out in bony tissue; in this site no limiting membrane forms and the c.

grows in an uncontrolled fashion, eroducing cancellous structures and inducing fracture, followed by spread to new sites.

**ovarian c.,** a cystic tumor of the ovary, either non-neoplastic (follicle, lutein, germinal inclusion, or endometrial) or neoplastic; either benign (pseudomucinous or serous cystadenoma, or dermoid) or malignant (carcinoma).

**paradental c.,** a c. developing in direct relation to a tooth.

**paraphysial c.'s,** c.'s arising from vestigial remnants of the paraphysis; they are the possible origin of some third ventricular colloid c.'s.

**parasitic c.,** one formed by the larva of a metazoan parasite, such as a hydatid or trichinal c.

**parent c.,** mother c.

**paroophorit'ic c.,** a c. arising from the parovarium (epoophoron, organ of Rosenmüller).

**parvilocular c.,** a tumor composed of multiple small c.'s.

**pearl c.,** a solid tumor of the iris caused by penetrating injury.

**pilar c.,** sebaceous c.

**pilif'erous c.,** a dermoid c. containing hair.

**pil'onid'al c.,** see pilonidal *sinus.*

**pineal c.,** a c. of the pineal gland; it rarely is of clinical importance.

**posttraumatic leptomeningeal c.,** a persistent cystic accumulation of cerebrospinal fluid with progressive loss of bone and dura, occurring at the site of a previous fracture.

**prolifera'tion c., prolif'erative c., prolif'erous c.,** a mother c. containing daughter c.'s; a c. with tumorous formation at one portion of the sac.

**prolig'erous c.,** adenocarcinoma.

**protozoan c.,** infectious form of many protozoan parasites such as *Entamoeba histolytica, Giardia lamblia, Balantidium coli,* etc., usually passed in the feces and protected by a highly condensed cytoplasm and resistant cell wall.

**pseudomu'cinous c.,** one containing a gelatinous (pseudomucinous) material, and, as a result of rupture or leakage, causing implants upon the peritoneum.

**radicular c.,** root c.; periapical c.; a dental c. developing from the peridontal membrane around the root of a nonvital tooth.

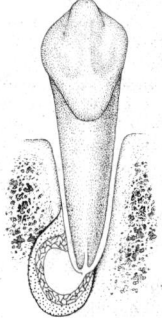

**Radicular Cyst**

**Rathke's cleft c.,** a simple intrasellar c. lined by cuboidal epithelium and believed to arise from remnants of Rathke's pouch.

**rete c. of ovary,** a c. derived from the germinal cords of the ovary.

**retention c.,** dilation, distention, or secretory c.; a c. resulting from some obstruction to the excretory duct of a gland.

**Sampson's c.,** chocolate c.

**sanguin'eous c.,** hemorrhagic c.

**seba'ceous c.,** atheromatous c.; pilar c. (2); steatocystoma (2); talpa; trichilemmal c.; wen; a keratinous c. of the skin, especially of the scalp; formerly believed to arise from subcutaneous glands by retention of excretion, but more recently thought to be derived from the outer hair root sheath.

**secondary c.,** daughter c.

**secre'tory c.,** retention c.

**seminal c.,** a c. of the testicle.

**sequestra'tion c.,** a cystic tumor arising from a portion of skin which was imprisoned in one of the lines of fusion during the growth of the embryo.

**serous c.,** a c. containing clear serous fluid; see also hygroma.

**soap c.,** butter c.

**solitary bone c.,** unicameral bone c.; osteocystoma; a unilocular c. containing serous fluid and lined with a thin layer of connective tissue, occurring usually in the shaft of a long bone in a child.

**sterile c.,** a hydatid c. without brood capsules.

**sublingual c.,** ranula.

**subsyno'vial c.,** distention of a synovial follicle.

**suprasellar c.,** craniopharyngioma.

**syno'vial c.,** thecal c.

**Tarlov's c.,** a perineural c. found in the proximal radicles of the lower spinal cord; it is usually productive of symptoms.

**tarry c.,** a c. or collection of old blood having a tarry or black, sticky appearance; usually due to endometriosis.

**tarsal c.,** chalazion.

**teratom'atous c.,** one containing structures derived from all three of the primary germ layers of the embryo.

**thecal c.,** synovial c.; ganglion (2); circumscribed distention of a tendon sheath.

**Thornwaldt's c.,** *bursa* pharyngea.

**thyroglos'sal duct c.,** thyrolingual c.; a c. in the midline of the neck resulting from nonclosure of a segment of the ductus thyroglossus.

**thyrolin'gual c.,** thyroglossal duct c.

**trichilemmal c.,** sebaceous c.

**tubular c.,** tubulocyst.

**umbil'ical c.,** vitellointestinal c.

**unicameral c.,** unilocular c.

**unicameral bone c.,** solitary bone c.

**uniloc'ular c.,** a simple c. having a single sac.

**unilocular hydatid c.,** the commonest form in man, caused by *Echinococcus granulosus;* found in liver, lungs, or any other site where the hexacanth embryo may settle if it passes the hepatic or pulmonary capillary filters; characterized by large, balloon-like forms lined internally with a germinative membrane, enclosed externally in a laminated membrane within a host-parasite capsule; filled with fluid (hydatid fluid) and infectious scoleces of the young tapeworms (hydatid sand).

**u'rachal c.,** allantoic c.

**urinary c.,** one containing extravasated urine.

**vitellointes'tinal c.,** umbilical c.; a small red sessile or pedunculated tumor at the umbilicus in an infant; it is due to the persistence of a segment of the vitellointestinal duct.

**Wolffian c.,** a c. arising from any mesonephric structure.

---

**cyst-.** See cysto-.

**cystad'enocarcino'ma.** A malignant neoplasm derived from glandular epithelium, in which cystic accumulations of retained secretions are formed; the neoplastic cells manifest varying degrees of anaplasia and invasiveness, and local extension and metastases occur. C.'s develop more frequently in the ovaries, where pseudomucinous and serous types are recognized.

**cyst'adeno'ma.** Cystoadenoma; a histologically benign neoplasm derived from glandular epithelium, in which cystic accumulations of retained secretions are formed; in some instances, considerable portions of the neoplasm, or even the entire mass, may be cystic. There is no evidence of invasion, and the neoplasms do not metastasize.

**c. adamanti'num,** an incorrect term for ameloblastoma or adamantinoma.

**papillary c. lymphomato'sum,** adenolymphoma; Warthin's tumor; a benign solid or cystic tumor composed of lymphoid tissue with germinal centers and epithelial cells forming two rows, believed to result from proliferation of the epithelium of parotid ducts included within lymph nodes that lie within or adjacent to the parotid gland.

**c. partim simplex partim papillif'erum,** a c. consisting of a combination of simple and papillary types of neoplastic epithelium.

**cystal'gia** [ cyst- + G. *algos,* pain ]. Pain in the bladder, especially the urinary bladder.

**cyst'amine.** Decarboxycystine; $(H_2NCH_2CH_2)_2S_2$; forms when cystine is distilled. See cysteamine.

**cystathi'onase.** Cystathionine $\gamma$-lyase.

**$\beta$-cystathionase.** Cystathionine $\beta$-lyase.

**$\gamma$-cystathionase.** Cystathionine $\gamma$-lyase.

**cystathi'onine.** $HOOC—CH(NH_2)CH_2—S—CH_2CH_2-$ $CH(NH_2)COOH$; an intermediate in the conversion of methionine to cysteine. Cleaved by cystathionase to yield cysteine.

**cystathionine $\beta$-lyase** (EC 4.4.1.8). $\beta$-Cystathionase; enzyme catalyzing cleavage of cystathionine to pyruvate, homocysteine, and $NH_3$. See also cystathionine $\gamma$-lyase.

**cystathionine $\gamma$-lyase** (EC 4.4.1.1). $\gamma$-Cystathionase; cystathionase; homoserine deaminase; homoserine dehydratase; cystine (and cysteine) desulfhydrase; a liver enzyme, requiring pyridoxal phosphate as coenzyme, that catalyzes the hydrolysis of cystathionine to cysteine and 2-ketobutyrate, releasing $NH_3$. Also catalyzes formation of 2-ketobutyrate from homoserine, of pyruvate (and $NH_3$ and $H_2S$) from cysteine, and of thiocysteine, pyruvate, and $NH_3$ from cystine. See also cystathionine $\beta$-lyase.

**cystathionine $\beta$-synthase** (EC 4.2.1.22). Serine sulfhydrase; cysteine synthase; methylcysteine synthase; $\beta$-thionase; enzyme catalyzing hydrolysis of cystathionine to serine and homocysteine. See also cystathionine $\gamma$-synthase.

**cystathionine $\gamma$-synthase** (EC 4.2.99.9). Enzyme catalyzing reaction between cystathionine and succinate to form cysteine and O-succinylhomoserine.

**cys'tathi'oninu'ria.** Heritable disorder characterized by inability to metabolize cystathionine normally; elevated concentrations of the amino acid develop in blood, tissue and urine; mental retardation is an associated condition.

**cystauchenitis** (sis-taw-ken-i'tis) [ cyst- + G. *auchēn,* neck, + suffix -*itis,* inflammation ]. Inflammation of the neck of the bladder.

**cystauchenotomy** (sis-taw-ken-ot'o-mī) [ cyst- + G. *auchēn,* neck, + *tomē,* incision ]. Cystidotrachelotomy; incision into the neck of the bladder.

**cystauxe** (sis-tawk'se) [ cyst- + G. *auxe,* growth ]. Dilation of the bladder, usually from chronic obstruction.

**cyste'amine.** 2-Aminoethanthiol; decarboxylated cysteine; $\beta$-mercaptoethylamine; $HS(CH_2)_2NH_2$; part of coenzyme A; used as a reducing agent in biochemical experiments and has been used for radiation sickness and chronic leukemia.

**cystectasia, cystectasy** (sist-ek-ta'sī-ah, sis-tek'ta-sī) [ cyst- + G. *ektasis,* a stretching ]. Dilation of the bladder.

**cystec'tomy** [ cyst- + G. *ektomē,* excision ]. 1. Excision of the gallbladder or of a portion of the urinary bladder. 2. Removal of a cyst.

**Bartholin's c.,** vulvovaginal c.; removal of a cyst of a major vestibular gland.

**vulvovaginal c.,** Bartholin's c.

**cyste'ic acid.** $HOOC—CH(NH_2)CH_2—SO_3H$; oxidation product of cysteine; a precursor of taurine and isethionic acid.

**cysteine** (sis'te-in). 2-Amino-3-mercaptopropionic acid; $HS—CH_2CH(NH_2)COOH$; an $\alpha$-amino acid found in most proteins; especially abundant in keratin.

**c. desulfhydrase,** cystathionine $\gamma$-lyase.

**c. synthase,** cystathionine $\beta$-synthase.

**cysteinesulfinic acid.** $HO_2S—CH_2CH(NH_2)COOH$; a natural oxidation product of cysteine; an intermediate in the formation of taurine (via cysteic acid).

**cysteinyl.** Aminoacyl radical of cysteine.

**cystelcosis, cystelcosia** (sis'tel-ko'sis, -ko'sī-ah) [ cyst- + G. *helkōsis,* ulceration ]. Ulceration of the bladder.

**cyst'elminth** [ cyst- + *helmins,* worm ]. Rarely used term for hydatid *cyst.*

**cystencephalus** (sis-ten-sef'al-us) [ cyst- + G. *enkephalos,* brain ]. A fetus with extreme internal hydrocephalus, so that the brain is little more than a sac distended with fluid.

**cystendesis** (sis-ten'de-sis) [ cyst- + G. *endesis,* a binding together ]. Suture of a wound in a bladder.

**cysti-.** See cysto-.

**cystic** (sis'tik). 1. Relating to the urinary bladder or gallbladder. 2. Relating to a cyst. 3. Containing cysts.

**cysticercoid** (sis'ti-sur-koyd) [ cysti- + G. *kerkos*, tail, + *eidos*, resemblance ]. A larval tapeworm resembling a cysticercus but having a smaller bladder, containing little or no fluid, in which scolex of the future adult tapeworm is found; the larval form is typically found in insect intermediate hosts.

**cysticercosis** (sis-tī-sur-ko'sis). Disease caused by cysticercus encystment of larvae ( *Cysticercus cellulosae* ) of *Taenia solium* in subcutaneous, muscle, or central nervous system tissues; it results from the hatching of the eggs in the intestines or by accidental ingestion of eggs from human feces. C. is typically developed in swine, producing measly pork; in man, encystment in the brain may cause serious nervous damage and encystment in the eye (usually the rear chamber) may cause ophthalmic damage.

**Cysticercus** (sis'tī-sur'kus) [ cysti- + G. *kerkos*, tail ]. Originally described as a genus of bladderworms, now known to be the encysted larvae of various taenioid tapeworms; the generic name is, however, retained as a convenience in referring to these larval encysted forms. C. is typically found in muscles of mammalian intermediate hosts that serve as prey of various predators, including man.

    **C. bo'vis,** the cysticercus larva of *Taenia saginata* in cattle; the cause of measly beef.

    **C. cellulo'sae,** the cysticercus larva of *Taenia solium* that causes cysticercosis.

    **C. fasciola'ris,** the strobilocercus larva of *Taenia taeniaeformis;* it is found in the liver of mice, rats, and other rodents.

    **C. multilocula'ris,** hydatid cyst of *Echinococcus multilocularis* (see alveolar hydatid *cyst*); very irregular in shape; sometimes found at the base of the brain and not encysted.

    **C. pisifor'mis,** the larva of *Taenia pisiformis;* it occurs in the liver and abdominal cavity of rabbits and hares.

    **C. tenuicol'lis,** the cystic form of *Taenia hydatigena;* it is found in the liver and peritoneal cavity of sheep, cattle, pigs, and wild ruminants.

**cysticolithectomy** (sis'tī-ko-lī-thek'to-mī) [ cystic (duct) + G. *lithos*, stone, + *ektomē*, excision ]. Operative removal of an impacted gallstone from the cystic duct.

**cys'ticolith'otripsy** [ cystic (duct) + G. *lithos*, stone, + *tripsis*, rubbing or crushing ]. Procedure of crushing a stone in the cystic duct.

**cysticorrhaphy** (sis-tī-kor'rä-fī) [ cystic (duct) + G. *raphē*, a stitching ]. Suture of the cystic bile duct.

**cysticot'omy** [ cystic (duct) + G. *tomē*, incision ]. An incision of the cystic bile duct.

**cys'tidoceliot'omy** [ G. *kystis*, bladder, + *koilia*, belly, + *tomē*, incision ]. Incision of the bladder through an incision in the abdominal wall.

**cystidolaparotomy** (sis'tī-do-lap'ar-ot'o-mī) [ G. *kystis*, bladder, + *lapara*, flank, + *tomē*, incision ]. Incision into the bladder after a preliminary abdominal section.

**cystidotrachelotomy** (sis'tī-do-trä-ke-lot'o-mī) [ G. *kystis*, bladder, + *trachēlos*, neck, + *tomē*, incision ]. Cystautrachenotomy.

**cystifelleotomy** (sis'tī-fel-e-ot'-omī) [ cysti- + L. *felleus*, pertaining to bile, + G. *tomē*, incision ]. Cholecystotomy.

**cys'tiform.** Cystoid.

**cystigerous** (sis-tij'er-us). Cystopherous.

**cys'tine.** Dicysteine; 3,3'-dithiobis(2-aminopropionic acid); $HOOC—CH(NH_2)—CH_2—S—S—CH_2—CH(NH_2)COOH$; an α-amino acid occurring in protein, notably keratin and insulin, sometimes occurring as a deposit in the urine, or forming a vesical calculus. An oxidation product of cysteine in which two —SH groups become one —S—S— group.

    **c. desulfhydrase,** cystathionine γ-lyase.

*meso-***cystine.** An isomer of cystine in which the configuration about one of the α-carbons is D, about the other, L, so that the molecule as a whole possesses a plane of symmetry and is optically inactive.

**cystinemia** (sis'tī-ne'mī-ah) [ cystine + G. *haima*, blood ]. The presence of cystine in blood.

**cystinosis** (sis'tī-no'sis). Abderholden-Fanconi syndrome; De Toni-Fanconi syndrome; Lignac-Fanconi syndrome; the most common of a group of diseases with tubular dysfunction, termed collectively Fanconi's syndrome ( *q. v.* ). C. is a recessive hereditary disease of early childhood characterized by widespread deposits of cystine crystals throughout the body, including bone marrow and other tissues which may be examined during life, with slight increase in the level of plasma cystine and cystinuria. This apparent abnormality in cystine metabolism is associated with a marked generalized aminoaciduria, glycosuria, polyuria, chronic acidosis, hypophosphatemia with vitamin D-resistant rickets, and often with hypokalemia The latter abnormalities are probably due to deficient tubular reabsorption and are accompanied by a characteristic abnormality of the proximal convoluted tubule, shown by microdissection to be narrowed at the glomerular junction ("swan-neck" deformity).

**cystinuria** (sis'tī-nu'rī-ah) [ cystine + G. *ouron*, urine ]. Excessive urinary excretion of cystine, along with lysine, arginine, and ornithine. It arises from defective transport systems for these acids in kidney and intestine, and renal function is sometimes compromised by cystine crystalluria. C. occurs in certain heritable diseases, such as the Fanconi syndrome (cystinosis) and hepatolenticular degeneration.

    **familial c.,** an inborn defect in renal tubular reabsorption of cystine, lysine, arginine and ornithine, with recurrent cystine calculus formation. Intestinal absorption of these four amino acids is also impaired.

**cystinyl.** The aminoacyl radical of cystine.

**cystiphorous** (sis-tif'or-us). Cystopherous.

**cystis,** pl. **cys'tides** (sis'tis) [ G. *kystis* ]. 1. Bladder; vesica. 2. A cyst.

    **c. fel'lea,** *vesica* fellea.

    **c. urina'ria,** *vesica* urinaria.

**cystistax'is** [ cysti- + G. *staxis*, trickling ]. Cystostaxis; oozing of blood from the mucous membrane of the bladder.

**cystitis** (sis-ti'tis) [ cyst- + G. suffix *-itis*, inflammation ]. Inflammation of a bladder, especially the urinary bladder.

    **c. colli,** inflammation of the neck of the bladder.

    **c. cys'tica,** c. characterized by the formation of cysts derived from glandlike invaginations of transitional epithelium.

    **follicular c.,** chronic c. characterized by small mucosal nodules due to lymphocytic infiltration with formation of lymphoid follicles.

    **c. glandula'ris,** chronic c. with glandlike invaginations of transitional epithelium.

    **interstitial c.,** Hunner's ulcer; chronic inflammation of the tunica propria with fibrosis in the muscularis of the bladder; occurs especially in women in the dome of the bladder, which is reduced in capacity.

**cystitome** (sis'tī-tōm). Capsulotome; cystotome; a delicate instrument used for incising the capsule of a cataractous lens.

**cystit'omy** [ cysti- + G. *tomē*, incision ]. 1. Capsulotomy. 2. Cystotomy. 3. Cholecystotomy.

**cysto-, cysti-, cyst-** [ G. *kystis*, bladder ]. Combining forms relating to (1) the bladder, (2) the cystic duct, and (3) a cyst.

**cystoadenoma** (sis'to-ad-e-no'mah). Cystadenoma.

**cystocarcino'ma.** A carcinoma in which cystic degeneration has occurred. Sometimes used as an incorrect term for cystadenocarcinoma.

**cystocele** (sis'to-sēl) [ cysto- + G. *kēlē*, hernia ]. Hernia of the bladder.

**cys'tochromos'copy.** Chromocystoscopy.

**cystocolos'tomy** [ cysto- + G. *kolon*, colon, + *stoma*, mouth ]. Cholecystocolostomy.

**cystodiaphanoscopy** (sis'to-di-ä-fan-os'ko-pī) [ cysto- + diaphanoscopy, *q.v.* ]. Transillumination of the abdomen by means of an electric light in the bladder.

**cystodiverticulum** (sis'to-di-ver-tik'u-lum). Vesical *diverticulum*.

**cystoduodenostomy** (sis'to-du'o-de-nos'to-mī) [ cysto- + duodenum, + G. *stoma*, mouth ]. Drainage of cyst into duodenum.

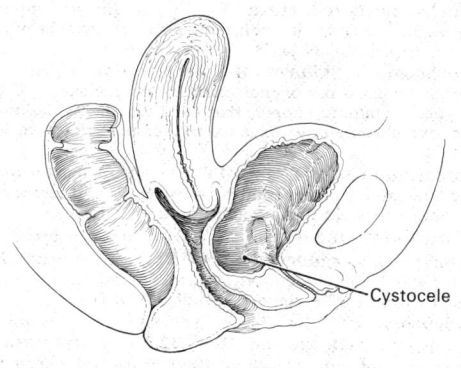

Cystocele

**Cystocele**

**cystoelytroplasty** (sis-to-el'ĭ-tro-plas-tĭ) [ cysto- + G. *elytron*, sheath, + *plassō*, to form ]. Operation for the repair of vesicovaginal fistula.

**cystoenterocele** (sis-to-en'ter-o-sēl) [ cysto- + G. *enteron*, intestine, + *kēlē*, hernia ]. Hernial protrusion of portions of the bladder and of the intestine.

**cystoenterostomy** (sis'to-en-ter-os'to-mĭ) [ cysto- + G. *enteron*, intestine, + *stoma*, mouth ]. Usually applies to internal drainage of pancreatic pseudocysts into some portion of intestinal tract.

**cystoepiplocele** (sis-to-ē-pip'lo-sēl) [ cysto- + G. *epiploon*, omentum, + *kēle*, tumor ]. Hernial protrusion of portions of the bladder and of the omentum.

**cystoepithelioma** (sis'to-ep-ĭ-the-lĭ-o'mah). Cystocarcinoma.

**cystofibro'ma.** A fibroma in which cysts or cystlike foci have formed.

**cystogastrostomy** (sis'to-gas-tros'to-mĭ) [ cysto- + G. *gastēr*, stomach, + *stoma*, mouth ]. Drainage of cyst into stomach.

**cys'togram.** An x-ray picture of the bladder.

**cystog'raphy** [ cysto- + G. *graphō*, to write ]. Roentgenography of the bladder following injection of a radiopaque substance.

**cystoid** [ cysto- + G. *eidos*, appearance ]. 1. Cystiform; bladder like; resembling a cyst. 2. A tumor resembling a cyst, with fluid, granular, or pultaceous contents, but without capsule.

**cystojejunostomy** (sis'to-je-ju-nos'to-mĭ) [ cysto- + G. *jejunum*, + G. *stoma*, mouth ]. Drainage of cyst into jejunum.

**cys'tolith** [ cysto- + G. *lithos*, stone ]. Vesical *calculus*.

**cystolithectomy** (sis'to-lĭ-thek'to-mĭ) [ cysto- + G. *lithos*, stone, + *ektomē*, excision ]. Cystolithotomy; removal of a stone from the bladder, expecially of a calculus from the gallbladder.

**cystolithiasis** (sis-to-lĭ-thi'a-sis) [ cysto- + G. *lithos*, stone, + suffix -*iasis*, condition ]. Stone in the bladder; the presence of a vesical calculus.

**cystolith'ic.** Relating to a vesical calculus.

**cys'tolithot'omy** [ cysto- + G. *lithos*, stone, + *tomē*, incision ]. Cystolithectomy.

**cystoma** (sis-to'mah) [ cyst- + G. suffix -*oma*, tumor ]. A cystic tumor; a new growth containing cysts.

   **myxoid c.,** myxocystoma.

**cystometer** (sis-tom'ĕ-tur) [ cysto- + G. *metron*, measure ]. A device by means of which, water being pumped into the bladder, a record is obtained of the amount of fluid passed in, and of the changing pressure reactions of the bladder (desire to void, sense of fullness, and the pain of overdistention) caused thereby.

**cys'tomet'rogram** [ cysto- + G. *metron*, measure, + *gramma*, a writing ]. A graphic record of pressure within the urinary bladder.

**cys'tometrog'raphy.** Measurement of pressure within the bladder.

**cystomor'phous** [ cysto- + G. *morphē*, form ]. Cystoid; bladder-like; cystlike.

**cys'tomyo'ma.** A myoma in which cysts or cystlike foci have developed.

**cystomyxoadenoma** (sis'to-mik'so-ad-e-no'mah). An adenoma in which there are cysts or cystlike foci in association with myxomatous change in the stroma.

**cystomyxoma** (sis'to-mik-so'mah). A myxoma in which cysts or cystlike foci have formed.

**cystoparal'ysis.** Paralysis of the bladder.

**cys'topexy** [ cysto- + G. *pēxis*, fixation ]. Ventrocystorrhaphy; surgical attachment of the gallbladder or of the urinary bladder to the abdominal wall.

**cystopherous** (sis-tof'er-us) [ cysto- + G. *phoreō*, to carry ]. Cystigerous; cystiphorous; cystic; containing cysts.

**cys'tophotog'raphy.** Photographing the interior of the bladder.

**cys'toplasty** [ cysto- + G. *plassō*, to form ]. Surgical repair of a defect in the bladder.

**cystoplegia** (sis-to-ple'jĭ-ah) [ cysto- + G. *plēgē*, a stroke ]. Paralysis of the bladder.

**cys'toproctos'tomy** [ cysto- + G. *prōktos*, anus, + *stoma*, mouth ]. The operative establishment of an opening between the bladder and the rectum.

**cystoptosis, cystoptosia** (sis-top'to-sis, sis-top-to'zĭ-ah) [ cysto- + G. *ptōsis*, a falling ]. Prolapse of the vesical mucous membrane into the urethra.

**cystopyelitis** (sis-to-pi-el-i'tis) [ cysto- + G. *pyelos*, trough (pelvis), + suffix -*itis*, inflammation ]. Inflammation of both the bladder and the pelvis of the kidney.

**cystopyelonephritis** (sis-to-pi'el-o-ne-fri'tis) [ cysto- + G. *pyelos*, trough (pelvis), + *nephros*, kidney, + suffix -*itis*, inflammation ]. Inflammation of the bladder, the pelvis of the kidney, and the kidney substance.

**cys'toradiog'raphy.** Radiography of the urinary bladder.

**cystorectostomy** (sis'to-rek-tos'to-mĭ) [ cysto- + rectum + G. *stoma*, mouth ]. Cystoproctostomy.

**cystorrhagia** (sis-to-ra'je-ah) [ cysto- + G. *rhēgnymi*, to burst forth ]. Hemorrhage from the bladder.

**cystorrhaphy** (sis-tor'ă-fĭ) [ cysto- + G. *raphē*, a sewing ]. Suture of a wound in the bladder.

**cystorrhea** (sis-to-re'ah) [ cysto- + G. *rhoia*, a flow ]. A mucous discharge from the bladder.

**cys'tosarco'ma.** A sarcoma in which the formation of cysts or cystlike foci has occurred.

   **c. phyllo'des,** adenomyxoma; giant fibroadenoma; telangiectatic c.; a very large or small circumscribed or infiltrating fibroadenomatous breast tumor that may be partly cystic; the stroma is cellular and resembles a fibrosarcoma, but the tumor is usually benign. The neoplasms occasionally metastasize as sarcomas; they are then termed malignant c. phyllodes.

   **telan'giectat'ic c.,** c. phyllodes.

**cys'toscope** [ cysto- + G. *skopeō*, to examine ]. A lighted tubular instrument for examining the interior of the bladder.

**cystos'copy.** The inspection of the interior of the bladder by means of a cystoscope.

**cys'tospasm.** Spasmodic contraction of the bladder.

**cystostax'is.** Cystistaxis.

**cystostomy** (sis-tos'to-mĭ) [ cysto- + G. *stoma*, mouth ]. The formation of a more or less permanent opening into the urinary bladder or gallbladder.

**cys'totome.** 1. An instrument for incising the urinary bladder or gallbladder. 2. Cystitome.

**cystotomy** (sis-tot'o-mĭ) [ cysto- + G. *tomē*, incision ]. 1. Vesicotomy; incision into urinary bladder or gallbladder. 2. Capsulotomy.

   **suprapu'bic c.,** epicystotomy; laparocystotomy (2); opening into the bladder through an incision above the symphysis pubis.

**cystotrachelotomy** (sis-to-trak-el-ot'o-mĭ) [ cysto- + G. *trachēlos*, neck, + *tomē*, incision ]. Cystauchenotomy.

**cystoureteritis** (sis-to-u-re-ter-i'tis). Inflammation of the bladder and of one or both ureters.

**cystoureterogram** (sis'to-u-re'ter-o-gram). An x-ray of bladder and ureter.

**cystoureterography** (sis'to-u-re'ter-og'ră-fĭ). Radiography of the bladder and ureter.

**cystourethritis** (sis-to-u-re-thri'tis). Inflammation of the bladder and of the urethra.

**cystourethrocele** (sis'to-u-re'thro-sēl) [ cysto- + urethra + G. kēlē, hernia ]. Hernia of the urinary bladder and urethra.

**cystourethrography** (sis'to-u're-throg'rä-fī). Roentenography of the bladder and urethra after visualization by means of a radiopaque substance.

**cystourethroscope** (sis-to-u-re'thro-scope). An instrument combining the uses of a cystoscope and a urethroscope.

**cys'tous.** Cystic.

**Cyt.** Symbol for cytosine.

**cyt-.** See cyto-.

**cy'tarabine** (USP). Arabinosylcytosine.

**cy'tase.** Metchnikoff's term for alexin or complement, which he held to be a digestive secretion of the leukocyte.

**cy'tax** [ G. kytos, cell, + L. taxo, to estimate ]. An apparatus for counting automatically the red blood cells, leukocytes, and lymphocytes of the blood and registering their relative proportions.

**cythemolysis** (si-tēm-(thēm-)ol'i-sis) [ G. kytos, cell, + haima, blood, + lysis, dissolution ]. Destruction or solution of the red blood cells. See also hemolysis, hemocytolysis.

**cythemolyt'ic** (si-tēm(thēm)-o-lit'ik). Relating to the lysis of red blood cells.

**cy'tidine.** 1-β-D-Ribofuranosylcytosine; cytosine ribonucleoside.

   **c. deaminase** (EC 3.5.4.5), see deaminases.

   **c. diphosphate choline,** an intermediate in the formation of phosphatidylcholine (lecithin); formed by the action of cytidine triphosphate (CTP) on phosphocholine, linking the choline phosphate group to the α-phosphate of the CTP to give a pyrophosphate.

   **c. phoshate,** see cytidylic acid.

**cytidyl'ic acid.** Cytidine phosphate (five are possible, depending on the site of attachment of the phosphate to the ribosyl OH's); a constituent of ribonucleic acids.

**cy'tisine.** Ulexine.

**cyto-, cyt-** [ G. kytos, a hollow (cell) ]. Combining forms meaning cell; when used as a suffix, -cyte.

**cy'toan'alyzer** [ cyto- + analyzer ]. An electronic optical machine that screens smears containing cells suspected of malignancy.

**cytoarchitectonics** (si'to-ar-kī-tek-ton'iks) [ cyto- + G. architektonikē, architectural ]. Cytoarchitecture.

**cytoarchitectural** (si-to-ar-kī-tek'tur-al). Pertaining to cytoarchitecture.

**cytoarchitecture** (si'to-ar'kī-tek-chūr). Cytoarchitectonics; the arrangement of cells in a tissue; the term commonly refers to the arrangement of nerve-cell bodies in the brain, especially the cerebral cortex.

**cytobiology** (si-to-bi-ol'o-jī). Cellular biology; cytology.

**cytobiotaxis** (si'to-bi-o-tak'sis) [ cyto- + G. bios, life, + taxis, arrangement ]. Cytoclesis.

**cytocentrum** (si-to-sen'trum) [ cyto- + G. kentron, center ]. Cell center; centrosome; central body; microcentrum; kinocentrum; a zone of cytoplasm that contains one or two centrioles but is devoid of other organelles; it is usually located near the nucleus.

**cytochemistry** (si'to-kem'is-trī). Histochemistry; study of intracellular distribution of chemicals, reaction sites, enzymes, etc., often by means of staining reactions, radioactive isotope uptake, or other methods.

**cytochrome** (si'to-krōm) [ cyto- + G. chrōma, color ]. A class of hemoprotein whose principal biological function is electron and/or hydrogen transport by virtue of a reversible valency change of the heme iron. Cytochromes are classified in four groups, called a, b, c, and d, according to spectrochemical characteristics. Many variants exist, particularly among bacteria and in green plants and algae. One of these is a variant of the c-type cytochrome called cytochrome f. The mitochondrial system of cytochromes provides electron transport through cytochrome c oxidase (cytochrome $aa_3$) to molecular oxygen as terminal electron acceptor (respiration).

**cytochrome $aa_3$.** Cytochrome c oxidase.

**cytochrome $b_5$ reductase** (EC 1.6.2.2). Enzyme catalyzing reduction of ferricytochrome $b_5$ to ferrocytochrome $b_5$ at the expense of NADH.

**cytochrome c oxidase** (EC 1.9.3.1). Cytochrome $aa_3$; indophenolase; indophenol oxidase; a cytochrome of the a type, containing copper, that catalyzes the oxidation of ferrocytochrome c by molecular oxygen to ferricytochrome c.

**cytochrome c peroxidase** (EC 1.11.1.5). A hemoprotein enzyme catalyzing reaction between $H_2O_2$ and ferrocytochrome c to yield ferricytochrome c.

**cytochrome c reductase.** NADH dehydrogenase.

**cytochrome $c_2$ reductase (NADPH)** (EC 1.6.2.5). Enzyme catalyzing reduction of ferricytochrome $c_2$ to ferrocytochrome $c_2$ at the expense of NADPH.

**cytochrome cd.** Cytochrome oxidase (Pseudomonas).

**cytochrome hydrogenase** (EC 1.12.2.1). Hydrogenase (q.v.); enzyme catalyzing reduction of ferricytochrome $c_3$ by $H_2$ to ferrocytochrome $c_3$.

**cytochrome oxidase (Pseudomonas)** (EC 1.9.3.2). Cytochrome cd; enzyme with action identical to that of cytochrome c oxidase, but acting on ferrocytochrome $c_2$.

**cytochrome P-450.** A cytochrome pigment that serves as the terminal oxidase for many mixed function oxidases, such as steroid hydroxylases. It is present in mitochondrial and microsomal fractions of certain tissues, such as the adrenal cortex. Named for the absorption maximum (450 nm) that the CO compound of the reduced pigment exhibits.

**cytochrome reductase (NADPH)** (EC 1.6.2.4). Enzyme catalyzing reduction of a ferricytochrome by NADPH to a ferrocytochrome, or the reverse.

**cytochylema** (si-to-ki-le'mah) [ cyto- + G. chylos, juice ]. The more fluid portion of the cytoplasm.

**cytoci'dal** [ cyto- + L. caedo, to kill ]. Causing the death of cells.

**cy'tocide** [ cyto- + L. caedo, to kill ]. An agent that is destructive to cells.

**cytocinesis** (si-to-sin-e'sis). Cytokinesis.

**cytoclasis** (si-tok'lä-sis) [ cyto- + G. klasia, a breaking ]. Fragmentation of the cells.

**cytoclas'tic.** Relating to cytoclasis; destructive of cells.

**cytoclesis** (si'to-kle'sis) [ cyto- + G. klēsis, a call ]. Cytobiotaxis; the influence of one cell on another.

**cytocuprien** (si'to-ku'pre-in). Erythrocuprien; a copper-containing protein found in human erythrocytes; similar or identical to hemocuprein; now known to be the enzyme superoxide dismutase (q.v.).

**cytocyst** (si'to-sist) [ cyto- + G. kystis, bladder ]. The bladder-like remains of the red blood cell or tissue cell that encloses a mature schizont; a rarely used term.

**cytodiagno'sis.** Diagnosis of the type and, when feasible, the cause of a pathologic process by means of microscopic study of cells in an exudate or other form of body fluid.

**cytodieresis** (si-to-di-er'e-sis). [ cyto- + G. diairesis, division ]. Cytokinesis.

**cytogene** (si'to-jēn). Plasmagene; a determinant of an inherited character located in the cytoplasm.

**cytogenesis** (si-to-jen'ē-sis) [ cyto- + G. genesis, origin ]. The origin and development of cells.

**cy'togenet'icist.** A specialist in cytogenetics.

**cy'togenet'ics.** The branch of genetics concerned with the structure and function of the cell, especially the chromosomes.

**cytogen'ic.** Relating to cytogenesis.

**cytogenous** (si-toj'en-us). Cell-forming.

**cy'toglucope'nia** [ cyto- + glucose + G. penia, poverty ]. Intracellular deficiency of glucose.

**cy'togram.** Microscopic findings of a smear of cells according to the Papanicolaou technique or a modification thereof.

**cytohet** (si'to-het) [ cyto- + heterozygous ]. Contraction designating a cell that, in a sense, is heterozygous in having cytoplasmic genetic elements from different parental types.

**cytohy'aloplasm.** Hyaloplasm.

**cytoid** (si'toyd) [ cyto- + G. eidos, resemblance ]. Resembling a cell.

**cytokinesis** (si-to-kin-e′sis) [ cyto- + G. *kinēsis*, movement ]. Cytocinesis; cytodieresis; the changes occurring in the protoplasm of the cell outside of the nucleus during cell division.

**cytoki′nins.** Term proposed in 1965 for a group of natural or synthetic chemicals that in certain plant systems have specific growth effects resembling the effects of the first known cytokinin, kinetin (6-furfurylaminopurine). To date, all or nearly all known c.'s are adenine derivatives with substituents in the N⁶ position.

**cytolemma** (si′to-lem′mah) [ cyto- + G. *lemma*, husk ]. Plasma *membrane*.

**cytolip′in.** A glycosphingolipid, specifically a ceramide oligosaccharide. Cytolipin H is a lactosylceramide, and may display immunological properties under certain conditions. Cytolipin K is the ceramide tetrasaccharide, globoside (*q.v.*).

**cytolog′ic.** Relating to cytology.

**cytol′ogist.** One who specializes in cytology.

**cytology** (si-tol′o-ji) [ cyto- + G. *logos*, study ]. The anatomy, physiology, pathology, and chemistry of the cell.

exfo′liative c., the examination, for diagnostic purposes, of cells denuded from a neoplasm (or other type of lesion) and recovered from the sediment of the exudate, secretions, or washings from the tissue, *e.g.*, sputum, vaginal secretion, gastric washings, urine, and so on.

**cytolymph** (si′to-limf). Hyaloplasm.

**cytol′ysin.** An antibody that, in association with complement, effects partial or complete destruction of an animal cell.

**cytolysis** (si-tol′ĭ-sis) [ cyto- + G. *lysis*, loosening ]. The dissolution of a cell.

**cytolysome** (si′to-li′sōm). Autophagic vacuole; a variety of secondary lysosome that contains mitochondria, ribosomes, or other organelles.

**cytolyt′ic.** Pertaining to cytolysis; possessing a solvent or destructive action on cells.

**cyto′ma** [ cyto- + G. suffix -*ōma*, tumor ]. An undesirable, general term to indicate any neoplasm composed almost entirely of neoplastic cells, with virtually no stroma or formation of histologic structures, such as glands, squamous epithelium, and so on.

**cytomegalic** (si′to-meg′ă-lik) [ cyto- + G. *megas*, big ]. Characterized by markedly enlarged cells. See cytomegalic inclusion *disease*.

**cytomeg′alovi′rus.** See under virus.

**cytomem′brane.** Plasma *membrane*.

**cytomere** (si′to-mēr) [ cyto- + G. *meros*, part ]. The structure separating the portions of the contents of a large schizont in the course of schizogony, as in some of the sporozoans undergoing exoerythrocytic asexual division. C.'s are caused by complex invaginations of the surface of the schizont, which isolates them; ultimately, c.'s complete the budding process in the formation of large numbers of merozoites.

**cytometaplasia** (si′to-met-ă-pla′zĭ-ah) [ cyto- + G. *metaplasis*, transformation, PLAS- ]. Change of form or function of a cell, other than that related to neoplasia.

**cytom′eter** [ cyto- + G. *metron*, measure ]. A standardized, usually ruled glass slide or small glass chamber of known volume, used in counting and measuring cells, especially blood cells.

**cytomicrosome** (si-to-mi′kro-sōm) [ cyto- + G. *mikros*, small, + *sōma*, body ]. See microsome.

**cytomi′tome** [ cyto- + G. *mitos*, thread ]. An obsolete term formerly used by cytologists to designate what appeared to be a fibrillar network in the cytoplasm of fixed cells.

**cytomorphology** (si′to-mor-fol′o-ji). The study of the structure of cells.

**cytomorphosis** (si′to-mor-fo′sis) [ cyto- + G. *morphōsis*, a shaping ]. The changes that the cell undergoes during the various stages of its existence. See also prosoplasia.

**cy′ton.** Obsolete term for perikaryon.

**cytopath′ic.** Pertaining to a diseased condition of a cell. See also cytopathic *effect*.

**cytopathogenic** (si′to-path-o-jen′ik). Pertaining to an agent or substance that causes a diseased condition in cells,

in contrast to histologic changes; used especially with reference to effects observed in cells in tissue cultures.

**cy′topathol′ogist.** A physician, usually skilled in anatomical pathology, who is specially trained and experienced in cytopathology.

**cytopathology** (si′to-pă-thol′o-ji). 1. The medical science and subspecialty that deals with studies and diagnoses of health and disease by microscopic examination and evaluation of cellular specimens; see also cytologic *examination;* exfoliative *cytology*. 2. Sometimes used as a synonym for cellular *pathology, q.v.*

**cytopemphis** (si′to-pem′fis). Transport of substances through cytoplasm, especially within vesicles formed from the cell membrane, being utilized by the cell.

**cytope′nia** [ cyto- + G. *penia*, poverty ]. A reduction, *i.e.*, hypocytosis, or a lack of cellular elements in the circulating blood.

**cytophagous** (si-tof′ă-gus). Devouring, or destructive to, cells.

**cytophagy** (si-tof′ă-ji) [ cyto- + G. *phagein*, to devour ]. The devouring of other cells by the phagocytes.

**cytopharynx** (si′to-făr-inks). An organelle in certain flagellates and ciliates that serves as a gullet through which food material passes from the cytostome to the cell interior; food passed is collected in food vacuoles, into which digestive enzymes are secreted.

**cytophil, cytophile** (si′to-fil, si′to-fil) [ cyto- + G. *philos*, fond ]. Having an affinity for cells; attracted by cells.

**cy′tophylac′tic.** Relating to cytophylaxis.

**cytophylaxis** (si-to-fi-lak′sis) [ cyto- + G. *phylaxis*, a guarding ]. Protection of the cells against lytic agents.

**cytophyletic** (si-to-fi-let′ik) [ cyto- + G. *phylē*, a tribe ]. Relating to the genealogy of a cell.

**cytopipette** (si′to-pī-pet′). A slightly curved, blunt end pipette usually made of glass and fitted with a rubber bulb to provide gentle negative pressure for the collection of vaginal secretions for cytological examination.

**cytoplasm** [ cyto- + G. *plasma*, thing formed ]. The substance of a cell exclusive of the nucleus. It contains various organelles and inclusions within a colloidal protoplasm.

**cytoplas′mic.** Relating to the cytoplasm.

**cytopoiesis** (si-to-poy-e′sis) [ cyto- + G. *poiēsis*, a making ]. Formation of cells.

**cy′toprepara′tion.** Laboratory preparation of a cellular specimen for cytologic examination.

**cytopyge** (si-to-pi′je) [ cyto- + G. *pygē*, buttocks ]. The anal orifice (cell "anus") found in certain structurally complex protozoa, such as the rumen-dwelling ciliates of herbivores, through which waste matter is ejected.

**cytoryctes, cytorrhyctes** (si-to-rik′tēz) [ cyto- + G. *oryktēs*, a digger ]. An old term for inclusion bodies (*e.g.*, Guarnieri bodies) now known to be the result of disease caused by filtrable viruses. The c.'s were erroneously presumed to be some form of protozoan parasite.

**cy′tosides.** *Ceramide* disaccharides.

**cytosine** (si′to-sēn). 2-Keto-4-aminopyrimidine; a pyrimidine base found in nucleic acids.

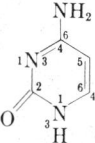

Cytosine

*Inner numbering,* official international (IUPAC); *outer numbering,* original Fischer (abandoned).

c. arabinoside, incorrect term for arabinosylcytosine.
c. deaminase (EC 3.5.4.1), see deaminases.
c. ribonucleoside, cytidine.

**cytosis** (si-to′sis) [ cyto- + G. suffix -*osis*, condition ]. 1. A condition in which there is more than the usual number of cells, as the c. of spinal fluid in acute leptomeningitis. 2.

Frequently used with a prefixed combining form as a means of describing certain features pertaining to cells; *e.g.,* isocytosis, equality in size; polycytosis, abnormal increase in number.

**cy'toskel'eton.** The tonofibrils, keratin, or other filaments serving to act as supportive cytoplasmic elements, especially of certain epithelial cells.

**cytosmear** (si'to-smēr). Cytologic *smear.*

**cytosol** (si'to-sol) [ cyto- + "sol," abbrev. of soluble ]. The cytoplasm minus the mitochondria and endoplasmic reticulum components.

**cy'tosome** [ cyto- + G. *sōma,* body ]. 1. The cell body exclusive of the nucleus. 2. Multilamellar body; one of the osmiophilic bodies which are 1 $\mu$ or less in diameter, have concentric lamellae, and occur in the great alveolar cells of the lung.

**cytostasis** (si-tos'tă-sis) [ cyto- + G. *stasis,* standing ]. The slowing of movement and accumulation of blood cells, especially polymorphonuclear leukocytes, in the capillaries, as in a region of inflammation; obstruction of a capillary as the result of accumulated leukocytes.

**cytostat'ic.** Characterized by cytostasis.

**cytostome** (si'to-stōm) [ cyto- + G. *stoma,* mouth ]. The cell "mouth" of certain complex protozoa, usually with a short gullet or cytopharynx leading food into the organism, where it is collected into food vacuoles, then circulated inside the body, eventually excreted through the cytopyge.

**cytotac'tic.** Relating to cytotaxis.

**cytotaxis, cytotaxia** (si-to-tak'sis, -tak'sĭ-ah) [ cyto- + G. *taxis,* arrangement ]. The attraction (positive c.) or repulsion (negative c.) of cells for one another.

**cytothesis** (si-toth'ĕ-sis) [ cyto- + G. *thesis,* a placing ].

The repair of injury in a cell; the restoration of cells.

**cytotox'ic.** Cytolytic; destructive to cells; pertaining to the effect of noncytophilic antibody on specific antigen, frequently, but not always, mediating the action of complement (*e.g.,* autoimmune hemolytic anemia).

**cytotoxin** (si'to-tok'sin) [ cyto- + G. *toxikon,* poison ]. A specific substance, usually with reference to antibody, that inhibits or prevents the functions of cells, or causes destruction of cells, or both. A cytolysin, for example, not only prevents function, but also leads to dissolution of the cell.

**cytotrophoblast** (si-to-trof'o-blast). Langhans' layer; the inner layer of the trophoblast, *q.v.*

**cytotropic** (si-to-trop'ik). Having an affinity for cells.

**cytotropism** (si-tot'ro-pizm) [ cyto- + G. *tropos,* a turning ]. 1. Affinity for cells. 2. Affinity for specific cells, especially the ability of viruses to localize in and damage specific cells.

**cytozo'ic.** Living in a cell; denoting certain parasitic protozoa.

**cytozoon** (si-to-zo'on) [ cyto- + G. *zōon,* animal ]. A protozoan cell parasite.

**cy'tozyme** [ cyto- + G. *zymē,* leaven ]. An obsolete term for thromboplastin.

**cy'tula** [ Mod. L. dim. of G. *kytos,* a hollow (cell) ]. The impregnated ovum.

**cytu'ria** [ G. *kytos,* cell, + *ouron,* urine ]. The passage of cells in unusual numbers in the urine.

**Czaplewski** (chă-plev'ske), Eugen, Polish bacteriologist, *1865. See C.'s *stain.*

**Czerny** (cher'ne), Vincenz, Heidelberg surgeon, 1842–1916. See C.'s *suture,* C.-Lembert *suture.*

# D

**D.** 1. Abbreviation in prescription writing for *da*, give, *detur, dentur*, let there be given. 2. Symbol for the vitamin D potency of cod liver oil, multiples of which (5D, 100D, etc.) are used to designate the vitamin D potency of irradiated ergosterol (viosterol) or other substances. 3. Chemical symbol for deuterium, $^2$H, heavy hydrogen. 4. Abbreviation, in optics, for diopter and for dexter (right). 5. Abbreviation, in electrodiagnosis, for duration, the current flowing and the circuit being closed. 6. Abbreviation, in dental formulas, for deciduous. 7. Symbol for dihydrouridine in nucleic acids. 8. Symbol for diffusing capacity. 9. As a subscript, refers to dead space.

**D-.** A prefix, printed as a small capital letter, indicating a chemical compound to be sterically related to D-glyceraldehyde, the basis of stereochemical nomenclature.

***d-.*** A prefix, printed as a lower case italicized letter, indicating a chemical compound to be dextrorotatory.

**-*d*.** Suffix, written in lower case italic, indicating a deuterium-containing compound. Subscripts ($d_2$, $d_3$, etc.) indicate the number of such atoms.

**2,4-D.** 2,4-Dichlorophenoxyacetic acid.

**Daae's disease.** See under disease.

**daboia, daboya** (dă-boy'ah) [ Hindu fr. *dabnā*, to lurk ]. *Vipera russellii;* the large, extremely deadly viper of the East Indies. The venom is coagulant in action and is used locally in a 1:10,000 solution for the arrest of hemorrhage in hemophilia.

**dacnoma'nia** [ G. *daknein*, to bite, + *mania*, insanity ]. An impulse to kill.

**DaCosta,** Jacob M., American surgeon, 1833–1900. See DaC.'s *syndrome.*

**d'Acosta,** José, 1539–1600. Jesuit priest who traveled in Peru in 1590 and observed Acosta's disease (*q. v.* under disease).

**dacry-.** See dacryo-.

**dacryadenitis** (dak'rī-ad-ē-ni'tis). Dacryoadenitis.

**dac'ryad'enoscir'rhus** [ dacryo- + G. *aden*, gland, + scirrhus ]. Obsolete term for cancer of lacrimal gland.

**dacryagogatresia** (dak-rī-ă'go-gă-tre'zĭ-ah) [ dacy- + G. *agōgos*, drawing forth, + atresia, *q. v.* ]. Obsolete term meaning obstruction or closure of a lacrimal duct.

**dacryagogue** (dak'rī-ă-gog) [ dacry- + G. *agōgos*, drawing forth ]. 1. Lacrimal duct. 2. Promoting the flow of tears. 3. An agent that stimulates the lacrimal gland to secretion.

**dacryo-, dacry-** (dak'rī-o-) [ G. *dakryon*, tear ]. Combining forms relating to tears, or to the lacrimal sac or duct.

**dacryoadenalgia** (dak-rī-o-ad-en-al'jĭ-ah) [ dacryo- + G. *adēn*, gland, + *algos*, pain ]. Pain in one of the lacrimal glands.

**dacryoadenitis** (dak-rī-o-ad-ē-ni'tis) [ dacryo- + G. *adēn*, gland, + suffix *-itis*, inflammation ]. Dacryadenitis; inflammation of the lacrimal gland.

**dacryoblennorrhea** (dak-rī-o-blen-or-re'ah) [ dacryo- + G. *blenna*, mucus, + *rhoia*, flow ]. Dacryocystoblennorrhea; a chronic discharge of mucus from a lacrimal sac.

**dacryocele** (dak'rī-o-sēl). Dacryocystocele.

**dacryocyst** (dak'rī-o-sist) [ dacryo- + G. *kystis*, sac ]. *Saccus* lacrimalis.

**dacryocystalgia** (dak-rī-o-sis-tal'jĭ-ah) [ dacryocyst + G. *algos*, pain ]. Pain in the lacrimal sac.

**dacryocystectomy** (dak'rī-o-sis-tek'to-mī) [ dacryocyst + G. *ektomē*, excision ]. Surgical removal of the lacrimal sac.

**dacryocystitis** (dak'rī-o-sis-ti'tis) [ dacryocyst + G. suffix *-itis*, inflammation ]. Inflammation of the lacrimal sac.

**dacryocys'titome.** Dacryocystotome.

**dacryocystoblennorrhea** (dak-rī-o-sis'to-blen-or-re'ah). Dacryoblennorrhea.

**dacryocystocele** (dak'rī-o-sis'to-sēl) [ dacryocyst + G. *kēlē*, hernia ]. Dacryocele; protrusion of the lacrimal sac.

**dacryocystoethmoidostomy** (dak'rī-o-sis'to-eth-moyd-os'to-mī). A simplified variation of dacryocystorhinostomy.

**dacryocystogram** (dak'rī-o-sis'to-gram) [ dacryocyst + G. *gramma*, a writing ]. An x-ray of the lacrimal apparatus obtained (after injection of radiopaque dyes) for the purpose of localizing site of obstruction; similar information is obtainable by means of a scintiphoto from a gamma camera after instilling a minute drop of technetium-99m.

**dacryocystoptosis, dacryocystoptosia** (dak'rī-o-sis'-top-to'sis, -to'sī-ah) [ dacryocyst + G. *ptōsis*, a falling ]. Downward displacement of the lacrimal sac.

**dacryocystorhinostenosis** (dak'rī-o-sis'to-ri'no-stě-no'-sis). Obstruction to the nasolacrimal duct.

**dacryocystorhinostomy** (dak'rī-sis'tor-ri-nos'to-mī) [ dacryocyst + G. *rhis* (*rhin-*), nose, + *stoma*, mouth ]. An operation effecting drainage of tears through a short circuit made in lacrimal bone and nasal mucosa.

**dacryocys'totome.** Dacryocystitome; a small knife for incising the lacrimal sac.

**dacryocystot'omy** (dak'rī-o-sis-tot'o-mī) [ dacryocyst + G. *tomē*, incision ]. Incision of the lacrimal sac.

**dacryohelco'sis** [ dacryo- + G. *helkōsis*, ulceration ]. Rarely used term for ulceration of the lacrimal sac or duct.

**dacryohemorrhea** (dak'rī-o-hem-o-re'ah) [ dacryo- + G. *haima*, blood, + *rhoia*, flow ]. The shedding of bloody tears.

**dacryolith** (dak'rī-o-lith) [ dacryo- + G. *lithos*, stone ]. Lacrimal calculus; tear stone; ophthalmolith; a concretion in the lacrimal apparatus.

  **Desmarre's d.'s,** white pseudoconcretions, composed of masses of *Nocardia* species found in the lacrimal canal.

**dacryolithiasis** (dak'rī-o-lĭ-thi'a-sis). The formation and presence of dacryoliths.

**dacryoma** (dak'rī-o'mah) [ dacryo- + G. suffix *-ōma*, tumor ]. 1. A cyst formed by the accumulation of tears in an obstructed lacrimal duct. 2. A tumor of the lacrimal apparatus.

**dacryon** (dak'rī-on) [ G. a tear ]. The point of junction of the frontomaxillary and lacrimomaxillary sutures on the medial wall of the orbit. See fig. under craniometric *point.*

**dacryops** (dak'rī-ops) [ dacryo- + G. *ōps*, eye ]. 1. Excess of tears in the eye. 2. A cyst of a tear duct of the lacrimal gland.

**dacryopyorrhea** (dak'rī-o-pi-ŏ-re'ah) [ dacryo- + G. *pyon*, pus, + *rhoia*, flow ]. The discharge of tears containing pus.

**dacryopyosis** (dak-rī-o-pi-o'sis) [ dacryo- + G. *pyōsis*, suppuration ]. Suppuration in the lacrimal sac or duct.

**dacryorhinocystotomy** (dak'rī-o-ri'nos-sis-tot'o-mī). Dacryocystorhinostomy.

**dacryorrhea** (dak'rī-o-re'ah) [ dacryo- + G. *rhoia*, flow ]. An excessive flow of tears.

**dacryosolenitis** (dak-rī-o-so-len-i'tis) [ dacryo- + G. *sōlēn*, a channel, + suffix *-itis*, inflammation ]. Inflammation of the lacrimal or nasal duct.

**dacryostenosis** (dak'rī-o-stě-no'sis) [ dacryo- + G. *stenōsis*, narrowing ]. Stricture of a lacrimal or nasal duct.

**dacryosyrinx** (dak'rī-o-sīr'inks) [ dacryo- + G. *syrinx*, pipe ]. Lacrimal *fistula.*

**dac'tinomycin** (USP). COSMEGEN; actinomycin D; produced by several species of *Streptomyces*, for example *S. parvulus;* used as an antineoplastic agent especially for Wilms' tumor in children and trophoblastic disease in women. It is highly irritating and must be administered intravenously with great care; skin eruptions, bone marrow depression, and other side effects may occur. See also actinomycin.

**dactyl** (dak'til) [ G. *daktylos* ]. A finger or toe.

**dactyl-.** See dactylo-.

**dactylagra** (dak-tī-lag'rah) [ dactyl- + G. *agra*, seizure ]. Obsolete word meaning gout in the fingers.

**dactylalgia** (dak-tī-lal'jĭ-ah) [ dactyl- + G. *algos*, pain ]. Dactylodynia; pain in the fingers.

**dactyledema** (dak'til-e-de'mah) [ dactyl- + G. *oidema*, swelling ]. Edema of the finger.

**dactyl'ia.** Syndactyly.

**dactyl'ion.** Obsolete synonym for syndactyly.

**dactylitis** (dak-til-i'tis). Inflammation of one or more fingers.

**sickle cell d.,** hand-and-foot *syndrome*.

**dactyl'ium.** Syndactyly.

**dactylo-, dactyl-** (dak'tĭ-lo-) [ G. *daktylos,* finger ]. Combining forms relating to the fingers, and sometimes to the toes.

**dactylocampsis** (dak'tĭ-lo-kamp'sis) [ dactylo- + G. *kampsis,* bending ]. Permanent flexion of the fingers.

**dactylocampsodynia** (dak'tĭ-lo-kamp'so-din'ĭ-ah) [ dactylo- + G. *kampsis,* a bending, + *odynē,* pain ]. Painful contraction of one or more fingers.

**dac'tylodyn'ia.** Dactylalgia.

**dactylogryposis** (dak-tĭ-lo-grĭ-po'sis) [ dactylo- + G. *gryposis,* a crooking ]. Contraction of the fingers.

**dactylology** (dak'tĭ-lol'o-jĭ) [ dactylo- + G. *logos,* word ]. Cheirology; chirology; the use of the finger alphabet in talking.

**dactylol'ysis sponta'nea** [ dactylo- + G. *lysis,* a loosening; L. *spontaneus,* willing ]. Ainhum.

**dactylomegaly** (dak'tĭ-lo-meg'ă-lĭ) [ dactylo- + G. *megas,* large ]. Megadactyly.

**dactyloscopy** (dak'tĭ-los'ko-pĭ) [ dactylo- + G. *skopeō,* to examine ]. An examination of the markings in prints made from the fingertips; employed as a method of personal identification. See Galton's system of classification of fingerprints (under fingerprint).

**dac'tylospasm.** Spasmodic contraction of the fingers.

**dactylosymphysis** (dak-tĭ-lo-sim'fĭ-sis) [ dactylo- + G. *symphysis,* a growing together ]. Obsolete synonym for syndactyly.

**dactylus,** pl. **dac'tyli** (dak'tĭ-lus) [ G. *daktylos* ]. Dactyl; a finger or a toe. See also digitus.

**dacuronium** (dak'u-ro'nĭ-um). A nondepolarizing steroid neuromuscular blocking agent with more rapid onset and shorter duration of action than pancuronium.

**dagga** (dag'ah) [ aborigines' term ]. Leaves of *Leonotis leonurus,* a plant found in South Africa, where it is smoked like tobacco with mild sedative effect. Term mistakenly applied to Indian hemp, *Cannabis sativa.*

**Dagnini,** Giuseppe, Italian physician, 1866–1928. See Aschner-D. *reflex.*

**DAH.** Abbreviation for disordered action of heart (soldier's heart; irritable heart; effort syndrome; cardiac neurosis).

**Dahl,** Andreas, Swedish botanist, 1751–1789. Gave his name to dahlin.

**dah'lin** [ dahlia, after *A. Dahl* ]. Inulin.

**dahllite** (dah'lit). Podolite; $CaCO_3 \cdot 2Ca_3(PO_4)_2$; a naturally occurring calcium phosphate, similar in structure to the mineral portions of bones and teeth.

**daisy.** A colloquial term for the segmented forms (merozoites) of the mature schizont of *Plasmodium malariae.*

**Dakin,** Henry D., New York chemist, 1880–1952. See D.-Carrel *treatment.*

**Dale,** Sir Henry H., English pharmacoligist, 1875–1968. Nobel laureate 1936 with Otto Loewi for investigations on the transmission of nerve impulses by chemical substances. See D.-Feldberg *law,* D. *reaction,* Schultz-D. *reaction.*

**Dalrymple,** John, English oculist, 1804–1852. See D.'s *disease, sign.*

**Dalton,** John, eminent English chemist, mathematician, and natural philosopher, 1766–1844. Founder of the atomic theory which he set forth in a work entitled *A New System of Chemical Philosophy* (1810). See D.'s *law,* D.-Henry *law.*

**dalton** (dawl'ton). Term unofficially used to indicate a unit of mass equal to $^1/_{12}$ the mass of a carbon-12 atom; 1.0000 in the atomic mass scale. Numerically, but not dimensionally, equal to molecular weight.

**Dalto'nian.** 1. Relating to John Dalton. 2. A color-blind person.

**daltonism** (dawl'ton-izm) [ J. *Dalton* ]. Color blindness, especially red blindness.

**Dam,** C. P. Henrik, Danish biochemist, *1895. Nobel laureate, 1943, with Edward A. Doisy, for their discovery of the chemical nature of vitamin K. See D. *unit.*

**dam** [ A.S. *fordemman,* to stop up ]. Any barrier to the flow of fluid; especially, in surgery and dentistry, a sheet of thin rubber arranged so as to shut off the part operated upon from the access of fluid. Rubber d. is frequently used in thin strips as a surgical drain.

**coffer d.,** rubber d.; in dentistry, a thin sheet of rubber adjusted around the neck of a tooth to prevent the access of saliva to the part operated upon.

**post d.,** postdam; posterior palatal *seal.*

**rubber d.,** (1) see d.; (2) coffer d.

**Damalinia** (dam-ă-lin'ĭ-ah). A genus of biting lice containing a number of species found on domestic and wild animals. These lice are all highly host-specific, one species being confined to each species of mammal. See also *Bovicola* and *Trichodectes.*

**dam'mar** [ Hind. *dāmar,* resin ]. A resin resembling copal, obtained from various species of *Shorea* (family Dipterocarpaceae) in the East Indies. It is used, dissolved in chloroform, for mounting microscopic specimens.

**damp.** 1. Humid; moist. 2. Atmospheric moisture. 3. Foul air in a mine; air charged with carbonic oxide or with various explosive hydrocarbon vapors.

**after d.,** see afterdamp.

**black d.,** choke d.

**choke d.,** black d., carbonic dioxide or anhydride, $CO_2$; air with a high percentage of carbon dioxide and a low percentage of oxygen; formed in coal mines; due to the slow oxidation of coal.

**fire d.,** methane.

**Dana,** Charles L., New York neurologist, 1852–1935. See D.'s *operation,* Putnam-D. *syndrome.*

**da'nazol** (USAN). 17α-Pregna-2,4-dien-20-yno[ 2,3-*d* ]isoxazol-17-ol; anterior pituitary suppressant.

**Dance,** Jean B. H., French physician, 1797–1832. See D.'s *sign.*

**dance.** Abnormal, histrionic movements related to brain damage.

**hilar d.,** vigorous pulmonary arterial pulsations due to increased blood flow often seen fluoroscopically in patients with congenital left-to-right shunts, especially septal defects.

**Saint Anthony's d.,** chorea.

**Saint John's d.,** chorea.

**Saint Vi'tus' d.,** Sydenham's *chorea.*

**Saint With's d.,** chorea.

**dandelion** (dan'de-li-on) [ Fr. *dent de lion,* lion's tooth ]. Taraxacum.

**dan'der.** Scales of the scalp.

**dan'druff.** Seborrhea sicca (2); pityriasis sicca, capitis, or furfuracea; scurf; the presence, in varying amounts, of white or gray scales in the hair of the scalp, due to the normal branny exfoliation of the epidermis.

**Dandy,** Walter E., American surgeon, 1886–1946. See D. *operations,* D.-Walker *syndrome.*

**Dane,** D. S. See D.'s *particles.*

**Danforth,** William Clark, U. S. obstetrician-gynecologist, 1878–1949. See D.'s *sign.*

**Danielssen,** Daniel C., Norwegian physician, 1815–1894. See D.'s *disease,* D.-Boeck *disease.*

**Danlos,** Henri A., French dermatologist, 1844–1912. See Ehlers-D. *syndrome.*

**dan'syl.** 5-Dimethylaminonaphthalene-1-sulfonyl radical; a blocking agent for $NH_2$ groups, used in peptide synthesis; abbreviated Dns or DNS.

**dan'thron.** Chrysazin; 1,8-dihydroxyanthraquinone; DORBANE; ISTIN; ISTIZIN. An anthraquinone laxative.

**Danysz** (dan'is), Jean, Polish pathologist in France, 1860–1928. See D. *phenomenon.*

**dap'sone** (USP, BP). DDS; diaminodiphenylsulfone; AVLOSULFONE; used in the treatment of leprosy and certain cutaneous diseases such as dermatitis herpetiformis, and is active against the tubercle bacillus; also used in the treatment of bovine coccidiosis and streptococcal mastitis. Dapsone, other sulfones, or long-acting sulfonamides enhance the chemoprophylactic action of quinine (or of a combination of chloroquine-primaquine, as well as of other antimalarials) against malaria.

**d'Arcet's metal.** See under metal.

**Darier** (dar-e-a'), Jean F., French dermatologist, 1856-1938. See D.'s *disease.*

**Darkschewitsch (Darkshevich),** Liverij O., Russian neurologist, 1858-1925. See *nucleus* of D.

**Darling,** Samuel Taylor, U. S. physician in Panama, 1872-1925. See D.'s *disease.*

**Darrow,** Mary A., U. S. stain technologist, 1894-1973. See Darrow red.

**Darrow red.** A basic oxazin dye, $C_{18}H_{14}N_3O_2Cl$, used as a stain for Nissl bodies.

**d'Arsonval,** Jacques A., French physiologist, 1851-1940. See d'A. *current.*

**darto'ic, dar'toid** [ G. *dartos,* flayed ]. Resembling tunica dartos in its slow, involuntary contractions.

**dar'tos** [ G. skinned or flayed, fr. *derō,* to skin ]. See *tunica* dartos.

  **d. mulieb'ris,** a very thin layer of smooth muscle in the integument of the labia majora; less well developed than the tunica dartos of the scrotum.

**Darwin,** Charles R., celebrated English biologist and evolutionist, 1809-1882. Advanced the theory of the origin of species through natural selection (survival of the fittest in the struggle for existence) and of the evolution of man from an ancestor common to himself and the ape. After collecting scientific data for over twenty years, published his great works, *The Origin of Species by Natural Selection* (1859) and *The Descent of Man* (1871). See Darwinian *ear, reflex, tubercle.*

**Dastre,** Jules Albert Francois, French physician, 1844-1917. See D.-Morat *law.*

**Dasyprocta** (das'ĭ-prok'tah) [ G. *dasyprōktos,* having hairy buttocks ]. A genus of rodents, the agoutis, a reservoir host of *Trypanosoma cruzi.*

**Dasypus** (das'ĭ-pus) [ G. *dasypous,* hairy-footed ]. The ninebanded armadillo of North and South America; Texas armadillo; mulita; cachicamo.

**Datura** (dă-tu'rah) [ Hindu ]. A genus of solanaceous plants, from a species of which stramonium is obtained.
  **D. fastuo'sa,** the seeds are used in India by the Thugs to produce unconsciousness.
  **D. metel,** *D. fastuosa* L. var. *alba;* contains scopolamine as its chief alkaloid and traces of hyoscyamine and atropine.
  **D. sanguin'ea** is used in Peru to produce unconsciousness, as are **D. fer'ox** and **D. arbore'a** in Brazil.
  **D. stramonium,** thorn apple; Jamestown weed; jimson weed; stink weed; apple of Peru; the dried leaf and flowering or fruiting tops with branches are known as stramonium.
  **D. tatula,** the dried leaf and flowering or fruiting tops with branches are known as stramonium.

**daturine** (dă-tu'rin, -rēn). Hyoscyamine.

**Daubenton** (do-bahn-tawn'), Louis J. M., French physician, 1716-1799. See D.'s *angle, line.*

**Dauerschlaf** [ Ger. ]. Prolonged sleep *treatment.*

**daunomycin.** An antibiotic of the rhodomycin group, obtained from *Streptomyces peucetius;* may be of value in the treatment of acute leukemia.

**Davaine,** Casimir J., French physician, 1812-1882. See D.'s *bacillus.*

**Davai'nea madagascarien'sis.** *Taenia demerariensis; Taenia madagascariensis;* a tapeworm found in man in Madagascar and elsewhere; the intermediary host is not known, but is presumed to be an arthropod.

**Davidoff,** M. von, German histologist, †1904. See D.'s *cells.*

**Davidsohn,** Hermann, German physician, 1842-1911. See D.'s *sign.*

**Davidson,** Edward C., American surgeon, 1894-1933. See D. *syringe.*

**Daviel** (dă-ve-el'), Jacques, French oculist, 1696-1762. See D.'s *operation, spoon,*

**Davis,** John Staige, Baltimore surgeon, 1872-1946. See D. *grafts.*

**Davis-Crowe mouth gag.** See under gag.

**Davy,** Edmund W., Irish physician, 1826-1899. See D.'s *test.*

**Davy,** Sir Humphry, English chemist, 1778-1829. Discovered the anesthetic properties of nitrous oxide, experimenting upon himself, and recognized its possibilities as an anesthetic in surgical operations; he separated from their salts: sodium, potassium, barium, calcium, and strontium; he invented a safety lamp for coal miners.

**Dawbarn,** Robert Hugh Mackay, American surgeon, 1860-1915. See D.'s *sign.*

**Dawson,** J. R., U. S. pathologist. See D.'s *encephalitis.*

**Day,** Richard H., American physician, 1813-1892. See D.'s *test.*

**Day,** Richard L. See Riley-D. *syndrome.*

**dazz'ling.** The consequence of illumination too intense for adaptation by the eye; in contrast to glare (*q.v.*), d. is alleviated by appropriate tinted glasses.

**DC.** Abbreviation of Dental Corps.

**D.C.** Abbreviation of Doctor of Chiropractic.

**dCMP deaminase** (EC 3.5.4.12). See deaminases.

**D.D.S.** Abbreviation for Doctor of Dental Surgery.

**DDT.** Abbreviation for dichlorodiphenyltrichloroethane.

**de-** [ L. *de,* from, away ]. Prefix carrying often a private or negative sense; denoting away from, cessation; it has sometimes an intensive force.

**deacidification** (de-ă-sid'ĭ-fĭ-ka'shun). The removal or neutralization of acid.

**deacon** (de'kon). Bob *veal.*

**deactivation** (de-ak-tĭ-va'shun). The process of rendering or of becoming inactive.

**deacylase** (de-as'il-ās). A member of the subclass of hydrolases (EC class 3) known as esterases, lipases, lactonases, and hydrolases (EC subclass 3.1); enzymes catalyzing the hydrolytic cleavage of an acyl group (R—CO—) in an ester linkage. Also includes enzymes cleaving amide linkages (EC subclass 3.5) and similar acyl compounds.

**dead** (ded). 1. Without life; see also death. 2. Numb.

**DEAE-cellulose.** See under cellulose.

**deaf** (def) [ A.S. *deáf* ]. Unable to hear; hearing indistinctly; hard of hearing.

**deafferentation** (de-af-er-ent-a'shun) [ L. *de,* from, + afferent, *q.v.* ]. A loss of the sensory nerve fibers from a portion of the body.

**deaf-mute** (def'mūt). An individual with deafmutism. One whose speech has never developed because of congenital or early acquired profound deafness.

**deafmutism** (def'mu'tizm). Inability to speak, due to congenital deafness or that occurring in early life.
  **endem'ic d.,** d. of goiter regions, due to severe thyroid deficiency.

**deaf'ness.** Loss of the ability to hear without designation of the degree of loss or the cause. For the sake of clarity the otologist usually prefers terms with clearer definitions. See: acusis, hearing, threshold shift, hypoacusis, anacusis, dysacusis, auditory agnosia, presbyacusis, diplacusis. The terms nerve d. or perceptive d. are no longer considered acceptable.
  **acoustic trauma d.,** boilermaker's d.,; industrial d.; occupational d.; loss of hearing due to changes in the organ of Corti secondary to overexposure to high intensity noise levels.
  **boiler-maker's d.,** acoustic trauma d.
  **central d.,** d. due to disease in the auditory area of the brain.
  **conductive d.,** hearing impairment caused by interference with sound or vibratory energy in the external canal, middle ear, or ossicles.
  **cortical d.,** d. resulting from a lesion of the cerebral cortex.
  **functional d.,** psychogenic d.
  **high frequency d.,** selective loss of hearing acuity for high frequencies, usually associated with neurosensory damage, common in acoustic trauma.
  **hysterical d.,** psychogenic d.
  **industrial d.,** acoustic trauma d.
  **low tone d.,** low frequency hearing loss; inability to hear low notes or frequencies.

**nerve d., neural d.,** retrocochlear d; d. due to dysfunction or disease in the auditory pathway or nerve.

**occupational d.,** acoustic trauma d.

**perceptive d.,** term formerly used to denote impaired hearing resulting from disease of or injury to the inner ear or the central mechanism involved in hearing.

**psychic d.,** psychogenic d.

**psychogenic d.,** functional d.; hysterical d.; psychic d.; sensory d.; hearing loss of a hysterical or functional type without evidence of organic cause or malingering; often follows severe psychic shock.

**retrocochlear d.,** nerve d.

**sensorineural d.,** term formerly called nerve d., inner ear d., and perceptive d.; hearing loss due to lesions or dysfunction of the cochlea or retrocochlear tracts and centers as opposed to conductive d.

**sensory d.,** psychogenic d.

**word d.,** auditory *aphasia.*

**dealbation** (de-al-ba'shun) [ L. *de-albo,* pp. *-atus,* to whiten ]. The act of whitening, bleaching, or blanching.

**dealcoholization** (de-al'ko-hol-ĭ-za'shun). The removal of alcohol from a fluid; in histologic technique, the removal of alcohol from a specimen that has been previously immersed in this fluid.

**deallergize** (de-al'ler-jīz). To reduce or remove allergic sensitivity.

**de Almeida,** F. P. See Almeida, F. P. de.

**deamidase** (de-am'ĭ-dās). See amidohydrolases.

**deamidation, deamidization** (de-am-ĭ-da'shun, de-am'ĭ-dĭ-za'shun). The hydrolytic removal of an amide group.

**deamidize** (de-am'ĭ-dīs). To remove the amide group of a compound, usually by hydrolysis.

**deaminases** (de-am'ĭ-na-sez). Enzymes catalyzing simple hydrolysis of C—NH₂ bonds of purines, pyrimidines, and pterins, usually named in terms of the substrate, *e.g.,* cytosine d. (EC 3.5.4.1), adenine d. (EC 3.5.4.2), guanine d. (EC 3.5.4.3), adenosine d. (EC 3.5.4.4), cytidine d. (EC 3.5.4.5), AMP d. (EC 3.5.4.6), ADP d. (EC 3.5.4.7), pterin d. (EC 3.5.4.11), dCMP d. (EC 3.5.4.12). Not generally used for deamination of noncyclic amides. Deaminases (EC group 3.5.4) are distinguished from ammonia-lyases (EC 4.3.1) in that the latter produce an unsaturation at the point of NH₃ removal.

**deamination, deaminization** (de-am-ĭ-na'shun, de-am'ĭ-nĭ-za'shun). Removal, usually by hydrolysis, of the NH₂ group from an amino compound.

**deaminize** (de-am'ĭ-nīz). To remove, usually by hydrolysis, the amino group from an amino compound.

**deamino-oxytocin.** An analogue of oxytocin in which the free amino group is absent. On a molar basis, it is more potent than oxytocin in stimulating uterine contractions at term and causing milk ejection in women and in various animal bioassays.

**de'anol acetam'idoben'zoate.** DEANER; the *p*-acetamidobenzoic acid salt of 2-dimethylaminoethanol; a central nervous system stimulant proposed to alleviate abnormally shortened attention spans in children with learning difficulties and behavioral problems. It is contraindicated in patients with grand mal epilepsy.

**deaquation** (de-ă-kwa'shun) [ L. *de,* from, + *aqua,* water ]. Dehydration.

**dearterialization** (de-ar-te'rĭ-al-i-za'shun). Changing the character of arterial blood to that of venous blood; deoxygenation of the blood.

**dearticulation** (de-ar-tik-u-la'shun). 1. Dislocation. 2. Disarticulation.

**death** (deth) [ A.S. *dēath* ]. 1. The cessation of life. 2. In multicellular organisms, d. is a gradual process at the cellular level, with tissues varying in their ability to withstand deprivation of oxygen. In higher organisms, d. is a cessation of integrated tissue and organ functions. 3. In man, d. is manifested by the loss of heart beat, by the absence of spontaneous breathing, and by cerebral death (*q. v.*).

**black d.,** term applied to the worldwide epidemic of the 14th century, of which some 60 million persons are said to have died; the descriptions indicate that it was pneumonic plague.

**cerebral d.,** irreparable brain damage manifested clinically by absence of purposive responsiveness to external stimuli, absence of cephalic reflexes, apnea, and an isoelectric electroencephalogram for at least 30 minutes in the absence of hypothermia and poisoning by central nervous system depressants.

**crib d.,** jargon for sudden and usually inexplicable d. in an apparently healthy infant; such infants are commonly found in a face-down position; autopsy findings rarely indicate a possible cause of d. See also sudden death *syndrome.*

**fetal d.,** d. *in utero* of a fetus which at birth weighs 500 gm. or more, irrespective or gestational age.

**infant d.,** d. of a liveborn infant (see liveborn *infant*); further classified as (1) early neonatal d., d. of a liveborn infant occurring less than 7 completed days (168 hours) from the time of birth; (2) late neonatal d., occurring after 7 completed days of age but before 28 completed days.

**local d.,** necrosis; gangrene; d. of a part of the body or of a tissue.

**maternal d.,** d. of a woman while she is pregnant or within 42 days after the termination of gestation, irrespective of the site and duration of pregnancy and of the cause of d.; the 42-day period is divided into period 1 (1 to 7 days following termination of cyesis) and period 2 (8 to 42 days following termination of cyesis). Maternal d.'s are further classified as direct or indirect. Direct maternal d. is that resulting from obstetric complications of the gestation, labor, or puerperium, and from interventions, omissions, incorrect treatment, or a chain of events caused by any of the above. Indirect maternal d. is an obstetric d. resulting from previously existing disease or from a disease that developed during pregnancy, labor, or the puerperium; it is not directly due to obstetric causes, but to conditions aggravated by the physiological effects of pregnancy.

**somatic d.,** d. of the entire body, as distinguished from local d.

**systemic d.,** somatic d.

**death-adder.** *Acanthopis antarcticus;* a poisonous Australian snake with a viper-like body form, wide head, and short tail; one of the most feared venomous snakes.

**death-rattle.** A respiratory gurgling or rattling in the throat of a dying person, caused by the loss of the cough reflex and accumulation of mucus; a rare and overdramatized sign.

**Deaver,** John B., U. S. surgeon, 1855–1931. See D.'s *incision.*

**debil'itant.** 1. Weakening; causing debility. 2. Obsolete term for a quieting agent or one that subdues excitement.

**debil'ity** [ L. *debilitas,* fr. *debilis,* weak, fr. *de-* priv. + *habilis,* able, fr. *habeo,* to have. ]. Weakness.

**de Bordeau** or **de Bordeu** (bor-do'), Théophile, French physician, 1722–1776. See de B. *theory.*

**debouch** (dĕ-boosh') [ Fr. *bouche,* mouth ]. To open or empty into another part.

**débouchement** (da-boosh-moń') [ Fr. ]. Opening or emptying into another part.

**Débove** (dĕ-buv'), Maurice Georges, Paris physician, 1845–1920. See D.'s *disease.*

**Debré phenomenon.** See under phenomenon.

**débridement** (da-brēd-moń') [ Fr. *débris,* waste ]. Excision of contused and devitalized tissue from a wound surface.

**debrisoquine sulfate** (dĕ-bris'o-kwin) (USAN). DE-CLINAX; 3-4-dihydro-2(1*H*)-isoquinoline carboxamidine sulfate; antihypertensive agent.

**debt** (det) [ L. *debitum,* debt ]. That which is owed; a liability or obligation to be rendered.

**alactic oxygen d.,** that part of the oxygen d. that is not lactacid oxygen d.; during recovery, stores of ATP and creatine phosphate must be replenished by oxidative metabolism, and a small amount of oxygen is also needed to restore the normal oxyhemoglobin levels throughout the circulating blood.

**lactacid oxygen d.,** that part of an oxygen d. represented by the production of lactic acid by anaerobic glycolysis during exercise and, therefore, by the need to eliminate it by oxidative metabolism during recovery.

**oxygen d.,** the extra oxygen, taken in by the body during recovery from exercise, beyond the resting needs of the body; sometimes used as if synonymous with oxygen *deficit, q.v.*

**deca-** (dek'ah-) [ G. *deka,* ten ]. A prefix used in the metric system to signify ten; also spelled deka-.

**dec'agram** (dek'ah-gram). A weight of 10 grams, equivalent to 154.32349 grains, or, roughly, 2.5 drams, apothecaries' weight.

**decalcifica'tion** [ L. *de-,* away, + *calx (calc-),* lime, + *facio,* to make ]. 1. The removal of lime salts, chiefly tricalcium phosphate, from bones and teeth, either *in vitro* or as a result of a pathologic process. 2. Precipitation of calcium from blood as by oxalate or fluoride, or the conversion of blood calcium to an un-ionized form as by citrate, thus preventing or delaying coagulation.

**decal'cify.** To remove lime or calcium salts, especially from bones or teeth.

**decal'cifying.** 1. Relating to an agent, measure, or process that removes calcium salts from bones or teeth. 2. Relating to a chemical, *e.g.,* oxalate, fluoride, or citrate, that renders blood incoagulable by removing calcium ion, necessary for the clotting mechanism.

**decaliter** (dek'ă-le-ter). A measure of 10 liters, the equivalent of 610.2 cubic inches, or, roughly, 10 quarts or 2.5 gallons.

**decal'vant** [ L. *decalvare,* to make bald ]. Removing the hair; making bald.

**dec'ame'ter.** Ten meters.

**dec'ametho'nium bromide** (NF). SYNCURINE; decamethylene-1,10-bis-trimethylammonium dibromide; a synthetic drug that blocks myoneural transmission and is used clinically to produce muscular relaxation during general anesthesia.

**dec'ane.** A paraffin hydrocarbon, $C_{10}H_{22}$.

**decano'ic acid.** *N*-Capric acid; see under capric.

**decano'in.** Caprin.

**decanormal** (dek-ă-nor'mal). Rarely used term denoting a solution 10 times the strength of a normal one; the usual usage is its symbol, 10 N.

**decant'** [ Mediev. L. *decantho,* fr. *de-* + *canthus,* the beak of a jug, fr. G. *kanthos,* corner of the eye ]. To pour off gently the upper clear portion of a fluid, leaving the sediment in the vessel.

**decantation** (de-kan-ta'shun). Pouring off the clear upper portion of a fluid.

**de'capacita'tion.** Prevention of capacitation by spermatozoa, and thus of their ability to fertilize ova. See also d. *factor.*

**decapitate** (de-kap'ĭ-tāt) [ L. *de-,* away, + *caput,* head ]. 1. To remove the head; specifically, to cut off the head of a fetus to facilitate delivery in cases of irremediable dystocia; or to cut off the head of an animal to prepare it for certain physiologic experiments. 2. Relating to an experimental animal with the head removed.

**decapitation** (de-kap-ĭ-ta'shun). The removal of a head; see decapitate.

**decap'itator.** 1. An instrument for removing the head of the fetus in embryotomy in cases of irremedial dystocia such as neglected shoulder presentation. 2. One who decapitates.

**decapsulation** (de-kap-su-la'shun). Depriving of a capsule or enveloping membrane.

**d. of the kidney,** stripping off the capsule of the kidney, a remedial measure in certain cases of chronic nephritis.

**decar'boniza'tion.** The process of arterialization of the blood by oxygenation and the removal of carbon dioxide in the lungs.

**decarbox'ylase.** An enzyme that removes a molecule of carbon dioxide from a carboxylic group (*e.g.,* from an α-amino acid, converting it into an amine). The d.'s are members of EC subclass 4.1.1 (EC class 4.1 comprises the carbon-carbon lyases).

**decarboxyla'tion.** A reaction involving the removal of a molecule of carbon dioxide from an organic compound, usually a carboxylic acid.

**decay** (de-ka') [ L. *de,* down, + *cado,* to fall ]. 1. The destruction of an organic substance by slow combustion, or gradual oxidation. 2. Putrefaction. 3. To deteriorate; to undergo slow combustion or putrefaction. 4. See caries.

**backward d.,** in dentistry, backward *caries.*

**deceleration** (de-sel'er-a'shun). 1. The act of decelerating. 2. The rate of decrease in velocity per unit of time.

**decentra'tion.** Removal from the center.

**decerebrate** (de-sĕr'ĕ-brāt). 1. To cause decerebration. 2. Denoting an animal so prepared, or a patient whose brain has suffered an injury which renders him in his neurologic behavior comparable to a decerebrate animal.

**decerebration** (de-sĕr'ĕ-bra'shun). Removal of the brain above the lower border of the corpora quadrigemina, or a complete section of the brain at this level or somewhat below.

**bloodless d.,** destroying the function of the cerebrum by tying the common carotid arteries and the basilar artery at about the middle of the pons.

**decer'ebrize.** To remove the brain.

**de Chauliac,** Guy. See Chauliac.

**dechloridation** (de-klo'rī-da'shun). Dechlorination; dechloruration; reducing sodium chloride in the tissues and fluids of the body by reducing its intake or increasing its excretion.

**dechlorina'tion.** Dechloridation.

**dechlorura'tion.** Dechloridation.

**de'cholest'eroliza'tion.** The reduction therapeutically of the cholesterol concentration of the blood.

**deci-** [ L. *decimus,* tenth ]. A prefix used in the metric system to signify one-tenth (10-1).

**decibel** (des'ĭ-bel) [ L. *decimus,* tenth, + bel, *q.v.* ]. Abbreviated db; one-tenth of a bel; unit for expressing the relative loudness of sound on a logarithmic scale.

**decidentia** (des'ĭ-den'shĭ-ah) [ L. coinage from *decidere,* to fall ]. Epilepsy.

**decidua** (de-sid'u-ah) [ L. *deciduus,* falling off (qualifying *membrana,* membrane, understood). CAD- ]. *Membrana* decidua.

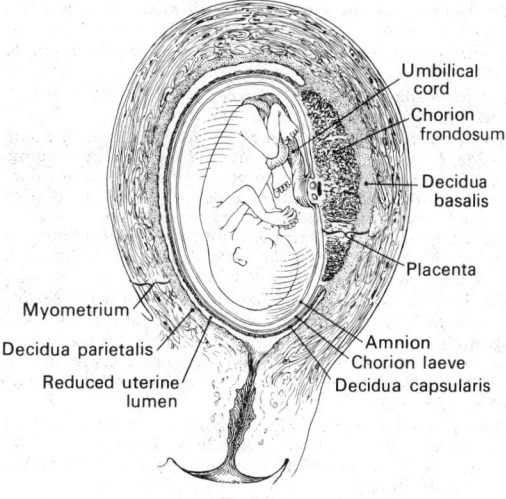

**Decidua**

Parts of the decidual complex as they appear early in the 5th month of pregnancy. (Slightly modified from Williams, J. W.: *Amer. J. Obstet. Gynec. 13:* 1-16, 1927.)

**d. basa'lis** [ NA ], d. serotina; the area of endometrium between the implanted chorionic vesicle and the myometrium. It becomes the maternal part of the placenta.

**d. capsula'ris** [ NA ], d. reflexa; membrana adventitia (2); the layer of endometrium overlying the implanted chorionic vesicle. It becomes progressively more attenuated as the chorionic vesicle enlarges. About the 4th month it is squeezed against the d. parietalis and thereafter undergoes rapid regression.

**ectopic d.,** deciduosis.

**d. menstrua'lis,** the succulent mucous membrane of the nonpregnant uterus at the menstrual period.

**d. parieta'lis** [ NA ], d. vera; uteroepichorial membrane; the altered mucous membrane lining the main cavity of the pregnant uterus elsewhere than at the site of attachment of the chorionic vesicle.

**d. polypo'sa,** d. parietalis showing polypoid projections of the endometrial surface.

**d. reflex'a,** d. capsularis.

**d. serot'ina,** d. basalis.

**d. spongio'sa,** the portion of the d. basalis attached to the myometrium.

**d. vera,** d. parietalis.

**decidual** (de-sid'u-al). Relating to the decidua.

**deciduation** (de-sid'u-a'shun) [ L. *deciduus,* falling off ]. The shedding of endometrial tissue during menstruation.

**deciduitis** (de-sid-u-i'tis). Inflammation of the decidua.

**deciduoma** (de-sid'u-o'mah). An intrauterine mass of decidual tissue, probably the result of hyperplasia of decidual cells retained in the uterus. It is doubtful that d. is a true neoplasm.

**Loeb's d.,** a mass of decidual tissue produced in the uterus, in the absence of a fertilized ovum, by means of mechanical or hormonal stimulation.

**d. malig'num,** a term formerly used for chorioadenoma.

**deciduosis** (de-sid'u-o'sis). Ectopic decidua; changes in tissues other than in the body of the uterus resembling those which occur in the endometrium during pregnancy.

**deciduous** (de-sid'u-us) [ L. *deciduus,* falling off. CAD- ]. 1. That which eventually falls off; not permanent. 2. In dentistry, often used to designate the first or primary dentition; see *dens* deciduus.

**deciduus** [ L. ] [ NA ]. 1. Decidual. 2. Deciduous.

**dec'igram.** A weight of 0.1 gm., the equivalent of 1.54 grain.

**deciliter** (des'ĭ-le-ter). A measure of 0.1 liter, equivalent to 6.1028 cubic inches or 3.38 American, 3.52 English fluid ounces.

**dec'imeter.** A linear measure of 0.1 meter, equivalent to 3.937 inches.

**dec'inor'mal.** One-tenth of normal; denoting a solution of this strength; abbreviation N/10 or 0.1 N.

**decipara** (dĕ-sip'ă-rah) [ L. *decem,* ten, + *pario,* to bear ]. A woman who has borne ten children.

**declination** (dek-lĭ-na'shun) [ L. *declinatio,* a bending aside, fr. *de-clino,* to bend aside. CLIM- ]. 1. A bending, sloping, or other deviation from a normal vertical position. 2. In ophthalmology, deflection of the vertical meridian of the eye to one or the other side in consequence of rotation of the eyeball in its anteroposterior axis; **negative d.** occurs when the upper pole of the vertical diameter approaches the nose; **positive d.,** when it turns toward the temple.

**dec'linator.** A form of retractor by means of which certain parts are kept out of the way during an operation.

**decline** (de-klin'). 1. A chronic progressive disease. 2. The stage of subsidence of the symptoms of an acute disease. 3. The period of catabolism or involution, coincident with beginning old age.

**declive** (de-kliv') [ L. *declivis,* sloping downward, fr. *clivus,* a slope, CLIM- ] [ NA ]. Declivis; lobulus clivi; the posterior sloping portion of the monticulus of the vermis of the cerebellum.

**decli'vis.** Declive.

**decoction** (de-kok'shun) [ L. *decoctio,* fr. *de-coquo,* pp. -*coctus,* to boil down ]. 1. The process of boiling. 2. The pharmacopeial name for preparations made by boiling crude vegetable drugs, and then straining, in the proportion of 50 gm. of the drug to 1000 ml. of water.

**décollement** (da-kul-mon') [ Fr. ungluing ]. The operation of separating tissues or organs which are adherent, either normally or pathologically.

**de'compensa'tion.** 1. A failure of compensation in heart disease. 2. The appearance or exacerbation of a mental disorder due to failure of defense mechanisms.

**schizophrenic d.,** the development of schizophrenia related to increased stress which cannot be mastered.

**decompose** (de'kom-pōz) [ L. *de,* from, down, + *com-pono,* pp. -*positus,* to put together ]. 1. To resolve a compound into its component parts; to disintegrate. 2. To decay.

**decomposition** (de'kom-po-zish'un). Decay; disintegration; lysis.

**decompression** (de'kom-presh'un) [ L. *de-,* from, down, + *com-primo,* pp. -*pressus,* to press together, fr. *premo,* to press ]. The removal of pressure.

**cardiac d.,** pericardial d.; incision into the pericardium for the relief of pressure due to the presence of blood or other fluid in the pericardial sac.

**cerebral d.,** removal of a piece of the cranium, usually in the subtemporal region, with incision of the dura, to relieve intracranial pressure.

**explosive d.,** rapid d.

**internal d.,** removal of intracranial tissue to relieve pressure.

**nerve d.,** the release of pressure on a nerve trunk by the surgical widening of the bony canal.

**orbital d.,** removal of a portion of the bony orbit, usually superior (Naffziger operation) or lateral (Krönlein operation).

**pericardial d.,** cardiac d.

**rapid d.,** sudden severe expansion of gases due to a reduction in ambient pressure.

**spinal d.,** the removal of pressure upon the spinal cord as by a tumor, cyst, hematoma, or bone.

**suboccipital d.,** d. of the posterior fossa by occipital craniectomy and opening of the dura.

**subtemporal d.,** d. of the brain by temporal craniectomy and opening of the dura over the inferolateral surface of the temporal lobe.

**trigeminal d.,** d. of the trigeminal nerve root.

**decongestant** (de-kon-jes'tant). 1. Decongestive. 2. An agent that possesses this action.

**decongestive** (de-kon-jes'tiv). Having the property of reducing congestion.

**de'contamina'tion.** Removal or neutralization of poisonous gas or other injurious agent from ground, buildings, clothing, etc., especially relating to war gases.

**decortica'tion** (de-kor-tĭ-ka'shun) [ L. *decortico,* pp. -*atus,* to deprive of bark, fr. *de,* from, + *cortex,* rind, bark ]. 1. Removal of the cortex, or external layer, beneath the capsule from any organ or structure. 2. An operation for removal of the residual clot and newly organized scar tissue that form after a hemothorax.

**cerebral d.,** destruction of the cerebral cortex, usually due to anoxia.

**reversible d.,** a temporary loss of function of the cerebral cortex.

**decortiza'tion.** Decortication.

**decrement** (dek're-ment) [ L. *decrementum,* fr. *decresco,* to decrease ]. 1. Decrease. 2. Decrease in conduction velocity at a particular point in a fiber; a result of altered properties at that point; see also decremental *conduction.*

**decrepitation** (de-krep'ĭ-ta'shun) [ L. *de,* from, + *crepo,* pp. *crepitus,* to crackle ]. Crackling; the snapping of certain salts when heated.

**decrudescence** (de'kroo-des'ens) [ L. *de,* from, + *crudesco,* to become worse, fr. *crudus,* crude ]. Abatement of the symptoms of disease.

**decubation** (de-ku-ba'shun) [ L. *de,* from, + *cubo,* to lie down ]. The final period of an infectious disease from the disappearance of the specific symptoms to complete restoration of health and the end of the infectious period.

**decubital** (de-ku'bĭ-tal). Relating to a decubitus ulcer.

**decubitus** (de-ku'bĭ-tus) [ L. *decumbo,* to lie down ]. 1. The position of the patient in bed, as dorsal d., lateral d. 2. Sometimes used to denote a decubitus ulcer.

**Andral's d.,** position assumed by the patient who lies on the sound side in cases of beginning pleurisy.

**decur'rent** [ L. *de-curro,* pp. -*cursus,* to run down ]. Extending downward.

**decus'sate** [ L. *decusso,* pp. -*atus,* to make in the form of an X, fr. *decussis,* the number ten (X) ]. 1. To cross. 2. Crossed like the arms of an X.

**decussatio,** pl. **decussatio'nes** (de-kus-sa'shĭ-o) [ L. (see decussate) ]. [ NA ]. Decussation. 1. In general, any crossing over or intersection of parts. 2. The intercrossing of two homonymous fiber bundles as each crosses over to the opposite side of the brain in the course of its ascent or descent through the brainstem or spinal cord.

**d. bra'chii conjuncti'vi,**   d. pedunculorum cerebellarium superiorum.

**d. fontina'lis,**   see *decussationes* tegmenti.

**d. lemnisco'rum** [ NA ], d. sensoria [ NA ]; decussation of medial lemniscus or fillet; sensory decussation of the medulla oblongata; the intercrossing of the fibers of the left and right medial lemniscus ascending from the nuclei gracilis and cuneatus, immediately rostral to the level of the decussation of the pyramidal tracts in the medulla oblongata.

**d. moto'ria** [ NA ], official alternative for d. pyramidum.

**d. nervo'rum trochlear'ium** [ NA ], decussation of trochlear nerves; the crossing of the two trochlear nerves at their exit through the velum medullare anterius.

**d. pedunculo'rum cerebella'rium superio'rum** [ NA ], decussation of superior cerebellar peduncles; decussation of the brachia conjunctiva; d. brachii conjunctivi; Wernekinck's decussation; the decussation of the left and right superior cerebellar peduncles in the tegmentum of the mesencephalon.

**d. pyram'idum** [ NA ], d. motoria [ NA ]; pyramidal or motor decussation; the intercrossing of the bundles of the pyramidal tracts at the lower border region of the medulla oblongata.

**d. senso'ria** [ NA ], official alternative for d. lemniscorum.

**decussatio'nes tegmen'ti** [ NA ], tegmental decussations; collective term denoting (1) the dorsal tegmental decussation (fountain decussation of Meynert, d. fontinalis) of the left and right tectospinal and tectobulbar tracts, and (2) the ventral tegmental decussation (decussation of Forel) of the left and right rubrospinal and rubrobulbar tracts; both decussations are located in the mesencephalon.

**decussation** (de-kus-sa'shun) [ L. *decussatio* ]. Decussatio.

**d. of brachia conjunctiva,**   *decussatio* pedunculorum cerebellarium superiorum.

**dorsal tegmental d.,**   see *decussationes* tegmenti.

**d. of the fillet,**   *decussatio* lemniscorum.

**Forel's d.,**   see *decussationes* tegmenti.

**fountain d.,**   see *decussationes* tegmenti.

**Held's d.,**   the crossing of some of the fibers arising from the cochlear nuclei to form the lateral lemniscus.

**d. of medial lemniscus,**   *decussatio* lemniscorum.

**Meynert's d.,**   see *decussationes* tegmenti.

**motor d.,**   *decussatio* pyramidum.

**optic d.,**   *chiasma* opticum.

**pyram'idal d.,**   *decussatio* pyramidum.

**rubrospinal d.,**   ventral tegmental d.; see *decussationes* tegmenti.

**sensory d. of medulla oblongata,**   *decussatio* lemniscorum.

**d. of superior cerebellar peduncles,**   *decussatio* pedunculorum cerebellarium superiorum.

**tectospinal d.,**   dorsal tegmental d.; see *decussationes* tegmenti.

**tegmental d.'s,**   *decussationes* tegmenti.

**d. of trochlear nerves,**   *decussatio* nervorum trochlearium.

**ventral tegmental d.,**   see *decussationes* tegmenti.

**Wernekinck's d.,**   *decussatio* pedunculorum cerebellarium superiorum.

**decussatio'nes.**   Plural of decussatio.

**dedentition** (de-den-tish'un). Obsolete term formerly used to denote loss of teeth.

**de'differentia'tion.**   1. The return of parts to a more homogeneous state; regression. 2. A term sometimes used to indicate the process by which mature, differentiated cells or tissues are the sites of origin of immature, undifferentiated elements of the same type, as in a fibroma that becomes a fibrosarcoma.

**dedolation** (de-do-la'shun) [ L. *de-dolo*, pp. *-atus*, to hew away ]. A slicing wound made by a sharp instrument grazing the surface.

**deDuve,** Christian, British-born biochemist, *1917. Nobel laureate, 1974, with Albert Claude and George Palade, for their discoveries concerning the structural and functional organization of the cell.

**de-efferentation** (de-ef-er-ent-a'shun) [ L. *de*, from, + efferent, *q.v.* ]. A loss of the motor nerve fibers to an area of the body.

**de-epicar'dializa'tion.**   Surgical destruction of the epicardium, usually by the application of phenol, designed to promote collateral circulation to the myocardium.

**Deetjen** (dāt'yen), Hermann, German physician, 1867–1915. See D.'s *bodies*.

**DEF.**   Abbreviation for decayed, extracted, or filled; a designation used in tooth examination.

**defatiga'tion** [ L. *de-fatigo*, pp. *-atus*, to tire out ]. Weariness; exhaustion; extreme fatigue.

**defecation** (def'e-ka'shun) [ L. *defaeco*, pp. *-atus*, to remove the dregs, purify, fr. *faex* (*faec-*), dregs ]. The discharge of excrement from the rectum.

**de'fect.**   Imperfection; malformation.

**aortic septal d.,**   a small congenital opening between the aorta and pulmonary artery about 1 cm. above the semilunar valves.

**atrial septal d.,**   a d. in the septum between the atria of the heart, due to failure of the ostium primum or secundum to close normally.

**congenital ectodermal d.,**   incomplete development of the epidermis and skin appendages. The skin is smooth and hairless, the facies abnormal, and teeth and nails may be affected; sweating may be deficient.

**coupling d.,**   see familial *goiter*.

**endocardial cushion d.,**   persistent atrioventricular *canal*.

**fibrous cortical d.,**   a common small d. in the cortex of a bone, usually the lower femoral shaft of a child, filled with fibrous tissue.

**filling d.,**   abnormal contour of any part of the gastrointestinal tract, seen by x-ray after contrast medium is introduced, indicating tumor or foreign body.

**iodide transport d.,**   see familial *goiter*.

**iodotyrosine deiodinase d.,**   see familial *goiter*.

**luteal phase d.,**   luteal phase deficiency; a condition characterized by inadequate secretion of progesterone during the luteal phase of the menstrual cycle, with resultant sterility; subnormal luteal function commonly attributed to abnormal pituitary gonadotropin secretion.

**organification d.,**   see familial *goiter*.

**ventricular septal d.,**   a congenital d. in the septum between the cardiac ventricles, usually resulting from failure of the bulbar septum to close the interventricular foramen.

**defective** (de-fek'tĭv) [ L. *defectivus;* fr. *deficio*, pp. *-fectus*, fr. *facio*, to do, to fail, to lack ]. 1. Imperfect. 2. A person lacking in some physical or mental quality.

**defemination** (de-fem-ĭ-na'shun) [ L. *de-*, away, + *femina*, woman ]. A weakening or loss of feminine characteristics.

**defense** (de-fens') [ L. *defendo*, to ward off ]. The methods used to control anxiety.

**screen d.,**   the use of falsified or incomplete memories or affects to cover repressed but associated memories and affects.

**ur-d.'s,**   see *ur-defenses*.

**defen'sive** [ L. *defendo*, pp. *-fensus*, to ward off ]. Defending; preserving from injury.

**def'erens** [ L. ] [ NA ]. Deferent.

**def'erent** [ L. *deferens*, pres. p. of *defero*, to carry away ]. Carrying away.

**def'erentec'tomy** [ (ductus) deferens, + G. *ektomē*, excision ]. Vasectomy.

**deferential** (def'er-en'shal). Relating to the ductus deferens.

**def'erenti'tis.**   Vasitis; spermatitis; inflammation of the ductus deferens.

**de'ferox'amine mes'ylate** (USP). DESFERAL; desferrioxamine mesylate; methanesulfonate of 30-amino-3,14,25-trihydroxy-3,9,14,20,25-penta-azatriacontane-2,10,13,21,24-pentaone; an iron chelate used in treatment of iron poisoning. Instillation of 10 per cent lyophilized deferoxamine mesylate in solution or ointment dissolves rust stains on the cornea after removal of an iron particle.

**defervescence** (de-fer-ves'ens) [ L. *de-fervesco*, to cease boiling, fr. *de-* neg. + *fervesco*, to begin to boil ]. Falling of an elevated temperature; abatement of fever.

**defibrillation** (de-fi-brĭ-la'shun). The arrest of fibrillation of the cardiac muscle (atrial or ventricular) with restoration of the normal rhythm.

**defi′brillator.** 1. Any agent or measure, *e.g.*, an electric shock, that arrests fibrillation of the ventricular muscle and restores the normal beat. 2. The machine designed to administer a defibrillating electric shock.

**external d.,** a d. that delivers its defibrillating shock through the unopened chest wall.

**defibrination** (de-fi-brĭ-na′shun). Removal of fibrin from blood, usually by means of constant agitation while the blood is collected in a container with glass beads or chips.

**deficiency** (de-fish′en-sĭ) [ L. *deficio,* to fail, fr. *facio,* to do ]. A lacking; something wanting. See also deficiency *disease;* for individual d.'s or d. diseases not listed here, see the name of the disease or the name of the substance (*e.g.,* enzyme) involved.

**antitrypsin d.,** d. of $\alpha_1$-antitrypsin, a glycoprotein of the postalbumin region of human serum, which may be moderate (40 to 60 per cent of normal activity) or severe (less than 10 per cent of normal) and is gene-determined. A heritable disorder that, in the severe form, is often associated with pulmonary emphysema.

**familial high density lipoprotein d.,** Tangier *disease.*

**immunological, immune,** or **immunity d.,** immunodeficiency.

**LCAT d.,** a rare condition characterized by corneal opacities, anemia, proteinuria, and very low levels of LCAT (lecithin cholesteral acyltransferase) activity.

**luteal phase d.,** luteal phase *defect.*

**mental d.,** mental *retardation.*

**pseudocholinesterase d.,** a heritable disorder manifested by exaggerated responses to drugs ordinarily hydrolyzed by serum pseudocholinesterase (*e.g.,* suxamethonium); believed to entail production of a variant enzyme that is less active than the normal enzyme in hydrolyzing appropriate substrates, but also abnormally resistant to the effects of anticholinesterases.

**pyruvate kinase d.,** a disorder in which essentially no pyruvate kinase is formed; characterized by hemolytic anemia of varying degree from one patient to another; autosomal recessive inheritance.

**riboflavin d.,** ariboflavinosis; properly, hyporiboflavinosis.

**secondary antibody d.,** secondary *hypogammaglobulinemia.*

**taste d.,** reduced or absent ability to detect a bitter taste in a group of compounds of which phenylthiourea is the prototype, due to the homozygous state of a recessive gene of high frequency; see also phenylthiourea.

**deficit** (def′ĭ-sit) [ L. *deficio,* to fail ]. The result of temporarily using up something faster than it is being replenished.

**oxygen d.,** the difference between oxygen uptake of the body during early stages of exercise and during a similar duration in a steady state of exercise; sometimes considered as the formation of the oxygen *debt, q.v.*

**pulse d.,** (1) the absence of palpable pulse waves in a peripheral artery for every heart beat, as is often seen in atrial fibrillation; (2) the number of such missing pulse waves (usually expressed as heart rate minus pulse rate per minute).

**definition** (def′ĭ-nish′un) [ L. *de-finio,* pp. *-finitus,* to bound, fr. *finis,* limit ]. In optics, the power of a lens to give a distinct image; see also resolving *power.*

**operational d.,** in the behavorial sciences, a d. in terms of observable conditions or operations under which an event occurs, and which can be used by other investigators to advance the art of their science.

**deflection** (de-flek′shun) [ L. *de-flecto,* pp. *-flexus,* to bend aside ]. 1. A moving to one side. 2. The bending of the light rays toward an opaque body. 3. In the electrocardiogram, a deviation of the curve from the isoelectric base line; any wave or complex of the electrocardiogram.

**intrinsic d.,** with the electrode in direct contact with the muscle fiber, a rapid downward d. from the peak of maximum positivity, signifying that the activation front has reached the subjacent muscle.

**intrinsicoid d.,** the abrupt downstroke from maximum positivity when the electrode is placed not directly on the muscle but at a distance, as in the unipolar chest leads in clinical electrocardiography.

**deflora′tion** [ L. *defloro,* pp. *-atus,* to deflower, fr. *de-* + *flos*(*flor-*), flower ]. Deflowering; depriving of virginity; the rupturing of the hymen, either in coitus or in vaginal examination.

**deflores′cence** [ L. *de-floresco,* to fade, wither, fr. *flos* (*flor-*), flower ]. Disappearance of the eruption in scarlet fever or other of the exanthemas.

**deflu′vium** [ L. fr. *de-fluo,* pp. *-fluxus,* to flow down ]. A flowing or falling; see also defluxio; defluxion.

**d. capillo′rum,** defluxio capillorum; a falling (or loss) of hair.

**d. ung′uium,** a falling (or loss) of nails.

**defluxio** (de-fluk′shĭ-o) [ L. ]. Defluxion.

**d. capillo′rum,** *defluvium* capillorum.

**d. cilio′rum,** Deplumation.

**defluxion** (de-fluk′shun) [ L. *defluxio, de-fluo,* pp. *-fluxus,* to flow down ]. Defluvium. 1. A falling down or out, as of the hair. 2. A flowing down or discharge of fluid.

**de′forma′tion** [ L. *de-formo,* pp. *-atus,* to deform, fr. *forma,* form ]. 1. A change of form from the normal. 2. A deformity. 3. In rheology, the change in the physical shape of a mass by applied stress.

**deform′ing.** Causing a deviation from the normal form.

**deform′ity.** A deviation from the normal shape or size, resulting in disfigurement; may be congenital or acquired.

**Akerlund d.,** indentation (incisura) with niche of duodenal cap as seen by x-ray.

**Arnold-Chiari d.,** Arnold-Chiari malformation or syndrome; cerebellomedullary malformation syndrome; malformation of the cerebellum (elongation of the cerebellar tonsils, and drawing of the cerebellum into the fourth ventricle) together with smallness of the medulla and pons and internal hydrocephalus; frequently associated with spina bifida (meningomyelocele or syringomyelocele).

**Erlenmeyer flask d.,** a d. at the end of certain long bones when there is a failure of the shaft of the bone to model to its normal tubular shape with the result that the bone stays wide for a much longer distance up the shaft than it usually does. This gives it the appearance of an Erlenmeyer flask, which is shaped like a truncated, somewhat blunted cone.

**gunstock d.,** a d. resulting from condylar fracture at the elbow in which the axis of the extended forearm is not continuous with that of the arm but is displaced to one side.

**J-sella d.,** pear-shaped or J-shaped d. of sella turcica caused by increased pressure on growing sphenoid bone; noted in the mucopolysaccharide storage diseases.

**lobster-claw d.,** a hand or foot, with the medial digits missing or fused so that it suggests the shape of a lobster claw. When only the 1st and 5th digits are present, also called bidactyly. Usually autosomal dominant inheritance.

**Madelung's d.,** carpus curvus; radius curvus; an inferior radioulnar subluxation due to a curvature of the lower extremity of the radius with concavity anterior.

**mermaid d.,** sirenomelia.

**pseudolobster-claw d.,** a condition resembling lobster-claw d. but with less complete suppression of the medial digits.

**reduction d.,** a congenital skeletal shortening or deficiency of one or more limbs.

**seal-fin d.,** deflection outward of the fingers in rheumatoid arthritis.

**silver fork d.,** the d. resembling the curve of the back of a fork seen in Colles' fractures.

**Sprengel's d.,** scapula elevata; congenital elevation of the scapula.

**torsional d.,** detortion; detorsion; distortion; distorsion; in orthopaedics, a d. caused by rotation of a portion of an extremity with relationship to the long axis of the entire extremity.

**Velpeau's d.,** rarely used eponym for silver-fork d.

**Volkmann's d.,** congenital luxation of the tibiotarsal joint.

**defur′fura′tion** [ L. *de,* away from, + *furfur,* bran ]. Branny desquamation; the shedding of the epidermis in the form of fine scales.

**deganglionate** (de-gang′glĭ-on-āt). To deprive of ganglia.

**degeneracy** (de-jen′er-ă-sĭ) [ L. *de,* from, + *genus,* (*gener-*), race ]. A condition marked by deterioration of the mental, physical, or moral processes.

**degen'erate.** 1. To pass to a lower level of mental or physical qualities; to fall below the normal type or state. 2. Below the normal; that has fallen to a lower level. 3. A person whose moral characteristics are below those of his society.

**degeneratio** (de-jen-er-a'shĭ-o) [ L. *degenero,* pp. *-atus,* fr. *de,* from, + *genus,* race ]. Degeneration.

    **d. mi'cans** [ L. *micare,* to glitter ], the formation of glistening hyaline masses from degenerating glia cells.

**degeneration** (de-jen-er-a'shun) [ L. *degeneratio, q.v.* ]. 1. Deterioration; sinking from a higher to a lower level of type. 2. A worsening of physical or mental qualities. 3. A retrogressive pathologic change in cells or tissues in consequence of which the functions may be inhibited or destroyed and the protoplasm is altered in such a manner that necrosis results; at some stages, the degenerative process is reversible.

    **Abercrombie's d.,** obsolete eponym for amyloid d.

    **ad'ipose d.,** fatty d.

    **adiposogen'ital d.,** *dystrophia* adiposogenitalis.

    **albuminoid d., albuminous d.,** cloudy *swelling.*

    **am'yloid d.,** waxy d. (1); infiltration of amyloid between cells and fibers of tissues and organs; see also amyloid.

    **angiolith'ic d.,** calcareous d. of the walls of the blood vessels.

    **ascending d.,** centripetal Wallerian d.

    **athero'matous d.,** focal accumulation of lipid material (atheroma) in the intima and subintimal portion of arteries, eventually resulting in fibrous thickening or calcification.

    **ballooning d.,** ballooning colliquation; a phenomenon observed especially in cells that are infected with certain viruses, resulting in conspicuous swelling of the cell, edema of the cytoplasm, and vacuolation; in some instances, the cell seems to have no cytoplasm, and the nucleus (or its remnants) "floats" in an empty space enclosed by the cell membrane.

    **basophilic d.,** blue staining of connective tissues when the hematoxylin-eosin stain is used. It is found in such conditions as lupus erythematosus, senile skin, and actinic dermatitis.

    **calca'reous d.,** in a precise sense, not a degenerative process *per se,* but the deposition of insoluble calcium salts in tissue that has degenerated and become necrotic, as in dystrophic calcification.

    **carneous d.,** red d.

    **ca'seous d.,** caseous *necrosis.*

    **colliquative d.,** liquefaction d.

    **colloid d.,** a d. similar to mucoid d., in which the material is inspissated.

    **colloid d. of the skin,** actinic *elastosis.*

    **Crooke's hyaline d.,** Crooke's hyaline *change.*

    **cystic heredomacular d.,** a form of heredomacular d. in which the lesion appears to be cystic; a form of Best's disease.

    **descending d.,** centrifugal Wallerian d.

    **elas'toid d.,** (1) elastosis; (2) hyaline d. of the elastic tissue of the arterial wall, seen during involution of the uterus.

    **elastotic d.,** d. of collagen fibers, with altered staining properties partly resembling elastic tissue; particularly, d. in the skin caused by chronic irradiation.

    **familial pseudoinflammatory macular d.,** familial pseudoinflammatory maculopathy; Sorsby's macular d.; macular d. that occurs during the fifth decade of life, with sudden development of a central scotoma in one eye followed rapidly by a similar lesion in the opposite eye; autosomal dominant inheritance.

    **fascicular d.,** neurogenic atrophy; muscular d. due to atrophy of motor neurons in the cord or brainstem.

    **fatty d.,** adipose d.; steatosis (2); abnormal formation of microscopically visible droplets of fat in the cytoplasm of cells, as a result of injury; fatty d. was previously believed to result from phanerosis, but this is now doubted, and the term fatty d. is used as a synonym for fatty metamorphosis.

    **fibrinoid d.,** a process resulting in poorly defined, deeply acidophilic, homogeneous, refractile deposits with some staining reactions that resemble fibrin, occurring in connective tissue, blood vessel walls, and other sites. Fibrinoid is usually metachromatic with toluidine blue, whereas fibrin usually is not; on the other hand, fibrin is ordinarily digested by trypsin, whereas fibrinoid resists the action of that enzyme.

    **fibrinous d.,** a process resulting in accumulation of material that has staining properties identical to those of fibrin; it is not known whether or not the material is actually fibrin.

    **fibroid d., fibrous d.,** not a d. *per se,* but rather a reparative process; cells and foci of tissue previously affected with degenerative processes, and necrosis, are replaced by cellular fibrous tissue; the fibrosis is morphologically identical to that in the early phase of so-called sclerotic d.

    **floccular d.,** cloudy *swelling.*

    **glassy d.,** hyaline d.

    **granular d.,** cloudy *swelling.*

    **granulovacuolar d.,** d. of hippocampal brain cells in elderly persons, characterized by the presence of Simchowicz *granules, q.v.*

    **gray d.,** d. of the white substance of the spinal cord, the fibers of which lose their myelin sheaths and become darker in color.

    **hepatolentic'ular d.,** lenticular progressive d.; Wilson's syndrome or disease; characterized by cirrhosis, d. in the basal ganglia of the brain, and deposition of green pigment in the periphery of the cornea; the plasma levels of ceruloplasmin and copper are decreased, urinary excretion of copper is increased, and the amounts of copper in the liver, brain, kidneys, and lenticular nucleus are unusually high; autosomal recessive inheritance.

    **heredomacular d.,** macular d.; tapetoretinal d.; a group of conditions characterized by bilateral progressive d. of the retina, centering about the macula lutea; central vision is progressively lost; autosomal dominant inheritance in some families, and autosomal recessive in others; strong intrafamily resemblance in age of onset, rate of progression, and ophthalmoscopic appearance of lesions. Various types are described, depending on age of onset (infantile, juvenile, adult) and morphology of lesions.

    **hy'aline d.,** a group of several degenerative processes that affect various cells and tissues, resulting in the formation of rounded masses ("droplets") or relatively broad bands of substances that are homogeneous, translucent, refractile, and moderately to deeply acidophilic. Hyaline d. may occur in the collagen of old fibrous tissue, smooth muscle of arterioles or the uterus, and as droplets in parenchymal cells.

    **hyaloideoretinal d.,** Wagner's disease; a progressive d. of the vitreous body and retina, associated with patchy choroid atrophy, myopic astigmatism, and development of cataracts and detachment of the retina; autosomal dominant inheritance.

    **hydrop'ic d.,** a condition in which the cell absorbs water and becomes vacuolated and swollen, sometimes to such a degree that it bursts; this change, occurring in a number of cells, results in the formation of a vesicle.

    **Kuhnt-Junius d.,** Kuhnt-Junius disease; disciform d. of macula retinae, characterized by subretinal exudate, hemorrhage, and ultimately a localized mass of organized tissue.

    **larda'ceous d.,** former term for amyloid d.

    **lenticular progressive d.,** hepatolenticular d.

    **liquefaction d.,** colliquative d.; the type of dissolution of the basal layer observed in lichen planus, lupus erythematosus, and other dermatologic conditions.

    **macular d.,** heredomacular d.

    **Mönckeberg's d.,** Mönckeberg's *arteriosclerosis.*

    **mu'cinoid d.,** a term suggested by Greenfield and Lyon to include both mucoid and colloid d., the essential cellular changes in both being similar, the only difference being that, in colloid d., the substance is firmer and more inspissated than in mucoid d., in which it is thin and jelly-like.

    **mucoid d.,** myxoid or myxomatous d.; a conversion of any of the connective tissues into a gelatinous or mucoid substance.

    **mucoid medial d.,** cystic medial *necrosis.*

    **myelin'ic d.,** formation of myelin figures in the cytoplasm of cells, possibly by degradation or hydration of lipoprotein of self-digested organelles.

    **myxoid d.,** mucoid d.

    **myxomatous d.,** mucoid d.

    **neurofibrillary d.,** formation of coarse, argentophilic, intracytoplasmic fibers, often in complex tangles within intracranial nerve cells that are undergoing aging; see also Alzheimer's *disease.*

**Nissl d.,** reaction at a distance; d. of the cell body occurring after division of the axon.

**olivopontocerebellar d.,** olivopontocerebellar *atrophy.*

**orthograde d.,** Wallerian d.

**parenchy'matous d.,** cloudy *swelling.*

**pol'ypoid d.,** an obsolete term, formerly used to describe the formation of thick, usually edematous papilliform projections from the mucous membrane.

**primary progressive cerebellar d.,** a familial ataxic condition related to cerebellar d.

**pseudotu'bular d.,** an advanced form of d. frequently observed in adrenal glands, especially those of patients with febrile infectious disease; the shrunken, lipid-depleted cells of the zona fasciculata (and sometimes the zona glomerulosa) are arranged in a circular pattern about spaces that may be empty or partly filled with fibrin, nicrotic cells, or amorphous material; the arrangement probably results from accumulation of fluid in spaces where cells have become necrotic.

**reaction of d.,** abbreviated DeR, D.R. or R.D.; the electrical reaction in a degenerated nerve and the muscles supplied by it; it consists in absence of response to both galvanic and faradic stimulus in the nerve and to faradic stimulus in the muscles. Muscle still may respond to galvanic stimulation, but the cathodal closing contraction is greater than the anodal closing contraction, the reverse of normal.

**red d.,** carneous d.; necrosis, with staining by hemoglobin, which may occur in uterine myomas, especially during pregnancy; marked by softening and a red color resembling partly cooked meat.

**reticular d.,** reticulating colliquation; severe epidermal edema resulting in multilocular bullae and ballooning d.

**retrograde d.,** d. with chromatolysis of nerve cells after division of their axons.

**sclerotic d.,** not a d. *per se,* in a strict sense, but the formation of irregular foci and plaques of densely cellular fibrous tissue, or collagenous and hyaline material in sites where a degenerative process is occurring, as in arteriosclerosis and certain other conditions.

**secondary d.,** d. of a nerve, affecting always the end which is cut off from its trophic center.

**senile d.,** (1) the process of involution occurring in old age; (2) senile *elastosis.* 3. Senile and presenile macular d. of the retina.

**Sorsby's macular d.,** familial pseudoinflammatory macular d.

**spongy d.,** Canavan's disease or sclerosis; a rare, recessively transmitted, fatal brain disease of infancy characterized by progressive paralysis, blindness, and megalencephaly; pathologically, there is extensive spongiform demyelination of the cerebral hemispheres.

**subacute combined d. of the spinal cord,** a subacute or chronic disorder of the spinal cord, such as that occurring in certain patients with pernicious anemia, characterized by a slight to moderate degree of gliosis in association with spongiform degeneration of the posterior and lateral columns; also termed combined system disease; funicular myelitis (2); funicular myelosis; Putnam-Dana syndrome; vitamin $B_{12}$ neuropathy; syndrome neuroanémique.

**tapetoretinal d.,** heredomacular d.

**transsynaptic d.,** transsynaptic chromatolysis; an atrophy of nerve cells sometimes following damage to the axons that make synaptic connection with them.

**tubular d.,** a misnomer for pseudotubular d.

**Türck's d.,** secondary d. of a nerve.

**vac'uolar d.,** formation of nonlipid vacuoles in cytoplasm, most frequently due to accumulation of water (hydropic d.).

**vitelliform d. of the macula,** a form of heredomacular d. in which the lesion is vitelliform in appearance; such a lesion may be found in Best's disease.

**vitelliruptive macular d.,** a later stage of vitelliform d. of the macula in which the lesion is vitelliruptive in appearance; such a lesion may be found in Best's disease.

**vitreous d.,** an obsolete term for hyaline d. producing a glassy appearance.

**Wallerian d.,** orthograde d.; d of a nerve fiber separated from its trophic center; the nerve cell is characterized by

proliferation of the nucleus of the interannular segment and by segmentation of the myelin, ending in atrophy and destruction of the axon.

**waxy d.,** (1) amyloid d.; (2) Zenker's d.

**Zenker's d.,** waxy d. (2); Zenker's necrosis; a form of hyaline d. in skeletal muscle, occurring in fairly long-continued febrile illnesses, and also in certain forms of anemia and toxic conditions.

**degen'erative.** Relating to degeneration.

**deglov'ing.** Intraoral surgical exposure of the bony mandibular anterior region; this procedure can be performed in the posterior region if necessary.

**deglut.** Abbreviation for Latin, *deglutiatur,* let it be swallowed.

**deglutition** (de-glu-tish'un) [ L. *de-glutio,* to swallow ]. The act of swallowing.

**deglu'titive.** Relating to deglutition.

**Degos,** R., French dermatologist. See D.'s *acanthoma, syndrome.*

**de Grandmont's operation.** See under operation.

**degree** [ Fr. *degré;* L. *gradus,* a step ]. 1. One of the divisions on the scale of a thermometer, barometer, etc. 2. $1/360$ part of the circumference of a circle. 3. A position or rank within a graded series.

**d.'s absolute, Celsius, centigrade, Fahrenheit, Kelvin, Rankine, Réamur,** see scale, also appendix 8.

**d.'s of freedom,** in psychology, the number of observations (*e.g.,* subjects, test items and scores, trials, conditions) minus the number of independent restrictions in the sampling undertaken.

**degusta'tion** [ L. *degustatio,* fr. *de-gusto,* pp. *-atus,* to taste ]. Tasting; the sense of taste.

**dehal'ogenase.** Any enzyme (EC subclass 3.8) removing halogen atoms from organic halides; see also iodide peroxidase.

**dehematize** (de-hem'ă-tīz) [ L. *de-,* from, + G. *haima* ( *haimat-*), blood ]. To deprive of blood, locally by pressure or generally by bleeding.

**Dehio** (da'he-o), Karl K., Russian physician, 1851–1927. See D.'s *test.*

**dehiscence** (de-his'ens) [ L. *dehiscere,* to split apart or open ]. A bursting open, splitting or gaping by the divergence of parts.

**root d.,** a loss of the buccal or lingual bone overlaying the root portion of a tooth leaving that area covered by soft tissue only.

**wound d.,** disruption of apposed surfaces of a wound.

**dehumaniza'tion** [ *de-* + *humanus,* human, fr. *homo,* man ]. Loss of human characteristics; brutalization by either mental or physical means; stripping one of his self-esteem.

**dehy'drase.** Former name for dehydratase.

**dehy'dratases.** Enzymes removing H and OH as $H_2O$ from a substrate, leaving a double bond, or adding a group to a double bond by the elimination of water from two substances to form a third. A class (EC 4.2.1) of lyase (hydro-lyases), *e.g.,* citrate dehydratase. Formerly called dehydrase. The term "synthase" is sometimes used when the synthetic aspect of the reaction is emphasized (*e.g.,* tryptophan synthase). Some trivial names of enzymes in this subclass bear the generic term hydratase, emphasizing the reverse reaction.

**dehy'drate** [ L. *de,* from + G. *hydōr* (*hydr-*), water ]. 1. To extract water from. 2. To lose water.

**dehydration** (de-hi-dra'shun). 1. Deprivation of water. 2. The reduction of water content. 3. Exsiccation (2). 4. Desiccation.

**absolute d.,** actual water deficit as measured by a difference from the normal or from a given water content.

**relative d.,** water deficit relative to content of solutes contributing effective osmotic pressure; state of increased effective osmotic pressure of body fluids.

**voluntary d.,** that physiologic lag or deficit that results when sensations of thirst are not strong enough to bring about complete replacement of water loss, as in rapid sweating.

**dehydro-** (de-hi'dro-). A prefix used in the names of those chemical compounds that differ from other and more familiar compounds in the absence of two hydrogen atoms;

*e.g.,* dehydroascorbic acid, which resembles ascorbic acid in all structural features except for its lack of two hydrogen atoms that are present in the ascorbic acid molecule.

**dehydroace'tic acid.** 3-Acetyl-6-methyl-2*H*-pyran- 2,4-(3*H*)-dione; renal blocking agent.

**dehy'droandros'terone.** Obsolete trivial name for dehydro-3-epiandrosterone.

**dehy'droascor'bic acid.** The reversibly oxidized form of ascorbic acid. Antiscorbutic, but is converted in the body to diketogulonic acid, which has no vitamin C activity.

**dehy'drobiliru'bin.** Biliverdin.

**dehydrocholate** (de-hi-dro-ko'lāt). A salt or ester of dehydrocholic acid.

**7-dehy'drocholes'terol.** Provitamin D₃; 5,7-cholestadien-3β-ol; a sterol in skin and other animal tissues that upon activation by ultraviolet light (activated 7-d.) becomes antirachitic and is then referred to as vitamin D₃. For cholestane structure, see steroids.

**24-dehydrocholesterol.** 5,24-Cholestadien-3β-ol.

**dehy'drochol'ic acid** (NF). 3,7,12-Trioxo-5β-cholan-24-oic acid; has a stimulating effect upon the secretion of bile by the liver (choleretic), and improves the absorption of essential food materials in states associated with deficient bile formation.

**dehy'drocor'ticosterone.** Obsolete and inaccurate trivial name for 11-deoxycortisol.

**11-dehydrocorticosterone.** Kendall's compound A; 21-hydroxy-4-pregnene-3,11,20-trione (for pregnene structure, see steroids); found in the adrenal cortex; principally a metabolite of corticosterone.

**dehydroemetine** (de-hi'dro-em-ĕ-tēn). A synthetic derivative of emetine; used in the treatment of intestinal amebiasis.

**d. resinate,** MEBADINE; a derivative of emetine effective orally in the treatment of leishmaniasis.

**dehydro-3-epiandrosterone.** Androstenolone; dehydroisoandrosterone; 3β-hydroxy-5-androstene-17-one (for structure of androstene, see steroids). A weakly androgenic steroid secreted largely by the adrenal cortex, but also by the testes; found also in urine; one of the principal components of urinary 17-ketosteroids.

**dehydrogenase** (de-hi'dro-jen-ās). Trivial name for those enzymes that catalyze removal of hydrogen from certain metabolites (hydrogen donors) and transfer it to other substances (hydrogen acceptors); the first metabolite is oxidized, the second reduced. Most of the oxidative enzymes (oxidoreductases, EC class 1) perform their oxidations in this manner, hence the name. For individual d.'s, see the specific names.

**aerobic d.,** an enzyme catalyzing the transfer of hydrogen from some metabolite to oxygen, forming hydrogen peroxide in the process; usually a metalloflavoenzyme; examples: xanthine oxidase (dehydrogenase) (EC 1.2.3.2) and others in classes EC 1.1.3, 1.2.3, 1.3.3, 1.4.3, 1.5.3, 1.7.3, 1.8.3, 1.9.3, 1.10.3.

**anaerobic d.,** an enzyme catalyzing transfer of hydrogen from some metabolite to some acceptor molecule (*e.g.,* NAD, cytochrome) other than oxygen; usually a pyridinoenzyme; *e.g.,* lactate d.'s (EC 1.1.1.27, 28; 1.1.2.3, 4) and isocitrate d.'s (EC 1.1.1.41, 42), and others in EC group 1, excluding those listed under aerobic d.

**Robison ester d.,** glucose-6-phosphate dehydrogenase.

**dehy'drogena'tion.** 1. The removal of a pair of hydrogen atoms from a compound, by the action of enzymes (dehydrogenases) or other catalysts. 2. The removal of hydrogen from the lungs by breathing oxygen in a semiclosed or nonrebreathing system for several minutes prior to the induction of inhalation anesthesia.

**dehy'drogenize.** Dehydrogenate; to subject to dehydrogenation.

**dehy'droi'soandros'terone.** Dehydro-3-epiandrosterone.

**dehydromor'phine.** Pseudomorphine.

**dehy'dropep'tidase II.** Aminoacylase.

**dehy'dropipecol'ic acid.** See pipecolic acid. The Δ¹ and Δ⁶ d.'s are intermediates in the catabolism of lysine.

**5-dehy'droquin'ic acid.** See quinic acid.

**dehy'droret'inal.** Dehydroretinaldehyde.

**dehy'droretinal'dehyde.** 3-Dehydroretinaldehyde; dehydroretinal; retinene-2; vitamin A₂ aldehyde; the same as dehydroretinol, but with —CHO instead of —CH₂OH at the terminal carbon of the side chain; *cf.* retinaldehyde.

**dehy'droretino'ic acid.** 3-Dehydroretinoic acid; the same as dehydroretinol, but with —COOH in place of —CH₂OH at the terminal carbon of the side chain; *cf.* retinoic acid.

**dehy'droret'inol.** 3-Dehydroretinol; vitamin A₂; the same as retinol, but with additional double bond in the 3-4 position of the cyclohexane ring.

**dehy'droshikim'ic acid.** An intermediate in the formation of aromatic compounds from glucose in plants and microorganisms. See *shikimic* acid.

**dehydrotestos'terone.** 17β-Hydroxyandrosta-1,4-dien-3-one; anabolic and androgenic agent.

**de'hyp'notize.** To bring out of the hypnotic state.

**deiminase** (de-im'ĭ-nās). An enzyme removing the imine (=NH) group, as in arginine d., which converts arginine to citrulline. Classified in EC group 3.5.3 (iminohydrolases).

**deiodase** (de-i'o-dās). Dehalogenase.

**Deiters** (di'ters), Otto F. K., German anatomist, 1834–1863. See D.'s *cells,* terminal *frames, nucleus, process.*

**dejec'ta** [ L. *dejicere,* to throw down ]. Ejecta (2); the matter passed from the bowel; *e.g.,* or excrementitious material.

**dejection** (de-jek'shun) [ L. *dejectio,* fr. *de-jicio,* pp. *-jectus,* to cast down, fr. *jacio,* to throw. JAC- ]. 1. Melancholy; mental depression. 2. Matter passed from the bowels. 3. Defecation; the passage of matter from the bowels.

**Déjérine** (da-zhĕ-rēn'), Joseph J., Paris neurologist, 1849–1917. See D.'s *disease,* hand *phenomenon,* peripheral *neurotabes, reflex, sign,* D.-Lichtheim *phenomenon,* D.-Roussy *syndrome,* D.-Sottas *disease,* Klumpke-D. *syndrome,* Landouzy-D. *dystrophy.*

**deka-** [ G. *deka,* ten ]. A prefix used in the metric system to signify ten. For words beginning thus, see deca-.

**delacerate** (de-las'er-āt) [ L. *de-lacero,* to tear in pieces, destroy, fr. *lacer,* mangled ]. To tear; to lacerate badly.

**delacrimation** (de'lak-rĭ-ma'shun) [ L. *delacrimation,* fr. *lacrimo,* pp. *-atus,* to weep ]. Excessive secretion of tears.

**de'lacta'tion.** Weaning.

**Delafield,** Francis, New York physician and pathologist, 1841–1915. See D.'s *hematoxylin.*

**de'lamina'tion** [ L. *de,* from, + *lamina,* a thin plate ]. A division into separate layers.

**Delaney,** James Joseph, U. S. congressman. See D. *clause.*

**de Lange,** Cornelia, Dutch pediatrician. See de L. *syndrome.*

**Delbet** (del-ba'), Paul, French surgeon, 1866–1924. See D.'s *sign.*

**Delbrück,** Max, U. S. biologist, *1906. Nobel laureate, 1969, with Alfred Hershey and Salvador Luria for their contributions to the understanding of the molecular biology of bacteriophage.

**Del Castillo,** E. B., Argentinian physician. See Ahumada-D. C. *syndrome,* Argonz-D. C. *syndrome.*

**de-lead** (de-led'). To cause the mobilization and excretion of lead deposited in the bones and other tissues, as by the administration of a chelating agent or acid salts.

**DeLee,** Joseph B., U. S. obstetrician and gynecologist, †1942. See D.'s *operation.*

**deleterious** (de-le-te'rĭ-us) [ G. *dēlētērios,* fr. *dēleomai,* to injure ]. Injurious; noxious; harmful.

**deletion of chromosomes.** See under chromosome.

**del'icate** [ L. *delicatus,* soft, luxurious, fr. *de,* from, + *lacio,* to entice ]. Of feeble resisting power.

**deligation** (de-li-ga'shun) [ L. *de-ligo,* pp. *-atus,* to tie together ]. Ligation.

**Delille,** A., French physician, 1876–1950. See Rénon-D. *syndrome.*

**delimitation** (de-lim'ĭ-ta'shun) [ L. *de-limito,* pp. *-atus,* to bound, fr. *limes,* boundary ]. Putting bounds or limits; marking off; preventing the spread of a morbid process in the body or of a disease in the community.

**deliquesce** (del-ĭ-kwes'). To become damp or liquid by absorbing water from the atmosphere, said of certain salts, for example, $CaCl_2$.

**deliquescence** (del'ĭ-kwes'ens) [ L. *de-liquesco*, to melt or become liquid ]. The process of deliquescing.

**deliques'cent.** Denoting a solid substance that readily absorbs water from the air, becoming damp or liquid; for example, $CaCl_2$.

**deliquium** (de-lik'wĭ-um). 1 [ L. fr. *de*, down, + *liqueo*, to be fluid ]. Deliquescence. 2 [ L. (a diff. word with same form) fr. *de-linquo*, to fail ]. A faint; a syncope.
    **d. an'imi,** syncope.

**delir'iant.** 1. Causing delirium. 2. A toxic agent that produces delirium. 3. One who is delirious.

**delirifacient** (de-lir-ĭ-fa'shent) [ L. *facio*, to make ]. 1. Causing delirium; deliriant. 2. A deliriant (2).

**delir'ious.** In a state of delirium.

**delir'ium** [ L. fr. *deliro*, to be crazy, fr. *de-* + *lira*, a furrow (*i.e.*, go out of the furrow) ]. A condition of extreme mental, and usually motor, excitement, marked by a rapid succession of confused and unconnected ideas, often with illusions and hallucinations.
    **active d.,** d. with motor excitement.
    **acute d.,** grave d.
    **d. alcohol'icum,** d. tremens.
    **anxious d.,** a condition of mild psychomotor disturbance in which the prominent note is a sort of incoherent apprehension or anxiety.
    **Bell's d.,** specific febrile d. of Dercum; a very intense d. associated with high fever but no physical signs of pneumonia, any exanthema, or other general disease.
    **collapse d.,** one caused by extreme physical depression induced by a shock, profuse hemorrhage, exhausting labor, et ·.
    **d. cordis,** atrial *fibrillation.*
    **d. grandiosum,** d. of grandeur; d. in which the subject is filled with ideas of his own importance, wealth, or power.
    **grave d.,** acute d.; a very pronounced and severe form of d. usually presaging the death of the patient.
    **low d.,** a form in which there is little excitement, either mental or motor, the ideas being confused and incoherent, but following each other slowly.
    **d. mussitans,** muttering d.; a form common in low fevers in which the subject is unconscious, but constantly mutters incoherently.
    **organic d.,** d. due to illness or injury to the central nervous system, *e.g.*, from head injury or poisoning.
    **d. of persecution,** d. in which the subject has the delusion that he is being persecuted.
    **posttraumatic d.,** a form of posttraumatic neuropsychologic disorder with disturbed consciousness, agitation, hallucinations, delusions, and/or disorientation.
    **senile d.,** the mental feebleness of extreme old age; dotage.
    **d. si'ne delir'io** [ d. without d. ], an abortive form of d. tremens, in which all the symptoms of tremor, precordial distress, dyspepsia, anxiety, restlessness, and sweating are present, but in which mental confusion and hallucinations do not supervene.
    **toxic d.,** d. caused by the action of a poison.
    **d. tre'mens** [ L. *tremere*, to dread ], d. alcoholicum; tromomania; a form of acute insanity due to alcoholic poisoning, marked by sweating, tremor, atonic dyspepsia, restlessness, anxiety, precordial distress, mental confusion, and hallucinations.

**delitescence** (del-ĭ-tes'ens) [ L. *delitesco*, to lie hidden away ]. 1. The sudden subsidence of symptoms; disappearance of a tumor or a cutaneous lesion. 2. Period of incubation of an infectious disease.

**deliv'er** [ thru O. Fr. fr. L. *de-* + *liber*, free ]. 1. To assist a woman in childbirth. 2. To extract from an enclosed place, as the child from the womb, a tumor from its capsule or surroundings, the crystalline lens in case of cataract, etc.

**deliv'ery.** Childbirth; accouchement; parturition; the passage of the baby from the genital canal into the external world. See also labor.
    **breech d.,** extraction or expulsion of a fetus that presents by the buttocks or feet.
    **cephalic d., assisted,** extraction of a fetus that presents by the head.

    **cephalic d., spontaneous,** unassisted expulsion of a fetus that presents by the head.
    **forceps d.,** assisted birth of the child by an instrument designed to grasp the child.
    **high forceps d.,** d. by forceps applied to fetal head before engagement has taken place.
    **low forceps d.,** d. by forceps to fetal head after it is clearly visible, the skull has reached the perineal floor and the sagittal suture is in the anteroposterior diameter of the pelvis.
    **midforceps d.,** d. by forceps to fetal head before the criteria of low forceps have been met, but after engagement has taken place.
    **postmortem d.,** the extraction of the fetus after the death of its mother.
    **premature d.,** the birth of a fetus before its proper time.

**delle** (del'eh). The central, lighter-colored portion of the erythrocyte, as observed in a stained film of blood.

**del'len** [ D. *delle*, low ground, pit ]. Shallow, saucer-like clearly defined excavations at the margin of the cornea, parallel to the limbus, about 1.5 by 2 mm., due to localized dehydration.

**delomorphous** (del'o-mor'fus) [ G. *dēlos*, manifest, + *morphē*, form ]. Of definite form and shape; a term applied in the past to the parietal cells of the gastric glands.

**delouse** (de-lows'). To remove lice from; to free from infestation with lice; a term used especially of prophylaxis of typhoid fever, trench fever, and other louse-borne diseases.

**Delpech** (del-pek'), Jacques M., French orthopedic surgeon, 1777–1832. See D.'s *abscess.*

**delphinine** (del'fin-ēn). An alkaloid, $C_{33}H_{45}NO_9$, from *Delphinium staphisagria* (family Ranunculaceae). Formerly used in neuralgia, palpitation, and chronic rheumatism, and externally in pediculosis. It resembles aconitine in its action.

**Delphin'ium** [ G. *delphinion*, larkspur ]. A genus of plants of the family Ranunculaceae.
    **D. aja'cis,** larkspur; knight's spur. The dried ripe seeds have been used externally as a parasiticide in pediculosis; rarely used now because of its toxicity. It contains the alkaloids ajacine and ajaconine.

**del Rio Hortega.** See Hortega.

**delta** [ the G. letter d, written as Δ (capital) or δ (lower case) ]. 1. Denoting the fourth in a series (usually δ). 2 [ NA ]. In anatomy, a triangular surface. 3. In chemistry, the capital Δ is used to denote an unsaturated (double) bond between carbon atoms, with superscripts indicating the positional number of the lower-numbered carbon atom (*e.g.*, $\Delta^5$ indicates a double bond between C-5 and C-6, but $\Delta^{9:11}$ one between C-9 and C-11); it is also used to indicate application of heat in a chemical reaction (*e.g.*, $A \xrightarrow{\Delta} B$), and as ⚡, the absence of heat treatment. The lower case δ is used to indicate the position of a substituent located on the fourth atom from the carboxyl or other primary functional group (*e.g.*, δ-guanidino-α-aminovaleric acid for arginine.
    **d. for'nicis,** *commissura* fornicis.
    **Galton's d.,** (1) a more or less well marked triangle, in a fingerprint, on either side where the straight ridges near the joint of the distal phalanx are succeeded by arches, loops, or whorls; see also Galton's system of classification of fingerprints (under fingerprint); (2) triradius.
    **d. mesoscap'ulae,** the flat triangular surface at the vertebral extremity of the spine of the scapula over which glides the tendon for the lower fibers of the trapezius muscle.

**deltoid** (del'toyd) [ G. *deltoeidēs*, shaped like the letter *delta* ]. 1. Resembling the Greek letter delta (Δ); triangular. 2. *Musculus* deltoideus.

**delusion** (de-lu'zhun) [ L. *de-ludo*, pp. *-lusus*, to play false, deceive, fr. *ludo*, to play ]. A false belief or wrong judgment.
    **depressive d.,** one connected with sad or distressing ideas.
    **expansive d.,** d. of grandeur.
    **d. of grandeur,** expansive d.; one in which the subject believes himself possessed of great wealth, intellect, importance, power, etc.

**d. of negation,** nihilistic d.; a depressive d. in which the victim imagines that the world and all that relates to it have ceased to exist.

**nihilistic d.,** d. of negation.

**d. of persecution, persecutory d.,** a false notion that one is being persecuted; characteristic symptom of paranoid schizophrenia.

**d. of reference,** idea of reference.

**somatic d.,** one having reference to an nonexistent lesion or alteration of some organ or part of the body; sometimes indistinguishable from hypochondriasis.

**systematized d.,** a d. that is logically founded upon a false premise and embraces a specific sector of the patient's life.

**unsystematized d.,** one of a group of apparently discrete, disconnected d.'s.

**delu'sional.** Relating to a delusion or delusions.

**demagnetize** (de-mag'ně-tīz). To take away or destroy magnetism.

**demarcation** (de-mar-ka'shun) [ Fr. fr. L. *de*, from, + Mediev. L. *marco*, to mark ]. A setting of limits; determining a boundary.

**line of d.,** a zone of inflammatory reaction separating a gangrenous area from healthy tissue.

**surface d.,** the line between paralyzed and functioning muscle.

**Demarquay** (dě-mar-ka'), Jean N., French surgeon, 1811–1875. See D.'s *symptom.*

**demas'culinizing.** Depriving of male characteristics or inhibiting development of such characteristics.

**Dematiaceae** (de-mat-ī-a'se-e). A family of imperfect fungi, order Moniales, that produce simple conidiophores.

**dematiaceous** (de-mat-ī-a'shus). Pertaining to fungi of the family Dematiaceae.

**dem'eca'rium bromide** (USP). HUMORSOL; a potent cholinesterase inhibitor used in the treatment of glaucoma and accommodative esotropia. It is stable in aqueous solution.

**demeclocycline** (dem-ek-lo-si'klēn) (NF). DECLOMYCIN; 7-chloro-6-demethyltetracycline; a broad spectrum antibiotic that is more slowly excreted and more stable in acid and alkali than other forms of the tetracyclines. Also available (NF) as the hydrochloride.

**demecolcine.** COLCEMID; *N*-desacetyl-*N*-methylcolchicine; an alkaloid from *Colchicum autumnale* (family Liliaceae) similar chemically to colchicine except that acetyl group is replaced by a methyl group. It is used for gout and leukemia, is said to be less toxic than colchicine, and has an action upon mitosis similar to that of colchicine.

**dement'ed.** Suffering from dementia or loss of reason.

**dementia** (de-men'she-ah) [ L. fr. *de-*priv. + *mens*, mind ]. A general mental deterioration due to organic or psychological factors.

**acute d.,** short, self-limited d.

**catatonic d.,** catatonic *schizophrenia.*

**chronic d.,** d. precox; schizophrenia.

**epileptic d.,** d. occurring in an individual afflicted with epilepsy, a result of the effects of repeated seizures over long periods.

**hebephren'ic d.,** hebephrenic *schizophrenia.*

**d. paralytica,** paralytic d.; general paresis.

**d. paranoi'des,** paranoid *schizophrenia.*

**posttraumatic d.,** a form of posttraumatic neuropsychologic disorder with mental impairment; see also neuropsychologic *disorder.*

**d. precox** [ L. precocious ], any of a group of psychotic disorders, particularly the schizophrenias; formerly used to describe schizophrenia as a single entity.

**d. preseni'lis,** d. developing at middle age.

**primary d.,** d. occurring independently of other forms of psychosis.

**secondary d.,** terminal d.; chronic d. following and due to a psychosis.

**senile d.,** an organic brain syndrome associated with aging and marked by progressive mental deterioration, loss of recent memory, lability of affect, difficulty with novel experience, self-centeredness, and childish behavior.

**terminal d.,** secondary d.

**toxic d.,** d. due to chemical poisoning, as in severe forms of drug addiction.

**dement'ing.** Tending to dementia.

**demeth'ylase.** *N*-Methylaminoacid oxidase (EC 1.5.3.2); a flavoenzyme catalyzing the dehydrogenation and subsequent hydrolytic cleavage of methyl groups from *N*-methylamino acids, producing formaldehyde and the free amino acid. Sarcosine oxidase (EC 1.5.3.2) acts similarly.

**demi-** [ Fr.; L. *dimidius*, half, fr. *di-* apart, + *medius*, middle ]. Semi-; hemi-; a prefix denoting half.

**dem'igaunt'let.** A glovelike bandage for the fingers and hand.

**dem'ilune.** [ Fr. half-moon ]. 1. A small body with a form similar to that of a half-moon or a crescent. 2. Term frequently used for the gametocyte of *Plasmodium falciparum.*

**Giannuzzi's d.'s,** serous d.'s.

**Heidenhain's d.'s.,** serous d.'s.

**serous d.'s,** Gianuzzi's crescents, cells, or d.'s; Heidenhain's crescents or d.'s; the serous cells at the distal end of a mucous, tubuloalveolar secretory unit of certain salivary glands.

**dem'imonstros'ity.** A congenital deformity in which the malformation is not so extreme as to render life impossible.

**demin'eraliza'tion.** A loss or decrease of the mineral constituents of the body or individual tissues, especially of bone.

**coefficient of d.,** the proportion of mineral compounds to the total dry residue of the urine; the average is 30 per cent.

**dem'ipen'niform.** Penniform on one side only; denoting certain muscles with fibers running at an acute angle from one side of a tendon.

**Democ'ritus** of Abdera, Greek philosopher, 460–360 B.C. Originated the theory that all matter was made up of minute particles or atoms and that all bodily activities were caused by the movements of such particles.

**Demodex** (dem'o-deks) [ G. *dēmos*, tallow, + *dēx*, a woodworm ]. A genus of very minute follicle mites (0.1 to 0.4 mm) of the family Demodicidae that invade the skin and are usually found in the sebaceous glands and hair follicles of mammals, including man. See demodectic *mange.*

**D. bo'vis,** a species that causes large swellings in the skin, filled with fluid or a cheezy material containing mites, which damages the hide of cattle.

**D. ca'nis,** causes red or demodectic mange, common, perhaps universal, in dogs; it is typically associated with the bacteria *Staphylococcus, Pyrogenes albus,* or allied forms, which are probably responsible for hair loss.

**D. ca'ti,** a species causing mange in cats.

**D. folliculo'rum,** follicular mite; mange mite;parasitizes the hair follicles and sebaceous glands of man and large domestic animals, commonly around the nose and scalp but sometimes on the scalp or elsewhere on the body; it is very common, universally distributed, and probably nonpathogenic.

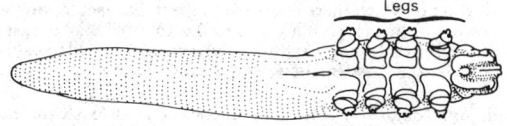

*Demodex folliculorum*

The follicle mite of man (×200). (From Najarian, H. H.: *Textbook of Medical Parasitology,* The Williams & Wilkins Co., Baltimore, 1967.)

**demography** (de-mog'ră-fī) [ G. *demos,* people, + *graphō,* to write ]. The study of groups of people, their environment, and their geographic distribution.

**dynamic d.,** a study of the functioning of a community, including statistical records.

**Demoivre's formula.** See under formula.

**de Mondeville,** Henri. See Mondeville, Henri de.

**demoniac** (de-mo'nī-ak) [ G. *daimōn,* a spirit ]. 1. Frenzied. 2. One said to be possessed of evil spirits; a lunatic.

**dem'onstrator** [ L. *de-monstro,* pp. *-atus,* to point out ]. An assistant to a professor of anatomy, surgery, etc., who prepares for the lecture by dissections, collection of patients, etc., or who instructs small classes supplementary to the regular lectures; a d. corresponds in a general way to the Dozent of a German university.

**De Morgan,** Campbell, English physician, 1811–1876. See De M.'s *spots.*

**demorphinization** (de-mor-fin-ĭ-za'shun). 1. Removal of morphine from an opiate. 2. The gradual withdrawal of morphine as a method of overcoming morphine dependence.

**demucosa'tion.** Excision of the mucosa of any part.

**demulcent** (de-mul'sent) [ L. *de-mulceo,* pp. *-mulctus,* to stroke lightly, to soften ]. Soothing; relieving irritation. 2. An agent, such as a mucilage or oil, that soothes and relieves irritation, especially of the mucous surfaces.

**demyelination, demyelinization** (de-mi'ĕ-lĭ-na'shun, de-mi'ĕ-lĭnĭ-za'shun). Destruction or loss of myelin from the medullary sheath of Schwann (peripheral nerve d.) or of myelin associated with oligodendroglia (central d.).

**denarcotize** (de-nar-ko-tīz). To remove narcotic properties from an opiate; to deprive of narcotic properties.

**de'nato'nium benzoate** (NF). BITREX; benzyldiethyl [ (2,6-xylylcarbamoyl)methyl ]ammonium benzoate; an alcohol denaturant.

**dena'tured.** Made unnatural; changed from the normal in any of its characteristics; adulterated, as by addition of methyl alcohol to ethyl alcohol. Often applied to proteins or nucleic acids heated to the point where tertiary structural characteristics are altered.

**dendrax'on** [ G. *dendron,* tree, + *axōn,* axis ]. Obsolete term for telodendron.

**den'driform** [ G. *dendron,* tree, + L. *forma,* form ]. Dendritic (1); dendroid; arborescent, tree-shaped, or branching.

**den'drite** [ G. *dendrītēs,* relating to a tree ]. 1. Dendron; dendritic process; neurodendrite; neurodendron; one of the two types of branching protoplasmic processes of the nerve cell (the other being the axon). 2. A crystalline, treelike structure formed during the freezing of an alloy.

　**apical d.,** apical *process.*

**dendrit'ic.** 1. Dendriform. 2. Relating to the dendrites of nerve cells.

**dendroid** (den'droyd) [ G. *dendron,* tree, + *eidos,* appearance ]. Dendriform.

**den'dron** [ G. a tree ]. Dendrite (1).

**denematize** (de-ne'mă-tīz). To free from infection with *Nematoda.*

**denervate** (de-ner'vāt). To cut off the nerve supply of a part by incision, excision, or blocking.

**dengue** (den'ga) [ Sp. a corruption of "dandy" fever ]. A disease of tropical and subtropical regions, occurring epidemically, and marked by intense aching in the head, muscles, and joints, and fever. There are usually two paroxysms, separated by a quiescent interval, during the second of which there is a scarlatiniform or maculopopular rash. The disease is thought to be due to protozoan parasite transmitted by a mosquito of the genus *Aedes.* Also called dandy, date, Aden, bouquet, breakbone, polka, or solar fever.

**denial** (de-ni'al). Negation; unconscious defense mechanism used to allay anxiety by denying the existence of important conflicts or troublesome impulses.

**denidation** (den-ĭ-da'shun) [ L. *de,* from, + *nidus,* nest ]. The exfoliation of the superficial portion of the mucous membrane of the uterus; stripping off of the menstrual decidua.

**Denis-Browne splint.** See under splint.

**de'nitra'tion.** Denitrification.

**denitrification** (de-ni'trĭ-fĭ-ka'shun). Removal of nitrogen from any material or chemical compound, especially from the soil, by certain (denitrifying) bacteria that, by converting soluble nitrates into insoluble nitrites, render the nitrogen unavailable for plant growth, chiefly when the oxygen supply is insufficient; withdrawal of nitrogen from the soil by plant growth.

**denitrify** (de-ni'trĭ-fi). To remove nitrogen from any material or chemical compound; see denitrification.

**denitrogenation** (de-ni'tro-jĕ-na'shun). Elimination of nitrogen from lungs and body tissues by breathing gases devoid of nitrogen.

**Denman,** Thomas, English obstetrician, 1733–1815. See D.'s spontaneous *evolution.*

**Denonvilliers** (dĕ-nawṅ-ve-ya), Charles P., Paris surgeon, 1808–1872. See D.'s *aponeurosis, ligament.*

**denop'terin.** DIMETFOL; *N*-{ *p*-{[ 1-(2-amino-4-hydroxy-6-pteridinyl)-ethyl ]methylamino} benzoyl} glutamic acid; used for treatment of leukemia.

**dens,** pl. **den'tes** (dens) [ L. ]. 1 [ NA ]. *Tooth.* 2 [ *NA* ]. The odontoid process; a strong toothlike process projecting upward from the body of the axis, or epistropheus, around which the atlas rotates. See also tooth, and figs. and subentries under tooth.

　**dentes acus'tici** [ NA ], auditory teeth of Huschke or Corti; tooth-shaped formations or ridges occurring on the vestibular lip of the limbus lamina spiralis of the cochlear duct.

　**d. angula'ris,** d. caninus.

　**d. bicus'pidus,** pl. **dentes bicuspidi,** d. premolaris.

　**d. caninus,** pl. **dentes canini** [ NA ], canine tooth; d. angularis; d. cuspidatus; cuspid; a tooth having a crown of thick conical shape and a long, slightly flattened conical root; there are two canine teeth in each jaw, one on either side adjacent to the distal surface of the lateral incisors, in both the deciduous and the permanent dentition.

　**d. cuspida'tus,** pl. **dentes cuspidati,** d. caninus.

　**d. decid'uus,** pl. **dentes decidui** [ NA ], d. lacteus; baby tooth; milk tooth; deciduous dentition; first dentition; primary dentition; primary tooth; temporary tooth; a tooth of the first set of teeth, comprising 20 in all, that erupts between the mean ages of 6 and 28 months of life.

　**d. incisivus,** pl. **dentes incisivi** [ NA ], incisor tooth; a tooth with a chisel-shaped crown and a single conical tapering root; there are four of these teeth in the anterior part of each jaw, in both the deciduous and the permanent dentitions.

　**d. in dente,** a developmental disturbance in tooth formation; the result of invagination of the epithelium associated with coronal development into the area which was destined to be pulp space. After calcification there is an invagination of enamel and dentin into the pulp space and a distortion of this space and the root contour to accommodate this invagination.

　**d. lacteus,** d. deciduus.

　**d. mola'ris,** pl. **dentes molares** [ NA ], molar; molar tooth; multicuspid tooth; cheek tooth; a tooth having a somewhat quadrangular crown with four or five cusps on the grinding surface; the root is bifid in the lower jaw, but there are three conical roots in the upper jaw; there are six molars in each jaw, three on either side behind the premolars in the permanent dentition; in the deciduous denture there are but four molars in each jaw, two on either side behind the canines. See also subentries under molar.

　**d. per'manens,** pl. **dentes permanentes** [ NA ], d. succedaneus; succedaneous tooth; second or permanent tooth; secondary dentition; succedaneous dentition; one of the 32 teeth belonging to the second or permanent dentition; the eruption of the permanent teeth begins from the 5th to the 7th year, and is not completed until the 17th to the 23rd year, when the last of the wisdom teeth appears.

　**d. premola'ris,** pl. **dentes premolares** [ NA ], premolar tooth; d. bicuspidus; a bicuspid tooth having two tubercles or cusps on the grinding surface and a flattened root, single in the lower jaw and upper second premolar and furrowed in the upper first premolar. There are four premolars in each jaw, two on either side between the canine and the molars; there are no premolars in the deciduous dentition.

　**d. sapien'tiae** [ L. *sapientia,* wisdom ], wisdom tooth; third molar.

　**d. seroti'nus** [ NA ], wisdom tooth; late tooth; the third molar tooth on each side in each jaw; the wisdom teeth erupt from the 18th to the 25th year; the root fangs are often fused, the separation being marked only by grooves.

　**d. succeda'neus,** d. permanens.

**densim'eter** [ L. *densitas,* density, + G. *metron,* measure ]. An instrument for measuring the density of a fluid.

**densitom'eter** [ L. *densitas,* density, + G. *metron,* measure ]. A special form of densimeter for measuring, by virtue of relative turbidity, the growth of bacteria in broth; useful in microbiological assay of nutrients and antibiotics, phage studies, etc.

**density** (den'sĭ-tĭ) [ L. *densitas*, fr. *densus*, thick ]. 1. The compactness of a substance; the ratio of mass to volume, usually expressed as gm. per cc. 2. The quantity of electricity on a given surface or in a given time per unit of volume. 3. Concentration.

**count d.,** photon d.

**flux d.,** flux (4).

**optical d.,** absorbance.

**photon d.,** count d.; a term used to describe the number of counted events recorded in radioisotope scanning per square centimeter or per square inch of imaged area.

**vapor d.,** the ratio of the weight of a gas or vapor to the weight of an equal volume of hydrogen measured under the same conditions of temperature and pressure.

**dent-, denti-, dento-** [ L. *dens*, tooth ]. Combining forms relating to the teeth.

**den'tal** [ L. *dens*, tooth ]. Relating to the teeth.

**dentalgia** (den-tal'jĭ-ah) [ L. *dens*, tooth, + G. *algos*, pain ]. Toothache.

**den'tate** [ L. *dentatus*, toothed ]. Notched; toothed; cogged.

**dentatum** (den-tah'tum) [ L. neut. of *dentatus*, toothed ]. *Nucleus* dentatus cerebelli.

**dentes** (den'tēz) [ L. ]. Plural of dens.

**denti-.** See dent-.

**den'ticle** [ L. *denticulus*, a small tooth ]. 1. A small tooth. 2. A pulpstone. 3. A slight projection from a hard surface.

**dentic'ulate, dentic'ulated.** 1. Finely dentated, notched, or serrated. 2. Having small teeth.

**den'tiform** [ denti- + L. *forma*, form ]. Tooth-shaped; pegged; odontoid.

**dentifrice** (den'tĭ-fris) [ L. *dentifricium*, fr. *dens*, tooth, + *frico*, pp. *frictus*, to rub ]. A tooth powder, toothpaste, tooth wash; any preparation used in the cleansing of the teeth.

**dentigerous** (den-tij'er-us) [ denti- + L. *gero*, to bear ]. Having or containing teeth, as a d. cyst.

**den'tila'bial** [ denti- + L. *labium*, lip ]. Relating to the teeth and lips.

**dentilingual** (den-tĭ-ling'gwal) [ denti- + L. *lingua*, tongue ]. Relating to the teeth and tongue.

**den'tin** [ L. *dens*, tooth ]. Dentinum.

**hereditary opalescent d.,** *dentinogenesis* imperfecta.

**hypersensitive d.,** exposed d. at cervical portion of tooth, painful to touch, sweetness, or temperature changes.

**primary d.,** d. which forms until the root is completed.

**secondary d.,** d. formed after tooth eruption as a result of irritation from caries, abrasion, injury, or simply due to age.

**sensitive d.,** the area of d. exposed to external stimuli due to attrition, abrasion, trauma, or loss of enamel.

**vascular d.,** vasodentin.

**den'tinal.** Relating to dentin.

**dentinal'gia** [ dentin + G. *algos*, pain ]. Pain or tenderness of the dentin.

**dentine** (den-tēn). Dentinum.

**den'tinocemen'tal.** Cementodentinal; relating to the dentin and cementum of teeth.

**dentinoenamel** (den'tĭ-no-e-nam'el). Amelodentinal; relating to the dentin and enamel of teeth.

**dentinogenesis** (den'tĭ-no-jen'ĕ-sis) [ dentin + G. *genesis*, production ]. The process of dentin formation in the development of teeth.

**d. imperfec'ta,** Capdepont's disease; dentinal dysplasia; hereditary opalescent dentin; a hereditary defect of dentin formation characterized by low mineral and high water and organic content, irregular direction of dentin tubules in a granular matrix, translucent or opalescent color of teeth, easy fracturing of enamel, wearing of occlusal surfaces and staining of exposed dentin, and obliteration of pulp chambers and canals; both deciduous and permanent teeth are affected.

**den'tinoid** [ dentin + G. *eidos*, resembling ]. 1. Resembling dentin. 2. Dentinoma.

**dentinoma** (den'tĭ-no'mah) [ dentin + G. suffix -*oma*, tumor ]. An odontogenic tumor in which dentin formation has been induced by invading epithelium.

**den'tinum** [ L. *dens*, tooth ] [ NA ]. Dentin; substantia eburnea; the ivory forming the mass of the tooth. About 20 per cent is organic matrix, mostly collagen, with some elastin and a small amount of mucopolysaccharide. The inorganic fraction (70 per cent) is mainly hydroxyapatite, with some carbonate, magnesium, and fluoride. The d. is traversed by a large number of fine tubules running from the pulp cavity outward. Within the tubules are processes from the odontoblasts (dentinal fibers).

**dentip'arous** [ denti- + L. *pario*, to bear ]. Tooth-bearing.

**den'tist.** One who practices dentistry. Legally, a d. is a person qualified by law to practice dentistry.

**den'tistry.** The healing science and art concerned with the care and health of all the tissues comprising the mouth. Emphasis is placed on (1) the prevention, diagnosis and treatment of diseases of the teeth and gingivae; (2) the replacement of missing teeth; (3) the correction of irregularities in the structure of the teeth and jaws; and (4) the study and care of nondental diseases affecting the superficial and deep structures of the oral cavity.

**community d.,** extramural practice, usually by students under university supervision, conducted for the benefit of inner city and other deprived or handicapped persons.

**forensic d.,** legal d.; dental jurisprudence; dentolegal science; forensic odontology; (1) the relation and application of dental facts to legal problems, as in using the teeth for identifying the dead; (2) the law in its bearing on the practice of dentistry.

**legal d.,** forensic d.

**operative d.,** restorative d.; usually refers to the individual restoration of teeth by means of amalgam, synthetic porcelain-like materials, or inlays.

**preventive d.,** principles and related dental and systemic procedures aimed at elimination or reduction of incidence of dental and oral disease and disorders.

**prosthetic d.,** prosthodontics.

**restorative d.,** operative d.

**dentition** (den-tish'un) [ L. *dentitio*, to teethe ]. The natural teeth, as considered collectively, in the dental arch; may be deciduous, permanent, or mixed.

**artificial d.,** denture.

**deciduous d.,** *dens* deciduus.

**delayed d.,** delayed eruption of the teeth.

**first d.,** *dens* deciduus.

**mandibular d.,** *arcus* dentalis inferior.

**maxillary d.,** *arcus* dentalis superior.

**natural d.,** see d.

**primary d.,** *dens* deciduus.

**retarded d.,** a d. in which growth phenomena such as calcification, elongation, and eruption occur later than in the average range of normal variation as a result of some systemic metabolic dysfunction (for example, hypothyroidism).

**secondary d.,** *dens* permanens.

**succedaneous d.,** *dens* permanens.

**dento-.** See dent-.

**den'toalve'olar.** Usually refers to that portion of the alveolar bone immediately about the teeth; refers also to the functional unity of teeth and alveolar bone.

**den'toid** [ dent- + G. *eidos*, resemblance ]. Odontoid; dentiform.

**den'tole'gal.** Relating to both dentistry and the law; see forensic dentistry.

**dentoliva** (den'to-li'vah) [ L. *dens*, tooth, + *oliva*, olive ]. Rarely used term for oliva, the inferior olive.

**dentulous** (den'tu-lus). Having natural teeth present in the mouth.

**denture** (den'tūr). 1. Artificial dentition; an artificial substitute for missing natural teeth and adjacent tissues. 2. Sometimes used to denote the dentition, *q.v.*, of animals.

**artificial d.,** d. (1).

**bar joint d.,** overlay d.

**complete d.,** full d.; a dental prosthesis which is a substitute for the lost natural dentition and associated structures of the maxillae or mandible.

**continuous gum d.,** a d. consisting of procelain teeth and tinted procelain d. material, fused to a platinum base.

**design d.,** a planned visualization of the form and extent of a dental prosthesis, arrived after a study of all factors involved.

**full d.,** complete d.

**immediate d.,** immediate insertion d.; a complete or partial d. constructed for insertion immediately following the removal of natural teeth.

**immediate insertion d.,** immediate d.

**implant d.,** a d. that receives its stability and retention from a substructure which is partially or wholly implanted under the soft tissues of the d. basal seat. See also implant d. *substructure* and implant d. *superstructure.*

**interim d.,** provisional d.; temporary d.; a dental prosthesis to be used for a short interval of time for reasons of esthetics, mastication, occlusal support, or convenience, or to condition the patient to the acceptance of an artificial substitute for missing natural teeth until more definite prosthetic dental treatment can be provided.

**overlay d.,** overdenture; telescopic d.; bar joint d.; hybrid prosthesis; a complete d. that is supported by both soft tissue and natural teeth that have been altered so as to permit the d. to fit over them. The altered teeth may have been fitted with short or long copings, locking devices, or connecting bars.

**partial d.,** bridgework; a dental prosthesis which restores one or more, but less than all, of the natural teeth and/or associated parts and which is supported by the teeth and/or the mucosa; it may be removable or fixed.

**partial d., distal extension,** a removal partial d. that is retained by natural teeth at one end of the d. base segments only, and in which a portion of the functional load is carried by the residual ridge.

**partial d., fixed,** bridge; a restoration of one or more missing teeth which cannot be readily removed by the patient or dentist; it is permanently attached to natural teeth or roots which furnish the primary support to the appliance.

**partial d., removable,** removable bridge; (1) a dental prosthesis which artificially supplies teeth and associated structures on a partially edentulous jaw, and which can be removed from the mouth and replaced at will; (2) a partial d. so designed that it may be removed from the mouth.

**provisional d.,** interim d.

**telescopic d.,** overlay d.

**temporary d.,** interim d.

**transitional d.,** a partial d. which is to serve as a temporary prosthesis and to which teeth will be added as more teeth are lost, and which will be replaced after postextraction tissue changes have occurred. A transitional d. may become an interim d. when all of the teeth have been removed from the dental arch.

**treatment d.,** a dental prosthesis used for the purpose of treating or conditioning the tissues which are called upon to support and retain a denture base.

**trial d.,** wax model d.; a setup of artificial teeth so fabricated that it may be placed in the patient's mouth to verify esthetics, for the making of records, or for any other operation deemed necessary before final commpletion of the d.

**wax model d.,** trial d.

**denture service.** Those procedures that are involved in the diagnosis, construction, and maintenance of artificial substitutes for missing natural teeth.

**den'turist.** A person other than a dentist (usually a technician), who engages in the practice of the denture phase of prosthodontics.

**Denucé** (dĕ-nü-sa'), Jean H. M., Bordeaux surgeon, 1859–1924. See D.'s *ligament.*

**denucleated** (de-nu'kle-a-ted). Deprived of a nucleus.

**denudation** (den'u-da'shun) [ L. *de-nudo,* to lay bare, fr. *de,* from, + *nudus,* naked ]. Depriving of a covering or protecting layer.

**denutrition** (de-nu-trish'un) [ L. *de,* from, + *nutrio,* pp. *nutritus,* to nourish ]. Rarely used or obsolete term meaning want or failure of nutrition.

**Denys** (den-ēs'), Joseph, Belgian bacteriologist, 1857–1932. See D.-Leclef *phenomenon.*

**deobstruent** (de-ob'stru-ent) [ L. *de-* priv. + *obstruo,* pp. *-structus,* to build against, obstruct ]. 1. Relieving or removing obstruction. 2. An agent that removes an obstruction to secretion or excretion.

**deo'dorant** [ L. *de-* priv. + *odoro,* pp. *-atus,* to give an odor to, fr. *odor,* a smell ]. 1. Removing a smell, especially an unpleasant smell. 2. An agent that destroys odors, especially disagreeable odors.

**deo'dorize.** To free from odor, especially from an unpleasant odor.

**deo'dorizer.** A substance that removes malodorous substances or converts them (especially products of decomposition) into odorless compounds, usually by a process of oxidation or absorption.

**deontology** (de'on-tol'o-jĭ) [ G. *deon* (*deont-*), that which is binding, pr. part. ntr. of *dei,* (impers.) it behooves, fr. *deō,* to bind, + *logos,* study ]. A study of the field of professional etiquette and duties.

**deoppilative** (de-op'pĭ-la-tiv) [ L. *de-* priv. + *op-pilo,* pp. *-atus,* to stop up, fr. *ob-* against, + *pilo,* to ram down ]. Deobstruent.

**deossification** (de-os'ĭ-fĭ-ka'shun) [ L. *de,* from, + *os,* bone, + *facio,* to make ]. Removal of the mineral constituents of bone.

**deoxida'tion.** Depriving a chemical compound of its oxygen.

**deox'idize.** To remove oxygen from its chemical combination.

**deoxy-.** Prefix (replacing desoxy-) to chemical names of substances containing carbohydrate moieties to indicate replacement of an —OH by an H; for example, the nucleosides and nucleotides comprised in DNA contain 2-deoxyribose units. The older spelling desoxy- is retained in some instances, and is official in the USP.

**deoxyaden'osine.** 2'-Deoxyribosyladenine, a constituent of DNA.

**deox'yadenyl'ic acid.** Adenine deoxyribonucleotide; deoxyadenosine phosphoric acid; a hydrolysis product of DNA, differing from adenylic acid in containing deoxyribose in place of ribose.

**deoxycholan'ic acid.** Deoxycholic acid; see cholic acid.

**deoxycho'late.** A salt or ester of deoxycholic acid.

**7-deoxycholic acid.** 3α,12α-Dihydroxy-5β-cholanic acid; a bile acid; used in biochemical preparations of ribosomes to solubilize lipoproteins of membranes (*i.e.,* as a detergent). Often abbreviated, in this context, DOC.

**deox'ycorticos'terone.** 11-Deoxycorticosterone; deoxycortone; Reichstein's substance Q; Kendall's desoxy compound B; 21-hydroxyprogesterone; 21-hydroxy- 4-pregnene-3,20-dione (for pregnene structure, see steroids). An adrenocortical steroid; principally a biosynthetic precursor of corticosterone, and possibly aldosterone; rarely appears in adrenocortical secretions. It is a potent mineralocorticoid, with no appreciable glucocorticoid activity.

**d. acetate,** desoxycorticosterone acetate (USP); deoxycortone acetate (BP); acetate salt used for intramuscular injection for replacement therapy of the adrenocortical steroid.

**d. pivalate,** desoxycorticosterone pivalate (NF); pivalate salt of the steroid.

**11-deoxycor'tisol.** Cortexolone; 11-deoxycortisone; Reichstein's substance S; 11-deoxy-17-hydroxycorticosterone; 17,21-dihydroxy-4-pregnene-3,20-dione; an adrenocortical steroid with weak biological activity; a biosynthetic precursor of cortisol.

**11-deoxycor'tisone.** 11-Deoxycortisol.

**deoxycor'tone.** Deoxycorticosterone.

**d. acetate implant** (BP), sterile cylinders prepared by fusion or heavy compression of the drug without the addition of any other substances.

**deoxycy'tidine.** 2'-Deoxyribosylcytosine, a constituent of DNA.

**deox'ycytidyl'ic acid.** Deoxycytidine phosphoric acid; a hydrolysis product of DNA.

**deoxydipyrimidine photolyase.** Dipyrimidine photolyase; photoreactivating enzyme; PR enzyme (2); an enzyme (EC 4.1.99.3) in yeast activated by light, whereupon it can reverse a previous photochemical reaction, cleaving the cyclobutane ring of the so-called thymine dimer.

**deoxyepineph'rine.** EPININE; 4- [ 2-(methylamino)-ethyl ]pyrocatechol; sympathomimetic amine used as a vasoconstrictor.

**deoxygenation** (de'ok-sī-jen-a'shun). The removing or depriving of oxygen.

**deoxyguan'osine.** 2'-Deoxyribosylguanine, a constituent of DNA.

**deoxyguanyl'ic acid.** Deoxyguanosine phosphoric acid, a hydrolysis product of DNA.

**deoxyhex'ose.** A hexose (6-carbon sugar) in which one OH is replaced by H.

**6-deoxyman'nose.** Rhamnose.

**deoxypen'tose.** A pentose (5-carbon sugar) in which one OH is replaced by H; 2-deoxyribose is the most important example.

**deoxypyridoxine** (de-ok'sī-pīr-ī-dok'sēn). 2,4-Dimethyl-3-hydroxy-5-hydroxymethylpyridine; a compound differing from pyridoxine in the presence of a methyl group rather than a hydroxymethyl group in position 4. A pyridoxine antagonist; it inhibits tyrosine decarboxylase.

**deoxyri'boal'dolase.** Deoxyribosephosphate aldolase.

**deoxyribonuclease** (de-ok'sī-ri-bo-nu'kle-ās). Abbreviated DNase, DNAase; an enzyme (a phosphodiesterase) hydrolyzing phosphodiester bonds in DNA. See also phosphodiesterase; nuclease; endonuclease.

   **d. I,** pancreatic d.; an endonuclease (EC 3.1.4.5) that produces a mixture of oligodeoxyribonucleotides, each ending in a 5'-phosphate.

   **d. II,** an endonuclease (EC 3.1.4.6) cleaving both strands of native DNA producing a mixture of oligodeoxynucleotides, each ending in a 3'-phosphate.

   **pancreatic d.,** d. I.

   **spleen d.,** spleen *endonuclease.*

**deoxyri'bonucle'ic acid.** DNA; the type of nucleic acid containing deoxyribose as the sugar component and found principally in the nuclei (chromatin, chromosomes) of animal and vegetable cells, usually loosely bound to protein (hence termed deoxyribonucleoprotein). Considered to be the autoreproducing component of chromosomes and of many viruses, and the repository of hereditary characteristics. Obsolete synonyms are thymus nucleic acid, thymonucleic acid, and deoxypentosenucleic acid.

   **DNA helix,** see under helix.

   **DNA polymerase,** see nucleotidyltransferase.

**deox'yri'bonu'cleopro'tein.** The complex of DNA and protein in which DNA is usually found upon cell disruption and isolation.

**deoxyri'bonu'cleoside.** A nucleoside containing 2-deoxyribose; condensation product of deoxyribose with purines or pyrimidines; component of DNA. See deoxyadenosine, deoxycytidine, etc.

**deoxyri'bonu'cleotide.** A nucleotide containing 2-deoxyribose; phosphate ester of deoxyribonucleosde; component of DNA.

**deoxyri'bose.** A deoxypentose; D-2-deoxyribose is the most common example, occurring in DNA and responsible for its name.

**deoxyribosephosphate aldolase.** Deoxyriboaldolase; enzyme (EC 4.1.2.4) catalyzing cleavage of deoxyribose 5-phosphate to glyceraldehyde 3-phosphate and acetaldehyde.

**deoxyri'boside.** Deoxyribose combined via its O-1 atom with a radical derived from an alcohol, in contradistinction to deoxyribosyl, in which the entire OH on C-1 is eliminated. Incorrectly used for the latter; deoxyribonucleosides are deoxyribosyl compounds, not deoxyribosides.

**deoxyri'botide.** A misnomer for deoxyribonucleotide, derived, by analogy with nucleoside-nucleotide, from the incorrect deoxyriboside (*q. v.*).

**deoxy sugars.** Sugars containing fewer oxygen atoms than carbon atoms and in which, consequently, one or more carbons in the molecule lack an attached hydroxyl group.

**deox'ythymidyl'ic acid.** Thymine deoxyribonucleotide; a component of DNA; originally called thymidylic acid, but the use of the deoxy-prefix is less ambiguous, as ribothymidylic acid is now known to exist.

**deoxyvi'rus.** See DNA viruses, under virus.

**deozonize** (de-o'zo-nīz). To deprive of ozone.

**depancreatize** (de-pan'kre-ā-tīz). To remove the pancreas by operation.

**depen'dence** [ L. *dependeo,* to hang from ]. The quality or condition of lacking independence by relying upon, being influenced by, or being subservient to a person or object reflecting a particular need.

   **alcohol d.,** alcoholism.

**deper'sonaliza'tion.** A state in which a person loses the feeling of his own identity in relation to others in his family or peer group, or loses the feeling of his own reality.

**dephos'phoryla'tion.** The removal of a phosphate group, usually hydrolytically and by enzyme action, from a compound.

**depigmenta'tion.** Loss of pigment; it may be partial or complete.

**depilate** (dep'ī-lāt) [ L. *de-pilo,* pp. *-atus,* to deprive of hair, fr. *de-* neg. + *pilo,* to grow hair ]. Epilate (*q. v.*); to remove hair by any means.

**depilation** (dep'ī-la'shun). Epilation; removal of hair.

**depilatory** (de-pil'ă-to-rī). Epilatory; decalvant; 1. Having the property of removing hair; relating to depilation. 2. An agent that causes the falling out of hair.

**deplete** (de-plēt) [ *de-pleo,* to empty, fr. L. *de-* priv. + *pleo,* to fill ]. 1. To remove; to empty; to cause evacuation. 2. To reduce the strength.

**depletion** (de-ple'shun). 1. The removal of accumulated fluids or solids. 2. A reduced state of strength from too free discharges. 3. Excessive loss of a constituent, usually essential, of the body, *e.g.,* salt, water, etc.

   **salt d., chloride d.,** excessive loss of sodium chloride from the body in urine, sweat, etc. Cause of secondary dehydration.

   **water d.,** reduction in the total volume of body water; dehydration.

**deplumation** (de'ploo-ma'shun) [ L. *de-* priv. + *plumo,* pp. *-atus,* to deprive of feathers, to pluck, fr. *pluma,* feather ]. Defluxio ciliorum; falling out (or loss) of the eyelashes.

**depolarization** (de-po'lar-ī-za'shun). The destruction, neutralization, or change in direction of polarity.

   **dendritic d.,** the loss of a negative charge in the dendrites of a nerve cell.

**depo'larize.** To deprive of polarity.

**depo'larizer.** A substance absorbing the liberated gases in an electric battery and so preventing polarization.

**depol'ymerases.** Name used originally, before hydrolytic action was understood, for enzymes catalyzing the hydrolysis of a macromolecule to simpler components; examples are nucleases and amylases.

**deposit** (de-poz'it) [ L. *de-pono,* pp. *-positus,* to lay down ]. A sediment; precipitate.

   **brick-dust d.,** a sediment of urates in the urine.

**depravation** (dep'ră-va'shun) [ L. *depravatio,* fr. *depravo,* pp. *-atus,* to corrupt, fr. *pravus,* corrupt ]. Depravity.

**depraved** (de-prāvd'). Deteriorated or degenerate; perverted; corrupt.

**deprav'ity.** Depravation; deterioration; degeneracy; perversion; a depraved act or the condition of being depraved.

**depres'sant** [ L. *de-primo,* pp. *-pressus,* to press down, fr. *premo,* to press ]. 1. Lowering the vital tone; reducing functional activity. 2. An agent that lowers nervous or functional activity; a sedative.

**depressed** (de-prest'). 1. Flattened from above downward. 2. Below the normal level or the level of the surrounding parts. 3. Below the normal functional level. 4. Dejected; lowered in spirits.

**depression** (de-presh'un). 1. A sinking below the surrounding level. 2. A hollow or sunken area. 3. Dejection; a sinking of spirits so as to constitute a clinically discernible condition; see also melancholia.

   **agitated d.,** melancholia agitata; d. with excitement and restlessness, usually considered a phase of manic-depressive psychosis or of involutional melancholia.

   **anaclitic d.,** impairment of an infant's physical, social, and intellectual development following separation from its mother or from a mothering influence; characterized by listlessness, withdrawal, and anorexia; precedes the stage called hospitalism (*q. v.*).

**endogenous d.**, a descriptive syndrome for a cluster of symptoms and features commonly occurring in middle life and in the absence of precipitants; *e.g.*, severe d. of mood, psychomotor agitation or retardation, diurnal mood variation with increased severity in the morning, early morning awakening and insomnia in the middle of the night, weight loss, self-reproach or guilt, and lack of reactivity to one's environment.

**Pacchionian d.'s**, *foveolae* granulares.

**pterygoid d.**, *fovea* pterygoidea.

**reactive d.**, a psychotic state occasioned directly by an intensely sad external situation (usually loss of a loved person), relieved by the removal of the external situation (*e.g.*, reunion with a loved person).

**spreading d.**, a decrease of activity evoked by local stimulation of the cerebral cortex and spreading slowly over the whole cortex.

**depres'sive.** Pushing down; causing depression, literally or figuratively.

**depres'somo'tor.** 1. Retarding motor activity. 2. An agent that slows or retards motion.

**depres'sor.** 1 [ NA ]. A muscle that flattens or lowers a part. 2. Anything that depresses or retards functional activity. 3. An instrument used to push certain structures out of the way during an operation. 4. Hypotensor; producing decreased blood pressure.

**tongue d.**, an instrument with broad flat extremity used for pressing down the tongue to facilitate examination of the fauces and pharynx.

**deprivation** (dep'ri-va'shun). Absence, loss, or withholding of something needed.

**emotional d.**, lack of adequate and appropriate interpersonal or environmental experiences, or both, usually in the early developmental years.

**sensory d.**, diminution or absence of usual external stimuli or perceptual opportunities, commonly resulting in psychological distress and aberrant functioning.

**depth.** Distance from the surface downward.

**anesthetic d.**, the degree of central nervous system depression produced by a general anesthetic agent; a function of potency of the anesthetic and the concentration in which it is administered.

**focal d.**, penetration (of a lens); the variation in image distance of a lens tolerable without objectionable blurring.

**depulization** (de-pu'li-za'shun) [ L. *de*, from, + *pulex* (*pulic-*), flea ]. Destruction of fleas which convey the plague bacillus from animals to man; a term used by those engaged in antiplague work.

**dep'urant** [ L. *de-*intens. + *puro*, pp. *-atus*, to make pure ]. 1. An agent or means used to effect purification. 2. An agent that promotes the excretion and removal of waste material.

**depuration** (dep'u-ra'shun). Purification; removal of waste products or foul excretions.

**dep'urative.** Tending to depurate; depurant.

**DePuy's splint.** See under splint.

**dequalin'ium acetate** (BP). MICRIN; 1,1'-decamethylene-bis[ 4-aminoquinaldinium acetate ]; antimicrobial agent.

**de Quervain** (dĕ-ker-van'), Fritz, Swiss surgeon, 1868 –1940. See de Q.'s *disease, fracture, thyroiditis.*

**DeR.** Abbreviation for reaction of *degeneration.*

**deradelphus** (dĕr-ă-del'fus) [ G. *derē*, neck, + *adelphos*, brother ]. Conjoined twins with a single head and neck and separate bodies below the thoracic level.

**deradenitis** (dĕr'ad-ĕ-ni'tis) [ G. *derē*, neck, + *adēn*, gland, + suffix *-itis*, inflammation ]. Obsolete term for inflammation of the lymph nodes in the neck (cervical adenitis).

**deradenoncus** (dĕr'ad-ĕ-nong'kus) [ G. *derē*, neck, + *adēn*, gland, + *onkos*, bulk. ONC- ]. An obsolete term for a swelling or palpable mass involving the cervical lymph nodes.

**derail'ment.** See tangentiality.

**deranencephaly, deranencephalia** (dĕr-an'en-sef'ă-li, -sĕ-fa'li-ah) [ G. *derē*, neck, + *an-*, priv., + *kephalē*, head ]. A congenital malformation in which the head is absent although there is a rudimentary neck.

**derangement** (de-rānj'ment) [ Fr. ]. 1. Disordering; a disturbance of the regular order or arrangement. 2. Mental disturbance; insanity.

**Hey's internal d.**, dislocation of the semilunar cartilages of the knee joint.

**Dercum,** Francis X., Philadelphia neurologist, 1856–1931. See D.'s *disease.*

**dereism** (de're-izm) [ L. *de*, away, + *res*, thing ]. Mental activity in fantasy in contrast to reality.

**dereistic** (de-re-is'tik). Living in imagination or fantasy.

**derencephalia** (der-en-sĕ-fa'li-ah). Derencephaly.

**derencephalocele** (der-en-sef'ă-lo-sēl) [ G. *derē*, neck, + *enkephalos*, brain, + *kēlē*, hernia ]. A fetus in which the cranium is defective and the very small brain partly extrudes through a defect in the upper cervical spinal canal.

**derencephalus** (der-en-sef'ă-lus). An individual with derencephaly.

**derencephaly** (der-en-sef'ă-li) [ G. *derē*, neck, + *enkephalos*, brain ]. Derencephalia; cervical rachischisis and anencephaly; a malformation involving an open cranial vault with a markedly defective brain usually crowded back toward bifid cervical vertebrae.

**derepression** (de're-presh'un). The process in which an inducer, usually a substrate of a specific enzyme pathway, combines with an active repressor (produced by a regulator gene) to deactivate the repressor; this results in activation of a previously repressed operator gene and activity of the structural genes controlled by the operator, followed by enzyme production; a homeostatic mechanism for regulating enzyme production in an inducible enzyme system.

**der'ic** [ G. *deros*, skin ]. Ectodermal; relating to the ectoderm, as distinguished from enteric.

**derivation** (der'i-va'shun) [ L. *derivatio*, fr. *derivo*, pp. *-atus*, to draw off, fr. *rivus*, a stream ]. 1. The drawing of blood or the body fluids to one part by means of cupping, blisters, etc., to relieve congestion in another. 2. Descent, with modifications; evolution.

**derivative** (de-riv'ă-tiv). 1. Relating to or producing derivation. 2. Something produced by modification of something preexisting. 3. Specifically, a chemical compound that may be produced from another compound of similar structure in one or more steps, as in replacement of H by an alkyl, acyl, amino groups, etc. See acetylation, for example.

**derm-, derma-, dermat-, dermato-, dermo-** [ G. *derma*, skin ]. Combining forms signifying skin.

**dermabrasion** (der-mă-bra'zhun). The operative procedure used to remove acne scars, farmer-sailor skin, and dermal nevi. It may be performed using sand paper, wire brushes, or other abrasive materials.

**Der'macen'tor** [ derm- + G. *kentōr*, a goader. CENT- ]. An ornate, characteristically marked genus of hard ticks (family Ixodidae) that possess eyes and festoons; members commonly attack dogs, man, and other mammals.

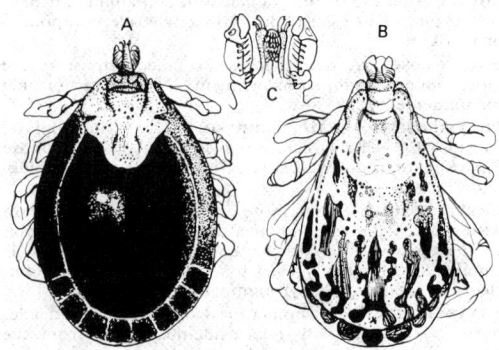

*Dermacentor andersoni* (**spotted fever tick**)

*A*, unengorged female; *B*, male; *C*, capitulum or mouthparts, showing palpi (outer pair of sensory structures), chelicerae (inner pair of cutting jaws), and hypostome (central spiny piercing and holding structure). (*A* and *B*, ×10; *C*, ×25.)

**D. albopic'tus,** horse tick; winter tick; found principally on horses, elk, moose, and deer in Canada and the western United States; it is a one-host tick, but man is sometimes attacked when skinning or dressing deer.

**D. anderso'ni,** Rocky Mountain tick; wood tick; formerly called *D. venustus;* it is the vector of spotted fever in the Rocky Mountain regions, and also transmits tularemia and causes tick paralysis; there are characteristic black and white markings on the large scutum of the male.

**D. ni'tens,** tropical horse tick; it is found on horses, cattle, sheep, pigs and other animals (usually on the ears of these hosts), chiefly in Florida, southern Texas, and Central America.

**D. occidenta'lis,** Pacific tick; wood tick; a species found on all domestic herbivores, deer, dogs, man, and other animals in California and western Oregon, and an important vector of bovine anaplasmosis.

**D. reticula'tus,** a common species attacking sheep, oxen, goats, and deer, and sometimes troublesome to man; it is found in Europe, Asia, and America.

**D. variabi'lis,** American dog tick; wood tick; common pest of dogs along the eastern seaboard of the United States from Massachusetts to Florida; a transmitter of tularemia and a principal vector of spotted fever in the central and eastern United States; it may also cause canine paralysis.

**der'mad** [ derm- + L. *ad,* to ]. In the direction of the outer integument.

**dermag'raphy.** Dermatographism.

**dermahe'mia** [ derma- + G. *haima,* blood ]. Hyperemia of the skin.

**der'mal.** Relating to the skin.

**dermalaxia** (der-mah-lak'sĭ-ah) [ derm- + G. *malaxis,* softening ]. Softening or relaxation of the skin.

**dermal'gia.** Dermatalgia.

**dermametropathism** (der'mah-me-trop'ă-thizm) [ derm- + G. *metron,* measure, + *pathos,* disease ]. A system of measurement of the intensity and nature of certain cutaneous disorders by observing the markings made by drawing a blunt instrument across the skin.

**dermamyiasis** (der-mah-mi-i'ă-sis). Myiasis of the skin.

**Dermanys'sus galli'nae** [ derm- + G. *nyssō,* to prick; L. *gallina,* hen ]. The red hen-mite, a parasite of chickens, pigeons, and other birds; it sometimes attacks man and causes an itching eruption, especially in sensitized individuals.

**dermat-** [ G. *derma,* skin ]. Combining form relating to the skin. For words beginning thus and not found here, see also derm-, dermato-, dermo-.

**dermatalgia** (der'mă-tal'jĭ-ah) [ dermat- + G. *algos,* pain ]. Dermalgia; dermatodynia; localized pain, usually confined to the skin.

**der'matan sulfate.** Formerly known as chondroitin sulfate B; a mucopolysaccharide containing L-iduronic acid and *N*-acetyl-D-galactosamine.

**dermat'ic.** Dermal.

**dermati'tis,** pl. **dermatit'ides** [ derm- + G. suffix *-itis,* inflammation ]. Inflammation of the skin.

**actinic d.,** eruption of sensitivity produced by exposure to sunlight, usually of specific electromagnetic energy; not a burn.

**d. aestiva'lis** [ L. *aestivus,* summer ], eczema recurring during the summer.

**d. ambustio'nis** [ L. *ambustio,* a scorching ], d. calorica; uritis; inflammation of the skin resulting from the action of heat.

**ancylostomiasis d.,** cutaneous *ancylostomiasis.*

**d. artefac'ta,** feigned eruption; d. autophytica; d. factitia; a self-induced eruption produced by self-inflicted trauma.

**atop'ic d.,** a. eczema; d. characterized by the distinctive phenomena of atopy.

**d. atroph'icans,** a diffuse idiopathic atrophy of the skin, involving the appendages.

**d. atrophicans lipoi'des diabet'ica,** see *necrobiosis* lipoidica.

**d. autophy'tica,** d. artefacta.

**berloque** or **berlock d.,** a type of photosensitization resulting in deep brown pigmentation on exposure to sunlight after exposure to bergamot oil and other essential oils in perfume.

**blastomyce'tic d., d. blastomycot'ica,** a cutaneous form of blastomycosis.

**bubble gum d.,** allergic contact d. developing about the lips in children who chew bubble gum. Caused by plastics in the gum substance.

**d. calor'ica,** d. ambustionis.

**caterpillar d.,** allergic contact d. caused by the larva of the browntail moth.

**chemical d.,** allergic contact d. or primary irritation d. due to application of chemicals; usually characterized by erythema, edema, and vesiculation of the exposed or contacted site.

**d. coccidioi'des,** coccidioidomycosis.

**d. combustio'nis,** inflammation of the skin following a burn.

**d. congelatio'nis,** frostbite.

**contact d.,** a delayed type of induced sensitivity (allergy) of the skin with varying degrees of erythema, edema, and vesiculation, resulting from cutaneous contact with a specific allergen.

**contact-type d.,** d. resembling contact d., but caused by an ingested or injected allergen (usually a drug, *e.g.,* quinine) and with a widespread or generalized distribution.

**contagious pustular d. of sheep,** contagious *ecthyma.*

**d. contusifor'mis** [ Mod. L. resembling contusions ], *erythema* nodosum.

**cosmetic d.,** a cutaneous eruption resulting from the application of a cosmetic, because of allergic sensitization or primary irritation.

**dhobie mark d.,** (do'bĭ) [ Hindi *dhobī,* washerman ], dhobie or washerman's mark; an allergic contact d. due to hypersensitivity to ingredients in laundry marking ink.

**diaper d.,** colloquially referred to as diaper, ammonia, or napkin rash; d. of thighs and buttocks supposedly due to ammonia produced in decomposing urine in infants' diapers.

**d. epidem'ica,** Saville's disease; d. exfoliative epidemica; an acute infectious disease marked by a vesicular d. followed by desquamation; it is accompanied by more or less severe constitutional symptoms, conjunctivitis, pharyngitis, and enlargement of the cervical glands; it may terminate fatally, especially when attacking the old and infirm.

**d. erythemato'sa,** erythema.

**d. exfoliati'va,** exfoliative d.

**d. exfoliati'va epidem'ica,** d. epidemica.

**d. exfoliativa infan'tum** or **neonato'rum,** keratolysis neonatorum; Ritter's disease (1); impetigo neonatorum (1); pemphigus neonatorum; a generalized pyoderma accompanied by exfoliative d., with constitutional symptoms, affecting young infants; frequently fatal.

**exfoliative d.,** d. exfoliativa; pityriasis rubra; Wilson's disease (2); generalized exfoliation with scaling of the skin and usually with erythema (erythroderma); may be associated with various benign dermatoses or with lymphomas.

**exudative discoid and lichenoid d.,** Sulzberger-Garbe *disease.*

**d. facti'tia,** d. artefacta.

**d. gangreno'sa infan'tum,** rupia escharotica; pemphigus gangrenosus (1); ecthyma gangrenosum; disseminated cutaneous gangrene; more or less extensive gangrene of the skin in infants, rarely following chickenpox or other infectious disease.

**d. herpetifor'mis,** d. multiformis; Duhring's disease; herpes circinatus bullosus; hydroa herpetiforme; a chronic disease of the skin marked by a severe, extensive, itching eruption of vesicles and papules which occur in groups; spontaneous healing rarely occurs except in children; relapses are common.

**d. hiema'lis** [ L. *hiems,* winter ], winter itch; frost itch; lumberman's itch; pruritus hiemalis; a recurrent eczema appearing with the advent of cold weather.

**industrial d.,** dermatosis industrialis; d. produced by some agent contacted in industry, or a previously existing eruption aggravated by some agent handled during the course of work.

**infectious eczematoid d.,** inflammatory reaction of skin adjacent to site of pyogenic infection, such as purulent otitis, the area around a colostomy, intranasal infection;

thought to be due to a local sensitization to the resident organisms.

**d. linearis migrans,** (1) cutaneous *larva migrans;* (2) the presence of botfly larvae in the skin.

**livedoid d.,** reddish blue mottled condition of skin due to affection of cutaneous vascular apparatus.

**mango d.,** a sensitization reaction; perioral d. caused by the resinous coating on the peel of the mango fruit.

**meadow d., meadow grass d.,** phytophlyctodermatitis; a phototoxic reaction to contact with a plant in which the bizarre configuration of the eruption is that of the streaky pattern of the plant contact; often occurs after sunbathing.

**d. medicamento'sa,** drug *eruption.*

**d. multifor'mis,** d. herpetiformis.

**nickel d.,** allergic d. due to nickel or other metals containing nickel as a diluent (gold, stainless steel, etc.).

**d. nodosa,** a papular eruption on legs, related to craw-craw.

**d. nodula'ris necrot'ica,** a recurrent eruption of vesicles, papules, and papulonecrotic lesions on the back, hands, feet, etc.

**occupational d.,** eruption of the skin, either as a response of allergic sensitization to substances encountered in an occupation, or as a reaction of primary irritation; also, the cutaneous changes resulting from exposure to factors of irritation inherent to the occupation (*e.g.,* friction, hydration, heat, cold, etc.).

**d. papilla'ris capillit'ii,** acne *keloid.*

**d. pediculoi'des ventrico'sus,** straw *itch.*

**plant d.,** d. venenata.

**primary irritant d.,** reaction of irritation on exposure of the skin to substances which are toxic to epidermal or connective tissue cells; lesions are usually erythematous, papular, but can be purulent or necrotic, depending on the nature of the toxic material applied.

**proliferative d.,** a contagious disease of sheep in which extensive scabs appear on the legs and feet. Beneath the scabs the underlying tissue is reddened and exhibits whitish points, which causes the surface to resemble that of a strawberry. The condition is caused by *Dermatophilus pedis.*

**rat mite d.,** an eruption of wheals, papules, or vesicles caused by the rat mite.

**d. re'pens** [ L. creeping ], *acrodermatitis* continua.

**rhus d.,** d. venenata.

**sandal strap d.,** allergic contact on the dorsal surfaces of the feet, caused by synthetic rubber sandal straps.

**Schamberg's d.,** progressive pigmentary *dermatosis.*

**schis'tosome d.,** Swimmer's itch (2); water itch (2); a sensitization response to repeated cutaneous invasion by cercariae of bird, mammal, or human schistosomes.

**seborrheic d.,** d. seborrheica; seborrheic dermatosis; seborrheic eczema; seborrhea corporis; Unna's disease; dyssebacia; a scaly macular eruption that occurs primarily on the face, scalp, interscapular area, pubic area, and about the anus. The lesions are covered with a slightly adherent oily scale.

**shoe dye d.,** allergic contact d. of the feet, caused by sensitivity to shoe dye.

**d. simplex,** *erythema* simplex.

**d. skiagraph'ica,** x-ray d.; inflammation of the skin due to the action of roentgen rays.

**solar d.,** a d. caused by exposure to the sun's rays in photosensitive persons.

**stasis d.,** erythema and scaling of the lower extremities due to impaired circulation and other factors, such as nutritional edema.

**subcorneal pustular d.,** subcorneal pustular *dermatosis.*

**traumatic d.,** any d. caused by an irritant substance or by a physical agent.

**trefoil d.,** trifoliosis.

**d. veg'etans,** pyoderma vegetans; a benign fungating granulomatous mass caused by chronic pyogenic infection.

**d. venena'ta** [ L. *veneum,* poison ], plant d.; rhus d.; a cutaneous eruption due to contact with a sensitizing agent such as poison ivy, resins, chemicals, cosmetics, etc. The eruption is edematous, erythematous, and vesicular.

**d. verruco'sa,** chromoblastomycosis.

**x-ray d.,** d. skiagraphica.

**dermatitogenic.** Rarely used term denoting a substance prone to produce a dermatitis.

**dermato-** [ G. *derma,* skin ]. Combining form relating to the skin. For words beginning thus and not found here, see also those beginning derm- and dermo-.

**der'matoal'loplasty.** Dermatohomoplasty.

**dermatoarthritis** (der'mă-to-ar-thri'tis). Associated skin disease and arthritis.

**lipoid d.,** a rare disease in which cutaneous papules composed of histiocytes containing glycolipids are associated with polyarthritis, often leading to shortening of the fingers.

**dermatoautoplasty** (der'mă-to-aw'to-plas-tĭ) [ dermato- + G. *autos,* self, + *plassō,* to form ]. Skin grafting with material taken from another part of the patient's own body; autografting of skin.

**Dermato'bia** [ dermato- + G. *bios,* way of living ]. A genus of flies of the family Oestridae, found in tropical America.

**D. cyaniven'tris,** *D. hominis.*

**D. hom'inis,** *D. cyaniventris;* human botfly; skin botfly; warble botfly; a large, blue, brown-winged fly whose larvae develop in boil-like cysts in the skin of man, many domestic animals, and some fowl. It is a very serious and damaging cattle parasite and frequently attacks small children. The eggs of this fly are laid on the legs or abdomen of another insect, such as the mosquito; the eggs later hatch, when stimulated by warmth or other factors, to release the botfly larvae on the skin of the mosquito's bloodmeal host, and the larvae quickly invade the skin to initiate dermatobial myiasis.

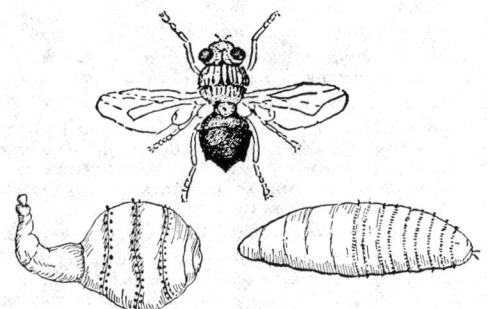

*Dermatobia hominis (Dermatobia cyaniventris)*
*Top,* adult female; *bottom,* larvae, early and late stages.

**dermatocele** (der'mă-to-sēl) [ dermato- + G. *kēlē,* hernia ]. A localized atrophy or herniation of skin that may result from a neurofibroma or a congenital defect.

**d. lipomato'sa,** a pedunculated lipoma undergoing cystic degeneration.

**dermatocellulitis** (der'mă-to-sel'u-li'tis). Inflammation of the skin and subcutaneous connective tissue.

**dermatochalasis** (der'mă-to-kă-la'sis) [ dermato- + G. *chalaō,* to loosen ]. *Cutis* laxa.

**dermatoconiosis** (der'mă-to-ko-nĭ-o'sis) [ dermato- + G. *konis,* dust, + suffix *-osis,* condition ]. An occupational dermatitis caused by local irritation from dust.

**dermatocyst** (der'mă-to-sist). A cyst of the skin.

**der'matodyn'ia** [ dermato- + G. *odynē,* pain ]. Dermatalgia.

**der'matofibro'ma.** A slowly growing, benign skin nodule, consisting of poorly demarcated cellular fibrous tissue enclosing collapsed capillaries, with scattered hemosiderin-pigmented and lipid macrophages. The following terms are considered by some to be synonymous with, and by others to be varieties of, d.: sclerosing hemangioma, histiocytoma, cutaneous nodule, nodular subepidermal fibrosis, fibroxanthoma, fibrous xanthoma, fibrous histiocytoma.

**der'matofi'brosarco'ma protu'berans.** A relatively slowly growing dermal neoplasm consisting of one or several, small, firm nodules that are usually covered by dark red-blue skin, which tends to be fixed to the palpable masses; histologically the neoplasm resembles a cellular sclerosing hemangioma in some portions, or a low-grade fibrosarcoma in others. Metastases are unusual, but the incidence of recurrence is fairly high. The neoplasm occurs most frequently in the fifth decade, especially in men, but is also observed in young adults and children.

**dermatoglyphics** (der-mă-to-glif′iks) [ dermato- + *glyphē,* carved work ]. 1. The configurations of the characteristic ridge patterns of the volar surfaces of the skin; in the hand of man, the distal segment of each digit has three types of configurations—whorl, loop, and arch; see also fingerprint. 2. The science or study of these configurations or patterns.

**dermat′ograph.** The linear wheal made in the skin in dermatographism.

**dermatographism** (der′mă-tog′ră-fizm) [ dermato- + G. *graphō,* to write ]. A form of urticaria in which whealing occurs in the site and in the configuration of application of stroking (pressure, friction) of the skin; also called dermatography, dermagraphy, dermographia; autographism; skin writing; factitious urticaria; Ebbecke's reaction.

**dermatog′raphy.** Dermatographism.

**der′matohet′eroplasty** [ dermato- + G. *heteros,* another, + *plassō,* to form ]. Heterografting of skin; skin grafting in which the material is derived from an animal of another species.

**der′matoho′moplasty** [ dermato- + G. *homos,* same, + *plastos,* formed ]. Dermatoalloplasty; skin grafting in which the material is obtained from another member of the same species; homografting of skin.

**der′matoid.** 1. Dermoid; resembling skin. 2. Dermal; relating to skin.

**dermatol′ogist.** A physician who specializes in the diagnosis and treatment of cutaneous lesions and the related systemic diseases; a "skin specialist."

**dermatology** (der′mă-tol′o-jĭ) [ dermato- + G. *logos,* study ]. The branch of medicine that has to do especially with the study of the skin, its chemistry, physiology, histopathology, cutaneous lesions, and the relationship of cutaneous lesions to systemic disease.

**dermatolysis** (der′mă-tol′ĭ-sis) [ dermato- + G. *lysis,* a loosening ]. Dermolysis; loosening of the skin; atrophy of the skin by disease; a term erroneously used as a synonym for cutis laxa.

   **d. palpebra′rum,** blepharochalasis.

**dermatoma** (der-mă-to′mah) [ dermato- + G. suffix -*oma,* tumor ]. A circumscribed thickening or hypertrophy of the skin.

**der′matome** [ dermato- + G. *tomē,* a cutting ]. 1. An instrument for cutting thin slices of skin for grafting, or excising small lesions. 2. Cutis plate; the dorsolateral part of an embryonic somite. 3. The area of skin that is supplied by cutaneous branches from a single spinal nerve; neighboring d.'s overlap to a considerable extent. See color plate 24.

**dermatomegaly** (der′mă-to-meg′ă-lĭ) [ dermato- + G. *megas,* large ]. Essentially means large skin; a congenital defect in which the skin hangs in folds. Erroneously used as a synonym for cutis laxa.

**dermatomere** (der′mă-to-mēr) [ dermato- + G. *meros,* part ]. A metameric area of the embryonic integument.

**dermatomucosomyositis** (der′mă-to-mu-ko′so-mi-o-si′-tis). Inflammatory lesions in muscles of head and neck accompanied by lesions on the skin and mucous membranes.

**dermatomyces** (der′mă-to-mi′sēz). Dermatophyte.

**dermatomyco′sis.** Dermatophytosis.

   **blastomyce′tic d.,** a cutaneous form of blastomycosis.

   **d. pedis,** *tinea* pedis.

**dermatomyoma** (der′mă-to-mi-o′mah) [ dermato- + G. *mys,* muscle, + suffix -*oma,* tumor ]. Leiomyoma of the skin, frequently multiple, originating from arrector pili muscles; occasionally solitary, from the muscle walls of small blood vessels.

**dermatomyositis** (der′mă-to-mi′o-si′tis) [ dermato- + G. *mys,* muscle, + suffix -*itis,* inflammation ]. A condition characterized by muscular weakness with a nonspecific eczematous skin eruption or urticaria. The muscles are tender, and owing to weakness the patient is unable to perform normal tasks. The condition is progressive: it commences with erythema and swelling of the eyelids, face, and parts of the limbs; muscular weakness follows the skin changes. The pathologic changes in the muscles are diagnostic, but the histopathologic skin changes are nonspecific.

**dermatoneurosis** (der′mă-to-nu-ro′sis). Dermoneurosis; any cutaneous eruption due to emotional stimuli; a cutaneous neurosis.

**dermatonosology** (der′mă-to-no-sol′o-jĭ) [ dermato- + G. *nosos,* disease, + *logos,* treatise ]. Dermonosology; the science of the nomenclature and classification of diseases of the skin.

**der′matono′sus.** Obsolete term for dermatosis.

**dermatopath′ia.** Dermatopathy.

   **d. pigmento′sa reticula′ris,** *livedo* reticularis.

**der′matopathol′ogy.** Histopathology of skin lesions.

**dermatopathy** (der′mă-top′ă-thĭ) [ dermato- + G. *pathos,* suffering ]. Dermopathy; dermatopathia (see subentries under both); any disease of the skin.

**Dermatophagoides pteronyssinus.** A common cosmopolitan sarcoptiform mite commonly found in house dust accumulation and thought to be a contributory cause of atopic house dust asthma.

**dermatophiliasis** (der′mă-to-fĭ-li′ă-sis). Infestation with *Tunga penetrans,* or chigoe, formerly called *Dermatophilus penetrans.*

**Dermatoph′ilus pen′etrans.** Former name for *Tunga penetrans.*

**der′matopho′bia** [ dermatosis + G. *phobos,* fear ]. A morbid fear of acquiring a skin disease.

**der′matophone.** An instrument used for listening to blood flow in the skin.

**dermatophylaxis** (der′mă-to-fi-lak′sis) [ dermato- + G. *phylaxis,* protection ]. Protection of the skin against infection.

**dermatophyte** (der′mă-to-fīt) [ dermato- + G. *phyton,* plant ]. Dermatomyces; dermophyte; cutaneous fungus; a fungus pathogenic for the skin.

**dermatophytid** (der′mă-tof′ĭ-tid) [ dermatophyte + suffix -*id* (1), *q.v.* ]. An allergic eruption, usually of small vesicles, that may develop on the hands or other areas in association with dermatophytosis.

**dermatophytosis** (der′mă-to-phi-to′sis). Dermatomycosis; dermomycosis; dermophytosis; epidermatophytosis; epidermatomycosis; epidermomycosis; an eruption caused by any one of the superficial dermatophytes (fungi); the lesions, which occur most commonly on the feet (athlete's foot) and in the groins, are characterized by erythema, small papular vesicles, fissures, and scaling.

**der′matoplas′tic.** Relating to dermatoplasty, or skin grafting.

**der′matoplas′ty** [ dermato- + G. *plassō,* to form ]. Dermoplasty; repair of defects of the skin; skin grafting.

   **septal d.,** an operation to graft the septum and turbinates with skin; used in hereditary hemorrhagic telangiectasia.

**dermatopolyneuritis** (der′mă-to-pol-ĭ-nu-ri-tis). Acrodynia (1).

**dermatorrhagia** (der′mă-to-ra′jĭ-ah) [ dermato- + G. *rhēgnymi,* to break forth ]. Hemorrhage from or into the skin.

   **d. parasit′ica,** a disease of the horse marked by numerous localized hemorrhages into and through the skin from small nodules, due to the presence of the parasitic filarial nematode, *Parafilaria multipapillosa.*

**dermatorrhea** (der′mă-to-re′ah) [ dermato- + G. *rhoia,* flow ]. An excessive secretion of the sebaceous or sweat glands of the skin.

**dermatorrhexis** (der′mă-to-rek′sis) [ dermato- + G. *rhēxis,* rupture ]. Rupture of the skin, such as is seen in striae cutis distensae or in the Ehlers-danlos syndrome.

**dermatosclerosis** (der′mă-to-skle-ro′sis) [ dermato- + G. *sclērō,* to harden ]. Scleroderma.

**dermatoscopy** (der-mă-tos′ko-pĭ) [ dermato- + G. *skopeō,* to view ]. Inspection of the skin, usually with the aid of a lens.

**dermato′sis,** pl. **dermatoses** [ dermato- + G. suffix -*osis,* condition ]. Any cutaneous lesion or group of lesions. A nonspecific term used to embrace eruptions of any type.

**acarine d.** [ G. *akari*, a mite ], an eruption caused by one of the acarine parasites.

**chick nutritional d.**, d. in chicks, with eruptions about the eyes, mouth, and feet; responds to pantothenic acid.

**dermolytic bullous d.**, epidermolysis bullosa dystrophica; a form of epidermolysis bullosa in which scarring develops after separation of the entire epidermis with blistering; it may be acquired or inherited as a dominant or recessive type.

**filarial d.**, sorehead; a disease of sheep on high mountain ranges during the summer caused by larvae of the filarial worm, *Elaeophora schneider*, which localize chiefly on the head, causing intense itching and loss of wool.

**d. industria'lis**, industrial *dermatitis*.

**Kaposi's d.**, *xeroderma* pigmentosum.

**lichenoid d.**, chronic skin eruption, eczematous in character; could be from any cause.

**d. medicamento'sa**, drug *eruption*.

**d. papulo'sa ni'gra**, brownish papular lesions, observed in Negroes, on the face and upper trunk. Histologically and clinically they resemble seborrheic keratoses.

**pigmented purpuric lichenoid d.**, Gougerot and Blum disease; an eruption comprised of lichenoid papules variously pigmented from the hemosiderin of the associated purpura; found on the legs, usually in men over 40 years of age.

**progressive pigmentary d.**, Schamberg's disease; Schamberg's dermatitis; purpura, especially of the legs in men, spreading to form brownish patches; associated microscopically with capillary dilation, diapedesis, and hemosiderosis.

**seborrheic d.**, seborrheic *dermatitis*.

**subcorneal pustular d.**, subcorneal pustular dermatitis; Sneddon-Wilkinson disease; a pruritic chronic annular eruption of sterile vesicles and pustules beneath the stratum corneum; bears a considerable resemblance to dermatitis herpetiformis.

**dermatoskel'eton.** Exoskeleton (1).

**der'matother'apy.** Treatment of skin diseases.

**dermatothlasia** (der'mă-to-thla'zĭ-ah) [ dermato- + G. *thlasis*, a bruising ]. An uncontrollable impulse to pinch and bruise the skin.

**dermatotropic** (der'mă-to-trop'ik) [ dermato- + G. *trōpe*, a turning ]. Having an affinity for the skin.

**dermatoxerasia** (der'mă-to-ze-ra'zĭ-ah) [ dermato- + G. *xērasia*, a dryness. XER- ]. Xeroderma.

**dermatozoiasis** (der'mat-o-zo-i'ă-sis) [ dermato- + G. *zōon*, animal, + suffix -*iasis*, condition ]. Dermatozoonosis.

**dermatozoon** (der-mă-to-zo'on) [ dermato- + G. *zōon*, animal ]. An animal parasite of the skin.

**dermatozoonosis** (der'mă-to-zo-o-no'sis, -zo-on'o-sis) [ dermato- + G. *zōon*, animal, + nosos, disease ]. Dermatozoiasis; rarely used terms for an eruption caused by an animal parasite.

**dermatozooplasty** (der'mă-to-zo'o-plas-tĭ) [ dermato- + G. *zōon*, animal, + *plassō*, to form ]. Skin grafting attempted with the skin of an animal. See dermatoheteroplasty.

**dermatrophia, dermatrophy** (der'mă-tro'fĭ-ah, der-mat'ro-fĭ). Atrophy or thinning of the skin.

**dermenchysis** (der-men'kĭ-sis) [ derm- + G. *enchysis*, a pouring in. CHY- ]. The subcutaneous administration of remedies.

**der'mic.** Dermal; dermatic; cutaneous; relating to the skin in general or to the dermis.

**der'mis** [ G. *derma*, skin ] [ NA ]. Corium.

**dermi'tis.** Dermatitis.

**dermo-** [ G. *derma*, skin ]. Combining form relating to the skin. For words beginning with dermo- but not found here, see also those beginning with derm-, dermat- and dermato-.

**der'moblast** [ dermo- + G. *blastos*, germ ]. One of the mesodermal cells from which the corium is developed.

**dermocyma** (der'mo-si'mah) [ dermo- + G. *kyma*, fetus ]. Unequal conjoined twins in which the smaller (parasitic) twin is buried in the integument of the larger (host).

**dermograph'ia, dermog'raphism, dermog'raphy.** Dermatographism.

**dermoid** (der'moyd) [ dermo- + G. *eidos*, resemblance ]. 1. Dermatoid; resembling skin. 2. Dermoid tumor; a congenital cystic tumor, filled with fluid or sebaceous matter, the walls of which are of dermal origin, sometimes giving rise to teeth, hair, and other dermal appendages.

**implantation d.**, epidermal *cyst*.

**inclu'sion d.**, a congenital cyst lined by epidermis, with skin appendages in the dermis along a line of embryonic closure.

**sequestration d.**, epidermal *cyst*.

**dermoidectomy** (der-moy-dek'to-mĭ) [ dermoid + G. *ektome*, excision ]. Operative removal of a dermoid cyst.

**der'molipo'ma** [ dermo- + G. *lipos*, fat, + suffix -*oma*, tumor ]. A type of solid dermoid cyst, especially of the orbit, containing few or no epithelial structures and a disproportionate amount of fat.

**dermol'ysis.** Dermatolysis.

**der'momyco'sis.** Dermatophytosis.

**der'monecrot'ic.** Pertaining to any application or illness which may cause necrosis of the skin.

**der'moneu'sis.** Dermatoneurosis.

**der'monosol'ogy.** Dermatonosology.

**dermop'athy.** Dermatopathy.

**diabetic d.**, small macules and papules of the extensor surfaces of the extremities (most commonly the shins) which become atrophic, hyperpigmented, and occasionally undergo ulceration with scarring.

**dermophlebitis** (der'mo-flĕ-bi'tis) [ dermo- + G. *phleps*, vein, + suffix -*itis*, inflammation ]. Inflammation of the superficial veins and the surrounding skin.

**der'mophyte.** Dermatophyte.

**der'mophyto'sis.** Dermatophytosis.

**der'moplasty.** Dermatoplasty.

**dermoskel'eton.** Exoskeleton (1).

**der'mosteno'sis** [ dermo- + G. *stenōsis*, a narrowing ]. Pathologic contraction of the skin.

**der'mosto'sis** [ derm- + G. *osteon*, bone, + suffix -*osis*, condition ]. *Osteosis* cutis.

**dermosyphilopathy** (der'mo-sif'ĭ-lop'ă-thĭ). Cutaneous lesions of syphilis; any syphilid.

**dermotox'in.** A substance elaborated by a living agent, especially an exotoxin formed by bacteria and characterized by its ability to cause pathologic changes in skin, *e.g.*, erythema, degenerative changes, or necrosis.

**dermotrop'ic.** Dermatotropic.

**dermovas'cular** [ dermo- + L. *vasculus*, small vessel ]. Pertaining to the blood vessels of the skin.

**derodidymus** (der'o-did'ĭ-mus) [ G. *derē*, neck, + *didymos*, twin ]. A conjoined twin with separate heads and necks but with a single body. See also dicephalus.

**de'rota'tion** [ L. *de*, away, + *rotatio*, turning ]. 1. A turning back. 2. In orthopaedics, the correction of a torsional *deformity* (q.v.).

**derrengadera** (der-ren-gah-dar'ah) [ Sp. *derrengado*, crooked ]. Murrina, especially that form in which posterior paralysis is marked.

**des-.** See de-.

**N-desacetyl-N-methylcolchicine.** Demecolcine.

**desam'idize.** Deamidize.

**De Sanctis**, Carlo. See D. S.-Cacchione *syndrome*.

**Desault** (dĕ-so'), Pierre J., French surgeon, 1744–1795. See D.'s *bandage, ligature*.

**Descartes** (da-cart'), René, eminent French philosopher, mathematician, and physiologist, 1596–1650. The founder of modern philosophy and one of the foremost proponents of the mechanistic or iatromathematical school, *q.v.* He considered the body a machine governed by a sensitive soul residing in the pineal gland. See D.'s *law*, Cartesian *coordinates*.

**Descemet** (des-ma'), Jean, French physician, 1732–1810. See D.'s *membrane*.

**descemetitis** (des-ĕ-mĕ-ti'tis). Inflammation of Descemet's membrane on the posterior surface of the cornea; keratitis punctata; serous cyclitis.

**descemetocele** (des-ĕ-met'o-sēl) [ Descemet's membrane + G. *kēlē*, hernia ]. Hernia of Descemet's membrane.

**descen'dens** [ L. ] [ NA ]. Descending.

**d. cervica'lis,** *radix* inferior ansae cervicalis.

**d. hypoglos'si,** *radix* superior ansae cervicalis.

**descen'ding** [ L. *de-scendo*, pp. -*scensus*, to come down, fr. *scando*, to climb ]. Running downward or toward the periphery.

**descensus** (de-sen'sus) [ L. ]. Descent; falling; ptosis; procidentia.

   **d. ab'errans testis,** incomplete descent of the testis which comes to rest in the inguinal canal, femoral canal, or perineal region, or under the skin of the penis.

   **d. paradox'us testis,** the descent of the right testis to the left half of the scrotum and the left testis to the right half.

   **d. testis** [ NA ], descent of the testis from the abdomen into the scrotum during the seventh and eighth months of intrauterine life.

   **d. u'teri,** falling of the womb.

   **d. ventric'uli,** gastroptosis.

**descent** (de-sent') [ L. descensus, *q.v.* ]. 1. A moving downward; see descensus and subentries. 2. In obstetrics, the passage of the presenting part into and through the birth canal.

**Deschamps** (da-shahn'), Joseph F. L., French surgeon, 1740–1824. See D.'s *needle.*

**desen'sitiza'tion.** 1. The reduction or abolition of allergic sensitivity or reactions to the specific antigen (allergen). 2. The act of removing an emotional complex.

   **systemic d.,** reciprocal inhibition (2); a type of behavior therapy for eliminating phobias or anxieties. The patient and therapist construct a list of imagined scenes eliciting the phobia, ranked from the least to the most anxiety-producing. The patient then is trained in deep muscle relaxation, and is repeatedly asked to imagine himself in the presence of the least anxiety-producing scene on the list until he feels himself fully relaxed. The procedure is repeated for each scene on the list until the patient develops the capacity to feel relaxed with any of the anxiety-producing scenes. Real life scenes are then substituted for the imagined scenes.

**desen'sitize.** 1. To reduce or remove any form of sensitivity. 2. To abate susceptibility to the action of a foreign protein. 3. In dentistry, to eliminate or subdue the painful response of exposed, vital dentin to irritative agents or thermal changes.

**deser'pidine.** HARMONYL; 11-desmethoxyreserpine; ester alkaloid isolated from *Rauwolfia canescens* (family Apocynaceae); same actions and uses as reserpine; appears to be somewhat less potent, with a more rapid onset of action.

**des'ferriox'amine mes'ylate** (BP). Deferoxamine mesylate.

**desiccant** (des'ĭ-kant) [ L. *de-sicco*, pp. -*siccatus*, to dry up ]. 1. Drying. 2. An agent that absorbs moisture; a drying agent.

**desiccate** (des'ĭ-kāt). To dry.

**desiccative** (des'ĭ-ka'tiv). Desiccant (1).

**desiccator** (des'ĭ-ka'tor). 1. A desiccant (2). 2. An apparatus, such as a glass chamber containing calcium chloride, sulfuric acid, or other desiccant, in which a material is placed for drying.

   **vacuum d.,** one that can be evacuated.

**de Signeux's dilator.** See under dilator.

**desip'ramine hydrochloride** (NF, BP). PERTOFRANE; desmethylimipramine hydrochloride; norimipramine hydrochloride; a dibenzazepine derivative; an antidepressant with actions and uses similar to those of imipramine.

**desirabil'ity.** In sensorimotor theory, an individual's psychological disequilibrium resulting from some incomplete adaption.

**deslan'oside.** CEDILANID D; desacetyllanatoside C; a rapidly acting steroid glycoside obtained from lanatoside C *(Digitalis lanata)* by alkaline hydrolysis; a cardiotonic.

**desm-.** See desmo-.

**Desmarres** (da-mar'), Louis A., French ophthalmologist, 1810–1882. See D.'s *dacryolith.*

**desmectasis, desmectasia** (dez-mek'tă-sis, des-mek-ta'zĭ-ah) [ desm- + G. *ektasis,* a stretching ]. Ectasia of a ligament.

**desmitis** (dez-mi'tis) [ desm- + G. suffix -*itis,* inflammation ]. Inflammation of a ligament.

**desmo-, desm-** (dez-mo-) [ G. *desmos,* a band ]. Combining forms meaning fibrous connection or ligament.

**desmocranium** (dez'mo-kra'nĭ-um). The mesenchymal primordium of the cranium.

**desmocytoma** (dez'mo-si-to'mah) [ desmo- + G. *kytos,* call, + suffix -*oma,* tumor ]. A neoplasm composed of actively proliferating fibroblasts; an obsolete term.

**Desmodil'lus auricular'is.** A South African gerbil that is a source of human plague infection.

**Desmodus** (dez'mo-dus) [ desmo- + G. *odous,* tooth ]. A genus of Chiroptera known generally as vampire bats, a blood-feeding genus endemic in Trinidad, Mexico, and Central and South America. *D. artibaeus, D. rotundus,* and *D. rufus,* three species found in Trinidad and South America, are carriers of paralyssa (Trinidad disease), a paralytic form of rabies.

**desmodynia** (dez-mo-din'ĭ-ah) [ desmo- + G. *odynē,* pain ]. Pain in a ligament.

**desmoenzymes** (dez-mo-enz'imz). Intracellular *enzymes.*

**desmogenous** (dez-moj'ĕ-nus) [ desmo- + G. suffix -*gen,* producing ]. Of connective tissue or ligamentous origin or causation, denoting, *e.g.,* a deformity due to contraction of ligaments, fascia, or a cicatrix.

**desmography** (dez-mog'ră-fĭ) [ desmo- + G. *graphō,* to describe ]. A description of, or treatise on, the ligaments.

**desmoid** (dez'moyd) [ desmo- + G. *eidos,* appearance, form ]. 1. Fibrous or ligamentous. 2. Desmoid tumor; a nodule or relatively large mass of unusually firm scarlike connective tissue resulting from active proliferation of fibroblasts, occurring most frequently in the abdominal muscles of women who have borne children; the fibroblasts infiltrate surrounding muscle and fascia.

**desmolases** (dez'mo-la-sez). Enzymes catalyzing reactions other than those involving hydrolysis; *e.g.,* those involving oxidation and reduction, isomerization, the breaking of carbon-carbon bonds. A nonspecific term.

**desmology** (dez-mol'o-jĭ) [ desmo- + G. *logos,* study ]. The branch of anatomy dealing with the ligaments.

**desmoma** (dez-mo'mah) [ desmo- + G. suffix -*oma,* tumor ]. Undesirable term for a fibroma.

**desmon** (dez'mon) [ G. *desmos,* band, bond ]. An old term for complement-fixing antibody.

**desmopathy** (dez-mop'ă-thĭ) [ desmo- + G. *pathos,* suffering ]. A disease of ligaments.

**desmoplasia** (dez-mo-pla'zĭ-ah) [ desmo- + G. *plasis,* a molding ]. The hyperplasia of fibroblasts and disproportionate formation of fibrous connective tissue.

**desmoplas'tic.** 1. Causing or forming adhesions. 2. Causing fibrosis in the vascular stroma of a neoplasm.

**desmosome** (dez'mo-sōm) [ desmo- + G. *sōma,* body ]. Bridge corpuscle; macula adherens; a site of adhesion between two cells, consisting of a dense plate separated from a similar structure in the other cell by a thin layer of extracellular material believed to have cementing properties.

**desmosterol** (dez-mos'ter-ol). 24-Dehydrocholesterol; postulated intermediate in cholesterol biosynthesis; accumulates after prolonged administration of substances interfering with the latter.

**desmotomy** (dez-mot'o-mĭ) [ desmo- + G. *tomē,* incision ]. Section of a ligament, *e.g.,* the flexor retinaculum of the hand.

**desomor'phine.** Dihydrodeoxymorphine-D; a morphine derivative with a shorter duration of analgesic action but greater addiction liability than morphine.

**des'ose.** Deoxy sugar.

**desoxy-.** For words beginning thus see under deoxy-, which has officially replaced most uses of desoxy- as a prefix denoting less oxygen.

**despeciation** (de-spe'shĭ-a'shun). 1. Alteration of, or loss of species characteristics. 2. The removal of species-specific antigenic properties from a foreign protein.

**D'Espine** (des-pēn'), Jean H. A., French physician, 1844–1931. See D'E.'s *sign.*

**despumation** (des-pu-ma'shun) [ L. *de-spumo,* pp. -*atus,* to skim, fr. *spumo,* to foam, fr. *spuma,* foam ]. 1. The rising of impurities to the surface of a liquid. 2. The skimming off of impurities on the surface of a liquid.

**desquamate** (des'kwă-māt) [ L. *desquamo*, pp. *-atus*, to scale off, fr. *squama*, a scale ]. To shred, peel, or scale off, as the casting off of the epidermis in scales or shreds, or the shedding of the outer layer of any surface.

**desquamation** (des'kwă-ma'shun). The shedding of the cuticle in scales.

**desquamative** (des-kwam'ă-tiv). Relating to or marked by desquamation from the skin or other surface.

**dest.** Abbreviation for L. *destilla*, distil, or *destillatus*, distilled, fr. *de-stilla*, to trickle down, distil.

**desternalization** (de-ster'nal-ĭ-za'shun). Separation of the sternum from the costal cartilages.

**desthiobiotin** (des'thi-o-bi'o-tin). A compound derived from biotin by the removal of the sulfur atom; can substitute for biotin in some microorganisms, but is without effect on or is inhibitory to the growth of others.

**destrudo** (de-stru'do) [ an artificial coinage on the analogy of *libido* fr. L. *destruere*, to destroy ]. The energy associated with the death or destructive instinct; opposite of libido.

**desulf'hydrases.** Enzymes or groups of enzymes catalyzing the removal of a molecule of $H_2S$ or substituted $H_2S$ from a compound; an example is the conversion of cysteine to pyruvic acid by cysteine desulfhydrase, better known as cystathionine γ-lyase (EC 4.4.1.1).

**desul'finase.** Term sometimes applied to the enzyme(s) removing sulfite (1) from cisteinesulfinate, an intermediate in cysteine degradation, yielding alanine or, by additional enzyme action, pyruvate and $NH_3$; and (2) from sulfinylpyruvate, postulated to be formed by deamination of cysteinesulfinate, yielding pyruvate. See aspartate 4-decarboxylase, which, in bacteria, can degrade cysteinesulfinic acid to alanine and $SO_2$ (reaction 1). Reaction 2, the degradation of sulfinylpyruvate, is now considered to be spontaneous, not requiring an enzyme.

**desul'furase.** Desulfhydrase.

**det.** Abbreviation, used in prescriptions, of Lat. *detur*, let there be given.

**detach'ment.** 1. A voluntary or involuntary separation from normal associations or environment. 2. Separation of a structure from its support.

**retinal d., d. of retina,** ablatio retinae; amotio retinae; separation of more or less of the retina from the choroid.

**exudative retinal d.,** d. of the retina that occurs without retinal breaks; it stems from inflammatory disease of choroid, retinal tumors, and retinal angiomatosis.

**rhegmatogenous retinal d.,** retinal separation precipitated by a hole or tear in the retina.

**detergent** (de-ter'jent) [ L. *de-tergeo*, pp. *-tersus*, to wipe off ]. 1. Cleansing. 2. A cleansing or purging agent, usually salts of long chain aliphatic bases or acids such as quaternary ammonium or sulfonic acid compounds, which, through a surface action that depends on possessing both hydrophilic and hydrophobic properties, exert cleansing (oil-dissolving) and antibacterial effects. The acridine derivatives, *e.g.*, acriflavine and proflavine, as well as other dyes, *e.g.*, brilliant green and crystal violet, have detergent properties for the same reasons.

**anion'ic d.'s.,** d.'s such as soaps (alkali metal salts of long chain fatty acids) that carry a negative electric charge on a lipid-like molecule and exert a limited antibacterial effect.

**cation'ic d.'s,** d.'s, such as the amine salts or quaternary ammonium or pyridinium compounds of long chain fatty acids, that carry positive electric charges on their hydrophobic groups.

**deterioration** (de-tēr'ĭ-o-ra'shun) [ L. *deterior*, worse ]. 1. The process or condition of becoming worse. 2. In psychiatry, dementia.

**alcoholic d.,** emotional blunting, organic defects, and d. in the moral sphere, occurring in persons chronically addicted to the use of alcohol.

**senile d.,** a slowly progressing decline in physical and mental health, apparently due to natural causes attendant upon the processes of aging.

**deter'minant** [ L. *determans*, determining, limiting ]. The factor that determines any given quality.

**antigenic d.,** determinant group; the particular chemical group of a molecule that determines immunological specificity.

**deter'mina'tion** [ L. *de-termino*, pp. *-atus*, to limit, determine, fr. *terminus*, a boundary ]. 1. A change, for the better or for the worse, in the course of a disease. 2. A general move toward a given point. 3. The measurement or estimation of any quantity or quality in scientific investigation, *e.g.*, of the calcium or of the sugar concentration of the serum or blood.

**determinism** (de-ter'mĭ-nizm). The proposition that all behavior is dependent on genetic and environmental influences and independent of free will.

**psychic d.,** in psychoanalysis, the concept that all psychological phenomena result from antecedent, unconsciously operating causes.

**deter'sive.** Detergent.

**dethyroidism** (de-thi'roy-dizm). See athyroidism.

**De Toni,** G. See D. T.-Fanconi *syndrome*.

**detor'sion.** Detortion.

**detortion** (de-tor'shun) [ L. *de-torqueo*, pp. *-tortus*, to turn or twist aside ]. Detorsion; rarely used terms for (1) tortional *deformity*, and (2) *derotation*.

**detoxicate** (de-tok'sĭ-kāt) [ L. *de*, from, + *toxicum*, poison ]. Detoxify; to diminish or remove the poisonous quality of any substance; to lessen the virulence of any pathogenic organism.

**detoxica'tion.** 1. Recovery from the toxic effects of a drug. 2. Removal of the toxic properties from a poison. 3. Metabolic conversion of pharmacologically active principles to pharmacologically less active principles.

**detox'ify.** Detoxicate.

**detrition** (de-trish'un) [ L. *de-tero*, pp. *-tritus*, to rub off ]. A wearing away by use or friction.

**detri'tus** [ L. (see detrition) ]. Any broken-down material, carious or gangrenous matter, gravel, etc.

**detrothy'ronine.** Dextrothyroxine sodium.

**detruncation** (de'trung-ka'shun) [ L. *de-trunco*, pp. *-atus*, to lop off, mutilate, fr. *truncus*, the bare trunk (of a tree) ]. Decapitation; removal and delivery of the trunk of the fetus.

**detru'sor** [ L. *detrudo*, to drive away ] [ NA ]. A muscle that has the action of expelling a substance.

**d. uri'nae** *musculus* detrusor urinae.

**detumescence** (de-tu-mes'ens) [ L. *de*, from, + *tumesco*, to swell up, fr. *tumeo*, to swell ]. Subsidence of a swelling.

**deut-.** See deutero-.

**deutencephalon** (du'ten-sef'ă-lon) [ G. *deuteros*, second, + *enkephalos*, brain ]. Rarely used synonym for diencephalon.

**deu'teranolo'pia.** Deuteranomaly.

**deuteranomaly** (du'ter-ă-nom'ă-lĭ) [ G. *deuteros*, second, + *anōmalia*, anomaly ]. Subnormal appreciation of green.

**deuteranope** (du'ter-ă-nōp). A person affected with deuteranopia.

**deuteranopia** (du'ter-ă-no'pĭ-ah) [ G. *deuteros*, second, + *anopia* ]. Green blindness; achloropsia; a form of dichromatism in which red, orange, yellow and green cannot be differentiated when their brightness and saturations are equal.

**deu'terate.** 1. A substance containing heavy hydrogen. 2. To incorporate heavy hydrogen into a substance.

**deuterio-.** Prefix indicating "containing deuterium."

**deuterium** (du-tēr'ĭ-um) [ G. *deuteros*, second ]. Hydrogen-2.

**d. oxide,** heavy *water*.

**deu'terize.** Deuterate.

**deutero-, deuto-, deut-** [ G. *deuteros*, second ]. Combining forms meaning two, or second (in a series).

**deuteron** (du'ter-on). Deuton; diplon; the nucleus of $^2H$. Composed of one neutron and one proton, it thus has one positive charge.

**deuteropathic** (du'ter-o-path'ik). Relating to a secondary affection, or deuteropathy.

**deuteropathy** (du'ter-op'ă-thĭ) [ deutero- + G. *pathos*, suffering ]. A secondary disease or symptom.

**deuteroplasm** (du'ter-o-plazm) [ deutero- + G. *plasma*, thing formed ]. Deutoplasm.

**deu'teropor'phyrin.** A porphyrin derivative resembling the protoporphyrins except that the two vinyl side chains are replaced by hydrogen.

**deuteroproteose** (du'ter-o-pro'te-ōz). Secondary proteose, resembling peptone more nearly than native protein.

**deuterotocia** (du-ter-o-to'sĭ-ah) [ deutero- + G. *tokos*, childbirth ]. Deuterotoky; a form of parthenogenesis in which the female has offspring of both sexes.

**deuterotoky** (du-ter-ot'o-kī). Deuterotocia.

**deuterotoxin** (du'ter-o-tok'sin). A hypothetical form of toxin in certain bacterial cultures, which has less marked affinity for antitoxin than has prototoxin.

**deutiodide** (du-ti'o-dĭd). Diiodide.

**deutipara** (du-tip'ă-rah) [ deutero- + L. *pario*, to bear ]. Secundipara.

**deuto-** (du'to-). See deutero-.

**deutobro'mide.** Of two compounds of bromine with a particular element or atom grouping, the one containing the greater number of bromine atoms.

**deutochlo'ride.** Bichloride.

**deutogenic** (du'to-jen'ik) [ deuto- + G. suffix *-gen*, production ]. Of secondary origin following an inductive influence.

**deutoiodide** (du-to-i'o-dĭd). Diiodide.

**deutom'erite** [ deuto- + L. *meros*, part ]. The posterior nucleated portion of an attached cephalont, separated by an ectoplasmic septum from the anterior portion, or protomerite.

**deuton** (du'ton). Deuteron.

**deutoplasm** (du'to-plazm) [ deuto- + G. *plasma*, thing formed ]. Deuteroplasm; the yolk of a meroblastic egg; the nonliving material in the cytoplasm, especially that stored in the ovum as food for the developing embryo; the commonest types are lipoid droplets and yolk granules.

**deutoplas'mic.** Relating to the deutoplasm.

**deutoplasmigenon** (du'to-plaz-mĭ-jen'on) [ deutoplasm + G. *genos*, birth ]. That which produces or gives rise to deutoplasm.

**deutoplasmolysis** (du'to-plaz-mol'ĭ-sis) [ deutoplasm + G. *lysis*, dissolution ]. The disintegration of deutoplasm.

**Deutschländer** (doych'lahn-der), Carl E. W., German surgeon, 1872–1942. See D.'s *disease*.

**devas'culariza'tion** [ L. *de*, away, + *vasculus*, small vessel, + G. *izo*, to cause ]. The removal of all or most of the blood vessels from any part or organ.

**devel'opment.** The act or process of natural progression from a previous, lower, or embryonic stage to a later, more complex, or adult stage.

  **psychosexual d.,** maturation and development of the psychic phase of sexuality from birth to adult life through the oral, anal, phallic, latency, and genital phases.

**Deventer,** Hendrik van, Dutch obstetrician, 1651–1724. See D.'s *diameters, pelvis.*

**deviance** (de'vī-ans) [ see deviation ]. Departure from an accepted norm, role, or rule.

  **psychiatric d.,** departure from accepted norms of mental health; see also mental *illness.*

  **role d.,** social d.

  **sexual d.,** departure from accepted sexual norms, for example, exhibitionism, homosexuality; this is a more modern term for what used to be called perversion.

  **social d.,** role d.; departure from accepted social norms; for example, being a hobo.

**deviation** (de-vī-a'shun) [ L. *devio*, to turn from the straight path, fr. *de*, from, + *via*, way ]. 1. Deflection; a turning away or aside from the normal point or course. 2. An abnormality. 3. In psychiatry, deviance. 4. A statistical measure representing the difference between an individual value in a set of values and the mean value in that set.

  **axis d.,** deflection of the electrical axis of the heart to the right or left of the normal; see also left axis d., right axis d., and related subentries under axis.

  **conjugate d. of the eyes,** (1) the turning of eyes equally and simultaneously in the same direction, as occurs normally; (2) a condition in which both eyes are pathologically turned to the same side as a result of either paralysis or muscular spasm.

  **immune d.,** split tolerance; the process in which a soluble protein antigen in Freund'complete adjuvant induces a sensitivity of the cell-dependent (delayed) kind in a normal guinea pig, but induces sensitivity of the antibody-dependent (immediate) kind in a guinea pig on which sensitivity of that (immediate) kind has already been induced by a previous injection of the soluble antigen without adjunct.

  **d. to the left,** *shift* to the left.

  **left axis d.,** a mean electrical axis of the heart pointing above − 30°; see hexaxial reference *system.*

  **primary d.,** the direction of the squinting eye away from the object when the latter is fixed by the sound eye.

  **d. to the right,** *shift* to the right.

  **right axis d.,** a mean electrical axis of the heart pointing to the right of + 90°; see hexaxial reference *system.*

  **secondary d.,** the turning of the normal eye away from the object when the latter is fixed by the squinting eye.

  **skew d.,** a hypertropia in which the eyes move in opposite directions equally.

  **standard d.,** abbreviated SD; symbol $\sigma$; statistical index of the degree of d. from central tendency; namely, of the variability within a distribution. It is the square root of the average of the squared deviations from the mean.

  **Vulpian's conjugate d.,** a turning of the head and eyes toward one side, occasionally observed after an apoplectic attack.

**Devic,** Eugène, French physician, †1930. See D.'s *disease.*

**device** (de-vīs). A contrivance, usually mechanical, designed to perform a specific function.

  **central-bearing d.,** a d. which provides a central point of bearing, or support, between upper and lower record bases. It consists of a contacting point which is attached to one base and a plate attached to the other which provides the surface on which the bearing point rests or moves.

  **central-bearing tracing d.,** a central-bearing d. used for making a tracing and/or for support between upper and lower bases.

  **intrauterine d.'s,** intrauterine contraceptive d.'s; abbreviated IUD or IUCD; pieces of plastic or metal having various shapes, such as a coil, loop, or bow, inserted into the uterus to exert a contraceptive effect; the means by which conception is prevented is not known.

**devil's grip** (sometimes erroneously spelled **grippe**). Epidemic *pleurodynia.*

**Devine,** Sir Hugh B., Australian surgeon, \*1878. See D. *exclusion.*

**de'viom'eter.** A form of strabismometer.

**devisceration** (de-vis-er-a'shun). Evisceration.

**devitalization** (de-vi'tal-ĭ-za'shun). 1. Deprivation of vitality or of vital properties. 2. In dentistry, the process by which a pulp is destroyed; *e.g.,* by chemical means, by infection, or by extirpation.

**devi'talize.** To deprive of vitality or of vital properties.

**devi'talized.** Devoid of life; dead.

**devolution** (dev'o-lu'shun) [ L. *de-volvo*, pp. -*volutus*, to roll down ]. 1. Involution. 2. Catabolism. 3. Degeneration.

**De Vries' theory.** See under theory.

**Dewar** (du'ar), Sir James, English chemist, 1842–1923. See D. *flask.*

**de Wecker's scissors.** See under scissors.

**dex'ameth'asone** (USP, BP). DECADRON, DERONIL, GAMMACORTEN; 9α-fluoro-16α-methylprednisolone; a synthetic analogue of cortisol, with similar biological action. Used as an anti-inflammatory agent.

  **d. sodium phosphate** (USP), DECADRON phosphate; the water-soluble ester of d., with the same actions and uses.

**dex'brompheni'ramine maleate** (NF). DISOMER; *d*-2-[ *p*-bromo-α-(2-dimethylaminoethyl)benzyl ]pyridine maleate; the dextrorotatory isomer of brompheniramine. Its antihistaminic activity is twice that of the racemic mixture.

**dex'chlorpheni'ramine maleate** (NF). POLARAMINE maleate; dextro- (or *d*-) chlorpheniramine; *d*-2-[ *p*-chloro-α-(2-dimethylaminoethyl)benzyl ]pyridine maleate; the dextrorotatory isomer of chlorpheniramine. Its antihistaminic activity is twice that of the racemic mixture.

**dexiocar'dia.** Dextrocardia.

**dexiv'acaine** (USAN). DEXACAINE; $d$-1-methyl-2',6'-pipecoloxylidide; anesthetic.

**dexpan'thenol** (USAN). ILOPAN; D-(+)-2,4-dihydroxy-N-(3-hydroxypropyl)-3,3-dimethylbutyramide; a cholinergic drug that produces miosis.

**dexter** (deks'ter) [ L. f. *dextra*, neut. *dextrum* ] [ NA ]. Right (abbreviation, D.).

**dextr-.** See dextro-.

**dex'trad** [ L. *dexter*, right, + *ad*, to ]. Toward the right side.

**dex'tral.** A right-handed person.

**dextral'ity.** Right-handedness.

**dex'tran.** 1 (BP). EXPANDEX; GENTRAN; a water-soluble, high molecular weight glucose polymer produced by the action of *Leuconostoc mesenteroides* on sucrose; average molecular weight 75,000. Used in isotonic sodium chloride solution for the treatment of shock, and in distilled water for the relief of the edema of nephrosis. 2. Lower molecular weight dextran (average, 40,000); has been found to improve blood flow in areas of stasis by reducing cellular aggregation. 3. Poly($\alpha$-1,6-glucose); $\alpha$-1,6-glucan with branch points (1.2; 1.3; 1.4) and spacing of these characteristic of the species; used as plasma substitutes or expanders (see dextransucrase).

**d. 40** (NF, BP), GENTRAN-40; d. with average molecular weight of 40,000; used as a plasma volume extender and blood flow adjuvant.

**d. 70** (USAN), MACRODEX; d. with average molecular weight of 70,000; used as a plasma volume expander.

**d. 75** (NF), GENTRAN-75; d. with an average molecular weight of 75,000; used as a plasma volume extender.

**d. 110** (BP), d. with average molecular weight of 110,000, available as 5 per cent solution in water or saline solution; used as a plasma volume expander.

**animal d.,** glycogen.

**d. sulfate** (BP), the sodium salt of sulfuric acid esters of the polysaccharide d. It contains not less than 10 units per mg. and not less than 14 per cent of sulfate. An anticoagulant.

**dex'tranase** (EC 3.2.1.11). Enzyme hydrolyzing 1,6-$\alpha$-glucosidic linkages in dextran, similar to older amylopectin 1,6-glucosidase.

**dex'transu'crase.** A glucosyltransferase (EC 2.4.1.5) that builds poly(1,6-$\alpha$-D-glucosyl), *i.e.*, polyglucoses or dextrans or $\alpha$-glucans, from sucrose, releasing D-fructose residues.

**dex'trase.** Nonspecific term for the complex of enzymes that converts dextrose (glucose) into lactic acid.

**dex'trifer'ron.** ASTRAFER; a colloidal solution of ferric hydroxide in complex with partially hydrolyzed dextrin. Used in the treatment of iron-deficiency anemia; it is suitable for intravenous administration and contains 20 mg. of iron per ml.

**dex'trin.** British gum; starch gum; a mixture of oligo($\alpha$-1,4-glucose) molecules formed during the enzymic or acid hydrolysis of starch, amylopectin, or glycogen. On further hydrolysis they are converted into glucose. Dextrin (usually white dextrin) is used in pharmaceutical preparations. Dextrins are of much lower molecular weight than dextrans, hence are not suitable as plasma expanders; *cf.* dextran (3) and limit dextrin.

**limit d.,** also called dextrin limit; the polysaccharide fragments remaining at the end (limit) of exhaustive hydrolysis of amylopectin or glycogen by $\alpha$-1,4-glucan maltohydrolase, which cannot hydrolyze the $\alpha$-1,6 bonds at branch points (*cf.* dextrin).

**dex'trinase.** Any of the enzymes catalyzing the hydrolysis of dextrins; *cf.* dextranase.

**limit d.,** oligo-1,6-glucosidase.

**dextrin dextranase.** Dextrin 6-glycosyltransferase; dextrin 6-glucosyltransferase; dextrin → dextran transglucosidase; a glucosyltransferase (EC 2.4.1.2) transferring 1,4-$\alpha$-D-glucosyl residues, thus catalyzing the synthesis of dextrans (with 1,6 links between monosaccharide units) from dextrins (with 1,4 links) by glucose transfer.

**dextrin → dextran transglucosidase.** Dextrin dextranase.

**dextrin 6-$\alpha$-glucosidase.** Amylo-1,6-glucosidase.

**dextrin 6-glucosyltransferase.** Dextrin dextranase.

**dextrin glycosyltransferase.** 4-$\alpha$-Glucanotransferase.

**dextrin 6-glycosyltransferase.** Dextrin dextranase.

**dex'trinogen'ic.** Starch-liquefying; dextrin-producing.

**dex'trino'sis.** Glycogenosis.

**debrancher deficiency limit d.,** type 3 *glycogenosis*.

**limit d.,** type 3 *glycogenosis.*

**dextrin transglycosylase.** 4-$\alpha$-Glucanotransferase.

**dextrinu'ria.** The passage of dextrin in the urine.

**dextrism** (deks'trizm). Right-handedness.

**dextro-** (deks'tro-) [ L. *dexter*, right ]. 1. A prefix meaning right, or toward or on the right side. 2. Chemical prefix meaning dextrorotatory; see also *d-*.

**dex'troamphet'amine phosphate** (NF). $d$-Amphetamine phosphate; monobasic d. phosphate; monobasic $d$-$\alpha$-methylphenethylamine phosphate. Same actions and uses as dextroamphetamine sulfate.

**dex'troamphet'amine sulfate** (USP). $d$-Amphetamine sulfate; dexamphetamine (BP); DEXEDRINE sulfate; (+)-$\alpha$-methylphenethylamine sulfate; similar in action to racemic amphetamine sulfate, but is more stimulating to the central nervous system; sympathomimetic and appetite depressant.

**dextrocardia** (deks'tro-kar'di-ah) [ dextro- + G. *kardia*, heart ]. Displacement of the heart to the right. There are two types; one in which the heart is simply displaced to the right, and another (cardiac heterotaxia) in which there is complete transposition, the "left" cardiac chambers being on the right and the "right" chambers on the left; the heart thus presents a mirror picture of the normal.

**corrected d.,** false d.; type 3 d.; displacement and rotation of the heart into the right side of the chest but without mirror transposition of the cardiac chambers.

**false d.,** corrected d.

**isolated d.,** type 2 d.; d. with mirror transposition of the cardiac chambers but without displacement of the abdominal viscera.

**secondary d.,** dextroposition of the heart.

**d. with situs inversus,** displacement of the heart to the right side of the chest with mirror transposition of the cardiac chambers together with transposition of the abdominal viscera.

**type 1 d.,** d. with situs inversus.

**type 2 d.,** isolated d.

**type 3 d.,** corrected d.,

**type 4 d.,** dextroposition of the heart.

**dex'trocar'diogram.** That part of the electrocardiogram that is derived from the right ventricle.

**dextrocerebral** (deks'tro-ser'e-bral). Having a dominant right cerebral hemisphere.

**dextroclination** (deks'tro-kli-na'shun). Dextrotorsion (2).

**dextrocular** (deks-trok'u-lar) [ dextro- + L. *oculus*, eye ]. Right-eyed; denoting one who uses the right eye by preference in monocular work, such as the use of the microscope.

**dextroduction** (deks'tro-duk'shun) [ dextro- + L. *duco*, pp. *ductus*, to lead ]. Rotation of an eye toward the right.

**dex'trogas'tria** [ dextro- + G. *gaster*, stomach ]. A condition in which the stomach is displaced to the right; usually associated with dextrocardia.

**dex'troglu'cose.** Dextrose; glucose.

**dex'trogram.** Electrocardiographic record in experimental animal supposedly representing spread of impulse through the right ventricle alone.

**dextrogyration** (deks'tro-ji-ra'shun) [ dextro- + L. *gyro*, pp. *-atus*, to turn in a circle, fr. *gyrus*. circle ]. A twisting to the right.

**dextroman'ual** [ dextro- + L. *manus*, hand ]. Right-handed.

**dex'trometh'orphan hydrobromide** (NF, BP). ROMILAR hydrobromide; hydrobromide of $d$-racemethorphan; $d$-3-methoxy-N-methylmorphinan hydrobromide. A synthetic morphine derivative used as an antitussive agent. It has no central depressant or analgesic action. It appears to have no addiction liability.

**dextromoramide tartrate** (BP). PALFIUM; DIMORLIN; a narcotic analgesic related chemically and pharmacologically to methadone.

**dextrop'edal** [ dextro- + L. *pes* (*ped*-), foot ]. Right-footed; denoting one who uses the right leg in preference to the left, in hopping, for instance.

**dextroposition** (deks'tro-po-zish'un). Abnormal right-sided location or origin of a normally left-sided structure, *e.g.*, origin of the aorta from the right ventricle.

**d. of the heart,** displacement of the heart into the right side of the chest by some disease of lungs, pleura, or diaphragm.

**dex'tropropox'yphene hydrochloride** (BP). Propoxyphene hydrochloride.

**dex'tropropox'yphene napsylate** (BP). *d*-Propoxyphene napsylate (see propoxyphene hydrochloride).

**dextrorotation** (deks'tro-ro-ta'shun). A turning or twisting to the right, used in particular of the clockwise twist given the plane of plane-polarized light by solutions of certain optically active substances.

**dextrorotatory** (deks'tro-ro'tă-to-rī). Turning the plane of polarization to the right, or clockwise, denoting certain crystals, solutions of dextrose, etc., capable of so doing.

**dex'trose** (USP, BP). Glucose.

**d. monohydrate** (BP), medicinal glucose; purified glucose.

**dex'trosinis'tral** [ dextro- + L. *sinister*, left ]. In a direction from right to left.

**dextrosu'ria.** Obsolete term for glycosuria.

**dex'trothyrox'ine sodium** (NF). D-Thyroxine sodium salt (see thyroxine); detrothyronine; BIOTIRMONE; CHOLOXIN; DETYROXIN; DETHYRONA; DETROID; an antihypercholesterolemic agent.

**dextrotorsion** (deks'tro-tor'shun) [ dextro- + L. *torsio*, a twisting ]. 1. A twisting to the right. 2. In ophthalmology, dextroclination; extorsion of the right eye or intorsion of the left eye.

**dextrotropic** (deks'tro-trop'ik) [ dextro- + G. *tropos*, a turn ]. Turning to the right.

**dextroversion** (deks'tro-ver'zhun) [ dextro- + L. *verto*, pp. *versus*, to turn ]. 1. Version (a turning) toward the right. 2. In ophthalmology, binocular conjugate movement to the right.

**d. of the heart,** corrected *dextrocardia.*

**dezymotize** (de-zi'mo-tiz) [ L. *de*, from, + G. *zymē*, leaven ]. To disinfect; to free from or destroy ferments.

**d'Herelle** (der-el'), Felix H., Canadian physician and bacteriologist in U.S.S.R., 1873–1949. See d'H. *phenomenon*, Twort-d'H. *phenomenon.*

**D. Hy.** Abbreviation for Doctor of Hygiene.

**di-** [ G. *dis*, two ]. Prefix denoting two, twice.

**Di.** Abbreviation for Diego blood group; see in appendix 2.

**dia-** [ G. *dia*, through ]. Prefix meaning through, throughout, completely. Distinguish from di- (two, or twice), from G. *dis.*

**diabetes** (di-ă-be'tēz) [ G. *diabētēs*, a compass, a siphon, diabetes. BAS- ]. Either d. insipidus or d. mellitus, diseases having in common the symptom polyuria. When used without qualification, it means d. mellitus.

**alimentary d.,** alimentary *glycosuria.*

**al'loxan d.,** experimental d. produced in animals by the administration of alloxan. The drug damages the insulin-producing islet cells of the pancreas.

**azot'ic d.,** baruria resulting from increased nitrogenous constituents of the urine.

**d. of bearded women,** Achard-Thiers *syndrome.*

**brittle d.,** d. that is labile, in which tolerance for carbohydrate and the need for insulin oscillate in an unpredictable fashion.

**bronzed d.,** hemochromatosis, with iron deposits in the skin, liver, and other viscera, often with severe liver damage and glycosuria.

**calcinu'ric d.,** hypercalcuria.

**cerebral d.,** cerebrosuria.

**conjugal d.,** d. affecting husband and wife at the same time.

**d. decip'iens** [ L. *decipere*, to cheat ]. masked d.; d. mellitus without polyuria and consequent thirst to indicate the presence of the disease.

**galactose d.,** galactosemia.

**growth-onset d. mellitus,** juvenile d.

**idiohypophysial d.,** the initial and reversible phase of d. mellitus produced by large quantities of endogenous or exogenous pituitary growth hormone.

**d. in'nocens,** renal *glycosuria.*

**d. insip'idus,** the chronic excretion of very large amounts of pale urine of low specific gravity, accompanied by extreme thirst; it ordinarily results from inadequate output of pituitary antidiuretic hormone, though it may be mimicked as a result of excessive fluid intake in emotionally disturbed individuals. See also hysterical *polydipsia.*

**insulinopenic d.,** any form of d. mellitus resulting from inadequate secretion of insulin.

**d. intermittens,** d. mellitus in which there are periods of relatively normal carbohydrate metabolism followed by relapses to the previous diabetic state.

**juvenile d.,** juvenile d. mellitus; growth-onset d. mellitus; severe d. mellitus, usually of abrupt onset during the first two decades of life. It is a form of brittle d. that is difficult to control, and insulin and dietary regulation are mandatory.

**juvenile d. mellitus,** juvenile d.

**latent d.,** a mild form of d. mellitus in which the patient displays no overt symptoms, but displays certain abnormal responses to diagnostic procedures, such as an elevated fasting blood glucose concentration or reduced glucose tolerance.

**lipoatrophic d.,** d. associated with loss or disappearance of fatty tissue.

**lipog'enous d.,** d. and obesity combined.

**masked d.,** d. decipiens.

**maturity-onset d.,** an often mild form of d. mellitus, of gradual onset in obese individuals over the age of 35. Most such individuals respond well to dietary regulation and/or oral hypoglycemic agents, but nevertheless often develop diabetic vascular complications and degenerative changes.

**d. melli'tus** [ L. sweetened with honey ], a metabolic disease in which carbohydrate utilization is reduced and that of lipid and protein enhanced. It is caused by deficiency of insulin and is characterized, in more severe cases, by glycosuria, water and electrolyte loss, ketoacidosis, and coma. Chronic complications include neuropathy, retinopathy, nephropathy, and generalized degenerative changes in large and small blood vessels.

**metahypophysial d.,** (1) d. mellitus caused by large quantities of endogenous or exogenous pituitary growth hormone; (2) term used to designate the irreversible phase of d. in acromegaly.

**Mosler's d.,** inosituria with excretion of large quantities of water.

**nephrogenic d. insipidus,** vasopressin-resistant d.; d. insipidus (*q.v.*) due to inability of the kidney tubules to respond to antidiuretic hormone; X-linked inheritance, full expression in males, partial defect in heterozygous females.

**pancreatic d.,** d. demonstrably dependent upon a pancreatic lesion; d. following removal of the pancreas in an animal.

**phlor'idzin** or **phlor'izin d.,** marked glycosuria without hyperglycemia following the experimental administration of phloridzin, which impairs renal tubular reabsorption of glucose.

**phosphat'ic d.,** phosphaturia; polyuria associated with emaciation, furunculosis, and other symptoms of d. mellitus, with an abnormal excretion of phosphates, but without glycosuria.

**piqûre d.** [ Fr. ], puncture d.

**pregnancy d.,** see subclinical d.

**puncture d.,** experimental d. produced in animals by puncture of the floor of the fourth ventricle of the brain.

**renal d.,** renal *glycosuria.*

**skin d.,** a term devised by Urbach to designate chronic skin lesions; he claimed to find a high fasting skin sugar level.

**starvation d.,** after prolonged fasting, glycosuria follows the ingestion of carbohydrate or glucose, because of reduced output of insulin or reduced ability to form glycogen.

**steroid d.,** d. produced by pharmacological doses of steroid hormones, particularly glucocorticoids or estrogens; characterized by one or more of the typical manifestations of d. mellitus.

**subclinical d.,** pseudodiabetes; a form of d. mellitus that is evident only under certain circumstances, such as pregnancy or extreme stress. Patients so afflicted may, in time, progress to the latent or overt forms of the disease.

**thiazide d.,** impaired carbohydrate metabolism associated with the use of thiazide diuretic drugs. Most severe manifestations are seen in patients having d. mellitus; impairment is mild or absent in nondiabetic individuals. The mechanism of thiazide action in causing this disorder is unknown.

**vasopressin-resistant d.,** nephrogenic d. insipidus.

**diabet'ic.** 1. Relating to or suffering from diabetes. 2. A subject of diabetes.

**diabetogenic** (di-ă-bet'o-jen'ik, -be'to-jen'ik). Causing diabetes.

**diabetogenous** (di-ă-bĕ-toj'en-us). Caused by diabetes.

**diabetometer** (di'ă-bĕ-tom'e-ter) [ diabetes + G. *metron,* measure ]. A form of polariscope devised for the determination of the presence and of the amount of sugar in urine.

**diabrosis** (di'ă-bro'sis) [ G. *diabrōsis,* ulceration, fr. *diabibrō-skō,* to eat up, akin to *brōmo,* food ]. A corrosion; perforation by an ulcer.

**diabrot'ic.** 1. Corroding. 2. A corrosive.

**diacele** (di'ah-sēl) [ G. *dia-,* through, + *koilia,* a hollow ]. *Ventriculus* tertius.

**diacetate** (di-as'ē-tāt). A salt or ester of diacetic (acetoacetic) acid (improper usage), or a compound containing two acetate residues.

**diacetemia** (di-as-ē-te'mĭ-ah). A form of acidosis resulting from the presence of acetoacetic (diacetic) acid in the blood.

**diacetic acid** (di-ă-se'tik, -ă-set'ik). *Acetoacetic* acid.

**diacetonuria** (di-as'ē-to-nu'rĭ-ah). Diaceturia.

**diaceturia** (di-as-ē-tu'rĭ-ah). Diacetonuria; the urinary excretion of acetoacetic (diacetic) acid.

**diacetyl** (di-as'ē-til). 2,3-Butanedione; a yellow liquid, $(CH_3CO)_2$, having the pungent odor of quinone.

**diac'etylmonox'ime.** DAM; a 2-oxo-oxime that can reactivate phosphorylated acetylcholinesterase *in vitro* and *in vivo;* it penetrates the blood-brain barrier.

**diac'etylmor'phine.** Heroin.

**diacid** (di-as'id). Denoting a substance containing two ionizable hydrogen atoms per molecule; or, more generally, a base capable of combining with two hydrogen ions per molecule.

**diaclasis, diaclasia** (di-ak'lă-sis, di-ă-kla'zĭ-ah) [ G. *diaklasis,* a breaking up, fr. *dia,* through, + *klasis,* a breaking ]. A fracture produced intentionally, usually for the correction of a deformity.

**di'aclast.** An instrument for craniectomy of a fetus.

**diacrinous** (di-ak'rĭ-nus) [ G. *dia-krinō,* to separate one from another ]. Excreting by simple passage through a gland cell; distinguished from ptyocrinous or apocrine.

**diacrisis** (di-ak'rĭ-sis) [ G. *dia-,* through, + *krisis,* a judgment ]. Diagnosis.

**diacritic, diacritical** (di'ă-krit'ik, -krit'ĭ-kal) [ G. *diakritikos,* able to distinguish ]. Distinguishing; diagnostic; allowing of distinction.

**diactinic** (di'ak-tin'ik) [ G. *dia,* through, + *aktis,* ray ]. Having the property of transmitting light capable of bringing about chemical reactions.

**diacylglyc'erol lip'ase.** Lipoprotein lipase; enzyme (EC 3.1.1.34) responsible for clearing the milky plasma of alimentary hyperlipemia by hydrolyzing the fats; its activity is enhanced by heparin and inactivated by heparinase. See also clearing *factor.*

**di'ad.** 1. The transverse tubule and a cisterna in cardiac muscle fibers. 2. Dyad.

**di'ader'mic** [ G. *dia,* through, + *derma,* skin ]. Percutaneous.

**diadochocine'sia.** Diadochokinesia.

**diadochokinesia, diadochokinesis** (di-ad'o-ko-kĭ-ne'zĭ-ah, -kĭ-ne'sis) [ G. *diadochos,* working in turn, + *kinēsis,* movement ]. The normal power of alternately bringing a limb into opposite positions, as of flexion and extention or of pronation and supination.

**diadochokinetic** (di-ad'o-ko-kĭ-net'ik). Relating to diadochokinesia.

**diagnose** (di-ag-nōz') [ G. *diagignōskō,* to distinguish ]. To determine the nature of a disease; to make a diagnosis.

**diagnosis** (di-ag-no'sis) [ G. *diagnōsis,* a deciding. GNO- ]. The determination of the nature of a disease.

**clinical d.,** a d. made from a study of the signs and symptoms of a disease.

**differential d.,** differentiation (2); the determination of which of two or more diseases with similar symptoms is the one from which the patient is suffering.

**d. by exclusion,** a d. made by excluding those affections to which some of the symptoms belong, leaving only one to which all the symptoms point; usually unsatisfactory.

**laboratory d.,** a d. made by a chemical, microscopic, bacteriologic, or biopsy study of secretions, discharges, blood, or tissue.

**pathologic d.** (1) a d. (sometimes a postmortem d.) made from a study of the lesions present; (2) a d. of the pathologic conditions present, determined by a study and comparison of the symptoms.

**physical d.,** a d. made by means of physical measures, such as auscultation, percussion, palpation, and inspection.

**topographic d.,** the determination of the seat of a disease.

**diagnos'tic.** Relating to or aiding in diagnosis.

**diagnostician** (di-ag-nos-tish'an). One who is experienced in making diagnoses.

**diagnos'ticum.** A preparation to be used in the performance of an experiment or test.

**diakinesis** (di'ă-kĭ-ne'sis) [ G. *dia,* through, + *kinēsis,* movement ]. The final stage of prophase in meiosis in which the chiasmata present during the diplotene stage disappear and the chromosomes continue to shorten.

**di'al** [ L. *dies,* day ]. A clock face or instrument resembling a clock face.

**astigmat'ic d.,** a diagram of radiating lines, used as a rough test for astigmatism; see fig. under astigmatism.

**dial'icor hydrochloride.** RELICOR; 2'-[ 2-(diethylamino)ethoxy ]-3-phenylpropiophenone hydrochloride; coronary vasodilator.

**Dialis'ter.** *Bacteroides; D. pneumosintes,* the type species of *D.,* is a member of the genus *Bacteroides.*

**D. pneumosin'tes,** *Bacteroides pneumosintes;* the type species of *D.*

**diallyl** (di-al'il). Denoting a compound containing two allyl groups.

**dialysance** (di-al'ĭ-sans) [ fr. dialysis ]. The number of milliliters of blood completely cleared of any substance by an artificial kidney or by peritoneal dialysis in a unit of time; conventional clearance formulas are expressed as milliliters per minute.

**dialysate** (di-al'ĭ-sāt). That part of the mixture that passes through the dialyzing membrane.

**dialysis** (di-al'ĭ-sis) [ G. a separation, fr. *dia-lyo,* to separate. LY- ]. 1. The separation of crystalloid from colloid substances (or smaller molecules from larger ones) in a solution by interposing a semipermeable membrane between the solution and water; the crystalloid (smaller) substances pass through the membrane into the water on the other side, the colloids do not. 2. Rarely used term for a fracture or rupture of continuity of soft parts.

**equilibrium d.,** in immunology, a method for determination of association constants for hapten-antibody reactions in a system in which the hapten (dialyzable) and antibody (nondialyzable) solutions are separated by semipermeable membranes. Since at equilibrium the quantity of free hapten will be the same in the two compartments, quantitative determinations can be made of hapten-bound antibody, free antibody, and free hapten.

**d. retinae,** disinsertion (2).

**dial'yzator.** An apparatus for carrying out dialysis.

**di'alyze.** To perform dialysis; to separate a substance from a solution by means of dialysis.

**di'alyzer.** A membrane for use in dialysis.

**diam'eter** [ G. *diametros,* fr. *dia,* through, + *metron,* measure ]. 1. A straight line connecting two opposite points on the surface of a more or less spherical or cylindrical body, or at the boundary of an opening or foramen, passing through the center of such body or opening. 2. The distance measured along such a line.

**Baudelocque's d.,** external *conjugate.*

**biparietal d.,** the distance between the two parietal eminences.

**buccolingual d.,** the d. of the crown of a tooth measured from the buccal to the lingual surfaces.

**conjugate d.,** conjugata.

**Deventer's d.'s,** the oblique d.'s of the pelvic inlet.

**d.'s of fetal skull,** see fig. under skull.

**d. media'nus,** conjugata.

**d. obli'qua** [ NA ], oblique d.; a measurement across the pelvic inlet from the sacroiliac joint of one side to the opposite iliopectineal eminence.

**oblique d.,** d. obliqua.

**trachelobregmatic d.,** the d. of the fetal head from the middle of the anterior fontanelle to the neck.

**d. transver'sa** [ NA ], transverse d.; the transverse d. of the pelvic inlet, measured between the terminal lines.

**transverse d.,** d. transversa.

**zygomatic d.,** the extreme breadth of the skull at the zygomatic arches.

**diamide** (di'ă-mīd, di'ă-mid). A compound containing two amide groups.

**diam'idines.** 1. A group of drugs, including stilbamidine, propamidine, and pentamidine, used as chemotherapeutic agents in the treatment of protozoal diseases, especially trypanosomiasis and leishmaniasis, and in systemic fungus infections, *e.g.,* blastomycosis. 2. Compounds containing two amidine groups.

**diamine** (di'ă-mēn, di'ă-min). An organic compound containing two amine groups per molecule; *e.g.,* ethylenediamine, $NH_2CH_2CH_2NH_2$.

**d. oxidase,** amine oxidase (pyridoxal-containing).

**diamino oxyhydrase.** Amine oxidase (pyridoxal-containing).

**diaminu'ria.** The excretion of diamines in the urine.

**diam'ocaine cyclamate** (USAN). 1-(2-Anilinoethyl)-4-[ 2-(diethylamino)ethoxy ]-4-phenylpiperidine; a local anesthetic.

**Diamond,** Louis K., American physician, *1902. See D.-Blackfan *anemia.*

**diam'promide sulfate.** *N*-[ 2-(methylphenethylamino)-propyl ]propionanilide sulfate; analgesic.

**diam'thazole dihydrochloride.** ASTEROL dihydrochloride; 6-(2-diethylaminoethoxy)-2-dimethylaminobenzothiazole dihydrochloride; antifungal agent for topical use.

**diamy'celine hydrochloride.** FUTRICAN; 1-(*p*-chlorobenzyl)-2-methylbenzimidazole hydrochloride; antifungal agent.

**diam'ylene.** Dipentene.

**dianoetic** (di'ă-no-et'ik) [ G. *dia,* through, + *noein,* to think ]. Of or pertaining to reason or other intellectual functions.

**diap'amide** (USAN). VECTREN; 4-chloro-*N*-methyl-3-(methylsulfamoyl)benzamide; diuretic with antihypertensive action.

**diapause** (di'ă-pawz). A period of biological quiescence or dormancy; an interval in which development is arrested or greatly slowed.

**embryonic d.,** a d. in the course of embryogenesis; postulated to occur in instances of double parturition and possibly of delayed implantation.

**diapedesis** (di'ă-pĕ-de'sis) [ G. *dia,* through, + *pēdēsis,* a leaping ]. The passage of blood, or any of its formed elements, through the intact walls of blood vessels.

**diaphanometer** (di-af'ă-nom'e-ter) [ G. *diaphanēs,* transparent, + *metron,* measure ]. An instrument for testing fluids by means of measuring their varying degrees of transparency.

**diaphanometry** (di-af'ă-nom'e-trī) [ G. *diaphanēs,* transparent, + *metron,* measure ]. The determination of the degree of translucency of a fluid, such as the urine.

**diaphanoscope** (di-af'ă-no-skōp) [ G. *diaphanēs,* transparent, + *skopeō,* to examine ]. Polyscope; an instrument for illuminating the interior of a cavity in order to determine the translucency of its walls.

**diaphanoscopy** (di-af'ă-nos'ko-pī). Examination of a cavity, such as the antrum of Highmore, by means of the diaphanoscope.

**diaphemetric** (di'ă-fĕ-met'rik) [ G. *dia,* through, + *haphē,* touch, + *metron,* measure ]. Relating to the determination of the degree of tactile sensibility.

**di'aphen hydrochloride.** 2-Diethylaminoethyl α-chlorodiphenylacetate hydrochloride; antihistaminic agent with anticholinergic properties.

**diaph'orase.** Originally, a series of flavoproteins with reductase activity in mitochondria; now lipoamide dehydrogenase.

**diaphoresis** (di'ă-fo-re'sis) [ G. *diaphorēsis,* fr. *dia,* through, + *phoreō,* to carry. PHER- ]. Perspiration (1).

**diaphoret'ic.** 1. Relating to, or causing, perspiration. 2. An agent that increases the secretion of the sweat.

**diaphragm** (di'ah-fram) [ G. *diaphragma, q.v.* ]. 1. Diaphragma (2). 2. A thin disk pierced with a hole of definite size, used in a microscope, camera, or other optical instrument in order to shut out the marginal rays of light, thus giving a more direct illumination. 3. A flexible metal ring covered with a dome-shaped sheet of elastic material used in the vagina to prevent pregnancy.

**Bucky d.,** a d. with moving grids that avoid grid shadows in roentgenograms.

**pelvic d.,** *diaphragma* pelvis.

**d. of sella,** *diaphragma* sellae.

**urogenital d.,** *diaphragma* urogenitale.

**diaphragma,** pl. **diaphragmata** (di-ah-frag'mah) [ G. *diaphragma,* a partition wall, midriff. PHRAG- ] [ NA ]. 1. A thin partition separating adjacent regions. 2. Diaphragm; midriff; phren (1); the musculomembranous partition between the abdominal and thoracic cavities.

**d. pelvis** [ NA ], diaphragm of the pelvis; pelvic diaphragm; composed of the paired levator ani and coccygeus muscles together with the fascia above and below them.

**d. sel'lae** [ NA ], diaphragm of the sella; tentorium of the hypophysis; a fold of dura mater extending transversely across the sella turcica and roofing over the hypophysis; it is perforated in its center for the passage of the infundibulum.

**d. urogenita'le** [ NA ], urogenital diaphragm; a triangular sheet of muscle between the ischiopubic rami; composed of the sphincter urethrae, and the deep transverse perineal muscles.

**diaphragmalgia** (di'ah-frag-mal'jī-ah) [ diaphragm + G. *algos,* pain ]. Diaphragmodynia; pain in the diaphragm.

**diaphragmatic** (di'ah-frag-mat'ik). Relating to the diaphragm.

**diaphragmatitis** (di'ah-frag-mă-ti'tis). Inflammation of the diaphragm.

**diaphragmatocele** (di'ah-frag-mat'o-sēl) [ diaphragm + G. *kēlē,* hernia ]. Diaphragmatic *hernia.*

**diaphragmi'tis.** Diaphragmatitis.

**diaphysectomy** (di'ă-fī-sek'to-mī) [ diaphysis + G. *ektome,* excision ]. Removal of more or less of the shaft of a long bone.

**diaphysial** (di-ă-fiz'ī-al). Relating to the diaphysis.

**diaphysis,** pl. **diaph'yses** (di-af'ī-sis) [ G. a growing between. PHYS- ] [ NA ]. The shaft of a long bone, as distinguished from the epiphyses, or extremities, and apophyses, or outgrowths.

**diaphysitis** (di-af-ī-si'tis). Inflammation of the shaft of a long bone.

**diapiresis** (di'ă-pi-re'sis) [ G. *diapeirō,* to drive through, fr. *peirō,* to pierce ]. The passage of colloidal or other small particles of suspended matter through the unruptured walls of the blood vessels; see diapedesis.

**di'aplacen'tal.** Passing through or "across" the placenta.

**diaplasis** (di-ap'lă-sis) [ G. a putting in shape. PLAS- ]. Diorthosis; setting of a fracture or reduction of a dislocation.

**diaplas'tic.** Pertaining to diaplasis.

**diaplex'us** [ G. *dia,* through, + L. *plexus,* a plaiting. PLIC- ]. Rarely used term for *plexus* choroideus ventriculi tertii.

**diapnoic, diapnotic** (di-ap-no'ik, -not'ik). 1. Relating to, or causing perspiration, especially insensible perspiration. 2. A mild sudorific.

**diapophysis** (di'ă-pof'ĭ-sis) [ G. *dia*, through, + *apophysis*, an offshoot. PHYS- ]. The upper articular surface of the transverse process of a vertebra.

**Diaptomus** (di-ap'to-mus). A genus of copepod crustacea, chief intermediate host for *Diphyllobothrium latum* in North America.

**diapyesis** (di-ă-pi-e'sis) [ G. fr. *dia*, through, + *pyon*, pus ]. Suppuration.

**diapyet'ic** [ G. *diapyetikos*. See diapyesis ]. 1. Relating to, or causing suppuration. 2. Anything provoking suppuration.

**diarrhea** (di-ah-re'ah) [ G. *diarrhoia*, fr. *dia*, through, + *rhoia*, a flow, a flux. RHE- ]. An abnormally frequent discharge of more or less fluid fecal matter from the bowel.

   **d. ablacto'rum,** d. occurring in infants at the time of weaning.

   **d. al'ba,** (1) celiac *disease;* (2) pullorum *disease.*

   **bovine virus d.,** a specific infectious disease of cattle, caused by a virus; characterized by ulceration of the mouth, pharynx, esophagus, and sometimes the stomachs and intestines, usually accompanied by severe d.

   **cholera'ic d.,** summer d.

   **d. chylo'sa,** celiac *disease.*

   **Co'chin China d.,** tropical *sprue.*

   **colliquative d.,** wasting d. associated with excessive discharge of fluid.

   **dysenter'ic d.,** d. in bacillary or amebic dysentery.

   **fatty d.,** d. seen in malabsorption, sprue, and chronic pancreatic disease.

   **gastrog'enous d.,** a d. which may occur in achylia gastrica, relieved by the administration of hydrochloric acid or, contrariwise, a d. caused by the excess secretion of gastric and other intestinal juices.

   **hill d.,** a morning d., attended with tympanites, affecting Europeans resident in India when visiting the mountains. In many parts of the world, d. occurs in visitors who are unaccustomed to the often informal conditions of sanitation, and the visitor is likely to name the d. after the place or the country where he has it.

   **lienter'ic d.,** d. in which undigested food appears in the stools.

   **morning d.,** a form in which there are several loose stools in the early morning and during the forenoon, the bowels being quiet during the remainder of the day and night.

   **mucous d.,** mucomembranous enteritis; d. with the presence of considerable mucus in the stools.

   **nocturnal d.,** d. that occurs chiefly at night, seen usually in association with diabetic neuropathy and alleged to be caused by lesions of the autonomic nervous system.

   **pan'creatog'enous d.,** d. in which the stools are bulky, pale, foul, greasy, and oily.

   **serous d.,** d. characterized by watery stools.

   **summer d.,** choleraic d.; summer complaint; d. of infants in hot weather; usually an acute gastroenteritis due to the presence of a microorganism of the *Shigella* or *Salmonella* groups.

   **traveler's d.,** d. of sudden onset and uncertain cause, lasting 1 to 3 days, occurring sporadically in travelers in all parts of the world, usually during the first week of a trip.

   **tropical d.,** tropical *sprue.*

   **vicarious d.,** d. caused by an attempt on the part of the system to relieve itself of water or excrementitious matters normally excreted by other channels.

   **watery d.,** serous d.

   **white d.,** (1) celiac *disease;* (2) pullorum *disease.*

**diarrheal** (di-ah-re'al). Relating to diarrhea.

**diarrheic** (di-ah-re'ik). Diarrheal.

**diarthric** (di-ar'thrik) [ G. *di-,* two, + *arthron,* joint ]. Biarticular; diarticular; relating to two joints.

**diarthrosis,** pl. **diarthro'ses** (di-ar-thro'sis) [ G. articulation. ARTH- ]. *Junctura* synovialis.

**diarticular** (di-ar-tik'u-lar). Diarthric.

**diaschisis** (di-as'kĭ-sis) [ G. a splitting. SCHI- ]. A sudden inhibition of function produced by an acute focal disturbance in a portion of the brain at a distance from the original seat of injury, but anatomically connected with it through fiber tracts.

**diascope** (di'ă-skōp) [ G. *dia,* through, + *skopeō,* to view ]. A flat glass plate through which, by means of pressure, one can examine superficial lesions.

**diascopy** (di-as'ko-pī) [ G. *dia,* through, + *skopeō,* to see ]. Examination of superficial lesions by means of the diascope.

**diastalsis** (di-ă-stal'sis) [ G. an arrangement. STAL- ]. The type of peristalsis in which a region of inhibition precedes the wave of contraction, as seen in the intestinal tract.

**diastal'tic.** Pertaining to diastalsis.

**diastase** (di'as-tās). A mixture, obtained from malt, containing amylolytic enzymes, principally α- and β-amylases (*q.v.*), converts starch into dextrin and maltose. Used to make soluble starches, and to aid in digestion of starches in certain types of dyspepsia.

**diastasis** (di-as'tă-sis) [ G. a separation. STA- ]. 1. Any simple separation of normally joined parts. 2. Separation of an epiphysis from the shaft of a long bone, occurring in the young without fracture of the bone. 3. The latter part of diastole when the blood enters the ventricle slowly and the venous pressure tends to rise.

   **d. rec'ti,** separation of recti abdominis.

**diastasuria** (di-as'tās-u'rī-ah). Amylasuria.

**diastat'ic.** Relating to a diastasis.

**diastema,** pl. **diaste'mata** (di'ă-ste'mah) [ G. *diastēma,* an interval, fr. *di-istēmi,* to set apart, fr. *dia* + *histēmi,* cause to stand. STA- ]. 1 [ NA ]. A fissure or abnormal opening in any part, especially if congenital. 2. A space between two adjacent teeth in the same dental arch. 3. A cleft or space between the maxillary lateral incisor and canine teeth, into which the lower canine is received when the jaws are closed; abnormal in man but normal in dogs and many other animals.

**diastematocrania** (di-ă-ste'mă-to-kra'nī-ah) [ G. *diastēma,* an interval, + *kranion,* skull ]. Congenital sagittal fissure of the skull.

**diastematomyelia** (di-ă-ste'mă-to-mi-e'lī-ah) [ G. *diastēma,* interval, + *myelon,* marrow ]. Diplomyelia in the bony spur; complete or incomplete sagittal division of spinal cord by osseous or fibrocartilaginous septum.

**diastematopyelia** (di-ă-ste'mă-to-pi-e'lī-ah) [ G. *diastēma,* interval, + *pyelos,* a trough (pelvis) ]. Congenital separation between the pubic bones.

**di'aster** [ G. *di-,* two, + *astēr,* star ]. The double star figure in mitosis, formed just before the division of the nucleus.

**diastereoisomers** (di'ă-stēr'e-o-i'so-merz). Optically active isomers that are not mirror images (*i.e.,* enantiomorphs); *e.g.,* glucose and galactose.

**diastole** (di-as'to-le) [ G. *diastolē,* dilation. STAL- ]. The dilation of the heart cavities, during which they fill with blood; d. of the atria precedes that of the ventricles; d. alternates rhythmically with systole or contraction of the heart musculature.

   **cardiac d.,** auxocardia.

   **gastric d.,** a somewhat fanciful name for a phase of relaxation of stomach peristalsis seen fluoroscopically or with the gastroscope.

**diastol'ic.** Relating to diastole.

**dias'trophism** [ G. *diastrophē,* fr. *diastrephein,* distortion ]. The distortion that occurs in objects as a result of bending.

**diataxia** (di'ă-tak'sī-ah). Ataxia affecting both sides of the body.

   **cerebral d.,** the ataxic type of cerebral birth palsy.

**diatela** (di-ă-te'lah) [ G. *dia,* through, between, + L. *tela,* web ]. Rarely used term for *tela* choroidea ventriculi tertii.

**diather'mal** [ G. *dia,* through, + *thermē,* heat ]. Diathermic.

**diather'mancy.** The condition of being diathermic.

**diather'manous** [ G. *dia-thermaino,* to heat through, fr. *thermos,* hot ]. Transcalent; permeable by heat rays.

**diather'mic.** Diathermal; relating to, characterized by, or affected by diathermy.

**diathermocoagulation** (di-ă-ther'mo-ko-ag-u-la'shun). Surgical *diathermy.*

**diathermy** (di'ă-ther'mī) [ G. *dia,* through, + *thermē,* heat ]. Transthermia; local mild elevation of temperature deep within the tissues, produced by high frequency current, ultrasonic waves, or microwave radiation.

**medical d.,** thermopenetration; d. of mild degree causing no destruction of tissue.

**short wave d.,** therapeutic elevation of temperature in the tissues by means of an oscillating electric current of extremely high frequency (10 to 100 million cycles per sec.) and a short wavelength of 3 to 30 meters.

**surgical d.,** diathermocoagulation; electrocoagulation with a high frequency electrocautery.

**diathesis** (di-ath'ĕ-sis) [ G. arrangement, condition. THE- ]. The constitutional or inborn state disposing to a disease, group of diseases, or metabolic or structural anomaly.

**contractural d.,** a tendency to contractures in hysteria.

**cystic d.,** a condition in which multiple cysts form in the liver, kidneys, and other organs.

**ex'udative d.,** a disposition to interstitial and subcutaneous serous or fibrinous infiltrations; the subjects suffer from swollen lymph nodes, thickening of the tongue, pruritus, seborrhea, and gastric and cardiac crises; the condition is aggravated by pilocarpine, but favorably affected by atropine and epinephrine.

**gouty d.,** inherited hyperuricemia predisposing to gout, usually appearing after puberty in males and, rarely, after the menopause in women.

**hemorrhagic d.,** any state with a tendency to spontaneous bleeding or bleeding from trivial trauma caused by a defect in clotting or a flaw in the structure of blood vessels.

**inopectic d.,** a state of body marked by a tendency to coagulation of fibrin resulting in thrombosis or embolism.

**neuropathic d.,** (1) obsolete for neurasthenia; (2) an inherited or congenital tendency to emotional instability.

**oxalic acid d.,** chronic oxalemia, with abnormally large amounts of oxalic acid derivatives in the urine.

**spasmodic d.,** a constitutional tendency to convulsions, especially in childhood.

**spasmophilic d.,** spasmophilia; a condition in which there is an abnormal mechanical or electrical excitability of the motor nerves, shown by a tendency to tetany, laryngeal spasm, or general convulsions.

**uric acid d.,** a supposed tendency to the formation of uric acid in excess, with resulting rheumatic and gouty symptoms.

**diathet'ic.** Relating to a diathesis.

**diathymosul'fone.** DIATOX; thymol sulfone; [ sulfonylbis-(p-phenyleneazo) ]dithymol; tuberculostatic agent.

**diatom** (di'ă-tom) [ G. diatomos, cut in two ]. An individual of microscopic unicellular algae, the shells of which compose a sedimentary infusorial earth.

**diatom'ic.** 1. Denoting a compound with a molecule made up of two atoms. 2. Denoting any ion or atomic grouping composed of two atoms only.

**diatoric** (di'ă-tor'ik) [ G. diatoros, pierced ]. 1. The vertical, cylindric aperture formed in the base of artificial porcelain teeth and extending into the body of the tooth. It serves as a mechanical means of attaching the tooth to the denture base. 2. A term used to describe teeth containing a diatoric.

**diatrizoate sodium.** See under sodium.

**diazasterol hydrochloride.** Azacosterol hydrochloride.

**diazepam** (di-āz'ĕ-pam) (USP, BP). VALIUM; 7-chloro-1,3-dihydro-1-methyl-5-phenyl- 2H-1,4-benzodiazepin-2-one; a skeletal muscle relaxant, sedative, and antianxiety agent; used to induce anesthesia by intravenous injection; also used as an anticonvulsant, particularly in the treatment of status epilepticus.

**di'azines.** A group of synthetic tuberculostatic drugs, such as pyrazine carboxamide and pyridazine-3-carboxamide.

**diazo-** (di-az'o-, di-a'zo-) [ G. di-, two, + Fr. azote, nitrogen. ZO- ]. A prefix denoting a compound containing the —N=N— or —N≡N+ group.

**diazo compound.** Azo compound.

**diaz'otize.** To introduce the diazo group into a chemical compound, usually through the treatment of an amine with nitrous acid.

**diazox'ide** (USP). HYPERSTAT; 7-chloro-3-methyl-2H-1,2,4-benzothiadiazine-1,1-dioxide; an antihypertensive agent used in the treatment of hypoglycemic states.

**diba'sic.** Bibasic; having two replaceable hydrogen atoms, denoting an acid with two ionizable hydrogen atoms.

**dibenz'epin hydrochloride** (USAN). NOVERIL; 10-[ 2-(dimethylamino)ethyl ]-5,10-dihydro-5-methyl-11H-dibenzo[ b,e ][ 1,4 ]diazepin-11-one hydrochloride; antidepressant.

**dibenzhep'tropine citrate.** BRONTINE; 3-α[ (10,11-dihydro-5H-dibenzo[ a,d -cyclohepten-5-yl)oxy ]tropane citrate; antihistaminic agent with anticholinergic properties.

**diben'zopyr'idine.** Acridine.

**dibenzthi'one.** FUNGIPLEX; 3,5-dibenzyltetrahydro-2H-1,3,5-thiadiazine-2-thione; antifungal agent.

**Dibothriocephalus** (di-both'rĭ-o-sef'ă-lus) [ G. di-, two, + bothrion, dim. of bothros, a pit, + kephalē, head ]. A genus of Cestoidea or tapeworms; see Diphyllobothrium.

**dibromopropam'idine isethionate** (BP). BRULIDINE; 2-hydroxyethanesulfonic acid; compound with 4,4'-(trimethylenedioxy)bis(3-bromobenzamidine); antiseptic.

**dibrom'salan** (USAN). 4',5-Dibromosalicylamilide; component of DIAPHENE; a disinfectant.

**dibucaine hydrochloride.** CINCHOCAINE hydrochloride; NUPERCAINE hydrochloride; 2-n-butoxy-N-[ 2-(diethylamino)ethyl ]cinchoninamide monohydrochloride; local anesthetic (surface and spinal anesthesia). Official in the NF as dibucaine.

**dibucaine number.** Abbreviated DN; differentiates usual from atypical pseudocholinesterase in instances of abnormal response to succinylcholine by the percentage of inhibition of the enzyme by dibucaine; normal enzyme has a DN of 80, and homozygous atypical has a DN of 20.

**di'bunate sodium.** BECANTAL; mixture of 3,6- and 3,7-di-tert-butyl-1-napthalenesulfonic acid sodium salt; antitussive agent.

**dibu'pyrone.** (Antipyrinylisobutylamino)methanesulfonic acid sodium salt; analgesic.

**dibu'toline sulfate.** DIBULINE sulfate; dibutyl urethane of dimethylethyl-β-hydroxyethylammonium sulfate; an anticholinergic agent. Used as a mydriatic and cycloplegic, and as a gastrointestinal antispasmodic.

**dibu'tyl phthal'ate.** n-Butyl phthalate; di-n-butyl ester of benzene-o-dicarboxylic acid; insect repellent.

**dicarboxylic acid cycle.** See under cycle.

**dicelous, dicoelous** (di-se'lus) [ G. di-, two, + koilos, hollow ]. Having two cavities or excavations on opposite surfaces.

**dicen'tric.** Having two centromeres; see d. chromosome.

**diceph'alous.** Having two heads.

**dicephalus** (di-sef'ă-lus) [ G. di-, two, + kephalē, head ]. Bicephalus; diplocephalus; symmetrical conjoined twins with two separate heads.

**d. di'auchenos,** a d. with separate necks.

**d. di'pus dibra'chius,** a d. in which the merging of the bodies has obliterated the appendages on the side of the union, leaving only two arms and two legs for the double body.

**d. di'pus tetrabra'chius,** a d. with only two feet but four separate arms; duplicitas anterior.

**d. di'pus tribra'chius,** a d. with only two lower extremities but with three arms.

**d. dipygus,** a d. with body double below the umbilicus.

**d. mon'auchenos,** a d. in which fusion has involved the cervical region so that the two heads are on a single neck.

**dicheilia, dichilia** (di-ki'lĭ-ah) [ G. di-, two, + cheilos, lip ]. A lip appearing to be double because of the presence of an abnormal fold.

**dicheiria, dichiria** (di-ki'rĭ-ah) [ G. di-, two, + cheir, hand ]. Diplocheiria; complete or incomplete duplication of the digits of the hand; see also polydactyly.

**dicheirus, dichirus** (di-ki'rus). An individual with dicheiria.

**dichloralphenazone** (BP). Dichloralantipyrine; a complex of chloral hydrate and phenazone; sedative and hypnotic.

**dichloramine-T.** Dichloramine; p-toluenesulfonic acid dichloramide; $CH_3C_6H_4SO_2NCl_2$; used as an antiseptic in surgical dressings, but may cause irritation of wounds.

**dichlor'isone.** DISODERM; 9α,11β-dichloro-17α,21-dihydroxy-1,4-pregnadiene-3,20-dione; topical antipruritic agent.

*p*-dichlorobenzene. $ClC_6H_4Cl$; an insecticide used chiefly as a moth repellent.

dichlorodiethyl sulfide. See mustard gas.

dichlorodifluoromethane (NF). FREON 12; $CF_2Cl_2$; an easily liquefiable gas used as a refrigerant and aerosol propellant.

*p,p'*-dichlorodiphenyl meth'yl carbinol. A synthetic compound found effective as a miticide; abbreviated DMC.

dichlorodiphenyltrichloroethane. DDT; 1,1,1-trichloro-2,2-*bis*(*p*-chlorophenyl)ethane; dicophane; chlorophenothane; an insecticide that came into prominence during and after World War II. For a time it proved very effective, but insect populations rapidly developed tolerance for it, hence much of its original effectiveness has been lost.

dichloroeth'ane. See ethylidene chloride.

di(2-chloroethyl)sulfide. Mustard gas.

dichlorohydrin. Dichloroisopropyl alcohol; a colorless, odorless fluid prepared by heating anhydrous glycerin with sulfur monochloride. A solvent of resins.

2,6-dichlor'oindophe'nol. A reagent for the chemical assay of ascorbic acid depending upon the reducing properties of the latter. It is red in acid solution; in the presence of the vitamin it undergoes reduction and becomes colorless, the vitamin being oxidized to dehydroascorbic acid.

dichloroisopropyl alcohol. Dichlorohydrin.

dichloroisoproterenol. DCI; dichlorisoproterenol; *dl*-1-[ 3,4-dichlorophenyl ]-2-isopropylaminoethanol; the congener of the adrenergic beta receptor stimulant, isoproterenol; it blocks the responses, involving beta receptors, to epinephrine and other sympathomimetic drugs.

dichlor'ometh'ane. $CH_2Cl_2$; methylene bichloride; chloromethyl monochloromethane; methylene chloride; an anesthetic for minor operations, especially in dentistry. Vapor is flammable.

dichlorometh'otrex'ate. *N*-[ 3,5-Dichloro-4-{[ (2,4-diamino-6-pteridinyl)methyl ]methylamino}benzoyl ]glutamic acid; folic acid antagonist used for treatment of leukemia.

dichlor'ophen (BP). ANTIPHEN; 2,2'-dihydroxy-5,5'methylenebix(4-chlorophenol); used topically as a fungicide and bactericide, and internally in the treatment of infections by tapeworms of man and domestic animals.

dichlor'ophenars'ine hydrochloride. (3-Amino-4-hydroxyphenyl)dichloroarisine hydrochloride; an arsenical antisyphilitic agent.

(2,4-dichlorophenoxy)acetic acid. 2,4-D; a weed-killer; a compound more toxic to broad-leaved dicotyledonous plants (weeds) than to the monocotyledonous ones (grains and grass).

dichlorotetrafluoroethane (NF). FREON 114; cryofluorane; used as a refrigerant and aerosol propellant; may be irritating to the respiratory tract and mildly narcotic.

dichlor'ovos. Dichlorvos.

dichlorphenamide (USP, BP). DARANIDE; 4,5-dichloro-*m*-benzenedisulfonamide; a carbonic anhydrase inhibitor with actions somewhat similar to acetazolamide. Given orally, it produces increased urinary excretion of electrolytes. Used in the systemic treatment of glaucoma.

2,6-di'chlorphe'nol-in'dophe'nol. Common misnomer for 2,6-dichloroindophenol, *q. v.*

dichlorpro'mazine. 2,4-Dichloro-10-[ 3-(dimethylamino)-propyl ]phenothiazine; antipsychotic agent.

dichlor'vos (USP). ATGARD; dichlorovos; phosphoric acid 2,2-dichlorovinyldimethyl ester; used as an anthelmintic in veterinary and human medicine.

dichorial, dichorionic (di-ko'rī-al, di-ko-rī-on'ik) [ G. *di*-, two, + chorion ]. Showing evidence of two chorions, as the placenta of diovular twins.

dichotomous (di-kot'o-mus). Relating to dichotomy.

dichotomy (di-kot'o-mī) [ G. *dichotomia*, a cutting in two, fr. *dicha*, in two, + *tomē*, a cutting ]. Division into two parts.

dichroic (di-kro'ik). Relating to dichroism.

dichroism (di'kro-izm) [ G. *di*-, two, + *chrōa*, color ]. The property of seeming to be differently colored when seen from different directions.

circular d., the change from circular polarization to elliptical polarization of monochromatic circularly polarized light in the immediate vicinity of the absorption band of the substance through which the light passes; see also Cotton *effect.*

dichroma'sia [ G. *di*, two, + *chrōma*, color ]. Dichromatism.

dichro'masy. Dichromatism.

dichromat (di'kro-mat). An individual with dichromatism.

dichromate (di-kro'māt). Bichromate; a compound containing the radical $Cr_2O_7 =$.

dichromatic (di'kro-mat'ik). 1. Having or exhibiting two colors. 2. Relating to dichromatism (2).

dichromatism (di-kro'mǎ-tizm) [ G. *di*-, two, + *chrōma*, color ]. 1. State of being dichromatic (1). 2. A form of defective color vision in which only two primary colors are seen and the spectrum is separated by an achromatic band; may occur as protanopia, deuteranopia, tritanopia, or tetartanopia. Also called dichromatopsia, parachromatopsia, parachromatism, dyschromatopsia, partial color blindness.

dichromatopsia (di-kro'mǎ-top'sǐ-ah) [ G. *di*-, two, + *chrōma*, color, + *opsis*, vision ]. Dichromatism (2).

dichromic (di-kro'mik). Having, or relating to, two colors.

dichromophil, dichromophile (di-kro'mo-fil, di-kro'-mo-fīl) [ G. *di*-, two, + *chrōma*, color, + *philos*, fond ]. Taking a double stain; denoting a tissue or cell taking both acid and basic dyes in different parts.

Dick, George Frederick (1881–1967), and Gladys R. H. (1881–1947), Chicago internists. See D. *method, test,* test *toxin.*

Dickens, Frank, British biochemist, 20th century. See D. *shunt.*

dicloxacil'lin sodium (USP). DYNAPEN; sodium-3-(2,6-dichlorophenyl)-5-methyl-4-isoazolylpenicillin; antimicrobial agent.

dicophane (di'ko-fān) (BP). DDT; see dichlorodiphenyltrichloroethane.

dicoria (di-ko'rī-ah) [ G. *di*-, two, + *korē*, pupil ]. Diplocoria.

Dicrocoe'lium [ G. *dikroos*, forked, + *koilia*, belly ]. A genus of digenetic Trematoda, or flukes.

D. dentrit'icum, formerly called *D. lanceolatum, D. lanceolata, Fasciola lanceolata, Distomum lanceolatum;* lancet fluke inhabiting the bile ducts and the gallbladder of many herbivorous mammals; rarely found in man, but an important parasite of sheep in New York state and in northern and central Europe.

dicrot'ic [ G. *dikrotos*, double-beating ]. Relating to dicrotism.

dicrotism (di'kro-tizm) [ G. *di*-, two, + *krotos*, a beat ]. That form of the pulse in which a double beat can be felt at the wrist for each beat of the heart; due to accentuation of the dicrotic wave.

Dictyocaulus (dik'tī-o-kaw'lus) [ G. *diktyon*, net, + *kaulos*, stalk ]. A genus of thin, elongate metastrongylid nematodes (subfamily Dictyocaulinae) that inhabit the air passages of herbivorous animals; commonly called lungworms.

D. arnfiel'di, occurs in the bronchi of horses, mules, and donkeys; generally it produces few or no symptoms, except with heavy infection.

D. fila'ria, the large or thread lungworm; the common lungworm of sheep, goats, camels, and many wild ruminants; it causes much damage, especially in younger animals, which cough and suffer from dyspnea; emaciation and anemia often occur.

D. vivip'arus, the common lungworm of cattle, deer, and other ruminants, usually found in the trachea, bronchi, and bronchioles; the chronic cough caused by this parasite is sometimes called hoose or husk, especially in the British Isles; the only commercial anthelmintic vaccine, from x-ray irradiated larvae, has been developed in England.

dictyokinesis (dik'tī-o-kī-ne'sis) [ G. *diktyon*, net, + *kinēsis*, motion ]. Golgiokinesis; the process of division of the Golgi apparatus and its distribution to the two daughter cells in mitosis.

**dictyoma** (dik-tī-o'mah) [ G. *dikyton*, net (retina), + suffix *-oma*, tumor ]. A tumor of the retina.

**dictyosome** (dik'tī-o-sōm) [ G. *diktyon*, net, + *sōma*, body ]. One of the fragments into which the Golgi body breaks up in mitosis.

**dicu'marol** (USP). DICOUMAROL; DICOUMARIN; bishydroxycoumarin; a derivative of coumarin, 3,3'-methylene bis(4-hydroxycoumarin); an anticoagulant agent that inhibits the formation of prothrombin in the liver.

Dicumarol (bishydroxycoumarin)

**dicyclomine hydrochloride** (di-si'klo-mēn) (USP, BP). BENTYL hydrochloride; 2-diethylaminoethyl bicyclohexyl-1-carboxylate hydrochloride. Anticholinergic drug with atropine-like action on the gastrointestinal tract.

**didactic** (di-dak'tik) [ G. *didaktikos*, fr. *didaskō*, to teach ]. Instructive; denoting medical teaching by lectures or textbooks as distinguished from clinical demonstration with patients.

**didactylism** (di-dak'tī-lizm) [ G. *di-*, two, + *daktylos*, finger or toe ]. The congenital condition of having but two fingers on a hand or two toes on a foot.

**didelphic** (di-del'fic) [ G. *di-*, two, + *delphys*, womb ]. Having or relating to a double uterus.

**Didelphys** (di-del'fis) [ G. *di-*, two, + *delphys*, womb ]. A genus of marsupials commonly called opossums. *D. marsupialis* is the common North American variety; *D. paraguayensis* is a South American form. These animals may serve as reservoir hosts of *Trypanosoma cruzi* in South America.

**didym-, didymo-** [ G. *didymos*, twin ]. Combining form denoting relationship to the didymus, testis; *cf.* -didymus, -dymus.

**didymalgia** (did-ī-mal'jī-ah) [ G. *didymos*, twin, pl. *didymoi*, the testes, + *algos*, pain ]. Orchialgia.

**didymitis** (did-ī-mi'tis) [ G. *didymos*, twin, pl. *didymoi*, the testes, + suffix *-itis*, inflammation ]. Orchitis.

**didymium** (di-dim'ī-um) [ G. *didymos*, twin (*i.e.*, twin of lanthanum, discovered in same mineral ]. A substance thought at the time of its discovery to be an element, but later found to be a mixture of praseodymium and neodymium.

**-didymus, -dymus** [ G. *didymos*, twin ]. Terminations denoting a conjoined twin, the first element of the word designating the part or parts of the twins which have remained *unfused*. The more common usage is to designate, instead, the parts *fused*, by use of the suffix -pagus, which see. See also conjoined twins, under twin.

**didymus** (did'ī-mus) [ G. *didymos*, a twin, pl. *didymoi*, testes ]. Testis.

**die**. In dentistry, the positive reproduction of the form of a prepared tooth in any suitable hard substance, usually in metal or specially prepared artificial stone; see also counterdie.

**diechoscope** (di-ek'o-skōp) [ G. *di-*, two, + *ēchō*, a sound, + *skopeō*, to examine ]. A form of stethoscope by means of which two sounds in two different parts can be listened to at the same time. A variety, called the symballophone, was invented by William Kerr.

**diecious** (di-e'shus) [ G. *di-*, two, + *oikia*, house ]. Applied to animals or plants that are sexually distinct, the individuals being of one or the other sex.

**Dieffenbach** (dēf'en-bakh), Johann F., German surgeon, 1792–1847. See D.'s *amputation, method.*

**Diego blood group.** See appendix 2, Blood Groups.

**dieldrin** (di-el'drin). A chlorinated hydrocarbon used as an insecticide; may cause toxic effects in persons and animals exposed to its action through skin contact, inhalation, or food contamination.

**dielectrography** (di'-e-lek-trog'ra-fī). Rheocardiography.

**dielectrolysis** (di'e-lek-trol'ī-sis). Electrophoresis.

**Diels,** Otto, German chemist, 1876–1954. See D.'s *hydrocarbon.*

**diencephalohypophysial** (di-en-sef'ă-lo-hi-po-fiz'ī-al). Relating to the diencephalon and hypophysis.

**diencephalon,** pl. **dienceph'ala** (di-en-sef'ă-lon) [ G. *dia*, through, + *enkephalos*, brain ] [ NA ], thalamencephalon [ NA ]; that part of the forebrain that is composed of the thalamus, the subthalamus, and the hypothalamus; some obsolete or rarely used synonyms are: deutencephalon; thalamic brain; interbrain; between-brain; 'tween-brain.

**diener** (de'ner) [ Ger. *diener*, servant ]. A laboratory worker who assists in training.

**di'enes'trol** (NF). Dienoestrol (BP); estrodienol; 3,4-bis-(*p*-hydroxyphenyl)-2,4-hexadiene; an estrogenic agent.

**Dientamoeba frag'ilis** (di-ent-ă-me'bah). A very small ameba parasitic in the large intestine of man and certain monkeys; usually nonpathogenic, but believed to be capable of sometimes causing low grade inflammation with mucous diarrhea and gastrointestinal disturbance in man.

**dieresis** (di-er'e-sis) [ G. *diairesis*, a division, fr. *di-aireō*, to divide into parts, fr. *dia*, apart, + *haireō*, to take ]. *Solution of continuity.*

**dieretic** (di-er-et'ik). 1. Relating to dieresis. 2. Dividing; ulcerating; corroding.

**diesterase** (di-es'ter-ās). See phosphodiesterase.

**diestrus** (di-es'trus) [ G. *dia* between, + *oistros*, desire ]. A period of sexual quiescence intervening between two periods of estrus.

**di'et** [ G. *diaita*, a way of life; a diet ]. 1. Food and drink in general. 2. A prescribed course of eating and drinking, in which the amount and kind of food, as well as the times at which it is to be taken, are regulated by the physician for therapeutic purposes. 3. Reduction of caloric intake so as to lose weight. 4. To follow any prescribed or specific d.

**absolute d.,** complete fasting.

**acid-ash d.,** one consisting largely of meat or fish, eggs, and cereals, but containing a minimal quantity of milk, fruit, and vegetables which, when catabolized, leave an acid residue to be excreted in the urine.

**adequate d.,** this d. containing all of the sixty-some essential ingredients that cannot be synthesized in adequate quantities by the organism, contained in the proper proportions for growth, lactation, nitrogen equilibrium, and repair of wear and tear in normal health. This includes necessary trace minerals, vitamins, and perhaps as yet unidentified factors.

**alkaline-ash d.,** basic d.; one consisting mainly of fruits, vegetables, and milk, with minimal amounts of meat, fish, eggs, cheese, and cereals which, when catabolized, leave an alkaline residue to be excreted in the urine.

**an'tiketogen'ic d.,** one high in carbohydrate and low in fat.

**balanced d.,** see adequate d.

**basal d.,** (1) one having a caloric value equal to the basal heat production; (2) in experiments in nutrition, a d. from which a given constituent, *e.g.*, a vitamin, mineral, or amino acid, the nutritional value of which is to be determined, is omitted for a period and the effects observed. The animal is observed for a second period during which the ingredient being studied is added to the d.

**basic d.,** alkaline-ash d. (not to be confused with basal or controlled d.).

**bland d.,** one free from roughage or spicy foods, usually the same as a soft or a light d.

**Chittenden's standard d.,** a d. containing from 47 to 55 gm. of protein, said to be sufficient to maintain the nitrogenous equilibrium in an adult male.

**clear liquid d.,** a d., often used postoperatively, consisting usually of water, tea, coffee, gelatin preparations, and clear soups or broth.

**Coleman-Shaffer d.,** a soft d. for typhoid fever patients, with a relatively high protein content furnished mainly by eggs; it also contains cream, cocoa, bread, and butter.

**controlled d.,** d. designed for therapeutic or experimental purposes. Such d.'s may be partially or largely synthetic and consist of purified substances. See also basal d.

**convalescent d.,** light d.

diabetic d., one suitable for a diabetic patient; it varies very considerably in accordance with the predilection of the physician and whether or not the patient is receiving insulin.

elimination d., one designed to detect what ingredient of the food causes allergic manifestations in the patient. Food items to which the patient may be sensitive are withdrawn separately and successively from the d. until that which causes the symptoms is discovered.

full liquid d., a d. consisting only of liquids but including cream soups, ice cream, and milk.

gout d., one containing a minimal quantity of purine bases, meats; liver, kidney, and sweetbread especially are excluded and replaced by dairy products, fruits, and cereals; wines and liquors are also forbidden.

high calorie d., one containing upward of 4000 calories per day, as eaten by those doing heavy work.

high fat d., one containing large amounts of fat, such as is eaten by heavy workers in winter; or a ketogenic d.

high sodium d., one with a high sodium chloride content; used in the treatment of adrenocortical insufficiency.

inadequate d., one that does not furnish sufficient calories for the energy expended or lacks some essential constituent, vitamin, mineral, or amino acid.

Karell d., a d. for cardiac edema consisting mainly of skimmed milk six times a day and orange or lemon juice; now rarely used.

Kempner's rice-fruit d., a d. prescribed for arterial hypertension or chronic renal disease, consisting mainly of rice and fruits with the necessary vitamins and minerals added but sodium restricted.

ketogen'ic d., a high-fat, low-carbohydrate, and protein d. causing ketosis.

light d., one suitable for a bed patient or for one convalescing from an illness and taking little exercise.

low calorie d., one of 1200 calories or less per day.

low fat d., one containing minimal amounts of fat; antiketogenic d.

low potassium d., d. for adrenal insufficiency.

low sodium d.'s, various d.'s containing moderate or severe restriction of sodium chloride and other sources of sodium; used in the treatment of hypertension, congestive failure, and other conditions and edema from other causes.

microbiotic d., a d. based on grains and unprocessed foods.

nephritic d., for acute nephritis; one with a low content of nitrogen and free from spices, condiments, and alcohol.

purine-free d., see gout d.

reducing d., a d. in which caloric expenditure is greater than caloric intake.

rice d., a d. consisting mainly of rice and fruit, with vitamins and iron, prescribed for the treatment of arterial hypertension and chronic renal disease with edema. It is also a low-salt, low-cholesterol, and low-fat d.; see also Kempner's rice-fruit d.

salt-free d., incorrect term for low sodium or low salt d.

smooth d., one containing little roughage, as used in peptic ulcer. See Sippy's *method.*

soft d., one composed of milk, eggs, tapicoa or rice puddings, fruit juices, mashed potatoes, applesauce, custards, ice cream, etc.

sour-milk d., d. used in vast quantities by Metchinkoff, who died at 70 in his quest for immortality. The current yogurt d. is a variant of this whimsey.

vegetarian d., one in which all flesh food is replaced by dairy products (milk, eggs, cheese), vegetables, fruits, and cereals.

yogurt d., a d. containing large quantities of the derivatives of sour or soured milk; sometimes taken in large quantities by bemused citizens who think it favors their health.

dietary (di'ē-tĕr-ī). Relating to the diet.

dietetic (di'ē-tet'ik). 1. Relating to diet. 2. Descriptive of food that, naturally or through processing, has a low caloric content.

dietetics (di'ē-tet'iks). The branch of therapeutics treating of food and drink in relation to health and disease.

diethadione. DIOXONE; 5,5-diethyldihydro-2$H$-1,3-oxazine-2,4(3$H$)-dione; analeptic.

diethanol'amine (NF). 2,2'-Iminodiethanol; used as an emulsifier and as a dispersing agent in cosmetics and pharmaceuticals.

dieth'azine hydrochloride. DIPARCOL; 10-(2-diethylaminoethyl)phenothiazine hydrochloride; used as antiparkinsonian agent with anticholinergic properties.

diethenoid fatty acid. See under *fatty acid.*

dieth'yl. 1. Normal butane. 2. A prefix denoting the presence of two ethyl radicals in the molecule.

d. ether, ethyl ether; sulfuric ether; anesthetic ether; ethyl oxide; $CH_3CH_2OCH_2CH_3$; a pungent, volatile liquid the vapor of which produces inhalation anesthesia; introduced in 1846 as the first successful surgical anesthetic.

dieth'ylaminoeth'yl cel'lulose. DEAE-cellulose (see under cellulose).

dieth'ylbarbitu'ric acid. Barbital.

dieth'ylcarbam'azine citrate (USP, BP). HETRAZAN; BANOCIDE; N,N-diethyl-4-methyl-1-piperazinecarboxamide citrate; an effective microfilaricide, though relatively ineffective against the adult filariae. May provoke an encephalopathy in loiasis; in onchocerciasis, it may produce severe allergic reactions, believed to be due to the destruction of the microfilariae.

dieth'ylenedi'amine. Piperazine.

1,4-dieth'ylene dioxide. Dioxane; a colorless liquid used as a solvent for cellulose esters and in histology as a drying agent.

diethylenetriaminepentaacetic acid. Penthanil; DTPA; a pentaacetic acid triamine, with affinity for heavy metals; used as the calcium sodium chelate in the treatment of iron-storage disease and poisoning from heavy metals and radioactive metals. See also ethylenediaminetetraacetic acid.

diethylmalonylurea (di-eth'il-mal-o-nil-u-re'ah). Barbital.

dieth'ylpro'pion hydrochloride (NF). TENUATE, TEPANIL; 1-phenyl-2-diethylaminopropanone-1 hydrochloride; a sympathomimetic amine related chemically to amphetamine, used to suppress the appetite. Central nervous system stimulation appears to be less pronounced than with other anorexigenic drugs.

diethylstilbestrol (di-eth'il-stil-bes'trol) (USP). Stilboestrol (BP); stilbestrol; 4,4'-dihydroxy-α,β-diethylstilbene; a synthetic crystalline compound, not a steroid, possessing estrogenic activity when given orally or by injection. Also available as the diphosphate (USP) and the dipropionate (NF).

diethyltoluamide. *m*-Delphene; OFF; N,N-diethyl-*m*-toluamide; insect repellent.

dieth'yltryp'tamine. DET; N,N-diethyltryptamine; a hallucinogenic agent similar to dimethyltryptamine.

dietitian (di'ē-tish'un). An expert in dietetics; one versed in the practical application of diet in the prophylaxis and treatment of disease.

Dietl (de'tl), Józef, Polish physician, 1804–1878. See D.'s *crisis.*

di'etogenet'ics. The biologic field dealing with the interrelationship between genotype, diet, and various food requirements.

di'etother'apy. Sitotherapy; trophotherapy; the treatment of disease by regulation of the diet.

Dieulafoy (de-ē-lä-fwä'), Georges, Paris physician, 1839–1911. See D.'s *erosion, theory.*

difarnesyl group. A 30-carbon open chain hexaisoprenoid hydrocarbon radical occurring as a side chain in vitamin $K_2$.

difenox'in (USAN). 1-(3-Cyano-3,3-diphenylpropyl)-4-phenylisonipecotic acid; an antiperistaltic drug.

dif'ference. The magnitude or degree by which one quantity differs from another of the same kind.

arteriovenous carbon dioxide d., the d. in carbon dioxide content (in volumes per cent) between the arterial and venous bloods.

arteriovenous oxygen d., the d. in the oxygen content (in volumes per cent) between arterial and venous bloods.

individual d.'s, in clinical psychology, deviations of individuals from the group average or from each other.

light d., (1) the d. in light sensitivity of the two eyes; (2) brightness difference *threshold.*

**standard error of d.,** a statistical index of the probability that a difference between two sample means is greater than zero.

**differential** (dif′er-en′shal) [ L. *dif-fero,* to carry apart (intrans.), differ, fr. *dis,* apart ]. Relating to or characterized by a difference; distinguishing.
　**threshold d.,** d. *threshold.*

**differentiated** (dif′er-en′shī-a-ted). Having a different character or function from the surrounding structures or from the original type; said of tissues, cells, or portions of the cytoplasm.

**differentiation** (dif′er-en′shī-a′shun). 1. Specialization (2); the acquiring or the possession of character or function different from that of the original type. 2. Differential *diagnosis.* 3. Partial removal of a stain from a histologic section to accentuate the staining differences of tissue components.
　**correlative d.,** d. due to the interaction of different parts of an organism.
　**invisible d.,** chemodifferentiation.

**diffluence** (dif′lu-ens) [ L. *dif-fluo,* to flow in different directions, dissolve (*dis,* apart) ]. Deliquescence; the process of becoming fluid.

**diffraction** (dī-frak′shun) [ L. *dif-fringo,* pp. *-fractus,* to break in pieces. FRA- ]. The deflection of the rays of light from a straight line in passing by the edge of an opaque body.

**diffusate** (dī-fu′zāt) [ L. *dif-fundo,* pp. *-fusus,* to pour in different directions ]. Dialysate.

**diffuse** (dī-fūz′) [ L. *dif-fundo,* pp. *-fusus,* to pour in different directions ]. Spread about, not circumscribed or limited.

**diffu′sible.** Capable of diffusing; not bound.

**diffusion** (dī-fu′zhun). 1. The random movement of free molecules or ions or small particles in solution or suspension under the influence of Brownian (thermal) motion toward a uniform distribution throughout the available volume. The rate is relatively rapid among liquids and gases, but takes place very slowly among solids. 2. Dialysis.
　**gel d.,** d. in a gel, as in the case of gel diffusion precipitin tests (*q.v.*) in which the immune reactants diffuse in agar.

**diflu′anine hydrochloride** (USAN). 1-(2-Anilino-ethyl)-4-[ 4,4-bis(*p*-fluorophenyl)butyl ]piperazine trihydrochloride; an analeptic drug.

**diflucor′tolone** (USAN). 6α,9-Difluoro-11β,21-dihydroxy-16α-methylpregna-1,4-diene-3,20-dione; a glucocorticoid steroid.

**diflu′midone sodium** (USAN). 3′-Benzoyl-1,1-difluoromethanesulfonanilide sodium salt; anti-inflammatory drug.

**diflupred′nate** (USAN). 6α,9-Difluoro-11β,17,21-trihydroxypregna-1,4-diene-3,20-dione 21-acetate 17-butyrate; anti-inflammatory drug.

**digamet′ic** (di-gă-met′ik). Heterogametic.

**digastric** (di-gas′trik) [ G. *di,* two, + *gastēr,* belly ]. 1. Having two bellies; denoting especially a muscle with two fleshy parts separated by an intervening tendinous part. 2. *Musculus* digastricus. 3. Relating to the d. muscle; denoting a fossa or groove with which it is in relation and a nerve supplying its posterior belly.

**digas′tricus** [ L. ] [ NA ]. Digastric; denoting the *musculus* digastricus.

**Digenea** (di-je′ne-ah) [ G. *di,* two, + *genesis,* generation ]. Subclass of parasitic flatworms of the class Trematoda or flukes, characterized by a complex life cycle involving developmental multiplying stages in a mollusc intermediate host and adult stage in a vertebrate, often involving an additional transport or true intermediate host; includes all of the common flukes of man and other mammals.

**digenesis** (di-jen′ĕ-sis) [ G. *di,* two, + *genesis,* generation ]. Reproduction in different ways in different generations, as seen in the nonsexual, or vertebrate, and the sexual, or invertebrate, cycles of the malarial and other parasites.

**digenetic** (di-jĕ-net′ik). 1. Heteroxenous; pertaining to or characterized by digenesis. 2. Pertaining to the digenetic fluke.

**Di George,** Angelo M., U. S. pediatrician, *1921. See D. G. *syndrome.*

**digest** (dī-jest′) [ L. *digero,* pp. *-gestus,* to force apart, divide, dissolve. GEST- ]. 1. To soften by moisture and heat. 2. To hydrolyze or break up into simpler chemical compounds by means of hydrolyzing enzymes or chemical action; denoting the action of the secretions of the alimentary tract upon the food. 3 (di′gest). The materials resulting from digestion or hydrolysis.

**diges′tant** 1. Aiding digestion. 2. An agent that favors or assists the process of digestion.

**diges′ter.** One who or that which digests.
　**Papin's d.,** a metallic vessel with a hermetically tight lid, provided with a safety valve, used for subjecting substances to the action of water at a temperature above 212°F.; it was originally devised to prove that when the pressure on a liquid is raised its boiling point is also raised.

**digestion** (dī-jes′chun, di-jes′chun) [ L. *digestio,* see digest ]. 1. The process of making a digest. 2. The process whereby the ingested food is converted into material suitable for assimilation for synthesis of the tissues or the liberation of energy.
　**gastric d.,** that part of d., chiefly of the proteins, carried on in the stomach by the enzymes of the gastric juice.
　**intercellular d.,** d. in a cavity by means of secretions from the surrounding cells, such as occurs in the metazoa.
　**intestinal d.,** that part of d. carried on in the intestine; it affects all the foodstuffs: starches, fats, and proteins.
　**intracellular d.,** d. within the boundaries of a cell, such as occurs in the protozoa and in phagocytes.
　**pancreatic d.,** d. in the intestine by the enzymes of the pancreatic juice.
　**peptic d.,** gastric d.
　**primary d.,** d. in the alimentary tract.
　**salivary d.,** the conversion of starch into sugar by the action of salivary amylase.
　**secondary d.,** the change in the chyle effected by the action of the cells of the body, whereby the final products of d. are assimilated in the process of metabolism.

**digestive** (dī-jes′tiv). 1. Relating to digestion. 2. Digestant (2).

**digilanide A, B, and C.** See lanatoside A, B, and C.

**digin** (dij′in). Gitogenin.

**diginigenin** (dij′ī-nī-jen′in). 3β-Hydroxy-12α,20α-epoxy-14β,17α-pregn-5-ene-11,15-dione (for pregnene structure, see steroids); the steroid glycone derived from diginin by hydrolysis.

**diginin** (dij′ī-nin). An inactive steroid glycoside isolated from the leaves of *Digitalis purpurea* (the seeds of which are the source of digitonin); yields diginigenin and diginose upon hydrolysis.

**diginose** (dij′ī-nōs). 3-Methyl-2,6-dideoxy-D-glucose; a sugar obtained by acid hydrolysis of diginin.

**digit** (dij′it) [ L. *digitus* ]. A finger or toe; see digitus.
　**clubbed d.'s,** Hippocratic fingers; clubbed fingers; drumstick fingers; a bulbous enlargement of the terminal phalanges, with coarse, longitudinally curved nails, seen in heart disease, phthisis, pulmonary osteoarthropathy, and certain other pulmonary affections.

**digital** (dij′ī-tal). Relating to or resembling a digit or digits or an impression made by them.

**digitalin** (dij′ī-tal′in, -ta′lin). A mixture of glycosides obtained from digitalis.
　**Nativelle's d.,** digitoxin.
　**d. verum,** true d.; Schmiedeberg's d.; a glycoside, $C_{36}H_{56}O_{14}$, from the seeds of *Digitalis purpurea,* occurring as a white amorphous or granular powder.

**digita′lis** [ L. ] [ NA ]. Digital.

**digitalis** (dij′ī-tal′is, -ta′lis) [ L. *digitalis,* relating to the fingers; in allusion to the finger-like flowers ]. Foxglove, purple foxglove; fairy gloves; fairy gloves; a genus of perennial flowering plants of the family Schrophulariaceae. *D. lanata,* a European species, and *D. purpurea* are the main sources of cardioactive steroid glycosides used in the treatment of certain heart diseases, especially heart failure. The glycosides of *D. purpurea* are digitoxin, gitoxin, and gitalin; the aglycones are the steroids digitoxigenin, gitoxigenin, and gitaligenin (gitoxigenin hydrate). The glycosides of *D. lanata* are digitoxin, gitoxin, and digoxin, and the steroid aglycones are digitoxigenin, gitoxigenin, and digoxigenin. For the precursor glycosides, see purpurea glycosides, and lanatosides.

**digitalism** (dij'ĭ-tal-izm). The symptoms caused by digitalis poisoning or overdosage.

**digitalization** (dij-ĭ-tal-ĭ-za'shun). The administration of digitalis by any one of a number of schedules until sufficient amounts are present in the body to produce the desired therapeutic effects.

**digita'lose.** 6-Deoxy-3-$O$-methylgalactose; 3-methyl-D-fucose; a sugar obtained from *Digitalis purpurea*, in which it is combined with a steroid.

**digitate** (dij'ĭ-tāt). Marked by a number of finger-like processes or impressions.

**digitation** (dij'ĭ-ta'shun) [ Mod. L. *digitatio* ]. A process resembling a finger.

**digitatio'nes hippocam'pi** [ Mod. L. pl. of *digitatio* ]. Pes hippocampi.

**digiti** (dij'ĭ-ti) [ L. ]. Plural of digitus.

**digitigrade** (dij'ĭ-tĭ-grād) [ L. *digitus*, finger, + *gradior*, pp. *gressus*, to walk ]. Animals whose weight is borne on the digits only, such as the dog and cat. Contrasted with plantigrade, which are those whose heels touch the ground, such as man and the bear.

**digitin** (dij'ĭ-tin). Digitonin.

**digitonin** (dij-ĭ-to'nin). Digitin; a steroid glycoside obtained from *Digitalis purpurea* and composed of digitogenin 1, galactose 2, glucose 2, and xylose 1, the sugars attached at C-3 of the digitogenin. It has no cardiac action. Used as a reagent in the determination of cholesterol and steroids having a 3-hydroxyl group of the beta configuration.

**digitoxicity.** A convenient colloquialism for digitalis toxicity.

**digitoxigenin** (dij-ĭ-tok-sĭ-jen'in). 3$\beta$,14-Dihydroxy-5$\beta$,14$\beta$-card-20(22)-enolide; $\Delta^{20:22}$-3,14,21-trihydroxynorcholenic acid lactone; a cardanolide steroid making up part of the molecule of digitoxin. For structure of cardanolides, see steroids.

**digitoxin** (dij-ĭ-tok'sin) (USP, BP). A secondary cardioactive glycoside, composed of digitoxigenin and 3 molecules of digitoxose attached to C-3 of the genin; obtained from the leaves of *Digitalis purpurea*; it is more completely absorbed from the gastrointestinal tract than is digitalis.

**digitox'ose.** 2,6-Dideoxy-D-*ribo*-hexose; 2-deoxy-D-altromethylose; $CH_3CHOH—CHOH—CHOH—CH_2—CHO$; the sugar component of the glycosides digitoxin, gitoxin, and digoxin. Obtained by mild acid hydrolysis of the glycosides.

**digitus,** gen. and pl. **digiti** (dij'ĭ-tus) [ L. ] [ NA ]. Digit; dactyl; dactylus; a finger or toe.

   **d. anula'ris** [ NA ], ring or fourth finger.

   **d. auricula'ris,** d. minimus (the little or fifth finger); called auricular because used in scratching or cleaning the external acoustic meatus.

   **d. extensus,** backward deviation of a finger.

   **d. flexus,** permanent flexion of a finger.

   **digiti hippocrat'ici,** clubbed *digits*.

   **digiti manus** [ NA ], fingers.

   **d. medius** [ NA ], middle or third finger.

   **d. minimus** [ NA ], the little or fifth finger.

   **digiti mortui,** dead *fingers*.

   **digiti pedis** [ NA ], toes.

   **d. recel'lens,** trigger *finger*.

   **d. valgus,** permanent deviation of one or more fingers to the radial side.

   **d. varus,** permanent deviation of one or more fingers to the ulnar side.

**diglossia** (di-glos'sĭ-ah) [ G. *di-*, two, + *glōssa*, tongue ]. A condition in which the tongue is bifid, or split longitudinally.

**diglos'sus.** One with a congenitally bifid tongue.

**digly'cocoll hydroiodide-iodine.** Two moles of diglycocoll hydroiodide combined with two atomic weights of iodine; antibacterial agent used in tablet form for the disinfection of drinking water.

**dignathus** (di-nath'us) [ G. *di-*, two, + *gnathos*, jaw ]. A malformed fetus with double lower jaw.

**digoxigenin** (dĭ-jok'sĭ-jen-in) Lanadigenin; 3$\beta$,12$\beta$,14-trihydroxycard-20(22)-enolide (for structure of cardenolides, see steroids); the steroid aglycone of digoxin.

**digoxin** (dĭ-jok'sin) (USP, BP). LANOXIN; a cardioactive steroid glycoside obtained from *Digitalis lanata*. It is composed of digoxigenin and 3 molecules of digitoxose.

**Di Guglielmo** (de-gool-yel'mo), Giovanni, Italian physician, 1886–1961. See D.'s *disease, syndrome.*

**diheterozygote** (di-het'er-o-zi'gōt) [ G. *di-*, two, + heterozygote ]. An individual heterozygous for two different gene pairs at two different loci.

**dihybrid** (di-hi'brid) [ G. *di-*, two, + L. *hybrida* ]. The offspring of parents differing in two characters.

**dihydral'azine sulfate.** NEPRESOL; 1,4-dihydrazinophthalazine sulfate; antihypertensive agent.

**dihy'drate.** A compound with two molecules of water of crystallization, as in gypsum (calcium sulfate dihydrate, $CaSO_4 \cdot 2H_2O$).

**dihydro-.** Chemical prefix indicating the addition of two hydrogen atoms.

**dihy'droandros'terone.** Obsolete and inaccurate trivial name for 5$\alpha$-androstane-3$\alpha$,17$\beta$-diol (*cf.* androstanediol).

**dihydroco'deine tartrate** (BP). PARZONE; PARACODIN; 6-hydroxy-3-methoxy-$N$-methyl-4,5-epoxymorphinan bitartrate; analgesic derivative of codeine, about one-sixth as potent as morphine; a narcotic antitussive.

**dihydroco'deinone.** HYDROCODONE; DICODID; HYCODAN; a weak analgesic derivative of codeine used principally as an antitussive.

**dihy'drocor'tisol.** 11$\beta$,17,21-Trihydroxy-5$\beta$-pregnane-3,20-dione (for structure of pregnane, see steroids); a metabolite of cortisol, reduced at the 4-5 double bond.

**dihy'drocor'tisone.** 17,21-Dihydroxy-5$\beta$-pregnane-3,11,20-trione (for pregnane structure, see steroids); a metabolite of cortisone.

**dihy'drodeox'ymor'phine-D.** Desomorphine.

**dihy'droergocor'nine.** DHO 180; prepared by the hydrogenation of ergocornine. It is less toxic than the latter. See dihydroergotoxine mesylate.

**dihy'droergocris'tine.** Prepared by the hydrogenation of ergocristine. It is less toxic than the latter. See dihydroergotoxine mesylate.

**dihy'droergocryp'tine.** Prepared by the hydrogenation of ergocryptine. It is less toxic than the latter. See dihydroergotoxine mesylate.

**dihydroergot'amine.** DHE-45; prepared by the hydrogenation of ergotamine; used in the treatment of migraine, and is less toxic and less oxytocic than ergotamine.

**dihydroer'gotox'ine mesylate** (NF). HYDERGINE; mixture of dihydroergocornine methanesulfate, dihydroergocristine methanesulfate, and dihydroergocryptine methane sulfate; used as an $\alpha$-adrenergic blocking agent for relief of hypertension.

**dihy'drofo'lic acid.** Intermediate between tetrahydrofolic acid and folic acid, the reduction requiring NADPH and occurring in mammalian cells.

**dihy'drolipo'ic acid.** $HSCH_2CH_2CH(SH)CH_2CH_2CH_2$-$CH_2COOH$; reduced lipoic acid, formed by cleavage of the —S—S— bond within the ring, as a result of the acceptance of two hydrogens.

**dihydromor'phine hydrochloride.** Paramorphan; $C_{17}H_{21}NO_3 \cdot HCl$; a narcotic analgesic.

**dihydromor'phinone hydrochloride** (USP). Hydromorphone hydrochloride.

**dihydro-orotase.** Carbamoylaspartate dehydrase; enzyme (EC 3.5.2.3) catalyzing ring closure of $N$-carbamoyl-L-aspartate to form L-dihydro-orotate.

**dihy'droproges'terone.** Pregnane-3,20-dione (for pregnane structure, see steroids); progesterone reduced at the 4-5 double bond.

**dihydropteroic acid** (di-hi'dro-tēr-o'ik) Intermediate in the conversion of guanosine to hydrofolic acid, a compound of 6-methylpteridine and $p$-aminobenzoic acid. It is the combining of these two substances that is inhibited by sulfonamides.

**dihy'drostrep'tomycin.** Similar in antibiotic action to streptomycin; it may damage the cochlear branch of the eighth cranial nerve, resulting in partial or complete irreversible deafness.

**dihydrotachysterol** (di-hi′dro-tă-kis′tē-rol) (USP, BP). AT 10; HYTAKEROL; 9.10-secoergosta-5,7,22-triene-3-β-ol. Produced by the reduction of tachysterol, a derivative of irradiated ergosterol, with feeble antirachitic action; it enhances urinary phosphate excretion, which is followed by a reciprocal rise in serum calcium levels. Used in the treatment of hypocalcemia due to hypoparathyroidism and in vitamin D-resistant rickets.

**dihy′drotestos′terone.** 17β-Hydroxy-5α-androstan-3-one (for androstane structure, see steroids); testosterone reduced at the 4-5 double bond; a semisynthetic steroid with appreciable androgenic activity.

**dihydrothe′elin.** Obsolete term for estradiol.

**dihydrouracil** (di-hi′dro-u′ră-sil). 5,6-Dihydrouracil; a reduction product of uracil and one of the intermediates in uracil catabolism.

**dihydroxy-.** Chemical prefix denoting addition of two hydroxyl groups. As a suffix, becomes -diol.

**dihydrox′yac′etone.** HOCH₂—CO—CH₂OH; glyceroketone; the simplest ketose; as d. phosphate, one of the intermediates in the glycolytic pathway of glucose catabolism and fat synthesis.

**d. phosphate,** CH₂OHCOCH₂OPO₃H₂; one of the products of the cleavage of fructose 1,6-bisphosphate under the catalytic influence of the enzyme, fructose bisphosphate aldolase (EC 4.1.2.13).

**dihydrox′yalu′minum am′inoac′etate** (NF). ALGLYN; ALZINOX; DIMOTHYN; ROBALATE; dihydroxy-(glycinato)-aluminum; basic aluminum glycinate; a basic aluminum salt of aminoacetic acid containing small amounts of aluminum hydroxide and aminoacetic acid. Used as an antacid in hyperchlorhydria and peptic ulcer. Also available (NF) as a magma.

**dihydrox′yalu′minum sodium carbonate** (NF). MINICID; KOMPENSAN; aluminum sodium carbonate hydroxide; a gastric antacid.

**3,4-dihydrox′yphen′ylal′anine.** See dopa.

**dihysteria** (di-his-te′rī-ah) [G. di-, two, + hystera, uterus]. Obsolete term for uterus didelphys.

**diiodide** (di-i′o-dīd). A compound containing two atoms of iodine in its molecule.

**diiodo-** (di-i′o-do). Chemical prefix indicating two atoms of iodine.

**diiodohydroxyquin** (di-i′o-do-hi-drok′sĭ-kwin) (USP). Diodoquin; 5,7-diiodo-8-quinolinol; diiodohydroxyquinoline; C₉H₅I₂NO; an antiprotozoal agent, used in the treatment of intestinal amebiasis.

**diiodopyr′amine.** A radiopaque compound used in salpingography.

**diisopro′mine hydrochloride.** BILAGOL; N,N-diisopropyl-3,3-diphenylpropylamine; cholagogue.

**diisopro′pyl fluorophos′phate.** Isoflurophate.

**diketohydrindylidene-diketohydrindamine.** The colored product formed in the reaction of an α-amino acid and ninhydrin (triketohydrindene hydrate); a reaction used in the quantitative assay of α-amino acids.

**diketone** (di-ke′tōn). An organic compound containing two carbonyl groups, acetylacetone (CH₃COCH₂COCH₃) being an example.

**diketopiperazines** (di-ke′to-pi-pĕr-ă-zēnz). A class of organic compounds with a closed ring structure formed from two α-amino acids by the joining of the α-amino group of each to the carboxyl group of the other, with the loss of two molecules of water. See cyclol.

**dil.** Abbreviation for L. dilue (imperative of diluo, to wash away, dilute), dilute, or dilutus, -a, -um (pp. of di- luo), diluted.

**dilaceration** (di-las-er-a′shun) [L. di-lacero, pp. laceratus, to tear in pieces, fr. lacer, mangled]. 1. The formation of an aperature through a cataractous lens by piercing the center and prying apart the two halves. 2. A displacement of some portion of a developing tooth which is then further developed in its new relation. 3. A tooth with sharply angulated root(s).

**dilatancy** (di-la′tan-sĭ) [L. dilato, to dilate]. An increasing viscosity with increasing rate of shear accompanied by volumetric expansion.

**dilatation** (dil-ah-ta′shun). Dilation.

**dil′ata′tor.** Dilator.

**dilation** (di-la′shun) [L. dilato, pp. dilatatus, to spread out, dilate]. Dilatation. 1. Enlargement of a cavity, canal, blood vessel, or opening, occurring physiologically or pathologically or made artificially. 2. The act of dilating or enlarging.

**gastric d.,** an acute distention of the stomach following operation or trauma; when severe, the stomach may contain several liters of fluid and air; condition may lead to death from hypovolemia or aspiration of gastric contents, when not promptly relieved by nasogastric intubation.

**prognath′ian** or **prognath′ic d.,** d. of the pyloric end of the stomach out of proportion to that of the cardia or fundus, giving the undershot appearance of a bulldog's jaw in the roentgen picture.

**di′lator.** Dilatator. 1. An instrument designed for enlarging a cavity, canal, or opening. 2 [NA]. A muscle the function of which is to pull open any orifice. 3. A substance that causes dilation of a structure such as a blood vessel or the pupil.

**Barnes′ d.,** Barnes′ bag.

**Bossi′s d.,** an instrument for rapid dilation of the cervix uteri; it consists of three or four blunt-pointed metallic rods which can be separated by a registering screw apparatus.

**de Signeux′s d.,** a modification of Bossi's cervical d.

**Frommer′s d.,** a modification of Bossi's cervical d.

**Goodell′s d.,** a uterine d. used for dilating the cervix.

**Hanks d.′s,** uterine d.′s of solid metal construction.

**Hegar′s d.′s,** a series of cylindrical bougies of graduated sizes used to dilate the cervical canal.

**d. ir′idis,** musculus dilator pupillae.

**Plummer′s d.,** an instrument for dilating the lower end of the esophagus in cardiospasm. It consists of a rubber tube stiffened by fish bone and a dilatable elongated balloon near its lower end; the lower tip is of metal and perforated. In difficult cases the tube is threaded along a guiding wire which has been previously swallowed by the patient.

**d. tubae,** musculus tensor veli palatini.

**Tubbs′ d.,** a surgical instrument used to dilate the stenotic mitral valve.

**dil′do, dil′doe.** An artificial penis; an object having the approximate shape and size of an erect penis, and commonly made of wood, plastic, or rubber; utilized to produce sexual pleasure by vaginal insertion.

**dill oil.** A volatile oil distilled from the fruit of Anethum graveolens (family Umbelliferae); carminative.

**dilox′anide fu′roate** (BP). FURAMIDE; HISTOMIBAL; 2,2-dichloro-4′-hydroxy-N-methylacetanilide furoate; amebicide for treatment of dysentery.

**diluent** (dil′u-ent). 1. Diluting; making weaker or more watery. 2. An agent that dilutes the strength of a solution or mixture.

**dilution** (di-lu′shun) [L. di-luo, pp. -lutus, to wash away, dilute]. 1. The act of reducing the concentration of a mixture or solution. 2. A weakened (diluted) solution. 3. In microbiologic techniques, a method for counting the number of viable cells in a suspension; a sample is diluted to the point where an aliquot, when plated, yields a countable number of separate colonies.

**dim.** Abbreviation for L. dimidius, -a, -um, half; see also ss.

**dima′zon.** 4-o-Tolylazo-o-diacetotoluide; an azo compound occurring in red crystals. Used with petrolatum as an ointment to stimulate epithelial cell proliferation and thus promote the healing of superficial wounds.

**dimef′line hydrochloride** (USAN). REMEFLIN; 8-dimethylaminomethyl-7-methoxy-3-methylflavone hydrochloride; analeptic.

**dime′lia** [G. di-, two, + melos, limb]. Congenital duplication of the whole or a part of a limb.

**dime′lus.** A fetus with dimelia.

**di'menhy'drinate** (USP, BP). DRAMAMINE; an amine salt of a theophyllinic acid; an antihistaminic, antinauseant, and antiemetic, used for motion sickness.

**dimenox'adol.** LOKARIN; ethoxydiphenylacetic acid 2-dimethylaminoethyl ester; analgesic.

**dimension** (dī-men'shun). Scope, size, magnitude; denoting, in the plural, linear measurements of length, width, and height.

**buccolingual d.,** the diameter or d. of a bicuspid or molar tooth from buccal to lingual surface.

**occlusal vertical d.,** the vertical d. of the face when the teeth or occlusion rims are in contact in centric occlusion; *decrease* in occlusal vertical d. may result from modification of tooth form by attrition or grinding, drifting of teeth, or, in edentulous patients, by resorption of residual ridges; *increase* may result from modifications of tooth form, tooth position, height of occlusion rims, rebasing or relining, or occlusal splints.

**rest vertical d.,** the vertical d. of the face with the jaws in rest relation. *Decrease* in rest vertical d. may or may not accompany a decrease in occlusal vertical d.; it may occur without a decrease in occlusal vertical d. in patients with a preponderant activity of the jaw-closing musculature, as in patients with muscular hypertenseness or in chronic gum chewers. *Increase* in rest vertical d. may or may not accompany an increase in occlusal vertical d.; it sometimes occurs after the removal of remaining occlusal contacts, perhaps as a result of the removal of noxious reflex stimuli.

**vertical d.,** vertical opening; a vertical measurement of the face between any two arbitrarily selected points which are conveniently located, one above and one below the mouth, usually in the midline.

**dimephep'tanol.** METHADOL; bimethadol; 6-(dimethylamino)-4,4-diphenyl-3-heptanol; analgesic.

**di'mer** [ G. *di-*, two, + suffix -mer, *q.v.* ]. A compound or unit produced by the combination of two like molecules; in the strictest case, without loss of atoms (thus nitrogen tetroxide, $N_2O_4$, is the d. of nitrogen dioxide, $NO_2$), usually by elimination of $H_2O$ or a similar small molecule between the two (*e.g.,* a disaccharide), but often by simple noncovalent association (as of two identical protein molecules). Higher orders of complexity are called trimers, tetramers, oligomers, polymers.

**di'mercap'rol** (USP, BP). British anti-Lewisite; BAL; 2,3-dimercaptopropanol; $HSCH_2CH(SH)CH_2OH$; a chelating agent; developed as an antidote for lewisite and other arsenical poisons. It acts by competing for the metal with the essential —SH groups in the pyruvate oxidase system of the cells. It forms, with arsenic, a stable, relatively nontoxic cyclic compound, the metal having a greater affinity for it than for the —SH groups of the cell proteins. Also used as an antidote for antimony, bismuth, chromium, mercury, gold, and nickel.

**dimercurion** (di-mer'kūr-i'on). Mercuric ion. $Hg^{++}$.

**dimeric.** Consisting of two parts; denoting a dimer.

**dim'erous** [ G. *di-*, two, + *meros*, part ]. Consisting of two parts.

**dimeth'acrine tartrate.** ISTONIL; 10-[ 3-(dimethylamino)-propyl ]-9,9-dimethylacridan tartrate; antidepressant.

**dimethicone** (di-meth'ĭ-kōn) (NF). SILICOTE; a silicone oil consisting of dimethylsiloxane polymers. It is usually incorporated into a petrolatum base or a nongreasy preparation and used for the protection of normal skin against various, chiefly industrial, skin irritants. May also be used to prevent ammoniacal dermatitis.

**di'meth'indene maleate** (NF). FORHISTAL maleate; 2-[ 1-[ 2- (2-dimethylaminoethyl) inden-3-yl ]ethyl ]pyridine maleate; an antihistamine also used as an antipruritic.

**dimethisoquin hydrochloride** (NF). QUOTANE; PRURALGIN; 3-butyl-1-(2-dimethylaminoethoxy)isoquinoline; an active surface anesthetic used to relieve itching and pain.

**di'methis'terone** (BP, NF). SECROSTERON; 6α-methyl-17-(1-propynyl)testosterone; 17-ethynyl-6α,21-dimethyltestosterone; 6α,21-dimethylethisterone; a modified testosterone or ethisterone. An orally effective synthetic progestin used alone or in combination with ethynyl estradiol as a contraceptive agent.

**dimethothi'azine.** MIGRISTENE; 10-[ 2-(dimethylamino)-propyl ]-*N,N*-dimethylphenothiazine-2-sulfonamide; anal-gesic and antihistaminic drug with antiserotonin properties.

**di'methox'anate hydrochloride.** COTHERA; 2-dimethylaminoethoxyethyl phenothiazine-10-carboxylate hydrochloride; a non-narcotic antitussive agent, less effective than codeine.

**2,5-dimethoxy-4-methylamphetamine.** A long-acting psychedelic drug; abbreviated DOM: also abbreviated STP (for serenity, tranquility, and peace).

**dimeth'ylaminoazoben'zene.** Butter yellow.

**dimethylarsin'ic acid.** Cacodylic acid.

**5,6-dimethylbenzimidazole.** One of the hydrolysis products of vitamin $B_{12}$.

**dimethylcarbinol.** Isopropyl alchohol.

**dimethyl-1-carbomethoxy-1-propen-2-yl phosphate.** An organic phosphorus compound used as a systemic poison for the extermination of such pests as mites, aphids, and houseflies.

**$β,β$-dimethylcysteine.** Penicillamine.

**dimethyl ether.** Methyl ether.

**dimethylethylcarbinol.** Amylene hydrate.

**dimethylphenylpiperazinium.** DMPP; a highly selective stimulant of autonomic ganglionic cells; used experimentally.

**dimethylphthalate** (di-meth'il-thal'at) (BP). Dimethyl ester of phthalic acid; insect repellent.

**dimeth'ylpiper'azine tartrate.** LYCETOL; LUPETAZINE tartrate; diuretic; also used as a uric acid solvent.

**dimethylpropiothetin.** See thetins.

**dimethyl sulfoxide** (USAN). DMSO; DROMISOL; DERMASORB; methyl sulfoxide, $Me_2SO$; an industrial solvent. It is a penetrating solvent, enhancing absorption of therapeutic agents from the skin, and has been proposed as an effective analgesic and anti-inflammatory agent in arthritis and bursitis; however, medicinal use has been restricted because of change of refractive index and production of corneal opacities in experimental animals.

**dimethylthetin.** See thetins.

**dimeth'ylthiam'butene.** DIMETHIBUTIN; *N,N*-1-trimethyl-3,3-di-2-thienylallylamine; non-narcotic analgesic.

**dimethyltocol.** See tocopherol (2).

**$N,N$-dimeth'yltryp'tamine.** DMT; present in several South American snuffs (*e.g.,* cohoba snuff) and in the leaves of *Prestonia amazonica* (family Apocynaceae). It is a psychotomimetic agent that produces effects similar to those of LSD; the onset is more rapid, with greater likelihood of a panic reaction and a shorter duration (1 to 2 hours, "businessman's trip"). It produces pronounced autonomic effects, including a marked increase in blood pressure.

**dimethyl tubocurarine chloride.** MECOSTRIN chloride; dimethyl ether of *d*-tubocurarine chloride; a skeletal muscle relaxant. See tubocurarine.

**dimethyl tubocurarine iodide** (NF). METUBINE iodide; dimethyl ether of *d*-tubocurarine iodide; with the same actions and uses as dimethyl tubocurarine chloride.

**dime'tria** [ G. *di,* two, + *mētra,* womb ]. *Uterus* didelphys.

**dimid'ium bromide.** A phenanthridinium compound used as a trypanocidal agent, especially in *Trypanosoma congolense* infections in cattle.

**Dimmer,** Friedrich, Austrian ophthalmologist, 1855–1926. See D.'s *keratitis.*

**dimorphic** (di-mor'fik). Dimorphous.

**dimorphism** (di-mor'fizm) [ G. *di-,* two, + *morphē,* shape ]. Existence in two shapes or forms; denoting a difference of crystal form exhibited by the same substance, or a difference in form or outward appearance between individuals of the same species, whether of plants or animals.

**sexual d.,** the somatic differences between male and female individuals that arise as a consequence of sexual maturation; inclusive of, but not restricted to, the secondary sexual characters.

**dimorphol'amine.** AMIPAN T; *N,N'*-ethylenebis[ *N*-butyl-4-morpholinecarboxamide; analeptic.

**dimorphous** (di-mor'fus). Having the property of dimorphism.

**dimple** (dim'pl). 1. An indentation, usually circular and of small area, in the chin, cheek, or sacral region; it is probably due to some developmental fault in the subcutaneous connective tissue, or in underlying bone. 2. A depression of similar appearance to 1, resulting from trauma or the contraction of scar tissue. 3. To cause d.'s.

**dimp'ling.** 1. Causing dimples. 2. A condition marked by the formation of dimples, natural or artificial.

**dineric** (di-nĕr'ik) [ G. *dinē*, an eddy, whirlpool ]. Eddying or whirling; denoting the movement of a liquid.

**di'nitrocel'lulose.** Pyroxylin.

**dinitro-o-cresol.** 2-Methyl-4,6-dinitrophenol; an insecticide used against mites in the form of a spray or dust; also used as a weed-killer.

**dinitrophenol** (di-ni'tro-fe'nol). DNP; $N_2$ph-OH; a dye $(C_6H_3(NO_2)_2OH)$ chemically related to trinitrophenol, picric acid. It is a metabolic stimulant, at one time suggested for the treatment of obesity, hypothyroidism, and other depressed metabolic states; it is, however, dangerously toxic. Used extensively in biochemical studies of oxidative processes.

**dinitrophenylamino acids.** Condensation products of amino acids with Sanger's reagent (fluorodinitrobenzene, FDNB, $N_2$ph-F); useful in identifying the N-terminal amino acid in a peptide chain, which combines with the reagent with elimination of HF.

**dinoflagellate** (di'no-flaj'e-lat) [ G. *dinos*, whirling, + L. *flagellum*, a whip ]. A plantlike flagellate of the subclass Phytomastigophorea, some species of which (*e.g.*, *Gonyaulax cantanella*) produce a potent neurotoxin that may cause severe food intoxication following ingestion of parasitized shellfish.

**di'noprost** (USAN). Prostaglandin $F_{2\alpha}$; 7-[ 3α,5α-dihydroxy-2β-[ (3*S*)-hydroxy-*trans*-1-octenyl ]cyclopentyl ]-*cis*-5-heptenoic acid; an oxytocic agent.

**d. tromethamine** (USAN), prostaglandin $F_{2\alpha}$ tromethamine; stimulant of uterine smooth muscle.

**di'nopros'tone** (USAN). Prostaglandin $E_2$; 7-[ 3α-hydroxy-2β-[ (3*S*)-3-hydroxy-*trans*-1-octenyl ]-5-oxo-1α-cyclopentyl ]-5-heptenoic acid; an oxytocic agent.

**dinor'mocyto'sis.** Isonormocytosis.

**Di'ocles** of Carystus, Greek physician of Alexandria, circa 350 B.C. A follower of Hippocrates and one of the earliest of the anatomists and a student of embryology; was the first to teach the value of counting the pulse; wrote a treatise on hygiene.

**Dioctophyma** (di-ok-to-fi'mah) [ L. fr. G. *dionkoun*, to distend, + *phyma*, growth ]. A genus of nematode worms of very large size, infecting the kidney.

**D. rena'le,** formerly called *Eustrongylus gigas* or *E. visceralis;* a blood-red, giant nematode, 16 inches long in the male, 39 inches in the female; found in the pelvis of the kidney and the peritoneal cavity of the dog, and is fairly common in wild carnivores like the mink, but rarely found in man; the life cycle is via branchiobdellid leeches ectoparasitic on crayfish, which are then eaten by various fishes and finally by man or any of a number of other mammalian fish-eating hosts.

**dioctyl calcium sulfosuccinate** (NF). Dioctyl sulfosuccinate calcium; SURFAK; calcium salt of bis(2-ethylhexyl)-sulfosuccinic a wetting agent; used in the treatment of constipation as a nonlaxative fecal softener.

**dioctyl sodium sulfosuccinate** (USP). 1. A hemolytic agent used in determinations of oxygen content of blood. 2. COLACE; DOXINATE; bis-2-ethylhexyl sodium sulfosuccinate; a surface-active agent used as a dispersing agent in topically applied preparations. After oral administration it lowers the surface tension of the gastrointestinal tract and is used in the treatment of constipation.

**Di'odon** [ G. *di-,* two, + *odous* (*odont-*), tooth ]. A genus of porcupine fishes related to balloon fish, globefish, and puffers. Although the common puffer is widely eaten as "sea squab" in the United States, many puffers, especially in the Pacific, are poisonous because of the presence of a neurotoxin, tetrodotoxin, in liver and ovary.

**di'odone** (BP). Iodopyracet.

**diodoquin** (di-o'do-kwin) (BP). Diiodohydroxyquin.

**Diogenes** (di-oj'ĕ-nēz). Greek philisopher, 412–323 B.C. See D. *cup; poculum* diogenis.

**-diol.** Suffix form of the prefix dihydroxy-.

**diolamine** (di-ōl'ă-mēn). USAN-approved contraction for diethanolamine, $NH(CH_2CH_2OH)_2$.

**diopsim'eter.** An instrument (obsolete) for measuring visual fields.

**diopter** (di-op'ter) [ G. *dioptra*, a leveling instrument. OPO- ]. The unit of refracting power of lenses, denoting a lens whose principal focus is at a distance of 1 meter (39.3 inches).

**prism d.,** the unit of measurement of the deviation of light in passing through a prism, being a deflection of 1 cm. at a distance of 1 meter.

**dioptos'copy.** Dioptroscopy.

**diop'tric.** 1. Relating to dioptrics. 2. Refractive. 3. Obsolete term for diopter.

**diop'trics.** The branch of optics that deals with the refraction of light.

**dioptrometer** (di-op-trom'e-ter) [ diopter + G. *metron,* measure ]. An instrument (obsolete) for measuring ocular refraction.

**dioptroscopy** (di-op-tros'ko-pĭ) [ diopter + G. *skopeō,* to examine ]. Dioptroscopy; determination of the degree of refraction by means of the ophthalmoscope.

**diop'try.** Obsolete term for diopter.

**diorthosis** (di'or-tho'sis) [ G. a making straight, fr. *di-orthoō,* to make straight, fr. *orthos,* straight ]. Diaplasis.

**Dioscorides** (di'os-kor-i'dēs), Pedacius, Greek surgeon in the Roman army, 54–68 A.D. Credited as the originator of materia medica. In his work on medical botany, which was considered authoritative for sixteen centuries, some 600 different plants or their derivatives were described.

**di'ose.** Glycolaldehyde; CHO—$CH_2OH$; theoretically the simplest sugar.

**diosgenin** (di'os-jen'in). A sapogenin derived from the saponins dioscin and trillin found in the roots of plants such as the yam; its steroid portion, 5-spirostene (see steroids for structure) serves as a source from which pregnenolone and progesterone can be prepared.

**diospyros** (di-os'pi-ros) [ G. *Dios pyros,* Jupiter's wheat (*Dios,* gen. of Zeus, L. Jupiter) ]. Persimmon; the unripe fruit of *Diospyros virginiana.* Astringent.

**diovulatory** (di-o'vu-lă-to'rĭ). Releasing two ova in one ovarian cycle.

**diox'adrol hydrochloride** (USAN). RELANE; *d*-2-(2,2-diphenyl-1,3-dioxoban-4-yl)piperidine hydrochloride; antidepressant.

**dioxahex'adecane.** PRESTONAL; a short-acting neuromuscular blocking agent with both depolarizing and non-depolarizing activity.

**diox'amate.** (2-Methyl-2-nonyl-1,3-dioxolan-4-yl)methyl carbamic acid ester; anticonvulsant.

**diox'ane.** 1,4-Diethylene dioxide.

**dioxaphetyl butyrate.** AMIDALGON; α,α-diphenyl-4-morpholinebutyric acid ethyl ester; analgesic with antispasmodic properties.

**dioxide** (di-ok'sīde). A molecule containing two atoms of oxygen.

**2,8-dioxyadenine.** The toxic product resulting from the administration of massive doses of adenine; toxicity due to the deposition of large crystalline masses in the kidney.

**dioxyben'zone** (USP). Dihydroxy-4-methoxybenzophenone; ultraviolet screen for topical application to the skin.

**dipen'tene.** *dl*-Limonene.

**dipep'tidase.** An enzyme catalyzing the hydrolysis of a dipeptide to its constituent amino acids.

**dipep'tide.** A combination of two amino acids by means of a peptide link.

**dipep'tidyl pep'tidase.** Cathepsin C; dipeptidyltransferase; a hydrolase (EC 3.4.14.1) cleaving dipeptides from polypeptides.

**dipep'tidyltrans'ferase.** Dipeptidyl peptidase.

**diper'odon hydrochloride** (NF). DIOTHANE; 3-piperidino-1,2-propanediol dicarbanilate hydrochloride; a local anesthetic used topically on various mucous membranes and for ocular operations.

**Dipetalonema** (di-pet'ah-lo-ne'mah) [ G. *di-,* two, + *petalon,* leaf, + *nema,* thread ]. A large genus of nematode filariae (including the genus *Acanthocheilonema,* according to recent authors), with species in man and many other mammals; as with other filarial worms, it produces microfilariae in blood or tissue fluids, and adults in deep connective tissue, membranes, or visceral surfaces.

**D. per'stans,** *Acanthocheilonema perstans.*

**D. recondi'tum,** a filarial worm of dogs, often confused with the canine heartworm, *Dirofilaria immitis.*

**D. streptocer'ca,** a sheathless microfilaria commonly found in the corium of the skin of West African residents and transmitted by the biting midge, *Culicoides grahami;* it causes a lichenoid condition of the skin.

**diphallus** (di-fal'us) [ G. *di-,* two, + *phallos,* penis ]. Double penis; bifid penis; a rare congenital anomaly; the organs may be symmetrical, or one placed above the other; there are often associated urogenital or other anomalies.

**diphasic** (di-fa'zik) [ G. *di-,* two, + *phasis,* appearance. PHAN- ]. Occurring in or referring to two phases or stages.

**diphe'manil methylsulfate** (NF). PRANTAL methylsulfate; 4-diphenylmethylene-1,1-dimethyl piperidinium methyl sulfate; used for peptic ulcers and for gastric hyperacidity and motility.

**diphemethox'idine.** CLEOFIL; 2-(diphenylmethyl)-1-piperidineethanol; an anorexigenic drug.

**diphenadione** (NF). DIPAXIN; 2-diphenylacetyl-1,3-indandione. An orally effective anticoagulant with actions and uses similar to those of bishydroxycoumarin.

**di'phenane, di'phenan.** BUTOLAN; *p*-benzylphenylcarbamate; used as a vermicide in oxyuriasis.

**diphenhy'dramine hydrochloride** (USP, BP). BENADRYL; 2-(diphenylmethoxy)-*N,N*-dimethylethylamine hydrochloride; an antihistaminic agent; also used in the treatment of parkinsonism and drug-induced parkinsonism.

**diphenicil'lin sodium.** ANCILLIN; 6-(2-biphenylcarboxoamido)-3,3-dimethyl-7-oxo-4-thia-1-azabicyclo[ 3.2.0 ]heptane-2-carboxylic acid sodium salt; a semisynthetic form of penicillin with antimicrobial properties.

**diphen'idol** (NF). VONTROL; α,α-diphenyl-1-piperidinebutanol; antiemetic agent.

*o*-**diphenol.** Pyrocatechol.

*o*-**diphenol oxidase.** Monophenol monooxygenase.

*p*-**diphenol oxidase.** Monophenol monooxygenase.

**diphenox'ylate hydrochloride** (USP, BP). 1-(3-Cyano-3,3-diphenylpropyl)-4-phenylpiperidine-4-carboxylic acid ethyl ester hydrochloride; ingredient of LOMOTIL (with atropine); chemically related to meperidine. It inhibits rhythmic contraction of smooth muscle, and is used as an antidiarrheal agent; has some addiction liability.

**diphenylchlorarsine** (di-fen'il-klor-ar'sēn). Sternutator; sneezing gas; inhalation causes violent sneezing, cough, salivation, headache, and retrosternal pain.

**diphenylhydantoin** (di-fen'il-hi-dan'to-in) (USP). DILANTIN; 5,5-diphenylhydantoin; an anticonvulsant agent used in the treatment of grand mal epilepsy. Also available as d. sodium (USP) and phenytoin sodium (BP), with same uses as d.

2,5-**diphenyloxazole.** PPO; a scintillator used in radioactivity measurements by scintillation counting.

**diphenylpy'raline hydrochloride** (NF). DIAFEN; 4-diphenylmethoxy-1-methylpiperidine hydrochloride; an antihistaminic agent similar in action and use to diphenhydramine, with a low incidence of side effects.

**diphosgene** (di-fos'jēn). Trichlormethyl chloroformate; ClCOOCCl₃; one of the poison gases used in World War I.

2,3-**diphos'phoglyc'erate.** A salt or ester of 2,3-diphosphoglyceric acid, *q.v.*

2,3-**diphos'phoglycer'ic acid.** A major component of certain mammalian erythrocytes, involved in the release of O₂ from HbO₂; postulated intermediate in the conversion of 3- to 2-phosphoglyceric acid.

**diphos'phopyr'idine nucleotide.** DPN; former name for nicotinamide adenine dinucleotide.

**diphos'phothi'amin.** Thiamin pyrophosphate.

**diphtheria** (dif-the'rĭ-ah) [ G. *diphthera,* leather ]. Syriac ulcer; a specific infectious disease due to *Corynebacterium*

*diphtheriae* and its highly potent toxin; it is marked by inflammation, with formation of a fibrinous exudate, of the mucous membrane of the throat, the nose, and sometimes the tracheobronchial tree; the toxin produces degeneration in peripheral nerves, heart muscle, and other tissues.

**avian d.,** see fowl *pox.*

**calf d.,** a disease of young calves manifested by deep and shallow erosions and diphtheritic exudates on the mucous membranes of the mouth and pharynx, caused by infection with *Actinomyces necrophorus.* The disease is very acute and highly fatal.

**cutaneous d.,** d. resulting from infection of the skin by *Corynebacterium diphtheriae.*

**false d.,** diphtheroid (1).

**surgical d.,** the formation of a false membrane on the surface of a wound.

**diphthe'rial.** Diphtheritic.

**diphtheriaphor** (dif-the'rĭ-ă-fōr) [ diphtheria + G. *phoros,* bearing ]. A carrier of diphtheria bacilli.

**diphtherin** (dif'thĕ-rin). The toxin of diphtheria; diphtherotoxin.

**diphtheritic** (dif'thĕ-rit'ik). Relating in any way to diphtheria, or the membrane characteristic of this disease.

**diphtheritis** (dif'thĕ-ri'tis). Diphtheria.

**diphtheroid** (dif'thĕ-royd) [ diphtheria + G. *eidos,* resemblance ]. 1. Pseudodiphtheria; false diphtheria; Epstein's disease; one of a group of local infections, suggesting diphtheria, caused by various microorganisms other than the *Corynebacterium diphtheriae.* 2. Any of the species resembling *Corynebacterium diphtheriae.*

**diph'therotox'in.** The toxin of diphtheria.

**diphthong** (dif'thong) [ G. *di-,* two, + *phthongos,* voice, sound ]. Vowel-like sound made while the articulators are in rapid movement from the position for one vowel to that of another.

**diphyllobothriasis** (di-fil'o-both-ri'ă-sis). Infection with the cestode *Diphyllobothrium latum* or broad fish tapeworm. Human infection is caused by ingestion of raw, or inadequately cooked, fish infected with the plerocercoid larva. Leukocytosis and eosinophilia may occur. If the worm is high enough in the alimentary canal, it may preempt the supply of vitamin B₁₂ or alter its absorption, leading to hyperchromic macrocytic anemia resembling pernicious anemia; particularly common among Scandinavians infected with this parasite.

**Diphyllobothrium** (di-fil-lo-both'ri-um) [ G. *di-,* two, + *phyllon,* leaf, + *bothrion,* little ditch ]. Sometimes called *Dibothriocephalus;* a large genus of cestodes, or tapeworms (family Pseudophyllidea) containing several species found in man, although only one, *D. latum,* is of widespread importance.

**D. corda'tum,** a species found in dogs, sea mammals, and occasionally man, in Greenland.

**D. la'tum,** *Taenia lata;* broad or broad fish tapeworm; found in man and fish eating mammals in many parts of northern Europe, in Japan, and elsewhere in Asia, and in Finnish populations of the American north central states; it often has several thousand segments, broader than long; the head has no sucking discs, but two deep sucking grooves, or bothria, at the borders; it may produce a pernicious anemia-like syndrome from differential absorption of vitamin B₁₂.

**D. linguloi'des,** *Spirometra mansoni.*

**D. man'soni,** *Spirometra mansoni.*

**D. mansonoi'des,** *Spirometra mansonoides.*

**diphyodont** (dif'ĭ-o-dont) [ G. *di-,* two, + *phyō,* to produce, + *odous* (*odont-*), tooth ]. Developing two sets of teeth, as man and most mammals.

**dipip'anone hydrochloride** (BP). PIPADONE; PIPIDOL; phenylpiperone; *dl*-4,4-diphenyl-6-piperidinoheptan-3-one hydrochloride; a narcotic congener of methadone, less potent than methadone.

**dipiproverine dihydrochloride.** LEVOSPASMOL; α-phenyl-1-piperidineacetic acid 2-piperidinoethyl ester; intestinal antispasmodic.

**diplacusis** (dip-lă-ku'sis) [ G. *diplous,* double, + *akousis,* a hearing ]. A difference of perception of sound by the two ears, either in time or in pitch, so that one sound is heard as two.

**d. binaura'lis,** a condition in which the same sound is heard differently by the two ears.

**d. dysharmon'ica,** a condition in which the same sound is heard with a different pitch in each ear.

**d. echo'ica,** a condition in which sound heard in the affected ear is repeated.

**d. monaura'lis,** a condition in which one sound is perceived as two in the same ear.

**diplegia** (di-ple'jĭ-ah) [ G. *di-,* two, + *plēgē,* a stroke ]. Double hemiplegia; paralysis of corresponding parts on both sides of the body.

**facial d.,** double facial paralysis; see Möbius' *syndrome.*

**infantile d.,** birth *palsy.*

**mas'ticatory d.,** paralysis of all the muscles of mastication.

**spastic d.,** hypertonic double hemiplegia, usually congenital. Also called Erb-Charcot disease; Little's disease; spastic spinal paralysis; tabes spasmodica.

**diplo-** (dip'lo-) [ G. *diplous,* double ]. Combining form meaning double, or twofold.

**dip'loalbuminu'ria.** The coexistence of nephritic, or pathologic, and nonnephritic, or physiologic, albuminuria.

**diplobacillus** (dip'lo-bă-sil'us). Two bacilli linked end to end.

**diplobacteria** (dip'lo-bak-te're-ah). Bacteria linked together in pairs.

**diploblas'tic** [ diplo- + G. *blastos,* germ ]. Formed of two germ layers.

**diplocar'dia** [ diplo- + G. *kardia,* heart ]. A condition in which the two lateral halves of the heart are more or less separated by a central fissure.

**dip'loceph'alus.** Dicephalus.

**diplocheiria, diplochiria** (dip'lo-ki-rī-ah) [ diplo- + G. *cheir,* hand ]. Dicheiria.

**diplococcemia** (dip-lo-kok-se'mī-ah). The presence of diplococci in the blood; used especially in referring to *Neisseria meningitidis* (meningococci) in circulating blood.

**diplococcin** (dip'lo-kok'sin). An antibiotic crystalline substance isolated from cultures of lactic acid-producing cocci present in milk. Active against microorganisms of the *Lactobacillus* group and certain Gram-positive cocci, but inactive against Gram-negative bacteria.

**diplococcoid** (dip'lo-kok'oyd). Resembling a diplococcus.

**Diplococcus** (dip'lo-kok'us) [ diplo- + G. *kokkos,* berry ]. *Streptococcus; D. pneumoniae,* the type species of *D.,* is a member of the genus *Streptococcus.*

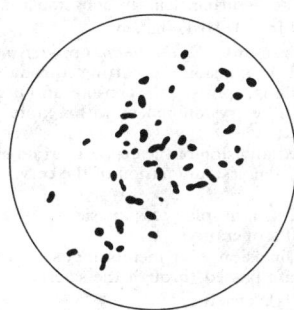

*Diplococcus pneumoniae*
(Original magnification, ×2400)

**diplococcus** (dip'lo-kok'us) [ diplo- + G. *kokkos,* berry ]. 1. Spherical or ovoid cells joined together in pairs. 2. Common name of any organism belonging to the bacterial genus *Diplococcus.*

**diplocoria** (dip'lo-ko'rī-ah) [ diplo- + G. *korē,* pupil ]. Dicoria; the presence of a double pupil in the eye.

**diploë** (dip'lo-e) [ G. *diploē,* fem. of *diplous,* double ] [ NA ]. The central layer of spongy bone between the two layers of compact bone, outer and inner plates or tables of the flat cranial bones.

**diplogenesis** (dip-lo-jen'ĕ-sis) [ diplo- + G. *genesis,* production ]. The production of a double fetus or of one with some parts doubled.

**Diplogonoporus** (dip'lo-go-nop'o-rus) [ diplo- + G. *gonos,* seed, + *poros,* pore ]. A genus of tapeworms found in Japan (*D. grandis*) and probably also in Roumania (*D. brauni*).

**dip'logram.** An x-ray with two exposures.

**diplo'ic.** Relating to the diploë.

**diploid** (dip'loyd) [ diplo- + G. *eidos* resemblance ]. Denoting the state of a cell containing twice the normal gametic number of chromosomes, one member of each chromosome pair derived from the father and one from the mother; the normal chromosome complement of somatic cells (in man, 46 chromosomes).

**diplois** [ L. fr G. *diploē, q.v.* ] [ NA ]. Diploic.

**diplokaryon** (dip'lo-kăr'ī-on) [ diplo- + G. *karyon,* nut (nucleus) ]. A cell nucleus containing twice the normal diploid number of chromosomes; *i.e.,* a tetraploid nucleus. See also polyploidy.

**diplomelituria** (dip-lo-mel-ĭ-tu'rī-ah) [ diplo- + G. *meli,* honey, + *ouron,* urine ]. The occurrence of diabetic and nondiabetic glycosuria in the same individual.

**diplomyelia** (dip-lo-mi-e'lĭ-ah) [ diplo- + G. *myelon,* marrow ]. A more or less complete doubling of the spinal cord; it may or may not be accompanied by a bony septum of the vertebral canal. See also diastematomyelia.

**dip'lon.** Deuteron.

**diplonema** (dip'lo-ne'mah) [ diplo- + G. *nema,* thread ]. The doubled form of the chromosome strand visible at the diplotene stage of meiosis.

**diploneural** (dip-lo-nu'ral) [ diplo- + G. *neuron,* nerve ]. Supplied by two nerves from different sources, said of certain muscles.

**diplopagus** (dip-lop'ă-gus) [ diplo- + G. *pagos,* something fixed ]. Cenadelphus; a general term for conjoined twins, each with fairly complete bodies, although one or more internal organs may be in common.

**diplopia** (dī-plo'pĭ-ah) [ diplo- + G. *ōps,* eye ]. Double vision; the condition in which a single object is perceived as two objects.

**binocular d.,** d. in which one image is seen by one eye and the other image by the other eye.

**crossed d.,** heteronymous d.

**direct d.,** homonymous d.

**heteron'ymous d.,** crossed d.; d. in which the false image is on the same side as the sound eye; d. due to divergent squint or paralysis of the internal rectus.

**homon'ymous d.,** simple d.; direct d.; d. in which the false image is on the same side as the affected eye; d. due to convergent squint or paralysis of the external rectus.

**mental d.,** awareness both of reality and also of one's illusions or hallucinations.

**monoc'ular d.,** monodiplopia; a form in which two objects are seen with the same eye, due to incomplete cataract, double pupil, etc.

**simple d.,** homonymous d.

**diplopiometer** (dip-lo-pī-om'e-ter). An instrument for determining the presence and the degree of diplopia.

**diplopo'dia** [ diplo- + G. *pous,* foot ]. Duplication of digits of the foot.

**diploscope** (dip'lo-skōp) [ diplo- + G. *skopeō,* to examine ]. An instrument for the study of binocular vision and of its anomalies.

**diplosome** (dip'lo-sōm) [ diplo- + G. *sōma,* body ]. The pair of centrioles of mammalian cells.

**diploso'mia** [ diplo- + G. *somā,* body, + suffix *-ia,* condition ]. A condition in which twins, seemingly functionally independent, are joined at one or more points.

**Dip'lospo'rium** [ diplo- + G. *sporos,* seed ]. A genus of rapidly growing fungi that are considered to be saprophytes; they are common contaminants in laboratory cultures.

**diplotene** (dip'lo-tēn) [ diplo- + G. *taenia,* band ]. The late stage of prophase in meiosis in which the paired homologous chromosomes begin to repel each other and move apart but are usually held together by regions of crossing or intertwining called chiasmata. The chiasmata are associated with breakage of two chromatids at corresponding points followed by refusion of the broken ends with exchange of segments between the chromatids; this is considered to be the cytologic basis for the genetic phenomenon of crossing-over, the exchange of blocks of genes between homologous chromosomes.

**diploteratology** (dip'lo-tĕr-ă-tol'o-jĭ). The division of teratology dealing with conjoined twins.

**dipodia** (di-po'dĭ-ah) [ G. *di-*, two, + *pous* (*pod-*), foot ]. 1. A developmental anomaly involving more or less complete duplication of a foot. 2. In conjoined twins a degree of fusion leaving two feet evident. 3. In sympus dipus a degree of fusion leaving two feet recognizable.

**di'pole.** A pair of separated electrical charges, one positive and one negative; doublet.

**dipropyltryptamine.** DPT; *N,N*-dipropyltryptamine; a hallucinogenic agent similar to dimethyltryptamine.

**diprosopus** (di-pros'o-pus, di-pro-so'pus) [ G. *di-*, two + *prosōpon*, face ]. Conjoined twins with almost complete fusion of the bodies but with duplication of the face or any part of it. See fig. under opodidymus.

    **d. parasit'icus,** a d. in which one of the faces is small and poorly developed.

**dipse'sis** [ G. *dipsein*, to thirst ]. Dipsosis; abnormal or excessive thirst, or a craving for certain unusual forms of drink.

**dip'sogen** [ G. *dipsa*, thirst, + suffix *-gen*, producing ]. A thirst-provoking agent.

**dipsoma'nia** [ G. *dipsa*, thirst, + *mania*, madness ]. Alcoholism; posiomania; a recurring compulsion to drink to excess of alcoholic beverages.

**dipso'sis** [ G. *dipsa*, thirst, + suffix *-osis*, condition ]. Dipsesis.

**dipsotherapy** (dip'so-thĕr-ă-pĭ). Treatment of certain diseases by abstention, as far as possible, from liquids.

**dip'teryx** [ G. *di-*, two, + *pteryx*, wing. PTER- ]. Tonka; tonka bean; snuff bean; the prepared seed of *Dipteryx* (*Coumarouna*) *odorata* or *appositifolia* (family Leguminosae), trees of N. Brazil and Guiana. The active constituent is coumarin.

**di'pus** [ G. *di-*, two, + *pous* (*pod-*), foot ]. An individual exhibiting dipodia.

**Dipus sagit'ta.** A small rodent of Southern Russia that serves as a vector, through fleas, of *Pasteurella pestis* (plague bacillus).

**dipygus** (di-pi'gus, dip'ĭ-gus) [ G. *di-*, two, + *pyge*, buttocks ]. Conjoined twins with the head and thorax completely merged, and the pelvis and lower extremities duplicated; when the duplications of the lower parts are symmetrical, usually called duplicitas posterior.

    **d. parasit'icus,** d. in which one of the components is poorly developed and "parasitic" on the larger.

**Dipylid'ium cani'num** [ G. *dipylos*, with two entrances; L. ntr. of *caninus*, pertaining to *canis*, dog ]. The commonest species of dog tapeworm, the double-pored tapeworm, the larvae of which are harbored by dog fleas or lice; the worm occasionally infects man, especially children licked by dogs that have recently nipped infected fleas.

**di'pyrid'amole** (USAN). PERSANTIN; 2,2',2'',2''-[ 4,8-dipiperidinopyrimidino[ 5,4-d ]pyrimidine-2,6-diyldinitrilo ]tetraethanol. It is a potent coronary vasodilator when administered intravenously; however, there is no convincing evidence that it has therapeutic effects when administered orally.

**dipyrimidine photolyase.** Deoxydipyrimidine photolyase.

**dipyrithione** (USAN). OMADINE disulfide; 2,2'-dithiopyridine-1,1'-dioxide; an antibacterial and antifungal agent.

**direc'tor** [ L. *dirigo*, pp. *-rectus*, to arrange, set in order. REG- ]. Staff (1).

**dirigation** (dĭr'ĭ-ga'shun) [ L. *dis-*, apart, + *rigare*, to draw off, sleuce off ]. The development of voluntary control over functions that are ordinarily involuntary.

**dirigomotor** (dĭr'ĭ-go-mo'tor). Directing muscular movement.

**Dirofilaria** (di-ro-fĭ-la'rĭ-ah) [ L. *dirus*, dread, + *Filaria* ]. A genus of filaria (family Onchocercidae, superfamily Filarioidea); *D.* species are usually found in mammals

other than man, but rare examples of human infection are known, *e.g.,* by *D. magalhaesi, D. repens,* and *D. louisianensis.*

    **D. conjuncti'vae,** a filarial worm found chiefly in horses; characterized by adult forms that live in the subcutaneous tissues, especially in the loose areolar type such as that about the eye; also reported from cystlike tumors in man.

    **D. immit'is,** the dog heartworm; a filarial worm found chiefly in the right ventricle pulmonary arteries of dogs; *D. immitis* and its canine host have been used to test chemotherapeutic agents; an extract of *D. immitis* may be used as a relatively nonspecific intradermal antigen in the diagnosis of human filariasis and in complement-fixation tests. See also *Dipetalonema reconditum.*

**dis-** [ L. an inseparable particle denoting separation, taking apart, sundering in two ]. Prefix having the same force as the original Latin preposition. Not to be confused with *dys-, q. v.*

**disabil'ity.** Medicolegal term signifying loss of function and earning power.

**disa'blement.** Medicolegal term signifying loss of function without loss of earning power.

**disaccharide** (dis-sak'ă-rīd). A condensation product of two monosaccharides by elimination of water (usually between an alcoholic OH and a hemiacetal OH); examples are sucrose, lactose, and maltose.

**disaggregation** (dis-ag'gre-ga'shun) [ L. *dis-*, separating, + *ag-grego* (*adg-*), pp. *-gregatus*, to add to something, fr. *grex*, a flock ]. 1. A breaking up into the component parts. 2. An inability to coordinate the various sensations and failure to observe their mutual relations.

**disarticula'tion** [ L. *dis-*, apart, + *articulus*, joint ]. Amputation in contiguity; aparthrosis (2); exarticulation; amputation of a limb through a joint, without cutting of bone.

**disassimila'tion.** Destructive or retrograde metabolism.

**disc.** See disk; also discus.

**disc-.** See disco-.

**discectomy** (dis-sek'to-me) [ G. *diskos*, disk, + *ektomē*, excision ]. Discotomy; excision, in part or whole, of an intervertebral disk.

**dis'charge.** 1. That which is emitted or evacuated, as an excretion or a secretion. 2. The activation or firing of a neuron.

    **after-d.,** see afterdischarge.

**Dische,** Zacharias, U. S. biochemist. See D. *reaction.*

**dischronation** (dis-kro-na'shun) [ L. *dis-*, apart, + G. *chronos,* time ]. A disturbance in the consciousness of time.

**disciform** (dis'ĭ-form). Disk-shaped.

**discission** (dis-sish'un) [ L. *di-scindo*, pp. *-scissus*, to tear asunder. SCHI- ]. Incision or cutting through a part; specifically needling, splitting the capsule, and breaking up the substance of the crystalline lens with a knife needle, in cases of soft cataract.

    **d. of the cervix,** division of the cervix uteri on either side for the relief of stenosis; an incision of the cervix to widen the canal.

    **d. of the pleura,** multiple cross incisions, for empyema, as in Ransohoff's operation.

    **posterior d.,** incision of a membranous cataract from behind by a knife passed through the sclera.

**discitis** (disk-i'tis). Diskitis.

**dis'clina'tion.** Extorsion (2).

**disco-, disc-** (dis'ko-) [ G. *diskos*, disk ]. Combining forms indicating relation to, or similarity to, a disk.

**discoblas'tic.** Relating to a discoblastula.

**discoblastula** (dis'ko-blas'tu-lah). A blastula of the type produced by the meroblastic discoidal cleavage of a large yolked ovum.

**discogastrula** (dis'ko-gas'tru-lah). A gastrula of the type formed after the discoidal cleavage of a large-yolked ovum.

**discogenic** (dis'ko-gen'ik). Denoting a disorder originating in or from the intervertebral disc.

**discography** (dis-kog'ră-fĭ) [ disco- + G. *graphō,* to write ]. Radiographic visualization of intervertebral disk space by injection of contrast media.

**discoid** (dis'koyd) [ disco- + G. *eidos*, appearance ]. 1. Resembling a disk. 2. In dentistry a disk-shaped excavator or carving tool.

**Discomyces** (dis-ko-mi'sēz) [ disco- + G. *mykēs*, fungus ]. A generic name used synonymously with the actinomycetes.

**discop'athy** (dis-kop'ă-thĭ) [ disco- + G. *pathos*, disease ]. Disease of a disk, particularly of the discus intervertebralis.

**traumatic cervical d.,** an injury characterized by fissuration, laceration and/or fragmentation of the disc or surrounding ligaments, with or without displacement of fragments against spinal cord, nerve roots, or ligaments.

**dis'coplacen'ta.** A placenta of discoid shape.

**disco'ria** [ G. *dis*, double, + *korē*, pupil ]. Diplocoria.

**discostroma** (dis'ko-stro'mah) [ disco- + stroma, *q.v.* ]. The stroma of a red blood cell.

**discotomy** (dis-kot'o-mĭ) [ disco- + G. *tomē*, incision ]. Discectomy.

**discrete** (dis-krēt) [ L. *dis-cerno*, pp. -*cretus*, to separate. CRET- ]. Separate; distinct; not joined to or incorporated with another; denoting certain lesions of the skin especially.

**discrimina'tion.** In conditioning, responding differentially, as when an organism makes one response to a reinforced stimulus and another response to an unreinforced stimulus.

**discus,** pl. **dis'ci** (dis'kus) [ L. fr. G. *diskos*, a quoit, disk ] [ NA ]. Disk, *q.v.;* any approximately flat circular surface.

**d. articula'ris** [ NA ], articular disk; intraarticular cartilage; interarticular fibrocartilage; a plate or ring of fibrocartilage attached to the joint capsule and separating the articular surfaces of the bones for a varying distance, sometimes completely; it serves to adapt two articular surfaces that are not entirely congruent.

**d. articula'ris acromioclavicula'ris** [ NA ], acromioclavicular disk; the articular disk of fibrocartilage usually found between the acromial end of the clavicle and the medial border of the acromion.

**d. articula'ris radioulna'ris** [ NA ], radioulnar articular disk; triquetrous cartilage (1); triangular disk or cartilage; radioulnar disk; the disk that holds together the distal ends of the radius and ulna. It is attached by its apex to a depression between the styloid process and distal surface of the head of the ulna, and by its base to the ridge separating the ulnar notch from the carpal surface of the radius.

**d. articula'ris sternoclavicula'ris** [ NA ], sternoclavicular articular disk; sternonavicular disk; the fibrocartilaginous disk that subdivides the sternoclavicular joint into two cavities.

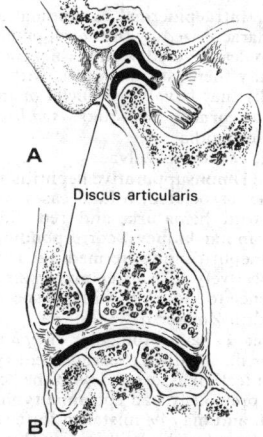

A
Discus articularis

B

**Articular Disks**
*A,* temporomandibular joint; *B,* distal radioulnar joint. See also fig. under joint.

**d. articula'ris temporomandibula'ris** [ NA ], temporomandibular articular disk; mandibular disk; the fibrocartilaginous plate that separates the joint into upper and lower cavities.

**d. interpu'bicus** [ NA ], interpubic disk; lamina fibrocartilaginea interpubica; the disk of fibrocartilage that unites the pubic bones at the pubic symphysis.

**d. intervertebra'lis** [ NA ], intervertebral disk or cartilage; fibrocartilago intervertebralis; a disk interposed between the bodies of adjacent vertebrae. It is composed of an outer fibrous part (anulus fibrosus) that surrounds a central gelatinous mass (nucleus pulposus).

**d. lentifor'mis,** Rarely used synonym for *nucleus* subthalamicus.

**d. nervi op'tici** [ NA ], blind spot (3); Mariotte's blind spot; papilla nervi optici; optic papilla; optic disk; porus opticus; a circular area of the retina, devoid of light receptors, toward which the optic nerve fibers converge to leave the eye.

**d. prolig'erus,** *cumulus* oophorus.

**discuss** (dis-kus') [ L. *dis-cutio*, pp. -*cussus*, to strike asunder, shatter, fr. *quatio*, to shake ]. To disperse; to cause to disappear or be absorbed.

**discus'sive.** Discutient.

**discutient** (dis-ku'she-ent) [ see discuss ]. 1. Scattering or dispersing a pathologic accumulation. 2. An agent that causes the dispersal of a tumor or pathologic collection of any sort.

**disdiaclast** (dis-di'ah-klast) [ G. *dis*, twice, + *dia*, through, + *klastos*, broken ]. A doubly refractive element in striated muscular tissue.

# DISEASE

**disease** (diz-ēz) [ Eng. *dis-* priv. + ease ]. 1. Morbus; illness; sickness; an interruption, cessation, or disorder of body functions, systems, or organs. 2. A disease *entity,* characterized usually by at least two of these criteria: a recognized etiologic agent (or agents); an identifiable group of signs and symptoms; consistent anatomical alterations.

**aaa d.,** endemic anemia of ancient Egypt, ascribed in the Papyrus Ebers to intestinal infestation, presumably with ancylostoma.

**ABO hemolytic d. of the newborn,** erythroblastosis fetalis due to maternal-fetal incompatibility with respect to an antigen of the ABO blood group; the fetus possesses A or B antigen which is lacking in the mother, and the mother produces immune type antibody which causes hemolysis of fetal erythrocytes.

**Acosta's d.,** hypobaropathy.

**acute d.,** an abnormal condition of the body or any of its parts, manifested by symptoms of a more or less violent character, and terminating, after a comparatively brief period, in recovery or death.

**Adams-Stokes d.,** Adams-Stokes *syndrome.*

**adaptation d.'s,** d.'s theoretically falling into Selye's concept of the general adaptation syndrome, *q.v.,* under syndrome.

**Addison's d.,** chronic adrenocortical *insufficiency.*

**Addison-Biermer d.,** pernicious *anemia.*

**adenoid d.,** (1) adenoids; (2) obsolete term for Hodgkin's d.

**akamushi d.** (ak-kah-moo'shĭ) [ Jap. *aka,* red, + *mushi,* bug ], tsutsugamushi d.

**Akureyri d.,** epidemic *neuromyasthenia.*

**Albers-Schönberg d.,** osteopetrosis.

**Albright's d.,** localized osteitis fibrosa; osteitis fibrosa circumscripta; osteitis fibrosa disseminata; polyostotic fibrous dysplasia with cutaneous pigmentation and endocrine disturbance, especially precocious puberty in girls.

**Aleutian d. of mink,** anorexia, diarrhea, weight loss, and death caused by a filterable agent resistant to formalin (0.3 per cent); occurs chiefly in mink homozygous for the recessive Aleutian gene; infection associated with greatly increased 6.4 S globulin.

**Alexander's d.,** a d. of the brain, of unknown cause, seen in children and characterized by rapid onset, mental deterioration, and paralysis, terminating fatally before the age of 5. Pathologic lesions include a widespread leukodystrophic change with eosinophilic deposits occurring at cerebral interfaces, all associated with megaloencephaly.

**Alibert's d.,** *mycosis* fungoides.

**alkali d.,** a term that has been applied by stockmen to various animal poisonings of plant and mineral origin in arid regions under the belief that they were caused by the ingestion of alkaline waters. A well known example is botulism of wild ducks, caused by feeding on decayed vegetation in nearly dried-up lakes.

**Almeida's d.,** South American *blastomycosis.*

**Alpers' d.,** *poliodystrophia* cerebri progressiva infantalis.

**Alzheimer's d.,** organic dementia occurring usually in persons under 50 years of age, associated with Alzheimer's sclerosis, neurofibrillary degeneration, and senile plaques.

**anarthritic rheumatoid d.,** rheumatoid d. without arthritis.

**Anders' d.,** *adiposis* dolorosa.

**Andersen's d.,** type 4 *glycogenosis.*

**antibody deficiency d.,** antibody deficiency *syndrome.*

**aorticorenal d.,** combined arteriosclerotic d. of both the abdominal aorta and one or both renal arteries.

**aortoiliac occlusive d.,** Leriche syndrome; obstruction of the abdominal aorta and its main branches by atherosclerosis.

**Aran-Duchenne d.,** progressive muscular *atrophy.*

**arc-welder's d.,** siderosis (1).

**Aujeszky's d.,** infectious bulbar paralysis; mad itch; pseudorabies; an acute d. affecting cattle, horses, dogs, and swine, caused by *Herpesvirus suis,* which has its reservoir in swine and is transmitted to wounds of other species by the nasal secretions. In species other than swine it is highly fatal. In very young swine it causes fatalities but in adult animals the disease is inapparent.

**Australian X d.,** Murray Valley *encephalitis.*

**autoimmune d.,** a d. resulting from an immune reaction produced by an individual's leukocytes or antibodies acting on the subject's own tissues or extracellular proteins. See also autoimmunization.

**aviator's d.,** term sometimes applied to aviation sickness in flying at high altitudes, analogous to the bends.

**Ayerza's d.,** a condition resembling polycythemia vera but resulting from primary pulmonary arteriosclerosis.

**Baelz' d.,** *cheilitis* glandularis.

**Balfour's d.,** chloroma.

**Ballet's d.,** *ophthalmoplegia* externa.

**Bal'me d.,** epidemic *pleurodynia.*

**Baló's d.,** encephalitis periaxialis concentrica.

**Bamberger's d.,** (1) saltatory *spasm;* (2) polyserositis.

**Bamberger-Marie d.,** (1) hypertrophic pulmonary *osteoarthropathy;* (2) see idiopathic Bamberger-Marie d.

**bamie d.,** epidemic *pleurodynia.*

**Bang's d.,** bovine *brucellosis.*

**Bannister's d.,** angioneurotic *edema.*

**Banti's d.,** Banti's *syndrome.*

**Barclay-Baron d.,** vallecular *dysphagia.*

**Barlow's d.,** infantile *scurvy.*

**Barraquer's d.,** progressive *lipodystrophy.*

**Basedow's d.,** Graves' d.

**Batten-Mayou d.,** late juvenile type of cerebral *sphingolipidosis, q.v.*

**Bayle's d.,** general paralysis of the insane.

**Bazin's d.,** *erythema* induratum.

**Bechterew's d.,** *spondylitis* deformans.

**Becker's d.,** an obscure South African cardiomyopathy leading to rapidly fatal congestive heart failure and idiopathic mural endomyocardial d.

**Begbie's d.,** (1) obsolete eponym for exophthalmic goiter; (2) localized chorea.

**Béguez César d.,** Chédiak-Steinbrink-Higashi *syndrome.*

**Behçet's d.,** Behçet's *syndrome.*

**Behr's d.,** adult or presenile form of heredomacular *degeneration.*

**Beigel's d.,** chignon; small brownish nodules or concretions on the hairs of wigs or toupees, possibly due to a fungus.

**Bennett's d.,** obsolete eponym for leukemia.

**Benson's d.,** asteroid *hyalosis.*

**Berlin's d.,** *concussion* of retina.

**Bernhardt's d.,** *meralgia* paraesthetica.

**Besnier-Boeck-Schaumann d.,** sarcoidosis.

**Best's d.,** heredomacular degeneration occurring during the first few years of life. See also vitelliform *degeneration* of the macula, and cystic heredomacular *degeneration.*

**Beurmann's d.,** the disseminated gummatous form of sporotrichosis, *q.v.*

**Bielschowsky's d.,** early juvenile type of cerebral *sphingolipidosis, q.v.*

**Biermer's d.,** pernicious *anemia.*

**Biett's d.,** *lupus* erythematosus.

**big liver d.,** see avian *lymphomatosis.*

**Binswanger's d.,** Binswanger's encephalopathy; encephalitis subcorticalis chronica; an organically caused dementia found in chronic hypertensives; it is characterized by recurrent edema of cerebral white matter, with secondary demyelination.

**bird-breeder's d.,** bird-breeder's *lung.*

**black d.,** infectious necrotic *hepatitis* of sheep.

**black-tongue d.,** a d. of dogs similar to human pellagra and due to niacin deficiency.

**blinding d.,** onchocerciasis.

**Bloch-Sulzberger d.,** *incontinentia* pigmenti.

**Blocq's d.,** astasia-abasia.

**Blount's d.,** Blount-Barber d.; nonrachitic bowlegs in children.

**Blount-Barber d.,** Blount's d.

**bluecomb d. of chickens,** housing d.; pullet d.; summer d.; avian monocytosis; an acute or subacute d. of young laying chickens characterized by lowered egg production, diarrhea, frequently cyanosis of the head, and pathologic changes involving chiefly the liver and kidney; the etiology is not definitely established, but may prove to be viral.

**bluecomb d. of turkeys,** transmissible enteritis; mud fever (2); an acute or chronic d. of young turkeys, with diarrhea, loss of weight, and often cyanosis of the head; the d. is caused by a reovirus.

**Boeck's d.,** sarcoidosis.

**Borna d.** [ *Borna,* a locality in Saxony where a severe epidemic occurred ], an infectious encephalomyelitis of horses, cattle, and sheep caused by Borna disease virus; it occurs in Germany and several other European countries; affected animals show depression, then excitment and spasms, and finally paralysis.

**Bornholm d.** [ *Bornholm,* an island in the Baltic where the d. appears to be endemic ], epidemic *pleurodynia.*

**Botkin's d.,** the Russian term for infectious hepatitis.

**Bouchard's d.,** myopathic dilation of the stomach.

**Bouillaud's d.,** acute rheumatic fever with carditis.

**Bourneville's d.,** tuberous *sclerosis.*

**Bourneville-Pringle d.,** tuberous sclerosis with adenoma sebaceum.

**Bowen's d.,** intraepidermal carcinoma; a precancerous dermatosis characterized by the development of pinkish or brownish papules covered with a thickened horny layer. Microscopically there is dyskeratosis with scattered giant epidermal cells that have large nuclei or mitotic figures.

**Bowen's d. of cornea,** Morquio's *syndrome.*

**Breda's d.,** espundia.

**Breisky's d.,** *kraurosis* vulvae.

**Bright's d.,** (1) nonsuppurative nephritis with albuminuria and edema, associated in fatal cases with large white kidneys; or with hematuria and red kidneys; or with contracted granular kidneys, corresponding to the stages of glomerulonephritis now termed subacute, acute, and chronic, respectively; (2) an eponym sometimes used in general reference to kidney d. without specifying the kind.

**Brill's d.,** Brill-Zinsser d.

**Brill-Symmer d.,** giant follicular *lymphoblastoma.*

**Brill-Zinsser d.,** Brill's d.; recrudescent typhus fever; an endogenous infection associated with the "carrier state" in persons who previously had epidemic typhus fever; it is a rather mild d. and may be mistaken for endemic (murine) typhus; first described by Brill in New York City but not recognized as a recrudescent form of epidemic typhus until after the work of Zinsser.

**Brinton's d.,** (1) *linitis* plastica; (2) infantile *scurvy.*

**brisket d.,** a d. of cattle, characterized by edematous swelling of the brisket and the tissues of the neck; the body cavities also contain large quantities of clear straw-colored transudate; this d. results from right heart failure as a consequence of increased pulmonary resistance, which is in some way associated with movement of animals to high altitudes.

**Brissaud's d.,** a tic or habit spasm.

**Brocq's d.,** a variety of parapsoriasis.

**Brodie's d.,** (1) Brodie's *knee;* (2) hysterical arthralgia; (3) hysterical spinal neuralgia, simulating Pott's disease, following a trauma.

**bronzed d.,** (1) Addison's d.; (2) hemochromatosis.

**Brooke's d.,** (1) trichoepithelioma; (2) *keratosis* follicularis contagiosa.

**Bruck's d.,** a d. marked by fragilitas ossium, ankylosis of the joints, and muscular atrophy.

**Brushfield-Wyatt d.,** nevoid amentia; mental retardation probably associated with Sturge-Weber syndrome.

**Buerger's d.,** *thromboangiitis* obliterans.

**Buhl's d.,** *icterus* neonatorum.

**Bury's d.,** *erythema* elevatum diutinum.

**Buschke's d.,** (1) *scleredema* adultorum; (2) cryptococcosis.

**Busquet's d.,** an osteoperiostitis of the metatarsal bones, leading to exostoses on the dorsum of the foot.

**buss d.,** bovine sporadic *encephalomyelitis.*

**Busse-Buschke d.,** cryptococcosis.

**Caffey's d.,** infantile cortical *hyperostosis.*

**caisson d.,** (ka'son) [ Fr. *caisson* (fr. *caisse,* a chest), a water-tight box or cylinder containing air under high pressure, used in sinking piers for bridges, etc. ], a symptom complex occurring in men working under high air pressures when too suddenly released to normal atmosphere (and in fliers suddenly going to high altitudes unprotected by counterpressure). It results from the escape from solution in the body fluids of bubbles—chiefly nitrogen—absorbed originally at high atmospheric pressure. It is characterized by headache, pain in the epigastrium, in the sinuses, and sometimes in a tooth socket, itching of the skin, vertigo, dyspnea, coughing, nausea, vomiting, sometimes paralysis. Additional symptoms may be "chokes" and severe peripheral circulatory collapse.

**California d.,** coccidioidomycosis.

**Calvé-Perthes d.,** epiphysial aseptic *necrosis* (*q.v.*) of the upper end of the femur.

**Canavan's d.,** spongy *degeneration.*

**Capdepont's d.,** *dentinogenesis* imperfecta.

**Carré's d.,** canine *distemper* (1).

**Carrión's d.,** Oroya *fever.*

**cat-bite d.,** cat-bite fever; same as rat-bite fever; presumably spread from rats to cats, and thus to man.

**cat-scratch d.,** an uleroglandular d. of man that frequently follows the scratch or bite of a cat, although some cases have occurred when there has been no contact with a cat; it is a seemingly specific infection, producing regional lymphadenitis, indolent reaction, and benign low grade infection; in some cases suppurated glands have to be drained surgically; the agent has not been isolated; diagnosis is based on the Foshay *test* (*q.v.*). Also called cat-scratch fever; benign inoculation reticulosis; nonbacterial regional lymphadenitis; benign inoculation lymphoreticulosis.

**Cazenave's d.,** *lupus* erythematosus.

**celiac d.,** nontropical sprue occurring in children; also called Gee's, or Gee-Herter, disease, syndrome, or infantilism; celiac syndrome; diarrhea chylosa; diarrhea alba (1) white diarrhea (1); intestinal infantilism; white flux (1).

**central core d.,** a heritable d. of skeletal muscle characterized by slowly progressive or chronic nonprogressive weakness; postulated to arise from a deficiency of phosphorylase *b* or a reduced ability to convert it to active phosphorylase. On biopsy the central core of muscle fibers stains abnormally.

**cerebrovas'cular d.,** symptoms of brain injury due to vascular insufficiency.

**Chagas' d., Chagas-Cruz d.,** South American *trypanosomiasis.*

**Championnière's d.,** fibrinous *bronchitis.*

**Charcot's d.,** (1) amyotrophic lateral *sclerosis;* (2) tabetic *arthropathy.*

**Charcot-Marie-Tooth d.,** peroneal muscular *atrophy.*

**Charlouis' d.,** yaws.

**Cheadle's d.,** infantile *scurvy.*

**Chédiak-Higashi d.,** Chédiak-Steinbrinck-Higashi *syndrome.*

**Chiari's d.,** Chiari's *syndrome.*

**Christensen-Krabbe d.,** *poliodystrophia* cerebri progressiva infantalis.

**Christian's d.,** (1) Hand-Schüller-Christian d.; (2) Weber-Christian d.

**Christmas d.** [ fr. *Christmas,* the name of a child suffering from the disease ], *hemophilia* B.

**chronic d.,** one of long continuance, marked usually by no very violent symptoms, sometimes ending in recovery, or else in death through cachexia or an intercurrent attack of acute d.

**chronic granulomatous d.,** congenital dysphagocytosis; a congenital defect in the killing of phagocytosed bacteria by polymorphonuclear leukocytes, resulting in increased susceptibility to severe infection; inheritance is usually by X-linked transmission to males.

**chronic hypertensive d.,** the presence of persistent hypertension, of whatever cause, before pregnancy or before the 20th week of gestation, or persistent hypertension beyond the 42nd postpartum day.

**chronic respiratory d.,** a common and serious d. of the respiratory tract of chickens; it is caused by a pleuropneumonia-like organism, *Mycoplasma gallinarum;* secondary infection with *Escherichia coli* is common.

**circling d.,** listeriosis.

**Civatte's d.,** *poikiloderma* of Civatte.

**clover d.,** trifoliosis.

**coal miners' d.,** anthracosis.

**Coats' d.,** exudative *retinitis.*

**Cockayne's d.,** Cockayne's *syndrome.*

**cold hemagglutinin d.,** autoallergic hemolytic anemia of the cold-antibody type; anemia associated with the hemagglutinating cold autoantibody.

**collagen d.'s,** collagenoses; a group of nonhereditary generalized d.'s affecting connective tissue and frequently characterized by fibrinoid necrosis or vasculitis. D.'s that have been included in this group are lupus erythematosus, scleroderma, rheumatoid arthritis, and rheumatic fever.

**combined system d.,** subacute combined *degeneration* of the spinal cord.

**communicable d.,** any d. that is transmissible by infection or contagion directly or through the agency of a vector.

**complicating d.,** a secondary or independent d. supervening in the course of an already existent affection.

**Concato's d.,** polyserositis.

**congenital d.,** one that is present in the infant at birth.

**Conradi's d.,** chondrodystrophia congenita punctata; congenital shortening of the humerus and femur, with stippled epiphyses, high arched palate, cataracts, erythroderma in the newborn, and scaling followed by follicular atrophoderma.

**constitutional d.,** d. related to diathesis, disposition, or constitution, often inherited as an inborn error of structure or metabolism.

**contagious d.,** an infectious d. transmissible by direct or indirect contact. Now more or less synonymous with communicable d.

**Cooper's d.,** chronic inflammation of the mamma, with the formation of cysts.

**Cori's d.,** type 3 *glycogenosis.*

**corn-meal d.,** see *Besnoitia tarandi.*

**corridor d. of cattle,** a tick-borne disease of cattle in Rhodesia and the Union of South Africa caused by *Theileria lawrenci,* lesions and symptoms similar to those of East Coast fever; buffaloes are reservoirs of infection, serving as sources of infection for cattle.

**Corrigan's d.,** aortic *regurgitation.*

**Corvisart's d.,** chronic hypertrophic myocarditis.

**Cotunnius' d.,** sciatica.

**crazy chick d.,** nutritional *encephalomalacia* of chicks.

**Creutzfeldt-Jakob d.,** spastic pseudosclerosis with corticostriatal-spinal degeneration; caused by one of the slow viruses.

**Crigler-Najjar d.,** Crigler-Najjar *syndrome.*

**Crocq's d.,** acrocyanosis.

**Crohn's d.,** regional *enteritis.*

**Crouzon's d.,** cranial dysostosis; craniofacial dysostosis; widening of the skull, with a high forehead, ocular hypertelorism, exophthalmos, beaked nose, and hypoplasia of the maxilla.

**Cruveilhier's d.,** progressive muscular *atrophy*.

**Cruveilhier-Baumgarten d.,** Cruveilhier-Baumgarten *syndrome*.

**Csillag's d.,** chronic atrophic and lichenoid dermatitis.

**Curschmann's d.,** frosted *liver*.

**Cushing's d.,** a designation sometimes reserved for those instances of Cushing's syndrome associated with a pituitary adenoma.

**cystic d.,** polycystic *kidney*.

**cystic d. of breast,** cystic *hyperplasia* of breasts.

**cystic d. of renal medulla,** microcystic d. of renal medulla; the presence of small cysts in the renal medulla associated with anemia, sodium depletion, and chronic renal failure; it is of two types: (1) autosomal recessive or juvenile type, begins at about age 10 and has an average duration of 6 to 8 years; it is also called familial juvenile nephrophthisis; (2) autosomal dominant or adult type, begins at about age 30 but has a more fulminant course.

**cystine storage d.,** cystinosis.

**cytomegalic inclusion d.,** inclusion body d.; the presence of large inclusion bodies within the cytoplasm and nuclei of enlarged cells of various organs of newborn infants dying with jaundice, hepatomegaly, splenomegaly, purpura, thrombocytopenia, and fever. The condition also occurs, at all ages, as a complication of other d.'s in which immune mechanisms are severely depressed, and has been found incidentally in salivary gland epithelium, apparently as a localized or mild infection (salivary gland virus d.).

**Daae's d.,** epidemic *pleurodynia*.

**Dalrymple's d.,** cyclokeratitis.

**dancing d.,** epidemic *chorea*.

**Danielssen's d.,** anesthetic *leprosy*.

**Danielssen-Boeck d.,** anesthetic *leprosy*.

**Darier's d.,** *keratosis* follicularis.

**Darling's d.,** histoplasmosis.

**Débove's d.,** obsolete eponym for idiopathic splenomegaly.

**decompression d.,** caisson d.

**deer-fly d.,** tularemia.

**deficiency d.,** a d. resulting from lack of calories, proteins, essential amino acids, fatty acids, vitamins, or trace minerals. Scurvy, beriberi, and rickets are examples.

**degenerative joint d.,** degenerative or hypertrophic arthritis; osteoarthritis; degeneration of articular cartilage, which may be primary or may be secondary to trauma or other conditions. Primary degenerative joint d. is very common in older persons, especially affecting weight-bearing joints; articular cartilage becomes soft, frayed, and thinned, with eburnation of subchondral bone and formation of marginal osteophytes.

**Déjérine's d.,** D.-Sottas d.

**Déjérine-Sottas d.,** Déjérine's d.; a dominantly inherited, progressive, chronic peripheral neuropathy associated with swelling and mucoid degeneration of peripheral nerves.

**demyelinating d.,** one of a group of d.'s of unknown cause in which there is extensive loss of the myelin sheaths of nerve fibers, as in multiple sclerosis and Schilder's disease.

**de Quervain's d.,** radial styloid tendovaginitis; fibrosis of the sheath of a tendon of the thumb.

**Dercum's d.,** *adiposis* dolorosa.

**Deutschländer's d.,** (1) march *foot*; (2) tumor of one of the metatarsal bones.

**Devic's d.,** *neuromyelitis* optica.

**diamond skin d.,** a form of swine erysipelas, caused by *Erysipelothrix rhusiopathiae*, in which rhomboidal erythematous areas appear on the skin.

**diffuse d.,** one that involves several or all of the spinal cord tracts; opposed to system d.

**Di Guglielmo's d.,** acute erythremic *myelosis*.

**disappearing bone d.,** Gorham's d.; extensive decalcification of a single bone; of unknown cause, sometimes associated with angioma.

**dog d.,** pappataci *fever*.

**Donohue's d.,** leprechaunism.

**drug d.,** a morbid condition resulting from the administration of a drug.

**Dubini's d.,** electric *chorea* (1).

**Dubois' d.,** Dubois' *abscess*.

**Duchenne's d.,** (1) *tabes* dorsalis; (2) childhood muscular *dystrophy*.

**Duchenne-Aran d.,** progressive muscular *atrophy*.

**Duhring's d.,** *dermatitis* herpetiformis.

**Dukes' d.,** fourth d.

**Duplay's d.,** scapulohumeral *periarthritis*.

**Dupuytren's d. of the foot,** plantar *fibromatosis*.

**Durante's d.,** *osteogenesis* imperfecta.

**Duroziez' d.,** congenital stenosis of the mitral valve.

**dust d.'s,** those pulmonary d.'s, *e.g.*, silicosis, anthracosis, etc., due to the inhalation of fine particles of coal, rock, or other material.

**Dutton's d.,** Dutton's fever; African tick-borne relapsing fever caused by *Borrelia duttoni* and spread by the soft tick, *Ornithodoros moubata*.

**dynamic d.,** functional d.

**Eales' d.,** recurrent retinal or intravitreous hemorrhages in young adults.

**Ebstein's d.,** Ebstein's *anomaly*.

**Eichstedt's d.,** *tinea* versicolor.

**Eisenmenger's d.,** Eisenmenger's *complex*.

**elevator d.,** a form of pneumonoconiosis occurring in workers in grain elevators.

**endemic d.,** one that prevails continuously or recurrently in a special locality.

**Engelmann's d.,** diaphysial *dysplasia*.

**English d.,** obsolete term for rickets.

**epidemic d.,** one that attacks simultaneously a large number of persons living in a particular locality.

**Epstein's d.,** diphtheroid (1).

**Erb's d.,** progressive bulbar *paralysis*.

**Erb-Charcot d.,** spastic *diplegia*.

**Eulenburg's d.,** congenital *paramyotonia*.

**exanthematous d.,** exanthema (1).

**extrapyramidal d.,** degenerative d. affecting the corpus striatum or other part of the extrapyramidal system, *e.g.*, parkinsonism, paralysis agitans, chorea, hepatolenticular degeneration.

**Fabry's d.,** angiokeratoma corporis diffusum; glycolipid lipidosis; an x-linked recessive disorder due to deficiency of the enzyme α-galactosidase and characterized by abnormal accumulations of neutral glycolipids in various tissues, purple skin lesions on thighs, buttocks, and genitalia, hypohidrosis, paresthesia in extremities, cornea verticillata, and spokelike posterior subcapsular cataracts; death results from renal, cardiac, or cerebrovascular complications.

**Fahr's d.,** progressive calcific deposition in the walls of cerebral blood vessels, occasionally associated with mental retardation and extrapyramidal symptoms.

**Favre-Durand-Nicolas d.,** *lymphogranuloma* venereum.

**Feer's d.,** Selter's d.; an affection marked by recurrent sweating, cyanosis of the extremities, motor weakness, tremor, rapid pulse, and insomnia.

**femoropopliteal occlusive d.,** obstruction of the femoral and popliteal arteries by atherosclerosis.

**Fenwick's d.,** idiopathic gastric atrophy; see atrophic *gastritis*.

**fibrocystic d. of the breasts,** cystic hyperplasia of the breast; chronic cystic mastitis; mammary dysplasia; cystic d. of the breast; Schimmelbusch's d.; Phocas' d.; Tillaux's d.; a benign d. common in women of the third, fourth, and fifth decades, characterized by formation, in one or both breasts, of small cysts containing fluid which may appear blue (see blue dome *cyst*), associated with stromal fibrosis and variable degrees of intraductal epithelial hyperplasia and sclerosing *adenosis* (*q.v.*). Some of these changes have been considered possibly premalignant and may in themselves be difficult to distinguish microscopically from carcinoma of the breast.

**fibrocystic d. of the pancreas,** see viscidosis.

**fifth d.,** *erythema* infectiosum.

**fifth venereal d.,** *granuloma* inguinale.

**Filatov's d.,** fourth d.

**Flatau-Schilder d.,** *encephalitis* periaxialis diffusa.

**flint d.,** chalicosis.

**Folling's d.,** phenylketonuria.

**foot and mouth d.,** aphthae epizooticae; contagious aphthae; epidemic stomatitis; aphthous fever; aphthosa; aftosa; a highly infectious disease of cattle, swine, and sheep caused by an RNA virus of the picornavirus group, and characterized by vesicular eruptions in the mouth and around and between the claws; man is affected only rarely.

**Forbes' d.,** type 3 *glycogenosis.*

**Fordyce's d.,** Fordyce's *spots.*

**Fothergill's d.,** (1) trigeminal *neuralgia;* (2) anginose *scarlatina.*

**Fournier's d.,** fulminating gangrene of the genitals.

**fourth d.,** Dukes' d.; Filatov's d.; scarlatinoid; scarlatinella; an exanthematous affection of childhood bearing a resemblance to scarlatina analogous to that of German measles to measles; it runs a mild course. Filatov (or Filatoff) subscribed to the existence of three primary specific fevers—scarlatina, morbilli, and rubella—and believed that there was a scarlatiniform type of rubella which constituted a distinct febrile illness; that was the fourth d. The etiology is unknown. There was also a disease called the "fifth d.": erythema infectiosum.

**fourth venereal d.,** (1) benign lymphogranulomatosis; (2) erosive and gangrenous balanitis.

**Fox-Fordyce d.,** apocrine miliaria; a rare chronic eruption of dry papules and distended ruptured apocrine glands, with follicular hyperkeratosis of the nipples, axillae, and pubic and sternal regions; pruritus is intense.

**Franklin's d.,** heavy chain d.

**Frei's d.,** *lymphogranuloma* venereum.

**Freiberg's d.,** epiphysial ischemic *necrosis,* of second metatarsal head.

**Friedländer's d.,** *endarteritis* obliterans.

**Friedmann's d.,** narcolepsy.

**Friedreich's d.,** *myoclonus* multiplex.

**Friend d.,** mouse leukemia caused by the Friend strain of virus.

**Fuerstner's d.,** pseudospastic paralysis with tremor.

**functional d.,** a dysfunction with no detectable anatomical lesion or physiological disturbance to explain its symptoms.

**fusospirochetal d.,** Vincent's d.

**Gairdner's d.,** angor pectoris; angina pectoris sine dolore; attacks of cardiac distress with mental apprehension.

**Gamna's d.,** a form of chronic splenomegaly characterized by conspicuous thickening of the capsule and the presence of multiple, small, rustlike, brown foci (Gamna-Gandy bodies, or sideretic nodules), which contain iron; this condition may be observed in fibrocongestive splenomegaly, sickle cell d., and some examples of hemochromatosis.

**Gandy-Nanta d.,** siderotic splenomegaly (splenogranulomatosis siderotica); probably the same as Gamna's d.

**garapata d.,** tick fever occurring in Spain.

**Garré's d.,** sclerosing *osteitis.*

**Gaucher's d.,** cerebrosidosis; cerebroside lipidosis; glycocerebroside accumulation in macrophages due to a genetic deficiency of glucocerebrosidase; it may occur in adults but occurs most severely in infants, in whom cerebroside also accumulates in neurons; it is marked by hepatosplenomegaly, lymphadenopathy, and bone destruction by characteristic cells containing cytoplasmic tubules.

**Gee's d.,** celiac d.

**Gerhardt's d.,** erythromelalgia.

**Gerlier's d.,** epidemic *vertigo.*

**germ d.,** any d. due to a microorganism.

**Gierke's d.,** type 1 *glycogenosis.*

**Gilbert's d.,** familial nonhemolytic *jaundice.*

**Gilchrist's d.,** North American *blastomycosis.*

**Gilles de la Tourette's d.,** Gilles de la Tourette's syndrome; Guinon's d.; Tourette's d.; motor incoordination with echolalia and coprolalia; a form of tic.

**Glanzmann's d.,** Glanzmann's *thrombasthenia.*

**Glasser's d.,** a d. of young pigs characterized by fibrinous arthritis, pleuritis, peritonitis, and pericarditis; it is caused by *Haemophilus suis.*

**glycogen storage d.,** glycogenosis.

**Goldflam d.,** *myasthenia* gravis.

**Goldscheider's d.,** *epidermolysis* bullosa simplex.

**Gorham's d.,** disappearing bone d.

**Gougerot and Blum D.,** pigmented purpuric lichenoid *dermatosis.*

**Gougerot-Sjögren d.,** Sjögren's *syndrome.*

**Gowers' d.,** (1) saltatory *spasm;* (2) a distal type of progressive muscular dystrophy.

**Graefe's d.,** *ophthalmoplegia* progressiva.

**graft versus host d.,** graft versus host reaction; H. d.; a kind of incompatibility reaction (which may be fatal) in a subject (host) of low immunological competence (deficient lymphoid tissue) who has been the recipient of immunologically competent lymphoid tissue from a donor who lacks at least one antigen possessed by the recipient host; the reaction, or disease, is the result of action of the transplanted cells against those host tissues that possess the antigen not possessed by the donor.

**Graves' d.,** Basedow's d.; Parry's d.; toxic goiter characterized by diffuse hyperplasia of the thyroid gland; a form of hyperthyroidism. Exophthalmos is a common, but not invariable, concomitant.

**greasy pig d.,** a generalized exudative epidermitis of young pigs, thought to be caused by *Staphylococcus hyicus;* it has a high incidence of mortality.

**Greenfield's d.,** late infantile form of metachromatic leukodystrophy.

**Greenhow's d.,** parasitic *melanoderma.*

**Griesinger's d.,** bilious typhoid of Griesinger, a severe form of louse-borne relapsing fever caused by *Borrelia recurrentis* and causing high fever, epistaxis, dyspnea, intense jaundice, purpura, and splenomegaly.

**grinder's d.,** pneumonoconiosis.

**Guinon's d.,** Gilles de la Tourette's d.

**Gull's d.,** myxedema.

**Gull-Sutton d.,** arteriolar *nephrosclerosis.*

**Günther's d.,** congenital erythropoietic *porphyria.*

**G. vs. H. d.,** graft *versus* host d.

**H d.,** Hartnup d.

**Haff d.** [ *Haff,* an arm of the Baltic Sea in East Prussia ], hemoglobinuria, muscular weakness, and pains in the limbs, occurring in persons living in the vicinity of the inlet, caused by arsenic poisoning from waste in a celluloid factory.

**Hailey and Hailey d.,** familial benign chronic *pemphigus.*

**Hall's d.,** cerebral anemia in infants, marked by symptoms simulating those of hydrocephalus.

**Hallopeau's d.,** (1) *acrodermatitis* continua; (2) *pemphigus* vegetans (2); (3) *lichen* sclerosus et atrophicus.

**Hamman's d.,** Hamman's *syndrome.*

**hand-foot-and-mouth d.,** An exanthematous eruption of small, pearl-gray vesicles of the fingers, toes, palms, and soles, accompanied by often painful vesicles and ulceration of the buccal mucous membrane and the tongue and by slight fever; the d. lasts 4 to 7 days; it is usually caused by Coxsackie virus type A-16, but others, including A-5, have been identified with this d.

**Hand-Schüller-Christian d.,** Schüller's d. or syndrome; Christian's syndrome; generalized lipid histiocytosis of bones, especially the skull, with bone destruction by accumulation of cells containing cholesterol esters, and eosinophil leukocytes; it may cause loosening and exfoliation of the teeth.

**Hansen's d.,** leprosy.

**Harada's d.,** Harada's *syndrome.*

**hard pad d.,** a common d. of young dogs manifested by general symptoms followed by foot soreness and excessive cornification of epithelial structures, especially those of the foot pads and nose. Such animals make a clacking sound when walking on hard surfaces. The d. also involves the nervous system in most instances. Most authorities now believe that this d. is a form of canine distemper caused by the virus of Carré.

**Hartnup d.,** Hartnup syndrome; a congenital metabolic disorder inherited as a Mendelian recessive character, consisting of aminoaciduria due to a defect in renal tubular absorption, and urinary excretion of tryptophan derivatives because defective intestinal absorption leads to bacterial degradation of unabsorbed tryptophan in the gut. The d. is characterized by a pellagra-like skin rash with temporary cerebellar ataxia.

**Hashimoto's d.,** Hashimoto's struma or thyroiditis; struma lymphomatosa; lymphadenoid goiter; infiltration of the thyroid gland with lymphocytes, resulting in progressive destruction of the parenchyma and hypothyroidism.

**Hayem's d.,** apoplectiform *myelitis.*

**heavy chain d.,** Franklin's d.; a term used for a group of d.'s, the paraproteinemias, characterized by abnormal $\gamma$-globulins and associated with malignant disorders of the plasmacytic and lymphoid cell series. Globulin fragments resembling, but not identical with, Fc fragment of IgG occur in large quantities in serum and urine.

**Hebra's d.,** (1) *erythema* multiforme; (2) familial non-hemolytic *jaundice.*

**Heerfordt's d.,** uveoparotid fever; now thought to be part of the syndrome of sarcoidosis.

**Heine-Medin d.,** acute anterior *poliomyelitis.*

**hemoglobin C d.,** homozygous state of hemoglobin C (*q.v.*).

**hemoglobin H d.,** see *hemoglobin* H.

**hemolyt'ic d. of newborn,** *erythroblastosis* fetalis.

**hemorrhagic d. of the newborn,** syndrome characterized by spontaneous internal or external bleeding accompanied by hypoprothrombinemia, slightly decreased platelets, markedly elevated bleeding and clotting times, usually occurring between the third and sixth days of life and effectively treated with vitamin K.

**hepatic storage d.,** see glycogen storage d.

**hepatolenticular d.,** hepatolenticular *degeneration.*

**hereditary d.,** one transmitted by genetic mechanisms from parents to offspring.

**Hers' d.,** type 6 *glycogenosis.*

**Heubner's d.,** syphilitic endarteritis obliterans of the cerebral vessels.

**hidebound d.,** scleroderma; usually applied to extensive involvement.

**Hippel's d.,** Lindau's d.

**Hippel-Lindau d.,** Lindau's d.

**Hirschsprung's d.,** congenital *megacolon.*

**Hjärre's d.,** coli granuloma; a granulomatous d. of the intestines and liver of chickens, due to coliform organisms.

**Hodgkin's d.,** anemia lymphatica; Trousseau's syndrome (1); a d. marked by chronic enlargement of the lymph nodes, often cervical at the onset and then generalized, together with enlargement of the spleen and often of the liver; there is no pronounced leukocytosis, but anemia and remittent or continuous fever are common. Hodgkin's d. is considered to be a malignant neoplasm of reticulum cells, of which bizarre and pathognomonic forms are found (Reed-Sternberg cells), associated with inflammatory infiltration of lymphocytes and eosinophilic leukocytes and fibrosis.

**Hodgson's d.,** dilation of the arch of the aorta associated with insufficiency of the aortic valve.

**hoof-and-mouth d.,** an incorrect but often used term for foot-and-mouth d.

**hookworm d.,** ancylostomiasis.

**Hoppe-Goldflam d.,** *myasthenia* gravis.

**housing d.,** bluecomb d. of chickens.

**Huchard's d.,** continued arterial hypertension, believed by Huchard to be the main cause of arteriosclerosis.

**Hurler's d.,** Hurler's *syndrome.*

**Hutchinson's d.,** (1) senile guttate *choroidopathy;* (2) *angioma* serpiginosum; (3) melanotic *whitlow.*

**Hutchinson-Gilford d.,** progeria.

**hyaline membrane d. of the newborn,** a d. seen especially in premature neonates with respiratory distress, characterized post mortem by atelectasis and an eosinophilic membrane lining alveolar ducts and associated with reduced amounts of lung surfactant.

**Hyde's d.,** *prurigo* nodularis.

**Iceland d.,** epidemic *neuromyasthenia.*

**I cell d.,** *mucolipidosis* II.

**idiopathic d.,** one of which we are ignorant of the cause.

**idiopathic Bamberger-Marie d.,** acropachyderma.

**immune complex d.,** d. evoked by the deposition of antigen-antibody or antigen-antibody-complement complexes on cell surfaces.

**inclusion cell d.,** *mucolipidosis* II.

**inclusion body d.,** cytomegalic inclusion d.

**infectious d., infective d.,** one resulting from the presence and activity of a microbial agent.

**inherited d.,** hereditary d.

**insufficiency d.,** deficiency d.

**intercurrent d.,** complicating d.

**interstitial d.,** one affecting chiefly the connective-tissue framework of an organ, the parenchyma suffering secondarily.

**iron storage d.,** the storage of excess iron in the parenchyma of many organs, in conditions such as idiopathic hemochromatosis or transfusion hemosiderosis.

**island d.,** tsutsugamushi d.

**Jaffe-Lichtenstein d.,** fibrous *dysplasia* of bone.

**Jaksch's d.,** *anemia* infantum pseudoleukemica.

**Jansky-Bielschowsky d.,** early juvenile type of cerebral *sphingolipidosis, q.v.*

**Jensen's d.,** *retinochoroiditis* juxtapapillaris.

**Johne's d.,** a d. occurring in cattle and sheep, usually manifested by thickening of the wall of the intestine, particularly of the ileum; caused by infection with *Mycobacterium paratuberculosis* (*M. johnei*).

**jumper d. of Maine,** a condition, probably neurotic, characterized by palmus; usually found in isolated communities such as certain parts of Maine.

**Jüngling's d.,** *osteitis* tuberculosa multiplex cystica.

**Kahler's d.,** multiple *myeloma.*

**Kashin-Bek d.,** a form of generalized osteoarthrosis limited to areas of Asia, including the Urov river; believed to result from ingestion of wheat infected with the fungus *Fusoria sporotrichiella.*

**Katayama d.** (kah-tah-yah'mah) [ Jap. *Katayama,* Mountainside, a town in Japan where the d. is common ], *schistosomiasis* japonicum.

**keda'ni d.** [ Jap. *kedani,* head louse ], tsutsugamushi d.

**Kienböck's d.,** lunatomalacia; osteolysis of the lunate bone following trauma to the wrist.

**Kimmelstiel-Wilson d.,** Kimmelstiel-Wilson syndrome; diabetic, intercapillary, or nodular glomerulosclerosis; a nodular hyaline deposit in tufts of the glomeruli of the kidneys associated with diabetes, albuminuria, hypertension, and edema of the nephrotic type.

**kinky-hair d.,** Menkes' syndrome; a congenital metabolic defect (x-linked recessive) manifest in short, sparse, poorly pigmented kinky hair; associated with failure to thrive, physical and mental retardation, and progressive severe deterioration of the brain.

**Klippel's d.,** arthritic general *pseudoparalysis.*

**Köhler's d.,** epiphysial aseptic *necrosis* (*q.v.*) of (1) the tarsal navicular bone, or (2) the patella.

**Krabbe's d.,** diffuse infantile familial *sclerosis.*

**Kufs' d.,** adult type of cerebral *sphingolipidosis, q.v.*

**Kugelberg-Welander d.,** juvenile muscular *atrophy.*

**Kuhnt-Junius d.,** Kuhnt-Junius *degeneration.*

**kukuru'ku d.,** occurs in Nigeria and is marked by jaundice and fever; not due to yellow fever virus but it resembles this d.; probably infective hepatitis.

**Kümmell's d.,** Kümmell-Verneuil d.; Kümmell's spondylitis; traumatic spondylopathy; rarefying osteitis of the vertebra, following an injury.

**Kümmell-Verneuil d.,** Kümmell's d.

**Kussmaul's d.,** *polyarteritis* nodosa.

**Kyasanur forest d.,** a d. occurring in the Kyasanur forest and in Mysore, India, caused by a group B arbovirus that is transmitted by a tick (*Haemaphysalis spinigera*). Symptoms include fever, headache, back and limb pains, diarrhea, and intestinal bleeding; central nervous system symptoms do not occur.

**Kyrle's d.,** *hyperkeratosis* follicularis et parafollicularis.

**Lafora's d.,** myoclonus *epilepsy.*

**Lane's d.,** *erythema* palmare hereditarium.

**Larrey-Weil d.,** Weil's disease.

**Lasègue's d.,** mania of persecution.

**laughing d.,** a disabling state of hypnosis or narcosis characterized by involuntary laughing induced by witch doctors; also the compulsive mirthless laughter of schizophrenics; also called kuru.

**Leber's d.,** Leber's hereditary optic *atrophy.*

**Legg's d.,** epiphysial aseptic *necrosis* (*q.v.*) of the upper end of the femur.

**Legg-Calvé-Perthes d.,** epiphysial aseptic *necrosis* (*q.v.*) of the upper end of the femur.

**Legg-Perthes d.,** epiphysial aseptic *necrosis* (*q.v.*) of the upper end of the femur.

**Leiner's d.,** *erythroderma* desquamativum.

**Leloir's d.,** *lupus* vulgaris erythematoides.

**Leroy's d.,** *mucolipidosis* II.

Letterer-Siwe d., nonlipid *histiocytosis.*

Leyden's d., periodical vomiting; attacks of nausea and vomiting recurring at regular intervals of weeks or months, lasting for a few hours or several days, the intervals being free from any gastric symptoms whatever.

Lindau's d., von Hippel-Lindau disease; Hippel's disease; retinocerebral angiomatosis; a type of phacomatosis, consisting of hemangiomas of the retina, which may be multiple and bilateral, associated with hemangiomas or hemangioblastomas primarily of the cerebellum and walls of the fourth ventricle, occasionally involving the spinal cord; sometimes associated with cysts or hamartomas of kidney, adrenal, or other organs; autosomal dominant inheritance.

Little's d., spastic *diplegia.*

Lobo's d., lobomycosis.

local d., one in which the morbid changes are confined to a single part or organ, usually without marked constitutional disturbance.

locoweed d., loco.

Löffler's d., Löffler's *endocarditis.*

loin d., botulism.

Lorain's d., idiopathic *infantilism.*

Lucas-Championnière d., fibrinous *bronchitis.*

lumpy skin d., an infectious d. of cattle in Africa, manifested by an acute febrile illness followed by the appearance of lumps and plaques under the skin and on some of the mucous membranes; a poxvirus and a herpesvirus have been associated with thid d.

lunger d., pulmonary *adenomatosis* of sheep.

Lutz-Splendore-Almeida d., South American *blastomycosis.*

Lyell's d., toxic epidermal *necrolysis.*

MacLean-Maxwell d., a chronic enlargement of the posterior third of the os calcis accompanied by pain on pressure and in walking.

Madelung's d., diffuse symmetrical lipomatosis, or deposit of fatty tissue, on the upper part of the back, shoulders, and neck.

Magitot's d., osteoperiostitis of the dental alveoli.

Maher's d., paracolpitis.

Majocchi's d., *purpura* annularis telangiectodes.

Malherbe's d., Malherbe's calcifying *epithelioma.*

Manson's d., *schistosomiasis* mansoni.

maple bark d., pneumonitis caused by spores of *Coniosporium corticale,* lurking under the bark of maple logs.

maple syrup urine d., maple syrup d.; maple sugar d.; branched chain ketonuria; branched chain ketoaciduria; a disorder caused by deficient oxidative decarboxylation of α-keto acid metabolites of leucine, isoleucine, and valine. These amino acids and their α-keto acid metabolites are present in blood and urine in elevated concentrations. Urine has an odor similar to that of maple syrup. Neonatal death is common; survivors usually exhibit gross brain damage. Autosomal recessive inheritance.

marble bone d., osteopetrosis.

Marchiafava-Bignami d., a degenerative process involving the corpus callosum that occurs in persons who drink excessive amounts of crude red wine.

Marek's d., a type of avian *lymphomatosis, q.v.*

Marfan's d., Marfan's *syndrome.*

margarine d., a toxic multiform erythema caused by a substance used in the manufacture of margarine.

Marie's d., (1) acromegaly; (2) hypertrophic pulmonary *osteoarthropathy;* (3) hereditary cerebellar *ataxia;* (4) ankylosing *spondylitis.*

Marie-Strümpell d., ankylosing *spondylitis.*

Marion's d., a congenital obstruction of the posterior urethra.

Martin's d., a periosteoarthritis of the foot from excessive walking.

McArdle's d., type 5 *glycogenosis.*

McArdle-Schmid-Pearson d., type 5 *glycogenosis.*

Medin's d., poliomyelitis.

Mediterranean-hemoglobin E d., thalassemia with hemoglobin E in the blood.

Meige's d., hereditary *lymphedema.*

Menétrièr's d., Menétrièr's syndrome; giant hypertrophic gastritis; erosive gastritis with pseudohyperplasia of the mucosa of the stomach related to giant hypertrophy of the gastric rugae.

Ménière's d., Ménière's syndrome; endolymphatic hydrops; an affection characterized clinically by vertigo, nausea, vomiting, tinnitus, and progressive deafness.

mental d., see mental *illness.*

Merzbacher-Pelizaeus d., hereditary cerebral leukodystrophy; aplasia axialis extracorticalis; familial degenerative d. of the brain marked by progressive sclerosis of white substance of the frontal lobes, mental deficiency, and vasomotor disorders.

Meyenburg's d., relapsing *perichondritis.*

Meyer's d., adenoids.

mianeh d., Persian relapsing *fever.*

Mibelli's d., porokeratosis.

microcystic d. of renal medulla, cystic d. of renal medulla.

midland d., botulism.

Mikulicz' d., benign swelling of the lacrimal, and usually also of the salivary glands in consequence of an infiltration of, and replacement of the normal gland structure by lymphoid tissue; also known as Mikulicz-Sjögren syndrome, since Sjögren's syndrome is thought to be a variant of Mikulicz' d. See also Mikulicz' *syndrome.*

Milian's d., ninth-day *erythema.*

Mills' d., ascending *hemiplegia.*

Milroy's d., hereditary *lymphedema.*

Milton's d., angioneurotic *edema.*

Minamata d. [ *Minamata* Bay, Japan ], toxic d., described in Japan, caused by eating fish contaminated with mercury; a neurological disorder resulting from poisoning by organic mercury compounds and characterized by peripheral paresthesia, dysarthria, ataxia, and loss of peripheral vision; it is usually severe and permanent, and may result in death.

miner's d., (1) miner's *anemia;* ancylostomiasis; (2) miner's *nystagmus.*

Mitchell's d., erythromelalgia.

Möbius' d., ophthalmoplegic migraine or periodic oculomotor paralysis.

molecular d., a d. in which there is a single alteration affecting only a particular molecule.

Mondor's d., thrombophlebitis of the thoracoepigastric vein of the breast and chest wall.

Morgagni's d., Adams-Stokes *syndrome.*

Morquio's d., Morquio's *syndrome.*

Morquio-Ullrich d., Morquio's *syndrome.*

Mortimer's d., nonulcerating multiple lupus vulgaris.

Morvan's d., syringomyelia.

Moschcowitz' d., thrombotic thrombocytopenic *purpura.*

motor neuron d., a general term including progressive muscular atrophy (infantile, juvenile, and adult), amyotrophic lateral sclerosis, progressive bulbar paralysis, and primary lateral sclerosis; frequently a familial d.

Mucha-Habermann d., *pityriasis* lichenoides et varioliformis acuta.

mucosal d.'s, sometimes called the mucosal d. complex; formerly considered to be a distinct d. entity, it is now considered identical to virus diarrhea of cattle.

Myà's d., congenital *megacolon.*

Nairobi d., a d. of sheep in East Africa; it is caused by a virus that is transmitted by a tick, *Rhipicephalus appendiculatus,* and is characterized by a hemorrhagic gastroenteritis, which causes death losses varying from 30 to 70 per cent of the lamb crop.

navicular d., navicular arthritis; podotrochilitis; a common cause of lameness in horses, especially light racing animals. It is essentially a chronic osteitis of the navicular bone associated with bursitis and inflammation of the plantar aponeurosis. It occurs most frequently in the forefeet. It is believed to be due to damage from frequent and severe strain.

Neftel's d., paresthesia of the head and trunk, and extreme discomfort in any but the recumbent position.

Nettleship's d., *urticaria* pigmentosa.

Neumann's d., *pemphigus* vegetans (1).

Newcastle d., an acute, febrile, and contagious d. of fowls resembling fowl plague, caused by an RNA virus, and grouped with the paramyxoviruses. It is characterized by high infectivity, respiratory and nervous symptoms. It is readily transmissible to man, in whom it causes a severe but transient conjunctivitis. The name "Newcastle" was applied by an English worker (Doyle) in 1927 to the d., which had appeared near Newcastle-on-Tyne. It was only later that it was identified as the same as the d. "Ranikhet" of India and other parts of Asia.

**Nicolas-Favre d.,** *lymphogranuloma* venereum.

**Niemann-Pick d.,** sphingomyelin lipidosis; lipid histiocytosis with accumulation of phospholipid (sphingomyelin) in histiocytes in the liver, spleen, lymph nodes and bone marrow. The d. occurs most commonly in Jewish infants and leads to early death; a more benign form may occur rarely in adults. Cerebral involvement may occur at a late stage, with red macular spots less common than in Tay-Sachs d. Autosomal recessive inheritance.

**nodular d.,** esophagostomiasis; a d. of herbivores and primates characterized by the presence of nodules, filled with caseous material, in the wall of the large intestine and cecum (occasionally a few may be present in the ileum); these nodules result from injury to the bowel wall from the encystment of the larvae of *Oesophagostomum;* the d. is generally not harmful, but the nodules reduce the value of intestine for use as catgut and sausage casings.

**Nonne-Milroy d.,** hereditary *lymphedema.*

**Norrie's d.,** atrophia bulborum hereditaria; congenital bilateral masses of tissue arising from the retina or vitreous and resembling glioma (pseudoglioma), usually with atrophy of iris and development of cataract; X-linked recessive inheritance.

**occupational d.,** one caused by damage produced by the occupation of the victim.

**Oguchi's d.,** congenital nonprogressive night blindness with yellow or gray coloration of fundus; after 2 or 3 hours in total darkness, normal color of fundus returns; autosomal recessive inheritance.

**Ollier's d.,** enchondromatosis.

**Oppenheim's d.,** *amyotonia* congenita.

**organic d.,** one in which there is anatomical change in some bodily tissue or organ.

**Ormond's d.,** idiopathic retroperitoneal *fibrosis.*

**Osgood-Schlatter d.,** epiphysial aseptic *necrosis (q. v.)* of the tibial tubercle.

**Osler's d.,** (1) erythremia; (2) hereditary hemorrhagic *telangiectasia.*

**Osler-Vaquez d.,** erythremia.

**Otto's d.,** Otto pelvis; arthrokatadysis; protrusio acetabuli; a d. resembling, in some respects, rheumatoid arthritis, but marked by an inward bulging of the acetabulum in consequence of which the prominence of the femur is reduced instead of being increased as in rheumatoid arthritis.

**overeating d.,** a d. of lambs, usually causing trouble when lambs are brought in from pasture and begin grain feeding. It is an acute, highly fatal intoxication originating in the gastrointestinal tract where type D of *Clostridium perfringens* has multiplied; enterotoxemia; pulpy kidney disease.

**Owren's d.,** parahemophilia; a condition in which there is congenital deficiency of factor V, resulting in prolongation of prothrombin time and coagulation time.

**Paas' d.,** a familial, and perhaps also hereditary, skeletal deformation, marked by coxa valga, double patella, shortening of the middle and terminal phalanges of fingers and toes, deformities of the elbows, scoliosis, and spondylitis deformans of the lumbar vertebrae, all these unilateral or bilateral.

**Paget's d.,** 1. osteitis deformans; a generalized skeletal disease, frequently familial, of older persons in which bone resorption and formation are both increased, leading to thickening and softening of bones, as in the skull, and bending of weight-bearing bones. 2. A d. of elderly women, characterized by an infiltrated, somewhat eczematous lesion surrounding and involving the nipple and areola, and associated with subjacent intraductal cancer of the breast and infiltration of the lower epidermis by malignant cells.

**Paltauf-Sternberg d.,** an old term for a condition now regarded as a form of Hodgkin's d.

**pandemic d.,** one that prevails more or less over the entire world.

**Panner's d.,** epiphysial aseptic *necrosis (q. v.)* of the capitellum of the humerus.

**parasitic d.,** one due to the presence and vital activity of animal or vegetable parasites; when the parasites are

unicellular and microscopic the d. is called infectious or infective.

**Parkinson's d.,** parkinsonism (1).

**paroxys'mal d.,** one characterized by explosive seizures, as epilepsy.

**parrot d.,** (1) psittacosis; (2) ornithosis.

**Parrot's d.,** (1) pseudoparalysis in infants, due to syphilitic osteochondritis; (2) achondroplasia; (3) marasmus.

**Parry's d.,** Graves' d.

**Pauzat's d.,** osteoplastic periostitis of the metatarsal bones, caused by excessive marching.

**Pavy's d.,** cyclic or recurrent physiologic albuminuria.

**Paxton's d.,** *trichomycosis* axillaris.

**pearl d.** [ Ger. *perlsucht* ], a form of tuberculosis in cattle in which tuberculous tissue takes the form of pearl- or grapelike bodies attached to the surface of the pleura or peritoneum.

**pearl-worker's d.,** inflammatory hypertrophy of the bones affecting grinders of mother of pearl.

**Pel-Ebstein d.,** Hodgkin's d. with periodic pyrexia.

**Pelizaeus-Merzbacher d.,** Merzbacher-Pelizaeus d.

**Pellegrini's d.,** a calcific density in the medial collateral ligament and/or bony growth at the internal condyle of the femur; a sequel of Stieda's fracture.

**pelvic inflammatory d.,** acute or chronic inflammation in the pelvic cavity; particularly, suppurative lesions of the female genital tract, such as salpingitis and its complications.

**periodic d.,** any d. in which attacks tend to recur at regular intervals, such as periodic abdominalgia, periodic arthralgia, periodic neutropenia, periodic fever, and periodic paralysis. The cause of the periodicity is still completely unknown.

**perna d.** (*per*chlor na*p*hthalin), halogen or chloric acne occurring in workers in perchlornaphthalin.

**Perthes d.,** epiphysial aseptic *necrosis (q. v.)* of the upper end of the femur.

**Pette-Döring d.,** nodular *panencephalitis.*

**Peyronie's d.,** van Buren's d.; fibrous cavernitis; d. of unknown cause in which there are plaques or strands of dense fibrous tissue surrounding the corpus cavernosum of the penis, causing deformity and painful erection; often associated with Dupuytren's contracture.

**Pfeiffer's d.,** glandular *fever.*

**Phocas' d.,** fibrocystic d. of the breasts.

**Pick's d.,** (1) [ F. Pick ], Pick's syndrome; a form of multiple serositis (or polyserositis) characterized by chronic congestive hepatomegaly, persistent or recurrent ascites, sometimes recurrent pleural effusion, peritonitis, and pleuritis, occurring in a patient with previous (or concurrent) hyalinizing pericarditis; also termed pericardial pseudocirrhosis of the liver; (2) [ A. Pick ], Pick's *atrophy.*

**pink d.,** acrodynia (1).

**Pinkus' d.,** *lichen* nitidus.

**plaster of Paris d.,** atrophy of bone in a limb which has been encased for some time in a plaster of Paris splint.

**Plummer's d.,** a name sometimes applied to hyperthyroidism resulting from a nodular toxic goiter; occasionally accompanied by exophthalmos.

**polycystic d. of kidneys,** see polycystic *kidney.*

**Pompe's d.,** type 2 *glycogenosis.*

**Posadas' d., Posadas-Wernicke d.,** coccidioidomycosis, especially the pulmonary granulomatous form.

**Pott's d.,** tuberculous *spondylitis.*

**Potter's d.,** Potter's *facies.*

**Poulet's d.,** rheumatic osteoperiostitis.

**pregnancy d. of sheep,** hypoglycemia; ketosis; lambing paralysis; lambing sickness; a highly fatal d. of well nourished ewes in the late stages of pregnancy. It is especially common in ewes carrying twin lambs. A metabolic d., it is caused by carbohydrate depletion of the blood and tissues. It is characterized by hypoglycemia, ketonuria, fatty infiltration of the liver, rapid emaciation, coma, and a high death rate.

**Pringle's d.,** *adenoma* sebaceum.

**Profichet's d.,** *calcinosis* circumscripta.

**pullet d.,** bluecomb d. of chickens.

**pullor'um d.,** diarrhea alba (2); white flux (2); white diarrhea (2); an infectious d. of chicks and other young birds caused by *Salmonella pullorum*, which is carried in the ovaries of adult hens and appears in the eggs; in incubator-hatched birds, the d. usually involves the lungs and air sacs, but often spreads in flocks of young birds as an alimentary tract infection manifested by severe diarrhea followed by septicemia and death.

**pulpy kidney d.,** overeating d.

**pulseless d.,** Takayashu's syndrome or disease; a progressive obliterative arteritis of the vessels arising from the arch of the aorta. See also aortic arch *syndrome.*

**Purtscher's d.,** traumatic retinal angiopathy following skull trauma or compression injuries to body; fundi show large white patches associated with the retinal veins about the disk or macula, hemorrhages and retinal edema; condition is transient, usually with full recovery.

**quiet hip d.,** epiphysial aseptic *necrosis (q.v.)* of the upper end of the femur.

**Quincke's d.,** angioneurotic *edema.*

**Quinquaud's d.,** *folliculitis* decalvans.

**rag-sorter's d.,** pulmonary anthrax, commonly called wool-sorter's d.

**Ranikhet d.,** Newcastle d.

**Rayer's d.,** biliary *xanthomatosis.*

**Raynaud's d.,** idiopathic paroxysmal bilateral cyanosis of the digits, due to arterial and arteriolar contraction, brought on by cold or emotion. See also Raynaud's *phenomenon.*

**Recklinghausen's d.,** neurofibromatosis.

**Recklinghausen's d. of bone,** *osteitis* fibrosa cystica.

**Refsum's d.,** Refsum's syndrome; heredopathia atactica polyneuritiformis; a rare degenerative disorder, transmitted as an autosomal recessive trait and caused by an absence of phytanic acid α-hydroxylase; it is clinically characterized by retinitis pigmentosa, polyneuritis, deafness, nystagmus, and cerebellar signs.

**Reiter's d.,** Reiter's *syndrome.*

**Rendu-Osler-Weber d.,** hereditary hemorrhagic *telangiectasia.*

**reversible d.,** d. that in its natural course or under therapy may be reversed.

**rheumatic d.,** rheumatism.

**rheumatic heart d.,** d. of the heart resulting from rheumatic fever, chiefly manifested by abnormalities of the valves.

**rheumatoid d.,** rheumatoid *arthritis,* referring particularly to nonarticular lesions such as subcutaneous nodules.

**Riedel's d.,** Riedel's *struma.*

**Riga's d.,** erosion or ulceration of the frenum of the tongue, with induration and the formation of a grayish membrane; it occurs in infants during dentition and is thought to be due to the habit of putting out the tongue, the frenum of which is irritated by rubbing against the new lower incisor teeth.

**Riggs' d.,** periodontitis.

**Ritter's d.,** (1) *dermatitis* exfoliativa infantum; (2) *icterus* neonatorum.

**Robinson's d.,** hidrocystoma(s) occurring in the skin of the face, especially in the region of the eyes.

**Roble's d.,** ocular *onchocerciasis.*

**Roger's d.,** maladie de Roger; a congenital cardiac anomaly consisting of a small isolated defect of the interventricular septum.

**Rokitansky's d.,** (1) acute yellow *atrophy* of the liver; (2) Chiari *syndrome.*

**Romberg's d.,** facial *hemiatrophy.*

**Rosenbach's d.,** (1) Heberden's *nodes;* (2) erysipeloid.

**Roth's d.,** *meralgia* paresthetica.

**Roth-Bernhardt d.,** *meralgia* paresthetica.

**Rougnon-Heberden d.,** *angina* pectoris.

**Roussy-Lévy d.,** Roussy-Lévy syndrome; a type of cerebellar ataxia regularly associated with wasting of the calves and intrinsic muscles of the hands and with absent tendon reflexes; pes cavus and claw toes develop; autosomal dominant inheritance.

**Rubarth's d.,** infectious canine *hepatitis.*

**runt d.,** wasting d.; a graft *versus* host reaction in mice first observed following intravenous injection of allogeneic spleen cells into newly born animals.

**Rust's d.,** tuberculosis of the two upper cervical vertebrae and their articulations.

**sacred d.,** epilepsy, referred to as such by Hippocrates.

**Saint Agatha's d.,** any d. of female breast.

**Saint Aignan's d.,** tinea.

**Saint Avertin's d.,** epilepsy.

**Saint Blaize's d.,** sore throat, especially tonsillitis.

**Saint Claire's d.,** conjunctivitis or any inflammatory d. of the eye.

**Saint Dymphna's d.,** any mental disease or disorder, or insanity.

**Saint Erasmus' d.,** colic.

**Saint Fiacre's d.,** hemorrhoids.

**Saint Gervasius' d.,** rheumatism.

**Saint Gete's d.,** leprosy, cancer, syphilis, or any phagedenic d.

**Saint Gile's d.,** cancer.

**Saint Guy's d.,** chorea.

**Saint Hubert's d.,** hydrophobia.

**Saint Mathurin's d.,** epileptic psychosis.

**Saint Modes'tus' d.,** chorea.

**Saint Roch's d.,** bubonic *plague.*

**Saint Rose's d.,** pellagra.

**Saint Valentine's d.,** epilepsy.

**Saint Zachary's d.,** mutism.

**Samoan eye d.,** *epitheliosis* desquamativa.

**sandworm d.,** an inflammatory eruption on the inner side of the sole, observed in certain parts of Australia, marked by a patch of erythema spreading in spirals, and disappearing spontaneously; probably a form of creeping eruption similar to larva migrans.

**Savill's d.,** *dermatitis* epidemica.

**Schamberg's d.,** progressive pigmentary *dermatosis.*

**Schenck's d.,** the gummatous lymphangitic form of sporotrichosis, *q.v.*

**Scheuermann's d.,** epiphysial aseptic *necrosis (q.v.)* of vertebral bodies.

**Schilder's d.,** *encephalitis* periaxialis diffusa.

**Schimmelbusch's d.,** fibrocystic d. of the breasts.

**Schlatter's d., Schlatter-Osgood d.,** Osgood-Schlatter d.

**Scholz' d.,** (1) familial demyelinating encephalopathy characterized by progressive spasticity and dementia in childhood; (2) juvenile form of metachromatic *leukodystrophy.*

**Schönlein's d.,** Henoch-Schönlein *purpura.*

**Schottmüller's d.,** paratyphoid *fever.*

**Schröder's d.,** a thickening of the uterine mucous membrane with uterine hemorrhage.

**Schüller's d.,** Hand-Schüller-Christian d.

**scle'rocystic d. of the ovary,** polycystic ovary *syndrome.*

**Scyth'ian d.,** atrophy of the external genitals with impotence, due to excessive and unnatural venery. Conceptually inaccurate; obsolete.

**secondary d.,** (1) a d. that follows and results from an earlier disease, injury, or event; (2) a wasting disorder that follows successful transplantation of bone marrow into lethally irradiated host; it is frequently severe and is usually associated with fever, anorexia, diarrhea, dermatitis, and desquamation.

**Selter's d.,** Feer's d.

**Senear-Usher d.,** *pemphigus* erythematosus.

**serum d.,** serum *sickness.*

**shimamushi d.** (she-mah-moo'she) [ Jap. *shima,* island, + *mushi,* bug ], tsutsugamushi d.

**sickle cell C d.,** a d. resulting from abnormal sickle-shaped erythrocytes in response to a lowering of the partial pressure of oxygen; it includes anemia, crises due to hemolysis or vascular occlusion, chronic leg ulcers and bone deformities, and infarcts of bone or of the spleen; sudden death occurs in individuals with sickle cell anemia or sickle cell trait.

**sickle cell-thalassemia d.,** microdrepanocytic *anemia.*

**silo-filler's d.,** pulmonary lesion produced by oxides of nitrogen produced by fresh silage. In its acute form it may kill from pulmonary edema or go on to a subacute or chronic proliferative pulmonary disease sometimes leading to chronic pulmonary invalidism.

**Simmonds' d.,** anterior pituitary insufficiency; commonly the result of a tumor or vascular occlusion; marked weight loss is possible, but not invariable, finding. Such patients are sometimes said to have a pituitary or hypophysial cachexia (older term, cachexia hypophysea).

**Simon's d.,** progressive *lipodystrophy.*

sixth d., *exanthema* subitum.

sixth veneral d., *lymphogranuloma* venereum.

Sjögren's d., Sjögren's *syndrome*.

skinbound d., scleroderma; see also hidebound d.

slipped tendon d., a perosis in the young chick, which allows the tendons on the caudal aspect of the tarsus to displace medially and laterally, so that the chick squats and walks on the plantar surface of the limbs, due to a deficiency of manganese.

slow virus d., a d. that follows a long, unremitting course, owing to lack of immune response; slow virus d.'s include scrapie in sheep, kuru, some cases of chronic hepatitis, and subacute inclusion body encephalitis related to measles; less definite possibilities include multiple sclerosis and some neoplasms.

Sneddon-Wilkinson d., subcorneal pustular *dermatosis*.

social d.'s, a term incorrectly used to designate venereal d.'s, especially gonorrhea and syphilis.

soil d., a d. supposed to be caused by emanation from the soil.

specific d., one produced by the action of a special pathogenic microorganism.

Spielmeyer-Stock d., retinal atrophy in amaurotic familial idiocy.

Spielmeyer-Vogt d., late juvenile type of cerebral *sphingolipidosis, q. v.*

sporadic d., one occurring in isolated cases in a locality.

Stargardt's d., a juvenile type of heredomacular degeneration.

steel-grinder's d., siderosis (1).

Steinert's d., myotonic *dystrophy*.

Sternberg's d., an old term for a condition now regarded as a form of Hodgkin's d.

Sticker's d., *erythema* infectiosum.

stiff lamb d., a muscular dystrophy occurring in young lambs fed on ewe's milk or on feed that is deficient in vitamin E or selenium, or both; see also white muscle d. of calves.

Still's d., juvenile rheumatoid *arthritis*.

Stokes-Adams d., Adams-Stokes *syndrome*.

stone-masons' d., silicosis.

storage d., accumulation of a specific substance within tissues, generally because of congenital deficiency of an enzyme necessary for further metabolism of the substance; for example, glycogen storage d.'s.

Strümpell's d., (1) *spondylitis* deformans; (2) acute epidemic leukoencephalitis.

Strümpell-Marie d., ankylosing *spondylitis*.

Strümpell-Westphal d., a diffuse form of pseudolenticular degeneration or Wilson's syndrome; Westphal's pseudosclerosis.

Sturge's d., Sturge-Weber *syndrome*.

Sturge-Weber d., Sturge-Weber *syndrome*.

Stuttgart d., the uremic form of canine leptospirosis, usually caused by *Leptospira canicola*.

subacute d., a d. marked by signs and symptoms less active than in an acute but more active than in a chronic disease.

subchronic d., a subacute d., but one with more of the characteristics of a chronic affection.

Sulzberger-Garbe d., Sulzberger-Garbe syndrome; exudative discoid and lichenoid dermatitis; a type of disseminated lichenified eczema.

summer d., bluecomb d. of chickens.

Sutton's d. [ R. L. Sutton ], *leukoderma* acquisitum centrifugum.

Sutton's d. [ R. L. Sutton, Jr. ], *periadenitis* mucosa necrotica recurrens.

Swediauer's d., Albert's d.

sweet clover d., a hemorrhagic d., due to dicumarol which causes marked reduction in prothrombin, occurring in cattle fed on sweet clover fodder, spoiled during curing.

Swift's d., acrodynia (1).

swine edema d., a clinical entity of unknown etiology but thought to be due to *Escherichia coli* toxins; it is characterized by edema of various parts of the body but particularly of the walls of the stomach and intestines.

swineherd's d., a leptospirosis occurring in those who attend swine or who are occupied in the slaughtering or processing of pork, characterized by aches and pains

throughout the body, fever, headache, dizziness, and nausea; due to *Leptospira pomona*.

Sydenham's d., Sydenham's *chorea*.

Sylvest's d., epidemic *pleurodynia*.

Takahara's d., acatalasemia.

Takayushi's d. (alternative spellings: Takayasu or Takayoshu), pulseless d.

Talma's d., *myotonia* acquisita.

Tangier d. [ named for an island in the Chesapeake Bay, the home of the family of first cases described ], analphalipoproteinemia; familial high density lipoprotein deficiency; a heritable disorder of lipid metabolism characterized by almost complete absence from plasma of high density lipoproteins, and by storage of cholesterol esters in foam cells, tonsillar enlargement, an orange or yellow-gray color of the pharyngeal and rectal mucosa, hepatosplenomegaly, lymph node enlargement, corneal opacity, and peripheral neuropathy. Autosomal recessive inheritance.

Taussig-Bing d., Taussig-Bing *syndrome*.

Tay's d., senile guttate *choroidopathy*.

Tay-Sachs d., infantile type of cerebral *sphingolipidosis, q. v.*

Taylor's d., diffuse idiopathic cutaneous atrophy.

Teschen d. [ *Teschen,* Silisia ], infectious porcine encephalomyelitis; a picornavirus infection of hogs resembling human poliomyelitis and occurring in various parts of the world. See also Teschen disease *virus*.

Theiler's d., (1) mouse *encephalomyelitis;* (2) equine serum *hepatitis*.

third d., rubella.

Thomsen's d., *myotonia* congenita.

thunder d., apoplexy.

thyrocar'diac d., heart d. resulting from hyperthyroidism.

Tillaux's d., fibrocystic d. of the breasts.

Tommaselli's d., hemoglobinuria supposed to be due to quinine intoxication.

Tornwaldt's d., inflammation or obstruction of the pharyngeal bursa or an adenoid cleft with the formation of a cyst containing pus.

Tourette's d., Gilles de la Tourette's d.

trembling d. of sheep and goats, scrapie.

Trinidad d., paralyssa.

tsutsugamu'shi d., an acute infectious disease, caused by *Rickettsia tsutsugamushi* and transmitted by *Trombicula akamushi* and *Trombicula deliensis,* that occurs in harvesters of hemp in some parts of Japan and is characterized by fever, painful swelling of the lymphatic glands, a small blackish scab on the genitals, neck, or axilla, and an eruption of large, dark red papules; it is often fatal, but in favorable cases lasts about 2 weeks; also called scrub, mite, or tropical typhus; tsutsugamushi, flood, Japanese river, kedani, or island fever; shimamushi, akamushi, kedani, or island disease.

tunnel d., (1) caisson d.; (2) ancylostomiasis.

Tzaneen d., a relatively mild theileriosis of cattle in Africa, caused by *Theileria mutans*.

Underwood's d., *sclerema* neonatorum.

Unna's d., seborrheic *dermatitis*.

Unverricht's d., myoclonus *epilepsy*.

Urbach-Wiethe d., lipid *proteinosis*.

vagabond's d., parasitic *melanoderma*.

vagrant's d., parasitic *melanoderma*.

van Buren's d., Peyronie's d.

Vaquez' d., erythremia.

vene'real d., syphilis, gonorrhea, chancroid, or other d. acquired in general through sexual intercourse.

veno-occlusive d. of the liver, obliterating endophlebitis of small hepatic vein radicles, described in Jamaican children, associated with ingestion of toxic plant substances in bush tea; causes ascites which may progress to cirrhosis.

Vidal's d., *lichen* simplex chronicus.

Vincent's d., an inflammatory condition with necrosis of gingival tissue as one of its main features. The necrotizing process has a distinct predilection for the interproximal papilla. Pain is a characteristic feature; other signs that may or may not be present are fetor oris, salivation, malaise and a slight rise in temperature. A symbiotic infection caused by *Borrelia, Treponema,* and fusiform bacilli which are normal inhabitants of the mouth. Also called necrotizing ulcerative gingivitis; Vincent's infection; Vincent's stomatitis; Vincent's angina; ulceromembranous angina; Plaut's angina; Plaut's ulcer; trench mouth; pharyngitis ulcerosa; fusospirochetal disease.

**Virchow's d.,** (1) acute congenital encephalitis; (2) *leontiasis* ossea.

**virus X d.,** a term applied to a number of virus d.'s of obscure etiology, *e.g.,* Australian X d.

**Vogt-Spielmeyer d.,** Spielmeyer-Vogt d.

**Voltolini's d.,** d. of the labyrinth, leading to deafmutism, in young children.

**von Economo's d.,** encephalitis lethargica; epidemic encephalitis; polioencephalitis infectiva; the basis for postencephalic parkinsonism, suspected to be of viral origin.

**von Gierke's d.,** see Gierke's d.

**von Hippel-Lindau d.,** Lindau's d.

**von Meyenburg's d.,** relapsing *perichondritis.*

**von Recklinghausen's d.,** see Recklinghausen's d.

**von Willebrand's d.,** angiohemophilia; hereditary pseudohemophilia; constitutional thrombopathy (1); vascular hemophilia; a hemorrhagic diathesis characterized by tendency to bleed primarily from mucous membranes, prolonged bleeding time, normal platelet count, normal clot retraction, partial and variable deficiency of factor VIII, and possibly a morphologic defect of platelets; autosomal dominant inheritance with reduced penetrance and variable expressivity.

**Voorhoeve's d.,** *osteopathia* striata.

**Wagner's d.,** hyaloideoretinal *degeneration.*

**Wardrop's d.,** *onychia* maligna.

**wart-hog d.,** African swine *fever.*

**wasting d.,** runt d.

**Weber-Christian d.,** nodular nonsuppurative *panniculitis.*

**Wegner's d.,** congenital syphilitic osteochondritis.

**Weil's d.,** infectious icterus; infectious jaundice (1); leptospirosis caused by *Leptospira icterohemorrhagiae* and believed to be acquired by contact with the urine of infected rats; characterized clinically by fever, jaundice, muscular pains, conjunctival congestion, and albuminuria; agglutinins regularly appear in the serum.

**Werdnig-Hoffmann d.,** infantile muscular *atrophy.*

**Werlhof's d.,** idiopathic thrombocytopenic *purpura.*

**Werner-His d.,** Volhynia *fever.*

**Wernicke's d.,** Wernicke's *syndrome.*

**Westphal's d.,** pseudosclerosis (3).

**Whipple's d.,** intestinal lipodystrophy; lipodystrophia intestinalis; lipophagic intestinal granulomatosis; a rare d. characterized by steatorrhea, frequently generalized lymphadenopathy, arthritis, fever, and cough. There are many "foamy" macrophages in the jejunal lamina propria, and lymph nodes that contain periodic acid-Schiff positive particles that appear bacilliform by electron microscopy.

**White's d.,** *keratosis* follicularis.

**white muscle d.,** a nutritional myopathy of young animals, manifested by stiffness and soreness; cardiac muscle damage is frequent, and affected muscles exhibit whitish, chalklike streaks, which are degenerated fibers; it is due to a deficiency of vitamin E or selenium, or both, and is seen most frequently in calves and lambs but has also been reported in other species.

**white spot d.,** *morphea* guttata.

**Whytt's d.,** internal *hydrocephalus.*

**Wilkie's d.,** superior mesenteric artery *syndrome.*

**Wilson's d.,** (1) [ Samuel A. Kinnier Wilson ], hepatolenticular *degeneration;* (2) [ Sir William J. E. Wilson ], exfoliative *dermatitis.*

**Winckel's d.,** *icterus* neonatorum.

**Windscheid's d.,** the nervous symptoms related to arteriosclerosis.

**Winiwarter-Buerger d.,** *thromboangiitis* obliterans.

**Winkelman's d.,** progressive pallidal degeneration.

**Winkler's d.,** *chondrodermatitis* nodularis chronica helicis.

**winter-vomiting d.,** see epidemic *vomiting.*

**Wohlfart-Kugelberg-Welander d.,** juvenile muscular *atrophy.*

**Wolman's d.,** a lipidosis characterized by xanthomatosis, adrenal calcification, hepatosplenomegaly, foam cells in bone marrow and other tissues, and vacuolated lymphocytes in peripheral blood; autosomal recessive inheritance.

**wool-sorter's d.,** pulmonary *anthrax.*

**X d. of cattle,** bovine *hyperkeratosis.*

**yellow d.,** xanthochromia; ochrodermatosis; jaundice.

**Ziehen-Oppenheim d.,** *dystonia* musculorum deformans.

**zymot'ic d.,** an old term for infectious d., due to the action of a living ferment.

---

**disengagement** (dis-en-gāj'ment) [ Fr. ]. The act of setting free or extricating; specifically, the emergence of the head from the vulva during childbirth, or ascent of the presenting part from the pelvis after the inlet has been negotiated.

**disequilibrium** (dis-e'kwĭ-lib'rĭ-um). A lack of equilibrium in any sense; specifically, a lack of proper adjustment between the moral and intellectual faculties.

**disgermino'ma.** Dysgerminoma.

**dish.** A shallow container, usually concave.

**Dappen d.,** trade name for a small glass receptacle with cone-shaped interior for holding a small quantity (1 or 2 ml.) of medicament.

**Petri d.,** a small, shallow, circular d. (usually 100 mm. in diameter with edges 15 mm. high) made of thin glass or clear plastic with a loosely fitting, overlapping cover used especially in microbiology for the cultivation of microorganisms on solid media; it is frequently referred to as a plate.

**Stender d.,** a flat shallow vessel used in staining sections.

**dishar'mony.** The state of being deranged or lacking in orderliness.

**occlusal d.,** (1) contacts of opposing occlusal surfaces of teeth which are not in harmony with other tooth contacts and with the anatomic and physiologic control of the mandible; (2) occlusions which do not coincide with their respective jaw relations. See also deflective occlusal *contact.*

**disimpaction** (dis'im-pak'shun). Withdrawal of impaction in a fractured bone.

**disinfect** (dis'in-fekt'). To destroy pathogenic microorganisms in or on any substance or to inhibit their growth and vital activity.

**disinfectant** (dis'in-fek'tant). 1. Destroying the germs of putrefaction or disease, or inhibiting their activity. 2. An agent that possesses this property.

**complete d.,** one that kills both vegetative forms and spores.

**incomplete d.,** one that kills only the vegetative forms, leaving the spores uninjured.

**disinfection** (dis'in-fek'shun). The destruction of pathogenic microorganisms or their toxins or vectors.

**Fuerbringer's hand d.,** brushing the hands and arms with warm soap and water for 3 minutes; the same repeated after cleaning the nails; rubbing with 70 per cent alcohol 2 minutes; brushing with a 2 per cent Lysol solution 2 minutes.

**disinhibition** (dis'in-hĭ-bish'un). The inhibition of an inhibition; the removal of an inhibitory effect by a stimulus, as when a conditioned reflex has undergone extinction, it may be restored by some extraneous stimulus.

**disinsertion** (dis-in-ser'shun). 1. Rupture of a tendon at its point of insertion into a bone. 2. Dialysis retinae; retinodialysis; separation of the retina from its insertion at the ora serrata.

**disintegration** (dis-in'tĕ-gra'shun). 1. Loss or separation of the component parts of a substance, such as occurs in catabolism or decay. 2. Disorganization of psychic processes.

**disinvagination** (dis'in-vaj-ĭ-na'shun). Relieving an invagination.

**disjugate** (dis'ju-gāt) [ L. *dis-,* apart, + *jugatus,* yoked ]. Not paired in action or joined together; the opposite of conjugate; see disjugate *movement.*

**disjunction** (dis-junk'shun) [ L. *dis-,* apart, + *junctura,* juncture ]. The separation of pairs of chromosomes at the anaphase stage of cell division.

**disk, disc** [ L. *discus;* G. *diskos,* a quoit, disk ]. 1. Discus. 2. In dentistry, a d.-shaped piece of thin paper or other material, coated with emery or other abrasive substance, used for cutting and polishing teeth and fillings. 3. Lamella (2).

**A d.'s,** A *bands.*

**acro′mioclavic′ular d.,** *discus* articularis acromioclavicularis.

**Amici's d.,** Z *line.*

**anisotropic d.,** A *band.*

**artic′ular d.,** *discus* articularis.

**blastoder′mic d.,** the aggregation of blastomeres of a telolecithal ovum after cleavage has occurred.

**blood d.,** platelet.

**Bowman's d.'s,** d.'s resulting from transverse segmentation of striated muscular fiber treated with weak acids, certain alkaline solutions, or freezing.

**Burlew d.,** an abrasive-impregnated rubber wheel used in dentistry for polishing.

**choked d.,** papilledema.

**ciliary d.,** *orbiculus* ciliaris.

**cuttlefish d.,** a circle of paper or thin plastic coated with ground cuttlefish bone; used, when attached to a mandrel and rotated by a dental handpiece, for fine smoothing and finishing of dental materials and tooth.

**diamond d.,** a steel d. with the cutting surface(s) covered with fine diamond chips, for use in a dental handpiece.

**embryonic d.,** germinal d.

**emery d.'s,** d.'s of paper or other materials coated with emery powder used in surfacing teeth or fillings.

**ger′minal d.,** germ d.; embryonic d.; the point in a telolecithal ovum where the embryo begins to be formed.

**H d.,** H *band.*

**Hensen's d.,** H *band.*

**herniated d.,** protruded d.; ruptured d.; protrusion of a degenerated or fragmented intervertebral d. into the intervertebral foramen compressing the nerve root.

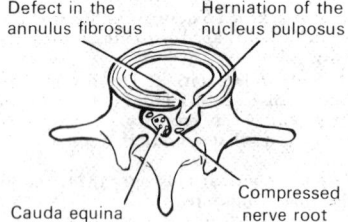

Defect in the annulus fibrosus    Herniation of the nucleus pulposus

Cauda equina    Compressed nerve root

**Herniated Disk**

Horizontal section of posterolateral herniation of the intervertebral disk. (From Salter, R. B.: *Textbook of Disorders and Injuries of the Musculoskeletal System,* The Williams & Wilkins Co., Baltimore, 1970.)

**I d.,** I *band.*

**intercalated d.,** an undulating double membrane separating adjacent cells in cardiac muscle fibers.

**intermediate d.,** Z *line.*

**interpu′bic d.,** *discus* interpubicus.

**intervertebral d.,** *discus* intervertebralis.

**isotropic d.,** I *band.*

**mandib′ular d.,** *discus* articularis temporomandibularis.

**Merkel's tactile d.,** *meniscus* tactus.

**Newton's d.,** a cardboard d. on which are seven colored sectors, each occupying proportionally the same space as the corresponding primary color in the spectrum; when the disk is rapidly rotated it appears white.

**optic d.,** *discus* nervi optici.

**Placido's d.,** keratoscope.

**prolig′erous d.,** *cumulus* oophorus.

**protruded d.,** herniated d.

**Q d.,** A *band.*

**radioulnar d.,** *discus* articularis radioulnaris.

**Ranvier's d.'s,** tactile nerve endings, of cupped disklike form, in the skin.

**Rekoss d.,** the rotating device for changing the lenses quickly and accurately in hand ophthalmoscopes.

**ruptured d.,** herniated d.

**sa′crococcyg′eal d.,** a thin plate of fibrocartilage interposed between the sacrum and coccyx.

**sandpaper d.'s,** d.'s of paper coated with various grits of silica; used for surfacing teeth or dental materials.

**spinning d.,** an aerosol generator designed for producing monodisperse aerosols.

**stenopeic d., stenopaic d.,** a metallic or other opaque d. with a narrow slit through which one looks; used as a test for astigmatism.

**ster′noclavic′ular d.,** *discus* articularis sternoclavicularis.

**straboscopic d.,** a lens or d., used in visual testing, that distorts objects.

**stroboscopic d.,** a revolving d. that gives successive views of a moving object.

**tactile d.,** *meniscus* tactus.

**transverse d.,** one of the dark transverse bands seen on examining a striated muscular fiber under the microscope.

**triangular d. of wrist,** *discus* articularis radioulnaris.

**Z d.,** Z *line.*

**diskitis** (disk-i′tis). Discitis; meniscitis; inflammation of any disk, especially of an interarticular cartilage.

**disko-.** For words beginning thus, see disco-.

**dis′locate.** To luxate; to put out of joint.

**dislocatio** (dēs-lo-kah′te-o, dis-lo-ka′shyo) [ L. ]. Dislocation.

   **d. erecta,** a subglenoid dislocation of the shoulder in which the arm is held vertically with the hand on top of the head; the head of the humerus is inferiorly placed.

**dislocation** (dis-lo-ka′shun) [ L. *dislocatio,* fr. *dis-,* apart, + *locatio,* a placing ]. Luxation; displacement of an organ or any part; specifically a disturbance or disarrangement of the normal relation of the bones entering into the formation of a joint.

   **d. of articular processes, vertebral, cervical,** jumped process complex; locked facets; complete d. of one or both articular processes, usually with overriding of the inferior articular process of the vertebra above into a position anterior to the superior articular process of the vertebra below.

   **compound d.,** one complicated by a wound opening from the surface down to the affected joint.

   **Kienböck's d.,** d. of semilunar bone.

   **Nélaton's d.,** wedging of the astragalus between the widely separated tibia and fibula, usually complicated with fracture.

   **simple d.,** one not complicated by an external wound.

   **vertebral, cervical d.,** a complete and persistent displacement of adjacent articular surfaces; see also vertebral subluxation.

**dismem′ber.** To amputate an arm or leg.

**dis′mutase.** A generic name for enzymes catalyzing the reaction of two identical molecules to produce two molecules in differing states of oxidation (*e.g.,* superoxide dismutase), phosphorylation (glucose 1-phosphate phosphodismutase), etc.

**dismutation** (dis′mu-ta′shun). An oxidation-reduction reaction involving a single substance; thus, two molecules of acetaldehyde may react, producing an oxidation product (acetic acid) and a reduction product (ethyl alcohol).

**disomic** (di-so′mik). Relating to disomy.

**disomy** (di′so-mī) [ G. *dis,* two, + *sōma,* body ]. The state of an individual or cell having two members of a pair of homologous chromosomes; the normal state in man, in contrast to monosomy and trisomy; can also apply to an abnormal chromosome represented twice in a single cell.

**di′sopyr′amide** (USAN). NORPACE; α-[ 2-(diisopropylamino)ethyl ]-α -phenyl-2-pyridineacetamide; an antiarrhythmic drug.

**disor′der.** A disturbance of function, structure, or both resulting from a genetic or embryologic failure in development, or from exogenous factors as poison, injury or disease. It may be inborn or acquired.

   **affective d.,** manic-depressive *psychosis.*

   **autonomic d.,** standard nomenclature used in reference to psychosomatic d.

   **behavior d.,** a general term used to denote mental illness, specifically those mental, emotional, or behavioral sub-

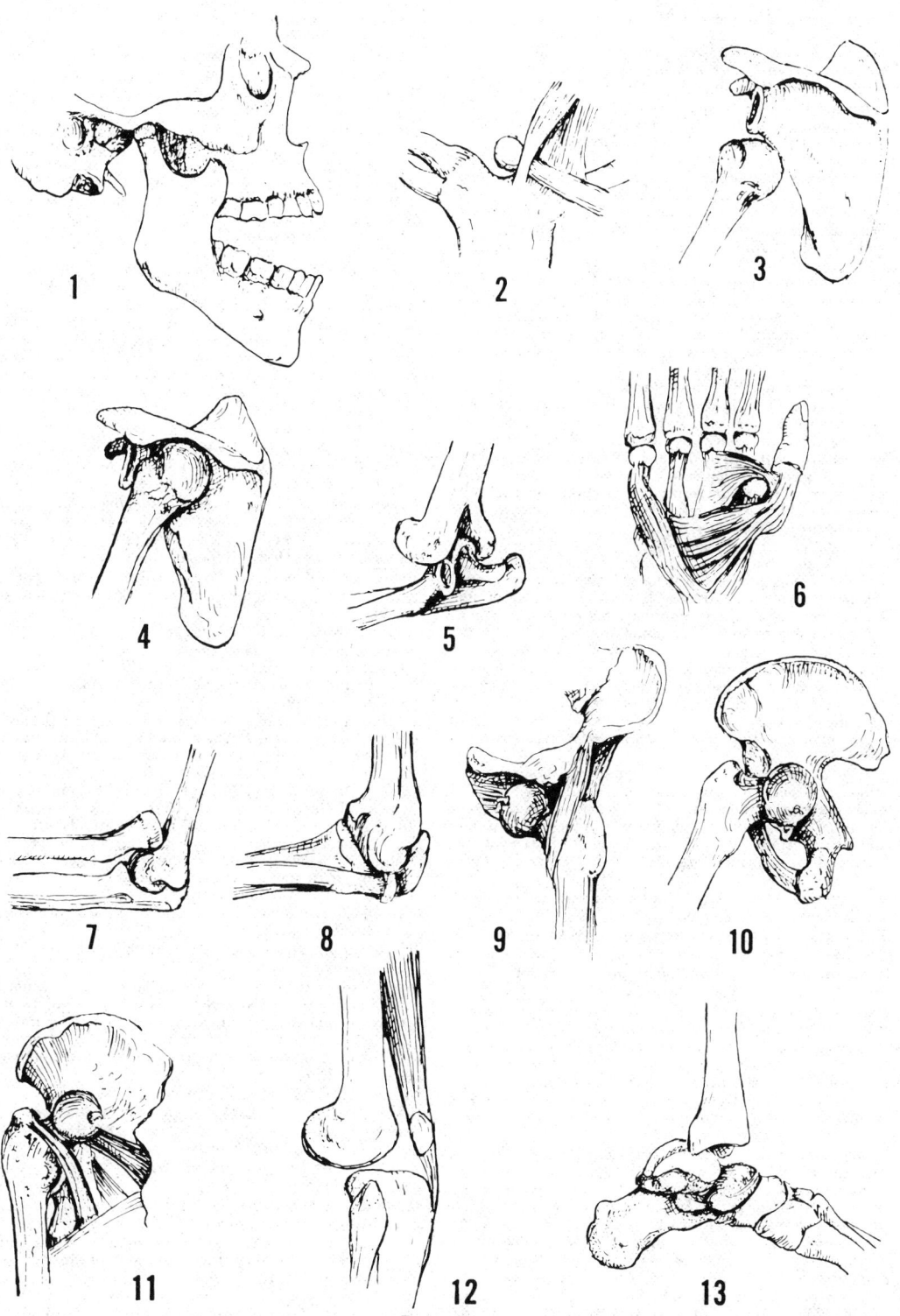

**Dislocations**

*1*, Dislocation of the lower jaw; *2*, upward dislocation of the sternal end of the clavicle; *3*, subglenoid dislocation of the head of the humerus; *4*, subspinous dislocation of the head of the humerus; *5*, dislocation backward of the bones of the forearm; *6*, dislocation backward of the phalanx of the thumb; *7*, dislocation of the radius forward; *8*, dislocation of the radius backward; *9*, anterior (obturator) dislocation of the hip; *10*, anterior (pubic) dislocation of the hip; *11*, posterior (dorsal) dislocation of the hip; *12*, forward dislocation of the knee; *13*, backward dislocation of the foot.

classes of mental illness for which organic correlates do not exist.

**character d.,** a term referring to a group of behavioral d.'s which has been replaced by a more general term, personality d. *q.v.*), of which character d.'s are now a subclass.

**emotional d.,** see mental *illness*.

**functional d.,** those with no known organic basis, dependent upon learning and past experience.

**immunoproliferative d.'s,** d.'s in which there is a continuing proliferation of cells of the immunocyte complex associated with autoallergic disturbances and γ-globulin abnormalities such as in chronic lymphocytic leukemia, "macroglobulinemias," and multiple myeloma, with the implication that the etiologic factor concerned might be immunologic (allergic).

**neuropsychologic d.,** acute or chronic brain syndrome; disturbance of mental function due to trauma, associated with one or more of the following manifestations: psychotic, neurotic, behavioral, psychophysiologic, and mental impairment; see also subentries under manifestation, and mental *impairment*.

**neuropsychologic d., acute,** brain *syndrome*, acute.

**neuropsychologic d., chronic,** brain *syndrome*, chronic.

**personality d.,** a general term for a group of behavioral d.'s, each characterized by usually lifelong, ingrained, maladaptive patterns of deviant behavior, life style, and social adjustment that are different in quality from psychotic and neurotic symptoms; former designations for these personality d.'s were psychopath and sociopath; see also subentries under personality.

**personality d., posttraumatic,** a form of neuropsychologic d., posttraumatic, characterized in adults by irritability, emotional lability, loss of initiative and sense of responsibility; and in children by hyperkinesis, emotional lability, and disobedient, impulsive, egocentric behavior.

**plasma iodoprotein d.,** see familial *goiter*.

**psychophysiologic d.,** standard nomenclature used in reference to psychosomatic d.

**psychosomatic d.,** a d. characterized by physical symptoms of psychic origin, usually involving a single organ system innervated by the autonomic nervous system; physiological and organic changes stem from a sustained disturbance.

**sleep d.,** (1) somnipathy; (2) hypnotic somnambulism.

**thought process d.,** an intellectual function symptom of schizophrenia, manifested by irrelevance and incoherence of verbal productions ranging from simple blocking and mild circumstantiality to total loosening of associations.

**visceral d.,** nomenclature used in reference to psychosomatic d.

**disor'ganiza'tion.** Destruction of an organ or tissue with consequent loss of function.

**disorientation** (dis-o'rī-en-ta'shun). Loss of the sense of familiarity with one's surroundings; loss of one's bearings.

**disparate** (dis'pǎ-rāt) [ L. *dis-paro*, pp. *-atus*, to separate, fr. *paro*, to prepare ]. Unequal; not alike.

**disparity** (dis-pǎr'ī-tĭ) [ L. *disparis*, dissimilar ]. The condition of being disparate.

**conjugate d.,** difference in the sizes of the retinal images in each eye, caused by asymmetrical convergence.

**fixation d.,** a condition in which retinal images, because of over- or underconvergence, do not fall on corresponding points; a measure of muscular imbalance while fusion is maintained.

**dispen'sary** [ L. *dis-penso*, pp. *-atus*, to distribute by weight, fr. *penso*, to weigh ]. 1. A physician's office, especially the office of one who dispenses his own medicines. 2. The office of a hospital apothecary, where medicines are given out on the physicians' orders. 3. An out-patient department of a hospital. 4. A public institution where the sick poor receive gratuitous treatment.

**dispen'satory** [ L. *dispensator*, a manager, steward; see dispensary ]. A work originally intended as a commentary on the Pharmacopeia, but now rather a supplement to that work. It contains an account of the sources, mode of preparation, physiologic action, and therapeutic uses of most of the agents, official and nonofficial, used in the treatment of disease.

**dispense.** To give out medicine and other necessities to the sick; to fill a medical prescription.

**di'spermy.** Entrance of two sperms into one ovum.

**disper'sal.** Dispersion (1).

**flash d.,** the property of rapid disintegration of a tablet when placed on the tongue.

**disperse** (dis-pers'). To dissipate, to cause disappearance of, to scatter, to dilute.

**dispersion** (dis-per'zhun). [ L. *dispersio* ]. 1. The act of dispersing or of being dispersed. 2. The more or less intimate incorporation of the particles of one substance into the mass of another, including solutions, suspensions, and colloidal dispersions. 3. Specifically, what is usually called a colloidal solution.

**coarse d.,** suspension (4).

**colloid'al d.,** colloid *solution*.

**molec'ular d.,** one in which the dispersed phase consists of individual molecules; if these molecules are of less than colloidal size, the result is a true solution.

**optical rotatory d.,** abbreviated ORD; the change in optical rotation with the wavelength of the incident monochromatic polarized light; the displacement of the former from zero within the absorption band is known as the Cotton effect (*q.v.*), from its discoverer.

**temporal d.,** asynchronous repolarization of myocardial fibers that predisposes to abnormal current flow and ectopy (especially with bradyarrhythmias).

**disper'sity.** The extent to which the dimensions of particles have been reduced in colloid formation.

**disper'soid.** A colloid solution in which the dispersed phase can be concentrated by centrifugation; called also molecular dispersed solution.

**disper'sonaliza'tion.** Depersonalization.

**dispireme** (di-spi'rēm) [ G. *di-,* twice, + *speirēma*, coil, convolution ]. The double chromatin skein in the telophase of mitosis.

**displaceability** (dis-plās'ă-bil'ī-tĭ). The capability of, or susceptibility to, displacement.

**tissue d.,** compression of tissue; the property of tissue that permits it to be moved from an initial or relaxed position or form.

**displacement** (dis-plās'ment). 1. Removal from the normal location or position. 2. The adding to a fluid (particularly a gas) in an open vessel one of greater density whereby the first is expelled. 3. In chemistry, a change in which one element, radical, or molecule is replaced by another, or in which one element exchanges electric charges with another by reduction or oxidation. 4. The d. of impulses from one expression to another, as from fighting to talking.

**affect d.,** a shift of feeling from the object originally arousing it to some associated object.

**mesial d.,** mesioplacement.

**tissue d.,** the change in the form or position of tissues as a result of pressure.

**Disse** (dis'ē), Josef, German anatomist, 1852–1912. See D.'s *spaces*.

**dissect** (dī-sekt') [ L. *dis-seco*, pp. *-sectus*, to cut asunder ]. 1. To cut apart or separate the tissues of the body in the study of anatomy. 2. In an operation, to separate the different structures along natural lines by cutting or tearing the connective tissue framework, instead of making a wide incision.

**dissection** (dī-sek'shun). The act of dissecting.

**dissem'inated** [ L. *dis-semino*, pp. *-atus*, to scatter seed, fr. *semen* (*-min-*), seed ]. Widely scattered throughout an organ, tissue, or the body.

**dissep'iment** [ L. *dis-sepio*, pp. *-septus*, to divide by a fence. SEPT- ]. Partition.

**dissimilation** (dis-sim-ī-la'shun). Disassimilation.

**dissimulation** (dis-sim-u-la'shun). The act of dissembling, especially of a state of health on the part of a sick person; the opposite of malingering or simulating illness.

**dissociation** (dis-so'sī-a'shun, -shī-a'shun) [ L. *dis-socio*, pp. *-atus*, to disjoin, separate, fr. *socius*, partner, ally ]. 1. Disassociation; separation; dissolution of relations. 2. The change of a complex into a more simple chemical compound by any lytic reaction or by ionization. 3. An unconscious process by which a group of mental processes is separated from the rest of the thinking processes, resulting in an independent functioning of these processes and a loss of the usual relationships.

**albu′minocytolog′ic d.,** increased protein in the cerebrospinal fluid without increase in cell count, characteristic of the Guillain-Barré syndrome; it is also associated with spinal block and with intracranial neoplasia, and is seen in the last phases of poliomyelitis.

**atrial d.,** mutually independent beating of the two atria or of parts of the atria.

**atrioventric′ular d.,** (1) any situation in which atria and ventricles are activated and contract independently, as in complete A-V block; (2) more specifically, the d. between atria and ventricles which results from slowing of the atrial pacemaker or acceleration of the ventricular pacemaker; interference-d.

**complete A-V d.,** (1) A-V d. not interrupted by ventricular captures; (2) complete A-V *block.*

**electrolytic d.,** see Arrhenius′ *doctrine.*

**incomplete A-V d.,** A-V d. interrupted by ventricular captures.

**electromechanical d.,** persistence of electrical activity in the heart without associated mechanical contraction; often a sign of cardiac rupture.

**interference d.,** d. with interference; A-V d. interrupted from time to time by ventricular captures.

**isorhythmic d.,** a-v d. characterized by equal or closely similar atrial and ventricular rates.

**longitudinal d.,** d. between parallel chambers of the heart, as between one atrium and the other or between one ventricle and the other, in contrast to d. between atria and ventricles.

**sleep d.,** sleep *paralysis.*

**syringomyelic d.,** loss of pain and temperature sensation with relative retention of tactile sensation, related to a cavity in the central portion of the cord interrupting the decussation of nerve fibers.

**tabetic d.,** loss of sensation of proprioceptive type due to involvement of the posterior columns of the spinal cord.

**dissolution** (dis′o-lu′shun) [ L. *dis-solvo,* pp. -*solutus,* to loose asunder, dissolve ]. 1. A dissolving. 2. Autolysis.

**gestalt d.,** a psychological phenomenon in which, after a short period of inspection, the whole of a picture seems scattered into fragments.

**dissolve** (dĭ-zolv′). To change or cause to change from the solid to a dispersed form by immersion in a fluid of suitable character.

**dissonance** (dis′so-nans) [ L. *dissonus,* discordant, confused ]. In social psychology and attitude theory, an aversive state which arises when an individual is aware of inconsistency or conflict within himself.

**dissymmetry** (dis-sim′ĕtrĭ) [ dis- + symmetry ]. 1. The absence of symmetry. 2. Symmetry in opposite directions; *e.g.,* hands.

**dis′tad.** Toward the periphery; in a distal direction.

**dis′tal** [ L. *distalis* ]. 1. Situated away from the center of the body, or from the point of origin; specifically applied to the extremity or distant part of a limb or organ. 2. In dentistry, away from the median sagittal plane of the face, following the curvature of the dental arch. 3. In a dorsal direction from any given point of reference.

**dista′lis** [ NA ]. Distal (1).

**distance** (dis′tans) [ L. *distantia,* fr. *di-sto,* to stand apart, be distant ]. The measure of space between two objects.

**focal d.,** the d. from the center of a lens to its focus.

**infinite d.,** infinity; the limit of distant vision, the rays entering the eyes from an object at that point being practically parallel.

**interarch d.,** interridge d.; interalveolar space; (1) the vertical d. between the maxillary and mandibular arches under conditions of vertical dimensions which must be specified; (2) the vertical d. between maxillary and mandibular ridges.

**interarch d., large** a large d. between the maxillary and mandibular arches; may also imply an excessive vertical dimension.

**interarch d., reduced,** closed bite; an occluding vertical dimension which results in an excessive interocclusal distance when the mandible is in rest position, and in a reduced interridge distance when the teeth are in contact.

**interarch d., small,** close bite; a small d. between the maxillary and mandibular arches.

**interocclusal d.,** interocclusal clearance; free-way space; interocclusal gap; interocclusal rest space; (1) vertical d. between the opposing occlusal surfaces; rest relation is assumed unless otherwise designated; (2) the d. between the occluding surfaces of the maxillary and mandibular teeth when the mandible is in its physiologic rest position.

**interridge d.,** interarch d.

**pupillary d.,** the d. between the major reference points in measuring for fitting of spectacle frames and lenses.

**sociometric d.,** some measurable degree of mutual or social perception; hypothetically, greater sociometric d. is associated with more inaccuracy in evaluating a relationship.

**distem′per** [ L. *dis*-priv. + *tempero,* to qualify, temper, fr. *tempus,* time ]. 1. Canine: Carre's disease; a specific disease of young dogs that is highly contagious, highly fatal, and caused by a virus. 2. Feline: panleukopenia.

**distensibility** (dis-ten′sĭ-bil′ĭ-tĭ) [ L. *dis-tendo,* to stretch apart. TEN- ]. The capability of being distended or stretched.

**distention, distension** (dis-ten′shun) [ L. *dis-tendere,* to stretch apart ]. The act or state of being distended or stretched.

**distichia, distichiasis** (dis-tik′ĭ-ah; dis-tĭ-ki′a-sis) [ G. *di-,* double, + *stichos,* row ]. The presence of two rows of eyelashes on one lid.

**distill** (dis-til′) [ L. *de-stillo* (*or di*-), pp. -*atus,* to drop down, fr. *stilla,* a drop ]. To extract a substance by volatilization and condensation (distillation).

**dis′tillate.** The product of distillation.

**distillation** (dis′tĭ-la′shun). The volatilization of a liquid by heat and the subsequent condensation of the vapor; a means of separating the volatile from the nonvolatile, or the more volatile from the less volatile, part of a liquid mixture.

**destructive d.,** dry d.

**dry d.,** destructive d.; the submission of an organic substance to heat in a closed vessel so that oxygen is absent and combustion prevented, with the object of effecting its decomposition with release of volatile constituents and the formation of new substances.

**fractional d.,** the d. of a compound liquid at varying degrees of heat whereby the components of different boiling points are collected separately.

**molecular d.,** d. in high vacuum, intended to make possible use of low temperatures to minimize damage to thermally labile molecules that would be decomposed by boiling at higher temperatures.

**distobuccal** (dis′to-buk′kal). Relating to the distal and buccal surfaces of a tooth; denoting the angle formed by their junction.

**dis′tobuc′co-occlu′sal.** Relating to the distal, buccal, and occlusal surfaces of a bicuspid or molar tooth; denoting especially the angle formed by the junction of these surfaces.

**dis′tobuc′copul′pal.** Relating to the point (trihedral) angle formed by the junction of a distal, buccal, and pulpal wall of a cavity (see point *angle*).

**distocervical** (dis′to-ser′vĭ-kal). Relating to the line angle formed by the junction of the distal and cervical (gingival) walls of a class V cavity (see line *angle*).

**distoclu′sal.** 1. Relating to or characterized by distocclusion. 2. Denoting a compound cavity or restoration involving the distal and occlusal surfaces of a tooth. 3. Denoting the line angle formed by the distal and occlusal walls of a (class V) cavity (see line *angle*).

**distoclusion** (dis′to-klu′zhun). Disto-occlusion; distal occlusion; a malocclusion in which the mandibular arch articulates with the maxillary arch in a position distal to normal; an Angle class II malocclusion.

**distogingival** (dis′to-jin′jĭ-val). Relating to the junction of the distal surface with the gingival line of a tooth.

**distoincisal** (dis′to-in-si′zal). Relating to the line (dihedral) angle formed by the junction of the distal and incisal walls of a (class V) cavity in an anterior tooth.

**distola′bial.** Relating to the distal and labial surfaces of a tooth; denoting the angle formed by their junction.

**dis'tola'biopul'pal.** Relating to the point (trihedral) angle formed by the junction of distal, labial and pulpal walls of the incisal part of a class IV (mesioincisal) cavity.

**distolingual** (dis-to-ling'gwal). Relating to the distal and lingual surfaces of a tooth; denoting the angle formed by their junction.

**distolinguo-occlusal** (dis'to-ling'gwo-ŏ-klu'zal). Relating to the distal, lingual, and occlusal surfaces of a bicuspid or molar tooth; denoting especially the angle formed by the junction of these surfaces.

**Dis'toma, Dis'tomum** [ G. *di*-, two, + *stoma*, mouth ]. An obsolete term for a group of trematode worms or flukes, the members of which are now usually referred to other genera, as *Fasciola, Fasciolopsis, Paragonimus, Opisthorchis, Cotylogonimus, Clonorchis, Dicrocoelium,* and *Schistosoma.*

**distomato'sis.** Distomiasis.

**distomiasis** (dis-to-mi'ă-sis). Distomatosis; an obsolete term denoting the presence in any of the organs or tissues of a worm formerly known as Distoma or Distomum; in general, infection by any parasitic trematode or fluke.
  **hemic d.,** schistosomiasis.
  **pulmonary d.,** paragonimiasis.

**distomolar** (dis'to-mo'lar). A supernumerary tooth located in the region the third molar tooth.

**dis'to-occlu'sal.** Distoclusal.

**dis'to-occlu'sion.** Distoclusion.

**dis'toplace'ment.** Malposition of a tooth in a posterior direction following the curvature of the dental arch.

**dis'topul'pal.** Relating to the line (dihedral) angle formed by the junction of the distal and pulpal walls of a cavity.

**distor'sion.** Distortion (3).

**distortion** (dis-tor'shun). 1. A prime mechanism that helps to repress or disguise unacceptable thoughts. 2. In dental impressions, the permanent deformation of the impression material after the registration of an imprint. 3. Distorsion; in orthopaedics, a torsional *deformity, q.v.*
  **parataxic d.,** an attitude toward another person based on a distorted evaluation of him, usually because of an identification of that person with emotionally significant figures in the patient's past life.

**distoversion** (dis'to-ver-zhun). Malposition of a tooth with its long axis inclined distal to normal.

**distrac'tibil'ity.** Disorder of the attention in which the mind is easily diverted by inconsequential occurrences.

**distraction** (dis-trak'shun) [ L. *dis-traho*, pp. *-tractus*, to pull in different directions ]. 1. Mental confusion; impossibility of concentration or fixation of the mind. 2. Extension of a limb made in a direction to draw apart the joint surfaces.

**distress** (dis-tres') [ L. *distringo*, to draw asunder ]. Mental or physical suffering or anguish.
  **fetal d.,** a threatening or adverse condition of the fetus, caused by stress; some of the criteria for recognition of fetal d. are cardiac arrhythmia, bradycardia, tachycardia, passage of meconium.

**distribution** (dis'trĭ-bu'shun) [ L. *dis-tribuo*, pp. *-tributus*, to distribute, fr. *tribus*, a tribe ]. 1. The passage of the branches of arteries or nerves to the several tissues and organs. 2. The area in which the branches of an artery or a nerve terminate, or the area supplied by such artery or nerve. 3. The relative numbers of individuals in various categories or populations.
  **binomial d.,** a d. obtained by expansion of the binomial $(q + p)^n$, where $p$ is the probability of an event occurring in one of two possible ways, $q$ is the alternative probability, and $n$ is the number of occurrences.
  **d. coefficient,** see under coefficient.
  **countercurrent d.,** A method of separation of two or more substances by repeated distribution between two immiscible liquid phases that move past each other in opposite directions; a form of liquid-liquid chromatography.
  **frequency d.,** a statistical description of raw data in terms of the number or frequency of items characterized by each of a series or range of values of a continuous variable.
  **Gaussian d.,** normal d.
  **normal d.,** Gaussian d.; a specific bell-shaped frequency d. commonly assumed by statisticians to represent the

infinite population of measurements from which a sample has been drawn; it is characterized by two parameters, the mean (x) and the standard deviation ($\sigma$) in the equation:

$$y = \frac{1}{\sigma\sqrt{2\pi}}\, e^{-\frac{(x - \bar{x})^2}{2\sigma^2}}$$

  **Poisson d.,** a discontinuous d. important in statistical work and defined by the equation $p(x) = (\mu^x / x\ !)\ e^{\text{-}\mu}$, where $x$ is the series of integers, $\mu$ is the mean, and $x\ !$ represents the factorial of $x$.

**districhiasis** (dis-trĭ-ki'ă-sis) [ G. *dis*, double, + *thrix* (*trich*-), hair ]. Growth of two hairs in a single follicle.

**dis'trix** [ G. *dis*, twice, + *thrix*, hair ]. Splitting of the hairs at their ends.

**distur'bance.** Deviation from, interruption of, or interference with a normal state.
  **emotional d.,** a behavioral d. or mental illness.
  **psychographic d.'s,** the use of a bombastic and inflated style as a symptom of a psychoneurosis.

**disulf'amide.** DISAMIDE; 5-chlorotoluene-2,4-disulfonamide; diuretic.

**disul'fate.** Bisulfate.

**disul'fide.** 1. Bisulfide (1); a molecule containing two atoms of sulfur to one of the other element, *e.g.*, $CS_2$, carbon disulfide. 2. A compound containing the —S—S— group, as in cystine.

**disulf'iram** (NF). ANTABUSE; tetraethylthiuram disulfide; bis(diethylthiocarbamyl)disulfide; an antioxidant that interferes with the normal metabolic degradation of alcohol in the body, resulting in increased acetaldehyde concentrations in blood and tissues. Used in the treatment of chronic alcoholism; when a small quantity of alcohol is consumed an unpleasant reaction ("Antabuse reaction") results. Also used as a chelator in copper and nickel poisoning.

**dita bark.** Alstonia.

**di'taine.** Echitamine.

**diterpenes** (di'ter'pēnz). Hydrocarbons or their derivatives built up out of 4 isoprene units, hence containing 20 carbon atoms and 4 branched methyl groups; notable examples are vitamin A and retinene.

**di'thiaz'anine iodide.** ALMINTHIC; DELVEX; 3-ethyl-2-[ 5-(3-ethyl-2-benzothiozolinylidene)-1,3-pentadienyl ]benzothiazolium iodide. A broad spectrum anthelmintic, effective against *Strongyloides,* but toxic.

**dithi'o.** A term applied to compounds containing two sulfur atoms. See also disulfide (2).

**dithranol** (BP). Anthralin.

**Dittrich,** Franz, German pathologist, 1815–1859. See D.'s *plugs, stenosis.*

**diuresis** (di'u-re'sis) [ G. *dia*, throughout, completely, + *ourēsis*, urination ]. Excretion of urine; commonly denotes production of unusually large volumes of urine.
  **alcohol d.,** d. following the ingestion of alcoholic beverages; due, in part, to inhibition of the output of antidiuretic hormone by the neurohypophysis.
  **osmotic d.,** d. due to a high concentration of osmotically active substances in the renal tubules, *e.g.*, urea, sodium sulfate, etc., which limit the reabsorption of water.
  **water d.,** the d. that follows water drinking; due to reduced secretion of the antidiuretic hormone of the neurohypophysis in response to the lowered osmotic pressure of the blood.

**diuret'ic.** 1. Promoting the excretion of urine. 2. An agent that increases the amount of urine.
  **cardiac d.,** a d. which acts through primary effect upon the heart, and thereby improves renal perfusion.
  **direct d.,** a d. whose primary effect is on renal tubular cells.
  **indirect d.,** one that acts by strengthening the heart or relieving renal congestion.

**diurgin disodium.** *N*-{[ 3-(Carboxymethylthiomercuri)-2-methoxypropyl ]carbamoyl}succinamic acid disodium salt; an organic mercurial compound used as diuretic.

**diurnal** (di-ur'nal) [ L. *diurnus*, of the day ]. 1. Pertaining to the daylight hours; opposite of nocturnal. 2. Repeating once each 24 hours, *e.g.*, a d. variation or a d. rhythm; *cf.* circadian.

**diurnule** (di-er'nūl) [ L. *diurnus*, daily, fr. *dies*, day ]. A pill, tablet, or capsule containing the maximum daily dose of a drug.

**div.** Abbreviation, used in prescriptions, of Lat. *divide*, divide, or *dividetur*, let it be divided.

**di'vaga'tion** [ L. *divagare*, to wander about ]. Rambling speech or thought.

**divalence, divalency** (di-va'lens, di-va'len-sī). Bivalence.

**divalent** (di-va'lent, div'ā-lent). Bivalent.

**divarication** (di-vār-ĭ-ka'shun) [ L. *divaricare*, to spread asunder ]. Separation; diastasis.

    **d. of recti**, diastasis recti; separation of the rectus muscles of the abdomen away from the midline, sometimes seen during or following pregnancy.

**divergence** (di-ver'jens) [ L. *di-*, apart, + *vergo*, to incline ]. 1. A moving or spreading apart or in different directions. 2. The spreading of branches of the neuron to form synapses with several other neurons.

**diver'gent.** Moving in different directions; radiating.

**diverticula** (di'ver-tik'u-lah). Plural of diverticulum.

**diverticu'lar.** Relating to a diverticulum.

**diverticulectomy** (di-ver-tik'u-lek'to-mī). The excision of a diverticulum.

**diverticulitis** (di-ver-tik'u-li'tis). Inflammation of a diverticulum, especially of the small pockets in the wall of the colon that fill with stagnant fecal material and become inflamed. Rarely they may cause obstruction, perforation, or bleeding.

**di'vertic'ulogram.** An x-ray of a diverticulum.

**diverticuloma** (di-ver-tik'u-lo-mah) [ diverticulum + G. suffix *-oma*, tumor ]. The development of a granulomatous mass in the wall of the colon which is the seat of diverticulitis.

**diverticulopexy** (di-ver-tik'u-lo-pek'sī) [ diverticulum + G. *pēxis*, fixation ]. A plastic operation to obliterate a diverticulum.

**diverticulo'sis.** The presence of a number of diverticula of the intestine. D. of the colon is very common in middle age; the lesions are acquired pulsion diverticula.

**diverticulum,** pl. **divertic'ula** (di-ver-tik'u-lum) [ L. *deverticulum* (or *di-*), a by-road, fr. *de-verto*, to turn aside ] [ NA ]. A pouch or sac opening from a tubular or saccular organ, such as the gut or bladder.

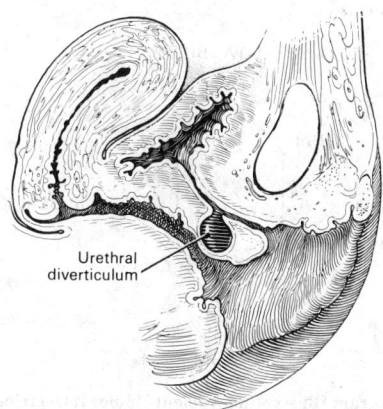

**Urethral Diverticulum**

    **allan'toenter'ic d.,** allantoic d.

    **allantoic d.,** allantoenteric d.; an entodermally lined outpouching of the hindgut of a very young embryo. It is the primordium of the allantois which in most amniotes later grows into the extraembryonic celom. In man the

distal part of the allantoic lumen is rudimentary, not extending beyond the belly stalk.

    **d. ampullae ductus deferentis** [ NA ], diverticula of the ampulla of the ductus deferens; the irregular sacculations of the ampullary part of the ductus deferens near its termination in the ejaculatory duct.

    **cervical d.,** a d. in the neck derived from retention of part of one of the pharyngeal pouches (entodermal) or branchial grooves (ectodermal) of the embryo.

    **duodenal d.,** a d. of the duodenum, often of large size, that is occasionally found projecting from the duodenum near the duodenal papilla.

    **epiphrenic d.,** d. which originates just above the cardioesophageal junction and usually protrudes to the right side of the lower meadiastinum.

    **false d.,** a term denoting a d. of the intestine that passes through a defect in the muscular wall of the gut and thus does not include a layer of muscle in its wall.

    **Heister's d.,** *bulbus* venae jugularis superior.

    **hypopharyngeal d.,** Zenker's d.; a d. of the hypopharynx, that part of the pharynx that lies below the aperture of the larynx.

    **Meckel's d.,** a blind sac or pouch, the remains of the omphaloenteric duct of the embryo; when, abnormally, it persists in the adult it is located on the ileum a short distance above the cecum.

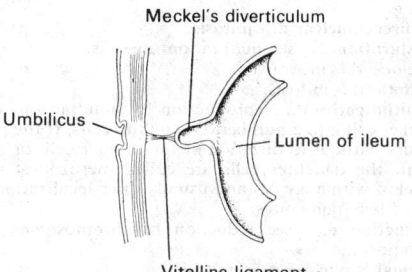

**Meckel's Diverticulum**
Combined with fibrous cord (vitelline ligament). (From Langman, J.: *Medical Embryology*, Ed. 2, The Williams & Wilkins Co., Baltimore, 1969.)

    **metaneph'ric d.,** an outgrowth from the caudal portion of the mesonephric duct on either side, which grows cephalodorsally to make contact with the masses of metanephrogenous tissue giving rise to the tubules of the permanent kidney. It gives rise to the epithelial lining of the ureter, the pelvis, and the collecting tubules of the kidney.

    **Nuck's d.,** *processus* vaginalis peritonei.

    **pancreatic diverticula,** the ventral and dorsal entodermal buds from the embryonic foregut which constitute the primordia of the parenchyma of the pancreas.

    **Pertik's d.,** an abnormally deep Rosenmüller's fossa, or recessus pharyngeus.

    **pharyngoesophageal d.,** a d. of the posterior pharyngeal wall opening just behind the cricoid cartilage.

    **pitu'itary d.,** a tubular outgrowth of ectoderm from the stomodeum of the embryo. It grows dorsad toward the infundibular process of the diencephalon, around which it forms a more or less cup-shaped mass, giving rise to the pars distalis and pars juxtaneuralis of the hypophysis. Also called Rathke's d., pocket, or pouch; craniopharyngeal canal.

    **pulsion d.,** a d. formed by pressure from within, frequently causing herniation of mucosa through the muscularis.

    **Rathke's d.,** pituitary d.

    **Rokitansky's d.,** traction d. of esophagus.

    **thyroglossal d.,** thyroid d.

    **thyroid d.,** thyroglossal d.; the entodermal bud from the floor of the embryonic pharynx which is the primordium of the parenchyma of the thyroid gland.

    **traction d.,** a d. formed by the pulling force of contracting bands of adhesion, occurring mainly in the esophagus.

    **true d.,** a term denoting a diverticulum that includes all the layers of the wall from which it protrudes.

**ventricular d.,** a congenital outpouching of the right or left ventricle.

**vesical d.,** cystodiverticulum; a d. of the bladder wall; may be either true or false type.

**Zenker's d.,** hypopharyngeal d.

**divicine** (di-vis-ēn). A base with alkaloidal properties present in *Lathyrus sativus* which is responsible, in part at least, for the latter's poisonous action. See lathyrism.

**divi-divi** (div'e-div'e) [ Native ]. The pods of several species of *Coesalpinia* (family Leguminosae), Central South American plants, containing much tannin. Used as an astringent in diarrhea.

**divi'nyl ether.** VINETHENE; DIVETHENE; vinyl ether; $CH_2CHOCHCH_2$; a rapidly acting inhalation anesthetic used principally for induction of anesthesia; prolonged administration is associated with adverse side effects on liver and central nervous system.

**division** (dĭ-vĭzh'un). Separation.

**cleavage d.,** the rapid mitotic d. of the zygote with decrease in size of individual cells or blastomeres and the formation of a morula; see also cleavage (1).

**equation d.,** nuclear d. in which each chromosome divides equally.

**heterotypic d.,** the first of the two d.'s of a maturing sex cell during which reduction of the chromosomes occurs.

**homotypic d.,** the second of the two d.'s of a maturing sex cell during which reduction of the chromosomes occurs.

**indirect nuclear d.,** mitosis.

**maturation d.,** see maturation; meiosis.

**meiotic d.,** meiosis.

**mitotic d.,** mitosis.

**multiplicative d.,** reproduction by simultaneous d. of a mother cell into a number of daughter cells. If the process occurs without fertilization of the mother cell, or encystment, the daughter cells are called merozoites; if they develop within a cyst, and usually after fertilization, they are called sporozoites.

**reduction d.,** see reduction of chromosomes, under chromosome.

**Remak's nuclear d.,** amitosis.

**divulse** (dĭ-vuls') [ L. *di-vello,* pp. *-vulvus,* to pull apart ]. To tear away or apart.

**divulsion** (dĭ-vul'shun). The removal of a part by tearing instead of by cutting or dissection. 2. The forcing apart of the walls of a cavity or canal; forcible dilation.

**divul'sor.** An instrument for forcible dilation of the urethra or other canal or cavity.

**dixyrazine.** ESUCOS; 2-{2-[ 4-(2-methyl-3-phenothiazin-10-ylpropyl-1-piperazinyl ]ethoxy}ethanol; a phenothiazine compound used as antipsychotic agent.

**dizygotic** (di'zi-got'ik) [ G. *di-,* two, + *zygotos,* yoked together ]. Relating to a twin pair derived from two separate zygotes.

**diz'ziness** [ A. S. *dyzig,* foolish ]. An imprecise term commonly used by patients in an attempt to describe various peculiar subjective symptoms such as faintness, giddiness, light-headedness, or unsteadiness; see also vertigo.

**diz'zy.** Giddy; suffering from dizziness or vertigo.

**djenkol** (jeng'kol). Jenghol *poisoning.*

**djenkolic acid** (jeng-kol'ik). $CH_2[ S—CH_2CH(NH_2)-COOH ]_2$; a sulfur-containing amino acid, resembling cystine but with a methylene bridge between the two sulfur atoms, first isolated in the djenkol bean.

**DL-.** Chemical prefix, written in small capital letters, characterizing a substance consisting of equal quantities of the two enantiomorphs, D and L. Replaces the older *dl-* (printed in lower case italics) as a more exact definition of structure.

**D.M.D.** Abbreviation of Doctor of Dental Medicine.

**DMF.** Decayed, missing, or filled; a designation used in tooth examination.

**DMPP.** Abbreviation for dimethylphenylpiperazinium.

**DMSO.** Abbreviation for dimethyl sulfoxide.

**DMT.** Abbreviation for dimethyltryptamine.

**DNA.** Abbreviation for deoxyribonucleic acid. For terms bearing this abbreviation, see subentries under deoxyribonucleic acid.

**DNase.** Abbreviation for deoxyribonuclease.

**DNP.** Abbreviation for the dinitrophenyl radical, $N_2ph—$.

**Dnp.** Abbreviation for deoxyribonucleoprotein.

**Dns, DNS.** Abbreviations for the dansyl radical.

**D.O.** Abbreviation for Doctor of Osteopathy.

**Dobie,** William M., English anatomist, 1828–1915. See D.'s line.

**DOC.** Abbreviation for (1) deoxycorticosterone; (2) 7-deoxycholic acid or deoxycholate.

**d'Ocagne,** Philbert M., French mathematician, 1862–1938. See d'Ocagne *nomogram.*

**docimasia, docimasy** (dos'ĭ-ma'zĭ-ah, dos'ĭ-ma-sĭ) [ G. *dokimasia,* fr. *dokimazō,* to assay (metals) ]. 1. An assay. 2. Examination of newborn infant's lungs to determine whether the baby has breathed or expanded its lungs with air and was therefore born alive.

**docimastic** (dos'ĭ-mas'tik). Relating to an assay.

**dock.** 1. The amputation of a part of the tail of horses, sheep, or dogs. 2. The base of the tail left after docking.

**n-docosanoic acid.** Behenic acid; $CH_3(CH_2)_{20}COOH$; a constituent of most fats and fish oils. Large amounts are found in jamba, mustard seed, and rape oils.

**doc'oseno'ic acid.** An unsaturated docosanoic acid contained in certain seed fats.

**doctor** [ L. a teacher, fr. *doceo,* pp. *doctus,* to teach ]. 1. A title conferred by a university on one who has followed a prescribed course of study, or given as a mark of distinction; as d. of medicine, d. of laws, philosophy, etc. 2. A physician, especially one upon whom has been conferred the degree of M.D. by a university or medical school. 3. To treat medically (popular). 4. To be treated by a d. (popular).

**doctrine** (dok'trin) [ L. *doceo,* to teach ]. Thing taught.

**Arrhenius' d.,** the theory of electrolytic dissociation (1887); in an electrically conductive solution (*e.g.,* acid, base, or salt), free ions are present before electrolysis, and the proportion of molecules dissociated into ions can be calculated from measurements of electrical conductivity as well as of osmotic pressure. The basis of modern understanding of electrolytes.

**humoral d.,** the ancient Greek theory of the four body humors (blood, yellow and black bile, and phlegm) that determined the bodily state in health and disease. The humors were associated with the four elements (air, fire, earth, and water), which in turn corresponded each to a pair of the qualities (hot, cold, dry, and moist). A proper and evenly balanced mixture of the humors was characteristic of health of body and mind; an imperfect balance resulted in disease. Thus also was temperament—sanguine (blood), choleric (yellow bile), melancholic (black bile), or phlegmatic (phlegm)—of body or mind supposed to be determined.

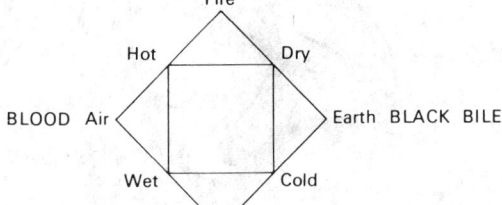

**Diagram Illustrating Ancient Humoral Doctrine**

**Monro's d., Monro-Kellie d.,** states that the cranial cavity is a closed rigid box and that therefore a change in the quantity of intracranial blood can occur only through the displacement of or replacement by cerebrospinal fluid.

**zymotic d.,** the obsolete d. that an infectious disease is in its nature essentially a fermentative process.

**dodecanoic acid** (do-dek'ă-no'ik). Lauric acid.

**dodecarbo'nium chloride.** STRAMINOL; UROLOCIDE; benzyl[ (dodecycarbamoylmethyl)dimethyl ]ammonium chloride; antiseptic.

**dodecyl** (do'dĕ-sil). The radical of *n*-dodecane.

    **d. gallate** (BP), dodecyl 3,4,5-trihydroxybenzoate; an antioxidant.

    **d. sulfate,** see sodium dodecyl sulfate.

**Döderlein** (dĕ'der-lin), Albert, S.G., Munich obstetrician, 1860–1941. See D.'s *bacillus.*

**Doerfler-Stewart test.** See under test.

**Doering** (dĕ'ring), Hans, German physician, *1886. See Neisser-D. *phenomenon.*

**dog'bane.** *Apocynum.*

**dog'fish.** 1. Sandshark; a small-toothed shark in the genus *Squalus,* family Squalidae, found on all coasts of the United States; includes both oviparous and viviparous forms; the young are called pups. 2. The bowfin, *Amia calva,* a freshwater ganoid fish of the United States.

**dog-grass.** Triticum.

**Dogiel** (do-zhe-el'), Alexander S., Russian histologist, 1852–1922. See D.'s *corpuscle.*

**Dogiel,** Jan von, Russian anatomist and physiologist, 1830–1905. See D.'s *cells.*

**dogmat'ic** [ G. *dogmatikos,* concerning opinions; *d. iatroi,* physicians who go by general principles; fr. *dogma,* an opinion ]. See dogmatic *school.*

**dogmatist** (dog'mă-tist). A follower of the dogmatic school.

**dog'wood.** Cornus.

**Döhle** (dĕ'leh), Karl G. P., German histologist and pathologist, 1855–1928. See D.'s *bodies, inclusions.*

**Doisy,** Edward A., American biochemist, *1893. Nobel laureate, 1943, with Henrik Dam for their discovery of the chemical nature of vitamin K. See Allen-D. *test, unit.*

**dol** [ L. *dolor,* pain ]. A unit measure of pain.

**dolicho-** (dol'ĭ-ko-) [ G. *dolichos,* long ]. Combining form meaning long.

**dolichocephalic** (dol-ĭ-ko-se-fal'ik) [ dolicho- + G. *kephalē,* head ]. Having a disproportionately long head; denoting a skull with a cephalic index below 75, or an individual with such a skull.

**dolichocephalous** (dol-ĭ-ko-sef'ă-lus). Dolichocephalic.

**dolichocephaly, dolichocephalism** (dol-ĭ-ko-sef'ă-lĭ, sef'ă-lizm). The condition of being dolichocephalic.

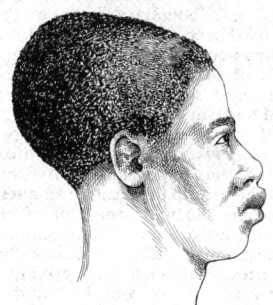

Dolichocephaly

**dolichocolon** (dol-ĭ-ko-ko'lon) [ dolicho- + G. *kolon,* colon ]. An excessively long colon.

**dolichocranial** (dol'ĭ-ko-kra'nĭ-al). Dolichocephalic.

**dolichoderus** (dol'ĭ-ko-dēr-us) [ G. *dolichodeiros,* person with long neck ]. A person having a disproportionately long neck.

**dolichofacial** (dol-ĭ-ko-fa'shal). Dolichoprosopic.

**dolichopel'lic, dolichopel'vic** [ dolicho- + G. *pellis,* bowl (pelvis) ]. Having a disproportionately long pelvis.

**dolichoprosopic, dolichoprosopous** (dol-ĭ-ko-pros-o'-pik, dol-ĭ-ko-pros'o-pus) [ dolicho- + G. *prosōpikos,* facial ]. Dolichofacial; having a disproportionately long face.

**dolichostenomelia** (dol-ĭ-ko-sten-o-me'lĭ-ah) [ dolicho- + G. *stenos,* narrow, + *melos,* limb ]. Arachnodactyly.

**dolichouranic** (dol-ĭ-ko-u-ran'ik) [ dolicho- + G. *ouranos,* vault of the palate ]. Dolichuranic; having a palatal index below 110.

**dolichuranic** (dol'ik-u-ran'ik). Dolichouranic.

**Döllinger** (dĕ'ling-er), Johann I. J., German physician, 1770–1841. See D.'s *tendinous ring.*

**do'lor** [ L. ]. Pain, one of the classic signs of inflammation.

    **d. cap'itis,** headache; especially pain due to changes in the scalp or bones rather than in the intracranial structures.

**do'lorif'ic.** Pain-producing.

**do'lorim'etry** [ L. *dolor,* pain, + G. *metron,* measure ]. The art and science of measuring pain.

**DOM.** Abbreviation for 2,5-dimethoxy-4-methylamphetamine.

**Domagk,** Gerhard J. P., German biochemist, 1895–1964. Nobel laureate, 1939, for the discovery of the antibacterial effects of the first sulfonamide drug.

**Dombrock blood group.** See appendix 2, Blood Groups.

**dom'inance.** The state of being dominant.

    **d. of genes,** see under gene.

**dom'inant** [ L. pres. p. of *dominor,* pp. *-atus,* to rule, fr. *dominus,* a master ]. 1. Ruling or controlling. 2. In genetics, denoting a character possessed by one of the parents of a hybrid which appears in the latter to the exclusion of a contrasted character (the recessive) from the other parent.

**Dominici** (dū-min-e-se'), Henri, French physician, 1867–1919. See D. *tube.*

**do'miphen bromide** (BP, USAN). BRADOSOL bromide; dodecyldimethyl(2-phenoxyethyl)ammonium bromide; antiseptic.

**Donath,** Julius, German physician, *1849. See D.-Landsteiner *phenomenon,* D.-Landsteiner cold *autoantibody,* Landsteiner-D. *test.*

**Donders,** Franz C., Dutch ophthalmologist, 1818–1889. See D.'s *glaucoma, law, pressure, rings, test.*

**Donders' space.** 38 See under space.

**Don Juan** (wahn) [ legendary Spanish nobleman ]. In psychiatry, a term used to denote males with compulsive sexual overactivity, usually with a succession of female partners.

**Donnan,** Frederick G., English physical chemist, 1870–1956. See D. *equilibrium,* Gibbs-D. *equilibrium.*

**Donné** (don-na'), Alfred, French physician, 1801–1878. See D.'s *corpuscles.*

**Donohue,** W. L., Canadian pathologist. See D.'s *disease.*

**do'nor** [ L. *dono,* pp. *donatus,* to donate, to give ]. 1. A person from whom the blood is drawn in the performance of blood transfusion. 2. A compound that will transfer an atom or a radical (H, $CH_2$, $NH_2$, etc.) to an acceptor. Methionine, for instance, is a methyl d. Used also for atoms that readily yield electrons to an acceptor (for example, nitrogen, which will donate both electrons to a shared pool in forming a coordinate bond).

    **universal d.,** in blood grouping, a person belonging to group O; *i.e.,* one whose corpuscles do not contain either agglutinogen A or B and are, therefore, not agglutinated by serum containing either of the ordinary isoagglutinins, alpha or beta.

**Donovan,** Charles, Irish surgeon, 1863–1951. See D. *bodies,* Leishman-D. *body.*

**don'ovano'sis.** Granuloma inguinale, caused by *Calymmatobacterium granulomatis,* which are observed intracellularly (in macrophages in the lesion) as Donovan bodies.

**dopa** (sometimes written Dopa or DOPA). 3,4-Dihydroxyphenylalanine; an intermediate in the catabolism of phenylalanine and tyrosine, and a precursor of norepinephrine, epinephrine, and melanin.

    **d. decarboxylase,** aromatic L-amino-acid decarboxylase (see under aromatic).

    **decarboxylated d.,** dopamine.

    **d. oxidase,** provisional name given the enzyme(s) catalyzing the formation of melanins from dopa. It now appears that the copper-containing monophenol monooxygenases are responsible for the oxidation of tyrosine to dopa and dopa quinone.

**d. quinone,** an oxidation product of d. and an intermediate in the formation of melanin from tyrosine.

*l*-**dopa.** Levodopa (USP); LARODOPA; used for the treatment of Parkinsonian disease.

**dopamine.** *o*-Hydroxytyramine; decarboxylated dopa; an intermediate in tyrosine metabolism and the precursor of norepinephrine and epinephrine. It is present in the central nervous system and is localized in the basal ganglia (caudate and lentiform nuclei), suggesting that d. may have functions other than as a precursor of norepinephrine.

**d. hydrochloride,** (USAN), a biogenic amine and neural transmitter substance, used as a vasopressor agent for treatment of shock.

**dopamine β -hydroxylase.** Dopamine β -monooxygenase.

**dopamine β -monooxygenase** (EC 1.14.17.1). Dopamine β -hydroxylase; enzyme catalyzing oxidation of ascorbate and dihydroxyphenylethylamine simultaneously by $O_2$ to yield norepinephrine and dehydroascorbate.

**dope** [ Dutch, *doop*, sauce ]. 1. Any drug, either stimulating or depressing; (*a*) administered to man or animal for its temporary effect, or (*b*) taken habitually. 2. To administer d.

**Doppler,** Christian J., Austrian mathematician and physicist in U. S., 1803–1853. See D. *effect, phenomenon, shift.*

**doraphobia** (do-rah-fo′bi-ah) [ G. *dora*, hide, skin, + *phobos*, fear ]. A morbid fear of touching the skin or fur of animals.

**Dorello,** P., Italian anatomist, \*1872. See D's *canal.*

**Dor′endorf,** H., German physician, \*1866. See D.'s *sign.*

**Döring,** G., German physician. See Pette-D. *disease.*

**dor′nase.** Obsolete term for deoxyribonuclease (*q. v.*); see also streptodornase.

**pancreatic d.,** DORNAVAC; a stabilized deoxyribonuclease preparation from beef pancreas; used by inhalation in form of aerosols to reduce thick mucopurulent secretions in certain bronchopulmonary infections.

**Dorno,** Carl, Swiss climatologist, 1865–1942. See D. *rays.*

**doromania** (do′ro-ma′ni-ah) [ G. *doron*, gift, + *mania*, insanity ]. An abnormal desire to give presents.

**dorsa** (dor′sah). Plural of dorsum.

**dorsabdom′inal.** Relating to the back and the abdomen.

**dor′sad** [ L. *dorsum*, back, + *ad*, to ]. Toward or in the direction of the back.

**dorsal** [ Mediev. L. *dorsalis*, fr. *dorsum*, back ]. Relating to the back; posterior.

**dorsal′gia** [ L. *dorsum*, back, + G. *algos*, pain ]. Dorsodynia; pain in the upper back.

**dorsa′lis** [ L. ] [ NA ]. Dorsal; posterior.

**Dorset,** Marion, American bacteriologist, \*1872. See D.'s culture *medium, stain.*

**dor′sicor′nu** [ L. *dorsum*, back, + *cornu*, horn ]. *Cornu* posterius.

**dor′siduct** [ L. *dorsum*, back, + *duco*, pp. *ductus*, to draw ]. To draw backward or toward the back.

**dorsiflexion** (dor′si-flek′shun). Turning of the foot or the toes upward.

**dorsiscapular** (dor′si-skap′u-lar). Relating to the dorsal surface of the scapula.

**dorsispinal** (dor′si-spi′nal). Relating to the spinal column, especially to its dorsal aspect.

**dorsocephalad** (dor′so-sef′ă-lad) [ L. *dorsum*, back, + G. *kephalē*, head, + L. *ad*, to ]. Toward the occiput, or back of the head.

**dorsodynia** (dor-so-din′i-ah) [ L. *dorsum*, back, + G. *odynē*, pain ]. Dorsalgia.

**dorsolat′eral.** Relating to the back and the side.

**dorsolum′bar.** Referring to the back in the region of the lower thoracic and upper lumbar vertebrae.

**dorsoven′trad.** In a direction from the dorsal to the ventral aspect.

**dor′sum,** gen. **dor′si,** pl. **dor′sa** [ L. back ]. 1 [ NA ]. The back of the body. 2 [ NA ]. The upper or posterior surface, or the back, of any part.

**d. ephip′ii,** d. sellae.

**d. linguae** [ NA ], the back of the tongue; the upper surface of the tongue.

**d. manus** [ NA ], the back of the hand.

**d. nasi** [ NA ], the ridge of the nose, looking forward and upward.

**d. pedis** [ NA ], the back, or upper surface, of the foot.

**d. penis** [ NA ], the aspect of the penis opposite to that of the urethra.

**d. scap′ulae,** the posterior surface of the scapula.

**d. sellae** [ NA ], d. ephipii; a square portion of bone on the body of the sphenoid posterior to the sella turcica or hypophysial fossa.

**dosage** (do′sij). 1. The giving of medicine or other therapeutic agent in prescribed amounts. 2. The determination of the proper dose of a remedy. Often incorrectly used for the word dose.

**dose** [ G. *dosis;* see dosis ]. The quantity of a drug or other remedy to be taken or applied all at one time or in fractional amounts within a given period.

**booster d.,** a d. given at some time after an initial d. to enhance the effect, said usually of antigens for the production of antibodies.

**broken d.,** refractive d.

**curative d.,** the quantity of any substance required to effect the cure of a disease or that will correct the manifestations of a deficiency of a particular factor in the diet, *e.g.,* vitamin, amino acid, or mineral.

**daily d.,** the total amount of a remedy that is to be taken within 24 hours.

**depth d.,** the amount of radiation received beneath the surface in proportion to the amount recorded at the surface.

**divided d.,** refractive d.

**effective d.,** see ED, and $ED_{50}$.

**epilation d.,** erythema d.

**erythema d.,** the minimal amount of x-rays or other form of radiation sufficient to produce an erythema in 10 days to 2 weeks after the application. It is regarded as the full d. that is safe to give at one time, and is not to be repeated until the expiration of 3 weeks to 1 month. This d. is indicated by the Sabouraud meter as the B tint, the Holzknecht as 5(5H), the Hampson as 4, and the Kienbock as 10.

**exit d.,** the amount of radiation leaving a body opposite the area of entry.

**fractional d.,** refractive d.

**initial d.,** a comparatively large d. given at the beginning of treatment to get the patient under the influence of the drug.

**L d.'s,** a group of terms that indicate the relative activity or potency of diphtheria toxin; the L is an abbreviation for Limes (li′mēz), *i.e.,* a boundary, limit, or threshold; the capital letter is used in combination with a lower case letter or a plus sign (or a subscript letter or plus sign) as a symbol for various d.'s of toxin, as indicated in the individual definitions. The L d.'s are distinctly different from the MLD and MRD, inasmuch as the latter two represent the *direct effects of toxin,* whereas the L d.'s pertain to the *combining power of toxin* with specific antitoxin.

**$L^+$, $L_+$ d.,** alternate symbol for $L^+$the limes tod [ Ger. death ] d. of diphtheria toxin, *i.e.,* the smallest amount of toxin that, when mixed with one unit of antitoxin and injected subcutaneously into a 250-gm. guinea pig, results in death of the animal within 96 hours (based on the average in a series). On theoretical grounds, one might expect that the difference between the L and $L_0$ d.'s would be identical to one MLD, but this is not so in actual practice; with various toxic filtrates, the difference may range from several to more than 100 MLD's, indicating that the toxin-antitoxin combination is *not* a firm chemical union that occurs in constant proportions.

**lethal d.,** one likely to cause death; see LD.

**Lf, $L_f$ d.,** symbol for the limes flocculation d. of diphtheria toxin, *i.e.,* the smallest amount of toxin that, when mixed with one unit of antitoxin, yields the most rapid flocculation in the Ramon test (*in vitro*). In general, the $L_f$ d. is slightly less than the $L_r$ d.

**Lo, $L_0$ d.,** symbol for the limes nul d. of diphtheria toxin, *i.e.,* the largest amount of toxin that, when mixed with one unit of antitoxin and injected subcutaneously into a 250-gm. guinea pig, yields no recognizable reaction in the average of a series; actually, the $L_0$ d. is usually recorded as the one that causes a barely perceptible local edema at the site of inoculation.

**Lr, $L_r$ d.,** symbol for the limes reacting d. of diphtheria toxin, *i.e.,* the smallest amount of toxin that, when mixed with one unit of antitoxin and injected intracutaneously in the shaved skin of a susceptible guinea pig, yields a minimal, positive reaction and inflammation localized to the region of the injection. The $L_r$ d. closely approximates the $L_0$ d., as would be expected, inasmuch as a slight excess of unneutralized toxin results in a reaction.

**maintenance d.,** see maintenance drug *therapy.*

**maximal d.,** the largest amount of a drug that an adult can take with safety.

**maximal permissible d.,** abbreviated MPD; the greatest d. of radiation to which members of a population may be exposed without harmful effects. The d. would include background, fallout, and medical or occupational exposure and the effects include genetic effects. This is defined in terms of acute or chronic exposure to organs, systems, regions of, and/or the whole body.

**minimal d.,** the smallest amount of a drug that will produce a physiologic effect in an adult.

**minimal infecting d.,** abbreviated M.I.D.; the smallest quantity of infectious material regularly producing infection; usually expressed as I.D.$_{50}$, the quantity causing infection in 50 per cent of a suitable series of animals or cells (cell cultures).

**MLD, mld,** abbreviation for the minimal lethal d. of a toxic substance, as assayed in various experimental animals; referring to diphtheria toxin, for example, the MLD is the least amount that, on an average, kills a 250-gm. guinea pig within 96 hours after subcutaneous inoculation.

**MLD$_{50}$, mld$_{50}$,** abbreviation for the minimal d. that is lethal for 50 per cent of the test animals in series being used for assay of a toxic substance, performed under conditions identical to those for determining the MLD.

**MRD, mrd,** abbreviation for the minimal reacting d. of a toxic substance, as manifested in the skin of a series of susceptible test animals; the assay is based on the development of a characteristic, minimal but definite, "standard," focal inflammation (congestion and edema, induration, degenerative changes, and desquamation of epidermal cells), becoming apparent in 18 to 24 hours after intracutaneous injection of the toxin, and attaining a peak in approximately 96 hours.

**optimum d.,** the d. of a drug (or rad or other radiation dose unit) that will produce the desired effect without any untoward symptoms.

**preventive d.,** the smallest amount, usually referring to a vitamin, amino acid, or mineral, that will prevent consequences of a lack of a particular food factor.

**refractive d.,** broken d.; divided d.; fractional d.; dosis refracta; a definite fraction of a full dose of a remedy; it is given repeatedly at short intervals, so that the full dose is taken within a specified period.

**sensitizing d.,** in experimental anaphylaxis, the antigenic inoculum that renders an animal susceptible (sensitive) to anaphylactic shock following a subsequent inoculum (shocking d.) of the same antigen (anaphylactogen).

**shocking d.,** in experimental anaphylaxis, the inoculum of antigen that causes anaphylactic shock in an animal sensitized by a previous inoculum (sensitizing d.) of the same antigen.

**skin d.,** the quantity of radiation delivered to the skin surface.

**therapeutic ratio of d.,** see under ratio.

**tolerance d.,** dosis tolerata; the largest dose of a remedy that the animal organism will accept without the production of injurious symptoms.

**dosim′etry** [ G. *dosis,* dose, + *metron,* measure ]. The accurate determination of dosage.

**thermoluminescence d.,** the calculation of a radiation dose by measuring the light output after heating a special absorbent material (*e.g.,* lithium fluoride) that had been placed in the radiation beam; the light output is proportional to the amount of radiation exposure.

**do′sis** [ G. a giving, a dose, fr. *didōmi,* fut. *dōsō,* to give ]. Dose; the amount of a medicine or other therapeutic agent that is to be taken at one time or within a stated period.

　　**d. curati′va,** curative *dose.*

　　**d. refrac′ta,** refractive *dose.*

　　**d. tolera′ta,** tolerance *dose.*

**dot.** Small spot.

　　**Gunn's d.'s,** Marcus Gunn's d.'s; minute, highly glistening, white or yellowish specks usually seen in the posterior part of the fundus; nonpathological.

　　**Maurer's d.'s,** Maurer's clefts; finely granular precipitates or irregular, tiny particles that usually occur diffusely (but sometimes as a band about the parasite) in the cytoplasm of red blood cells infected with malarial parasites; the particles are stained red by means of the Romanovsky dyes, and are characteristic of *Plasmodium falciparum* infections, although they are occasionally observed in *P. malariae* infections.

　　**Trantas' d.'s,** pale, grayish red, uneven nodules of gelatinous aspect at the limbal conjunctiva in vernal conjunctivitis.

**do′tage.** Senility; dotardness; the loss of previously intact mental powers, common in extreme old age.

**doublet** (dub′let). 1. A combination of two lenses designed to correct the chromatic and spherical aberration. 2. Dipole.

　　**Wollaston's d.,** a combination of two planoconvex lenses in the eyepiece of a microscope designed to correct the chromatic aberration.

**douche** (doosh) [ Fr. fr. *doucher,* to pour ]. 1. A current of water, gas, or vapor directed against the surface or projected into a cavity. 2. An instrument for giving a d. 3. To apply a d.

**Douglas,** Beverly, Nashville surgeon, *1891. See D. *graft.*

**Douglas,** Claude G., English physiologist, 1882–1963. See D. *bag.*

**Douglas,** James, Scottish anatomist in London, 1675–1742. See D.'s *abscess, cul–de–sac, fold, line, pouch, cavum douglasi.*

**Douglas,** John C., Irish obstetrician, 1777–1850. See D.'s spontaneous *evolution,* D.'s *mechanism.*

**dourine** (doo′rēn) [ Fr. ]. Mal de coit; equine syphilis; a venereally transmitted trypanosomiasis of horses caused by *Trypanosoma equiperdum* and characterized by inflammation of the genitals, glandular swelling, and paralysis of the hind quarters; virulence varies with the strain, and is especially severe in the European strain.

**dove′tail.** A form given to a cavity preparation to enable the restoration to withstand forces tending to displace it laterally. The name derives from the fact that the side walls diverge in the direction opposite to the displacing force and so resemble the tail of a dove. Frequently referred to as a lock with the name of the surface of the tooth on which it is placed (occlusal; lingual).

**dow′el.** 1. A cast gold or preformed metal pin placed into a root canal for the purpose of providing retention for a crown. 2. A preformed metal pin placed in a copper-plated die to provide a die stem.

**down.** Fine, soft hair.

　　**malignant d.,** *hypertrichosis* lanuginosa.

**Down,** John L. H., London physician, 1828–1896. See D.'s *syndrome.*

**Downes,** Andrew J., American physician. See D. separate-urine *siphon.*

**dox′apram hydrochloride** (NF). STIMULEXIN; DOPRAM; 1-ethyl-4- (2-morpholinoethyl)-3,3-diphenyl-2-pyrrolidone monohydrochloride (or hydrochloride hydrate); a central nervous system stimulant, used as a respiratory stimulant in anesthesia.

**dox′epin hydrochloride** (NF). SINEQUAN; ADAPIN; CURATIN; *N,N*-dimethyldibenz[ *b,e* ]oxepin-Δ$^{11(6}$*H* $^{),\gamma}$-propylamine hydrochloride; antidepressant and antipruritic agent.

**doxycy′cline** (USP). VIBRAMYCIN; 4-(dimethylamino)-de; tetracycline antibiotic with antimicrobial properties.

**doxyl′amine succinate** (NF). DECAPRYN succinate; 2-[ α- (2-dimethylaminoethoxy)-α-methylbenzyl ]pyridine succinate; an antihistaminic agent.

**Doyère** (dwa-yair'), Louis, French physiologist, 1811–1863. See D.'s *eminence*.

**Doyne,** Robert Walter, English ophthalmologist, 1857–1916. See D.'s honeycomb *choroidopathy*.

**D.P.** Abbreviation for Doctor of Podiatry.

**D.P.H.** Abbreviation of Doctor or Diploma of Public Health.

**D.P.M.** Abbreviation for Doctor of Podiatric Medicine.

**DPN.** Abbreviation for diphosphopyridine nucleotide, now more officially known as nicotinamide adenine dinucleotide (NAD).

**DPNH.** Abbreviation for reduced diphosphopyridine nucleotide. See DPN.

**DPNH → aldehyde transhydrogenase.** Aldehyde reductase.

**DPT.** Abbreviation for dipropyltryptamine.

**D.R.** or **R.D.** Abbreviation for reaction of *degeneration*.

**dr.** Abbreviation for dram.

**drachm** (dram) [ G. *drachmē*, an ancient Greek weight, equivalent to about 60 gr. ]. Dram.

**dracontiasis** (dra-kon-ti'ă-sis) [ G. *drakōn* (*drakont-*), dragon ]. Infection with *Dracunculus medinensis, q.v.*

**dracun'culi'asis.** Dracontiasis.

**dracun'culo'sis.** Dracontiasis.

**Dracunculus** (dră-kung'ku-lus) [ L. dim. of *draco*, serpent ]. A genus of the superfamily Dracunculoidea, nematodes that have some resemblances to true filaria worms, but adult forms are larger (females being as long as 1 meter), and the intermediate host is a crustacean (rather than an insect).

    **D. loa,** old incorrect term for *Loa loa.*

    **D. medinen'sis** [ L. of Medina ], skin-infecting, yard-long nematode worms, formerly incorrectly classed as a *Filaria* species; popularly known as guinea worm, Medina worm, serpent worm, and dragon worm, and frequently thought to be the "fiery serpent" that plagued the Israelites; adult worms live anywhere in the body of man (and also various fur-bearing animals), and the females migrate along fascial planes to subcutaneous tissues, where troublesome chronic ulcers are formed in the skin; when the host contacts water (as in bathing), larvae are discharged and may be ingested by *Cyclops* species (crustaceans), the intermediate host. Man and various animals contract the infection as a result of ingesting the crustaceans that contain infective larvae. The disease is known as dracunculosis, dracunculiasis, or dracontiasis.

    **D. oc'uli,** old incorrect term for *Loa loa,* a true filaria worm.

    **D. persa'rum** [ L. of the Persians ], old term for *D. medinensis.*

**draft, draught** (draft). 1. A current of air in a confined space. 2. A quantity of liquid medicine ordered as a single dose.

**drag.** 1. The lower or cast side of a denture flask. 2. Any tendency for one moving thing to pull something else along with it.

    **solvent d.,** the influence exerted by a flow of solvent through a membrane on the simultaneous movement of a solute through the membrane.

**dragée** (dră-zha') [ Fr. ]. A sugar-coated pill or capsule.

**Dragendorff,** Georg J. N., German physician and pharmaceutical chemist, 1836–1898. See D.'s *test*.

**Drager,** Glenn A., U. S. neurologist, *1917. See Shy-D. *syndrome*.

**Drager respirometer.** See under respirometer.

**dragon's blood.** Red resinous material obtained from several species of plants; used as antistringent and coloring agent.

**drain** [ A. S. *drehnian,* to draw off ]. 1. To draw off the fluid from a cavity, especially to provide for its exit as soon as it is formed. 2. An arrangement, in the shape of a tube or wick, for removing the fluid as it collects in a cavity, especially a wound cavity.

    **cigarette d.,** a wick of gauze wrapped in rubber tissue, providing capillary drainage.

    **Mikulicz' d.,** a d. made of several strings of gauze held together by a single layer of the same material.

    **Mosher d.,** consists of copper mesh in the form of a truncated cone; used in wounds or suppurating lesions of the brain.

    **Penrose d.,** a cigarette d. composed of rubber tubing containing a length of absorbent gauze.

    **stab d.,** a d. passed into the cavity through a puncture made at a dependent part away from the wound of operation, designed to prevent infection of the wound.

    **sump d.,** a d. consisting of an outer tube resembling in size and shape an ordinary test tube, and a more slender tube within it which is attached to a suction pump. The outer tube is pierced at its blind end to allow fluid to pass into its interior and be carried away through the suction tube.

    **Wylie's d.,** an instrument resembling a stem pessary with enlarged, but not bulbous, extremity, on the lateral surface of which is a deep longitudinal groove, forming a gutter for drainage of the uterine cavity.

**drain'age.** The continuous withdrawal of pus and other fluids from a wound or other cavity.

    **capillary d.,** d. by means of a wick of gauze, horsehair, or other material.

    **closed d.,** d. of chest to prevent entrance of air.

    **dependent d.,** downward d.; d. from the lowest part.

    **open d.,** d. without sealing off the outside air.

    **through d.,** d. obtained by the passage of a perforated tube, open at both extremities, through a cavity; in addition to providing for the escape of fluids, this allows for the washing out of the cavity by the forcing of a solution through the tube.

    **tidal d.,** d. of a paralyzed urinary bladder by means of an irrigation apparatus.

    **ves'icocelo'mic d.,** the d. of ascitic fluid into the bladder through a catheter.

**dram** [ see drachm ]. Drachm; a unit of weight; $1/8$ oz., 60 gr., apothecaries' weight; $1/16$ oz., avoirdupois weight.

**Draper,** John W., English chemist, 1811–1882. See D.'s *law.*

**drap'etoma'nia** [ G. *drapetēs,* runaway, + *mania,* insanity ]. Dromomania.

**draught** (draft). Draft.

**draw-sheet.** A narrow sheet placed crosswise on the bed under the patient's buttocks, with a rubber sheet of the same width beneath it; when soiled that part is drawn from under the patient, leaving the next dry section for him to lie upon.

**dream.** The ideas or images formed in the mind during sleep.

    **anxiety d.,** a d. (or nightmare) of which anxiety forms an important part.

    **wet d.,** oneirogmus; a true physiologic orgasm during sleep including, in males, a nocturnal seminal emission usually accompanying a d. with sexual content.

**dream-work.** In psychoanalysis, the process by which the change from latent to manifest content of a dream is effected.

**drench.** 1. The pouring of a liquid medicinal agent from a bottle into the mouth of an animal while holding its head high, thus forcing it to swallow. 2. The liquid medicinal agent intended for giving to an animal by drenching.

**drepanidium** (drep'ă-nid'ĭ-um) [ G. *drepanē,* a sickle ]. A young, sickle-shaped or crescentic form of a gregarine.

**drepanocyte** (drep'ă-no-sīt) [ G. *drepanē,* sickle, + *kytos,* a hollow (cell) ]. Sickle *cell.*

**drepanocythemia** (drep'ă-no-si-the'mĭ-ah) [ drepanocyte + G. *haima,* blood ]. Sickle cell *anemia.*

**drepanocytic** (drep-ă-no-sit'ik). Relating to, or resembling a sickle cell.

**drep'anocyto'sis** [ drepanocyte + suffix *-osis,* condition ]. Sickle cell *anemia.*

**dresser.** In Great Britain, a surgical extern or intern, one whose duty it is to dress wounds, etc.

**dressing.** The material applied to a wound for the purpose of excluding the air, absorbing drainage, etc.

    **antiseptic d.,** a d. of gauze impregnated with bichloride of mercury, carbolic acid, or other antiseptic.

    **fixed d.,** a bandage stiffened with sodium silicate, plaster of Paris, or starch in order to secure immobilization when it dries.

**Lister's d.,** an antiseptic d. of gauze impregnated with carbolic acid.

**occlu'sive d.,** one that hermetically seals a wound.

**water d.,** an application of gauze, cotton, or other material that is kept wet with sterilized water.

**Dreyer,** Georges, Oxford pathologist, 1873–1934. See D.'s *formula.*

**dribble.** To drool, slaver, drivel; to fall in drops, as the urine from a distended bladder.

**drifting.** Random movement of a tooth to a position of greater stability.

**mesial d.,** the gradual movement of a tooth or teeth anteriorly.

**Drigalski** (dre-gahl'ske), Wilhelm von, German bacteriologist, 1871–1950. See D.-Conradi *agar*, Conradi-D. *agar*.

**drill.** 1. To make a hole in bone or other hard substance. 2. An instrument for making or enlarging a hole in bone or in a tooth.

**bur d.,** see bur.

**dental d.,** a rotary, power-driven instrument, usually called a dental handpiece, into which cutting points may be inserted; see bur.

**Drinker,** Philip, American industrial hygienist, *1894. See D. *respirator.*

**drip.** 1. To fall a drop at a time. 2. A falling in drops.

**intrave'nous d.,** the slow but continuous introduction of glucose and saline solution, specific serums, etc., by intravenous injection of a drop at a time.

**Murphy d.,** see Murphy's *method* (1).

**postnasal d.,** term sometimes used to describe sensation of excessive mucoid or mucopurulent discharge from the posterior nares.

**drip-sheet.** A cool sheet wrapped around the body, the patient standing in a basin of warm water.

**drive.** 1. A basic compelling urge. 2. In psychology, classified as either innate (*e.g.,* hunger) or learned (*e.g.,* hoarding) and appetitive (*e.g.,* hunger, thirst, sex) or aversive (*e.g.,* fear, pain, grief). See also motive, motivation, and their subentries.

**acquired d.'s,** secondary d.'s.

**exploratory d.,** the d. to investigate the unfamiliar or unknown; it has not been determined whether this d. is innate or acquired.

**kinetic d.,** excessive excitation of the kinetic system.

**learned d.,** motive.

**physiological d.'s,** primary d.'s; those d.'s which stem from the biological needs of an organism.

**primary d.'s,** physiological d.'s.

**secondary d.'s,** acquired d.'s; those d.'s not directly related to biological needs; a secondary d. can be learned as an offshoot of a primary d., in which case it is often referred to as a motive (*q. v.*).

**driving.** The induction of a frequency in the electroencephalogram by sensory stimulation at this frequency.

**photic d.,** a change in the alpha frequency corresponding to a flicker.

**drocar'bil** (NF). NEMURAL; *N*-acetyl-4-hydroxy-*m*-arsanilic acid compounded with arecoline minus its hydrobromide; used as a veterinary anthelmintic.

**dro'mic** [ G. *dromos,* a running, race-course ]. Relating to nerve impulses that are conducted in the normal direction; *cf.* antidromic.

**drom'ograph** [ G. *dromos,* a running, + *graphō,* to record ]. An instrument for recording the rapidity of the blood circulation.

**drom'omania** [ G. *dromos,* a running, + *mania,* insanity ]. Drapetomania; uncontrollable impulse to wander or travel.

**dro'mostan'olone propionate** (NF). DROLBAN; 17β-hydroxy-2α-methyl-5α-androstan-3-one propionate; antineoplastic agent, used in metastatic carcinoma of the breast.

**dromotropic** (drom'o-trop'ik) [ G. *dromos,* a running, + *tropikos,* relating to *tropē,* a turn ]. Influencing the conductivity of nerves.

**negatively d.,** diminishing nerve conductivity.

**positively d.,** increasing nerve conductivity.

**drop** [ A. S. *droppan* ]. 1. To fall in globules. 2. To pour liquid from a container in separate globules, not in a continuous stream. 3. A globule of liquid that falls from a

container. 4. Gutta; a volume of liquid regarded as a unit of measure; equivalent in the case of water to about 1 minim; see also drops. 5. A liquid medicine dosed in d.'s. 6. A solid confection in globular form, usually directed to be allowed to dissolve in the mouth.

**hanging d.,** a d. of liquid on the undersurface of the object glass for examination under the microscope.

**dropacism** (drop'ă-sizm) [ G. *dropakizein,* to apply a depilatory ]. Epilation of hair by use of wax or plaster.

**droperidol** (dro-pĕr'ĭ-dol) (NF). INAPSINE; a butyrophenone drug used in neuroleptanalgesia and preanesthetic medication; it causes mental detachment, absence of voluntary movements (catatonia), a specific inhibitory effect on the chemoreceptor trigger zone controlling nausea and vomiting, and α-adrenergic receptor block.

**drop'let.** A small drop.

**kinoplasmic d.,** a small mass of membrane-bound cytoplasm passing backward over the head of the sperm during ripening in the male genital tract of some animals.

**drops.** A popular term for a medicine taken in doses measured by d.'s, usually a tincture, or applied by dropping, as a collyrium.

**eye d.,** see ophthalmic *solution.*

**knock-out d.,** a popular name for chloral alcoholate given with criminal intent to produce unconsciousness rapidly; it is formed by adding chloral hydrate to beer or some stronger alcoholic liquor.

**stomach d.,** a stomachic tonic, usually tincture of gentian, alone or with other stomachics.

**drop'sical.** Relating to or suffering from dropsy.

**dropsy** (drop'sĭ) [ G. *hydrōps.* HYDR- ]. An old term for hydrops.

**epidemic d.,** a disease causing occasional epidemics in India and Mauritius; marked by d., anemia, eruptive angiomatosis, and mild fever, with a mortality ranging up to 10 per cent. Contaminated mustard has been suggested as a causative agent but the disease seems to be associated with nutritional deficiency.

**famine d.,** famine *edema.*

**drowsiness.** See consciousness.

**drug.** 1. A therapeutic agent; any substance, other than food, used in the prevention, diagnosis, alleviation, treatment, or cure of disease in man and animal; for types or classifications of d.'s, see the specific name; see also subentries under agent. 2. To give or take a d., in this sense usually implying an overly large quantity. 3. To narcotize.

**crude d.,** an unrefined preparation, usually of plant origin, that occurs either in the entire, nearly entire, broken, cut, or powdered state.

**drug-fast.** Pertaining to microorganisms that resist or become tolerant to an antibacterial agent.

**drum, drumhead.** *Membrana* tympani.

**Drummond,** Sir David, English physician, 1852–1932. See D.-Morison *operation,* D.'s *sign.*

**drunk'eness.** Intoxication, usually alcoholic.

**sleep d.,** somnolentia; a half-waking condition in which the faculty of orientation is in abeyance, and under the influence of nightmare-like ideas the person may become actively excited and violent.

**drusen** (droo'sen) [ Ger. pl. of *druse,* bump, body ]. Hyaline or colloid bodies that contain sialomuccin and cerebroside and are formed from degenerated retinal pigment cells in the inner collagenous zone of Bruch's membrane.

**Drysdale,** Thomas M., Philadelphia gynecologist, 1831–1904. See D.'s *corpuscles.*

**D.t.** Abbreviation for duration *tetany.*

**DT-diaphorase.** NAD(P)H dehydrogenase (quinone).

**dTMP.** Abbreviation for thymidine 5'-phosphate.

**DTPA.** Abbreviation for diethylenetriaminepentaacetic acid.

**du'alism** [ L. *dualis,* relating to two, fr. *duo,* two ]. 1. In chemistry, a theory advanced by Berzelius that every compound, no matter how many elements enter into it, is composed of two parts, one electrically negative, the other positive; still applicable, with modification, to polar compounds, but inapplicable to nonpolar compounds. 2. In hematology, the concept that blood cells have two origins, *i.e.,* lymphogenous or myelogenous. 3. The theory that the mind and body are two distinct systems, independent and different in nature.

**Duane,** Alexander, New York ophthalmologist, 1858–1926. See D.'s *syndrome, test.*

**Dubin,** I. N., U. S. pathologist, *1913. See D.-Johnson syndrome.

**Dubini** (doo-be'ne), Angelo, Milan physician, 1813–1902. See D.'s *disease.*

**DuBois,** Eugene F., American physiologist, 1882–1959. See D.'s *formula,* Aub-D. *table* of basal metabolic rates.

**Dubois** (dü-bwah'), Paul, Paris obstetrician, 1795–1871. See D.'s *abscess, disease, shears.*

**duboisia** (du-boy'sĭ-ah). The leaves of *Duboisia myoporoides* (family Solanaceae), corkwood elm, a tree of Australia. Properties are similar to those of belladonna and hyoscyamus.

**duboisine** (du-boy'sēn). An alkaloid obtained from duboisia; see hyoscyamine.

**Du Bois-Reymond,** Emil H., German physiologist, 1818–1896. See D. B.-R.'s *law.*

**Duboscq** (du-bosk), Jules, Paris optician, 1817–1886. See D.'s *colorimeter.*

**Dubreuil-Chambardel** (du-brë-e-sham-bar-del'), Louis, French dentist, 1879–1927. See D.-C. *syndrome.*

**Dubreuilh,** M. W., French dermatologist. See precancerous *melanosis* of D.

**Duchenne** (dü-shen'), Guillaume B. A., French neurologist, 1806–1875. See D.'s *disease,* D.-Aran *disease,* Aran-D. *disease,* D.'s *dystrophy,* D.'s *paralysis,* D.-Erb *paralysis,* D.'s *sign,* D.'s *syndrome.*

**Duckworth's phenomenon.** See under phenomenon.

**Ducrey** (doo-kra'e), Augusto, Italian dermatologist, 1860–1940. See D.'s *bacillus.*

# DUCT

**duct** [ L. *duco,* pp. *ductus,* to lead ]. 1. To turn; to vert; denoting the revolving movement of a limb or other part. 2. To lead; to draw from or to a fixed point. 3. A tubular structure giving exit to the secretion of a gland, or conducting any fluid. For the anatomical names of the d.'s, see ductulus and ductus. See also canal.

**aberrant d.,** *ductulus* aberrans.

**aber'rant bile d.'s,** small d.'s occasionally present in the ligaments of the liver or originating from the surface of the liver.

**accessory pancreat'ic d.,** *ductus* pancreaticus accessorius.

**alve'olar d.,** (1) *ductulus* alveolaris; (2) the smallest of the intralobular d.'s in the mammary gland; the secretory alveoli open into them.

**amniot'ic d.,** the transitory opening between the seroamniotic folds just before they fuse to form the seroamniotic raphe.

**d. of Aran'tius,** *ductus* venosus.

**arte'rial d.,** *ductus* arteriosus.

**Bartholin's d.,** *ductus* sublingualis major.

**Bellini's d.'s,** straight collecting tubules of the kidney.

**Bernard's d.,** *ductus* pancreaticus accessorius.

**bile d.,** biliary d.; gall d.; any of the d.'s conveying bile between the liver and the intestine, including hepatic, cystic, and common bile d. See fig. under *vesica* fellea.

**biliary d.,** bile d.

**Blasius' d.,** *ductus* parotideus.

**Botallo's d.,** *ductus* arteriosus.

**branchial d.,** the lumen of one of the pharyngeal pouches of the young embryo, elongated and narrowed by later differential growth.

**bucconeu'ral d.,** craniopharyngeal d.

**d. of bulbourethral gland,** *ductus* glandulae bulbourethralis.

**canalic'ular d.'s,** (1) *ductus* lactiferi; (2) *ductuli* biliferi.

**carotid d.,** *ductus* caroticus.

**cervical d.,** see branchial d. and cervical *diverticulum.*

**choledoch d.,** *ductus* choledochus.

**coch'lear d.,** *ductus* cochlearis.

**common bile d.,** *ductus* choledochus.

**common gall d.,** *ductus* choledochus.

**common hepatic d.,** *ductus* hepaticus communis.

**cra'niopharyn'geal d.,** bucconeural d.; hypophysial d.; the slender tubular part of the hypophysial diverticulum; the stalk of Rathke's pocket.

**Cuvier's d.'s,** old term for the common cardinal veins.

**cystic d.,** *ductus* cysticus.

**cystic gall d.,** *ductus* cysticus.

**def'erent d.,** *ductus* deferens.

**efferent d.,** *ductulus* efferens testis.

**ejaculatory d.,** *ductus* ejaculatorius.

**endolymphat'ic d.,** *ductus* endolymphaticus.

**d. of epididymis,** *ductus* epididymidis.

**d. of the epooph'oron,** *ductus* epoophori longitudinalis.

**excre'tory d.,** ductus excretorius; a d. carrying the secretion from a gland or a fluid from any reservoir.

**excretory d. of seminal vesicle,** *ductus* excretorius vesiculae seminalis.

**fron'tona'sal d.,** the passage that leads downward from the frontal sinus to open into the infundibulum of the middle meatus of the nasal cavity.

**galactoph'orous d.'s,** *ductus* lactiferi.

**gall d.,** bile d.

**Gartner's d.,** *ductus* epoophori longitudinalis.

**genital d.,** the genital *tract.*

**gut'tural d.,** *tuba* auditiva.

**hemithoracic d.,** ductus hemithoracicus; an accessory thoracic duct, usually emptying into the thoracic duct but sometimes discharging independently into the right subclavian vein.

**Hensen's d.,** *ductus* reuniens.

**hepatic d.,** *ductus* hepaticus.

**hep'atocys'tic d.,** *ductus* hepaticus communis.

**His' d.,** *ductus* thyroglossus.

**Hoffmann's d.,** *ductus* pancreaticus.

**hypophysial d.,** craniopharyngeal d.

**incisive d.,** *ductus* incisivus.

**intercalated d.'s,** the minute d.'s of glands, such as the salivary and the pancreas, that lead from the acini; they are lined by flat cells.

**in'terlo'bar d.,** a d. draining the secretion of the lobe of a gland and formed by the junction of a number of interlobular d.'s.

**in'terlob'ular d.,** any d. leading from a lobule of a gland and formed by the junction of the fine d.'s draining the acini.

**lacrimal d.,** *canaliculus* lacrimalis.

**lactif'erous d.'s,** *ductus* lactiferi.

**left d. of caudate lobe,** *ductus* lobi caudati sinister.

**left hepatic d.,** *ductus* hepaticus sinister.

**Leydig's d.,** *ductus* mesonephricus.

**longitudinal d. of epoophoron,** *ductus* epoophori longitudinalis.

**Luschka's d.'s,** glandlike tubular structures in the wall of the gallbladder, especially in the part covered with peritoneum.

**lymphat'ic d.,** one of the two large lymph channels, *ductus* lymphaticus dexter, or *ductus* thoracicus.

**major sublingual d.,** *ductus* sublingualis major.

**mamillary d.'s,** *ductus* lactiferi.

**mammary d.'s,** *ductus* lactiferi.

**mesoneph'ric d.,** *ductus* mesonephricus.

**metaneph'ric d.,** the slender tubular portion of the metanephric diverticulum; it is the primordium of the epithelial lining of the ureter.

**milk d.'s,** *ductus* lactiferi.

**minor sublingual d.'s,** *ductus* sublinguales minores.

**Müller's d., Müller'ian d.,** *ductus* paramesonephricus.

**nasal d.,** *ductus* nasolacrimalis.

**nasolac'rimal d.,** *ductus* nasolacrimalis.

**nephric d.,** pronephric d.

**om'phalomesenter'ic d.,** yolk *stalk.*

**pancreat'ic d.,** *ductus* pancreaticus.

**pap'illary d.'s,** the principal straight excretory d.'s in the kidney medulla and papillae whose openings form the area cribrosa.

**par'amesoneph'ric d.,** *ductus* paramesonephricus.

**par'aure'thral d.'s,** *ductus* paraurethrales.

**parotid d.,** *ductus* parotideus.

**Pecquet's d.,** *ductus* thoracicus.

**perilymphat'ic d.,** *ductus* perilymphaticus.

**pharyngobranchial d.'s,** see *ductus* pharyngobranchialis III and IV.

**proneph'ric d.,** the d. of the pronephros.

**prostatic d.'s,** *ductuli* prostatici.

**right d. of caudate lobe,** *ductus* lobi caudati dexter.

**right hepatic d.,** *ductus* hepaticus dexter.

**right lymphatic d.,** *ductus* lymphaticus dexter.

**Rivinus' d.'s,** *ductus* sublinguales.

**salivary d.,** a type of intralobular d. found in salivary glands which contributes to the secretion; also called secretory or striated d.

**Santorini's d.,** *ductus* pancreaticus accessorius.

**Schüller's d.'s,** *ductus* paraurethrales.

**semicircular d.'s,** *ductus* semicirculares.

**sem'inal d.,** any one of the d.'s conveying semen from the epididymis to the urethra, ductus deferens, d. of the seminal vesicles, or ejaculatory d.

**d. of seminal vesicle,** *ductus* excretorius vesiculae seminalis.

**d.'s of Skene's glands,** *ductus* paraurethrales.

**spermat'ic d.,** *ductus* deferens.

**Stensen's d., d. of Steno,** *ductus* parotideus.

**submandib'ular d.,** *ductus* submandibularis.

**submaxil'lary d.,** *ductus* submandibularis.

**sudoriferous d.,** *ductus* sudoriferus.

**sweat d.,** *ductus* sudoriferus.

**testicular d.,** *ductus* deferens.

**thoracic d.,** *ductus* thoracicus.

**thyroglos'sal d.,** *ductus* thyroglossus.

**thyrolin'gual d.,** *ductus* thyroglossus.

**umbilical d.,** archaic term for yolk-stalk.

**uniting d.,** *ductus* reuniens.

**utric'ulosac'cular d.,** *ductus* utriculosaccularis.

**venous d. of Arantius,** *ductus* venosus.

**vitelline d., vitellointestinal d.,** archaic terms for yolk-stalk.

**Walther's d.'s,** *ductus* sublinguales minores.

**Wharton's d.,** *ductus* submandibularis.

**Wirsung's d.,** *ductus* pancreaticus.

**Wolffian d.,** *ductus* mesonephricus.

---

**ductal** (duk'tal). Relating to a duct.

**ductile** (duk'til) [ L. *ductilis*, capable of being led or drawn ]. Pertaining to the property of a material that allows it to be bent, drawn out (as a wire), or otherwise deformed without breaking.

**duction** (duk'shun) [ L. *duco*, to lead ]. 1. The act of leading, bringing, conducting. 2. The monocular action of the oculorotatory muscles; usually additionally designating direction of movement of the eye, *e.g.*, movement toward nose, adduction; toward temple, abduction; upward supraduction; downward, deorsumduction.

**F d.,** sexduction; the transfer of chromosomal fragments from one bacterium to another by means of F' carriers.

**passive d.,** a maneuver to determine whether a mechanical obstruction is present in the eye; with forceps grasping an eye muscle, an attempt is made to passively move the eyeball in the direction of restricted rotation.

**duct'less.** Having no duct; denoting certain glands having only an internal secretion.

**ductular** (duk'tu-lar). Relating to a ductule.

**ductule** (duk'tūl). Ductulus.

**aberrant d.,** *ductulus* aberrans.

**biliary d.'s,** *ductuli* biliferi.

**excretory d.'s of lacrimal gland,** *ductuli* excretorii glandulae lacrimalis.

**interlobular d.'s,** *ductuli* interlobulares.

**prostatic d.'s,** *ductuli* prostatici.

**transverse d.'s of epoophoron,** *ductuli* transversi epoophori.

**ductulus,** pl. **duc'tuli** (duk'tu-lus) [ Mod. L. dim. of L. *ductus*, duct ] [ NA ]. Ductule; a minute duct.

**d. aber'rans,** pl. **ductuli aberran'tes** [ NA ], aberrant ductule; aberrant duct; vas aberrans; one of the diverticula of the epididymis. The **d. aberrans superius** is a diverticulum from the head of the epididymis; the **d. aberrans inferius,** vas aberrans of Haller, extends from the tail of the epididymis.

**d. alveola'ris,** pl. **ductuli alveolares** [ NA ], alveolar duct (1); the part of the respiratory passages beyond a respiratory bronchiole; from it arise alveolar sacs and alveoli.

**ductuli bilif'eri** [ NA ], biliary ductules; ductus biliferi; canalicular ducts (2); the excretory ducts of the liver that connect the interlobular ductules to the right (or left) hepatic duct.

**d. ef'ferens testis,** pl. **ductuli efferen'tes testis** [ NA ], efferent duct; one of a number (12 to 14) of small seminal ducts leading from the testis to the head of the epididymis.

**ductuli excreto'rii glan'dulae lacrima'lis** [ NA ], excretory ductules of the lacrimal gland; the multiple (6 to 10) excretory ducts of the lacrimal gland that open into the superior fornix of the conjunctival sac.

**ductuli interlobula'res** [ NA ], interlobular ductules; bile ductules occupying portal canals between hepatic lobules which open into the ductuli biliferi.

**ductuli parooph'ori,** tubuli paroophori; the tubular remnants of the embryonic mesonephros which form the paroophoron.

**ductuli prostat'ici** [ NA ], prostatic ductules; prostatic ducts; ductus prostatici; about 20 minute canals which receive the prostatic secretion from the glandular tubules and discharge it through openings on either side of the urethral crest in the posterior wall of the urethra.

**ductuli transver'si epooph'ori** [ NA ], transverse ductules of the epoophoron; a series of 10 to 15 short tubules that open into the longitudinal duct of the epoophoron.

---

# DUCTUS

---

**ductus,** gen. and pl. **duc'tus** (duk'tus) [ L. a leading, fr. *duco,* pp. *ductus,* to lead ] [ NA ]. Duct (3).

**d. aber'rans,** *ductulus* aberrans.

**d. aran'tii,** d. venosus.

**d. arterio'sus** [ NA ], Botallo's duct; arterial canal or duct; a fetal vessel connecting the left pulmonary artery with the descending aorta. During the first two months after birth, it normally becomes changed into a fibrous cord, the ligamentum arteriosum. Its occasional failure to close postnatally causes a definite cardiovascular handicap that can be dealt with surgically.

**d. bilif'eri,** *ductuli* biliferi.

**d. carot'icus,** carotid duct; a portion of the embryonic dorsal aorta between positions at which it is joined by the third and fourth arch arteries; it disappears early in development.

**d. choled'ochus** [ NA ], common bile or gall duct; choledoch duct; choledoch; choledochus; formed by the union of the hepatic and cystic ducts; it discharges at the duodenal papilla.

**d. cochlea'ris** [ NA ], cochlear duct; Löwenberg's scala or canal; membranous cochlea; scala media; a spirally arranged membranous tube suspended within the cochlea, occupying the lower portion of the vestibular scala; it begins by a blind extremity, *cecum vestibulare,* in the cochlear recess of the vestibule, terminating in another blind extremity, *cecum cupulare* or lagena, at the cupola of the cochlea; it contains endolymph and communicates with the sacculus by the ductus reuniens. The organum spirale (organ of Corti), the neuroepithelial receptor organ for hearing, occupies the floor of the duct.

**d. cys'ticus** [ NA ], cystic duct; cystic gall duct; the d. leading from the gallbladder; it joins the hepatic duct to form the common bile duct.

**d. def'erens** [ NA ], deferent duct; vas deferens; spermatic duct; testicular duct; the secretory duct of the testicle, running from the epididymis, of which it is the continuation, to the prostatic urethra where it terminates as the ejaculatory duct. See figs. under scrotum and *vesicula seminalis.*

**d. dorsopancreat'icus,** d. pancreaticus accessorius.

**d. ejaculato'rius** [ NA ], ejaculatory duct; the duct formed by the union of the deferent duct and the excretory duct of the seminal vesicle, which opens into the prostatic urethra.

**d. endolymphat'icus** [ NA ], endolymphatic duct; a small membranous canal, connecting with both saccule and utricle of the membranous labyrinth, passing through the aqueductus vestibuli, and terminating in a dilated blind extremity, the saccus endolymphaticus, on the posterior surface of the petrous portion of the temporal bone beneath the dura mater.

**d. epidid'ymidis** [ NA ], duct of the epididymis; a convoluted tube into which the efferent ductules open and which itself terminates in the deferent duct.

**d. epoophori longitudina'lis** [ NA ], longitudinal duct of epoophoron; Gartner's duct or canal; Malpighian canal; rudimentary vestige of the mesonephric duct in the female into which the tubules of the epoophoron open; it is located in the broad ligament of the uterus, parallel with the lateral part of the uterine tube.

**d. excreto'rius,** excretory *duct.*

**d. excreto'rius vesic'ulae semina'lis** [ NA ], excretory duct of the seminal vesicle; the passage leading from a seminal vesicle to the ejaculatory duct.

**d. glan'dulae bulbourethra'lis** [ NA ], duct of the bulbourethral gland; the long slender duct on each side passes down through the inferior fascia of the urogenital diaphragm to enter the bulb of the penis and course forward 2 or 3 cm. before terminating in the urethra.

**d. hemithorac'icus,** hemithoracic *duct.*

**d. hepat'icus commu'nis** [ NA ], common hepatic duct; hepatocystic duct; the part of the biliary duct system that is formed by the confluence of right and left hepatic ducts. At the porta hepatis it is joined by the cystic duct to become the common bile duct.

**d. hepat'icus dexter** [ NA ], right hepatic duct; the duct that transmits bile to the common hepatic duct from the right half of the liver.

**d. hepat'icus sinister** [ NA ], left hepatic duct; the duct that drains bile from the left half of the liver, including the left quadrate and caudate lobes.

**d. incisi'vus** [ NA ], incisive duct; a rudimentary duct, or protrusion of the mucous membrane into the incisive canal, on either side of the anterior extremity of the nasal crest.

**d. lactif'eri** [ NA ], lactiferous ducts; milk ducts; galactophorous canals or ducts; canalicular ducts (1); mammary ducts; galactophores; the ducts, numbering 15 or 20, which drain the lobes of the mammary gland. They open at the nipple.

**d. lingua'lis,** a pit on the upper surface of the tongue at the apex of the sulcus terminalis. It marks the point of origin of the d. thyroglossus of the embryo. Known more commonly as the foramen cecum.

**d. lo'bi cauda'ti dex'ter** [ NA ], right duct of the caudate lobe; the bile duct from the right half of the caudate lobe, a tributary to the right hepatic duct.

**d. lo'bi cauda'ti sinis'ter** [ NA ], left duct of the caudate lobe; a tributary to the left hepatic duct draining bile from the left half of the caudate lobe.

**d. lymphat'icus dexter** [ NA ], right lymphatic duct; d. thoracicus dexter; one of the two terminal lymph vessels, a short trunk somewhat less than an inch in length, formed by the union of the right jugular lymphatic vessel and vessels from the lymph nodes of the right superior limb, thoracic wall, and both lungs; it lies on the right side of the root of the neck and empties into the right brachiocephalic vein.

**d. mesoneph'ricus** [ NA ], mesonephric duct; Wolffian duct; Leydig's duct; a duct in the embryo draining the mesonephric tubules; in the male it becomes the ductus deferens; in the female it becomes vestigial. See also *ductus* epoophori longitudinalis.

**d. nasolacrima'lis** [ NA ], nasolacrimal duct; nasal duct; the passage leading downward from the lacrimal sac on each side to the anterior portion of the inferior meatus of the nose, through which tears are conducted into the nasal cavity. See fig. under *apparatus* lacrimalis.

**d. om'phalomesenter'icus,** yolk *stalk.*

**d. pancreat'icus** [ NA ], pancreatic duct; Wirsung's canal or duct; Hoffmann's duct; the excretory duct of the pancreas which extends through the gland from tail to head where it empties into the duodenum at the greater duodenal papilla.

**d. pancreat'icus accesso'rius** [ NA ], accessory pancreatic duct; d. dorsopancreaticus; Bernard's or Santorini's canal

or duct; the excretory duct of the head of the pancreas, one branch of which joins the pancreatic duct, the other opening independently into the duodenum at the lesser duodenal papilla.

**d. paramesonephricus** [ NA ], paramesonephric duct; Müller's duct; Müllerian duct; Müller's canal; one of the embryonic tubes extending along the mesonephros roughly parallel to the mesonephric duct and emptying into the cloaca. In the female the upper parts of the ducts form the uterine tubes; more caudally the right and left ducts fuse to form the uterus and vagina. In the male they disappear, except for the vestigial vagina masculina and the appendix testis.

**d. paraurethra'les** [ NA ], paraurethral ducts; Schüller's ducts; ducts of Skene's (paraurethral) glands.

**d. parotid'eus** [ NA ], parotid duct; Steno's or Stensen's duct; Blasius' duct; the duct of the parotid gland opening from the cheek into the vestibule of the mouth opposite the neck of the superior second molar tooth.

**patent d. arteriosus,** see d. arteriosus.

**d. perilymphat'icus** [ NA ], perilymphatic duct; cochlear aqueduct; aqueductus cochleae; a fine canal connecting the perilymphatic space of the cochlea with the subarachnoid space.

**d. pharyngobranchia'lis III,** a narrow communication between the third branchial pouch and the pharynx in the embryo.

**d. pharyngobranchia'lis IV,** a narrow communication between the fourth branchial pouch and the pharynx in the embryo.

**d. prostat'ici,** *ductuli* prostatici.

**d. reuniens** [ NA ], uniting canal or duct; Hensen's canal or duct; canaliculus or canalis reuniens; a short membranous tube passing from the lower end of the saccule to the cochlear duct of the membranous labyrinth.

**d. semicircula'res** [ NA ], semicircular ducts; three small membranous tubes that lie within the bony labyrinth and form loops of about two-thirds of a circle. The three (**d. semicircularis anterior, d. semicircularis lateralis,** and **d. semicircularis posterior**) lie in planes at right angles to each other and open into the vestibule by five openings of which one is common to two ducts. Each duct has an ampulla at one end within which filaments of the vestibular nerve terminate.

**d. sublingua'lis major** [ NA ], major sublingual duct; duct of Bartholin; the duct that drains the anterior portion of the sublingual gland. It opens at the sublingual papilla.

**d. sublingua'les minores** [ NA ], minor sublingual ducts; Walther's canals or ducts; from 8 to 20 small ducts of the sublingual salivary gland which open into the mouth on the surface of the sublingual fold; a few join the submandibular ducts.

**d. submandibula'ris** [ NA ], submandibular duct; d. submaxillaris; submaxillary duct; Wharton's duct; the duct of the submandibular salivary gland; it opens at the sublingual papilla near the frenulum of the tongue.

**d. submaxilla'ris,** d. submandibularis.

**d. sudorif'erus** [ NA ], sudoriferous duct; sweat duct; the superficial portion of the sweat gland which passes through the corium and epidermis, opening on the surface by the porus sudoriferus or sweat pore.

**d. thoracicus** [ NA ], thoracic duct; van Hoorne's canal; Pecquet's duct; the largest lymph vessel in the body, beginning at the cisterna chyli at about the level of the second lumbar vertebra, it passes through the aortic opening of the diaphragm, crosses the posterior mediastinum, and discharges into the left brachiocephalic vein at its origin.

**d. thoracicus dexter** [ NA ], *ductus* lymphaticus dexter.

**d. thyroglos'sus** [ NA ], thyroglossal duct; His' canal or duct; thyrolingual duct; a transitory entodermal tube in the embryo, carrying thyroid forming tissue at its caudal end. Normally the duct disappears after the thyroid has moved to its definitive location in the neck. Its point of origin is regularly marked on the root of the adult tongue by the foramen cecum; occasionally its incomplete regression results in the formation of cysts along its embryonic course. A pyramidal lobe on the thyroid isthmus, when present, marks the original point of continuity of the thyroglossal duct with the thyroid gland.

**d. utric'ulosaccula'ris** [ NA ], utriculosaccular duct; a duct that is given off from the inner aspect of the utricle and joins the endolymphatic duct a short distance from its origin from the saccule.

**d. veno'sus** [ NA ], Arantius' duct or canal; venous duct or venous canal of Arantius; ductus venosus arantii; the continuation, in the fetus, of the umbilical vein through the liver to the vena cava inferior; after birth its lumen becomes obliterated, forming the ligamentum venosum.

**d. venosus arantii,** d. venosus.

**Duddell,** Benedict, English oculist, 18th century. See D.'s *membrane.*

**Dudley,** Emilius C., Chicago gynecologist, 1850–1928. See D.'s *operation.*

**Duffy blood group.** See appendix 2, Blood Groups.

**Dugas,** Louis A., American physician, 1806–1884. See D.'s *test.*

**Duhring** (dür'ing), Louis A., Philadelphia dermatologist, 1845–1913. See D.'s *disease.*

**Dührssen** (dür'sen), Alfred, German obstetrician-gynecologist, 1862–1933. See D.'s *incisions, operation.*

**duipara** (du-ip'ah-rah) [ L. *duo,* two, + *pario,* to bear ]. Secundipara.

**Dukes,** Clement, English physician, 1845–1925. See D.'s *disease.*

**Dukes,** Cuthbert E., English pathologist, *1890. See D.'s *classification.*

**dulcamara** (dul'kah-mah'rah) [ L. *dulcis,* sweet, + *amarus,* bitter ]. Bittersweet; poisonberry; wolfgrape; the dried young branches of *Solanum dulcamara* (family Solanaceae), a climbing plant of the north temperate zone. Diuretic, diaphoretic, sedative, and narcotic.

**dulcam'arin.** Dulcarin; a glucoside, $C_{22}H_{34}O_{10}$, obtained from dulcamara.

**dul'carin.** Dulcamarin.

**dul'cin.** Sucrol.

**dul'cite.** Galactitol.

**dul'citol.** Galactitol.

**dul'cose.** Galactitol.

**dull.** Not sharp or acute, in any sense; qualifying a surgical instrument, the action of the mind, pain, a sound (especially the percussion note), etc.

**dull'ness, dul'ness.** The character of the sound obtained by percussing over a solid part which is incapable of vibrating.

    **area of cardiac d.,** see under area.

    **Gerhardt's d.,** a narrow rectangular area of d. on percussion in the second and third left interspaces overlying the dilated pulmonary artery in cases of patent ductus arteriosus.

    **shifting d.,** the movement of the sign elicited by percussion when fluid free, usually in the abdominal cavity, changes its position as the patient is moved.

**Dulong** (dü-lawn'), Pierre L., French chemist, 1785–1838. See D.-Petit *law.*

**dumas.** Pink parangi (Ceylon); foot yaws.

**dumb** [ A.S. ]. Mute; speechless; unable to speak.

**dum'miness.** Mental dullness and apathy occurring as a sequel of acute encephalitis in the horse.

**dum'my.** See pontic.

**Dumontpallier** (dü-mawn-pal-ya'), Alphonse, French physician, 1826–1898. See D.'s *pessary.*

**dumping.** See dumping *syndrome.*

**Duncan,** James M., Scottish gynecologist, 1826–1890. See D.'s *folds, mechanism, ventricle.*

**duocrinin.** A postulated gastrointestinal hormone that is liberated by the contact of gastric contents with the intestine and that stimulates the secretory activity of the duodenal glands (Brunner's glands). Existence of this hormone has not been clearly demonstrated.

**duodenal** (du'o-de'nal, du-od'ĕ-nal). Relating to the duodenum.

**duodenectomy** (du-o-dĕ-nek'to-mĭ) [ duodenum + G. *ek-tomē,* excision ]. Exsection of the duodenum.

**duode'nin.** A substance supposedly contained in duodenal extracts that causes hypoglycemia. Original observations not confirmed by other investigators.

**duodenitis** (du-od-ĕ-ni'tis). Inflammation of the duodenum.

**duodeno-** (du-o-de'no-, du-od'ĕ-no-) [ L. *duodenum, q.v.* ]. Combining form relating to the duodenum.

**duodenocholangitis** (du-o-de'no-ko-lan-ji'tis) [ duodeno- + G. *cholē,* bile, + *angeion,* vessel, + suffix *-itis,* inflammation ]. Inflammation of the duodenum and common bile duct.

**duodenocholecystostomy** (du-o-de'no-ko-le-sis-tos'to-mĭ) [ duodeno- + G. *cholē,* bile, + *kystis,* bladder, + *stoma,* mouth ]. Duodenocystostomy; the operative formation of a fistula between duodenum and gallbladder.

**duodenocholedochotomy** (du-o-de'no-ko-led-o-kot'o-mĭ) [ duodeno- + G. *cholēdochus,* bile duct, + *tomē,* incision ]. Incision into the common bile duct and the adjacent portion of the duodenum.

**duodenocystostomy** (du-o-de'no-sis-tos'to-mĭ). Duodenocholecystostomy.

**duodenoenterostomy** (du-o-de'no-en'ter-os'to-mĭ) [ duodeno- + G. *enteron,* intestine, + *stoma,* mouth ]. The operative establishment of communication between the duodenum and another part of the intestinal tract.

**duodenojejunostomy** (du-o-de'no-jē-ju-nos'to-mĭ) [ duodeno- + jejunum, + G. *stoma,* mouth ]. The operative formation of an artificial communication between the duodenum and the jejunum.

**duodenolysis** (du-o-dĕ-nol'ĭ-sis) [ duodeno- + G. *lysis,* a freeing ]. The operation in which adhesions of the duodenum are cut and the bowel freed from surrounding structures.

**duodenorrhaphy** (du-o-de-nor'ă-fĭ) [ duodeno- + G. *rhaphē,* a seam ]. The operation for repairing by suture a tear or incision in the duodenum.

**duodenoscopy** (du-o-de-nos'ko-pĭ) [ duodeno- + G. *skopeō,* to examine ]. Observation of the interior of the duodenum by means of an endoscope.

**duodenostomy** (du-o-de-nos'to-mĭ) [ duodeno- + G. *stoma,* mouth ]. The operative establishment of a fistula into the duodenum.

**duodenotomy** (du-o-de-not'o-mĭ) [ duodeno- + G. *tomē,* incision ]. A cutting into the duodenum.

**duodenum,** gen. **duodeni,** pl. **duodena** (du-o-de'num, du-od'ĕ-num) [ Mediev. L. fr. L. *duodeni,* twelve ] [ NA ]. The first division of the small intestine, about 11 inches or 12 fingerbreadths (hence the name) in length, extending from the pylorus to the junction with the jejunum at the level of the first or second lumbar vertebra on the left side. It is divided into the pars superior, the first part of which is the duodenal cap, the pars descendens, into which the bile and pancreatic ducts open, the pars horizontalis (inferior) and the pars ascendens, terminating at the duodenojejunal junction.

**Duplay** (dü-pla-e'), Simon, French surgeon, 1836–1924. See D.'s *disease.*

**duplication** (du'plĭ-ka'shun). A doubling; see also reduplication.

    **d. of chromosomes,** see under chromosome.

**duplicitas** (du-plis'e-tahs) [ L. a being double, fr. *duplex* (*duplic-*), two-fold. PLIC-]. Doubling of a part.

    **d. anterior,** conjoined twins in which fusion has united the pelvis and lower extremities, leaving the thoraces and head separate. See also cephalodidymus.

    **d. posterior,** iliadelphus; conjoined twins in which the heads and upper parts of the bodies have become fused, leaving the buttocks and legs separate. See also dipygus and dipygus parasiticus. See fig. on p. 428.

**du'plitized.** Term used to describe an x-ray film that has been double-coated.

**dupp.** Syllable used to imitate the heart's second sound as heard on auscultation, being sharper and higher pitched than the first sound (*lubb*).

**Dupré's muscle.** See under muscle.

**Dupuy-Dutemps,** Louis, Paris ophthalmologist, *1871. See D.-D. *operation.*

**Dupuytren** (dü-püe-trahn'), Guillaume, French surgeon

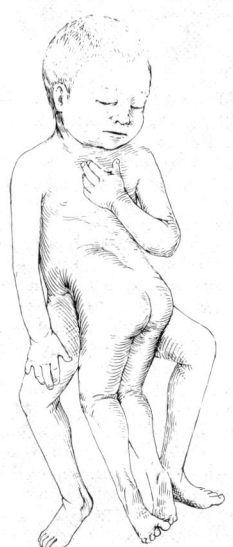

**Duplicitas Posterior**

and surgical pathologist, 1777–1835. See D.'s *amputation, canal, contracture, disease* (of foot), *enterotome, fascia, fracture, hydrocele, sign, suture, tourniquet.*

**dura** (du′rah) [ L. fem. of *durus,* hard ]. Dura mater.

**du′ral.** Duramatral; relating to the dura mater.

**dural′umin.** An alloy of aluminum (aluminium) slightly heavier than this metal but nearly as strong as steel and noncorrodible; used in the manufacture of surgical and orthopaedic appliances.

**dura mater** (du′rah ma′ter) [ L. hard mother ]. Dura; pachymeninx (as distinguished from leptomeninx, the combined pia mater and arachnoidea); a tough, fibrous membrane forming the outer envelope of the brain (the d. mater encephali) and the spinal cord (the d. mater spinalis).

  **d. mater enceph′ali** [ NA ], the intracranial dura, consisting of two layers, the outer one of which adheres to the periosteum of the cranial bones; the inner layer is fused with the outer except that locally the two layers separate to enclose large venous ducts, the sinus durae matris.

  **d. mater spina′lis** [ NA ], the d. mater of the spinal cord; it does not (in contrast to the d. mater encephali) adhere to the enveloping bony structures (vertebrae), and it is separated from the latter by a considerable space, the epidural space, containing the plexus venosi vertebrales interni and variable amounts of fatty tissue.

**durama′tral.** Dural.

**Durand,** J., French physician, *1876. See Favre-D.-Nicolas *disease.*

**Duran-Reynals,** Francisco, American bacteriologist, 1899–1958. See D.-R.'s *factor.*

**Durante's disease.** See under disease.

**duraplasty** (du′rah-plas-tĭ) [ dura (mater) + G. *plassō,* to form ]. A plastic or reconstructive operation on the dura mater.

**duration** (du-ra′shun). A continuous period of time.

  **half amplitude pulse d.,** the time, in milliseconds, required for a wave form to reach half of its full magnitude.

  **pulse d.,** the interval between the leading and trailing edges of an output pulse.

**Dürck,** Hermann, Munich pathologist, *1869. See D.'s *nodes.*

**Duret** (du-rā′), Henri, French neurosurgeon, 1849–1921. See D.'s *lesion.*

**Durham,** Arthur E., English surgeon, 1834–1895. See D.'s *tube.*

**Durham rule.** See under rule.

**Duroziez** (dü-ro-ze-a′), Paul L., Paris physician, 1826 –1897. See D.'s *disease, murmur, symptom.*

**Dutton,** Joseph Everett, English physician, 1877–1905. See D.'s *disease,* relapsing *fever.*

**Duverney** (dü-ver′na), Joseph G., French anatomist, 1648–1730. See D.'s *fissure, foramen, gland, muscle.*

**D.V.M.** Abbreviation for Doctor of Veterinary Medicine. This degree is now standard in the United States. The University of Pennsylvania uses the abbreviation V.M.D.

**dwarf** [ A.S. *dweorh* ]. Nanus; pigmy; a markedly undersized person. See also subentries under dwarfism.

  **achondroplastic d.,** see achondroplasia.

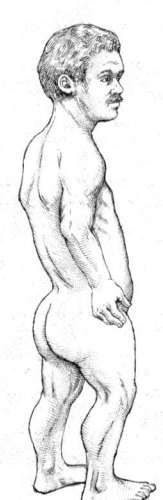

**Achondroplastic Dwarf**

  **asexual d.,** a d. with deficient sexual development who is beyond the age of puberty.

  **ateliotic d.,** idiopathic d.; a normally proportioned individual of unusually short stature; such d.'s are functionally normal, by currently available criteria, and the cause of this condition is not known.

  **Fröhlich's d.,** an individual with Fröhlich's syndrome; see also *dystrophia* adiposogenitalis.

  **hypothyroid d.,** cretin.

  **idiopathic d.,** ateliotic d.

  **infantile d.,** a subject of infantilism.

  **micromel′ic d.,** one whose limbs are unduly small.

  **normal d.,** physiologic d.

  **phocomelic d.,** one in whom the diaphyses of the long bones are extremely short, or in whom the intermediate parts of the limbs are absent.

  **physiologic d.,** an undersized person, not deformed, whose development has been symmetrical and at a normal rate, but less in extent than that of members of other races, members of other families, or other members of the same family.

  **primordial d.,** see primordial *dwarfism.*

  **senile d.,** a d. with craniofacial anomalies; progeroid in appearance.

  **sexual d.,** an adult primordial d. with perfect sexual development.

  **true d.,** nanosome; either a primordial or sexual d., or an infantile or asexual d.

**dwarf′ishness.** Dwarfism.

**dwarf′ism.** Dwarfishness; nanism; nanosoma; nanosomia; abnormal smallness; the condition of being undersized. See also subentries under dwarf.

  **aortic d.,** underdevelopment associated with severe aortic stenosis.

  **camptomelic d.,** d. with shortening of the lower limbs, due to anterior bending of the femur and tibia.

  **chondrodystrophic d.,** see chondrodystrophy.

**diastrophic d.,** hereditary skeletal dysplasia, with clubfoot, deformity of the thumbs and fingers, and neonatal hematoma of the pinna.

**Laron type d.,** d. associated with an absence of somatomedin and with high plasma levels of somatotropin.

**lethal d.,** d. leading to intrauterine or neonatal death.

**Lorain-Lévi d.,** primordial d.

**mesomelic d.,** d. with shortness of the midsegments (forearms, forelegs) of the extremities.

**metatropic d.,** a congenital skeletal dysplasia characterized by a changing pattern of d. in which there is a lengthening of the trunk (relative to the limbs) at birth but with a subsequent shortening.

**pituitary d.,** Lorain-Lévi infantilism or syndrome; pituitary nanism; a rare form of d. caused by the absence of a functional anterior pituitary gland; it may be present at birth or may develop during early childhood.

**polydystrophic d.,** Maroteaux-Lamy *syndrome.*

**primordial d.,** Lorain-Lévi d.; growth retardation that begins during intrauterine life and is present at birth; pituitary hormone levels are normal.

**pseudometatropic d.,** a congenital skeletal dysplasia similar to metatropic dwarfism but not fulfilling the rigid diagnostic criteria.

**thanatophoric d.,** a lethal d. characterized by micromelia, bowed long bones, enlarged head, and flattened vertebral bodies.

**tryptophanuria with d.,** see under tryptophanuria.

**Dy.** Chemical symbol of the element dysprosium.

**dy′ad** [ G. *dyas,* the number two, duality ]. 1. Diad (2); a pair. 2. In chemistry, a bivalent element. 3. A pair of persons in an interactional situation, *e.g.,* patient and therapist, husband and wife.

**dyclonine hydrochloride** (di′klo-nēn). DYCLONE; 4′-butoxy-3-piperidino-propiophenone hydrochloride. A topical local anesthetic with rapid onset of low systemic toxicity in concentrations under 1 per cent. It does not contain the ester or amide linkage typical of local anesthetic agents.

**dydrogesterone** (di′dro-jes′ter-ōn) (NF, BP). DUPHASTON; 9β ,10α-pregna-4,6-diene-3,20-dione (for pregnane structure, see steroids). A synthetic steroid derived from retroprogesterone. It exerts its progestational effects in therapeutic doses largely on the endometrium; has not been observed to inhibit ovulation or to raise body temperature.

**dye** (di) [ A.S. *deah, deag* ]. A stain; coloring matter; a compound consisting of chromophore and auxochrome groups attached to one or more benzene rings, its color being due to the chromophore and its dyeing affinities to the auxochrome. D.'s are used in the laboratory for staining tissues and microorganisms, clinically as antiseptics and germicides, and some as stimulants of epithelial growth. Individual d.'s and classes of d.'s are listed under their chemical, color, eponymic, or otherwise specific names.

**salt d.,** neutral *stain.*

**-dymus** [ G. *-dymos,* fold ]. 1. A suffix to be combined with number roots, as didymus, tridymus, tetradymus, etc. (two-, three-, fourfold). 2. An occasionally used shortened form for -didymus, which see.

**dynamics** (di-nam′iks) [ G. *dynamis,* force ]. 1. The science of forces and their laws. 2. In psychiatry, the determination of how behavior patterns and emotional reactions 3. In the behavioral sciences, any of the numerous intrapersonal and interpersonal influences or phenomena associated with personality development and interpersonal processes.

**group d.,** a term used to represent the study of underlying features of group behavior, *e.g.,* motives, attitudes; it is concerned with group change rather than with static characteristics.

**dynamo-** (di′nă-mo-) [ G. *dynamis,* force ]. Combining form relating to force or energy.

**dynamogenesis** (di′nă-mo-jen′ĕ-sis) [ dynamo- + G. *genesis,* production ]. Dynamogeny; the production of force, especially of muscular or nervous energy.

**dynamogen′ic.** Producing power or force, especially nervous or muscular power or activity.

**dynamogeny** (di′nă-moj′ĕ-nī). Dynamogenesis.

**dynamograph** (di-nam′o-graf) [ dynamo- + G. *graphō,* to write ]. An instrument for recording the degree of muscular power.

**dynamometer** (di-nă-mom′e-ter) [ dynamo- + G. *metron,* measure ]. Ergometer; an instrument for measuring the degree of muscular power.

**dynamoscope** (di-nam′o-skōp) [ dynamo- + G. *skopeō,* to examine ]. A modified stethoscope for auscultation of the muscles.

**dynamoscopy** (di-nă-mos′ko-pī). Auscultation of a contracting muscle.

**dynatherm** (di′nă-therm) [ G. *dynamis,* force, + *thermē,* heat ]. An apparatus for inducing diathermy.

**dyne** (dīn) [ G. *dynamis,* force ]. The unit of force in the CGS system, replaced in the SI system by the newton (1 newton = $10^5$ dynes). A dyne is the force that gives a body of 1 g mass an acceleration of 1 cm/sec²; force in dynes equals mass in grams time acceleration expressed as cm/sec², or $F$ (dynes) = $m$ (grams) $\times$ $a$ (cm/sec²).

**dyphylline** (di-fil′in). NEOTHYLLINE; 7-(2,3-dihydroxypropyl) theophylline; exhibits characteristic peripheral vasodilator and bronchodilator actions of other theophylline compounds; used in angina pectoris and coronary disease whenever myocardial stimulation would not be harmful.

**dys-** [ G. ]. Prefix conveying the idea of bad or difficult. Not to be confused with dis-, *q.v.*

**dysacousia, dysacusia** (dis-ă-koo′sī-ah). Dysacusis.

**dysacusis** (dis-a-koo′sis) [ dys- + G. *akousis,* hearing ]. Dysacousia; dysacusia. 1. Any impairment of hearing that is not primarily a loss of ability to perceive sound. Loss of discrimination for words, syllables, or phonemes, or loss of discrimination in terms of the understanding of words or in terms of pitch; involving difficulty in processing details of sound as opposed to lack of sensitivity to sound. 2. Pain or discomfort in the ear from exposure to sound.

**dys′adapta′tion.** Dysaptation.

**dys′adrenocort′icism.** Clinical state produced by deranged function of the adrenal cortex and its hormones.

**dysantigraphia** (dis′an-tī-graf′ī-ah) [ dys- + G. *antigraphō,* to write back ]. A form of agraphia in which the subject is unable to copy writing or print.

**dysaphia** (dis-a′fī-ah, dis-af′ī-ah) [ dys- + G. *haphē,* touch ]. An impairment in the sense of touch.

**dysaphic** (dis-a′fik). Relating to impaired tactile sensibility.

**dysaptation** (dis′ap-ta′shun). Dysadaptation; inability of the retina and iris to accommodate well to varying intensities of light.

**dysarteriotony** (dis-ar-te-rī-ot′o-nī) [ dys- + G. *artēria,* artery, + *tonos,* tension ]. Abnormal blood pressure, either too high or too low.

**dysarthria** (dis-ar′thrī-ah) [ dys- + G. *arthroō,* to articulate ]. Disturbance of articulation due to emotional stress or to paralysis, incoordination, or spasticity of the muscles used for speaking.

**d. litera′lis,** stammering.

**d. syllaba′ris spasmod′ica,** stuttering.

**dysar′thric.** Relating to difficulty in articulating.

**dysarthrosis** (dis-ar-thro′sis) [ dys- + G. *arthrōsis,* joint ]. 1. Dysarthria. 2. Malformation of a joint. 3. A false joint.

**dysautonomia** (dis-aw-to-no′mī-ah) [ dys- + G. *autonomia,* self-government ]. Abnormal functioning of the autonomic nervous system.

**familial d.,** Riley-Day syndrome; a congenital syndrome with specific disturbances of the nervous system and aberrations in autonomic nervous system function such as indifference to pain, diminished lacrimation, poor vasomotor control, motor incoordination, labile cardiovascular reactions, hyporeflexia, frequent attacks of bronchial pneumonia, hypersalivation with aspiration and trouble in swallowing, hyperemesis, emotional instability, and an intolerance for anesthetics. Autosomal recessive inheritance.

**dysbarism** (dis′bar-izm) [ dys- + G. *baros,* weight ]. The symptom complex resulting from exposure to decreased or changing barometric pressure, including the effects of rapid decompression. a general term that includes all physiologic effects resulting from changes in barometric pressure with the exception of hypoxia.

**dysbasia** (dis-ba'zĭ-ah) [ dys- + G. *basis*, a step ]. 1. Difficulty in walking. 2. The difficult or distorted walking that occurs in mental patients.

    **d. angiosclerot'ica, d. angiospas'tica,** obsolete terms meaning intermittent difficulty in walking due to peripheral vascular causes.

    **d. intermittens,** intermittent difficulty in walking.

    **d. lordot'ica progressi'va,** torsion neurosis, an affection characterized by lordoscoliosis of the lower portion of the vertebral column, occurring when the patient stands or walks and usually disappearing when he lies down.

    **d. neurasthen'ica intermittens,** intermittent difficulty in walking occurring in persons with mental disorders.

**dysbolism** (dis'bo-lizm) [ dys- + G. *bolē*(*metabolē*), + -*ismos*, metabolism ]. Abnormal, but not necessarily morbid, metabolism, as in alkaptonuria.

**dysbu'lia** [ dys- + G. *boulē*, will ]. Weakness and uncertainty of will power.

**dysbu'lic.** Relating to dysbulia.

**dyscephalia** (dis'sĕ-fa'lĭ-ah) [ dys- + G. *kephalē*, head ]. Dyscephaly; malformation of the head and face.

    **d. mandib'ulo-oculofacia'lis,** a syndrome of bony anomalies of the calvaria, face and jaw, with birdlike face, narrow curved nose, multiple eye defects including microphthalmia, microcornea and cataract, often with alopecia overlying skull sutures or alopecia areata and hypoplasia or absence of eyebrows. Has also been referred to as congenital sutural alopecia; congenital cataract with cranial malformation; progeria with cataract; progeria with microphthalmia; bird-face and congenital cataract; congenital ectodermal dysplasia; mandibulofacial or mandibulo-oculofacial dysmorphia; oculomandibulodyscephaly; Hallermann-Streiff syndrome.

**dyscephaly** (dis-sef'ă-lĭ). Dyscephalia.

**dyscheiral, dyschiral** (dis-ki'ral). Relating to dyscheiria.

**dyscheiria, dyschiria** (dis-ki'rĭ-ah) [ dys- + G. *cheir*, hand ]. A disorder of sensibility in which, although there is no apparent loss of sensation, the patient is unable to tell which side of the body has been touched (acheiria), or refers it to the wrong side (allocheiria), or to both sides (syncheiria).

**dyschezia** (dis-ke'zĭ-ah) [ dys- + G. *chezō*, to defecate ]. Difficulty in defecation.

**dyschiria** (dis-ki'rĭ-ah). Dyscheiria.

**dyschondrogenesis** (dis-kon-dro-jen'ĕ-sis) [ dys- + G. *chondros*, cartilage, + *genesis*, production ]. Abnormal development of cartilage.

**dyschondroplasia** (dis-kon-dro-pla'zĭ-ah) [ dys- + G. *chondros*, cartilage, + *plasis*, a forming ]. Enchondromatosis.

    **d. with hemangiomas,** Maffuci's *syndrome.*

**dyschondrosteosis** (dis-kon-dros'te-o'sis) [ dys- + G. *chondros*, cartilage, + *osteon*, bone, + suffix -*osis*, condition ]. Leri-Weill syndrome; a bone dysplasia characterized by bowing of the radius, dorsal dislocation of the distal ulna and proximal carpal bones, and mesomelic dwarfism; autosomal dominant inheritance.

**dyschroia, dyschroa** (dis-kroy'ah, dis-kro'ah) [ dys- + G. *chroia, chroa,* color. CHROM- ]. A bad complexion; discoloration of the skin.

**dyschromatopsia** (dis-kro-mă-top'sĭ-ah) [ dys- + G. *chrōma,* color, + *opsis,* vision ]. Dichromatism.

**dyschromatosis** (dis-kro'mă-to'sis) [ dys- + G. *chrōma,* color, + suffix -*osis,* condition ]. An asymptomatic anomaly of pigmentation occurring among the Japanese. May be localized or diffuse.

**dyschro'mia** (dis-kro'mĭ-ah). Any abnormality in the color of the skin.

**dyscinesia** (dis'sĭ-ne'zĭ-ah). Dyskinesia.

**dyscoimesis** (dis-koy-me'sis) [ dys- + G. *koimēsis,* a sleeping, fr. *koimaō,* to put to sleep ]. A form of insomnia marked by difficulty or delay in falling asleep.

**dyscoria** (dis-ko'rĭ-ah) [ dys- + G. *korē,* pupil of eye ]. Abnormality in the shape of the pupil.

**dyscrasia** (dis-kra'zhĭ-ah) [ G. bad temperament, fr. dys- + *krasis,* a mixing ]. 1. A morbid general state resulting from the presence of abnormal material in the blood. 2. An old term to indicate disease.

    **blood d.,** a diseased state of the blood; usually refers to abnormal cellular elements of more or less permanent character.

    **lymphatic d.,** obsolete term for Hodgkin's disease.

**dyscra'sic, dyscrat'ic.** Pertaining to or affected with dyscrasia.

**dyscrinism** (dis-kri'nizm) [ dys- + G. *krinō,* to separate, secrete ]. An obsolete word denoting a condition resulting from an altered secretion of any of the glands, especially of the endocrines.

**dysdiadochocinesia** (dis-di-ad'o-ko-sĭ-ne'zĭ-ah). Dysdiadochokinesia.

**dysdiadochokinesia** (dis-di-ad'o-ko-kĭ-ne'zĭ-ah) [ dys- + diadochokinesia, *q. v.* ]. Impairment of the power of alternately moving a limb in opposite directions, as of flexion and extension.

**dysdiemorrhysis** (dis'di-e-mor'ĭ-sis) [ dys- + G. *dia,* through, + *haima,* blood, + *rhysis,* a flowing. RHE- ]. Sluggishness of the capillary circulation.

**dys'ekpne'a** [ dys- + G. *ek,* out, + *pnoia,* breathing ]. The clinical state of protracted or difficult expiration.

**dysembryoma** (dis-em'brĭ-o'mah). A teratoid tumor with its tissues showing more irregular arrangement than the typical embryomas.

**dysembryoplasia** (dis-em'brĭ-o-pla'zĭ-ah) [ dys- + G. *embryon,* fetus, + *plasis,* a molding ]. Prenatal malformation.

**dysemia** (dis-e'mĭ-ah) [ dys- + G. *haima,* blood ]. Any abnormal condition or disease of the blood.

**dysencepha'lia splanchnocys'tica.** Gruber's syndrome; a congenital polycystic disease of the liver and kidneys, associated with meningoencephalocele.

**dysendocrinism** (dis-en-dok'rin-izm). Dysendocrinia; dysendocriniasis; obsolete terms denoting faulty or deficient action of the endocrine glands, and the disorders resulting therefrom.

**dyseneia** (dis'e-ne'ah) [ dys- + G. *ania,* bridle; *dysēnios,* refractory ]. Defective articulation secondary to deafness.

**dysenteric** (dis'en-tĕr'ik). Relating to or suffering from dysentery.

**dysentery** (dis'en-tĕr-ĭ) [ G. *dysenteria,* fr. *dys-,* bad, + *entera,* bowels ]. A disease marked by frequent watery stools, often with blood and mucus, and characterized clinically by pain, tenesmus, fever, and dehydration.

    **ame'bic d.,** diarrhea resulting from ulcerative inflammation of the colon, caused by *Entamoeba hystolytica* or other amoebae; may be mild or severe and associated with systemic infestation by amebas.

    **bac'illary d.,** infection with *Shigella dysenteriae, Shigella flexneri,* or other organisms.

    **balantid'ial d.,** a type of colitis resembling in many respects amebic d.; caused by the parasite *Balantidium coli.*

    **bilhar'zial d.,** d. due to infection with *Schistosoma japonica, S. mansoni,* or *S. haematobium.*

    **chronic d. of cattle,** Johne's *disease.*

    **ful'minating d.,** malignant d.

    **helmin'thic d.,** due to infection with vermiform parasites in the intestine.

    **Japanese d.,** bacillary d.

    **lamb d.,** a specific d. of lambs in Scotland and certain other countries caused by type B toxins of *Clostridium perfringens;* see also enterotoxemia.

    **lying-down d.,** term applied to bacillary d., as opposed to amebic or "walking d."

    **malig'nant d.,** d. in which the symptoms are intensely acute, leading to prostration, collapse, and often death.

    **Sonne d.,** d. due to *Shigella sonnei.* Sometimes milder than other types of bacterial (*Shigella*) d.

    **spiril'lar d.,** a form of d. or diarrhea, described as occurring in the south of France, believed to be caused by a spirillum present in great numbers in the intestinal epithelia.

    **swine d.,** an acute hemorrhagic colitis of swine, often accompanied by gastritis; the small intestines usually are not involved; it is thought to be caused by *Treponema hyodysenteriae* and has a high mortality rate, especially among feeder pigs.

    **viral d.,** profuse watery diarrhea due to, or thought to be due to, a virus.

**winter d. of cattle,** a specific, highly contagious and severe disease of unknown origin; the disease is seen in the cold months of the year, outbreaks generally abate after a few days; the death rate is low, but the loss in flesh and milk is often high.

**dyserethism** (dis-ěr'e-thizm) [ dys- + G. *erethismos,* irritation ]. A condition of slow response to stimuli.

**dysergia** (dis-er'jĭ-ah) [ dys- + G. *ergon,* work ]. A lack of harmonious action between the muscles concerned in executing any definite voluntary movement.

**dysesthesia** (dis-es-the'zĭ-ah) [ G. *dysaisthesia,* fr. *dys-,* hard, difficult, + *aisthēsis,* sensation ]. 1. Impairment of sensation short of anesthesia. 2. A condition in which a disagreeable sensation is produced by ordinary stimuli.

**dysfibrinogenemia** (dis'fi-brin'o-jĕ-ne'mĭ-ah). A familial disorder of qualitatively abnormal fibrinogens. Various types are classified as follows: Amsterdam, Bethesda II, Cleveland, Los Angeles, Saint Louis, Zurich I and II: major defect, aggregation of fibrin monomers; thrombin time prolonged; inhibitory effect on normal clotting; asymptomatic. Bethesda I and Detroit: major defect, fibrinopeptide release; thrombin time prolonged; inhibitory effect on normal clotting; abnormal bleeding. Baltimore: major defect, fibrinopeptide release; thrombin time prolonged; no inhibitory effect on normal clotting; bleeding and thrombosis. Leuven: major defect, questionable aggregation of fibrin monomers; thrombin time prolonged; slight inhibitory effect on normal clotting; abnormal bleeding. Metz: major defect unreported; thrombin time infinite; effect on normal clotting unreported; abnormal bleeding. Nancy: major defect, aggregation of fibrin monomers; thrombin time prolonged; slight inhibitory effect on normal clotting; asymptomatic. Oklahoma: major defect unreported; thrombin time normal; no effect on normal clotting; abnormal bleeding. Oslo: major defect unreported; thrombin time shortened; effect on normal clotting unreported; abnormal thrombosis. Parma: major defect unreported; thrombin time infinite; no inhibitory effect on normal clotting; abnormal bleeding. Paris I: major defect unreported; thrombin time infinite; inhibitory effect on normal clotting; asymptomatic. Paris II: major defect unreported; thrombin time prolonged; inhibitory effect on normal clotting; asymptomatic. Troyes: major defect unreported; thrombin time prolonged; effect on normal clotting unreported; asymptomatic. Vancouver: major defect unreported; thrombin time prolonged; no effect on normal clotting; abnormal bleeding. Wiesbaden: major defect, aggregation of fibrin monomers; thrombin time prolonged; inhibitory effect on normal clotting; bleeding and thrombosis.

**dysfunction** (dis-funk'shun). Difficult or abnormal function.

**constitu'tional hepatic d.,** familial nonhemolytic *jaundice.*

**dental d.,** abnormal functioning of dental structures.

**papillary muscle d.,** papillary muscle syndrome; impaired function of a papillary muscle, usually due to ischemia or infarction, with resulting incompetence of the mitral valve.

**dysgam'maglob'uline'mia.** A disturbance of the percentage distribution of γ-globulins.

**dysgenesis** (dis-jen'ĕ-sis) [ dys- + G. *genesis,* generation ]. Defective embryonic development.

**gonadal d.,** defective gonadal development; varying types and degrees have been identified; gonadal aplasia or agenesis, rudimentary gonads, congenitally defective gonads, and true hermaphroditism. The character of the external genitalia, genital ducts, and secondary sexual development are only sometimes uniquely related to a given type of gonadal d.

**iridocorneal mesodermal d.,** Rieger's anomaly or syndrome; mesodermal d. of cornea and iris, producing pupillary anomalies, posterior embryotoxon, and secondary glaucoma.

**seminiferous tubule d.,** germinal aplasia; a disorder in which the seminiferous tubules exhibit an abnormal cyto-architecture and extensive hyalinization. The testes are small, and few spermatozoa are formed. The body habitus may be eunuchoid, gynecomastia may be present, and urinary gonadotropin output is usually elevated. The incidence of mental deficiency and illness is above normal.

Sex chromatin may be male or female. Androgen secretion ranges from subnormal to normal. Seminiferous tubule d. is a constant feature of (and is often used synonymously with) Klinefelter's *syndrome, q.v.*

**dysgen'ic.** Applying to factors that have a detrimental effect upon hereditary qualities, physical or mental. The opposite of eugenic.

**dysgerminoma** (dis-jer'mĭ-no'mah) [ dys- + L. *germen,* a bud or sprout, + G. suffix -*ōma,* tumor ]. A rare malignant neoplasm of the ovary, a counterpart of seminoma of the testis. D.'s are composed of undifferentiated gonadal germinal cells, and occur more frequently in patients less than 20 years of age. The neoplasms are gray-yellow and firm, contain foci of necrosis and hemorrhage, and tend to be encapsulated; characteristically, they spread by way of lymphatic vessels, but widespread metastases also occur.

**dysgeusia** (dis-gu'sĭ-ah) [ dys- + G. *geusis,* taste ]. Impairment or perversion of the gustatory sense.

**dysglycemia** (dis-gli-se'mĭ-ah). A condition of abnormal carbohydrate metabolism, marked by the excretion of sugar in the urine, but differing from diabetes by its benign evolution and prognosis; a syndrome rather than a disease. Obsolete.

**dysgnathia** (dis-na'thĭ-ah) [ dys- + G. *gnathos,* jaw ]. Designation for those abnormalities that extend beyond the teeth and include the maxilla or mandible, or both.

**dysgnosia** (dis-no'sĭ-ah) [ G. *dysgnōsia,* difficulty of knowing. GNO- ]. Any cognitive disorder, *i.e.,* any mental disorder or disease.

**dysgon'ic** [ dys- + G. *gonikos,* relating to the seed or offspring ]. A term used to indicate that the growth of a bacterial culture is slow and relatively poor; used especially in reference to the growth of cultures of the bovine tubercle bacillus (*Mycobacterium bovis*). See also eugonic.

**dysgraphia** (dis-graf'ĭ-ah) [ dys- + G. *graphē,* writing ]. 1. Difficulty in writing. 2. Writer's *cramp.*

**dyshematopoiesia** (dis-he'mă-to-poy-e'sĭ-ah) [ dys- + G. *haima* (*haimat-*), blood, + *poiēsis,* making ]. Imperfect formation of blood.

**dyshidria** (dis-hid'rĭ-ah). Dyshidrosis.

**dyshidrosis, dysidrosis** (dis-ĭ-dro'sis) [ dys- + G. *hidrōs,* sweat ]. Pompholyx; cheiropompholyx; a vesicular or vesicopustular eruption that occurs primarily on the hands and feet; the lesions spread peripherally but have a tendency to central clearing.

**dyshormonism** (dis-hor'mo-nizm). Obsolete term, denoting deficiency in any of the internal secretions, or hormones.

**dyshypophysia, dyshypophysism** (dis-hi-po-fiz'ĭ-ah, dis-hi-pof'ĭ-sizm). Obsolete terms denoting perverted action of the anterior lobe of the hypophysis cerebri, and the symptoms resulting therefrom.

**dysidria** (dis-id'rĭ-ah). Dyshidrosis.

**dysinsulinism** (dis-in'su-lin-izm). Disordered secretion of insulin, resulting in irregular attacks of hyperglycemia and hypoglycemia, due to disease of the pancreas involving the islands of Langerhans. Obsolete usage.

**dyskaryosis** (dis-kăr-ĭ-o'sis) [ dys- + G. *karyon,* nucleus, + suffix -*ōsis,* condition ]. Abnormal maturation seen in exfoliated cells which have normal cytoplasm but hyperchromatic nuclei, or irregular chromatin distribution; d. may be followed by the development of a malignant neoplasm.

**dyskaryotic** (dis-kăr-ĭ-ot'ik). Pertaining to or characterized by dyskaryosis.

**dyskeratoma** (dis-kĕr-ă-to'mah) [ dys- + G. *keras,* horn, + suffix -*oma,* tumor ]. A skin tumor showing dyskeratosis.

**warty d.,** a benign solitary tumor of the skin, usually of the scalp, face, or neck, with a central keratotic plug; it appears to arise from a hair follicle, and microscopically resembles a lesion of keratosis follicularis but is larger, with more extensive epithelial downgrowth.

**dyskeratosis** (dis-kĕr-ă-to'sis) [ dys- + G. *keras,* horn, + suffix -*osis,* condition ]. A defect in keratin formation in which some cells of the epidermis undergo premature or atypical keratinization. It may be benign or malignant.

**dyskinesia** (dis-kĭ-ne′zĭ-ah) [ dys- + G. *kinēsis,* movement ]. Difficulty in performing voluntary movements.

 **d. al′gera,** a hysterical condition in which active movement causes pain.

 **extrapyramidal d.'s,** movement disorders attributed to pathological states of one or the other part of the extrapyramidal motor system (see extrapyramidal) and generally characterized by insuppressible, stereotyped, automatic movements that cease only during sleep; examples are Parkinson's disease, chorea, athetosis, and hemiballism.

 **d. intermittens,** intermittent limping.

 **tardive oral d.,** (1) a syndrome marked by involuntary movement of the lips or jaw and other dystonic gestures; (2) an extrapyramidal effect of certain psychotropic drug treatments.

 **tracheobronchial d.,** degeneration of elastic and connective tissue of bronchi and trachea.

**dyslalia** (dis-la′lĭ-ah, -lal′ĭ-ah) [ dys- + G. *lalia,* talking ]. Disorder of articulation due to structural abnormalities of the articulatory organs or impaired hearing.

**dyslexia** (dis-lek′sĭ-ah) [ dys- + G. *lexis,* word, phrase ]. Incomplete alexia; a level of reading ability markedly below that expected on the basis of the individual's level of over-all intelligence or ability in skills.

**dyslipidosis** (dis-lip-ĭ-do′sis). An inborn disorder of lipid metabolism.

**dyslochia** (dis-lo′kĭ-ah) [ dys- + G. *lochia, q.v.* ]. Abnormal puerperal discharge.

**dyslogia** (dis-lo′jĭ-ah) [ dys- + G. *logos,* speaking, reason ]. 1. Impairment in the power of speech in consequence of a central lesion. 2. Impairment of the reasoning faculty.

**dysmasesis** (dis-mă-se′sis) [ dys- + G. *masēsis,* chewing ]. Difficulty in mastication.

**dys′mature.** 1. Denoting faulty development or ripening; often connotes structural or functional abnormalities, or both. 2. In obstetrics, denotes an infant whose birth weight is inappropriately low for its gestational age.

**dysmegalopsia** (dis-meg′ă-lop′sĭ-ah) [ dys- + G. *megas,* great, + *opsis,* vision ]. Difficulty in appreciation of the size of objects; a condition in which objects appear larger than they are.

**dysme′lia** [ dys- + G. *melos,* limb ]. A congenital abnormality characterized by missing or foreshortened extremities, sometimes with associated spine abnormalities; caused by metabolic disturbance at the time of limb anlage development.

**dysmenorrhea** (dis-men-o-re′ah) [ dys- + G. *mēn,* month, + *rhoia,* a flow ]. Difficult and painful menstruation.

 **essential d.,** primary d.

 **functional d.,** primary d.

 **intrinsic d.,** primary d.

 **mechanical d.,** d. due to an obstruction to the escape of the menstrual blood, as in cervical stenosis.

 **mem′branous d.,** d. accompanied by an exfoliation of the menstrual decidua.

 **obstructive d.,** mechanical d.

 **ova′rian d.,** d. due to disease of an ovary; secondary d.

 **primary d.,** d. due to a functional disturbance and not to inflammation, new growths, or anatomic factors; intrinsic d.; functional d.; essential d.

 **secondary d.,** d. due to inflammation, infection, tumor, or anatomical or orthopaedic factors.

 **spasmod′ic d.,** d. accompanied by painful contractions of the uterus.

 **tubal d.,** d. due to stenosis or other abnormal condition of the Fallopian tubes; secondary d.

 **ureter′ic d.,** pain due to spasm of the ureter occurring at the time of the menses; secondary d.

 **u′terine d.,** d. resulting from disease of the uterus; secondary d.

 **vag′inal d.,** d. due to obstruction or other abnormal condition in the vagina; secondary d.

**dysmentia** (dis-men′shĭ-ah) [ dys- + L. *mens* (*ment*-), mind ]. A disturbance in intellectual functioning which may be temporary.

**dysmetria** (dis-me′trĭ-ah, -met′rĭ-ah) [ dys- + G. *metron,* measure ]. A form of dysergia in which the subject is unable to arrest a muscular movement at the desired point.

**dysmim′ia** [ dys- + G. *mimeomai,* to mimic ]. 1. Impairment of the power of expression by gestures. 2. Imperfect power of imitation.

**dysmnesia** (dis-ne′zĭ-ah) [ dys- + G. *mnēmē* (in compounds *mnēsi*-), memory. MN- ]. A naturally poor or an impaired memory.

**dysmor′phia.** Dysmorphism.

 **mandibulo-oculofacial d.,** *dyscephalia* mandibulo-oculofacialis.

**dysmorphism** (dis-mor′fizm) [ G. *dysmorphia,* badness of form ]. 1. Abnormality of shape. 2. Allomorphism.

**dysmorphophobia** (dis-mor-fo-fo′bĭ-ah) [ dys- + G. *morphē,* form, + *phobos,* fear ]. A morbid fear of deformity.

**dysmyelination** (dis-mi-ĕ-lĭ-na′shun). Breakdown of a myelin sheath of a nerve fiber, caused by abnormal myelin metabolism.

**dysmyotonia** (dis-mi-o-to′nĭ-ah) [ dys- + G. *mys,* muscle, + *tonos,* tension, tone ]. Abnormal muscular tonicity (either hyper- or hypo-); see dystonia.

**dysnystaxis** (dis-nis-tak′sis) [ dys- + G. *nystaxis,* , drowsiness ]. Light sleep; a condition of half sleep.

**dysodontiasis** (dis-o-don-ti′ă-sis) [ dys- + G. *odous,* tooth, + suffix -*iasis,* condition ]. Difficulty or irregularity in the eruption of the teeth.

**dysontogenesis** (dis-on′to-jen′ĕ-sis) [ dys- + G. *ōn,* being, + *genesis,* generation ]. Defective development of the individual.

**dysontogenetic** (dis-on-to-jĕ-net′ik). Marked by defective development of the individual.

**dysopia, dysopsia** (dis-o′pĭ-ah, dis-op′sĭ-ah) [ G. *dysōpia,* fr. *dys-,* bad, + *opsis,* vision ]. Impaired sight.

**dysorexia** (dis-o-rek′sĭ-ah) [ dys- + G. *orexis,* appetite ]. Diminished or perverted appetite.

**dysosmia** (dis-oz′mĭ-ah) [ dys- + G. *osmē,* smell ]. Impaired sense of smell.

**dysosteogenesis** (dis-os-te-o-jen′ĕ-sis) [ dys- + G. *osteon,* bone, + *genesis,* production ]. Dysostosis; defective bone formation.

**dysostosis** (dis-os-to′sis) [ dys- + G. *osteon,* bone, + suffix -*osis,* condition ]. Dysosteogenesis.

 **acrofacial d.,** acrofacial syndrome; mandibulofacial d. associated with malformations of the extremities.

 **cleidocranial (or clidocranial) d.,** a development defect characterized by absence or rudimentary development of the clavicles, abnormal shape of the skull with depression of the sagittal suture, frontal bosses, and many Wormian bones, and aplasia or hypoplasia of teeth. Autosomal dominant inheritance.

 **cranial d.,** Crouzon's *disease.*

 **craniofacial d.,** Crouzon's *disease.*

 **mandibulofacial d.,** a variable syndrome of malformations primarily of derivatives of the first branchial arch; the palpebral fissures slope outward and downward with notches or coloboma in the outer third of the lower lids, there are bony defects or hypoplasia of malar bones and zygoma, hypoplasia of the mandible, macrostomia with high or cleft palate and malposition and malocclusion of teeth, low-set malformed external ears, atypical hair growth, occasional pits or clefts between mouth and ear. Called Franceschetti's syndrome if complete or nearly complete; Treacher Collins syndrome if limited to orbit and malar region. This plus certain other facial defects called first arch syndrome by Francois and others.

 **metaphysial d.,** a rare developmental abnormality of the skeleton in which metaphyses of tubular bones are expanded by deposits of cartilage.

 **d. multiplex,** Hurler's *syndrome.*

 **orodigitofacial d.,** an inherited syndrome with varying combinations of defects of the oral cavity, face, and hands, including lobulated or bifid tongue, cleft or pseudocleft palate, tongue tumors, missing or malpositioned teeth, pug-nose, depressed nasal bridge, brachydactyly, clinodactyly, incomplete syndactyly, and frequently mental retardation; it is found only in females, with X-linked dominant inheritance from mother to daughter, and is probably lethal in male fetuses; also known as oral-facial-digital

(OFD), orodigitofacial, Papillon-Léage and Psaume syndrome.

**otomandibu'ular d.,** hypoplasia of the mandible, often with malformation of the temporomandibular joint, associated with malformations of the ear but not eye or malar defects.

**dysox'idative.** Caused by difficult or deficient oxidation.

**dysoxidi'zable.** Not readily oxidized.

**dyspal'lia** [ dys- + L. *pallium,* cloak ]. Developmental distortion of the brain mantle.

**dyspancreatism** (dis-pan'kre-ă-tizm). A condition of disturbed functioning of the pancreas. Obsolete.

**dyspareunia** (dis-pă-ru'nĭ-ah) [ dys- + G. *pareunos,* lying beside, fr. *para,* beside, + *eunē,* a bed ]. The occurrence of pain in the sexual act.

**dyspep'sia** [ dys- + G. *pepsis,* digestion. PEP- ]. Indigestion or upset stomach.

**adhesion d.,** pain, d., and other symptoms alleged to result from perigastric adhesions.

**acid d.,** d. associated with undue gastric acidity.

**aton'ic d.,** d. with impaired tone in the muscular walls of the stomach.

**fermen'tative d.,** d. accompanied by fermentation of the contents of the stomach, usually occurring in gastric dilation.

**flat'ulent d.,** d. with frequent eructations of swallowed air, sometimes without underlying organic disease.

**functional d.,** (1) atonic d.; (2) nervous d.

**gastric d.,** impairment of gastric digestion.

**intestinal d.,** alleged to result from impaired digestive power of the intestines.

**mastoid d.,** d. occurring as the main symptomatic expression of mastoiditis.

**nervous d.,** d. associated with nervousness, tension, or neurosis.

**reflex d.,** nervous d. excited by reflex irritation from disease in some other part.

**dyspep'tic.** Relating to or suffering from dyspepsia.

**dysper'matism, dysper'mia.** Dysspermatism.

**dysphagia, dysphagy** (dis-fa'jĭ-ah, dis-fa'jĭ) [ dys- + G. *phagein,* to eat. PHAG- ]. Aglutition; aphagia; odynophagia; difficulty in swallowing.

**d. luso'ria** [ coinage from L. *lusus naturae,* a sport of nature ], d. said to be due to compression by the right subclavian artery arising abnormally from the thoracic aorta and passing behind or in front of the esophagus.

**d. nervo'sa, nervous d.,** esophagism.

**sideropenic d.,** Plummer-Vinson *syndrome.*

**vallecular d.,** d. caused by food becoming lodged above the epiglottis.

**dysphag'ocyto'sis.** Disordered phagocytosis, especially failure of cells to ingest and digest bacteria.

**congenital d.,** chronic granulomatous *disease.*

**dysphasia** (dis-fa'zĭ-ah) [ dys- + G. *phasis,* speaking ]. Lack of coordination in speech, and failure to arrange words in an understandable way; related to cortical damage.

**dysphemia** (dis-fe'mĭ-ah) [ dys- + G. *phēmē,* speech ]. Disorder of phonation, articulation, or hearing due to emotional or intellectual deficits.

**dysphonia** (dis-fo'nĭ-ah) [ dys- + G. *phōnē,* voice ]. Hoarseness; difficulty or pain in speaking.

**d. plicae ventricula'ris,** phonation with the ventricular bands rather than with the vocal cords, one of the causes of hoarseness.

**d. pu'berum,** the breaking of the voice in boys at puberty.

**d. spas'tica,** phonic spasm; a spasmodic contraction of the adductor muscles of the larynx excited by attempted phonation, occurring chiefly in public speakers and analogous seemingly to writer's cramp.

**dysphoria** (dis-fo'rĭ-ah) [ G. extreme discomfort, fr. *dys-,* difficult, bad, + *phora,* a bearing ]. A feeling of unpleasantness or discomfort.

**dysphrasia** (dis-fra'zĭ-ah) [ dys- + G. *phrasis,* speaking ]. Dysphasia.

**dysphylaxia** (dis-fi-lak'sĭ-ah) [ dys- + G. *phylaxis,* watching ]. A form of insomnia marked by too early awakening.

**dys'pigmenta'tion.** Any abnormality in the formation or distribution of pigment, especially in the skin; usually applied to an abnormal reduction in pigmentation (depigmentation).

**dyspinealism** (dis-pin'e-al-izm). The syndrome supposed to result from the deficiency of pineal gland secretion.

**dyspituitarism** (dis-pĭ-tu'ĭ-těr-izm). The complex of phenomena due to abnormal secretion, either excessive or deficient, of the pituitary body.

**dysplasia** (dis-pla'zĭ-ah) [ dys- + G. *plasis,* a molding ]. Abnormal tissue development; see also heteroplasia.

**anhidrotic ectodermal d.,** hereditary ectodermal d.; Christ-Siemens syndrome; congenital absence of sweat glands resulting in heat intolerance, malformed and missing teeth, sparse fragile hair; sometimes with deformed nails, absent breast tissue, mental retardation or syndactyly; X-linked recessive inheritance.

**anteroposterior d.,** anteroposterior facial d.; anterofacial d.; abnormal growth of the face or cranium in an anteroposterior direction as seen and measured from a cephalogram.

**asphyxiating thoracic d.,** hereditary hypoplasia of the thorax, associated with pelvic skeletal abnormality.

**atriodigital d.,** Hold-Oram *syndrome.*

**cervical d.,** d. of the uterine cervix; epithelial d. of cervical squamous epithelium, occurring most often in young women; appears to regress frequently, but may progress over a long period to carcinoma.

**chondroectodermal d.,** Ellis-van Crevald syndrome; triad of chondrodysplasia (dwarfism due to short extremities but normal trunk, characteristic changes of epiphyses and ossification centers), ectodermal dysplasia (dysplasia or hypoplasia of teeth and nails), and polydactyly, with congenital heart defects in over half of patients; autosomal recessive inheritance.

**congenital ectodermal d.,** *dyscephalia* mandibulo-oculofacialis.

**craniometaphysial d.,** syndrome of metaphysial d. associated with severe sclerosis and overgrowth of bones of the skull (leontiasis ossea).

**cretinoid d.,** see cretinism.

**dentinal d.,** *dentinogenesis* imperfecta.

**diaphysial d.,** Engelmann's disease; progressive, symmetrical fusiform enlargement of the shafts of long bones characterized by the formation of excessive new periosteal and endosteal bone and irregular conversion of this cortical bone into cancellous bone. Anemia does not occur as a rule. See also osteopetrosis.

**ectodermal d.,** a congenital defect of the ectodermal tissues, including the skin and its appendages, manifested in dry skin, thin hair, deformities of the nails and teeth, bossing of the frontal bones, and marked diminution of sweat glands with an intolerance to heat; see also anhidrotic ectodermal d. and hidrotic ectodermal d.

**enamel d.,** *amelogenesis* imperfecta.

**d. epiphysia'lis hemime'lia,** tarsomegaly.

**d. epiphysialis multiplex,** multiple epiphysial d.; a developmental error of epiphyses characterized by difficulty in walking, pain and stiffness of joints, stubby fingers and often dwarfism of short-limb type; on x-ray the epiphyses are mottled and irregular, ossification centers are late in appearance and may be multiple, but the vertebrae are normal.

**d. epiphysia'lis puncta'ta** chondrodystrophia calcificans congenita; stippled epiphysis; a developmental error of the epiphyses characterized by severe deformities, the epiphyses are ossified from several discrete centers and have a stippled appearance, the shafts of the long bones are thick; congenital cataract and mental retardation are often present.

**epithelial d.,** nonmalignant disorders of differentiation of epithelial cells.

**familial fibrous d. of jaws.,** cherubism.

**familial white folded d., oral,** a benign, hereditary abnormality with clinical characteristics of grayish white oral mucosal lesions of soft consistency, presenting as deep folds with a corrugated appearance.

**fibromuscular d.,** idiopathic, nonatherosclerotic disease leading to stenosis of arteries, usually the renal arteries. Fibromuscular d. of one or both renal arteries is one cause of hypertension (especially in relatively young women) that can be treated surgically. See also fibromuscular *hyperplasia* and perimuscular *fibrosis.*.

**fibrous d. of bone,** Jaffe-Lichtenstein disease; a disturbance of medullary bone maintenance in which bone undergoing physiologic lysis is replaced by abnormal proliferation of fibrous tissue, resulting in asymmetric distortion and expansion of bone; may be confined to a single bone (monostotic fibrous d.) or involve multiple bones (polyostotic fibrous d.).

**hereditary ectodermal d.,** anhidrotic ectodermal d.

**hereditary renal-retinal d.,** a disorder characterized by retinitis pigmentosa, nephrogenic diabetes insipidus, and progressive azotemia; histologically, the kidneys exhibit hyalinization of some, but not all, glomeruli, focal tubular atrophy, vascular sclerosis, a fibrotic interstitium, thickening of tubular basement membranes, and an absence of tubular cysts in the cortex and medulla. Autosomal recessive inheritance of this disorder appears probable.

**hidrotic ectodermal d.,** congenital dystrophy of the nails and hair, often associated with keratoderma of the palms and soles.

**lymphopenic thymic d.,** thymic *alymphoplasia.*

**mammary d.,** fibrocystic *disease* of the breasts.

**mandibulofacial d.,** mandibulofacial *dysostosis.*

**metaphysial d.,** a failure of remodeling to normal tubular structure of new bone at the metaphyses of long bones; the ends of long bones appear to be expanded and porotic, with thin cortex. There may be an associated overgrowth of head bones (craniometaphysial d.).

**monostotic fibrous d.,** see fibrous d. of bone.

**multiple epiphysial d.,** d. epiphysialis multiplex.

**oculoauriculovertebral d.,** Goldenhar's syndrome; characterized by epibulbar dermoids, preauricular appendages, micrognathia, and vertebral and other anomalies.

**oculodentodigital d.,** Meyer-Schwickerath and Weyers syndrome; oculodentodigital syndrome; microphthalmia, coloboma or anomalies of the iris associated with malformed and malpositioned teeth, and anomalies of the fingers including syndactyly, camptodactyly, or absent phalanges.

**oculovertebral d.,** oculovertebral syndrome; Weyers-Thier syndrome; d. oculovertebralis; microphthalmia, colobomas or anophthalmia with small orbit, twisted face due to unilateral dysplasia of maxilla, macrostomia with malformed teeth and malocclusion, vertebral malformations, and branched and hypoplastic ribs.

**polyostotic fibrous d.,** multifocal osteitis fibrosa; the occurrence of lesions of fibrous d. in multiple bones, commonly on one side of the body; may occur with other abnormalities in Albright's disease. See also fibrous d. of bone.

**pseudoachondroplastic spondyloepiphysial d.,** severe dwarfism with onset at 2 to 4 years of age; it is characterized by short limbs, a relatively long trunk, and a normal skull and facies.

**retinal d.,** an overgrowth of glial tissue compensating for aplasia of neural elements.

**spondyloepiphysial d.,** a group of conditions characterized by growth insufficiency of the vertebral column, with flattening of vertebrae, and often involving the epiphyses at the hip and shoulder; results in dwarfism of the short trunk type, often also with short extremities, sometimes with other malformations; types with dominant, recessive, and X-linked recessive inheritance have been described in different families.

**ventriculoradial d.,** a congenital syndrome consisting of a ventricular septal defect with associated absence of thumb or radius.

**dysplas′tic.** Pertaining to or marked by dysplasia.

**dyspnea** (disp-ne′ah) [ G. *dyspnoia,* fr. *dys-,* bad, + *pnoē,* breathing ]. Shortness of breath; subjective difficulty or distress in breathing, frequently rapid breathing, usually associated with serious disease of the heart or lungs.

**paroxysmal nocturnal d.,** acute d. appearing suddenly at night, usually waking the patient after an hour or two of sleep; caused by pulmonary congestion and edema which result from left-sided heart failure.

**Traube's d.,** inspiratory d. with maximal expansion of the chest and a slow respiratory rhythm.

**dyspneic** (disp-ne′ik). Out of breath; relating to or suffering from dyspnea.

**dyspnoeneurosis** (disp-ne-nu-ro′sis). A nervous shortness of breath.

**dyspragia** (dis-pra′jĭ-ah) [ G. lack of success, fr. *prassō,* to do ]. Dyspraxia.

**d. intermit′tens,** intermittent limping.

**dyspraxia** (dis-prak′sĭ-ah) [ dys- + G. *praxis,* a doing ]. Impaired or painful functioning in any organ.

**dysprosium** (dis-pro′sĭ-um). A metallic element of the lanthanide (rare earth) series, symbol Dy, atomic No. 66, atomic weight 162.51.

**dysproteinemia** (dis-pro′tēn-e′mĭ-ah, -pro′te-in-e′mĭ-ah). An abnormality in plasma proteins, especially among the albumin and globulin fractions, resulting from a metabolic disorder.

**dysraphia** (dis-raf′ĭ-ah). Dysraphism.

**dysraphism** (dis′rǎ-fizm) [ dys- + G. *raphē,* suture ]. Dysraphia. 1. Defective fusion. 2. Incomplete raphe formation.

**dysrhythmia** (dis-rith′mĭ-ah) [ dys- + G. *rhythmos,* rhythm ]. Defective rhythm. See also entries and fig. under rhythm.

**electroencephalographic d.,** a diffusely irregular brain wave tracing.

**paroxys′mal cer′ebral d.,** a diffusely abnormal electroencephalogram considered by some to indicate epilepsy.

**dyssebacia** (dis′sĕ-ba′shĭ-ah) [ dys- + L. *sebum,* grease ]. Seborrheic *dermatitis.*

**dysspermatism, dysspermia** (dis-sper′mǎ-tizm, dis-sper′mĭ-ah) [ dys- + G. *sperma,* seed ]. The occurrence of pain or discomfort in the discharge of the seminal fluid.

**dysspondylism** (dis-spon′dĭ-lizm) [ dys- + G. *spondylos,* vertebra ]. An abnormality of development of the spine or vertebral column.

**dysstasia** (dis-sta′sĭ-ah) [ dys- + G. *stasis,* standing ]. Difficulty in standing.

**dysstatic** (dis-stat′ik). Marked by difficulty in standing.

**dyssyllabia** (dis-sil-la′bĭ-ah) [ dys- + G. *syllabē,* syllable ]. Syllable-stumbling.

**dyssynergia** (dis-sin-er′jĭ-ah) [ dys- + G. *syn,* with, + *ergon,* work ]. Ataxia.

**d. cerebella′ris myoclon′ica,** an affection with symptoms similar to d. cerebellaris progressive, with the addition of myoclonus and epilepsy.

**d. cerebellar′is progressi′va,** Hunt's *syndrome* (1).

**dyssystole** (dis-sis′to-le). A defective cardiac systole; *cf.* asystole.

**dystaxia** (dis-tak′sis) [ dys- + G. *taxis,* order ]. A mild degree of ataxia.

**dysthymia** (dis-thi′mĭ-ah) [ dys- + G. *thymos,* mind, emotion. THYM-2 ]. Any mental disorder or disease.

**dysthy′reo′sis.** Dysthyroidea.

**dysthyroidea, dysthyroidism** (dis-thi-roy′de-ah, dis-thi′-roy-dizm). Obsolete terms for thyroid dysfunction, thought by Plummer to result from the production of a hormone deficient in iodine.

**dystocia** (dis-to′sĭ-ah) [ G. *dystokia,* fr. *dys-,* difficult, + *tokos,* childbirth ]. Difficult childbirth. It is called **fetal d.** if the cause is some abnormality of the fetus, and **maternal d.** if the cause is maternal.

**placen′tal d.,** retention or difficult delivery of the placenta.

**dystonia** (dis-to′nĭ-ah) [ dys- + G. *tonos,* tension ]. A state of abnormal (either hypo- or hyper-) tonicity in any of the tissues.

**d. lenticula′ris,** d. musculorum deformans.

**d. musculo′rum defor′mans,** d. lenticularis; Ziehen-Oppenheim disease; progressive torsion spasm of childhood; an affection, occurring especially in children, marked by muscular contractions producing most peculiar distortions of the spine and hips; the musculature is hypertonic when in action, hypotonic when at rest.

**dyston′ic.** Pertaining to dystonia.

**dystopia** (dis-to′pĭ-ah) [ dys- + G. *topos,* place ]. Malposition.

**d. canthorum,** Waardenburg's *syndrome.*

**d. transver′sa externa testis,** crossing over of the testis under the skin of the dorsum of the penis to the contralateral half of the scrotum; see also *descensus paradoxus testis.*

**d. transver′sa inter′na tes′tis,** the passage of the testes each into a contralateral inguinal canal within the pelvis and coming to lie in the corresponding half of the scrotum; see also *descensus* paradoxus testis.

**dystop'ic.** Malplaced; ectopic; out of place.

**dystrophia** (dis-tro'fĭ-ah) [ L. fr. G. *dys-*, bad, + *trophē*, nourishment ]. Dystrophy.

**d. adipo'sogenita'lis,** adiposogenital dystrophy; adiposogenital syndrome; hypophysis syndrome; adiposis orchica; an imperfectly understood and often misdiagnosed disorder. It is called Fröhlich's syndrome when caused by an adenohypophysial tumor; may also be caused by hypothalamic lesions in areas regulating appetite and gonadal development. It is characterized primarily by obesity and genital hypoplasia. Dwarfism is rare; when present, it is thought to reflect hypothyroidism.

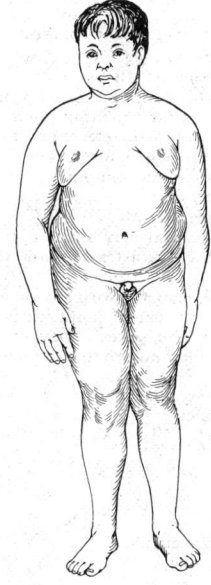

**Dystrophia Adiposogenitalis,. Juvenile Type**

(From Goldzieher, M. A.: *The Endocrine Glands*, Appleton-Century-Crofts, Inc., New York, 1939.)

**d. brevicollis** (brev-ĭ-kol'lis), a condition marked by symptoms of d. adiposogenitalis together with a deforming shortness of the neck, but without synostosis of the cervical vertebrae seen in Klippel-Feil syndrome.

**d. endothelia'lis cor'neae,** cornea guttata (Vogt); droplike corneal endothelial prominences.

**d. epithelia'lis cor'neae,** Fuchs' epithelial *dystrophy*.

**d. myoton'ica,** myotonic *dystrophy*.

**d. un'guium,** dystrophy of the nails.

**dystrophic** (dis-trof'ik). Relating to dystrophy.

**dystrophoneurosis** (dis-trof'o-nu-ro'sis) [ dys- + G. *trophē*, nourishment, + *neuron*, nerve, + suffix *-osis*, condition ]. Any nervous disease associated with faulty nutrition.

**dystrophy** (dis'tro-fĭ) [ dys- + G. *trophē*, nourishment ]. Dystrophia; defective nutrition.

**adiposogenital d.,** *dystrophia* adiposogenitalis.

**Barnes' d.,** a rare type of muscular d., with muscles often hypertrophic and stronger than normal early, but later becoming weak and atrophic.

**childhood muscular d.,** a heritable disorder primarily afflicting boys. Between the ages of 2 and 6 years, muscular weakness first appears in the pelvic girdle and spreads with relative rapidity to the musculature of the pectoral girdle, trunk, and extremities; muscular pseudohypertrophy (enlarged, weakened, inelastic masses) is a common finding, as are contractures of muscle and tendon. Also called pseudohypertrophic d.; pseudomuscular hypertrophy;

pseudohypertrophic muscular paralysis; Duchenne's d., disease, or paralysis.

**craniocarpotarsal d.,** Freeman-Sheldon syndrome; whistling face syndrome; congenital association of skeletal defects (ulnar deviation of hands with camptodactyly, talipes equinovarus, and frontal bone defects) and characteristic facies (protrusion of lips as in whistling, sunken eyes with hypertelorism, and small nose); autosomal dominant inheritance.

**Duchenne's d.,** childhood muscular d.

**elastic d.,** elastic tissue degeneration as observed in chronic actinic effect, senile elastosis, etc.

**facioscapulohumeral muscular d.,** Landouzy-Déjèrine d.; a relatively benign type of d. commencing in childhood and characterized by wasting and weakness, mainly of the muscles of the face, shoulder girdle, and arms; autosomal dominant inheritance.

**fleck d. of cornea,** a bilateral condition characterized by the presence of subtle spots in the corneal stroma; the spots vary in size and shape, and have sharp margins and clear centers; photophobia or increased sensitivity may or may not be present; autosomal dominant inheritance.

**Fuchs' epithelial dystrophy,** dystrophia epithelialis corneae; a condition dependent on a prior endothelial d. of the cornea; it begins with a fine spreading central edema, is eventually bilateral, and occurs predominantly in elderly women.

**Groenouw's corneal d.,** (1) a granular type, with autosomal dominant inheritance; (2) a macular type, with autosomal recessive inheritance.

**gutter d. of cornea,** keratoleptynsis; a marginal furrow usually inferiorly about 1 mm. from limbus and sometimes bilateral; an occasional complication of keratoconjunctivitis sicca and rheumatoid arthritis.

**Landouzy-Déjèrine d.,** facioscapulohumeral muscular d.

**lattice corneal d.,** a reticular type of d. with autosomal dominant inheritance; it is manifest at puberty and progresses slowly; eventually useful vision is lost.

**Leyden-Möbius muscular d.,** limb-girdle muscular d.

**limb-girdle muscular d.,** Leyden-Möbius muscular d.; pelvofemoral muscular d.; a progressive disorder that usually begins in the preadolescent period; manifestations include those of childhood and facioscapulohumeral muscular d.; commonly, the pelvic girdle is most severely involved; autosomal recessive inheritance.

**muscular d.,** myodystrophia; myodystrophy; inborn abnormality of muscle associated with dysfunction and ultimately with deterioration.

**myotonic d.,** dystrophia myotonica; myotonia atropica or dystropica; Steinert's disease; a familial, chronic, and slowly progressive disease inherited as autosomal dominant, with onset usually in the third decade, and marked by atrophy of the muscles, failing vision, lenticular opacities, ptosis, slurred speech, and general muscular weakness; there may be atelectasis of the lungs and cyanosis due to involvement of the diaphragm.

**pelvofemoral muscular d.,** limb-girdle muscular d.

**progressive muscular d.,** Erb's atrophy; a form of progressive muscular atrophy in which the disease begins in the muscle and not in the spinal centers.

**progressive tapetochoroidal d.,** choroideremia (2).

**pseudohypertrophic muscular d.,** childhood muscular d.

**Salzmann's nodular corneal d.,** large and prominent nodules of a solid, opaque material that stands out from the surface of the cornea. Occurs occasionally in persons previously affected by phlyctenular keratitis.

**sympathetic reflex d.,** an illness consisting of superficial and deep pain of a spreading and burning character, vasomotor disturbances, trophic changes, and limitation of movement, occurring in an extremity after some physical disturbance in that extremity.

**dystropy** (dis'tro-pĭ) [ dys- + G. *tropos*, a turning ]. Abnormal or eccentric behavior.

**dysuria** (dis-u'rĭ-ah) [ dys- + G. *ouron*, urine ]. Difficulty or pain in urination.

**dysuric** (dis-u'rik). Relating to or suffering from dysuria.

**dysury** (dis'u-rĭ). Dysuria.

**dysversion** (dis-ver'zhun) [ dys- + L. *verto*, to turn ]. A turning in any direction, less than inversion; particularly d. of the optic nerve head (situs inversus of the optic desk).

# E

**E.** 1. Abbreviation for emmetropia or emmetropic. 2. Abbreviation for extraction *ratio*. 3. As a subscript, refers to expired *gas*.

**E₀⁺, E₀.** Symbols for oxidation-reduction *potential;* see also quinhydrone *electrode*.

**Eagle,** Harry, U. S. physician and cell biologist, \*1905. See E.'s *medium*.

**Eales,** Henry, English physician, 1852–1913. See E.'s *disease*.

**ear** [ A.S. *eáre* ]. 1. The organ of hearing: composed of the **external e.,** which includes the auricle and the external acoustic, or auditory, meatus; the **middle e.,** or the tympanic cavity with its ossicles; and the **internal** or **inner e.,** or labyrinth, which includes the semicircular canals, vestibule, and cochlea. 2. The pinna or auricle (see auricle).

    **aviator's e.,** *aerotitis* media.

    **Aztec e.,** an auricle with the lobule absent.

    **Blainville e.'s,** asymmetry in size or shape of the auricles.

    **boxer's e.,** cauliflower e.

    **Cagot e.,** (kȧ-go′) [ name of a degenerate race in the Pyrenees among whom physical stigmata are common ], an auricle having no lobulus.

    **cauliflower e.,** boxer's e.; thickening and induration of the e. with distortion of contours following extravasation of blood within its tissues.

    **Darwinian e.,** an auricle in which the upper border is not rolled over to form the helix, but projects upward as a flat, sharp edge.

    **lop e.,** see *lop-ear*.

    **Morel's e.,** a large, misshapen, outstanding auricle, with obliterated grooves and thinned edges.

    **Mozart e.,** a deformity of the pinna where the two crura of the antihelix and the crus of the helix are fixed, giving a bulging appearance of the superior part of the pinna. The composer Mozart is said to have possessed this deformity.

    **scroll e.,** a deformity of the external e. in which the pinna is rolled forward.

    **Stahl's e.,** a deformed external e., in which the fossa ovalis and upper portion of the scaphoid fossa are covered by the helix; regarded as a stigma of degenerate constitution.

    **Wildermuth's e.,** an e. in which the helix is turned backward and the anthelix is prominent.

**ear′ache.** Otalgia; otodynia; pain in the ear.

**ear′drum.** *Membrana* tympani.

**Earle,** Wilton R., U. S. pathologist, 1902–1962. See Earle L *fibrosarcoma*.

**Earle's solution** See under solution.

**earth** (urth) [ A.S. *eorthe* ]. 1. The globe; world. 2. Soil; dirt; the loose material on the surface of the earth. 3. An insoluble oxide of aluminum or of certain other elements characterized by a high melting point.

    **alkaline e.'s,** any of the elements in the family Be, Mg, Ca, Sr, Ba, Ra, the hydroxides of which are highly ionized, hence alkaline in water solution.

    **bone e.,** bone *ash*.

    **diatomic e.,** see diatom.

    **fuller's e.,** a refined clay sometimes used as a dusting powder or applied moistened with water as a form of poultice.

    **rare e.'s,** those elements with atomic numbers from 57 to 71, inclusive, often called lanthanides (after lanthanum, first member of the series); they closely resemble one another chemically and are thus difficult to separate from each other.

**earth-eating.** Geophagia.

**ear′wax.** Cerumen.

**eat** [ A.S. *etan* ]. 1. To take solid food. 2. To chew and

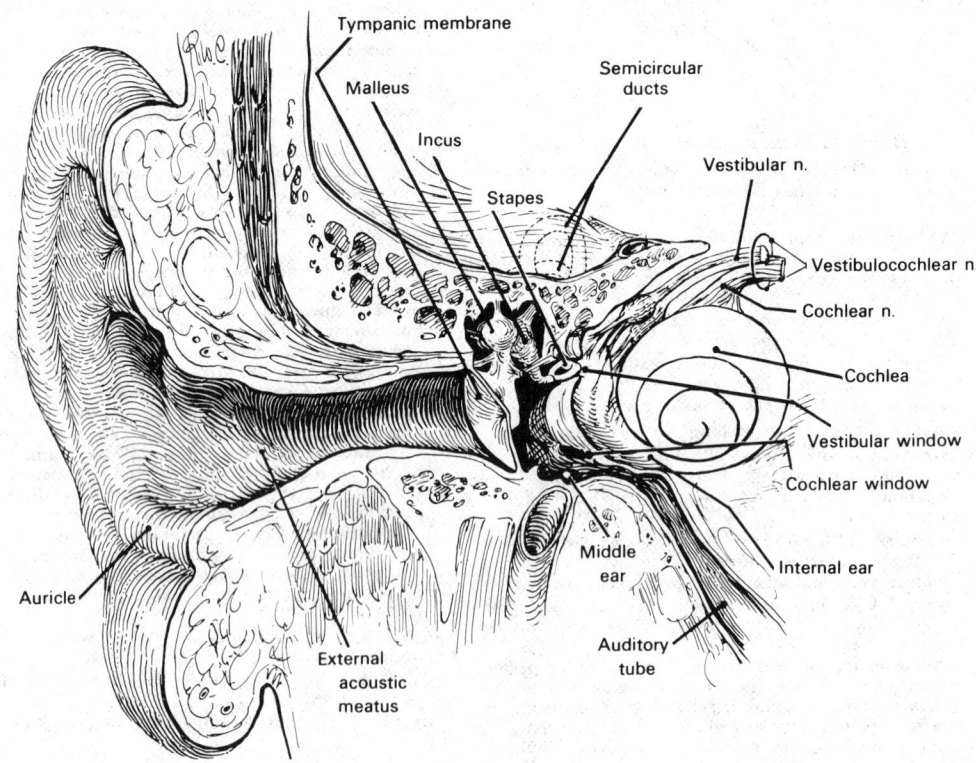

**Ear**
Section through the petrous part of the temporal bone to show the outer, middle, and inner ear

swallow any substance as one would food. 3. To corrode.

**Eaton agent, Eaton agent pneumonia.** See under agent and pneumonia.

**E.B., EB.** Abbreviation for elementary body.

**ebb.** The gradual decline in the opsonic index at the end of the positive phase.

**Ebbecke's reaction.** See under reaction.

**Ebbinghaus,** Hermann, German, 1850–1909. See E. *test.*

**Eberth** (a'bairt), Karl J., German physician, 1835–1926. Gave his name to *Eberthella.* See E.'s *lines, perithelium.*

**Eberthella** (a-ber-tel'lah) [ K. J. *Eberth* ]. An obsolete name of a genus of bacteria. The type species, *E. typhi,* is a member of the genus *Salmonella* (*S. typhi*), and the name *E.* is therefore no longer in use.

**Ebner,** A. G. Victor von, Vienna histologist, 1842–1925. See E.'s *glands, reticulum.*

**ebonation** (e-bo-na'shun). Removal of loose fragments of bone from a wound.

**ébranlement** (ā-brahn-luh-mahnt') [ Fr. ]. Twisting a polyp on its stalk to cause atrophy.

**ebri'etas, ebriety** [ L. fr. *ebrius,* drunk ]. Inebriety; drunkenness.

**Ebstein,** Wilhelm, German physician, 1836–1912. See E.'s *anomaly, disease, sign,* Pel-E. *disease, symptom.*

**eb'ullism** [ L. *ebullire,* to boil out ]. The formation of water vapor bubbles in the tissues brought on by an extreme reduction in barometric pressure. This occurs if the body is exposed to pressures which are found above an altitude of 63,000 feet.

**ebur** (e'bur) [ L. *ivory* ]. A tissue resembling ivory in outward appearance or structure.
  **e. dentis,** dentin; substantia eburnea.

**eburnation** (e-bur-na'shun) [ L. *eburneus,* of ivory ]. A change in exposed subchondral bone in degenerative joint disease in which it is converted into a dense, smooth substance like ivory.

**eburneous** (e-bur'ne-us). Resembling ivory, especially in color.

**EC.** Abbreviation for Enzyme Commission of the International Union of Biochemistry. This abbreviation is used in conjunction with a unique number to define a specific enzyme in the Enzyme Commission's list (*Enzyme Nomenclature,* Elsevier Publishing Co., 1965; see *Science 150:* 719, 1965). For example, EC 1.1.1.1 defines an alcohol dehydrogenase; EC 6.4.1.2 defines acetyl-CoA carboxylase. EC numbers are selectively used in *Stedman* entries.

**ec-.** Prefix fr. G. preposition meaning out of, away from.

**écarteur** (a-kar-tër') [ Fr. *écarter,* to separate ]. A retractor.

**ecaudate** (e-kaw'dāt) [ L. *e-* priv. + *cauda,* tail ]. Tailless.

**ecbolic** (ek-bol'ik) [ G. *ekbolē,* a throwing out, abortion. BALL- ]. 1. Accelerating childbirth; oxytocic; producing abortion. 2. An agent that hastens delivery or produces abortion.

**ecboline** (ek'bō-lēn). Ergotoxine.

**eccentric** (ek-sen'trik) [ G. *ek,* out, + *kentron,* center ]. 1. Abnormal or peculiar in ideas, actions, or speech. 2. Proceeding from a center. 3. Peripheral. (In the second and third meanings often written excentric.)

**eccentrochondroplasia** (ek-sen'tro-kon-dro-pla-zī'ah) [ G. *ek,* out + *kentron,* center, + *chondros,* cartilage, + *plasis,* a molding ]. Abnormal epiphysial development from eccentric centers of ossification.

**eccentropiesis** (ek-sen-tro-pi-e'sis) [ G. *ek,* out, + *kentron,* center, + *piesis,* pressure ]. Pressure exerted from within outward.

**eccephalosis** (ek'sef-al-o'sis) [ G. *ek,* out, + *kephalē,* head ]. Excerebration.

**ecchondroma** (ek-kon-dro'mah) [ G. *ek,* from, + *chondros,* cartilage, + suffix *-oma,* tumor ]. 1. A cartilaginous neoplasm arising as an overgrowth from normally situated cartilage, as a mass protruding from the articular surface of a bone, in contrast to enchondroma (or chondroma proper), which occurs within the bone, or in other structures. 2. An enchondroma which has burst through the shaft of a bone and become pedunculated.

**ecchondrosis** (ek-kon-dro'sis). Ecchondroma.
  **e. physalifor'mis,** e. physaliphora.

**e. physaliph'ora,** e. physaliformis; a notochordal rest of the cranial clivus which may form a small tumor.

**ecchondrotome** (ek-kon'dro-tōm) [ G. *ek,* out, + *chondros,* cartilage, + *tomē,* incision ]. Chondrotome.

**ecchymoma** (ek-ī-mo'mah) [ G. *ek,* out, + *chymos,* juice (CHY-), + suffix *-oma,* tumor ]. A slight hematoma following a bruise.

**ecchymosed** (ek'ī-mōzd). Characterized by or affected with ecchymosis.

**ecchymosis,** pl. **ecchymo'ses** (ek-ī-mo'sis) [ G. *ekchymōsis,* ecchymosis, fr. *ek,* out, + *chymos,* juice ]. A purplish patch caused by extravasation of blood into the skin; ecchymoses differ from petechiae only in size.
  **Bayard's e.,** subpleural and subpericardial hemorrhages in infants who have been suffocated *in utero,* see Tardieu's ecchymoses.
  **H-shaped e.,** the e. observed in cases of rupture of the tendo Achillis.
  **Roederer's ecchymoses,** minute ecchymoses on the pleura and pericardium sometimes seen in stillborn infants, thought to be due to an attempt of the fetus to breathe while in the uterus (anoxic capillary injury).
  **Tardieu's ecchymoses,** Tardieu's spots; subpleural and subpericardial petechiae or ecchymoses (or both), as observed in the tissues of persons who have been strangled, or otherwise asphyxiated; the same pathologic process as that resulting in Bayard's ecchymoses.

**ecchymotic** (ek-ī-mot'ik). Relating to an ecchymosis.

**Eccles** (ek'lz), John C., Australian physiologist, *1903. Nobel laureate, 1963, with Alan L. Hodgkin and Andrew F. Huxley, for their studies of nervous system functions, especially of nerves and synapses.

**eccoprotic** (ek-o-prot'ik) [ G. *ek,* out, + *kopros,* dung ]. Laxative; cathartic.

**eccrine** (ek'rin) [ G. *ek-krino,* to secrete ]. 1. Exocrine. 2. Denoting the flow of sweat.

**eccrinology** (ek'rī-nol'o-jī) [ G. *ek-drino,* to secrete, + *logos,* study ]. The branch of physiology and of anatomy that treats of the secretions and the secreting (exocrine) glands.

**eccrisis** (ek'rī-sis) [ G. separation ]. 1. The removal of waste products. 2. Any waste product; excrement.

**eccritic** (ek-krit'ik). 1. Promoting the expulsion of waste matters. 2. An agent that promotes excretion.

**eccyclomastoma** (ek-si'clo-mas-to'mah). Eccyclomastopathy.

**eccyclomastopathy** (ek-si'clo-mas-top'ā-thī) [ G. *ek,* from, out, + *kyklos,* circle, + *mastos,* breast, + *pathos,* suffering ]. Eccyclomastoma; the occurrence of isolated masses of the same connective tissue or epithelial accumulation as found in cyclomastopathy.

**eccyesis** (ek-si-e'sis) [ G. *ek,* out, + *kyēsis,* pregnancy. CYES- ]. Ectopic *pregnancy.*

**ecdemic** (ek-dem'ik) [ G. *ekdēmos,* foreign, from home, fr. *dēmos,* people ]. Denoting a disease brought into a region from without, not epidemic or endemic.

**ecderon** (ek'dĕ-ron) [ G. *ek,* out, + *deros,* skin. DER- ]. The outer portion of the general integument, as distinguished from enderon.

**ecdysiasm** (ek-diz'ī-azm) [ G. as from *ekdysiazesthai,* to remove one's clothes ]. A morbid tendency to undress to produce sexual desire in others.

**ecdysiotropin** (ek-dī'zī-o-tro'pin). Brain *hormone.*

**ecdysis** (ek'dī-sis) [ G. *ekdysis,* shedding ]. Desquamation; sloughing; molting; a necessary phenomenon to permit growth in arthropods and skin renewal in amphibians and reptiles; see also ecdysone.

**ecdysones** (ek'dī-sōnz) [ see ecdysis ]. Molting hormone; a hormone produced by the prothoracic glands of insects after stimulation by brain hormone; important in the developmental process of flies, beetles, and moths which pass through one or more larval stages before pupating and metamorphosing into an adult. (See also ecdysial *glands,* and *corpora* allata). At least four varieties of ecdysone are known, all derivatives of α-ecdysone (2β, 3β, 14α, 22R, 25-pentahydroxy-5β-cholest-7-en-6-one) by virtue of hydroxyl groups at 20 and/or 26, and thus called α-ecdysone,

20-hydroxyecdysone, 20,26-dihydroxyecdysone, and 26-hydroxyecdysone.

**ECG.** Abbreviation for electrocardiogram; also abbreviated EKG.

**ecgonine** (ek'go-nēn, -nin). 3β-Hydroxy-2β-tropanecarboxylic acid; the important part of the cocaine molecule.

**echeosis** (ek'e-o'sis) [ G. *echein*, to suffer from noises in ears ]. Mental disturbance caused by long-continued, disturbing noises.

**Echidnoph'aga gallina'cea.** The sticktight flea, a serious pest of poultry in subtropical America. It also frequently attacks domestic animals and man.

**echin-.** See echino-.

**echinate** (ek'ī-māt). Echinulate.

**echinenone** (ē-kin'ē-nōn). β-Caroten-4-one.

**echino-, echin-** (ē-ki'no-, ek'ī-no-) [ G. *echinos*, hedgehog, sea urchin ]. Combining forms meaning prickly or spiny.

**Echinochasmus** (ē-ki'no-kaz'mus) [ echino- + G. *chasma*, open mouth ]. A genus of digenetic flukes (family Echinostomatidae), particularly common in wading and fish-eating birds.

   **E. perfolia'tus** var. **japon'icus,** infects (rarely) the intestine of man in Japan.

**echinococcosis** (ē-ki'no-kok-ko'sis). Infection with *Echinococcus.*

**Echinococcus** (ē-ki'no-kok'us) [ echino- + G. *kokkos*, a berry ]. A genus of taeniid tapeworms of very small size, two to three segments in adult worms; adults are found in dogs and various wild canids and other Carnivora, and larvae are found in hydatid cysts in rodents, ruminants, and man.

   **E. granulo'sus,** hydatid tapeworm; a species infecting the dog and cat; the larval form (hydatid cyst) may occur in man, giving rise to a massive tumor in the liver and other organs and tissues.

   **E. multilocula'ris,** a species occurring in foxes; the larva (multiloculate hydatid cyst) is found in the liver of microtine rodents and (rarely) in herbivores and man; it produces a proliferative (but sometimes slow-growing) multiloculate cyst in the liver that is usually fatal.

**Echinodermata** (ē-ki'no-der'mah-tah) [ echino- + G. *derma*, skin ]. A phylum of Metazoa which includes starfish, sea urchins, sea lilies, and other classes. All but the sea cucumbers (Holothuroidea) are basically radially symmetrical and most possess a calcareous endoskeleton with external spines. They inhabit the sea bottom, some near shore, others in deep water.

**Echinoidea** (ek'ī-noy'de-ah) [ echino- + G. *eidos*, form ]. Sea urchins; a class of marine forms of the phylum Echinodermata.

**Echinorhynchus** (ē-ki'no-ring'kus) [ echino- + G. *rhynchos*, snout ]. A genus of acanthocephalid worms; originally included species now contained in *Macracanthorhynchus, Gigantorhynchus,* and other genera.

   **E. hom'inis,** a form described from the small intestine of a Bohemian boy; it was possibly the same as *Macracanthorhynchus hirudinaceus,* normally of swine.

**echinosis** (ek'ī-no'sis) [ echino- + G. suffix *-osis*, condition ]. Condition in which the red blood cells have lost

their smooth outlines, resembling an echinus or sea urchin.

**Echinostoma** (ē-ki'no-sto'mah, ek'ī-nos'to-mah) [ echino- + G. *stoma*, mouth ]. A genus of digenetic flukes (family Echinostomatidae) with characteristic oral spines; it is widely distributed and parasitic in a broad range of bird and mammal hosts; several species have been reported from man.

   **E. iloca'num,** a species reported from man in the Philippines.

   **E. malay'anum,** a species typically found in the pig, but reported from man in Malaya; infection results from ingestion of snails with infective cysts (metacercariae).

**echinulate** (ē-kin'u-lāt) [ Mod. L. *echinulus*, dim. of L. *echinus*, hedgehog ]. Echinate; prickly or spinous.

**echis** (ek'is, e'kis) [ G. *echis*, a viper ]. Carpet viper; a genus of vipers that produces a deadly venom. They occur in Africa and Arabia.

**echitamine** (ē-kit'ä-min, -mēn). Ditaine; an alkaloid obtained from the bark of *Alstonia;* has curare-like and antimalarial action.

**echo** (ek'o) [ G. ]. A reverberating sound sometimes heard in auscultation of the chest.

**echoacousia** (ek'o-ă-koo'zī-ah) [ echo + G. *akouō,* to hear ]. A subjective disturbance of hearing in which a sound heard appears to be repeated.

**echoaortography** (ek'o-a-or-tog'rä-fī) [ echo + aortography ]. The application of ultrasound techniques to the diagnosis and study of the aorta, particularly the abdominal aorta.

**echocardiography** (ek'o-kar-dī-og'rä-fī) [ echo + cardiography ]. 1. The use of ultrasound in the diagnosis of cardiovascular lesions, especially mitral disease, pericardial effusion, and abdominal aortic aneurysm. 2. The ultrasonic record of the size, motion, and composition of various cardiac structures.

**echoencephalography** (ek'o-en-sef-ă-log'rä-fī) [ echo + encephalography ]. The use of reflected ultrasound in the diagnosis of intracranial processes.

**echographia** (ek'o-graf'ī-ah) [ echo + G. *graphō,* to write ]. A form of agraphia in which one can write from dictation or copy but cannot do original writing.

**echography** (ē-kog'rä-fī) [ echo + G. *graphō,* to write ]. A method of measuring the variations in echoes reflected by ultrasonic vibrations exceeding 20,000 per second from tissues or foreign bodies of varying density. This method has some analogies to radar.

**echokinesis, echokinesia** (ek'o-kī-ne'sis, -ne'zī-ah) [ echo + G. *kinēsis,* movement ]. Echopraxia.

**echolalia** (ek'o-la'lī-ah) [ echo + G. *lalia,* a form of speech ]. Echophrasia; echo reaction; the involuntary repetition of a word or sentence just spoken by another person.

**ech'oloca'tion.** Term applied to the method by which bats direct their flight and avoid solid objects. The creatures emit high-pitched cries which, though inaudible to human ears, are heard by the bats themselves as reflected sounds (echoes) from objects in their path.

**echomatism** (ē-ko'mă-tizm) [ echo + G. *matizō,* to strive to do ]. Echopraxia.

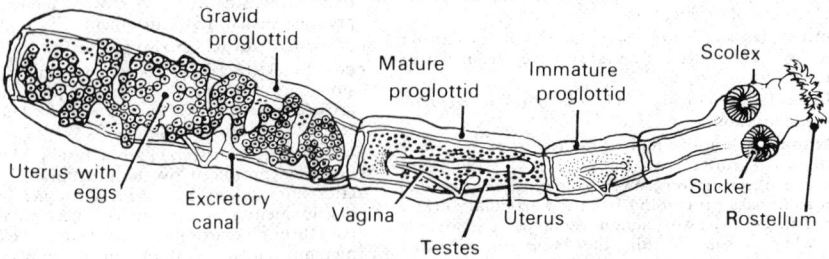

*Echinococcus granulosus*
(Magnification, ×20)

**echomimia** (ek'o-min'ĭ-ah) [ echo + G. *mimēsis*, imitation ]. Echopathy.

**echomotism** (ek'o-mo'tizm) [ echo + L. *motio*, motion ]. Echopraxia.

**echopathy** (ĕ-kop'ă-thĭ) [ echo + G. *pathos*, suffering ]. A mental disorder in which the words or actions of another are imitated and repeated by the patient.

**echophony, echophonia** (ĕ-kof'o-nĭ, ek'o-fo'nĭ-ah) [ echo + G. *phōnē*, voice ]. A duplication of the voice sound occasionally heard in auscultation of the chest.

**echophotony** (ek'o-fot'o-nĭ) [ echo + G. *phōs* (*phōt-*), light, + *tonos*, tone ]. The mental association of sound tones with particular colors.

**echophrasia** (ek-o-fra'zĭ-ah) [ echo + *phrasis*, speech ]. Echolalia.

**echopraxia** (ek'o-prak'sĭ-ah) [ echo + G. *praxis*, action ]. Echokinesia; echomatism; echomotism; the involuntary imitation of movements made by another.

**echothiophate iodide** (ek'o-thi'o-fāt) (USP, BP). PHOSPHOLINE iodide; 217 MI; diethoxyphosphorylthiocholine iodide; a potent organophosphorus compound and cholinesterase inhibitor, used in the treatment of glaucoma.

**Eck,** Nikolai V., Russian physiologist, 1847–1917. See E. *fistula,* reverse E. *fistula.*

**Ecker,** Alexander, Freiburg anatomist, 1816–1887. See E.'s *convolution, fissure.*

**Ecker,** Enrique E., U. S. bacteriologist, 1887–1966. See Rees-E. *fluid.*

**eclabium** (ek-la'bĭ-um) [ G. *ek*, out, + L. *labium*, lip ]. Eversion of a lip.

**eclampsia** (ek-lamp'sĭ-ah) [ G. *eklampsis*, a shining forth ]. The occurrence of one or more convulsions, not attributable to other cerebral conditions such as epilepsy or cerebral hemorrhage, in a patient with preeclampsia.

**puer'peral e.,** convulsions and coma associated with hypertension, edema, or proteinuria occurring in a woman following delivery.

**eclampsism** (ek-lamp'sizm). A state in which the general signs point to the early occurrence of puerperal eclampsia, but convulsions do not take place.

**eclamp'tic.** Relating to eclampsia.

**eclamptogenic** (ek-lamp'to-jen'ik). Eclamptogenous; causing eclampsia.

**eclamptogenous** (ek-lamp-toj'en-us). Eclamptogenic.

**eclectic** (ek-lek'tik) [ G. *eklektikos*, selecting, fr. *ek*, out, + *lego*, to select ]. Picking out from different sources what appears to be the best.

**eclecticism** (ek-lek'tĭ-sizm). Practice of eclectic medicine, *q. v.*

**eclipse.** See eclipse *period.*

**ecmnesia** (ek-ne'zĭ-ah) [ G. *ek*, out, + *mnēsios*, relating to memory. MN- ]. Loss of memory for recent events.

**eco-** (e'ko-) [ G. *oikos*, house, household, habitation ]. Combining form denoting relationship to environment (*e.g.*, the ecology).

**ecoid** (e'koyd) [ eco- + G. *eidos*, resemblance ]. The framework of a red blood cell.

**ecology** (e-kol'o-jĭ) [ eco- + G. *logos*, study ]. Bionomics (2); the branch of biology that deals with the mutual relations of living organisms and their environments, or the relations of organisms to each other.

**human e.,** the relations of persons to their total (biologic and social) environment.

**ecomania** (e'ko-ma'nĭ-ah) [ eco- + G. *mania*, frenzy ]. Oikomania; any neurotic disorder supposed to result from something unpleasant or dreadful in one's home environment.

**Economo** (a-kon'o-mo), Constantin von. See von Economo, Constantin.

**economy** (e-kon'o-mĭ) [ G. *oikonomia*, management of the house, fr. *oikos*, house, + *nomos*, usage, law ]. The system; the body regarded as an aggregate of functioning organs.

**ecoparasite** (e'ko-păr'ă-sī t) [ eco- + parasite ]. Ecosite.

**ecosite** (e'ko-sīt) [ eco- + G. *sitos*, food ]. Ecoparasite; a microparasite to which its host is immune under normal conditions.

**ecospecies** (e'ko-spe'shēz) [ eco- + species ]. Two or more populations of a species isolated by ecological barriers but able to exchange genes freely; species partially separated from one another by differences in habitat or behavior.

**ecosystem** (e'ko-sis-tem) [ eco- + system ]. An ecological system; a stipulated functional unit of organisms, which interact with one another and with the nonliving portions of their environment; commonly delimited in terms of a geographical entity, such as the e. of a small watershed.

**parasite-host e.,** parasitocenose.

**écouteur** (a-koo-tēr') [ Fr. a listener-in ]. One who obtains erotic gratification through listening to sexual accounts.

**écouvillon** (ā-koo-vee-yōhn') [ Fr., cleaning brush ]. A brush with firm bristles for freshening sores or the interior of a cavity.

**ecphoria** (ek-fo'rĭ-ah) [ G. *ek*, out, + *phora*, a carrying ]. The recall of memory.

**ecphorize** (ek'fo-rīz) [ see ecphoria ]. To revive a memory.

**ecphyadectomy** (ek-fi-ă-dek'to-mĭ) [ G. *ekphyas*, an appendage, + *ektomē*, excision ]. Appendectomy.

**ecphyaditis** (ek-fi-ă-di'tis) [ G. *ekphyas*, an appendage, + suffix *-itis*, inflammation ]. Appendicitis.

**ecphylactic** (ek-fi-lak'tik). Relating to ecphylaxis.

**ecphylaxis** (ek-fi-lak'sis) [ G. *ek*, out of, + *phylaxis*, protection ]. A condition in which the antibodies or phylactic agents in the blood have become inactivated or are excluded from the focus of infection.

**ecphy'ma** [ G. a pimply eruption. PHYS- ]. A warty growth or protuberance.

**écraseur** (a-krah-zēr') [ Fr. *écraser*, to crush ]. A snare, especially one of great strength for cutting through the base or pedicle of a tumor.

**Chassaignac's é.,** a strong steel chain snare used for crushing through the pedicle of a tumor.

**ecstasy** (ek'stă-sĭ) [ G. *ekstasis*. STA- ]. Mental exaltation, with more or less sensory anesthesia and a rapturous expression.

**ecstatic** (ek-stat'ik). Relating to or marked by ecstasy.

**ecstrophe** (ek'stro-fe). Exstrophy.

**ECT.** Abbreviation for electroconvulsive (electroshock) therapy; see under therapy.

**ect-.** See ecto-.

**ectaco'lia** [ G. *ektasis*, a stretching, + *kolon*, colon ]. Colectasia.

**ectad** (ek'tad) [ G. *ektos*, outside, + L. *ad*, to ]. Outward.

**ectal** (ek'tal) [ G. *ektos*, outside ]. Outer; external.

**-ecta'sia, -ec'tasis** [ G. *ektasis*, a stretching. TEN- ]. Combining form in suffix position used to denote dilation or expansion.

**ecta'sia, ec'tasis** (ek-ta'zĭ-ah, ek'tă-sis) [ G. *ektasis*, a stretching ]. Dilation of a tubular structure.

**e. cordis,** dilation of the heart.

**diffuse arterial e.,** spontaneous enlargement with dilation of the vessels in a circumscribed area; see also cirsoid aneurysm.

**hypostatic e.,** dilation of a blood vessel, usually a vein, in a dependent portion of the body, as in varicose veins of the leg.

**mammary duct e.,** dilation of mammary ducts by lipid and cellular debris in older women. Rupture of ducts may result in granulomatous inflammation and infiltration by plasma cells. See also plasma cell *mastitis.*

**pap'illary e.,** senile *hemangioma.*

**senile e.,** senile *hemangioma.*

**e. ventric'uli paradoxa,** hourglass *stomach.*

**ectatic** (ek-tat'ik). Relating to or marked by ectasis.

**ectental** (ek-ten'tal) [ G. *ektos*, outside, + *entos*, within ]. Ectoental; relating to both ectoderm and entoderm; denoting the line where these two layers join.

**ECTEOLA-cellulose.** See under cellulose.

**ecterograph** (ek-tĕr'o-graf) [ G. *ektos*, outside, + *graphō*, to write ]. A modified pneumatograph used in making graphic records of the movements of the intestine.

**ectethmoid** (ekt-eth'moyd) [ G. *ektos*, outside, + ethmoid ]. Ectoethmoid; either of the lateral areas of the ethmoid bone in which the ethmoid cells are located.

**ecthyma** (ek-thi'mah) [ G. a pustule ]. A pyogenic infection due to staphylococci or streptococci. The ulcers may be single or multiple, and heal with scar formation.

**contagious e.,** orf; soremouth; contagious pustular stomatitis; a specific virus disease of sheep and goats caused by a virus and characterized by vesiculation and ulceration of the lips; the disease is transmissible to man.

**e. gangreno'sum,** *dermatitis* gangrenosa infantum.

**ecthymat'iform, ecthy'miform.** Resembling ecthyma.

**ecthyreosis** (ek-thi-re-o'sis). Removal of the thyroid gland and the presence of symptoms resulting therefrom. Obsolete.

**ectiris** (ekt-i'ris) [ G. *ektos,* outside, + iris ]. The outer layer of the iris.

**ecto-, ect-** (ek'to-) [ G. *ektos,* outside ]. Combining forms denoting outer, on the outside. See also exo-.

**ectoantigen** (ek-to-an'ti-jen). 1. Exoantigen; any toxin or other exciter of antibody formation, separate or separable from its source. 2. An antigen presumed to be derived chiefly from the ectoplasm of bacterial cells.

**ectoblast** (ek'to-blast) [ ecto- + G. *blastos,* germ ]. 1. The ectoderm. 2. Term used by some experimental embryologists to mean the original outer cell layer from which the primary germ layers are formed; in this sense it would be synonymous with protoderm.

**ectocardia** (ek-to-kar'di-ah) [ ecto- + G. *kardia,* heart ]. Exocardia; congenital misplacement of the heart.

**ectocar'diac, ectocar'dial.** Relating to ectocardia.

**ectocervical** (ek'to-ser'vi-kal). Pertaining to the pars vaginalis of the cervix uteri lined with stratified squamous epithelium.

**ectochoroidea** (ek'to-ko-roy'de-ah). The outer layer of the choroid coat of the eye.

**ectocolostomy** (ek'to-ko-los'to-mi) [ ecto- + colostomy ]. The formation of an opening into the colon through the abdominal wall.

**ectocornea** (ek'to-kor'ne-ah). The outer layer of the cornea.

**ectocrine** (ek'to-krin) [ ecto- + G. *krino,* to separate ]. 1. Relating to substances, either synthesized or arising by decomposition of organisms, that affect plant life. 2. A compound with ectocrine properties. 3. An ectohormone.

**ecological e.,** a chemical substance that undergoes biosynthesis in one species and that exerts an effect on the function of another species through mechanisms of the external environment; the biosynthesis of vitamins by ruminants and their subsequent ingestion by other animals is an example. Ectohormones (*q.v.*) are also examples of ecological e.'s.

**ectocyst** (ek'to-sist). The outer layer of a hydatid cyst.

**ectoderm** (ek'to-derm) [ ecto- + G. *derma,* skin ]. Epiblast; the outer layer of cells in the embryo, after the establishing of the primary germ layers.

**epithelial e.,** superficial e.; that part of the e. that separates from the neuroectoderm at about the fourth week of embryonic life; it gives rise to the epidermis and its specialized derivatives.

**superficial e.,** epithelial e.

**ectoder'mal, ectoder'mic.** Relating to the ectoderm.

**ec'todermato'sis.** Ectodermosis.

**ec'todermo'sis.** Ectodermatosis; a disorder of any organ or tissue developed from the ectoderm.

**e. erosiva plu'riorificia'lis,** *erythema* multiforme exudativum.

**ectoentad** (ek-to-en'tad). From without inward.

**ectoental** (ek-to-en'tal). Ectental.

**ectoenzyme** (ek'to-en'zim). An enzyme that is excreted externally.

**ectoethmoid** (ek-to-eth'moyd). Ectethmoid.

**ectogenous** (ek-toj'en-us) [ ecto- + G. suffix *-gen,* producing ]. Originating outside of the organism; applied to an infectious disease, a parasite, etc.

**ectoglobular** (ek-to-glob'u-lar). Not within a globular body; specifically not within a red blood cell.

**ectohormone** (ek'to-hor'mōn). A parahormonic chemical mediator of ecological significance. E.'s are secreted, largely by invertebrate animals, by an organism into its immediate environment (air or water). Acting through a distance, an e. can alter the behavior or functional activity of a second organism, often, though not always, of the same species as that secreting the e. See also ecological *ectocrine.*

**ectoloph** (ek'to-lof) [ ecto- + G. *lophos,* crest ]. The external ridge on an upper molar tooth in most ungulates.

**ectomeninx** (ek'to-me'ningks, -men'ingks) [ ecto- + G. *mēninx,* membrane ]. A primitive condensation of mesenchyme surrounding the embryonic brain.

**ectomere** (ek'to-mēr) [ ecto- + G. *meros,* part ]. One of the blastomeres destined to take part in forming the ectoderm.

**ectomerogony** (ek'to-mĕ-rog'o-ni) [ ecto- + G. *meros,* part, + *gonē,* generation ]. The production of merozoites in the asexual reproduction of sporozoan parasites on the surface of schizonts and of blastophores, or by infolding into the schizont, as contrasted with endomerogony; e. has been observed in various species of *Eimeria.*

**ectomesenchyme** (ek'to-mes'en-kim) [ ecto- + G. *mesos,* middle, + *enkyma,* infusion ]. Mesectoderm.

**ectomorph** (ek'to-morf) [ ecto- + G. *morphē,* form ]. Longitype; a constitutional body type or build (biotype or somatotype) in which tissues that originated from the ectoderm prevail; from the morphological standpoint, the members predominate over the trunk.

**ectomorph'ic.** Relating to ectomorphs.

**-ectomy** (-ek'to-mi) [ G. *ektomē,* excision ]. Combining form used as a suffix to denote operative removal of any organ or gland.

**ectopagia** (ek'to-pa'ji-ah) [ ecto- + G. *pagos,* something fixed, + suffix *-ia,* condition ]. The condition in conjoined twins in which the bodies are joined laterally.

**ectopagus** (ek-top'ă-gus). Conjoined twins with ectopagia.

**ectopar'asite.** A parasite that lives on the surface of the body.

**ectoparasit'icide.** An agent that is applied directly to the human host to kill ectoparasites.

**ec'topar'asitism.** Infestation.

**ectoperitcnitis** (ek'to-pĕr-ĭ-to-ni'tis). Inflammation beginning in the deeper layer of the peritoneum which is next to the viscera or the abdominal wall.

**ectophyte** (ek'to-fit) [ ecto- + G. *phyton,* plant ]. A vegetable parasite of the skin.

**ectopia** (ek-to'pi-ah) [ G. *ektopos,* out of place, fr. *ektos,* outside, + *topos,* place ]. Ectopy; congenital displacement of any organ or part of the body.

**e. cloacae,** *exstrophy* of the cloaca.

**e. cor'dis,** congenital condition in which the heart is exposed on the chest wall because of maldevelopment of the sternum and pericardium.

**e. len'tis,** displacement of the lens of the eye.

**e. pupil'lae congen'ita,** marked excentric congenital displacement of the pupil.

**e. re'nis,** displacement of the kidney.

**e. tes'tis,** see ectopic *testis.*

**e. ves'icae,** *exstrophy* of bladder.

**ectopic** (ek-top'ik) [ see ectopia ]. 1. Aberrant; heterotopic; out of place; said of an organ which is not in its proper position, or of a pregnancy occurring elsewhere than in the cavity of the uterus. 2. In cardiography, denoting a heart beat that has its origin in some abnormal focus; arising from a focus other than the sinoatrial node. 3. In neuropathology, denoting displaced gray matter, typically in the deep cerebral white matter.

**ec'toplacen'tal.** 1. Outside, beyond, or surrounding the placenta; referring especially to the parts of the trophoblast in primates not directly involved in the formation of the placenta. 2. Referring to the actively growing part of the trophoblast involved in the formation of the placenta in rodents.

**ectoplasm** (ek'to-plazm) [ ecto- + G. *plasma,* something formed ]. A condensation of the cytoplasm at the periphery of a cell.

**ectoplasmat'ic.** Ectoplasmic.

**ectoplasmic** (ek'to-plaz'mik). Ectoplasmatic; ectoplastic; relating to the ectoplasm.

**ectoplas'tic.** Ectoplasmic.

**ectopy** (ek'to-pi). Ectopia.

**ectoretina** (ek′to-ret′ĭ-nah). The outer layer of the retina.

**ectosarc** (ek′to-sark) [ ecto- + G. *sarx*, flesh ]. The outer membrane, or ectoplasm, of a protozoon.

**ectoscopy** (ek-tos′ko-pĭ) [ ecto- + G. *skopeō*, to examine ]. A method of diagnosis of disease of any of the internal organs by a study of movements of the abdominal wall or thorax caused by phonation.

**ectosteal** (ek-tos′te-al) [ ecto- + G. *osteon* bone ]. Relating to the external surface of a bone.

**ectostosis** (ek′tos-to′sis) [ ecto- + G. *osteon*, bone, + suffix -*osis*, condition ]. Ossification in cartilage beneath the perichondrium, or the formation of bone beneath the periosteum.

**ec′tothrix** [ ecto- + G. *thrix*, hair ]. Literally, upon hair shafts; usually applied to certain species of fungi which affect the surface of hair shafts and sometimes skin.

**ectotox′in.** Extracellular *toxin.*

**ectozo′on** [ ecto- + G. *zōon*, animal ]. An animal parasite living on the surface of the body.

**ectro-** (ek′tro-) [ G. *ektrōsis*, miscarriage ]. Combining form denoting congenital absence of a part.

**ectrocheiry, ectrochiry** (ek-tro-ki′rĭ) [ ectro- + G. *cheir*, hand ]. Total or partial absence of a hand.

**ectrodactyly, ectrodactyl′ia, ectrodact′ylism** (ek′-tro-dak′tĭ-lĭ) [ ectro- + G. *daktylos*, finger ]. Congenital absence of one or more fingers or toes.

**ectrogen′ic.** Relating to ectrogeny.

**ectrogeny** (ek-troj′en-ĭ) [ ectro- + G. suffix -*gen*, producing ]. Congenital absence of any part.

**ectropody** (ek-trop′o-dĭ) [ ectro- + G. *pous*, foot ]. Total or partial absence of a foot.

**ectromelia** (ek-tro-me′lĭ-ah) [ see ectromelus ]. 1. A congenital lack of one or more of the limbs. 2. Mousepox; infectious e.; a poxlike virus disease of mice, characterized by gangrene and loss of a foot or feet and by necrotic areas in the internal organs; in laboratory mouse colonies it usually causes a high mortality.

**ectromel′ic.** Relating to an ectromelus.

**ectromelus** (ek-trom′ĕ-lus) [ ectro- + G. *melos*, limb ]. An individual with one or more limbs absent or malformed.

**ectro′pion, ectro′pium** [ G. *ek*, out, + *tropē*, a turning ]. A rolling outward of the margin of a part; *e.g.*, an eyelid.
    **flaccid e.,** paralytic e.; e. of the lower lid due to relaxation of the skin and orbicularis muscle.
    **paralytic e.,** flaccid e.
    **e. u′veae,** a forward curling eversion of the pigment layer and sphincter of the iris.

**ectrosyndactyly** (ek-tro-sin-dak′tĭ-lĭ) [ ectro- + G. *syn*, together, + *daktylos*, finger ]. A congenital deformity marked by the absence of one or more digits and the fusion of others.

**ectrot′ic** [ G. *ektrōtikos*, relating to abortion, fr. *ektrōsis*, miscarriage ]. Abortive (3).

**ectylurea** (ek′til-u-re′ah). LEVANIL; NOSTYN; 2-ethyl-*cis*-crotonylurea; a mild sedative used in the treatment of nervous tension and anxiety.

**ectype** (ek′tĭp) [ G. *ek*, out, + *typos*, stamp, model ]. Extreme somatotype, such as ectomorph (longitype) or endomorph (brachytype).

**ecuresis** (ek′u-re′sis) [ G. *ek*, out, + *ourēsis*, urination ]. A condition in which urinary excretion and intake of water act to produce an absolute dehydration of the body. See also emuresis.

**eczema** (ek′zĕ-mah, eg′zĕ-mah, eg-ze′mah) [ G. fr. *ekzeō*, to boil over. ZE- ]. Generic term for acute or chronic inflammatory conditions of the skin, typically erythematous, edematous, papular, vesicular, and crusting; followed often by lichenification and scaling and occasionally by duskiness of the erythema and, infrequently, hyperpigmentation; often accompanied by sensations of itching and burning; sometimes referred to colloquially as tetter, dry tetter, scaly tetter.
    **allergic e.,** macular, papular, or vesicular eruption due to an allergic reaction.
    **atopic e.,** atopic *dermatitis.*
    **baker's e.,** an allergic eruption due to hypersensitivity on contact with flour, yeast, or other ingredients handled by bakers.

    **e. diabetico′rum,** e. occurring in diabetes.
    **e. ep′ilans,** e. with hair loss.
    **e. erythemato′sum,** a dry form of e. marked by more or less extensive areas of redness with scaly desquamation.
    **facial e.,** a photosensitivity disease of sheep in New Zealand associated with ingestion of plants during periods when autumn rains produce lush growth following seasons of dryness and close grazing; hepatic disease, caused by toxins of *Pithomyces chartarum*, which grows on the plants, is the predisposing cause.
    **flexural e.,** e. of skin at the flexures of elbow, knees, wrists, etc.
    **hand e.,** e. that predominantly and persistently affects the hands; of multiple causation, including allergic, industrial, dyshidrotic, and atopic mechanisms.
    **e. herpet′icum,** herpes simplex complicating e.; Kaposi's varicelliform eruption; pustulosis vacciniformis acuta; a febrile condition occurring most commonly in children, consisting of a widespread eruption of vesicles rapidly becoming umbilicated pustules; clinically indistinguishable from a generalized vaccinia; it has been suggested that vaccinia virus is the etiologic agent.
    **e. hypertroph′icum,** e. marked by papillary hypertrophy of the skin.
    **e. infan′tile,** e. in infants; the clinical appearance is identical to e. in adults.
    **e. intertri′go,** see intertrigo.
    **lichenoid e.,** chronic e.; thickening of skin in e.
    **e. mad′idans,** weeping e.; humid, moist, or wet tetter; a moist eczematous eruption.
    **e. margina′tum,** *tinea* cruris.
    **e. nummula′re,** discrete, coin-shaped patches of e.
    **e. papulo′sum,** a dermatitis marked by an eruption of discrete or aggregated reddish excoriated papules.
    **e. parasit′icum,** eczematous eruption precipitated by parasite infestation.
    **e. pustulo′sum,** impetigo eczematodes; a later stage of vesicular e., in which the vesicles have become secondarily infected. The lesions become covered with pus crusts.
    **e. rubrum,** a stage of vesicular e., presenting red, excoriated, weeping areas.
    **seborrheic e.,** seborrheic *dermatitis.*
    **e. squamo′sum,** a form of dry, scaly e.
    **stasis e.,** eczematous eruption on legs due to or aggravated by vascular stasis.
    **tropical e.,** e. occurring in plaques on extensors of the extremities; of common occurrence and unknown etiology.
    **e. tylot′icum,** eczematous eruption of palms and soles with marked hyperkeratosis.
    **e. vaccina′tum,** a form of generalized vaccinia supervening upon an existing atopic e.; it is characterized by crops of vesicles and vesicopustules appearing on the face, neck, extremities, and trunk, with even minimal atopic involvement; it is accompanied by a high fever, malaise, and enlargement of the lymph nodes.
    **varicose e.,** e. occurring over varicose veins of the legs.
    **e. verruco′sum,** e. with hyperkeratosis; chronic lichenified e.
    **e. vesiculo′sum,** dermatitis marked by an eruption of vesicles upon erythematous patches that rupture and exude serum.
    **weeping e.,** e. madidans.
    **winter e.,** e. resulting from accelerated evaporation of moisture (including insensitive sweat) from the cutaneous surface; occurs as dry, crackled plaques, usually on the extremities, but not infrequently also on the trunk in any season under circumstances (occupational, environmental) of excessively rapid drying out of skin.

**eczematization** (ek-zem′ă-tī-za′shun). 1. The formation of an eruption resembling eczema. 2. The occurrence of eczema secondary to a preexisting dermatosis.

**eczematous** (ek-sem′ă-tus). Marked by or resembling eczema.

**ED.** Abbreviation for an effective dose of a chemical or therapeutic agent; see also dose.

**ED$_{50}$.** Abbreviation for the dose which produces the desired effect in 50 per cent of the test animals.

**edathamil.** Ethylenediaminetetraacetic acid.

**ede′a** [ G. *aidoia*, genitals ]. The external genitals.

**Edebohls** (ed'e-bölz), George M., New York surgeon, 1853–1908. See E.'s *operation, position.*

**edeitis** (e-de-i'tis) [ G. *aidoia,* genitals, + suffix -*itis,* inflammation ]. Vulvitis.

**Edelman,** Gerald M., U. S. molecular immunologist, *1929. Nobel laureate, 1972, with Rodney R. Porter, for their studies in the basic structure of antibodies.

**edema** (e-de'mah) [ G. *oidēma,* a swelling ]. An accumulation of an excessive amount of fluid in cells, tissues, or serous cavities.

  **angioneurotic e.,** periodically recurring episodes of noninflammatory swelling of skin, mucous membranes, viscera and brain of sudden onset and lasting hours to days, occasionally with arthralgia, purpura or fever; cerebral or glottal e. may cause death; dominant autosomal inheritance with reduced penetrance. Also called Bannister's disease; circumscribed, periodic, or Quincke's e.; giant urticaria or hives; urticaria gigans; u. tuberosa; hydrops hypostrophos.

  **Berlin's e.,** see *concussion* of retina.

  **blue e.,** the swelling and cyanosis of an extremity in hysterical paralysis.

  **brain e.,** a type of brain swelling characterized by increased volume of the extravascular compartment; see also brain *swelling.*

  **brown e.,** e. of the lungs associated with chronic passive congestion.

  **bullous e.,** a reddened, swollen appearance of the ureteral orifice in the bladder wall, frequently observed in tuberculosis of the ureter.

  **cachec'tic e.,** e. occurring in diseases characterized by hypoproteinemic hydremia.

  **cardiac e.,** e. resulting from congestive heart failure.

  **cerebral e.,** swelling of neuropile and white matter following disruption of blood-brain barrier and disturbance of cortical electrolyte balance; frequently associated with passage of proteinaceous material into gray or white substance.

  **circumscribed e.,** angioneurotic e.

  **concussion e.,** see *concussion* of retina.

  **e. ex vac'uo,** an increase of fluid in a cavity with unyielding walls, such as the skull or spinal canal, when part of the contents has become atrophied.

  **famine e.,** war e.; hunger e.; nutritional e. resulting from many factors, chief of which is hypoalbuminemia.

  **e. frigidum,** obsolete term for noninflammatory e.

  **gestational e.,** cyesedema; the occurrence of a generalized and excessive accumulation of fluid in the tissues of greater than 1+ pitting edema after 12 hours' rest in bed, or of a weight gain of 5 pounds or more in 1 week due to the influence of pregnancy.

  **e. glottidis,** laryngeal e.

  **heat e.,** e. caused by excessively high external temperature.

  **hydre'mic e.,** marantic e.; e. occurring in states marked by pronounced hydremia.

  **inflammatory e.,** a swelling due to effusion of fluid in the soft parts surrounding a focus of inflammation.

  **lymphatic e.,** leukophlegmasia; e. due to stasis in the lymph channels.

  **malignant e.,** a form of anthrax in which the eyelids, lips, and other parts of the face, the neck, and the upper extremities are the seats of marked e., with an eruption of vesicles and bullae, which is prone to become gangrenous; the constitutional symptoms are those characteristic of extreme sepsis.

  **maran'tic e.,** hydremic e.

  **menstrual e.,** the retention of water and increase in weight, which occurs during or preceding menstruation.

  **e. neonato'rum,** a diffuse, firm e. occurring in the newborn; it begins usually in the legs and spreads upward, and is commonly fatal.

  **noninflammatory e.,** simple e. due to mechanical or other causes, not marked by inflammation or congestion.

  **nutritional e.,** a form of swelling resulting apparently from insufficient protein intake together with excess ingestion of fluid and salt. See also famine e.

  **e. of the optic disk,** papilledema.

  **periodic e.,** angioneurotic e.

  **pitting e.,** e. that retains for a time the indentation produced by pressure.

  **premenstrual e.,** see menstrual e.

  **pulmonary e.,** e. of lungs usually resulting from mitral stenosis or left ventricular failure.

  **Quincke's e.,** angioneurotic e.

  **rheumatismal e.,** in rheumatic fever, a red, painful swelling of the extremities.

  **salt e.,** e. from sodium chloride retention.

  **solid e.,** infiltration of the subcutaneous tissues by mucoid material, as in myxedema.

  **war e.,** famine e.

  **Yangtze e.,** gnathostomiasis.

**edematization** (e-dem'ă-tī-za'shun). Making edematous.

**edem'atous.** Marked by edema.

**Edenta'ta** [ L. *edentatus,* toothless ]. An order of placental mammals which includes the armadillo, sloth, and ant-eater. Only the latter lacks teeth, thus the ordinal name is a misnomer for the homodont toothed armadillo and the leaf-eating well toothed sloth; formerly, the aardvark and pangolin were included in this order.

**eden'tate.** Toothless.

**edentulate** (e-den'tu-lāt). Edentulous.

**edentulous** (e-den'tu-lus) [ L. *edentulus,* toothless ]. Toothless; without teeth.

**edeocephalus** (e'de-o-sef'ă-lus) [ G. *aidoia,* genitals, + *kephalē,* head ]. Aidoiocephalus; a malformed fetus with cyclopia, a more or less cylindrical proboscis in the nasal region, and a defectively formed mouth.

**e'deoma'nia** [ G. *aidoia,* genitals, + *mania,* insanity ]. Aidoiomania; strong and abnormal sexual interest.

**edes'tin.** A globulin derived from the castor oil bean, hemp seed, and other seeds.

**ed'etate.** 1. Salt of edetic acid (*i.e.,* of ethylenediaminetetraacetic acid *q.v.,* for uses and pharmacologic action). 2. USAN-approved contraction for ethylenediaminetetraacetate.

  **e. calcium disodium** (USP), sodium calcium e. (BP); calcium disodium VERSENATE; a mixture of the dihydrate and trihydrate of the calcium disodium salt of ethylenediaminetetraacetic acid (*q.v.*).

  **disodium e.** (USP, BP), ENDRATE disodium; chelating agent that binds calcium.

  **ferric sodium e.,** FERROSTRANE; FERROSTRENE; SYBRON; ferric monosodium ethylenediaminetetraacetate; used in iron deficiency anemia.

  **e. trisodium** (USAN), trisodium hydrogen salt; a chelating agent.

**edet'ic acid** (USP). Ethylenediaminetetraacetic acid.

**edge.** Margin; border.

  **cutting e.,** (1) the beveled, knifelike, sharpened working angle of a dental hand instrument; (2) *margo* incisalis.

  **denture e.,** denture *border.*

  **leading e.,** the initial part of a wave form at maximum slope.

  **incisal e.,** *margo* incisalis.

  **shearing e.,** *margo* incisalis.

**Edinger** (ed'in-ger), Ludwig, German anatomist, 1855–1918. See E.'s *fibers,* E.-Westphal *nucleus.*

**edis'ylate.** USAN-approved contraction for 1,2-ethanedisulfonate, $^-O_3S(CH_2)_2SO_3^-$.

**Ed'lefsen,** Gustav J. F., German physician, 1842–1910. See E.'s *reagent.*

**Edman's method** or **reagent.** See phenylisothiocyanate.

**Edridge-Green,** F. W., English ophthalmologist, 1863–1953. See E.-G. *theory.*

**edropho'nium chloride** (USP, BP). TENSILON; dimethylethyl (3-hydroxyphenyl)ammonium chloride; a competitive antagonist of skeletal muscle relaxants (curare derivatives and gallamine triethiodide). Used as an antidote for curariform drugs, as a diagnostic agent in myasthenia gravis, and in myasthenic crisis.

**EDTA.** Abbreviation for ethylenediaminetetraacetic acid.

**educated** (ed'u-ka-ted) [ L. *educo,* pp. -*atus,* to educate, fr. *e-duco,* pp. -*ductus,* to lead out ]. So modified as to be insusceptible to the poison of a specific infection; denoting the condition of the phagocytes in cases of acquired immunity.

**e'duct.** An extract.

**eduction** (e-duk'shun) [ L. *eductio,* a drawing out ]. Emergence from general anesthesia.

**edul'corant.** Sweetening.

**edul'corate** [ L. *e-*intens, + *dulcoro,* to sweeten, fr. *dulcor,* sweetness, fr. *dulcis,* sweet ]. To sweeten or render less acrid.

**Edwards,** J. H., British physician. See E.'s *syndrome.*

**EEG.** Abbreviation for electroencephalogram.

**effect** (ĕ-fekt') [ L. *ef-ficio,* pp. *effectus,* to accomplish, fr. *facio,* to do ]. The result or consequence of an action.

**additive e.,** an effect wherein two substances or actions used in combination produce a total e. the same as the sum of the individual e.'s.

**after-e.,** see aftereffect.

**Arias-Stella e.,** Arias-Stella phenomenon; focal, unusual, decidual changes in endometrial glandular epithelium, consisting of intraluminal budding, and nuclear enlargement and hyperchromatism with cytoplasmic swelling and vacuolation.

**autokinetic e.,** in psychology, the apparent drifting about of a small, fixed, spot of light which is being observed in a dark room.

**Bernoulli e.,** production of small droplets when a gas is passed rapidly across a narrow, fluid-filled orifice; a technique of humidification.

**Bohr e.,** the influence exerted by carbon dioxide ($CO_2$) on the oxygen dissociation curve of blood, *i.e.,* the curve is shifted to the right, which means a reduction in the affinity of hemoglobin for oxygen.

**clasp-knife e.,** clasp-knife *spasticity.*

**Compton e.,** in electromagnetic radiations of medium energy, this denotes a change in wavelength of the bombarding photon with the dislodgement of an orbital electron, usually from an outer shell.

**Cotton e.,** the positive and negative displacement from zero of the rotation of plane polarized monochromatic light and the change of monochromatic circularly polarized light into elliptically polarized light in the immediate vicinity of the absorption band of the substance through which the light passes. See also optical rotatory *dispersion.*

**Crabtree e.,** inhibition of cellular respiration of isolated systems by high concentrations of glucose; "reciprocal" of Pasteur e.

**cumulative e.,** cumulative action; the condition in which repeated administration of a drug may produce e.'s that are more pronounced than the e.'s produced by the first dose. A cumulative e. can be avoided by administering the maintenance dose at intervals that balance the rate of absorbtion with the rate of excretion and inactivation.

**cytopathic e.** degenerative changes in cells (especially in tissue culture) associated with the multiplication of certain viruses; when, in tissue culture, spread of virus is restricted by an overlay of agar (or other suitable substance) the cytopathic e. may lead to formation of plaque.

**Doppler e.,** Doppler phenomenon; a change in frequency is observed when the sound and observer are in relative motion away from or toward each other. See also Doppler *shift.*

**electrophonic e.,** the sensation of hearing produced when an alternating current of suitable frequency and magnitude is passed from an external source through a person.

**experimenter e.'s,** the influence of the experimenter's behavior, personality traits, or expectancies on the results of his own research.

**Fahraeus-Lindqvist e.,** sigma e.; the decrease in apparent viscosity that occurs when a suspension, such as blood, is made to flow through a tube of smaller diameter; observed in tubes less than about 0.3 mm. in diameter.

**Haldane e.,** the promotion of carbon dioxide dissociation by oxygenation of hemoglobin.

**mutase e.,** the simultaneous oxidation and reduction of a substrate by an enzyme in an oxidation-reduction system.

**Orbeli e.,** the fatigue of a muscle stimulated by its nerve (*i.e.,* indirectly) is reduced by concurrent stimulation of sympathetic fibers to the muscle; thought to be caused by norepinephrine diffusing from adrenergic fibers which innervate blood vessels in the muscle.

**Pasteur's e.,** the inhibition of fermentation by oxygen, first observed by Pasteur.

**photechic e.,** the ability of an agent, instead of light, to make possible the development of a photographic film.

**photoelectric e.,** the loss of electrons from the surface of a metal upon exposure to light.

**position e.,** a change in the phenotypic expression of one or more genes due to a change in position with respect to other genes; may result from change in chromosome structure or from crossing-over.

**Russell e.,** photechic e.

**second gas e.,** when a constant concentration of an anesthetic like halothane is inspired, the rise in alveolar concentration is accelerated by concomitant administration of nitrous oxide, because alveolar uptake of the latter creates a potential subatmospheric intrapulmonary pressure that leads to increased tracheal inflow.

**side-e.,** see *side-effect.*

**sigma e.,** Fahraeus-Lindqvist e.

**Somogyi e.,** reactive hyperglycemia followed by hypoglycemia; the hypoglycemia may be subclinical and difficult to detect.

**Staub-Traugott e.,** in normal persons, a drop in blood glucose follows a second oral dose of glucose given 30 minutes or so after the first.

**Stiles-Crawford e.,** when light reacts on the retinal cones straight-on, it produces a greater visual stimulation than when coming in obliquely.

**Venturi e.,** term applied to the operation of a Venturi tube and similar systems.

**Vulpian's e.,** after section and degeneration of the hypoglossal nerve, stimulation of the chorda tympani going to the tongue causes a slow and prolonged contraction of the lingual muscles and vasodilation.

**Zeeman e.,** the splitting of spectral lines into three or more symmetrically placed lines when the light source is subjected to a magnetic field.

**effec'tor** [ L. producer ]. Sherrington's term for a peripheral tissue that receives nerve impulses and reacts by contraction (muscle), secretion (gland), or a discharge of electricity (electric organ of certain bony fishes).

**effemination** (ef-fem-ĭ-na'shun) [ L. *ef-femino,* pp. *-atus,* to make feminine, fr. *ex,* out, + *femina,* woman ]. Acquisition of feminine characteristics, either physiologically by women, or pathologically by individuals of either sex.

**ef'ferens** [ L. ] [ NA ]. Efferent.

**ef'ferent** L. *efferens,* fr. *effero,* to bring out ]. Centrifugal (1); exodic; conducting (fluid or a nerve impulse) outward from a given organ or part thereof; *e.g.,* the efferent connections of a group of nerve cells, efferent blood vessels, or excretory duct of an organ.

**gamma e.,** the thin axon of a gamma motor neuron innervating the intrafusal muscle fibers of a muscle spindle.

**effervesce** (ef'er-ves') [ L. *ef-fervesco,* to boil up, from *ferveo,* to boil ]. To boil up or form bubbles rising to the surface of a fluid in large numbers, as in the evolution of $CO_2$ from aqueous solution when the pressure is reduced.

**effervescent** (ef-er-ves'ent). 1. Boiling; bubbling; effervescing. 2. Causing to effervesce, as an e. powder. 3. Tending to effervesce when freed from pressure, as an e. solution.

**efficiency** (ĕ-fish'en-sĭ). 1. The production of the desired effects or results with minimum waste of time, effort, or skill. 2. A measure of effectiveness; specifically, the useful work output divided by the energy input.

**visual e.,** a rating used in computing compensation for ocular injuries, incorporating measurements of central acuity, visual field, and ocular motility.

**effleurage** (ef-flĕr-azh') [ Fr. *effleurer,* to touch lightly ]. A stroking movement in massage.

**effloresce** (ef-flor-es') [ L. *ef-floresco (exf-),* to blossom, fr. *flos (flor-),* flower ]. To become powdery by losing the water of crystallization on exposure to a dry atmosphere.

**efflores'cence.** The process of efflorescing.

**efflores'cent.** Denoting a crystalline body that gradually changes to a powder by losing its water of crystallization when exposed to the air.

**effluvium, pl. efflu'via** (ĕ-flu'vĭ-um) [ L. a flowing out, fr. *ef-fluo,* to flow out ]. An exhalation, especially one of bad odor or injurious influence.

**effort.** Deliberate exertion of physical or mental power.

**distributed e.,** in psychology, learning that involves small units of work and interpolated rest periods, as contrasted with massed learning, in which the individual works continually until the skill is mastered.

**effuse** (ĕ-fūs') [ L. *ef-fundo,* pp. *-fusus;* to pour out. FUN- ]. Thin and widely spread; denoting the surface character of a bacterial culture.

**effusion** (ĕ-fu'zhun) [ L. *effusio,* a pouring out. FUN- ]. 1. The escape of fluid from the blood vessels or lymphatics into the tissues or a cavity. 2. The fluid effused.

**egersis** (e-ger'sis) [ G. a waking ]. Extremely alert wakefulness.

**egest** (e-jest') [ L. *e-gero,* pp. *-gestus,* to carry out, discharge. GEST- ]. To discharge unabsorbed food residues from the digestive tract.

**egesta** (e-jes'tah) [ L. ntr. pl. of pp., see egest ]. Excreta; dejecta.

**egg** [ A.S. *aeg* ]. The female sexual cell or gamete; after fertilization and fusion of the pronuclei it is a zygote and no longer an egg, although some authors refer to a 2-celled or 4-celled "egg." In the reptile and bird the egg is provided with a protective shell, membranes, albumin, and yolk for the nourishment of the embryo. See also oocyte, ovum.

**cen'trolec'ithal e.,** one in which the yolk is concentrated near the center of the e. cell, as is the case in many of the insects.

**ho'molec'ithal e.,** one in which the total amount of yolk is small and fairly uniformly distributed throughout the cytoplasm.

**isolec'ithal e.,** homolecithal e.

**microlec'ithal e.,** one containing a small amount of deutoplasm.

**telolec'ithal e.,** one containing a relatively large quantity of deutoplasm concentrated at the abapical pole; *e.g.,* e.'s of reptiles and birds.

**white of e.,** albumen.

**Eggleston,** Cary, American physician, *1884. See E. *method.*

**egg'shell.** Testa (1); the calcareous envelope of a bird's egg.

**egilops** (e'jĭ-lops) [ G. *aigilops,* a lacrimal fistula, fr. *aix* (*aig-*), goat, + *ops,* eye ]. A swelling, abscess, or fistula at the inner canthus of the eye.

**eglandulous** (e-glan'du-lus) [ L. *e,* without, + gland or glandula, *q.v.* ]. Without glands.

**Egli's glands.** See under gland.

**e'go** [ L. I ]. In psychoanalysis, one of the three components of the psychic apparatus in the Freudian structural framework, the other two being the id and superego. Although the e. has some conscious components, many of its functions are learned and automatic. It occupies a position between the primal instincts (pleasure principle) and the demands of the outer world (reality principle), and therefore mediates between the person and external reality by performing the important functions of perceiving the needs of the self, both physical and psychological, and the qualities and attitudes of the environment. It evaluates, coordinates, and integrates these perceptions so that internal demands can be adjusted to external requirements, and is also responsible for certain defensive functions to protect the person against the demands of the id and superego.

**egobronchophony** (e'go-brong-kof'o-nĭ) [ G. *aix* (*aig-*), goat, + *bronchos,* bronchus, + *phōnē,* voice ]. Egophony with bronchophony.

**egocentric** [ ego + G. *kentron,* center ]. Marked by extreme concentration of attention upon oneself; selfish; self-centered.

**egocentricity** (e'go-sen-tris'ĭ-tĭ). The condition of being egocentric.

**ego-dystonic** (e'go-dis-ton'ik) [ ego + G. *dys,* bad, + *tonos,* tension ]. Repugnant to or at variance with the aims of the ego.

**egomania** (e'go-ma'nĭ-ah) [ ego + G. *mania,* frenzy ]. Extreme self-appreciation or self-content.

**egophonic** (e-go-fon'ik). Relating to egophony, as e. resonance.

**egophony** (e-gof'o-nĭ) [ G. *aix* (*aig-*), goat, + *phōnē,* voice ]. Tragophony; capriloquism; a peculiar broken quality of the voice sounds, like the bleating of a goat, heard about the upper level of the fluid in cases of pleurisy with effusion.

**ego-syntonic** (e'go-sin-ton'ik) [ ego + G. *syn,* together, + *tonos,* tension ]. Acceptable to the aims of the ego.

**egotropic** (e'go-trop'ik) [ ego + G. *tropē,* a turning ]. Introspective; self-centered.

**Eh, eH.** Symbol for oxidation-reduction *potential.* Now more commonly used are the symbols $E_0{}^+$, $E^0$.

**Ehlers** (a'lairs), Edward L., Danish dermatologist, 1863–1937. See E.-Danlos *syndrome.*

**Ehrenritter** (a'ren-rit-er), Johann, Austrian anatomist, †1790. See E.'s *ganglion.*

**Eh'ret,** Heinrich, German physician, *1870. See E.'s *phenomenon.*

**Ehrlich** (air'lich), Paul, German bacteriologist and immunologist, 1854–1915. Nobel laureate, 1908, with Elie Metchnikoff, for their work on immunity. See E.'s *anemia, body, hematoxylin, phenomenon, postulate, reactions, stains, theorem, theory,* Koch-E. *stain.*

**Eichhorst** (īkh'horst), Hermann L., Swiss physician, 1849–1921. See E.'s *corpuscles, neuritis.*

**Eichstedt** (īkh'stet), Karl F., German dermatologist, 1816–1892. See E.'s *disease.*

**Eicken** (i'ken), Karl v., German laryngologist, 1873–1960. See E.'s *method.*

**eicosanoic acid.** Arachidic acid.

**eidetic** (i-det'ik) [ G. *eidon,* saw (aorist of verb with no pres. in use) ]. 1. Relating to the power of visualization of objects previously seen or imagined. 2. A person possessing this power in high degree.

**eidoptometry** (i-dop-tom'e-trī) [ G. *eidos,* form, + *optikos,* referring to vision, + *metron,* measure ]. The measurement of the acuteness of form vision.

**Eijkman** (ik'man), Christiaan, Dutch physiologist and bacteriologist, 1858–1930. Nobel laureate, 1929, with Frederick G. Hopkins, for early vitamin studies and discovery of the cause of beriberi.

**eikonometer, eiconometer** (i-ko-nom'e-ter) [ G. *eikon,* image, + *metron,* measure ]. 1. An instrument for determining the magnifying power of a microscope, or the size of a microscopic object. 2. An instrument for determining the degree of aniseikonia.

**eiloid** (i'loyd) [ G. *eilō,* to roll up, + *eidos,* appearance ]. Resembling a coil or roll.

**Eimeria** (i-me'rĭ-ah) [ Theodor *Eimer* ]. The largest, most economically important, and most widespread genus of the coccidial protozoan parasites (family Eimeriidae, class Sporozoa); the mature oocyst contains four sporocysts, each of which contains two sporozoites. E. is highly pathogenic, especially in young hosts. Many species infect wild vertebrates; domesticated mammals and birds commonly are infected with one or more species.

**E. ana'tis,** found in the small intestine of wild ducks.

**E. or coccidia of cattle,** *E. zuernii* is the species most often associated with clinical cases of coccidiosis in calves and young adults; found in cecum and lower bowel, and sometimes in small intestine. *E. bovis* occurs principally in the small intestine and causes clinically recognizable disease. Less common species are *E. ellipsoidalis, E. bukidnonensis, E. cylindrica, E. canadensis, E. auburnensis, E. subspherica, E. alabamensis, E. brasiliense, E. ildefonsoi,* and *E. wyomingensis.*

**E. or coccidia of chickens,** *E. tenella* produces cecal coccidiosis of young chicks; *E. necatrix* produces severe disease in small intestine and ceca; *E. acervulina, E. hagani,* and *E. praecox* localize in the duodenum; *E. mitis* localizes in the small intestine; *E. brunetti* localizes in the lower small intestine and rectum; *E. maxima* localizes in the lower small intestine.

**E. or coccidia of geese,** *E. truncata* occurs in the kidney tubules where it causes much damage and considerable mortality in young birds; *E. anseris, E. nocens,* and *E. parvula* occur in the small intestine; the pathogenicity of the intestinal forms in geese is in doubt.

**E. or coccidia of pheasants,** *E. phasiani* and *E. dispersa* infect the small intestine; coccidiosis of pheasants in captivity may be very destructive.

**E.** or **coccidia of rabbits,** *E. stiedae* is the most common form in rabbits and affects the bile ducts; *E. perforans* affects the small intestine and cecum; *E. media, E. magna,* and *E. irresidua* affect the small intestine.

**E.** or **coccidia of sheep and goats,** *E. ovina (arloingi)* is the most common and most destructive coccidium of sheep; principal losses are in young lambs. *E. minakolyakimovae* is another highly pathogenic parasite of sheep. *E. parva* and *E. pallida* are frequently found but are believed to be of low virulence. *E. faurei, E. intricata, E. granulosa, E. ahsata, E. hawkins, E. gilruthi, E. gonzalezi, E. christenseni, E. punctata, E. crandallis,* and *E. honessi* are species found in sheep or goats; their pathogenicity is believed to be low. All of these species involve the epithelium of the small intestine.

**E.** or **coccidia of swine,** *E. debliecki* is the most common and most pathogenic. and involves the small intestine, cecum, and colon; *E. scabra* involves the small intestine; *E. perminuta, E. spinosa, E. scrofae, E. suis, E. cerdonis, E. porci,* and *E. neodebliecki* are believed to have little pathogenicity. See *Isospora* for other species.

**E.** or **coccidia of turkeys,** *E. meleagrimitis* localizes in the jejunum; *E. meleagridis* localizes in the cecum; *E. dispersa* and *E. innocua* localize in the small intestine; *E. adenoeides* localizes in lower ileum, cecum, and rectum; *E. gallopavonis* localizes in the ileum and rectum.

**E. sardinae,** occurs in sardines and herring, and has been found in the feces of men who had eaten these fish; it was once erroneously believed to be a coccidium of man.

**Eimeriidae** (i-mer-i'e-de). A family of sporozoan parasites of animals generally known under the common name, coccidia. The important genera, from a veterinary and medical standpoint, are *Eimeria* and *Isospora;* infections with *Eimeria* are by far the most common and the most serious in domesticated animals.

**Einhorn** (in'horn), Max, New York gastroenterologist, 1862–1953. See E.'s *saccharimeter.*

**Einstein,** Albert, American theoretical physicist, 1879–1955. Gave his name to the einstein and to einsteinium.

**einstein** [ A. *Einstein* ]. A unit of energy equal to 1 mol quantum, hence to $6.02 = 10^{23}$ quanta.

**einsteinium** (in-stin'i-um) [ A. *Einstein* ]. Radioactive element, artificially prepared in 1955, atomic no. 99, atomic symbol at first E, then changed officially to Es.

**Einthoven** (int'ho-fen), Willem, Dutch physiologist, 1860–1927. Nobel laureate, 1924, for devising a galvanometer used in investigations of electrocardiography.

**Eisenlohr** (i'zen-lor), Carl, German physician, 1847–1896. See E.'s *syndrome.*

**Eisenmenger** (i'zen-meng-er), Victor, German physician, 1864–1932. See E.'s *complex, disease, syndrome, tetralogy.*

**eisodic** (i-sod'ik) [ G. *eis,* into, + *hodos,* a way ]. Afferent.

**ejaculatio** (e-jak-u-la'shi-o) [ L. see JAC- ]. Ejaculation.
  **e. deficiens** absence of ejaculation.
  **e. pre'cox,** premature *ejaculation.*
  **e. retarda'ta,** unusually delayed ejaculation, constituting one of the symptoms of impotence.

**ejaculation** (e-jak-u-la'shun) [ L. *ejaculatio* ]. Emission of seminal fluid.
  **premature e.,** ejaculatio precox; prospermia; during sexual intercourse, too rapid achievement of climax and e. in the male relative to his own or his partner's wishes.

**ejac'ulatory.** Relating to an ejaculation.

**ejecta** (e-jek'ta) [ L. ntr. pl. of *ejectus,* pp. of *ejicio,* to throw out. JAC- ]. 1. Material that is ejected. 2. Dejecta.

**ejection** (e-jek'shun) [ L. *ejectio,* from *ejicio,* to cast out ]. 1. The act of driving or throwing out by physical force from within. 2. That which is ejected.

**ejec'tor.** A device used for forcibly expelling (ejecting) a substance.
  **saliva e.,** a hollow, perforated suction tube used in the evacuation of saliva or liquid debris from the oral cavity.

**eka-cesium.** Francium.

**eka-iodine.** Astatine.

**eka-manganese.** Technetium.

**Ekbom,** K. A., Swedish physician. See E. *syndrome.*

**EKG.** Abbreviation for electrocardiogram; also abbreviated ECG.

**ekiri** (e-ki'ri) [ Jap. ]. An acute, toxic form of dysentery of infants seen in Japan and due to the Sonne bacillus.

**EKY.** Abbreviation for electrokymogram.

**elabora'tion** [ L. *e-laboro,* pp. *-atus,* to labor, endeavor, fr. *labor,* toil, to work out ]. The process of working out in detail by labor and study.
  **secondary e.,** the mental process occurring partly during dreaming and partly during the recalling or telling of a dream by means of which the latent (relatively organized) content of the dream is brought into increasingly more coherent and logical order, resulting in the manifest content of the dream; as aspect of dream work.

**Elaeoph'ora schnei'deri.** The bloodworm of sheep; a nematode causing filarial dermatosis.

**elaidic acid** (el-a-id'ik). $CH_3(CH_2)_7CH=CH(CH_2)_7-COOH;$ *trans-*9-octadecenoic acid; an unsaturated monobasic *trans*-isomer of oleic acid.

**elaidin** (e-la'i-din). The elaidic acid triester of glycerol; found in certain nondrying oils; an isomer of olein.

**elaiopathia** (el'a-o-path'i-ah) [ G. *elaion,* oil, + *pathos,* suffering ]. Eleopathy.

**Elapidae** (e-lap'i-de) [ G. *elops,* a serpent ]. A snake family characterized by two short fixed fangs and a potent neurotoxic venom. It includes cobra, krait, mamba, and coral snakes.

**Elasmobranchii** (e-las'mo-brang'ke-i) [ G. *elasmos,* a metal plate, + *branchia,* gills ]. Elasmobranchs; the cartilaginous fishes, sharks, rays, and skates. Class *Chondrichthyes.*

**elas'tance.** A measure of the tendency of a structure to return to its original form after removal of a deforming force. In medicine and physiology, usually a measure of the tendency of a hollow viscus (*e.g.* lung, urinary bladder, gall bladder) to recoil toward its original dimensions upon removal of a distending or compressing force, the recoil pressure resulting from a unit distention on compression of the viscus. E. is the reciprocal of compliance, *q.v.* The relationship between elasticity and e. is of the same nature as that between the specific inductive capacity of an insulator material and the capacitance of a particular condenser made from that material.

**elas'tase.** Pancreatopeptidase E; elastinase; a hydrolase (EC 3.4.21.11, formerly 3.4.4.7) hydrolyzing elastin. It is formed from proelastase and is structurally homologous with trypsin and other serine proteinases.

**elas'tic** [ G. *elastreō,* epic form of *elaunō,* drive, push ]. Having the property of returning to the original shape after being compressed, bent, or otherwise distorted.

**elas'tica.** 1. The elastic layer in the wall of an artery. 2. Elastic *tissue.*

**elas'ticin.** Elastin.

**elasticity** (e-las-tis'i-ti). The quality or condition of being elastic.
  **physical e. of muscle,** the quality of muscle that enables it to yield to passive physical stretch.
  **physiologic e. of muscle,** the biologic quality, unique for muscle, of being able to change and resume size under neuromuscular control.
  **total e. of muscle,** the combined effect of physical and physiologic e. of muscle.

**elas'tin.** The major connective tissue protein of elastic structures (*e.g.,* large blood vessels); a yellow, elastic, fibrous mucoprotein.

**elas'tinase.** Elastase.

**elastofibro'ma.** A nonencapsulated mass of poorly cellular, collagenous, fibrous tissue and elastic tissue; occurs usually in subscapular adipose tissue of old persons (where it is termed e. dorsi), and may not be a neoplasm but may result from friction between the scapula and ribs.

**elastoidin.** A complex collagen.

**elasto'ma.** *Pseudoxanthoma* elasticum.

**elastom'eter.** A device for measuring the elasticity of any body or of the animal tissues.

**elastomu'cin.** Mucoprotein of connective tissue; see elastin.

**elastorrhexis** (e-las'to-rek'sis) [ G. *rhēxis,* rupture. RHAG- ]. Fragmentation of elastic tissue in which the normal wavy strands appear shredded and clumped, and take the basophilic stain.

**elasto'sis.** Degenerative change in elastic tissue.

   **actinic e.,** colloid milia; colloid degeneration of the skin that takes place in the elastic tissue of the dermis in persons who are repeatedly or constantly exposed to sunlight over a period of many years.

   **e. dystroph'ica,** angioid streaks of the retina due to rupture of Bruch's membrane; a manifestation of pseudoxanthoma elasticum.

   **e. per'forans serpigino'sa,** circinate groups of asymptomatic keratotic papules; the epidermis is thickened around a central plug of keratin, overlying an accumulation of elastic tissue.

   **senile e.,** senile degeneration (2); elastic tissue degeneration seen histologically in the skin of the elderly or in those who have chronic actinic effect.

**elastra'tion.** Use of a strong rubber band for the purpose of castrating male lambs. Although it is effective for the purpose, many of the victims fall prey to tetanus infections.

**elation** (e-la'shun) [ L. *elatio,* fr. *ef-fero,* pp. *e-latus,* to lift up ]. The exaggerated feeling or expression of excitement or gaiety.

**Elaut** (a'lout), Leon J. S., Belgian anatomist. See E.'s *triangle.*

**elbow** (el'bo) [ A.S. *elnboga* ]. 1. Ancon; cubitus; the joint between the arm and the forearm. 2. An angular body resembling a flexed e.

   **bend of the e.,** *fossa cubitalis.*

   **capped e.,** shoe *boil.*

   **gunstock deformity of the e.,** see under deformity.

   **e. lameness,** lameness in the horse most commonly due to disease of the joint, sprain of the lateral ligaments, or rupture of the triceps.

   **miner's e.,** inflammation with fluid distention of the olecranon bursa.

   **point of the e.,** olecranon.

   **tennis e.,** condition characterized by pain in or near lateral epicondyle of humerus, or in extensor muscle mass of forearm, as a result of unusual strain (not necessarily tennis). Also called epicondylalgia externa.

**elbowed** (el'bōd). Angular; kneed.

**el'der.** Sambucus; the dried flowers of *Sambucus canadensis* (family Caprifoliaceae).

**Eldridge-Green lamp.** See under lamp.

**elecampane** (el'e-kam-pān') [ Mediev. L. *inula campana,* elacampane, fr. L. *inula,* e. + *campus,* field ]. Inula; elfwort; horseheal; scabwort; the rhizome and roots of *Inula helenium* (family Compositae); a source of inulin.

**electriza'tion.** 1. The act of electrifying. 2. Treatment by means of electricity.

**electro-** [ G. *ēlektron,* amber (electricity) ]. Prefix denoting electric or electricity.

**elec'troanal'ysis.** Quantitative analysis of metals by electrolysis.

**electroanesthesia** (e-lek'tro-an-es-the'zī-ah). Anesthesia produced by an electric current.

**electroaxonography** (e-lek'tro-ak-son-og'rä-fī). Axonography.

**elec'troba'sograph** [ electro- + G. *basis,* walking, + *graphō,* to write ]. Apparatus for recording the gait.

**elec'trobiol'ogy.** The science concerned with electrical phenomena in living organisms.

**elec'trobios'copy** [ electro- + G. *bios,* life, + *skopeō,* to examine ]. The use of electricity as a means of determining whether life is extinct or not.

**electrocar'diogram** [ electro- + G. *kardia,* heart, + *gramma,* a drawing ]. The graphic record of the heart's action currents obtained with the electrocardiograph. Abbreviated ECG or EKG.

   **unipolar e.,** one taken with the exploring electrode placed on the chest overlying the heart or upon a single limb, the indifferent electrode being the central terminal.

**elec'trocar'diograph.** An instrument for recording the potential of the electrical currents that traverse the heart and initiate its contraction.

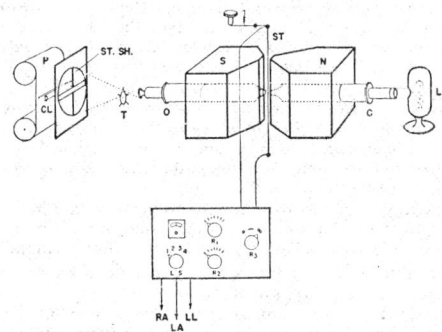

**Electrocardiograph**

Diagram of the principal parts of original string galvanometer model. *P,* roll of photographic paper moving behind the lens, *CL,* which narrows the shadow, *ST.SH,* of the string, *ST,* to a thin, vertical line and focuses it upon the sensitive paper. By means of ruled etchings upon the lens, horizontal lines 1 mm. and ⅕ mm. apart are thrown upon the record; the heights of the waves in the electrocardiogram can thus be measured and the electromotive force in each wave calculated. *T* is a rotating toothed disk that breaks the light beam at regular intervals of 1/50 or 1/25 second and, by throwing vertical shadow lines upon the record, serves as a time marker. *O* and *C* indicate the positions of the lenses in the projection system; *S* and *N* are the poles of the electromagnet; *L* is the source of light. The current from the subject passes through the control box below. Switches on the dial enable a record from any lead to be taken. *RA, LA,* and *LL* represent the three standard leads, right arm, left arm, and left leg. (Courtesy of Dr. L. N. Katz.)

   **e. of amplifier type,** one in which the current is increased by a radioamplifying tube and then recorded.

**elec'trocardiog'raphy.** 1. A method of recording electrical currents traversing the heart muscle just previous to each heart beat; the machine used is an electrocardiograph, and the result obtained is an electrocardiogram. 2. The study and interpretation of electrocardiograms.

   **fetal e.,** recording the electrocardiogram of the fetus *in utero.*

   **intrabronchial e.,** the taking of an electrocardiogram with the exploring electrode inserted into a bronchus.

**electrocardiophonography** (e-lek'tro-kar-dī-o-fo-nog'rä-fī) [ electro- + G. *kardia,* heart, + *phōnē,* sound, + *graphō,* to write ]. A method of recording the heart sounds, the record being an electrocardiophonogram, or, more simply, an electrophonogram.

**elec'trocar'dioscope.** An oscilloscope for the continuous monitoring of the electrocardiogram.

**electrocatalysis** (e-lek'tro-kă-tal'ī-sis). Catalysis, or chemical decomposition, produced by electricity.

**electrocauterization** (e-lek'tro-caw'ter-i-za'shun). 1. Cauterization by passage of high frequency current through tissue. 2. Cauterization by metal that has been heated by a current of electricity.

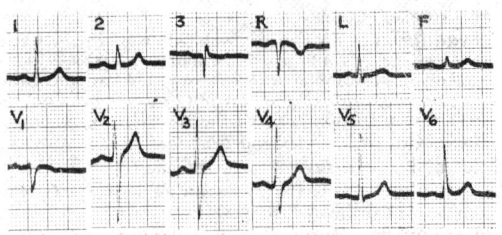

**Normal 12-Lead Electrocardiogram**

**electrocautery** (e-lek'tro-caw'ter-ĭ). 1. An instrument for directing a high frequency current through a local area of tissue. 2. A metal cauterizing instrument heated by an electric current.

**elec'trochem'ical.** Relating to electrochemistry.

**elec'trochem'istry.** The study of those chemical reactions effected by means of electricity and the mechanisms involved; the study of the electrical aspects of chemical reactions.

**electrocholecystectomy** (e-lek'tro-ko'le-sis-tek'to-mĭ). Removal of gallbladder by electrosurgery.

**electrocholecystocausis** (e-lek'tro-ko-le-sis'to-kaw'sis). Cauterization of gallbladder by electrosurgery.

**electrocoagulation** (e-lek'tro-ko-ag-u-la'shun). Coagulation produced by an electrocautery.

**elec'trocontractil'ity.** The power of contraction of muscular tissue in response to an electrical stimulus.

**elec'troconvul'sive.** Denoting a convulsive response to an electrical stimulus; see electroshock *therapy.*

**elec'trocor'ticogram.** A record of electrical activity derived from the cerebral cortex.

**elec'trocorticog'raphy.** The technique of surveying the electrical activity of the cerebral cortex.

**electrocute** (e-lek'tro-kūt) [ electro- + execute ]. To cause death by the passage of an electric current through the body, either accidentally or in carrying out a legal death sentence.

**electrocution** (e-lek-tro-ku'shun). Death caused by electricity; see electrocute.

**electrocystography** (e-lek'tro-sis-tog'ră-fĭ). Recording of electric currents from the urinary bladder.

**elec'trode** [ electro- + G. *hodos,* way ]. 1. One of the two extremities of an electric circuit; one of the two poles of an electric battery or of the end of the conductors connected thereto. 2. An electrical terminal specialized for a particular electrochemical reaction.

  **active e.,** therapeutic e.

  **calomel e.,** an e. in which the wire is connected through a pool of mercury to a paste of mercurous chloride ($Hg_2Cl_2$, calomel) in a potassium chloride solution covered by more potassium chloride solution; commonly used as a reference electrode.

  **carbon dioxide e.,** Severinghaus e.; a glass e. in a film of bicarbonate solution covered by a thin plastic membrane permeable to carbon dioxide but impermeable to water and electrolytes; the carbon dioxide pressure of a gas or liquid sample quickly equilibrates through the membrane and is measured in terms of the resulting pH of the bicarbonate solution, as sensed by the glass electrode; commonly used to analyze arterial blood samples.

  **central terminal e.,** in electrocardiography, one in which connections from the three limbs (right arm, left arm, and left leg) are joined and led to the electrocardiograph to form the indifferent e.

  **Clark e.,** an oxygen e. consisting of the tip of a platinum wire exposed to a thin film of electrolyte covered by a plastic membrane permeable to oxygen but not to water or the electrolyte. When a certain voltage is applied, oxygen is destroyed at the platinum surface; the flow of current is then proportional to the rate at which oxygen can diffuse to the platinum surface from the gas or liquid sample outside the membrane, and is thus a measure of the oxygen pressure in the sample; commonly used to measure oxygen pressure in arterial blood samples.

  **dispersing e.,** indifferent e.

  **exciting e.,** therapeutic e.

  **exploring e.,** one which is on or near an excitable tissue; in unipolar electrocardiography it is on the chest in the region of the heart and is paired with an indifferent electrode.

  **glass e.,** a thin-walled glass bulb filled with some standard buffer solution and a little quinhydrone (see quinhydrone e. below) and a platinum wire. When it is immersed in an unknown solution, a potential difference develops that varies with the pH of the unknown solution; this difference can be made to give the pH. Most pH meters in common use contain a glass e.

  **hydrogen e.,** the ultimate standard of reference in all pH determinations, but limited and technically difficult to use.

It consists of a piece of spongy platinum black partly immersed in a solution in a small glass tube. The tube above the solution is filled with hydrogen gas that is bubbled through the solution and that is absorbed by the platinum. The electrode thus measures the potential between $H_2$ and $H^+$, the "standard" potential of which (1 atmosphere, 1 molar) is taken as zero; hence the hydrogen e. potential measures [ $H^+$ ] or pH.

  **indifferent e.,** dispersing e.; silent e.; in unipolar electrocardiography, a remote e. placed either upon a single limb or connected with the central terminal and paired with an exploring e.; the indifferent e. is supposed to contribute little or nothing to the resulting record.

  **lo'calizing e.,** therapeutic e.

  **negative e.,** cathode.

  **oxygen e.,** an e., usually consisting of a platinum wire or dropping mercury, used to measure the oxygen concentration in a solution by polarography.

  **positive e.,** anode.

  **quinhydrone e.,** one of several oxidation-reduction e.'s ("redox" e.'s) in which the ratio of the two forms (quinone-quinhydrone), determined by the hydrogen ion concentration, sets up a potential that can be measured and converted to a pH value; fails above pH 8.

  **reference e.,** an e. expected to have a constant potential, such as a calomel e., and used with another electrode to complete an electrical circuit through a solution; *e.g.,* when a reference e. is used with a glass e. for pH measurement, changes in voltage between the two e.'s can be attributed to the effects of pH on the glass e. alone.

  **Severinghaus e.,** carbon dioxide e.

  **silent e.,** indifferent e.

  **therapeutic e.,** localizing e.; the e. by means of which the therapeutic action of the electricity is obtained.

**electroder'mal** [ electro- + G. *derma,* skin ]. Pertaining to electric properties of the skin, usually referring to altered resistance.

**elec'trodesicca'tion** [ electro- + L. *desicco,* to dry up ]. Destruction of growths (usually of the skin but also of available surfaces of mucous membrane) by monopolar electric current or Ouidin current.

**electrodiagno'sis.** Determination of the nature of a disease through observation of changes in electrical irritability.

**electrodial'ysis.** The removal in an electric field of ions from larger molecules and particles.

**electroencephalogram** (e-lek'tro-en-sef'ă-lo-gram). The record, obtained by means of the electroencephalograph, of the brain potentials derived from scalp electrodes.

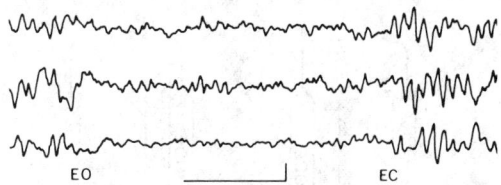

**Electroencephalogram**

EEG from left occipital, midline occipital, and right occipital leads to show the effect of opening (*EO*) and closing (*EC*) the eyes on the alpha rhythm; the horizontal line at the base indicates a time interval of 1 second and the vertical arm a calibration of 50 microvolts.

  **flat e.,** isoelectric e.

  **isoelectric e.,** flat e.; a record indicating the absence of electric potentials of cerebral origin of over 2 microvolts during a period of, at least, 30 minutes, when recording from symmetrically placed electrode pairs 10 or more cm. apart and with interelectrode resistances between 100 and 10,000 ohms.

**electroencephalograph** (e-lek'tro-en-sef'ă-lo-graf) [ electro- + G. *encephalon,* brain, + *graphō,* to write ]. An apparatus consisting of amplifiers and a write-out system for recording the electric potentials of the brain derived from leads of the scalp. It is useful in localizing intracranial lesions and brain tumors, and distinguishing between diffuse and focal brain lesions in epilepsy.

**electroencephalography** (e-lek'tro-en-sef'ă-log'ră-fĭ). The registration of the electrical potentials recorded by an electroencephalograph; the record is called an electroencephalogram.

**electroendosmosis** (e-lek'tro-en'dos-mo'sis). Endosmosis produced by means of an electric field.

**elec'trogas'trogram.** The record obtained with the electrogastrograph.

**elec'trogas'trograph.** An instrument for recording the electrical phenomena associated with gastric secretion and motility.

**elec'trogastrog'raphy.** The recording of the electrical phenomena associated with gastric secretion and motility.

**elec'trogram.** 1. Any record on paper or film made by an electrical event. 2. In electrophysiology, a recording taken directly from the surface by unipolar or bipolar leads.

**electrography** (e-lek-trog'ră-fĭ) [ electro- + G. *graphō*, to write ]. The technique of making a graphic record by electrical means.

His bundle e., the science of recording electrograms from the bundle of His, either in the experimental animal or in man during cardiac catheterization.

**electrohemostasis** (e-lek'tro-hĕ-mos'tă-sis, -he'mo-sta'sis) [ electro- + G. *haima*, blood, + *stasis*, halt ]. The arrest of hemorrhage by means of the electrocautery.

**electrohysterograph** (e-lek'tro-his'ter-o-graf) [ electro- + G. *hystera*, womb, + *graphō*, to write ]. Instrument that records uterine electrical activity.

**electroky'mogram.** The graphic record of the heart's movements produced by the electrokymograph. Abbreviated EKY.

**elec'troky'mograph.** [ electro- + G. *kyma*, wave, + *graphō*, to write ]. An apparatus for recording, from changes in the x-ray silhouette, the movements of the heart and great vessels. It consists of a fluoroscope, x-ray tube, and a photomultiplier tube together with an electrocardiograph.

**electrokymography** (e-lek-tro-ki-mog'ră-fĭ). 1. The registration of the movements of the heart and great vessels by means of the electrokymograph. 2. The science and technique of interpreting electrokymograms.

**electrolithotrity** (e-lek'tro-lĭ-thot'rĭ-tĭ) [ electro- + G. *lithos*, stone, + L. *tero*, pp. *tritus*, to rub ]. Electrolysis of a vesical calculus.

**electrolysis** (e-lek-trol'ĭ-sis) [ electro- + G. *lysis*, dissolution ]. 1. Decomposition of a salt or other chemical compound by means of an electric current. 2. Decomposition of certain of the body tissues by means of electricity.

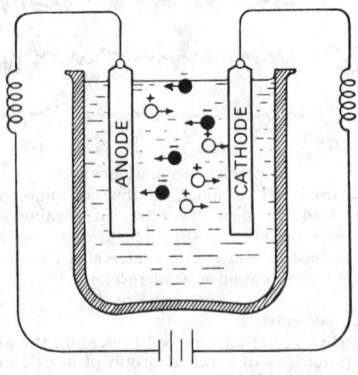

**Chemical Electrolysis**

The liquid contains a crystalloid such as sodium chloride. The circles represent anions (*black*) and cations (*clear*).

**electrolyte** (e-lek'tro-lit) [ electro- + G. *lytos*, soluble ]. Any compound that, in solution, conducts a current in electricity and is decomposed by it; an ionizable substance in solution.

**amphoter'ic e.,** an e. that can either give up or take on a hydrogen ion and can thus behave as either an acid or a base; ampholyte.

**electrolytic** (e-lek'tro-lit'ik). Referring to or caused by electrolysis.

**theory of e. dissociation,** see Arrhenius' *doctrine.*

**electrolyzable** (e-lek'tro-li'za-bl). Capable of being decomposed by means of an electric current.

**elec'trolyze.** To decompose chemically by means of an electric current.

**elec'trolyzer.** An apparatus for the treatment of strictures, fibromas, etc., by electrolysis.

**electromag'net.** A bar of soft iron rendered magnetic by an electric current encircling it.

**electromassage** (e-lek'tro-mas-sazh'). Massage combined with the application of electricity.

**electromy'ogram.** A graphic representation of the somatic electric currents associated with muscular action; abbreviated EMG.

**electromy'ograph.** An instrument for recording electrical currents generated in an active muscle.

**electromyography** (e-lek'tro-mi-og'ră-fĭ) [ electro- + G. *mys*, muscle, + *graphō*, to write ]. A method of recording the electrical currents generated in an active muscle.

**elec'tron.** One of the negatively charged subatomic particles that, distributed about the positive nucleus, constitute the atom; when emitted from inside the nucleus of a radioactive substance the e.'s are called beta particles; in mass they are estimated to be $1/_{1838}$ of the hydrogen atom.

**emis'sion e.,** beta particle or similar electron resulting from radioactive decay.

**speeding e.,** beta *particle.*

**va'lence e.,** one of the e.'s that take part in the chemical reaction of the atom.

**elec'tronarco'sis.** Production of insensibility to pain by the use of electrical current.

**electroneg'ative.** Relating to or charged with negative electricity; referring to an element whose uncharged atoms have a tendency to ionize by adding electrons, thus becoming anions (*e.g.,* oxygen, fluorine, or chlorine).

**electroneurography** (e-lek'tro-nu-rog'ră-fĭ). A method of recording the electrical changes and nerve conduction velocities associated with the passing of impulses along peripheral nerves.

**electroneurolysis** (e-lek'tro-nu-rol'ĭ-sis). Destruction of nerve tissue by electricity.

**electroneuromyography** (e-lek'tro-nu'ro-mi-og'ră-fĭ). A method of measuring changes in a peripheral nerve by combining electromyography of a muscle with electrical stimulation of the nerve trunk carrying fibers to and from the muscle.

**electron'ic.** Pertaining to electrons.

**electronization** (e-lek'tron-ĭ-za'shun). Chemical reduction; the addition of an electron to a compound.

**electron-volt.** Abbreviated ev; the energy imparted to an electron by a potential of 1 volt; equal to $1.6 \times 10^{-12}$ erg in the CGS system, or $1.6 \times 10^{-19}$ joule in the SI system.

**electronystagmography** (e-lek'tro-ni-stag-mog'ră-fĭ) [ electro- + nystagmus + G. *graphō*, to write ]. A method of nystagmography based on electro-oculography; skin electrodes are placed at outer canthi to register horizontal nystagmus; above and below each eye for vertical nystagmus. Abbreviated ENG.

**electro-oculogram** (e-lek-tro-ok'u-lo-gram). A record on paper or film of electric currents in electro-oculography.

**electro-oculography** (e-lek-tro-ok'u-log'ră-fĭ). Abbreviated EOG; oculography using electrodes placed on the skin adjacent to the lateral canthi to detect a standing potential difference between the front and the back of the eyeball; a sensitive electrical test for detection of retinal dysfunction.

**elec'tro-osmo'sis.** The diffusion of a substance through a membrane in an electric field.

**electropathol'ogy.** The study of pathologic conditions in their relation to electrical reactions.

**elec'tropher'ogram.** Electrophoretogram; ionogram; ionopherogram; the densitometric or colorimetric pattern obtained from filter paper strips on which substances have been separated by electrophoresis; may also refer to the strips themselves.

**electrophil, electrophile** (e-lek'tro-fil, -fīl) [ electro- + G. *philos*, fond ]. 1. The electron-attracting atom or agent in an organic reaction; the opposite of nucleophil. 2. Electrophilic; relating to an electrophil.

**electrophilic** (elek'tro-fil'ik). Electrophil (2).

**electropho'bia** [ electro- + G. *phobos*, fear ]. Morbid fear of electricity.

**electrophore** (e-lek'tro-fōr). An appliance for obtaining electricity by induction; electrophorus.

**electrophoresis** (e-lek-tro-fo-re'sis) [ electro- + G. *phorēsis*, a carrying ]. The movement of particles in an electric field toward one or other electric pole, anode or cathode.

  **disc e.,** a modification of gel e. in which a discontinuity (pH, gel pore size) is introduced near the origin to produce a lamina (disc) of the materials being separated. The separating bands retain their disc-like shape as they move through the gel. The term "disc" was originally proposed by the inventor primarily to express the idea of *discontinuity*, secondarily to reflect the *disc*oid shape of the separate bands.

  **gel e.,** e. through a gel, usually contained in a cylindrical tube.

  **thin-layer e.,** abbreviated TLE; electrophoretic migrations (separations) through a thin layer of inert material, such as cellulose, supported on a glass or plastic plate.

**elec'trophoret'ic.** Relating to electrophoresis, as an e. separation.

**elec'trophoret'ogram.** Electropherogram.

**electroph'orus.** Electrophore.

**elec'tropho'tother'apy.** Phototherapy in which the source of the rays is the electric light.

**electrophrenic** (e-lek'tro-fren'ik). Denoting electrical stimulation of the phrenic nerve usually at its motor point in the neck. See also e. *respiration.*

**elec'trophysiol'ogy.** The branch of science which treats of electrical phenomena that are associated with physiologic processes. Electrical phenomena are prominent in neurons and effectors.

**elec'troplate.** To plate or coat with a metal by means of electrolysis. Dental impressions are sometimes plated with copper or silver to produce a die with a metal surface. Since impression materials are nonconductors, they are first coated with a metallizing agent in order that they may be plated.

**electroplexy** (e-lek'tro-plek'sī) [ electro- + G. *plessō*, to strike ]. Striking with electric current, as in electric shock therapy, or accidentally by lightning or electrocution.

**electropneumograph** (e-lek'tro-nu'mo-graf). An electric apparatus used for recording breathing.

**elec'tropos'itive.** Relating to or charged with positive electricity; referring to an element whose atoms tend to lose electrons; *e.g.,* sodium, potassium, or calcium.

**electropunc'ture.** The passage of an electrical current through needle electrodes piercing the tissues.

**elec'troradiol'ogy.** The use of electricity and x-ray in treatment.

**electroradiometer** (e-lek'tro-ra-dī-om'e-ter) [ electro- + L. *radius*, ray, + G. *metron*, measure ]. A modified electroscope designed for the differentiation of radiant energy.

**electroretinogram** (e-lek'tro-ret'ī-no-gram) [ electro- + retina + G. *gramma*, something written ]. A record of retinal action currents, registered by a galvanometer, from

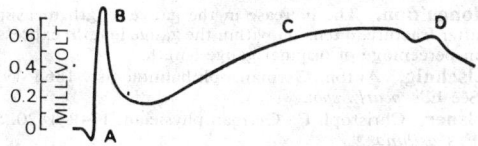

**Electroretinogram**
The waves *A, B,* and *C* are inscribed when light is thrown into the eye; the *D* wave occurs when the light is shut off.

the surface of the eyeball and originated by a pulse of light. Abbreviation, ERG.

**electroretinography** (e-lek'tro-ret'ī-nog'rǎ-fī). The recording and study of the retinal action currents.

**electrosalivogram** (e-lek'tro-sǎ-li'vo-gram). A record of electrical activity in the salivary glands during secretion.

**electroscission** (e-lek'tro-sī-shun) [ electro- + L. *scissio,* to cleave ]. Division of the tissues by means of an electrocautery knife.

**elec'troscope** [ electro- + G. *skopeō,* to examine ]. An instrument for the detection of electrical charges or gaseous ions (*e.g.,* from β-rays or x-rays). It consists of two strips of gold leaf, suspended from an insulated conductor and enclosed in an airtight container.

**elec'troshock.** See electroshock *therapy.*

**elec'trosol.** Colloidal *metal.*

**elec'trospectrog'raphy.** The recording of electroencephalographic wave patterns, their study and interpretation.

**elec'trospi'nogram.** Record of electrical activity of the spinal cord.

**elec'trostenol'ysis.** The precipitation of metals in membrane pores in the course of electrolysis.

**electrostethograph** (e-lek'tro-steth'o-graf) [ electro- + G. *stēthos,* chest, + *graphō,* to record ]. An electrical instrument that amplifies or records the respiratory and cardiac sounds of the chest.

**electrostriction** (e-lek'tro-strik'shun). The contraction in volume in a protein solution during proteolysis due to the formation of new charged groups.

**electrosur'gery.** The use of electricity in surgery.

**electrosyn'thesis.** Forming a compound by means of electrical action.

**electrotax'is** [ electro- + G. *taxis,* orderly arrangement ]. Electrotropism; galvanotaxis; galvanotropism; reaction of plant or animal protoplasm to either an anode or a cathode; see also tropism.

  **negative e.,** e. by which an organism is attracted toward an anode or repelled from a cathode.

  **positive e.,** e. by which an organism is attracted toward a cathode or repelled from an anode.

**electrothanasia** (e-lek'tro-thǎ-na'zī-ah) [ electro- + G. *thanatos,* death ]. Electrocution.

**electrotherapeutics, electrotherapy** (e-lek'tro-thěr-ǎ-pu'tiks, e-lek'tro-thěr'ǎ-pī). The use of electricity in the treatment of disease.

**elec'trotherm** [ electro- + G. *thermē,* heat ]. A flexible sheet of resistance coils, covered with felt, used for applying heat to the surface of the body.

**elec'trotome.** An electric scalpel.

**electrotomy** (e-lek-trot'o-mī) [ electro- + G. *tomē,* incision ]. Noncoagulating diathermy excision of tissue.

**electroton'ic.** Relating to electrotonus.

**electrotonus** (e-lek-trot'o-nus, e-lek-tro-to'nus) [ electro- + G. *tonos,* tension ]. The changes in excitability and conductivity in a nerve or muscle cell caused by the passage of a constant electric current. See also catelectrotonus and anelectrotonus.

**electrotropism** (e-lek-trot'ro-pizm, e-lek'tro-tro'pizm) [ electro- + G. *tropē,* a turning ]. Electrotaxis.

**electuary** (e-lek'chu-a-rī) [ G. *eleikton,* a medicine that melts in the mouth, fr. *ekleichō,* to lick up ]. Confection.

**eledoisin.** An undecapeptide formed in the venom gland of cephalopods of the genus *Eledone.* Causes vasodilation and contraction of extravascular smooth muscle. Over a hundred derivatives and fragments, constituting the eledoisins, have been made and investigated.

**eleidin** (e-le'ī-din). A refractile substance related to keratin present in the stratum lucidum of the epidermis.

**el'ement** [ L. *elementum,* a rudiment, beginning ]. 1. A substance composed of atoms of only one kind, *i.e.,* of identical atomic number, that therefore cannot be decomposed into two or more substances, and that can lose its chemical property only by union with some other e. (For a list of e.'s, see appendix 9.) 2. An indivisible structure or entity.

  **acid'ulous e.,** an e. whose oxides unite with water to form acids only, never bases (*e.g.,* sulfur, phosphorus).

**amphoter'ic e.,** an e. one or more of whose oxides unite with water to form hydroxides that may act as acids or as bases (*e.g.,* aluminum).

**anatom'ical e.,** any anatomical unit, such as a cell.

**bas'ylous e.,** an e. whose oxides unite with water to form bases only, never acids (*e.g.,* sodium, barium).

**electroneg'ative e.,** an e. whose atoms have a tendency to accept electrons and form negative ions (*e.g.,* oxygen).

**electropos'itive e.,** an e. whose atoms have a tendency to lose electrons and form positive ions (*e.g.,* sodium).

**labile e.'s,** tissue cells, as of epithelium, connective tissue, etc., that continue to multiply by mitosis during the life of the individual.

**morpholog'ic e.,** anatomical e.

**neutral e.,** an e. of the zero group of the periodic system comprising the rare gases, He, Ne, Kr, etc.

**noble e.,** noble *metal.*

**rare earth e.'s,** see rare *earths.*

**trace e.'s.,** e.'s present in minute amounts in the body; many, *e.g.,* iodine, zinc, copper, cobalt, manganese, molybdenum, etc., are essential in metabolism or for the manufacture of essential compounds, *e.g.,* the thyroid hormone, insulin, cyanocobalamin, enzymes such as carbonic anhydrase, xanthine dehydrogenase, etc.

**elemen'tary.** Relating to an element; simple, not compounded.

**élément constant** [ Fr. ]. Term sometimes used to describe the fraction of phospholipid in a particular tissue or organ that remains relatively constant in amount under varying conditions.

**eleo-** [ G. *elaion,* oil ]. Combining form relating to oil; see also oleo-.

**eleoma** (el-e-o'mah) [ G. *elaion,* oil, + suffix *-oma,* tumor ]. Lipogranuloma.

**eleometer** (el-e-om'e-ter) [ G. *elaion,* oil, + *metron,* measure ]. Oleometer.

**eleopathy** (el-e-op'ă-thī). Elaiopathia; a boggy swelling of the joints said to be due to a fatty deposit following contusion; or possibly a condition resulting from the injection of paraffin oil as a form of malingering.

**eleoptene** (el-e-op'tēn). The fluid or volatile portion of a volatile oil, as distinguished from its crystallizable portion, or stearoptene.

**eleostearic acid** (el-e-o-stēr'ik, -ste-ăr'ik). An 18-carbon fatty acid with three double bonds (at carbons 9, 11, and 13), isomeric with linolenic acid. Found in plant fats.

**eleotherapy** (el-e-o-thěr'ă-pi) [ G. *elaion,* oil ]. Oleotherapy.

**eleothorax** (el-e-o-tho'raks) [ G. *elaion,* oil ]. Oleothorax.

**elephantiac** (el-e-fan'tī-ak). Relating to elephantiasis.

**elephantiasis** (el-e-fan-ti'ă-sis) [ G. fr. *elephas,* elephant ]. Barbados leg; elephant leg; pachyderma; lepra orientalis; Malabar leprosy; pes febricitans; hypertrophy or fibrosis following long-term sensitization of the skin and subcutaneous tissue due to obstructed circulation in the blood or lymphatic vessels, often by the presence of the filarial worms *Wuchereria bancrofti* or *Brugia malayi.*

**e. chirur'gica,** swelling of a part due to obliteration, following a surgical operation, of the lymphatics draining it.

**e. congen'ita angiomato'sa,** Klippel-Trenaunay-Weber *syndrome.*

**congen'ital e.,** congenital enlargement of one or more of the limbs or other parts, due to dilation of the lymphatics; see also hereditary *lymphedema.*

**gingival e.,** fibrous hyperplasia of gingiva.

**e. graeco'rum,** leprosy.

**e. ital'ica,** pellagra.

**e. neuromato'sa,** enlargement of a limb due to diffuse neurofibromatosis of the skin and subcutaneous tissue; see also neurofibromatosis.

**nevoid e.,** thickening of skin, usually unilateral, involving a small area or the entire extremity, due to congenital enlargement of lymph vessels and lymph vessel obstruction.

**e. nostras,** a solid, persisting edema of the eyelids and face that follows recurrent erysipelas or, sometimes, results from injury.

**e. telangiecto'des,** hypertrophy of the skin and subcutaneous tissues accompanied by and dependent upon dilation of the blood vessels.

**e. vul'vae,** chronic hypertrophic *vulvitis.*

**eleutheromania** (el-u-ther-o-ma'nī-ah) [ G. *eleutheros,* free, + *mania,* madness ]. Excessive passion for freedom.

**eleva'tion.** Raised place; eminence.

**tactile e.'s,** *toruli* tactiles.

**el'evator** [ L. fr. *e-levo,* pp. *-atus,* to lift up ]. 1. An instrument for prying up a sunken part, as the depressed fragment of bone in fracture of the skull. 2. Dental lever; a surgical instrument used to luxate and remove teeth and roots that cannot be engaged by the beaks of a forceps, or to loosen teeth and roots prior to forceps application.

**perios'teal e.,** a strong steel instrument used for prying up periosteum from the bone.

**screw e.,** a dental instrument with a threaded extremity used for extracting the root of a broken tooth.

**elf'wort.** Elecampane.

**elim'inant.** 1. Evacuant promoting excretion or the removal of waste. 2. An agent that increases excretion.

**elimina'tion** [ L. *elimino,* pp. *-atus,* to turn out of doors, fr. *limen,* threshold ]. Expulsion; removal of waste material from the body; the getting rid of anything.

**carbon dioxide e.,** symbol $\dot{V}CO_2$; the rate at which carbon dioxide enters the alveolar gas from the blood, equal in the steady state to the metabolic production of carbon dioxide by tissue metabolism throughout the body; units: ml/min STPD.

**elinguation** (e-ling-gwa'shun) [ L. *e,* out, + *lingua,* tongue ]. Glossectomy.

**elixir** (e-lik'ser) [ Mediev. L. fr. Ar. *al-iksir,* the philosopher's stone ]. A clear, sweetened, hydroalcoholic liquid intended for oral use. E.'s contain flavoring substances and are used either as vehicles or for the therapeutic effect of the active medicinal agents.

**Elliot,** John W., Boston surgeon, 1852–1925. See E.'s *position.*

**Elliot,** Robert H., British ophthalmologist, 1864–1936. See E.'s *operation.*

**Elliott's law.** See under law.

**ellip'sis** [ G. *ek-,* out, + *leipsis,* leaving ]. The omission of words or ideas, leaving the whole to be completed by the reader or listener.

**ellip'soid** [ G. *ellips,* oval, + *eidos,* form ]. 1. An oval condensation of reticular cells surrounding the second part of the penicillate artery of the spleen. 2. The outer end of the inner segment of the retinal rod. 3. Having the shape of an ellipse or oval.

**ellipsoideus** [ L. ] [ NA ]. Ellipsoid (3).

**elliptocyte** (ē-lip'to-sīt) [ G. *elleipsis,* a leaving out, an ellipse, + *kytos,* cell ]. Ovalocyte; an elliptical red blood corpuscle found normally in the lower vertebrates with the exception of Cyclostomata. In mammals it occurs normally only among the camels (family Camelidae), hence cameloid cell.

**elliptocytosis** (e-lip'to-si-to'sis). A relatively rare herditary abnormality of hemopoiesis in which 50 to 90 per cent of the red blood cells consist of rod forms and elliptocytes, frequently with an associated hemolytic anemia. See also elliptocytic *anemia.*

**Ellis,** Richard W. B., English physician, 20th century. See E.-van Creveld *syndrome.*

**Ellis types 1 and 2 nephritis or glomerulonephritis.** See under glomerulonephritis.

**Ellison,** E. H., American physician. See Zollinger-E. *syndrome, tumor.*

**Ellsworth,** R. See E.-Howard *test.*

**elonga'tion.** The increase in the gauge length measured after fracture in tension within the gauge length, expressed in percentage of original gauge length.

**Elschnig,** Anton, German ophthalmologist, 1863–1939. See E.'s *pearls, spots.*

**Elsner,** Christoph F., German physician, 1749–1820. See E.'s *asthma.*

**eluant** (el'u-ant). Eluent.

**el'uate** [ see elution ]. The material washed out of paper or out of a column of adsorbent in chromatography.

**el'uent** [ see elution ]. Eluant; a liquid used in the process of elution.

**elute** (e-lūt'). To perform or accomplish an elution.

**elution** (e-lu'shun) [ L. *e-luo*, pp. *lutus*, to wash out ]. 1. The separation, by washing, of one solid from another. 2. The removal, by means of a suitable solvent, of one material from another that is insoluble in that solvent.

**elutriation** (e-lu-trī-a'shun) [ L. *elutrio*, pp. *-atus*, to wash out, decant, fr. *e-luo*, to wash out ]. 1. The separation of a coarse insoluble powder from a finer one by suspending them in water and pouring off the finer powder from the upper part of the fluid, the coarser one sinking first to the bottom. 2. Elution.

**elytritis** (el'ī-trī'tis) [ G. *elytron*, sheath (vagina), + suffix *-itis*, inflammation ]. Vaginitis.

**elytro-** (el'ī-tro-) [ G. *elytron*, sheath (vagina) ]. Combining form denoting the vagina. See also colpo-, vagino-.

**elytrocele** (el'ī-tro-sēl) [ elytro- + G. *kēlē*, tumor ]. Colpocele (1).

**elytroclasia** (el'ī-tro-kla'zī-ah) [ elytro- + G. *klasis*, a breaking ]. Rupture of the vagina.

**elytroplasty** (el'ī-tro-plas'tī) [ elytro- + G. *plassō*, to form ]. Vaginoplasty.

**elytroptosia** (el'ī-trop-to'zī-ah) [ elytro- + G. *ptōsis*, a falling ]. Colpoptosis.

**elytrorrhaphy** (el-ī-tror'ă-fī) [ elytro- + G. *raphē*, a sewing ]. Colporrhaphy.

**elytrostenosis** (el'ī-tro-stĕ-no'sis) [ elytro- + G. *stenōsis*, a narrowing ]. Colpostenosis.

**elytrotomy** (el'ī-trot'o-mī) [ elytro- + G. *tomē*, incision ]. Vaginotomy.

**em-.** See en-.

**emaciation** (e-ma-sī-a'shun) [ L. *e-macio*, pp. *-atus*, to make thin ]. Extreme loss of flesh; a growing lean.

**emaculation** (e-mak'u-la'shun) [ L. *emaculo*, pp. *-atus*, to clear from spots, fr. *e-*, out, + *macula*, spot ]. The removal of spots or other blemishes from the skin.

**emailloid** (em'ĭ-loyd, e-ma'loyd) [ Fr. *émail*, enamel, + G. *eidos*, resemblance ]. Obsolete term for a tumor arising from the enamel of a tooth.

**emanation** (em-ă-na'shun) [ L. *e-mano*, pp. *-atus*, to flow out ]. Exhalation; effluvium; the radiation from a radioactive element.

    **actinium e.,** radon-219.

    **radium e.,** radon-222.

    **thorium e.,** radon-220.

**em'anator'ium.** An institution where treatment is applied by radioactive waters and the inhalation of radium emanations.

**eman'cipa'tion.** In embryology, the delimiting of a specific area in an organ-forming field, giving definite shape and limits to the organ primordium.

**em'anon.** Radon; archaic term once used to denote all radon isotopes collectively, when radon itself is restricted to the isotope radon-222, the naturally occurring intermediate of the uranium-238 radioactive series; so called because original names for radon-219, radon-220, and radon-222 were, respectively, "actinium emanation," "thorium emanation," and "radium emanation."

**em'another'apy.** Treatment of various diseases by means of radium emanation (radon), or other emanation.

**emarginate** (e-mar'jĭ-nāt) [ L. *emargino*, to deprive of its edge, fr. *e-* priv. + *margo* (*margin-*), edge ]. Nicked; with broken margin.

**emasculation** (e-mas-ku-la'shun) [ L. *emasculo*, pp. *-atus*, to castrate, fr. *e-* priv. + *masculus*, masculine, fr. *mas*, male ]. Castration.

**emas'culator.** An instrument used to castrate animals by crushing and cutting the spermatic cord.

**Embadomonas** (em-bă-dom'o-nus, em'bă-do-mo'nus) [ G. *embadon*, surface, + *monas*, unit, monad ]. Old name for *Retortamonas*.

**embalm** (em-bahm') [ L. *in*, in, + *balsamum*, balsam ]. To treat a dead body with balsams or antiseptics to preserve it from decay.

**Embden,** Gustav G., German biochemist, 1874–1933. See E. *ester*, Robinson-E. *ester*, E.-Meyerhof *pathway*, E.-Meyerhof-Parnas *pathway*.

**embed'.** Imbed; to surround a pathological or histological specimen with a firm and sometimes hard medium such as paraffin, wax, celloidin, or a resin, in order to make possible the cutting of thin sections for microscopic examination.

**embe'lia.** The dried fruit of *Embelia ribes* and *E. robusta* (family Myrsinaceae), small trees of India; contains embolin, 2,5-dihydroxy-3-undecyl-*p*-benzoquinone. Has been used as a teniacide.

**emboitement** (ahm-bwaht-mahn') [ Fr., encasement ]. See preformation *theory*.

**embola'lia.** Embololalia.

**embole** (em'bo-le) [ G. *embolē*, insertion. BALL- ]. 1. An operation, not used in present day orthopaedics, for the reduction of a dislocation. 2. Formation of the gastrula by invagination.

**embolectomy** (em'bo-lek'to-mī) [ G. *embolos*, a plug (embolus), + *ektomē*, excision ]. Excision of an embolus.

**embole'mia** [ G. *embolos*, a plug (embolus), + *haima*, blood ]. The presence of septic emboli in the circulating blood, leading to the formation of abscesses and pyemia.

**em'boli.** Plural of embolus.

**embo'lia.** Embole.

**embol'ic.** Relating to an embolus or to embolism.

**embol'iform** [ G. *embolos*, plug (embolus), + L. *forma*, form ]. Shaped like an embolus.

**embolism** (em'bo-lizm) [ G. *embolisma*, a piece or patch, lit. something thrust in. BALL- ]. Obstruction or occlusion of a vessel by a transported clot or vegetation, a mass of bacteria, or other foreign material.

    **air e.,** gas e.; the presence of bubbles of air in the heart or vessels, most commonly in the veins near the heart, or the right atrium or ventricle, which may obstruct pulmonary blood flow; occurrence is related to the entry of air into the venous circulation following trauma or operations, especially when large veins are opened, as with radical neck dissection, radical mastectomy, amputations, extracorporeal circulation.

    **amniotic fluid e.,** obstruction of small blood vessels by epithelial squames in amniotic fluid entering the maternal circulation, causing obstetric shock; see also amniotic fluid *syndrome*.

    **atheroma e.,** cholesterol e.

    **bland e.,** simple, nonseptic e.

    **cholesterol e.,** atheroembolism; atheroma e.; e. of lipid debris from an ulcerated atheromatous deposit, generally from a large artery to small arterial branches; it is usually small and rarely causes infarction.

    **crossed e.,** paradoxical e.

    **direct e.,** e. occurring in the direction of the blood current.

    **fat e.,** oil e.; the occurrence of fat globules in the circulation following fractures of a long bone, in burns, in parturition, and in association with fatty degeneration of the liver. The emboli most commonly block pulmonary or cerebral vessels when symptoms referable to either or both of these regions appear.

    **gas e.,** air e.

    **hematog'enous e.,** e. occurring in a blood vessel.

    **infective e.,** pyemic e.

    **lymph e., lymphog'enous e.,** e. occurring in a lymphatic vessel.

    **mil'iary e.,** multiple e.; e. occurring simultaneously in a number of capillaries.

    **multiple e.,** (1) miliary e.; (2) e. caused by the arrest of a number of small emboli.

    **oil e.,** fat e.

    **paradox'ical e.,** crossed e.; plugging of a systemic artery by an embolus derived from the venous system which, when it reaches the right side of the heart, is diverted through a septal defect or patent foramen ovale to the arterial side, thus bypassing the pulmonary circulation.

    **pulmonary e.,** e. of pulmonary arteries, most frequently by detached fragments of thrombus from a leg vein, especially when thrombosis has followed an operation or confinement to bed.

**pye′mic e.,** infective e.; plugging of an artery by an embolus detached from a suppurating thrombus.

**retinal e.,** e. of central artery of retina.

**retrograde e.,** venous e.; the plugging of a vein by a mass carried in a direction opposite to that of the normal blood current.

**venous e.,** retrograde e.

**emboliza′tion.** Therapeutic introduction of various substances into the circulation for the purpose of occluding vessels, usually for carotid cavernous fistula or arteriovenous malformation.

**embolola′lia** [ G. *embolos,* something thrown in, fr. *em-ballo,* to throw in (BALL-), + *lalia,* speaking ]. Embolalia; embolophasia; embolophrasia; the interjection of meaningless words in the sentence when speaking.

**embolomycotic** (em′bo-lo-mi-kot′ik) [ G. *embolos,* a plug (embolus), + *mykēs,* fungus ]. Relating to or caused by an infective embolus.

**embolophasia** (em′bo-lo-fa′zī-ah) [ G. *embolos,* something thrown in, + *phasis,* a saying ]. Embololalia.

**embolophrasia** (em′bo-lo-fra′zī-ah) [ G. *embolos,* something thrown in, + *phrasis,* phrase ]. Embololalia.

**embolus,** pl. **em′boli** (em′bo-lus) [ G. *embolos,* a plug, wedge or stopper. BALL- ]. 1. A plug, composed of a detached clot, mass of bacteria, or other foreign body, occluding a blood vessel. 2. *Nucleus emboliformis.*

**air e.,** a bubble of air plugging a small vessel; see air *embolism.*

**bland e.,** a simple e., not septic in character.

**capillary e.,** a minute e. that lodges in a capillary.

**catheter e.,** a peculiar, coiled worm-shaped e. composed of tortuous platelet and fibrin aggregates produced during vascular catheterization, originating on the catheter or its guide wire.

**cel′lular e.,** an e. composed of a mass of cells transported from disintegrating tissue.

**crossed e.,** pardoxical e.; an e. which, originating in the venous system, passes through a septal defect or patent foramen ovale to the arterial side; or a minute e. that passes through the pulmonary capillaries from venous to arterial system.

**fat e.,** oil e.; an e. of oil or fatty matter.

**ob′turating e.,** an e. completely closing the lumen of a vessel.

**oil e.,** fat e.

**pantaloon e.,** saddle e.

**paradox′ical e.,** crossed e.

**ret′rograde e.,** one which, traveling in the venous blood toward the heart, is sidetracked into a smaller vein, such as a hepatic or renal vein, and, moving in a direction opposite to the blood flow, lodges in the vessel.

**riding or straddling e.,** an e. arrested at the point of bifurcation of an artery and blocking more or less completely both branches of the vessel.

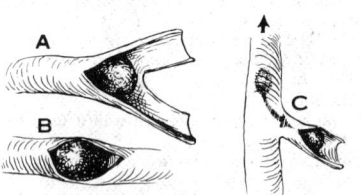

**Embolus**

*A,* riding embolus; *B,* obturating embolus; *C,* retrograde embolus; *shaded arrow* indicates path of embolus; *solid arrow,* direction of blood flow.

**saddle e.,** pantaloon e.; a large e. that straddles the bifurcation of the aorta and so occludes both common iliac arteries.

**tumor e.,** an e., comprised of neoplastic tissue, which is transported and lodged in a blood or lymphatic vessel and which may grow as a metastasis.

**em′boly.** Embole.

**embouchement** (ahm-boosh-mon) [ Fr. ]. The opening of one blood vessel into another.

**embrasure** (em-bra′zhūr) [ Fr. an opening in a wall for cannon ]. In dentistry, denoting an opening that widens outwardly or inwardly; that part of the interproximal space gingival to the contact point that spreads out toward the labial, lingual, or buccal aspect.

**buccal e.,** a space existing on the facial side of the contact points between two adjacent teeth.

**labial e.,** a space formed by the contours of two adjacent teeth from their point or area of contact to their labial or facial aspects.

**occlusal e.,** a space existing on the occlusal side of the contact points between two adjacent teeth.

**embrocation** (em′bro-ka′shun) [ G. *embrochē,* a fomentation ]. Rarely used term meaning (1) liniment, or (2) the application of a liniment.

**embry-.** See embryo-.

**embryatrics** (em′brī-at′riks) [ embryo- + G. *iatros,* physician ]. Fetology.

**embryectomy** (em-brī-ek′to-mī) [ embryo- + G. *ektomē,* excision ]. The operative removal of the product of conception, especially in ectopic pregnancy.

**embryo** (em′brī-o) [ G. *embryon,* fr. *en,* in, + *bryō,* to be full, swell ]. 1. An organism in the early stages of

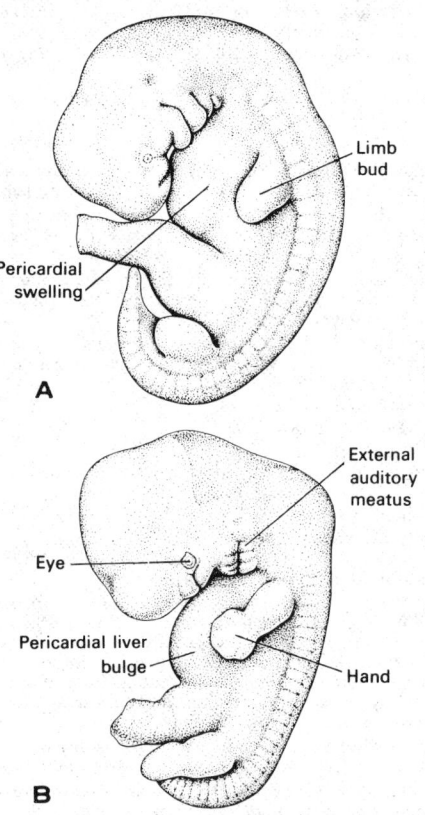

**A**

Limb bud

Pericardial swelling

**B**

External auditory meatus

Eye

Pericardial liver bulge

Hand

**Embryo (Schematic Drawing)**

*A,* a 5-week human embryo seen from the left, showing the paddle-shaped limb buds and the pharyngeal arches; crown-rump length is approximately 7 mm. *B,* a 6-week human embryo seen from the left; crown-rump length is approximately 13 mm.; the upper limb buds show a flattened terminal portion with four radial grooves; note the formation of the eye and the external auditory meatus flanked on each side by three hillocks derived from the mandibular and hyoid arches. (Modified after Streeter, from Langman, J.: *Medical Embryology,* Ed. 2, The Williams & Wilkins Co., Baltimore, 1969.)

development. 2. [ NA ]. In man, the developing organism from conception until approximately the end of the second month; developmental stages from this time to birth are commonly designated as fetal. 3. A primordial plant within a seed.

**heterogametic e.,** a male embryo with XY sex chromosomes.

**hexacanth e.,** the e. of tapeworms such as *Taenia saginata* which have three pairs of hooks.

**homogametic e.,** a female e. with XX sex chromosomes.

**presomite e.,** an e. prior to the appearance of the first pair of somites, about 20 to 21 days after fertilization in humans.

**previllous e.,** the e. of a placental mammal prior to the formation of chorionic villi.

**embryo-, embry-** [ G. *embryon*, embryo ]. Combining forms relating to the embryo.

**em′bryocar′dia** [ embryo- + G. *kardia*, heart ]. A condition in which the cadence of the heart sounds resembles that of the fetus, the first and second sounds becoming alike and evenly spaced; a sign of serious myocardial disease; also called tic-tac rhythm; tic-tac sounds, pendulum rhythm.

**ju′gular e.,** atrial *flutter.*

**embryoctony** (em′brī-ok′to-nī) [ embryo- + G. *kteinō*, to destroy ]. Feticide.

**embryogenesis** (em′brī-o-jen′ē-sis) [ embryo- + G. *genesis*, production ]. That phase of prenatal development involved in the establishing of the characteristic configuration of the embryonic body; e. is usually regarded, in humans, as extending from the end of the 2nd week, when the embryonic disk is formed, to the end of the 8th week, after which the conceptus is usually spoken of as a fetus.

**embryogen′ic, embryogenet′ic.** Producing an embryo; relating to the formation of an embryo.

**embryogeny** (em′brī-oj′ē-nī). The origin and growth of the embryo.

**embryography** (em′brī-og′rā-fī) [ embryo- + G. *graphō*, to write ]. A treatise describing the formation and development of the embryo.

**embryoid** (em′brī-oyd). Embryonoid.

**embryol′ogist.** One who makes a special study of embryology.

**embryology** (em′brī-ol′o-jī) [ embryo- + G. *logos*, study ]. The science of the origin and development of the organism from the fertilization of the ovum to the period of extrauterine or extraovular life.

**embryo′ma.** Embryonal *tumor.*

**e. of the kidney,** Wilms′ *tumor.*

**embryomorphous** (em′brī-o-mor′fus) [ embryo- + G. *morphē*, shape ]. 1. Relating to the formation and structure of the embryo. 2. Applied to structures or tissues in the body similar to those in the embryo, or embryonal rests.

**embryonal** (em′brī-o-nal). Relating to an embryo.

**embryonate** (em′brī-o-nāt). 1. Embryonal. 2. Containing an embryo.

**embryonic** (em-brī-on′ik). In the condition of an embryo; rudimentary.

**embryoniform** (em-brī-on′ī-form). Embryonoid.

**embryonization** (em′brī-on-ī-za′shun). Reversion of a cell or a tissue to an embryonic form.

**embryonoid** (em′brī-o-noyd) [ embryo- + G. *eidos*, appearance ]. Embryoid; resembling an embryo or a fetus.

**embryony** (em′brī-o-nī). The condition of being an embryo.

**embryopathy** (em′brī-op′ā-thī) [ embryo- + G. *pathos*, disease ]. A morbid condition in the embryo or fetus.

**embryophore** (em′brī-o-fōr) [ embryo- + G. *phoros*, bearing ]. A membrane or thickened wall around the hexacanth embryo of tapeworms, forming the inner portion of the eggshell. In the genus *Taenia* the e. is exceptionally thick, with radial striations, and forms the usual eggshell or capsule, a highly protective structure.

**embryoplas′tic** [ embryo- + G. *plassō*, to form ]. Relating to the formation of an embryo.

**embryoscope** (em′brī-o-skōp) [ embryo- + G. *skopeō*, to examine ]. An instrument for examining the embryos in hens′ eggs at different stages of development.

**embryotocia** (em′brī-o-to′sī-ah) [ embryo- + G. *tokos*, childbirth ]. Abortion.

**em′bryotome.** Any instrument used in embryotomy.

**embryotomy** (em-brī-ot′o-mī) [ embryo- + G. *tomē*, cutting ]. Any mutilating operation on the fetus to make possible its removal when delivery is impossible by natural means.

**embryotoxon** (em′brī-o-tok′son) [ embryo- + G. *toxon*, bow ]. A congenital opacity of the periphery of the cornea.

**anterior e.,** *arcus* juvenilis.

**posterior e.,** a developmental atavistic trait marked by a prominent white ring of Schwalbe and iris strands that partially obscure the chamber angle.

**embryotroph** (em′brī-o-trōf) [ embryo- + G. *trophē*, nourishment ]. 1. Histotroph; the nutritive material supplied to the embryo during development. 2. In the implantation stages of deciduate placental mammals, the fluid adjacent to the blastodermic vesicle; this fluid is a mixture of the secretion of the uterine glands, cellular debris resulting from the trophoblastic invasion of the endometrium, and exudated plasma.

**embryotrophic** (em′brī-o-trof′ik). Relating to any process or agency directed to the nourishment of the embryo.

**embryotrophy** (em′brī-ot′ro-fī) [ embryo- + G. *trophē*, nourishment ]. The nutrition of the embryo.

**embryulcia** (em-brī-ul′sī-ah) [ G. *embryoulkia*, extraction of the embryo, fr. *helcō*, to draw, drag ]. Mechanical extraction of the embryo or fetus from the uterus.

**embryul′cus** [ G. *embryoulkos*, a midwife′s forceps ]. A hook-shaped instrument for use in extracting the dead embryo or fetus retained in the uterus, or in cases of abortion.

**emdabol.** 17β-Hydroxy-1α,7α-dimercapto-17-methylandrost-4-en-3-one 1,7-diacetate; a synthetic steroid anabolic agent.

**emed′ullate** [ L. *e-*, from, + *medulla*, marrow ]. To extract the marrow or pith of anything.

**emergence** (e-mer′jens). Recovery of normal brain function following a period of unconsciousness.

**emergency** (e-mer′jen-sī) [ L. *e-mergo*, pp. *-mersus*, to rise up, emerge, fr. *mergo*, to plunge into, dip ]. An unlooked-for contingency or happening; a sudden demand for action.

**emergent** (e-mer′jent). 1. Arising suddenly and unexpectedly and calling for quick judgment and prompt action. 2. Coming out; leaving a cavity or other part.

**Emerson method.** See under method.

**em′ery.** An abrasive containing aluminum oxide and iron.

**em′esis** [ G. fr. *emeō*, to vomit ]. Vomiting. Also used as a combining form in a suffix position.

**emet′ic** [ G. *emetikos*, producing vomiting, fr. *emeō*, to vomit ]. 1. Relating to or causing vomiting. 2. An agent that causes vomiting.

**emet′icol′ogy.** Emetology.

**em′etine.** Cephaeline methyl ether; $C_{29}H_{40}N_2O_4$; principal alkaloid of ipecac; emetic. Salts of e. are used in amebiasis. Available as e. hydrochloride (USP, BP).

**emetocathartic** (em′ē-to-hā-thar′tik). 1. Both emetic and cathartic. 2. An agent that causes vomiting and purging.

**emetology** (em′ē-tol′o-jī) [ G. *emetos*, a vomiting, + *logos*, study ]. Study of vomiting in all its aspects.

**emetomania** (em′ē-to-ma′nī-ah) [ G. *emetos*, vomiting, + *mania*, frenzy ]. Morbid desire to vomit; formerly, although now rarely seen, a common symptom of hysteria.

**emetophobia** (em′ē-to-fo′bī-ah) [ G. *emetos*, vomiting, + *phobos*, fear ]. Morbid fear of vomiting; formerly, although now rarely seen, a common symptom of hysteria.

**emex.** 5,6-Dihydro-1-methyl-5,6-dioxo-3-indolinesulfonic acid 5-semicarbazone sodium salt; hemostatic agent.

**EMF.** Abbreviation for electromotive *force.*

**EMG.** Abbreviation for electromyogram.

**-emia** [ G. *haima*, blood ]. Suffix meaning blood.

**emiction** (e-mik′shun). Urination.

**emigra′tion** [ L. *e-migro*, pp. *-atus*, to emigrate ]. The passage of white blood cells through the endothelium and wall of small blood vessels.

**em'inence** [ L. *eminentia, q.v.* ]. A circumscribed area raised above the general level of the surrounding surface; see eminentia.

**arcuate e.,** *eminentia* arcuata.

**artic'ular e.,** *tuberculum* articulare.

**canine e.,** an elevation on the maxilla corresponding to the socket of the canine tooth.

**collateral e.,** *eminentia* collateralis.

**e. of concha,** *eminentia* conchae.

**cruciate or cruciform e.,** *eminentia* cruciformis.

**deltoid e.,** *tuberositas* deltoidea.

**Doyère's e.,** the slightly elevated area of the striated muscle fiber's surface that corresponds to the site of the motor *endplate, q.v.*

**facial e.,** *colliculus* facialis.

**frontal e.,** *tuber* frontale.

**genital e.,** in very young embryos, the vaguely outlined median elevation immediately cephalic to the proctoderm. Its central part develops into the genital tubercle.

**hy'pobranch'ial e.,** the copula linguae; His' copula; a median elevation in the floor of the embryonic pharynx caudal to the tuberculum impar. It merges laterally with the ventral part of the second and third branchial arches; in later development it is incorporated in the root of the tongue.

**hypoglossal e.,** *trigonum* nervi hypoglossi.

**hypothe'nar e.,** the elevation on the medial side of the palm produced by the short muscles of the little finger.

**ileocecal e.,** *valva* ileocecalis.

**iliopectineal e.,** *eminentia* iliopubica.

**iliopu'bic e.,** *eminentia* iliopubica.

**intercon'dylar** or **intercon'dyloid e.,** *eminentia* intercondylaris.

**medial e.,** *eminentia* medialis.

**median e.,** *eminentia* mediana; the slightly prominent lower segment of the infundibulum of the hypothalamus, immediately proximal to the hypophysial stalk; the region is characterized by the capillary tufts of the infundibular arteries, from which the hypothalamohypophysial portal *system (q.v.)* of veins arises.

**olivary e.,** oliva.

**orbital e.,** *eminentia* orbitalis.

**parietal e.,** *tuber* parietale.

**pyramidal e.,** *eminentia* pyramidalis.

**radial e. of wrist,** eminentia carpi radialis; a rather large flat e. on the radial side of the palmar aspect of the wrist, due to the tuberosity of scaphoid and the ridge on the trapezium.

**restiform e.,** *eminentia* restiformis.

**round e.,** *eminentia* medialis.

**e. of the scapha,** *eminentia* scaphae.

**thenar e.,** the swelling on the lateral part of the palm of the hand caused by the short muscles of the thumb.

**thyroid e.,** *prominentia* laryngea.

**e. of the triangular fossa,** *eminentia* fossae triangularis.

**ulnar e. of wrist,** eminentia carpi ulnaris; an e. smaller than the radial, on the ulnar side of the palmar aspect of the wrist, due to presence of the pisiform bone.

# EMINENTIA

**eminentia,** pl. **eminentiae** (em-ĭ-nen'shĭ-ah) [ L. prominence, fr. *e-mineo,* to stand out, project ] [ NA ]. Eminence; a circumscribed, elevated area.

**e. abducen'tis,** *colliculus* facialis.

**e. arcua'ta** [ NA ], arcuate eminence; a prominence on the anterior surface of the petrous portion of the temporal bone indicating the position of the superior semicircular canal.

**e. articula'ris,** *tuberculum* articulare.

**e. carpi radia'lis,** radial *eminence* of the wrist.

**e. carpi ulna'ris,** ulnar *eminence* of the wrist.

**e. collatera'lis** [ NA ], collateral eminence; a longitudinal elevation of the floor of the collateral trigone of the lateral ventricle of the brain, between the hippocampus and the calcar avis, caused by the proximity of the bottom of the collateral fissure.

**e. conchae** [ NA ], eminence of the concha; apophysis conchae; the prominence on the cranial surface of the auricle corresponding to the concha.

**e. crucifor'mis** [ NA ], cruciate or cruciform eminence; a figure on the internal surface of the occipital bone formed by ridges running forward and backward from the protuberance and by the margins of the groove for the transverse sinus on either side; it divides the surface of the bone into four fossae, a cerebral and a cerebellar on each side.

**e. facia'lis,** *colliculus* facialis.

**e. fossae triangula'ris** [ NA ], eminence of the triangular fossa; e. triangularis; agger perpendicularis; the prominence on the cranial surface of the auricle corresponding to the triangular fossa.

**e. fronta'lis,** *tuber* frontale.

**e. hypoglos'si,** *trigonum* nervi hypoglossi.

**e. iliopu'bica** [ NA ], iliopubic or iliopectineal eminence; a rounded elevation on the superior surface of the hip bone at the junction of the ilium and the superior ramus of the pubis.

**e. intercondyla'ris** [ NA ], e. intercondyloidea; intercondylar or intercondyloid eminence; spinous process of the tibia; an elevation on the proximal extremity of the tibia between the two articular surfaces.

**e. intercondyloid'ea,** e. intercondylaris.

**e. media'lis** [ NA ], medial eminence; round eminence; e. teres; funiculus teres; longitudinal elevation of the floor of the fossa rhomboidea or fourth ventricle, extending along either side of the midline throughout the length of the rhombencephalon.

**e. media'na,** median *eminence.*

**e. orbitalis,** orbital eminence or tubercle; Whitnall's orbital tubercle; a constant (about 90 per cent of the cases) elevation on the orbital aspect of the zygomatic bone, 1 cm. below the zygomaticofrontal suture, also palpable in the living subject.

**e. parieta'lis,** *tuber* parietale.

**e. pyramida'lis** [ NA ], pyramidal eminence; pyramid of the tympanum; a conical projection posterior to the vestibular window in the middle ear; it is hollow and contains the stapedius muscle.

**e. restifor'mis,** restiform eminence; a prominence of the dorsolateral surface of the medulla oblongata corresponding to the inferior cerebellar peduncle.

**e. scaphae** [ NA ], eminence of the scapha; the prominence on the cranial surface of the auricle corresponding to the scapha.

**e. sym'physis,** *tuberculum* mentale.

**e. te'res,** e. medialis.

**e. triangula'ris,** e. fossae triangularis.

**e'miocyto'sis** [ L. *emitto,* to send forth, + G. *kytos,* cell, + suffix -*osis,* condition ]. Exocytosis (2).

**emissarium** (em-ĭ-sa'rĭ-um) [ L. an outlet, fr. *e-mitto,* pp. -*missus,* to send out ]. *Vena* emissaria.

**e. condyloid'eum,** *vena* emissaria condylaris.

**e. mastoid'eum,** *vena* emissaria mastoidea.

**e. occipita'le,** *vena* emissaria occipitalis.

**e. parieta'le,** *vena* emissaria parietalis.

**emissa'rius** [ L. ] [ NA ]. Emissary.

**em'issary** [ see emissarium ]. 1. Relating to, or providing, an outlet or drain. 2. *Vena* emissaria.

**emission** (e-mish'un) [ L. *emissio;* fr. *e-mitto,* to send out ]. A discharge; referring usually to a seminal discharge occurring during sleep.

**emissiv'ity.** The giving off of heat rays. A perfect "black body" has an e. of 1, a highly polished metallic surface may have an e. as low as 0.02.

**emmenagogic** (ĕ-men'ă-goj'ik). Relating to or acting as an emmenagogue.

**emmenagogue** (ĕ-men'ă-gog) [ G. *emmēnos,* monthly, fr. *en,* in, + *mēn,* month (MEN-), + *agōgos,* leading ]. 1. Promoting or increasing the menstrual flow. 2. An agent that induces or increases menstruation.

**emmenia** (ĕ-men'ĭ-ah, ĕ-me'nĭ-ah) [ G. *emmēnos,* monthly ]. Menses.

**emmenic** (ĕ-men'ik). Relating to the menses.

**em'menin.** Unofficial name given to an estrogenic substance once isolated from the placenta; probably the glucuronide of estriol.

**emmeniopathy** (ĕ-men'ĭ-op'ă-thĭ) [ G. *emmēnos*, monthly, + *pathos*, suffering ]. A disorder of menstruation.

**emmenology** (em-e-nol'o-jĭ) [ G. *emmēnos*, monthly, + *logos*, study ]. The branch of medicine that has to do especially with the physiology and pathology of menstruation.

**Emmens' S/L test.** See under test.

**Emmet,** Thomas A., New York gynecologist, 1828–1919. See E.'s *method, needle, operation.*

**emmetrope** (em'e-trōp). A person with emmetropia.

**emmetro'pia** [ G. *emmetros*, according to measure, + *ōps*, eye ]. The state of refraction of the eye in which parallel rays, when the eye is at rest, are focused exactly on the retina.

**em'odin.** 1,3,8-Trihydroxy-6-methylanthraquinone; frangula e., rheum e., frangulic acid; archin; a crystalline substance found in rhubarb, senna, cascara sagrada, and other purgative drugs; see also aloe-emodin.

**emollient** (e-mol'yent) [ L. *emolliens*, pres. p. of *e-mollio, emollire*, to soften. MOLL- ]. Malactic. 1. Soothing to skin or mucous membrane. 2. An agent that softens the skin or soothes irritation in skin or mucous membrane.

**emotion** (e-mo'shun) [ L. *e-moveo*, pp. *-motus*, to move out, agitate ]. A strong feeling, aroused mental state, or intense state of drive or unrest directed toward a definite object and evidenced in both behavior and in psychologic changes.

**emotional** (e-mo'shun-al). Relating to any of the emotions.

**emotiovascular** (e-mo'shī-o-vas'ku-lar). Relating to the vascular changes, such as pallor and blushing, caused by emotions of various kinds.

**emp.** Abbreviation of L. *emplastrum,* plaster.

**empasm, empasma** (em'pazm, em-paz'mah) [ G. *empasma*, fr. *em-passo*, to sprinkle on ]. A dusting powder.

**empath'ic.** Relating to or marked by empathy.

**em'pathize.** To feel empathy in relation to another person; to enter into another's feelings, to put oneself in another's place.

**empathy** (em'pă-thĭ) [ G. *en (em)*, in, + *pathos*, feeling ]. 1. The intellectual and occasionally emotional identification with another person's mental and emotional states, as distinguished from sympathy. 2. The anthropomorphization or humanizing of objects and feeling oneself as in and part of them.

    **generative e.,** the inner experience of sharing in and comprehending the momentary psychologic state of another person.

**Empedocles** (em-ped'ō-klēs), Greek philosopher, poet, physician, and statesman, *circa* 460 B.C. See humoral *doctrine* of which he was a proponent.

**emperipolesis** (em-pĕr'ĭ-po-le'sis) [ G. *en (em)*, inside, + *peri*, around, + *poleomai*, to wander about ]. Active penetration of one cell by another, which remains intact; e. has been observed in tissue cultures in which polymorphonuclear leukocytes have entered macrophages and subsequently left.

**emphlysis** (em'flĭ-sis) [ G. *en*, in, + *phlysis*, an eruption, fr. *phlyō*, to boil over ]. A vesicular eruption, such as pemphigus.

**emphrac'tic.** Relating to emphraxis.

**emphraxis** (em-frak'sis) [ G. a stoppage. PHRAG- ]. 1. A clogging of the mouths of the sweat glands. 2. An impaction.

**emphysema** (em-fī-se'mah) [ G. inflation of stomach, etc. fr. *en*, in, + *physēma*, a blowing, fr. *physa*, bellows ]. 1. The presence of air in the interstices of the connective tissue of a part. 2. Increase in the size of air spaces distal to the terminal bronchioles, either from dilation or from destruction of their walls.

    **atroph'ic e.,** substantive e.

    **centrilobular e.,** small rounded foci of e. in the center of the secondary pulmonary lobules; formed by dilation of respiratory bronchioles and destruction of adjacent lung tissue.

    **com'pensating** or **compen'satory e.,** increase in the air capacity of a portion of the lung when another portion is consolidated or unable to perform its respiratory function.

    **cuta'neous e.,** subcutaneous e.

    **ectat'ic e.,** pulmonary e. in which the alveoli are dilated beyond their full normal capacity, yet without atrophy of their walls and blood vessels.

    **glass blower's e.,** e. supposed to result from stretching of the alveolar portions of the lung in glass blowers.

    **interlob'ular e.,** interstitial e. in the connective tissue septa between the pulmonary lobules.

    **intersti'tial e.,** (1) the presence of air in the pulmonary tissues consequent upon rupture of the air cells; (2) the presence of air or gas in the connective tissue.

    **intest'inal e.,** *pneumatosis* cystoides intestinalis.

    **Jenner's e.,** senile e. associated with loss of elasticity of the lung.

    **medias'tinal e.,** deflection of air, usually from a ruptured emphysematous bleb in the lung, into the mediastinal tissue.

    **paracinar e.,** paralobular e., enlargement of air spaces in any part of the pulmonary lobules, mainly by atrophy or destruction of alveolar walls.

    **paralobular e.,** paracinar e.

    **paraseptal e.,** e. involving the periphery of the pulmonary lobules.

    **pul'monary e.,** emphysema (2).

    **scalp e.,** presence of gas in the interstices of the subcutaneous tissues.

    **senile e.,** substantive e. consequent upon the physiologic atrophy of old age.

    **subcuta'neous e.,** aerodermectasia; the presence of air or gas in the subcutaneous tissues.

    **subgaleal e.,** extracranial *pneumatocele.*

    **sub'stantive e.,** increase in size of the pulmonary vesicles through atrophy of their walls and breaking down of the septa between adjacent air cells.

    **surgical e.,** subcutaneous e. following operation or injury.

    **vesic'ular e.,** emphysema (2).

**emphysematous** (em'fī-sem'ă-tus). Relating to or affected with emphysema.

**empiric** (em-pĭr-ik) [ see empirical ]. 1. Empirical. 2. A member of a school of Graeco-Roman physicians, late B.C. to early A.D., who placed their confidence in and their practice purely on experience, avoiding all speculation, theory, or abstract reasoning; they were little concerned with causes or with correlating symptoms in order to gain a true understanding of a disease; they even held basic knowledge, physiology, pathology, and anatomy in low esteem and of no value in practice.

**empirical** (em-pĭr-ĭ-kal) [ G. *empeirikos;* fr. *empeiria*, experience, fr. *en*, in, + *peira*, a trial ]. 1. Empiric (1); founded on practical experience but not proved scientifically. 2. Relating to an empiric (2).

**empiricism** (em-pĭr'ĭ-sizm). A looking to experience as a guide to practice or to the therapeutic use of any remedy.

**emplas'trum** [ G. *emplastron*, plaster. PLAS- ]. See plaster.

**emporiat'rics** [ G. *emporos*, traveler, + *iatros*, physician ]. The science of the health of travelers visiting foreign countries.

**emprosthotonos** (em'pros-thot'o-nus) [ G. *emprosthen*, forward, + *tonos*, tension ]. Tetanus anticus; a tetanic contraction of the flexor muscles, curving the back with concavity forward.

**emptysis** (emp'tĭ-sis) [ G. a spitting, fr. *ptyō*, fut. *ptysō*, to spit ]. Hemoptysis.

**empyema** (em'pi-e'mah, em'pī-e'mah) [ G. *empyēma*, suppuration, fr. *en*, in, + *pyon*, pus ]. Pus in a body cavity; when used without qualification, refers to pyothorax (pus in the pleural cavity).

    **e. articuli,** suppurative *arthritis.*

    **e. benig'num,** latent e.; chronic purulent sinusitis or pyothorax with mild or no constitutional symptoms.

    **e. of the chest,** pyothorax.

    **extradural e.,** epidural *abscess.*

    **latent e.,** the presence of pus in a cavity, especially one of the accessory sinuses, unattended by subjective symptoms.

**loc'ulated e.,** pyothorax in which pleural adhesions form one or more pockets containing pus.

**mastoid e.,** mastoiditis.

**e. necessita'tis,** a form of e. of the chest in which the pus burrows to the outside, producing a subcutaneous abscess which finally ruptures. It may result in spontaneous recovery without the necessity of operation.

**e. of the pericar'dium,** pyopericardium.

**pul'sating e.,** a large, tense collection of pus in the pleural cavity through which the cardiac pulsations are transmitted to the chest wall.

**subdural e.,** subdural *abscess.*

**empyemic** (em-pi-e'mik). Relating to empyema.

**empyesis** (em-pi-e'sis) [ G. suppuration. PYO- ]. A pustular eruption.

**empyocele** (em'pi-o-sēl) [ G. *en,* in, + *pyon,* pus, + *kēlē,* tumor ]. A suppurating hydrocele; a collection of pus in the scrotum.

**empyreuma** (em-pi-ru'mah) [ G. a banked fire. PYR- ]. The characteristic odor given off by organic substances when charred or subjected to destructive distillation in closed vessels.

**empyreumatic** (em'pi-ru-mat'ik). Produced by charring or destructive distillation of wood or other organic substance; referring to the characteristic odor (empyreuma) of charred organic matter.

**emu.** Abbreviation for electromagnetic *units.*

**emul.** Abbreviation for L. *emulsum,* emulsion.

**emulgent** (e-mul'jent) [ L. *e-*mulgeo, pp. *-mulsus,* to milk out, drain out ]. Denoting a straining, extracting, or purifying process.

**emul'sifier.** An agent, such as gum arabic or the yolk of an egg, used to make an emulsion of a fixed oil.

**emul'sify.** To make in the form of an emulsion.

**emul'sin.** 1. A preparation, derived from almonds, that contains β-glucosidase. 2. Sometimes used as a synonym for β-glucosidase; "emulsin" was one of the earliest enzymes to be studied (*ca.* 1830).

**emulsion** (e-mul'shun) [ Mod. L. fr. *e-mulgeo,* pp. *-mulsus,* to milk or drain out ]. A system containing two immiscible liquids in which one is dispersed, in the form of very small globules, throughout the other. That in the form of globules is called the "dispersed" or "discontinuous" phase; the second liquid is referred to as the "dispersion medium" or the "continuous phase."

**emul'sive.** 1. Denoting a substance that can be made into an emulsion. 2. Denoting a substance, such as a mucilage, by which a fat or resin can be emulsified. 3. Making soft or pliant. 4. Affording a fixed oil on pressure.

**emulsoid** (e-mul'soyd). Emulsion colloid; hydrophilic or lyophilic colloid; a colloidal dispersion in which the dispersed particles are more or less liquid and exert a certain attraction on and absorb a certain quantity of the fluid in which they are suspended.

**emure'sis** [ G. *en(em),* in, + *ourēsis,* urination ]. A condition in which urinary excretion and intake of water act to produce an absolute hydration of the body. See also ecuresis.

**emylcamate.** STRIATRAN; NUNCITAL; 1-ethyl-1-methylpropyl carbamate; mild sedative, used to control tension and anxiety and to relieve pain and muscular spasm.

**en-.** Prefix fr. G. preposition meaning in; appears as em- before b, p, or m.

**enallylpropymal.** 56 NORCONUMAL; 5-allyl-5-isopropyl-1-methylbarbituric acid; hypnotic with intermediate duration of action.

**enam'el.** Enamelum.

**mottled e.,** alterations in e. formation due to excessive fluoride ingestion during tooth formation. Varies in appearance from small white opacities to yellow and black spotting.

**nanoid e.,** dwarfed e.; a condition of abnormal thinness of the e.

**whorled e.,** e. in which the rods assume a spiral or twisting course.

**enam'elogen'esis.** Amelogenesis.

**e. imperfecta,** *amelogenesis* imperfecta.

**enam'elo'ma.** Enamel pearl; a developmental anomaly in which there is a small nodule of enamel below the cementoenamel junction, usually at the bifurcation of molar teeth.

**enam'elum** [ NA ]. Enamel; substantia adamantina; the hard, glistening substance covering the exposed portion of the tooth. It is composed of an inorganic portion (about 96 per cent) made up of hydroxyapatite with small amounts of carbonate, magnesium, fluoride, and an organic matrix of glycoprotein and a keratin-like protein. Structurally, it is made up of oriented rods each of which consists of a stack of rodlets encased in an organic prism sheath.

**enan'thate.** USAN-approved contraction for heptanoate, $CH_3(CH_2)_5COO^-$.

**enanthem, enanthema** (en-an'them, en'an-the'mah) [ G. *en,* in, + *anthēma* (found only in compounds), bloom, eruption, fr. *antheō,* to bloom ]. A mucous membrane eruption, especially one occurring in connection with one of the exanthemas.

**en'anthem'atous.** Relating to an enanthem.

**enanthesis** (en'an-the'sis) [ G. *en,* in, + *anthēsis,* full bloom ]. The skin eruption of a general disease, such as scarlatina or typhoid fever.

**enanthrope** (en'an-thrōp) [ G. *en,* in, + *anthrōpos,* man ]. A disease originating within the organism; an autoinfection.

**enantio-** [ G. *enantios,* opposite ]. Combining form meaning opposite, opposed, or opposing.

**enantiobiosis** (e-nan'tī-o-bi-o'sis) [ enantio- + G. *biōsis,* way of living ]. Antagonistic symbiosis.

**enantiomer** (e-nan'tī-o-mer) [ enantio- + G. *meros,* part ]. One of a pair of molecules that are mirror images of each other. Also called antimer; enantiomorph; optical antipode.

**enantiomer'ic.** Pertaining to enantiomerism.

**enantiom'erism.** In chemistry, isomerism in which the molecules in their configuration are related to one another like an object and its mirror image; consequently not superimposable. Such isomerism entails optical activity, both enantiomers rotating the plane of plane polarized light equally, but in opposite directions.

**enan'tiomorph.** 1. A crystal whose structure is related to that of another, like an object and its nonsuperimposable mirror image. 2. Enantiomer.

**enantiomorphic, enantiomorphous** (e-nan'tī-o-mor'fic, -mor'fus) [ enantio- + G. *morphē,* form ]. 1. Relating to two objects, *e.g.,* crystals or right- and left-handed gloves, each of which is the mirror image of the other. 2. In chemistry, relating to isomers, the optical activities of which are equal in magnitude but opposite in sign.

**enantiomorphism** (e-nan'tī-o-mor'fizm) [ enantio- + G. *morphē,* form ]. The relation of two objects similar in form, but not superposable, as the two hands, or an object and its mirror image.

**enan'tiopath'ia.** Enantiopathy.

**enan'tiopath'ic.** 1. Mutually antagonistic or antidotal, referring to morbid states. 2. Allopathic.

**enantiopathy** (e-nan'tī-op'ă-thī) [ enantio- + G. *pathos,* suffering ]. 1. Antipathy; treating with antidotes; a method of treatment in which the remedy produces symptoms that are the direct opposite of those of the treated disease. 2. Mutual antagonism of two morbid states, yielding a cancelling out of signs and symptoms.

**enantiothamnosis** (e-nan'tī-o-tham-no'sis) [ enantio- + G. *thamnos,* bush, + suffix *-osis,* condition ]. A condition marked by the occurrence of variously sized nodules, having a central opening giving exit to pus, due to infection by a fungus *Enantiothamnus braulti.*

**enarthro'dial.** Relating to an enarthrosis.

**enarthro'sis** [ G. *en-arthrōsis,* a jointing where the ball is deep set in the socket ]. *Articulatio* spheroidea.

**encanthis** (en-kan'this) [ G. *en,* in, + *kanthos,* canthus ]. A minute tumor or excrescence at the inner angle of the eye.

**encapsulated** (en-kap'su-la'ted). Enclosed in a sheath or capsule.

**encapsulation** (en-kap-su-la'shun) [ L. *in* + *capsula,* dim. of *capsa,* box ]. Enclosure in a capsule or sheath.

**Encapsula'tus.** *Klebsiella.*

**encap′suled.** Encapsulated.

**encardi′tis.** Endocarditis.

**encatarrhaphy** (en-kat-ar′ră-fī) [ G. *enkatarrhaptō*, to sew in. RAPH- ]. The artificial implantation of an organ or tissue in a part where it does not naturally occur.

**enceinte** (on-sant′) [ Fr. ]. Pregnant.

**encelitis, enceliitis** (en-se-li′tis, en-se-le-i′tis) [ G. *en*, in, + *koilia*, belly ]. Inflammation of any of the abdominal viscera.

**encephal-.** See encephalo-.

**encephalalgia** (en-sef′ă-lal′jī-ah) [ encephalo- + G. *algos*, pain ]. Cephalalgia; headache.

**encephalatroph′ic.** Relating to encephalatrophy.

**encephalatrophy** (en-sef′ă-lat′ro-fī) [ encephalo- + G. *a-* priv. + *trophē*, nourishment ]. Atrophy of the brain.

**encephalauxe** (en-sef′ă-lawk′se) [ encephalo- + G. *auxē*, increase ]. Hypertrophy of the brain.

**encéphale isolé** (ahn-sef-al′ē-so-la′) [ Fr. isolated brain ]. An experimental animal with transection of the midbrain. It never becomes conscious, and its brain wave pattern is that of sleep.

**encephalemia** (en-sef′ă-le′mī-ah) [ encephalo- + G. *haima*, blood ]. Brain *congestion*.

**encephalic** (en′sĕ-fal′ik). Relating to the brain, or to the structures within the cranium.

**encephalit′ic.** Relating to encephalitis.

**encephalitides** (en-sef′ă-lit′ī-dēz). Plural of encephalitis.

**encephalitis,** pl. **encephalitides** (en-sef′ă-li′tis, en-sef′ă-lit′ī-dēz) [ G. *enkephalos*, brain, + suffix -*itis*, inflammation ]. Cephalitis; inflammation of the brain.

  **acute hemorrhag′ic e.,** e. hemorrhagica.

  **acute necrotizing e.,** an acute form of e., usually caused by herpes simplex virus and affecting largely the temporal lobes and limbic system.

  **Australian X e.,** Murray Valley e.

  **Coxsackie e.,** an inflammation of the brain, seen mainly in infants and involving principally the gray matter of the medulla and cord; it is caused by Coxsackie (B) virus.

  **Dawson's e.,** inclusion body e.

  **epidemic e.,** von Economo's *disease*.

  **equine e.,** equine *encephalomyelitis*.

  **Far East Russian e.,** tick-borne e. (Eastern subtype).

  **fox e.,** a disease of foxes caused by the infectious canine hepatitis virus (fox encephalitis virus).

  **e. hemorrhag′ica,** acute hemorrhagic e.; e. of apoplectiform character due to blood extravasation.

  **herpes e.,** e. caused by the herpes simplex virus.

  **hyperergic e.,** e. as a result of an immunologic allergic reaction of the nervous system to antigenic stimuli.

  **Ilhéus e.,** an arbovirus (group B) e. caused by the Ilhéus virus and endemic to eastern Brazil and other parts of South and Central America.

  **inclusion body e.,** Dawson's e.; subacute inclusion body e.; a usually fatal disease, seemingly of viral origin, that causes varying types of inflammatory reaction in both the white and gray matter and is characterized by the presence of inclusion bodies (usually nuclear); the clinical course progresses from personality change to mental deterioration and progressive paralysis.

  **Japanese B e.,** e. japonica; Russian autumn e.; an epidemic e. or encephalomyelitis of Japan, Russia (Siberia), and other parts of Asia; it is due to the Japanese B e. virus (a group B arbovirus).

  **e. japon′ica,** Japanese B e.

  **lead e.,** lead *encephalopathy*.

  **e. lethar′gica,** von Economo's *disease*.

  **Mengo e.,** an e. occurring in Africa, due to Mengo virus, a strain of encephalomyocarditis virus.

  **Murray Valley e.,** Australian X disease; Australian X e.; a severe e. with a high mortality rate reported as occurring in the Murray Valley of Australia; the disease is most severe in children, and is ushered in by headache, fever, malaise, drowsiness or convulsions, and rigidity of the neck; extensive brain damage may result. It is caused by the Murray Valley encephalitis *virus, q.v.*

  **necrotizing e.,** an e. with extensive necrosis in the cerebral cortex, and with lesser damage in the basal ganglia and brainstem.

  **e. neonato′rum,** e. of the newborn, described by Virchow as marked by the presence of numbers of fat-laden cells in the brain.

  **opossum e.,** e. of opossum caused by *Chlamydia psittaci*.

  **e. periaxia′lis concen′trica,** Baló's disease; clinically similar to e. periaxialis diffusa, but pathologically characterized by concentric globes or circles of demyelination of cerebral white matter separated by normal tissue.

  **e. periaxia′lis diffu′sa,** diffuse sclerosis; Flatau-Schilder disease; Schilder's disease; an affection occurring chiefly in children, marked by progressive dementia, convulsions, failure of hearing, and spastic paralysis followed by rapidly increasing speech defect, gradual loss of sight, and death; the white matter of the brain is confluently demyelinated and degenerated, having a gelatinous appearance, but the cortex and meninges are not involved.

  **postvaccinal e.,** demyelinating e. following vaccination.

  **purulent e.,** e. pyogenica.

  **e. pyogen′ica,** suppurative or purulent e.; a form marked by the occurrence of numerous miliary abscesses (disseminated cerebral microabscesses) and minute blood extravasations in the brain substance).

  **Russian autumn e.,** Japanese B e.

  **Russian spring-summer e. (Eastern subtype),** tick-borne e. (Eastern subtype).

  **Russian spring-summer e. (Western subtype),** tick-borne e. (Central European subtype).

  **Russian tick-borne e.,** tick-borne e. (Eastern subtype).

  **secondary e.,** e. following vaccination for smallpox or during convalescence from measles, mumps, varicella, and certain other infectious diseases, usually of the demyelinating kind.

  **subacute inclusion body e.,** inclusion body e.

  **e. subcortica′lis chron′ica,** Binswanger's *disease*.

  **suppurative e.,** e. pyogenica.

  **tick-borne e. (Central European subtype),** biundulant meningoencephalitis; Central European tick-borne fever; diphasic milk fever; Russian spring-summer e. (Western subtype); tick-borne meningoencephalitis caused by a group B arbovirus closely related to the virus causing the Far Eastern type; it is transmitted by *Ixodes ricinus*, also by infected raw milk, especially that of goats.

  **tick-borne e. (Eastern subtype),** a severe form of e. caused by a group B arbovirus, and transmitted by ticks (*Ixodes pertulcatus* and *I. ricinus*); also known as Far East Russian e.; Russian spring-summer e. (Eastern subtype); Russian tick-borne e.; vernal e.; woodcutter's e.

  **van Bogaert's e.,** subacute sclerosing *leukoencephalitis*.

  **varicella e.,** occurring as a complication of chickenpox.

  **vernal e.,** tick-borne e. (Eastern subtype).

  **woodcutter's e.,** tick-borne e. (Eastern subtype).

**encephalitogen** (en-sef′ă-li-to′jen) [ encephalitis + G. suffix -*gen*, producing ]. An agent which evokes encephalitis, particularly with reference to the antigen which produces experimental allergic encephalomyelitis.

**encephalitogenic** (en-sef′ă-lī-to-jen′ik). Encephalitis-producing; typically by hypersensitivity mechanisms; see encephalitogen.

**Encephalitozoon** (en-sef′ă-lī-to-zo′on) [ encephalitis + G. *zōon*, animal ]. A genus of protozoan parasites of the family Toxoplasmatidae, class Sporozoa. *E. cuniculi* occurs in brain, liver, kidneys, speen and other organs of dogs, rabbits, rats and mice, sometimes causing encephalitis and systemic disturbances in puppies and rabbits.

**encephalization** (en-sef′ă-lī-za′shun). Corticalization.

**encephalo-, encephal-** (en-sef′ă-lo-) [ G. *enkephalos*, brain ]. Combining forms indicating the brain or some relationship thereto.

**encephalocele** (en-sef′ă-lo-sēl) [ encephalo- + G. *kēlē*, hernia ]. Craniocele; cranium bifidum; congenital gap in the skull, usually with herniation of brain substance or meninges.

**encephalodynia** (en-sef′ă-lo-din′ī-ah) [ encephalo- + G. *odynē*, pain ]. Headache.

**encephalodysplasia** (en-sef′ă-lo-dis-pla′zī-ah) [ encephalo- + G. *dys*, bad, + *plasis*, a molding ]. Congenital abnormality of the brain.

**enceph′alogram** [ encephalo- + G. *gramma*, a drawing ]. A roentgenogram of the contents of the skull.

**encephalography** (en-sef'ă-log'ră-fĭ) [ encephalo- + G. *graphō,* to write ]. Roentgenography of the brain.

**encephaloid** (en-sef'ă-loyd) [ encephalo- + G. *eidos,* resemblance ]. Resembling brain substance; denoting a carcinoma of brainlike consistence, with reference to gross features.

**encephalolith** (en-sef'ă-lo-lith) [ encephalo- + G. *lithos,* stone ]. Cerebral calculus; a concretion in the brain or one of its ventricles.

**encephalology** (en-sef-ă-lol'o-jĭ) [ encephalo- + G. *logos,* study ]. The branch of medicine dealing with the brain in all its relations.

**encephalo'ma.** Cerebroma; herniation of brain substance.

**encephalomalacia** (en-sef'ă-lo-mă-la'shĭ-ah) [ encephalo- + G. *malakia,* softness ]. Cerebromalacia; softening of the brain; infarction of brain tissue, usually caused by vascular insufficiency.

   **nutritional e. of chicks,** crazy chick disease; a d. of young chicks caused by vitamin E deficiency.

**encephalomeningitis** (en-sef'ă-lo-men-in-ji'tis) [ encephalo- + G. *mēninx,* suffix *-itis,* inflammation ]. Meningoencephalitis.

**encephalomeningocele** (en-sef'ă-lo-mĕ-nin'go-sēl) [ encephalo- + G. *mēninx,* membrane, + *kēlē,* hernia ]. Meningoencephalocele.

**encephalomeningopathy** (en-sef'ă-lo-men-in-gop'ă-thĭ). Meningoencephalopathy.

**encephalomere** (en-sef'ă-lo-mēr) [ encephalo- + G. *meros,* a part ]. A neuromere.

**encephalom'eter** [ encephalo- + G. *metron,* measure ]. An apparatus for indicating on the skull the location of the cortical centers.

**encephalomyelitis** (en-sef'ă-lo-mi'ĕ-li'tis) [ encephalo- + G. *myelon,* + suffix *-itis,* inflammation ]. An acute inflammation of the brain and spinal cord.

   **acute disseminated e.,** a diffuse inflammation of the brain and spinal cord usually caused by a perivascular hypersensitivity response.

   **avian infectious e.,** epidemic *tremor.*

   **benign myalgic e.,** epidemic *neuromyasthenia.*

   **bovine sporadic e.,** buss disease; an acute, septic e., pleuritis, and peritonitis of cattle caused by *Chlamydia psittaci;* it occurs in the north central states of the United States and perhaps elsewhere.

   **eastern equine e.,** abbreviated EEE; a form of equine e. seen in the eastern United States and caused by the eastern equine e. virus; initial fever and viremia are followed by signs of central nervous system involvement (excitement, then somnolence, paralysis, and death); mortality in horses may reach 90 per cent; the incidence of clinical infection in man is low but mortality may be high.

   **epidemic myalgic e.,** epidemic *neuromyasthenia.*

   **equine e.,** equine encephalitis; an acute, often fatal virus disease of horses and mules characterized by central nervous system disturbances; in the United States, this disease may be caused by any one of three arthropod-borne viruses, and their resulting diseases are designated western equine e. (WEE), eastern equine e. (EEE), or Venezuelan equine e. (VEE); certain birds are reservoirs for these viruses, which also may cause neurologic disease in man; in Germany, a similar disease caused by a different virus is known as Borna disease.

   **experimental allergic e.,** a demyelinating allergic e. produced by the injection of brain tissue, usually with an adjuvant.

   **granulomatous e.,** a disease causing necrosis and granulomas in the substance of the brain.

   **infectious porcine e.,** Teschen *disease.*

   **mouse e.,** Theiler's disease (1); mouse poliomyelitis; due to the mouse encephalomyelitis virus, which is not pathogenic in monkeys or in man, but attacks mouse colonies and causes a flaccid paralysis, usually of the hind limbs.

   **Venezuelan equine e.,** abbreviated VEE; a form of equine e. found in parts of South America, Panama, and Trinidad, and caused by the Venezuelan equine e. virus; it is characterized by less central nervous system involvement than occurs in either eastern or western equine e., but fever, diarrhea, and depression are common; in man, there is fever and severe headache after an incubation period of 2

to 5 days, and in a few cases there has been central nervous system involvement.

   **virus e.,** an acute e. due to a neurotropic virus.

   **western equine e.,** an equine e. found in the western United States and parts of South America and caused by the western equine e. virus; the infection is similar to but milder than eastern equine e., mortality being no greater than 20 to 30 per cent; infection in man is, as a rule, inapparent, but about 10 per cent of cases with central nervous system involvement are fatal.

   **zoster e.,** inflammation of the brain and spinal cord caused by the virus of herpes zoster-varicella.

**encephalomyelocele** (en-sef'ă-lo-mi'ĕ-lo-sēl) [ G. *enkephalos,* brain, + *myelon,* marrow, + *kēlē,* hernia ]. A congenital defect in the occipital region with herniation of the meninges, medulla, and spinal cord.

**encephalomyeloneuropathy** (en-sef'ă-lo-mi'ĕ-lo-nu-rop'ă-thĭ). A disease involving the brain, spinal cord and peripheral nerves.

**enceph'alomyelop'athy** [ G. *enkephalos,* brain, + *myelon,* marrow, + *pathos,* suffering ]. Any disease of both brain and spinal cord.

   **epidemic myalgic e.,** a disease superficially resembling poliomyelitis, characterized by diffuse involvement of the nervous system associated with myalgia.

**enceph'alomy'eloradiculi'tis.** Inflammation involving the brain, spinal cord, and peripheral nerves; see also Guillain-Barré *syndrome.*

**enceph'alomy'eloradiculop'athy.** A disease process involving the brain, spinal cord, and spinal roots.

**encephalomyocarditis** (en-sef'ă-lo-mi'o-kar-di'tis). Associated encephalitis and myocarditis.

**encephalon,** pl. **encephala** (en-sef'ă-lon) [ G. *enkephalos,* brain, fr. *en,* in, + *kephalē,* head ] [ NA ]. The brain; that portion of the cerebrospinal axis contained within the cranium.

**encephalonarcosis** (en-sef'ă-lo-nar-ko'sis) [ encephalo- + G. *narkē,* stupor ]. Stupor or coma from brain disease.

**enceph'alopath'ia.** Encephalopathy.

   **e. addiso'nia,** apathy, somnolence, or rarely psychic irritative symptoms, occurring in the course of Addison's disease, probably related to electrolyte imbalance.

**encephalopathy** (en-sef'ă-lop'ă-thĭ) [ encephalo- + G. *pathos,* suffering ]. Cerebropathy; any disease of the brain.

   **bilirubin e.,** e. due to the toxic effects of bilirubin; see also *icterus* neonatorum; kernicterus.

   **Binswanger's e.,** Binswanger's *disease.*

   **demy'elinating e.,** progressive subcortical e.; extensive idiopathic loss of myelin sheaths in the brain, as occurs in Scholz's disease, Krabbe's disease, encephalitis periaxialis concentrica, encephalitis periaxialis diffusa, and leukodystrophy.

   **familial e.,** a progressive form of e. occurring in young members of the same family; characterized by headache, vertigo, ataxia, drowsiness and stupor, and sometimes convulsions.

   **hepatic e.,** portal-systemic e.

   **hypernatremic e.,** subarachnoid and subdural effusions in infants with hypernatremic dehydration.

   **hypertensive e.,** cerebral symptoms such as headache, somnolence, convulsions, and vomiting, occurring in advanced stages of arterial hypertension.

   **lead e.,** lead encephalitis; saturnine e.; a rapidly developing e., caused by the ingestion of lead compounds and seen particularly in early childhood; it is characterized pathologically by extensive cerebral edema, status spongiosus, neurocytolysis, and some reactive inflammation; clinical manifestations are convulsions, delirium, hallucinations, and other cerebral symptoms due to chronic lead poisoning; see also lead *poisoning.*

   **palindromic e.,** recurrent e.; a relatively mild form which tends to recur.

   **pancreatic e.,** an e. associated with extensive pancreatic necrosis; the cerebral lesions consist of capillary necrosis, perivascular bleeding, and focal gliosis.

   **portal-systemic e.,** hepatic e.; an e. associated with cirrhosis of the liver, and cerebral manifestations may include coma; attributed to the passage of toxic nitrogenous substances from the portal to the systemic circulation.

**progressive subcortical e.,** demyelinating e.

**recurrent e.,** palindromic e.

**saturnine e.,** lead e.

**thyrotoxic e.,** a rare condition arising in severe cases of thyrotoxicosis, marked by bulbar symptoms (disturbances in deglutition, mastication, and speech) and loss of consciousness merging into deep coma.

**traumatic e.,** disturbance of structure or function (or both) of nerve cells, glia, or intracranial vessels resulting from injury.

**traumatic progressive e.,** chronic brain damage resulting from multiple brain injuries.

**Wernicke's e.,** Wernicke's *syndrome*.

**Wernicke-Korsakoff e.,** see Wernicke's *syndrome* and Korsakoff's *syndrome*.

**encephalopsy** (en-sef'ă-lop'sī) [ encephalo- + G. *opsis*, sight ]. The association of special colors with words or other sensory data.

**encephalopsychosis** (en-sef'ă-lo-si-ko'sis). Organic psychosis; a psychosis related to demonstrable brain damage.

**encephalopuncture** (en-sef'ă-lo-punk'chūr). Puncture of the brain substance.

**encephalopyosis** (en-sef'ă-lo-pi-o'sis) [ encephalo- + G. *pyōsis*, suppuration ]. Purulent inflammation of the brain.

**encephalorrhachidian** (en-sef'ă-lo-ră-kid'ī-an) [ encephalo- + G. *rhachis*, spine ]. Cerebrospinal.

**encephalorrhagia** (en-sef'ă-lo-ra'jī-ah) [ encephalo- + G. *rhēgnymi*, to burst forth ]. Cerebral hemorrhage; apoplexy.

**encephaloschisis** (en-sef'ă-los'kī-sis) [ encephalo- + G. *schisis*, fissure ]. Developmental failure of closure of the rostral part of the neural tube.

**encephalosclerosis** (en-sef'ă-lo-skle-ro'sis) [ encephalo- + G. *sklērōsis*, hardening ]. Cerebrosclerosis; a sclerosis, or hardening, of the brain.

**encephaloscope** (en-sef'ă-lo-skōp) [ encephalo- + G. *skopeō*, to view ]. Cerebroscope (1); any instrument used to view the interior of a brain abscess or other cerebral cavity through an opening in the skull.

**encephaloscopy** (en-sef'ă-los'ko-pī). Cerebroscopy; examination of the brain or the cavity of a cerebral abscess by direct inspection.

**encephalosis** (en-sef'ă-lo'sis). Cerebrosis; any organic disease of the brain.

**enceph'alospi'nal.** Cerebrospinal.

**encephalothlipsis** (en-sef'ă-lo-thlip'sis) [ encephalo- + G. *thlipsis*, pressure ]. Compression of the brain.

**enceph'alotome.** An instrument for use in performing encephalotomy.

**encephalotomy** (en-sef'ă-lot'o-mī) [ encephalo- + G. *tomē*, incision ]. Dissection or incision of the brain.

**enchondral** (en-kon'dral). Endochondral.

**enchondroma** (en-kon-dro'mah) [ Mod. L. fr. G. *en*, in, + *chondros*, cartilage, + suffix -*oma*, tumor ]. A benign cartilaginous growth starting within the medullary cavity of a bone originally formed from cartilage. E.'s may distend the cortex, especially of small bones, and may be solitary or occur in endochondromatosis.

**enchondromato'sis.** Dyschondroplasia; Ollier's disease; nonfamilial hamartomatous proliferation of cartilage in the metaphyses of several bones, most commonly of the hands and feet, causing distorted growth in length or pathological fractures.

**enchondromatous** (en-kon-dro'mă-tus). Relating to or having the elements of enchondroma.

**enchondrosarcoma** (en-kon-dro-sar-ko'mah). A malignant neoplasm of cartilage cells derived from an enchondroma, or occurring in the same locations.

**enclave** (en-klāv, ahn-klahv') [ Fr. fr. L. *clavis*, key ]. An enclosure; a detached mass of tissue enclosed in tissue of another kind; seen especially in the case of isolated masses of gland tissue detached from the main gland.

**enclavoma** (en-klă-vo'mah). Mixed tumor of salivary gland; see under tumor.

**enclit'ic** [ G. *enkilitikos*, leaning on, fr. *en*, on, + *klinō*, to make recline ]. Inclined; denoting especially the relation of the planes of the fetal head to those of the pelvis of the mother.

**encopre'sis** [ G. *kopros*, ordure ]. Involuntary passage of feces.

**encra'nial.** Endocranial.

**encranius** (en-kra'nī-us) [ G. *en*, in, + *kranion*, skull ]. A form of fetal inclusion in which the smaller of the conjoined twins (parasite) lies partly or wholly within the cranial cavity of the larger (autosite).

**encyopyelitis** (en-si'o-pi-ĕ-li'tis) [ G. *enkyesis*, pregnancy, + pyelitis, *q.v.* ]. Pyelitis occurring during pregnancy.

**encys'ted** [ G. *kystis*, bladder ]. Encapsuled; surrounded by a closed membranous bag.

**encyst'ment.** The condition of being or becoming encysted.

**end.** An extremity, or the most remote point of an extremity.

**distal e.,** heel (2); the posterior extremity of a dental appliance.

**root e.,** root *apex*.

**end-.** See endo-.

**endadelphus** (en'dă-del'fus) [ G. *en*, in, + *adelphos*, brother ]. Conjoined twins in which the smaller (parasite) is within the body of the larger (autosite).

**Endamoeba** (end'ă-me'bah). A genus of amebae parasitic in invertebrates.

**endangeitis** (end-an-je-i'tis). Endangiitis.

**endangiitis** (end-an-jī-i'tis) [ endo- + G. *angeion*, vessel, + suffix -*itis*, inflammation ]. Endoangitis; endangeitis; endovasculitis; inflammation of the intima or inner coat of a blood vessel.

**e. obliterans,** inflammation of the intima of a vessel with resulting occlusion of its lumen.

**endaortitis** (end-a-or-ti'tis). Inflammation of the intima, or inner coat, of the aorta.

**endarterectomy** (end-ar-ter-ek'to-mī) [ endarterium, *q.v.*, + G. *ektomē*, excision ]. Excision of the lining of an artery and occluding atheromatous deposits.

**coronary e.,** the coronary artery is entered through a terminal branch, and occluding material, including intima, is avulsed.

**endarteritis** (end'ar-ter-i'tis) [ endo- + arteritis, *q.v.* ]. Endoarteritis; inflammation of the inner coat of an artery.

**bacterial e.,** implantation and growth of bacteria with formation of vegetations on the arterial wall, such as may occur in a patent ductus arteriosus or arteriovenous fistula.

**e. defor'mans,** e. with atheromatous patches and calcareous deposits.

**e. oblit'erans,** obliterating e.; Friedländer's disease; an extreme degree of e. proliferans closing the lumen of the artery.

**e. prolif'erans,** chronic e. accompanied by a marked increase of fibrous tissue in the intima.

**endaural** (end-aw'ral) [ endo- + L. *auris*, ear ]. Within the ear.

**end'brain.** Telencephalon.

**end-bulb.** See under bulb.

**end-brush.** Telodendrion.

**end-diastol'ic.** 1. Occurring at the end of diastole, immediately before the next systole, as in end-diastolic pressure. 2. Interrupting the final moments of diastole, barely premature, as in end-diastolic extrasystole.

**ende'mia.** An endemic disease.

**ende'mial.** Endemic (1).

**endem'ic** [ G. *endēmos*, native, fr. *en*, in, + *dēmos*, the people ]. Present in a community or among a group of people; said of a disease prevailing continually in a region; *cf.* epidemic.

**endemoepidemic** (en-dem'o-ep-ī-dem'ik). Denoting a temporary large increase in the number of cases of an endemic disease.

**endergonic** (end'er-gon'ik) [ endo- + G. *ergon*, work ]. Referring to a chemical reaction that takes place with absorption of energy from its surroundings (*i.e.*, becomes cool); *cf.* exergonic.

**endermic, endermatic** (en-der'mik, en-der-mat'ik) [ G. *en*, in, + *derma* (*dermat-*), skin ]. In or through the skin; denoting a method of treatment, as by inunction; the remedy produces its constitutional effect when absorbed through the skin surface to which it is applied.

**endermism** (en-der'mizm). Endermic medication; see endermic.

**endermosis** (en'der-mo'sis). Any eruptive disease of the mucous membrane.

**en'deron** [ G. *en,* in, + *deros,* skin ]. Corium.

**enderon'ic.** Relating to the enderon.

**Enders,** John F., U. S. microbiologist, *1897. Nobel laureate, 1954, with Thomas H. Weller and Frederick G. Robbins, for their discovery of the ability of poliomyelitis viruses to grow in cultures of various types of tissue.

**end-feet.** axon *terminals.*

**end'gut.** Hindgut.

**end'ing.** 1. A termination or conclusion. 2. A nerve e.

**annulospiral e.,** the termination of a large-caliber sensory nerve fiber within a muscle spindle (neuromuscular spindle). After entering the muscle spindle the fiber divides into two flat, ribbon-like branches that wind themselves in rings or spirals about the intrafusal muscle fibers. See fig. under neuromuscular *spindle.*

**calyciform e., caliciform e.,** a synaptic e. in relation to certain neuroepithelial hair cells of the inner ear.

**epilemmal e.,** a nerve e. in close relation to the outer surface of the sarcolemma.

**flower-spray e.,** flower-spray organ of Ruffini; one of the two types of sensory nerve e. associated with the muscle spindle (the other being the annulospiral e.). In this type, the fiber branches spread out upon the surface of the intrafusal fibers like a spray of flowers. See fig. under neuromuscular *spindle.*

**free nerve e.'s,** *terminationes* nervorum liberae.

**grape e.'s,** an autodescriptive term applied to synaptic terminals at the ends of short, stalklike axon branches.

**hed'eriform e.,** a type of free sensory ending in the skin.

**nerve e.,** any one of the specialized terminations of peripheral sensory or motor nerve fibers; see motor *end-plate,* and various listings under corpuscle and bulb.

**sole-plate e.,** motor *endplate.*

**synaptic e.'s,** axon *terminals.*

**Endo,** Shigeru, Japanese bacteriologist, 1869–1937. See E.'s *agar, medium.*

**endo-, end-** [ G. *endon,* within ]. Prefix indicating within, inner, absorbing, containing; see also ento-.

**en'doabdom'inal.** Within the abdomen.

**endoaneurysmoplasty** (en'do-an-u-riz-mo-plas'tĭ). Aneurysmoplasty.

**endoaneurysmorrhaphy** (en'do-an'u-riz-mor'ă-fĭ) [ endo- + G. *aneurysma,* aneurysm, + *raphe,* suture ]. Aneurysmoplasty.

**endoangiitis** (en-do-an-jĭ-i'tis). Endangiitis.

**endoantitox'in.** An antibody contained within the cell that elaborates it, and normally not released into the surrounding plasma during the life of the cell.

**endo-aortitis** (en'do-a-or-ti'tis). Endaortitis.

**endoappendicitis** (en'do-ă-pen-dĭ-si'tis). Simple catarrhal inflammation, limited more or less strictly to the mucosal surface of the vermiform appendix.

**endoarteritis** (en'do-ar-ter-i'tis). Endarteritis.

**endoauscultation** (en'do-aws-kul-ta'shun). Auscultation of the thoracic organs, especially the heart, by means of a stethoscopic tube passed into the esophagus or into the heart.

**endoben'ziline bromide.** ULCYN; choline bromide α-phenyl-5-norbornene-2-glycolate; intestinal antispasmodic.

**endobiot'ic.** Living as a parasite within the host.

**en'doblast** [ endo- + G. *blastos,* germ ]. Entoderm.

**endobronchial** (en-do-brong'kĭ-al). Intrabronchial.

**endocar'diac, endocar'dial.** 1. Intracardiac; within the heart. 2. Relating to the endocardium.

**endocardiography** (en'do-kar-dĭ-og'ră-fĭ). Electrocardiography with the exploring electrode within the chambers of the heart. See also intracardiac *catheter.*

**en'docardit'ic.** Relating to endocarditis.

**endocarditis** (en'do-kar-di'tis). Inflammation of the endocardium, or lining membrane of the heart. It may involve only the membrane covering the valves (valvular e.) or the general lining of the chambers of the heart (mural e.).

**abacterial thrombotic e.,** nonbacterial thrombotic e.

**atypical verrucous e.,** Libman-Sacks e.

**bacteria-free stage of bacterial e.,** described prior to the antibiotic era and presumably due to spontaneous healing of the bacterial vegetations.

**bacterial e.,** e. caused by the direct invasion of bacteria and leading to deformity of the valve leaflets; **acute bacterial e.** is caused by pyogenic organisms such as hemolytic streptococci or staphylococci; **subacute bacterial e.** is usually due to *Streptococcus viridans* or *S. fecalis.*

**cachectic e.,** nonbacterial thrombotic e.

**e. chorda'lis,** e. affecting particularly the chordae tendineae.

**constrictive e.,** endomyocardial fibroelastosis producing a clinical picture identical with constrictive pericarditis.

**infectious e., infective e.,** e. due to infection by microorganisms, including bacteria, fungi, and *Coxiella burnetii.*

**isolated parietal e.,** fibrous thickening of the endocardium of the left ventricle without valvular involvement.

**Libman-Sacks e.,** atypical verrucous e.; Libman-Sacks syndrome; nonbacterial verrucous e. sometimes associated with disseminated lupus erythematosus.

**Löffler's e.,** Löffler's syndrome (2) or disease; fibroplastic parietal endocarditis with eosinophilia; an e. of obscure cause characterized by progressive congestive heart failure, multiple systemic emboli, and eosinophilia.

**Löffler's fibroplastic e.,** Löffler's e.

**malignant e.,** septic e.; acute bacterial e., usually secondary to suppuration elsewhere and running a fulminating course.

**marantic e.,** nonbacterial thrombotic e. associated with cancer and other debilitating diseases.

**mural e.,** inflammation of the endocardium other than valvular.

**nonbacterial thrombotic e.,** abacterial thrombotic e.; cachectic e.; terminal e.; thromboendocarditis; verrucous endocardial lesions occurring in the terminal stages of many chronic infectious and wasting diseases.

**nonbacterial ver'rucous e.,** Libman-Sacks *syndrome.*

**pol'ypous e.,** bacterial e. with the formation of pedunculated masses of fibrin, or thrombi, attached to the ulcerated valves.

**rheumatic e.,** endocardial involvement as part of the acute rheumatic process, recognized clinically by valvular involvement.

**septic e.,** malignant e.

**terminal e.,** nonbacterial thrombotic e.

**val'vular e.,** inflammation confined to the endocardium of the valves.

**vegetative e.,** verrucous e.; e. associated with the presence of fibrinous clots (vegetations) forming on the ulcerated surfaces of the valves.

**verrucous e.,** vegetative e.

**endocar'dium,** pl. **endocar'dia** [ endo- + G. *kardia,* heart ]. [ NA ]. The innermost tunic of the heart, which includes endothelium and subendothelial connective tissue. In the atrial wall smooth muscle and numerous elastic fibers also occur.

**endoceliac** (en-do-se'lĭ-ak) [ endo- + G. *koilia,* cavity, ventricle ]. Intracelial; within one of the body cavities.

**endocervical** (en'do-ser'vĭ-kal). 1. Intracervical; within any cervix, specifically within the cervix uteri. 2. Relating to the endocervix.

**endocervicitis** (en'do-ser-vĭ-si'tis). Endotrachelitis; inflammation of the mucous membrane of the cervix uteri.

**endocervix** (en'do-ser'viks). The mucous membrane of the cervical canal.

**endochondral** (en-do-kon'dral) [ endo- + G. *chondros,* cartilage ]. Intracartilaginous.

**endocolitis** (en'do-ko-li'tis). Simple catarrhal inflammation of the colon.

**endocolpitis** (en'do-kol-pi'tis) [ endo- + G. *colpos,* vagina, + suffix -*itis,* inflammation ]. Inflammation of the vaginal mucous membrane.

**endocom'plement.** A complement once assumed to be present within a certain species of cell, which enhanced the hemolytic action of snake venom.

**endocra'nial.** 1. Within the cranium. 2. Relating to the endocranium.

**endocrani'tis.** Inflammation of the endocranium; cerebral pachymeningitis.

**endocranium** (en'do-kra'nĭ-um). The lining membrane of the cranium, or dura mater of the brain.

**endocrine** (en'do-krin) [ endo- + G. *krino*, to separate. CRIN- ]. 1. Secreting internally, most commonly into the systemic circulation; of or pertaining to such secretion. 2. The internal or hormonal secretion of a ductless gland. 3. Denoting a gland that furnishes an internal secretion; see also endocrine *gland*.

**endocrin'ic.** Obsolete term for endocrine (1).

**endocrinism** (en-dok'rĭ-nizm). Obsolete term for endocrinopathy.

**endocrinology** (en'do-krī-nol'o-jĭ) [ endocrine + G. *logos*, study ]. The science dealing with the internal secretions and their physiologic and pathologic relations.

**endocrinoma** (en'do-krī-no'mah). A tumor with endocrine tissue that retains the function of the parent organ, usually to an excessive degree.

**endocrinopathic** (en-do-krin'o-path'ik). Relating to or suffering from an endocrinopathy.

**endocrinopathy** (en'do-krī-nop'ă-thĭ). A disorder in the function of an endocrine gland and the consequences thereof.

   **multiple e.,** endocrine polyglandular *syndrome*.

**en'docrin'other'apy.** Treatment of disease by the administration of extracts of endocrine glands.

**endocrinous** (en-dok'rĭ-nus). Obsolete term for endocrine (1).

**endocyclic** (en'do-si'klik, sik'lik). Within a cycle or ring; for example, the 6 C atoms of the benzene ring in toluene; opposite of exocyclic.

**endocyma** (en-do-si'mah) [ endo- + G. *kyma*, fetus ]. A teratoma, or possibly an included parasitic twin, in a visceral location.

**endocyst** (en'do-sist). The inner layer of a hydatid cyst.

**endocystitis** (en'do-sis-ti'tis) [ endo- + G. *kystis*, bladder, + suffix -*itis*, inflammation ]. Inflammation of the mucous membrane of the bladder; see cystitis.

**endocytosis** (en'do-si-to'sis) [ endo- + G. *kytos*, cell, + suffix -*osis*, condition ]. The process, including pinocytosis and phagocytosis, whereby materials are taken into a cell by the invagination of the plasma membrane, which it breaks off as a boundary membrane of the part engulfed.

**en'doderm.** Entoderm.

**Endodermophyton** (en'do-der-mof'ĭ-ton) [ endo- + G. *derma*, skin, + *phyton*, plant ]. A genus of fungi (Hyphomycetes) several species of which cause forms of tinea in man; the fungus grows in the epidermis between the superficial and deep layers but does not attack the hairs or hair follicles. The form produced in man is typically tinea imbricata.

**endodiascope** (en'do-di'ă-skōp). An x-ray tube that may be placed within a cavity of the body.

**endodiascopy** (en'do-di-as'ko-pĭ) [ endo- + G. *dia*, through, + *skopeō*, to view ]. X-ray by means of an endodiascope.

**endodontia** (en-do-don'shĭ-ah). Endodontics.

**endodon'tics** [ endo- + G. *odous*, tooth ]. Endodontia; a field of dentistry concerned with the diagnosis and treatment of diseases and injuries of the dental pulp and periapical tissues of teeth.

**endodon'tist.** One who specializes in the practice of endodontics.

**endodontol'ogist.** An endodontist.

**endodontol'ogy.** Endodontics.

**endodyocyte** (en'do-di'o-sīt) [ endo- + G. *dys*, two, + *kytos*, cell ]. Merozoite.

**endodyogeny** (en'do-di-oj'ē-nĭ) [ endo- + G. *dys*, two, + *genesis*, creation ]. The pattern of internal budding characteristic of members of the coccidian genus *Frankelia*, in which the crescent-shaped trophozoite parasites form two organisms within the parent cell or membrane; the two parasites are freed by rupture of the parent cell; *cf.* endopolygeny.

**en'doenteri'tis** [ endo- + G. *enteron*, intestine, suffix -*itis*, inflammation ]. Inflammation of the intestinal mucous membrane.

**en'doen'zyme.** Intracellular *enzyme*.

**endoesophagitis** (en'de-e-sof'ă-ji'tis). Inflammation of the internal lining of the esophagus.

**endofaradism** (en'do-făr-ă-dizm). The application of faradic electricity to the interior of any cavity of the body.

**endogal'vanism.** The application of a galvanic current to the interior of any cavity of the body.

**endogamy** (en-dog'ă-mĭ) [ endo- + G. *gamos*, marriage ]. Reproduction by conjugation between sister cells, the descendants of one original cell.

**endogas'tric.** Within the stomach.

**en'dogastri'tis** [ endo- + G. *gastēr*, stomach, + suffix -*itis*, inflammation ]. Inflammation of the mucous membrane of the stomach; see gastritis.

**endogenic** (en'do-jen'ik). Endogenous.

**endogenote** (en'do-je'nōt). In microbial genetics, the original genome of a merozygote.

**endogenous** (en-doj'ē-nus) [ endo- + G. suffix -*gen*, production ]. Endogenic; originating or produced within the organism or one of its parts.

**endoglo'bar.** Endoglobular.

**endoglob'ular.** Within a globular body; specifically, within a red blood cell.

**endognathion** (en-dog-nath'ĭ-on, en-do-na'thĭ-on) [ endo- + G. *gnathos*, jaw ]. The medial of the two segments constituting the incisive bone; see mesognathion.

**endoherniotomy** (en'do-her-nĭ-ot'o-mĭ). Closure, by sutures, of the interior lining of a hernial sac.

**en'dointoxica'tion.** Poisoning by an endogenous toxin.

**endolaryngeal** (en'do-lă-rin'je-al). Within the larynx.

**Endolimax** (en-do-li'maks) [ endo- + G. *leimax*, a meadow or garden ]. A genus of amebae parasitic in the large intestine of man and other animals, not generally considered to be pathogenic.

   **E. ca'viae,** occurs in the cecum of guinea pigs.

   **E. gregarinifor'mis,** found in the ceca of chickens, turkeys, guinea fowls, pheasants, ducks, and many other birds.

   **E. na'na,** a species of worldwide distribution found in the large intestine of man, other primates, and pigs.

**endolymph** (en'do-limf). Endolympha.

**endolympha** (en'do-lim'fah) [ endo- + L. *lympha*, a clear fluid ]. [ NA ]. Endolymph; the fluid contained within the membranous labyrinth of the inner ear.

**endolym'phic.** Relating to the endolymph.

**endolysin** (en-dol'ĭ-sin). Leukin.

**endomeninx** (en'do-me'ningks, -men'ingks) [ endo- + G. *meninx*, membrane ]. The inner membrane surrounding the embryonic neural tube; it is concerned with the formation of the leptomeninges.

**endomerogony** (en'do-mĕ-rog'o-nĭ) [ endo- + G. *meros*, part, + *gonē*, generation ]. Production of merozoites in the asexual reproduction of sporozoan protozoa by a process originating in the interior of the schizont (as contrasted with ectomerogony); observed in species of *Eimeria*.

**endometrial** (en'do-me'trĭ-al). Relating to or composed of endometrium.

**endometrioma** (en'do-me'trĭ-o'mah). A circumscribed mass of ectopic endometrial tissue in endometriosis.

**endometriosis** (en-do-me-trĭ-o'sis). The ectopic occurrence of endometrial tissue, frequently forming cysts containing altered blood.

   **stromal e.,** see endometrial stromal *sarcoma*.

**endometritis** (en-do-me-tri'tis). Inflammation of the endometrium.

   **decid'ual e.,** inflammation of the decidual mucous membrane of the gravid uterus.

   **diphtherit'ic e.,** inflammation of the uterine mucous membrane, with a dirty brownish exudate, not necessarily due to the presence of the Klebs-Loeffler bacillus.

   **e. dis'secans,** e. with ulceration and exfoliation of the mucous membrane.

**endometrium,** pl. **endome'tria** (en'do-me'trĭ-um) [ endo- + G. + *mētra*, uterus ]. [ NA ]. Tunica mucosa uteri [ NA ]; the mucous membrane comprising the inner layer of the uterine wall; it consists of a simple columnar epithelium and a lamina propria that contains simple tubular uterine glands.

**Swiss cheese e.,** cystic-glandular hyperplasia of the e.; glandular hyperplasia of the e. with cyst formation, associated with pathologic uterine bleeding (as in metropathia hemorrhagica); due to excess estrogenic stimulation. See also *metropathia* hemorrhagica.

**endometropic** (en'do-me-trop'ik) [ endo- + G. *metra*, uterus, + *trope̅,* a turning ]. Denoting an external stimulus capable of producing a response of the uterus, specifically the endometrium.

**endomitosis** (en'do-mi-to'sis). Endopolyploidy.

**endomorph** (en'do-morf) [ endo- + G. *morphe̅,* form ]. Brachytype; a constitutional body type or build (biotype or somatotype) in which tissues that originated in the endoderm prevail. From the morphological standpoint, the trunk predominates over the members.

**endomorphic** (en'do-mor'fik). Relating to, or having the characteristics of, an endomorph.

**endomotorsonde** (en'do-mo'tor-sond') [ endo- + L. *motor,* mover, + Fr. *sonde,* sounding line ]. Radiotelemetering capsule for studying the interior of the gastrointestinal tract.

**endomy'cin.** Helixin.

**endomyocardial** (en'do-mi'o-kar'di̅-al). Relating to the endocardium and the myocardium.

**en'domy'ocardi'tis.** Inflammation of both endocardium and myocardium.

**endomysium** (en'do-miz'i̅-um, -mis'i̅-um) [ endo- + G. *mys,* muscle ]. The fine connective tissue sheath surrounding a muscle fiber.

**endoneuritis** (en-do-nu-ri'tis). Inflammation of the endoneurium.

**endoneurium** (en-do-nu'ri̅-um) [ endo- + G. *neuron,* nerve ]. Henle's sheath; sheath of Key and Retzius; the delicate connective tissue enveloping individual nerve fibers within a peripheral nerve.

**endonuclease** (en'do-nu'kle-a̅s). A nuclease (phosphodiesterase) that cleaves polynucleotides (nucleic acids) at interior bonds, thus producing poly- or oligonucleotide fragments of varying size (contrast exonuclease). Deoxyribonucleases I and II, ribonucleases I and II, and guanyloribonuclease (ribonuclease T₁) are endonucleases.

**nucleate e.** (EC 3.1.4.9), azotobacter nuclease; mung bean nuclease; a nuclease (a nucleate nucleotidohydrolase) that forms oligonucleotides ending in 5'-phosphates from RNA and DNA.

**spleen e.,** spleen deoxyribonuclease; spleen phosphodiesterase; micrococcal nuclease; enzyme (EC 3.1.4.7) cleaving nucleic acids to oligonucleotides terminating in 3'-phosphates.

**endonucleolus** (en'do-nu-kle'o-lus). A minute unstainable spot near the center of a nucleolus.

**endopar'asite.** A parasite living within the body of its host; see parasite.

**endopar'asitism.** Infection.

**endopep'tidase.** An enzyme catalyzing the hydrolysis of a peptide chain at points well within the chain, not near termini (*e.g.,* pepsin, trypsin, and ribonuclease).

**endoperiarteritis** (en'do-per̅'ĭ-ar-ter-i'tis) [ endo- + G. *peri,* around, + arteritis ]. Inflammation of the inner and outer (and all) the coats of an artery.

**endopericarditis** (en'do-per̅'ĭ-kar-di'tis) [ endo- + G. *peri,* around, + *kardia,* heart, + suffix -*itis,* inflammation ]. Simultaneous inflammation of the endocardium and pericardium.

**endoperimyocarditis** (en'do-per̅'i-mi'o-kar-di'tis) [ endo- + G. *peri,* around, + *mys,* muscle, + *kardia,* heart, + suffix -*itis,* inflammation ]. Simultaneous inflammation of the heart muscle and of its inner and outer membranes, or endocardium and pericardium.

**endoperineuritis** (en'do-per̅'ĭ-nu-ri'tis). Inflammation of both endoneurium and perineurium.

**endoperitonitis** (en'do-per̅'ĭ-to-ni'tis). Superficial inflammation of the peritoneum; see peritonitis.

**endophlebitis** (en'do-fle̅-bi'tis) [ endo- + G. *phleps* (*phleb-*), vein, + suffix -*itis,* inflammation ]. Inflammation of the intima, or lining membrane, of a vein.

**endophthalmitis** (en-dof-thal-mi'tis) [ endo- + G. *ophthalmos,* eye, + suffix -*itis,* inflammation ]. Inflammation

of the internal structures of of the tissues in the eyeball.

**mycotic e.,** e. following ocular injury or surgery (*e.g.,* cataract extraction); it is characterized by gradual onset, infiltration of the vitreous with conglomerate opacities, aqueous flare, microcystic edema of the corneal epithelium, and negative bacterial cultures.

**e. phacoanaphylac'tica,** inflammation of the uveal tract occurring in cataractous eyes spontaneously or after operation as a result of sensitization by loose lens material in one eye; simulates sympathetic ophthalmia, and is relieved by intracapsular extraction of cataract in affected eye.

**starch e.** a postoperative sterile e. caused by the inadvertent entrance into the open eye (during cataract surgery) of starch granules from surgical gloves or drapes; prompt corticosteroid therapy produces a rapid and favorable response.

**endophyte** (en'do-fit) [ endo- + G. *phyton,* plant ]. A parasite living inside another organism.

**endophytic** (en-do-fit'ik). 1. Pertaining to an endophyte. 2. In dentistry, term used in reference to the growth pattern of oral lesions that invade the lamina propria and submucosa.

**en'doplasm.** In certain cells, especially protozoa, the inner or medullary part of the cytoplasm as opposed to the ectoplasm.

**en'doplast** [ endo- + G. *plastos,* formed ]. Former name for endosome.

**endoplas'tic.** Relating to the endoplasm.

**endopolygeny** (en'do-po-lij'ĕ-ni̅) [ endo- + G. *polys,* many, + *genesis,* creation ]. Asexual reproduction in which more than two offspring are formed within the parent organism and in which two or possibly more nuclear divisions occur before merozoite formation begins; a form of internal budding observed in *Toxoplasma gondii;* cf. endodyogeny.

**endopolyphosphatase.** Polyphosphate depolymerase; metaphosphatase; polyphosphatase; enzyme (EC 3.6.1.10) hydrolyzing polyphosphate to pentaphosphate.

**en'dopol'yploid.** Relating to endopolyploidy.

**endopolyploidy** (en'do-pol'i̅-ploy-di̅) [ endo- + polyploidy, *q.v.* ]. Endomitosis; the process or state of duplication of the chromosomes without accompanying spindle formation or cytokinesis, resulting in a polyploid nucleus.

**en'doradiog'raphy.** Study of organs or cavities by use of x-ray and a radiopaque substance.

**endoreduplication** (en'do-re-du'pli̅-ka'shun). A form of polyploidy or polysomy characterized by redoubling of chromosomes giving rise to four-stranded chromosomes at prophase and metaphase.

**end organ.** See under organ.

**endorrhachis** (en-do-ra'kis) [ endo- + G. *rhachis,* the spine ]. Lining membrane of the spinal canal; spinal dura mater.

**en'dosalpingio'sis.** Adenomyosis involving the interior of a uterine tube or aberrant mucous membrane in the ovary representing tubal mucosa rather than endometriosis.

**endosalpingitis** (en'do-sal-pin-ji'tis) [ endo- + G. *salpinx* (*salping-*), tube, + -*itis* ]. Inflammation of the lining membrane of the Eustachian or of the Fallopian tube.

**endosarc** (en'do-sark) [ endo- + G. *sarx* (*sark-*), flesh ]. Entosarc; the endoplasm of a protozoan.

**en'doscope** [ endo- + G. *skopeo̅,* to examine ]. An instrument for the examination of the interior of a canal or hollow viscus.

**endoscopy** (en-dos'ko-pi̅) [ see endoscope ]. Examination of the interior of a canal or hollow viscus.

**endosep'sis.** Autosepticemia.

**endoskel'eton.** The internal bony framework of the body; the skeleton in its usual context as distinguished from exoskeleton.

**endosmometer** (en'dos-mom'e-ter) [ endosmosis + G. *metron,* measure ]. A device for determining the velocity of endosmosis.

**endosmosis** (en'dos-mo'sis). Osmosis in a direction toward the interior of a cell or a cavity.

**endosmot'ic.** Relating to endosmosis.

**en'dosome** [ endo- + G. *soma,* body ]. A more or less central body in the vesicular nucleus of certain Feulgen-negative (DNA −) protozoa (*e.g.,* trypanosomes, parasitic amebae, and phytoflagellates), with the chromatin (DNA +) lying between the nuclear membrane and the e.; formerly also called endoplast; *cf.* nucleolus.

**en'dospore** [ endo- + G. *sporos,* seed ]. 1. A resistant body formed within the vegetative cells of some bacteria, particularly those belonging to the genera *Bacillus* and *Clostridium.* 2. A spore borne within a cell, such as a sporangiospore, or borne within the tubular end of a sporophore, as in certain fungi.

**endosteal** (en-dos'te-al). Relating to the endosteum.

**endosteitis, endostitis** (en'dos-te-i'tis, en'dos-ti'tis). Perimyelitis; inflammation of the endosteum or of the medullary cavity of a bone.

**endosteoma** (en-dos'te-o'mah) [ endo- + G. *osteon,* bone, + suffix -*ōma,* tumor ]. Endostoma; a benign neoplasm of bone tissue in the medullary cavity of a bone.

**endostethoscope** (en'do-steth'o-skōp) [ endo- + G. *stēthos,* chest, + *skopeō,* to examine ]. A tube for passage into the esophagus, used in endoauscultation.

**endosteum** (en-dos'te-um) [ endo- + G. *osteon,* bone ]. Medullary membrane; perimyelis; thin membrane lining the inner surface of bone in the central medullary cavity.

**endosto'ma.** Endosteoma.

**en'dotendin'eum** [ endo- + L. *tendon,* tendon, + -*eus,* adj.; the whole, in its neuter form, used substantively ]. The fine connective tissue surrounding secondary fascicles of a tendon.

**endothelial** (en'do-the'lī-al). Relating to the endothelium.

**endotheliochorial** (en'do-the'lī-o-ko'rī-al). See endotheliochorial *placenta.*

**endotheliocyte** (en-do-the'lī-o-sīt). Endothelial *leukocyte.*

**endothelioid** (en-do-the'lī-oyd). Resembling endothelium.

**endothelioma** (en'do-the-lī-o'mah). A generic term for a group of neoplasms derived from the endothelial tissue of blood vessels or lymphatic channels; e.'s may be benign or malignant, although angiosarcoma is a better term for the latter.

**endotheliosis** (en'do-the-lī-o'sis). Proliferation of endothelium.

**endothelium,** pl. **endothe'lia** (en'do-the'lī-um) [ endo- + G. *thēlē,* nipple ] [ NA ]. A layer of flat cells lining especially blood and lymphatic vessels; it corresponds to the mesothelium of the serous cavities.

**e. cam'erae anterio'ris** [ NA ], endothelium of the anterior chamber; a single layer of large, squamous cells that covers the posterior surface of the cornea and anterior surface of the iris.

**endother'mic.** Denoting a chemical reaction during the progress of which there is absorption of heat; *cf.* endergonic.

**en'dother'my.** Diathermy.

**en'dothrix** [ endo- + G. *thrix,* hair ]. A trichophyton (notably *Trichophyton violaceum* and *T. tonsurans)* whose spores and mycelia characteristically invade the interior of hair; there is no conspicuous external sheath of spores (as with ectothrix).

**endothyroidopexy** (en'do-thi-roy'do-pek'sī). Endothyropexy.

**endothyropexy** (en-do-thi'ro-pek-sī) [ endo- + thyroid + G. *pēxis,* a fixing ]. Operative dislocation of the thyroid gland and its fixation in the side of the neck.

**endotoxemia** (en'do-tok-se'mī-ah). The presence in the blood of endotoxins, which, if derived from Gram-negative bacilli, may cause a generalized Shwartzman phenomenon with shock.

**endotoxicosis** (en'do-tok-sī-ko'sis). Poisoning by an endotoxin.

**endotox'in.** 1. A bacterial toxin not freely liberated into the surrounding medium, in contrast to exotoxin. 2. The complex phospholipid-polysaccharide macromolecules which form an integral part of the cell wall of a variety of relatively avirulent as well as virulent strains of Gram-negative bacteria including the enterobacteria, vibrios, *Brucella,* and *Neisseria;* they are released only when the integrity of the cell wall is disturbed, are relatively heat-stable, are less potent than most exotoxins, and are less specific; they do not form toxoids; when injected in sufficient quantities, they cause a state of shock accompanied by severe diarrhea, and, in smaller doses, fever and leukopenia followed by leukocytosis; they have the capacity of eliciting the Shwartzman and the Sanarelli-Shwartzman phenomena.

**endotracheal** (en'do-tra'ke-al). Within the trachea.

**endotrachelitis** (en'do-trak-el-i'tis). Endocervicitis.

**endovaccination** (en'do-vak'sī-na'shun). Oral administration of vaccines.

**endovasculitis** (en'do-vas'ku-li'tis). Endangiitis.

**endovenous** (en'do-ve'nus). Intravenous.

**end'plate, end-plate.** The ending of a motor nerve fiber in relation to a skeletal muscle fiber.

**motor e.,** myoneural junction; sole-plate ending; the large and complex end-formation by which the axon of a motor neuron establishes synaptic contact with a striated muscle fiber (cell). Several terminal branches of a motor axon end in irregular, club-shaped synaptic end-formations which are bedded in a single trough-like depression of the muscle fiber's surface. The postsynaptic membrane, the sarcolemma that forms the bottom of the trough, is greatly increased in surface area by deep infoldings protruding into the underlying cytoplasm of the muscle fiber; the subsynaptic interval between the plasma membrane of the axon terminals and the sarcolemma is filled with an amorphous substance. The trough is closed off toward the surface by the Schwann sheath which peels away from the axons as the latter enter the trough, and thus forms a lid over the trough; the slight bulge of this closure plate corresponds to Doyère's eminence.

**endyma** (en'dī-mah) [ G. a garment ]. Ependyma.

**-ene.** A suffix applied to a chemical name indicating the presence of a carbon-carbon double bond; *e.g.,* propene (unsaturated propane, $CH_3$—$CH = CH_2$).

**enediol** (ēn-di'ōl). A substance formed by proton migration from a —CHOH group α to an aldehyde or a ketone to the oxygen of the aldehyde or ketone, usually induced by alkali, giving rise to doubly bonded carbon atoms (the -ene group) each bearing a —CHOH group (a diol); a special case of enolization; —CH(OH)—CO— → —C(OH)= C(OH)—.

**enema** (en'e-mah) [ G. ]. Clyster; rectal injection; lavement; a fluid injected into the rectum for the purpose of clearing out the bowel, or of administering drugs or food.

**analep'tic e.,** an e. of a pint of lukewarm water with one-half teaspoonful of table salt.

**barium e.,** administration of barium, a radiopaque medium, for x-ray study of the lower intestinal tract.

**blind e.,** the introduction into the rectum of a rubber tube to facilitate the expulsion of flatus.

**contrast e.,** barium e.

**double contrast e.,** after evacuation of a barium e. and injection of a small amount of air into rectum, x-ray study will show finer details of mucosa.

**flatus e.,** an e. of magnesium sulfate in glycerin and warm water.

**high e.,** an e. thrown high up into the colon.

**nutrient e.,** a rectal injection of predigested food.

**soapsuds e.,** an e. of shredded or powdered soap in warm water.

**thirst e.,** analeptic e.

**turpentine e.,** an e. of turpentine and olive oil in soapsuds.

**enem'ator.** An appliance for use in giving an enema.

**enemi'asis.** The use of enemas.

**energetics** (en'er-jet'iks). The study of the energy changes involved in physical and chemical changes.

**energom'eter** [ G. *energeia,* energy, + *metron,* measure ]. An apparatus for measuring blood pressure.

**energy** (en'er-jī) [ G. *energeia,* fr. *en,* in, + *ergon,* work ]. Activity; the exertion of power; dynamic force; the capacity to do work, taking the forms of kinetic e., potential e., chemical e., electrical e., surface e., etc.

**e. of activation,** the quantity of e. that must be added to that already possessed by a molecule or molecules in order to initiate a reaction. Usually expressed in the Arrhenius equation relating a velocity constant to absolute temperature.

**binding e.,** the e. that would be released if a particular atomic nucleus were formed through the combination of individual protons and neutrons.

**chemical e.,** e. liberated by a chemical reaction or absorbed in the formation of a chemical compound.

**conservation of e.,** the principle that the total amount of e. remains always the same, none being lost or created in any chemical or physical process or in the conversion of one kind of energy into another.

**free e.,** a thermodynamic function symbolized as *F* or *G* (Gibbs' free e.); defined as $H - \bar{E} \cdot TS$, where *H* is the enthalpy of a system, *T* the absolute temperature, and *S* the entropy; chemical reactions proceed spontaneously in the direction that involves a net decrease in the free e. of the system.

**Gibbs' free e.,** see free e.

**high e. compounds,** see under compound.

**high e. phosphate,** see under phosphate.

**kinetic e.,** the e. of motion.

**latent e.,** potential e.

**nerve e.,** potential e.

**nuclear e.,** e. given off in the course of nuclear reaction or stored in the formation of an atomic nucleus.

**e. of position,** potential e.

**potential e.,** latent e.; nerve e.; e. of position; the e., existing in a body by virtue of its position or state of existence, which is not being exerted at the time.

**psychic e.,** in psychoanalysis, a hypothetical mental force regarded as analogous to the physical concept of e.; e. enabling and vitalizing an individual's psychological activity; see also libido.

**radiant e.,** the e. contained in light rays or any other form of radiation.

**solar e.,** the e. of sunlight.

**total e.,** the sum of kinetic and potential e.'s.

**enervation** (en'er-va'shun) [ L. *enervo,* pp. *-atus,* to enervate, fr. *e-* priv. + *nervus,* nerve ]. Failure of nerve force; weakening.

**en'flurane** (USAN). ETHRANE; 2-chloro-1,1,2-trifluoroethyl difluoromethyl ether; a potent volatile inhalation anesthetic; nonflammable and nonexplosive; side effects include abnormal electroencephalographic activity.

**engagement** (en-gaj'ment). In obstetrics, the mechanism by which the biparietal diameter of the fetal head enters the plane of the inlet.

**engastrius** (en-gas'tri-us) [ G. *en,* in, + *gaster,* belly ]. Unequal conjoined twins in which the smaller (parasite) is wholly or partly within the abdomen of the larger (host or autosite).

**Engel,** Rudolph C., Alsatian biochemist, 1850–1916. See E.'s *alkalimetry.*

**Engelmann,** Guido, *1876. See E.'s disease.

**Engelmann** (eng'el-mahn). Theodor W., German physiologist, 1843–1909. See E.'s basal *knobs.*

**engine** (en'jin). An apparatus or machine that produces mechanical energy or force.

**dental e.,** the motive power of the dental handpiece which causes the bur to rotate; usually a fractional horsepower motor, but recently an air- or water-impelled turbine, or an ultrasonic generator.

**en'gineer'ing.** The practical application of physical, mechanical, and mathematical principles.

**biomedical e.,** the application of e. principles to obtain solutions to biomedical problems; usually involves collaboration of engineers and biological scientists.

**dental e.,** the application of e. principles to dentistry.

**Englisch** (eng'lish), Josef, Vienna physician, 1835–1915. See E.'s *sinus.*

**englobe** (en-glōb). To take in by a spheroidal body; said of the ingestion of bacteria and other foreign bodies by the phagocytes.

**englobe'ment.** The process of inclusion by a spheroidal body, such as a leukocyte.

**engorged** (en-gorjd') [ O. Fr. fr. Mediev. L. *gorgia,* throat, narrow passage, fr. L. *gurges,* a whirlpool ]. Congested; hyperemic; absolutely filled; distended with fluid.

**engorgement** (en-gorj'ment). Distention with fluid or other material; congestion.

**en'gram** [ G. *en,* in, + *gramma,* mark ]. In the mnemic hypothesis (*q.v.*), a physical habit or memory trace made on the protoplasm of an organism by the repetition of stimuli.

**engraphia** (en-graf'i-ah). The formation of engrams.

**enhance'ment.** 1. The act of augmenting. 2. In immunology, the prolongation of a process or event by suppressing an opposing process.

**immunological e.,** the phenomenon of humoral antibody having an opposing effect upon cell-mediated immunity in tissue transplantation (tumor or other); rejection of an allograft (homograft) in an animal rendered immune by a previous transplant can be delayed by first immunizing the animal with dead tissue and thus eliciting humoral antibodies of the same kind.

**enhem'atospore, enhem'ospore** [ G. *en,* in, + *haima,* blood, + *sporos,* seed ]. Obsolete terms for merozoite.

**enkatar'rhaphy.** Encatarrhaphy.

**enlargement.** 1. An increase in size. 2. An intumescence or swelling.

**cervical e. of spinal cord,** *intumescentia* cervicalis.

**gingival e.,** an overgrowth (localized or diffuse) of gingival tissue, nonspecific in nature. See also gingival *hyperplasia,* gingival *hypertrophy.*

**lumbar e. of spinal cord,** *intumescentia* lumbalis.

**e'nol.** A compound possessing a hydroxyl group (alcohol) attached to a doubly bonded (ethylenic) carbon atom (—CH = CH(OH)—); the prefix or infix, properly italicized when attached to an otherwise complete name, is derived as an abbreviation of ethyl*ene* alcoh*ol.* Example: phospho*enol*pyruvate.

**e'nolase.** (EC 4.2.1.11). Phosphopyruvate hydratase; an enzyme catalyzing the dehydration of 2-phospho-D-glycerate to phospho*enol*pyruvate.

**enoliza'tion.** The conversion of a keto to an enol form; *e.g.,* $CH_3COCOOH \rightarrow CH_2 = C(OH)COOH$.

**enology** (e-nol'o-ji) [ G. *oinos,* wine, + *logos,* study ]. A branch of enzymology that is concerned with the specific application of the fermentative process in making wine.

**e'nolpyru'vate.** $CH_2 = C - COO^-$, the form of pyruvate

HO

encountered in the biologically important phospho*enol*pyruvate (or *enol*pyruvate phosphate), not in the free form.

**enophthal'mia.** Enophthalmos.

**enophthalmos** (en'of-thal'mos) [ G. *en,* in, + *ophthalmos,* eye ]. Enophthalmia; recession of the eyeball within the orbit.

**enorgan'ic.** Occurring as an innate characteristic of the organism.

**enosimania** (en'o-si-ma'ni-ah) [ G. *enosis,* a quaking, + *mania,* insanity ]. Obsessive belief of having committed an unpardonable offense.

**enostosis** (en'os-to'sis) [ G. *en,* in, + *osteon,* bone, + suffix *-osis,* condition ]. A mass of proliferating bone tissue within a bone.

**enox'idase.** A presumed oxidase causing the souring of wines.

**enoyl** e'no-il) [ *-ene,* for unsaturation, + *-oyl,* for an acid radical ]. The acyl radical of an unsaturated aliphatic acid.

**enoyl-ACP reductase.** Crotonyl-ACP reductase; enzyme (EC 1.3.1.9) catalyzing hydrogenation of acyl-ACP complexes to 2,3-dehydroacyl-ACP's, with NAD$^+$ as hydrogen acceptor, reactions of importance in fatty acid metabolism.

**enoyl-ACP reductase (NADPH).** Acyl-ACP dehydrogenase; acyl-ACP reductase; enzyme (EC 1.3.1.10) carrying out the same reaction as enoyl-ACP reductase, but with NADP$^+$ as hydrogen acceptor.

**enoyl-CoA hydratase** (EC 4.2.1.17). Enoyl hydrase; crotonase; enzyme catalyzing reversible reaction between an L-3-hydroxyacyl-CoA and a 2,3 (or 3,4)-*trans*-enoyl-CoA.

**enoyl-CoA reductase.** Acyl-CoA dehydrogenase (NADP$^+$).

**enoyl hydrase.** Enoyl-CoA hydratase.

**Enroth's sign.** See under sign.

**en'siform** [ L. *ensis*, sword, + *forma*, appearance ]. Xiphoid; sword-shaped.

**en'sister'num** [ L. *ensis*, sword, + sternum, *q. v.* ]. Processus xiphoideus.

**ens mor'bi** [ L. the entity of a disease ]. The actual nature or quintessence of a disease.

**ensomphalus** (en-som'fă-lus) [ G. *en*, in, + *sōma*, body, + *omphalos*, umbilicus ]. Conjoined twins that are practically independent, vitally, but are united by bands in the abdominal region or side.

**enstrophe** (en'stro-fe) [ G. *en*, in, + *strophē*, a turning ]. Entropion (2).

**ent-.** See ento-.

**en'tad** [ G. *entos*, within, + L. *ad*, to ]. Toward the interior.

**en'tal** [ G. *entos*, within ]. Relating to the interior; inside.

**entamebiasis** (ent-ă-me-bi'ă-sis). Infection with *Entamoeba histolytica;* see amebiasis and amebic *dysentery.*

**Entamoeba** (ent-ă-me'bah) [ G. *entos*, within + *amoibe*, change ]. A genus of ameba parasitic in the digestive tract of man and other primates and many domestic and wild mammals and birds. With the exception of the pathogenic large race of *E. histolytica*, members of the genus appear to be relatively harmless inhabitants of the host. Some E. species not defined individually in the subentries below are: *E. anatis* in ducks; *E. caviae* in guinea pigs; *E. chattoni* in monkeys and probably man; *E. cuniculi* in rabbits; *E. equi* and *E. equibuccalis* in horses; *E. gallinarum* in chickens, turkeys, guinea fowl, ducks and geese; *E. muris* in rodents; *E. ovis* in sheep and goats; *E. suis* in pigs and possibly man; *E. suigingivalis* in pigs; *E. wenyoni* in goats.

    **E. bo'vis,** found in the large intestine of cattle.

    **E. bucca'lis,** former name for *E. gingivalis.*

    **E. co'li,** occurs in the large intestine of man, other primates, dogs and possibly pigs.

    **E. gingiva'lis,** formerly called *E. buccalis;* found in the oral cavity of man, other primates, dogs, and cats; in man, it is frequently associated with, but probably does not cause, dental caries.

    **E. hartman'ni,** found in the large intestine of man, other primates, and dogs; often confused with *E. histolytica,* but considered to be a distinct strain or species that is nonpathogenic and smaller than *E. histolytica* but otherwise indistinguishable from it; formerly called the small race of *E. histolytica.*

    **E. histoly'tica,** the only distinct pathogen of the genus, the so-called large race of *E. histolytica,* causing tropical or amebic dysentery in man in warmer parts of the world and sporadic cases of dysentery in dogs; in man, the organism penetrates the epithelial tissues of the colon, causing ulceration, and may reach the liver by the portal blood

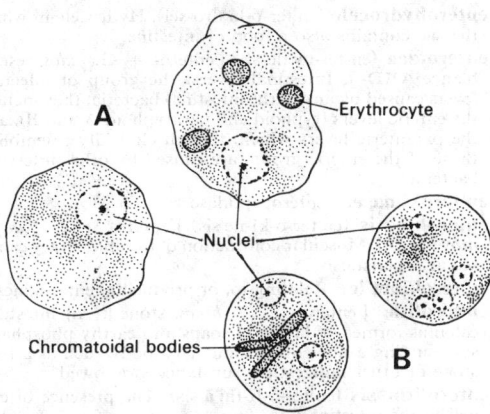

*Entamoeba histolytica*
    *A*, trophozoites, one ameba having ingested erythrocytes (×1000); *B*, cysts, one of which has chromatoidal bodies (×1500). (From Najarian. H. H.: *Textbook of Medical Parasitology*, The Williams & Wilkins Co, Baltimore, 1967.)

stream, producing abscesses, and (rarely) may spread to other organs, such as the lungs, brain, kidney, including the skin; these extraintestinal infections are frequently fatal.

**entasia, entasis** (en'ta'zī-ah, en'tă-sis) [ G. distention ]. Tonic *spasm.*

**entat'ic** [ G. *enteinein*, to stretch; metaphorically, to intensify ]. 1. Pertaining to entasia. 2. Invigorating; aphrodisiac.

**enter-.** See entero-.

**en'teral.** Within the intestine, as distinguished from parenteral.

**enteralgia** (en'ter-al'jī-ah) [ entero- + G. *algos*, pain ]. Cramps; colic; severe abdominal pain, accompanying spasm of the bowel.

**en'teram'ine.** Serotonin.

**enterectasis** (en'ter-ek'tă-sis) [ entero- + G. *ektasis*, a stretching ]. Dilation of the bowel.

**enterectomy** (en'ter-ek'to-mĭ) [ entero- + G. *ektomē*, excision ]. Resection of a segment of the intestine.

**enterelcosis** (en'ter-el-ko'sis) [ entero- + G. *helkos*, ulcer ]. Ulceration of the bowel.

**enterepiplocele** (en'ter-e-pip'lo-sēl) [ entero- + G. *epiploon*, omentum, + *kēlē*, hernia ]. Enteroepiplocele; a hernia of the omentum as well as of the intestine.

**enteric** (en-tĕr'ik) [ G. *enterikos*, from *entera*, bowels ]. Relating to the intestine.

**enter'icus** [ L. ] [ NA ]. Enteric.

**enterischiocele** (en-ter-is'kĭ-o-sēl) [ entero- + G. *ischion*, hip joint, + *kēlē*, hernia ]. Sciatic *hernia.*

**enteritis** (en-ter-i'tis) [ entero- + suffix -*itis*, inflammation ]. Inflammation of the intestine.

    **e. anaphylac'tica,** a hemorrhagic and necrotizing inflammation developing in the ileum (and also the colon) of sensitized dogs when they are fed a second dose of the sensitizing material.

    **chronic cicatrizing e.,** regional e.

    **e. colostra'lis,** diarrhea in the nursing infant caused by the persistence of colostrum corpuscles in the mother's milk.

    **diphtheritic e.,** e. with the formation of a membrane or a false membrane.

    **feline infectious e.,** panleukopenia.

    **e. of mink,** a disease of mink similar to feline infectious agranulocytosis (e.) and caused by strains of the same virus.

    **mucous e.,** an affection of the intestinal mucous membrane characterized by constipation or diarrhea, sometimes alternating, colic, and the passage of pseudomembranous shreds or incomplete casts of the intestine.

    **phleg'monous e.,** severe acute inflammation of the intestine, with walls edematous and infiltrated with pus.

    **e. polypo'sa,** e. associated with polyp formation.

    **pseudomem'branous e.,** pseudomembranous *enterocolitis.*

    **regional e.,** Crohn's disease; regional or terminal ileitis; granulomatous, segmented e. of unknown cause, involving the terminal ileum and less frequently other parts of the gastrointestinal tract. Regional e. is characterized by patchy, deep ulcers that may cause fistulas, and narrowing and thickening of the bowel by fibrosis and lymphocytic infiltration, with noncaseating tuberculoid granulomas which may also be found in regional lymph nodes.

    **transmissible e.,** bluecomb *disease* of turkeys.

**entero-, enter-** [ G. *enteron*, intestine ]. Combining form relating to the intestines.

**en'teroanastomo'sis.** Enteroenterostomy.

**enteroan'thelone.** Enterogastrone.

**enteroapocleisis** (en'ter-o-ap'o-kli'sis) [ entero- + G. *apokleisis*, exclusion, fr. *apo*, from, + *kleiō*, to close ]. The shutting out of a segment of the intestine by forming an anastomosis between the parts above and below.

**Enterobacter** (en'ter-o-bak'ter). A genus of aerobic, facultatively anaerobic, nonsporeforming, motile bacteria (family Enterobacteriaceae) containing Gram-negative rods. The cells are peritrichous, and some strains have encapsulated cells. Glucose is fermented with the production of acid and gas. The Voges-Proskauer test is usually positive. Gelatin is slowly liquefied by the most commonly occurring forms (*E. clocae*). These organisms occur in the feces of man and other animals and in sewage, soil, water, and dairy products; occasionally they are found in urine and pus, and in other pathological materials from animals. The type species is *E. cloacae.*

**E. aerog'enes,** a species found in water, soil, sewage, dairy products, and the feces of man and other animals. Organisms previously identified as motile strains of *Aerobacter aerogenes* are now placed in this species.

**E. clo'acae,** *Aerobacter cloacae;* a species found in the feces of man and other animals and in sewage, soil, and water; it is occasionally found in urine and pus, and in other pathological materials from animals. This is the type species of the genus *E.*

**Enterobacteriaceae** (en'ter-o-bak-te-rī-a'se-e). A family of aerobic, facultatively anaerobic, nonsporeforming bacteria (order Eubacteriales) containing Gram-negative rods. Some species are nonmotile, and nonmotile variants of motile species occur; the motile cells are peritrichous. These organisms grow well on artificial media. They reduce nitrates to nitrites and utilize glucose fermentatively with the production of acid or acid and gas. Indophenol oxidase is not produced by these organisms. They do not liquefy alginate, and pectate is liquefied only by members of one genus, *Pectobacterium.* This family includes many animal parasites and some plant parasites causing blights, galls, and soft rots. Some of these organisms occur as saprophytes which decompose carbohydrate-containing plant materials. The type genus is *Escherichia.*

**en'terobacte'rium.** A member of the family Enterobacteriaceae.

**enterobiasis** (en'ter-o-bi'ǎ-sis). Infection with *Enterobius vermicularis,* the human pinworm.

**Enterobius** (en-ter-o'bī-us) [ entero- + G. *bios,* life ]. A genus of nematode worms, formerly called *Oxyuris,* that includes the pinworms of man and primates.

**E. vermicula'ris,** seat worm; the pinworm of man, formerly called *Oxyuris vermicularis.*

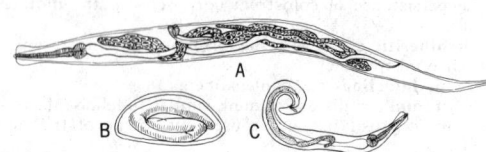

***Enterobius vermicularis***

*A,* gravid female; *B,* egg; *C,* male (original magnification, *A* and *C,* ×15; *B,* ×500).

**enterobrosis, enterobrosia** (en'ter-o-bro'sis, -bro'jĭ-ah) [ entero- + G. *brōsis,* corrosion ]. Perforation of the intestine.

**enterocele** (en'ter-o-sēl). 1 [ entero- +G. *kēlē,* hernia ]. An intestinal hernia. 2 [ entero- +G. *koilia,* a hollow ]. *Cavum abdominis.*

**partial e.,** parietal *hernia.*

**enterocentesis** (en'ter-o-sen-te'sis) [ entero- + G. *kentēsis,* puncture ]. Puncture of the gut with a hollow needle in order to give exit to gas, or to withdraw fluids distending the bowel.

**enterochirurgia** (en'ter-o-ki-rur'jĭ-ah). Intestinal surgery.

**enterocholecystostomy** (en'ter-o-ko-le-sis-tos'to-mī) [ entero- + G. *cholē,* bile, + *kystis,* bladder, + *stoma,* mouth ]. Cholecystenterostomy.

**enterocholecystotomy** (en'ter-o-ko'le-sis-tot'o-mī) [ entero- + G. *tomē,* a cutting ]. Cholecystenterotomy; incision of both intestine and gallbladder.

**enterocleisis** (en-ter-o-kli'sis) [ entero- + G. *kleisis,* a closing ]. Occlusion of the lumen of the alimentary canal.

**omental e.,** use of omentum to aid closure of an opening in intestine.

**enteroclysis** (en-ter-ok'lĭ-sis) [ entero- + G. *klysis,* a washing out ]. A high *enema.*

**enterococcus** (en'ter-o-kok'us) [ entero- + G. *kokkos,* a berry ]. A streptococcus which inhabits the intestinal tract.

**enterocolitis** (en'ter-o-ko-li'tis) [ entero- + G. *kolon,* colon, + suffix *-itis,* inflammation ]. Inflammation of the mucous membrane of a greater or lesser extent of both small and large intestines.

**antibiotic e.,** e. caused by oral administration of broad spectrum antibiotics, resulting from antibiotic-resistant staphylococci or the overgrowth of yeasts and fungi, when the normal fecal Gram-negative organisms are absent.

**pseudomem'branous e.,** pseudomembranous colitis; e. with the formation and passage in the stools of pseudomembranous material; occurs most commonly as a postoperative complication due to shock or as a sequel to prolonged antibiotic therapy. The pathogen is usually the staphylococcus.

**regional e.,** the changes of regional *enteritis* (*q.v.*) involving both the colon and the small intestine.

**enterocolostomy** (en'ter-o-ko-los'to-mī) [ entero- + G. *kōlon,* colon, + *stoma,* mouth ]. Operation for establishing an artifical opening between the small intestine and some portion of the colon.

**enterocyst** (en'ter-o-sist) [ entero- + G. *kystis,* bladder ]. A cyst of the wall of the intestine.

**enterocystocele** (en'ter-o-sis'to-sēl) [ entero- + G. *kystis,* bladder, + *kēlē,* hernia ]. A hernia of both intestine and bladder wall.

**enterocysto'ma.** Enterocyst.

**enterodynia** (en'ter-o-din'ĭ-ah) [ entero- + G. *odynē,* pain ]. Enteralgia.

**en'teroenteros'tomy.** Enteroanastomosis; intestinal anastomosis; the establishment of a communication between two noncontinuous segments of intestine.

**enteroepiplocele** (en'ter-o-ĕ-pip'lo-sēl). Enterepiplocele.

**en'terogastri'tis** [ entero- + G. *gastēr,* belly, + suffix *-itis,* inflammation ]. Gastroenteritis.

**en'terogas'trone.** Anthelone E; enteroanthelone; a hormone, obtained from intestinal mucosa, that inhibits gastric secretion and motility. Secretion of e. is stimulated by exposure of duodenal mucosa to dietary lipids.

**enterogenous** (en-ter-oj'ĕ-nus) [ entero- + G. suffix *-gen,* producing ]. Of intestinal origin.

**en'terograph.** An instrument designed for making a graphic record of the intestinal movements.

**enterography** (en-ter-og'rǎ-fī) [ entero- + G. *graphō,* to write ]. 1. A description of the intestines. 2. The making of a graphic curve delineating the intestinal movements.

**en'terohepati'tis** [ entero- + G. *hēpar* (*hēpat-*), liver, + suffix *-itis,* inflammation ]. Inflammation of both the intestine and the liver.

**infectious e.,** histomoniasis.

**enterohepatocele** (en'ter-o-hep'ǎ-to-sēl) [ entero- + G. *hēpar* (*hēpat-*), liver, + *kēlē,* hernia ]. Congenital umbilical hernia containing intestine and liver.

**enterohydrocele** (en'ter-o-hi'dro-sēl). Hydrocele in which the sac contains also a loop of intestine.

**enteroidea** (en-ter-oy'de-ah) [ entero- + G. *eidos,* resemblance. OID- ]. Intestinal fevers; the group of infection fevers caused by any of the intestinal bacteria; they include the enteric fevers (typhoid and paratyphoid A and B), and the parenteric fevers which, though clinically resembling those of the enteric group, are caused by other intestinal bacteria.

**en'teroki'nase.** Enteropeptidase.

**enterokinesis** (en'ter-o-kī-ne'sis) [ entero- + G. *kinēsis,* movement ]. Muscular contraction of the alimentary canal; see also peristalsis.

**en'terokinet'ic.** Relating to, or producing, enterokinesis.

**en'terolith** [ entero- + G. *lithos,* stone ]. An intestinal calculus formed of layers of soaps and earthy phosphates surrounding a nucleus of some hard body such as a fruit stone or other indigestible substance swallowed.

**enterolithiasis** (en'ter-o-lī-thi'ǎ-sis). The presence of calculi in the intestine.

**enterology** (en-ter-ol'o-jī) [ entero- + G. *logos,* study ]. The branch of medical science dealing especially with the intestinal tract.

**enterolysis** (en-ter-ol'ĭ-sis) [ entero- + G. *lysis,* dissolution ]. Eradication of intestinal adhesions.

**enteromeg'aly, enteromega'lia** [ entero- + G. *megas*, great ]. Megaloenteron.

**enterome'nia** [ entero- + G. *emmēnos*, monthly ]. Vicarious menstruation in the intestine.

**enteromerocele** (en'ter-o-me'ro-sēl) [ entero- + G. *mēros*, thigh, + *kēlē*, hernia ]. Femoral *hernia.*

**enterom'eter** [ entero- + G. *metron*, measure ]. An instrument used in measuring the diameter of the intestine.

**Enteromonas** (en'ter-o-mo'nas, en-ter-om'o-nas) [ entero- + G. *monas*, monad ]. A genus of flagellate protozoa, one species of which, *E. hominis*, is found as a rare nonpathogenic resident in the human intestine.

**enteromycosis** (en'ter-o-mi-ko'sis) [ entero- + G. *mykēs*, fungus, + suffix -*osis*, condition ]. An intestinal disease of fungal origin.

**en'teroni'tis** [ entero- + suffix -*itis*, inflammation ]. Enteritis; inflammation of the small intestine.

    **polyt'ropous e.,** acute infectious gastroenteritis; an affection marked by the sudden onset of nausea or vomiting, diarrhea, abdominal distress, and a dull headache.

**enteroparesis** (en'ter-o-pă-re'sis, -păr'ĭ-sis) [ entero- + G. *paresis*, slackening, relaxation ]. A state of diminished or arrested peristalsis with flaccidity of the intestinal walls.

**en'teropath'ogen'ic.** Pathogenic for the alimentary canal.

**enterop'athy** [ entero- + G. *pathos*, suffering ]. An intestinal disease.

    **protein-losing e.,** increased fecal loss of serum protein, especially albumin, causing hypoproteinemia.

**enteropep'tidase** (EC 3.4.4.8). Enterokinase; an intestinal proteolytic enzyme that converts trypsinogen into trypsin.

**en'teropexy** [ entero- + G. *pēxis*, fixation ]. Fixation of a segment of the intestine to the abdominal wall.

**en'teroplasty** [ entero- + G. *plassō*, to mold ]. Plastic surgery of the intestine, *e.g.*, closure of perforation, relief of constrictions.

**enteroplegia** (en'ter-o-ple'jĭ-ah) [ entero- + G. *plēgē*, stroke ]. See ileus.

**en'teroplex.** An instrument for use in effecting union of the divided ends of the intestine.

**en'teroplexy** [ entero- + G. *plexis*, weaving ]. Joining of the divided ends of the intestine.

**enteroproctia** (en'ter-o-prok'shĭ-ah) [ entero- + G. *prōktos*, anus ]. The presence of an artifical anus.

**enteroptosis, enteroptosia** (en-ter-op-to'sis, -to'sĭ-ah) [ entero- + G. *ptōsis*, a falling ]. The abnormal descent of the intestines in the abdominal cavity, usually associated with falling of the other viscera.

**enteroptot'ic** (en'ter-o-tot'ik). Relating to or suffering from enteroptosia, prolapse of the abdominal viscera.

**en'terore'nal.** Relating to both the intestines and the kidneys.

**enterorrhagia** (en-ter-o-ra'jĭ-ah) [ entero- + G. *rhēgnymi*, to burst forth ]. Intestinal *hemorrhage.*

**enterorrhaphy** (en'ter-or'ă-fĭ) [ entero- + G. *rhaphē*, suture ]. Suture of the intestine in case of perforation or in the operation of anastomosis.

**enterorrhexis** (en'ter-o-rek'sis) [ entero- + G. *rhēxis*, rupture ]. Rupture of the gut or bowel.

**en'teroscope** [ entero- + G. *skopeō*, to view ]. A form of speculum for aid in inspecting the inside of the intestine in operative cases.

**en'terosep'sis** [ entero- + G. *sēpsis*, putrefaction ]. Sepsis occurring in or derived from the alimentary canal.

**enterospasm** (en'ter-o-spazm) [ entero- + G. *spasmos*, spasm ]. Increased, irregular, and painful peristalsis.

**enterostasis** (en-ter-os'tă-sis) [ entero- + G. *stasis*, a standing ]. Intestinal stasis; a retardation or arrest of the passage of the intestinal contents.

**enterostax'is** [ entero- + G. *staxis*, a dripping ]. Oozing of blood from the mucous membrane of the intestine.

**en'terosteno'sis** [ entero- + G. *stenōsis*, narrowing ]. Narrowing of the lumen of the intestine.

**enteros'tomy** [ entero- + G. *stoma*, mouth ]. The establishment of an artificial anus or fistula into the intestine through the abdominal wall.

**gun-barrel e.,** a double-barrel e. in which both proximal and distal openings of divided intestine are sutured to the exterior of the abdomen wall.

**enterotome** (en'ter-o-tōm) [ entero- + G. *tomē*, a cutting ]. An instrument for incising the intestine, especially in the operation for artificial anus.

    **Dupuytren's e.,** a cutting forceps used in making an artificial anus.

**enterot'omy.** Incision into the intestine.

**en'terotoxe'mia** [ entero- + toxemia, *q.v.* ]. Acute, highly fatal diseases, chiefly of cattle and sheep, caused by toxins produced in the intestine by various types of *Clostridium perfringens;* also called lamb dysentery; milk colic, hemorrhagic enterotoxemia; pulpy kidney diesase; overeating disease; infectious enterotoxemia of sheep.

**en'terotoxica'tion.** Autointoxication.

**enterotox'in.** A cytotoxin specific for the cells of the mucous membrane of the intestine.

    **Escherichia coli e.,** e. produced by certain strains (serotypes) of *Escherichia coli*, seemingly associated with a transferable episome.

    **staphylococcal e.,** a soluble exotoxin produced by some strains of *Staphylococcus aureus*, and a cause of outbreaks of food poisoning (*q.v.*); three immunologically different staphylococcal e.'s are recognized, but only one (type B) has been well studied.

**enterotox'ism.** Autointoxication.

**en'terotrop'ic** [ entero- + G. *tropikos*, turning ]. Attracted by or affecting the intestine.

**enterovi'rus.** See under virus.

**enterozo'ic.** Relating to an enterozoon.

**enterozoon** (en'ter-o-zo'on) [ entero- + G. *zōon*, animal ]. An animal parasite in the intestine.

**en'thalpy** [ G. *enthalpein*, to warm in ]. Heat content, symbolized as *H*. A thermodynamic function, defined as $E + PV$, where $E$ is the internal energy of a system, $P$ the pressure, and $V$ the volume.

**en'thesis** [ G. an insertion, fr. *en*, in, + *thesis*, a placing. THE- ]. The insertion of metallic or other nonvital material to take the place of lost tissue.

**enthesitis** (en'the-si'tis) [ G. *enthetos*, implanted, + suffix -*itis*, inflammation ]. Traumatic disease occurring at the insertion of muscles where recurring concentration of muscle stress provokes inflammation with a strong tendency toward fibrosis and calcification.

**enthet'ic.** 1. Relating to enthesis. 2. Exogenous.

**enthlasis** (en'thlă-sis) [ G. a dent, fr. *en*, in, + *thlaō*, to crush ]. Depressed fracture of the skull.

**entire.** Denoting the margin of a bacterial colony which is smooth and continuous, without indentations or projections.

**entity** (en'tĭ-tĭ) [ L. *ens* (*ent*-), being, pres. p. of *esse*, to be ]. An independent thing; that which contains in itself all the conditions essential to individuality; that which forms of itself a complete whole; denoting a separate and distinct disease or condition; see also disease (2).

**ento-, ent-** [ G. *entos*, within ]. Prefixes meaning inner, or within; see also endo-.

**en'toblast** [ ento- + G. *blastos*, germ ]. Entoderm.

**entocele** (en'to-sēl) [ ento- + G. *kēlē*, hernia ]. An internal hernia.

**entochoroidea** (en'to-ko-roy'de-ah) [ ento- + G. *chorioeidēs*, choroid ]. The inner layer of the choroid coat of the eye.

**en'tocone** [ ento- + G. *kōnos*, cone ]. The mesiolingual cusp of a maxillary molar tooth.

**entoco'nid** [ ento- + G. *kōnos*, cone ]. The inner posterior cusp of a mandibular molar tooth.

**entocor'nea.** *Lamina* limitans posterior corneae.

**en'tocra'nial.** Endocranial.

**en'tocra'nium.** Endocranium.

**en'toderm** [ ento- + G. *derma*, skin ]. Endoderm; hypoblast; endoblast; entoblast; the innermost of the three primary germ layers of the embryo. It gives rise to the epithelial lining of the primitive gut tract, its glands, and the epithelial component of structures arising as outgrowths from the gut.

**entoectad** (en-to-ek'tad) [ G. *entos*, within, + *ektos*, without, + L. *ad*, to ]. From within outward.

**entoma** [ G. incision ]. The vulvar slit formed by the approximation of the labia majora.

**entomion** (en-to'mī-on) [ G. *entomē*, notch. TOM- ]. The tip of the mastoid angle of the parietal bone.

**entomology** (en'to-mol'o-jī) [ G. *entomon*, insect, + *logos*, study ]. The study of insects.

**entomophobia** (en'to-mo-fo'bī-ah) [ G. *entomon*, insect, + *phobos*, fear ]. Morbid fear of insects.

**Entomophthora** (en-to-mof'tho-rah) [ G. *entomē*, insect, + *phthora*, destruction ]. A genus of fungi belonging to the class Zygomycetes; the members of the genus are chiefly parasitic on insects. Asexual reproduction occurs by modified sporangia functioning as conidia, which are forcibly discharged. Such organisms have caused phycomycosis (zygomycosis) in animals, and a closely related species, *Basidiobolus ranarum*, has been reported to cause phycomycosis in man.

**entop'ic** [ G. *en*, within, + *topos*, place ]. Placed within; occurring or situated in the normal place; opposed to ectopic.

**en'toplasm.** Endoplasm.

**entop'tic** [ ento- + G. *optikos*, relating to vision ]. Within the eyeball.

**entoptoscopy** (en-top-tos'ko-pī) [ ento- + G. *optos*, visible, + *skopeō*, to view ]. Examination of the interior of the eyeball.

**entoret'ina.** Henle's nervous layer; the layers of the retina from the outer plexiform to the nerve fiber layer inclusive.

**entorhinal** (en-to-ri'nal). Within the rhinencephalon, medial to the sulcus rhinalis (rhinal sulcus); the term specifically denotes the entorhinal *area, q.v.*

**en'tosarc.** Endosarc.

**Entozo'a.** A branch of the subkingdom Metazoa, whose members possess a digestive cavity or tract; includes all higher animals as well as many invertebrate forms.

**entozo'on**, pl. **entozoa** [ ento- + G. *zōon*, animal ]. An animal parasite the habitat of which is any of the internal organs or tissues.

**en'trails.** The viscera of an animal.

**entro'pion, entro'pium** [ G. *en*, in, + *tropē*, a turning ]. 1. Inversion or turning inward of a part. 2. Enstrophe; the infolding of the margin of an eyelid.

  **e. u'veae,** inversion of the pupillary margin.

**entro'pionize.** To invert a part.

**entropy** (en'tro-pī) [ G. *entropia*, a turning towards. TREP- ]. That fraction of heat (energy) content not available for the performance of work, usually because (in a chemical reaction) it has gone to increasing the random motion of the atoms or molecules in the system. Thus e. is a measure of randomness or disorder. It occurs in the free energy ($F$) equation, $F = H - TS$ ($H$ = enthalpy or heat content, $T$ = absolute temperature, $S$ = entropy), which, applied to the free energy available in a reaction at a given temperature ($\Delta F$) becomes $\Delta F = \Delta H - T\Delta S$. At equilibrium, $\Delta H = T\Delta S$. See also second *law.*

**en'typy** [ G. *entypē*, pattern ]. The condition in an early mammalian embryo in which the entoderm covers the embryonic and amniotic ectoderm. Part of the preplacental trophoblast may, also, be covered.

**enucleate** (e-nu'kle-āt). To remove entirely; to shell out like a nut, as in the removal of an eye from its socket.

**enucleation** (e-nu-kle-a'shun) [ L. *enucleo*, to remove the kernel, fr. *e*, out, + *nucleus*, nut, kernel ]. 1. The removal of a tumor or other body (such as the eyeball) entire, without rupture, as one shells out the kernel of a nut. 2. The removal or destruction of the nucleus of a cell.

**enuresis** (en'u-re'sis) [ G. *en-oureō*, to urinate in ]. Bed-wetting; involuntary passage of urine, usually occurring at night or during sleep.

**en'velope.** In anatomy, a structure that encloses or covers.

  **nuclear e.,** nuclear membrane; karyotheca; caryotheca; the double membrane at the boundary of the nucleoplasm. A space or cisterna about 150 Å wide occurs between the two layers. The outer membrane is continuous at intervals with the endoplasmic reticulum. Regularly spaced pores, which are closed by a thin diaphragm, occur in the envelope.

**envenomation** (en-ven'om-a'shun). The act of injecting a poisonous material (venom) by sting, spine, bite, or other venom apparatus.

**envi'ronment** [ Fr. *environ*, around ]. The milieu; the aggregate of all of the external conditions and influences affecting the life and development of an organism.

**en'vy.** One's feeling of discontent or jealousy resulting from comparison with another person.

  **penis e.,** the psychoanalytic concept in which a female envies male characteristics or capabilities, especially the possession of a penis.

**enzootic** (en-zo-ot'ik) [ G. *en*, in, + *zōon*, animal ]. Denoting a disease of animals which is indigenous to a certain locality, analogous to an endemic disease among men.

**enzygotic** (en-zi-got'ik) [ G. *eis* (*en*), one, + zygote ]. Derived from a single fertilized ovum, denoting twins so derived.

**enzymatic** (en-zi-mat'ik). Enzymic; relating to an enzyme.

**enzyme** (en'zim) [ G. *en*, in, + *zymē*, leaven. ZE- ]. Ferment; a protein, secreted by cells, that acts as a catalyst to induce chemical changes in other substances, itself remaining apparently unchanged by the process. Enzymes, with the exception of those discovered long ago (*e.g.*, pepsin, emulsin), are generally named by adding -ase to the name of the substrate on which the enzyme acts (*e.g.*, glucosidase, nuclease) or the substance activated (*e.g.*, hydrogenase) and/or the type of reaction (*e.g.*, oxidoreductase, transferase, hydrolase, lyase, isomerase, ligase or synthetase—these being the six main groups in the Enzyme Nomenclature recommendations of the International Union of Biochemistry, 1964, 1965, 1973). For individual enzymes not listed as subentries here, see the specific name.

  **acetyl-activating e.,** acetyl-CoA synthetase; see under acetyl-CoA.

  **adaptive e.,** an e. that can be detected in a growing culture of a microorganism, after the addition of a particular substance (inducer) to the culture medium, that can act on the inducer, and was not detectable prior to the addition. See induced e.

  **autolyt'ic e.,** an e. capable of causing autolysis of the cell forming it.

  **brancher e., branching e.,** 1,4-α-glucan branching enzyme; see under glucan.

  **β-carotene cleavage e.,** β-carotene 15,15′-dioxygenase.

  **clotting e.'s,** see thrombin and rennin.

  **condensing e.,** citrate synthase.

  **D e.,** 4-α-glucanotransferase.

  **deam'idizing e.,** amidohydrolase.

  **deaminating e.'s,** deaminases.

  **debrancher e.'s, debranching e.'s,** debranching factors; e.'s that bring about destruction of branches in glycogen; formerly considered to be one enzyme (R-enzyme, etc.), now known to be a mixture of transferases (4α -glucanotransferase) and hydrolases (amylo-1,6-glucosidase). See also isoamylase; pullulanase.

  **disproportionating e.,** 4-α-glucanotransferase.

  **extracellular e.,** exoenzyme; lyoenzyme; an e. performing its functions outside a cell, *e.g.*, the various digestive e.'s.

  **hydrolyzing e.'s,** hydrolases.

  **induced e.,** "induced enzyme synthesis" has generally replaced the older term, "adaptive enzyme formation," to describe the appearance *de novo* of an enzyme activity in response to the addition of its substrate (or an analogue thereof) to cells not normally metabolizing that substrate. A prototype is the β-galactosidase of *Escherichia coli*, synthesized upon the addition of various galactosides, whether or not these are good substrates.

  **inducible e.,** one that is produced only in response to demand created by accumulation or addition of a substrate compound; see also induced e., and derepression.

  **intracel'lular e.,** endoenzyme; one that performs its functions within the cell. Most e.'s are intracellular e.'s.

  **lab-e.,** rennin.

  **methionine-activating e.,** methionine adenosyltransferase.

  **new yellow e.,** D-amino acid oxidase (EC 1.4.3.3); a flavoenzyme found in yeast, so called to distinguish it from Warburg's "old yellow e." (NADPH dehydrogenase, EC

1.6.99.1); contains FAD as coenzyme, instead of FMN as does the old yellow e.

**old yellow e.,** NADPH dehydrogenase.

**P e.,** phosphorylase (2).

**photoreactivating e.,** deoxydipyrimidine photolyase.

**PR e.,** (1) phosphorylase-rupturing e. (see phosphorylase phosphatase); (2) photoreactivating enzyme (see deoxydipyrimidine photolyase.

**pyridinoprotein e.,** nicotinamide adenine dinucleotide.

**Q e.,** see 1,4-α-glucan branching enzyme (under glucan).

**R e.,** see amylopectin 1,6-glucosidase; pullulanase.

**reducing e.,** reductase.

**repressible e.,** one that is produced continuously unless production is repressed by excess of a product (corepressor); see also inactive *repressor.*

**respiratory e.,** one of those e.'s in tissues that is a part of an oxidation-reduction system accomplishing the conversion of substrates to $CO_2$ and $H_2O$ and the transfer of the electrons removed to $O_2$.

**scavenger e.,** catalase.

**Schardinger e.,** xanthine oxidase.

**splitting e.'s,** e.'s that, like aldolases, catalyze the conversion of a molecule into two smaller molecules without the addition or subtraction of any atoms.

**T e.,** 1,4-α-glucan 6-α-glucosyltransferase.

**transferring e.'s,** transferases.

**Warburg's old yellow e.,** NADPH dehydrogenase.

**Enzyme Commission.** See EC.

**enzymic** (en-zi'mik). Enzymatic.

**enzymoids.** Enzymes that have been slightly altered chemically and can still bind substrate, although they can no longer catalyze the appropriate reaction; *e.g.,* the methyl ester of lysozyme.

**enzymol'ogist.** Zymologist; one versed in the science of enzymology, or fermentation.

**enzymology** (en'zi-mol'o-jī) [ enzyme + G. *logos,* study ]. Zymology; the branch of chemistry that deals with fermentation.

**enzymolysis** (en-zi-mol'ĭ-sis) [ enzyme + G. *lysis,* dissolution ]. Fermentation. Obsolete term for fermentation (enzymic digestion).

**enzymopathy** (en-zi-mop'ă-thī) [ enzyme + G. *pathos,* disease ]. Disturbance of enzyme function, including genetic deficiency of specific enzymes.

**enzymosis** (en-zi-mo'sis) [ enzyme + G. suffix -*osis,* condition ]. Obsolete term for fermentation (enzymic digestion).

**EOG.** Abbreviation for electro-oculography.

**eonism** (e'o-nizm) [ after chevalier d'Eon de Beaumont, 1728–1810 ]. Male *transvestism.*

**e'osin** [ G. *ēōs,* dawn ]. Sodium salts of 2',4',5',7'-tetrabromofluorescein or 4',5'-dibromo-2',7'-dinitrofluorescein, also known as eosin Y (for yellowish) or eosin YS, or eosin I Bluish, respectively; solution in water or alcohol is red with greenish yellow fluorescence. The eosins are acid dyes with important uses as cytoplasmic and counterstains in histology.

**ethyl e.,** see under ethyl.

**eosin'oblast.** A myeloblast that later becomes an eosinophil.

**eosin'ocyte.** Eosinophilic *leukocyte.*

**eosin'ope'nia** [ eosino(phil) + G. *penia,* poverty ]. The presence of eosinophils in an abnormally small number in the peripheral blood stream.

**eosinophil, eosinophile** (e-o-sin'o-fil, e-o-sin'o-fīl) [ eosin + G. *philos,* fond ]. Eosinophilic *leukocyte.* See color plate 14.

**eosinophil'ia.** Eosinophilic *leukocytosis.*

**tropical e.,** e. associated with cough and asthma, caused by occult filarial infection and occurring most frequently in India and southeast Asia.

**eosinophil'ic.** Staining readily with eosin dyes; denoting such cell or tissue elements.

**eosinotactic** (e-o-sin-o-tak'tik) [ eosino(phile) + G. *taktikos,* in orderly arrangement. TAX- ]. Exerting a force of attraction or repulsion on eosinophile cells.

**eosinotax'is.** Movement of eosinophils with reference to a chemical which attracts or repels them.

**eosophobia** (e-o'so-fo'bī-ah) [ G. *ēōs,* dawn, + *phobos,* fear ]. Morbid fear of the dawn.

**epactal** (e-pak'tal) [ G. *epaktos,* imported, fr. *epagō,* to bring on or in. ACT- ]. Supernumerary.

**epamniotic** (ep'am-nī-ot'ik) [ G. *epi,* upon, + amnion ]. Upon or above the amnion.

**ep'arsal'gia.** Epersalgia.

**eparterial** (ep'ar-tēr-ī-al) [ G. *epi,* upon, + *artēia,* artery ]. Upon or over an artery.

**epax'ial** [ G. *epi,* upon, + L. *axis,* axis ]. Above or behind any axis, such as the spinal axis or the axis of a limb.

**ependyma** (ep-en'dī-mah) [ G. *ependyma,* an upper garment ] [ NA ]. Endyma; the cellular membrane lining the central canal of the spinal cord and the brain ventricles.

**ependymal** (ep-en'dī-mal). Relating to the ependyma.

**ependymitis** (ep-en-dī-mi'tis). Inflammation of the ependyma.

**ependymoblast** (ep-en'dī-mo-blast) [ ependyma + G. *blastos,* germ ]. An embryonic ependymal cell.

**ependymoblastoma** (ep-en'dī-mo-blas-to'mah) [ ependymoblast + G. suffix -*oma,* tumor ]. A gliogenous neoplasm of the central nervous system, occurring typically in childhood; the prototype tumor cells resemble ependymoblasts.

**ependymocyte** (ep-en'dī-mo-sit) [ ependyma + G. *kytos,* cell ]. An ependymal cell.

**ependymoma** (ep-en'dī-mo'mah). A glioma or neoplasm of the brain derived from ependymal cells; they are relatively undifferentiated and comprise approximately 1 to 3 per cent of all intracranial neoplasms. E.'s occur in all age groups, and may originate from the lining of any of the ventricles or (more commonly) the central canal of the spinal cord. Histologically, the neoplastic cells tend to be arranged radially about blood vessels, to which they are attached by means of fibrillary processes.

**epersalgia** (ep-er-sal'jī-ah) [ G. *epairō,* to lift up, + *algos,* pain ]. Pain and soreness from overuse or unaccustomed use of a part, as a joint or muscle.

**Eperythrozoon** (ep'e-rith'ro-zo'on) [ G. *epi,* upon + *erythros,* red, + *zoōn,* animal ]. A genus of minute rickettsia-like parasites of animals occurring upon the surface of erythrocytes and in the plasma. They appear as rings, coccoids, and short rods when clustered on the surface of the red cells in stained films. Some species cause anemia and icterus. They are currently classified in the family Bartonellaceae (order Rickettsiales).

**E. coccoi'des,** commonly present in mice, but splenectomy is usually required to reveal infections; rats and hamsters may be artifically infected; bloodsucking arthropods, especially lice, have been implicated as biological vectors, and mechanical transmission by bloodsucking flies has been demonstrated; the pathogenic effect is slight except when combined with other disease-producing agents.

**E. o'vis,** causes disease in sheep in South Africa.

**E. suis,** produces icterus and anemia in young pigs, and icteroanemia of swine.

**E. wenyo'ni,** found in blood of cattle; significance not known.

**eperythrozoonosis** (ep'e-rith'ro-zo-o-no'sis). Infection with any species of eperythrozoon.

**ephapse** (ef'aps) [ G. *ephapsis,* contact ]. A place where two or more nerve cell processes (axons, dendrites) touch without forming a typical synaptic contact; the possibility of some form of neural transmission at such nonsynaptic contact sites has often been suggested.

**ephaptic** (e-fap'tik). Relating to an ephase.

**ephebiatrics** (ē-fe'bī-at'riks) [ G. *ephebos,* Athenian youth of military age ]. Hebiatrics; the branch of medicine devoted to the treatment of individuals in the approximate age range of 13 to 21 years; sometimes termed adolescent medicine.

**ephe'bic** [ G. *ephēbikos,* relating to youth, fr. *hēbē,* youth ]. Pubertal; relating to the period of puberty or to a youth.

**ephebology** (ef'e-bol'o-jī) [ G. *ephēbos,* puberty, + *logos,* study ]. The branch of science relating to the morphologic and other changes incidental to puberty.

**Eph'edra** [ G. the plant horsetail, fr. *epi*, upon, + *hedra*, seat ]. A genus of shrubs of the family *Gnetaceae*.

**E. antisyphilit'ica, E. nevadensis,** mountain rush; tepopote; teamster's tea; a shrub of the southwestern U. S. and Mexico, the stems were formerly used in the treatment of venereal and urinary diseases. Contains little or no ephedrine.

**E. equiseti'na,** Ma huang; *E. sinica;* the major sources of natural *l*-ephedrine and *d*-pseudoephedrine.

**E. vulga'ris** var. **helve'tia,** the plant that Nagai claimed to have used when he first isolated ephedrine in pure form. Probably not a valid name.

**ephedrine** (ef-ed'rin) (NF). 1-Phenyl-2-methylamino-1-propanol; an alkaloid from the leaves of *Ephedra equisetina, E. sinica,* and other species of *Ephedra,* or produced synthetically. An adrenergic (sympathomimetic) agent with actions similar to those of epinephrine. Used as a bronchodilator in bronchial asthma, mydriatic, pressor agent, and topical vasoconstrictor. Official salts are e. hydrochloride (NF, BP) and e. sulfate (USP).

**ephelis,** pl. **ephelides** (ef-e'lis, ef-e'lĭ-dēz) [ G. ]. A freckle.

**ephidrosis** (ef'ĭ-dro'sis) [ G. superficial perspiration ]. 1. Moderate sweating. 2. Localized hyperhidrosis; profound localized sweating.

**epi-.** G. preposition, used as a prefix, meaning upon, following, or subsequent to.

**epiandros'terone.** 3β-Hydroxy-5α-androstan-17-one (for androstane structure, see steroids); isoandrosterone; an inactive isomer (3β instead of 3α) of androsterone; found in urine and testicular and ovarian tissue.

**ep'iblast** [ epi- + G. *blastos,* germ ]. Ectoderm.

**epiblas'tic.** Relating to the epiblast.

**epiblepharon** (ep'ĭ-blef'ar-on) [ epi- + G. *blepharon,* eyelid ]. A congenital horizontal skin near the margin of the eyelid, due to abnormal insertion of muscle fibers. In the upper lid it simulates blepharochalasis; in the lower lid its presence causes an innocuous, and spontaneously disappearing, turning inward of the lashes.

**epiboly, epibole** (ē-pib'o-le) [ G. *epibolē,* a throwing or laying on. BALL- ]. A process involved in the gastrulation of telolecithal eggs in which, as a result of differential growth, some of the cells of the primordial outer layer (protoderm) move over the surface toward the lips of the blastopore. When these cells have arrived at the blastopore margins by e. they move inward (undergo involution), forming entoderm and mesoderm.

**epibul'bar.** Upon a bulb of any kind; specifically, upon the eyeball.

**epican'thus** [ epi- + G. *kanthos,* canthus ]. Plica palpebronasalis; a fold of skin extending from the root of the nose to the inner termination of the eyebrow, overlapping the medial canthus. Its presence is normal in the Mongolian.

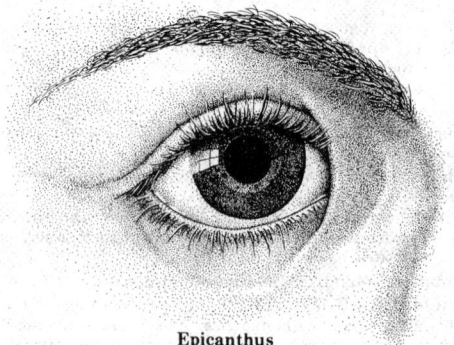

**Epicanthus**

**e. inversus,** a crescentic upward fold of skin from the lower eyelid at the inner canthus; frequent in congenital blepharoptosis.

**epicar'dia** [ epi- + cardia, *q. v.* ]. The aboral portion of the esophagus from where it passes through the diaphragm to the stomach; the abdominal portion of the esophagus.

**epicar'dium** [ epi- + G. *kardia,* heart ]. [ NA ]. The visceral layer of the pericardium; lamina visceralis; the serous membrane that immediately envelopes the heart.

**epicholes'tanol.** 3α-Hydroxycholestane (for structure of cholestane, see steroids).

**epicholes'terol.** 5-Cholesten-3α-ol; an isomer of cholesterol, in which the 3-hydroxyl group has the alpha rather than the beta configuration.

**epichordal** (ep-ĭ-kor'dal) [ epi- + G. *chordē,* a chord ]. On the dorsal side of the notochord; applicable particularly to that part of the brain developing dorsal to the cephalic part of the notochord.

**epicomus** (ep-ĭ-ko'mus, e-pik'o-mus) [ epi- + G. *komē,* hair of the head ]. Unequal conjoined twins in which the smaller (parasite) is joined to the larger (autosite) at the occiput. See also *craniopagus* parasiticus.

**epicondylalgia** (ep'ĭ-kon'dĭ-lal'jĭ-ah) [ epicondyle + G. *algos,* pain ]. Pain in an epicondyle of the humerus or in the tendons or muscles attached thereto.

**e. externa,** tennis *elbow.*

**epicondyle** (ep-ĭ-kon'dĭl) [ epi- + G. *kondylos,* a knuckle ]. Epicondylus.

**epicondylian** (ep-ĭ-kon-dil'ĭ-an). Epicondylic.

**epicondylic** (ep-ĭ-kon-dil'ik). Epicondylian; relating to an epicondyle or to the part above a condyle.

**epicondylitis** (ep'ĭ-kon-dĭ-li'tis). Infection or inflammation of an epicondyle.

**epicondylus,** pl. **epicon'dyli** (ep-ĭ-kon'dĭ-lus) [ L. ] [ NA ]. Epicondyle; a projection from a long bone near the articular extremity above or upon the condyle.

**e. latera'lis** [ NA ], lateral epicondyle; (*a*) of the humerus; situated at the lateral side of the distal end of the bone; (*b*) of the femur, located proximal to the lateral condyle.

**e. media'lis** [ NA ], medial epicondyle; (1) of the humerus; epitrochlea; situated proximal and medial to the condyle; (2) of the femur, located proximal to the medial condyle.

**epicoracoid** (ep-ĭ-kor'ă-koyd). Upon or above the coracoid process.

**epicorneascleritis** (ep-ĭ-kor'ne-ah-skle-ri'tis). A superficial transient inflammatory infection of the cornea and sclera.

**epicra'nium** [ epi- + G. *kranion,* skull ]. The scalp; galea capitis; the muscle, aponeurosis, and skin covering the cranium.

**epicrisis** (ep-ĭ-kri'sis). A secondary crisis; a crisis terminating a recrudescence of morbid symptoms following a primary crisis.

**epicrit'ic** [ G. *epikritikos,* adjudicatory, fr. *epi,* on, + *krinō,* to separate, judge ]. Term introduced by Henry Head to denote that component of the somatic sensory modality by which one is enabled to discriminate the finer degrees of touch and temperature stimuli, and to localize these stimuli on the body surface; distinguished from protopathic.

**epicystitis** (ep-ĭ-sis-ti'tis) [ epi- + G. *kystis,* bladder, + suffix *-itis,* inflammation ]. Inflammation of the cellular tissue above the bladder.

**epicystotomy** (ep'ĭ-sis-tot'o-mĭ) [ epi- + G. *kystis,* bladder, + *tomē,* incision ]. Suprapubic *cystotomy.*

**epicyte** (ep'ĭ-sit) [ epi- + G. *kytos,* cell ]. A cell membrane, especially of protozoa.

**epicyto'ma** [ epi- + G. *kytos,* cell, + suffix *-oma,* tumor ]. Undesirable term for squamous or basal cell carcinoma.

**epidem'ic** [ epi- + G. *dēmos,* the people ]. 1. A disease attacking many people in a community simultaneously; distinguished from endemic, since the disease is not continuously present but has been introduced from outside. 2. The extensive prevalence in a community of a disease brought from without, or a temporary increase in number of cases of an endemic disease.

**epidemicity** (ep-ĭ-dem-is'ĭ-tĭ). The state of prevailing disease in epidemic form.

**epidemiography** (ep-ĭ-dem-ĭ-og'ră-fĭ) [ G. *epidēmios,* epidemic, + *graphē,* a writing ]. A descriptive treatise of epidemic diseases or of any particular epidemic.

**epidemiology** (ep-ĭ-dem-ĭ-ol'o-jĭ) [ G. *epidēmios,* epidemic, + *logos,* study ]. The study of the prevalence and spread of disease in a community, especially infectious and epidemic diseases.

**ep'iderm, epider'ma.** Epidermis.

**epider'mal, epidermat'ic, epider'mic.** Relating to the epidermis.

**epider'matomyco'sis.** Dermatomycosis.

**epider'matoplas'ty** [ epidermis + G. *plassō*, to form ]. Skin grafting by means of strips (Thiersch's) or small patches (Reverdin's) of epidermis with the underlying outer layer of the corium.

**epider'mic.** Epidermal.

**ep'ider'midaliza'tion.** The change from columnar to stratified squamous epithelium.

**epidermido'sis.** Epidermosis.

**epidermis** (ep'ĭ-der'mis) [ G. *epidermis*, the outer skin, fr. *epi*, on, + *derma*, skin ] [ NA ]. Cuticle; cuticula; epiderm; epiderma; the outer epithelial portion of the skin (cutis). The e. of the palms and soles has the following strata: stratum corneum (horny layer), stratum lucidum (clear layer), stratum granulosum (granular layer), stratum spinosum (prickle cell layer), stratum basale (basal cell layer). In other parts of the body the stratum granulosum and the stratum lucidum may be absent.

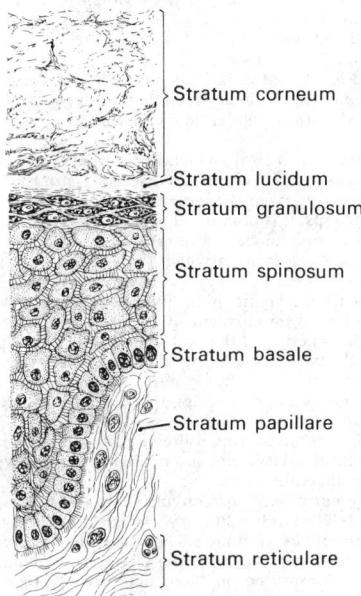

Stratum corneum

Stratum lucidum
Stratum granulosum

Stratum spinosum

Stratum basale

Stratum papillare

Stratum reticulare

**Epidermis**

Microscopic section of epidermis of thick skin and a small part of the corium. See also fig. under corium.

**ep'idermi'tis.** Inflammation of the epidermis or superficial layers of the skin.

**epidermiza'tion.** 1. Skin grafting. 2. The covering of an area with epidermis.

**epidermodysplasia** (ep'ĭ-der'mo-dis-pla'zĭ-ah) [ epidermis + G. *dys-*, bad, + *plasis*, a molding ]. Faulty growth or development of the epidermis.

  **e. verrucifor'mis,** a genodermatosis characterized by the development of flat warts on the hands and feet.

**epider'moid** [ epidermis + G. *eidos*, appearance ]. 1. Resembling epidermis. 2. A cholesteatoma or other tumor arising from aberrant epidermic cells.

**epidermol'ysis** [ epidermis + G. *lysis*, loosening ]. A condition in which the epidermis is loosely attached to the corium, readily exfoliating or forming blisters.

  **e. bullo'sa,** a group of inherited chronic noninflammatory skin diseases in which large bullae and erosions result from slight mechanical trauma.

  **e. bullo'sa dystroph'ica,** dermolytic bullous *dermatosis*.

  **e. bullo'sa sim'plex,** Goldscheider's disease; e. bullosa in which lesions heal rapidly without scarring and there is degeneration of basal epidermal cells; inherited as a dominant autosomal trait.

  **e. necrot'icans combustifor'mis,** toxic epidermal *necrolysis*.

**epider'momyco'sis.** Dermatophytosis.

**Epidermophyton** (ep'ĭ-der-mof'ĭ-ton, -der'mo-fi'ton) [ epidermis + G. *phyton*, plant ]. A genus of fungi, separated by Sabouraud from *Trichophyton* on the ground that it never invades the hair follicles.

  **E. flocco'sum,** the only species in the genus; it is anthropophilic, pathogenic, and a common cause of epidermophytosis (tinea pedis).

**epider'mophyto'sis.** Dermatophytosis.

  **e. in'terdigita'lis pedum,** *tinea* pedis.

**epidermo'sis.** Epidermidosis; a skin disease affecting only the epidermis.

**epidiascope** (ep-ĭ-di'ah-skōp) [ epi- + G. *dia*, through, + *skopeō*, to view ]. A projector by which images are reflected by a mirror through a lens, or lenses, onto a screen, using reflected light for opaque objects and transmitted light for translucent or transparent ones.

**epididymal** (ep-ĭ-did'ĭ-mal). Relating to the epididymis.

**epididymectomy** (ep-ĭ-did'ĭ-mek'to-mĭ) [ epididymis + G. *ektomē*, excision ]. Epididymidectomy; operative removal of the epididymis.

**epididymidectomy** (ep-ĭ-did-ĭ-mid-ek'to-mĭ). Epididymectomy.

**epidid'ymis,** gen. **epididym'idis,** pl. **epididym'ides** (ep-ĭ-did'ĭ-mis) [ Mod. L. fr. G. *epididymis*, fr. *epi*, on, + *didymos*, twin, in pl. testes ] [ NA ]. The first, convoluted, portion of the excretory duct of the testis, passing from above downward along the posterior border of this gland; at the lower extremity of the testis it turns upward and gradually merges into the ductus deferens. The cauda epididymidis and the beginning of the ductus deferens are the reservoir of the spermatozoa. See fig. under scrotum.

**epididymisoplasty** (ep'ĭ-did'ĭ-mis-o-plas'tĭ). Epididymoplasty.

**epididymitis** (ep-ĭ-did-ĭ-mi'tis). Inflammation of the epididymis.

**epididymo-orchitis** (ep-ĭ-did-ĭ-mo-or-ki'tis) [ epididymis + G. *orchis*, testis ]. Simultaneous inflammation of both epididymis and testis.

**epididymoplasty** (ep'ĭ-did'ĭ-mo-plas'tĭ) [ epididymis + G. *plassō*, to form ]. Epididymisoplasty; surgical repair of the epididymis.

**epididymotomy** (ep'ĭ-did-ĭ-mot'o-mĭ) [ epididymis + G. *tomē*, a cutting ]. Incision into the epididymis, usually for the relief of pain and tension in epididymitis.

**epididymovasostomy** (ep'ĭ-did'ĭ-mo-vă-sos'to-mĭ) [ epididymis + vasostomy ]. Surgical anastomosis of the vas deferens to the epididymis.

**epidu'ral.** Peridural; upon (or outside) the dura mater.

**epidurog'raphy.** Radiographic visualization of the epidural space following the regional instillation of a radiopaque contrast medium.

**16-epiestriol** (ep'ĭ-es'trĭ-ol). 1,3,5(10)-Estratriene-3,16β,17β-triol; epimer, C-16, of estriol (for structure of estrane, see steroids); an estrogenic metabolite found in urine, bile, and the placenta.

**16,17-epiestriol.** 1,3,5(10)-Estratriene-3,16β,17α-triol; double epimer (at 16 and 17) of estriol (for estrane structure, see steroids); an estrogenic metabolite found in urine.

**17-epiestriol.** 1,3,5(10)-Estratriene-3,16α,17α-triol; epimer, at C-17, of estriol (for estrane structure, see steroids); an estrogenic metabolite found in urine during pregnancy.

**epifascial** (ep-ĭ-fash'ĭ-al). Upon the surface of a fascia, denoting a method of injecting drugs in which the solution is put on the fascia lata instead of injected into the substance of the muscle.

**epigastral'gia** [ epigastrium + G. *algos*, pain ]. Pain in the epigastric region.

**epigas'tric.** Relating to the epigastrium.

**epigas'trium** [ G. *epigastrion* ] [ NA ]. Regio epigastrica.

**epigas′trius.** Unequal conjoined twins in which the smaller (parasite) is attached to the larger (host) in the epigastric region.

**epigastrocele** (ep-ī-gas′tro-sēl) [ epigastrium + G. *kēlē*, hernia ]. A hernia in the epigastric region.

**epigastrorrhaphy** (ep′ī-gas-tror′ă-fī) [ epigastrium + G. *rhaphē*, suture ]. Suture of a wound of the abdominal wall in the epigastric region.

**epigenesis** (ep-ī-jen′ĕ-sis) [ epi- + G. *genesis*, creation ]. The theory that the offspring is developed as a result of the union of the ovum and sperm. It is in antithesis to the old preformation theory that a new individual existed in miniature encased in the ovum (as believed by the ovists) or in the sperm (as believed by the homunculists), and merely unfolded and enlarged in the body of the female parent.

**ep′igenet′ic.** Relating to epigenesis.

**epiglot′tic, epiglottid′ean.** Relating to the epiglottis.

**epiglottidectomy** (ep′ī-glot′ī-dek′to-mī) [ epiglottis + G. *ektomē*, excision ]. Excision of the epiglottis.

**epiglottiditis** (ep-ī-glot-id-i′tis). Epiglottitis.

**epiglot′tis** [ G. *epiglōttis*, fr. *epi*, on, + *glōttis*, the mouth of the windpipe ] [ NA ]. A leaf-shaped plate of elastic cartilage, covered with mucous membrane, at the root of the tongue, which folds back over the aperture of the larynx, covering it, during the act of swallowing.

**epiglottitis** (ep-ī-glot-i′tis). Epiglottiditis; inflammation of the epiglottis, which may cause respiratory obstruction, especially in children; frequently due to infection by *Haemophilus influenzae* type b.

**epignathus** (ĕ-pig′nă-thus) [ epi- + G. *gnathos*, jaw ]. Unequal conjoined twins in which the smaller incomplete one (the parasite) is attached to the larger one (the autosite) at the lower jaw.

**epihyal** (ep-ī-hi′al). Above the hyoid arch.

**epihy′oid.** Upon the hyoid bone; denoting certain accessory thyroid glands lying above the geniohyoid muscle.

**epilamellar** (ep′ī-lă-mel′ar) [ epi- + L. *lamella*, dim. of *lamina*, a thin metal plate ]. Upon or above a basement membrane.

**epilate** (ep′ī-lāt) [ L. *e*, out, + *pilus*, a hair ]. Depilate; to extract a hair; remove the hair from a part by forcible extraction, electrolysis, or loosening at the root by chemical means.

**epilation** (ep′ī-la′shun). The act or result of removing hair.

**epil′atory.** Depilatory.

**epilem′ma** [ epi- *lemma*, husk ]. The connective tissue sheath of nerve fibers near their termination.

**epilepidoma** (ep-ī-lep-ī-do′mah) [ epi- + G. *lepis*, rind, + suffix -*oma*, tumor ]. A tumor resulting from hyperplasia of tissue derived from the true epiblast.

**epilep′sia** [ G. ]. Epilepsy.

   **e. nu′tans,** head nodding attacks in children.

   **e. partia′lis contin′ua,** Kojewnikoff's epilepsy; a form of epilepsy marked by repetitive clonic muscular contractions with or without major convulsions.

   **e. rotato′ria,** attacks in which the body spins or rotates.

**epilepsy** (ep′ī-lep′sī) [ G. *epilēpsia*, seizure. LAB- ]. "Falling sickness"; a chronic disorder characterized by paroxysmal attacks of brain dysfunction usually associated with some alteration of consciousness. The attacks may remain confined to elementary or complex impairment of behavior or may progress to a generalized convulsion.

   **abortive e.,** (1) short attacks which, at times, may progress to convulsions; (2) absence.

   **accel′erative e.,** procursive e.

   **acquired e.,** an e. related causally to a postnatal factor such as cerebral infection or injury.

   **activated e.,** iatrogenically induced seizures.

   **akinetic e.,** epileptic manifestations without movement, usually with loss of consciousness.

   **atonic e.,** e. characterized by loss of muscular tone.

   **automatic e.,** psychomotor e.

   **autonomic diencephalic e.,** vasomotor e.; episodes of autonomic dysfunction presumably due to diencephalic irritation.

   **centrencephalic e.,** e. characterized electroencephalographically by bilateral synchronous discharges, and clinically by petit or grand mal.

   **cor′tical e.,** focal e.

   **delayed e.,** an e. beginning in adult life.

   **ether e.,** ether fit; e. precipitated by hyperventilation during induction of ether anesthesia.

   **focal e.,** cortical e.; partial e.; an epileptic attack beginning with an isolated disturbance of cerebral function such as a twitching of a limb, a somatosensory or special sense phenomenon, or a disturbance of higher mental function.

   **generalized e.,** grand mal e.; major e.; idiopathic e. (2); a seizure characterized by loss of consciousness and tonic spasm of the musculature, and usually followed by repetitive generalized clonic jerking.

   **grand mal e.,** generalized e.

   **idiopath′ic e.,** (1) an e. without evident cause; (2) generalized e.

   **Jacksonian e.,** focal e. with a "march" of the attack usually from distal to proximal limb musculature.

   **Kojewnikoff's e.,** *epilepsia* partialis continua.

   **larval e.,** (1) abortive e.; (2) masked e.; (3) latent e.; epileptic brain wave patterns without a clinical history of e.

   **laryn′geal e.,** e. precipitated by violent coughing due to hyperventilation.

   **latent e.,** larval e. (3).

   **major e.,** generalized e.

   **masked e.,** larval e. (2); a form of e. characterized by a paroxysmal disturbance such as headache or vomiting associated with an epileptic electroencephalographic pattern.

   **matu′tinal e.,** a form which occurs on awakening.

   **myoclonus e.,** Unverricht's disease; Lafora's disease; a seizure characterized by sporadic or continuous clonus of muscle groups; it is of familial origin and is associated with progressive mental deterioration.

   **nocturnal e.,** a form in which the attacks occur at night.

   **partial e.,** focal e.

   **petit mal e.,** petit mal; pyknoepilepsy; pyknolepsy; attacks of brief impairment of consciousness often associated with flickering of the eyelids and mild twitching of the mouth; electroencephalographically characterized by a 3 per second spike and dome pattern.

   **photogenic e.,** e. precipitated by intermittent light stimulation.

   **pleural e.,** convulsions following puncture or irrigation of the pleural cavity; they are probably due to hyperventilation or air embolism.

   **posttraumatic e.,** a convulsive state following and causally related to head injury. Because the term is loosely used without discrimination between mere temporal and actual causal relationships, the Congress of Neurological Surgeons Committee on Nomenclature of Head Injuries has suggested the following criteria: (1) the individual should have had no history of pretraumatic convulsive manifestations; (2) he should have no other systemic or cerebral condition that might reasonably be associated with convulsions; (3) the alleged trauma must have been of such magnitude that, with reasonable certainty, brain damage resulted; (4) the alleged attacks must be bona fide epilepsy; (5) the location of the injury must be related to the type of seizure; (6) the electroencephalogram must be consistent with the type of seizure.

   **posttraumatic e., early,** convulsions beginning a few minutes to one month after injury; recurrent attacks are unlikely.

   **posttraumatic e., late,** convulsive attacks beginning more than a month after head injury.

   **procur′sive e.,** accelerative e.; a psychomotor attack initiated by whirling or running.

   **psychic e.,** (1) the occurrence of attacks of maniacal excitement, coming on alone or following minor attacks (petit mal); (2) somnambulic e.; (3) epileptoid convulsions of a purely emotional origin; (4) psychomotor e. attacks of complex psychic disturbances such as déjà vu, hallucinations, etc.

   **psychomotor e.,** automatic e.; temporal lobe e.; attacks characterized clinically by impairment of consciousness and amnesia for the episode, often associated with semipurposeful movements of the arms or legs and sometimes with psychic disturbances such as hallucinations; spike discharges in the temporal region are usually seen during light sleep.

**reflex e.,** a form in which the attacks are excited by peripheral irritation.

**ret'inal e.,** focal e. with temporary blindness.

**secondary generalized e.,** e. with focal manifestations progressing to a generalized convulsion.

**sensory e.,** focal e. initiated by a somatosensory phenomenon.

**sleep e.,** narcolepsy.

**somnam'bulic e.,** psychomotor e. followed by a state resembling somnambulism in which the patient performs complicated acts naturally and well but of which he has no subsequent remembrance.

**symptomat'ic e.,** a form of e., usually focal, due to obvious brain disease.

**tardy e.,** delayed e.

**temporal lobe e.,** psychomotor e.

**thalam'ic e.,** sensory e. in which attacks of temporary mental disturbance are marked by delusions of sensation.

**tonic e.,** a convulsive attack in which the body is rigid.

**tornado e.,** attacks with an aura of severe vertigo and a feeling of being drawn up into space.

**un'cinate e.,** a form of psychomotor e. initiated by a dreamy state and hallucinations of smell and taste.

**vasomotor e.,** autonomic diencephalic e.

**vasovagal e.,** autonomic attacks due to hypothalamic or midbrain irritation.

**visceral e.,** e. in which there are visceral symptoms or visceral sensations in the aura. Most cases have their focus in the temporal lobe of the brain.

**epilep'tic.** 1. Relating to or suffering from epilepsy. 2. A sufferer from epilepsy.

**epilep'tiform.** Epileptoid.

**epileptogenic, epileptogenous** (ep-ĭ-lep-to-jen'ik, ep-ĭ-lep-toj'ĕ-nus). Causing epilepsy.

**epileptoid** (ep-ĭ-lep'toyd) [ G. epilēpsia, seizure, epilepsy, + eidos, resemblance ]. Resembling epilepsy; epileptiform; denoting certain convulsions, especially of functional nature.

**epiloia** (ep-ĭ-loy'ah) [ a contrived term, i.e., invented by Sherlock, 1911, without classical or other etymological roots ]. Tuberous sclerosis.

**epimandib'ular** [ epi- + L. mandibulum, mandible ]. Upon the lower jaw.

**ep'imas'tigote** [ epi- + G. mastix, whip ]. Term replacing "crithidial stage," to avoid confusion with the insect-parasitizing flagellates of the genus Crithidia. In the e. stage the flagellum arises from the kinetoplast alongside the nucleus and emerges from the anterior end of the organism. An undulating membrane is present.

**epimenorrhagia** (ep-ĭ-men-o-ra'jĭ-ah). Too prolonged and too profuse menstruation occurring at any time during menstrual life, but most frequent at the beginning and end of this period.

**epimenorrhea** (ep-ĭ-men-o-re'ah). Too frequent menstruation, occurring at any time during menstrual life, but particularly at the menarche or preclimacterium.

**ep'imer** [ epi- + G. meros, part ]. One of two molecules differing only in the spatial arrangement about a single carbon atom; e.g., glucose and galactose (with respect to carbon 4); cf. anomer, also sugars, for formulas.

**epimerase** (ep'ĭ-mer-ās). A class of enzymes (EC 5.1) catalyzing epimeric changes.

**epimere** (ep'ĭ-mēr) [ epi- + G. meros, part ]. The dorsal part of the myotome; see myotome (3).

**epimerite** (ep'ĭ-mēr'ĭt) [ epi- + G. meros, part ]. The hooklike anchoring structure at the anterior end of a cephaline gregarine sporozoan. It is left embedded in tissues when the rest of the cephalont is freed in the lumen of the intestine.

**epimes'trol** (USAN). STIMOVUL; 3-methoxyestra-1,3,5(10)-triene-16α,17α-diol; anterior pituitary activating agent.

**epimicroscope** (ep'ĭ-mi'kro-skōp). Opaque microscope; a microscope with a condenser built around the objective;

used for the investigation of opaque, or only slightly translucent, minute specimens.

**epimorpho'sis** (ep'ĭ-mor'fo-sis, -mor-fo'sis) [ epi- + G. morphē, shape ]. Regeneration of a part of an organism by growth at the cut surface.

**epimysium** (ep-ĭ-miz'ĭ-um) [ epi- + G. mys, muscle ]. Perimysium externum; the fibrous envelope surrounding a skeletal muscle.

**epinephrectomy** (ep-ĭ-nĕ-frek'to-mī) [ epi- + G. nephros, kidney, + ektomē, excision ]. Obsolete term for adrenalectomy.

**epinephrine** (ep'ĭ-nef'rin) (USP). ADRENALIN; adrenaline (BP); 3,4-dihydroxy-α-(methylaminomethyl)benzyl alcohol; a catecholamine; the chief neurohormone of the adrenal medulla of most species. It is the most potent stimulant (sympathomimetic) of adrenergic α- and β-receptors, resulting in increased heart rate and force of contraction, vasoconstriction or vasodilation, relaxation of bronchiolar and intestinal smooth muscle, glycogenolysis, lipolysis, and other metabolic effects. It is used in the treatment of bronchial asthma (status asthmaticus), acute allergic disorders, open-angle glaucoma, and heart block, and as a topical and local vasoconstrictor.

$$HO-\hspace{-4pt}\langle\text{ring}\rangle\hspace{-4pt}-CHCH_2-NH-CH_3$$

Epinephrine

**e. bitartrate** (USP), SUPRARENIN; adrenaline acid tartrate (BP), crystalline powder that slowly darkens on exposure to light and air.

**e. reversal,** adrenaline reversal; the fall in blood pressure produced by e. when given following blockade of α-adrenergic receptors by an appropriate drug such as phenoxybenzamine. The vasodilation reflects the ability of e. to activate β-adrenergic receptors which, in vascular smooth muscle, are inhibitory. In the absence of α-receptor blockade, the β-receptor activation by e. is masked by its predominant action on vascular α-receptors, which causes vasoconstriction.

**epinephritis** (ep-ĭ-nĕ-fri'tis) [ epi- + G. nephros, kidney, + suffix -itis, inflammation ]. Obsolete term for inflammation of the adrenal gland.

**epinephros** (ep'ĭ-nef'ros) [ epi- + G. nephros, kidney ]. Glandula suprarenalis.

**epineural** (ep-ĭ-nu'ral). On a neural arch of a vertebrae.

**epineurial** (ep-ĭ-nu'rĭ-al). Relating to the epineurium.

**epineurium** (ep-ĭ-nu'rĭ-um) [ epi- + G. neuron, nerve ]. The connective tissue encapsulating a nerve trunk and binding together the fascicles; it contains the blood vessels and lymphatics supplying the nerves.

**epino'sic.** Relating to epinosis.

**epinosis** (ep'ĭ-no'sis) [ epi- + G. nosos, disease ]. An imaginary feeling of illness following a real illness.

**epionychium** (ep-ĭ-ŏ-nik'ĭ-um). Eponychium.

**epiotic** (ep'ĭ-ot'ik, -o'tik) [ epi- + G. ous, ear ]. One of the components of the otic capsule of some vertebrates; in the mammal the petrosal or petrous temporal bone incorporates the various otic elements seen in lower vertebrates.

**epipas'tic** [ G. epi-passō, to sprinkle over ]. 1. Usable as a dusting powder. 2. A dusting powder.

**epipericardial** (ep'ĭ-pĕr-ĭ-kar'dĭ-al). Upon or about the pericardium.

**epipharynx** (ep'ĭ-făr'ingks) [ G. epi, on, over, + pharynx ]. Pars nasalis pharyngis.

**epiphenomenon** (ep'ĭ-fe-nom'e-non). A symptom appearing during the course of a disease, which is not of usual occurrence and not necessarily associated with the disease.

**epiphora** (e-pif'o-rah) [ G. a sudden flow, fr. epi, on, + pherō, to bear. PHER- ]. Watery eye; an overflow of tears upon the cheek, due to narrowing of any part of the tear-conducting apparatus.

**epiphrenic, epiphrenal** (ep'ĭ-fren'ik, -fre'nal) [ epi- + G. phrēn, diaphragm ]. Upon or above the diaphragm.

**epiphylaxis** (ep-ĭ-fi-lak′sis) [ epi- + G. *phylaxis*, protection ]. Reinforcement of normal phylaxis; increase of the protective powers of the blood and other fluids.

**epiphysial, epiphyseal** (ep-ĭ-fiz′ĭ-al). Relating to an epiphysis.

**epiphysiodesis** (ep-ĭ-friz′ĭ-od′ĕ-sis) [ epiphysis + G. *desis*, bind ]. Premature union of the epiphysis with the diaphysis, resulting in cessation of growth.

**epiphysiolysis** (ep-ĭ-fiz-ĭ-ol′ĭ-sis) [ epiphysis + G. *lysis*, loosening ]. Loosening or separation of an epiphysis from the shaft of a bone.

**epiphysiopathy** (ep-ĭ-fiz-ĭ-op′ă-thĭ) [ epiphysis + G. *pathos*, suffering ]. Any disorder of an epiphysis, either that of the long bones or of the cerebrum (the pineal gland).

**epiphysis**, pl. **epiph′yses** (e-pif′ĭ-sis) [ G. an excrescence, fr. *epi*, upon, + *physis*, growth ] [ NA ]. A part of a long bone developed from a center of ossification distinct from that of the shaft and separated at first from the latter by a layer of cartilage.

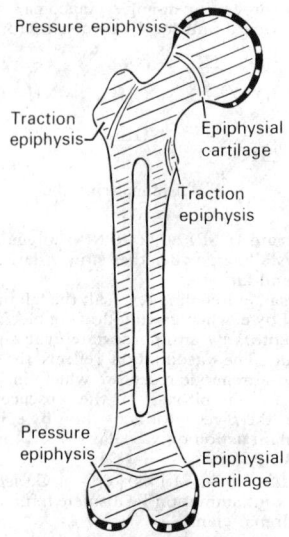

**Epiphyses of the Femur**

(Slightly modified from Salter, R. B.: *Textbook of Disorders and Injuries of the Musculoskeletal System*, The Williams & Wilkins Co., Baltimore, 1970.)

    **atavistic e.,** a bone that is independent phylogenetically but is now fused with another bone, *e.g.,* coracoid process of the scapula.

    **e. cer′ebri,** *corpus* pineale.

    **pressure e.,** a secondary center of ossification in the articular end of a long bone.

    **stippled e.,** *dysplasia* epiphysialis punctata.

    **traction e.,** a secondary center of ossification at the site of attachment of a tendon.

**epiphysitis** (e-pif′ĭ-si′tis). Inflammation of an epiphysis.

**ep′iphyte** (ep′ĭ-fīt) [ epi- + G. *phyton*, a plant ]. A parasitic fungus on the skin.

**epipial** (ep′ĭ-pi′al). On the pia mater.

**epiplo-** (e-pip′lo-, ep′ĭ-plo-) [ G. *epiploon*, omentum ]. Combining form relating to the omentum. See also omento-.

**epiplocele** (e-pip′lo-sēl) [ epiplo- + G. *kēlē*, hernia ]. Hernia of the omentum.

**epiploectomy** (ep′ĭ-plo-ek′to-mĭ) [ epiplo- + G. *ektomē*, excision ]. Omentectomy; resection or excision of omentum.

**epiploenterocele** (e-pip′lo-en′ter-o-sēl) [ epiplo- + G. *enteron*, intestine, + *kēlē*, hernia ]. Herniation of omentum and intestine.

**epiploic** (ep′ĭ-plo′ik). Omental; relating to the epiploon, or omentum.

**epiplomerocele** (ep′ĭ-plo-me′ro-sēl) [ epiplo- + G. *mēros*, thigh, + *kēlē*, hernia ]. A femoral hernia containing omentum.

**epiplomphalocele** (ep-ĭ-plom-fal′o-sēl) [ epiplo- + G. *omphalos*, umbilicus, + *kēlē*, hernia ]. An umbilical hernia containing omentum.

**epiploon** (e-pip′lo-on) [ G. ]. *Omentum* majus.

**epip′lopexy** [ epiplo- + G. *pēxis*, fixation ]. Omentopexy.

**epip′loplas′ty** [ epiplo- + G. *plassō*, to form ]. Omentoplasty.

**epiplorrhaphy** (ep′ĭ-plor′ă-fĭ) [ epiplo- + G. *rhaphē*, stitching ]. Omentorrhaphy.

**epiploscheocele** (ep-ĭ-plos′ke-o-sēl) [ epiplo- + G. *oscheon*, scrotum, + *kēlē*, hernia ]. Scrotal hernia containing omentum.

**epipro′pidine** (USAN). 1,1′-Bis(2,3-epoxypropyl)-4,4′-bipiperidine; antineoplastic agent.

**epipteric** (ep′ip-tēr′ik). In the neighborhood of the pterion.

**epipygus** (ep′ĭ-pi′gus) [ epi- + G. *pygē*, buttocks ]. Unequal conjoined twins in which the smaller, incomplete one (parasite) is attached to the buttock of the larger one (the host or autosite).

**epirhamnose** (ep′ĭ-ram′nōz). 6-Deoxyglucose; a methylpentose that is a constituent of the glycoside, convolvulin.

**episclera** (ep′ĭ-skle′rah) [ epi- + sclera, *q.v.* ]. The connective tissue between the sclera and the conjunctiva.

**episcle′ral.** 1. Upon the sclerotic coat of the eye. 2. Relating to the episclera.

**episcleritis** (ep-ĭ-skle-ri′tis). Inflammation of the episcleral or subconjunctival connective tissue.

**episio-** (ĕ-pis′ĭ-o-, ĕ-pe′ze-o-) [ G. *episeion*, pudenda ]. Combining form relating to the vulva.

**episioclisia, episiocleisis** (ĕ-pis-ĭ-o-kli′sĭ-ah) [ episio- + G. *kleisis*, closure ]. Operative occlusion of the vulva.

**episioelytrorrhaphy** (ĕ-pis-ĭ-o-el-ĭ-tror′ă-fĭ) [ episio- + G. *elytron*, sheath (vagina), + *rhaphē*, stitching ]. Narrowing the vulva and vagina by suturing a longitudinal fold in the canal, in order to give better support to the uterus in cases of a tendency to prolapse.

**episioperineoplasty** (ĕ-pis′ĭ-o-pĕr-ĭ-ne′o-plas′tĭ) [ episio- + G. *perinaion*, perineum, + *plassō*, to form ]. Plastic surgery on vulva and perineum.

**episioperineorrhaphy** (ĕ-pis′ĭ-o-pĕr′ĭ-ne-or′ă-fĭ) [ episio- + G. *perinaion*, perineum, + *rhaphē*, a stitching ]. Repair of a ruptured perineum and lacerated vulva or repair of a surgical incision of the vulva and perineum; made for obstetrical purposes.

**episioplasty** (ĕ-pis′ĭ-o-plas′tĭ) [ episio- + G. *plassō*, to form ]. Repair of a defect of the vulva by means of a plastic operation.

**episiorrhagia** (ĕ-pis′ĭ-o-ra′jĭ-ah) [ episio- + G. *rhēgnymi*, to burst forth ]. Hemorrhage from the vulva.

**episiorrhaphy** (ĕ-pis-ĭ-or′ă-fĭ) [ episio- + G. *rhaphē*, a stitching ]. Repair of a lacerated vulva or an episiotomy.

**episiostenosis** (ĕ-pis′ĭ-o-stĕ-no′sis) [ episio- + G. *stenōsis*, narrowing ]. Narrowing of the vulvar orifice.

**episiotomy** (ĕ-pis-ĭ-ot′o-mĭ) [ episio- + G. *tomē*, incision ]. Surgical incision of the vulva to prevent laceration at the time of delivery or to facilitate vaginal surgery.

**ep′isome** [ epi- + G. *sōma*, body (chromosome) ]. In microbial genetics, one of a class of genetic elements that can exist either as chromosomal segments or as freely replicating extrachromosomal fragments; important in relation to development of bacterial resistance to antibiotics, and also to pathogenicity (as in the case of *Escherichia coli* enterotoxin.

    **resistance-transfer e.'s,** R *factors.*

**epispa′dia.** Epispadias.

**epispad′ial.** Relating to an epispadias.

**epispadias** (ep-ĭ-spa′dĭ-as, -spad′ĭ-as) [ epi- + G. *spadōn*, a rent. SPA- ]. A malformation in which the urethra opens on the dorsum of the penis.

**epispas′tic.** Vesicant.

**epispi′nal.** Upon the vertebral column or spinal cord, or upon any structure resembling a spine.

**episplenitis** (ep-ĭ-sple-ni′tis). Inflammation of the capsule of the spleen.

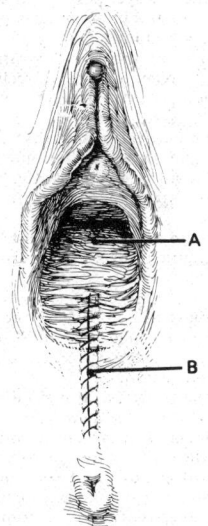

**Episiotomy**

*A*, vagina; *B*, median episiotomy closed by continuous suture.

**epis'tasis** [ G. scum; epi- + G. *stasis*, a standing ]. 1. Scum; a pellicle forming on the surface of urine after it has stood for a time. 2. A form of gene interaction whereby one gene masks or interferes with the phenotypic expression of one or more genes at other loci; the gene whose phenotype is expressed is said to be "epistatic," while the gene or genes whose phenotype is altered or suppressed is said to be "hypostatic."

**epistat'ic.** Relating to epistasis.

**epistaxis** (ep'ĭ-stak'sis) [ G. fr. *epistazō*, to bleed at the nose, fr. *epi*, on, + *stazō*, to fall in drops ]. Nosebleed; nasal hemorrhage.

   **renal e.,** hematuria occurring without evidence of any lesion; angioneurotic hematuria; renal hemophilia.

**epistemophilia** (ĕ-pis'te-mo-fil'ĭ-ah) [ G. *epistēmē*, knowledge, + *philos*, fond ]. The love, or excessive love, of knowledge.

**epis'temophil'iac.** One who has an excessive or unusual love of knowledge.

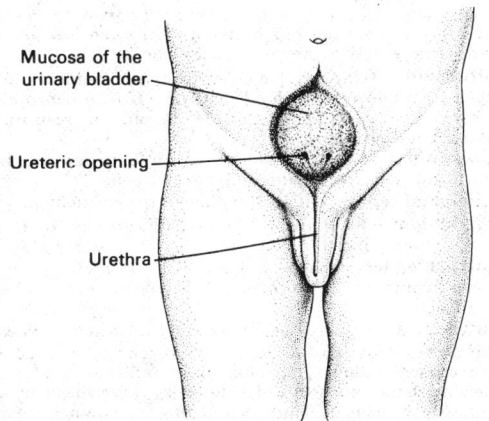

**Epispadias and Ectopia of the Bladder**

(From Langman, J.: *Medical Embryology*, Ed. 2, The Williams & Wilkins Co., Baltimore, 1969.)

**epister'nal.** Suprasternal; over or on the sternum; relating to the episternum.

**epister'num** [ epi- + L. *sternum*, chest ]. *Manubrium sterni*.

**epistropheus** (ep-ĭ-stro'fe-us) [ G. the pivot. STREP- ]. Axis (5).

**epitar'sus** [ epi- + G. *tarsos*, flat mat, edge of eyelid ]. A fold of conjunctiva arising on the tarsal surface of the lid and losing itself in the skin close to the medial canthus.

**epitax'y** [ epi- + G. *taxis*, arrangement ]. The growth of one crystal in one or more specific orientations on the substrate of another kind of crystal with a close geometric fit between the networks in contact. Examples are see in the alternating layers of different composition in stones from the kidney and gallbladder, indicating an abrupt change of composition during formation.

**epitendineum** (ep'ĭ-ten-din'e-um) [ L. ]. Epitenon; the white fibrous sheath surrounding a tendon.

**epitenon** (ĕ-pit'ĕ-non). Epitendineum.

**17-epitestos'terone.**	17α-Hydroxy-4-androsten-3-one; 17α epimer of testosterone (for testosterone structure, see steroids); a biologically inactive steroid found in testes and ovaries; may be a metabolite of 4-androstene-3,17-dione and a precursor of 17α-estradiol.

**epithalamus** (ep'ĭ-thal'ă-mus) [ epi- + thalamus ] [ NA ]. A small dorsal area of the thalamus correspoding to the habenula.

**ep'ithalax'ia** [ epithelium + G. *allaxis*, exchange ]. Shedding of any surface epithelium, but especially of that lining the intestine.

**epithe'lia.** Plural of epithelium.

**epithe'lial.** Relating to or consisting of epithelium.

**epithe'lializa'tion.** Epithelization; the formation of epithelium over a denuded surface.

**epithe'lialize.** To accomplish epithelialization.

**epitheliocyte** (ep'i-the'li-o-sit) [ epithelium + G. *kytos*, cell ]. One of the three tissue culture cell types; the others are mechanocytes and amebocytes.

**epithe'liofi'bril.** Tonofibril.

**epithe'lioglan'dular.** Relating to glandular epithelium.

**epithelioid** (ep-ĭ-the'lĭ-oyd) [ epithelium + G. *eidos*, resemblance ]. Resembling or having some of the characteristics of epithelium.

**epitheliolysin** (ep-ĭ-the-li-ol'ĭ-sin). A specific lysin in blood serum, acting upon epithelial cells; it destroys the cells of an animal of the same species as the one from which the epithelial cells (used as antigen) were derived.

**epitheliolytic** (ep-ĭ-the'lĭ-o-lit'ik). Destructive to epithelium.

**epithelioma** (ep-ĭ-the'lĭ-o'mah) [ epithelium + G. suffix *-oma*, tumor ]. 1. An epithelial neoplasm or hamartoma of the skin, especially of skin appendage origin. 2. A carcinoma of the skin derived from squamous, basal, or adnexal cells.

   **e. adenoi'des cys'ticum,** trichoepithelioma.

   **basal cell e.,** basal cell *carcinoma*.

   **benign cystic e.,** trichoepithelioma.

   **Borst-Jadassohn type intraepidermal e.,** lesions clinically suggestive of seborrheic keratosis or nevus with nests of immature or abnormal cells within the epidermis.

   **e. contagio'sum,** fowl *pox*.

   **Malherbe's calcifying e.,** Malherbe's disease; pilomatrixoma; a benign tumor occurring beneath the skin, consisting of basal cells of skin appendage or epidermal origin, together with necrotic epithelium that may be calcified. Foreign body giant cells are seen in the surrounding fibrous tissue.

**epithelio'matous.** Pertaining to epithelioma.

**epitheliopathy** (ep-ĭ-the'lĭ-op'ă-thĭ) [ epithelium + G. *pathos*, suffering ]. Disease involving epithelium.

   **pigment e.,** pigment *epithelium*.

**epitheliosis** (ep-ĭ-the-lĭ-o'sis). Proliferation of epithelial cells, as seen in the conjunctiva in Paul's reaction and in ducts of the breast in fibrocystic disease.

   **bovine e.,** malignant catarrhal *fever*.

   **e. desquamati'va,** Samoan eye disease; an e. occurring endemically in certain islands of the Pacific; trachoma granules do not develop, but atrophy of the conjunctiva occurs; caused by inclusion bodies formerly called *Lyozoon atrophicans.*

**epithe'lite.** A skin lesion resulting from excessive irradiation.

**epithelium,** pl. **epithelia** (ep-ĭ-the'lĭ-um) [ G. *epi,* upon, + *thēlē,* nipple, a term applied originally to the thin skin covering the nipples and the papillary layer of the border of the lips ] [ NA ]. The purely cellular, avascular layer covering all the free surfaces, cutaneous, mucous, and serous, including the glands and other structures derived therefrom.

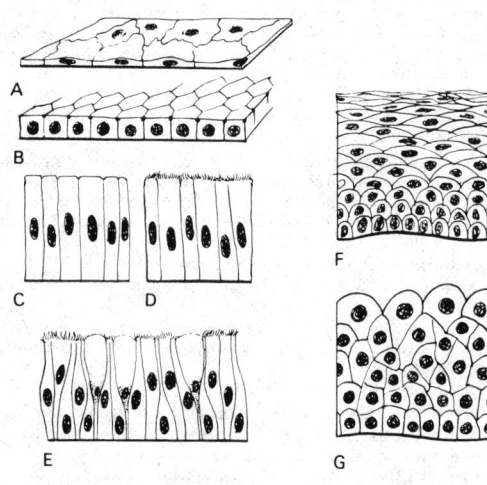

**Types of Epithelium**
*A,* simple squamous; *B,* simple cuboidal; *C,* simple columnar; *D,* ciliated columnar; *E,* pseudostratified ciliated columnar with goblet cells; *F,* stratified squamous; *G,* transitional.

**e. ante'rius cor'neae** [ NA ], anterior e. of the cornea; the stratified squamous e. covering the outer surface of the cornea. It is smooth, consists usually of five layers of cells, and contains numerous free nerve endings.

**cil'iated e.,** any e. having motile cilia on the free surface.

**colum'nar e.,** e. formed of a single layer of prismatic cells taller than they are wide.

**crevicular e.,** sulcular e.; the stratified squamous e. lining the inner aspect of the soft tissue wall of the gingival sulcus.

**cuboidal e.,** simple e. with cells appearing as cubes in a vertical section but as polyhedra in surface view.

**cylindrical e.,** columnar e.

**e. duc'tus semicircula'ris** [ NA ], the simple squamous e. of the semicircular ducts.

**enamel e.,** usually referred to as reduced enamel e.; term used to denote the several layers of the enamel organ remaining on the enamel surface after formation of enamel is completed.

**external enamel e.,** the cuboidal cells of the outer layer of an enamel organ of a developing tooth.

**germinal e.,** (1) a layer of celomic epithelial cells covering the gonadial ridges as they are formed on the mesial border of the mesonephroi near the root of the mesentery; (2) the mesothelial covering of the adult ovary.

**gingival e.,** a stratified squamous e. that undergoes some degree of keratinization and is connected to the enamel or cementum of the tooth and to connective tissue beneath it.

**glandular e.,** e. composed of secretory cells.

**laminated e.,** stratified e.

**e. of lens,** e. lentis.

**e. len'tis** [ NA ], e. of the lens; the layer of cuboidal cells lying on the anterior surface of the crystalline lens inside the lens capsule. At the equator the cells elongate and give rise to the lens fibers.

**mesenchymal e.,** the flat e. derived from mesenchymal cells found lining certain connective tissue spaces such as

the anterior chamber of eye, perilymph spaces in the ear, and subdural and subarachnoid spaces.

**muscle e.,** myoepithelium.

**olfactory e.,** an e. of the pseudostratified type which contains olfactory, receptor, nerve cells whose axons extend to the olfactory bulb of the brain.

**pavement e.,** simple squamous e.

**pigment e.,** pigment epitheliopathy; an acute disease manifested by rapid loss of vision, and multifocal, cream-colored placoid lesions of the retinal pigment epithelium; resolves spontaneously with return of visual function.

**pigmented e.,** e. composed of cells containing granules of pigment as in the pigment layer of the retina or on the back of the iris.

**pseudostratified e.,** an e. which gives a superficial appearance of being stratified because the cell nuclei are at different levels, but in which all cells reach the basement membrane, hence it is classed as a simple e.

**reduced enamel e.,** enamel e.

**respiratory e.,** the pseudostratified ciliated e. that lines the conducting portion of the airway, including part of the nasal cavity and larynx, the trachea, and bronchi.

**seminiferous e.,** the e. lining the convoluted tubules of the testis where spermatogenesis and spermiogenesis occur.

**simple e.,** an e. having one layer of cells.

**simple squamous e.,** pavement e.; e. composed of a single layer of flattened scalelike cells, such as mesothelium, endothelium, and that in the pulmonary alveoli.

**strat'ified e.,** a type composed of a series of layers, the cells of each varying in size and shape. It is named more specifically according to the type of cells at the surface, *e.g.,* stratified squamous e., stratified columnar e., stratified ciliated columnar e.

**stratified ciliated columnar e.,** an e. consisting of several layers of cells with the deeper cells being polyhedral in form and the surface ones columnar with motile cilia. The fetal esophagus is lined with this type.

**stratified squamous e.,** an e. consisting of several layers in which the surface cells are flattened and scalelike and the deeper cells are polyhedral in form; the surface may be cornified and dry, or noncornified and moist.

**sulcular e.,** crevicular e.

**tesselated e.,** a term formerly used to designate a simple e. having the appearance of a mosaic, in surface view.

**transitional e.,** stratified e. of several layers, each of which is formed by a transformation of the cells from the layer below; it occurs in the kidney, ureter, and bladder.

**epithelization** (ep-ĭ-the-lĭ-za'shun). Epithelialization.

**ep'ithem** [ G. *epithēma,* a cover ]. An external application, such as a poultice, but not a plaster or ointment.

**epithesis** (e-pith'e-sis) [ epi- + G. *tithenai,* to place ]. 1. Orthopaedic correction of a deformed extremity. 2. A splint or other apparatus applied to an extremity.

**ep'ithet** [ G. *epithetos,* added, fr. epi- + *tithenai,* to place ]. A characterizing term or name.

**specific e.,** in bacteriology, the second part of the name of a species; the name of a bacterial species consists of two parts, the generic name and the specific e.

**epithi'azide** (USAN). THIAVER; 6-chloro-3,4-dihydro-3-{[ (2,2,2-trifluoroethyl)-thio ] methyl}-2$H$-1,2,4-benzothiadiazine-7-sulfonamide 1,1-dioxide; diuretic for treatment of essential hypertension.

**epitox'oid.** A toxoid that has less affinity for specific antitoxin than that manifested by the toxin.

**epitrichial** (ep-ĭ-trik'ĭ-al). Relating to the epitrichium.

**epitrichium** (ep-ĭ-trik'ĭ-um) [ epi- + G. *trichion,* dim, of *thrix,* (*trich-*), hair ]. Periderm.

**epitrochlea** (ep-ĭ-trok'le-ah) [ epi- + L. *trochlea,* a pulley, block, contr. fr. G. *trochilia* ]. *Epicondylus medialis humeri.*

**epitrochlear** (ep-ĭ-trok'le-ar). Relating to the epitrochlea.

**epituberculosis** (ep-ĭ-tu-ber-ku-lo'sis). The occurrence of glandular swelling and pulmonary infiltration in the neighborhood of a focus of pulmonary tuberculosis or of enlarged bronchial glands, simulating caseation but not always tuberculous in essence. The sputum often contains no bacilli, though the tuberculin test may be positive. The affection, which is usually apyretic, occurs most often in the young. Recovery is the rule.

**epitympan'ic.** Above, or in the upper part of, the tympanum.

**epitympanum** (ep'ĭ-tim'pă-num). *Recessus* epitympanicus.

**epityphlitis** (ep'ĭ-tif-li'tis) [ epi- + G. *typhlon*, cecum, + suffix -*itis*, inflammation ]. Appendicitis.

**epivaginitis** (ep-ĭ-vaj-ĭ-ni'tis) [ epi- + L. *vagina*, sheath, + G. suffix -*itis*, inflammation ]. A chronic veneral disease of cattle long known in certain areas in Africa and recognized recently in California. It is believed to be of viral origin, and is characterized by vaginitis and sterility in females, and epididymitis and sterility in males.

**epizo'ic.** Living as a parasite on the skin surface.

**epizoology** (ep-ĭ-zo-ol'o-jĭ) [ epi- + G. *zōon*, animal, + *logos*, study ]. Epizootiology.

**epizoon,** pl. **epizoa** (ep-ĭ-zo'on, ep-ĭ-zo'ah) [ epi- + G. *zōon*, animal ]. An animal parasite living on the body surface.

**epizootic** (ep'ĭ-zo-ot'ik) [ epi- + G. *zōon*, animal ]. 1. Denoting a disease attacking a large number of animals simultaneously. 2. Denoting the prevalence of a disease among animals, similar to an epidemic among humans.

**epizootiology** (ep-ĭ-zo-ot'ĭ-ol-o-jĭ) [ epi- + G. *zōon*, animal, + *logos*, study ]. Epizoology; the science that deals with epidemics of disease among animals.

**épluchage** (a-plü-shazh') [ F. picking, cleaning ]. The removal of all contaminated tissue in infected wounds.

**eponychia** (ep-o-nik'ĭ-ah). Infection involving the proximal nail fold.

**eponychium** (ep-on-nik'ĭ-um) [ G. *epi*, upon, + *onyx* (*onych*-), nail ]. Epionychium. 1. The condensed eleidin-rich areas of the epidermis preceding the formation of the nail in the embryo. 2 [ NA ]. Perionychium; the epidermis forming the ungual wall behind and at the sides of the nail. 3. The thin skin adherent to the nail at its proximal portion. See fig. under unguis.

**eponym** (ep'o-nim) [ G. *epōnymos*, named after ]. The name of a disease, structure, operation, or procedure, supposedly derived from the name of the person who discovered or described it first.

**eponym'ic.** 1. Relating to an eponym. 2. An eponym.

**epon'ymous.** Eponymic.

**epoophorectomy** (ep-o-of'o-rek'to-mĭ) [ G. *epi*, upon, + *ōophoros*, bearing eggs, + *ektomē*, excision ]. Removal of the epoophoron.

**epoophoron** (ep'o-of'o-ron) [ epi- + G. *ōophoros*, egg-bearing ]. [ NA ]. Organ of Rosenmüller; pampiniform body; a collection of rudimentary tubules in the mesosalpinx between the ovary and the uterine tube; it is the remains of the tubules of the Wolffian body and is the analogue of the paradidymis in the male.

   **duct of e.,** *ductus* epoophori longitudinalis.

**epornitic** (ep'or-nit'ik). Relating to epornosis.

**epornosis** (ep'or-no'sis) [ *epi* + G. *ornis*, bird, + suffix -*osis*, condition ]. Term for epizootic when applied to birds.

**epox'y.** Chemical term describing an oxygen atom bound to two linked carbon atoms, *e.g.*, —CH—CH—. Produced

                                   O

from peracids acting on alkenes. Important chemical intermediates; basis of epoxy resins (polymers) formed from epoxy monomers.

**Epsom salt.** Magnesium sulfate.

**EPSP.** Abbreviation for excitatory postsynaptic *potential*.

**Epstein,** Alois, German pediatrician, 1849–1918. See E.'s *cysts, disease, pearls*.

**Epstein,** B., German physician. See E.'s *symptom*.

**epulis** (ep-u'lis) [ G. *epoulis*, a gumboil. UL-2 ]. Peripheral fibroma; persisting inflammatory hyperplasia of the gingiva.

   **e. fissura'tum,** inflammatory fibrous *hyperplasia*.

   **e. gravida'rum,** gingival tumors of pregnancy.

   **pigmented e.,** melanotic neuroectodermal *tumor*.

**ep'uloid.** A nodule or mass (in the gingival tissue) that resembles an epulis.

**epulosis** (ep'u-lo'sis) [ G. *epoulōsis*, a scarring over ]. Cicatrization.

**epulot'ic.** 1. Cicatrizing. 2. An agent that promotes cicatrization.

**equation** (e-kwa'zhun) [ L. *aequare*, to make equal ]. A statement expressing the equality of two things, usually with the use of mathematical or chemical symbols.

   **Arrhenius' e.,** an e. relating chemical reaction rate ($k$) to the absolute temperature ($T$) by the equation ($d \ln k / dT$) $= (\Delta E / RT^2)$.

   **Bohr's e.,** an e. to calculate the respiratory dead space from the fact that gas expired from the lungs is a mixture of gas from the dead space and gas from the alveoli, *i.e.*, the dead space volume divided by the tidal volume equals the difference between alveolar and mixed expired gas composition, divided by the difference between alveolar and inspired gas composition; gas composition can be expressed in any consistent units of concentration or partial pressure of oxygen or carbon dioxide.

   **chemical e.,** an e. on one side of which are the reactants and on the other side the products of a chemical reaction; the two halves may be separated by an equals sign or by arrows.

   **constant field e.,** Goldman e.

   **Einthoven's e.,** Einthoven's *law*.

   **Gibbs-Helmholtz e.,** expresses the relationship in a galvanic cell between the chemical energy transformed and the maximal electromotive force obtainable.

   **Goldman e.,** constant field e.; Goldman-Hodgkin-Katz (GHK) e.; an e. derived to predict membrane potentials in terms of the membrane's permeability to ions and their concentrations on either side.

   **Goldman-Hodgkin-Katz (GHK) e.,** Goldman e.

   **Hasselbalch's e.,** Henderson-Hasselbalch e.

   **Henderson-Hasselbalch e.,** Hasselbalch's e.; a formula relating the pH of a solution to the ratio of bicarbonate ion concentration to free carbon dioxide in solution: pH = pK' + log ([ $HCO_3^-$ ]/[ $CO_2$ ]). The value of pK' for blood plasma is 6.10 and includes the first dissociation constant of $H_2CO_3$, the relation between [ $H_2CO_3$ ] and [ $CO_2$ ], and other corrections. The partial pressure of $CO_2$ multiplied by its solubility (0.0301 mM/liter/mm Hg) is commonly substituted for [ $CO_2$ ]. Example: When the plasma bicarbonate concentration is 24 mEq/liter and the $P_{CO_2}$ is 40 mm Hg, the pH = 6.10 + log (24/0.0301 × 40) = 7.40.

   **Hill's e.,** $y/100 = (Kx^n/1 + Kx^n)$, where $y$ is the per cent saturation of blood, $x$ the oxygen pressure, and $K$ and $n$ are constants; this represents the shape of the oxygen dissociation curve of hemoglobin, which would be hyperbolic if $n$ equaled 1, but which becomes increasingly sigmoid with higher values of $n$; for human blood, $n$ equals 2.5.

   **Hufner's e.,** an e. expressing the relationship between myoglobin dissociation and oxygen partial pressure: ([ $MBO_2$ ]/[ Mb ]) = ($K × pO_2$).

   **Lineweaver-Burk e.,** a rearrangement of the Michaelis-Menten equation, $K_m = [ S ](V_{max} - V)/V$, to $[ S ]/V = [ S ]/V_{max} + K_m/V_{max}$, in which form a plot of $[ S ]/V$ versus $[ S ]$ gives a straight line of slope $1/V_{max}$ and intercept $K_m$. See also Michaelis-Menten *constant*.

   **Michaelis-Menten e.,** see Michaelis-Menten *constant*.

   **Nernst e.,** the e. relating the equilibrium potential of electrodes to ion concentrations; the e. relating the electrical potential and concentration gradient of an ion across a permeable membrane at equilibrium: $E = [ RT/nF ] [ \ln (C_1/C_2) ]$, where $E$ = potential, R = absolute gas constant, $T$ = absolute temperature, $n$ = valence, $F$ = the Faraday, ln = the natural logarithm, and $C_1$ and $C_2$ are the ion concentrations on the two sides; in nonideal solutions, concentration should be replaced by activity; see also Nernst theory, activity (2).

   **personal e.,** a slight error in judgment, perceptual response, or action peculiar to the individual and so constant that it is usually possible to allow for it in accepting the person's statements or conclusions, thus arriving at approximate exactness.

**equa'tor** [ Mediev. L. *aequator*, fr. L. *aequo*, to make equal ] [ NA ]. A line encircling a globular body, equidistant at all points from the two poles; the periphery of a plane cutting a sphere at the midpoint of, and at right angles to, its axis.

**e. bulbi oc'uli** [ NA ], e. of the eyeball; an imaginary line encircling the globe of the eye equidistant from the anterior and posterior poles.

**e. of the crystalline lens,** e. lentis.

**e. of the eyeball,** e. bulbi oculi.

**e. lentis** [ NA ], e. of the crystalline lens; the periphery of the lens lying between the two layers of the zonula ciliaris.

**equatorial** (e-kwa-to'rī-al). Situated, like the earth's equator, equidistant from each end.

**equiaxial** (e'kwī-ak'sī-al). Having axes of equal length.

**e'quicalor'ic** [ L. *aequus,* equal, + *calor,* heat ]. Equal in heat value; see also isodynamic.

**equilenin** (e'kwī-len'in). 3-Hydroxy-1,3,5(10),6,8-estrapentaen-17-one; an estrogenic steroid isolated from pregnant mare's urine. For structure of parent estrane, see steroids.

**equilibration** (e'kwī-lī-bra'shun). 1. The act of maintaining an equilibrium or balance. 2. The act of exposing a liquid, *e.g.,* blood or plasma, to a gas at a certain partial pressure until the partial pressures of the gas within and without the liquid are equal. 3. In dentistry, the equalization of pressure, as in occlusal e., *q.v.*

**occlusal e.,** the modification of occlusal forms of teeth by grinding with the intent of equalizing occlusal stress, or producing simultaneous occlusal contacts, or of harmonizing cuspal relations.

**equilibrium** (e'kwī-lib'rī-um) [ L. *aequilibrium,* a horizontal position, fr. *aequus,* equal, + *libra,* a balance ]. Poise; the condition of being evenly balanced; A state of repose between two or more antagonistic forces that exactly counteract each other, or (more often in chemistry) a state of apparent repose created by two reactions proceeding in opposite directions at equal speed—this being termed dynamic e. In chemical equations, these opposite directions are sometimes indicated by two opposing arrows ( ⇌ ) instead of the equal sign. See also equilibrium *constant.*

**acid-base e.,** acid-base *balance.*

**Donnan e.,** Gibbs-Donnan e.; when a semipermeable membrane or its equivalent (*e.g.,* a solid ion-exchanger) separates a nondiffusible substance, such as protein, from diffusible substances, the diffusible anions and cations are distributed on the two sides of the membrane so that (1) the products of their concentrations are equal, and (2) the sum of the diffusible and nondiffusible anions on either side of the membrane is equal to the sum of the concentrations of diffusible and nondiffusible cations. The unequal distribution of diffusible ions causes a potential difference between two sides of the membrane (membrane potential).

**Gibbs-Donnan e.,** Donnan e.

**homeostatic e.,** see homeostasis.

**nitrog'enous e.,** a condition in which the amount of nitrogen excreted from the body equals that taken in with the food; nutritive e. so far as protein is concerned.

**nutritive e.,** physiologic e.; condition in which there is a perfect balance between intake and excretion of nutritive material, so that there is no increase or loss in weight.

**physiologic e.,** nutritive e.

**radioactive e.,** a situation (not a true equilibrium) in which a particular atom is being produced by the radioactive breakdown of a precursor while it is itself breaking down, the two breakdowns matching so that the temporary amount of the atom in question remains constant.

**equilin** (ek'wī-lin). 3-Hydroxy-1,3,5(10),7-estratraen-17-one (for estrane structure, see steroids); an estrogenic steroid occurring in the urine of pregnant mares.

**equimolecular** (e'kwī-mo-lek'u-lar). Containing an equal number of molecules; referring, for example, to two or more solutions.

**equination** (e'kwī-na'shun). Inoculation of man with the virus of horsepox, as a means of protection against smallpox.

**equine** (ē'kwin) [ L. *equinus,* fr. *equus,* horse ]. Relating to, derived from, or resembling the horse, mule, ass, or other members of the genus *Equus.*

**equinovalgus** (e-kwi'no-val'gus, ek'wī-no-). *Talipes* equinovalgus.

**equinovarus** (e-kwi'no-va'rus, ek'wī-no-). *Talipes* equinovarus.

**equinus** [ L. ] [ NA ]. Equine.

**equipax.** Carbamic acid 1-cyclohexylpropyl ester; antianxiety agent.

**equiseto'sis.** A toxicosis in horses caused by eating equisetum.

**equitoxic** (e'kwī-tok'sik). Of equivalent toxicity.

**equivalence, equivalency** (e-kwiv'ā-lens, -len-sī) [ L. *aequus,* equal, + *valentia,* strength (valence) ]. 1. The property of an element or radical of combining with or displacing, in definite and fixed proportion, another element or radical in a compound. 2. Valence.

**equivalent** (e-kwiv'ā-lent) [ see equivalence ]. 1. Equal in any respect. 2. Something that is equal in size, weight, force, or any other quality to something else.

**chemical e.,** gram e.

**combustion e.,** the heat value of a gram of carbohydrate or fat oxidized outside the body.

**epileptic e.,** usually in a psychomotor epileptic, instead of a typical seizure some other manifestation occurs, such as cough, abdominal pain, severe headache, etc. See also epileptic *temper.*

**gold e.,** see under gold.

**gram e.,** chemical e.; combining weight; equivalent weight; (1) the weight in grams of an element that combines with or replaces 1 gm. of hydrogen; (2) the atomic or molecular weight in grams of an atom or group of atoms involved in a chemical reaction divided by the number of electrons donated, taken up, or shared by the atom or group of atoms in the course of that reaction; (3) the weight of a substance contained in 1 liter of 1 normal solution (a variant of (1)).

**Joule's e.,** the dynamic e. of heat; the amount of work that, if converted into heat, will raise the temperature of 1 pound of water 1°F. is 778 foot-pounds; in metric units, 1 calorie, which raises 1 gm water 1°C., equals $4.18 \times 10^7$ dynecentimeters.

**nitrogen e.,** see under nitrogen.

**psychic e.,** a transitory mental obscuration manifested by amnesia, fugue, sleepwalking, or the like, taking the place of an ordinary epileptic or hysterical attack.

**starch e.,** see under starch.

**toxic e.,** the amount of toxin or other poison per kilogram of weight necessary to kill an animal.

**Er.** Chemical symbol of the element erbium.

**ER.** Abbreviation for endoplasmic *reticulum.*

**erasion** (e-ra'zhun) [ L. *eradere,* to erase ]. The scraping away of tissue, especially of bone.

**Erasistratus** (er-ā-sist'rā-tus), Greek physician, surgeon, anatomist, and physiologist of the Alexandrian School, circa 300 B.C. He was one of the first to dissect and describe different parts of the human body, including the trachea, atria, and valves of the heart with the chordae tendineae. He opposed the humoral doctrine and has been called the Father of Physiology.

**Erb,** Wilhelm H., German neurologist, 1840–1921. See E.'s *atrophy,* E.'s *disease,* E.-Charcot *disease,* E.'s *palsy,* E.'s *paralysis,* E.'s spinal *paralysis,* Duchenne-E. *paralysis,* E.'s *point,* E.'s *sign,* E.-Westphal *sign,* Westphal-E. *sign.*

**Erben,** Siegmund, Vienna physician, *1863. See E.'s *phenomenon.*

**ERBF.** Abbreviation for effective renal blood *flow.*

**er'bium.** A rare earth (lanthanide) element, symbol Er, atomic no. 68, atomic weight 167.27.

**Erdheim,** Jakob, 1874–1937. See E. *tumor.*

**Erdmann,** Hugo, German chemist, 1862–1910. See E.'s *reagent.*

**erec'tile.** Capable of erection; see e. *tissue.*

**erection** (e-rek'shun) [ L. *erectio,* fr. *erigo,* pp. *erectus,* to set up ]. The condition of erectile tissue when filled with blood, which then becomes hard and unyielding; denoting especially this state of the external genital organs.

**persistent e. of penis,** priapism.

**erector** [ Mod. L. ]. 1. One who or that which raises or makes erect. 2 [ NA ]. Denoting specifically certain muscles having such action.

**eremacausis** (ĕr'e-mā-kaw'sis) [ G. *ērema,* softly, gently, + *kausis,* a burning ]. Slow combustion or oxidation, as by exposure to air.

**eremiopho'bia.** Eremophobia.

**eremophilia** (ĕr'e-mo-fil'ĭ-ah) [ G. *erēmia*, solitude, + *philia*, affection for ]. Morbid desire to be alone.

**eremophobia** (ĕr'e-mo-fo'bĭ-ah) [ G. *erēmia*, solitude, + *phobos*, fear ]. Eremiophobia; morbid fear of deserted places or of solitude.

**erep'sin.** Obsolete term for peptidases secreted in the intestinal juice.

**erep'tase.** Erepsin.

**erethism** (ĕr'ĕ-thizm) [ G. *erethismos*, irritation ]. An abnormal state of excitement or irritation, either general or local.

**erethis'mic, erethis'tic, erethit'ic.** Marked by or causing erethism; excited; irritable.

**erethizophrenia** (ĕr-ĕ-thiz'o-fre'nĭ-ah) [ G. *erethizō*, to excite, + *phrēn*, the mind ]. Exaggerated mental irritability.

**ereuthophobia** (ĕr'u-tho-fo'bĭ-ah) [ G. *ereuthos*, blushing, + *phobos*, fear ]. A morbid fear of blushing.

**ERG.** Abbreviation for electroretinogram.

**erg** [ G. *ergon*, work. ERG- ]. The unit of work in the cgs system; the amount of work done by 1 dyne acting through 1 cm.; 1 gm. cm.²/sec.² One erg equals $10^{-7}$ joule, the SI unit of work.

**ergasia** (er-ga'zĭ-ah) [ G. work. ERG- ]. 1. Any form of activity, especially mental. 2. The total of functions and reactions of an individual.

**ergasiodermatosis** (er-gas'ĭ-o-der-mă-to'sis). An occupational dermatosis.

**ergasiomania** (er-gas-ĭ-o-ma'nĭ-ah) [ G. *ergasia*, work, + *mania*, insanity ]. A morbid or obsessive need to work.

**ergasiophobia** (er-gas-ĭ-o-fo'bĭ-ah) [ G. *ergasia*, work, + *phobos*, fear ]. An aversion to work of any kind.

**ergasthenia** (er-gas-the'nĭ-ah) [ G. *ergasia*, work, + *astheneia*, weakness, disease ]. Debility or any morbid symptoms due to overwork.

**ergastoplasm** (er-gas'to-plazm) [ G. *ergastēr*, a workman, + *plasma*, something formed ]. Granular cytoplasmic reticulum.

**ergin** (er'jin). A hypothetical substance in the blood or tissue fluids presumed to lead to the allergic phenomenon, as a result of the union of the e. with allergen. See also reagin.

**erg'ine.** Lysergic acid amide.

**ergo-** [ G. *ergon*, work ]. Combining form relating to work.

**ergoba'sine.** Ergonovine.

**er'gocalcif'erol** (USP, BP). D₂; calciferol; viosterol; v. D of plant origin; 9,10-secocholesta-5,7,10(19),22-ergostatet-raen-3β-ol; arises from ultraviolet irradiation of ergosterol, which is cleaved at the 9,10 bond and develops a double bond between C-10 and C-19. Used in prophylaxis and treatment of vitamin D deficiency.

**er'gocor'nine.** $C_{31}H_{39}N_5 O_5$; an alkaloid isolated from ergot; isomeric with ergocorninine.

**er'gocris'tine.** $C_{35}H_{39}N_5O_5$; an alkaloid isolated from ergot; isomeric with ergocristinine.

**er'gocryp'tine.** $C_{32}H_{41}N_5O_5$; an alkaloid isolated from ergot; isomeric with ergocryptinine.

**ergodynamograph** (er'go-di-nam'o-graf) [ ergo- + G. *dynamis*, force, + *graphō*, to write ]. An instrument for recording both the degree of muscular force and the amount of the work accomplished by muscular contraction.

**ergoesthesiograph** (er'go-es-the'zĭ-o-graf) [ ergo- + G. *aisthēsis*, sensation, + *graphō*, to record ]. An apparatus for recording graphically muscular aptness as shown in the ability to counterbalance variable resistances.

**ergogenic** (er-go-jen'ik). Tending to increase work.

**ergograph** (er'go-graf) [ ergo- + G. *graphō*, to write ]. An instrument for recording the amount of work done by muscular contractions, or the amplitude of contraction.

  **Mosso's e.,** an instrument consisting of pulleys, weights, and a recording lever, which is used to obtain a graphic record of flexion of a finger, hand, or arm.

**ergographic** (er-go-graf'ik). Relating to the ergograph and the record made by it.

**ergom'eter** (er-gom'e-ter) [ ergo- + G. *metron*, measure ]. Dynamometer.

**ergomet'rine.** Ergonovine.

  **e. maleate** (BP), ergonovine maleate.

**ergonom'ics** [ ergo- + G. *nomos*, law ]. A branch of ecology dealing with human factors in the design and operations of machines and the physical environment.

**ergonovine** (er-go-no'vēn, -vin). Ergometrine, ergobasine, ergostetrine; an alkaloid from ergot; on hydrolysis it yields D-lysergic acid and L-2-aminopropanol.

  **e. maleate,** ergometrine maleate (BP); a powerful oxytocic agent. This action is more prominent, and other actions of ergot (vasoconstriction, central nervous system stimulation, adrenergic blockade, etc.) are less prominent than for other ergot alkaloids. Effective orally and parenterally.

**ergophore** (er'go-fōr) [ ergo- + G. *phoros*, bearing ]. Denoting the reactive group of the antigen or antibody molecule upon which its specific action (toxic, lytic, etc.) depends, in contrast to the haptophore or combining group.

**ergosine** (er'go-sēn, -sin). An alkaloid from ergot with actions similar to those of ergotamine.

**er'gostat** [ ergo- + G. *statos*, standing, placed. STA- ]. A form of machine for exercising the muscles.

**ergos'terin.** Ergosterol.

**ergos'terol.** 5,7,22-Ergostatrien-3β-ol (for structure of ergostene, see steroids); most important of the provitamins D₂; ultraviolet irradiation converts e. to lumisterol, tachysterol, and vitamin D₂.

**ergostetrine** (er-go-stet'rēn, -rin). Ergonovine.

**er'got.** Secale cornutum or clavatum; spurred rye; rye smut; the sclerotium of the fungus *Claviceps purpurea;* a horny, elongated, blackish purple mass of peculiar disagreeable odor, which replaces the grain of rye (*Secale cereale*) attacked by this fungus. It causes contraction of the muscular coat of the arteries, raising blood pressure, and contraction of the uterine muscle.

**ergotamine** (er-got'am-ēn). $c_{33}H_{35}N_5O_5$; an alkaloid from ergot. It is a potent stimulant of smooth muscle, particularly of the blood vessels and the uterus, and produces adrenergic blockade (chiefly of the alpha receptors). Used for the relief of migraine. The hydrogenated e., dihydroergotamine, is less toxic and has fewer side-effects.

  **e. tartrate** (USP, BP), GYNERGEN; has same action as e.

**ergotaminine** (er-got-am'ĭ-nēn). An isomer of ergotamine but practically inert.

**ergother'apy** [ G. *ergon*, work, + *therapeia*, therapy ]. Treatment of disease by muscular exercise.

**ergothio'neine.** Thioneine; 2'-thiolhistidine betaine; the betaine of a sulfur-containing derivative of histidine, present in blood and other mammalian tissue and in ergot.

**ergot'inine.** A mixture (1:1:1) of ergocorninine, ergocristidinine, and ergocryptimine, isomeric with ergotoxine but devoid of pharmacologic activity.

**ergotism** (er'got-izm). Poisoning by a toxic substance contained in the sclerotia of the fungus, *Claviceps purpurea*, which grows on many grasses and on some grains, especially rye. The symptoms are identical with those of fescue foot, *i.e.,* lameness and necrosis of the extremities due to contraction of the peripheral vascular bed.

**er'gotized.** 1. Said of rye attacked by *Claviceps purpurea*. 2. Under the therapeutic or toxic influence of ergot.

**ergotoxine** (er'go-tok'sēn, -sin). Ecboline; a mixture of alkaloids obtained from ergot, consisting of a 1:1:1 mixture of ergocristine, ergocornine and ergokryptine. This mixture is a potent stimulant of smooth muscle, particularly of the blood vessels and uterus. It produces adrenergic blockade (chiefly of the alpha receptors). It is more toxic than the other natural and semisynthetic ergot alkaloids.

**ergotropic** (er'go-trop'ik) [ ergo- + G. *tropos*, a turning ]. The term introduced by W. R. Hess to denote those mechanisms and the functional status of the nervous system that favor the organism's capacity to expend energy, as distinguished from the trophotropic mechanisms promoting rest and reconstitution of energy stores. In general, the balance between ergotropic and trophotropic nervous mechanisms corresponds in large part to that between the sympathetic and parasympathetic subdivisions of the autonomic nervous system.

**Erichsen,** John E., London surgeon, 1818–1896. See E.'s *sign.*

**Erina'ceus europae'us** [ L. *erinaceus,* hedgehog ]. A European hedgehog very susceptible to yellow fever.

**eriodictin** (ĕr-ĭ-o-dik'tin). Eriodictyol-L-rhamnoside; a glycoside associated with hesperidin in citrin or vitamin P.

**eriodictyol** (ĕr-ĭ-o-dikt'ĭ-ol). The aglycone of eriodictin, a 3′,4′,5,7-tetrahydroxyflavanone (*cf.* catechin); used for treatment of Ménière's disease.

**er'iodic'tyon** (NF). Mountain balm; yerba santa; the dried leaves of *Eriodictyon californicum* (family Hydrophyllaceae). The fluidextract and the syrup have been used as an expectorant and to mask the taste of bitter substances.

**eris'iphake, eris'ophake.** Erysiphake.

**Erlanger,** Joseph, U. S. physiologist, *1874. Nobel laureate, 1944, with Herbert S. Gasser for their discoveries relating to the highly differentiated functions of single nerve fibers.

**Erlenmeyer** (air'len-mi-er), Emil, German chemist, 1825–1909. See E. *flask,* E. flask *deformity.*

**Ernst,** Paul, German pathologist, 1859–1937. See Babès-E. *bodies.*

**erode** (e-rōd') [ L. *erodere,* to gnaw away ]. To wear away; to corrode; to remove by ulceration.

**erogenous** (e-roj'ĕ-nus). Capable of producing sexual excitement when stimulated.

**eros** (e'ros, ĕr'os) [ G. love ]. In psychoanalysis, the life principle representing all instinctual tendencies toward procreation and life, as opposed to thanatos (*q. v.*). See also subentries under instinct.

**erose** (e-rōs') [ L. *erodo,* pp. *erosus,* to gnaw away ]. Denoting an edge or margin which is irregularly notched or indented, as if gnawed away; used especially in reference to bacterial colonies.

**erosion** (e-ro'zhun) [ L. *erosio,* fr. *erodo,* to gnaw away ]. 1. A wearing away; a state of being worn away. 2. A shallow ulcer; in the stomach and intestine, an ulcer limited to the mucosa, with no penetration of the muscularis mucosa. 3. Odontolysis; the wearing away of the surface of a tooth by chemical action; when the cause is unknown, it is referred to as idiopathic e.

  **Dieulafoy's e.,** acute ulcerative gastroenteritis complicating pneumonia, possibly caused by overproduction of cortisone.

**ero'sive.** 1. Having the property of eroding or wearing away. 2. An eroding agent.

**erot'ic** [ G. *erōtikos,* relating to love, fr. *erōs,* love ]. Relating to sexual passion; lustful; having the quality to arouse sexual drive.

**eroticism** (ĕ-rot'ĭ-sizm). Erotism.

**erotism** (ĕr'o-tizm). Eroticism; a condition of sexual excitement.

  **anal e.,** pleasurable experience centered around the anal zone, especially during the anal phase in children.

**er'otization.** Libidinization; the act of erotizing or the state of being erotized.

**erotogen'esis.** The origin or genesis of sexual impulses.

**erotogenic** (ĕr'o-to-jen'ik) [ G. *erōs,* love, + suffix *-gen,* production ]. Causing sexual excitement.

**erotomania** (ĕr'o-to-ma'nĭ-ah) [ G. *erōs,* love, + *mania,* frenzy ]. Excessive or morbid inclination to erotic thoughts and behavior.

**ero'topath.** A subject of erotopathy.

**erotopath'ic.** Relating to erotopathy.

**erotopathy** (ĕr'o-top'ă-thĭ) [ G. *erōs,* love, + *pathos,* suffering ]. Any abnormality of the sexual impulse.

**erotophobia** (ĕr'o-to-fo'bĭ-ah) [ G. *erōs,* love, + *phobos,* fear ]. A morbid aversion to the thought of sexual love and to its physical expression.

**erotopsychic** (ĕr'o-to-si'kik) [ G. *erōs,* love, + *psychē,* the mind ]. Erotopathic.

**ERPF.** Abbreviation for effective renal plasma *flow.*

**erratic** (ĕr-rat'ik) [ L. *erro,* pp. *erratus,* to wander ]. 1. Eccentric. 2. Denoting pains or other symptoms that change their seat, wandering from one part of the body to another.

**erubes'cence** [ L. *erubescere,* to redden ]. A blush, or reddening of the skin.

**erubescent** (ĕr-u-bes'ent). Denoting a flushing or reddening of the skin.

**eru'cic acid.** *cis-*13-Docosenoic acid; a 22-carbon unsaturated fatty acid present in the seeds of nasturtium (Indian cress) and of several *Cruciferae* species (rape, mustard, and wallflower).

**eructation** (e-ruk-ta'shun) [ L. *eructo,* pp. *-atus,* to belch ]. Belching; the raising of gas or of a small quantity of acid fluid from the stomach.

**eruption** (e-rup'shun) [ L. *e-rumpo,* pp. *-ruptus,* to break out ]. 1. A breaking out, especially the appearance of lesions on the skin. 2. A rapidly developing dermatosis of the skin or mucous membranes, especially when appearing as a local manifestation of a general disease, such as typhoid fever or one of the exanthemata; an e. is characterized, according to the nature of the lesion, as macular, papular, vesicular, pustular, bullous, nodular, erythematous, etc. 3. The passage of a tooth through the alveolar process and perforation of the gums; cutting of a tooth.

  **accelerated e.,** refers to a dental e. pattern which is advanced chronologically, in comparison with the average pattern of dental e. It is marked by e. of the first tooth at an earlier age than the average, with the intervals of time between subsequent dental e.'s shorter than in the average e. pattern.

  **butterfly e.,** butterfly (2).

  **clinical e.,** development of the crown of a tooth that can be observed clinically.

  **continuous e.,** the e. of a tooth into the mouth and its continuous movement in a vertical direction.

  **creeping e.,** cutaneous *larva* migrans.

  **delayed e.,** refers to a dental e. pattern which is later chronologically in comparison with the average pattern of dental e. It is marked by e. of the first tooth at a later age than the average, with the intervals of time between subsequent dental e.'s longer than in the average e. pattern.

  **drug e.,** dermatitis medicamentosa; dermatosis medicamentosa; drug or medicinal rash; medicinal eruption; any e. caused by the ingestion, injection, inhalation, or insertion of a drug, most often the result of allergic sensitization; reactions to drugs applied to the cutaneous surface are not generally designated as drug e., but rather as contact type dermatitis.

  **fixed drug e.,** a type of drug e. that recurs at a fixed site (or sites) following the administration of a particular drug; the lesions usually consist of intensely erythematous and purplish, sharply demarcated macules, and occasionally of herpetic vesicles; the affected areas undergo gradual involution, but flare and enlarge on readministration of the offending drug.

  **iodine e.,** an acneform or follicular e. or granulomatous lesion caused by a reaction to systemic iodine or iodide administration.

  **Kaposi's varicel'liform e.,** *eczema* herpeticum.

  **medicinal e.,** drug *eruption.*

  **polymorphic light e.,** a papular, sometimes eczematous, e. appearing in a few hours and lasting up to several days on skin exposed to shortwave ultraviolet light; the exact mechanism is not known.

  **serum e.,** serum *sickness.*

  **surgical e.,** the uncovering of an unerupted tooth to permit its further e. into the oral cavity by surgically removing overlying soft tissue, bone, and sometimes teeth.

**erup'tive.** Characterized by eruption.

**ERV.** Abbreviation for expiratory reserve *volume.*

**erysimum** (ĕ-ris'ĭ-mum) [ G. *erysimon,* hedgemustard ]. E. *helveticum* and E. *crepidifolium* (family Cruciferae); contains a β-glycoside, helvetocoside, which is one mole strophanthidin and one mole d-digitoxose.

**erysipelas** (ĕr-ĭ-sip'ĕ-las) [ G. from *erythros,* red, + *pella,* skin ]. Rose (1); a specific, acute, inflammatory disease caused by a hemolytic streptococcus. The eruption, limited to the skin and sharply defined, is usually accompanied by severe constitutional symptoms.

  **coast e.,** onchocerciasis.

  **e. inter'num,** an erysipelatous eruption in the vagina, uterus, and peritoneum, occurring in the puerperium.

  **e. mi'grans,** ambulant e.; wandering e.; a widely spreading form involving the entire face, or even the surface of the body.

**e. perstans faciei,** chronic, dusky red eruption of erysipelas on the face.

**phleg′monous e.,** a form marked by invasion of the subcutaneous tissues, with the formation of deep-seated abscesses.

**e. pustulo′sum,** development of pustules over the area of e.

**surgical e.,** e. caused by infection of the wound following a surgical procedure.

**swine e.,** a destructive disease of swine, occurring in both acute and chronic forms, caused by a bacterium, *Erysipelothrix rhusiopathiae.*

**e. verruco′sum,** development of verrucous or warty lesions on the area of e.

**erysipelatous** (ĕr′ĭ-sĭ-pel′ă-tus). Relating to erysipelas.

**erysip′elococ′cus.** *Streptococcus pyogenes.*

**erysip′eloid** [ G. *erysipelas* + *eidos,* resemblance ]. Rosenbach's disease (2); pseudoerysipelas; a specific cellulitis of the hand, caused by *Erysipelothrix rhusiopathiae.* It occurs most commonly in persons handling fish or meat.

**Erysipelothrix** (ĕr-ĭ-sip′ĕ-lo-thriks, -sĭ-pel′o-thriks) [ erysipelas + G. *thrix,* hair ]. A genus of bacteria (family Corynebacteriaceae) containing nonmotile, Gram-positive, rod-shaped organisms which have a tendency to form long filaments; older cells tend to become Gram-negative. They produce acid but no gas from glucose. They are facultatively anaerobic and catalase-negative. Members of this genus are parasitic on mammals, birds, and fish. The type species is *E. rhusiopathiae.*

    **E. insidio′sa,** *E. rhusiopathiae.*

    **E. rhusiopath′iae** (roo-sĭ-o-path′ĭ′ē), *E. insidiosa;* a species which causes swine erysipelas, human erysipeloid, and mouse septicemia; it commonly infects fish handlers. It is the type species of the genus *E.*

**erysip′elotox′in.** A toxin produced by types of *Streptococcus pyogenes* (group A hemolytic streptococci), the bacterial cause of erysipelas.

**erysiphake** (ĕ-ris′ĭ-fāk) [ G. *erysis,* a drawing, + *phakos,* lentil ]. A suction cup attached to an aspiration apparatus which holds the lens by the anterior surface and extracts it by suction.

**erythema** (ĕr-ĭ-the′mah) [ G. *erythēma,* flush ]. Dermatitis erythematosa; redness of the skin; inflammation.

    **e. ab ig′ne** [ L. *ignis,* fire ], e. caloricum.

    **acrodynic e.,** acrodynia (1).

    **e. annula′re,** rounded or ringed lesions.

    **e. annulare centrif′ugum,** a chronic recurring erythematous eruption consisting of small and large annular lesions, both discrete and confluent; there is usually a scant marginal scale.

    **e. annulare rheumat′icum,** a variant of e. multiforme associated with rheumatic fever.

    **e. arthrit′icum epidem′icum,** see Haverhill *fever.*

    **e. bullo′sum,** e. multiforme with formation of large vesicles or bullae.

    **e. calor′icum** [ L. *calor,* heat ], e. ab igne; toasted shins; a reticulated, pigmented, macular eruption that occurs, mostly on the shins, of bakers, stokers, and others exposed to radiant heat.

    **e. centrif′ugum,** *lupus* erythematosus.

    **e. circina′tum,** e. multiforme in which the lesions are grouped in more or less circular fashion.

    **e. dyschro′mium per′stans,** variously sized gray or red, slightly elevated, macular lesions that tend to coalesce on the trunks, extremities, and face, clinically resembling pinta gut with no demonstrable treponema, with negative serology, and no benefit from penicillin.

    **e. eleva′tum diu′tinum** [ L. lasting ], Bury's disease; a chronic eruption of flattened nodules, of a pinkish or purplish color, occurring in plaques on the buttocks and extensors of wrists, elbows, and knees, becoming fibrotic and finally scarring.

    **e. endem′icum,** pellagra.

    **e. exfoliati′va,** *keratolysis* exfoliativa.

    **e. fugax,** a diffuse e. of the face, trunk, and extremities occurring in erethistic persons during the excitement caused by a medical examination.

    **e. gyra′tum,** e. circinatum in which the various rings overlap each other.

    **hemorrhagic exudative e.,** Henoch-Schönlein *purpura.*

    **e. indura′tum,** tuberculosis cutis indurativa; Bazin's disease; hard subcutaneous nodules that frequently break down, forming necrotic ulcers. They occur usually on the calves, less frequently on the thighs or arms, and are associated with tuberculosis.

    **e. infectio′sum,** fifth disease; a mild infectious disease characterized by an erythematous maculopapular eruption, accompanied by little or no fever; probably of viral etiology.

    **e. intertri′go,** see intertrigo.

    **e. iris,** herpes iris (1); concentric rings of e. varying in intensity, characteristic of e. multiforme.

    **Jaquet's e. infan′tum,** an eruption in infants, occurring beneath the diaper and involving the buttocks, thighs, and abdomen.

    **e. kerato′des,** keratodermia with an erythematous border.

    **mac′ular e.,** roseola.

    **e. margina′tum,** a variant of e. multiforme seen in rheumatic fever.

    **e. migrans,** geographical *tongue.*

    **e. migrans linguae,** geographical *tongue.*

    **Milian's e.,** ninth-day e.

    **e. multifor′me,** Hebra's disease (1); herpes iris (2); e. polymorphe; an eruption of macules, papules, or vesicles, presenting a multiform appearance. Its origin may be allergic, seasonal, or drug sensitivity. The characteristic lesion is the target or iris lesion. The condition is acute in onset, and may run a severe course with fatal termination. The eruption can be recurrent.

    **e. multiforme bullosum,** e. multiforme exudativum.

    **e. multiforme exudati′vum,** e. multiforme bullosum; ectodermosis erosiva pluriorificialis; referred to also as Stevens-Johnson syndrome; a bullous eruption which may be extensive, involving the mucous membranes and large areas of the body. The condition may produce serious subjective symptoms, and may have a fatal termination. See also ocular-mucous membrane *syndrome.*

    **e. necrot′icans combustifor′mis,** toxic epidermal *necrolysis.*

    **ninth-day e.,** Milian's e. or disease; a nontoxic eruption which simulates measles or a toxic erythema, occurring usually on the ninth day of a course of medication. First described as a reaction to arsenical treatment of syphilis.

    **e. nodo′sum,** dermatitis contusiformis; nodal fever; a dermatosis marked by the formation of painful nodes on the extensor surfaces of the lower extremities. It may be associated with rheumatic fever, or it may be evidence of drug sensitivity. The lesions are self-limiting, but tend to recur.

    **e. nodo′sum syphilit′icum,** gumma of skin of lower extremities.

    **e. palma′re heredita′rium,** Lane's disease; a condition characterized by asymptomatic symmetrical palmer e.; autosomal dominant inheritance.

    **e. papula′tum,** the papular form of e. multiforme.

    **e. paratrim′ma,** e. due to stasis over pressure points.

    **e. pernio,** chilblain.

    **e. per′stans,** probably a chronic form of e. multiforme in which the relapses recur so persistently that the eruption is almost permanent.

    **e. polymorphe,** e. multiforme.

    **scarlatin′iform e.,** e. scarlatinoides; an erythematous macular eruption accompanied by slight constitutional symptoms and followed by desquamation.

    **e. simplex,** dermatitis simplex; blushing or redness of the skin caused by a toxic reaction or a neurovascular phenomenon.

    **e. solare** [ L. *sol,* sun ], sunburn.

    **symptomatic e.,** a general term applied to various e.'s associated with systemic disease, fevers, allergic states, etc.

    **e. tox′icum,** flushing of the skin due to allergic reaction to some toxic substance.

    **e. toxicum neonato′rum,** a common transient eruption of erythema, small papules, and occasionally pustules filled with eosinophil leukocytes overlying hair follicles of the newborn.

    **e. tubercula′tum,** e. multiforme in which the papules are of large size.

    **e. venena′ta,** e. due to contact with some sensitizing substance.

**erythematous** (ĕr-ĭ-them′ă-tus, -the′mă-tus). Relating to or marked by erythema.

**erythe′matovesic′ular.** Denoting a condition characterized by edema, erythema, and vesiculation, as in allergic contact dermatitis.

**erythr-.** See erythro-.

**erythralgia** (ĕr-ĭ-thral′jĭ-ah) [ erythro- + G. *algos*, pain ]. Painful redness of the skin; see also erythromelalgia.

**erythrasma** (ĕr-ĭ-thraz′mah) [ G. *erythrainō*, to redden ]. An eruption of reddish brown patches, in the axillae and groins especially, due to the presence of *Corynebacterium minutissimum.*

**erythredema** (ĕ-rith′re-de′mah) [ erythro- + G. *oidēma*, swelling ]. Acrodynia (1).

**erythremia** (ĕr′ĭ-thre′mĭ-ah) [ erythro- + G. *haima*, blood ]. Polycythemia of unknown cause; a chronic disease characterized by bone marrow hyperplasia, an increase in blood volume as well as in the number of red cells, redness or cyanosis of the skin, and splenomegaly. Also called Osler's disease (1); Vaquez' disease; Osler-Vaquez disease; polycythemia rubra; polycythemia vera; polycythemia rubra vera.

**erythrism** (ĕr′ĭ-thrizm) [ G. *erythros*, red ]. Redness of the hair with a ruddy, freckled complexion.

**erythristic** (ĕr-ĭ-thris′tik). Rufous; relating to or marked by erythrism; having a ruddy complexion and reddish hair.

**eryth′ritol.** Erythrite; erythrol; tetrahydroxybutane; the 4-carbon sugar alcohol obtained by the reduction of erythrose; found in lichens, algae, and fungi; notable for its sweetness, which is twice that of sucrose.

**eryth′rityl tetrani′trate** (USAN). CARDILATE; erythrol tetranitrate; tetranitrol; vasodilator used in angina pectoris and hypertension. It is very explosive and must be mixed with a diluent, such as lactose. Listed in NF as erythrityl tetranitrate, diluted.

**erythro-, erythr-** [ G. *erythros*, red ]. 1. Combining forms meaning red or denoting relationship to redness. 2. Prefix indicating the structure of erythrose in a larger sugar; used as such, it is italicized (for example, 2-deoxy-D-*erythro*-pentose is the systematic name of the 2-deoxyribose found in DNA).

**erythroblast** (ĕ-rith′ro-blast) [ erythro- + G. *blastos*, germ ]. As originally used by Ehrlich, referred to all forms of human red blood cells that contained a nucleus, pathologic as well as normal. The normal series of maturation was called normoblastic, and the pathologic series, megaloblastic; the pathologic series is observed in pernicious anemia in relapse. This original nomenclature has been followed by Naegele, Ferrata, Downey, Jones, Wintrobe, and others. Doan, Cunningham, and Sabin have used the term megaloblast in a different sense, to indicate the first generation of cells in the red blood cell series which can be distinguished from precursor endothelial cells, hence with this usage, megaloblast denotes both a normal and an abnormal cell. Probably most modern workers use the nomenclature of Ehrlich; however, there is much confusion as to usage of terms. In the **normoblastic series** of maturation four stages of development can be recognized: (1) *pronormoblast* (rubriblast, macroblast of Naegeli, proerythroblast of Ferrata, megaloblast of Sabin, and lymphoid hemoblast of Pappenheim), the youngest precursor of the erythrocyte, possessing a relatively large nucleus with a thin rim of basophilic cytoplasm; (2) *basophilic normoblast* (prorubricyte, basophilic erythroblast of Ferrata, and early erythroblast of Sabin); it differs from the pronormoblast in that the nucleoli are absent and the cytoplasm is more densely basophilic; (3) *polychromatic normoblast* (rubricyte or late erythroblast of Sabin), designates a wide range of maturation from the beginning of recognizable hemoglobin in the cytoplasm to the complete disappearance of basophilia; (4) *orthochromatic normoblast* (metarubricyte, acidophilic normoblast), connotes a nucleated erythrocyte with most of the complement of hemoglobin. In the **megaloblastic series** of maturation, stages similar to those found in the normoblastic series are seen, namely: (1) *promegaloblast* (pernicious anemia type rubriblast), in which chromatin is uniformly distributed, with no tendency to clump, and 3 to 5 nucleoli usually present; (2) *basophilic megaloblast* (pernicious anemia type proru-

bricyte), similar to the promegaloblast, with an intensely blue cytoplasm and no nucleoli; (3) *polychromatic megaloblast* (pernicious anemia type rubricyte), in which cytoplasm is multicolored as a result of the beginning development of hemoglobin; and (4) *orthochromatic megaloblast* (pernicious anemia type metarubricyte), in which cytoplasm manifests the fairly uniform eosinophilia that is characteristic of fully developed hemoglobin. In the **normal series** of maturation, after loss of the nucleus, the young erythrocytes are called *reticulocytes;* these cells may be recognized with supravital stains such as brilliant cresyl blue; ultimately the reticulocytes become erythrocytes, or mature red blood cells. See color plates 14-16.

**erythroblastemia** (ĕ-rith′ro-blas-te′mĭ-ah) [ erythroblast + G. *haima*, blood ]. The presence of nucleated red cells in the peripheral blood.

**eryth′roblas′tope′nia** [ erythroblast + G. *penia*, poverty ]. A primary deficiency of erythroblasts seen in aplastic anemia; a deficiency of erythroblasts in bone marrow.

**erythroblastosis** (ĕ-rith′ro-blas-to′sis) [ erythroblast + suffix -*osis*, condition ]. The presence in considerable number of erythroblasts in the blood.

   **avian e.,** fowl e.; an expression of disease of the avian leukosis-sarcoma complex; characterized by severe anemia and large numbers of erythroblasts in the blood; chickens are most susceptible but fatal natural infections have been reported in guinea fowl.

   **e. feta′lis,** fetal e.; hemolytic disease of the newborn; a grave hemolytic anemia that, in most instances, results from development in the mother of anti-Rh antibody in response to the Rh factor in the (Rh-positive) fetal blood; it is characterized by many erythroblasts in the circulation, and often generalized edema (*hydrops foetalis*) and enlargement of the liver and spleen. The disease is sometimes caused by antibodies for blood factors other than Rh, and, in rare examples, the cause is not conclusively known.

   **fowl e.,** avian e.

**eryth′roblastot′ic.** Pertaining to erythroblastosis (especially erythroblastosis fetalis).

**erythrocatalysis** (ĕ-rith′ro-kă-tal′ĭ-sis) [ erythro- + G. *katalysis*, dissolution ]. Phagocytosis of the red blood cells.

**erythrochloropia** (ĕ-rith′ro-klo-ro′pĭ-ah) [ erythro- + G. *chlōros*, green, + *ōps*, eye ]. Partial color blindness with ability to distinguish correctly only red and green.

**eryth′rochlorop′sia.** Erythrochloropia.

**erythrochromia** (ĕ-rith′ro-kro′mĭ-ah) [ erythro- + G. *chrōma*, color ]. A red coloration or staining.

**erythroclasis** (ĕr′ith-rok′lă-sis) [ erythro- + G. *klasis*, breaking ]. Fragmentation of the red blood cells.

**erythroclastic** (ĕ-rith′ro-klas′tik). Pertaining to erythroclasis; destructive to red blood cells.

**erythrocruorin** (ĕ-rith′ro-ku-or′in). Large, hemoglobin-like molecules occurring in dissolved form in the blood of certain annelid worms and molluscs.

**erythrocuprein** (ĕ-rith′ro-ku′pre-in). Cytocuprein.

**eryth′rocyano′sis** [ erythro- + G. *kyanos*, blue, + suffix -*osis*, condition ]. A condition seen in children, girls, and women particularly, in which exposure of the limbs to cold causes them to become swollen and dusky red; it results from direct exposure to cold but not freezing temperatures.

**erythrocyte** (ĕ-rith′ro-sīt) [ erythro- + G. *kytos*, cell ]. Red corpuscle; a mature red blood cell. See color plates 15 and 16.

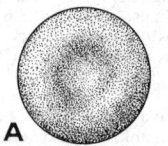 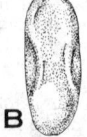 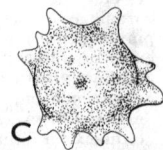

**Erythrocyte**

Erythrocytes in 0.9 per cent sodium chloride solution. A, viewed from broad surface; B, profile; C, crenated. (After Broderson.)

**erythrocythemia** (ĕ-rith'ro-si-the'mĭ-ah) [ erythro- + G. *kytos*, cell, + *haima*, blood ]. Abnormal increase in the number of red blood cells; see also polycythemia; erythremia.

**erythrocytic** (ĕ-rith'ro-sit'ik). Pertaining to a red blood cell (erythrocyte).

**erythrocytoblast** (ĕ-rith'ro-si'to-blast) [ erythro- + G. *kytos*, cell, + *blastos*, germ ]. Erythroblast.

**erythrocytolysin** (ĕ-rith'ro-si-tol'ĭ-sin). Hemolysin; any substance that has a lytic effect on red blood cells.

**erythrocytolysis** (ĕ-rith'ro-si-tol'ĭ-sis) [ erythrocyte + G. *lysis*, loosening ]. Hemolysis.

**eryth'rocytom'eter** [ erythrocyte + G. *metron*, measure ]. An instrument for counting the red blood cells. Hayden uses this term for an instrument to measure the diameter of red blood cells.

**erythrocytopenia** (ĕ-rith'ro-si'to-pe'nĭ-ah). Erythropenia.

**erythrocytopoiesis** (ĕ-rith'ro-si'to-poy-e'sis). Erythropoiesis.

**erythrocytorrhexis** (ĕ-rith'ro-si'to-rek'sis) [ erythrocyte + G. *rhēxis*, rupture ]. Plasmorrhexis; a partial erythrocytolysis, in which particles of protoplasm escape from the red blood cells, which then become crenated and deformed.

**erythrocytoschisis** (ĕ-rith'ro-si-tos'kĭ-sis) [ erythrocyte + G. *schisis*, a splitting ]. Plasmoschisis; a breaking up of the red blood cells into small particles that resemble platelets, morphologically.

**erythrocytosis** (ĕ-rith'ro-si-to'sis). Polycythemia, especially that which occurs in response to some known stimulus.

**erythrocyturia** (ĕ-rith'ro-si-tu'rĭ-ah). Red blood cells in urine.

**ery'throdegen'erative.** Pertaining to or characterized by degeneration of the red blood cells.

**erythroderma** (ĕ-rith'ro-der'mah) [ erythro- + G. *derma*, skin ]. Erythrodermatitis; erythema (reddish color) caused by an inflammatory reaction. The term is nonspecific and must be modified by a descriptive term.

   **congenital ichthyosiform e.,** ichthyosiform e.; keratoma malignum; a genodermatosis characterized by diffuse chronic erythema and scale formation with hyperkeratosis of palms and soles, and associated in varying degrees with other defects, including ocular and neural changes.

   **e. desquamati'vum,** Leiner's disease; severe, extensive seborrheic dermatitis in the newborn. Frequently occurs in undernourished, cachectic children.

   **e. exfoliati'va,** *keratolysis* exfoliativa.

   **ichthyosiform e.,** congenital ichthyosiform e.

   **maculopapular e.,** pityriasis lichenoides; lichen variegatus; an eruption of macules and papules of reddish color.

   **e. psoriat'icum,** extensive exfoliative dermatitis simulating psoriasis.

**eryth'rodermati'tis.** Erythroderma.

**eryth'rodex'trin.** A modified dextrin which is turned red by iodine.

**erythrodontia** (ĕ-rith'ro-don'shĭ-ah) [ erythro- + G. *odous*, tooth ]. Reddish discoloration of the teeth, as may occur in porphyria.

**erythrogen'esis imperfec'ta.** Congenital hypoplastic *anemia.*

**erythrogenic** (ĕ-rith'ro-jen'ik) [ erythro- + suffix -*gen*, producing ]. 1. Producing red, as causing an eruption or a red color sensation. 2. Pertaining to the formation of red blood cells.

**erythrogonium,** pl. **erythrogo'nia** (ĕ-rith'ro-go'nĭ-um) [ erythro- + G. *gonē*, generation ]. The precursor of an erythrocyte; occasionally refers to the erythropoietic tissue as a whole.

**erythroid** (ĕr'ĭ-throyd, ĕ-rith'royd). Reddish in color.

**erythroidine** (ĕ-rith'roy-dēn, -din). An alkaloid obtained from *Erythrina* (family Leguminosae). It has a curare-like action.

**erythrokeratoderma** (ĕ-rith'ro-kĕr'ă-to-der'mah). The association of erythroderma and hyperkeratosis.

   **e. variabi'lis,** keratosis rubra figurata; a dermatosis characterized by hyperkeratotic plaques of bizarre, geographic configuration, associated with erythrodermic areas that may vary remarkably in size, shape, and position from

day to day; onset is usually in the first year of life; autosomal dominant inheritance.

**eryth'rokinet'ics** [ erythro- + G. *kinēsis*, movement ]. A consideration of the kinetics of erythrocytes from their generation to destruction; erythrokinetic studies are sometimes made in cases of anemia to evaluate the balance between erythrocyte production and destruction.

**erythrol.** Erythritol.

**eryth'rolabe.** One of two postulated pigments in the cones of the eye, absorbing most actively in the red; *cf.* chlorolabe.

**erythroleukemia** (ĕ-rith'ro-lu-ke'mĭ-ah). Simultaneous neoplastic proliferation of erythroblastic and leukoblastic tissues; see also Di Guglielmo's *disease.*

**erythroleukosis** (ĕ-rith'ro-lu-ko'sis). Leukanemia; panmyelosis; a condition resembling leukemia in which the erythropoietic tissue is affected in addition to the leukopoietic tissue.

**erythrolysin** (ĕr'ĭ-throl'ĭ-sin). Erythrocytolysin; hemolysin.

**erythrolysis** (ĕr'ĭ-throl'ĭ-sis). Hemolysis.

**erythromelalgia** (ĕ-rith'ro-mel-al'jĭ-ah) [ erythro- + G. *melos*, limb, + *algos*, pain ]. Paroxysmal throbbing and burning pain in the skin, affecting one or both legs and feet, sometimes one or both hands, accompanied by a dusky mottled redness of the parts; associated with polycythemia vera, thrombocythemia, gout, neurological disease, or heavy-metal poisoning. Also called Mitchell's disease; Gerhardt's disease; red neuralgia; rodonalgia.

**erythromelia** (ĕ-rith'ro-me'lĭ-ah) [ erythro- + G. *melos*, limb ]. Diffuse idiopathic erythema and atrophy of the skin of the lower limbs.

**erythrometer** (ĕr'ĭ-throm'e-ter) [ erythro- + G. *metron*, measure ]. Instrument for measuring degrees of redness.

**eryth'romy'cin** (USP, BP). ILOTYCIN; an antibiotic agent obtained from cultures of a strain of *Streptomyces erythreus* found in soil; it is active against *Corynebacterium diphtheriae* and several other species of *Corynebacterium*, Group A hemolytic streptocci, *Diplococcus pneumoniae*, and *Hemophilus pertussis*. Gram-positive bacteria are in general more sensitive to its action than the Gram-negative, though the *Neisseria* and *Brucella* groups are susceptible to its action.

   **e. B,** berythromycin.

   **e. estolate** (BP, USAN), ILOSONE; same therapeutic uses as e. It is acid-stable and may be given orally; jaundice may occur.

   **e. ethylcarbonate,** the ethylcarbonate of e.; administered orally for the same purposes as e.

   **e. ethylsuccinate** (NF), PEDIAMYCIN; effective orally, with same therapeutic uses as e.; no hepatic toxicity has been noted.

   **e. gluceptate** (USP), has the same actions as e., but used for intravenous administration.

   **e. lactobi'onate** (USP), a water-soluble salt of e. used intravenously or intramuscularly.

   **e. stearate** (USP, BP), same uses and action as e. base.

**erythron** (ĕr'ĭ-thron). The total mass of circulating red blood cells, and that part of the hematopoietic tissue from which they are derived.

**erythroneocytosis** (ĕ-rith'ro-ne'o-si-to'sis) [ erythrocyte + G. *neos*, new, + *kytos*, cell, + suffix -*osis*, condition ]. Presence in the peripheral circulation of regenerative forms of red blood cells.

**erythropenia** (ĕ-rith'ro-pe'nĭ-ah) [ erythrocyte + G. *penia*, poverty ]. Erythrocytopenia; deficiency in the number of red blood cells.

**erythrophage** (ĕ-rith'ro-fāj) [ erythrocyte + G. *phagein*, to eat ]. A phagocyte that englobes and destroys red blood cells.

**erythrophagia** (ĕ-rith'ro-fa'jĭ-ah). Phagocytic destruction of red blood cells.

**erythrophagocytosis** (ĕ-rith'ro-fag'o-si-to'sis). Phagocytosis of erythrocytes.

**erythrophil** (ĕ-rith'ro-fil) [ erythro- + G. *philos*, fond ]. 1. Erythrophilic; staining readily with red dyes. 2. A cell or tissue element that stains red.

**eryth'rophil'ic.** Erythrophil (1).

**erythrophleine** (ĕ-rith'ro-fle'in). An alkaloid with digitalis-like action extracted from the bark of *Erythrophloeum guineense.*

**erythrophleum** (ĕ-rith'ro-fle'um) [ erythro- + G. *phloios,* bark ]. The dried bark of *Erythrophloeum guineense* (*E. judiciale*) (family Leguminosae); an African ordeal poison; also called ordeal bark; sassy bark; grigri; mancona bark; red-water tree bark.

**erythrophore** (ĕ-rith'ro-fōr) [ erythro- + G. *phoros,* bearing ]. Allophore; a chromatophore containing granules of a red or brown pigment.

**erythrophose** (ĕ-rith'ro-fōz, ĕr'ī-thro-fōz) [ erythro- + G. *phōs,* light ]. A red phose.

**erythro'pia.** Erythropsia.

**erythroplasia** (ĕ-rith'ro-pla'zĭ-ah) [ erythro- + G. *plassō,* to form ]. Erythema and dysplasia of the epithelium.
　**e. of Queyrat,** intraepithelial carcinoma (carcinoma *in situ*) of the glans penis.

**erythropoiesis** (ĕ-rith'ro-poy-e'sis) [ erythrocyte + G. *poiēsis,* a making ]. Erythrocytopoiesis; the formation of red blood cells.

**erythropoietic** (ĕ-rith'ro-poy-et'ik). Pertaining to or characterized by erythropoiesis.

**erythropoietin** (ĕ-rith'ro-poy'ĕ-tin). A sialic acid-containing protein that enhances erythropoiesis by stimulating formation of proerythroblasts and release of reticulocytes from bone marrow. Secreted by the kidney and possibly by other tissues. Can be detected in human plasma and urine.

**erythroprosopalgia** (ĕ-rith'ro-pros-o-pal'jĭ-ah) [ erythro- + G. *prosōpon,* face, + *algos,* pain ]. A disorder similar to erythromelalgia, but with the pain and redness occurring in the face.

**erythropsia** (ĕ-rith-rop'sĭ-ah) [ erythro- + G. *ōps,* eye ]. Erythropia; red vision; a condition in which all objects appear to be tinged with red.

**erythropsin** (ĕr'ī-throp'sin). Rhodopsin.

**erythropyknosis** (ĕ-rith'ro-pik-no'sis) [ erythro- + G. *pyknos,* dense ]. Alteration of the red blood cells to the condition called "brassy bodies," under the influence of the malarial parasite.

**erythrorrhexis** (ĕr'ī-thro-rek'sis, ĕ-rith'ro-rek'sis) [ erythrocyte + G. *rhēxis,* rupture ]. Fragmentation of the red blood cells.

**er'ythrose.** A tetrose; an isomer of threose. For structure, see sugars.

**eryth'rosin B.** Tetraiodofluorescein; a fluorescent red acid dye, $C_{20}H_6O_5I_4Na_2$, used as a counterstain in histology.

**erythrothrombomonoblastosis** (ĕ-rith'ro-throm'bo-mon-o-blas-to'sis) [ erythro- + G. *thrombos,* a clot, + mono(cyte) + *blastos,* germ ]. A leukemia-like disorder of the hemopoietic system characterized by: (1) initial splenomegaly; (2) various changes in the blood, including thrombocythemia, erythroblastemia, hypochromic anemia, atypical or immature monocytes, increased bone marrow activity; (3) increased metabolic rate; (4) bone atrophy not unlike Gaucher type.

**er'ythrox'yline.** The name by which cocaine was called by its discoverer, Gaedeke, in 1855.

**er'ythrox'ylon co'ca** [ erythro- + G. *xylon,* wood ]. Coca; a tree (family Erythroxylaceae) indigenous in Bolivia, Chile, and Peru from which cocaine is obtained.

**eryth'rulose.** The 2-keto analog of erythrose.

**erythruria** (ĕr'ī-thru'rĭ-ah) [ erythro- + G. *ouron,* urine ]. The passage of red urine.

**Esbach,** Georges H., Paris physician, 1843–1890. See E.'s *reagent.*

**escape.** Occurs when a higher pacemaker defaults or A-V conduction fails and a lower pacemaker comes to the rescue and assumes the function of pacemaking for one or more beats.
　**nodal e.,** e. with the A-V node as pacemaker.
　**ventricular e.,** e. with an ectopic ventricular focus as pacemaker.

**eschar** (es'kar) [ G. *eschara,* a fireplace, a scab caused by burning ]. A thick, coagulated crust or slough which develops following a thermal burn or chemical or physical cauterization of the skin.

**escharotic** (es-kă-rot'ik). Caustic; corrosive.

**escharotomy** (es-kă-rot'o-mĭ) [ eschar + G. *tomē,* incision ]. A surgical incision in a burn eschar to lessen constriction of a distal part.

**Escherich,** Theodor, German physician, 1857–1911. Gave his name to *Escherichia.* See E.'s *sign.*

**Escherichia** (esh-er-ik'ĭah) [ T. *Escherich* ]. A genus of aerobic, facultatively anaerobic bacteria which contains short, motile or nonmotile, Gram-negative rods. Motile cells are peritrichous. Glucose and lactose are fermented with the production of acid and gas. These organisms are found in feces; occasionally they are pathogenic to man, causing enteritis, peritonitis, cystitis, etc. It is the type genus of the family Enterobacteriaceae. The type species is E. coli.
　**E. au'rescens,** a species commonly found in fecal matter; also found in an infected eye and in contaminated water supplies.
　**E. co'li,** a species that occurs normally in the intestines of man and other vertebrates and is widely distributed in nature; a frequent cause of infections of the urogenital tract and of diarrhea in infants. Enteropathogenic strains (serotypes) of *E. coli* cause diarrhea due to enterotoxin, the production of which seems to be associated with a transferable episome. *E. coli* is the type species of the genus.
　**E. freundii,** *Citrobacter freundii.*
　**E. intermedia,** *Citrobacter intermedius.*

**eschrolalia** (es-kro-la'lĭ-ah) [ G. *aischros,* shameful, + *lalia,* talking ]. Coprolalia.

**escor'cin.** Escorcinol; a brown powder derived from esculetin; used for the detection of defects in the cornea and conjunctiva, which it marks by a red coloration.

**Escula'pian.** Aesculapian.

**esculent** (es'ku-lent) [ L. *esculentus,* edible ]. Edible.

**escu'letin.** 6,7-Dihydroxycoumarin; cichorigenin; the aglucone of esculin; used in the manufacture of escorcin, and in filters for absorption of ultraviolet light.

**es'culin** [ L. *aesculus,* the Italian oak ]. 6,7-Dihydroxycoumarin 6-glucoside; a glucoside from horse-chestnut bark; used as a sunburn protective.

**escutcheon** (es-kuch'un) [ through Old Fr. fr. L. *scutum,* shield ]. The region of the skin in quadrupeds (usually cattle) between the hind legs above the udder and below the anus; the hair in this region generally grows upward.

**eser'idine.** GENESERINE; eserine aminoxide; eserine oxide; $C_{15}H_{21}N_3O_3$; an alkaloid from the seed of *Physostigma;* a parasympathomimetic agent.

**es'erine.** Physostigmine.

**-esis** [ G. suffix *-esis,* condition or process ]. Suffix meaning condition, action, or process.

**Esmarch** (es'markh), Johann F. A. von, German surgeon, 1823–1908. See E.'s *bandage.*

**esocataphoria** (es'o-kat-ă-fo'rĭ-ah) [ G. *esō,* inward, + *kata,* down, + *phora,* a carrying ]. Convergent squint combined with cataphoria, the eye turning down and in.

**es'odevia'tion.** Esophoria or esotropia.

**esodic** (ĕ-sod'ik) [ G. *esō,* inward, + *hodos,* way ]. Afferent.

**esoethmoiditis** (es'o-eth-moy-di'tis) [ G. *esō,* within, + ethmoid, *q.v.,* + suffix *-itis,* inflammation ]. Inflammation of the lining membrane of the ethmoid cells.

**es'ogastri'tis** [ G. *esō,* within, + *gastēr,* stomach, + suffix *-itis,* inflammation ]. Catarrhal inflammation of the mucous membrane of the stomach.

**esophagalgia** (e-sof'ă-gal'jĭ-ah) [ esophagus + G. *algos,* pain ]. Esophagodynia; pain in the esophagus.

**esophageal** (e-sof'ă-je'al, e'-sō-faj'e-al). Relating to the esophagus.

**esophagectasia** (e-sof-ă-jek-ta'zĭ-ah). Esophagectasis.

**esophagectasis** (e-sof-ă-jek'tă-sis) [ esophagus + G. *ektasis,* a stretching ]. Esophagectasia; dilation of the esophagus.

**esophagectomy** (e-sof'ă-jek'to-mĭ) [ esophagus + G. *ektomē,* excision ]. Excision of any part of the esophagus.

**esophagi** (e-sof'ă-je). Plural of esophagus.

**esophagism** (e-sof'ă-jizm). Spasmodic stricture of the esophagus.

**esophagitis** (e-sof-ă-ji'tis). Inflammation of the esophagus.
　**peptic e.,** inflammation of the lower esophagus from regurgitation of acid gastric contents, producing subster-

nal pain. Heartburn and regurgitation of acid juice also may result.

**esophagocardioplasty** (e-sof'ă-go-kar'dī-o-plas-tī). A plastic operation on the esophagus and cardiac end of the stomach.

**esophagocele** (e-sof'ă-go-sēl) [ esophagus + G. *kēlē,* hernia ]. Protrusion of the mucous membrane of the esophagus through a rent in the muscular coat.

**esophagodynia** (e-sof'ă-go-din'ī-ah) [ esophagus + G. *odynē,* pain ]. Esophagalgia.

**esophagoenterostomy** (e-sof'ă-go-en-ter-os'to-mī) [ esophagus + G. *enteron,* intestine, + *stoma,* mouth ]. The operative formation of a direct communication between the esophagus and intestine.

**esoph'agogastrec'tomy.** Removal of a portion of the lower esophagus and proximal stomach; operation used for treatment of neoplasms or strictures of the lower esophagus and proximal stomach, especially those lesions located at or near the cardioesophageal junction.

**esoph'agogas'troanas'tomo'sis.** An anastomosis between esophagus and stomach.

**esophagogastromyotomy** (e-sof'ă-go-gas'tro-mi-ot'o-mī). Esophagomyotomy.

**esoph'agogas'troplas'ty.** Cardioplasty.

**esophagogastrostomy** (e-sof'ă-go-gas-tros'to-mī) [ esophagus + G. *gastēr,* stomach, + *stoma,* mouth ]. Anastomosis of esophagus to stomach following esophagogastrectomy.

**esophagomalacia** (e-sof'ă-go-mă-la'shī-ah) [ esophagus + G. *malakia,* softness ]. Softening of the walls of the esophagus.

**esophagomycosis** (e-sof'ă-go-mi-ko'sis) [ esophagus + G. *mykēs,* fungus, + suffix -*osis,* condition ]. Any fungous disease of the esophagus.

**esophagomyotomy** (e-sof'ă-go-mi-ot'o-mī) [ esophagus + G. *mys,* muscle, + *tomē,* incision ]. Cardiomyotomy; esophagogastromyotomy; Heller operation; treatment of esophageal achalasia by longitudinal division of the lowest part of the esophageal muscle; some muscle fibers of the cardia may also be divided.

**esophagoplasty** (e-sof'ă-go-plas'tī) [ esophagus + G. *plassō,* to form ]. Repair of a defect in the wall of the esophagus by a plastic operation.

**esophagoplication** (e-sof'ăgo-pli-ka'shun) [ esophagus + L. *plico,* to fold ]. Reduction in size of a dilated esophagus or of a pouch in the same by making longitudinal folds or tucks in its wall.

**esophagoptosis, esophagoptosia** (e-sof'ă-gop-to'sis, -to'-sī-ah) [ esophagus + G. *ptōsis,* a falling ]. Relaxation and downward displacement of the walls of the esophagus.

**esoph'agoscope** [ esophagus + G. *skopeō,* to examine ]. A form of endoscope for inspecting the esophagus.

**esophagoscopy** (e-sof'ă-gos'ko-pī) [ esophagus + G. *skopeō,* to examine ]. Inspection of the interior of the esophagus.

**esophagospasm** (e-sof'ă-go-spazm). Spasm of the walls of the esophagus.

**esophagostenosis** (e-sof'ă-go-stē-no'sis) [ esophagus + G. *stenōsis,* a narrowing ]. Stricture or a general narrowing of the esophagus.

**esophagostomiasis** (e-sof'ă-go-sto-mi'ă-sis) [ esophagus + G. *stoma,* mouth, + suffix -*iasis,* condition ]. Nodular *disease.*

**esophagostomy** (e-sof'ă-gos'to-mī) [ esophagus + G. *stoma,* mouth ]. The operative formation of an opening directly into the esophagus from without.

**esophagotomy** (e-sof-ă-got'o-mī) [ esophagus + G. *tomē,* an incision ]. An incision through the wall of the esophagus.

**esoph'agram.** A roentgenogram of the esophagus.

**esophagus,** pl. **esoph'agi** (e-sof'ă-gus) [ G. *oisophagos,* gullet. PHAG- ] [ NA ]. The gullet; the swallow; the portion of the digestive canal between the pharynx and stomach. It consists of a *pars cervicalis, pars thoracica,* and *pars abdominalis,* and extends from the lower border of the cricoid cartilage, opposite the sixth cervical vertebra, to the cardiac orifice of the stomach opposite the eleventh thoracic vertebra, a distance of about 25 cm. (10 inches).

**esophoria** (es-o-fo'rī-ah) [ G. *esō,* inward, + *phora,* a carrying ]. A tendency of one eye to deviate inward.

**esophoric** (es-o-for'ik). Relating to or marked by esophoria.

**esophylaxis** (es'o-fi-lak'sis) [ G. *eso,* within, + *phylaxis,* a guarding ]. Protection against disease by the biologic action of the cells and fluids of the body; see also exophylaxis.

**esosphenoiditis** (es'o-sfe'noyd-i'tis) [ G. *esō,* within, + sphenoid, *q.v.,* + suffix -*itis,* inflammation ]. Osteomyelitis of the sphenoid bone.

**esotro'pia** [ G. *esō,* inward, + *tropē,* turn ]. Convergent strabismus; the form of strabismus in which the visual axes converge; may be paralytic or concomitant, monocular or alternating. Also called cross-eye, or internal or convergent squint. See fig. under strabismus.

**A-e.,** convergent strabismus greater in upward than in downward gaze.

**V-e.,** convergent strabismus greater in downward than in upward gaze.

**X-e.,** increasing convergence from primary position in both upward and downward gaze.

**esotrop'ic.** Relating to or marked by esotropia.

**ESP.** Abbreviation for extrasensory *perception.*

**espundia** (es-poon'dī-ah). Bubas braziliana; Breda's disease; a type of American leishmaniasis caused by *Leishmania braziliensis* that effects the mucous membranes, particularly in the nasal and oral region, resulting in grossly destructive changes; particularly common in Brazil where a significant proportion of persons infected with *L. braziliensis* develop this condition. May develop metastatically from sores originally found elsewhere on the body.

**esquillectomy** (es-kil-ek'to-mī, es-kwil-lek'to-mī) [ Fr. *esquille,* fragment, + G. *ektomē,* excision ]. Operation for the removal of detached bony fragments in cases of comminuted fracture.

**esquinan'cea** [ Fr. *esquinancie,* quinsy ]. Sense of suffocation caused by an inflammatory swelling in the throat, *e.g.,* suppurative tonsillitis.

**ESR.** Abbreviation for (1) erythrocyte sedimentation *rate;* (2) electron spin *resonance.*

**es'sence** [ L. *essentia,* fr. *esse,* to be ]. 1. The true characteristic or substance of a body. 2. An element. 3. A fluid extract. 4. An alcoholic solution, or spirit, of the volatile oil of a plant. 5. Any volatile substance responsible for odor or taste of the organism (usually a plant) producing it; by extension, synthetic perfumes or flavors.

**essential** (ē-sen'shal). 1. Necessary, indispensable (*e.g.,* amino acids). 2. Characteristic of. 3. Determining. 4. Idiopathic, inherent. 5. Relating to an essence (*e.g.,* e. oil).

**Esser,** Johannes F. S., Dutch surgeon, 1877–1946. See E.'s *operation.*

**Essig splint.** See under splint.

**es'ter.** An organic compound containing the grouping, —$X(O)_n$—O— ($X$ = carbon, sulfur, phosphorus, etc.), formed by the elimination of $H_2O$ between the —OH of an acid group and the —OH of an alcohol group. Usually written as in ethyl acetate (from acetic acid and ethyl alcohol), $CH_3CO_2C_2H_5$.

**Cori e.,** glucose 1-phosphate.

**Embden e.,** hexosephosphate; an equilibrium mixture of glucose 6-phosphate and fructose 6-phosphate.

**Harden-Young e.,** fructose 1,6-bisphosphate.

**Robison e., Robison-Embden e.,** D-glucose 6-phosphate.

**es'terase.** A generic term for enzymes (EC class 3.1, hydrolases) that catalyze the hydrolysis of esters, *e.g.,* acetylcholinesterase (cholinesterase).

**C1 e.,** the activated first component of complement (C1); see component of *complement.*

**C1 e. inhibitor,** an $\alpha_2$-neuraminoglycoprotein that inhibits the enzymatic activity of the activated first component of complement (C1 esterase); see also component of *complement.*

**esterification** (es'tĕr'ĭ-fĭ-ka'shun). The process of forming an ester, as in the reaction of ethanol and acetic acid to form the ester, ethyl acetate.

**es'terol'ysis.** The splitting of a chemical bond with the addition of the elements of an ester at the point of splitting.

**Estes,** William L., Jr., American surgeon, 1885–1940. See E. *operation*.

**esthematology** (es-the-mă-tol'o-jĭ) [ G. *aisthēma*, perception, + *logos*, study ]. The science of the senses and sense organs.

**esthesia** (es-the'zĭ-ah) [ G. *aisthesis*, sensation ]. Perception; sensitivity.

**esthe'sic** [ G. *aisthēsis*, sensation ]. Relating to the mental perception of the existence of any part of the body.

**esthesio-** (es-the'zĭ-o-) [ G. *aesthēsis*, sensation ]. Combining form relating to sensation or perception.

**esthesiodic** (es-the'zĭ-od'ik) [ esthesio- + G. *hodos*, way ]. Esthesodic; sensory; conveying sensory impressions.

**esthesiogenesis** (es-the'zĭ-o-jen'e-sis) [ esthesio- + G. *genesis*, generation ]. The production of sensation, especially of nervous erethism.

**esthesiogen'ic.** Producing a sensation.

**esthesiography** (es-the'zĭ-og'ră-fĭ) [ esthesio- + G. *graphē*, a writing ]. 1. A description of the organs of sense and of the mechanism of sensation. 2. Mapping out on the skin the areas of tactile and other forms of sensibility.

**esthesiology** (es-the'zĭ-ol'o-jĭ) [ esthesio- + G. *logos*, study ]. Science in relation to sensory phenomena.

**esthesiometer** (es-the-zĭ-om'e-ter) [ esthesio- + G. *metron*, measure ]. Tactometer; an instrument for determining the state of tactile and other forms of sensibility.

**esthesiom'etry.** Measurment of the degree of tactile or other sensibility.

**esthe'sioneu'rocyto'ma.** A neoplasm composed of nearly mature neuron-like cells believed to arise from a spinal ganglion.

　**olfactory e.,** olfactory *neuroblastoma*.

**esthesioneurosis** (es-the'zĭ-o-nu-ro'sis). Any sensory neurosis, such as anesthesia, hyperesthesia, paresthesia, etc.

**esthesionosus** (es-the'zĭ-on'o-sus) [ esthesio- + G. *nosos*, disease ]. Esthesioneurosis.

**esthe'siophysiol'ogy.** The physiology of sensation and the sense organs.

**esthesioscopy** (es-the-zĭ-os'ko-pĭ) [ esthesio- + G. *skopeō*, to view ]. Examination into the degree and extent of tactile and other forms of sensibility.

**esthesodic** (es'the-zod'ik). Esthesiodic.

**esthet'ic** [ G. *aisthēsis*, sensation ]. 1. Pertaining to the sensations. 2. Pertaining to esthetics (*i.e.,* beauty).

**esthet'ics.** The branch of philosophy dealing with beauty, especially with the components thereof, *viz.,* color and form.

　**denture e.,** (1) the cosmetic effect produced by a dental prosthesis; (2) the qualities involved in the appearance of a given restoration.

**esthiomene** (es-thĭ-om'e-ne) [ G. *esthiomenos*, eaten, eroded, pr. part. pass. of *esthiō*, to eat ]. An ulcerative lesion of the vulva surrounded by fibrous induration and edema, associated with lymphogranuloma inguinale.

**esthiom'enous** [ see esthiomene ]. Corroding; ulcerating; phagedenic.

**es'tival** [ L. *aestivus*, summer (adj.) ]. Aestival; relating to or occurring in the summer.

**estiva'tion.** Living through the summer in a quiescent, torpid state; as opposed to hibernation.

**estivoautumnal** (es'tĭ-vo-aw-tum'nal) [ L. *aestivus*, summer (adj.), + *autumnalis*, autumnal ]. Relating to or occurring in summer and autumn.

**Estlander,** Jakob A., Finnish surgeon, 1831–1881. See E.'s *operation*.

**es'tolate.** USAN-approved contraction for propionate lauryl sulfate.

**estradiol** (es'tră-di'ol) (NF). 17β-Estradiol; 1,3,5(10)-estratriene-3,17β-diol (for structure, see steroids). The most potent naturally occurring estrogen in mammals (17α-estradiol exhibits considerably less biological activity). It is formed by the ovary, the placenta, the testis, and possibly the adrenal cortex. The therapeutic indications for estradiol are those typical of an estrogen.

　**e. benzoate** (NF), oestradiol benzoate (BP); fatty acid esters of 17β-estradiol usually dissolved in oil for injection

purposes. Such esters exhibit a longer duration of action than does the unesterified steroid.

　**e. cypionate** (USP), DEPO-estradiol; has the same actions and uses as e. but has a prolonged duration of action; administered in oil by intramuscular injection.

　**e. dipropionate** (NF), OVOCYCLIN; an esterfied natural estrogen for parenteral use.

　**ethinyl e.** (USP), ethynyl e.

　**ethynyl e.,** ethinyl e.; oestradiol ethinyl (BP); 17α-ethynyl-1,3,5-estratriene-3,17-diol (for structure of estrane, see steroids); a semisynthetic derivative of 17β-estradiol. Active by mouth, it is among the most potent of known estrogenic compounds.

　**e. undecylate** (USAN), DELESTREE; an esterfied natural estrogen for parenteral use.

　**e. valerate** (USP), DELESTROGEN; estradiol 17-valerate; estra-1,3,5(10)-triene-3,17β-diol 17-valerate; same actions and uses as e., but has a prolonged duration of action. Administered in sesame oil by intramuscular injection.

**α-estradiol.** 17α-Estradiol; the relatively inert stereoisomer (at C-14) of 17β-estradiol. According to the system of notation used prior to 1948, α-estradiol was the potent stereoisomer. Found in the placenta and urine during pregnancy.

**β-estradiol.** Estradiol.

**es'tragon oil.** Tarragon oil.

**es'trane.** Parent hydrocarbon of the (steroid) estrogenic compounds (estradiol, estrone, estriol); conceived for the purpose of establishing systematic nomenclature. For structure, see steroids.

**estratriene** (es'tră-tri'ēn). 1,3,5(10)-Estratriene; the unsaturated estrane that is the nucleus of most naturally occurring estrogenic steroids in animals. For estrane structure, see steroids.

**estra'zinol hydrobromide** (USAN). *dl*-3-Methoxy-8-aza-17-nor-17α-pregna-1,3,5-(10)-trien-20-yn-17-ol hydrobromide; an estrogenic substance.

**es'trin.** Estrogen.

**es'trinase.** An enzyme in the liver that inactivates estrogens.

**estriol** (es'trĭ-ol). Theelol; folliculin hydrate; trihydroxyestrin; 1,3,5(10)-estratriene-3,16α,17β-triol for estrane structure, see steroids). A metabolite of, and considerably less potent than, 17β-estradiol; it is usually the predominant estrogenic metabolite found in urine.

**estrogen** (es'tro-jen). Generic term for any substance, whether naturally occurring or synthetic, that exerts biological effects characteristic of estrogenic hormones, such as estradiol; named for its ability to induce estrus in lower mammals. E.'s are formed by the ovary, placenta, testes, and possibly the adrenal cortex, as well as certain plants. Besides stimulation of secondary sexual characteristics, they also exert systemic effects, such as growth and maturation of long bones. The e.'s are used therapeutically in any disorder attributable to e. deficiency, to prevent or stop lactation, to suppress ovulation, and to ameliorate carcinoma of the breast and of the prostate.

　**conjugated e.** (USP), PREMARIN; ESTRIFOL; CONESTRON; AMNESTROGEN; an amorphous preparation of naturally occurring, water-soluble, conjugated forms of mixed e.'s obtained from the urine of pregnant mares; the principal e. present is sodium estrone sulfate. Suitable for parenteral, oral, and topical administration, and used in conditions responsive to e. therapy.

　**esterified e.'s** (USP), mixture of esters for oral administration.

**estrogen'ic.** 1. Causing estrus in animals. 2. Having an action similar to that of an estrogen.

**estroma'nia** [ G. *oistros*, mad desire, + *mania*, insanity ]. Nymphomania.

**estromimetic** (es'tro-mĭ-met'ik). Obsolete term for estrogenic.

**estrone** (es'trōn) (NF). Theelin; folliculin; follicular hormone; ketohydroxyestrin; 3-hydroxy-1,3,5(10)-estratrien-17-one (for structure of estrane, see steroids). A metabolite of 17β-estradiol, commonly found in urine; has considerably less biological activity than the parent hormone. Suggested for the treatment of menopausal symptoms and other conditions related to estrogen deficiency, and for gonorrheal vaginitis in children. Also available (NF) as e. sodium sulfate.

**estrous** (es'trus). Estrual; to estrus.

**estrual** (es'tru-al). Estrous.

**es'trum.** Estrus.

**es'trus** [ G. *oistros*, mad desire. EST- ]. Estrum; heat (2); that portion or phase of the sexual cycle of female animals characterized by willingness to permit coitus; readily detectable behavioral and other signs are exhibited by animals during this period. See estrous *cycle* for a table of estrous cycles of common domesticated animals.

   **postpartum e.,** e. with ovulation and corpus luteum production which occurs in some species (*e.g.*, the fur seal) immediately following the birth of the young.

**estua'rium** [ L. *aestus*, heat ]. A vapor bath.

**esu.** Abbreviation for electrostatic *unit*.

**es'ylate.** USAN-approved contraction for ethanesulfonate, $CH_3CH_2SO_3{}^-$.

**etafed'rine hydrochloride** (USAN). NOVEDRIN; *l*-*N*-ethylephedrine hydrochloride; sympathomimetic drug for treatment of bronchial asthma.

**état** (a-tah') [ Fr. state ]. A condition or state.

   **e. criblé** [ Fr. sieve ], in neuropathology, a term describing perivascular atrophy of cerebral tissue.

   **e. mamelonné** [ Fr. knobby, tubercular ], the condition of the gastric mucous membrane in chronic inflammation, when it presents numerous nodular projections.

**ethac'ridine lactate.** ETHODIN; RIVANOL; acrinol; 6,9-diamino-2-ethoxyacridine lactate; antiseptic for treatment of wounds.

**ethacry'nate sodium** (USP). Sodium salt of ethacrynic acid for parenteral use.

**ethacrynic acid** (eth'ă-krin'ik) (USP, BP). EDECRIN; [ 2,3-dichloro-4-(2-methylenebutyryl)phenoxy]acetic acid; an unsaturated ketone derivative of aryloxyacetic acid; a potent diuretic and a weak antihypertensive; used in the treatment of severe edema in heart failure or cirrhosis.

**ethadione.** DIDIONE; 3-ethyl-5,5-dimethyl-2,4-oxazolidinedione; anticonvulsant.

**ethambutol hydrochloride** (eth-am'bu-tol) (USP). MYAMBUTOL; (+)-2,2'-(ethylenedimino)-di(1-butanol) dihydrochloride; tuberculostatic, effective against organisms resistant to other tuberculostatic drugs; a serious reaction is visual impairment which, however, appears to be reversible.

**ethamivan** (eth-am'ĭ-van) (NF). EMIVAN; *N*,*N*-diethylvanillamide; 3-methoxyl-4-hydroxybenzoic acid diethylamide; a central nervous system stimulant and analeptic, used as an adjunctive agent in the treatment of severe respiratory depression due to barbiturates and carbon dioxide retention.

**ethamoxytriphetol.** MER-25; 1-[ *p*-(2-diethylaminoethoxy)phenyl ]-2-(*p*-methoxyphenyl)-1-phenylethanol; an estrogen antagonist under investigation as an antifertility agent.

**etham'sylate** (USAN). DICYNONE; cyclonamine; 1-hydroxyl-4-oxo-2,5-cyclohexadiene-1-sulfonic acid compound with diethylamine; hemostatic agent.

**eth'anal.** Acetaldehyde.

**eth'ane.** $CH_3CH_3$; a constituent of natural and "bottled" gases.

**ethanediamine** (eth'ăn-di'am-ēn). Ethylenediamine.

**ethanoic acid** (eth'ă-no'ik). Acetic acid.

**eth'anol.** See alcohol (2).

**ethanol'amine.** β-Hydroxyethylamine; colamine; 2-aminoethanol; $HO(CH_2)_2NH_2$; used to prepare e. oleate injection; a sclerosing agent for varicose veins.

   **e. oleate,** ESCLEROSIMA; sclerosing agent used for treatment of varicose veins.

**ethav'erine hydrochloride.** PAPETHERINE; ethylpapaverine hydrochloride; 6,7-diethoxy-1-(3,4-diethoxybenzyl) isoquinoline hydrochloride; smooth muscle relaxant.

**ethchlorvynol** (eth-klōr-vi'nol) (NF, BP). PLACIDYL; ethyl β-chlorovinyl ethynyl carbinol. Hypnotic and anticonvulsant; used for the induction of sleep in simple insomnia and as a daytime sedative.

**eth'ene.** Ethylene.

**eth'enyl.** Vinyl.

**ether** (e'ther) [ G. *aithēr*, the pure upper air ]. Any organic compound in which two carbon atoms are linked to a common oxygen atom: —C—O—C—; loosely used to refer to diethyl ether or anesthetic ether. A large number of ethers have anesthetic properties. For individual ethers, see the specific name, *e.g.*, cyclopropyl ethyl ether, diethyl ether, divinyl ether, enflurane, ethyl vinyl ether, fluroxene, isoflurane, methoxyflurane.

   **anesthetic e.,** (1) diethyl ether; (2) increasingly regarded as a general designation for many ethers.

   **solvent e.** (BP), a fairly pure form of e. ($C_4H_{10}O$) but not sufficiently pure for anesthesia; used as a solvent.

**ethereal** (e-the're-al) [ G. *aitherios*, etherial, fr. *aithēr*, the upper air ]. Relating to or containing ether.

**ether'ifica'tion.** Conversion of an alcohol into ether.

**ether'ify.** To convert into ether.

**etherization** (e'ther-ĭ-za'shun). The administration of ether to produce anesthesia.

**e'therize.** To produce anesthesia by the administration of ether.

**ethi'azide.** HYPERTANE; 6-chloro-3-ethyl-3,4-dihydro-2 *H*-1,2,4-benzothiadiazine-7-sulfonamide 1,1-dioxide; diuretic.

**ethical** (eth'ĭ-kal). Relating to ethics; in conformity with the rules governing personal and professional conduct.

**ethics** (eth'iks) [ G. *ethikos*, arising from custom, fr. *ethos*, custom ]. The science of morality.

   **medical e.,** the principles of proper professional conduct concerning the rights and duties of the physician himself, his patients, and his fellow practitioners.

**eth'idene.** Ethylidene.

**ethin'amate** (NF). VALMID; 1-ethynylcyclohexyl carbamate. A mild central nervous system depressant used for induction of sleep in simple insomnia and as a daytime sedative.

**ethindrone.** Ethisterone.

**eth'inyl.** Ethynyl.

**ethinylestrenol.** Lynestrenol.

**ethiodized oil** (eth-i'o-dīzd) (USP). An iodine addition product of the ethyl ester of the fatty acid of poppyseed oil; a sterile radiopaque medium.

   **e. oil I 131** (USAN), radioactive substance with antineoplastic activity.

**ethionamide** (ē-thi'on-ă-mid) (USP, BP). TRECATOR; 2-ethylthioisonicotinamide; used in the treatment of pulmonary tuberculosis. When the drug is administered alone, bacterial resistance develops rapidly; it should be given only with other antituberculous agents.

**ethi'onine.** A methionine analogue, differing in the presence of an S—ethyl group in the molecule in place of an S—methyl group; a methionine antagonist.

**ethis'terone** (BP). Ethindrone: pregneninolone; 17α-ethynyltestosterone; an orally effective, semisynthetic steroid that has biological effects similar to those of progesterone.

**ethmo-** [ G. *ēthmos*, sieve ]. Combining form (1) meaning ethmoid; (2) relating to the ethmoid bone.

**eth'mocardi'tis** [ ethmo- + G. *kardia*, heart, + suffix -*itis*, inflammation ]. Cardiosclerosis.

**ethmocephalus** (eth'mo-sef'ă-lus) [ ethmo- + G. *kephalē*, head ]. A congenitally malformed individual with a rudimentary nose which is proboscis-shaped. It may show traces of imperforate nostrils at its distal end. A variety of cebocephalus.

**ethmocra'nial.** Relating to the ethmoid bone and the cranium as a whole.

**ethmofron'tal.** Relating to the ethmoid and the frontal bones.

**ethmoid** (eth'moyd) [ G. *ēthmos*, sieve, + *eidos*, resemblance ]. 1. Resembling a sieve; cribriform. 2. Relating to the e. bone, *os* ethmoidale.

**ethmoid'al.** Ethmoid.

**ethmoidectomy** (eth-moy-dek'to-mī) [ ethmo- + G. *ektomē*, excision ]. Removal of more or less of the mucosal lining and bony partitions between the ethmoid sinuses.

**ethmoiditis** (eth-moy-di'tis). Inflammation of the ethmoid sinuses.

**ethmolac′rimal.** Relating to the ethmoid and the lacrimal bones.

**ethmomax′illary.** Relating to the ethmoid and the maxillary bones.

**ethmona′sal.** Relating to the ethmoid and the nasal bones.

**ethmopal′atal.** Relating to the ethmoid and the palate bones.

**ethmosphenoid** (eth-mo-sfe′noyd). Relating to the ethmoid and sphenoid bones.

**ethmotur′binals.** The conchae of the ethmoid bone; the superior and middle conchae; occasionally a third exists.

**ethmovomerine** (eth′mo-vo′mer-in). Relating to the ethmoid bone and the vomer.

**ethmyphitis** (eth-mī-fi′tis) [ ethmo- + G. *hyphe,* web, + suffix -*itis,* inflammation ]. Obsolete term for cellulitis.

**ethnocentrism** (eth-no-sen′trizm) [ G. *ethnos,* race, tribe, + *kentron,* center of a circle, + ism ]. The tendency to evaluate other groups according to the values and standards of one's own ethnic group, especially with the conviction that one's own ethnic group is superior to the other groups.

**eth′ohep′tazine citrate.** ZACTANE citrate; ethyl hexahydro-1-methyl-4-phenylazepinecarboxylate citrate. An analgesic related to meperidine but devoid of addiction liability. It is approximately as effective as codeine but it may be less effective than aspirin in some conditions such as postpartum pain.

**ethohexadiol** (eth′o-heks′ā-di′ol, -heks-a′dī-ol). 2-Ethyl-1,3-hexanediol; used as an insect repellant, in compound dimethyl phthalate solution.

**ethologist** (e-thol′o-jist). A specialist in ethology.

**ethology** (e-thol′o-jī) [ G. *ethos,* character, habit, + *logos,* study ]. The study of animal behavior.

**ethomox′ane hydrochloride.** Ethoxybutamoxane hydrochloride; 2-(butylaminomethyl)-8-ethoxy-1,4-benzodioxan hydrochloride; antianxiety agent.

**ethopro′pazine hydrochloride** (USP, BP). PARSIDOL hydrochloride; profenamine hydrochloride; 10-(2-diethylaminopropyl)-phenothiazine hydrochloride; an anticholinergic agent with some antihistaminic and ganglionic blocking activity; used in the symptomatic treatment of paralysis agitans, and experimentally for the inhibition of pseudocholinesterase.

**ethosuximide** (eth′o-suks′ī-mid) (USP, BP). ZARONTIN; 2-ethyl-2-methylsuccinimide; α,α-ethylmethylsuccinimide; an anticonvulsant used in the control of petit mal epilepsy; bone marrow damage and aplastic anemia may occasionally occur.

**ethotoin** (ĕ-tho′to-in) (BP). PEGANONE; 3-ethyl-5-phenylhydantoin. An anticonvulsant used in the treatment of grand mal epilepsy.

**ethox′azene hydrochloride** (USAN). SERENIUM; 4-[ (*p*-ethoxyphenyl)azo ]-*m*-phenylenediamine monohydrochloride; an azo compound used as a urinary antiseptic; changes the color of the urine to orange or red; an acid-base indicator.

**ethox′y.** The monovalent radical, $CH_3CH_2O$—.

**ethoxybu′tamox′ane hydrochloride.** Ethomoxane hydrochloride.

**ethoxycaf′feine.** 1,3,7-Trimethyl-2,6-dioxo-8-ethoxypurine; has been used in neuralgia and migraine.

**2-ethoxyeth′anol.** CELLOSOLVE; OXITOL; ethylene glycol monoethyl ether; $HOCH_2CH_2OC_2H_5$; an industrial solvent.

**ethoxyzol′amide** (USP). CARDRASE; 6-ethoxy-2-benzothiazolesulfonamide. A diuretic related chemically and pharmacologically to acetazolamide. Also used as an adjunct in the treatment of glaucoma and epilepsy.

**ethybenztro′pine hydrochloride.** PONALID; 3-diphenylmethoxy-8-ethylnortropane hydrochloride; anticholinergic agent.

**eth′yl.** The hydrocarbon radical, $CH_3CH_2$—.
  **e. alcohol,** alcohol (USP, BP); ethanol; grain alcohol; wine spirit; $C_2H_5$—OH; the alcohol of wine, whiskey, and other spirituous beverages. See also alcohol.
  **e. aminobenzoate,** benzocaine.
  **e. biscoumac′etate,** TROMEXAN; 3,3′-carboxymethylene bis-(4-hydroxycoumarin)ethyl ester; ethyl 4:4′-dihydroxydicoumarin-3:3′-yl-acetate. An anticoagulant chemically related to bishydroxycoumarin.
  **e. butyrate,** $CH_3CH_2CH_2COOCH_2CH_3$; used in perfumery.
  **e. carbamate,** urethan.
  **e. carbanilate,** phenylurethan.
  **e. chloride** (NF, BP), KELENE; chloroethane; chlorethyl; a very volatile liquid (under increased pressure); used to produce local anesthesia by superficial freezing, and as a general anesthetic by inhalation.
  **e. eosin,** the e. ester of tetrabromofluorescein, $C_{22}H_{11}O_5Br_4Na$, also known as alcohol soluble eosin; a fluorescent red acid dye used as a counterstain in histology.
  **e. ether,** diethyl ether.
  **e. formate,** a volatile, flammable liquid used as a fumigant, agricultural larvicide, and fungicide; also used as a flavor.
  **e. nitrite,** nitrous ether.
  **e. oleate** (NF, BP), used as an alternative vehicle in BP injections of deoxycorticosterone acetate, menaphthone, etc.
  **e. oxide,** diethyl ether.
  **e. salicylate,** the salicylic acid ester of e. alcohol, with the same action as oil of wintergreen (methyl salicylate).
  **e. vanillate,** ethyl-4-hydroxy-3-methoxybenzoate. Used in the treatment of disseminated histoplasmosis and coccidioidomycosis. Toxic effects are frequent.
  **e. vanillin** (NF), 3-ethoxy-4-hydroxybenzaldehyde; a homologue of vanillin, four times as strong in flavor; used as a flavor, and in perfumery.

**eth′ylate.** A compound in which the hydrogen of the hydroxyl group of an alcohol is replaced by a metallic atom, usually sodium or potassium, *e.g.,* $C_2H_5ONa$.

**eth′ylcar′binol.** Propyl alcohol.

**eth′ylcarbon′ic acid.** Propionic acid.

**eth′ylcel′lulose** (NF). ETHOCEL; an ethyl ether of cellulose, used as a tablet binder.

**eth′ylene.** Ethene; olefiant gas; $CH_2CH_2$; a constituent of ordinary illuminating gas; explosive; used as an inhalation anesthetic slightly more potent than nitrous oxide.
  **e. oxide** (USP), used for sterilizing surgical instruments.

**eth′ylenedi′amine** (USP). Ethanediamine; $H_2N(CH_2)_2$-$NH_2$; a volatile colorless liquid of ammoniacal odor and caustic taste.
  **e. dihydrochloride,** used as a urinary acidifier.

**eth′ylenedi′aminetet′raace′tic acid.** Abbreviated EDTA; edetic acid; edathamil; VERSENE; ($HOOC$—$CH_2)_2N(CH_2)_2N(CH_2$—$COOH)_2$; a chelating agent used to remove multivalent cations from solution as chelates; used in biochemical research to remove $Mg^{++}$, $Fe^{++}$, etc., from reactions affected by such ions. As the sodium salt, it is used as a water softener, to stabilize drugs rapidly decomposed in the presence of traces of metal ions, and as anticoagulant. As the sodium calcium salt, used to remove radium, lead, strontium, plutonium, and cadmium from the skeleton, forming a stable, un-ionized soluble compound that is excreted by the kidneys; renal toxicity (tubular destruction) may occur.

**eth′ylenehy′drin sulfonic acid.** Isethionic acid.

**eth′yles′trenol** (USAN). MAXIBOLIN; ORGABOLIN; 17α-ethyl-4-estren-17β-ol; a semisynthetic, orally effective, anabolic steroid; used to accelerate anabolism or to retard excessive catabolism; in addition, it can exert typically androgenic effects.

**ethylhex′edrine.** Cyclexedrine.

**ethylhydrocupreine** (eth-il-hi′dro-ku′prēn). OPTOQUINE; hydrocupreine ethyl ether; a synthetic compound closely related to quinine; active against pneumococcal infections. Used locally in such infections of the eye, but given orally it injures the optic nerve. Also available as e. hydrochloride.

**ethyl′idene.** Ethidene; the radical $CH_3CH$= (*cf.* ethyl).
  **e. chloride,** 1,1-dichloroethane; $Cl_2CHCH_3$; a highly potent, rapidly acting inhalation anesthetic with viscerotoxic potential.

**ethyl′idyne.** The radical $CH_3C\equiv$ (*cf.* ethylidene).

**ethylisobu′trazine.** DIQUEL; SERGETYL; 10-(3-dimethylamino-2-methylpropyl)-2-ethylphenothiazine; antihistaminic.

**eth′ylmeth′ylcar′binol.** Secondary butyl alcohol.

**ethylmethylthiambutene.** EMETHIBUTIN; *N*-ethyl-*N*-1-di-methyl-3,3-di-2-thienylallylamine; analgesic.

**eth′ylmor′phine hydrochloride.** DIONIN; the ethyl ether of morphine; an antispasmodic, antitussive, and analgesic, used locally as an irritant lymphagogue in chronic catarrhal middle ear disease, atrophic rhinitis, and painful ocular diseases (iritis, corneal ulcer, etc.).

**ethylnorepinephrine hydrochloride** (eth′il-nor-ep′ī-nef′-rin). ENE; BRONKEPHRINE hydrochloride; BUTANEFRINE hydrochloride; α-(1-aminopropyl)-3,4-dihydroxybenzyl alcohol hydrochloride; sympathomimetic, used in asthma; it does not raise the blood pressure.

**eth′ylpar′aben** (USP). Ethyl *p*-hydroxybenzoate; an antifungal preservative.

**ethylphenacemide.** BENURIDE; (2-phenylbutyryl)urea; anticonvulsant.

**ethylphenylephrine hydrochloride.** EFFORTIL; α-[(ethylamino)methyl]-*m*-hydroxybenzyl alcohol hydrochloride; a sympathomimetic amine vasopressor agent.

**eth′ylstib′amine.** NEOSTIBOSAN; Fourneau 693; a synthetic organic compound of antimony. Used in the treatment of several protozoal diseases, and for the relief of pain in multiple myeloma.

**eth′ylvi′nyl ether.** VINAMAR; vinylethyl ether; $CH_3CH_2OCHCH_2$; a flammable inhalation anesthetic of moderate potency.

**ethynerone** (ĕ-thin′er-ōn) (USAN). 21-Chloro-17-hydroxy-19-nor-17-pregna-4,9-dien-20-yn-3-one; progestational agent.

**ethynodiol** (ĕ-thin′o-di-ōl). 17α-Ethynyl-4-estrene-3β,17β-diol (for estrane structure, see steroids); a semisynthetic, orally effective steroid with biological effects that largely resemble those of progesterone; in addition, it is weakly estrogenic and androgenic. Administered in combination with an estrogen as an oral contraceptive.

   **e. diacetate** (BP, USP), OVULEN; METRULIN; 3,17-diacetate of ethynodiol; an antifertility agent, usually used in combination with mestranol.

**ethynyl** (eth′ī-nil). Ethinyl; acetenyl; the monovalent radical $HC≡C—$.

   **e. estradiol,** see under estradiol.

**ethyser′pine.** *dl*-17-Demethoxy-17α-ethylreserpine; a neuron-blocking agent used for the treatment of essential hypertension.

**etiane.** 5β-Androstane.

**etianic acids.** Androstane-17-carboxylic acids; see etio-.

**etidocaine.** DURANEST; (+)-2-(ethylpropylamino)-2′,6′-butyroxylidide; a local anesthetic drug.

**etidron′ic acid** (USAN). (1-Hydroxyethylidene)diphosphoric acid; a substance that regulates bone calcium.

**etio-** (e′tī-o-). 1. Prefix used with (for example) cholane to indicate replacement of the C-17 side chain by H; thus, etiocholane is 5β-androstane. See also etianic acids. 2 [ G. *aitia*, cause ]. Combining form meaning cause.

**etioallocholane** (e′tī-o-al-o-ko-lān). 5α-Androstane.

**etiocholane** (e′tī-o-ko′lān). 5β-Androstane.

**etiocholanolone** (e′tī-o-ko-lan′o-lōn). 3α-Hydroxy-5β-androstan-17-one (for androstane structure, see steroids); a metabolite of adrenocortical and testicular hormones; an important urinary 17-ketosteroid; produces fever when given to human beings, but no other biological effects.

**etiogenic** (e′tī-o-jen′ik) [ G. *aitia*, cause, + *genesis*, production ]. Causal.

**e′tiolated.** Subjected to, or characterized by, etiolation.

**e′tiolation** [ Fr. *étioler*, to blanch ]. 1. Paleness or pallor resulting from absence of light, as in persons confined because of illness or imprisoned, or in plants bleached by being deprived of light. 2. The process of blanching, bleaching, or making pale by withholding light.

**etiologic** (e′tī-o-loj′ik) Relating to etiology.

**etiologist** (e′tī-ol′o-jist). A student of etiology.

**etiology** (e′tī-ol′o-jī) [ G. *aitia*, cause, + *logos*, treatise, discourse ]. Causation; the doctrine of causes, the study of causes; specifically, the cause of disease.

**e′tiopath′ic** [ G. *aitia*, cause, + *pathos*, disease ]. Relating to specific lesions concerned with the cause of a disease.

**e′tiopor′phyrin.** A porphyrin derivative characterized by the presence on each of the four pyrrole rings of one methyl group and one ethyl group. Four isomeric forms are thus possible (see porphin).

**etiotropic** (e-tī-o-trop′ik) [ G. *aitia*, cause, + *tropē*, a turning ]. Directed against the cause; denoting a remedy that attenuates or destroys the causal factor of a disease; opposed to nosotropic.

**etonitazene.** 1-[ (2-Diethylamino)ethyl ]-2-(*p*-ethoxybenzyl)-5-nitrobenzimidazole; analgesic.

**etophylate.** ETAPHYLLINE; piperazine theophylline-7-acetate; diuretic and smooth muscle relaxant.

**etorphine hydrochloride.** Tetrahydro-7α-(1-hydroxy-1-methylbutyl)-6,14-endo-ethenooripavine hydrochloride; narcotic analgesic.

**etox′adrol hydrochloride** (USAN). D-2-(2-Ethyl-2-phenyl-1,3-dioxolan-4-yl)-piperidine hydrochloride; local anesthetic.

**etozolin.** 3-Methyl-4-oxo-5-piperidino-2,α-thiazolidine-acetic acid ethyl ester; diuretic.

**etrot′omy** [ G. *ētron*, abdomen, + *tomē*, incision ]. Suprapubic incision.

**etymide.** Carbiphene hydrochloride.

**Eu.** Chemical symbol of the element europium.

**eu-.** G. particle, used as a prefix, meaning good, well.

**Eu′bacteria′les.** An obsolete order of bacteria which contained simple, undifferentiated, rigid cells which were either spheres or straight rods. It contained motile (peritrichous) and nonmotile, Gram-negative and Gram-positive, and sporeforming and nonsporeforming species. The order contained 13 families: Achromobacteraceae, Azotobacteraceae, Bacillaceae, Bacteroidaceae, Brevibacteriaceae, Brucellaceae, Corynebacteriaceae, Enterobacteriaceae, Lactobacillaceae, Micrococcaceae, Neisseriaceae, Propionibacteriaceae, and Rhizobacteriaceae.

**Eubacterium** (u-bak-tēr′ī-um) A genus of anaerobic, nonsporeforming, nonmotile bacteria containing straight or curved Gram-positive rods which usually occur singly, in pairs, or in short chains. Usually these organisms attack carbohydrates. They may be pathogenic. The type species is *E. foedans.*

   **E. aerofa′ciens,** a species infrequently found in human intestines; pathogenic for mice.

   **E. bifor′me,** a species that occurs infrequently in human intestines; pathogenic for rabbits but not for mice.

   **E. combe′si,** *Cillobacterium combesi;* a species from forest soil from French West Africa; it is not pathogenic for guinea pigs or mice.

   **E. contor′tum,** *Catenabacterium contortum;* a species found in cases of putrid, gangrenous appendicitis and in the intestines.

   **E. crispa′tum,** a species found in pus from a dental abscess.

   **E. discifor′mans,** a species found in cases of fetid suppurations in empyema, pulmonary gangrene, liver abscess, and dermatosis; occurs commonly in the respiratory system, the liver, and the skin; pathogenic for man, rabbits, guinea pigs, and mice.

   **E. ethylicum,** a species found in a case of gastritis; occurs infrequently in the human stomach.

   **E. filamento′sum,** *Catenabacterium filamentosum;* a species found in the intestines of rats; it is also found in cases of acute appendicitis, lung abscess, putrid pleurisy, and uterine suppuration.

   **E. foedans,** a species found in spoiled, salted ham; it is the type species of the genus.

   **E. lentum,** a species occurring commonly in the feces of normal persons.

   **E. limo′sum,** a species that occurs in human feces and presumably in the feces of other warm-blooded animals.

   **E. minu′tum,** a species that occurs infrequently in the intestines of breast-fed infants; it was originally found in a case of infant diarrhea; it is pathogenic for mice.

   **E. monilifor′me,** *Cillobacterium moniliforme;* a species found rarely in the human respiratory systems; it is pathogenic for guinea pigs, causing death in eight days.

   **E. multifor′me,** *Cillobacterium multiforme;* a species isolated from the feces of a dog and from soil from Equatorial Africa; it is not pathogenic for guinea pigs.

**E. nio'sii,** a species that occurs in the respiratory tract; pathogenic for rabbits and guinea pigs.

**E. par'vum,** a species found in the large intestine of a horse and in a case of acute appendicitis; it occurs infrequently in the intestines of foals and of humans, and is not pathogenic for laboratory animals.

**E. poeciloi'des,** a species infrequently found in human intestines; originally found in a case of intestinal occlusion. It is pathogenic for guinea pigs and rabbits.

**E. pseudotortuo'sum,** a species found in a case of purulent, acute appendicitis; occurs uncommonly in the intestines.

**E. quar'tum,** a species found in cases of infantile diarrhea; occurs in the intestines of children, but is rather uncommon.

**E. quin'tum,** a species found in cases of infantile diarrhea; pathogenic for guinea pigs.

**E. recta'le,** a species found in association with a rectal ulcer; occurs in the rectum.

**E. tenue,** *Cillobacterium tenue;* a species isolated from dog feces; its pathogenicity is unknown.

**E. tortuo'sum,** a species found infrequently in the intestines of humans.

**eubiotics** (u-bi-ot'iks) [ eu- + G. *biotikos,* relating to life ]. The science of hygienic living.

**eu'bolism.** Obsolete word meaning normal body metabolism.

**eu'caine hydrochloride.** β-Eucaine hydrochloride; 2,2,6-trimethyl-4-piperidinol benzoate hydrochloride; local anesthetic for surface anesthesia.

**eucalyp'tol.** Cineole.

**eucalyp'tus.** The dried leaves of *Eucalyptus globulus* (family Myrtaceae), blue gum tree; Australian fever tree; used in the treatment of malaria, bronchitis, asthma, and chronic gonorrhea.

**e. gum,** see under gum.

**e. oil** (NF, BP), the volatile oil distilled with steam from the fresh leaf of *Eucalyptus globulus* or some other species of *Eucalyptus;* contains not less than 70 per cent of eucalyptol; used as an antiseptic, stimulant, and expectorant.

**eucapnia** (u-kap'ni-ah) [ eu- + G. *kapnos,* vapor ]. A state in which the arterial carbon dioxide pressure is optimal; see also normocapnia.

**eucaryote** (u-kăr'ĭ-ot) [ eu- + G. *karyon,* kernel, nut ]. Eukaryote; an organism whose cells contain a limiting membrane around the nuclear material; *cf.* procaryote.

**eu'caryot'ic.** Eukaryotic; pertaining to a eucaryote.

**euca'sin.** Ammonium caseinate; prepared by passing ammonia gas over finely powdered dry casein. Added as a concentrated food to bouillon, chocolate, etc.

**eucatropine hydrochloride** (u-kat'ro-pēn) (USP). EUPHTHALMINE hydrochloride; 1,2,2,6-tetramethyl-4-piperidinol mandelate hydrochloride; a mydriatic; produces no anesthesia, pain, or increased intraocular tension.

**Eucestoda** (u'ses-to'dah). Cestoda.

**euchlorhydria** (u'klor-hi'drĭ-ah). Normal chlorhydria; a condition in which free hydrochloric acid exists in normal amount in the gastric juice.

**eucholia** (u-ko'lĭ-ah) [ eu- + G. *cholē,* bile ]. A normal state of the bile as regards quantity and quality.

**euchromatic** (u'kro-mat'ik). Orthochromatic.

**euchromatin** (u-kro'mă-tin). That portion of the chromosome found by ultraviolet microspectrophotometry to be relatively rich in nucleic acid.

**euchro'mosome.** Autosome.

**eucort'icalism.** Normal functioning of the adrenal cortex.

**eucrasia** (u-kra'zhĭ-ah) [ G. *eukrasia,* good temperament, fr. *eu,* well, + *krasis,* a mixing ]. 1. The normal balance in the body of the qualities, functions, and chemical and physical states. 2. A condition of reduced susceptibility to certain drugs, articles of diet, etc.; see also orthocrasia, idiosyncrasy.

**eucupine** (u'ku-pēn). Isopentylhydrocupreine; hydrocupreine isopentyl ether; a derivative of quinine; antiseptic and local anesthetic.

**eudemonia** (u'de-mo'nĭ-ah) [ eu- + G. *daimon,* destiny ]. A feeling of well-being or happiness.

**eudiaphoresis** (u'di-ah-fo-re'sis) [ eu- + G. *diaphorēsis,* perspiration ]. Normal, free sweating.

**eudiemorrhysis** (u-di-ĕ-mor'ĭ-sis) [ eu- + G. *dia,* through, + *haima,* blood, + *rhysis,* a flowing ]. A free normal capillary circulation.

**eudiometer** (u-dī-om'e-ter) [ G. *eudios,* fine, clear (of air and weather), + *metron,* measure ]. A graduated glass vessel used to test the purity of air and in the volumetric analysis of gases.

**eudip'sia** [ eu- + G. *dipsa,* thirst ]. Ordinary mild thirst.

**euergasia** (u'er-ga'zĭ-ah) [ eu- + G. *ergasia,* work ]. Good mentality.

**Euflagellata** (u-flaj'ĕ-la'tah). Flagellata.

**Eugenia** (u-je'nĭ-ah) [ after Prince *Eugene* of Savoy ]. A genus of trees of the family Myrtaceae. *E. caryophyllata* furnishes cloves; *E. jambolana,* jambul; *E. pimenta,* pimenta or allspice.

**eugenic** (u-jen'ik). Relating to the science of eugenics; tending to racial improvement through breeding from stock possessing the most desirable characteristics.

**e. acid,** eugenol.

**eugenics** (u-jen'iks) [ G. *eugeneia,* nobility of birth, fr. *eu,* well, + *genesis,* production ]. Aristogenics; the science which deals with the influences, especially prenatal influences, that tend to better the innate qualities of man and to develop them to the highest degree.

**eugenism** (u'jen-izm). "The aggregate of the most favorable conditions for healthy and happy existence" (Galton).

**eu'genol** (USP, BP). Eugenic acid; 4-allyl-2-methoxyphenol; obtained from oil of cloves; used in dentistry with zinc oxide as a sedative temporary restoration and as a base for impression materials; also used in perfumery as a substitute for oil of cloves.

**eugenothenics** (u-jen-o-then'iks) [ eu- + G. *genos,* race, + *theinai,* to place ]. The study of population improvement by regulation of both genetic and environmental factors.

**Euglena** (u-gle'nah) [ eu- + G. *glēnē,* eyeball ]. A genus of the family Euglenidae.

**E. grac'ilis,** sometimes used in assaying vitamin $B_{12}$ concentrations of serum and urine in various types of anemia.

**E. vir'idis,** inhabits stagnant pools, often in great numbers.

**Euglenidae** (u-gle'nĭ-de). A family of green (phytomonad) flagellates.

**euglobulin** (u-glob'u-lin). That fraction of the serum globulin less soluble in $(NH_4)_2SO_4$ solution than the pseudoglobulin fraction.

**euglycemic** (u-gli-se'mik) [ eu- + G. *glykys,* sweet, + *haima,* blood ]. Denoting an agent that produces a normal blood glucose concentration.

**eugnathia** (u-na'thĭ-ah, -nath'ĭ-ah) [ eu- + G. *gnathos,* jaw ]. Eugnathic anomaly; designation for those abnormalities that are limited to the teeth and their immediate alveolar supports.

**eugnosia** (u-no'sĭ-ah) [ eu- + G. *gnōsis,* perception ]. Normal perception related to the ability to synthesize sensory stimuli.

**eugonic** (u-gon'ik) [ G. *eugonos,* productive, fr. *eu,* well, + *gonos,* seed, offspring. GEN- ]. A term used to indicate that the growth of a bacterial culture is rapid and relatively luxuriant; used especially in reference to the growth of cultures of the human tubercle bacillus (*Mycobacterium tuberculosis*). See also dysgonic.

**Eugregarinida** (u'greg-ă-rin'ĭ-dah) [ eu- + L. *gregarius,* gregarious ]. An order of gregarines (subclass Gregarinia), reproducing only by sporogeny in which schizogeny is absent. They are parasites of annelids and arthropods.

**euhydration** (u'hi-dra'shun). Normal state of body water content; absence of absolute or relative hydration or dehydration.

**euka'ryote.** Eucaryote.

**eu'karyot'ic.** Eucaryotic.

**eukeratin** (u-kĕr'ă-tin). Hard keratin present in hair, wool, horn, nails, etc.

**eukinesia** (u'kĭ-ne'zĭ-ah) [ eu- + G. *kinēsis,* movement ]. Normal movement.

**Eulenburg** (oi'len-boorg), Albert, German neurologist, 1840–1917. See E.'s *disease*.

**Euler,** Ulf von, Swedish physiologist, *1905. Nobel laureate, 1970, with Julius Axelrod and Bernard Katz for their work on humoral transmitter substances and mechanisms at nerve terminals.

**eulicin.** Antibiotic produced by a species of *Streptomyces* similar to *Streptomyces parvus;* possesses antifungal activity.

**eumetria** (u-me'trī-ah) [ G. moderation, goodness of meter ]. Graduation of the strength of nerve impulses.

**eumorphism** (u-mor'fizm) [ eu- + G. *morphē,* shape ]. Preservation of the natural form of a cell.

**eumycetes** (u'mi-se'tēz) [ eu- + G. *mykēs,* fungus ]. True fungi.

**eunoia** (u-noy'ah) [ G. goodwill, fr. *eu,* well, + *nous,* mind ]. A normal mental state.

**eunuch** (u'nuk) [ G. *eunouchos,* fr. *eunē,* bed, + *echein,* to have, because used as chamberlain ]. One whose testes have been removed or have never developed.
 **pitu'itary e.,** see *dystrophia* adiposogenitalis.

**eunuchism** (u'nuk-izm). 1. Absence of the testes and the consequences hereof; the state of being a eunuch. 2. Eunuchoidism.

**eunuchoid** (u'nuk-oyd) [ G. *eunouchos,* eunuch, + *eidos,* resembling ]. Partially resembling, or having the general characteristics of, a eunuch.

**eunuchoidism** (u'nuk-oyd-izm). Male hypogonadism; a state in which testes are present but fail to function; may be of gonadal or pituitary origin.
 **hy'pergonadotrop'ic e.,** e. of gonadal origin; commonly accompanied by enhanced excretion of urinary gonadotropins. One example of this kind of disorder is Klinefelter's syndrome, *q.v.*
 **hy'pogonad'otrop'ic e.,** hypogonadotropic *hypogonadism.*

**euonymus** (u-on'ĭ-mus) [ G. *euōnymos,* from *eu,* well, + *onyma,* name, having a good name, lucky ]. The dried root bark of *Euonymus atropurpureus (family Celastraceae);* wahoo; burning bush; arrow wood; has been used as a laxative.

**euosmia** (u-oz'mĭ-ah) [ eu- + G. *osmē,* smell ]. 1. A pleasant odor. 2. Normal olfaction.

**eupancreatism** (u-pan'kre-ā-tizm). The state of normal pancreatic digestive function.

**euparal** (u'par-al). A medium for mounting histologic specimens, composed of sandarac, eucalyptol, paraldehyde, camphor, and phenyl salicylate.

**Euparyphium** (u'pă-rif'ĭ-um) [ eu- + G. *paryphē,* a border ]. A genus of rare and nonpathogenic flukes (family Echinostomatidae), several species of which have been reported from the intestine of man.

**eupath'eoscope.** A device, resembling a thermointegrator, for measuring environmental warmth.

**eupat'orin.** 3',5-Dihydroxy-4',6,7-trimethoxyflavone (*cf.* catechin); obtained from several species of *Eupatorium.* Emetic.

**Eupatorium** (u-pă-to'rĭ-um) [ G. *eupatorion,* agrimony, named after Mirthridates *Eupator*]. A genus of composite herbs, several species of which are used medicinally and as popular household remedies.
 **E. aromat'icum,** smaller white snakeroot. Used as a sedative and antispasmodic.
 **E. perfolia'tum,** boneset; thoroughwort; sweating herb; the dried leaves and flowering tops have formerly been official under the title "eupatorium," the drug being used as a diaphoretic and as a bitter tonic.

**eupav'erin hydrochloride.** SORBOSAN; 1-benzyl-3-ethyl-6,7-dimethoxyisoquinoline hydrochloride; smooth muscle relaxant.

**eupepsia** (u'pep'sĭ-ah) [ G. fr. *eu,* well, + *pepsis,* digestion ]. Good digestion.

**eupep'tic.** Digesting well; having a good digestion.

**euphenics** (u-fe'niks) [ eu- + G. *phainō,* to show forth ]. Changes in the phenotype of an organism by means other than controlled breeding, as, for example, by altering intracellular composition of nucleic acids.

**Euphorbia** (u-for'bĭ-ah) [ G. *euphorbion,* an African plant, spurge ]. A genus of plants, the spurges (family Euphor-

biaceae), mostly shrubs, though some are bushes or trees, some species of which are used in medicine.
 **E. pilulif'era,** asthma-weed; the dried herb, used in asthma, coryza, and other respiratory affections, in angina pectoris, and as an antispasmodic.
 **E. resinif'era,** a species from which is obtained the gum resin euphorbium.

**euphoria** (u-fo'rī-ah) [ eu- + G. *pherō,* to bear ]. A feeling of well-being, commonly exaggerated and not necessarily well founded.

**euphoriant** (u-fo'rī-ant). Euphoretic. 1. Having the capability to produce a sense of well-being (euphoria). 2. An agent with such a capability.

**euphoretic** (u-fo-ret'ik). Euphoriant.

**Euphrac'tus sexcinc'tus** [ eu- + G. *phraktos,* protected; L. *sex,* six, + *cinctus,* girdled ]. A species of armadillo (Brazil), a reservoir host of *Trypanosoma cruzi.*

**euplasia** (u-pla'zī-ah) [ eu- + G. *plassō, to form* ]. The state of cells or tissue which is normal or typical for that particular type.

**euplas'tic** [ G. *euplastos,* easily molded; *eu,* well, + *plassō,* to form ]. 1. Relating to euplasia. 2. Healing readily and well.

**euploid** (u'ployd). Relating to euploidy.

**euploidy** (u'ploy-dī) [ eu- + G. *-ploos, -fold* ]. The state of a cell whose number of chromosomes is an exact multiple of the haploid number normal for the species.

**eupnea** (ūp-ne'ah) [ G. *eupnoia,* fr. *eu,* well, + *pnoia,* breath ]. Easy, free respiration; the type observed in the normal subject under resting conditions.

**eupraxia** (u-prak'sī-ah) [ eu- + G. *praxis,* a doing ]. Normal ability to perform coordinated movements.

**Euproc'tis chrysorrhoe'a** [ eu- + G. *prōktos,* rump; *chrysos,* gold, + *rhoia,* flow ]. The brown-tail moth, the hairs of the cocoon and caterpillar of which cause a troublesome dermatitis.

**eurhythmia** (u-rith'mĭ-ah) [ eu- + G. *rhythmos,* rhythm ]. Harmonious body relationships of the separate organs.

**europium** (u-ro'pĭ-um) [ L. *Europa,* Europe ]. An element of the rare earth (lanthanide) group, symbol Eu, atomic no. 63, atomic weight 152.0.

**Eurotium** (u-ro'shī-um) [ G. *eurōs,* mold ]. An ascomycetous genus of fungi.

**eury-** (u'rī-) [ G. *eurys,* wide ]. Combining form meaning wide or broad.

**eurycephalic, eurycephalous** (u'rī-sĕ-fal'ik, -sef'ă-lus) [ eury- + G. *kephalēs,* head ]. Brachycephalic.

**eurygnathic** (u-rig-nath'ik). Eurygnathous; having a wide jaw.

**eurygnathism** (u-rig'nă-thizm) [ eury- + G. *gnathos,* jaw ]. The condition of having a wide jaw.

**eurygnathous** (u-rig'nă-thus). Eurygnathic.

**euryon** (u'rī-on) [ G. *eurys,* broad ]. The extremity, on either side, of the greatest transverse diameter of the head; a point used in craniometry.

**euryopia** (u'rī-o'pī-ah) [ eury- + G. *ops,* eye ]. A wide interorbital distance; a normal variation as seen in the Chinese and not due to a pathological condition as in hypertelorism.

**eurysomatic** (u'rī-so-mat'ik) [ eury- + G. *soma,* body ]. Having a thick-set body.

**euscope** (u'skōp) [ eu- + G. *skopeō,* to view ]. An instrument for showing on a screen an enlarged image from a microscope.

**Eusimulium** (u'sī-mu'lī-um). *Simulium.*

**Eustachian** (u-sta'kī-an, u-sta'shī-an). Described by or attributed to Bartolonmeo E. Eustachio.

**Eustachio,** Bartolommeo E., Italian anatomist, 1520–1574. See Eustachian *catheter, cushion, tonsil, tube, tuber, valve.*

**eustachitis** (u-sta-ki'tis). Inflammation of the mucous membrane of the Eustachian tube.

**eusthenia** (u-sthe'nī-ah) [ eu- + G. *sthenos,* strength ]. Normal strength.

**Eustrongylus** (u-stron'jī-lus) [ eu- + G. *strongylos,* rounded ]. A genus of Nematoda of the family Strongylidae, parasitic in pigs and other domestic animals.

**E. gigas,** *Dioctophyma renale.*

**E. viscera'lis,** *Dioctophyma renale.*

**eusystole** (u-sis'to-le) [ eu- + systole, *q.v.* ]. A condition in which the cardiac systole is normal in force and time.

**eusystolic** (u-sis-tol'ik). 1. Relating to eusystole. 2. One whose heart beats normally.

**eutectic** (u-tek'tik). 1. Easily melted; denoting specifically mixtures of certain chemical compounds that have a lower melting point than any of their ingredients; denoting, for instance, a solid such as menthol that, when triturated with another solid of the same class, such as camphor, unites with it to form a liquid, the mixture having a lower melting point than either of its components. 2. The alloy that freezes at a constant temperature; the lowest of the series.

**eutexia** (u-tek'sĭ-ah) [ eu- + G. *tēxis*, a melting away, dissolution ]. The formation of a eutectic.

**euthanasia** (u'thă-na'zĭ-ah) [ eu- + G. *thanatos*, death ]. 1. A quiet, painless death. 2. The intentional putting to death by artificial means of persons with incurable or painful disease.

**euthen'ics** [ G. *euthenein*, to thrive ]. The science that deals with establishing optimum living conditions for plants, animals, or humans, especially through care for proper provisioning and environment.

**eutherapeutic** (u'thĕr-ă-pu'tik). Having excellent curative properties.

**Eutheria** (u-the'rĭ-ah) [ eu- + G. *thērion*, animal ]. A subclass of mammals, excluding monotremes and marsupials, having a placenta through which the young are nourished.

**euthermic** (u-ther'mik) [ eu- + G. *thermos*, warm ]. At an optimal temperature.

**euthymia** (u-thi'mĭ-ah) [ eu- + G. *thymos*, mind. THYM-2 ]. Joyfulness; mental peace and tranquility.

**euthyroidism** (u-thi'roy-dizm). A condition in which the thyroid gland is functioning normally, its secretion being of proper amount and constitution.

**euthyscope** (u'thĭ-skōp) [ G. *euthys*, straight, + *skopeō*, to view ]. A modified ophthalmoscope with which the site of excentric fixation may be dazzled by a bright light while the true fovea is simultaneously shielded by an opaque disk in the center of this light bundle. Used in pleoptics.

**euthyscopy** (u-this'ko-pĭ). Examination with the euthyscope.

**eutocia** (u-to'sĭ-ah) [ eu- + G. *tokos*, childbirth ]. Easy, normal childbirth.

**eutonic** (u-ton'ik) [ eu- + G. *tonus*, tone ]. Normotonic (1).

**eutrichosis** (u-trĭ-ko'sis) [ eu- + G. *thrix*, hair ]. A normal growth of healthy hair.

**eutrophia** (u-tro'fĭ-ah) [ G. fr. *eu*, well, + *trophē*, nourishment ]. A state of normal nourishment and growth.

**eutroph'ic.** Relating to, characterized by, or promoting eutrophia.

**eutrophy** (u'tro-fĭ). Eutrophia.

**euvo'lia.** Normal water content or volume of a given compartment; *e.g.*, extracellular e.

**eV, ev.** Abbreviation for electron-volt.

**evacuant** (e-vak'u-ant). 1. Promoting an excretion, especially of the bowels. 2. An agent that increases excretion, especially a cathartic.

**evacuate** (e-vak'u-āt) [ L. *e-vacuo*, pp. *-vacuatus*, to empty out ]. To accomplish evacuation.

**evacuation** (e-vak'u-a'shun). 1. Removal of waste material, especially from the bowels. 2. Stool; material discharged from the bowels. 3. Removal of air from a closed vessel; production of a vacuum.

**evacuator** (e-vak'u-a-tor). A mechanical evacuant; an instrument for the removal of impacted feces from the rectum.

**evadol hydrochloride.** EVACLIN; 2-amino-1,2-bis(*p*-methoxyphenyl)ethanol; analgesic with sedative properties.

**evagination** (e-vaj-ĭ-na'shun) [ L. *e*, out, + *vagina*, sheath ]. The protrusion of some part or organ from its normal position.

**evanescent** (ev-ă-nes'sent) [ L. *e*, out, + *vanescere*, to vanish ]. Of short duration.

**Evans,** Herbert M., American anatomist, 1882–1971. See *Evans* blue.

**Evans blue** (USP). C.I. Direct Blue 53; tetrasodium salt of 4,4'-bis[ 7-(1-amino-8-hydroxy-2,4-disulfo)naphthylazo ]-3,3'-bitolyl; $C_{34}H_{24}N_6Na_4O_{14}S_4$; a diazo dye used for the determination of the blood volume on the basis of the dilution of a standard solution of the dye in the plasma after its intravenous injection.

**evap'ora'tion** [ L. *e*, out, + *vaporare*, to emit vapor ]. Volatilization. 1. A change from liquid to vapor form. 2. Loss of volume of a liquid by conversion into vapor.

  **heat of e.,** see under heat.

**eventration** (e'ven-tra'shun) [ L. *e*, out, + *venter*, belly ]. 1. Protrusion of omentum and/or intestine through an opening in the abdominal wall. 2. Removal of the contents of the abdominal cavity.

  **e. of the diaphragm,** extreme elevation of a half or part of the diaphragm, which is usually atrophic and abnormally thin.

**eversion** (e-ver-zhun) [ L. *e-everto*, pp. *-versus*, to overturn ]. A turning outward, as of the eyelid.

**evert** [ L. *e-verto*, to overturn ]. To turn outward.

**evidement** (a-vēd-moń') [ Fr. *évider*, to scoop out ]. The scraping out of morbid tissue from a natural or pathologic cavity.

**e'vil.** Disease; illness.

  **quarter e.,** blackleg.

  **joint e.,** (1) anesthetic *leprosy*, (2) joint *ill.*

  **king's e.,** scrofula, which was formerly thought to be curable by the touch of a king.

  **poll e.,** suppurative inflammation of the cranial nuchal (atlantal) bursa that lies between the atlas and the cranial end of the ligamentum nuchae in the horse.

  **Saint John's e.,** epilepsy.

  **Saint Main's e.,** the itch.

  **Saint Martin's e.,** chronic alcoholism.

**eviration** (ev-ĭ-ra'shun, e-vi-ra'shun) [ L. *e*, out, + *vir*, man ]. 1. Castration. 2. Loss or absence of the masculine, with acquirement of feminine characteristics; a type of effemination.

**evisceration** (e-vis-er-a'shun) [ L. *eviscero*, pp. *-atus*, to disembowel. VISC- ]. 1. Exenteration. 2. Removal of the contents of the eyeball, leaving only the sclera. 3. Disembowelling. 4. Protrusion of the abdominal viscera, *e.g.*, through a defect created by wound dehiscence.

**evisceroneurotomy** (e-vis'er-o-nu-rot'o-mĭ) [ L. *eviscero*, to disembowel, + G. *neuron*, nerve, + *tomē*, a cutting ]. Evisceration of the eye with division of the optic nerve.

**E-viton.** The unit of quantity of ultraviolet radiation which is effective biologically.

**evocation** (ev'o-ka-shun, e'vo-ka'shun) [ L. *evoco*, pp. *evocatus*, to call forth, evoke ]. The induction of a particular tissue produced by the action of an evocator during embryogenesis.

**ev'oca'tor.** The substance discharged from an organizer which is a factor in the control of morphogenesis in the early embryo.

**evolu'tion** [ L. *e-volvo*, pp. *-volutus*, to roll out ]. A continuing process of change from one state, condition or form to another.

  **bathmic e.,** orthogenic e.; a change of type due to something inherent in the constitution, independent of the environment.

  **biologic e.,** organic e.; the doctrine that all forms of animal or plant life have been derived by gradual changes from simpler forms or from a single cell.

  **convergent e.,** the evolutionary development of similar structures in two or more species, often widely separated phylogenetically, in response to similarities of environment.

  **Denman's spontaneous e.,** a mechanism of spontaneous molding of the fetus and impaction of the shoulder with prolapse of the arm noted in some cases of transverse lie, whereby vaginal delivery is achieved with the breech appearing at the vulva immediately after the prolapsed shoulder.

  **Douglas' spontaneous e.,** mechanism whereby molding of the fetus and impaction of the shoulder and prolapsed arm occurs in transverse lie, which allows vaginal delivery whereby the lateral aspect of the thorax follows the prolapsed shoulder.

emergent e., a character appearing suddenly due to a mutation.

organic e., biologic evolution.

orthogenic e., bathmic e.

saltatory e., the theory that e. of a new species from an older one may occur as a large "jump," such as a major repatterning of chromosomes, rather than by gradual accumulation of small "steps" or mutations.

spontaneous e., the unaided delivery of the fetus from a transverse lie.

evulsion (e-vul'shun) [ L. *evulsio*, fr. *e-vello*, pp. - *vulsus*, to pluck out ]. A forcible pulling out or extraction; *cf.* avulsion.

Ewart (yoo'art), William, English physician, 1848–1929. See E.'s *procedure, sign.*

ewe (yew). A female sheep of breeding age.

Ewing, James, American pathologist, 1866–1943. See E.'s *sarcoma, tumor.*

Ewing, James H., 1798–1827. See E.'s *sign.*

ex- [ L. and G. out of ]. Prefix denoting out of, from, away from.

exacerbation (eks-as-er-ba'shun) [ L. *ex-acerbo*, pp. - *auts*, to exasperate, increase, fr. *acerbus*, sour. AC- ]. An increase in the severity of a disease or any of its signs or symptoms.

examina'tion. Any investigation made for the purpose of diagnosis.

cytologic e., Papanicolaou e.; the microscopic evaluation of a cellular specimen for cancer detection and diagnosis, for evaluation of the endocrine status, and for clinical or investigative study of other dsease or health processes or states. First developed by Papanicolaou and made clinically valuable in the female genital tract by Papanicolaou and Traut, it is also useful in other areas, such as respiratory tract, urinary tract, body cavities, breast. See also cytopathology.

Papanicolaou e., cytologic e.

postmortem e., autopsy.

exam'iner [ L. *examino*, to weigh, examine ]. One who performs an examination.

medical e., (1) a physician who examines a patient, or an applicant for insurance, and reports upon his physical condition to the company or individual at whose request the examination was made; (2) in states where the office of coroner has been abolished, a physician appointed to investigate all cases of sudden or violent death; (3) one who examines a candidate for a degree or makes a test of the knowledge of a student for advancement to a higher grade in a teaching institution.

exan'them [ G. *exanthēma*, efflorescence; an eruption, fr. *anthos*, flower. ANTH- ]. Exanthema.

exanthe'ma [ G. ]. Exanthem. 1. A skin eruption occurring as a symptom of an acute viral or coccal disease; *e.g.*, scarlet fever or measles. 2. An acute disease, *e.g.*, scarlet fever or measles, accompanied by an eruption on the skin.

Boston e., [ after the city in which an epidemic occurred ], a viral disease resembling e. subitum, with the e. appearing after the fever has subsided; it is caused by strain 16 of ECHO virus.

coital e., a virus disease of cattle and horses, characterized by vesicles, later by pustules, on the mucous membranes of the genital tract; it is transmitted by coitus.

keratoid e., a symptom occurring in the secondary stage of yaws: patches of fine, light colored, furfuraceous desquamation, scattered irregularly over limbs and trunk.

e. subi'tum, pseudorubella; rose rash of infants; roseola infantilis or infantum; sixth disease; a viral disease of infants and young children, marked by sudden onset with fever lasting several days (sometimes with convulsions) and followed by a fine macular (sometimes maculopapular) rash that appears within a few hours to a day after the fever has subsided.

vesicular e., a viral disease of swine that closely resembles foot-and-mouth disease.

exanthem'atous. Relating to an exanthema.

exanthe'sis [ G. ]. 1. A rash or exanthem. 2. The coming out of a rash or eruption.

e. arthro'sia, dengue.

exanthrope (eks'an-throp) [ G. *ex*, out of, + *anthrōpos*, man ]. An external cause of disease, one not originating in the body.

exanthrop'ic. Originating outside of the human body.

exarteritis (eks-ar-ter-i'tis). Periarteritis.

exarticula'tion [ L. *ex*, out, + *articulus*, joint ]. Disarticulation.

excalation (eks'kă-la'shun) [ G. *ex*, from, + *chalān*, to abate, release ]. The absence, suppression or failure of development of one of a series of things; for example, the e. (absence) of a digit.

excavatio (eks-kă-va'shi-o) [ L. fr. *ex-cavo*, pp. -*cavatus*, to hollow out, fr. *ex*, out, + *cavus*, hollow ] [ NA ]. Excavation; pouch.

e. disci [ NA ], excavation of the disk of the optic nerve; e. papillae; physiologic excavation; the normally occurring depression or pit in the center of the optic disk.

e. papil'lae e. disci.

e. rectouteri'na [ NA ], rectouterine pouch; rectovaginouterine pouch; cavum Douglasi; Douglas' cul-de-sac; Douglas' pouch; a pocket formed by the deflection of the peritoneum from the rectum to the uterus.

e. rectovesica'lis [ NA ], rectovesical pouch; the fold of peritoneum that extends between the rectum and the bladder in the male.

e. vesicouteri'na [ NA ], uterovesical or vesicouterine pouch; cavum vesicouterina; the fold of peritoneum that extends down between the bladder and the uterus.

excavation (eks-kă-va'shun). 1. The formation of a cavity; hollowing out. 2. A natural cavity or recess; excavatio. 3. A cavity formed artificially or as the result of a pathologic process.

atroph'ic e., an exaggeration of the normal or physiologic cupping of the optic disk (excavatio disci) caused by atrophy of the optic nerve.

e. of disk of optic nerve, *excavatio* disci.

glauco'matous e., glaucomatous *cup.*

physiologic e., *excavatio* disci.

ex'cavator. 1. An instrument like a large sharp spoon or scoop, used in scraping out pathologic tissue. 2. In dentistry, a tool, generally a small spoon or curette, for cleaning out and shaping a carious cavity preparatory to filling.

hatchet e., see hatchet.

hoe e., a single-bevelled instrument, used in dentistry, with the blade at an angle to the axis of the handle and the cutting edge perpendicular to the plane of the angle. If the angle approaches 90° the instrument is used with a pull stroke; if it is small it may be used as a chisel.

excel'sin. A protein of the Brazil nut, *Bertholletia excelsa.*

excementosis (ek'se-men-to'sis). Outgrowth of cementum or root surface; corresponds to exostosis on bone surface.

excentric (ek-sen'trik). Efferent; eccentric; away from the center.

excerebration (ek'ser-e-bra'shun). Eccephalosis; removal of the brain in the operation of embryotomy.

excern (ek-sern') [ L. *ex-cerno*, to sift out ]. To excrete.

excernent (ek-ser'nent). 1. Excretory; excreting; promoting excretion. 2. An agent that promotes excretion or causes an evacuation.

excipient (ek-sip'ĭ-ent) [ L. *excipiens;* pres. p. of *ex-cipio*, to take out. CAP- ]. A more or less inert substance added in a prescription as a diluent or vehicle or to give form or consistency when the remedy is given in pill form; simple syrup, aromatic powder, honey, and various elixirs are examples of e.'s.

excise (ek-sīz). To cut out; see also resect.

excision (ek-sizh'un) [ L. *excidere*, to cut out ]. The act of cutting out; the operative removal of a portion of a limb or organ; see also resection.

total e., total biopsy; e. of tissue for gross and microscopic examination in such a manner that the entire lesion is removed rather than only a portion of it.

excitability (ek-si'tă-bil'ĭ-tĭ). Having the capability of being excitable.

exci'table. Irritable (1); capable of quick response to a stimulus; potentiality for emotional arousal.

**exci′tant** [ L. *excito*, pp. -*atus*, pres. p. -*ans*, to arouse ]. 1. Stimulating. 2. A stimulant.

**excitation** (ek-si-ta′shun). Stimulation; increasing the rapidity or intensity of the physical or mental processes.

**exci′tatory.** Tending to produce excitation.

**excite′ment.** An emotional state characterized by its potential for impulsive or poorly controlled activity.

**catatonic e.,** catatonic *schizophrenia*.

**manic e.,** a mental state resembling acute delirium, from which it differs, however, in that there are less confusion and incoherence of ideas and sometimes the patient has a measure of control over his actions.

**exci′toglan′dular.** Increasing the secretory activity of a gland.

**exci′tometabol′ic.** Increasing the activity of the metabolic processes.

**exci′tomo′tor.** Centrokinetic (2); causing or increasing the rapidity of motion.

**exci′tomus′cular.** Causing muscular activity.

**exci′tor.** A stimulant; that which excites to increased action.

**exci′tose′cretory.** Stimulating to secretion.

**exci′tovas′cular.** Increasing the activity of the circulation.

**exclave** (eks-klāv′) [ L. *ex*, out, + -*clave* (in enclave, *q.v.*) ]. An outlying, detached portion of a gland or other part, such as the thyroid or pancreas; an accessory gland.

**exclusion** (eks-klu′zhun) [ L. *ex-cludo*, pp. -*clusus*, to shut out. CLAUS- ]. Shutting out; disconnecting from the main portion.

**Devine e.,** e. of pylorus, followed by gastrojejunostomy, for cure of duodenal ulcer.

**excochleation** (eks-kok-le-a′shun) [ L. *ex*, out, + *cochlear*, to spoon ]. Scraping out the contents of a cavity.

**excon′jugant.** A member of a conjugating pair of protozoan ciliates after separation and prior to the subsequent mitotic division of each of the e.'s; see also conjugation (3).

**excoriate** (eks-ko′rī-āt). To scratch.

**excoriation** (eks-ko′rī-a′shun) [ L. *excorio*, to skin, strip, fr. *corium*, skin, hide ]. A scratch mark. A linear break in the skin surface, usually covered with blood or serous crusts.

**excrement** (eks′kre-ment) [ L. *ex-cerno*, pp. -*cretus*, to separate. CRET- ]. Waste matter or any excretion cast out of the body; feces.

**excrementitious** (eks-kre-men-tish′us). Relating to any cast out waste material.

**excrescence** (eks-kres′ens) [ L. *ex-cresco*, pp. -*cretus*, to grow forth. CRES- ]. Any outgrowth from the surface.

**cauliflower e.,** *condyloma* acuminatum.

**excreta** (eks-kre′tah) [ L. neut. pl. of *excretus*, pp. of *ex-cerno*, to separate ]. Excreted material; cast out waste matter.

**excrete** (eks-krēt′). To separate from the blood and cast out; denoting the function of structures the product of whose activity is waste matter and not utilized in the body.

**excre′ter.** A person who is a carrier of pathogenic organisms, and who excretes them in the urine or feces.

**excretion** [ see excrement ]. 1. The process whereby the undigested residue of food and the waste products of metabolism are eliminated. 2. The product of a tissue or organ that is waste material to be passed out of the body.

**ex′cretory.** Relating to excretion.

**excursion** (eks-kur′zhun). Any movement from one point to another, usually with the implied idea of returning again to the original position.

**lateral e.,** movement of the mandible to the right or left side.

**protrusive e.,** movement of the mandible to a position forward or forward and lateral of the centric position.

**excurva′tion.** Excurvature.

**excur′vature.** A curving outward.

**excystation** (ek′sis-ta′shun) [ L. *ex-halo*, pp. -*halatus*, to denoting the action of certain encysted organisms in escaping from their envelope.

**exemia** (eks-e′mī-ah) [ G. *ex*, out of, + *haima*, blood ]. A condition in which a considerable portion of the blood is temporarily removed from the general circulating mass, as in shock, when there is a great accumulation within the abdomen.

**exencepha′lia.** Exencephaly.

**exencephalic** (eks′en-sē-fal′ik). Exencephalous; relating to exencephaly.

**exencephalocele** (eks′en-sef′ă-lo-sēl) [ *ex*, out, + G. *enkephalos*, brain, + *kēlē*, tumor ]. Herniation of the brain.

**exenceph′alous.** Exencephalic.

**exencephalus** (eks′en-sef′ă-lus). A congenitally malformed fetus with exencephaly.

**exencephaly** (eks′en-sef′ă-lī) [ G. *ex*, out, + *enkephalos*, brain ]. Exencephalia; a condition in which the skull is defective, the brain being exposed or extruding.

**exenteration** (eks-en′ter-a′shun) [ G. *ex*, out, + *enteron*, bowel ]. Evisceration (1); removal of an organ or organs.

**anterior pelvic e.,** removal of the bladder, lower parts of the ureters, vagina, uterus, adnexa, and adjacent lymph nodes; a urinary diversion is necessary.

**pelvic e.,** removal of all or a portion of the pelvic viscera; usually performed to surgically ablate cancer involving urinary bladder, uterine cervix, or rectum.

**posterior pelvic e.,** removal of the vagina, uterus, adnexa, rectum, anus, and adjacent lymph nodes; a colostomy is necessary.

**total pelvic e.,** Brunschwig's operation (2); removal of the bladder, lower parts of the ureters, vagina, uterus, adnexa, rectum, anus, and adjacent lymph nodes; a colostomy and urinary diversion are necessary.

**exenteri′tis** (eks-en-ter-i′tis) [ G. *exō*, on the outside, + enteritis ]. Inflammation of the peritoneal covering of the intestine.

**exercise** (eks′er-siz). 1. *Active:* bodily exertion for the sake of restoring the organs and functions to a healthy state or keeping them healthy. 2. *Passive:* motion of limbs without effort by the patient.

**exeresis** (eks-er′e-sis) [ G. *exairesis*, a taking out, fr. *haireō*, to take, grasp ]. Excision, or surgical removal of any part or organ. Also used as combining form in suffix position.

**exergon′ic** [ exo- + G. *ergon*, work ]. Referring to a reaction that takes place with release of energy to its surroundings (*e.g.*, the dilution of $H_2SO_4$, the oxidation of carbon). The opposite of endergonic.

**exfeta′tion** [ L. *ex*, out, + fetus ]. Obsolete term for extrauterine pregnancy.

**exflagellation** (eks-flaj′ē-la′shun). The extrusion of rapidly waving flagellum-like microgametes from microgametocytes. In the case of human malaria parasites, this occurs in the blood meal taken by the proper anopheline vector within a few minutes after migration of the infected blood by the mosquito.

**exfoliatio** (eks-fo′lī-a′shī-o) [ Mod. L. fr. L. *ex*, out, + *folium*, leaf ]. Exfoliation.

**e. area′ta, e. areata linguae,** geographical *tongue*.

**exfoliation** (eks-fo′lī-a′shun) [ L. *exfolatio, q.v.* ]. 1. Detachment of superficial cells of an epithelium or surface layer of a structure. 2. Scaling or desquamation of the horny layer of epidermis, which varies in amount from minute quantities to shedding the entire integument. 3. Loss of deciduous teeth following physiological loss of root structure. 4. Extrusion of permanent teeth as a result of disease or loss of their antagonists.

**e. of the lens,** sheetlike separation of the capsule of the lens; it may occur if the eyes are exposed to intense heat.

**lamellar e. of the newborn,** see collodion *baby*.

**exfoliative** (eks-fo′lī-a′tiv) [ Mod. L. *exfoliativus* ]. Marked by exfoliation, desquamation, or profuse scaling.

**exhalation** (eks-ha-la′shun) [ L. *ex-halo*, pp. -*halatus*, to breathe out ]. 1. Expiration; breathing out. 2. The giving forth of gas or vapor. 3. Emanation; any exhaled or emitted gas or vapor.

**ex′hale.** 1. To breathe out or expire. 2. To emit a gas or vapor or odor.

**exhaustion** (eg-zos′chun) [ L. *ex-haurio*, pp. -*haustus*, to draw out, empty ]. 1. Extreme fatigue; inability to respond to stimuli. 2. Removal of contents; using up of a supply of anything. 3. Extraction of the active constituents of a drug by treating with water, alcohol, or other solvent.

**heat e.,** a form of reaction to heat, marked by prostration, weakness, and collapse, resulting from unrecognized or unavoidable dehydration.

**nervous e.,** obsolete term for neurasthenia or mental illness generally.

**exhibitionist** (ek'sĭ-bish'un-ist). One who has a morbid compulsion to expose the genitals to a person of the opposite sex.

**exhilarant** (eg-zil'ar-ant) [ L. *ex-hilero*, pp. *-atus*, pres. p. *-ans*, to gladden ]. Mentally stimulating.

**exhumation** (eks-hu-ma'shun) [ L. *ex*, out of, + *humus*, earth ]. Disinterment.

**exitus** (ek'sĭ-tus) [ L. fr. *ex-eo*, pp. *-itus*, to go out ]. 1. Exit; outlet. 2. Death.

**Exner,** Siegmund, Vienna physiologist, 1846–1926. See Call-E. *bodies*, E.'s *plexus*.

**exo-** (ek'so-) [ G. *exō*, outside ]. Prefix meaning exterior, external, or outward. See also ecto-.

**exoantigen** (ek'so-an'tĭ-jen). Ectoantigen.

**exobiol'ogy.** The science dealing with life on other planets.

**exocar'dia.** Ectocardia.

**exocataphoria** (ek'so-kat'ă-fo'rī-ah) [ exo- + G. *kata*, downward, + *phora*, a carrying ]. A tendency of the eye to deviate outward and downward.

**exochorion** (ek'so-ko'rī-on). Archaic term for trophectoderm.

**exocrine** (ek'so-krin) [ exo- + G. *krinō*, to separate. CRIN- ]. 1. Eccrine; denoting glandular secretion that is delivered to a surface; opposed to endocrine. 2. Pertaining to a gland that secretes outwardly through excretory ducts.

**exocyclic** (ek'so-si'klik, -sik'lik). Relating to atoms or groups attached to a cyclic structure but not themselves cyclic (*e.g.,* the —CH₃ group of toluene is exocyclic). Opposite of endocyclic.

**exocyto'sis** [ exo- + G. *kytos*, cell, + suffix *-osis*, condition ]. 1. The appearance of migrating inflammatory cells in the epidermis. 2. Emiocytosis; the process whereby secretory granules or droplets are released from a cell; the membrane around the granule fuses with the cell membrane, which ruptures, and the secretion is discharged.

**ex'odevia'tion.** Exophoria or exotropia.

**exod'ic** [ exo- + G. *hodos*, way ]. Efferent.

**exodontia** (eks-o-don'shī-ah) [ exo- + G. *odous*, tooth ]. Tooth extraction; the branch of dental practice that deals with extraction of teeth.

**exodontist** (eks-o-don'tist). One who specializes in the extraction of teeth.

**ex'oen'zyme.** Extracellular *enzyme*.

**exogamy** (eks-og'ă-mĭ) [ exo- + G. *gamos*, marriage ]. Sexual reproduction by means of conjugation of two gametes of different ancestry, as in certain protozoan species.

**ex'ogas'trula.** An abnormal embryo in which the primitive gut has been everted.

**exogenet'ic.** Exogenous.

**exogenote** (ek'so-je'nōt). In microbial genetics, the fragment of genetic material that has been transferred from a donor to the recipient and is homologous for a region of the recipient's original genome (endogenote), producing in the homologous region a condition analogous to diploidy.

**exogenous** (eks-oj'ĕ-nus) [ exo- + G. suffix *-gen*, production ]. Exogenetic; originating or produced outside.

**exo-1,4-α-glucosidase.** Glucoamylase; amyloglucosidase; γ-amylase; acid maltase; hydrolase (EC 3.2.1.3) removing terminal 1,4-linked glucose residues from nonreducing ends of chains with release of β-glucose.

**exolever** (eks'o-le'ver) [ exo- + L. *levare*, to raise ]. A modified elevator for the extraction of tooth roots.

**exom'eter.** [ exo- + G. *metron*, measure ]. A device for recording the fluorescence of x-ray as compared to candle power.

**exomphalos** (eks-om'fă-lus) [ G. *ex*, out, + *omphalos*, umbilicus ]. Exumbilication. 1. Protrusion of the umbilicus. 2. Umbilical *hernia*.

**exonuclease** (eks-o-nu'kle-ās). A nuclease that releases one nucleotide at a time, serially, beginning at one end of a polynucleotide (nucleic acid). Several have been prepared

from *Escherichia coli*, designated e. I, e. II, etc.; *cf.* endonuclease.

**exopath'ic.** Denoting a disease that originates is outside the body.

**exop'athy** [ exo- + G. *pathos*, suffering ]. A disease produced by some cause outside the body.

**exopep'tidase.** An enzyme that catalyzes the hydrolysis of the terminal amino acid of a peptide chain; *e.g.,* carboxypeptidase.

**exophoria** (ek'so-fo'rī-ah) [ exo- + G. *phora*, a carrying ]. A tendency of one eye to deviate outward.

**exophor'ic.** Relating to exophoria.

**exophthalmic** (eks-of-thal'mik). Relating to exophthalmos; marked by prominence of the eyeball.

**exophthalmometer** (eks-of-thal-mom'e-ter) [ exophthalmos + G. *metron*, measure ]. Statometer; an instrument for measuring the amount of protrusion of the eyeball.

**exophthalmos, exophthalmus** (eks-of-thal'mos) [ G. *ex*, out, + *ophthalmos*, eye ]. Protrusion of the eyeballs.

**malig'nant e.,** severe protrusion of the eyeballs; unresponsive to treatment, often leading to blindness.

**exophylaxis** (ek'so-fi-lak'sis) [ exo- + G. *phylaxis*, a guarding ]. Protection against the entrance of disease into the body from without, such as afforded by the skin; see also esophylaxis.

**ex'ophyte** (ek'so-fīt) [ exo- + G. *phyton*, plant ]. An exterior or external parasite.

**exophytic** (ek'so-fit'ik). 1. Pertaining to an exophyte. 2. In dentistry, term used in reference to the growth pattern of oral lesions that project into the oral cavity.

**ex'oplasm.** Ectoplasm.

**exopneumopexy, exopneumonopexy** (ek'so-nu'mo-pek'sĭ, -nu-mo'no-pek'sĭ) [ exo- + pneumonopexy, *q.v.* ]. Fixation of lung outside of the chest cavity.

**exorbitism** (eks-or'bĭ-tizm). Obsolete term for exophthalmos.

**ex'osero'sis.** Serous exudation from the skin surface, as in eczema or abrasions.

**exoskel'eton.** 1. Dermoskeleton; dermatoskeleton; all hard parts, such as hair, teeth, nails, feathers, dermal plates, scales, etc., developed from the ectoderm or mesoderm in vertebrates. 2. The outer chitinous envelope of an insect, or the chitinous or calcareous covering of certain Crustacea and other invertebrates.

**exosmosis** (eks-os-mo'sis). Osmosis from within outward, as from the interior of a blood vessel.

**exosplenopexy** (ek'so-splē'no-pek-sĭ) [ exo- + G. *splēn*, spleen, + *pēxis*, fastening ]. Suturing the spleen to an opening in the abdominal wall.

**ex'ospore** [ exo- + G. *sporos*, seed ]. Exogenous spore, not encased in a sporangium.

**exospo'rium.** The outer envelope of a spore.

**exostectomy** (eks-os-tek'to-mĭ) [ exostosis + G. *ektomē*, excision ]. Exostosectomy; removal of an exostosis.

**exostosec'tomy.** Exostectomy.

**exostosis,** pl. **exosto'ses** (eks-os-to'sis) [ exo- + G. *osteon*, bone, + suffix *-osis*, condition ]. A bony tumor springing from the surface of a bone, most commonly in the form of ossification of muscular attachments.

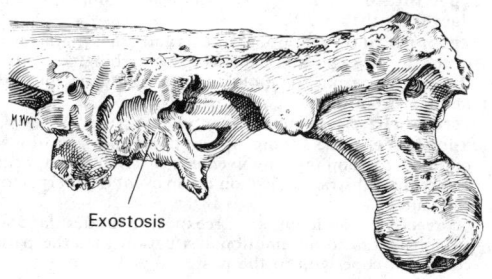

**Exostosis**
Found on femur of *Pithecanthropus erectus* (Java man)

**e. bursa'ta,** an e. springing from the joint surface of a bone and covered with cartilage and a synovial sac.

**e. cartilagin'ea,** an e. springing from the epiphysis or joint surface of a bone; an ossified chondroma; see also hereditary multiple exostoses.

**dental e.,** a bonelike growth springing from the root of a tooth.

**diaphysial juxtaepiphysial e.,** see diaphysial *aclasis*.

**hereditary multiple exostoses,** hereditary deforming chondrodysplasia; osteochondromatosis; a disturbance of enchondral bone growth in which multiple osteochondromas of long bones appear during childhood, with shortening of the radius and fibula; autosomal dominant inheritance. See also diaphysial *aclasis*.

**ivory e.,** a small, rounded, eburnated tumor springing from a bone, usually one of the cranial bones.

**multiple e.,** hereditary multiple exostoses.

**solitary osteocartilaginous e.,** osteochondroma.

**exoteric** (ek-so-tĕr'ik) [ G. *exōterikos*, outer ]. Of external origin; arising outside the organism.

**ex'other'mic** [ exo- + G. + *thermē*, heat ]. 1. Denoting a chemical reaction attended by the development of heat; *cf.* exergonic. 2. Relating to the external warmth of the body.

**exotox'ic.** 1. Relating to an exotoxin. 2. Relating to the introduction of an exogenous poison or toxin.

**exotox'in.** Extracellular *toxin*.

**exotro'pia** [ exo- + G. *trope*, turn ]. Divergent strabismus; external squint or strabismus the form of strabismus in which the visual axes diverge; may be paralytic or concomitant, monocular or alternating; see fig. under strabismus.

**A-e.,** divergent strabismus greater in downward than in upward gaze.

**V-e.,** divergent strabismus greater in upward than in downward gaze.

**X-e.,** increasing divergence from primary position in both upward and downward gaze.

**expan'sion** [ L. *ex-pando*, pp. *-pansus*, to spread out ]. 1. An increase in size as of chest or lungs. 2. The spreading out of any structure, as a tendon. 3. An expanse; a wide area.

**hygroscopic e.,** (1) e. due to the absorption of moisture; (2) in dental casting, the addition of water to the surface of the casting investment during setting to increase the size of the mold.

**perceptual e.,** development of an ability to recognize and interpret sensory stimuli through associations with past similar stimuli; perceptual e. by relaxation of defenses is a goal of psychotherapy.

**setting e.,** the dimensional increase that occurs concurrently with the hardening of various materials, such as plaster of Paris.

**wax e.,** in dentistry, a method of expanding wax patterns to compensate for the shrinkage of gold during the casting process.

**expan'siveness.** In psychiatry, megalomania; greatly exaggerated sense of importance.

**expectorant** (eks-pek'to-rant) [ L. *ex*, out, + *pectus*, chest ]. 1. Promoting secretion from the mucous membrane of the air passages or facilitating its expulsion. 2. An agent that increases bronchial secretion and facilitates its expulsion.

**expec'torate.** 1. To spit; to eject saliva, mucus, or other fluid from the mouth.

**expectora'tion.** 1. Sputum; mucus and other fluids formed in the air passages and expelled by coughing. 2. Spitting; the expelling from the mouth of saliva, mucus, and other material from the air passages.

**prune-juice e.,** prune-juice *sputum*.

**exper'ience.** The feeling of emotions and sensations as opposed to thinking; involvement in what is happening rather than abstract reflection on an event or interpersonal encounter.

**corrective emotional e.,** reexposure under favorable circumstances to an emotional situation that the patient could not cope with in the past.

**exper'iment.** A test or trial.

**control e.,** an e., chemical or animal, used to check another, to verify the result, or to demonstrate what would

have occurred had the factor under study been omitted. See also control, and control *animal*.

**delayed reaction e.,** a method of measuring memory; a stimulus is presented and removed before the organism is permitted to respond to it; the interval during which the stimulus is absent, providing the organism responds correctly, is an indication of the length of memory.

**double blind e.,** an e. conducted with neither experimenter nor subjects knowing which e. is the control; prevents bias in recording results.

**factorial e.'s,** an experimental design in which two or more series of treatments are tried in all combinations.

**Goltz' e.,** reflex inhibition of the heart in the frog by taps upon the abdomen.

**Hertzian e.'s,** e.'s demonstrating that electromagnetic induction is propagated in waves, analogous to waves of light but not affecting the retina.

**Küss' e.'s,** to show that the epithelium is impermeable; injections into the bladder of solutions of belladonna or of opium are followed by no symptoms of poisoning.

**Mariotte's e.,** one looks fixedly with one eye (the other being closed), at a black dot on a card, on which is also marked a black cross; as the card is moved to or from the eye, at a certain distance the cross becomes invisible but appears again as the card is moved further; this proves the existence of the blind spot where the optic nerve enters the eye.

**Müller's e.,** Müller's maneuver (2); after a forced expiration, an attempt at inspiration is made with closed mouth and nose or closed glottis, whereby the negative pressure in the chest and lungs is made very subatmospheric; the reverse of Valsalva *maneuver* (2).

**Nussbaum's e.,** exclusion of the glomeruli of the kidney from the circulation by ligation of the renal artery in animals, like the frog, that have a renal portal system to maintain circulation to the tubules.

**Römer's e.,** the instillation of abrin into the conjunctiva, demonstrating the local formation of antitoxins.

**Scheiner's e.,** a demonstration of accommodation; through two minute holes in a card, separated from each other by less than the diameter of the pupil, one looks at a pin; at a short distance from the eye the pin appears double; as it is moved from the eye a point is found where it appears single, and beyond which it remains single for the normal eye, but for the myopic eye it soon again becomes double.

**Stensen's e.,** compression of the abdominal aorta of an animal very promptly causes paralysis of the posterior portions of the body since the blood supply to the lumbar cord is almost entirely shut off.

**Toynbee's e.,** swallowing when the mouth and nose are closed causes rarefaction of air in the tympanum.

**Valsalva's e.,** Valsalva *maneuver* (1).

**Weber's e.,** if the peripheral end of the divided vagus nerve is stimulated the heart is arrested in diastole.

**expiration** (eks'pī-ra'shun) [ L. *expiro* or *ex-spiro*, pp. *-atus*, to breathe out ]. Exhalation (1); breathing out.

**expi'ratory.** Relating to expiration.

**expire** (eks-pīr'). 1. To breathe out; to exhale. 2. To die.

**explant** (eks-plant'). Living tissue transferred from an organism to an artificial medium for culture.

**explantation** (eks-plan-ta'shun). The act of transferring an explant.

**explode** (eks-plōd'). To cause or to undergo explosion.

**explora'tion** [ L. *ex-ploro*, pp. *-ploratus*, to explore ]. Examination; investigation; a search for symptoms to aid in diagnosis.

**explor'atory.** Relating to or with a view to exploration.

**explo'rer.** A sharp, pointed probe used to investigate natural or restored teeth surfaces in order to detect caries or other defects.

**explosion** (eks-plo'zhun) [ L. *explosio*, fr. *explodo*, to drive away by clapping ]. 1. A bursting. 2. A sudden increase or outbreak, as an epidemic or a population explosion. 3. Chemical change or disintegration accompanied by noisy violence, as in the rapid conversion of an inflammable solid or liquid to a gas. 4. A sudden discharge of force.

**expo'nent.** A symbol, written as a superscript, indicating the number of times a factor is to be involved in a repeated multiplication.

**expose** (eks-pōz'). Applied to the dental pulp; to uncover; to bring into view.

**express** [ L. *ex-premo*, pp. -*pressus*, to press out ]. To press or squeeze out.

**expres'sion.** 1. Squeezing out; expelling by pressure. 2. Mobility of the features giving liveliness to the face.

**expul'sive** [ L. *ex-pello*, pp. -*pulsus*, to drive out ]. Tending to expel.

**exsanguinate** (ek-sang'gwĭ-nāt) [ L. *ex*, out, + *sanguis* (-*guin*), blood ]. 1. To deprive of blood; to make bloodless. 2. Exsanguine.

**exsanguination** (ek-sang'gwĭ-na'shun). Depriving of blood; making exsanguine.

**exsanguine** (ek-sang'gwin). Bloodless; anemic.

**exsect** (ek-sekt') [ L. *ex-seco*, pp. -*sectus*, to cut out. SEC- ]. Excise.

**exsection** (ek-sek'shun). Excision.

**exsiccant** (ek-sik'ant) [ L. *ex-sicco*, pp. -*siccatus*, to dry up, fr. *siccus*, dry ]. 1. Drying; absorbing. 2. A dusting or drying powder.

**exsiccate** (ek'sĭ-kāt). To dry; to absorb moisture.

**exsiccation** (ek'sĭ-ka'shun). 1. The process of drying. 2. Dehydration; the removal of water of crystallization.

**exsiccosis** (ek'sĭ-ko'sis) [ L. *ex*, out, + *siccus*, dry, + -*osis* ]. The process of thoroughly drying out.

**exsomatize** (ek-so'mă-tiz) [ G. *ex*, out of, + *sōma*, body ]. To remove from the body.

**exsorption** (ek-sorp'shun) [ G. *ex*, out, + *sorbēre*, to suck ]. Movement of substances from the blood into the lumen of the gut.

**exstrophy** (ek'stro-fī) [ G. *ex*, out, + *strophē*, a turning ]. A congenital turning out or eversion of a hollow organ.

  **e. of the bladder,** ectopia vesicae; a congenital gap in the anterior wall of the bladder and the abdominal wall in front of it, the posterior wall of the bladder being exposed.

  **e. of the cloaca,** ectopia cloacae; a developmental anomaly in which an area of intestinal mucosa is interposed between two separate areas of the urinary bladder.

**ext.** Abbreviation for L. *extractum*, extract.

**extend** [ L. *ex-tendo*, pp. -*tensus*, to stretch out. TEN- ]. To straighten a limb, to diminish or extinguish the angle formed by flexion; to place the distal segment of a limb in such a position that its axis is continuous with that of the proximal segment.

**exten'sion** [ L. *extensio*, to stretch out ]. 1. The act of bringing the distal portion of a joint in continuity (though only parallel) with the long axis of the proximal portion. 2. A pulling or dragging force exerted on a limb in a direction away from the body; see also traction, and relevant subentries.

  **Buck's e.,** an apparatus for applying a tensile force on the leg through a tape applying force to the skin; friction between the tape and skin permits application of force, which is mediated through a cord over a pulley, suspending a weight.

  **Codivilla's e.,** skeletal e.; a weight pulling from calipers or a pin passed through lower end of bone; the direction of force is in line with the long axis of the proximal portion.

  **e. per contiguita'tem,** extending through contact and touch.

  **e. per continuita'tem,** extending through direct spread or invasion and in continuity.

  **nail e.,** e. by a weight on a nail or pin in the distal fragment of a fracture.

  **ridge e.,** an intraoral surgical operation for deepening the labial, buccal, and/or lingual sulci; it is performed to increase the intraoral height of the alveolar ridge in order to assist denture retention.

  **skeletal e.,** Codivilla's e.

**exten'sor** [ L. one who stretches, fr. *ex-tendo*, to stretch out ] [ NA ]. A muscle the contraction of which tends to straighten a limb; the antagonist of a flexor; see under muscle.

**exte'rior** [ L. ]. Outside; external.

**exte'riorize.** 1. To direct a patient's interests, thoughts, or feelings into a channel leading outside himself, to some definite aim or object. 2. To expose an organ temporarily for observation, or permanently for purposes of physiologic experiment, *e.g.*, fixation of the spleen or segment of bowel with blood supply intact to the outer aspect of the abdominal wall.

**ex'tern** [ F. *externe*, outside, a day scholar ]. An advanced student or recent graduate who assists in the medical or surgical care of hospital patients, but who lives outside of the institution.

**exter'nal** [ L. *externus* ]. Exterior; on the outside or farther from the center; often incorrectly used to mean lateral.

**exter'nus** [ NA ]. External.

**exteroceptive** (eks'ter-o-sep'tiv) [ L. *exterus*, outside, + *capere*, to take. CAP-2 ]. Relating to the exteroceptors; denoting the surface of the body containing the end organs adapted to receive impressions or stimuli from without.

**exteroceptor** (eks'ter-o-sep'tor) [ L. *exterus*, external, + *receptor*, receiver. CAP-2 ]. One of the peripheral end organs of the afferent nerves in the skin or mucous membrane, which respond to stimulation by external agents.

**exterofective** (eks'ter-o-fek'tiv) [ L. ab. *extero*, from outside, + *affectus*, affected, + -*ivus*, adj. ending ]. Pertaining to the response of the nervous system to external stimuli.

**extima** (eks'tĭ-mah) [ L. fem. of *extimus*, outermost ]. Rarely used term for the adventitia (outer coat) of a blood vessel.

**extinction** (eks-tingk'shun) [ L. *extinguo*, to quench ]. 1. A progressive reduction in the strength of the conditioned response in successive conditioning trials during which only the conditioned stimulus is presented and the unconditioned stimulus is deliberately omitted. 2. Absorbance.

  **specific e.,** specific absorption *coefficient.*

**extinguish** (eks-ting'wish) [ L. *extinguo*, to quench ]. 1. To quench, as a flame; to abolish; to cause loss of identity; to destroy. 2. In psychology, to progressively abolish a previously conditioned response.

**extirpation** (eks-tir-pa'shun) [ L. *extirpo*, pp. -*atus*, to root out, fr. *stirps*, a stalk, root ]. The entire removal of an organ or part or of a pathologic structure.

**Exton,** William G., American physician, 1876–1943. See E. *reagent*, E.-Rose *test.*

**extorsion** (eks-tor'shun) [ L. *extorsio*, fr. *ex-torqueo*, pp. -*tortus*, to twist out ]. 1. Outward rotation of a limb or of an organ. 2. Disclination; rotation of the eye temporally around its anteroposterior axis.

**extor'tor.** Outward rotator.

**extra-.** Prefix fr. L. preposition meaning without, outside of.

**extra-artic'ular.** Outside of a joint.

**extrabuc'cal.** Outside of the cheek.

**extrabul'bar.** Outside of or unrelated to any bulb, such as the bulb of the urethra, or the medulla oblongata.

**extracaliceal** (eks'tra-kă-lis'e-al). Outside of a calix.

**ex'tracap'sular.** Outside of the capsule of a joint.

**extracar'pal.** 1. Outside of, having no relation to, the carpus. 2. On the outer side of the carpus.

**extracel'lular.** Outside of the cells.

**extracorporeal** (eks'trah-kor-po're-al). Outside of, or unrelated to, the body or any anatomical "corpus."

**extracorpuscular** (eks-trah-kor-pus'ku-lar). Outside of the corpuscles, especially the blood corpuscles.

**extracra'nial.** Outside of the cranial cavity.

**ex'tract.** 1. A concentrated preparation of a vegetable or animal drug obtained by removing the active constituents of the drug with suitable solvents, evaporating all or nearly all of the solvent, and adjusting the residual mass or powder to the prescribed standard. 2. To remove part of a mixture with a solvent.

  **alcoholic e.,** a solid e. obtained by extracting the alcohol-soluble principles of a drug, followed by the evaporation of the alcohol.

  **allergenic e.'s, allergic e.'s,** e. (usually containing protein) from various sources, *e.g.*, food, bacteria, pollen, and the like, suspected of specific action in stimulating manifestations of allergy.

**allergic e.,** allergenic e.

**Buchner e.,** a cell-free e. of yeast; such was prepared by the two Buchner brothers in the 1890's and observed by them to catalyze alcoholic fermentation. This observation essentially eliminated "vitalism" as being responsible for biological chemical reactions and set the stage for the beginnings of modern biochemistry in the subsequent studies of Harden and Young on Buchner e.'s.

**equivalent e.,** valoid; a fluidextract of the same strength, weight for weight, as the original drug.

**fluid e.,** see fluidextract.

**hydroalcoholic e.,** a solid e. obtained by extracting the soluble principles of the drug with alcohol and water, followed by evaporation of the solution.

**liquid e.,** the BP equivalent of the USP fluidextract.

**pollen e.,** liquid obtained by extracting the protein from the pollen of plants with a liquid consisting of 5 per cent of dextrose or an appropriate salt solution and 0.5 per cent of phenol in distilled water.

**extrac'tant.** An agent used to isolate or extract a substance from a mixture or combination of substances, from the tissues, or from a crude drug. etc.

**extraction** (eks-trak'shun) [ L. *ex-traho,* pp. -*tractus,* to draw out ]. 1. The act of luxating and removing a tooth from its alveolus. 2. The partitioning of material (solute) into a solvent. 3. The active portion of a drug; the making of an extract. 4. Surgical removal by pulling out. 5. In obstetrics, the pulling out of the baby.

**breech e.,** obstetrical e. of the baby by the buttocks.

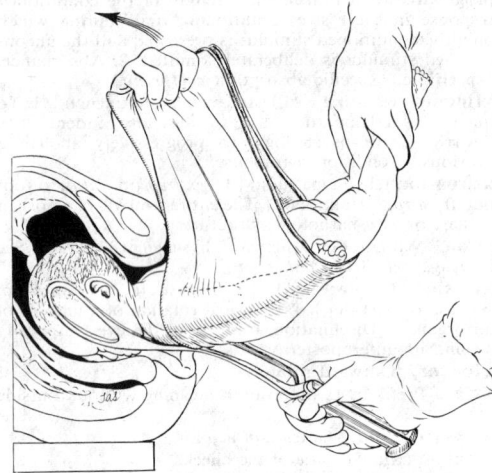

**Breech Extraction**
Management of fetal arms to facilitate the application of the Piper forceps to the aftercoming head. (From Savage, J. E.: Management of the fetal arms in breech extraction. *Obstet. Gynec. 3:* 55, 1954. Used with permission.)

**flap e.,** e. of a cataract through a limbal incision with a flap of conjunctiva.

**podalic e.,** obstetrical e. of the baby by the feet; see fig. under version.

**extrac'tive.** Substances present in vegetable or animal tissue that can be separated by successive treatment with alcohol and/or water and recovered by evaporation of the solution.

**extrac'tor.** An instrument for use in drawing or pulling out any natural part, as a tooth, or a foreign body.

**Murless head e.,** a fenestrated curved blade with an S-shaped handle for lifting the fetal head in lower segment cesarean section.

**vacuum e.,** a device for producing traction upon the head of a fetus by means of a soft cup held by a vacuum.

**extracystic** (eks-trah-sis'tik). Outside of, or unrelated to, the gallbladder or urinary bladder or any cystic tumor.

**extradu'ral.** 1. On the outer side of the dura mater. 2. Unconnected with the dura mater.

**extraembryonic** (eks-trah-em'brī-on'ik). Outside the embryonic body; pertaining, for example, to membranes which are concerned with the embryo's protection and nutrition and which are discarded at birth without being incorporated in the body of the embryo.

**extraepiphysial** (eks'trah-ep-ĭ-fiz'ĭ-al). Not relating to, or connected with, an epiphysis.

**extragenital** (eks'trah-jen'ĭ-tal). Outside of, away from, or unrelated to, the genital organs.

**extrahepat'ic.** Outside of, or unrelated to, the liver.

**extrajec'tion** [ L. *ex,* out of, + *jacio,* to cast ]. Attributing or projecting one's own psychic process to another person.

**ex'traligamen'tous.** Outside of, or unconnected with, a ligament.

**extramalle'olus.** *Malleolus* lateralis.

**extramedullary** (eks'trah-med'ul-ēr-ĭ). Outside of, or unrelated to, any medulla, especially the medulla oblongata.

**extramu'ral** [ extra- + L. *murus,* wall ]. Outside, not in the substance, of the wall of a part.

**extraneous** (eks-tra'ne-us) [ L. *extraneus* ]. Outside of the organism and not belonging to it.

**extranuclear** (eks-trah-nu'kle'ar). Located outside of, or not involving, a cell nucleus.

**extraocular** (eks-trah-ok'u-lar). Adjacent to but outside the eyeball.

**extraoral** (eks-trah-o'ral). Outside of the oral cavity; external to the oral cavity. In its usual use it includes anything external to the lips and cheeks also.

**extrapapillary** (eks-trah-pap'ĭ-lĕ-rĭ). Unconnected with any papillary structure.

**extraparenchymal** (eks-trah-pă'reng-ki'mal). Unrelated to the parenchyma of an organ.

**extraperineal** (eks-trah-pĕr'ĭ-ne'al) Not connected with the perineum.

**extraperiosteal** (eks-trah-pĕr'ĭ-os'te-al). Not connected with, or unrelated to, the periosteum.

**extraperitoneal** (eks-trah-pĕr-ĭ-to-ne'al). Outside of the peritoneal cavity.

**extraphysiologic** (eks-trah-fiz-ĭ-o-loj'ik). Outside of the domain of physiology; more than physiologic, therefore pathologic.

**extraplacen'tal.** Unrelated to the placenta.

**extraprostatic** (eks-trah-pros-tat'ik). Outside of, or independent of, the prostate gland.

**extraprostati'tis.** Paraprostatitis.

**extrapulmonary** (eks-trah-pul'mo-nĕr-ĭ). Outside of the lungs, having no relation to the lungs.

**extrapyramidal** (eks-trah-pī-ram'ĭ-dal). See extrapyramidal motor *system.*

**extrasen'sory.** Outside or beyond the ordinary senses; not limited to the senses; *e.g.,* clairvoyance or thought transference.

**extrase'rous.** Outside of a serous cavity.

**extrasomat'ic.** Outside of, or unrelated to, the body.

**extrasystole** (eks'trah-sis'to-le). Premature beat; premature systole; an ectopic, usually premature, contraction of the heart; such beats arise from the atrium, the A-V node, or the ventricle and interrupt the dominant, usually sinus, rhythm; they are in some way dependent on the preceding beat and are therefore "forced" beats.

**atrial e.,** auricular e.; a premature contraction of the heart arising from an ectopic atrial focus.

**auric'ular e.,** atrial e.

**A-V e.,** junctional e.; an e. arising from the "junctional" tissues, either the A-V node or A-V bundle.

**A-V nodal e.,** atrioventricular nodal e.; nodal e.; a premature beat arising from the atrioventricular (A-V) node and leading to a simultaneous or almost simultaneous contraction of atria and ventricles.

**infrano'dal e.,** ventricular e.

**inter'polated e.,** a ventricular e. which, instead of being followed by a compensatory pause, is sandwiched between two consecutive sinus cycles.

**junctional e.,** A-V e.

**lower nodal e.,** a nodal e. supposed to arise from the lower part of the A-V node, recognized in the electrocar-

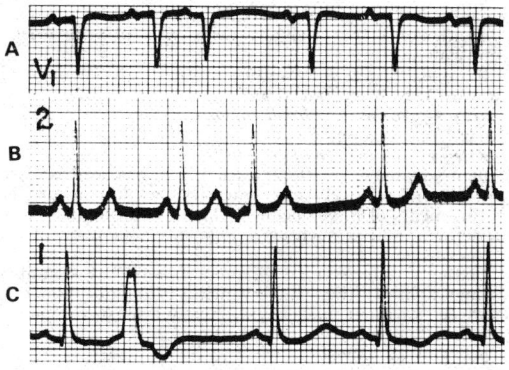

**Extrasystoles**
*A*, atrial; *B*, A-V nodal; *C*, ventricular

diogram by the retrograde P wave that follows the QRS complex.

**midnodal e.,** a nodal e. supposed to arise from the midportion of the A-V node and recognized in the electrocardiogram by absence of the P wave that is lost within the normal QRS complex.

**nodal e.,** A-V nodal e.

**return e.,** a form of reciprocal rhythm in which the impulse having arisen in the ventricle ascends toward the atria, but before reaching the atria is reflected back to the ventricles to produce a second ventricular contraction.

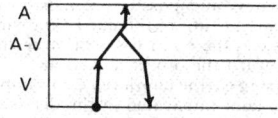

**Return Extrasystole**

**supraventric'ular e.,** an e. arising from a center above the ventricle, *i.e.,* atrium or A-V node.

**upper nodal e.,** a nodal e. supposed to arise from the upper part of the A-V node; recognized in the electrocardiogram by a retrograde P wave preceding the QRS complex by an abnormally short P-R interval.

**ventricular e.,** infranodal e.; a premature contraction of the ventricle.

**extratar'sal.** 1. Outside of, having no relation to, the tarsus. 2. On the outer side of the tarsus.

**extratracheal** (eks-trah-tra'ke-al). Outside of the trachea.

**extratu'bal.** Outside of any tube; specifically, not in the auditory (Eustachian) or uterine (Fallopian) tubes.

**extrauterine** (eks-trah-u'ter-in). Outside of the uterus.

**extravaginal** (eks-trah-vaj'ĭ-nal). Outside of the vagina.

**extravasate** (eks-trav'ă-sāt) [ L. *extra,* out of, + *vas,* vessel ]. 1. To exude from or pass out of a vessel into the tissues, said of blood, lymph, or urine. 2. Extravasation (2); the material thus extruded.

**extravasation** (eks-trav'ă-sa'shun). 1. The act of extravasating. 2. Extravasate (2).

**extravas'cular.** Outside of the blood vessels or lymphatics or of any special blood vessel.

**extraventric'ular.** Outside of any ventricle, especially of one of the ventricles of the heart.

**ex'traver'sion.** Extroversion.

**extravisual** (ek-strah-vizh'u-al). Outside the field of vision, or beyond the visible spectrum.

**extrem'ital.** Relating to an extremity; distal.

**extrem'itas** [ L. from *extremus,* last, outermost ]. 1. Extremity; limb; member; one of the arms or legs. 2 [ NA ] One of the ends of an oval or elongated organ, such as the kidney or ovary.

**e. acromia'lis clavic'ulae** [ NA ], acromial extremity of the clavicle; the flattened lateral extremity of the clavicle that articulates with the acromion and is anchored to the coracoid process by the conoid and trapezoid ligaments.

**e. anterior** [ NA ], anterior extremity; specifically, the anterior pole of the spleen (polus lienalis inferior).

**e. inferior** [ NA ], inferior extremity; inferior pole; the rounded inferior end of either the kidney (polus renalis inferior) or the testis.

**e. posterior** [ NA ], posterior extremity; specifically, the posterior pole of the spleen (polus lienalis superior).

**e. sterna'lis clavic'ulae** [ NA ], sternal extremity of the clavicle; the enlarged medial end of the clavicle that articulates with the manubrium sterni.

**e. superior** [ NA ], superior extremity; superior pole; the rounded superior end of either the kidney (polus renalis superior) or the testis.

**e. tuba'ria** [ NA ], tubal extremity; lateral pole; the rounded lateral end of the ovary.

**e. uteri'na** [ NA ], uterine extremity; medial pole; the rounded medial end of the ovary.

**extrem'ity.** Extremitas.

**anterior e.,** *extremitas* anterior.

**anterior e. of caudate nucleus,** *caput* nuclei caudati.

**distal e. of ulna,** *caput* ulnae.

**inferior e.,** *extremitas* inferior.

**lower e.,** *membrum* inferius.

**posterior e.,** *extremitas* posterior.

**superior e.,** *extremitas* superior.

**tubal e.,** *extremitas* tubaria.

**upper e.,** *membrum* superius.

**upper e. of fibula,** *caput* fibulae.

**uterine e.,** *extremitas* uterina.

**extrinsic** (eks-trin'sik) [ L. *extrinsecus,* from without ]. Originating outside of the part where found or upon which it acts; denoting especially a muscle.

**ex'trogastrula'tion.** See exogastrula.

**ex'trospec'tion.** Constant examination of the skin because of fear of parasites or dirt.

**extroversion** (eks'tro-ver'zhun, -shun) [ incorrectly formed fr. L. *extra,* outside, + *verto,* pp. *versus,* to turn ]. 1. A turning outward. 2. A trait involving social intercourse, in contrast to introversion (*q.v.*).

**ex'trovert.** A gregarious person whose chief interests lie outside himself, and who is involved in the affairs of others, in contrast to an introvert (*q.v.*).

**extrude** (eks-trood'). To thrust forth or to force out; to protrude.

**extrusion** (eks-troo'zhun). A forcing out of a normal position.

**e. of a tooth,** elongation of a tooth; movement of a tooth in an occlusal or incisal direction.

**extubate** (eks'tu-bāt). To accomplish extubation.

**extubation** (eks'tu-ba'shun) [ L. *ex,* out, + *tuba,* tube ]. The removal of a tube from an organ, structure, or orifice; specifically, the removal of the tube after intubation of the larynx or trachea.

**exudate** (eks'u-dāt) [ L. *ex,* out, + *sudare,* to sweat ]. Exudation (2).

**inflammatory e.,** fluid with a relatively high content of serum proteins and leukocytes, formed as a reaction to injury of tissue and blood vessels.

**exudation** (eks-u-da'shun). 1. The act of exuding. 2. Exudate; passage of fluid, often coagulable, or blood cells into tissues or cavities, especially as a result of increased vascular permeability.

**exudative** (eks-u'dă-tiv). Relating to the process of exudation or to an exudate.

**exude** (eks-ūd') [ L. *ex,* out, + *sudare,* to sweat ]. To ooze or pass out gradually through the tissues; said of a fluid or semisolid that may become encrusted or infected.

**exulcerans** (eks-ul'ser-anz). Ulcerating.

**ex'umbilica'tion** [ L. *ex,* out, + *umbilicus,* navel ]. Exomphalos.

**exuviae** (ex-u've-e) [ L. clothing, etc., stripped from the body, fr. *exuo*, pp. *exutus*, to strip off ]. Any cast off parts, as desquamated epidermis.

**eye** [ A.S. *eāge* ]. Oculus; ophthalmos; the organ of vision.

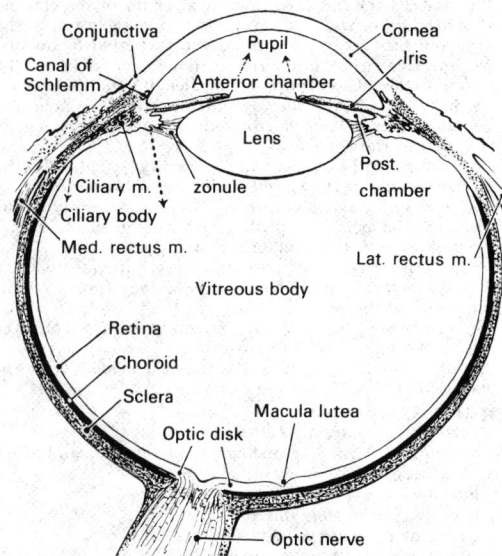

**The Human Eye (Right)**

**amaurot'ic cat's e.**, a yellow reflex from the dilated pupil in cases of glioma (retinoblastoma) or pseudoglioma.

**artificial e.**, a curved disk of opaque glass or plastic, with an imitation iris and pupil in the center, inserted beneath the eyelids and supported by the stump left after evisceration or enucleation; it may be ready-made (stock) or custom-made.

**black e.**, ecchymosis of the lids and their surroundings.

**blear e.**, lippitude; blepharitis accompanied by a viscid discharge that tends to cause the lid edges to cling together.

**bovine cancer e.**, a common malady of cattle, especially of the Hereford breed. It occurs principally in animals that have unpigmented skin around the e.'s. It is a malignant, squamous cell carcinoma originating in the conjunctival mucous membranes or the surrounding skin. It occurs most commonly in range cattle living in regions of intense sunlight.

**brassy e.**, a conjunctivitis that occurs in brass workers and is caused by brass dust or indirect contact by rubbing the e.'s after handling objects made of brass.

**cinema e.**, actinic *conjunctivitis*.

**compound e.**, the eye of arthropods, most highly developed in insects and crustaceans; the e. consists of a group of functionally related visual elements (ommatidia) whose corneal surfaces collectively form a segment of a sphere.

**crossed e.'s**, cross-eye; the e.'s in esotropia or exotropia.

**cyclope'an e.**, see cyclopia.

**dark-adapted e.**, scotopic e.; an e. that has been in darkness or semidarkness for some time and has undergone regeneration of visual purple and dilation of the pupil, which renders it more sensitive to low illumination—a function of the rods.

**dominant e.**, the one that primarily subserves orientation and is usually used in testing the e.'s with monocular instruments.

**epiphy'sial e.**, pineal e.

**exciting e.**, the originally diseased e. in sympathetic ophthalmia.

**fixing e.**, the e., in cases of strabismus, that is directed toward the object looked at.

**gray e.**, see avian *lymphomatosis*.

**hare's e.**, lagophthalmos.

**Klieg e.**, actinic *conjunctivitis*.

**light-adapted e.**, photopic e.; an e. that has been exposed to light of relatively high intensity and has undergone adjustments of photochemical change and pupillary constriction. Sight in such an e. is mainly a function of the retinal cones.

**Listing's reduced e.**, a representation that simplifies calculations of retinal imagery: radius of anterior refracting surface, 5.1 mm.; total length, 20 mm.; distance of nodal point to retina, 15 mm.

**pari'etal e.**, pineal e.

**photop'ic e.**, light-adapted e.

**pin'eal e.**, epiphysial e.; parietal e.; an e. in or near the median line in certain crustacea and lower vertebrates; homologue of pineal gland in higher forms. A median eye of different origin and significance may occur as a maldevelopment in man; see cyclopia.

**pink e.**, see pinkeye.

**reduced e.**, a simplified design of the ocular optical system, represented as having a single refracting surface and a uniform index of refraction; a model based on this concept is used in retinoscopy and ophthalmoscopy.

**schematic e.**, the representation of the optical system of an ideal normal eye in which are listed the curvatures and indices of refraction of the refracting elements and their intervening distances.

**scotop'ic e.**, dark-adapted e.

**shipyard e.**, a type of epidemic keratoconjunctivitis.

**Snellen's reform e.**, an artificial e. formed of two concavoconvex plates with a hollow space between them.

**spectacle e.'s**, a condition in rats caused by pantothenic acid deficiency, and possibly of inositol lack as well, in which a hairless ring of inflamed skin surrounds the e.'s.

**squinting e.**, the e., in cases of strabismus, that is not directed toward the object looked at.

**sympathizing e.**, the uninjured e. in sympathetic ophthalmia that is later implicated in the disease process.

**watery e.**, (1) epiphora; (2) excessive lacrimation.

**web e.**, pterygium (1).

**white e.**, see avian *lymphomatosis*.

**white of the e.**, the visible portion of the sclera.

**eye'ball.** *Bulbus* oculi.

**eye'brow.** Supercilium.

**eye'grounds.** The fundus of the eye as seen with the ophthalmoscope.

**eye'lash.** Cilium; one of the stiff hairs projecting from the tarsal margin of the eyelid.

**eye'lid.** Palpebra.

**lower e.**, *palpebra* inferior.

**third e.**, *plica* semilunaris conjunctivae (2).

**upper e.**, *palpebra* superior.

**eye'piece.** The compound lens at the end of the microscope tube nearest the eye; it magnifies the image made by the objective; see cut under microscope.

**eye'spot.** 1. A colored spot or plastid (chromatophore) in a unicellular organism. 2. Ocellus.

**eye'stone.** A small smooth shell or other object that is inserted beneath the eyelid for the purpose of removing a foreign body.

**eye'strain.** Asthenopia; fatigue of the ciliary muscle or of some of the extrinsic muscles of the eyeball, due to errors of refraction or to imbalance of the ocular muscles; the symptoms are, in different cases, pain in the eyes, lacrimation, headache, and various other reflex symptoms.

# F

**F.** Chemical symbol for the element fluorine; abbreviation or symbol for fractional *concentration,* followed by subscripts indicating location and chemical species; free *energy;* Fahrenheit; faraday; force; visual *field;* and filial *generation;* symbol for free *energy.*

**F₁, F₂, F₃, F₄, etc.** Symbols for first, second, third, and fourth filial generations, etc.; see filial *generation.*

**f.** Symbol for respiratory *frequency.*

**Fab (portion, piece, or fragment).** See immunoglobulin.

**fabella** (fă-bel'lah) [ Mod. L. dim of *faba,* bean ]. A small sesamoid bone in the tendon of the lateral head of the gastrocnemius muscle.

**Faber,** Knud H., Danish physician, 1862–1956. See F.'s *anemia, syndrome.*

**fabia'na.** The dried leaves and twigs of *Fabiana imbricata* (*Solanaceae*); pichi; a shrub of Chile. Has been used in the treatment of renal calculi and chronic cystitis.

**fabrica'tion.** Confabulation; the malingering of symptoms or illness.

**Fabric'ius,** Hieron'ymus ab Aquapenden'te, Italian anatomist and embryologist, 1533–1619. Succeeded Fallopius as professor of anatomy at Padua; taught William Harvey, who no doubt was inspired by and owed much to his teachings; described the valves of the veins in his work *De Venarum Ostiolis;* studied the development of the embryo, publishing a work *De Formato Foetu. See bursa* fabricii, F.'s ship.

**Fabry,** Johannes, German dermatologist, 1860–1930. See F.'s *disease.*

**fabulation** (fab'u-la'shun) [ L. *fabulatio,* fr. *fabulor,* pp. *-atus,* to speak ]. Confabulation.

**F.A.C.D.** Abbreviation for Fellow of the American College of Dentists.

**face.** The front portion of the head; countenance.
  **bird f.,** brachygnathia.
  **cow f.,** *facies* bovina.
  **dish f.,** *facies* scaphoidea.
  **frog f.,** the appearance caused by broadening of the nose which occurs in certain cases of nasal polypus.
  **Hippocrat'ic f.,** Hippocratic *facies.*
  **mask-like f.,** Parkinson's *facies.*
  **moon f.,** the round, usually red face, with large jowls, seen in Cushing's disease or in hyperadrenocorticalism.

**face-bow.** Hinge-bow; a caliper-like device used to record the relationship of the jaws to the temporomandibular joints; the record may then be used to orient the maxillary cast to the opening and closing axis of the articulator.
  **adjustable axis f.-b.,** kinematic f.-b.; hinge-bow; a f.-b. whose caliper ends can be adjusted to permit location of the axis of rotation of the mandible.
  **kinematic f.-b.,** adjustable axis f.-b.

**facet, facette** (fas'et, fă-set') [ Fr. *facette* ]. 1. A small smooth area on a bone or other firm structure. 2. A worn spot on a tooth, produced by chewing.

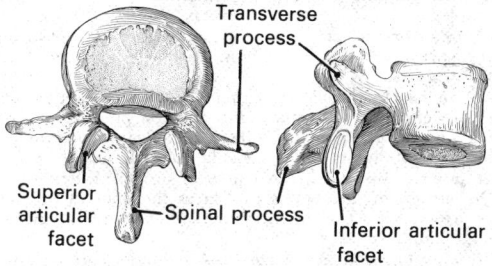

**Facets of a Lumbar Vertebra**

**Lenoir's f.,** a f. on the medial surface of the patella.
**locked f.'s,** see dislocation of articular processes (vertebral, cervical), under dislocation.

**squatting f.,** a f. on the anterior surface of the lower extremity of the tibia seen in certain tribes whose members habitually assume a squatting position.

**facetectomy** (fas'ē-tek'to-mī) [ facet + G. *ektomē,* excision ]. Excision of a facet.

**facial** (fa'shal). Relating to the face.

**facia'lis** [ L. ] [ NA ]. Facial.

**-facient** [ L. *facio,* to make ]. Suffix meaning one who or that which brings about.

---

# FACIES

---

**facies,** pl. **facies** (fa'she-ēz, fash'e-ēz) [ L. ]. 1 [ NA ]. Face; countenance. 2 [ NA ]. Surface. 3. Expression.
  **acromial articular f. of the clavicle,** *facies* articularis acromialis claviculae.
  **adenoid f.,** the open-mouthed and often stupid appearance in children with adenoid hypertrophy, associated with a pinched nose and narrow nares.
  **f. ante'rior** [ NA ], anterior surface; the surface of a structure or part of the body that faces forward.
  **f. ante'rior maxil'lae** [ NA ], anterior surface of the maxilla; that portion of the body of the maxilla lying below the orbit and lateral to the nasal fossa. The infraorbital foramen opens onto this surface.
  **f. ante'rior palpebra'rum** [ NA ], anterior surface of the eyelid; the external surface of the lid, covered with thin skin.
  **f. ante'rior par'tis petro'sae** [ NA ], anterior surface of the petrous part of the temporal bone.
  **f. anterior patel'lae** [ NA ], anterior surface of the patella; the convex, vertically ridged anterior aspect of the patella covered by part of the tendon of insertion of the quadriceps femoris.
  **f. antoni'na,** a facial expression due to alteration in the lids and anterior segment of the eye, as found in leprosy.
  **aortic f.,** the pale sallow complexion of one suffering from incompetence of the aortic valve.
  **f. artic'ular'is** [ NA ], any articular surface.
  **f. articula'ris acromia'lis clavic'ulae** [ NA ], acromial articular surface of the clavicle; the small oval articular facet on the lateral end of the clavicle for union with the acromion.
  **f. articula'ris acro'mii** [ NA ], surface of the acromion; the small oval articular facet on the medial border of the acromion that articulates with the lateral end of the clavicle.
  **f. articula'ris ante'rior den'tis** [ NA ], anterior articular surface of the dens; the curved articular facet on the anterior aspect of the dens that articulates with the anterior arch of the atlas.
  **f. articula'ris arytenoi'dea** [ NA ], arytenoidal articular surface; one of two oval facets on the superior margin of the cricoid lamina for articulation with the arytenoid cartilages.
  **f. articula'ris calca'nea ta'li** [ NA ], calcaneal articular surface of the talus; divided into three parts, the *f. articularis calcanea posterior* is an oval facet on the under side of the talus for union with the calcaneus in the subtalar joint, the *f. articularis calcanea media* and *f. articularis calcanea anterior* underlie the head of the talus and contribute to the talocalcaneonavicular joint.
  **f. articula'ris cap'itis cos'tae** [ NA ], articular surface of the head of a rib; an articular surface on the head of a rib that articulates with the body of a vertebra.
  **f. articula'ris cap'itis fibulae** [ NA ], articular surface of the head of the fibula; the flat circular surface on the head of the fibula for articulation with the corresponding facet on the lateral condyle of the tibia.
  **f. articula'ris car'pea ra'dii** [ NA ], carpal articular surface of the radius; the biconcave distal surface of the

radius for articulation with the scaphoid bone laterally and the lunate medially.

**f. articula'ris cuboi'dea calca'nei** [ NA ], cuboidal articular surface of the calcaneus; the saddle-shaped surface on the anterior end of the calcaneus for articulation with the cuboid bone.

**f. articula'ris fibula'ris tib'iae** [ NA ], fibular articular surface of the tibia; the flat circular articular surface on the inferior and lateral aspect of the lateral condyle of the tibia for articulation with the head of the fibula.

**f. articula'ris infe'rior tib'iae** [ NA ], inferior articular surface of the tibia; the quadrilateral surface on the distal end of the tibia for articulation with the talus; it is concave anteroposteriorly and broader anteriorly.

**f. articula'ris malle'oli fib'ulae** [ NA ], malleolar articular surface of the fibula; the surface on the medial aspect of the lateral malleolus that articulates with the talus.

**f. articula'ris malle'oli tib'iae** [ NA ], malleolar articular surface of the tibia; the articular facet on the lateral surface of the medial malleolus for articulation with the side of the talus; it is continuous with the inferior articular surface of the tibia.

**f. articula'ris navicula'ris ta'li** [ NA ], navicular articular surface of the talus; the large convex surface on the head of the talus for articulation with the navicular bone.

**f. articula'ris patel'lae** [ NA ], articular surface of the patella; the posterior surface of the patella, covered with hyaline cartilage and subdivided by a vertical ridge into a larger lateral and a smaller medial surface for articulation with the corresponding condyles of the femur.

**f. articula'ris poste'rior den'tis** [ NA ], posterior articular surface of the dens; the surface that articulates with the transverse ligament of the atlas.

**f. articula'ris sterna'lis clavic'ulae** [ NA ], sternal articular surface of the clavicle; the articular surface on the sternal end of the clavicle that articulates with the fibrocartilaginous disk of the sternoclavicular joint as well as with the first costal cartilage.

**f. articula'ris supe'rior tib'iae** [ NA ], superior articular surface of the tibia; it is divided into medial and lateral portions for articulation with the condyles of the femur.

**f. articula'ris tala'ris calca'nei** [ NA ], talar articular surface of the calcaneus; one of three facets that articulate with the overlying talus; the f. articularis talaris anterior and f. articularis talaris media contribute to the talocalcaneonavicular joint and are separated by the tarsal canal from the f. articularis talaris posterior which enters into the subtalar joint.

**f. articula'ris thyroi'dea** [ NA ], thyroidal articular surface; one of two small circular facets on the cricoid cartilage near the inferior margin of the junction of the arch and lamina for articulation with the inferior horns of the thyroid cartilage.

**f. articula'ris tuber'culi cos'tae** [ NA ], articular surface of the tubercle of a rib; an oval facet on the inferomedial part of the tubercle of a rib for articulation with a pit on the transverse process of a vertebra.

**f. auricula'ris os'sis il'ii** [ NA ], auricular surface of the ilium; the irregular, L-shaped articular surface on the medial aspect of the ilium that articulates with the sacrum.

**f. auricula'ris os'sis sac'ri** [ NA ], auricular surface of the sacrum; the rough articular surface on the lateral aspect of the sacrum that articulates with the ilium on each side.

**f. bovi'na**, cow face; the cowlike face of ocular hypertelorism.

**f. bucca'lis**, f. vestibularis.

**f. cerebra'lis**, cerebral surface; the internal surface of a cranial bone.

**f. cerebra'lis alae majoris** [ NA ], cerebral surface of the greater wing of the sphenoid.

**f. cerebra'lis partis squamo'sae** [ NA ], cerebral surface of the squamous part of the temporal bone.

**cherubic f.**, the characteristic f. seen in cherubism (familial fibrous *dysplasia, q.v.*); also seen in glycogenosis, particularly type 2.

**f. co'lica** [ NA ], colic surface; one of the visceral surfaces of the spleen; see f. visceralis lienis.

**f. contac'tus** [ NA ], contact surface; the surface of a tooth that faces the adjacent tooth in the dental arch. Opposing contact surfaces are f. distalis and f. mesialis.

**Corvisart's f.**, the f. of cardiac insufficiency.

**f. costa'lis pulmo'nis** [ NA ], costal surface of the lung; the surface of each lung that lies in contact with the costal pleura.

**f. costa'lis scap'ulae** [ NA ], costal surface of the scapula; the concave aspect of the body of the scapula that faces the thorax and that principally lodges the subscapularis muscle.

**f. diaphragmat'ica cor'dis** [ NA ], diaphragmatic surface of the heart; the surface facing the diaphragm; it is formed by both right and left ventricles.

**f. diaphragmat'ica hep'atis** [ NA ], diaphragmatic surface of the liver; the smooth, convex surface of the liver that conforms to the diaphragm; posteriorly it presents a sizable bare area devoid of peritoneum.

**f. diaphragmat'ica pulmo'nis** [ NA ], diaphragmatic surface of the lung; the concave inferior surface that faces the diaphragm.

**f. dista'lis** [ NA ], distal surface; surface of the f. contactus of a tooth that is directed away from the median plane of the dental arch; opposite to f. mesialis.

**f. doloro'sa**, facial expression of a sick or unhappy person.

**f. dorsa'lis os'sis sac'ri** [ NA ], dorsal surface of the sacrum; the posterosuperior aspect of the sacrum marked by a median and two lateral sacral crests between which four dorsal sacral foramina are located on each side.

**f. dorsa'lis scap'ulae** [ NA ], dorsal surface of the scapula; the outer aspect of the body of the scapula, subdivided by the prominent spine of the scapula into a smaller supraspinous fossa and a larger infraspinous fossa.

**elfin f.**, f. characterized by a short, upturned nose, wide mouth, widely spaced eyes, and full cheeks; it may be associated with hypercalcemia, supravalvular aortic stenosis, and mental retardation.

**f. exter'na os'sis fronta'lis** [ NA ], external surface of the frontal bone; the convex outer surface of the frontal bone.

**f. exter'na os'sis parieta'lis** [ NA ], external surface of the parietal bone; the convex outer surface of the parietal bone.

**f. facia'lis** [ NA ], f. vestibularis.

**f. fibula'ris** [ NA ], fibular surface; an alternate term for f. lateralis when referring to the leg or foot or to structures therein.

**f. gas'trica** [ NA ], gastric surface; one of the visceral surfaces of the spleen; see f. visceralis lienis.

**f. glu'tea os'sis il'ii** [ NA ], gluteal surface of the ilium; the external surface of the ala marked by the anterior, posterior and inferior gluteal lines that separate the origins of the gluteal muscles.

**Hall's f.**, the disproportion of forehead to face seen in hydrocephalus.

**Hippocratic f., f. hippocratica**, Hippocratic face; a pinched expression of the face, with sunken eyes, hollow cheeks and temples, relaxed lips, and leaden complexion, observed in one dying after an exhausting illness.

**hound-dog f.**, the facial appearance in cutis laxa, with loose facial skin hanging in folds.

**Hurloid f.**, the coarse gargoyle-like facial appearance characteristically seen in the mucopolysaccharidoses and mucolipidoses.

**Hutchinson's f.**, the peculiar facial expression produced by the drooping lids and motionless eyeballs of ophthalmoplegia.

**f. infe'rior cer'ebri** [ NA ], basis cerebri; base of brain; the surface of the entire brain visible when seen from below.

**f. infe'rior hemisphe'rii cerebel'li** [ NA ], inferior surface of the cerebellar hemisphere; it rests in the posterior cranial fossa and overlies the medulla; it includes the semilunaris inferior, lobulus biventer, tonsilla cerebelli, and flocculus.

**f. infe'rior lin'guae** [ NA ], inferior surface of the tongue; the surface of the tongue that faces the floor of the oral cavity, its mucosa being thin, smooth and devoid of papillae.

**f. infe'rior par'tis petro'sae** [ NA ], inferior surface of the petrous part of the temporal bone; the portion of the petrous part of the temporal bone that contributes to the external base of the skull.

**f. infratempora'lis maxil'lae** [ NA ], infratemporal surface of the maxilla; the posterolateral surface of the body of the maxilla that faces the infratemporal fossa.

**f. interloba′res pulmo′nis** [ NA ], interlobar surfaces of the lung; the pulmonary surfaces in the interlobar fissures of the lung.

**f. inter′na os′sis fronta′lis** [ NA ], internal surface of the frontal bone; the surface of the frontal bone that contributes to the boundary of the cranial cavity.

**f. inter′na os′sis parieta′lis** [ NA ], internal surface of the parietal bone; the concave surface of the parietal bone forming part of the wall of the cranial cavity.

**f. intestina′lis u′teri** [ NA ], intestinal surface of the uterus; the posterosuperior peritonealized surface with which loops of intestine come in contact.

**f. labia′lis,** f. vestibularis.

**f. latera′lis** [ NA ], lateral surface; the surface of a part of the body that faces away from the midline.

**le′onine f.,** leontiasis.

**f. lingua′lis** [ NA ], lingual surface; the surface of a tooth that faces the tongue.

**f. luna′ta acetab′uli** [ NA ], lunate surface of the acetabulum; the curved articular surface that surrounds the acetabular fossa and articulates with the head of the femur.

**f. malleola′ris latera′lis** [ NA ], lateral malleolar surface; that surface of the trochlea of the talus that articulates with the lateral malleolus of the fibula.

**f. malleola′ris media′lis** [ NA ], medial malleolar surface; the surface of the trochlea of the talus that articulates with the medial malleolus of the tibia.

**f. masticato′ria,** f. occlusalis.

**f. maxilla′ris os′sis palati′ni** [ NA ], maxillary surface of the palatine bone; the lateral surface of the perpendicular lamina of the palatine bone.

**f. maxilla′ris os′sis sphenoida′lis** [ NA ], maxillary surface of the sphenoid bone; that part of the anterior surface of the greater wing of the sphenoid that is perforated by the foramen rotundum and forms the posterior boundary of the pterygopalatine fossa.

**f. media′lis** [ NA ], medial surface; the surface of a part of the body that faces toward the midline.

**f. media′lis cer′ebri** [ NA ], medial surface of the cerebral hemisphere, facing, above as well as anterior and posterior to the corpus callosum, the falx cerebri, below it the mesencephalon and the dura-covered medial wall of the middle cerebral fossa.

**f. media′lis pulmo′nis** [ NA ], medial surface of the lung; it consists of a vertebral part posteriorly and a mediastinal part facing the mediastinal pleura.

**f. mesia′lis** [ NA ], mesial surface; surface of the f. contactus of a tooth that is directed toward the median plane of the dental arch; opposite to the f. distalis.

**mitral f.,** the pink, slightly cyanosed cheeks of patients with mitral valve disease.

**myasthen′ic f.,** the facial expression in myasthenia gravis, caused by drooping of the eyelids and weakness of the muscles of the face.

**myopath′ic f.,** a peculiar facial appearance characterized by protrusion of the lips, drooping of the lids, and general relaxation of the muscles of the face; caused by muscular weakness.

**f. nasa′lis maxil′lae** [ NA ], nasal surface of the maxilla; it forms part of the lateral nasal wall with a large defect (*hiatus maxillaris*) posteriorly and the lacrimal sulcus in its midportion.

**f. occlusa′lis** [ NA ], occlusal surface (1); f. masticatoria; masticating, masticatory, or grinding surface; the surface that occludes with or contacts an opposing surface of a tooth in the opposing jaw.

**f. orbita′lis maxil′lae** [ NA ], orbital surface of the maxilla; the triangular surface of the maxilla forming most of the floor of the orbit; it articulates posteriorly with the palatine bone, medially with the ethmoid and laterally with the zygomatic bone and is marked by the infraorbital sulcus and canal.

**f. ovar′ica,** Wells′ f.; the pinched, drawn face of a woman with ovarian tumor.

**f. palati′na** [ NA ], palatine surface; the inferior surface of the horizontal plate of the palatine bone.

**f. palma′ris** [ NA ], palmar surface; the anterior surface of a finger.

**Parkinson's f.,** the expressionless or masklike f. characteristic of parkinsonism (1).

**f. patella′ris fem′oris** [ NA ], patellar surface of the femur; the depression between the femoral condyles anteriorly that accommodates the patella.

**f. pelvi′na os′sis sa′cri** [ NA ], pelvic surface of the sacrum; the surface of the sacrum that faces downward and forward forming part of the posterior wall of the pelvic cavity; it is marked by four pelvic sacral foramina on each side.

**f. planta′ris** [ NA ], plantar surface; the inferior surface of a toe.

**f. poplit′ea fem′oris** [ NA ], popliteal plane or surface of the femur; planum popliteum; the posterior surface of the lower end of the femur between the diverging lips of the linea aspera.

**f. poste′rior** [ NA ], posterior surface; the surface of a part of the body that faces toward the posterior part of the body.

**f. poste′rior palpebra′rum** [ NA ], posterior surface of the eyelid; the internal surface of the lid, covered with conjunctiva.

**f. poste′rior par′tis petro′sae** [ NA ], posterior surface of the petrous part of the temporal bone; the surface of the petrous part of the temporal bone that contributes to the posterior cranial fossa.

**Potter's f.,** Potter's disease; characteristic f. seen in bilateral renal agenesis and other severe renal malformations, exhibiting ocular hypertelorism, low-set ears, receding chin, and flattening of the nose.

**f. pulmona′lis cor′dis** [ NA ], pulmonary surface of the heart; the left surface of the heart formed by the left ventricle.

**f. radia′lis** [ NA ], radial surface; an alternate term for f. lateralis when referring to the forearm or hand or structures therein.

**f. rena′lis** [ NA ], renal surface; (1) the surface of the suprarenal gland in contact with the kidney; (2) one of the visceral surfaces of the spleen, see f. visceralis lienis.

**f. sacropelvi′na os′sis il′ii** [ NA ], sacropelvic surface of the ilium; the medial surface of the ilium behind and below the iliac fossa; it includes the iliac tuberosity, the auricular surface and the smooth pelvic surface below and in front of the auricular surface.

**f. scaphoi′dea,** dish face; a facial malformation characterized by protuberant forehead, depressed nose and upper jaw, with prominence of the chin.

**f. sternocosta′lis cor′dis** [ NA ], sternocostal surface of the heart; the anterior aspect of the heart, formed mostly by the right ventricle and to a lesser extent the left ventricle.

**f. supe′rior** [ NA ], superior surface; the surface of the trochlea of the talus in contact with the inferior articular surface of the tibia.

**f. supe′rior hemisphe′rii cerebel′li** [ NA ], superior (upper) surface of the cerebellar hemisphere; it lies against the under surface of the tentorium and includes the ala lobuli centralis, lobulus quadrangularis, lobulus simplex, and lobulus semilunaris superior.

**f. superolatera′lis cer′ebri** [ NA ], superolateral surface of the cerebrum; cortical convexity; the aspect of the cerebral hemisphere that lies in contact with the flat bones of the skull; it includes parts of the frontal, parietal, temporal, and occipital lobes.

**f. symphy′sialis** [ NA ], symphysial surface of the pubis.

**f. tempora′lis** [ NA ], temporal surface; the name given to the surface of a bone which contributes to the temporal fossa; the following have a f. temporalis: greater wing of the sphenoid, squamous part of the temporal, frontal, and zygomatic bones.

**f. tibia′lis** [ NA ], tibial surface; an alternate term for f. medialis when referring to the leg or foot or to structures therein.

**f. ulna′ris** [ NA ], ulnar surface; an alternate term for f. medialis when referring to the forearm or hand or to structures therein.

**f. urethra′lis pe′nis** [ NA ], urethral surface of the penis; the surface opposite to the dorsum penis.

**f. vesica′lis u′teri** [ NA ], vesical surface of the uterus; the surface facing the bladder and separated from it by the uterovesical pouch of peritoneum.

**f. vestibula′ris** [ NA ], vestibular surface; facial surface; f. facialis; buccal surface (1); f. buccalis; labial surface (1);

f. labialis; the surface of a tooth that faces the vestibule of the mouth; opposite to the f. lingualis.

**f. viscera′lis hep′atis** [ NA ], visceral surface of the liver; the posteroinferior surface of the liver that faces adjacent abdominal organs. The porta hepatis and gallbladder are located on this surface.

**f. viscera′lis lie′nis** [ NA ], visceral surface of the spleen; the surface of the spleen in contact with adjacent viscera; f. colica (colic surface), f. gastrica (gastric surface), and f. renalis (renal surface) are the visceral surfaces of the spleen. **Wells′ f.,** f. ovarica.

---

**facilitation** (fă-sil′ĭ-ta′shun) [ L. *facilitas*, fr. *facilis*, easy. FAC- ]. The enhancement or reinforcement of a reflex or other nervous activity by the arrival at the reflex center of impulses having their origin elsewhere.

**facing** (fās′ing). A tooth-colored material (usually plastic or porcelain) used to hide the buccal or labial surface of a gold crown to give the outward appearance of a natural tooth.

**facio-** (fa′shi-o-) [ L. *facies*, face ]. Combining form relating to the face.

**faciobrachial** (fa′shĭ-o-bra′kĭ-al). Relating to the face and the arm; denoting a form of juvenile muscular dystrophy.

**faciocephalalgia** (fa′shĭ-o-sef′ă-lal′jĭ-ah). Neuralgic pain in the face.

**faciocervical** (fa′shĭ-o-ser′vĭ-kal). Relating to the face and neck; denoting a form of progressive dystrophy of the muscles of these regions.

**faciolingual** (fa′shĭ-o-ling′gwal). Relating to the face and the tongue, often denoting a paralysis affecting these parts.

**fa′cioplas′ty** [ facio- + G. *plastos*, formed ]. Reparative or reconstructive surgery of the facial soft tissues.

**facioplegia** (fa′shĭ-o-ple′jĭ-ah) [ facio- + G. *plēgē*, a stroke ]. Facial *palsy.*

**facioscapulohumeral** (fa′shĭ-o-skap′u-lo-hu′mer-al). Relating to the face, the scapula, and the upper arm; denoting a form of muscular dystrophy, or infantile progressive muscular atrophy.

**F.A.C.O.G.** Fellow of the American College of Obstetricians and Gynecologists.

**F.A.C.P.** Abbreviation for Fellow of the American College of Physicians.

**F.A.C.R.** Abbreviation for Fellow of the American College of Radiologists.

**F.A.C.S.** Abbreviation for Fellow of the American College of Surgeons.

**facteur** [ Fr. ]. Factor.
**f. antihemophilique A,** *factor* VIII.
**f. antihemophilique B,** *factor* IX.

**F-actin.** See under actin.

**factitious** (fak-tish′us) [ L. *factitius*, made by art, fr. *facio*, to make ]. Artificial; self-induced; not natural. A f. dermatitis (for example) is one induced by the patient because of a variety of psychiatric mechanisms.

# FACTOR

---

**factor** (fak′ter) [ L. maker, causer, fr. *facio*, to make ]. 1. One of the contributing causes in any action. 2. One of the components which by multiplication makes up a number or expression. 3. Gene. 4. Vitamin or other essential element.

**f. I,** in the clotting of blood, fibrinogen.

**f. II,** (1) in the clotting of blood, prothrombin; (2) lipoic *acid.*

**f. III,** in the clotting of blood, tissue *thromboplastin.*

**f. IV,** in the clotting of blood, calcium ions.

**f. V,** in the clotting of blood, known by several terms: proaccelerin (Owren), labile f. (Quick), plasma ac-globulin (Ware and Seegars), thrombogene (Nolf), prothrombinase (Owren), prothrombokinase (Milstone), plasmin prothrombins conversion f. or PPCF (Stefanini), component A

of prothrombin (Quick), prothrombin accelerator (Fantl and Nance), and cofactor of thromboplastin (Honorato). Deficiency of this f. leads to a rare hemorrhagic tendency known as parahemophilia or hypoproaccelerinemia, with autosomal recessive inheritance; heterozygous individuals are recognized by reduced levels of f. V but have no bleeding tendency. See also prothrombinase.

**f. V$_{1a}$,** cobyric acid.

**f. VII,** in the clotting of blood, known by several terms: proconvertin (Owren), serum prothrombin conversion accelerator or SPCA (de Vries, Alexander), stable f. (Stefanini), cofactor V (Owren), serozyme (Bordet), kappa f. (Sorbye and Dam), prothrombinogen (Quick), cothromboplastin (Mann and Hurn), serum accelerator (Jacox). F. VII is known to be involved in: (1) the congenital deficiency of f. VII, with purpura and bleeding from mucous membranes, autosomal recessive inheritance; (2) the acquired deficiency of f. VII in association with a deficiency of vitamin K, the neonatal period, and the administration of prothrombinopenic drugs; and (3) the acquired excess of f. VII in some patients with thromboembolism. F. VII accelerates the conversion of prothrombin to thrombin, in the presence of tissue thromboplastin, calcium, and f. V.

**f. VIII,** in the clotting of blood, known by the following synonyms: antihemophilic globulin (Patek and Taylor), antihemophilic globulin A (Cramer), antihemophilic f. or AHF (Brinkhous), plasma thromboplastin f. or PTF (Ratnoff), plasma thromboplastin f. A (Aggeler), thromboplastic plasma component or TPC (Shinowara), facteur antihemophilique A (Soulier), thromboplastinogen (Quick), prothrombokinase (Feissly), platelet cofactor (Johnson), plasmokinin (Laki), and thrombokatilysin (Leggenhager). Deficiency of f. VIII is associated with classic hemophilia A, an X-linked hemorrhagic tendency that occurs almost exclusively in males; clotting time is prolonged, less thromboplastin is formed, and the conversion of prothrombin is diminished.

**f. IX,** in the clotting of blood, also known as: Christmas f. (Biggs and Macfarlane), plasma thromboplastin component or PTC (Aggeler), antihemophilic globulin B (Cramer), plasma thromboplastin f. B (Aggeler), plasma f. X (Shulman), and facteur antihemophilique B (Soulier). Deficiency of this f. causes hemophilia B or Christmas disease, which resembles hemophilia A, and is an inherited defect that leads to a severe hemorrhagic disorder. F. IX is required for the formation of intrinsic blood thromboplastin, and affects the amount formed (rather than the rate).

**f. X,** in the clotting of blood, also known as Stuart f. or Stuart-Prower f.; it is required for prothrombin conversion in the presence or absence of tissue extract. Deficiency may be congenital, resulting in a hemorrhagic tendency conditioned by an incompletely recessive autosomal gene, or acquired as a result of anticoagulant therapy with coumarin type drugs.

**f. X for Haemophilus,** hemin.

**f. XI,** in the clotting of blood, also known as plasma thromboplastin antecedent or PTA f.; it is a component of the contact system and is absorbed from plasma and serum by glass and similar surfaces. Deficiency of f. XI results in a hemorrhagic tendency and is caused by an autosomal recessive gene.

**f. XII,** in the clotting of blood, also known as glass f. and Hageman f. Deficiency of f. XII results in great prolongation of the clotting time of venous blood, but only rarely in a hemorrhagic tendency. Deficiency is caused by an autosomal recessive gene.

**f. XIII,** in the clotting of blood; thrombin catalyzes the conversion of f. XIII into its active form, fibrinase (also called fibrin-stabilizing f., Laki-Lorand f., or L-F f.), which cross-links subunits of the fibrin clot to form insoluble fibrin.

**f. 3,** (1) operational name given to an incompletely characterized selenium-containing natural product which, in minute amounts, prevents liver damage in rats due to deficiency of vitamin E; (2) f. III in the vitamin B$_{12}$ series, 5-hydroxybenzimidazole, analogue of the usual B$_{12}$ nucleotide components; also known as f. I (capital letter I).

**f. A,** see properdin factor A, under properdin.

**ABO f.'s,** see ABO blood group, appendix 2.

**accelerator f.,** f. V.

**acetate replacement f.,** lipoic acid.

**adrenal weight f.,** a postulated substance of adenohypophysial origin responsible for maintenance of the weight of the adrenal cortex.

**alpha f.,** an obsolete term for the female sex hormone, $17\beta$-estradiol.

**anhydrocitrovorum f.,** anhydroleucovorin.

**animal protein factor (APF),** vitamin $B_{12}$ plus unidentified factors.

**antiacrodynia f.,** vitamin $B_6$.

**an'tialope'cia f.,** inositol.

**antianemia f.,** folic acid.

**antiberiberi f.,** thiamin.

**anti-black-tongue f.,** nicotinic acid.

**anticomplementary f.,** zymosan.

**anti-egg-white-injury f.,** biotin.

**antifertility f.,** phosphorylated *hesperidin.*

**anti-gizzard erosion f.,** vitamin U.

**anti-gray-hair f.,** *p*-aminobenzoic acid; see under aminobenzoic.

**antihemophilic f. A,** f. VIII.

**antihemophilic f. B,** f. IX.

**antihemorrhagic f.,** vitamin K.

**antineuritic f.,** thiamin.

**antinuclear f.,** ANF; a f. present in serum with strong affinity for nuclei and detected by fluorescent antibody technique; present in lupus erythematosus, rheumatic arthritis, and certain other conditions.

**antiophthalmic f.,** vitamin A.

**antipellag'ra f.,** nicotinic acid.

**an'tipernic'ious anemia f.,** vitamin $B_{12}$.

**antisterility f.,** vitamin E.

**anti-stiffness f.,** stigmasterol (*q.v.*); a fat-soluble vitamin that influences calcium and phosphorus metabolism. Deficiency of this f. is associated with muscular degeneration, calcinosis and stiffness of the muscles, and other signs and symptoms of the collagen diseases.

**antixerophthal'mic f., antixerotic f.,** vitamin A.

**augmenting f.,** a supposed principle of the anterior lobe of the pituitary which enhances the action of the luteinizing hormone (LH). Its existence has been denied.

**f. B,** see properdin factor B, under properdin.

**$B_T$ f.,** carnitine.

**bacteriocin f.'s,** bacteriocinogens.

**beta f.,** a postulated hormone that controls the progestational phase of the female sexual cycle. It remains to be identified and defined.

**bi'fidus f.,** an unidentified substance associated with *Lactobacillus bifidus* var. *Penn.*, present in mammalian milk.

**biotic f.'s,** environmental f.'s or influences resulting from the activities of living organisms, as contrasted to those resulting from climatic, geological, or other f.'s.

**Bittner's milk f.,** mammary cancer *virus* of mice.

**blood f.,** see under blood; see also appendix 2, Blood Groups.

**branching f.,** 1,4-$\alpha$-glucan-branching enzyme; see under glucan.

**C f.,** a protein restoring phosphorylation and loss of water from mitochondria caused to swell by glutathione, a process releasing C factor into the medium.

**Castle's extrinsic f.,** vitamin $B_{12}$; formerly also thought to be a separate erythrocyte-maturing f. of the liver.

**Castle's intrinsic f.,** a f. secreted by the neck cells of gastric glands; required for adequate absorption of vitamin $B_{12}$; secretion is inadequate in patients with pernicious anemia. The chemical structure of this f. is unknown; it appears to be a relatively small protein or polypeptide or to be secreted as an attachment to such a molecule.

**chick antidermati'tis f.,** pantothenic acid.

**chick antipellag'ra f.,** pantothenic acid.

**Christmas f.,** f. IX.

**citrovor'um f.,** folinic acid.

**clearing f.'s,** lipoprotein lipases that appear in plasma during lipemia and catalyze hydrolysis of triglycerides only when the latter are bound to protein and when an acceptor (*e.g.*, serum albumin) is present, thus "clearing" the plasma.

**clotting f.,** various plasma components involved in the clotting process, including, notably, fibrinogen (f. I),

prothrombin (f. II), thromboplastin (f. III), and calcium ion (f. IV).

**coagulation f.,** clotting f.

**cobra venom f.,** a component of cobra venom that activates C3 proactivator (cobra venom cofactor; properdin factor B) of the properdin system (*q.v.*, under properdin), leading to activation of other components of complement and lysis of unsensitized erythrocytes. See also component of *complement.*

**coen'zyme f.,** diaphorase.

**complement chemotactic f.,** see under complement.

**contraceptive f.,** phosphorylated *hesperidin.*

**corticotropin-releasing f.,** CRF; corticotropin-releasing hormone; a substance of hypothalamic origin capable of accelerating pituitary secretion of corticotropin; found in the vicinity of the median eminence in the form of several polypeptides. It has been postulated that neurohypophysial vasopressin can exert a similar effect.

**coupling f.'s,** proteins that restore phosphorylating ability to mitochondria that have lost it, that is, have become "uncoupled" so that oxidation no longer produces ATP.

**f. D,** see properdin factor D, under properdin.

**debranching f.,** debranching *enzyme.*

**decapacitation f.,** a f., postulated to be present in epididymal fluid and seminal plasma, that prevents the capacitation of spermatozoa.

**diabetogen'ic f.,** a f. in crude extracts of the anterior lobe of the hypophysis that produces degenerative changes in the islet cells of the pancreas and causes permanent diabetes. The chronic administration of purified pituitary growth hormone produces similar results.

**Duran-Reynals' permeability f., Duran-Reynals' spreading f.,** see hyaluronidases.

**f. E,** see properdin f. E, under properdin.

**epidermal growth f.,** a heat-stable, antigenic protein isolated from the submaxillary glands of male mice; when injected into newborn animals it accelerates eyelid opening and tooth eruption; it stimulates epidermal growth and keratinization; in larger doses it inhibits body growth and hair development and produces fatty livers.

**eryth'rocyte maturation f.,** vitamin $B_{12}$.

**essential food f.'s,** those substances required in the diet: certain amino acids and unsaturated fatty acids, vitamins, essential minerals, etc.

**extrinsic f.,** dietary vitamin $B_{12}$.

**f. f,** a chemical (postulated by T. Lewis), formed in ischemic skeletal or cardiac muscle, held to be responsible for the pain of intermittent claudication and angina pectoris.

**F f.,** F *agent.*

**F' f.,** F' *agent.*

**fermentation Lactobacillus casei f.,** pteropterin.

**fertility f.,** F *agent.*

**fibrin-stabilizing f.,** see f. XIII.

**filtrate f.** pantothenic acid.

**follicle-stimulating hormone-releasing f.,** FRF; FSH-RF; FSH-releasing hormone; a substance of hypothalamic origin capable of accelerating pituitary secretion of follicle--stimulating hormone. It appears to be formed in the vicinity of the median eminence. Little is known about its chemical structure.

**G f.,** the single common variance or f. that is common to (*i.e.*, empirically intercorrelates) different intelligence tests (general).

**galact'agogue f.,** a f. in extracts of the posterior lobe of the hypophysis which, by stimulating the smooth muscle of the lobulo-alveolar system of the mammary gland, causes a flow of milk from the nipple. Oxytocin is capable of producing an identical effect.

**galact'opoiet'ic f.,** prolactin.

**glass f.,** f. XII.

**gly'cotrop'ic f.,** a principle in extracts of the anterior lobe of the hypophysis that raises the blood sugar and antagonizes the action of insulin. Purified pituitary growth hormone has been shown to produce an identical effect.

**f. Gm,** a f. that determines certain of the allotypes of human immunoglobulins; found only on the $\gamma$ chains of IgG ($\gamma$-globulin).

**growth f.,** any f., mineral, vitamin, or hormone, that promotes growth in young organisms.

growth hormone-releasing f., somatoliberin.

f. H, (1) biotin; (2) vitamin B$_{12}$ analogue or precursor.

H f. of Lewis, histamine-like substance present in the deeper layers of the skin. It is probably histamine itself, and is responsible for inflammatory vascular reactions of the human skin.

Hageman f., f. XII.

HG f., glucagon.

human antihemophilic f. (USP), human antihemophilic fraction (BP); antihemophilic globulin; HEMOFIL; a lyophilized concentrate of f. VIII, obtained from fresh normal human plasma; used as a hemostatic agent in hemophilia.

hyperglycemic-glycogenolytic f., glucagon.

f. I (letter I), see f. 3.

inhibition f., migration-inhibitory f.

insulin-antagonizing f., glycotropic f.

intrinsic f., see Castle's intrinsic f.

f. Inv, a f. that determines certain of the allotypes of human immunoglobulins; found on the κ chains of IgG, IgA, IgM, and Bence Jones protein.

kappa f., f. VII.

labile f., f. V.

Lac'tobacil'lus bulgar'icus f., pantetheine.

Lac'tobacil'lus ca'sei f., folic acid.

lactogen'ic f., prolactin.

Laki-Lorand f., see f. XIII.

L.E. f.'s, antinuclear immunoglobulins in plasma of persons with disseminated lupus erythematosus, associated with positive L.E. tests.

lethal f., a gene mutation or chromosomal structural change which, when expressed, causes death prior to sexual maturity.

leu'kocyto'sis-promoting f., a substance obtained by Menkin from inflammatory exudates; it stimulates leukocytosis.

leukope'nic f., a principle obtained by Menkin from inflammatory exudates; it causes leukopenia when injected into normal animals.

lipotropic f., choline.

liver filtrate f., pantothenic acid.

liver Lactobacil'lus ca'sei f., folic acid.

liver residue f., molybdenum.

L-L f., see f. XIII.

luteinizing hormone-releasing f., LRF; LH-RF; LH-releasing hormone; a substance of hypothalamic origin capable of accelerating pituitary secretion of luteinizing hormone. It and a decapeptide amide and appears to be formed in the vicinity of the median eminence.

lymph node permeability f., abbreviated LNPF; a substance, released by lymphocytes when stimulated or damaged, that increases capillary permeability and the accumulation of mononuclear cells.

mam'mogenic f., prolactin.

maturation f., vitamin B$_{12}$.

migration-inhibitory f., inhibition f.; a soluble, nondialyzable substance that is produced by sensitized lymphocytes (i.e., lymphocytes from a sensitized animal) when exposed to the specific antigen, and that causes adherence and inhibition of migration of macrophages.

milk f., mammary cancer virus of mice.

monkey antianemia f., folic acid.

mouse antialope'cia f., inositol.

nerve growth f., abbreviated NGF; a protein that controls the development of sympathetic postganglionic neurons and possibly also sensory (dorsal root) ganglion cells in mammals; it has been isolated from the submaxillary glands of male mice. When injected into newborn animals, sympathetic ganglia become hyperplastic and hypertrophic. Similar, but not identical, factors have been isolated from the venoms of several species of snakes.

P f., (1) vitamin P; (2) see P blood group, appendix 2.

pellagra-preventing f., P-P f., nicotinic acid.

plasma labile f., f. V.

plasma thromboplastin f. (PTF); f. VIII.

plasma thromboplastin f. B, f. IX.

plasmin prothrombins conversion f. (PPCF), f. V.

platelet f. 3, a blood coagulation factor derived from platelets; chemically, a phospholipid lipoprotein. Acts with certain plasma thromboplastin f.'s to convert prothrombin to thrombin.

platelet tissue f., thromboplastin.

f. PP, vitamins B$_6$.

prolactin-inhibiting f., PIF; a substance of hypothalamic origin capable of inhibiting the synthesis and release of prolactin by the anterior pituitary gland.

properdin f.'s, see under properdin.

protein f., see under protein.

prothrombin conversion f., prothrombin converting f., f. VII.

PTA f., f. XI.

PTC f., f. IX.

pyruvate oxidation f., lipoic acid.

f. R, folic acid.

R f.'s, resistance f.'s; resistance-transfer episomes; extrachromosomal elements (episomes) responsible for rapid spread of drug resistance among bacteria, notably the Enterobacteriaceae. There are two general types with respect to bacteria carrying the F agent (q. v.): those that are epistatic (fertility-inhibiting, fi$^+$) and those that are not (fi$^-$). R f.'s consist of two components that can be transferred independently: the genetic determinants for drug resistance, per se, and the element that confers transferability (transfer f.).

relaxation f., substance presumably involved in the return of muscle fibrils to the resting state after nervous stimulation ceases, postulated to act by withdrawing Ca$^{++}$ from myosin-ATPase sites.

releasing f., RF; releasing hormone; a substance of hypothalamic origin capable of accelerating the rate of secretion of a given hormone by the anterior pituitary gland; the chemical nature and factors influencing the rate of secretion are only partially known. See also corticotropin-releasing f., follicle-stimulating hormone releasing f., growth hormone releasing f., luteinizing hormone releasing f., thyrotropin-releasing f.

resistance f.'s, R f's.

resistance-inducing f., an agent from normal chick embryos that interferes with multiplication of the avian leukosis-sarcoma virus, and is seemingly an avirulent leukosis virus antigenically related to the avian leukosis-sarcoma virus.

resistance-transfer f., transfer f.

Reynals' f., see hyaluronidases.

rheumatoid f.'s, globulins in the serum of patients with rheumatoid arthritis that enhance agglutination of suspended particles (see latex test and Rose-Waaler test) coated with pooled human γ-globulin.

S f., the individual variables, or empirically most minute subclusters of intercorrelations or common variance, found in different intelligence tests (specific).

secretor f., an inherited capacity to secrete antigens of the ABO blood group in saliva and other body fluids, controlled by a pair of allelic genes designated Se and se (or S and s), with Se dominant to se. The saliva of secretors (genotype SeSe or Sese) contains the blood group substances A, B or H found in their erythrocytes. The saliva of nonsecretors (genotype sese) contains no blood group substance. In most populations about 75 per cent of persons are secretors. Tests for ABH secretion are useful in genetic linkage and population studies. The secretor phenomenon is also closely associated with the Lewis blood group (see also Lewis blood group, in appendix 2, Blood Groups).

sex f., F agent.

skin f., biotin.

S. lactis R f., folic acid.

Slater f., coenzyme Q.

somatotropin release-inhibiting f., somatostatin.

somatotropin-releasing f., somatoliberin.

spreading f., see hyaluronidases.

stable f., f. VII.

Stuart f., Stuart-Prower f., f. X.

sulfation f., somatomedin.

f. T, vitamin T.

thymic lymphopoietic f., thymosin; a glycoprotein with molecular weight of less than 10,000, that has been extracted from thymus; there is ground for the belief that this thymus-produced humoral factor(s) or hormone(s) confers immunological competence on thymus-dependent cells and induces lymphopoiesis.

thyrotoxic complement-fixation f., a form of thyrotoxin; an antigen found most readily in thyroid tissue from thyrotoxic individuals; known to be chemically and immunologically distinct from thyroglobulin, and fixes complement when combined with antibody related to the γ-globulin fraction of serum. With the exception of extremely small concentrations, the antigen is rarely found in normal glands or in diseased glands that are not associated with thyrotoxicosis; it is probably an intracellular substance (possibly a constituent of the "microsomal fraction"), and does not contain iodine in significant quantity. Not related to the complement-fixation reaction occurring with serum in Hashimoto's disease, in which the antigen is thyroglobulin.

**thyrotropin-releasing f.,** TRF; TSH-RF; thyrotropin-releasing hormone; a substance of hypothalamic origin capable of accelerating pituitary secretion of thyrotropin; chemically, it is pyroglutamyl-histidyl-proline amide (at least for the procine and ovine species).

**transfer f.,** abbreviated TF; (1) resistance-transfer f. (RTF); the component of the R f. that confers transferability of genetic determinants such as drug resistance and colicinogeny; (2) a substance, free of nucleic acid and antibody, that is obtained from the leukocytes of a person with a delayed-type sensitivity and that will, following injection into the skin of a nonsensitive person, transfer the specific sensitivity to the recipient.

**transforming f.,** the DNA responsible for bacterial transformation; see also transformation (5).

**transmethylation f.,** choline.

**f. U,** folic acid.

**ulcer-preventive f.,** vitamin U.

**uncoupling f.,** uncoupler.

**W f.,** biotin.

**Y f.,** pyridoxine.

**yeast el'uate f.,** pyridoxine.

**facto'rial.** 1. Pertaining to a statistical factor or factors. 2. Of an integer, that integer multiplied by each smaller integer in succession down to one; e.g., 5 ! equals 5 × 4 × 3 × 2.

**facultative** (fak'ul-ta'tiv). Able to live under more than one specific set of environmental conditions; with an alternative pathway; see facultative *parasite*.

**faculty** (fak'ul-tĭ). A natural or specialized power of a living organism.

**FAD.** Abbreviation for *flavin* adenine dinucleotide.

α **-fagarine.** α-Allocryptopine; one of two modifications of allocryptopine.

**Faget** (fă-zha'), Jean C., French physician, 1818–1884. See F.'s *sign*.

**fagin, fagine** (fa'jin, -jĕn). See choline.

**fagopyrism, fagopyris'mus** (fag'o-pi'rizm, fă-gop'ĭ-rizm) [ L. *fagus*, beech, + G. *pyros*, wheat ]. Poisoning by buckwheat, St. John's wort, clover, etc., an idiosyncrasy marked by nausea and vomiting, urticaria, photosensitization, and irritation of the conjunctiva and nasal mucous membrane.

**Fahr,** Theodore, German physician, 1877–1945. See F.'s *disease*.

**Fahraeus,** Robert (Robin) Sanno, Swedish pathologist, *1888. See F.-Lindqvist *effect*.

**Fahrenheit** făr'en-hīt, fahr'en-hīt), Gabriel D., German physicist, 1686–1736. See F. *scale*.

**fail'ure.** The state of being lacking or insufficient.

**backward heart f.,** the theory of backward f. maintains that the phenomena of congestive heart f. result from passive engorgement of the veins caused by a "backward" rise in pressure proximal to the failing cardiac chambers.

**cardiac f.,** heart f.

**congestive f.,** heart f. (1).

**coronary f.,** acute coronary insufficiency.

**forward heart f.,** the theory of forward f. maintains that the phenomena of congestive heart f. result from the inadequate cardiac output, and especially from the consequent inadequacy of renal blood flow with resulting retention of sodium and water.

**heart f.,** (1) congestive f.; cardiac f. or insufficiency; myocardial insufficiency; mechanical inadequacy of the heart so that as a pump it fails to maintain the circulation of blood, with the result that congestion and edema

develop in the tissues; see also forward f., backward f., right and left ventricular f.; (2) the resulting clinical syndrome consisting of shortness of breath, pitting edema, enlarged tender liver, engorged neck veins, and pulmonary rales.

**high output f.,** heart f. in which, despite relative myocardial insufficiency and consequent congestive f., the cardiac output is maintained at normal or supernormal levels, as is sometimes seen in emphysema, thyrotoxicosis, etc.

**left ventricular f.,** congestive heart f. manifested by signs of pulmonary congestion and edema, *i.e.*, dyspnea, basal rales, pulmonary edema, etc.

**low output f.,** heart f. in which the cardiac output is subnormal, as is usually seen in f. due to coronary, hypertensive, or rheumatic heart disease.

**pacemaker f.,** f. of an artificial pacemaker to generate or deliver effective stimuli to the myocardium.

**power f.,** pump f.

**pump f.,** power f.; a term used to emphasize default of the heart as a mechanical pump in contrast with electrical f. in which the cardiac inadequacy is secondary to disturbance of the electrical impulse (arrhythmia); in acute myocardial infarction, pump f. signifies congestive heart failure, pulmonary edema, or cardiogenic shock.

**right ventricular f.,** congestive heart f. manifested by distention of the neck veins, enlargement of the liver, and dependent edema.

**secondary f.,** decreasing responsiveness to an oral hypoglycemic agent after an initial satisfactory response; usually occurs several months after initiation of treatment; also termed a relapse.

**faint.** 1. Extremely weak; threatened with syncope. 2. An attack of syncope.

**fal'cate.** Falciform.

**fal'ces.** Plural of falx.

**falcial** (fal'shal). Relating to the falx cerebelli or falx cerebri.

**falciform** (fal'sĭ-form) [ L. *falx*, sickle, + *forma*, form ]. Falcate; falcular; crescentic or sickle-shaped.

**falcula** (fal'ku-lah) [ L. dim. of *falx* ]. Falx cerebelli.

**fal'cular.** 1. Relating to the falx cerebelli. 2. Falciform.

**fal'icain.** 3-Piperidino-4'-propoxypropiophenone hydrochloride; local anesthetic.

**fallacia** (fal-la'ke-ah) [ L. deceit, deception ]. A visual illusion or hallucination.

**Fallo'pius (Fallo'pio),** Gabriele, Italian anatomist, 1523–1562. See Fallopian *aqueduct, arch, canal, hiatus, ligament, neuritis, pregnancy, tube*.

**Fallot** (fal-o'), Étienne-Louis A., French physician, 1850–1911. See *pentalogy* of F., F.'s *tetrad, triad, tetralogy*.

**fal'sifica'tion.** The deliberate act of misrepresentation so as to deceive.

**retrospective f.,** unconscious distortion of past experience to conform to present psychological needs.

**Falta,** Wilhelm, Vienna physician, 1875–1950. See Kahn and F.'s *sign*.

**falx,** pl. **fal'ces** [ L. sickle ] [ NA ]. A sickle-shaped structure.

**f. aponeurot'ica,** f. inguinalis.

**f. cerebel'li** [ NA ], falcula; a short process of dura mater projecting forward from the internal occipital crest below the tentorium; it occupies the posterior cerebellar notch and the vallecula, and bifurcates below into two diverging limbs passing to either side of the foramen magnum.

**f. cer'ebri** [ NA ], the scythe-shaped fold of dura mater in the longitudinal fissure between the two cerebral hemispheres; it is attached anteriorly to the crista galli of the ethmoid bone and behind to the upper surface of the tentorium.

**f. inguina'lis** [ NA ], tendo conjunctivus [ NA ]; inguinal aponeurotic fold; conjoined or conjoint tendon; f. aponeurotica; common tendon of insertion of the transversus and obliquus internus muscles into the crest and spine of the pubis and iliopectineal line. It is frequently muscular rather than aponeurotic and may be poorly developed.

**f. septi,** *valvula* foraminis ovalis.

**fames** (fa'mēz) [ L. ]. Hunger.

**f. cani'na, f. bovi'na,** bulimia.

**famil′ial** [ L. *familia*, family ]. Affecting several members of the same family, usually within a single sibship.

**fam′ily** [ L. *familia* ]. 1. A group of blood relatives, or, more strictly, the parents and their children. 2. In biologic classification, a division between the order and the tribe or genus.

**fam′otine hydrochloride** (USAN). 1-[ (*p*-Chlorophenoxy)methyl ]-3,4-dihydroisoquinoline hydrochloride; an antiviral agent.

**Fañanas,** J., Spanish physician. See F. *cell.*

**Fanconi** (fahn-ko′ne), Guido, Swiss pediatrician, *1882. See F.'s *anemia*, F.'s *pancytopenia*, F.'s *syndrome*, Abderhalden-F. *syndrome*, De Toni-F. *syndrome*, Lignac-F. *syndrome.*

**fang** [ A.S. *fōhan*, to seize ]. 1. A long tooth or tusk, usually a canine. 2. The hollow tooth of a snake through which the venom is ejected.

**fango** (fang′go) [ IT. mud ]. Mud from the Battaglio thermal springs in Italy, applied externally in the treatment of rheumatism and other diseases of the joints and muscles.

**Fan′nia.** A genus of flies of the family Muscidae.

**F. canicularis,** the lesser housefly; resembles the common housefly, *Musca domestica*, though somewhat smaller; said to be a cause of intestinal myiasis in Europe, but erroneous conclusions may result from contamination of feces after passage.

**F. scalaris,** latrine fly; commonly lays eggs in liquid feces of man and animals, which hatch in 1 to 2 days; distinguished from *F. canicularis* by two rather than three brown stripes on thorax of adult fly.

**fan′tasy** [ G. *phantasia*, idea, image ]. Imagery that is more or less coherent, as in dreams and daydreams, yet unrestricted by reality.

**fan′tridone hydrochloride** (USAN). 5-[ 3-(Dimethylamino)propyl ]-6(5*H*)-phenanthridinone monohydrochloride monohydrate; antidepressant.

**Farabeuf** (far-ă-bĕf′), Louis H., Paris surgeon, 1841–1910. See F.'s *amputation, operation, triangle.*

**farad** (făr′ad) [ M. *Faraday* ]. A practical unit of electrical capacity, being the capacity of a condenser having a charge of 1 coulomb under an electromotive force of 1 volt.

**farada′ic.** Faradic.

**Faraday,** Michael, English physicist and chemist, 1791–1867. Gave his name to farad and faraday. See F.'s *cage, constant, laws, space.*

**faraday** (făr′ă-da) [ M. *Faraday* ]. 96,500 coulombs; the amount of electricity required to reduce one equivalent of (*e.g.*) silver ion.

**faradic** (fă-rad′ik). Faradaic; relating to induced electricity.

**faradism** (făr′ă-dizm). Faradic (induction) electricity.

**surging f.,** a current of gradually increasing and decreasing amplitude obtained by interposing a rhythmic resistance to the alternating current produced by the induction coil.

**far′adiza′tion.** The therapeutic application of the faradic, or induced, electrical current.

**far′adocontractil′ity.** The contractility of the muscles under the stimulus of a faradic current.

**far′adomus′cular.** Denoting the effect of applying a faradic current directly to a muscle.

**far′adopalpa′tion.** Galvanopalpation.

**far′adother′apy.** Treatment of disease or paralysis by means of the faradic or induced electric current.

**farcin du boeuf** (far-sań′dü-büf′) [ Fr. cattle farcy ]. A cattle disease in Guadaloupe, characterized by suppurative lymphadenitis and lymphangitis, the glands discharging a creamy pus containing *Nocardia farcinica.*

**farcy** (far′sĭ) [ L. *farcio*, to stuff ]. The skin form of glanders.

**farfara** (far′far-ah) [ L. *farfarus*, coltsfoot ]. Coltsfoot leaves; tussilago leaves; the dried leaves of *Tussilago farfara* (family Compositae).

**farina** (fă-re′nah) [ L. ]. Flour; meal.

**f. ave′nae,** oatmeal prepared from the grain of *Avena sativa*. In the form of gruel it is used as a laxative article of diet and also externally as a poultice.

**f. trit′ici,** wheaten flour; the ground and sifted grain of *Triticum sativum*, wheat. An article of diet; sometimes used externally, moistened with hot milk or water, as a poultice.

**farinaceous** (făr′ĭ-na′shus). 1. Relating to farina or flour. 2. Starchy.

**far′nesene.** 2,6,10-Trimethyl-2,6,9,11-dodecatetraene; a straight open chain hydrocarbon, built up of three isoprene units, obtained by the reduction of farnesol.

**f. alcohol,** farnesol.

**far′nesol.** Farnesene alcohol; found in oil of citronella; a difarnesyl group occurs in the side chain of vitamin $K_2$ and constitutes squalene. (Compare carotenoids.)

**Farnesol**

(Dotted lines indicate formal division into isoprenyl groups)

**Farr,** William, English medical statistician, 1807–1883. See F.'s *law.*

**Farrant's fluid.** See under fluid.

**Farre,** Arthur, English obstetrician and gynecologist, 1811–1887. See F.'s *line.*

**Farre,** John R., English physician, 1775–1862. See F.'s *tubercles.*

**farrow** (făr′o). The act of a sow in giving birth to pigs.

**far′sight′edness.** Hyperopia.

# FASCIA

**fascia,** pl. **fasciae** (fash′ĭ-ah, fash′ĭ-e) [ L. a band or fillet. FASC- ]. 1 [ NA ]. A sheet of fibrous tissue which envelops the body beneath the skin, and also encloses the muscles and groups of muscles, and separates their several layers or groups. 2. In surgery, a bandage.

**Abernethy's f.,** a layer of subperitoneal areolar tissue in front of the external iliac artery.

**anal f.,** f. diaphragmatis pelvis inferior.

**antebrachial f.,** f. antebrachii.

**f. antebrachii** [ NA ], antebrachial f.; the deep f. of the forearm; it is continuous with the brachial f.; in the region of the wrist it forms two thickened bands, the extensor and flexor retinacula.

**f. axilla′ris** [ NA ], axillary f.; the f. that forms the floor of the axilla. It is continuous with the pectoral and clavipectoral f. anteriorly, with the brachial f. laterally, and with the f. of the latissimus dorsi and serratus anterior muscles posteriorly and medially.

**axillary f.,** f. axillaris.

**bicip′ital f.,** *aponeurosis* musculi bicipitis brachii.

**brachial f.,** f. brachii.

**f. brachii** [ NA ], brachial f.; the deep f. of the arm; it is continuous proximally with the pectoral f. and the f. covering the deltoid; distally it is continuous with the antebrachial f.

**broad f.,** f. lata.

**f. buc′copharyn′gea** [ NA ], buccopharyngeal f.; the f. that covers the muscular layer of the pharynx and is continued forwards onto the buccinator muscle.

**buccopharyngeal f.,** f. buccopharyngea.

**Buck's f.,** f. penis profunda.

**f. bulbi,** *vagina* bulbi.

**Camper's f.,** superficial layer of the tela subcutanea of the abdomen.

**cervical f.,** f. cervicalis.

**f. cervica′lis** [ NA ], cervical f.; the f. of the neck. It is divided into an external or investing layer (*lamina superficialis*) that surrounds the neck and encloses the trapezius and sternocleidomastoid muscles, a pretracheal or middle layer (*lamina pretrachealis*) in relation to the infrahyoid muscles, and a prevertebral layer (*lamina prevertebralis*) applied to the vertebrae and axial muscles.

**f. cine′rea,** *gyrus* fasciolaris.

**clavipectoral f.,** f. clavipectoralis.

**f. clavipectora′lis** [ NA ], clavipectoral f.; a f. that extends between the coracoid process, the clavicle, and the thoracic wall. It envelops the subclavius and pectoralis minor muscles and forms a strong membrane in the interval between them.

**f. clitoridis** [ NA ], the f. of the clitoris, comparable to the f. of the penis.

**f. of clitoris,** f. clitoridis.

**Colles′ f.,** f. perinei superficialis.

**Cooper′s f.,** f. cremasterica.

**cremasteric f.,** f. cremasterica.

**f. cremasterica** [ NA ], cremasteric f.; Cooper′s f.; Scarpa′s sheath; one of the coverings of the spermatic cord, formed of delicate connective tissue and of muscular fibers derived from the internal oblique muscle.

**cribriform f.,** f. cribrosa.

**f. cribro′sa** [ NA ], cribriform f.; Hesselbach′s f.; the part of the superficial f. of the thigh that covers the saphenous opening.

**f. cruris** [ NA ], the deep f. of the leg; it is continuous with the f. lata and is attached proximally to the patella, ligamentum patellae, the tubercle and condyles of the tibia, and the head of the fibula; distally it is thickened to form the flexor and extensor retinacula.

**Cruveilhier′s f.,** f. perinei superficialis.

**deep f.,** a thin fibrous membrane, devoid of fat, that invests the muscles, separating the several groups and the individual muscles, forms sheaths for the nerves and vessels, becomes specialized around the joints to form or strengthen ligaments, envelops various organs and glands, and binds all the structures together into a firm compact mass.

**deep f. of arm,** f. brachii.

**deep f. of forearm,** f. antebrachii.

**deep f. of leg,** f. cruris.

**f. denta′ta hippocam′pi,** *gyrus* dentatus.

**dentate f.,** *gyrus* dentatus.

**f. diaphragma′tis pelvis inferior** [ NA ], inferior f. of the pelvic diaphragm; anal fascia; the f. that covers the inferior aspect of the levator ani and coccygeus muscles.

**f. diaphragma′tis pelvis superior** [ NA ], superior f. of the pelvic diaphragm; the f. on the superior aspect of the levator ani and coccygeus muscles.

**f. diaphragma′tis urogenita′lis infe′rior** [ NA ], membrana perinei [ NA ]; inferior f. of the urogenital diaphragm; Camper′s ligament; ligamentum triangulare; triangular ligament; perineal membrane; the layer of f. extending between the ischiopubic rami inferior to the sphincter urethrae and the deep transverse perineal muscles.

**f. diaphragma′tis urogenita′lis superior** [ NA ], superior f. of the urogenital diaphragm; the layer of f. extending between the ischiopubic rami superior to the sphincter urethrae and the deep transverse perineal muscles.

**dorsal f. of foot,** f. dorsalis pedis.

**f. dorsa′lis ma′nus** [ NA ], f. of the dorsum of the hand; it consists of an outer, supratendinous layer continuous with the dorsal antebrachial f., an infratendinous layer deep to the long extensor tendons, and a dorsal interosseous fascia. The first two layers fuse to the second and fifth metacarpals.

**f. dorsa′lis pe′dis** [ NA ], dorsal fascia of the foot; the f. that encloses the extensor tendons of the toes and blends with the inferior extensor retinaculum.

**f. of dorsum of hand,** f. dorsalis manus.

**Dupuytren′s f.,** *aponeurosis* palmaris.

**endopelvic f.,** f. pelvis visceralis.

**endothoracic f.,** f. endothoracica.

**f. endothora′cica** [ NA ], endothoracic f.; the extrapleural f. that lines the wall of the thorax. It extends over the cupula of the pleura as the suprapleural membrane and also forms a thin layer between the diaphragm and pleura f. phrenicopleuralis).

**external spermatic f.,** f. spermatica externa.

**f. of extraocular muscles,** f. muscularis musculorum bulbi.

**extraperitoneal f.,** f. subperitonealis.

**f. of forearm,** f. antebrachii.

**Godman′s f.** an extension of the pretracheal f. into the thorax and on to the pericardium.

**Hesselbach′s f.,** f. cribrosa.

**iliac f.,** f. iliaca.

**f. ili′aca** [ NA ], iliac f.; the f. covering the iliacus and psoas muscles.

**iliopectineal f.,** a f. formed by the union of the iliac and the pectineal fasciae covering the floor of the iliopectineal fossa.

**inferior f. of pelvic diaphragm,** f. diaphragmatis pelvis inferior.

**inferior f. of urogenital diaphragm,** f. diaphragmatis urogenitalis inferior.

**in′fraspina′tus f.,** f. infraspinata; it is attached to the borders of the infraspinous fossa and covers the infraspinatus muscle; it is continuous with f. covering the deltoid.

**infundibuliform f.,** f. spermatica interna.

**intercolum′nar fasciae,** *fibrae* intercrurales.

**internal spermatic f.,** f. spermatica interna.

**interosseous f.,** the f. covering the interosseous muscles of the hand or foot; it consists of a dorsal layer and a palmar or plantar layer.

**lac′rimal f.,** that part of the periorbita that bridges across the fossa for lacrimal sac.

**f. lata** [ NA ], broad f.; the strong f. enveloping the muscles of the thigh.

**f. of leg,** f. cruris.

**lumbodorsal f.,** f. thoracolumbalis.

**masseteric f.,** f. masseterica.

**f. massete′rica** [ NA ], masseteric f.; the f. that covers the lateral surface of the masseter muscle.

**middle cervical f.,** *lamina* pretrachealis.

**f. muscula′ris musculorum bulbi** [ NA ], the f. of the extraocular muscles; it is thin posteriorly but becomes thicker close to the eye where it is continued into the bulbar sheath.

**f. of neck,** f. cervicalis.

**f. nuchae** [ NA ], nuchal f.; the f. that encloses the posterior muscles of the neck.

**nuchal f.,** f. nuchae.

**obturator f.,** f. obturatoria.

**f. obturato′ria** [ NA ], obturator f.; the portion of the pelvic f. that covers the obturator internus muscle.

**orbital fasciae** fasciae orbitales.

**fasciae orbita′les** [ NA ], orbital f.; the fascial layers in the orbit consisting of periorbita, septum orbitale, f. muscularis musculorum bulbi, and vagina bulbi.

**palmar f.,** *aponeurosis* palmaris.

**parotid f.,** f. parotidea.

**f. parotid′ea** [ NA ], parotid f.; the part of the deep cervical f. that ensheaths the parotid gland and is fixed above to the zygomatic arch.

**f. parotid′eomasseter′ica,** a dense membrane covering both the lateral and medial surfaces of the parotid gland, continuous anteriorly with the f. covering the masseter muscle. See f. parotidea and f. masseterica.

**pectoral f.,** f. pectoralis.

**f. pectora′lis** [ NA ], pectoral f.; the f. that covers the pectoralis major muscle; it is attached to the sternum and to the clavicle; laterally and below it is continuous with the f. of the shoulder, axilla, and thorax.

**f. pelvis** [ NA ], f. of the pelvis; it includes parietal and visceral components. The **f. pelvis parietalis,** including the f. obturatoria, covers the muscles that pass from the interior of the pelvis to the thigh. The **f. pelvis visceralis,** often called endopelvic f., covers the pelvic organs and surrounds vessels and nerves in the subperitoneal space.

**f. penis** [ NA ], f. of the penis; it is divided into two layers, superficial (**f. penis superficialis**) continuous with f. perinei superficialis, and deep (**f. penis profunda**) also known as Buck′s f., which surrounds the three cavernous bodies of the penis.

**f. perine′i superficia′lis** [ NA ], superficial f. of the perineum; Colles′ f.; the membranous layer of the subcutaneous tissue in the urogenital region attaching posteriorly to the border of the urogenital diaphragm, at the sides to the ischiopubic rami, and continuing anteriorly onto the abdominal wall.

**perirenal f.,** renal f.

**pharyngobasilar f.,** f. pharyngobasilaris.

**f. pharyngobasila'ris** [ NA ], pharyngobasilar f.; tela submucosa pharyngis; aponeurosis pharyngea; the fibrous coat of the pharyngeal wall situated between the mucous and muscular coats; it is attached above to the basilar part of the occipital bone, and the petrous part of the temporal bone.

**f. phrenicopleura'lis** [ NA ], phrenicopleural f.; the thin layer of endothoracic f. intervening between the diaphragmatic pleura and the diaphragm.

**plantar f.**, *aponeurosis* plantaris.

**poplite'al f.**, the f. that covers the popliteal fossa.

**Porter's f.**, *lamina* pretrachealis.

**pretracheal f.**, *lamina* pretrachealis.

**prevertebral f.**, *lamina* prevertebralis.

**f. pros'tatae** [ NA ], f. of the prostate; the condensation of pelvic visceral f. that encloses the prostate gland.

**f. of prostate**, f. prostatae.

**rectoves'ical f.**, *septum* rectovesicale.

**renal f.**, perirenal f.; Gerota's capsule; the condensation of the fibroareolar tissue and fat surrounding the kidney to form a sheath for the organ.

**Scarpa's f.**, the deeper, membranous or lamellar part of the subcutaneous tissue of the lower abdominal wall; it is continuous with the superficial perineal (Colles') f.

**semilu'nar f.**, *aponeurosis* musculi bicipitis brachii.

**Sibson's f.**, *membrana* suprapleuralis.

**f. spermat'ica exter'na** [ NA ], external spermatic f.; the outer fascial covering of the spermatic cord. It is continuous at the superficial inguinal ring with the facia covering the external oblique muscle.

**f. spermatica interna** [ NA ], internal spermatic f.; infundibuliform f.; the inner covering of the spermatic cord, continuous above the deep inguinal ring with transversalis f.

**subperitoneal f.**, f. subperitonealis.

**f. subperitonea'lis** [ NA ], subperitoneal f.; extraperitoneal f.; the thin layer of f. and adipose tissue between the peritoneum and f. transversalis.

**superficial f.**, *tela* subcutanea.

**superficial f. of perineum**, f. perinei superficialis.

**superior f. of pelvic diaphragm**, f. diaphragmatis pelvis superior.

**superior f. of urogenital diaphragm**, f. diaphragmatis urogenitalis superior.

**Tarin's f.**, *gyrus* dentatus.

**temporal f.**, f. temporalis.

**f. tempora'lis** [ NA ], temporal f.; temporal aponeurosis; the f. covering the temporal muscle; it is attached above to the superior temporal line and below it splits to enclose a space containing veins and fat above the zygomatic arch.

**f. thoracolumba'lis** [ NA ], thoracolumbar f.; thoracolumbar aponeurosis; lumbodoral f.; the f. which covers the deep muscles of the back; it is attached to the angles of the ribs and to the spines of the thoracic, lumbar, and sacral vertebrae, to the transverse processes of the lumbar vertebrae, to the lower border of the 12th rib and to the iliac crest, as well as to the lumbocostal, iliolumbar, intertransverse, and supraspinous ligaments.

**Toldt's f.**, continuation of Treitz's f. behind the body of the pancreas.

**f. transversa'lis** [ NA ], transversalis f.; the lining f. of the abdominal cavity, between the inner surface of the abdominal musculature and the peritoneum.

**Treitz's f.**, f. behind the head of the pancreas.

**f. triangula'ris abdom'inis**, *ligamentum* reflexum.

**Tyrrell's f.**, *septum* rectovesicale.

**umbilical prevesical f.**, the thin fascial layer interposed between the transversalis f. and the umbilicovesical f. It extends between the medial umbilical ligaments from the umbilicus downward in front of the bladder, forming the posterior boundary of the retropubic space.

**umbil'icoves'ical f.**, a thin fascial layer that extends between the medial umbilical ligaments and is continuous with f. enclosing the bladder.

**Zuckerkandl's f.**, a f. in relation to the posterior aspect of the kidney.

---

**fascial** (fash'ĭ-al). Relating to any fascia.
**fascicle** (fas'ĭ-kl). Fasciculus.

**muscle f.**, a bundle of muscle fibers surrounded by perimysium.

**nerve f.**, a bundle of nerve fibers surrounded by perineurium.

**fascicular** (fă-sik'u-lar). Relating to a fasciculus; arranged in the form of a bundle or collection of rods.

**fascic'ulate, fascic'ulated.** Fascicular.

**fasciculation** (fă-sik-u-la'shun). 1. An arrangement in the form of fasciculi. 2. Involuntary contractions, or twitchings, of groups (fasciculi) of muscle fibers, a coarser form of muscular contraction than fibrillation.

**fasciculi** (fa-sik'u-li). Plural of fasciculus.

**fascic'uli'tis op'tica.** An inflammation of both the bulbar and the retrobulbar part of the optic fasciculus. The concept fasciculitis optica contains inflammatory, demyelinizing and degenerative lesions.

# FASCICULUS

**fasciculus**, gen. and pl. **fasciculi** (fă-sik'u-lus, fă-sik'u-li) [ L. dim. of *fascis*, bundle ] [ NA ]. Fascicle; a band or bundle of fibers, usually of muscle or nerve fibers.

**f. ante'rior pro'prius**, anterior ground bundle; the ground bundle of the anterior column of the spinal cord; see fasciculi proprii.

**arcuate f.**, (1) f. longitudinalis superior; (2) f. uncinatus.

**f. at'rioventricula'ris** [ NA ], truncus atrioventricularis [ NA ]; bundle of His; atrioventricular trunk, bundle, or band; Gaskell's bridge; ventriculonector; Keith's, Kent's, or Kent-His bundle; the bundle of modified cardiac muscle fibers that begins at the atrioventricular node and passes through the right atrioventricular anulus fibrosis to the membranous part of the interventricular septum; its right and left branches extend to the lower, muscular area of the septum and ramify in the subendocardium of the right and left ventricles.

**Burdach's f.**, f. cuneatus.

**cal'carine f.**, a group of short association fibers beneath the calcarine fissure of the occipital lobe of the cerebrum.

**central tegmen'tal f.**, *tractus* tegmentalis centralis.

**f. cir'cumoliva'ris pyram'idis**, an anomalous bundle of nerve fibers on the anterior surface of the medulla oblongata that emerges from the pyramid and curves forward and dorsalward over the lower pole of the olive; it is variously interpreted as an aberrant bundle of (1) pontocerebellar fibers or (2) corticopontine fibers.

**f. corticospina'lis ante'rior**, *tractus* pyramidalis anterior.

**f. corticospina'lis latera'lis**, *tractus* pyramidalis lateralis.

**cuneate f.**, f. cuneatus.

**f. cunea'tus** [ NA ], cuneate or wedge-shaped f.; Burdach's f., column, or tract; cuneate funiculus; the larger lateral subdivision of the funiculus posterior (*q.v.*).

**dorsal longitudinal f.**, f. longitudinalis dorsalis.

**dorsolateral f.**, f. dorsolateralis.

**f. dorsolatera'lis** [ NA ], tractus dorsolateralis [ NA ]; dorsolateral f. or tract; f. marginalis; Lissauer's f., bundle, tract, or marginal zone; Spitzka's marginal tract or zone; Waldeyer's tract or zonal layer; a longitudinal bundle of thin, unmyelinated and poorly myelinated fibers capping the apex of the posterior horn of the spinal gray matter, composed of posterior root fibers and short association fibers that interconnect neighboring segments of the posterior horn.

**Flechsig's fasciculi**, f. anterior proprius and f. lateralis proprius; see fasciculi proprii.

**Foville's f.**, *stria* terminalis.

**fronto-occip'ital f.**, f. occipitofrontalis.

**f. grac'ilis** [ NA ], slender f.; column or tract of Goll; funiculus gracilis; the smaller medial subdivision of the funiculus posterior, *q.v.*

**hooked f.**, f. uncinatus.

**inferior longitudinal f.**, f. longitudinalis inferior.

**interfascicular f.**, f. semilunaris.

**f. interfascicula'ris** [ NA ], official alternative term for f. semilunaris.

intersegmental fasciculi, fasciculi proprii.

**f. latera'lis plex'us brachia'lis** [ NA ], lateral cord of the brachial plexus; formed by the anterior divisions of the superior and middle trunks, this cord gives off the lateral pectoral nerve and terminates by dividing into the musculocutaneous nerve and the lateral root of the median nerve.

**f. latera'lis pro'prius,** lateral ground bundle; see fasciculi proprii.

**f. lenticula'ris,** see *ansa* lenticularis.

**f. longitudina'lis dorsa'lis** [ NA ], dorsal longitudinal f.; bundle or tract of Schütz; a bundle of thin, poorly myelinated nerve fibers reciprocally connecting the periventricular zone of the hypothalamus with ventral parts of the central gray substance of the midbrain.

**f. longitudina'lis inferior** [ NA ], inferior longitudinal f.; a well marked bundle of long association fibers running the whole length of the occipital and temporal lobes of the cerebrum, in part parallel with the inferior horn of the lateral ventricle.

**f. longitudina'lis media'lis** [ NA ], medial longitudinal f.; posterior longitudinal bundle; Collier's tract; a longitudinal bundle of fibers extending from the upper border of the mesencephalon into the cervical segments of the spinal cord, located close to the midline and ventral to the central gray matter; it is composed largely of fibers from the vestibular nuclei ascending to the motor neurons innervating the external eye muscles (abducens, trochlear, and oculomotor nuclei), and descending to spinal cord segments innervating the musculature of the neck.

**fascic'uli longitudina'les pon'tis,** the massive bundles of corticofugal fibers passing longitudinally through the pontine gray matter (pars basilaris pontis); they are composed of corticopontine, corticobulbar, and corticospinal fibers.

**f. longitudina'lis superior** [ NA ], superior longitudinal f.; arcuate f. (1); a bundle of long association fibers in the lateral portion of the centrum ovale of the cerebral hemisphere, connecting the frontal, occipital, and temporal lobes; the fibers pass from the frontal lobe through the operculum to the posterior end of the Sylvian fissure, where many fibers radiate into the occipital lobe and others turn downward and forward around the putamen and pass to the anterior portion of the temporal lobe.

**f. macula'ris,** the collection of fibers in the optic nerve directly connected with the macula lutea.

**mamillotegmental f.,** f. mamillotegmentalis.

**f. mamillotegmenta'lis** [ NA ], mamillotegmental f.; a small bundle of fibers that passes dorsalward from the mamillary body for a short distance with the mamillothalamic tract, then turns down the brainstem to reach the dorsal and ventral tegmental nuclei of the mesencephalon.

**mamillothalamic f.,** f. mamillothalamicus.

**f. mamillothalam'icus** [ NA ], mamillothalamic tract or f.; f. thalamomamillaris; bundle of Vicq d'Azyr; a compact, thick bundle of nerve fibers that passes dorsalward from the mamillary body on either side to terminate in the anterior nucleus of the thalamus.

**f. margina'lis,** *fasciculus* dorsolateralis.

**medial longitudinal f.,** f. longitudinalis medialis.

**f. media'lis plex'us brachia'lis** [ NA ], medial cord of the brachial plexus; formed by the anterior division of the inferior trunk, it gives off the medial pectoral nerve, the medial brachial cutaneous, medial antebrachial cutaneous, ulnar, and the medial root of the median nerves.

**Meynert's f.,** f. retroflexus.

**f. obli'quus pontis,** oblique bundle of the pons; a bundle of fibers in the ventral surface of the pons running from the anterior mesial portion outward and backward.

**occipitofrontal f.,** f. occipitofrontalis.

**f. occip'itofronta'lis,** occipitofrontal f.; fronto-occipital f.; a bundle of association fibers extending from the frontal to the occipital lobes of the cerebrum.

**oval f.,** see f. semilunaris.

**f. pedun'culomamilla'ris,** *pedunculus* corporis mamillaris.

**perpendicular f.,** a bundle of association fibers running vertically and interconnecting regions of the temporal, occipital, and parietal lobes.

**f. poste'rior plex'us brachia'lis** [ NA ], posterior cord of the brachial plexus; formed by the posterior divisions of the

upper, middle and lower trunks, it gives rise to the subscapular, thoracodorsal, axillary, and radial nerves.

**proper fasciculi,** fasciculi proprii.

**fasciculi pro'prii** [ NA ], proper fasciculi; ground bundles; Flechsig's fasciculi or ground bundles (f. anterior proprius and f. lateralis proprius); intersegmental fasciculi; ascending and descending association fiber systems of the spinal cord. These lie deep in the anterior, lateral, and posterior funiculi adjacent to the gray matter.

**f. pyramida'lis ante'rior,** *tractus* pyramidalis anterior.

**f. pyramida'lis latera'lis,** *tractus* pyramidalis lateralis.

**retroflex f.,** f. retroflexus.

**f. retroflex'us** [ NA ], retroflex f.; Meynert's f. or retroflex bundle; habenulointerpeduncular tract; tractus habenulopeduncularis; a compact bundle of fibers arising in the habenula and passing ventralward to the interpeduncular nucleus at the base of the midbrain; part of its fibers bypass this nucleus and terminate in the raphe nuclei of the caudal mesencephalic tegmentum.

**f. rotun'dus,** *tractus* solitarius.

**fasciculi rubroreticula'res** [ NA ], bundles of fibers that connect the red nucleus to the pontine and midbrain reticular nuclei.

**semilunar f.,** f. semilunaris.

**f. semiluna'ris** [ NA ], f. interfascicularis [ NA ]; semilunar or interfascicular f.; comma bundle or comma tract of Schultze; a compact bundle composed of descending branches of posterior root fibers located near the border between the fasciculi gracilis and cuneatus of the cervical and thoracic spinal cord; it corresponds to the septomarginal f., Hoche's tract, or oval area of Flechsig in the lumbar, and to the triangle of Philippe-Gombault in the sacral spinal segments; like these, it can be demonstrated only in cases of demyelination resulting from dorsal root lesions.

**septomarginal f.,** f. septomarginalis; see f. semilunaris.

**f. septomargina'lis** [ NA ], septomarginal f. or tract; see f. semilunaris.

**slender f.,** f. gracilis.

**f. solita'rius,** *tractus* solitarius.

**subcallosal f.,** f. subcallosus.

**f. subcallo'sus** [ NA ], subcallosal f.; a bundle of thin nerve fibers running longitudinally beneath the corpus callosum in the angle between the latter and the caudate nucleus; it forms an anterior continuation of the tapetum of the temporal lobe and appears to consist largely of fibers projecting from the cerebral cortex to the caudate nucleus.

**superior longitudinal f.,** f. longitudinalis superior.

**f. thalam'icus,** see *fields* of Forel.

**f. thal'amomamilla'ris,** f. mamillothalamicus.

**transverse fasciculi,** fasciculi transversi.

**fasciculi transver'si** [ NA ], transverse fasciculi; the transversely directed fibers in the distal portions of the palmar and plantar aponeuroses.

**unciform f.,** f. uncinatus.

**uncinate f.,** f. uncinatus.

**f. uncina'tus** [ NA ], uncinate, unciform, or hooked f.; arcuate f. (2); frontotemporal or temporofrontal tract; a band of long association fibers reciprocally connecting the frontal and temporal lobes of the cerebrum, running caudalward through the white matter of the frontal lobe, sharply curving ventrally under the stem of the Sylvian fissure, and then fanning out to the cortex of the anterior half of the superior and middle temporal gyri.

**wedge-shaped f.,** f. cuneatus.

---

**fasciectomy** (fă-shĭ-ek'to-mĭ) [ fascia + G. *ektomē,* excision ]. Excision of strips of fascia.

**fasciitis** (fash'ĭ-i'tis). 1. Inflammation in fascia. 2. Reactive proliferation of fibroblasts in fascia.

**nodular f.,** proliferative f.; pseudosarcomatous f.; a tumor-like proliferation of fibroblasts, with mild inflammatory exudation occurring in fascia. The fibrosis may infiltrate surrounding tissue but does not progress indefinitely or metastasize. The cause is not known but the condition is not thought to be neoplastic.

**proliferative f.,** nodular f.

**pseudosarcomatous f.,** nodular f.

**fascio-** (fash'ĭ-o-, fas'ĭ-o-) [ L. *fascia,* a band or fillet ]. Combining form relating to a fascia.

**fasciodesis** (fash'ĭ-od'ē-sis) [ fascio- + G. *desis*, a binding together ]. The operative attachment of a fascia to another fascia or a tendon.

**Fasciola** (fā-se'o-lah, fā-si'o-lah) [ L. dim. of *fascia* ]. The genus of large, leaf-shaped, digenetic liver flukes (class Trematoda) of mammals.

**F. gigan'tica**, a species, resembling *F. hepatica* but of larger size, found in herbivores, especially in Africa.

**F. hepat'ica**, formerly called *Distomum hepaticum;* liver fluke; sheep liver fluke; the common liver fluke inhabiting the bile ducts of sheep and cattle; the intermediate host is a snail (*Limneus truncatulus, L. humilis, L. viator*) from which the cercaria escape and become encysted on watercress, lettuce, and other vegetables by means of which they gain access to the intestinal canal; rarely, this fluke is reported from man, where it may cause considerable biliary damage; adult worms accidently ingested in uncooked infected liver may lodge in the throat, causing a condition known as halzoun.

**fasciola**, pl. **fasci'olae** (fā-se'o-lah, fā-si'o-lah) [ L. dim. of *fascia*, band, fillet ]. A small band or group of fibers.

**f. cine'rea**, *gyrus* fasciolaris.

**fasci'olar.** Relating to the gyrus fasciolaris.

**fascioliasis** (fā-se'o-li'ă-sis, fas'ĭ-o-li'ă-sis). Infection with a species of *Fasciola*. See also halzoun.

**Fascioloides america'na.** Previously called *F. magna; Distomum magnum;* a fluke found in the lungs and liver of deer and sometimes cattle in North America; it is not known to infest man.

**fas'ciolopsi'asis.** Parasitization by any of the flukes of the genus *Fasciolopsis.*

**Fasciolopsis** (fas'ĭ-o-lop'sis, fash'ĭ-o-) [ *Fasciola* + G. *opsis*, form, appearance ]. A genus of very large intestinal flukes.

**F. bus'ki**, formerly called *Distomum buski; D. crassum;* a species found in the intestine of man in eastern and southern Asia; transmitted via ingestion of water chestnut

or other vegetation contaminated with infective metacercariae.

**F. rathoui'si** reported in a few cases in the intestine or liver in Chinese.

**fascioplasty,** (fash'ĭ-o-plastĭ). A plastic operation on fascia.

**fasciorrhaphy** (fash-ĭ-or'ră-fĭ) [ fascio- + G. *raphē*, suture ]. Aponeurorrhaphy; suture of a fascia or aponeurosis.

**fasciotomy** (fash-ĭ-ot'o-mĭ) [ fascio- + G. *tomē*, incision ]. Incision through a fascia; used in the treatment of certain vascular disorders when marked swelling is anticipated which could compromise blood flow; f. is often combined with embolectomy in the treatment of acute arterial embolism.

**fascitis** (fā-si'tis). Fasciitis.

**fast** [ A.S. *foest*, firm, fixed ]. Durable; resistant to change; applied to stained microorganisms which cannot be decolorized. See acid-fast.

**fastid'ium cib'i** [ L. ]. A fickle or finicky appetite, caused by distaste for food.

**fastiga'tum** [ L. *fastigatus*, pointed ]. *Nucleus* fastigii.

**fastigium** (fas-tij'ĭ-um) [ L. top, as of a gable; a pointed extremity ]. 1. Summit of the roof of the fourth ventricle of the brain, an angle formed by the union of the anterior and posterior medullary vela pushing up into the substance of the vermis. 2. The acme or height of a fever or any acute disease; the period of full development of an infectious disease.

**fast'ness.** The state of tolerance exhibited by bacteria to a drug or other agent; see fast.

**fat** [ A.S. *faet* ]. 1. Adipose *tissue*. 2. Obese; adipose; corpulent. 3. Oily; greasy. 4. A greasy, soft-solid material, found in animal tissues and many plants, composed of a mixture of glycerides; together with oils these make up that class of foodstuffs known as simple lipids.

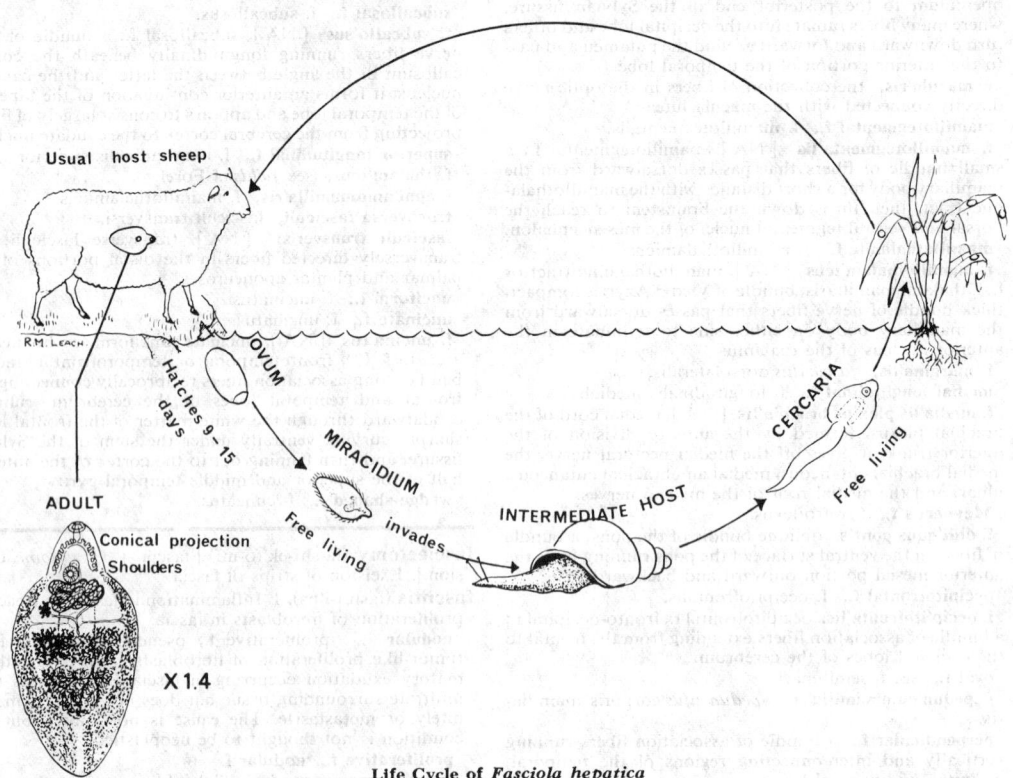

**Life Cycle of *Fasciola hepatica***

(Modified after Jeffrey, H. D. and Leach, R. M.: *Atlas of Medical Helminthology and Protozoology*, Churchill Livingstone, Edinburgh, 1966.)

**brown f.,** thermogenic tissue that is composed of cells containing numerous small fat droplets. Lobular masses are found in the interscapular and mediastinal regions and other locations. Although found most frequently in certain hibernating animals, it is also found in pigs, rodents, and the newborn of man. Also called hibernating gland; interscapular gland; interscapular hibernoma; multilocular f.; multilocular adipose tissue.

**caul f.,** the f. contained in the caul.

**multilocular f.,** brown f.

**neutral f.,** a triester of one or more of the fatty acids and glycerol; same as f. (3).

**saturated f.,** see saturated *fatty acid.*

**swine f.,** lard; adeps.

**unilocular f.,** white fat (2); adipose tissue in which the fat is present in a single droplet within the fat cells.

**unsaturated f.,** see unsaturated *fatty acid.*

**white f.,** (1) adipose *tissue;* (2) unilocular f.

**fa'tal** [ L. *fatalis,* of or belonging to fate ]. 1. Inevitable. 2. Mortal; causing death.

**fatal'ity.** A condition, disease, or disaster ending in death.

**fatigability** (fat'ĭ-gă-bil'ĭ-tĭ). Condition in which fatigue is easily induced.

**fatigable** (fat'ĭ-gă-bl) [ L. *fatigabilis,* easily tired, fr. *fatigo,* to tire ]. Tiring on very slight exertion.

**fatigue** (fă-tēg) [ Fr. fr. L. *fatigo,* to tire ]. 1. That state following a period of mental or bodily activity character- ized by a lessened capacity for work and reduced efficiency of accomplishment, usually accompanied by a feeling of weariness, sleepiness, or irritability; it may also supervene when from any cause energy expenditure outstrips restor- ative processes, *e.g.,* lack of sleep or food. 2. Sensation of boredom and lassitude due to absence of stimulation, monotony, or lack of interest in one's surroundings. F. may be purely physical and confined to a single organ, *e.g.,* of muscles or gland after a period of prolonged activity.

**auditory f.,** temporary shift of threshold sensitivity following exposure to sound.

**fat-pad.** An accumulation of somewhat encapsulated adi- pose tissue.

**Bichat's f.-p.,** *corpus* adiposum buccae.

**Imlach's f.-p.,** fat surrounding the round ligament of the uterus in the inguinal canal.

**fat'ty.** Relating in any sense to fat.

**fatty acid.** Any acid derived from fats by hydrolysis (*e.g.,* oleic, palmitic, or stearic acids); any long chain monobasic organic acid.

**diethenoid f. acid,** a f. acid containing two double bonds, *e.g.,* linoleic acid.

**f. acid oxidation cycle,** see under cycle.

**saturated f. acid,** a fatty acid, the carbon chain of which contains no ethylenic or other unsaturated linkages be- tween carbon atoms; the most common examples are stearic acid and palmitic acid; called saturated because it is not capable of absorbing any more hydrogen; see hydrogenation.

**f. acid thiokinase,** see (1) acyl-CoA synthetase, and (2) butyryl-CoA synthetase.

**unsaturated f. acid,** a fatty acid, the carbon chain of which possesses one or more double or triple bonds; the most common examples are: oleic acid, with one double bond in the molecule, and linoleic acid, with two; called unsaturated because it is capable of absorbing additional hydrogen; see hydrogenation.

**fauces,** gen. **fau'cium** (faw'sēz) [ L. the throat ] [ NA ]. The space between the cavity of the mouth and the pharynx.

**faucial** (faw'shal). Relating to the fauces.

**faucitis** (faw-si'tis). Inflammation of the fauces.

**fauna** (faw'nah) [ Mod. L. application of *Fauna,* sister of *Faunus,* a rural deity ]. The animal forms of a continent, district, locality, or habitat.

**faveolate** (fa-ve'o-lāt). Pitted.

**faveolus,** pl. **fave'oli** (fa-ve'o-lus) [ Mod. L. dim of *favus,* honeycomb ]. A small pit or depression.

**fa'vid.** An allergic reaction in the skin observed in patients who have favus.

**fa'vism** [ Ital. *favismo,* from *fava,* bean ]. Fabism; an acute condition, seen chiefly in Italy, following the ingestion of certain species of beans, *e.g., Vicia faba,* or inhalation of the pollen of its flower; it is characterized by fever, headache, abdominal pain, severe anemia, prostration, and coma; apparently caused by sensitivity reactions. Treated by blood transfusion.

**Favre** (fä'vr), Maurice, French physician, *1876. See Gamna-F. *bodies,* F.-Durand-Nicolas *disease,* Nicolas-F. *disease.*

**favus** (fa'vus, fah'vus) [ L. honeycomb ]. Tinea favosa or vera; mycosis favosa; porrigo scutulata, favosa, or lupinosa; crusted or honeycomb ringworm; a persistent and scarring fungal infection of scalp and nails caused by *Trichophyton schönleinii.*

**Fc (portion, piece, or fragment).** See immunoglobulin.

**FDA.** Abbreviation for Food and Drug Administration of the United States Department of Health, Education and Welfare.

**FDNB.** Abbreviation for fluoro-2,4-dinitrobenzene.

**F-duction.** See under duction.

**Fe.** Chemical symbol of the element iron.

**fear** [ A.S. *faer* ]. Apprehension; dread; alarm. F. has an identifiable stimulus, and thus is differentiated from anxiety which has no easily identifiable stimulus.

**morbid f.,** phobia.

**feath'er.** 1. A characteristic integumental derivative of birds. 2. The long hair on the caudal aspect of the limbs of certain breeds of horses (Belgians, shires) and dogs (setters, retrievers).

**fea'tures** [ through Old Fr. fr. L. *factura,* a making, fr. *facio,* to do ]. The various parts of the face, forehead, eyes, nose, mouth, chin, cheeks, and ears, that give to it its individuality and character.

**feb'ricant.** Febrifacient.

**febricula** (fē-brik'u-lah) [ L. dim. of *febris,* fever ]. Simple continued fever; a mild fever of short duration, of indefinite origin, and without any distinctive pathology.

**febrifacient** (feb'rĭ-fa'shent) [ L. *febris,* fever, + *facio,* to make ]. 1. Fabrific; causing fever. 2. Anything that produces fever.

**febrif'erous** [ L. *febris,* fever, + *fero,* to bear, + *-ous* ]. Causing or favoring the development of fever.

**febrif'ic.** Febrifacient.

**febrif'ugal.** Febrifuge (1).

**febrifuge** (feb'rĭ-fūj) [ L. *febris,* fever, + *fugo,* to put to flight ]. 1. Febrifugal; alexipyretic; antipyretic; reducing fever. 2. A remedy for fever.

**febrile** (feb'ril, fe'bril). Feverish; pyretic; relating to fever.

**fe'bris** [ L. ]. Fever.

**fecal** (fe'kal). Relating to feces.

**fe'calith** [ L. *faeces,* feces, + G. *lithos,* stone ]. Coprolith; a fecal concretion.

**fe'caloid** [ L. *faeces,* feces, + G. *eidos,* resemblance ]. Resembling feces.

**fe'calo'ma.** Coproma.

**fecaluria** (fe'kă-lu'rĭ-ah) [ L. *faeces,* feces, + G. *ouron,* urine ]. The commingling of feces with urine passed from the urethra in persons with a fistula connecting the rectum and bladder, often noticed most dramatically by the passage of flatus through the urethra.

**feces** (fe'sēz) [ L., pl. of *faex* (*faec-*), dregs ]. Excrement; the matter discharged from the bowel during defecation, consisting of the undigested residue of the food, epithe- lium, the intestinal mucus, bacteria, and waste material from the food. See fig. on p. 514.

**f. cruen'tae,** Melena; bloody stools.

**Fechner** (fekh'ner), Gustav T., German physicist, 1801-1887. See Weber-F. *law,* F.-Weber *law.*

**fec'ula** [ L. *faecula,* tartar, dim. of *faex,* dregs. FEC- ]. Starch.

**fec'ulent.** Excrementitious; fecal; foul.

**fecund** (fe'kund, fek'und) [ L. *fecundus,* fruitful ]. Produc- tive; fertile; capable of producing offspring.

**fecundate** (fe'kun-dāt) [ L. *fecundo,* pp. *-atus,* to make fruitful, fertilize ]. To impregnate; to make fertile.

**fecundation** (fe'kun-da'shun). Rendering fertile; see also fertilization, impregnation.

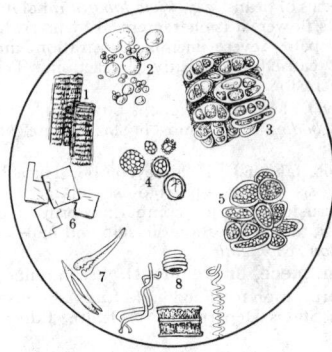

### Feces

Microscopic appearance of common objects in the feces; original magnification ×800, *1*, Muscle fibers (meat); *2*, casein and fat droplets; *3*, portions of cereal husks; *4*, spores of fungi; *5*, endosperm of rice; *6*, cholesterol crystals; *7*, hairs of wheat grain; *8*, vegetable spirals. (Redrawn from Manson-Bahr, P. H.: *Manson's Tropical Diseases*, Ed. 16, © Ballière, Tindall & Cassell, Ltd., London, 1966. Used with permission.)

**fecun'dity.** Pronounced fertility; capability of repeated fertilization.

**feedback** 1. In a given system, the return, as input, of some of the output, as a regulatory mechanism; *e.g.*, the regulation of a furnace by a thermostat. 2. An explanation for the learning of motor skills: sensory stimuli set up by the motor act produce correction in the nervous system. 3. The feeling evoked by another person's reaction to oneself. 4. The regulation of the output of a hormone by the results of the hormone's own actions. 5. A process whereby a part of the output of an amplifier or transcriber is returned to the input.

  **negative f.,** occurs if the sign or sense of the returned signal is such as to reduce amplification.

  **positive f.,** occurs when the sign or sense is such as to increase amplification or lead to instability.

**feed'ing.** Giving food or nourishment.

  **forced f., forcible f.,** (1) giving liquid food through a nasal tube passed into the stomach; (2) forcing a person to eat more food than he desires.

  **nasal f.,** the giving of milk or other fluid food through a flexible rubber tube passed through the nostril into the stomach.

  **sham** or **fictitious f.,** a procedure used in the study of the psychic phase of gastric secretion. In experiments on dogs, the food, after being eaten, does not enter the stomach but issues from an esophageal fistula made in the neck. The chewing and swallowing of food causes an abundant secretion of gastric juice.

**feel'ing.** 1. Any kind of conscious experience of sensation. 2. The mental perception of a sensory stimulus. 3. A quality of any mental state, whereby it is recognized as pleasurable or the reverse.

  **ambivalent f.'s,** emotions of opposite character, such as love and hate, concurrently experienced toward the same person.

  **chirognostic f.,** the sense of "sidedness"; the power to recognize, with eyes closed, which side is touched.

  **positive f.,** warm friendly f., as opposed to hostility.

  **f. of unreality,** the f. that things are not real; see also depersonalization.

**Feer** (fare), Emil, Swiss pediatrician, 1864–1955. See F.'s *disease.*

**Fehling** (fa'ling), Hermann von, German chemist, 1812–1885. See F.'s *reagent, solution.*

**Feil** (fāl), André, French physician, *1884. See Klippel-F. *syndrome.*

**Feiss** (fis), Henry O., American orthopedic surgeon, 20th century. See F. *line.*

**fel,** gen. **fellis** [ L. ]. Bile.

**Feldberg,** Wilhelm, English physiologist, *1900. See Dale-F. *law.*

**Felidae** (fe'lǐ-de) [ L. *felis,* cat ]. A family of carnivora embracing the cats, tigers, lions, etc.

**feline** (fe'lin) [ L. *felis,* cat ]. Pertaining or relating to cats.

**felinine.** HOCH₂CH₂C(CH₃)₂SCH₂CH(NH₂)COOH; an S-alkyl derivative of cysteine, found in cat urine.

**Felix,** Arthur, Prague bacteriologist, 1887–1956. See Weil-F. *reaction.*

**Félix,** Jules, French physician, 1838–1912. See F.'s *antiserum.*

**fella'tio** [ L. ]. Fellation; fellatorism; irrumation; oral-genital intercourse; the act of taking the penis of another person into the mouth.

**fellation** (fĕ-la'shun). Fellatio.

**fellator** (fel'ă-tor, fĕ-la'ter) [ L. ]. A male who takes the oral part in fellatio.

**fellatorism** (fel'ă-to-rizm). Fellatio.

**fellatrix** (fel-ă-triks'). A female who takes the oral part in fellatio.

**fel'on** [ M.E. *feloun,* malignant ]. Whitlow; a purulent infection or abscess involving the bulbous distal end of a finger.

**felt'work.** 1. Fibrous network. 2. A close plexus of nerve fibrils; see neuropile.

**Felty,** Augustus R., American physician, *1895. See F.'s *syndrome.*

**felypressin** (fel'ǐ-pres'in) (USAN). Lysine vasopressin with phenylalanine at position 2.

**fe'male.** In zoology, denoting the sex that bears the young or the sexual cell which develops into a new organism.

  **genetic f.,** (1) an individual with a normal female karyotype, including two X chromosomes; (2) an individual whose cell nuclei contain Barr sex chromatin bodies, which are normally present in f.'s and absent in males; patients with ambiguous sexual development or Turner's syndrome are classed as genetic males or genetic f.'s by absence or presence of Barr bodies even though their sex chromosome complement may be abnormal.

**feminism** (fem'ǐ-nizm) [ L. *femina,* woman ]. Possession of feminine characteristics by the male.

**feminization** (fem'ǐ-nǐ-za'shun). The acquisition of female characteristics by the male.

**fem'oral.** Relating to the femur or thigh.

**femorocele** (fem'o-ro-sēl) [ L. *femur,* thigh, + G. *kēlē,* hernia ]. Femoral hernia.

**fem'orotib'ial.** Relating to the femur and the tibia.

**femto-** [ Danish *femten,* fifteen ]. A prefix used in the metric system to signify one-quadrillionth (10⁻¹⁵) of any unit. Symbol, f.

**fe'mur,** pl. **fem'ora,** gen. **fem'oris** [ L. thigh ] [ NA ]. 1. Thigh bone; the long bone of the thigh, articulating with the hip bone proximally and the tibia and patella distally. 2. The thigh.

**fenal'amide** (USAN). Ethyl *N*-[ 2-(diethylamino)ethyl ]-2-ethyl-2-phenylmalonamate; a smooth muscle relaxant.

**fen'camine hydrochloride.** EUVITOL hydrochloride; *N*-ethyl-3-phenyl-2-norbornanamine hydrochloride; central nervous system stimulant.

**fen'clonine** (USAN). DL-3-(*p*-Chlorophenyl)alanine; a serotonin inhibitor.

**fenestra,** pl. **fenes'trae** (fĕ-nes'trah) [ L. window ] 1 [ NA ]. An anatomical aperture, often closed by a membrane. 2. An opening left in a plaster of Paris or other form of fixed dressing in order to permit access to a wound or inspection of the part. 3. The opening in one of the blades of a forceps.

  **f. choled'ocha,** a surgical opening in the wall of the duodenum at the entrance of common bile and pancreatic ducts.

  **f. coch'leae** [ NA ], f. of the cochlea; cochlear window; f. rotunda; round window; an opening on the medial wall of the middle ear leading into the cochlea, closed in life by the secondary tympanic membrane.

  **f. nonova'lis,** artificial opening through the otic capsule of the lateral semicircular canal connecting the membranous labyrinth with the mastoid cavity produced during fenestration surgery.

**f. ova′lis,**  f. vestibuli.

**f. rotun′da,**  f. cochleae.

**f. vestib′uli** [ NA ], f. of the vestibule; vestibular window; f. ovalis; oval window; an oval opening on the medial wall of the tympanic cavity leading into the vestibule, closed in life by the foot of the stapes.

**fenes′trated.**  Having fenestrae or window-like openings.

**fen′estra′tion.** 1. The presence of openings or fenestrae in a part; see fenestration *operation.* 2. Making openings in a dressing to allow inspection of the parts. 3. Artifistulation; in dentistry, a surgical perforation of the mucoperiosteum and alveolar plate to expose the root tip of a tooth to permit drainage of tissue exudate.

**tracheal f.,**  a surgical procedure to create an epithelialized mucocutaneous opening from the neck into the trachea.

**fenes′trel**  (USAN). 5-Ethyl-6-methyl-4-phenyl-3-cyclohexene-1-carboxylic acid; an estrogenic substance.

**feneth′azine.**  ANERGAN; 10-(2-dimethylaminoethyl)-phenothiazine; antihistaminic.

**feneth′ylline hydrochloride**  (USAN). CAPTAGON; 7-{2-[ (α-methylphenethyl)amino ]ethyl}theophylline hydrochloride; analeptic agent.

**fenflu′ramine hydrochloride**  (USAN). PONDEREX; *N*-ethyl-α-methyl-*m*-(trifluoromethyl)phenethylamine hydrochloride; anorexigenic agent.

**fen′nel** [ through Old Fr. fr. L. *faeniculum*, fennel, dim. of *faenum*, hay ]. Fennel seed; foeniculum; the dried ripe fruit of cultivated varieties of *Foeniculum vulgare* (family Umbelliferae); a herb native to Southern Europe and Asia. Diaphoretic and carminative.

**f. oil,**  a volatile oil distilled from the fruit of *Foeniculum vulgare*; a flavor.

**fenpip′ramide methobromide.**  RESANTIN; 1-(3-carbamoyl-3,3-diphenylpropyl)-1-methylpiperidinium bromide; intestinal antispasmodic.

**fenpiprane.**  ASPASAN; 1-(3,3-diphenylpropyl)piperidine; antiallergic agent with antispasmodic properties.

**fen′tanyl citrate**  (USP). SUBLIMAZE; phentanyl; *N*-(1-phenethyl-4-piperidyl)propionanilide citrate; a narcotic analgesic about 100 times as potent as morphine; used as supplementary analgesic agent in general anesthesia.

**fen′ticlor**  (USAN). 2,2′-Thiobis[ 4-chlorophenol ]; a topical anti-infective agent.

**fenugreek** (fen′u-grēk) [ L. *faenum graecum*, fenugreek, fr. *faenum*, hay, + *Graecus*, Greek ]. *Trigonella faenumgraecum* (Leguminosae); an annual plant indigenous to West Asia and cultivated in Africa and parts of Europe. The mucilaginous seeds are used as food and in the preparation of culinary spices (curry).

**Fenwick,**  Samuel, English physician, 1821–1902. See F.'s *disease.*

**Féréol**  (fa-ra-ol′), Louis H. F., Paris physician, 1825–1891. See F.'s *nodes.* F.-Graux *palsy.*

**Fergusson,**  Sir William, British surgeon, 1808–1877. See F.'s *incision, speculum.*

**ferment** (fer-ment′). To cause or to undergo fermentation.

**ferment** (fer′ment) [ L. *fermentum*, leaven ]. Obsolete synonym for enzyme.

**protective f.,**  Abderhalden *test.*

**ferment′able.**  Capable of undergoing fermentation.

**fer′menta′tion** [ L. *fermento*, pp. -*atus*, to ferment ]. Enzymolysis; a chemical change induced in a complex organic compound by the action of an enzyme, whereby the substance is split up into more simple compounds.

**acetous f.,**  f. of wine or beer whereby the alcohol is oxidized to form acetic acid.

**amylic f.,**  f. of potato or corn mash, or other starchy material, by which fusel oil is produced.

**lactic acid f.,**  the production of lactic acid in milk, or other carbohydrate-containing media, caused by the presence of any one of a number of lactic acid bacteria.

**ferment′ative.**  Causing or having the ability to cause fermentation.

**fermium** (fer′mĭ-um). Radioactive element, artificially prepared in 1955, atomic no. 100, atomic symbol Fm.

**fern** [ A.S. fearn ]. A cryptogamic (flowerless) plant of the class *Filicineae.*

**lady f.,**  female f.; *Athyrium filix–femina.*

**male f.**  (BP), aspidium.

**male f. oleoresin,**  aspidium oleoresin.

**sweet f.,**  comptonia.

**Fernbach,**  Auguste, French microbiologist, 1860–1939. See F. *flask.*

**fern′ing.**  A term used to describe the pattern of arborization produced by cervical mucus, secreted at midcycle, upon crystallization, which resembles somewhat a fern or a palm leaf.

**fer′ratin.**  Sodium iron albuminate; a hematinic.

**fer′redox′in.**  An iron-containing protein that has been considered, largely because of its low redox potential (−0.42 volt), to accept the light-produced electron from chlorophyll at the initiation of photosynthesis. Because of the lower potential of the primary photochemical act, several substances (inorganic iron, another iron-containing protein, "ferredoxin reducing substance," pteridines) may function prior to the reduction of ferredoxin. Ferredoxin is involved in several oxidation-reduction reactions in living organisms.

**f. hydrogenase,**  see hydrogenase.

**Ferrein**  (fer-rań′; fer-rīn′), Antoine, French anatomist, 1693–1769. See F.'s *canal, cords, foramen, ligament, pyramid, tube, vasa* aberrentia, *processus* Ferreini.

**Ferri,**  Alphonse, Italian surgeon, 1515–1595. Gave his name to alphonsin.

**ferri-** (fĕr′ĭ-) [ L. *ferrum*, iron ]. Prefix designating the presence in a compound of a ferric ion, Fe .

**ferric** (fĕr′ik). 1. Relating to iron; ferruginous. 2. Denoting a salt containing iron in its higher (triad) valence; $Fe^{+++}$.

**f. alum,**  f. ammonium sulfate.

**f. ammonium citrate**  (BP), soluble f. citrate; brown f. ammonium citrate; used in hypochromic anemia; it is relatively free of astringent and irritant action.

**f. ammonium citrate, green,**  used in hypochromic anemia.

**f. ammonium sulfate**  (USP), iron alum; ferric alum; ammonium ferric sulfate; an astringent and styptic.

**f. chloride**  (USP), iron trichloride; iron perchloride; astringent and styptic.

**f. citrate,**  used in anemia.

**f. fructose**  (USAN), FERRITOSE; fructose-iron complex with potassium; a hematinic drug.

**f. glycerophosphate,**  a tonic and a source of iron.

**f. hydroxide,**  hydrated iron oxide; used, freshly prepared, as an antidote to arsenic poisoning.

**f. oxide, red,**  used as a coloring material (together with yellow f. oxide) for preparations designed for application to the skin.

**f. oxide, yellow,**  same use as red f. oxide.

**f. phosphate,**  used as a feed and as a food supplement.

**f. phosphate, soluble,**  f. phosphate with sodium citrate; used for iron deficiency anemia.

**f. sodium edetate,**  see under edetate.

**f. sulfate,**  iron persulfate; iron tersulfate; iron sesquisulfate; astringent and styptic.

**ferrichromes** (fĕr′ĭ-krōmz). Growth factors for various fungi; naturally occurring ferric hydroxamates, based on a cyclic hexapeptide containing serine, glycine, and (5-*N*-hydroxy)ornithine, and complexed with one ferric atom.

**fer′ricy′anide.**  Salt of the anion $Fe(CN)_6{}^{3-}$.

**fer′ricy′tochrome.**  Cytochrome *c* (oxidized).

**ferricytochrome *c*₃.**  See hydrogenase.

**fer′riheme.**  See hemin.

**fer′rihemoglo′bin.**  Methemoglobin.

**fer′ripor′phyrin.**  The compound formed between ferric ion and a porphyrin; ferriprotoporphyrin (hemin) is the best known example.

**fer′ripro′topor′phyrin.**  Hemin.

**fer′ritin.**  An iron protein complex containing up to 23 per cent of iron, formed by the union of ferric iron with apoferritin; found in the intestinal mucosa, spleen, liver.

**ferro-** (fĕr′o-) [ L. *ferrum*, iron ]. A prefix designating the presence of metallic iron or of the divalent ion $Fe^{++}$ in a compound, *e.g.*, potassium ferrocyanide.

**ferrocholinate** (fĕr'o-ko'lĭ-nāt). CHEL-IRON; FERROLIP; iron choline citrate chelate. Used for oral administration in the treatment and prevention of iron deficiency anemias.

**fer'rocy'anide.** A compound containing the negative ion $Fe(CN)_6^{4-}$.

**fer'rocyan'ogen.** Ferrocyanide.

**fer'rocy'tochrome.** Cytochrome *c* (reduced).

**ferrom'eter** [ L. *ferrum,* iron, + G. *metron,* measure ]. A device for estimating the proportion of iron in the blood.

**fer'ropor'phyrin.** The compound formed between ferrous ion and a porphyrin; ferroprotoporphyrin (heme) is the best known example.

**fer'ropro'teins.** Proteins containing iron in a prosthetic group, *e.g.,* heme, cytochrome.

**fer'ropro'topor'phyrin.** Heme.

**fer'rosil'icon.** An alloy of iron and silicon.

**ferrosoferric** (fĕr-o'so-fĕr'ik). Relating to a combination of a ferrous with a ferric compound, as in $Fe_3O_4$.

**fer'rother'apy** [ L. *ferrum,* iron ]. The use of iron in treatment.

**fer'rous.** 1. Relating to iron; ferruginous. 2. Denoting a salt containing iron in its lowest valence ($Fe^{2+}$), *e.g.,* ferrous chloride, $FeCl_2$.

  **f. bromide,** iron bromide; has been used in the treatment of chorea.

  **f. citrate,** occurs in several forms, two of which are monoferrous acid citrate monohydrate and triferrous dicitrate decahydrate; used in iron deficiency anemia. USP lists the radiopharmaceutical, ferrous citrate $^{59}Fe$ (FER-RUTOPE).

  **f. fumarate** (USP, BP), iron fumarate; a hematinic.

  **f. glu'conate** (NF, BP), used in the treatment of anemia.

  **f. lactate,** a relatively nonastringent chalybeate.

  **f. succinate** (BP), used in the prevention and treatment of iron deficiency anemia.

  **f. sulfate** (USP, BP), iron sulfate; green or iron vitriol; copperas; used in anemia; the commercial impure variety (copperas) is used as a deodorant and disinfectant.

  **f. sulfate, dried** (USP, BP), exsiccated iron sulfate; a hematinic.

**ferrugination** (fĕ-ru'jĭ-na'shun) [ L. *ferrugo,* iron-rust ]. The deposition of ferric salts in the walls of small blood vessels, typically within the basal ganglia and cerebellum.

**ferruginous** (fĕ-ru'jĭ-nus). Chalybeate (1); relating to or containing iron.

**ferrule** (fĕr'ul) [ corrupted through Old F. and Medieval L. fr. L. *viriola,* a small bracelet ]. See coping.

**fer'rum** [ L. ]. Iron.

**Ferry,** Erwin S., U. S. physicist, *1868. See F.-Porter *law.*

**fer'tile** [ L. *fertilis; fero,* to bear ]. 1. Fruitful; capable of conceiving and bearing young. 2. Impregnated; fertilized.

**fertil'ity.** The state of being fertile; specifically, the ability to produce young.

**fer'tiliza'tion.** The process that begins with the penetration of the secondary oocyte by the spermatozoon and is completed with the fusion of the male and female pronuclei.

**fertil'izin.** Name applied to an ectohormone secreted by echinoderm ova that stimulates activation and agglutination of spermatozoa of the same species; f. represents one type of gamone.

**Ferula** (fĕr'u-lah) [ L. the plant fennel giant ]. A genus of plants of the family Umbelliferae; of the various species *F. assa-foetida, F. rubricaulis* and *F. foetida* furnish asafetida; *F. galbaniflua* and *F. rubricaulis,* galbanium; and *F. sumbul* furnishes sumbul.

**fervescence** (fer-ves'ens) [ L. *fervesco,* to begin to boil, fr. *ferveo,* to boil ]. An increase of fever.

**fes'ter** [ L. *fistula* ]. 1. To ulcerate. 2. An ulcer. 3. To form pus or putrefy.

**fes'tinant** [ L. *festino,* to hasten ]. Rapid; quick; hastening; accelerating.

**festina'tion** [ L. *festino,* to hasten ]. The peculiar acceleration of gait noted in parkinsonism (1) and some other nervous affections.

**festoon'** [ thr. Fr. fr. L. *festum,* festival, hence festive decorations ]. 1. A carving in the base material of a denture that simulate the contours of the natural tissue that is being replaced by the denture. 2. A distinguishing characteristic of certain hard tick species, consisting of small rectangular areas separated by grooves along the posterior margin of the dorsum of both males and females.

  **gingival f.,** an arcuate enlargement of the marginal gingiva.

  **McCall's f.,** a gingival f. that may be caused by occlusal trauma.

**fe'tal.** Relating to a fetus.

**fe'talism.** The presence of certain fetal structures or characteristics in the body after birth.

**fetation** (fe-ta'shun). Pregnancy.

**feticide** (fe'tĭ-sīd) [ L. *fetus* + *caedo,* to kill ]. Induced abortion; embryectony; the destruction of the embryo or fetus in the uterus.

**fetid** (fet'id, fe'tid) [ L. *foetidus* ]. Foul-smelling.

**fetish** (fet'ish, fe'tish) [ Fr. *fétiche,* fr. L. *factitius,* made by art, artificial, fr. *facio,* pp. *factus,* to make ]. An inanimate object or nonsexual body part that is regarded as endowed with magic or erotic qualities; *e.g.,* an article of underwear or other clothing, or hair or foot.

**fetishism** (fet'ish-izm, fe'tish-izm). The act of worshipping or using for sexual arousal and gratification that which is regarded as a fetish.

**fet'lock.** The metacarpophalangeal and metatarsophalangeal joints of ungulates; also the cushion-like caudal projection above the hoof of the horse and similar animals, and the tuft of hair in this region.

**fetography** (fe-tog'ră-fī) [ L. *fetus* + G. *graphō,* to write ]. Roentgenography of the fetus *in utero.*

**fetology** (fe-tol'o-jī) [ L. *fetus* + G. *logos,* study ]. Embryatrics; the branch of medicine concerned with the study, diagnosis and treatment of the fetus *in utero.*

**fetometry** (fe-tom'e-trī) [ L. *fetus* + G. *metron,* measure ]. Estimation of the size of the fetus, especially of its head, prior to delivery.

**fe'toplacen'tal.** Relating to the fetus and its placenta.

**fe'tor** [ L. an offensive smell, fr. *feteo,* to stink ]. A very offensive odor.

  **f. ex o're** [ L. from the mouth ], halitosis.

  **f. hepat'icus,** a peculiar odor to the breath in persons with severe liver disease; caused by volatile aromatic substances that accumulate in the blood and urine.

**fetox'ylate hydrochloride** (USAN). 2-Phenoxyethyl 1-(3-cyano-3,3-diphenylpropyl)-4-phenylisonipecotate monohydrochloride; a smooth muscle relaxant.

**fetuin** (fe'tu-in). An $\alpha$-globulin obtained from fetal and newborn calf serum; molecular weight 40,000; 22 per cent carbohydrate (*N*-acetylmuramic acid; galactose).

**fe'tus,** pl. **fe'tuses** [ L. offspring ]. 1. The unborn young of a viviparous animal after it has taken form in the uterus. 2 [ NA ]. In man, it represents the product of conception from the end of the eighth week to the moment of birth. See color plate 23, and figs. under amnion, decidua, embryo, skull, and uterus.

  **f. anid'eus,** anideus.

  **har'lequin f.,** a newborn infant, usually premature, with a form of ichthyosis vulgaris characterized by encasement of the body in grayish brown, often fissured plaques and by grotesque deformity of the face, hands, and feet.

  **f. in fe'tu,** a double f. in which the small imperfectly formed parasite is contained within the autosite.

  **f. papyra'ceus,** one of twin f.'s that has died and been pressed flat against the uterine wall by the growth of the living f.

  **f. sanguinolen'tus,** a dark colored, partly macerated f.

**Feulgen** (foil'gen), Robert, German biochemist, 1884–1955. See F. *count, reaction, test.*

**FEV.** Abbreviation for forced expiratory *volume.*

# FEVER

**fe′ver** [ A.S. *fefer*]. 1. Pyrexia; febris; a bodily temperature above the normal of 98.6°F. (37°C.); a disease in which there is an elevation of the body temperature above the normal.

**abortus f.,** brucellosis.

**absorption f.,** an elevation of temperature often occurring, without other untoward symptoms, shortly after childbirth, assumed to be due to the absorption of the discharges through abrasions of the vaginal wall.

**accli′mating f.,** elevated temperature with malaise that occurs upon working in a very hot environment.

**acmastic f.** [ G. *akmastikos*, in full bloom ], continued f.

**A′den f.,** dengue.

**aestivoautumnal f.,** falciparum *malaria.*

**African swine f.,** a highly fatal disease of European swine in East Africa caused by a virus having its reservoir in wild wart hogs and bush pigs. The disease resembles hog cholera (swine f.) very closely but the viruses of these diseases do not cross immunize.

**algid pernicious f.,** a pernicious malarial attack in which the patient presents all the symptoms of collapse.

**f. and ague,** malaria.

**aph′thous f.,** foot and mouth *disease.*

**Archibald's f.,** a disease occurring in the Sudan, characterized by drowsiness, caused by microorganisms of the *Bacillus cloacae* group.

**ardent f.,** heat apoplexy; a term sometimes applied to hyperpyrexia occurring in intermittent malarial f.

**Argentinian hemorrhagic f.,** a form of hemorrhagic f. observed in South America, seemingly transmitted by contact from rodents to man and caused by an RNA virus (Junin virus).

**aseptic f.,** pyrexia accompanied with malaise due to the absorption of dead but not putrefactive tissue following an injury.

**Assam f.,** visceral *leishmaniasis.*

**autumn f.,** seven-day f.; (1) a f. resembling dengue occurring at the end of the summer in India; (2) hasamiyami.

**biliary f. of dogs,** a form of babesiosis (piroplasmosis) of the dog characterized by fever and icterus and caused by *Babesia canis.*

**biliary f. of horses,** equine *babesiosis.*

**bilious remittent f.,** (1) an old term for relapsing f.; (2) malarial "bilious" vomiting associated with marked increase of bilirubin in severe subtertian f.

**black f.,** Rocky Mountain spotted f.

**blackwater f.,** malarial *hemoglobinuria.*

**blue f.,** Rocky Mountain spotted f.

**Bolivian hemorrhagic f.,** similar to Argentinian hemorrhagic f., and caused by the Machupo virus, serologically related to the Junin virus.

**bouquet f.,** dengue.

**boutonneuse f.,** tick typhus in tropical and South Africa, and Asia, caused by *Rickettsia conorii.*

**bovine ephemeral f.,** ephemeral f. of cattle.

**bovine milk f.,** milk f. (2).

**brain f.,** an inexact term for encephalitis of unknown etiology.

**breakbone f.,** dengue.

**bullous f.,** *pemphigus* acuta.

**burdwan f.,** visceral *leishmaniasis.*

**cachec′tic f.,** visceral *leishmaniasis.*

**camp f.,** typhus.

**canefield f.,** field f.

**canic′ola f.,** a disease of man, caused by *Leptospira canicola,* acquired usually from dogs but rarely from cattle and swine. The disease is transmitted by infective urine.

**Carter's f.,** an Asiatic relapsing f. caused by *Borrelia cartere.*

**cat f.,** panleukopenia.

**cat-bite f.,** cat-bite *disease.*

**cat-scratch f.,** cat-scratch *disease.*

**catarrhal f.,** an old term for the group embracing the common cold, influenza, and lobular and lobar pneumonia.

**catheter f.,** urinary f.

**Central European tick-borne f.,** tick-borne *encephalitis* (Central European subtype).

**cerebrospinal f.,** meningococcal *meningitis.*

**Chagres f.,** Panama f.; a pernicious malarial f. from which the laborers building the Panama railroad suffered.

**Charcot's intermittent f.,** f., chills, right upper quadrant pain, and jaundice associated with intermittently obstructing common duct stones.

**childbed f.,** puerperal f.

**coastal f.,** East Coast f.

**Colorado tick f.,** tick f. (5); an arbovirus infection transmitted to man by a tick (*Dermacentor andersoni*). The symptoms are mild, there is no rash, the temperature is not excessive, and the disease is very rarely, if ever, fatal; the prodromes are similar to those of Rocky Mountain spotted f., and it is possible that it is merely an attenuated form of that disease.

**Congolian red f.,** murine *typhus.*

**continued f.,** acmastic f.; a f. of some duration in which there are no intermissions or marked remissions in the temperature.

**cotton-mill f.,** byssinosis.

**Crimean hemorrhagic f.,** a form of hemorrhagic f. occurring in central Russia; distinct from Omsk hemorrhagic, and transmitted by species of the tick *Hyalomma;* caused by an ungrouped arbovirus.

**Cyprus f.,** brucellosis.

**dandy f.,** dengue.

**date f.,** dengue.

**deer-fly f.,** tularemia.

**deer hemorrhagic f.,** a hemorrhagic disease of certain deer of the central and eastern United States; virus is present in the blood and infection is thought to be arthropod-borne.

**dehydration f.,** thirst f.

**dengue f.,** dengue.

**desert f.,** coccidioidomycosis, benign form.

**digestive f.,** a slight rise of body temperature occurring during the period of digestion.

**diphasic milk f.,** tick-borne *encephalitis* (Central European subtype).

**double quotidian f.,** malaria in which two paroxysms occur daily.

**Dumdum f.,** visceral *leishmaniasis.*

**Dutton's relapsing fever,** Dutton's *disease.*

**East Coast f.,** a serious disease of cattle chiefly in East Africa caused by the protozoan *Theileria parva* and characterized by high fever, swelling of the lymph nodes, and high mortality (90 to 100 per cent, less in endemic areas) and transmitted by *Rhipicephalus appendiculatus* and other ticks of the genera *Rhipicephalus* and *Hyalomma;* also called bovine theileriosis, Rhodesian tick f., amakebe, and coastal f.

**elephan′toid f.,** lymphangitis and an elevation of temperature marking the beginning of endemic elephantiasis (filariasis).

**English sweating f.,** *anglicus* sudor.

**enter′ic f.,** (1) typhoid f.; (2) the group of typhoid and paratyphoid A and B f.'s.

**entericoid f.,** a f., neither paratyphoid nor typhoid, but resembling the latter; *cf.* parenteric f.

**ephem′eral f.,** a febricula lasting no more than a day or two.

**ephem′eral f. of cattle,** bovine ephemeral f.; three-day sickness; stiff sickness; an acute febrile disease of cattle in Africa and other warm countries of the eastern hemisphere caused by a virus and characterized by low mortality, high temperature, stiffness and lameness.

**epidemic hemorrhag′ic f.,** hemorrhagic f.

**epimastical f.** [ G. *epakmastikos,* coming to a height ], a f. increasing steadily until its acme is reached, then declining by crisis or lysis.

**equine biliary f.,** equine *babesiosis.*

**equine swamp f.,** swamp f. (1).

**eruptive f.,** tick *typhus.*

**essential f.,** f. without known infectious disease.

**exanthematous f.,** fever associated with an exanthem.

**exsicca'tion f.,** thirst f.

**falciparum f.,** falciparum *malaria.*

**familial Mediterranean f.,** familial paroxysmal *polyserositis.*

**famine f.,** relapsing f.

**fatigue f.,** an elevation of the body temperature, lasting sometimes several days, following excessive and long continued muscular exertion.

**f. in the feet,** laminitis in the horse.

**field f.,** canefield f.; a leptospirosis caused by *Leptospira australis* A.

**five-day f.,** Volhynia f.

**flood f.,** tsutsugamushi *disease.*

**food f.,** a disorder of childhood consisting of a sudden rise of temperature accompanied by more or less marked digestive disturbances, continued for a few days to several weeks; believed to be a form of food poisoning.

**Fort Bragg f.,** pretibial f.

**Gambian f.,** [ *Gambia,* a British colony on the West Coast of Africa ], an irregular relapsing f., lasting one to four days with intermissions of two to five days, marked by enlargement of the spleen, frequent pulse, and rapid breathing; due to the presence in the blood of *Trypanosoma gambiense,* the pathogenic microorganism of sleeping sickness.

**gastric f.,** catarrhal *gastritis.*

**gastric remittent f.,** brucellosis.

**glandular f.,** infectious *mononucleosis.*

**Hav'erhill f.** [ *Haverhill,* Mass., where an epidemic of the affection occurred in 1926 ], erythema arthriticum epidemicum; an infection by *Streptobacillus moniliformis* marked by initial chills and high f., gradually subsiding, by arthritis usually in the larger joints and spine, and by a rash occurring chiefly over the joints and on the extensor surfaces of the extremities; the duration of the disease was from two to three weeks. The term Haverhill f. is used to indicate *Streptobacillus moniliformis* infections not associated with rat bite, in contradistinction to rat-bite f.

**hay f.,** autumnal catarrh; an acute irritative inflammation of the mucous membranes of the eyes and upper respiratory passages accompanied by itching and profuse watery secretion, followed occasionally by bronchitis and asthma; the individual attack recurs annually at the same or nearly the same time of the year, either spring, summer, or late summer and autumn, caused by the pollen of trees, grasses, and flowering shrubs, respectively.

**hectic f.,** hectic (3).

**hematu'ric bilious f.,** hematuria due to renal lesions caused by the malarial hematozoon, *Plasmodium falciparum.*

**hemoglobinu'ric f.,** malarial *hemoglobinuria.*

**hemorrhag'ic f.,** Manchurian hemorrhagic f.; Korean hemorrhagic f.; epidemic hemorrhagic f.; a condition characterized by an acute onset of headache, chills and high f., sweating, thirst, photophobia, coryza, cough, myalgia, arthralgia, and abdominal pain with nausea and vomiting. This phase lasts for from three to six days and is followed by capillary hemorrhages, edema, oliguria, and shock. The cause of the disease is unknown, but it is suspected of being arthropod-borne; first known to Western medicine during Korean war, when soldiers were affected. Has also been observed in Manchuria.

**hepat'ic intermittent f.,** ague-like paroxysms occurring in cases of calculus in the common bile duct.

**herpet'ic f.,** a disease, apparently infectious, marked by chills, nausea, elevation of temperature, sore throat, and a herpetic eruption on the face and other parts; it is of short duration, three or four days, and so far as known never fatal.

**hospital f.,** classical endemic typhus.

**Ilhéus f.,** febrile illness caused by the Ilhéus virus, an arborvirus of group B; it is transmitted by the mosquito; see also Ilhéus *encephalitis.*

**inani'tion f.,** thirst f.

**intermenstrual f.,** an elevation of temperature sometimes observed in tuberculous women between the menstrual periods.

**intermittent malarial f.,** see intermittent *malaria.*

**inundation f.,** tsutsugamushi *disease.*

**island f.,** tsutsugamushi *disease.*

**jail f.,** typhus.

**Japanese river f.,** tsutsugamushi *disease.*

**jungle f.,** malaria.

**jungle yellow f.,** a form occurring in South America, transmitted by *Aedes leucocloenus* and various treetop mosquitoes of the Haemagogus complex; transmitted normally to primates, occasionally by chance to man to set off a human outbreak of classical yellow fever transmitted by *Aedes aegypti.*

**kedani f.,** tsutsugamushi *disease.*

**Kew garden f.,** rickettsial *pox.*

**Kinkiang f.,** *schistosomiasis* japonicum.

**Korean hemorrhagic f.,** hemorrhagic f.

**laurel f.,** an affection of the same nature as hay f., occurring at the time of flowering of laurel.

**lechuguilla f.,** lechuguilla *poisoning.*

**low f.,** one associated with a depressed state of the nervous system and dulling of mental processes.

**malarial f.,** see malaria, and subentries there.

**malignant catarrhal f.,** malignant catarrh of cattle; malignant head catarrh; bovine epitheliosis; a severe, sporadic virus disease of cattle characterized by catarrhal inflammation of the mucous membranes, enlargement of the lymphatic glands, and involvement of the central nervous system. The mortality rate is very high.

**malignant tertian f.,** falciparum *malaria.*

**Malta f.,** brucellosis.

**Manchurian f.,** a f. closely resembling typhus that prevails from September to December in South Manchuria; the probable pathogen is *Rickettsia manchuriae.*

**Manchurian hemorrhagic f.,** hemorrhagic f.

**Marseilles f.,** tick *typhus.*

**marsh f.,** malaria.

**Mediterranean f.,** (1) brucellosis; (2) familial paroxysmal *polyserositis.*

**Mediterranean exanthem'atous f.,** an affection occurring sporadically in the Mediterranean littoral marked by a severe chill with abrupt rise of temperature, pains in the joints, tonsillitis, diarrhea, and vomiting; on the 3rd to 5th day a rash of elevated nonconfluent macules beginning on the thighs and spreading to the entire body; the disease lasts from ten days to a fortnight and then disappears by rapid lysis without desquamation.

**meningotyphoid f.,** typhoid f. marked by symptoms of more or less irritation or inflammation of the cerebral or spinal meninges.

**metal fume f.,** brass founder's *ague;* zinc chills.

**mian'eh f.,** the form of relapsing f. occurring in Iran, due to *Borrelia persica.*

**miliary f.,** (1) an infectious desease characterized by f., profuse sweating, and the production of sudamina, occurring formerly in severe epidemics; (2) miliaria.

**milk f.,** (1) a slight elevation of temperature following childbirth, said to be due to the establishment of the secretion of milk, but probably the same as absorption f.; (2) bovine milk f.; parturient paresis; parturient paralysis; an afebrile disease, occurring shortly after parturition in dairy cattle, manifested by loss of consciousness and general paralysis; it is a disease of metabolism in which a hypocalcemia is characteristic.

**mill f.,** byssinosis.

**miniature scarlet f.** [ L. *minio,* pp. *atus,* to color with *minium,* red-lead ], a reaction consisting of f., nausea, vomiting, and a transient scarlatiniform rash which appears in a susceptible person when injected with the toxin of *Streptococcus pyogenes.*

**monolep'tic f.,** denoting a f. having but one seizure; a continued f.; distinguished from polyleptic f.

**Mossman f.,** a f., noted especially among sugar cane cutters in the Mossman District of North Queensland; caused by *Leptospira australia.*

**mountain f.,** altitude *sickness.*

**mud f.,** (1) a leptospirosis caused by *Leptospira grippotyphosa;* (2) bluecomb *disease* of turkeys.

**mumu f.,** Samoan term for elephantoid f.

**nine mile f.,** Q f.

**nodal f.,** *erythema* nodosum.

**North Queensland tick f.,** a mild form of tick typhus with eschar, adenopathy, rash and fever; caused by *Rickettsia australis.* thought to be transmitted by the tick, *Ixodes holocyclus.*

**Omsk hemorrhagic f.,** a tick-borne group B arbovirus infection of central Russia, associated with gastrointestinal symptoms and hemorrhages but little or no central nervous system involvement.

**Oro'ya f.,** Carrion's disease; a specific, acute, febrile, endemic disease of the Peruvian Andes, caused by *Bartonella bacilliformis;* marked by high fever, rheumatic pains, progressive, severe anemia, and albuminuria. See also bartonellosis.

**Pahvant Valley f.,** tularemia.

**pal'udal f.,** malaria.

**Panama f.,** Chagres f.

**pappataci f.** (pap-pah-tah'sī), phlebotomus f.; sandfly f.; Pym's f.; three-day f.; an infectious, not contagious, disease occurring in the Balkan Peninsula and other parts of southern Europe; its symptoms resemble those of dengue but are less severe and of shorter duration; the pathogenic organism is apparently introduced by the bite of a sandfly, *Phlebotomus papatasi.*

**pap'ular f.,** an affection characterized by mild f., rheumatoid pains, and a maculopapular eruption.

**paraty'phoid f.,** Schottmüller's disease; an acute infectious disease with symptoms and lesions resembling those of typhoid f., though milder in character; it is associated with the presence of the paratyphoid bacillus, of which at least three varieties (types A, B, and C) have been described; see *Salmonella paratyphi, S. schotmülleri,* and *S. hirschfeldii.*

**parenter'ic f.,** one of a group of f.'s clinically resembling typhoid and paratyphoid A and B, but caused by bacteria differing specifically from those of either of these diseases.

**parrot f.,** psittacosis.

**Persian relapsing f.,** mianeh disease; a tick-borne relapsing f., occurring in the Middle East, caused by *Borrelia persica* and transmitted by *Ornithodoros tholozani* and possibly by *Ornithodoros lahorensis.*

**petechial f.,** (1) an old term for meningococcal meningitis with petechiae; (2) *purpura* hemorrhagica (2).

**pharyn'goconjuncti'val f.,** an epidemic disease characterized by f., pharyngitis, and conjunctivitis; due to adenovirus, usually type 3, but occasionally other types.

**phlebot'omus f.,** pappataci f.

**polka f.,** dengue.

**polylep'tic f.,** denoting a f. occurring in two or more paroxysms, *e.g.,* smallpox, relapsing f., or intermittent f.; distinguished from monoleptic f.

**pol'ymer fume f.,** a condition marked by f., pain in the chest, and cough caused by the inhalation of fumes given off by a plastic, polytetrafluorethylene, when heated; workers engaged in molding this material or shaping it with high speed cutting or grinding tools are exposed to the toxic fumes.

**Pomona f.,** leptospirosis, mostly of hogs and cattle, spread by contact with the urine of animals, caused by *Leptospira pomona.*

**pretib'ial f.,** Fort Bragg f.; a mild disease first observed at Fort Bragg, N. C., characterized by f., moderate prostration, splenomegaly, and a rash on the anterior aspects of the legs; due to *Leptospira autumnalis.*

**protein f.,** f. produced by the injection of foreign protein, such as milk.

**puerperal f.,** childbed f.; f. occurring after childbirth.

**Pym's f.,** pappataci f.

**pyogenic f.,** pyemia.

**Q f.,** a disease caused by a rickettsial organism, *Coxiella burneti* (*Rickettsia burneti*) The "Q" is an abbreviation for "query," so named because the etiologic agent was not known; it is not named (as many think) after Queensland, Australia, where the disease was first recognized in 1935. It was soon found to occur in the United States, where it had been known as "nine mile f." The organism is propagated in sheep and cattle, where it produces no symptoms. Human infections occur as a result of contact with such animals, also human contact, air infection, and other sources.

**quartan f.,** malariae *malaria.*

**quotidian f.,** quotidian *malaria.*

**rabbit f.,** tularemia.

**rat-bite f.,** headache, f., lymphangitis, and lymphadenitis following the bite of a rat or other rodent; due either to *Spirillum minus* or to *Streptobacillus moniliformis;* the latter resembles Haverhill f., but is contracted from a rat bite.

**recurrent f.,** relapsing f.

**red f., red f. of the Congo,** murine *typhus.*

**redwater f.,** (1) bovine *babesiosis;* (2) a disease of cattle and occasionally of sheep caused by infection with *Clostridium hemolyticum;* it is highly fatal.

**relapsing f.,** recurrent f.; an acute infectious disease caused by any one of a number of strains of *Borrelia.* It is marked by a number of febrile attacks lasting about six days and separated from each other by apyretic intervals of about the same length; the microorganism is found in the blood during the febrile periods but not during the intervals, the disappearance being associated with specific antibodies and previously evoked antibodies. From an epidemiologic viewpoint there are two varieties: louse-borne (European or cosmopolitan relapsing f.) occurs chiefly in Europe, northern Africa, and India, and is caused by strains of *B. recurrentis;* the tick-borne variety occurs in Africa, Asia, North and South America, and is caused by a variety of species of *Borrelia,* each of which is transmitted by a different species of the soft tick, *Ornithodorus.*

**remittent malarial f.,** see remittent *malaria.*

**rheumatic f.,** f. occurring during recovery from infection, usually of the throat, with group A streptococci; it occurs in children and young adults, and is variably associated with acute migratory polyarthritis, Sydenham's chorea, subcutaneous nodules over bony prominences, myocarditis with formation of Aschoff bodies, which may cause acute cardiac failure, and endocarditis which is frequently followed by scarring of valves, causing stenosis or incompetence.

**Rhodesian tick f.,** East Coast f.

**ricefield f.,** a disease occurring in Indonesia, caused by *Leptospira bataviae.*

**Rift Valley f.** [ *Rift Valley* in Kenya, British East Africa ], enzootic hepatitis; a fatal endemic disease of sheep, the virus of which is pathogenic also for man and for cattle.

**Rio Grande f.,** brucellosis.

**rock f.,** brucellosis.

**Rocky Mountain spotted f.,** tick f. (4); black f.; blue f.; an acute infectious disease, of high mortality, characterized by arthritic and muscular pains, a moderately high continuous f., and a profuse petechial eruption. It occurs in the spring of the year in several of the states in the Rocky Mountain region. The pathogenic organism is not definitely determined (see Rickett's *organism* and *Babesia hominis*), but it is transmitted by two or more species of tick of the genus *Dermacentor, D. andersoni* and *D. modestus* both being implicated; it has also been found in the body of the American dog tick (*D. variabilis*).

**Roman f.,** malignant tertian, falciparum, or aestivoautumnal f., formerly prevalent in the Roman Campagna and in the city of Rome; caused by *Plasmodium falciparum.*

**saku'shu f.,** hasamiyami.

**Salonica** or **Saloniki f.,** a type of trench f. affecting the allied troops in Greece during World War I.

**salt f.,** elevated temperature in an infant, following a rectal injection of a salt solution; see also thirst f.

**sandfly f.,** pappataci f.

**San Joaquin f.** (wah-kēn'), coccidioidomycosis, benign form.

**scarlet f.,** scarlatina.

**septic f.,** septicemia.

**seven-day f.,** autumn f.

**shank f.,** synonym for trench f. caused by *Rickettsia quintana.*

**sheep f.,** heartwater.

**ship f.,** typhus.

**shipping f.,** (1) in horses this term is synonymous with pinkeye or influenza; (2) in cattle the term refers to a common syndrome seen especially during or after shipping in cold weather, manifested by acute inflammation of the upper respiratory tract usually terminating in pneumonia; some cases of shipping f. are caused by *Pasteurella* organisms (hemorrhagic septicemia), others are of unknown etiology.

**show f.,** feline *panleukopenia.*

**simple continued f.,** febricula.

**slow f.,** a continued f. of long duration.

**snail f.,** schistosomiasis.

**solar f.,** (1) dengue; (2) sunstroke.

**South African tick-bite f.,** a typhus-like fever of South Africa in the area bounded by Capetown, Southern Rhodesia, and Mozambique, caused by the *Rickettsia rickettsii;* usually there are primary eschar and regional atonitis, rigors, and emaculopapular rash on the fifth day, often with severe central nervous system symptoms.

**spirillum f.,** relapsing f.

**splenic f.,** anthrax (2).

**spotted f.,** (1) an old term for meningococcal meningitis with petechiae; (2) tick typhus caused by *Rickettsia rickettsii* in North and South America and Siberia.

**steroid f.,** f. presumably caused by elevated plasma concentrations of certain pyrogenic steroids; can be produced by administration of etiocholanolone.

**stiffneck f.,** (1) dengue; (2) cerebrospinal *meningitis.*

**swamp f.,** (1) equine infectious *anemia;* (2) malaria.

**swine f.,** hog *cholera.*

**symptomatic f.,** traumatic f.

**syphilitic f.,** the elevation of temperature often present in the early roseolous stage of secondary syphilis.

**tertian f.,** vivax *malaria.*

**Texas cattle f.,** bovine *babesiosis.*

**therapeutic f.,** pyretotherapy (1).

**thermic f.,** heatstroke.

**thirst f.,** dehydration f.; exsiccation f.; inanition f.; an elevation of temperature in infants after reduction of fluid intake, diarrhea or vomiting, probably caused by reduced blood water and consequently a heat loss by evaporation. An analogous condition in adults is seen when active work is persisted in in the face of dehydration.

**three-day f.,** pappataci f.

**tick f.,** (1) any infectious disease of man or the lower animals caused by a protozoan blood parasite transmitted through the agency of a tick; (2) the tick-borne variety of relapsing f.; (3) bovine *babesiosis;* (4) Rocky Mountain spotted f.; (5) Colorado tick f.

**Transcaucasian f.,** a disease similar to East Coast f., caused by *Theileria annulata.*

**traumatic f.,** symptomatic f.; traumatopyra; wound f.; elevation of temperature following an injury.

**trench f.,** a specific infectious f. of a relapsing type observed among the troops in World War I and caused by *Rickettsia quintana.* It is normally transmitted by infected lice (*Pediculus*).

**trypan'osome f.,** the febrile stage of sleeping sickness.

**tsutsugamu'shi f.,** tsutsugamushi *disease.*

**typh f.,** a term proposed to include all low f.'s of the type of typhus or typhoid.

**typhoid f.,** enteric f.; abdominal typhoid; an acute infectious disease caused by *Salmonella typhi.* It is characterized by a continued f., rising in a steplike curve the first week, great physical and mental depression, an eruption of rose-colored spots on the chest and abdomen, meteorism, often diarrhea, sometimes intestinal hemorrhage or perforation of the bowel; the average duration is four weeks, though aborted forms and relapses are not uncommon. The lesions are located chiefly in the lymph follicles of the intestines, the mesenteric glands, and the spleen. The antibody titer of the Widal test rises during the infection, and positive blood and urine cultures become negative. Treatment with chloramphenicol is usually fairly effective.

**typhus f.,** typhus.

**undulant f.,** [ referring to the wavy appearance of the long temperature curve ], brucellosis.

**ure'thral f.,** urinary f.

**urinary f.,** catheter f.; urethral f.; an elevation of temperature, usually slight and transitory, following catheterization of the urethra, or the passage of blood clots, gravel, or a calculus.

**urtica'rial f.,** schistosomiasis japonicum.

**u'veoparot'id f.,** chronic enlargement of the parotid glands and inflammation of the uveal tract accompanied by a long-continued f. of low degree; now recognized as a form of sarcoidosis.

**Uzbekistan hemorrhagic f.,** a f. in Central Asia probably transmitted by *Hyalomma anatolicum.*

**valley f.,** coccidioidomycosis, benign form.

**vernal f.,** a malarial f.

**vivax f.,** vivax *malaria.*

**Volhyn'ia f.** [ *Volhynia,* in Poland and Russia ], five-day f., Werner-His disease; perhaps the same as trench f.

**war f.,** typhus.

**West African f.,** malarial *hemoglobinuria.*

**West Nile f.,** febrile illness caused by the group B arborvirus as characterized by headache, fever, maculopapular rash, myalgia, lymphadenopathy, and leukopenia; spread by *Culex* mosquitoes from a reservoir in birds.

**wound f.,** traumatic f.

**Yangtze Valley f.,** schistosomiasis japonicum.

**yellow f.,** a tropical mosquito-borne viral hepatitis, due to a group B arbovirus; an urban form is believed to be transmitted by *Aedes aegypti* and a rural, jungle, or sylvatic form from tree-dwelling mammals by various mosquitos. Yellow f. is characterized clinically by fever, slow pulse, albuminuria, jaundice, congestion of the face, and hemorrhages, especially hematemesis (hence the synonym, "black vomit"); it is fatal in 5 to 10 per cent of the cases, otherwise recovery is complete.

**Zika f.,** a f. named for a forest in Uganda where the Chikungunya virus has been isolated. Infection is characterized by the sudden onset of high f. This is a severe prostrating illness with symptoms analogous to dengue.

---

**Fevold test.** See under test.

**FF.** Abbreviation for filtration *fraction.*

**fi'ant.** Plural of *fiat,* "let there be made."

**fi'at,** pl. **fi'ant** [ L. 3 pers. sing. pres. subj. (used in the sense of the imperative) of *fieri,* to be made ]. A term used in prescription writing, meaning, "let there be made."

---

# FIBER

**fi'ber** [ L. *fibra* ]. Fibra [ NA ]; fibre; a slender thread or filament. In anatomy, the term refers to (1) extracellular filamentous structures such as collagenic or elastic connective tissue fibers; (2) the nerve cell axon with its glial envelope; (3) certain elongated, hence threadlike cells such as muscle cells and the epithelial cells composing the major part of the eye lens.

**A f.'s,** myelinated nerve f.'s in somatic nerves, measuring 1 to 22 $\mu$ in diameter, conducting nerve impulses at a rate of 6 to 120 meters per second.

**accelerator f.'s,** augmentor f.'s; postganglionic sympathetic nerve f.'s originating in the superior middle and inferior cervical ganglia of the sympathetic trunk, conveying nervous impulses to the heart that tend to increase the rapidity and force of the cardiac pulsations.

**adrenergic f.'s,** nerve f.'s that transmit nervous impulses to other nerve cells (or smooth muscle or gland cells) by the medium of the adrenaline-like transmitter substance norepinephrine (noradrenaline).

**afferent f.'s,** those that convey impulses to a ganglion or to a nerve center in the brain or spinal cord.

**alpha f.'s,** large somatic motor or proprioceptive nerve f.'s conducting impulses at rates near 100 meters per second.

**anastomosing f.'s, anastomotic f.'s,** individual f.'s passing from one nerve trunk or muscle bundle to another.

**arcuate f.'s,** nervous or tendinous f.'s passing in the form of an arch from one part to another; see subentries under *fibrae* arcuatae.

**argyrophilic f.'s,** reticular connective tissue f.'s that react with silver salts and appear black microscopically. See also reticular f.'s.

**association f.'s,** intrinsic f.'s; endogenous f.'s; nerve f.'s interconnecting individual subdivisions of a given brain structure; for example, different regions of the cerebral cortex, different segments of the spinal cord. See also *fasciculus* occipitofrontalis, *fasciculi* proprii, *fasciculus* longitudinalis superior, *fasciculus* uncinatus, *fibrae* arcuatae.

**augmentor f.'s,** accelerator f.'s.

**B f.'s,** myelinated nerve f.'s in autonomic nerves, of a diameter of 2 $\mu$ or less, conducting at a rate of 3 to 15 meters per second.

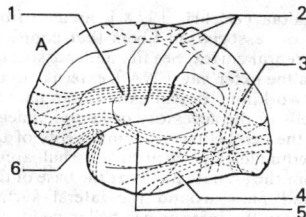

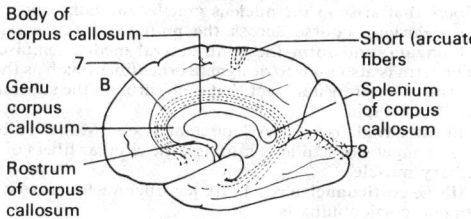

Body of
corpus callosum
7—
Genu
corpus B
callosum—
Rostrum
of corpus
callosum

Short (arcuate)
fibers
Splenium
of corpus
callosum
8

**Association Fibers of the Cerebrum**

*A*, projected onto the lateral surface of the hemisphere; *B*, onto the medial surface; *1*, superior longitudinal fasciculus; *2*, short association bundles; *3*, vertical occipital fasciculus; *4*, inferior longitudinal fasciculus; *5*, occipitofrontal fasciculus; *6*, uncinate fasciculus; *7*, cingulum; *8*, calcarine fasciculus. (After Dr. Murray Barr, modified.)

**Bergmann's f.'s,** filamentous glia f.'s traversing the cerebellar cortex perpendicular to the surface.

**beta f.'s,** nerve f.'s having conduction velocities of about 40 meters per second.

**C f.'s,** unmyelinated f.'s, 0.4 to 1.2 $\mu$ in diameter, conducting nerve impulses at a velocity of 0.7 to 2.3 meters per second.

**cholinergic f.'s,** nerve f.'s that transmit impulses to other nerve cells or to muscle fibers or gland cells by the medium of the transmitter substance acetylcholine.

**chromatic f.,** chromonema.

**circular f.'s,** *fibrae* circulares.

**climbing f.'s,** nerve f.'s in the cerebellar cortex that synapse with the principal dendrites or Purkinje cells.

**collagen f., collagenous f.'s,** white f.; an individual f. that varies in diameter from less that 1 $\mu$ to about 12 $\mu$ and is composed of fibrils and interfibrillar cement. The f.'s, which are usually arranged in bundles, undergo some branching and are of indefinite length. Chemically the f. is a scleroprotein, collagen, which yields gelatin upon boiling. They make up the principal element of irregular connective tissue, tendons, aponeuroses and most ligaments, and occur in the matrix of cartilage and osseous tissue.

**commissural f.'s,** nerve f.'s crossing the midline and connecting the two symmetrical halves of the nervous system.

**cone f.'s,** fine, tortuous f.'s extending from each cone in the fovea of the retina to its cell body, the cone cell, in the outer nuclear layer.

**corticobular f.'s,** nerve f.'s projecting from the motor and somatic sensory cortex to the rhombencephalon; included in this corticofugal f. system are corticoreticular f.'s terminating in the reticular formation of the rhombencephalon, and corticonuclear f.'s to the motor nuclei innervating the musculature of the face, tongue, and jaws, and to some of the rhombencephalic sensory nuclei. See also *tractus* corticobulbaris.

**corticonuclear f.'s,** *fibrae* corticonucleares; see *tractus* corticobulbaris.

**corticopontine f.'s,** *fibrae* corticopontinae.

**corticoreticular f.'s,** *fibrae* corticoreticulares.

**corticospinal f.'s,** *fibrae* corticospinales.

**dentinal f.'s, dental f.'s,** (1) Tomes' f.'s; the processes of the pulpal cells, the odontoblasts, which extend in radial fashion through the dentin to the dentoenamel junction and are contained within the dentinal tubules; (2) the intertubular fine collagenous f.'s which with the dentinal

ground substance infiltrated with calcium salts constitutes the dentinal matrix.

**depressor f.'s,** sensory nerve f.'s having pressure-sensitive nerve endings in the wall of certain arteries, and capable of activating blood pressure-lowering brainstem mechanisms when stimulated by an increase in intraarterial pressure.

**Edinger's f.'s,** f.'s in the cerebrum of amphibia forming part of the optic pathway.

**ef'ferent f.,** see efferent.

**elastic f.'s,** yellow f.'s; f.'s that are 0.2 to 2 $\mu$ in diameter but may be larger in some ligaments; they branch and anastomose to form networks and fuse to form fenestrated membranes; the f.'s and membranes consist of microfibrils about 130 Å wide and an amorphous substance containing elastin.

**enamel f.'s,** *prismata* adamantina.

**endog'enous f.'s,** association f.'s.

**exog'enous f.'s,** nerve f.'s by which a given region of the central nervous system is connected with other regions; the term applies to both afferent and efferent fiber connections.

**external arcuate f.'s,** *fibrae* arcuatae externae.

**gamma f.'s,** nerve f.'s that have a conduction rate of about 20 meters per second; see also gamma *efferent.*

**Gerdy's f.'s,** *ligamentum* metacarpeum transversum superficiale.

**Gratiolet's f.'s,** *radiatio* optica.

**gray f.'s,** unmyelinated f.'s.

**inhibitory f.'s,** nerve f.'s that inhibit the activity of the nerve cells with which they have synaptic connections, or of the effector tissue (smooth muscle, heart muscle, glands) in which they terminate.

**intercolumnar f.'s,** *fibrae* intercrurales.

**intercrural f.'s,** *fibrae* intercrurales.

**internal arcuate f.'s,** *fibrae* arcuatae internae.

**intrafusal f.'s,** muscle f.'s forming a neuromuscular spindle.

**intrinsic f.'s,** association f.'s.

**Korff's f.'s,** argyrophilic f.'s that pass between odontoblasts at the periphery of the dental pulp and fan out into the dentin.

**Kühne's f.,** artificial muscle f. made by filling the intestine of an insect with a growth of myxomycetes; used to demonstrate the contractility of protoplasm.

**f.'s of lens,** *fibrae* lentis.

**Mauthner's f.,** an axon extending from the metencephalon to the caudal end of the spinal cord of fishes and amphibians. It provides the final common path for impulses to muscles of the tail.

**medullated nerve f.,** myelinated nerve f.

**meridional f.'s,** *fibrae* meridionales.

**mossy f.'s,** highly branched nerve f.'s in the cerebellar cortex that synapse with granule cell dendrites.

**motor f.'s,** the filaments in a mixed nerve that transmit motor impulses.

**Müller's f.'s,** (1) *fibrae* circulares; (2) Müller's radial cells; sustentacular f.'s; sustenacular neuroglial cells of the retina, running through the thickness of the retina from the internal limiting membrane to the bases of the rods and cones where they form a row of junctional complexes.

**myelinated nerve f.,** medullated nerve f.; an axon enveloped by a myelin sheath formed by oligodendroglia cells (in brain and spinal cord) or Schwann cells (in peripheral nerves).

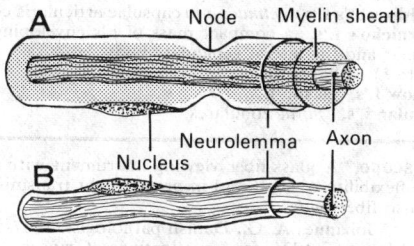

A Node Myelin sheath

B Neurolemma Axon
Nucleus

**Nerve Fibers**

*A*, myelinated; *B*, unmyelinated

**Nélaton's f.'s,** Nélaton's *sphincter.*

**nerve f.,** the axon of a nerve cell, ensheathed by oligodendroglia cells in brain and spinal cord, and by Schwann cells in peripheral nerves.

**nonmedullated f.'s,** unmyelinated f.'s.

**oblique f.'s of stomach,** *fibrae* oblique ventriculi.

**osteocollagenous f.'s,** fine collagenous f.'s in the matrix of osseous tissue.

**osteogenetic f.'s,** the f.'s in the osteogenetic layer of the periosteum.

**pectinate f.'s,** *musculi* pectinati.

**perforating f.'s,** Sharpey's f.'s; bundles of collagenous f.'s that pass into the outer circumferential lamellae of bone or the cementum of teeth.

**periodontal membrane f.'s,** the collagen f.'s, running from the cementum to the alveolar bone, that suspend a tooth in its socket; they include apical, oblique, horizontal, and alveolar crest f.'s, indicating that the orientation of the f.'s varies at different levels.

**periventricular f.'s,** *fibrae* periventriculares.

**pilomotor f.'s,** nerve f.'s to the arrectores pilorum muscles of hair follicles responsible for piloerection.

**precollagenous f.'s,** immature, argyrophilic f.'s.

**pressor f.'s,** sensory nerve f.'s that cause vasoconstriction and rise of blood pressure on stimulation.

**projection f.'s,** nerve f.'s connecting the cerebral cortex with other centers in the brain or spinal cord.

**Prussak's f.'s,** elastic and connective tissue f.'s bounding the pars flaccida membranae tympani.

**Purkinje's f.'s,** interlacing f.'s formed of modified cardiac muscle cells with central granulated protoplasm containing one or two nuclei and a transversely striated peripheral portion; they are found beneath the endocardium; see also conducting system of the heart, under *system.*

**pyramidal f.'s,** *fibrae* pyramidales.

**Reissner's f.,** a rodlike, highly refractive f. running from the subcommissural organ down throughout the length of the central canal of the brainstem and spinal cord.

**Remak's f.'s,** unmyelinated f.'s.

**reticular f.'s,** argyrophilic, small, branching intercellular f. elements which may be continuous with collagen f.'s.

**Retzius' f.'s,** stiff f.'s in Deiters' cells.

**Sappey's f.'s,** nonstriated muscular f.'s in the check ligament of the eyeball.

**Sharpey's f.'s,** perforating f.'s.

**skeletal muscle f.'s,** multinucleated, contractile tissue elements varying from less that 10 μ to 100 μ in diameter and from less than 1 mm. to several cm. in length. The f. consists of sarcoplasm and cross-striated myofibrils which in turn consist of myofilaments.

**spindle f.,** traction f.; a fibril of the astrosphere that extends from the centrosome to the centromere of a chromosome and is concerned with movement of the chromosome toward the pole of the cell during cell division.

**Stilling's f.'s,** *formatio* reticularis.

**sudomotor f.'s,** postganglionic sympathetic nerve f.'s innervating the sweat glands.

**sustentacular f.'s of retina,** Müller's f.'s (2).

**tautomeric f.'s,** see tautomeric.

**Tomes' f.'s,** dentinal f.'s (1).

**traction f.,** spindle f.

**transverse f.'s of pons,** *fibrae* pontis transversae.

**unmyelinated f.'s,** Remak's f.'s; gray f.'s; nonmedullated f.'s; nerve f.'s (axons) lacking a fatty sheath but in common with others enveloped by a sheath of Schwann cells.

**Weitbrecht's f.'s,** *retinaculum* capsulae articularis coxae.

**Wernicke's f.'s,** a compact mass of f.'s enveloping the pulvinar and the lateral geniculate body.

**white f.,** collagen f.

**yellow f.'s,** elastic f.'s.

**zonular f.'s,** *fibrae* zonulares.

**fi'berscope.** A glass-fiber viewing instrument with complete flexibility of shaft and improved light transmission. See also fiber *optics.*

**Fibiger,** Johannes A. G., Danish pathologist, 1867–1928. Nobel laureate, 1926, for investigations of cancer.

**fibr-.** See fibro-.

**fibra,** pl. **fibrae** (fi'brah, fi'bre) [ L. ] [ NA ]. Fiber.

**fibrae arcua'tae cer'ebri** [ NA ], arcuate fibers of the cerebrum; short association fibers that connect adjacent gyri in the cerebral cortex. See fig. under association *fibers.*

**fibrae arcua'tae exter'nae** [ NA ], external arcuate fibers; they are of two kinds, dorsal external arcuate fibers that arise from cells in the accessory or lateral cuneate nucleus and pass to the cerebellum as components of the inferior cerebellar peduncle, and ventral external arcuate fibers that arise from the arcuate nuclei at the base of the medulla oblongata and pass around the lateral surface of the medulla to enter the inferior cerebellar peduncle.

**fibrae arcua'tae inter'nae** [ NA ], internal arcuate fibers; fibers that arise in the nucleus gracilis and cuneatus, pass in a curving course across the midline of the medulla oblongata, and form the contralateral medial lemniscus. The term is also used to designate other fibers such as those of the olivocerebellar tract that arch through the substance of the medulla.

**fibrae circula'res** [ NA ], circular fibers; Müller's fibers (1); Rouget's or Müller's muscles; the circular fibers of the ciliary muscle.

**fibrae corticonuclea'res** [ NA ], corticonuclear fibers; see *tractus* corticobulbaris.

**fibrae corticopon'tinae,** corticopontine fibers; the fibers that compose the *tractus* corticopontini.

**fibrae corticoreticula'res** [ NA ], corticoreticular fibers; corticofugal fibers distributed to the reticular formation of the mesencephalon and rhombencephalon. See also corticobulbar *fibers.*

**fibrae corticospina'les** [ NA ], corticospinal fibers; the nerve fibers composing the tractus corticospinales (tractus pyramidales).

**fibrae intercrura'les** [ NA ], intercrural fibers; intercolumnar fibers; horizontal arched fibers that pass from the inguinal ligament across the superficial inguinal ring.

**fibrae len'tis** [ NA ], fibers of the lens; the elongated cells of ectodermal origin forming the substance of the crystalline lens of the eye.

**fibrae meridiona'les** [ NA ], meridional fibers; the longitudinal fibers of the ciliary muscle.

**fibrae obli'quae ventric'uli** [ NA ], oblique fibers of the stomach; the smooth muscle fibers of the innermost layer of the tunica muscularis of the stomach; the fibers occur chiefly at the cardiac end of the stomach and spread over the anterior and posterior surfaces.

**fibrae periventricula'res** [ NA ], periventricular fibers; a heterogeneous system of thin nerve fibers in the periventricular gray matter of the hypothalamus; the dorsal longitudinal fasciculus is a caudal continuation of the system.

**fibrae pon'tis transver'sae** [ NA ], transverse fibers of the pons; fibers arising from the nuclei pontis that decussate and pass into the cerebellum as the middle cerebellar peduncles.

**fibrae pyramida'les,** pyramidal fibers; fibers of the corticospinal (pyramidal) tracts; see *tractus* pyramidalis.

**fibrae zonulares** [ NA ], zonular fibers; delicate fibers that pass from the equator of the lens to the ciliary body, collectively known as the zonula ciliaris or suspensory ligament of the lens; see *zonula* ciliaris.

**fibre** (fi'ber). Fiber.

**fibremia** (fi-bre'mi-ah) [ fibrin + G. *haima,* blood ]. Inosemia (2); fibrinemia; presence of formed fibrin in the blood, causing thrombosis or embolism.

**fi'bril** [ Mod. L. *fibrilla, q.v.* ]. A minute fiber.

**muscular f.,** myofibril.

**subpellicular f.,** subpellicular *microtubule.*

**unit f.'s,** the f.'s which together with an interfibrillar cementing substance comprise a collagen fiber. They range from 20 to 200 mμ and average about 100 mμ in diameter.

**fibrilla,** pl. **fibrillae** (fi-bril'lah, fi-bril'le) [ Mod. L. dim. of L. *fibra,* a fiber ]. Fibril.

**fibrillar, fibrillary** (fi'brĭ-lar, -lēr-ĭ). Relating to a fibril, or to fine rapid contractions or twitchings of fibers or of small groups of fibers in skeletal or cardiac muscle.

**fi'brillate.** 1. To make or to become fibrillar. 2. Fibrillated. 3. To be in a state of fibrillation (3).

**fi'brillated.** Fibrillar; fibrous; composed of fibrils.

**fibrillation** (fi'brĭ-la'shun). 1. The condition of being fibrillated. 2. The formation of fibrils. 3. Exceedingly rapid contractions or twitching of muscular fibrils, but not of the muscle as a whole. 4. Vermicular twitching, usually slow, of individual muscular fibers. Commonly occurs in atria or ventricles of the heart as well as in recently denervated skeletal muscle fibers.

**atrial f., auricular f.,** ataxia cordis; delirium cordis; in which the normal rhythmical contractions of the cardiac atria are replaced by rapid irregular twitchings of the muscular wall; the ventricles respond irregularly to the dysrhythmic bombardment from the atria.

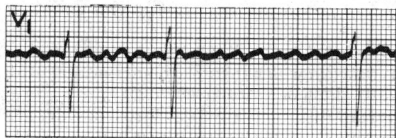

**Atrial Fibrillation**

**ventricular f.,** fine, rapid, fibrillary movements of the ventricular muscle that replace the normal contraction.

**fibrillogenesis** (fi-bril'o-jen'ĕ-sis). The development of fine fibrils (as seen with the electron microscope) normally present in collagenous fibers of connective tissue. The fibrils are from 700 to 1400 Ångstrom units in diameter, show cross-striations which average 640 Ångstrom units, and are embedded in a cement substance.

**fi'brin** [ L. *fibra*, fiber ]. An elastic filamentous protein derived from fibrinogen by the action of thrombin, which releases fibrinopeptides A and B (also termed cofibrins A and B) from fibrinogen, in coagulation of the blood.

**fi'brinase.** 1. See *factor* XIII. 2. Synonym for plasmin.

**fi'brina'tion.** 1. The formation of fibrin. 2. Fibrinosis; the capability of forming fibrin in abnormally great amount in the process of coagulation, or in an exudate; denoting a state of the blood in certain inflammatory conditions.

**fi'brine'mia.** Fibremia.

**fibrino-** [ L. *fibra*, fiber ]. Combining form relating to fibrin.

**fi'brinocel'lular.** Composed of fibrin and cells, as in certain types of exudates resulting from acute inflammation.

**fibrinogen** (fi-brin'o-jen). Factor I (blood clotting); a globulin of the blood plasma that is converted into the coagulated protein, fibrin, by the action of thrombin in the presence of ionized calcium; it is this change that produces coagulation of the blood.

**human f.** (USP, BP), prepared from normal human plasma; a coagulant (clotting factor), used as an adjunct in the management of acute, congenital, or acquired chronic hypofibrinogenemia.

**fibrin'ogenase.** Thrombin.

**fibrinogenic, fibrinogenous** (fi'bri-no-jen'ik, fi'bri-noj'ĕ-nus). Pertaining to fibrinogen; producing fibrin.

**fibrin'ogenope'nia** [ fibrinogen + G. *penia*, poverty ]. A concentration of fibrinogen in the blood that is less than the normal.

**fibrinoid** (fi'brĭ-noyd) [ fibrin + G. *eidos*, resemblance ]. 1. Resembling fibrin. 2. A deeply or brilliantly acidophilic, homogeneous, refractile, proteinaceous material that (1) is frequently formed in the walls of blood vessels and in connective tissue of patients with such diseases as disseminated lupus erythematosus, polyarteritis nodosa, scleroderma, dermatomyositis, and rheumatic fever, and (2) is sometimes observed in healing wounds, chronic peptic ulcers, the placenta, necrotic arterioles of malignant hypertension, and other unrelated conditions. Although f. resembles fibrin in certain morphologic features, there are also differences. F. is resistant to digestion by means of trypsin, whereas fibrin is easily digested. The original concept, that f. represents a degeneration or necrosis of collagen fibers, is probably not correct, inasmuch as more recent studies (by means of electron microscopy and other techniques) indicate that collagen may remain. The composition is variable in different conditions, and may include fibrin, γ-globulin, DNA, and acid mucopolysaccharide.

**fi'brinol'ysin.** Plasmin.

**fibrinolysis** (fi'brī-nol'ĭ-sis) [ fibrino- + G. *lysis*, dissolution ]. The hydrolysis of fibrin.

**fi'brinopep'tide.** One of two peptides (termed A and B) released from fibrinogen by the action of thrombin; they contain 18 and 20 aminoacyl residues, respectively.

**fi'brinoplas'tin.** One of the components of globulin in blood plasma.

**Schmidt's f.,** archaic term for a globulin in blood plasma, thought by Schmidt to combine with fibrinogen and result in the formation of fibrin.

**fi'brinopu'rulent.** Pertaining to pus or suppurative exudate that contains a relatively large amount of fibrin.

**fibrinoscopy** (fi'brī-nos'ko-pī) [ fibrino- + G. *skopeō*, to view ]. The chemical and physical examination of the fibrin of exudates, blood clots, etc.

**fibrinosis** (fi'brī-no'sis). Fibrination (2).

**fi'brinous.** Pertaining to or composed of fibrin.

**fi'brinu'ria.** The passage of urine that contains fibrin.

**fibro-, fibr-** [ L. *fibra*, fiber ]. Combining forms denoting fiber.

**fibroadenia** (fi-bro-ă-de'nĭ-ah) [ fibro- + G. *adēn*, gland ]. An obsolete designation for fibrous degeneration of glandular tissue.

**fibroadenoma** (fi'bro-ad-ĕ-no'ma). Adenoma fibrosum; fibroid adenoma; a benign neoplasm derived from glandular epithelium, in which there is a conspicuous stroma of proliferating fibroblasts and connective tissue elements.

**giant f.,** *cystosarcoma* phyllodes.

**intracanalicular f.,** a f. of the breast consisting of nodules of fibrous tissue which invaginate and compress the ducts.

**pericanalicular f.,** a f. of the breast consisting of an increased number of small ducts surrounded by concentric bands of fibrous tissue.

**fibroadipose** (fi'bro-ad'ĭ-pōz). Fibrofatty; relating to or containing both fibrous and fatty structures.

**fibroareolar** (fi'bro-ă-re'o-lar). Denoting connective tissue that is both fibrous and areolar in character.

**fi'broblast.** An elongated cell with cytoplasmic processes present in connective tissue, capable of forming collagen fibers. In chronic inflammatory states f.'s may arise from reticuloendothelial elements. An inactive f. is sometimes called a fibrocyte.

**fi'broblas'tic.** Relating to fibroblasts.

**fi'brocarcino'ma.** Scirrhous *carcinoma*.

**fi'brocar'tilage.** Fibrocartilago; a variety of cartilage that contains visible collagenic fibers. A strongly basophilic ground substance is present in the territory of the chondrocytes. See also entries under fibrocartilago.

**circumferen'tial f.,** a ring of f. around the articular end of a bone, serving to deepen the joint cavity.

**external semilunar f.,** *meniscus* lateralis.

**interartic'ular f.,** *discus* articularis.

**internal semilunar f. of knee joint,** *meniscus* medialis.

**semilu'nar f.,** *meniscus* medialis.

**strat'iform f.,** a layer of f. in the bottom of a groove in a bone through which a tendon runs.

**fibrocartilaginous** (fi'bro-kar-tĭ-laj'ĭ-nus). Relating to or composed of fibrocartilage.

**fi'brocartila'go** [ NA ]. Fibrocartilage.

**f. basa'lis,** basilar cartilage; the cartilage that fills the foramen lacerum of the skull.

**f. interarticula'ris,** *discus* articularis.

**f. intervertebra'lis,** *discus* intervertebralis.

**fi'brocel'lular.** Both fibrous and cellular.

**fibrocementoma** (fi'bro-se'men-to'mah). See cementoma.

**fibrochondritis** (fi'bro-kon-dri'tis). Inflammation of a fibrocartilage.

**fibrochondroma** (fi'bro-kon-dro'mah). A benign neoplasm of cartilaginous tissue, in which there is a relatively unusual amount of fibrous stroma.

**fi'broconges'tive.** Term sometimes used to indicate the general condition of an organ or tissue in which acute or chronic, persistent congestion has resulted in degeneration and necrosis of cells and replacement with connective tissue elements, as in chronic congestive splenomegaly.

**fi'brocyst** (fi'bro-sist). Any cystic lesion that is circumscribed by or situated within a conspicuous amount of fibrous connective tissue.

**fi′brocys′tic.** Pertaining to or characterized by the presence of fibrocysts.

**fibrocystoma** (fi′bro-sis-to′mah). A benign neoplasm, usually derived from glandular epithelium, characterized by cysts within a conspicuous fibrous stroma.

**fibrocyte** (fi′bro-sit) [ fibro- + G. *kytos,* cell ]. Fibroblast (designation sometimes applied to a fibroblast that is inactive).

**fibrodysplasia** (fi′bro-dis-pla′zī-ah). Abnormal development of fibrous connective tissue.

  **f. ossif′icans progres′siva,** a generalized heritable disorder of connective tissue in which bone replaces tendons, fasciae, and ligaments; see also fibrous *dysplasia* of bone.

**fi′broelas′tic.** Composed of collagen and elastic fibers.

**fi′broelasto′sis.** See endomyocardial f.

  **endocard′ial f.,** endomyocardial f.

  **endomyocardial f.,** endocardial sclerosis; a congenital condition characterized by thickening of the ventricular mural endocardium (chiefly due to fibrous and elastic tissue), thickening and malformation of the cardiac valves, subendocardial changes in the myocardium, and hypertrophy of the heart. The chief symptoms are cyanosis, dyspnea, anorexia, and irritability. Recent studies suggest that virus infection may play a role in some cases.

**fibroenchondroma** (fi′bro-en-kon-dro′mah). An enchondroma in which the neoplastic cartilage cells are situated within an abundant fibrous stroma.

**fibroepithelioma** (fi′bro-ep-ī-the-lī-o′mah). A skin tumor composed of fibrous tissue intersected by thin anastomosing bands of basal cells of the epidermis, first described by Pinkus; transformation to basal cell carcinoma may occur. Also called premalignant f., and f. of Pinkus.

**fi′brofat′ty.** Fibroadipose.

**fibrogliosis** (fi′bro-glī-o′sis) [ fibro- + G. *glia,* glue, + suffix *-osis,* condition ]. A cellular reaction within the brain, usually in response to a penetrating injury, in which both astrocytes and fibroblasts participate and which culminates in a fibrous and glial scar.

**fi′broid** [ fibro- + G. *eidos,* resemblance ]. 1. Resembling or composed of fibers or fibrous tissue; fibrous. 2. An old term for certain types of leiomyoma, especially those occurring in the uterus. 3. Fibroleiomyoma.

**fibroidectomy** (fi′broyd-ek′to-mī) [ fibroid + G. *ektomē,* excision ]. Fibromectomy; the removal of a fibroid tumor.

**fibroin** (fi′bro-in). A white, insoluble protein forming the main pportion (70 per cent) of cobweb and silk.

**fi′brokerato′ma.** A keratotic cutaneous polyp containing abundant connective tissue.

**fibroleiomyoma** (fi-bro-li′o-mi-o′mah). Leiomyofibroma; fibroid; a leiomyoma containing non-neoplastic collagenous fibrous tissue, which may make the tumor hard; f.'s usually arise in the myometrium, and the proportion of fibrous tissue increases with age.

**fi′brolipo′ma.** Lipoma fibrosum; a lipoma with an abundant stroma of fibrous tissue.

**fi′brolipo′matous.** Pertaining to or of the nature of a fibrolipoma.

**fibroma** (fi-bro′mah) [ fibro- + G. suffix *-oma,* tumor ]. A benign neoplasm derived from fibrous connective tissue.

  **ameloblastic f.,** ameloblastofibroma; a variety of ameloblastoma; a histologically benign neoplasm characterized by ameloblasts and fairly dense stroma (mesenchymal tissue) derived from odontogenic tissues.

  **cementifying f.,** cementoblastoma; cementoma (2); an isolated mass of cementum containing a variable amount of fibrous stroma, situated within a jawbone.

  **chondromyxoid f.,** chondrofibroma; chondromyxoma; an uncommon benign bone tumor, occurring most frequently in the tibia of adolescents and young adults.

  **concentric f.,** a benign neoplasm, actually a leiomyoma, that occupies the entire circumference of the wall of the uterus.

  **f. fungoi′des,** *mycosis* fungoides.

  **f. lipomato′des,** xanthoma.

  **f. mollus′cum,** (1) neurofibroma; (2) skin *tag.*

  **f. mollus′cum gravida′rum,** molluscum fibrosum gravidarum; skin that develop on women during pregnancy and subsequently disappear.

  **multiple f.,** neurofibromatosis.

  **f. myxomato′des,** myxofibroma.

  **nonossifying f.,** a loculated osteolytic focus of cellular fibrous tissue, slightly expanding a bone, usually near the end of a long bone in older children.

  **f. pen′dulum,** molluscum pendulum; a large, pendulous, fibrous tumor of the skin.

  **f. sarcomato′sum,** fibrosarcoma.

  **senile f.,** skin *tag.*

  **Shope f.,** a connective tissue tumor of cottontail rabbits found by Shope to be transmissible with cellular suspensions or Berkefeld filtrates. It is related to myxomatosis, and is used in Europe as a vaccine to protect against the myxoma virus.

  **telangiectat′ic f.,** angiofibroma; a benign neoplasm of fibrous tissue in which there are numerous, small and large, frequently dilated, vascular channels.

**fibromatoid** (fi-bro′mă-toyd). A focus, nodule, or mass (of proliferating fibroblasts) that resembles a fibroma, but is not regarded as neoplastic.

**fibromatosis** (fi-bro-mă-to′sis). 1. A condition characterized by the occurrence of multiple fibromas, with a relatively large distribution. 2. Abnormal hyperplasia of fibrous tissue.

  **palmar f.,** nodular fibroblastic proliferation in the palmar fascia of one or both hands, preceding or associated with Dupuytren's contracture.

  **plantar f.,** Dupuytren's disease of the foot; nodular fibroblastic proliferation in plantar fascia of one or both feet; rarely associated with contracture.

**fibro′matous.** Pertaining to, or of the nature of, a fibroma.

**fi′bromec′tomy.** Fibroidectomy.

**fi′bromus′cular.** Both fibrous and muscular; relating to both fibrous and muscular tissues.

**fibromyectomy** (fi′bro-mi-ek′to-mī). Excision of a fibromyoma.

**fibromyitis** (fi-bro-mi-i′tis). Fibromyositis.

**fibromyoma** (fi′bro-mi-o′mah). A leiomyoma that contains a relatively abundant amount of fibrous tissue.

  **telangiectatic f.,** vascular *leiomyoma.*

**fibromyositis** (fi′bro-mi′o-si′tis) [ fibro- + G. *mys,* muscle, + suffix *-itis,* inflammation ]. Chronic inflammation of a muscle with an overgrowth, or hyperplasia, of the connective tissue.

**fibromyxoma** (fi′bro-mik-so′mah) [ fibro- + G. *myxa,* mucus, + suffix *-oma,* tumor ]. A myxoma that contains a relatively abundant amount of mature fibroblasts and connective tissue.

**fi′broneuro′ma.** A neuroma with relatively abundant stroma of fibrous tissue.

**fibro-osteo′ma.** An osteoma in which the neoplastic bone-forming cells are situated within a relatively abundant stroma of fibrous tissue.

**fi′bropapillo′ma.** A papilloma characterized by a conspicuous amount of fibrous connective tissue at the base and forming the cores upon which the neoplastic epithelial cells are massed.

**fibroplasia** (fi′bro-pla′zī-ah) [ fibro- + G. *plasis,* a molding ]. Production of fibrous tissue, usually implying an abnormal increase of non-neoplastic fibrous tissue.

  **retrolen′tal f.,** abnormal growth of fibrous tissue behind the crystalline lens. Often used as a synonym for *retinopathy* of prematurity, *q.v.*

**fibroplas′tic** fibro- + G. *plastos,* formed ]. Producing fibrous tissue.

**fi′broplate.** An articular disk of fibrocartilage.

**fibropolypus** (fi-bro-pol′ī-pus). A polypus composed chiefly of fibrous tissue.

**fibropsammoma** (fi′bro-sam-mo′mah). A psammoma that has an unusually abundant, dense stroma of fibrous tissue; a form of meningioma.

**fi′broretic′ulate.** Relating to or consisting of a network of fibrous tissue.

**fi′brosarco′ma.** Fibroma sarcomatosum; a malignant neoplasm derived from fibrous connective tissue, characterized by immature, proliferating fibroblasts or undifferentiated, anaplastic spindle cells; f.'s tend to invade locally and metastasize widely, although some forms manifest a relatively low degree of malignancy.

**Earle L f.,** a transplantable f. derived from subcutaneous tissue of a mouse of C3H strain, grown in tissue culture to which 20-methylcholanthrene had been added.

**fi'brose.** 1. To form fibrous tissue. 2. Fibrous.

**fi'brose'rous.** Composed of fibrous tissue with a serous surface; denoting any serous membrane.

**fibrosis** (fi-bro'sis). The formation of fibrous tissue, usually as a reparative or reactive process; the term is not used with reference to the formation of fibrous tissue that is a normal constituent of an organ or tissue.

**arteriocap'illary f.,** sclerosis involving the walls of the smaller arteries, arterioles, and the capillaries; diffuse arteriosclerosis.

**cystic f. of pancreas,** see viscidosis.

**endomyocardial f.,** thickening of the ventricular endocardium by f., involving the subendocardial myocardium, and sometimes the atrioventricular valves, with mural thrombosis; occurs in adults and is endemic in parts of Africa.

**hepatolienal f.,** see Banti's *syndrome.*

**idiopathic retroperitoneal f.,** Ormond's disease; idiopathic fibrous retroperitonitis; periureteritis plastica; a sclerosing, fibrosing disorganization of retroperitoneal structures commonly involving and often obstructing the ureters.

**leptomeningeal f.,** a fibrous reaction within the subarachnoid space; sometimes a sequel to infectious or chemical meningitis; see also adhesive *arachnoiditis.*

**nodular subepidermal f.,** see dermatofibroma.

**perimuscular f.,** subadventitial f.; f. in the outer media of arteries, usually the renal arteries of young women, where it causes segmental stenosis and hypertension. Perimuscular f. is a variety of fibromuscular *dysplasia.*

**replacement f.,** the formation of fibrous tissue that occupies sites where various other cells and tissues have become atrophied, or degenerated and necrotic.

**retroperitoneal f.,** idiopathic retroperitoneal f.

**subadventitial f.,** perimuscular f.

**fi'brosi'tis** [ fibro- + G. suffix -*itis,* inflammation ]. 1. Inflammation of fibrous tissue. 2. Term used to denote aching, soreness, or stiffness in the absence of objective abnormalities.

**cervical f.,** see posttraumatic neck *syndrome.*

**fi'brotho'rax,** Fibrosis of the pleural space, sometimes with captive lung.

**fibrot'ic.** Pertaining to or characterized by fibrosis.

**fi'brous.** Composed of or containing fibroblasts, and also the fibrils and fibers of connective tissue formed by such cells.

**fibroxanthoma** (fi'bro-zan-tho'mah). See dermatofibroma.

**fibula** (fib'u-lah) [ L. *fibula* (contr. fr. *figibula*), that which fastens, a clasp, buckle, fr. *figo,* to fix, fasten ] [ NA ]. Calf bone; peroneal bone; splint bone (2); lateral and smaller of the two bones of the leg; it articulates with the tibia above and the tibia and talus below.

**fib'ular** [ L. *fibularis* ]. Relating to the fibula.

**fibula'ris** [ Mod. L. ] [ NA ]. Fibular.

**fibulocalcaneal** (fib'u-lo-kal-ka'ne-al). Relating to the fibula and the calcaneus, or os calcis.

**fi'cin.** A proteolytic enzyme (EC 3.4.22.3) isolated from figs (*Ficus carica, globata,* and *doliaria*). It is used as an anthelmintic (digests *Trichinella* and *Ascaris*), and in industry as a protein digestant.

**Fick,** Adolf, German physician, 1829–1901. See F. *principle.*

**fico'sis** [ L. *ficus,* fig ]. Sycosis.

**fi'cus** [ L. ]. Fig.

**Fiedler,** Carl L. A., German physician, 1835–1921. See F.'s *myocarditis.*

**field** (feld) [ A.S. *feld* ]. A definite area of plane surface, considered in relation to some specific object.

**auditory f.,** the space included within the limits of hearing of a definite sound, as of a tuning fork.

**Broca's f.,** Broca's *center.*

**Cohnheim's f.'s,** Cohnheim's *areas.*

**f. of consciousness,** see under consciousness.

**f. of fixation,** see under fixation.

**f.'s of Forel,** tegmental f.'s of Forel; campi foreli; three circumscript, myelin-rich regions ("Haubenfelder" or H-fields) of the subthalamus; (1) *field H₁,* corresponding to the fasciculus thalamicus, a horizontal fiber stratum marking the border between the caudal half of the subthalamus and the overlying thalamus, composed of pallidothalamic fibers of the ansa lenticularis and cerebellothalamic fibers of the brachium conjunctivum, and separated by the zona incerta from the more ventrally placed (2) *field H₂* formed by the fasciculus lenticularis, a fiber sheet over the dorsal border of the subthalamic nucleus composed largely of pallidothalamic fibers; (3) *field H* or prerubral field, a large field of intermingling gray and white matter immediately rostral to the red nucleus, uniting fields H₁ and H₂ around the medial margin of the zona incerta; its gray matter forms the prerubral nucleus. See also *ansa* lenticularis.

**free f.,** a f. (three-dimensional space) in a homogeneous, isotropic medium free from boundaries. In practice, a f. in which boundary effects are negligible.

**H f.'s,** see f.'s of Forel.

**individuation f.,** the f. within which an organizer can bring about the rearrangement of primordial tissues in such a manner that a complete embryo is formed.

**Krönig's f.,** Krönig's *area.*

**magnetic f.,** the sphere of influence of a magnet.

**microscopic f.,** the area whithin which objects are visible with microscope oculars and objectives of various magnifying powers.

**prerubral f.,** see f.'s of Forel.

**surplus f.,** part of the visual f. in cases of nontotal hemianopsia that passes beyond the point of fixation, thus encroaching upon the blind area.

**tegmental f.'s of Forel,** f.'s of Forel.

**visual f.,** the area within which objects are more or less distinctly seen by the eye in a fixed position.

**Wernicke's f.,** Wernicke's *center.*

**Fielding,** George H., English anatomist, 1801–1871. See F.'s *membrane.*

**field-vole.** A species of field mouse (*Microtus montebelloi*), normal host of *Leptospira hebdomadis,* the cause of seven-day fever or nanukayami fever (Japan).

**fig** [ L. *ficus;* A.S. *fic* ]. Ficus; the partially dried fruit of *Ficus carica* (family Moraceae); used as a nutrient, mild laxative, and demulcent.

**FIGLU.** Abbreviation for formiminoglutamic acid.

**Figueira** (fe-ga'e-rah), Fernandes, Brazilian pediatrician, †1928. See F.'s *syndrome.*

**figura'tus** [ L. *figuro,* pp -*atus,* to form, fashion ]. Figured; a term descriptive of certain skin lesions.

**fig'ure.** 1. A form or shape. 2. A person representing the essential aspects of a particular role.

**authority f.,** a real or projected person in a position of power; during the transference phase of psychoanalysis, the psychoanalyst becomes an authority f.

**fortification f.'s,** visual hallucinations that often accompany an attack of migraine, taking the form of scintillating colored lights or zigzag luminous bands, suggestive of the top of the wall of a turret.

**mitotic f.,** the microscopic appearance of a cell undergoing mitosis; a cell whose chromosomes are visible with the light microscope.

**myelin f.,** myelin body; a minute structure with concentric or parallel layers resembling those of the myelin sheath of a nerve; see myelin.

**Purkinje's f.'s,** shadows of the retinal vessels, seen as dark lines on a yellowish field when a candle or small electric light is held to the side of the eye in a dark room.

**Stifel's f.,** a black disk with a central white spot, used to determine the position and diameter of the blind spot in the human eye.

**figure and ground.** That aspect of perception wherein the perceived is separated into at least two parts, each with different attributes but influencing one another. Figure is the most distinct; ground the least formed; *e.g.,* a bird (figure) seen against the sky (ground).

**fila** (fi'lah) [ L. ]. Plural of filum.

**filaceous** (fi-la'shus) [ L. *filum,* a thread ]. Filamentous.

**fil'ament** [ L. *filamentum,* fr. *filum,* a thread ]. 1. Filamentum. 2. In bacteriology, a fine threadlike form, unsegmented or segmented without constrictions.

**axial f.,** the central f. of a flagellum or cilium; with the electron microscope it is seen as a complex of nine peripheral pairs of fibrils or microtubules and a central pair.

**parabasal f.,** term formerly used for rhizoplast.

**root f.'s,** *fila* radicularia.

**spermat'ic f.,** a spermatozoon, especially the tail of a spermatozoon.

**filamen'tous.** 1. Threadlike in structure. 2. Composed of filaments or threadlike structures.

**filamen'tum,** pl. **filamen'ta** [ L. ] [ NA ]. Filament (1); a fibril, fine fiber, or threadlike structure.

**fi'lar** [ L. *filum,* a thread ]. Fibrillar; filamentous.

**Filaria,** pl. **filariae** (fĭ-lăr'ĭ-ah, fĭ-lăr'ĭ-e) [ L. *filum,* a thread ]. Old generic term for a group of onchocercid parasites that live as adults in the tissues of body cavities of many vertebrates. The females lay partially embryonated eggs; the embryos uncoil (sheathed or not sheathed by a shell membrane) and circulate in blood or tissue fluids as microfilariae. If ingested by an appropriate bloodsucking arthropod, larval stages will develop and, some days later, the infective larvae may be deposited on another vertebrate host's skin when the arthropod seeks another blood meal. Species parasitic in man are *Wuchereria bancrofti, Brugia malayi, Onchocerca volvulus, Acanthocheilonema perstans, Dipetalonema streptocerca, Mansonella ozzardi,* and *Loa loa.*

**F. ban'crofti,** old term for *Wuchereria bancrofti.*

**F. demarquay'i,** old term for *Mansonella ozzardi.*

**F. diur'na,** a postulated species in which the microfilariae are found in circulating blood during the daytime only; probably identical to *Wuchereria bancrofti.*

**F. extraocula'ris,** a species found in a fibrous tumor of the eye of a Caucasian girl; possibly the same as *Loa loa.*

**F. hom'inis o'ris,** a species found once in the mouth of a child. Correct identification uncertain.

**F. labia'lis,** a species of which one specimen was extracted from a pustule of the lip. Correct identification uncertain.

**F. lentis, F. loa,** old terms for *Loa loa.*

**F. magalha'esi,** a postulated species that morphologically resembles *Wuchereria bancrofti;* found at autopsy in the left ventricle of a Brazilian. Some observers think the organism is a species of *Dirofilaria.*

**F. mala'ya,** old term for *Wuchereria malayi.*

**F. medinen'sis,** old term for *Dracunculus medinensis.*

**F. noctur'na,** old term for *Wuchereria bancrofti.*

**F. oc'uli humani,** old term for *Loa loa.*

**F. oz'zardi,** old term for *Mansonella ozzardi.*

**F. perstans,** old term for *Acanthocheilonema* (or *Dipetalonema*) *perstans.*

**F. philippinen'sis,** a species of *F.* described from man in the Philippine Islands; identification uncertain.

**F. restifor'mis,** a form obtained once from the urethra of a young man; identification uncertain.

**F. san'guinis hom'inis,** old term for *Acanthocheilonema* (or *Dipetalonema*) *perstans.*

**F. tanigu'chii,** a species recovered from a lymphatic gland in a Japanese; identification uncertain.

**F. vol'vulus,** old term for *Onchocerca volvulus.*

**fila'rial.** Pertaining to a filaria (or filariae), including the microfilaria stage.

**filariasis** (fil'ă-ri'ă-sis). The presence of filariae in the blood (microfilariasis) and tissues of the body; the disease occurs in tropical and subtropical regions. Filariasis may be asymptomatic, and living worms cause minimal tissue reaction. Death of the adult worms causes marked inflammation and lymphatic obstruction. Elephantiasis, lymph scrotum, and chyluria are manifestations of the disease.

**filaricide** (fi-lăr'ĭ-sīd) [ L. *caedo,* to kill ]. 1. Fatal to filariae. 2. An agent that kills filariae.

**filar'iform.** 1. Resembling filariae or other types of small nematode worms. 2. Thin or hairlike.

**Filarioidea** (fi-lăr'ĭ-oyd'e-ah). A superfamily of filarial nematodes parasitic in many animal species, including man. See *Filaria,* also *Acanthocheilonema, Dipetalonema, Dirofilaria, Loa, Mansonella, Onchocerca, Wuchereria,* and *Brugia.*

**Filaroides** (fil'ă-roy'dēz). A genus of nematode parasites occurring in the lungs, bronchi, and trachea of dogs.

**F. milksi,** occurs in the trachea and bronchi of dogs in the United States.

**F. osleri,** a small, widely distributed nematode that occurs in small nodules in the trachea and bronchi and, rarely, in the lungs of the dog. The nodules are gray-white or pink, usually less than 1 cm. in diameter. The disease is chronic and usually not fatal. The most marked symptom is a harsh cough.

**Filatov** (fe-lah'tawf), Nil F., Russian pediatrician, 1847–1902. See F.'s *disease, spots.*

**Filatov** (fe-lah'tawf), Vladimir P., Russian ophthalmologist, 1875–1956. See F.-Gillies tubed *pedicle.*

**file.** A tool for smoothing, grinding, or cutting.

**Hedström f.,** a coarse root canal f. similar to a rasp.

**root canal f.,** a pointed, flexible, steel intracanal instrument used in rasping canal walls.

**fil'ial** [ L. *filialis,* fr. *filius,* son, *filia,* daughter ]. Denoting the relationship of offspring to parents. See filial *generation.*

**filicic acid** (fĭ-lis'ik). Filixic acid.

**filicin** (fil'ĭ-sin). Filixic acid.

**filicinic acid** (fil-ĭ-sin'ik). 3,5-Dihydroxy-4,4-dimethyl-2,5-cyclohexadiene-1-one; a constituent of filixic acid.

**fil'iform** [ L. *filum,* thread ]. 1. Filamentous; hairlike; threadlike. 2. In bacteriology, denoting an even growth along the line of inoculation, either stroke or stab.

**filimar'isin.** FILIPIN; 14-deoxylagosin; an antibiotic substance produced by *Streptomyces filipinensis;* possesses antifungal properties.

**fil'ioparen'tal.** Pertaining to child-parent relationship.

**fil'ipunc'ture** [ L. *filum,* thread ]. Treatment of an aneurysm by the insertion of a coil of slender wire to induce coagulation.

**filix'ic acid.** Filicin; filicic acid; a mixture of several closely related substances, each comprising three substituted filicinic acid molecules; obtained from male fern; anthelmintic.

**fil'let** [ Fr. *filet,* a band ]. 1. Lemniscus. 2. A skein or loop of cord or tape used for making traction on a part of the fetus.

**lateral f.,** *lemniscus* lateralis.

**medial f.,** *lemniscus* medialis.

**fil'ling.** Plug; stopping; any substance, such as gold, amalgam, etc., used for restoring the portion missing from a tooth as a result of drilling out of decay in the tooth.

**combination f.,** a tooth f. of two or more materials applied in layers.

**compound f.,** a restoration that involves more than one surface of a tooth.

**direct acrylic f.,** direct resin f. of autopolymerizing acrylic.

**direct composite resin f.,** direct resin f. composed of an autopolymerizing epoxy resin and methacrylic acid matrix with as much as 78 per cent of reinforcing fillers such as glass beads, rods, quartz, or lithium aluminum silicate.

**direct resin f.,** a restoration made by inserting a plastic mix of autopolymerizing resin(s) in a cavity prepared in a tooth, as opposed to curing a nonautopolymerizing resin in a matrix and cementing the completed restoration in the cavity.

**overhanging f.,** one with excessive material at the junction of the f. margin and the tooth.

**permanent f.,** one designed to endure for as long a period as possible, in contradistinction to a temporary or provisional f.

**plastic f. material,** in dentistry, a material that may be shaped directly to the tooth cavity, such as amalgam, cement or resin.

**root canal f.,** a gutta percha, silver, or plastic cone that has been carried into a root canal, either alone or in conjunction with a cement, paste, or solvent, for the purpose of eliminating the canal space.

**silicate f.'s,** restorations of lost tooth structures made with silicate cement.

**temporary f.,** in dentistry, an interim filling.

**film.** A light-sensitive substance used in taking photographs.

**bite wing f.,** a special packaging of roentgenographic f. that allows an appendage of one f. package to be held between the occlusal surfaces of the teeth.

**precorneal f.,** a protective film, 7 to 9 $\mu$ thick, consisting of external oily, intermediate watery, and deep mucoprotein layers.

**filopodium,** pl. **filopo'dia** (fi'lo-po'dĭ-um) [ L. *filum*, thread, + G. *pous*, foot ]. A slender, filamentous pseudopodium of certain free-living amebae.

**fi'lopres'sure** [ L. *filum*, thread ]. Temporary pressure on a blood vessel by a ligature, which is removed when the flow of blood has ceased.

**filovaricosis** (fi'lo-văr-ĭ-ko'sis) [ L. *filum*, thread, + *varix*, dilation of vein ]. A series of swellings along the course of the axon of a nerve fiber.

**fil'ter** [ Mediev. L. *filtro*, pp -*atus*, to strain through felt, fr. *filtrum*, felt ]. 1. To pass a fluid through a porous substance that arrests suspended solid particles; see also percolate. 2. An apparatus provided with a porous substance through which a fluid is passed in order to separate it from any solids it may contain. 3. A translucent screen, used in radiotherapy, that permits the passage of certain rays and inhibits the passage of others which have a lower and less desirable energy.

**Berkefeld f.,** a f. of diatomaceous earth through which ordinary bacteria do not pass, so that the filtrate is bacteriologically sterile. There are three grades: W, fine; N, normal; V, coarse.

**Chamberland f.,** Pasteur-Chamberland f.; one of unglazed porcelain through which liquid is forced under pressure; microorganisms not ultramicroscopic do not pass. There are various grades, numbered L$_1$, L$_2$, etc.; L$_5$(F) and L$_7$(B) are the usual types for f. purposes; F permits only particles smaller than 0.2 $\mu$ to pass, the bacteriophage (estimated size 0.03 $\mu$) passes all grades, even the finest.

**Coors f.,** an unglazed porcelain f.

**Gooch f.,** a porcelain cup with a perforated bottom. A layer of asbestos fibers over the perforations acts as the filtering agent.

**Kitasato's f.,** an unglazed porcelain tube (closed at one end) through which fluid is drawn by means of suction; may be used for removal of microorganisms from specimens that are suitable for such filtration.

**Pasteur-Chamberland f.,** Chamberland f.

**f. press,** a machine consisting of two plates between which a canvas bag containing the liquid or semiliquid substance is held and can be subjected to pressure, which facilitates filtration through the pores of the canvas.

**fil'trable, fil'terable.** Capable of passing a filter; frequently applied to smaller viruses and some bacteria.

**fil'trate** [ see filter ]. Liquid that has passed through a filter.

**filtration** (fil-tra'shun). The process of passing a liquid through a filter.

**gel f.,** the separation of molecular sizes by passage of a mixture through columns of beads of cross-linked dextrans (Sephadex is the prototype) or similar relatively inert material of a well defined pore size range; the larger the molecule, the less time it spends in the interior of the beads, thus emerging earlier from the column than smaller molecules.

**fil'trum** [ Mediev. L. ]. A filter.

**Merkel's f. ventric'uli,** f. ventriculi.

**f. ventric'uli,** Merkel's f.; a groove between the two prominences, in each lateral wall of the vestibule of the larynx, formed by the cuneiform and the arytenoid cartilages.

**fi'lum,** pl. **fi'la** [ L. thread ] [ NA ]. A structure of filamentous or threadlike appearance.

**f. durae matris spinalis** [ NA ], the termination of the spinal dura mater, surrounding the f. terminale of the cord, and attached to the deep dorsal sacrococcygeal ligament.

**fila olfacto'ria,** nervi olfactorii; see under nervus.

**fila radicula'ria** [ NA ], root filaments; nerve rootlets; the small, individual fiber fascicles into which the roots of all of the spinal nerves and several cranial nerves (hypoglossus, vagus, oculomotorius) divide in fanlike fashion before entering or leaving the spinal cord or brainstem; the spinal dorsal root may divide into 8 to 12 such rootlets.

**terminal f.,** f. terminale.

**f. termina'le** [ NA ], terminal f.; terminal thread; nervus impar; a long, slender connective tissue strand extending from the extremity of the conus medullaris to the termination of the spinal canal.

**fimbria,** pl. **fimbriae** (fim'brĭ-ah, fim'brĭ-e) [ L. fringe ]. 1 [ NA ]. Any fringelike structure. 2. Pilus (2).

**f. hippocam'pi** [ NA ], corpus fimbriatum (1); tenia hippocampi; a narrow, sharp-edged crest of white matter, continuous with the alveus, attached to the medial border of the hippocampus; it is composed of (1) efferent fibers of the hippocampus that eventually come to form the fornix, (2) fibers of the hippocampal commissure, and (3) septohippocampal fibers.

**f. ova'rica** [ NA ], the longest of the fimbriae at the distal end of the uterine tube.

**fimbriae tubae uteri'nae** [ NA ], the irregularly branched or fringed processes surrounding the abdominal opening of the uterine tube; most of the epithelial cells have cilia which beat toward the uterus.

**fim'briate, fim'briated.** Having fimbriae.

**fimbriectomy** (fim'brĭ-ek'to-mĭ) [ L. *fimbria*, fringe, + G. *ektomē*, excision ]. Excision of fimbriae.

**fimbriocele** (fim'brĭ-o-sēl) [ *fimbria*, fringe, + G. *kēlē*, hernia ]. A hernia of the corpus fimbriatum of the oviduct.

**fim'brioplasty** [ L. *fimbria*, fringe, + G. *plastos*, formed ]. A corrective operation upon the tubal fimbriae.

**Finckh,** Johann, German psychiatrist, 1873. See F. *test*.

**fine'ness.** A designator used to indicate gold content of an alloy, 1000 fine being 24-carat or pure gold.

**fin'ger** [ A.S. ]. One of the digits of the hand; *digitus* manus.

**baseball f.,** (1) dislocation of the terminal phalanx dorsally, the flexor tendons holding it in the false position by wrapping themselves around the head of the second phalanx; the latter is buttonholed through the capsule of the joint; (2) another term used for hammer f.; implies causation rather than description of f.

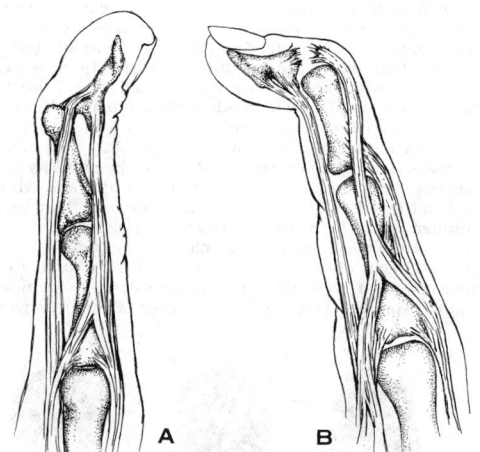

Baseball Finger (*A*) and Hammer Finger (*B*)

**bolster f.,** monilial infection of nail fold.

**clubbed f.'s,** clubbed *digits*.

**dead f.'s,** waxy f.'s; acroasphyxia; impaired digital circulation, possibly a mild form of Raynaud's disease, marked by a purplish or waxy white color of the f.'s, with subnormal local temperature and paresthesia.

**drop f.,** flexion of the terminal phalanx of a f., with loss of the power of extension, due to rupture of the extensor tendon near its insertion at the base of the distal phalanx, or to paralysis of the extensor muscle.

**drumstick f.'s,** clubbed *digits*.

**fifth f.,** *digitus* minimus.

**first f.,** thumb; pollex.

**fourth f.,** *digitus* anularis.

**hammer f.,** mallet f.; flexion at the distal interphalangeal joint of a f. due to detachment of the extensor tendon as a result of a blow on the tip of the f. when extended. See fig. under baseball f.

**Hippocratic f.'s,** clubbed *digits.*

**index f.,** index (1).

**jerk f.,** trigger f.

**little f.,** *digitus* minimus.

**lock f.,** trigger f.

**mallet f.,** hammer f.

**middle f.,** *digitus* medius.

**Morse f.,** telegrapher's *cramp.*

**ring f.,** *digitus* anularis.

**sausage f.'s,** the thick, short f.'s of acromegaly.

**second f.,** index (1).

**snap f.,** trigger f.

**spade f.'s,** the course, thick f.'s of acromegaly or myxedema.

**spider f.,** arachnodactyly.

**spring f.,** trigger f.

**stuck f.,** trigger f.

**third f.,** *digitus* medius.

**trigger f.,** an affection in which the movement of the f. is arrested for a moment in flexion or extension and then continues with a jerk. Also variously known as jerk f., lock f., snap f., spring f., stuck f., and digitus recellens.

**waxy f.'s,** dead f.'s.

**webbed f.'s,** two or more f.'s united and enclosed in a common sheath of skin.

**white f.'s,** an occupational disease occurring in operators of pneumatic hammers who are exposed to cold, affecting usually the f.'s of the left hand.

**fingeragnosia** (fing'ger-ag-no'sĭ-ah) [ finger + agnosia, *q.v.* ]. The inability to recognize the individual fingers of the hand or distinguish the one that is being tactually stimulated.

**fin'gernail.** See unguis.

**fin'gerprint.** An impression of the inked bulb of the distal phalanx of a finger, showing the configuration of the ridges, used as a means of identification; see also dermatoglyphics, Galton's system of classification of f.'s. 2. Terms sometimes used, informally, with reference to any analytical method capable of making fine distinctions between similar compounds. Thus, the pattern of an infrared absorption curve or of a two-dimensional paper chromatograph may be so referred to.

**Galton's system of classification of f.'s,** a system of classification based on the variations in the patterns of the ridges, which are grouped into arches, loops, and whorls; called the A.L.W. or arch-loop-whorl system. "Arches are formed when the ridges run from one side to the other of the bulb of the digit, without making any backward turn, but no twist; whorls, when there is a turn through at least one complete circle; they are also considered to include all duplex spirals." The abbreviations used in making a record

**Fingerprints**

*1* and *2,* loops showing Galton's delta; *3,* arches; *4,* whorls; *5,* circles; *6,* showing the mark of a scar.

of f.'s are: *a,* arch; *l,* loop; *w,* whorl; *i,* loop with an inner (thumb side) slope; *o,* loop with an outer (little-finger side) slope. The ten digits are registered in four groups as follows; distinguished by capital letters: *A,* the fore, middle, and ring fingers of the right hand; *C,* the thumb and little finger of the right hand; *D,* the thumb and little finger of the left hand.

**Finkeldey,** W. See Wharthin-F. *cells.*

**Finney,** John M. T., Baltimore surgeon, 1863–1942. See F.'s *operation, pyloroplasty.*

**Finsen,** Niels R., Danish physician, 1860–1904. Nobel laureate, 1903, for his contribution to the treatment of diseases, especially lupus vulgaris, with concentrated light radiation. See F. *light.*

**Finsterer's operation.** See under operation.

**Fiocca,** Rufino, Italian physician, 19th century. See F.'s *stain.*

**fir.** Abies.

**fire.** In dermatology, erysipelas.

**St. Francis' f.,** erysipelas.

**fire'damp.** Methane (marsh gas) or other light hydrocarbons forming an explosive mixture with the oxygen of the air.

**first aid.** Immediate assistance given in the case of injury or sudden illnes by a bystander or other lay person, before the arrival of the physician.

**Fischer,** Emil, German chemist, 1852–1919. See F. projection formulas of sugars (under *sugars*).

**Fischer,** Louis, New York pediatrician, 1864–1944. See F.'s cerebral *murmur, symptom, sign.*

**Fischer's needle.** See under needle.

**Fisher's syndrome.** See under syndrome.

**fission** (fish'un) [ L. *fissio,* a cleaving, fr. *findo,* pp. *fissus,* to cleave. FIS- ]. 1. The act of splitting, *e.g.,* amitotic division of a cell or its nucleus. 2. Splitting of the nucleus of an atom.

**bi'nary f.,** simple f. in which the two new cells are approximately equal in size.

**bud f.,** gemmation.

**multiple f.,** sporulation; division of the nucleus, simultaneously or successively, into a number of daughter nuclei, followed by division of the cell body into an equal number of parts, each containing a nucleus.

**simple f.,** division of the nucleus and then the cell body into two parts; see also binary f.

**fissiparity** (fis'ĭ-păr'ĭ-tĭ) [ L. *findo,* pp. *fissus,* split; + *pario,* pp. *paritus,* to bring forth ]. Schizogenesis.

**fissip'arous** [ L. *fissus; findere,* to cleave, + *pario,* to produce ]. Reproducing or propagating by fission.

**Fissipe'dia** [ L. *fissus,* cloven, + *pes* (*ped*-), foot ]. A suborder of the carnivora with separated toes, *e.g.,* dogs, cats, bears.

# FISSURA

**fissura,** pl. **fissur'ae** (fis-su'rah) [ L. fr. *findo,* to cleave. FIS- ] [ NA ]. Fissure (*q.v.*); a deep cleft; in neuroanatomy, a particularly deep sulcus of the surface of the brain or spinal cord.

**f. antitragohelici'na** [ NA ], antitragohelicine fissure; a fissure in the auricular cartilage between the cauda helicis and the antitragus.

**f. calcari'na,** *sulcus* calcarinus.

**fissurae cerebel'li** [ NA ], cerebellar fissures; the deep furrows between the lobules of the cerebellum. See also postcentral *fissure;* f. prima; f. secunda.

**f. cer'ebri latera'lis,** *sulcus* lateralis cerebri.

**f. choroi'dea** [ NA ], choroid fissure (1); the narrow cleft along the medial wall of the lateral ventricle along the margins of which the choroid plexus is attached; it lies between the upper surface of the thalamus and lateral edge of the fornix in the central part of the ventricle and between the stria terminalis and fimbria hippocampi in the inferior horn.

**f. collatera'lis,** *sulcus* collateralis.

**f. dentata,** *sulcus* hippocampi.

**f. hippocampi,** *sulcus* hippocampi.

**f. horizonta'lis cerebel'li** [ NA ], horizontal fissure of the cerebellum; great horizontal fissure; a deep cleft encircling the circumference of the cerebellum.

**f. horizonta'lis pulmonis dextri** [ NA ], horizontal fissure of right lung; the deep fissure that separates the upper and middle lobes of the right lung.

**f. ligamen'ti tere'tis** [ NA ], fissure of the round ligament; fissure for ligamentum teres; umbilical fissure; a shallow groove on the inferior surface of the liver, running from the inferior border to the left extremity of the porta hepatis. It lodges the ligamentum teres.

**f. ligamen'ti veno'si** [ NA ], fissure of the venous ligament; a deep cleft on the posterior surface of the liver between the left lobe and the caudate lobe; it lodges the ligamentum venosum—the remnant of the ductus venosus.

**f. longitudina'lis cer'ebri** [ NA ], longitudinal fissure of the cerebrum; great longitudinal fissure; a deep cleft separating the two hemispheres of the cerebrum, but bridged by the corpus callosum and hippocampal commissure.

**f. media'na ante'rior medul'lae oblonga'tae** [ NA ], anterior median fissure or anteromedian groove of the medulla oblongata; the longitudinal groove in the midline of the anterior aspect of the medulla oblongata; it is continuous with the f. mediana anterior of the spinal cord. It ends at the lower border of the pons in the foramen cecum. Its lower part is largely obliterated by the decussation of the pyramids.

**f. media'na ante'rior medul'lae spina'lis** [ NA ], anterior median fissure or anteromedian groove of the spinal cord; sulcus ventralis; a deep fissure in the median line of the anterior surface of the spinal cord.

**f. obliqua** [ NA ], oblique fissure; the deep fissure in each lung that runs obliquely downward and forward. It divides the upper and lower lobes of the left lung and separates the upper and middle lobes from the lower lobe of the right lung.

**f. orbita'lis inferior** [ NA ], inferior orbital fissure; sphenomaxillary fissure; a cleft between the greater wing of the sphenoid and the orbital plate of the maxilla, through which pass the maxillary division of the fifth nerve, the orbital branch of the same, fibers from pterygopalatine (Meckel's) or sphenopa ganglion, and the infraorbital vessels.

**f. orbita'lis superior** [ NA ], superior orbital fissure; sphenoidal fissure; foramen lacerum anterius; a cleft between the greater and the lesser wing of the sphenoid establishing a channel of communication between the middle cranial fossa and the orbit, through which pass the third, fourth, ophthalmic division of the fifth, and the sixth cranial nerves, and the ophthalmic veins.

**f. parietooccipita'lis,** *sulcus* parietooccipitalis.

**f. petrooccipita'lis** [ NA ], occipital fissure; Ecker's fissure; a fissure passing backward from the foramen lacerum between the outer side of the basioccipital and the posterior and medial border of the petrous portion of the temporal bone.

**f. petrosquamo'sa** [ NA ], petrosquamous fissure; a shallow fissure indicating externally the line of fusion of the petrous and squamous portions of the temporal bone.

**f. petrotympan'ica** [ NA ], petrotympanic fissure; Glaserian fissure; a fissure between the tympanic and petrous portions of the temporal bone; it transmits the chorda tympani nerve.

**f. posterolatera'lis** [ NA ], posterolateral fissure; the earliest fissure to appear in the development of the cerebellum; it separates the flocculus and nodulus from the uvula and tonsil.

**f. pri'ma cerebel'li** [ NA ], primary fissure; a deep V-shaped fissure that marks the superior surface of the cerebellum and demarcates the anterior lobe from the rest of the cerebellum.

**f. pterygoid'ea,** *incisura* pterygoidea.

**f. pterygomaxilla'ris** [ NA ], pterygomaxillary fissure; the narrow gap between the lateral pterygoid plate and the maxilla through which the infratemporal fossa communicates with the pterygopalatine fossa.

**f. pterygopalati'na,** f. pterygomaxillaris.

**f. puden'di,** *rima* pudendi.

**f. secun'da cerebel'li** [ NA ], secondary fissure; a fissure that separates the uvula of the inferior vermis of the cerebellum from the pyramid.

**f. sphenopetro'sa** [ NA ], sphenopetrosal fissure; a narrow fissure between the under surface of the great wing of the sphenoid and the petrous portion of the temporal bone.

**f. transver'sa cerebel'li,** transverse fissure of the cerebellum; the cleft caused by the protrusion of the anterior lobe of the cerebellum over the superior and middle cerebellar peduncles.

**f. transver'sa cer'ebri** [ NA ], transverse fissure of the cerebrum; the space between the corpus callosum and fornix above, and the dorsal surface of the thalamus below, bounded laterally by the choroid fissure of the lateral ventricle, lined by pia mater, and opening caudally below the splenium of the corpus callosum into the cisterna ambiens of the subarachnoid space.

**f. tympanomastoid'ea** [ NA ], tympanomastoid fissure; a fissure separating the tympanic portion from the mastoid portion of the temporal bone; it transmits the auricular branch of the vagus nerve.

**f. tympanosquamo'sa** [ NA ], tympanosquamous fissure; the fissure separating the tympanic part of the temporal bone from the squamous part. It is continuous medially with the petrotympanic fissure and the petrosquamous fissure.

**fissural** (fish'ur-al). Relating to a fissure.

**fissuration** (fish'ur-a'shun). State of being fissured.

# FISSURE

**fissure** (fish'ur) [ L. *fissura* ]. 1. A deep furrow, cleft, or slit. For the normal anatomical f.'s, see fissura; for most of the brain f.'s, see sulcus. 2. In dentistry, a developmental break or fault in the enamel of a tooth.

**abdominal f.,** congenital failure to close the ventral body wall; see also celosomia.

**anal f.,** fissure-in-ano; a crack or slit in the mucous membrane of the anus, very painful and difficult to heal.

**anterior median f. of medulla oblongata,** *fissura* mediana anterior medullae oblongatae.

**anterior median f. of spinal cord,** *fissura* mediana anterior medullae spinalis.

**antitragohel'icine f.,** *fissura* antitragohelicina.

**ape f.,** *sulcus* lunatus cerebri.

**auricular f.,** *fissura* tympanomastoidea.

**Bichat's f.,** the nearly circular f. corresponding to the medial margin of the cerebral (pallial) mantle, marking the hilus of the cerebral hemisphere, consisting of the fissura (sulcus) callosomarginalis and fissura choroidea along the hippocampus, both of which are continuous with the stem of the f. of Sylvius at the anterior extremity of the temporal lobe.

**branchial f.,** a persistent branchial cleft.

**Broca's f.,** the f. surrounding Broca's convolution.

**calcarine f.,** *sulcus* calcarinus.

**callosomarginal f.,** *sulcus* cinguli.

**cerebellar f.'s,** *fissurae* cerebelli.

**cerebral f.'s,** see separately named f.'s, also sulci.

**choroid f.,** (1) *fissura* choroidea; (2) in the embryo the temporary gap in the ventral margin of the developing optic cup.

**Clevenger's f.,** *sulcus* temporalis inferior.

**collateral f.,** *sulcus* collateralis.

**decidual f.,** a cleft in the decidua basalis or placenta.

**dentate f.,** *sulcus* hippocampi.

**Duverney's f.,** *incisura* cartilaginis meatus acustici externi.

**Ecker's f.,** *fissura* petrooccipitalis.

**enamel f.,** a deep cleft between adjoining cusps affording retention to caries-producing agents.

**Glaserian f.,** *fissura* petrotympanica.

**great horizontal f.,** *fissura* horizontalis cerebelli.

**great longitudinal f.,** *fissura* longitudinalis cerebri.

**Henle's f.'s.** minute spaces filled with connective tissue between the muscular fasciculi of the heart.

**hippocampal f.,** *sulcus* hippocampi.

**horizontal f. of cerebellum,** *fissura* horizontalis cerebelli.

**horizontal f. of right lung,** *fissura* horizontalis pulmonis dextri.

**inferior orbital f.,** *fissura* orbitalis inferior.

**lateral cerebral f.,** *sulcus* lateralis cerebri.

**f. for ligamentum teres,** *fissura* ligamenti teretis.

**linguogingival f.,** a f. sometimes occurring on the lingual surface of one of the upper incisors and extending into the cementum.

**f.'s of liver,** five in number: (1) umbilical; (2) of the ductus venosus (these two constituting the left sagittal f.); (3) portal or porta hepatis; (4) for the vena cava; (5) for the gallbladder (these two constituting the right sagittal f.); see also under fossa and porta hepatis.

**longitudinal f. of cerebrum,** *fissura* longitudinalis cerebri.

**lunate f.,** *sulcus* lunatus cerebri.

**f.'s of lung,** see *fissura* horizontalis and *fissura* obliqua.

**oblique f.,** *fissura* obliqua.

**occipital f.,** *fissura* petrooccipitalis.

**oral f.,** *rima* oris.

**palpebral f.,** *rima* palpebrarum.

**Pansch's f.,** a cerebral f. running from the lower extremity of the central f. nearly to the end of the occipital lobe.

**paracentral f.,** a curved f. on the medial surface of the cerebral hemisphere, bounding the paracentral gyrus and separating it from the precuneus and the gyrus cinguli.

**parietooccipital f.,** *sulcus* parietooccipitalis.

**petrosquamous f.,** *fissura* petrosquamosa.

**petrotympanic f.,** *fissura* petrotympanica.

**postcentral f.,** a f. on the superior surface of the cerebellum that separates the culmen (lobulus culminis) from the central lobule.

**posterior median f. of the medulla oblongata,** *sulcus* medianus posterior medullae oblongatae.

**posterior median f. of spinal cord,** *sulcus* medianus posterior medullae spinalis.

**posterolateral f.,** *fissura* posterolateralis.

**posthippocampal f.,** *sulcus* calcarinus.

**postlingual f.,** a transverse f. on the superior vermis of the cerebellum separating the lingula from the central lobule.

**postlunate f.,** a transverse f. on the superior vermis of the cerebellum separating the posterior lunate lobule in front from the ansiform lobule behind.

**postpyramidal f.,** a f. that separates the pyramid of the cerebellum from the tuber.

**postrhinal f.,** a f. separating the hippocampal from the collateral gyrus.

**primary f.,** *fissura* prima cerebelli.

**pterygoid f.,** *incisura* pterygoidea.

**pterygomaxillary f.,** *fissura* pterygomaxillaris.

**rhinal f.,** *sulcus* rhinalis.

**Rolando's f.,** *sulcus* centralis.

**f. of round ligament,** *fissura* ligamenti teretis.

**Santorini's f.'s,** *incisura* cartilaginis meatus acustici externi.

**secondary f.,** *fissura* secunda cerebelli.

**simian f.,** *sulcus* lunatus cerebri.

**sphenoidal f.,** *fissura* orbitalis superior.

**sphenomaxillary f.,** *fissura* orbitalis inferior.

**sphenopetrosal f.,** *fissura* sphenopetrosa.

**squamotympanic f.,** *fissura* tympanosquamosa.

**superior orbital f.,** *fissura* orbitalis superior.

**supertemporal f.,** *sulcus* temporalis superior.

**f. of Sylvius,** *sulcus* lateralis cerebri.

**temporal f.,** *sulcus* temporalis.

**transverse f. of cerebellum,** *fissura* transversa cerebelli.

**transverse f. of cerebrum,** *fissura* transversa cerebri.

**transverse f. of the lung,** *fissura* horizontalis pulmonis dextri.

**tympanomastoid f.,** *fissura* tympanomastoidea.

**tympanosquamous f.,** *fissura* tympanosquamosa.

**umbilical f.,** *fissura* ligamenti teretis.

**f. of venous ligament,** *fissura* ligamenti venosi.

**vestibular f. of cochlea,** in the lower part of the first turn of the cochlea, a fine f. formed by a spiral lamina which projects from the outer wall of the cochlea but does not quite reach the osseous spiral lamina, thus leaving a narrow gap.

**zygal f.,** a figure formed by two nearly parallel cerebral f.'s connected by a short f. at right angles, forming an H.

# FISTULA

**fistula,** pl. **fistulae** or **fistulas** (fis'tu-lah) [ L. a pipe, a tube. FIS- ]. A pathologic sinus or abnormal passage leading from an abscess cavity or a hollow organ to the surface, or from one abscess cavity or organ to another.

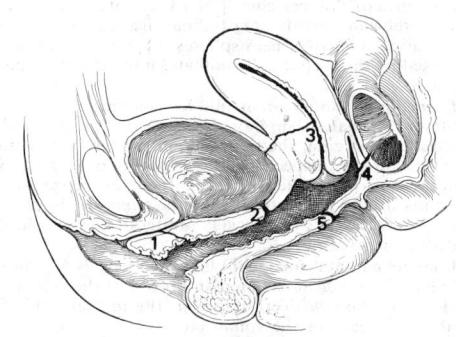

**Fistulas**
*1,* Urethrovaginal; *2,* vesicovaginal; *3,* vesicouterine; *4,* enterovaginal; *5,* rectovaginal.

**abdominal f.,** a tract leading from one of the abdominal viscera to the external surface.

**amphibol'ic f., amphib'olous f.,** a complete f.; an anal f. opening both externally and internally.

**anal f.,** a f. opening at or near the anus; usually, but not always, opening into the rectum above the internal sphincter.

**arteriovenous f.,** an abnormal communication between an artery and a vein, usually resulting in the formation of an arteriovenous aneurysm.

**f. au'ris congen'ita,** a congenital f. resulting from a defect in the formation of the auricle of the ear.

**biliary f.,** a f. leading to the gallbladder or other portion of the biliary tract.

**f. bimuco'sa,** (1) a complete f., both ends of which open on the mucous surface; (2) perforation into two neighboring intestinal coils in certain cases of peritonitis.

**blind f.,** incomplete f.; one that ends in a cul-de-sac, being open at one extremity only.

**bran'chial f.,** a congenital f. in the neck resulting from incomplete closure of a branchial cleft.

**bronchoesophageal f.,** communication between a bronchus and the esophagus; may occur in association with either infection or tumors involving a bronchus or the esophagus.

**bronchopleural f.,** communication between a bronchus and a collection of pus in the pleural cavity; usually results from rupture of a neglected pleural collection into the lung substance.

**carotid-cavernous f.,** arteriovenous communication resulting from rupture of the intracavernous portion of the carotid artery.

**cervical f.,** a f. that opens in the midline of the neck and is caused by suppuration and rupture of a thyroglossal cyst.

**f. cer'vicovagina'lis laquea'ta** [ L. *laqueatus*, paneled ]. a fistulous communication between the uterine cervical canal and the vagina.

**cholecystoduodenal f.,** communication between gallbladder and duodenum secondary to severe cholecystitis with perforation and abscess formation; stones erode through adjacent duodenal wall; x-rays may show air in biliary passages; large stones may cause obstruction of the small intestine (*i.e.*, "gallstone ileus").

**coccyg'eal f.,** a fistulous opening of a dermoid cyst in the coccygeal region.

**f. colli congen'ita,** a congenital f. of the neck leading to the pharynx, larynx, or trachea.

**co'locuta'neous f.,** one between colon and skin.

**co'loil'eal f.,** one between colon and ileum.

**colonic f.,** (1) internal, between colon and a hollow viscus; (2) external, between colon and skin.

**co'lovag'inal f.,** a f. between colon and vagina.

**co'loves'ical f.,** vesicocolonic f.; a f. between colon and urinary bladder.

**complete f.,** one that is open at both ends.

**f. cor'neae,** a f. resulting from an unhealed wound in the cornea, the external opening usually being covered with conjunctiva.

**craniosinus f.,** one between the cerebral space and a nasal sinus.

**dental f.,** f. gingivalis.

**duodenal f.,** an opening through the duodenal wall leading into the peritoneal cavity, into another organ, or through the abdominal wall, due to disease or disruption of a surgical closure.

**Eck f.,** shutting off the liver of an experimental animal from the portal circulation by making an anastomosis between the vena cava and portal vein and then ligating the latter close to the liver.

**enterocutaneous f.,** a f. between intestine and skin of abdomen.

**enterovag'inal f.,** a fistulous passage connecting some portion of the intestine and the vagina.

**enteroves'ical f.,** a f. connecting the intestine and the bladder.

**external f.,** a f. between a hollow viscus and the skin.

**fecal f.,** an intestinal f.

**gastric f.,** a fistulous tract leading from the abdominal wall into the stomach.

**gastrocol'ic f.,** a fistulous communication between the stomach and the colon; usually resulting from penetration of a gastrojejunal ulcer recurrent at the site of a retrocolic gastrojejunostomy.

**gastrocuta'neous f.,** one between stomach and skin.

**gastroduode'nal f.,** an abnormal opening between the stomach and the duodenum.

**gastrointes'tinal f.,** a fistulous tract connecting the stomach with any portion of the intestine.

**genitou'rinary f.,** urogenital f.; a fistulous opening into any portion of the urogenital tract.

**gingival f.,** f. gingivalis.

**f. gingiva'lis,** dental f.; gingival f.; a tract leading from a chronic apical abscess to a gingival surface.

**hepatic f.,** a f. leading to the liver.

**hep'atopleu'ral f.,** a f. between liver and pleura.

**horseshoe f.,** an anal f. partially encircling the anus and opening at both extremities on the cutaneous surface.

**incomplete f.,** blind f.

**internal f.,** a f. between hollow viscera.

**intestinal f.,** fecal f.; stercoral f.; a tract leading from the lumen of the bowel to the exterior; may develop following any process which produces a perforation of the intestine, *i.e.*, regional enteritis, carcinoma, diverticulitis, foreign bodies.

**lacrimal f.,** fistula lacrimalis; dacryosyrinx; a f. opening into a tear duct or the lacrimal sac.

**lacteal f.,** mammary f.; a fistulous opening into one of the lacteal ducts.

**lymphatic f.,** fistula lymphatica; a congenital f. in the neck connecting with a lymphatic vessel and giving exit to lymph.

**Mann-Bollman f.,** used in experimental investigations. A loop of ileum is isolated, the distal (aboral) end is anastomosed laterally to and communicating with the duodenum or other part of the small intestine; the open proximal (oral) end is sutured to the abdominal wall. Peristaltic waves travel from oral to aboral end; leakage to the exterior is thus reduced to a minimum.

**met'roperitone'al f.,** uteroperitoneal f.

**oroantral f.,** communication between the maxillary antrum and the mouth, most common over the first or second upper molar tooth; usually a complication of dental extraction or maxillary sinus infection.

**orofacial f.,** an opening between the cutaneous surface of the face and the oral cavity.

**oronasal f.,** an opening between the nasal cavity and the oral cavity.

**pari'etal f.,** thoracic f.; a f., either blind or complete, opening on the wall of the thorax or abdomen.

**perineovag'inal f.,** a f. through the perineum, opening into the vagina.

**pharyn'geal f.,** a form of f. colli congenita.

**piloni'dal f.,** pilonidal *sinus*.

**pul'monary f.,** a parietal f. communicating with the lung.

**rectola'bial f.,** rectovulvar f.; one opening into the rectum and on the surface of a labium majus.

**rectoure'thral f.,** one connecting the rectum and the urethra.

**rectovag'inal f.,** a fistulous opening between the rectum and the vagina.

**rectoves'ical f.,** a fistulous communication between the rectum and the bladder.

**rectovestib'ular f.,** a f. between rectum and vestibule.

**rectovul'var f.,** rectolabial f.

**reverse Eck f.,** anastomosis of the portal vein with the inferior vena cava and ligation of the latter above the anastomosis but below the hepatic veins. The blood from the lower part of the body is thus directed through the hepatic circulation.

**sal'ivary f.,** an opening between a salivary duct or gland and the cutaneous surface, or into the oral cavity through other than the normal anatomical pathway.

**sigmoidovesical f.,** a f. between sigmoid colon and urinary bladder.

**spermat'ic f.,** a f. communicating with the testis or any of the seminal passages.

**ster'coral f.,** intestinal f.

**Thiry's f.,** an artificial f. for collecting the intestinal juice of a dog or other animal for experimental purposes. A loop of intestine is isolated, its vascular and nervous connections being preserved, the continuity of the intestinal tract being restored by anastomosis; one end of the isolated segment is closed, the other attached to the skin of the abdomen.

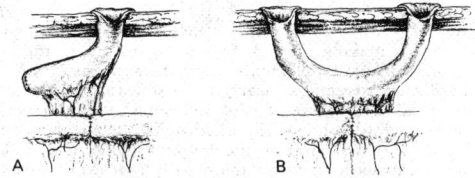

**Fistulas for the Study of Intestinal Motility**
*A*, Thiry; *B*, Thiry-Vella; see also fig. under Biebl *loop*. (From Youmans, W. B., *Nervous and Neurohumoral Regulation of Intestinal Motility*, Monographs in the Physiological Sciences, Interscience Publishers, Inc., New York, 1949. Used with permission.)

**Thiry-Vella f.,** Vella's f.; experimental isolation of a segment of intestine in a dog or other animal, the mesenteric attachment being preserved; the divided ends of the intestine at each end of the segment are joined by anastomosis, and the ends of the segment itself are stitched to openings in the abdominal wall.

**thorac'ic f.,** parietal f.

**tra'cheal f.,** a form of f. colli congenita.

**tracheobiliary f.,** a rare congenital anastomosis between an accessory bronchus and aberrant biliary duct system.

**tracheoesophageal f.,** congenital abnormality involving a communication between the trachea and esophagus; often associated with esophageal atresia; may also be acquired; in the adult the etiology is similar to that of bronchoesophageal f.

**umbilical f.,** a f. of intestine or urachus at the umbilicus.

**u'rachal f.,** a f. connecting the urachus with the rectum or other hollow organ.

**u'rinary f.,** f. urinaria; a f. of any part of the urinary tract.

**urogen'ital f.,** genitourinary f.

**uteroperitoneal f.,** metroperitoneal f.; a fistulous tract through the uterine wall opening into the peritoneal cavity.

**Vella's f.,** Thiry-Vella f.

**vesical f.,** one from the urinary bladder.

**vesicocolonic f.,** colovesical f.

**vesicointestinal f.,** a f. between urinary bladder and small intestine.

**vesicovaginal f.,** f. between bladder and vagina.

**vesicovaginorectal f.,** an abnormal opening between the vagina and the bladder and rectum; obstetrical trauma, malignant lesions of the lower generative tract, or radiotherapy may be antecedent causal factors.

**vitelline f.,** a f. between the umbilicus and the terminal ileum along the course of a persistent vitelline cord.

---

**fistula'tion, fistuliza'tion.** Formation of a fistula in a part; becoming fistulous.

**fis'tulatome** [ fistula + G. *tomē*, a cutting ]. Syringotome; fistula knife; a long, thin-bladed, probe-pointed knife for slitting up a fistula.

**fistulat'omy.** Fistulotomy.

**fistulectomy** (fis'tu-lek'to-mĭ) [ fistula + G. *ektomē*, excision ]. Syringectomy; excision of the walls of a fistula.

**fistuloenterostomy** (fis'tu-lo-en'ter-os'to-mĭ) [ fistula + G. *enteron*, intestine, + *stoma*, mouth ]. An operation connecting a fistula with the intestine.

**fistulotomy** (fis'tu-lot'o-mĭ) [ fistula + G. *tomē*, incision ]. Fistulatomy; syringotomy; incision or surgical enlargement of a fistula.

**fis'tulous.** Relating to or containing a fistula.

**fit** [ A.S. *fitt* ]. 1. An attack of an acute disease, or the sudden appearance of some symptom, such as coughing. 2. A convulsion. 3. In dentistry, the adaptation of any dental restoration, *viz.*, of an inlay to the cavity preparation in a tooth, or of a denture to its basal seat.

**ether f.,** ether *epilepsy.*

**fit'ness.** 1. Well-being. 2 Suitability.

**physical f.,** a state of well-being in which performance is optimal.

**Fitz-Hugh,** T., Jr., U. S. physician, 1894–1963. See F.-H. and Curtis *syndrome.*

**fixa'tion** [ L. *figo*, pp. *fixus*, to fix, fasten ]. 1. The condition of being fixed or firmly attached or set. 2. The art of fixing or making firm. 3. Fixing; in histology, the rapid killing of tissue elements and their preservation and hardening, to retain as nearly as possible the same relations they had in the living body. 4. In chemistry, the conversion of a gas into solid or liquid form by chemical reactions either with or without the help of living tissue. Thus nitrogen can be fixed by union with hydrogen under heat and pressure to form first ammonia and then solid ammonium salts; or by more complex reactions under the influence of nitrogen fixing bacteria, to form amino acids. 5. In psychoanalysis, the quality of being firmly attached or fixed to a particular person or object; the arrest of development at a particular psychosexual stage. 6. A close and paralyzing attachment to another person, such as mother or father. 7. In ophthalmology and neurology, the coordinated positioning and accommodation of both eyes that results in bringing or maintaining a sharp image of a stationary or moving object on the fovea of both eyes.

**binocular f.,** both eyes directed to the same target at the same time.

**complement f.,** see under complement.

**elastic band f.,** the stabilization of fractured segments of the jaws by means of intermaxillary elastics applied to splints or appliances.

**external pin f.,** in oral surgery, stabilization of fractures with pins drilled into the bony part through the overlying skin and connected by a metal bar.

**external pin f., biphase,** pin f. by replacing the rigid metal bar connector with an acrylic bar adapted at the time of the reduction.

**field of f.,** the angular distance around which the line of f. can be turned.

**Freudian f.,** see fixation (5).

**intermaxillary f.,** maxillomandibular f.

**internal f.,** f. of fractured bone by metallic substances applied directly to the bone.

**intraosseous f.,** stabilization of fractured bony parts by direct f. to one another with surgical wires, screws, pins, or plates.

**line of f.,** a line joining the object or the f. point) with the fovea and passing through the nodal point.

**mandibulomaxillary f.,** maxillomandibular f.

**maxillomandibular f.,** intermaxillary f.; mandibulomaxillary f.; the f. of fractures of the maxillae or mandible in a functional relationship with the opposing dental arch by using elastics, wire ligatures, arch bars, or other splints.

**mother f.,** inordinate attachment of child to mother.

**nasomandibular f.,** mandibular immobilization, especially for edentulous jaws, with maxillomandibular splints, attached by connecting a circum-mandibular wire with an intraoral interosseous wire passed through a hole drilled into the anterior nasal spine of the maxillae.

**fix'ative.** 1. Serving to fix, bind, or make firm or stable. 2. A substance used for the preservation of gross and histologic specimens of tissue, or individual cells, usually by denaturing and precipitating or cross-linking the protein constituents; see also fluid and solution.

**Park-Williams f.,** for spirochetes; expose for a few seconds to the fumes of a 2 per cent solution of osmic acid.

**Schaudinn's f.,** a solution especially useful in fixing and staining protozoa in small "bulk" specimens: saturated mercuric chloride in 0.85 per cent aqueous solution of sodium chloride 2 parts, plus 95 per cent or absolute alcohol 1 part; immediately prior to use, glacial acetic acid is added, to a final concentration of 1 per cent.

**van Gehuchten's f.,** a solution consisting of water 250, osmic acid 0.5, potassium dichromate 6.

**fix'ing.** Fixation (3).

**flaccid** (flak'sid, flas'id) [ L. *flaccidus* ]. Relaxed; flabby; without tone.

**Flack,** Martin, English physiologist, 1882–1931. See F.'s *node*, Keith and F. *node.*

**flagecidin.** Anisomycin.

**flagella** (fla-jĕl'ah). Plural of flagellum.

**flagellar** (flă-jel'ar). Relating to a flagellum or to the extremity of a protozoan.

**Flagellata** (flaj'ĕ-la'tah). Flagellate protozoans (commonly termed flagellates) or Mastigophora; a class (or superclass) of protozoans provided with one or more flagella; includes parasitic forms such as the trypanosomes and the leishmaniae.

**flagellate** (flaj'ĕ-lāt). 1. Possessing one or more flagella. 2. Common name for a member of the Flagellata.

**collared f.,** one of the choanoflagellates.

**flagellated** (flaj'ĕ-la-ted). Possessing one or more flagella.

**flagellation** (flaj'ĕ-la'shun) [ L. *flagellatus*, fr. *flagellāre*, to whip or scourge ]. Whipping either one's self or another as a means of arousing or heightening sexual feeling.

**flagellin** flaj'el-lin). A protein with a molecular weight of about 20,000 and containing the amino acid, $\epsilon$ -$N$-methyllysine; found in the flagella of bacteria.

**flagellosis** (flaj'ĕ-lo'sis). Infection with flagellated protozoa in the intestinal or genital tract, *e.g.*, trichomoniasis.

**flagellum,** pl. **flagella** (flă-jel'um) [ L. a whip, dim. of *flagrum*, a whip ]. A whiplike locomotory organelle of constant structural arrangment consisting of nine double peripheral microtubules and two single central microtubules (as seen under the electron microscope). The f. arises from a deeply staining basal granule, often connected to the nucleus by a fiber, the rhizoplast. Though characteristic of the protozoan class Mastigophora, comparable structures are commonly found in many other groups, *e.g.*, in spermatozoa.

**flammabil'ity.** Inflammability; the property of burning readily and quickly; to be differentiated from explosibility, the property of detonating.

**flange.** That part of the denture base which extends from the cervical ends of the teeth to the border of the denture.

**buccal f.,** the portion of the f. of a denture that occupies the buccal vestibule of the mouth.

**denture f.,** (1) the essentially vertical extension from the body of the denture into one of the vestibules of the oral cavity. Also, on the lower denture, the essentially vertical extension along the lingual side of the alveololingual sulcus; (2) the buccal and labial vertical extension of upper or lower denture base, and the lingual vertical extension of the lower one. The buccal and labial denture f.'s have two surfaces: the buccal or labial surface and the basal seat surface. The lower lingual f. also has two surfaces: the basal seat surface and the lingual surface.

**labial f.,** the portion of the f. of a denture which occupies the labial vestibule of the mouth.

**lingual f.,** the portion of the f. of a mandibular denture that occupies the space adjacent to the tongue.

**flank.** Latus.

**flap.** 1. A tongue or lip of tissue, cut away from the underlying parts but attached at one end; used in plastic surgery for filling a defect in a neighboring region, or to cover the cut end of the bone after amputation. 2. A peculiar flapping movement of the hands; see asterixis.

**bone f.,** in neurosurgery, attached *craniotomy.*

**cellulocutaneous f.,** a f. of skin and subcutaneous tissue.

**envelope f.,** a f. of mucoperiosteal tissues retracted from a horizontal linear incision (as long as the free gingival margin) with no vertical component of that incision.

**free bone f.,** in neurosurgery, detached *craniotomy.*

**gingival f.,** a portion of the gingiva whose coronal margin is surgically detached from the tooth and the alveolar process.

**island f.,** full thickness f. with pedicle.

**jump f.,** a f. transferred to a desired location by stages; see also tubed pedicle f.

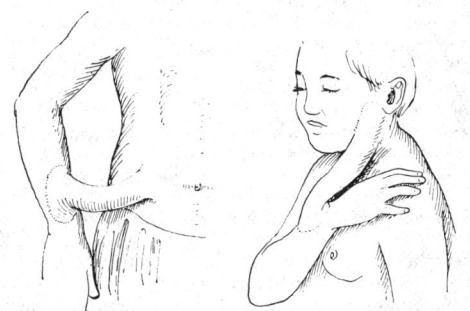

**Jump Flap of Skin from Abdomen to Face**
(From Converse, J. M.: *Kazanjian and Converse's Surgical Treatment of Facial Injuries,* Ed. 3, The Williams & Wilkins Co., Baltimore, 1974.)

**lingual tongue f.,** a f. used to repair fistulae of the hard palate; combines the raising of a palatal f. to form the floor of the nose, and a f. taken from the back or edge of the tongue to form the palatal surface.

**liver f.,** asterixis.

**mucoperiosteal f.,** a f. of mucosal tissue, including the periosteum, reflected from a bone.

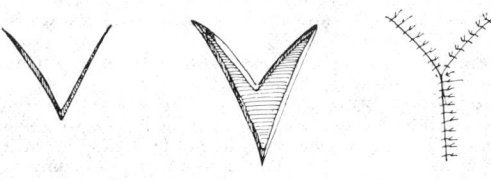

**A Sliding Flap**
(From Converse, J. M.: *Kazanjian & Converse's Surgical Treatment of Facial Injuries,* Ed. 3, The Williams & Wilkins Co., Baltimore, 1974.)

**pedicle f.,** a detached mass of tissues containing cutaneous and subcutaneous components, with an adequate blood supply being maintained at its base.

**pericoronal f.,** tissue around the crown of a tooth, mostly used to designate the portion of tissue covering the partially erupted tooth.

**sliding f.,** a f. in which the incision is shaped like a V and, after closure, like a Y; used either to lengthen or shorten a localized area of tissue.

**tubed pedicle f.,** a f. of skin and subcutaneous tissue formed as a tube attached at both ends, moved by transferring alternate ends at time intervals adequate for revascularization; see also jump f.

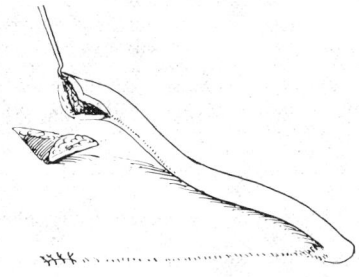

**Transfer of Tubed Pedicle Flap**
(From Converse, J. M.: *Kazanjian and Converse's Surgical Treatment of Facial Injuries,* Ed. 3, The Williams & Wilkins Co., Baltimore, 1974.)

**flare.** A diffuse redness of the skin extending beyond the local reaction to the application of an irritant; it is due to dilation of the arterioles and capillaries; depends upon an axon reflex set up by the liberation of a histamine-like substance in skin when injured. See also triple *response.*

**flarim'eter.** A modified spirometer by means of which one is able to make observations on the relative values of and comparisons between vital capacity, breath-holding ability, systolic and diastolic blood pressures, the heart rate and stroke volume.

**flash.** 1. A sudden and brief burst of light or heat. 2. Excess material extruded between the sections of a flask in the process of molding denture bases or other dental restorations.

**hot f.,** (1) one of the vasomotor symptoms of the climacterium. Occurs less frequently than hot flushes, and may involve the whole body as a f. of heat; (2) this term is also used interchangeably with hot *flush, q. v.*

**flash'blindness.** A temporary loss of vision produced when retinal light-sensitive pigments are bleached by light more intense than that to which the retina is physiologically adapted at that moment.

**flask.** A small receptacle, usually of glass, used for holding liquids, powder, or gases.

**casting f.,** refractory f.

**crown f.,** denture f.

**denture f.,** crown f.; a sectional metal boxlike case in which a sectional mold is made of plaster of Paris or artificial stone for the purpose of compressing and curing dentures or other resinous restorations.

**Dewar f.,** vacuum f.; a glass vessel, often silvered, with two walls, the space between which is evacuated; used for maintaining materials at constant temperature or, more usually, at low temperature.

**Erlenmeyer f.,** one with a conical body and broad base and a narrow neck.

**Fernbach f.,** a f. used in microbial fermentations where a large surface area of the liquid substrate is required.

**Florence f.,** a globular long-necked bottle of thin glass used for holding water or other liquid in laboratory work.

**injection f.,** a denture f. designed so as to permit the forced flow of denture base material from a reservoir into the mold after the flask is closed and during curing.

**refractory f.,** casting f.; casting ring; a metal tube in which a refractory mold is made for casting metal dental restorations or appliances.

**vacuum f.,** Dewar f.

**volumetric f.,** a f. calibrated to contain or to deliver a definite amount of liquid.

**flask'ing.** The process of investing the cast and a wax denture in a flask preparatory to molding the denture-base material into the form of the denture.

**Flatau** (flä′tow), Edward, Warsaw neurologist, 1869–1932. See F.-Schilder *disease*, F.'s *law.*

**flat'foot.** *Talipes* planus.

**flatulence** (flat′u-lens) [ Mod. L. *flatulentus,* fr. L. *flatus,* a blowing, fr. *flo,* pp. *flatus,* to blow ]. The presence of an excessive amount of gas in the stomach and intestines.

**flat'ulent.** Relating to or suffering from flatulence.

**fla'tus** [ L. a blowing ]. 1. Expired air (rare). 2. Gas in the stomach or intestine. 3. Eructation.

**f. vagina'lis,** expulsion of gas from the vagina.

**flat'worm.** A member of the phylum Platyhelminthes, including the tapeworms and flukes.

**flavacidin.** Amylpenicillin sodium.

**fla'vanone.** 2,3-Dihydroflavone; 2-phenyl-4-chromanone (*cf.* flavone).

**flave'do** [ L. *flavus,* yellow ]. Yellowness or sallowness of the skin.

**flavianic acid** (fla′vī-an′ik). A naphthol derivative, 7-hydroxy-4,6-dinitronaphthalene-sulfonic acid, useful in the precipitation (and subsequent determination) of arginine and other basic substances; a dye.

**fla'vicid.** 3-Amino-6-dimethylamino-2,7,10-trimethylacridinium hydrochloride; a topical antiseptic.

**fla'vicin.** Amylpenicillin sodium.

**flavin, flavine** (fla′vin, -vēn, flav′in, -ēn). [ L. *flavus,* yellow ]. 1. Riboflavin (vitamin B₂). 2. A yellow acridine dye, preparations of which are used as antiseptics; see acriflavine, flavicid, and proflavine.

**f. adenine dinucleotide,** a condensation product of riboflavin and adenosine diphosphate; the coenzyme of various aerobic dehydrogenases, *e.g.,* D-amino acid oxidases (EC 1.4.3.3).

**f. mononucleotide,** riboflavin 5′-phosphate; a coenzyme involved in the action of various aerobic dehydrogenases, notably L-amino acid oxidase (EC 1.4.3.2).

**Flavobacterium** (fla-vo-bak-te′rĭ-um) [ L. *flavus,* yellow ]. A genus of aerobic to facultatively anaerobic, non-sporeforming, motile and nonmotile bacteria (family Achromobacteraceae) containing Gram-negative rods; motile cells are peritrichous. These organisms characteristically produce yellow, orange, red, or yellow-brown pigments. They are found in soil and fresh and salt water. Some species are pathogenic. The type species is *F. aquatile.*

**F. aquati'le,** a species found in water containing a high percentage of calcium carbonate; it is the type species of *F.*

**F. breve,** a species found in sewage; pathogenic for laboratory animals.

**F. piscicida,** a species pathogenic for fish.

**flavoenzyme** (fla′vo-en′zīm). Any enzyme that possesses a flavin nucleotide as coenzyme; *e.g.,* xanthine oxidase (EC 1.2.3.2), succinate dehydrogenase (EC 1.3.99.1).

**fla'voki'nase.** Riboflavin kinase.

**fla'vone.** 2-Phenyl-4H-1-benzopyran-4-one or 2-phenyl-chromone; a plant pigment, basis of the flavonoids. See quercetin, rutin; *cf.* catechol.

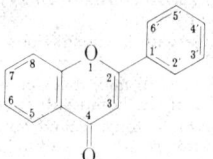

Flavone

**fla'vonoids.** Substances of plant origin containing flavone in various combinations (anthoxanthins, apigenins, flavones, quercitins, etc.) with varying biological activities.

**fla'vopro'tein.** A compound protein (enzyme) possessing a flavin as prosthetic group.

**fla'vor.** 1. The quality affecting the taste or odor of any substance. 2. A therapeutically inert substance added to a prescription to give an agreeable taste to the mixture.

**flavox'ate hydrochloride** (USAN). URIPAS; 2-piperidino-ethyl 3-methyl-4-oxo-2-phenyl-4H-1-benzopyran-8-carboxylate hydrochloride; a smooth muscle relaxant for the urinary tract.

**fla'vus** [ L. ] [ NA ]. Yellow.

**flax** [ A.S. *fleax* ]. A plant of the genus *Linum* (family Linaceae), from which is obtained linseed oil and textile linen.

**flax'seed.** Linseed.

**f. oil,** linseed oil.

**flea.** An insect of the order Siphonaptera, marked by lateral compression, sucking mouthparts, extraordinary jumping powers, and ectoparasitic adult life in the hair and feathers of warm-blooded animals.

**cat f.,** *Ctenocephalides felis.*

**chigger f.,** common name for *Tunga penetrans.*

**dog f.,** *Ctenocephalides canis.*

**human f.,** common name for *Pulex irritans.*

**rat f.,** a f. parasitic on the rat; among those involved in transmitting bubonic plague, the chief vector is *Xenopsylla cheopis,* though *X. braziliensis* and *X. astia* are also efficient vectors.

**sand f.,** common name for *Tunga penetrans.*

**sticktight f.,** *Echidnophaga gallinacea.*

**water f.'s,** Copepoda.

**fleam** [ a corruption thru Old Fr. fr. G. *phlebotomon,* a lancet, fr. *phleps,* vein, + *temnō,* to cut ]. A lancet, especially one for phlebotomy or a gum lancet.

**Flechsig** (flek′zig), Paul E., German neurologist, 1847–1929. See F.'s *areas,* oval *area, bundles, fasciculus, nucleus semilunaris, tract,* oval *tract.*

**flec'tion.** Flexion.

**fleece of Stilling.** The white fibers surrounding the nucleus dentatus of the cerebellum.

**Fleisch,** Alfred, Swiss physician and physiologist, *1892. See F. *pneumotachograph.*

**Fleischer** (flī′sher), Richard, German physician, 1848–1909. See F.'s *ring,* Kayser-F. *ring.*

**Fleischl** (flīsh′l), Ernst von (von Marxow), Vienna pathologist, 1846–1891. See F.'s *hemometer.*

**Fleischmann** (flīsh′mahn), Gottfried, German anatomist, 1777–1850. See F.'s *bursa.*

**Fleischner lines.** See under line.

**Fleitmann** (flīt′mahn), Theodore, German chemist, 19th century. See F.'s *test.*

**Fleming,** Sir Alexander, Scottish bacteriologist in London, 1881–1955. Nobel laureate, 1945, with Ernst B. Chain and Sir Howard Florey for the discovery in 1928 of penicillin and its curative effect in various infectious diseases.

**Flemming,** Walther, German anatomist, 1943–1905. See intermediate *body* of F., germinal *center* of F., F.'s *fluid, solution,* triple *stain.*

**flesh** [ A.S. *flaesc* ]. 1. The meat of animals used for food. 2. Muscular tissue. 3. Stoutness (popular).

**goose f.,** *cutis* anserina.

**proud f.,** exuberant granulations at the site of a wound surface or ulcer.

**Fletcher,** Horace, American dietitian, 1849–1919. Gave his name to fletcherism and fletcherize.

**fletch'erism.** Paltophagy; a dietary system advocated by Horace Fletcher, consisting in most complete mastication, carried to the point where all taste of the food is lost, and in abstention from food until driven thereto by hunger.

**fletch'erize.** To practice fletcherism.

**flex** [ L. *flecto,* pp. *flexus,* to bend ]. To bend; to move a joint in such a direction as to approximate the two parts which it connects.

**flexibil'itas ce'rea** [ L. waxy flexibility ]. The peculiar rigidity of catalepsy which may be overcome by slight external force, but which returns at once, holding the limb firmly in the new position.

**flexim′eter.** An instrument for measuring the degree of flexion possible in a joint.

**flexion** (flek′shun) [ L. *flecto,* pp. *flectus,* to bend. FLECT- ]. Flection. 1. The act of flexing or bending *e.g.,* bending of a joint so as to approximate the parts it connects; bending of the spine so that the concavity of the curve looks forward. 2. The condition of being flexed or bent.

    **plantar f.,** turning the foot or toes downward.

**Flexner,** Simon, New York pathologist, 1863–1946. See F.'s *bacillus.*

**flex′or** [ NA ]. A muscle the action of which is to flex a joint.

**flexura,** pl. **flexu′rae** (flek-shoor′ah) [ L. a bending. FLECT- ] [ NA ]. Flexure; a bend, as in an organ or structure.

    **f. co′li dex′tra** [ NA ], right colic flexure; hepatic flexure; the bend of the colon at the juncture of its ascending and transverse portions.

    **f. co′li sinis′tra** [ NA ], left colic flexure; splenic flexure; the bend at the junction of the transverse and descending colon.

    **f. duode′ni infe′rior** [ NA ], inferior flexure of the duodenum; the bend at the junction of the descending and horizontal parts of the duodenum. Occasionally a bend, the left inferior duodenal flexure, occurs at the junction of the horizontal and ascending parts.

    **f. duode′ni supe′rior** [ NA ], superior flexure of the duodenum; the flexure at the junction of the superior and descending parts of the duodenum.

    **f. duode′nojejuna′lis** [ NA ], duodenojejunal flexure or angle; an abrupt bend in the small intestine at the junction of the duodenum and jejunum.

    **f. perinea′lis recti** [ NA ], perineal flexure of the rectum; the anteroposterior curve with convexity anteriorward of the last portion of the rectum.

    **f. sacra′lis recti** [ NA ], sacral flexure of the rectum; the anteroposterior curve with concavity anteriorward of the first portion of the rectum.

    **f. sigmoid′ea,** *colon* sigmoideum.

**flexural** (flek′shur-al). Relating to a flexure.

**flexure** (flek′shur) [ L. *flexura* ]. Flexura.

    **caudal f.,** sacral f.; the bend in the lumbosacral region of the embryo.

    **cephalic f.,** cranial f.; cerebral f.; mesencephalic f.; the sharp, ventrally concave bend in the developing midbrain of the embryo.

    **cerebral f.,** cephalic f.

    **cervical f.,** the ventrally concave bend at the juncture of the brainstem and spinal cord in the embryo.

    **cranial f.,** cephalic f.

    **dorsal f.,** a f. in the mid-dorsal region in the embryo.

    **duodenojejunal f.,** *flexura* duodenojejunalis.

    **hepatic f.,** *flexura* coli dextra.

    **inferior f. of duodenum,** *flexura* duodeni inferior.

    **left colic f.,** *flexura* coli sinistra.

    **lumbar f.,** normal ventral curve of vertebral column in the lumbar region.

    **mesencephalic f.,** cephalic f.

    **perineal f. of rectum,** *flexura* perinealis recti.

    **pontine f.,** the dorsally concave curvature of the rhombencephalon in the embryo.

    **right colic f.,** *flexura* coli dextra.

    **sacral f.,** caudal f.

    **sacral f. of rectum,** *flexura* sacralis recti.

    **sigmoid f.,** *colon* sigmoideum.

    **splenic f.,** *flexura* coli sinistra.

    **superior f. of duodenum,** *flexura* duodeni superior.

    **telencephalic f.,** a f. appearing in the embryonic forebrain region.

**flick′er.** The visual sensation caused by stimulation of the retina by a series of intermittent light flashes occurring at a certain rate. See also flicker *fusion,* critical flicker-fusion *frequency.*

**Flieringa,** H. J., Dutch ophthalmologist. See F.'s *ring.*

**flight into disease.** Gain through falling ill or assuming the sick role; see epinosic *gain.*

**flight into health.** In psychoanalysis, the early but often only temporary disappearance of the symptoms that ostensibly brought the patient into therapy; a defense against the anxiety engendered by the prospect of further psychoanalytic exploration of the patient's conflicts.

**Flint,** Austin, American physician, 1812–1886. See F.'s *murmur.*

**Flint,** Austin, Jr., American physiologist, 1836–1915. See F.'s *arcade.*

**flip.** A burn occurring on one side only of the wound of entrance in a pistol wound of the soft parts.

**float** (flōt). 1. A metal instrument used for filing down sharp points and ridges on the molar teeth of old horses. 2. The process of filing such teeth.

**float′ing.** 1. Free; unattached; denoting the last two pairs of ribs, the cartilages of which are free. 2. Out of the normal position; unduly movable; wandering; denoting an occasional abnormal condition of certain organs, as the kidneys, liver, spleen, etc.

**floc** (flok). A colloquial term for the product of a flocculation, *i.e.,* the separation of the disperse phase of a colloidal suspension into discrete, usually visible particles, as in certain serologic precipitin tests.

**floccilegium** (flok-sī-le′jī-um) [ L. *floccus,* a tuft of wool, + *lego,* to gather together ]. Floccillation.

**floccillation** (flok-sī-la′shun) [ Mod. L. *flocculus* ]. Carphologia; crocidismus; floccilegium; tilmus; an aimless plucking at the bedclothes, as if one were picking off threads or tufts of cotton, occurring in the delirium of a fever.

**floccose** (flok′ōs) [ L. *floccus,* a flock of wool ]. In bacteriology, applied to a growth of short curving filaments or chains, closely but irregularly disposed.

**floc′culable.** Capable of undergoing flocculation.

**floc′cular.** Relating to a flocculus of any sort; specifically to the flocculus of the cerebellum.

**floc′culate.** To become flocculent.

**floc′cula′tion.** Flocculence; precipitation from solution in the form of fleecy masses; the process of becoming flocculent.

**floccule** (flok′ūl). Flocculus.

**floc′culence.** Flocculation.

**flocculent** (flok′u-lent). 1. Resembling tufts of cotton or wool; denoting a fluid, such as the urine, containing numerous shreds or fluffy particles of gray-white or white mucus or other material. 2. In bacteriology, denoting a fluid culture in which there are numerous colonies either floating in the fluid medium or loosely deposited at the bottom.

**flocculonodular** (flok′u-lo-nod′u-lar). See flocculonodular *lobe.*

**flocculus,** pl. **floc′culi** (flok′u-lus) [ Mod. L. dim. of L. *floccus,* a tuft of wool ]. Floccule. 1. A tuft or shred of cotton or wool or anything resembling it. 2 [ NA ]. A small lobe of the cerebellum at the posterior border of the brachium pontis anterior to the lobulus biventer; it is associated with the nodulus of the vermis; together, these two structures compose the vestibular part of the cerebellum.

    **accessory f.,** an occasional small lobule of the cerebellum in the immediate neighborhood of the flocculus.

**flock.** A group of animals that live or travel together; applied especially to sheep and domestic birds.

**Flocks.** Milton, San Francisco physician. See Harrington-F. *test.*

**Flood,** Valentine, Irish surgeon, 1800–1847. See F.'s *ligament.*

**flood** (flud) [ A.S. *flōd* ]. 1. To bleed profusely from the uterus, as after childbirth or in cases of menorrhagia. 2. A profuse menstrual discharge (lay terminology).

**flood′ing.** 1. Bleeding profusely from the uterus, especially after childbirth or in severe cases of menorrhagia. 2. A profuse uterine hemorrhage. 3. A type of behavior therapy in which the patient, at the beginning of therapy as the therapeutic strategy, imagines the most anxiety-producing scene and fully immerses (floods) himself in it, as opposed to systemic desensitization (*q. v.*).

**floor** (flōr). The lower inner surface of an open space or hollow organ.

**flora** (flo'rah) [ L. *Flora*, goddess of flowers, fr. *flos* (*flor-*), a flower ]. 1. Plant life, usually of a certain locality or district. 2. The various bacterial and other microscopic forms of life inhabiting the individual, for example the intestines (intestinal f.), the mouth (oral f.).

**floran'tyrone.** ZANCHOL; γ-oxy-γ-(8-fluoranthene)butyric acid. Used in chronic cholecystitis and cholangitis. It increases the volume of bile without increasing the quantity of bile solids or stimulating evacuation of the gallbladder.

**Florence,** Albert, French physician, 1851–1927. See F.'s *crystals, reaction, test.*

**Florence flask.** See under flask.

**Florey,** Sir Howard W., English pathologist, 1898–1968. Nobel laureate, 1945, with Sir Alexander Fleming and Ernst B. Chain, for the discovery of penicillin and its curative effect in various infectious diseases. See F. *unit.*

**florid** (flōr'id) [ L. *floridus*, flowery ]. Of a bright red color; denoting certain cutaneous lesions.

**florigen** (flor'ĭ-jen) [ L. *flora*, flower, + suffix -*gen*, production ]. Any substance that promotes the flowering of plants; the term is used to designate plant hormones believed to be formed in the leaves and transmitted through plants to the buds.

**Florschütz,** Georg, German physician, *1859. See F.'s *formula.*

**Flory,** Paul J., U. S. physical chemist, *1910. Nobel laureate, 1974, for his theories on the physical chemistry of polymers.

**floss.** Any silky, filamentous or threadlike material.

**dental f.,** floss silk; an untwisted thread made from fine, short, silk fibers, frequently waxed; used for cleansing interproximal spaces and between poor contact areas of teeth, for ligating teeth under the rubber dam, and, less frequently, in combination with a few cotton fibers, for slow separation.

**flota'tion.** A process for separating solids by the tendency to float upon or sink into a liquid.

**Flourens** (floo-rahn'), Marie J. P., French physiologist, 1794–1867. See F.'s *theory.*

**flow** [ A.S. *flōwan* ]. 1. To bleed from the uterus less profusely than in flooding. 2. The menstrual discharge. 3. The movement of a fluid or gas; specifically, the volume of fluid or gas passing a given point per unit of time. In respiratory physiology, the symbol for gas flow is *V* and for blood flow is *Q,* followed by subscripts denoting location and chemical species. 4. In rheology, a permanent deformation of a body which proceeds with time.

**Bingham f.,** the f. characteristics exhibited by a Bingham *plastic, q.v.*

**effective renal blood f.,** the amount of blood flowing to the parts of the kidney that are concerned with production of constituents of urine. Abbreviated ERBF.

**effective renal plasma f.,** the amount of plasma flowing to the parts of the kidney that have a function in the production of constituents of urine; the clearance of substances such as Diodrast and *p*-aminohippuric acid, assuming that the extraction ratio in the peritubular capillaries is 100 per cent; abbreviated ERPF.

**laminar f.,** the relative motion of elements of a fluid along smooth parallel paths.

**Newtonian f.,** the type of f. characteristic of a Newtonian *fluid, q.v.*

**shear f.,** a f. of a material in which parallel planes in the material are displaced in a direction parallel to each other.

**Flower,** Sir William H., English surgeon and anatomist, 1831–1899. See F.'s *bone,* dental *index.*

**flower basket of Bochdalek.** Part of the plexus choroideus of the fourth ventricle protruding through Luschka's foramen and resting on the dorsal surface of the glossopharyngeal nerve.

**flower of paradise.** *Catha edulis.*

**flowers.** A mineral substance in a powdery state after sublimation.

**f. of ben'zoin,** benzoic acid.

**f. of sulfur,** sublimed sulfur.

**f. of zinc,** zinc oxide.

**flow'meter.** A device for measuring velocity or volume of flow of liquids or gases.

**floxuridine** (floks-u'rĭ-dēn) (USAN). 5-FUDR; 5-fluoro-2'-deoxyuridine; the deoxynucleoside of fluorouracil; appears to be effective in the treatment of gastrointestinal cancer. Fluorouracil is metabolized to f. and this, in turn, to 5-fluoro-2'-deoxyuridine 5'-monophosphate. The latter agent inhibits thymidylic synthetase; uridine phosphatase is also inhibited.

**flu'anisone.** SEDALANDE; haloanisone; 4'-fluoro-4-[ 4-(*o*-methoxyphenyl)-1-piperazinyl ]butyrophenone; antianxiety agent.

**flu'crylate** (USAN). 2,2,2-Trifluoro-1-methylethyl-2-cyanoacrylate; a tissue adhesive used in surgery.

**fluctuate** (fluk'tu-āt) [ L. *fluctuo,* pp. -*atus,* to flow in waves ]. 1. To move in waves. 2. To vary, to change from time to time, as in referring to any quantity or quality, *e.g.,* height of blood pressure, concentration of substance in urine or blood, secretory activity, etc.

**fluctuation** (fluk'tu-a'shun). A wavelike motion felt on palpating a cavity with nonrigid walls, *e.g.,* the abdomen, when containing fluid.

**flucy'tosine** (USAN). ANCOBON; 5-fluorocytosine; an antifungal drug.

**flu'dorex** (USAN). β-Methoxy-*N*-methyl-*m*-(trifluoromethyl)phenethylamine; an anorexic, also with antiemetic activity.

**flu'drocor'tisone.** ALFLORONE; FLORINEF; F-CORTEF; FLUDROCORTONE; FLUOHYDRISONE; 9α-fluorohydrocortisone; 9α-fluorocortisol; 9α-fluoro-17-hydroxycorticosterone; 9α-fluoro-11β, 17α,21-trihydroxy-4-pregnene-3,20-dione (for pregnene structure, see steroids). Used as the acetate, *q.v.*

**f. acetate** (USP, BP), F-CORTEF acetate; FLURINEF acetate; fludrocortisone 21-acetate. Too potent a mineralocorticoid for systemic use, except in cases of adrenocortical insufficiency; otherwise used only topically.

**flufenam'ic acid** (USAN). ARLEF; *N*-(α,α,α-trifluoro-*m*-tolyl)anthranilic acid; anti-inflammatory agent for treatment of arthritis.

**flufen'isal** (USAN). 4'-Fluoro-4-hydroxy-3-biphenylcarboxylic acid acetate; analgesic.

**flu'id** [ L. *fluridus,* fr. *fluo,* to flow ]. 1. Flowing; liquid; gaseous. 2. A nonsolid substance, either liquid or gas.

**allantoic f.,** the f. within the allantoic cavity.

**Altmann's f.,** a fixing f. containing equal parts of a 5 per cent potassium bichromate solution and a 2 per cent osmic acid solution.

**amniotic f.,** liquor amnii; a liquid within the amnion that surrounds the fetus and protects it from injury.

**Berthollet's f.,** a mixture of the solutions of sodium chloride and sodium hypochlorite.

**Bouin's f.,** Bouin's solution; a histologic fixing f. consisting of glacial acetic acid 5, formalin 25, saturated solution of picric acid 75.

**Brodie f.,** an aqueous salt solution used in manometers designed for testing gas evolution or uptake as in cell respiration.

**Callison's f.,** a diluting f. for counting red blood cells. One milliliter of Loeffler's alkaline methylene blue, 1 ml. of formalin, 10 ml. of glycerol, 1 gm. of neutral ammonium oxalate, and 2.5 gm. of sodium chloride are added to 90 ml. of distilled water, mixed well, and permitted to stand until the solids are dissolved and the reagent is clear; the preparation is filtered prior to use.

**cerebrospinal f.,** *liquor* cerebrospinalis.

**ex'tracel'lular f.,** (1) the interstitial f. and the plasma, constituting about 20 per cent of the weight of the body; (2) sometimes used to mean all f. outside of cells, usually excluding transcellular f.

**ex'travas'cular f.,** all f. outside the blood vessels, *i.e.,* interstitial, intracellular, and transcellular f.'s; it constitutes about 48 to 58 per cent of the body weight.

**Farrant's f.,** a f. containing gum arabic, glycerin, and arsenic, for the preservation of delicate anatomical specimens.

**Flemming's f.,** Flemming's solution; a cytologic fixative f. containing chromic acid, osmic acid, and acetic acid.

**formol-Müller f.,** Müller's f. containing 2 per cent of commercial formalin.

**formol-Zenker f.,** Zenker's f. in which the glacial acetic acid has been replaced by 5 or 10 ml. of formalin. See Helly's f.

**Helly's f.,** potassium bichromate, 2.5 gm.; mercuric chloride, 5 gm.; distilled water, 100 ml.; formalin, added at time of fixation, 5 ml.

**Hermann's f.,** a hardening f. of glacial acetic acid 4,2 per cent aqueous solution of osmic acid 8,1 per cent acqueous solution of platinum chloride 60.

**infranatant f.,** clear f. which, after the settling out of an insoluble liquid or solid by the action of normal gravity or of centrifugal force, takes up the lower portion of the contents of a vessel.

**interstitial f.,** tissue f.; the f. in spaces between the tissue cells, constituting about 16 per cent of the weight of the body; closely similar in composition to lymph.

**in'tracel'lular f.,** the f. within the tissue cells; it constitutes about 30 to 40 per cent of the body weight.

**in'traoc'ular f.,** the f. within the anterior and posterior chambers of the eye.

**Marchi's f.,** 2 parts Müller's f. mixed with 1 part 1 per cent osmium tetroxide. Used to demonstrate degenerating myelin. See M.'s method.

**Müller's f.,** a hardening f., composed of potassium bichromate 2.5, sodium sulfate 1, distilled water 100.

**Newtonian f.,** a f. in which flow and rate of shear are always proportional to the applied stress; such f. precisely obeys Poiseuille's law; cf. non-Newtonian f.

**non-Newtonian f.,** a f. in which flow and rate of shear are not always proportional to the applied stress and which does not obey Poiseuille's law; for examples, see also anomalous *viscosity*, Fahraeus-Lindqvist *effect*, Bingham *plastic*; compare Newtonian f.

**Orth's f.,** formalin (35 to 37 per cent formaldehyde) 1 part, plus 10 parts of Müller's f.

**Parker's f.,** a hardening f. of formaldehyde 1, in 70 per cent alcohol 100.

**pleural f.,** the thin film of f. between the visceral and parietal pleurae.

**prostatic f.,** succus prostaticus; a whitish secretion that is one of the constituents of the semen.

**pseudoplastic f.,** a f. which exhibits shear thinning, *q.v.*

**Rees-Ecker f.,** an aqueous solution of sodium citrate, sucrose and brilliant cresyl blue used in platelet counts.

**Scarpa's f.,** endolymph.

**seminal f.,** semen (1).

**supernatant f.,** clear f. which, after the settling out of an insoluble liquid or solid by the action of normal gravity or of centrifugal force, takes up the upper portion of the contents of a vessel.

**syno'vial f.,** synovia.

**testicular f.,** spermine.

**Thoma's f.,** nitric acid 1, 95 per cent alcohol 25; a f. for decalcifying bone in the preparation of histologic specimens.

**tissue f.,** interstitial f.

**transcellular f.'s,** the f.'s that are not inside cells, but are separated from plasma and interstitial f. by cellular barriers; *e.g.,* cerebrospinal f., synovial f., pleural f.

**uterine f.,** f. providing nutrition for the embryo; it is secreted by the endometrial glands during the menstrual cycle.

**ventricular f.,** the portion of the cerebrospinal f. that is contained in the ventricles of the brain.

**Zenker's f.,** a fixative consisting of mercuric chloride 5 gm., potassium bichromate 2.5 gm., sodium sulfate 1 gm., glacial acetic acid 5 ml., water 100 ml.

**flu'idex'tract.** A pharmacopeial liquid preparation (termed liquid extract in the BP) of vegetable drugs, containing alcohol as a solvent or as a preservative, or both, and so made that each milliliter contains the therapeutic constituents of 1 gm. of the standard drug that it represents. F.'s are made by percolation; the required menstruum, the time of maceration, and the rate of flow during percolation are specified in the monographs.

**fluidglycerates** (flu'id-glis'er-āts). Pharmaceutical preparations formerly official in the National Formulary, containing approximately 50 per cent by volume of glycerin but no alcohol, and of the same drug strength as fluidextracts.

**fluidism** (flu'ĭ-dizm). Humoralism; see humoral *doctrine*.

**fluid'ity.** The reciprocal of viscosity; unit: rhe = poise$^{-1}$.

**fluidounce** (flu'id-owns'). A measure of capacity containing 8 fluidrams. The imperial f. is a measure containing 1 avoirdupois ounce, 437.5 grains, of distilled water at 15.6°C.; the U.S. f. is $1/128$ gallon and contains 454.6 grains of distilled water at 25°C. The imperial f. equals 28.4 ml.; the U.S. f. equals 29.57 ml.

**fluidrachm, fluidram** (flu'ĭ-dram'). A measure of capacity; $1/8$ of a fluidounce; a teaspoonful. The imperial f. contains 54.8 grains of distilled water, and is equal to 3.55 ml.; the U.S. f. contains 57.1 grains of distilled water and equals 3.70 ml.

**fluke** (flook) [ A.S. *flōc*, flatfish ]. The common name for members of the class Trematoda (phylum Platyhelminthes). All f.'s of mammals are internal parasites in the adult stage (order Digenea) and are characterized by complex digenetic life cycles involving a snail initial host, in which larval multiplication occurs, and the release of swimming larvae (cercariae) which directly penetrate the skin of the final host, as in schistosomes, encyst on vegetation, as in *Fasciola*, or encyst in another intermediate, as in *Clonorchis* and other fish-borne f.'s. F.'s of lower vertebrates, especially fish, are frequently monogenetic ectoparasites or gill parasites (order Monogenea).

**blood f.,** one that lives in the mesenteric-portal blood stream and the associated vesical and pelvic venous plexuses; *Schistosoma haematobium*, the vesical blood f.; *S. mansoni*, Manson's intestinal blood f.; *S. japonicum*, the Oriental blood f.

**bronchial f.,** *Paragonimus westermani.*

**cat liver f.,** *Opisthorchis felineus.*

**Chinese liver f.,** *Clonorchis sinensis.*

**digenetic f.,** trematode in the subclass Digenea.

**Egyptian intestinal f.,** *Heterophyes heterophyes.*

**intestinal f.,** usually refers to large form, *Fasciolopsis buski* (formerly termed *Distoma crassum*); the small intestinal f. is *Heterophyes heterophyes,* or Egyptian intestinal f.

**lancet f.,** *Dicrocoelium dendriticum.*

**liver f.,** *Fasciola hepatica.*

**lung f.,** *Paragonimus westermani.*

**Oriental f.,** *Clonorchis sinensis.*

**rumen f.,** *Paramphistomum.*

**sheep liver f.,** *Fasciola hepatica.*

**flu'men,** pl. **flu'mina** [ L. ]. A flowing, or stream.

**flumina pilo'rum** [ NA ], hair streams; the curved lines along which the hairs are arranged on the head and various parts of the body, especially noticeable in the fetus.

**flumeth'asone** (USAN). FLUCORT; $6\alpha,9\alpha$-difluoro-$11\beta,17\alpha,21$-trihydroxy-$16\alpha$-methylpregna-1,4-diene-3,20-dione; a synthetic corticosteroid. The 21-pivalate salt is available as LOCORTEN.

**flu'methi'azide.** ADEMOL; 6-trifluoromethyl-7-sulfamoyl-4*H*-1,2,4-benzothiadiazine 1,1-dioxide; an orally effective diuretic agent, related chemically to chlorothiazide and with similar pharmacologic actions and uses.

**flumet'ramide** (USAN). DURAFLEX; 6-($\alpha,\alpha,\alpha$-trifluoro-*p*-tolyl)-3-morpholinone; skeletal muscle relaxant.

**flu'mina.** Plural of flumen.

**flunar'izine hydrochloride** (USAN). (*E*)-1-[ bis-*p*-Fluorophenyl)methyl ]-4-cinnamylpiperazine dihydrochloride; a vasodilator agent.

**fluni'dazole** (USAN). 2-(*p*-Fluorophenyl)-5-nitroimidazol-1-ethanol; an antiprotozoal agent.

**fluo-** [ L. *fluo,* pp. *fluxus,* to flow ]. Combining form denoting flow (contrast fluor-, fluoro-).

**flu'ocin'olone acetonide** (USP). SYNALAR; DERMALAR; JELLIN; SYNANDONE; $6\alpha,9\alpha$-difluoro-$11\beta,16\alpha,17\alpha,21$-tetrahydroxy-1,4-pregnadiene-3,20-dione; cyclic 16,17-acetal with acetone; $6\alpha,9\alpha$-difluoro-$16\alpha$-hydroxyprednisolone 16,17'-acetonide (for structure, see steroids). A fluorinated corticosteroid for topical use in the treatment of selected dermatoses.

**flu'ocor'tolone** (USAN). $6\alpha$-Fluoro-$11\beta,21$-dihydroxy-$16\alpha$-methylpregna-1,4-diene-3,20-dione (for pregnane structure, see steroids); a glucocorticoid used as an anti-inflammatory agent.

**f. hexanoate** (BP), salt used topically in the treatment of skin diseases.

**f. pivalate** (BP), alternate salt used topically.

**fluor-, fluoro-.** Prefixes denoting fluorine.

**flu'or albus** [ L. white flow ]. Leukorrhea.

**fluorapatite** (flu'or-ap'ă-tīt). $3Ca_3(PO_4)_2 \cdot CaF_2$; a naturally occurring fluorophosphate of calcium.

**9 H-flu'orene.** Diphenylenemethane; occurs in coal tar; parent of 2-acetylaminofluorene, a carcinogenic compound.

9H-Fluorene

**fluorescein** (flu'or-es'e-in). Resorcinolphthalein; 9-(o-Carboxyphenyl)-6-hydroxy-3 H-xanthen-3-one; D&C Yellow No. 7; an orange-red crystalline powder that yields a bright green fluorescence in solution; it is reduced to fluorescin.

    **f. dyes,** f. and its derivatives, the more important being eosin, phloxine, rose bengal, and merbromin.

    **f. isothiocyanate,** a derivative of f., used as a fluorescent label for specific proteins to permit histologic observation of their distribution. See immunofluorescence *methods.*

    **f. sodium** (USP, BP), resorcinolphthalein sodium; uranine; a dye used for diagnosis of certain ocular diseases and for differentiation or delineation of organ parts in surgery; also used to determine circulation time.

**fluorescence** (flu-or-es'ens). The re-emission of light following upon absorption of it, the reemitted light being generally of lower frequency than that absorbed; f. is most noticeable when the absorbed light is in the (invisible) ultraviolet range and the re-emitted light in the visible range; the term is also applied to the re-emitted light itself. Distinguished from phosphorescence in that in f. re-emission ceases when light absorption ceases while in phosphorescence re-emission persists for a perceptible period of time thereafter.

**fluorescent** (flu-or-es'ent). Possessing the quality of fluorescence.

**flu'orescin.** Reduced fluorescein; resorcinolphthalein; similar uses as fluorescein.

**fluoridate** (flu'or-ĭ-dāt). Fluorinate; to perform fluoridation.

**fluoridation** (flu'or-ĭ-da'shun). Fluorination; the addition of fluorides to the drinking water, usually 1 p.p.m., to reduce incidence of dental decay.

**flu'oride.** A compound of fluorine with a metal, a nonmetal, or an organic radical.

**fluoridization** (flu'or-ĭ-dī-za'shun). The use of fluorine any any form to reduce incidence of dental decay.

**fluoridize** (flu'or-ĭ-dīz). To perform fluoridization.

**fluorimeter** (flu'or-im'e-ter). Fluorometer.

**fluorinate** (flu'or-ĭ-nāt). Fluoridate.

**fluorination** (flu'or-ĭ-na'shun). Fluoridation.

**fluorine** (flu'or-ēn). A gaseous chemical element, symbol F, atomic no. 9, atomic weight 19.00.

**fluoro-.** See fluor-.

**fluorochrome** (flu'or-o-krōm). Any fluorescent dye, used to stain tissues and cells for examination by ultraviolet fluorescence microscopy.

**fluorochroming.** The tagging or "labeling" of antibody with a fluorescent dye in order that it may be observed with a microscope (using ultra-violet light), as a means of studying the origin, distribution, and sites of reaction (with antigen) in tissues.

**9α -flu'orocor'tisol.** Fludrocortisone.

**fluoro-2,4-dinitrobenzene.** FDNB; $N_2$ph-F; Dnp-F; Sanger's reagent; used to combine with the free $NH_2$ group of the $NH_2$-terminal amino acid residue in a peptide, thus marking this residue. The combined forms are known as DNP-proteins, Dnp-aminoacyl, etc., the fluorine having been replaced to leave a dinitrophenyl residue (DNP, Dnp, or $N_2$ph-).

**fluorography** (flu'or-og'ră-fī). Photofluorography.

**9α -flu'orohy'drocor'tisone.** Fludrocortisone.

**flu'orom'eter.** A device for interpreting the shadows in an x-ray projection on the screen; fluorimeter.

**flu'orometh'olone** (NF). OXYLONE; 9α- fluoro-11β,17α-dihydroxy-6α -methyl-1,4-pregnadiene-3,20-dione(for pregnane structure, see steroids); a glucocorticoid for topical use.

**fluororoentgenography** (flu'or-o-rent'gen-og'ră-fī). Photofluorography.

**fluoroscope** (flu-or'o-skōp) [ fluorescence + G. *skopeō,* to examine ]. An apparatus for rendering visible the shadows of the x-rays which, after passing through the body examined, are projected on a fluorescent screen of calcium tungstate.

**fluoroscopic** (flu'or-o-skop'ik). Relating to or effected by means of fluoroscopy.

**fluoroscopy** (flu-or-os'ko-pī). Examination of the inner parts of the body by means of the fluoroscope.

**flu'oro'sis.** 1. A condition caused by an excessive intake of fluorine (2 or more p.p.m. in drinking water). Characterized mainly by mottling of the enamel of the teeth. 2. Chronic poisoning of livestock with fluorides. These sometimes are contained in rock phosphates used as feed supplements, but more often are ingested as forage contaminants near large aluminum plants, the fluorides being deposited from the factory fumes. The disease blackens and softens developing teeth and reduces bones to brittle chalky structures.

    **chronic endemic f.,** enamel f.; endemic dental f.; f. caused by excessive fluorine in the natural water supply, as seen in parts of India; osteosclerosis with ankylosis of the spine may develop.

    **enamel f.,** chronic endemic f.

    **endemic dental f.,** chronic endemic f.

**fluorouracil** (flu'or-o-u'ră-sil) (USP). 5-Fluorouracil; a pyrimidine analogue effective in the treatment of gastrointestinal cancer; it has shown some effectiveness in other types of carcinomas. The cells of certain neoplasms incorporate uracil into ribonucleic acid more readily than do normal tissue cells. See also floxuridine.

**flu'oxymes'terone** (BP, USP). HALOTESTIN; ULTANDREN; 9α -fluoro-11β, 17β -dihydroxy-17α -methyl-4-androstene-3-one (for androstene structure, see steroids). An orally effective synthetic halogenated steroid, related in chemical structure and pharmacologic action to methyltestosterone, but more potent.

**flupenthixol dihydrochloride.** FLUANOXOL; 4-{3-[ 2-(trifluoromethyl)thioxanthen-9-ylidene ]propyl}-1-piperazineethanol dihydrochloride; neuroleptic agent.

**fluper'olone acetate** (USAN). METHRAL; 9α -fluoro-11β,17α,21- trihydroxy-21-methylpregna-1,4-diene-3,20-dione 21-acetate; synthetic corticosteroid used as an anti-inflammatory agent.

**flu'phen'azine.** 4-[ 3-[ 2-(Trifluoromethyl)phenothiazin-10-yl ]propyl ]-1-piperazine ethanol; a phenothiazine-piperazine compound.

    **f. enanthate** (USP), PROLIXIN enanthate; a potent, long-acting (10 to 14 days) antipsychotic agent, used parenterally.

    **f. hydrochloride** (USP, BP), PROLIXIN; PERMITIL; an antipsychotic agent, used in the management of acute and chronic schizophrenia, involutional, senile, and toxic psychoses, and the manic phase of manic-depressive psychosis.

**flu'prednis'olone** (USAN). ALPHADROL; 6α -fluoro-11β,17α,21-trihydroxy-1,4-pregnadiene-3,20-dione (for pregnane structure, see steroids); a glucocorticoid with anti-inflammatory activity and toxicity similar to those of cortisol.

**flurandrenolone** (floor'an-dren'o-lōn) (USAN). CORDRAN; 6α -fluoro-16α -hydroxyhydrocorticosterone; a fluorinated corticosteroid for topical use in the treatment of dermatoses.

**fluraz'epam hydrochloride** (NF). DALMANE; 7-chloro-1-[ 2-(diethylamino)ethyl ]-5-(o-fluorophenyl)-1,3-dihydro-2 H-1,4-benzodiazepin-2-one dihydrochloride; hypnotic.

**fluroges'tone acetate** (USAN). CRONOLONE; 9-fluoro-11β,17-dihydroxypregn-4-ene-3,20-dione 17-acetate; progestational agent.

**flurothyl** (floor'o-thil) (NF). INDOKLON; bis(2,2,2-trifluoroethyl) ether; a convulsant, administered by inhalation for the same indications as electroconvulsive therapy; produces grand mal convulsions.

**fluroxene** (floor-ok'sēn) (NF). FLUOROMAR; 2,2,2-trifluoroethyl vinyl ether; a volatile, halogenated hydrocarbon anesthetic agent for inhalation anesthesia, used to fortify nitrous oxide anesthesia and for minor surgical procedures not requiring profound relaxation.

**Flury strain vaccines.** See under vaccine.

**flush.** 1. To wash out a wound or a cavity with a full stream of water. 2. A transient erythema due to heat, exertion, stress, or disease.

  **hectic f.,** redness of the face associated with a rise of temperature in various fevers.

  **hot f.,** a vasomotor symptom of the climacterium; sudden vasodilation with a sensation of heat, usually involving the face and neck, and upper part of the chest; sweats, often profuse, frequently follow the f.

  **malar f.,** localized hectic f. of the malar eminences, often occurring in tuberculosis, and sometimes seen in rheumatic fever.

**fluti'azin** (USAN). 8-(Trifluoromethyl)phenothiazine-1-carboxylic acid; an anti-inflammatory drug for veterinary use.

**flut'ter** [ A.S. *flotorian,* to float about ]. Agitation; tremulousness.

  **atrial f., auricular f.,** jugular embryocardia; rapid regular atrial contractions occurring usually at rates between 250 and 400 per minute and often producing "saw-tooth" waves in the electrocardiogram.

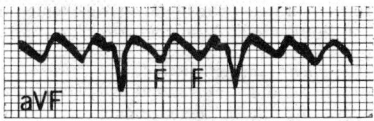

**Atrial Flutter**

  **di'aphragmat'ic f.,** rapid rhythmical contractions (average, 150 per minute) of the diaphragm, simulating atrial f. clinically and sometimes electrocardiographically.

  **impure f.,** mixture of atrial flutter (FF) and fibrillation (ff) waves in the electrocardiogram.

  **ocular f.,** a spontaneous, brief, intermittent, horizontal oscillation of the eyes occurring during fixation; it often coexists with ocular dysmetria in cerebellar syndromes associated with hydrocephalus or cerebral atrophy.

  **ventricular f.,** a form of rapid ventricular tachycardia in which the electrocardiographic complexes assume a regular undulating pattern with an absence of distinct QRS and T waves.

**flutter-fibrillation.** An electrocardiographic pattern of atrial activity with features of both fibrillation and flutter.

**flux** [ L. *fluxus,* a flow, fr. *fluo,* pp. *fluxus,* to flow ]. 1. The discharge of more or less fluid material in large amount from a cavity or surface of the body; a diarrhea. 2. Material discharged from the bowels. 3. A material used to remove oxides from the surface of molten metal and to protect it when casting; it serves a similar purpose in soldering operations. Also, an ingredient in dental porcelain which by its lower melting temperature helps to bond the silica particles. 4. Flux density; symbol J; the moles of a substance crossing through a unit area of a boundary layer or membrane per unit of time.

  **alvine f.,** simple diarrhea.

  **bloody f.,** dysentery.

  **luminous f.,** the quantity of light emitted from a point source in a given time; its unit is the lumen.

  **monthly f.,** the menses.

  **net f.,** the difference between the two unidirectional f.'s.

  **seba'ceous f.,** steatorrhea.

  **unidirectional f.,** the f. of a substance from one surface of a boundary layer or membrane to the other, disregarding any counterbalancing f. in the other direction, as measured by tracer technique.

  **white f.,** (1) celiac *disease;* (2) pullorum *disease.*

**fly** [ A.S. *fleóge* ]. A two-winged insect in the order Diptera; typical flies of the housefly type and similar forms are in the family Muscidae. For some types of flies not listed as subentries here (usually written as one word), see the full name (*e.g.,* blowfly, botfly, gadfly, horsefly, housefly).

  **black f.,** a species of *Simulium, q. v.*

  **bluebottle f.,** *Calliphora.*

  **caddis f.,** a member of the insect order Trichoptera, *q. v.*

  **cheese f.,** *Piophila casei.*

  **deer f.,** *Chrysops.*

  **flesh flies,** Diptera whose larvae (maggots) develop in putrifying or living tissues. Maggots of the latter group produce myiasis; these include screwworms (both primary and secondary invaders); wool maggots of sheep (cause of "strike"); botflies or skin maggots of man and domestic animals (including warble or heel flies); head or nasal bots of sheep and goats, horses, camels, and deer; and horse bots (or gadflies) whose larvae develop in the stomach, duodenum, or rectum of horses.

  **heel f.,** see botfly.

  **horn f.,** *Siphona irritans.*

  **latrine f.,** *Fannia scolaris.*

  **louse f.'s,** pupiparous, dorsoventrally flattened dipterous ectoparasites of the family Hippoboscidae. See also *Hippobosca* and *Melophagus.*

  **mangrove f.,** species of *Chrysops* in Africa, vectors of *Loa loa;* for example, *Chrysops silacea.*

  **nose f.,** *Oestrus ovis.*

  **Russian f.,** cantharis.

  **sand f.,** a small, biting, dipterous midge of the genus *Phlebotomus;* vectors of leishmaniasis.

  **screw worm f.,** *Callitroga hominivorax; C. macellaria.*

  **Spanish f.,** cantharis.

  **stable f.,** *Stomoxys calcitrans.*

  **tsetse f.,** see *Glossina.*

  **warble f.,** see botfly.

**Flynn,** P. See F.-Aird *syndrome.*

**FMN.** Abbreviation for flavin mononucleotide.

**foal** (fōl). 1. A newborn horse. In show ring classification, a foal is an animal born on or after January 1 of the year shown. 2. The act of giving birth to a foal.

**foam** (fōm). 1. Masses of small bubbles on the surface of a liquid. 2. To produce such bubbles. 3. Also applied to masses of air cells in a solid or semisolid, *e.g.,* f. rubber.

  **human fibrin f.** (BP), a dry artificial sponge of human fibrin prepared by clotting with thrombin a f. of a solution of human fibrinogen. The clotted f. is dried from the frozen state and heated. Used as a topical anticoagulant.

**fo'cal.** Relating to a focus.

**foci** (fo'si). Plural of focus.

**focim'eter.** An instrument for finding the vergence power of a lens or system of lenses.

**focus,** pl. **foci** (fo'kus, fo'si) [ L. a hearth ]. 1. The point at which the light rays meet after passing through a convex lens, such as the crystalline lens of the eye. 2. The center, or the starting point, of a disease process.

  **con'jugate foci,** two points in relation to a lens or concave mirror, so that the rays from a light at one point are focused at the other, and *vice versa.*

  **Ghon's f.,** Ghon's *tubercle.*

  **principal f.,** the real or virtual meeting point of rays passing into a lens parallel to its axis.

  **real f.,** the point of meeting of convergent rays.

  **virtual f.,** the point from which divergent rays seem to proceed, or that at which they would meet if prolonged backward.

**fog.** A haze, mist, or cloud that obscures vision.

  **mental f.,** a clouding of consciousness, usually with more or less complete loss of memory for the past life or a part of it.

**Fogarty,** T. J., American surgeon. See F.'s *catheter.*

**fog'ging.** Dimness of vision; nephelopia.

**foil.** An extremely thin, pliable sheet of metal.

  **gold f.,** pure gold rolled into extremely thin sheets; used in the restoration of carious or fractured teeth. See also cohesive *gold* and noncohesive *gold.*

  **platinum f.,** pure platinum rolled into extremely thin sheets; its high fusing point makes it suitable as a matrix for various soldering procedures in dentistry, and also suitable for providing internal form to porcelain restorations during their fabrication.

**tinfoil,** (1) tin rolled into extremely thin sheets; (2) a base metal f. used as a separating material, as between the cast and denture-base material during flasking and curing procedures.

**Foix,** C. See F.-Alajouanine *myelitis*.

**fo'lacin.** Folic acid.

**fo'late.** A salt or ester of folic acid.

# FOLD

**fold.** 1. Plica (*q.v.*); a ridge or margin apparently formed by the doubling back of a lamina. 2. In the embryo, a transient elevation or reduplication of tissue in the form of a lamina.

**alar f.'s,** *plicae* alares.

**amniotic f.,** Schultze's f.; a f. of amniotic membrane enclosing the vitelline duct; it extends from the point of insertion of the umbilical cord to the yolk sac. In reptiles and birds it is the reflected edge of the amnion where it folds over to cover the embryo during early development.

**ar'yepiglot'tic** or **aryt'enoepiglottide'an f.,** *plica* aryepiglottica.

**axillary f.,** *plica* axillaris.

**caval f.,** a f. near the base of the dorsal mesentery on its right side, in which a primordial segment of the inferior vena cava is developed between the right subcardinal vein and vessels within the liver.

**cecal f.'s,** *plicae* cecales.

**f. of chorda tympani,** *plica* chordae tympani.

**ciliary f.'s,** *plicae* ciliares.

**circular f.'s,** *plicae* circulares.

**Douglas' f.,** *plica* rectouterina.

**Duncan's f.'s,** the f.'s on the peritoneal surface of the uterus immediately after delivery.

**duodenojejunal f.,** *plica* duodenalis superior.

**duodenomesocolic f.,** *plica* duodenalis inferior.

**epigastric f.,** *plica* umbilicalis lateralis.

**falciform retinal f.,** a congenital f. from disk to ciliary region in inferior temporal quadrant of the retina.

**fimbriated f.,** *plica* fimbriata.

**gastric f.'s,** *plicae* gastricae.

**gastropancreatic f.'s,** *plicae* gastropancreaticae.

**genital f.,** urogenital *ridge*.

**glossopalatine f.,** *arcus* palatoglossus.

**gluteal f.,** a prominent f. that marks the upper limit of the thigh from the lower limit of the buttock; it coincides with the lower border of the gluteus maximus muscle.

**Guérin's f.,** *valvula* fossae navicularis.

**Hasner's f.,** *plica* lacrimalis.

**head f.,** a ventral folding of the cephalic extremity in the embryonic disk, so that the brain lies rostrad to the mouth and pericardium.

**Houston's f.'s,** *plicae* transversales recti.

**ileocecal f.,** *plica* ileocecalis.

**incudal f.,** *plica* incudis.

**inferior duodenal f.,** *plica* duodenalis inferior.

**infrapatellar f.,** *plica* synovialis infrapatellaris.

**inguinal f.,** *plica* inguinalis.

**inguinal aponeurotic f.,** *falx* inguinalis.

**interureteric f.,** *plica* interureterica.

**f.'s of iris,** *plicae* iridis.

**Kerckring's f.'s,** *plicae* circulares.

**labioscrotal f.'s,** lateral f.'s at either side of the embryonic cloacal membrane that develop into either the scrotum or the labia majora.

**lacrimal f.,** *plica* lacrimalis.

**lateral f.'s,** ventral foldings of the lateral margins of the embryonic disk, thus establishing the definitive embryonic body form.

**lateral glossoepiglottic f.,** *plica* glossoepiglottica lateralis.

**lateral nasal f.,** lateral nasal process; an ectodermally covered mesenchymal swelling separating the embryonic olfactory pit from the developing eye.

**lateral umbilical f.,** *plica* umbilicalis lateralis.

**f. of left vena cava,** *plica* venae cavae sinistrae.

**longitudinal f. of duodenum,** *plica* longitudinalis duodeni.

**mallear f.,** *plica* mallearis.

**mammary f.,** mammary *ridge*.

**Marshall's vestigial f.,** *plica* venae cavae sinistrae.

**medial nasal f.'s,** medial nasal processes; ectodermally covered mesenchymal swellings lying medial to the olfactory placodes in the embryo.

**medial umbilical f.,** *plica* umbilicalis medialis.

**mesonephric f.,** urogenital *ridge*.

**middle glossoepiglottic f.,** *plica* glossoepiglottica mediana.

**middle umbilical f.,** *plica* umbilicalis mediana.

**mucobuccal f.,** the line of flexure of the mucous membrane as it passes from the mandible or maxillae to the cheek.

**mucosal f.'s of gallbladder,** *plicae* tunicae mucosae vesicae felleae.

**nail f.,** a groove in the cutis in which lie the margins and proximal edge of the nail.

**neural f.'s,** The elevated margins of the neural groove.

**opercular f.,** tissue forming a bridge or an adhesion between the tonsil and the anterior pillar of the fauces.

**palmate f.'s,** *plicae* palmatae.

**paraduodenal f.,** *plica* paraduodenalis.

**pericardiopleural f.,** a f. formed in the embryonic pericardiopleural opening; it eventually closes off the pleural from the pericardial cavity.

**pharyn'goepiglot'tic f.'s** f.'s formed by the reflection of the mucous membrane of the epiglottis on the lateral wall of the pharynx.

**pleuroperitoneal f.,** pleuroperitoneal *membrane*.

**presplenic f.,** a fan-shaped f. of peritoneum that passes from the gastrosplenic ligament near the lower end of the spleen to the phrenicocolic ligament with which it blends. It contains branches of the splenic or the left gastroepiploic artery.

**rectal f.,** *plica* transversalis recti.

**rectouterine f.,** and **rectovaginal f.,** *plica* rectouterina.

**rectovesical f.,** the f. of peritoneum in the male that bounds the rectovesical pouch laterally.

**retrotarsal f.,** *fornix* conjunctivae.

**Rindfleisch's f.'s,** semilunar f.'s of the serous surface of the pericardium, embracing the beginning of the aorta.

**sacrogenital f.'s,** peritoneal f.'s that extend backward from the sides of the bladder, on either side of the rectum, to the sacrum; they form the lateral boundaries of the rectovesical pouch.

**salpingopalatine f.,** *plica* salpingopalatina.

**salpingopharyngeal f.,** *plica* salpingopharyngea.

**Schultze's f.,** amniotic f.

**semilunar f.,** *plica* semilunaris.

**semilunar f. of colon,** *plica* semilunaris coli.

**semilunar conjunctival f.,** *plica* semilunaris conjunctivae.

**spiral f. of cystic duct,** *plica* spiralis ductus cystici.

**stapedial f.,** *plica* stapedis.

**sublingual f.,** *plica* sublingualis.

**superior duodenal f.,** *plica* duodenalis superior.

**synovial f.,** *plica* synovialis.

**tail f.,** the ventral folding of the caudal extremity of the embryonic disk.

**transverse f.'s of rectum,** *plicae* transversales recti.

**Treves' f.,** *plica* ileocecalis.

**triangular f.,** *plica* triangularis.

**Tröltsch's f.,** *plica* mallearis.

**urachal f.,** *plica* umbilicalis mediana.

**ureteric f.,** *plica* interureterica.

**urorectal f.,** urorectal *septum*.

**uterovesical f.,** vesicouterine *ligament*.

**vascular f. of the cecum,** *plica* cecalis vascularis.

**Vater's f.,** a f. of mucous membrane in the duodenum just above the greater duodenal papilla.

**ventricular f.,** *plica* vestibularis.

**vestibular f. of larynx,** *plica* vestibularis.

**vestigial f.,** *plica* venae cavae sinistrae.

**vocal f.,** *plica* vocalis.

**Foley,** Frederic E. B., American urologist, 1891–1966. See F. *catheter*, F.'s *operation*.

**fo'lia.** Plural of folium.

**foliaceous** (fo-lĭ-a′shus). Leaflike; foliate.

**fo′liar.** Foliate.

**fo′liate.** Pertaining to or resembling a leaf or leaflet.

**fo′lic acid.** Collective term for pteroylglutamic acids and their oligoglutamic acid conjugates; used specifically for pteroyl(mono)glutamic acid; also known as folacin, liver *Lactobacillus casei* factor, vitamin M, vitamin $B_{10}$, $B_{11}$, $B_c$; factor U; factor R; a member of the vitamin B complex; growth factor for *L. casei* and *Streptococcus faecalis* (*S. lactis* R). It is isolated from green leaves and from liver; has also been synthesized. Involved (as 5,6,7,8-tetrahydro derivatives) in many one-carbon transfer reactions, notably in synthesis of thymidylic acid (methyl group) required for DNA synthesis. It is the precursor of folinic acid (citrovorum factor). The normal human daily requirement is 0.1 to 0.2 mg.; deficiency causes inadequate nucleic acid synthesis, with megaloblastic anemia, growth failure, and abnormal intestinal epithelium. It is used in the treatment of megaloblastic anemias not due to vitamin $B_{12}$ deficiency, and for anemias of sprue; it will not correct the metabolic effect permitting gliadin toxicity in nontropical sprue. It stimulates the production of leukocytes, and has been used in the treatment of leukopenia and agranulocytosis. Folic acid is official in the USP and BP.

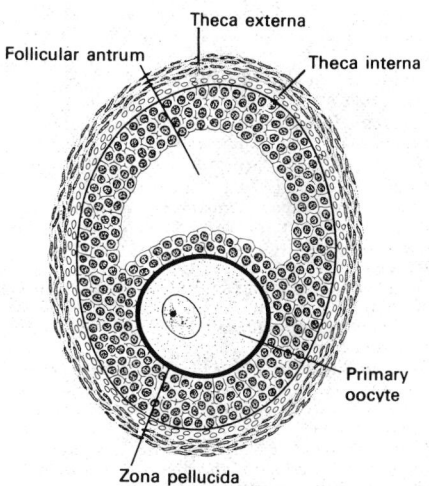

I

pteroic acid (pteroyl)          glutamic acid (glutamyl)

**Folic acid**

**f. acid antagonists,** compounds, such as aminopterin and amethopterin, that neutralize the action of folic acid and thus produce a folic acid deficiency. They have been used in treating acute lymphatic leukemia.

**f. acid conjugate,** folate compounds with three molecules of glutamic acid instead of one (pteroyltriglutamic acid or *Lactobacillus casei* factor), or with seven (pteroylheptaglutamic acid or vitamin $B_c$ conjugate).

**folie** (fo-le′) [ Fr. folly ]. Old term for madness or insanity.

**f. à deux** (ă-dü) [ Fr. *deux,* two ], double insanity; identical or similar mental disorders affecting two individuals, usually members of the same family living together.

**f. du doute** (doot), doubting mania; an excessive doubting about all the affairs of life and a morbid scrupulosity in regard to minutiae.

**f. gémellaire** (zha-mel-air′) [ Fr. relating to twins ], a psychosis appearing simultaneously, or nearly so, in twins, who are not necessarily living together or intemately associated at the time.

**f. musculaire,** severe chorea.

**f. de pourquoi** (poor-kwah′) [ Fr. *pourquoi,* why ], a psychopathologic tendency to ask questions.

**f. raisonnante** (ra-zŭ-nahnt′), delusional insanity; paranoia.

**Folin,** Otto K. O., American biochemist, 1867–1934. See F.'s *test, reaction,* F.-Looney *test.*

**folin′ic acid.** 5-Formyl-5,6,7,8-tetrahydrofolic acid; citrovorum factor; leucovorin; the compound that acts as formyl group carrier in transformylation reactions. The calcium salt is used to counteract toxic effects of folic acid antagonists, for the treatment of megaloblastic anemias, and as an adjunct to cyanocobalamin in pernicious anemia.

**fo′liose.** Foliate.

**folium,** pl. **folia** (fo′lī-um, fo′lī-ah) [ L. a leaf ] [ NA ]. A broad, thin, leaflike structure.

**folia cerebel′li** [ NA ], folia of the cerebellum; the narrow, leaf-like gyri of the cerebellar cortex. Also see f. vermis.

**folia lin′guae,** four or five vertical folds on the border of the tongue just in front of the palatoglossal arch; see *papilla* foliata.

**f. ver′mis** [ NA ], a small posterior subdivision of the superior vermis of the cerebellum.

**Folius.** See Folli.

**Folli** (fol-e′) (**Folius**), Cecilio, Venice anatomist, 1615–1660. See F.'s *process.*

**follicle** (fol′ĭ-kl) [ L. *folliculus,* a small sac, dim. of *follis,* a pair of bellows ]. 1. Folliculus. 2. An ovarian f.; one of the spheroidal cell aggregations in the ovary containing an ovum.

**aggregated f.'s,** *folliculi* lymphatici aggregati.

**anovular ovarian f.,** a f. that does not contain an ovum.

**atretic ovarian f.,** corpus atreticum; a f. that degenerates before coming to maturity; great numbers of such atretic f.'s occur in the ovary before puberty, and even in the sexually mature woman several are formed each month.

**dental f.,** the dental sac with its enclosed developing tooth.

**gastric f.'s,** *glandulae* gastricae.

**gastric lymphatic f.,** *folliculus* lymphaticus gastricus.

**Graafian f.,** vesicular ovarian f.

**growing ovarian f.,** a f. having several layers of proliferating follicular cells surrounding the ovum.

**hair f.,** *folliculus* pili.

**intestinal f.'s,** *glandulae* intestinales.

**Lieberkühn's f.'s,** *glandulae* intestinales.

**lingual f.'s,** *folliculi* linguales.

**lymph f., lymphatic f.,** *folliculus* lymphaticus.

**lymphatic f.'s of larynx,** *folliculi* lymphatici laryngei.

**lymphatic f.'s of rectum,** *folliculi* lymphatici recti.

**mature ovarian f.,** a f. ready for ovulation; in the human ovary its antrum attains a diameter of 6 to 8 mm. and presents a surface bulge; a first maturation division usually occurs just prior to the rupture of the f.

Theca externa

Follicular antrum          Theca interna

Primary oocyte

Zona pellucida

**Schematic Representation of a Maturing Follicle**

The oocyte surrounded by the zona pellucida is eccentrically located and the follicular antrum has developed by coalescence of intercellular spaces. (From Langman, J.: *Medical Embryology,* Ed. 2, The Williams & Wilkins Co., Baltimore, 1969.)

**Montgomery's f.,** *glandula* areolaris.

**Nabothian f.,** Nabothian *cyst.*

**ovarian f.,** see follicle (2).

**polyovular ovarian f.,** a f. containing more than one ovum.

**primary ovarian f.,** folliculus ovaricus primarius; an ovarian f. before the appearance of an antrum; marked by developmental changes in the oocyte and follicular cells so that the latter form one or more layers of cuboidal or columnar cells; the f. becomes surrounded by a sheath of stroma, the theca.

**primordial ovarian f.,** a f. in which the primordial oocyte is surrounded by a single layer of flattened follicular cells.

**sebaceous f.,** *glandula* sebacea.

**secondary f.,** vesicular ovarian f.

**solitary f.'s,** *folliculi* lymphatici solitarii.

**splenic lymph f.'s,** *folliculi* lymphatici lienales.

**thyroid f.'s,** *folliculi* glandulae thyroideae.

**vesicular ovarian f.,** folliculus ovaricus vesiculosa; secondary f.; a f. in which the oocyte attains its full size and is surrounded by a thickened oolema (zona pellucida) at the periphery of the fluid-filled antrum. The follicular cells proliferate and form a dense layer called the membrana granulosa. The theca of the f. develops into internal and external layers.

**folliclis** (fol-e-klēs) [ Fr. ]. Papulonecrotic *tuberculid.*

**follicular** (fŏ-lik′u-lar). Relating to a follicle or follicles.

**follic′ulin.** Estrone.

**folliculitis** (fŏ-lik-u-li′tis). An inflammatory reaction in hair follicles. The lesions may be papules or pustules.

**f. absce′dens et suffo′diens,** a chronic progressive follicular-pustular eruption in the scalp.

**ag′minate f.,** *granuloma* trichophyticum.

**f. bar′bae,** *tinea* sycosis.

**f. decal′vans** [ L. *decalvo,* make bald ], alopecia follicularis; Quinquaud's disease; a papular or pustular inflammation of the hair follicles of the scalp, resulting in scarring and loss of hair in the affected area.

**f. keloida′lis,** acne *keloid.*

**f. na′res per′forans,** inflammation of a hair follicle in the nose. The infection perforates through the nose to the outside.

**f. ulerythemato′sa reticula′ta,** atrophoderma reticulatum symmetricum faciei; atrophoderma vermiculatum; erythematous "ice-pick" or pitted scars on the cheeks; a scarring type of folliculitis.

**folliculoid** (fŏ-lik′u-loyd). An obsolete term used (1) to describe an action similar to that of estradiol, the follicular hormone, and (2) as a name for any principle having this action.

**folliculoma** (fŏ-lik′u-lo′mah). 1. Granulosa cell *tumor.* 2. Cystic enlargement of a Graafian follicle.

**folliculosis** (fŏ-lik′u-lo′sis). The presence of lymph follicles in abnormally great numbers.

**folliculus, pl. follic′uli** (fŏ-lik′u-lus) [ L. a small sac, dim. of *follis,* bellows ]. [ NA ]. Follicle (*q.v.*). 1. A more or less spherical mass of cells sometimes containing a cavity. 2. A crypt or minute cul-de-sac or lacuna, such as the depression in the skin, from which the hair emerges.

**folliculi glan′dulae thyroi′deae** [ NA ], follicles of the thyroid gland; the small spherical vesicular components of the thyroid gland lined with epithelium and containing colloid in varying amounts. The colloid serves for storage of thyroid hormones.

**follic′uli lingua′les** [ NA ], lingual follicles; collections of lymphoid tissue in the mucosa of the pharyngeal part of the tongue posterior to the terminal sulcus collectively forming the lingual tonsil.

**f. lymphaticus** [ NA ], nodulus lymphaticus; lymph nodule or follicle; one of the spherical masses of lymphoid cells frequently having a more lightly staining center.

**folliculi lymphat′ici aggrega′ti** [ NA ], aggregated nodules or follicles; Peyer's patches or glands; agmen peyerianum; collections of many lymphoid nodules closely packed together, forming oblong elevations on the mucous membrane of the small intestine.

**folliculi lymphat′ici aggrega′ti appen′dicis vermifor′mis** [ NA ], masses of lymphoid tissue in the submucous coat of the vermiform appendix.

**f. lymphat′icus gastricus** [ NA ], gastric lymphatic follicle; one of the numerous small masses of lymphoid tissue in the gastric mucosa.

**folliculi lymphat′ici laryn′gei** [ NA ], lymphatic follicles of the larynx; small follicles located on the posterior aspect of the epiglottis and in the ventricle of the larynx.

**folliculi lymphat′ici liena′les** [ NA ], splenic lymph follicles or nodules; splenic corpuscles; Malpighian corpuscles or bodies; small nodular masses of lymphoid tissue

attached to the sides of the smaller arterial branches.

**follic′uli lymphat′ici rec′ti** [ NA ], lymphatic follicles of the rectum; scattered collections of lymphoid tissue in the wall of the rectum.

**folliculi lymphat′ici solita′rii** [ NA ], solitary follicles; solitary nodules of the intestine; minute nodules of lymphoid tissue projecting from the mucous membrane of the small and large intestines, being especially numerous in the cecum and appendix.

**f. ovar′icus prima′rius** [ NA ], primary ovarian *follicle.*

**f. ovaricus vesiculo′sus** [ NA ], vesicular ovarian *follicle.*

**f. pili** [ NA ], hair follicle; a deep, narrow pit, formed by invagination of the epidermis and corium; it contains the root of the hair and into it the ducts of the sebaceous glands open; the follicle is lined by a fibrous sheath derived from the corium, and by the outer and inner root sheaths derived from the epidermis.

**Folling,** I. A. See F.'s *disease.*

**fol′ly.** Early 19th century term for madness or insanity; see folie.

**Foltz,** Jean C. E., French ophthalmologist, 1822–1876. See F.'s *valvules.*

**fomentation** (fo′men-ta′shun) [ L. *fomento,* pp. *-atus,* to foment, fr. *fomentum,* a poultice, fr. *foveo,* to keep warm ]. 1. Poultice; stupe; a warm application. 2. Polticing; the application of warmth and moisture in the treatment of disease.

**fomes, pl. fomites** (fo′mēz, fo′mĭ-tēz) [ L. tinder, fr. *foveo,* to keep warm ]. A substance, such as clothing, capable of absorbing and transmitting the contagium of disease; usually used in the plural.

**fo′nazine mesylate** (USAN). PROMAQUID; 10-[ 2-(dimethylamino)propyl ]-*N,N*-dimethylphenothiazine-2-sulfonamide monomethanesulfonate; a serotonin inhibitor.

**Fo′nio,** Anton, Bern physician, *1889. See F.'s *solution.*

**Fonsecaea** (fon-se-se′ah). A genus of dematiaceous fungi which contain species, such as *F. compactum, F. dermatitidis,* and *F. pedrosoi,* that are causative agents of chromoblastomycosis.

**fontac′toscope.** An electroscope for estimating the radioactivity of waters and gases.

**Fontana,** Arturo, Italian dermatologist, 1873–1950. See F.'s *stain.*

**Fontana,** Felice, Italian physiologist, 1720–1805. See F.'s *canal, space.*

**fontanel, fontanelle** (fon′tă-nel′) [ Fr. dim. of *fontaine,* fountain, spring ]. Fonticulus.

**anterior f.,** *fonticulus* anterior.

**anterolateral f.,** *fonticulus* sphenoidalis.

**bregmatic f.,** *fonticulus* anterior.

**Casser's f.,** *fonticulus* mastoideus.

**cranial f.'s,** *fonticuli* cranii.

**frontal f.,** *fonticulus* anterior.

**Gerdy's f.,** sagittal f.

**mastoid f.,** *fonticulus* mastoideus.

**occipital f.,** *fonticulus* posterior.

**posterior f.,** *fonticulus* posterior.

**posterolateral f.,** *fonticulus* mastoideus.

**sag′ittal f.,** an occasional f.-like defect in the sagittal suture in the newborn.

**sphenoidal f.,** *fonticulus* sphenoidalis.

**fonticulus, pl. fontic′uli** (fon-tik′u-lus) [ L. dim. of *fons* ( *font-*), fountain, spring ] [ NA ]. Fontanel; one of several membranous intervals at the angles of the cranial bones in the infant. There are normally six, corresponding to the pterion and asterion, on either side, and to the bregma and lambda, in the median line, in the adult.

**f. ante′rior** [ NA ], anterior fontanel; frontal fontanel; bregmatic fontanel; a diamond-shaped membranous interval at the junction of the coronal, sagittal and metopic sutures where the frontal angles of the parietal bones meet the two ununited halves of the frontal.

**fonticuli cra′nii** [ NA ], cranial fontanels; the membranous intervals between the angles of the cranial bones in the infant. They include the *f. anterior, f. posterior, f. sphenoidalis* and *f. mastoideus.*

**f. mastoideus** [ NA ], mastoid fontanel; posterolateral fontanel; the membranous interval on either side between the mastoid angle of the parietal bone, the mastoid portion of the temporal bone and the occipital bone.

**f. poste'rior** [ NA ], posterior fontanel; occipital fontanel; a triangular interval at the union of the lambdoid and sagittal sutures where the occipital angles of the parietal bones meet the occipital.

**f. sphenoida'lis** [ NA ], sphenoidal fontanel; anterolateral fontanel; an irregularly shaped interval on either side where the frontal, sphenoidal angle of the parietal, squamous portion of the temporal and greater wing of the sphenoid meet.

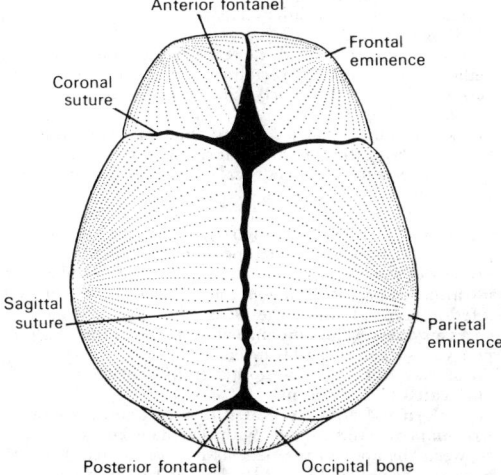

**Fonticuli (Fontanels) in Skull of Newborn**
Seen from above. (From Langman. J.: *Medical Embryology*, Ed. 2, The Williams & Wilkins Co., Baltimore, 1969.)

**food** [ A.S. *fōda* ]. Aliment; nourishment; what is eaten to supply the necessary nutritive elements.

**foot** [ A.S. *fōt* ]. 1. Pes; the lower, pedal, podalic, extremity of the leg. 2. A unit of length, containing 12 inches, equal to 30.48 cm.

**athlete's f.,** *tinea* pedis.

**broad f.,** *metatarsus* latus.

**buttress f.,** a condition of the horse's f. in which there is exostosis of the extensor process of the third phalanx, with swelling and chronic inflammation at the coronary band on the anterior surface of the f.

**claw f.,** a condition of the f. characterized by hyperextension at the metatarsophalangeal joint and flexion at the interphalangeal joints, as a fixed contracture.

**cleft f.,** a congenital deformity in which the division between the toes, especially the third and fourth, extends more or less into the metatarsal region.

**club f.,** talipes.

**contracted f.,** (1) *talipes* cavus; (2) a condition of the horse in which a part of the foot, often a heel, is contracted and shrunken as a result of loss of moisture in the hoof; see also hoof-bound.

**crooked f.,** lack of symmetry in the two sides of a horse's hoof, due usually to bad shoeing.

**cross f.,** *talipes* varus.

**drop f.,** see foot-drop.

**fescue f.,** fescue poisoning; poisoning by a toxic principle in tall fescue grass. It is mainly a disease of cattle, but sheep are sometimes affected. Lameness in the hind feet is first noticed, followed by necrosis of the extremities.

**flat f.,** flatfoot; see *talipes* planus.

**Friedreich's f.,** a form of talipes cavus occurring in Friedreich's disease.

**fungous f.,** maduromycosis.

**f. of hippocampus,** *pes* hippocampi.

**hollow f.,** *talipes* cavus.

**Hong Kong f.,** *tinea* pedis.

**immersion f.,** trench f.; a condition resulting from prolonged exposure to damp and cold; the extremity is initially cold and anesthetic, but on rewarming becomes

hyperemic, paresthetic, and hyperhidrotic; recovery is often slow.

**Madu'ra f.,** maduromycosis.

**march f.,** Deutschländer's disease (1); a painful condition of one f. or both feet as a result of unaccustomed prolonged stress; march fracture(s) may be present or develop subsequently.

**Morand's f.,** a f. having eight toes.

**mossy f.,** lymphedematous keratoderma; lymphostatic verrucosis; a profuse velvety papillomatous growth that develops large warty projections; caused by chronic lymphedema and stasis.

**pumiced f.,** a condition of the horse's hoof, frequently associated with chronic laminitis, in which the sole is level with or extends beyond the bearing surface of the hoof wall, causing lameness particularly when the animal moves on hard surface. The sole becomes thick and flaky.

**reel f.,** clubfoot; see talipes.

**shuffle f.,** a popular term applied to the gait in spastic paralysis and to steppage in foot-drop.

**spastic flat f.,** eversion of the f. due to tautness of the tendons (peroneal) on the outer side; often associated with abnormal bars of bone between the calcaneum and the navicular (scaphoid) or between the navicular and the talus.

**splay f.,** *talipes* planus.

**split f.,** cleft f.

**spread f.,** *metatarsus* latus.

**stump f.,** clubfoot; see talipes.

**swell f.,** swelling and redness of the metatarsus, with pain and disability due to sprain of the ligaments (syndesmitis metatarsea), and frequently detachment of them from the bones, chips of bone being torn off with the rupture. The trouble results from jumping or the strain of dancing or long marches, being especially produced, it is said, by the goose-step method of marching practiced in certain armies.

**tip f.,** *talipes* equinus.

**trench f.,** immersion f.

**weak f.,** an incipient flatfoot.

**foot'candle.** Illumination or brightness equivalent to 1 lumen per square foot. Replaced in the SI system by the candela (1 lumen per square meter).

**foot-drop.** Paralysis of the dorsiflexor muscles of the foot and ankle, as a consequence of which the foot falls, the toes dragging on the ground in walking.

**foot'plate, foot-plate.** 1. *Basis* stapedis. 2. Pedicel.

**foot-pound.** The energy expended, or work done, in raising a mass of 1 pound a height of 1 foot, vertically against gravitational force.

**foot-poundal.** Energy exerted, or work done, when a force of 1 poundal displaces a body 1 foot in the direction of the force.

**forage** (fo-rahzh') [ F. boring ]. The operation of cutting a channel by surgical diathermy through an enlarged prostate.

# FORAMEN

**foramen,** pl. **foramina** (fo-ra'men, fo-ram'ĭ-nah) [ L. an aperture, fr. *foro*, to pierce ] [ NA ]. An aperture or perforation through a bone or a membranous structure.

**alveolar foramina,** foramina alveolaria.

**foramina alveolaria** [ NA ], alveolar foramina; openings of the posterior dental canals on the posterolateral surface of the body of the maxilla.

**anterior con'dyloid f.,** *canalis* hypoglossi.

**anterior palatine foramina,** foramina palatina minora.

**aor'tic f.,** *hiatus* aorticus.

**apical f.,** f. apicis dentis.

**f. apicis dentis** [ NA ], apical dental f.; the opening at the apex of the root of a tooth that gives passage to the nerve and blood vessels.

**arach'noid f.,** *apertura* mediana ventriculi quarti.

**Bichat's f.,** *cisterna* venae magnae cerebri.

**blind f. of frontal bone,** f. cecum ossis frontalis.

blind f. of tongue, f. cecum linguae.

Bochdalek's f., pleuroperitoneal *hiatus.*

Botallo's f., the orifice of communication between the two atria of the fetal heart.

Bozzi's f., *macula* retinae.

f. bursae omenta'lis major'is, a f. produced by two folds of peritoneum that encroach upon and constrict the lesser sac of peritoneum; it forms a communication between the superior recess of the lesser sac which lies above it and the inferior recess below.

carot'id f., the opening at each extremity of the carotid canal in the petrous portion of the temporal bone; the external carotid f. is one the inferior surface of the pyramid; the internal is at the apex.

cecal f. of frontal bone, f. cecum ossis frontalis.

cecal f. of tongue, f. cecum linguae.

f. cecum linguae [ NA ], blind f. of the tongue; Morgagni's f. (1); a median pit on the dorsum of the posterior part of the tongue, from which the limbs of a V-shaped furrow run forward and outward. It is the site of origin of the thyroid gland in the embryo.

f. cecum of medulla oblongata, Vicq d'Azyr's f.; small triangular depression at the lower boundary of the pons that marks the upper limit of the median fissure of the medulla oblongata.

f. cecum ossis frontalis [ NA ], blind f. of the frontal bone; the f. formed by a notch at the lower end of the frontal crest and its articulation with the ethmoid bone.

conjugate f., a f. formed by the notches of two bones in apposition.

f. costotransversa'rium [ NA ], costotransverse f.; an opening between the neck of a rib and the transverse process of a vertebra, occupied by the costotransverse ligament.

costotransverse f., f. costotransversarium.

f. diaphrag'matis sellae, a hole in the center of the diaphragm of the sella giving passage to the infundibulum.

Duverney's f., f. epiploicum.

emissary sphenoidal f., a small f. situated in the sphenoid bone between the f. ovale and the scaphoid fossa; it transmits an emissary vein from the cavernous sinus.

epiploic f., f. epiploicum.

f. epiplo'icum [ NA ], epiploic f.; Duverney's f.; aditus ad saccum peritonaei minorum; f. of Winslow; the passage, below and behind the portal fissure of the liver, connecting the two sacs of the peritoneum.

ethmoidal f., f. ethmoidale.

f. ethmoida'le [ NA ], ethmoidal f.; one of two foramina, anterior (f. ethmoidale anterius) and posterior (f. ethmoidale posterius), formed by grooves on either edge of the ethmoidal notch of the frontal bone, and completed by similar grooves on the ethmoid bone.

external auditory f., *meatus* acusticus externus.

Ferrein's f., *hiatus* canalis nervi petrosi majoris.

f. fronta'le [ NA ], an occasional small opening in the supraorbital margin of the frontal bone medial to the supraorbital foramen. See also *incisura* frontalis.

great f., f. magnum.

greater palatine f., f. palatinum majus.

Huschke's f., an opening in the floor of the bony meatus acusticus, usually closed in the adult.

Hyrtl's f., *porus* crotaphytico-buccinatorius.

incisive f., f. incisivum.

f. incisi'vum [ NA ], incisive f.; incisor f.; f. of Stensen; one of several (usually four) openings of the incisive canals into the incisive fossa.

incisor f., f. incisivum.

inferior dental f., f. mandibulae.

infraorbital f., f. infraorbitale.

f. infraorbita'le [ NA ], infraorbital f.; the external opening of the infraorbital canal, on the anterior surface of the body of the maxilla.

interatrial f. primum, ostium primum; f. subseptale; (1) in the embryonic heart the temporary opening between right and left atria situated between the lower margin of the septum primum and the atrioventricular canal cushions; (2) in an adult heart the abnormal persistence of the so-named communication which is normal in young embryos.

interatrial f. secundum, ostium secundum; a secondary opening appearing in the upper part of the septum primum in the sixth week of embryonic life, just prior to the closure of the interatrial f. primum.

internal auditory f., *porus* acusticus internus.

interventricular f., f. interventriculare.

f. interventricula're [ NA ], interventricular f.; f. of Monro; porta (2); the short, often slitlike passage that, on both the left and right side, connects the third brain ventricle (in the diencephalon) with the lateral ventricle (in the cerebral hemisphere); the passage is bounded anteriorly by the columna fornicis and posteriorly by the anterior pole of the thalamus.

intervertebral f., f. intervertebrale.

f. intervertebra'le [ NA ], intervertebral f.; one of a number of openings into the spinal canal bounded by the pedicles of adjoining vertebrae above and below, the vertebral bodies anteriorly, and the articular processes posteriorly.

f. ischiad'icum [ NA ], sciatic f.; one of two foramina, the f. i. majus and the f. i. minus, formed by the sacrospinous and sacrotuberous ligaments crossing the sciatic notches of the hip bone.

jugular f., f. jugulare.

f. jugula're [ NA ], jugular f.; a passage between the petrous portion of the temporal bone and the jugular process of the occipital, sometimes divided into two by the intrajugular processes; it contains the internal jugular vein, inferior petrosal sinus, the glossopharyngeal, vagus, and accessory nerves, and meningeal branches of the ascending pharyngeal and occipital arteries.

f. of Key-Retzius, *apertura* lateralis ventriculi quarti.

lacerated f. f. lacerum.

f. lac'erum [ NA ], lacerated f.; f. lacerum medium; an irregular aperture filled with cartilage in the living, between the apex of the petrous part of the temporal, the body of the sphenoid, and the basilar part of the occipital bones. Several structures pass along the margins of the f. but no structures pass through.

f. lac'erum ante'rius, *fissura* orbitalis superior.

f. lac'erum medium, f. lacerum.

f. lac'erum posterius, f. jugulare.

Lannelongue's foramina, venous openings into the right atrium, probably identical with f. venae minimae (Thebesian f.).

f. latera'lis ventric'uli quar'ti, *apertura* lateralis ventriculi quarti.

lesser palatine foramina, f. palatina minora.

f. of Luschka, *apertura* lateralis ventriculi quarti.

Magendie's f., *apertura* mediana ventriculi quarti.

f. mag'num, great f.; the large opening in the basal part of the occipital bone through which the spinal cord becomes continuous with the medulla oblongata.

malar f., f. zygomaticofaciale.

f. mandib'ulae [ NA ], mandibular f.; inferior dental f.; the opening into the mandibular canal on the medial surface of the ramus of the mandible.

mandibular f., f. mandibulae.

mastoid f., f. mastoideum.

f. mastoideum [ NA ], mastoid f.; an opening at the posterior portion of the mastoid process, transmitting a small artery to the dura and an emissary vein to the lateral sinus.

mental f., f. mentale.

f. menta'le [ NA ], mental f.; mental canal; the anterior opening of the mandibular canal on the body of the mandible lateral to and above the mental tubercle.

Monro's f., f. interventriculare.

Morgagni's f., (1) f. cecum linguae; (2) parasternal hernia; congenital defect in the fusion of sternal and costal elements of the diaphragmatic anlage.

nasal f., vascular f. opening on the outer surface of each nasal bone.

foramina nervo'sa [ NA ], habenulae perforata; zona perforata; the perforations along the tympanic lip of the spiral lamina giving passage to the cochlear nerves.

f. nutricium [ NA ], nutrient f.; the external opening of the canalis nutricius in a bone.

nutrient f., f. nutricium.

obturator f., f. obturatum.

f. obtura'tum [ NA ], obturator f.; a large, oval or irregularly triangular aperture in the hip bone, the margins of which are formed by the pubis and the ischium; it is closed in the natural state by the obturator membrane, except for a small opening for the passage of the obturator vessels and nerve.

**olfac'tory f.,** one of the openings in the cribriform plate of the ethmoid bone, transmitting the olfactory nerves.

**optic f.,** *canalis* opticus.

**f. opticum,** *canalis* opticus.

**f. ova'le,** (1) [ NA ], in the fetal heart, the oval opening in septum secundum; the persistent part of septum primum acts as a valve for this interatrial communication during fetal life and postnatally becomes fused to septum secundum to close it; (2) [ NA ], a large oval opening in the greater wing of the sphenoid bone, transmitting the nerve and a small meningeal artery; (3) valvular incompetence of the f. ovale of the heart; a condition contrasting with probe patency of the f. ovale in that the valvula foraminis ovalis has abnormal perforations in it or is of insufficient size to afford adequate valvular action at the f. ovale prenatally, or effect a complete closure postnatally.

**Pacchionian f.,** *incisura* tentorii.

**foramina palatina minora** [ NA ], lesser palatine foramina; anterior palatine foramina; openings on the hard palate of palatine canals passing vertically through the tuberosity of the palate bone and transmitting the smaller palatine nerves and vessels.

**f. palatinum majus** [ NA ], greater palatine f.; an opening in the posterolateral corner of the hard palate opposite the last molar tooth, marking the lower end of the pterygopalatine canal.

**foramina papilla'ria re'nis** [ NA ], papillary foramina of the kidney; numerous minute openings, the apertures of the secreting tubules, in the summit of each renal papilla.

**papillary foramina of kidney,** foramina papillaria renis.

**parietal f.,** f. parietale.

**f. parieta'le** [ NA ], parietal f.; a f. in the parietal bone near the sagittal margin posteriorly; it transmits an emissary vein to the superior sagittal sinus.

**posterior con'dyloid f.,** *canalis* condylaris.

**posterior pal'atine f.,** f. palatinum majus.

**postgle'noid f.,** a small f. that is sometimes present in the temporal bone immediately in front of the external acoustic meatus.

**f. quadra'tum,** f. venae cavae.

**Retzius' f.,** *apertura* lateralis ventriculi quarti.

**Rivinus' f.,** obsolescent eponym for pleuroperitoneal *hiatus.*

**root f.,** opening at or near the apex of the root of a tooth through which nerves and blood vessels are conducted.

**f. rotun'dum** [ NA ], round f.; an opening in the great wing of the sphenoid bone, transmitting the maxillary nerve.

**round f.,** f. rotundum.

**sacral f.,** f. sacrale.

**f. sacra'le** [ NA ], sacral f.; one of the foramina sacralia, the openings between the fused sacral vertebrae transmitting the sacral nerves. The anterior foramina, **foramina sacralia pelvina,** transmit ventral branches of the sacral nerves. The posterior foramina, **foramina sacralia dorsalia,** give passage to dorsal branches of the sacral nerves.

**Scarpa's foramina,** two openings in the line of the intermaxillary suture; the anterior f. transmits the left nasopalatine nerve, the posterior the right.

**sciatic f.,** f. ischiadicum.

**f. singula're** [ NA ], solitary f.; a f. in the internal acoustic meatus, behind the area cochlearis, that transmits the nerves to the ampulla of the posterior semicircular duct.

**Soemmering's f.,** *fovea* centralis, which was thought at one time to be an opening.

**solitary f.,** f. singulare.

**sphenopalatine f.,** f. sphenopalatinum.

**f. sphenopalati'num** [ NA ], sphenopalatine f.; the f. formed from the sphenopalatine notch of the palate bone when closed in by articulation with the under surface of the sphenoid bone.

**sphenotic f.,** f. lacerum.

**f. spino'sum** [ NA ], an opening in the great wing of the sphenoid bone, anterior to the spine, transmitting the middle meningeal artery.

**Stensen's f.,** f. incisivum.

**stylomastoid f.,** f. stylomastoideum.

**f. stylomastoid'eum** [ NA ], stylomastoid f.; an opening on the inferior surface of the petrous portion of the temporal bone, between the styloid and mastoid processes; it transmits the facial nerve and stylomastoid artery.

**f. subsepta'le,** interatrial f. primum.

**supraorbital f.,** f. supraorbitale.

**f. supraorbita'le** [ NA ], supraorbital f.; a f. in the supraorbital margin of the frontal bone at the junction of the medial and intermediate thirds. See also *incisura* supraorbitalis.

**Tarin's f.,** *canalis* facialis.

**Thebesian f.,** f. venae minimae.

**thyroid f.,** (1) f. thyroideum; (2) an obsolete term for f. obturatum.

**f. thyroid'eum** [ NA ], thyroid f.; an opening occasionally existing in one or both of the plates of the thyroid cartilage.

**f. transversa'rium** [ NA ], transverse f.; vertebroarterial f.; the f. in the transverse process of a cervical vertebra for the passage of the vertebral artery and vein and sympathetic nerve plexus.

**transverse f.,** f. transversarium.

**f. of vena cava,** f. venae cavae.

**f. venae cavae** [ NA ], f. of the vena cava; f. quadratum; an opening in the right lobe of the central tendon of the diaphragm which transmits the inferior vena cava and branches of the right phrenic nerve.

**f. venae min'imae** [ NA ], one of the foramina venarum minimarum or foramina of the smallest veins; Thebesian f.; one of a number of fossae in the wall of the right auricle, or atrium, containing the openings of minute veins.

**vert'ebral f.,** f. vertebrale.

**f. vertebra'le,** [ NA ], vertebral f.; the f. formed by the union of the vertebral arch with the body.

**vertebroarte'rial f.,** f. transversarium.

**Vesalius' f.,** a minute, in constant opening in the sphenoid bone, anterior and medial to the f. ovale, transmitting a small emissary vein from the cavernous sinus.

**Vicq d'Azyr's f.,** f. cecum of medulla oblongata.

**Vieussens' foramina,** foramina venarum minimarum.

**Weitbrecht's f.,** an opening in the capsular ligament of the shoulder joint, communicating with a bursa beneath the tendon of the subscapularis muscle.

**Winslow's f.,** f. epiploicum.

**zygomaticofacial f.,** f. zygomaticofaciale.

**f. zygomaticofacia'le** [ NA ], zygomaticofacial f.; malar f.; the opening on the outer surface of the zygomatic bone below the orbital margin that transmits the zygomaticofacial nerve.

**zygomaticoorbital f.,** f. zygomaticoorbitale.

**f. zygomat'icoorbita'le** [ NA ], zygomaticoorbital f.; the common opening on the orbital surface of the zygomatic bone of the canals transmitting the zygomaticofacial and zygomaticotemporal nerves; sometimes each of these canals has a separate opening on the orbital surface.

**zygomaticotemporal f.,** f. zygomaticotemporale.

**f. zygomat'icotempora'le** [ NA ], zygomaticotemporal f.; the opening, on the temporal surface of the zygomatic bone, of the canal that gives passage to the zygomaticotemporal nerve.

---

**foram'ina.** Plural of foramen.

**Foraminifera** (fo-ram'ĭ-nif'er-ah, for'ă-mĭ-nif'er-ah) [ L. *foramen,* aperture, + *fero,* to carry ]. A subclass of Rhizopoda having anastomosing pseudopodia; these form a network around the cell which usually develops into a complex calcareous shell; important component of ocean bottom and rockbeds overlying oil deposits.

**foraminiferous** (fo-ram'ĭ-nif'er-us, for'ă-mĭ-nif'er-us). 1. Having openings or foramina. 2. Relating to the Foraminifera.

**for'aminot'omy** [ L. *foramen,* aperture, + G. *tomē,* a cutting ]. Surgical enlargement of the intervertebral foramen.

**foraminulum,** pl. **foramin'ula** (for'ă-min'u-lum) [ Mod. L. dim. of *foramen* ]. A very minute foramen.

**Forbes,** A. P. See F.-Albright *syndrome.*

**Forbes,** Gilbert B., American pediatrician, *1915. See F. *disease.*

**Forbes,** Thomas R. See Hooker-F. *test.*

force [ L. *fortis*, strong ]. Power; strength; that which tends to produce motion in a body.

**animal f.,** muscular power.

**anterior component of f.,** see under component.

**chewing f.,** the degree of force applied by the muscles of mastication during the mastication of food; see also masticatory f.

**component of f.,** see under component.

**electromotive f.,** abbreviated EMF; the f. (measured in volts) that causes the flow of electricity from one point to another.

**G f.,** inertial f. produced by accelerations or gravity, expressed in gravitational units; one G is equal to the pull of gravity at the earth's surface at sea level and 45° latitude (32.2 ft./sec.$^2$; 980.6 cm./sec.$^2$); see also G. (1) and *g*.

**London f.'s,** interactions between atoms caused by dipoles created by electron distribution; the same as Van der Waal's f.'s, *q.v.*

**f. of mastication,** masticatory f.; biting strength; the motive f. created by the dynamic action of the muscles during the physiologic act of mastication.

**masticatory f.,** f. of mastication.

**nerve f., nervous f.,** the property of nerve tissue to conduct stimuli.

**occlusal f.,** the result of muscular f. applied on opposing teeth.

**psychic f.,** psychic *energy*.

**reserve f.,** the energy residing in the organism or any of its parts above that required for its normal functioning.

**van der Waals' f.'s,** first postulated by van der Waals in 1873 to explain deviations from ideal gas behavior seen in real gases; the attractive f.'s between atoms or molecules other than electrostatic (ionic) or covalent (sharing of electrons) or hydrogen bonding (sharing a proton); generally ascribed to dipolar and dispersion effects, $\pi$-electrons, etc. These relatively nondescript f.'s contribute to socalled hydrophobic binding or organophilicity, the attraction of nonpolar substances (organic molecules) to each other.

**vital f.,** see vitalism.

**for'ceps** [ L. a pair of tongs ]. 1. An instrument for seizing anything and making compression or traction. 2 [ NA ]. Bands of white fibers in the brain, f. major and f. minor.

**alligator f.,** see fig.

**Allis f.,** a grasping or tissue f.; see fig. under culdocentesis.

**f. anterior,** f. minor.

**Arruga's f.,** a popular f. for the intracapsular extraction of a cataract.

**artery f.,** a locking f. with sloping blades for grasping the end of an artery until a ligature is applied.

**axis-traction f.,** obstetrical f. provided with a second handle so attached that traction can be made in the line in which the head must move in the axis of the pelvis.

**Babcock f.,** grasping f. used in handling delicate tissues.

**Barton's f.,** f. with one fixed curved blade and a lunged anterior blade for application to a high transverse head.

**bone f.,** a strong f. used for seizing and removing fragments of bone.

**bulldog f.,** a f. for holding a bleeding vessel.

**bullet f.,** f. with thin curved blades with serrated grasping surface, used for extracting a bullet from tissues.

**capsule f.,** a fine, strong f. used for removing the capsule of the lens in cataract.

**Chamberlen f.,** the original obstetrical f., and without a curve.

**clamp f. (rubber dam),** rubber dam clamp f.; a f. with pronged jaws designed to engage the jaws of a rubber dam clamp so that they may be separated to pass over the widest buccolingual contour of a tooth.

**clip f.,** a small f. with spring catch to hold a bleeding vessel.

**dental f.,** extracting f.; f. used to luxate teeth and remove them from the alveolus.

**dressing f.,** a f. for general use in dressing wounds, removing fragments of necrosed tissue, small foreign bodies, etc.

**extracting f.,** dental f.

**hemostatic f.,** f. with a catch for locking the blades, used for seizing the cut end of an artery to control hemorrhage.

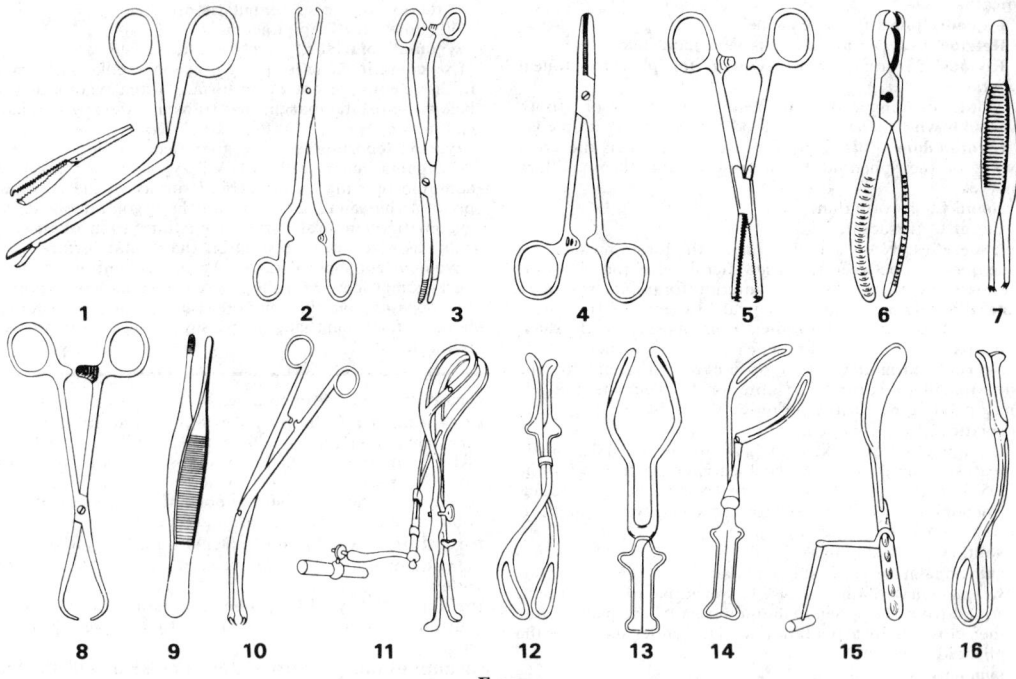

**Forceps**

Types of forceps: *1*, alligator; *2*, bullet; *3*, dressing; *4*, hemostatic; *5*, Kocher's; *6*, lion-jaw bone-holding (osteophore); *7*, mouse-tooth; *8*, tenaculum; *9*, thumb; *10*, vulsella. Types of obstetrical forceps: *11*, Tarnier's axis traction; *12*, Kjelland's; *13*, Simpson's; *14*, Barton's; *15*, Tucker-McLean, Bill's axis traction handle; *16*, Piper's.

**Hodge's f.,** a form of obstetrical f.

**Kjelland's f.,** f. having a sliding lock, and little pelvic curve.

**Knapp's f.,** roller f.; trachoma f.; a small f., the blades of which are formed of rollers, used to express trachomatous granulations on the palpebral conjunctiva.

**Kocher's f.,** a f. for grasping the tissues in a surgical operation or for making compression of bleeding structures.

**Koeberlé's f.,** a hemostatic f.

**Lahey f.,** thyroid f. useful in delivering the uterus at vaginohysterectomy.

**Laplace's f.,** a f. for approximating intestine during surgical anastomosis.

**Levret's f.,** a modification of the Chamberlen f., curved to correspond to the curve of the parturient passage.

**lion-jaw bone-holding f.,** see fig.

**Liston's f.,** a bone-cutting f.

**Löwenberg's f.,** f. with short curved blades ending in rounded grasping extremities devised for the removal of adenoid growths in the nasopharynx.

**f. ma'jor** [ NA ], f. posterior; pars occipitalis; occipital part of the radiation of the corpus callosum; that part of the fiber radiation of the corpus callosum which bends sharply backward into the occipital lobe of the cerebrum.

**f. mi'nor** [ NA ], f. anterior; pars frontalis; frontal part of the radiation of the corpus callosum; that part of the fiber radiation of the corpus callosum which bends forward toward the frontal pole of the cerebrum.

**mosquito f.,** a very small f. for holding tissue.

**mouse-tooth f.,** f. with one or two fine points at the tip of each blade, fitting into hollows between the points on the opposite blade.

**nonfenestrated f.,** obstetrical f. without fenestrae or openings in the blades, thus facilitating rotation of the head.

**obstetrical f.,** f. used for grasping and making traction on or rotation of the fetal head. They are introduced separately into the genital canal, permitting the fetal head to be grasped firmly but with minimal compression, and then are articulated after being placed in correct position. Each branch is made up of four portions: blade, handle, shank, and lock.

**O'Hara f.,** two slender clamp f. held together by a serrefine, used in the technique of intestinal anastomosis.

**Péan's f.,** a clamp for obtaining hemostasis by forcipressure.

**Piper's f.,** obstetrical f. used to facilitate delivery of the head in breech presentation; see figs. under forceps and under breech *extraction.*

**f. posterior,** f. major.

**roller f.,** Knapp's f.

**Simpson's f.,** an obstetrical f.

**speculum f.,** a slender f. for use through a speculum, a form of tubular f.

**Tarnier's f.,** f. used in axis *traction, q.v.*

**tenac'ulum f.,** f. with jaws armed each with a sharp, straight hook like a tenaculum.

**thumb f.,** spring f. used by compression with thumb and forefinger.

**torsion f.,** f. used for making torsion on an artery to arrest hemorrhage.

**tracho'ma f.,** Knapp's f.

**tubular f.,** a long slender f. intended for use through a cannula or other tubular instrument.

**Tucker-McLean f.,** see fig.

**vulsella f., vulsel'lum f.,** volsella; f. with vulsellum hooks at the tip of each blade.

**Walsham f.,** one used in rhinoplasty for straightening irregularities of the nasal septum.

**Wells' f.,** a hemostatic f.

**Willett's f.,** willet's clamp; a scalp traction f. used to treat placenta previa by pulling fetal head down against the placenta.

**Forchheimer** (for'shi-mur), Frederick, Cincinnati physician, 1853–1913. See F.'s *sign.*

**for'cipate.** Shaped like a forceps.

**for'cipressure.** A method of arresting hemorrhage by compressing the artery with forceps.

**Fordyce,** John A., New York dermatologist, 1858–1925. See F.'s *angiokeratoma, disease, granules, spots,* Fox-F. *disease.*

**fore'arm.** Antebrachium; the segment of the superior limb between the elbow and the wrist.

**fore'brain.** Prosencephalon.

**fore'conscious.** Denoting memories, not at present in the consciousness, which can be evoked from time to time; or an unconscious mental process which becomes conscious only on the fulfillment of certain conditions.

**fore'finger.** Index (1).

**fore'foot.** A front foot of a quadruped.

**fore'gut.** Headgut; the cephalic portion of the primitive digestive tube in the embryo. From its entoderm arises the epithelial lining of the pharynx, trachea, lungs, esophagus, and stomach; the first part and cranial half of the second part of the duodenum; and the parenchyma of the liver and pancreas.

**forehead** (for'ed, fōr'hed). Frons.

**Olympian f.,** the abnormally prominent, high, and broad f. in hereditary syphilis.

**fore'kidney.** Pronephros.

**Forel,** Auguste H., Swiss neurologist, 1848–1931. See F.'s *decussation, fields,* tegmental *fields.*

**fore'milk.** 1. Colostrum. 2. The first portion of milk obtained from the cow's udder at milking.

**forensic** (fo-ren'sik) [ L. *forensis,* of a forum ]. Pertaining to, or used in, legal proceedings. See also forensic *dentistry, medicine; psychiatry, psychology.*

**fore'play.** The stimulative sexual play preceding sexual intercourse.

**fore'pleasure.** The sexual pleasure resulting from the foreplay that precedes the final genital-orgastic pleasure in sexual intercourse.

**fore'skin.** Preputium.

**fore'stomach.** *Antrum* cardiacum.

**fore'top.** The tuft of a horse's main, covering the forehead.

**fore'waters.** Bulging membranes filled with amniotic fluid presenting in front of the fetal head.

**forging** (for'jing). A defect of the horse's gait in which the under surface of the front foot (or shoe) is struck with the toe of the rear foot (or shoe) of the same side while trotting.

**fork.** 1. A pronged instrument used for holding or lifting. 2. An instrument resembling a f. in that it has tines or prongs.

**bite f.,** face-bow f.

**face-bow f.,** bite f.; that part of the face-bow assemblage used to attach the maxillary trial base to the face-bow proper.

**tuning f.,** a steel or magnesium instrument roughly resembling a two-pronged f., the vibrations of the prongs of which, when struck, give a musical note; used to test the hearing, especially bone conduction.

**form** [ L. *forma* ]. Shape; structure; mold.

**accolé f.'s,** appliqué f.'s.

**appliqué f.'s,** accolé f.'s; a term applied to the manner in which the ring stage of *Plasmodium falciparum* parasitizes the marginal portion of erythrocytes.

**arch f.,** the shape of the dental arch.

**boat f.,** the less stable of two conformations assumed by 6-membered cyclic sugars (pyranoses); opposed to chair f. See also Haworth conformational formulas, under sugars.

**chair f.,** the more stable of two conformations assumed by 6-membered cyclic sugars (*e.g.,* the pyranoses); opposed to boat f. See also Haworth conformational formulas, under sugars.

**convenience f.,** a step in the preparation of a cavity in a tooth, designed to make the operative procedure easier.

**face f.,** (1) the outline f. of the face; (2) the outline f. of the face from an anterior view.

**half-chair f.,** see Haworth conformational formulas, under sugars.

**involution f.,** an irregular or atypical bacterial cell produced as a result of exposure to unfavorable conditions.

**L. f.,** L-phase *variant.*

**occlusal f.,** occlusal pattern; the f. of the occlusal surface of a tooth or a row of teeth.

**posterior tooth f.,** the distinguishing contours of the occlusal surface of the various posterior teeth.

**replicative f.,** RF; the altered, double-stranded f. to which single-stranded coliphage DNA is converted after infection of a susceptible bacterium, formation of the complementary ("minus") strand being mediated by enzymes that were present in the bacterium before entrance of the viral ("plus") strand.

**resistance f.,** in dentistry, the orientation given the seat of a cavity so that no shear between it and the base of the restoration may result under the force of mastication. This is brought about by placing the seat at right angles to this force. Usually thought of in connection with retention f., to which it is intimately related.

**retention f.,** in dentistry, the modification of shape of a cavity (as a dove-tailed lock or undercuts) for the purpose of preventing the restoration from being displaced by lateral compo.;ents of force due to cusp and ridge inclines. Usually thought of in connection with resistance f., to which it is intimately related.

**sickle f.,** malarial *crescent.*

**skew f.,** see Haworth conformational formulas, under sugars.

**tooth f.,** dental anatomy; the characteristics of the curves, lines, angles, and contours of various teeth which permit their identification and differentiation.

**twist f.,** see Haworth conformational formulas, under sugars.

**wave f.,** waveshape; the f. of a pulse; *e.g.,* of the pacemaker pulse as demonstrated on the oscilloscope under a specified load.

**wax f.,** wax *pattern.*

**formal′dehyde** [ form(ic) + aldehyde ]. Formic aldehyde, methyl aldehyde; a pungent gas, H—CHO; used as an antiseptic and disinfectant.

**f. dehydrogenase** (EC 1.2.1.1), enzyme catalyzing the exidation of formaldehyde to formic acid.

**formalin.** Formol; a 37 per cent aqueous solution of formaldehyde.

**formalinize.** To add formalin solution to inactivated vaccines without destroying their immunizing power.

**formamidase** (EC 3.5.1.9). Formylase; kynurenine formamidase; an enzyme catalyzing the hydrolysis of formylkynurenine to kynurenine and formate—a reaction of significance in tryptophan catabolism.

**for′mate.** A salt or ester of formic acid; contains the monovalent radical HCOO—.

**f. dehydrogenases,** bacterial enzymes catalyzing breakdown of formic acid (formate) to $CO_2$ and a reduced hydrogen acceptor, either NAD (EC 1.2.1.2) or cytochrome *b* (EC 1.2.2.1).

**formatio** (for-ma′shī-o) [ L. fr. *formo,* pp. *-atus,* to form ] [ NA ]. A formation; a structure of definite shape or cellular arrangement.

**f. hippocampa′lis,** hippocampal formation; see hippocampus.

**f. reticula′ris** [ NA ], reticular formation; reticular substance (2); substantia reticularis; Stilling's fibers; a massive but vaguely delimited neural apparatus composed of closely intermingled gray and white matter and extending throughout the length of the spinal cord and upward into the diencephalon. The term is vague and refers by-and-large to the large neuronal population of the brainstem and spinal cord that does not compose motoneuronal cell groups or cell groups forming part of specific sensory conduction systems. Its neurons generally have long dendrites and heterogeneous afferent connections, the reason why the formation is often called "nonspecific." The f. reticularis has extremely complex, largely polysynaptic ascending and descending connections that play a dominant role in the central control of autonomic (respiration, blood pressure, thermoregulation, etc.) and endocrine functions, as well as in bodily posture, skeletomuscular reflex activity, and general behavioral states such as alertness and sleep. See also reticular activating *system.*

**formation** (for-ma′shun). 1. Formatio. 2. That which is formed. 3. The act of giving form and shape.

**concept f.,** in psychology, the learning to conceive and respond in terms of abstract ideas based upon an action or object.

**personality f.,** the life history associated with the development of individual patterns and of one's individuality.

**reaction f.,** in psychoanalysis, the development of conscious attitudes and interests that are the opposites of certain unconscious or infantile trends; *e.g.,* excessive cleanliness as a reaction to anal interests.

**reticular f.,** *formatio* reticularis.

**rouleaux f.** [ Fr. pl. of *rouleau,* a roll ], the arrangement of red blood cells in fluid blood (or in diluted suspensions) with their biconcave surfaces in apposition, thereby forming groups that resemble stacks of coins.

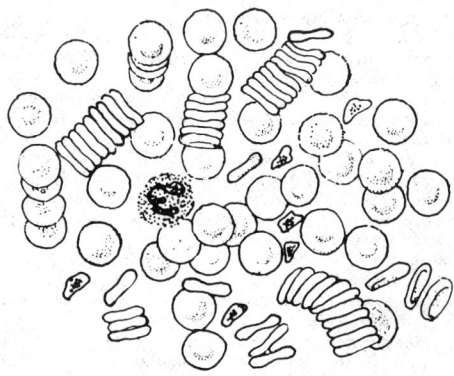

**Red Blood Cells in Rouleaux Formation**

**symptom f.,** symptom *substitution.*

**for′mazan.** A water-insoluble colored compound of the general structure, $RNH—N=CR'—N=NR''$, formed by reduction of a tetrazolium salt (*q.v.*) in the histochemical demonstration of oxidative enzymes. The R's are usually phenyl groups.

**form′board.** A board containing cut-outs in various shapes, into which blocks of corresponding shape are to be fitted; an intelligence test.

**forme fruste,** pl. **formes frustes** (form früst) [ Fr. from L. *forma,* form; *frustra,* without effect ]. A partial or arrested form of disease.

**for′mic** [ L. *formica,* ant ]. Relating to ants; pertaining to f. acid.

**f. acid,** H—COOH; the smallest carboxylic acid. A strong caustic; used as an astringent and counterirritant.

**f. aldehyde,** formaldehyde.

**f. hydrogenylase,** see formate dehydrogenase.

**formication** (for′mĭ-ka′shun) [ L. *formica,* ant ]. A form of paresthesia in which there is a sensation as of ants running over the skin.

**formiminoglutamic acid.** $HN=CH—NH—CH(COOH)CH_2CH_2COOH$; an intermediate in histidine catabolism. An intermediate metabolite in the conversion of histidine to glutamic acid; f. acid may appear in the urine of patients with folic acid or vitamin $B_{12}$ deficiency, or liver disease. Sometimes abbreviated FIGLU.

**formini′trazole.** AROXINE; *N*-(5-nitro-2-thiazolyl)formamide; antitrichomonal agent administered intravaginally.

**formol.** Formalin.

**formononetin.** Neochanin; 7-hydroxy-4′-methoxyisoflavone; diuretic.

**formosulfathi′azole.** INTRAFORMAZOL; *N*′-(2-thiazyl)sulfanilamide condensation product with formaldehyde; antimicrobial agent for treatment of intestinal infections.

# FORMULA

**for'mula,** pl. **formulas** or **formulae** [ L. dim. of *forma,* form ]. 1. A recipe or prescription containing directions for the compounding of a medicinal preparation. 2. In chemistry, a symbol or collection of symbols expressing the number of atoms of the element or elements forming one molecule of a substance, together with, on occasion, information concerning the arrangement of the atoms within the molecule, their electronic structure, their charge, the nature of the bonds within the molecule, and so on.

**Arneth f.,** the normal, approximate ratio of polymorphonuclear neutrophils, based on the number of lobes in the nuclei, as follows: 1 lobe, 5 per cent; 2 lobes, 35 per cent; 3 lobes, 41 per cent; 4 lobes, 17 per cent; 5 lobes, 2 per cent.

**Bazett's f.,** a f. for correcting the observed Q-T interval in the electrocardiogram for cardiac rate: corrected Q-T = Q-T sec/$\sqrt{\text{R-R}}$ sec.

**Bernhardt's f.,** used to calculate the ideal weight, in kilograms, for an adult. It is the height in centimeters times the chest circumference in centimeters divided by 240.

**Bird's f.,** the third and fourth figures in a 4-digit value for the specific gravity of urine are also an approximate indication of the number of grains of solids per ounce.

**Black's f.,** a translation of Pignet's f. into British measurements: $F = (W + C) - H;$ $F$ is the empirical factor, $W$ is the weight in pounds, $C$ the chest girth in inches at full inspiration, and $H$ the height in inches; a man is classed as very strong when $F$ is over 120, strong between 110 and 120, good 100 to 110, fair 90 to 100, weak 80 to 90, very weak under 80.

**Broca's f.,** a fully developed man (30 years old) should weigh as many kilograms as he is centimeters in height over and above 1 meter.

**chemical f.,** a statement of the structure of a molecule expressed in chemical symbols.

**Christison's f.,** Häser's f.

**constitutional f.,** structural f.

**Demoivre's f.,** a f. for calculating life expectancy. It is two-thirds of the difference between the age of the person and 80.

**dental f.,** a statement in tabular form of the number of each kind of teeth in the jaw; the dental f. for man is, for the deciduous teeth:

$$\text{i.} \ \frac{2\text{-}2}{2\text{-}2}, \ \text{c.} \ \frac{1\text{-}1}{1\text{-}1}, \ \text{m.} \ \frac{2\text{-}2}{2\text{-}2} = 20$$

for the permanent teeth:

$$\text{i.} \ \frac{2\text{-}2}{2\text{-}2}, \ \text{c.} \ \frac{1\text{-}1}{1\text{-}1}, \ \text{bic.} \ \frac{2\text{-}2}{2\text{-}2}, \ \text{m.} \ \frac{3\text{-}3}{3\text{-}3} = 32.$$

**Dreyer's f.,** a f. indicating relationship between vital capacity and body surface area.

**DuBois' f.,** a f. for calculating body surface area from height and weight. Tables derived from this f. are available and can be used to express metabolism in terms of calories produced per hour per square meter of body surface. See also Aub-DuBois *table.*

**electrical f.,** a graphic representation by means of symbols of the reaction of a muscle to an electrical stimulus.

**empirical f.,** molecular f.; in chemistry, a f. indicating the kind and number of atoms in the molecules of a substance, or its composition, but not the relation of the atoms to each other or the intimate structure of the molecule, *i.e.,* its constitution.

**Fischer's projection f.'s,** see under sugars.

**Florschütz' f.,** indicating the correct relation of height to the abdominal circumference — $L : (2B - L)$, $L$ representing the individual's height, and $B$ the circumference of the abdomen; the correct figure so determined would be 5, and any below that would indicate an increase in adiposity.

**Gorlin f.,** a f. for calculating the area of the orifice of a cardiac valve, based on flow across the valve and the mean pressures in the chambers on either side of the valve.

**graphic f.,** structural f.

**Haines' f.,** the last two figures of the specific gravity of a specimen of urine multiplied by 1.1 indicates the number of grains of solids in each fluid ounce.

**Häser's f.,** Christison's f.; Trapp-Häser f.; the figure 2.33 multiplied by the last two figures of the specific gravity of the urine gives the number of grams of urinary solids per liter.

**Haworth perspective and conformational f.'s,** see under sugars.

**Long's f.,** f. for estimating from the specific gravity of a specimen of urine the approximate amount of solids in grams per liter; the last two figures of the value for specific gravity are multiplied by 2.6.

**Mall's f.,** the age (in days) of an embryo is indicated by the square root of its length (measured from vertex to breech) in millimeters multiplied by 100.

**McLean's f.,** a modification of Ambard's coefficient, giving the result in terms per cent: The index of urea excretion =

$$\frac{\text{gm. urea}/24 \text{ hr.} \ \sqrt{\text{gm. urea per liter urine}} \times 8.96}{\text{weight in kg.} \times (\text{gm. urea per liter blood})^2}$$

**Meeh-Dubois f.,** a f. for calculating a man's surface area where his height and weight are known: $A = W\,0.425 \times H\,0.725 \times 71.84$ (a constant) where $A$ = surface area in sq. cm., $W$ = wt. in kg. and $H$ = height in cm.

**molec'ular f.,** empirical f.

**official f.,** a f. contained in the Pharmacopeia or the National Formulary.

**Pignet's f.,** see Black's f.

**Poiseuille's f.,** Poiseuille's *coefficient.*

**Poisson-Pearson f.,** a f. to determine the statistical error in calculating the endemic index of malaria: let $N$ = total number of children under 15 years in a locality; $n$ = total number examined for the spleen-rate; $x$ = number found with enlarged spleen; $(x/n)\,100$ = spleen-rate; $e\%$ = percentage of error; then the percentage error will be, by this f.:

$$e\% = \frac{200}{n} \ \sqrt{\frac{2x(n-x)}{n}} \ \sqrt{1 - \frac{n-1}{N-1}}.$$

**Ranke's f.,** $A$ = grams of albumin per liter of a serous fluid: then, $A$ = (sp. gr. − 1000) × 0.52 − 5.406.

**rational f.,** in chemistry, a f. that indicates more or less completely the constitution as well as the composition of a substance.

**Reuss' f.,** a means of estimating the approximate amount of albumin in a transudate or exudate; $3/8$ (sp. gr. − 1.000) − 2.8 results in a value that is a practicable indication of the percentage of albumin in the fluid.

**Runeberg's f.,** a f. for estimating the percentage of albumin in a serous fluid, similar to Reuss' f. except that, instead of 2.8, 2.73 is subtracted in the instance of a transudate, and 2.88 in that of an inflammatory exudate.

**spatial f.,** stereochemical f.

**stereochemical f.,** spatial f.; a chemical f. in which the distribution of the atoms or atomic groupings in space are indicated.

**structural f.,** graphic f.; one in which the connections of the atoms and groups of atoms, as well as their kind and number, are indicated.

**Trapp's f., Trapp-Häser f.,** Häser's f.

**typical f.,** in chemistry, a f. constructed after that of one of the three types, hydrogen, water, and ammonia, and indicating partially the constitution of a substance.

**Van Slyke's f.,** a f. for calculating the urinary coefficient in relation to various substances: $D/(Bl \times \sqrt{Wt} \times V)$;

$D$ = daily output of the substance in the urine expressed in gm.; $Bl$ = gm. of the same substance per liter in the blood; $Wt$ = weight of the patient in kg.; $V$ = amount of total urine excreted in 24 hours.

**vertebral f.,** a f. indicating the number of vertebrae in each segment of the spinal column; for man it is C. 7, T. 12, L. 5, S. 5, Co. 4 = 33, the letters standing for cervical, thoracic, lumbar, sacral, and coccygeal.

**Worm-Mueller's f.,** a f. for the quantitative estimation of sugar in the urine.

---

**for'mulary.** A collection of formulas for the compounding of medicinal preparations. See *National Formulary; Pharmacopeia.*

**formulation, Haworth.** See Haworth formulas, under sugars.

**formyl** (for'mil). The radical, H—CO—.

**active f.,** the 1-carbon fragment; the f. group taking part in transformylation reactions with a folic acid derivative in the role of carrier.

**formylase** (for'mĭ-lās). Formamidase.

**for'mylkynur'enine.** The product of the oxidative cleavage of the indole ring in tryptophan, possibly the intermediate first formed in tryptophan catabolism.

**for'nicate.** 1 [ L. *fornicatus,* arched, fr. *fornix,* vault, arch ]. Vaulted or arched; resembling a fornix. 2 [ see fornication ]. To commit fornication.

**fornication** (for'nĭ-ka'shun) [ L. *fornicatio,* an arched or vaulted basement (brothel). FORN- ]. Sexual intercourse, especially between unmarried partners.

**for'nicator.** The male who engages in fornication.

**for'nicatrix.** The female who engages in fornication.

**fornices** (for'nĭ-sēz). Plural of fornix.

**fornix, gen. for'nicis, pl. for'nices** (for'niks) [ L. arch, vault ]. 1 [ NA ]. In general, an arch-shaped structure; often the arch-shaped roof (or roof portion) of an anatomical space. 2 [ NA ]. Trigonum cerebrale; the compact, white fiber bundle by which the hippocampus of each cerebral hemisphere projects to the septum, anterior nucleus of the thalamus, and mamillary body. Arising largely from pyramidal cells of Ammon's horn, the fibers of the f. first accumulate in the fimbria hippocampi, and in their further course compose, sequentially, the crus fornicis, corpus fornicis, and columna fornicis.

**f. conjuncti'vae** [ NA ], conjunctival cul-de-sac; the space formed by the junction of the bulbar and palpebral portions of the conjunctiva, that of the upper lid being the **f. conjunctivae superior** and that of the lower lid the **f. conjunctivae inferior.**

**f. pharyn'gis** [ NA ], vault of the pharynx; the upper end of the nasopharynx roofed over by the posterior wall arching forward to join the borders of the posterior nares.

**f. sac'ci lacrima'lis** [ NA ], fornix of the lacrimal sac; the upper, blind end of the lacrimal sac that extends above the openings of the lacrimal canaliculi.

**transverse f.,** *commissura* fornicis.

**f. u'teri,** f. vaginae.

**f. vagi'nae** [ NA ], the recess at the vault of the vagina, anterior, posterior, or lateral to the cervix uteri.

**Forsmann** (fors'man), Werner T. O., German surgeon, *1904. Nobel laureate, 1956, with André F. Cournand and Dickinson W. Richards for their discoveries concerning heart catheterization and pathological changes in the circulatory system.

**Forssell,** Gösta, Swedish radiologist, 1876–1950. See F.'s *sinus.*

**Forssman,** Hans, Swedish physician. See Börjeson-F.-Lehman *syndrome.*

**Forssman,** John, Swedish pathologist, 1868–1947. See F. *antibody, antigen, reaction,* F. antigen-antibody *reaction.*

**Förster** (fër'ster), Richard, German ophthalmologist, 1825–1902. See F.'s *phenomenon, photometer, uveitis.*

**Foshay,** Lee, U. S. physician, *1896. See F. *test.*

**fospirate** (fos'pĭ-rāt) (USAN). TORELLE; dimethyl 3,5,6-trichloro-2-pyridyl phosphate; anthelmintic for veterinary use.

# FOSSA

---

**fossa, gen. and pl. fossae** (fos'ah, fos'e) [ L. a trench or ditch ] [ NA ]. A depression usually more or less longitudinal in shape below the level of the surface of a part.

**acetabular f.,** f. acetabuli.

**f. acetab'uli** [ NA ], acetabular f.; a depressed area in the floor of the acetabulum above the acetabular notch.

**adipose fossae,** subcutaneous spaces containing accumulations of fat in the mamma.

**amyg'daloid f.,** the hollow between the pillars of the fauces that contains the tonsil.

**anconal f.,** f. olecrani.

**anterior cranial f.,** see f. cranii.

**f. anthel'icis** [ NA ], f. of the anthelix; the depression on the medial surface of the auricle that corresponds to the anthelix.

**f. of anthelix,** f. anthelicis.

**artic'ular f. of temporal bone,** f. mandibularis.

**f. axilla'ris** [ NA ], axillary fossa; armpit; the depression between the medial side of the arm and the chest wall, bounded by the anterior and posterior axillary folds. See also axilla.

**axillary f.,** f. axillaris.

**Bichat's f.,** f. pterygopalatina.

**Biesiadecki's f.,** iliacosubfascial f.

**Broesike's f.,** parajejunal f.; a recess in the peritoneum in the mesentery of the upper part of the jejunum.

**f. canina** [ NA ], canine f.; a depression on the anterior surface of the maxilla below the infraorbital foramen and on the lateral side of the canine eminence; it is the site of origin of the levator anguli oris muscle.

**canine f.,** f. canina.

**f. carot'ica,** *trigonum* caroticum.

**Claudius' f.,** ovarian f.

**condylar f.,** f. condylaris ossis occipitalis.

**f. condyla'ris ossis occipita'lis** [ NA ], condylar f.; a depression behind the condyle of the occipital bone in which the posterior margin of the superior facet of the atlas lies in extension.

**coronoid f.,** f. coronoidea.

**f. coronoi'dea** [ NA ], coronoid f.; a hollow on the anterior surface of the distal end of the humerus, just above the trochlea, in which the coronoid process of the ulna rests when the elbow is flexed.

**cranial f.,** f. cranii.

**f. cranii** [ NA ], cranial f.; one of three hollows (anterior, middle, and posterior) on the internal base of the skull that lodge the cerebrum (fossa cranii anterior and media) and the cerebellum (f. cranii posterior).

**crural f.,** *fovea* femoralis.

**Cruveilhier's f.,** f. scaphoidea ossis sphenoidalis.

**cubital f.,** f. cubitalis.

**f. cubita'lis** [ NA ], cubital f., bend of the elbow; chelidon; antecubital space; the f. in front of the elbow.

**digastric f.,** f. digastrica.

**f. digas'trica** [ NA ], digastric f.; a hollow on the posterior surface of the base of the mandible, on either side of the median plane, giving attachment to the anterior belly of the digastric muscle.

**digital f.,** f. trochanterica.

**digital f. of the fibula,** f. malleoli lateralis.

**f. ductus veno'si** [ NA ], fissure on the undersurface of the liver posteriorly, between the Spigelian, or caudate, and the left lobes, lodging a fibrous band, the remains of the ductus venosus of the fetus.

**duodenal fossae,** *recessus* duodenales.

**duodenojejunal f.,** *recessus* duodenalis superior.

**epigastric f.,** f. epigastrica.

**f. epigas'trica** [ NA ], epigastric f.; scrobiculus cordis; pit of the stomach; the region, usually a slight depression, just inferior to the xiphoid process of the sternum.

**fem'oral f.,** *fovea* femoralis.

**floc'cular f.,** f. subarcuata.

**gallbladder f.,** f. vesicae felleae.

**Gerdy's hyoid f.,** *trigonum* caroticum.

**f. glandulae lacrima'lis** [ NA ], f. of the lacrimal gland; lacrimal f.; a hollow in the orbital plate of the frontal bone, formed by the overhanging margin and zygomatic process, lodging the lacrimal gland.

**glenoid f.,** *cavitas* glenoidalis.

**greater supraclavicular f.,** f. supraclavicularis major.

**Gruber-Landzert f.,** *recessus* duodenalis inferior.

**hyaloid f.,** f. hyaloidea.

**f. hyaloidea** [ NA ], hyaloid f.; lenticular f.; a depression on the anterior surface of the vitreous body in which lies the lens.

**hypophysial f.,** f. hypophysialis.

**f. hypophysia'lis** [ NA ], hypophysial f.; pituitary f.; f. of the sphenoid bone housing the pituitary gland.

**iliac f.,** f. iliaca.

**f. iliaca** [ NA ], iliac f.; the smooth inner surface of the ilium above the arcuate line, giving attachment to the iliacus muscle.

**iliacosubfascial f.,** f. iliacosubfascialis; a depression on the inner surface of the abdomen between the psoas muscle and the crest of the ilium.

**iliopectineal f.,** a hollow between the iliopsoas and pectineus muscles in the center of the femoral (Scarpa's) triangle, lodging the femoral vessels and nerve.

**f. incisi'va** [ NA ], incisive fossa; the depression in the midline of the bony palate behind the central incisors into which the incisive canals open.

**incisive f.,** f. incisiva.

**incudal f.,** f. incudis.

**f. in'cudis** [ NA ], incudal f.; f. for the incus; a small depression in the lower and posterior part of the epitympanic recess that lodges the short limb of the incus.

**f. for incus,** f. incudis.

**inferior duodenal f.,** *recessus* duodenalis inferior.

**infraclavicular f.,** *regio* infraclavicularis.

**infraduodenal f.,** f. infraduodenalis; a peritoneal recess sometimes found extending laterally a distance of $^3/_4$ to $^1/_2$ inch below the third portion of the duodenum. See fig. under *recessus* duodenalis.

**f. infraspina'ta** [ NA ], infraspinous f.; the hollow on the dorsal aspect of the scapula inferior to the spine, giving attachment chiefly to the infraspinatus muscle.

**infraspinous f.,** f. infraspinata.

**infratemporal f.,** f. infratemporalis.

**f. infratempora'lis** [ NA ], infratemporal f.; zygomatic f.; the cavity on the side of the skull bounded laterally by the zygoma and ramus of the mandible, medially by the lateral pterygoid plate, anteriorly by the zygomatic process of the maxilla, posteriorly by the articular eminence of the temporal bone and the posterior border of the lateral pterygoid plate, and above by the squama of the temporal bone and the infratemporal crest on the greater wing of the sphenoid bone.

**inguinal f.,** f. inguinalis.

**f. inguina'lis latera'lis** [ NA ], lateral inguinal f.; a depression on the peritoneal surface of the anterior abdominal wall lateral to the ridge formed by the inferior epigastric artery; it corresponds to the position of the deep inguinal ring.

**f. inguina'lis media'lis** [ NA ], medial inguinal f.; fovea inguinalis interna; a depression on the peritoneal surface of the anterior abdominal wall between the ridges formed by the inferior epigastric and the obliterated hypogastric arteries.

**innominate f.,** f. innominata; a shallow depression between the false vocal cord and the arytenoepiglottic fold on either side.

**intercondylar f. of femur,** f. intercondylaris femoris.

**f. intercondyla'ris femoris** [ NA ], intercondylar f. of the femur; the deep f. between the femoral condyles in which the cruciate ligaments are attached.

**intercondyloid f., intercondylic f.,** (1) *area* intercondylaris tibiae; (2) f. intercondylaris femoris.

**f. intermesocol'ica transver'sa,** a f. occupying the position of the duodenojejunal f., extending transversely from right to left for about the length of a finger. See fig. under *recessus* duodenalis.

**interpeduncular f.,** f. interpeduncularis.

**f. interpeduncula'ris** [ NA ], interpeduncular f.; Tarin's f.; deep depression on the inferior surface of the mesencephalon, between the two cerebral peduncles, the floor of which is formed by the posterior perforated substance.

**intrabul'bar f.,** the dilated commencement of the spongy part of the male urethra lying within the bulb of the penis.

**ischiorectal f.,** f. ischiorectalis.

**f. ischiorecta'lis** [ NA ], ischiorectal f.; a wedge-shaped space with its base towards the perineum between the tuberosity of the ischium and the obturator internus muscle laterally and the external anal sphincter and the levator ani muscle medially.

**Jobert de Lamballe's f.,** the hollow formed by the adductor magnus and the sartorius and gracilis.

**Jonnesco's f.,** *recessus* duodenalis superior.

**jugular f.,** f. jugularis.

**f. jugula'ris,** jugular f.; (1) [ NA ]; an oval depression near the posterior border of the petrous portion of the temporal bone, medial to the styloid process, in which lies the beginning of the internal jugular vein; (2) the depression in the anterior part of the neck just superior to the jugular notch of the manubrium sterni.

**lac'rimal f.,** f. glandulae lacrimalis.

**f. of lacrimal sac,** f. sacci lacrimalis.

**Landzert's f.,** a f. formed by two peritoneal folds, enclosing the left colic artery and the inferior mesenteric vein, respectively, at the side of the duodenum; it is smaller than the f. paraduodenalis which is sometimes found in the same region.

**lateral f. of brain,** f. lateralis cerebri.

**lateral cerebral f.,** f. lateralis cerebri.

**lateral inguinal f.,** f. inguinalis lateralis.

**f. of lateral malleolus,** f. malleoli lateralis.

**f. latera'lis cer'ebri** [ NA ], lateral cerebral f.; lateral f. of the brain; f. of Sylvius; vallecula sylvii; the deep depression of the basal surface of the forebrain that corresponds in position to the anterior perforated substance. Bounded medially by the optic tract and rostrally by the orbital surface of the frontal lobe, it extends laterally around the overhanging pole of the temporal lobe into the Sylvian fissure (sulcus lateralis).

**lenticular f.,** f. hyaloidea.

**lesser supraclavicular f.,** f. supraclavicularis minor.

**Malgaigne's f.,** *trigonum* caroticum.

**f. malle'oli fib'ulae,** f. malleoli lateralis.

**f. malle'oli latera'lis** [ NA ], f. of the lateral malleolus; a large rough depression on the medial aspect of the lower end of the fibula just behind the articular facet for the talus giving attachment to the posterior talofibular and the transverse tibiofibular ligaments.

**mandibular f.,** f. mandibularis.

**f. mandibula'ris** [ NA ], mandibular f.; glenoid f. or cavity; a deep hollow in the squamous portion of the temporal bone at the root of the zygoma, in which rests the condyle of the mandible.

**mastoid f.,** f. mastoidea; a depression on the mastoid portion of the temporal bone, behind the suprameatal spine; its floor is marked by numerous small openings for blood vessels.

**medial inguinal f.,** f. inguinalis medialis.

**Merkel's f.,** a depression between the ventricles of the larynx.

**mesentericoparietal f.,** parajejunal f.

**middle cranial f.,** see f. cranii.

**Mohrenheim's f.,** *regio* infraclavicularis.

**Morgagni's f.,** f. navicularis urethrae.

**mylohyoid f.,** *sulcus* mylohyoideus.

**navicular f. of urethra,** f. navicularis urethrae.

**f. navicula'ris auric'ulae,** f. triangularis.

**f. navicula'ris auris,** scapha.

**f. navicula'ris cruveilhier,** f. scaphoidea ossis sphenoidalis.

**f. navicula'ris ure'thrae** [ NA ], navicular f. of the urethra; f. of Morgagni; the terminal dilated portion of the urethra in the glans penis.

**f. navicula'ris vestibulae vaginae,** f. vestibuli vaginae.

**f. olecrani** [ NA ], olecranon f.; a hollow on the dorsum of the distal end of the humerus, just above the trochlea, in which the olecranon process of the ulna rests when the elbow is extended.

**olecranon f.,** f. olecrani.

**oval f.,** f. ovalis.

**f. ova'lis,** (1) [ NA ], oval f.; an oval depression on the lower part of the septum of the atrium; its floor corresponds to the septum primum of the fetal heart; (2) hiatus saphenus.

**ovarian f.,** Claudius' f.; a depression on the lateral wall of the pelvis; it is bounded in front by the obliterated umbilical artery, and behind by the ureter and the uterine vessels. It lodges the ovary.

**paraduodenal f.,** *recessus* paraduodenalis.

**parajejunal f.,** f. parajejunalis; mesentericoparietal f. or recess; a peritoneal f. that has been seen in a few cases in which the jejunum has no mesentery but is attached to the posterior parietal peritoneum; the f. begins at the point where the mesentery ends, and is seen on raising up the knuckle of free intestine.

**pararect'al f.,** a depression on either side of the rectum formed by the reflection of the peritoneum to the posterior pelvic wall.

**paraves'ical f.,** a depression formed by the peritoneum on each side of the urinary bladder.

**peritone'al f.'s,** depressions or pouches formed between various peritoneal folds; they may be the sites of internal hernias.

**petrosal f.,** *fossula* petrosa.

**pir'iform f.,** *recessus* piriformis.

**pitu'itary f.,** f. hypophysialis.

**pituitary f. of sphenoid bone,** f. hypophysialis.

**f. poplit'ea** [ NA ], popliteal f. or space; the lozenge-shaped space posterior to the knee joint bounded superiorly by the biceps femoris and the semimembranosus muscle and inferiorly by the two heads of the gastrocnemius muscle.

**popliteal f.,** f. poplitea.

**posterior cranial f.,** see f. cranii.

**f. provesica'lis,** Hartmann's *pouch.*

**pterygoid f.,** f. pterygoidea.

**f. pterygoi'dea** [ NA ], pterygoid f.; the f. formed by the divergence posteriorly of the plates of the pterygoid process of the sphenoid bone; it lodges the medial pterygoid and the tensor palati muscles.

**pterygomaxillary f.,** f. pterygopalatina.

**f. pterygopalati'na** [ NA ], pterygopalatine f.; a small depression between the front of the root of the pterygoid process of the sphenoid bone and the back of the maxilla.

**pterygopalatine f.,** f. pterygopalatina.

**radial f.,** f. radialis.

**f. radia'lis** [ NA ], radial f.; a shallow depression above the capitulum of the humerus in front, in which the margin of the head of the radius rests when the elbow is in extreme flexion.

**retroduodenal f.,** *recessus* retroduodenalis.

**retromandibular f.,** f. retromandibularis; the depression beneath the auricle behind the angle of the jaw.

**retromolar f.,** a triangular depression in the mandible posterior to the third molar tooth.

**rhomboid f.,** f. rhomboidea.

**f. rhomboi'dea** [ NA ], rhomboid f.; the floor of the fourth ventricle of the brain, formed by the ventricular surface of the rhombencephalon.

**Rosenmüller's f.,** *recessus* pharyngeus.

**f. sacci lacrima'lis** [ NA ], f. of the lacrimal sac; a f. formed by the lacrimal grooves of the lacrimal bone and of the frontal process of the maxilla, lodging the lacrimal sac.

**f. sagitta'lis dextra,** a sagittal groove on the liver formed by the combined f. vesicae felleae anteriorly, and f. venae cavae posteriorly, separated by the caudate process of the liver.

**f. sagitta'lis sinis'tra,** a sagittal groove on the liver formed by the combined f. venae umbilicalis anteriorly, and f. ductus venosi posteriorly.

**scaphoid f. of sphenoid bone,** f. scaphoidea ossis sphenoidalis.

**f. scaphoid'ea ossis sphenoida'lis** [ NA ], scaphoid f. of the sphenoid bone; Cruveilhier's f.; a hollow on the posterior surface of the medial lamina of the pterygoid process; it gives origin to the tensor muscle of the soft palate.

**f. scarpae major,** *trigonum* femorale.

**sigmoid f.,** *sulcus* sinus sigmoidei.

**sphenomaxillary f.,** f. pterygopalatina.

**f. subarcuata** [ NA ], subarcuate f.; floccular f.; an irregular depression on the posterior surface of the petrous portion of the temporal bone, above and a little lateral to the internal acoustic meatus.

**subarcuate f.,** f. subarcuata.

**subcecal f.,** Treitz's f.

**subinguinal f.,** the depression on the anterior surface of the thigh beneath the groin.

**sublingual f.,** *fovea* sublingualis.

**submandib'ular f.,** *fovea* submandibularis.

**f. submandibula'ris,** *fovea* submandibularis.

**submaxillary f.,** *fovea* submandibularis.

**subscapular f.,** f. subscapularis.

**f. subscapula'ris** [ NA ], subscapular f.; the concave ventral aspect of the body of the scapula giving attachment to the subscapularis muscle.

**superior duodenal f.,** *recessus* duodenalis superior.

**supraclavicular f.,** f. supraclavicularis.

**f. supraclavicula'ris major** [ NA ], the greater supraclavicular f.; an alternate term for *trigonum* omoclaviculare.

**f. supraclavicula'ris minor** [ NA ], lesser supraclavicular f.; Zang's space; triangular space between the two heads of origin of the sternocleidomastoid muscle.

**supramastoid f.,** f. supramastoidea; a small f. at the junction of the posterior and superior margins of the external auditory canal.

**f. supraspina'ta** [ NA ], supraspinous f.; the hollow on the dorsal aspect of the scapula above the spine, lodging the supraspinatus muscle.

**supraspinous f.,** f. supraspinata.

**supratonsillar f.,** f. supratonsillaris.

**f. supratonsilla'ris** [ NA ], supratonsillar f. or recess; the interval between the anterior and posterior pillars of the fauces above the tonsil.

**supraves'ical f.,** f. supravesicalis.

**f. supravesica'lis** [ NA ], supravesical f.; the depression on the peritoneal surface of the anterior abdominal wall between the median and medial umbilical folds.

**f. of Sylvius,** f. lateralis cerebri.

**Tarin's f.,** f. interpeduncularis.

**temporal f.,** f. temporalis.

**f. tempora'lis** [ NA ], temporal f.; the space on the side of the cranium bounded by the temporal lines and terminating below at the level of the zygomatic arch.

**f. termina'lis ure'thrae,** f. navicularis urethrae masculinae.

**tonsillar f.,** f. tonsillaris.

**f. tonsilla'ris** [ NA ], tonsillar fossa; the depression between the palatoglossal and palatopharyngeal arches occupied by the palatine tonsil.

**Treitz's f.,** subcecal f.; an inconstant depression in the peritoneum extending posterior to the cecum.

**triangular f.,** f. triangularis.

**f. triangula'ris** [ NA ], triangular f.; the depression at the upper part of the auricle between the two crura of the antihelix.

**trochanteric f.,** f. trochanterica.

**f. trochanter'ica** [ NA ], trochanteric f.; digital f.; a depression at the root of the neck of the femur beneath the curved tip of the great trochanter; it gives insertion to the tendon of the obturator externus.

**troch'lear f.,** *fovea* trochlearis.

**f. trochlea'ris,** *fovea* trochlearis.

**umbilical f.,** *fissura* ligamenti teretis.

**Velpeau's f.,** f. ischiorectalis.

**f. venae cavae,** *sulcus* venae cavae.

**f. venae umbilica'lis,** *fissura* ligamenti teretis.

**f. veno'sa,** *recessus* paraduodenalis.

**ver'mian f.,** a small depression near the lower part of the internal occipital crest which lodges part of the inferior vermis of the cerebellum.

**f. vesi'cae fel'leae** [ NA ], f. for the gallbladder; a depression on the under surface of the liver anteriorly, between the quadrate and the right lobes, lodging the gallbladder.

**vestib'ular f.,** f. vestibuli vaginae.

**f. of vestibule of vagina,** f. vestibuli vaginae.

**f. vestib'uli vagi'nae** [ NA ], f. of the vestibule of the vagina; the portion of the vestibule of the vagina between the frenulum of the pudendal lips and the posterior commissure of the vulva.

**Waldeyer's fossae,** *recessus* duodenales.
**zygomatic f.,** f. infratemporalis.

**fossette** (fŏ-set') [ Fr. dim. of *fosse,* a ditch ]. 1. A small fossa. 2. A small but deep corneal ulcer.

**fos'sula, pl. fos'sulae** [ L. dim. of *fossa,* ditch ]. 1 [ NA ]. A fossette; a small fossa. 2. A minor fissure or slight depression on the surface of the cerebrum.

  **f. fenes'trae coch'leae** [ NA ], little fossa of the fenestra of the cochlea; a depression on the medial wall of the middle ear at the bottom of which is the cochlear window.

  **f. fenes'trae vestib'uli** [ NA ], little fossa of the fenestra of the vestibule; a depression on the medial wall of the middle ear at the bottom of which is the vestibular window.

  **f. petro'sa** [ NA ], petrosal fossa; a small and often only faintly marked depression on the inferior surface of the petrous portion of the temporal bone, between the jugular fossa and the opening of the carotid canal; here opens the canaliculus tympanicus transmitting the tympanic nerve.

  **f. rotun'da,** f. fenestrae cochleae.

**fos'sulae tonsilla'res** [ NA ], tonsillar fossulae; the small pits at the openings of the tonsillar crypts onto the medial surface of the tonsil.

**fos'sulate.** Containing a fossula or small fossa; grooved; hollowed out.

**Foster frame.** See under frame.

**Fothergill's sign.** See under sign.

**Fothergill,** John, English physician, 1712–1780. See F.'s *disease, neuralgia.*

**Fothergill,** William E., English gynecologist, 1865–1926. See F.'s *operation.*

**Fouchet** (foo-sha') A., French physician, *1894. See F.'s *reagent.*

**foudroyant** (foo-droy'ant) [ Fr. *foudroyer,* to strike by lightning ]. Fulminant.

**foulage** (foo-lahzh') [ Fr. impression ]. Kneading and pressure of the muscles, constituting a form of massage.

**fouls.** foot rot (2); a necrotizing infection of the skin between the claws of cattle, causing severe lameness. *Actinomyces necrophorus* is always found in the lesions and is believed to play an important role in the disease.

**founda'tion.** A base; a supporting structure.

  **denture f.,** denture-supporting area; basal seat; stress-bearing area; supporting area; tissue-bearing area; that portion of the oral structures which is available to support a denture. See also denture f. *area* and *surface;* mean f. *plane.*

**found'er.** Laminitis (2).

**fourchette** (foor-shet') [ Fr. dim. of *fourché,* fr. L. *furca,* fork ]. *Frenulum* labiorum pudendi.

**Fourneau** (foor-no'), Ernest F. A., French chemist, 1872–1949. See *Fourneau 710, Fourneau 933.*

**Fourneau 710.** RHONDOQUIN; PLASMOCID; a synthetic quinoline; antimalarial agent.

**Fourneau 933.** Piperoxan hydrochloride.

**Fournier** (foor-ne-a'), Jean A., Paris syphilographer, 1832–1914. See F.'s *disease.*

**fout-ta-ta-rou.** Duroziez' onomatope to imitate the cadence of the auscultatory findings in mitral stenosis (*fout-,* first sound; *ta-,* second sound; *ta-,* opening snap; *rou-,* diastolic rumble).

**fovea, pl. foveae** (fo've-ah, fo've-e) [ L. a pit ] [ NA ]. A cup-shaped depression or pit.

  **f. ante'rior,** f. superior.

  **f. articula'ris infe'rior atlan'tis** [ NA ], inferior articular pit of the atlas; one of the two concave surfaces on the lateral masses of the atlas that articulate with corresponding surfaces on the axis.

  **f. articula'ris supe'rior atlan'tis** [ NA ], superior articular pit of the atlas; one of the two concave articular surfaces on the superior aspect of the lateral masses of the atlas that articulate with the occipital condyles.

  **f. cap'itis fem'oris** [ NA ], pit of the head of the femur; a depression on the extremity of the head of the femur giving attachment to the ligamentum teres.

  **f. cardi'aca,** anterior intestinal portal; the opening of the foregut into the midgut.

  **f. centra'lis ret'inae** [ NA ], central pit; a depression in the center of the macula retinae where only cones are present and blood vessels are lacking.

  **f. coc'cygis,** postnatal pit of a newborn; it marks the site where the embryonic spinal cord attaches to the skin.

  **f. costa'lis inferior** [ NA ], inferior costal pit; demifacet on the lower edge of the body of a vertebra articulating with the head of a rib.

  **f. costa'lis superior** [ NA ], superior costal pit; a demifacet on the upper edge of the body of a vertebra articulating with the head of a rib; a single rib articulates with the f. costalis inferior and f. costalis superior of the adjacent vertebrae.

  **f. costa'lis transversa'lis** [ NA ], costal pit of the transverse process; a facet on the transverse process of a vertebra for articulation with the tubercle of a rib.

  **f. dentis atlan'tis** [ NA ], a circular facet on the posterior (inner) surface of the anterior arch of the atlas which articulates with the dens of the axis.

  **f. ellip'tica,** *recessus* ellipticus.

  **f. femora'lis,** femoral or crural fossa; a depression on the peritoneal surface of the abdominal wall, posterior to the inguinal ligament, corresponding to the situation of the femoral ring.

  **f. hemiellip'tica,** *recessus* ellipticus.

  **f. hemisphe'rica,** *recessus* sphericus.

  **f. infe'rior** [ NA ], a triangular area of the rhomboidal fossa below the striae medullares of either side.

  **f. inguina'lis interna,** *fossa* inguinalis medialis.

**Morgagni's f.,** *fossa* navicularis urethrae.

  **f. oblon'ga cartilag'inis arytenoid'eae** [ NA ], oblong pit of the arytenoid cartilage; a broad shallow depression on the anterolateral surface of the arytenoid cartilage, separated from the f. triangularis above by the arcuate crest.

  **f. pterygoid'ea** [ NA ], pterygoid pit or depression; a depression on the medial side of the neck of the condylar process of the mandible, giving attachment to the lateral pterygoid muscle.

  **f. sphe'rica,** *recessus* sphericus.

  **f. sublingua'lis** [ NA ], sublingual pit; a shallow depression on either side of the mental spine, on the inner surface of the body of the mandible, superior to the mylohyoid line, lodging the sublingual gland.

  **f. submandibula'ris** [ NA ], submandibular fossa; submaxillary fossa; the depression on the medial surface of the body of the mandible inferior to the mylohyoid line in which the submandibular gland is lodged.

  **f. submaxilla'ris,** f. submandibularis.

  **f. supe'rior** [ NA ], f. anterior; a slight depression on either side of the rhomboidal fossa, above the striae medullares.

  **f. supravesica'lis,** *fossa* supravesicalis.

  **temporal f.,** a depression in the retina of several unrelated species of birds. It is thought to function chiefly in binocular vision when a central f. is also present; owls have only a temporal f. in contrast to bifovate hawks, humming birds, and swallows; gannets have only a central f.

  **f. triangula'ris cartilag'inis arytenoid'eae** [ NA ], a deep depression in the upper portion of the anterolateral surface of the arytenoid cartilage, separated from the f. oblonga below by a ridge, the arcuate crest.

  **f. trochlea'ris** [ NA ], trochlear pit; a shallow depression in the roof of the orbit and close to the medial margin to which is attached the pulley for the superior oblique tendon.

**foveate, foveated** (fo'-ve-āt, fo've-ā-ted). Pitted; having foveas or depressions on the surface.

**foveation** (fo-ve-a'shun) [ L. *fovea,* a pit ]. Pitted scar formation as in smallpox, chickenpox, or vaccina.

**foveola, pl. foveolae** (fo-ve'o-lah, fo-ve'o-le) [ Mod. L. dim. of L. *fovea,* pit ] [ NA ]. A minute fovea or pit.

  **f. coccyge'a** [ NA ], coccygeal f.; a depression over the coccyx.

  **coccygeal f.,** f. coccygea.

  **f. gas'trica** [ NA ], gastric pit; one of the numerous small pits in the mucous membrane of the stomach at the bottom of which are the mouths of the gastric glands.

  **f. granula'ris** [ NA ], granular pit; Pacchionian depressions or pits on the inner surface of the skull, along the course of the superior sagittal sinus, in which are lodged the arachnoidal granulations.

**f. papilla′ris,** the minute depression sometimes seen at the apex of a papilla of the kidney where the excretory tubes open into a calyx.

**foveolar** (fo-ve′o-lar). Pertaining to a foveola.

**foveolate** (fo′ve-o-lāt, fo-ve′o-lāt). Having minute pits (foveolae) or small depressions on the surface.

**Foville** (fo-vēl′), Achille L., French neurologist, 1799–1878. See F.'s *fasciculus.*

**Foville,** Achille L. Francois, French psychiatrist, 1831–1887. See F.'s *syndrome.*

**Fowler,** George R., New York surgeon, 1848–1906. See F.'s *position.*

**Fox,** B. W. See Goldman-F. *knife.*

**Fox,** George H., New York dermatologist, 1846–1937. See F.-Fordyce *disease.*

**Fox,** William T., English dermatologist, 1836–1879. See F.'s *impetigo.*

**fox′glove.** Digitalis.

**Fox′ia.** An obsolete term for a genus of fungi identified as a cause of tinea nigra.

**Fr.** Chemical symbol of the element francium.

**Fracasto′rius or Fracas′toro,** Girolamo of Verona, Italian physician and poet, 1478–1553. Noted mainly for his poem *Syphilis sive Morbus Gallicus* in which the name Syphilus and the disease were connected; he emphasized the therapeutic value of mercury.

**Fraccaro,** M. See Schmid-F. *syndrome.*

**fraction** (frak′shun). Quotient of two quantities; an aliquot portion.

    **amorphous f. of adrenal cortex,** noncrystalline residue of an acetone extract of the adrenal cortex after crystalline steroids, *e.g.,* corticosterone, deoxycorticosterone, etc., have been isolated.

    **blood plasma f.'s,** portions of the blood plasma as separated by electrophoresis or other technique.

    **ejection f. (systolic),** the ratio of cardiac stroke volume to end-diastolic volume.

    **filtration f.,** abbreviated FF; the f. of the plasma entering the kidney that filters into the lumen of the renal tubules; it is determined by dividing the glomerular filtration rate by the renal plasma flow; normally, it is around 0.17.

    **human antihemophilic f.** (BP), human antihemophilic *factor.*

    **mole f.,** the ratio of the moles of one component of a system to the total moles of all the components present.

    **plasma protein f.,** see under protein.

**fractionation** (frak′shun-a′shun). The protraction of a total therapeutic radiation dose over a period of time, ordinarily days or weeks, in order to minimize untoward radiation effects on normal contiguous tissue.

# FRACTURE

**fracture** (frak′cher) [ L. *fractura,* a break. FRA- ]. 1. To break. 2. A break, especially the breaking of a bone or cartilage.

    **apophysial f.,** separation of apophysis from bone.

    **artic′ular f.,** intra-articular f.; one involving the joint surface of a bone.

    **atrophic f.,** spontaneous f. due to atrophy.

    **avulsion f.,** a tearing away of a part of a bone, usually by tendon, ligament or capsule.

    **Barton's f.,** f. of the lower articular extremity of the radius.

    **basal skull f.,** see skull f., basal.

    **Bennett's f.,** f. of the proximal end of the first metacarpal bone, passing obliquely through the base of the bone, and detaching the greater part of the articular facet; it simulates a dislocation of the thumb. Also called stave of the thumb.

    **bent f.,** green-stick f.

    **blow-out f.,** a f. of the floor of the orbit by a blow producing sudden increase in intraorbital pressure.

    **boxer's f.,** f. of first metacarpal bone.

    **bucket-handle f.,** rarely used term for bucket-handle *tear.*

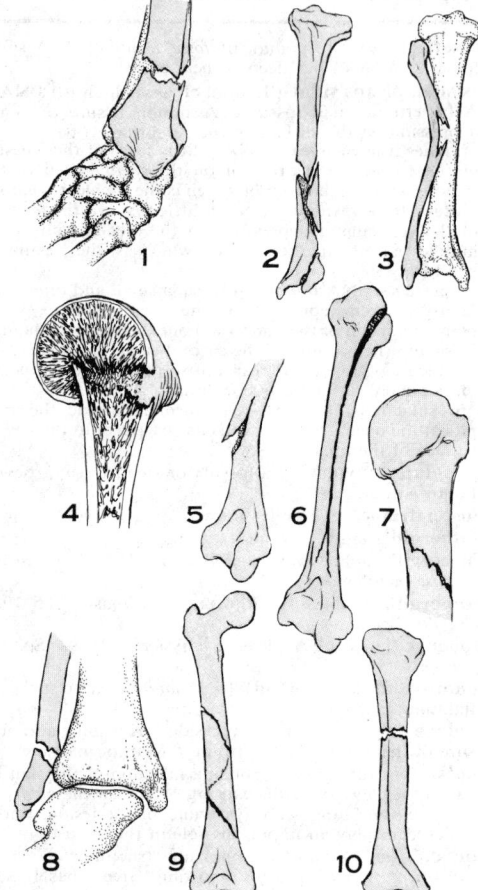

**Types of Fractures**

*1,* Colles'; *2,* comminuted; *3,* green-stick; *4,* impacted; *5,* incomplete; *6,* linear; *7,* oblique; *8,* Pott's; *9,* spiral; *10,* transverse.

    **butterfly f.,** a comminuted f. in which there are two doubly wedge-shaped lateral fragments split off, one from each of the main fragments.

    **buttonhole f.,** perforation of a bone with loss of substance, as in a gunshot wound.

    **cap′illary f.,** pilation; a f. without separation of the fragments, the line of break being hairlike, as seen sometimes in the skull.

    **chisel f.,** a f. of the head of the radius in which a segment is obliquely detached, though usually held by periosteum at its lower end.

    **closed f.,** one in which skin is unbroken at site of f.

    **closed skull f.,** see skull f., closed.

    **Colles' f.,** a f. of the lower end of the radius with displacement of the hand backward and outward, an extension f.; a flexion f. in the same location is sometimes called a reversed Colles' f. and also Smith's f.

    **com′minuted f.,** thrypsis; a f. in which the bone is broken into a number of pieces.

    **complicated f.,** a f. with significant soft tissue injury besides the bone (in neurovascular injury).

    **composite f.,** multiple f.

    **compound f.,** open f.; one in which there is an open wound of the soft parts leading down to the seat of f.

    **compound skull f.,** see skull f., open.

    **f. by contrecoup,** f. of skull opposite impact.

**cough f.,** f. of a rib, usually the 5th or 7th, caused by vigorous coughing.

**craniofacial dysjunction f.,** LeFort III f.; transverse facial f.; a complex f. in which the facial bones are separated from the cranial bones.

**dentate f.,** one in which the opposing surfaces are rough, with toothed or serrate projections fitting into corresponding indentations.

**depressed f.,** see skull f., depressed.

**de Quervain's f.,** f. of navicular bone with dislocation of lunar bone.

**derby hat f.,** see skull f., depressed.

**diastatic skull f.,** see skull f., diastatic.

**direct f.,** a f., especially of the skull, occurring at the point of injury.

**dish-pan f.,** see skull f., depressed.

**dislocation f.,** a f. of a bone near an articulation with its concomitant dislocation from that joint.

**double f.,** the occurrence of two f.'s in different bones at the same time, or in two parts of the same bone.

**Dupuytren's f.,** f. of lower part of fibula, with dislocation of ankle.

**dyscrasic f.,** a f. occurring in general malnutrition.

**epiphys'ial f.,** separation of the epiphysis of a long bone, caused by trauma.

**expressed skull f.,** see skull f., expressed.

**extracap'sular f.,** a f. at the articular extremity of a bone, but outside of the line of attachment of the capsular ligament of the joint.

**fatigue f.,** f. that occurs in bone subject to repeated (or unusual) small endogenous stress, for example, stress f. of metatarsal in new soldiers unaccustomed to long hikes; most often transverse in configuration.

**fissured f.,** linear f.

**Galeazzi's f.,** f. of distal end of radius with dislocation of distal end of ulna.

**Gosselin's f.,** v-shaped f. of distal end of tibia.

**green-stick f.,** bent f.; hickory-stick f.; willow f.; the bending of a bone with incomplete f. involving the convex side of the curve only.

**Guérin's f.,** LeFort I f.; horizontal f.; a f. of the facial bones in which there is a horizontal f. at the base of the maxillae above the apices of the teeth.

**gutter f.,** a long, narrow, depressed f. of the skull.

**hickory-stick f.,** green-stick f.

**horizontal f.,** Guérin's f.

**impacted f.,** one in which one of the fragments is driven into the cancellar tissue of the other fragment.

**incomplete f.,** one in which the line of f. does not include the entire bone.

**indirect f.,** a f., especially of the skull, that occurs at a point not at the site of impact.

**intra-artic'ular f.,** articular f.

**intracap'sular f.,** one at the articular extremity of a bone within the line of insertion of the capsular ligament of the joint.

**intraperios'teal f.,** a f. in which the periosteum is not ruptured.

**intrau'terine f.,** fetal f.; a f. of one or more bones of a fetus occurring before birth.

**lead pipe f.,** compression at point of impact with a linear f. on opposite side.

**LeFort I f.,** Guérin's f.

**LeFort II f.,** pyramidal f.

**LeFort III f.,** craniofacial dysjunction f.

**lin'ear f.,** fissured f.; a f. running parallel with the long axis of the bone.

**linear skull f.,** see skull f., linear.

**longitu'dinal f.,** one involving the bone in the line of its axis.

**loose f.,** complete f. with wide separation of the broken ends.

**march f.,** f. of tibia or femur, without obvious displacement, occurring during a march, usually of a fatiguing character; see also march *foot.*

**Monteggia's f.,** f. of the ulna with dislocation of the head of the radius.

**Moore's f.,** f. of distal end of radius with luxation of distal end of ulna.

**multiple f.,** composite f.; a f. of several bones occurring simultaneously or one involving several different parts of the same bone.

**neurogenic f.,** a f. in bone weakened by disease of the nerve supply.

**oblique f.,** one the line of which runs obliquely to the axis of the bone.

**occult f.,** a condition in which there are clinical signs of f. but no x-ray evidence; after 3 or 4 weeks x-ray shows new bone formation.

**open f.,** compound f.

**open skull f.,** see skull f., open.

**parry f.,** rarely used term denoting f. of ulna with dislocation of radius when arm is raised to protect against a blow aimed at the head.

**pertrochanteric f.,** a f. through great trochanter of femur.

**ping-pong f.,** see skull f., depressed.

**pond f.,** circular depressed skull fracture.

**Pott's f.,** f. of the lower part of the fibula and of the malleolus of the tibia, with outward displacement of the foot.

**pressure f.,** one caused by force of malignant growth.

**pyramidal f.,** LeFort II f.; a f. of the midfacial skeleton with the principal f. lines meeting at an apex at or near the superior aspect of the nasal bones.

**secondary f.,** one occurring as a consequence of necrosis or some other disease of the bone.

**Shepherd's f.,** a f. of the external tubercle (posterior process) of the talus, sometimes mistaken for a displacement of the os trigonum.

**silver-fork f.,** a Colles' f. of the wrist in which the deformity has the appearance of a fork in profile.

**simple f.,** an uncomplicated, not compound f.

**simple skull f.,** see skull f., closed.

**Skillern's f.,** f. of distal radius with green-stick f. of neighboring portion of ulna.

**skull f.,** a break of the cranium resulting from trauma.

**skull f., basal,** one involving the base of the cranium.

**skull f., closed,** or **simple,** one with intact overlying scalp and/or mucous membranes.

**skull f., comminuted,** a f. with fragmentation of bone.

**skull f., depressed,** a f. with inward displacement of a part of the calvarium; the so-called "dish-pan," "derby hat," and "ping-pong" f.'s consist of regular cranial concavity in infants and may or may not be associated with f.

**skull f., diastatic,** (1) separation of cranial bones at a suture; (2) f. with marked separation of bone fragments.

**skull f., expressed,** one with outward displacement of a part of the cranium.

**skull f., linear,** a f. resembling a line.

**skull f., open,** or **compound,** a f. with laceration of overlying scalp and/or mucous membrane.

**skull f., stellate,** multiple radiating linear f.'s.

**Smith's f.,** reversed Colles' f.; f. of the radius near its lower articular surface with displacement of the fragment toward the palmar aspect.

**spiral f.,** one in which the line of break runs obliquely up one side of the bone.

**splintered f.,** a comminuted f. in which the fragments are long and sharp-pointed.

**spontaneous f.,** one occurring without any external injury.

**sprain f.,** f. in which a ligament, capsule, or tendon tears off a portion of bone.

**sprain f. (vertebral, cervical),** a sprain in which a small portion of adjacent bone has been pulled or pushed off; the teardrop f. is an example.

**stellate f.,** one in which the lines of break radiate from a central point.

**stellate skull f.,** see skull f., stellate.

**Stieda's f.,** f. of the internal condyle of the femur; a bony outgrowth from that region is called Pellegrini's disease.

**strain f.,** the tearing off, by a sudden force, of a piece of bone attached to a tendon, ligament, or capsule; the force may be exogenous or endogenous.

**stress f.,** f. occurring usually from sudden, strong, violent, endogenous force (e.g., a simple f. of fibula in a runner); distinct from strain f., in that stress f. is not at the point of connective tissue attachment, but usually at the point of muscular attachment.

**subcapital f.,** intracapsular f.; f. of a bone, such as the femur, just below its head.

**subperiosteal f.,** a f. occurring beneath the periosteum, and without displacement.

**supracondylar f.,** a f. of the distal end of the humerus.

**teardrop f.,** see sprain f. (vertebral, cervical).

**torsion f.,** one resulting from twisting of the limb.

**torus f.,** folding f.; a deformity caused by a force applied at each extremity of a long bone in a child; this is not a true f., but a local bulging caused by the longitudinal compression of the soft bone; it occurs in the radius or ulna or both.

**transcervical f.,** a f. through the neck of the femur.

**transcondylar f.,** a f. through condyles of the humerus.

**transverse f.,** one the line of which forms a right angle with the axis of the bone.

**transverse facial f.,** craniofacial dysjunction f.

**trimalleolar f.,** a f. through both malleoli and the posterior tip of the tibia.

**trophic f.,** one due to disturbance of nutrition of the bone.

**ununi'ted f.,** one in which union fails to occur, the ends of the bone becoming rounded and more or less eburnated, a false joint resulting.

**Wagstaffe's f.,** f., with displacement, of the inner malleolus.

**willow f.,** green-stick f.

---

**Fraenkel,** Albert, Berlin physician, 1848–1916. See F.'s *pneumococcus*, F.-Weichselbaum *pneumococcus*.

**Fraenkel,** Bernhard, Berlin laryngologist, 1836–1911. See F.'s *speculum*.

**Fraenken,** Carl, German bacteriologist, 1861–1915. See F.-Gabbet *stain*.

**fragilitas** (frä-jil'ĭ-tas) [ L. ]. Fragility.

**f. crin'ium** [ L. gen. pl. of *crinis*, hair ], brittleness of the hair; a condition in which the hair of the head or face tends to split or break off.

**f. os'sium,** Osteogenesis imperfecta (*q.v.*); brittleness of the bones; a pathologic condition in which the bones break readily.

**f. san'guinis,** *fragility* of the blood.

**fragility** (frä-jil'ĭ-tī) [ L. *fragilitas*. FRA- ]. Brittleness; liability to break, burst, or disintegrate.

**f. of the blood,** fragilitas sanguinis; increased susceptibility of the red blood cells to break down when the proportion of the saline content of the fluid is altered.

**fragilocyte** (frä-jil'o-sit) [ L. *fragilis*, brittle, + G. *kytos*, hollow (cell) ]. A red blood cell that is unusually fragile when subjected to a hypotonic salt solution.

**fragilocytosis** (frä-jil'o-si-to'sis). A condition of the blood in which the red blood cells are abnormally fragile.

**frag'ment.** A small part.

**Fab f.,** also called Fab portion or piece; see immunoglobulin.

**Fc f.,** also called Fc portion or piece; see immunoglobulin.

**fraise** (fraze) [ Fr. strawberry ]. A burr in the shape of a hemispherical button with cutting edges, used to enlarge a trephine opening in the skull or to cut osteoplastic flaps; the smooth convexity of the button prevents injury to the dura.

**frambesia** (fram-be'zĭ-ah) [ Fr. *framboise*, raspberry ]. Yaws.

**frambesiform** (fram-be'zĭ-form). Resembling the lesion of frambesia.

**frambesioma** (fram-be-zĭ-o'mah) [ frambesia + suffix -*oma*, tumor ]. Yaw; the primary individual lesion of frambesia or yaws.

**frame.** A structure made of parts fitted together.

**Balkan f.,** Balkan beam or splint; an overhead pole or f., supported on uprights attached to the bed posts or to a separate stand, from which a splinted limb is slung in the treatment of fracture or joint disease.

**Bradford f.,** an oblong rectangular f. made of pipe, over which are stretched transversely two strips of canvas; permits trunk and lower extermities to move as a unit.

**Deiters' terminal f.'s,** platelike structures in the organ of Corti uniting the outer phalangeal cells with Hensen's cells.

**Foster f.,** a reversible bed similar to a Stryker f.

**occluding f.,** see articulator.

**Stryker f.,** a f. that holds the patient and permits turning in various planes without individual motion of parts.

**trial f.,** a type of spectacle f. having variable adjustments, for holding trial lenses during retinoscopy or refraction.

**Whitman's f.,** similar to the Bradford f., but with curved sides.

**frame'work.** 1. Stroma. 2. In dentistry, the skeletal prosthesis (usually metal) around which and to which are attached the remaining portions of the prosthesis to produce the finished appliance (partial denture).

**Franceschetti,** A., Swiss ophthalmologist. See F.'s *syndrome*.

**Francisella** (fran'sĭ-sel'la). A genus of nonmotile, non-sporeforming, aerobic bacteria which contains small, Gram-negative cocci and rods. Capsules are rarely produced and the cells may show bipolar staining. These organisms are highly pleomorphic. They do not grow on plain agar or in liquid media without special enrichment. These organisms are pathogenic and cause laremia in man. The type species is *F. tularensis*.

**F. tularen'sis,** *Pasteurella tularensis;* a species which causes tularemia in man; it is transmitted to man from wild animals by bloodsucking insects, by contact with infected animals, or by drinking water. This organism penetrates unbroken skin to cause infection. It is infectious for man and most rodents. It is the type species of the genus *F.*

**francium** (fran'sĭ-um) [ *France,* native country of Mlle. M. Perey, the discoverer ]. Radioactive element of the alkali metal series; symbol Fr, atomic no. 87; half life of most stable known isotope (f.-223) is 21 minutes; discovered in 1939 among the decay products of uranium-235.

**Francke** (frahn'keh), Karl E., German physician, 1859–1920. See F.'s *needle*.

**frangula** (frang'gu-lah). The bark of *Rhamnus frangula* (family Rhamnaceae); laxative or cathartic.

**f. emodin,** emodin.

**frangulic acid.** Emodin.

**fran'gulin.** Rhamnoxanthin; emodine-*l*-rhamnoside; $C_{21}H_{20}O_9$; a glycoside from frangula. Has been used as a purgative.

**Frank,** Alfred E., German physician, *1884. See F.'s capillary *toxicosis.*

**Frankenhäuser** (frahn'ken-hoy-zer), Ferdinand, German gynecologist, †1894. See F.'s *ganglion.*

**Frankfort horizontal plane.** See under plane.

**Frankfort mandibular plane angle.** See under angle.

**frankincense** (frangk'in-sens) [ Mediev. L. *francum incensum,* pure incense ]. Olibanum.

**Franklin,** Benjamin, American physicist and statesman, 1706–1790. Gave his name to franklinism and franklinization. See F. *spectacles.*

**Franklin,** E. C. See F.'s *disease.*

**franklin'ic.** Denoting static or frictional electricity.

**frank'linism** [ B. *Franklin* ]. Static or frictional electricity.

**frank'liniza'tion.** The therapeutic use of static electricity.

**Fräntzel's murmur.** See under murmur.

**Fraser,** G. R., British geneticist. See F.'s *syndrome.*

**Fraunhofer,** Joseph von, German optician, 1787–1826. See F.'s *lines.*

**Frazier,** Charles H., U. S. surgeon, 1870–1936. See F.'s *needle*, F.-Spiller *operation.*

**FRC.** Abbreviation for functional residual *capacity.*

**F.R.C.P.** Abbreviation for Fellow of the Royal College of Physicians (London).

**F.R.C.P.C.** Abbreviation for Fellow of the Royal College of Physicians (Canada).

**F.R.C.P.E.** Abbreviation for Fellow of the Royal College of Physicians (Edinburgh).

**F.R.C.P.I.** Abbreviation for Fellow of the Royal College of Physicians (Ireland).

**F.R.C.S.** Abbreviation for Fellow of the Royal College of Surgeons.

**F.R.C.S.C.** Abbreviation for Fellow of the Royal College of Surgeons (Canada).

**F.R.C.S.E.** Abbreviation for Fellow of the Royal College of Surgeons (Edinburgh).

**F.R.C.S.I.** Abbreviation for Fellow of the Royal College of Surgeons (Ireland).

**freckle** (frek'l) [ O. Eng. *freken* ]. Ephelis; yellowish or brownish macules developing on the exposed parts of the skin, especially in persons of sandy complexion. The lesions increase in number on exposure to the sun. The epidermis is microscopically normal except for increased melanin. See also lentigo.

   **Hutchinson's f.,** *melanosis* circumscripta precancerosa.

   **melanotic f.,** *melanosis* circumscripta precancerosa.

**Fredet** (frĕ-da'), Pierre, French surgeon, 1870–1946. See F.-Ramstedt *operation.*

**Freeman,** E. A. See F.-Sheldon *syndrome.*

**freemartin** [ etym. uncert.; possibly from Sc. *fear* or *fearr,* a sterile and dry cow, + *martin,* fr. Martinmas (in November) when cattle, especially the sterile and those unproductive of milk, were slaughtered ]. A masculinized, female twin calf, caused by the twin fetuses being of opposite sexes. The chorionic blood vessels become fused at a very early stage of embryonic development with the result that the hormones of the male are conveyed in the circulation to the female twin and influences its sexual development. A f. is sterile, its uterus is undeveloped, and the clitoris is enlarged and penis-like; there may be structures resembling the ductus deferens and seminal vesicles. F.'s are a type of hermaphrodite.

**freeze-drying.** Lyophilization.

**freezing.** Congelation (1); congealing, stiffening, or hardening by exposure to cold.

   **gastric f.,** treatment for peptic ulcer designed to reduce or eliminate the production of acid gastric juice by freezing the secretory cells with a supercooled fluid introduced into a balloon.

**Frei** (fri), Wilhelm S., German dermatologist, 1885–1943. See F.''s *bubo, disease,* F.-Hoffman *reaction,* F. *test.*

**Freiberg,** Albert Henry, U. S. surgeon, 1869–1940. See F.'s *disease.*

**Frejka pillow.** See under pillow.

**fremitus** (frem'ĭ-tus) [ L. a dull roaring sound, fr. *fremo,* pp. -*itus,* to roar, resound ]. A vibration imparted to the hand resting on the chest or other part of the body. See also thrill.

   **bronchial f.,** bronchial rales perceptible to the hand resting on the chest, as well as by the ear.

   **hydatid f.,** hydatid *thrill.*

   **pericar'dial f.,** vibration in the chest wall produced by the friction of opposing roughened surfaces of the pericardium.

   **pleural f.,** vibration in the chest wall produced by the rubbing together of the roughened opposing surfaces of the pleura.

   **rhonchal f.,** f. produced by vibrations from the passage of air in the bronchial tubes partially obstructed by mucous secretion.

   **subjective f.,** vibration felt within the chest by the patient himself, when humming with the mouth closed; or f. felt when there is a rough, pericardial or pleural friction rub, particularly when pain is minimal.

   **tactile f.,** vibration felt with the hand on the chest during vocal f.

   **tussive f.,** a form of f. similar to the vocal, produced by a cough.

   **vocal f.,** the vibration in the chest wall, felt on palpation, produced by the spoken voice.

**fre'na.** Plural of frenum.

**fre'nal.** Relating to any frenum.

**frenectomy** (fre-nek'to-mi) [ frenum + G. *ektomē,* excision ]. The removal of any frenum.

**Frenkel,** Heinrich S., Swiss neurologist, 1860–1931. See F.'s *method, symptom.*

**Frenkel,** Henri, French ophthalmologist, 1864–1934. See F.'s anterior ocular traumatic *syndrome.*

**frenoplasty** (fre'no-plas'tĭ) [ frenum + G. *plassō,* to fashion ]. The correction of an abnormally attached frenum by surgically repositioning it.

**frenotomy** (fre-not'o-mĭ) [ frenum + G. *tomē,* a cutting ]. Division of any frenum, especially of the frenum linguae for the relief of tongue-tie.

**fren'ulum,** pl. **frenula** [ Mod. L. dim. of L. *frenum,* bridle ] [ NA ]. A small frenum or bridle.

   **f. cerebell'i,** f. veli medullaris superius.

   **f. clitor'idis** [ NA ], f. or bridle of the clitoris; the line of union of the inner portions of the labia minora on the under surface of the glans clitoridis.

   **f. of clitoris,** f. clitoridis.

   **f. epiglot'tidis,** *plica* glossoepiglottica mediana.

   **f. of Giacomini,** uncus *band* of Giacomini.

   **f. of ileocecal valve,** f. valvae ileocecalis.

   **f. la'bii inferio'ris, f. la'bii superio'ris** [ NA ], f. of the lower lip, f. of the upper lip; the folds of mucous membrane extending from the gum to the middle line of the lower and upper lips, respectively.

   **f. labio'rum** [ NA ], f. of the pudendal lips; f. laborium minorum; f. pudendi; the fourchette; the fold connecting the two labia minora posteriorly.

   **f. lin'guae** [ NA ], f. of the tongue; vinculum linguae; a fold of mucous membrane extending from the floor of the mouth to the midline of the under surface of the tongue.

   **frenula of lips,** f. labii inferioris and superioris.

   **f. of Macdowel,** tendinous fasciculi passing from the tendon of insertion of the pectoralis major muscle across the bicipital groove.

   **f. of Morgagni,** f. valvae ileocecalis.

   **f. of prepuce,** f. preputii.

   **f. prepu'tii** [ NA ], f. of the prepuce; vinculum preputii; a fold of mucous membrane passing from the undersurface of the glans penis to the deep surface of the prepuce.

   **f. prepu'tii clitor'idis,** f. clitoridis.

   **f. of pudendal lips,** f. labiorum pudendi.

   **f. puden'di,** f. labiorum pudendi.

   **f. of superior medullary velum,** f. veli medullaris superius.

   **synovial frenula,** *vincula* tendinum.

   **f. of tongue,** f. linguae.

   **f. valvae ileoceca'lis** [ NA ], f. of the ileocecal valve; frenum or f. of Morgagni; a fold more evident in cadavers running from the junction of the two commissures of the ileocecal valve on either side along the inner wall of the cecocolic junction.

   **f. ve'li medulla'ris supe'rius** [ NA ], f. of the superior medullary velum; a band passing from the longitudinal groove between the corpora quadrigemina on to the superior medullary velum.

**fre'num,** pl. **frena, frenums** [ L. a bridle, curb ]. Frenulum [ NA ]. 1. A narrow reflection or fold of mucous membrane passing from a more fixed to a movable part, as from the gum to the deep surface of the lip, serving in a measure to check undue movement of the part. 2. An anatomical structure resembling such a fold.

   **Morgagni's f.,** *frenulum* valvae ileocecalis.

   **synovial f.,** *vincula* tendinum.

**frenzy** (fren'zĭ) [ thr. Old Fr. and L. fr. G. *phrenēsis,* inflammation of the brain, fr. *phrēn,* mind ]. Violent delirium; mania.

**frequency** (fre'kwen-sĭ) [ L. *frequens,* repeated, often, constant ]. The number of regular recurrences in a given time, *e.g.,* heart beats, sound vibrations.

   **critical flicker fusion f.,** the minimal number of flashes of light per second at which a light stimulus no longer gives a continuing visual sensation.

   **dominant f.,** the particular f. in an electroencephalogram that occurs most of the time.

   **f. of micturition,** micturition at short intervals; it may result from increased urine formation or decreased bladder capacity.

   **respiratory f.,** symbol $f$; the number of breaths per minute.

**frequen'tin.** An antibiotic aldehyde, $C_{14}H_{20}O_4$, obtained from cultures of *Penicillium frequentans.*

**Frerichs** (fra'rikhs), Friedrich T. von, German pathologist and clinician, 1819–1885. See F.'s *theory.*

**fresh'ening.** The beginning of a new lactation period by a dairy cow or a goat. Practically synonymous with calving and kidding.

**Fresnel,** Augustin Jean, French physicist, 1788–1827. See F. *lens.*

**fress'reflex** [ Ger. ]. Sucking and chewing movements elicited by stimulation of the face and lips.

**fre'tum,** pl. **fre'ta** [ L. ]. A strait; a constriction.

**Freud** (froyd), Sigmund, Austrian neurologist and psychiatrist, 1856–1939, founder of psychoanalysis, *q. v.*

**Freudian** (froy'dī-an). Having reference to the theories of Sigmund Freud.

**Freudian slip** [ Sigmund *Freud* ]. A mistake which presumably suggests some underlying motive, often sexual or aggressive in nature.

**Freund,** Jules, U. S. bacteriologist, born in Hungary, 1890–1960. See F.'s complete *adjuvant,* F.'s incomplete *adjuvant.*

**Freund** (froynt), Wilhelm A., German gynecologist, 1833–1918. See F.'s *anomaly, law, operation.*

**Frey,** L. See F.'s *syndrome.*

**Frey** (fri), Max von, German physician, 1852–1932. See F.'s irritation *hairs.*

**Freyer** (fri'er), Sir Peter Johnston, British physician, 1851–1921. See F.'s *operation.*

**FRF.** Abbreviation for follicle-stimulating hormone releasing *factor.*

**fri'able** [ L. *friabilis,* fr. *frio,* to crumble ]. 1. Easily reduced to powder. 2. In bacteriology, denoting a dry and brittle culture falling into powder when touched or shaken.

**fric'ative.** Speech sound made by forcing the air stream through a narrow orifice.

**Fricke** (frik'eh), Johann K., German surgeon, 1790–1841. See F.'s *bandage.*

**Fridenberg** (fre'den-berg), Percy H., New York ophthalmologist, 1868–1960. See F.'s stigmometric card *test.*

**Friderichsen,** Carl, Danish physician, *1886. See Waterhouse-F. *syndrome,* F.-Waterhouse *syndrome.*

**Friedländer** (frēd'lĕn-der), Carl, German pathologist, 1847–1887. See F.'s *bacillus, pneumonia, stain* (for capsules).

**Friedländer** (frēd'lĕn-der), Max, German physician, *1841. See F.'s *disease.*

**Friedman,** E. A. See F.'s *curve.*

**Friedman,** Maurice H., American physician, *1903. See F.-Lapham *test,* F. *test.*

**Friedmann's disease.** See under disease.

**Friedreich** (frēd'rikh), Nikolaus, German neurologist, 1825–1882. See F.'s *ataxia, disease, foot, phenomenon, sign.*

**Friend disease.** See under disease.

**Friend virus.** See under virus.

**friente** (fre-en'te). An erythematous dermatitis attributed to the fungus *Ustilago hypodytes;* occurs among wood cutters and field workers.

**frigid** (frij'id) [ L. *frigidus,* cold ]. 1. Cold. 2. Temperamentally, especially sexually, cold or irresponsive.

**frigidity** (frī-jid'ĭ-tī). Anaphrodisia; the state of being frigid.

**frigolabile** (frig'o-la'bil) [ L. *frigus,* cold, + *labilis,* perishable ]. Subject to destruction by cold.

**frigorific** (frig'o-rif'ik) [ L. *frigus,* cold, + *facio,* to make ]. Producing cold.

**frigorism** (frig'o-rizm) [ L. *frigus,* cold ]. A pathologic condition resulting from the action of extreme cold upon the body.

**frig'ory** [ L. *frigus,* cold ]. The cold required for cooling 1 gm. of water 1°C.

**frigostabile, frigostable** (frig'o-sta'bil, -sta'bl) [ L. *frigus,* cold, + *stabilis,* stable ]. Not subject to destruction by a low temperature.

**frig'other'apy.** Cryotherapy.

**fringe.** Fimbria.

cervical f., hairlike wisps or linear strands of blood vessels seen on the neck.

costal f., the "zona corona"; an irregularly disposed collection of visible veins seen in the skin of people usually of or past middle age. Has no specific connection with any deep structure, such as the diaphragm, and no necessary connection with underlying pulmonary or cardiac disease.

Richard's f.'s, *fimbriae* tubae uterinae.

synovial f., *villi* synoviales.

**fringing** (frin'jing). A bulbous deformation of the calyx of the kidney together with a tortuous elongation of the stem, sometimes seen in the x-ray picture in early stages of tuberculosis of the kidney.

**frit** [ Fr. *frit,* fried ]. In dentistry, (*a*) the material from which the glaze for artificial teeth is made; (*b*) a powdered pigment material used in coloring the porcelain of artificial teeth.

**Fritsch,** Heinrich, German gynecologist, 1844–1915. See Bozeman-F. *catheter.*

**Froehde's reagent.** See under reagent.

**frog** [ A.S. *frogge* ]. 1. An amphibian in the order Anura, which includes the toads; the old name of the class was Batrachia. The commonest frog genera are *Rana* (grass frogs) and *Hyla* (tree frogs). 2. A specialized portion of the hoof of the horse. It is a wedge-shaped, horny mass lying between the bars and the sole on the ground surface of the foot.

f. in the throat, a collection of mucus in the larynx causing hoarseness and an inclination to hawk.

**Fröhlich** (frē'likh), Alfred, Vienna neurologist and pharmacologist, 1871–1953. See F.'s *dwarf, syndrome.*

**Frohn,** Damianus, German physician, *1843. See F.'s *reagent.*

**Froin** (fro-an'), Georges, French physician, *1874. See F.'s *syndrome.*

**frôlement** (frol-mon') [ Fr. ]. 1. Light friction or massage with the palm of the hand. 2. A rustling sound heard in auscultation.

**Froment,** Jules, Lyon physician, *1878. See F.'s *sign.*

**Frommel,** Richard, German gynecologist, 1854–1912. See F.'s *operation,* Chiari-F. *syndrome.*

**Frommer's dilator.** See under dilator.

**frons,** gen. **frontis** [ L. ] [ NA ], Forehead; brow; metopon; the part of the face between the eyebrows and the hairy scalp.

**fron'tad.** Toward the front.

**fron'tal.** 1. In front; relating to the anterior part of a body. 2. Frontalis.

**fronta'lis** [ L. ] [ NA ]. Frontal; referring to the frontal (coronal) plane or to the frontal bone or forehead.

**fron'toma'lar.** Frontozygomatic.

**fron'tomax'illary.** Relating to the frontal and the maxillary bones.

**fron'tona'sal.** Relating to the frontal and the nasal bones.

**frontooccipital** (fron'to-ok-sip'ĭ-tal). Relating to the frontal and the occipital bones, or to the forehead and the occiput.

**frontoparietal** (fron'to-pă-ri'e-tal). Relating to the frontal and the parietal bones.

**fron'totem'poral.** Relating to the frontal and the temporal bones.

**frontozygomatic** (fron'to-zi'go-mat'ik). Frontomalar; relating to the frontal and zygomatic bones.

**Froriep** (fro'rēp), August von, German anatomist, 1849–1917. See F.'s *ganglion, induration.*

**Frost,** William A., English ophthalmologist, 1853–1935. See F.-Lang *operation.*

**frost'bite.** Congelation (2); dermatitis congelationis; local tissue destruction resulting from exposure to extreme cold or contact with extremely cold objects; in mild cases, it results in erythema and slight pain; in severe cases, it can be painless or paresthetic and result in blistering, deep-seated destruction, and gangrene.

**frottage** (fro-tahzh') [ F., a rubbing ]. 1. The rubbing movement in massage. 2. Production of sexual excitement by rubbing against someone.

**frotteur** (fro-tuhr'). One who gets sexual excitement through frottage.

**F.R.S.** Abbreviation for Fellow of the Royal Society.

**F.R.S.C.** Abbreviation for Fellow of the Royal Society (Canada).

**Fru.** Abbreviation for fructose.

**fructo-** (fruk'to-) [ L. *fructus,* fruit ]. Prefix (indicating the fructose configuration) to suffixes -furanose, -pyranose, -syl, -side, -san, etc.

**fruc'tofu'ranose.** D-Fructose in furanose form. See structures under sugars.

**β-fructofuranosidase** (EC 3.2.1.26). Invertase; invertin; saccharase; sucrase; β-*h*-fructosidase; an enzyme converting β-D-fructofuranosides (*e.g.,* sucrose) to an alcohol (glucose) and D-fructose (invert sugar; see inversion (2)).

**fruc′toki′nase** (EC 2.7.1.4). A liver enzyme that catalyzes the reaction of ATP and D-fructose to form fructose 6-phosphate.

**fruc′tosan.** A polyfructose (*e.g.*, inulin) containing small amounts of other sugars; present in certain tubers. Also called levan, levulin, levulan, levulosan.

**fructose** (fruk′tōs) (NF, BP). See D-fructose.

**D-fructose.** (fruk′tōs) Fructose; levulose; laevulose; fruit sugar; D-*arabino*-2-hexulose, a 2-ketohexose; for structure, see sugars. Physiologically (in D form), the most important of the ketohexoses, and one of the two products of sucrose hydrolysis. Used intravenously when either oral carbohydrate or fluid intake requires replacement or supplement. It is metabolized or converted to glycogen in the absence of insulin.

**fructose bisphosphate aldolase** (EC 4.1.2.13). Fructose diphosphate aldolase; ketose-1-phosphate aldolase; 1-phosphofructaldolase; zymohexase; enzyme cleaving fructose 1,6-bisphosphate to dihydroxyacetone (glyceroketone) phosphate and glyceraldehyde 3-phosphate; also acts on certain ketose 1-phosphates.

**fructose diphosphate aldolase** Fructose bisphosphate aldolase.

**fruc′toside.** Fructose in —C—O— linkage where the —C—O— group is the original 2 group of the fructose (R usually C).

**fructosuria** (fruk′to-su′rī-ah) [ G. *ouron*, urine ]. The excretion of fructose in the urine.

    **essential f.,** a benign, asymptomatic metabolic abnormality due to deficiency of fructokinase, the first enzyme in the specific fructose pathway; fructose appears in the blood and urine, but is simply excreted unchanged; autosomal recessive inheritance. See also hereditary fructose *intolerance.*

**fructosyl-** (fruk′to-sil-). Prefix indicating fructose in —C—R— (not —C—O—R— ) linkage through its carbon-2 (R usually C).

**frusemide** (BP). Furosemide.

**frustration** (frus′tra′shun) [ L. *frustro,* pp. -*atus,* to deceive, disappoint, fr. *frustra* (adv.), in vain ]. Used as a physiologic, psychologic, or psychiatric term to indicate the thwarting of or inability to gratify a desire or to satisfy an urge or need.

**FSH.** Abbreviation for follicle-stimulating *hormone.*

**FSH-RF.** Abbreviation for follicle-stimulating hormone releasing *factor.*

**ft.** An abbreviation of the Latin *fiat* (sing.), *fiant* (pl.), meaning "let there be made"; a term used in prescription writing.

**Fuchs** (fooks), Ernst, German ophthalmologist, 1851–1930. See F.'s *adenoma, coloboma, dystrophy, stomas, syndrome.*

**Fuchs** (fooks), Leonhard, German botanist, 1501–1566. Gave his name to fuchsin.

**fuchsin** (fook′sin) [ L. *Fuchs* ]. A nonspecific term referring to any of several red rosanilin dyes used as stains in histology and bacteriology.

    **acid f.,** a mixture of the sodium salts bi- and trisulfonic acids of rosanilin and pararosanilin.

    **basic f.,** diamond f.; a mixture of rosanilin and pararosanilin chlorides.

    **carbolic f.,** Ziehl's *solution.*

    **diamond f.,** basic f.

**fuchsinophil** (fook′sī-no-fil) [ fuchsin + G. *philos,* fond ]. 1. Fuchsinophilic; staining readily with fuchsin dyes. 2. A cell or histologic element that stains readily with fuchsin.

**fuchsinophilia** (fook′sī-no-fil′ī-ah). The property of staining readily with fuchsin.

**fuchsinophil′ic.** Fuchsinophil (1).

**fucose** (fu′kōs). 6-Deoxygalactose; a methylpentose, the L-configuration of which occurs in the mucopolysaccharides of the blood group substances, in human milk (as a polysaccharide), and elsewhere in nature. For structure, see sugars.

**fucosidosis** (fu′ko-si-do′sis). A metabolic storage disease characterized by accumulation of fucose-containing glycolipids and deficiency of the enzyme alpha fucosidase; progressive neurologic deterioration begins after the first

year of life, accompanied by spasticity, tremor, and mild skeletal changes; autosomal recessive inheritance.

**fucosterol** (fu-kos′ter-ol). 5,24(28)-Stigmastadiene-3β-ol; 24-ethylidene-5-cholesten-3β-ol (for structure, see steroids); a sterol obtained from seaweed, of the genus *Fucus.*

**Fucus** (fu′kus) [ L. rock-lichen, fr. G. *phykos,* seaweed ]. A genus of seaweeds, family Fucaceae.

    **F. crispus,** chondrus (2).

    **F. vesiculo′sus,** *Quercus marina;* bladder wrack; cutweed; kelp; a seaweed of the northern Atlantic and Pacific coasts.

**FUDR.** See floxuridine.

**Fuerbringer** (für′bring-er), Paul, Berlin physician, 1849–1930. See F.'s hand *disinfection.*

**Fuerstner** (fürst′ner), C., German psychiatrist, 1848–1906. See F.'s *disease.*

**fugacity** (fu-gas′ĭ-tī) [ L. *fuga,* flight ]. The tendency of a fluid, as a result of all forces acting on it, to leave a given site in the body; the escaping tendency of a fluid.

**-fuge** [ L. *fuga,* flight ]. Suffix meaning flight, denoting that which causes flight (*e.g.,* centrifuge).

**fugitive** (fu′jĭ-tĭv) [ L. *fugitivus,* fleeing, fr. *fugio,* pp. *fugitus,* to flee ]. 1. Temporary; transient. 2. Wandering; flying; denoting certain inconstant symptoms.

**fugue** (fūg) [ Fr. fr. L. *fuga,* flight ]. A period in his past for which a person alleges almost complete amnesia. Habits and skills are usually unaffected. He leaves home and starts a new life with different conduct. Afterward, earlier events are remembered but those of the f. period are alleged to be forgotten. Validation of the reality of this phenomenon is extremely difficult.

**fu′gutoxin.** Term applied to the poison derived from the ovaries and skin of the Pacific pufferfish.

**Fukala** (foo-kah′lah), Vinzenz, Vienna ophthalmologist, 1847–1911. See F.'s *operation.*

**ful′crum,** pl. **ful′cra, ful′crums** [ L. a bedpost, fr. *fulcio,* to prop up ]. A prop, or the point on which a lever turns.

**ful′gurant** [ L. *fulguro,* pres. p. -*ans,* to lighten ]. Fulminant; foudroyant; sudden, like a flash of lightning.

**ful′gurating.** 1. Fulgurant. 2. Relating to fulguration.

**fulguration** (ful-gu-ra′shun) [ L. *fulgur,* lightning stroke ]. Destruction of tissue by means of sparks from a d'Arsonval current or other apparatus.

**Füllkörper** (fül′ker-per) [ Ger. fill-bodies ]. Degenerated glia cells.

**ful′minant** [ L. *fulmino,* pp. -*atus,* to hurl lightning, fr. *fulmen* (*fulmin*-), lightning ]. Fulgurant; foudroyant; occurring with lightning-like rapidity; applied to certain pains, as those of tabes dorsalis.

**ful′minating.** Fulgurating; running a speedy course, with rapid worsening.

**fumagillin** (fu′mă-jil′in). A crystalline antibiotic obtained from *Aspergillus fumigatus.* Has little antibacterial, antifungal, or antiviral activity but is highly potent as an amebicide, having a direct lethal effect on the intestinal form of *Entamoeba histolytica.*

**fu′marase.** Fumarate hydratase.

**fu′marate hydratase** (EC 4.2.1.2). Fumarase; an enzyme (a hydro-lyase) catalyzing the interconversion of fumaric acid and malic acid, a reaction of importance in the tricarboxylic acid cycle.

**fumarate reductase (NADH).** An oxidoreductase (EC 1.3.1.6) catalyzing reduction of fumarate to succinate.

**fumaric acid** (fu-măr′ik). *Trans*-butenedioic acid; an unsaturated dicarboxylic acid occurring as an intermediate in the tricarboxylic acid cycle.

$$\text{HC—COOH}$$
$$\text{HOOC—CH}$$

Fumaric acid

**fu′marine.** Protopine.

**fu′marylace′toace′tic acid.** HOOC—CH = (CO—CH₂)₂—COOH; one of the intermediates in the later stages in the catabolism of phenylalanine and tyrosine.

**fu'miga'cin.** Helvolic acid.

**fu'migant** [ see fumigate ]. Any vaporous substance used as a disinfectant or pesticide.

**fu'migate** [ L. *fumigo* pp. *-atus*, to fumigate, fr. *fumus*, smoke, + *ago*, to drive ]. To expose to the action of smoke or of fumes of any kind, as of sulfur, as a means of disinfection.

**fu'miga'tin.** A substituted benzoquinone; an antibiotic principle isolated from cultures of *Aspergillus fumigatus*. Moderately active against Gram-positive bacteria.

**fumiga'tion.** The act of fumigating; the use of a fumigant.

**fu'ming** [ L. *fumus*, smoke ]. Giving forth a visible vapor, a property of concentrated nitric, sulfuric, and hydrochloric acids, and certain other substances.

**functio laesa** [ L. ]. Loss of function; a fifth sign of inflammation added by Galen to those enunciated by Celsus (rubor, tumor, calor, and dolor).

**function** (fungk'shun) [ L. *functio*, fr. *fungor*, pp. *functus*, to perform ]. 1. The special action or physiologic property of an organ or other part of the body. 2. To perform its special work or office, said of an organ or other part of the body. 3. The general properties of any substance, depending on its chemical character and relation to other substances, according to which it may be grouped among acids, bases, alcohols, esters, etc. 4. A particular reactive grouping in a molecule. A functional group, *e.g.*, is the —OH group of an alcohol.

**allomer'ic f.,** the combined f. of the several segments of the spinal cord and medulla, communicating with each other by means of the white matter.

**arousal f.,** the ability of a sensory event to arouse the cortex to vigilance or readiness. See also discriminant *stimulus*.

**atrial transport f.,** the role of the atria in filling and stretching the ventricles by their presystolic contraction, without which the force of ventricular contraction and the cardiac output may significantly decrease.

**isomer'ic f.,** the individual f. of an isolated segment of the spinal cord.

**modulation transfer f.,** see under modulation.

**func'tional.** 1. Relating to a function or the functions. 2. Used in the sense of nonorganic; *i.e.*, a î. ailment is one that is not caused by a structural defect.

**functionalism** (funk'shun-al-ism). A branch of psychology primarily interested in the function of mental processes in man and animals, especially the role of the mind, intellect, emotions, and behavior in an individual's adaptation to his environment, as contrasted with structuralism, *q.v.*

**fun'dal.** Relating to a fundus.

**fun'dament** [ L. *fundamentum*, foundation, fr. *fundus*, bottom ]. 1. A foundation. 2. The anus.

**fundectomy** (fun-dek'to-mĭ) [ fundus + G. *ektomē*, excision ]. Fundusectomy.

**fun'dic.** Relating to a fundus.

**fun'diform** [ L. *funda*, a sling, + *forma*, shape ]. Looped; sling-shaped.

**fundoplication** (fun'do-pli-ka'shun) [ fundus + L. *plico*, to fold ]. Nissen's operation; suture of the fundus of the stomach around the esophagus to prevent regurgitation, in operations for hiatal hernia.

**Fun'dulus** [ Mod. L. fr. L. *fundus*, bottom ]. A genus of marine and fresh-water fish, of many species, native to the United States; commonly called killifish, mumichog, or mudfish. They are widely used as bait fish, experimental fish, or in mosquito-control programs.

**fun'dus,** pl. **fun'di** [ L. bottom ] [ NA ]. Bas-fond; the bottom or lowest part of a sac or hollow organ; that part farthest removed from the opening or exit.

**f. flavimacula'tus,** a genetic disorder of the pigment epithelium manifested by yellowish white flecks.

**leopard f.,** tesselated f.

**f. mea'tus acus'tici inter'ni** [ NA ], f. of the internal acoustic (auditory) meatus; the thin plate of bone separating the cochlea and vestibule from the internal acoustic meatus; it is divided by the transverse crest into a superior and an inferior fossa; the former is pierced by the facial canal and foramina for nerves to the utricle and ampullae of the superior and lateral semicircular ducts; the latter by foramina giving passage to the cochlear nerves, nerve fibers to the vestibule, and by nerves to the ampulla of the posterior semicircular duct.

**f. oc'uli,** the portion of the interior of the eyeball around the posterior pole; the part exposed to view through the ophthalmoscope; see eyegrounds.

**tesselated f.,** f. tigré, leopard or tigroid f. or retina; a normal f. to which a deeply pigmented choroid gives the appearance of dark polygonal areas between the choroidal vessels, especially in the periphery.

**f. tigré** (te-gra'), tesselated f.

**tigroid f.,** tesselated f.

**f. tym'pani,** *paries* jugularis tympani.

**f. u'teri** [ NA ], f. of the uterus; the upper rounded extremity of the uterus above the openings of the uterine (Fallopian) tubes.

**f. ventric'uli** [ NA ], f. of the stomach; greater cul-de-sac; the portion of the cardiac part of the stomach that lies above the cardiac notch.

**f. vesi'cae fel'leae** [ NA ], f. of the gallbladder; the wide closed end of the gallbladder situated at the inferior border of the liver.

**f. vesi'cae urina'riae** [ NA ], f. of the urinary bladder; the base of the bladder, formed by the posterior wall which is somewhat convex.

**funduscope** (fun'dus-skōp) [ L. *fundus*, bottom, + G. *skopeō*, to view ]. Ophthalmoscope.

**fun'duscop'ic.** Relating to the visualization of the eyegrounds with the ophthalmoscope.

**fundus'copy.** Ophthalmoscopy.

**fundusec'tomy** [ L. *fundus*, cardia, + G. *ektomē*, excision ]. Fundectomy; excision of the uterine or gastric fundus.

**fungal** (fung'gal). Relating to a fungus; fungoid; fungous.

**fungate** (fung'gāt). To grow exuberantly like a fungus or spongy growth.

**fungemia** (fun-je'mĭ-ah). Fungal infection disseminated by way of the blood stream.

**fungi** (fun'ji). Plural of fungus.

**Fungi** (fun'-ji) [ L. *Fungus*, a mushroom ]. A division of plantlike organisms, growing in irregular masses, without roots, stems, or leaves and devoid of chlorophyll or other pigments capable of photosynthesis. Each organism (thallus) usually possesses filamentous, branched somatic structures (hyphae) surrounded by cell walls containing cellulose or chitin or both, and containing true nuclei. The organisms reproduce sexually or asexually (spore formation). Such organisms may obtain nutrition from other living organisms as parasites or from dead organic matter as saprophytes.

**F. Imperfecti,** a class or group of fungi in which the members reproduce by asexual means and a sexual method is either unknown or has been lost permanently.

**fungicidal** (fun-jĭ-si'dal) [ fungus + L. *caedo*, to kill ]. Having a destructive (killing) action on fungi.

**fungicide** (fun'jĭ-sīd). Mycocide; any substance that has a destructive (killing) action upon fungi.

**fungicidin** (fun'jĭ-si'din). Nystatin.

**fungiform** (fun'jĭ-form). Fungilliform; shaped like a fungus or mushroom; applied to any structure with a broad, often branched, free portion and a narrower base.

**fungilliform** (fun-jil'-ĭ-form) [ Mod L. *fungillus*, dim. of L. *fungus* ]. Fungiform.

**fungistatic** (fun-jĭ-stat'ik) [ fungus + G. *statos*, standing ]. Mycostatic; having an inhibiting action upon the growth of fungi.

**fungitoxic** (fun'jĭ-tok'sik). Poisonous or in any way deleterious to the growth of fungi; fungicidal.

**fungitoxicity** (fun'jĭ-tok-sis'ĭ-tĭ). The property of being fungitoxic.

**fungoid** (fung'goyd). Resembling a fungus; denoting an exuberant morbid growth on the surface of the body.

**fungosity** (fung-gos'ĭ-tĭ). A fungoid growth.

**fungous** (fung'gus). Relating to a fungus.

**fungus,** pl. **fungi** (fung'gus, fun'ji) [ L. *fungus*, a mushroom ]. 1. A member of the Fungi; a plantlike organism feeding on organic matter; such are mushrooms, yeasts, and molds. See also Fungi. 2. A fungosity, or fungoid growth.

**alpha f.,** term applied by Quincke to the f. of favus herpetiformis, now called *Trichophyton schönleinii.*

**beta f.,** term applied by Quincke to a strain of *Trichophyton schönleinii,* the favus f.

**f. cer'ebri,** an ulcerated cerebral hernia with granulation tissue protruding from scalp wound.

**cuta'neous f.,** dermatophyte.

**fission f.,** a schizomycete (bacterium).

**gamma f.,** term applied by Quincke to a strain of *Trichophyton schönleinii,* the favus f.

**f. haemato'des,** an obsolete term; formerly denoted a soft, fungating, easily bleeding, malignant neoplasm.

**mosaic f.,** a pseudofungus in which intercellular deposits of cholesterol are obtained in scrapings from the lesions.

**ray f.,** a bacterium which is a member of the order Actinomycetales.

**slime f.,** mycetozoa.

**thread f.,** a general term for various fungi, such as those causing favus, tinea tonsurans, etc.

**thrush f.,** *Candida albicans;* also improperly termed *Monilia albicans,* and formerly *Oidium* or *Saccharomyces albicans.*

**umbil'ical f.,** a mass of granulation tissue on the stump of the umbilical cord in the newborn.

**yeast f.,** saccharomyces.

**fu'nic.** Relating to the funis, or umbilical cord.

**fu'nicle.** Funiculus.

**funicular** (fu-nik'u-lar). 1. Relating to a funiculus. 2. Funic.

**funiculitis** (fu-nik'u-li'tis) [ funiculus + G. suffix *-itis,* inflammation ]. 1. Inflammation of a funiculus, especially of the spermatic cord. 2. Inflammation of that portion of a spinal nerve that lies within the intervertebral canal.

**endemic f.,** filarial f.

**filarial f.,** endemic f.; cellulitis of the spermatic cord due to filariasis; occurs endemically in Cylon and Egypt, and probably elsewhere in the East.

**funiculopexy** (fu-nik'u-lo-pek'sĭ) [ funiculus + G. *pēxis,* a fixing. PECT- ]. The procedure by which the spermatic cord is sutured to the surrounding tissue in the operation for undescended testicle.

**funiculus,** pl. **funic'uli** (fu-nik'u-lus) [ L. dim. of *funis,* cord ] [ NA ]. A small, cordlike structure, such as (1) one of the bundles of nerve fibers the aggregate of which compose the nerve trunk; (2) f. spermaticus; (3) f. umbilicalis.

**f. am'nii,** amniotic cord found in several domestic animals.

**anterior f.,** f. anterior.

**f. ante'rior** [ NA ], anterior f.; anterior white column of spinal cord; a column or bundle of white matter on either side of the anterior median fissure, between that and the anterolateral sulcus.

**cuneate f.,** *fasciculus* cuneatus.

**f. dorsa'lis,** f. posterior.

**f. gra'cilis,** *fasciculus* gracilis.

**lateral f. of spinal cord,** f. lateralis.

**f. latera'lis** [ NA ], lateral f. of spinal cord; anterolateral column of spinal cord; the lateral white column of the spinal cord between the lines of exit and entrance of the anterior and posterior nerve roots.

**funiculi medu'lae spinalis** [ NA ], any of the columns of the spinal cord.

**posterior f.,** f. posterior.

**f. poste'rior** [ NA ], posterior f.; f. dorsalis posterior white column of the spinal cord; the large, wedge-shaped, fiber bundle lying between the posterior gray column and the posterior midplane, and composed largely of dorsal root fibers.

**f. sep'arans,** an oblique ridge in the floor of the fourth ventricle of the brain, separating the area postrema from the ala cinerea, or trigonum vagi.

**f. solita'rius,** *tractus* solitarius.

**f. spermat'icus** [ NA ], spermatic cord; chorda spermatica; testicular cord; the cord formed by the ductus deferens and its associated structures extending from the deep inguinal ring through the inguinal canal into the scrotum.

**f. te'res,** *eminentia* medialis.

**f. umbilica'lis** [ NA ], umbilical cord; chorda umbilicalis; funis (1); the definitive connecting stalk between the embryo or fetus and the placenta; at birth it consists of

loose mesenchyme (Wharton's jelly) in which are embedded the umbilical vessels.

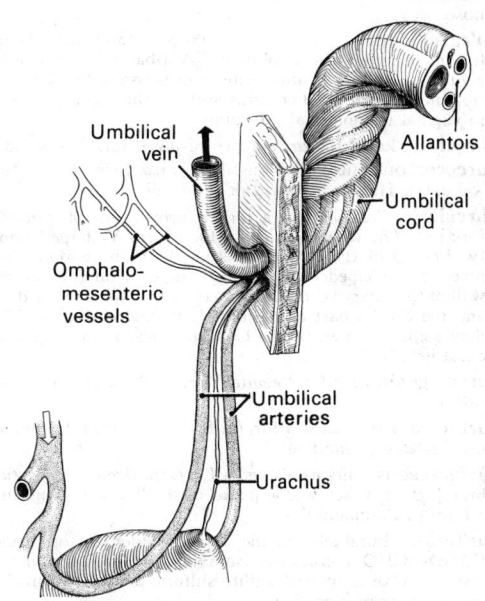

**Funiculus Umbilicalis (Umbilical Cord)**

**fu'niform** [ L. *funis,* cord, + *forma,* shape ]. Ropelike.

**fu'nis** [ L. a rope, cord ]. 1. *Funiculus* umbilicalis. 2. A cordlike structure.

**Funkenstein,** Daniel H., American physiologist. See F. *test.*

**fun'nel.** 1. A hollow conical vessel with a tube of variable length proceeding from its apex, used in pouring fluids from one container to another, in filtering, etc. 2. In anatomy, infundibulum.

**Buchner f.,** a porcelain f. the upper part of which has vertical walls; at the junction of this part with the conical part of f. is a perforated porcelain plate upon which filter paper can be laid.

**Martegiani's f.,** Martegiani's area; the funnel-shaped dilation of the posterior extremity of the hyaloid canal.

**pial f.,** the pia-lined channel in which each blood vessel entering the brain lies suspended; essentially, the pial f.'s are perivascular extensions of the subarachnoid space.

**FUO.** Abbreviation for fever of unknown origin.

**fur.** 1. The coat of soft, fine hair of some mammals. 2. A layer of epithelium, mucus, and debris on the dorsum of the tongue. Its relation to underlying disease or disturbance of the alimentary canal is not proved.

**furaltadone** (fu-ral'tă-dōn). ALTAFUR; a complex morpholino-furfuryl-oxazolidone; used in the treatment of trypanosomiasis, particularly the meningoencephalitic stage; in veterinary medicine, used for the treatment of bovine mastitis and certain bacterial infections of poultry.

**furamterene.** FUTERENE; 2,4,7-triamino-6-(2-furyl)pteridine; diuretic.

**fu'ran.** A cyclic compound found, usually in saturated form, in those sugars with an oxygen bridge between carbon atoms 1 and 4, or 2 and 5, or 3 and 7, for which reason they are known as furanoses (furan + -ose for sugar).

$$HC \overset{O}{\underset{\underset{H}{C}-\underset{H}{C}}{\diagdown}} CH$$

**Furan**

**fu′ranose.** A saccharide unit or molecule containing the furan grouping; specific examples are preceded by prefixes indicating the configuration, *e.g.*, fructofuranose, ribofuranose.

**fu′razol′idone** (NF). FUROXONE; 3-(5-nitro-2-furfurylideneamino)-2-oxazolidine. Antibacterial and antiprotozoal activity against enteric organisms. Used in the treatment of bacterial enteritis and diarrhea, and topically in vaginal trichomonal infections.

**furcal** (fur′kal) [ L. *furca*, a two-pronged fork ]. Forked.

**furcocercous** (fur-ko-ser′kus) [ L. *furca*, fork, + G. *kerkos*, tail ]. Having a forked or bifid tail.

**furcula** (fur′ku-lah) [ L. a forked prop, dim. of *furca*, a fork ]. 1. The fused clavicles which form V-shaped bone (wishbone) of the bird's skeleton. 2. In the embryo, an inverted U-shaped elevation that appears on the ventral wall of the pharynx, being formed by the two linear ridges and the caudal part of the hypobranchial eminence. The depression enclosed by the U is known as the laryngotracheal groove.

**fureur genitale** [ Fr. "genital rage" ]. Nymphomania or satyriasis.

**furfur,** pl. **furfures** (fur′fur, fur′fu-rēz) [ L. bran ]. Epidermal scale; *e.g.*, dandruff.

**furfuraceous** (fur-fu-ra′shus) [ L. *furfuraceus*, fr. *furfur*, bran ]. Branny; scaly; composed of small scales; denoting a form of desquamation.

**fur′fural.** Furaldehyde; the 2-carboxaldehyde of furan; $C_4H_3O$—CHO; a colorless aromatic fluid obtained in the distillation of bran with dilute sulfuric acid. Used in the manufacture of medicinal agents.

**fur′furol.** 2-Carbinol derivative of furan; $C_4H_3O$—$CH_2OH$.

**furfuryl** (fur′fu-ril). The monovalent radical derived from furfurol by loss of the OH group.
   **f. trimeth′ylammo′nium i′odide,** furtrethonium iodide.

**fur′nace.** A stovelike apparatus containing a chamber for heating, melting, or fusing, by means of a heat source such as gas or electricity.
   **dental f.,** (1) a f. used to eliminate the wax pattern from the investment mold prior to casting in gold or semiprecious metal; (2) a f. used to fuse and glaze dental porcelains.
   **muffle f.,** (1) an electric f. heated by direct transfer of heat from a resistant muffle; (2) a dental f. heated by a muffle.

**fu′ror** [ L. ]. Rage; madness; fury.
   **f. epilep′ticus,** attacks of anger to which epileptics are occasionally subject, occurring without apparent provocation and without disturbance of consciousness.

**furosemide** (fu-ro′sĕ-mid) (USP). LASIX; frusemide; 4-chloro-*N*-furfuryl-5-sulfamoylanthranilic acid; an orally effective diuretic resembling organic mercurials in its effects on the renal excretion of electrolytes.

**fu′rostan.** A 16β,22-epoxycholestane (for structure, see steroids).

**furrow** (fur′ro) [ A.S. *furh* ]. A groove or sulcus.
   **digital f.,** one of the grooves on the palmar surface of a finger, at the level of an interphalangeal joint.
   **genital f.,** a groove on the genital tubercle in the embryo, appearing toward the end of the second month.
   **gluteal f.,** *sulcus* gluteus.
   **mentolabial f.,** *sulcus* mentolabialis.
   **primitive f.,** the groove in the primitive streak.
   **Schmorl's f.,** a focal linear depression in the apical portion of the lung, resulting from defective development of the first rib; some observers think that such pulmonary tissue is more susceptible to the effects of tubercle bacilli.

**fur′salan** (USAN). 3,5-Dibromo-*N*-(tetrahydrofurfuryl)-salicylamide; disinfectant.

**Fürth,** Otto von, German physician, *1867. See F.'s *myosin*.

**fur′tretho′nium iodide.** Furfuryl trimethylammonium iodide; parasympathetic stimulating drug, suggested for the treatment of atonic or hypotonic bladder.

**furuncular** (fu-rung′ku-lar). Furunculous; relating to a boil or furuncle.

**furuncle** (fu′rung-kl) [ L. *furunculus*, a petty thief ]. Furunculus; boil; a localized pyogenic infection originating in a hair follicle.

**furunculoid** (fu-rung′ku-loyd) [ furunculus + G. *eidos*, resemblance ]. Resembling a boil.

**furunculosis** (fu-rung′ku-lo′sis). A condition marked by the presence of furuncles or boils.
   **f. orienta′lis,** the boil or sore of cutaneous leishmaniasis.

**furunculous** (fu-rung′ku-lus). Furuncular.

**furunculus,** pl. **furun′culi** (fu-rung′ku-lus) [ L. a petty thief, a boil, dim. of *fur*, a thief ]. Furuncle.

**furze.** *Ulex europaeus.*

**Fusarium** (fu-za′rī-um) [ L. *fusus*, spindle ]. A genus of rapidly growing saprophytic fungi producing characteristic sickle-shaped, multiseptate macroconidia; one of the causative agents of corneal ulcer and mycotic keratitis.

**fuscin** (fus′in) [ L. *fuscus*, dusky ]. A benzodipyran derivative; the melanin-like pigment of the retinal pigment epithelium.

**fus′cus** [ L. ] [ NA ]. Dark or dusky in color.

**fusel oil** (fu′zel). A mixture, in varying proportions, of amyl, butyl, hexyl, and propyl alcohols; present in newly distilled spirits.

**fu′sidate sodium** (USAN). Sodium fusidate (BP); FUCIDINE; the sodium salt of fusidic acid, *q.v.*; possesses antimicrobial properties.

**fusid′ic acid.** Ramycin; 3,11,16-trihydroxy-4,8,10,14-tetramethyl-17-(1′-carboxyisohept-4′-enylidene) cyclopenta[ *a* ]phenanthrene 16-acetate (a steroid derivative); a fermentation product of *Fusidium coccineum*, a parasitic fungus on the plant *Veronica*. See fusidate sodium.

**fusiform** (fu′zĭ-form, fu′sī-) [ L. *fusus*, a spindle, + *forma*, form ]. Spindle-shaped; tapering at both ends.

**Fu′sifor′mis** [ see fusiform ]. An obsolete generic name sometimes used for the anaerobic, fusiform bacteria found in the human mouth. These organisms are closely related to the anaerobic organisms found in the human intestine and placed in the genus *Fusobacterium*. The type species is *F. termitidis*, an organism believed to be a myxobacter.

**fusimotor** (fu′zĭ-mo′tor) [ L. *fusus*, spindle, + *movere*, to move ]. Pertaining to the efferent innervation of intrafusal muscle fibers by gamma motor neurons. See also neuromuscular *spindle*.

**fusion** (fu′zhun) [ L. *fusio*, a pouring, fr. *fundo*, pp. *fusus*, to pour ]. 1. Liquefaction by heat; melting. 2. Uniting; joining together. 3. The blending of the images seen by the two eyes into one perfect image, producing binocular vision. 4. The growth together, as one, of two or more teeth, in consequence of the abnormal union of their formative organs.
   **flicker f.,** the blending of the separate images of the two eyes into one while illuminated by intermittent flashes of light; see also critical flicker-fusion *frequency*.
   **nuclear f.,** the formation of more complex atomic nuclei from less complex; as in the formation of helium nuclei from hydrogen nuclei (hydrogen f.).
   **spinal f.,** spine f.; spondylosyndesis; an operative procedure to accomplish bone ankylosis between two or more vertebrae.
   **vertebral f.,** spondylosyndesis; surgical ankylosis of the spine.

**Fusobacterium** (fu-zo-bak-te′rī-um) [ L. *fusus*, a spindle, + bacterium, *q.v.* ]. A genus of bacteria (family Bacteroidaceae) containing Gram-negative, nonsporeforming, obligately anaerobic rods which produce butyric acid as a major metabolic product. Nonmotile and motile organisms occur; motile cells are peritrichous. These organisms are found in cavities of man and other animals; some species are pathogenic. The type species is *F. nucleatum*.
   **F. fusiforme,** fusiform bacillus; a species found in the mouth and in infections of the mouth, upper respiratory tract, and wounds.
   **F. mortiferum,** *Sphaerophorus mortiferus;* a species found in various infections in man.
   **F. necropho′rum,** *Fusiformis necrophorus; Necrobacterium necrophorum; Sphaerophorus necrophorus;* necrosis bacillus; a species which probably occurs as a normal inhabitant of the mucous membranes of man and other animals but which appears to be responsible for several

necrotic and gangrenous lesions in animals, such as calf diphtheria, labial necrosis of rabbits, and foot rot of sheep, and occasionally for necrotic lesions in man. It is the type species of *Sphaerophorus*.

**F. nuclea'tum,** a species found in the mouth and infections of the upper respiratory tract and pleural cavity, occasionally of the lower intestinal tract. It is the type species of the genus *F.*

**F. plauti,** a species found in the buccal cavity; also found in cultures of *Entamoeba histolytica.*

**fusocellular** (fu'zo-sel'u-lar). Spindle-celled.

**fusospirochetal** (fu-zo-spi-ro-ke'tal). Referring to the associated fusiform and spirochetal organisms such as those found in the lesions of Vincent's angina.

**fustigation** (fus'tĭ-ga'shun) [ L. *fustigo,* pp. -*atus,* to beat with a cudgel ]. A form of massage consisting in beating the surface with light rods.

**fus'tin** [ L. *fustis,* a stick, cudgel, in Mediev. L. a tree ]. 3,3',4',7-Tetrahydroxyflavanone; a yellow dye from fustic, *Rhus cotinus,* or Venetian sumac.

**Fy blood group.** See Duffy blood group, appendix 2.

# G

**G.** Abbreviation or symbol for (1) Newtonian *constant* of gravitation or gravitational *unit;* (2) glucose, as in UDPG; and (3) guanylic acid residues in polynucleotides, as in poly(G).

**G.** Symbol for Gibbs' free *energy.*

**g.** Abbreviation for gram; also abbreviated gm.

**g.** A mathematical constant expressing acceleration of a body due to gravity; for example, 100,000 × *g* means 100,000 times the acceleration due to gravity. The value of *g* is approximately 980 cm. (9.8 meters) or 32 feet per second, per second.

**Ga.** Chemical symbol for the element gallium.

**GABA.** Abbreviation for γ-*aminobutyric* acid.

**Gabbet,** Henry S., English physician, 19th century. See Fraenken-G. *stain,* G.'s *solution, stain.*

**G acid.** 2-Naphthol-6,8-disulfonic acid.

**G-actin.** See under actin.

**Gaddum,** John H., English biochemist, *1900. See G.-Schild *test.*

**gad′fly.** See *Tabanus.*

**Gadidae** (gad′ĭ-de). A family of fishes that includes the burbot and cod (genus *Gadus*), from livers of which an oil rich in vitamins A and D is obtained.

**gadole′ic acid.** 9-Eicosenoic acid; an unsaturated fatty acid from cod liver oil and other sources; *cf.* arachidic acid.

**Gadolin,** Johan, Finnish chemist, 1760–1852. Gave his name to gadolinium.

**gad′olin′ium** [ *J. Gadolin* ]. An element of the lanthanide group, symbol Gd, atomic no. 64, atomic weight 157.26.

**Ga′dus** [ Mod. L. fr. G. *gados,* a fish, probably cod ]. A genus of fishes including the burbot and the cod, *G. morrhua,* from the liver of which is obtained cod liver oil.

**Gaenslen,** Frederick J., U. S. surgeon, 1877–1937. See G.'s *sign.*

**Gaffky,** Georg T. A., German hygienist, 1850–1918. See G. *scale, table.*

**gag.** 1. To retch; to cause to retch or heave. 2. To prevent from talking. 3. An instrument adjusted between the teeth to keep the mouth from closing during operations in the mouth or throat.

    **Davis-Crowe mouth g.,** instrument used for opening the mouth, depressing the tongue, maintaining the airway, and transmitting volatile anesthetics during tonsillectomy or oropharyngeal surgery.

**gage** (gāj). Gauge.

**gain.** Increase; profit.

    **epino′sic g.,** secondary g.

    **parano′sic g.,** primary g.

    **primary g.,** paranosic g.; the alleviation of anxiety derived from the conversion of emotional concerns into demonstrably organic illnesses (*e.g.,* hysterical blindness or paralysis), as contrasted with the secondary g.

    **secondary g.,** epinosic g.; the interpersonal or social advantages (*i.e.,* assistance, attention, and sympathy) gained indirectly from organic illness, as contrasted with the primary g.

**Gairdner,** Sir William T., Scottish physician, 1824–1907. See G.'s *disease.*

**Gaisböck,** F. See G.'s *syndrome.*

**gait** (gāt). Manner of walking.

    **atax′ic g.,** an unsteady, staggering, or irregular g.

    **cerebel′lar g.,** a staggering g., often with a tendency to fall to one or other side, forward or backward.

    **Charcot's g.,** the g. of hereditary ataxia.

    **equine g.,** a high steppage g. necessitated by foot drop of peroneal nerve paralysis.

    **festinating g.,** see festination.

    **gluteus maximus g.,** compensatory backward propulsion of trunk to maintain center of gravity over support.

    **gluteus medius g.,** compensatory list of body (or throw of trunk) to weak gluteal side, to put center of gravity over the femur.

    **goose g.,** a peculiar waddling g. seen in some cases of arthritis.

    **helicopod g.,** helicopodia; a g. in which the feet are thrown in half circles, as in hemiplegia.

    **hemiple′gic g.,** the walk of hemiplegics characterized by swinging the affected leg in a half circle.

    **high steppage g.,** a g. in which the foot is raised higher than is necessary and brought down suddenly in a flapping manner; often seen in peroneal nerve palsy and tabes.

    **Oppenheim's g.,** the g. of disseminated sclerosis; a swinging motion of head, body, and extremities.

    **scissor g.,** one leg crosses in front of the other, so that the imprint of the left foot is on the right and *vice versa.*

    **spastic g.,** a g. characterized by stiffness of legs, feet and toes.

    **steppage g.,** see high steppage g.

**Gal.** Symbol for galactose.

**galact-.** See galacto-.

**galactacrasia** (gă-lak′tă-kra′zĭ-ah) [ galact- + G. *akrasia,* bad mixture, fr. *a-* priv. + *krasis,* a mixing ]. Abnormal composition of mother's milk.

**galactagogue** (gă-lak′tă-gog) [ galact- + G. *agōgos,* leading, ACT- ]. Galactopoietic. 1. Increasing the secretion of milk. 2. An agent that promotes the secretion and flow of milk.

**galac′tan.** 1. Gelose; a polysaccharide (galactosan; polygalactose) found in the cell walls of algae. It yields galactose upon hydrolysis. 2. *β*-D-1,6-anhydrogalactopyranose; an internal (cyclic) anhydride of galactose.

**galac′tans.** Pectic acids; a group of carbohydrates in citrus pectins, hemicelluloses, and mucilages, containing galacturonic acid and other sugars. See also galactosans.

**galactaric acid.** Mucic acid.

**galac′tic.** Pertaining to milk; promoting the flow of milk.

**galactidrosis** (gă-lak′tĭ-dro′sis) [ galact- + G. *hidrōs,* sweat ]. Sweating of a milky fluid.

**galac′tin.** Obsolete term for prolactin.

**galactischia** (gal′ak-tis′kĭ-ah) [ galact- + G. *ischō,* to check ]. Galactoschesia.

**galac′titol.** Dulcitol; dulcite; dulcose; melampyrin; the hexitol of galactose, found naturally in various species of *Euonymus* and *Melampyrum.*

**galacto- galact-** (gă-lak′to-) [ G. *gala,* milk ]. Combining forms indicating milk.

**galac′toblast** [ galacto- + *blastos,* germ ]. Colostrum *corpuscle.*

**galactobolic** (gă-lak′to-bol′ik) [ galacto- + G. *bole,* throwing ]. Causing the release or ejection of milk from the breast.

**galactocele** (gălak′to-sēl) [ galacto- + G. *kēlē,* tumor ]. A retention cyst caused by occlusion of a lactiferous duct.

**galactogen** (gă-lak′to-jen) [ galacto- + G. suffix *-gen,* producing ]. A polysaccharide containing galactose in various forms.

**galac′toki′nase.** An enzyme (a phosphotransferase, EC 2.7.1.6) that, in the presence of ATP, catalyzes the phosphorylation of galactose to galactose 1-phosphate.

**galac′tolip′id.** Cerebroside.

**galac′tolip′in.** Cerebroside.

**galactometastasis** (gă-lak′to-mē-tas′tă-sis). Galactoplania; the supposed metastasis of milk, or its secretion elsewhere than by the mammary glands.

**galactometer** (gal′ak-tom′e-ter) [ galacto- + G. *metron,* measure ]. Lactometer; a form of hydrometer for determining the specific gravity of milk as an indication of its fat content.

**galactopathy** (gal′ak-top′ă-thī). Galactotherapy.

**galactophagous** (gal′ak-tof′ă-gus) [ galacto- + G. *phagein,* to eat ]. Subsisting on milk.

**galactophagy** (gal′ak-tof′ă-jī) [ galacto- + G. *phagein,* to eat ]. Milk diet.

**galactophore** (gă-lak′to-fōr) [ galacto- + G. *phoros,* bearing ]. A milk duct; see *ductus* lactiferi.

**galactophoritis** (gă-lak′to-fo-ri′tis). Inflammation of the milk ducts.

**galactophorous** (gal-ak-tof'o-rus). Conveying milk.

**galactophthisis** (gal'ak-tof'thĭ-sis) [ galact- + G. + *phthisis*, a wasting ]. A loss of flesh and strength assumed to be caused by unduly prolonged lactation.

**galactophygous** (gal'ak-tof'ĭ-gus) [ galacto- + G. *phygē*, flight, banishment ]. Lactifuge (1).

**galac'topla'nia** [ galacto- + G. *planē*, wandering ]. Galactometastasis.

**galactopoiesis** (gă-lak'to-poy-e'sis) [ galacto- + G. *poiesis*, forming ]. Milk production.

**galactopoietic** (gă-lak'to-poy-et'ik). Pertaining to galactopoiesis.

**galac'topy'ranose.** D-Galactose in pyranose form. See structures under sugars.

**galactorrhea** (gă-lak'to-re'ah) [ galacto- + G. *rhoia*, a flow ]. A continued discharge of milk from the breasts in the intervals of nursing or after the child has been weaned.

**galac'tosam'ine.** Chondrosamine; the 2-amino 2-deoxy derivative of galactose, $NH_2$ replacing the 2-OH group; it occurs in various mucopolysaccharides, notably of chondroitin sulfuric acid and of B blood group substance.

**galac'tosans.** Polysaccharides of galactose; polygalactose; *e.g.,* agar.

**galactoschesia, galactoschesis** (gă-lak'to-ske'zĭ-ah, gal'-ak-tos'ke-sis) [ galacto- + G. *schesis*, a checking ]. Galactischia; galactostasia; a checking of the secretion of milk.

**galac'toscope** [ galacto- + G. *skopeō*, to examine ]. Lactoscope; an instrument for judging of the richness and purity of milk by the translucency of a thin layer.

**galac'tose.** A hexose found (in D form) as a constituent of lactose, cerebrosides, mucoproteins, etc., in galactoside or galactosyl combination. For structure, see sugars.

**galactosemia** (gă-lak'to-se'mĭ-ah) [ galactose + G. *haima*, blood ]. An inborn error of galactose metabolism due to congenital deficiency of the enzyme galactosyl-1-phosphate uridylyltransferase, resulting in tissue accumulation of galactose 1-phosphate; patients exhibit nutritional failure, hepatosplenomegaly with cirrhosis, cataracts, mental retardation, galactosuria, aminoaciduria, and albuminuria; manifestations regress or disappear if galactose is removed from the diet; autosomal recessive inheritance.

**galactose-1-phosphate uridylyltransferase.** Enzyme (EC 2.7.7.10) catalyzing the reaction of UTP and α-D-galactose 1-phosphate to form UDPgalactose.

**α-galactosidase** (EC 3.2.1.22). Melibiase; an enzyme (a hydrolase) catalyzing the hydrolysis of α-D-galactosides to D-galactose.

**β-galactosidase** (EC 3.2.1.23). Lactase; a sugar-splitting enzyme that catalyzes the hydrolysis of milk sugar, or lactose, into glucose and galactose, and that of other β-D-galactosides; it also catalyzes galactotransferase reactions; a decreased concentration or an absence of this enzyme is believed to be the basis for $G_{M1}$ gangliosidosis.

**galac'tosides.** Glycosides of galactose.

**galactosis** (gal'ak-to'sis) [ galacto- + G. suffix -*osis*, condition ]. The formation of milk by the lacteal glands.

**galactostasia, galactostasis** (gă-lak'to-sta'sĭ-ah, gal'-ak-tos'tă-sis) [ galacto- + G. *stasis*, a standing ]. Galactoschesia.

**galac'tosu'ria** [ galactose + G. *ouron*, urine ]. The excretion of galactose in the urine.

**galac'tosyl.** The glycosyl radical of galactose.

**galac'tosylglu'cose.** Lactose.

**galac'tother'apy.** 1. Treatment of disease by means of an exclusive or nearly exclusive milk diet; milk cure. 2. Medicinal treatment of a nursing infant by giving to the mother a drug that is excreted in part by the milk.

**galac'totox'icon.** A toxic substance of unknown composition found in poisonous milk.

**galac'totox'in.** A poison in stale milk, probably different from galactotoxicon.

**galac'towal'denase.** UDPglucose epimerase.

**galactozymase** (gă-lak'to-zi'mās). A starch-hydrolyzing enzyme (amylase) in milk.

**galacturia** (gal'ak-tu'rĭ-ah) [ galacto- + G. *ouron*, urine ]. The passage of turbid, milklike urine; see also chyluria.

**galac'turon'ic acid.** Pectic acid; an oxidation product of galactose, in which the 6-$CH_2OH$ group has become a —COOH group.

**galacturonose.** Galacturonic acid.

**gal'alith** [ G. *gala*, milk, + *lithos*, stone ]. Paracasein hardened by formalin; used in the manufacture of absorbable intestinal anastomosis buttons, and for other purposes.

**galan'gal** [ Mediev. L. *galanga*, mild ginger, fr. Chinese ]. Galanga; galingal; Chinese ginger; the rhizome of *Alpinia offcinarum* (family Zingiberaceae); aromatic stimulant and carminative.

**galan'thamine.** NIVALIN; $C_{17}H_{21}NO_3$; a naturally occurring anticholinesterase isolated from the Caucasian snowdrop, *Galanthus woronowii* (family Amaryllidaceae); used as an antagonist to nondepolarizing muscle relaxants.

**Galant's reflex.** See under reflex.

**Galassi's pupillary phenomenon.** See under phenomenon.

**Galbiati** (gahl-be-ah'te), Gennaro, Italian obstetrician, 1776–1844. See G.'s *operation*.

**galea** (ga'le-ah) [ L. a helmet ]. 1 [ NA ]. A structure shaped like a helmet. 2. The g. aponeurotica. 3. A form of bandage covering the head. 4. Caul (1).

  **g. aponeurot'ica** [ NA ], epicranial aponeurosis; the aponeurosis connecting the frontalis and occipitalis muscles to form the epicranius.

  **g. cap'itis**, acrosomal vesicle; a double-layered membranous covering of the nucleus in the spermatic head.

**Galeati** (gah-la-ah'te), Domenicao, Italian physician, 1686–1775. See G.'s *glands*.

**galeatomy** (ga-le-at'o-mī) [ galea + G. *tomē*, incision ]. Cutting of the galea aponeurotica.

**Galeazzi,** Riccardo, Milan surgeon, 1886–1952. See G.'s *fracture*.

**Galen,** or **Galenasi,** Claudius, Greek physician and medical scientist born at Pergamus in Asia Minor, c. 130–201 A.D. Practiced medicine in Rome; wrote voluminously, theorized, and dogmatized on many medical subjects: anatomy, physiology, pathology, symptomatology, and treatment. For nearly fifteen centuries his teachings were accepted as the infallible authority on all medical questions; to oppose them or even doubt them was looked upon almost as heresy. He supported the humoral doctrine, and G.'s theory of the movement of the blood was held until Harvey's discovery of the circulation was accepted. See also G.'s *anastomosis, bandage,* innominate *gland, nerve, vein,* and great *vein* of G.

**gale'na.** Lead sulfide.

**Galen'ic.** Relating to Galen or to his theories.

**galenicals** (ga-len'ĭ-kalz). 1. Herbs and other vegetable drugs, as distinguished from the mineral or chemical remedies. 2. Crude drugs and the tinctures, decoctions, and other preparations made from them, as distinguished from the alkaloids and other active principles. 3. Remedies prepared according to an official formula.

**galeropia, galeropsia** (gal'er-o'pī-ah, -op'sī-ah) [ G. *galeros*, cheerful, + *ōps*, eye ]. A pathological condition in which objects appear abnormally clear.

**Gall,** Franz J., German anatomist, 1758–1828. See G.'s *craniology.*

**gall** (gawl) [ A.S. *gealla* ]. 1. The bile. 2. An excoriation or erosion. 3. Nutgall.

**gal'la** [ L. ]. Nutgall.

**Gallais,** Alfred, French physician. See Cooke-Apert-G. *syndrome.*

**gal'lamine tri'ethi'odide** (USP, BP). FLAXEDIL triethiodide; [ ν-phenenyltris(oxyethylene) ]tris[ triethylammonium iodide ]; a triple quaternary ammonium compound used as a skeletal muscle relaxant for the same purposes as curare; unlike curare it has no effect on ganglionic transmission.

**Gallavardin,** Louis, French physician, *1875. See G.'s *phenomenon.*

**gallbladder** (gawl'blad-der). *Vesica fellea.*

  **sandpaper g.,** a roughened condition of the mucous membrane of the g., due to the deposit of cholesterin crystals, associated usually with the presence of gallstones.

**strawberry g.,** a g. of which the mucosa is dotted with yellowish cholesterol deposits contrasting with the red hyperemic background.

**gallein** (gal'e-in). Pyrogallolphthalein; a tetrahydroxyfluoran, structurally related to fluorescein; an indicator of the reaction of a fluid, its alcoholic solution being turned rose-red above pH 6.6, yellowish brown below pH 4.

**gal'lic acid.** 3,4,5-Trihydroxybenzoic acid; usually made from tannic acid or nutgalls. Used locally as an astringent, for the same purpose as tannic acid.

**gal'licin.** Methyl gallate; gallic-acid methyl ester; used as an astringent antiseptic in conjunctivitis and keratitis, and as an antioxidant.

**Gallie,** William E., Canadian surgeon, 1882–1959. See G.'s *transplant.*

**Galliformes** (gal'ĭ-for'mēz) [ L. *gallus,* a cock, + *forma,* form ]. An order of birds embracing the pheasant, turkey, and chicken.

**Galli-Mainini,** Carlos, Buenos Aires physician. See G.-M. *test.*

**gallinaceous** (gal'ĭ-na'shus) [ L. *gallinaceus,* fr. *gallina,* a hen ]. Pertaining to the order Galliformes.

**gallium** (gal'ĭ-um) [ L. *Gallia,* France ]. A rare metal, symbol Ga, atomic no. 31, atomic weight 69.7, melting point 30°C.

**gal'lium-67.** 67Ga; a cyclotron-produced radionuclide with a physical half-life of 78 hours and major gamma ray emmisions of 93, 184, and 296 kiloelectron volts; it is used in the citrate form as a tumor- and inflammation-localizing radiotracer.

**gallium-68.** 68Ga; a positron emitter with a physical half-life of 1.13 hour; used in brain scanning.

**gallocy'anin.** A blue oxazin dye, $C_{15}H_{13}N_2O_5Cl$, used as a stain for ribonucleic acid.

**gal'lon.** A measure of liquid capacity containing 4 quarts, 231 cubic inches, or 8.3389 pounds of distilled water; it is the equivalent of 3.7853 liters. The British imperial g. contains 277.274 cubic inches.

**gal'lop.** 1. A gait of horses; a fast, leaping gait. The weight is borne alternately by both forefeet and by both hindfeet. 2. Gallop rhythm; Traube's bruit; a triple cadence to the heart sounds at rates of 100 beats per minute or more; due to an abnormal third or fourth heart sound being heard in addition to the first and second sounds, and usually indicative of a serious disease.

**atrial g.,** presystolic g.

**presystolic g.,** atrial g.; g. rhythm in which the g. sound occurs in late diastole and is an audible fourth heart sound.

**protodiastolic g.,** g. rhythm in which the g. sound occurs in early diastole and is an abnormal third heart sound.

**summation g.,** g. rhythm in which the g. sound is due to superimposition of third and fourth heart sounds; sometimes heard in normal subjects with tachycardia, but usually indicative of myocardial disease.

**systolic g.,** a triple cadence to the heart sounds in which the extra sound occurs during systole, usually in the form of a systolic "click."

**gal'lows hu'mor.** Humorous or jesting behavior in the face of disaster or death.

**gall'sickness.** Anaplasmosis.

**mild g.,** benign bovine *theileriosis.*

**gall'stone.** Cholelith; a concretion in the gallbladder or a bile duct, composed chiefly of cholesterol crystals.

**opacifying g.'s,** g.'s becoming roentgenographically opaque after prolonged exposure to cholecystographic contrast mediums.

**silent g.'s,** g.'s that cause no symptoms and are discovered incidentally by x-ray, at operation, or post mortem.

**Gal'lus** [ L. *gallus,* a cock ]. A genus of gallinaceous birds including *G. domestica,* the domestic chicken.

**galsiekte** (gahl'sek-teh) [ D. *gal,* bile, + *siekte,* sickness, bilious fever ]. Galziekte. 1. Anaplasmosis. 2. General term applied by South African farmers to a variety of diseases including anthrax, heartwater, rinderpest, East Coast fever, etc.

**Galton,** Francis, English scientist, 1822–1911. See G.'s *delta,* system of classification of fingerprints (under *fingerprint*), *law, whistle.*

**Galvani,** Luigi, Italian physician and anatomist, 1737–1798. Gave his name to galvanism.

**galvan'ic.** Pertaining to galvanism.

**galvanism** (gal'vă-nizm) [ L. *Galvani* ]. 1. Direct current electricity produced by chemical action, as in a galvanic, or voltaic, or chemical cell. 2. Oral manifestations sometimes occurring when dental restorations of dissimilar metals, such as silver and gold, are placed in close proximity to one another.

**gal'vaniza'tion.** The application of direct current, or galvanic electricity, as in galvanizing (electroplating).

**galvano-.** Prefix meaning electrical, denoting primarily direct current (*e.g.,* galvanometer, galvanization).

**gal'vanocau'tery.** An actual cautery made by heating a wire by a galvanic current.

**gal'vanochem'ical.** Electrochemical.

**gal'vanocontractil'ity.** The capability of a muscle of contracting under the stimulus of a galvanic (direct) current.

**galvanofaradization** (gal'vă-no-făr'ad-ĭ-za'shun). The simultaneous application of a galvanic and a faradic current.

**galvanolysis** (gal'vă-nol'ĭ-sis). Electrolysis.

**gal'vanom'eter.** An instrument for measuring the strength of an electric current.

**Einthoven's string g.,** string g.

**string g.,** Einthoven's string g.; thread g.; a g. designed by Einthoven and introduced by him in 1901 for recording variations in electrical potentials generated in the heart; it is the forerunner of the modern electrocardiograph.

**thread g.,** string g.

**gal'vanomus'cular.** Denoting the effect of the application of a galvanic (direct) current to a muscle.

**gal'vanoner'vous.** Denoting the effect of the application of the constant current to a nerve trunk.

**gal'vanopalpa'tion.** Faradopalpation; esthesiometry by means of a sharp-pointed electrode through which a feeble current passes to the cathode applied to an indifferent part.

**gal'vanoscope** [ galvano- + G. *skopeō,* to view ]. An instrument for detecting the presence of a galvanic current.

**gal'vanosur'gery.** Operation with direct electric current.

**gal'vanotax'is.** Electrotaxis.

**gal'vanother'apy.** Treatment of disease by applications of the galvanic current.

**galvanotonus** (gal'vă-not'o-nus) [ galvano- + G. *tonos,* tension ]. 1. Electrotonus. 2. Tonic muscular contraction in response to a galvanic stimulus.

**galvanotropism** (gal'vă-not'ro-pizm) [ galvano- + G. *tropē,* a turning ]. Electrotaxis.

**galziekte** (gahl'zēk-teh). Galsiekte.

**gamabufagin** (gam'ă-bu'fă-jin). Gamabufotalin.

**gamabufogenin** (gam'a-bu'fo-jen-in). Gamabufotalin.

**gamabufotalin** (gam'ă-bu'fo-tal-in). Gamabufagin; gamabufogenin; a trihydroxybufadienolide (for structure, see steroids); a steroid glucoside of the class of bufagins present in the venoms of tropical toads of the family Bufonidae; chemically and in its pharmacologic action resembles digitalis.

**gambir** (gam'bĭr). Catechu; pale catechu; an extract from the leaves of *Uncaria* (*Ourouparia*) gambier (family Rubiaceae); used as an astringent. The commercial g. is known as terra japonica.

**game.** A contest, physical or mental, conducted according to set rules, played for amusement or for a stake.

**language g.,** in philosophy, all the operations and behaviors contained in and expressed by symbols, language rules, and the social customs concerning language use.

**model g.,** the use of g.'s, especially of g.'s of strategy, for the explanation of human behavior (both normal and abnormal).

**gamete** (gam'ēt) [ G. *gametēs,* husband; *gametē,* wife, GAM- ]. 1. One of two cells undergoing karyogamy or true conjugation. 2. In heredity, any germ cell, whether ovum, spermatozoon, or pollen cell.

**gameto-** [ see gamete ]. Combining form relating to a gamete.

**gametocide** (gă-me'to-sīd) [ gameto- + L. *caedo*, to kill ]. An agent that is destructive to gametes, specifically the malarial gametocytes.

**gametocyte** (gă-me'to-sīt) [ gameto- + G. *kytos*, cell ]. Gamont; a cell capable of dividing to produce gametes; a spermatocyte or oocyte.

**gametogenesis** (gam'e-to-jen'ĕ-sis) [ gameto- + G. *genesis*, production ]. The process of formation and development of gametes.

**gametogonia** (gam'e-to-go'nĭ-ah). Gametogony.

**gametogony** (gam'e-tog'o-nĭ) [ gameto- + G. *gonus*, a begetting ]. Gametogonia; a stage in the sexual cycle of *Plasmodium* species and certain other protozoa, in which male and female gametocytes are formed; in the case of malarial parasites, this stage occurs in the blood of man, and the gametocytes are infective for mosquitoes.

**gametoid** (gam'e-toyd). Pertaining to certain biologic features that resemble those characteristic of gametes or reproductive cells.

**gametokinetic** (gam'e-to-kĭ-net'ik) [ gameto- + G. *kinēsis*, movement ]. Moving toward, or causing, karyogamy or true conjugation.

**gametophagia** (gam-e-to-fa'jĭ-ah) [ gameto- + G. *phagein*, to eat ]. The disappearance of the male or female element in zygosis or true conjugation.

**Gamgee** (gam'je), Sampson, British surgeon, 1828–1886. See G. *tissue*.

**ga'mic** [ G. *gamikos*, pert. to marriage ]. Relating to or derived from sexual union; usually used as a suffix.

**gamma** (gam'ah) [ G. ]. The third letter of the Greek alphabet, γ. Used as a symbol for: (1) the third in a series (*e.g.*, γ-globulin); (2) the fourth carbon atom in an aliphatic acid; (3) the position two removed from the alpha-position in the benzene ring; (4) microgram (obsolete); (5) $10^{-4}$ gauss. For chemical compounds having this prefix, see the specific names.

**gamma-benzene hexachloride** (USP, BP). Lindane.

**gam'magram.** Photoscan.

**gammopathy** (gă-mop'ă-thĭ). A primary disturbance in immunoglobulin (γ-globulin) synthesis.

**Gamna,** Carlos, Italian physician, *1896. See G.-Favre *bodies*, Gandy-G. *bodies*, G.-Gandy *bodies*, *nodules*, G.'s *disease*.

**gam'ogen'esis** [ G. *gamos*, marriage, + *genesis*, production ]. Sexual reproduction.

**gam'one.** Chemotactic sexual hormone; a chemical substance (ectohormone) secreted by plus gametes of certain algae whereby they attract minus gametes to effect fertilization.

**gam'ont** [ G. *gamos*, marriage, + *ōn* (*ont*-), being ]. Gametocyte.

**gamophagia** (gam-o-fa'jĭ-ah). Gametophagia.

**gamophobia** (gam'o-fo'bĭ-ah) [ G. *gamos*, marriage, + *phobos*, fear ]. Fear of marriage.

**gampsodactyly, gampsodactylia** (gamp'so-dak'tĭ-lĭ, -dak-til'ĭ-ah) [ G. *gampsos*, curved, crooked, + *daktylos*, finger, toe ]. Rarely used term for clawfoot.

**Gandy,** Charles, French physician, *1872. See Gamna-G. *bodies*, *nodules*, G.-Gamna *bodies*, G.-Nanta *disease*.

**ganga** (gang'gah). An extract of the flowers of *Cannabis sativa* (Indian hemp or hasheesh) which grows in India, Persia, and Arabia. See also cannabis.

**ganglia** (gang'glĭ-ah). Plural of ganglion.

**ganglial** (gang'glĭ-al). Ganglionic; relating to a ganglion.

**gangliate, gangliated** (gang'glĭ-āt, gang'glĭ-a-ted). Ganglionated; having ganglia.

**gangliec'tomy.** Ganglionectomy.

**gangliform** (gang'glĭ-form). Ganglioform; having the form or appearance of a ganglion.

**gangliitis** (gang-glĭ-i'tis). Ganglionitis.

**ganglioblast** (gang'glĭ-o-blast) [ ganglion + G. *blastos*, germ ]. An embryonic cell giving rise to ganglion cells.

**gangliocyte** (gang'glĭ-o-sit). Ganglion *cell*.

**gangliocytoma** (gang'glĭ-o-si-to'mah). Ganglioneuroma.

**gan'glioform.** Gangliform.

**ganglioglioma** (gang'glĭ-o-glī-o'mah). Central *ganglioneuroma*.

**ganglioma** (gang'lĭ-o'mah). Ganglioneuroma.

# GANGLION

**ganglion,** pl. **ganglia, ganglions** (gang'glĭ-on) [ G. a swelling or knot ]. 1 [ NA ]. Neural g.; nerve g.; neuroganglion; originally (but now obsolete), any group of nerve cell bodies, whether in the central or peripheral nervous system; currently, an aggregation of nerve cell bodies located in the peripheral nervous system. 2. A cyst containing mucopolysaccharide-rich fluid within fibrous tissue or, occasionally, muscle or a semilunar cartilage; usually attached to a tendon sheath in the hand or foot.

**aberrant g.,** a collection of nerve cells sometimes found on a posterior spinal nerve root between the spinal g. and the spinal cord.

**acousticofacial g.,** a primordial ganglionic cell mass in young embryos which later separates into the acoustic or spiral g. of the 8th nerve and the geniculate g. of the 7th (facial) nerve.

**Acrel's g.,** (1) pseudoganglion on the posterior interosseous nerve on the dorsal aspect of the wrist joint; (2) a cyst on a tendon of an extensor muscle at the level of the wrist.

**Andersch's g.,** g. inferius nervi glossopharyngei.

**aorticorenal ganglia,** ganglia aorticorenalia.

**ganglia aorticorena'lia** [ NA ], aorticorenal ganglia; a semidetached portion of the celiac or semilunar ganglia, at the origin of each renal artery; contains the sympathetic neurons innervating the vasculature of the kidney.

**Arnold's g.,** (1) g. oticum; (2) a neural g. in the intercarotid sympathetic plexus surrounding the internal carotid artery.

**auditory g.,** g. spirale cochleae.

**Auerbach's ganglia,** collections of parasympathetic nerve cells in the myenteric plexus; see *plexus* myentericus.

**auricular g.,** g. oticum.

**autonomic ganglia,** visceral ganglia; see *systema* nervosum autonomicum.

**ganglia of autonomic plexus,** ganglia plexuum autonomicorum.

**basal ganglia,** originally, all of the large masses of gray matter at the base of the cerebral hemisphere; currently, the corpus striatum (caudate and lentiform nuclei) and cell groups associated with the corpus striatum, such as the subthalamic nucleus and substantia nigra.

**Bezold's g.,** an aggregation of nerve cells in the interatrial septum.

**Bochdalek's g.,** a g. of the plexus of the dental nerve lying in the maxilla just above the root of the canine tooth.

**Bock's g.,** carotid g.

**Böttcher's g.,** g. on the cochlear nerve in the internal acoustic meatus.

**cardiac ganglia,** ganglia cardiaca.

**ganglia cardi'aca** [ NA ], cardiac ganglia; Wrisberg's ganglia; parasympathetic ganglia of the cardiac plexus lying between the arch of the aorta and the bifurcation of the pulmonary artery.

**carotid g.,** Laumonier's g.; Bock's g.; a small ganglionic swelling on filaments from the internal carotid plexus, lying on the under surface of the carotid artery in the cavernous sinus.

**celiac ganglia,** ganglia celiaca.

**ganglia celia'ca** [ NA ], celiac ganglia; solar ganglia; Willis' centrum nervosum; the largest and highest group of sympathetic prevertebral ganglia, located on the upper part of the abdominal aorta, composed of the paired semilunar, aorticorenal, and superior mesenteric ganglia, and containing the sympathetic neurons whose unmyelinated postganglionic axons innervate the stomach, liver, gallbladder, spleen, kidney, small intestine, and ascending and transverse colon.

**g. cervica'le me'dium** [ NA ], middle cervical g.; a sympathetic g., of small size and sometimes absent; located at the level of the cricoid cartilage.

**g. cervica'le supe'rius** [ NA ], superior cervical g.; the uppermost and largest of the ganglia of the sympathetic trunk, lying near the base of the skull between the internal carotid artery and the internal jugular vein.

**cervicothoracic g.,** g. cervicothoracicum.

**g. cer'vicothora'cicum** [ NA ], g. stellatum [ NA ]; cervicothoracic g.; stellate g.; inferior cervical g.; a sympathetic trunk g. lying behind the subclavian artery near the origin of the vertebral artery, at the level of the seventh cervical vertebra, close to the first thoracic g. with which it is sometimes fused.

**g. cilia're** [ NA ], ciliary g.; lenticular g.; Schacher's g.; a small parasympathetic g. lying in the orbit behind the eye, between the optic nerve and the lateral rectus muscle. It receives its preganglionic innervation from the nucleus of Edinger-Westphal in the midbrain by way of the oculomotor nerve, and in turn gives rise to postganglionic fibers that innervate the ciliary muscle and the sphincter (narrowing) muscle of the pupil.

**ciliary g.,** g. ciliare.

**Cloquet's g.,** a g. described as attached to the nasopalatine nerve; of questionable existence.

**coccygeal g.,** g. impar.

**Corti's g.,** g. spirale cochleae.

**diffuse g.,** a cystic swelling due to inflammatory effusion into one or several adjacent tendon sheaths.

**dorsal root g.,** g. spinale.

**Ehrenritter's g.,** g. superius nervi glossopharyngei.

**g. extracrania'le,** g. inferius nervi glossopharyngei.

**g. of facial nerve,** g. geniculi.

**Frankenhäuser's g.,** *plexus* uterovaginalis.

**Froriep's g.,** a temporary collection of nerve cells on the dorsal aspect of the hypoglossal nerve in the embryo; it represents a rudimentary sensory g.

**Gasserian g.,** g. trigeminale.

**geniculate g.,** g. geniculi.

**g. genic'uli** [ NA ], geniculate g.; intumescentia ganglioformis; g. of the facial nerve, more specifically, of the intermediate nerve; a g. containing the sensory neurons innervating the taste buds on the anterior two-thirds of the tongue.

**Gudden's g.,** *nucleus* interpeduncularis.

**g. haben'ulae,** *nucleus* habenulae.

**Huber's g.,** a g. sometimes found on the 1st cervical nerve.

**hypogastric ganglia,** ganglia pelvina.

**g. im'par** [ NA ], coccygeal g.; Walther's g,; the most inferior, unpaired g. of the sympathetic trunk.

**inferior cervical g.,** g. cervicothoracicum.

**inferior g. of glossopharyngeal nerve,** g. inferius nervi glossopharyngei.

**inferior mesenteric g.,** g. mesentericum inferius.

**inferior g. of vagus,** g. inferius nervi vagi.

**g. infe'rius ner'vi glossopharyn'gei** [ NA ], inferior g. of the glossopharyngeal nerve; petrosal or petrous g.; g. extracraniale; Andersch's g.; the lower of two sensory g.'s on the glossopharyngeal nerve as it traverses the jugular foramen.

**g. inferius nervi vagi** [ NA ], inferior g. of the vagus; nodose g.; g. of the trunk of the vagus; a large sensory g. of the vagus, at the level of the transverse processes of the first and second cervical vertebrae.

**intercrural g.,** *nucleus* interpeduncularis.

**ganglia interme'dia** [ NA ], intermediate ganglia; small sympathetic ganglia most commonly found on the rami communicantes in the cervical and lumbar region.

**intermediate ganglia,** ganglia intermedia.

**g. of intermediate nerve,** g. geniculi.

**interpeduncular g.,** *nucleus* interpeduncularis.

**intervertebral g.,** g. spinale.

**intracranial g.,** g. superius nervi glossopharyngei.

**g. isth'mi,** *nucleus* interpeduncularis.

**jugular ganglia,** see g. superius nervi glossopharyngei and g. superius nervi vagi.

**Laumonier's g.,** carotid g.

**Lee's g.,** *plexus* uterovaginalis.

**lenticular g.,** g. ciliare.

**Lobstein's g.,** an inconstant enlargement on the greater splanchnic nerve a little above the diaphragm.

**Ludwig's g.,** a small collection of parasympathetic nerve cells in the interatrial septum.

**ganglia lumba'lia trun'ci sympath'ici** [ NA ], lumbar ganglia; four or more ganglia on the medial border of the psoas major muscle on either side; they form, with the sacral and coccygeal ganglia and their connecting cords, the abdominopelvic sympathetic trunk.

**lumbar ganglia,** ganglia lumbalia trunci sympathici.

**Meckel's g.,** g. pterygopalatinum.

**g. mesenter' icum infe'rius** [ NA ], inferior mesenteric g.; the lowest of the sympathetic prevertebral ganglia, located at the origin of the inferior mesenteric artery from the aorta and containing the sympathetic neurons innervating the descending and sigmoid colon.

**g. mesenter'icum supe'rius** [ NA ], superior mesenteric g.; a paired sympathetic g. located at the origin of the superior mesenteric artery from the aotra, forming part of the g. celiacum of the celiac plexus.

**middle cervical g.,** g. cervicale medium.

**nasal g.,** g. pterygopalatinum.

**nerve g.,** g. (1).

**neural g.,** ganglion (1).

**nodose g.,** g. inferius nervi vagi. vagi).

**otic g.,** g. oticum.

**g. o'ticum** [ NA ], otic g.; auricular g.; Arnold's g. (1); otoganglion; an autonomic g. situated just below the foramen ovale medial to the mandibular nerve.

**parasympathetic ganglia,** those ganglia of the autonomic nervous system that are composed of cholinergic neurons receiving afferent fibers originating from preganglionic visceral motor neurons in either the brainstem or the middle sacral segments (S2 to S4) of the spinal cord. On the basis of their location with respect to the organs they innervate, parasympathetic ganglia can be categorized as juxtamural ganglia and intramural ganglia; see also *systema* nervosum autonomicum.

**paravertebral ganglia,** the ganglia of the sympathetic trunk, strung out segmentally along the side of the vertebral column.

**pelvic ganglia,** 12 ganglia pelvina.

**ganglia pelvi'na** [ NA ], pelvic ganglia; hypogastric ganglia; the parasympathetic ganglia scattered through the pelvic plexus on either side.

**periosteal g.,** serous abscess; albuminous periostitis; a flattened subperiosteal cavity containing clear, yellow, viscid synovia-like fluid.

**petrosal g., petrous g.,** g. inferius nervi glossopharyngei.

**phrenic ganglia,** ganglia phrenica.

**ganglia phren'ica** [ NA ], phrenic ganglia; several small sensory ganglia contained in the phrenic plexuses.

**ganglia plex'uum autonomico'rum** [ NA ], ganglia of the autonomic plexuses; autonomic ganglia lying in plexuses of autonomic fibers, *e.g.*, the celiac and inferior mesenteric ganglia of the sympathetic, and the small parasympathetic ganglia of the myenteric plexus.

**prevertebral ganglia,** the sympathetic ganglia (semilunar, aorticorenal, superior and inferior mesenteric) lying in front of the vertebral column, as distinguished from the paravertebral ganglia of the sympathetic trunk strung out along each side of the vertebral column.

**pterygopalatine g.,** g. pterygopalatinum.

**g. pterygopalati'num** [ NA ], pterygopalatine g.; sphenopalatine g.; nasal g.; Meckel's g.; a small g. in the upper part of the pterygopalatine fossa.

**Remak's ganglia,** (1) groups of nerve cells in the wall of the venous sinus where it joins the right atrium of the heart; (2) autonomic ganglia in nerves of the stomach.

**renal ganglia** ganglia renalia.

**ganglia rena'lia** [ NA ], renal ganglia; small scattered ganglia along the renal plexus.

**Ribes' g.,** the uppermost sympathetic g., situated on the anterior communicating artery of the brain.

**sacral ganglia,** ganglia sacralia trunci sympathici.

**ganglia sacra'lia trun'ci sympath'ici** [ NA ], sacral ganglia; three or four ganglia on either side constituting, with the g. impar and the connecting cords, the pelvic portion of the sympathetic trunk.

**Scarpa's g.,** g. vestibulare.

**Schacher's g.,** g. ciliare.

**semilunar g.,** g. trigeminale.

**sensory g.,** a cluster of primary sensory neurons forming a usually visible swelling in the course of a peripheral nerve or its dorsal root; such nerve cells establish the sole afferent neural connection between the sensory periphery (skin, mucous membranes of the oral and nasal cavities, muscle tissue, tendons, joint capsules, special sense organs, blood vessel walls, tissues of the internal organs) and the central nervous system; they are the cells of origin of all sensory fibers of the peripheral nervous system. Examples of sensory ganglia are the dorsal root ganglia of the segmental spinal nerves, the large semilunar ganglion of the trigeminal nerve, and the ganglion spirale of the cochlear nerve.

**Soemmering's g.,** *substantia* nigra.

**solar ganglia,** ganglia celiaca.

**sphenopalatine g.,** g. pterygopalatinum.

**spinal g.,** g. spinale.

**g. spina′le** [ NA ], spinal g.; dorsal root g.; intervertebral g.; the g. of the posterior root of each spinal segmental nerve, containing the cell bodies of the pseudounipolar primary sensory neurons whose peripheral axon branch becomes part of the mixed segmental nerve, while the central axon branch enters the spinal cord as a component of the sensory posterior root.

**spiral g. of cochlea,** g. spirale cochleae.

**g. spira′le coch′leae** [ NA ], spiral g. of the cochlea; Corti's g.; auditory g.; an elongated g. of bipolar sensory nerve cell bodies on the cochlear branch of the auditory nerve in the spiral canal of the modiolus; each g. cell issues a peripheral axon that passes between the layers of the lamina spiralis ossea to the organ of Corti, and a central axon that enters the hindbrain as a component of the auditory nerve.

**splanchnic g.,** g. splanchnicum.

**g. splanch′nicum** [ NA ], splanchnic g.; a g. not infrequently present in the course of the greater splanchnic nerve.

**stellate g.,** g. cervicothoracicum.

**g. stella′tum** [ NA ], an official alternate term for g. cervicothoracicum.

**sublingual g.,** g. sublinguale.

**g. sublingua′le,** sublingual g.; a small parasympathetic g. just anterior to the submandibular g.; it innervates the sublingual gland.

**submandibular g.,** g. submandibulare.

**g. submandibula′re** [ NA ], submandibular g.; submaxillary g.; a small parasympathetic g. suspended from the lingual nerve; its postganglionic branches go to the submandibular gland and the submandibular duct; its preganglionic fibers come from the nucleus salivatorius by way of the chorda tympani.

**submaxillary g.,** g. submandibulare.

**superior cervical g.,** g. cervicale superius.

**superior g. of glossopharyngeal nerve,** g. superius nervi glossopharyngei.

**superior mesenteric g.,** g. mesentericum superius.

**g. supe′rius ner′vi glossopharyn′gei** [ NA ], superior g. of the glossopharyngeal nerve; Ehrenritter's g.; intracranial g.; the upper and smaller of two ganglia on the glossopharyngeal nerve as it traverses the jugular foramen.

**g. supe′rius ner′vi va′gi** [ NA ], superior g. of the vagus nerve; a small sensory g. on the vagus as it traverses the jugular foramen.

**sympathetic ganglia,** those ganglia of the autonomic nervous system that are composed of adrenergic neurons receiving afferent fibers originating from preganglionic visceral motor neurons in the lateral horn of the thoracic and upper lumbar segments of the spinal cord (Th 1–L 2). On the basis of their location, the sympathetic ganglia can be classified as paravertebral ganglia (ganglia trunci sympathici) and prevertebral ganglia (ganglia celiaca). See also *systema* nervosum autonomicum.

**ganglia of sympathetic trunk,** ganglia trunci sympathici.

**terminal g.,** g. terminale.

**g. termina′le** [ NA ], terminal ganglion; (1) the scattered postganglionic autonomic neurons located in or close to the wall of the organ innervated; they are usually parasympathetic; (2) cells located along the nervi terminales.

**thoracic ganglia,** ganglia thoracica trunci sympathici.

**ganglia thorac′ica trun′ci sympath′ici** [ NA ], thoracic ganglia 11 or 12 ganglia; on either side, at the level of the head of each rib, constituting with the connecting nerve cords the thoracic portion of the sympathetic trunk.

**trigeminal g.,** g. trigeminale.

**g. trigemina′le** [ NA ], trigeminal g.; semilunar g.; Gasserian g.; the large flattened sensory g. of the trigeminal

nerve lying in close relation to the cavernous sinus along the medial part of the middle cranial fossa.

**Troisier's g.,** historic term for a supraclavicular lymph node that is palpably enlarged as the result of a metastasis from a malignant neoplasm; the presence of such a node indicates that the probable site of primary involvement is in a thoracic or abdominal organ or tissue. See also signal *node.*

**ganglia trun′ci sympath′ici** [ NA ], ganglia of the sympathetic trunk; the clusters of postganglionic nerve cell bodies located at intervals along the sympathetic trunks, including the superior cervical g., middle cervical g., cervicothoracic (stellate) g., thoracic ganglia, lumbar ganglia, sacral ganglia, and the g. impar.

**g. of trunk of vagus,** g. inferius nervi vagi.

**tympanic g.,** g. tympanicum.

**g. tympan′icum** [ NA ], tympanic g.; a small g. on the tympanic nerve during its passage through the petrous portion of the temporal bone.

**Valentin's g.,** a g. on the superior alveolar nerve.

**vertebral g.,** g. vertebrale.

**g. vertebra′le** [ NA ], vertebral g.; a small g. located along the sympathetic trunk between the middle cervical g. and the cervicothoracic g.; its occurrence is inconstant.

**vestibular g.,** g. vestibulare.

**g. vestibula′re** [ NA ], vestibular g., Scarpa's g.; a collection of bipolar nerve cell bodies forming a swelling on the vestibular nerve in the internal auditory meatus. It is subdivided into a pars superior and a pars inferior, associated with the utriculoampullar and saccular branches.

**Vieussens' g.,** *plexus* celiacus.

**Walther's g.,** g. impar.

**Wrisberg's ganglia,** ganglia cardiaca.

**wrist g.,** cystic protrusion of a part of a tendon sheath or joint capsule on dorsum of wrist.

---

**gan′gliona′ted.** Gangliate.

**ganglionectomy** (gang′lĭ-o-nek′to-mĭ) [ ganglion + G. *ektomē,* excision ]. Gangliectomy; excision of a ganglion.

**ganglioneuroma** (gang-glĭ-o-nu-ro′mah). Gangliocytoma; ganglioma; neuroma verum; neurocytoma; a benign neoplasm composed of mature ganglionic neurons, in varying numbers, scattered singly or in clumps within a relatively abundant and dense stroma of neurofibrils and collagenous fibers. G.'s are firm and encapsulated, and frequently contain foci of calcification; most of them are found in young persons less than 20 years old, usually in the posterior mediastinum and retroperitoneum, sometimes in relation to the adrenal glands.

**central g.,** ganglioglioma; a rare form of glioma composed of nearly mature, slowly growing neuron-like cells; found in the optic chasm or cerebral white matter.

**dumbbell g.,** one in which the gross configuration resembles a dumbbell, *e.g.,* two spheroidal masses connected by a narrow portion, usually the result of the neoplasm being somewhat molded by a resistant structure such as two ribs.

**ganglioneuromatosis** (gang′glĭ-o-nu′ro-mă-to′sis). State of having many widespread ganglioneuromas.

**ganglionic** (gang-glĭ-on′ik). Relating to a ganglion in any sense.

**ganglionitis** (gang′glĭ-o-ni′tis). Gangliitis. 1. Inflammation of a lymphatic ganglion. 2. Inflammation of a nerve ganglion.

**ganglionostomy** (gang′glĭ-o-nos′to-mĭ) [ ganglion + G. *stoma,* mouth ]. Making an opening into a ganglion (2).

**ganglioplegic** (gang′glĭ-o-ple′jik) [ ganglion + G. *plēgē,* stroke, shock ]. A pharmacologic compound that paralyzes an autonomic ganglion, usually for a relatively short period of time.

**ganglioside** (gang′glĭ-o-sĭd). A glycosphingolipid chemically similar to cerebrosides but containing additional carbohydrate moieties, N-acetylglucosamine and N-acetylneuraminic acid (a sialic acid) (in some species, N-glycolylneuraminic acid). Found principally in nerve tissue and spleen.

**gangliosidosis** (gang′glĭ-o-si′do′sis). Ganglioside lipidosis; any disease characterized, in part, by the abnormal accumulation within the nervous system of specific gangliosides. Such gangliosides normally are present only in trace quantities.

$G_{M1}$ g., generalized g.; characterized by accumulation of a specific monosialoganglioside, designated $G_{M1}$. Resembles Tay-Sachs disease, except that visceral mucopolysaccharidosis is also present.

$G_{M2}$ g., Tay-Sachs disease; see cerebral *sphingolipidosis*.

generalized g., $G_{M1}$ g.

**gango'sa** [ Sp. *gangoso*, snuffling; fem. to agree with *emfermedad*, disease ]. Rhinopharyngitis mutilans; now generally regarded as a sequel to yaws; a destructive ulceration beginning on the soft palate and extending thence to the hard palate, nasopharynx, and nose, resulting in mutilating cicatrices. The disease, so far as is known, occurs only in certain portions of the tropics, especially the islands of the Pacific.

**gangrene** (gang'grēn) [ G. *gangraina*, an eating sore, fr. *grao*, to gnaw ]. Necrosis due to obstruction of blood supply; may be localized to a small area or involve the entire extremity or, rarely, bilateral; may be wet or dry.

angiosclerot'ic g., dry g. resulting from sclerotic changes in the arteries, with subsequent occlusion, as in the aged due to arteriosclerosis.

cold g., dry g.

cutaneous g., g. of the skin characterized by sloughing; may occur in shingles or in any acute infection that interferes with superficial circulation.

decu'bital g., decubitus *ulcer*.

diabet'ic g., g. resulting from vascular pathology associated with diabetes.

dissem'inated cuta'neous g., *dermatitis* gangrenosa infantum.

dry g., cold g.; mummification necrosis; a form of g. in which the involved part is dry and shriveled.

embol'ic g., g. resulting from the plugging of an artery by an embolus.

emphysem'atous g., gas g.

gas g., emphysematous g.; progressive emphysematous necrosis; g. occurring in a wound infected with various anaerobic, spore-forming bacteria (*Clostridium*), especially *C. welchii* (*C. perfringens*) and *C. oedematiens*. There is crepitation of the surrounding tissues due to gas liberated by bacterial fementation and constitutional septic symptoms. See also gas *phlegmon*.

hemorrhagic g., g. occurring rarely in meningococcal septicemia.

hospital g., decubitus *ulcer*.

hot g., g. following inflammation of the part.

Meleney's synergistic g., g. of the skin and subcutaneous tissues, usually following an operation, caused by an interaction between microaerophilic nonhemolytic streptococci and aerobic hemolytic staphylococci; produces extensive tissue necrosis, with undermining ulcers.

moist g., a form in which the necrosed part is moist and soft.

neurotic g., g. developing on a neurotically induced excoriation of the skin.

nosoco'mial g., decubitus *ulcer*.

Pott's g., senile g.

prese'nile spontaneous g., g. occurring in middle life as a result of thromboangiitis obliterans.

pressure g., decubitus *ulcer*.

progressive bacterial synergistic g., superficial death of tissue due to bacterial infection.

senile g., Pott's g.; dry g. occurring in the aged in consequence of occlusion of an artery; it affects especially the extremities.

spontaneous g. of the newborn, g. due to vascular occlusion of unknown cause, usually in marasmic or dehydrated infants.

static g., venous g.; moist g. due to obstruction in the return circulation.

symmet'rical g., g. affecting the two sides of the body; it is seen particularly in severe arteriosclerosis, myocardial infarction, and ball valve thrombus.

thrombot'ic g., g. due to occlusion of an artery by a thrombus.

trophic g., g. due to disorder of the trophic nerves of the part.

venous g., static g.

wet g., ischemic necrosis of an extremity with bacterial infection; it produces cellulitis adjacent to the necrotic areas.

white g., leukonecrosis; death of a part accompanied by the formation of grayish white sloughs.

**gan'grenous.** Relating to or affected with gangrene; mortified.

**gan'oblast.** Adamantoblast.

**Ganong,** W. F. See Lown-G.-Levine *syndrome*.

**Ganser,** Sigbert J. M., German psychiatrist, 1853–1931. See G.'s *commissures, nucleus* basalis of G., G.'s *syndrome*.

**Gant,** Samuel G., U. S. surgeon, 1870–1944. See G. *clamp*.

**Gantzner's muscle** or **accessory bundle.** See under muscle.

**gap.** 1. A hiatus or opening in a structure. An interval or discontinuity in any series or sequence.

air-bone g., the difference between the threshold for hearing acuity by bone conduction and by air conduction.

auscultatory g., silent g.; a silent interval sometimes perceived during the determination of the blood pressure, at a point some millimeters below the systolic pressure; failure to raise the pressure high enough may give a false idea of the systolic pressure if this phenomenon is present.

Bochdalek's g., a variable, triangular opening in the diaphragm on either side above the arcus lumbocostalis.

interocclusal g., interocclusal distance.

silent g., auscultatory g.

**gapes** (gāps). A disease of young chickens, turkeys and other birds caused by the gapeworm, *Syngamus trachea*, which localizes in the trachea and causes gasping and choking.

**gape'worm.** *Syngamus trachea.*

**Garbe,** William. See Sulzberger-G. *disease, syndrome.*

**Garden,** Alexander, British physician and naturalist, 1728–1791. Gave his name to *Gardenia.*

**Garde'nia** [ A. *Garden* ]. A genus of shrubs of the family Rubicaceae. The fruits of *G. florida*, *G. grandiflora*, and *G. radicans* are demulcent and refrigerant, and also furnish a yellow dye, gardenin.

**Gardner,** Eldon J., U. S. geneticist, *1909. See G. 's *syndrome.*

**Garel,** Jean, French physician, 1852–1931. See G.'s *sign.*

**garget** (gahr'jet). Bovine *mastitis.*

**gar'gle** [ thru Old Fr. fr. L. *gurgulio*, gullet, windpipe ]. 1. To rinse the fauces by taking fluid in the mouth and forcing the expired breath through it while the head is held far back. 2. A medicated fluid used for gargling; a throat wash.

**gargoylism** (gar'goyl-izm) [ gargoyle, fr. L. *gurgulio*, gullet ]. The gargoyle-like facies and related characteristics of Hurler's syndrome and Hunter's syndrome; see both.

autosomal recessive g., Hurler's *syndrome*.

X-linked recessive g., Hunter's *syndrome*.

**Gariel** (gă-re-el'), Maurice, Paris physician, 1812–1878. See G.'s *pessary.*

**Garland,** Hugh. See Marinesco-G. *syndrome.*

**gar'lic.** Allium.

g. oil, a volatile oil from the bulb or entire plant of *Allium sativum* (family Liliaceae); contains diallyl disulfide and allyl propyl disulfide; has been used as an anthelmintic and rubefacient.

**Garré,** Carl, Swiss surgeon, 1857–1928. See G.'s *disease.*

**garrulity** (gă-ru'lĭtĭ) [ L. *garrulitas*, fr. *garrio*, to chatter ]. Loquacity; talkativeness.

**Gärtner** (gairt'ner), August, German physician, 1848–1934. See G.'s *bacillus, method,* vein *phenomenon, tonometer.*

**Gartner,** Herman T., Danish anatomist, 1785–1827. See G.'s *canal, cyst, duct.*

**gas** [ a word coined by Van Helmont, a Belgian chemist of the seventeenth century ]. 1. A thin fluid, like air, capable of indefinite expansion, but convertible by compression and cold into a liquid and, eventually, solid. 2. To subject to the action of a g.

alveolar g., alveolar air; symbol subscript A; the g. in the pulmonary alveoli, where $O_2$-$CO_2$ exchange with pulmonary capillary blood occurs.

**anesthetic g.,** a compound above its boiling point at room temperature capable of producing general anesthesia upon inhalation.

**asphyx′iating g.,** carbon monoxide.

**carbonic acid g.,** carbon dioxide.

**Clayton g.,** a g. chiefly sulfurous acid with some sulfuric acid, used to kill the vermin in the hold of a ship.

**expired g.,** (1) any g. that has been expired from the lungs; (2) often used synonymously with mixed expired g.

**hemolyt′ic g.,** a poisonous g. (arsine), inhalation of which causes hemolysis with hemoglobinuria, jaundice, gastroenteritis, and nephritis.

**ideal alveolar g.,** the uniform composition of g. that would exist in all alveoli for a given total respiratory exchange if all alveoli had identical ventilation-perfusion ratios and achieved perfect equilibrium with the blood leaving the pulmonary capillaries.

**inert g.,** noble g.

**inspired g.,** symbol subscript $I$; (1) any g. that is being inhaled; (2) specifically, that g. after it has been humidified at body temperature.

**laughing g.** [ so called because its inhalation sometimes excites a hilarious delirium preceding insensibility ], nitrous oxide.

**marsh g.,** methane.

**mephitic g.,** carbon dioxide.

**mixed expired g.,** one or more complete breaths of expired g. coming thoroughly mixed from the dead space and the alveoli.

**mustard g.,** see under mustard.

**noble g.'s,** rare g.'s; zero group in the periodic series: helium, neon, argon, krypton, xenon, and radon.

**olef′iant g.,** ethylene.

**premixed g.,** g. in a cylinder containing 50 or 60 per cent nitrous oxide with oxygen.

**sneezing g.,** sternutator; see diphenylchlorarsine.

**suffocating g.,** a g. that causes intense irritation of the bronchial tubes and lungs, resulting in pulmonary edema; among g.'s so used are chlorine, phosgene, diphosgene, and oxychlorcarbon.

**tear g.,** a g., such as acetone, benzene bromide, and xylol, that causes irritation of the conjunctiva and profuse lacrimation; see also lacrimator.

**ves′icating g.,** dichlorodiethyl sulfide; see *mustard* gas.

**vomiting g.,** chloropicrin.

**water g.,** an illuminating and fuel g. produced by passing steam over red-hot coal; consists chiefly of hydrogen, hydrocarbons, and carbon monoxide.

**gaseous** (gas′e-us). Of the nature of gas.

**Gasis,** Demetrius, Athens physician. See G.'s *stain.*

**Gaskell,** Walter H., English physiologist, 1847–1914. See G.'s *bridge, clamp, nerves.*

**gas′kin.** That part of the hindlimb of the horse between the stifle (knee) and the hock (ankle).

**gasom′eter.** A calibrated instrument or vessel for measuring the volumes of gases. Used in clinical and physiologic investigation for measuring respiratory gases.

**gasome′tric.** Relating to gasometry.

**gasom′etry.** The measurement of gases; the determination of the relative proportion of gases in a mixture.

**Gasser,** Herbert S., U. S. physiologist, 1888–1963. Nobel laureate, 1944, with Joseph Erlanger, for their discoveries relating to the highly differentiated functions of single nerve fibers.

**Gasser (Gasserio),** Johann L., Vienna anatomist, 18th century. See Gasserian *ganglion.*

**gasserec′tomy.** Excision of the Gasserian ganglion.

**Gasse′rian.** Relating to or described by Johann L. Gasser.

**gas′sing.** Poisoning by irrespirable or otherwise noxious gases.

**gas′ter** [ G. *gastēr,* belly ]. [ NA ]. Stomach.

**gastr-.** See gastro-.

**gastradenitis** (gas′trä-dē-ni′tis) [ gastr- + G. *adēn,* gland, + suffix -*itis,* inflammation ]. Gastroadenitis; inflammation of the glands of the stomach.

**gastral′gia** [ gastr- + G. *algos,* pain ]. Stomachache.

**gastrectasis, gastrectasia** (gas-trek′tä-sis, gas-trek-ta′zī-ah) [ gastr- + G. *ektasis,* extension ]. Dilation of the stomach.

**gastrectomy** (gas-trek′to-mī) [ gastr- + G. *ektomē,* excision ]. Excision of a part or all of the stomach.

**Belcher g.,** one similar to Billroth g. See Billroth's *operations.*

**Pólya g.,** Pólya's *operation.*

**gas′tric.** Relating to the stomach.

**gastricsin** (gas-trik′sin) (EC 3.4.4.22). A peptidase, found in close association with pepsin.

**gas′tricus** [ L. ] [ NA ]. Gastric.

**gas′trin.** A hormone, secreted in the pyloric-antral mucosa of the stomach, that stimulates secretion of HC1 by the parietal cells of the gastric glands. G. is a heptadecapeptide, the terminal tetrapeptide (Trp-Met-Asp-Phe-$NH_2$) being as active as the whole molecule. G. was formerly thought to be histamine, which has a similar effect.

**gastri′tis** [ gastr- + G. suffix -*itis,* inflammation ]. Inflammation of the stomach.

**atroph′ic g.,** chronic g. with atrophy of the mucous membrane and more or less destruction of the peptic glands.

**catarrhal g.,** gastric fever; g. with excessive secretion of mucus.

**exfoliative g.,** g. with excessive cellular exfoliation.

**g. fibroplas′tica,** g. with fibrosis and sclerosis.

**giant hypertrophic g.,** Ménétrier's *disease.*

**hypertroph′ic g.,** thickening of the gastric mucous membrane and hyperplasia of the peptic glands, found in the Zollinger-Ellison syndrome.

**interstitial g.,** inflammation of the stomach involving the submucosa and muscle coats.

**phleg′monous g.,** severe inflammation, chiefly of the submucous coat, with purulent infiltration of the wall of the stomach.

**pol′ypous g.,** a form of chronic g., in which there is irregular atrophy of the mucous membrane with cystic degeneration giving rise to a knobby or polypous appearance of the surface.

**pseudomembranous g.,** g. characterized by the formation of a false membrane.

**sclerot′ic g.,** sclerosis ventriculi; a fibrous thickening of the walls of the stomach with diminution in the capacity of the organ.

**traumatic g.,** "hardware disease"; a condition of cattle, caused by the penetration of the stomach wall, usually the reticulum, by any kind of sharp object (usually metallic) which has been swallowed.

**gastro-, gastr-** [ G. *gastēr,* stomach ]. Combining forms denoting the stomach.

**gastroacephalus** (gas′tro-ä-sef′ä-lus) [ gastro- + G. *a*-priv. + *kephalē,* head ]. Unequal conjoined twins in which an acephalous parasite is attached to the abdomen of the autosite.

**gas′troadeni′tis.** Gastradenitis.

**gastroalbumorrhea** (gas′tro-al-bu′mo-re′ah) [ gastro- + albumin, + G. *rhoia,* flow ]. Loss of albumin into the stomach.

**gastroamorphus** (gas′tro-ä-mor′fus) [ gastro- + G. *amorphos,* unshapely ]. An included amorphous parasitic twin within the abdomen of the autosite.

**gas′troanastomo′sis.** Gastrogastrostomy; the formation of an artificial communication between the cardiac and pyloric extremities of the stomach, in cases of nearly impermeable hourglass contraction of that organ.

**gastroatonia** (gas′tro-ä-to′nī-ah) [ gastro- + G. *atonia,* languor ]. Loss of tone in the stomach.

**gastroblennorrhea** (gas′tro-blen-o-re′ah) [ gastro- + blennorrhea, *q.v.* ]. Excessive proliferation of mucus by the stomach.

**gas′trocar′diac.** Relating to both the stomach and the heart.

**gastrocele** (gas′tro-sēl) [ gastro- + G. *kēlē,* hernia ]. Gastrocoele. 1. Archenteron. 2. Hernia of a portion of the stomach.

**gastrochronorrhea** (gas′tro-kron-o-re′ah) [ gastro- + G. *chronos,* time (chronic), + *rhoia,* a flow ]. Excessive, continuous gastric secretion.

**gastrocnemius** (gas-trok-ne′mī-us) [ G. *gastroknēmia,* calf of the leg, fr. *gaster*(gastr-), belly, + *knēmē,* leg ]. *Musculus gastrocnemius.*

**gastrocoele** (gas'tro-sēl). Gastrocele.

**gastrocolic** (gas'tro-kol'ik). Relating to the stomach and the colon.

**gastrocolitis** (gas'tro-ko-li'tis). Inflammation of both stomach and colon.

**gastrocoloptosis** (gas'tro-kol-op-to'sis) [ gastro- + G. *kōlon*, colon, + *ptōsis*, a falling ]. Displacement downward of stomach and colon.

**gastrocolostomy** (gas'tro-ko-los'to-mī) [ gastro- + G. *kōlon*, colon, + *stoma*, mouth ]. The formation of a communication between stomach and colon.

**gastrocolotomy** (gas'tro-ko-lot'o-mī) [ gastro- + G. *kōlon*, colon, + *tome*, incision ]. Incision into stomach and colon.

**gastrodialysis** (gas'tro-di-al'ī-sis). Dialysis across the mucous membrane of the stomach.

**gastrodiaphane** (gas-tro-di'ah-fān) [ gastro- + G. *dia*, through, + *phanē*, a light ]. A small electric light bulb passed through an esophageal tube into the stomach.

**gas'trodiaphanos'copy.** Gastrodiaphany.

**gastrodiaphany** (gas-tro-di-af'a-nī). Examination of the anterior wall of the stomach by means of the lights and shadows cast by a gastrodiaphane.

**Gastrodiscoi'des hom'inis** [ gastro- + G. *diskos*, disk; L. *homo*, gen. *hominis*, man ]. A trematode sometimes found in the intestinal canal of man, in India, the Malay States, and China. Its normal host is the pig.

**Gastrodis'cus hom'inis.** *Gastrodiscoides hominis.*

**gastroduodenal** (gas'tro-du'o-de'nal, -du-od'ē-nal). Relating to the stomach and duodenum.

**gas'trodu'odeni'tis.** Inflammation of both stomach and duodenum.

**gas'trodu'odenos'copy** [ gastro- + duodenum, + *skopeō*, to view ]. Visualization of the interior of the stomach and duodenum by means of a gastroscope.

**gas'trodu'odenos'tomy** [ gastro- + duodenum + G. *stoma*, mouth ]. Operative establishment of a communication, other than the natural one, between the stomach and the duodenum.

**gastrodynia** (gas-tro-din'ī-ah) [ gastro- + G. *odynē*, pain ]. Stomachache.

**gastroenteric** (gas'tro-en-tĕr'ik). Gastrointestinal.

**gastroenteritis** (gas'tro-en-ter-i'tis) [ gastro- + G. *enteron*, intestine, + suffix -*itis*, inflammation ]. Inflammation of the mucous membrane of both stomach and intestine.

   **transmissible g. of swine,** abbreviation TGE; a rapidly spreading virus disease of swine, characterized by severe diarrhea and vomiting. The mortality of pigs younger than 10 days is high; of older pigs it is low.

**gas'troen'teroanastomo'sis.** An artificial opening between the stomach and some noncontinuous portion of the intestine.

**gastroenterocolitis** (gas'tro-en'ter-o-ko-li'tis) [ gastro- + G. *enteron*, intestine, + *kōlon*, colon, + suffix -*itis*, inflammation ]. Inflammatory disease involving the stomach and intestines.

**gas'troen'terocolos'tomy** [ gastro- + G. *enteron*, intestine, + *kōlon*, colon + *stoma*, mouth ]. The operative formation of direct communication between the stomach and the large and small intestines.

**gas'troenterol'ogist.** A specialist in diseases of the stomach and intestine.

**gas'troenterol'ogy** [ gastro- + G. *enteron*, intestine, + *logos*, study ]. The branch of medical science that has to do with the function and disorders of the stomach and intestines.

**gas'troenterop'athy** [ gastro- + G. *enteron*, intestine, + *pathos*, suffering ]. Any disorder of the alimentary canal.

**gas'troen'teroplas'ty** [ gastro- + G. *enteron*, intestine, + *plassō*, to form ]. Operative repair of defects in the stomach and intestine.

**gastroenteroptosis** (gas'tro-en'ter-op-to'sis) [ gastro- + G. *enteron*, intestine, + *ptōsis*, a falling ]. Downward displacement of the stomach and a portion of the intestine.

**gas'troenteros'tomy** [ gastro- + G. *enteron*, intestine, + *stoma*, mouth ]. Establishment of an artificial opening between the stomach and the intestine, either anterior or posterior to the mesocolon.

**gas'troenterot'omy** [ gastro- + G. *enteron*, intestine, + *tome*, incision ]. Section into both stomach and intestine.

**gastroepiploic** (gas'tro-ep'ī-plo'ik). Relating to the stomach and the greater omentum (epiploon).

**gastroesophageal** (gas'tro-e-sof'ah-je'al) [ gastro- + G. *oisophagos*, gullet (esophagus) ]. Relating to both stomach and esophagus.

**gastroesophagitis** (gas'tro-e-sof'ah-ji'tis). Inflammation of the stomach and esophagus.

**gas'troesoph'agos'tomy** [ gastro- + G. *oisophagos*, gullet (esophagus), + *stoma*, mouth ]. The making of a new opening between esophagus and stomach for stricture of distal end of esophagus.

**gas'trogastros'tomy.** Gastroanastomosis.

**gastrogavage** (gas-tro-gă-vahzh'). Gastrostogavage; artificial feeding through an opening in the wall of the stomach. Usually shortened to gavage.

**gas'trogen'ic.** Deriving from or caused by the stomach.

**gas'trograph** [ gastro- + G. *graphē*, a writing ]. Gastrokinesograph; an instrument for recording graphically the movements of the stomach.

**gas'trohepat'ic** [ gastro- + G. *hēpar* (*hēpat*-), liver ]. Relating to the stomach and the liver.

**gastrohydrorrhea** (gas'tro-hi'dro-re'ah) [ gastro- + G. *hydōr*, water, + *rhoia*, a flow ]. An excretion into the stomach of a large amount of watery fluid containing neither hydrochloric acid nor rennet nor pepsin ferments.

**gastroileitis** (gas-tro-il-e-i'tis). Inflammation of the alimentary canal in which the stomach and ileum are preponderantly involved.

**gastroileostomy** (gas'tro-il-e-os'to-mī). A surgical joining of stomach to ileum; a technical error in which the ileum instead of jejunum is selected for the site of a gastrojejunostomy.

**gas'trointes'tinal.** Gastroenteric; relating to the stomach and intestines.

**gastrojejunocolic** (gas'tro-je-ju'no-kol'ik). Referring to the stomach, jejunum, and colon.

**gastrojejunostomy** (gas'tro-je-ju-nos'to-mī) [ gastro- + jejunum G. *stoma*, mouth ]. Gastronesteostomy; establishment of a direct communication between the stomach and the jejunum.

**gastrokinesograph** (gas'tro-kĭ-ne'so-graf) [ gastro- + G. *kinēsis*, motion, + *graphē*, a writing ]. Gastrograph.

**gastrolavage** (gas-tro-lă-vahzh'). Lavage of the stomach.

**gastrolienal** (gas-tro-li'e-nal) [ gastro- + L. *lien*, spleen ]. Gastrosplenic.

**gas'trolith** [ gastro- + G. *lithos*, stone ]. A concretion in the stomach; a gastric calculus.

**gastrolithiasis** (gas'tro-lī-thi'ă-sis). The presence of one or more calculi in the stomach, with the symptoms associated therewith.

**gastrol'ogist.** A specialist in diseases of the stomach.

**gastrol'ogy** [ gastro- + G. *logos*, study ]. The branch of medical science that has to do with the stomach and its diseases. Usually gastroenterology is implied and employed.

**gastrolysis** (gas-trol'ī-sis) [ gastro- + G. *lysis*, loosening ]. Separation of perigastric adhesions.

**gastromalacia** (gas'tro-mă-la'shī-ah) [ gastro- + G. *malakia*, softness ]. Softening of the walls of the stomach.

**gastromegaly** (gas'tro-meg'ă-lī) [ gastro- + G. *megas* (*megal*-), large ]. 1. Enlargement of the abdomen. 2. Enlargement of the stomach.

**gastromelus** (gas-trom'ē-lus) [ gastro- + G. *melos*, a limb ]. An individual having a supernumerary limb attached to the abdomen.

**gastromycosis** (gas'tro-mi-ko'sis) [ gastro- + G. *mykēs*, fungus, + suffix -*osis*, condition ]. A fungous growth in the stomach.

**gastromyxorrhea** (gas'tro-mik'so-re'ah) [ gastro- + G. *myxa*, mucus, + *rhoia*, a flow ]. Excessive secretion of mucus in the stomach.

**gastronesteostomy** (gas'tro-ne-ste-os'to-mī) [ gastro- + G. *nēstis*, jejunum, + *stoma*, mouth ]. Gastrojejunostomy.

**gastropagus** (gas-trop'ă-gus) [ gastro- + -pagus, *q.v.* ]. Conjoined twins united at the abdomen.

**gas'troparal'ysis.** Paralysis of the muscular coat of the stomach.

**gas'troparasi'tus.** Unequal conjoined twins in which the incomplete parasite is attached to, or within, the abdomen of the autosite.

**gastroparesis** (gas'tro-pă-re'sis, -păr'e-sis) [ gastro- + G. *paresis,* a letting go, paralysis. ES- ]. A slight degree of gastroparalysis.

 **g. diabeticorum,** dilation of the stomach with gastric retention in diabetics, commonly seen in association with severe acidosis or coma.

**gastropath'ic.** Relating to a disease of the stomach.

**gastropathy** (gas-trop'ă-thī) [ gastro- + G. *pathos,* disease ]. Any disease of the stomach.

**gastropexy** (gas'tro-pek'sī) [ gastro- + G. *pēxis,* fixation ]. Attachment of the stomach to the abdominal wall.

**Gastrophilus** (gas-trof'ī-lus) See botfly.

 **G. hemorrhoidalis,** the nose fly; a botfly of the horse.

 **G. intestina'lis,** the common horse botfly or nit fly; the larvae, known as bots, develop in the stomach of the horse.

 **G. nasalis,** a botfly of the horse; chin fly; throat fly.

**gastrophore** (gas'tro-fōr) [ gastro- + G. *phoros,* bearing ]. An appliance for holding the stomach during an operation upon that organ.

**gastrophotor** (gas'tro-fo'tor). An apparatus for photographing the interior of the stomach, consisting of a tubular camera attached to the end of a rubber tube.

**gastrophrenic** (gas'tro-fren'ik) [ gastro- + G. *phrēn,* diaphragm ]. Relating to the stomach and the diaphragm.

**gas'troplasty** [ gastro- + G. *plassō,* to form ]. Operative treatment of a defect of any kind in the stomach, such as an hourglass contraction.

**gastroplication** (gas'tro-pli-ka'shun) [ gastro- + L. *plicare,* to fold. PLIC- ]. Gastroptyxis; gastrorrhapy (2); stomach reefing; an operation for reducing the size of the stomach by making a longitudinal fold with the peritoneal surfaces in apposition.

**gastropneumonic** (gas'tro-nu-mon'ik) [ gastro- + G. *pneumōn,* lung ]. Relating to the stomach and the lungs.

**Gastropoda** (gas-trop'o-dah) [ gastro- + G. *pous* (*pod-*), foot ]. A class of the *Mollusca* that includes the snails, whelks, slugs, and limpets.

**gastroptosis, gastroptosia** (gas'trop-to'sis, -to'sī-ah) [ gastro- + G. *ptosis,* a falling ]. Ventroptosis; downward displacement of the stomach.

**gastroptyxis** (gas'trop-tik'sis) [ gastro- + G. *ptyxis,* a fold ]. Gastroplication.

**gastropul'monary.** Gastropneumonic; pneumogastric.

**gastropylorectomy** (gas'tro-pi'lo-rek'to-mī). Pylorectomy.

**gastropyloric** (gas'tro-pi-lor'ik). Relating to the stomach as a whole and to the pylorus.

**gastrorrhagia** (gas-tro-ra'jī-ah) [ gastro- + G. *rhēgnymi,* to burst forth ]. Hemorrhage from the stomach.

**gastrorrhaphy** (gas-tror'ă-fī) [ gastro- + G. *rhaphē,* a stitching ]. 1. Suture of a perforation of the stomach. 2. Gastroplication.

**gastrorrhea** (gas-tror-re'ah) [ gastro- + G. *rhoia,* a flow ]. Excessive secretion of gastric juice (gastrosuccorrhea) or of mucus (gastromyxorrhea) by the stomach.

**gastrorrhexis** (gas'tro-rek'sis) [ gastro- + G. *rhēxis,* a bursting ]. A tear or bursting of the stomach.

**gastroschisis** (gas-tros'kī-sis) [ gastro- + G. *schisis,* a fissure ]. Celoschisis; a congenital defect in the abdominal wall, usually with protrusion of the viscera.

**gas'troscope** [ gastro- + G. *skopeō,* to examine ]. An endoscope for inspecting the inner surface of the stomach.

**gastroscop'ic.** Relating to gastroscopy.

**gastros'copy.** Inspection of the inner surface of the stomach through an endoscope.

**gas'trospasm.** Spasmodic contraction of the walls of the stomach.

**gastrosplen'ic.** Relating to the stomach and the spleen.

**gastrostaxis** (gas'tro-stak'sis) [ gastro- + G. *staxis,* trickling ]. Oozing of blood from the mucous membrane of the stomach.

**gas'trosteno'sis** [ gastro- + G. *stenosis,* narrowing ]. Diminution in size of the cavity of the stomach.

**gastrostogavage** (gas-tros'to-gă-vahzh') [ gastrostomy + gavage ]. Gastrogavage.

**gastrostolavage** (gas-tros'to-lă-vahzh'). Lavage of the stomach through a gastric fistula.

**gastrostomo'sis.** Gastrostomy.

**gastrostomy** (gas-tros'to-mī) [ gastro- + G. *stoma,* mouth ]. The establishment of an artificial opening into the stomach.

**gas'trother'apy.** 1. Treatment of diseases of the stomach. 2. Treatment of pernicious anemia by an extract of the mucous membrane of the stomach of the hog.

**gastrothoracopagus** (gas'tro-tho-ră-kop'ă-gus) [ gastro- + G. *thōrax,* chest, + *pagos,* something fixed ]. Conjoined twins united at thorax and abdomen.

**gas'trotome.** A knife for incising the stomach.

**gastrot'omy** [ gastro- + G. *tomē,* incision ]. Incision into the stomach.

**gas'trotonom'eter.** An apparatus used in gastrotonometry.

**gastrotonometry** (gas'tro-to-nom'e-trī) [ gastro- + G. *tonos,* tension, + *metron,* measure ]. The measurement of intragastric pressure.

**gastrotox'ic.** Poisonous to the stomach.

**gastrotox'in.** A cytotoxin specific for the cells of the mucous membrane of the stomach.

**gastrotropic** (gas'tro-trop'ik) [ gastro- + G. *tropikos,* turning ]. Affecting the stomach.

**gastrox'ia** [ gastro- + G. *oxys,* keen, acid (see oxy-) ]. Gastroxynsis.

**gastroxynsis** (gas-trok-sin'sis) [ gastro- + G. *oxynō,* to make sharp, acid, OX- ]. Gastroxia; intermittent excessive secretion of the gastric juice.

**gastrula** (gas'tru-lah) [ Mod. L. dim. of G. *gastēr,* belly ]. The embryo in the stage of development following the blastula; in lower forms with minimal yolk is a simple double-layered structure consisting of ectoderm and entoderm enclosing a central cavity, called the archenteron or gastrocele, which opens to the outside by way of the blastopore. In forms with considerable yolk the configuration of the g. is greatly modified.

**gastrula'tion.** The formation of the gastrula by transformation of the blastula.

**Gatch,** Willis D., American surgeon, 1878–1961. See G. *bed, method.*

**Gaucher** (go-sha'), Philippe C. E., French physician, 1854–1918. See G. *cells,* G.'s *disease.*

**gauge** (gāj). A measuring device.

 **bite g.,** gnathodynamometer.

 **Boley g.,** a caliper-type g. graduated in millimeters used to measure the thickness of various dental materials.

 **catheter g.,** a metal plate with holes of graduated diameter used to determine the size of a catheter.

 **strain g.,** a device, employing the Wheatstone bridge principle, used for accurate measurement of forces such as strain, stress, or pressure.

 **undercut g.,** a device, used with a surveyor, to precisely locate areas for the placement of the retentive components of clasps when designing removable partial dentures.

**gaultheria** (gawl-the'rī-ah). Any plant of the genus *Gaultheria* (family Ericaceae), evergreen shrubs.

 **g. oil,** checkerberry oil; wintergreen oil; a volatile oil distilled from the leaves of *Gaultheria procumbens;* see also methyl salicylate.

**gaul'therin.** A glycoside from the bark of several species of *Betula,* birch; it yields methyl salicylate, d-glucose, and d-xylose on hydrolysis.

**Gaultier** (gōl-te-a'), Jean F., Canadian physician and botanist, 1708–1756. Gave his name to *Gaultheria.*

**gauntlet** (gawnt'let). A glove; see under bandage.

**gauss** (gows) [ J. K. F. *Gauss* ]. A unit of magnetic field intensity.

**Gauss,** Johann K. F., German physicist, 1777–1855. Gave his name to gauss. See also Gaussian *curve, distribution.*

**Gauss,** Karl J., German gynecologist, 1875–1957. See G.'s *sign.*

**Gaussel** (go-sel'), A., French physician, 1871–1937. See Grasset-G. *phenomenon.*

**gauze** (gawz). A bleached cotton cloth of plain weave, used for dressings, bandages, and absorbent sponges.

**petrolatum g.,** g. saturated with petrolatum.

**gavage** (gă-vahzh') [ Fr. *gaver,* to gorge fowls ]. Feeding by the stomach tube.

**Gavard** (gă-var'), Hyacinthe, French anatomist, 1753–1802. See G.'s *muscle.*

**Gay,** Alexander H., Russian anatomist, 1842–1907. See G.'s *glands.*

**Gay-Lussac** (ga-lü-sak'), Joseph L., Paris naturalist, 1778–1850. See G.-L.'s *law.*

**gaze.** The act of looking steadily in one direction for a period of time.

**conjugate g.,** movement of the eyes with the visual axes parallel.

**Gd.** Chemical symbol of the element gadolinium.

**GDP.** Abbreviation for guanosine 5'-diphosphate.

**GDPmannose phosphorylase.** Mannose-1-phosphate guanylyltransferase.

**Ge.** Chemical symbol of the element germanium.

**Gee,** Samuel J., British physician, 1839–1911. See G.'s *disease,* G.-Herter *infantilism,* G.-Herter *syndrome.*

**geeldikkop** (gēl-dik'kop) [ Dutch, "yellow, thick head" ]. A hepatogenous photosensitivity of sheep caused by eating the plant, *Tribulus terrestris.*

**Geigel,** Richard, German physician, 1859–1930. See G.'s *reflex.*

**Geiger,** Hans, German physician, 1882–1945. See G.-Müller *tube, counter.*

**Geissler** (gis'ler), Ernst, German physician, *1866. See G. *test.*

**gel** (jel) [ Mod. L. *gelatum* ]. 1. A jelly or the solid or semisolid phase of a colloidal solution. 2. To form a g. or jelly; to convert a sol into a g. 3. Pharmacopeial g.'s are suspensions, in a water medium, of insoluble drugs in hydrated form wherein the particle size approaches or attains colloidal dimensions.

**colloidal g.,** a colloid that has developed resistance to flow because of chemical or thermal change.

**gelasmus** (jĕ-laz'mus) [ Gr. *gelasma,* a laugh, fr. *gelaō,* to laugh ]. Spasmodic, hysterical laughter.

**gelate** (jel'āt). Gelatinize.

**gelatin** (jel'ă-tin) [ L. *gelo,* pp. *gelatus,* to freeze, congeal ] (USP, BP). A derived protein formed from the collagen of the tissues by boiling in water. Glue, size, and isinglass are forms of g. It swells up when put in cold water, but dissolves only in hot water. Used as a hemostatic, plasma substitute, and protein food adjunct in malnutrition.

**absorbable g. film,** a sterile, nonantigenic, absorbable, water-insoluble, thin sheet of g. prepared by drying a g.-formaldehyde solution on plates. It is used in the closure and repair of defects in membranes such as the dura mater or the pleura; it undergoes absorption in from 1 to 6 months.

**g. film** (NF), hemostatic agent.

**glyc'erinated g.,** glycerogelatin; glycogelatin; glycerin jelly; made of equal parts of g. and glycerin; a firm mass liquefying at gentle heat. It is used as a vehicle for suppositories and urethral bougies.

**Irish moss g.,** extracted from Irish moss. Used to make the mucilage of Irish moss that is used as a substitute for gum arabic in making emulsions.

**vegetable g.,** a substance similar to g., obtained from gluten.

**zinc g.** see under zinc.

**gelatiniferous** (jel'ă-tĭ-nif'er-us) [ gelatin + L. *fero,* to bear ]. Producing or containing gelatin.

**gelatinization** (jĕ-lat'ĭ-nĭ-za'shun). Conversion into gelatin or a substance resembling it.

**gelatinize** (jĕ-lat'ĭ-nīz). Gelate. 1. To convert into gelatin. 2. To become gelatinous.

**gelatinoid** (jĕ-lat'ĭ-noyd). Resembling gelatin.

**gelatino'sus** [ L. ] [ NA ]. Gelatinous.

**gelatinous** (jĕ-lat'ĭ-nus). 1. Relating to gelatin. 2. Jelly-like; resembling gelatin.

**gelation** (jĕ-la'shun). In colloidal chemistry, the transformation of a sol into a gel.

**gelatum** (jĕ-la'tum) [ Mod. L. ]. Jelly; gel.

**geld'er.** One who castrates male horses, *i.e.,* makes geldings.

**gelding** (gel'ding). A castrated male horse.

**Gélineau** (zhel-in-ō'), Jean B. E., French physician, *1859. See G.'s *syndrome.*

**Gell,** P. G., British immunologist. See G. and Coombs *reactions.*

**Gellé** (zhel-a'), Marie-Ernst, Paris otologist, 1834–1923. See G. *test.*

**gelose** (jel'ōs). Galactan.

**gelo'sis** (je-lo'sis) [ L. *gelo,* to freeze, congeal, + G. suffix *-osis,* condition ]. An extremely firm mass in tissue (especially in a muscle), with a consistency resembling that of frozen tissue.

**gelotripsy** (jel'o-trip-sī) [ gelosis + G. *tripsis,* a rubbing, fr. *tribō,* to rub ]. Nerve point massage; rubbing away an indurated swelling or tender point in neuralgia and myalgia.

**gelsemine** (jel'sē-mēn). A crystallizable alkaloid derived from gelsemium; mydriatic and central nervous system stimulant.

**gelsemium** (jel-se'mī-um, gel-sem'ī-um) [ Mod. L. fr. Pers. *yāsmin,* jasmine ]. The rhizome and roots of *Gelsemium sempervirens* (family Loganiaceae), yellow jasmine or jessamine.

**Gély** (zha-le'), Jules A., French surgeon, 1806–1861. See G.'s *suture.*

**gem-** [ shortened form of L. *geminus,* twin ]. Chemical prefix denoting twin substitutions on a single atom (*e.g.,* the *gem*-dimethyl substitution on carbon-4 of lanosterol.

**gemellipara** (jem-el-lip'ă-rah) [ L. *gemellus,* twin, + *pario,* to bear ]. A woman who has given birth to twins.

**gemellology** (jem'el-ol'o-jī) [ L. *gemellus,* twin-born, + G. *logos,* study ]. The study of twins and the phenomenology of twinning.

**gemellus** (jĕ-mel'us) [ L. dim. of *geminus,* twin ]. *Musculus* gemellus.

**geminate** (jem'ī-nāt) [ L. *gemino,* pp. *-atus,* to double, fr. *geminus,* twin ]. Occurring in pairs.

**gemination** (jem'ī-na'shun) [ L. *geminatio,* a doubling ]. Embryologic partial division of a primordium, as, *e.g.,* of a single tooth germ, resulting in two partially or completely separated crowns.

**gem'inous.** Referring to gemination.

**gemistocyte** (jĕ-mis'to-sīt). Protoplasmic *astrocyte* (1).

**gemistocytoma** (jĕ-mis'to-si-to'mah). Protoplasmic *astrocytoma.*

**gemma** (jem'ah) [ L. bud ]. Any budlike or bulblike body, especially a taste bud or end bulb.

**gemmation** (jem-ma'shun) [ L. *gemma,* a bud ]. Budding; bud fission; a form of fission in which the parent cell does not divide, but puts out a budlike process (daughter cell) of small size, containing its proportion of chromatin, which then separates and begins an independent existence.

**gemmule** (jem'ūl) [ L. *gemmula,* dim. of *gemma,* bud ]. 1. A small bud that projects from the parent cell, and finally becomes detached, forming a cell of a new generation. 2. Dendritic *spine.* 3. Hypothetical particles which, according to Darwin's theory of inheritance, were transferred from the body cells to germ cells of the parent organism; thus characters were transmitted to the offspring.

**Hoboken's g.'s,** Hoboken's *nodules.*

**gen-, -gen** [ G. *genos,* birth. GEN- ]. 1. Combining form, used in the prefix or suffix position, meaning "producing" or "coming to be." 2. In chemistry, its use as a suffix indicates "precursor of," as in zymogen (precursor of an enzyme); see also pro-.

**gena** (je'nah) [ L. ]. Cheek; the side of the face.

**genal** (je'nal). Relating to the gena, or cheek.

**gender** (jen'der). The anatomical sex of an individual.

**gene** (jēn) [ G. *genos*, birth. GEN- ]. The functional unit of heredity. Each g. occupies a specific place or locus on a chromosome, is capable of reproducing itself exactly at each cell division, and is capable of directing the formation of an enzyme or other protein. The g. as a functional unit probably consists of a discrete segment of a giant deoxyribonucleic acid (DNA) molecule containing the proper number of purine (adenine and guanine) and pyrimidine (cytosine and thymine) bases in the correct sequence to code the sequence of amino acids needed to form a specific peptide. Protein synthesis is mediated by molecules of messenger ribonucleic acid (messenger-RNA) formed on the chromosome with the g. unit of DNA acting as a template, which then pass into the cytoplasm and become oriented on the ribosomes where they in turn act as templates to organize a chain of amino acids to form a peptide. G.'s normally occur in pairs in all cells except gametes as a consequence of the fact that all chromosomes are paired except the sex chromosomes (X and Y) of the male.

**allelic g.,** see allele; also dominance of g.'s.

**autosomal g.,** one located on any chromosome other than a sex chromosome (X or Y).

**control g.,** operator g. or regulator g.

**crossing over of g.'s,** the reciprocal exchange of material between two paired chromosomes during meiosis, resulting in the transfer of a block of g.'s from each chromosome to its homologue.

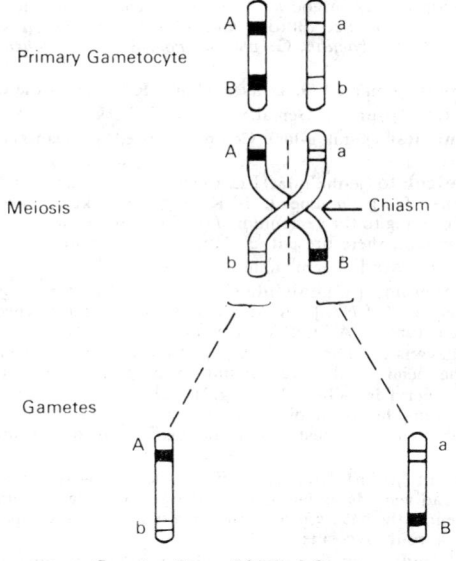

Primary Gametocyte

Meiosis ← Chiasm

Gametes

**Crossing Over of Linked Genes**

**dominance of g.'s,** an expression of the apparent physiologic relationship existing between two or more g.'s that may occupy the same chromosome locus (alleles). At a specific paired locus there are three possible combinations of two allelic g.'s *A* and *a*. The pair may consist of both g.'s of one type, *AA*, both of contrasting type, *aa*, or one of each, *Aa*. If both are alike, *AA* or *aa*, the individual or cell is homozygous with respect to the gene concerned. If they are different, *Aa*, the individual or cell is heterozygous. If a heterozygous individual presents only the hereditary characteristic determined by g. *A*, while the effect of g. *a* is not apparent, g. *A* is said to be dominant and g. *a* is said to be recessive. In this case the dominant homozygote, *AA*, and the heterozygote, *Aa*, should be indistinguishable. If both g.'s produce a recognizable or intermediate effect in the heterozygote the three classes, *AA*, *Aa* and *aa*, are distinguishable each from the others, and there is intermediate dominance or no dominance between the alleles. Dominance relationships may in some cases be modified by environmental factors. In a series of

multiple alleles complex dominance relationships may exist.

**histocompatibility g.,** a g. (in laboratory animals), whose product can elicit an immune response and thereby cause rejection of a homograft when tissue is transplanted from one individual to another.

**holandric g.,** g. located on a Y chromosome; Y-linked g.

**lethal g.,** one that causes death of the organism when in a specified condition, homozygous or heterozygous.

**mimic g.'s,** nonallelic (independent) g.'s with closely similar effects.

**mosaicism of g.'s,** see mosaic (2).

**operator g.,** a g. with the function of activating the production of messenger-RNA by one or more adjacent structural g.'s; part of the feedback system for determining the rate of production of an enzyme. See fig. under protein.

**recessive g.,** see dominance of g.'s.

**regulator g.,** a g. with the function of producing a repressor substance capable of combining with an operator g. and inhibiting the ability of the operator g. to activate one or more structural g.'s, thus preventing the production of a specific enzyme; when the enzyme is again demanded, a specific regulatory metabolite combines with the repressor substance and removes its inhibiting effect on the operator gene, and thus starts production of the enzyme. See fig. under protein.

**segregation of g.'s,** the separation of the paired state of g.'s which occurs at the reduction division of meiosis. Only one member of each somatic g. pair is included in each sperm or ovum. An individual heterozygous for a g. pair, *Aa*, will form gametes half containing g. *A* and half containing g. *a*.

**sex-linked g.,** one located on a sex chromosome, in usual usage the X chromosome.

**structural g.,** a g. with the function of determining the structure (amino acid sequence) of a specific protein or peptide. See fig. under protein.

**X-linked g.,** one located on an X chromosome.

**Y-linked g.,** one located on a Y chromosome.

**genealogy** (je-ne-al'o-jī) [ G. *genea*, descent, + *logos*, study ]. The history of the descent of a person or family.

**geneogenous** (je-ne-oj'ĕ-nus) [ G. *genea*, descent, + suffix *-gen*, producing ]. Of parental origin; congenital.

**gen'era.** Plural of genus.

**gen'eralist.** A general physician or family physician; a physician trained to take care of the majority of nonsurgical diseases, sometimes including obstetrics.

**gen'eraliza'tion.** 1. The rendering or becoming general, diffuse, or widespread, as when a primarily local disease becomes systemic. 2. The reasoning by which a basic conclusion is reached which applies to different items, each having some common factor.

**stimulus g.,** in conditioning, the eliciting of a conditioned response by stimuli similar to a particular conditioned stimulus.

**gen'erate** [ L. *genero*, pp. *-atus*, to beget. GEN- ]. 1. To produce. 2. To procreate.

**genera'tion** [ L. *generatio*, fr. *genero*, pp. *-atus*, to beget. GEN- ]. 1. Procreation; reproduction. 2. A stage in succession of descent; *e.g.*, father, son, and grandson are three g.'s.

**alternation of g.'s,** a succession of g.'s of individuals like and unlike the original parents, or an alternation of sexual and nonsexual g.'s.

**asex'ual g., nonsexual g.,** reproduction by fission, gemmation, or in any other way without union of the male and female cell, or conjugation; see also parthenogenesis.

**filial g.,** the offspring resulting from a genetically specified mating: first filial g. (symbol $F_1$), the offspring resulting from mating of parents of contrasting genotypes; second filial g. ($F_2$), the offspring resulting from the mating of two $F_1$ individuals; third filial g. ($F_3$), fourth filial g. ($F_4$), etc., the offspring in succeeding g.'s of continued inbreeding of $F_1$ descendents.

**parental g.** (symbol $P_1$), the parents of a mating, usually experimental, involving contrasting genotypes; the original mating of a genetic experiment; parents of the $F_1$ g.

**sexual g.,** reproduction by conjugation, or the union of male and female cells.

**spontaneous g.,** heterogenesis (2); the supposed origin of living matter *de novo,* or from the vitalization of nonliving matter. See also biogenesis.

**virgin g.,** parthenogenesis.

**gen′erative.** Relating to generation.

**gen′erator.** An apparatus in which a vapor, gas, or aerosol is formed from a liquid or solid by heat, chemical, or other process.

**aerosol g.,** a device for producing airborne suspensions of small particles for inhalation therapy or experimental work. See also La Mer g.; spinning *disk;* vibrating *reed.*

**asynchronous pulse g.,** fixed rate pulse g.; one in which the rate of discharge is independent of the natural activity of the heart.

**atrial synchronous pulse g.,** atrial triggered pulse g.; a ventricular stimulating pulse whose rate of discharge is directly determined by the atrial rate.

**atrial triggered pulse g.,** atrial synchronous pulse g.

**demand pulse g.,** ventricular inhibited pulse g.

**fixed rate pulse g.,** asynchronous pulse g.

**La Mer g.,** a condensation aerosol g. designed for producing monodisperse aerosols.

**pulse g.,** the electronic assembly within a pacemaker that includes power source and pulse-forming elements and may include circuitry for additional functions.

**radionuclide g.,** a column containing a large amount of a particular radionuclide that decays down to a second radionuclide of shorter physical half-life. The daughter radionuclide is separated from the parent by the process of elution and affords a continuing supply of relatively short-lived radionuclides for laboratory use. The elution is loosely termed "milking" and the generator is loosely referred to as a "radioactive cow."

**standby pulse g.,** ventricular inhibited pulse g.

**ventricular inhibited pulse g.,** demand pulse g.; standby pulse g.; one which suppresses its output in response to natural ventricular activity but which, in the absence of such activity, functions as an asynchronous pulse.

**ventricular synchronous pulse g.,** ventricular triggered pulse g.; a pulse which delivers its output synchronously with naturally occurring ventricular activity but which, in the absence of such activity, functions as an asynchronous pulse.

**ventricular triggered pulse g.,** ventricular synchronous pulse g.

**gener′ic** [ L. *genus* (*gener-*), birth. GEN- ]. 1. Relating to or denoting a genus. 2. General. 3. Characteristic or distinctive. 4. See *generic name.*

**generic name.** 1. In chemistry, a noun that indicates the class or type of a single compound, *i.e.,* a class name. "Class" is more appropriate and more often used than is generic in chemistry. Salt, saccharide (sugar), hexose, alcohol, aldehyde, lactone, acid, amine, alkane, steroid, vitamin D, etc., are examples. 2. In the drug and commercial fields, generic names are synonymous with, albeit a misnomer for, nonproprietary names. Nonproprietary names apply to individual substances regardless of manufacturer, whereas proprietary or trademark names usually apply to preparations (which usually incorporate several substances) and are often limited to use by one manufacturer. Nonproprietary names, like trademarks, are almost always coined designations and are derived in many different ways. Nonproprietary names often have an "official" connotation, since they are recognized or recommended by governmental agencies (*e.g.,* Federal Food and Drug Administration) as well as by quasi-official organizations (National Formulary, U. S. Pharmacopeia, U. S. Adopted Names Council, or the World Health Organization); similar names coined without official sanction are sometimes referred to as trivial names.

**gene′sial.** Relating to generation.

**genesiology** (jen-e-sī-ol′o-jī) [ G. *genesis,* generation, + *logos,* study ]. The branch of science that has to do with generation or reproduction.

**genesis** (jen′ē-sis) [ G. ]. Generation; procreation; production; origin. Also used as combining form in suffix position.

**genesistron** (jen′ē-sis′tron). A postulated primitive genome unit of about 500 million daltons, such as is found in mycoplasma.

**genetic** (jĕ-net′ik). Relating to (1) genetics, and (2) ontogenesis.

**geneticist** (jĕ-net′ĭ-sist). A student of genetics.

**genetics** (jĕ-net′iks) [ G. *genesis,* origin or production ]. The branch of science that deals with heredity.

**behavior g.,** a field of psychology concerned with the influence of heredity on behavior.

**biochemical g.,** the study of the application of biochemistry to genetics, as in the elucidation of the manner in which deoxyribonucleic acid (DNA) molecules replicate and control the synthesis of specific enzymes by way of the genetic code.

**microbial g.,** the study of hereditary mechanisms in organisms in which the hereditary material (DNA and/or RNA) is not suspended in karyolymph within a nuclear membrane and is not regulated, during division, by a mitotic mechanism.

**statistical g.,** the study of the applications of principles of statistics to problems in genetics.

**genetotrophic** (jĕ-net′o-trof′ik) [ G. *genesis,* origin, + *trophē,* nourishment ]. Relating to inherited individual distinctions in nutritional requirements.

**Geneva Convention.** An international agreement formed at meetings in Geneva, Switzerland, in 1864 and 1906, relating (among medical subjects) to the safeguarding of the wounded in battle, of those having the care of them, and of the buildings in which they are being treated. The direct outcome of the first of these meetings was the establishment of the Red Cross Society.

**Gengou** (zhon-goo′), Octave, French bacteriologist 1875–1957. See Bordet and G.'s potato blood *agar,* Bordet-G. *bacillus,* G. *phenomenon,* Bordet-G. *phenomenon.*

**genial** (je-ni′al) [ G. *geneion,* chin ]. Relating to the chin.

**genian** (je-ni′an). Genial.

**genicular** (jĕ-nik′u-lar). Commonly used to mean genual, *q. v.*

**geniculate** (je-nik′u-lāt) [ L. *geniculo,* pp. -*atus,* to bend the knee, fr. *genu,* knee ]. 1. Kneed; bent like a knee. 2. Referring to the geniculum of the facial nerve, denoting the ganglion there present. 3. *Corpus* geniculatum.

**genic′ulated.** Geniculate (1).

**geniculum,** pl. **genic′ula** (je-nik′u-lum) [ L. dim. of *genu,* knee ]. 1 [ NA ]. A small genu or angular kneelike structure. 2. A knotlike structure.

**g. cana′lis facia′lis** [ NA ], g. of facial canal; the bend in the facial canal corresponding to the g. nervi facialis.

**g. nervi facia′lis** [ NA ], g. (knee) of the facial nerve; a rectangular bend of the facial nerve in the facial canal where it turns posterior in the medial wall of the middle ear.

**-genin** (jen′in). Used as a suffix in such terms as bufogenin (toad venoms, bufanolides), gitoxigenin (a plant genin) to denote the basic steroid unit of the toxic substance, usually a steroid glycoside.

**ge′niogloss′us** [ G. *geneion,* chin, + *glōssa,* tongue ]. *Musculus* genioglossus.

**geniohyoid** (je′nī-o-hi′oyd). *Musculus* geniohyoideus.

**geniohyoideus** (je′nī-o-hi-o-id′e-us) [ G. *geneion,* chin, + *hyoeidēs,* y-shaped, hyoid ]. *Musculus* geniohyoideus.

**genion** (je-ni′on) [ G. *geneion,* chin ]. The tip of the mental spine, a point in craniometry.

**ge′nioplasty** [ G. *geneion,* chin, cheek, + *plassō,* to form ]. Genyplasty; a surgical procedure whereby the mental prominence is built outward by means of bone, cartilage, tantalum mesh, or alloplastic materials.

**genistein** (jĕ-nis′ta-in). 4′,5,7-Trihydroxyisoflavone; prunetol; the aglucon of genistin and of sophoricoside; a coumarin derivative, with appreciable estrogenic activity, found in subterranean clover.

**genis′tin.** Genistein 7-glucoside.

**gen′ital.** 1. Relating to reproduction, or generation. 2. Relating to the organs of reproduction (the genitals). 3. Relating to or characterized by genitality.

**genitalia** (jen′ĭ-ta′lĭ-ah) [ L. neut. pl. of *genitalis,* genital ]. The genitals.

**ambiguous external g.,** external g. not clearly of either sex; most commonly designates external g. that are incompletely masculinized.

**external g.,** the vulva, and the penis and scrotum.

**genitality** (jen'ī-tal'ī-tī). In psychoanalysis, a term referring to the genital components of sexuality (*i.e.*, the penis and vagina), as opposed, for example, to orality and anality.

**gen'itals.** The organs of generation; the reproductive organs.

**gen'itocru'ral.** Genitofemoral.

**gen'itofem'oral.** Genitocrural; relating to the genitalia and the thigh; denoting the g. nerve.

**genitourinary** (jen-ĭ-to-u'rī-na-rī). Urogenital; relating to reproduction and to urination; denoting the organs concerned in these functions.

**genius** (jēn'yus) [ L. ]. 1. Markedly superior intellectual or artistic abilities or exceptional creative power. 2. A person so endowed.

**ge'nius epidem'icus** [ Mod. L. ]. The influence, atmospheric, telluric, or cosmic, or the combination of any two or three, anciently regarded as the cause of epidemic and endemic diseases.

**Gennari** (jen-nah're), Francisco, Italian anatomist, 18th century. See G.'s *band, line, stria, stripe.*

**gen'odermatol'ogy** [ G. *genos*, birth, descent, + *derma*, skin, + *logos*, theory ]. Study of the hereditary aspects of cutaneous disorders.

**gen'odermato'sis.** A skin condition of genetic origin.

**genome** (je'nōm, -nom) [ gene + chromosome ]. 1. A complete set of chromosomes derived from one parent, the haploid number of a gamete. 2. The total gene complement of a set of chromosomes found in higher life forms, or the functionally similar but simpler linear arrangements found in bacteria and viruses; see also chromosome; nucleus (2).

**genote** (je'nōt). In microbial genetics, an element of recombination when one of the pair is not a complete chromosome; commonly used as a suffix (*e.g.*, endogenote, exogenote, F genote).

    **F g. (F-genote),** F' *agent.*

**genotype** (jen'o-tip) [ G. *genos*, birth, descent, + *typos*, type ]. The genetic constitution of an individual; may be used with respect to gene combination at one specified locus or with respect to any specified combination of loci. For specific blood group genotypes, see appendix 2, Blood Groups.

**genotypical** (jen'o-tip'ī-kal). Relating to the genotype.

**Gensoul's disease.** See under disease.

**gentamicin** (jen'tă-mi'sin). GARAMYCIN; gentamycin; a broad spectrum antibiotic obtained from *Micromonospora purpurea* and *M. echinospora;* it inhibits the growth of both Gram-positive and Gram-negative bacteria. It is almost completely excreted, in unchanged form, by glomerular filtration. Irreversible vestibular damage may occur. Official (USP), as g. sulfate.

**gentian** (jen'shan). (BP). Gentian root; the dried rhizome and roots of *Gentiana lutea* (family Gentianaceae), a herb of southern and central Europe. A simple bitter.

    **g. violet** (USP), methylrosaniline chloride.

**gentianophil, gentianophile** (jen'shan-o-fil, -fil) [ gentian + G. *philos*, fond ]. Staining readily with gentian violet.

**gentianophilous** (jen'shan-of'ĭ-lus). Gentianophil.

**gentianophobic** (jen'shan-o-fo'bik) [ gentian + G. *phobos*, fear ]. Not taking a gentian violet stain, or taking it poorly.

**gentianophobous** (jen'shan-of'o-bus) Gentianophobic.

**gentiobiase** (jen'shī-o-bi'ās). β-Glucosidase.

**gentiobiose** (jen'shī-o-bi'ōs). Amygdalose; a constituent of the naturally occurring glycoside, amygdalin; a disaccharide consisting of two glucose residues bound by a 1,6 linkage, rather than the 1,4 of maltose and cellobiose.

**gentiopicrin** (jen'shī-o-pik'rin). A glucoside of a substituted pyrancarboxylic lactone, obtained from gentian. Formerly used as an antimalarial drug.

**gen'tisin.** Gentianin; gentianic acid; substituted xanthenone; obtained from gentian.

**genu,** gen. **ge'nus,** pl. **gen'ua** (je'nu) [ L. ]. 1 [ NA ]. The knee. 2 [ NA ]. Any structure of angular shape resembling a flexed knee.

**g. cap'sulae inter'nae** [ NA ], g., or knee, of the internal capsule; the obtuse angle, opening laterally in the horizontal plane, formed by the union of the two limbs (crus anterius and crus posterius) of the internal capsule.

**g. cor'poris callo'si** [ NA ], g. or knee of the corpus callosum; the anterior extremity of the corpus callosum that here folds downward and backward on itself, terminating in the rostrum.

**g. of corpus callosum,** g. corporis callosi.

**g. extror'sum,** obsolete term for g. varum with the center of curvature at the knee.

**g. of facial nerve,** g. nervi facialis.

**g. impres'sum,** obsolete term denoting a deformity marked by bending of the knee laterally with dragging of the patella away from its femoral contact, a flattening of the superficial strata of the cartilage, and consequent resistance to the motion of the joint.

**g. of internal capsule,** g. capsulae internae.

**g. intror'sum,** obsolete term for g. valgum.

**g. ner'vi facial'lis** [ NA ], g. of the facial nerve; the curve which the fibers of the root of the facial nerve describe around the abducens nucleus in the pontine tegmentum.

**g. recurva'tum,** back-knee; a condition of hyperextension of the knee, the lower extremity making a curve with concavity looking forward.

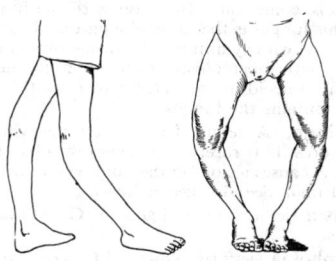

**Genu Recurvatum (*left*) and Genu Varum (*right*)**

**g. val'gum,** knock-knee; tibia valga; a deformity marked by abduction of the leg in relation to the thigh.

**g. va'rum,** bowleg; bandy-leg; g. extrorsum; an outward bowing of the legs.

**genual** (jen'u-al) [ L. *genu*, knee ]. Genicular; relating to the knee.

**ge'nucu'bital** [ L. *genu*, knee, + *cubitum*, elbow ]. Relating to the knees and the elbows; denoting the knee-elbow *position.*

**genupectoral** (je-nu-pek'to-ral) [ G. *genu*, knee, + *pectus* (*pector*-), breast, sternum ]. Relating to the knees and the chest; denoting the knee-chest *position.*

**genus,** pl. **genera** (je'nus, jen'er-ah) [ L. birth, descent ]. In natural history classification, the division between the family, or tribe, and the species. A group of species alike in the broad features of their organization but different in detail.

**genyantrum** (jen-e-an'trum) [ G. *genys*, cheek, + *antron*, cave ]. *Sinus* maxillaris.

**genychiloplasty** (jen-ī-ki'lo-plas-tī) [ G. *genys*, cheek, + *cheilos*, lip, + *plassō*, to form ]. Reparative surgery of the cheek and lip.

**gen'yplasty** [ G. *genys*, jaw, cheek, + *plassō*, to form ]. Genioplasty.

**geo-** (je'o-) [ G. *gē*, earth ]. Combining form relating to the earth, or to soil.

**ge'omed'icine.** Nosochthonography; nosogeography; the science that deals with the influence of climatic and environmental conditions on health and disease.

**geomy'cin.** Antibiotic substance produced by *Streptomyces xanthophaeus;* possesses antimicrobial activity.

**geopathol'ogy.** The study of disease in relation to regions, climates, and so on, including the effects of types of land, water, air, and other forms of life in the environment.

**geophagia, geophagism, geophagy** (je-o-fa'jĭ-ah) [ geo- + G. *phagein*, to eat ]. The practice of eating dirt or clay;

also variously referred to as earth eating; dirt eating; chthonophagia; geotragia; African cachexia.

**geophagist** (je-of'ă-jist). One who practices geophagia.

**geophilic** (je'o-fil'ik) [ geo- + G. *phileō*, to love ]. Soil seeking or soil preferring; designates preference of a parasite for soil rather than a human or animal host.

**Geophilus** (je-of'ĭ-lus). A genus of centipedes, characterized by very large numbers of legs (47 to 67 pairs); includes *G. californius, G. rubens,* and *G. umbraticus,* in the United States.

**Georgi** (gha-or'ge), Walter, German bacteriologist, 1889–1920. See Sachs-G. *reaction, test.*

**Geosciurus** [ geo- + G. *skiouros,* squirrel ]. A ground squirrel of southern Africa sometimes considered a subgenus of Xerus. These small rodents tame readily and are frequently kept as pets. They may contract bubonic plague, as do several other rodents, and thus constitute a potential danger to human health.

**geotaxis** (je-o-tak'sis) [ geo- + G. *taxis,* orderly arrangement ]. Geotropism; a form of positive barotaxis in which there is a tendency to growth or movement toward or into the earth.

**geotragia** (je-o-tra'jĭ-ah) [ geo- + G. *tragein,* to munch ]. Geophagia.

**geotrichosis** (je'o-trī-ko'sis) [ geo- + G. *thrix,* hair, + suffix *-osis,* condition ]. Infection with the fungus *Geotrichum;* this fungus is the cause of a chronic bronchopulmonary disease with symptoms of chronic bronchitis; may be confused with tuberculosis or pneumonitis; the sputum is white and mucoid in character, has a yeastlike odor, and usually contains the fungus.

**Geot'richum.** A genus of yeastlike fungi which produce arthrospores but rarely blastospores. One species, *G. candidum,* causes lesions in the pulmonary and alimentary tracts of man. See also geotrichosis.

**geotropism** (je-ot'ro-pizm) [ geo- + G. *tropē,* a turning ]. Geotaxis.

**gephyrophobia** (je-fi'ro-fo'bĭ-ah) [ G. *gephyra,* bridge, + *phobos,* fear ]. Fear of crossing a bridge or walking along a river bank.

**Geraghty** (ger'ah-tĭ), John T., American physician, 1876–1924. See G.'s *test,* Rowntree and G.'s *test.*

**geraniol** (jĕ-ra'nĭ-ol). *trans*-3,7-Dimethyl-2,6-octadienol; lemonol; a terpene alcohol found in oils of rose, geranium, sassafras, lavender, etc. Used in perfume manufacture.

**Gerard** of Cremona, Italian translator, 1114–1187. Made available in Latin important Arabic medical works of Avicenna, Rhazes, Albucasis, and the Greek texts of Hippocrates, Galen, and others.

**geratology** (jĕr-ă-tol'o-jĭ). Geriatrics.

**gerbil** (jer'bil) [ Mod. L. *gerbillus,* fr. Arab. ]. A name applied to any of 13 genera of small rodents from Africa and Asia in the subfamily Gerbillinae. They resemble jerboas or kangaroo rats and can survive without drinking water. The jird (*Meriones*) is often confused with the gerbil (*Gerbillus*) in pet shops.

**Gerdy** (zher-de'), Pierre N., Paris surgeon, 1797–1856. See G.'s *fibers, fontanel,* hyoid *fossa, ligament,* interauricular *loop, tubercle.*

**Gerhardt** (gär'hart), Carl J., Berlin physician, 1833–1902. See G.'s *disease, dullness,* G.-Semon *law,* G.'s *reaction, sign, test* (for acetoacetic acid).

**Gerhardt** (zher-hart'), Charles F., Paris chemist, 1816–1856. See G.'s *test* (for urobilin).

**geriat'ric.** Relating to old age or to geriatrics.

**geriatrics** (jĕr'ĭ-at'riks) [ G. *gēras,* old age, + *iatrikos,* healing ]. Geratology; gerontology; presbytiatrics; the science of old age; old people in their physiologic and pathologic aspects.

**dental g.,** gerodontics; gerodontology; treatment of dental problems peculiar to advanced age.

**Gerlach** (ger'lahkh), Andreas C., German veterinary surgeon, 1811–1877. See G.'s *valvula.*

**Gerlach** (ger'lahkh), Joseph, German anatomist, 1820–1896. See G.'s annular *tendon, tonsil, valve.*

**Gerlier** (zher-le-a'), Felix, Swiss physician, 1840–1914. See G.'s *disease.*

**germ** (jerm) [ L. *germen,* sprout, bud, germ ]. 1. A microbe; a microorganism. 2. A primordium; the earliest trace of a structure within an embryo.

**enamel g.,** one of a series of knoblike projections from the dental lamina, later becoming bell-shaped and receiving in its hollow the dental papilla; the enamel organ of a developing tooth.

**reserve tooth g.,** enamel organ and papilla of a permanent tooth.

**tooth g.,** the enamel organ and dentin papilla, constituting the developing tooth.

**germa'nium** [ L. *Germania,* Germany ]. A grayish white metallic element, symbol Ge, atomic no. 32; atomic weight 72.60.

**germici'dal.** Germicide (1).

**ger'micide** [ germ + L. *caedo,* to kill ]. 1. Germicidal; destructive to germs or microbes. 2. An agent with this action.

**germinal** (jer'mĭ-nal). Relating to a germ or (botany) to germination.

**ger'mine diacetate.** A semisynthetic veratrum alkaloid that antagonizes nondepolarizing muscle relaxants; used in the treatment of myasthenia gravis.

**germinoma** (jer'mĭ-no'mah). Neoplasm of germinal tissue that normally differentiates to form sperm cells or ova; for example, teratoma of the testis.

**gero-, geront-, geronto-** [ G. *gerōn,* old man ]. Combining forms relating to old age.

**geroderma** (jer-o-der'mah) [ gero- + G. *derma,* skin ]. 1. The atrophic skin of the aged. 2. Any condition in which the skin is thinned and wrinkled, resembling the integument of old age.

**gerodon'tics, gerodontol'ogy.** [ gero- + G. *odous,* tooth ]. Dental *geriatrics.*

**geromarasmus** (jer'o-mă-raz'mus) [ gero- + G. *marasmos,* a wasting ]. Senile atrophy or wasting.

**geromorphism** (jer'o-mor'fizm) [ gero- + G. *morphē,* form ]. A condition of premature senility.

**gerontal** (jĕ-ron'tal). Senile; relating to an old man.

**geronto-.** See gero-.

**gerontology** (jĕr'on-tol'o-jĭ) [ geronto- + G. *logos,* study ]. Geriatrics.

**gerontophilia** (jĕ-ron'to-fil'ĭ-ah) [ geronto- + G. *philos,* fond ]. Morbid love for old persons.

**gerontophobia** (jĕ-ron'to-fo'bĭ-ah) [ geronto- + G. *phobos,* fear ]. Morbid fear of old persons.

**gerontopia** (jĕr'on-to'pĭ-ah) [ geronto- + G. *ōps,* eye ]. Second *sight.*

**geron'totherapeu'tics.** The science dealing with treatment of the aged.

**geron'tother'apy.** Geriatric therapy; the treatment of disease in the elderly and the aged.

**gerontoxon** (jĕr'on-tok'son) [ geronto- + G. *toxon,* bow ]. *Arcus* senilis.

**Gerota** (ga-ro'tah), Dumitru, Roumanian surgeon, 1867–1939. See G.'s *capsule, method.*

**Gersh,** Isidore, U. S. histologist, *1907. See Altmann-G. *method.*

**Gerstmann** (gairst'mahn), Josef, Vienna neurologist, *1887. See G. *syndrome.*

**gestagen** (jes'tă-jen). Inclusive term used to denote any one of several gestagenic substances, which are usually steroid hormones.

**gestagen'ic.** Inducing progestational effects in the uterus.

**gestalt** (gĕ-stahlt) [ Ger. shape ]. A system of phenomena so integrated as to constitute a functional unit with properties not derivable from its parts.

**gestalt'ism** [ see gestalt ]. The theory in psychology that the objects of mind come as complete forms or configurations which cannot be split into parts; *e.g.,* a square is perceived as such rather than as four discrete lines.

**gestation** (jes-ta'shun) [ L. *gestatio,* from *gesto,* pp. *gestatus,* to bear ]. Pregnancy. There is considerable breed variation within the species, as well as individual variation, in the length of the g. period.

*Gestation periods of common domesticated animals (in days)*

| Species | Range | Average |
|---|---|---|
| Ass | 365–375 | 370 |
| Horse | 329–346 | 340 |
| Cow | 273–291 | 282 |
| Sheep | 143–152 | 148 |
| Goat | 148–156 | 148 |
| Swine | 111–116 | 114 |
| Dog | 58–63 | 60 |
| Cat | 56–65 | 63 |
| Rabbit | 30–32 | 32 |
| Guinea pig | 67–68 | 68 |
| Rat | 21–22 | 22 |
| Mouse | 18–20 | |

**gestosis,** pl. **gestoses** (jes-to'sis) [ L. *gesto,* to carry, to bear, + G. suffix *-osis,* condition ]. A disorder of pregnancy.

**gesture.** (jes'chur) [ L. *gestus,* movement, gesture ]. Any movement expressive of an idea, opinion, or emotion.

**suicide g.,** an apparent attempt at suicide by someone wishing to attract attention, gain sympathy, or achieve some goal other than self-destruction.

**Getsowa's adenoma.** See under adenoma.

**Gey's solution.** See under solution.

**GFR.** Abbreviation for glomerular filtration *rate.*

**GH.** Abbreviation for growth hormone (somatotropin, *q. v.*).

**ghee** (ge) [ English spelling of Hindu *ghi* ]. A clarified butter in India made from cow or buffalo milk that has been coagulated before churning. An emollient, a dressing for wounds, and a food. Also used as an unguent by the Brahmins in religious ceremonies.

**Gheel colony.** See under colony.

**Ghon,** Anton, Prague pathologist, 1866–1936. See G. and Sachs *bacillus,* G.'s *focus,* primary *lesion, tubercle.*

**GHRF, GH-RF.** Abbreviation for growth hormone-releasing factor (somatoliberin, *q. v.*).

**GHRH, GH-RH.** Abbreviation for growth hormone-releasing hormone (somatoliberin, *q. v.*).

**Giacomini** (jah-ko-me'ne), Carlo, Italian anatomist, 1841–1898. See *band of* G., *frenulum of* G., uncus *band of* G.

**Giannuzzi** (jahn-noot'tse), Italian anatomist, 1839–1876. See G.'s *cells, crescents, demilunes.*

**Gianotti,** F. See G.-Crosti *syndrome.*

**giantism** (ji'an-tizm). Gigantism.

**Giard** (je-ar'), Alfred, French biologist, 1846–1908. Gave his name to *Giardia.*

**Giardia** (je-ar'de-ah) [ A. *Giard* ]. A genus of parasitic flagellates that parasitize the small intestine of many mammals, including most domestic animals and man. Many species have been described, but recent workers have suggested that these should be reduced to only two or three species.

**G. bo'vis,** occurs in the small intestine of cattle.

**G. ca'nis,** occurs in the small intestine of dogs.

**G. ca'ti,** occurs in the small and large intestines of cats.

**G. lam'blia,** formerly called *G. intestinalis, G. mesnili,* and *Lamblia intestinalis;* a flattened, heart-shaped organism (10 to 20 μ in length) with eight flagella; it attaches itself to the intestinal mucosa by means of a pair of sucking organs; it is usually asymptomatic except in heavy infections, when it may interfere with absorption of fats and produce flatulence, steatorrhea, and acute discomfort; it is the common species of *G.* in man, but is also found in pigs.

**giardiasis** (je'ar-di'ā-sis). Lambliasis; infection with *Giardia lamblia,* giving rise to diarrheic or dysenteric symptoms.

**chinchilla g.,** an intestinal infection of chinchilla characterized by diarrhea, anorexia, lassitude, and frequently death, believed to be caused by the presence of large numbers of *Giardia.*

**gibberellins** (jib'er-el'inz). Substances produced by the fungus *Gibberella fujikuroi,* which behave as plant growth hormones.

**gibberish** (jib'er-ish, gib'er-ish). Unintelligible and incoherent language.

**gibbon** (gib'on) [ Fr. ]. A genus of anthropoid apes, *Hylobates,* of the superfamily Hominoidea.

**gibbous** (gib'us) [ L. *gibbosus* ]. Humped; humpbacked.

**Gibbs,** J. Willard, American mathematician and physicist, 1839–1903. See G.-Donnan *equilibrium,* G.-Helmholtz *equation,* Helmholtz-G. *theory,* G.'s *theorem,* G.'s *free energy.*

**gibbus** (gib'us) [ L. a hump ]. Extreme kyphosis, hump, or hunch; a deformity of spine in which there is a sharply angulated segment, the apex of the angle being posterior.

**giblets** (jib'lets) [ O. E. *gibelet* ]. Edible viscera of fowl.

**Gibney,** Virgil P., American orthopedist, 1847–1927. See G.'s fixation *bandage.*

**Gibson,** George A., Scottish physician, 1854–1913. See G. *murmur.*

**Gibson,** Kasson C., U. S. dentist, 1849–1925. See G.'s *bandage.*

**gid.** Staggers (2).

**Giemsa** (gēm'zah), Gustav, Hamburg bacteriologist, 1867–1948. See G. *stain.*

**Gierke** (gēr'keh), Edgar von, German pathologist, *1877. See G.'s *disease.*

**Gierke** (gēr'keh), Hans P. B., German anatomist, 1847–1886. See G.'s respiratory *bundle.*

**Giffard,** W., English midwife, †1731. See G.'s *maneuver.*

**Gifford,** Harold, American ophthalmologist, 1858–1929. See G.'s *operation, reflex, sign.*

**giga-** (gi'gah-) [ G. *gigas,* giant ]. A prefix used in the metric system to signify one billion ($10^9$).

**gigantism** (ji'gan-tizm) [ G. *gigas,* giant ]. Giantism; gigantosoma; a condition of abnormal size, or overgrowth, of the entire body or of any of its parts.

**acromegalic g.,** g. in which the signs of acromegaly are present along with the abnormally great height; a form of pituitary g., *q. v.*

**cerebral g.,** a syndrome characterized by increased birth weight and length (above 90th percentile); accelerated growth rate for the first 4 or 5 years without elevation of serum growth hormone levels, then reversion to normal growth rate; characteristic facies with prognathism, hypertelorism, antimongoloid slant, and dolichocephalic skull; moderate mental retardation; and impaired coordination.

**eunuchoid g.,** g. with deficient development of sexual organs; may be of pituitary or gonadal origin.

**pituitary g.,** a form of g. caused by hypersecretion of pituitary growth hormone; a rare disorder commonly the result of a pituitary adenoma; the life span ordinarily does not exceed three decades.

**primor'dial g.,** unusually large size from birth due to familial or genetic factors and not to hyperpituitarism.

**giganto-** (ji-gan'to-) [ G. *gigas,* giant ]. Combining form meaning huge, or gigantic.

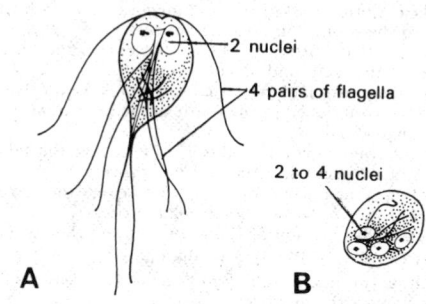

*Giardia lamblia*

A, trophozoite; B, cyst. (From Najarian, H. H.: *Textbook of Medical Parasitology,* The Williams & Wilkins Co., 1967.)

**gigantoblast** (ji-gan'to-blast) [ giganto- + G. *blastos*, germ ]. Gigantochromoblast; an unusually large erythroblast, or nucleated immature red blood cell.

**gigantochromoblast** (ji-gan'to-kro'mo-blast) [ giganto- + G. *chrōma*, color, + *blastos*, germ ]. Gigantoblast.

**gigantocyte** (ji-gan'to-sit) [ giganto- + G. *kytos*, cell ]. 1. A giant cell. 2. An abnormally large erythrocyte; macrocyte.

**gigantomastia** (ji-gan'to-mas'tī-ah) [ giganto- + G. *mastos*, breast ]. Massive hypertrophy of the breast.

**Gigantorhynchus** (ji-gan'to-ring'kus) [ giganto- + G. *rhynchos*, snout ]. See *Macracanthorynchus* and *Moniliformis*.

**gigantosoma** (ji-gan-to-so'mah) [ giganto- + G. *sōma*, body ]. Gigantism.

**Gigli** (jēl'ye), Leonardo, Italian gynecologist, 1863–1908. See G.'s *operation, saw*.

**Gilbert**, Nicholas A., French physician, 1858–1927. See G.'s *disease*.

**Gilbert**, William, English physicist, 1544–1603. Gave his name to gilbert.

**gilbert** [ W. *Gilbert* ]. The unit of magnetomotive force or magnetic potential.

**Gilchrist**, Thomas C., American physician, 1862–1927. See G.'s *disease, mycosis*.

**Gilford**, Hastings, English physician, 1861–1941. See Hutchinson-G. *disease, syndrome*.

**Gill**, A. Bruce, American surgeon, *1876. See G.'s bone-block *operation*.

**Gilles de la Tourette** (zhēl-dē-lă-too-ret'), Georges, Paris physician, 1857–1904. See G. de la T.'s *disease, syndrome*.

**Gillette** (ge'let), Eugène P., French surgeon, 1836–1886. See G.'s suspensory *ligament*.

**Gilliam**, David Tod, American gynecologist, 1844–1923. See G.'s *operation*.

**Gillies** (gil'lēs), Sir Harold D., English surgeon, 1882–1960. See G.'s *operation*, Filatov-G. tubed *pedicle*.

**Gillmore needle.** See under needle.

**Gill Wylie.** See Wylie.

**gilt.** A young sow, usually under one year of age and before she has farrowed a litter.

**Gimbernat**, Antonio de, Spanish surgeon, 1734–1816. See G.'s *ligament*.

**ginger** (jin'jer) (BP). Zingiber; the dried rhizome of *Zingiber officinale* (family Zingiberaceae), known in commerce as Jamaica g., African g., and Cochin g. The outer cortical layers are often either partially or completely removed. Carminative and flavoring agent.
  **Chinese g.,** galangal.
  **Indian g.,** *Asarum canadense*.
  **g. oleoresin,** carminative, stimulant, and flavoring agent.
  **wild g.,** *Asarum canadense*.

**gingili oil.** Sesame oil.

**gingiva**, gen. and pl. **gingi'vae** (jin'jī-vah) [ L. ] [ NA ]. The gum; the dense fibrous tissue, covered by mucous membrane, that envelops the alveolar processes of the upper and lower jaws and surrounds the necks of the teeth.
  **alveolar g.,** gingival tissue supplied to the alveolar bone.
  **attached g.,** that part of the oral mucosa which is firmly bound to the tooth and alveolar process.
  **buccal g.,** that portion of the g. that covers the buccal surfaces of the teeth and alveolar process.
  **free g.,** that portion of the g. that surrounds the tooth and is not directly attached to the tooth surface; the outer wall of the gingival sulcus.
  **labial g.,** that portion of the g. that covers the labial surfaces of the teeth and the alveolar process.
  **lingual g.,** that portion of the g. that covers the lingual surfaces of the teeth and the alveolar process.
  **septal g.,** that portion of the g. that covers the septum.

**gingival** (jin'jī-val). Relating to the gums.

**gingivalgia** (jin'jī-val'jī-ah) [ gingiva + G. *algos*, pain ]. Diffuse pain in the gingiva.

**gingivectomy** (jin'jī-vek'to-mī) [ gingiva + G. *ektomē*, excision ]. Surgical resection of unsupported gingival tissue.

**gingivitis** (jin-jī-vi'tis) [ gingiva + G. suffix -*itis*, inflammation ]. Inflammation of the gingival tissue.
  **acute necrotizing ulcerative g.,** Vincent's *disease*.
  **afunctional g.,** inflammation of the gingiva caused by lack of function.
  **chronic g.,** a low grade inflammation of the marginal gingiva without resorption of underlying alveolar bone.
  **chronic desquamative g.,** chronic desquamative gingivosis; a diffuse or patchy, often painful erythematous area of the gingiva with loss of stippling. It is frequently seen in females and histologically represents an alteration in the connective tissue associated with epithelial atrophy, and is of hormonal etiology.
  **cotton-roll g.,** ulcerous or membranoulcerous lesions of the gingiva produced by the desquamative trauma of removing cotton rolls from the mouth.
  **diabetic g.,** inflammation of gingiva frequently seen in uncontrolled diabetes.
  **Dilantin hyperplastic g.,** hyperplastic gingivae caused by ingestion of diphenylhydantoin.
  **fusospirillary g.,** ulceromembranous g.
  **hormonal g.,** enlargement of the gingiva, especially during pregnancy and puberty, due to a hormonal disturbance.
  **leukemic hyperplastic g.,** enlarged gingiva due to infiltration of leukemic cells.
  **marginal g.,** inflammation of marginal gingiva (not involving bone).
  **necrotizing ulcerative g.,** Vincent's *disease*.
  **pregnancy g.,** inflammatory changes in the gingiva which appear during gestation.
  **proliferative g.,** inflammatory changes in the gingiva characterized by proliferation of the gingival components.
  **suppurating g.,** a chronic inflammation of the gingival tissues characterized by a suppurative exudate.
  **ul'ceromem'branous g.,** Vincent's *disease*.

**gingivo-** (jin'jī-vo-) [ L. *gingiva, q.v.* ]. Combining form relating to the gingivae.

**gingivoaxial** (jin'jī-vo-ak'sī-al). Pertaining to the line angle formed by the gingival and axial walls of a cavity (see line *angle*).

**gingivoectomy** (jin'jī-vo-ek'to-mī). Gingivectomy.

**gingivoglossitis** (jin'jī-vo-glos-si'tis). Uloglossitis; inflammation of both the tongue and gingival tissues. See also stomatitis.

**gin'givola'bial.** Refers to the line angle formed by the junction of the gingival and labial walls of a (class III or IV) cavity (see line *angle*).

**gingivolinguax'ial.** Refers to the point (trihedral) angle formed by gingival, lingual, and axial walls of a cavity (see point *angle*).

**gingivo-osseous** (jin'jī-vo-os'e-us). Referring to the gingiva and its underlying bone.

**gin'givoplas'ty.** A surgical procedure that reshapes and recontours the gingival tissue in order to attain esthetic, physiologic, and functional form.

**gingivosis** (jin'jī-vo'sis). A dystrophic gingival disease observed in malnourished and chronically ailing hospitalized children in postwar Italy. The course of the disease is cyclic and passes through three definite stages. Recent investigators have included cases of chronic desquamative gingivitis under the over-all classification of g.
  **chronic desquamative g.,** chronic desquamative *gingivitis*.

**gingivostomatitis** (jin'jī-vo-sto'mă-ti'tis) [ gingivo- + G. *stoma*, month, + suffix -*itis*, inflammation ]. Inflammation of the gingival tissues of the oral cavity.
  **herpetic g.,** g. due to herpes simplex virus.

**gingivostomatosis** (jin'jī-vo-sto'mă-to'sis) [ gingivo- + G. *stoma*, mouth, + suffix -*osis*, condition ]. Any disease of both the gingiva and portions of the oral mucosa.
  **white folded g.,** (1) familial white folded *dysplasia*; (2) *nevus* spongiosus albus mucosae.

**ginglyform** (jing'glī-form, ging-) [ G. *ginglymos*, a hinge joint, + L. *forma*, form ]. Ginglymoid.

**ginglymoarthrodial** (jing'glī-mo-ar-thro'dī-al, ging-). Denoting a joint having the form of both ginglymus and arthrodia, or hinge joint and sliding joint.

**ginglymoid** (jing'glī-moyd, ging-) [ G. *ginglymos*, a hinge joint, + *eidos*, resembling ]. Relating to or resembling a hinge joint.

**ginglymus** (jing'glī-mus, ging-) [ G. *ginglymos* ] [ NA ]. Hinge joint; a uniaxial joint in which a broad, transversely cylindrical convexity on one bone fits into a corresponding concavity on the other, allowing of motion in one plane only, as in the elbow. See fig. under joint.

**hel'icoid g.,** *articulatio* trochoidea.

**lateral g.,** *articulatio* trochoidea.

**ginseng** (jin'seng) [ Ch. ]. The roots of several species of *Panax* (family Araliaceae), esteemed as of great medicinal virtue by the Chinese, but not used in western medicine.

**Girard,** A. See G.'s *reagent.*

**gir'dle** [ A.S. *gyrdel* ]. 1. A belt; a zone. 2. Cingulum.

**Hitzig's g.,** an analgesic cuirass at the level of the mammae, in the region supplied by the third to sixth dorsal nerves, observed in tabes dorsalis.

**Neptune's g.,** a wet pack applied around the abdomen.

**pelvic g.,** *cingulum* membri inferioris.

**shoulder g.,** *cingulum* membri superioris.

**thoracic g.,** *cingulum* membri superioris.

**Girdner,** John H., New York physician, 1856–1933. See G.'s *probe.*

**girth.** The measure around the body of an animal a little behind the forelegs.

**gitalin** (jit'ă-lin). Amorphous gitalin; GITALIGIN; an extract of *Digitalis purpurea* containing a mixture of glycosides (digitoxin, gitoxin, gitaloxin, and others) and genins; action and uses are similar to those of digitalis, but a more favorable therapeutic index has been claimed for gitalin as compared to other digitalis preparations. Its duration of action is intermediate between that of digitoxin and digoxin.

**githagism** (gith'ă-jism) [ L. *gith*, a plant, Roman coriander, + *ago*, to drive ]. A disease similar to lathyrism, believed to be due to poisoning by seeds of the corn cockle, *Lychnis githago.*

**gitogenin** (jit'o-jen-in). Digin; (25 *R*)-5α-spirostane-2α,3β -diol; the genin of gitonin. A cardiotonic agent.

**gitoxigenin** (jī-tok'sī-jen-in). 3β,14,16β-Trihydroxy-5β,14β-card-20(22)-enolide; 3β,14β,16β-tetrahydroxy-24-nor-20(22)-cholen-23:21-lactone (for cardanolide and cholane structures, see steroids); the aglycone, or genin, of gitoxin.

**gitoxin** (jī-tok'sin). Anhydrogitalin; bigitalin; pseudodigitoxin; a C-3 tridigitoxoside of gitoxigenin; a secondary cardiac glycoside from *Digitalis purpurea* and *D. lanata.*

**git'terzelle** [ Ger. fr. *gitter*, lattice, + *zelle*, cell ]. Compound granule *cell.*

**Giuffrida-Ruggieri** (joof-fre'dah-rood-jer'e), Vincenzo, Italian anthropologist, 1872–1922. See G.-R. *stigma.*

**giz'zard.** The ventriculus, or muscular portion, of the stomach of a bird in which food is ground and mixed with the gastric juice secreted by the proventriculus.

**glabella** (glă-bel'ah) [ L. *glabellus*, hairless, smooth, dim. of *glaber* ]. 1 [ NA ]. A smooth prominence, most marked in the male, on the frontal bone above the root of the nose. 2. The most forward projecting point of the forehead in the midline at the level of the supraorbital ridges; see fig. under craniometric *point.*

**glabel'lad.** Toward the glabella.

**gla'brate.** Glabrous.

**glabrif'icin** [ L. *glaber*, smooth, + *facio*, to make ]. Obsolete term for a variety of antibody that is assumed to cause disintegration of the envelope of a capsulated bacterium.

**gla'brous** [ L. *glaber*, smooth ]. Smooth; hairless; term applied to areas of body where hair does not normally grow, *i.e.*, palms or soles.

**glad'iate** [ L. *gladius*, a sword ]. Sword-shaped; ensiform; xiphoid.

**gladiolus** (glă-di'o-lus, glad'ī-o'lus) [ L. dim. of *gladius*, a sword ]. *Corpus* sterni.

**glair'y.** Mucoid; viscous; resembling the white of egg.

# GLAND

**gland** [ L. *glans*, acorn. GLAN- ]. A secreting organ. The secretion may be poured out upon the surface or into a cavity, or it may be at once taken into the blood without appearing externally; it may be of service to the economy, in digestion, as a lubricant, etc., or it may be purely excrementitious, removing waste and poisonous material from the body.

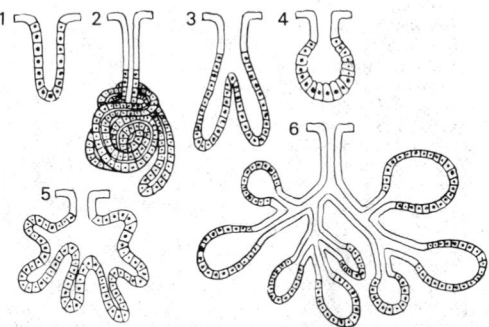

**Types of Glands**

*1,* Simple tubular; *2,* simple coiled tubular; *3,* branched tubular; *4,* simple alveolar; *5.* branched alveolar; *6,* compound alveolar.

**accessory g.,** a small mass of glandular structure, detached from but lying near another and larger g., to which it is similar in structure and probably in function.

**accessory lacrimal g.'s,** *glandulae* lacrimales accessoriae.

**accessory parotid g.,** *glandula* parotis accessoria.

**accessory suprarenal g.'s,** *glandulae* suprarenales accessoriae.

**accessory thyroid g.,** *glandula* thyroidea accessoria.

**acid g.,** oxyntic g.; one of the gastric g.'s secreting the acid of the gastric juice; see *glandulae* gastricae.

**acinotubular g.,** tubuloacinar g.

**acinous g.** (as'in-us), one in which the secretory unit (or units) has a grapelike shape and a very small lumen; *e.g.,* the exocrine part of the pancreas.

**admax'illary g.,** *glandula* parotis accessoria.

**adre'nal g.,** *glandula* suprarenalis.

**aggregate g.'s,** *folliculi* lymphatici aggregati.

**agminate** or **agminated g.'s,** *folliculi* lymphatici aggregati.

**Albarran's g.'s,** Albarran y Dominguez' tubles; minute submucosal glands or branching tubules in the subcervical region of the prostate g., emptying for the most part into the posterior portion of the urethra.

**albu'minous g.,** one that secretes a watery fluid.

**alve'olar g.,** one in which the secretory unit (or units) has a saclike form and an obvious lumen; *e.g.,* the active mammary gland.

**a'nal g.,** (1) one of a number of large sudoriferous g.'s in the mucous membrane of the anus; (2) an incorrect synonym for anal *sac, q. v.*

**anterior lingual g.,** *glandula* lingualis anterior.

**ap'ical g.,** *glandula* lingualis anterior.

**ap'ocrine g.,** a coiled, tubular g. the cells of which were formerly believed to contribute part of their protoplasmic substance to their secretion.

**are'olar g.'s,** *glandulae* areolares.

**arteriococcygeal g.** (ar-te'rī-o-kok-sij'e-al), *corpus* coccygeum.

**aryt'enoid g.'s,** *glandulae* laryngeae.

**Aselli's g.'s,** *nodi* lymphatici mesenterici.

**Avicenna's g.,** an encapsulated tumor.

**ax'illary g.'s,** *nodi* lymphatici axillares.

ax'illary sweat g.'s, glandulae sudoriferae axillares, many of which differ from those of the surface of the body generally in undergoing enlargement at puberty and having an apocrine structure.

**Bartholin's g.,** *glandula* vestibularis major.

**Bauhin's g.,** *glandula* lingualis anterior.

**g.'s of biliary mucosa,** *glandulae* mucosae biliosae.

**Blandin's g.,** *glandula* lingualis anterior.

**Boerhaave's g.'s,** *glandulae* sudoriferae.

**Bowman's g.,** see *glandula* olfactoria.

**bra'chial g.,** one of the lymph nodes of the arm.

**bron'chial g.'s,** (1) *nodus* lymphaticus tracheobronchialis; (2) *nodus* lymphaticus bronchopulmonalis; (3) glandulae bronchiales.

**Bruch's g.'s,** trachoma g.'s; lymph nodes in the palpebral conjunctiva.

**Brunner's g.'s,** *glandulae* duodenales.

**buccal g.'s,** *glandulae* buccales.

**bul'boure'thral g.,** *glandula* bulbourethralis.

**cardiac g.,** a coiled tubular g. located in the cardiac region of the stomach.

**celiac g.'s,** *nodi* lymphatici celiaci.

**ceru'minous g.'s,** *glandulae* ceruminosae.

**cer'vical g.'s,** (1) *nodus* lymphaticus cervicales (2) *glandulae* cervicales uteri.

**Ciaccio's g.'s,** *glandulae* lacrimales accessoriae.

**ciliary g.'s,** *glandulae* ciliares.

**circuma'nal g.'s,** *glandulae* circumanales.

**coccyg'eal g.,** *corpus* coccygeum.

**coil g.,** convoluted g.; a g. whose secretory part is convoluted.

**compound g.,** one whose larger excretory ducts branch repeatedly into smaller ducts which ultimately drain secretory units.

**conjunctival g.'s,** *glandulae* conjunctivales.

**convoluted g.,** coil g.

**Cowper's g.,** *glandula* bulbourethralis.

**crop g.,** cells in the crop of male and female pigeons and doves that secrete a caseous or milklike material with which the bird feeds its young. It is stimulated to secrete by prolactin, the lactogenic hormone of the anterior hypophysis, and is used as a test object for assaying the activity of this hormone.

**ductless g.'s,** *glandulae* sine ductibus.

**duodenal g.,** *glandula* duodenalis.

**Duverney's g.,** *glandula* vestibularis major.

**Ebner's g.'s,** serous g.'s of the tongue opening in the bottom of the trough surrounding the circumvallate papillae.

**eccrine g.,** a coiled tubular sweat g. (other than apocrine g.'s) that occurs on almost all parts of the body.

**ecdysial g.'s,** prothoracic g.'s; thoracid g.'s; peritracheal g.'s; ventral g.'s; insect structures that originate from the ectoderm of the ventrocaudal part of the head and serve as a source of ecdysone.

**Egli's g.'s,** small, inconstant mucous g.'s of the ureter and renal pelvis.

**en'docrine g.'s,** *glandulae* sine ductibus.

**esopha'geal g.'s,** *glandulae* esophageae.

**excre'tory g.,** a g. separating excrementitious or waste material from the blood.

**exocrine g.,** a g. from which secretions reach a free surface of the body by ducts.

**external salivary g.,** *glandula* parotis.

**follic'ular g.,** a g. consisting of follicles.

**fundus g.'s,** *glandulae* gastricae.

**Galeati's g.'s,** *glandulae* intestinales.

**Galen's innominate g.,** pars palpebralis glandulae lacrimalis; see *glandula* lacrimalis.

**gastric g.'s,** *glandulae* gastricae.

**Gay's g.'s,** *glandulae* circumanales.

**genal g.'s,** *glandulae* buccales.

**gen'ital g.,** (1) testis; (2) ovarium.

**Gley's g.'s,** *glandulae* parathyroideae.

**glomiform g.'s,** *glandulae* glomiformes.

**greater vestibular g.,** *glandula* vestibularis major.

**Guérin's g.'s,** *glandulae* urethrales urethrae femininae.

**Harder's g., Harderian g.,** (1) the deep g. of the semilunar conjunctival fold or "third eyelid" found in animals such as pig and deer; (2) a misnomer for the superficial g. of the semilunar conjunctival fold in the dog. Not present in man.

**Havers' g.'s,** synovial g.'s; collections of adipose tissue in the hip, knee, and other joints, covered by synovial membrane, thought by Havers to be g.'s secreting the synovia.

**hemal g.,** hemal *node*.

**hematopoiet'ic g.,** a blood-forming organ, such as the spleen.

**he'molymph g.,** hemal *node*.

**hi'bernating g.** brown *fat*.

**holocrine g.,** a g. whose secretion consists of disintegrated cells of the g. itself; *e.g.,* a sebaceous g., opposed to merocrine g.

**in'guinal g.,** *nodus* lymphaticus inguinalis.

**internal salivary g.,** the sublingual and submandibular g.'s regarded as one.

**g.'s of internal secretion,** *glandulae* sine ductibus.

**in'terre'nal g.,** interrenal *body*.

**interscap'ular g.,** brown *fat*.

**intersti'tial g.,** see interstitial *cells*.

**intestinal g.'s,,** *glandulae* intestinales.

**intraepithelial g.'s,** accumulations of glandular cells that lie within an epithelium, as those of the urethra.

**jugular g.,** signal *node*.

**Knoll's g.'s,** g.'s in the ventricular folds of the larynx (false vocal cords).

**Kölliker's g.'s,** *glandulae* olfactoriae.

**Krause's g.'s,** (1) *glandulae* lacrimales accessoriae; (2) g.'s in the mucous membrane of the tympanic cavity.

**labial g.'s,** *glandulae* labiales.

**lac'rimal g.,** *glandula* lacrimalis.

**lactif'erous g.,** *glandula* mammaria.

**laryngeal g.'s,** *glandulae* laryngeae.

**lesser vestibular g.'s,** *glandulae* vestibulares minores.

**Lieberkühn's g.'s,** *glandulae* intestinales.

**Littre's g.'s,** *glandulae* urethrales urethrae masculinae.

**Luschka's g.,** (1) *tonsilla* pharyngea; (2) *corpus* coccygeum.

**Luschka's cystic g.'s,** minute glandular lobules occupying little oval depressions in the wall of the gallbladder near the neck.

**lymph g.,** *nodus* lymphaticus.

**Malpighian g.'s,** *folliculi* lymphatici lienales.

**mam'mary g.,** *glandula* mammaria.

**marrow-lymph g.,** a type of hemal node, resembling the bone marrow in structure and probable function.

**master g.,** *hypophysis* cerebri.

**max'illary g.,** *glandula* submandibularis.

**Mehlis' g.,** a petal-like arrangement of glandular projections that surround the trematode (fluke) or cestode (tapeworm) ootype in the center of the ovarian complex; function is uncertain; it is not the "shell gland" as once thought, but may serve a lubricatory or hormonal function.

**Meibomian g.'s,** *glandulae* tarsales.

**merocrine g.,** a g. that is repeatedly functional, not destroyed while secreting; opposite of holocrine g.

**Méry's g.,** *glandula* bulbourethralis.

**mesenter'ic g.,** *nodus* lymphaticus mesentericus.

**me'trial g.,** collections of granular epithelial cells in the uterine muscle beneath the placenta that develop during pregnancy in certain animals (*e.g.,* mouse, rat). The cells are thought to disintegrate and pass (as a holocrine secretion) into the afferent placental vessels to furnish nutriment for the embryo.

**mil'iary g.'s,** *glandulae* sudoriferae.

**milk g.,** *glandula* mammaria.

**mixed g.,** (1) a g. that contains both serous and mucous secretory units; (2) a g. that is both exocrine and endocrine, *e.g.,* the pancreas.

**molar g.'s,** *glandulae* molares.

**Moll's g.'s,** *glandulae* ciliares.

**Montgomery's g.'s,** *glandulae* areolares.

**g.'s of mouth,** *glandulae* oris.

**mucilag'inous g.,** one of the synovial villi, supposed by Havers to secrete the synovia.

**mucip'arous g.,** *glandula* mucosa.

**mucous g.,** *glandula* mucosa.

**mucous g.'s of auditory tube,** *glandulae* tubariae.

**Nabothian g.,** Nabothian *cyst*.

**nasal g.'s,** *glandulae* nasales.

**Nuhn's g.,** *glandula* lingualis anterior.

**odorif'erous g.,** (1) a g., such as Tyson's g., the secretion of which has a strong odor; (2) see scent g.'s.

**oil g.'s,** (1) *glandulae* sebaceae; (2) uropygial g.

**olfactory g.'s,** *glandulae* olfactoriae.

**optic g.'s,** paired structures in cephalopod brain that secrete a gonadotropic principle.

**oxyn'tic g.,** acid g.

**Pacchionian g.'s,** *granulationes* arachnoideales.

**palatine g.'s,** *glandulae* palatinae.

**pal'pebral g.'s,** *glandulae* tarsales.

**parathy'roid g.,** *glandulae* parathyroideae.

**paraurethral g.'s,** *glandulae* urethrales urethrae femininae.

**parotid g.,** *glandula* parotis.

**pec'toral g.'s,** see *nodi* lymphatici axillares.

**peptic g.,** a pepsin-secreting g., see *glandulae* gastricae.

**perianal odoriferous g.'s,** see scent g.'s.

**peritracheal g.'s,** ecdysial g.'s.

**perspi'ratory g.'s,** *glandulae* sudoriferae.

**Peyer's g.'s,** *folliculi* lymphatici aggregati.

**pharyn'geal g.'s,** *glandulae* pharyngeae.

**Philip's g.'s,** enlarged deep g.'s just above the clavicle, found always in children with pulmonary tuberculosis and occasionally in others.

**pilous g.,** a sebaceous g. emptying into the hair follicle.

**pin'eal g.,** *corpus* pineale.

**pitu'itary g.,** hypophysis.

**Poirier's g.,** a lymph node on the uterine artery where it crosses the ureter.

**preen g.,** uropygial g.

**prehyoid g.,** *glandula* thyroidea accessoria.

**preputial g.'s,** *glandulae* preputiales.

**prostate g.,** prostata.

**prothoracic g.'s,** ecdysial g.'s.

**pylor'ic g.'s,** *glandulae* pyloricae.

**rac'emose g.,** one in which the g. has the appearance of a bunch of grapes if viewed as a three-dimensional reconstruction, *e.g.,* a compound acinous or alveolar g.

**Rivinus' g.,** *glandulae* sublingualis.

**Rosenmüller's g.,** *node* of Cloquet.

**sac'cular g.,** a single alveolar g.

**sal'ivary g. of abdomen,** pancreas.

**scent g.'s,** cutaneous g.'s producing odoriferous secretions (pheromones or recognition odors); they may be located on different parts of the body, *e.g.,* under the chin (rabbit); between the digits (goat); on the medial surface of the metatarsus (deer), in the preorbital fold (antelope); in the occipital region (camel); on the flank (hamster); in the perianal region and on the dorsum of the tail base (carnivores).

**seba'ceous g.'s,** *glandulae* sebaceae.

**sen'tinel g.,** a single enlarged lymph node in the omentum that may be an indication of an ulcer opposite to it in the greater or lesser curvature of the stomach.

**seromucous g.,** *glandula* seromucosa.

**serous g.,** *glandula* serosa.

**Serres' g.'s,** epithelial cell rests found in the subepithelial connective tissue in the palate of the newborn, similar to those found in the gingivae.

**sexual g.,** (1) testis; (2) ovary. See also gonad.

**Skene's g.'s,** *glandulae* urethrales urethrae femininae.

**solitary g.,** one of the lymphatic follicles of the intestine.

**sublingual g.,** *glandula* sublingualis.

**submandibular g.,** *glandula* submandibularis.

**submax'illary g.,** *glandula* submandibularis.

**sudoriferous g.'s,** *glandulae* sudoriferae.

**suprahy'oid g.,** *glandula* thyroidea accessoria.

**suprarenal g.,** *glandula* suprarenalis.

**Suzanne's g.,** a small mucous g. in the floor of the mouth.

**sweat g.'s,** *glandulae* sudoriferae.

**synovial g.'s,** Havers' g.'s.

**target g.,** the effector that functions when stimulated by the internal secretion of another gland or by some other stimulus.

**tarsal g.'s,** *glandulae* tarsales.

**Terson's g.'s,** *glandulae* conjunctivales.

**Theile's g.'s,** glandular structures in the walls of the cystic duct and, in small numbers, in the pelvis of the gallbladder.

**thoracic g.'s,** ecdysial g.'s.

**thymus g.,** thymus.

**thyroid g.,** *glandula* thyroidea.

**Tiedemann's g.,** *glandula* vestibularis major.

**tracheal g.'s,** *glandulae* tracheales.

**tracho'ma g.'s,** Bruch's g.'s.

**g.'s of tube,** *glandulae* tubariae.

**tu'bular g.,** one composed of one or more tubules ending in a blind extremity.

**tubuloacinar g.,** acinotubular g.; one whose secretory elements are elongated acini.

**tubuloalveolar g.,** one that has secretory units of short tubules.

**tympan'ic g.,** tympanic body; (1) one of the mucous g.'s in the mucosa of the tympanic cavity; (2) a small, reddish, ganglionic mass lying on the tympanic nerve in the tympanic canal.

**Tyson's g.'s,** *glandulae* preputiales.

**unicellular g.,** a single secretory cell such as a mucous goblet cell.

**urethral g.'s,** *glandulae* urethrales.

**uropygial g.,** glandula uropygius; oil g. (2); preen g.; a compound alveolar g. of birds located on the dorsum of the tail or pygostyle; the secretion of this g. (fatty acids and wax) exits from a papilla on the dorsal surface at the base of the tail feathers; the bird applies the substance to its feathers by means of the bill when preening. The uropygial g. is lacking in some species but its waterproofing ability is essential to water birds.

**uterine g.'s,** *glandulae* uterinae.

**vag'inal g.,** one of the mucous g.'s in the mucous membrane of the vagina.

**vascular g.** hemal *node.*

**ventral g.'s,** ecdysial g.'s.

**ves'ical g.,** one of a number of mucous follicles, not true g.'s, in the mucous membrane near the neck of the bladder.

**vestib'ular g.,** *glandula* vestibularis.

**vulvovag'inal g.,** *glandula* vestibularis major.

**Waldeyer's g.'s,** coil g.'s near the margins of the eyelids.

**Wasmann's g.'s,** *glandulae* gastricae.

**Weber's g.'s,** muciparous g.'s at the border of the tongue on either side posteriorly.

**Wepfer's g.'s,** *glandulae* duodenales.

**Wölfler's g.,** *glandula* thyroidea accessoria.

**Wolfring's g.'s,** *glandulae* lacrimales accessoriae.

**Zeis' g.'s,** sebaceous g.'s opening into the follicles of the eyelashes.

---

**glan'derous.** Relating to glanders.

**glan'ders** [ O. Fr. *glandres,* glands ]. A chronic debilitating disease of horses and other equids, as well as some members of the cat family, caused by *Actinobacillus mallei.* G. is transmissible to man. It attacks the mucous membranes of the nostrils of the horse, attended with an increased and vitiated secretion and discharge of mucus, and enlargement and induration of the glands of the lower jaw.

**glandilem'ma** [ L. *glandula,* gland, + G. *lemma,* sheath ]. The capsule of a gland.

**glandula,** pl. **glan'dulae** (glan'du-lah) [ L. gland, dim. of *glans,* acorn. GLAN- ] [ NA ]. A glandule or small gland.

**glandulae areola'res** [ NA ], areolar glands; Montgomery's glands; a number of cutaneous glands forming small, rounded projections from the surface of the areola of the mamma.

**g. atrabilia'ris** [ so called because in the 17th and 18th centuries the suprarenal glands were believed by some to be the source of black bile ], g. suprarenalis.

**g. basila'ris,** hypophysis.

**glandulae bronchia'les** [ NA ], bronchial glands; mucous and seromucous glands whose secretory units lie outside of the muscle of the bronchi.

**glandulae bucca'les** [ NA ], buccal glands; genal glands; numerous racemose, mucous, or serous glands in the submucous tissue of the cheeks.

**g. bulbourethra'lis** [ NA ], bulbourethral gland; antiparastata; antiprostate; Cowper's gland; Méry's gland; one of two small compound racemose glands, which produce a mucoid secretion, lying side by side along the membranous urethra just above the bulb of the corpus spongiosum; they discharge through a small duct into the spongy portion of the urethra.

**glandulae cerumino'sae** [ NA ], ceruminous glands; apocrine sudoriferous glands in the external acoustic meatus.

**glandulae cervica'les uteri** [ NA ], cervical glands of the uterus; branched mucus-secreting glands in the mucosa of the cervix.

**glandulae cilia'res** [ NA ], ciliary glands; glands of Moll; a number of modified apocrine sudoriferous glands in the eyelids, with ducts that usually open into the follicles of the eyelashes.

**glandulae circumana'les** [ NA ], circumanal glands; Gay's glands; large apocrine sweat glands surrounding the anus.

**glandulae conjunctiva'les** [ NA ], conjunctival glands; Terson's glands; clusters of mucous cells in the conjunctival epithelium, most numerous on the bulbar conjunctiva.

**glandulae cu'tis** [ NA ], any of the glands of the skin.

**glandulae duodena'les** [ NA ], duodenal glands; glands of Brunner; Wepfer's glands; small, branched, coiled tubular glands which occur mostly in the submucosa of the first part of the duodenum. They secrete a mucoid substance.

**glandulae esopha'geae** [ NA ], esophageal glands; a variable number of small compound mucous glands in the submucosa of the esophagus, similar to the cardiac glands.

**glandulae gas'tricae** [ NA ], glandulae propriae [ NA ]; gastric glands; gastric follicles; fundus glands; Wasmann's glands; branched tubular glands lying in the mucosa of the fundus and body of the stomach. Such glands contain parietal cells which secrete hydrochloric acid, zymogen cells which produce pepsin and mucous cells.

**glandulae glomifor'mes** [ NA ], glomiform glands; tubular glands of the skin, the blind extremity of which, the secretory part, *glomerulus*, is coiled in the form of a ball.

**glandulae intestina'les** [ NA ], intestinal glands or follicles; follicles or crypts of Lieberkühn; Galeati's glands; the tubular glands in the mucous membrane of the small and large intestines.

**glandulae labia'les** [ NA ], labial glands; mucous or serous glands in the submucous tissue of the lips.

**g. lacrima'lis** [ NA ], lacrimal gland; the gland that secretes tears; it consists of 6 to 12 separate compound tubuloalveolar serous glands which are located in the upper lateral part of the orbit and is partially divided into a smaller *pars palpebralis* (Galen's innominate gland) and a larger *pars orbitalis* by the lateral horn of the aponeurosis of the levator palpebrae muscle. See fig. under *apparatus* lacrimalis.

**glandulae lacrima'les accesso'riae** [ NA ], accessory lacrimal glands; Krause's glands (1); Wolfring's glands; Ciaccio's glands; minute glands in the subconjunctiva of the eyelid, secreting a watery fluid.

**glandulae laryn'geae** [ NA ], laryngeal glands; a large number of mixed glands in the mucous membrane of the larynx; they are called, according to their situation, anterior, middle, and posterior.

**g. lingua'lis ante'rior** [ NA ], anterior lingual gland; apical gland; gland of Nuhn, Bauhin, or Blandin; one of the small mixed glands deeply placed near the apex of the tongue on each side of the frenulum.

**g. mamma'ria** [ NA ], mammary gland; lactiferous gland; milk gland; the compound alveolar gland that forms the breast. It consists of 15 to 24 lobes separated by adipose tissue and fibrous septa; each lobe consists of many lobules. The parenchyma of the resting gland consists of ducts and the alveoli develop only during pregnancy. See also mamma.

**glandulae mola'res** [ NA ], molar glands; four or five large buccal glands in the neighborhood of the last molar tooth.

**g. muco'sa** [ NA ], mucous gland; muciparous gland; a gland that secretes mucus.

**glandulae muco'sae bilio'sae** [ NA ], glands of the biliary mucosa; small, mucous, tubuloalveolar glands in the mucosa of the larger bile ducts and especially in the neck of the gallbladder.

**glandulae nasa'les** [ NA ], nasal glands; seromucous glands in the respiratory region of the nasal mucous membrane.

**glandulae olfacto'riae** [ NA ], olfactory glands; Kölliker's glands; branched tubuloalveolar serous secreting glands (of Bowman) in the mucous membrane of the olfactory region of the nasal cavity.

**glandulae oris,** [ NA ], glands of the mouth; glands that empty into the oral cavity.

**glandulae palati'nae** [ NA ], palatine glands; a number of racemose mucous glands in the posterior half of the submucous tissue covering the hard palate.

**g. parathyroi'dea** [ NA ], parathyroid gland; epithelial body; one of Gley's glands or Sandström's bodies; one of two small paired endocrine glands, *superior* and *inferior*, usually found embedded in the connective tissue capsule on the posterior surface of the thyroid gland; they are concerned with the metabolism of calcium and phosphorus. The parenchyma is composed of chief and oxyphilic cells arranged in anastomosing cords.

**g. paro'tis** [ NA ], parotid gland; external salivary gland; the largest of the salivary glands; one of two glands situated below and in front of the ear, on either side, extending from the angle of the jaw to the zygoma and backward to the sternocleidomastoid muscle. It is subdivided into a *pars superficialis* and a *pars profunda* by emerging branches of the facial nerve. It discharges through the parotid duct. The parotid gland is a compound, acinous gland the secretory units of which are all serous in the adult human.

**g. parotis accesso'ria** [ NA ], accessory parotid gland; an occasional islet of parotid tissue separate from the mass of the gland, lying anteriorly just above the commencement of the parotid duct.

**glandulae pharyn'gea** [ NA ], pharyngeal glands; racemose mucous glands beneath the mucous membrane of the pharynx.

**g. pituita'ria** [ NA ], hypophysis.

**glandulae preputia'les** [ NA ], preputial glands; Tyson's glands; sebaceous glands of the corona glandis and inner surface of the prepuce.

**glandulae pro'priae** [ NA ], alternate term for glandulae gastricae.

**g. prostatica,** prostata.

**glandulae pylor'icae** [ NA ], pyloric glands; the coiled, tubular glands of the pylorus whose cells secrete mucus.

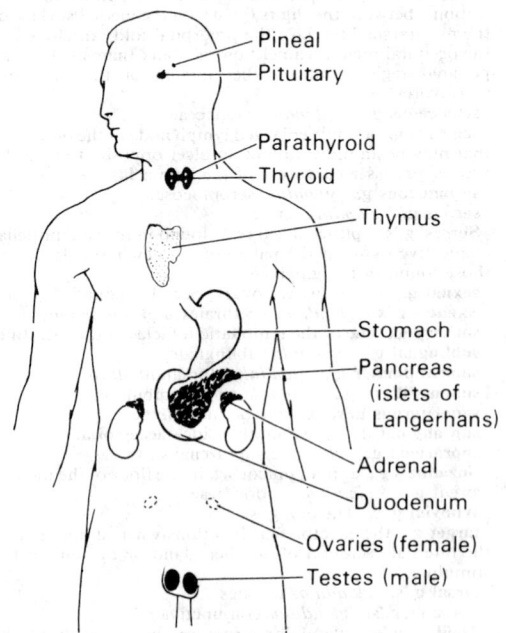

**Positions of the Endocrine Glands**
(From Moment, G. B., and Habermann, H. M.: *Biology: A Full Spectrum*, The Williams & Wilkins Co., Baltimore, 1973.)

**glandulae seba'ceae** [ NA ], sebaceous glands or crypts; oil glands; numerous holocrine glands in the corium that usually open into the hair follicles and secrete an oily, semifluid substance, sebum cutaneum.

**g. seromuco'sa** [ NA ], seromucous gland; (1) a gland in which some of the secretory cells are serous and some mucous; (2) a gland whose cells secrete a fluid intermediate between a watery and a viscous, mucoid substance.

**g. serosa** [ NA ], serous gland; a gland that secretes a watery substance that may or may not contain an enzyme.

**glandulae sine duc'tibus** [ NA ], ductless glands; endocrine glands; glands of internal secretion; glands that have no ducts, their secretions being absorbed directly into the blood.

**g. sublingua'lis** [ NA ], sublingual gland; Rivinus' gland; one of two salivary glands in the floor of the mouth beneath the tongue, discharging through the sublingual ducts. Most of the secretory units in the human gland are mucus-secreting with serous demilunes.

**g. submandibula'ris** [ NA ], submandibular gland; submaxillary gland; one of two salivary glands in the neck, located in the space bounded by the two bellies of the digastric muscle and the angle of the mandible; it discharges through the submandibular duct (Wharton). The secretory units are predominantly serous although a few mucous alveoli, some with serous demilunes, occur.

**glandulae sudoriferae** [ NA ], sudoriferous glands; sweat, miliary, or perspiratory glands; Boerhaave's glands; the coil glands of the skin that secrete the sweat.

**g. suprarena'lis** [ NA ], suprarenal gland or body; adrenal gland, body, or capsule; glandula atrabiliaris (*q.v.*); atrabiliary or suprarenal capsule; epinephros; butterfly adrenal; a flattened, roughly triangular body resting upon the upper end of each kidney; it is one of the ductless glands furnishing internal secretions (epinephrine and norepinephrine from the medulla and steroid hormones from the cortex).

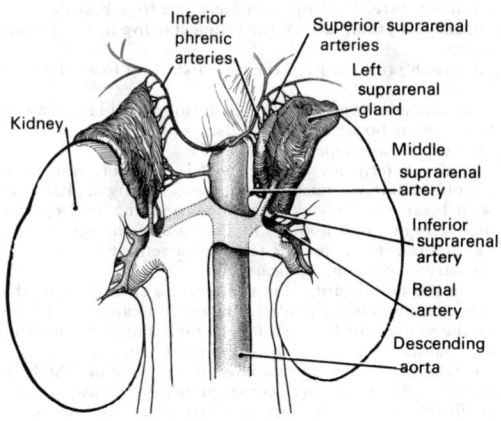

**Glandula Suprarenalis**

**glandulae suprarena'les accesso'riae** [ NA ], accessory suprarenal glands; isolated, often minute, masses of suprarenal tissue sometimes found near the main glands or in the broad ligament or the epididymis.

**glandulae tarsa'les** [ NA ], tarsal or palpebral glands; Meibomian glands; sebaceous glands embedded in the tarsal plate of each eyelid, discharging at the edge of the lid near the posterior border.

**g. thyroi'dea** [ NA ], thyroid gland or body; a ductless gland, consisting of irregularly spheroidal follicles, lying in front and to the sides of the upper part of the trachea. It is of horseshoe shape, with two lateral lobes connected by a narrow central portion, the isthmus; occasionally an elongated offshoot, the pyramidal lobe, passes upward from the isthmus in front of the trachea. It is supplied by branches from the external carotid and subclavian arteries, and its nerves are derived from the middle cervical and cervicothoracic ganglia of the sympathetic system.

**g. thyroi'dea accesso'ria**, pl. **glandulae thyroideae accessoriae** [ NA ], accessory thyroid gland; prehyoid gland; an isolated mass, or one of several such masses, of thyroid tissue, sometimes present in the side of the neck, or just above the hyoid bone (suprahyoid accessory thyroid gland), or even as low down as the arch of the aorta.

**glandulae trachea'les** [ NA ], tracheal glands; numerous tubuloalveolar mixed glands located principally in the submucosa of the trachea; they open into the tracheal lumen through short ducts.

**glandulae tuba'riae** [ NA ], glands of the tube; mucous glands of the auditory tube, located principally near the pharyngeal end of the tube.

**glandulae urethra'les urethrae femini'nae** [ NA ], urethral glands of female urethra; paraurethral glands; Skene's glands; Guérin's glands; numerous mucous glands in the wall of the urethra.

**glandulae urethra'les urethrae masculi'nae** [ NA ], urethral glands of male urethra; Littre's glands; numerous mucous glands in the wall of the pars cavernosa urethrae.

**g. uropy'gius**, uropygial *gland*.

**glandulae uteri'nae** [ NA ], uterine glands; numerous tubular glands in the uterine mucosa.

**g. vestibula'ris major** [ NA ], greater vestibular gland; Bartholin's, Tiedemann's, or Duverney's gland; vulvovaginal gland; one of two mucoid-secreting tubuloalveolar glands on either side of the lower part of the vagina, the equivalent of the bulbourethral glands in the male.

**glandulae vestibula'res mino'res** [ NA ], lesser vestibular glands; a number of minute mucous glands opening on the surface of the vestibule between the orifices of the vagina and urethra.

**glan'dular.** Relating to a gland.

**glandule** (glan'dūl) [ L. *glandula, q.v.* ]. A small gland.

**glan'dulous.** Glandular.

**glans**, pl. **glan'des** [ L. acorn ] [ NA ]. A conical acorn-shaped structure.

**g. clitor'idis** [ NA ], a small mass of erectile tissue capping the body of the clitoris.

**g. penis** [ NA ], balanus; the conical expansion of the corpus spongiosum which forms the head of the penis.

**Glanzmann,** Eduard, Swiss clinician, 1887–1959. See G.'s *disease, thrombasthenia.*

**glaphenine.** GLIFANAN; *N*-(7-chloro-4-quinolyl)anthanilic acid 2,3-dihydroxypropyl ester; anti-inflammatory agent with analgesic properties.

**glare.** A visual disturbance caused by uneven distribution of illumination in the visual field.

**central g.**, g. produced in night driving by the bright lights of an oncoming car; it causes transient peripheral blindness.

**peripheral g.**, g. occurring when there is more light on the eye than on the work; it diminishes visual acuity.

**veiling g.**, g. from light scattered over the retina by opacities in lens or vitreous; this reduces contrasts and thus lessens visibility.

**glarom'eter.** An instrument that measures sensitivity to central glare from the headlights of an approaching vehicle.

**Glaser,** Johann H., Swiss anatomist, 1629–1675. See Glaserian *artery, fissure.*

**Glasgow,** William C., American physician, 1845–1907. See G.'s *sign.*

**glass** [ A.S. *glaes* ]. A transparent brittle substance, a compound of silica with oxides of various bases.

**cover g.**, a thin g. disk or plate covering an object examined under the microscope.

**crown g.**, a compound of lime, potash, alumina, and silica; commonly used in lenses; has a low dispersion (52.2) relative to index of refraction (1.523).

**cupping g.**, a g. vessel, from which the air has been exhausted by heat or a special suction apparatus, applied to the skin in order to draw blood to the surface. See also cupping, and entries under cup.

**flint g.**, contains lead oxide in place of lime and is more refractive than crown g. but softer and heavier; used in reading segments of fused bifocal lenses.

**object g.**, objective.

**quartz g.**, a transparent, colorless crystal made by fusing pure quartz sand. It transmits ultraviolet light.

**soluble g.,** water g.; a silicate of potassium or sodium, soluble in hot water but solid at ordinary temperatures; used for fixed dressings.

**vita g.,** a specially prepared g. that is transparent to antirachitic (ultraviolet) rays of the spectrum.

**water g.,** soluble g.

**Wood's g.,** a g. containing nickel oxide, used in the diagnosis of ringworm of the scalp due to *Microsporum audouini* or *M. canis;* the infected hairs are brilliantly fluorescent when viewed in ultraviolet light filtered through this g. (Wood's light).

**Glasser's disease.** See under disease.

**glasses.** 1. Spectacles. 2. Lenses for correcting refractive errors in the eyes. See lens and spectacles.

**Glauber,** Johann R., Dutch chemist, 1604–1668. See G.'s *salt.*

**glaucarubin** (glaw'kǎ-ru'bin). GLARUBIN; a crystalline glycoside isolated from the fruit of *Simarouba glauca* (family Simarubaceae), a tropical plant found in Central America and northern South America. Used as an intestinal amebicide.

**glaucoma** (glaw-ko'mah) [ G. *glaukōma,* opacity of the crystalline lens, fr. *glaukos,* bluish green ]. A disease of the eye characterized by increased intraocular pressure due to restricted outflow of the aqueous through the aqueous veins and Schlemm's canal, excavation and degeneration of the optic disk, and nerve fiber bundle damage producing arcuate defects in the field of vision.

**absolute g.,** the final stage of blindness in g.

**congenital g.,** buphthalmos.

**Donders' g.,** g. simplex.

**g. ful'minans,** acute congestive g. rapidly followed by blindness.

**narrow (closed) angle g.,** g. in which the space between the base of the iris and the cornea at the trabecular meshwork is narrowed or obliterated.

**open angle g.,** g. in which the trabecular meshwork is free from encroachment by the base of the iris.

**phacolytic g.,** g. secondary to hypermature cataract and due to plugging of the trabecular spaces by permuted cortical material.

**pigmentary g.,** open angle g. caused by accumulation of pigment particles in the trabecular zone.

**pseudoexfoliative capsular g.,** secondary g. incident to a degenerative cyclitis producing deposits on anterior lens capsule.

**secondary g.,** g. occurring as a sequel of preexisting ocular disease or injury.

**g. simplex,** Donders' g.; noncongestive, open angle g.

**glaucomatocyclitic** (glaw-ko'mǎ-to-sǐ-klit'ik). Denoting increased intraocular tension associated with evidences of cyclitis. See also glaucomatocyclitic *crisis.*

**glaucomatous** (glaw-ko'mǎ-tus). Relating to glaucoma.

**glaucosuria** (glaw'ko-su'rǐ-ah) [ G. *glaukos,* bluish green, + *ouron,* urine ]. Obsolete term for indicanuria.

**GLC.** Abbreviation for gas-liquid *chromatography.*

**Glc, GlcA, GlcN, GlcNAc, GlcUA.** Symbols for the radicals of glucose, gluconic acid, glucosamine, *N*-acetylglucosamine, and glucuronic acid.

**gleet.** A slight chronic discharge of thin mucus from the urethra, following gonorrhea.

**gleety.** Relating to gleet.

**gle'nohu'meral.** Relating to the glenoid cavity and the humerus.

**glenoid** (gle'noyd, glen'oyd) [ G. *glēnoeidēs,* fr. *glēnē,* pupil of eye, socket of joint, honeycomb, + *eidos,* appearance ]. Resembling a socket; denoting the articular depression of the scapula entering into the formation of the shoulder joint.

**Glenospora** (gle-nos'po-rah) [ G. *glēnē* (see glenoid), + *sporos,* seed ]. A genus of polymorphous fungi, several species of which have been found in cases of otomycosis or mycetoma.

**glenosporosis** (gle-no-spo-ro'sis). An affection caused by the presence of a species of fungus of the genus *Glenospora.*

**Gley** (gla), Marcel E., French physiologist, 1857–1930. See G.'s *cells, glands.*

**glia** (gli'ah) [ G. glue ]. Neuroglia.

**Alzheimer's g.,** a degenerative alteration of neuroglial cells, noted in patients with extensive hepatic disease.

**gli'acyte** [ G. *glia,* glue, + *kytos,* cell ]. A neuroglia cell; see neuroglia.

**gli'adin.** Glutin; a protein separable from wheat and rye glutens. A member of a group of simple proteins, the prolamins, insoluble in water, absolute alcohol, and neutral solvents, but soluble in 70 to 80 per cent alcohol.

**gli'al.** Pertaining to glia or neuroglia.

**glide.** A smooth, or effortless, continuous movement.

**mandibular g.,** the side-to-side, protrusive, and intermediate movement of the mandible occurring when the teeth or other occluding surfaces are in contact.

**glio-** [ G. *glia,* glue ]. Combining form meaning glue or gluelike, relating specifically to the neuroglia.

**gli'oblasto'ma multifor'me** [ G. *glia,* glue, + *blastos,* germ, sprout, + suffix -*oma,* tumor ]. Grade IV astrocytoma; a rapidly growing, malignant tumor of the cerebral hemispheric white matter; it is composed of primitive glial cells, most commonly of astrocytic origin.

**gli'oblasto'sis cer'ebri.** Astrocytosis cerebri; a diffuse intracranial neoplasm of astrocytic origin.

**Glioclad'ium.** A genus of rapidly growing, saprophytic fungi that colonially resembles *Penicillium* but is distinguished from it by clustering of the conidia in large masses.

**glioma** (gli-o'mah) [ G. *glia,* glue, + suffix -*oma,* tumor ]. Any neoplasm derived from one of the various types of cells that form the parenchyma of the brain, pineal gland, posterior pituitary gland, and retina; *e.g.,* astroblastoma, astrocytoma, glioblastoma multiforme, ganglioglioma, spongioblastoma polare, medulloblastoma, ependymoma, oligodendroglioma, pinealoma, and so on. G.'s rarely metastasize to sites outside of the central nervous system, but occasionally spread by means of implantation on the meninges of the brain and spinal cord. Most g.'s are malignant as a result of their location or their invasive and destructive tendencies. Neoplasms of the spinal cord are relatively rare, but approximately one-fourth are g.'s.

**g. endoph'ytum,** a g. of the retina starting from the inner layers.

**g. exoph'ytum,** a g. of the retina starting from the outer layers.

**gigantocellular g.,** a histologic form of glioblastoma with large, often bizarre, tumor cells.

**mixed g.,** astroependymoma.

**nasal g.,** term for a lesion that is probably not a true neoplasm, but an unusual anomaly consisting of glial tissue with bizarre astrocytes, ganglionic neurons, and ependymal cells in small nodules at the base of the nose.

**g. of the retina,** former term for a retinoblastoma.

**g. sarcomato'sum,** gliosarcoma.

**g. of the spinal cord,** almost always an ependymoma that originates in some site along the central canal; neoplasms of the spinal cord are relatively rare, but g.'s constitute approximately one-fourth of the total.

**g. telangiecto'des,** a telangiectatic g., one in which the stroma has numerous, conspicuous, frequently dilated small blood vessels and capillaries, as well as large, endothelium-rimmed "lakes" of blood.

**gliomato'sis.** The presence of a glioma, especially one that involves a relatively large portion of the brain, as a solitary mass or as mutiple foci.

**glio'matous.** Pertaining to or characterized by a glioma.

**gliomyxoma** (gli'o-mik-so'mah). A myxoma that contains a considerable amount of proliferating glial cells and fibers.

**glioneuroma** (gli'o-nu-ro'mah). A ganglioneuroma derived from neurons, with numerous glial cells and fibers in the matrix.

**gli'osarco'ma.** Glioma sarcomatosum; a glioma consisting of immature, undifferentiated, pleomorphic, spindle-shaped cells with relatively large, hyperchromatic, frequently bizarre nuclei and poorly formed fibrillary processes. Sometimes used as a term for a malignant neoplasm derived from connective tissue (*e.g.,* that associated with blood vessels in the brain), in which there is a considerable amount of proliferating glial cells. See also spongioblastoma.

**glio'sis.** A condition marked by the occurrence of overgrowth or tumors of the neuroglia.

**isomorphous g.,** a scar in which the previous arrangement of neuroglial fibers is preserved. See also brain *cicatrix*.

**piloid g.,** an area of chronic, reactive astrocytosis composed of thin, hairlike cells in vaguely parallel array.

**gli′otoxin.** $C_{13}H_{14}O_4N_2S_2$; an antibiotic agent active against Gram-positive but not against Gram-negative bacteria; it is also strongly fungicidal. It has been isolated from various species of *Trichoderma*; it attacks and destroys the pathogenic fungus of plants *Rhyzoctonia solani*. It is toxic to animal tissues.

**glischruria** (glis-kru′rĭ-ah) [ G. *glischros,* gluey, + *ouron,* urine ]. The presence of glischrin in the urine.

**Glisson,** Francis, English physician, anatomist, physiologist and pathologist, 1597–1677. See G.'s *capsule, cirrhosis, sphincter.*

**glissoni′tis.** Inflammation of Glisson's capsule, or the connective tissue surrounding the portal vein and the hepatic artery and bile ducts.

**Gln.** Symbol for the radical of glutamine (glutaminyl).

**glo′bal.** The complete, generalized, overall, or total aspect.

**globe.** Globus.

**glo′bi.** 1. Plural of globus, *q. v.* 2. Brown, bodies sometimes found in the granulomatous lesions of leprosy, in addition to the macrophages that contain the acid-fast bacilli; g. are thought to be degenerate forms of such cells, in which the organisms are no longer viable and have become granular or amorphous.

**Globid′ium.** See *Besnoitia.*

**glo′bin.** The protein of hemoglobin.

**glo′binom′eter.** An instrument for determining the relative proportions of hemoglobin.

**Globoceph′alus.** A genus of hookworm (subfamily Uncinariinae, family Ancylostomatidae) consisting of about five species, chiefly found in the small intestine of pigs.

**G. urosubula′tus,** a common hookworm of wild and domestic pigs; it is distributed worldwide.

**glo′boside.** A glycosphingolipid, specifically a ceramide tetrasaccharide (tetraglycosylceramide), isolated from kidney and erythrocytes, probably identical with cytolipin K, of the structure *N*-acetylgalactosaminyl($\beta 1 \rightarrow 3$)galactosyl($\beta 1 \rightarrow 4$)glucosylceramide.

**globule** (glob′ūl) [ L. *globulus,* dim. of *globus,* a ball ]. 1. A small spherical body of any kind. 2. A fat droplet in milk.

**dentin g.,** calcospherites formed by calcification or mineralization of the dentin occurring in globular areas.

**directing g.,** archaic for polar *body.*

**extrusion g.,** archaic for polar *body.*

**Morgagni's g.'s,** Morgagni's spheres; drops of fluid beneath the capsule and between lens fibers in early cataract.

**polar g.,** polar *body.*

**globulicidal** (glob′u-lĭ-si′dal) [ L. *globulus,* + *caedo,* to kill ]. Hemolytic; globulicide (1); destructive to the blood cells, especially the erythrocytes.

**globulicide** (glob′u-lĭ-sīd). 1. Globulicidal. 2. An agent destructive to the red and white blood cells.

**globuliferous** (glob-u-lif′er-us) [ L. *globulus,* globule, + *fero,* to bear ]. Containing globules or corpuscles, especially red blood cells.

**globulim′eter** [ L. *globulus,* globule, + G. *metron,* measure ]. Hemocytometer.

**glob′ulin** [ L. *globulus,* globule ]. Name for a family of proteins precipitated from plasma (or serum) by half-saturation with ammonium sulfate (*i.e.,* addition of an equal volume of saturated ammonium sulfate). The g.'s may be further fractionated by solubility and other separation methods into many subgroups, the main groups being known as α-, β-, and γ-g.; these differ with respect to associated lipids or carbohydrates and in their content of many physiologically important factors. Among the latter are immunoglobulins (antibodies) in the β and γ fractions, lipoproteins in the α and β fractions (see acanthocytosis), gluco- or mucoproteins (orosomucoid, haptoglobin), and metal-binding and metal-transporting proteins (transferrin, siderophilin, ceruloplasmin). Other substances found in g. fractions are: macroglobulin, plasminogen, prothrombin, euglobulin, antihemophilic g., fibrinogen, cryoglobulin.

$\beta_{1C}$ **g.,** the third component (C3) of complement; see component of *complement.*

$\beta_{1E}$ **g.,** the fourth component (C4) of complement; see component of *complement.*

$\beta_{1F}$ **g.,** the fifth component (C5) of complement; see component of *complement.*

**ac-g.,** accelerator g.

**accelerator g.,** ac-g.; accelerin; a g. in blood; a substance in serum that hastens the conversion of prothrombin to thrombin in the presence of thromboplastin and ionized calcium. See *factor* V (plasma accelerator g.) and serum accelerator g.

**antihemophilic g.,** *factor* VIII.

**corticosteroid-binding g.,** transcortin.

**human gamma g.,** human normal immunoglobulin (BP); a preparation of the proteins of liquid human plasma, containing the antibodies of normal adults. It is obtained from pooled liquid human plasma from a number of donors and may be prepared by precipitation with organic solvents under controlled conditions of pH, ionic strength and temperature.

**immune serum g.** (USP), immune serum g. (human); a sterile solution of g.'s that contains many antibodies normally present in adult human blood. It contains not less than 15 gm. and not more than 18 gm. of protein per 100 ml., not less than 90 per cent of which is γ-g. Each lot of immune serum g. is derived from an original plasma or serum pool (venous and placental blood) from at least 1000 individuals. A passive immunizing agent.

**measles immune g.** (USP), measles immune g. (human); a sterile solution of g.'s derived from the blood plasma of normal, adult human donors. It is prepared from immune serum g. that complies, after dilution if necessary, with the measles antibody requirement of the U. S. Public Health Service. It contains not less than 10 gm. and not more than 18 gm. of protein per 100 ml., of which not less than 90 per cent is γ-g. A passive immunizing agent.

**pertussis immune g.** (USP); a sterile solution of g.'s derived from the plasma of adult human donors who have been immunized with pertussis vaccine. It is used both prophylactically and therapeutically.

**plasma accelerator g.,** see *factor* V.

**poliomyelitis immune g. (human),** a sterile solution of g.'s that contains those antibodies normally present in adult human blood. It is a passive immunologic agent that attenuates or prevents poliomyelitis, measles, and infectious hepatitis. It confers temporary but significant protection against paralytic polio.

**Rh₀ (D) immune g.,** a globulin fraction of antibody specific for the most common antigen, $Rh_0$ (D), of the Rh group (see appendix 2); used to prevent Rh-sensitization of an Rh-negative woman after delivery of an Rh-positive fetus.

**serum accelerator (Ac)-g.,** a substance in serum that accelerates the conversion of prothrombin to thrombin in the presence of thromboplastin and calcium. It is produced by the action of traces of thrombin upon plasma accelerator g.

**tetanus immune g.** (USP); a sterile solution of g.'s derived from the blood plasma of adult human donors who have been immunized with tetanus toxoid. It contains not less than 10 gm. and not more than 18 gm. of protein per 100 ml., of which not less than 90 per cent is γ-g. A passive immunizing agent.

**thyroxine-binding g.,** TBG; thyroxine-binding protein (TBP); an α-globulin of blood with a strong binding affinity for thyroxine. Triiodothyronine is bound to it much less firmly.

**g. zinc insulin,** see under insulin.

**globulinuria** (glob′u-lin-u′rĭ-ah). The excretion of globulin in the urine, usually, if not always, in association with serum albumin.

**globulolysis** (glob′u-lol′ĭ-sis) [ globule + G. *lysis,* solution ]. Dissolution of blood cells, especially with reference to erythrocytes, *i.e.,* hemolysis.

**glob′ulus** [ L. ]. Globule.

**glo′bus,** pl. **glo′bi** [ L. ]. 1 [ NA ]. A round body; sphere; ball; globe. 2. See globi.

**g. hyster′icus,** apopnixis; a sensation as of a ball in the throat or as if the throat were compressed; a symptom of hysteria.

**g. major,** *caput* epididymidis.

**g. minor,** *cauda* epididymidis.

**g. pal'lidus** [ NA ], pale globe; pallidum; the inner and lighter gray portion of the lentiform or lenticular nucleus; see also paleostriatum.

**glo'mal.** Relating to or involving a glomus.

**glomangioma** (glo-man'jī-o'mah). Glomus *tumor.*

**glomangiosis** (glo-man'jī-o'sis). The occurrence of multiple complexes of small vascular channels, each resembling a glomus.

**pulmonary g.,** g. occurring within small pulmonary arteries in severe pulmonary hypertension and congenital heart disease.

**glome.** Glomus.

**glomectomy** (glo-mek'to-mī) [ L. *glomus* + G. *ektomē,* cutting out ]. Excision of a glomus tumor.

**glomerular** (glo-mēr'u-lar). Relating to a glomerulus; affecting the glomeruli; clustered; glomerulate.

**glomerule** (glom'er-ūl). Glomerulus.

**glomerulitis** (glo-mēr'u-li'tis). Inflammation of a glomerulus, specifically of the renal glomeruli; see also glomerulonephritis.

**glomerulonephritis** (glo-mēr'u-lo-nĕ-fri'tis) [ glomerulus + G. *nephros,* kidney, + suffix -*itis,* inflammation ]. Renal disease characterized by bilateral inflammatory changes in glomeruli which are not the result of infection of the kidneys.

**acute g.,** g. that frequently occurs as a late complication of pharyngitis, especially due to type 12 β-hemolytic streptococci, characterized by abrupt onset of hematuria, edema of the face, oliguria, and variable azotemia and hypertension. The renal glomeruli usually show cellular proliferation or infiltration by polymorphonuclear leukocytes.

**acute hemorrhagic g.,** acute g.

**chronic g.,** g. that presents with persisting proteinuria, chronic renal failure, and hypertension, of insidious onset or as a late sequel of acute g.; the kidneys are symmetrically contracted and granular, with scarring and loss of glomeruli and the presence of tubular atrophy and interstitial fibrosis.

**chronic hypocomplementemic g.,** membranoproliferative g.

**diffuse g.,** g. affecting most of the renal glomeruli; it may lead to azotemia.

**Ellis type 1 g.,** Ellis type 1 nephritis; g. presenting as acute g., followed by complete recovery in most cases, or the development of rapidly progressive g., or incomplete remission with persistent proteinuria and subsequent development of chronic g.

**Ellis type 2 g.,** Ellis type 2 nephritis; g. which is usually not related to preceding bacterial infection; characterized by an insidious onset of the nephrotic syndrome, failure of complete remission, and eventual development of chronic renal failure. The kidneys usually show membranous g.

**exudative g.,** g. with infiltration of glomeruli by polymorphonuclear leukocytes, occurring in acute g.

**focal g.,** g. affecting a small proportion of renal glomeruli, not associated with azotemia. Focal g. commonly presents with hematuria and may be associated with acute upper respiratory infection in young males, not usually due to streptococcus.

**focal embolic g.,** g. associated with subacute bacterial endocarditis, frequently producing microscopic hematuria without azotemia. There is no direct evidence that the focal lesions in the glomeruli are due to embolism from vegetations on the heart valves.

**induced g.,** serum *nephritis.*

**lobular g.,** membranoproliferative g.

**local g.,** segmental g.

**membranoproliferative g.,** exudative g.; chronic hypocomplementemic g.; lobular g.; chronic g. characterized by mesangial cell proliferation, increased lobular separation of glomeruli, thickening of glomerular capillary walls by nodular subendothelial deposits and increased mesangial matrix, and low serum levels of complement; it occurs mainly in older girls with a very slow course, episodes of hematuria or edema, and hypertension.

**membranous g.,** g. characterized by diffuse thickening of glomerular capillary basement membranes, due in part to deposits of immunoglobulins, and clinically by an insidious onset of the nephrotic syndrome and failure of disappearance of proteinuria.

**proliferative g.,** g. with hypercellularity of glomeruli due to proliferation of endothelial or mesangial cells, occurring in acute g. and membranoproliferative g.

**rapidly progressive g.,** g. usually presenting insidiously, without preceding streptococcal infection, with increasing renal failure leading to death within a few months. At autopsy the kidneys are normal in size and show numerous glomerular capsular epithelial crescents.

**segmental g.,** local g.; g. affecting only part of a glomerulus or glomeruli; see also focal g.

**subacute g.,** subacute nephritis; g. with proteinuria, hematuria and azotemia persisting for many weeks. The renal changes are variable, including those of rapidly progressive and membranoproliferative g.

**glomerulopathy** (glo-mer'u-lop'ă-thī) [ glomerulus + G. *pathos,* suffering ]. Glomerular disease of any type.

**focal sclerosing g.,** focal, segmental glomerulosclerosis reported in adults and children with normal serum complement, progressing to chronic glomerulonephritis.

**glomerulosclerosis** (glo-mēr'u-lo-skle-ro'sis) [ glomerulus + G. *sklērōsis,* hardness ]. Hyaline deposits or scarring within the renal glomeruli, a degenerative process occurring in association with renal arteriosclerosis or diabetes.

**diabetic g.,** Kimmelstiel-Wilson *disease.*

**intercap'illary g.,** Kimmelstiel-Wilson *disease.*

**nodular g.,** Kimmelstiel-Wilson *disease.*

**glomerulose** (glo-mēr'u-lōs). Glomerular.

**glomerulus,** pl. **glomer'uli** (glo-mēr'u-lus) [ Mod. L. dim. of L. *glomus,* a ball of yarn. GLO- ] [ NA ]. 1. A plexus of capillaries. 2. Malpighian g., tuft formed of capillary loops at the beginning of each uriniferous tubule in the kidney; this tuft with its capsule (Bowman's capsule) constitutes the corpusculum renis (Malpighian body). 3. The twisted secretory portion of a sweat gland. 4. A cluster of dendritic ramifications and axon terminals in often complex synaptic relationship with each other, surrounded by a glial sheath.

**Malpighian g.,** g. (2).

**g. of mesonephros,** one of the tufts of capillary vessels within the mesonephros derived from a lateral branch of the primary aorta. Each g. is connected to a tubule.

**olfactory g.,** one of the small spherical territories in the olfactory bulb in which dendrites of mitral and tufted cells synapse with axons of olfactory receptor cells.

**g. of pronephros,** one of the tufts of capillary vessels in the pronephros derived from a lateral branch of the aorta.

**glo'mus** [ L. *glomus* (*glomer-*), pl. *glomera,* a ball ]. 1 [ NA ]. A small globular body. 2. A highly organized arteriolovenular anastomosis between a small artery and a venule, forming a tiny nodular focus in the nailbed, pads of the fingers and toes, ears, hands, and feet and many other organs of the body. The afferent arteriole enters the connective tissue capsule of the g., becomes devoid of an internal elastic membrane, and develops a relatively thick epithelioid muscular wall and small lumen; the anastomosis may be branched and convoluted, richly innervated with sympathetic and myelinated nerves, and connected with a short, thin-walled vein that drains into a periglomic vein and then into one of the veins of the skin. The g. functions as a shunt or bypass regulating mechanism in the flow of blood, temperature, and conservation of heat in the part as well as in the indirect control of the blood pressure and other functions of the circulatory system.

**g. aor'ticum,** aortic body; one of the small bilateral structures, similar to the glomus caroticum, attached to a small branch of the aorta near its arch; they contain chemoreceptors that respond primarily to decreases in blood oxygen tension; less sensitive to decreases in blood pH or increases in carbon dioxide tension.

**g. carot'icum** [ NA ], carotid body; intercarotid body; nodulus caroticus; a small epithelioid structure located just above the bifurcation of the common carotid artery on each side. It consists of granular principal cells and nongranular supporting cells, a sinusoidal vascular bed and a rich network of sensory fibers of the glossopharyngeal nerve. It serves as a chemoreceptor organ responsive to oxygen lack, carbon dioxide excess, and increased hydrogen ion concentration.

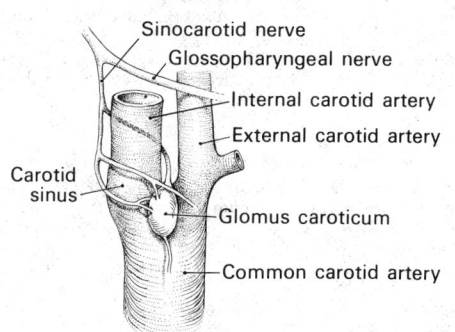

**Glomus Caroticum**

**choroid g.,** g. choroideum.

**g. choroide'um** [ NA ], choroid g.; choroid skein; a marked enlargement of the choroid plexus of the lateral ventricle at the junction of the central part with the inferior horn.

**g. coccyge'um,** *corpus* coccygeum.

**g. intravaga'le,** a minute collection of chemoreceptor cells on the auricular branch of the vagus nerve. A tumor of this g. may cause deafness and tinnitus.

**g. jugula're,** a microscopic collection of chemoreceptor tissue in the adventitia of the jugular bulb; a tumor of this g. may cause paralysis of the vocal cords and attacks of dizziness, blackout, and nystagmus.

**g. pulmona'le,** a structure similar to the g. caroticum, found in relation to the pulmonary artery.

**glonoin** (glo'no-in). Nitroglycerin.

**gloss-.** See glosso-.

**glos'sa** [ G. ]. Lingua; tongue.

**glossagra** (glos-ag'rah) [ gloss- + G. *agra,* a seizure ]. Glossalgia of gouty origin.

**glos'sal.** Relating to the tongue.

**glossalgia** (glos-al'jī-ah) [ gloss- + G. *algos,* pain ]. Glossodynia.

**glossan'thrax** [ gloss- + G. *anthrax* a carbuncle. ANTHR- ]. Carbuncle of the tongue.

**glossec'tomy** [ gloss- + G. *ektomē,* excision ]. Elinguation; lingulectomy; excision or amputation of the tongue.

**Glossi'na** [ G. *glōssa,* tongue ]. A genus of bloodsucking Diptera (tsetse flies) confined to Africa; they serve as intermediate hosts of the pathogenic trypanosomes that cause various forms of African sleeping sickness in humans and domestic animals.

**G. mor'sitans,** (1) originally thought to be the sole transmitter of *Trypanosoma brucei,* the cause of nagana in central Africa. This species in some regions transmits this disease but it is not the sole or even the principal transmitting agent; (2) the vector of *T. rhodesiense,* one of the pathogenic agents of East African, Rhodesian, or acute sleeping sickness.

**G. pallid'ipes,** the principal transmitter of nagana; it also transmits *Trypanosoma rhodesiensi.*

**G. palpa'lis,** a species of *G.* that transmits *Trypanosoma gambiense,* one of the pathogenic parasites of West African, Gambian, or chronic sleeping sickness.

**glossi'tis** [ gloss- + G. suffix *-itis,* inflammation ]. Inflammation of the tongue.

**g. area'ta exfoliati'va,** geographical *tongue.*

**atroph'ic g.,** bald tongue; smooth, glistening tongue with atrophic papillae, observed in pernicious anemia and in the late stages of chronic recurrent pellagra.

**benign migratory g.,** geographical *tongue.*

**g. desic'cans,** a painful affection of the tongue, of unknown origin, in which the surface becomes raw and fissured.

**Hunter's g.,** g. of pernicious anemia.

**Moeller's g.,** a chronic painful form of superficial g.

**g. parasit'ica,** black *tongue.*

**glosso-, gloss-** [ G. *glōssa,* tongue ]. Combining forms relating to the tongue.

**glossocele** (glos'o-sēl) [ glosso- + G. *kēlē,* tumor, hernia ]. Protrusion of the tongue from the mouth, owing to its excessive size. See also macroglossia.

**glos'socinesthet'ic.** Glossokinesthetic.

**glossodontotropism** (glos'o-don'to-tro-pizm) [ glosso- + G. *odous (odont-),* tooth, + *tropos,* a turning ]. A manifestation of tension or anxiety in which the tongue is attracted to the teeth or to dental faults.

**glossodynamometer** (glos'o-di'nā-mom'e-ter) [ glosso- + G. *dynamis,* power, + *metron,* measure ]. An apparatus for estimating the contractile force of the tongue muscles.

**glossodynia** (glos-o-din'ī-ah) [ glosso- + G. *odynē,* pain ]. Glossalgia; glossopyrosis; a condition characterized by burning or painful tongue.

**glossodyniotropism** (glos'o-din'ī-o-tro-pizm) [ glosso- + G. *odynē,* pain, + *tropos,* a turning ]. Apparent satisfaction from subjecting the tongue to a pain-inducing dental fault; considered by some to be a masochistic behavior or manifestation.

**glossoepiglottic, glossoepiglottidean** (glos'o-ep-ī-glot'-ik, glos'o-ep-ī-glō-tid'e-an). Relating to the tongue and the epiglottis.

**glos'sograph** [ glosso- + G. *graphō,* to write ]. An instrument for recording the movements of the tongue in speaking.

**glossohyal** (glos-o-hi'al). Hyoglossal.

**glossokinesthetic** (glos'o-kin-es-thet'ik) [ glosso- + G. *kinēsis,* movement, + *aisthētikos,* perceptive ]. Denoting the subjective sensation of the movements of the tongue.

**glossola'lia** [ glosso- + G. *lalia,* talk, chat ]. Unintelligible jargon.

**glossology** (glos-ol'o-jī) [ glosso- + G. *logos,* study ]. Glottology; the branch of medical science dealing with the tongue and its diseases.

**glossolysis** (glos-ol'ī-sis) [ glosso- + G. + *lysis,* a loosening ]. Glossoplegia; paralysis of the tongue.

**glossoncus** (glos-ong'kus) [ glosso- + G. *onkos,* mass, tumor ]. Any swelling (*i.e.,* tumor in the broad sense) involving the tongue, including neoplasms.

**glossopalati'nus** [ glosso- + Mod. L. *palatinus,* fr. L. *palatum,* palate ]. *Musculus* palatoglossus.

**glossopathy** (glos-op'ā-thī) [ glosso- + G. *pathos,* suffering ]. A disease of the tongue.

**glossopharyngeal** (glos'o-fā-rin'je-al). Relating to the tongue and the pharynx.

**glossopharyngeus** (glos'o-fā-rin'je-us, -fār'in-je'us). *Musculus* glossopharyngeus.

**glossophytia** (glos'o-fi'tī-ah) [ glosso- + G. *phyton,* plant ]. Black *tongue.*

**glossophyton** (glos'o-fi'ton) [ glosso- + G. *phyton,* plant ]. A fungus observed in the dark patches of hypertrophied filiform papillae and desquamated epithelial cells in certain instances of nigrities linguae (black tongue) and thought by some observers to be the etiologic agent.

**glossoplasty** (glos'o-plas'tī) [ glosso- + G. *plassō,* to form ]. Reparative or plastic surgery of the tongue.

**glossoplegia** (glos'o-ple'jī-ah) [ glosso- + G. *plēgē,* stroke ]. Glossolysis.

**glossoptosis, glossoptosia** (glos'op-to'sis, -op-to'sī-ah) [ glosso- + G. *ptōsis,* a falling ]. Downward displacement of the tongue.

**glossopyrosis** (glos-o-pi-ro'sis) [ glosso- + G. *pyrosis,* a burning ]. Glossodynia.

**glossorrhaphy** (glos-sor'ā-fī) [ glosso- + G. *rhaphē,* suture ]. Suture of a wound of the tongue.

**glossoscopy** (glos-os'ko-pī) [ glosso- + G. *skopeō,* to view ]. Examination of the tongue.

**glossospasm** (glos'o-spazm). Spasmodic contraction of the tongue.

**glossostere'sis.** Glossectomy.

**glossot'omy** [ glosso- + G. *tomē,* incision ]. Any cutting operation on the tongue.

**glossotrichia** (glos-o-trik'ī-ah) [ glosso- + G. *thrix,* hair ]. Hairy *tongue.*

**glot'tic.** Relating to (1) the tongue or (2) the glottis.

**glottiditis** (glot'ĭ-di'tis). Glossitis.

**glottidospasm** (glot'ĭ-do-spazm). Laryngospasm.

**glottis**, pl. **glottides** (glot'is, glot'ĭ-dēz) [ G. *glōttis*, aperture of the larynx ] [ NA ]. The vocal apparatus of the larynx, consisting of the vocal folds of mucous membrane investing the vocal ligament and vocal muscle on each side, the free edges of which are the vocal cords, and of a median fissure, the rima glottidis.

  **false g.**, *rima* vestibuli.

  **g. respirato'ria,** *pars* intercartilaginea rimae glottidis.

  **g. spu'ria,** *rima* vestibuli.

  **true g.**, *rima* glottidis.

  **g. vera,** *rima* glottidis.

  **g. voca'lis,** *pars* intermembranacea rimae glottidis.

**glotti'tis.** Glossitis.

**glottol'ogy** [ G. *glōssa, glōtta,* tongue, + *logos,* study ]. Glossology.

**Glu.** Abbreviation for glutamic acid or glutamyl.

**glucagon** (glu'kă-gon) (USP). Hyperglycemic-glycogenolytic factor; HG factor; HGF; a hormone consisting of a straight chain polypeptide of 29 residues (bovine g.), extracted from pancreatic alpha cells. Parenteral administration of 0.5 to 1 mg. results in prompt mobilization of hepatic glycogen, thus elevating blood glucose concentration. It activates hepatic phosphorylase, thereby increasing glycogenolysis; decreases gastric motility and gastric and pancreatic secretions; and increases urinary excretion of nitrogen and potassium; it has no effect on muscle phosphorylase. It is used, as the hydrochloride, in the treatment of glycogen storage disease (von Gierke's), and hypoglycemia, particularly hypoglycemic coma due to exogenously administered insulin (the subsequent use of oral or parenteral glucose is recommended).

  **gut g.,** a substance of intestinal origin that is secreted into the blood following ingestion of glucose; it is a potent stimulus to the secretion of insulin. Its chemical structure and the biologic effects that it produces are different from those of g.; this substance does cross-react, however, with antibodies to g.

**glucal** (glu'kal). Glycal; an unsaturated sugar derivative in which the adjacent hydroxyl groups are removed, one of which is that upon the carbon-1 of the aldose (or carbon-2 of the ketose), yielding a CH=CH between these two positions.

**glucan** (glu'kan). A polyglucose (*e.g.*, callose, cellulose, starch amylose, glycogen amylose).

**1,4-α-glucan branching enzyme** (EC 2.4.1.18). α-Glucan branching glycosyltransferase; an enzyme (glucanotransferase) in muscle and in plants that cleaves α-1,4 linkages in glycogen or starch, transferring the fragments into α-1,6 linkages, creating branches in the polysaccharide molecules (whence the terms "branching enzyme" and "branching factor"); in plants, converts amylose to amylopectin. Deficiency (hereditary) causes type 4 glycogenosis. The plant enzyme has been termed Q enzyme.

**α-glucan branching glycosyltransferase.** 1,4-α-Glucan branching enzyme.

**1,4-α-glucan 6-α-glucosyltransferase** (EC 2.4.1.24). Amylo-1-4,1-6-transglucosidase; amylo-(1,4 → 1,6)-transglucosylase; oligoglucan-branching glycosyltransferase; T enzyme; a glucosyltransferase that transfers an α-glucosyl residue in a 1,4-α-glucan to the primary hydroxyl group of glucose in a 1,4-α-glucan. See also 1,4-α-glucan branching enzyme.

**4-α-glucanotransferase** (EC 2.4.1.25). Dextrin transglycosylase; dextrin glycosyltransferase; D enzyme; disproportionating enzyme; amylomaltase; a 4-glycosyltransferase converting maltodextrins into amylose and glucose by transferring parts of 1,4-glucan chains to new 4-positions on glucose or other 1,4-glucans.

**α-glucan phosphorylase.** Glycogen phosphorylase.

**glucaric acid.** Saccharic acid.

**glu'cases.** Obsolete term for enzymes cleaving starch to glucose (see amylase).

**glucemia** (glu-se'mĭ-ah). Obsolete term for glycemia.

**glucep'tate.** USAN-approved contraction for glucoheptonate.

**glucide** (glu'sid). Obsolete term at one time suggested to embrace the carbohydrates and the glucosides; modern equivalent is saccharide.

**gluciphore** (glu'sĭ-fōr) [ G. *glykys,* sweet, + *phoros,* bearing ]. The chemical group believed to be responsible for sweet taste.

**gluco-** (glu'ko-). Combining form denoting relationship to glucose; see also glyco-.

**glu'coam'ylase.** Exo-1,4-α-glucosidase.

**glucoascorbic acid** (glu'ko-as-kor'bik). 3-Keto-D-glucoheptonofuranolactone; a compound resembling ascorbic acid but with an additional —CHOH— between the 5 and 6 carbon atoms of ascorbic acid; shows toxic effects on addition to diet but these are not, apparently, caused by ascorbic acid antagonism.

**glu'cocer'ebroside.** Glucosylceramide.

**glucocinin** (glu-ko-sin'in). Glucokinin.

**glu'cocoid.** Obsolete term for glucocorticoid.

**glu'cocor'ticoid.** 1. Any steroid-like compound capable of significantly influencing intermediary metabolism, such as promotion of hepatic glycogen deposition, and of exerting a clinically useful anti-inflammatory effect. Cortisol is the most potent of the naturally occurring g.'s; most semisynthetic g.'s are cortisol derivatives. 2. Used as an adjective to designate this type of biological activity.

**glu'cocorticotroph'ic.** Indicating a principle of the anterior hypophysis that stimulates the production of glucocorticoid hormones of the adrenal cortex. No hormone exerting only this effect has been identified.

**glucocy'amine.** Glycocyamine.

**glu'cofu'ranose.** D-Glucose in furanose form (see sugars).

**glucogen'ic.** Giving rise to glucose; used particularly in connnection with those amino acids that result in glycosuria when fed to pancreatectomized animals; opposed in this case to ketogenic.

**glucohe'mia.** Obsolete term for glycemia.

**glucoinvertase.** α-Glucosidase.

**glucoki'nase** (EC 2.7.1.2). A hexokinase or phosphotransferase that, in the presence of ATP, catalyzes the conversion of glucose to glucose 6-phosphate.

**glu'cokinet'ic.** Mobilizing glucose.

**glucokin'in.** A substance extractable from plant tissues and yeasts and occurring in animal feedstuffs; it exerts a hypoglycemic action when injected into or ingested by animals; it acts by damaging the liver and depressing its function in producing and liberating glucose into the bloodstream.

**glucolip'ids.** Those cerebrosides that contain glucose as part of the molecule.

**glucol'ysis.** Glycolysis.

**gluconeogenesis** (glu'ko-ne'o-jen'ĕ-sis). Glyconeogenesis.

**glucon'ic acid.** The hexonic (aldonic) acid derived from glucose by oxidation of the —CHO group to —COOH.

**gluconolac'tonase.** Lactonase; an enzyme (EC 3.1.1.17) catalyzing the hydrolysis of gluconolactone to gluconic acid.

**glucope'nia.** Hypoglycemia.

**glu'copro'tein.** Glycoprotein.

**glu'copy'ranose.** D-Glucose in its pyranose form. See structures under sugars.

**glucosaccharic acid** (glu'ko-să-kăr'ik). *Saccharic* acid.

**gluco'samine.** Chitosamine; 2-amino-2-deoxy-D-glucose; an amino sugar found in chitin, cell membranes, and mucopolysaccharides generally.

**glu'cosans.** Anhydrides of glucose; polysaccharides, *e.g.,* cellulose, glycogen, starch, dextrins, yielding glucose upon hydrolysis.

**glu'cose.** d-glucose (for structure, see sugars); dextrose (USP and BP); blood sugar; corn sugar; grape sugar; starch sugar; GLUCOLIN; DEXTROPUR; DEXTROSOL; a dextrorotatory monosaccharide (hexose) found in the free state in fruits and other parts of plants, and combined in glucosides, disaccharides (often with fructose), oligosaccharides, and polysaccharides; it is the product of complete hydrolysis of cellulose, starch, and glycogen. Free g. occurs in the blood (normal human concentration, 80 to 120 mg. per 100 ml.); in diabetes mellitus, it appears in the urine. It is the principal source of energy for man and many other organisms.

**g. dehydrogenase** (EC 1.1.1.47), converts $\beta$-D-glucose to D-glucono-$\delta$-lactone, transferring hydrogen to NAD or NADP; cf. g. oxidase.

**liquid g.** (USP), consists of dextrose, dextrins, maltose, and water; obtained by the incomplete hydrolysis of starch. A pharmaceutic necessity.

**g. oxidase** (EC 1.1.3.4), notatin; glucose aerodehydrogenase; penatin; penicillin B; corylophyline; an antibacterial flavoprotein enzyme produced by *Penicillum notatum;* it is antibacterial only in the presence of glucose and oxygen, its effect being due to the oxidation of glucose to glucono-$\delta$-lactone, with conversion of $O_2$ to $H_2O_2$.

**g. transport maximum,** see under maximum.

**glucose-6-phosphatase** (EC 3.1.3.9). A liver enzyme catalyzing the hydrolysis of glucose 6-phosphate to glucose and inorganic phosphate; inherited deficiency of this enzyme is thought to be responsible for the glycogen storage disease known as type I or von Gierke's disease.

**glucose-6-phosphate dehydrogenase** (EC 1.1.1.49). Zwischenferment; Robison ester dehydrogenase; a pyridinoenzyme (NADP as coenzyme) catalyzing the dehydrogenation (oxidation) of glucose 6-phosphate to 6-phosphogluconolactone, the reaction initiating the Dickens shunt.

**glucosephosphate isomerase** (EC 5.3.1.9). Phosphohexose isomerase; phosphohexomutase; hexosephosphate isomerase; an isomerizing enzyme that catalyzes the interconversion of fructose 6-phosphate and glucose 6-phosphate.

**glucose-1-phosphate kinase.** Phosphoglucokinase.

**glucose-1-phosphate phosphodismutase** (EC 2.7.1.41). A phosphotransferase catalyzing the transfer of a phosphate residue from one glucose-1-phosphate to another, yielding glucose 1,6-bisphosphate.

$\alpha$**-glucosidase** (EC 3.2.1.20). Maltase; glucoinvertase; a glucohydrolase removing terminal nonreducing 1,4-linked $\alpha$-glucose residues by hydrolysis, yielding $\alpha$-glucose.

$\beta$**-glu'cosidase** (EC 3.2.1.21). Gentiobiase; cellobiase; amygdalase; a glucohydrolase similar to $\alpha$-glucosidase, but it attacks $\beta$-glucosides and releases $\beta$-glucose. Some $\beta$-glucosidases attack $\beta$-D-galactosides, $\alpha$-L-arabinosides, $\beta$-D-xylosides.

**glu'cosidases.** Enzymes that hydrolyze glucosides to glucose; e.g., $\alpha$- and $\beta$-glucosidases.

**glu'coside.** A compound of glucose with an alcohol or other R—OH compound involving loss of the H atom of the 1-OH (hemiacetal) group of the glucose, yielding a —C—O—R link from the carbon 1 of the glucose; a glycoside of glucose.

**glu'cosone.** A 2-dehydrogenation product (2-keto) of glucose; a possible intermediate in the formation of glucosamine from glucose.

**glucosul'fone sodium.** PROMIN sodium; sodium $p,p'$-sulfonylbis(aniline-$N$-glucoside sulfonate); chemotherapeutic agent used in the treatment of leprosy. Parenteral administration is better tolerated than oral administration.

**glucosuria** (glu'ko-su'rĭ-ah). The urinary excretion of glucose, usually in enhanced quantities.

**glu'cosylcer'amide.** Glucocerebroside; a neutral glycolipid containing equimolar amounts of fatty acid, glucose, and sphingosine.

**glu'cosyltrans'ferase.** Transglucosylase; any enzyme transferring glucosyl groups from one compound to another. Glucosyltransferases are found in EC subclass 2.4 (the glycosyltransferases).

**glucuronate** (glu-ku'ro-nāt). A salt or ester of glucuronic acid.

**glu'curone.** D-Glucuronolactone.

**glucuron'ic acid.** The uronic acid of glucose in which carbon 6 is oxidized to a carboxyl group. Detoxicates or inactivates various substances, e.g., benzoic acid, phenol, camphor, and the female sex hormones, undergoing conjugation with such substances in the liver. The glucuronides so formed are excreted in the urine.

$\beta$**-glucuronidase.** An enzyme (a hydrolase, EC 3.2.1.31) catalyzing the hydrolysis of various $\beta$-D-glucuronides, liberating free glucuronic acid.

**glucu'ronide.** A glycoside of glucuronic acid (q. v.). Many foreign chemicals, as well as catabolic products of normal body constituents (such as the steroid hormones), are commonly excreted in the urine as g.'s, the conjugation taking place in the liver.

**D-glucuronolactone.** Glucurone; lactone of D-glucofuranuronic acid; used as a means of administering orally glucuronic acid in the management of collagen and joint diseases. Its usefulness in such conditions has not been established.

**g. isonicotinoylhydrazone,** GLYCONIAZIDE; tuberculostatic agent.

**glucu'ronose.** Glucuronic acid.

**glue-sniffing.** Inhalation of fumes from plastic cements; the solvents, which include toluene, xylene, and benzene, induce central nervous system stimulation followed by depression. See also solvent *inhalation.*

**Gluge** (gloo'geh), Gottlieb, German histologist, 1812–1898. See G.'s *corpuscles.*

**glu'mito'cin.** 4-Serine, 8-glutamine oxytocin; a neurohypophysial hormone formed by some cartilaginous fishes, such as sharks and rays; its physiological effects in these animals are unknown.

**glu'tamate.** A salt or ester of glutamic acid.

**g. acetyltransferase,** ornithine acetyltransferase; enzyme (EC 2.3.1.35) catalyzing transfer of acetyl from $\alpha$-$N$-acetylornithine to glutamate.

**g. dehydrogenases,** glutamic acid dehydrogenases; pyridinoenzymes (EC 1.4.1.2, 3, and 4) catalyzing the deamination of glutamic acid to $\alpha$-ketoglutaric acid (2-oxoglutarate) with reduction of $NAD^+$ or $NADP^+$.

**glutamate** $\gamma$**-carboxypeptidase.** Conjugase; $\gamma$-glutamate carboxypeptidase; carboxypeptidase G; $N$-pteroyl-L-glutamate hydrolase; $\gamma$-peptidyl-L-glutamate hydrolase; a hydrolase (EC 3.4.12.10) cleaving glutamate residues from peptidyl glutamates or pteridine glutamates.

$\gamma$**-glutamate carboxypeptidase.** Glutamate $\gamma$-carboxypeptidase.

**glutam'ic acid.** An amino acid, HOOC—$CH_2$—$CH_2$—CH($NH_2$)COOH, occurring in proteins; symbol, Glu.

**g. acid dehydrogenases,** glutamate dehydrogenases.

**g. acid hydrochloride,** ACIDULIN; MURIPSIN; a gastric acidifier alleged to aid in digestion; also used for gastric HCl replacement therapy.

**glutam'ic-ox'aloace'tic transam'inase.** Aspartate aminotransferase.

**glutam'ic-pyru'vic transam'inase.** Alanine aminotransferase.

**glutam'inase** (EC 3.5.1.2). An enzyme in kidney and other tissues that catalyzes the breakdown of glutamine to ammonia and glutamic acid.

**glutamine** (glu'tă-mēn (-min), glu-tam'in). Glutaminic acid; the $\delta$-amide of glutamic acid. Derived by oxidation from proline in the liver or by the combination of glutamic acid with ammonia; it is present in proteins, in blood and other tissues; it is an important source of urinary ammonia, being broken down in the kidney by the action of the enzyme glutaminase. Symbol, Gln or Glu($NH_2$).

**g. synthetase** (EC 6.3.1.2), an enzyme that catalyzes the amination of glutamic acid to g. with the concomitant hydrolysis of ATP to ADP and $P_i$.

**glutamin'ic acid.** Glutamine.

**glutamoyl** (glu-tam'o-il). The radical of glutamic acid from which both $\alpha$- and $\delta$-hydroxyl groups have been removed.

**glutamyl** (glu-tam'il, glu'tă-mil). The radical of glutamic acid from which the $\alpha$- or the $\delta$-hydroxyl group has been removed.

**glutar'ic acid.** $HOOCCH_2CH_2CH_2COOH$; a dicarboxylic acid, an intermediate in tryptophan catabolism.

**glutaryl-CoA synthetase** (EC 6.2.1.6). Similar to acyl-CoA synthetase (q. v. under acylcoenzyme A), but splits ATP or GTP or ITP to the diphosphate in acting on glutarate.

**glutathione** (glu-tă-thi'ōn). $\gamma$-L-Glutamyl-L-cysteinylglycine; a tripeptide of glycine, cystine, and glutamic acid, the glutamic acid being attached by way of its $\gamma$-carboxyl group, a mode of attachment differing from its usual connection by way of the $\alpha$-carboxyl (peptide link) in protein molecules. In the oxidized form (abbreviated GSSG) it acts in cells as a hydrogen acceptor and, in the reduced form (abbreviated GSH), as a hydrogen donor. The oxidized form is reduced by glutathione reductase (EC 1.6.4.2). It appears to be a ubiquitous reducing agent, involved in many redox reactions.

**gluteal** (glu'te-al) [ G. *gloutos,* buttock ]. Relating to the buttocks.

**glu'telins.** A class of simple proteins occurring in the seeds of grain, soluble in dilute acids and alkalies, but not in neutral solutions (*e.g.,* glutenin from wheat).

**glu'ten** [ L. *gluten,* glue ]. Wheat gum; the insoluble protein constituent of wheat and other grains, a mixture of gliadin, glutenin, and other proteins.

**g. casein,** a protein resembling casein, present in g.

**glu'tenin.** A glutelin in wheat.

**glu'teofem'oral.** Relating to the buttocks and the thigh.

**gluteo-inguinal** (glu'te-o-ing'gwĭ-nal). Relating to the buttock and the groin.

**gluteth'imide** (NF, BP). DORIDEN; 2-ethyl-2-phenyl-glutarimide. A central nervous system depressant used as a hypnotic in simple insomnia and as a preoperative and daytime sedative.

**glute'us.** *Musculus* gluteus.

**glu'tin.** 1. Gliadin. 2. Gelatin.

**glutinosin.** Antibiotic substance produced by *Metarrhizium glutinosum;* an antifungal agent.

**glu'tinous.** Adhesive; sticky.

**glutitis** (glu-ti'tis) [ G. *gloutos,* buttock, + suffix *-itis,* inflammation ]. Inflammation of the muscles of the buttock.

**glu'toscope** [ L. *gluten,* glue, + G. *skopeō,* to view ]. An apparatus devised by Bevan for the diagnosis of *Brucella abortus* infection in man by means of the agglutination test.

**glu'tose.** A 3-ketohexose similar in stereochemical arrangement to glucose.

**Glx.** Symbol for the radical of Glu and/or Gln; denotes uncertainty as between Glu and Gln.

**Gly.** Symbol for the radical of glycine (glycyl).

**gly'buride** (USAN). DIABETA; 1-[ [ *p*-[ 2-(5-chloro-*o*-anisamido)ethyl ]phenyl ]sulfonyl ]-3-cyclohexylurea; an oral hypoglycemic drug.

**glybuthi'azol.** GLIPASOL; *N*'-(5-*tert*-butyl-1,3,4-thiadiazol-2-yl)-sulfanilamide; oral hypoglycemic agent for the treatment of diabetes mellitus.

**gly'cal.** Glucal.

**gly'can.** Polysaccharide.

**glycanohydrolases** (EC group 3.2.1). Hydrolases acting on glycans; chitinase and hyaluronoglucosidase are glycanohydrolases.

**glycemia** (gli-se'mĭ-ah) [ G. *glykys,* sweet, + *haima,* blood ]. The presence of glucose in the blood.

**glyceraldehyde** (glis'er-al'de-hid). Glyceric aldehyde; glycerose; HOCH₂CHOHCHO; a triose; the simplest optically active monosaccharide. The dextrorotatory isomer is taken as the structural reference point for all D compounds; the levorotatory isomer for all L compounds.

**glyceraldehyde 3-phosphate.** CHOCHOHCH₂OPO₃H₂; an intermediate in the glycolytic breakdown of glucose; one of the products of the splitting of fructose 1,6-bisphosphate under the catalytic influence of fructose-bisphosphate aldolase.

**glyceric acid** (glĭ-sĕr'ik, glis'er-ik). CH₂OHCHOH-COOH; the fatty acid analogue of glycerol; occurring, particularly in the form of phosphorylated derivatives, as an intermediate in glycolysis.

**L-glyceric aciduria.** Excretion of L-glyceric acid in the urine; a primary metabolic error due to deficiency of D-glyceric dehydrogenase resulting in excretion of L-glyceric and oxalic acids, leading to the clinical syndrome of oxalosis with frequent formation of oxalate renal calculi.

**glyceric aldehyde.** Glyceraldehyde.

**glyceridases** (glis'er-ĭ-dās-ez). A general term for enzymes catalyzing the hydrolysis of glycerol esters (glycerides); *e.g.,* triacylglycerol lipase (EC 3.1.1.3).

**glyceride** (glis'er-id, -id). An ester of glycerol. The term is usually used in combination with phospho- (phosphoglyceride). The use of mono-, di-, and triglyceride is being

replaced by the more precise terms mono-, di-, and triacylglycerol, respectively.

**mixed g.'s,** g.'s which, on hydrolysis, yield more than one variety of fatty acid.

**glycerin** (glis'er-in) (USP, BP). Glycerol.

**g. jelly,** glycerinated *gelatin.*

**glyc'erite.** 1. Glycerol. 2. A pharmaceutical preparation made by triturating the active medicinal substance with glycerol.

**starch g.** (NF), contains starch 100 gm., benzoic acid 2 gm., purified water 200 ml., and glycerin 700 gm., in each 1000 gm. Topical emollient.

**tannic acid g.,** g. of tannin; contains tannic acid 20, sodium citrate 1, exsiccated sodium sulfite 0.2, and glycerin 78.8. Astringent.

**glyc'erogel'atin.** Glycerinated *gelatin.*

**glyc'eroki'nase.** Glycerol kinase.

**glycerol** (glis'er-ol). 1,2,3-Propanetriol; glycerin; glycerite (1); glyceryl alcohol; C₃H₅(OH)₃; a sweet, oily fluid, obtained by the saponification of fats and fixed oils. It is used as a solvent, as an application to roughened and chapped skin, by injection or in the form of suppository for constipation, orally to reduce ocular tension, and as a vehicle and sweetening agent. It is a pharmaceutical necessity for several official preparations.

**g. ether,** a phosphatidate in which the fatty acid at the α' position of the glycerol is replaced by A,β unsaturated alcohol residue in ether linkage to the glycerol.

**iodinated g.,** ORGANIDIN; isomeric mixture of 67–75 per cent of 2-(1-iodoethyl)-1,3-dioxolane-4-methanol and 33–25 per cent of 2-(2-iodoethyl)-1,3-dioxolane-4-methanol; a mucolytic agent.

**g. kinase** (EC 2.7.1.30), glycerokinase; catalyzes reaction between ATP and glycerol to yield glycerol phosphate and ADP.

**glycerophosphates** (glis'er-o-fos'fāts). Salts or esters of glycerophosphoric acids; some are used therapeutically.

**glycerophosphocholine.** Glycerylphosphorylcholine; HOCH₂CHOHCH₂OP(O₂H)OCH₂CH₂N⁺(CH₃)₃; a component of phosphatidylcholines (lecithins), in which the 2 OH's of glycerophosphocholine are esterified with fatty acids.

**glyc'erophosphor'ic acids.** Phosphoric esters of glycerol.

**glycerose** (glis'er-ōz). Glyceraldehyde.

**glyceryl** (glis'er-il) [ G. *hylē,* stuff ]. The trivalent radical, C₃H₅, of glycerol; often used in error for glycero- or glyceryl.

**g. alcohol,** glycerol.

**g. borate,** boroglycerin.

**g. ether,** an aliphatic alcohol in ether linkage to the α carbon of glycerol; three such compounds (chimyl, batyl, and selachyl alcohols) have been isolated from shark oil.

**g. guaiacolate** (NF), guaiacol glyceryl (glycerol) ether; GUAIAMAR; 3-(*o*-methoxyphenoxy)-1,2-propanediol; an expectorant that reduces the viscosity of sputum.

**g. monostearate** (NF), MONOSTEARIN; the ester of glycerol and one molecule of stearic acid; used in the manufacture of cosmetic creams and dermatologic preparations.

**g. triac'etate,** triacetin; triacetylglycerol; used as a solvent of basic dyes, and as a fixative in perfumery.

**g. trinitrate,** nitroglycerin.

**glyc'erylphos'phorylcho'line.** Glycerophosphocholine.

**gly'cine.** Aminoacetic acid, NH₂—CH₂—COOH. Used as a nutrient and dietary supplement, and in solution for irrigation. Symbol, Gly.

**g. amidinotransferase** (EC 2.1.4.1), g. transamidinase; an enzyme catalyzing the transfer of an amidine group from arginine to glycine, forming glycocyamine and ornithine; an important reaction in creatine synthesis.

**g. dehydrogenase,** an enzyme (EC 1.4.1.10) that catalyzes the conversion of glycine to glyoxylic acid and ammonia.

**g. succinate cycle,** see under cycle.

**g. transamidinase,** g. amidinotransferase.

**glycinemia** (gli'si-ne'mĭ-ah). Hyperglycinuria with hyperglycinemia; see under hyperglycinuria.

**glycineamide ribonucleotide.** Intermediate in purine biosynthesis, in which the amide N of glycineamide is linked to the C-1 of a ribosyl moiety.

**glycine-rich β-glycoprotein.** See cobra venom *cofactor,* and *properdin* factor B.

**glycinuria** (gli'sĭ-nu'rĭ-ah). The excretion of glycine in the urine.

    **familial g.,** a metabolic disorder believed to be due to defective renal glycine reabsorption; it may or may not be accompanied by oxalate urolithiasis; autosomal dominant inheritance.

**glyco-** (gli'ko-) [ G. *glykys,* sweet ]. Combining form denoting relationship to sugars in general; see gluco-, fructo-, etc., for individual sugars.

**glycoaldehydetransferase.** Transketolase.

**glycobi'arsol** (NF). MILIBIS; (hydrogen *N*-glycoloylarsanilato)oxobismuth; a pentavalent arsenical containing bismuth; used in the treatment of milder forms of intestinal amebiasis or as subsequent therapy.

**glycocalyx** (gli'ko-ka'liks) [ glyco- + G. *kalyx,* husk, shell ]. An outer coating of carbohydrate-rich molecules detected, with the electron microscope, on the free surface of certain cells.

**glycocholate** (gli'ko-ko'lāt). A salt or ester of glycocholic acid.

    **g. sodium,** a normal constituent of bile of man and herbivora; glycocholate sodium from herbivora is purified and used as a choleretic and cholagogue.

**glycocholic acid** (gli'ko-ko'lik). One of the major bile acid conjugates; cholylglycine, formed by condensation of the —COOH group of cholic acid and the NH₂ group of glycine; water-soluble and a powerful detergent.

**gly'cocin.** Glycine.

**gly'cocoll.** Glycine.

**gly'cocor'ticoid.** Glucocorticoid.

**glycocy'amine.** 2-Guanidinoacetic acid; glucocyamine; $HN = C(NH_2)NHCH_2COOH$; formed by the transfer of the amidine group from arginine to glycine.

**glycogel'atin.** Glycerinated *gelatin.*

**glycogen** (gli'ko-jen). Animal dextran; a glucosan of high molecular weight, resembling amylopectin in structure, but even more highly branched; found in most of the tissues of the body, especially those of the liver and muscular tissue; the principal carbohydrate reserve, it is readily converted into glucose.

    **g. phosphorylase** phosphorylase (2).

    **g. synthase,** a glucosyltransferase (EC 2.4.1.11) catalyzing the incorporation of glucose from UDPglucose into 1,4-α-D-glucosyl chains.

**glycogenase** (gli'ko-jĕ-nās'). An enzyme catalyzing the breakdown of glycogen to glucose 1-phosphate (*e.g.,* phosphorylase); amylo-1,6-glucosidase, 4-α-glucanotransferase, and α- and β-amylase.

**glycogenesis** (gli-ko-jen'e-sis) [ glyco- + G. *genesis,* production ]. The formation of glycogen from glucose by means of glycogen synthase and dextran dextranase. The first enzyme catalyzes formation of a polyglucose with α—1,4 links from UDPglucose; the second cleaves fragments from one chain and transfers them to an α-1,6 linkage in another.

**glycogenet'ic, glycogen'ic.** Relating to glycogenesis.

**glycogenolysis** (gli'ko-jĕ-nol'ĭ-sis). The hydrolysis of glycogen to glucose; see glycogenesis.

**glycogenosis** (gli'ko-jĕ-no'sis). Glycogen storage disease; any of the glycogen deposition diseases characterized by accumulation of glycogen of normal or abnormal chemical structure in tissue. There may be enlargement of the liver, heart, or striated muscle, including the tongue, with progressive muscular weakness. Six types (Cori classification) are recognized, depending on the enzyme deficiency involved; see types 1 to 6, below.

    **generalized g.,** type 2 g.

    **glucose 6-phosphatase hepatorenal g.,** type 1 g.

    **hepatophosphorylase deficiency g.,** type 6 g.

    **myophosphorylase deficiency g.,** type 5 g.

    **type 1 g.,** von Gierke's disease; glucose 6-phosphatase hepatorenal g.; g. due to glucose 6-phosphatase deficiency resulting in accumulation of excessive amounts of glycogen of normal chemical structure, particularly in liver and kidney.

    **type 2 g.,** generalized g.; Pompe's disease; g. due to lysosomal α-1,4-glucosidase deficiency resulting in accumulation of excessive amounts of glycogen of normal chemical structure in heart, muscle, liver and nervous system.

    **type 3 g.,** Cori's disease; Forbes' disease; limit dextrinosis; debrancher deficiency limit dextrinosis; g. due to amylo-1,6-glucosidase (debrancher enzyme) deficiency resulting in accumulation of abnormal glycogen with short outer chains in liver and muscle.

    **type 4 g.,** Andersen's disease; brancher deficiency amylopectinosis; familial cirrhosis of the liver with storage of abnormal glycogen; g. due to brancher enzyme deficiency resulting in accumulation of abnormal glycogen with long inner and outer chains in liver, kidney, muscle, and other tissues.

    **type 5 g.,** McArdle's disease; McArdle-Schmid-Pearson disease; myophosphorylase deficiency g.; g. due to muscle glycogen phosphorylase deficiency resulting in accumulation of glycogen of normal chemical structure in muscle.

    **type 6 g.,** hepatophosphorylase deficiency g.; Hers' disease; g. due to hepatic glycogen phosphorylase deficiency resulting in accumulation of glycogen of normal chemical structure in liver and leukocytes.

**glycogenous** (gli-koj'ĕ-nus). Glycogenetic.

**glycogeny** (gli-koj'ĕ-nĭ). Glycogenesis.

**glycogeusia** (gli-ko-gu'sĭ-ah) [ glyco- + G. *geusis,* taste ]. A subjective sweet taste.

**glycoglycinuria** (gli'ko-gli-sĭ-nu'rĭ-ah). A metabolic disorder characterized by glucosuria and hyperglycinuria; autosomal dominant inheritance.

**glycol** (gli'kol). 1. A compound containing adjacent alcohol groups. 2. Ethylene glycol; the simplest glycol, $CH_2OHCH_2OH$.

**glycolacria** (gli'ko-lak'rĭ-ah) [ glyco- + L. *lacrima,* tear, + suffix -*ia,* condition ]. An abnormally high concentration of glucose in tears; associated with hyperglycemia.

**gly'colal'dehyde.** $CH_2OHCHO$; diose; the simplest possible sugar; the aerobic deamination product of ethanolamine; a probable intermediate in the interconversion of serine and glycine.

**glycol'ic acid.** $HOCH_2COOH$; an intermediate in the interconversion of glycine and ethanolamine.

**glycolic aciduria.** Excessive excretion of glycolic acid in the urine; a primary metabolic defect due to deficiency of 2-hydroxy-3-oxoadipate carboxylase, resulting in excretion of glycolic and oxalic acids, leading to the clinical syndrome of oxalosis.

**gly'colip'id.** Glycosphingolipid.

**glycolyl** (gli'ko-lil). The —CO—CH₂OH radical, replacing acetyl in some sialic acids; the products are sometimes referred to as *N*-glycolylneuraminic acids.

**glycolysis** (gli-kol'ĭ-sis) [ glyco- + G. *lysis,* a loosening ]. The energy-yielding conversion of glucose to lactic acid in various tissues, notably muscle; since molecular oxygen is not consumed in the process, this is frequently referred to as "anaerobic g."

**glycolyt'ic.** Relating to glycolysis.

**glyconeogenesis** (gli'ko-ne-o-jen'e-sis) [ glyco- + G. *neos,* new, + *genesis,* production ]. The formation of glycogen from noncarbohydrates, such as protein or fat, by conversion of the latter to glucose. See glycogenesis.

**glycopenia** (gli'ko-pe'nĭ-ah) [ glyco- + G. *penia,* poverty ]. A deficiency of any or all sugars in an organ or tissue.

**glycopexis** (gli-ko-pek'sis) [ glyco- + G. *pēxis,* fixation ]. The storing of glycogen in the liver; obsolete.

**Glycophagus** (gli-kof'ă-gus) [ glyco- + G. *phagein,* to eat ]. A common genus of grain mites, frequently implicated in dermatitis among food handlers. See also *Tyrophagus putrescentiae.*

**glycophilia** (gli-ko-fil'ĭ-ah) [ glyko- + G. *phileō,* to love ]. A condition in which there is a distinct tendency to develop hyperglycemia, even after the ingestion of a relatively small quantity of glucose.

**glycopolyuria** (gli'ko-pol-ĭ-u'rĭ-ah) [ glyco- + G. *polys,* much, + *ouron,* urine ]. Obsolete term for diabetes mellitus in which the polyuria is more marked than the glycosuria.

**gly'copro'tein.** Glucoprotein. 1. One of a group of protein-carbohydrate compounds (conjugated proteins), among which the most important are the mucins, mucoid, and amyloid. 2. Sometimes restricted to proteins containing small amounts of carbohydrate, in contrast to mucoids or mucoproteins, usually measured as hexosamine. Such conjugated proteins are found in many places, notably γ-globulins, $α_1$-globulins, $α_2$-globulins, transferrin, etc., and are contained in mucus and mucins. See also mucoprotein.

**$β_2$-glycoprotein II.** See cobra venom *cofactor*, and *properdin* factor B.

**glycoptyalism** (gli'ko-ti'ă-lizm) [ glyco- + G. *ptyalon*, saliva ]. Glycosialia.

**glycopyr'rolate** (NF). ROBINUL; 3-hydroxy-1,1-dimethylpyrrolidinium bromide α-cyclopentylmandelate; a cholinergic blocking agent used as an adjunct in the treatment of peptic ulcer; contraindicated in patients with glaucoma, cardiospasm, and prostatic hypertrophy.

**glycorrhachia** (gli-kŏra'kĭ-ah, -rak-ĭ-ah) [ glyco- + G. *rhachis*, spine ]. The presence of sugar in the cerebrospinal fluid.

**glycorrhea** (gli-ko-re'ah) [ glyco- + G. *rhoia*, a flow ]. A discharge of sugar from the body, as in glucosuria, especially in unusually large quantities.

**glycosecretory** (gli'ko-se-kre'to-rĭ). Causing or involved in the secretion of glycogen.

**glycosialia** (gli'ko-si-al'ĭ-ah, -a'lĭ-ah) [ glyco- + G. *sialon*, saliva ]. Glycoptyalism; the presence of sugar in the saliva.

**glycosialorrhea** (gli'ko-si'ă-lo-re'ah) [ glyco- + G. *sialon*, saliva, + *rhoia*, a flow ]. An excessive secretion of saliva that contains sugar.

**gly'coside.** The condensation product of a sugar with any other radical involving the loss of the H of the hemiacetal OH of the sugar, thus leaving the O of this OH as the link. Thus, the condensation through the O-1 with an alcohol, which loses its OH, yields an alcohol-glycoside. Links involving loss of the 1-OH, as with a purine or pyrimidine, yield glycosyl compounds.

***N*-glycoside.** Misnomer for glycosyl.

**glycosometer** (gli'ko-som'e-ter) [ glyco- + G. *metron*, measure ]. An instrument for determining the approximate proportion of sugar in the urine in glycosuria.

**glycosphingolipid** (gli'co-sfing-o-lip'id). Ceramide saccharide; a ceramide linked to one or more sugars *via* the terminal OH group. Included as g.'s are cerebrosides (monoglycosylceramides, ceramide monosaccharides), gangliosides (g.'s containing neuraminic acid) and ceramide oligosaccharides (oligoglycosylceramides). The prefix glyc- may be replaced by gluc-, galact-, lact-, etc.

**gly'costat'ic.** Indicating the property of certain extracts of the anterior hypophysis that permits the body to maintain its glycogen stores in muscle, liver, and other tissues. Purified pituitary growth hormone exerts such an effect in skeletal muscle.

**glycosuria** (gli-ko-su'rĭ-ah) [ glyco- + G. *ouron*, urine ]. 1. Glucosuria. 2. The urinary excretion of carbohydrates.

**alimentary g.**, that developing after the ingestion of a moderate amount of sugar or starch, which normally is disposed of without appearing in the urine.

**benign g.**, g. not associated with diabetes mellitus but resulting from a low renal threshold for sugar.

**digestive g.**, alimentary g.

**negligible g.**, *diabetes* innocens.

**nervous g.**, g. produced by a localized lesion of the medulla or stimulation of splanchnic nerves.

**normoglyce'mic g.**, the excretion of sugar in the urine when the amount in the blood is not in excess of normal; renal g.

**pathologic g.**, chronic excretion of relatively large amounts of sugar in the urine.

**phlor'idzin** or **phlor'izin g.**, the presence of sugar in the urine after the experimental administration of phloridzin, which results in a lower renal threshold for reabsorption of glucose.

**renal g.**, the recurring or persistent excretion of glucose in the urine, in association with blood levels that are in the normal range; results from the failure of renal tubules to reabsorb glucose at a normal rate from the glomerular filtrate. Diabetes innocens.

**glycosu'ric acid.** Homogentisic acid.

**gly'cosyl.** The radical resulting from detachment of the OH of the hemiacetal of a saccharide. Contrast glycoside.

**g. compound**, the compound formed between a sugar and another organic substance in which the OH of the reducing (hemiacetal) group of the former is removed; the natural nucleosides, in which a heterocyclic N becomes linked directly to the C-1 of ribose (or deoxyribose) to yield ribosyl compounds, are well known examples. Such compounds were formerly known as *N*-glycosides (*N*-ribosides).

**gly'cosyltrans'ferase.** Transglycosylase; any enzyme (EC subclass 2.4) transferring glycosyl groups from one compound to another.

**glycotropic, glycotrophic** (gli'ko-trop'ik, -trof'ik) [ glyco- + G. *trophē*, nourishment; *tropē*, a turning ]. Pertaining to a principle in extracts of the anterior lobe of the pituitary that antagonizes the action of insulin and causes hyperglycemia. See glycotropic *factor*.

**glycuresis** (gli-ku-re'sis) [ glyco- + G. *ourēsis*, urination ]. Glycosuria.

**glycu'ronate.** A salt or ester of a uronic acid (*e.g.*, glucuronate).

**glycuron'ic acid.** A uronic acid (*e.g.*, glucuronic acid).

**glycuron'idase.** Glucuronidase.

**glycu'ronide.** A glycoside of a uronic acid (*e.g.*, glucuronide).

**glycuronu'ria.** The presence of glucuronic acid in the urine.

**glycyl** (gli'sil). Univalent acid radical derived from glycine.

**g. betaine**, betaine.

**g. chain**, see under chain.

**glycyrrhetinic** or **glycyrrhetic acid** (glis'ĭ-re-tin'ik, -re'tik). The aglycone of glycyrrhizic acid; $C_{30}H_{46}O_4$; a pentacyclic terpene.

**glycyrrhiza** (glis-ĭ-ri'zah) [ G. fr. *glykys*, sweet, + *rhiza*, root ] (USP). Liquorice (BP); glycyrrhizae radix; licorice root; the dried rhizome and root of *Glycyrrhiza glabra* (family Leguminoseae) and allied species; demulcent, slightly laxative, and expectorant, and also used to disguise the taste of other remedies. BP. Its action appears to depend upon glycyrrhizic acid, a salt-retaining principle that mimics the action of aldosterone. Patients ingesting licorice show hypertension, alkalosis, and suppressed plasma renin activity. Aldosterone secretion, however, is also suppressed as a result of volume expansion.

**glycyrrhizic** or **glycyrrhizinic acid** (glis'ĭ-ri'zik, -ri-zin'-ik). Glycyrrhizin; a very sweet glycoside present in glycyrrhiza; $C_{42}H_{62}O_{16}$. On hydrolysis it yields 2 mols of glucuronic acid and 1 of glycyrrhetinic acid.

**glycyrrhizin** (glis'ĭ-ri'zin). Glycyrrhizic acid.

**glyox'al.** CHO—CHO; the simplest dialdehyde.

**glyox'alase.** Lactoyl-glutathione lyase (glyoxalase I) or hydroxyacylglutathione hydrolase (glyoxalase II); an enzyme in red cells and other tissues that converts glyoxal and substituted glyoxals into the corresponding hydroxy acids.

**g. I**, lactoyl-glutathione lyase.

**g. II**, hydroxyacylglutathione hydrolase.

**glyox'aline.** Imidazole.

**glyox'ylate transac'etase.** Malate synthase.

**glyoxyldiureide.** Allantoin.

**glyoxyl'ic acid.** CHO—COOH; produced by the action of glycine oxidase upon glycine or sarcosine, or from allantoic acid by allantoicase.

**g. acid cycle**, see under cycle.

**Glyptocra'nium gasteracanthoi'des** [ G. *glyptos*, carved, + *kranion*, skull; *gastēr*, belly, + *akantha*, thorn ]. Pruning spider; Peruvian tarantula; a poisonous Peruvian spider whose bite causes local gangrene, hematuria, and neurotoxic symptoms.

**gm.** Abbreviation for gram; also abbreviated g.

**Gmelin** (mel'in), Leopold, German physiologist and chemist, 1788–1853. See G.'s *test*, Rosenbach-G. *test*.

**GMP.** Abbreviation for guanosine 5'-phosphoric acid.

**gnashing** (nash'ing). The grinding together of the teeth as a nonmasticatory function; usually associated with emotional tension; see also bruxism; bruxomania.

**gnat** (nat) [ A.S. *gnaet* ]. A general term applied to several species of minute insects; a midge; a "no-see-um." British authors sometimes include mosquitoes in this group, but this is not done in America.

**buffalo g.,** a species of *Simulium, q. v.*

**eye g.,** see *Hippolates.*

**gnath-.** See gnatho-.

**gnathalgia** (nă-thal'jĭ-ah) [ G. *gnathos,* jaw, + *algos,* pain ]. Gnathodynia.

**gnathic** (nath'ik) [ G. *gnathos,* jaw ]. Relating to the jaw or alveolar process.

**gnathion** (nath'ĭ-on) [ G. *gnathos,* jaw ]. The most inferior point of the mandible in the midline. See fig. under craniometric *point.*

**gnathitis** (nă-thi'tis) [ G. *gnathos,* jaw, + suffix *-itis,* inflammation ]. Inflammation of the jaw.

**gnatho-, gnath-** (nath'o-) [ G. *gnathos,* jaw ]. Combining form relating to the jaw.

**gnathocephalus** (nath-o-sef'al-us) [ *gnatho-* + G. *kephalē,* head ]. A malformed fetus with little of the head except the jaws.

**gnathodynamics** (nath-o-di-nam'iks) [ gnatho- + G. *dynamis,* power ]. Refers to the relationship during function of the opposing occlusal (and incisal) surfaces of the teeth in contact (see occlusion) and of the mandibular condyles to the skull. It is also concerned with the tensive forces of the muscles of mastication, their magnitude, direction, and point of application; the components of forces due to cuspal inclines and resulting stresses in the supporting structures; the motions of the mandible.

**gnathodynamometer** (nath'o-di'nah-mom'e-ter) [ gnatho- + dynamometer ]. Bite gauge; occlusometer; a device for measuring biting pressure.

**Bimeter g.,** manufacturer's designation for a g. equipped with a central-bearing point of adjustable height and used in prosthodontics to determine the "power point" as an aid in establishing the occlusal vertical dimension.

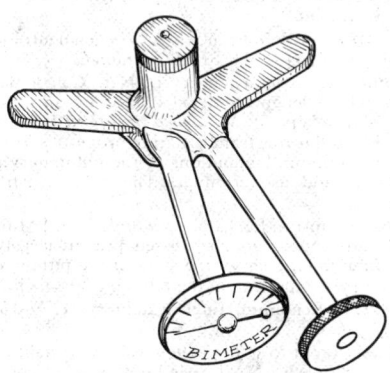

**Bimeter Gnathodynamometer**

**gnathodynia** (nath-o-din'ĭ-ah) [ G. gnatho- + G. *odynē,* pain ]. Gnathalgia; pain in the jaw.

**gnathography** (nă-thog'ră-fĭ). The recording of the action of the masticatory apparatus in function.

**gnathological** (nath'o-loj'ĭ-kal). Pertaining to gnathodynamics.

**gnathology** (nă-thol'o-jĭ). The science of gnathodynamics.

**gnathopalatoschisis** (nath'o-pal-a-tos'kĭ-sis). Clefts of prepalate and palate.

**gnathoplasty** (nath'o-plas-tĭ) [ gnatho- + G. *plassō,* to form ]. Reparative surgery of the jaw.

**gnathoschisis** (nă-thos'kĭ-sis) [ gnatho- + G. *schisis,* a cleaving ]. Developmental cleft of alveolar process.

**gnathostatics** (nath'o-stat'iks) [ gnatho- + G. *statikos,* causing to stand ]. In orthodontic diagnosis, a technical procedure for orienting the dentition to certain cranial landmarks.

**Gnathostoma** (nă-thos'to-mah) [ gnatho- + G. *stoma,* mouth ]. A genus of spiruroid nematode worms characterized by several rows of cuticular spines about the head and by multiple-host aquatic life cycles; it includes pathogenic parasites of cats, cattle, and swine.

**G. siamen'se,** invalid name for *G. spinigerum.*

**G. spinig'erum,** a parasite of cats, dogs, and wild carnivores, but has occasionally been found in man in the Far East; it is transmitted via copepods and fish; human infection is usually confined to the skin, but several cases have been reported of infection of the human eye or brain with wandering larvae of this species.

**gnathostomiasis** (nath-o-sto-mi'ăsis). Yangtze edema; a migrating edema, or creeping eruption, caused by cutaneous infection by larvae of *Gnathostoma spinigerum.*

**gnoscopine** (nos'ko-pēn). α-Gnoscopine; *dl*-narcotine; an opium alkaloid, $C_{22}H_{23}NO_7$, obtained by racemization of noscapine (*q. v.*); antitussive.

**gnosia** (no'sĭ-ah) [ G. *gnōsis,* knowledge ]. The perceptive faculty enabling one to recognize the form and the nature of persons and things.

**gnotobiology** (no'to-bi-ol'o-jĭ) [ G. *gnotos,* known, + *bios,* life, + *logos,* study ]. The study of animals in the absence of bacteria, viruses, fungi, and so on, throughout the life of an animal; *i.e.,* of a "germ-free" animal in which there is no other form of life.

**gnotobiota** (no'to-bi-o'tah) [ G. *gnotos,* known, + L. *biota, q. v.* ]. Living colonies or species, assembled from pure isolates.

**gnotobiote** (no'to-bi'ōt). An individual organism from a group assembled from pure isolates.

**gnotobiotics** (no-to-bi-ot'iks). Gnotobiology.

**goal** (gōl). In psychology, any object or objective that an organism seeks to attain or achieve.

**go'a powder.** Araroba.

**Godélier** (go-da-le-a'), Charles P., French physician, 1813–1877. See G.'s *law.*

**Godman,** John D., American anatomist, 1794–1830. See G.'s *fascia.*

**Goeckerman treatment.** See under treatment.

**Goethe** (gë'tē), Johann W. von, German poet, philosopher, and scientist, 1749–1832. See G.'s *bone.*

**Gofman,** Moses, German physician, *1887. See G. *test.*

**Goggia** (gah'jah), Carlo P., Italian physician, 20th century. See G.'s *sign.*

**gog'gle.** 1. A screen cover for the eye. 2. A kind of spectacle with auxiliary shields for protecting the eyes.

**plethysmographic g.,** a specially designed g. to serve as an ophthalmodynamometer while permitting subjective visual and objective ocular changes during transient increased intraocular pressure.

**goiter** (goy'ter) [ Fr. from L. *guttur,* throat ]. Struma; a chronic enlargement of the thyroid gland, not due to a neoplasm, occurring endemically in certain localities, especially mountainous regions, and sporadically elsewhere.

**aber'rant g.,** enlargement of a supernumerary thyroid gland.

**acute g.,** one that develops very rapidly.

**adeno'matous g.,** an enlargement of the thyroid gland due to the growth of one or more encapsulated adenomas or multiple nonencapsulated colloid nodules within its substance.

**cabbage g.,** g. due to cabbage or other goitrogenic item of the diet.

**colloid g.,** adenoma gelatinosa; a form in which the contents of the follicles increase greatly, causing pressure atrophy of the epithelium so that the gelatinous matter predominates in the tumor.

**cystic g.,** an enlargement in the thyroid region due to the presence of one or more cysts within the gland.

**diffuse g.,** g. in which the morbid process involves the whole gland, as opposed to nodular g. or thyroid adenoma.

**diver g.,** wandering g.; a freely movable g. that is sometimes above and sometimes below the sternal notch.

**endem'ic g.,** g., usually of simple type, that is prevalent in certain regions, *e.g.,* Alps, where dietary intake of iodine is suboptimal.

**exophthal'mic g.,** any of the various forms of hyperthyroidism in which the thyroid gland is enlarged and exophthalmos is present.

**familial g.,** a group of heritable thyroid disorders in which g. is commonly apparent first during childhood; they are often associated with skeletal and/or mental retardation and other signs of hyperthyroidism may develop with age. Various types of familial g. have been identified: (1) iodide transport defect, in which the gland is unable to concentrate iodide; (2) organification defect, in which the iodination of tyrosine is defective; (3) Pendred's *syndrome;* (4) coupling defect, in which cretinism results from defective coupling of iodotyrosines to form iodothyronines; (5) iodotyrosine deiodinase defect, in which deiodination of iodotyrosine is defective and there is considerable glandular loss of these hormonal precursors and cretinism may be present; and (6) plasma iodoprotein disorder, in which an abnormal iodinated serum protein is present that is insoluble in acidic butanol.

**familial g. and deafmutism,** Pendred's *syndrome.*

**fibrous g.,** a firm hyperplasia of the thyroid and its capsule.

**follic'ular g.,** parenchymatous g.

**lingual g.,** a tumor of thyroid tissue involving the embryonic rudiment at the base of the tongue.

**lymphadenoid g.,** Hashimoto's *disease.*

**mi'crofollic'ular g.,** g. in which the glandular tissue consists of unusually small colloid filled follicles and areas of undifferentiated tissue with indistinct follicle formation.

**multinod'ular g.,** adenomatous g. with several colloid nodules.

**nontox'ic g.,** g. not accompanied by hyperthyroidism.

**parenchy'matous g.,** follicular g.; a form in which there is a great increase in the follicles with proliferation of the epithelium.

**simple g.,** thyroid enlargement unaccompanied by constitutional effects, *e.g.,* hypo- or hyperthyroidism. Commonly caused by inadequate dietary intake of iodine.

**subster'nal g.,** enlargement of the thyroid gland, chiefly of the lower part of the isthmus, palpable with difficulty or not at all.

**suf'focative g.,** one that by pressure causes extreme dyspnea.

**thorac'ic g.,** enlargement of accessory thyroid tissue in the thorax with or without hyperthyroidism.

**toxic g.,** one that forms an excessive secretion, causing signs and symptoms of hyperthyroidism.

**wandering g.,** diver g.

**goitrin** (goy'trin). 5-Vinyl-2-thiooxazolidone; the antithyroid or goitrogenic compound obtained from turnips and the seeds of cruciferous plants; only trace quantities of it are found in cabbage.

**goitrogen** (goy'tro-jen). Any substance that induces goiter, *e.g.,* cabbage, rapeseed, etc.

**goitrogenic** (goy-tro-jen'ik). Causing goiter.

**gold.** Aurum; a yellow metallic element, symbol Au, atomic no. 79, atomic weight 197.2.

**cohesive g.,** nearly pure g. so treated that it will weld cold.

**colloidal radioactive g.,** radiogold colloid.

**g. equivalent,** g. number; a unit of power of the protective colloids; the number of milligrams of protective colloid just sufficient to prevent the precipitation of 10 ml. of a 0.0053 to 0.0058 per cent gold solution by the action of 1 ml. of a 10 per cent sodium chloride solution.

**g. foil,** see cohesive g. and noncohesive g.

**mat g.,** powdered g. formed by electrolytic precipitation, compressed into strips, and sintered.

**noncohesive g.,** the condition of a pure g. foil which prevents welding. It may be temporary or permanent, depending on the chemical used in its treatment. Temporary treatment is for the purpose of protecting the foil from atmospheric contaminants. Foil so treated may be rendered cohesive by heating (annealing). Permanently noncohesive foil requires a different technique and instruments. It is most generally used in large tooth cavities with strong lateral walls.

**powdered g.,** g. formed by atomizing or by chemical precipitation, lightly precondensed, and wrapped with gold foil so as to form pellets.

**g. sodium thiom'alate** (USP), sodium aurothiomalate; disodium aurothiomalate; used in the treatment of rheumatoid arthritis.

**g. sodium thiosulfate,** sodium aurothiosulfate; used in the treatment of lupus erythematosus and some cases of rheumatoid arthritis.

**soft g.,** a type I casting g. alloy (American Dental Association specification no. 5).

**Goldberg,** Minnie Berelson, San Francisco internist, *1900. See G.-Maxwell *syndrome.*

**Goldblatt,** Harry, Cleveland pathologist, *1891. See G.'s *clamp, hypertension, kidney, phenomenon.*

**Goldenhar,** M., French physician. See G.'s *syndrome.*

**golden seal.** Hydrastis.

**Goldflam,** Samuel V., Polish neurologist, 1852–1932. See G. *disease,* Hoppe-G. *disease.*

**Goldhorn's stain.** See under stain.

**Goldman,** David E., U. S. physiologist, *1911. See G. *equation.*

**Goldman,** H. M. See G.-Fox *knife.*

**Goldmann,** Hans, Swiss ophthalmologist, *1899. See G. *perimeter,* G.'s applanation *tonometer.*

**Goldscheider** (gōlt'shi-der), J. K. A. E. Alfred, German neurologist, 1858–1935. See G.'s *disease, test.*

**Goldstein,** Hyman I., American physician, 1887–1954. See G.'s toe *sign.*

**Goldthwait,** Joel E., Boston surgeon, 1866–1961. See G.'s *sign.*

**Golgi** (gol'je), Camillo, Italian histologist, 1843–1926. Nobel laureate, 1906, with Santiago Ramon y Cajal, in recognition of their work in the structure of the nervous system. See G. *apparatus,* Holmgren-G. *canals,* G.'s *cells,* G. *complex,* G.-Mazzoni *corpuscle,* G.'s tendon *organ,* internal *reticulum, solution, stain, zone.*

**golgiokinesis** (gol'jī-o-kī-ne'sis). Dictyokinesis.

**Goll,** Friedrich, Swiss anatomist, 1829–1903. See G.'s *column, nucleus, tract.*

**Goltz,** Friedrich L., German physiologist, 1834–1902. See G.'s *experiment.*

**Gombault** (gom-bo'), Francois A., French neurologist and pathologist, 1844–1904. See G.'s *triangle.*

**go'menol** [ *Gomen,* a locality in New Caledonia, + L. *oleum,* oil ]. Oleogomenol; oil of niaouli; an ethereal oil obtained from a plant, *Melaleuca viridiflora.* It has germicidal action and is free from irritating properties. It has been used in chronic inflammations of the pulmonary mucous membrane and as vermifuge. The chief constituent is cineole.

**gomitoli** (gom-ī'to-lī) [ Ital. *gomitolo,* coil ]. Intricately coiled and looped capillary vessels present largely in the upper fundibular stem of the stalk of the pituitary gland; they comprise a portion of the pituitary portal circulation.

**Gompertz,** Benjamin, English actuary, 1779–1865. See G.'s *hypothesis.*

**gomphosis** (gom-fo'sis) [ G. *gomphos,* bolt, nail, + suffix *-osis,* condition ] [ NA ]. Peg and socket articulation; gompholic joint; a form of fibrous joint in which a peglike process fits into a hole, as the root of a tooth into the socket in the alveolus.

**gonacratia** (gon'ā-kra'shī-ah) [ G. *gonē,* seed, + *akrateia,* debility, fr. *a-* priv. + *kratos,* strength ]. Obsolete term meaning spermatorrhea.

**gon'ad** [ Mod. L. fr. G. *gonē,* seed ]. An organ that produces sex cells; the testis of a male or the ovary of a female.

**female g.,** ovary.

**indifferent g.,** the primordial organ in an embryo before its differentiation into testis or ovary.

**male g.,** testis.

**gonad-.** See gonado-.

**gon'adal.** Relating to a gonad.

**gon'adec'tomy** [ gonado- + G. *ektomē,* excision ]. Excision of ovary or testis.

**gonado-, gonad-** [ G. *gonē,* seed ]. Combining forms relating to the gonads.

**gon'adop'athy** [ gonado- + G. *pathos,* suffering ]. Disease affecting the gonads.

**gonadotroph** (go-nad'o-trof, -gon'ä-do-). A cell of the adenohypophysis that affects certain cells of the ovary or testis.

**gonadotrophic** (gon'ä-do-trof'ik). Gonadotropic.

**gonadotrophin** (gon'ä-do-tro'fin) [ gonado- + G. *trophē*, nourishment ]. Gonadotropin.

**gonadotropic** (gon'ä-do-trop'ik) [ gonado- + G. *tropē*, a turning ]. Gonadotrophic. 1. Descriptive of or relating to the actions of a gonadotropin. 2. Promoting the growth and/or function of the gonads.

**gonadotropin** (gon'ä-do-tro'pin). Gonadotrophin; gonadotrotropic hormone; a hormone capable of promoting gonadal growth and function; such effects, as exerted by a single hormone, are usually limited to discrete functions or histological components of a gonad, such as stimulation of follicular growth or of androgen formation. Most g.'s exert their effects in both sexes, although the effect of a given g. will be very different usually in males and in females. 2. Any substance capable of producing the biological effects described above.

   **anterior pitu'itary g.,** any g. of hypophysial origin. This phrase was formerly used to designate a single hormone, because it was thought that the anterior hypophysis secreted only one g.

   **chorion'ic g.** (USP), anterior pituitary-like substance; a glycoprotein with a carbohydrate fraction composed of galactose and hexosamine, prepared from the urine of pregnant women; a hormone that is produced by the placental trophoblastic cells. Its most important role appears to be stimulation, during the first trimester, of ovarian secretion of the estrogen and progesterone required for the integrity of conceptus. It appears to play no significant role in the last two trimesters of pregnancy, as these steroid hormones are then formed by the placenta. Used in the treatment of cryptorchidism and as an aid to conception in women by substituting for endogenous luteinizing hormone,

   **equine g.,** pregnant mare's serum g.; PMSG; formed by the equine placenta. Its activity in animals is similar to that of the follicle-stimulating hormone; relatively ineffective in human beings.

   **human chorionic g.,** HCG; see chorionic g.

   **human menopausal g.,** HMG; an injectable preparation obtained from the urine of menopausal women; biological activity is similar to that of follicle-stimulating hormone, but also weakly mimics the effects of luteinizing hormone. Used in conjunction with human chorionic gonadotropin to induce ovulation. See also menotropins.

   **pregnant mare's serum g.,** abbreviated PMSG; see equine g.

**gon'aduct** [ gonado- + duct ]. 1. Seminal *duct.* 2. Oviduct.

**gonag'ra.** Gonatagra.

**gonalgia** (go-nal'jï-ah) [ G. *gony*, knee, + *algos*, pain ]. Pain in the knee.

**gonane.** The hypothetical parent hydrocarbon molecule of the gonadal steroid hormones, such as estrane or androstane (*cf.* sterane). Term was conceived to achieve forms of systematic nomenclature; see steroids.

**gonangiectomy** (gon-an-jï-ek'to-mï) [ G. *gonē*, seed, + *angeion*, vessel, + *ektomē*, excision ]. Vasectomy.

**gonarthritis** (gon-ar-thri'tis) [ G. *gony*, knee, + *arthron*, joint, + suffix *-itis*, inflammation ]. Inflammation of the knee joint.

**gonarthrocace** (gon'ar-throk'ä-sē) [ G. *gony*, knee, + *arthron*, joint, + *kakē*, vice ]. White swelling; tuberculosis of the knee joint.

**gonarthromeningitis** (gon-ar'thro-men-in-ji'tis) [ G. *gony*, knee, + *arthron*, joint, + *mēninx*, membrane, + suffix *-itis*, inflammation ]. Synovitis of the knee.

**gonarthrotomy** (gon'ar-throt'o-mï) [ G. *gony*, knee, + *arthron*, joint, + *tomē*, incision ]. Incision into the knee joint.

**gonatagra** (gon'ä-tag'rah) [ G. *gony*, knee, + *agra*, seizure ]. Gonagra; gout in the knee.

**gonatocele** (go-nat'o-sēl) [ G. *gony*, knee, + *kēlē*, tumor ]. White swelling; tumor of the knee.

**gonecyst, gonecystis** (gon'e-sist, gon-e-sis'tis) [ G. *gonē*, seed, + *kystis*, bladder ]. *Vesicula seminalis.*

**gonecystolith** (gon-e-sis'to-lith) [ gonecyst + G. *kystis*, bladder, + *lithos*, stone ]. A concretion or calculus in a seminal vesicle.

**gonepoiesis** (gon-e-poy-e'sis) [ G. *gonē*, seed, + *poiēsis*, a producing ]. Obsolete term for spermatogenesis.

**gonepoietic** (gon-e-poy-et'ik). Obsolete term for spermatogenic.

**Gongylonema** (gon'jï-lo-ne'mah) [ Gr. *gongylos*, round, + *nēma*, thread ]. An important genus of spiruroid nematodes that parasitize birds (6 species) and mammals (24 species). Several species are of veterinary importance; one is of medical importance.

   **G. ingluvic'ola,** parasitic in the mucosa of the crop, esophagus, and proventriculus of chickens, turkeys, and quail and transmitted by infected beetles; it tunnels into the crop wall but is relatively nonpathogenic.

   **G. neoplas'ticum,** parasitic in the stomach or esophagus epithelium of various rodents, rabbits, and sheep and transmitted by coprophagous beetles; this species is often associated with neoplasms in the stomach and esophagus of infected rats.

   **G. pul'chrum,** the gullet worm of cattle; it penetrates the submucosa of the esophagus or rumen of many domestic and wild ruminants, and of pigs, bears, and man (human cases are chiefly caused by immature worms); it is transmitted by coprophagous beetles and is distributed worldwide.

**Gonin** (go-nan'), Jules, Swiss ophthalmologist, 1870–1935. See G. *operation.*

**gonio-** [ G. *gōnia*, angle ]. Combining form meaning angle.

**goniocraniometry** (go'nï-o-kra-nï-om'e-trï) [ G. *gōnia*, angle, + *kranion*, skull, + *metron*, measure ]. Measurement of the angles of the cranium.

**goniodysgenesis** (go'nï-o-dis-jen'ē-sis) [ G. *gōnia*, angle, + dysgenesis ]. Developmental aberration of the mesodermal portion of the anterior ocular segment.

**gonioma** (gon'ï-o'mah) [ G. *gonē*, seed, + suffix *-oma*, tumor ]. Former term for a malignant neoplasm of the testis thought to be derived from the first stages of spermatogenetic cells; probably the same as embryonal carcinoma of the testis.

**goniometer** (go-nï-om'e-ter) [ G. *gōnia*, angle, + *metron*, measure ]. 1. An instrument for measuring angles, as of crystals. 2. An appliance for the static test of labyrinthine disease. It consists of a plank, one end of which may be raised to any desired height. The patient stands upon the plank as one end is gradually raised, and the point is noted at which he can no longer preserve his balance.

**gonion,** pl. **go'nia** (go'nï-on) [ G. *gōnia*, an angle ]. The point of the angle of the mandible. See fig. under craniometric *point.*

**go'niopuncture.** An operation for congenital glaucoma in which a puncture is made in the filtration angle of the anterior chamber.

**gonioscope** (go'nï-o-skōp) [ G. *gōnia*, angle, + *skopeō*, to examine ]. An optical instrument for examining the filtration angle of the anterior chamber.

**gonios'copy.** Examination of the angle of the anterior chamber of the eye with a gonioscope or with a contact prism lens and beam illumination from the slitlamp. See fig. on p. 598.

**goniosynechia** (go'nï-o-sï-nek'ï-ah) [ G. *gōnia*, angle, + *synechis*, holding together ]. Adhesion of the iris to the posterior surface of the cornea in the angle of the anterior chamber; associated with angle-closure glaucoma.

**goniotomy** (go'nï-ot'o-mï) [ G. *gōnia*, angle, + *tomē*, incision ]. Surgical opening of Schlemm's canal by way of the angle of the anterior chamber in congenital glaucoma.

**gonitis** (go-ni'tis) [ G. *gony*, knee, + suffix *-itis*, inflammation ]. Inflammation of the knee.

**gonoblennorrhea** (gon'o-blen-o-re'ah) [ G. *gonē*, seed, + *blennos*, mucus, + *rhoia*, a flow ]. Gonorrhea.

**gonocele** (gon'o-sēl) [ G. *gonē*, seed, + *kēlē*, tumor ]. A cystic lesion of the epididymis or rete testis, resulting from obstruction and containing secretions from the testis; g.'s that contain spermatozoa are termed spermatoceles.

**gonochorism, gonochorismus** (gon-ok'o-rizm, gon-ok-o-riz'mus) [ G. *gonē*, seed, sex, + *chōrizō*, to separate ]. Normal gonadal differentiation appropriate to the sex.

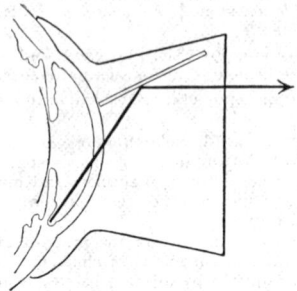

**Optics of the Goldmann Gonioscopic Mirror**
The mirror in the special contact lens makes an angle of 64 degrees with the front surface of the contact lens. The rays of light which emanate from the angle of the anterior chamber are reflected by the mirror into the observer's eye. The lower chamber angle is seen when the mirror is placed above, and *vice versa*. (From Gorin, G., and Posner, A.: *Slit-Lamp Gonioscopy*, Ed. 3, The Williams & Wilkins Co., Baltimore, 1967.)

**gonocide** (gon'o-sid). Gonococcicide. 1. Destructive to the gonococcus. 2. An agent that kills gonococci.

**gonococcal** (gon'o-kok'al). Gonococcic; relating to the gonococcus.

**gonococcemia** (gon-o-kok-se'mĭ-ah) [ gonococcus + G. *haima*, blood ]. The presence of gonococci in the circulating blood.

**gonococcic** (gon'o-kok'sik). Gonococcal.

**gonococcicide** (gon-o-kok'sĭ-sīd) [ gonococcus + L. *caedo*, to kill ]. Gonocide.

**gonococcin** (gon-o-kok'sin). A glycerin extract of gonococci, used in the cutireaction test for gonorrheal infection.

**gonococcus,** pl. **gonococ'ci** (gon-o-kok'us) [ G. *gonē*, seed, + *kokkos*, berry ]. *Neisseria gonorrhoeae.*

**gonocyte** (gon'o-sit) [ G. *gonē*, seed, + *kytos*, hollow (cell) ]. Primordial germ *cell.*

**gonohe'mia.** Gonococcemia.

**gonom'ery** [ G. *gonē*, seed, + *meros*, part ]. Condition in which paternal and maternal chromosomes remain in two distinct groups in the zygote.

**gono-opsonin.** A specific gonococcal opsonin.

**gonophage** (gon'o-fāj). A gonocidal bacteriophage.

**gon'ophore, gonoph'orus** [ G. *gonē*, seed, + *phoros*, bearing. PHER- ]. Any structure serving to store up or conduct the sexual cells; oviduct, spermatic duct, uterus, or seminal vesicle; an accessory generative organ.

**gon'opod** [ G. *gonos*, offspring, + *podos*, foot ]. A modified anal fin found in some fishes. It is a male secondary sexual character under androgenic control.

**gonorrhea** (gon'o-re'ah) [ G. *gonorrhoia*, fr. *gonē*, seed, + *rhoia*, a flow ]. Gonoblennorrhea; specific urethritis; urethritis venera; a contagious catarrhal inflammation of the genital mucous membrane, transmitted chiefly by coitus, and due to *Neisseria gonorrhoeae*. It may involve the lower or upper genital tract, especially the uterine tubes, or spread to the peritoneum and rarely to the heart, joints, or other structures by way of the blood stream.

**gonorrhe'al.** Relating to gonorrhea.

**gonotoxe'mia.** Toxic condition resulting from the hematogenous dissemination of gonococci and the effects of the absorbed endotoxin.

**gonotox'in.** The endotoxin elaborated by the gonococcus, *Neisseria gonorrhoeae.*

**gonotyl** (gon'o-til) [ G. *gonos*, offspring, + *tylē*, knob ]. A sucker-like structure enclosing the genital pore of flukes of the family Heterophyidae, *q. v.*

**Gonyaulax catanella.** A marine dinoflagellate protozoan that produces a powerful toxin which accumulates in the tissues of mussels and other shellfish and may cause fatal mussel poisoning in man.

**gon'ycamp'sis** [ G. *gony*, knee, + *kampsis*, a bending or curving ]. Ankylosis or any abnormal curvature of the knee.

**gonyocele** (gon'ĭ-o-sel) [ G. *gony*, knee, + *kēlē*, tumor ]. White *swelling.*

**gonyoncus** (gon'ĭ-ong'kus) [ G. *gony*, knee, + *onkos*, mass ]. White *swelling.*

**Gooch filter.** See under filter.

**Goodell,** William, U. S. gynecologist, 1829–1894. See G.'s *dilator, sign.*

**Goodpasture,** Ernest W., American pathologist, 1886 –1960. See G.'s *stains, syndrome.*

**Goormaghtigh,** Norbert, Belgian physician, 1890–1960. See G.'s *cells.*

**goose'flesh.** *Cutis* anserina.

**Gordius** (gor'dĭ-us) [ L. fr. G. *Gordios*, king of Gordium in Phrygia; an allusion to the knotlike twistings of these worms ]. An old name for the nematode genus *Dracunculus*, properly applied to members of the Gordiacea or Nematomorpha, the hair worms of horses.

**Gordon,** Alfred, Philadelphia neurologist, 1874–1953. See G.'s *reflex, sign, symptom.*

**Gordon's splint.** See under splint.

**Gorgas,** William C., American army surgeon, 1854–1920. Freed Havana and later the Panama Canal zone of yellow fever and malaria by screening patients with these diseases and instituting measures to destroy and prevent the breeding of mosquitoes.

**gorge.** Throat; guttur; gullet.

**gorget** (gor'jet). A director or guide with wide groove for use in lithotomy.

   **probe g.,** a g. with a probe-pointed tip.

**Gorham,** Lemuel W., U. S. physician, 1885–1968. See G.'s *disease.*

**Goriaew's rule.** See under rule.

**Gorlin,** Robert J., U. S. oral pathologist, *1923. See G.'s *sign*, G.-Chaudhry-Moss *syndrome.*

**Gorlin's formula.** See under formula.

**goron'dou.** Goundou.

**gorse.** *Ulex europaeus.*

**Gosselin,** Léon Athanese, French surgeon, 1815–1887. See G.'s *fracture.*

**gos'sypine.** Obsolete name for choline.

**GOT.** Abbreviation for glutamic oxaloacetic transaminase, which is now known as aspartate aminotransferase.

**Göthlin** (gët'lin), Gustaf F., Swedish physiologist, *1874. See G.'s *test.*

**Gottron,** H. A., German physician. See Arndt-G. *syndrome.*

**gouge** (gowj). A strong, longitudinally curved chisel used in operation on bone.

**Gougerot** (goo-jer-o'), Henri, French physician, 1881–1955. See G.-Sjögren's *disease*, G. and Blum *disease.*

**Gould,** Sir Alfred P., English surgeon, 1852–1922. See G.'s *suture.*

**Gould,** George M., American ophthalmologist and medical lexicographer, 1848–1922. See G.'s *sign.*

**goundou** (goon'doo) [ native name ]. Henpuye; gorondou; gros nez; anákhré; a disease, endemic in West Africa, characterized by exostoses from the nasal processes of the maxillary bones, producing a symmetrical swelling on each side of the nose; it is generally believed to be an osteitis connected in some way with yaws.

**gout** (gowt) [ L. *gutta*, drop ]. Arthritis uratica; an inherited metabolic disorder occurring especially in men, characterized by a raised but variable blood uric acid level, recurrent acute arthritis of sudden onset, deposition of crystalline sodium urate in connective tissues and articular cartilage, and progressive chronic arthritis.

   **abartic'ular g.,** irregular g.; g. involving structures other than the joints.

   **artic'ular g.,** arthrolithiasis; the usual form of g. attacking one or more of the joints.

   **calcium g.,** the presence of tophi-like depositions of calcium in the neighborhood of joints which become painful, swollen, and tender, occurring sometimes in persons consuming large quantities of calcium, usually in the form of milk. The serum calcium may be raised above normal but the inorganic phosphorus of the blood, the serum phosphatase, the urinary excretion of calcium, and the calcium of the bones are all at normal levels; the condition therefore differs from the disturbances of calcium metabolism occurring in hyperparathyroidism; there is usually some degree of impairment of renal function.

**interval g.,** an asymptomatic phase between acute attacks of g.

**irregular g.,** abarticular g.

**latent g.,** masked g.; goutiness; uric acid diathesis; a condition marked by scaly eruptions of the skin, twinges in the joints, and so forth, without frank arthritis.

**lead g.,** saturnine g.

**masked g.,** latent g.

**poor man's g.,** g. occurring in persons subject to exposure and privation and distinctly not attributable to dietetic excess.

**retroce′dent g.,** the occurrence of severe gastric, cardiac, or cerebral symptoms during an attack of g., especially when the joint symptoms at the same time suddenly subside.

**sat′urnine g.,** g. occurring in a subject with lead poisoning.

**secondary g.,** g. resulting from increased nucleoprotein metabolism and uric acid production, in patients with diseases of the blood and bone marrow, and in lead poisoning.

**topha′ceous g.,** g. in which deposits of uric acid occur in the joints and in tophi, especially of cartilaginous areas.

**goutiness** (gowt′ĭ-nes). Gouty diathesis; latent gout; a state in which one is prone to suffer from various scaly skin diseases, gastric disturbances, arteriosclerosis, and acute inflammations of the ocular structures which are attributable to a disturbance of metabolism, allied to gout, occurring in families in which there is a history of articular or regular gout.

**gouty** (gow′tĭ). Relating to gout.

**Gowers,** Sir William R., London neurologist, 1845–1915. See G.'s *column, contraction, disease, syndrome, tract.*

**Goyrand's injury.** See under injury.

**GPT.** Abbreviation for glutamic pyruvic transaminase, which is now known as alanine aminotransferase.

**gr.** Abbreviation for grain, a measure of weight.

**Graaf** (grahf), Reijnier de, Dutch physiologist and histologist, 1641–1673. See Graafian *follicle.*

**gracilis** (gras′ĭ-lis) [ L. ] [ NA ]. Slender; denoting a thin or slender structure.

**Gradenigo** (grah-den-e′go), Giuseppe, Italian physician, 1859–1926. See G.'s *syndrome.*

**gra′dient.** Rate of change of temperature, pressure, or other variable as a function of distance.

**at′rioventric′ular g.,** the diastolic pressure difference between the atrium and ventricle.

**concentration g.,** density g.; a solution in which the concentration of a solute increases in a continuous fashion from top to bottom, or end to end, of a container (*e.g.*, the centrifuge tube in density gradient centrifugation).

**density g.,** concentration g.; see also density g. *centrifugation.*

**electrochemical g.,** a measure of the tendency of an ion to move passively from one point to another, taking into consideration the differences in its concentration and in the electrical potentials between the two points; commonly expressed as the additional voltage needed to achieve equilibrium.

**mitral g.,** the diastolic pressure difference between the left atrium and left ventricle.

**systolic g.,** the difference in pressure during systole between two communicating cardiovascular chambers, *e.g.*, between the left ventricle and left atrium in mitral insufficiency.

**ventricular g.,** the algebraic sum of (*i.e.*, the net electrical difference between) the area enclosed within the QRS complex and that within the T wave in the electrocardiogram.

**grad′uate** [ Mediev. L. *graduatus,* fr. L. *gradus,* step ]. A vessel, usually of glass, suitably marked, used for measuring the volume of liquids.

**grad′uated.** Marked by lines or in other ways to denote capacity, degrees, percentages, etc.; applied to a thermometer, barometer, etc.

**Graefe** (gra′feh), Albrecht von, German ophthalmologist, 1828–1870. See G.'s *disease, knife, operation, sign,* pseudo-G. *sign,* G.'s *spots, test.*

**Graefenberg,** Ernst, German gynecologist in America, *1881. See G. *ring.*

**graft** [ A.S. *graef* ]. 1. Anything inserted into something else so as to become an integral part of the latter; specifically, a bit of epidermis, strip of skin, piece of bone, tooth, etc., inserted into a part in order to supply a defect. 2. The performance of a grafting procedure.

**accordion g.,** a g. which, by means of multiple slits, can be stretched to cover a large area.

**allogeneic g.,** homograft, other than isogeneic.

**anastomosed g.,** one in which circulation is established by surgical anastomoses of blood vessels.

**animal g.,** zooplastic g.

**autodermic g.,** a skin g. from one part of the body to another.

**autogenous bone g.,** a bone g. from one part of the body to another.

**autologous g.,** autograft.

**autoplastic g.,** autograft.

**Blair-Brown g.,** split-thickness g.

**Braun g.,** full-thickness g.

**Braun-Wangensteen g.,** g.'s of skin taken from large g.

**brephoplastic g.,** transplantation of tissue from an embryo or newborn to the adult.

**cable g.,** a multiple strand nerve g. arranged as a pathway for regeneration of axons.

**chessboard g.'s,** postage stamp g.'s.

**chorioallantoic g.,** transplanting of living material to the chorioallantoic membrane of the embryonic chick.

**cutis g.,** g. of true skin, from which epidermis and subcutaneous tissue have been separated, used in plastic surgery in place of fascia.

**Davis g.'s,** small, deep skin g.'s.

**delayed g.,** one postponed until after elimination of infection and formation of a bed of healthy granulation tissue.

**dermoepidermic g.,** see Thiersch's *method.*

**Douglas g.,** sieve g.

**fascia g.,** g. of fibrous tissue, usually the fascia lata.

**fat g.,** one used to fill a cavity or depression.

**filler g.,** a g. used for the filling of defects, *e.g.*, filling a cyst with bone chips.

**free g.,** a g. separated from its normal attachments.

**full-thickness g.,** Braun g.; a g. of full thickness of skin and subcutaneous tissue.

**heterodermic g.,** a g. of skin from one person to another.

**heterologous g.,** heterograft.

**heteroplastic g.,** heterograft.

**heterospecific g.,** heterograft.

**heterotopic g.,** transplantation of a tissue or organ into a position it normally does not occupy.

**homologous g.,** homograft.

**homoplastic g.,** homograft.

**hyperplastic g.,** one in active proliferation.

**implantation g.,** one in which small sections of skin are placed into granulation tissue.

**infused g.,** transplantation by injection of a suspension of cells.

**interspecific g.,** heterograft.

**isogeneic g.,** isograft.

**isologous g.,** isograft.

**isoplastic g.,** isograft.

**jump g.,** a pedicle g. transferred from one position to another.

**Kiel g.,** denatured calf bone used to fill defects or restore facial contour; often used for chin and nasal augmentation.

**Krause's g.,** Krause's *method.*

**mesh g.,** thick-split g. of skin which has been incised in several places to allow covering a larger area and to prevent accumulation of serum beneath the g.

**mucosal g.,** a split-thickness g. involving the mucosa.

**nerve g.,** the insertion of nerve substance to fill a gap between the divided ends of a nerve; the grafted tissue acts as a bridge and does not form part of the new tissue.

**Ollier's g.,** see Thiersch's *method.*

**orthotop'ic g.,** transplantation of a tissue or organ into its normal anatomical position.

**pedicle g.,** one in which the transplant retains a blood supply from the donor site, at least temporarily.

**periosteal g.,** a g. of periosteum, placed on bare bone.

**pinch g.,** small bits of skin removed from healthy area and seeded in site to be covered.

**postage stamp g.'s,** chessboard g.'s; multiple, small thick-split g.'s of skin.

**rope g.,** a pedicle or tube g. temporarily attached at both ends.

**sieve g.,** Douglas g.; a g. with small circular pieces removed; only the ring of the tissue is used.

**skin g.,** a piece of skin removed from one part of the body to another to cover a denuded area (autograft), or taken from one person and used on another (homograft, allograft).

**sleeve g.,** a g. for repairing a severed nerve by connecting central and peripheral ends with a sleevelike structure.

**split-thickness g.,** Blair-Brown g.; a skin g. employing only a superficial layer of the dermis.

**sponge g.,** Hamilton's method; a thin bit of sponge laid on an ulcerated surface with the object of stimulating the growth of epidermis.

**syngeneic g.,** isograft.

**tendon g.,** tendon *transplantation.*

**Thiersch's g.,** Thiersch's *method.*

**thick-split g.,** one with a thickness of about three-quarters of the skin.

**Wolfe's g.,** a dermal g. involving the entire thickness of the skin but without any subcutaneous fat; see also Wolfe's *method.*

**xenogeneic g.,** a term sometimes used to denote grafts between animals from phylogenically widely separated species.

**zooplas'tic g.,** animal g.; a g. taken from one of the lower animals; a heterograft in man.

**graft'ing.** Inserting a graft.

**Graham,** Thomas, English chemist, 1805–1869. See G.'s *law.*

**Grahamel'la** [ G. S. *Graham-Smith* ]. A genus of aerobic, nonmotile microorganisms (order Rickettsiales) containing long or short, rod-shaped, Gram-negative cells which resemble those of *Bartonella* but which are less pleomorphic. These organisms occur within the erythrocytes of lower mammals, but they appear to be nonpathogenic and do not affect the health of the host. The type species is *G. talpae.*

**G. peromysci,** a species that occurs naturally in the deer mouse.

**G. talpae,** a species found in the erythrocytes of moles; it is the type species of the genus *G.*

**Graham Steell,** Manchester physician, 1851–1942. See G. S.'s *murmur.*

**grain** [ L. *granum* ]. 1. Cereal plants, corn, wheat, rye, etc. 2. A seed of one of the cereal plants. 3. A minute, hard particle of any substance, as of sand. 4. A unit of weight, $1/60$ dram, $1/437.5$ avoirdupois ounce, $1/480$ Troy ounce, $1/5760$ Troy pound, $1/7000$ avoirdupois pound; the equivalent of 0.0648 gm. 5. See grains.

**g. alcohol,** see alcohol (2).

**grains.** Hyaline bodies within the horny layer of epidermis, found in keratosis follicularis.

**Gram,** Hans C. J., Danish bacteriologist, 1853–1938. See G.'s *stain,* Weigert-G. *stain.*

**gram.** A unit of weight in the metric or centesimal system, the equivalent of 15.432 grains. Abbreviated gm. or g.

**g. equivalent,** see under equivalent.

**-gram** [ G. *gramma,* character, mark ]. Suffix denoting recording of many sorts.

**gram-centimeter.** The energy exerted, or work done, when a mass of 1 gm. is raised a height of 1 cm.

**gramici'din** (NF). A One of a group of polypeptides produced by *Bacillus brevis.* Its natural mixture with tyrocidin is known as tyrothricin. It is active against Gram-positive cocci and bacilli. It is mainly bacteriostatic in action, having little bacteriocidal effect, and is used topically.

**graminivorous** (grā-mǐ-niv'o-rus) [ L. *gramen* (*gramin-*), grass, + *voro,* to eat ]. Grass-eating; herbivorous.

**gram'meter.** A unit of energy; the force required to raise a weight of 1 gm. (15 gr.) to a height of 1 meter (39 in.).

**gram-molecule.** The amount of a substance with a mass of the number of grams of its molecular weight; thus a g.-m. of hydrogen weighs 2 gm.; of water 18 gm.

**Gram-negative.** See Gram's *stain.*

**Gram-positive.** See Gram's *stain.*

**gra'na** [ pl. of L. *granum,* grain ]. Bodies within the chloroplasts of plant cells that contain layers composed of chlorophyll and phosphatides.

**grana'tum** [ L. *granatus,* having many seeds ]. Pomegranate; pomegranate bark; the bark of the root and stem of *Punica granatum* (family Punicaceae). Anthelmintic.

**gran'diose.** A term pertaining to feelings of great importance, expansiveness, or delusions of grandeur.

**grand mal.** See generalized *epilepsy.*

**Grandry** (grahṅ-dre'), French anatomist, 19th century. See G.'s *corpuscles.*

**Granger's line.** See under line.

**Granit,** Ragnar A., Finnish neurophysiologist, *1900. Nobel laureate, 1967, with Haldan K. Hartline and George Wald, for their studies in visual physiology. See G.'s *loop.*

**gran'ular.** 1. Composed of or resembling granules or granulations. 2. Particles with strong affinity for nuclear stains, seen in many bacterial species.

**granula'tio,** pl. **granulatio'nes** [ L. ]. Granulation.

**granulationes arachnoidea'les** [ NA ], arachnoidal granulations or villi; Pacchionian bodies; numerous villuslike projections of the cranial arachnoid through the dura into the superior sagittal sinus or its lateral venous lacunae.

**granula'tion** (gran'u-la'shun) [ L. *granulatio* ]. 1. Formation into grains or granules; the state of being granular. 2. A granular mass in or on the surface of any organ or membrane; or one of the individual granules forming the mass. 3. The formation of minute, rounded, fleshy connective tissue projections on the surface of a wound, ulcer, or inflamed tissue surface in the process of healing; one of the fleshy granules composing this surface; see also granulation *tissue;* 4. In pharmacy, the formation of crystals by constant agitation of a supersaturated solution of a salt.

**arachnoidal g.'s,** *granulationes* arachnoideales.

**Bayle's g.'s,** miliary tubercles.

**Pacchionian g.'s,** *granulationes* arachnoideales.

**Virchow's g.,** granulations made up of ependyma and glial cells in the brain ventricles in neurosyphilis.

**granulatio'nes.** Plural of granulatio.

**granule** (gran'ūl) [ L. *granulum,* dim. of *granum,* grain ]. 1. A grain; a granulation; a minute discrete mass. 2. A very small pill, usually gelatin coated or sugar coated, containing a drug to be given in small dose; pellet.

**acid'ophil g.,** oxyphil g.; one staining with an acid dye such as eosin.

**acrosomal g.,** the proacrosomal g. after adherence to the nuclear surface.

**alpha g.,** a g. of an alpha cell which was named as the first of several kinds or because it was acidophilic.

**Altmann's g.,** fuchsinophil g.

**am'phophil g.,** one that stains with both acid and basic dyes.

**argentaffin g.'s,** g.'s that reduce silver ions in staining solution.

**azu'rophil g.,** kappa g.; one that stains a reddish purple color with an azure dye; such g.'s are seen in dry smears of certain mature and developing blood cells; the g.'s are membrane-bound primary lysosomes containing enzymes.

**basal g.,** basal *body.*

**bas'ophil g.,** one that stains readily with a basic dye.

**Bensley's specific g.'s,** g.'s in the cells of the islands of Langerhans in the pancreas.

**beta g.,** a g. of a beta cell.

**Birbeck's g.,** Langerhans' g.

**Bollinger g.'s,** (1) relatively small, but frequently microscopically visible, pale yellow or yellow-white g.'s observed in the granulomatous lesion, or the exudate, in botryomycosis; the g.'s consist of irregular aggregates or colonizations of Gram-positive cocci, usually staphylococci; (2) term sometimes incorrectly used synonymously with Bollinger bodies.

**chromatic g.,** a g. of chromophil *substance.*

**chro′mophil g.,** (1) any readily stainable g.; (2) a g. of chromophil *substance.*

**chro′mophobe g.'s,** those that do not stain or stain poorly with the ordinary dyes; such g.'s are present in some cells in the anterior lobe of the pituitary.

**cone g.,** nucleus of a retinal cell connecting with one of the cones.

**Crooke's g.'s,** lumpy masses of basophilic material in the basophil cells of the anterior lobe of the pituitary, associated with Cushing's disease, or following the administration of ACTH.

**delta g.,** a g. of a delta cell.

**elementary g.,** a particle of blood dust, or hemoconia.

**eosin′ophil g.,** one that stains with eosin.

**Fordyce's g.'s,** Fordyce's *spots.*

**fuchsin′ophil g.,** Altmann's g.; a g. that has an affinity for fuchsin.

**iodophil g.,** one of the g.'s, taking on a brown stain with iodine, found in many of the polymorphonuclear leukocytes in pneumonia, erysipelas, scarlet fever, and various other acute diseases.

**kappa g.,** azurophil g.

**Langerhans' g.,** Birbeck's g.; a g. with characteristic platelet-like ultrastructure; first reported in Langerhans' cells of the epidermis.

**Langley's g.'s,** g.'s in serous secreting cells.

**metachromat′ic g.'s,** (1) g.'s that stain a color different from that of the dye used; see also metachromasia; (2) sometimes used as a synonym for volutin.

**mucin′ogen g.'s,** g.'s that produce mucin, as in cells of the salivary glands and in the gastric and intestinal mucosae.

**Neusser's g.'s,** tiny basophilic g.'s sometimes observed in an indistinct zone about the nucleus of a leukocyte.

**neu′trophil g.,** one stainable with the neutral component of stains; e.g., the Romanovsky type for blood.

**Nissl g.,** a g. of chromophil *substance.*

**ox′yphil g.,** acidophil g.

**Palade g.,** ribosome.

**Plehn's karyochromatophil g.'s,** Schuegner's g.'s; basophilic g.'s frequently observed in the conjugating form of malarial parasites.

**proacrosomal g.,** precursor of the acrosome; located within the acroblast. Acrosome formation begins when this g. migrates from the acroblast to adhere to the nucleus; see also acrosomal g.

**prosecretion g.'s,** g.'s in the cytoplasm of a cell indicative of a preliminary step in the formation of a secretory product.

**rod g.,** the nucleus of a retinal cell connecting with one of the rods.

**Schuegner's g.'s,** Plehn's g.'s.

**Schüffner's g.'s,** fine, round, uniform, red or red-yellow g.'s (as colored with Romanovsky stains) frequently observed in erythrocytes infected with *Plasmodium vivax* and *P. ovale,* but only seldom in *P. malariae* and *P. falciparum* infections; at first, the g.'s are distributed fairly evenly throughout the stroma of the erythrocyte; later they become larger and more conspicuous, sometimes seeming to fill the cell, and eventually may surround the maturing schizont with a narrow, stippled margin. The granules tend to be well preserved in thick sections, and provide a means of recognizing the probability of *P. vivax* (tertian) malaria.

**sem′inal g.,** one of the minute granular bodies present in the spermatic fluid.

**Simchowicz g.'s,** multiple basophilic cytoplasmic g.'s, each surrounded by a clear vacuole; noted in the hippocampal brain cells of elderly persons and a characteristic of granulovacuolar degeneration.

**volutin g.'s,** small, fairly regular g.'s or globule-like particles of refractile, metachromatic, probably nucleoprotein material in the cytoplasm of various microorganisms, e.g., certain bacteria, protozoa, yeasts and yeastlike fungi.

**Zimmermann's g.,** platelet.

**zy′mogen g.,** a term applied to various g.'s in enzyme-secreting cells, such as those of salivary glands, pancreas, and gastric glands; believed to be the source of zymogen.

**granulo-** [ L. *granulum,* granule ]. Combining form meaning granular, or denoting relationship to granules.

**gran′uloblast** [ granulo- + G. *blastos,* germ ]. Myeloblast; an immature hematopoietic cell capable of giving rise to granulocytes.

**gran′uloblasto′sis.** A leukemic form of leukosis in the chicken characterized by an increase of immature, granular blood cells in the circulating blood and frequently infiltration of the parenchymatous organs.

**granulocyte** (gran′u-lo-sit) [ granulo- + G. *kytos,* cell ]. A mature granular leukocyte, including neutrophilic, acidophilic, and basophilic types of polymorphonuclear leukocytes, *i.e.,* respectively, neutrophils, eosinophils, and basophils.

**immature g.,** see immature neutrophil. The same cell as described under immature neutrophil, except that it may be neutrophilic, acidophilic, or basophilic in character.

**granulocytopenia** (gran-u-lo-si-to-pe′ni-ah) [ granulocyte + G. *penia,* poverty ]. Granulopenia; hypogranulocytosis; less than the normal number of granular leukocytes in the blood.

**granulocytopoietic** (gran′u-lo-si-to-poy-et′ik) [ granulocyte + G. *poieō,* to make ]. Granulopoietic.

**granulocytosis** (gran′u-lo-si-to′sis). A condition characterized by more than the normal number of granulocytes in the circulating blood or in the tissues.

**granulo′ma** [ granulo- + G. suffix -*oma,,* tumor ]. An indefinite term applied to nodular inflammatory lesions, usually small or granular, firm, persistent, and containing proliferated macrophages.

**ame′bic g.,** ameboma.

**g. annula′re,** lichen annularis; heloderma simplex et annularis; a papular eruption prone to develop on the distal portions of the extremities and over prominences. Other areas may be involved; the condition may be generalized. The waxy papules tend to form annular lesions characterized microscopically by foci of dermal necrosis bordered by fibroblasts and lymphocytes. The eruption is chronic. The cause is unknown.

**apical g.,** dental g.

**beryllium g.,** a sarcoid-like granulomatous reaction to exposure to beryllium.

**canine venereal g.,** transmissible venereal tumor; a rapidly growing, infectious, soft, easily bleeding, connective tissue tumor occurring in the vagina of the female dog and on the penis and sheath of the male; ordinarily transmitted by coitus.

**coccidioid′al g.,** coccidioidomycosis.

**co′li g.,** Hjärre's *disease.*

**g. cryptogenet′icum, g. cryptogen′icum,** obsolete terms for Hodgkin's disease.

**dental g.,** apical g.; a small collection of granulation tissue occurring at the apex of a tooth.

**g. endem′icum,** the oriental boil of cutaneous leishmaniasis.

**eosinophilic g.,** a lesion observed more frequently in children and adolescents, but occasionally in young adults; occurs chiefly as a solitary lesion in one bone, but multiple involvement is sometimes observed, and similar foci may develop in the lung. Eosinophilic g. is characterized by numerous histiocytes (which may be in almost solid sheets), numerous eosinophils (in irregular aggregates or diffusely scattered), and occasional foci of necrosis. There is evidence that the condition may be related to Hand-Schüller-Christian disease, possibly representing a different clinical form of the same disease.

**g. gangrenes′cens,** lethal midline g.

**g. gravida′rum,** pregnancy tumor; a gingival swelling composed of vascular connective tissue appearing during pregnancy; it may subside and reappear in subsequent pregnancies, or may persist as a benign fibrous tissue mass.

**infectious g.,** any granulomatous lesion known to be caused by a living agent, *e.g.,* bacteria, fungi, helminths, and so on.

**g. inguinale,** g. pudendi; ulcerating g. of pudenda; one of the venereal diseases; a specific g., caused by *Donovania granulomatis.* The ulcerating granulomatous lesions occur in the inguinal regions and the genitalia. Peripheral extension of the lesions produces extensive destruction.

**g. inguina′le trop′icum,** groin ulcer; an elongated ulcer, with elevated papillary edges, sometimes occurring in the groin in persons in the tropics.

**laryngeal g.,** a polypoid granulomatous projection of granulomatous tissue into the lumen of the larynx, commonly following a traumatic tracheal intubation.

**lethal midline g.,** g. gangrenescens; malignant g.; destructive granulomatous lesion usually arising in the nose or paranasal sinuses and ending fatally. It may be distinguished from Wegener's granulomatosis by the absence of angiitis and of involvement of other organs.

**lipoid g.,** one characterized by aggregates or accumulations of fairly large mononuclear phagocytes that contain lipid; the typical cells are derived from the reticuloendothelial system, and are frequently termed foam cells, xanthoma cells, and so on.

**lipophagic g.,** a lesion formed as a result of the inflammatory reaction provoked by foci of necrosis in subcutaneous fat, as in certain types of traumatic injury; the central focus of necrotic material is surrounded by an irregular zone of numerous macrophages, many of which become laden with tiny globules of lipid; the peripheral portion consists of an indistinct rim of newly formed capillaries and proliferating fibroblasts, sometimes with a few lymphocytes and macrophages.

**malignant g.,** lethal midline g.

**g. malig'num,** obsolete term for lymphogranuloma venereum.

**oily g.,** reaction to inclusion of bulky, insoluble liquid (often oily substance); the reaction occurs several months, but sometimes years, after injection of the material.

**par'acoccidioid'al g.,** South American *blastomycosis.*

**parasit'ic g.,** cutaneous leishmaniasis manifested as warty papules affecting primarily the lower limbs.

**g. pudendi,** g. inguinale.

**g. pyogen'icum, pyogenic g.,** a small, spheroidal or ovoid mass of inflamed, highly vascular, granulation tissue (not actually a g.), frequently with an ulcerated surface, projecting from the skin; occurs also in the gingiva, usually on the labial or lingual surface; in some instances, staphylococci (or a mixture of bacteria) may be isolated. Histologically, the mass resembles a capillary hemangioma.

**reparative giant cell g.,** giant cell epulis; a non-neoplastic, fibrovascular lesion containing multinucleated giant cells and hemosiderin, occurring in the gums (peripheral giant cell reparative g.) or jawbones (central or intraosseous g.).

**g. sarcomato'des,** *mycosis* fungoides.

**sea urchin g.,** granulomatous nodules, either foreign-body type or sarcoidal, from the retention of the spin of the sea urchin, occurring several months after the wounding of the skin.

**sil'icon g.,** eruption of granulomatous lesions due to traumatic inoculation of the skin with sand, or materials that contain silicon. This condition may follow dermabrasion using sandpaper technique.

**swimming pool g.,** chronic, low grade, infectious, verrucous lesion most commonly seen on the knees. Although due to an acid-fast bacillus of the genus *Mycobacterium,* it is not tuberculous.

**g. trichophyt'icum,** hypertrophic ringworm; agminate folliculitis; inflammatory ringworm of the body, attended with edema and dilated follicles, discharging pus.

**g. trop'icum,** yaws.

**ulcerating g. of the pudenda,** g. inguinale.

**g. vene'reum,** sometimes used as a synonym for g. inguinale.

**zirconium g.,** g. from zirconium salts, usually occurring in the axillae, from antiperspirants containing this material; may also be caused by intradermal injection of antigens containing the lactate salt (*e.g.,* Kvein antigen).

**granulomatosis** (gran'u-lo-mă-to'sis). Any condition characterized by multiple granulomas.

**lipoid g., lipid g.,** xanthomatosis.

**lipopha'gic intestinal g.,** Whipple's *disease.*

**malignant g.,** undesirable term sometimes used for Hodgkin's disease, or for lymphogranuloma venereum.

**g. siderot'ica,** a form in which firm, brown foci that contain iron pigment, Gamna nodules, are present in an enlarged spleen.

**Wegener's g.,** a rare, fatal disease of young or middle-aged men, in which progressive ulceration of the upper respiratory tract, including the nose and paranasal sinuses,

is accompanied by necrotizing arteritis; pulmonary infarction and glomerulonephritis may occur.

**granulom'atous.** Having the characteristics of a granuloma.

**granulomere** (gran'u-lo-mēr) [ granulo- + G. *meros,* a part ]. The central part of a blood platelet.

**gran'ulope'nia.** Granulocytopenia.

**gran'uloplasm.** The inner substance of an ameba, or other unicellular organism, within the ectoplasm and surrounding the necleus.

**gran'uloplas'tic.** Forming granules.

**granulopoiesis** (gran'u-lo-poy-e'sis) [ granulo(cyte) + G. *poiēsis,* a making ]. Granulocytopoiesis; production of granulocytes. In adults, granulocytes are produced chiefly in the red bone marrow of flat bones.

**granulopoietic** (gran'u-lo-poy-et'ik). Pertaining to granulopoiesis.

**granulo'sa.** *Stratum* granulosum folliculi ovarici vesiculosi.

**granulosarcoid** (gran'u-lo-sar-koyd) [ granulo- + G. *sarx,* flesh, + *eidos,* resemblance ]. *Mycosis* fungoides.

**gran'ulosarco'ma.** *Mycosis* fungoides.

**granulo'sis.** Granulosity; a mass of minute granules of any character.

**g. ru'bra na'si,** erythema, papules, and occasional vesicles of the tip of the nose and extending upward and laterally to the cheeks, resulting from occlusion of sweat ducts.

**granulos'ity.** Granulosis.

**gra'num,** pl. **gra'na** [ L. ]. Grain; see grana.

**grape** [ O. Fr. *grappe,* a cluster ]. 1. The fruit of *Vitis vinifera* (family Vitaceae). 2. A structure or growth resembling a g. or bunch of g.'s.

**Carswell's g.'s,** masses of tubercles, in pulmonary tuberculosis, clustered around the finer bronchioles like a bunch of g.'s.

**-graph** [ G. *graphō,* to write ]. Combining form (suffix) designating the instrument that makes the recording, *e.g.,* "electrocardiograph."

**graph** (graf) [ G. *graphō,* to write ]. A line or tracing denoting varying values of commodities, temperatures, urinary output, etc.; more generally, any geometric or pictorial representation of measurements that might otherwise be expressed in tabular form.

**graphanesthesia** (graf'an-es-the'zī-ah) [ G. *graphē,* writing + *anaisthēsia,* fr. *an-* priv. + *aisthēsis,* sensation ]. The inability to recognize figures written on the skin; this inability is observed in some forms of organic brain disease.

**graphesthesia** (graf'es-the'zī-ah) [ G. *graphē,* writing, + *aisthēsis,* perception ]. Ability to recognize figures written on the skin.

**graph'ite.** Plumbago; black lead; a crystallizable, soft black form of carbon.

**Graph'ium.** A genus of slow-growing, polymorphic, saprophytic fungi in which several spore types are found.

**grapho-, -graphy** [ G. *graphō,* to write ]. Combining forms denoting a writing or description.

**graphology** (grā-fol'o-jī) [ grapho- + G. *logos,* study ]. The study of handwriting as an indication of temperament or character.

**graphoma'nia** [ grapho- + G. *mania,* insanity ]. Morbid and excessive impulse to write.

**graphomotor** (graf'o-mo'tor) [ grapho- + L. *motus,* fr. *movere,* to move ]. Relating to the movements concerned in writing.

**graph'opathol'ogy** [ grapho- + pathology ]. Interpretation of personality disorders from a study of handwriting.

**graphopho'bia** [ grapho- + G. *phobos,* fear ]. Morbid fear of writing.

**graphorrhea** (graf-o-re'ă) [ grapho- + G. *rhoia,* flow ]. The writing of long lists of meaningless words.

**graphospasm** (graf'o-spazm). Writer's *cramp.*

**grasp.** Grip.

**pen g.,** a method, similar to that of holding a pen in writing, of grasping an instrument, *cf.* palm g.

**palm g.,** holding an object by wrapping the palm and the fingers around it.

**Grasset** (grah-sa'), Joseph, French physician, 1849–1918. See G.'s *law,* Landouzy-G. *law,* G.'s *phenomenon,* G.-Gaussel *phenomenon,* G.'s *sign.*

**Gratiolet** (grä-se-o-la'), Louis P., Paris anatomist, 1815–1865. See G.'s *fibers, radiation.*

**grattage** (grä-tazh') [ Fr. scraping ]. The scraping or brushing of an ulcer or surface with sluggish granulations, to stimulate the healing process.

**Gräupner** (groyp'ner), Sigurd C., German physician, 1861–1916. See G.'s *method.*

**grave** [ L. *gravis,* heavy, grave ]. Denoting symptoms of a serious or dangerous character.

**grav'el.** Small concretions, usually of uric acid, calcium oxalate, or phosphates, formed in the kidney and passed through the ureter, bladder, and urethra.

**Graves,** Robert J., Irish physician, 1797–1853. See G.'s *disease.*

**grav'id.** Pregnant.

**grav'ida** [ L. *gravidus* (adj.), fem. *gravida,* fr. *gravis,* heavy ]. A pregnant woman.

**gravid'ic.** Relating to pregnancy or a pregnant woman.

**grav'idism.** Pregnancy.

**graviditas** [ L. ]. Pregnancy.

    g. **examnia'lis,** extraamniotic *pregnancy.*

    g. **exochoria'lis,** extrachorial *pregnancy.*

**gravidity** (grä-vid'ĭ-tĭ) [ L. *graviditas,* pregnancy ]. Number of pregnancies.

**grav'idocar'diac.** Relating to an affection of the heart during pregnancy.

**gravimeter** (grä-vim'e-ter) [ L. *gravis,* heavy, + G. *metron,* measure ]. Hydrometer.

**gravimet'ric.** Relating to or determined by weight.

**gravireceptors** (grav'ĭ-re-sep'tors). Highly specialized receptor organs and nerve endings in the inner ear, joints, tendons, and muscles, that give the brain information about body position, equilibrium, direction of gravitational forces, and the sensation of "down" or "up."

**gravitation** (grav-ĭ-ta'shun) [ L. *gravitas,* weight ]. The force of attraction between any two bodies in the universe, varying directly as the product of their masses and inversely as the square of the distance between their centers.

    **Newtonian constant of g.,** see under constant.

**gravity** (grav'ĭ-tĭ) [ L. *gravitas* ]. Weight; gravitational force.

    **specific g.,** density; the weight of any body compared with that of another body of equal volume regarded as the unit; usually the weight of a liquid compared with that of distilled water.

    **zero-g.,** see zerogravity.

**Grawitz** (grah'vits), Paul, German pathologist, 1850–1932. See G.'s *basophilia, cachexia,* slumbering *cells, tumor.*

**gray-out.** A partial loss of consciousness and impaired vision due to decreased cerebral blood flow as may occur in pilots experiencing an acceleration force operating in the head to foot direction; see also blackout and red-out.

**Greeff** (gräf), C. Richard, German ophthalmologist, 1862–1938. See Prowazek-G. *bodies.*

**green.** Of the color of grass or leaves; a color between blue and yellow in the spectrum. For individual green dyes not listed below see specific name.

    **brilliant g.,** the sulfate of di-(*p*-diethylamino)-triphenyl carbinolanhydride. An indicator dye that changes from yellow to g. at pH 0.0 to 2.6; also used as a topical antiseptic and a bacteriostatic agent in culture media.

    **fast g. FCF,** an acid arylmethane dye, $C_{37}H_{34}N_2O_{10}S_3Na_2$, used as a cytoplasmic and collagen stain in histology.

    **light g. SF yellowish,** an acid arylmethane dye, $C_{37}H_{34}N_2O_9S_3Na_2$, used as a plasma stain in plant and animal histology.

    **Scheele's g.,** cupric arsenite.

**Greenfield,** J. Godwin, British neuropathologist, 1884–1958. See G.'s *disease.*

**Greenhow,** Edward H., English physician, 1814–1888. See G.'s *disease.*

**Greenough microscope.** See under microscope.

**gref'fotome** [ Fr. *greff,* graft, + G. *tōme,* incision ]. An instrument for slicing off bits of epidermis to use in grafting.

**greg'aloid** [ L. *grex* (*greg*-), a flock ]. Denoting a colony of protozoa formed by the chance union of independent cells.

**Gregarina** (greg'ä-ri'nah) [ L. *gregarius,* gregarious, fr. *grex* (*greg*-), a flock ]. A genus of sporozoan protozoa, parasitic in annelids and arthropods, and lacking schizogeny in the life cycle.

**greg'arine.** An organism in the order Gregarinida.

**Gregarinida** (greg'ä-rin'ĭ-dah) [ see gregarina ]. An order of Telosporidia in the Sporozoa, in which reproduction is usually be sporulation only, lacking schizogeny, and parasitic in annelids and arthropods.

**gregarinosis** (greg'ä-rĭ-no'sis). A disease due to the presence of gregarines.

**Greig,** D. M. See G.'s *syndrome.*

**gression** (gres'shun) [ L. *grador,* pp. *gressus,* to walk, fr. *gradus,* a step ]. Displacement of a tooth backward.

**Greville bath.** See under bath.

**Grey Turner,** George, English surgeon, 1877–1951. See G. T.'s *sign.*

**grid.** A chart with horizontal and perpendicular lines for plotting curves.

    **Wetzel g.,** chart of growth, plotting height, weight, physical fitness and related aspects of young and adolescent children during growth.

**grief.** A normal emotional response to an external loss. It is distinguished from depression since it subsides after a reasonable time.

**Griesinger** (gre'zing-er), Wilhelm, German neurologist, 1817–1868. See G.'s *disease, symptom,* bilious *typhoid of* G.

**grif'fin-claw.** See griffin-claw *hand.*

**Grindel,** David H., German botanist, 1776–1836. Gave his name to grindelia.

**grindelia** (grin-de'le-ah) [ H. *Grindel* ]. The dried leaves and flowering tops of *Grindelia camporum, G. humilius,* and *G. squarrosa* (family Compositae); California gum-plant; g. robusta. Used as an expectorant; a fluidextract has been used externally in the treatment of rhus poisoning.

**grind'ing.** Abrasion (3).

    **selective g.,** the modification of the occlusal forms of teeth by g. according to a plan or by g. at selected places marked by articulating ribbon or paper.

**grinding-in.** A term used to denote the act of correcting occlusal disharmonies by grinding the natural or artificial teeth.

**grip.** 1. Gripppe. 2. Grasp.

    **devil's g.,** epidemic *pleurodynia.*

    **Pawlik's g.,** a method of determining the progress of labor by grasping the fetus through the abdominal wall and thus ascertaining what part still lies above the pelvic rim.

**gripe** [ A.S. *gripan,* to seize ]. Colic; tormina; a sharp pain in the bowels.

**grippal** (grip'al). Influenzal.

**grippe** (grip) [ Fr. *gripper,* to seize ]. Influenza.

**grisein** (gris'e-in). An antibiotic of a reddish color containing iron; obtained from cultures of *Streptomyces griseus.*

**gris'eoful'vin** (USP, BP). FULVICIN; GRIFULVIN; GRIFULVIN V; GRISACTIN; an antibiotic produced by *Penicillium griseofulvin* and *Penicillium patulum.* Used in the systemic treatment of superficial fungal infections caused by the dermatophytes *Microsporum, Trichophyton,* and *Epidermophyton.* It is fungistatic and not fungicidal. Serious side-effects occur infrequently.

**griseomy'cin.** Lomycin; an antibiotic substance produced by a fungus related to *Streptomyces griseolus.*

**gris'eus** [ L. ] [ NA ]. Gray.

**Grisolle** (gre-zol'), Augustin, French physician, 1811–1869. See G.'s *sign.*

**Grisonel'la ratelli'na.** A South American weasel, a reservoir host of *Trypanosoma cruzi.*

**gristle** (gris'l) [ A.S. ]. Cartilage.

**Gritti,** Rocco, Italian surgeon, 1828–1920. See G.'s *amputation.*

**Grocco,** Pietro, Italian clinician, 1857–1916. See Orsi-G. *method*, G.'s *sign*, *triangle*.

**Groenouw** (grë'now), Arthur, German ophthalmologist, 1862–1945. See G.'s corneal *dystrophy*.

**groin.** *Regio inguinalis*.

**Grönblad,** Ester E., Swedish ophthalmologist, *1898. See G.-Strandberg *syndrome*.

# GROOVE

**groove.** Furrow; sulcus; a narrow, elongated depression on any surface.

**abomasal g.,** *sulcus* abomasi.

**alveolobuccal g.,** alveolobuccal sulcus; gingivobuccal g. or sulcus; the upper and lower half of the buccal vestibule on each side.

**alve'olola'bial g.,** alveololabial sulcus; gingivolabial g. or sulcus; (1) the upper and lower half of the labial vestibule; (2) in the embryo, the g. formed by the deepening of the primary labial g.; its inner wall becomes incorporated with the alveolar process of the mandible or the maxilla, and its outer wall with the lips and cheeks.

**alveololingual g.,** alveololingual sulcus; gingivolingual g. or sulcus; (1) that part of the oral cavity proper, on each side of the frenulum linguae, between the tongue and the mandibular alveolar process or ridge; (2) in the embryo, the g. on each side between the lingual primordium and the alveolar elevations of the mandible.

**anterior auricular g.,** *incisura* anterior auris.

**anterior parame'dian g.,** *sulcus* intermedius anterior.

**anterolateral g.** *sulcus* lateralis anterior.

**anteromedian g.,** (1) *fissura* mediana anterior medullae oblongatae; (2) *fissura* mediana anterior medullae spinalis.

**arterial g.'s,** *sulci* arteriosi.

**at'rioventric'ular g.,** *sulcus* coronarius.

**g. for auditory tube,** *sulcus* tubae auditivae.

**auric'uloventric'ular g.,** *sulcus* coronarius.

**bicip'ital g.,** *sulcus* intertubercularis.

**Blessig's g.** or **lacuna**, obsolescent eponym referring to a local modification of the configuration of the inner layer of the embryonic cup indicating the position of the ora serrata, or anterior edge of the retina.

**branchial g.,** an external embryonic g. between contiguous branchial arches; see also branchial *clefts*.

**carot'id g.,** *sulcus* caroticus.

**carpal g.,** *sulcus* carpi.

**cav'ernous g.,** *sulcus* caroticus.

**costal g.,** *sulcus* costae.

**g. of crus helix,** *sulcus* cruris helicis.

**dental g.,** a transitory depression in the gingival surface of the embryonic jaw along the line of ingrowth of the dental lamina.

**esophageal g.,** *sulcus* reticuli.

**ethmoidal g.,** *sulcus* ethmoidalis.

frontal g.'s, see entries under *sulcus* frontalis.

**gastric g.,** *sulcus* ventriculi.

**gingivobuccal g.,** alveolobuccal g.

**gingivolabial g.,** alveololabial g.

**gingivolingual g.,** alveololingual g.

**g. of greater petrosal nerve,** *sulcus* nervi petrosi majoris.

**Harrison's g.,** a deformity of the ribs which results from the pull of the diaphragm on ribs weakened by rickets or other softening of the bone.

**inferior petrosal g.,** *sulcus* sinus petrosi inferioris.

**infraorbital g.,** *sulcus* infraorbitalis.

**interos'seous g.,** (1) *sulcus* calcanei; (2) *sulcus* tali.

**intertubercular g.,** *sulcus* intertubercularis.

**interventricular g.'s,** *sulcus* interventricularis anterior and *sulcus* interventricularis posterior.

**lac'rimal g.,** *sulcus* lacrimalis.

**laryng'otra'cheal g.,** the depression in the floor of the posterior part of the pharynx, continued downward on the ventral wall of the foregut. From it are developed the lower part of the larynx and the trachea, bronchi, and lungs.

**lateral bicipital g.,** *sulcus* bicipitalis lateralis.

**g. of lesser petrosal nerve,** *sulcus* nervi petrosi minoris.

**linguogingival g.,** a g. separating the embryonic mandibular portion of the tongue from the remainder of the mandibular process.

**Lucas' g.,** *stria* spinosa.

**mastoid g.,** *incisura* mastoidea.

**medial bicipital g.,** *sulcus* bicipitalis medialis.

**med'ullary g.,** neural g.

**musculospi'ral g.,** *sulcus* nervi radialis.

**mylohy'oid g.,** *sulcus* mylohyoideus.

**g. of nail matrix,** *sulcus* matricis unguis.

**nasolabial g.,** *sulcus* nasolabialis.

**nasopal'atine g.,** a g. on the vomer lodging the nasopalatine nerve.

**nasopharyn'geal g.,** an indistinct line marking the boundary between the nasal cavities and the rhinopharynx.

**neural g.,** medullary g.; the gutter-like g. formed in the midline of the embryo's dorsal surface by the progressive elevation of the lateral margins of the neural plate; the ultimate fusion of the left with the right margin results in the formation of the neural tube.

**ob'turator g.,** *sulcus* obturatorius.

**occip'ital g.,** *sulcus* arteriae occipitalis.

**olfactory g.,** *sulcus* olfactorius.

**omasal g.,** *sulcus* omasi.

**optic g.,** *sulcus* chiasmatis.

**pal'atine g.,** *sulcus* palatinus.

**palatovaginal g.,** *sulcus* palatovaginalis.

**paraglenoid g.,** preauricular g.

**pharyngeal g.'s,** embryonic entodermal or ectodermal g.'s between successive pharyngeal arches.

**pharyng'otympan'ic g.,** a g. formed by the spine and the posterior border of the greater wing of the sphenoid bone together with the posteromedial side of the petrous part of the temporal bone; it lodges the cartilaginous part of the pharyngotympanic tube.

**poplit'eal g.,** sulcus popliteus; a g. on the lateral condyle of the femur between the epicondyle and the articular margin. Its anterior end gives origin to the popliteus muscle; its posterior end lodges the tendon of the muscle when the knee is fully flexed.

**posterior auricular g.,** *sulcus* auriculae posterior.

**posterior intermediate g.,** *sulcus* intermedius posterior.

**posterior parame'dian g.,** *sulcus* intermedius posterior.

**posterolateral g.,** *sulcus* lateralis posterior.

**primitive g.,** the median depression in the primitive streak flanked by the primitive ridges.

**pterygopal'atine g.,** *sulcus* palatinus major.

**g. for radial nerve,** *sulcus* nervi radialis.

**retention g.,** retention *area*.

**reticular g.,** *sulcus* reticuli.

**rhombic g.'s,** seven pairs of transverse furrows in the floor of the embryonic hindbrain.

**sagittal g.,** *sulcus* sinus sagittalis superioris.

**Sibson's g.,** a g. occasionally seen on the outer side of the thorax formed by the prominent lower border of the pectoralis major muscle.

**sigmoid g.,** *sulcus* sinus sigmoidei.

**skin g.'s,** *sulci* cutis.

**g. for spinal nerve,** *sulcus* nervi spinalis.

**spiral g.,** *sulcus* nervi radialis.

**subcla'vian g.,** a shallow g. on the clavicle lodging the subclavius muscle.

**g. for subclavian artery,** *sulcus* arteriae subclaviae.

**g. for subclavian vein,** *sulcus* venae subclaviae.

**subcos'tal g.,** *sulcus* costae.

**g. for tendon of flexor hallucis longus,** *sulcus* tendinis musculi flexoris hallucis longi.

**g. for tendon of long peroneal muscle,** *sulcus* tendinis musculi peronei longi.

**tracheobronchial g.,** a median ventral diverticulum of the embryonic foregut that gives rise to the epithelial component of the respiratory system.

**tympanic g.,** *sulcus* tympanicus.

**g. for ulnar nerve,** *sulcus* nervi ulnaris.

**urethral g.,** the g. on the undersurface of the embryonic penis which ultimately is closed to form the penile portion of the urethra.

**venous g.'s,** *sulci* venosi.

**ver'tebral g.,** the depression bounded by the spinous processes and laminae of the vertebrae, in which lie the deep muscles of the back.

**vomerovaginal g.,** *sulcus* vomerovaginalis.

---

**group.** 1. A number of similar or related objects. 2. In chemistry, a radical; for individual chemical groups, see the specific name.

**characterizing g.,** a g. of atoms in a molecule that distinguishes the class of substances in which it occurs from all other classes; thus carbonyl (CO) is the characterizing g. of ketones; COOH, of organic acids, etc.

**connective tissue g.,** a collective name for mucous tissue, dentin, bone, cartilage, and ordinary connective tissue, all derived from the mesenchyme.

**control g.,** a g. of subjects participating in the same experiment as another g. of subjects except for the inclusion of the variable under investigation. See also control (1 and 2).

**cytophil g.,** the atom g. in the antibody (amboceptor) that binds it to the cell.

**determinant g.,** antigenic *determinant.*

**encounter g.,** A form of psychological sensitivity training that emphasizes the experiencing of individual relationships within the g. and minimizes intellectual and didactic imput. The g. focuses on the present rather than concerning itself with the past or outside problems of its members. See also sensitivity training g.

**experimental g.,** task-oriented g.; a g. of subjects participating in the variable of an experiment, as opposed to the control g. (*q.v.*).

**functional g.,** see function (4).

**matched g.'s,** a method of experimental control in which subjects in one g. are matched on a one-to-one basis with subjects in other g.'s concerning all organism variables (*e.g.,* age, sex, height, weight) which the experimenter deems important.

**partial g.'s,** an old, infrequently used term for the sum of the different antibodies (in an immune serum) that correspond to various antigenic fractions of the microorganism.

**prosthetic g.,** a non-amino acid compound attached to a protein, usually in a reversible fashion, that confers new properties upon the conjugated protein thus produced; *e.g.* enzyme activity (see apoenzyme, holoenzyme), oxygen transport ability (heme + globin → hemoglobin).

**sensitivity training g.,** a g. in which members seek to develop self-awareness and an understanding of g. processes rather than to obtain therapy for an emotional disturbance. See also encounter g.; personal growth *laboratory.*

**symptom g.,** (1) syndrome; (2) complex (1).

**T g.,** abbreviation for training g.

**task-oriented g.,** experimental g.

**therapeutic g.,** any g. of patients meeting together for mutual psychotherapeutic goals.

**training g.,** T g.; any g. emphasizing training in self-awareness and group dynamics.

**growth.** The increase in size of a living being or any of its parts occurring in the process of development.

**accretionary g.,** g. by an increase of intercellular material.

**appositional g.,** g. accomplished by the addition of new layers on those previously formed; *e.g.,* the addition of lamellae in the formation of bone. It is the characteristic method of g. when rigid materials are involved.

**auxetic g.,** intussusceptive g.; g. by increase in the size of component cells.

**differential g.,** different rates of g. in associated tissues or structures. Used especially in embryology when the differences in g. rates result in changing the original proportions or relations.

**interstitial g.,** g. from a number of different centers within an area. In contrast with appositional g., it can occur only when the materials involved are nonrigid.

**intussusceptive g.,** auxetic g.

**multiplicative g.,** g. by an increase in the number of cells.

**new g.,** neoplasm.

**grub.** Wormlike larva or maggot of certain insects, particularly in the orders Coleoptera, Hymenoptera, and Diptera.

**cattle g.,** the larva or maggot of *Hypoderma bovis* and *H. lineatum,* often called heel flies, ox warble flies, or bomb flies; see *Hypoderma* and ox *bots.*

**Gruber,** George B., German physician. See G.'s *syndrome.*

**Gruber,** Josef, Austrian otologist, 1827–1900. See G.'s *method.*

**Gruber,** Max von, Munich hygienist, 1853–1927. See G.'s *reaction,* G.-Widal *reaction.*

**Gruber,** Wenaslaus L., Russian anatomist, 1814–1890. See G.'s *cul-de-sac,* G.-Landzert *fossa.*

**gru'el** [ thru O. Fr. fr. Mediev. L. *grutum,* meal ]. A semiliquid food of oatmeal or other cereal boiled in water; thin porridge.

**grunt.** A deep, short, guttural sound.

**expiratory g.,** a sound caused by mid-duction of the ventricular ligaments of the larynx as a result of surgical manipulations in the subdiaphragmatic areas; this traction relfex can usually be diminished by deepening anesthesia, but it may persist even in the third plane and necessitate endotracheal intubation.

**grunt'ing.** A laryngeal sound sometimes made by a horse suffering from laryngeal hemiplegia (roaring) when struck or moved suddenly.

**Grütz,** O. See Bürger-G. *syndrome.*

**Grynfeltt,** Joseph C., French surgeon, 1840–1913. See G.'s *triangle.*

**gryochrome** (gri'o-krōm) [ G. *gry,* something insignificant, + *chrōma,* color ]. A term applied by Nissl to nerve cells in which the stainable portion is present in the form of minute granules without definite arrangement.

**gryposis** (grī-po'sis) [ G. *grypos,* hooked, + suffix -*osis,* condition ]. An abnormal curvature.

**g. unguium,** onychogryposis.

**GSH.** Abbreviation for reduced *glutathione.*

**GSR.** Abbreviation for galvanic skin *response.*

**GSSG.** Abbreviation for oxidized *glutathione.*

**gt.** Abbreviation of L. *gutta,* drop.

**GTP.** Abbreviation for guanosine 5'-triphosphate.

**gtt.** Abbreviation of L. *guttae,* drops.

**guaiac** (gwi'ak) [ Sp. *guayaco,* imitating the native Carib name ] (USP). Guaiac gum; the resin of *Guiacum* wood; nauseant, diaphoretic, stimulant, and alterative.

**guaiacin** (gwi'ă-sin). A brownish, amorphous powder obtained from guaiac wood. Used as a reagent for oxidases, with which it gives a blue color.

**guaiacol** (gwi'ă-kol). *o*-Methoxyphenol; 2-*O*-methyl-pyrocatechol; catechol-monomethyl ether; $C_6H_4(OH)(OCH_3)$; has been used as an expectorant and intestinal disinfectant.

**g. carbonate,** DUOTAL; a white crystalline powder, insoluble in water; same uses as g.

**g. glyceryl ether,** glyceryl guaiacolate.

**g. phosphate,** phosphoric guaiacyl ether; a white crystalline powder, insoluble in water. Used as an intestinal antiseptic and in fever.

**guaiacum wood** (gwi'ă-kum). Lignum vitae; lignum benedictum; lignum sanctum; the heartwood of *Guaiacum officinale* or of *G. sanctum* (family Zygophyllaceae); a small tree of the West Indies and the Caribbean coast of South America. This wood is remarkable for its hardness and density and is the source of guaiac.

**guaithylline** (gwi'thĭ-lin) (USAN). ECLABRON; 3-(*o*-methoxyphenoxy)-1,2-propanediol compound with theophylline; smooth muscle relaxant for treatment of bronchial asthma.

**guanacline sulfate** (gwahn'ă-klēn) (USAN). [ 2-(3,6-Dihydro-4-methyl-1(2*H*)-pyridyl)ethyl ]guanidine sulfate dihydrate; an antihypertensive drug.

**guan'adrel sulfate** (USAN). ANAREL; (1,4-dioxaspiro [ 4,5 ]dec-2-ylmethyl)guanidine sulfate; an antihypertensive drug.

**guanase** (gwah'nās). Guanine deaminase.

**guanazolo** (gwah'nă-zo'lo). 8-Azaguanine.

**guanethidine sulfate** (USP, BP). ISMELIN; [ 2-(octahydro-1-azocinyl)-ethyl ]-guanidine sulfate; a potent antihypertensive agent. It appears to interfere with the release of the chemical mediator (norepinephrine) at the sympathetic neuroeffector junction; it does not produce ganglionic or parasympathetic blockade with recommended doses. In ophthalmology, it is used topically for the treatment of glaucoma and to counteract eyelid retraction in Graves' disease.

**guanidine** (gwah'nĭ-den, -din). $NH_2$—$C(NH)$—$NH_2$; strongly basic, usually found (in some plants and lower animals) as the hydrochloride. Formed in putrefying nitrogenous matter.

**guan'idinoac'etate meth'yltrans'ferase** (EC 2.1.1.2). Guanidinoacetate methylpherase; the enzyme catalyzing the transfer of a methyl group from S-adenosylmethionine ("active methionine") to guanidinoacetate (glycocyamine), forming creatine.

**guan'idinoace'tic acid.** Glycocyamine.

**guanine** (gwah'nen, -nin). 2-Amino-6-oxypurine; one of the two major purines occurring in nucleic acid.

Guanine

  **g. deaminase** (EC 3.5.4.3), guanase; a deaminase of the liver that catalyzes the conversion of guanine into xanthine.

  **g. deoxyribonucleotide,** deoxyguanylic acid.

  **g. ribonucleotide,** guanylic acid.

**guanochlor sulfate** (gwahn'o-klor) (USAN). VATENSOL; ‖[ 2-(2,6-dichlorophenoxy)ethyl ]amino‖guanidine sulfate; used as α-adrenergic blocking agent for treatment of essential hypertension.

**guanophores** (gwahn-o-forz) [ guanine + G. *phoros,* bearing ]. Cells in the skin of some cold-blooded vertebrates (particularly fishes) which contain granules composed of guanine and give the creatures a metallic (gold or silver) luster.

**guanosine** (gwah'no-sen, -sin). 9-β-D-Ribosylguanine (guanine combined through its N-9 with the C-1 of β-D-ribose); a major constituent of RNA and of guanine nucleotides.

  **g. phosphorylase** (EC 2.4.2.15), a phosphorylase that phosphorylyzes guanosine to guanine and ribose 1-phosphate.

**guanosine 5′-triphosphate.** GTP; similar to ATP; immediate precursor of guanine nucleotides in RNA.

**guanox'an sulfate** (USAN). ENVACAR; (1,4-benzodioxan-2-ylmethyl)guanidine sulfate; antihypertensive agent.

**guanyl** (gwah'nil). 1. Radical of guanine. 2. Mistakenly used for guanylyl, the radical of guanylic acid. 3. An obsolete term for the amidino radical (from amidine), $H_2N$—$C(NH)$—.

**guanylate cyclase** (EC 4.6.1.2). Guanylyl cyclase; analogous to adenylate (adenylyl) cyclase, but cyclizing guanosine triphosphate to guanosine 3′:5′-cyclic phosphate.

**guanylic acid** (gwah-nil'ik). Guanosine 5′-phosphate; guanine ribonucleotide.

**guan'ylori'bonu'clease** (EC 3.4.1.8). A nuclease cleaving ribonucleic acids at the 3′-5′link of a guanosine 3′-phosphate residue, producing oligonucleotides terminating in this nucleotide, a transferase (endonuclease) in the first (cyclizing) step, a phosphodiesterase in the second (hydrolyzing) step. Also called ribonuclease $T_1$; takadiastase $T_1$.

**guanylyl cyclase.** Guanylate cyclase.

**guarana** (gwah-rah-nah') [ Native Brazilian word ]. A dried paste of the crushed seeds of *Paullinia cupana* (family Sapindaceae), a vine extensively cultivated in Brazil. It contains guaranine (caffeine), saponin, a volatile oil, and paullinitannic acid. Has been used for the relief of headache.

**guar'anine.** Caffeine.

**Guarnieri** (gwar-ne-a're), Giuseppi, Italian physician, 1856–1918. See G.'s gelatin *agar,* G.'s *bodies.*

**gubernaculum** (gu'ber-nak'u-lum) [ L. a helm ]. A fibrous cord connnecting two structures.

  **g. den'tis,** a connective tissue band uniting the tooth sac with the gum.

  **Hunter's g.,** g. testis.

  **g. tes'tis** [ NA ], Hunter's g.; a mesenchymal column of tissue that connects the fetal testis to the developing scrotum; it appears to play a significant role in testicular descent.

**Gubler,** Adolphe, Paris physician, 1821–1879. See G.'s *hemiplegia, icterus, line, paralysis, syndrome,* Millard-G. *syndrome,* G.'s *tumor.*

**Gudden,** Bernhard A. von, German alienist, 1824–1886. See G.'s *commissure, ganglion,* tegmental *nuclei.*

**Guéneau de Mussy** (ga-no'de-mü-se'). Noël F. O., Paris physician, 1813–1885. See G. de M.'s *point.*

**Guenther's stain.** See under stain.

**Guérin** (ga-ran'), Alphonse F. M., Paris surgeon, 1816–1895. See bacille bilié de Calmette-G., G.'s *fold, fracture, gland, sinus,* Calmette-G. *vaccine,* G.'s *valve.*

**guidance** (gi'dans). 1. A guide, *q.v.* 2. The act of guiding.

  **condylar g.,** condylar guide; the mechanical device on an articulator which is intended to produce g. in an articulator movement similar to those produced by the paths of the condyles in the temporomandibular joints. See also condylar guidance *inclination.*

  **incisal g.,** incisal path; the influence on mandibular movements caused by the contacting surfaces of the mandibular and maxillary anterior teeth during eccentric excursions.

**guide** (gīd). 1. Staff (1). 2. To lead in a set course. 3. Any device or contrivance that sets a course. See also subentries under guidance.

  **anterior g.,** incisal g.

  **anterior g., adjustable,** an incisal g. with a superior surface that may be changed to provide variations in the incisal g. angle.

  **condylar g.,** condylar *guidance.*

  **incisal g.,** anterior g.; in dentistry, that part of an articulator on which the anterior g. pin rests to maintain the vertical dimension of occlusion and the incisal g. angle as established by the incisal guidance.

  **mold g.,** a g. used to specify the shape of artificial teeth, or of an artificial tooth.

**guideline** (gid'lin). A marking in the form of a line that serves as a guide or reference.

  **clasp g.,** survey *line.*

  **Cummer's g.,** survey *line.*

**Guillain,** Georges, French neurologist, 1876–1961. See G.-Barré *reflex, syndrome.*

**guillotine** (gil'o-ten) [ Fr. an instrument for the decapitation of condemned criminals ]. An instrument in the shape of a metal ring through which runs a sliding knifeblade, used in cutting off an enlarged tonsil.

**guinea green** (gin'ĭ). A diaminotriphenylmethane dye, used as an indicator for H-ion determinations, changing at pH 6.0 from magenta to green.

**guinea pig** (gin'ĭ). *Cavia porcellus.*

**Guinon** (ge-nawn'), Georges, Paris physician, 1859–1929. See G.'s *disease.*

**gula,** gen. **gulae** [ L. ]. Throat; gullet.

**Guldberg-Waage law.** See under law.

**Gull,** Sir William W., English physician, 1816–1890. See G.'s *disease,* G.-Sutton *disease.*

**gul'let** [ L. *gula,* throat ]. Pharynx and esophagus, used in swallowing.

**Gullstrand** (gool'strahnd), Allvar, Swedish ophthalmologist, 1862–1930. Nobel laureate, 1911, for his work on the dioptrics of the eye.

**L-gulonic acid.** Oxidation product (—CHO → COOH) of L-gulose; reduction product of glucuronic acid (—CHO → $CH_2OH$); a precursor (except in primates and guinea pigs) of ascorbic acid via L-gulonolactone.

**L-gulonolactone.** Dihydroascorbic acid; the immediate precursor of ascorbic acid in those animals capable of ascorbic acid biosynthesis.

**gu'losacchar'ic acid.** Saccharic acid.

**gu′lose.** One of the eight pairs (D and L) of aldoses. For structure, see sugars.

**gum** [ A.S. *gōma*, jaw ]. Gingiva.

    **blue g.,** see blue *line.*

**gum.** 1 [ L. *gummi* ]. The dried exuded sap from a number of trees and shrubs, forming an amorphous bittle mass; it forms usually a mucilaginous solution in water.

    **animal g.,** a gumlike polysaccharide derived from mucin.

    **g. arabic,** see arabin and acacia.

    **Basso′ra g.,** a g. resembling tragacanth, acacia, and the gummy exudate of cherry and plum trees; it comes from Persia and Turkey; used in making storax.

    **g. benjamin, g. benzoin,** benzoin.

    **blue g. tree,** *Eucalyptus.*

    **British g.,** dextrin.

    **Cape g.,** a g. (resembling acacia) from *Acacia horrida* of South Africa.

    **eucalyptus g.,** eucalyptus kino; red g.; a dried gummy exudation from *Eucalyptus rostrata* and other species of *Eucalyptus* (family Myrtaceae); used as an astringent (in gargles and troches) and antidiarrheal agent.

    **ghatti g.,** Indian g.

    **g. guai′ac,** guaiac.

    **guar g.** (NF), the ground endosperms of *Cyamopsis tetragonolobus;* used in pharmaceutical jelly formulations.

    **Indian g.,** ghatti g.; an exudation from *Anogeisus latifolia* (family Combrettaceae); the mucilage is used as a substitute for acacia mucilage.

    **karaya g.,** sterculia g.

    **red g.,** eucalyptus g.

    **g. resin,** see under resin.

    **sen′egal g.,** the g. of *Acacia senegal.*

    **starch g.,** dextrin.

    **stercu′lia g.,** karaya g.; the dried gummy exudation from *Sterculia urens, S. villosa, S. tragacantha,* or other species of *Sterculia,* or from *Cochlospermum gossypium* or other species of *Cochlospermum* (family Bixaceae). Used as a hydrophilic laxative and in the manufacture of lotions and pastes.

    **g. thus,** see (1) olibanum, and (2) turpentine.

    **g. trag′acanth,** tragacanth.

    **wattle g.,** a g. resembling acacia, from a species of *Acacia* growing in Australia.

**gum′boil.** Gingival *abscess.*

**gumma,** pl. **gummas** or **gum′mata** (gum′ah) [ L. *gummi,* gum, fr. G. *kommi* ]. Gummatous syphilid; nodular syphilid; tubercular syphilid; syphiloma; an infectious granuloma that is characteristic of tertiary syphilis, but does not develop with regularity and is observed only infrequently. G.'s may be solitary (as large as 8 to 10 cm. in diameter) or multiple and diffusely scattered (1 mm. or less in diameter). G.'s are characterized by an irregular central portion that is firm, sometimes partially hyalinized, and consisting of coagulative necrosis in which "ghosts" of structures may be recognized; a poorly defined middle zone of epithelioid cells, with occasional multinucleated giant cells; and a peripheral zone of fibroblasts and numerous capillaries, with infiltrated lymphocytes and plasma cells. As g.'s become older, an irregular scar or rounded fibrous nodule persists.

**gummatous** (gum′ă-tus). Pertaining to or characterized by the features of a gumma.

**gum′my.** 1. Viscous; mucilaginous; resembling a gum. 2. Pertaining to the gross consistency of or resembling a gumma.

**Gumprecht** (goom′prekt), Ferdinand, German physician, *1864. See Klein-G. shadow *nuclei,* G.'s *shadows.*

**Gunn,** Robert Marcus, English ophthalmologist, 1850–1909. See G.'s *dots, phenomenon, sign, syndrome.*

**Günning,** Jan W., Dutch chemist, 1827–1901. See G.'s *reaction.*

**Gunning splint.** See under splint.

**Günther,** Hans, German physician, 1884–1956. See G.'s *disease.*

**Günz** (günts), Justus G., German anatomist, 1714–1789. See G.'s *ligament.*

**Guo.** Abbreviation for guanosine.

**gurgulio** (goor-goo′lĭ-o) [ L. gullet, windpipe ]. Uvula.

**Gussenbauer** (goos′en-bow-er), Carl, German surgeon, 1842–1903. See G.'s *suture.*

**gusta′tion** [ L. *gustatio,* fr. *gusto,* pp. *-atus,* to taste ]. The act of tasting; the sense of taste.

**gus′tatory.** Relating to gustation, or taste.

**gut** [ A.S. ]. 1. The intestine. 2. Embryonic digestive tube. 3. Abbreviated term for catgut.

    **blind g.,** cecum.

    **end-g.,** hindgut.

    **fore-g.,** see foregut.

    **head-g.,** foregut.

    **hind-g.** see hindgut.

    **mid-g.,** see midgut.

    **postanal g.,** postcloacal g.; tailgut; an extension of the hindgut caudal to the point at which the anal opening is formed.

    **postcloacal g.,** postanal g.

    **preoral g.,** Seessel's *pocket.*

    **silkworm g.,** a suture material obtained by drawing out in a single thread the fluid silk in a silkworm just ready to spin its cocoon.

    **surgical g.,** surgical *suture.*

    **tail-g.,** postanal g.

**Guthrie,** George J., London surgeon, 1785–1856. See G.'s *muscle.*

**Guthrie test.** See under test.

**Gutmann,** C. See Michaelis-G. *body.*

**gutta** (gut′ah) [ L. ]. A drop; see drop (4), and drops.

    **g. sere′na,** amaurosis.

**gutta-percha** (gut′ah-per′chah) [ Malay *gatah,* gum, + *percha,* the name of a tree ] (USP). The coagulated, purified, dried, milky juice of trees of the genera *Palaguium* and *Payena* (family Sapotaceae). Used as a temporary filling material in dentistry, and in the manufacture of splints and electrical insulators; a solution is used as a substitute for collodion, as a protective and to seal incised wounds.

    **g.-p. cone,** a cone-shaped, semirigid root canal filling material composed of g.-p. and zinc oxide.

    **g.-p. spreader,** an instrument used in dentistry for condensing g.-p. laterally in a root canal.

**gut′tate.** Of the shape of, or resembling, a drop, characterizing certain cutaneous lesions.

**gutta′tim** [ L. ]. Drop by drop.

**gut′tur** [ L. ]. Throat.

**guttural** (gut′er-al). Throaty; relating to the throat.

**gutturotetany** (gut′ur-o-tet′ă-nĭ) [ L. *guttur,* throat, + G. *tetanos,* convulsive tension ]. Laryngeal spasm causing a temporary stutter.

**Gutzeit** (goot′sit), Max A. G., German chemist, 1847–1915. See G.'s *test.*

**Guy de Chauliac.** See Chauliac, Guy de.

**Guyon** (gü-yawn′), Felix J. C., Paris surgeon, 1831–1920. See G.'s *amputation, isthmus, method, sign.*

**Gymnamoebida** (jim-nă-me′bĭ-dah) [ G. *gymnos,* naked, + *amoibē,* change (ameba) ]. An order of Amoebea, in which there is no shell, though there may be an enveloping layer of condensed ectoplasm; the genus *Amoeba* is in this order.

**gymnastics** (jim-nas′tiks) [ G. *gymnos,* naked ]. Muscular exercise, performed indoors, as distinguished from athletics, and usually by means of special apparatus.

    **Swedish g.,** Swedish *movements.*

**gymnema** (jim-ne′mah) [ G. *gymnos,* naked, + *nēma,* thread ]. The leaves of *Gymnema sylvestre* (family Asclepiadaceae), a tree of tropical Africa; contains gymnemic acid.

**gymné′mic acid.** $C_{32}H_{55}O_{12}$; an acid of glycosidal character occurring in the leaves of *Gymnema sylvestre,* or *Asclepias geminata.* Completely dulls taste for bitter or sweet for several hours.

**gymnocolon** (jim′no-ko′lon). See gymnocolon *bath.*

**gymnocyte** (jim′no-sit) [ G. *gymnos,* naked, + *kytos,* hollow (cell) ]. Obsolete term referring to a cell without limiting membrane.

**gymnophobia** (jim-no-fo′bĭ-ah) [ G. *gymnos,* naked, + *phobos,* fear ]. Morbid fear of the sight of a naked person or of an uncovered part of the body.

**gymnosperms** (jim'no-spermz) [ G. *gymnos*, naked, + *sperma*, seed ]. A subdivision of the spermatophytes, or seed-bearing plants, comprising approximately 700 living species. The seeds are not covered by a carpel or ovary wall, *i.e.*, the ovule is naked and the pollen is brought directly into contact with its surface.

**gyn-.** See gyno-.

**Gynaecophorus** (jin'e-kof'o-rus, gi'ne-, ji'ne-) [ gyne- + G. *phoros*, bearing ]. Old name for *Schistosoma*.

**gynaminic acid** (jin'ă-min'ik). Pyrrole form of aldol condensation product of pyruvate and *N*-acetylglucosamine; reported in human milk; apparently identical with sialic acid from other sources.

**gynandrism** (jī-nan'drizm, gi'-nan-drizm, ji-) [ gyn- + G. *anēr* (*andr*-), man ]. A developmental abnormality characterized by hypertrophy of the clitoris and union of the labia majora, simulating in appearance the penis and scrotum.

**gynan'droblasto'ma.** 1. Arrhenoblastoma. 2. A rare variety of arrhenoblastoma of the ovary, containing theco-granulomatous elements and producing simultaneous androgenic and estrogenic effects.

**gynandroid** (jī-nan'droyd, gi-, ji-) [ gyn- + G. *anēr* (*andr*-), man, + *eidos*, resemblance ]. An individual exhibiting gynandrism.

**gynandromorph** (jī-nan'dro-morf, gi-, ji-) [ gyn- + G. *anēr* (*andr*-), man, + *morphē*, form ]. An abnormal individual of which some portions of the body have male characteristics and others female.

**gynandromorphism** (jī-nan-dro-mor'fizm) [ gyn- + G. *anēr* (*andr*-), man, + *morphē*, form ]. A combination of male and female characteristics.

**gynan'dromor'phous.** Having both male and female characteristics.

**gynatresia** (jin'ă-tre'zī-ah, gi-, ji-) [ gyn- + G. *a*- priv. + *trēsis*, a hole ]. Occlusion of some part of the female genital tract, especially occlusion of the vagina by a more or less thick membrane.

**gyne-, gyneco-** (gi'ne-, jin'e-, ji'ne-). See gyno-.

**gynecic** (jī-ne'sik). Relating to the diseases peculiar to women.

**gynecogen** (jin'e-ko-jen, gi-) [ gyneco- + suffix -*gen*, producing ]. A substance that produces or stimulates female characteristics. Obsolete.

**gynecogenic** (jin'e-ko-jen'ik, -gi'ne-ko-, ji'ne-ko-). 1. Giving birth predominantly to females. 2. Obsolete term meaning productive of female characteristics.

**gynecography** (gi'ne-kog'ră-fī, jin'e-) [ gyne- + G. *graphō*, to write ]. Hysterosalpingography.

**gynecoid** (gi'ne-koyd, jin'e-koyd) [ gyneco- + G. *eidos*, resemblance ]. Resembling a woman in form and structure.

**gyn'ecolog'ic, gyn'ecolog'ical.** Relating to gynecology.

**gynecology** (gi'ne-kol-o-jī, jin'e-) [ gyneco- + G. *logos*, study ]. The branch of medicine which has to do with the diseases peculiar to women, primarily those of the genital tract, as well as female endocrinology and reproductive physiology.

**gynecomania** (gi'ne-ko-ma'nī-ah, jin'e-) [ gyneco- + G. *mania*, frenzy ]. Morbid or excessive desire for women.

**gynecomastia, gynecomasty** (gi'ne-ko-mas'tī-ah, jin'e-). [ gyneco- + G. *mastos*, breast ]. Excessive development of the male mammary glands, sometimes secreting milk; a common, transient occurrence in normal adolescence.

**gy'necoma'zia** [ gyneco- + G. *mazos*, breast ]. Obsolete synonym for gynecomastia.

**gy'necos'mics** [ gyneco- + G. *kosmeo*, to decorate ]. Obsolete term for female secondary sex characteristics.

**gynephobia** (gi'ne-fo'bī-ah, jin'e-) [ gyne- + G. *phobos*, fear ]. A morbid fear of women.

**gyniatrics** (jin'ī-at'riks, gi-, ji-) [ gyn- + G. *iatrikos*, of medicine or surgery ]. Gyniatry; treatment of the diseases of women.

**gyniat'ry.** Gyniatrics.

**gyno-, gyn-, gyne-, gyneco-** (jin'o-, gi'no-, ji'no-) [ G. *gynē*, woman ]. Combining forms relating to woman.

**gynocar'dia oil.** Chaulmoogra oil.

**gynogamones** (gi'no-gam'ōnz, jin'o-) [ gyno- + G. *gamos*, marriage ]. Gamones produced by the ovum of marine invertebrate organisms; g. I is believed to play a part in stimulating the swimming movements of the spermatozoa; g. II appears to be a factor in the adherence of the sperm head to the surface of the ovum as a step toward penetration.

**gynogenesis** (gi'no-jen'ē-sis, jin'o-) [ gyno- + G. *genesis*, production ]. Egg development activated by a spermatozoon, but to which the male gamete contributes no genetic material.

**gyn'omas'tia.** Obsolete alternative spelling for gynecomastia.

**gynopathy** (jī-nop'ă-thī, gi-) [ gyno- + G. *pathos*, suffering ]. Any disease peculiar to women.

**gynoplastics** (jin'o-plas'tiks, gi'no-, ji'no-) [ gyno- + G. *plassō*, to form ]. Reparative or plastic surgery of the female genital organs.

**gypsum** (jip'sum) [ L. fr. G. *gypsos* ]. Calcium sulfate.
    **dried g.,** *plaster* of Paris.

**gyrate** (ji'rāt) [ L. *gyro*, pp. *gyratus*, to turn round in a circle, *gyrus* ]. 1. Of convoluted or ring shape. 2. To revolve.

**gyra'tion.** 1. Revolution; circular motion. 2. Arrangement of convolutions or gyri in the brain.

**gyre** (jir). Gyrus; convolution.

**gyrectomy** (ji-rek'to-mī) [ G. *gyros*, ring (gyrus), + *ektomē*, excision ]. Excision of a cerebral gyrus.
    **frontal g.,** topectomy.

**gyrencephalic** (ji'ren-sē-fal'ik) [ G. *gyros*, ring (gyrus), + *enkaphalē*, brain ]. Denoting brains, such as that of man, in which the cerebral cortex has convolutions, in contrast to the lissencephalic (smooth) brains of small mammals such as the rodents.

**gyri** (ji'ri) [ L. ]. Plural of gyrus.

**gyrochrome** (ji'ro-krōm) [ G. *gyros*, a ring, circle, + *chrōma*, a color ]. Denoting a nerve cell in which the chromophil substance is arranged roughly in rings.

**gyromele** (ji'ro-mēl) [ G. *gyros*, circle, + *mēlē*, a probe ]. An instrument used for cleansing the stomach; it consists of a sponge at the end of a revolving rod, which is passed through a stomach tube.

**gyrosa** (ji-ro'sah) [ L. ]. Sham-movement *vertigo*.

**gyrose** (ji'rōs) [ G. *gyros*, circle ]. Marked by irregular curved lines like the surface of a cerebral hemisphere.

**gyrospasm** (ji'ro-spazm) [ G. *gyros*, circle, + *spasmos*, spasm. SPA- ]. Spasmodic rotary movements of the head.

# GYRUS

**gyrus,** gen. and pl. **gy'ri** (ji'rus) [ L. fr. G. *gyros*, circle ] [ NA ]. Convolution; one of the prominent rounded elevations that form the cerebral hemispheres. Each gyrus consists of the exposed superficial portion and a portion hidden from view in the wall and floor of the sulcus.
    **angular g.,** g. angularis.
    **g. angula'ris** [ NA ], angular g. or convolution; a folded convolution in the inferior parietal lobule formed by the united posterior ends of the superior and middle temporal gyri.
    **annectant g.,** transitional g.
    **anterior central g.,** g. precentralis.
    **anterior pyriform g.,** prepyriform g.
    **ascending frontal g.,** g. precentralis.
    **ascending parietal g.,** g. postcentralis.
    **gyri bre'ves in'sulae** [ NA ], short gyri of insula; several short, radiating gyri converging toward the base of the insula, composing the anterior two-thirds of the insular cortex.
    **callosal g.,** g. cinguli.
    **central gyri,** the gyri precentralis and postcentralis.
    **gyri cer'ebri** [ NA ], the gyri or convolutions of the cerebral cortex.
    **cingulate g.,** g. cinguli.
    **g. cin'guli** [ NA ], cingulate g. or convolution; callosal g. or convolution; falciform lobe; lobus falciformis; a long,

curved convolution of the medial surface of the cortical hemisphere, arched over the corpus callosum from which it is separated by the deep sulcus corporis callosi; together with the g. parahippocampalis, with which it is continuous behind the corpus callosum, it forms the g. fornicatus.

**deep transitional g.,** the transverse g. of the embryo which in development becomes buried in the depth of the central sulcus of the cerebral hemisphere.

**dentate g.,** g. dentatus.

**g. denta'tus** [ NA ], dentate g. or fascia; Tarin's fascia; fascia dentata hippocampi; one of the two interlocking gyri composing the hippocampus, the other one being the cornu ammonis (Ammon's horn).

**fasciolar g.,** g. fasciolaris.

**g. fasciola'ris** [ NA ], fasciolar g.; fascia cinerea; fasciola cinerea; a small paired band that passes around the splenium of the corpus callosum from the lateral longitudinal stria to the g. dentatus.

**g. fornica'tus,** the horse-shaped cortical convolution bordering the hilus of the cerebral hemisphere; its upper limb is formed by the g. cinguli, its lower by the g. parahippocampalis.

**g. fronta'lis infe'rior** [ NA ], inferior frontal g. or convolution; a broad convolution on the convexity of the frontal lobe of the cerebrum between the inferior frontal sulcus and the fissure of Sylvius; it is divided by branches of the lateral (Sylvian) fissure into three parts: pars basilaris (opercularis), pars triangularis, and pars orbitalis; the first two constitute a portion of the frontal operculum.

**g. fronta'lis me'dius** [ NA ], middle frontal g. or convolution; a convolution on the convexity of each frontal lobe of the cerebrum running in an anteroposterior direction between the superior and inferior frontal sulci.

**g. fronta'lis supe'rior** [ NA ], superior frontal g. or convolution; marginal g.; a broad convolution running in an anteroposterior direction on the inner edge of the convex surface and on the mesial surface of each frontal lobe.

**fusiform g.,** g. fusiformis.

**g. fusifor'mis,** g. occipitotemporalis lateralis [ NA ]; fusiform g.; lateral occipitotemporal g.; lobulus fusiformis; an extremely long convolution extending lengthwise over the ventral aspect of the temporal and occipital lobes, demarcated medially by the sulcus collateralis from the lingual g. and the anterior part of the parahippocampal g., laterally by the sulcus temporalis inferior from the inferior temporal g.

**Heschl's gyri,** gyri temporales transversi.

**hippocampal g.,** g. parahippocampalis.

**inferior frontal g.,** g. frontalis inferior.

**inferior occipital g.,** a g. situated below the lateral occipital sulcus on the lower part of the lateral surface of the occipital lobe.

**inferior parietal g.,** lobulus parietalis inferior.

**inferior temporal g.,** g. temporalis inferior.

**gyri in'sulae** [ NA ], the gyri breves insulae and g. longus insulae.

**interlocking gyri,** several small gyri in the walls of the central sulcus of the hemisphere; the opposed gyri interlock with one another.

**lateral occipitotemporal g.** g. fusiformis.

**lingual g.,** g. lingualis.

**g. lingua'lis** [ NA ], g. occipitotemporalis medialis [ NA ]; lingual g.; medial occipitotemporal g.; a relatively short, horizontal convolution on the inferomedial aspect of the occipital and temporal lobes, demarcated from the lateral occipitotemporal or fusiform g. by the deep sulcus collateralis, from the cuneus by the calcarine sulcus; its anterior extreme abuts the isthmus of the parahippocampal g. The medial or upper strip of the g. forming the lower bank of the calcarine sulcus corresponds to the inferior half of the area striata or primary visual cortex and represents the contralateral upper quadrant of the binocular field of vision.

**long g. of insula,** g. longus insulae.

**g. lon'gus in'sulae** [ NA ], long g. of the insula; the most posterior and longest of the slender and relatively straight gyri that compose the insula.

**marginal g.,** g. frontalis superior.

**medial occipitotemporal g.,** g. lingualis.

**middle frontal g.,** g. frontalis medius.

**middle temporal g.** g. temporalis medius.

**occipital gyri,** see inferior occipital g. and superior occipital g.

**g. occip'itotempora'lis latera'lis** [ NA ], g. fusiformis.

**g. occip'itotempora'lis media'lis** [ NA ], g. lingualis.

**orbital gyri,** gyri orbitales.

**gyri orbita'les** [ NA ], orbital gyri; a number of small, irregular convolutions occupying the concave inferior surface of each frontal lobe of the cerebrum.

**parahippocampal g.,** g. parahippocampalis.

**g. par'ahippocampa'lis** [ NA ], parahippocampal g.; hippocampal g. or convolution; a long convolution on the medial surface of the temporal lobe, forming the lower part of the g. fornicatus, extending from behind the splenium corporis callosi forward along the g. dentatus of the hippocampus from which it is demarcated by the hippocampal fissure. The anterior extreme of the g. curves back upon itself, thus forming the uncus, the major location of the olfactory cortex. See also entorhinal *area*.

**paraterminal g.,** g. paraterminalis.

**g. paratermina'lis** [ NA ], g. subcallosus.

**postcentral g.,** g. postcentralis.

**g. postcentra'lis** [ NA ], postcentral g.; posterior central g. or convolution; ascending parietal g. or convolution; the anterior convolution of the parietal lobe, bounded in front by the central sulcus (fissure of Rolando) and posteriorly by the interparietal sulcus.

**posterior central g.,** g. postcentralis.

**precentral g.,** g. precentralis.

**g. precentra'lis** [ NA ], anterior central g. or convolution; ascending frontal g. or convolution; the posterior convolution of the frontal lobe bounded posteriorly by the central sulcus (fissure of Rolando) and anteriorly by the precentral sulcus; motor cortex.

**prepyriform g.,** anterior pyriform g.; covers deeply placed amygdaloid nucleus; concerned with olfactory function.

**g. rec'tus** [ NA ], straight g.; a g. running along the medial part of the orbital surface of the frontal lobe of the cerebral hemisphere. It is bounded laterally by the olfactory sulcus.

**Retzius' g.,** the intralimbic g. in the cortical portion of the rhinencephalon.

**short gyri of the insula,** gyri breves insulae.

**splenial g.,** the band of cortex on the medial surface of the cerebral hemisphere which passes around the splenium of the corpus callosum, narrowing anteriorly and finally blending with the indusium griseum.

**straight g.,** g. rectus.

**subcallosal g.,** g. subcallosus.

**g. subcallo'sus** [ NA ], g. paraterminalis [ NA ]; pedunculus corporis callosi [ NA ]; area subcallosa [ NA ]; subcallosal g. or area; peduncle of the corpus callosum; paraterminal g. or body; corpus paraterminale; Zuckerkandl's convolution; a slender, vertical, whitish band immediately anterior to the lamina terminalis and anterior commissure. Contrary to its name, it is not a cortical convolution, but, instead, the ventral continuation of the septum pellucidum: precommissural septum or anterior limb of the diagonal band of Broca. See also septal *area;* diagonal *band* of Broca.

**superior frontal g.,** g. frontalis superior.

**superior occipital g.,** a g. lying above the lateral occipital sulcus on the lateral surface of the occipital lobe.

**superior parietal g.,** lobulus parietalis superior.

**superior temporal g.,** g. temporalis superior.

**supracallosal g.,** indusium griseum.

**supramarginal g.,** g. supramarginalis.

**g. supramargina'lis** [ NA ], supramarginal g. or convolution; a folded convolution capping the posterior extremity of the lateral (Sylvian) sulcus; together with the g. angularis, it forms the inferior half of the parietal lobe.

**g. tempora'lis infe'rior** [ NA ], inferior temporal g. or convolution; third temporal convolution; a sagittal convolution on the inferolateral border of the temporal lobe of the cerebrum, separated from the middle temporal g. by the inferior temporal sulcus. On the inferior surface of the temporal lobe it is separated from the medial occipitotemporal g. by the occipitotemporal sulcus. It includes the lateral occipitotemporal g.

**g. tempora'lis me'dius** [ NA ], middle temporal g. or convolution; second temporal convolution; a longitudinal

g. on the lateral surface of the temporal lobe, between the superior and inferior temporal sulci.

**g. tempora'lis supe'rior** [ NA ], superior temporal g. or convolution; first temporal convolution; a longitudinal g. on the lateral surface of the temporal lobe between the lateral (Sylvian) fissure and the superior temporal sulcus.

**gyri tempora'les transver'si** [ NA ], transverse temporal gyri or convolutions; Heschl's gyri; two or three convolu-

tions running transversely on the upper surface of the temporal lobe bordering on the lateral (Sylvian) fissure, separated from each other by the transverse temporal sulci.

**transitional g.,** annectant g.; transitional convolution; a small convolution connecting two lobes or two main gyri in the depth of a sulcus.

**transverse temporal gyri,** gyri temporales transversi.
**uncinate g.,** uncus (2).

# H

**H.** Abbreviation or symbol for (1) hyperopia or hyperopic; (2) horizontal; (3) Hauch; (4) Holzknecht unit; (5) inductance in henries; (6) the element hydrogen; (7) the Fraunhofer line at λ 3968 due to calcium; (8) oersted.

**H⁺.** Symbol for hydrogen ion, the proton.

**²H.** Hydrogen isotope of mass 2; deuterium (also abbreviated D or *d*).

**³H.** Hydrogen isotope (artificial; radioactive) of mass 3; tritium (also abbreviated T or *t*).

**h.** Symbol for Planck's *constant*.

**HA.** Abbreviation for an acid.

**HAA.** Abbreviation for hepatitis-associated *antigen*.

**Haab** (hahb), Otto, Zurich ophthalmologist, 1850–1931. See H.'s *magnet, reflex.*

**Haase's rule.** See under rule.

**Habel test.** See under test.

**habena,** pl. **habe'nae** (hä-be'nah) [ L. strap. HAB- ]. 1. A frenum or restricting fibrous band. 2. Habenula (2). 3. A restraining bandage.

**hab'enal, habe'nar.** Relating to a habena.

**habenula,** pl. **haben'ulae** (hä-ben'u-lah) [ L. See HAB- ]. 1. A frenulum. 2. In neuroanatomy, the term originally denoted the stalk of the pineal gland (pineal habenula; pedunculus of pineal body), but gradually came to refer to a neighboring group of nerve cells with which the pineal gland was believed to be associated, the "ganglion habenulae." Currently, the term habenula [ NA ], exclusively refers to this circumscript cell mass in the dorsomedial thalamus, embedded in the posterior end of the stria medullaris from which it received most of its afferent fibers. By way of the fasciculus retroflexus (habenulointerpeduncular tract) it projects to the interpeduncular nucleus and other paramedian cell groups of the midbrain tegmentum. The habenula is also known as the epithalamus. Despite its proximity to the pineal stalk, no habenulopineal fiber connection is known to exist.

**h. of cecum,** extension of the posteromedial colic tenia, dorsal or ventral to the terminal ileum.

**Haller's h.,** Scarpa's h.; the cordlike remains of the vaginal process of the peritoneum.

**habenulae perfora'ta,** *foramina* nervosa.

**pineal h.,** the peduncle or stalk of the pineal gland; see habenula (2).

**Scarpa's h.,** Haller's h.

**h. urethra'lis,** one of two fine, whitish lines running from the meatus urethrae to the clitoris in girls and young women; they are the vestiges of the anterior part of the corpus spongiosum.

**haben'ular.** Relating to a habenula, especially the stalk of the pineal body.

**Habermann,** R. See Mucha-H. *disease.*

**hab'it** [ L. *habeo*, pp. *habitus*, to have. HAB- ]. 1. An act, behavioral response, practice, or custom established by frequent repetition of the same act; see also addiction. 2. A basic variable in the study of conditioning and learning used to designate a new response learned either by association or by being followed by a reward or reinforced event.

**h. of body,** habitus.

**drug h.,** drug *addiction.*

**enteroptotic h.,** *habitus* enteroptoticus.

**opium h.,** opium *addiction.*

**habit'uation.** 1. The process of forming a habit, referring generally to psychological dependence on the continued use of a drug to maintain a sense of well-being, which can result in drug addiction. 2. The method by which the nervous system reduces or inhibits responsiveness during repeated stimulation.

**hab'itus** [ L. habit ]. The physical characteristics of a person. Correlations have been attempted between various types of h. and altered susceptibilities to the development of certain disorders.

**h. apoplec'ticus,** thickset and corpulent appearance with short bull neck, red face, and tortuous temporal arteries, supposed to indicate a disposition towards apoplexy.

**Chvostek's h.,** a combination of hypotrichosis of the trunk, axilla, and pubis, dense hair on the brows and a full beard, enlargement of the pineal gland, small thyroid, atrophy of the testes; said to favor the development of cirrhosis of the liver, Dupuytren's contracture, and other diseases of "fibrous tissue."

**h. enteroptot'icus,** linear build, with long narrow thorax and abdomen, and costal angle below 90°. The viscera tend to sag from their mesenteric moorings under the influence of gravity. At one time this was interpreted to signify disease.

**fetal h.,** fetal attitude; relationship of one fetal part to another.

**gracile h.,** a frail, underweight appearance, characteristic of the child with an atrial septal defect.

**habromania** (hab'ro-ma'ni-ah) [ G. *habros*, graceful, + *mania,* insanity ]. Morbid impulse toward gaiety.

**Habrone'ma** [ G. *habros,* graceful; delicate, + *nēma,* a thread ]. A genus of spiruroid nematodes inhabiting the stomach of horses. The larvae develop in housefly and stable fly maggots living in manure, become infective when the fly larvae pupates, and are carried by adult flies to open wounds on horses, where they leave the flies and cause summer sores, bursatti, or cutaneous habronemiasis. Reinfection of the horse's stomach by H. occurs by accidental ingestion of infected flies or from licking wounds in which infective larvae are found.

**H. ma'jus, H. micros'toma,** two species similar in appearance, hosts, distribution, and life cycle to *H. muscae;* the intermediate host is the stable fly, *Stomoxys calcitrans.*

**H. megas'toma,** causes tumors in the gastric mucosa that contain large numbers of the small nematodes; the larvae cause cutaneous habronemiasis; the intermediate host is the common housefly, *Musca domestica.*

**H. mus'cae,** occurs in the stomach of the horse, mule, ass, or zebra; the intermediate host is the common housefly, *Musca domestica,* or related flies.

**habronemiasis** (hab'ro-ne-mi'ă-sis). Infection of horses with any species of *Habronema;* commonly denotes wound infections that contain the larvae of this worm.

**cutaneous h.,** summer sores; draschiosis; chronic granulomatous sores on the skin of horses caused by fly-borne release and penetration of the larvae of *Draschia megastoma* (primarily), *Habronema muscae,* and *H. majus* into skin wounds, followed by feeding or migrating of the larvae therein; it persists for long periods as pulpy lesions, but the sores usually regress spontaneously in the winter.

**hack'ing.** A chopping stroke made with the edge of the hand in massage.

**Hadfield,** G. See Clarke-Hadfield *syndrome.*

**Hadrurus** (hă-dru'rus) A genus of scorpions found in southwestern United States, characterized by numerous setae on the stinger; the commonest species is *H. arizonensis,* the olive hairy scorpion. See also Scorpionida.

**Haeckel,** Ernest H., German naturalist, 1834–1919. See H.'s gastrea *theory,* H.'s *law.*

**haem-** [ G. *haima,* blood ]. For words so beginning, and not found here, see under hem-.

**haem.** Heme.

**Haemadip'sa ceylon'ica** [ G. *haima,* blood, + *dipsa,* thirst ]. A species of land leech found in Ceylon; it attaches itself to the skin of animals or man. Its bite is painful, and numerous bites may cause anemia.

**Haemamoeba** (hem-ă-me'bah). An old term for ameboid protozoa now classified in the order Haemosporidia, blood parasites that include the genus *Plasmodium.*

**Haemaphysalis** (hem'ă-fi'să-lis, he'mă-) [ G. *haima,* blood, + *physaleos,* full of wind ]. A genus of small, eyeless, inornate ticks that have festoons and a characteristic basis capituli; the sexes are similar. As larvae and nymphs, they are found chiefly on small mammals and birds; as adults, they are found on larger mammals and some birds. They are important as vectors of disease and especially of viruses that may be carried long distances on migrating birds.

**H. chordei'lis,** bird tick; a common tick of turkeys and upland game birds in North America and a possible vector of wildlife diseases.

**H. cinnabar'ina** [ G. *kinnabarinos,* like cinnabar, vermilion ], a tick that occurs chiefly in the dry district of British Columbia; strains of this species can cause ascending paraplegia or tick paralysis in both man and animals.

**H. cinnabar'ina puncta'ta,** a race of *H.* in Europe, North Africa, and Japan; larvae and nymphs feed on terrestrial reptiles, and adults on various domestic herbivores, rabbits, and hedgehogs; it transmits bovine babesiosis and anaplasmosis.

**H. leach'i,** a species of Africa, Asia, and Australia; it occurs on domestic and wild carnivores, on small rodents, and occasionally on cattle; it transmits canine babesiosis.

**H. leporispalus'tris** [ L. fem. of *paluster,* marshy ], rabbit tick; occurs in all species of rabbits, and on many wild birds, in all parts of North America from Alaska to Mexico, and is important in the spread of Rocky Mountain spotted fever and tularemia among rabbits; it does not attack man or most domestic animals, and does not spread these diseases to them, but serves to maintain the infection in reservoir hosts.

**haemastrontium** (hem-ă-stron'shĭ-um). A stain used in histology, made by adding strontium chloride to a solution of hematein and aluminum chloride in citric acid and alcohol.

**Haematopinus** (hem'ă-to-pi'nus, he'mă-to-). An important genus of sucking lice (family Haematopinidae) affecting swine and other domestic and wild animals; it is normally nonpathogenic. It is similar to *Eperythrozoon,* except that *H.* is not found free in the plasma and no ring forms are seen.

**H. asi'ni,** the sucking louse of horses, mules, and asses.

**H. euryster'nus,** the cosmopolitan short-nose sucking louse of cattle.

**H. quadripertusus,** the cattle tail louse or tail switch louse.

**H. su'is,** the very large "blue louse" of swine; the common pig louse.

**Haemobartonella** (he'mo-bar-to-nel'ah). A genus of microorganisms (order Rickettsiales) which are parasites found in and on the surface of erythrocytes. They rarely produce disease in animals without splenectomy, and are markedly influenced by arsenical compounds. They are identical to *Eperythrozoon* species, except that *H.* species are not found free in the plasma nor are ring forms seen on the surface of infected erythrocytes. Species are found in laboratory rats, and in dogs, cats, cattle, goats, pigs, and other domestic and wild animals. The type species is *H. muris.*

**H. blari'nae,** a species found in the blood of the short-tailed shrew (*Blarina brevicauda*).

**H. bo'vis,** a species found in cattle, in which it appears to cause little damage.

**H. ca'nis,** a species found in dog fleas (*Ctenocephalides* sp.) and in the erythrocytes of infected animals; it is widespread, occurring in Europe, India, North and South Africa, and North and South America.

**H. fe'lis,** produces an acute febrile illness or chronic anemia in cats; it is believed to be relatively common.

**H. micro'ti,** a species occurring in the blood of the mole (*Microtus pennsylvanicus pennsylvanicus*).

**H. mu'ris,** a species found in ectoparasites such as the rat louse (*Polyplax spinulosus*), the flea (*Xenopsylla cheopsis*), and possibly the bedbug (*Cimex lectularis*); it is the type species of *H.*

**H. peromys'ci,** a species found in the blood of deer mice (*Peromyscus leucopus novaboracensis*).

**H. sciu'ri,** a species found in the blood of gray squirrels (*Sciurus carolinensis leucotis*); it is slightly pathogenic for the gray squirrel and nonpathogenic for normal white mice.

**H. sturman'ii,** a species found in the blood of buffaloes in Palestine.

**H. tryzze' ri,** a species occurring in the blood of the Peruvian guinea pig (*Cavia porcellus*); it has also been found in the blood of native guinea pigs in Colombia.

**Haemococcidium** (he'mo-kok-sid'ĭ-um). An old name for *Plasmodium* species.

**Haemodip'sus ventrico'sus** [ G. *haima,* blood, + *dipsos,* thirst; L. *venter* (*ventr-*), belly ]. The rabbit louse, a transmitter of *Pasteurella tularensis.*

**Haemogregarina** (he'mo-greg-ă-ri'nah) [ G. *haima,* blood, + L. *grex,* a flock ]. A sporozoan protozoan genus (family Haemogregarinidae) that usually parasitizes the blood cells of cold-blooded animals and the digestive system of invertebrate primary hosts.

**Haemonchus** (he-mong'kus) [ G. *haima,* blood, + *onchos,* spear ]. An economically important genus of nematode parasites (family Trichostrongylidae) occurring in the abomasum of ruminant animals and causing severe anemia, especially in younger or previously unexposed animals.

**H. contor'tus,** the large stomach worn, barberpole worm, or twisted stomach worm of cattle, sheep, goats, and other ruminants; white filamentous ovaries that spiral around the straight, blood-filled gut are characteristic in the female nematode; this species causes a serious and common form of anemia, particularly in sheep; a few cases have been reported from man.

**H. pla'cei,** occurs in the abomasum of cattle, sheep, and goats.

**H. simil'is,** found in the abomasum of cattle and sheep.

**Haemophilus** (he-mof'ĭ-lus) [ G. *haima,* blood, + *philos,* fond ]. *Hemophilus;* a genus of aerobic to facultatively anaerobic, nonmotile bacteria (family Brucellaceae) containing minute, Gram-negative rod-shaped cells which sometimes form threads and are pleomorphic. These organisms are strictly parasitic, growing best, or only, on media containing blood. They may or may not be pathogenic and occur in various lesions and secretions, as well as in normal respiratory tracts, of vertebrates. The type species is *H. influenzae.*

**H. aegyptius,** a species that causes acute or subacute infectious conjunctivitis in areas with warm climates.

**H. aprophilus,** a species found in the blood and on the heart valve in a case of endocarditis.

**H. citreus,** a species found in genital secretions from acute and chronic cases of vesicular exanthema (exanthema coitale) in cattle.

**H. ducrey'i,** Ducrey's bacillus; a species which causes soft chancre (chancroid).

**H. gallina'rum,** a species that causes fowl coryza.

**H. haemoglobinophilus,** a species which occurs in large numbers in preputial secretions of dogs.

**H. haemolyt'icus,** a species which is usually nonpathogenic but which, on rare occasions, causes subacute endocarditis.

**H. influen'zae,** the influenza bacillus; Pfeiffer's bacillus; Koch-Weeks bacillus; a species found in the respiratory tract. Causes acute respiratory infections, acute conjunctivitis, and purulent meningitis in children, rarely in adults. Originally considered to be the cause of influenze. It is the type species of the genus *H.*

**H. influenzae-murium,** a species that causes conjunctivitis and respiratory infections in mice.

**H. ovis,** a species that causes bronchial pneumonia and generalized hemorrhagic involvement in sheep.

**H. parahaemoly'ticus,** a species found in the upper respiratory tract, and associated frequently with pharyngitis; occasionally causes subacute endocarditis.

**H. parainfluen'zae,** a species which is usually nonpathogenic but which occasionally causes subacute endocarditis.

**H. piscium,** a species that causes ulcer disease in trout.

**H. putoriorum,** a species found in the respiratory tracts of ferrets.

**H. su'is,** a species which, with a filtrable virus, causes Glasser's disease.

**Haemoproteus** (he'mo-pro'te-us, -hem'o-) [ G. *haima,* blood, + *Proteus,* a sea god who had the power of assuming different shapes ]. A genus of Haemosporidia parasitic in birds and reptiles; combined with *Leucocytozoon* and *Hepatocystis* in the family Haemoproteidae. Schizogony occurs in endothelial cells of blood vessels, especially in the lungs, while halter-shaped gametocytes are found in the red blood cells. Infection is transmitted by pupiparous Diptera, such as louse flies (Hippoboscidae) and midges (*Culicoides*).

**Haemosporidia** (he'mo-spo-rid'ĭ-um, hem'o-) [ G. *haima*, blood, + *sporos*, seed. SPER- ]. Name for an order of sporozoa in the class Telosporidia, now equivalent to the order Eucoccida (or Eucoccidiorida) in the class Telosporea (or Sporozoasida), in which are included many of the most important pathogens of man, domestic animals, and birds; these pathogens are chiefly the malarial parasites of the genus *Plasmodium* and related members of the family Plasmodiidae.

**Haemostrongylus vaso'rum** (he'mo-stron'jĭ-lus). *Angiostrongylus vasorum.*

**Haenel** (ha'nel), Heinrich G., German neurologist, *1874. See H.'s *symptom.*

**Haffkine,** Waldemar M. W., Russian physician, 1860–1930. See H.'s *vaccine.*

**hafnium** (haf'nĭ-um) [ L. *Hafniae,* Copenhagen ]. A rare chemical element, symbol Hf, atomic no. 72, atomic weight 178.50.

**Hagedorn** (hah'geh-dorn), Werner, German surgeon, 1831–1894. See H. *needle.*

**Hageman factor.** See under factor.

**hagiotherapy** (ha'jĭ-o-thĕr'ă-pĭ) [ G. *hagios,* sacred ]. Treatment of the sick by means of contact with relics of the saints, visits to shrines, and other religious observances.

**Hahn's oxine reagent.** See under reagent.

**Hahnemann** (hah'ne-mahn), Samuel C. F., German physician, 1755–1843. Founder of homeopathy.

**Hahnemannian** (hah-ně-mahn'ĭ-an). Relating to Hahnemann or to the doctrine he taught.

**Haidinger** (hi'ding-er), Wilhelm von, Austrian mineralogist, 1795–1871. See H.'s *brushes.*

**Hailey,** Howard. See Hailey and Hailey *disease.*

**Hailey,** Hugh. See Hailey and Hailey *disease.*

**Haines,** Walter S., American chemist and toxicologist, 1850–1923. See H.'s *formula, reagent.*

**hair** [ A.S. *haer* ]. 1. Pilus. 2. One of the fine, hairlike processes of the auditory cells of the labyrinth, and of other sensory cells, called auditory h.'s, sensory h.'s, etc.

  **auditory h.'s,** cilia on the free surface of the auditory cells.

  **bamboo h.,** trichorrhexis invaginata; h. with nodules along the shaft caused by intermittent fracturing and telescoping of the h., with intervening lengths of normal h., giving the appearance of bamboo; seen in Netherton's syndrome.

  **bayonet h.,** a spindle-shaped developmental defect occurring at the tapered end of the hair.

  **beaded h.,** monilethrix.

  **burrowing h.'s,** ingrown h.'s.

  **club h.,** a h. in resting state, prior to shedding, in which the bulb has become a club-shaped mass.

  **exclamation point h.,** the type of h. found at margins of patches of alopecia areata; the bulb is absent.

  **Frey's irritation h.'s,** short h.'s of varying degrees of stiffness, set at right angles into the end of a light wooden handle; used for determining the presence and degree of irritability of pressure points in the skin.

  **ingrown h.'s,** burrowing h.'s; pili cuniculati; pili incarnati; most commonly found in men on bearded portion of face and neck; the h.'s grow at more acute angles than is normal, and in all directions; they incompletely clear the follicle, turn back in, and cause formation of pustules and papules.

  **kinky h.,** tightly curled or bent hair.

  **lanugo h.,** lanugo.

  **monil'iform h.,** monilethrix.

  **nettling h.'s,** sharp-pointed barbed h.'s of certain caterpillars which cause a dermatitis when brought in contact with the skin.

  **ringed h.,** thrix annulata; pili annulati; leukotrichia annularis; trichonosus versicolor; a condition in which the h. shows alternate pigmented and white segments.

  **Schridde cancer h.'s,** thick, lusterless h.'s, growing here and there in the beard and the temporal region, said to occur in cancerous patients, but found also in persons with other cachectic conditions.

  **stellate h.,** h. split in several strands at free end.

  **tactile h.,** the vibrissae or whiskers of animals such as rats and cats which have especially well developed touch endings in the follicular wall.

  **taste h.'s,** hairlike projections of gustatory cells of taste buds. Electron micrographs show them to be condensations of secretion rather than true h.'s.

  **terminal h.,** adult h.

  **twisted h.'s,** pili torti; see under pilus.

  **vellus h.,** soft, downy h.

  **woolly h.,** tightly coiled h. with the texture of wool.

**hair'ball.** Trichobezoar.

**hair'less.** Glabrous.

**hairy.** 1. Hairlike. 2. Covered with hair. 3. Pertaining to hair.

**halation** (hă-la'shun). Blurring of the visual image by irradiation of light.

**hal'azone.** *p*-(*N,N*-Dichlorosulfamyl)benzoic acid; a chloramine used for the sterilization of drinking water.

**Halbeisen,** W. A. See Stryker-H. *syndrome.*

**Halberg,** G. P., U. S. ophthalmologist, *1915. See H. *tonometer.*

**Halberstaedter,** Ludwig, German physician, 1876–1949. See H.-Prowazek *bodies.*

**Haldane,** John S., Scottish physiologist at Oxford, 1860–1936. See H. *apparatus, chamber, effect, transformation, tube.*

**Hales,** Stephen, English physiologist, 1677–1761. See H.'s *piesimeter.*

**halethazole.** EPISOL; 5-chloro-2-[ *p*-(diethylaminoethoxy)phenyl ]benzothiazole; antiseptic with antifungal properties.

**half-life.** 1. The period during which the radioactivity of a radioactive substance, due to disintegration, is reduced to half of its original value; it ranges from quadrillions of years to quadrillionths of a second, depending on the particular nuclide being considered. 2. See half-time.

  **biological h.-l.,** the time taken for one-half of an administered radioactive substance to be lost through biological processes.

  **effective h.-l.,** the time required for one-half of an administered dose of radioactivity to be dissipated through a combination of physical decay and biological turnover.

  **physical h.-l.,** the time required for a given number of atoms, of a specific radionuclide, to undergo disintegration.

**half-moon.** The lunula.

  **red h.-m.,** irregular red discoloration of the usually pale demilunes at the base of the fingernails; may be seen in congestive failure, malignant disease, or liver disease, but not specific for any.

**half-time.** The time, in a first-order chemical (or enzymic) reaction, for half of the substance (substrate) to be converted or to disappear; see also half-*life.*

**half'way house.** A facility for patients who no longer require the complete facilities of a hospital but are not yet prepared to return to their communities, *e.g.,* psychiatric patients, narcotic addicts, alcoholics.

**hal'ibut liver oil** (BP). The fixed oil obtained from the fresh or suitably preserved livers of halibut species of the genus *Hippoglossus* (family Pleuronectidae); a supplementary source of vitamins A and D.

**halide** (hal'id). A salt or compound of a halogen.

**haliphagia** (hal'ĭ-fa'jĭ-ah) [ G. *hals,* salt, + *phagein,* to eat ]. The ingestion of an excessive quantity of a salt or salts, especially of sodium chloride, calcium, magnesium, or potassium salts, or of sodium bicarbonate.

**halisteresis** (hă-lis'ter-e'sis) [ G. *hals,* salt, + *steresis,* privation, fr. *stereō,* to deprive ]. Halosteresis; a deficiency of lime salts in the bones; see also osteomalacia.

**halis'teret'ic.** Relating to or marked by halisteresis.

**halito'sis** [ L. *halitus,* breath, + G. suffix -*osis,* condition ]. Fetor ex ore; offensive breath.

**hal'itus** [ L. fr. *halo,* to breathe ]. Any exhalation, as of a breath or vapor.

**Hall,** Marshall, English physician and physiologist, 1790–1857. See H.'s *disease, facies.*

**hallachrome** (hal'ă-krōm). A quinone intermediate, derived from dopa, in the formation of melanin from tyrosine.

**Hallé,** Adrien J. M. N., Paris physician, 1859–1947. See H.'s *point.*

**Haller,** Albrecht v., Swiss physiologist, 1708–1777. See H.'s *ansa, anulus, arches, circle, cones, habenula, insula, line, plexus, rete,* vascular *tissue, tripod, tunica, unguis, vas aberrans.*

**Hallermann,** Wilhelm, German ophthalmologist. See H.-Streiff *syndrome.*

**Hallervorden,** Julius, German neurologist, 1882–1965. See H. *syndrome.*

**hallex,** pl. **hal'lices** (hal'eks) [ L. ]. Hallux.

**Hallion** (al-yawn'), L. French physiologist, 1862–1940. See H.'s *test.*

**Hallopeau** (al-o-po'), Franc-ois H., Paris dermatologist, 1842–1919. See H.'s *acrodermatitis, disease.*

**hal'lucal.** Relating to the hallux.

**hallucination** (hă-lu'sĭ-na'shun) [ L. *alucinari,* to wander in mind ]. A strongly experienced false perception which has a compulsive sense of the reality of the object or event, although relevant and adequate stimuli for such a perception by others is lacking.

**gustatory h.,** h. of taste.

**hypnagogic h.,** h. occurring in the period between wakefulness and sleep.

**Lilliputian h.,** h. of diminutive objects or persons.

**olfactory h.,** h. of smell.

**stump h.,** the sensation as of the continual presence of a limb or a portion of a limb after its amputation; see also phantom *limb.*

**hallucinogen** (hă-lu'sĭ-no-jen) [ G. suffix *-gen,* producing ]. A hallucinatory chemical, drug, or agent, specifically a chemical whose most prominent pharmacologic action is on the central nervous system (*e.g.,* mescaline). It elicits, in normal subjects, optical or auditory hallucinations, depersonalization, perceptual disturbances, and disturbances of thought processes.

**hallucinogenic** (hă-lu'sĭ-no-jen'ik). Relating to a hallucinogen.

**hallucinosis** (hă-lu'sĭ-no'sis). A psychosis marked especially by more or less persistent hallucinations.

**hal'lus.** Hallux.

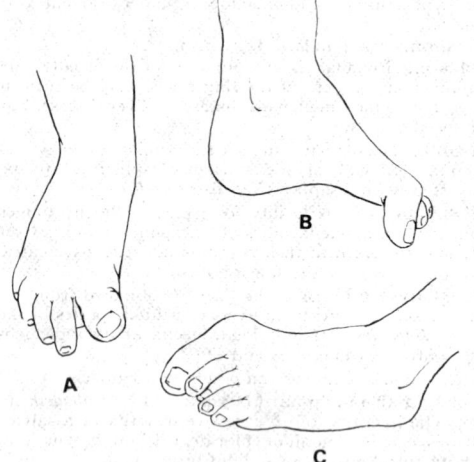

**Malformations of the Hallux**
*A,* hallux varus; *B,* hallux flexus; *C,* hallux valgus

**hallux,** pl. **hal'luces** (hal'uks) [ a Mod. L. form for L. *hallex* (*hallic-*), great toe ] [ NA ]. The great toe; the first digit of the foot.

**h. doloro'sus,** painful toe; a condition, usually associated with flatfoot, in which walking causes severe pain in the metatarsophalangeal joint of the great toe.

**h. exten'sus,** a deformity in which the great toe is held rigidly in the extended position.

**h. flexus,** hammer toe involving the first toe.

**h. malleus,** hammer toe involving the first toe.

**h. rig'idus,** stiff toe; a condition in which there is stiffness in the first metatarsophalangeal joint; the joint may be the site of a hypertrophic arthritis.

**h. valgus,** a deviation of the tip of the first toe, or main axis of the toe, toward the outer or lateral side of the foot.

**h. varus,** deviation of the main axis of the great toe to the inner side of the foot away from its neighbor.

**halmatogenesis** (hal'mă-to-jen'ĕ-sis) [ G. *halma,* a spring, leap, + *genesis,* production, generation ]. Saltatory variation; a sudden change of type from one generation to the other.

**ha'lo** [ G. *halōs,* threshing floor on which oxen trod a circle; the halo round the sun or moon ]. 1. A reddish yellow ring surrounding the optic disk, due to a widening out of the scleral ring permitting the deeper structures to show through. 2. An annular flare of light surrounding a luminous body. 3. An areola.

**anemic h.,** pale, relatively avascular areas in the skin seen around vascular spiders, cherry angiomas, and sometimes in acute macular eruptions.

**glauco'matous h.,** glaucomatous ring; rainbow symptom; a yellowish white ring, indicating atrophy of the choroid, surrounding the optic disk in glaucoma.

**haloan'isone.** Fluanisone.

**hal'oderma** [ halogen + G. *derma,* skin ]. Dermatosis caused in ingestion of injection of halogens, most notably bromides and iodides.

**halogen** (hal'o-jen) [ G. *hals,* salt, + suffix *-gen,* producing ]. One of the chlorine group (fluorine, chlorine, bromine, iodine) of elements; they form monobasic acids with hydrogen, and their hydroxides (fluorine forms none) are also monobasic acids. The radioactive element, astatine, also belongs to the h. group.

**halogenation** (hal'o-jĕ-na'shun). Incorporation of one or more halogen atoms in a molecule to alter physical properties and pharmacological action.

**Haloge'ton.** A genus of plants (family Chenopodiaceae) on range lands in western United States and other arid regions of the world. It causes poisoning in cattle and sheep because of the presence of soluble oxalates in the plant.

**hal'oid.** Resembling a halogen.

**halom'eter.** 1. An instrument used to measure the diffraction halo of a red blood cell. (It is claimed that the halo of the large erythrocyte of pernicious anemia is smaller than that of the normal cell; the hazy colorless halo of normal size is characteristic of secondary anemia.) 2. An instrument for measuring the ocular halos.

**haloper'idol** (USP, BP). HALDOL; SERENASE; a butyrophenone chemically related to meperidine; an antipsychotic agent that produces extrapyramidal effects in many patients; also used in Huntington's chorea and Gilles de la Tourette's disease.

**halophil, halophile** (hal'o-fil, -fīl) [ G. *hals,* salt, + *philos,* fond ]. A microorganism whose growth is enhanced by or dependent on a high salt concentration.

**halophil'ic.** Requiring a high concentration of salt for growth.

**ha'loproges'terone** (USAN). PROHALONE; 17α-bromo-6α-gluoroprogesterone; progestational agent.

**haloprogin** (ha-lo-pro'jin) (USAN). POLIK; 3-iodo-2-propynyl 2,4,5-trichlorophenyl ether; antifungal agent.

**halopro'pane.** 3-Bromo-1,1,2,2-tetrafluoropropane; a potent inhalation anesthetic of limited usefulness because of arrhythmogenic potential.

**halostere'sis.** Halisteresis.

**hal'othane** (USP, BP). FLUOTHANE; 2-bromo-2-chloro-1,1,1-trifluoroethane; a potent inhalation anesthetic; nonflammable and nonexplosive; rapid onset and rapid reversal plus benign odor contribute to its wide popularity; side-effects include respiratory and cardiovascular depression, sensitization to epinephrine-induced arrhythmias, and rare development of hepatic damage.

**Halsted,** William S., Baltimore surgeon, 1852–1922. See H.'s *incision, law, operation, suture.*

**Halterid'ium** [ G. *haltēres,* weights held in the hand in leaping ]. A former name for *Haemoproteus.*

**halzoun** (hal'zun). The local name of a buccopharyngeal infection occurring in Lebanon, caused by adults of the liver fluke *Fasciola hepatica*, that wander into the throat after ingestion of infected cattle liver by the human host.

**Ham,** T. H. See H.'s *test*.

**ham** [ A.S. ]. 1. Poples. 2. The buttock and back part of the thigh.

**hamamelis,** gen. **hamamel'idis** (ham'ah-me'lis) [ Mod. L. fr. G. *hama-mēlis*, gen. *-mēlidos*, a tree with fruit like a pear, fr. *hama*, together with, + *mēlon*, apple ]. Witch hazel; spotted hazel; a shrub or small tree, *Hamamelis virginiana* (family Harmarmelidaceae), growing in damp, rocky soil in the eastern and central parts of North America.

 **h. bark,** witch hazel bark; used for the same purpose as the leaves.

 **h. leaf,** witch hazel leaf; the dried leaves collected in the autumn. Used externally as a application to contusions and other injuries, in headache and for the cure of noninflammatory hemorrhoids. The water, popularly known as "extract of witch hazel," is made from the bark.

**hamartia** (ham-ar'shi-ah) [ G. *hamartion*, a bodily defect ]. A localized developmental disturbance characterized by abnormal arrangement and/or combinations of the tissues normally present in the area.

**hamar'toblasto'ma** [ hamartoma + blastoma ]. A malignant neoplasm of undifferentiated anaplastic cells thought to be derived from a hamartoma.

**hamartochondromatosis** (ham-ar'to-kon'dro-mă-to'sis) [ G. *hamartion*, bodily defect, + *chondros*, cartilage, + suffix *-osis*, condition ]. Neoplasm-like foci of cartilaginous tissue in sites where cartilage is a normal constituent, but in which the growth of cartilage cells is out of proportion to the other elements of the organ.

**hamartoma** (ham'ar-to'mah) [ G. *hamartion*, a bodily defect, + suffix *-oma*, tumor ]. A focal malformation that resembles a neoplasm, grossly and even microscopically; h.'s result from faulty development in an organ, and they are composed of an abnormal mixture of tissue elements, or an abnormal proportion of a single element, normally present in that site. They develop and grow at virtually the same rate as normal components, and are not likely to result in compression of adjacent tissue (in contrast to neoplastic tissue).

**hamartophobia** (ham'ar-to-fo'bī-ah) [ G. *hamartia*, fault, + *phobos*, fear ]. Morbid fear of error or sin.

**hama'tum** [ L. neut. of *hamatus*, hooked, fr. *hamus*, a hook ]. *Os* hamatum.

**hama'tus** [ L. ] [ NA ]. Hooked; possessing a hook.

**hamax'opho'bia.** Amaxophobia.

**Hamburger,** Hartog J., Dutch physiologist, 1859-1924. See H.'s *law, phenomenon*.

**Hamilton,** David J., Scottish pathologist, 1849-1909. See H.'s *method*.

**Hamilton,** Frank H., American surgeon, 1813-1886. See H.'s *pseudophlegmon, test*.

**Hamilton-Swartz test.** See under test.

**Hamman,** Louis, American physician, 1877-1946. See H.'s *disease, sign, syndrome*, H.-Rich *syndrome*.

**Hammarsten,** Olof, Swedish physiological chemist, 1841-1932. See H.'s *reagent*.

**ham'mer.** Malleus.

**Hammerschlag** (hahm'er-shlahg), Albert, Austrian physician, 1863-1935. See H.'s *method*.

**Hampson unit.** See under unit.

**Hampton,** Aubrey Otis, American radiologist, 1900-1955. See H. *hump, line, maneuver, technique*.

**ham'ster.** The name given to any of four genera of small rodents widely used in research and as pets: *Cricetus cricetus*, the common or black-bellied hamster of Europe and eastern Russia, has a gestation period of 16 to 20 days and gives birth to 6 to 12 young. *Mesocricetus auratus*, the golden hamster, is native to Rumania, Bulgaria, and the Middle East; it was introduced to the United States in 1938. The dwarf hamster, *Phodopus sungorus*, of Siberia, Manchuria, and China is the smallest of the four. The long-tailed hamster of southeastern Europe and Asia Minor is ratlike in appearance and is rarely seen in the United States. All hamster are seed and plant feeders, store food, hibernate in winter, and breed throughout the year under laboratory conditions.

**ham'string.** 1. One of the tendons bounding the popliteal space on either side; the medial h. comprises the tendons of the semimembranosus, semitendinosus, gracilis, and sartorius muscles; the lateral h. is the tendon of the biceps femoris. 2. In domestic animals, the combined tendons of the superficial digital flexors, triceps aurae, biceps femoris, and semitendinosus which are referred to as the common calcanean tendon (tendo calcaneus communis); it is attached to the tuber calcis of the hock.

**ham'ular** [ L. *hamulus, q.v.* ]. Hook-shaped; unciform.

**ham'ulus,** gen. and pl. **ham'uli** [ L. dim. of *hamus*, hook ] [ NA ]. Any hooklike structure.

 **h. coch'leae,** h. laminae spiralis.

 **h. lacrima'lis** [ NA ], lacrimal h.; hamular process of the lacrimal bone; the hooklike lower end of the lacrimal crest, curving between the frontal process and orbital surface of the maxilla to form the upper aperture of the bony portion of the nasolacrimal canal.

 **h. lam'inae spira'lis** [ NA ], hook of the spiral lamina; the upper hooklike termination of the bony spiral lamina of the cochlea.

 **h. ossis hama'ti** [ NA ], the hook of the hamate bone; a hooklike process on the distal and medial part of the palmar surface of the hamate bone.

 **h. pterygoid'eus** [ NA ], pterygoid h.; hamular process of the sphenoid bone; the inferior, hook-shaped extremity of the medial plate of the pterygoid process.

**Hancock,** Henry, London surgeon, 1809-1880. See H.'s *amputation*.

**Hand,** Alfred, American pediatrician, 1868-1949. See H.-Schüller-Christian *disease*.

**hand** [ A.S. ]. 1. Manus. 2. A unit of measurement used in expressing height of horses. A h. equals 4 inches. The measurement is made from the highest point of the withers to the ground. A height of 15-3 means 15 h.'s plus 3 inches, or 63 inches.

 **accoucheur's h.,** obstetrical h.; position of the h. in tetany or in muscular dystrophy, said by the imaginative to resemble the position assumed by physician's h. in making a vaginal examination. The fingers are flexed at the metacarpophalangeal points and extended at the phalangeal joints, with the thumb flexed and adducted into the palm.

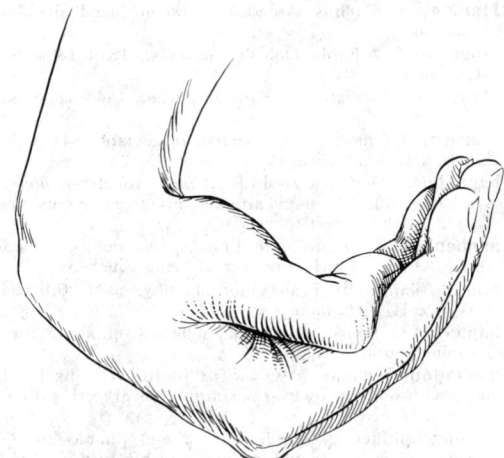

**Accoucheur's Hand**
Produced by spasm in tetany

 **ape h.,** a deformity marked by extension of the thumb at nearly a right angle with the axis of the h.

 **claw h.,** see clawhand.

 **cleft h.,** split h.; main fourché; a congenital deformity in which the division between the fingers, especially between the third and fourth, extends into the metacarpal region. See also lobster-claw *deformity*.

**club h.,** talipomanus.

**crab h.,** erysipeloid.

**drop h.,** wrist-drop.

**flat h.,** *manus* plana.

**ghoul h.,** a condition seen in African Negroes, probably a manifestation of tertiary yaws, marked by depigmentation of the palms and contraction of the skin which give a clawlike and corpselike appearance to the h.'s.

**griffin-claw h.,** Griffin-claw; main en griffe; atrophy of the interosseous muscles of the h. with extension of metacarpophalangeal joints and flexion of the phalangeal joints.

**lobster-claw h.,** lobster-claw *deformity.*

**Marinescu's succulent h.,** edema of the h. with coldness and lividity of the skin, observed in syringomyelia.

**obstetrical h.,** accoucheur's h.

**opera-glass h.,** main en lorgnette; a deformity of the h. seen in chronic absorptive arthritis, the fingers and wrists being shortened and the covering skin wrinkled into transverse folds; the phalanges appear to be retracted into one another like an opera glass or miniature telescope.

**skeleton h.,** extension of fingers with atrophy of muscles; occurs in progressive muscular atrophy.

**spade h.,** the coarse, thick, square h. of acromegaly or myxedema.

**split h.,** cleft h.

**trench h.,** frostbite of the h.

**trident h.,** a h. in which the fingers are of nearly equal length and deflected at the first interphalangeal joint, so as to give a forklike shape; seen in achondroplasia and other conditions.

**writing h.,** a contraction of the h. muscles in paralysis agitans, bringing the fingers somewhat in the position of holding a pen.

**hand'piece.** A hand instrument provided with a chuck for holding tools used for removing tooth structure, polishing, condensing, etc. Usually has rotary, may have vibratory motion. Rotary type is driven by a belt (rarely a flexible cable) from the source of power or, in case of air or water, is driven by turbines with a turbine in the h. itself.

**hang'nail.** Agnail; a loose tag of epidermis attached at the proximal portion in the medial or lateral nail fold.

**Hanhart,** Ernst. See H.'s *syndrome.*

**Hanks,** Horace Tracy, 1837–1900. See H. *dilators.*

**Hanks' solution.** See under solution.

**Hanlon,** C. Rollins, American surgeon. See Blalock-H. *operation.*

**Hannover,** Adolph, Danish anatomist, 1814–1894. See H.'s *canal.*

**Hanot** (ă-no'), Victor C., Paris physician, 1844–1896. See H.'s *cirrhosis.*

**Hansen,** Gerhard A., Norwegian physician, 1841–1912. See H.'s *bacillus, disease.*

**haphalgesia** (haf-al-je'zĭ-ah) [ G. *haphē,* touch, + *algēsis,* sense of pain ]. Pain or an extremely disagreeable sensation caused by the merest touch.

**haphephobia** (haf-e-fo'bĭ-ah) [ G. *haphē,* touch, + *phobos,* fear ]. A morbid dislike or fear of being touched.

**Hapke** (hahp'keh), Franz, German physician, 20th century. See H.'s *phenomenon.*

**haplo-** [ G. *haplous,* simple, single ]. Combining form meaning simple or single.

**hap'lodont** [ haplo- + G. *odous,* tooth ]. Having molar teeth with simple crowns, *i.e.,* simple conical teeth without ridges or tubercles.

**Haplographiaceae** (hap-lo-graf-ĭ-a'se-e) [ haplo- + G. *grapheion,* pencil, stylus ]. A family of blastosporic fungi with hyphae distinct from the conidia, the latter being in chains or, when parasitic in man, in grapelike masses.

**haploid** (hap'loyd) [ haplo- + -ploid, *q.v.* ]. Monoploid; denoting the number of chromosomes in sperm or ova, which is half the number in somatic (diploid) cells; the h. number in man is 23.

**haplology** (hap-lol'o-jĭ) [ haplo- + G. *logos,* study ]. The omission of syllables because of excessive speed of utterance.

**haplopia** (hap-lo'pĭ-ah) [ haplo- + G. *ōps,* eye ]. Single, normal vision, as distinguished from diplopia.

**haploscope** (hap'lo-skōp) [ haplo- + G. *skopeō,* to view ]. An instrument for presenting separate views to the two eyes so that they may be seen as one.

**mirror h.,** a h. using mirrors to displace the field of view of the two eyes, as in Worth's amblyoscope and the synoptophore.

**haploscopic** (hap-lo-skop'ik). Relating to a haploscope.

**Haplosporidia** (hap'lo-spo-rid'ĭ-ah) [ haplo- + G. *sporos,* seed ]. An order of Sporozoa which reproduces asexually by schizogeny; spores are produced; there are no flagellae, though pseudopodia may be present. Little is known about the life histories.

**hap'lotype** [ haplo- + G. *typos,* impression, model ]. The genetic constitution of an individual with respect to one member of a pair of allelic genes; individuals are of the same h. (but of different genotypes) if alike with respect to one allele of a pair but different with respect to the other allele of a pair.

**hap'ten** [ G. *haptō,* to fasten, bind ]. Partial antigen; an incomplete antigen being incapable alone of causing the production of antibodies but capable of combining with specific antibodies; a h. may cause the production of antibodies when it has been covalently linked to protein. See also hapten inhibition of *precipitation.*

**Rh h.,** h. extracted from Rh-positive erythrocytes.

**haptics** [ G. *haptō,* to grasp, touch. HAP- ]. The science of the tactile sense.

**hap'tin** [ G. *haptō,* to fasten, bind ]. According to the side chain theory, a castoff receptor.

**haptodysphoria** (hap'to-dis-fo'rĭ-ah) [ G. *haptō,* to touch, + dysphoria, *q.v.* ]. An unpleasant sensation derived from touching certain objects.

**hap'toglo'bin.** An $\alpha_2$-globulin in human serum, so called because of its ability to combine with hemoglobin, whereupon it becomes a weak peroxidase. Genetically controlled as to type (3), the h. level is diminished in hemolytic conditions and in acute hepatitis.

**haptometer** (hap-tom'e-ter) [ G. *haptō,* to touch, + *metron,* measure ]. Instrument for measuring sensitivity to touch.

**haptophil, haptophile** (hap'to-fil, -fil) [ G. *haptō,* to fasten, bind, + *phileō,* to love ]. Formerly denoting the atom group of a receptor that unites with the haptophore group of a toxin.

**haptophore** (hap'to-fōr) [ G. *haptō,* to bind, + *phoros,* bearing ]. The atom group of an antigen or antibody molecule by means of which the molecule can combine with a cell or with its corresponding antibody or antigen, respectively.

**haptophor'ic, haptoph'orous.** Relating to or denoting the action of a haptophore.

**Harada,** E., Japanese ophthalmologist. See H.'s *disease, syndrome.*

**Harden,** Sir Arthur, British biochemist, 1865–1940. See H.-Young *ester.*

**Harder,** Johann J., Swiss anatomist, 1656–1711. See H.'s *gland.*

**Harding,** Harold E., British pathologist. See H.-Passey *melanoma.*

**hard'ness.** The degree of firmness of a solid. The degree of h. of a substance is shown by its resistance to deformation, scratching or abrasion. See also hardness *scale,* and relevant subentries under *number.*

**indentation h.,** a number related to the size of the impression made by an indenter (or tool) of specific size and shape under a known load.

**hare'lip.** Cleft *lip.*

**ha'rem.** A group of mares kept together for breeding purposes.

**har'maline.** Harmidine; 4,9-dihydro-7-methoxy-1-methyl-3*H*-pyrido[ 3,4-*b* ]indole; 3,4-dihydroharmine; obtained from seeds of *Peganum harmala* (Zygophyllaceae) and from *Banisteria caapi* (Malpighiaceae). It is an amine oxidase inhibitor and a central nervous system stimulant; has been tried in parkinsonism.

**har'midine.** Harmaline.

**harmine** (har'mēn). Banisterine; yageine; telepathine; leucoharmine; 7-methoxy-1-methyl-9H-pyrido[ 3,4-*b* ]indole; obtained from *Peganum harmala* (family Zygophyllaceae) and *Banisteria caapi* (family Malpighaceae). It is a central nervous system stimulant and potent monoamine oxidase inhibitor. Psychic effects resemble those of LSD, but sedative and depressive qualities may predominate over hallucinatory manifestations.

**harmo′nia** [ L. and G. a joining ]. *Sutura* plana.

**harmon′ic.** Components of complex sound whose frequencies are multiples of the fundamental frequency of the sound. The fundamental frequency is called the first harmonic; the second harmonic has twice the frequency of the fundamental, and so forth.

**har′mony.** Agreement; accord; in dentistry, denotes occlusal h., *q.v.*

   **occlusal h.,** denotes occlusions without deflective or interceptive occlusal contacts in centric jaw relation as well as eccentric movements.

   **occlusal h., functional,** such occlusal relationship of opposing teeth in all functional ranges and movements as will provide the greatest masticatory efficiency without causing undue strain or trauma upon the supporting tissues.

**harpaxophobia** (har′paks-o-fo′bĭ-ah) [ G. *harpax,* robber, + *phobos,* fear ]. Morbid fear of robbers.

**harpoon′.** A small, sharp-pointed instrument with a barbed head used for extracting bits of muscular and other tissue for microscopic examination.

**Harrington,** David O., U. S. ophthalmologist, *1904. See H.-Flocks *test.*

**Harris,** Henry A., English anatomist, *1886. See H.'s *lines.*

**Harris,** Malcolm L., American surgeon, 1862–1936. See H. *segregator, separator.*

**Harris,** Wilfred, English physician, 1869–1960. See H.'s *migraine.*

**Harris′ hematoxylin.** See under hematoxylin.

**Harris-Ray test.** See under test.

**Harrison′s groove.** See under groove.

**Hartel,** F., German surgeon, 20th century. See H.'s *technique.*

**Hartline,** Haldan K., U. S. biophysicist, *1903. Nobel laureate, 1967, with Ragnar Granit and George Wald, for their studies in visual physiology.

**Hartman,** LeRoy L., American dentist, 1893–1951. See H.'s *solution.*

**Hartmann,** Arthur, Berlin laryngologist, 1849–1931. See H.'s *curette.*

**Hartmann,** Robert, German anatomist, 1831–1893. See H.'s *pouch.*

**Hartnup disease** or **syndrome.** See under disease.

**harts′horn.** Ammonia water; any volatile ammonium salt, such as the carbonate.

**harvest bug.** The larva of *Trombicula* species.

**Harvey,** William, English physician, 1578–1657. The discoverer of the circulation of the blood. The book announcing this discovery was entitled *Exercitatio anatomica de motu cordis et sanguinis in animalibus,* published in Frankfort in 1628. He studied anatomy and medicine at Padua, being a student under Fabricius. He also undertook researches in embryology, publishing an important work on the subject, *De Generatione Animalium.*

**hasamiyami.** Autumn fever (2); akiyami; sakushu fever; a fever occurring in Japan in the autumn; it resembles Weil's disease but is milder and is caused by *Leptospira autumnalis.*

**Häser,** Heinrich, German physician, 1811–1885. See H.'s *formula,* Trapp-H. *formula.*

**hash′eesh.** Hashish.

**Hashimoto,** H., Japanese surgeon, 1881–1934. See H.'s *disease, struma, thyroiditis.*

**hash′ish, hash′eesh** [ Arabic, hay ]. A form of cannabis that consists largely of resin from the flowering tops and sprouts of cultivated female plants; contains the highest concentration of cannabinols among the preparations derived from cannabis.

**Hasner,** Joseph R., Prague oculist, 1819–1892. See H.'s *fold, valve.*

**Hassall,** Arthur H., English physician, 1817–1894. See H.'s *bodies,* H.-Henle *bodies;* H.'s concentric *corpuscles,* Virchow-H. *bodies.*

**Hasselbalch,** Karl, Danish biochemist and physician, *1874. See H. *equation,* Henderson-H. *equation.*

**Hastings,** Thomas W., U. S. physician, 1873–1942. See H.'s *stain.*

**Hata** (hah′tah), Sahachiro, Japanese physician and chemist, 1873–1938. See H.'s *phenomenon.*

**hatch′et.** A tool used in dentistry, that has an end cutting blade at an angle to the axis of the handle. May have one or two bevels, in the former case made in pairs, right and left, and referred to as enamel h.'s. Used for removing enamel and dentin, usually on posterior teeth where access with a chisel is difficult.

**Hau′benfel′der** [ Ger. ]. H fields; see *fields* of Forel.

**Hauch** (howkh) [ Ger. breath ]. Symbol H; a term used to designate the flagellar antigen of bacteria. See also H *antigen.*

**Haudek** (how′dek), Martin, Vienna roentgenologist, 1880–1931. See H.'s *niche.*

**Hauser's stain for spores.** See under stain.

**haustorium,** pl. **hausto′ria** (haw-sto′rĭ-um) [ Mod. L. fr. L. *haustus,* a drinking ]. An organ for the absorption of nutriment.

**haustra** (haw′strah) [ L. ]. Plural of haustrum.

**haustral** (haw′stral). Relating to a haustrum.

**haustration** (haw-stra′shun). An increase in prominence of the haustra.

**haustrum,** pl. **haus′tra** (haw′strum) [ L. a machine for drawing water, fr. *haurio,* pp. *haustus,* to draw up, drink up ] [ NA ]. Cellula coli; h. coli [ NA ]; one of the sacculations of the colon, caused by the fact that the teniae, or longitudinal bands, are slightly shorter than the gut so that the latter is thrown into tucks or pouches.

**haustus** (haw′stus) [ L. a drink, draft ]. A potion or medicinal draft.

**Haverhil′lia multifor′mis.** An organism regarded as identical with *Streptobacillus moniliformis.*

**Havers,** Clopton, English anatomist, 1650–1702. See H.'s (Haversian) *canals, glands, lamellae, spaces, system.*

**Haversian** (ha-ver′shan). Relating to Clopton Havers and the various osseous structures described by him.

**haw.** The third eyelid, or nictitating membrane, of the horse.

**Hawley,** C. A. See H. *appliance.*

**Haworth,** Walter Norman, British chemist, 1883–1950. See H. perspective formulas and conformational formulas of cyclic sugars, under *sugars.*

**Hayem** (a-yahn′), Georges, Paris physician, 1841–1933. See H.-Widal *anemia,* H.-Widal *syndrome,* H's *disease, hematoblast, solution.*

**Haygarth,** John, English physician, 1740–1827. See H.'s *nodes, nodosities.*

**Haynes,** Irving S., U. S. surgeon, 1861–1946. See H.'s *operation.*

**ha′zelwort.** *Asarum europaeum.*

**Hb.** Abbreviation for hemoglobin.

**HB₄Ag.** Abbreviation for hepatitis B core *antigen.*

**HB₄Ag.** Abbreviation for hepatitis B surface *antigen.*

**HbCO.** Abbreviation for carboxyhemoglobin.

**HbO₂.** Abbreviation for oxyhemoglobin.

**Hb S.** Abbreviation for sickle cell *hemoglobin.*

**HCG.** Abbreviation for human chorionic *gonadotropin.*

**Hct.** Abbreviation for hematocrit (2).

**He.** Chemical symbol of the element helium.

**Head,** Sir Henry, English neurologist, 1861–1940. See H.'s *areas, lines, zones.*

**head** (hed) [ A.S. *heáfod* ]. 1. Caput; the upper or anterior extremity of the animal body, containing the brain and the organs of sight, hearing, taste, and smell. 2. The upper, anterior, or larger extremity of any body or structure. 3. The rounded extremity of a bone. 4. That end of a muscle which is attached to the less movable part of the skeleton.

   **absorber h.,** see under absorber.

   **big-h.,** see big-head.

**bulldog h.,** the broad h. with high vault occurring in achondroplasia.

**dynamite h.,** see dynamite *headache*.

**h. of epididymis,** *caput* epididymidis.

**h. of femur,** *caput* femoris.

**h. of fibula,** *caput* fibulae.

**hourglass h.,** the skull with depressed coronal suture in hereditary syphilis.

**h. of humerus,** *caput* humeri.

**h. of malleus,** *caput* mallei.

**h. of mandible,** *caput* mandibulae.

**Medusa h.,** *caput* medusae.

**h. of metacarpal bone,** *caput* ossis metacarpalis.

**h. of phalanx,** *caput* phalangis.

**powder h.,** dynamite *headache*.

**h. of radius,** *caput* radii.

**saddle h.,** clinocephaly.

**sore-h.,** see sorehead.

**h. of stapes,** *caput* stapedis.

**swell-h.,** see swellhead.

**swelled h.,** Paget's disease of the skull.

**h. of talus,** *caput* tali.

**h. of ulna,** *caput* ulnae.

**white h.,** witkop.

**head′ache.** Cephalalgia; cephalea; cephalodynia; cerebralgia; diffuse pain in various parts of the head, not confined to the area of distribution of any nerve.

**bilious h.,** migraine.

**blind h.,** migraine.

**cluster h.,** probably a migraine variant, precipitated by the injection of histamine; characterized by recurrent, severe, unilateral orbitotemporal h.'s associated with conjunctival injection; also called histaminic h. or cephalalgia; Horton's h. or cephalgia.

**dynamite h.,** powder head; an intense throbbing h. affecting workmen and others handling high explosives.

**fibrosit′ic h.,** h. centered in the occipital region due to fibrositis of the occipital muscles; tender areas are present and commonly tender nodules are found in the scalp in the lower occipital region.

**histaminic h.,** cluster h.

**Horton′s h.,** cluster h.

**migraine h.,** see migraine.

**nodular h.,** radiating pain in the head accompanied by nodular swellings in the splenius, frontalis, trapezius, and other muscles.

**organic h.,** h. due to disease of the brain or its coverings.

**reflex h.,** symptomatic h.

**sick h.,** migraine.

**spinal h.,** h. following spinal anesthesia in 3 to 20 per cent of patients; it is usually frontal or occipital, precipitated by sitting or upright posture, relieved by lying down; postulated to be due to leakage of cerebrospinal fluid from subarachnoid space through the site of the puncture.

**symptomatic h.,** h. due to disease or abnormality in some organ more or less distant from the brain; one due to eyestrain, for example.

**tension h.,** h. associated with nervous tension, anxiety, etc., often related to chronic contraction of the scalp muscles.

**vacuum h.,** h. due to closure of the frontal sinus.

**vascular h.,** migraine.

**head′gut.** Foregut.

**head-tilt.** A tilt of the head commonly associated with paralysis of vertical ocular muscles.

**heal** (hēl) [ A.S. *healan* ]. 1. To restore to health, especially to cause an ulcer or wound to cicatrize or unite. 2. To become well, to be cured; to cicatrize or close, said of an ulcer or wound.

**heal′er.** 1. A physician; one who heals or cures. 2. One who claims to cure by Christian Science, mental healing, new thought, or other form of suggestion.

**heal′ing.** 1. Curing; restoring to health; promoting the closure of wounds and ulcers. 2. The process of a return to health. 3. The closing of a wound; see also union.

**h. by first intention,** etc., see under intention.

**health** (helth) [ A.S. *haelth* ]. The state of the organism when it functions optimally without evidence of disease or abnormality.

**bill of h.,** a certificate issued by a public h. official indicating that passengers of a public conveyance are free from infectious disease and may be admitted without detention.

**Board of H.,** a committee, appointed by the public authority, whose duty it is to formulate rules for the guidance of the public h. officials.

**Department of H.,** the division of a municipal or state government which executes measures for the protection of the h. of the community.

**mental h.,** emotional, behavioral, and social maturity; normality; the absence of mental or behavioral disorder; a state of psychological well-being in which a person has achieved a satisfactory integration of his instinctual drives acceptable to both himself and his social milieu.

**Public H. Service,** a bureau of the U. S. Department of Health, Education, and Welfare, served by a corps of medical officers presided over by a surgeon general; the h. work of the Service consists in scientific research, domestic and insular quarantine, care of the marine hospitals, publication of sanitary reports and statistics; associated with it is the Hygienic Laboratory, among the duties of which is the inspection of all vaccines and therapeutic or diagnostic serums offered for sale.

**health′y.** Well; in a state of normal functioning; free from disease.

**Heaney,** Noble Sproat, U. S. gynecological surgeon and obstetrician, 1880–1955. See H.'s *operation*.

**hear** (hēr) [ A.S. *hēran* ]. To perceive sounds; denoting the function of the ear.

**hearing** (hēr′ing). The ability to perceive sound; the sensation of sound as opposed to vibration.

**after-h.,** aftersound.

**color h.,** pseudochromesthesia; a subjective color sensation produced by certain sounds.

**conductive h. impairment,** that attributable to interference with the apparatus conducting sound to the inner ear.

**h. impairment,** reduction in the ability to perceive sound. If on the basis of interference with the conduction of sound to the end organ, it is conductive h. impairment; if on the basis of malfunction of the end organ or neural elements involved in the conduction of or interpretation of nerve impulses originating in the cochlea, it is sensorineural h. impairment.

**h. level,** a term used in otology to describe a deviation in decibels from a standard value for zero on audiometers. The measure of the status of h. as read directly on the h. loss scale of an audiometer.

**h. loss,** a term used in otology to describe the symptom of reduced auditory sensitivity. The measurement of the degree of h. loss in terms of a deviation in decibels from an individual's previous audiogram is referred to as a threshold shift, *q. v.*

**low tone h. loss,** low tone *deafness*.

**noise-induced h. loss,** acoustic trauma *deafness*.

**normal h.,** acusis.

**sensorineural h. loss,** a type of h. loss resulting from dysfunction of the end organ or nerve fiber, or both.

**heart** (hart) [ A.S. *heorte* ]. Cor; a hollow muscular organ which receives the blood from the veins and propels it into the arteries. It is divided by a musculomembranous septum into two halves—right or venous and left or arterial—each of which consists of a receiving chamber (atrium) and an ejecting chamber (ventricle).

**alternation of the h.,** see under alternation.

**armored h.,** Panzerherz; calcareous deposits in the pericardium occurring in subacute or chronic inflammation.

**athletic h.,** hypertrophy of the h. supposedly due to overindulgence in athletics.

**beer h.,** beer-drinker's *cardiomyopathy*.

**bony h.,** the presence of more or less extensive calcareous patches in the pericardium and walls of the h.

**dextroposition of the h.,** see under dextroposition.

**dextroversion of the heart.,** corrected dextrocardia.

**drop h.,** cardioptosia.

**fatty h.,** (1) fatty degeneration of the myocardium; (2) cor adiposum; an overaccumulation of adipose tissue on the external surface of the h. with sometimes an infiltration of fat between the muscle bundles of the h. wall.

**frosted h.,** hyaloserositis (*q.v.*) involving the pericardium.

**hairy h.,** fibrinous *pericarditis.*

**hanging h.,** suspended h.

**horizontal h.,** description of the h.'s electrical axis when this is directed at approximately − 30°; recognized in the electrocardiogram when the QRS in lead aVL is positive while that in aVF is negative.

**h. hurry,** tachycardia.

**hypoplastic h.,** a small h., as seen in Addison's disease.

**icing h.,** hyaloserositis (*q.v.*) involving the pericardium.

**intermediate h.,** description of the h.'s electrical axis when this is directed at approximately + 30°; recognized in the electrocardiogram when the QRS complexes in both aVL and aVF are mainly positive.

**irritable h.,** neurocirculatory *asthenia.*

**left h.,** term used to embrace both left atrium and left ventricle.

**luxus h.,** a German term for combined dilation and hypertrophy of the h., especially of the left ventricle.

**movable h.,** *cor* mobile.

**myxedema h.,** the enlarged h. associated with severe hypothyroidism.

**parchment h.,** right ventricular hypoplasia; a congenital or acquired condition in which there is thinning of the right ventricular myocardium.

**pendulous h.,** *cor* pendulum.

**pulmonary h.,** the right atrium and ventricle, receiving the venous blood and propelling it to the lungs; see also *cor* pulmonale.

**right h.,** term used to embrace both right atrium and right ventricle.

**sabot h.,** *coeur* en sabot.

**semihorizontal h.,** description of the h.'s electrical axis when this is directed at approximately 0°; recognized in the electrocardiogram when the QRS complex in lead aVL is positive while that in aVF is isodiphasic.

**semivertical h.,** description of the h.'s electrical axis when this is directed at approximately + 60°; recognized in the electrocardiogram when the QRS complex in lead aVF is positive while that in aVL is isodiphasic.

**skin h.,** the peripheral blood vessels.

**soldier's h.,** neurocirculatory *asthenia.*

**suspended h.,** hanging h.; a h. which gives the appearance on x-ray of being suspended from the great vessels, its lower surface not resting upon the diaphragm.

**systemic h.,** the left atrium and ventricle, receiving the aerated blood from the lungs and propelling it throughout the body.

**tear-drop h.,** h. presenting a symmetrical vertically elongated appearance on x-ray.

**tiger h.,** a fatty, degenerated h. in which the fat is disposed in the form of broken stripes.

**tobacco h.,** cardiac irritability marked by irregular action, palpitation, and sometimes pain, occurring as a result of the excessive use of tobacco.

**venous h.,** the right side (atrium and ventricle) of the h.

**vertical h.,** description of the h.'s electrical axis when this is directed at approximately + 90°; recognized in the electrocardiogram when the QRS complex in aVL is negative while that in aVF is positive.

**waist of the h.,** in the chest x-ray, the middle segment of the cardiac silhouette, containing the pulmonary salient.

**wooden-shoe h.,** *coeur* en sabot.

**heart′burn.** Pyrosis.

**heart′mobile.** A modified ambulance or van used to transport to hospital the victims of real or suspected heart attacks.

**heart′water.** A disease of south and central Africa occurring in cattle, sheep, and goats. It is caused by a rickettsial organism, *Cowdria ruminantium,* which is transmitted by the "bont" tick, *Amblyomma hebraeum.*

**heart′worm.** *Dirofilaria immitis.*

**heat** (hēt) [ A.S. *haete* ]. 1. The opposite of cold; a high temperature; the sensation produced by proximity to fire or an incandescent object. The basis of h. is the kinetic energy of atoms, which becomes zero at absolute zero. 2. Estrus.

**atomic h.,** the amount of h. required to raise an atom from 0° to 1°C. Approximately the same for all elements (about 6 Cal. per gram-atom).

**h. of combustion,** the quantity of h. liberated per gram-molecule when a substance undergoes complete oxidation.

**h. of compression,** the h. produced when a gas is compressed.

**conductive h.,** h. transmitted by direct contact as by an electric pad or hot water bottle.

**convective h.,** h. conveyed by a warm medium, such as air or water, in motion from its source.

**conversive h.,** h. produced in a body by the absorption of waves which are not in themselves hot, such as the sun's rays or infrared radiation.

**h. of crystallization,** the quantity of h. liberated or absorbed per mol when a substance passes into the crystalline state.

**h. of dissociation,** the h. (expressed in calories) expended in the dissociation of 1 mole of a substance into specified products.

**h. of evaporation,** the h. absorbed in the evaporation of water, sweat or other liquid; for water it amounts to 540 calories per gram at 100°C.

**h. of formation,** the h. (expressed in calories) absorbed or liberated during the reaction in which a mole of a compound forms from the necessary elements.

**initial h.,** the first burst of h. produced after the beginning of a muscle twitch, described by A. V. Hill.

**innate h.,** in ancient Greek medicine the h. of the heart, sustained by the pneuma and distributed by the arteries throughout the body.

**latent h.,** the amount of h. which a substance may absorb without an increase in temperature, as in conversion from solid to liquid state, or from liquid to gaseous state; opposed to sensible h.

**molecular h.,** the product of the specific h. of a body multiplied by its molecular weight.

**prickly h.,** *miliaria* rubra.

**radiant h.,** the h. given off from any body in the form of waves, similar to the light waves, but of greater wavelength.

**sensible h.,** the h. which, when absorbed by a substance, causes a rise in temperature; opposed to latent h.

**h. of solution,** the quantity of h. absorbed or evolved when a solid is dissolved in a liquid.

**specific h.,** the h. required to raise any substance through 1° of temperature, compared with that raising the same volume of water 1°.

**h. of vaporization,** h. of evaporation.

**heaves** (hēvz). A chronic pulmonary emphysema of horses. Symptoms include a wheezy cough and dyspnea, especially when exercised. The precise cause is not known.

**hebeosteotomy** (he′be-os′te-ot′o-mi, heb′e-) [ G. *hēbē,* pubes, + *osteon,* bone, + *tomē,* incision ]. Pubiotomy.

**hebephrenia** (he-be-fre′nĭ-ah, heb′e-) [ G. *hēbē,* puberty, + *phrēn,* the mind ]. Hebephrenic schizophrenia; a type of schizophrenia characterized by shallow and inappropriate affect, giggling, and silly, regressive behavior and mannerisms.

**Heberden,** William, London physician, 1710–1801. See H.'s *asthma,* Rougnon-H. *disease,* H.'s *nodes, nodosity.*

**hebet′ic** [ G. *hēbētikos,* youthful, fr. *hēbē,* youth ]. Pertaining to youth.

**hebet′omy** [ G. *hēbē,* pubes, + *tomē,* incision ]. Pubiotomy.

**hebetude** (heb′e-tūd) [ L. *hebetudo,* fr. *hebeo,* to be dull ]. Dullness; lethargy.

**hebiatrics** (he′bĭ-at′riks) [ G. *hēbē,* youth, + *iatrio,* to heal ]. Ephebiatrics.

**he′bin** [ G. *hēbe,* puberty ]. An obsolete term, once used to designate a hormone (gonadotrophin), secreted by the anterior lobe of the hypophysis, which stimulates the sex glands.

**hebosteotomy** (he-bos′te-ot′o-mi) [ G. *hēbē,* pubes, + *osteon,* bone, + *tomē,* a cutting ]. Pubiotomy.

**hebot′omy** [ G. *hēbē,* pubes, + *tomē,* cutting ]. Pubiotomy.

**Hebra** (ha′brah), Ferdinand von, Vienna dermatologist, 1816–1880. See H.'s *disease, prurigo.*

**hecateromeric** (hek′ă-ter-o-mer′ik) [ G. *hekateros,* each of two, + *meros,* part ]. Hecatomeric; hecatomeral; denoting a spinal neuron whose axon divides and gives off processes to both sides of the cord; usually the same as a heteromeric neuron.

**hecatom′eral, hec′atomer′ic.** Hecateromeric.

**Hecker,** Karl v., Munich obstetrician, 1827–1882. See H.'s *law.*

**hectic** (hek′tik) [ G. *hektikos,* habitual, hectic, consumptive, fr. *hexis,* habit. ECT- ]. 1. Constitutional. 2. Denoting an afternoon rise of temperature, accompanied by a flush on the cheeks, occurring in active tuberculosis. 3. Denoting flush accompanying h. fever.

**hecto-** [ G. *hekaton,* one hundred ]. A prefix used in the metric system to signify one hundred ($10^2$).

**hec′togram.** One hundred grams, the equivalent of 1543.7 grains.

**hec′toliter.** One hundred liters, the equivalent of 105.7 quarts or 26.4 American (22 imperial) gallons.

**hedaquin′ium chloride.** TEOQUIL; hexadecamethylene-1,16-bis(isoquinolinium chloride); topical antifungal agent.

**hedeoma** (he-de-o′mah). See pennyroyal.

**hederiform** (hed′er′ĭ-form) [ L. *hedera,* ivy, + *forma,* shape ]. Ivy-shaped; a term used for certain sensory endings in the skin.

**hedonophobia** (he′do-no-fo′bĭ-ah) [ G. *hēdonē,* delight, + *phobos,* fear ]. Morbid fear of pleasure.

**hedrocele** (hed′ro-sēl) [ G. *hedra,* a seat, the fundament, + *kēlē,* hernia ]. Prolapse of the intestine through the anus; proctocele.

**Hedström file.** See under file.

**heel** [ A.S. *hēla* ]. 1. Calx (2); the posterior, rounded extremity of the foot. 2. In dentistry, distal *end.*

**contracted h.,** contracted *foot.*

**cracked h.,** *keratoderma* plantare sulcatum.

**grease h.,** (1) initially, lesions of horsepox occurring in the skin of the flexor surface of the fetlock of the horse; (2) scratches; now frequently applied to any weeping, eczematous condition of that area.

**painful h.,** calcodynia; calcaneodynia; a condition in which bearing the weight on the h. causes more or less severe pain.

**prominent h.,** a condition marked by a tender swelling on the os calcis due to a thickening of the periosteum or fibrous tissue covering the back of the os calcis.

**Heerfordt** (hehr′fort), C. F., Danish oculist, *1871. See H.'s *disease.*

**Hegar** (ha′gar), Alfred, German gynecologist, 1830–1914. See H.'s *dilators, method, sign.*

**Hegglin's anomaly.** See under anomaly.

**Hehner** (hay′ner), Otto, English chemist, 1853–1924. See H. *number.*

**Heidenhain** (hi′den-hin), Rudolph P., German histologist and physiologist, 1834–1897. See H.'s *crescents, demilunes, law, pouch, stain,* Biondi-H. *stain.*

**height** (hit). Vertical measurement.

**anterior facial h.,** abbreviated AFH; in cephalometrics, the linear measurement along a line extending from the nasion to the point menton.

**h. of contour,** the line encircling a tooth or other structure at its greatest bulge or diameter with respect to a selected path of insertion.

**cusp h.,** (1) the shortest distance between the tip of a cusp and its base plane; (2) the shortest distance between the deepest part of the central fossa of a posterior tooth and a line connecting the points of the cusps of the tooth.

**facial h.,** the superior-inferior dimension of the face.

**nasal h.,** the distance between the nasion and the lower border of the nasal aperture.

**orbital h.,** the distance between the midpoints of the upper and lower margins of the orbit.

**Heilbronner** (hil′bron-er), Karl, Dutch physician, 1879–1914. See H.'s *thigh.*

**Heile,** B., German surgeon. See H. *operation.*

**Heim** (him), Friedrich L. K., German physician, 1770–1839. See H.-Kreysig *sign.*

**Heine** (hi′neh), Jacob, German physician, 1800–1879. See H.-Medin *disease.*

**Heine** (hi′neh), Leopold, German ophthalmologist, 1870–1940. See H.'s *operation.*

**Heineke** (hi′nek-eh), Walter H., German surgeon, 1834–1901. See H.-Mikulicz *pyloroplasty.*

**Heinz** (hints), Roberts, German pathologist, 1865–1924. See H. *bodies.*

**Heisrath** (his-raht), Friedrich, German ophthalmologist, 1850–1904. See H.'s *operation.*

**Heister** (hi′ster), Lorenz, German anatomist, 1683–1758. See H.'s *diverticulum, valves.*

**helcomenia** (hel′ko-me′nĭ-ah) [ G. *helkos,* ulcer, + *emmēnos,* monthly ]. The occurrence of ulcers at the time of a menstruation.

**helcoplasty** (hel′ko-plas′tĭ) [ G. *helkos,* ulcer, + *plassō,* to mold ]. The reparative or plastic surgery of ulcers; skin grafting for the cure of ulcers.

**Held,** Hans, German anatomist, *1866. See H.'s *bundle, decussation, end-feet.*

**hel′enin.** Alantolactone.

**he′lian′thine.** See methyl orange.

**Helian′thus.** A genus of plants, the sunflower of the family Compositae.

**H. an′nuus,** a species the seeds of which are the source of sunflower seed oil.

**hel′ical.** [ G. *helix,* a coil ]. 1. Relating to a helix. 2. Resembling a helix.

**hel′icine** [ G. *helix,* a coil ]. 1. Relating to a helix. 2. Resembling a helix.

**helicoid** (hel′ĭ-koyd) [ G. *helix,* a coil, + *eidos,* resemblance ]. Resembling a helix.

**hel′icopo′dia** [ G. *helix,* a coil, + *pous,* foot ]. Helicopod *gait.*

**helicoru′bin.** A respiratory pigment (chromoprotein) found in the certain mollusks, consisting of hematin and a nitrogenous component of unknown chemical constitution. Similar to hemoglobin in structure and function.

**hel′icotre′ma** [ G. *helix,* a spiral, + *trēma,* a hole ] [ NA ]. Scarpa's hiatus; a semilunar opening at the apex of the cochlea between the free curved edge of the lamina of the modiolus and the hamulus of the lamina spiralis ossea, through which the scala vestibuli and the scala tympani of the cochlea communicate with one another.

**heliencephalitis** (he-lĭ-en-sef-al-i′tis) [ G. *helios,* sun, + *enkephalos,* brain, + suffix *-itis,* inflammation ]. Inflammation of the brain following sunstroke.

**helio-** [ G. *hēlios,* sun ]. Combining form relating to the sun.

**helioaerotherapy** (he′lĭ-o-a′er-o-thēr-ă-pī). Treatment with sunshine and air.

**Heliodorus** (he′lĭ-o-do′rus). Greek surgeon in Rome, the second century A.D. He was the first to ligate blood vessels and to treat stricture by internal urethrotomy.

**heliopathy** (he′lĭ-op′ă-thī) [ helio- + G. *pathos,* suffering ]. Injury from exposure to sunlight.

**he′liopho′bia** [ helio- + G. *phobos,* fear ]. A morbid fear of exposure to the sun's rays.

**helio′sis** [ helio- + G. suffix *-osis,* condition ]. Sunstroke.

**heliotaxis** (he-lĭ-o-tak′sis) [ helio- + G. *taxis,* orderly arrangement ]. Heliotropism; a form of phototaxis, and perhaps of thermotaxis, in which there is a tendency to growth or movement toward (positive h.) or away from (negative h.) the sun or the sunlight.

**he′liother′apy.** Treatment of a patient by exposure to direct sunlight.

**heliot′ropin.** Piperonal.

**heliotropism** (he-lĭ-ot′ro-pizm) [ helio- + G. *tropē,* a turning ]. Heliotaxis.

**Heliozoa** (he′lĭ-o-zo′ah) [ helio- + G. *zoōn,* animal ]. An order of the class Sarcodina, in the phylum Protozoa; distinguished by stiff, radiating filaments, usually naked, though some have a skeleton of siliceous scales and spines. They are mostly fresh water dwellers, and colonial forms are common.

**he′lium** [ G. *hēlios,* the sun ]. A gaseous element present in minute amounts in the atmosphere. Symbol He, atomic no. 2, atomic weight 4.003. H. (USP, BP) is used as a diluent of medicinal gases, to facilitate breathing in certain types of respiratory obstruction and in caisson disease.

**helium-3.** ³He; tralphium; the rare stable isotope of h. (1 part in a million of ordinary h.); produced by the beta-decay of tritium.

**helium-4.** ⁴He; the common h. isotope, making up 99.999 per cent of natural h.; it is emitted in the form of alpha rays (which are h. nuclei), from a variety of radioactive nuclides.

**helix,** pl. **helices** (he'liks, hel'ĭ-sēz) [ L. fr. G. *helix,* a coil. HELIC- ]. 1 [ NA ]. The margin of the auricle; a folded rim of cartilage forming the upper part of the anterior, the superior, and the greater part of the posterior edges of the auricle. 2. A snail. 3. A line in the shape of a coil (or a spring, or the threads on a bolt), each point being equidistant from a straight line that is the axis of the cylinder in which each point of the h. lies; often, mistakenly, applied to a spiral.

α **h.,** the right-handed helical form assumed by many proteins, deduced by Pauling and Corey from x-ray diffraction studies of collagen; the h. is stabilized by =CO·HN= hydrogen bonds (the dot represents the H bond).

**DNA h.,** see Watson-Crick h.

**double h.,** see Watson-Crick h.

**Pauling-Corey h.,** see α h.

**twin h.,** see Watson-Crick h.

**Watson-Crick h.,** the helical structure assumed by two strands of deoxyribonucleic acid, held together throughout their length by hydrogen bonds between bases on opposite strands. See also hydrogen *bond.*

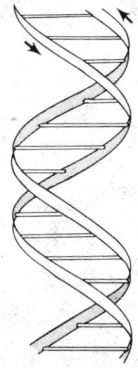

**Diagrammatic Drawing of the Watson-Crick or Double Helix of DNA**
Horizontal bands indicate the hydrogen-bonded base pairs (adenine to thymine, and guanine to cytosine) that bridge the gap between strands. Vertical ribbons indicate the deoxyribose-phosphate-deoxyribose-phosphate . . . strands, or backbone, the deoxyriboses lying at the junction of the bases and holding them, the phosphates lying between these junctions. Arrows indicate that the bonds between deoxyriboses and phosphates are in opposite sequences in the two strands (3′ → 5′ in one, 5′ → 3′ in the other).

**helix'in.** Endomycin; an antifungal antibiotic produced by a species of *Streptomyces;* it contains four active components, h.'s A, B, C, and D. Endomycin A and B are identical to h. A and h. B.

**hellebore** (hel'e-bōr) [ G. *helleboros* ]. A plant of the genus *Helleborus,* especially *H. niger,* and of other (unrelated) genera.

**American h.,** *Veratrum viride.*

**black h.,** helleborus.

**European h.,** *Veratrum album.*

**false h.,** adonis.

**green h.,** *Veratrum viride.*

**white h.,** *Veratrum album.*

**helleborin** (hel-leb'o-rin, hel'e-bo'rin). A toxic glycoside from green hellebore; narcotic.

**helleborism** (hel'e-bor-izm). A condition resulting from poisoning by veratrum.

**helleb'orus** [ G. *helleboros* ]. 1. Black hellebore; Christmas (or New Year) rose; the dried rhizome and roots of *Helleborus niger* (family Ranunculaceae). Cardiac and arterial tonic, diuretic, and cathartic.

**hellebrin.** Helebrigenin glucorhamnoside; a cardiotonic (digitalis-like) glycoside from *Helleborus niger;* it is irritating to the mucous membranes.

**Heller,** Arnold L. G., German pathologist, 1840–1913. See H.'s *plexus.*

**Heller,** Ernst, Leipzig surgeon, 1877–1964. See H. *operation.*

**Hellin,** Dyonizy, Polish pathologist, 1867–1935. See H.'s *law.*

**Helly's fluid.** See under fluid.

**Helmholtz,** Hermann L. F. von, German physician, physicist, and physiologist, 1821–1894. See Gibbs-H. *equation,* H.'s axis *ligament, H. theories,* Young-H. *theory* of color vision.

**hel'minth** [ G. *helmins,* worm ]. An intestinal vermiform parasite. See fig. on p. 622, showing ova of h.'s.

**helminthagogue** (hel-minth'ă-gog) [ G. *helmins,* worm, + *agōgos,* leading ]. Anthelmintic.

**helminthemesis** (hel-min-them'e-sis) [ G. *helmins,* a worm, + *emesis,* vomiting ]. The vomiting or expulsion through the mouth of intestinal worms.

**helminthiasis** (hel'min-thi'ă-sis). The condition of having intestinal vermiform parasites.

**helmin'thic, helmin'tic.** Anthelmintic.

**hel'minthism.** Helminthiasis.

**helminthochorton** (hel-min-tho-kor'ton) [ G. *helmins,* worm, + *chortos,* cattle fodder, grass ]. Corsican moss; a mixture of various marine plants. Used as a vermifuge.

**helmin'thoid** [ G. *helminthōdēs,* wormlike, fr. *helmins,* worm, + *eidos,* resemblance ]. Wormlike.

**helminthol'ogy** [ G. *helmins,* worm, + *logos,* study ]. The branch of science that treats of worms; especially the branch of zoology and of medicine that has to do with intestinal vermiform parasites.

**helmintho'ma** [ G. *helmins,* worm, + suffix *-oma,* tumor ]. A discrete nodule of granulomatous inflammation (including the healed stage) caused by a helminth or its products, so termed on the basis of certain gross resemblances to a neoplasm.

**Helminthospor'ium.** A genus of rapidly growing, saprophytic fungi that are common laboratory contaminants.

**helmin'tic.** Helminthic.

**Heloderma** (he'lo-der'mah) [ G. *hēlos,* nail, + *derma,* skin ]. The only genus of poisonous lizards, such as the Gila monster, so named because of the tubercular scales which cover their bodies. They are native to Mexico and the southwestern United States.

**heloderma simplex et annularis.** *Granuloma* annulare.

**heloma** (he-lo'mah) [ G. *hēlos,* nail, + suffix *-oma,* tumor ]. Clavus; a corn.

**h. durum,** hard *corn.*

**h. mol'le,** soft *corn.*

**helo'sis** [ G. *hēlousthai,* to become callous ]. Corns.

**helot'omy** [ heloma + G. *tomē,* cutting ]. Cutting a corn; the surgical treatment of corns.

**helvol'ic acid.** Fumigacin; an antibiotic principle (a steroid derivative similar in structure to fusidic acid) isolated from cultures of *Aspergillus fumigatus.* It is markedly bacteriostatic against Gram-positive bacteria.

**Helweg** (hel'veg), Hans K. S., Danish physician, 1847–1901. See H.'s *bundle.*

**hem-, hema-** [ G. *haima,* blood ]. Combining forms meaning blood. See also the terms beginning with hemat-, hemato-, and hemo-.

**he'mabarom'eter** [ hema- + G. *baros,* weight, + *metron,* measure ]. An instrument for determining the specific gravity of the blood.

**hemachromatosis** (he'mă-kro-mă-to'sis). Hemochromatosis.

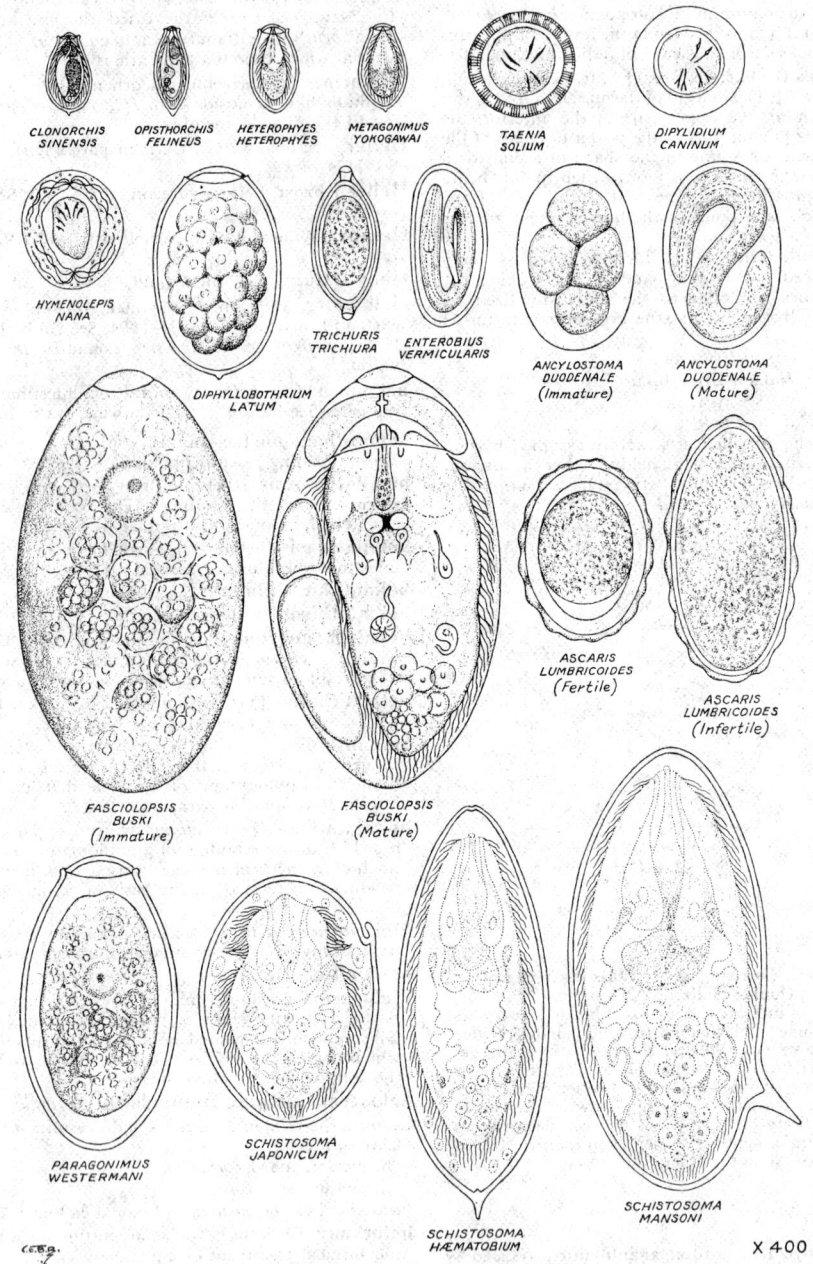

CLONORCHIS SINENSIS    OPISTHORCHIS FELINEUS    HETEROPHYES HETEROPHYES    METAGONIMUS YOKOGAWAI    TAENIA SOLIUM    DIPYLIDIUM CANINUM

HYMENOLEPIS NANA    DIPHYLLOBOTHRIUM LATUM    TRICHURIS TRICHIURA    ENTEROBIUS VERMICULARIS    ANCYLOSTOMA DUODENALE (Immature)    ANCYLOSTOMA DUODENALE (Mature)

FASCIOLOPSIS BUSKI (Immature)    FASCIOLOPSIS BUSKI (Mature)    ASCARIS LUMBRICOIDES (Fertile)    ASCARIS LUMBRICOIDES (Infertile)

PARAGONIMUS WESTERMANI    SCHISTOSOMA JAPONICUM    SCHISTOSOMA HÆMATOBIUM    SCHISTOSOMA MANSONI

X 400

**Ova of Common Helminths of Man**

(From Belding, D. L.: *Textbook of Parasitology*, Ed. 3, © Appleton-Century-Crofts, New York, 1965. Used with permission.)

**hemachrome** (he'mă-krōm) [ hema- + G. *chrōma*, color ]. The coloring matter of the blood, hemoglobin or hematin.

**hemachrosis** (he'mă-kro'sis) [ hema- + G. *chrōsis*, coloration ]. An intensified redness of the blood.

**he'macytom'eter.** Hemocytometer.

**he'macytozo'on.** Hemocytozoon.

**hem'adosteno'sis** [ G. *haimas* (*haimad-*), a stream of blood, + *stenōsis*, a narrowing ]. Contraction of the arteries.

**hemadrom'eter.** Hemodromometer.

**he'madro'mograph** [ hema- + G. *dromos*, a course + *graphō*, to record ]. Hemodromograph.

**he'madromom'eter.** Hemodromometer.

**hemadsorption** (hem'ad-sorp'shun). A phenomenon manifested by an agent or substance adhering to or being adsorbed on the surface of a red blood cell, as tuberculin (for example) can be adsorbed on red blood cells under certain conditions.

**he'madynamom'eter.** Hemodynamometer.

**hemafa'cient.** Hemopoietic.

**hemagglutination** (he'mă-glu'tĭ-na'shun, hem-). Hemoagglutination; the agglutination of red blood cells; may be immune as a result of specific antibody either for red blood cell antigens *per se* or other antigens which coat the red blood cells, or may be nonimmune as in h. caused by viruses or other microbes.

**passive h.,** a kind of passive agglutination in which erythrocytes, usually modified by mild treatment with tannic acid or other chemicals, are used to adsorb soluble antigen onto their surface, and which then agglutinate in the presence of antiserum specific for the adsorbed antigen.

**viral h.,** the nonimmune agglutination of suspended red blood cells by certain of a wide range of otherwise unrelated viruses, usually by the virion itself but in some instances by products of viral growth, the species of erythrocyte agglutinated differing with the different viruses; see also hemagglutination *inhibition.*

**hemagglutinin** (he'mă-glu'tĭ-nin, hem-). Hemoagglutinin; a substance, antibody or other, that causes hemagglutination.

**hemagogic** (he'mă-goj'ik, hem-). Hemagogue (1).

**hemagogue** (he'mă-gog, hem-) [ hem- + G. *agogos*, leading ]. 1. Promoting a flow of blood. 2. An agent that promotes a flow of blood. 3. Emmenagogue.

**he'mal** [ G. *haima*, blood ]. 1. Relating to the blood or blood vessels. 2. Referring to the ventral side of the spinal axis where the heart and great vessels are located; opposed to neural.

**hemal'um.** A solution of hematoxylin and alum, used as a nuclear stain in histology, especially with eosin as a counterstain.

**Hemame'ba.** See *Haemamoeba.*

**hem'amebi'asis.** Any infection with ameboid forms of parasites in red blood cells, as in malaria.

**hemanalysis** (hem'ă-nal'ĭ-sis) [ G. *haima*, blood, + analysis ]. Analysis of the blood; an examination of blood, especially with reference to chemical methods.

**hemangiectasis, hemangiectasia** (he-man'jĭ-ek'tā-sis, -ek-ta'zĭ-ah) [ G. *haima*, blood, + *angeion*, vessel, + *ektasis*, a stretching ]. Dilation of blood vessels.

**hemangio-** (he-man'jĭ-o-) [ G. *haima*, blood, + *angeion*, vessel ]. Combining form relating to the blood vessels.

**hemangioameloblastoma** (he-man'jĭ-o-am'ē-lo-blas-to'mah). Undesirable term for a very highly vascular ameloblastoma.

**hemangioblast** (he-man'jĭ-o-blast) [ hemangio- + G. *blastos*, germ ]. A primitive embryonic cell of mesodermal origin which produces cells giving rise to vascular endothelium, to reticuloendothelial elements and to blood-forming cells of all types.

**hemangioblastoma** (he-man'jĭ-o-blas-to'mah). Angioblastoma; Lindau's tumor; a benign cerebellar neoplasm composed of capillary vessel-forming endothelial cells; a slowly growing tumor that affects, primarily, middle-aged individuals.

**hemangioendothelioblastoma** (he-man'jĭ-o-en-do-the'-lĭ-o-blas-to'mah) [ hemangio- + endothelium + G. *blastos*, germ, + suffix *-oma*, tumor ]. Hemangioendothelioma

in which the endothelial cells seem to be especially immature forms.

**hemangioendothelioma** (he-man'jĭ-o-en-do-the-lĭ-o'mah) [ hemangio- + endothelium + G. suffix *-oma*, tumor ]. Hemendothelioma; a neoplasm derived from blood vessels, and characterized by numerous, prominent endothelial cells that occur singly, in aggregates, and as the lining of congeries of vascular tubes or channels. H.'s in the elderly may be malignant (hemangiosarcoma), but those that occur in children are benign and probably represent a growing stage of capillary hemangioma.

**h. tubero'sum mul'tiplex,** an eruption of pinkish papules, caused by hyperplasia of the endothelium of the superficial blood vessels.

**hemangiofibroma** (he-man'jĭ-o-fi-bro'mah). A hemangioma with an abundant fibrous tissue framework.

**juvenile h.,** juvenile *angiofibroma.*

**hemangioma** (he-man'jĭ-o'mah) [ hemangio- + G. suffix *-oma*, tumor ]. Not actually a true neoplasm, but a congenital anomaly; proliferation of vascular endothelium leads to a mass that resembles neoplastic tissue. It can occur anywhere in the body but is most frequently noticed in the skin and subcutaneous tissues.

**capillary h.,** arterial h.; h. congenitale or simplex; a congenital lesion consisting of numerous, variably sized but predominantly small, closely packed capillaries that are usually separated only by a thin network of reticulin; the endothelial cells lining the capillaries are relatively large and prominent, frequently resulting in an extremely small lumen or only a potential space as a lumen; see also *nevus vascularis.*

**cavernous h.,** cavernous angioma; nevus cavernosus; cavernoma; a vascular erectile tumor containing large blood-filled spaces, due apparently to dilation and thickening of the walls of the capillary loops.

**h. con'genita'le,** capillary h.

**h. pla'num exten'sum,** a benign, flat, cutaneous hemangioma of considerable size.

**racemose h.,** cirsoid *aneurysm.*

**sclerosing h.,** see dermatofibroma.

**senile h.,** a red papule due to weakening of the capillary wall, seen in most persons over 30 years of age; termed also cherry angioma; papillary ectasia; senile ectasia; De Morgan's spots; ruby spots.

**h. simplex,** capillary h.

**hemangiomatosis** (he-man'jĭ-o-mă-to'sis). A condition in which there are numerous hemangiomas.

**hemangiopericytoma** (he-man'jĭ-o-pĕr'ĭ-si-to'mah) [ hemangio- + pericyte + G. suffix *-oma*, tumor ]. A rare vascular neoplasm composed of round and spindle cells that are presumably derived from the pericytes; the vascular nature of h.'s is not always clinically or grossly apparent, inasmuch as the neoplastic cells tend to be irregularly and closely packed among numerous small capillaries; the latter are frequently obscure, or occult, and difficult to recognize without the study of reticulum stains. H.'s are variable in their clinical effects, some being benign, whereas others are malignant.

**hemangiosarcoma** (he-man'jĭ-o-sar-ko'mah). A rare malignant neoplasm characterized by rapidly proliferating, extensively infiltrating, anaplastic cells derived from blood vessels and lining blood-filled spaces.

**hemapheic** (hem-ă-fe'ik). Pertaining to or containing hemaphein.

**hemaphein** (hem-ă-fe'in) [ G. *haima*, blood, + *phaios*, dusky ]. A brown pathologic pigment derived from hemoglobin; it is said to be a combination of indican and urobilin.

**hemapheism** (hem'ă-fe'izm). The presence of hemaphein in the blood plasma and urine.

**hemar'thron, hemar'thros.** Hemarthrosis.

**hemarthrosis** (hem'ar-thro'sis) [ G. *haima*, blood, + *arthron*, joint ]. Hemarthron; hemarthros; hemophilic joint; blood in a joint.

**hemat-** (he'mat-, hem'at-) [ G. *haima* (*haimat-*), blood ]. Combining form meaning blood.

**hematachometer** (he'mă-tă-kom'e-ter). Hemotachometer.

**hemataerometer** (he'mat-a'er-om'e-ter) [ hemat- + G. *aēr*, air, + *metron*, measure ]. An instrument for estimating the relative partial pressures of gases in the blood.

**hematapostasis** (he'mat-ă-pos'tă-sis) [ hemat- + G. *apostasis*, departure ]. Vicarious *menstruation*.

**hematapostema** (he'mat-ă-pos-te'mah, hem'at-) [ hemat- + G. *apostēma*, abscess ]. An abscess into which blood has effused.

**hematein** (he'mă-te'in, hem'ă-te'in) An oxidation product of hematoxylin.

**hematemesis** (he'mă-tem'e-sis) [ hemat- + G. *emesis*, vomiting ]. Vomiting of blood.

**hematencephalon** (he'mat-en-sef'ă-lon, hem'at-) [ hemat- + G. *enkephalos*, brain ]. Cerebral *hemorrhage*.

**hemather'apy.** Hemotherapeutics.

**hematherm** (he'mă-therm) [ G. *haima*, blood, + *thermos*, warm ]. Warm-blooded animal; any of the animals, including mammals and birds, which tend to maintain a constant body temperature.

**hemather'mal** [ G. *haima*, blood, + *thermos*, warm ]. Hemathermous; hematothermal; warm-blooded; denoting a mammal or bird whose blood is of a constant temperature; *cf.* poikilothermal.

**hemather'mous.** Hemathermal.

**hemathidrosis** (he'mat-ĭ-dro'sis). Hematidrosis.

**hematho'rax.** Hemothorax.

**hemat'ic.** 1. Hemic; relating to blood. 2. A hematinic.

**hem'atid** [ hemat- + suffix -*id, q.v.* ]. 1. A red blood cell. 2. Infrequently used as a term for a cutaneous eruption presumed to be caused by a substance in the circulating blood.

**hematidrosis** (he'mat-ĭ-dro'sis, hem'at-) [ hemat- + G. *hidrōs*, sweat ]. Hemathidrosis; hemidrosis (1); sudor sanguineus; excretion of blood or blood pigment in the sweat; an extremely rare disorder.

**hematim'eter.** Hemocytometer.

**hem'atin.** An iron-protoporphyrin differing from heme in that the central iron atom is in the ferric ($Fe^{2+}$) rather than the ferrous ($Fe^{3+}$) state; the prosthetic group of methemoglobin.

**hematinemia** (hem'ă-tin-e'mĭ-ah) [ hematin + G. *haima*, blood ]. The presence of heme in the circulating blood.

**hematinic** (hem'ă-tin'ik). 1. Improving the condition of the blood. 2. An agent that improves the quality of blood by increasing the number of erythrocytes and/or the hemoglobin concentration.

**hem'atinom'eter.** Hemoglobinometer.

**hematinuria** (hem'ă-tin-u'rĭ-ah) [ hematin + G. *ouron*, urine ]. The presence of heme in the urine.

**hemato-** (hem'ă-to-, he'mă-to-) [ G. *haima* (*haimat-*), blood ]. Combining form meaning blood. For words beginning with this prefix but not found here, see those beginning with hemo-.

**hematoaerometer** (hem'ă-to-a'er-om'e-ter). Hemataerometer.

**hematobium** (he'mă-to'bĭ-um) [ hemato- + G. *bios*, life ]. Any microorganism that is parasitic in the blood, especially an animal form or hematozoon.

**hematoblast** hem'ă-to-blast) [ hemato- + G. *blastos*, germ ]. A primitive, undifferentiated form of blood cell from which erythroblasts, lymphoblasts, myeloblasts, and other immature blood cells are derived; probably identical or closely similar to hemocytoblast and hemohistioblast. H.'s are present only in small numbers in normal bone marrow, and are difficult to identify in smears, inasmuch as they are fragile and easily disintegrated; when marrow is hyperplastic, the h.'s may be observed in small groups.
  **Hayem's h.,** platelet.

**hematocele** (hem'ă-to-sēl) [ hemato- + G. *kēlē*, tumor ]. 1. A blood cyst. 2. An effusion of blood into a canal or a cavity of the body; hematocelia. 3. A swelling due to effusion of blood into the tunica vaginalis testis.
  **pelvic h.,** an intraperitoneal effusion of blood into the pelvis.
  **puden'dal h.,** an effusion of blood into the labium majus.

**hematocelia** (hem'ă-to-se'lĭ-ah). Hematocele (2).

**hematocephalus** (hem'ă-to-sef'ă-lus) [ hemato- + G. *kephalē*, head ]. Intracranial effusion of blood, commonly in a fetus.

**hematochezia** (hem'ă-to-ke'zĭ-ah) [ hemato- + G. *chezō*, to go to stool ]. The passage of bloody stools, in contradistinction to melena, or tarry stools.

**hematochlorin** (hem'ă-to-klo'rin). A green coloring matter derived from hemoglobin obtained from the placenta.

**hematochyluria** (hem'ă-to-ki-lu'rĭ-ah) [ hemato- + G. *chylos*, juice, + *ouron*, urine ]. The presence of blood as well as chyle in the urine.

**hematocolpometra** (hem'ă-to-kol'po-me'trah) [ hemato- + G. *kolpos*, vagina, + *mētra*, womb ]. An accumulation of blood in the uterus and vagina resulting from an imperforate hymen or other lower vaginal obstruction.

**hematocolpos** (hem'ă-to-kol'pos) [ hemato- + G. *kolpos*, vagina ]. An accumulation of menstrual blood in the vagina in consequence of imperforate hymen or other obstruction.

**hematocrit** (hem'ă-to-krit) [ hemato- + G. *krinō*, to separate ]. 1. A centrifuge or device for separating the cells and other particulate elements of the blood from the plasma. 2. The percentage of the volume of a blood sample occupied by cells, as determined by a h.; abbreviated Hct.

**hematocryal** (hem'ă-tok'rĭ-al) [ hemato- + G. *kryos*, cold ]. Poikilothermal.

**hem'atocrys'tallin.** Hemoglobin.

**hematocyst** (hem'ă-to-sist). Hemorrhagic *cyst*.

**hematocystis** (hem'ă-to-sis'tis) [ hemato- + G. *kystis*, bladder ]. An effusion of blood into the bladder.

**hem'atocyte.** Hemocyte.

**hem'atocy'toblast.** Hemocytoblast.

**hem'atocytol'ysis.** Hemocytolysis.

**hem'atocytom'eter.** Hemocytometer.

**hematocytozoon** (hem'ă-to-si'to-zo'on). Hemocytozoon.

**hematocyturia** (hem'ă-to-si-tu'rĭ-ah) [ hemato- + G. *kytos*, cell, + *ouron*, urine ]. The presence of red blood cells in the urine; true hematuria as distinguished from hemoglobinuria.

**hem'atodyscra'sia.** Hemodyscrasia.

**hem'atodys'trophy.** Hemodystrophy.

**hematogenesis** (hem'ă-to-jen'ĕ-sis) [ hemato- + G. *genesis*, production ]. Hemopoiesis.

**hematogenic, hematogenous** (hem'ă-to-jen'ik, hem-ă-toj'en-us). 1. Forming blood; hemopoietic. 2. Pertaining to anything produced from, derived from, or transported by the blood.

**hem'atoglo'bin, hem'atoglob'ulin.** Hemoglobin.

**hem'atohis'tioblast.** Hemohistioblast.

**hem'atohis'ton.** Globin.

**he'matoid** [ hemato- + G. *eidos*, resemblance ]. Sanguineous; bloody; resembling blood.

**hematoidin** (hēm-ă-toy'din). Blood crystals; h. crystals; a pigment derived from hemoglobin which contains no iron but is closely related to or similar to bilirubin. H. is formed intracellularly presumably within reticuloendothelial cells, but is often found extracellularly after 5 to 7 days in foci of previous hemorrhage. it occurs as refractile, yellow-brown and orange-red granules, but more characteristically as rhomboid plates arranged in a radial pattern, so-called h. burrs.

**hematol'ogist.** A physician trained and experienced in hematology, *i.e.,* skilled in performing diagnostic examinations of blood and bone marrow, or in treatment of such diseases, or both.

**hematology** (he'mă-tol'o-jĭ, hem'ă-tol'o-jĭ) [ hemato- + G. *logos*, study ]. Hemology; the medical specialty that pertains to the anatomy, physiology, pathology, symptomatology, and therapeutics related to the blood and blood-forming tissues.

**hematolymphangioma** (hem'ă-to-limf'an-jĭ-o'-mah). A congenital anomaly consisting of numerous, closely packed, variably sized lymphatic vessels and larger channels, in association with a moderate number of blood vessels of a similar type.

**hematol'ysis.** Hemolysis.

**hematolyt'ic.** Hemolytic.

**hematoma** (he'mă-to'mah, hem'ă-to'mah) [ hemato- + G. suffix *-oma*, tumor ]. A localized mass of extravasated blood that is relatively or completely confined within an organ or tissue, a space, or a potential space; the blood is usually clotted (or partly clotted), and, depending on how long it has been there, may manifest various degrees of organization and decolorization.

**h. auris,** othematoma.

**epidural h.** extradural *hemorrhage.*

**intracranial h.,** see intracranial *hemorrhage,* and related entries under hemorrhage.

**intramural h.,** a h. of the duodenum, usually resulting from trauma; the blood clot in the wall of the duodenum may expand and cause obstruction of the bowel lumen.

**subdural h.,** subdural *hemorrhage.*

**he'matom'ancy** [ hemato- + G. *manteia,* divination ]. Diagnosis by means of various types of examination of the blood or bone marrow, or both.

**hem'atomanom'eter.** Hemomanometer.

**he'matom'eter** [ hemato- + G. *metron,* measure ]. Hemocytometer.

**hematometra** (hem'ă-to-me'trah) [ hemato- + G. *mētra,* uterus ]. Hemometra; a collection or retention of blood in the uterine cavity.

**he'matom'etry** [ hemato- + G. *metron,* measure ]. Hemometry; examination of the blood in order to determine any or all of the following: (1) the total number, types, and relative proportions of various blood cells; (2) the number or proportion of other formed elements; (3) the percentage of hemoglobin. In some instances, h. is used to include a determination of blood pressure.

**hematomphalocele** (hem'at-om-fal'o-sēl) [ hemato- + G. *omphalos,* umbilicus, + *kēlē,* hernia ]. An umbilical hernia into which an effusion of blood has taken place.

**hematomyelia** (hem'ă-to-mi-e'lĭ-ah) [ hemato- + G. *myelos,* marrow ]. Hematorrhachis interna; myelapoplexy; myelorrhagia; hemorrhage into the substance of the spinal cord; it is usually a posttraumatic lesion but may also be encountered in instances of spinal cord capillary telangiectases.

**hematomyelopore** (hem'ă-to-mi'ĕ-lo-pōr) [ hemato- + G. *myelos,* marrow, + *poros,* a pore ]. The formation of porosities in the spinal cord as a result of hemorrhages.

**hematon'ic.** Hematinic.

**hem'atopathol'ogy** [ hemato- + G. *pathos,* suffering, + *logos,* study ]. Hemopathology; the medical science dealing with diseases and abnormal conditions of the blood and hemopoietic tissues.

**hematop'athy.** Hemopathy.

**hematopenia** (hem'ă-to-pe'nĭ-ah) [ hemato- + G. *penia,* poverty ]. Deficiency of blood, including hypocytosis or cytopenia.

**hematophagia** (hem'ă-to-fa'jĭ-ah) [ hemato- + G. *phagein,* to eat ]. Hemophagia. 1. Living on the blood of another animal, as does the vampire bat or a leech. 2. The drinking of blood as a therapeutic measure.

**hematophagocyte** (hem'ă-to-fag'o-sīt). Hemophagocyte.

**hematophagous** (hem'ă-tof'ă-gus) [ hemato- + G. *phagein,* to eat ]. Subsisting on blood.

**hematophagus** (hem'ă-tof'ă-gus) [ hemato- + G. *phagein,* to eat ]. A blood eater; referring especially to bloodsucking insects.

**hematophyte** (hem'ă-to-fīt) [ hemato- + G. *phyton,* plant ]. Any microorganism of the plant kingdom, *e.g.,* a bacterium or fungus, living in the blood.

**hem'atopla'nia** [ hemato- + G. *planē,* a wandering ]. Vicarious *menstruation.*

**hem'atoplas'tic** [ hemato- + G. *plassō,* to form ]. Hemopoietic.

**hematopoiesis** (hem'ă-to-poy-e'sis). Hemopoiesis.

**hematopoietic** (hem'ă-to-poy-et'ik). Hemopoietic.

**hematopoietine** (hem'ă-to-poy'ĕ-tin). Erythropoietin.

**hematoporphyria** (hem'ă-to-por-fĭ-rĭ-ah, -por-fi'rĭ-ah) [ hemato- + G. *porphyra,* purple ]. Older term for any disorder of prophyrin metabolism, regardless of the cause.

**hem'atopor'phyrin.** 1,3,5,8-Tetramethyl-2,4-bis(α-hydroxyethyl)porphine-6,7-bispropionic acid; a dark red, almost purple substance resulting from the decomposition of hemoglobin; the chemical composition is that of heme with the iron removed and the two vinyl (—CH=CH₂) groups hydrated to hydroxyethyl (—CHOH—CH₃).

**hem'atopor'phyrine'mia.** Older term used to designate the occurrence of hematoporphyrin in the circulating blood.

**hem'atopor'phyrinu'ria.** Older term used to designate enhanced urinary excretion of porphyrins.

**hem'atopo'sia** [ hemato- + G. *posis,* a drinking ]. Hematophagia (2).

**hematop'sia** [ hemato- + G. *opsis,* vision ]. Hemorrhage into the eye.

**hematorrhachis** (hem-ă-tor'ă-kis) [ hemato- + G. *rhachis,* spine ]. Spinal apoplexy; spinal hemorrhage.

**h. externa,** extradural or subdural h.; hemorrhage into the spinal canal external to the cord, either within or outside the dura.

**h. interna,** hematomyelia.

**hem'atosal'pinx** [ hemato- + G. *salpinx,* a trumpet ]. Hemosalpinx; a collection of blood in a tube, often associated with a tubal pregnancy.

**hematoscheocele** (hem'ă-tos'ke-o-sēl) [ hemato- + G. *oscheon,* scrotum, + *kēlē,* hernia, tumor ]. An accumulation of blood in the scrotal cavity.

**hem'atoscope** [ hemato- + G. *skopeō,* to examine ]. Hemoscope. 1. An electric photometer used for estimating the number of red blood cells suspended in blood (or other fluid), by means of measuring the dispersion of light. 2. A spectrophotometer for determining the percentage of hemoglobin in blood (or other fluid).

**hematos'copy.** The analysis of blood by means of a hematoscope.

**hem'atosep'sis.** Septicemia.

**hemato'sin.** Hematin.

**hemato'sis.** 1. Hemopoiesis. 2. Oxygenation of the venous blood in the lungs.

**hem'atospec'troscope.** A spectroscope especially adapted to examination of the blood.

**hematospectroscopy** (hem'ă-to-spek-tros'ko-pī). Examination of blood by means of a spectroscope.

**hematospermatocele** (hem'ă-to-sper'mă-to-sēl). A spermatocele that contains blood.

**hem'atostat'ic.** 1. Hemostatic. 2. Due to stagnation or arrest of blood in the vessels of the part.

**hematostaxis** (hem'ă-to-stak'sis) [ hemato- + G. *staxis,* a dripping ]. Spontaneous bleeding due to a disease of the blood.

**hematos'teon** [ hemato- + G. *osteon,* bone ]. Bleeding in the medullary cavity of a bone.

**hem'atother'mal.** Hemathermal.

**hem'atotox'in.** Hemotoxin.

**hematotrachelos** (hem'ă-to-trā-ke'lus) [ hemato- + G. *trachēlos,* neck ]. Distention of the cervix uteri with accumulated blood.

**hem'atotrop'ic.** Hemotropic.

**hematox'ic.** Hemotoxic.

**hematox'in.** Hemotoxin.

**he'matox'ylin.** A dark yellow or orange crystalline compound, $C_{16}H_{14}O_6 \cdot 3H_2O$, containing the coloring matter of *Haematoxylon campechianum,* or logwood, from which it is obtained by extraction with ether; used as a dye in histology, especially for cell nuclei. Its staining properties depend upon its oxidation to hematein. Also used as an indicator: red to yellow at pH 0.0 to 1.0, yellow to violet at pH 5.0 to 6.0.

**Boehmer's h.,** two solutions are prepared: (a) 1 gm. of h. crystals in 10 ml. of absolute alcohol, and (b) 20 gm. of potassium alum in 200 ml. of distilled water; after standing for 24 hours, the two solutions are mixed and "aged" by means of exposure to air for a week; the stain should be filtered before use.

**Delafield's h.,** a stain for histologic specimens: h. 4, ammonia-alum 25, absolute alcohol 25, methyl alcohol 100, glycerin 100, water 400.

**Ehrlich's h.,** h. 2, glacial acetic acid 10, alum 31, glycerin, absolute alcohol, and water 100 of each. Can be ripened immediately by adding 0.2 gm. of sodium iodate.

**Harris' h.,** h. 1, ammonium alum 20, absolute alcohol 10, water 200, mercuric chloride 0.5. Heat to 100°C. for a few minutes. Glacial acetic acid (8 cc.) can be added.

**he'matox'ylon** [ hemato- + G. *xylon,* wood ]. Logwood; the heart wood of *Haematoxylon campechianum* (family Leguminosae), a tree of Central America. Used as an astringent and tonic and occasionally in diarrhea, but used chiefly as a source of hematoxylin.

**hematozo'ic.** Hemozoic.

**hematozo'on.** Hemozoon.

**hemature'sis.** Hematuria, especially with reference to unusually large amounts.

**hematu'ria** [ hemato- + G. *ouron,* urine ]. Any condition in which the urine contains blood or red blood cells.

**angioneurotic h.,** renal *epistaxis.*

**Egyptian h.,** *schistosomiasis* haematobium.

**endemic h.,** *schistosomiasis* haematobium.

**essential h.,** that in which the cause and source are not recognized.

**false h.,** pseudohematuria.

**microscopic h.,** that recognized only by means of microscopic examination of urine or urinary sediment.

**renal h.,** that resulting from extravasation of blood into the glomerular spaces, or tubules, or pelves of the kidneys.

**urethral h.,** that in which the site of bleeding is in the urethra.

**vesical h.,** that in which the site of bleeding is in the urinary bladder.

**hemautograph** (hēm-aw'to-graf) [ G. *haima,* blood, + *autos,* self, + *graphō,* to write ]. A tracing made on a moving strip of paper by a minute spurt from a punctured artery.

**hem'bra.** Ulcerative cutaneous leishmaniasis.

**heme** (hēm). Reduced hematin; ferroprotoporphyrin; protoheme; ferroheme; 1,3,5,8-tetramethyl-2,4-bis(vinyl)-porphine-6,7-bispropionic acid, ferrous complex; the prosthetic, oxygen-carrying, color-furnishing constituent of hemoglobin. For structure, see porphine.

**hemelytrometra** (hēm-el'ĭ-tro-me'-trah) [ G. *haima,* blood, *elytron,* sheath (vagina), + *mētra,* uterus ]. An accumulation of blood in both uterus and vagina in cases of imperforate hymen.

**hemen'dothelio'ma.** Hemangioendothelioma.

**hemeralopia** (hem'er-al-o'pi-ah) [ G. *hēmera,* day, + *alaos,* obscure, + *ōps,* eye ]. Day blindness; inability to see as distinctly in a bright light as in a dim one.

**hemerythrins** (hēm'e-rith'rinz). Iron-containing, oxygen-binding compounds in some worms, with molecular weights approximately that of hemoglobin but differing from hemoglobin in that the molecules do not contain porphyrin groups.

**hemi-** [ G. ]. A prefix signifying one-half.

**hemiablepsia** (hem'ĭ-ă-blep'sĭ-ah) [ hemi- + G. *a-* priv. + *blepō,* to see ]. Obsolete synonym for hemianopsia.

**hemiacardius** (hem'ĭ-ă-kar'dĭ-us) [ hemi- + G. *a-* priv. + *kardia,* heart ]. One of twin fetuses, in which only a part of the circulation is effected by its own heart, the rest being moved by the heart of the other twin.

**hemiacetal** (hem'ĭ-as'e-tal). A hydrated aldehyde, RCH(OH)OR', in which one of the hydroxyl groups is esterified with an alcohol (in an acetal, both hydroxyl groups are so esterified). In the aldose sugars, the esterification is internal (R is R') and labile, brought about by the migration of the H of the 4-OH or 5-OH to the carbonyl O, yielding the furanose or pyranose structures (see sugars for these structures). The hemiacetal forms of the sugars are involved in all polysaccharides, as glycosyls or glycosides. See also hemiketal.

**hemiachromatopsia** (hem'ĭ-ă-kro-mă-top'sĭ-ah) [ hemi- + G. *a-* priv. + *chrōma,* color, + *opsis,* vision ]. Color *hemianopsia.*

**hemiacrosomia** (hem'ĭ-ak'ro-so'mĭ-ah) [ hemi- + G. *akron,* extremity, *akros,* extreme, + *sōma,* body ]. A congenital form of hemihypertrophy.

**hemiageusia** (hem'ĭ-ă-gu'sĭ-ah) [ hemi- + G. *a-* priv. + *geusis,* taste ]. Hemiageustia; hemigeusia; loss of taste from one side of the tongue.

**hemialgia** (hem-ĭ-al'jĭ-ah) [ hemi- + G. *algos,* pain ]. Pain affecting one entire half of the body.

**hemiamblyopia** (hem'ĭ-am-blĭ-o'pĭ-ah). Amblyopia affecting one-half of the visual field of one or both eyes.

**hemiamyosthenia** (hem'ĭ-ă-mi'os-the'nĭ-ah) [ hemi- + G. *a-* priv. + *mys* (*myo-*), muscle, + *stheneia,* strength ]. Hemiparesis.

**hemianalgesia** (hem'ĭ-an'al-je'zĭ-ah). Analgesia, or loss of sensibility to pain, affecting one side of the body.

**hemianencephaly** (hem'ĭ-an'en-sef'ă-lĭ). Anencephaly on one side only, or involving one side much more extensively than the other.

**hemianesthesia** (hem'ĭ-an-es-the'-zĭ-ah). Anesthesia, or loss of tactile sensibility, on one side of the body.

**alternate h.,** crossed h.; h. affecting the head on one side and the body and extremities on the other side.

**crossed h.,** alternate h.

**hemiano'pia.** Hemianopsia.

**hemianopsia** (hem'ĭ-an-op'sĭ-ah) [ hemi- + G. *an-* priv. + *opsis,* vision ]. Hemianopia; loss of vision for one half of the visual field of one or both eyes.

**absolute h.,** h. in which the affected field is totally blind to all visual stimuli.

**altitudinal h.,** a defect in the visual field in which the upper or lower half is lost; may be unilateral or bilateral.

**bilateral h.,** binocular h.; h. affecting both eyes.

**binasal h.,** blindness in the nasal field of vision of both eyes.

**binocular h.,** bilateral h.

**bitemporal h.,** blindness in the temporal field of vision of both eyes.

**color h.,** hemiachromatopsia; loss of color perception in half of each visual field.

**complete h.,** h. involving a full half of the visual field.

**congruous h.,** h. in which the visual field defects in both eyes are completely symmetrical in every respect.

**crossed h.,** altitudinal h. involving the upper field of one eye and the lower field of the other.

**heteronymous h.,** crossed h.

**homonymous h.,** lateral h.; loss of sight in the corresponding (right or left) lateral halves of the eyes.

**incomplete h.,** h. involving less than half the visual field of each eye.

**incongruous h.,** an incomplete or asymmetric homonymous h.

**lateral h.,** homonymous h.

**quadrantic h.,** quadrantanopsia; loss of vision in a quarter section of the visual field of one or both eyes; if bilateral, it may be homonymous or heteronymous, binasal or bitemporal, or crossed, *i.e.,* involving the upper quadrant in one eye and the lower quadrant in the other.

**relative h.,** h. regarding only the color sense or form sense or both, the light sense remaining.

**unilateral h., uniocular h.,** loss of sight in half the visual field of one eye only.

**hem'ianop'tic.** Pertaining to hemianopsia.

**hemianosmia** (hem'ĭ-an-oz'mĭ-ah) [ hemi- + G. *an-* priv. + *osmē,* smell ]. Loss of the sense of smell on one side.

**hemiaplasia** (hem'ĭ-a-pla'zĭ-ah) [ hemi- + aplasia, *q.v.* ]. Absence of one lobe of a bilobed organ; used especially with reference to the thyroid gland.

**hemiapraxia** (hem'ĭ-ă-prak'sĭ-ah). Apraxia affecting one side of the body.

**hemiasynergia** (hem'ĭ-ă-sin-er'jĭ-ah). Asynergia affecting one lateral of the body.

**hem'iatax'ia.** Ataxia affecting one side of the body.

**hemiathetosis** (hem'ĭ-ath'e-to'sis). Athetosis affecting one hand, or one hand and foot, only.

**hemiatrophy** (hem-ĭ-at'ro-fĭ). Atrophy of one lateral half of a part or of an organ, as the face or tongue.

**facial h.,** Romberg's disease, trophoneurosis, or syndrome; facial trophoneurosis; atrophy, usually progressive, affecting the tissues of one side of the face; saber-cut depression on forehead, heterochromia iridis, or bullous keratopathy may be present.

**progressive lingual h.,** lingual trophoneurosis; atrophy of one lateral half of the tongue.

**hemiballism** (hem'ĭ-bal'izm) [ hemi- + G. *ballismos,* jumping about ]. Violent athetoid and choreic movements involving one side of the body; related to damage to the subthalamic nucleus of the opposite side of the brain.

**hem'iblock.** Arrest of the impulse in one of the two main divisions of the left branch of the bundle of His; *i.e.*, in either the anterior (superior) division or the posterior (inferior) division.

**he'mic.** Hemal; relating to the blood.

**hem'icar'dia** [ hemi- + G. *kardia*, heart ]. 1. One lateral half, including atrium and ventricle, of the heart. 2. A congenital malformation of the heart in which only two of the usual four chambers are formed.
  **h. dextra,** the right *heart*.
  **h. sinistra,** the left *heart*.

**hem'icar'dius.** An individual with hemicardia (2).

**hem'icel'lulose.** Plant cell-wall polysaccharides closely associated with cellulose (xylans, mannans, galactans, and others).

**hem'icen'trum** [ hemi- + G. *kentron*, center ]. One of the two lateral halves of the body of the vertebra.

**hemicephalalgia** (hem'ĭ-sef'ă-lal'jĭ-ah) [ hemi- + G. *kephalē*, head, + *algos*, pain ]. Hemicrania (2); the unilateral headache characteristic of typical migraine.

**hemicephalia** (hem'ĭ-sē-fa'lĭ-ah) [ hemi- + G. *kephalē*, head ]. Partial anencephaly; congenital failure of the cerebrum to develop normally. Usually the cerebellum and basal ganglia are represented at least in rudimentary form.

**hemicephalus** (hem'ĭ-sef'ă-lus). A malformed fetus exhibiting hemicephalia.

**hemicerebrum** (hem'ĭ-sĕr'e-brum). A cerebral hemisphere.

**hemicholin'ium chloride.** A synthetic quaternary ammonium compound that impairs neuromuscular transmission by inhibiting the release or synthesis of acetylcholine.

**Hemichorda** (hem'ĭ-kor'dah). Hemichordata.

**Hemichordata** (hem'ĭ-kor-da'tah). Hemichorda; a group comprised of large, wormlike marine animals with gill-slits to the pharynx and a conical proboscis; a ciliated larval stage (tonaria) resembles that of echinoderms.

**hemichorea** (hem'ĭ-ko-re'ah). Chorea dimidiata; hemilateral chorea; chorea involving the muscles on one side only.

**hemichromosome** (hem'ĭ-kro'mo-sŏm). A lateral half of a chromosome.

**hem'icolec'tomy** [ hemi- + G. *kolon*, colon, + *ektomē*, excision ]. Removal of part of the colon.

**hemicrania** (hem-ĭ-kra'nĭ-ah). [ hemi- + G. *kranion*, skull ]. 1. Migraine. 2. Hemicephalalgia.

**hem'icraniec'tomy** [ hemi- + G. *kranion*, skull, + *ektome*, excision ]. Hemicraniotomy.

**hem'icranio'sis.** Enlargement of one side of the cranium.

**hem'icraniot'omy** [ hemi- + G *kranion*, skull, + *tome*, cut ]. Hemicraniectomy; separation and reflection of the greater part or all of one-half of the cranium, as a preliminary to an operation upon the brain.

**hemidiaphoresis** (hem'ĭ-di-ă-fo-re'sis). Hemihidrosis; hemidrosis (2); diaphoresis, or sweating, on one side of the body.

**hemidrosis** (hem-ĭ-dro'sis). 1. Hematidrosis. 2. Hemidiaphoresis.

**hemidysesthesia** (hem'ĭ-dis-es-the'-zĭ-ah). Dysesthesia affecting one lateral half of the body.

**hemidystrophy** (hem-ĭ-dis'tro-fĭ) [ hemi- + G. *dys-*, ill, + *trophē*, nourishment, growth ]. A condition of underdevelopment of one lateral half of the body.

**hemiectromelia** (hem'ĭ-ek-tro-me'lĭ-ah) [ hemi- + ectromelia, *q.v.* ]. Defective development of the limbs on one side of the body.

**hemiencephalus** (hem'ĭ-en-sef'ă-lus). Hemicephalus.

**hem'iep'ilepsy.** One-sided epilepsy, the convulsive movements occurring on one side of the body only.

**hemifa'cial.** Pertaining to one side of the face.

**hem'igastrec'tomy.** Excision of one-half of the stomach.

**hemigeusia** (hem'ĭ-gu'sĭ-ah). Hemiageusia.

**hem'iglo'bin.** Methemoglobin. See also hemoglobin.

**hem'iglos'sal** [ hemi- + G. *glōssa*, tongue ]. Hemilingual.

**hem'iglossec'tomy** [ hemi- + G. *glōssa*, tongue, + *ektome*, excision ]. Surgical removal of one-half of the tongue.

**hem'iglossi'tis** [ hemi- + G. *glōssa*, tongue, + suffix *-itis*, inflammation ]. A vesicular eruption on one side of the tongue and the corresponding inner surface of the cheek, probably herpetic.

**hemignath'ia** (hem'ĭ-nath'ĭ-ah) [ hemi- + G. *gnathos*, jaw ]. Defective development of one side of the lower jaw.

**hem'ihep'atec'tomy.** Surgical removal of one-half or a lobe of the liver.

**hemihidro'sis.** Hemidiaphoresis.

**hemihydranencephaly** (hem'ĭ-hi'dran-en-sef'ă-lĭ). A unilateral form of hydranencephaly.

**hemihypalgesia** (hem'ĭ-hi-pal-je'zĭ-ah). A partial loss of sensibility to pain, or hypalgesia, affecting one lateral half of the body.

**hemihyperesthesia** (hem'ĭ-hi'per-es-the'zĭ-ah). Hyperesthesia, or increased tactile and painful sensibility, affecting one side of the body.

**hemihyperidrosis** (hem'ĭ-hi-per-i-dro'sis) [ hemi- + G. *hyper*, over, + *hidrōsis*, sweating ]. Excessive sweating confined to one side of the body.

**hem'ihyperto'nia** [ hemi- + G. *hyper*, over, + *tonos*, tone ]. Hemitonia; exaggerated muscular tonicity on one lateral half of the body.

**hemihypertrophy** (hem'ĭ-hi-per'tro-fĭ). Muscular hypertrophy of one side of the face or body.

**hemihypesthesia** (hem'ĭ-hi-pes-the'zĭ-ah). Hemihypoesthesia.

**hemihypoesthesia** (hem'ĭ-hi-po-es-the'zĭ-ah) [ hemi- + G. *hypo*, under, + *aisthēses*, sensation ]. Diminished sensibility in one lateral half of the body.

**hem'ihypoto'nia** [ hemi- + G. *hypo*, under, + *tonos*, tone ]. A partial loss of muscular tonicity on one side of the body.

**hemikaryon** (hem'ĭ-kăr'ĭ-on) [ hemi- + G. *karyon*, nut (nucleus) ]. A cell nucleus containing the haploid number of chromosomes.

**hemike'tal.** A hydrated ketone, $R_2C(OH)OR'$, in which one of the hydroxyl groups is esterified with an alcohol (in a ketal, both hydroxyl groups are so esterified). In the ketose sugars, migration of an alcoholic H from the δ or ε OH to the keto O leads to intramolecular cyclization (furanose or pyranose), R and R' thus being the same carbon chain. The hemiketal forms of the sugars are involved in polysaccharide formation, as glycosyls or glycosides. See also hemiacetal.

**hem'ilaminec'tomy** [ hemi- + L. *lamina*, layer, + G. *ektome*, excision ]. Removal of a portion of a vertebral lamina, usually performed for exploration of, access to, or decompression of the intraspinal contents; often used to denote unilateral laminectomy.

**hemilaryngectomy** (hem'ĭ-lăr-in-jek'to-mĭ) [ hemi- + G. *larynx* (*laryng-*), larynx, + *ektome*, excision ]. Excision of one lateral half of the larynx.

**hemilat'eral.** Relating to one lateral half.

**hemilesion** (hem-ĭ-le'zhun). Unilateral lesion.

**hemilin'gual** [ hemi- + L. *lingua*, tongue ]. Relating to one lateral half of the tongue.

**hem'imac'roglos'sia** [ hemi- + G. *makros*, large, + *glōssa*, tongue ]. Enlargement of half the tongue.

**hem'imandibulec'tomy.** Resection of one-half of the mandible.

**hemimelia** (hem'ĭ-me'lĭ-ah) [ hemi- + G. *melos*, limb ]. A condition marked by defects in the limbs.

**hemimelus** (hem'ĭ-me'lus, hem-im'e-lus). An individual with hemimelia.

**he'min.** The chloride of heme in which $Fe^+$ has become $Fe^{3+}$ (hematin is the hydroxide). Also termed hematin chloride; chlorohemin; ferriheme chloride, ferriprotoporphyrin; ferriporphyrin chloride; Teichman's crystals; factor X for *Haemophilus*.

**heminephrectomy** (hem'ĭ-ne-frek'to-mĭ) [ hemi- + G. *nephros*, kidney, + *ektome*, excision ]. Excision of part of a kidney.

**hemiopalgia** (hem'ĭ-o-pal'jĭ-ah) [ hemi- + G. *ōps*, eye, + *algos*, pain ]. Pain in one eye, usually accompanied by hemicrania.

**hemiopia** (hem-ĭ-o'pĭ-ah) [ hemi- + G. *ōps*, eye ]. Obsolete term for hemianopsia.

**hemipagus** (hem-ip'ă-gus) [ hemi- + G. *pagos*, something fixed ]. Conjoined twins united laterally at the thorax, or at the thorax and neck, and sometimes also at the jaws.

**hemiparanesthesia** (hem'ĭ-păr-an-es-the'zĭ-ah). Anesthesia of one lower extremity, or of the lower part of one side of the body.

**hemiparaplegia** (hem'ĭ-păr'ah'ple'jĭ-ah). Paralysis of one leg.

**hemiparesis** (hem'ĭ-pă-re'sis, -păr'e-sis). Slight paralysis affecting one side only.

**hem'ipelvec'tomy** [ hemi- + L. *pelvis*, basin (pelvis), + G. *ektomē*, excision ]. Amputation of an entire leg together with the os innominatum.

**hemiplegia** (hem'ĭ-ple'jĭ-ah) [ hemi- + G. *plēgē*, a stroke ]. Paralysis of one side of the body.

**alternate h.**, paralysis of facial muscles on one side and of the extremities on the other, due to a unilateral lesion of the brain stem; also called Gubler's h., paralysis, or syndrome, crossed h. or paralysis, and stauroplegia.

**ascending h.**, Mills' disease; ascending paralysis affecting one lateral half of the body.

**contralateral h.**, paralysis occurring on the side opposite to the causal central lesion.

**crossed h.**, alternate h.

**double h.**, diplegia.

**facial h.**, paralysis of one side of the face, the muscles of the extremities being unaffected.

**Gubler's h.**, alternate h.

**hereditary h.**, h. with atrophy, present at birth.

**infantile h.**, birth *palsy*.

**spastic h.**, a h. with increased tone in the antigravity muscles of the affected side.

**hemiplegic** (hem-ĭ-ple'jik). Relating to hemiplegia.

**Hemiptera** (hem-ip'ter-ah) [ hemi- + G. *pteron*, wing ]. An arthropod order of the class Insecta that includes many plant lice and other true bugs; only a few are bloodsuckers and¹ of medical importance. The best known species is *Cimex lectularius*, the common bedbug. The triatomine bloodsucking bugs, vectors of Chagas' disease, are the most important disease vectors in the order.

**hemipyonephrosis** (hem'i-pi'o-ne-fro'sis). Unilateral pyonephrosis, or pyonephrosis of half a kidney.

**hemiscotosis** (hem'ĭ-sko-to'sis) [ hemi- + G. *skotōsis*, a darkening ]. Obsolete term for hemianopsia.

**hemisec'tion.** The surgical removal of a root of a multi-rooted tooth and its related coronal portion.

**hemisep'tum.** A lateral half of any septum.

**hemiso'mus** [ hemi- + G. *sōma*, body ]. An individual with one side of the body imperfectly developed.

**hem'ispasm.** A spasm affecting one or more muscles of one side of the face or body only.

**hemisphere** (hem'ĭ-sfēr) [ hemi- + G. *sphaira*, ball, globe ]. 1. Hemispherium, *q.v.* 2. Half of a spherical structure.

**cerebellar h.**, *hemispherium* cerebelli.

**cerebral h.**, *hemispherium* cerebri.

**dominant h.**, that cerebral hemisphere that (1) contains the representation of speech, and (2) controls the arm and leg used preferentially in skilled movements.

**hemispherectomy** (hem'i-sfēr-ek'to-mĭ). Excision of one cerebral hemisphere; undertaken for malignant tumors, infantile hemiplegia due to birth injury, and other cerebral conditions.

**hemispherium** (hem'ĭ-sfe'rĭ-um) [ G. *hemisphairion* ] [ NA ]. Hemisphere. 1. H. cerebri. 2. H. cerebelli.

**h. bul'bi ure'thrae**, one of the lateral halves of the bulb of the urethra that are separated by a median groove on the posterior part of the undersurface.

**h. cerebel'li** [ NA ], cerebellar hemisphere; hemispherium (2); the large part of the cerebellum lateral to the vermis cerebelli.

**h. cer'ebri** [ NA ], cerebral hemisphere; hemispherium (1); the large mass of the endbrain, or telencephalon, on either side of the midline, consisting of the cerebral cortex and its associated fiber systems, together with the deeper-lying corpus striatum.

**Hemispora** (hem'ĭ-spo'rah) [ hemi- + G. *sporos*, seed ]. Generic name for certain species of *Fungi imperfecti* in which chains of conidia develop from tubular structures that form as the result of a constriction at the end of each of a series of short hyphal branches; close septations divide the contents of the tube into relatively square, thick-walled, deeply staining segments that eventually

separate and become rounded, thick-walled spores with rough surfaces. *H.* organisms occur fairly frequently as contaminants in cultures for other fungi; they are usually regarded as nonpathogenic forms, but there are a few reported instances in which they were apparently the causal agents of disease.

**hem'isporo'sis.** Chronic infection thought to be caused by *Hemispora stellata*, and characterized by granulomatous inflammation that tends to resemble the gummatous lesion of tertiary syphilis. The disease is relatively rare, and only a few examples of osteitis, periosteitis, "cold abscess" of subcutaneous tissue and muscle, and chronic ulcer of the skin have been described as being caused by *Hemispora* organisms. Cutaneous lesions are said to resemble those observed in sporotrichosis.

**hemistrumectomy** (hem'ĭ-stru-mek'to-mĭ) [ hemi- + L. *struma, q.v.*, + G. *ektomē*, excision ]. Excision of approximately one-half of a goitrous tumor.

**hemisulfur mustard.** See under mustard.

**hemisyndrome** (hem'ĭ-sin-drōm). A condition in which one-half of the body is atrophied or hypertrophied.

**hemisystole** (hem'ĭ-sis'to'le). Systole alternans; contraction of the left ventricle following every second atrial contraction only, so that there is but one pulse beat to every two heart beats.

**hemiterata** (hem-ĭ-tĕr'ah-tah) [ hemi- + G. *terata*, pl. of *teras*, a monster ]. Persons with congenital malformations which are not so marked or so disabling as to merit the term "monster" for their possessors.

**hemiterat'ic.** Relating to hemiterata.

**hemiter'pene.** Isoprene.

**hemithermoanesthesia** (hem'ĭ-ther'mo-an-es-the'zĭ-ah). Loss of sensibility to heat and cold affecting one side of the body.

**hemitho'rax.** One side of the thorax.

**hemito'mias** [ hemi- + G. *tomias*, eunuch, fr. *tomē*, a cutting ]. A man with but one testis.

**hemito'nia.** Hemihypertonia.

**hemitox'in.** A toxin of half the normal strength.

**hemitremor** (hem'ĭ-trem'or, -tre'mor). Tremor affecting the muscles of one side of the body.

**hemiver'tebra.** A congenital defect of the spine in which one side of a vertebra more or less completely fails to develop.

**hemizygos'ity.** The state of having unpaired genes in an otherwise diploid cell; males are normally hemizygous for genes on the X chromosome.

**hemizy'gote** [ hemi- + G. *zygōtos*, yoked (see zygote) ]. An individual hemizygous with respect to one or more specified genes (*e.g.*, a hemophilic male is a h. with respect to the gene for hemophilia).

**hemizy'gous.** Relating to hemizygosity.

**hem'lock.** 1. Conium. 2. *Abies canadensis.*

**hemo-** (he'mo-, hem'o-) [ G. *haima*, blood ]. A prefix signifying blood. For words not found under hemo- see hemato-. For official taxonomic names denoting genera, see Haemo-.

**he'moagglu'tination.** Hemagglutination.

**he'moagglu'tinin.** Hemagglutinin.

**he'moalkalim'eter.** A device for determining the degree of alkalinity of the blood.

**he'moan'titoxin.** An antibody that neutralizes the effects of a hemotoxin, such as the hemolytic material in cobra venom.

**He'mobartonel'la.** See *Haemobartonella.*

**he'mobil'ia.** Bleeding into the biliary passages, usually as a result of hepatic trauma.

**he'moblast.** Hemocytoblast.

**lymphoid h. of Pappenheim**, pronormoblast; see discussion under erythroblast.

**he'moblasto'sis.** A proliferative condition of the hematopoietic tissues in general.

**hemocatharsis** (he'mo-kă-thar'sis) [ hemo- + G. *katharsis*, a cleansing ]. Cleansing the blood.

**he'mocatheret'ic** [ hemo- + G. *kathairetikos*, destructive ]. Having the power, as possessed by the spleen, to destroy fragile erythrocytes.

**hemocele** (he'mo-sēl) [ hemo- + G. *koilōma,* cavity ]. The system of blood-containing spaces pervading the body in arthropods.

**he'moce'lom** [ hemo- + G. *koilōma,* cavity ]. Archaic designation for pericardial *cavity* (2).

**hemocholecyst** (he'mo-ko'le-sist, -kol'e-sist) [ hemo- + G. *cholē,* bile, + *kystis,* bladder ]. 1. A cyst containing blood and bile. 2. Nontraumatic hemorrhage or old blood accumulated in the gallbladder.

**hemocholecystitis** (he'mo-ko'le-sis-ti'tis). Hemorrhagic cholecystitis.

**hemochorial** (he'mo-ko'rī-al). See hemochorial *placenta.*

**hemochromatosis** (he'mo-kro-mă-to'sis) [ hemo- + G. *chrōma,* color, + suffix -*osis,* condition ]. A disease of older men with excessive iron intake, possibly due to inherited excessive absorption of iron; characterized by pigmentation of the skin and hemosiderin deposits in the liver, pancreas, and other organs, often associated with cirrhosis, glycosuria and bronze diabetes.

  **exogenous h.,** hemosiderosis due to repeated blood transfusions; it may progress to pigmentary cirrhosis.

**hemochrome** (he'mo-krōm). Hemochromogen.

**hemochromogen** (he'mo-kro'mo-jen) [ hemo- + G. *chrōma,* color, + suffix -*gen,* producing ]. Hemochrome; term originally used for combinations of ferro- or ferriporphyrins with 2 moles of a nitrogenous base, *e.g.,* pyridine ferroporphyrin.

  **h. of hemoglobin,** derived from hemoglobin by treating it with alkali, the globin being thereby denatured.

**hemochromometer** (he'mo-kro-mom'e-ter) [ hemo- + G. *chrōma,* color, + *metron,* measure ]. An apparatus for determining the percentage of hemoglobin in the blood by means of comparing the properly treated specimen with a standard solution of an appropriate compound, *e.g.,* ammonium picrocarminate.

**he'mochromom'etry.** The determination of the percentage of hemoglobin in the blood, by means of a hemochromometer.

**hemoclasis, hemoclasia** (he-mok'lă-sis, he'mo-kla'zī-ah) [ hemo- + G. *klasis,* a breaking ]. Rupture, dissolution (hemolysis), or other type of destruction of red blood cells.

**he'moclas'tic.** Pertaining to hemoclasis.

**he'moconcentra'tion.** Decrease in the volume of plasma in relation to the number of red blood cells; increase in the

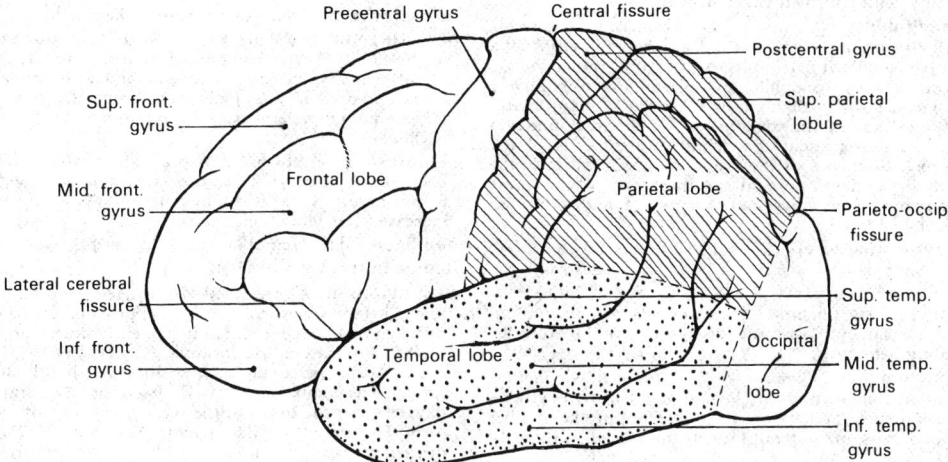

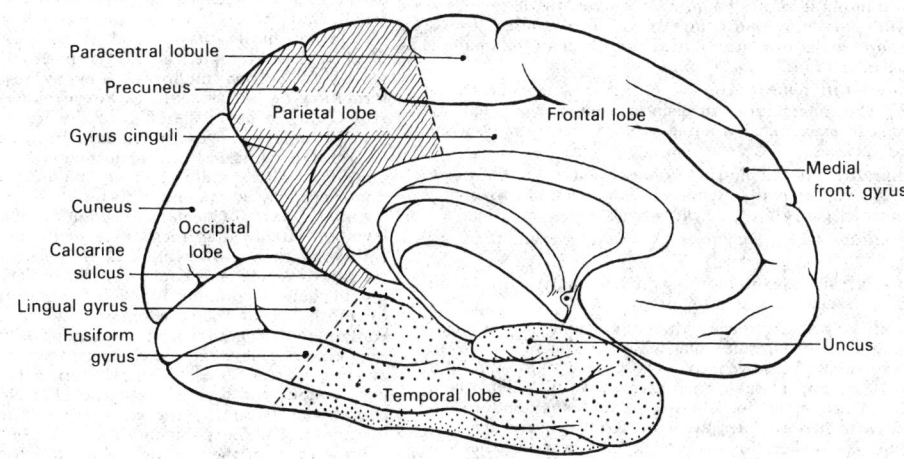

**Cerebral Hemispheres**
The lateral (*A*) and medial (*B*) aspects of the cerebral hemispheres with principal gyri

concentration of red blood cells in the circulating blood.

**hemoconia** (he'mo-ko'nĭ-ah) [ hemo- + G. *konis*, dust ]. Blood dust; dust corpuscle; blood motes; small refractive particles in the circulating blood, probably lipid material associated with fragmented stroma from red blood cells.

**hemoconiosis** (he'mo-ko-nĭ-o'sis). A condition in which there is an abnormal amount of blood dust, or hemoconia, in the blood.

**hemocriny** (he-mok'rĭ-nĭ) [ hemo- + G. *krino*, to separate ]. Obsolete term used to designate the process whereby an endocrine organ secretes its hormone directly into the blood stream, *e.g.*, the anterior lobe of the hypophysis.

**hemocryoscopy** (he'mo-kri-os'ko-pĭ) [ hemo- + G. *kryos*, cold, + *skopeō*, to examine ]. Determination of the freezing point of blood.

**hemocrys'tallin.** Hemoglobin.

**hemocuprein** (he'mo-ku'pre-in). A copper-containing protein found in the erythrocytes of several mammals; similar or identical to cytocuprein (erythrocuprein); now known to be the enzyme superoxide dismutase (*q.v.*).

**he'mocy'anin.** An oxygen-carrying substance (molecular weight approximately $6 \times 10^6$) of lower sea animals in which copper is an essential component.

**he'mocyte** [ hemo- + G. *kytos*, a hollow (cell) ]. Hematocyte; any cell or formed element of the blood.

**he'mocy'toblast** [ hemo- + G. *kytos*, cell, + *blastos*, germ ]. Stem cell; mesameboid cell (2); hematocytoblast; a primitive blood cell derived from embryonic mesenchyme, characterized by basophilic cytoplasm and a relatively large nucleus with a spongy, loose network of chromatin and several nucleoli; mitochondria are extremely fine and delicate. H.'s represent the primitive stem cells of the monophyletic theory of the origin of blood and have the potentiality of developing into erythroblasts, young forms of the granulocytic series, megakaryocytes, and so on. See color plate 15.

**hemocytocatheresis** (he'mo-si'to-kă-thĕr'e-sis) [ hemo- + G. *kytos*, a hollow (cell), + *kathairesis*, destruction ]. Hemolysis, or other type of destruction of red blood cells.

**he'mocytol'ysis** [ hemo- + G. *kytos*, cell, + *lysis*, dissolution ]. Hematocytolysis; the dissolution of blood cells, including hemolysis.

**he'mocytom'eter** [ hemo- + G. *kytos*, cell, + *metron*, measure ]. Hemacytometer; hematimeter; hematocytometer; hematometer; an apparatus for estimating the number of blood cells in a quantitatively measured volume of blood.

**Thoma-Zeiss h.,** Thoma's counting chamber; an apparatus for counting the blood cells; it consists of a glass pipette, provided with an ampulla for collecting the blood and diluting it, and a counting chamber; the latter has a depth of $1/10$ mm. and is marked off into squares of $1/400$ sq. mm., so that the space indicated by each of the smallest squares contains $1/4000$ cu. mm.

**he'mocy'totrip'sis** [ hemo- + G. *kytos*, + *tripsis*, a grinding ]. The fragmentation or disintegration of blood cells by means of mechanical trauma, *e.g.*, compression between hard surfaces.

**hemocytozoon** (he'mo-si'to-zo'on) [ hemo- + G. *kytos*, cell, + *zōon*, animal ]. Hemacytozoon; hematocytozoon; a protozoon parasite of the blood cells.

**he'modiagno'sis.** Diagnosis by means of examination of the blood.

**hemodialysis** (he'mo-di-al'ĭ-sis). The dialysis of blood against a semipermeable membrane.

**hemodi'alyzer.** Artificial kidney; a machine for hemodialysis in acute or chronic renal failure. Toxic substances in the blood are removed by exposure to dialyzing fluid across a semipermeable membrane. Excess water which accumulates in the body between dialyses is removed, by positive hydrostatic pressure in the Kolff twin coil artificial kidney and by suction across the membrane in the Kül dialyzer.

**ultrafiltration h.,** a h. that uses fluid pressure differentials to bring about loss (usually) of protein-free fluid from the blood to the bath, as in certain edematous conditions.

**he'modi'astase.** Blood amylase.

**he'modilu'tion.** Increase in the volume of plasma in relation to red blood cells; reduced concentration of red blood cells in the circulation.

**he'modro'mograph** [ hemo- + G. *dromos*, course, + *graphō*, to record ]. Hemadromograph; an instrument for recording the rapidity of the blood circulation.

**he'modromom'eter** [ hemo- + G. *dromos*, course, + *metron*, measure ]. Hemadrometer; hemadromometer; an instrument for measuring the rapidity of the blood circulation.

**he'modynam'ic.** Relating to the physical aspects of the blood circulation.

**he'modynam'ics** [ hemo- + G. *dynamis*, power ]. The study of the dynamics of the blood circulation.

**hemodynamometer** (he'mo-di'nă-mom'e-ter) [ hemo- + G. *dynamis*, force, + *metron*, measure ]. Hemadynamometer; an instrument for determining the blood pressure.

**hemodyscrasia** (he'mo-dis-kra'ze-ah) [ hemo- + dyscrasia, *q.v.* ]. Any abnormal condition or disorder of the blood and hemopoietic tissue, used especially with reference to those resulting in changes in the formed elements.

**hemodystrophy** (hēm-o-dis'tro-fĭ). Any disease or abnormal condition of the blood and hemopoietic tissues, exclusive of simple transitory changes.

**he'moendothe'lial.** See hemoendothelial *placenta*.

**he'mofer'rum.** The iron content of hemoglobin.

**hemoflagellates** (he'mo-flaj'ĕ-lāts). Protozoan flagellates in the family Trypanosomatidae that are parasitic in the blood of many species of domestic and wild animals and birds, and of man. They include the genera *Leishmania* and *Trypanosoma*, several species of which are important pathogens.

**hemofuscin** (he-mo-fus'in). A brown pigment derived from hemoglobin; occurs in urine occasionally along with hemosiderin. Such a finding is usually indicative of increased red blood cell destruction.

**hemogen'esis.** Hemopoiesis.

**hemogen'ic.** Hemopoietic.

**he'moglo'bin.** Abbreviated Hb; the red, respiratory protein of erythrocytes, consisting of approximately 6 per cent heme and 94 per cent globin (a protein); molecular weight, 68,000; typical empiric formula, $(C_{738}H_{1166}FeN_{203}O_{208}S_2)_4$; the values for percentage composition are slightly different for various animal species. H. (symbol, Hb) transports oxygen from the lungs to the tissues, and this oxygenated form is termed oxyhemoglobin (symbol, $HbO_2$). The oxygen is readily released in the tissues, where $HbO_2$ becomes Hb. The latter combines with carbon dioxide (resulting from cellular respiration) and forms h. carbamate, the chief form in which carbon dioxide is transported to the lungs. The carbamate then becomes converted to $HbO_2$, and the cycle continues. When h. is exposed to certain chemicals, its normal respiratory function is blocked. For example, the oxygen in $HbO_2$ is easily displaced by carbon monoxide, thereby resulting in the formation of fairly stable carboxyhemoglobin (symbol, HbCO), as in asphyxiation resulting from inhalation of exhaust fumes from gasoline engines. In addition, when the iron in h. is oxidized from the ferrous to ferric state, as in poisoning with nitrates and certain other chemicals, a nonrespiratory compound is formed, *i.e.*, methemoglobin (symbol, MetHb), which is sometimes termed hemiglobin (symbol, Hi). In man there are four kinds of normal h.: embryonic (Hb Gower-2), fetal (Hb F), and two adult types (Hb A, Hb $A_2$). Each of these consists of two alpha globin chains containing 141 amino acid residues, and two of another kind (beta, gamma, delta or epsilon) each containing 146 amino acid residues. The production of each kind of globin chain is controlled by a structural gene of similar Greek letter designation; normal individuals are homozygous for the normal gene at each of five loci. Mutations, resulting in the substitution of one amino acid for another in the polypeptide chain, can occur at any codon in any of the five loci. Mutations have resulted in production of more than 100 types of abnormal h., most of no known clinical significance. In addition, deletions of one or more amino acid residues are known, and gene rearrangements due to unequal crossing over between homologous chromosomes. The listing of h. types below includes only the abnormal types known to be of clinical significance. Newly discovered abnormal h. types are first assigned a name, usually the location where discovered; a molecular formula is added when determined. The formula consists of Greek letters to designate the basic chains, with subscript 2 if there are two identical chains; a superscript letter ($^A$ if normal for adult h., etc.) is added, or the superscript may designate the site of amino acid substitution (numbering amino acid residues from the N terminus of the polypeptide) and specifying the change, using standard abbreviations for the amino acids.

**h. A,** normal adult h. (Hb A) with molecular formula $\alpha_2{}^A\beta_2{}^A$.

**h. A₂,** the normal h. (Hb A₂) of the molecular formula $\alpha_2{}^A\delta_2$, which makes up approximately 1.5 to 3 per cent of the total h. concentration.

**h. Barts,** a h. homotetramer (all four polypeptides identical) of molecular formula $\gamma_4$, found in the early embryo; this type is not effective in oxygen transport.

**bile pigment h.,** choleglobin.

**h. C,** an abnormal h. with substitution of lysine for glutamic acid at the 6th position of the beta chain, of molecular formula $\alpha_2{}^A\beta_2{}^{6\ Glu\ -Lys}$; this type reduces the normal plasticity of erythrocytes. Heterozygotes: Hb C trait, about 28 to 44 per cent of total h. is Hb C, no anemia. Homozygotes: nearly all h. is Hb. C, moderate normocytic hemolytic anemia. Individuals heterozygous for both Hb C and Hb S (Hb SC disease) and for Hb C and thalassemia are known, and have atypical hemolytic anemias.

**h. C$_{Georgetown}$** and **h. C$_{Harlem}$,** two abnormal h.'s, both with the substitution of valine for glutamic acid at the 6th position of the beta chain as in Hb S, and in addition each has a second substitution; Hb C$_{Harlem}$ has substitution of asparagine for aspartic acid at position 73 of the beta chain; Hb C$_{Georgetown}$ has a second substitution in one of the core residues (positions 83 through 120); both types cause sickling of erythrocytes similar to Hb S (q.v.).

**carbon monoxide h.,** carboxyhemoglobin.

**h. Chesapeake,** an abnormal h. with a single alpha chain substitution, molecular formula $\alpha_2{}^{92\ Arg\ -Leu}\beta_2{}^A$; heterozygotes have polycythemia, apparently to compensate for the increased oxygen affinity of this h., resulting in decreased liberation of oxygen in the tissues.

**h. D$_{Punjab}$,** an abnormal h. with a single beta chain substitution, molecular formula $\alpha_2{}^A\beta_2{}^{121\ Glu\ -Gln}$; heterozygotes are asymptomatic, homozygotes have mild hemolytic anemia.

**h. E,** an abnormal h. with a single beta chain substitution, molecular formula $\alpha_2{}^A\beta_2{}^{26\ Glu\ -Lys}$, common in southeast Asia, especially Thailand; heterozygotes are asymptomatic with 35 to 45 per cent Hb E; homozygotes have mild to moderate hemolytic anemia with 90 to 100 per cent Hb E and remainder Hb F.

**h. F,** normal fetal h. (Hb F) of molecular formula $\alpha_2{}^A\gamma_2{}^F$, which is the major h. component during intrauterine life, then decreases rapidly during infancy to reach a concentration of less than 0.5 per cent in normal children and adults. The concentration of Hb F is increased in some hemoglobinopathies and in some cases of hypoplastic anemia, pernicious anemia, and leukemia.

**h. F (hereditary persistence of),** a condition due to a gene that depresses synthesis of beta and delta chains (as in thalassemia), but this is fully compensated by increased gamma chain synthesis and there is no anemia; three types: African, no beta or delta chain synthesis by the chromosome with the abnormal gene, heterozygotes have 20 to 30 per cent Hb F and Hb A₂ slightly decreased, homozygotes form no Hb A or Hb A₂; Greek type, reduced beta and delta chain synthesis, heterozygotes have 10 to 20 per cent Hb F and normal Hb A₂; Swiss type, heterozygotes have only 1 to 3 per cent Hb F and normal Hb A₂.

**fetal h.,** h. F.

**h. Gower-1,** a h. homotetramer (all four polypeptides identical) of molecular formula $\epsilon_4$, found in the early embryo; this type is not effective in oxygen transport.

**h. Gower-2,** a normal h. of molecular formula $\alpha_2{}^A\epsilon_2$, that is a major h. component of the early embryo, but production of epsilon chains normally ceases at about the third month of fetal development.

**green h.,** choleglobin.

**h. H,** a h. homotetramer (all four polypeptides identical) of molecular formula $\beta_4$, found only when alpha chain synthesis is depressed; it is not effective in oxygen transport. Hb H disease is a thalassemia-like syndrome in individuals heterozygous for both severe and mild genes for alpha thalassemia; moderate anemia and red cell abnormalities with 25 to 35 per cent Hb Barts at birth, but with Hb Barts later replaced by Hb H and with Hb A₂ decreased.

**h. I,** an abnormal h. with a single alpha chain substitution, molecular formula $\alpha_2{}^{16\ Lys\ -Glu}\beta_2{}^A$ a thalassemia-like syndrome has been found in individuals heterozygous for both Hb I and alpha thalassemia genes, with formation of about 70 per cent Hb I.

**h. J$_{Capetown}$,** an abnormal h. with a single alpha chain substitution, molecular formula $\alpha_2{}^{92\ Arg\ -Gln}\beta_2{}^A$; heterozygotes have polycythemia because of increased oxygen affinity of this h. (see h. Chesapeake).

**h. Kansas,** an abnormal h. of molecular formula $\alpha_2{}^A\beta_2{}^{102\ Asn\ -Thr}$; found in association with familial cyanosis due to decreased oxygen affinity of this h.

**h. Lepore,** a group of abnormal h.'s with normal alpha chains but the non-alpha chains consist of the N-terminal portion of the delta chain joined to the C-terminal portion of the beta chain, apparently as the result of nonhomologous pairing and crossing over between the genes for beta and delta chains. The major types are Hb Lepore $_{Boston}$, Hb Lepore $_{Hollandia}$, and Hb Lepore $_{Baltimore}$, which differ in the region of crossing over. Heterozygotes form about 10 per cent Hb Lepore, normal amounts of Hb A2, and moderately increased amounts of Hb F and usually have mild anemia, microcytosis, and hypochromia. Homozygotes form only Hb Lepore and Hb F and have severe anemia (thalassemia major syndrome).

**h. M,** a group of abnormal h.'s in which a single amino acid substitution favors the formation of methemoglobin in spite of normal quantities of methemoglobin reductase enzyme; heterozygotes have congenital methemoglobinemia; the homozygous state of these genes is unknown and is presumably lethal. Specific types include: Hb M$_{Iwate}$, $\alpha^{87\ His\ -Tyr}$ (alpha chain, position 87, histidine replaced by tyrosine); Hb M$_{Hyde\ Park}$, $\beta^{92\ His\ -Tyr}$; Hb M$_{Boston}$, $\alpha^{58\ His\ -Tyr}$; Hb M$_{Saskatoon}$, $\beta^{63\ His\ -Tyr}$; Hb M$_{Milwaukee-1}$, $\beta^{67\ Val\ -Glu}$.

**muscle h.,** myoglobin.

**ox'ygenated h.,** oxyhemoglobin.

**h. Rainier,** an abnormal h. of the molecular formula $\alpha_2{}^A\beta_2{}^{145\ Tyr\ -His}$; heterozygotes have polycythemia because of increased oxygen affinity of this h. (see h. Chesapeake).

**reduced h.,** the form of h. in red blood cells after the oxygen of oxyhemoglobin is released in the tissues.

**h. S,** an abnormal h. with substitution of valine for glutamic acid at the 6th position of the beta chain, of the molecular formula $\alpha_2{}^A\beta_2{}^S$, or more specifically $\alpha_2{}^A\beta_2{}^{6\ Glu\ -Val}$. Heterozygous state: sickle cell trait, no anemia, Hb S 20 to 45 per cent of total, rest Hb A. Homozygous state: sickle cell anemia, Hb S 75 to 100 per cent total, rest Hb F or Hb A₂.

**sickle cell h.,** h. S.

**h. Yakima,** an abnormal h. of the molecular formula $\alpha_2{}^A\beta_2{}^{99\ Asp\ -His}$; heterozygotes have polycythemia because of increased oxygen affinity of this h. (see h. Chesapeake).

**unstable h.'s,** a group of rare h.'s with amino acid substitutions (or amino acid deletions in three types) that alter the three-dimensional shape of the globin in a manner that renders the molecule unstable; these h.'s have an increased but variable tendency to auto-oxidation and Heinz body formation and are associated with congenital nonspherocytic hemolytic anemia. The unstable beta chain abnormalities include h.'s Freiburg, Genova, Gun Hill, Hammersmith, Köln, Philly, Sabine, Santa Ana, Sidney, Wien, Zürich; unstable alpha chain abnormalities include h.'s Bibba, Sinai, Torino.

**he'moglobine'mia.** The presence of free hemoglobin in the blood plasma, as when intravascular hemolysis occurs.

**h. paralytica,** azoturia of horses.

**puerperal h.,** postparturient hemoglobinuria.

**hemoglobinocholia** (he'mo-glo'bĭ-no-ko'lī-ah) [ hemoglobin + G. cholē, bile ]. The presence of hemoglobin in the bile.

**he'moglo'binol'ysis** [ hemoglobin + G. lysis, dissolution ]. Destruction or chemical splitting of hemoglobin.

**he′moglo′binom′eter.** Hematinometer; an instrument for estimating the amount of hemoglobin in the blood, indicated in percentages of the normal.

**hemoglobinopathy** (he′mo-glo-bī-nop′ă-thī) [ hemoglobin + G. *pathos,* disease ]. A disorder or disease caused by or associated with the presence of hemoglobins in the blood, *e.g.,* sickle cell disease, thalassemia, hemoglobin C, D, E, H, or I disorders. Occasionally, combinations of abnormal hemoglobins are seen in hemoglobinopathies.

**he′moglo′binopep′sia** [ hemoglobin + G. *pepsis,* digestion ]. Hemoglobinolysis.

**he′moglo′binophil′ic** [ hemoglobin + G. *phileō,* to love ]. Relating to certain microorganisms that cannot be cultured except in the presence of hemoglobin.

**hemoglobinuria** (he′mo-glo-bī-nu′rī-ah) [ hemoglobin + G. *ouron,* urine ]. The presence of hemoglobin in the urine, including certain closely related pigments that are formed from slight alteration of the hemoglobin molecule; when present in sufficient quantities, they result in the urine being colored varying shades from light red-yellow to fairly dark red; due to the Donath-Lansteiner cold autoantibody.

  **bovine h.,** bovine *babesiosis.*

  **epidemic h.,** the presence in the urine of young infants of hemoglobin or of pigments derived from it, and attended with cyanosis, jaundice, etc., in the infant. Epidemic h. may be due to secondary methemoglobinemia.

  **malarial h.,** blackwater fever; bilious remittent fever; hemoglobinuric fever; West African fever; a condition now uncommon, caused by malignant tertian malaria, *Plasmodium falciparum,* frequently seen in Caucasians after interrupted treatment with quinine; possibly an autoimmune disease.

  **march h.,** a form occurring after marathon races, protracted marching, or heavy physical exercise.

  **paroxysmal nocturnal h.,** Marchiafava-Micheli syndrome or anemia; an infrequent disorder with insidious onset and chronic course, characterized by signs of hemolytic anemia, hemoglobinuria (chiefly at night), pallor, icterus or bronzing of the skin, a moderate degree of splenomegaly, and sometimes hepatomegaly. Both sexes are affected, usually in the third or fourth decade; the red blood cells are usually macrocytic and vary considerably in size, but there is no evidence of spherocytosis, erythrophagocytosis, or abnormal leukocytes.

  **postparturient h.,** puerperal h.; puerperal hemoglobinemia; a sudden, severe hemolytic disease that appears sporadically in well nourished dairy cows 2 to 4 weeks after claving, and usually occurs in stabled animals in the winter and early spring; the mortality rate is 10 to 40 per cent; the cause is not known, although the disease is often associated with hypophosphatemia.

  **puerperal h.,** postparturient h.

  **toxic h.,** h. occurring after the ingestion of various poisons, in certain blood diseases, and in certain infections.

**he′moglobinu′ric.** Relating to or marked by hemoglobinuria.

**he′moglob′ulin.** Hemoglobin.

**he′mogram** [ hemo- + G. *gramma,* a drawing ]. A complete, detailed record of the findings in a thorough examination of the blood, especially with reference to the numbers, proportions, and morphologic features of the formed elements.

**he′mohis′tioblast** [ hemo- + G. *histion,* web, + *blastos,* germ ]. Hematohistioblast; a primitive mesenchymal cell believed to be capable of developing into all types of blood cells, including monocytes, and into histiocytes.

**hemoleukocyte** (he′mo-lu′ko-sit). Obsolete term for leukocyte.

**he′molip′ase.** Blood lipase.

**he′molith** [ hemo- + G. *lithos,* stone ]. A concretion in the wall of a blood vessel.

**hemol′ogy.** Hematology.

**he′molymph** [ hemo- + L. *lympha,* clear water ]. 1. The blood and lymph, in the sense of a "circulating tissue." 2. The nutrient fluid of certain invertebrates.

**hemolysate** (he-mol′ī-sāt). Preparation resulting from the lysis of erythrocytes.

**hemolysin** (he-mol′ī-sin). 1. Any substance elaborated by a living agent and capable of causing destruction (*i.e.,* lysis)

of red blood cells and liberation of their hemoglobin. 2. A sensitizing (complement-fixing) antibody that combines with red blood cells of the antigenic type that stimulated formation of the h., affecting the cells in such a manner that complement fixes with the antibody-cell union and causes dissolution of the cells, with liberation of their hemoglobin; sometimes termed amboceptor.

  *α* **h.,** see *α hemolysis.*

  *α′* **h.,** see *α′ hemolysis.*

  *β* **h.,** see *β hemolysis.*

  **bacterial h.,** any hemolytic agent elaborated by various species of bacteria, or by certain strains within a species.

  **cold h.,** the Donath-Landsteiner cold autoantibody; h. which combines with erythrocytes at temperatures below 20°C.

  **heterophil h.,** a sensitizing antibody that can combine with red blood cells of various species (in addition to those used as the antigen in stimulating the formation of the h.), resulting in hemolysis when the proper amount of complement is present.

  **immune h.,** a sensitizing, complement-fixing, hemolytic antibody formed in an animal as the result of parenteral administration of red blood cells or whole blood from another species; immune h. may also be formed in human beings who are transfused with human blood that is antigenic in the recipient, *e.g.,* the formation of anti-Rh antibody in an Rh-negative person who is treated with Rh-positive red blood cells.

  **natural h.,** one occurring in the plasma of an animal of one species, *e.g.,* a dog, which fixes complement with the red blood cells of some other species, *e.g.,* a rabbit, thereby causing hemolysis of the cells of the rabbit, although the dog was not previously exposed to antigenic stimulation with such cells.

  **specific h.,** a sensitizing, complement-fixing, hemolytic antibody that reacts totally or completely with red blood cells of the antigenic type used to stimulate the formation of the h.

  **warm-cold h.,** h. which combines with red blood cells at temperatures below 20°C. and are eluted at warmer temperatures, *e.g.,* 30 to 37°C. See Donath-Landsteiner cold *autoantibody* and hemagglutinating cold *autoantibody.*

**hemolysinogen** (he′mo-li-sin′o-jen). The antigenic material in red blood cells that stimulates the formation of hemolysin.

**hemolysis** (he-mol′ī-sis) [ hemo- + G. *lysis,* destruction ]. Erythrolysis; erythrocytolysis; hematolysis; the alteration, dissolution, or destruction of red blood cells in such a manner that hemoglobin is liberated into the medium in which the cells are suspended. H. may be caused by specific complement-fixing antibodies, toxins, various chemical agents, tonicity, freezing and thawing, heating, and so on.

  *α* **h.,** an incomplete type of h. observed in blood agar, with many erythrocytes being destroyed (*i.e.,* no longer recognizable) in an irregular, indistinctly outlined, comparatively narrow zone (*e.g.,* 1 or 2 mm.) immediately surrounding a bacterial colony, whereas moderate numbers of erythrocytes remain apparently intact; the agar and recognizable erythrocytes are usually discolored, green to relatively dark green-brown; around the discolored zone, there is a second, irregular, vaguely delimited, narrow, peripheral zone of fairly clear agar in which there are only a few intact erythrocytes, the others having been lysed. When the typical discoloration occurs, the process is termed viridans h., and this is the usual form of *α* hemolysis; on the other hand, *α* hemolysis may occur without the greening change.

  *α′* **h.,** observed infrequently in blood agar cultures of occasional strains of streptococci; the zone of h. about the colony is not as clear, or wide, or distinctly outlined as it is in *β* hemolysis; there are a few, apparently intact erythrocytes throughout the zone, but they are more numerous in the immediate vicinity of the colony, and there is no discoloration (as there is in viridans h.); the unique feature is that the zone becomes wider, *i.e.,* the process is stimulated, when the culture is incubated at refrigerator temperatures (not true for *β* hemolysis). Some strains of streptococci that are *α′*-hemolytic on horse blood agar cause typical viridans h. on rabbit blood agar.

$\beta$ **h.,** complete or "true" h. observed in blood agar cultures of various bacteria, especially hemolytic streptococci and staphylococci; virtually all of the erythrocytes are destroyed in a relatively wide, regularly circumscribed, circular zone about the colony, thereby resulting in a clear "halo" of transparent agar; the zone of h. is frequently much wider than the diameter of the colony. The degree of change varies with species of erythrocytes, *e.g.*, those of sheep and rabbits are usually more easily hemolyzed than those of man, and so on. The hemolysin acts extracellularly (in the absence of the bacterial cells) and may be quantitatively estimated by means of tube-dilution tests of a bacteria-free filtrate (containing the hemolytic substance) with a suspension of erythrocytes.

$\gamma$ **h.,** a term sometimes used to indicate that there is no h. in relation to bacterial colonies in or on blood agar; thus, nonhemolytic organisms may be referred to as producing $\gamma$ h.

**biologic h.,** h. caused by agents elaborated by various animal and plant forms.

**conditioned h.,** immune h.

**immune h.,** conditioned h.; h. caused by complement when erythrocytes have been sensitized by specific complement-fixing antibody.

**venom h.,** that caused by hemolytic material in the venom of various species of snakes or other venomous animals.

**viridans h.,** see $\alpha$ h.

**hemolysoid** (he-mol′ĭ-soyd) [ hemolysin + G. *eidos*, resemblance ]. A nonhemolyzing hemolysin, *i.e.*, sensitizing antibody altered in such a manner that it combines with erythrocytes (the specific antigen), but complement cannot fix with the antigen-antibody union, and hemolysis does not occur. In accordance with the Ehrlich side chain theory (now generally discarded), h. was regarded as a hemolysin that had lost its toxophore group, although the haptophore group remained.

**he′molyt′ic.** Hematolytic; globulicidal; hemotoxic (2); destructive to blood cells, resulting in liberation of hemoglobin.

**he′molyza′tion.** The production or occurrence of hemolysis.

**hemolyze** (he′mo-liz). To produce hemolysis or liberation of the hemoglobin from red blood cells.

**he′momanom′eter.** Hematomanometer; a manometer constructed and calibrated in such a manner that it is suitable for determining blood pressure.

**hemomediastinum** (he′mo-me′dĭ-ă-sti′num). Hematomediastinum; effusion of blood into the mediastinum.

**hemom′eter** [ hemo- + G. *metron*, measure ]. Hemoglobinometer; also used infrequently as a term for hemocytometer.

**Fleischl's h.,** an instrument for estimating the percentage of hemoglobin in the blood, by comparing a definite dilution of a drop of blood with a wedge-shaped piece of ruby glass under water.

**he′mome′tra.** Hematometra.

**hemom′etry.** Hematometry.

**hemonchosis** (he-mong-ko′sis). Infection of sheep or other ruminants with *Haemonchus contortus.*

**hemonephrosis** (he′mo-ne-fro′sis) [ hemo- + G. *nephros*, kidney ]. An accumulation of blood in the pelvis of the kidney.

**he′monor′moblast.** Erythroblast.

**he′mopathol′ogy.** Hematopathology.

**hemopathy** (he-mop′ă-thi) [ hemo- + G. *pathos*, suffering ]. Hematopathy; any abnormal condition or disease of the blood or hemopoietic tissues.

**he′mopericar′dium.** An effusion of blood into the pericardial sac; hematopericardium.

**hemoperitoneum** (he′mo-pĕr′ĭ-kar′dĭ-um). Hematoperitoneum; effusion of blood into the peritoneal cavity.

**he′mopex′in.** A serum protein related to $\beta$-globulins, with molecular weight around 70,000, containing 20 per cent carbohydrate, consisting of sialic acid, mannose, galactose, fructose, and hexosamine. Important in binding heme and porphyrins, perhaps regulating heme in drug metabolism.

**hemophagia** (he′mo-fa′je-ah). Hematophagia.

**hemophagocyte** (he′mo-fag′o-sit) [ hemo- + phagocyte, *q.v.* ]. Hematophagocyte; a phagocytic cell that engulfs and

usually destroys blood cells, especially erythrocytes and others of the erythroid series.

**hemophagocytosis** (he′mo-fag′o-si-to′sis). The process of engulfment (and usually destruction) of blood cells by the various types of phagocytic cells; used especially with reference to the engulfment of erythrocytes and others of the erythroid series.

**hemophil, hemophile** (he′mo-fil, -fil) [ hemo- + G. *philos*, fond ]. Applied to microorganisms growing preferably in media containing blood.

**hemophilia** (he′mo-fil′ĭ-ah) [ hemo- + G. *philos*, fond ]. Hematophilia; angiostaxis; an inherited disorder of the blood marked by a permanent tendency to hemorrhages, spontaneous or traumatic, due to a defect in the coagulating power of the blood.

**h. A.,** h. due to deficiency of factor VIII (see under factor); a sex-linked recessive condition affecting males.

**h. B.,** Christmas disease; a clotting disorder caused by the hereditary deficiency of plasma thromboplastic component (clotting factor IX).

**renal h.,** renal *epistaxis.*

**vascular h.,** von Willebrand's *disease.*

**he′mophil′iac.** A person suffering from hemophilia.

**hemophilic** (he-mo-fil′ik). Relating to hemophilia.

**Hemoph′ilus.** *Haemophilus.*

**he′mopho′bia** [ hemo- + G. *phobos*, fear ]. A morbid fear of blood or of bleeding.

**hemophoresis** (he′mo-fo-re′sis) [ hemo- + G. *phoreō*, to bear ]. Blood convection or irrigation of tissues.

**hemophthalmia** (he′mof-thal′mĭ-ah) [ hemo- + G. *ophthalmos*, eye ]. An effusion of blood into the eyeball.

**he′mophthal′mus.** Hemophthalmia.

**hemophthisis** (he-mof′thĭ-sis, he′mof-thi′sis) [ hemo- + G. *phthisis*, a wasting away ]. Anemia resulting from (1) abnormal degeneration or destruction, or (2) a deficiency in the formation of red blood cells.

**hemopiezometer** (he′mo-pi′e-zom′e-ter) [ hemo- + G. *piezein*, to press, + *metron*, measure ]. Any apparatus for measuring blood pressure.

**he′moplas′tic.** Hemopoietic.

**hemoplasty** (he′mo-plas′ti) [ hemo- + G. *plassō*, to form ]. The formation or elaboration of blood by the hemopoietic tissues.

**hemopneumopericardium** (he′mo-nu′mo-pĕr-ĭ-kar-dī′um). Pneumohemopericardium; the occurrence of blood and air in the pericardium, resulting from disease or injury.

**hemopneumothorax** (he′mo-nu′mo-tho′raks) [ hemo- + G. *pneuma*, air, + thorax ]. Accumulation of air and blood in the pleural cavity.

**hemopoiesis** (he′mo-poy-e′sis) [ hemo- + G. *poiēsis*, a making ]. Hematopoiesis; hematosis (1); sanguification; the process of formation and development of the various types of blood cells and other formed elements.

**hemopoietic** (he′mo-poy-et′ik). Hemafacient; hematopoietic; hematoplastic; sanguifacient; pertaining to or related to the formation of blood cells.

**hemopoietin** (hēm-o-poy′ē-tin). Erythropoietin.

**hemoporphyrin** (he′mo-por′fĭ-rin). The prophyrin component of heme.

**he′moprecip′itin.** An antibody that combines with and precipitates soluble antigenic material from erythrocytes.

**he′mopro′tein.** Protein linked to a metal-porphyrin compound; hemoglobins, catalases, peroxidases (iron), chlorophyll (magnesium) are examples.

**hemop′sonin.** An antibody that combines with erythrocytes (the specific antigen) and sensitizes the cells in such a manner that they are more susceptible to phagocytosis; erythrocytopsonin; hemotropin.

**hemoptysis** (he-mop′tĭ-sis) [ hemo- + G. *ptysis*, a spitting ]. Pulmonary hemorrhage; the spitting of blood derived from the lungs or bronchial tubes.

**cardiac h.,** h. secondary to heart disease or tachycardia.

**endemic h.,** paragonimiasis.

**parasitic h.,** paragonimiasis.

**hemopyelectasis, hemopyelectasia** (he′mo-pi′ē-lek′tă-sis, -pi′ē-lek-ta′zi-ah) [ hemo- + pyelectasia, *q.v.* ]. Dilation of the pelvis of the kidney with blood and urine.

**he′morepel′lant.** 1. A substance or surface that discourages the adherence of blood. 2. Having such an action.

**hemorheology** (hem′o-re-ol′o-ji) [ hemo- + G. *rheō*, to flow, + *logos*, study ]. The science of rheology of the blood; the relation of pressures, flow, volumes, and resistances in blood vessels.

**hemorrhachis** (he-mor′ă-kis). Hematorrhachis.

**hemorrhage** (hem′ō-rij) [ G. *haimorrhagia*, fr. *haima*, blood, + *rhēgnymi*, to burst forth. RHAG- ]. Bleeding; a flow of blood, especially if it is very profuse.

   **accidental h.,** term used principally by British obstetricians as a synonym for abruptio placentae.

   **brainstem h.,** a secondary form of intracranial h. caused by brainstem compression exerted from above in instances of rapidly expanding intracranial lesions.

   **bronchial h.,** hemoptysis.

   **cerebral h.,** h. into the substance of the cerebrum, usually in the region of the internal capsule by the rupture of the lenticulostriate artery.

   **concealed h.,** internal h.

   **extradural h.,** epidural hematoma; an accumulation of blood between the skull and the dura mater.

   **gastric h.,** hemorrhage into the stomach.

   **intermediate h.,** h. that is recurrent.

   **internal h.,** concealed h.; bleeding into one of the organs or cavities of the body.

   **intestinal h.,** enterorrhagia; any bleeding within the intestinal tract.

   **intracerebral h.,** extravasation of blood within the brain substance.

   **intracranial h.,** escape of blood within the cranium due to loss of integrity of vascular channels, frequently leading to formation of hematoma (localized accumulation of blood).

   **intrapartum h.,** h. occurring in the course of normal labor and delivery.

   **intraventricular h.,** extravasation of blood into the ventricular system of the brain.

   **nasal h.,** epistaxis.

   **parenchymatous h.,** an escape of blood into the substance of an organ.

   **h. per rhex′is,** h. due to the rupture of a blood vessel.

   **petechial h.,** punctate h.; capillary h. into the skin, forming petechiae.

   **pontine h.,** h. occurring in the substance of the pons, typically in hypertensive patients.

   **postpartum h.,** h. from the birth canal in excess of 500 ml. during the first 24 hours after birth.

   **primary h.,** h. occurring immediately upon receipt of the injury, distinguished from intermediate or secondary h.

   **pulmonary h.,** hemoptysis.

   **punctate h.,** petechial h.

   **renal h.,** hematuria.

   **secondary h.,** h. occurring at a more or less considerable interval after an injury or an operation.

   **serous h.,** profuse transudation of plasma through the walls of the capillaries, as in serous diarrhea.

   **splinter h.,** linear subungual h. typically seen in but not diagnostic of bacterial endocarditis.

   **subarachnoid h.,** extravasation of blood into the subarachnoid space, usually spreading throughout the cerebrospinal fluid pathways.

   **subdural h.,** subdural hematoma; hemorrhagic pachymeningitis; extravasation of blood between the dural and arachnoidal membranes; chronic hematomas may become encapsulated by neomembranes.

   **subgaleal h.,** collection of blood beneath the galea aponeurotica.

   **unavoidable h.,** h. occurring during labor in cases of placenta previa, distinguished from accidental h. (British).

**hemorrhagenic** (hem-ō-ră-jen′ik) [ hemorrhage + G. *genesis*, production ]. Causing hemorrhage.

**hemorrhagic** (hem-ō-raj′ik). Relating to or marked by hemorrhage.

**hemorrhagins** (hem′o-raj′inz, -ra′jins). A group of toxins found in certain venoms and poisonous material from some plants, *e.g.*, rattlesnake venom and ricin; h. causes degeneration and lysis of endothelial cells in capillaries and small vessels, thereby resulting in numerous small hemorrhages in the tissues.

**hemorrhagiparous** (hem′ō-ră-jip′ă-rus) [ hemorrhage + L. *pario*, to produce ]. Hemorrhagenic.

**hemorrhea** (hem′o-re′ah) [ G. *haimorrhoia*, fr. *haima*, blood, + *rhoia*, a flow ]. Hemorrhage.

**hemorrhoid** (hem′o-royd) [ see hemorrhoids ]. Denoting one of the tumors or varices constituting piles or hemorrhoids; see hemorrhoids.

**hemorrhoidal** (hem-o-roy′dal). 1. Relating to hemorrhoids. 2. Applied to certain arteries supplying the region of the rectum and anus; see *arteria rectalis*.

**hemorrhoidectomy** (hem′o-roy-dek′to-mi) [ hemorrhoids + G. *ektomē*, excision ]. An operation for the cure of hemorrhoids.

**hem′orrhoidol′ysis** [ hemorrhoids + G. *lysis*, destruction ]. The dissolution of hemorrhoids.

**hemorrhoids** (hem′o-roydz) [ G. *haimorrhois*, pl. *haimorrhoides*, veins likely to bleed, fr. *haima*, blood, + *rhoia*, a flow ]. Piles; a varicose condition of the external hemorrhoidal veins causing painful swellings at the anus. When the dilated veins form tumors to the outer side of the external sphincter, or are covered by the skin of the anal canal, the condition is called **external h.**; when the swollen veins are beneath the mucous membrane within the sphincter it is called **internal h.**

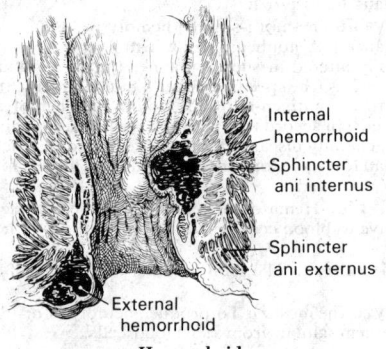

Internal hemorrhoid
Sphincter ani internus
Sphincter ani externus
External hemorrhoid

**Hemorrhoids**

   **cuta′neous h.,** hyperplasia of the connective tissue in one or more of the normal radiating folds of the skin immediately surrounding the anus.

**he′mosal′pinx.** Hematosalpinx.

**he′moscope.** Hematoscope.

**he′mosen′sitin.** Antigenic material that may be adsorbed on the surface of red blood cells, by means of mixing and incubating the reagents at 37°C.; cells treated with a h. may be used in identifying specific antibody in a serum, inasmuch as the latter (in various proportions) causes lysis or agglutination of the coated cells.

**he′mosi′alem′esis** [ hemo- + G. *sialon*, saliva, + *emesis*, vomiting ]. Vomiting of blood and saliva.

**he′mosid′erin.** Golden yellow or yellow-brown insoluble product of phagocytic digestion of hematin; it contains up to 37 per cent dry weight of iron and stains blue with potassium ferrocyanide.

**he′mosidero′sis.** The accumulation of hemosiderin in tissue.

   **nutritional h.,** a disease seen in native Africans; it results from an unbalanced diet that is deficient in maize and probably in protein, and perhaps also contains toxic materials; there is excessive absorption of iron. The liver is chiefly affected.

   **pulmonary h.,** usually associated with mitral stenosis; marked by an accumulation of macrophages loaded with hemosiderin within the alveoli.

**he′mosper′mia** [ hemo- + G. *sperma*, seed ]. Hematospermia; the presence of blood in the seminal fluid.

   **h. spuria,** h. occurring in the prostatic urethra.

   **h. vera,** h. in which the bleeding is from the seminal vesicles.

**he′mosporid′ium.** A blood parasite of the order Haemosporidia.

**he′mosporines.** Common term for members of the order Haemosporidia.

**he′mosta′sia.** Hemostasis.

**hemostasis** (he-mos′tă-sis, he′mo-sta′sis) [ hemo- + G. *stasis*, a standing ]. Hemostasia. 1. The arrest of bleeding. 2. The arrest of the circulation in the blood vessels of a part. 3. Stagnation of blood.

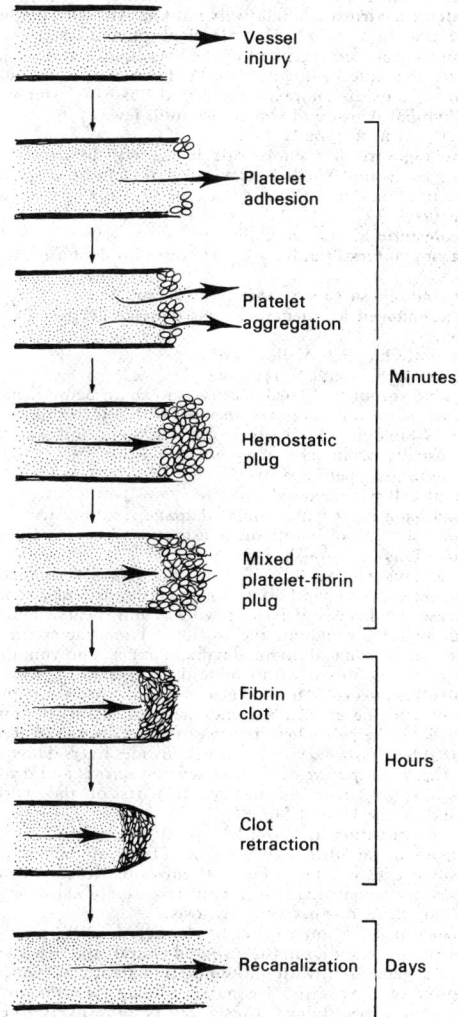

**Hemostasis**

Morphological events of hemostasis. (Modified after Harker, L. A.: *Hemostasis Manual*, University of Washington, Seattle, 1969.)

**he′mostat.** 1. Any agent that arrests, chemically or mechanically, the flow of blood from an open vessel. 2. An instrument for arresting hemorrhage by compression of the bleeding vessel.

**he′mostat′ic.** 1. Arresting the flow of blood within the vessels. 2. Arresting hemorrhage; styptic.

**he′mostyp′tic** [ hemo- + G. *styptikos*, astringent ]. Styptic.

**hemotachometer** (he′mo-tă-kom′e-ter) [ hemo- + G. *tachos*, swiftness, + *metron*, measure ]. Hematachometer; an instrument for measuring the rapidity of the flow of blood in the arteries.

**hemotherapeutics** (he′mo-thĕr-ă-pu′tiks). The use of blood (either transfusion from a human or drinking the blood of animals) in the treatment of disease.

**he′mother′apy.** Hemotherapeutics.

**he′motho′rax.** Hematothorax; an effusion of blood into the pleural cavity.

**he′mothy′mia** [ hemo- + G. *thymos*, desire, anger ]. Passion for blood; an insane impulse to murder.

**he′motox′ic.** Hematotoxic. 1. Causing blood poisoning. 2. Hemolytic.

**he′motox′in.** Any substance that causes destruction of red blood cells, including various hemolysins; usually used with reference to substances of biologic origin, in contrast to chemicals, such as acids, alkalies, and so on.
  **cobra h.,** the constituent in cobra venom that hemolyzes the red blood cells of various species.

**hemotroph, hemotrophe** (he′mo-trof) [ hemo- + G. *trophē*, food ]. The materials supplied to the embryos of placental mammals through the maternal blood stream.

**he′motrop′ic** [ hemo- + G. *tropos*, a turning ]. Pertaining to the mechanism by which a substance in or on blood cells, especially the erythrocytes, attracts phagocytic cells; the latter change direction and migrate toward the h. cells.

**hemot′ropin.** A substance that manifests a hemotropic effect on phagocytic cells, including hemopsonin and erythrocytopsonin.

**he′motym′panum.** The presence of blood in the middle ear.

**he′mozo′ic.** Parasitic in the blood of vertebrates; denoting certain protozoa.

**he′mozo′in.** Name given to a mixture of degradation products of hemoglobin brought about by microorganisms, involving denaturation of hemoglobin, oxidation of the iron, and partial digestion of the protein moiety (globin). It may accumulate in conspicuous quantities in the spleen, liver, and brain of persons with malaria, particularly falciparum malaria.

**he′mozo′on** [ hemo- + G. *zoön*, animal ]. Hematozoon; a protozoan or metazoan parasite that lives in the circulating blood of the host during a part or all of its life cycle.

**hemp** [ A.S. *henep* ]. The herbaceous plants of the genus *Cannabis.*
  **American h.,** *Cannabis sativa* var. *americana.*
  **Canadian h.,** *Apocynum cannabinum.*
  **Indian h.,** *Cannabis sativa* var. *indica.*

**HEMPAS.** See HEMPAS *cells.*

**hemuresis** (hem-u-re′sis). Hematuria.

**hen′bane.** Hyoscyamus.

**Hench,** Philip S., U. S. physician *1896. Nobel laureate, 1950, with Edward C. Kendall and Tadeus Reichstein, for their discoveries relating to the hormones of the adrenal cortex.

**Henderson,** Lawrence J., U.S. biochemist, 1879–1942. See H.-Hasselbalch *equation.*

**Henke,** Wilhelm, German anatomist, 1834–1896. See H.'s *space.*

**Henle,** Friedrich G. J., German anatomist, pathologist, and histologist, 1809–1885. See Hassall-H. *bodies,* H.'s *ampulla, ansa, fissures, layer,* nervous *layer,* outer fiber *layer* of H., H.'s *loop, membrane,* fenestrated *membrane, reaction, sheath, spine, tubules, warts.*

**henna** (hen′ah) [ Ar. *hennā* ]. The leaves of Egyptian privet, *Lawsonia inermis.* Used as a cosmetic and hair dye.

**Henoch,** Eduard H., German pediatrician, 1820–1910. See H.'s *angina,* H.-Schönlein *purpura.*

**henpu′ye** [ native term on the Gold Coast meaning "dog-nose" ]. Goundou.

**Henry,** Joseph, American physicist, 1797–1878. Gave his name to the henry. See Dalton-H. *law.*

**Henry,** William, English chemist, 1775–1837. See H.'s *law.*

**henry** (hen′rī) [ J. *Henry* ]. The unit of electrical induction; symbol *H.*

**Henseleit,** K. See Krebs-H. *cycle.*

**Hensen,** Victor, German anatomist and physiologist, 1835–1924. See H.'s *canal, cell, disk, duct, knot, line, node, stripe.*

**Hensing,** Friedrich W., German anatomist, 1719–1745. See H.'s *ligament*.

**he′par,** gen. **he′patis** [ L. borrowed fr. G. *hēpar*, gen. *hēpatos*, the liver ] [ NA ]. The liver.

**h. lobatum,** a fissured liver, from the scars of healed syphilitic gummas.

**hep′aran sulfate.** Heparitin sulfate.

**hep′arin.** A complex anticoagulant principle first isolated from canine liver, then from bovine liver and lung, and now known to be a constituent of various tissue (especially liver and lung) and mast cells in several mammalian species. The principle and active constituent is a mucopolysaccharide comprised of D-glucuronic acid and D-glucosamine, both sulfated, in 1,4-α linkage, molecular weight approximately 17,000. In conjunction with a serum protein cofactor (the so-called heparin cofactor), h. is an antithrombin and an antiprothrombin; it prevents platelet agglutination and thus prevents thrombus formation. H. also enhances activity of "clearing factors" (lipoprotein lipases). H. is destroyed by h. lyase, *q.v.*

**h. eliminase,** h. lyase.

**h. lyase** (EC 4.2.2.7), formerly heparinase (EC 3.3.1.19); h. eliminase; enzyme eliminating Δ-4,5-D-glucuronate residues from heparin and similar 1,4-linked polyglucuronates.

**h. sodium** (USP, BP), a mixture of active principles (usually obtained from various tissues of domestic animals) having the properties of prolonging the clotting time of human blood; used in the treatment of angina pectoris, intermittent claudication, coronary thrombosis, and similar conditions.

**hep′arinase** Heparin lyase.

**hep′arine′mia.** The presence of demonstrable levels of heparin in the circulating blood.

**hep′arinize.** A colloquial term pertaining to the therapeutic administration of heparin.

**hep′aritin sulfate.** Heparan sulfate; a heteropolysaccharide resembling heparin, consisting of a repeating disaccharide of sulfated D-glucuronate and D-glucosamine; found in tissues of individuals with Hurler's disease.

**hepat-, hepatico-, hepato-** [ G. *hēpar* (*hēpat-*), liver ]. Combining forms denoting the liver.

**hepatalgia** (hep′ă-tal′jĭ-ah) [ hepat- + G. *algos*, pain ]. Hepatodynia; pain in the liver.

**hepatatrophia, hepatatrophy** (hep′ă-tă-tro′fĭ-ah, hep′ă-tat′ro-fĭ). *Atrophy* of the liver.

**hepatectomy** (hep′ă-tek′to-mĭ) [ hepat- + G. *ektomē*, excision ]. Removal of a part of the liver in man; or complete removal of the liver in an experimental animal. See also reverse Eck *fistula*.

**hepat′ic** [ G. *hēpatikos* ]. Relating to the liver.

**hepatico-.** See hepat-.

**hepaticodochotomy** (he-pat′ĭ-ko-do-kot′o-mĭ). Combined choledochotomy and hepaticotomy.

**hepaticoduodenostomy** (he-pat′ĭ-ko-du′o-de-nos′to-mĭ) [ hepatico- + duodenostomy ]. Establishment of artificial communication between the hepatic duct and the duodenum.

**hepaticoenterostomy** (he-pat′ĭ-ko-en-ter-os′to-mĭ) [ hepatico- + enterostomy ]. Hepatocholangioenterostomy; establishment of an artificial communication between the hepatic duct and the intestine.

**hepaticogastrostomy** (he-pat′ĭ-ko-gas-tros′to-mĭ) [ hepatico- + gastrostomy ]. Establishment of a communication between the hepatic duct and the stomach.

**hepat′icolithot′omy** [ hepatico- + G. *lithos*, stone, + *tomē*, a cutting ]. Removal of a stone from a hepatic duct.

**hepaticolithotripsy** (he-pat′ĭ-ko-lith′o-trip-sĭ) [ hepatico- + G. *lithos*, stone, + *tripsis*, a rubbing ]. The crushing of a biliary calculus in the hepatic duct.

**hepat′icopul′monary.** Hepatopneumonic.

**hepaticostomy** (he-pat′ĭ-kos′to-mĭ) [ hepatico- + G. *stoma*, mouth ]. The operative establishment of a permanent opening into the hepatic duct.

**hepaticotomy** (he-pat′ĭ-kot′o-mĭ) [ hepatico- + G. *tomē*, incision ]. Incision into the hepatic duct.

**hep′atin.** Glycogen.

**hepatit′ic.** Relating to hepatitis.

**hepatitis** (hep′ă-ti′tis) [ hepat- + G. suffix -*itis*, inflammation ]. Inflammation of the liver, usually from a viral infection, sometimes from toxic agents.

**h. A,** viral h. type A.

**active chronic h.,** subacute h.; juvenile cirrhosis; posthepatitic cirrhosis; liver disease that evolves from a persisting h. and usually progresses to a coarsely nodular postnecrotic cirrhosis; see also plasma cell h. and lupoid h.

**acute parenchy′matous h.,** acute yellow atrophy of the liver; see under atrophy.

**anicter′ic virus h.,** a relatively mild h., without jaundice, and due to a virus. The principal physical signs and symptoms are enlargement of the liver, lymph nodes, and often the spleen, together with headache, continuous fatigue, nausea, anorexia, sudden distaste for smoking, abdominal pains, and sometimes mild fever.

**h. B,** viral h. type B.

**cholangiolitic h.,** cholestatic h.; h. with inflammatory changes around small bile ducts, producing mainly obstructive jaundice. The disease may be due to viral infection.

**cholestatic h.,** cholangiolitic h.

**chronic intersti′tial h.,** obsolete term for cirrhosis of the liver.

**h. contagio′sa ca′nis,** infectious canine h.

**drug-induced h.,** hepatocellular damage produced by a drug.

**enzootic h.,** Rift Valley *fever*.

**epidemic h.,** viral h. type A.

**equine serum h.,** Theiler's disease (2); an acute hepatic disease of the horse, often associated with prior administration of biological products; neurologic signs and jaundice are usually prominent signs; etiology is unknown.

**h. exter′na,** perihepatitis.

**giant cell h.,** neonatal h.

**halothane h.,** hepatocellular damage resulting from the administration of halothane anesthesia.

**infectious h.,** viral h. type A.

**infectious canine h.,** h. contagiosa canis; Rubarth's disease; a specific viral disease of dogs; the virus also causes disease in foxes, wolves, coyotes, and bears, and is widespread throughout the world; it is characterized by fever, leukopenia, abdominal pain, diarrhea, and vomiting; frequently confused with canine distemper in the past.

**infectious necrotic h. of sheep,** black disease (so named because of the extensive hemorrhages seen on the inner surface of the pelt when it is removed); a disease of sheep caused by *Clostridium novyi*, which invades livers damaged by *Fasciola hepatica* and causes severe necrosis and death; this disease occurs in nearly all parts of the world, including the United States.

**long incubation h.,** viral h. type B.

**lupoid h.,** jaundice with evidence of liver cell damage and positive L.E. cell tests, but without evidence of systemic lupus erythematosus. Liver biopsies usually show active chronic h. or postnecrotic cirrhosis.

**neonatal h.,** giant cell h.; h. characterized by onset of obstructive jaundice in the neonatal period, and hepatocellular degeneration with multinucleated giant cell transformation of liver cells. Neonatal h. may be difficult to distinguish from biliary atresia, but is more likely to end with recovery, although cirrhosis may develop. The cause is unknown.

**peliosis h.,** purpura with hepatitis sometimes resulting from hypoprothrombinemia.

**plasma cell h.,** active chronic h. with plasma cell infiltration of the liver, occurring mostly in women and children; characterized by amenorrhea, arthritis, high γ-globulins, and sometimes with positive L.E. cell tests.

**serum h.,** viral h. type B.

**short incubation h.,** viral h. type A.

**subacute h.,** active chronic h.

**suppurative h.,** h. with abscess formation; often amebic in origin.

**transfusion h.,** viral h. type B.

**viral h.,** either viral h. type A or viral h. type B; in the acute stage both types are characterized by necrosis of scattered liver cells and periportal inflammation, mainly by lymphocytes.

**viral h. type A,** infectious h.; virus A h.; h. A; epidemic h.; short incubation h.; a virus disease with a short incubation period (usually 15 to 40 days), caused by hepatitis virus A (infectious hepatitis virus); the disease may be inapparent, mild, severe, and occasionally fatal; it is commonly seen in epidemics, and transmission is by the fecal-oral route; necrosis of liver cells is characteristic and jaundice is a common symptom; γ-Globulin may be preventive.

**viral h. type B,** serum h.; virus B h.; h. B; transfusion h.; long incubation h.; a virus disease with a long incubation period (usually 60 to 160 days); the disease is caused by hepatitis virus B (serum hepatitis virus), which usually is transmitted by injection of infected blood or blood derivatives or merely by use of contaminated needles, lancets, or other instruments; Clinically and pathologically, the disease is similar to viral h. type A (infectious h.); however, there is no cross-protective immunity.

**virus A h.,** viral h. type A.

**virus B h.,** viral h. type B.

**virus h. of ducks,** a virus disease of very young ducklings, manifested by an acute illness of several days followed by death; the principal lesions are an enlarged liver filled with ecchymotic hemorrhages.

**hepatization** (hep'ă-tī-za'shun). The conversion of a loose tissue into a firm mass like the substance of the liver; denoting especially such a change in the lungs in the consolidation of pneumonia.

**gray h.,** the second stage of h. in pneumonia, when the exudate is beginning to degenerate prior to breaking down; the color is a yellowish gray or mottled.

**red h.,** the first stage of h. in which the exudate is blood-stained.

**yellow h.,** the final stage of h. in which the exudate is becoming purulent.

**hepato-.** See hepat-.

**hep'atoblasto'ma.** A malignant neoplasm occurring in children, primary in the liver, composed of tissue resembling fetal or mature liver cells or bile ducts.

**hep'atocarcino'ma.** Malignant *hepatoma.*

**hepatocele** (hep'ă-to-sēl, he-pat'o-sēl) [ hepato- + G. *kēlē,* hernia ]. Hernia of the liver; protrusion of part of the liver through the abdominal wall or the diaphragm.

**hep'atocer'ebral.** Indicating a relationship between the liver and the brain, particularly such as prevails in hepatic coma, with neurologic abnormalities.

**hepatocholangioenterostomy** (hep'ă-to-ko-lan'jī-o-en-ter-os'to-mĭ) [ hepato- + G. *cholē,* bile, + *angeion,* vessel, + *enteron,* intestine, + *stoma,* mouth ]. Hepaticoenterostomy.

**hepatocholangiojejunostomy** (hep'ă-to-ko-lan'jī-o-je-ju-nos'to-mĭ) [ hepato- + G. *cholē,* bile, + *angeion,* vessel, + *jejunostomy* ]. Implantation of hepatic duct into the jejunum.

**hepatocholangiostomy** (hep-ă-to-ko-lan-jī-os'to-mĭ). Opening into the common bile duct to establish free drainage.

**hepatocholangitis** (hep'ă-to-ko-lan-ji'tis). Inflammation of the liver and biliary tree.

**hepatocirrhosis** (hep'ă-to-sĭ-ro'sis). *Cirrhosis* of the liver.

**hepatocuprein** (hep'ă-to-ku'pre-in). A copper-containing protein found in ox liver.

**hep'atocys'tic** [ hepato- + G. *kystis,* bladder ]. Relating to the gallbladder, or to both liver and gallbladder.

**Hepatocystis** (hep'ă-to-sis'tis) [ hepato- + G. *kystis,* bladder ]. A genus of blood-parasitizing sporozoans in the family Plasmodiidae with gametocytes in red cells and cystlike exoerythrocytic schizonts in the liver parenchyma; parasitic in lower primates, rodents, bats, and hippopotami.

**hep'atocyte.** A parenchymal liver cell.

**hep'atoduodenos'tomy.** Hepaticoduodenostomy.

**hep'atodyn'ia** [ hepato- + G. *odynē,* pain ]. Hepatalgia.

**hep'atodys'entery.** Dysentery associated with liver disease.

**hep'atodys'trophy.** Dystrophy of the liver.

**hepatoenteric** (hep'ă-to-en-tĕr'ik) [ hepato- + G. *enteron,* intestine ]. Relating to the liver and the intestine.

**hep'atogas'tric.** Relating to the liver and the stomach.

**hepatogenic, hepatogenous** (hep-ă-to-jen'ik, hep-ă-toj'-en-us). Of hepatic origin; formed in the liver.

**hepatog'raphy** [ hepato- + G. *graphē,* a writing ]. 1. Roentgenography of the liver. 2. A treatise on the liver.

**hepatohemia** (hep'ă-to-he'mĭ-ah) [ hepato- + G. *haima,* blood ]. Congestion of the liver.

**hepatoid** (hep'ă-toyd) [ hepato- + G. *eidos,* resemblance ]. Resembling or like the liver.

**hep'atojug'ularom'eter** [ hepato- + L. *jugulum,* throat, + G. *metron,* measure ]. An apparatus for the quantitative control and measurement of the pressure and force applied over the liver in the hepatojugular reflux test.

**hepatolienography** (hep'ă-to-li-en-og'ră-fī) [ hepato- + L. *lien,* spleen, + G. *graphē,* a writing ]. 1. Hepatosplenography. 2. A treatise on the liver and spleen.

**hep'atolie'nomeg'aly.** Hepatosplenomegaly.

**hep'atolith** [ hepato- + G. *lithos,* stone ]. A biliary calculus; concretion in the liver.

**hepatolithectomy** (hep'ă-to-lī-thek40 to-mĭ) [ hepato- + G. *lithos,* stone, + *ektomē,* excision ]. Operative removal of a calculus from the liver.

**hepatolithiasis** (hep'ă-to-lī-thi'ă-sis) [ hepato- + G. *lithiasis,* presence of a calculus ]. The presence of calculi in the liver.

**hepatol'ogist.** One skilled in a knowledge of the diseases of the liver.

**hepatology** (hep'ă-tol'o-jī) [ hepato- + G. *logos,* study ]. The branch of medical science treating especially of the liver.

**hepatolysin** (hep-ă-tol'ĭ-sin). A cytolysin that destroys parenchymal cells of the liver.

**hepato'ma** [ hepato- + G. suffix -*oma,* tumor ]. See malignant h.

**malignant h.,** hepatocellular carcinoma; hepatocarcinoma; hepatoma; liver cell carcinoma; a carcinoma derived from parenchymal cells of the liver.

**hepatomalacia** (hep'ă-to-mă-la'shī-ah) [ hepato- + G. *malakia,* softening ]. Softening of the liver.

**hep'atomega'lia.** Hepatomegaly.

**hepatomegaly** (hep'ă-to-meg'ă-lī) [ hepato- + G. *megas,* large ]. Hepatomegalia; megalohepatia; enlargement of the liver.

**hepatomelanosis** (hep'ă-to-mel'ă-no'sis) [ hepato- + G. *melas,* black, + suffix -*osis,* condition ]. Deep pigmentation of the liver.

**hepatomphalocele** (hep'ă-tom-fal'o-sēl, -tom'fă-lo-sēl) [ hepato- + omphalocele, *q.v.* ]. Umbilical hernia with involvment of the liver.

**hep'atom'phalos.** Hepatomphalocele.

**hepatonecrosis** (hep'ă-to-ne-kro'sis). Death of liver cells leading to gangrene or acute yellow atrophy.

**hepatonephric** (hep'ă-to-nef'rik). Relating to the liver and the kidney.

**hepatonephromegaly** (hep'ă-to-nef'ro-meg'ă-lī) [ hepato- + G. *nephros,* kidney, + *megas,* great ]. Enlargement of both liver and kidney or kidneys.

**hep'atopath'ic.** Damaging the liver.

**hepatopathy** (hep'ă-top'ă-thī) [ hepato- + G. *pathos,* suffering ]. A disease of the liver.

**hepatoperitonitis** (hep'ă-to-pĕr'ĭ-to-ni'tis). Perihepatitis.

**hep'atopex'y** [ hepato- + G. *pēxis,* fixation ]. The anchoring of a movable liver to the abdominal wall.

**hepatophyma** (hep'ă-to-fi'mah) [ hepato- + G. *phyma,* tumor ]. Rounded or nodular tumor of the liver.

**hepatopneumonic** (hep'ă-to-nu-mon'ik) [ hepato- + G. *pneumonikos,* pulmonary ]. Relating to the liver and the lungs.

**hep'atopor'tal.** Relating to the portal system of the liver.

**hepatoptosis** (hep'ă-top-to'sis, hep'ă-to-to'sis) [ hepato- + G. *ptōsis,* a failing ]. Downward displacement of the liver.

**hep'atopul'monary.** Hepatopneumonic.

**hepatore'nal** [ hepato- + L. *renalis,* renal, fr. *renes,* kidneys ]. Hepatonephric.

**hepatorrhagia** (hep'ă-to-ra'jī-ah) [ hepato- + G. *rhēgnymi,* to burst forth ]. Hemorrhage into or from the liver.

**hepatorrhaphy** (hep'ă-tor'ă-fĭ) [ hepato- + G. *rhaphē,* a suture ]. Suture of a wound of the liver.

**hepatorrhea** (hep'ă-to-re'ah) [ hepato- + G. *rhoia,* a flow ]. Cholorrhea.

**hepatorrhexis** (hep'ă-to-rek'sis) [ hepato- + G. *rhēxis,* rupture ]. Rupture of the liver.

**hepatoscopy** (hep'ă-tos'ko-pĭ) [ hepato- + G. *skopeō,* to examine ]. Examination of the liver.

**hepatosplenitis** (hep'ă-to-sple-ni'tis). Inflammation of the liver and spleen.

**hepatosplenography** (hep'ă-to-sple-nog'ră-fĭ). The use of contrast dyes to outline or depict the liver and spleen roentgenographically.

**hepatosplenomegaly** (hep'ă-to-sple-no-meg'ă-lĭ) [ hepato- + G. *splēn,* spleen, + *megas,* large ]. Enlargement of the liver and spleen.

**hepatosplenopathy** (hep'ă-to-sple-nop'ă-thĭ). Disease of the liver and spleen.

**hepatostomy** (hep'ă-tos'to-mĭ) [ hepato- + G. *stoma,* mouth ]. The establishment of a fissure into the liver.

**hep'atother'apy.** 1. Treatment of disease of the liver. 2. The therapeutic use of liver extract or of the raw substance of the liver.

**hep'atothrom'bin.** A clotting factor formed in the liver and existing in blood.

**hepatotomy** (hep'ă-tot'o-mĭ) [ hepato- + G. *tomē,* incision ]. Incision into the liver substance.

**hepatotoxemia** (hep'ă-to-tok-se'mĭ-ah) [ hepato- + G. *toxikon,* poison, + *haima,* blood ]. Autointoxication assumed to be due to improper functioning of the liver.

**hep'atotox'ic.** Relating to an agent that damages the liver or pertaining to any such action.

**hep'atotox'in.** A toxin that is destructive to parenchymal cells of the liver.

**Hep'atozo'on** [ hepato- + G. *zōon,* animal ]. A genus of protozoan parasites of the family Haemogregarinidae, in which schizogony occurs in the visceral organs and gametogony in the leukocytes or erythrocytes of vertebrate animals, and sporogony in certain ticks and other blood-sucking invertebrates. *H. canis* occurs in dogs, cats, jackals and hyenas, but is most pathogenic in dogs in which it may cause serious disease and death. Other species have been described from rats, mice, rabbits, and squirrels.

**hepta-** [ G. *hepta,* seven ]. Prefix denoting seven.

**hep'tabar'bital.** MEDOMIN; 5-(1-cyclohepten-1-yl)-5-ethylbarbituric acid; a short-acting barbiturate, producing sedation, hypnosis, or anesthesia, depending upon the dose administered.

**heptachromic** (hep'tah-kro'mik) [ G. *hepta,* seven, + *chrōma,* color ]. 1. Pertaining to or exhibiting the seven colors of the spectrum. 2. Having normal color vision.

**hep'tad.** A septivalent chemical element or radical.

**heptam'inol hydrochloride.** HEPTAMYL; 6-amino-2-methyl-2-heptanol hydrochloride; myocardial stimulant.

**hep'tazone hydrochloride.** Phenadoxone hydrochloride.

**hep'tose.** A sugar with 7 carbon atoms in its molecule.

**hep'tulose.** A ketoheptose.

D-*altro*-2-**heptulose.** Sedoheptulose.

D-*manno*-**heptulose.** A ketoheptose of the mannose configuration, occurring in the urine of individuals who have eaten a large quantity of avocados.

**hep'tylpenicil'lin.** Heptylpenicillinic acid; see penicillin K.

**Heraclitus** (her-ă-kli'tus), Greek philosopher born at Ephesus, 556–460 B.C. Believed that fire was the essential and fundamental principle in the universe and that all Nature owing to this essence was in a constant state of flow (flux); in all things, even in those which to our senses seemed permanent and motionless, there was perpetual movement and a state of ceaseless change.

**Herbert,** Herbert, English ophthalmic surgeon, 1865–1942. See H.'s *operation.*

**herbivorous** (her-biv'o-rus) [ L. *herba,* herb, + *voro,* to devour ]. Feeding on plants.

**Herbst** (hairpst), Ernst F. G., German anatomist, 1803–1893. See H.'s *corpuscles.*

**hereditary** (hĕ-red'ĭ-tĕr-ĭ) [ L. *hereditarius;* fr. *heres* (*hered-*), an heir ]. Transmitted from parent to offspring; derived from ancestry; obtained by inheritance.

**heredita'tion.** The influence of heredity.

**heredity** (hĕ-red'ĭ-tĭ) [ L. *hereditas,* inheritance, fr. *heres* (*hered-*), heir ]. The transmission of characters from parent to offspring.

**heredo-** (hĕr'e-do-) [ L. *heres,* an heir ]. A prefix denoting heredity.

**heredoataxia** (hĕr'e-do-ă-tak'sĭ-ah). Hereditary spinal *ataxia.*

**heredodegeneration** (hĕr'e-do-de-jen-er-a'shun). Retrogressive pathologic change, of genetic etiology, in cells or tissues.

**heredofamilial** (hĕr'e-do-fă-mil'ĭ-al). Denoting an inherited condition present in more than one member of a family.

**heredoimmunity** (hĕr'e-do-im-mu'nĭ-tĭ). Hereditary immunity.

**heredolues** (hĕr'e-do-lu'ēz) [ heredo- + L. *lues,* a plague (syphilis) ]. Heredosyphilis.

**heredoluetic** (hĕr'e-do-lu-et'ik). Heredosyphilitic.

**her'edopath'ia atac'tica polyneuri'tifor'mis.** Refsum's *disease.*

**her'edoret'inopath'ia congen'ita.** *Amaurosis* congenita of Leber.

**heredosyphilis** (hĕr'e-do-sif'ĭ-lis). Syphilis acquired *in utero.*

**heredosyphilitic** (hĕr'e-do-sif'ĭ-lit'ik). Congenitally syphilitic.

**Herellea.** A bacterial generic name which has been rejected by international action because its type species, *H. vaginicola,* is unrecognizable.

**herelleo'sis.** A septic infection, sometimes severe but rarely fatal, caused by widespread, usually harmless commensal bacteria identified as belonging to the genus *Herellea.*

**Hering,** Heinrich Ewald, German physiologist, 1866–1948. See H.'s sinus *nerve,* H.-Breuer *reflex,* Traube-H. *curve.*

**Hering,** Karl Ewald Konstantin, German physiologist, 1834–1918. See *canal* of H., Traube-H. *curves, waves,* H.'s *test,* H.'s *theory,* Semon-H. *theory.*

**heritage** (hĕr'ĭ-tij) [ O. Fr. See heredity ]. The total of all the inherited characters.

**Hermann,** Friedrich, German anatomist, 1859–1920. See H.'s *fluid.*

**hermaph'rodism.** Hermaphroditism.

**hermaphrodite** (her-maf'ro-dit) [ G. *Hermaphroditus,* the son of *Hermēs,* Mercury, + *Aphroditē,* Venus. HERM- ]. An individual with hermaphroditism.

**hermaphroditism** (her-maf'ro-dit-izm). The presence in one individual of both ovarian and testicular tissue, *i.e.,* true h.

   **adre'nal h.,** altered sexual characters due to disorders in adrenocortical function, most often female virilization; not an example of true h.

   **bilateral h.,** true h. with ovotestis on both sides.

   **dimid'iate h.** lateral h.

   **false h.,** pseudohermaphroditism.

   **female h.,** more correctly designated as female pseudohermaphroditism, as the term is commonly used; however, it can designate an instance of true h., in which bodily characteristics are predominantly female.

   **lateral h.,** dimidiate h.; a form in which a testis is present on one side and an ovary on the other.

   **male h.,** more correctly designated as male pseudohermaphroditism, as the term is commonly used; however, it can designate an instance of true h. in which bodily characteristics are predominantly male.

   **transverse h.,** pseudohermaphroditism, in which the external genital organs are characteristic of one sex and the gonads are characteristic of the other sex.

   **true h.,** h. in which both ovarian and testicular tissue are present.

   **unilateral h.,** h. in which the doubling of sex characteristics occurs only on one side; ovotestis on one side and either ovary or testis on the other.

**hermet'ic.** Airtight; denoting a vessel closed or sealed in such a way that air can neither enter it nor issue from it.

# HERNIA

**hernia** (her'nĭ-ah) [ L. rupture ]. Rupture; the protrusion of an organ or part of an organ or other structure through the wall of the cavity normally containing it. See color plate 9.

**abdominal h.,** laparocele; a h. protruding through or into any part of the abdominal wall; see color plate 9.

**antevesical h.,** an interstitial h. projecting medially from the internal inguinal ring.

**Barth's h.,** engagement of a loop of intestine between a persistent vitelline duct and the abdominal wall.

**Béclard's h.,** h. through the opening for the saphenous vein.

**h. en bissac',** preperitoneal inguinal h.

**Bochdalek's h.,** a dorsolateral diaphragmatic h. probably due to a defect in the development of the pleuroperitoneal membrane.

**h. of the broad ligament of the uterus,** a coil of intestine contained in a pouch projecting into the substance of the broad ligament.

**cecal h.,** a h. containing cecum.

**cerebral h.,** protrusion of brain substance through a defect in the skull.

**Cloquet's h.,** a femoral h. perforating the aponeurosis of the pectineus and insinuating itself between this aponeurosis and the muscle, lying therefore behind the femoral vessels.

**complete h.,** an indirect inguinal h. in which the contents extend into the tunica vaginalis.

**concealed h.,** one not found on inspection or palpation.

**Cooper's h.,** femoral h. with two sacs, the second passing through a defect in the superficial fascia and appearing immediately beneath the skin, the first being in the femoral canal.

**crural h.,** femoral h.

**diaphragmat'ic h.,** diaphragmatocele; protrusion of an abdominal viscus or viscera into the chest through a defect in the respiratory diaphragm; the most common type is the hiatal h.

**double loop h.,** "w" h.

**dry h.,** one with adherency of sac and contents.

**duodenojejunal h.,** Treitz' h.; retroperitoneal h.; a h. in the subperitoneal tissues.

**epigastric h.,** h. through the linea alba above the navel.

**extrasaccular h.,** sliding h.

**fascial h.,** a bulging of muscle through a defect in its fascia.

**fatty h.,** pannicular h., or a fascial h., in which a mass of adipose tissue escapes through a gap in a fascia or aponeurosis.

**fem'oral h.,** enteromerocele; femorocele; crural h.; h. through the femoral ring.

**gastroesophageal h.,** a hiatal h. into the thorax.

**glu'teal h.,** sciatic h.

**Hesselbach's h.,** h. with diverticula through the cribriform fascia, presenting a lobular outline.

**Hey's h.,** bilocular femoral h., one sac being in the canal, the other passing through a defect in the superficial fascia and lying beneath the skin.

**hiatal h., hia'tus h.,** h. of a part of the stomach through the esophageal hiatus of the diaphragm.

**Holthouse's h.,** inguinal h. with extension of the loop of intestine along Poupart's ligament.

**ili'acosubfas'cial h.,** a h. the sac of which passes through the iliac fascia and lies in the iliac fossa in contact with the iliacus muscle.

**incar'cerated h.,** irreducible h.

**incisional h.,** h. occurring through a surgical scar.

**infantile h.,** a form in which an intestinal loop descends behind the tunica vaginalis, having, therefore, three peritoneal layers in front of it.

**in'guinal h.,** h. of the intestine at the inguinal region; a direct inguinal h. passes directly through the abdominal wall between the deep epigastric artery and the edge of the rectus muscle; an indirect inguinal h. passes through the inguinal canal.

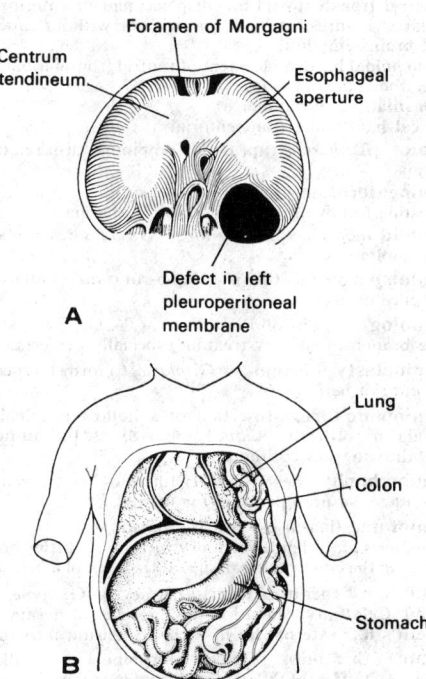

**Congenital Diaphragmatic Hernia**

*A,* caudal surface of the diaphragm, showing a large defect of the pleuroperitoneal membrane on the left side. *B,* hernia of the intestinal loops and part of the stomach into the left pleural cavity; the heart and mediastinum are frequently pushed to the right, while the left lung is compressed. (From Langman, J.: *Medical Embryology,* Ed. 2, The Williams & Wilkins Co., Baltimore, 1969.)

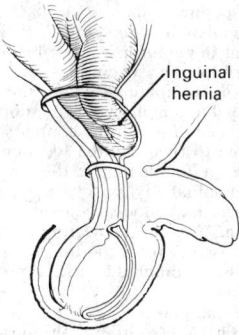

**Inguinal Hernia**
(See also color plate 9)

**in'guinocru'ral h., in'guinofem'oral h.,** a bilocular or double h., both inguinal and (more or less completely) femoral.

**inguinolabial h.,** an inguinal hernia descending into the labium.

**in'guinoproperitone'al h.,** properitoneal inguinal h.

**inguinoscrotal h.,** an inguinal h. descending into the scrotum alongside the tunica vaginalis testis.

**inguinosuperficial h.,** an inguinal h. that has turned cephalad away from the scrotum and lies subcutaneously on the abdominal muscles.

**internal vaginal testicular h.,** a h. the pouch of which is subperitoneal, the testicle and vaginal pouch not having descended through the inguinal canal.

**intersig'moid h.,** one into the intersigmoid fossa on the under surface of the root of the mesosigmoid near the inner border of the psoas magnus muscle.

**intersti'tial h.,** one in which the knuckle of intestine is between any two of the layers of the abdominal wall.

**intraepiplo'ic h.,** a coil of intestine incarcerated in an omental sac.

**intrailiac h.,** an interstitial h. projecting from the internal inguinal ring.

**intrapelvic h.,** an interstitial h. projecting into the pelvis from the internal inguinal ring.

**irredu'cible h.,** incarcerated h.; one which, as a result of adhesions or for any other reason, cannot be reduced without operation.

**ischiatic h.,** a h. through the sacrosciatic foramen.

**Krönlein's h.,** properitoneal inguinal h.

**labial h.,** one into a labium majus.

**lateral ventral h.,** spigelian h.

**Laugier's h.,** a h. passing through an opening in Gimbernat's ligament.

**levator h.,** pudendal h.

**Littré's h.,** (1) parietal h.; (2) h. of Meckel's diverticulum.

**lumbar h.,** a protrusion between the last rib and the iliac crest where the aponeurosis of the transversus muscle is covered only by the latissimus dorsi.

**Malgaigne's h.,** infantile inguinal h. prior to the descent of the testis.

**Maydl's h.,** retrograde strangulated h., the intestine having descended into the sac in the form of a W, the two external loops being connected by an internal or intraabdominal loop.

**meningeal h.,** herniation of meninges through a spina bifida.

**mesenteric h.,** h. through a hole in the mesentery.

**obturator h.,** h. through the obturator foramen.

**pannic'ular h.,** the escape of a mass of subcutaneous fat through a gap in a fascia or an aponeurosis; fatty h.

**paraesophageal h.,** h. through the esophageal hiatus of the diaphragm.

**paraperitone'al h.,** a vesical h. in which only a part of the protruded organ is covered by the peritoneum of the sac.

**parasaccular h.,** sliding h.

**parasternal h.,** Morgagni's *foramen (2)*.

**pari'etal h.,** Richter's h.; Littré's h. (1); partial enterocele; h. in which only a portion of the wall of the intestine is engaged.

**perineal h.,** perineocele.

**Petit's h.,** lumbar h., occurring in Petit's triangle.

**properitone'al in'guinal h.,** h. en bissac; Kronlein's h.; inguinoproperitoneal h.; a complicated h. having a double sac, one part in the inguinal canal, the other projecting from the internal inguinal ring in the subperitoneal tissues.

**reducible h.,** one in which the contents of the hernia sac can be returned to their normal location.

**ret'rograde h.,** a double loop h. the central loop of which lies in the abdominal cavity.

**retroperitone'al h.,** duodenojejunal h.

**retropu'bic h.,** a h. projecting downward, in the subperitoneal tissues, from the internal inguinal ring.

**retrosternal h.,** a diaphragmatic h. protruding through Morgagni's foramen.

**Richter's h.,** parietal h.

**Rokitansky's h.,** a separation of the muscular fibers of the bowel allowing protrusion of a sac of the mucous membrane or one of the peritoneum.

**sciat'ic h.,** gluteal h.; ischiocele; enterischiocele; protrusion of intestine through the great sacrosciatic foramen.

**scrotal h.,** oscheocele; complete inguinal h., with abode in the scrotum.

**sliding h., slipped h.,** extrasaccular or parasaccular h.; a h. in which an abdominal viscus forms part of the sac.

**sliding esophageal hiatal h.,** displacement of the cardioesophageal junction and a portion of the fundus of the stomach through the esophageal hiatus into the posterior mediastinum.

**sliding hiatal h.,** h. of the esophagus through the diaphragm into the posterior mediastinum, with partial peritoneal sac anteriorly.

**slipped h.,** sliding h.

**Spigelian h.,** lateral ventral h.; abdominal h. through the semilunar line.

**strangulated h.,** one that is both irreducible and incarcerated and in which the blood circulation is also arrested, gangrene occurring unless speedy relief is afforded.

**synovial h.,** protrusion of a fold of the stratum synoviale through a rent in the stratum fibrosum of a joint capsule.

**Treitz' h.,** duodenojejunal h.

**umbil'ical h.,** exomphalos; a h. in which bowel or omentum protrudes through the abdominal wall under the skin at the umbilicus.

**vaginal h., posterior,** downward displacement of the pouch of Douglas.

**Velpeau's h.,** femoral h. in which the intestine is in front of the blood vessels.

**ventral h.,** an abdominal incisional h.

**"w" h.,** double loop h.; the presence of two loops of intestine in a hernial sac.

---

**her'nial.** Relating to hernia.

**her'niated.** 1. Relating to any structure protruded through a hernial opening. 2. Suffering from hernia.

**herniation** (her'nĭ-a'shun). The process of formation of a protrusion.

**caudal transtentorial h.,** uncal h.; displacement of medial temporal structures into incisura, with or without rostrocaudal brainstem shift.

**cingulate h.,** displacement of the cingulate gyrus beneath the falx.

**foraminal h.,** tonsillar h.; displacement of cerebellar tonsils through the foramen magnum.

**rostral transtentorial h.,** displacement of anterior cerebellar structures into incisura, with or without caudorostral brainstem shift.

**sphenoidal h.,** displacement of ventral frontal lobar tissue over the sphenoid ridge.

**tonsillar h.,** foraminal h.

**uncal h.,** caudal transtentorial h.

**hernio-** [ L. *hernia,* rupture ]. Combining form relating to hernia.

**hernioenterotomy** (her'nĭ-o-en-ter-ot'mĭ). Opening of the intestine following the reduction of a hernia.

**hernioid** (her'nĭ-oyd) [ hernio- + G. *eidos,* resemblance ]. Resembling hernia.

**herniolaparotomy** (her'nĭ-o-lap-ă-rot'o-mĭ). Laparotomy for cure of hernia.

**herniology** (her'nĭ-ol'o-jĭ) [ hernio- + G. *logos,* study ]. The branch of surgery treating especially of hernia.

**her'nioplasty** [ hernio- + G. *plassō,* to form ]. Operation for cure of hernia.

**her'niopunc'ture.** Insertion of a hollow needle into a hernia in order to reduce the size of the tumor by withdrawing gas or liquid.

**herniorrhaphy** (her'nĭ-or'ă-fĭ) [ hernio- + G. *rhaphē,* a seam ]. A suture operation for hernia.

**herniotome** (her'nĭ-o-tōm). Hernia *knife.*

**Cooper's h.,** a slender bistoury with short cutting edge for dividing the constricting tissues at the neck of a hernial sac.

**herniotomy** (her'nĭ-ot'o-mĭ) [ hernio- + G. *tomē,* a cutting ]. Celotomy; operation for the relief of hernia.

**Petit's h.,** external h.; h. without incision into the sac.

**heroin** (hĕr'o-in). Diacetylmorphine; an alkaloid, $C_{17}H_{17}(OC_2H_3O)_2ON$, prepared from morphine by acetylation; formerly used for the relief of cough. Because of the danger of addiction, its manufacture and importation into the United States is prohibited by Federal law.

**Herophilus** (hĕ-rof'ĭ-lus). Greek physician and anatomist of the Alexandrian school, circa 300 B.C. One of the first to dissect the human body; described the brain noting cerebrum and cerebellum and distinguished nerves from tendons and blood vessels. He described the cerebral sinus (torcular herophili), and named the duodenum and prostate gland. He counted the pulse with a water clock and described various pulse rhythms. See *torcular* herophili.

**herpangina** (herp-an'jĭ-nah, herp-an-ji'nah). A disease caused by types of Coxsackie virus and marked by a sudden onset of fever, loss of appetite, dysphagia, pharyngitis, and sometimes abdominal pain, nausea, and vomiting. Vesiculopapular lesions about 1 to 2 mm. in diameter are present around the fauces; these soon break down to form grayish yellow ulcers.

**herpes** (her'pēz) [ G. *herpēs*, a spreading skin eruption, shingles, fr. *herpō*, to creep ]. Serpigo (2); an eruption of groups of deep-seated vesicles on erythematous bases.

  **h. catarrha'lis,** h. simplex.

  **h. circina'tus bullo'sus,** *dermatitis* herpetiformis.

  **h. cor'neae,** herpetic *keratitis.*

  **h. desquamans,** *tinea* imbricata.

  **h. digita'lis,** h. simplex.

  **h. facia'lis,** h. simplex.

  **h. febri'lis,** h. simplex.

  **h. generalisa'tus,** generalized h. simplex virus infection.

  **h. genita'lis,** h. simplex.

  **h. gestatio'nis,** hydroa gestationis; a polymorphous, bullous eruption, more common on the extremities than on the trunk, with the appearance of pemphigoid or dermatitis herpetiformis; recurrent during each subsequent pregnancy after onset.

  **h. iris,** (1) *erythema* iris; (2) *erythema* multiforme.

  **h. labia'lis,** h. simplex of the lips.

  **h. menta'lis,** h. simplex.

  **h. preputia'lis,** h. simplex.

  **h. progenita'lis,** h. simplex of the genitalia.

  **h. simplex,** an infection by h. simplex virus, marked by the eruption of one or more groups of vesicles on the vermilion border of the lips, at the external nares, or on the glans, prepuce, or vulva. Such infection is commonly recrudescent and reappears during other febrile illnesses or even physiologic states such as menstruation. Also called, according to site, fever blister, cold sore, h. digitalis, h. catarrhalis, h. facialis, h. febrilis, h. genitalis, h. labialis, mentalis, h. preputialis, h. progenitalis.

  **h. ton'surans,** *tinea* tonsurans.

  **h. zoster** [ G. *zōster,* girdle ], zona (2); zoster; shingles; an infection caused by *Herpesvirus varicellae,* characterized by an eruption of groups of vesicles on one side of the body following the course of a nerve. The condition is self-limited but may be accompanied by or followed by severe postherpetic pain.

  **h. zoster ophthalmicus,** a herpetic involvement of the ophthalmic branch of the trigeminal nerve.

  **h. zoster varicello'sus,** h. zoster associated with disseminated varicelliform lesions.

**herpesvirus** (her'pēz-vi'rus). See under *virus.*

**herpet'ic.** 1. Relating to or characterized by herpes. 2. Relating to the herpesvirus.

**herpet'iform.** Resembling herpes.

**herpetism** (her'pĕ-tizm). A supposed herpetic diathesis, described chiefly by French writers.

**Herpetomonas** (her'pĕ-tom'o-nas) [ G. *herpeton,* a reptile (fr. *herpō,* to creep), + *monas,* unit (one of the *Monadidae*) ]. A genus of asexual, monogenetic flagellates (family Trypanosomatidae), strictly insect parasites, with a variety of body forms including leptomad, crithidial, leishmanial, and trypanosome-like. Infective forms are passed in the host feces.

  **H. muscae domes'ticae,** the type species of *H.,* found in the common housefly.

  **H. sarcoph'agae,** a species found in the flesh fly, *Sarcophaga haemorrhoidalis.*

**Herring,** Percy T., English physiologist, *1872. See H. *bodies.*

**Hers,** H. G. See H.'s *disease.*

**hersage** (ār-sahzh') [ Fr. (from L. *hirpex,* a large rake), a harrowing ]. Separating the individual fibers of a nerve trunk.

**Hershey,** Alfred, U. S. virologist, *1908. Nobel laureate, 1969, with Max Delbrück and Salvador Luria for their contributions to the understanding of the molecular biology of bacteriophage.

**Herter,** Christian A., American physician, 1865–1910. See H.'s *infantilism,* Gee-H. *infantilism,* Gee-H. *syndrome.*

**Hertwig,** Richard, German zoologist, 1850–1937. See Magendie-H. *sign, syndrome.*

**Hertwig,** Wilhelm A. O., German embryologist, 1849–1922. See H.'s *sheath.*

**Hertz,** Heinrich R., German physicist, 1857–1894. See Hertzian *experiments, rays.*

**hertz** [ H. R. *Hertz* ]. Abbreviated Hz; a unit of frequency equivalent to 1 cycle per second; used officially in audiometry.

**Herxheimer** (herks'hi-mer), Karl, German dermatologist, *1861. See H.'s *reaction,* Jarisch-H. *reaction.*

**Her'yng,** Théodor, Warsaw laryngologist, 1847–1925. See H.'s *sign,* Voltolini-H. *sign.*

**herzstoss** (hārz'stos) [ Ger. ]. Cardiac systole characterized by a massive diffuse precordial heave without any definite point of maximal impulse.

**Heschl** (hesh'l), Richard L., Austrian pathologist, 1824–1881. See H.'s *gyrus.*

**hesitancy** (hez'ĭ-tăn-sĭ). An involuntary delay or inability in starting the urinary stream.

**hes'perano'pia** [ G. *hespera,* evening, + *an-* priv. + *ōps,* eye ]. Rarely used term for nyctalopia.

**hesper'etin.** The aglycone of hesperidin; 3',5,7-trihydroxy-4'-methoxyflavanone (flavone, which see for structure).

**hesper'idin.** Hesperetin 7-rutinoside; hesperetin 7-rhamnoglucoside; a flavone diglycoside obtained from unripe citrus fruit. It reputedly possesses vitamin P activity.

  **phosphor'ylated h.,** suggested as an antifertility agent; supposedly active when orally administered. This compound is an inhibitor of hyaluronidase and the contraceptive action claimed for it (but probably unwarranted) is prevention of the destruction of the cells of the corona radiata surrounding the ovum, a barrier to the penetration of the spermatozoon which is normally removed by the action of hyaluronidase(s).

**Hess,** Alfred F., U. S. physician, 1875–1933. See H.'s *test.*

**Hess,** Walter R., Swiss physiologist, *1881. Nobel laureate, 1949, with Antonio Egas Moniz, for the discovery of the functional organization of the interbrain as a coordinator of the activities of the internal organ. See trophotropic *zone* of H.

**Hesselbach** (hes'el-bahkh), Franz K., German surgeon, 1759–1816. See H.'s *fascia, hernia, ligament, triangle.*

**hetacil'lin** (USAN). VERSAPIN; 6-(2,2-dimethyl-5-oxo-4-phenyl-1-imidazolidinyl)penicillanic acid; a semisynthetic penicillin compound with antimicrobial properties.

**heter-.** See hetero-.

**heteradelphus** (het'er-ă-del'fus) [ heter- + G. *adelphos,* brother ]. Unequal conjoined twins with the smaller incomplete one (the parasite) attached to the larger more nearly normal one (the autosite).

**het'era'kid.** Common name for members of the genus *Heterakis.*

**Het'era'kis.** A genus of nematode parasites of poultry (family Heterakidae, order Ascaroidea). *H. gallinarum* is the cecal worm of chickens, turkeys, and many gallinaceous birds. It plays a role in the transmission of *Histomonas meleagridis,* which causes histomoniasis. Other species are *H. brevispiculum, H. dispar, H. isolonche,* and *H. spumosa,* the latter a cecal parasite of rats and other rodents.

**hetera'lius** [ heter- + G. *halios,* useless ]. Unequal conjoined twins in which the parasite is so undeveloped as to be scarcely recognizable as such, appearing as little more than an excrescence on the autosite.

**heterax'ial.** Having mutually perpendicular axes of unequal length.

**heterecious** (het-er-e'shĭ-us) [ heter- + G. *oikion,* home ]. Metoxenous; having more than one host; said of a parasite passing different stages of its existence in different animals.

**heterecism** (het'er-e-sizm) [ heter- + G. *oikion,* home ]. Metoxeny; the occurrence, in a parasite, of two cycles of existence, passed in two different hosts.

**heteresthesia** (het-er-es-the'zĭ-ah) [ heter- + G. *aisthēsis,* sensation ]. A change occurring in the degree (either plus or minus) of the sensory response to a cutaneous stimulus as the latter crosses a certain line on the surface.

**hetero-, heter-** [ G. *heteros*, other ]. Combining form meaning other, or different.

**het'eroagglu'tinin.** A form of hemagglutinin, one that agglutinates the red blood cells of species other than that in which the h. occurs. See also hemagglutinin.

**heteroantibody** (het'er-o-an'tĭ-bod-ĭ). Antibody that is heterologous with respect to antigen, in contradistinction to isoantibody; see also heterologous (2).

**het'eroat'om.** An atom, other than carbon, located in the ring structure of an organic compound, as the N in pyridines or pyrimidines (heterocyclic compounds).

**heteroauxin** (het'er-o-awk'sin). β-Indoleacetic acid; one of the plant growth hormones.

**het'eroblas'tic** [ hetero- + G. *blastos*, germ ]. Developing from more than a single type of tissue; distinguished from homoblastic.

**het'erocel'lular.** Formed of cells of different kinds.

**het'erocen'tric.** 1. Having different centers, said of rays that do not meet at a common focus. 2. Interested in others, rather than in one's self; the opposite of egocentric.

**het'eroceph'alus** [ hetero- + G. *kephalē*, head ]. A conjoined twin with heads of unequal size.

**heterocheiral, heterochiral** (het-er-o-ki'ral) [ hetero- + G. *cheir*, hand ]. Relating to or referred to the other hand.

**heterochromatin** (het'er-o-kro'mă-tin). A chromosome or segment of a chromosome that remains condensed during interphase and thus stains deeply, or exhibits positive heteropyknosis.

**heterochromia** (het-er-o-kro'mĭ-ah) [ hetero- + G. *chrōma*, color ]. A difference in coloration in two structures or two parts of the same structure which are normally alike in color.

   **binocular h.**, congenital defects of pigmentation, with or without extraocular pigmentary defects.

   **h. i'ridis**, a difference in coloration in the structure of the irides, or different parts of the same iris. See binocular h. and monocular h.

   **monocular h.**, nevi of the iris; variegated iris.

**heterochromosome** (het'er-o-kro'mo-sōm). Allosome.

**heterochromous** (het'er-o-kro'mus). Having an abnormal difference in coloration.

**heterochron** (het'er-o-kron) [ hetero- + G. *chronos*, time ]. Having varying chronaxies.

**heterochronia** (het-er-o-kro'nĭ-ah) [ hetero- + G. *chronos*, time ]. The origin or development of tissues or organs at an unusual time or out of the regular sequence; opposed to synchronia.

**heterochronic** (het'er-o-kron'ik). Heterochronous.

**heterochronous** (het-er-ok'ro-nus). Heterochronic; relating to heterochronia; referring especially to tissue occurring in a given locality at a time when it should not normally be found there.

**het'eroclad'ic** [ hetero- + G. *klados*, a twig ]. Denoting an anastomosis between branches of different arterial trunks, as distinguished from homocladic.

**heterocrine** (het'er-o-krin) [ hetero- + G. *krino*, to separate ]. Allocrine; denoting the secretion of two or more kinds of material.

**het'erocri'sis.** An irregular crisis, one occurring at an abnormal time or with unusual symptoms.

**heterocyclic compound** (het'er-o-si'klik, -sik'lik). See under compound.

**heterocytotropic** (het'er-o-si'to-tro'pik, -trop'ik) [ hetero- + G. *kytos*, cell, + *trope*, a turning toward ]. Having an affinity for cells of a different species.

**het'eroder'mic** [ hetero- + G. *derma*, skin ]. Denoting the method of skin grafting in which the grafts are taken from the skin of another animal (dermatoheteroplasty); the term formerly was used at times for grafts from another person (homograft or allograft). The prefix hetero- is now used to indicate different species when reference is to tissue transplants.

**het'erodisperse.** Of varying size; term used to describe aerosols of which the particles are nonuniform in size.

**het'erodont** [ hetero- + G. *odous*, tooth ]. Having teeth of varying shapes, such as those of man and the majority of mammals; opposed to homodont.

**Heterodoxus spiniger.** A biting louse of the dog; sometimes called the kangaroo louse.

**heterodromus** (het-ĕr-ŏd'ro-mus) [ hetero- + G. *dromos*, running ]. Moving in the opposite direction.

**heterodymus** (het'er-od'ĭ-mus) [ hetero- + G. *didymos*, twin ]. Unequal conjoined twins in which the incomplete parasite, consisting of head and neck and more or less thorax, is attached to the anterior surface of the autosite.

**heteroerotic** het'er-o-e-rot'ik). Relating to the attachment of sexual interest to objects outside of the self, as opposed to autoerotic.

**het'erogamet'ic** [ hetero- + G. *gametikos*, connubial ]. Digametic; relating to production of gametes of contrasting types with respect to sex chromosomes; human males are heterogametic.

**heterog'amous.** Relating to heterogamy.

**heterogamy** (het'er-og'ă-mĭ) [ hetero- + G. *gamos*, marriage ]. 1. Conjugation of unlike gametes. 2. Alternation of generations in which two kinds of sexual generation alternate. 3. Bearing different types of flowers. 4. Reproduction by indirect methods of pollination.

**het'erogene'ic, het'erogen'ic.** Pertaining to different gene constitutions, especially with respect to different species.

**heterogeneity** (het'er-o-jĕ-ne'ĭ-tĭ). Heterogeneous state or quality.

**heterogeneous** (het'er-o-je'ne-us). Composed of parts having various and dissimilar characteristics or properties.

**heterogenesis** (het-er-o-jen'ĕ-sis) [ hetero- + G. *genesis*, production ]. 1. The production of offspring unlike the parents. 2. Spontaneous *generation*.

**heterogenetic** (het'er-o-jĕ-net'ik). Relating to heterogenesis.

**heterogenote** (het'ĕ-ro-je'nōt). In microbial genetics, an organism that contains an exogenous piece of genetic material that differs somewhat from the corresponding region of its own original genome, in a very limited way resembling a heterozygote.

**heterogenous** (het-er-oj'ĕ-nus). Having a different or dissimilar origin.

**het'erograft.** heterotransplant; heterologous, heteroplastic, heterospecific, or interspecific graft; a graft transferred from one species to another.

**het'erohypno'sis.** Hypnosis induced by or in another; as opposed to autohypnosis.

**heteroimmune** (het'er-o-ĭ-mūn). Pertaining to an immune state induced by heterologous antigen; see also immune (2); heterologous (2); heteroantibody.

**het'eroinfec'tion.** The usual form of infection from outside the body; distinguished from autoinfection or autoinoculation.

**heteroinoculation** (het'er-o-in-ok-u-la'shun). Inoculation with virus originating outside the body; distinguished from autoinoculation.

**het'erointoxica'tion.** See intoxication; in contradistinction to autointoxication.

**heterokeratoplasty** (het'er-o-kĕr'ă-to-plas'tĭ). Keratoplasty in which the cornea from one species of animal is grafted to the eye of an animal of a different species.

**heterokinesia** (het'er-o-kĭ-ne'zĭ-ah) [ hetero- + G. *kinēsis*, movement ]. Heterokinesis (2); executing movements the reverse of those one is told to make.

**heterokinesis** (het'er-o-kĭ-ne'sis). 1. Differential distribution of X and Y chromosomes during meiotic cell division. 2. Heterokinesia.

**het'erola'lia** [ hetero- + G. *lalia*, speech ]. Heterophasia; heterophemia; the habitual substitution of meaningless or inappropriate words for those intended; a form of aphasia.

**het'erolat'eral** [ hetero- + L. *latus*, side ]. Contralateral; on, or relating to, the opposite side.

**het'erolip'ids.** Lipids containing in their molecules N and P atoms in addition to the usual C, H, and O; compound lipids (*e.g.*, lecithins).

**het'erolit'eral** [ hetero- + L. *litera*, letter ]. Relating to stammering or the substitution of one letter for another in the pronunciation of certain words.

**heterologous** (het'er-ol'o-gus) [ hetero- + G. *logos*, ratio, relation ]. 1. Pertaining to cytologic or histologic elements that do not normally occur in that part or region of the body. 2. Derived from an animal of a different species, as the serum of a horse is h. for a rabbit.

**heterology** (het'er-ol'o-jī). A departure from the normal in structure, arrangement, or mode or time of development.

**heterol'ysin.** A lysin that is formed in one species of animal and manifests lytic activity on the cells of a different species.

**heterolysis** (het-er-ol'ī-sis) [ hetero- + G. *lysis*, a loosening ]. Dissolution or digestion of cells or protein components from one species by a lytic agent from a different species.

**het'erolyt'ic.** Pertaining to heterolysis or to the effect of a heterolysin.

**heteromastigote** (het-er-o-mas'tī-gōt). A mastigote having two flagella, one anterior and one posterior.

**heterom'eral.** Heteromeric (2).

**heteromeric** (het'er-o-mĕr'ik) [ hetero- + G. *meros*, part ]. 1. Having a different chemical composition. 2. Heteromeral; heteromerous; denoting spinal neurons that have processes passing over to the opposite side of the cord.

**heterom'erous.** Heteromeric (2).

**heterometaplasia** (het'er-o-met-ă-pla'zī-ah). Tissue transformation resulting in the production of a tissue foreign to the part where produced.

**heterometric** (het'er-o-met'rik) [ hetero- + G. *metron*, measure ]. Involving or depending upon a change in size.

**het'erometro'pia** [ hetero- + G. *metron*, measure, + *ōps*, eye ]. A condition in which the degree of refraction is unlike in the two eyes.

**het'eromorph'ism** [ hetero- + G. *morphē*, shape ]. In cytogenetics, a difference in shape or size between the two members of a pair of mataphase chromosomes (*i.e.*, between homologous chromosomes).

**heteromorphosis** (het'er-o-mor-fo'sis) [ hetero- + G. *morphōsis*, a molding ]. 1. The development of one tissue from a tissue of another kind or type. 2. Embryonic development of tissue or an organ inappropriate to its site.

**het'eromor'phous.** Differing from the normal type.

**hetero'nium bromide** (USAN). HETRUM bromide; 3-hydroxy-1,1-dimethylpyrrolidinium bromide α-phenyl-2-thiopheneglycolate; an anticholinergic agent.

**heteronomous** (het-er-on'o-mus) [ hetero- + G. *nomos*, law ]. 1. Different from the type; abnormal. 2. Subject to the direction or law of another; not self-governing.

**heteronomy** (het-er-on'o-mī) [ hetero- + G. *nomos*, law ]. The condition or state of being heteronomous; the opposite of autonomy.

**heteronymous** (het-er-on'ī-mus) [ G. *heterōnymos*, having a different name, fr. *onyma*, or *onoma*, name ]. Having different names or expressed in different terms.

**het'ero-os'teoplas'ty.** Osteoplasty with the use of bone transplanted from another animal; formerly used, at times, for transplants from another person.

**heteropagus** (het'er-op'ā-gus) [ hetero- + G. *pagos*, fixed ]. Unequal conjoined twins in which the imperfectly developed parasite is attached to the ventral portion of the autosite. See also epigastrius.

**heteropathy** (het'er-op'ā-thī) [ hetero- + G. *pathos*, suffering ]. 1. Abnormal sensitivity to stimuli. 2. Allopathy.

**heterophasia** (het-er-o-fa'zī-ah) [ hetero- + G. *phasis*, speech ]. Heterolalia.

**heterophemia, heterophemy** (het-er-o-fe'mī-ah, het-er-of'e-mī) [ hetero- + G. *phēmē*, a speech ]. Heterolalia.

**heterophil, heterophile** (het'er-o-fil, -fil) [ hetero- + G. *philos*, fond ]. The neutrophil leukocyte in man; in some animals the granules vary in size and staining reaction. 2. Pertaining to heterogenetic antigens and related antibody; for example, parenteral administration of a suitably prepared emulsion of guinea pig kidney, in a rabbit, results in antibody that reacts not only with guinea pig antigen, but also lyses the red blood cells of sheep. See also under antigen and antibody.

**het'eropho'nia** [ hetero- + G. *phōnē*, voice ]. 1. The change of voice at puberty. 2. Any abnormality in the voice sounds.

**het'eropho'ria** [ hetero- + G. *phora*, movement. PHER- ]. A tendency of one eye to deviate in one or another direction in consequence of imperfect balance of the ocular muscles.

**heterophthalmus** (het'er-of-thal'mus) [ hetero- + G. *ophthalmos*, eye ]. Allophthalmia; a difference in the appearance of the two eyes, usually due to heterochromia of one or both of the irises.

**heterophthongia** (het-er-of-thon'jī-ah) [ G. *heterophthongos*, fr. *heteros*, different, + *phthongos*, sound, voice ]. Heterophonia.

**Heterophyes** (het'er-of'ī-ēz) [ hetero- + G. *phyē*, stature, form ]. A genus of digenetic flukes (family Heterophyidae) that are parasitic in fish-eating birds and mammals, including man. Cercariae from infected snails penetrate fish, which are eaten by the final hosts.

   **H. heteroph'yes,** Egyptian intestinal fluke; small intestinal fluke; a species infecting the small intestine and cecum in man and other fish-eating mammals in Egypt and the Far East.

   **H. katsura'dai,** a species, somewhat smaller than *H. heterophyes*, found in Japan.

**heterophyiasis** (het'er-o-fi-i'ah-sis). Infection with a heterophyid trematode, particularly *Heterophyes heterophyes*.

**Heterophyidae** (het'er-o-fi'ī-de). A family of tiny fishborne trematodes, including the genus *Heterophyes*, with its common human parasite, *H. heterophyes*.

**het'eropla'sia** [ hetero- + G. *plasis*, a forming ]. Alloplasia. 1. The development of cytologic and histologic elements that are not normal for the organ or part in question, as the growth of bone in a site where there is normally fibrous connective tissue. 2. The malposition of tissue or a part that is otherwise normal, as a ureter that develops at the lower pole of a kidney.

**het'eroplas'tic.** 1. Pertaining to or manifesting heteroplasia. 2. Relating to heteroplasty.

**het'eroplas'tid.** The graft in heteroplasty.

**het'eroplasty** [ hetero- + G. *plassō*, to form ]. Surgical grafting with tissue derived from an animal of another species; formerly, but no longer, used to indicate a graft other than an autograft.

**het'eroploid.** Relating to heteroploidy.

**heteroploidy** (het'er-o-ploy'dī) [ hetero- + -ploid, *q.v.* ]. The state of an individual or cell possessing a chromosome number other than the normal diploid number (in man, 46).

**heteropolysaccharide** (het'er-o-pol-ī-sak'ar-id). A polysaccharide yielding on hydrolysis two or more different kinds of monosaccharides, or substances derived from them.

**heteropsia** (het-er-op'sī-ah) [ hetero- + G. *opsis*, vision ]. Inequality of vision in the two eyes.

**heteropsychologic** (het'er-o-si-ko-loj'ik). Relating to ideas developed from without or derived from another's consciousness.

**heterop'tics** [ hetero- + G. *optikos*, optic ]. Visual hallucinations; perverted vision.

**heteropyknosis** (het'er-o-pik-no'sis) [ hetero- + G. *pyknos*, dense ]. Any state of variable density; refers usually to differences in degree of density between chromosomes of different cells, or between individual chromosomes.

**het'erosac'charide.** A glycoside in which a sugar group is attached to a nonsugar group; *e.g.*, amygdalin.

**heteroscope** (het'er-o-skōp) [ hetero- + G. *skopeō*, to view ]. An apparatus for determining the range of vision of a strabismic eye.

**heteros'copy.** The determination of the range of vision of the eyes in strabismus.

**het'erosexual'ity.** Erotic attraction, predisposition, or sexual congress between persons of the opposite sex; the normal sexual inclination, as opposed to homosexuality.

**hetero'sis.** The beneficial effect of crossing (hybridization) upon growth, vigor, and physical or mental qualities in a strain of plants or in animal stock, as measured by the midparent mean and $F_1$.

**het'erosome** [ hetero- + G. *sōma*, body ]. In genetics, the chromosomes that are different in the two sexes; sex chromosomes.

**het′erospecif′ic.** Heterologous, as pertains to grafts.

**het′erosugges′tion.** Suggestion received from another person; opposed to autosuggestion.

**het′erotax′ia** [ hetero- + G. *taxis*, arrangement ]. Heterotaxis; heterotaxy; abnormal arrangement of organs or parts of the body in relation to each other.

  **cardiac h.,** dextrocardia in which the heart gives a mirror picture of the normal.

**heterotax′ic.** Abnormally placed or arranged.

**heterotax′is, het′erotaxy.** Heterotaxia.

**het′erothal′lic** [ hetero- + G. *thallos*, a young shoot ]. In fungi, pertaining to the mating of two different thalli for sexual reproduction, as contrasted with homothallic.

**heterotic** (het′er-ot′ik). Relating to heterosis.

**het′eroto′nia** [ hetero- + G. *tonos*, tension ]. Abnormality or variation in tension or tonus.

**het′eroto′pia** [ hetero- + G. *topos*, place ]. Ectopia; a displacement of parts; local heterology. 1. The occurrence of masses of gray matter of the brain or spinal cord in abnormal situations. 2. The presence of any material in a part from which it is normally absent.

**het′erotop′ic.** Ectopic; misplaced; relating to heterotopia.

**heterotopous** (het-er-ot′o-pus). Heterotopic; referring especially to teratomas composed of tissues that are out of place in the region where found.

**het′erotrans′plant.** Heterograft.

**het′erotransplanta′tion.** Heterografting; the performance of a heterograft.

**heterotrichosis** (het′er-o-trī-ko′sis) [ hetero- + G. *trichōsis*, growth of hair ]. A condition characterized by hair growth of variegated color.

**heterotroph** (het′er-o-trof, -trōf) [ hetero- + G. *trophē*, nourishment ]. A microorganism that obtains its carbon, as well as its energy, from organic compounds; see also autotroph.

**heterotrophia** (het′er-o-tro′fī-ah) [ hetero- + G. *trophē*, nourishment ]. 1. An unusual or abnormal mode of obtaining nourishment. 2. Perverted nutrition.

**heterotrophic** (het′er-o-trof′ik). 1. Relating to a heterotroph. 2. Relating to or characterized by heterotrophia.

**heterotrophy** (het′er-ot′ro-fī). Heterotrophia.

**het′erotro′pia, heterot′ropy** [ hetero- + G. *tropē*, a turning ]. Strabismus.

**heterotypic** (het′er-o-tip′ik). Of a different or unusual type or form.

**heteroxanthine** (het′er-o-zan′thin). 7-Methylxanthine; 7-methyl-2,6-oxypurine; one of the alloxuric bases in urine, representing end products of purine metabolism.

**heteroxenous** (het′er-ok′sē-nus) [ hetero- + G. *xenos*, stranger ]. Digenetic (1).

**heterozoic** (het-er-o-zo′ik) [ hetero- + G. *zōikos*, relating to an animal ]. Relating to another animal or another species of animal.

**heterozygosis** (het′er-o-zi-go′sis). Heterozygosity.

**heterozygosity** (het′er-o-zi-gos′ī-tī) [ hetero- + G. *zygon*, a yoke ]. The state of having different allelic genes at one or more paired loci in homologous chromosomes.

**heterozygote** (het-er-o-zi′gōt) [ hetero- + G. *zygotos*, yoked ]. A heterozygous individual.

**heterozygous** (het′er-o-zi′gus). Relating to heterozygosity.

**hettocyrtosis** (het-o-sur-to′sis) [ G. *hettōn*, less, irreg. compar. of *mikros*, small, + *kyrtōsis*, a being hump-backed, fr. *kyrtos*, curved ]. A rarely used term denoting a minor degree of curvature of the spine or of one of the long bones.

**Heubner** (hoyb′ner), Johann O. L., Berlin pediatrician, 1843–1926. See H.'s *disease*.

**Heuser**, Chester, U. S. embryologist, *1885. See H.'s *membrane*.

**Hewlett**, Richard T., American bacteriologist, 1865–1940. See H.'s *stain* (for capsules).

**hexa-, hex-** [ G. *hex*, six ]. Prefixes meaning six.

**hexaben′din dihydrochloride.** USTIMON dihydrochloride; 3,4,5-trimethoxybenzoic acid diester with 3,3′-[ ethylenebis(methylimino) ]-di-1-propanol dihydrochloride; coronary and cerebral vasodilator.

**hexacanth** (hek′sah-kanth) [ hexa- + G. *akantha*, hook or thorn ]. Oncosphere; the motile six-hooked first-stage larva

of certain cyclophyllidean cestodes; it emerges from the egg and actively claws its way through the intermediate host's intestine prior to development into the next larval stage; for example, the h. of *Taenia saginata*, which penetrates the intestine of a cow that ingested the egg, then forms a cysticercus or bladder worm in the muscles of the intermediate host.

**hexacarbacho′line bromide.** IMBRETIL; hexabiscarbacholine bromide; choline bromide hexamethylenedicarbamate; hexamethylene-1,6-bis(carbamoylcholine bromide); a neuromuscular blocking agent with depolarizing and nondepolarizing actions.

**hexachlo′rocyclohex′ane.** Lindane.

**hex′achlorophene** (USP). Hexachlorophane (BP); PHISOHEX; 2,2′-methylenebis(3,4,6-trichlorophenol). Antibacterial; used in soaps and detergents to inhibit bacterial growth; excessive use causes neurological lesions.

**hexachromic** (hek′sah-kro′mik) [ hexa- + G. *chromō*, color ]. 1. Exhibiting six of the seven spectral colors. 2. Lacking the ability to perceive one of the seven spectral colors, usually violet.

**hexacy′clonate sodium.** GEVILON; 1-(hydroxymethyl)cyclohexaneaceticacid salt; psycholeptic agent.

**hex′ad.** A sexivalent element or radical.

**hexadactyly, hexadactylism** (hek′sah-dak′tī-lī, -lizm) [ hexa- + G. *daktylos*, finger ]. The presence of six fingers or six toes on one or both hands or feet.

**hex′adecano′ic acid.** Palmitic acid.

**hex′adec′anol.** Cetyl alcohol.

**hex′adimeth′rine bro′mide.** POLYBRENE; a polymer of $N,N,N′,N′$-tetramethylhexamethylenediamine and trimethylene bromide; a highly basic compound that neutralizes the anticoagulant action of heparin *in vitro* and *in vivo* by forming a stable salt with the acidic heparin.

**hexadi′phane.** NORBILINE; 1-(3,3-diphenylpropyl)hexameihyleneimine; intestinal antispasmodic with choleretic properties.

**hexafluorenium bromide** (hek′sah-flu-o-re′nī-um) (NF). MYLAXEN; IN 117; hexamethylene-bis[ fluoren-9-yldimethylammonium bromide ]; acts as a potentiator for succinylcholine in anesthesiology by producing a mild nondepolarizing neuromuscular blockade; also inhibits plasma cholinesterase.

**hexamer** (hek′să-mer) [ hexa- + G. *meros*, part ]. See virion.

**hex′ametho′nium chlo′ride.** BISTRIUM chloride; HEXAMETON chloride; C-6; hexamethylene-bis(trimethylammonium chloride); a ganglionic blocking agent used in the treatment of hypertension, usually in combination with other hypotensive drugs. Hexamethonium is also used as the bromide (Gangliostat; Vagolysin), and as the tartrate (in BP, the dihydrogen tartrate).

**hexam′idine isethionate.** HEXOMEDINE; *p,p′*-(hexamethylenedioxy)dibenzamidine; topical antiseptic.

**hex′amine.** Methenamine.

**Hexamita** (hek-sam′ī-tah) [ hexa- + G. *mitos*, thread ]. A protozoan genus of flagellates having a symmetrical body, two anterior nuclei, six anterior and two posterior flagella, and two separate axostyles; they are parasitic in the small intestine of many gallinaceous birds and of certain mammals.

  **H. meleagridis**, occurs in the turkey, peafowl, pheasant, quail and Chukkar partridge; it is most pathogenic in turkeys, causing outbreaks of hexamitiasis.

**hexamitiasis** (hek-sam′ī-ti′ă-sis). Hexamitosis; an infectious catarrhal enteritis of turkeys, quail, Chukkar partridges, and other gallinaceous birds caused by *Hexamita meleagridis* and manifested by diarrhea. Adult birds are symptomless carriers, but poults under 10 weeks often are severely affected.

**hexamitosis** (hek-sam′ī-to′sis). Hexamitiasis.

**hex′ane.** A saturated hydrocarbon, $C_6H_{14}$, of the paraffin series.

**hex′ano′ic acid.** *N*-Caproic acid; see under caproic.

**hex′aploi′dy.** See polyploidy.

**Hexapoda** (hek-sap′o-dah) [ hexa- + G. *pous*, foot ]. Six-legged arthropods forming the class Insecta.

**hex'avac'cine.** A polyvalent vaccine containing six different antigens.

**hex'edine** (USAN). STERISOL; 2,6-bis(2-ethylhexyl)hexahydro-7α-methyl-1*H*-imidazol[1,5-*c*]imidazole; antimicrobial agent.

**Hexenmilch** (hek'sen-milkh) [ Ger. *hex,* witch, + *milch,* milk ]. Witch's *milk.*

**hexes'trol.** CYCLOESTROL; *p,p'*-(1,2-diethylethylene)diphenol; dihydrodiethylstilbestrol; a synthetic compound with estrogenic activity.

**hex'ethal sodium.** ORTAL sodium; sodium 5-ethyl-5-hexylbarbiturate; a barbiturate sedative and hypnotic of short duration.

**hexet'idine.** STERILATE; 5-amino-1,3-bis-(2-ethylhexyl)-hexahydro-5-methylpyrimidine; local anti-infective agent used in the treatment of vaginitis and cervicitis due to fungal and protozoan organisms.

**hex'itol.** The polyol (sugar alcohol) obtained on the reduction of a hexose.

**hexobar'bital sodium** (NF). EVIPAL sodium; sodium 5-(1-cyclohexen-1-yl)-1,5-dimethylbarbiturate. A barbiturate sedative and hypnotic of short duration.

**hex'ocyc'lium methylsulfate** (NF). TRAL; *N*⁴-(β-cyclohexyl-β-hydroxy-β-phenylethyl)-*N*¹- methylpiperazine dimethylsulfate; an anticholinergic quaternary ammonium compound used for the adjunctive management of peptic ulcers, hyperacidity and hypermotility of the gastrointestinal tract.

**hex'oki'nase** (EC 2.7.1.1). A phosphotransferase present in yeast, muscle, and other tissues that catalyzes the phosphorylation of glucose and other hexoses to form hexose 6-phosphate (phosphate is transferred from ATP, which is converted to ADP).

**hex'one bases.** See under base.

**hexon'ic acid.** The aldonic acid obtained on the oxidation of the aldehyde group of an aldohexose to a carboxylic acid (*e.g.,* gluconic acid from glucose).

**hex'osam'ine.** The amine derivative ($NH_2$ replacing OH) of a hexose; *e.g.,* glucosamine.

**hex'osamin'idase.** General term for enzymes cleaving *N*-acetylhexose (glucose or galactose) residues from ganglioside-like oligosaccharides. At least four specific enzymes carrying out this type of reaction are known, α-*N*-acetylgalactosaminidase (EC 3.2.1.49), α-*N*-acetylglucosaminidase (EC 3.2.1.50), β-*N*-acetylhexosaminidase (EC 3.2.1.52), and β-*N*-acetylgalactosaminidase (EC 3.2.1.53), each being specific for the configuration and type of sugar included in the name. The absence of h. forms the basis for Tay-Sachs disease and other gangliosidoses.

**hex'osans.** Polyhexoses; polysaccharides with the general formula $(C_6H_{10}O_5)_x$ which, on hydrolysis, yield hexoses. Included are glucosans, mannosans, galactosans, and fructosans.

**hex'ose.** A monosaccharide containing six carbon atoms in the molecule ($C_6H_{12}O_6$); glucose is the principal hexose in nature.

**hexosebisphosphatase** (EC 3.1.3.11). Hexosediphosphatase; hydrolase removing the 1-phosphate from D-fructose-1,6-bisphosphate.

**hexosediphosphatase.** Hexosebisphosphatase.

**hexose phosphatase.** An enzyme catalyzing the hydrolysis of a hexose phosphate to a hexose (*e.g.,* glucose-6-phosphate, EC 3.1.3.9).

**hexosephosphate isomerase.** Glucosephosphate isomerase.

**hexose-1-phosphate uridylyltransferase** (EC 2.7.7.12). Uridyltransferase; phosphogalactoisomerase; an enzyme system that catalyzes the interconversion of glucose 1-phosphate and galactose 1-phosphate with simultaneous interconversion of UDPglucose and UDPgalactose. See also UDPglucose epimerase.

**hexulose** (heks'u-lōs). A ketohexose; *e.g.,* fructose.

**hexuron'ic acid.** The uronic acid of a hexose.

**hex'yl.** The radical of hexane, $CH_3(CH_2)_4CH_2—$.

**hex'ylcaine hydrochloride** (NF). CYCLAINE; cyclohexylamino-2-propylbenzoate hydrochloride. A local anesthetic with an ester linkage; suitable for surface application,

infiltration, spinal anesthesia, or nerve block. It is about twice as potent as procaine.

**hex'ylresor'cinol** (NF, BP). 4-Hexyl-1,3-dihydroxybenzene; a broad spectrum anthelmintic, fairly effective but highly caustic; it is the drug of choice in infections produced by *Trichuris trichiura* (whipworm) and *Fasciolopsis buski* (large intestinal fluke); useful also in infestations by other trematodes (*Heterophyes heterophyes* and *Metagonimus yokogawai*), various tapeworms, *Ascaris lumbricoides* (roundworm), and *Necator americanus* (hookworm).

**hexyltheobro'mine.** COSALDON; 1-hexyl-3,7-dimethylxanthine; vasodilator.

**Hey** (hā), William, English surgeon, 1736–1819. See H.'s *amputation,* internal *derangement, hernia, ligament, operation.*

**Heymans** (hi'mens), Corneille J. F., Belgian pharmacologist, *1892. Nobel laureate 1938, for his discovery of the role of the carotid sinus in the regulation of respiration.

**Heynsius** (hin'se-oos), Adrian, Dutch physician, 1831–1885. See H.'s *test.*

**Hf.** Chemical symbol of the element hafnium.

**Hg.** Chemical symbol of the element mercury (hydrargyrum).

**HGF.** Abbreviation for hyperglycemic-glycogenolytic factor (glucagon).

**hiatal** (hi-a'tal). Relating to a hiatus.

**hiatus,** pl. **hiatus** (hi-a'tus) [ L. an aperture, fr. *hio,* pp. *hiatus,* to yawn ] [ NA ]. 1. An aperture or fissure. 2. A foramen.

  **h. adducto'rius** [ NA ], an alternate term for h. tendineus.

  **h. aor'ticus** [ NA ], aortic opening; the opening in the diaphragm bounded by the two crura, the vertebral column, and the middle arcuate ligament, through which pass the aorta and thoracic duct.

  **Breschet's h.,** helicotrema.

  **h. cana'lis facia'lis,** h. canalis nervi petrosi majoris.

  **h. cana'lis nervi petro'si majo'ris** [ NA ], h. of the canal for the greater petrosal nerve; h. of the facial canal; Ferrein's foramen; the opening on the anterior aspect of the petrous part of the temporal bone which leads to the facial canal and gives passage to the greater petrosal nerve.

  **h. cana'lis nervi petro'si mino'ris** [ NA ], h. of the canal of the lesser petrosal nerve; the small opening in the petrous bone lateral to the h. for the greater petrosal nerve that gives passage to the lesser petrosal nerve.

  **h. esophage'us** [ NA ], esophageal opening; the opening in the diaphragm, between the central tendon and the h. aorticus, through which pass the esophagus and the two vagus nerves.

  **h. ethmoida'lis,** h. semilunaris.

  **Fallopian h.,** h. canalis nervi petrosi majoris.

  **h. maxilla'ris** [ NA ], maxillary h.; the opening into the maxillary sinus on the nasal surface of the maxilla.

  **pleuropericardial h.,** an opening connecting the pleural and pericardial cavities; usually the result of incomplete development of the pleuropericardial fold of the embryo.

  **pleuroperitoneal h.,** Bochdalek's foramen; an opening through the diaphragm, connecting pleural and peritoneal cavities; usually the result of defective development of the pleuroperitoneal membrane in the embryo. If the defect is extensive there may be herniation of digestive organs into the pleural cavity. See also diaphragmatic *hernia.*

  **h. sacra'lis** [ NA ], sacral h.; a gap at the lower end of the sacrum, exposing the spinal canal, due to failure of the laminae of the last sacral segment to coalesce.

  **h. saphenus** [ NA ], saphenous opening; fossa ovalis (2); the opening in the fascia lata below the medial part of the inguinal ligament through which the saphenous vein passes to enter the femoral vein.

  **Scarpa's h.,** helicotrema.

  **h. semiluna'ris** [ NA ], semilunar h.; h. ethmoidalis; a deep, narrow groove in the lateral wall of the middle meatus of the nasal fossa, into which the maxillary sinus, the frontonasal duct, and the middle ethmoid cells open.

  **h. subarcua'tus,** *fossa* subarcuata.

  **h. tendin'eus** [ NA ], tendinous opening; h. adductorius; femoral opening; the aperture in the tendon of insertion of the adductor magnus that transmits the femoral artery and vein from the adductor canal to the popliteal space.

**h. tota′lis sacra′lis,** incomplete development of sacral vertebrae.

**Hibbs,** Russell A., American surgeon, 1869–1932. See H.'s *operation.*

**hibernation** (hi′ber-na′shun) [ L. *hibernus,* relating to winter ]. Winter sleep; a torpid condition in which certain animals pass the cold months. True hibernators, such as woodchucks, ground squirrels, dormice, and some others, have body temperatures reduced to near the freezing point, with a very slow heartbeat, low metabolism, and infrequent respirations. Partial hibernators, such as bears, skunks, and raccoons, have reduced physiologic activity during the cold months, but they are not comatose.

**artificial h.,** the use of a mixture of drugs, including antihistamines, narcotics, hypnotics, and adrenolytic compounds, to induce sleep or a dormant state analogous to that observed in hibernating animals; once used as an adjuvant to anesthesia.

**hibernoma** (hi′ber-no′mah) [ L. *hibernus,* pertaining to winter, + G. suffix *-oma,* tumor ]. A rare type of benign neoplasm in human beings, consisting of brown fat that resembles the fat in certain hibernating animals; individual tumor cells contain multiple lipid deposits. See also *brown fat.*

**interscapular h.,** brown *fat.*

**hiccup, hiccough** (hik′up). A diaphragmatic spasm causing a sudden inhalation which is interrupted by a spasmodic closure of the glottis, producing a noise.

**epidemic h.,** a persistent h. occurring as a complication of influenza.

**Hicks,** John Braxton, English gynecologist, 1823–1897. See H.'s *sign, version.*

**hidradenitis** (hi-drad′e-ni′tis) [ G. *hidrōs,* sweat, + *adēn,* gland, + suffix *-itis,* inflammation ]. Inflammation of the sweat glands; more specifically, of the apocrine glands.

**h. axilla′ris of Verneuil,** an axillary abscess.

**h. suppurati′va,** spiradenitis; inflammation of the apocrine sweat glands of the perianal, axillary, and genital areas or under the breasts, producing chronic abscesses or sinuses.

**hidradenoma** (hi-drad-e-no′mah) [ G. *hidrōs,* sweat, + *adēn,* gland, + suffix *-oma,* tumor ]. A relatively infrequent, benign neoplasm derived from epithelial cells of sweat glands; may be solid or cystic, and sometimes increase to fairly large masses; two histologic types are recognized, nodular h. and papillary h.

**clear cell h.,** nodular h.

**nodular h.,** solid or clear cell h.; myoepithelioma; eccrine spiradenoma; mixed tumor of the skin; a solid, benign tumor of the skin believed to originate from epithelial cells of sweat glands.

**papillary h.,** adenoma hidroadenoides of vulva; apocrine a.; a solitary tumor occurring usually in the labia majora, cystic and papillary, and composed of epithelium resembling that of apocrine glands.

**solid h.,** nodular h.

**hidro-, hidr-** [ G. *hidrōs,* sweat ]. Combining forms relating to sweat or sweat glands.

**hidro′a.** Hydroa.

**hidrocystoma** (hi′dro-sis-to′mah) [ hidro- + G. *kystis,* bladder, + suffix *-oma,* tumor ]. A cystic form of hidradenoma.

**hidropoiesis** (hi-dro-poy-e′sis) [ hidro- + G. *poiēsis,* formation ]. The formation of sweat.

**hidropoietic** (hi′dro-poy-et′ik). Relating to hidropoiesis.

**hi′drosadeni′tis.** Hidradenitis.

**hidroschesis** (hi-dros′ke-sis) [ hidro- + G. *schesis,* a checking ]. Suppression of sweating.

**hidro′sis** [ G. *hidrōs,* sweat, + suffix *-osis,* condition ]. Excessive sweating.

**hidrot′ic.** Relating to or causing hidrosis; sudorific.

**hieralgia** (hi-er-al′ji-ah) [ G. *hieros,* sacred (sacrum), + *algos,* pain ]. Sacralgia.

**hierarchy** (hi′er-ar′kī, hi-rar′kī) [ G. *hierarchia,* rule or power of the high priest ]. 1. Any system of persons or things ranked one above the other. 2. In psychology and psychiatry, an organization of habits or concepts in which simpler components are combined to form increasingly complex integrations.

**dominance h.,** a social situation in which one organism dominates all below it, the next all below it, and so on down to the organism dominated by all; *e.g.,* the pecking order in barnyard hens.

**Maslow's h.,** a ranking of needs which man presumably fills successively in the order of lowest to highest; they are physiological needs, love and belonging, self-esteem, and self-actualization.

**response h.,** alternative reactions or modes of adjustment to a given situation arranged in the probable order of prior effectiveness; *e.g.,* a mother attempting to discipline an unruly child may first cajole, then plead, scold, and finally punish. Her behaviors can be ordered along a response h. for further monitoring of effectiveness.

**hierolisthesis** (hi′er-o-lis-the′sis) [ G. *heiros,* sacred (sacrum), + *olisthainein,* to slip ]. Sacrolisthesis.

**hieromania** (hi-er-o-ma′ni-ah) [ G. *hieros,* holy, + *mania,* insanity ]. Religious insanity.

**hierophobia** (hi-er-o-fo′bi-ah) [ G. *hieros,* holy, + *phobos,* fear ]. Morbid fear of religious or sacred objects.

**hierotherapy** (hi′er-o-thĕr′ă-pī) [ G. hieros, holy, + *therapeia,* therapy ]. Faith healing; treatment of disease by prayer and religious practices.

**Higashi,** O. See Chédiak-H. *disease,* Chédiak-Steinbrinck-H. *anomaly, syndrome.*

**Highmore,** Nathaniel, English anatomist, 1613–1685. See *antrum* of H., H.'s *body.*

**hi′lar.** Pertaining to a hilus.

**hilitis** (hi-li′tis). Inflammation of the lining membrane of any hilus.

**Hill,** Archibald V., English biophysicist, *1886. Nobel laureate, 1922, with Otto Meyerhof, for the discovery relating to the production of heat in muscle. See H.'s *equation.*

**Hill reaction.** See under reaction.

**Hill's sign.** See under sign.

**Hillis,** David S. See H.'s *maneuver.*

**hil′lock.** In anatomy, any small elevation or prominence.

**axon h.,** implantation cone; the conical area of origin of the axon from the nerve cell body; it contains parallel arrays of microtubules and a dense undercoating.

**facial h.,** *colliculus* facialis.

**sem′inal h.,** *colliculus* seminalis.

**Hilton,** John, English surgeon, 1804–1878. See H.'s *law,* white *line, method, sac.*

**hi′lum** [ L. a small bit or trifle ]. 1. Obsolete synonym for hilus. 2. The pedicle of the flap in a plastic operation.

**hi′lus,** pl. **hi′li** (the [ an E. variant of L. *hilum* ] [ NA ]. 1. Porta (1); the part of an organ where the nerves and vessels enter and leave. 2. A depression or slit resembling the h. in the olivary nucleus of the brain.

**h. of dentate nucleus,** h. nuclei dentati.

**h. of kidney,** h. renalis.

**h. li′enis** [ NA ], h. of spleen; a fissure on the gastric surface of the spleen, giving passage to the splenic vessels and nerves.

**h. of lung,** h. pulmonis.

**h. of lymph node,** h. nodi lymphatici.

**h. no′di lymphat′ici** [ NA ], h. of a lymph node; the depressed area of the surface of a lymph node through which the efferent lymphatics emerge from the medulla and through which blood vessels enter and leave the node.

**h. nu′clei denta′ti** [ NA ], h. of dentate nucleus; the mouth of the flasklike dentate nucleus of the cerebellum, directed inward, and giving exit to many of the fibers which compose the pedunculus cerebellaris superior or brachium conjunctivum.

**h. nu′clei oliva′ris** [ NA ], h. of the olivary nucleus; the medially oriented opening in the folded cell layer composing the inferior olivary nucleus through which the efferent fibers of the nucleus make their exit.

**h. of olivary nucleus,** h. nuclei olivaris.

**h. ova′rii** [ NA ], h. of ovary; the depression along the mesovarian margin, at the insertion of the mesovarium, where vessels and nerves enter or leave the ovary.

**h. of ovary,** h. ovarii.

**h. pulmo′nis** [ NA ], h. of lung; a wedge-shaped depression on the mediastinal surface of each lung, where the bronchus, blood vessels, nerves, and lymphatics enter or leave the viscus.

**h. rena'lis** [ NA ], h. of kidney; the depression on the medial border of the kidney through which pass the vessels and nerves and which contains the apex of the renal pelvis.

**h. of spleen,** h. lienis.

**hi'manto'sis** [ G. *himas,* strap, + *-osis,* morbid condition ]. Long uvula.

**hind'brain.** Rhombencephalon.

**Hindenlang,** Karl, German physician, 1854–1884. See H.'s *test.*

**hind'gut.** Endgut. 1. The large intestine, rectum, and anal canal. 2. The caudal or terminal part of the embryonic gut.

**hind'water.** 1. *Hydrorrhea* gravidarum. 2. Liquor amnii in utero behind the presenting part of the fetus.

**Hines,** Marion, American neurologist, *1889. See strip *area* of H.

**hinge-bow.** Face-bow.

**hin'ney.** A hybrid resulting from the mating of a male horse (stallion) with a female ass (jennet).

**Hinton,** William A., American physician, 1883–1959. See H. *test.*

**hip** [ A.S. *hype* ]. Coxa; the lateral prominence of the pelvis from the waist to the thigh; more strictly the h. joint.

**snapping h.,** a condition in which a tendon under tension, moving over a protuberance of the proximal end of the femur, causes a click.

**Hippel,** Eugen von. See von Hippel, Eugen.

**Hippelates** (hip'ĕ-la'tēz). The eye gnats; a genus of flies in the family Chloropidae (fruit flies) that are attracted to the body secretions and fluids of animals and man, particularly of the eyes. *H.* is suspected of transmitting certain types of conjunctivitis (such as pinkeye), bovine mastitis, and yaws (frambesia tropica).

**Hippobosca** (hip-o-bos'kah) [ G. *hippos,* horse, + *boskein,* to feed ]. A genus of pupiparous louse flies (family Hippoboscidae) related to the tsetse flies; they are ectoparasites on birds and mammals; see also *Melophagus.*

**Hippobos'cidae.** A family of winged and wingless flies (order Diptera) that are parasitic on birds and mammals; it includes the genera *Hippobosca* and *Melophagus.*

**hippocam'pal.** Relating to the hippocampus.

**hippocampus** (hip-po-kam'pus) [ G. *hippocampos,* seahorse. HIPP- ] [ NA ]. Hippocampus major; the complex, internally convoluted structure that forms the medial margin ("hem") of the cortical mantle of the cerebral hemisphere, bordering the choroid fissure of the lateral ventricle, and composed of two gyri (Ammon's horn and the dentate gyrus), together with their white matter, the alveus and fimbria hippocampi. In monkeys, apes, and man the h. is confined to the temporal lobe by the massive development of the corpus callosum. Cytoarchitecturally a unique form of allocortex (archicortex), the h. forms part of the limbic system (formerly rhinencephalon). Its major afferent connections are with the entorhinal area of the parahippocampal gyrus, and septum pellucidum; by way of the fornix it projects to the septum, anterior nucleus of the thalamus, and mamillary body.

**h. major,** hippocampus.

**h. minor,** *calcar* avis.

**Hippocrates** (hip-pok'ra-tēz), Greek physician, called the "Father of Medicine," born in the island of Cos about 460 B.C. and died about 377 B.C. He placed medicine on a scientific foundation, freeing it from superstition, philosophy, and religious rites; gave sound and shrewd descriptions of many diseases and raised the ethical standards of medical practice; his physiology, pathology, and therapeutics were based largely upon the humoral doctrines of his predecessors. See (in addition to subentries below) H.'s *bandage, cap,* Hippocratic *facies, fingers, nails, school, succussion.*

**aph'orisms of H.,** a number of medical observations, rules, and pithy expressions of clinical wisdom found in Books I to III of the Hippocratic writings.

**Hippocratic collections,** the written works of H., his predecessors and contemporaries. Only a portion are genuine compositions of the "Father of Medicine." Those thought to be genuine are, *Prognostic; Regimen in Acute Diseases; Epidemics; Airs, Waters, Places; The Aphorisms;*

*Fractures; Wounds in the Head;* and probably, *On the Sacred Disease.*

**Hippocratic oath,** an oath demanded of the young physician about to enter upon the practice of his profession, the composition of which, though usually attributed to H., is probably an ancient oath of the Asclepiads. It appears in a book of the Hippocratic collections as follows: "I swear by Apollo the physician, by Aesculapius, Hygeia, and Panacea, and I take to witness all the gods, all the goddesses, to keep according to my ability and my judgment the following Oath:

"To consider dear to me as my parents him who taught me this art; to live in common with him and if necessary to share my goods with him; to look upon his children as my own brothers, to teach them this art if they so desire without fee or written promise; to impart to my sons and the sons of the master who taught me and the disciples who have enrolled themselves and have agreed to the rules of the profession, but to these alone, the precepts and the instruction. I will prescribe regimen for the good of my patients according to my ability and my judgment and never do harm to anyone. To please no one will I prescribe a deadly drug, nor give advice which may cause his death. Nor will I give a woman a pessary to procure abortion. But I will preserve the purity of my life and my art. I will not cut for stone, even for patients in whom the disease is manifest; I will leave this operation to be performed by practitioners (specialists in this art). In every house where I come I will enter only for the good of my patients, keeping myself far from all intentional ill-doing and all seduction, and especially from the pleasures of love with women or with men, be they free or slaves. All that may come to my knowledge in the exercise of my profession or outside of my profession or in daily commerce with men, which ought not to be spread abroad, I will keep secret and will never reveal. If I keep this oath faithfully, may I enjoy my life and practice my art, respected by all men and in all times; but if I swerve from it or violate it, may the reverse be my lot."

**Hippocrat'ic.** Relating to Hippocrates.

**hippoc'ratism.** The imitation of nature's efforts in the therapeutic management of disease.

**hip'pulin.** A urinary product of estrogen metabolism in the mare; tentatively identified as 8-dehydro-14-isoestrone.

**hip'purate.** A salt or ester of hippuric acid.

**hippu'ria.** The excretion of an abnormally large amount of hippuric acid in the urine.

**hippu'ric acid.** *N*-Benzoylglycine; an acid found in the urine of many herbivorous animals; used therapeutically in the form of its salts (hippurates of calcium and ammonium).

**hippu'ricase.** Aminocylase.

**hip'pus** [ G. *hippos,* horse, from a fancied suggestion of galloping movements. HIPP- ]. Spasmodic, rhythmical movements of the pupil, independent of illumination, convergence, or psychic stimuli.

**respiratory h.,** dilation of the pupils occurring during inspiration, and contraction during expiration.

**hir'ci.** Plural of hircus.

**hircismus** (hur-siz'mus) [ L. *hircus,* goat ]. Offensive odor of the axillae.

**hircus,** gen. and pl. **hir'ci** (hur'kus) [ L. he-goat ]. 1. The odor of the axillae. 2 [ NA ]. One of the hairs growing in the axillae. 3. Tragus.

**Hirschberg,** Julius, German oculist, 1843–1925. See H.'s *method.*

**Hirschberg,** Leonard K., Baltimore physician, *1877. See H.'s *reflex.*

**Hirschfeld's canals.** See under canal.

**Hirschsprung,** Harold, Copenhagen physician, 1830–1916. See H.'s *disease.*

**hirsute** (hur-sūt') [ L. *hirsutus,* shaggy ]. Hairy; relating to or characterized by hirsutism.

**hirsuties** (hur-su'te-ēz) [ a Mod. L. form fr. L. *hirsutus,* shaggy ]. Hirsutism.

**hirsutism** (hur'su-tizm) [ L. *hirsutus,* shaggy ]. Hirsuties; presence of excessive bodily and facial hair, especially in women; may be present in normal adults as an expression of an ethnic characteristic or may develop in children or adults as the result of a metabolic disorder, usually endocrine in nature.

**Apert's h.,** h. caused by a virilizing disorder of adrenocortical origin.

**constitutional h.,** mild to moderate degree of h. present in an individual exhibiting otherwise normal endocrine and reproductive function; it appears to be a heritable form of h. and commonly is an expression of an ethnic characteristic.

**idiopathic h.,** hirsutism of uncertain origin in women; some such patients may additionally exhibit menstrual abnormalities and sterility. Some authorities believe the hirsutism reflects hypersecretion of adrenocortical androgens.

**hirtellous** (hur'tel-lus) [ L. *hirtus*, hairy, shaggy ]. Having or resembling fine hairs; term describing the filamentous protein polysaccharide coating of microvilli.

**hirudicide** (hi-ru'di-sid) [ L. *hirudo*, leech, + *caedo*, to kill ]. An agent that kills leeches.

**hir'udin** [ L. *hirudo*, leech ]. A substance extracted from the salivary glands of the leech that has the property of preventing coagulation of the blood. An antithrombin.

**Hirudinea** (hir'u-din'e-ah) [ L. *hirudo*, leech ]. Leeches, *q.v.*; a class of worms (phylum Annelida) with flat, segmented bodies, a sucker at the posterior end, and often a smaller sucker at the anterior pole; they are predatory on invertebrate tissues, or feed on blood and tissue exudates of vertebrates.

**hirudiniasis** (hir'u-di-ni'ă-sis). A condition resulting from attack by leeches.

**external h.,** h. due to aquatic or land leeches attaching themselves to the skin.

**internal h.,** h. due to aquatic leeches being accidently taken into the mouth or nose in drinking.

**Hirudo** (hi-ru'do) [ L. leech ]. A genus of leeches (class Hirudinea, family Gnathobdellidae); the species most commonly used in medicine are: *H. australis*, Australian leech; *H. decora*, American leech; *H. interrupta* or *H. troctina*, a leech of Northern Africa; *H. medicinalis*, speckled, Swedish, or German leech, the species in most general use; *H. officinalis*, a variety of the preceding; *H. provincialis*, the green or Hungarian leech; *H. quinquestriata*, five-striped leech. See also leech.

**His.** Symbol for histidyl.

**His,** Wilhelm, Sr., Swiss anatomist and embryologist in Germany, 1831–1904. See H.'s *canal, copula, duct, isthmus, rule, spaces.*

**His,** Wilhelm, Jr., German physician, 1863–1934. See H.'s *band, bundle,* Kent-H. *bundle,* Werner-H. *disease,* H.'s *spindle,* H.-Tawara *system.*

**Hiss,** Philip H., U. S. bacteriologist, 1868–1913. See H.'s *stain.*

**histaffine** (his'tă-fēn) [ G. *histos*, web, + L. *affinis*, related ]. 1. Manifesting a tendency to combine with or adhere to tissues. 2. A hypothetical substance thought by some to occur in the blood of certain persons with trypanosomiasis or syphilis, and postulated to combine with specific constituents in tissues in such a manner that complement fixation occurs.

**histam'inase.** Amine oxidase (pyridoxal-containing).

**histamine** (his'tă-mēn). 2-(4-Imidazolyl)ethylamine; a depressor amine derived from histidine by decarboxylation. Present in ergot and in animal tissues, also formed from histidine by putrefaction; powerful stimulant of gastric secretion and constrictor of bronchial smooth muscle. When pricked into the skin in high dilution, it causes the triple response. It is a vasodilator (capillaries and arterioles) and causes a fall in blood pressure. It, or a substance indistinguishable in action from it, is liberated in the skin as a result of injury. See also histamine *shock.*

**h. acid phosphate** (BP), same action and use as h. phosphate.

**h. azopro'tein,** h. conjugated with despeciated horse serum globulin which at one time was proposed for active "immunization" against h. in certain idiosyncratic allergies, with the view that the resulting antibodies would neutralize h. upon their release.

**h. liberators,** substances, such as the compound produced by condensation of *p*-methoxyphenylethylmethyla-

mine with formaldehyde, which cause the release of endogenous h. and the induction of a variety of reactions, *e.g.,* erythema, vasodilation, hypotension, itching, gastric secretion, shocklike manifestations, and an increase in the histamine content of the plasma. Their effects are neutralized by antihistamine drugs.

**h. phosphate** (USP), used in the treatment of certain allergies, cephalalgia, and acute multiple sclerosis with varying results; also used to test gastric secretory function, in the diagnosis of pheochromocytoma and in the treatment of Ménière's disease.

**histamine-fast.** Indicating the absence of the normal response to histamine, especially in speaking of true gastric anacidity.

**his'tamine'mia.** The presence of histamine in the circulating blood.

**his'taminu'ria.** The excretion of histamine in the urine.

**histangic** (his-tan'jik). Histoangic.

**his'tidase.** Histidine ammonia-lyase.

**histidinal.** The aldehyde analogue of histidine (—CHO replacing —COOH).

**his'tidinase.** Histidine ammonia-lyase.

**his'tidine.** α-Amino-β-4-imidazolylpropionic acid; a basic amino acid in proteins.

**Histidine**

**h. ammonia-lyase** (EC 4.3.1.3), histidase; h. deaminase; enzyme catalyzing deamination of histidine to urocanate.

**h. deaminase,** h. ammonia-lyase.

**h. decarboxylase** (EC 4.1.1.22), an enzyme catalyzing the decarboxylation of histidine to histamine. a Requires pyridoxal phosphate.

**his'tidine'mia.** Ahistidasia; elevation of blood histidine level and excretion of histidine and related imidazole metabolites in urine due to deficiency of histidase activity; speech defect, mild mental retardation are associated conditions in about half of the patients; growth retardation in some; autosomal recessive inheritance.

**his'tidinol.** The alcohol analogue of histidine (—COOH becomes —CH₂OH).

**his'tidinu'ria.** The excretion of considerable amounts of histidine in the urine; frequently observed in later months of pregnancy, and in histidinemia.

**his'tidyl.** Symbol, His; the radical of histidine.

**histio-** [ G. *histion*, web (tissue) ]. Combining form relating to tissue.

**his'tioblast** [ histio- + G. *blastos*, germ ]. Histoblast; a tissue-forming cell.

**histiocyte** (his'tī-o-sīt) [ histio- + G. *kytos*, cell ]. A macrophage present in connective tissue; see reticuloendothelial *system.*

**cardiac h.,** caterpillar cell; Anitschkow cell or myocyte; a large mononuclear cell found in connective tissue of the heart wall in inflammatory conditions, especially in the Aschoff body. The ovoid nucleus contains a central chromatin mass appearing as a wavy bar in longitudinal section.

**histiocytoma** (his'tī-o-si-to'mah) [ histio- + G. *kytos*, cell, + suffix *-ōma*, tumor ]. A tumor composed of histiocytes.

**fibrous h.,** dermatofibroma.

**his'tiocyto'sis.** A generalized multiplication of histiocytes.

**kerasin h.,** Gaucher's *disease.*

**lipid h.,** h. with cytoplasmic accumulation of lipid, either cholesterol (Hand-Schüller-Christian disease), phospholipid (Niemann-Pick disease), or kerasin (Gaucher's disease).

**nonlipid h.,** Letterer-Siwe disease; an acute progressive generalized disease in young children, characterized by a purpuric rash, enlargement of lymph glands and spleen, and invasion of the spleen, liver, and bone marrow by histiocytes.

**h. X,** histiocytic proliferation of undetermined type, possibly Hand-Schüller-Christian d. or eosinophilic granuloma of bone.

**histiogenic** (his′tĭ-o-jen′ik). Histogenous.

**histioid** (his′tĭ-oyd). Histoid.

**histio′ma.** Histoma.

**histionic** (his′tĭ-on′ik). Relating to any tissue.

**histo-** [ G. *histos*, web (tissue) ]. Combining form denoting relationship to tissue.

**histoangic** (his′to-an′jik) [ histo- + G. *angeion*, vessel ]. Histangic; relating to the structure of blood vessels, especially in terms of their function.

**his′toblast.** Histioblast.

**his′tochem′istry.** Cytochemistry.

**his′tocompat′ibil′ity.** State of immunologic similarity or identity of tissues sufficient to permit successful homograft (allograft) transplantation; implies identity of histocompatibility genes in donor and recipient with respect to the particular tissue.

**histocyte** (his′to-sīt). Histiocyte.

**his′tocyto′sis.** Histiocytosis.

**his′todifferen′tia′tion.** The morphologic appearance of tissue characteristics during development.

**histofluorescence** (his-to-flu-or-es′ens). Fluorescence of the tissues under exposure to ultraviolet rays following the injection of a fluorescent substance.

**histogenesis** (his′to-jen′ĕ-sis) [ histo- + G. *genesis*, origin ]. Histogeny; the origin of a tissue; the formation and development of the tissues of the body.

**his′togenet′ic.** Relating to histogenesis.

**histogenous** (his-toj′ĕ-nus) [ histo- + G. suffix -*gen*, producing ]. Formed by the tissues; *e.g.*, the h. cells in an exudate arising from proliferation of the fixed tissue cells.

**histogeny** (his-toj′ĕ-nĭ). Histogenesis.

**his′togram** [ histo- + G. *gramma*, a writing ]. The graphic columnar or bar representation of the relationship of two factors—usually time and frequency—to an event.

**histoid** (his′toyd) [ histo- + G. *eidos*, resemblance ]. 1. Resembling in structure one of the tissues of the body. 2. Sometimes used with reference to the histologic structure of a neoplasm derived from and consisting of a single, relatively simple type of neoplastic tissue that closely resembles the normal, as in certain fibromas, leiomyomas, and the like.

**his′toincompatibil′ity.** State of immunologic dissimilarity of tissues sufficient to cause rejection of homograft when tissue is transplanted from one individual to another; implies a difference in histocompatibility genes in donor and recipient.

**histolog′ic, histolog′ical.** Pertaining to histology.

**histologist** (his-tol′o-jist). One who specializes in the science of histology.

**histology** (his-tol′o-jĭ) [ histo- + G. *logos*, study ]. The science that deals with the minute structure of cells, tissues, and organs in relation to their function; see microscopic anatomy.

**histolysis** (his-tol′ĭ-sis) [ histo- + G. *lysis*, dissolution ]. Disintegration of tissue.

**histo′ma** histo- + G. suffix -*oma*, tumor ]. Histioma; a benign neoplasm in which the cytologic and histologic elements are closely similar to those of normal tissue from which the neoplastic cells are derived.

**his′tometaplas′tic.** Exciting tissue metaplasia.

**Histomo′nas meleag′ridis.** A flagellate parasitizing the intestine and liver of turkeys, chickens, and many other domestic and wild gallinaceous birds; it is nearly ubiquitous but rarely pathogenic in chickens; in the turkey, it causes histomoniasis. It is now considered to be in a family (Monocercomonadidae) related to the trichomonads.

**histomoniasis** (his′to-mo-ni′ă-sis). Blackhead (2); infectious enterohepatitis; a disease chiefly affecting turkeys; it is caused by *Histomonas meleagridis* and is characterized by acute onset, a high mortality rate, and ulcerative and necrotic lesions of the liver and cecum. It is transmitted

inside the eggs of *Heterakis gallinae*, which is primarily responsible for maintaining and spreading the infection.

**his′tone.** One of a number of simple proteins containing a high proportion of basic amino acids; soluble in water and in dilute acids and alkalies; not coagulable by heat; examples are, globin in hemoglobin, and the proteins associated with nucleic acids (so-called nucleoproteins) in nucleic plant and animal tissues.

**h. base,** see under base.

**h. nucleate,** (1) nucleohistone; (2) nucleoprotein.

**his′tonec′tomy** [ histo- + G. *ektomē*, excision ]. Periarterial *sympathectomy*.

**histoneurology** (his-to-nu-rol′o-jĭ). Neurohistology.

**histon′omy** [ histo- + G. *nomos*, law ]. The law of the development and structure of the tissues of the body.

**histonu′ria.** The excretion of histone in the urine, as observed in certain instances of leukemia, febrile illnesses, and wasting diseases.

**his′topath′ogen′esis.** [ histogenesis + pathogenesis ]. Abnormal embryonic development or growth of tissue.

**his′topathol′ogy.** Pathologic histology; the science or study dealing with the cytologic and histologic structure of abnormal or diseased tissue.

**his′tophysiol′ogy.** The microscopic study of tissues in relation to their functions.

**Histoplasma** (his′to-plaz′mah) [ histo- + G. *plasma*, something formed ]. A genus of yeastlike fungi, of which the species *H. capsulatum* and *H. duboisii* are the causative agents of histoplasmosis and African histoplasmosis, respectively; see also histoplasmosis.

**hist′oplas′min** (USP). A concentrate of soluble growth products of *Histoplasma capsulatum;* used as a dermal reactivity indicator.

**histoplasmoma** (his′to-plaz-mo′mah) [ *Histoplasma* + G. suffix -*oma*, tumor ]. An infectious granuloma caused by the fungus *Histoplasma capsulatum.*

**histoplasmosis** (his′to-plaz-mo′sis). Darling′s disease; an infectious disease usually caused by *Histoplasma capsulatum* and occasionally by *H. duboisii.* Cases of h. due to *H. duboisii* have thus far been limited to tropical Africa. Human infection with *H. capsulatum* is widely distributed in the world; however, the population of certain regions, such as the Mississippi-Missouri-Ohio river valleys, shows a high incidence of infection as measured by the histoplasmin skin test. The natural habitat of *H. capsulatum* is the soil, particularly soils contaminated by the dejecta of fowl, birds, or bats; numerous epidemics have followed visits to, or work in, such areas. The infection is normally acquired by inhalation of spores of the fungus in dust. In the vast majority of persons infected, a primary, benign, pneumonitis is produced, similar in clinical features to primary tuberculosis. In occasional persons infected, the primary disease progresses to produce localized lesions in lung, such as pulmonary cavitation, or the typical disseminated disease of the reticuloendothelial system which is manifested by fever, emaciation, splenomegaly, leukopenia, etc.

**African h.,** a distinct, large-sized variant due to *Histoplasma duboisii,* growing chiefly in giant cells, causing lesions localized to skin, bone or lacrimal gland; or disseminated with multiple foci of osteomyelitis and visceropathy. Generalized forms produce lesions in lymph nodes, spleen, liver, bone, and lungs, though lung involvement is uncommon. Responds to surgery and amphotericin B.

**his′toradiog′raphy.** Roentgenography of tissue; refers specifically to microscopic sections of tissue.

**historrhexis** (his-to-rek′sis) [ histo- + G. *rhēxis*, rupture ]. Breakdown of tissue by some agency other than infection.

**Histosporid′ium carcinomato′sum.** A presumed intracellular sporozoan parasite formerly postulated as a causal agent of cancer.

**his′tothrom′bin.** A thrombin derived from connective tissue.

**his′totome** [ histo- + G. *tomē*, cut ]. Microtome.

**histot′omy.** Microtomy.

**histotox′ic.** Relating to poisoning of the respiratory enzyme system of the tissues.

**histotroph** (his′to-trof). Embryotroph (1).

**histotroph'ic** [ histo- + G. *trophē,* nourishment ]. Providing nourishment for or favoring the formation of tissue.

**histotrop'ic** [ histo- + G. *tropikos,* turning ]. Attracted toward the tissues; denoting certain parasites, stains, and chemical compounds.

**histozo'ic** [ histo- + G. *zōikos,* relating to an animal ]. Living in the tissues outside of a cell body; denoting certain parasitic protozoa.

**Hitzig.** Eduard, German psychiatrist, 1838–1907. See H.'s *girdle.*

**hives.** Urticaria.

**Hjärre,** A., German pathologist, 1897–1958. See H.'s *disease.*

**Hl.** Abbreviation for latent *hyperopia.*

**Hm.** Abbreviation for manifest *hyperopia.*

**HMG.** Abbreviation for human menopausal *gonadotropin.*

**HN2.** Abbreviation for nitrogen mustard; see under mustard.

**Ho.** Chemical symbol of the element holmium.

**hoar'hound** [ A.S. *hār hune* ]. Marrubium.

**hoarse** [ A.S. *hās* ]. Having a rough, harsh voice.

**hoarse'ness.** An unnaturally deep and harsh quality of the voice.

**Hobo'ken,** Nicholas v., Dutch anatomist and physician, 1632–1678. See H.'s *gemmules, nodules, valves.*

**Hoche** (ho'kĕ), Alfred E., German psychiatrist, 1865–1943. See H.'s *bundle, tract.*

**Hochsinger** (hŏkh'zing-er), Karl, Vienna pediatrician, *1860. See H.'s *phenomenon.*

**hock.** The tarsus in the horse and other quadrupeds; the joint of the hind limb between the stifle and the fetlock. Corresponds to the ankle in man.

   **capped h.,** calcaneal *bursitis.*

   **cow h.,** a faulty conformation of the hind legs in horses in which the h.'s are too close together and the feet too wide, the leg axis being directed outward and forward instead of straight forward.

   **curby h.,** curb.

**Hodge,** Hugh L., Philadelphia gynecologist, 1796–1873. See H.'s *forceps, pessary.*

**Hodgen,** John T., American surgeon, 1826–1882. See H.'s *splint.*

**Hodgkin,** Alan L., English physiologist, *1914. Nobel laureate, 1963, with Andrew F. Huxley and John C. Eccles for their studies of nervous system functions, especially of nerves and synapses. See Goldman-H.-Katz *equation.*

**Hodgkin,** Thomas, English physician, 1798–1866. See H.'s *disease, paragranuloma.*

**Hodgkin-Key murmur.** See under murmur.

**Hodgson** (hoj'son), Joseph, English physician, 1788–1869. See H.'s *disease.*

**hodi-potsy** (ho'dī-pot'sī). A dermatosis encountered in Madagascar resembling tinea flava.

**hodoneuromere** (ho-do-nu'ro-mēr) [ G. *hodos,* path, + *neuron,* nerve, + *meros,* part ]. In embryology, a metameric segment of the neural tube with its pair of nerves and their branches. Rarely used term.

**hodopho'bia** [ G. *hodos,* path, + *phobos,* fear ]. Morbid fear of traveling.

**Hoechst's peptone.** See under peptone.

**Hoeppli,** Reinhard. See H. *phenomenon.*

**hof** [ Ger. court ]. The hollow in the cytoplasm of a cell that lodges the nucleus.

**Hofacker** (hof'ak-ur), Johann D., German obstetrician, 1788–1828. See H.-Sadler *laws.*

**Hofbauer,** J. Isfred I., American gynecologist, *1878. See H. *cell.*

**Hoffa,** Albert, German surgeon, 1859–1908. See H.'s *operation.*

**Hoffmann,** G. P. Wellenhof von, Austrian bacteriologist, *1843. See H.'s *bacillus.*

**Hoffmann,** Johann, German neurologist, 1857–1919. See H.'s muscular *atrophy,* Werdnig-H. *disease,* H.'s *phenomenon, reflex, signs.*

**Hoffmann,** Moritz, German anatomist, 1622–1698. See H.'s *duct.*

**Hofmeister,** F., German biochemist, 1850–1922. See H. *series.*

**Hofmeister,** Franz von, German surgeon, 1867–1926. See H.'s *operation,* H.-Pólya *anastomosis.*

**Hogben,** L. T. See H. *test.*

**hogg.** English term for a young sheep which has never been shorn, generally one 10 to 14 months of age. See also hogget.

**hog'get.** English term for a yearling sheep of either sex. It is sometimes used for a yearling colt or boar.

**holandric** (hol-an'drik) [ G. *holos,* entire, + *aner,* man ]. Related to genes located on the Y chromosome.

**hol'arthrit'ic.** Relating to holarthritis.

**holarthritis** (hol'ar-thri'tis) [ G. *holos,* entire, + *arthron,* joint, + suffix *-itis,* inflammation ]. Inflammation of all or a great number of the joints.

**Holden,** Luther, English anatomist, 1815–1905. See H.'s *line.*

**holiat'ric.** Concerning holiatry.

**ho'liatry** [ G. *holos,* whole, + *iatreia,* medical treatment ]. Whole treatment; care of the entire patient in all aspects.

**holism** (ho'lizm) [ G. *holos,* entire ]. Holistic *psychology.*

**holistic** (ho-lis'tik). Relating to holism.

**Holl,** Mortiz, Austrian surgeon, 1852–1920. See H.'s *ligament.*

**Hollander,** Franklin, U. S. physiologist, *1899. See H.'s *test.*

**Hollenhorst** Robert W., U. S. ophthalmologist, *1913. See H. *plaques.*

**Holley,** Robert W., U. S. biochemist, *1922. Nobel laureate, 1968, with Marshall W. Nirenberg and Har Gobind Khorana, for their interpretation of the genetic code and its function in protein synthesis.

**hol'low.** Concavity; depression.

   **Sebileau's h.,** depression between the inferior aspect of the tongue and the sublingual glands.

**Holm,** Gillis E. A., Swedish geologist, 1891–1927. Gave his name to holmium.

**Holmes,** Eric G., British neurologist, *1897. See Stewart-H. *sign.*

**Holmes,** Gordon M., London neurologist, 1876–1965. See H.-Adie *syndrome.*

**Holmes,** Oliver Wendell, American physician, author and poet, 1809–1894. Professor of anatomy and physiology at Harvard. Notable in medicine for his recognition of the contagious nature of puerperal fever (septicemia). His views, which met bitter opposition from some of his contemporaries, were published in a paper in 1843, *On the Contagiousness of Puerperal Fever.* His works in the field of literature are among the American classics.

**Holmgrén,** Alarik F., Swedish physiologist, 1831–1897. See H.'s *test.*

**Holmgrén,** Emil A., Danish histologist, 1866–1922. See H.-Golgi *canals.*

**holmium** (hol'mī-um) [ G. *Holm* ]. An element of the lanthanide group, symbol Ho, atomic no. 67, atomic weight 164.94.

**holo-** (hol'o-, ho'lo-) [ G. *holos,* whole, entire, complete ]. Combining form denoting entirety or relationship to a whole.

**holoacardius** (hol'o-ă-kar'dī-us) [ holo- + G. *a-* priv. + *kardia,* heart ]. A separate, grossly defective twin lacking a heart of its own, its blood supply being dependent on a shunt from the placental circulation of a more nearly normal twin; a placental parasitic twin or omphalosite.

   **h. aceph'alus,** a h. also lacking a head.

   **h. acor'mus,** a h. in which little more than the head is represented.

   **h. amor'phus,** a h. in which the body of the parasite is represented by only a shapeless mass.

**holo-ACP synthase** (EC 2.7.8.7). Enzyme catalyzing transfer of 4'-phosphopantetheinyl residue from CoA to a serine of apo-ACP to form holo-ACP.

**holoacrania** (hol'o-ă-kra'nī-ah) [ holo- + G. *a-* priv. + *kranion,* skull ]. A congenital skull defect in which bones of the vault are absent.

**holoanencephaly** (hol'o-an-en-sef'ă-lī) [ holo- + G. *an-priv.* + *enkephalos*, brain ]. Complete absence of cranium and brain.

**hol'oblas'tic** [ holo- + G. *blastos*, germ ]. Denoting the involvement of the entire (isolecithal or moderately telolecithal) ovum in cleavage.

**holocephalic** (hol'o-sĕ-fal'ik) [ holo- + G. *kephalē*, head ]. Denoting a fetus deficient in certain parts, but with the head complete.

**holocrine** (hol'o-krin) [ holo- + G. *krinō*, to separate ]. See holocrine *gland.*

**hol'odiastol'ic.** Relating to or occupying the entire diastole.

**holoendemic** (hol'o-en-dem'ik). Endemic in the entire population, as trachoma in the villages of Saudi Arabia.

**holoenzyme** (hol'o-en'zim). The complete enzyme *i.e.*, apoenzyme plus coenzyme.

**hologastroschisis** (hol'o-gas-tros'kī-sis) [ holo- + G. *gastēr*, belly, + *schisis*, cleaving ]. A congenital malformation involving a cleft which extends the entire length of the abdomen.

**hol'ogram** [ holo- + G. *gramma*, something written ]. A three-dimensional image.

**hologynic** (hol'o-jin'ik) [ holo- + G. *gynē*, woman ]. Related to sex-limited characters manifest only in females.

**hol'omas'tigote** [ holo- + G. *mastix*, whip ]. Having flagella over the entire surface.

**holomorphosis** (hol'o-mor-fo'sis) [ holo- + G. *morphosis*, shaping ]. Attainment or reestablishment of physical wholeness.

**holomy'cin.** 6-Acetamido-1,2-dithiolo[ 4,3-*b* ]pyrrol-5-(4 *H*)-one; antibiotic produced by a strain of *Streptomyces griseus*; possesses antimicrobial properties.

**holophytic** (hol-o-fit'ik) [ holo- + G. *phyton*, plant ]. Exactly like a plant in metabolism or mode of obtaining nourishment; denoting certain protozoans.

**holoprosencephaly** (hol'o-pros'en-sef'ă-lī) [ holo- + G. *prosō*, forward, + *enkephalos*, brain ]. Failure of the forebrain to divide into hemispheres or lobes.

**holorachischisis** (hol'o-rā-kis'kī-sis) [ holo- + G. *rhachis*, spine, + *schisis*, fissure ]. Rachischis totalis; spina bifida of the entire spinal column.

**hol'osystol'ic.** Pansystolic.

**holotelencephaly** (hol'o-tel-en-sef'ă-lī) [ holo- + telencephalon, *q.v.* ]. Congenital absence of one cerebral ventricle with no separation of the cerebral hemispheres; associated with arrhinencephaly.

**holothurigenin** (hol'o-thu'ri-jen-in). A sapogenin obtained from the sea cucumber, *Holothuria vagabunda*; it is the steroid aglycon of the holothurins.

**holothurin** (hol'o-thu'rin). A mixture of toxic, membrane-active, steroid glycosides (saponins) obtained from sea cucumbers (order Echinodermata, class Holothuroidea); the steroid component is holothurigenin.

**hol'otoxin.** A substance isolated from various species of sea cucumbers (*Holothuria*); it appears to be a steroid glycoside. It exhibits a potent antifungal action against a variety of such organisms, including pathogenic fungi of vegetable origin; the antibacterial activity of h. appears to be negligible.

**Holotrichida** (hol-o-trik'ī-dah) [ holo- + G. *thrix*, hair ]. An order of Ciliata in which cilia are distributed over the entire body.

**holotrichous** (hol-ot'rī-kus) [ holo- + G. *thrix*, hair ]. Having cilia over the entire surface.

**holozoic** (hol-o-zō'ik) [ holo- + G. *zōon*, animal ]. Resembling exactly an animal in its metabolism or mode of obtaining nourishment; denoting certain protozoans in distinction to others which are holophytic.

**Holt,** M. See H.-Oram *syndrome.*

**Holt'house,** Carsten, English surgeon, 1810–1901. See H.'s *hernia.*

**Holzknecht unit.** See under unit.

**Holzmann,** Walter, German physician. See Much-H. *reaction.*

**homalocephalous** (hom'ă-lo-sef'ă-lus) [ G. *homalos*, level, + *kephalē*, head ]. Having a flattened head.

**Homalomyia** (hom'ă-lo-mi'yah) [ G. *homalos*, even, + *myia*, a fly ]. A genus of flies the larvae of which sometimes infest human or animal intestines.

**homaluria** (hom'ă-lu'rī-ah) [ G. *homalos*, level, + *ouron*, urine ]. Normal urine flow.

**Homans,** John, American surgeon, 1877–1954. See H.'s *sign.*

**homat'ropine.** Tropine mandelate; mandelytropine; an anticholinergic agent used in the treatment of hyperchlorhydria and gastrointestinal spasm; also a mydriatic and cycloplegic. Available as the hydrobromide (USP, BP), and as the methylbromide (NF).

**homaxial** (ho-mak'sī-al) [ G. *homos*, the same, + *axis* ]. Having all the axes alike, as a sphere.

**Home,** Sir Everard, English surgeon, 1756–1832. See H.'s *lobe.*

**homeo-** [ G. *homoios*, like ]. Combining form meaning the same, or alike. For some words so beginning but not found here see also those beginning homo-.

**homeocyte** (ho'me-o-sit) [ homeo- + G. *kytes*, cell ]. An obsolete term for a lymphocyte.

**homeometric** (ho'me-o-met'rik) [ homeo- + G. *metron*, measure ]. Without change in size.

**homeomorphous** (ho'me-o-mor'fus) [ homeo- + G. *morphē*, shape ]. Of similar shape, but not necessarily of the same composition.

**ho'meopath.** Homeopathist.

**homeopathic** (ho'me-o-path'ik). Relating to homeopathy.

**homeopathist** (ho'me-op'ă-thist). A medical practitioner of the homeopathic school.

**homeopathy** (ho-me-op'ă-thī) [ homeo- + G. *pathos*, suffering ]. A system of therapy developed by Samuel Hahnemann on the theory that large doses of a certain drug given to a healthy person will produce certain conditions which, when occurring spontaneously as symptoms of a disease, are relieved by the same drug in small doses. This was called the "law of similia," from the aphorism, *similia similibus curantur*—a sort of "fighting fire with fire" therapy. Many different ideas, such as the theory of dynamization (that repeated trituration, or dilution with agitation, enhanced the power of a drug) characterized the cult. The real value of h. was to demonstrate the healing powers of nature and the therapeutic virtue of placebos.

**homeoplasia** (ho-me-o-pla'zī-ah) [ homeo- + G. *plasis*, a molding ]. The formation of new tissue of the same character as that already existing in the part.

**homeoplas'tic.** Relating to or characterized by homeoplasia.

**homeostasis** (ho'me-os'tă-sis) [ homeo- + G. *stasis*, a standing ]. 1. The state of equilibrium (balance between opposing pressures) in the body with respect to various functions and to the chemical compositions of the fluids and tissues, *e.g.*, temperature, heart rate, blood pressure, water content, blood sugar, etc. 2. The processes through which such bodily equilibrium is maintained.

**homeostat'ic.** Relating to homeostasis.

**homeotherapeutic** (ho'me-o-thĕr-ă-pu'tik). 1. Homeopathic. 2. Relating to homeotherapy.

**homeother'apy.** Treatment or prevention of a disease by means of a product similar to, but not identical with, the active causal agent, as in Jennerian vaccination.

**ho'meother'mal.** Homothermal.

**homeotypical** (ho'me-o-tip'ī-kal). Of or resembling the usual type.

**homergy** (hom'er-jī) [ G. *homos*, same, + *ergon*, work ]. Obsolete term meaning normal metabolism and its results.

**homicidal** (hom'ī-si'dal). Having a tendency toward homicide.

**hom'icide** [ L. *homo*, man, + *caedo*, to kill ]. 1. The killing of one human being by another. 2. One who takes the life of another.

**homid'ium bro'mide.** Ethidium bromide; a phenanthridinium derivative useful in treating nagana caused by either *Trypanosoma congolense* or *T. vivax.*

**homigrade.** See homigrade *scale.*

**Homin'idae.** The Primate family which includes modern man (*Homo sapiens*) and several groups of fossil men; *e.g.*, Neanderthals, Pithecanthropines, and Australopithecines.

**Hominoidea** (hom'ĭ-noy'de-ah) [ L. *homo* (*homin-*), man, + G. *eidos*, form ]. A superfamily of the Primates including the anthropoid apes and man. Divided into the families Pongidae (anthropoid apes) and Hominidae (man).

**Ho'mo** [ L. man ] [ NA ]. The genus of Primates that includes man.

**H. sapiens** [ L. wise man ], modern man.

**homo-** (ho'mo-) [ G. *homos*, the same ]. A combining form meaning the same or alike.

**ho'mobi'otin.** A compound resembling biotin except for the substitution of an oxygen atom for the sulfur and the presence of an additional $CH_2$ group in the side chain; an active biotin antagonist.

**ho'moblas'tic** [ homo- + G. *blastos*, germ ]. Developing from a single type of tissue.

**ho'mocam'fin.** CYCLOSAL; HEXETONE; 3-isopropyl-5-methyl-cyclohexanone; a central nervous system stimulant.

**ho'mocar'nosine.** $N^2$-(γ-Aminobutyryl)histidine; brain contains 10 times as much h. as carnosine. H. in brain is formed from γ-aminobutyric acid, which in turn comes from glutamic acid.

**ho'mocen'tric.** Having the same center; concentric; denoting rays that meet at a common focus; opposed to heterocentric.

**homochlorcy'clizine dihydrochloride.** HOMOCLOMIN; 1- (*p*-chloro-α-phenylbenzyl) hexahydro-4-methyl-1*H*-1,4-diazepine; antihistaminic agent with antiserotonin properties.

**homochronous** (ho-mok'ro-nus) [ homo- + G. *chronos*, time ]. 1. Occurring at the same time; synchronous. 2. Occurring at the same age in each generation.

**homoclad'ic** [ homo- + G. *klados*, a branch ]. Denoting an anastomosis between branches of the same arterial trunk; opposed to heterocladic.

**homocyclic compound** (ho'mo-si'klik, -sik'lik). Isocyclic *compound*.

**homocysteine** (ho'mo-sis'te-ēn). $HSCH_2CH_2CHNH_2$-COOH; a sulfur-containing amino acid, a homologue of cysteine; produced by the demethylation of methionine, and an intermediate in the biosynthesis of cysteine from methionine via cystathionine.

**homocystine** (ho'mo-sis'tēn). The disulfide resulting from the mild oxidation of homocysteine. An analogue of cystine.

**ho'mocys'tinu'ria.** A heritable (autosomal recessive) disorder characterized by excretion of homocystine in urine, mental retardation, ectopia lentis, sparse blond hair, genu valgum, convulsive tendency, failure to thrive, thrombo-embolic episodes, and fatty changes of liver; associated with defective formation of cystathionine synthetase.

**homocytotropic** (ho'mo-si'to-tro'pik, -trop'ik) [ homo- + G. *kytos*, cell, + *tropē*, a turning toward ]. Having an affinity for cells of the same or a closely related species.

**ho'modont** [ homo- + G. *odous*, tooth ]. Having teeth all alike in form, as those of the lower vertebrates; opposed to heterodont.

**homodromous** (ho-mod'ro-mus) [ homo- + G. *dromos*, running ]. Moving in the same direction.

**homoeroticism** (ho-mo-ē-rot'ĭ-sizm). Homoerotism.

**homoerotism** (ho-mo-er'o-tizm) [ homo- + G. *erōs*, love ]. Homoeroticism; homosexuality.

**ho'mogamet'ic** [ homo- + G. *gametikos*, connubial ]. Monogametic; producing only one type of gamete with respect to sex chromosomes; in man and most animals the female is the h. sex.

**homogamy** (ho-mog'ă-mī) [ homo- + G. *gamos*, marriage ]. Similarity of husband and wife in a specific trait.

**homogenate** (ho-moj'ĕ-nāt). That which is made homogeneous; specifically, in biochemistry, tissue ground into a creamy consistency in which the cell structure is disintegrated (so-called "cell-free"). See also brei.

**homogeneous** (ho-mo-je'ne-us) [ homo- + G. *genos*, race ]. Of uniform structure or composition throughout.

**homogenesis** (ho-mo-jen'e-sis) [ homo- + G. *genesis*, production ]. Homogeny; reproduction in which the offspring is similar to the parents; opposed to heterogenesis.

**homogenization** (ho-moj'ĕ-nī-za'shun). The process by which a material is made homogeneous.

**homogenize** (ho-moj'ĕ-nīz). To make homogeneous.

**homogenous** (ho-moj'ĕ-nus) [ homo- + G. *genos*, family, kind ]. Having a structural similarity because of descent from a common ancestor.

**homogen'tisate 1,2-diox'ygenase** (EC 1.13.11.5). Homogentisicase; homogentisic acid oxidase; an iron-containing enzyme that catalyzes the oxidative cleavage of the benzene ring by $O_2$ in homogentisic acid, forming maleylacetoacetic acid. Congenital lack of this enzyme results in the disorder of metabolism known as alkaptonuria.

**ho'mogentis'ic acid.** Alkapton; (2,5-dihydroxyphenyl)acetic acid: an acid occurring in the urine in alkaptonuria; it is an intermediate in tyrosine catabolism, accumulating in those persons suffering a congenital deficiency of the enzyme homogentisase. It oxidizes rapidly in air if made alkaline, to a quinone that polymerizes to a melanin-like material.

**h. acid oxidase,** Homogentisate 1,2-dioxygenase.

**ho'mogen'tisicase.** Homogentisate 1,2-dioxygenase.

**homogentisuria** (ho'mo-jen'tĭ-su'rĭ-ah). Alkaptonuria.

**homogeny** (ho-moj'ĕ-nī). Homogenesis.

**ho'mograft.** Allogeneic graft; homologous graft; homoplastic graft; homotransplant; a piece of tissue or an organ transferred from one member to another member of the same species, not identical twins; used generally or with respect to animal strains not isogeneic for histocompatibility genes.

**allogeneic h.,** allograft.

**isogeneic h.,** isograft.

**h. rejection,** see rejection.

**syngeneic h.,** isograft.

**homoioplasia** (ho-moy-o-pla'sĭ-ah). Homeoplasia.

**homoiothermal** (ho-moy-o-ther'mal). Homothermal.

**homokeratoplasty** (ho'mo-kĕr'ă-to-plas'tĭ). Keratoplasty in which the cornea from one person is grafted to the eye of another; the donor can be living, dead, or a stillbirth.

**ho'molat'eral** [ homo- + L. *latus*, side ]. Ipsilateral; on or relating to the same side.

**ho'molip'ids.** Lipids with molecules containing only C, H, and O; simple lipids.

**homologous** (ho-mol'o-gus) [ see homologue ]. Corresponding or alike in certain critical attributes: (1) in biology or zoology, of organs or parts corresponding in evolutionary origin and similar to some extent in structure, but not necessarily similar in function; (2) in chemistry, of a single chemical series, differing by fixed increments; (3) in genetics, of chromosomes or chromosome parts identical with respect to their genetic loci; (4) in immunology, of serum or tissue derived from members of a single species; (5) in mathematics, of certain geometric properties.

**homologue** (hom'o-log) [ homo- + G. *logos*, word, ratio, relation ]. A member of a homologous pair or series.

**homol'ogy.** The state of being homologous.

**homol'ysin.** A sensitizing, hemolytic antibody (hemolysin) formed as the result of stimulation by an antigen derived from an animal of the same species; isolysin or isohemolysin, as distinguished from heterolysin and autolysin. See also hemolysin.

**homol'ysis.** Isolysis or isohemolysis; lysis of red blood cells by a homolysin and complement.

**homomorphic** (ho-mo-mor'fik) [ homo- + G. *morphē*, shape, appearance ]. Denoting two or more structures of similar size and shape.

**homonomous** (ho-mon'o-mus) [ G. *homonemos*, under the same laws, fr. *homos*, same, + *nomos*, law ]. Denoting parts, having similar form and structure, arranged in a series, as the fingers or toes.

**homonomy** (ho-mon'o-mī). The condition of being homonomous.

**homonymous** (ho-mon'ĭ-mus) [ G. *homōnymous*, of the same name, fr. *onyma*, name ]. Having the same name or expressed in the same terms, *e.g.*, the corresponding halves (right or left, superior or inferior) of the retinas.

**ho'mophenes.** Words in which the visible organs of speech behave the same, *e.g.*, tug, tongue, tuck.

**ho'mophil** [ homo- + G. *philos*, fond ]. Denoting an antibody that reacts only with the specific antigen.

**ho'moplas'tic.** Similar in form and structure, but not in origin.

**ho'moplas'ty.** Repair of a defect by a homograft.

**homopolymer** (ho'mo-pol'ĭ-mer). A polymer yielding a single substance on hydrolysis, or composed of a series of identical radicals. Polylysine, poly(adenylic acid), polyglucose are homopolymers; homopolysaccharides, homopolynucleotides, homopolypeptides are homopolymer types.

**homopolysaccharide** (ho'mo-pol-ĭ-sak'ar-id). See homopolymer.

**homoprotocatechuic acid** (ho'mo-pro'to-kat-ĭ-chu'ik). (3,4-Dihydroxyphenyl)acetic acid; an isomer of homogentisic acid found in urine; a degradation product of tyrosine, dopa, and hydroxytyramine.

**ho'moqui'nine.** Apoquinine.

**homorganic** (hom'or-gan'ik). Produced by the same organs, or by homologous organs.

**homosal'ate** (USAN). HELIOPHAN; 3,3,5-trimethylcyclohexyl salicylate; an ultraviolet screening agent for topical application to the skin.

**ho'moser'ine.** HOCH$_2$CH$_2$CH(NH$_2$)COOH; a hydroxyamino acid differing from serine in the possession of an additional CH$_2$ group; formed in the conversion of methionine to cysteine.

    **h. deaminase,** cystathionine γ-lyase.

    **h. dehydratase,** cystathionine γ-lyase.

**homosexual** (ho'mo-sek'shu-al). 1. Relating to or possessing erotic attraction toward the same sex. 2. A person who prefers to engage in sexual behavior with others of the same sex.

**homosexuality** (ho'mo-sek-shu-al'ĭ-tĭ). Homoerotism; sexual behavior, including sexual congress, between individuals of the same sex, especially past puberty.

    **female h.,** lesbianism.

    **latent h.,** unconscious h.; an erotic inclination toward members of the same sex not consciously experienced or expressed in overt action; opposite of overt h. Use of this term is disappearing because of both its potentially iatrogenic effect and the inability to validate the phenomenon by techniques outside of psychoanalytic theory.

    **overt h.,** homosexual inclinations consciously experienced and expressed in actual homosexual behavior, as opposed to latent h.

    **unconscious h.,** latent h.

**D-ho'moster'oid.** A steroid in which the D ring is made up of six carbon atoms instead of the usual five. See steroids for structure.

**4-ho'mosulfanil'amide hydrochloride.** Mafenide.

**ho'mothal'lic** [ homo- + G. *thallos*, a young shoot ]. Among fungi, the capacity to reproduce on the same thallus, without involving heterothallic fusion, as in the production of progeny from a single ascospore; *cf.* heterothallic.

**ho'mother'mal** [ homo- + G. *thermē*, heat ]. Homeothermal; homothermic; homothermous; having always the same temperature; denoting the warm-blooded animals.

**ho'moton'ic.** Of uniform tension or tonus.

**ho'motop'ic** [ homo- + G. *topos*, place ]. Pertaining to or occurring at the same place or part of the body.

**ho'motrans'plant.** Homograft.

**ho'motype** [ homo- + G. *typos* type ]. Any part or organ of the same structure or function as another, especially as one on the opposite side of the body.

**homotyp'ic, homotyp'ical.** Of the same type or form; corresponding to the other one of two paired organs or parts.

**ho'movanil'lic acid.** A phenol found in human urine; arising through the methylation of homoprotocatechuic acid on the meta-OH group.

**homozoic** (ho'mo-zo'ik) [ homo- + G. *zōikos*, relating to an animal ]. Relating to the same animal or the same species of animal.

**ho'mozygo'sis.** Homozygosity.

**homozygosity** (ho'mo-zi-gos'ĭ-tĭ) [ homo- + G. *zygon*, yoke ]. The state of having identical genes at one or more paired loci in homologous chromosomes.

**homozygote** (ho-mo-zi'gōt) [ homo- + G. *zygōtos*, yoke ]. A homozygous individual.

**homozygous** (ho-mo-zi'gus). Relating to homozygosity.

**homunculus** (ho-mungk'u-lus) [ L. dim. of *homo*, man ]. An exceedingly minute body which, according to the views of development held by medical scientists of the 16th and 17th centuries, was contained in a sex cell. From this preformed but infinitely small structure the human body was supposed to be developed. See also preformation *theory*, and epigenesis.

**Hondu'ras bark.** Cascara amara.

**hon'ey** [ A.S. *hunig* ]. Clarified h.; mel; a saccharine substance deposited in the honeycomb by the honeybee, *Apis mellifera*. Used as an excipient, as a flavor in gargles and cough remedies, and as a food.

**honk.** A sound similar to that of a goose.

    **systolic h.,** systolic whoop; a somewhat musical systolic murmur likened to the honking of a goose; sometimes of innocent but unexplained origin, at other times a sign of mitral insufficiency.

**hood** [ O.E. *hōd*, hat ]. The anterior part of the integument of soft ticks (family Argasidae) that extends over the capitulum and forms part of the camerostome.

**hood'ed.** Having darkly pigmented hair on the anterior part of the body and white hair on the posterior part; characteristic of some types of rats.

**hoof** [ A.S. *hōf* ]. The horny covering of the ends of the digits or feet in many animals; it consists, like nails and horns, of thickened and modified epidermis or cuticle.

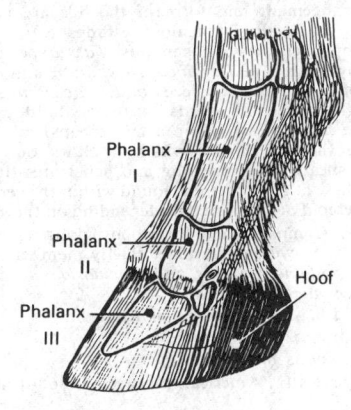

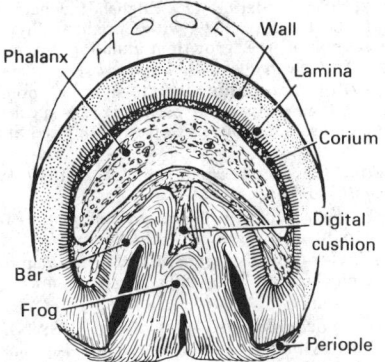

**Horse's Hoof**

**hoof-bound.** A condition of dryness and contraction of the h. of a horse; it results in pain and lameness.

**hook** [ A.S. *hōk* ]. An instrument curved or bent near its tip, used for fixation of a part or traction.

**blunt-h.,** (1) a strong, hook-shaped bar that is passed between abdomen and thigh to make traction in cases of difficult breech presentation; (2) a dull h. used in the performance of embryotomy.

**Braun's h.,** a steel h. with sharp concavity, used for decapitation of the fetus.

**calvarial h.,** an instrument used in prying off the top of the skull after it has been sawed around, at autopsies and dissections.

**h. of hamate bone,** *hamulus* ossis hamati.

**Malgaigne's h.'s,** h.'s that seize the upper and lower fragments of a fractured patella and are then approximated by screws.

**Pajot's h.,** a h. used in decapitation of the fetus; it has a groove which carries a strong cord, the decapitation being effected by a sawing movement of the string.

**palate h.,** an instrument for pulling forward the soft palate in order to facilitate posterior rhinoscopy.

**squint h.,** a surgical instrument used in operations on muscles of the eye.

**tracheotomy h.,** right-angled h. used in holding the trachea steady during tracheotomy.

**Tyrrell's h.,** a slender blunt h. used for drawing out the iris in iridectomy.

**Hooke,** Robert, English experimental physicist, 1635 –1703. See Hookean *behavior*, H.'s *law.*

**Hooker,** Charles W. See H.-Forbes *test.*

**hook'lets.** 1. Clawlike, retractile chitinous hooks that encircle or line the rostellum of the scolex of certain taenioid tapeworms and form part of the anchoring capacity of the scolex by which the tapeworm attaches to the intestinal mucosa, with the additional aid of suckers. The h.'s can be withdrawn and the rostellum inverted when the tapeworm moves. Arrangement and form of the h.'s are used to characterize the families of taenioid cestodes; *e.g.*, there are two overlapping circlets of h.'s in most *Taenia* species, and multiple rows of h.'s in *Davainea, Dipylidium,* and others. 2. Those of degenerated scoleces of *Echinococcus* species found in the tissues or fluids of the hydatid cyst. 3. Oncosphere h.'s, the six (10 in a few groups) h.'s of the oncosphere (hexacanth) by which it claws out of its membrane sheath after hatching and penetrates the host gut wall. These h.'s can often be found within the cercomer of the procercoid or cysticercoid (depending on the group).

**hook'worm.** Common name for bloodsucking nematodes of the family Ancylostomatidae, chiefly members of the genera *Ancylostoma, Necator,* and *Uncinaria.*

**dog h.,** see *Ancylostoma caninum.*

**New World h.,** see *Necator americanus.*

**Old World h.,** see *Ancylostoma.*

**hoose.** Verminous *bronchitis.*

**Hoover,** Charles F., American physician, 1865–1927. See H.'s *signs.*

**Hopkins,** Sir Frederick G., English biochemist, 1861 –1947. Nobel laureate, 1929, with Christiaan Eijkman, for his discovery of the growth-stimulating vitamins. See Benedict-H.-Cole *reagent*, H.-Cole *test.*

**Hoplopsyllus anomalus** (hop'lo-sil'us ah-nom'ah-lus) [ G. *hoplo,* tool, weapon, + *psyll,* flea ]. A species of flea parasitic on ground squirrels of western United States and a vector of plague.

**Hopmann,** Carl M., German rhinologist, 1849–1925. See H.'s *papilloma, polyp.*

**Hoppe** (hop'e), Johann I., Swiss physiologist, 1811–1891. See H.-Goldflam *disease.*

**Hoppe-Seyler** (hop'e-si'ler), Ernst F. I., German physiologist and biochemist, 1825–1895. See H.-S. *test.*

**hops.** Humulus.

**hoquizil hydrochloride** (ho'kwĭ-zil) (USAN). 2-Hydroxy-2-methylpropyl 4-(6,7-dimethoxy-4-quinazolinyl)-1-piperazinecarboxylate monohydrochloride; bronchodilator.

**hordenine** (hor'dĕ-nēn) [ L. *hordeum,* barley ]. *p*-(2-Dimethylaminoethyl)phenol; an alkaloid, developed in barley

during the process of germination; sympathomimetic agent.

**hordeolum** (hor-de'o-lum) [ Mod. L. fr. L. *hordeolus,* a sty in the eye, dim. of *hordeum,* barley ]. A suppurative infection of a marginal gland of the eyelid.

**h. externum,** sty; inflammation of the sebaceous gland of an eyelash.

**h. inter'num, h. meibomia'num,** Meibomian sty; an acute purulent infection of a Meibomian gland.

**hor'deum.** Barley.

**hore'hound** [ A.S. *hār hūnd* ]. Marrubium.

**Horgan,** Edmund, American physician, *1884. See Lyon and H. *method.*

**horismascope** (ho-riz'mă-skōp) [ G. *horisma,* a boundary, + *skopeō,* to examine ]. A U-shaped test tube, used in the acid test for albumin in the urine; one arm of the tube has a black background against which a faint cloud of albumin may be fairly easily recognized at and adjacent to the interface between acid and urine.

**horizocardia** (ho-ri'zo-kar'dī-ah) [ G. *horizōn,* the bounding line, horizon, + *kardia,* heart ]. A horizontal position of the heart on the diaphragm, due to marked eccentric hypertrophy or to dilation of both ventricles.

**horizons, Streeter.** Developmental stages in young human embryos. Streeter defined 23 "horizons" from fertilization through the first 2 months on the basis of the degree of advancement of certain selected structural features in addition to size measurement.

**horizonta'lis** [ L. ] [ NA ]. Horizontal, referring to the plane of the body, perpendicular to the vertical plane, at right angles both to the median and coronal planes, that separates the body into upper and lower parts.

**hor'mion** [ G. *hormos,* cord, chain, necklace ]. The point of junction of the posterior border of the vomer with the sphenoid bone.

**Hormoden'drum** [ G. *hormos,* chain, + *dendron,* tree ]. A genus of fungi; *H. pedrosoi* and *H. compactum* cause chromoblastomycosis. Synonymous with *Cladosporium.*

**H. fontoynon'ti,** a species found in the scales of hodi-potsy.

**hor'monal.** Pertaining to hormones.

# HORMONE

**hormone** (hor'mōn) [ G. *hormōn,* pres. part. of *hormaō,* to rouse or set in motion ]. A chemical substance, formed in one organ or part of the body and carried in the blood to another organ or part. Depending on the specificity of their effects, h.'s can alter the functional activity, and sometimes the structure, of just one organ or of various numbers of them. A number of h.'s are formed by ductless glands, but secretin and pancreozymin, formed in the gastrointestinal tract, by definition are also h.'s. For h.'s not listed below, see specific names.

**adipokinetic h.,** Adipokinin.

**adrenocortical h.'s,** h.'s secreted by the human adrenal cortex; the principal ones are cortisol, aldosterone, and corticosterone; others include several weakly androgenic h.'s.

**adrenocorticotropic (-trophic) h.,** abbreviated ACTH; corticotrophin; adrenocorticotropin; adrenocorticotrophin; adrenotropic h.; the h. of the anterior lobe of the hypophysis; it governs the nutrition and growth of the adrenal cortex, stimulates it to functional activity, and also possesses extraadrenal adipokinetic activity; this h. is a polypeptide containing 39 amino acids, but exact structure varies from one species to another; see also big *ACTH,* little *ACTH.*

**adrenotropic (-trophic) h.,** adrenocorticotropic h.

**androgen'ic h.,** any h. that produces a masculinizing effect; of the naturally occurring androgenic h.'s, testosterone is the most potent.

**anterior pitu'itary-like h.,** chorionic *gonadotropin.*

**antidiuretic h.,** vasopressin.

**antigonadotropic (-trophic) h.'s,** postulated antihormones produced by the pituitary body that inhibit the action of gonadotropic h.'s; now thought to be antibodies either to endogenous or to exogenous gonadotropins.

**atret'ic h.,** a principle present in anterior lobe extracts which is believed by some to cause atresia of Graafian follicles and to inhibit the production of gonadotrophins. Satisfactory evidence for the existence of such a h. has not been obtained.

**h. B,** an ectohormone of unknown structure secreted by male strains of several species of the genus *Achyla,* an aquatic fungus; h. B. initiates formation of oogonia in female strains of *Achyla.*

**brain h.,** ecdysiotropin; prothoracotropic h.; a substance formed in neurosecretory cells of insect brain and secreted into the hemolymph *via* the corpora cardiaca; acts on the prothoracic gland to stimulate ecdysone secretion.

**chemotactic sexual h.,** gamone.

**chorionic gonadotropic (-trophic) h.,** chorionic *gonadotropin.*

**chorionic "growth hormone-prolactin,"** human placental *lactogen.*

**chromatophorotropic (-trophic) h.,** see melanocyte-stimulating h.

**corpus luteum h.,** progesterone.

**cortical h.'s,** the steroid h.'s produced by the adrenal cortex.

**corticotropic (-trophic) h.,** adrenocorticotropic h.

**diabetogen'ic h.,** a postulated h. in crude extracts of the anterior lobe of the hypophysis that causes exhaustion, atrophy of the islands of Langerhans, and the symptoms of diabetes. Such effects can be produced by large quantities of pituitary growth h.

**erythropoietic h.,** any h. that stimulates the formation of red blood cells, *e.g.,* testosterone.

**estrogen'ic h.,** estradiol.

**female h.,** estradiol.

**follicle-stimulating h.,** FSH; a glycoprotein h. of the anterior pituitary gland; it stimulates the Graafian follicles of the ovary and assists subsequently in follicular maturation and the secretion of estradiol. In the male, it stimulates the epithelium of the seminiferous tubules and is partially responsible for inducing spermatogenesis.

**follicular h.,** estradiol.

**galactopoietic h.,** prolactin.

**gametokinet'ic h.,** follicle-stimulating h.

**gastrointestinal h.,** any secretion of the gastrointestinal mucosa affecting the timing and quantity of various digestive secretions; *e.g., secretin.*

**glycoprotein h.'s,** those anterior pituitary h.'s that are glycoproteins; *e.g.,* thyrotrophic h., interstitial cell-stimulating h., and follicle-stimulating h.

**glycotropic (-trophic) h.,** a postulated h. of the anterior lobe of the pituitary which antagonizes the action of insulin and causes hyperglycemia. Such effects can be produced by pituitary growth h.

**gonadotropic (-trophic) h.,** a gonadotropin (*q.v.*); by usage, it connotes a h. of pituitary origin.

**growth h.,** somatotropin.

**growth hormone-releasing h.,** somatoliberin.

**heart h.,** herz h.

**herz h.,** heart h.; cardiac h.; a substance present in extracts of cardiac tissue that augments cardiac contraction; possibly adenosine, a catecholamine, or some nonspecific stimulant present generally in tissues.

**hypophysiotropic (-trophic) h.,** a h. that stimulates the rate of secretion of hypophysial h.'s, as do, for example, the releasing factors.

**interstitial cell-stimulating h.** (ICSH), luteinizing h.

**intracellular h.,** an incorrect term sometimes applied to a substance that influences the differentiation of cells in its immediate neighborhood; see evocator.

**juvenile h.,** a substance formed in the corpora allata of insects; however, it may also be found in other insect tissues and in various plants; it favors synthesis of larval structures, is gonadotropic in insects, and activates the prothoracic gland.

**ketogenic h.,** a postulated principle in extracts of the anterior lobe of the pituitary that causes ketonemia and ketonuria in animals on a fat diet or fasting.

**lactogenic h.,** prolactin.

**luteinizing h.** (LH), interstitial cell-stimulating h. (ICSH); lutein-stimulating h. (LSH); a glycoprotein h. stimulating the final ripening of the follicles and the secretion of progesterone by them, their rupture to release the egg, and the conversion of the ruptured follicle into the corpus luteum.

**luteotropic (-trophic) h.,** luteotropin; an anterior pituitary h. (probably prolactin), whose action maintains the function of the corpus luteum; such an effect can be demonstrated in only a few species, most notably the rat.

**male h.,** (1) testosterone; (2) androgen.

**mammogenic h.'s,** mammogens I and II; h.'s thought by some to be liberated from the anterior lobe of the pituitary, that stimulate development of the breasts. Mammogen I stimulates the growth of the ducts and is liberated by the action of estradiol, whereas mammogen II stimulates the growth of the alveoli and is liberated by the action of progesterone. There is no satisfactory evidence for the existence of these h.'s.

**mammotropic (-trophic) h.,** prolactin.

**melanocyte-stimulating h.,** MSH; intermedin; melanophore-expanding principle; a peptide h. secreted by the intermediate lobe of the pituitary gland. It causes dispersion of melanin with melanophores (chromatophores), resulting in darkening of the skin; this effect is readily demonstrated in some lower vertebrates, such as frogs and fishes. It causes skin darkening in human beings, presumably by promoting melanin synthesis with melanocytes. It is uncertain whether MSH is identical with chromatophorotropic h.

**molting h.,** ecdysone.

**morphogenic h.,** a term not in good usage but sometimes used to mean evocator.

**natriuretic h.,** a postulated h., believed to be a polypeptide formed in the posterior hypothalamus and to promote urinary sodium.

**ovarian h.'s,** h.'s secreted by the human ovary; the principal ones are 17β-estradiol and progesterone; in addition, the ovary secretes h.'s having androgenic activity; it is not yet clearly known whether the human ovary secretes relaxin.

**pancreatic h.'s,** see insulin, lipocaic, kallikrein, and glucagon.

**pancreatic hyperglycemic h.,** glucagon.

**parathyroid h.,** a peptide h. formed by the parathyroid glands; it raises the serum calcium when administered parenterally by causing bone resorption. Only preparations of animal origin are available for therapeutic use, to the effects of which patients usually become refractory within several months.

**parathyrotropic (-trophic) h.,** a postulated h. of the anterior lobe of the pituitary which supposedly influences the growth and function of the parathyroid glands. There is no satisfactory evidence for the existence of such h.'s.

**pituitary gonadotropic (-trophic) h.,** anterior pituitary *gonadotropin.*

**pituitary growth h.,** somatotropin.

**placental h.,** any of the h.'s elaborated by the placenta, namely, chorionic gonadotropin, estrogen, progesterone, and human placental lactogen.

**placental growth h.,** human placental *lactogen.*

**plant h.'s,** auxins.

**progestational h.,** progesterone.

**prothoracic gland h.,** ecdysone.

**prothoracotropic h.,** brain h.

**releasing h.,** abbreviated RH; releasing *factor.*

**saliva~y gland h.,** parotin.

**salivary taste h.'s,** specific activating substances suggested as being present in saliva and essential for taste perception. There is no satisfactory evidence for their existence.

**sex h.'s,** a general term covering those steroid h.'s that are formed by testicular, ovarian, and adrenocortical tissues, and that are androgens or estrogens.

**somatotropic (-trophic) h.,** somatotropin.

**steroid h.'s,** those h.'s possessing the cyclopentanoperhydrophenanthrene ring system (steroid nucleus) in their molecules, including androgens, estrogens, and the adrenocortical h.'s.

**sympathetic h.,** sympathin.

**testicular h.'s,** h.'s secreted by the human testis, the principal one being testosterone. In addition, the testis secretes androstenedione and one or more steroid h.'s having estrogenic activity.

**thyroid h.,** a term that commonly refers to thyroxine, but may also include triiodothyronine.

**thyrotropic (-trophic) h.,** thyrotropin.

**tropic h.'s, trophic h.'s,** those h.'s of the anterior lobe of the pituitary that affect the growth, nutrition, or function of other endocrine glands, *e.g.,* luteinizing h., adrenocorticotropic h., etc.

**wound h.,** see traumatic acid.

**hormonogenesis** (hor'mo-no-jen'ĕ-sis). Hormonopoiesis; the formation of hormones.

**hormonogenic** (hor'mo-no-jen'ik). Hormonopoietic; pertaining to the formation of a hormone.

**hormonopoiesis** (hor'mo-no-poy-e'sis) [ hormone + G. *poiēsis,* production ]. Hormonogenesis.

**hormonopoietic** (hor'mo-no-poy-et'ik). Hormonogenic.

**hormonoprivia** (hor'mo-no-priv'ĭ-ah) [ hormone + G. *privus,* deprived of ]. Obsolete term meaning partial or total deprivation of hormones.

**hor'monother'apy.** Treatment with hormones.

**horn** [ A.S. ]. Cornu.

**Ammon's h.** [ G. *Ammōn,* the Egyptian deity *Amūn* ], see hippocampus.

**anterior h.,** *cornu anterius.*

**cicatricial h.,** a keratinous h. projecting outward from a scar.

**h. of the clit'oris,** a horny excrescence sometimes occurring beneath the prepuce of the clitoris.

**cutaneous h.,** cornu cutaneum; cornu humanum; warty h.; a protruding keratotic growth of the skin; the base may show changes of senile keratosis or carcinoma.

**dorsal h.,** *cornu posterius.*

**frontal h.,** see *ventriculus* lateralis.

**greater h.,** *cornu majus.*

**iliac h.,** bony spur of posterior part of ilium, often found in arthro-onychodysplasia.

**inferior h.,** *cornu inferius.*

**inferior h. of saphenous opening,** *cornu* inferius (2).

**inferior h. of thyroid cartilage,** *cornu* inferius (1).

**lateral h.,** *cornu laterale.*

**lesser h.,** *cornu minus.*

**nail h.,** overgrown nail.

**occipital h.,** see *ventriculus* lateralis.

**posterior h.,** *cornu posterius.*

**pulp h.,** a prolongation of the pulp extending toward the cusp of a tooth.

**sacral h.,** *cornu sacrale.*

**sebaceous h.,** a solid outgrowth from a sebaceous cyst.

**superior h. of saphenous opening,** *cornu* superius (2).

**superior h. of thyroid cartilage,** *cornu* superius (1).

**temporal h.,** see *ventriculus* lateralis.

**ventral h.,** *cornu anterius.*

**warty h.,** cutaneous h.

**Horner,** Johann F., Zurich ophthalmologist, 1831–1886. See H.'s *syndrome,* Bernard-H. *syndrome.*

**Horner,** William E., U. S. anatomist, 1793–1853. See H.'s *muscle.*

**Horner's teeth.** See under tooth.

**hor'nifica'tion.** Cornification.

**horny.** Corneous; of the nature or structure of horn.

**horopter** (ho-rop'ter) [ G. *horos,* limit, + *optēr,* one who sees, fr. *ops,* eye ]. The sum of the points in space, the images of which for a given distance fall on corresponding retinal points. If the fixation point is 2 meters, the horopter is a straight line; if less, a curve concave to the face; if more, a convex curve.

**horripilation** (hor-rip'ĭ-la'shun) [ L. *horreo,* to bristle, + *pilus,* hair ]. Erection of short hairs.

**hor'ror** [ L. ]. Dread; fear.

**h. autotox'icus** [ L., dread of self-poisoning ]. A term introduced by Ehrlich, meaning that immunity is directed against foreign materials but not against the constituents of one's own body; exceptions to this concept are the autoallergic reactions and diseases.

**h. feminae,** morbid dread of women.

**h. fusio'nis** [ L., dread of intermingling ], inability to obtain binocular fusion.

**horse'fly.** See *Tabanus;* also *Anthomyia canalicularis.*

**horse'power.** A unit of power, 550 foot-pounds per second, or 746 watts per second.

**horse'pox.** Equine contagious pustular stomatitis; usually appears as typical eruptions in the mouth, sometimes on the skin of the fetlocks. The virus of h. is indistinguishable from that of vaccinia and is believed to be the same.

**Horsley,** Sir Victor A. H., London surgeon, 1857–1916. See H.'s *operation, test,* bone *wax.*

**horseradish** (hors'rad-ish). Armoracia.

**Hortega** (hor-tā'gah), Pio del Rio, Spanish neurohistologist in South America, 1882–1945. See H. *cell.*

**hor'tobe'zoar** [ L. *hortus,* garden, + bezoar ]. Phytobezoar.

**Horton,** Bayard T., U. S. physician, *1895. See H.'s *cephalalgia,* headache.

**hospital** [ L. *hospitalis,* for a guest, fr. *hospes* (*hospit-*), a host, a guest ]. Nosocomion; an institution for the treatment, care, and cure of the sick and wounded, for the study of disease, and for the training of physicians and nurses.

**base h.,** a large h., at a large military base, that cares for sick and wounded received from smaller units nearer the front.

**camp h.,** station h.

**closed h.,** one in which only members of the attending or consulting staff may admit and treat patients.

**cottage h.,** a small h. with a very small nursing staff and usually no resident physician.

**day h.,** a special facility, or an arrangement within a h. setting, that enables the patient to come to the h. for treatment during the day and return home at night; see also night h.

**evacuation h.,** a mobile h. of the U.S. Army that receives patients from aid stations and cares for them until they can be evacuated to a general h.

**field h.,** an aid station.

**general h.,** a large h. (1000 beds) of the U.S., British, or Canadian Army, with fixed location, receiving patients from an evacuation h.; or any large civilian h. that is equipped to care for medical, surgical, or maternity cases and has a resident medical staff.

**government h.,** state h.; one controlled by officials of the city, county, state, or nation.

**group h.,** a private h. organized and controlled by a group of physicians for the reception and care of their own patients only.

**isolation h.,** one for the care of patients with contagious diseases.

**maternity h.,** a special h. for the care of women in childbirth.

**mental h.,** a medical institution for the care and treatment of persons with psychiatric disorders.

**municipal h.,** a government h. controlled by city officials.

**night h.,** a special facility, or an arrangement within a h. setting, providing treatment and lodging at night for patients able to work in the community during the day; see also day h.

**open h.,** any h. in which reputable practitioners, not members of the regular staff, are permitted to send their own patients and control their treatment.

**philanthropic h.,** voluntary h.

**private h.,** the same as group h. except that it is controlled by a single practitioner or by him and the associates in his office.

**proprietary h.,** private h.

**public h.,** government h.

**special h.,** one for the medical and surgical care of sufferers from special diseases (of the ear, nose, throat, eyes, etc.).

**state h.,** a h. supported by taxpayers through their state government.

**station h.,** a small h. (250 beds) of the U.S. army with a fixed location, serving the local needs of a camp or permanent military post.

**surgical h.,** a mobile h. of the U.S. Army for immediate surgical aid to the more serious casualties; it is located close to a h. station, but is not a part of the division which it serves.

**Veterans Administration h.,** a h. erected at government expense, supported by the Veterans Administration for care of veterans of U.S. wars and retired service men and women.

**voluntary h.,** a h. (often a closed h.) supported by voluntary contributions and under the control of a (usually self appointed) board of managers.

**weekend h.,** a special facility, or an arrangement within a h. setting, which enables a patient to work in the community during the work week and receive treatment in the hospital during the weekend.

**hospitalism** (hos′pī-tal-ism). The second stage of a depression observed in the first year of human life, following anaclitic depression (*q.v.*), characterized by stupor and ultimately wasting away; usually caused by prolonged hospitalization in which an infant is separated from its mother or a mothering influence.

**hos′pitaliza′tion.** Confinement in a hospital as a patient for diagnostic study and treatment.

**host** [ L. *hospes*, a host, a guest ]. The organism at the expense of which a parasite lives.

**definitive h.,** final h.; one in which a parasite reaches the adult or sexually mature stage.

**final h.,** definitive h.

**intermediate h.,** intermediary h., secondary h., one in which larval or developmental stages occur.

**paratenic h.,** transport h.; an intermediate h. in which no development of the parasite occurs, though presence of a paratenic h. may be required as an essential link in the completion of the parasite's life cycle (*e.g.,* the successive fish h.'s that carry the plerocercoid of *Diphyllobothrium latum*, the broad fish tapeworm, to larger food fish eaten by man).

**reservoir h.,** the h. of an infection that can also infect man, hence one that serves as a potential source of human reinfection and as a means of sustaining the parasite when it is not infecting man.

**secondary h.,** intermediate h.

**transport h.,** paratenic h.

**hott′entotism** [ Hottentot, a South African race, so named by the Dutch (D. *hateren* to stammer, and *tateren* to stutter) because of the peculiar sounds of their speech ]. A form of stammering.

**Hotz,** Ferdinand Carl, American opthalmologist, 1843–1908. See H.-Anagnostakis *operation.*

**Houghton,** E. M., American physician, 1867–1937. See H.'s *test.*

**house′fly.** See *Musca domestica* (common housefly), and *Fannia canicularis* (lesser housefly).

**Houssay** (oo-si′), Bernardo A., Argentine physiologist, 1887–1971. Nobel laureate, 1947, with Carl F. Cori and Gerty T. Cori, for the discovery of the part played by the hormone of the anterior pituitary lobe in the metabolism of sugar. See H. *animal, phenomenon, syndrome.*

**Houston,** John, Dublin physician, 1802–1845. See H.'s *folds, muscle, valves.*

**ho′ven.** Bloating in cattle.

**Howard,** John Eager. See Ellsworth-H. *test.*

**Howe,** Percy. U. S. dentist. See H.'s silver precipitation *method.*

**Howell,** William H., American physiologist, 1860–1945. See H.-Jolly *bodies,* H.'s *unit.*

**Howship,** John, London surgeon, 1781–1841. See H.'s *lacunae,* H.'s *symptom,* Romberg-H. *symptom.*

**Hoyer,** Heinrich F., Polish anatomist and histologist, 1834–1907. See H.'s *canals.*

**HPL.** Abbreviation for human placental *lactogen.*

**Ht.** Abbreviation for total *hyperopia.*

**5-HT.** Abbreviation for 5-hydroxytryptamine. See serotonin.

**H-tet′anase.** Behring's term for the hemolytic constituent of tetanus toxin.

**Huber,** Johann J., Swiss anatomist, 1707–1778. See H.'s *ganglion.*

**Hubrecht** [ hoo′brekt), Ambrosius A. W., Dutch zoologist and comparative anatomist, 1858–1915. See H.'s protocordal *knot.*

**Huchard** (ü-shar′), Henri, Paris physician, 1844–1910. See H.'s *disease.*

**Hucker-Conn solution.** See under solution.

**Hudson,** Arthur Cyril, British ophthalmologist, 1875–1962. See H.'s *line,* H.-Ståhli *line.*

**hue.** One of the three qualities of color; it is determined by the wavelength or a combination of wavelengths of light; other two qualities are saturation and brightness.

**Hueck** (hük), Alexander F., German anatomist, 1802–1842. See H.'s *ligament.*

**Huët,** G. J., Amsterdam physician. See Pelger-H. nuclear *anomaly.*

**Hueter** (hüt′er), Karl, German surgeon, 1838–1882. See H.'s *maneuver,* Vogt-H. *point,* H.'s *sign.*

**Huffman,** John William, U. S. obstetrician and gynecologist. See H. *speculum.*

**Hufnagel,** Charles A., American surgeon, \*1916. See H. *valve.*

**Hufner's equation.** See under equation.

**Huggins,** Charles B., U. S. surgeon, \*1901. Nobel laureate, 1966, with Peyton Rous, for their investigations of cancer. See H.'s *operation, test.* H. Miller-Jensen *test.*

**Huguenin** (ü-gĕ-naṅ), Gustave, Swiss psychiatrist, 1841–1920. See H.'s *edema.*

**Huguier** (ü-ge-a′), Pierre C., Paris surgeon, 1804–1873. See H.'s *canal, circle, sinus, theory.*

**Huhner** (hoo′ner), Max, U. S. urologist, 1873–1947. See H. *test.*

**Hull's triad.** See under triad.

**hum.** A low continuous murmur.

**venous h.,** nun's murmur; a musical murmur, usually continuous, heard on auscultation over the large veins at the base of the neck when an anemic patient is upright and looks to the opposite side. The h. may also be heard over the umbilicus with large portal anastomotic veins.

**humectant** (hu-mek′tant). Moist.

**humectation** (hu-mek-ta′shun) [ L. *humecto,* pp. *-mectus,* to moisten, fr. *humeo,* to be damp ]. 1. The therapeutic application of moisture. 2. Serous infiltration of the tissues. 3. The soaking of a crude drug in water preparatory to the making of an extract.

**hu′meral.** Relating to the humerus.

**hu′merora′dial.** Relating to both humerus and radius; denoting especially the ratio of length of one to the other.

**hu′meroscap′ular.** Relating to both humerus and scapula.

**hu′meroul′nar.** Relating to both humerus and ulna; denoting especially the ratio of length of one to the other.

**hu′merus,** gen. and pl. **hu′meri** [ L. shoulder. HUMER- ] [ NA ]. The bone of the arm, articulating with the scapula above and the radius and ulna below.

**humid′ity** [ L. *humiditas,* dampness ]. Moisture or dampness, as of the air.

**absolute h.,** the amount of water vapor present per unit volume of gas or air when saturated at a given temperature.

**relative h.,** the actual amount of water vapor present in the air or in a gas, divided by the amount necessary for saturation at the same temperature and pressure; expressed as a percentage.

**hu′min.** An insoluble brownish residue obtained upon acid hydrolysis of protein, probably involving carbohydrate impurities.

**hu′mor,** gen. **humo′ris** [ L. correctly, *umor,* liquid ]. 1. The extracellular fluids of the body: blood and lymph. 2 [ NA ]. Any clear fluid or semifluid hyaline anatomical substance. 3. A substance, such as a soluble food material (extractive), which is absorbed and carried in the blood to act upon a gland or other tissue. 4. A substance formed in the body but acting locally, *e.g.,* acetylcholine liberated at nerve terminals. 5. One of the elemental body fluids that were the basis of the physiologic and pathologic teachings of the Hippocratic school: blood, yellow bile, black bile, and phlegm; see also humoral *doctrine.*

**aqueous h.,** h. aquosus.

**h. aquo′sus** [ NA ], aqueous h.; the watery fluid that fills the anterior and posterior chambers of the eye. It is formed by the ciliary processes, passes through the posterior chamber and the pupil into the anterior chamber where it is reabsorbed into the venous system at the iridocorneal angle by way of the sinus venosus (canal of Schlemm).

**crys'talline h.,** obsolete term for the lens of the eye.

**Morgagni's h.,** Morgagni's *liquor.*

**oc'ular h.,** any one of the three h.'s of the eye: aqueous, crystalline, and vitreous.

**peccant h.'s,** based on the historic humoral theory of disease, such h.'s or deranged fluids in the body were regarded as the direct causes of various illnesses.

**thunder h.,** an obstinate skin eruption.

**vitreous h.,** h. vitreus.

**h. vit'reus** [ NA ], vitreous h.; the fluid component of the corpus vitreum.

**hu'moral.** Relating to a humor in any sense.

**hu'moralism, hu'morism** [ L. *umor, humor,* moisture ]. Humoral *doctrine.*

**hump.** A rounded protuberance or bulge.

**Hampton h.,** a pleura-based density usually at the costophrenic angles and convex toward the pulmonary hilum, seen in pulmonary infarct.

**hump'back.** Nonmedical term for kyphosis.

**Humphry,** Sir George M., English surgeon, 1820–1896. See H.'s *ligament.*

**hu'mulin.** Lupulin.

**humulus** (hu'mu-lus) [ Mediev. L. ]. Hops; the dried fruits (strobiles) of *Humulus lupulus* (family Moraceae), a climbing herb of central and northern Asia, Europe, and North America. Aromatic bitter, mildly sedative, and diuretic. A hop poultice is applied in cases of superficial inflammation. Primarily used in the brewing industry for giving aroma and flavor to beer.

**hunch'back.** Nonmedical term for kyphosis.

**Hung's method.** See under method.

**hun'ger** [ A.S. ]. 1. A desire or need for food. 2. Any appetite, strong desire, or craving.

**affect h.,** emotional h. for maternal love and feelings of protection and care implied in the mother-child relationship.

**air h.,** dyspnea characterized by deep labored respiration, such as may occur in acidosis; see also Kussmaul *respiration.*

**diminished h.,** anorexia.

**excessive h.,** bulimia.

**narcotic h.,** the physiological craving for narcotics.

**Hunner,** Guy L., U. S. surgeon, 1868–1957. See H.'s *stricture, ulcer.*

**Hunt,** James Ramsay, U. S. neurologist, 1872–1937. See H.'s *atrophy, neuralgia,* paradoxical *phenomenon,* syndromes, Ramsay H.'s *syndromes.*

**Hunter,** Charles. See H.'s *syndrome.*

**Hunter,** John, Scottish surgeon, anatomist, physiologist, and pathologist, 1728–1793. See H.'s *canal, chancre, induration, operation.*

**Hunter,** William, London anatomist and obstetrician, 1718–1783. See H.'s *gubernaculum, ligament, line, membrane.*

**Hunter,** William, London pathologist, 1861–1937. See H.'s *glossitis.*

**Huntington,** George, U. S. physician, 1850–1916. See H.'s *chorea.*

**Hurler,** Gertrud, Austrian pediatrician. See H.'s *disease, syndrome,* Hurloid *facies,* Pfaundler-H. *syndrome.*

**Hürthle** (hërt'l), Karl W., German histologist, 1860–1945. See H. *cell,* H. cell *adenoma, carcinoma, tumor.*

**Huschke** (hoosh'ke) Emil, German anatomist, 1797–1858. See H.'s *cartilages, foramen, valve,* H.'s auditory *teeth* (under tooth).

**Hutchinson,** Sir Jonathan, English surgeon, 1828–1913. See H.'s *disease,* H.-Gilford *disease, syndrome,* H.'s *facies, freckle, mask,* crescentic *notch, patch, pupil, teeth,* (see under tooth), *triad.*

**Hutchison,** Robert, English pediatrician, 1871–1960. See H.'s *syndrome.*

**Huxley,** Andrew F., English physiologist, *1917. Nobel laureate, 1963, with John C. Eccles and Alan L. Hodgkin,

for their studies of nervous system functions, especially of nerves and synapses.

**Huxley,** Thomas H., English biologist, physiologist, and comparative anatomist, 1825–1895. See H.'s *layer.*

**Huygens** (hi'gens), Christian, Dutch physicist, 1629–1695. See H.'s *ocular.*

**hyal-.** See hyalo-.

**hyalin** (hi'ä-lin) [ G. *hyalos,* glass ]. A clear, eosinophilic, homogeneous substance occurring in degeneration; for example, in arteriolar walls in arteriolar sclerosis and in glomerular tufts in diabetic glomerulosclerosis.

**alcoholic h.,** Mallory *bodies.*

**hyaline** (hi'ä-lin, -lēn) [ G. *hyalos,* glass ]. Of a glassy, homogeneous, translucent appearance. The term refers to a characteristic gross and microscopic appearance, not to a chemically specific substance.

**hy'aliniza'tion.** The formation of hyalin.

**hyalino'sis.** Hyaline *degeneration,* especially that of relatively extensive degree.

**hyalinu'ria.** The excretion of hyalin or casts of hyaline material in the urine.

**hyalinus** [ L. ] [ NA ]. Hyaline.

**hyalitis** (hi-al-i'tis). Inflammation of the vitreous; the inflammatory changes extend into the avascular vitreous from adjacent structures. For degenerative changes of the vitreous, see hyalosis.

**suppurative h.,** purulent vitreous humor due to exudation from adjacent structures, as in panophthalmitis.

**hyalo-, hyal-** (hi'ä-lo-) [ G. *hyalos,* glass ]. Combining forms meaning glassy, or relating to hyalin.

**hy'alobi'uron'ic acid.** A disaccharide made up of *N*-acetylglucosamine and glucuronic acid in a 1,3-linkage; occurring in hyaluronic acid as the repeating unit. (See hyaluronic acid.)

**hyal'ogens.** Substances related to mucoids found in many animal structures, such as cartilage, vitreous humor, hydatid cysts, etc., and yielding sugars on hydrolysis.

**hy'aloid** [ hyalo- + G. *eidos,* resemblance ]. Glassy in appearance; hyaline.

**hyalo'ma** [ hyalo- + G. suffix, *-oma,* tumor ]. Colloid milium; a circumscribed, papular, colloid degeneration of the skin; the occurrence of small white papules in the skin of the cheeks and forehead.

**hyalomere** (hi'ä-lo-mēr) [ hyalo- + G. *meros,* part ]. The clear periphery of a blood platelet.

**hyalomitome** (hi-al-om'it-ōm) [ hyalo- + G. *mitos,* thread ]. Hyaloplasm.

**Hyalomma** (hi-ä-lom'mah) [ hyalo- + G. *omma,* eye ]. An Old World genus (about 20 species) of large ixodid ticks with submarginal eyes, coalesced festoons, an ornate scutum, and a long rostrum. Adults parasitize all domestic animals and a wide variety of wild animals; larvae or nymphs may parasitize small mammals, birds, and reptiles. Species of *H.* harbor a great variety of pathogens of man and animals, and also cause considerable mechanical injury.

**H. anato'licum,** a tick of cattle, horses, and other ruminants; it is a probable vector of Uzbekistan hemorrhagic fever and of a Near Eastern variety of equine encephalomyelitis from horses, donkeys, and sheep in Egypt and Syria.

**H. margina'tum,** a particularly common tick carried by birds migrating between Europe and Asia and Africa, and the probable vector of the virus of Crimean hemorrhagic fever.

**H. variega'tum,** vector of the viral agent of lymphocytic choriomeningitis in Ethiopia.

**hy'alomu'coid.** The mucoid present in the vitreous humor.

**hyalonyxis** (hi'ä-lo-nik'sis) [ hyalo- + G. *nyxis,* puncture ]. Surgical puncture of the vitreous humor.

**hyalophagia, hyalophagy** (hi'ä-lo-fa'jī-ah, hi'ä-lof'ä-jī) [ hyalo- + G. *phagein,* to eat ]. The eating or chewing of glass.

**hyalophobia** (hi'ä-lo-fo'bī-ah) [ hyalo- + G. *phobos,* fear ]. Morbid fear of glass or of touching glass.

**hyaloplasm, hyaloplasma** (hi'ä-lo-plazm, -plaz-mah) [ hyalo- + G. *plasma,* thing formed ]. The protoplasmic fluid substance of a cell; some older (obsolescent or obsolete) synonyms are: hyalomitome; cytohyaloplasm; cytolymph; paraplasm.

**nuclear h.,** karyolymph.

**hyaloserositis** (hi'ă-lo-se-ro-si'tis) [ hyalo- + Mod. L. *serosa*, serous membrane, + suffix *-itis*, inflammation ]. Inflammation of a serous membrane with a fibrinous exudate that eventually becomes hyalinized, resulting in a relatively thick, dense, opaque, glistening, white or gray-white coating; when the process involves the visceral serous membranes of various organs, the grossly apparent condition is sometimes colloquially termed icing liver, sugar-coated spleen, frosted heart, and so on, depending on the site.

**hyalo'sis** [ hyalo- + suffix *-osis*, condition ]. Degenerative changes in the vitreous humor.

**asteroid h.,** Benson's disease; numerous small spherical bodies ("snowball" opacities) in solid vitreous, visible ophthalmoscopically; a senile change, usually unilateral, and not affecting vision.

**punctate h.,** a condition marked by minute opacities in the vitreous.

**hyalosome** (hi-al'o-sōm) [ hyalo- + G. *sōma*, body ]. An oval or round structure within a cell nucleus that stains faintly but otherwise resembles a nucleolus.

**hyal'urate.** Hyaluronate.

**hyalu'ronate.** Hyalurate; a salt or ester of hyaluronic acid.

**h. lyase,** hyaluronic lyase; a lyase (EC 4.2.2.1) cleaving hyaluronic acids; see also hyaluronidases.

**hyaluronic acid** (hi'al-u-ron'ik). A mucopolysaccharide made up of alternating residues of glucuronic acid and *N*-acetylglucosamine (hyalobiuronic acid), forming a gelatinous material in the tissue spaces, and an intercellular cement substance generally throughout the body, *e.g.*, in the vitreous humor, in and around joints, and in many other situations. It is hydrolyzed to a disaccharide or tetrasaccharide unit by the action of the enzyme, hyaluronidase.

Hyaluronic acid (repeating unit)

**hy'aluron'ic ly'ase** Hyaluronate lyase.

**hyaluron'idase** 1 (BP). ALIDASE; soluble enzyme product prepared from mammalian testes. Used to increase the effect of local anesthetics and to permit wider infiltration of subcutaneously administered fluids; also suggested in the treatment of certain forms of arthritis to promote resolution of redundant tissue; also to speed the resorption of traumatic or postoperative edema and hematoma. 2. See hyaluronidases.

**hyaluron'idases.** Term used, loosely, for any of three enzymes (hyaluronoglucosidase, EC 3.2.1.35; hyaluronoglucuronidase, EC 3.2.1.36; hyaluronate lyase, EC 4.2.2.1) that hydrolyze hyaluronic acid; one or more of them are present in testis, sperm, bee and snake venoms, type II pneumococci, certain hemolytic streptococci, etc. Some common synonyms for the hyaluronidases are spreading factor, Reynals' factor; Duran-Reynals' spreading factor or permeability factor; mucinase; invasin. See also hyaluronidase.

**hyaluronoglucosidase.** Enzyme (EC 3.2.1.35) hydrolyzing 1,4 linkages in hyaluronates; see also hyaluronidases.

**hyaluronoglucuronidase.** Enzyme (EC 3.2.1.36) hydrolyzing 1,3 linkages in hyaluronates; see also hyaluronidases.

**hybaroxia** (hi'bă-rok'sĭ-ah) [ G. *hyper*, above, + *baros*, pressure, + *oxys*, acute ]. Oxygen therapy with pressures greater than 1 atmosphere or ambient oxygen pressure applied in a chamber or room rather than through or applied only for positive pressure breathing.

**hyben'zate.** USAN-approved contraction for *o*-(4-hydroxybenzoyl)benzoate.

**hy'brid** [ L. *hybrida*, offspring of a tame sow and a wild boar ]. Crossbreed; an individual (plant or animal) whose parents are different varieities of the same species or belong to different but closely allied species.

**hy'bridism.** The state of being hybrid.

**hy'bridiza'tion.** Crossbreeding; the process of breeding a hybrid.

**hycan'thone** (USAN). ESTRENOL; 1-[ [ 2-(diethyl )amino)-ethyl ]-4-(hydroxymethyl)thioxanthen-9-one; an antischistosomal drug.

**hy'clate.** USAN-approved contraction for monohydrochloride hemiethanolate hemihydrate, HCl·$1/_2$ C$_2$H$_5$OH·$1/_2$ H$_2$O.

**hydantoin** (hi-dan'to-in). Glycocolyl-urea; 2,4-(3$H$,5$H$)-imidazoledione; derived from urea or from allantoin.

$$\text{NH—CO—NH—CO—CH}_2$$

**hydanto'inate.** A salt of hydantoin.

**hydatid** (hi'dă-tid) [ G. *hydatis*, a drop of water, a hyatid. HYDR- ]. 1. A hydatid *cyst*. 2. A vesicular structure resembling an echinococcus cyst.

**Morgagni's h.,** *appendix* vesiculosa.

**nonpedun'culated h.,** *appendix* testis.

**pedun'culated h.,** *appendix* epididymidis.

**sessile h.,** *appendix* testis.

**stalked h.,** *appendix* vesiculosus.

**hydatidiform** (hi'dă-tid'ĭ-form). Having the form or appearance of a hydatid.

**hydatidocele** (hi-dă-tid'o-sēl) [ hydatid + G. *kēlē*, tumor ]. A cystic mass composed of one or more hydatids formed in the scrotum.

**hydatidoma** (hi'dă-tĭ-do'mah) [ hydatid + G. suffix *-oma*, tumor ]. A benign neoplasm in which there is prominent formation of hydatids.

**hydatidosis** (hi'dă-tĭ-do'sis). The morbid state caused by the presence of hydatid cysts.

**hydatidostomy** (hi'dă-tĭ-dos'to-mĭ) [ hydatid + G. *stoma*, mouth ]. The surgical evacuation of a hydatid cyst.

**Hy'datig'era taeniaefor'mis.** *Taenia taeniaeformis*.

**hydatoid** (hi'dă-toyd) [ G. *hydōr* (*hydat*-), water, + *eidos*, resemblance ]. 1. The aqueous humor. 2. The hyaloid membrane. 3. Relating to the aqueous humor.

**Hyde,** James N., American dermatologist, 1840–1910. See H.'s *disease*.

**Hydnocarpus** (hid'no-kar'pus) [ G. *hydneō*, to nourish, + *karpos*, fruit ]. A genus of trees (family Flacourtiaceae) of India and Burma.

**H. wightiana,** a species the ripe seed of which is a source of chaulmoogra and chaulmoogra oil.

**hydnocarpus oil** (hid'no-kar'pus). Chaulmoogra oil.

**hydr-.** See hydro-.

**hydrab'amine penicillin.** See under penicillin.

**hydracetin** (hi-dras'ĕ-tin). Pure form of acetylphenylhydrazine.

**hy'dradeni'tis.** Hidradenitis.

**hydradeno'ma.** Hidradenoma.

**hydragogue** (hi'dră-gog) [ hydr- + G. *agōgos*, drawing forth ]. Producing a discharge of watery fluid; denoting a class of cathartics that retain fluids in the intestine and aid in the removal of edematous fluids, *e.g.*, saline cathartics.

**hydral'azine hydrochloride** (USP). APRESOLINE hydrochloride; 1-hydrazinophthalazine hydrochloride; an adrenergic blocking agent used in hypertension, usually in combination with rauwolfia alkaloids, or ganglionic blocking agents. It also increases renal blood flow.

**hy'dramine.** A hydroxylamine.

**hydrami'trazine tartrate.** MELADRAZINE tartrate; LISIDONIL; 2,4-bis(diethylamino)-6-hydrazino-*s*-triazine tartrate; intestinal antispasmodic.

**hydramnion, hydramnios** (hi-dram'nĭ-on, -nĭ-os) [ G. *hydōr*, water, + amnion ]. The presence of an excessive amount of amniotic fluid; dropsy of the amnion.

**hydranencephaly** (hi'dran-en-sef'ă-lī) [ hydro- + G. *an*-priv. + *enkephalos*, brain ]. Congenital absence of cerebral hemispheres; the basal ganglia and remnants of mesencephalon are covered by leptomeninges, dura, skull bones, and skin, in contrast to anencephaly.

**hydran'gea** [ hydr- + G. *angeion*, vessel ]. Seven-barks; the dried root of *Hydrangea arborescens* (family Saxifragaceae), a shrub common in the Ohio Valley. Used at one time as a diuretic in the treatment of cystitis. Popularly regarded as antilithic.

**hydran'gin.** Umbelliferone.

**hydrargaphen.** HYDRAPHEN; Phenylmercuric methylenet is(2-naphthyl-3-sulfonic acid); antibacterial and antimyc,tic agent.

**hydrargyria** (hi-drar-jīr'ī-ah) [ L. *hydrargyrum*, mercury ]. Mercurial *poisoning*.

**hydrargyrism** (hi-drar'jī-rizm). Mercury *poisoning*.

**hydrargyrum**, gen. **hydrargyri** (hi-drar'jī-rum) [ G. *hydrargyros*, quicksilver, fr. *hydōr*, water, + *argyros*, silver ]. Mercury.

**hy'drarthro'dial.** Relating to hydrarthrosis.

**hydrarthron** (hi-drar'thron). Hydrarthrosis.

**hydrarthrosis** (hi-drar-thro'sis) [ hydr- + G. *arthron*, joint ]. Hydrops articuli; effusion of a serous fluid into a joint cavity.

   **intermit'tent h.,** an affection characterized by a periodically recurring serous effusion into the cavity of a joint; the articulation may be the seat of a chronic arthritis or may apparently be normal in the intervals of the attacks.

**hydrar'thrus.** Hydrarthrosis.

**hy'drase.** Hydratase.

**hydrastine** (hi-dras-tēn). An alkaloid of hydrastis; an isoquinoline chemically related to narcotine. As the hydrochloride, used locally in the treatment of catarrhal inflammation of the mucous membranes, and internally in the treatment of gastric inflammation, as a uterine stimulant, and to check uterine hemmorrhage.

**hydrastinine** (hi-dras'tī-nēn). A semisynthetic alkaloid prepared from hydrastine; the hydrochloride has been used in uterine hemorrhage and as an oxytocic; in large does it is a powerful depressant of the entire motor tract (motor cortex, nerve, and muscle).

**hydras'tis** [ Mod. L. fr. G. *hydōr* (hydro-), water, + *draō*, to accomplish ]. Golden seal; yellow root; Indian turmeric; jaundice root; the dried rhizome of *Hydrastis canadensis*, (family Ranunculaceae), a native of the eastern United States; used in the treatment of chronic catarrhal states of the mucous membranes and in metrorrhagia.

**hy'dratase.** Trivial name applied, together with dehydratase, to certain hydro-lyases (EC class 4.2.1), enzymes catalyzing hydration-dehydration of certain C—O linkages. The hydro-lyases, in turn, belong to class 4, the lyases, enzymes removing groups nonhydrolytically. Example, fumarate hydratase (EC 4.2.1.2).

**hy'drate.** An aqueous solvate (in older terminology, a hydroxide); a compound crystallizing with one or more molecules of water; *e.g.*, CuSO$_4$.5H$_2$O.

**hy'drated.** Combined with water, forming a hydrate.

**hydra'tion.** 1. The addition of water. To be differentiated from hydrolysis, where the union with water is accompanied by a splitting of the original molecule and the water molecule. 2. Clinically, the taking in of water; used much more commonly in the sense of reduced h. or dehydration.

   **absolute h.,** actual water excess as measured by a difference between the normal or from a given water content.

**hy'drazid, hy'drazide.** An organic compound of the general formula RCO—NHNH$_2$; an acyl derivative of hydrazine.

**hydrazine** (hi'dră-zēn). Diamine; H$_2$N—NH$_2$, from which phenylhydrazine and similar products are derived.

**hy'drazinol'ysis.** Cleavage of chemical bonds by hydrazine (NH$_2$—NH$_2$), applied in protein and nucleic acid degradations.

**hydrazone** (hi'dră-zōn). A substance derived from aldehydes and ketones by reaction with hydrazine or a hydrazine derivative, to give the grouping $>$C=N—NH$_2$.

**hydremia** (hi-dre'mī-ah) [ hydr- + G. *haima*, blood ]. Dilution anemia; polyplasmia; a condition in which the blood

volume is increased as a result of an increase of plasma, with or without a reduction in the concentration of protein; there elements, an excess of plasma in proportion to the formed elements, and a corresponding decrease in hematocrit.

**hydrencephalocele** (hi'dren-sef'ă-lo-sēl) [ hydr- + G. *enkephalos*, brain, + *kēlē*, tumor ]. Hydrocephalocele; hydroencephalocele; protrusion, through a cleft in the skull, of brain substance expanded into a sac containing fluid.

**hydrencephalomeningocele** (hi'dren-sef'ă-lo-mē-nin'go-sēl). A protrusion through a defect in the skull of a sac containing meninges, brain substance, and spinal fluid.

**hydrencephalus** (hi'dren-sef'ă-lus) [ hydr- + G. *enkephalos*, brain ]. Rarely used term for internal *hydrocephalus*.

**hydriatic** (hi-drī-at'ik). Hydriatric.

**hydriatric** (hi-drī-at'rik) [ hydr- + G. *iatrikos*, relating to medicine ]. Hydrotherapeutic; hydriatic; relating to the use of water in the treatment of disease.

**hy'dric.** Relating to hydrogen in chemical combination.

**hydride** (hi'drid, hi'drīd). A compound of hydrogen in which it assumes a formal negative charge, *e.g.*, sodium borohydride, NaBH$_4$.

   **h. ion,** the H· ion, transferred to acceptor molecules in some biological oxidations.

**hydrindantin.** The reduced form of ninhydrin.

**hydro-, hydr-** [ G. *hydōr*, water ]. Combining forms denoting (1) water or association with water; (2) hydrogen.

**hydro'a** [ hydro + G. *ōon*, egg ]. Hidroa; any bullous eruption.

   **h. aestiva'le** [ L. *aestivus*, summer ], h. vacciniforme.

   **h. febrile,** *herpes* simplex.

   **h. gestatio'nis,** *herpes* gestationis.

   **h. herpetifor'me,** *dermatitis* herpetiformis.

   **h. puero'rum** [ L. gen. pl. of *puer*, a boy ], h. vacciniforme.

   **h. vaccinifor'me,** h. aestivale; h. puerorum; a hereditary recurrent eruption of umbilicated bullae, occurring on exposure to the sun and affecting chiefly male children or young men.

   **h. vesiculosum,** erythema multiforme with iris or vesicular lesions.

**hydroadip'sia** [ hydro- + G. *a*- priv. + *dipsa*, thirst ]. Absence of thirst for water.

**hy'droappen'dix.** Distention of the vermiform appendix with a serous fluid.

**hydrobilirubin** (hi'dro-bil-ī-ru'bin). A dark brown-red pigment that may be formed when bilirubin is reduced.

**hydrobleph'aron** [ hydro- + G. *blepharon*, eyelid ]. Edematous swelling of the eyelid.

**hydrobro'mate.** A salt of hydrobromic acid.

**hydrobro'mic acid.** An aqueous solution of hydrogen bromide; used as a substitute for the bromides.

**hydrocalycosis** (hi'dro-kal'ī-ko'sis) [ hydro- + G. *kalyx*, cup of a flower ]. A rare symptomless anomaly of the renal calix which is dilated from obstruction of the infundibulum; usually discovered incidentally at pyelography or autopsy.

**hydrocar'bon.** A compound containing only hydrogen and carbon.

   **carcinogenic h.,** a h., usually aromatic and polycyclic, capable of inducing cancer; *e.g.*, 20-methylcholanthrene. When injected or ingested, carcinogenic h.'s may cause sarcomas in subcutaneous tissue or carcinomas in many organs.

   **Diels' h.,** 3'-methyl-1,2-cyclopentenophenanthrene; a phenanthrene derivative obtained by the dehydrogenation of various steroids.

   **saturated h.,** a h. that contains the greatest possible number of hydrogen atoms, so that the molecule contains neither rings nor multiple bonds.

**hydrocar'dia.** Hydropericardium.

**hydrocele** (hi'dro-sēl) [ hydro- + G. *kēlē*, hernia ]. A collection of serous fluid in a sacculated cavity; specifically, such a collection in the tunica vaginalis testis.

   **cervical h.,** h. colli; a cyst formed by secretion into a persistent duct or fissure of the neck.

   **h. colli,** cervical h.

   **congenital h.,** a collection of fluid in the unobliterated

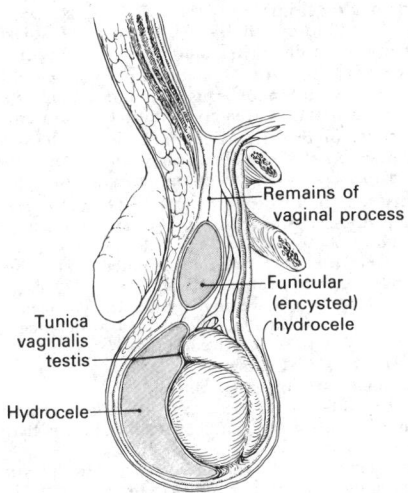

Hydrocele

canal leading from the abdominal cavity to the investing sac of the testis.

**Dupuytren's h.,** bilocular h. in which the sac fills the scrotum and also extends into the abdominal cavity beneath the peritoneum.

**h. fem'inae,** h. muliebris; Nuck's h.; an accumulation of serous fluid in the labium majus or in the canal of Nuck.

**filarial h.,** h. due to microfilaria (chiefly of *Wuchereria bancrofti*) in the tunica vaginalis.

**funicular h.,** fluid in a portion of the tunica vaginalis shut off from both testis and abdominal cavity.

**h. mulie'bris,** h. feminae.

**Nuck's h.,** h. feminae.

**h. spina'lis,** *spina* bifida.

**hydrocelectomy** (hi'dro-se-lek'to-mi) [ hydrocele + G. *ektomē*, excision ]. Excision of a hydrocele.

**hydrocephalic** (hi'dro-sĕ-fal'ik). Relating to or suffering from hydrocephalus.

**hydrocephalocele** (hi-dro-sef'ă-lo-sēl). Hydrencephalocele.

**hydroceph'aloid.** 1. Resembling hydrocephalus. 2. A condition in infants suffering from diarrhea or other exhausting disease, in which there are general symptoms resembling those of hydrocephalus without, however, any abnormal accumulation of cerebrospinal fluid.

**hydrocephalus** (hi'dro-sef'ă-lus) [ hydro- + G. *kephalē*, head ]. 1. A condition marked by an excessive accumulation of fluid dilating the cerebral ventricles, thinning the brain, and causing a separation of cranial bones. 2. In infants, an accumulation of fluid in the subarachnoid or subdural space.

**communicating h.,** h. in which there is a connection between ventricles and lumbar cerebrospinal fluid.

**congenital h.,** primary h.; h. due to developmental defect of brain.

**external h.,** (1) accumulation of fluid in the subarachnoid spaces of the brain; (2) accumulation of fluid in the subdural space due to a persistent communication between the subarachnoid and subdural spaces.

**h. ex vacuo,** h. due to loss or atrophy of brain tissue.

**internal h.,** hydrencephalus; Whytt's disease; h. in which the accumulation of fluid is confined to the ventricles.

**noncommunicating h.,** obstructive h.

**obstructive h.,** noncommunicating h.; h. with ventricular block.

**otitic h.,** a form of thrombotic h. associated with otitis media and thrombosis of one or both lateral intracranial sinuses.

**postmeningitic h.,** ventricular dilation following meningitis and secondary to obstruction of cerebrospinal fluid pathways.

**posttraumatic h.,** ventricular dilation following injury, and due either to impaired circulation and/or absorption of cerebrospinal fluid or to loss of brain substance (h. ex vacuo).

**primary h.,** congenital h.

**secondary h.,** an accumulation of fluid in the cranial cavity, due to meningitis or obstruction to the venous flow.

**thrombot'ic h.,** increase in cerebrospinal fluid and of intracranial pressure following thrombosis of the cerebral veins or sinuses; caused by septic infection, dehydration, tuberculosis, typhoid, leukemia, and other conditions.

**toxic h.,** thrombotic h. associated with some general infection or toxic state.

**hydrochlorbenzethylamine dimaleate.** INDUMOX; 2-{2-{2-[4-(*p*-chloro-α-phenylbenzyl)-1-piperazinyl]ethoxy}ethoxy}ethanol dimaleate; hypnotic.

**hydrochlo'ric acid** (USP, BP). HCl; muriatic acid; the acid of gastric juice; the commercial product is used as an escharotic and internally for achlorhydria. The gas and the concentrated solution are strong irritants.

**diluted h. acid** (USP), dilute h. acid (BP); contains, in each 100 ml., 10 gm. of HCl.

**hydrochlo'ride.** A compound formed by the addition of a hydrochloric acid molecule to an amine or related substance, *e.g.,* guanine hydrochloride.

**hy'drochlo'rothi'azide** (USP, BP). ESIDRIX; HYDRO-DIU-RIL; ORETIC; 6-chloro-3,4-dihydro-2 *H*-1,2,4-benzothiadiazine-7-sulfonamide 1,1-dioxide; a potent, orally effective diuretic agent related to chlorothiazide.

**hydrocholecystis** (hi-dro-ko-le-sis'tis) [ hydro- + G. *cholē*, bile, + *kystis*, bladder ]. An effusion of serous fluid into the gallbladder.

**hydrocholeresis** (hi'dro-ko'ler-e'sis, -kol'er-e'sis) [ hydro- + G. *cholē*, bile, + *hairesis*, a taking ]. Increased output of a watery bile of low specific gravity, viscosity, and solid content.

**hy'drocholeret'ic.** Pertaining to hydrocholeresis.

**hydrocinchonidine** (hi-dro-sin-kon'i-dēn). Dihydrocinchonidine; cinchamidine; an alkaloid of cinchona; toxic in large doses and therapeutically no more efficient than quinine.

**hydrociachonine** (hi-dro-sin'ko-nēn). Cinchotine; cinconifine; pseudocinchonine; a stereoisomer of hydrocinchonidine.

**hydrocirsocele** (hi-dro-sur'so-sēl) [ hydro- + G. *kirsos*, varix, + *kēlē*, tumor ]. Hydrocele complicated with varicocele.

**hydroco'done bitartrate** (USAN). HYCODAN; DICODID; dihydrocodeinone bitartrate; a narcotic analgesic and

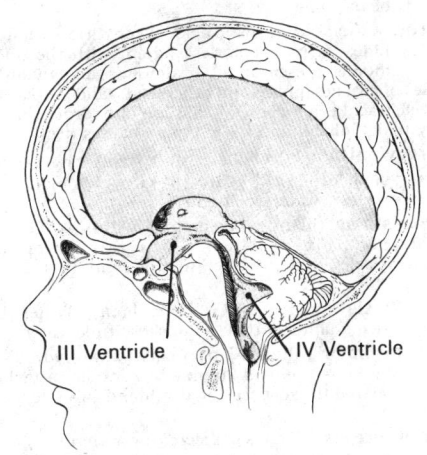

**Hydrocephalus**

Hydrocephalus due to a block at the foramen of Magendie. The thin wall of the fourth ventricle is herniated into the upper spinal canal, owing to the pressure within the fourth ventricle.

antitussive, similar in action to other salts of codeine but more active and more liable to cause addiction.

**hydrocol′loid.** A gelatinous colloid in unstable equilibrium with its contained water, useful in dentistry for impressions because of its dimensional stability under controlled conditions.

    **irreversible h.,** a h. whose physical state is changed by an irreversible chemical reaction when water is added to a powder and insoluble calcium alginate is formed.

    **reversible h.,** a h. composed of an agar-agar base whose physical state may be changed to that of a liquid by the application of heat and then changed to that of an elastic gel by cooling.

**hydrocolpocele, hydrocolpos** (hi′dro-kol′po-sēl, -kol′-pos) [ hydro- + G. *kolpos,* bosom (vagina) ]. An accumulation of mucus or other nonsanguineous fluid in the vagina.

**hydrocor′tamate hydrochloride** (NF). MAGNACORT; 17-hydroxycorticosterone-21-diethylaminoacetate hydrochloride; cortisol 21-(*N,N*-diethyl)glycinate hydrochloride; an ester-salt of hydrocortisone, used topically in the treatment of acute and chronic dermatoses.

**hy′drocor′tisone** (USP, BP). Cortisol; Kendall's compound F; Reichstein's substance M; 17α-hydroxycorticosterone; 11β,17,21-trihydroxy-4-pregnene-3,20-dione (for pregnene structure, see steroids); a reduction product (at C-11) of cortisone. It is a steroid hormone secreted by the adrenal cortex (the active hormone secreted in the greatest quantity by the adrenals) and is the most potent of the naturally occurring glucocorticoids. Manufactured under various trade names, *e.g.,* CORTEF, CORTIFAN, CORTRIL, HYCORTOLE, HYDROCORTONE.

    **h. acetate** (USP, BP), Cortisol acetate; hydrocortisone 21-acetate; CORTEF acetate; CORTRIL acetate; HYDROCORTONE acetate; similar actions and uses as hydrocortisone.

    **h. cyclopentylpropionate,** CORTEF fluid; an ester of hydrocortisone.

    **h. cypionate** (NF), salt of cortisone for oral administration.

    **h. hydrogen succinate** (BP), administered intravenously.

    **h. sodium phosphate** (USP), hydrocortisone 21-(disodium phosphate); an anti-inflammatory agent for intravenous or intramuscular administration.

    **h. sodium succinate** (USP, BP), SOLU-CORTEF; a very soluble ester salt of hydrocortisone (cortisol). Used parenterally in the management of emergencies resulting from acute adrenal insufficiency.

**hydrocotar′nine.** 5,6,7,8-Tetrahydro-4-methoxy-6-methyl-1,3-dioxolo[ 4,5-*g* ]isoquinoline; an alkaloidal principle derived from cotarnine; it is the basic hydrolytic product of narcotine; also obtained from the mother liquors of thebaine.

**hy′drocyan′ic acid.** Prussic acid, cyanhydric acid; hydrogen cyanide; HCN; a colorless liquid, with the odor of bitter almonds, present in bitter almonds (amygdalin), the stones of peaches, plums and other fruits, and laurel leaves. Scheele's acid is a 4 per cent solution of hydrocyanic acid. Very toxic; inhalation of 300 p.p.m. causes death.

**hy′drocy′anism.** Poisoning with hydrocyanic acid.

**hydrocyst** (hi′dro-sist) [ hydro- + G. *kystis,* bladder ]. A cyst with clear, watery contents.

**hydrocystoma** (hi′dro-sis-to′mah) [ hydro- + G. *kystis,* bladder, + suffix -*oma,* tumor ]. An eruption of deeply seated vesicles, due to retention of fluid in the sweat follicles.

**hy′drodip′sia** [ hydro- + G. *dipsa,* thirst ]. Water thirst, characterizing animals that ordinarily drink water.

**hydrodipsomania** (hi′dro-dip′so-ma′nĭ-ah) [ hydro- + G. *dipsa,* thirst, + *mania,* frenzy ]. Periodic attacks of uncontrollable thirst, occasionally found in epileptic patients.

**hy′drodi′ure′sis.** Diuresis effected by water.

**hydrodynamics** (hi′dro-di-nam′iks) [ hydro- + G. *dynamis,* force ]. The branch of physics that deals with the flow of liquids.

**hy′droelec′tric.** Relating to a combination of electricity and water, as the electric bath.

**hy′droenceph′alocele.** Hydrencephalocele.

**hydroflu′methi′azide** (NF, BP). SALURON; 3,4-dihydro-6-(trifluoromethyl)-2*H*-1,2,4-benzothiadiazine-7-sulfonamide 1,1-dioxide; a diuretic and antihypertensive.

**hy′drofluor′ic acid.** A solution of hydrogen flouride gas in water; a poisonous, caustic, foaming liquid that is used to clean metals; extremely irritating to skin and lungs.

**hydrogel** (hi′dro-jel). A colloid in which the particles are in the external or dispersion phase and water in the internal or dispersed phase; see fig. under hydrosol.

**hydrogen** (hi′dro-jen) [ hydro- + G. suffix -*gen,* producing ]. A gaseous element, symbol H, atomic no. 1, atomic weight 1.0080.

    **h. accep′tor,** (1) h. carrier; (2) a metabolite attaching and transporting h. in metabolism.

    **activated h.,** h. removed by a dehydrogenase, *e.g.,* a flavoprotein, from a metabolite for transference to another substance with which it combines.

    **arseniureted h.,** arsine.

    **h. bond,** see under bond.

    **h. bromide,** a colorless gas with a very irritating odor. Fumes in moist air. In aqeous solution, it is hydrobromic acid.

    **car′bureted h., h. car′bide,** archaic terms for gaseous compounds of carbon and h. "Light carbureted h." usually refers to methane.

    **h. carrier,** a molecule that, in conjunction with a tissue enzyme system, carries hydrogen from one metabolite (oxidant) to another (reductant) or to molecular oxygen to form $H_2O$.

    **h. chloride,** HCl; a very soluble gas which, in solution, forms hydrochloric acid.

    **h. cy′anide,** hydrocyanic acid.

    **h. dehydrogenase,** see dehydrogenase.

    **h. diox′ide,** h. peroxide.

    **h. donor,** metabolite from which h. is removed (by a dehydrogenase system) and transferred by an h. carrier to another metabolite, which is thus reduced.

    **h. exponent,** the logarithm of the h. ion concentration in blood or other fluid; its negative is the pH of that fluid.

    **heavy h.,** hydrogen-2.

    **h. ion,** a h. atom minus its electron and therefore carrying a unit positive charge. It is a bare proton and does not exist as such in solution; in water, the h. ion combines with a water molecule to form hydronium or oxonium ion, $OH_3{}^+$; it is this ion that is usually being dealt with when we talk of h. ion.

    **h. number,** the quantity of h. that 1 gm. of fat will absorb; it is a measure of the amount of unsaturated fatty acids in the fat; see also *iodine* number.

    **h. perox′ide,** h. dioxide; hydroperoxide; $H_2O_2$; an unstable compound readily broken down to water and oxygen, a reaction catalyzed by various powdered metals and by the enzyme, catalase. A 3 per cent solution is used as a mild antiseptic for skin and mucous membranes.

    **h. phosphide,** phosphine.

    **phosphureted h.,** phosphine.

    **h. sulfide,** sulfureted h.; $H_2S$; a colorless, flammable, toxic gas with a familiar "rotten egg" odor, formed in the decomposition of organic matter containing sulfur; used as a reagent, and in the manufacture of chemicals.

    **sul′fureted h.,** h. sulfide.

    **h. transport,** the transfer of h. through the action of an enzyme system from one metabolite (h. donor) to another (h. acceptor); the former is thus oxidized and the latter reduced.

**hydrogen-1.** ¹H; protium; the common h. isotope, making up 99.985 per cent of the h. atoms occurring in nature.

**hydrogen-2.** ²H; heavy hydrogen; deuterium (symbol D); the isotope of h. of atomic weight 2; the less common stable isotope of h. making up 0.015 per cent of the h. atoms occurring in nature. See also deuterio- and -*d.*

**hydrogen-3.** ³H; tritium (symbol T); a hydrogen isotope of mass number 3; weakly radioactive, emitting beta particles to become the stable helium-3; half-life, 12.5 years.

**hydrogenase** (hi′dro-jě-nās) Any enzyme that abstracts molecular hydrogen (H₃) from NADH (hydrogen dehydrogenase, EC 1.12.1.2), or adds it to ferricytochrome c₃ (cytochrome hydrogenase, EC 1.12.2.1) or to ferredoxin(s) (ferredoxin hydrogenase, EC 1.12.99.1). The last-named has also been called hydrogenlyase.

**hydro'gena'tion.** The addition of hydrogen to a compound, especially to an unsaturated fat or fatty acid; thus soft fats or oils are solidified or "hardened."

**hydrogenlyase.** Ferredoxin hydrogenase (see hydrogenase).

**hy'drokinet'ic.** Pertaining to the motion of fluids and the forces giving rise to such motion.

**hy'drokinet'ics.** That branch of kinetics dealing with fluids in motion.

**hy'drola'bile.** Unstable in the presence of water.

**hy'drolabil'ity.** State in which the fluid in the tissues readily changes in amount.

**hy'drolab'yrinth.** Hydrops labyrinthi; excess of endolymph in the inner ear.

**hy'drolases.** Hydrolyzing enzymes (EC class 3); enzymes cleaving substrates with addition of $H_2O$ at the point of cleavage. Esterases, phosphatases, nucleases, peptidases, etc., are all h.'s.

**hydro-lyases.** A class of lyases (EC 4.2.1) comprising enzymes removing H and OH as water, leading to formation of new double bonds within the affected molecule; the trivial names usually contain dehydratase or hydratase (e.g., carbonate dehydratase catalyzes the breakdown of $H_2CO_3$ to $CO_2$ and $H_2O$; citrate dehydratase catalyzes the conversion of citrate to cis-aconitate).

**hy'drolymph.** The circulating fluid in many of the invertebrates.

**hydrolysate** (hi-drol'ĭ-sāt). A solution containing the products of a hydrolysis.

**hydrolysis** (hi-drol'ĭ-sis) [ hydro- + G. lysis, dissolution ]. A chemical process whereby a compound is cleaved into two (or more) simpler compounds with the uptake of the H and OH parts of a water molecule on either side of the chemical bond cleaved. Hydrolysis is effected by the action of acids, alkalies, or enzymes.

**hydrolyt'ic.** Referring to or causing hydrolysis.

**hy'drolyze.** To subject to hydrolysis.

**hydro'ma.** Hygroma.

**hydromassage** (hi'dro-mă-sahzh). Massage produced by streams of water.

**hydromeningocele** (hi-dro-men-in'go-sēl) [ hydro- + G. mēninx, membrane, + kēlē, hernia ]. Protrusion of the meninges of brain or spinal cord through a defect in the bony wall, the sac so formed containing fluid.

**hydrom'eter** [ hydro- + G. mēron, measure ]. Gravimeter; an instrument for determining the specific gravity of a liquid.

**hydrometra** (hi'dro-me'trah) [ hydro- + G. mētra, uterus ]. An accumulation of thin mucus or other watery fluid in the cavity of the uterus.

**hydromet'ric.** Relating to hydrometry or the hydrometer.

**hydrometrocolpos** (hi'dro-me'tro-kol'pos) [ hydro- + G. mētra, uterus, + kolpos, bosom (vagina) ]. Distention of uterus and vagina by fluid other than blood or pus.

**hydrom'etry.** The determination of the specific gravity of a fluid by means of a hydrometer.

**hydromicrocephaly** (hi'dro-mi'kro-sef'ă-lī). Microcephaly associated with an increased amount of cerebrospinal fluid.

**hydromor'phone hydrochloride** (NF). DILAUDID; dihydromorphinone or dimorphone hydrochloride; a synthetic derivative of morphine, with analgesic potency about 10 times that of morphine.

**hydromphalus** (hi-drom'fă-lus) [ hydro- + G. omphalos, umbilicus ]. A cystic tumor at the umbilicus, most commonly a vitellointestinal cyst.

**hydromyelia** (hi-dro-mi-e'lī-ah) [ hydro- + G. myelos, marrow ]. An increase of fluid in the dilated central canal of the spinal cord, or in congenital cavities elsewhere in the cord substance.

**hydromyelocele** (hi'dro-mi'ē-lo-sēl) [ hydro- + G. myelos, marrow, + kēlē, tumor, hernia ]. The protrusion of a portion of cord, thinned out into a sac distended with cerebrospinal fluid, through a spina bifida.

**hy'dromyo'ma.** A leiomyoma that contains cystlike foci of proteinaceous fluid; h.'s occur more frequently in leiomyomas of the uterus, as a result of degenerative changes.

**hydronephrosis** (hi'dro-ne-fro'sis) [ hydro- + G. nephros, kidney, + suffix -osis, condition ]. Dilation of the pelvis and calices of one or both kidneys resulting from obstruction to the flow of urine.

**hy'dronephrot'ic.** Relating to hydronephrosis.

**hydro'nium ion.** The hydrated proton, $OH^+_3$, the form in which hydrogen ion ($H^+$) actually exists in water.

**hydroparasalpinx** (hi'dro-păr-ah-sal'pinks) [ hydro- + G. para, beside, + salpinx, trumpet ]. An accumulation of serous fluid in the accessory tubes of the oviduct.

**hydropath'ic.** 1. Relating to hydropathy. 2. Hydrotherapeutic.

**hydropathy** (hi-drop'ă-thī). The use of water in the treatment of disease.

**hydropenia** (hi'dro-pe'nĭ-ah) [ hydro- + G. penia, poverty ]. Reduction or deprivation of water.

**hy'drope'nic.** Pertaining to or characterized by hydropenia.

**hydropericarditis** (hi'dro-pĕr-ĭ-kar-di'tis). Pericarditis with a large serous effusion.

**hydropericardium** (hi'dro-pĕr-ĭ-kar'dĭ-um). Cardiac dropsy; hydrocardia; a noninflammatory accumulation of fluid in the pericardial sac.

**hydroperion** (hi'dro-pĕr'ĭ-on) [ hydro- + G. peri, about, + ōon, egg ]. A fluid present, in the early stages of pregnancy, between the decidua parietalis and the decidua capsularis.

**hydroperitoneum, hydroperitonia** (hi'dro-pĕr'ĭ-to-ne'um, -pĕr'ĭ-to'nĭ-ah) [ hydro- + peritoneum, q.v. ]. Ascites.

**hy'droperox'idases.** Those oxidoreductases that require $H_2O_2$ as hydrogen acceptors; e.g., peroxidases, catalase.

**hydrophagocytosis** (hi'dro-fag'o-si-to'sis). The engulfing or absorption of droplets of plasma by phagocytic cells.

**hy'drophil, hy'drophile.** Hydrophilic.

**hydrophilia** (hi-dro-fil'ĭ-ah) [ hydro- + G. philos, fond ]. A tendency of the blood and tissues to absorb fluid.

**hydrophilic** (hi-dro-fil'ik). Hydrophil; hydrophile; hydrophilous; denoting the property of attracting or associating with water molecules, possessed by polar radicals or ions. Opposed to hydrophobic.

**hydrophilous** (hi-drof'ĭ-lus). 1. Hydrophilic. 2. Lyophilic.

**hydrophobia** (hi-dro-fo'bĭ-ah) [ hydro- + G. phobos, fear ]. Rabies in man.

**hydropho'bic.** 1. Relating to or suffering from hydrophobia. 2. Repelling water; the alkyl side chains in amino acids are hydrophobic, tending to leave the water phase and congregate in another. Opposite of hydrophilic.

**hydrophorograph** (hi'dro-fōr'o-graf) [ G. hydrophoros, carrying water, + graphō, to record ]. An instrument for recording the flow or pressure of a fluid; e.g., the flow of urine or the pressure of spinal fluid.

**hydrophthalmia, hydrophthalmos, hydrophthalmus** (hi'drof-thal'mĭ-ah, -thal'mos) [ hydro- + G. ophthalmos, eye ]. Buphthalmos.

**hydrophysometra** (hi'dro-fi'so-me'trah) [ hydro- + G. physa, bellows, wind, + metra, uterus ]. The presence of fluid and gas in the uterine cavity.

**hydrop'ic.** Dropsical; relating to dropsy.

**hydropneumatosis** (hi-dro-nu-mă-to'sis) [ hydro- + G. pneuma, breath, spirit, PN- ]. Combined emphysema and edema; the presence of liquid and gas in the tissues.

**hydropneumogony** (hi'dro-nu-mo'go-nĭ) [ hydro- + G. pneuma, air, + gony, knee ]. Injection of air into a joint to determine the amount of effusion.

**hydropneumopericardium** (hi-dro-nu'mo-pĕr-ĭ-kar'dĭ-um) [ hydro- + G. pneuma, air, + pericardium, q.v. ]. Pneumohydropericardium; the presence of a serous effusion and of gas in the pericardial sac.

**hydropneumoperitoneum** (hi-dro-nu'mo-pĕr-ĭ-to-ne'um) [ hydro- + G. pneuma, air, + peritoneum, q.v. ]. The presence of gas and serous fluid in the peritoneal cavity.

**hydropneumothorax** (hi'dro-nu'mo-tho'raks) [ hydro- + G. *pneuma*, air, + 'thorax, *q.v.* ]. The presence of both gas and fluids in the pleural cavity.

**hy'dropo'sia** [ hydro- + G. *posis*, drinking ]. Water-drinking, characterizing animals that ordinarily drink water.

**hy'drops** [ G. *hydrōps* ]. Dropsy; an excessive accumulation of clear, watery fluid in any of the tissues or cavities of the body; synonymous, according to its character and location, with ascites, anasarca, edema, etc.

    **h. abdom'inis,** ascites.

    **h. artic'uli,** hydrarthrosis.

    **endolymphatic h.,** Ménière's *disease.*

    **fetal h.,** h. fetalis; abnormal accumulation of serous fluid in the fetal tissues, as in erythroblastosis fetalis.

    **h. feta'lis,** fetal h.

    **h. follic'uli,** accumulation of fluid in a Graafian follicle.

    **h. hypos'trophos,** angioneurotic *edema.*

    **h. labyrin'thi,** hydrolabyrinth.

    **h. ovarii,** hydrovarium.

    **h. spurius,** *pseudomyxoma* peritonei.

    **h. tubae,** hydrosalpinx.

    **h. tubae pro'fluens,** intermittent hydrosalpinx; an intermittent discharge of watery fluid from the oviduct.

**hydropyonephrosis** (hi'dro-pi'o-ne-fro'sis) [ hydro- + G. *pyon*, pus, + nephrosis, *q.v.* ]. The presence of purulent urine in the pelvis and calices of the kidney following obstruction of the ureter.

**hydroquin'one** (USP). *p*-Dihydroxybenzene; an antioxidant used in ointment.

**hydrorchis** (hi-dror'kis) [ hydro- + G. *orchis*, testicle ]. A collection of water (hydrocele) in the testis, as in the tunica vaginalis or along the spermatic cord.

**hydrorheostat** (hi'dro-re'o-stat). A rheostat in which resistance to the flow of electric current is provided by water.

**hydrorrhea** (hi-dro-re'ah) [ hydro- + G. *rhoia*, flow ]. A profuse discharge of watery fluid from any part.

    **h. grav'idae, h. gravida'rum,** discharge of a watery fluid from the vagina during pregnancy.

**hydrosal'pinx** [ hydro- + G. *salpinx*, trumpet ]. An accumulation of serous fluid in the Fallopian tube, often an end result of pyosalpinx.

**hydrosar'ca** [ hydro- + G. *sarx*, flesh ]. Anasarca.

**hydrosarcocele** (hi-dro-sar'ko-sēl) [ hydro- + G. *sarx*, flesh, + *kēlē*, tumor ]. A chronic swelling of the testis complicated with hydrocele.

**hydroscheocele** (hi-dros'ke-o-sēl) [ hydro- + G. *oscheon*, scrotum, + *kēlē*, hernia ]. A scrotal hernia complicated with a serous effusion in the sac.

**hy'drosol.** A colloid in aqueous solution, the particles being in the dispersed or internal phase, with water in the external or dispersion phase; see also hydrogel.

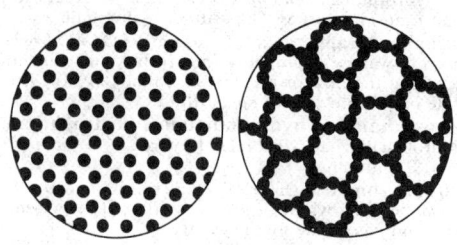

Hydrosol (*left*); Hydrogel (*right*)

**hydrosphygmograph** (hi-dro-sfig'mo-graf). A sphygmograph in which the pulse beat is transmitted to the recorder through a column of water.

**hy'drospirom'eter.** A spirometer in which the force of the expired air is indicated by the rise of a column of water.

**hy'drostat** [ hydro- + G. *statikos*, causing to stand ]. A device for regulating water level.

**hydrostat'ic.** Relating to the pressure of fluids or to their properties when in equilibrium.

**hydrosudopathy** (hi'dro-su-dop'ā-thī) [ hydro- + L. *sudor*, sweat, + G. *pathos*, suffering ]. Hydrosudotherapy.

**hy'drosu'dother'apy.** Hydrosudopathy; hydrotherapy combined with induced sweating, as in the Turkish bath.

**hydrosyringomyelia** (hi'dro-sīr-in'go-mi-e'lī-ah) [ hydro- + G. *hydōr*, water, + *syrinx*, a tube, + *myelos*, marrow ]. Syringomyelia.

**hydrotax'is** [ hydro- + G. *taxis*, arrangement ]. The movement of cells or organisms in relation to water.

**hydrotherapeu'tics.** Hydrotherapy.

**hydrotherapy** (hi'dro-thěr'ā-pī) [ hydro- + G. *therapeia*, therapy ]. Use of water by external application; either for its pressure effect or as a means of applying physical energy to the tissues.

**hy'drother'mal** [ hydro- + G. *thermē*, heat ]. Relating to hot water.

**hydrothionemia** (hi-dro-thi-o-ne'mī-ah) [ hydro- + G. *theion*, sulfur, + *haima*, blood ]. The presence of hydrogen sulfide in the circulating blood.

**hydrothionuria** (hi-dro-thi-o-nu'rī-ah) [ hydro- + G. *theion*, sulfur, + *ouron*, urine ]. The excretion of hydrogen sulfide in the urine.

**hydrotho'rax.** Pleurorrhea; the presence of serous fluid in one or both pleural cavities, usually resulting from cardiac failure and passive congestion of the lungs, venous obstruction, hydremia, and so on. In a precise sense, the term h. does not include conditions in which the effusion is associated with inflammatory reactions.

    **chylous h.,** the presence of chyle in a pleural cavity, resulting from a defect in the thoracic duct.

**hydrot'omy** [ hydro- + G. *tomē*, a cutting ]. Tearing apart the tissue elements in histology, by the injection of water.

**hydrotropism** (hi-drot'ro-pizm, hi'dro-tro'pizm) [ hydro- + G. *tropos*, a turning ]. The property in growing organisms of turning toward a moist surface (positive h.) or away from a moist surface (negative h.).

**hydroureter** (hi'dro-u-re'ter, -ūr'e-ter). Distention of the ureter with urine, due to blockage from any cause.

**hy'drous.** Hydrated.

**hydrovarium** (hi'dro-va'rī-um). A collection of fluid in the ovary.

**hydroxam'ic acids.** R—CO—NH—OH; hydroxylamine derivatives of carboxylic acids, including amino acids, formed by the action of hydroxylamine.

**hydrox'ide.** A compound containing a hydroxyl group; particularly a compound that liberates OH⁻ upon dissolving in water.

**hydrox'ocobal'amin.** (NF, BP). Vitamin $B_{12a}$ or $B_{12b}$, differing from cyanocobalamin (vitamin $B_{12}$) in the presence of a hydroxyl ion in place of the cyanide ion. See also aquacobalamin, and vitamin $B_{12}$.

**hydroxy-.** Prefix indicating addition or substitution of the —OH group to or in the compound whose name follows (*e.g.,* hydroxyproline). See also oxy-, oxo-, oxa-.

**hydrox'y acid.** An organic acid containing both OH and COOH groups; *e.g.,* lactic acid.

**3-hydroxyacyl-CoA dehydrogenase** (EC 1.1.1.35). $\beta$-Ketoreductase; $\beta$-ketohydrogenase; $\beta$-hydroxyacyl dehydrogenase; enzyme catalyzing the oxidation of a 3-hydroxyacylcoenzyme A to a 3-ketoacylcoenzyme A with reduction of NAD; one of the enzymes of the fatty acid oxidation cycle.

**hydrox'yac'ylglu'tathi'one hy'drolase.** Glyoxalase II; an enzyme (EC 3.1.2.6) with catalytic activity similar to that of lactoyl-glutathione lyase (glyoxalase I), but more general.

**hydrox'yamphet'amine hydrobromide.** PAREDRINE hydrobromide; *p*-(2-aminopropyl)phenol hydrobromide; sympathomimetic; decongestant and mydriatic. It is devoid of central nervous system stimulation.

**hydrox'yap'atite.** $3Ca_3(PO_4)_2 \cdot Ca(OH)_2$, a natural mineral structure that the crystal lattice of bones and teeth closely resembles; used in chromatography of nucleic acids.

***p*-hydroxybenzylpenicillin.** Penicillin X.

**$\gamma$-hydroxybutyric acid.** $CH_2OH(CH_2)_2COOH$; a potent hypnotic, also used as an intravenous anesthetic.

**hydrox'ychlo'roquine sulfate** (USP, BP). PLAQUENIL sulfate; a quinoline derivative; an antimalarial agent whose actions and uses resemble those of chloroquine phosphate. The incidence of untoward effects is lower. Also used in the treatment of lupus erythematosus and rheumatoid arthritis.

**25-hydrox'ychol'ecalcif'erol.** A metabolite of cholecalciferol (vitamin D$_3$) produced largely in the liver; it is more potent than the parent vitamin in promoting intestinal absorption of calcium and in curing rickets; it promotes decalcification of bone in much the same fashion as parathyroid hormone.

**hydrox'ydi'one sodium succinate.** VIADRIL; sodium 21-hydroxypregnane-3,20-dione succinate (for structure, see steroids); a steroid (with no endocrine effects) that produces a nonselective central nervous system depression similar to, but slower than, thiopental. It is used intravenously as a basal anesthetic or for the induction of general anesthesia prior to maintenance with gaseous anesthetic agents; does not produce adequate analgesia and muscular relaxation for most surgical procedures.

**hydroxyephed'rine.** SUPRIFEN; $p$-hydroxy-α[ 1-(methylamino)ethyl ]benzyl alcohol; sympathomimetic agent for treatment of shock.

**hydrox'yhe'min.** Hematin.

**hydrox'yl.** The atom group or radical, OH.

**hydroxylamine** (hi-droks'il-ă'měn). NH$_2$OH; oxammonium; a partially oxidized derivative of ammonia; reacts with carbonyl groups to produce oximes. Forms acid salts, e.g., h. hydrochloride, HONH$_2$·HCl.

**h. reductase** (EC 1.7.7.1), enzyme catalyzing reduction of hydroxylamine to ammonia with a variety of donors (e.g., methylene blue, flavin); see also NADH-hydroxylamine reductase.

**hydrox'ylami'no.** The monovalent group, —NHOH.

**hydrox'ylap'atite.** Hydroxyapatite.

**hydrox'ylases.** Enzymes catalyzing formation of hydroxyl groups by addition of an oxygen atom, hence oxidizing the substrate. Most are found in EC subclass 1.14. See steroid hydroxylases.

**hydroxylation** (hi-drok'sī-la'shun). The placing of a hydroxyl group on another compound in a position where one did not exist before.

**hydrox'yner'vone.** A cerebroside containing α-hydroxynervonic acid.

**hydrox'yphen'amate** (USAN). LISTICA; 2-hydroxy-2-phenylbutyl carbamate; a tranquilizer.

**hydroxyphenyluria** (hi-drok'sī-fen'il-u'rī-ah). Urinary excretion of tyrosine and phenylalanine, as a result of ascorbic acid deficiency; occurs notably in those premature infants who lack this vitamin.

**hydroxypro'caine.** OXYCAINE; OXYPROCAIN; 2-hydroxyprocaine; diethylaminoethyl $p$-aminosalicylate; a synthetic local anesthetic used for regional nerve blocks.

**17α-hydrox'yproges'terone.** PRODOX; 17α-hydroxy-4-pregnen-3,20-dione (for pregnane structure, see steroids). Medical use is similar to that of progesterone.

**17α-hydroxyprogesterone acetate.** PRODOX acetate; useful in conditions in which parenterally administered progesterone or 17α-hydroxyprogesterone caproate is indicated. Possesses some androgenic potency, and may cause virilizing changes in a female fetus. Effective orally.

**17α-hydroxyprogesterone caproate** (USP). DELALUTIN; hydroxyprogesterone hexanoate; essentially the same actions and uses as progesterone, but more potent and with longer duration of action.

**hydroxyproges'terone hexanoate** (BP). 17α-Hydroxyprogesterone caproate.

**hydrox'ypro'line.** 4-Hydroxy-2-pyrrolidinecarboxylic acid; an imino acid found among the hydrolysis products of collagen; not found in proteins other than those of connective tissue.

**hydrox'yproline'mia.** A metabolic disorder characterized by enhanced plasma concentrations and urinary excretion of free hydroxyproline; associated with severe mental retardation.

**hydrox'ypro'pyl meth'ylcel'lulose** (USP). The propylene glycol ether of methylcellulose; used as a suspending agent.

**15-hydroxyprostaglandin dehydrogenase.** An enzyme (EC 1.1.1.141) that catalyzes the oxidation of prostaglandins, rendering them inactive, by converting the 15-hydroxyl group to a keto group.

**8-hydrox'yquin'oline sulfate.** CHINOSOL; QUINOSOL; antiseptic, antiperspirant, and deodorant.

**hydroxystilbamidine isethionate** (USP). 2-Hydroxy-4,4'-stilbenedicarboxamidine di-β-hydroxyethanesulfonate. Antifungal and antiprotozoan agent used in the treatment of North American blastomycosis and coccidioidomycosis.

**hydrox'ystrep'tomy'cin.** Reticulin; a natural analogue of streptomycin, differing by an —OH in place of —H in the CH$_3$ group of the streptose moiety; produced by Streptomyces griseo-carneus; similar in action to streptomycin, but reported to be highly toxic in man.

**2-hydroxytetracaine hydrochloride.** SALICAIN; RHENOCAIN; $p$-butylaminosalicylic acid-2-dimethylaminoethyl ester hydrochloride; a potent synthetic local anesthetic effective by topical application and by injection.

**5-hydrox'ytryp'tamine.** Serotonin.

**hydroxytryptophan decarboxylase.** Aromatic L-amino-acid decarboxylase.

**o-hydrox'yty'ramine.** Dopamine.

**hydrox'yure'a** (USP). HYDREA; CH$_4$N$_2$O$_2$; antineoplastic agent.

**hydrox'yzine pamoate** (NF). ATARAX; VISTARIL; a substituted naphthoic ester of a substituted piperazine; a mild sedative and minor tranquilizer used in neuroses. Hydroxyzine is also available (NF) as the hydrochloride.

**Hydrozoa** (hi'dro-zo'ah) [ hydro- + G. zōon, animal ]. A class of the coelenterates including the aquatic forms Hydra a freshwater polyp; Physalia, the "Portuguese man-of-war," a syphonophore; and Millepora, a stinging coral.

**hydru'ria** [ hydro- + G. ouron, urine ]. Polyuria.

**hydru'ric.** Relating to polyuria.

**hygieiolatry** (hi-je-yol'ă-trī) [ G. hygieia, health, + latreia, worship ]. An extreme observance of the laws of health.

**hygieiology** (hi-je-yol'o-jī) [ G. hygieia, health, + -logia ]. 1. The science of hygiene. 2. The sum of all measures for the spread and popularization of public health knowledge.

**hygieist** (hi'je-ist) [ G. hygieia, health ]. Hygienist.

**hygiene** (hi'jēn, hi'jī-ēn) [ G. hygieinos, healthful, fr. hygiēs, healthy ]. The science of health.

**criminal h.,** the branch of mental h. or penology devoted to the study of the causes and prevention of criminality and the treatment of criminals.

**mental h.,** the science and practice of maintaining and restoring mental health; a branch of psychiatry which has become an interdisciplinary field attracting subspecialists in psychology, nursing, social work, law, and other professions.

**oral h.,** the cleaning of the mouth by means of brushing, flossing, irrigating, massaging, or the use of other devices. See also oral physiotherapy.

**hygienic** (hi-je'nik, hi-jī-en'ik). Healthful; relating to hygiene; tending to preserve health.

**hygienist** (hi-je'nist, hi'jī-en-ist). Hygiest; one who is skilled in the science of health.

**dental h.,** a professional auxiliary in denistry, licensed in 50 states. A dental health educator permitted by law to give dental prophylaxis and other preventive treatment. Professional education, 2 years for certificate, 4 years for B.S. degree.

**hygric** (hi'grik) [ G. hygros, moist ]. Relating to moisture.

**h. acid,** 1-methylproline; 1-methyl-2-pyrrolidinecarboxylic acid.

**hy'grine.** 2-Acetonyl-1-methylpyrrolidine; N-methyl-2-acetonylpyrrolidine; an alkaloid derived from coca leaves.

**hygro-, hygr-** (hi'gro-) [ G. hygros, moist ]. Combining forms meaning moist, relating to moisture or humidity.

**hygrobleph'aric** (hi'gro-blě-fär'ik) [ hygro- + G. blepharon, eyelid ]. Pertaining to abnormal moistening of the eyelids.

**hygro'ma** [ hygro- + G. suffix -oma, tumor ]. Hydroma; a cystic swelling containing a serous fluid, such as cystic lymphangioma, housemaid's knee, etc.

**h. axilla're,** h. of the axillary region.

**h. colli cys'ticum,** cervical h.; a benign neoplastic cystic tumor of the neck, of lymphatic origin.

**subdural h.,** accumulation in the subdural space of proteinaceous fluid, usually derived from serum.

**hygrom'eter** [ hygro- + G. *metron,* measure ]. Psychrometer.

**hygrom'etry.** Psychrometry.

**hygrophobia** (hi'gro-fo'bĭ-ah) [ hygro- + G. *phobos,* fear ]. Morbid fear of dampness or moisture.

**hy'groscop'ic.** Capable of readily absorbing and retaining moisture, as is true of NaOH, CaCl₂, etc. Sometimes "hydroscopic" is incorrectly substituted.

**hygrostomia** (hi'gro-sto'mĭ-ah) [ hygro- + G. *stoma,* mouth ]. Sialism.

**Hyl.** Symbol for the hydroxylysine radical.

**hyla** (hi'lah). A lateral extension of the cerebral aqueduct (Sylvius).

**hylephobia** (hi'lĕ-fo'bĭ-ah) [ G. *hylē,* forest, + *phobos,* fear ]. Hylophobia; morbid fear of forests.

**hyloma** (ni-lo'mah) [ G. *hylē,* stuff, crude matter, + suffix *-oma,* tumor ]. Hylic tumor; a neoplasm of hylic or pulp tissue, resulting from proliferation of elements derived from the embryonic pulp of epiblastic origin.

**mesenchymal h.,** a neoplasm of tissue derived from the mesoblastic pulp or mesenchyme.

**mesothe'lial h.,** a neoplasm derived from tissue of mesothelial origin.

**hylopathism** (hi-lop'ă-thizm) [ G. *hylē,* matter, + *pathos,* feeling ]. The notion that inanimate matter is endowed with sensation.

**hylopho'bia.** Hylephobia.

**hy'men** [ G. *hymēn,* membrane ] [ NA ]. Claustrum virgin-

ale; virginal membrane; a thin crescentic or annular membranous fold partly occluding the vaginal external orifice in the virgin.

**h. bifenestra'tus, h. bifo'ris,** one in which there are two openings separated by a wide septum; see h. septus.

**h. cribrifor'mis,** one with a number of small perforations.

**h. denticula'tus,** one with markedly serrated edges.

**h. imperfora'tus,** one in which there is no opening, the membrane completely occluding the vagina.

**h. infundibulifor'mis,** a projecting, funnel-shaped h. with a central opening with sloping edges.

**h. sculpta'tus,** one with markedly uneven and ragged edges.

**h. septus,** one in which there are two openings separated by a narrow band of tissue; see h. bifenestratus.

**h. subsep'tus,** one in which the opening is partly closed by a septum.

**vertical h.,** one in which the opening is perpendicular.

**hy'menal.** Relating to the hymen.

**hymenectomy** (hi'mĕ-nek'to-mĭ) [ G. *hymēn,* membrane, + *ektomē,* excision ]. Excision of the hymen.

**hymenitis** (hi'mĕ-ni'tis). Inflammation of the hymen.

**hymenoid** (hi'mĕ-noyd). Membranous; resembling the hymen.

**hymenolepiasis** (hi'mĕ-no-lĕ-pi'ă-sis). Illness produced by infection with *Hymenolepis.*

**hy'menolep'idid.** Common name for tapeworms of the family Hymenolepididae.

**Hy'menolep'ididae.** A family of tapeworms (order Cyclophyllidea) that includes the medically important genus *Hymenolepis.*

**Hymenolepis** (hi'mĕ-nol'e-pis) [ G. *hymēn,* membrane, + *lepis,* rind. LEP- ]. The largest genus (family Hymenolepididae) of tapeworms in the order Cyclophyllidea.

**H. diminu'ta,** a tapeworm of rats and mice, seldom found in man; its cysticercoid larvae are harbored by beetles, fleas, caterpillars, and other insects.

**H. lanceola'ta,** a tapeworm of aquatic birds, rarely found in man.

**H. na'na, H. na'na frater'na,** *Taenia diminuta; Taenia minima;* the dwarf mouse tapeworm; a very small tapeworm of man, sometimes found in great numbers in the intestine; the cysticercoid can develop through all its stages in a single host, or it can pass through a two-host cycle, as *H. diminuta* and most other cestodes necessarily must do.

**hymenology** (hi'mĕ-nol'o-jĭ) [ G. *hymēn,* membrane, + *logos,* study ]. The branch of anatomy and physiology dealing with the membranes of the body.

**Hymenoptera** (hi'mĕ-nop'ter-ah) [ G. *hymēn,* membrane, + *pteron,* wing ]. An order of insects, including bees, wasps, and ants, characterized by locked pairs of membranous wings.

**hymenorrhaphy** (hi-men-or'ă-fĭ) [ G. *hymēn,* membrane, + *raphē,* a suture ]. Suture of the hymen in order to close the vagina.

**hymenotome** (hi-men'o-tōm). A knife used in dividing the hymen or other membranes.

**hymenotomy** (hi'mĕ-not'o-mĭ) [ G. *hymēn,* membrane, + *tomē,* incision ]. Division of a hymen.

**hyo-** (hi'o-) [ G. *hyoeides,* shaped like the letter upsilon, υ ]. Combining form meaning U-shaped, or hyoid.

**hyodeoxychol(an)ic acid.** $3\alpha,6\alpha$-Dihydroxy-$5\beta$-cholanic acid (for structure of cholanic acid, see steroids).

**hyoepiglottic** (hi'o-ep-ĭ-glot'ik). Relating to the hyoid bone and the epiglottis; denoting the elastic h. ligament connecting the two structures.

**hyoepiglottidean** (hi'o-ep-ĭ-glot-id'e-an). Hyoepiglottic.

**hyoglossal** (hi'o-glos'al). Relating to the hyoid bone and the tongue.

**hy'oglos'sus.** *Musculus* hyoglossus.

**hyoid** (hi'oyd) [ G. *hyoeides,* shaped like the letter upsilon, υ ]. U-shaped or V-shaped; denoting the *os* hyoideum and the *apparatus* hyoideus.

**hyoi'deus** [ L. ] [ NA ]. Hyoid.

**hyopharyngeus** (hi'o-făr-in-je'us). See *musculus* constrictor pharyngis medius.

**Various Forms of the Hymen**

*1,* Bifenestratus; *2,* cribriformis; *3,* denticulatus; *4,* imperforatus; *5,* infundibuliformis; *6,* sculptatus; *7,* septus; *8,* subseptus.

**hyoscine** (hi'o-sēn). Scopolamine.

**h. hy'drobro'mide** (BP), scopolamine hydrobromide.

**hyoscyamine** (hi-o-si'a-mēn) (NF). Daturine; duboisine; *l*-tropine tropate; an alkaloid found in hyoscyamus, belladonna, duboisia, and stramonium; it is the levorotatory component of the racemic mixture; atropine; used as an antispasmodic, analgesic, and sedative.

**h. hy'drobro'mide** (NF), used for the same purposes as the alkaloid.

**h. sulfate** (NF), used as an antispasmodic, hypnotic, sedative and in parkinsonism to relieve tremor, rigidity, and excessive salivation.

*dl*-**hyoscy'amine.** Atropine.

**hyoscyamus** (hi'o-si'ă-mus) [ G. *hyoskyamos*, henbane or hog's bean, fr. *hys*, gen. *hyos*, a hog, + *kyamos*, a bean ] (BP). Henbane; insane root; poison tobacco; stinking nightshade; the leaves and flowering tops of *Hyoscyamus niger* (family Solanaceae); it contains hyoscyamine and hyoscine (scopolamine). Anodyne and antispasmodic. Powdered h. is official in the BP.

**Hyostrongylus rubidus** (hi'o-stron'jĭ-lus ru'bĭ-dus). The red stomach worm of swine; a small reddish trichostrongyle nematode that burrows into the mucosa of the fundus of the pig stomach and sucks blood; moderate numbers appear to cause little damage unless the animal's resistance is lowered by other factors.

**hyothyroid** (hi'o-thi'royd). See *membrana* thyrohyoidea.

**Hyp.** Symbol for the hypoxanthine radical.

**hyp-.** Variation of the combining form hypo-, often used before a vowel. For words beginning with hyp- and not found here, see those beginning with hypo-.

**hypacidity** (hi-pă-sid'ĭ-tĭ). Subacidity.

**hy'pacu'sia.** Hypacusis.

**h. hysterica,** partial psychogenic deafness.

**hypacusis** (hi-pă-ku'sis) [ hypo- + G. *akousis*, hearing ]. Hypacusia; hypoacusis; reduction in ability to perceive sound; hearing impairment attributable to deficiency in the peripheral organs of hearing; may be on a conductive or neurosensory basis.

**hy'palbumine'mia** [ G. *hypo*, under, + albuminemia ]. Hypoalbuminemia.

**hy'palbumino'sis** [ G. *hypo*, under, + albuminosis ]. An abnormally low content of albumin in the fluids of the body.

**hypalgesia** (hi-pal-je'zĭ-ah) [ G. *hypo*, under, + *algēsis*, sense of pain ]. Decreased sensibility to pain.

**hypalgesic, hypalgetic** (hi-pal-je'sik, -jet'ik). Relating to hypalgesia; having diminished sensitiveness to pain.

**hypalgia** (hi-pal'jĭ-ah) [ G. *hypo*, under, + *algos*, pain ]. Hypalgesia.

**hypamnion, hypamnios** (hi-pam'nĭ-on, hi-pam'nĭ-os) [ G. *hypo*, under, + amnion ]. The presence of an abnormally small amount of amniotic fluid.

**hy'panacine'sia.** Hypanakinesia.

**hypanakinesia, hypanakinesis** (hi-pan'ă-kin-e'sĭ-ah, hi-pan'ă-kin-e'sis) [ G. *hypo*, under, + *anakinēsis*, a to-and-fro movement. CIN- ]. A diminution in the normal gastric or intestinal movements.

**hypaphorine** (hi-paf'o-rin). The betaine of tryptophan, from *Erythrina americana* and other species of *Erythrina* (family Leguminosae); produces convulsions.

**hyparterial** (hi'par-tēr'ĭ-al, hip'-) [ G. *hypo*, beneath, + *artēria*, artery ]. 1. Below or beneath an artery. 2. The bronchi that pass below the pulmonary arteries.

**hypax'ial** [ G. *hypo*, beneath, + axis ]. Below any axis, such as the spinal axis or the axis of a limb.

**hypazoturia** (hi'paz-o-tu'rĭ-ah). Hypoazoturia.

**hypencephalon** (hi'pen-sef'ă-lon) [ G. *hypo*, under, + *enkephalos*, brain ]. The midbrain, pons, and medulla.

**hypengyophobia** (hi-pen'je-o-fo'bĭ-ah) [ G. *hypengyos*, responsible, + *phobos*, fear ]. Morbid fear of responsibility.

**hyper-** [ G. *hyper*, above, over ]. A prefix denoting excessive, above the normal. See also super-.

**hyperacanthosis** (hi'per-ă-kan-tho'sis). Hypertrophy of the prickle cell layer of the epidermis.

**hyperacid** (hi-per-as'id). Superacid; excessively acid.

**hyperacidity** (hi'per-ă-sid'ĭ-tĭ). An abnormal degree of acidity.

**hyperacusis, hyperacusia** (hi'per-ă-ku'sis, -ku'sĭ-ah) [ hyper- + G. *akousis*, a hearing ]. Abnormal acuteness of hearing, auditory hyperesthesia, due to increased irritability of the sensory neural mechanism.

**hy'peradeno'sis** [ hyper- + G. *adēn*, gland, + suffix -*ōsis*, condition ]. Glandular enlargement; especially enlargement of the lymphatic glands.

**hy'peradipo'sis, hyperadipos'ity.** An extreme degree of adiposis or fatness.

**hy'peradrenalcor'ticalism.** Hyperadrenocorticalism.

**hyperadrenalemia** (hi'per-ă-dre'nal-e'mĭ-ah) [ hyper- + adrenal secretion + G. *haima*, blood ]. Hyperadrenia.

**hy'peradre'nalism.** Hyperadrenia.

**hyperadrenia** (hi'per-ad-re'nĭ-ah). Hyperadrenalemia; obsolete terms formerly used in referring to the symptoms from overactivity of adrenal secretions or from diminished antagonistic secretions.

**hy'peradrenocor'ticalism.** Hypercortisonism; hyperadrenalism; hyperadrenalcorticalism; excessive secretion of adrenocortical hormones, usually cortisol.

**hyperalbuminosis** (hi'per-al-bu'mĭ-no'sis). The presence of an abnormally large amount of albumin in the fluids of the body.

**hy'peralcohole'mia.** An abnormally high content of alcohol in the circulating blood, usually in reference to ethyl alcohol.

**hyperaldosteronism** (hi'per-al-dos'ter-on-izm). Aldosteronism.

**hyperalgesia** (hi-per-al-je'zĭ-ah) [ hyper- + G. *algos*, pain ]. Hyperalgia; extreme sensitiveness to painful stimuli.

**auditory h.,** painful reaction to noises not ordinarily unpleasant.

**hy'peralge'sic, hy'peralget'ic.** Relating to hyperalgesia.

**hy'peral'gia.** Hyperalgesia.

**hy'peralimenta'tion.** superalimentation; overfeeding; the administration or consumption of food beyond normal requirements.

**parenteral h.,** administration of fluids containing essential nutrients through a venous catheter positioned in the superior vena cava; therapy is continuous and permits total replacement of nutritional needs at a slow rate, which minimizes overloading and excessive renal losses.

**hy'peralkales'cence.** Superalkalinity.

**hyperallantoinuria** (hi'per-ă-lan'to-in-u'rĭ-ah). Increased excretion of allantoin in the urine.

**hyperaminoaciduria** (hi'per-am'ĭ-no-as'ĭ-du'rĭ-ah). Aminoaciduria.

**hy'perammone'mia.** See ammoniemia.

**hyperamylasemia** (hi'per-am'ĭ-la-se'mĭ-ah) [ hyper- + amylase, + G. *haima*, blood ]. Elevated serum amylase, seen as one of the features of acute pancreatitis.

**hy'peranacine'sia.** Hyperanakinesia.

**hyperanakinesia, hyperanakinesis** (hi'per-an'ă-kĭ-ne'zĭ-ah, -e'sis) [ hyper- + G. *anakinēsis*, to-and-fro movement ]. Excessive to-and-fro movement, *e.g.*, of the stomach or intestine.

**hyperaphia** (hi'per-a'fĭ-ah) [ hyper- + G. *haphē*, touch ]. Tactile hyperesthesia; oxyaphia; extreme sensitiveness to touch.

**hyperaph'ic.** Marked by hyperaphia.

**hyperasialadenism** (hi'per-a-si-al'ad-en-izm) [ hyper- + G. *a*- priv. + *sialon*, saliva, + *adēn*, gland ]. A postulated state resulting from excessive secretion of parotin.

**hyperazotemia** (hi'per-az'o-te'mĭ-ah). An abnormally large amount of nonprotein nitrogenous matter, especially urea, in the circulating blood.

**hyperazoturia** (hi'per-az'o-tu'rĭ-ah) [ hyper- + Fr. *azote*, nitrogen, + G. *ouron*, urine ]. The excretion of an abnormally large amount of nonprotein nitrogenous matter, especially urea, in the urine.

**hyperbaric** (hi'per-băr'ik) [ hyper- + G. *baros*, weight ]. Pertaining to pressure of ambient gases greater than 1 atmosphere.

**hyperbarism** (hi'per-băr'izm) [ hyper- + G. *baros*, weight, + suffix -*ismos*, condition ]. Disturbances in the body resulting from the pressure of ambient gases at greater than 1 atmosphere. Examples include nitrogen *narcosis* and oxygen *toxicity, q.v.*

**hy′perbetalip′oproteine′mia.** Enhanced concentration of β-lipoproteins in the blood.
  **familial h.,** see familial *hyperlipoproteinemia.*

**hy′perbilirubine′mia.** An abnormally large amount of bilirubin in the circulating blood, resulting in clinically apparent icterus or jaundice when the concentration is sufficient.

**hyperbrachycephaly** (hi′per-brak-ĭ-sef′ă-lĭ) [ hyper- + G. *brachys,* short, + *kephalē,* head ]. An extreme degree of brachycephaly, with a cephalic index of over 85.

**hyperbulia** (hi′per-bu′lĭ-ah) [ hyper- + G. *boulē,* will ]. Excessive wilfulness.

**hypercalcemia** (hi′per-kal-se′mĭ-ah). An abnormally high concentration of calcium compounds in the circulating blood; commonly used to indicate an elevated concentration of calcium ions in the blood.
  **idiopath′c h. of infants,** persistent h. of unknown cause in very young children, associated with osteosclerosis, renal insufficiency, and sometimes hypertension. There may be a wide mouth, thick upper lip, and receding chin, with low mentality and general debility.

**hy′percalcinu′ria.** Hypercalciuria.

**hypercalciuria** (hi′per-kal-sĭ-u′rĭ-ah). Hypercalcinuria; hypercalcuria; the excretion of abnormally large amounts of calcium in the urine, as in hyperparathyroidism.

**hy′percalcu′ria.** Hypercalciuria.

**hypercapnia** (hi′per-kap′nĭ-ah) [ hyper- + G. *kapnos,* smoke, vapor ]. Hypercarbia; the presence of an abnormally large amount of carbon dioxide in the circulating blood, *i.e.,* an increased arterial carbon dioxide tension.

**hy′percar′bia.** Hypercapnia.

**hy′percar′dia** [ hyper- + G. *kardia,* heart ]. Hypertrophy of the heart.

**hypercatharsis** (hi′per-kă-thar′sis) [ hyper- + G. *katharsis,* a cleansing ]. Excessive movements of the bowels.

**hy′percathar′tic.** 1. Causing excessive purgation. 2. An agent having an excessive purgative action.

**hypercathexis** (hi′per-kă-thek′sis) [ hyper- + cathexis, *q.v.* ]. In psychoanalysis, the excessive investment of an object with libido or interest.

**hy′percedemo′nia** [ hyper- + G. *kēdemonia,* solicitude as guardian ]. Excessive grief, anxiety, or protectiveness about someone or something confided to one's care.

**hypercementosis** (hi′per-se′men-to′sis) [ hyper- + L. *caementum,* a rough quarry stone, + suffix *-osis,* condition ]. Cementum hyperplasia; an overgrowth of cementum on the root of a tooth which may be caused by localized trauma or inflammation, metabolic dysfunction, or developmental defect.

**hyperchloremia** (hi′per-klo-re′mĭ-ah). An abnormally large amount of chloride ions in the circulating blood.

**hyperchlorhydria** (hi′per-klōr-hid′rĭ-ah) [ hyper- + chlorhydric (acid) ]. Hyperhydrochloria; the presence of an abnormal amount of hydrochloric acid in the stomach.

**hy′perchlo′ride.** Perchloride.

**hyperchloruria** (hi′per-klōr-u′rĭ-ah). Increased excretion of chloride ions in the urine.

**hypercholesteremia** (hi′per-ko-les′ter-e′mĭ-ah). Hypercholesterolemia.

**hy′percholes′terine′mia.** Hypercholesterolemia.

**hypercholesterolemia** (hi′per-ko-les′ter-ol-e′mĭ-ah). Hypercholesteremia; hypercholesterinemia; the presence of an abnormally large amount of cholesterol in the cells and plasma of the circulating blood.
  **familial h.,** type II familial *hyperlipoproteinemia.*
  **familial h. with hyperlipemia,** type III familial *hyperlipoproteinemia.*

**hypercholesterolia** (hi′per-ko-les′ter-o′lĭ-ah). The presence of an abnormally large quantity of cholesterol in the bile.

**hypercholia** (hi-per-ko′lĭ-ah) [ hyper- + G. *cholē,* bile ]. A condition in which an abnormally large amount of bile is formed in the liver.

**hyperchromasia** (hi′per-kro-ma′sĭ-ah). Hyperchromatism.

**hyperchromatic** (hi′per-kro-mat′ik) [ hyper- + G. *chrōma,* color ]. Abnormally highly colored, excessively stained, or overpigmented.

**hyperchromatism** (hi′per-kro′mă-tizm) [ hyper- + G. *chrōma,* color ]. 1. Excessive pigmentation. 2. Increased staining capacity, especially of cell nuclei for hematoxylin. 3. An increase in chromatin in cell nuclei.

**hyperchromemia** (hi′per-kro-me′mĭ-ah) [ hyper- + G. *chrōma,* color, + *haima,* blood ]. Abnormally high color index of the blood.

**hy′perchro′mia.** Hyperchromatism.
  **macrocytic h.,** so-called hyperchromatic macrocythemia; inasmuch as the red blood cells are larger than normal, the *total amount* of hemoglobin per cell is increased, but the *percentage* of hemoglobin per cell is usually in the normochromic range.

**hy′perchro′mic.** 1. Hyperchromatic. 2. Denoting increase in light absorption.

**hyperchylia** (hi-per-ki′lĭ-ah) [ hyper- + G. *chylos,* juice ]. An excessive secretion of gastric juice.

**hyperchylomicronemia** (hi′per-ki-lo-mi-kro-ne′me-ah). Increased plasma concentrations of chylomicrons.
  **familial h.,** type I familial *hyperlipoproteinemia.*
  **familial h. with hyperprebetalipoproteinemia,** type V familial *hyperlipoproteinemia.*

**hypercinesis, hypercinesia** (hi′per-sĭ-ne′sis, -sĭ-ne′zĭ-ah). Hyperkinesis.

**hypercorticoidism** (hi′per-kor′tĭ-koyd-izm) [ hyper- + corticoid ]. Excessive secretion of one or more steroid hormones of the adrenal cortex; sometimes used also to designate the state produced by administration of large quantities of steroids having glucocorticoid activity.

**hy′percor′tisonism.** Hyperadrenocorticalism.

**hypercrinism** (hi-per-kri′nizm) [ hyper- + G. *krinō,* to separate (secrete) ]. Obsolete term, once used in referring to a condition resulting from an excessive secretion of any of the glands, especially of the endocrine glands.

**hypercryalgesia** (hi′per-kri-al-je′zĭ-ah) [ hyper- + G. *kryos,* cold, + *algēsis,* the sense of pain ]. Hypercryesthesia.

**hypercryesthesia** (hi′per-kri-es-the′zĭ-ah) [ hyper- + G. *kryos,* cold, + *aisthēsis,* sensation ]. Hypercryalgesia; extreme sensibility to cold.

**hypercupremia** (hi′per-ku-pre′mĭ-ah) [ hyper- + L. *cuprum,* copper, + G. *haima,* blood ]. An abnormally high level of plasma copper.

**hypercyanotic** (hi′per-si′ă-not′ik). Marked by extreme cyanosis.

**hypercyesis, hypercyesia** (hi′per-si-e′sis, -e′zĭ-ah) [ hyper- + G. *kyēsis,* pregnancy ]. Superfetation.

**hypercythemia** (hi′per-si-the′mĭ-ah) [ hyper- + G. *kytos,* cell, + *haima,* blood ]. Hypererythrocythemia; the presence of an abnormally high number of red blood cells in the circulating blood.

**hypercytochromia** (hi′per-si′to-kro′mĭ-ah) [ hyper- + G. *kytos,* cell, + *chrōma,* color ]. Increased intensity of staining of a cell, especially with reference to blood cells.

**hypercytosis** (hi′per-si-to′sis). Any condition in which there is an abnormal increase in the number of cells in the circulating blood or the tissues; frequently used synonymously with leukocytosis.

**hyperdactyly, hyperdactylia, hyperdactylism** (hi′per-dak′tĭ-lĭ, -dak-til′ĭ-ah, -dak′tĭ-lizm) [ hyper- + G. *daktylos,* finger or toe ]. The presence of supernumerary fingers or toes.

**hyperdiastole** (hi-per-di-as′to-le). Extreme cardiac diastole.

**hyperdicrotic** (hi′per-di-krot′ik). Pronouncedly dicrotic; superdicrotic.

**hyperdicrotism** (hi′per-dik′ro-tizm, -di′kro-tizm). Extreme dicrotism.

**hyperdiemorrhysis** (hi′per-di′ē-mor′ĭ-sis) [ hyper- + G. *dia,* through, + *haima,* blood, + *rhysis,* a flowing ]. Capillary hyperemia.

**hy′perdip′sia** [ hyper- + G. *dipsa,* thirst ]. Intense thirst; thirst that is relatively temporary. See also polydipsia.

**hy′perdisten′tion.** Superdistention; extreme distention.

**hyperdiuresis** (hi'per-di'u-re'sis). Obsolete term for extreme diuresis, or polyuria.

**hyperdynamia** (hi'per-di-na'mĭ-ah, -nam'ĭ-ah) [ hyper- + G. *dynamis*, force ]. Extreme violence or muscular restlessness.

   **h. u'teri,** excessive uterine contractions in childbirth.

**hy'perdynam'ic.** Marked by hyperdynamia.

**hyperechema** (hi'per-e-ke'mah) [ hyper- + G. *ēchēma*, sound ]. Auditory magnification or exaggeration.

**hyperemesis** (hi'per-em'e-sis) [ hyper- + G. *emesis*, vomiting ]. Excessive vomiting.

   **h. gravida'rum,** pernicious vomiting in pregnancy.

   **h. hi'emis,** Zahorsky's term for polytropous enteronitis.

   **h. lacten'tium,** the vomiting of nurslings with pyloric stenosis.

**hy'peremet'ic.** Marked by excessive vomiting.

**hy'pere'mia** [ hyper- + G. *haima*, blood ]. The presence of an increased amount of blood in a part; see also congestion.

   **active h.,** h. due to an increased afflux of arterial blood in the dilated capillaries.

   **arterial h.,** active h.

   **Bier's h.,** Bier's *method* (2).

   **collateral h.,** the increased blood flow through collateral channels when the circulation through the main artery to a part is arrested, as when the blood supply to one lung or to a portion of it is occluded the blood flow to the other lung or portion of a lung is increased.

   **constriction h.,** Bier's *method* (2).

   **flux'ionary h.,** active h.

   **passive h.,** h. due to an obstruction in the flow of blood from the affected part, the venous radicles being distended.

   **peristatic h.,** peristasis.

   **reactive h.,** that which follows when the blood supply to a part has been arrested for a time and is then restored.

   **venous h.,** passive h.

**hy'pere'mic.** Showing hyperemia; having an excessive quantity of blood.

**hyperemization** (hi'per-e'mĭ-za'shun). Artificially produced hyperemia; see also Bier's *method* (2).

**hyperencephalus** (hi'per-en-sef'ă-lus) [ hyper- + G. *enkephalos*, brain ]. A fetus with the vault of the cranium deficient, exposing the poorly formed brain.

**hyperendocrinism** (hi'per-en-dok'rĭ-nizm) [ hyper- + G. *endon*, within, + *krinō*, to separate ]. Obsolete term once used in referring to abnormal increase in any of the internal secretions.

**hyperenzymemia** (hi'per-en-zim-e'mĭ-ah). An increase in the level of an enzyme (or enzymes) in the blood, as the greater amount of amylolytic enzyme in acute pancreatitis.

**hypereosinophilia** (hi'per-e'o-sin'o-fil'ĭ-ah). A greater degree of abnormal increase in the number of eosinophilic granulocytes in the circulating blood or the tissues; for example, in diseases where the degree of eosinophilia usually ranges from 10 to 30 per cent, an increase to 50 or 60 per cent (or more) might be regarded as h.

**hyperephidrosis** (hi'per-ef-ĭ-dro'sis) [ hyper- + G. *ephidrōsis*, perspiration ]. Hyperhidrosis.

**hyperepithymia** (hi'per-ep'ĭ-thi'mĭ-ah) [ hyper- + G. *epithymia*, yearning ]. Inordinate desire.

**hyperequilibrium** (hi-per-e'kwĭ-lib'rĭ-um). A tendency to vertigo on slight rotary movement.

**hyperergasia** (hi-per-er-ga'zĭ-ah) [ hyper- + G. *ergasia*, work ]. Increased or excessive functional activity.

**hyperergia** (hi'per-er'jĭ-ah). Allergic hypersensitivity.

**hyperergic** (hi-per-er'jik). Relating to hyperergia; hypergic.

**hypererythrocythemia** (hi'per-e-rith'ro-si-the'mĭ-ah). Hypercythemia.

**hyperesophoria** (hi'per-es'o-fo'rĭ-ah) [ hyper- + G. *esō*, inward, + *phora*, movement ]. A tendency of one eye to deviate upward and inward in consequence of muscular insufficiency.

**hyperesthesia** (hi'per-es-the'zĭ-ah) [ hyper- + G. *aisthēsis*, sensation ]. Oxyesthesia; abnormal acuteness of sensitivity to touch, pain, or other sensory stimuli.

   **cer'ebral h.,** h. due to some central lesion in the brain.

   **cervical h.,** the hypersensitivity of teeth in the cervical area due to exposure of the dentin.

   **gus'tatory h.,** hypergeusia.

   **muscular h.,** hypermyesthesia; sensitiveness of the muscles to pressure.

   **h. olfactoria, olfactory h.,** hyperosmia.

   **h. optica,** extreme sensitiveness of the eyes to light.

   **tactile h.,** hyperaphia.

**hy'peresthet'ic.** Marked by hyperesthesia.

**hy'peres'trinism.** Obsolete term meaning excessive production of estrogen.

**hyperestrogenemia** (hi'per-es-tro-jen-e'mĭ-ah) [ hyper- + estrogen + G. *haima*, blood ]. Obsolete term, referring to a condition in which the estrogenic hormone is present in undue proportion in the blood.

**hyperexophoria** (hi'per-ek'so-fo'rĭ-ah) [ hyper- + G. *exō*, outward, + *phora*, movement ]. A tendency of one eye to deviate upward and outward, due to muscular insufficiency.

**hy'perexten'sion.** Superextension; extension of a limb or part beyond the normal limit.

**hy'perferre'mia.** High serum iron level; found in hemochromatosis.

**hyperfibrinogenemia** (hi'per-fi-brin'o-jĕ-ne'mĭ-ah). An increased level of fibrinogen in the blood.

**hy'perflex'ion.** Superflexion; flexion of a limb or part beyond the normal limit.

**hy'perfollic'uline'mia.** Obsolete term referring to the presence of an excessive amount of estrogen in the blood.

**hy'perfollic'uloidism.** Excessive production of estradiol, as seen in new growths derived from the Graafian follicles, a cause of abnormal uterine bleeding, *e.g.,* metropathia hemorrhagica.

**hy'pergalacto'sis** [ hyper- + G. *gala*, milk, + suffix *-osis*, condition ]. Excessive secretion of milk.

**hy'pergammaglob'uline'mia.** An increased amount of the γ-globulins in the plasma, such as that frequently observed in chronic infectious diseases.

**hypergasia** (hi'per-ga'zĭ-ah) [ G. *hypo* (*hyp-*), under, + *ergasia*, work ]. Diminished functional activity.

**hypergenesis** (hi'per-jen'ĕ-sis) [ hyper- + G. *genesis*, production ]. Excessive development or redundant production of parts or organs of the body.

**hy'pergenet'ic.** Relating to hypergenesis.

**hypergenitalism** (hi'per-jen'ĭ-tă-lizm). 1. Abnormally overdeveloped genitalia for age of individual. 2. Abnormally large genitalia in adults.

**hypergeusia** (hi-per-gu'sĭ-ah, -ju'sĭ-ah) [ hyper- + G. *geusis*, taste ]. Gustatory hyperesthesia; oxygeusia; abnormal acuteness of the sense of taste.

**hypergia** (hi-per'jĭ-ah). Hyperergia.

**hyper'gic.** Hyperergic.

**hypergigantosoma** (hi'per-ji-gan'to-so'mah) [ hyper- + G. *gigas* (*gigant-*), giant, + *sōma*, body ]. Obsolete term for excessive bodily development or gigantism.

**hy'perglan'dular.** Characterized by overactivity or increased size of gland.

**hyperglobu'lia, hyperglob'ulism** [ hyper- + L. *globulus*, globule ]. Hypercythemia; polycythemia; erythrocytosis.

**hyperglobulinemia** (hi'per-glob'u-lin-e'mĭ-ah). An abnormally large amount of globulins in the circulating blood plasma.

**hyperglycemia** (hi'per-gli-se'mĭ-ah) [ hyper- + G. *glykys*, sweet, + *haima*, blood ]. An abnormally high concentration of glucose in the circulating blood, especially with reference to a fasting level.

   **anacidotic h.,** nonketotic h.; a syndrome characterized by severe h., plasma hyperosmolality, dehydration, and, in some cases, focal motor seizures; no ketoacidosis is present.

   **nonketotic h.,** anacidotic h.

**hyperglyceridemia** (hi'per-glis'er-id-e'mĭ-ah). Elevated plasma concentration of glycerides, that are usually present within chylomicrons; a normal condition if transiently present after absorption of a meal containing lipids, but abnormal if it is a persistent state.

   **exogenous h.,** persistent h. due to retarded rate of removal from plasma of chylomicrons of dietary origin;

occurs in alcoholism, hypothyroidism, insulinopenic diabetes mellitus, types I and V hyperlipoproteinemia, and during acute pancreatitis.

**hyperglycinemia** (hi'per-gli'sin-e'mĭ-ah). Elevated plasma glycine concentration; see also *hyperglycinuria* with hyperglycinemia.

**hyperglycinuria** (hi'per-gli'sin-u'rĭ-ah). Enhanced urinary excretion of glycine.

**h. with hyperglycinemia**, glycinemia; a metabolic disorder generally appearing in the neonatal period and commonly fatal; characterized by vomiting, metabolic acidosis, ketonuria, osteoporosis, periodic thrombocytopenia, and neutropenia; the nature of the metabolic abnormality is unknown; autosomal recessive inheritance.

**hy'pergly'coder'mia.** The presence of excessive glucose in the skin.

**hyperglycogenolysis** (hi'per-gli'ko-jĕ-nol'ĭ-sis). Excessive glycogenolysis.

**hyperglycorrhachia** (hi'per-gli-ko-rak'ĭ-ah) [ hyper- + G. *glykys*, sweet, + *rhachis*, spine ]. An excessive amount of sugar in the cerebrospinal fluid.

**hyperglycosemia** (hi'per-gli'ko-se'mĭ-ah). Hyperglycemia.

**hyperglycosuria** (hi'per-gli-ko-su'rĭ-ah). Persistent excretion of unusually large amounts of glucose in the urine; *i.e.*, an extreme degree of glucosuria.

**hyperglyoxylemia** (hi'per-gli-ok'sil-e'mĭ-ah). Enhanced plasma (and possibly tissue) concentrations of glyoxylate; may develop during thiamine deficiency.

**hypergnosis** (hi'per-no'sis) [ hyper- + G. *gnosis*, knowledge ]. 1. The projection of inner conflicts into the environment. 2. Exaggerated perception such as the expansion of an isolated thought.

**hypergonadism** (hi'per-gon'ă-dizm). Enhanced secretion of the gonadal hormones.

**hypergonadotropic (-trophic)** (hi'per-gon'ă-do-trop'ik, -trof'ik). Indicating an increased production or excretion of gonadotropic hormones.

**hypergranulo'sis.** Increased thickness of the granular layer of the epidermis, associated with hyperkeratosis.

**hyperguanidinemia** (hi'per-gwan-ĭ-dĭ-ne'mĭ-ah). A condition in which there is an abnormally large amount of guanidine in the circulating blood.

**hypergynecosmia** (hi'per-jĭ-ne-koz'mĭ-ah) [ hyper- + G. *gyne*, woman, + *kosmeō*, to decorate ]. The overdevelopment of secondary sex characteristics of the mature female or their precocious development in the young girl.

**hyperhedonia, hyperhedonism** (hi'per-he-do'nĭ-ah, -he'don-izm) [ hyper- + G. *hēdonē*, pleasure ]. 1. The feeling of an abnormally great pleasure in any act or from any happening. 2. Sexual erethism.

**hy'perhe'moglobine'mia.** An unusually large amount of hemoglobin in the circulating blood plasma; *i.e.*, much more than that ordinarily observed in most examples of hemoglobinemia.

**hyperheparinemia** (hi'per-hep'ar-ĭn-e'mĭ-ah). Elevated plasma concentration of heparin; believed to be the cause of a heritable bleeding tendency.

**hyperhidrosis** (hi'per-hi-dro'sis) [ hyper- + hidrosis ]. Hyperidrosis; hyperephidrosis; polyhidrosis; polyidrosis; excessive or profuse sweating.

**h. oleo'sa**, *seborrhea* oleosa.

**hy'perhor'monal.** Obsolete term referring to increased secretion of hormones.

**hy'perhor'monism.** Obsolete term for the state characterized by increased secretion of hormones.

**hy'perhydra'tion.** Excess water content of the body; water retention; may result from the intravenous administration of unduly large amounts of glucose solution; water intoxication.

**hyperhydrochloria** (hi'per-hi'dro-klo'rĭ-ah). Hyperchlorhydria.

**hy'perhy'dropex'y, hy'perhy'dropex'is** [ hyper- + G. *hydōr*, water, + *pēgnynai*, to fasten ]. Increased fixation of water in tissues.

**hyper'icin.** A photosensitizing substance present in hypericum, a pigment with red fluorescence. It produces tonic and tranquilizing effects.

**hyper'icum** [ L. fr. G. *hyperikon*, St. John's wort, fr. *hypo*, under, + *erikē*, heather ]. Rosin rose; St. John's wort; touch-and-heal; the herb *Hypericum perforatum* (family Hyperiaceae) which contains hypericin; has been used as a vulnerary and astringent, and internally as an emmenagogue and diuretic.

**hyperidrosis** (hi'per-ĭ-dro'sis). Hyperhidrosis.

**hyperindicanemia** (hi'per-in'dĭ-kan-e'mĭ-ah). An unusually large amount of indican in the circulating blood; *i.e.*, greater than that observed in most instances of indicanemia.

**hyperinosemia** (hi'per-i'no-se'mĭ-ah) [ hyper- + G. *is* (*in-*), fiber, + *haima*, blood ]. A greatly increased quantity of fibrinogen in the circulating blood; under certain conditions, unusually large amounts of fibrin may be formed, thereby resulting in a greater degree of coagulability of the blood.

**hyperino'sis.** Hyperinosemia.

**hyperinsulinism** (hi'per-in'su-lin'izm). A condition resulting from an excessive secretion of insulin by the islets of Langerhans, resulting in hypoglycemia; the symptoms are those of insulin shock, though more chronic in character.

**hyperinvolution** (hi'per-in'vo-lu'shun). Superinvolution.

**hyperisotonic** (hi'per-i'so-ton'ik). Hypertonic.

**hy'perkale'mia** [ hyper- + Mod. L. *kalium*, potash, + G. *haima*, blood ]. A greater than normal concentration of potassium ions in the circulating blood; may be due to tissue destruction, renal failure, and Addison's disease; may cause bradycardia with hypotension and changes in the electrocardiogram, including elevation of the T wave, and muscle weakness.

**hyperkaliemia** (hi'per-kal'ĭ-e'mĭ-ah). Hyperkalemia.

**hyperkaluresis** (hi'per-kal'u-re'sis) [ hyper- + Mod. L. *kalium*, potassium, + G. *oureō*, to urinate ]. Excessive urinary excretion of potassium.

**hy'perker'atiniza'tion.** Hyperkeratosis.

**hyperkeratomycosis** (hi'per-kĕr'ă-to-mi-ko'sis). Thickening of the horny layer of the skin due to mycotic infection.

**hyperkeratosis** (hi'per-kĕr'ă-to'sis). 1. Hyperkeratinization; hypertrophy of the horny layer of the epidermis; see also keratoderma and keratosis. 2. A mouth disease with clinical characteristics usually of variously sized and shaped, grayish or grayish white, flat, adherent patches; having diffuse borders, a soft and almost normal consistency, peripheral margins that gradually fuse with surrounding normal tissue, and a smooth surface with no papillary projections, fissures, erosions, or ulcerations.

**bovine h.**, X disease of cattle; a specific disease characterized by thickening and hardening of the skin and proliferation of the epithelium of some of the mucous membranes; caused by poisoning from processed feed grains contaminated with certain highly chlorinated naphthalenes used as wood preservatives and constituents of lubricating greases.

**h. congen'ita**, *ichthyosis* vulgaris.

**h. eccen'trica**, porokeratosis.

**epidermolytic h.**, ichthyosis hystrix or spinosa; porcupine skin; a bullous form of congenital ichthyosiform erythroderma inherited as an autosomal dominant and present at birth; characterized by coarse, verruciform scaling most prominent in the flexural areas, and associated with blister formation; histologically, there is hyperkeratosis, bizarre granular reticular spaces in the epidermis, acanthosis, and rapid epidermal cell turnover.

**h. figura'ta centrif'uga atroph'ica**, porokeratosis.

**h. follicula'ris et parafollicula'ris**, Kyrle's disease; h. penetrans; discrete and confluent horny plugs on crateriform base, usually occurring on the arms and legs.

**h. pen'etrans**, h. follicularis et parafollicularis.

**h. subungua'lis**, h. affecting the nailbeds of the fingers or toes.

**hyperketonemia** (hi'per-ke'to-ne'mĭ-ah). Elevated concentrations of ketone bodies in blood.

**hyperketonuria** (hi'per-ke'to-nu'rĭ-ah). Increased urinary excretion of ketonic compounds.

**hyperkinemia** (hi'per-kĭ-ne'mĭ-ah) [ hyper- + G. *kineō*, to move, + *haima*, blood ]. Increased volume flow through the circulation; increased circulation rate; supernormal cardiac output.

**hyperkinesis, hyperkinesia** (hi'per-kĭ-ne'sis, -ne'zĭ-ah) [ hyper- + G. *kinēsis*, motion ]. Hypercinesis; 1. Excessive motility; supermotility. 2. Excessive muscular activity.

**hy'perkinet'ic.** Pertaining to or characterized by hyperkinesia.

**hy'perlacta'tion.** Superlactation.

**hyperleukocytosis** (hi'per-lu'ko-si-to'sis). An unusually great increase in the number and proportion of leukocytes in the circulating blood or the tissues; *i.e.*, much more than that ordinarily observed in most instances of leukocytosis.

**hyperlipemia** (hi'per-lip-e'mĭ-ah) [ hyper- + G. *lipos*, fat, + *haima*, blood ]. Lipemia.
   **carbohydrate-induced h.,** see types III and IV familial *hyperlipoproteinemia.*
   **combined fat- and carbohydrate-induced h.,** type V familial *hyperlipoproteinemia.*
   **familial fat-induced h.,** type I familial *hyperlipoproteinemia.*
   **idiopathic h.,** type I familial *hyperlipoproteinemia.*
   **mixed h.,** type V familial *hyperlipoproteinemia.*

**hyperlipidemia** (hi'per-lip'ĭ-de'mĭ-ah). Lipemia.

**hyperlipoidemia** (hi'per-lip'oy-de'mĭ-ah). Lipemia.

**hyperlipoproteinemia** (hi'per-lip'o-pro'te-in-e'mĭ-ah, -pro'tēn-). An increase in the lipoprotein concentration of the blood.
   **acquired h.,** nonfamilial h.; h. that develops as a consequence of some primary disease, such as thyroid deficiency.
   **familial h.,** a group of diseases characterized by changes in concentration of β-lipoproteins and pre-β-lipoproteins and the lipids associated with them. See types I through V familial h.
   **type I familial h.,** Bürger-Grütz syndrome; familial fat-induced hyperlipemia; familial hyperchylomicronemia; idiopathic hyperlipemia; characterized by the presence of large amounts of chylomicrons and triglycerides on a normal diet, and disappearance of these on a fat-free diet; low α- and β-lipoproteins on a normal diet, with increase on fat-free diet; decreased plasma postheparin lipolytic activity; low tissue lipoprotein lipase activity. Patients have bouts of abdominal pain, hepatosplenomegaly, and eruptive xanthomas; autosomal recessive inheritance.
   **type II familial h.,** familial hyperbetalipoproteinemia; familial hypercholesterolemia; familial hypercholesteremic xanthomatosis; characterized by increased plasma levels of β-lipoproteins, cholesterol, and phospholipids, but normal triglycerides; autosomal inheritance; heterozygotes have mild lipid changes and are susceptible to coronary atherosclerosis in middle age, homozygotes have severe changes often with generalized xanthomatosis and coronary atherosclerosis as young adults.
   **type III familial h.,** familial hyperbetalipoproteinemia and hyperprebetalipoproteinemia; familial hypercholesterolemia with hyperlipemia; carbohydrate-induced hyperlipemia; characterized by increased plasma levels of β-lipoproteins, pre-β-lipoproteins, cholesterol, phospholipids, and triglycerides; hypertriglyceridemia is endogenous, induced by high carbohydrate diet; abnormal glucose tolerance; patients frequently have eruptive xanthomas and atheromatosis, particularly coronary artery disease; autosomal recessive inheritance.
   **type IV familial h.,** familial hyperprebetalipoproteinemia; carbohydrate-induced hyperlipemia; plasma levels of pre-β-lipoproteins and triglycerides are increased while on a normal diet, but β-lipoproteins, cholesterol, and phospholipids are normal; hypertriglyceridemia is endogenous, induced by high carbohydrate diet; some patients have abnormal glucose tolerance and susceptibility to ischemic heart disease; probably autosomal recessive inheritance.
   **type V familial h.,** familial hyperchylomicronemia with hyperprebetalipoproteinemia; mixed hyperlipemia; combined fat- and carbohydrate-induced hyperlipemia; characterized by increased plasma levels of chylomicrons, pre-β-lipoproteins, and triglycerides, with slight elevation of cholesterole while on a normal diet, with β-lipoproteins normal; patients may have bouts of abdominal pain, hepatosplenomegaly, susceptibility to atherosclerosis; abnormal glucose tolerance; probably autosomal recessive inheritance.

**hy'perlipo'sis** [ hyper- + G. *lipos*, fat ]. 1. Excessive adiposity. 2. An extreme degree of fatty degeneration.

**hyperlithuria** (hi'per-lĭ-thu'rĭ-ah). An excessive excretion of uric (lithic) acid in the urine.

**hyperlogia** (hi'per-lo'jĭ-ah) [ hyper- + G. *logios*, eloquent ]. Morbid loquacity.

**hy'perlordo'sis.** Extreme lordosis.

**hyperlysinemia** (hi'per-li'sin-e'mĭ-ah). Abnormal increase of the amino acid lysine in the circulating blood; associated with mental retardation, convulsions, anemia and asthenia; autosomal recessive inheritance.

**hyperlysinuria** (hi'per-li'sin-u'rĭ-ah). The presence of abnormally high concentrations of lysine in the urine; a form of aminoaciduria that occurs in cystinuria, hepatolenticular degeneration, and the Fanconi syndrome.

**hy'permas'tia** [ hyper- + G. *mastos*, breast ]. Polymastia.

**hy'permegaso'mia** [ hyper- + G. *megas*, great, + *sōma*, body ]. Obsolete term for excessive bodily development or gigantism.

**hypermenorrhea** (hi'per-men'o-re'ah) [ hyper- + G. *mēn*, month, + *rhoia*, flow ]. Menorrhagia; prolonged or profuse menses.

**hy'permetab'olism.** Heat production by the body above normal, as in thyrotoxicosis.

**hy'permet'amor'phosis** [ hyper- + G. *metamorphōsis*, transformation ]. Excessive change; specifically, rapid change of ideas occurring in mental disorder.
   **h. of Wernicke,** after removal of both temporal lobes a monkey will pick up, over and over again, any object that is within its field of vision.

**hy'perme'tria** [ hyper- + G. *metron*, measure ]. A manifestation of ataxia characterized by overreaching a desired object or goal.

**hypermetrope** (hi-per-met'rōp). Hyperope.

**hypermetropia** (hi'per-me-tro'pĭ-ah) [ hyper- + G. *metron*, measure, + *ōps*, eye ]. Hyperopia.

**hypermi'croso'mia** [ hyper- + G. *mikros*, small, + *sōma*, body ]. Obsolete term for extreme smallness of body; dwarfism; nanism.

**hy'permim'ia** [ hyper- + G. *mimeia*, farce ]. Excessive mimetic movements.

**hypermnesia** (hi-perm-ne'zĭ-ah) [ hyper- + G. *mnēmē*, memory ]. 1. Extreme power of memory. 2. A capacity under hypnosis for immediate registration and precise recall of many more individual items than is thought possible under ordinary circumstances.

**hy'permorph** [ hyper- + G. *morphē*, form ]. One whose sitting height is low in proportion to the standing height, owing to great length of limb. See also hypomorph and mesomorph.

**hypermyesthesia** (hi'per-mi'es-the'zĭ-ah) [ hyper- + G. *mys*, muscle, + *aisthēsis*, feeling ]. Muscular *hyperesthesia*.

**hypermyotonia** (hi'per-mi-o-to'nĭ-ah) [ hyper- + G. *mys*, muscle, + *tonos*, tension ]. Extreme muscular tonus.

**hypermyotrophy** (hi-per-mi-ot'ro-fĭ) [ hyper- + G. *mys*, muscle, + *trophē*, nourishment ]. Muscular hypertrophy.

**hypernatremia** (hi'per-nă-tre'mĭ-ah) [ hyper- + *natrium* (*q.v.*), + G. *haima*, blood ]. An abnormally high plasma concentration of sodium ions.

**hypernea** (hi'per-ne'ah). Hypernoia.

**hyperneocytosis** (hi'per-ne'o-si-to'sis) [ hyper- + G. *neos*, new, + *kytos*, cell, + suffix -*osis*, condition ]. Hyperskeocytosis; hyperleukocytosis in which there are considerable numbers of immature and young cells (especially in the granulocytic series); *i.e.*, a "shift to the left" in the hemogram.

**hypernephroid** (hi'per-nef'royd) [ hyper- + G. *nephros*, kidney, + *eidos*, appearance ]. Resembling or of the type of the adrenal body.

**hypernephroma** (hi'per-ne-fro'mah) [ hyper- + G. *nephros*, kidney, + suffix -*oma*, tumor ]. Renal *adenocarcinoma*.
   **h. ova'rii,** obsolete term for arrhenoblastoma.

**hypernoia** (hi-per-noy'ah) [ hyper- + G. *noeō*, to think ]. Hypernea; hyperpsychosis. 1. Great rapidity of thought. 2. Excessive mental activity or imagination.

**hy'pernom'ic** [ hyper- + G. *nomos*, law ]. Uncontrolled on the side of excess.

**hypernutrition** (hi-per-nu-trish'un). Supernutrition.

**hyperoncotic** (hi'per-on-kot'ik). Indicating an oncotic pressure higher than normal, *e.g.*, of blood plasma.

**hyperontomorph** (hi-per-on'to-morf) [ hyper- + G. *on, being,* + *morphē,* form ]. An individual of the thin epithelial type, with a tendency to hyperthyroidism (a concept of uncertain validity).

**hyperonychia** (hi-per-o-nik'ī-ah) [ hyper- + G. *onyx, (onych-),* nail ]. Hypertrophy of the nails.

**hyperope** (hi'per-ōp). Hypermetrope; one suffering from hyperopia.

**hyperopia** (hi'per-o'pī-ah) [ hyper- + G. *ōps,* eye ]. Hypermetropia; farsightedness; a condition in which, in consequence of an error in refraction or flattening of the globe of the eye, parallel rays are focused behind the retina.

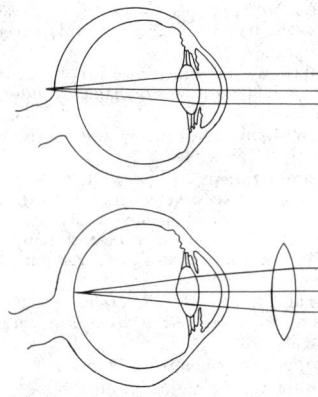

**Hyperopia**
*Top,* diagram showing course of parallel rays in the hyperopic eye; *bottom,* after correction by means of a convex lens.

**absolute h.,** manifest h. that cannot be overcome by an effort of accommodation.

**axial h.,** h. due to shortening of the anteroposterior diameter of the globe of the eye.

**h. of curvature,** h. due to diminution of convexity of the refracting media of the eye.

**facultative h.,** manifest h. that can be overcome by an effort of accommodation.

**latent h.,** the difference between total and manifest h.

**manifest h.,** the h. that can be measured by convex lenses without the use of a cycloplegic.

**total h.,** that which can be determined after complete paralysis of accommodation by means of a cycloplegic.

**hyperorality** (hi'per-o-ral'ī-tī) [ hyper- + L. *os (or-),* mouth ]. A condition in which unlikely objects are placed in the mouth.

**hyperorchidism** (hi'per-or'kī-dizm) [ hyper- + G. *orchis,* testis ]. Increased size or functioning of the testes.

**hyperorexia** (hi'per-o-rek'sī-ah) [ hyper- + G. *orexis,* appetite ]. Bulimia.

**hyperorthocytosis** (hi'per-or'tho-si-to'sis) [ hyper- + G. *orthos,* correct, + *kytos,* cell, + suffix *-osis,* condition ]. Hyperleukocytosis in which the relative percentages of the various types of white blood cells are within the normal range and immature forms are not observed.

**hyperosmia** (hi-per-oz'mī-ah) [ hyper- + G. *osmē,* sense of smell ]. Olfactory hyperesthesia; hyperosphresia; oxyosmia; oxyosphresia; an exaggerated or abnormally acute sense of smell.

**hyperosmolarity** (hi'per-os-mo-lăr'ī-tī). 1. An increase in the osmotic concentration of a solution expressed as osmols of solute per liter of solution. 2. Elevated osmolality of serum or plasma.

**hy'perosmot'ic.** Relating to increased osmosis.

**hyperosphresia, hyperosphresis** (hi'per-os-fre'sī-ah, hi'per-os-fre'sis) [ hyper- + G. *osphrēsis,* smell ]. Hyperosmia.

**hy'perosto'sis** [ hyper- + G. *osteon,* bone, + *-osis* ]. 1. Hypertrophy of bone. 2. Exostosis.

**flowing h.,** rheostosis.

**h. frontal'is interna,** abnormal deposition of bone on the inner aspect of the os frontale, visible by x-ray; may be a part of Morgagni's syndrome.

**generalized cortical h.,** Van Buchem's *syndrome.*

**infantile cortical h.,** Caffey's disease or syndrome; Caffey-Silverman syndrome; subperiosteal bone formation over many bones, especially the mandible and clavicles and the shafts of long bones; it follows fever, usually appearing before 6 months of age.

**streak h.,** rheostosis.

**hy'perova'ria.** Rarely used synonym for hyperovarianism.

**hyperovarianism** (hi'per-o-va'rī-an-izm). A condition of sexual precocity in young girls, due to premature development of the ovaries accompanied by the secretion of ovarian hormones.

**hyperoxaluria** (hi'per-ok'să-lu'rī-ah). An unusually large amount of oxalic acid or oxalates in the urine.

**primary h. and oxalosis,** a metabolic disorder characterized by calcium oxalate nephrocalcinosis and nephrolithiasis, plus extrarenal oxalosis; urinary output of oxalic and glycolic acids is greatly increased; usually evident clinically in the first decade of life; although life expectancy cannot with certainty be predicted, this disorder frequently produces progressive renal failure and terminal uremia; autosomal recessive inheritance.

**hyperoxia** (hi'per-ok'sī-ah). 1. An increased amount of oxygen in tissues and organs. 2. A greater oxygen tension than normal, such as that produced by breathing air or oxygen at pressures greater than 1 atmosphere.

**hy'peroxida'tion.** Excessive oxidation.

**hyperpancreatism** (hi'per-pan'kre-ă-tizm). A condition of increased activity of the pancreas, trypsin being in excess among the enzymes.

**hy'perpar'asite.** A secondary parasite capable of development within a previously existing parasite.

**hyperparasitism** (hi'per-păr'ă-sit-izm). Biparasitism; a condition in which a secondary parasite develops within a previously existing parasite.

**hyperparathyroidism** (hi'per-păr-ah-thi'roy-dizm). A condition due to an increase in the secretion of the parathyroids, causing generalized osteitis fibrosa cystica, elevated serum calcium, decreased serum phosphorus, and increased excretion of both calcium and phosphorus.

**primary h.,** h. due to neoplasms or idiopathic hyperplasia of the parathyroid glands.

**secondary h.,** h. that arises as a result of disordered metabolism, as in renal diseases characterized by hypercalciuria, rickets, or osteomalacia; associated with hyperplasia of the parathyroid glands.

**hyperparotidism** (hi'per-pă-rot'ī-dizm). Increased activity of the parotid glands.

**hy'perpath'ia** [ hyper- + G. *pathos,* suffering ]. Oxypathia; exaggerated subjective response to painful stimuli.

**hy'perpep'sia** [ hyper- + G. *pepsis,* digestion ]. 1. Abnormally rapid digestion. 2. Impaired digestion with hyperchlorhydria.

**hyperpepsinia** (hi-per-pep-sin'ī-ah). An excess of pepsin in the gastric juice.

**hyperperistalsis** (hi'pĕr'ī-stal'sis). Hyperprochoresis; peristaltic unrest; excessive rapidity of the passage of food through the stomach and intestine.

**hyperphagia** (hi'per-fa'jī-ah) [ hyper- + G. *phagein,* to eat ]. Gluttony; overeating.

**hyperphalangism** (hi'per-fă-lan'jizm). Polyphalangism; the presence of a supernumerary phalanx in a finger or toe.

**hyperphonesis** (hi'per-fo-ne'sis) [ hyper- + G. *phōnēsis,* sounding ]. An increase in the percussion sound, or of the voice sound in ausculation.

**hyperphonia** (hi'per-fo'nī-ah) [ hyper- + G. *phōnē,* sound, voice ]. Stammering or stuttering resulting from excessive tension of the vocal muscles.

**hyperphoria** (hi'per-fo'rī-ah) [ hyper- + G. *phora,* motion ]. A tendency of the visual axis of one eye to rise above that of its normal fellow.

**hyperphosphatasemia** (hi′per-fos′fă-tă-se′mĭ-ah). Abnormally high content of alkaline phosphatase in the circulating blood; see also hyperphosphatasia.

**hyperphosphatasia** (hi′per-fos′fă-ta′zĭ-ah). Osteoectasia; elevated alkaline phosphatase, with dwarfism, macrocranium, blue sclerae, and expansion of the diaphyses of tubular bones with multiple fractures; autosomal recessive trait.

**hyperphosphatemia** (hi′per-fos-fă-te′mĭ-ah). Abnormally high concentration of phosphates in the circulating blood.

**hy′perphos′phatu′ria.** An increased excretion of phosphates in the urine.

**hyperphrenia** (hi-per-fre′nĭ-ah) [ hyper- + G. *phrēn*, mind ]. Excessive degree of intellectual activity; a form of mania.

**hyperpiesis, hyperpiesia** (hi′per-pi-e′sis, -pi-e′zĭ-ah) [ hyper- + G. *piesis*, pressure ]. Essential *hypertension*.

**hyperpietic** (hi-per-pi-et′ik). Relating to or marked by extremely high blood pressure.

**hy′perpigmenta′tion.** An excess of pigment in a tissue or part.

**hyperpipecolatemia** (hi′per-pip-e-ko-la-te′mĭ-ah). A metabolic disorder in which serum concentrations of pipecolic acid are greatly increased; characterized by hepatomegaly and progressive, generalized demyelination of the nervous system.

**hyperpituitarism** (hi′per-pĭ-tu′ĭ-tă-rizm). Excessive production of anterior pituitary hormones, especially growth hormone; may result in gigantism or acromegaly.

**hyperplasia** (hi′per-pla′zĭ-ah) [ hyper- + G. *plasis*, a molding ]. An increase in number of cells in a tissue or organ, excluding tumor formation, whereby the bulk of the part or organ is increased. See also hypertrophy.

    **angiofollicular mediastinal lymph node h.,** benign mediastinal lymph node h.

    **basal cell h.,** increase in the number of cells in an epithelium resembling the basal cells; a variety of epithelial dysplasia.

    **benign mediastinal lymph node h.,** angiofollicular mediastinal lymph node h.; solitary masses of lymphoid tissue containing concentric perivascular aggregates of lymphocytes, occurring usually in the mediastinum or hilar region of young adults.

    **cementum h.,** hypercementosis.

    **congenital adrenal h.,** a group of diseases arising from specific enzymatic defects in corticosteroid biosynthesis; adrenal h. with excessive secretion of adrenal androgens develops as a result of these defects. The four major types (with clinical similarities but distinct genetic and biochemical differences) are: (1) simple virilizing form; (2) sodium-losing form; (3) hypertensive form; and (4) 3β-hydroxysteroid dehydrogenase defect; autosomal recessive inheritance.

    **congenital sebaceous gland h.,** *nevus* sebaceus.

    **cystic h.,** formation of multiple retention cysts from obstruction of ducts or glands by h. of the lining epithelium, as in fibrocystic disease of the breast and metropathia hemorrhagica.

    **cystic h. of the breasts,** fibrocystic *disease* of the breasts.

    **cystic-glandular h. of the endometrium,** Swiss cheese *endometrium*.

    **denture h.,** *epulis* fissuratum.

    **fibromuscular h.,** thickening of arterial media by fibrosis and muscular h., usually involving the renal arteries and causing multifocal stenosis and hypertension. Fibromuscular h. is a variety of fibromuscular dysplasia.

    **gingival h.,** a swelling of the gingiva due to cellular proliferation.

    **inflammatory fibrous h.,** epulis fissuratum; the enlargement and overgrowth of tissue in the mucobuccal or labial fold; produced by dentures that no longer exhibit an anatomical relationship to the alveolar ridges.

    **inflammatory papillary h.,** polypoid masses found in the center of the palate under ill-fitting dentures.

    **pseudoepitheliomatous h.,** a benign increase in epidermal cells, observed in chronic inflammatory dermatoses; microscopically, it resembles squamous cell carcinoma.

**hyperplasmia** (hi-per-plaz′mĭ-ah). 1. An excessive accumulation of white blood cells (especially of a single type) within various organs and tissues, but in association with a peripheral white blood cell count that is within the normal range; subleukemic or aleukemic leukemia. 2. An increase in the size of red blood cells as a result of imbibition.

**hy′perplas′tic.** Relating to hyperplasia.

**hy′perploid.** Relating to hyperploidy.

**hyperploidy** (hi′per-ploy′dĭ) [ hyper- + -ploid, *q.v.* ]. State of a cell or individual possessing one or more chromosomes in addition to the normal number.

**hyperpnea** (hi′perp-ne′ah) [ hyper- + G. *pnoē*, breathing ]. A condition in which the respiration is deeper and more rapid than normal.

**hy′perpo′lariza′tion.** An increase in polarization of membranes or nerves or muscle cells; the reverse change from that associated with excitatory action.

**hyperponesis** (hi′per-po-ne′sis) [ hyper- + G. *ponos,* toil ]. Exaggerated activity within the motor portion of the nervous system.

**hyperposia** (hi′per-po′zĭ-ah) [ hyper- + G. *posis,* drinking ]. Intense or forced drinking; drinking that is relatively temporary; see also polyposia.

**hy′perpotasse′mia.** Hyperkalemia.

**hyperpragia** (hi-per-pra′jĭ-ah) [ hyper- + G. *prassō,* to do, PRAG- ]. Excessive mental activity, as in the manic phase of manic-depressive insanity.

**hyperpraxia** (hi′per-prak′sĭ-ah) [ hyper- + G. *praxis,* action ]. Excessive activity.

**hyperprebetalipoproteinemia** (hi′per-pre-ba′tah-lip-o-pro′te-in-e′mĭ-ah, -pro′tēn-). Increased concentrations of pre-β-lipoproteins in the blood.

    **familial h.,** see types III and IV *hyperlipoproteinemia*.

**hyperprochoresis** (hi′per-pro-ko-re′sis) [ hyper- + G. *prochōreō,* to go forward ]. Hyperperistalsis.

**hy′perproline′mia.** A metabolic disorder characterized by enhanced plasma proline concentrations and urinary excretion of proline, hydroxyproline, and glycine; associated with mental retardation and renal anomalies and disease; autosomal recessive inheritance.

**hyperprosexia** (hi′per-pro-sek′sĭ-ah) [ hyper- + G. *prosexis,* attention, fr. *pros-echō,* fut. *-exō,* to hold to ]. Fixation of the mind on one idea.

**hyperproteinemia** (hi-per-pro′te-in-e′mĭ-ah, -pro′tēn-). An abnormally large concentration of protein in plasma.

**hyperproteosis** (hi′per-pro-te-o′sis). The condition due to an excessive amount of protein in the diet.

**hyperpselaphesia** (hi′perp-sel′ă-fe′zĭ-ah) [ hyper- + G. *psēlaphēsis,* touching ]. Hyperaphia.

**hyperpsychosis** (hi-per-si-ko′sis) [ hyper- + G. *psychōsis,* mental activity ]. Hypernoia.

**hyperpyretic** (hi-per-pi-ret′ik). Hyperpyrexial; relating to hyperpyrexia.

**hyperpyrexia** (hi′per-pi-rek′sĭ-ah) [ hyper- + G. *pyrexis,* feverishness ]. Extremely high fever.

    **h. figmenta′tica,** fabrication of fever.

    **fulminant h.,** malignant *hyperthermia.*

    **heat h.,** heat *stroke.*

**hy′perpyrex′ial.** Hyperpyretic.

**hyperreflexia** (hi′per-re-flek′sĭ-ah). A condition in which the deep tendon reflexes are exaggerated.

**hyperresonance** (hi′per-rez′o-nans). An extreme degree of resonance.

**hypersalemia** (hi-per-sal-e′mĭ-ah). An increase in the salt content of the circulating blood.

**hy′persa′line.** Marked by increased salinity.

**hy′persaliva′tion.** Increased salivation.

**hy′persecre′tion.** Excessive secretion.

**hy′persen′sitiveness.** Hypersensitivity. 1. Abnormal sensitiveness or sensitivity; a condition in which the response to a stimulus is excessive in degree. 2. Allergy; the state of induced sensitivity.

**hypersensitiv′ity.** Hypersensitiveness.

**hypersensitization** (hi′per-sen′sĭ-tĭ-za′shun). The immunological process by which hypersensitiveness (2) is induced.

**hy′perserotone′mia.** Unusually large amounts of serotonin in the circulating blood, probably a causal factor in the carcinoid syndrome.

**hypersialosis** (hi'per-si-ă-lo'sis) [ hyper- + G. *sialon*, saliva ]. Increased salivation.

**hyperskeocytosis** (hi'per-ske'o-si-to'sis) [ G. *skaios*, left, + *kytos*, cell, + suffix *-osis*, condition ]. Hyperneocytosis.

**hypersomatotropism** (hi'per-so'mă-to-tro'pizm). A state characterized by abnormally enhanced secretion of pituitary growth hormone (somatotropin).

**hy'perso'mia** [ hyper- + G. *sōma*, body ]. Gigantism.

**hy'persom'nia** [ hyper- + L. *somnus*, sleep ]. A condition, probably toxic, in which one sleeps for an excessively long time, but is normal in the intervals; it is distinguished from somnolence, in which one is always inclined to sleep.

**hy'person'ic** [ hyper- + L. *sonus*, sound ]. Pertaining to or characterized by supersonic speeds of Mach 5 or greater. While any speed above the speed of sound may be referred to as supersonic, speeds of Mach 5 or greater are specifically referred to as h.

**hypersphyxia** (hi-per-sfik'sī-ah) [ hyper- + G. *sphyxis*, pulse ]. A condition of high blood pressure and increased circulatory activity.

**hy'persple'nism.** A condition, or group of conditions, in which the hemolytic action of the spleen is greatly increased. Several blood disorders have been attributed to this condition, *e.g.*, chronic neutropenia and thrombocytopenic purpura.

**hypersteatosis** (hi'per-ste-ă-to'sis). Excessive sebaceous secretion.

**hyperstereoroentgenography** (hi'per-ster-e-o-rĕnt-gen-og'ră-fe). Roentgenography with the two positions from which the rays are projected rather widely separated.

**hypersthenia** (hi'per-sthe'nī-ah) [ hyper- + G. *sthenos*, strength ]. Excessive tension or strength.

**hy'persthen'ic.** Pertaining to or marked by hypersthenia.

**hypersthenuria** (hi'per-sthen-u'rī-ah) [ hyper- + G. *sthenos*, strength, + *ouron*, urine ]. Excretion of urine of unusually high specific gravity and concentration of solutes, resulting usually from loss or deprivation of water.

**hy'persusceptibil'ity.** Inordinate response to an infective, chemical, or other agent.

**hypersystole** (hi-per-sis'to-le). Abnormal force or duration of the cardiac systole.

**hy'persystol'ic.** 1. Relating to or marked by hypersystole. 2. One whose heart contracts with undue force.

**hypertarachia** (hi'per-tă-rak'ī-ah) [ hyper- + G. *tarachē*, disorder, confusion ]. Exaggerated irritability of the nervous system.

**hypertelorism** (hi'per-tel'or-izm) [ hyper- + G. *tele*, far off, + *horizō*, to separate, fr. *horos*, a boundary ]. Abnormal distance between two paired organs.

  **canthal h.,** telecanthus.

  **ocular h.,** Greig's syndrome; extreme width between the eyes due to an enlarged sphenoid bone; other congenital deformities and mental retardation may be associated.

**hy'perten'sinase.** Angiotensinase.

**hy'pertensin'ogen.** Angiotensinogen.

**hypertension** (hi'per-ten'shun) [ hyper- + L. *tensio*, tension ]. High arterial blood pressure.

  **adrenal h.,** h. due to a pheochromocytoma.

  **benign h.,** red h.; essential h. that runs a relatively long and symptomless course.

  **essential h.,** hyperpiesis; primary h.; idiopathic h.; h. without preexisting renal disease or known cause.

  **Goldblatt's h.,** Goldblatt *phenomenon*.

  **idiopathic h.,** essential h.

  **malignant h.,** severe h. that runs a rapid course, causing necrosis of arteriolar walls in kidney, retina, etc. Hemorrhages occur, and death most frequently is caused by uremia or of a cerebral vessel.

  **neuromuscular h.,** heightened tone of skeletal muscles with increased tendon reflexes.

  **pale h.,** h. with pallor of the skin, a severe form with pronounced constriction of peripheral vessels.

  **portal h.,** h. in the portal system as seen in cirrhosis of the liver and other conditions causing obstruction to the portal vein.

  **postpartum h.,** increased tension or blood pressure during the six weeks immediately following the completion of labor.

  **primary h.,** essential h.

  **pulmonary h.,** h. in the pulmonary circuit. It may be primary, or secondary to pulmonary or cardiac disease, *e.g.*, fibrosis of the lung or mitral stenosis.

  **red h.,** benign h.

  **renal h.,** h. secondary to renal disease.

  **renovascular h.,** h. produced by renal arterial obstruction.

  **transient h.,** development of hypertension during pregnancy, or within the first 24 hours postpartum, in a previously normotensive woman; no other evidence of preeclampsia or hypertensive vascular disease is present; the blood pressure returns to normotensive levels within 10 days following parturition.

**hy'perten'sive.** 1. Marked by an increased blood pressure. 2. A person suffering from high blood pressure.

**hy'perten'sor.** Pressor.

**hy'pertes'toidism.** Hypergonadism in the male; proliferation of Leydig cells with excessive production of testosterone.

**hyperthecosis** (hi'per-the-ko'sis) Diffuse hyperplasia of the theca cells of the Graafian follicles.

  **testoid h.,** hyperplasia of Leydig cells of the testis.

**hyperthelesia** (hi'per-thĕ-le'zī-ah) [ hyper- + G. *thelēsis*, will ]. Hyperbulia.

**hy'perthe'lia** [ hyper- + G. *thēlē*, nipple ]. The presence of supernumerary nipples, the number of breasts being two only.

**hypertherm** (hi-per-therm') [ hyper- + G. *thermē*, heat ]. A machine used to produce sustained high fever.

**hyperthermalgesia** (hi-per-ther'mal-je'zī-ah) [ hyper- + G. *thermē*, heat, + *algēsis*, pain ]. Extreme sensitivity to heat.

**hy'perther'mia** [ hyper- + G. *thermē*, heat ]. Therapeutically induced hyperpyrexia.

  **malignant h.,** fulminant hyperpyrexia; rapid onset of extremely high fever with muscle rigidity, precipitated in genetically susceptible persons by halothane or succinylcholine.

**hyperthermoesthesia** (hi-per-ther'mo-es-the'zī-ah) [ hyper- + G. *thermē*, heat, + *aisthēsis*, feeling ]. Extreme sensitiveness to heat.

**hyperthrombinemia** (hi'per-throm-bin-e'mī-ah). An abnormal increase of thrombin in the blood, frequently resulting in a tendency to intravascular coagulation.

**hy'perthy'mia** [ hyper- + G. *thymos*, soul, thought ]. Excessive emotivity.

**hy'perthy'mic.** Pertaining to (1) hyperthymia, and (2) hyperthymism.

**hy'perthy'mism.** Excessive activity of the thymus gland, postulated to be a causal factor in certain instances of unexpected and sudden death; *i.e.*, the controversial *status thymolymphaticus*.

**hyperthymization** (hi'per-thi-mī-za'shun). Hyperthymism.

**hyperthyrea** (hi-per-thi're-ah). Obsolete term for hyperthyroidism.

**hyperthyroidism** (hi'per-thi'royd-izm). An abnormality of the thyroid gland in which thyroid secretion is usually increased and is no longer under regulatory control of hypothalamic-pituitary centers.

  **latent h.,** a condition resembling Graves' disease in some respects, but actually not due to an excessive production of thyroid hormone; also variously known as parabasedoid disease, or a basedoid state. An obscure concept of uncertain validity.

  **ophthalmic h.,** hyperthyroidism with exophthalmos; serum concentrations of thyroid hormones may be elevated or normal, but in the latter case are not suppressed by exogenous triiodothyronine.

  **primary h.,** h. due to a disorder originating within the thyroid gland, in contrast to one of pituitary origin.

  **secondary h.,** h. due to stimulation of the thyroid gland by an excess of thyrotrophin secreted by the pituitary gland.

**hy'perthyro'sis.** Obsolete term for hyperthyroidism.

**hy'perthyrox'inemia.** An elevated thyroxine concentration in blood.

**hy'perto'nia** [ hyper- + G. *tonos,* tension ]. Hypertonicity (1); extreme tension of the muscles or arteries.

**h. polycythe'mica,** a form of polycythemia without a prominent degree of splenomegaly, but with increased blood pressure.

**sympathetic h.,** overfunction of the sympathetic system, often manifested as anxiety.

**hy'perton'ic.** 1. Having a greater degree of tension. 2. Having a greater osmotic pressure than a reference solution, which is ordinarily assumed to be blood plasma or interstitial fluid.

**h. salt solution,** see under solution.

**hypertonicity** (hi'per-to-nis'ĭ-tĭ). 1. Hypertonia. 2. An increased effective osmotic pressure of body fluids.

**hypertrichiasis** (hi'per-trĭ-ki'ă-sis). Hypertrichosis.

**hypertrichophrydia** (hi'per-trik'o-frĭ'dĭ-ah) [ hyper- + G. *thrix,* hair, + *ophrys,* eyebrow ]. Excessively thick eyebrows.

**hypertrichosis** (hi'per-trĭ-ko'sis) [ hyper- + G. *trichōsis,* a being hairy ]. Hypertrichiasis; growth of hair in excess of the normal.

**h. lanugino'sa,** malignant down; excessive growth of fine hair over entire body; a rare congenital condition; may also occur as an acquired condition in association with internal disorder.

**nevoid h.,** congenital growth of hair abnormal for site or in texture, color, or length; often associated with other nevoid abnormalities.

**h. partia'lis,** abnormally excessive hair growth in patches in unusual areas.

**h. universa'lis,** generalized excessive hair growth.

**hypertriglyceridemia** (hi'per-tri-glis'er-id-e'mĭ-ah). Elevated triglyceride concentration in blood.

**familial h.,** a heritable disease, of which two forms have been described: (1) exogenous, or fat-induced; occurs only after meals of normal or greater content of lipids, and believed to represent a congenital deficiency of lipoprotein lipase; (2) endogenous or carbohydrate-induced, especially evident after meals rich in carbohydrates; believed to result from abnormally great conversion of carbohydrate to triglycerides.

**hy'pertro'phia** Hypertrophy.

**hypertrophic** (hi'per-trof'ik). Relating to or characterized by hypertrophy.

**hypertrophy** (hi-per'tro-fĭ) [ hyper- + G. *trophē,* nourishment ]. Overgrowth; general increase in bulk of a part or organ, not due to tumor formation. Use of the term may be restricted to denote greater bulk through increase in size, but not in number, of the individual tissue elements. See also hyperplasia.

**adaptive h.,** thickening of the walls of a hollow organ, like the urinary bladder, when there is obstruction to outflow.

**compen'satory h.,** increase in size of an organ or part of an organ or tissue, when called upon to do the work of a disabled or destroyed synergist.

**compensatory h. of the heart,** thickening of the walls of the heart in cases of valvular disease.

**complemen'tary h.,** increase in size or expansion of part of an organ or tissue to fill the space left by the destruction of another portion of the same organ or tissue.

**concen'tric h.,** thickening of the walls of the heart or any cavity with apparent diminution of the capacity of the cavity.

**eccen'tric h.,** thickening of the wall of the heart or other cavity, with dilation.

**endem'ic h.,** h. of the os calcis ("big heel"); peculiar enlargement of the os calcis occurring on the Gold Coast, and in Formosa among the native population. It is preceded by fever and pain in the heel.

**false h.,** pseudohypertrophy.

**functional h.,** physiologic h.

**gingival h.,** non-neoplastic swelling of the gingiva.

**hemangiectatic h.,** Klippel-Trenaunay-Weber *syndrome.*

**numerical h.,** hyperplasia.

**physiologic h.,** functional h.; temporary increase in size of an organ or part to provide for a natural increase of function such as occurs in the walls of the uterus and in the mammae during pregnancy.

**pseudomuscular h.,** childhood muscular *dystrophy.*

**quantitative h.,** hyperplasia.

**simple h.,** increase in size of cells.

**simulated h.,** increased size of a part due to continued growth unrestrained by attritions, as is seen in the case of the teeth of certain animals when the opposing teeth have been destroyed.

**true h.,** an increase in size involving all the different tissues composing the part.

**vicarious h.,** h. of an organ following failure of another organ because of a functional relationship between them; enlargement of the pituitary gland, after destruction of the thyroid, is an example.

**hy'pertro'pia** [ hyper- + G. *tropē,* a turn ]. *Strabismus sursum vergens.*

**hy'perty'rosine'mia.** See tyrosinemia.

**hyperuresis** (hi'per-u-re'sis) [ hyper- + G. *oureō,* to urinate ]. Obsolete synonym for polyuria.

**hyperuricemia** (hi'per-u'rĭ-se'mĭ-ah). Enhanced blood concentrations of uric acid.

**hy'perurice'mic.** Relating to or characterized by hyperuricemia.

**hyperuricuria** (hi'per-u'rĭ-ku'rĭ-ah). Increased urinary excretion of uric acid.

**hy'pervaccina'tion.** Repeated inoculation of a person or animal already immunized; used as a means of preparing a highly potent antiserum.

**hypervalinemia** (hi'per-val-ĭ-ne'mĭ-ah). Abnormally high plasma concentrations of valine; a common finding in maple syrup urine *disease, q.v.*

**hyper'vascular** (hi'per-vas'ku-lar) [ hyper- + L. *vas,* a vessel ]. Abnormally vascular; containing an excessive number of blood vessels.

**hy'perven'tila'tion.** Overventilation; increased alveolar ventilation relative to metabolic carbon dioxide production, so that alveolar carbon dioxide pressure tends to fall below normal.

**hypervitaminosis** (hi'per-vi'tă-min-o'sis). A condition resulting from the ingestion of an excessive amount of a vitamin preparation, the symptoms varying according to the particular vitamin implicated. Serious effects may be caused by overdosage with vitamin A B or D and, and rarely, with water-soluble vitamins.

**hypervolemia** (hi'per-vo-le'mĭ-ah) [ hyper- + L. *volumen,* volume, + G. *haima,* blood ]. Plethora; abnormally increased volume of blood.

**hy'pervole'mic.** Pertaining to or characterized by hypervolemia.

**hypervolia** (hi'per-vo'lĭ-ah). Augmented water content or volume of a given compartment; *e.g.,* cellular h.

**hypesthesia** (hi-pes-the'zĭ-ah) [ G. *hypo,* under, + *aisthēsis,* feeling ]. Hypoesthesia; diminished sensibility.

**hypha,** pl. **hyphae** (hi'fah) [ G. *hyphē,* a web ]. One of the branching tubular filaments, usually septate, comprising the vegetative portion of the mycelium of fungi.

**spiral h.,** h. that end in a flat or helical coil, as in *Trichophyton.*

**hyphedonia** (hip-he-do'nĭ-ah) [ G. *hypo,* under, + *hēdonē,* pleasure ]. A habitually lessened or attenuated degree of pleasure caused by occurrences that should normally give great pleasure.

**hyphe'ma.** Hyphemia.

**hyphemia** (hi-fe'mĭ-ah) [ G. *hypo,* under, + *haima,* blood ]. Hyphema; hemorrhage into the anterior chamber of the eye.

**intertrop'ical** or **tropical h.,** ancylostomiasis.

**hyphidrosis** (hip-hi-dro'sis). Hypohidrosis.

**hyphomyco'sis.** Infection with Hyphomycetes, chiefly *Hyphomyces destruens* in horses; see also phycomycosis.

**hypinosis** (hip'ĭ-mo'sis) [ G. *hypo,* under, + *is (in-),* fiber, + suffix *-osis,* condition ]. Diminished coagulability of the blood, resulting from a reduction in the content of fibrinogen, to levels less than the physiologic mean of approximately 0.27 per cent.

**hyp'inot'ic.** Pertaining to or characterized by hypinosis.

**hypn-.** See hypno-.

**hypnagogic** (hip-nă-goj'ik) [ hypno- + G. *agōgos,* leading ]. 1. Denoting a transitional state, related to the hypnoidal, preceding the oncome of sleep; applied also to various hallucinations that may manifest themselves at that time. 2. Inducing sleep; hypnotic.

**hypnagogue** (hip'nă-gog) [ hypno- + G. *agōgos*, leading ]. 1. Inducing sleep; hypnotic. 2. An agent so acting.

**hypnalgia** (hip-nal'jĭ-ah) [ hypno- + G. *algos*, pain ]. Dream pain; pain occurring during sleep.

**hyp'nanalyt'ic.** Hypnoanalytic.

**hypnapagogic** (hip-nap-ă-goj'ik) [ hypno- + G. *apo*, from, + *agōgos*, leading ]. 1. Denoting a state similar to the hypnagogic, through which the mind passes in coming out of sleep; denoting also delusions experienced at such time. 2. Causing wakefulness; preventing sleep.

**hypnenergia** (hip'nen-er'jĭ-ah) [ hypno- + G. *energeia*, action ]. Somnambulism.

**hypnesthesia** (hip'nes-the'zĭ-ah) [ hypno- + G. *aisthēsis*, sensation ]. Drowsiness.

**hypnic** [ G. *hypnikos*, relating to sleep ]. 1. Relating to sleep. 2. Causing sleep; somnifacient; somniferous.

**hypno-, hypn-** [ G. *hypnos*, sleep ]. Combining forms relating to sleep or hypnosis.

**hyp'noanal'ysis.** Psychoanalysis or other psychotherapy which employs hypnosis as an adjunctive technique.

**hyp'noanalyt'ic.** Pertaining to hypnoanalysis.

**hyp'nobat.** Sleepwalker; somnambulist.

**hypnobatia** (hip-no-ba'she-ah) [ hypno- + G. *batio*, to walk, go, BAS- ]. Somnambulism (1).

**hyp'nocathar'sis** [ hypno- + catharsis, *q.v.* ]. Ventilation of emotions under hypnosis.

**hypnocinematograph** (hip-no-sin-e-mat'o-graf) [ hypno- + G. *kinēma*, movement, + *graphē*, a record ]. Somnocinematograph.

**hyp'nocyst** [ hypno- + G. *kystis*, bladder (cyst) ]. A quiescent or "sleeping" cyst; an encysted protozoon, the reproductive activity of which is in abeyance.

**hypnodon'tics** [ hypno- + G. *odous*, tooth ]. Hypnosis as applied to the practice of dentistry.

**hypnogenesis** (hip-no-jen'ĕ-sis) [ hypno- + G. *genesis*, production ]. The induction of sleep or of the hypnotic state.

**hypnogenic** (hip-no-jen'ik). Hypnogenous; relating to hypnogenesis; causing sleep or the hypnotic state.

**hypnogenous** (hip-noj'ĕ-nus). Hypnogenic.

**hypnoidal** (hip-noy'dal) [ hypno- + G. *eidos*, resemblance ]. Resembling hypnosis; denoting the subwaking state, a mental condition intermediate between sleeping and waking.

**hyp'nolepsy** [ hypno- + G. *lēpsis*, a seizing ]. Narcolepsy.

**hypnol'ogist.** 1. A student of hypnology. 2. Hypnotist.

**hypnology** (hip-nol'o-jĭ) [ hypno- + G. *logos*, study ]. The branch of scientific inquiry regarding sleep or hypnosis and its phenomena.

**hypnophobia** (hip'no-fo'bĭ-ah) [ hypno- + G. *phobos*, fear ]. Morbid fear of falling asleep.

**hyp'nopom'pic** [ hypno- + G. *pompē*, procession ]. Denoting the occurrence of visions or dreams during the drowsy state preceding or following sleep.

**hypnosis** (hip-no'sis) [ G. *hypnos*, sleep, + suffix -*osis*, condition ]. 1. Hypnotic state; an artificially induced trance-like state resembling sonambulism in which the subject is highly susceptible to suggestion, oblivious to all else, and responds readily to the commands of the hypnotist. Arguments concerning the validity of this phenomenon are still unresolved.

**lethargic h.,** trance coma; the deep sleep following major h.

**major h.,** a state of extreme suggestibility in h. in which the subject is insensible to all outside impressions except the commands or suggestions of the hypnotist.

**minor h.,** an induced state resembling normal sleep in which, however, the subject is obedient to suggestion, though not to the extent of catalepsy or somnambulism.

**hyp'nother'apy.** 1. The treatment of disease by inducing prolonged sleep. 2. Psychotherapeutic treatment by means of hypnotism.

**hypnotic** (hip-not'ik) [ G. *hypnōtikos*, causing one to sleep ]. 1. Causing sleep. 2. A remedy having this property.

3. Relating to hypnotism. 4. One who is under the influence of hypnotism, or who is readily hypnotized.

**hypnotism** (hip'no-tizm) [ G. *hypnos*, sleep ]. 1. The process or act of inducing hypnosis. 2. The practice or study of hypnosis.

**hyp'notist.** One who practices hypnotism.

**hyp'notize.** To induct one into hypnosis.

**hyp'notoid.** Resembling hypnosis.

**hyp'notox'in.** A substance, according to one theory of sleep, that is supposed to accumulate in the brain during waking hours and bring about sleep

**hypo-** [ G. *hypo*, under ]. A prefix, equivalent to sub-, denoting (1) a location beneath something else; (2) a diminution or deficiency; (3) the lowest, or least rich in oxygen, of a series of chemical compounds (*e.g.*, hypochlorite).

**hypoacidity** (hi'po-ă-sid'ĭ-tĭ). Lower acidity.

**hy'poacu'sis.** Hypacusis.

**hypoadenia** (hi'po-ă-de'nĭ-ah) [ hypo- + G. *adēn*, gland ]. Any deficiency in the function of a glandular organ or tissue.

**hypoadrenalemia** (hi'po-ad-ren'al-e'mĭ-ah) [ hypo- + adrenal + G. *haima*, blood ]. Abnormally small quantities of adrenal glandular secretions in the circulating blood, *i.e.*, various hormones elaborated by the cortical and medullary portions of the glands. An obsolete usage.

**hy'poadre'nalism.** Reduced adrenocortical function.

**hypoadre'nia.** An obsolete term referring to a deficiency of the adrenal glands, especially one developing after a relatively protracted period of exhaustive secretory activity such that frequently associated with fulminant infectious diseases.

**hy'poalbumine'mia.** An abnormally low concentration of albumin in blood.

**hypoalimentation** (hi'po-al-ĭ-men-ta'shun). Subalimentation.

**hy'poantu'itarism.** Obsolete term for idiopathic infantilism.

**hypoazoturia** (hi-po-az-o-tu'rĭ-ah) [ hypo- + Fr. *azote*, nitrogen, + G. *ouron*, urine ]. Excretion of abnormally small quantities of nonprotein nitrogenous material (especially urea) in the urine.

**hypobaric** (hi'po-băr'ik) [ hypo- + G. *baros*, weight ]. Characterized by pressure or weight of one substance which is less than the pressure or weight of another substance; *e.g.*, h. gases are those below 1 atmosphere; h. solutions are those lighter than the diluent to which they are added.

**hypobaropathy** (hi'po-băr-op'ă-thĭ) [ hypo- + G. *baros*, weight, + *pathos*, suffering ]. Aviators' sickness; altitude sickness; altitude anoxia; Acosta's disease; mountain sickness; the syndrome caused by greatly diminished air pressure and reduced oxygen intake.

**hy'poblast** [ hypo- + G. *blastos*, germ ]. Entoderm.

**hypoblas'tic.** Relating to or derived from the hypoblast.

**hypoblepharon** (hi'po-blef'ă-ron) [ hypo- + G. *blepharon*, eyelid ]. Obsolescent term meaning (1) a swelling beneath the eyelid; (2) an artificial eye.

**hypobranchial** (hi'po-brang'kĭ-al). Located beneath the gills (branchiae).

**hypobro'mite.** A salt of hypobromous acid.

**hypobro'mous acid.** An acid, HOBr, the aqueous solution of which possesses oxidizing and bleaching properties.

**hypobu'lia** [ hypo- + G. *boulē*, will ]. Deficient will power.

**hypocalcemia** (hi-po-kal-se'mĭ-ah). Abnormally low levels of calcium in the circulating blood; commonly denotes subnormal concentrations of calcium ions.

**hypocalcification** (hi-po-kal'sĭ-fĭ-ka'shun). Deficient calcification of bone or teeth.

**enamel h.,** a defect of enamel maturation, caused by local, systemic, or hereditary factors, and characterized by low mineral and high water content; the enamel may be chalky or cheesy in consistency, becomes stained from yellow to light brown, and breaks down rapidly; the teeth may become worn level with the gum line, and the exposed dentin stains heavily; both primary and secondary teeth are affected; a type of amelogenesis imperfecta. See also fluorosis.

**hypocapnia** (hi-po-kap'ni-ah) [ hypo- + G. *kapnos*, smoke ]. Hypocarbia; an abnormally low tension of carbon dioxide in the circulating blood; a relatively slight to moderate degree of acapnia.

**hypocar'bia.** Hypocapnia.

**hypocelom** (hi-po-se'lom) [ hypo- + G. *koilos*, hollow ]. The ventral portion of the celom, or body cavity, of the embryo.

**hypochloremia** (hi'po-klo-re'mi-ah). An abnormally low level of chloride ions in the circulating blood.

**hypochlore'mic.** Pertaining to or characterized by hypochloremia.

**hypochlorhydria** (hi'po-klor-hid'ri-ah). Hypohydrochloria; the presence of an abnormally small amount of hydrochloric acid in the stomach (less than 0.14 per cent).

**hypochlo'rite.** A salt of hypochlorous acid.

**hypochlo'rous acid.** An acid, HOCl, having oxidizing and bleaching properties.

**hypochloruria** (hi'po-klor-u'ri-ah). Excretion of abnormally small quantities of chloride ions in the urine.

**hypocholestere'mia.** Hypocholesterolemia.

**hypocholesterine'mia.** Hypocholesterolemia.

**hypocholesterolemia** (hi'po-ko-les'ter-ol-e'mi-ah). Hypocholesteremia; hypocholesterinemia; the presence of abnormally small smounts of cholesterol in the circulating blood.

**hypocholia** (hi'po-ko'li-ah). Oligocholia.

**hypochondria** (hi-po-kon'dri-ah). Hypochondriasis.

**hypochondriac** (hi'po-kon'dri-ak). 1. Hypochondriacal. 2. A victim of hypochondriasis. 3. Beneath the ribs, relating to the hypochondrium.

**hypochondriacal** (hi-po-kon-dri'ă-kal). Relating to or suffering from hypochondriasis.

**hypochondriasis** (hi-po-kon-dri'ă-sis) [ hypochondrium (*q.v.*), regarded as the site of hypochondria, + suffix -*iasis*, condition ]. Hypochondria; a morbid concern about one's own health and exaggerated attention to any unusual bodily or mental sensations; a false belief that one is suffering from some disease.

**hypochondrium,** pl. **hypochon'dria** (hi-po-kon'dri-um) [ L. fr. G. *hypochondrion*, abdomen, belly, from *hypo*, under, + *chondros*, cartilage (of ribs) ]. *Regio* hypochondriaca.

**hypochordal** (hi-po-kor'dal) [ hypo- + G. *chordē*, cord ]. On the ventral side of the spinal cord.

**hypochoresis** (hi'po-ko-re'sis) [ G. *hypochōrēsai*, to evacuate downward ]. Defecation.

**hypochromasia** (hi'po-kro-ma'zi-ah). Hypochromia.

**hypochromatic** (hi-po-kro-mat'ik) [ hypo- + G. *chrōma*, color ]. Containing a small amount of pigment, or less than the normal amount for the individual tissue.

**hypochromatism** (hi-po-kro'mă-tizm). 1. The condition of being hypochromatic. 2. Hypochromia.

**hypochromatosis** (hi-po-kro-mă-to'sis). Chromatolysis.

**hypochromemia** (hi-po-kro-me'mi-ah) [ hypo- + G. *chrōma*, color, + *haima*, blood ]. Anemia characterized by a color index that is less than unity.

**hypochromia** (hi-po-kro'mi-ah) [ hypo- + G. *chrōma*, color ]. Hypochromasia; an anemic condition in which the percentage of hemoglobin in the red blood cells is less than the normal range.

**hypochromic** (hi-po-kro'mik). 1. Hypochromatic. 2. Denoting decrease in light absorption.

**hypochrosis** (hi-po-kro'sis) [ hypo- + G. *chrōsis*, a tinting ]. Hypochromia.

**hypochylia** (hi-po-ki'li-ah) [ hypo- + G. *chylos*, juice ]. Oligochylia.

**hypocine'sia.** Hypokinesia.

**hy'pocomplemente'mia.** Acomplementemia; a hereditary or acquired condition of the blood in which one or another component of complement is lacking or reduced in amount; the first to be recognized in man was a hereditary incomplete deficiency of the second component of complement (C2), but deficiencies in other components have since been reported.

**hy'pocone** [ hypo- + G. *kōnos*, pine cone ]. The distolingual cusp of an upper molar tooth.

**hy'pocon'id.** The distobuccal cusp of a lower molar tooth.

**hy'pocon'ule** [ hypo- + Mod. L. dim. of L. *conus*, cone ]. The distal, fifth, cusp of an upper molar tooth.

**hy'pocon'ulid** [ hypo- + Mod. L. dim. of *conus*, cone ]. The distal, fifth, cusp of a lower molar tooth.

**hypocorticoidism** (hi'po-kor'ti-koyd-izm). Adrenocortical insufficiency.

**hypocrinism** (hi-po-kri'nizm) [ hypo- + G. *krinō*, to separate ]. See hypoendocrinism.

**hypocupremia** (hi'po-ku-pre'mi-ah) [ hypo- + L. *cuprum*, copper, + G. *haima*, blood ]. Reduced copper content of the blood; found in Wilson's disease because ceruloplasmin is depressed, even though serum albumin-attached copper is increased.

**hypocystotomy** (hi'po-sis-tot'o-mi). Perineal cystotomy.

**hypocythemia** (hi'po-si-the'mi-ah) [ hypo- + G. *kytos*, cell, + *haima*, blood ]. Hypocytosis of the circulating blood, such as that observed in aplastic anemia.

    **progressive h.,** refractory anemia.

**hypocytosis** (hi'po-si-to'sis) [ hypo- + G. *kytos*, cell, + suffix -*osis*, condition ]. Cytopenia; pancytopenia; oligocythemia; varying degrees of abnormally low numbers of red and white cells and other formed elements of the blood. In some instances, the term is also used to indicate a paucity of component cells of any tissue.

**hy'podac'tyly, hy'podactyl'ia, hypodac'tylism** [ hypo- + G. *daktylos*, finger, + -*ia*, condition ]. Less than the full normal complement of digits.

**hy'poderm** [ hypo- + G. *derma*, skin ]. *Tela* subcutanea.

**Hypoderma** (hi'po-der'mah) [ hypo- + G. *derma*, skin ]. A genus of botflies whose larvae are the cause of the tropical form of myiasis linearis (larva migrans) of man; occasionally they invade the interior of the eye.

    **H. bo'vis,** one of the botflies of cattle; the ova are deposited on hairs of the legs, and the larvae penetrate the skin and migrate through the tissues to the skin of the back, where they appear during late winter as the common warbles; these ulcerate to the surface and mature larvae escape in early summer, fall to the ground, pupate, and give rise to a new generation of flies.

    **H. linea'tum,** a species of botfly of cattle.

**hy'podermat'ic.** Hypodermic.

**hypodermatoclysis** (hi-po-der-mă-tok'li-sis). Hypodermoclysis.

**hypodermatomy** (hi'po-der-mat'o-mi) [ hypo- + G. *derma*, skin, + *tomē*, incision ]. Subcutaneous division of a tendon or other structure.

**hypoder'mic.** 1. Subcutaneous; beneath the skin. 2. Hypodermic *injection.* 3. Hypodermic *syringe.*

**hy'poder'mis.** *Tela* subcutanea.

**hypodermoclysis** (hi'po-der-mok'li-sis) [ hypo- + G. *derma*, skin, + *klysis*, a washing out ]. The subcutaneous injection of a saline or other solution.

**hy'poder'molithi'asis** [ hypo- + G. *derma*, skin, + lithiasis ]. Subcutaneous deposits of calcium; see also *calcinosis* cutis.

**hypodip'sia** [ hypo- + G. *dipsa*, thirst ]. Insensible, twilight, or subliminal thirst; a physiologic condition, perhaps of hypertonicity of body fluids, insufficient to initiate drinking but at times sufficient to sustain drinking when started; loosely, oligodipsia.

**hypodontia** (hi'po-don'shi-ah) [ hypo- + G. *odous*, tooth ]. Partial anodontia; oligodontia (2); a condition of congenitally absent teeth; usually the secondary teeth are missing.

**hypodynamia** (hi'po-di-na'mi-ah, -di-nam'i-ah) [ hypo- + G. *dynamis*, force ]. Diminished power.

    **h. cordis,** diminished force of cardiac contraction.

**hy'podynam'ic.** Possessing or exhibiting subnormal power or force.

**hypoeccrisis** (hi'po-ek'ri-sis) [ hypo- + eccrisis, *q.v.* ]. Reduced excretion of waste matter.

**hypoeccritic** (hi'po-ĕ-krit'ik). Characterized by hypoeccrisis.

**hypoemia** (hi'po-e'mi-ah) [ hypo- + G. *haima*, blood ]. Ischemia; a subnormal amount of blood in a tissue or part.

**hypoendocrinism** (hi'po-en-dok'rĭ-nizm) [ hypo- + G. *endon*, within, + *krinō*, to separate ]. Hypocrinism; hypocrisia; obsolete terms meaning insufficiency of internal secretion from one or more glands.

**hypoendocrisia** (hi'po-en-do-kriz'ĭ-ah). See hypoendocrinism.

**hypoeosinophilia** (hi'po-e'o-sin'o-fil'ĭ-ah). Eosinopenia.

**hypoequilibrium** (hi-po-e'kwĭ-lib-rĭ-um) [ hypo- + equilibrium ]. Absence of a tendency to vertigo after long continued rotary movements.

**hypoergia, hypoergy** (hi-po-er'jĭ-ah, hi-po-er'jĭ) [ hypo- + G. (*en*)*ergeia*, from *ergon*, work ]. Hyposensitiveness.

**hypoesophoria** (hi-po-es-o-fo'rĭ-ah) [ hypo- + G. *esō*, within, + *phoros*, bearing ]. Combined downward and inward deviation of the eyeball.

**hypoesthesia** (hi-po-es-the'zĭ-ah). Hypesthesia.

**hypoexophoria** (hi-po-ek'so-fo'rĭ-ah) [ hypo- + G. *exō*, without, + *phoros*, bearing ]. Combined outward and downward deviation of the eyeball.

**hypoferre'mia.** A deficiency of iron in the circulating blood.

**hypofibrinogenemia** (hi'po-fi-brin'o-jĕ-ne'mĭ-ah). Abnormally low concentration of blood clotting factor I, *i.e.*, fibrinogen, in the circulating blood plasma.

**hypofunction** (hi'po-funk'shun). Reduced, low, or inadequate function.

**hypogalactia** (hi'po-gă-lak'shĭ-ah) [ hypo- + G. *gala*, milk ]. State of insufficient milk production.

**hypogalac'tous.** Producing insufficient milk.

**hypogammaglobinemia** (hi'po-gam'ah-glo'bin-e'mĭ-ah). Hypogammaglobulinemia.

**hy'pogam'maglob'uline'mia.** See agammaglobulinemia; also secondary h.

  **primary h.,** primary *agammaglobulinemia.*

  **secondary h.,** secondary agammaglobulinemia; secondary antibody deficiency; an unusually small amount of γ-globulin in the plasma protein, in association with (1) idiopathic hypoproteinemia—levels of 200 to 400 mg. per 100 ml., or (2) a nephrotic syndrome—levels of 200 to 300 mg. per 100 ml. In both categories, there are usually no significant, probably related pathologic changes in the lymphoid tissues, and the h. is thought to result from increased catabolism of protein; in addition, increased excretion of globulin (in the urine) is observed in various instances of the nephrotic syndrome.

**hypogas'tric.** Relating to the hypogastrium.

**hypogastrium** (hi'po-gas'trĭ-um) [ G. *hypogastrion*, lower belly, fr. *hypo*, under, + *gastēr*, belly ] [ NA ]. *Regio pubica.*

**hypogastrocele** (hi'po-gas'tro-sēl) [ hypogastrium + G. *kēlē*, hernia ]. Hernia of the lower part of the abdomen.

**hypogastropagus** (hi'po-gas-trop'ă-gus) [ hypogastrium + G. *pagos*, fr. *pēgnynai*, to fasten ]. Twins joined at the hypogastrium.

**hypogastroschisis** (hi'po-gas-tros'kĭ-sis) [ hypogastrium + G. *schisis*, cleaving ]. Congenital fissure in the hypogastric region.

**hypogenesis** (hi'po-jen'ĕ-sis) [ hypo- + G. *genesis*, origin ]. General underdevelopment of parts or organs of the body.

  **polar h.,** less than normal degree of development at the cephalic or caudal extremity of the embryo.

**hypogenet'ic.** Relating to deficient development.

**hypogenitalism** (hi-po-jen'ĭ-tal-izm). Partial or complete failure of maturation of the genitalia; commonly, a consequence of hypogonadism.

**hypogeusia** (hi-po-gu'sĭ-ah) [ hypo- + G. *geusis*, taste ]. A blunting of the sense of taste.

**hy'poglan'dular.** Marked by inadequate function of glands. An obsolete usage.

**hypoglobu'lia** [ hypo- + G. *globulus*, globule ]. Abnormally low numbers of red blood cells in the circulating blood; also used infrequently with reference to abnormally decreased proportions of erythroid elements in the bone marrow.

**hypoglos'sal** [ L. *hypoglossus* fr. hypo- + *glossus*, tongue ]. Below the tongue.

**hypoglos'sis.** Hypoglottis.

**hypoglos'sus** [ L. ] [ NA ]. Hypoglossal.

**hypoglot'tis** [ G. *hypoglōssis*, or -*glōttis*, under surface of tongue, fr. *hypo*, under, + *glōssa*, tongue ]. The undersurface of the tongue.

**hypoglycemia** (hi-po-gli-se'mĭ-ah). An abnormally small concentration of glucose in the circulating blood, *i.e.*, less than the minimum of the normal range.

  **leucine h.,** reduction in blood glucose concentration produced by administration of leucine; believed to reflect the ability of this amino acid to stimulate insulin secretion.

**hypoglyce'mic.** Pertaining to or characterized by hypoglycemia.

**hypoglycemosis** (hi'po-gli'se-mo'sis). Hypoglycemia, but especially with reference to the syndrome characterized by a low level of glucose in the blood, hunger, nervousness, alternating pallor and flushing of the face, sweating, and dizziness. An obsolete usage.

**hypoglycogenolysis** (hi'po-gli'ko-jĕ-nol'ĭ-sis). Deficient glycogenolysis.

**hypoglycorrhachia** (hi'po-gli-ko-rak'ĭ-ah) [ hypo- + G. *glykys*, sweet, + *rhachis*, spine ]. Depressed concentration of sugar in the cerebrospinal fluid; noted particularly in bacterial meningitis.

**hypognathous** (hi'po-nath'su, hi-pog'nă-thus) [ hypo- + G. *gnathos*, jaw ]. Having a congenitally defectively developed lower jaw.

**hypognathus** (hi'po-nath'us, hi-pog'nă-thus) [ hypo- + G. *gnathos*, jaw ]. Unequal conjoined twins in which the rudimentary parasite is attached to the mandible of the autosite.

**hypogonad'ia.** Obsolete synonym for hypogonadism.

**hypogonadism** (hi'po-go'nad-izm). Inadequate gonadal function, as manifested by deficiencies in gametogenesis and/or the secretion of gonadal hormones.

  **h. with anosmia,** Kallmann's syndrome; failure of sexual development secondary to inadequate secretion of pituitary gonadotropins, associated with anosmia due to agenesis of the olfactory lobes of the brain; probably X-linked inheritance.

  **familial hypogonadotropic h.,** a disorder characterized by failure of sexual development, owing to inadequate secretion of pituitary gonadotropins; probably autosomal recessive inheritance.

  **hypogonadotropic h.,** hypogonadotropic eunuchoidism; secondary h.; defective gonadal development or function (or both) resulting from inadequate secretion of pituitary gonadotropins.

  **primary h.,** defective gonadal development or function, or both, due to some abnormality within the gonad itself.

  **secondary h.,** hypogonadotropic h.

**hypogonadotropic (-trophic)** (hi'po-gon'ă-do-trop'ik, -trof'ik). Indicating inadequate secretion of gonadotrophins and the consequence thereof.

**hypogranulocytosis** (hi-po-gran-u-lo-si-to'sis). Granulocytopenia.

**hypohepatia** (hi-po-he-pat'ĭ-ah) [ hypo- + G. *hēpar*, liver ]. Underfunctioning of the liver.

**hypohidrosis** (hi'po-hi-dro'sis). Hypoidrosis; hyphidrosis; diminished perspiration.

**hy'pohidrot'ic.** Characterized by diminished sweating.

**hypohydremia** (hi'po-hi-dre'mĭ-ah) [ hypo- + G. *hydōr*, water, + *haima*, blood ]. Any deficiency in the amount of fluid in the blood.

**hypohy'drochlo'ria.** Hypochlorhydria.

**hypohyloma** (hi'po-hi-lo'mah) [ hypo- + G. *hylē*, substance, + suffix -*oma*, tumor ]. A neoplasm resulting from abnormal proliferation of tissue derived from the embryonic pulp of hypoblastic origin.

**hypohypnot'ic** [ hypo- + G. *hypnos*, sleep ]. Denoting incomplete or light slumber.

**hypoidrosis** (hi'po-id-ro'sis). Hypohidrosis.

**hypoinsulinism** (hi-po-in'su-lin-izm). Obsolete term for diabetes mellitus.

**hypoiodite** (hi'po-i'o-dīt). Salt of hypoiodous acid.

**hypoiodous acid.** HOI; exists only in solution and decomposes rapidly even then; can be used as an oxidizing agent.

**hypoisotonic** (hi'po-i'so-ton'ik). Hypotonic.

**hy'pokale'mia** [ hypo- + Mod. L. *kalium*, potassium, + G. *haima*, blood ]. The presence of an abnormally small concentration of potassium ions in the circulating blood; occurs in familial periodic paralysis and in potassium depletion due to excessive loss from the gastrointestinal tract or kidneys. Increased urinary loss may be due to renal disease, diabetic ketosis, aldosteronism, Cushing's syndrome, and the use of diuretics. The changes of h. may include vacuolation of renal tubular epithelial cytoplasm with impairment of urinary concentrating power and acidification, flattening of the T wave of the electrocardiogram, and muscle weakness.

**hypokinemia** (hi'po-kī-ne'mī-ah) [ hypo- + G. *kineo*, to move, + *haima*, blood ]. Reduced volume flow through the circulation; reduced circulation rate; subnormal cardiac output.

**hypokinesis, hypokinesia** (hi'po-kī-ne'sis, -kī-ne'zī-ah) [ hypo- + G. *kinēsis*, movement ]. Hypomotility; diminished or slow movement.

**hypokinet'ic.** Relating to or characterized by hypokinesis.

**hypolepidoma** (hi'po-lep'ī-do'mah) [ hypo- + G. *lepis*, rind, + suffix *-oma*, tumor ]. A neoplasm resulting from abnormal proliferation of one of the tissues derived from the hypoblast.

**hypoleukemia** (hi'po-lu-ke'mī-ah). A term infrequently used for a condition interpreted as intermediate between (1) classic leukemia (with numerous abnormal cells in the tissues and in the circulating blood), and (2) subleukemic or aleukemic leukemia (with numerous abnormal cells in the tissues, but not in the circulating blood).

**hypoleukocytosis** (hi'po-lu'ko-si-to'sis). Leukocytopenia; less than the minimal number of white blood cells ordinarily regarded as within the normal range for circulating blood, *e.g.*, less than 6000 per cu. mm.

**hypoleydigism** (hi-po-li'dig-ism). Subnormal secretion of androgens by the cells of Leydig; hypogonadism in the male.

**hypolipo'sis.** The presence of an abnormally small amount of fat in the tissues.

**hypolo'gia** [ hypo- + G. *logos*, word ]. Lack of ability for speech.

**hypolymphemia** (hi'po-lim-fe'mī-ah). Abnormally small numbers of lymphocytes in the circulating blood.

**hy'pomagnese'mia.** Subnormal plasma concentration of magnesium; may cause convulsions and concurrent hypocalcemia.

**hypoma'nia.** A mild degree of mania.

**hypomas'tia** [ hypo- + G. *mastos*, breast ]. Hypomazia; atrophy or congenital smallness of the breasts.

**hypoma'zia.** Hypomastia.

**hypomelancholia** (hi'po-mel-an-ko'lī-ah). A mild degree of mental depression.

**hypomelanosis** (hi'po-mel-ă-no'sis) [ hypo- + melanosis, *q. v.* ]. Leukoderma.

**hypomenorrhea** (hi'po-men-o-re'ah) [ hypo- + G. *mēn*, month, + *rhoia*, flow ]. A diminution of the flow or a shortening of the duration of menstruation.

**hypomere** (hi'po-mēr) [ hypo- + G. *meros*, part ]. 1. The portion of the myotome that extends ventrolaterally to form body-wall muscle, innervated by the primary ventral ramus of a spinal nerve. 2. Less commonly, the somatic and splanchnic layers of the lateral mesoderm which give rise to the lining of the celom.

**hy'pometab'olism.** Reduced metabolism; see also hypometabolic *state.*

**euthyroid h.,** an unusual condition resembling myxedema but with an apparently normal thyroid gland.

**hy'pome'tria** [ hypo- + G. *metron*, measure ]. A manifestation of ataxia characterized by underreaching an object or goal.

**hypomnesia** (hi-pom-ne'zī-ah) [ hypo- + G. *mnēmē*, memory ]. Impaired memory.

**hy'pomorph** [ hypo- + G. *morphē*, form ]. A person whose standing height is short in proportion to the sitting height, owing to shortness of limb. See also hypermorph and mesomorph.

**hypomotil'ity.** Hypokinesis.

**hypomyelinogenesis** (hi-po-mi'ĕ-lin-o-jen'ĕ-sis). Defective formation of myelin in the spinal cord and brain; the basis for a number of demyelinating diseases.

**hypomyotonia** (hi-po-mi-o-to'nī-ah) [ hypo- + *mys* (*myo-*) muscle, + *tonos*, tension ]. A condition of diminished muscular tonus.

**hypomyxia** (hi-po-mik'sī-ah) [ hypo- + G. *myxa*, mucus ]. A condition in which the secretion of mucus is diminished.

**hyponanosoma** (hi'po-na'no-so'mah) [ hypo- + G. *nanos*, dwarf, + *sōma*, body ]. Obsolete term meaning extreme dwarfism.

**hyponatremia** (hi'po-nă-tre'mī-ah) [ hypo- + *natrium* (*q.v.*), + G. *haima*, blood ]. Abnormally low concentrations of sodium ions in the circulating blood.

**hyponea** (hi-po-ne'ah). Hyponoia.

**hyponeocytosis** (hi'po-ne'o-si-to'sis) [ hypo- + G. *neos*, new, + *kytos*, cell, + suffix *-osis*, condition ]. Hyposkeocytosis; leukopenia associated with the presence of immature and young leukocytes (especially in the granulocytic series), *i.e.*, a "shift to the left" in the hemogram.

**hyponoia** (hi'po-noy'ah) [ hypo- + G. *noeō*, to think ]. Hypopsychosis; hyponea; deficient or sluggish mental activity or imagination.

**hyponychial** (hy-po-nik'ī-al). Beneath the (finger or toe) nail; subungual.

**hyponychium** (hy-po-nik'ī-um) [ hypo- + G. *onyx*, nail ] [ NA ]. The thickened cornified layer of the epidermis beneath the free border of the nail.

**hyponychon** (hi-pon'ī-kon) [ hypo- + G. *onyx*, nail ]. A subungual ecchymosis.

**hypooncotic** (hi'po-on-kot'ik). Indicating an oncotic pressure less than normal, *e.g.*, of blood plasma.

**hypoorchidism** (hi'po-or'kī-dizm) [ hypo- + G. *orchis*, testis ]. Obsolete term meaning reduced testicular function.

**hypoorthocytosis** (hi'po-or'tho-si-to'sis) [ hypo- + G. *orthos*, correct, + *kytos*, cell, + suffix *-osis*, condition ]. Leukopenia in which the relative numbers of the various types of white blood cells are within the normal range, and no immature cells are found in the circulating blood.

**hypoovaria** (hi'po-o-va'rī-ah). Rarely used synonym for hypoovarianism.

**hypoovarianism** (hi'po-o-va'rī-an-izm). Inadequate ovarian function; commonly refers to reduced secretion of ovarian hormones.

**hypopancreatism** (hi'po-pan'kre-ă-tizm). A condition of diminished activity of the pancreas.

**hypopancreorrhea** (hi'po-pan'kre-o-re'ah) [ hypo- + pancreas, + G. *rhoia*, flow ]. Reduced delivery of pancreatic secretions.

**hypoparathyroidism** (hi'po-păr-ah-thi'roy-dizm). A condition due to diminution or absence of the secretion of the parathyroid hormones. See also pseudohypoparathyroidism and pseudo-pseudohypoparathyroidism.

**familial h.,** idiopathic h. in members of the same family, with low serum calcium and tetany, and sometimes with increased bone density.

**hypopep'sia** [ hypo- + G. *pepsis*, digestion ]. Oligopepsia; impaired digestion, especially that due to a deficiency of pepsin.

**hy'poperistal'sis.** Reduced or inadequate peristalsis.

**hypophalangism** (hi'po-fă-lan'jizm). Congenital absence of one or more of the phalanges of a finger or toe.

**α-hypoph'amine.** Oxytocin.

**β-hypophamine.** Vasopressin.

**hypopharyngoscope** (hi'po-fă-ring'o-skōp). Instrument used for examination of the hypopharynx.

**hypopharynx** (hi'po-făr'inks). *Pars laryngea pharyngis.*

**hypophonesis** (hi-po-fo-ne'sis) [ hypo- + G. *phōnēsis*, a sounding ]. A sound that is diminished or fainter than usual, in percussion or auscultation.

**hypopho'nia** [ hypo- + G. *phōnē*, voice ]. An abnormally weak voice due to incoordination of the muscles concerned in vocalization.

**hypopho'ria** [ hypo- + G. *phora*, motion ]. A tendency of the visual axis of one eye to sink below that of its normal fellow.

**hypophosphatasemia** (hi′po-fos′fā-tā-se′mĭ-ah). Hypophosphatasia.

**hypophosphatasia** (hi′po-fos′fā-ta′zĭ-ah). Hypophosphatasemia; an abnormally low content of alkaline phosphatase in the circulating blood.

  **congenital h.,** a rare disorder associated with a low level of serum alkaline phosphatase, excretion of phosphoethanolamine, hypercalcemia, skeletal abnormalities, pathologic fractures, craniostenosis, and often early death; eyes may show blue sclerae, lid retraction, band keratopathy, cataracts, papilledema, and optic atrophy.

**hypophosphatemia** (hi′po-fos-fā-te′mĭ-ah). Abnormally low concentrations of phosphates in the circulating blood.

**hy′pophos′phatu′ria.** Oligophosphaturia; reduced urinary excretion of phosphates.

**hy′pophos′phorous acid** (NF). Contains 31 per cent $HPH_2O_2$. Used as a stabilizing reducing agent in pharmaceutical preparations.

**hypophrasia** (hi-po-fra′zĭ-ah) [ hypo- + G. *phrasis,* speaking ]. Slowness or lack of speech associated with a psychosis.

**hypophysec′tomize.** To remove the hypophysis cerebri.

**hypophysectomy** (hi-pof′ĭ-sek-to-me). Excision or destruction of the pituitary gland by means of craniotomy or stereotaxy.

**hypophysial, hypophyseal** (hi-po-fiz′ĭ-al). Relating to a hypophysis.

**hypoph′ysin.** PITUITRIN; an aqueous extract of the posterior lobe of the fresh hypophysis of cattle; contains oxytocin and vasopressin.

**hypophysioprivic** (hi′po-fiz′ĭ-o-priv′ik) [ hypophysis + L. *privus,* deprived of ]. Hypophyseoprivic, hypophysoprivus; denoting the condition in which the pituitary gland may be functionally inactive or may be absent, as after hypophysectomy.

**hypophysis** (hi-pof′ĭ-sis) [ G. an undergrowth. PHYS- ] [ NA ], glandula pituitaria [ NA ]; pituitary gland; h. cerebri; an unpaired, compound gland suspended from the base of the hypothalamus by a short, cordlike extension of the infundibulum, the hypophysial (or pituitary) stalk. The h. consists of two major subdivisions: (1) a posterior lobe (lobus posterior hypophyseos; neurohypophysis) which (a) appears as the bulbous end of the stalk, (b) like the latter, develops in ontogeny as a downgrowth from the brain, hence is part of the central nervous system, and (c) is composed of modified glia cells (pituicytes), blood vessels, and unmyelinated nerve fibers originating largely in the large-celled supraoptic and paraventricular nuclei of the hypothalamus and conveying to the lobe for storage and release the hormones vasopressin and oxytocin; (2) the larger anterior lobe (lobus anterior hypophyseos; adenohypophysis) which (a) consists of cords of epithelial cells of various types interspersed with sinusoid capillaries, (b) develops from the roof of the embryonic oral cavity and thus, despite its adherence to the posterior lobe, is not a true part of the brain, and (c) unlike the posterior lobe receives no direct innervation from the hypothalamus but, instead, is governed by the hypothalamus by the medium of chemical transmitter agents ("releasing factors") elaborated by hypothalamic neurons and transported by a system of blood vessels (the hypothalamohypophysial portal system) to the anterior lobe which in response releases into the systemic circulation any one (or combination) of a variety of tropic (thyrotropic, gonadotropic, adrenocorticotropic, and other) hormones, each of which activates the corresponding endocrine gland, triggering the release of its hormone. With the exception of the adrenal medulla and the parathyroid gland, the function of all peripheral endocrine organs depends heavily upon the functional integrity of the hypothalamus and anterior lobe of the h.; in the absence of a functioning anterior lobe these organs undergo a profound atrophy. Destruction of the posterior lobe or of the supraoptic nuclei, by contrast, causes excessive diuresis: diabetes insipidus. The function of two small, histologically distinct subdivisions of the anterior lobe, the pars intermedia and pars tuberalis, is still unclear. See also hypothalamus; hypothalamohypophysial portal *system.*

  **h. cerebri,** hypophysis.

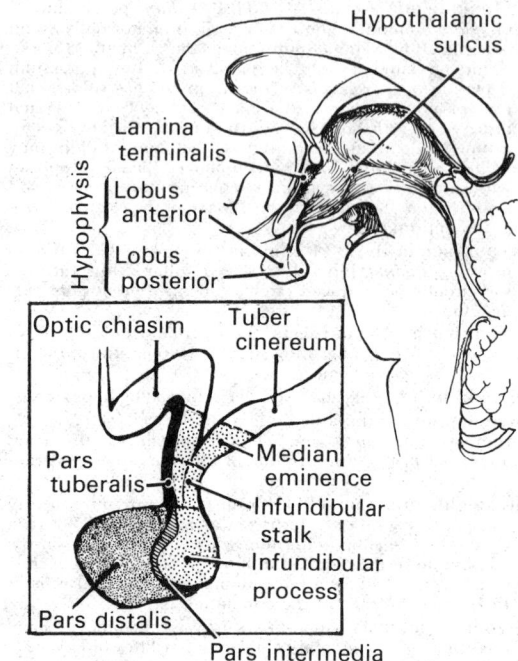

*Hypophysis and Hypothalamus*

  **pharyn′geal h.,** *pars* pharyngea lobi anterioris hypophyseos.

  **h. sicca,** desiccated h.; see posterior *pituitary.*

**hypophysoprivus** (hi-pof′ĭ-so-pri′vus). Hypophysioprivic.

**hypopiesis** (hi′po-pi-e′sis) [ hypo- + G. *piesis,* pressure ]. Hypotension.

  **orthostatic h.,** orthostatic *hypotension.*

**hypopituitarism** (hi′po-pĭ-tu′ĭ-tā-rizm). A condition due to diminished activity of the anterior lobe of the hypophysis; entails inadequate secretion, to varying degrees, of one or more anterior pituitary hormones.

**hypoplasia** (hi′po-pla′zĭ-ah) [ hypo- + G. *plasis,* a molding ]. 1. Underdevelopment of tissue or an organ, usually due to a decrease in the number of cells. 2. Atrophy due to destruction of some of the elements and not merely to their general reduction in size.

  **cartilage-hair h.,** an inherited form of dwarfism characterized by shortness of the extremities without skull defects, and with sparse, brittle hair of light color.

  **enamel h.,** a hereditary defect of enamel matrix formation, with deficiency of enamel rods and cementing substance; enamel is hard but thin, teeth may be conical or cylindrical in shape, with lack of contact between teeth, occlusal surfaces become worn, and yellow staining appears where the dentin is exposed; both deciduous and permanent teeth are affected. A type of amelogenesis imperfecta.

  **focal dermal h.,** a rare congenital condition characterized by scattered areas of thinning of the skin, and by pigmentation.

  **optic nerve h.,** congenitally small optic disk due to failure of maturation of retinal ganglion cells, with a reduced number of normal nerve fibers; visual impairment may be marked.

  **right ventricular h.,** parchment *heart.*

**hypoplas′tic.** Pertaining to or characterized by hypoplasia.

**hy′poploid.** Characterized by hypoploidy.

**hypoploidy** (hi′po-ploy′dī) [ hypo- + -ploid, *q.v.* ]. State of having lost one or more chromosomes.

**hypopnea** (hi-pop′ne-ah) [ hypo- + G. *pnoē,* breathing ]. Decrease in amount of air breathed per minute. Depth of breathing, rather than rate, usually is decreased. See also eupnea; hyperpnea.

**hypoporosis** (hi-po-po-ro'sis) [ hypo- + G. *pōros*, callus, + suffix -*osis*, condition ]. Deficient formation of callus after fracture of a bone.

**hypopo'sia** [ hypo- + G. *posis*, drinking ]. Hypodipsia, with emphasis on tendency to drink rather than on the reduced sensation of thirst.

**hy'popotasse'mia.** Hypokalemia.

**hy'poprax'ia** [ hypo- + G. *praxis*, action, + suffix -*ia*, condition ]. Deficient activity.

**hypoproaccelerinemia** (hi'po-pro-ak-sel'er-in-e'mi-ah). Abnormally low concentration of blood-clotting factor V, *i.e.*, proaccelerin, in the circulating blood; a deficiency leads to a rare hemorrhagic tendency known as parahemophilia.

**hy'popro'convert'ine'mia.** Abnormally low concentration of blood-clotting factor VII, *i.e.*, proconvertin, in the circulating blood; a deficiency causes a quantitative prolongation of the prothrombin time.

**hypoproteinemia** (hi-po-pro'te-in-e'mi-ah, -pro'tēn-). Abnormally small amounts of total protein in the circulating blood plasma.

**hypoproteinosis** (hi-po-pro'te-in-o'sis, -pro'tēn-). A condition, especially in children, due to a dietary deficiency of protein. It consists of anorexia, vomiting, retardation of growth, anemia, and increased susceptibility to infections. Kwashiorkor is a disease in which protein undernutrition is a major etiologic factor.

**hypoprothrombinemia** (hi'po-pro-throm'bin-e'mi-ah). Abnormally small amounts of blood-clotting factor II, *i.e.*, prothrombin, in the circulating blood.

**hypopselaphesia** (hi-pop-sel'ă-fe'zi-ah) [ hypo- + G. *psēlaphēsis*, touch ]. Diminished tactile sensibility; tactile hypesthesia.

**hypopsychosis** (hi-po-si-ko'sis). Hyponoia.

**hypoptyalism** (hi'po-ti'ă-lizm) [ hypo- + G. *ptyalon*, saliva ]. Reduced secretion of saliva.

**hypopyon** (hi-po'pi-on) [ hypo- + G. *pyon*, pus ]. The presence of a puslike fluid in the anterior chamber of the eye. See also onyx (2).

**hyporeflexia** (hi'po-re-flek'si-ah). A condition in which the reflexes are weakened.

**hy'pori'boflavino'sis.** A deficiency disease caused by an inadequate intake of riboflavin. This word should be used instead of the more commonly used ariboflavinosis.

**hyposalemia** (hi-po-sal-e'mi-ah) [ hypo- + L. *sal*, salt, + G. *haima*, blood ]. Obsolete term meaning abnormally small amounts of various salts in the circulating blood; was sometimes used as a synonym for hypochloremia.

**hy'posal'iva'tion.** Reduced salivation.

**hyposarca** (hi'po-sar'kah) [ hypo- + G. *sarx* (*sark*-), flesh ]. Extreme anasarca or dropsy of the subcutaneous connective tissue.

**hyposcheotomy** (hi-pos-ke-ot'o-mi) [ hypo- + G. *oscheon*, scrotum, + *tomē*, incision ]. Incision or puncture into a hydrocele at its most dependent point.

**hyposcle'ral.** Beneath the sclerotic coat of the eyeball.

**hyposecre'tion.** Diminished secretion.

**hyposen'sitiveness.** Subnormal sensitiveness or sensitivity; a condition in which the response to a stimulus is unusually delayed or lessened in degree.

**hyposen'sitize.** To reduce sensitivity usually with reference to allergy (induced sensitivity).

**hyposialadenitis** (hi'po-si'al-ad-en-i'tis) [ hypo- + G. *sialon*, saliva, + *adēn*, gland, + suffix -*itis*, inflammation ]. Inflammation of the submaxillary salivary glands.

**hyposkeocytosis** (hi'po-ske'o-si-to'sis) [ hypo- + *skaios*, left, + *kytos*, cell, + suffix -*osis*, condition ]. Hyponeocytosis.

**hyposmia** (hi-poz'mi-ah) [ hypo- + G. *osmē*, smell ]. Hyposphresia; olfactory hypesthesia; diminished sense of smell.

**hyposmosis** (hi'pos-mo'sis). A reduction in the rapidity of osmosis.

**hyposomatotropism** (hi'po-so'mă-to-tro'pizm). A state characterized by deficient secretion of pituitary growth hormone (somatotropin).

**hyposo'mia** [ hypo- + G. *sōma*, body ]. Inadequate development of the body.

**hyposom'niac** [ hypo- + L. *somnus*, sleep ]. Pertaining to reduction in time of sleeping.

**hypospa'diac.** 1. Relating to hypospadias. 2. A sufferer from hypospadias.

**hypospadias** (hi-po-spa'di-as) [ G. one having the orifice of the penis too low, fr. *hypospaō*, to draw away from under. SPA- ]. A developmental anomaly characterized by a defect in the wall of the urethra so that the canal is open for a greater or lesser distance on the under surface of the penis; also a similar defect in the female in which the urethra opens into the vagina.

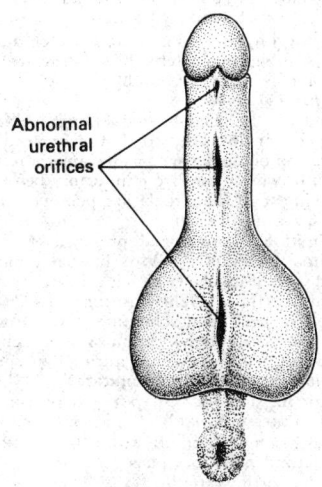

Abnormal urethral orifices

**Hypospadias**
Showing the various locations of abnormal urethral orifices. (From Langman, J.: *Medical Embryology*, Ed. 2, The Williams & Wilkins Co., Baltimore, 1969.)

    **balan'ic h.,** h. involving the male, or glans penis.

    **penoscrotal h.,** h. involving the penis and scrotum.

    **h. perinea'lis,** one in which a cleft runs forward from a little in front of the anus and into which the urethra opens; the scrotum is usually cleft as well, the testes undescended, and the penis rudimentary.

**hyposphresia** (hi'pos-fre'zi-ah) [ hypo- + G. *osphrēsis*, smell ]. Hyposmia.

**hyposphyxia** (hi-po-sfik'si-ah) [ hypo- + G. *sphyxis*, pulse, SPHYG- ]. Abnormally low blood pressure with sluggishness of the circulation.

**hypostasis** (hi-pos'tă-sis) [ G. *hypo-stasis*, a standing under, sediment. STA- ]. 1. A sediment; the matter rising to the surface, instead of sinking, is called epistasis. 2. Hypostatic congestion.

    **h. pulmonum,** hydrostatic congestion of the lung.

**hypostat'ic.** 1. Sedimentary; resulting from a dependent position. 2. Relating to epistasis.

**hyposthenia** (hi'pos-the'ni-ah) [ hypo- + G. *sthenos*, strength ]. Weakness.

**hypostheniant** (hi'pos-the'ni-ant). 1. Weakening. 2. An agent that reduces strength.

**hyposthenic** (hi'pos-then'ik). Weak.

**hyposthenuria** (hi'pos-thē-nu'ri-ah) [ hypo- + G. *sthenos*, strength, + *ouron*, urine ]. Secretion of urine of low specific gravity, due to inability of the tubules of the kidneys to produce a concentrated urine; it occurs chiefly in chronic nephritis.

    **tubular h.,** a synonym for h.

**hypostome** (hi'po-stōm) [ hypo- + G. *stoma*, mouth ]. The central unpaired holdfast organ of the tick capitulum; the

h. is covered with recurved spines that enable it to serve as an anchoring device while the tick feeds.

**hypostomia** (hi′po-sto′mi-ah) [ hypo- + G. *stoma*, mouth ]. A form of microstomia in which the oral opening is a small vertical slit.

**hyposto′sis** [ hypo- + G. *osteon*, bone, + suffix *-osis*, condition ]. Deficient development of bone.

**hypostypsis** (hi′po-stip′sis) [ hypo- + G. *stypsis*, astringence ]. A state of mild astringence.

**hypostyp′tic.** Mildly styptic or astringent.

**hy′posu′prare′nalism.** Obsolete synonym for hypoadrenalism.

**hyposystole** (hi-po-sis′to-le). A weak or incomplete cardiac systole.

**hypotax′ia** [ hypo- + G. *taxis*, order ]. A condition of weak or imperfect coordination.

**hy′potel′orism** [ hypo- + G. *tēle*, far off, + *horizō*, to separate, fr. *horos*, boundary ]. Abnormal closeness of eyes.

**hypoten′sion** [ hypo- + L. *tensio*, a stretching, TEN- ]. 1. Hypopiesis; subnormal arterial blood pressure. 2. Reduced pressure or tension of any kind.
   **arterial h.,** (1) above.
   **controlled h.,** induced h.; reduction of blood pressure during operation in order to diminish bleeding, by the administration of a drug such as hexamethonium bromide or by withdrawing blood from an artery before operation and returning it to the circulation postoperatively.
   **induced h.,** controlled h.
   **intracra′nial h.,** subnormal pressure of cerebrospinal fluid; it most commonly follows lumbar puncture and is associated with headache (which is relieved by recumbency but returns in the upright position), nausea, vomiting, stiffness of the neck, and sometimes fever. Intracranial h. may also result from dehydration or subarachnoid block, and may occur in diabetic coma, during hyperpnea, or after the injection of a hypertonic solution.
   **orthostatic h.,** orthostatic hypopiesis; postural h.; a form of low blood pressure that occurs when the subject stands.
   **positional h.,** h. that results from the position in which the anesthetized patient is placed.
   **postural h.,** orthostatic h.
   **spinal h.,** h. due to the vasodilation produced following the administration of extensive spinal anesthesia.

**hypoten′sive.** Characterized by low blood pressure or causing reduction in blood pressure.

**hy′poten′sor.** Depressor (4).

**hy′potes′toidism.** Obsolete term for male hypogonadism.

**hypothalamohypophysial** (hi′po-thal′ă-mo-hi′po-fiz′ī-al). Relating to both the hypothalamus and the hypophysis.

**hy′pothal′amus** [ hypo- + thalamus, *q.v.* ] [ NA ]. The ventral and medial region of the diencephalon forming the walls of the ventral half of the third ventricle, delineated from the thalamus by the hypothalamic sulcus, lying medial to the internal capsule and subthalamus, continuous with the precommissural septum anteriorly and with the mesencephalic midbrain tegmentum and central gray substance posteriorly. Its ventral surface is marked by, from before backward: (1) the optic chiasma, (2) the unpaired infundibulum which extends by way of the infundibular stalk into the posterior lobe of the hypophysis, and (3) the paired mamillary bodies. The nerve cells of the h. are grouped into a large number of nuclei: the large-celled supraoptic n. and paraventricular n., the lateral preoptic n., lateral hypothalamic n., and nuclei tuberis, the medially placed medial preoptic n., anterior hypothalamic n., ventromedial n., dorsomedial n., arcuate n., posterior hypothalamic n., premamillary nuclei, and mamillary body. It has afferent fiber connections with the midbrain and limbic system (hippocampus, amygdala, and septal area), efferent fiber connections with the same structures and with the posterior lobe of the hypophysis; its functional connection with the anterior lobe of the hypophysis is established by a system of hypothalamo-hypophysial blood vessels. The h. is prominently involved in the functions of the autonomic nervous system and, through its vascular link with the anterior lobe of the hypophysis, in endocrine mechanisms; it also appears to play a role in the nervous mechanisms underlying moods and motivational states. See also hypophysis, median *eminence;* fornix; medial forebrain *bundle;* septal *area;* and *stria* terminalis.

**hypothelesia** (hi′po-thě-le′zi-ah) [ hypo- + G. *thelēsis*, will ]. Weakness of will.

**hypothenar** (hi′po-the′nar, hi-poth′e-nar) [ hypo- + G. *thenar*, the palm ]. 1 [ NA ]. Antithenar; the fleshy mass at the medial side of the palm. 2. Denoting any structure in relation with this part.

**hypother′mal.** 1. Denoting a subnormal bodily temperature, one below 98.6°F. (37°C.). 2. Tepid.

**hypother′mia** [ hypo- + G. *thermē*, heat ]. A body temperature below 98.6°F. (37°C.).
   **accidental h.,** unintentional and dangerous fall in body temperature on exposure to a cold environment; may occur in infants and in the newborn, particularly during operations; may also occur in the elderly.
   **h. by body cavity cooling,** h. induced by instillation of chilled saline into the pleural cavity during thoracotomy, into the peritoneal cavity during laparotomy, into the bladder by catheter, into the rectum as an ice water enema, or into the stomach by gastric balloon.
   **h. by extracorporeal methods,** h. induced by removing blood from the circulation, cooling it by means of a heat exchanger in an extracorporeal circulation (venovenous or cardiopulmonary bypass), and then returning the cold blood to the body.
   **moderate h.,** h. induced by surface cooling to 23–32° C.; it is essential to maintain adequate spontaneous cardiac action.
   **profound h.,** a body temperature of 12–20° C. produced by use of a heat exchanger unit and a pump-oxygenator.
   **regional h.,** cooling an organ (*e.g.*, the brain) that is vulnerable to ischemia during occlusion of the circulation by cooling the blood entering that organ.
   **h. by surface cooling,** h. induced by any of several methods, including immersing the body in cold water and ice bath, air cooling, or use of ice bags packed around the body, refrigerated blankets, or cold water spray.
   **total body h.,** the deliberate reduction of total body temperature, in order to reduce the general metabolism of the tissues; accomplished by inactivation of the heat-regulating mechanism by administering a central nervous system depressant (any volatile anesthetic or nonvolatile basal narcotic) and exposing the body to a cold environment (water bath, cold air) just above freezing temperatures.

**hypothesis** (hi-poth′e-sis) [ L. fr. G. *hypotithenai*, to propose or suppose ]. A supposition or assumption advanced as a basis for reasoning or argument, or as a guide to experimental investigation; a tentative theory unsupported by the essential facts that would prove its truth.
   **Avogadro's h.,** Avogadro's *law.*
   **Bail's h.,** this states that, in any fluid culture of bacteria, there is a limiting density of population which cannot be exceeded. This is called the M-concentration.
   **frustration-aggression h.,** the theory that frustration may lead to aggression, but that aggression is always the result of some form of frustration.
   **Gompertz' h.,** a theory that the force of mortality increases in geometrical progression; being based on the assumption that the average exhaustion of a man's power to avoid death is such that at the end of equal infinitely small intervals of time he loses equal proportions of the power to oppose destruction which he had at the commencement of each of these intervals.
   **insular h.,** the theory of the origin of diabetes mellitus from destruction or loss of function of the islets of Langerhans in the pancreas.
   **Lyon h.,** the concept that one X-chromosome is inactive during interphase in normal females, and is represented in interphase cell nuclei as the sex chromatin body; as either X-chromosome may be inactivated, females heterozygous for an X-linked mutant gene may show patches of tissue expressing the phenotype of the mutant gene while the majority of tissue remains normal; see also sex *chromatin.*
   **Makeham's h.,** a development of Gompertz' h. as to the law of mortality following some mathematical law. Makeham assumed that death was the consequence of two generally coexisting causes: (1) chance, (2) a deterioration

or increased inability to withstand destruction. The first of these is constant, the second is an increasing geometrical progression.

**Michaelis-Menten h.,** that a complex is formed between an enzyme and its substrate, which complex then decomposes to yield free enzyme and the reaction products, the latter rate determining the over-all rate of substrate-product conversion. See also Michaelis-Menten *constant.*

**mnemic h.** (ne′mik), mnemism; the theory that stimuli or irritants leave definite traces (engrams) on the protoplasm of the animal or plant, and when these stimuli are regularly repeated they induce a habit which persists after the stimuli cease; assuming that the germ cells share with the nerve cells in the possession of engrams, acquired habits may thus be transmitted to the descendants.

**sequence h.,** that the amino acid sequence of a protein is determined by a particular sequence of nucleotides (the cistron) in the DNA of the organism producing the protein.

**sliding filament h.,** the theory that the contracting muscle shortens because two sets of filaments slide past each other.

**Starling's h.,** the principle that net filtration through capillary membranes is proportional to the transmembrane hydrostatic pressure difference minus the transmembrane oncotic pressure difference; although well established, it is called Starling's h. to distinguish it from Starling's law of the heart, *q.v.*

**zwitter h.** [ Ger. *Zwitter,* hermaphrodite, mongrel ], that an ampholytic molecule (*e.g.,* an amino acid) yields, at the isoelectric point, equal numbers of basic and acid ions, thus becoming an ion (zwitterion) with an equal number of negative and positive charges.

**hypothrombinemia** (hi′po-throm-bin-e′mī-ah). Abnormally small amounts of thrombin in the circulating blood, thereby resulting in bleeding tendency.

**hy′pothromboplastine′mia.** Abnormally small amounts of blood-clotting factor III, *i.e.,* thromboplastin, in the blood, as a result of deficient quantities being released from the tissues.

**hypothymia** (hi-po-thi′mī-ah) [ hypo- + G. *thymos,* mind, soul ]. Depression of spirits; the "blues."

**hy′pothy′mic.** Pertaining to (1) hypothymia, and (2) hypothymism.

**hy′pothy′mism.** Inadequate function of the thymus.

**hypothy′rea.** Obsolete synonym for hypothyroidism.

**hypothy′roid.** Marked by reduced thyroid function.

**hypothyroida′tion.** Obsolete term meaning the induction of hypothyroidism.

**hypothyroid′ea.** Obsolete synonym for hypothyroidism.

**hypothyroidism** (hi′po-thi′royd-izm) [ hypo- + G. *thyreoeidēs,* thyroid ]. Diminished production of thyroid hormone, leading to thyroid insufficiency. See also myxedema and cretinism.

**infantile h.,** cretinism.

**secondary h.,** h. that arises as a consequence of inadequate thyrotropin secretion by the anterior pituitary gland.

**hy′pothyro′sis.** Obsolete synonym for hypothyroidism.

**hypothyroxinemia** (hi′po-thi-rok′sin-e′mī-ah). A subnormal thyroxine concentration in blood.

**hypoto′nia** [ hypo- + G. *tonos,* tone ]. Hypotonicity; hypotonus; 1. Reduced tension in any part, as in the eyeball. 2. Relaxation of the arteries. 3. A condition in which there is a diminution or loss of muscular tonicity, in consequence of which the muscles may be stretched beyond their normal limits.

**hypoton′ic.** Hypoisotonic. 1. Having a lesser degree of tension. 2. Having a lesser osmotic pressure than a reference solution, which is ordinarily assumed to be blood plasma or interstitial fluid.

**hypotonicity** (hi′po-to-nis′ī-tī). 1. Hypotonia. 2. A decreased effective osmotic pressure.

**hypoto′nus, hypot′ony.** Hypotonia.

**hypotoxicity** (hi-po-toks-is′ī-tī). Reduced toxicity; the quality of being only slightly poisonous.

**hypotrichiasis** (hi′po-trī-ki′ă-sis). Hypotrichosis.

**hypotrichosis** (hi-po-trī-ko′sis) [ hypo- + G. *trichōsis,* hairiness ]. Oligotrichosis; oligotrichia; hypotrichiasis; a deficiency of hair on the head and body.

**hypotro′pia** [ hypo- + G. *trope,* turn ]. *Strabismus* deorsum vergens.

**hy′potympanot′omy** [ hypo- + G. *tympanon,* tympanum, + *tome,* incision ]. Operative procedure developed by Shambaugh for the complete surgical extirpation, without sacrifice of hearing, of small tumors confined to the lower tympanic cavity.

**hypotympanum** (hi′po-tim′pă-num). The lower part of the tympanic cavity. It is separated by a bony wall from the jugular bulb.

**hypouresis** (hi′po-u-re′sis). Reduced flow of urine.

**hypouricuria** (hi′po-u′rī-ku′rī-ah). Reduced excretion of uric acid in the urine.

**hypourocrinia** (hi′po-u′ro-krin′ī-ah) [ hypo- + G. *oureo,* to urinate, + *krino,* to separate ]. Obsolete term meaning scanty urine.

**hypovaria** (hi-po-va′rī-ah). Hypoovarianism.

**hy′pova′rianism.** Hypoovarianism.

**hy′poventila′tion.** Underventilation; reduced alveolar ventilation relative to metabolic carbon dioxide production, so that alveolar carbon dioxide pressure tends to rise above normal.

**hy′povitamino′sis.** A state characterized by insufficiency of one or more essential vitamins. It exists first as a humoral depletion, then functional changes occur, and finally morphologic lesions appear.

**hypovolemia** (hi-po-vo-le′mī-ah) [ hypo- + L. *volumen,* volume, + G. *haima,* blood ]. Oligemia.

**hypovolia** (hi′po-vo′lī-ah) [ hypo- + L. *volumen,* volume ]. Diminished water content or volume of a given compartment; *e.g.,* extracellular h.

**hypoxanthine** (hi-pok-san′thin). 6-Oxypurine; a purine present in the muscles and other tissues and formed during purine catabolism, by deamination of adenine.

**Hypoxanthine**

**h. oxidase,** xanthine oxidase.

**hypoxemia** (hi-pok-se′mī-ah) [ hypo- + oxygen, + G. *haima,* blood ]. Subnormal oxygenation of arterial blood short of anoxia.

**hypox′ia.** Decrease below normal levels of oxygen in air, blood, or tissue short of anoxia.

**hypsarhythmia** (hip′să-rith′mī-ah) [ G. *hypsi,* high, + a-priv. + *rhythmos,* rhythm ]. Hypsarrhythmia; the abnormal and characteristically chaotic electroencephalogram commonly found in patients with infantile spasms.

**hyp′sarrhyth′mia.** Correct alternative spelling for hypsarhythmia; the latter, however, is the spelling of the original coinage and is the one in general use.

**hypsi-, hypso-** [ G. *hypsos,* height ]. Combining forms meaning high or denoting relationship to height.

**hypsibrachycephalic** (hip-sī-brak′ī-sē-fal′ik) [ hypsi- + G. *brachys,* broad, + *kephale,* head ]. Having a high broad head, such as that of a Malay.

**hypsicephalic** (hip′sī-sē-fal′ik). Oxycephalic.

**hypsicephaly** (hip′sī-sef′ă-lī) [ hypsi- + G. *kephale,* head ]. Oxycephaly.

**hypsiconchous** (hip-sī-kon′kus) [ hypsi- + G. *konchos,* a shell, the upper part of the skull ]. Having a high orbit, with an orbital index above 85.

**hypsiloid** (hip′sī-loyd) [ G. *upsilon (ypsilon)* ]. Y-shaped; U-shaped.

**hypsistaphylia** (hip′sī-stă-fil′ī-ah) [ hypsi- + G. *staphyle,* uvula ]. A condition in which the palate is high and narrow.

**hypsistenocephalic** (hip-sī-sten'o-sē-fal'ik) [ hypsi- + G. *stenos,* narrow, + *kephalē,* head ]. Having a high, narrow head, such as that of an Abyssinian.

**hypso-.** See hypsi-.

**hypsocephaly** (hip'so-sef'ă-lī) [ hypso- + G. *kephalē,* head ]. Oxycephaly.

**hypsochromic** (hip'so-kro'mik) [ hypso- + G. *chroma,* color ]. Denoting the shift of an absorption spectrum maximum to a shorter wavelength.

**hypsodont** (hip'so-dont) [ hypso- + G. *odous,* tooth ]. Having long teeth.

**hypsopho'bia** [ hypso- + G. *phobos,* fear ]. Acrophobia.

**hypuresis** (hip'u-re'sis) [ hypo- + G. *oureō,* to urinate ]. Obsolete term for scanty urine.

**hypurgia** (hi-pur'ji-ah) [ G. *hypourgia,* help, service, fr. *hypo,* + *ergon,* work ]. Any of the minor factors modifying the course of a disease either for good or for ill, especially the former.

**Hyrtl** (her'tl), Joseph, Vienna anatomist, 1810–1894. See H.'s *anastomosis, foramen, loop,* epitympanic *recess, sphincter.*

**hyster-.** See hystero-.

**hysteralgia** (his'ter-al'ji-ah) [ hystero- + G. *algos,* pain ]. Hysterodynia; uteralgia; metralgia, metrodynia; neuralgic pain in the uterus.

**hysteratresia** (his'ter-ă-tre'zī-ah). Atresia of the uterine cavity, usually resulting from inflammatory endocervical adhesions.

**hysteraux'in.** Growth-stimulating portion of female sex hormone; an obsolete usage.

**hysterec'tomize.** To perform a hysterectomy.

**hysterectomy** (his-ter-ek'to-mī) [ hystero- + G. *ektomē,* excision ]. Removal of the uterus; unless otherwise specified, usually used to denote complete removal of the uterus (corpus and cervix).

**abdominal h.,** celiohysterectomy; abdominohysterectomy; laparohysterectomy; removal of the uterus through an incision in the abdominal wall.

**abdom'inovaginal h.,** a combined vaginal and abdominal surgical approach that allows partial or complete removal of vagina, vulva, rectum, and perineum (abdominoperineal approach), as well as pelvic organs; usually done in cases of advanced pelvic cancer.

**cesarean h.,** Porro h. or operation; cesarean section followed by h.

**modified radical h.,** TeLinde operation; an extended h. in which a portion of the upper vagina is removed; the ureters are exposed and pulled back laterally without dissection from the ureteral bed.

**paravaginal h.,** removal of the uterus through a perineal incision involving only the lower two-thirds of the vaginal wall.

**Porro h.,** cesarean h.

**radical h.,** complete removal of the uterus, upper vagina, and parametrium.

**subtotal h.,** supracervical h.

**supracervical h.,** subtotal h.; removal of the fundus of the uterus, leaving the cervix *in situ.*

**vaginal h.,** vaginohysterectomy; colpohysterectomy; removal of the uterus through the vagina without incising the wall of the abdomen.

**hystere'sis** [ G. *hysterēsis,* a coming later. HYST- 2 ]. 1. Failure of either one of two related phenomena to keep pace with the other; or any situation in which the value of one depends upon whether the other has been increasing or decreasing. 2. The lag of a magnetic effect behind its cause; magnetic inertia. 3. The temperature differential that exists when a substance, such as reversible hydrocolloid, melts at one temperature and solidifies at another.

**static h.,** the difference in the value reached by a dependent variable at a particular constant value of the independent variable, depending on whether the latter value had been approached from above or below; *e.g.,* in measuring the pressure volume relations of the lungs, if one completely expires and then inspires to a particular volume and holds it constant, the transpulmonary pressure required to maintain that lung volume is greater than if one had completely inspired and then expired to the same volume and held it constant.

**hystereurynter** (his'ter-u-rin'ter) [ hystero- + G. *eurynein,* to dilate ]. Metreurynter; an inflatable bag used inside the lower uterine segment and cervix to prevent cord prolapse or to tamponade a bleeding placental margin in placenta previa.

**hystereurysis** (his'ter-u'rī-sis) [ hystero- + G. *eurynein,* to dilate, fr. *eurys,* wide ]. Metreurysis; dilation of the lower segment and cervical canal of the uterus.

**hysteria** (his-tēr'ī-ah) [ G. *hystera,* womb, because formerly thought to be of uterine causation. HYST- ]. A diagnostic term, referable to a wide variety of psychogenic symptoms involving disorder of function which may be mental, sensory, motor, or visceral.

**anxiety h.,** h. characterized by manifest anxiety.

**conversion h.,** conversion h. neurosis; conversion reaction; h. characterized by the substituion through psychic transformation of physical signs or symptoms for anxiety; fainting under emotional stress (hysterical syncope) is a common example, but the term is generally restricted to such major symptoms as psychic blindness, deafness, or paralysis.

**major h.,** grande hysterie; a syndrome described at length by Charcot; characterized by a first stage of aura, a second stage of epileptoid convulsions, a third stage of tonic and clonic spasms; a fourth stage of dramatic behavior; and a fifth stage of delirium; the entire attack may last from a few minutes to half an hour. Sometimes used as a synonym for hysteroepilepsy.

**minor h.,** a mild form of h. characterized chiefly by subjective pains, nervousness, undue sensitiveness, and sometimes attacks of emotional excitement, but without paralysis or other stigmata.

**traumatic h.,** hysterotraumatism.

**hysteriac** (his-tēr'ī-ak). A hysterical person.

**hysteric** (his-tēr'ik). 1. Hysterical. 2. A hysterical person.

**hysterical** (his-tēr'ī-kal). Relating to or suffering from hysteria.

**hystericism** (his-tēr'ī-sizm). A tendency or predisposition to hysteria.

**hystericoneuralgic** (his-tēr'ī-ko-nu-ral'jik). Relating to neuralgic pains of hysterical origin.

**hysterics** (his-tēr'iks). An emotional explosion accompanied often by crying, laughing, and screaming.

**hysteritis** (his-ter-i'tis). Metritis.

**hystero-, hyster-.** 1 [ G. *hystera,* womb (uterus) ]. Combining forms denoting (1) the uterus (see also utero-, metr-), or (2) hysteria, *q.v.* 2 [ G. *hysteros,* later ]. Combining forms meaning late or following.

**hysterobubonocele** (his'ter-o-bu-bon'o-sēl) [ hystero- + G. *boubōn,* groin, + *kēlē,* hernia ]. An inguinal hernia containing the uterus.

**hys'terocat'alepsy.** Hysteria with cataleptic manifestations.

**hysterocele** (his'ter-o-sēl) [ hystero- + G. *kēlē,* hernia ]. Metrocele. 1. An abdominal or perineal hernia containing part or all of the uterus. 2. Protrusion of uterine contents into a weakened, bulging area of uterine wall.

**hysterocervicotomy** (his'ter-o-ser'vī-kot'o-mī) [ hystero- + L. *cervix,* neck + G. *tomē,* incision ]. Hysterotrachelotomy.

**hysterocleisis** (his'ter-o-kli'sis) [ hystero- + G. *kleisis,* closure ]. Operative occlusion of the uterus.

**hys'terocol'poscope** [ hystero- + G. *kolpos,* vagina, + *skopeō,* to view ]. An instrument for inspection of uterine cavity and vagina.

**hysterocystocleisis** (his'ter-o-sis'to-kli'sis) [ hystero- + G. *kystis,* bladder, + *kleisis,* closure ]. Bozeman's *operation.*

**hys'terocys'topexy** [ hystero- + G. *kystis,* bladder, + *pēxis,* fixation ]. Attachment of both uterus and bladder to the abdominal wall for the cure of prolapse.

**hysterodynia** (his'ter-o-din'ī-ah) [ hystero- + G. *odynē,* pain ]. Hysteralgia.

**hysteroepilepsy** (his'ter-o-ep'ī-lep-sī). Hysterical convulsions; see major *hysteria.*

**hysterofrenic** (his'ter-o-fren'ik) [ hystero- + L. *freno,* to curb ]. Arresting a hysterical attack; denoting certain areas pressure upon which has this effect.

**hysterogenic, hysterogenous** (his-ter-o-jen'ik, his-ter-oj'ē-nus). Causing hysterical symptoms or reactions.

**hys'terogram.** 1. An x-ray of the uterus, usually using contrast media. 2. A record of strength of uterine contractions.

**hys'terograph.** An apparatus for recording the strength of uterine contractions.

**hysterography** (his'ter-og'rä-fī) [ hystero- + G. *graphō*, to write ]. Metrography. 1. X-raying a uterine cavity filled with contrast medium. 2. The procedure of recording uterine contractions.

**hys'teroid** [ hystero- + G. *eidos*, resemblance ]. Resembling or simulating hysteria.

**hys'terolith** [ hystero- + G. *lithos*, stone ]. Uterine *calculus*.

**hysterology** (his'ter-ol'o-jī) [ hystero- + G. *logos*, study ]. The branch of medical science treating of the uterus in all its relations.

**hysteroloxia** (his'ter-o-lok'sī-ah) [ hystero- + G. *loxos*, slanting ]. Oblique version or flexion of the uterus.

**hysterolysis** (his-ter-ol'ī-sis) [ hystero- + G. *lysis*, dissolution ]. Breaking up of adhesions between the uterus and neighboring parts.

**hys'teroma'nia** [ hystero- + G. *mania*, madness ]. Metramania.

**hysterom'eter** [ hystero- + G. *metron*, measure ]. Uterometer; a graduated sound for measuring the depth of the uterine cavity.

**hysteromyoma** (his'ter-o-mi-o'mah) [ hystero- + G. *mys*, muscle, + suffix *-oma*, tumor ]. A myoma of the uterus.

**hysteromyomectomy** (his'ter-o-mi-o-mek'to-mī) [ hysteromyoma + G. *ektomē*, excision ]. Operative removal of a uterine myoma.

**hysteromyotomy** (his'ter-o-mi-ot'o-mī) [ hystero- + G. *mys*, muscle, + *tomē*, incision ]. Incision into the muscles of the uterus.

**hys'teronar'colepsy.** Narcolepsy of emotional origin.

**hystero-oophorectomy** (his'ter-o-o'of-o-rek'to-mī) [ hystero- + G. *ōon*, egg, + *phoros*, bearing, + *ektomē*, excision ]. Surgical removal of the uterus and ovaries.

**hysteropathy** (his'ter-op'ä-thī) [ hystero- + G. *pathos*, suffering ]. Any disease of the uterus.

**hys'teropexy** [ hystero- + G. *pēxis*, fixation ]. Uteropexy; uterofixation; the fixation of a misplaced or abnormally movable uterus.

    **abdominal h.,** laparohysteropexy; attachment of the uterus to the anterior abdominal wall.

    **vaginal h.,** attachment of the uterus to the peritoneal covering of the vagina.

**hysterophore** (his'ter-o-fōr) [ hystero- + G. *phoros*, bearing ]. A pessary or other support for a prolapsed or displaced uterus.

**hystero'pia** [ hystero- + G. *ōps* (*ōp-*), eye ]. A hysterical visual defect.

**hys'teroplas'ty.** Uteroplasty.

**hysteropsychosis** (his'ter-o-si-ko'sis). Hysterical *psychosis*.

**hysteroptosis, hysteroptosia** (his'ter-op-to'sis, -to'sī-ah) [ hystero- + G. *ptōsis*, a falling ]. Metroptosis.

**hysterorrhaphy** (his'ter-or'ä-fī) [ hystero- + G. *raphē*, suture ]. Sutural repair of a lacerated uterus.

**hysterorrhexis** (his'ter-o-rek'sis) [ hystero- + G. *rhēxis*, rupture ]. Metrorrhexis; rupture of the uterus.

**hysterosalpingectomy** (his'ter-o-sal-pin-jek'to-mī) [ hystero- + G. *salpinx*, a trumpet, + *ektomē*, excision ]. An operation for the removal of the uterus and one or both uterine tubes.

**hysterosalpingography** (his'ter-o-sal-ping-gog'rä-fī) [ hystero- + G. *salpinx*, a trumpet, + *graphō*, to write ]. Metrosalpingography; uterosalpingography; roentgenography of the uterus and oviducts after the injection of radiopaque material.

**hysterosalpingo-oophorectomy** (his'ter-o-sal-ping-go-o'of-o-rek'to-mī) [ hystero- + G. *salpinx*, trumpet, + *ōon*, egg, + *phoros*, bearing, + *ektomē*, excision ]. Excision of the uterus, oviducts, and ovaries.

**hysterosalpingostomy** (his'ter-o-sal-ping-gos'to-mī) [ hystero- + G. *salpinx*, trumpet, + *stoma*, mouth ]. An operation to restore patency of a tube.

**hysteroscope** (his'ter-o-skōp) [ hystero- + G. *skopeō*, to view ]. Uteroscope; metroscope; an endoscope used in direct visual examination of the uterine cavity.

**hysteroscopy** (his'ter-os'ko-pī). Uteroscopy; visual instrumental inspection of the uterine cavity.

**hys'terospasm.** Spasm of the uterus.

**hysterostomatocleisis** (his'ter-o-sto'mä-to-kli'sis) [ hystero- + G. *stoma*, mouth, + *kleisis*, closure ]. Closure of cervical canal, usually in vesicouterine fistula to prevent leakage of urine from cervix.

**hys'terosto'matome.** An instrument to incise the cervix uteri.

**hys'terostomat'omy, hys'terostomatot'omy** [ hystero- + G. *stoma*, mouth, + *tomē*, incision ]. Hysterotrachelotomy.

**hysterosystole** (his-ter-o-sis'to-le) [ G. *hysteros*, following, after, + *systolē*, a contracting. STAL- ]. A delayed contraction of the heart coming after its normal time; opposed to premature contraction or extrasystole.

**hys'terothermom'etry.** Measurement of uterine temperature.

**hys'terotome.** Uterotome; metrotome; metratome; an instrument for incising the uterus.

**hysterot'omy** [ hystero- + G. *tomē*, incision ]. Uterotomy; metrotomy; metratomy; incision of the uterus.

    **abdominal h.,** transabdominal incision into the uterus; also variously referred to as abdominohysterotomy, abdominouterotomy; celiohysterotomy, laparohysterotomy, laparouterotomy.

    **vaginal h.,** colpohysterotomy; incision into the uterus via the vagina.

**hys'teroto'nin** [ hystero- + G. *tonos*, tension ]. Pressor substance found in decidua and amniotic fluid of patients with toxemia of pregnancy.

**hysterotrachelectomy** (his'ter-o-trak'el-ek'to-mī) [ hystero- + G. *trachēlos*, neck, + *ektomē*, excision ]. Removal of cervix uteri.

**hysterotracheloplasty** (his'ter-o-trak'el-o-plas'tī) [ hystero- + G. *trachēlos*, neck, + *plastos*, formed, shaped ]. Plastic repair of the cervix uteri.

**hysterotrachelorrhaphy** (his'ter-o-trak-el-or'ä-fī) [ hystero- + G. *trachēlos*, neck, + *rhaphē*, a seam ]. Sutural repair of a lacerated cervix uteri.

**hysterotrachelotomy** (his'ter-o-trak'el-ot'o-mī) [ hystero- + G. *trachēlos*, neck, + *tomē*, incision ]. Hysterocervicotomy; hysterostomatotomy; incision of the cervix uteri.

**hys'terotraumat'ic.** Relating to hysterotraumatism.

**hysterotraumatism** (his'ter-o-traw'mä-tizm). Traumatic hysteria; hysteria following the shock of a severe injury.

**hysterotris'mus.** 1. Hysterical lockjaw; that is, symptoms of lockjaw on a functional or hysterical basis. 2. Spasm of the uterus.

**hysterotubography** (his'ter-o-tu-bog'rä-fī). Hysterosalpingography.

**hysterythrine.** Erythrine red; female sex hormone producing congestion.

**Hz.** Abbreviation for hertz.

# I

**I.** 1. Chemical symbol of the element iodine. 2. Symbol for luminous *intensity*. 3. Abbreviation for intensity of electrical current, expressed in amperes. 4. As a subscript, symbol for inspired *gas*. 5. Designation for I blood group (see appendix 2, Blood groups).

**-ia** [ G. *-ia*, a primitive substantive-forming suffix, denoting action or an abstract ]. Suffix denoting condition; used in formation of names of many diseases.

**IANC.** Abbreviation for International Anatomical Nomenclature Committee; see *Nomina Anatomica.*

**-iasis** [ G. ]. A suffix meaning a condition or state expressed by a verb terminating in *-aō* or *-iaō*, as psoriasis from *psōriaō*, to have the itch or mange. In medical neologisms it has the same value as, and is sometimes interchangeable with, *-osis*, as trichiniasis or trichinosis.

**iatraliptic** (i-ă-tră-lip'tik) [ G. *iatros*, physician, + *aleiptēs*, an anointer ]. Denoting treatment by inunction, or the epidermic method.

**iatralip'tics.** Method of treatment by inunction.

**iatric** (i-at'rik) [ G. *iatros*, physician ]. Medical; produced by a physician.

**iatro-** [ G. *iatros*, physician ]. Combining form denoting relation to physicians or to medicine.

**iatrochemical** (i-at'ro-kem'ĭ-kal). Denoting a school of medicine practicing iatrochemistry.

**iatrochemist** (i-at'ro-kem'ist). A member of the iatrochemical school.

**iatrochemistry** (i-at'ro-kem'is-trī). The study of chemistry in relation to physiologic and pathologic processes and the treatment of disease by chemical substance as practiced by a school of medical thought in the 17th century.

**iatrogenic** (i-at'ro-jen'ik) [ iatro- + G. suffix *-gen*, producing ]. Resulting from, or in the course of, professional activities of a physician or surgeon; often used to imply autosuggestion resulting from physician's discussion, examination, or suggestions.

**iatrology** (i'at-rol'o-jī) [ iatro- + G. *logos*, study ]. Medical science.

**iat'romathemat'ical.** Iatrophysical.

**iatromechanical** (i-at'ro-me-kan'ĭ-kal). Iatrophysical.

**iatrophysical** (i-at'ro-fiz'ĭ-kal). Denoting a school of medicine in the seventeenth century, which explained all physiologic and pathologic phenomena by the laws of physics; opposed to the iatrochemical school.

**iat'rophys'icist.** A member of the iatrophysical school.

**iat'rophys'ics.** Medical physics.

**iatrotechnique** (i-at'ro-tek-nēk') [ iatro- + G. *technē*, art ]. Medical and surgical art; the technique or mode of application of medical science.

**ibogaine** (i-bo'ga-ēn, -in). C$_{20}$H$_{26}$N$_2$O; an alkaloid containing the indolethylamine moiety, a characteristic of many psychotomimetic, hallucinogenic agents; obtained from the African plant, *Tabernanthe iboga* (family Apocynaceae). It is claimed to relieve fatigue, and is being tried as an antidepressant agent.

**ibrotamide.** NEODORM; α-bromo-α-isopropylbutramide; sedative.

**ibufenac** (i-bu'fe-nak) (USAN). DYTRANSIN; (*p*-isobutylphenyl)acetic acid; analgesic with anti-inflammatory properties.

**ibuprofen** (i-bu'pro-fen) (USAN). MOTRIN; *dl-p*-isobutylhydratropic acid; an anti-inflammatory agent.

**-ic.** 1. A suffix denoting that the element to the name of which it is attached is in combination in one of its higher valencies (*e.g.*, phosphoric ester). 2. A suffix indicating an acid (*e.g.*, carboxylic acid).

**ICD.** Abbreviation for *International Classification of Diseases of the World Health Organization.*

**ICDA.** Abbreviation for *International Classification of Diseases, Adapted for Use in the United States;* includes a classification of surgical operations and other therapeutic and diagnostic procedures.

**ice.** Water in its solid state.

**ichnogram** (ik'no-gram) [ G. *ichnos*, footstep, + *gramma*, a drawing, fr. *graphō*, to write ]. Imprint of the soles of the feet, taken standing.

**ichor** (i'kor) [ G. *ichōr*, serum. ICHOR- ]. A thin, watery discharge from an ulcer or unhealthy wound.

**ichoremia** (i'ko-re'mĭ-ah) Ichorrhemia.

**ichoroid** (i'ko-royd) [ G. *ichōr*, serum, + *eidos*, resemblance ]. Denoting a thin, purulent discharge.

**ichorous** (i'kor-us). Relating to or resembling ichor; serous.

**ichorrhea** (i'ko-re'ah) [ G. *ichōr*, serum, + *rhoia*, a flow ]. A profuse ichorous discharge.

**ichorrhemia** (i'ko-re'mĭ-ah) [ G. *ichōr*, serum, + *rhoia*, a flow, + *haima*, blood ]. Ichoremia; blood poisoning from the absorption of an ichorous discharge.

**ichthammol** (ik'tham-mol) (NF, BP). Ammonium ichthosulfonate; sulfonated bitumen; ammonium sulfoichthyolate; a viscous fluid, reddish brown to brownish black in color, with a strong, characteristic, empyreumatic odor, soluble in water and in glycerin; obtained by the destructive distillation of certain bituminous schists, sulfonating the distillate and neutralizing the product with ammonia. It is used in skin disorders; its beneficial effect is due to its mild irritant, stimulant, antiseptic, and analgesic action. Occasionally used as an expectorant.

**ichthulin** (ik'thu-lin). The globulin fraction of fish eggs analogous to the vitellin of birds' eggs; the i. of some fishes is toxic to warm-blooded animals.

**ichthyism** (ik'thĭ-izm) [ G. *ichthys*, fish ]. Ichthyismus; poisoning by eating stale or otherwise unfit fish.

**ichthyismus** (ik'thĭ-iz'mus) [ G. *ichthys*, fish ]. Ichthyism.
  **i. exanthemat'icus**, toxic erythematous eruption due to ingestion of spoiled fish.

**ichthyo-** (ik'thĭ-o-) [ G. *ichthys*, fish ]. Combining form relating to fish.

**ichthyoacanthotoxism** (ik'thĭi-o-ă-kan'tho-tok'sizm) [ ichthyo- + G. *akantha*, thorn, + *toxikon*, poison ]. Poisoning from the stings or spines of venomous fishes.

**ichthyocolla** (ik-thĭ-o-kol'ah) [ ichthyo- + G. *kolla*, glue ]. Isinglass: fish gelatin obtained from sounds or swim bladders of fish such as the hake, cod, and sturgeon; used as a glue, a food substitute, and a clarifying agent.

**ichthyohemotoxin** (ik'thĭ-o-he'mo-tok'sin) [ ichthyo- + G. *haima*, blood, + *toxikon*, poison ]. The toxic substance in the blood of certain fishes.

**ichthyohemotoxism** (ik'thĭ-o-he'mo-tok'sizm). Poisoning resulting from the ingestion of fish containing the toxic substance, ichthyohemotoxin.

**ichthyoid** (ik'thĭ-oyd) [ ichthyo- + G. *eidos*, resemblance ]. Fish-shaped.

**ichthyootoxin** (ik'thĭ-o-o-tok'sin) [ ichthyo- + G. *ōon*, egg, + *toxikon*, poison ]. Toxic substance restricted to the roe of fishes.

**ichthyophagous** (ik'thĭ-of'ă-gus) [ ichthyo- + G. *phagein*, to eat. PHAG- ]. Fish-eating; subsisting on fish.

**ichthyophagy** (ik'thĭ-of'ă-jī) [ ichthyo- + G. *phagein*, to eat ]. The habit of fish-eating.

**ichthyophobia** (ik'thĭ-o-fo'bĭ-ah) [ ichthyo- + G. *phobos*, fear ]. Morbid fear of fish.

**ichthyosarcotoxin** (ik'thĭ-o-sar'ko-tok'sin) [ ichthyo- + G. *sarx*, flesh, + *toxikon*, poison ]. Toxic substance found in the flesh or organs of fishes.

**ichthyosarcotoxism** (ik'thĭ-o-sar'ko-tok'sizm) [ ichthyo- + G. *sarx*, flesh, + *toxikon*, poison ]. Poisoning caused by the toxic substance (ichthyosarcotoxin) in the flesh or organs of fish.

**ichthyosis** (ik-thĭ-o'sis) [ ichthyo- + suffix *-osis*, condition ]. A congenital disorder of keratinization characterized by dryness and fishskin-like scaling of the skin; it is often associated with other defects, and is distinguishable genetically, clinically, and by epidermal cell kinetics; also known as alligator or fish skin; i. sauroderma; sauriasis; sauriderma; sauriosis; sauroderma.
  **acquired i.**, a thickening and scaling of the skin associated with some malignant diseases (*e.g.*, Hodgkin's

disease, lymphosarcoma), leprosy, and severe nutritional deficiencies.

**i. congenita neonatorum,** generalized i. with parchment-like skin seen in premature babies.

**i. cor′nea,** ocular complication of a congenital abnormality of the skin consisting of dryness, scaling and hypercornification.

**i. follicula′ris,** a form of autosomal dominant type of i., with horny follicular plugging of the extensor surfaces of the extremities; onset in early childhood.

**i. hys′trix** [ G. *hystrix,* hedgehog ], epidermolytic *hyperkeratosis.*

**i. intrauteri′na,** i. vulgaris.

**lamellar i.,** a dry form of congenital ichthyosiform erythroderma inherited as an autosomal recessive and present at birth; characterized by large, coarse scales over most of the body and thickened palms and soles, and associated with ectropion; histologically, there is hyperkeratosis, a prominent granular layer in the epidermis, slight acanthosis, many mitotic figures, and rapid epidermal cell turnover.

**i. linguae,** leukoplakia.

**nacreous i.,** dry pearly scales characteristic of this variant.

**i. palma′ris et planta′ris,** *keratosis* palmaris et plantaris.

**i. sauroder′ma** [ G. *sauros,* lizard, + *derma,* skin ], ichthyosis.

**i. scutula′ta** [ L. *scutulatus,* lozenge-shaped, checkered ], i. marked by diamond-shaped or shield-shaped lesions.

**i. seba′cea,** the presence of an unusual amount of vernix caseosa.

**i. seba′cea cornea,** a type of i. with vernix caseosa as seen in the newborn.

**i. sim′plex,** i. vulgaris.

**i. spino′sa,** epidermolytic *hyperkeratosis.*

**i. u′teri,** transformation of the columnar epithelium of the endometrium into stratified squamous epithelium.

**i. vulga′ris,** a form of i. inherited as an autosomal dominant with onset in childhood of fine scales on the trunk and extremities but not on the flexural areas, and associated with atopy and prominent palmar and plantar markings; histologically, there is hyperkeratosis, absence of a granular layer in the epidermis, and normal epidermal cell turnover; also known as hyperkeratosis congenita; i. intrauterina or simplex; keratoma diffusum; keratosis diffusa fetalis.

**x-linked i.,** a form of i. that appears at birth or in early infancy and affects only males; characterized by scaling predominantly on the neck and trunk but not on the palms and soles, and associated with small cataracts; histologically, there is hyperkeratosis, a granular layer in the epidermis, and normal epidermal cell turnover.

**ichthyotic** (ik-thī-ot′ik). Relating to ichthyosis.

**ichthyotocin** (ik′thī-o-to′sin). Isotocin; 4-serine,8-isoleucine oxytocin; a neurohypophysial hormone formed by many bony (teleostean and holostean) fishes; its physiological effect in these animals is unknown.

**ichthyotoxicology** (ik′thī-o-tok-sī-kol′o-jī) [ ichthyo- + G. *toxikon,* poison, + *logos,* study ]. The study of the poisons produced by fishes, their recognition, effects, and antidotes.

**ichthyotoxicon** (ik-thī-o-tok′sī-kon) [ ichthyo- + G. *toxikon,* poison ]. Fish poison; a toxic principle in certain fishes.

**ichthyotoxin** (ik′thī-o-tok′sin) [ ichthyo- + G. *toxicon,* poison ]. The hemolytic active principle of eel serum.

**ichthyotoxism** (ik′thī-o-tok′sizm) [ ichthyo- + G. *toxikon,* poison ]. Poisoning by fish.

**iconolagny** (i-kon-o-lag′nī) [ G. *eikōn,* image, + *lagneia,* lewdness ]. Nonmorbid sexual excitement aroused by the sight of suggestive pictures or sculptures.

**i′conoma′nia** [ G. *eikōn,* image, + *mania,* insanity ]. Morbid impulse to worship images.

**icosahedral** (i′ko-sā-he′dral) [ G. *eikosi,* twenty, + suffix *-edros,* having sides or bases ]. Having 20 equal triangular surfaces (*e.g.,* most viruses with cubic symmetry).

**-ics.** Suffix denoting science, practice, or treatment.

**ICSH.** Abbreviation of interstitial cell-stimulating *hormone.*

**ictal** (ik′tal) [ L. *ictus,* a stroke ]. Relating to or caused by a stroke or seizure (*e.g.,* epilepsy).

**icteric** (ik-tĕr′ik) [ G. *ikterikos,* jaundiced ]. Relating to or marked by icterus (jaundice).

**icteritious** (ik-ter-ish′us). Icteroid.

**ictero-** (ik′ter-o-) [ G. *ikteros,* icterus, jaundice ]. Combining form relating to icterus.

**icteroane′mia.** Hayem-Widal *syndrome.*

**swine i.,** an infectious disease of swine manifested by icterus, anemia, and emaciation; it is associated with, and believed to be caused by *Eperythrozoon suis.*

**ic′terogen′ic** [ ictero- + suffix *-gen,* producing ]. Causing jaundice.

**icterohematuric** (ik′ter-o-hem′ā-tu′rik) [ ictero- + G. *haima,* blood, + *ouron,* urine ]. Denoting jaundice with the passage of blood in the urine.

**ic′terohem′oglobinu′ria.** Jaundice with hemoglobin in the urine.

**ic′terohepati′tis** [ ictero- + G. *hēpar,* liver, + suffix *-itis,* inflammation ]. Inflammation of the liver with jaundice as a prominent symptom.

**icteroid** (ik′ter-oyd) [ ictero- + G. *eidos,* resemblance ]. Icteritious; yellow-hued, or seemingly jaundiced.

**icterus** (ik′ter-us) [ G. *ikteros* ]. Jaundice.

**acquired hemolytic i.,** Hayem-Widal *syndrome.*

**benign familial i.,** familial nonhemolytic *jaundice.*

**chronic familial i.,** hereditary *spherocytosis.*

**congenital hemolytic i.,** hereditary *spherocytosis.*

**cythemolytic i.,** i. caused by absorption of bile produced in excess through stimulation by free hemoglobin caused by the destruction of red blood corpuscles.

**i. gra′vis,** malignant jaundice; jaundice associated with high fever and delirium seen in acute yellow atrophy and other destructive diseases of the liver.

**Gubler's i.,** a form of hematogenous jaundice assumed by Gubler to be due to such rapid hemolysis that the liver is unable to dispose of the hemoglobin set free.

**infectious i.,** Weil's *disease.*

**maverohepatic i.** [ named after Samuel *Maverick,* who gave his name to unbranded cattle ]. Dubin-Johnson *syndrome.*

**i. mel′as,** black jaundice (2); a form in which the skin assumes a dirty dark brown color.

**i. neonato′rum,** Buhl's disease; Winckel's disease; Ritter's disease (2); jaundice of the newborn; black jaundice (1); pedicterus; it is either of a mild form and temporary, physiologic jaundice, or of severe and usually fatal form due to congenital occlusion of the common bile duct, erythroblastosis fetalis, congenital syphilitic cirrhosis of the liver, or septic pylephlebitis.

**physiologic i.,** physiologic jaundice; mild jaundice of the newborn due mainly to functional immaturity of the liver.

**i. pre′cox,** a relatively innocent but rapidly developing type of jaundice with mild anemia in the newborn, most frequently caused by ABO incompatibility between mother and fetus.

**spirochetal i.,** see Weil's *disease.*

**ictom′eter** [ L. *ictus,* stroke, + G. *metron,* measure ]. An apparatus for determining the force of the apex beat of the heart.

**ictus** (ik′tus) [ L. ]. 1. A stroke or attack. 2. A beat.

**i. cordis,** heart *beat.*

**i. epilep′ticus,** an epileptic convulsion.

**i. paralyt′icus,** a paralytic stroke.

**i. san′guinis,** apoplexy.

**i. solis,** sunstroke.

**id** [ L. *id* (3rd person demons. pronoun), that ]. 1. In psychoanalysis, a part of the "psychic or mental apparatus," which is completely in the unconscious realm, unorganized, the reservoir of psychic energy or libido, and under the influence of the primary processes. 2. A single term for the total of all psychic energy available from the innate drives and impulses in a newborn infant. Through socialization this diffuse, undirected energy becomes channeled in less egocentric and more socially responsive directions (development of the ego from the id).

**-id.** 1 [ G. *-eidēs,* resembling, through Fr. *-id* ]. A suffix indicating a state of sensitivity of the skin in which a part remote from the primary lesion reacts ("-id reaction") to substances of the pathogen, giving rise to a secondary inflammatory lesion. The lesion manifesting the reaction is designated by the use of -id as a suffix, *e.g.*, syphilid, tuberculid, microbid. 2 [ G. *-idio- n*, a diminutive ending ]. Suffix indicating a small or young specimen, *e.g.*, spermatid.

**-ide.** A suffix denoting a binary chemical compound; formerly denoted by the qualification, -ureted; as hydrogen sulfide, or sulfureted hydrogen. As suffix to a sugar name, indicates substitution for the H of the hemiacetal OH (*e.g.*, glycoside).

**idea** (i-de´ah) [ G. semblance ]. Any mental image or concept.

**autochthonous i.'s,** thoughts that suddenly burst into awareness as if they are terribly important, often as if they have come from an outside source.

**compulsive i.,** a fixed and inappropriate idea.

**dominant i.,** one that governs all the actions and thoughts of the individual.

**fixed i.,** (1) permanent dominant i.; idée fixe; an obsession; an exaggerated notion, belief, or delusion that persists, despite evidence to the contrary, and controls the mind. (2) the obstinate conviction of a psychotic person regarding the correctness of his delusion.

**hyperquantivalent i.,** an idea which dominates all thought and cannot easily be changed.

**i. of reference,** delusion of reference; the misinterpretation that other people's statements or acts pertain to one's self when, in fact, they do not.

**ideal** (i-de´al). A standard of perfection.

**ego i.,** the i. set by a person for himself; the part of the personality that comprises the goals and aims of the self; it usually refers to the emulation of significant persons with whom it has identified.

**ideation** (i-de-a´shun). The formation of ideas.

**idea´tional.** Relating to ideation, or the formation of ideas.

**idée fixe** (e-da´feks´) [ Fr. obsession ]. Fixed *idea*.

**identification** (i-den´tǐ-fǐ-ka´shun) [ Mediev. L. *identicus,* fr. L. *idem,* the same, + *facio,* to make ]. 1. In the behavioral sciences, an imitation, sense of oneness, or psychic continuity with another person or group. 2. In psychoanalysis, an unconscious defense mechanism in which a person incorporates into himself the mental picture of another person and then patterns himself after this person, and thus sees himself as like that person; distinguished from imitation, a conscious process.

**iden´tity.** The social role of the person and his perception of it.

**ego i.,** the ego's sense of its own identity.

**gender i.,** the anatomical-sexual i. of the person; opposite of gender role.

**masculine i.,** a well-developed sense of gender affiliation with males.

**sense of i.,** the person's sense of his own identity or selfhood.

**ideo-** (i´de-o-, id´e-o-) [ G. *idea,* form, notion ]. Combining form pertaining to ideas or ideation.

**i´deody´namism.** The neural mechanism which generates an idea.

**ideogenetic, ideogenous** (i´de-o-jě-net´ik, i´de-oj´ě-nus). Generated by the mind.

**ideoglandular** (i´de-o-glan´du-lar). Relating to secretion or glandular activity aroused by a mental image, as in the "watering of the mouth" excited by the thought of savory food.

**ideokinetic** (i´de-o-kǐ-net´ik, id´e-o-). Ideomotor.

**ideology** (i´de-ol´o-jǐ; id´e-ol´o-jǐ) [ ideo- + G. *logos,* study ]. The composite system of ideas, beliefs, and attitudes that constitutes an individual's or group's organized view of others.

**i´deometabol´ic.** Pertaining to metabolic changes produced by mental activity.

**ideometabolism** (i-de-o-mě-tab´o-lizm). Metabolism as influenced by the mental processes.

**ideomotion** (i-de-o-mo´shun). Muscular movement executed under the influence of a dominant idea, being practically automatic and not volitional.

**i´deomo´tor.** Ideokinetic; ideomuscular; relating to ideomotion.

**ideomuscular** (i´de-o-mus´ku-lar). Ideomotor.

**ideoplastia** (i-de-o-plas´tǐ-ah) [ ideo- + G. *plassō,* to form ]. The receptive condition in a hypnotized person in which he is thought to be completely open to suggestion.

**ideovascular** (i-de-o-vas´ku-lar). Relating to circulatory changes excited by a mental image or idea.

**idio-** (id´ǐ-o-) [ G. *idios,* one's own. IDIO- ]. Combining form meaning private, distinctive, peculiar to.

**idioagglutinin** (id´ǐ-o-ǎ-glu´tin-in). An agglutinin that occurs naturally in the blood of a person or an animal, without the injection of a stimulating antigen or the passive transfer of antibody.

**idiochromosome** (id´ǐ-o-kro´mo-sōm). Sex *chromosome*.

**idiocrasy** (id´ǐ-ok´rǎ-sǐ) [ G. *idiokrasia,* a peculiar temperament, fr. *idios,* individual, + *krasis,* a mixture, temperament ]. Idiosyncrasy.

**id´iocrat´ic.** Idiosyncratic.

**idiocy** (id´ǐ-o-sǐ) [ G. *idiōteria,* awkwardness, uncouthness. IDIO- ]. An obsolete term for a subclass of mental *retardation* (*q. v.*).

**amaurotic familial i.,** obsolete term for cerebral *sphingolipidosis.*

**Aztec i.,** microcephalic i., marked by receding forehead and chin, the profile having a triangular form.

**cre´tinoid i.,** cretinism.

**diple´gic i.,** paralytic i. in which the paralysis affects like extremities on both sides of the body.

**eclamptic i.,** i. resulting from the convulsive state.

**epileptic i.,** i. associated with epilepsy.

**gen´etous i.,** congenital i. of obscure causation.

**hemiple´gic i.,** paralytic i. in which the paralysis has the form of hemiplegia.

**hydrocephal´ic i.,** i. associated with chronic hydrocephalus.

**microcephal´ic i.,** i. occurring in a child with small skull and brain, without paralysis or other signs of a focal lesion.

**mongo´lian** or **mon´goloid i.,** Down's *syndrome.*

**paralytic i.,** i. due to cerebral lesions occurring in infancy and causing spastic or other forms of paralysis.

**paraple´gic i.,** paralytic i. in which the muscular affection has the form of a paraplegia.

**senso´rial i.,** mental deficiency dependent upon the loss in infancy, or congenital absence, of one or more of the special senses.

**traumatic i.,** mental deficiency assumed to be due to a fall, a blow, or other injury received at birth, in infancy, or in early childhood.

**id´iodynam´ic.** Independently active.

**idiogamist** (id´ǐ-og´ǎ-mist) [ idio- + G. *gamos,* marriage ]. One who is capable of sexual union with only one or a few individuals of the opposite sex, being impotent in the presence of any others.

**idiogenesis** (id´ǐ-o-jen´ě-sis) [ idio- + G. *genesis,* production ]. Origin without evident cause; denoting especially that of a so-called idiopathic disease.

**id´ioglos´sia** [ idio- + G. *glōssa,* tongue, speech ]. An extreme form of lalling or vowel or consonant substitution, by which the speech of a child may be made unintelligible and appear to be another language to one who has not the key to the literal changes.

**id´ioglot´tic.** Relating to idioglossia.

**id´iogram** [ idio- + G. *gramma,* something written ]. 1. Karyotype. 2. A diagrammatic representation of chromosome morphology characteristic of a species or population.

**id´iograph´ic** [ idio- + G. *graphō,* to write ]. Pertaining to the behavior of a particular individual as an individual, as opposed to nomothetic; i. analyses are of special interest in clinical psychology.

**idioheteroagglutinin** (id´ǐ-o-het´er-o-ǎ-glu´tin-in) [ idio- + G. *heteros,* another, + agglutinin ]. An idioagglutinin occurring in the blood of one animal, but capable of combining with the antigenic material from another species.

**id´ioheterol´ysin.** An idiolysin occurring in the blood of an animal of one species, but capable of combining with the red blood cells of another species, thereby causing hemolysis when complement is present.

**idiohypnotism** (id-ǐ-o-hip´no-tizm). Autohypnosis.

**idioisoagglutinin** (id'ĭ-o-i'so-ă-glu'tin-in) [ idio- + G. *isos*, equal, + agglutinin ]. An idioagglutinin occurring in the blood of an animal of a certain species, capable of agglutinating the cells from animals of the same species.

**idioisolysin** (id'ĭ-o-i-sol'ĭ-sin). An idiolysin occurring in the blood of an animal of a certain species, capable of combining with the red blood cells from animals of the same species, thereby causing hemolysis when complement is present.

**id'iola'lia** [ idio- + G. *lalia*, talk ]. The use of a language invented by the person himself.

**idiolysin** (id-ĭ-ol'ĭ-sin). A lysin that occurs naturally in the blood of a person or an animal, without the injection of a stimulating antigen or the passive transfer of antibody.

**idiometritis** (id-ĭ-o-me-tri'tis) [ idio- + G. *metra*, womb, + suffix *-itis*, inflammation ]. Uterine myositis; inflammation of the uterine musculature.

**idiomuscular** (id'ĭ-o-mus'ku-lar). Relating to the muscles alone, independent of the nervous control.

**idioneurosis** (id'ĭ-o-nu-ro'sis). A functional neurosis; one arising without apparent extrinsic cause.

**id'iono'dal.** Arising from the A-V node itself; applied to the ventricular rhythm in complete S-A or A-V block, or in other forms of A-V dissociation, when the A-V node rather than an ectopic ventricular focus controls the ventricles; see also idioventricular.

**id'iopathet'ic.** Idiopathic.

**id'iopath'ic** [ idio- + G. *pathos*, suffering ]. Denoting a disease of unknown cause.

**idiopathy** (id'ĭ-op'ă-thĭ) [ idio- + G. *pathos*, suffering ]. A primary disease; one arising without apparent extrinsic cause.

**idiophrenic** (id'ĭ-o-fren'ik) [ idio- + G. *phrēn*, mind ]. Relating to, or originating in, the mind or brain alone, not reflex or secondary.

**idiopsychologic** (id'ĭ-o-si-ko-loj'ik). Relating to ideas developed within one's own mind, independent of suggestion from without.

**idioreflex** (id-ĭ-o-re'fleks). A reflex due to a stimulus or irritation originating in the organ or part in which the reflex occurs.

**idiosome** (id'ĭ-o-sōm) [ idio- + G. *sōma*, body ]. 1. The attraction sphere of a spermatid or of an oocyte. 2. The indivisible element of living matter.

**idiospasm** (id'ĭ-o-spazm). A localized spasm.

**idiosyncrasy** (id'ĭ-o-sin'kra-sĭ) [ G. *idiosynkrasia*, fr. *idios*, one's own, + *synkrasis*, a mixing together ]. 1. Idiocrasy; an individual mental, behavioral, or physical characteristic of peculiarity. 2. Idiosyncratic sensitivity; an acquired (induced) sensitivity (allergy) to certain foods, drugs, etc., associated with the Prausnitz-Küstner (IgE class) antibody and marked by a strong familial (hereditary) tendency, rendering it peculiar to a relatively small portion of the total population. See also acquired (induced) *sensitivity*.

**id'iosyncrat'ic.** Idiocratic; relating to or marked by an idiosyncrasy.

**idiot** (id'ĭ-ot) [ G. *idiōtēs*, an ignorant, uncouth person. IDIO- ]. An obsolete term for a subclass of mental *retardation* (*q.v.*) or an individual classified therein.

  **mongolian i.,** a pejorative term for a person exhibiting mongolism (Down's syndrome).

  **pithecoid i.,** one having an apelike formation of the face.

**idiot-prodigy.** Idiot-savant.

**idiot-savant** [ Fr. ], Idiot-prodigy; a person of low general intelligence who possesses an unusual faculty in doing mental arithmetic, remembering dates or numbers, or in performing other mental tasks of which most normal persons are incapable.

**idiotrophic** (id'ĭ-o-trof'ik) [ idio- + G. *trophē*, food ]. Capable of choosing its own food.

**idiotropic** (id'ĭ-o-trop'ik) [ idio- + G. *tropē*, a turning ]. Turning inward upon one's self.

**idiovariation** (id-ĭ-o-va-rĭ-a'shun). The process of constant change in the hereditary qualities of a strain of organism; mutation.

**idioventricular** (id-ĭ-o-ven-trik'u-lar). Pertaining to or associated with the cardiac ventricles alone, when dissociated from the atria.

**iditol** (i'dĭ-tol). Reduction product of the hexose idose.

**i'dose.** One of the aldohexoses, isomeric with glucose and galactose. See formulas under sugar.

**idoxuridine** (i'doks-u'rĭ-dēn) (USP, BP). 2'-Deoxy-5-iodouridine; 5-iododeoxyuridine (IdUrd; IdU); a pyrimidine analogue that produces both antiviral and anticancer effects by interference with DNA synthesis; used locally in the eye for the treatment of keratitis from herpes simplex or vaccinia.

**IDP.** Abbreviation for inosine 5'-diphosphate.

**idro'sis** [ G. *hidrōs*, sweat ]. Hidrosis.

**iduron'ic acid.** The uronic acid of idose; a constituent of dermatan sulfate (formerly chondroitin sulfate B).

**Ig.** Abbreviation for immunoglobulin.

**ignatia** (ig-na'shĭ-ah) [ *St. Ignatius* ]. Ignatia amara; St. Ignatius' bean; the dried ripe seed of *Strychnos ignatii* (family Loganiaceae). It is similar in its properties to nux vomica and is a source of strychnine.

**ignipedites** (ig'nĭ-pĕ-di'tēz) [ L. *ignis*, fire, + *pes* (*ped-*), foot, + G. *itēs* ]. Hot-foot; burning pain in the soles of the feet, due to multiple neuritis.

**ig'nis** [ L. ]. Fire.

  **i. sa'cer** [ sacred fire ], obsolete term for herpes zoster.

**ig'notine.** Carnosine.

**IH.** Abbreviation for infectious *hepatitis*.

**iko'ta.** A neurosis, similar to latah, affecting married women among the Samoyeds of Siberia.

**ILA.** Abbreviation for insulin-like activity; see under insulin.

**Ile.** Symbol for the isoleucine radical (sometimes, incorrectly, Ilu or Ileu).

**ileac** (il'e-ak). Relating to (1) ileus, and (2) the ileum.

**ileadelphus** (il'e-ă-del'fus). Iliadelphus.

**ileal** (il'e-al). Of or pertaining to the ileum.

**ileectomy** (il-e-ek'to-mĭ) [ ileum + G. *ektomē*, excision ]. Removal of the ileum.

**ileitis** (il-e-i'tis). Inflammation of the ileum.

  **backwash i.,** term applied to involvement of the terminal ileum in the inflammatory and ulcerative changes seen in chronic ulcerative colitis; in some cases this may represent involvement of ileum and proximal colon by a granulomatous process (*i.e.*, Crohn's disease of terminal ileum and proximal colon).

  **distal i.,** regional *enteritis*.

  **regional i.,** regional *enteritis*.

  **terminal i.,** regional *enteritis*.

**ileo-** (il'e-o-) [ ileum, *q.v.* ]. Combining form denoting relationship to the ileum.

**ileocecal** (il'e-o-se'kal). Relating to both ileum and cecum.

**ileocecostomy** (il'e-o-se-kos'to-mĭ). Cecoileostomy; surgical anastomosis of ileum to cecum.

**ileocecum** (il-e-o-se'kum). The combined ileum and cecum.

**il'eocol'ic.** Relating to the ileum and the colon.

**ileocolitis** (il-e-o-ko-li'tis). Inflammation of the mucous membrane of a greater or lesser extent of both ileum and colon.

  **i. ulcero'sa chron'ica,** a chronic form of i. marked by mild intermittent fever, anorexia, anemia, slight diarrhea, dull pain in the inguinal (or iliac) region, and rapid pulse.

**il'eocolon'ic.** Ileocolic.

**ileocolostomy** (il'e-o-ko-los'to-mĭ) [ ileo- + colostomy ]. The establishment of a communication between the ileum and the colon.

**il'eocolot'omy.** Ileocolostomy.

**ileocystoplasty** (il'e-o-sis'to-plas'tĭ) [ ileo- + G. *kystis*, bladder, + *plastos*, molded ]. The use of an isolated intestinal segment to augment bladder capacity.

**ileoentectropy** (il'e-o-en-tek'tro-pĭ) [ ileo- + G. *entos*, within, + *ek*, out, + *tropē*, a turning ]. Eversion of a segment of the ileum.

**ileoileostomy** (il'e-o-il-e-os'to-mĭ) [ ileum + ileum + G. *stoma*, mouth ]. Establishment of a communication between two noncontinuous portions of the ileum.

**ileojejunitis** (il'e-o-jĕ-ju-ni'tis). A chronic inflammatory condition involving the jejunum and parts or most of the ileum. It takes different forms; a granulomatous state resembling regional ileitis may be present; pseudodiverticula may form, or cicatricial stenosis of the bowel may occur.

**ileopexy** (il'e-o-pek'sĭ) [ ileo- + G. *pēxis,* fixation ]. Surgical fixation of ileum in an unnatural position.

**ileoproctostomy** (il'e-o-prok-tos'to-mĭ) [ ileo- + G. *prŏktos,* anus (rectum), + *stoma,* mouth ]. Establishment of a communication between the ileum and the rectum.

**ileorectostomy** (il'e-o-rek-tos'to-mĭ) [ ileum + rectum + G. *stoma,* mouth ]. Ileoproctostomy.

**ileorrhaphy** (il'e-or'ă-fĭ) [ ileo- + G. *raphe,* suture ]. Suturing the ileum.

**ileosigmoidostomy** (il'e-o-sig'moyd-os'ko-pĭ) [ ileo- + sigmoid, + G. *stoma,* mouth ]. Establishment of a communication between the ileum and the sigmoid colon.

**ileostomy** (il'e-os'to-mĭ) [ ileo- + G. *stoma,* mouth ]. The establishment of a fistula leading from without into the ileum.

**ileotomy** (il'e-ot'o-mĭ) [ ileo- + G. *tomē,* incision ]. Cutting into the ileum.

**il'eotransversos'tomy** [ ileum + transverse colon, + G. *stoma,* mouth ]. Surgical anastomosis of ileum to transverse colon.

**il'eoty'phus.** Obsolete term for typhoid fever.

**ileum** (il'e-um) [ L. fr. G. *eileō,* to roll up, twist ] [ NA ]. The third portion of the small intestine, about 12 feet in length, extending from the junction with the jejunum to the orifice of the terminal ileum.

 **i. du'plex,** tubular or cystic segmental duplications of alimentary tract.

**ileus** (il'e-us) [ G. *eileos,* intestinal colic, from *eilō,* to roll up tight ]. Mechanical or adynamic obstruction of the bowel attended with severe colicky pain, vomiting, and often fever and dehydration.

 **adynam'ic i.,** paralytic i.

 **dynam'ic i.,** obstruction due to spastic contraction of a segment of the bowel.

 **gallstone i.,** obstruction of the small intestine produced by passage of a gallstone from the biliary tract (usually gallbladder) into the intestinal tract (usually duodenum); occurrence and site of obstruction depend upon size of the stone; however, the usual location is at or near the ileocecal junction.

 **mechanical i.,** obstruction of the bowel due to some mechanical cause, *e.g.,* volvulus, gallstone, adhesions, etc.

 **meconium i.,** intestinal obstruction in the newborn following inspissation of meconium due to lack of trypsin; associated with cystic fibrosis of pancreas.

 **occlusive i.,** complete mechanical blocking of the intestinal lumen.

 **paralyt'ic i.,** nonmechanical obstruction of the bowel from paralysis of bowel wall usually as a result of localized or generalized peritonitis or shock.

 **spastic i.,** dynamic i.

 **i. subpar'ta,** obstruction of the large bowel by pressure of the pregnant uterus.

 **terminal i.,** obstruction of the lower part of the small bowel.

 **verminous i.,** obstruction due to masses of intestinal parasites.

**iliac** (il'ĭ-ak). Relating to the ilium.

**ili'acus.** See *musculus* iliacus.

**iliadelphus** (il'ĭ-ă-del'fus) [ L. *ilium* + G. *adelphos,* brother ]. *Duplicitas* posterior.

**ilio-** (il'ĭ-o-) [ L. *ilium, q. v.* ]. Combining form denoting relationship to the ilium.

**iliococcygeal** (il'ĭ-o-kok-sij'e-al). Relating to the ilium and the coccyx.

**iliocolotomy** (il'ĭ-o-ko-lot'o-mĭ) [ ilio- G. *kolon,* colon, + *tomē,* incision ]. The operation of opening into the colon in the iliac, or inguinal, region.

**il'iocos'tal.** Relating to the ilium and the ribs; denoting muscles passing between the two parts.

**il'iocosta'lis.** See *musculus* iliocostalis.

**il'iofem'oral.** Relating to the ilium and the femur.

**il'iofem'oroplas'ty.** A method of securing a hip fusion by an extra-articular technique (a joint by-pass procedure) in which a turned down bone flap from the ilium is placed into a split in the greater trochanter.

**il'iohypogas'tric.** Relating to the iliac and the hypogastric regions.

**ilioinguinal** (il'ĭ-o-ing'gwĭ-nal). Relating to the iliac region and the groin.

**iliolumbar** (il-ĭ-o-lum'bar). Relating to the iliac and the lumbar regions.

**iliometer** (il'ĭ-om'e-ter) [ ilio- + G. *metron,* measure ]. An instrument for measuring exact position of iliac spines and lower vertebrae.

**iliopagus** (il'ĭ-op'ă-gus) [ ilio- + G. *pagos,* something fixed ]. Conjoined twins in which the fusion is restricted to the iliac region.

**iliopectineal** (il'ĭ-o-pek-tin'e-al). Relating to the ilium and the pubes.

**il'iopel'vic.** Relating to the iliac region and the cavity of the pelvis.

**il'iosa'cral.** Relating to the ilium and the sacrum.

**iliosciatic** (il'-ĭ-o-si-at'ik). Relating to the ilium and the ischium.

**il'iospi'nal.** Relating to the ilium and the spinal column.

**iliothoracopagus** (il'ĭ-o-tho-ră-kop'ă-gus) [ ilio- + G. *thorax,* chest, + *pagos,* fixed ]. Ischiothoracopagus; conjoined twins in which union occurs through the ilia and extends to involve the thoraces.

**il'iotib'ial.** Relating to the ilium and the tibia.

**iliotrochanteric** (il'ĭ-o-tro-kan-ter'ik). Relating to the ilium and the great trochanter of the femur.

**ilioxiphopagus** (il'ĭ-o-zi-fop'ă-gus) [ ilio- + xiphoid, + G. *pagos,* fixed ]. Conjoined twins in which the fusion extends from the xiphoid to the iliac region.

**ilium,** pl. **il'ia** (il'ĭ-um) [ L. groin, flank ] [ NA ]. *Os* ilium.

**ill.** In veterinary medicine, a term used to denote disease.

 **joint i.,** joint evil; a chronic suppurative inflammation of the joints of foals and other newly born animals, due to umbilical infection with pyogenic bacteria, one of the commonest being *Actinobacillus equuli.*

 **leaping i.,** louping i.

 **louping i.,** leaping i.; a highly virulent viral encephalomyelitis of sheep characterized by cerebellar ataxia and spread by ticks; it can also affect cattle and man.

 **navel i.,** a term applied to any kind of acute generalized infections of young mammals having their origin in a wound infection occurring in the stump of the umbilical cord; these infections generally are pyemic, and liver and lung abscesses and multiple acute arthritis are characteristic.

 **quarter i.,** blackleg.

**illaqueation** (il'ă-kwe-a'shun) [ L. *il-laqueo,* pp. -*atus,* to ensnare (*in* + *laqueo*) ]. Pulling away an inverted eyelash by passing a loop of thread behind it.

**illicium** (il-lis'e-um) [ L. an allurement, fr. *il-licio,* to allure ]. Chinese or star anise; the dried fruit of *Ilicium verum* (family Magnoliaceae), an evergreen shrub or small tree of southern China. Stimulating carminative.

**illinition** (il-in-ish'un) [ L. *il-lino,* pp. -*litus,* to smear on (*in* + *lino*) ]. Friction of the surface made after the application of an ointment, to facilitate absorption.

**ill'ness.** Disease.

 **functional i.,** functional *disorder.*

 **mental i.,** (1) also variously referred to as mental or emotional disease, disturbance, or disorder or behavioral disorder; a broadly inclusive term, generally denoting one or all of the following: (*a*) a disease of the brain, with predominant behavioral symptoms, as in paresis or acute alcoholism; (*b*) a disease of the "mind" or personality, evidenced by abnormal behavior, as in hysteria or schizophrenia; (*c*) a disorder of conduct, evidenced by socially deviant behavior, as in promiscuity or homosexuality; (2) any psychiatric illness listed in the *Standard Nomenclature of Diseases and Operations* of the American Medical Association, or in the *Diagnostic and Statistical Manual for Mental Disorders* of the American Psychiatric Association.

**illumination** (ĭ-lu'mĭ-na'shun) [ L. *il-lumino,* pp. -*atus,* to light up, fr. *lumen* (-*min*-), light ]. 1. Throwing light on the body or a part or into a cavity for diagnostic purposes. 2. Lighting an object under a microscope.

**ax'ial i.,** central i.; the transmission or reflection of light in the direction of the axis of the optical system in a microscope.

**central i.,** axial i.

**contact i.,** i. of the eye by means of an instrument in contact with the cornea or bulbar conjunctiva.

**critical i.,** the precise focusing of the light source directly upon the object being examined.

**dark-field i.,** a procedure in which a black circular shield is used to block the majority of the vertically directed rays of light (*i.e.*, the field is dark), and a circumferential, suitably angled, mirrored surface is used to direct the peripheral rays horizontally against the object, thereby reflecting the light vertically through the objective lens and along the optical axis; thus, the object is well illuminated in a contrasting dark background.

**dark-ground i.,** dark-field i.

**direct i.,** erect or vertical i.; that in which the rays of light are directed downward, almost perpendicularly onto the upper surface of the object, which reflects the rays upward into the optical system.

**erect i.,** direct i.

**Köhler i.,** i. of microscopic objects where the light source is focused on the condenser diaphragm and the diaphragm of the light is in focus with the object to be observed.

**lateral i.,** oblique i.; the rays of light are directed diagonally onto the upper surface of the object, from a source located to one side and slightly above the object.

**oblique i.,** lateral i.

**through i.,** transillumination.

**vertical i.,** direct i.

**illuminism** (ī-lu'mǐ-nizm). A state of exaltation shown by a psychotic patient in which he has delusions and hallucinations of communion with supernatural or exalted beings.

**illusion** (ī-lu'zhun) [ L. *illusio*, fr. *il-ludo*, pp. -*lusus*, to play at, mock (*in* + *ludo*, play) ]. A false perception; the mistaking of something for what it is not.

**optical i.,** a false interpretation of a visual sensation; Zöllner's lines (*q. v.* under line) illustrate one of the many geometrical optical i.'s.

**illusional** (ī-lu'zhun-al). Relating to or of the nature of an illusion.

**illyngophobia** (il-ling'o-pho'bī-ah) [ G. *illyngos*, dizziness, + *phobos*, fear ]. Fear of vertigo.

**I.M., i.m.** Abbreviation for intramuscular, or intramuscularly.

**ima** (i'mah) [ L. ]. Lowest; see also imus.

**image** (im'ij) [ L. *imago*, likeness ]. The representation or picture of an object made by the rays of light emanating or reflected from it.

**accidental i.,** afterimage.

**after-i.,** see afterimage.

**body i.,** body schema; (1) the cerebral representation of all body sensation organized in the parietal cortex; (2) the person's i. or concept of his own body, in contrast to his actual, anatomic body or to others' concept of it.

**direct i.,** a virtual i., such as the erect i. in direct ophthalmoscopy.

**eidetic i.,** vivid mental i. in the form of a dream, fantasy, or an unusual power of memory and visualization of objects previously seen or imagined.

**false i.,** the i. in the deviating eye in strabismus.

**heteronymous i.,** a double i. in physiological diplopia, when fixation is beyond the object; the right i. then comes from the left eye, while the left i. originates from the right eye.

**homonymous i.'s.,** double i.'s produced by stimuli arising from points proximal to the horopter.

**hypnagogic i.,** imagery occurring between wakefulness and sleep.

**hypnopompic i.,** imagery occurring after the sleeping state and before complete wakefulness; similar to hypnagogic imagery except for the time of occurrence.

**incidental i.,** afterimage.

**inverted i.,** real i.

**mental i.,** a picture of an object not present, produced in the mind by memory or imagination.

**mirror i.,** a representation of an object or part thereof as its reflected i. in a glass mirror.

**motor i.,** the cerebral i. of possible body movements.

**optical i.,** an i. formed by the refraction or reflection of light.

**Purkinje's i.'s,** three reflections of an i., noted by one looking at the pupil of another person, formed by the anterior surface of the cornea and the two surfaces of the crystalline lens; the first two are upright and virtual i.'s; that from the posterior surface of the crystalline lens is inverted and real; called also Purkinje-Sanson i.'s; Sanson's i.'s.

**Purkinje-Sanson i.'s,** Purkinje i.'s.

**real i.,** inverted i.; one formed by the convergence of the actual rays of light from an object.

**ret'inal i.,** a real i. formed on the retina.

**Sanson's i.'s,** Purkinje's i.'s.

**sensory i.,** based on one or more types of sensation.

**specular i.,** the i. of a source of light made visible by the relection from a mirror.

**tactile i.,** an i. of an object as perceived by the sense of touch.

**virtual i.,** an erect i. formed by the projection of rays by the eye; though perceptible to the eye it cannot be thrown on a screen. In direct ophthalmoscopy, the i. is virtual.

**visual i.,** a collection of foci corresponding to all the luminous points of an object.

**imaginal** (ī-maj'ǐ-nal). Relating to an image or to the process of imagining.

**imago** (ī-ma'go) [ L. image ]. 1. The last stage of an insect after it has completed all its metamorphoses through the egg, larva, and pupa; the adult insect form. 2. Archetype (2).

**imbal'ance** [ L. *in*- neg. + *bi-lanx* (-*lanc*-), having two scales, fr. *bis*, twice, + *lanx*, dish, scale of a balance ]. 1. Lack of equality in power between opposing forces. 2. Lack of equality in some aspect of binocular vision, such as strabismus, heterophoria, anisometropia, or aniseikonia.

**autonom'ic i.,** a lack of balance between sympathetic and parasympathetic nervous systems, especially in relation to the vasomotor disturbances.

**sex chromosome i.,** see under chromosome.

**sympathet'ic i.,** vagotonia.

**vasomo'tor i.,** autonomic i.

**imbecile** (im'bĕ-sil) [ L. *imbecillus*, weak, silly ]. An obsolete term for a subclass of mental *retardation* (*q. v.*).

**moral i.,** amoralis; an obsolete term for a person with pronounced mental defect who has strong criminal propensities little or not at all affected by punishment.

**imbed.** Embed.

**imbibition** (im'bĭ-bish'un) [ L. *im-bibo*, to drink in (*in* + *bibo*) ]. 1. The absorption of fluid by a solid body without resultant chemical change in either. 2. Taking up of water by a gel. This increases the size of the gel.

**imbricate, imbricated** (im'brĭ-kāt, im'brĭ-ka-ted) [ L. *imbricatus*, covered with tiles ]. Overlapping like shingles.

**imbrication** (im'brĭ-ka'shun) [ see imbricate ]. The operative overlapping of layers of tissue in the closure of wounds or the repair of defects.

**Imhotep, Iemhetep** (ēm-hō'tep, i-em-hē'tep). Ancient Egyptian demigod of medicine, corresponding to the Roman Aesculapius and the Greek Asclepios.

**imidazole** (im'id-az'ōl). Glyoxaline; 1,3-diazole; 1,3-diaza-2,4-cyclopentadiene; a five-membered heterocyclic compound occurring in histidine.

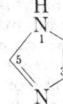

Imidazole

**imidazolyl** (im'id-az'o-lil). Iminazolyl; the radical of imidazole, as in imidazolylethylamine (histamine).

**imide** (im'īd). The radical or group, =NH, attached to two —CO— groups (as in succinimide).

**imido-** (im'ī-do-, ī-me'do-). Prefix denoting the radical of an imide, formed by the loss of the H of the =NH group (*e.g.*, succinimido-).

**im'idopep'tidase.** Proline dipeptidase.

**im'inaz'olyl.** Imidazolyl.

**-imine.** Suffix indicating the group $= NH$.

**imino-** (im'ĭ-no-, ĭ-me'no-). Prefix denoting an imine.

**im'ino acids.** Compounds with molecules containing both an acid group (usually the carboxyl, COOH) and an imino group ($= NH$); e.g., proline and hydroxyproline.

**im'inodipep'tidase** Prolyl dipeptidase.

**iminoglycinuria** (im'in-o-gli-sĭ-nu'rĭ-ah). A benign inborn error of amino acid transport; glycine, proline, and hydroxyproline are excreted in the urine.

**im'inohy'drolases.** Enzymes hydrolyzing imino groups (e.g.,arginine deiminase);distinct from amidinohydrolases.

**imipramine hydrochloride** (USP, BP). TOFRANIL; PRESA-MINE; 5-(3-dimethylaminopropyl)-10,11-dihydro-5H-dibenz(b,f)azepine hydrochloride; an antidepressant.

**Imlach** (im'lak), Francis, Scottish anatomist and surgeon, 1819–1891. See I.'s fat-pad, ring.

**immedicable** (im-med'ĭ-kă-bl) [ L. in- neg. + medicabilis, curable ]. Incurable; beyond the reach of remedies.

**immersion** (ĭ-mer'zhun) [ L. im-mergo, pp. -mersus, to dip in (in + mergo) ]. 1. The placing of a body under water or other liquid. 2. In microscopy, the use of a fluid medium (placed on the slide being examined) in order to exclude air from between the glass slide and the bottom lens of an immersion objective, which is brought into direct contact with the fluid; this procedure prevents much loss of light that results from diffusion when rays pass through glass (the slide) and into air.

  **homoge'neous i.,** the use of a fluid that has a refractive index virtually identical to that of glass.

  **oil i., water i.,** see immersion system.

**immiscible** (im-mis'ĭ-bl) [ L. im-misceo, to mix in (in + misceo ]. Incapable of mutual solution; e.g., oil and water.

**immobilization** (im-mo'bĭ-lĭ-za'shun) [ see immobilize ]. The act of making immovable.

**immobilize** (im-mo'bĭ-lĭz) [ L. in-neg. + mobilis, movable. MOV- ]. To render fixed or incapable of moving.

**immune** (ĭ-mūn') [ L. immunis, free from service, fr. in, neg., + munus (muner-), service ]. 1. Free from the possibility of acquiring a given infectious disease; resistant to an infectious disease. 2. Pertaining to the mechanism of sensitization (allergization) in which the reactivity is so altered by previous contact with an antigen that the responsive tissues respond quickly upon subsequent contact, or to in vitro reactions with antibody-containing serum from such sensitized (allergized) animals or persons.

**immunifacient** (im'mu-nĭ-fa'shent) [ L. immunis, exempt, + faciens, making, pr. part. of facio ]. Making immune; said of a semelincident disease or of a prophylactic serum or vaccine.

**immu'nitas** [ L. ]. Immunity.

  **i. non sterili'sans,** infection immunity, q.v., a condition in which a person has natural or acquired immunity to certain antigens, toxins, or noxious substances from microorganisms, although the latter persist in the body; for example, carriers may harbor large numbers of typhoid organisms, but have no signs or symptoms of illness caused by such bacteria.

**immunity** (ĭ-mu'nĭ-tĭ) [ L. immunitas (see immune) ]. The status or quality of being immune.

  **acquired i.,** resistance as the result of previous experience in the lifetime of the individual in question. It may be active and specific as a result of naturally acquired (apparent or inapparent) infection or of intentional vaccination (artificial active i.); or it may be passive, being acquired from transfer of antibodies from another person or from an animal, either naturally, as from mother to fetus, or by intentional inoculation (artificial passive i.), and, with respect to the particular antibodies transferred, it is specific.

  **active i.,** see acquired i.

  **antivi'ral i.,** i. resulting from virus infection, either naturally acquired or produced by intentional vaccination; compared to some bacterial i.'s, it is of relatively long duration, but this may be the result of infection-immunity rather than being peculiar to virus infection per se, since it occurs also in bacterial i. after infections such as typhoid fever.

  **artificial active i.,** see acquired i.

  **artificial passive i.,** see acquired i.

  **bacteriophage i.,** the state that is induced in a bacterium by lysogenization, the lysogenic bacterium being insusceptible to further lysogenization or to a lytic cycle by a superinfecting bacteriophage, in contradistinction to bacteriophage resistance, q.v.

  **cell-mediated i.,** cellular i.

  **cellular i.,** cell-mediated i.; i. associated with cellular elements, in contradistinction to humoral i., as originally proposed in Metchnikoff's phagocytic theory.

  **genetic i.,** innate i.

  **group** or **herd i.,** a concept that there is resistance or relative resistance to the spread of infectious disease in a herd or group, irrespective of the presence or absence of a significant degree of i. in the individual members of the herd or group.

  **humoral i.,** i. associated with circulating antibodies, in contradistinction to cellular i.

  **infection-i.,** the paradoxical immune status in which resistance to reinfection coincides with the persistence of the original infection.

  **inhe'rent i.,** innate i.

  **innate i.,** inherent, genetic, or natural, or nonspecific i.; autarcesis; resistance manifested by a species, or by races, families, and individuals in a species, although the groups or individuals had not been immunized (sensitized, allergized) by previous infection or vaccination. It results from body mechanisms that are poorly understood, but are different from those responsible for the altered reactivity (see immune (2)) associated with the specific nature of acquired i., and, in general, is nonspecific and is not stimulated by specific antigens.

  **local i.,** a natural or acquired i. to certain infectious agents, as manifested by some organs, tissues, or relatively large regions of the body.

  **natural i.,** innate i.

  **nonspecific i.,** innate i.

  **passive i.,** see acquired i.

  **relative i.,** a modified, not completely effective resistance that results when there is a sort of "fluctuating equilibrium" between the defense mechanisms of the host and the infective agent.

  **specific i.,** the immune status (see immune (2)) in which there is an altered reactivity directed solely against the antigenic determinants (infectious agent or other) that stimulated it; see acquired i.

  **specific active i.,** see acquired i.

  **specific innate i.,** see acquired i.

  **stress i.,** insusceptibility or resistance to the effects of emotional strain.

**immunization** (im'u-nĭ-za'shun). Vaccination; allergization; the process or procedure by which resistance is produced in a person, animal, or plant.

  **active i.,** the production of active immunity.

  **passive i.,** the production of passive immunity.

**immuno-** (im'u-no-, ĭ-mu'no-) [ L. immunis, immune, q.v. ]. Combining form meaning immune, or relating to immunity.

**im'munoagglutina'tion.** Specific agglutination effected by antibody.

**im'munoas'say.** Immunochemical assay; detection and assay of hormones, or other substances, by serological (immunological) methods; in most applications the hormones (or other substance) in question serves as antigen, both in antibody production and in measurement of antibody by the test substance. See also radioimmunoassay; radioimmunoelectrophoresis; immunological pregnancy test.

  **double antibody i.,** double antibody precipitation.

**immunochemistry** (im'u-no-kem'is-trĭ). The special field of chemistry that pertains to immunologic phenomena, e.g., chemical reactions related to antigen stimulation of tissues, chemical studies of antigens and antibody, and so on.

**im'munoconglu'tinin.** An autoantibody kind of immunoglobulin (IgM) formed in animals (or man) against their own complement following injection of complement-containing complexes or sensitized bacteria. To be distinguished from conglutinins, which are normal serum components of bovine species.

**immunocyte** (im'u-no-sīt) [ immuno- + G. *kytos*, cell ]. A leukocyte capable, actively or potentially, of producing antibodies.

**immunocytology** (im'mu-no-si-tol'o-jī) [ immuno- + G. *kytos*, cell, + *logos*, study ]. The study of cell constituents by immunologic methods, such as the use of fluorescent antibodies.

**immunodeficiency** (im'u-no-de-fish'en-si). Immunological d.; immunity or immune deficiency; a condition resulting from ineffective functioning of the immunological mechanism. I.'s may be *primary* (due to a defect in the immune mechanism *per se*), or they may be *secondary* (dependent upon another disease process). They may be *specific* (due to defect in either the B-lymphocyte or the T-lymphocyte system, or both), or they may be *nonspecific* (due to defect in one or another component of the nonspecific immune mechanism, e.g., the complement system).

   **combined i.,** i. of both the B-lymphocytes and T-lymphocytes.

**im'munodepres'sant.** An immunosuppressive *agent*.

**im'munodepres'sor.** An immunosuppressive *agent*.

**im'munodiagno'sis.** The process of determining specified immunologic characteristics of individuals or of cells, serum, or other biologic specimens.

**immunodiffusion** (im'u-no-dī-fu'zhun, ī-mu'no-). A technique of study of antigen-antibody reactions by observing precipitates formed by combination of specific antigen and antibodies which have diffused in a gel in which they had been separately placed.

**immunoelectrophoresis** (im'u-no-e-lek'tro-fo-re'sis, ī-mu'no-). A kind of precipitin test in which the components of one group of immunological reactants (usually a mixture of antigens) are first separated on the basis of electrophoretic mobility in agar or other medium, the separated components then being identified, by means of the technique of double diffusion, on the basis of precipitates formed by reaction with components of the other group of reactants (antibodies).

**im'munofer'ritin.** Antibody-ferritin conjugate, used to identify specific antigen by electron microscopy.

**immunofluorescence** (im'u-no-flu-or-es'ens, ī-mu'no-). The use of fluorescein-labeled antibodies to identify bacterial, viral, or other antigenic material specific for the labeled antibody. The specific binding of antibody can be determined microscopically by the production of a characteristic visible light by the application of ultraviolet rays to the preparation.

   **direct i.,** i. in which the antibody specific for the antigen being tested for is fluorescein-labeled.

   **indirect i.,** i. in which neither the antigen nor its specific antibody is fluorescein-labeled, but the combination of antibody with antigen is determined by the use of fluorescein-labeled antiglobulin; *e.g.*, antiserum prepared in rabbits is permitted to combine with the specific antigen being tested, and the presence of antibody is then determined by adding fluorescein-labeled antibody specific for rabbit globulin.

**immunogen** (ī-mu'no-jen). An antigen.

**im'munogenet'ics.** The branch of genetics concerned with inheritance of differences in antigens or antigenic responses.

**im'munogen'ic.** Antigenic.

**immunogenicity** (im'u-no-jē-nis'ī-tī). Antigenicity.

**im'munoglob'ulin.** Abbreviated Ig, by recommendation of WHO (replacing Greek letters). Ig's are a class of structurally related proteins consisting of two pairs of polypeptide chains, one pair of "light" (low molecular weight) chains ($\kappa$ or $\lambda$), one pair of "heavy" chains ($\gamma$, $\alpha$, or $\mu$), all four linked together by disulfide bonds (see fig.). On the basis of the structural and antigenic properties of the heavy chains, Ig's are classified (in order of relative amounts present in normal serum) as IgG (7 S in size, 80 per cent), IgA (10 to 15 per cent), IgM (19 S, 5 to 10 per cent), IgD (less than 0.1 per cent), and IgE (less than 0.01 per cent). Each class is subdivided on the basis of light chains ($\kappa$ and $\lambda$) common to heavy chain classes. Subclasses, based on differences in the heavy chains, are referred to as IgG-1, etc.

When split by papain, Ig's yield three pieces: the Fc piece, consisting of the C-terminal portion of the "heavy" (H) chains, with no antibody activity but capable of fixing complement, and crystallizable; and two identical Fab pieces, carrying the antigen-binding sites and each consisting of a "light" (L) chain bound to the remainder of a "heavy" (H) chain.

Antibodies are Ig's, and all Ig's probably function as antibodies. Patients with multiple myeloma excrete (urine) a protein known as Bence Jones protein, and this has been the key to much of what is known about Ig chemistry and structure. These patients have, in their serum, a large amount of an abnormal Ig, either IgG or IgA, resembling antibodies in structure and site of synthesis. Each patient's Ig has its own unique acid sequence. His Bence Jones protein is also unique but is identical to the light chain of his myeloma globulin. Macroglobulinemia patients produce large amounts of IgM; again, each patient's Ig is unique. In a rare condition known as heavy chain disease, the patient makes an incomplete immunoglobulin and excretes a defective heavy chain in the urine. A benign disorder known as hypergammaglobulinemia purpura results in antibodies of the IgG class. All of these classes are homogeneous and susceptible to amino acid sequence analysis.

From the study of Bence Jones proteins, it is known that all light chains are divided into a region of variable sequence ($V_L$) and one of constant sequence ($C_L$), each comprising about half the length of the light chain. The constant regions of all human light chains of the same type ($\kappa$ or $\lambda$) are identical except for a single amino acid substitution, under genetic controls. Heavy chains are similarly divided, although the $V_H$ region, while similar in length to the $V_L$ region, is only one-third or one-fourth the length of the $C_H$ region. Since there are no restrictions apparent on which light chains may combine with which heavy chains, many permutations in structure are possible, leading to the almost infinite number of antibodies found in nature.

Light chain ($\kappa$ or $\lambda$) $\equiv$ Bence Jones protein

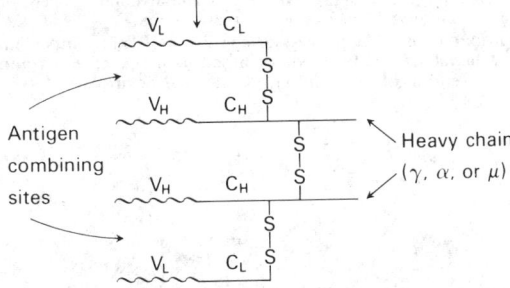

**immunohematology** (im'u-no-he-mă-tol'o-jī, ī-mu'no-). That division of hematology concerned with immune, or antigen-antibody, reactions, and with related changes in the blood.

**immunol'ogist.** One who pursues the science of immunology.

**immunology** (im'u-nol'o-jī) [ immuno- + G. *logos*, study ]. The science dealing with the various phenomena of immunity, induced sensitivity, and allergy.

**immunopathology** (im'u-no-pă-thol'o-jī, ī-mu'no-). The study of diseases or conditions resulting from reactions of immunity (antigen-antibody reactions).

**im'munoprecipita'tion.** Immune *precipitation*.

**immunoprotein** (im'u-no-pro'te-in, ī-mu'no-). Immunoglobulin.

**immunoreaction** (im'u-no-re-ak'shun). An immunologic reaction, especially *in vitro* between antigen and antibody.

**im'munoselec'tion.** Selective death or survival of fetuses of different genotypes depending on immunologic incompatibility with the mother (example: erythroblastosis fetalis, *q.v.*).

**im'munosuppres'sant.** Immunosuppressive *agent*.

**im'munosuppres'sion.** Suppression of immunologic response, usually with reference to grafts or organ transplants, by use of chemical, pharmocologic, physical, or immunologic agents.

**im'munosur'gery.** Surgery employing specific immune serum.

**immunosympathectomy** (im'u-no-sim'pă-thek'to-mĭ). Inhibition of development of sympathetic ganglia induced in newborn animals by injection of antiserum specific for the protein which selectively enhances growth of sympathetic neurons.

**im'munother'apy.** Treatment directed at the production of immunity.

**im'munotol'erance.** Immunological *tolerance.*

**im'munotox'in.** Any antitoxin.

**immunotransfusion** (im'u-no-trans-fu'zhun, ĭ-mu'no-). An indirect transfusion in which the donor is first immunized by means of injections of an antigen prepared from microorganisms isolated from the recipient; later, the donor's blood is collected, defibrinated, and then administered to the patient; the latter is then presumably passively immunized by means of antibody formed in the donor, *i.e.,* antibody that reacts with the microorganisms in the patient.

**imol'amine hydrochloride.** ANGOLON; 4-[ 2-(diethylamino)ethyl ]-5-imino-3-phenyl-Δ²-1,2,4-oxadiazoline hydrochloride; local anesthetic.

**IMP.** Abbreviation for inosine 5'-phosphate (inosine monophosphate, inosinic acid).

**im'pact.** The forcible striking of one body against another.

**impact'** [ L. *impingo,* pp. -*pactus,* to strike at (*in* + *pango*), fasten, drive in ]. To press closely together so as to render immovable.

**impac'ted.** 1. Pressed closely together so as to be immovable; said of a fracture in which the jagged ends of the broken bone are wedged together. 2. Denoting a fetus that, because of its large size or narrowing of the pelvic canal, has become wedged and incapable of spontaneous advance or recession. 3. Denoting a tooth so placed in the alveolus as to be incapable of eruption into normal position. 4. Denoting teeth being driven into the alveolar process or surrounding tissues as a result of trauma.

**impac'tion.** The process or condition of being impacted.
   **dental i.,** confinement of a tooth in the alveolus and prevention of its eruption into normal position.

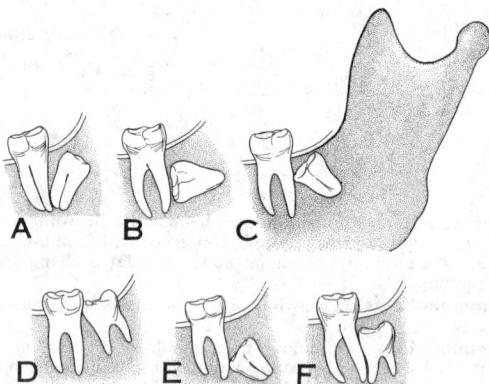

**Impacted Mandibular Third Molar**
*A,* distoangular; *B,* horizontal; *C,* mesioangular; *D,* high level; *E,* low level; *F,* vertical.

   **food i.,** the forcible wedging of food between adjacent teeth during mastication.

**impair'ment.** Weakening, damage, or deterioration; for example, as a result of injury or disease.
   **conductive hearing i., hearing i.,** see under hearing.
   **mental i.,** a disorder characterized by the display of an intellectual defect, as shown or determined by diminished cognitive interpersonal, social, and vocational effectiveness and by psychological examination and assessment. See also neuropsychologic *disorder.*

**impal'pable** [ L. *im-,* neg. + *palpabilis,* that can be felt. PALP- ]. Not capable of being felt; denoting a powder so fine as to be free from the slightest grittiness, or a pulse that cannot be detected by the finger pressing on the artery.

**impaludism** (im-pal'u-dizm) [ L. *in,* in, + *palus,* a marsh ]. Malaria.

**im'par** [ L. ] [ NA ]. Unpaired; azygous.

**imparidigitate** (im-par-ĭ-dij'ĭ-tāt) [ L. *impar,* unequal, + *digitus,* digit ]. Perissodactyl; perissodactylous; having an odd number of fingers or toes.

**impa'tent.** Not patent; closed.

**impe'dance.** 1. The total opposition to flow. When flow is steady, i. is simply the resistance, *i.e.,* the driving pressure per unit flow; when flow is changing, i. also includes the factors that oppose changes in flow. Thus, deviations of i., from simple ohmic resistance because of the effects of capacitance and inductance, become more important in alternating current as the frequency of oscillations increases. 2. In fluid analogies (*e.g.,* pulsatile flow of blood, to-and-fro flow of respiratory gas), i. depends not only on viscous resistance but also upon compressibility, compliance, inertance, and the frequency of imposed oscillations. 3. The resistance of an acoustic system of being set in motion.

**imperception** (im-per-sep'shun) [ L. *in-,* not, + *per-cipio,* pp. -*ceptus,* to perceive. CAP- ]. Inability to form a mental picture of an object by combining the sensations arising therefrom; insufficiency of perception.

**imper'forate** [ L. *im-* neg. + *per-foro,* pp. -*atus,* to bore through ]. Atretic; closed; without an opening.

**imperforation** (im-per'fo-ra'shun) [ see imperforate ]. The condition of being atretic, occluded, or closed; indicated in compound words by the prefix *atreto-* or the suffix -*atresia.*

**impermeable** (im-per'me-ă-bl) [ L. *im-permeabilis,* not to be passed through, fr. *in-* neg. + *per-meo,* to pass through (*meo,* go) ]. Impenetrable, impervious to fluids.

**impermeant** (im-per'me-ant) [ L. *im-,* neg. + *permano,* to penetrate ]. Unable to pass through a particular semipermeable membrane.

**impersistence** (im-per-sis'tens) [ L. *im-,* neg. + *persisto,* to persist ]. A transitory existence or occurrence, lasting only a short time.
   **motor i.,** inability to sustain a movement.

**impetiginization** (im'pe-tij'ĭ-nĭ-za'shun). The occurrence of impetigo in an area of preexisting dermatosis.

**impetiginous** (im-pe-tij'ĭ-nus). Relating to impetigo.

**impetigo** (im'pe-tigo) [ L. a scabby eruption, fr. *im-peto* (*inp-*), to rush upon, attack ]. Fox's i.; i. contagiosa; Corlett's pyosis; a contagious superficial pyoderma that begins with a superficial flaccid vesicle which ruptures and forms a thick yellowish crust, most commonly occurring on the face; caused by staphylococci or streptococci.
   **Bockhart's i.,** follicular i.
   **i. bullo'sa,** i. with lesions of large size, forming bullae.
   **bullous i. of the newborn,** i. neonatorum (2); pemphigus gangrenosus (2); usually widely disseminated bullous lesions, appearing soon after birth; staphylococcic infection, occasionally mixed with streptococci.
   **i. contagio'sa,** old synonym for i.
   **i. eczemato'des,** *eczema* pustulosum.
   **follic'ular i.,** Bockhart's i.; a follicular pustular eruption involving the scalp or other hairy area.
   **Fox's i.,** old eponym for i.
   **i. herpetifor'mis,** a rare pyoderma occurring most commonly in pregnant women; an eruption of small, closely aggregated pustules, developing upon an inflammatory base, accompanied by severe general symptoms.
   **i. neonato'rum,** (1) *dermatitis* exfoliativa infantum; (2) bullous i. of the newborn.

**im'petus** [ L. an onset, fr. *im-peto,* to attack ]. A psychoanalytical term denoting the motor element of an instinct; the amount of force of the individual's energy which the instinctive impulse demands.

**implant** [ L. *im-,* in, + *planto,* pp. -*atus,* to plant, fr. *planta,* a sprout, shoot ]. 1. To graft; to insert. 2. Material inserted or grafted into intact tissues of a host, *e.g.,* an insertor containing radium or radon. 3. In dentistry, a graft or insert set firmly or deeply or onto the alveolar recess prepared for its insertion; see also i. *denture*.

**carcinomatous i.'s,** transference of carcinoma cells from a primary tumor to adjacent tissues where growth continues.

**cochlear i.,** an electronic device implanted under the skin with electrodes to the cochlea or eighth nerve to create sound sensation in persons with total sensory deafness.

**endometrial i.'s,** fragments of endometrial mucosa implanted on pelvic structure following retrograde transference through the oviducts.

**endo-osseous i.,** an artificial root of variable form inserted into the alveolar bone and protruding through the mucosa to provide support on which a restoration can be placed.

**magnetic i.,** a tissue-tolerated, magnetized metal placed within the bone to aid in denture retention; a similar magnet is placed in the overlying denture to complete the field.

**pin i.,** a type of ventplant, usually rod-shaped, used in the area of the maxillary sinuses.

**post i.,** that portion of an i. substructure that protrudes through the mucosa to connect with the restoration.

**submucosal i.,** an i. resting beneath the mucosa; see also i. denture.

**subperiosteal i.,** an artificial metal appliance made to conform to the shape of a bone and placed on its surface beneath the periosteum; see implant denture *substructure*.

**triplant i.,** a combination of three pin i.'s to form a single abutment to support or retain a dental prosthesis.

**implanta'tion.** 1. The attachment of the fertilized ovum (blastocyst) to the endometrium, and its embedding in the compact layer, occurring six or seven days after fertilization of the ovum. 2. The insertion of a natural tooth into an artificially constructed alveolus. 3. Tissue grafting; see implant; graft; transplantation.

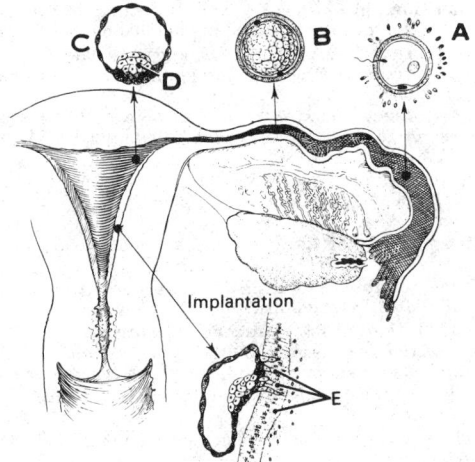

**Implantation**

A, sperm entering ovum; B, morula; C, blastocyst (enters uterus at about 5th day; D, inner cell mass of blastocyst; E, implantation, with trophoblastic cells penetrating between cells of uterine epithelium.

**central i.,** circumferential or superficial i.; that in which the blastocyst remains in the uterine cavity (*e.g.,* rhesus monkey, carnivores, rabbit).

**circumferential i.,** central i.

**cortical i.,** i. of blastocyst in the ovarian cortex, causing an ovarian pregnancy.

**delayed i.,** a phenomenon characterized by an interval ranging from a few weeks to approximately 6 months between the time an ovum is fertilized and subsequent i. of the zygote; exhibited by various animals, including the marten and the armadillo.

**eccentric i.,** i. in which the blastocyst lies in a uterine crypt (*e.g.,* mouse, rat, hamster).

**filigree i.,** McGavin method; the burying of a filigree, or network, of silver in the abdominal wall in order to close a large abdominal hernia.

**hypodermic i.,** injection of material under the skin.

**interstitial i.,** that in which the blastocyst lies within the substance of the endometrium (*e.g.,* man, guinea pig).

**nerve i.,** planting one nerve into the sheath of another nerve.

**pellet i.,** the insertion intramuscularly or subcutaneously of a hormone or other active therapeutic agent in pellet form, in order to provide protracted absorption at a rate slower than subcutaneous or intramuscular injection; a means of providing a sustained therapeutic effect with agents not active when ingested.

**periosteal i.,** insertion of a normal tendon into a periosteum as a replacement of a paralyzed tendon.

**superficial i.,** central i.

**impletion** (im-ple'shun) [ L. *implere*, to fill up ]. A term denoting the normal lack of awareness of the blind spot in the temporal field of each eye, even with one eye closed, due to cortical mediation.

**implosion** (im-plo'shun). A type of behavior therapy, similar to flooding, during which the patient is given massive exposure to extreme anxiety-arousing stimuli by being asked to describe, and thus relive in his imagination, those life events or situations typically producing these overwhelming emotional reactions. As the patient does so, the therapist attempts to extinguish the future influence of such unconscious material over the patient's behavior and feelings, and previous avoidance responses to the stimuli are replaced by more appropriate responses.

**im'potence, im'potency** [ L. *impotentia, q. v.* ]. 1. Weakness; lack of power. 2. Specifically, lack of power, in the male, to copulate; may involve inability to achieve penile erection or to achieve ejaculation, or both; a manifestation, usually, of a neurological or emotional dysfunction.

**atonic i.,** i. caused by paralysis of the motor nerves.

**orgastic i.,** the inability to achieve orgasm or the climax of the sexual act.

**paretic i.,** i. caused by a lesion of the central nervous system.

**psychic i.,** that caused by psychologic factors.

**symptomatic i.,** i. caused by disturbance of the sensory perineal reflexes.

**impotentia** (im-po-ten'shi-ah) [ L. inability, fr. *in-* neg. + *potentia*, power, fr. *potens (-ent-)*, powerful ]. Impotence.

**i. coeun'di,** inability to cohabit, especially of the male to perform the sexual act.

**i. erigen'di,** impotence due to absence of the power of erection.

**i. generandi,** inability to reproduce.

**impreg'nate** [ L. *im-*, in, + *praegnans*, with child. GEN- ]. 1. To fecundate; to cause to conceive. 2. To saturate; to permeate with another substance.

**impregna'tion.** 1. The act of making pregnant. 2. Saturation.

**impres'sio,** pl. **impressio'nes** [ L. ] [ NA ]. Impression; a mark seemingly made by pressure of one body on another.

**i. cardi'aca hep'atis** [ NA ], cardiac impression of liver; a depression on the superior area of the diaphragmatic surface of the liver corresponding to the position of the heart.

**i. cardi'aca pulmo'nis** [ NA ], cardiac impression of the lung; the depression on the medial surface of each lung produced by the presence of the heart. It is more pronounced on the left lung.

**i. col'ica** [ NA ], colic impression; a hollow on the undersurface of the right lobe of the liver anteriorly, corresponding to the situation of the right flexure and beginning of the transverse colon.

**impressiones digita'tae** [ NA ], digitate impressions; the depressions on the inner surface of the skull which correspond to the convolutions of the brain.

**i. duodena'lis** [ NA ], duodenal impression; a hollow on the undersurface of the right lobe of the liver alongside the gallbladder, marking the situation of the duodenum.

**i. esophage'a** [ NA ], esophageal impression; the marking of the esophagus on the back of the left lobe of the liver.

**i. gas'trica** [ NA ], gastric impression; a hollow on the undersurface of the left lobe of the liver corresponding to the location of the stomach.

**i. ligamenti costoclavicula'ris** [ NA ], impression for the costoclavicular ligament; rhomboid impression; tuberositas costalis; costal tuberosity; an irregular pitted area on the inferior surface of the clavicle at its sternal end, giving attachment to the costoclavicular ligament.

**i. petro'sa pal'lii**, petrosal impression of the pallium; a shallow impression on the inferior surface of the cerebral hemisphere made by the superior margin of the petrous part of the temporal bone.

**i. rena'lis** [ NA ], renal impression; a hollow on the undersurface of the right lobe of the liver, in which lies the right kidney.

**i. suprarena'lis** [ NA ], suprarenal impression; a hollow on the undersurface of the right lobe of the liver, adjoining the sulcus venae cavae, in which lies the right suprarenal gland.

**i. trigem'ini** [ NA ], trigeminal impression; a depression on the anterior surface of the petrous portion of the temporal bone, near the apex, lodging the trigeminal ganglion.

**impression** (im-presh'un) [ L. *impressio*, fr. *im-primo*, pp. -*pressus*, to press upon (*in* + *premo*) ]. 1. A mark seemingly made by pressure of one structure or organ upon another; see impressio. 2. An effect produced upon the mind by some external object acting through the organs of sense. 3. An imprint or negative likeness. 4. The negative form of the teeth and/or other tissues of the oral cavity, made in a plastic material which becomes relatively hard or set while in contact with these tissues. An i. is made in order to reproduce a positive form or cast of the recorded tissues. (I.'s are classified, according to the materials of which they are made, as reversible and irreversible hydrocolloid i., modeling plastic i., plaster i., wax i.)

**after-i.**, aftersensation.

**basilar i.**, an invagination of brain stem and cerebellar structures downward into the foramen magnum with compression of the basilar artery.

**cardiac i. of liver**, *impressio* cardiaca hepatis.

**cardiac i. of lung**, *impressio* cardiaca pulmonis.

**colic i.**, *impressio* colica.

**complete denture i.**, (1) an i. of an edentulous arch made for the purpose of constructing a complete denture; (2) a negative registration of the entire denture-bearing, stabilizing area of either the maxillae or mandible; (3) a negative registration of the entire denture foundation and border seal areas present in the edentulous mouth.

**i. for costoclavicular ligament**, *impressio* ligamenti costoclavicularis.

**deltoid i.**, *tuberositas* deltoidea.

**digitate i.'s**, *impressiones* digitatae.

**direct bone i.**, an i. of denuded bone, used in the construction of denture implants.

**duodenal i.**, *impressio* duodenalis.

**esophageal i.**, *impressio* esophagea.

**gastric i.**, *impressio* gastrica.

**maternal i.**, a strong emotion or shock, experienced by a pregnant woman, popularly supposed to be the cause of a malformation or surface marking of the fetus, also the lesion or malformation supposed to result from the mental i. of the mother. This concept is not based on fact. There are no nervous communications between mother and fetus.

**mental i.**, i. (2).

**partial denture i.**, an i. or negative copy of all or a part of the partially edentulous dental arch or area, made for the purpose of designing or constructing a partial denture.

**preliminary i.**, primary i.; in dentistry, one made for the purpose of diagnosis or the construction of a tray.

**primary i.**, preliminary i.

**renal i.**, *impressio* renalis.

**rhomboid i.**, *impressio* ligamenti costoclavicularis.

**sectional i.**, an i. that is made in sections.

**suprarenal i.**, *impressio* suprarenalis.

**trigeminal i.**, *impressio* trigeminalis.

**imprint'ing.** A particular kind of learning characterized by its occurrence in the first few hours of life, and which determines species-recognition behavior.

**impu'beral.** Relating to impuberism; obsolete term.

**impu'berism.** An obsolete term meaning the continuation of the prepubertal state into adolescent or adult life; was sometimes applied to the normal prepubertal period.

**im'pulse** [ L. *im-pello*, pp. -*pulsus*, to push against, impel (*inp-*) ]. 1. A sudden pushing or driving force. 2. A sudden, often unreasoning, determination to perform some act. 3. The action potential of a nerve fiber.

**cardiac i.**, movement of the chest wall produced by cardiac contraction.

**irresistible i.**, a compulsion to act that the individual feels or claims he cannot resist.

**morbid i.**, one that drives a person to commit some act, usually of a deviant or forbidden nature, notwithstanding his efforts to restrain himself.

**impulsion** (im-pul'shun). An abnormal urge to perform certain activity, often unpleasant.

**impul'sive.** Relating to or actuated by an impulse, rather than controlled by reason.

**i'mus** [ L. ] [ NA ]. Lowest; the most inferior or caudal of several similar structures.

**IMViC.** See IMViC *reaction*.

**In.** Chemical symbol of the element indium.

**in-** [ L. ]. 1. Prefix conveying a sense of negation; un-, not. 2. Prefix denoting in, within, inside. 3. A prefix denoting an intensive action. Appears as im- before b, p, or m.

**inac'tion.** Inactivity; rest; lack of response to a stimulus.

**inac'tivate.** To destroy the activity or the effects of an agent or substance, as the activity of complement is destroyed when serum is heated.

**inactiva'tion.** The process of destroying or removing the activity or the effects of an agent or substance; for example, the complementary effect of a serum may be destroyed by means of i. at 56°C. for 30 min.

**inan'imate.** Not alive.

**inanition** (in'ă-nish'un) [ L. *inanis*, empty ]. Exhaustion from lack of food or defect in assimilation.

**inapparent** (in'ă-păr'ent). Not apparent; latent; beneath the threshold of clinical recognition; as an inapparent infection.

**inappetence** (in-ap'ē-tens) [ L. *in-* neg. + *ap-peto*, pp. -*petitus*, to strive after, long for (*adp-*) ]. Lack of desire or of craving.

**inartic'ulate.** Not articulate. 1. Not in the form of intelligible speech. 2. Unable to satisfactorily express oneself in words.

**in articulo mor'tis** [ L. *articulus*, moment; *mors*, death. ARTIC- ]. At the moment of death.

**inassim'ilable.** Not assimilable; not capable of being appropriated for the nutrition of the body.

**inatten'tion.** Lack of attention; negligence.

**selective i.**, an aspect of attentiveness in which a person attempts to ignore or avoid that which generates anxiety.

**in'born.** Innate; inherited; implanted during development in utero.

**in'breed'ing.** A practice of mating animals that are closely related.

**coefficient of i.**, see under coefficient.

**incarcerated** (in-kar'ser-a-ted) [ L. *in*, in, + *carcero*, pp. -*atus*, to imprison, fr. *carcer*, prison ]. Confined; imprisoned; denoting, for example, an irreducible hernia.

**incarnant** (in-kar'nant) [ L. *incarno*, pp. -*atus*, fr. *in* + *caro* (*carn-*), flesh ]. Promoting or accelerating the granulation of a wound.

**incar'native.** Incarnant.

**incendiarism** (in-sen'dī-ă-rizm) [ L. *incendiarius*, causing a conflagration ]. Pyromania.

**incen'tive** [ LL. *incentivus*, provocative ]. In experimental psychology, an object or goal of motivated behavior.

**incest** (in'sest) [ L. *incestus*, unchaste, fr. *in-*, not, + *castus*, chaste ]. 1. Sexual relations between persons closely related by blood (especially between parents and children, brother and sister). 2. The crime of sexual relations between persons related by blood, where such cohabitation is prohibited by law.

**incestuous** (in-ses'tu-us). 1. Guilty of incest. 2. Pertaining to incest.

**incidence** (in′sĭ-dens) [ L. *incido*, to fall into or upon, to happen. CAD- ]. 1. The amount or extent of an occurrence, *e.g.*, the number of cases of a disease; see also rate. 2. In optics, the falling of a ray of light on a surface.

**incident** (in′sĭ-dent) [ L. *incido*, pp. -*casus*, to fall into, to meet with. CAD- ]. Going toward; impinging upon, as incident rays.

**incisal** (in-si′zal) [ L. *incido*, pp. -*cisus*, to cut into. CES- ]. Cutting; relating to the cutting edges of the incisor and cuspid teeth.

**incise** (in-sīz′). To cut with a knife.

**incision** (in-sizh′un) [ L. *incisio*. CES- ]. A cut; a surgical wound; a division of the soft parts made with a knife.

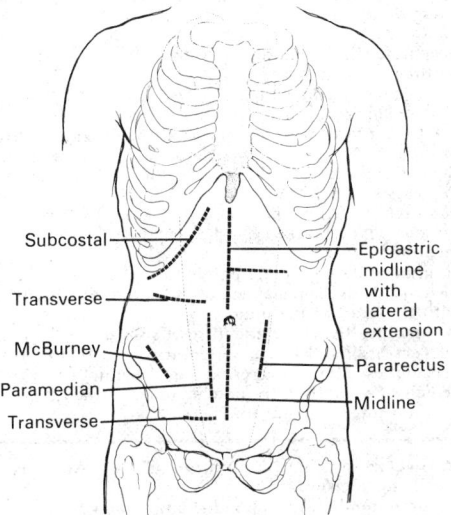

Subcostal
Epigastric midline with lateral extension
Transverse
McBurney
Pararectus
Paramedian
Midline
Transverse

**Abdominal Incisions**

**Agnew-Verhoeff i.,** i. for release of pus in the lacrimal sac in acute phlegmonous dacryocystitis; an angular keratome placed over the caruncle is plunged to the bone, after which large lacrimal probes are passed into the nasolacrimal duct.

**Bar's i.,** an i. in the median line of the abdomen above the umbilicus, in cesarean section; longitudinal i. of the uterus from the fundus to Bandl's ring.

**Battle's i.,** vertical i. of abdominal wall with retraction of rectus muscle medially.

**Bergmann's i.,** an i. in the flank for exposing the kidney.

**Bevan's i.,** an i. along the lateral border of the rectus abdominis, exposing the gallbladder.

**celiotomy i.,** an i. through the abdominal wall.

**Deaver's i.,** for appendectomy, an i. in right lower abdominal quadrant, with medial displacement of the rectus muscle.

**Dührssen's i.'s,** three surgical i.'s of an incompletely

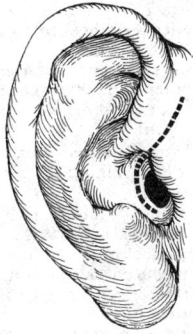

**Endaural Incision**

dilated cervix, corresponding roughly to 2, 6, and 10 o'clock, used as a means of effecting immediate delivery of the fetus.

**endaural i.,** i. through the external auditory canal to permit mastoid surgery.

**exploratory i.,** one made in order to ascertain the condition present.

**Fergusson's i.,** an i. for excision of maxillae.

**Halsted's i.,** see Halsted's *operation.*

**Kehr's i.,** an i. from xiphoid to pubis.

**Kocher's i.,** an i. parallel with right costal margin, for exposure of the gallbladder.

**Langenbeck's i.,** an i. through the linea semilunaris made in order to expose the spleen or tail of the pancreas.

**Mackenrodt's i.,** a transverse i. on the lower abdomen.

**McBurney's i.,** an i. parallel with the course of the external oblique muscle, one or two inches from the anterior superior spine of the ilium; used in the operation for appendicitis.

**paramedian i.,** one lateral to the midline.

**Parker's i.,** an oblique i. nearly parallel with Poupart's ligament over the area of dullness in appendiceal abscess.

**Perthes' i.,** one for exposure of organs in right upper abdominal quadrant.

**Pfannenstiel's i.,** an i. made transversely, down to and including the external sheath of the recti muscles, about an inch above the pubes, the muscles being split or separated in the direction of their fibers; advocated for operations on the pelvic organs.

**Wilde's i.,** an i. parallel to the pinna of the ear and about half an inch behind it, made to relieve tension in mastoid periostitis.

**inci′sive.** 1. Incisus; cutting; having the power to cut. 2. Relating to the incisor teeth.

**inci′sor** [ L. *incido*, to cut into. CES- ]. One of the cutting teeth, or i. teeth, four in number in each jaw at the apex of the dental arch.

**central i.,** the first tooth in the maxilla and mandible on either side of the midsagittal plane of the head.

**lateral i.,** the second i.

**scalpriform i.'s,** the cutting or gnawing i.'s of a rodent.

**second i.,** lateral i.; second maxillary or mandibular permanent or deciduous tooth on either side of the midsagittal plane of the head.

# INCISURA

**incisura,** pl. **incisu′rae** (in′si-su′rah, in′sĭ-su′rah) [ L. a cutting into. CES- ]. 1. Incision. 2 [ NA ]. Incisure; notch; emargination; an indentation at the edge of any structure.

**i. acetab′uli** [ NA ], acetabular notch; cotyloid notch; a gap in the lower part of the margin of the acetabulum.

**i. angula′ris** [ NA ], angular notch; sulcus angularis; a sharp angular depression in the lesser curvature of the stomach at the junction of the body with the pyloric canal.

**i. anterior au′ris** [ NA ], anterior notch of the ear; a notch between the tuberculum supratragicum and the crus helicis.

**i. ap′icis cordis** [ NA ], notch of the apex of the heart; a slight notch near the apex of the heart where the anterior interventricular sulcus reaches the diaphragmatic surface of the heart.

**i. cardi′aca** [ NA ], cardiac notch; a deep notch between the esophagus and fundus of the stomach.

**i. cardi′aca pulmo′nis sinis′tri** [ NA ], cardiac notch of the left lung; the notch in the anterior border of the superior lobe of the left lung which accommodates the pericardium.

**i. cartilag′inis mea′tus acus′tici exter′ni** [ NA ], notch in the cartilage of the external acoustic meatus; i. santorini; Santorini's incisure or fissure; Duverney's fissure; one of (usually) two vertical fissures in the anterior portion of the cartilage of the external auditory meatus, filled by fibrous tissue.

**i. cerebel′li ante′rior,** anterior notch of the cerebellum; semilunar notch (1); a wide, shallow notch on the anterior surface of the cerebellum occupied by the superior cerebellar peduncles and the inferior quadrigeminal bodies.

**i. cerebel'li poste'rior,** posterior notch of the cerebellum; marsupial notch; a narrow notch between the cerebellar hemispheres posteriorly, occupied by the falx cerebelli.

**i. clavicula'ris** [ NA ], the clavicular notch or facet; a hollow on either side of the upper surface of the manubrium sterni which articulates with the clavicle.

**i. costa'lis** [ NA ], costal notch; one of the notches or facets on the lateral edge of the sternum for articulation with a rib.

**i. ethmoida'lis** [ NA ], ethmoidal notch; an oblong gap between the orbital parts of the frontal bone in which the ethmoid bone is lodged.

**i. fibula'ris** [ NA ], fibular notch; a hollow on the lateral surface of the lower end of the tibia in which the fibula is lodged.

**i. fronta'lis** [ NA ], frontal notch; a small notch, sometimes a foramen, on the orbital margin of the frontal bone medial to the supraorbital notch.

**i. interarytenoid'ea** [ NA ], interarytenoid notch; the posterior portion of the aditus laryngis between the two arytenoid cartilages.

**i. intertrag'ica** [ NA ], intertragic notch; the deep notch in the lower part of the auricle between the tragus and antitragus.

**i. ischiad'ica ma'jor** [ NA ], greater sciatic notch; the deep indentation in the posterior border of the hip bone at the point of union of the ilium and ischium.

**i. ischiad'ica mi'nor** [ NA ], lesser sciatic notch; the notch in the posterior border of the ischium below the ischial spine.

**i. jugula'ris** [ NA ], jugular notch; (1) the notch in the occipital bone which forms one boundary of the jugular foramen; (2) the notch in the temporal bone which forms one boundary of the jugular foramen; (3) suprasternal notch; sternal notch; presternal notch; interclavicular notch; the large notch in the superior margin of the sternum.

**i. lacrima'lis** [ NA ], lacrimal notch; the notch on the frontal process of the maxilla into which the lacrimal bone fits.

**i. ligamen'ti tere'tis hep'atis** [ NA ], notch for the round ligament; the notch in the inferior border of the liver that accommodates the round ligament.

**i. mandib'ulae** [ NA ], mandibular notch; sigmoid notch; the deep notch between the condylar and coronoid processes of the mandible.

**i. mastoid'ea** [ NA ], mastoid notch; digastric notch; the groove medial to the mastoid process of the temporal bone from which the digastric muscle originates.

**i. nasa'lis** [ NA ], nasal notch; the notch in the medial border of the maxilla anteriorly which, with its fellow, forms the piriform opening of the nasal cavity.

**i. pancre'atis** [ NA ], pancreatic notch; a notch separating the uncinate process of the head of the pancreas from the neck.

**i. parieta'lis** [ NA ], parietal notch; the angle posteriorly between the squamous and petrous parts of the temporal bone.

**i. preoccipita'lis** [ NA ], preoccipital notch; an indentation in the ventrolateral border of the temporal lobe of the cerebral hemisphere.

**i. pterygoid'ea** [ NA ], pterygoid notch; pterygoid fissure; the cleft between the medial and lateral laminae of the pterygoid process of the sphenoid bone into which the pyramidal process of the palatine bone is fitted.

**i. radia'lis** [ NA ], radial notch; the concavity on the lateral aspect of the coronoid process of the ulna which articulates with the head of the radius.

**i. rivi'ni,** i. tympanica.

**i. santori'ni,** i. cartilaginis meatus acustici externi.

**i. scap'ulae** [ NA ], scapular or suprascapular notch; a notch on the superior border of the scapula through which the suprascapular nerve passes.

**i. semiluna'ris ulnae,** i. trochlearis.

**i. sphenopalati'na** [ NA ], sphenopalatine notch; the deep notch between the orbital and sphenoidal processes of the palate bone which is converted into the foramen of the same name by the under surface of the sphenoid bone.

**i. supraorbita'lis** [ NA ], supraorbital notch; a groove in the orbital margin of the frontal bone, about the junction of the inner and middle thirds, through which pass the supraorbital nerve and artery. See also *foramen* supraorbitale.

**i. tento'rii** [ NA ], notch of the tentorium; Pacchionian foramen; the triangular opening in the tentorium cerebelli through which the brainstem extends from the posterior into the middle cranial fossa.

**i. termina'lis auris** [ NA ], terminal notch of the auricle; a deep notch separating the lamina tragi and cartilage of the external auditory meatus from the main auricular cartilage, the two being connected below by the isthmus.

**i. thyroid'ea inferior** [ NA ], inferior thyroid notch; a shallow notch in the middle of the lower border of the thyroid cartilage.

**i. thyroid'ea superior** [ NA ], superior thyroid notch; a deep notch in the middle of the upper border of the thyroid cartilage.

**i. trag'ica,** i. intertragica.

**i. trochlea'ris** [ NA ], trochlear notch; semilunar notch (2); the large semicircular notch at the proximal extremity of the ulna between the olecranon and coronoid processes that articulates with the trochlea of the humerus.

**i. tympan'ica** [ NA ], tympanic notch; Rivinus' incisure or notch; i. rivini; the notch in the superior part of the tympanic ring bridged by the flaccid part of the tympanic membrane.

**i. ulna'ris** [ NA ], ulnar notch; the concave surface on the medial side of the distal end of the radius which articulates with the head of the ulna.

**i. umbilica'lis,** i. ligamenti teretis hepatis.

**i. vertebra'lis** [ NA ], vertebral notch; one of the two concavities above (superior) and below (inferior) the pedicle of a vertebra; the notches of two adjacent vertebrae form an intervertebral foramen.

---

**incisure** (in-si'zhūr) [ L. *incisura.* CES- ]. An incision or notch; see incisura.

    **Lantermann's i.'s,** Schmidt-Lantermann i.

    **Rivinus' i.,** *incisura* tympanica.

    **Santorini's i.,** *incisura* cartilaginis meatus acustici externi.

    **Schmidt-Lantermann i.'s,** Lantermann's i.'s; funnel-shaped interruptions in the regular structure of the myelin sheath of nerve fibers, formerly interpreted as actual breaks in the sheath but shown by electron microscopy to correspond each to a strand of cytoplasm locally separating the two otherwise fused oligodendroglial (or, in peripheral nerves, Schwann cell) membranes composing the myelin sheath.

    **tympanic i.,** *incisura* tympanica.

**inci'sus** [ L. ] [ NA ]. Incisive; incisor.

**inclinatio,** pl. **inclinatio'nes** (in'klī-na'shī-o) [ L. ]. Inclination.

    **i. pelvis** [ NA ], the inclination of the pelvis; the angle which the plane of the pelvic inlet makes with the horizontal plane.

**inclination** (in-klī-na'shun) [ L. *inclinatio,* a leaning. CLIM- ]. A leaning or sloping. In dentistry, the deviation of the long axis of a tooth from the perpendicular.

    **condylar guidance i.,** the angle of i. of the condylar guidance (*q.v.,* under guidance) to an accepted horizontal plane.

    **enamel rod i.,** the direction of the enamel rods with reference to the outer surface of the enamel of a tooth.

    **lateral condylar i.,** the direction of the lateral condyle path (*q.v.,* under path).

**in'clinom'eter** [ L. *in-clino,* pp. -*atus,* to incline (CLIM-) ]. An instrument for determining the direction of the ocular axes in astigmatism.

**inclusion** (in-klu'zhun) [ L. *inclusio,* a shutting in, fr. *includo,* pp. -*clusus,* to close in. CLAUS- ]. 1. Any foreign or heterogenous substance contained in a cell or in any tissue or organ, not introduced as a result of trauma. 2. The process by which a foreign or heterogenous structure is misplaced in another tissue.

    **cell i.'s,** (1) metaplasm; the nonliving elements of the cytoplasm which are metabolic products of the cell, *e.g.,* pigment granules or crystals; (2) storage materials such as glycogen or fat; (3) engulfed material such as carbon or other foreign substances. See also inclusion *body*.

**Döhle's i.'s,** Döhle's *bodies.*

**fetal i.,** unequal conjoined twins in which the incompletely developed parasite is wholly inclosed within the autosite.

**leukocyte i.'s,** Döhle's *bodies.*

**incoercible** (in-ko-er'sĭ-bl) [ L. *in-* neg. + *coerceo,* pp. *-ercitus,* to hold together, restrain, fr. *arceo,* to shut up ]. Impossible to control, to restrain, or to stop.

**incoherent** (in-ko-hēr'ent) [ L. *in-* neg. + *co-haereo,* pp. *-haesus,* to cling together, fr. *haereo,* to stick ]. Not coherent; disjointed; confused; denoting a lack of connectedness or organization of parts during verbal expression.

**incompatibility** (in'kom-pat-ĭ-bil'ĭ-tĭ). The quality of being incompatible.

**physiologic i.,** a form in which the substances in a mixture exert opposing physiologic actions.

**therapeutic i.,** physiologic i.

**incompatible** (in'kom-pat'ĭ-bl) [ L. *in-* neg. + *con-,* with, + *patior,* pp. *passus,* to suffer ]. 1. Not of suitable composition to be combined or mixed with another agent or substance, without resulting in an undesirable reaction (including chemical alteration or destruction); *e.g.,* certain reacting chemicals may not be used as ingredients in the same prescription, or the blood of a group B donor may not be administered to a group A recipient without unwanted reactions. 2. Denoting persons who can not freely associate together without resulting anxiety and conflict.

**incompetence, incompetency** (in-kom'pe-tens, in-kom'pe-ten-sĭ) [ L. *in-* neg. + *com-peto,* strive after together ]. 1. Insufficiency (2); the quality of being incompetent or incapable of performing the allotted function, especially failure of cardiac or venous valves to close completely. 2. In psychiatry, the mental ability to distinguish right from wrong or to manage one's affairs.

**aortic i.,** defective closure of aortic valve permitting regurgitation into left ventricle during diastole.

**cardiac i.,** inability of the ventricles to pump out the blood returning to the atria fast enough to prevent an abnormal rise in atrial pressure.

**mitral i.,** defective closure of mitral valve permitting regurgitation into left atrium during systole.

**muscular i.,** imperfect closure of an anatomically normal cardiac valve, in consequence of defective action of the papillary muscles.

**pulmonary i., pulmonic i.,** defective closure of pulmonic valve permitting regurgitation into right ventricle during diastole.

**pylor'ic i.,** a patulous state or want of tone of the pylorus that allows the passage of food into the intestine before gastric digestion is completed.

**relative i.,** imperfect closure of a cardiac valve, in consequence of excessive dilation of the corresponding cavity of the heart.

**tricuspid i.,** defective closure of tricuspid valve permitting regurgitation into right atrium during systole.

**val'vular i.,** a leaky state of one or more of the cardiac valves, the valve not closing tightly and blood therefore regurgitating through it.

**incon'stant.** 1. Variable; irregular. 2. In anatomy, denoting a structure, such as an artery, nerve, etc., that may or may not be present.

**incon'tinence** [ L. *in-continentia,* fr. *in-* neg. + *con-tineo,* to hold together, fr. *teneo,* to hold ]. Incontinentia. 1. Inability to prevent the discharge of any of the excretions, especially of urine or feces. 2. Lack of restraint of the appetites, especially the sexual appetite; *cf.* intemperance.

**active i.,** a discharge of urine or feces in the normal way at intervals, but involuntarily.

**i. of feces,** involuntary evacuation of feces, as in spinal cord lesions.

**i. of milk,** galactorrhea.

**i. with overflow,** continuous overdistention of the urinary bladder due to a nervous lesion, with dribbling of urine.

**paradoxical i.,** distention of urinary bladder, with dribbling of urine.

**passive i.,** dribbling of urine by reason of inability of the bladder to empty itself and of consequent overdistention.

**i. of pigment,** loss of melanin from the epidermis, and accumulation in melanophores in the upper dermis; seen in several inflammatory diseases of the skin and in *incontinentia* pigmenti, *q.v.*

**urinary exertional i.,** urinary stress i.

**urinary stress i.,** leakage of urine as a result of coughing, straining, or some sudden voluntary movement due to weakness of the muscles around the neck of the bladder and surrounding the vagina, resulting in an incompetent internal vesical sphincter; may occur in otherwise normal women.

**i. of urine,** involuntary passage of urine; enuresis.

**incontinentia** (in-kon'tĭ-nen'shĭ-ah) [ L. ]. Incontinence.

**i. alvi,** incontinence of feces.

**i. pigmen'ti,** Bloch-Sulzberger disease; an inherited developmental defect of the skin which may also involve other structures; i. pigmenti is characterized by pigmented lesions in linear, zebra-stripe, and other bizarre configurations, sometimes preceded by vesicles and bullae, and occasionally accompanied by other developmental abnormalities.

**incoordination** (in-ko-or-dĭ-na'shun) [ L. *in-* neg. + coordination, *q.v.* ]. Ataxia; lack of coordination, or of harmonious working together of the various muscles concerned in the execution of more or less complicated movements.

**incorporation** (in-kor'po-ra'shun) [ L. *in-,* in, + *corporare,* pp. *corporatus,* to make into a body ]. In psychoanalysis, a type of identification with another person; identification through oral incorporation or "eating" of the object.

**increment** (in'kre-ment) [ L. *incrementum,* increase ]. A change in the value of a variable; usually an increase, with "decrement" applied to a decrease, though "increment" can also correctly be applied to both.

**incretion** (in-kre'shun) [ L. *in,* within, + *secernere,* to separate. CRET- ]. Internal secretion. 1. The functional activity of an endocrine gland. 2. The product of the activity of an endocrine gland; hormone or chalone. This term (hence many other words with the prefix increto-) is no longer in common usage.

**increto-** [ L. *in,* within, + *secernere,* to separate ]. Combining form pertaining to internal secretion. Most words beginning thus are absolete or obsolescent; see incretion.

**incre'todi'agno'sis.** Obsolete term meaning the diagnosis of functional activity of endocrine glands.

**incretogenous** (in'kre-toj'e-nus). Favoring the proliferation of internal secretions. Obsolete.

**in'cretol'ogy.** Obsolete synonym for endocrinology.

**in'cretop'athy.** Obsolete term for endocrine disease.

**incretory** (in'kre-to-rĭ). Obsolete term relating to the process of incretion or to its products.

**incre'tother'apy.** Treatment of endocrine disease or with endocrine preparations. Obsolete usage.

**incrustation** (in'krus-ta'shun) [ L. *in-crusto,* pp. *-atus,* to incrust, fr. *crusta,* crust ]. 1. The formation of a crust or a scab. 2. A coating of some adventitious material or an exudate; a scab.

**incubation** (in'ku-ba'shun) [ L. *incubo,* to lie on ]. 1. The act of maintaining controlled environmental conditions for the purpose of favoring growth or development of microbial or tissue cultures. 2. The maintenance of an artificial environment for an infant, usually a premature or hypoxic one, by providing proper temperature, humidity, and, usually, oxygen. 3. The development without sign or symptom of an infection from the time it gains entry until the appearance of the first signs or symptoms.

**incubator** (in'ku-ba'tor). 1. A container in which controlled environmental conditions may be maintained; used for culturing microorganisms. 2. An apparatus for maintaining an infant (usually premature) in an environment of proper oxygenation, humidity, and temperature.

**incubus** (in'ku-bus) [ L. fr. *incubo,* to lie on. CUB- ]. 1. Originally, an evil spirit which lay upon and oppressed sleeping persons; esp., a male spirit which copulated with sleeping women, as contrasted with succubus. 2. Nightmare.

**in'cudal.** Relating to the incus.

**incudec'tomy** [ incus + G. *ektomē,* excision ]. Removal of the incus of the tympanum.

**incudes** (in-ku'dēz) [ L. ]. Plural of incus.

**incudiform** (in-ku′dĭ-form) [ L. *incus* (*incud*-), anvil ]. Shaped like an anvil.

**incu′domal′leal.** Relating to the incus and the malleus; denoting the articulation between the anvil and the hammer in the middle ear.

**incu′dostape′dial.** Relating to the incus and the stapes; denoting the articulation between the anvil and the stirrup in the middle ear.

**incurable** (in-kūr′ă-bl). Not curable.

**incurvation** (in′kur-va′shun). An inward curvature; a bending inward.

**incus,** gen. **incu′dis,** pl. **incu′des** (ing′kus) [ L. anvil ] [ NA ]. Anvil; the middle of the three ossicles in the middle ear; it has a body (*corpus incudis*) and two limbs or processes (crus longum incudis and crus breve incudis); at the tip of the long limb is a small knob, *processus lenticularis,* which articulates with the head of the stapes.

**indagation** (in-da-ga′shun) [ L. *indago,* pp. *-atus,* to search ]. An examination or investigation; specifically, the determination of the condition of the genital parts at the termination of the puerperium preliminary to the discharge of the patient.

**indeciduate** (in′de-sid′u-āt). Relating to the mammals (Indecidua) that do not shed any maternal uterine tissue when expelling the placenta at birth (horse, pig) in contrast to deciduate mammals (man, dog, rodent).

**indenization** (in-den-i-za′shun) [ *in-* + denizen ]. Innidiation.

**indenta′tion** [ Mediev. L. *in-dento,* pp. *-atus,* to make notches like teeth, fr. L. *dens* (*dent*-), tooth ]. 1. The act of notching or pitting. 2. A notch. 3. A state of being notched.

# INDEX

**index,** gen. **in′dicis,** (in′deks) [ L. one that points out, an informer, the forefinger, an index, fr. *in-dico,* pp. *-atus,* to declare ]. 1 [ NA ]. The second finger (the thumb being counted as the first); forefinger; pointing or index finger. 2. A guide, standard, indicator, symbol, or number denoting the relation in respect to size, capacity, or function, of one part or thing to another. 3. A core or mold used to record or maintain the relative position of a tooth or teeth to one another and/or to a cast. 4. A guide, usually made of plaster, used to reposition teeth, casts, or parts.

**absorbancy i.,** specific absorption *coefficient.*

**alve′olar i.,** (1) gnathic i.; (2) basilar i.

**anesthetic i.,** ratio of the number of units of anesthetic required for anesthesia to the number of units of anesthetic required to produce respiratory failure.

**antitryptic i.,** an obsolete term for the relative retardation in loss of viscosity of a solution of casein incubated with trypsin, to which a drop of abnormal blood serum (as from a cancerous patient) has been added, compared with that in a similar solution to which normal serum has been added; if the former drips through the tube of the viscosimeter in 100 seconds, and the latter in 104 seconds, the antitryptic i. is 4.

**Arneth i.,** an expression based on adding the percentages of polymorphonuclear neutrophils with 1 or 2 lobes in their nuclei, plus one-half the percentage with 3 lobes; the normal value is 60 per cent. See also Arneth *formula,* Arneth *count.*

**auric′ular i.,** relation of the width to the height of the auricle or pinna: (width of pinna × 100)/length of pinna.

**Ayala's i.,** Ayala's quotient; spinal quotient; the cerebrospinal i. when 10 ml. of cerebrospinal fluid have been removed.

**bas′ilar i.,** alveolar i. (2); ratio between the basialveolar line and the maximum length of the cranium, according to the formula: (basialveolar line × 100)/length of cranium.

**Bodecker i.,** a modification of the DMF caries i.

**buffer i.,** buffer value; see under buffer.

**cardiac i.,** the minute cardiac output per square meter of body surface.

**cardiothoracic i.,** the greatest transverse diameter of the heart shadow by x-ray compared with the greatest transverse diameter of the chest, normally less than 1/2.

**cephal′ic i.,** the ratio of the maximal breadth to the maximal length of the head, obtained by the formula: (breadth × 100)/length.

**cephalo-orbital i.,** the ratio of the cubic content of the two orbits to that of the cranial cavity multiplied by 100.

**cephalorrhachidian i.,** cerebrospinal i.

**cerebral i.,** the ratio of the transverse to the anteroposterior diameter of the cranial cavity multiplied by 100.

**cerebrospinal i.,** cephalorrhachidian i.; the figure obtained by multiplying the pressure of the cerebrospinal fluid, after fluid has been withdrawn by spinal puncture, by the quantity of fluid withdrawn and then dividing by the original pressure.

**chemotherapeutic i.,** the ratio of the minimal effective dose of a chemotherapeutic agent to the maximal tolerated dose. Originally used by Ehrlich to express the relative toxicity of a chemotherapeutic agent to a parasite and to its host.

**chest i.,** thoracic i.

**color i.,** blood quotient; "valeur globulaire"; globular value; C. I.: the ratio between the amount of hemoglobin and the number of red blood cells, obtained by means of dividing the concentration of hemoglobin (expressed as per cent of normal) by the relative number of red blood cells (expressed as per cent, on the basis of 5,000,000 per cu. mm. as normal); the average color i. is approximately 0.85.

**Colour Index,** abbreviated C.I.; a four-volume publication dealing with the chemistry of a vast number of dyes, in which each is identified by a unique five-digit C.I. number, *e.g.,* methylene blue, C.I. 52015.

**cranial i.,** the ratio of the maximal breadth to the maximal length of the skull, obtained by the formula: (breadth × 100)/length.

**degenerative i.,** the percentage of granulocytes that contain toxic granules in the cytoplasm, as compared with the total percentage of granulocytes.

**dental i.,** relation of the dental length (distance from the anterior surface of the first premolar to the posterior surface of the third molar) to the basinasal (basion to nasion) length: (dental length × 100)/basinasal length.

**DMF caries i.,** an i. of past caries experience; a technique for handling statistically the number of decayed, missing, and filled teeth in the mouth.

**effective temperature i.,** a composite i. of environmental comfort which is compared after exposure to different combinations of air temperature, humidity, and movement.

**empathic i.,** the degree of empathy experienced by one in respect of another person, more particularly of a sufferer from some morbid emotional or somatic condition.

**endem′ic i.,** the percentage of children infected with malaria or other endemic disease, in any given locality.

**i. of excursion of the uterus,** the distance, expressed in centimeters, that the uterus can be displaced upward and downward; the normal i. is 4 cm., 2 cm. in each direction, in nulliparae, and 6 to 8 cm. in multiparae.

**facial i.,** relation of the length of the face to its maximal width between the zygomatic prominences; to get the **superior facial i.,** the length is measured from the nasion to the alveolar point: (nasialveolar length × 100)/bizygomatic width; **total facial i.,** the length is measured from the nasion to the mental tubercle: (nasimental length × 100)/bizygomatic width.

**Flower's dental i.,** dental i.

**free thyroxine i.,** an arbitrary value obtained by multiplying the triiodothyronine uptake by the serum thyroxine concentration; it largely corrects for variations in thyroid-bound globulin concentration by providing a clinically valid estimate of the physiologically active free thyroxine; direct assay or laboratory measurement of free serum thyroxine yields a more accurate value.

**gnath′ic i.,** alveolar i. (1); relation between the basialveolar (basion to alveolar point) and basinasal (basion to nasion) lengths: (basialveolar length × 100)/basinasal length; the result indicates the degree of projection of the maxilla or upper jaw.

**height-length i.,** vertical i.

**hemore'nal salt i.,** the ratio of the quantity of inorganic salts in the urine to that of the inorganic salts in the blood; a figure obtained by means of dividing the electrical resistance of the blood by that of the urine; it varies from 3 to 5 in health.

**icteric i.,** see icterus i.

**ic'terus i.,** an obsolete test of historical interest only; a value that indicates the relative level of bilirubin in serum or plasma; calculated by comparing (in a colorimeter) the intensity of the color of the specimen with that of a standard solution (potassium dichromate, 0.05 gm., in 500 ml. of water, plus 0.2 ml. of sulfuric acid). The normal range is 3 to 5, and values greater than 15 are usually associated with clinically apparent jaundice; an i. less than 3 is observed in various examples of secondary anemia, aplastic anemia, and chlorosis. Sometimes erroneously called icteric i.: it is an i. of jaundice, not a jaundiced i.

**iron i.,** a figure obtained by means of dividing the figure for the average content of iron in normal blood (42.74 mg.) by the red cell count in millions; it normally varies between 8 and 9; in pernicious anemia, the i. is usually greater than 10, but it tends to be normal in chronic secondary anemia.

**length-breadth i.,** cephalic i.

**length-height i.,** vertical i.

**leukope'nic i.,** a significant decrease in the white blood count after ingestion of food to which a patient is thought to be hypersensitive; a count made during the normal fasting state is used as the basis for evaluation, and a postprandial count that is decreased by more than 1000 per cu. mm. is interpreted as a positive test for sensitivity to the food ingested.

**maturation i.,** an i. indicating the degree of maturation attained by the vaginal epithelium as adjudged by the cell types exfoliated therefrom. It represents the percentage of parabasal cells/intermediate cells/superficials, in that order. A shift to the left indicates more immature cells on the surface (atrophy) while a shift to the right represents more mature epithelium. The i. serves as an objective expression of one important facet in cytohormonal evaluation of a patient's response to her endocrine milieu.

**metacarpal i.,** the average ratio of length to breadth of metacarpals II to V; this ratio is increased in the Marfan syndrome.

**molar absorbancy i.,** molar absorption *coefficient.*

**nasal i.,** relation of the greatest width of the nasal aperture to the length of a line from the nasion to the lower border of the nasal aperture: (nasal width × 100)/nasal height.

**nucleoplasmic i.,** the quotient of the nuclear volume divided by the cytoplasmic volume.

**obesity i.,** body weight divided by body volume.

**opsonic i.,** a value that indicates the relative content of opsonin in the blood of a person with an infectious disease, as evaluated *in vitro* in comparison with presumably normal blood; the opsonic i. is calculated from the following equation: phagocytic i. of normal serum ÷ phagocytic i. of test serum $= 1 \div x$, where $x$ represents the opsonic i.

**or'bital i.,** relation of the height of the orbit to its width: (orbital height × 100)/orbital width.

**pal'atal** or **pal'atine i.,** palatomaxillary i.

**pal'atomax'illary i.,** relation of the palatomaxillary width, measured between the outer borders of the alveolar arch just above the middle of the second molar tooth, and the palatomaxillary length, measured from the alveolar point to the middle of a transverse line touching the posterior borders of the two maxillae = (palatomaxillary width × 100)/palatomaxillary length; it notes the varying forms of the dental arcade and palate.

**pelvic i.,** the ratio of the conjugate to the transverse diameter of the pelvis, a number obtained by multiplying the conjugate diameter of the pelvis by 100, and dividing by the greatest transverse width across the inlet.

**phagocytic i.,** the average number of bacteria observed in the cytoplasm of polymorphonuclear leukocytes after mixing and incubating, at 37°C., (1) a suspension of washed, presumably normal leukocytes, (2) the serum to be tested—for opsonin, and (3) a young culture of microorganisms that are causing disease in the patient. If specific opsonin is present in the serum, greater numbers of bacteria are ingested by the leukocytes.

**PMA i.,** a clinical i. used in epidemiologic studies of periodontal disease; based on the degree of the effect of the disease on the papillae and marginal and attached gingivae.

**ponderal i.,** cube root of body weight times 100 divided by stature.

**refrac'tive i.,** symbol, *n;* the relative velocity of light in another medium compared to the velocity in air; *e.g.,* in the case of air to crown glass, $n=1.52$; in the case of air to water, $n=1.33$. See also *law* of refraction.

**Röhrer's i.,** body weight in grams times 100 divided by the cube of height in centimeters.

**sa'cral i.,** a ratio obtained by multiplying the greatest breadth of the sacrum by 100 and dividing by the length.

**satura'tion i.,** an indication of the relative concentration of hemoglobin in the red blood cells, calculated as follows: grams of hemoglobin per 100 ml., expressed as per cent of normal ÷ hematocrit value, expressed as per cent of normal = saturation i. The normal i. for adults and infants is 0.97 to 1.02; in primary and secondary anemia, the i. is usually considerably less than 0.97.

**Schilling's i.,** Schilling's *blood count.*

**small increment sensitivity i.,** see SISI *test.*

**spiro-i.,** see *spiro-index.*

**splenic i.,** a rough indication of the salubrity, or the reverse, in regard to malaria of a particular district, judged by the relative absence or prevalence of enlarged spleens among the population.

**staph'ylo-opson'ic i.,** the opsonic i. calculated in relation to a staphylococcal infection, with a young culture of *Staphylococcus aureus* or the strain of staphylococcus from the patient being used in the test.

**therapeutic i.,** the ratio of $LD_{50}$ to $ED_{50}$, used in quantitative comparison of drugs.

**thorac'ic i.,** anteroposterior diameter of the thorax times 100 divided by the transverse diameter of the thorax.

**tibiofem'oral i.,** the ratio obtained by multiplying the length of the tibia by 100 and dividing by the length of the femur.

**transver'sover'tical i.,** vertical i.

**tuber'culo-opson'ic i.,** the opsonic i. calculated in relation to tuberculous infection, with an actively growing culture of *Mycobacterium tuberculosis* or the strain of tubercle bacillus from the patient being used in the test.

**urea i.,** Ambard's *coefficient* or *law.*

**uricolytic i.,** the percentage of uric acid oxidized to allantoin before being secreted.

**ventilation i.,** the figure obtained by dividing the ventilation test by the vital capacity.

**vertical i.,** the relation of the height to the length of the skull: (height × 100)/length.

**vital i.,** the ratio of births to deaths within a population during a given time.

**volume i.,** an indication of the relative size (*i.e.,* volume) of erythrocytes, calculated as follows: hematocrit value, expressed as per cent of normal ÷ red blood cell count, expressed as per cent of normal = volume i.

**zygomat'icoauric'ular i.,** the ratio between the zygomatic and the auricular diameters of the skull or head.

---

**in'dican.** 1. Plant i.; indoxyl β-D-glucoside, from *Indigofera* spp., a source of indigo. 2. Metabolic i.; the potassium salt of 3-indoxylsulfuric acid, a substance found in the sweat and in variable amount in the urine, indicative, when in quantity, of protein putrefaction in the intestine (urinary indican); see also Jaffe's *test.*

**in'dicanidro'sis** [ indican + G. *hidrōs*, sweat ]. Excretion of indican in the sweat.

**in'dicant** [ L. *in-dico*, pp. *-atus*, pres. p. *-ans* (*-ant*), to point out ]. 1. Pointing out; indicating. 2. An indication; especially a symptom indicating the proper line of treatment.

**indicanuria** (in'dĭ-kan-u'rĭ-ah). An increased urinary excretion of indican, a derivative of indol formed chiefly in the intestine when protein is putrefied; indol is also formed during the putrefaction of protein in other sites.

**indication** (in'dĭ-ka'shun) [ L. fr. *in-dico*, to point out, fr. *dico*, to proclaim ]. A suggestion or pointer as to the proper treatment of a disease; it may be furnished by a knowledge of the cause (**causal i.**), by the symptoms present ( **symptomatic i.**), or by nature of the disease (**specific i.**).

**in'dica'tor** [ L. one that points out ]. In chemical analysis a substance that changes color within a certain definite range of pH or oxidation potential, or in any way renders visible the completion of a chemical reaction; litmus, for example, shows red or blue if a solution to which it is added is acid or alkaline, respectively; phenol red is yellow at pH 7.1 but turns faintly pink at pH 7.2.

**oxidation-reduction i.,** redox i.; a substance that undergoes a definite color change at a specific oxidation potential.

**indicophose** (in'dĭ-ko-fōz) [ G. *indikon*, indigo, + *phōs*, light ]. A phose of blue color.

**Indiella** (in-dĭ-el'lah). An obsolete name for a genus of fungi, several species of which cause mycetoma. The several species are *I. mansoni, I reynier,* and *I. somaliensis. I. mansoni* appears to have been *Allescheria boydii* and *I. somaliensis* appears to have been *Streptomyces* (*Nocardia*) *somaliensis.*

**indigestion** (in'dĭ-jes'chun). Failure of proper digestion and absorption of food in the alimentary tract, and the consequences thereof.

**acid i.,** thought to represent hyperchlorhydria; term often used by the laity as a synonym for pyrosis.

**fat i.,** steatorrhea.

**gastric i.,** dyspepsia.

**nervous i.,** i. caused by emotional upsets.

**indigenous** (in-dij'ĕ-nus) [ L. *indigenus,* born in, fr. *indu,* within (old form of *in*), + suffix -*gen,* producing ]. Native; natural to the country where found.

**indigitation** (in-dij-ĭ-ta'shun) [ L. *in,* into + *digitus,* digit ]. Intussusception; invagination.

**indigo** (in'dĭ-go) [ L. *indicum,* fr. G. *indikon,* indigo, ntr. of *Indikos,* Indian ]. Indigo blue; indigotin; Δ²,²'-biindoline)-3,3'-dione; a blue dyestuff obtained from *Indigofera tinctoria,* and other species of *Indigofera* (family Leguminosae). Also made synthetically.

**i. blue,** indigo.

**i. carmine** (BP), sodium indigotindisulfonate (USP); sodium indigotin 5,5'-disulfonate; a blue dye used for measurement of kidney function.

**indigotin** (in-dig'o-tin, in'dĭ-go'tin). Indigo.

**indigouria, indiguria** (in'di-go-u'rĭ-ah, in-dĭ-gu'rĭ-ah). The excretion of indigo in the urine.

**indiru'bin.** Δ²,³'-Biindoline-2',3-dione, an isomer of indigo; see also urorosein.

**indisposition** (in-dis-po-zish'un) [ L. *in* neg. + *dispositio,* an arrangement, fr. *dis-pono,* pp. -*positus,* to place apart ]. A slight illness; malaise.

**indium** (in'dĭ-um) [ *indigo,* because it gives a blue line in the spectrum ]. A metallic element, symbol In, atomic no. 49, atomic weight 114.82.

**in'dium-111.** ¹¹¹In; a cyclotron-produced radionuclide with a physical half-life of 2.8 days and with gamma ray emissions of 173 and 247 kiloelectron volts. In a chloride form, it is used as a bone marrow and tumor-localizing tracer; in a chelate form, as a cerebrospinal fluid tracer.

**individuation** (in'dĭ-vid'u-a'shun). 1. The development of the individual from the specific. 2. In Jungian psychology, the process by which one's personality is differentiated, developed, and expressed.

**in'docy'anine green** (USP). CARDIO-GREEN; a tricarbocyanine dye used in blood volume determinations and in liver function tests.

**indocybin.** Psilocybin.

**indolaceturia** (in-dōl-as-ĕ-tu'rĭ-ah). The excretion of an appreciable amount of indolacetic acid in the urine; one manifestation of Hartnup disease.

**indol'amine.** A general term for an indole or indole derivative containing a primary, secondary, or tertiary amine group (*e.g.,* serotonin).

**indole** (in'dōl). 2,3-Benzopyrrole; basis of many biologically active substances (*e.g.,* serotonin, tryptophan).

**in'dolent** [ L. *in-* neg. + *doleo,* pr. p. *dolens* (-*ent-*), to feel pain ]. Inactive; sluggish; painless or nearly so.

**indo'lic acids.** Metabolites of tryptophan formed within the body or by intestinal microorganisms. The principal indolic acids encountered in urine are indoleacetic acid, indoleacetylglutamine, 5-hydroxyindoleacetic acid, and indolelactic acid.

**in'doline.** 2,3-Dihydroindole.

**indologenous** (in'do-loj'ĕ-nus). Producing or causing the production of indole.

**in'dolu'ria.** Excretion of indole in the urine; actual reference commonly is to indolic acids and indoxyl, as indole itself rarely appears in the urine.

**indolyl** (in'do-lil). The radical of indole, as in β-(3-indolyl)alanine, tryptophan.

**indometh'acin** (BP, NF). INDOCIN; 1-(*p*-chlorobenzoyl)-5-methoxy-2-methylindole-3-acetic acid; an analgesic, antipyretic, and anti-inflammatory nonsteroidal agent as effective as the salicylates in the management of rhematoid arthritis; also used in the treatment of osteoarthritis, ankylosing spondylitis, and gout. Untoward effects are common.

**indophe'nolase.** Cytochrome *c* oxidase.

**in'dophe'nol ox'idase.** Cytochrome *c* oxidase.

**indox'yl.** The 3-radical of 3-hydroxyindole; a product of intestinal bacterial degradation of indoleacetic acid, excreted in the urine as indoleaceturic acid (conjugated with glycine) or as sulfate (urinary indican) or glucuronide (glucosiduronate); increased amounts are excreted by phenylketonuric patients.

**indoxyluria** (in-dok'sil-u'rĭ-ah). The excretion of indoxyl, especially indoxyl sulfate, in the urine; i. may be associated with indicanuria, inasmuch as hydrolysis of indican results in formation of indoxyl.

**induce** (in'dūs'). To cause or bring about; see induction.

**indu'cer.** A molecule, usually a substrate of a specific enzyme pathway, that combines with active repressor (produced by a regulator gene) to deactivate the repressor; this results in activation of a previously repressed operator gene and initiates activity of the structural genes controlled by the operator, which in turn results in enzyme production; a homeostatic mechanism for regulating enzyme production in an inducible enzyme system. See fig. under protein.

**inductance** (in-duk'tans) [ see induction ]. The coefficient of electromagnetic induction. The unit of inductance is the henry, symbol H.

**induction** (in-duk'shun) [ L. *inductio,* a leading in ]. 1. Production or causation. 2. The period from the start of anesthesia to the establishment of a depth of anesthesia adequate for operation. 3. In embryology, the influence exerted by an organizer or evocator on the differentiation of adjacent cells or on the development of an embryonic structure. Spemann, in 1935, was awarded the Nobel Prize for development of this concept. 4. A modification imposed upon the offspring by the action of environment on the germ cells of one or both parents. 5. In microbiology, the change from probacteriophage (prophage) to vegetative phage that may occur spontaneously or after stimulation by certain physical and chemical agents. 6. In enzymology, the process of increasing the amount or the activity of an enzyme; see inducer. 7. One of the stages in the process of hypnosis.

**lysogenic i.,** i. that occurs when prophage is transferred to a nonlysogenic bacterium by conjugation or by transduction.

**spinal i.,** the manner in which one sensory stimulus lowers the threshold for another.

**induc'tor.** 1. An agent bringing about induction. 2. An evocator. 3. An organizer.

**inducto'rium.** An instrument used, especially in physiologic experiments, for generating currents of induced electricity as a means of stimulating nerve or muscle.

**induc'totherm** [ induction (2) + G. *thermē,* heat ]. A device for producing artificial fever by electric induction.

Indole

**induc'tother'my** [ induction (2) + G. *thermē*, heat ]. Artificial fever production by means of electromagnetic induction.

**in'dulin.** A blue dye used as a stain in histology and bacteriology.

**indulinophil, indulinophile** (in-du-lin'o-fil, -fĭl) [ indulin + G. *philos*, fond ]. Taking an indulin stain readily.

**in'durated** [ L. *in-duro*, pp. *-duratus*, to harden, fr. *durus*, hard ]. Hardened; in the field of medicine, usually used with reference to "soft tissues" becoming firm or extremely firm, but not as hard as bone.

**induration** (in'du-ra'shun) [ L. *induratio* (see indurated) ]. 1. The process of becoming extremely firm or hard, or having such physical features; see also indurated. 2. A focus or region of indurated tissue.

   **brown i. of the lung,** pigment i. of the lung; a condition characterized by firmness of the lungs, and a brown color associated with hemosiderin-pigmented macrophages in alveoli, consequent upon long-continued congestion due to heart disease.

   **cyanotic i.,** that related to persistent, chronic venous congestion in an organ or tissue, frequently resulting in fibrous thickening of the walls of the walls of the veins and eventual fibrosis of adjacent tissue; the affected tissue becomes firmer than normal, and tends to have an unusual, red-blue color.

   **fibroid i.,** cirrhosis.

   **Froriep's i.,** *myositis* fibrosa.

   **granular i.,** cirrhosis.

   **gray i.,** a condition occurring in lungs during and after pneumonic processes in which there is failure of resolution; there is a conspicuous increase in fibrous connective tissue in the walls of the alveoli, and also within the alveoli (*i.e.*, fibrous organization of exudate); in contrast to brown i., there is usually not a prominent degree of pigmentation, unless chronic passive congestion is also present.

   **Hunter's i.,** Hunter's *chancre.*

   **lam'inate i.,** a relatively narrow, but distinct, peripherally situated zone of numerous, fairly densely accumulated lymphocytes, plasma cells, and mononuclear macrophages in the corium; characteristically observed in the classic primary lesion of syphilis, *i.e.*, a chancre.

   **parchment i.,** a more advanced form of laminate i., *i.e.*, the zone of infiltrated cells is broader and more prominent.

   **pigment i. of the lung,** brown i. of the lung.

   **plastic i.,** sclerosis of corpus cavernosum of penis.

   **red i.,** a condition observed in lungs in which there is an advanced degree of acute passive congestion, or acute pneumonitis (sometimes termed interstitial pneumonia), or a similar pathologic process.

**in'durative.** Pertaining to, causing, or characterized by induration.

**indusium,** pl. **indu'sia** (in-du'zĭ-um) [ L. a woman's undergarment, fr. *induo*, to put on ]. 1. A membranous layer or covering. 2. The amnion.

   **i. gris'eum** [ NA ], supracallosal gyrus; a thin layer of gray matter on the dorsal surface of the corpus callosum in which the striae longitudinalis medialis and lateralis (striae lancisi) lie embedded. The i. griseum is a rudimentary component of the hippocampus, continuous caudally around the splenium of the corpus callosum with the gyrus fasciolaris or fasciola cinerea, a slender convolution in turn continuous with the dentate gyrus or fascia dentata of the hippocampus; rostrally the i. griseum curves around the genu and rostrum corporis callosi, and extends ventralward to the olfactory trigone as the tenia tecta or rudimentum hippocampi, hidden in the depth of the sulcus parolfactorius posterior that marks the anterior border of the gyrus subcallosus or precommissural septum.

**inebriant** (in-e'brĭ-ant) [ see inebriety ]. 1. Making drunk; intoxicating. 2. An intoxicant.

**inebriation** (in-e'brĭ-a'shun) [ see inebriety ]. Intoxication.

**inebriety** (in-e-bri'e-tĭ) [ L. *in*-intensive + *ebrietas*, drunkenness ]. The habitual indulgence in alcoholic beverages in excessive amounts.

**inert** (in-ert') [ L. *iners*, unskillful, sluggish, fr. *in*, neg. + *ars*, art ]. 1. Slow in action; sluggish. 2. Inactive. 3. Devoid of active chemical properties, as the inert gases. 4. Having no pharmacologic or therapeutic action; denoting a drug.

**inertia** (in-er'shĭ-ah, in-er'shah) [ L. want of skill, laziness ]. 1. The state of a physical body in which it "resists" any force tending to move it from a position of rest or to change its uniform motion. 2. Denoting inactivity or lack of force; lack of mental or physical vigor; sluggishness of thought or action.

   **psychic i.,** a psychiatric term denoting resistance to any change in ideas or to progress; fixation of an idea.

   **uterine i.,** absence of effective uterine contractions during labor. When the uterus fails to contract with sufficient force to effect continuous dilation or effacement of the cervix or descent or rotation of the fetal head, and the uterus is easily indentable at the acme of contraction, the i. is called primary or true uterine i.; when the uterine contractions are vigorous to start with but, as a result of the exhaustion or dehydration of the patient, decrease in vigor, and progress of labor ceases, the condition is called secondary uterine i.

**in extre'mis** [ L. *extremus*, last ]. At the point of death.

**in'fancy.** Babyhood; the earliest period of extrauterine life; roughly, the first 2 years of life.

**in'fant** [ L. *infans*, not speaking ]. 1. A child under the age of 2 years. 2. A newborn baby.

   **i. Her'cules,** term applied to young children with precocious sexual and muscular development due to a virilizing adrenocortical disorder.

   **liveborn i.,** the product of a livebirth; an i. who shows evidence of life after birth; life is considered to be present after birth if any one of the following is observed: if the infant breathes, if the infant shows beating of the heart, if pulsation of the umbilical cord occurs, or if there is definite movement of voluntary muscles.

   **post-term i.,** an i. with a gestational age of 42 completed weeks or more (294 days or more).

   **preterm i.,** an i. with gestational age of less than 37 completed weeks (259 completed days).

   **stillborn i.,** an i. who shows no evidence of life after birth; *cf.* liveborn i.

   **term i.,** an i. with gestational age of 37 completed weeks (259 completed days) to less than 42 completed weeks (less than 294 completed days).

**infan'ticide** [ infant + L. *caedo*, to kill ]. 1. The killing of an infant. 2. One who murders an infant.

**infan'ticul'ture.** Puericulture.

**in'fantile.** Relating to, or characteristic of, infants or infancy.

**infantilism** (in-fan'tĭ-lizm). 1. A state marked by extremely slow development of mind and body. 2. Childishness, as in a temper tantrum by an adolescent or adult.

   **angioplastic i.,** i. due to defective development of the vascular system.

   **Brissaud's i.,** cretinism.

   **cachec'tic i.,** a form of i., due apparently to chronic infection (malaria, tuberculosis, etc.), autointoxication, or chronic drug poisoning.

   **dysthyroi'dal i.,** cretinism.

   **Gee-Herter i.,** celiac *disease.*

   **hepat'ic i.,** a form associated with cirrhosis of the liver.

   **Herter's i.,** celiac *disease.*

   **hypothy'roid i.,** cretinism.

   **idiopath'ic i.,** Lorain's disease; proportionate i.; dwarfism generally associated with hypogonadism; may be caused by deficient secretion of anterior pituitary hormones.

   **intestinal i.,** celiac *disease.*

   **Lorain-Lévi i.,** pituitary *dwarfism.*

   **lymphat'ic i.,** Paltauf's i. or nanism; a form associated with lymphatism (obsolete usage).

   **myxedem'atous i.,** cretinism.

   **Paltauf's i.,** lymphatic i.

   **pancreat'ic i.,** a form associated with deficiency or absence of the pancreatic secretion. See fibrocystic *disease* of the pancreas.

   **partial i.,** obsolete term denoting arrested development affecting a special tissue or organ, such as cryptorchism, a patent foramen ovale, etc.

   **pitu'itary i.,** descriptive of a pituitary *dwarf.*

   **proportionate i.,** idiopathic i.

   **renal i.,** renal *rickets.*

   **sexual i.,** failure to develop secondary sexual characteristics after the normal time of puberty.

**static i.,** a condition observed in young children resembling spastic spinal paralysis; it is marked by hypotonia of the muscles of the trunk and hypertonia of the muscles of the extremities.

**tubal i.,** descriptive of a corkscrew-like Fallopian tube as seen in fetal life.

**universal i.,** idiopathic i.

**infarct** (in'farkt) [ L. *in-farcio,* pp. *-fartus* (*-ctus,* an incorrect form), to stuff into ]. Infarction (2); an area of necrosis resulting from local arrest or sudden insufficiency of arterial or venous blood supply.

**anemic i.,** white i. (1); pale i.; an i. in which little or no bleeding into tissue spaces occurs when the blood supply is obstructed.

**hemorrhag'ic i.,** red i.

**pale i.,** anemic i.

**red i.,** hemorrhagic i.; an area, red and swollen, the seat of infiltration of blood from collateral channels before coagulation has occurred.

**uric acid i.,** precipitates of uric acid distending renal collecting tubules in the newborn; there is no necrosis, therefore the term infarct is a misnomer.

**white i.,** (1) anemic i.; (2) in the placenta, intervillous fibrin with ischemic necrosis of villi.

**Zahn's i.,** a pseudoinfarct of the liver, consisting of an area of congestion with parenchymal atrophy but no necrosis; due to obstruction of a branch of the portal vein.

**infarction** (in-fark'shun). 1. Local arrest or sudden insufficiency of arterial or venous blood supply due to emboli, thrombi, vascular torsion, or pressure that produces a macroscopic area of necrosis; the heart, brain, spleen, kidney, intestine, lung, and testes are most affected, as are tumors, especially of the ovary or uterus. 2. Infarct.

**anterior myocardial i.,** involving the anterior wall of the heart, and producing indicative electrocardiographic changes in leads I and aVL and the anterior chest leads.

**anteroinferior myocardial i.,** one involving both anterior and inferior walls of the heart simultaneously.

**anterolat'eral myocardial i.,** extensive anterior i. producing indicative changes across the precordium as well as in leads I and aVL.

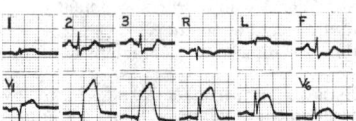

**Acute Anterolateral Myocardial Infarction**
(From Marriott, H. J. L.: *Practical Electrocardiography,* Ed. 4, The Williams & Wilkins Co., Baltimore, 1968.)

**anterosep'tal myocardial i.,** an anterior i. in which indicative electrocardiographic changes are confined to the right chest leads ($V_1$-$V_4$).

**cardiac i.,** myocardial i.

**diaphragmatic myocardial i.,** inferior myocardial i.

**inferior myocardial i.,** diaphragmatic myocardial i.; in which the inferior or diaphragmatic wall of the heart is involved, producing indicative changes in leads II, III, and aVF in the electrocardiogram.

**inferolat'eral myocardial i.,** involving the inferior and lateral surfaces of the heart and producing indicative changes in the electrocardiogram in leads II, III, aVF, V5, and V6.

**lateral myocardial i.,** one involving only the lateral wall of the heart, producing indicative electrocardiographic changes confined to leads I, aVL, V5, and V6.

**myocardial i.,** cardiac i.; i. of an area of the heart muscle usually as a result of occlusion of a coronary artery.

**myocardial i. in H-form,** i. involving the septum along with both inferior and anterior walls to make an H-shaped configuration.

**posterior myocardial i.,** in which the i. involves the posterior wall of the heart; also formerly used of i.'s involving the inferior or diaphragmatic surface of the heart.

**silent myocardial i.,** one that produces none of the characteristic symptoms and signs of myocardial i.

**subendocardial myocardial i.,** one that involves only the layer of muscle subjacent to the endocardium.

**through-and-through myocardial i.,** transmural myocardial i.

**transmural myocardial i.,** through-and-through myocardial i.; one that involves the whole thickness of the heart muscle from endocardium to epicardium.

**watershed i.,** cortical i. in an area of blood supply between two major cerebral arteries.

**infarc'toid.** Resembling an infarction.

**infect** (in-fekt') [ L. *in-ficio,* pp. *-fectus,* to dip into, dye, corrupt, infect, fr. *in* + *facio,* to make. FAC- ]. 1. To enter, invade, or inhabit another organism, causing infection or contamination. 2. To dwell internally, endoparasitically, as opposed to externally (infestation).

**infection** (in-fek'shun). Endoparasitism; multiplication of microorganisms in the body proper. Multiplication of bacteria of the "normal" flora of the intestinal tract is not usually viewed as being an i., whereas multiplication of other organisms, *e.g., Vibrio cholerae,* might be viewed as an i.

**agonal i.,** terminal i.

**apical i.,** the implantation of a microorganism at the apex of a tooth; usually the result of the migration of a microorganism from the pulp canal through the apical foramen.

**coli i.,** i. with the colon bacillus.

**cross i.,** i. spread from one source to another, person to person, animal to person, person to animal, animal to animal.

**cryptogenic i.,** bacterial, viral, or other i., the source of which is unknown.

**droplet i.,** i. acquired through the inhalation of droplets or aerosols of saliva or sputum containing virus or other microorganisms expelled by another person during sneezing, coughing, laughing, or talking.

**endog'enous i.,** i. caused by an infectious agent already present in the body, the previous i. having been inapparent.

**focal i.,** an old term which distinguishes local i.'s (focal) from generalized i.'s (sepsis).

**mass i.,** i. resulting from the entrance of a large number of pathogens into the circulation or tissues.

**mixed i.,** i. by more than one variety of pathogenic microorganisms.

**pyogenic i.,** i. characterized by local pus formation or pyemia.

**secondary i.,** an i., usually septic, occurring in a person or animal already suffering from an i. of another nature.

**superficial scalp i.,** an i. external to the galea; for example, folliculitis or cellulitis.

**terminal i.,** an acute i., commonly pneumonic or septic, occurring toward the end of any disease (usually a chronic disease), and often the cause of death.

**Vincent's i.,** Vincent's *disease.*

**zo'ogene'ic i.,** i. associated with animals.

**infection-immunity.** See under immunity.

**infectiosity** (in-fek-shī-os'ī-tī). Infectiousness.

**infectious** (in-fek'shus). 1. Capable of being transmitted by infection, with or without actual contact (see also contagious). 2. Producing an infection; infective. 3. Denoting a disease due to the action of a microorganism.

**infec'tive.** Relating to an infection; infectious.

**infecundity** (in-fe-kun'dī-tī) [ L. *infecunditas,* barrenness ]. Sterility in woman; barrenness.

**inferior** (in-fe'rī-or) [ L. lower ] [ NA ]. Lower; below in relation to another structure; caudal.

**infe'rior'ity.** The condition or state of being or feeling inadequate or inferior, especially to others similarly situated.

**in'fertil'ity.** [ L. *in-* neg. + *fertilis,* fruitful ]. Relative sterility; diminished or absent fertility; does not imply (either in the male or the female) the existence of as positive or irreversible a condition as sterility. In the female, it indicates adequate anatomical structures and equivocal function, with the possibility of pregnancy that may or may not proceed to term.

**infest** (in-fest') [ L. *infesto,* pp. *-atus,* to attack ]. 1. To infect, usually by macroscopic parasites; to invade parasitically. 2. To occupy a site and dwell ectoparasitically on the external surface, as opposed to dwelling within a host (infection).

**infesta′tion.** Ectoparasitism; the act or process of infesting.

**infibulation** (in-fib-u-la′shun) [ L. *in-fibulo,* pp. *-atus,* to buckle together, fr. *in,* in, + *fibula,* a clasp ]. Stitching together the lips of the vulva or of the prepuce in order to prevent copulation.

**infiltrate** (in-fil′trāt) [ L. *in* + Mediev. L. *filtro,* pp -atus, to strain through felt, fr. *filtrum,* felt ]. 1. To percolate; to enter or cause to enter the pores of a substance, denoting a liquid. 2. Material that has permeated or infiltrated into the tissues.

    **Assmann′s tuberculous i.,** infraclavicular i.

    **infraclavic′ular i.,** Assmann's early tuberculous i.; an incipient lesion of tuberculous infection.

**infiltration** (in′fil-tra′shun). 1. The act of passing into or interpenetrating a substance, cell, or tissue; said of gases, fluids, or matters held in solution. 2. The gas, fluid, or dissolved matter that has entered any substance, cell, or tissue.

    **ad′ipose i.,** growth of normal adult fat cells in sites where they are not usually present.

    **calcareous i.,** calcification.

    **cellular i.,** migration of cells from their sources of origin, or direct extension of cells as a result of unusual growth and multiplication, thereby resulting in (1) fairly well defined foci, or (2) irregular accumulations, or (3) diffusely distributed individual cells in the connective tissue and interstices of various organs and tissues; the term is used especially with reference to such changes associated with inflammations and certain types of malignant neoplasms.

    **epituberculous i.,** an i. superimposed upon a tuberculous lesion.

    **fatty i.,** abnormal accumulation of fat droplets in the cytoplasm of cells, particularly of fat derived from outside the cells; see also fatty *degeneration.*

    **gelat′inous i.,** gray i.

    **gray i.,** gelatinous i.; a term sometimes used for the relatively rapidly formed, semisolid, gray or gray-white exudate (chiefly necrotic cells and remnants of tissue, and macrophages) resulting from unusually acute, overwhelming, diffuse tuberculous infection in the lung, *i.e.,* tuberculous pneumonia.

    **paraneural i.,** i. around a nerve.

**infin′ity.** See infinite *distance.*

**infirm** (in-firm′) [ L. *in-firmus,* fr. *in-* neg. + *firmus,* strong ]. Weak or feeble because of old age or disease.

**infirmary** (in-fir′mā-rī) [ L. *infirmarium;* see infirm ]. A small hospital, especially in a school or college.

**infirmity** (in-fir′mī-tī). A weakness; an abnormal, more or less disabling, condition of mind or body.

**inflammabil′ity.** Flammability.

**inflammation** (in′flă-ma′shun) [ L. *inflammo,* pp. *-atus,* fr. *in,* in, + *flamma,* flame ]. A fundamental pathologic process consisting of a dynamic complex of cytologic and histologic reactions that occur in the affected blood vessels and adjacent tissues (of man and other animals) in response to an injury or abnormal stimulation caused by a physical, chemical, or biologic agent (or combinations of such agents), including (1) the local reactions and resulting morphologic changes, (2) the destruction or removal of the injurious material, and (3) the responses that lead to repair and healing. The so-called *cardinal signs* of i. are: *rubor*—redness, *calor*—heat (or warmth), *tumor*—swelling, and *dolor*—pain; a fifth sign, *i.e., functio laesa*—inhibited or lost function, is sometimes added. The redness and warmth result from an increased amount of blood in the affected tissue, which is usually congested; swelling ordinarily occurs from the congestion and exudation; pressure on (or stretching of) nerve endings, as well as changes in osmotic pressure and pH may lead to pain; the disturbance in function may result from discomfort of certain movements or the actual destruction of an anatomic part. All of the signs may be observed in certain instances, but no one of them is necessarily always present.

    **acute i.,** any i. that has a fairly rapid onset, and then relatively soon comes to a crisis; *i.e.,* there is resolution of the pathologic process and the patient recovers, or the patient dies from the condition. Acute i.'s are usually

manifest for only a few days, but, in some instances, they may persist for several days or even a few weeks; at any rate, the duration is relatively short, and the termination is clear and distinct. See also chronic i.

    **adhesive i.,** one in which the amount of fibrin in the exudate is sufficient to result in a slight or moderate degree of adherence of adjacent tissues, as in the healing of a wound by first intention.

    **allergic i.,** an inflammatory reaction occurring in tissue as the result of an increased or accelerated response to a specific antigen (or type of antigen), irrespective of the damage or benefit to the person whose tissues manifest the altered reactivity. Allergic i. in man is of two general types: (1) immediate, characterized by demonstrable specific antibody in the serum, and an *immediate response,* and with respect to certain allergens, such as pollens, occurs in greater incidence in certain families; (2) the delayed or bacterial type of allergic i., characterized by no eosinophilia of the peripheral blood and tissues, no demonstrable antibody in the serum, and the presence of a *delayed response.*

    **alterative i.,** a somewhat controversial term frequently used to designate a rather unique form of local reaction to injury, a response sometimes known as degenerative i., such as that occasionally observed in the walls of blood vessels and in parenchymal cells of various organs in reacting to certain chemicals, viruses, and other intracellular agents; the response is characterized by degenerative changes in the cytoplasm and nucleus, frequently resulting in necrosis, but exudation (if any) is ordinarily observed only in the wall of the affected vessel, or in the interstices immediately adjacent to the affected vessel or parenchymal cells.

    **atroph′ic i.,** fibroid i.; a form of chronic i. or repeated episodes of acute i. in which the continued or recurrent proliferation of fibroblasts results in the formation of fibrous tissue that eventually contracts and leads to compression and atrophy of parenchymal tissue.

    **catarrh′al i.,** an inflammatory process that is most frequent in the respiratory tract, but may occur in any mucous menbrane; characterized by hyperemia of the mucosal vessels, edema of the interstitial tissue, enlargement of the secretory epithelial cells (which proliferate and form conspicuous globules of mucus), and an irregular layer of viscous, mucinous material on the surface. As exudation progresses, variable numbers of neutrophils migrate into the affected tissue and are included in the exudate, along with fragments of degenerated and necrotic epithelial cells; thus, a catarrhal i. may frequently become mucopurulent.

    **chronic i.,** an i. that is the antithesis of acute i.; chronic i.'s may begin (1) with a relatively rapid onset, or (2) in a slow, insidious, and even unnoticed manner, but, in either event, they tend to persist for several months or years; the termination of the pathologic process is indefinite and frequently not recognizable, unless it causes the patient's death. Chronic i. results when the injuring agent (or products resulting from its presence) persist in the lesion, and the host's tissues respond in a manner (or to a degree) that is not sufficient to overcome completely the continuing effects of the injuring agent.

    **croupous i.,** an acute fibrinous i. in which a fairly tenacious pseudomembrane is formed in the larynx and frequently extends into the trachea and bronchi; the coagulated exudate may interfere with the passage of air and with the proper oxygenation of blood. See also pseudomembranous i.

    **degenerative i.,** alterative i.

    **ex′udative i.,** one in which the conspicuous or distinguishing feature is an exudate, which may be (1) chiefly serous, serofibrinous, fibrinous, or mucous (*i.e.,* relatively few cells are present), or may be (2) characterized by relatively large numbers of neutrophils, eosinophils, lymphocytes, monocytes, or plasma cells, frequently with one or two types being predominant. Exudative i. occurs not only as a separate and distinct pathologic process, but also frequently as a part of certain granulomatous i.'s.

    **fibrinopurulent i.,** a purulent i. in which the exudate (*i.e.,* pus) contains an unusually large amount of fibrin; also, a fibrinous or serofibrinous i. in which the accumulation of large numbers of polymorphonuclear leukocytes results in liquefactive necrosis of tissue and the formation of pus with a relatively large quantity of fibrin.

**fi'brinous i.,** an exudative i. in which there is a disproportionately large amount of fibrin.

**fibroid i.,** atrophic i.

**granulomatous i.,** a form of proliferative i.; see granuloma.

**hyperplast'ic i.,** proliferative i.

**immune i.,** (1) allergic i. of the delayed type; an inflammatory reaction in which the usual response of the tissues has been modified by various factors that have a significant role in immunity; increased activity, (2) any allergic i., whether of the immediate or delayed types.

**intersti'tial i.,** one in which the inflammatory reaction occurs chiefly in the supportive fibrous connective tissue or stroma of an organ.

**necrotic i., necrotizing i.,** usually an acute inflammatory reaction in which the predominant histologic change is fairly rapid necrosis that occurs diffusely or extensively in relatively large foci throughout the affected tissue, frequently with only little or no evidence of cells in the exudate.

**parenchy'matous i.,** alterative i.

**productive i.,** a vague term ordinarily used with reference to proliferative i., with or without an exudate; also sometimes used to indicate any i. in which grossly visible exudate is formed.

**proliferative i.,** hyperplastic i.; an inflammatory reaction in which the distinguishing feature is an actual increase in the number of tissue cells, especially the reticuloendothelial macrophages, in contrast to cells exuded from blood vessels; in addition, exudates of various types are likely to be observed in granulomas and other forms of proliferative i., but the latter may occur without an exudate being formed (as in certain infections caused by virus).

**pseudomembranous i.,** a form of exudative i. that involves mucous and serous membranes; relatively large quantities of fibrin in the exudate result in a rather tenacious membrane-like covering that is fairly adherent to the underlying acutely inflamed tissue; the pseudomembrane usually contains (in addition to the dense network of fibrin) varying quantities of plasma protein, degenerated and necrotic elements from the affected tissue, polymorphonuclear leukocytes, bacteria, and so on.

**purulent i.,** an acute exudative i. in which the accumulation of polymorphonuclear leukocytes is sufficiently great that their enzymes cause liquefaction of the affected tissues, focally or diffusely; the purulent exudate is frequently termed *pus*, and consists of plasma (and its constituents), end products of the enzymatic digestion of tissue, degenerated and necrotic cells and their debris, polymorphonuclear leukocytes and other white blood cells, the causal agent of the i., and so on. See also suppurative i.

**sclerosing i.,** i. leading to extensive formation of fibrous and scar tissue.

**serofibrinous i.,** one in which the exudate consists chiefly of serous fluid with an unusually large proportion of fibrin.

**serous i.,** an exudative i. in which the exudate is predominantly fluid (*i.e.,* exuded from the blood vessels), with the protein, electrolytes, and other material contained therein; relatively few (if any) cells are observed.

**subacute i.,** an i. that is intermediate in duration between that of an acute i. and that of a chronic i.; subacute i.'s usually persist longer than 3 or 4 weeks (this varies for individual diseases), but do not remain active sufficiently long to be regarded as chronic. See also acute i. and chronic i.

**suppurative i.,** basically the same process as that in purulent i., but suppuration (*i.e.,* liquefactive necrosis caused by the leukocytic enzymes) may occur in small foci without grossly visible quantities of pus being formed; in most instances, the two terms may be used synonymously.

**inflam'matory.** Pertaining to, characterized by, resulting from, or becoming affected by inflammation.

**infla'tion** [ L. *inflatio*, fr. *in-flo*, pp. *-flatus*, to blow into, inflate ]. Distention by a liquid or gas.

**infla'tor.** An instrument for injecting air.

**inflection, inflexion** (in-flek'shun) [ L. *in-flecto*, pp. *-flexus*, to bend ]. 1. An inward bending. 2. An obsolete term for diffraction.

**influenza** (in-flu-en'zah) [ It. fr. L. *in-fluo*, pr. p. *influens* ]. The grippe; the flu; epidemic rheum; an acute infectious disease known since 1933 to be due to a virus. The disease commonly occurs in epidemics or pandemics which develop quickly, spread rapidly, and involve sizable proportions of the population. The mortality rate is normally low. Influenza is fundamentally an acute respiratory disease in which the inhaled virus attacks the respiratory epithelial cells of susceptible persons and produces a catarrhal inflammation. The disease is characterized by sudden onset, chills, fever, severe prostration, headache, muscle aches, and a dry cough. Symptoms referrable to the gastrointestinal tract are uncommon; hence, the designation intestinal flu is a misnomer. The so-called nervous form probably refers to the severe prostration and and delerium which sometimes occur. Complications in the form of secondary bacterial infections are common, including bronchitis, sinusitis, otitis media, and pneumonia.

**Asian i.,** worldwide i., apparently originating in China in the summer of 1957, producing a much milder disease than the pandemic of 1917–1919.

**endem'ic i.,** i. nostras; acute catarrhal fever; winter grippe; a disease resembling in its general features pandemic i., but usually of less severe type, occurring with more or less regularity during the cold season, especially in the larger cities of the world.

**equine i.,** an upper respiratory infection of horses caused by either of two subtypes of type A influenza virus.

**i. lymphat'ica,** glandular *fever.*

**i. nostras,** endemic i.

**swine i.,** an acute respiratory disease caused by a virus which resembles very closely one of the types found in man; this disease is believed to have become adapted to swine in the United States during the great human pandemic in 1918.

**influen'zal.** Relating to, marked by, or resulting from, influenza.

**infold** (in-fōld'). To inclose within a fold, as in the operation of "infolding" an ulcer of the stomach, in which the walls of the organ on either side of the lesion are brought together and sutured.

**informational RNA.** Messenger RNA; see under ribonucleic acid.

**infra-** [ L. below ]. Prefix denoting a position below the part denoted by the word to which it is joined.

**infra-axillary** (in'frah-ak'sĭ-lěr-ĭ). Below the axilla.

**infrabulge** (in'frah-bulj). 1. That portion of the crown of a tooth gingival to the clasp guide or survey line, or height of contour. 2. That area of a tooth where the retentive portion of a clasp of a removable partial denture is placed.

**infracardiac** (in'frah-kar'dĭ-ak). Beneath the heart; below the level of the heart.

**infracerebral** (in'frah-sĕr'e-bral). Pertaining to that portion of the nervous system below the level of the cerebrum.

**in'fraclavic'ular.** Below the clavicle.

**infraclusion** (in'frah-klu'zhun). Infraocclusion; infraversion (3); the state wherein a tooth has failed to erupt to the maxillomandibular plane of interdigitation.

**infracor'tical.** Beneath the cortex of an organ, mainly the brain or kidney; subcortical.

**infracos'tal.** Below a rib or the ribs.

**infracotyloid** (in'frah-kot'ĭ-loyd). Below the acetabulum or cotyloid cavity.

**infracris'tal** [ infra- + L. *crista*, crest ]. Below the supraventricular crest; usually used in reference to ventricular septal defect.

**infraction** (in-frak'shun) [ L. *infractio*, a breaking, fr. *infringere*, to break ]. A fracture; especially one without displacement.

**infracture** (in-frak'chūr). Infraction.

**infradiaphragmatic** (in'frah-di'ah-frag-mat'ik). Subdiaphragmatic; below the diaphragm.

**infraglenoid** (in'frah-gle'noyd). Below the glenoid cavity of the scapula.

**infraglot'tic.** Below the glottis; subglottic.

**infrahepat'ic.** Below the liver.

**infrahyoid** (in'frah-hi'oyd). Below the hyoid bone; denoting especially a group of muscles: the sternohyoideus, sternothyroideus, thyrohyoideus, and omohyoideus.

**inframam'mary.** Below the mammary gland.

**inframandib'ular.** Beneath the mandible or lower jaw.

**inframar'ginal.** Below any margin or edge.

**inframax'illary.** Submaxillary; inframandibular.

**infranatant** (in'frah-na'tant) [ infra- + L. *natare*, to swim ]. See infranatant *fluid.*

**infraocclusion** (in'frah-ō-klu'zhun). See infraclusion.

**infraorbital** (in'frah-or'bĭ-tal). Beneath the orbit or in the floor of the orbit.

**infrapatel'lar.** Below the patella; denoting especially a bursa and a pad of fat, or plica synovialis patellaris.

**infrapsychic** (in'frah-si'kik). Automatic.

**infrared** (in'frah-red). Beyond the red end of the spectrum; denoting that section of the electromagnetic spectrum, invisible to the eye, with wavelengths from 7700 Å. units upward to about 10,000,000.

**infrascap'ular.** Below the scapula.

**infrasonic** (in'frah-son'ik) [ infra- + L. *sonus*, sound ]. See infrasonic *sound.*

**infraspina'tus.** See under musculus.

**infraspi'nous.** Below a spine or spinous process; specifically, the fossa infraspinata.

**infrasplenic** (in'frah-splen'ik, -sple'nik). Beneath or below the spleen.

**infraster'nal.** Below the sternum.

**infratem'poral.** Below the temporal fossa.

**infrathoracic** (in-frah-tho-ras'ik). Below or at the lower portion of the thorax.

**infraton'sillar.** Below the palatine tonsil.

**infratrochlear** (in'frah-trok'le-ar). Below the trochlea or pulley of the superior oblique muscle of the eye.

**infraumbilical** (in'frah-um-bil'ĭ-kal). Below the umbilicus.

**infraversion** (in'frah-ver'shun). 1. A turning (version) downward. 2. In ophthalmology, binocular conjugate movement downward. 3. In dentistry, infraclusion.

**infriction** (in-frik'shun) [ L. *in*, on, + *frictio*, a rubbing ]. The application of liniments or ointments combined with friction.

**infundibula** (in'fun'dib'u-lah). Plural of infundibulum.

**infundibular** (in-fun-dib'u-lar). Relating to an infundibulum.

**infundibulectomy** (in'fun-dib'u-lek'to-mĭ) [ infundibulum + G. *ektomē*, excision ]. Excision of the infundibulum, especially of hypertrophied myocardium encroaching on the ventricular outflow tract.

**infundibuliform** (in-fun-dib'u-lĭ-form) [ L. *infundibulum*, funnel, + *forma*, form ]. Funnel-shaped.

**infundibulin** (in-fun-dib'u-lin). A 20 per cent solution of an extract of the posterior lobe of the hypophysis cerebri.

**infundibuloma** (in-fun-dib'u-lo'mah) [ infundibulum + G. suffix -*oma*, tumor ]. A piloid astrocytoma arising in tissues adjacent to the third ventricle of the cerebrum.

**infundib'ulo-ova'rian.** Relating to the fimbriated extremity of a uterine tube and the ovary.

**infundib'ulopel'vic.** Relating to any two structures called infundibulum and pelvis, such as the expanded portion of a calyx and the pelvis of the kidney, or the fimbriated extremity of the uterine tube and the pelvis.

**infundib'uloventric'ular.** Between the conus arteriosus and the right ventricle; designating the i. crest (see *crista* supraventricularis).

**infundibulum,** pl. **infundib'ula** (in'fun-dib'u-lum) [ L. a funnel ]. 1 [ NA ]. A funnel or funnel-shaped structure or passage. 2. Free cephalic extremity of the uterine tube or oviduct. 3. Expanding portion of a calix as it opens into the pelvis of the kidney. 4 [ NA ]. Official alternative name for *conus* arteriosus. 5. Termination of a bronchiole in the alveolus. 6. Termination of the cochlear canal beneath the cupola. 7 [ NA ]. The funnel-shaped, unpaired prominence of the base of the hypothalamus behind the optic chiasm, enclosing the infundibular recess of the third ventricle and continuous below with the stalk of the hypophysis. 8. Mark (2); i. of teeth; the contact surface indentation in the incisor and cheek teeth of a horse.

**ethmoid i.,** i. ethmoidale.

**i. ethmoida'le** [ NA ], a passage from the middle meatus of the nose communicating with the anterior ethmoidal cells and frontal sinus.

**i. hypothal'ami** [ NA ], hypothalamic i.; the apical portion of the tuber cinereum extending into the stalk of the hypophysis.

**hypothalamic i.,** i. hypothalami.

**i. of lungs,** in the embryo, one of the expanded extremities of the subdivisions of the lung buds; in later development minute pouches (the air sacs) appear in its wall.

**i. of teeth,** i. (8).

**i. tubae uteri'nae** [ NA ], i. of the uterine tube; the funnel-like expansion of the abdominal extremity of the uterine (Fallopian) tube.

**i. of uterine tube,** i. tubae uterinae.

**infusible** (in-fu'zĭ-bl). 1. Incapable of being melted or fused. 2. Capable of being made into an infusion.

**infusion** (in-fu'zhun) [ L. *infusio*, fr. *in-fundo*, pp. -*fusus*, to pour in ]. 1. The process of steeping a substance in water, either cold or hot but below the boiling point, in order to extract its soluble principles; distinguished from decoction, which is effected with boiling water. 2. A medicinal preparation obtained by steeping the crude drug in water. 3. The introduction of fluid other than blood, *e.g.*, saline solution, into a vein.

**cold i.,** an i. prepared by steeping the drug in cold water.

**infusodecoction** (in-fu'zo-de-kok'shun). 1. Infusion followed by decoction. 2. A medicinal preparation made by steeping the crude drug first in cold water and then in boiling water.

**Infusoria** (in'fu-so'rĭ-ah) [ a Mod. L. use of the pl. of L. *infusorium*, a vessel for lamp oil, fr. *in-fundo*, to pour in ]. Former term for Ciliata, *q.v.*

**infuso'rian.** Archaic term for a member of the class Infusoria, or, properly, Ciliata.

**ingesta** (in-jes'tah) [ pl. of L. *ingestum*, ntr. pp. of *in-gero*, -*gestus*, to carry in. GEST- ]. Solid or liquid nutrients taken into the body.

**ingestion** (in-jes'chun) [ L. *ingestio*, a pouring in ]. The introduction of food and drink into the stomach.

**ingestive** (in-jes'tiv). Relating to ingestion.

**ingluvies** (in-glu'vĭ-ēz) [ L. ]. The crop of a bird.

**Ingrassia,** Giovanni F., Italian anatomist, 1510–1580. See I.'s *apophyses, wings.*

**ingravescent** (in'grā-ves'ent) [ L. *ingravesco*, to grow heavier, fr. *gravis*, heavy ]. Increasing in severity.

**inguen,** gen. **in'guinis,** pl. **in'guina** (ing'gwen) [ L. ] [ NA ]. Regio inguinalis.

**inguinal** (ing'gwĭ-nal). Relating to the groin.

**in'guinocru'ral.** Relating to the groin and the thigh; see i. *hernia.*

**inguinodynia** (ing'gwĭ-no-din'ĭ-ah) [ L. *inguen* (*inguin-*), groin, + G. *odynē*, pain ]. Pain in the groin.

**inguinola'bial.** Relating to the groin and the labium; see i. *hernia.*

**in'guinoscro'tal.** Relating to the groin and the scrotum; see i. *hernia.*

**inha'lant** [ see inhalation ]. 1. That which is inhaled; a remedy given by inhalation. 2. A drug (or combination of drugs) with high vapor pressure, carried by an air current into the nasal passage, where it produces its effect. 3. A group of products (also called insufflations) consisting of finely powdered or liquid drugs that are carried to the respiratory passages by the use of special devices such as low pressure aerosol containers. See also inhalation; aerosol.

**inhalation** (in-hā-la'shun) [ L. *in-halo*, pp. -*halatus*, to breathe at or in ]. 1. Drawing in the breath. 2. Drawing a medicated vapor in with the breath. 3. A solution of a drug or combination of drugs for administration as a nebulized mist intended to reach the respiratory tree. For full therapeutic effect the droplet size should not exceed a few microns.

**solvent i.,** for the purpose of self-intoxication, i. of volatile organic solvents used in glue, nail polish remover, lacquer thinners, cleaning fluid, lighter fluid, and gasoline. See also glue-sniffing.

**inhale** (in-hāl'). To draw in the breath; to inspire.

**inha'ler.** 1. A masklike apparatus over the nose and mouth, through which to breathe when the air is cold and raw or laden with dust or noxious vapors. 2. An apparatus for administering remedies by inhalation.

**inheritance** (in-hĕr'ĭ-tans) [ L. *heredito,* inherit, fr. *heres* (*hered*-), an heir ]. 1. Characters or qualities that are transmitted from parent to offspring. 2. That which is inherited. 3. The act of inheriting.

    **alternative i.,** (1) Mendelian i.; (2) Galton's term for an assumed form in which all the characters are derived from one parent.

    **blending i.,** Galton's term for that form in which the maternal and paternal characters appear to blend in the offspring.

    **collateral i.,** the appearance of characters in collateral members of a family group, as when an uncle and a niece show the same character inherited from a common ancestor; it occurs with recessive characters appearing irregularly, in contrast to dominant characters transmitted directly from one generation to the next.

    **criss-cross i.,** obsolete term for X-linked inheritance.

    **cytoplasmic i.,** transmission of characters dependent on self-perpetuating elements not nuclear in origin.

    **dominant i.,** see dominance of genes, under gene.

    **extrachromosomal i.,** transmission of characters dependent on some factor not connected with the chromosomes.

    **extranuclear i.,** cytoplasmic i.

    **holandric i.,** transmission of a trait determined by a gene on the Y chromosome.

    **hologynic i.,** transmission of a trait from mother to all daughters and no sons, attributed to attached (partially fused) X chromosomes, to cytoplasmic inheritance, or to sex limitation with abnormal segregation.

    **homochronous i.,** i. of characters that appear in the offspring at the same age as they appeared in the parent.

    **maternal i.,** transmission of characters that are dependent on peculiarities of the egg cytoplasm produced, in turn, by nuclear genes.

    **Mendelian i.,** see Mendel's *law.*

    **mosaic i.,** i. in which the paternal influence is dominant in one group of cells and the maternal in another.

    **partic'ulate i.,** Mendelian i.; that in which some characters are derived from one parent, others from the other.

    **recessive i.,** see dominance of genes, under gene.

    **sex-linked i.,** see sex *linkage.*

**inhib'in.** 1. A postulated testicular hormone that depresses the gonadotropic activity of the pituitary gland. Its existence has not been satisfactorily demonstrated. 2. A postulated proteinase inhibitor.

**inhib'it.** To curb or restrain.

**inhib'itine.** Carnosine.

**inhibition** (in'hĭ-bish'un) [ L. *in-hibeo,* pp. -*hibitus,* to keep back, fr. *habeo,* to have ]. 1. The depression or arrest of a function. 2. In psychoanalysis, the restraining of instinctual or unconscious drives or tendencies, especially if they conflict with one's conscience or with the demands of society. 3. In psychology, a generic term for a variety of processes associated with the gradual attenuation, masking, and extinction of a previously conditioned response.

    **allogeneic i.,** i. of allogeneic cells that occurs when they are cultured after having been mixed together with added phytohemagglutinin (which causes the cells to adhere to each other; plaques develop in which cell growth is inhibited, seemingly because allogeneic cells in contact cause death of each other.

    **central i.,** suppression or diminution of outgoing impulses from a reflex center.

    **competitive i.,** selective i.; blocking of the action of enzymes on its substrate by replacing the latter with a similar but inactive compound, one capable of combining with the active site of the enzyme but not being acted upon or split by it. The classic example is sulfonamide *vs.* *p*-aminobenzoic acid. See also antigenic *competition.*

    **feedback i.,** feedback mechanism; i. of activity by an end product of the action; for example, pituitary thyrotrophic hormone stimulates thyroglobulin production, and thyroglobulin decreases thyrotrophin formation.

    **hapten i. of precipitation,** see under precipitation.

    **hemagglutination i.,** i. of nonimmune hemagglutination by antibody specific for the nonspecific hemagglutinin; *e.g.,* viral hemagglutination (*q. v.*) will not occur if antibody specific for the virus is added before addition of red blood cells. The i. is specific and is widely used for virus identification and for antibody determination.

    **noncompetitive i.,** a type of enzyme i. in which the inhibiting compound does not compete with the natural substrate for the active site on the enzyme, but inhibits reaction by combining with the enzyme-substrate complex, once the latter has been formed.

    **potassium i.,** arrest of the heart in the fully relaxed state as a result of potassium intoxication.

    **proactive i.,** a type of interference or negative transfer, observed in memory experiments and other learning situations, when something learned previously interferes with present learning or recall, as compared with retroactive i.

    **reciprocal i.,** (1) reciprocal *innervation;* (2) systematic *desensitization.*

    **reflex i.,** a situation in which sensory stimuli decrease reflex activity.

    **retroactive i.,** the partial or complete obliteration of memory by a more recent event, particularly new learning, as compared with proactive i.

    **selective i.,** competitive i.

    **Wedensky i.,** a series of very rapidly repeated stimuli applied to the motor nerve fails to excite the muscle but a response results with a slower rate of stimulation.

**inhib'itor.** 1. An agent that restrains or retards physiologic, chemical, or enzymatic action. For individual inhibitors, see under specific name. 2. A nerve, stimulation of which represses activity.

    **calcification i.,** an acidic peptide of unknown structure, found in blood and urine, that inhibits the formation of hydroxylapatite crystals in osteoid cartilage.

**inhib'itory.** Restraining; tending to inhibit.

**inhomogeneity** (in'ho-mo-jĕ-ne'ĭ-tĭ). Heterogeneity.

**inhomogeneous** (in'ho-mo-je'ne-us). Heterogeneous.

**iniac, inial** (in'ĭ-ak, in'ĭ-al). Relating to the inion.

**iniad** (in'ĭ-ad) [ L. *ad,* to ]. In a direction toward the inion.

**iniencephalus** (in'ĭ-en-sef'ă-lus). An individual with iniencephaly.

**iniencephaly** (in'ĭ-en-sef'ă-lĭ) [ G. *inion,* back of the head, + *enkephalos,* brain ]. A malformation consisting of a cranial defect at the occiput, the brain being exposed. It is likely to be combined with a cervical rachischisis and retroflexion.

**inion** (in'ĭ-on) [ G. nape of the neck ] [ NA ]. The external occipital protuberance used as a fixed point in cephalometry and craniometry. See fig. under craniometric *point.*

**iniopagus** (in'ĭ-op'ă-gus) [ inion + G. *pagos,* fixed ]. *Craniopagus* occipitalis.

**iniops** (in'ĭ-ops) [ inion + G. *ōps,* eye, face ]. *Janiceps* asymmetrus.

**initis** (in-i'tis) [ G. *is* (*in-*), fiber, + suffix -*itis,* inflammation ]. 1. Inflammation of fibrous tissue. 2. Myositis.

**inject** (in-jekt') [ L. *injicio,* to throw in ]. To introduce into the body; denoting a fluid forced into one of the cavities, beneath the skin, or into a blood vessel; see also injection.

**injec'table.** 1. Capable of being injected into anything. 2. Capable of receiving an injection.

**injec'ted.** 1. Denoting a fluid introduced into the body. 2. Having the blood vessels visibly distended with blood; congested.

**injectio,** gen. **injectio'nis,** pl. **injectio'nes** (in-jek'she-o) [ L. *injicio,* pp. -*jectus,* to throw in ]. Injection.

**injection** (in-jek'shun) [ L. *injectio, q. v.* ]. 1. The introduction of a medicinal substance or nutrient material into the subcutaneous cellular tissue (subcutaneous or hypodermic), the muscular tissue (intramuscular), a vein (intravenous), the rectum (rectal i., clyster, or enema), the vagina (vaginal i., or douche), the urethra, or other canals or cavities of the body. 2. An injectable pharmaceutical preparation. 3. Congestion or hyperemia.

    **depot i.,** an i. of a substance in a vehicle which tends to keep it at the site of i. so that absorption occurs over a prolonged period.

**hypodermic i.,** the administration of a remedy in liquid form by i. into the subcutaneous connective tissues.

**intrathe'cal i.,** introduction of material for diffusion throughout the subarachnoid space by means of lumbar or ventricular puncture.

**jet i.,** the hypodermic i. of drugs, by a small, high-pressure apparatus, without the use of a needle.

**lactated Ringer's i.** (USP), a sterile solution of calcium chloride, potassium chloride, sodium chloride, and sodium lactate in water for injection; used intravenously as a systemic alkalizer and a fluid and electrolyte replenisher.

**Ringer's i.** (USP), a sterile solution of sodium chloride, potassium chloride, and calcium chloride; each 100 ml. contains between 820 and 900 mg. of sodium chloride, between 25 and 35 mg. of potassium chloride, and between 30 and 37 mg. of calcium chloride; used intravenously as a fluid and electrolyte replenisher.

**sensitizing i.,** one that sensitizes a person with an allergic response to subsequent exposure to the antigen (allergen).

**injec'tor.** A device for making injections.

**jet i.,** a machine that generates high pressure, causing liquid to be forced through a small orifice and enabling such liquid to attain a velocity sufficient to penetrate the skin or mucous membrane.

**in'jure.** To wound; to hurt.

**injury** (in'ju-rĭ) [ L. *injuria,* fr. *in-* neg. + *jus (jur-),* right ]. Damage; trauma; an accidental or inflicted wound.

**blast i.,** tearing of lung tissue or rupture of abdominal viscera without external i., caused by blast of air from explosion of shell or bomb.

**contrecoup i. of brain,** an i. occurring beneath the skull opposite to the area of impact.

**coup i. of brain,** direct i. of brain; an i. occurring directly beneath the area of impact.

**current of i.,** see under current.

**direct i. of brain,** coup i. of brain.

**egg-white i. syndrome,** see under syndrome.

**Goyrand's i.,** dislocation of head of radius beneath annular ligament.

**head i., closed,** a head i. in which continuity of the scalp and mucous membranes is maintained.

**head i., open,** a head i. in which there is loss of continuity of scalp or mucous membranes; the term is sometimes used to indicate a communication between the exterior and the intracranial cavity; see also penetrating *wound.*

**hyperextension-hyperflexion i.,** violence to the body causing the unsupported head to hyperextend and hyperflex the neck rapidly. The term should not be used to imply any specific resultant pathologic condition or syndrome.

**immersion blast i.,** i. to abdominal viscera which may amount to rupture or tears, by explosion under water (depth charge) while body is immersed.

**i. of intervertebral disk (cervical),** see traumatic cervical *discopathy.*

**whiplash i.,** a popular term for hyperextension-hyperflexion i.'s of the neck (see hyperextension-hyperflexion i.).

**in'lay.** 1. In dentistry, a prefabricated restoration sealed in the cavity with cement. 2. A graft of bone into a bone cavity. 3. A graft of skin into a wound cavity for epithelialization.

**direct** and **indirect methods for making i.'s,** see under method.

**epithelial i.,** Esser's operation; filling of a defect by wrapping a Thiersch graft around an accurately fitted mold which is then inserted into the opening, the edges of which are approximated by sutures; at the end of 10 days the mold is removed when the cavity is seen to be lined with epithelium.

**gold i.,** a gold restoration fabricated by casting in a mold made from a wax pattern. The restoration is sealed in the prepared cavity with dental cement.

**porcelain i.,** a fused porcelain restoration luted in a cavity prepared in a tooth that has been damaged, usually by dental caries.

**wax i.,** essentially a mixture of waxes and hydrocarbons of the paraffin series compounded to have properties best suited for forming i. patterns.

**in'let.** A passage leading into a cavity.

**pelvic i.,** *apertura* pelvis superior.

**innate** (in-nāt) [ L. *in-nascor,* pp. *-natus,* to be born in, pp. as adj. inborn, innate ]. Inborn.

**innervation** (in'er-va'shun) [ L. *in,* in, + *nervus,* nerve ]. The supply of nerve fibers functionally connected with a part.

**recip'rocal i.,** reciprocal inhibition (1); contraction in a muscle is accompanied by a loss of tone or by relaxation in the antagonistic muscle.

**innidiation** (in-nid-ĭ-a'shun) [ L. *in,* in, + *nidus,* nest ]. The growth and multiplication of abnormal cells in another location to which they have been transported by means of lymph or the blood stream, or both; metastasis; colonization, indenization.

**innocent** (in'o-sent) [ L. *innocens (-ent-),* fr. *in,* neg., + *noceo,* to injure ]. Benign.

**innocuous** (ĭ-nok'u-us) [ L. *innocuus* ]. Harmless; innoxious.

**innominatal** (in-nom'i-na-tal). Relating to the hip bone.

**innominate** (in-nom'in-āt) [ L. *innominatus,* fr. *in-* neg. + *nomen (nomin-),* name ]. Nameless.

**innoxious** (ĭ-nok'shus) [ L. *in-noxius,* fr. *in,* neg. + *noceo,* to injure ]. Harmless.

**Ino.** Symbol for the radical of inosine.

**ino-, in-** (in'o-) [ G. *is(in-),* fiber ]. Combining form relating to fiber, or meaning fibrous; in most terms (especially in pathology) the combining form fibro- has replaced this obsolescent or obsolete usage.

**inochondritis** (in'o-kon-dri'tis). Obsolete term for fibrochondritis.

**inochondroma** (in'o-kon-dro'mah). Obsolete term for fibrochondroma.

**inoc'ulabil'ity.** The quality of being inoculable.

**inoc'ulable.** 1. Transmissible by inoculation. 2. Susceptible to a disease transmissible by inoculation.

**inoculate** (in-ok'u-lāt) [ L. *inoculo,* pp. *-atus,* to ingraft. OCUL- ]. 1. To introduce the agent of a disease or other antigenic material into the subcutaneous tissue or a blood vessel or through an abraded or absorbing surface for preventive, curative, or experimental purposes. 2. To implant microorganisms or infectious material into or upon culture media. 3. To communicate a disease by transferring its virus.

**inoculation** (in-ok'u-la'shun). Introduction into the body of the causative organism of a disease.

**inoc'ulum.** The microorganism or other material introduced by inoculation.

**in'ocysto'ma.** Obsolete term for fibrocystoma.

**inocyte** (in'o-sīt). Obsolete term for fibroblast.

**inoepithelioma** (in'o-ep-ĭ-the-lĭ-o'mah). Obsolete term for a carcinoma with a densely fibrous stroma; see also fibroepithelioma.

**inogenesis** (in-o-jen'e-sis). Obsolete term meaning formation of fibrous or muscular tissue.

**inoglia** (in-og'lĭ-ah). Fibroglia.

**inohymenitis** (in-o-hi-men-i'tis) [ ino- + G. hymēn, membrane, + suffix *-itis,* inflammation ]. Obsolete term denoting inflammation of an aponeurosis or other fibrous membrane.

**inoleiomyoma** (in'o-li'o-mi-o'mah). Obsolete term for a leiomyoma (*i.e.,* benign neoplasm of smooth muscle) with an unusually prominent stroma of fibrous tissue elements.

**in'olith** [ ino- + G. *lithos,* stone ]. Obsolete term for a concretion composed chiefly of material formed by fibrous tissue.

**ino'ma.** Obsolete term for fibroma.

**inomyoma** (in-o-mi-o'mah). Obsolete term for fibromyoma.

**inomyositis** (in-o-mi-o-si'tis). Obsolete term for fibromyositis.

**inomyxoma** (in'o-mik-so'mah). Obsolete term for fibromyxoma.

**inopec'tic.** Relating to inopexia.

**inop'erable.** Denoting that which cannot be operated upon or cannot be removed by operation.

**inopexia** (in'o-pek'sĭ-ah) [ ino- + G. *pēxis,* fixation ]. Coagulation of the blood in the vessels during life.

**inophragma** (in'o-frag'mah) [ ino- + G. *phragma*, fence ]. Obsolete term for Z *line*.

**in'organ'ic.** 1. Originally, not organic; not formed by living organisms; 2. In chemistry, refers to compounds not containing covalent bonds between atoms.

**inosamine** (in-ōs'ā-min, -mēn). An inositol in which an —OH group is replaced by an —NH₂ group.

**inosclerosis** (in'o-skle-ro'sis). 1. Sclerosis resulting from a great increase in fibrous tissue. 2. Greatly increased density of fibrous tissue, usually as the result of large proportions of collagen. The term is obsolete for both usages.

**inoscopy** (in-os'ko-pī) [ ino- + G. *skopeō*, to look at ]. The microscopic examination of biologic materials (*e.g.*, tissue, sputum, clotted blood, and so on) after dissecting or chemically digesting the fibrillary elements and strands of fibrin.

**inosculate** (in-os'ku-lāt) [ L. *in*, in, + *osculum*, dim. of *os*, mouth ]. Anastomose.

**inosculation** (in-os'ku-la'shun). Anastomosis.

**in'ose.** Inositol.

**inosemia** (in-o-se'mī-ah) [ inose + G. *haima*, blood ]. 1. The presence of inositol in the circulating blood. 2. Fibremia.

**ino'sinate.** A salt or ester of inosinic acid.

**in'osine.** 9-β-D-Ribosylhypoxanthine; a nucleoside formed by the deamination of adenosine.
  **i. nucleosidase** (EC 3.2.2.2), see nucleosidases.

**in'osin'ic acid.** Inosine phosphate; a mononucleotide found in muscular and other tissues.

**inosinyl** (in-o'sī-nil). The radical of inosinic acid.

**in'osite.** Inositol.

**inositis** (in-o-si'tis). Obsolete term for fibrositis (1).

**inositol** (in-o'sī-tōl, in-os'ī-tōl, -tol). Hexahydroxycyclohexane; mouse antialopecia factor; a member of the B₂ complex necessary for growth of yeast and of mice, present in muscle and liver. Its absence from the diet causes alopecia and dermatitis in mice and "spectacle eyes" in rats. Occurs in a number of stereoisomeric forms (known as *cis-*, *epi-*, *allo-*, *neo-*, *myo-*, *muco-*, *chiro-*, and *scyllo-*inositols); the most abundant naturally occurring one is *myo*-inositol (usually meant when "inositol" occurs alone).
  **i. niacinate** (USAN), DILCIT; hexanicotinoyl inositol; peripheral vasodilator.

**meso-inositol.** 1. *Myo*-inositol. 2. Generic term for any isomer of inositol in which the hydroxyl groups are so arranged that the molecule as a whole possesses a plane of symmetry and is optically inactive.

**myo-inositol.** Myoinositol; 1,2,3,5/4,6-inositol (formerly termed *meso*-inositol); the best known inositol, widely distributed in microorganisms, higher plants, and animals. In plants, it is found fully phosphorylated (phytic acid) and as a Mg, Ca salt (phytin) of the hexaphosphate. Partially phosphorylated and free *myo*-inositols occur throughout nature, and in many tissues; *myo*-inositol is a constituent of certain phosphatides (the inositides).

*myo*-Inositol

**inosituria** (in'o-si-tu'rī-ah) [ inositol + G. *ouron*, urine ]. The excretion of inositol in the urine.

**in'osose.** An inositol in which the C-1 is a ketone rather than an alcohol; a 2,3,4,5,6-pentahydroxycyclohexanone.

**inosteatoma** (in-os'te-ā-to'mah). Obsolete term, denoting a benign neoplasm of fat cells (*i.e.*, a lipoma) with a prominent stroma of fibrous connective tissue.

**inosuria** (in'o-su'rī-ah). 1. Inosituria. 2. The occurrence of fibrin in the urine.

**inotropic** (in-o-trop'ik) [ ino- + G. *tropos*, a turning ]. Influencing the contractility of muscular tissue.

  **negatively i.,** weakening muscular action.
  **positively i.,** strengthening muscular action.

**inquest** (in'kwest) [ L. *in*, in, + *quaero*, pp. *quaisitus*, to seek ]. A legal inquiry into the cause of sudden, violent, or mysterious death.

**inquiline** (in'kwī-lin, -lin) [ L. *inquilinus*, an inhabitant of a place that is not his own, fr. *in*, in, + *colo*, to inhabit ]. An animal that lives habitually in the abode of some other species (an oyster crab within the shell of an oyster) causing little or no inconvenience to the host; see also commensal.

**insal'ivate.** To mix the food with saliva during mastication.

**insaliva'tion.** The mixing of the food with saliva.

**insalubrious** (in'sā-lu'brī-us) [ L. *in-salubris*, unwholesome ]. Unwholesome; unhealthful.

**insane** (in-sān') [ L. *in*- neg. + *sanus*, sound, sane ]. 1. Of unsound mind; deranged; crazy; non compos mentis; lunatic. 2. Relating to insanity.

**insanitary** (in-san'ī-tēr-ī) [ L. *in*- neg. + *sanus*, sound ]. Unhealthful; insalubrious; injurious to health.

**insanity** (in-san'ī-tī) [ L. *in*-neg. + *sanus*, sound ]. 1. Now outmoded term, more or less synonymous with severe mental illness or psychosis. 2. In law, has been used to denote that degree of mental illness which negates the individual's legal responsibility or capacity. See also mental *illness*; psychosis.
  **acute confusional i.,** psychosis of sudden onset characterized by confusion.
  **adolescent i.,** a schizophrenic episode in an adolescent.
  **affective i.,** manic-depressive *psychosis*.
  **alcoholic i.,** a form of toxic i., due to the immoderate indulgence in alcoholic beverages.
  **alternating i.,** manic-depressive *psychosis*.
  **Basedow'ian i.,** manic-depressive psychosis occurring in thyrotoxicosis.
  **chore'ic i.,** a psychosis, sometimes associated with chorea, which usually assumes a confusional form.
  **circular i.,** manic-depressive *psychosis*.
  **commu'nicated i.,** *folie* à deux.
  **compulsive i.,** a mental state marked by an obsession or fixed idea that often compels to acts against the will and despite the anxious resistance of the patient.
  **confu'sional i.,** infection-exhaustion *psychosis*.
  **criminal i.,** in forensic psychiatry, a term that is defined by such legal precedents as the American Law Institute rule, Durham rule, M'Naghten rule, and New Hampshire rule (*q.v.* under rule).
  **cyclic i.,** manic-depressive *psychosis*.
  **degenerative i.,** phrenasthenia or psychasthenia occurring in the degenerative period of life.
  **delusional i.,** any form of insanity in which delusions or hallucinations dominate the clinical picture; see also paranoia.
  **double i.,** *folie* à deux.
  **drug i.,** a toxic i. due to the use of some drug such as opium or cocaine.
  **hysterical i.,** hysterical *psychosis*.
  **idiophrenic i.,** i. related to organic brain disease.
  **impulsive i.,** a condition in which a sudden morbid impulse arises and drives the patient at once, without reflection or attempt at resistance, to the commission of some act.
  **induced i.,** *folie* à deux.
  **intermittent i.,** manic-depressive *psychosis*.
  **manic-depressive i.,** manic-depressive *psychosis*.
  **moral i.,** an irresistible impulse to commit wrong or immoral acts.
  **partial i.,** term sometimes used as a synonym for monomania.
  **periodic i.,** manic-depressive *psychosis*.
  **religious i.,** theomania.
  **senile i.,** degenerative i. in the aged.
  **simulta'neous i.,** *folie* à deux.
  **toxic i.,** a psychosis, usually confusional i., due to the action of some poison, such as alcohol, opium, etc., or to autotoxemia.

**inscriptio** (in-skrip'shī-o) [ L. fr. *in-scribo*, pp. -*scriptus*, to write on ]. Inscription.
  **i. tendin'ea,** *intersectio* tendinea.

**inscription** (in-skrip'shun) [ L. *inscriptio* ]. 1. The main part of a prescription; that which indicates the drugs and the quantity of each to be used in the mixture. 2. A mark, band, or line.

    **ten'dinous i.,** *intersectio* tendinea.

**Insecta** (in-sek'tah) [ L. pl. of *insectum*, insect, fr. *in-seco*, pp. *-sectus*, to cut into. SEC-2 ]. Insects. A class of animals with three pairs of jointed legs and usually two pairs of wings, belonging to the phylum Arthropoda. Many are parasitic, others serve as intermediate hosts for parasites that cause human diseases. Some are wingless, others have only one pair of wings. Respiration is by branched, cuticle-lined air tubes or tracheas that carry air from openings on the sides of the thorax directly to the tissues.

**insectarium** (in-sek-ta'rĭ-um) [ L. ]. Place for keeping and breeding insects for scientific purposes.

**insecticide** (in-sek'tĭ-sīd) [ insect + L. *caedō*, to kill ]. An agent that kills insects.

**insectifuge** (in-sek'tĭ-fūj) [ insect + L. *fugo*, to put to flight ]. Material that drives off insects.

**Insectivora** (in'sek-tiv'o-rah) [ insect + L. *voro*, to devour ]. An order of small, plantigrade, placental mammals that are extremely active and often highly predaceous; they feed mostly on insects and small rodents, although the jes or potomogale of Africa feeds on fish. Eight living families include the solenodons of Cuba and Haiti; tenrecs of Madagascar; hedgehog of Europe and Asia; shrews and moles of the United States, Africa, and Asia. Only Australia and parts of South America lack insectivores.

**insectivorous** (in'sek-tiv'o-rus) [ insect + L. *voro*, to devour ]. Insect-eating.

**insectology** (in'sek-tol'o-jĭ) [ insect + G. *logos*, study ]. Entomology; the science of insects, especially as it affects man.

**insecurity** (in'se-ku-rĭ'tĭ). A feeling of unprotectedness and helplessness.

**insemination** (in-sem'ĭ-na'shun) [ L. *in-semino*, pp. *-atus*, to sow or plant in, fr. *semen*, seed ]. The deposit of seminal fluid within the vagina; normally introduced during coitus.

    **artificial i.,** the introduction of semen of the husband (homologous i.) or of another (heterologous i.) into the vagina otherwise than through the act of coitus.

    **heterol'ogous i.,** artificial i. with semen from one who is not the woman's husband.

    **homol'ogous i.,** artificial i. with the husband's semen.

**insenescence** (in'sĕ-nes'ens) [ L. *insenescere*, to begin to grow old ]. The process of becoming senile.

**insensible** (in-sen'sĭ-bl) [ L. *in-sensibilis*, fr. *in*, neg. + *sentio*, pp. *sensus*, to feel ]. 1. Unconscious. 2. Not appreciable by the senses.

**insertion** (in-ser'shun) [ L. *insertio*, a planting in, fr. *inserto*, *-sertus*, to plant in ]. 1. A putting in. 2. The attachment of a muscle to the more movable part of the skeleton, as distinguished from origin. 3. In dentistry, the intraoral placing of a dental prosthesis.

    **parasol i.,** velamentous i.

    **path of i.,** the direction in which a prosthesis is inserted upon and removed from the abutment teeth.

    **velamen'tous i.,** parasol i.; a form of i. of the fetal blood vessels into the placenta, in which they separate before reaching that structure and make their way to it in a fold of amnion, somewhat like the ribs of an open parasol.

**insheathed** (in-shēthd'). Enclosed in a sheath or capsule; encysted.

**insidious** (in-sid'ĭ-us) [ L. *insidiosus*, cunning, fr. *insidioe* (pl.), an ambush, fr. *in* + *sedeo*, to sit ]. Treacherous; stealthy; denoting a disease that progresses with few or no symptoms to indicate its gravity.

**insight** (in'sīt). Self-understanding.

**in si'tu** [ L. *in*, in, + *situs*, site ]. In position.

**insola'tion** [ L. *insolare*, to place in the sun ]. 1. Exposure to the sun's rays. 2. Sunstroke.

**insoluble** (in-sol'u-bl). Not soluble.

**insomnia** (in-som'nĭ-ah) [ L. fr. *in-* priv. + *somnus*, sleep ]. Anhypnosis; wakefulness; inability to sleep, in the absence of external impediments, such as noise, a bright light, etc., during the period when sleep should normally occur; it may vary in degree from restlessness or disturbed slumber

to a curtailment of the normal length of sleep or to absolute wakefulness.

**insomniac** (in-som'nĭ-ak). 1. A sufferer from insomnia. 2. Exhibiting, tending toward, or producing insomnia.

**insorp'tion** [ L. *in*, in, + *sorbēre*, to suck ]. Movement of substances from the lumen of the gut into the blood.

**inspec'tionism.** Sexual pleasure from looking at genitals.

**inspersion** (in-sper'shun, -zhun) [ L. *inspersio*, fr. *in-spergo*, pp. *-spersus*, to scatter upon, fr. *spargo*, to scatter ]. Sprinkling with a fluid or a powder.

**inspiration** (in'spĭ-ra'shun) [ L. *inspiratio*, fr. *in-spiro*, pp. *-atus*, to breathe in ]. Inhalation; the act of breathing in.

    **crowing i.,** noisy breathing associated with respiratory obstruction usually at the larynx.

**inspirator** (in'spĭ-ra'tor) [ L. ]. 1. Inhaler. 2. Respirator.

**inspiratory** (in-spi'rä-to-rĭ). Relating to or timed during inhalation.

**inspire** (in-spīr'). To breathe in; to take a breath; to inhale.

**inspirometer** (in'spi-rom'e-ter) [ L. *in-spiro*, to breathe in, + G. *metron*, measure ]. An instrument for measuring the force, frequency, or volume of the inspirations.

**inspis'sated** [ L. *in-* intensive + *spisso*, pp. *-atus*, to thicken ]. Thickened by evaporation or absorption of fluid.

**inspissation** (in'spĭ-sa'shun). 1. The act of thickening by evaporation or by the absorption of fluid. 2. An increased thickness or diminished fluidity.

**inspis'sator.** An apparatus for evaporating fluids.

**instability** (in'stä-bil'ĭ-tĭ). The state of being unstable, or lacking stability.

    **vertebral, cervical i.,** excessive mobility of cervical vertebrae due to damage to ligaments; see also vertebral *subluxation*.

**in'star** [ L. form ]. Any of the successive stages in the metamorphosis of insects.

**in'step.** The arch, or highest part of the dorsum of the foot.

**instillation** (in'stĭ-la'shun) [ L. *instillatio*, fr. *in-stillo*, pp. *-atus*, to pour in by drops, fr. *stilla*, a drop ]. The dropping of a liquid on or into a part.

**instillator** (in'stĭ-la'tor). A dropper.

**in'stinct** [ L. *instinctus*, impulse ]. 1. An enduring disposition or tendency of an organism to act in an organized and biologically adaptive manner characteristic of its species. 2. The unreasoning impulse to perform some purposive action without an immediate consciousness of the end to which that action will lead. 3. The force which we assume to exist behind the tension caused by the needs of the id.

    **aggressive i.,** death i.

    **death i.,** aggressive i.; the i. of all living creatures toward self-destruction, death, or a return to the inorganic lifelessness from which they arose.

    **ego i.'s,** self-preservative needs and self-love, as opposed to object love; drives that are primarily erotic.

    **herd i.,** social i., the tendency or inclination to band together with and share the customs of others of a group, to conform to the opinions and adopt the views of the group.

    **life i.,** sexual i.; the i. of self-preservation and sexual procreation; the basic urge toward preservation of the species.

    **sexual i.,** life i.

    **social i.,** herd i.

**instinc'tive, instinc'tual.** Relating to instinct.

**instrument** (in'stru-ment) [ L. *instrumentum* ]. A tool or implement.

    **diamond cutting i.'s,** cylinders, disks, and other cutting i.'s to which numerous small diamond pyramids have been held by a plating of metal (usually chromium). The diamonds are locked on by plating to the base and up the side of the diamonds. Used in dentistry.

    **Krueger i. stop,** a mechanical device limiting the insertion of a root canal instrument into a canal.

    **Ohm's i.,** an i. for photographing simultaneously, on a moving sensitized film, the heart sounds and the tracings of the jugular and radial pulses; see also phonophotography.

    **plugging i.,** see plugger.

**Sabouraud-Noiré i.,** a device for measuring the quantity of x-rays by means of the change in color of a disk of barium platinocyanide which exposure to them produces; the unit used in this method is called teinte B, or tint B = erythema dose.

**stereotaxic i.,** an apparatus attached to the head, used to localize precisely an area in the brain.

**test handle i.,** a root canal i. the handle of which is similar to a mandrel; used for adjusting the length of a reamer or file in order to limit its insertion into a root canal.

**Wood's biopsy i.,** a flexible gastric biopsy tube.

**in'strumenta'rium.** A collection of instruments and other equipment for an operation or for a medical procedure.

**in'strumenta'tion.** 1. The use of instruments. 2. In dentistry, the application of armamentarium in a restorative procedure.

**insuccation** (in'suk-ka'shun) [ L. *insuco,* pp. *-atus,* to soak in, fr. *in* + *sucus,* juice, sap (improp. *succ-*) ]. Maceration; soaking; especially of a crude drug to prepare it for further pharmaceutical operation.

**insudate** (in'su-dāt) [ L. *in,* in, + *sudare,* to sweat ]. Fluid swelling within an arterial wall (ordinarily serous), differing from an exudate in that it does not come to lie extramurally.

**insufficiency** (in-sŭ-fish'en-sĭ) [ L. *in-* neg. + *sufficientia,* fr. *suf-ficio*(*sub-f*), to suffice. FAC- ]. 1. Lack of completeness of function or of power. 2. Incompetence (1).

**acute adrenocortical i.,** Addisonian or adrenal crisis; Bernard-Sergent syndrome; severe adrenocortical i. resulting from untreated chronic adrenocortical i.; characterized by nausea, vomiting, hypotension, and frequently hyperthemia, hyponatremia, hyperkalemia, and hypoglycemia; death results if untreated.

**adrenocortical i.,** loss, to varying degrees, of adrenocortical function.

**aortic i.,** see valvular i.

**capsular i.,** adrenal i.

**cardiac i.,** heart *failure.*

**chronic adrenocortical i.,** Addison's disease; caused by idiopathic atrophy or destruction of both adrenal glands by tuberculosis or other diseases; characterized by fatigue, decreased blood pressure, weight loss, melanin pigmentation of the skin and mucous membranes, anorexia, and nausea or vomiting; without appropriate replacement therapy, it leads to acute adrenocortical i.

**coronary i.,** inadequate coronary circulation leading to anginal pain.

**i. of the eyelids,** a condition in which the eyelids are closed only by conscious effort, and remain open during sleep.

**hepat'ic i.,** defective functional activity of the liver cells.

**latent adrenocortical i.,** partial adrenocortical i.

**mitral i.,** see valvular i.

**muscular i.,** failure of any muscle to contract with its normal force, especially such failure of any of the eye muscles.

**myocardial i.,** heart *failure.*

**parathyroid i.,** hypoparathyroidism.

**partial adrenocortical i.,** latent adrenocortical i.; normal basal adrenocortical function with failure of adrenocortical reserve to respond to ACTH stimulation.

**primary adrenocortical i.,** adrenocortical i. caused by disease, destruction, or surgical removal of the adrenal cortices.

**pulmonary i.,** see valvular i.

**pyloric i.,** patulousness of the pyloric outlet of the stomach.

**renal i.,** defective function of the kidneys.

**respiratory i.,** failure to provide oxygen to the cells of the body and to remove excess carbon dioxide from them.

**secondary adrenocortical i.,** adrenocortical i. caused by failure of ACTH secretion resulting from anterior pituitary disease, or by ACTH inhibition resulting from exogenous steroid therapy.

**thyroid i.,** hypothyroidism.

**tricuspid i.,** see valvular i.

**u'terine i.,** atony of the uterine musculature.

**val'vular i.,** failure of the cardiac valves to close perfectly, thus allowing regurgitation of blood past the closed valve;

named, according to the valve involved, aortic, mitral, pulmonary, or tricuspid i.

**velopharyngeal i.,** anatomical deficiency in the soft palate or superior constrictor muscle, resulting in the inability to achieve velopharyngeal closure.

**venous i.,** inadequate drainage of venous blood from a part, resulting in edema or dermatosis.

**insuf'flate** [ L. *in-sufflo,* pp. *-atus,* to blow on or into, fr. *sub,* under, + *flo,* to blow. FLAT- ]. To blow into; to fill the lungs of an asphyxiated person with air, either by means of an apparatus or from the lungs of the operator; or to blow a medicated vapor, powder, or anesthetic into the lungs or into any cavity of the body.

**in'suffla'tion.** 1. The act or process of insufflating. 2. An inhalant (3).

**perire'nal i.,** injection of air or carbon dioxide about the kidneys for roentgenographic visualization of the adrenal glands.

**tu'bal i.,** Rubin *test.*

**in'suffla'tor.** An instrument used in insufflation.

**insula,** gen. and pl. **in'sulae** (in'su-lah) [ L. island ]. 1 [ NA ]. Insular cortex or area; island of Reil; an oval region of the cerebral cortex overlying the capsula extrema, lateral to the lenticular nucleus, buried in the depth of the fissura lateralis cerebri (Sylvian fissure). 2. Island, *q. v.* 3. Any circumscribed body or patch on the skin.

**Haller's i.,** Haller's anulus; bifurcation of the thoracic duct at the 8th thoracic vertebra.

**in'sular.** Relating to any insula, especially the island of Reil.

**insulate** (in'su-lāt) [ L. *insulatus,* (adj.) made like an island ]. 1. To prevent the passage of electricity by the interposition of a nonconducting substance such as glass or rubber. 2. To interpose a material which is a poor conductor of heat between two bodies of different temperatures in order to prevent the passage of heat from one to the other.

**insulation** (in-su-la'shun). 1. The act of insulating. 2. The nonconducting substance which offers a barrier to the passage of heat or electricity. 3. The state of being insulated.

**in'sula'tor.** A nonconducting material by means of which insulation is effected.

**insulin** (in'su-lin). A peptide hormone of completely known chemical structure, secreted by the pancreatic islets of Langerhans. It promotes glucose utilization, protein synthesis, and the formation and storage of neutral lipids. Insulins, obtained from various animals and available in a variety of preparations, are used parenterally in the treatment of diabetes mellitus.

**i.-like activity,** a measure of substances, usually in plasma, that exert biological effects similar to those of i. in various bioassays. Sometimes used as a measure of plasma i. concentrations; always gives higher values than immunochemical techniques for the measurement of i. Abbreviated ILA.

**i. antagonist,** a serum factor in the plasma albumin fraction that opposes i.; found in larger amounts in diabetic persons than in normal persons.

**atypical i.,** an insulin-like material whose biological effects are not inhibited by i. antiserum; present in large amounts in the plasma of obese adult diabetics, but in low concentrations in juvenile and nonobese adult diabetics.

**biphasic i.** (BP), the specific antidiabetic principle of the pancreas of the ox in a solution of that from the pancreas of the pig.

**globin zinc i.** (USP, BP), a sterile solution of i. modified by the addition of zinc chloride and globin; it contains 40 or 80 units per ml.; duration of action is about 18 hours.

**immunoreactive i.,** abbreviated IRI; that portion of i. in blood measured by immunochemical methods for the hormone; presumed to represent the free (unbound) and biologically active fraction of total blood i.

**i. injection** (USP, BP), regular i. injection; the USP preparation contains 40, 80, 100, or 500 USP i. units per ml.; the BP preparations contains 20, 40, or 80 units per ml.; it is administered subcutaneously and occasionally intravenously; the onset of action is rapid, duration is brief (5 to 7 hours), and it is compatible for mixing with long-acting i. preparations; used in the treatment of diabetic acidosis and for insulin coma.

**isophane i.** (USP, BP), NPH i.; a modified form of i. composed of i., protamine, and zinc; an intermediately acting preparation used for the treatment of diabetes mellitus.

**NPH i.,** isophane i.

**protamine zinc i.** (USP, BP), i. modified by the addition of protamine and zinc chloride; it contains 40 or 80 units per ml.

**regular i.,** see i. injection.

**i. zinc suspension** (USP, BP), LENTE i.; a sterile, buffered suspension with zinc chloride, containing 40 or 80 units per ml.; the solid phase of the suspension consists of a mixture of 7 parts of crystalline i. and 3 parts of amorphous i.

**i. zinc suspension, amorphous** (BP), equivalent to i. zinc suspension, prompt (USP).

**i. zinc suspension, crystalline** (BP), equivalent to i. zinc suspension, extended (USP).

**i. zinc suspension, extended** (USP), ULTRALENTE i.; crystalline i. zinc suspension (BP); a long-acting i. suspension, obtained from beef, with an approximate time of onset of 7 hours and duration of action of 36 hours.

**i. zinc suspension, prompt** (USP), SEMILENTE i.; amorphous i. zinc suspension (BP); a sterile solution of i. in buffered water for injection, modified by the addition of zinc chloride such that the solid phase of the suspension is amorphous; it contains 40 or 80 units per ml.; the duration of action is equivalent to that of i. injection (regular i.).

**insulinase** (in'su-lin-ās). An enzyme (EC 3.4.99.10) in liver, kidney, and muscle, capable of inactivating insulin.

**insulinemia** (in-su-lin-e'mī-ah) [ insulin + G. *haima*, blood ]. Literally, insulin in the circulating blood, but the term usually connotes abnormally large concentrations of insulin in the circulating blood.

**in'sulin'ization.** Obsolete term meaning treatment with insulin.

**insulinogenesis** (in'su-lin-o-jen'ĕ-sis) [ insulin + G. *genesis*, production ]. Production of insulin.

**insulinogen'ic, insulogen'ic.** Relating to insulinogenesis.

**insulinoma** (in'su-lin-o'mah). Islet cell *adenoma.*

**in'sulism.** Obsolete synonym for hyperinsulinism.

**insulitis** (in'su-li'tis) [ L. *insula,* island, + suffix *-itis,* inflammation ]. A relatively unusual histologic change in which the islands of Langerhans are edematous and contain small numbers of leukocytes, *i.e.,* "inflammation" of the insular tissue.

**insulo'ma** [ L. *insula,* island, + suffix *-oma,* tumor ]. Islet cell *adenoma.*

**in'sult** [ L. *insultus* ]. 1. An injury or trauma. 2. See insultus.

**insul'tus** [ L. a reviling, insult, fr. *insulto,* to leap upon, abuse, fr. *salio,* to leap ]. Attack, as i. apoplectiform'is, i. epileptiform'is, i. syncopa'lis (fainting), etc.

**insusceptibility** (in'sus-sep'tĭ-bil'ĭ-tī) [ L. *suscipio,* pp. *-ceptus,* to take upon one, fr. *sub,* under, + *capio,* to take ]. Lack or absence of susceptibility; immunity.

**integration** (in'te-gra'shun) [ L. *integro,* pp. *-atus,* to make whole, fr. *integer,* whole ]. 1. The state of being combined, or the process of combining, into a complete and harmonious whole. 2. In physiology, building up by accretion; anabolism.

**personality i.,** the useful organization of old and new experience, data, and emotional capacities into the personality; the harmonious organization of the personality.

**integument** (in-teg'u-ment) [ L. *integumentum,* a covering, fr. *in-tego,* to cover ]. 1. The enveloping membrane of the body; integumentum commune. 2. The rind, capsule, or covering of any body or part.

**integumen'tary.** Relating to the integument; cutaneous; dermal.

**integumen'tum** [ L. ]. Integument.

**i. commu'ne** [ NA ], the integument in general; it includes in addition to the epidermis and dermis all of the derivatives of the epidermis, *i.e.,* hairs, nails, sudoriferous and sebaceous glands, and mammary glands.

**intellectualization** (in-tel-lek'chu-al-ĭ-za'shun) [ L. *intellectus,* perception, discernment ]. Thinking compulsion; an unconscious defense mechanism in which reasoning, logic,

or attention to intellectual minutiae is used in an attempt to avoid confrontation with an objectionable impulse, affect, or interpersonal situation.

**intel'ligence** [ L. *intelligentia* ]. 1. As used by laymen, an individual's aggregate capacity to act purposefully, think rationally, and deal effectively with his environment, especially in relation to the extent of his perceived effectiveness in meeting challenges. 2. As used by psychologists, an individual's relative standing on two quantitative indices, measured i. and effectiveness of adaptive behavior. A quantitative score or similar index on both indices constitutes the psychologist's operational definition of i.

**abstract i.,** the capacity to understand and manage abstract ideas and symbols.

**measured i.,** that i. which can be ranked relative to an age or peer group quantitative index through scores on i. tests.

**mechanical i.,** the capacity to understand and manage technical mechanisms.

**social i.,** the capacity to understand and manage human relations and social affairs.

**superior i.,** hyperphrenia.

**intem'perance** [ L. *intemperantia,* fr. *in-*neg. + *temperantia,* moderation ]. Acrasia; lack of proper self-control, usually in reference to the use of alcoholic beverages; *cf.* incontinence.

**intensim'eter.** An instrument for measuring intensity of radiation.

**intensity** [ L. *in-tendo,* pp. *-tensus,* to stretch out. TEN- ]. Marked tension; great activity; strength; *e.g.,* i. of light or sound; often used simply to denote a measure of the degree or amount of some quality.

**luminous i.,** symbol, I; candle-power; the luminous flux per unit solid angle in a given direction.

**inten'sive.** Relating to or marked by intensity; denoting a form of treatment by means of very large doses or of substances possessing great strength or activity.

**intention** (in-ten'shun) [ L. *intentio,* a stretching out; intention ]. 1. An objective. 2. In surgery, a process or operation.

**healing** or **union by first i.,** primary adhesion; immediate agglutination; healing by fibrinous adhesion without suppuration or granulation tissue formation.

**healing** or **union by second i.,** secondary adhesion; mediate agglutination; union of two granulating surfaces accompanied by more or less suppuration.

**healing by third i.,** the filling of a wound cavity or ulcer by granulations, with subsequent cicatrization.

**inter-** [ L. *inter,* between ]. A prefix conveying the meaning of between, among.

**interacinar** (in-ter-as'ĭ-nar). Interacinous.

**interacinous** (in-ter-as'in-us). Interacinar; between the acini of a gland.

**interalveolar** (in'ter-al-ve'o-lar). Between any alveoli, especially the alveoli of the lungs.

**interan'nular** [ inter- + L. *anulus,* ring ]. Between any two ringlike structures or constrictions.

**interarch** (in'ter-arch). See interarch *distance.*

**interartic'ular** [ inter- + L. *articulus,* joint ]. 1. Between two joints. 2. Between two joint surfaces.

**interarytenoid** (in'ter-ăr'ĭ-te'noyd). Between the arytenoid cartilages.

**interaster'ic.** Between the two asteria; see asterion.

**interatrial** (in-ter-a'trī-al). Between the atria of the heart.

**interauricular** (in'ter-aw-rik'u-lar). 1. Interatrial. 2. Between the auricles or pinnae.

**interbody.** Obsolete term for complement-fixing antibody; from Ehrlich's original noncommittal term "zwischen Körper," which he replaced with the more committal term amboceptor.

**interbrain.** Obsolete synonym for diencephalon.

**intercadence** (in-ter-ka'dens) [ inter- + L. *cado,* pr. p. *cadens* (*-ent-*), to fall ]. Extreme dicrotism; interpolated extrasystole; the occurrence of an extra beat between the two regular pulse beats.

**interca'dent.** Irregular in rhythm; characterized by intercadence.

**intercalary** (in-ter'kă-lĕr-ī, in'ter-kal'ă-rī) [ L. *intercalarius,* concerning an insertion, fr. *intercalo, -atus,* to insert (by proclamation) fr. *calo*, to proclaim ]. Occurring between two others; as in a pulse tracing, an upstroke interposed between two normal pulse beats.

**intercalated** (in-ter'kă-la-ted). Interposed; inserted between two others.

**intercala'tus** [ L. ] [ NA ]. Intercalated.

**intercanalic'ular.** Between canaliculi in any sense.

**intercap'illary.** Between or among capillary vessels.

**intercarot'ic, intercarot'id.** Between the internal and external carotid arteries.

**intercar'pal.** Between the carpal bones.

**intercartilaginous** (in'ter-kar-tĭ-laj'ĭ-nus). Between or connecting cartilages.

**intercavernous** (in'ter-kav'er-nus). Between two cavities.

**intercel'lular.** Between or among cells.

**intercen'tral.** Connecting or lying between two or more centers.

**intercen'trum,** pl. **intercen'tra.** In veterinary anatomy, an intervertebral disk between vertebrae, and the hemal arch beneath vertebrae of some reptiles, birds, and mammals; see also hemal *arch.*

**intercerebral** (in'ter-sĕr'ĕ-bral). Between the cerebral hemispheres.

**interchondral** (in-ter-kon'dral) [ inter- + L. *chondros*, cartilage ]. Intercartilaginous.

**intercil'ium** [ inter- + L. *cilium*, eyelid ]. Glabella.

**interclavic'ular.** Between or connecting the clavicles.

**intercoccygeal** (in'ter-kok-sij'ĭ-al). Situated between unfused segments of the coccyx.

**intercolumnar** (in-ter-kŏ-lum'nar). Between any two columns, as the columns or crura of the anulus inguinalis superficialis.

**intercon'dylar, intercondyl'ic, intercon'dyloid.** Between two condyles.

**intercos'tal** [ inter- + L. *costa*, rib ]. Between the ribs.

**intercostohumeral** (in'ter-kos'to-hu'mer-al). Relating to an intercostal space and the arm; denoting certain branches of the intercostal nerves supplying the skin of the arm.

**intercos'tohumera'lis.** See *nervi* intercostobrachiales.

**intercourse** (in'ter-kōrs) [ L. *intercursus*, a running between ]. Communication or dealings between or among people; interchange of ideas.

sexual i., coitus.

**in'tercri'cothyrot'omy.** Cricothyrotomy.

**intercris'tal.** Between two crests, as between the crests of the ilia, applied to one of the pelvic measurements.

**intercru'ral.** Between two crura in any sense, those of the jaw, the cerebral peduncles of the brain, the superficial inguinal ring, etc.

**intercur'rent** [ inter- + L. *curro*, pr. p. *currens* (*-ent*-), to run ]. Intervening; said of a disease attacking a person already ill of another malady.

**intercuspation** (in'ter-kus-pa'shun). The interdigitation of cusps of opposing teeth.

**intercusping** (in-ter-kus'ping) [ L. *inter*, among, mutually, + cusp ]. The normal fitting together of the occlusal surfaces of two opposing teeth.

**intercutaneomucous** (in'ter-ku-ta'ne-o-mu'kus). Between skin and mucous membrane, as in the cheek or lip or at the mucocutaneous border of the lips or anus.

**interdeferential** (in-ter-def-er-en'shal). Between the deferent ducts.

**interden'tal** [ inter- + L. *dens*, tooth ]. 1. Between the teeth. 2. Denoting the relationship between the proximal surfaces of the teeth of the same arch.

**interdentium** (in-ter-den'shĭ-um). The interval between any two contiguous teeth.

**interdigit** (in-ter-dij'it). That part of the sloping extremity of the hand or foot lying between any two adjacent fingers or toes.

**interdigital** (in-ter-dij'ĭ-tal). Between the fingers or toes.

**interdigitation** (in-ter-dij-ĭ-ta'shun) [ inter- + L. *digitus*, finger ]. 1. The mutual interlocking of toothed or tongue-like processes. 2. The processes thus interlocked. 3.

Infoldings or plicae of adjacent cell or plasma membranes. 4. Intercuspation.

**interdis'cipline** [ inter- + L. *disciplina*, knowledge ]. The overlapping interests of different fields of medicine and science.

**in'terface.** 1. A surface that forms a common boundary of two bodies. 2. In dentistry, a boundary: metal, between metal and nonsolvent solder, or between metal and surface oxide; crystalline, between adjacent crystals; structural, between tooth and restorative material.

dermoepidermal i., the line of meeting of the dermis and epidermis.

**interfa'cial.** Relating to an interface.

**interfascic'ular.** Between fasciculi.

**interfem'oral.** Between the thighs.

**interference** (in-ter-fēr'ens) [ inter- + L. *ferio*, to strike ]. 1. The coming together of waves in various media in such a way that the crests of one series correspond to the hollows of the other, the two thus neutralizing each other; or so that the crests of the two series correspond, thus increasing the excursions of the waves. 2. The collision within the myocardium of two waves of excitation, as is seen in fusion beats. 3. In A-V dissociation, the disturbance of the regular rhythm of the ventricles by a conducted impulse from the atria, *i.e.,* by a ventricular capture. 4. Superinfection, mutual extinction, or cell blockade; occurs when susceptible cells are exposed to two viruses in some instances at the same time and in other instances at different times.

cuspal i., defective occlusal contact.

**interfer'ing.** Brushing; in the horse, the striking of the fetlock or cannon bone by the opposite foot while in motion.

**interferom'eter.** An instrument for measuring minute distances or movements through the interference of light waves thereby produced.

electron i., an i. that employs an electron beam in place of a light beam.

**interferom'etry.** Measurement of minute distances or movements by the resulting interaction of light rays.

electron i., i. in which a beam of electrons is used instead of a beam of light.

**in'terfer'ons.** Macromolecules of molecular weight in the range of 20,000, produced in cell cultures or host tissues in response to infection with active or inactivated virus, capable of inducing a state of resistance to superinfection with related or unrelated virus; they are small proteins and interfere with viruses other than the one which evoked them, but are much more effective in the cells of the species of animal in which they were evoked than in others.

**interfibrillar, interfibrillary** (in'ter-fi'brĭ-lar, -fi-bril'ar, -fi'brĭ-lĕr-ĭ). Between fibrils.

**interfi'brous.** Between fibers.

**interfil'amen'tous.** Between filaments.

**interfron'tal.** Between the unfused halves of the frontal bone; denoting a suture there present.

**interganglionic** (in'ter-gang'lĭ-on'ik). Between or among or connecting ganglia.

**intergemmal** (in'ter-jem'al) [ inter- + L. *gemma*, bud ]. Between any two or more budlike or bulblike bodies such as the taste buds; denoting especially a nerve termination between two end bulbs.

**interglob'ular.** Between globules.

**intergluteal** (in-ter-glu'te-al) [ inter- + G. *gloutos*, buttock ]. Between the buttocks.

**intergo'nial** [ inter- + G. *gōnia*, angle ]. Between the two gonia; see gonion.

**intergyral** (in-ter-ji'ral). Between the gyri or convolutions of the brain.

**interhemicerebral** (in'ter-hem'ĭ-sĕr'ĕ-bral). Intercerebral; between the cerebral hemispheres.

**interictal** (in'ter-ik'tal) [ inter- + L. *ictus*, stroke ]. Denoting the interval between convulsions.

**inte'rior.** Relating to the inside; situated within.

**interischiadic** (in-ter-is-kĭ-ad'ic). Between the two ischia; especially, between the two tuberosities of the ischia.

**interkine'sis** [ inter- + G. *kinēsis*, movement ]. Interphase, particularly the interval between the first and second nuclear divisions in meiosis.

**interlamellar** (in'ter-lă-mel'ar, -lam'ē-lar). Between lamellae.

**interlo'bar.** Between the lobes of an organ or other structure.

**interlobitis** (in'ter-lo-bi'tis). Inflammation of the pleura separating two pulmonary lobes.

**interlob'ular.** Between the lobules of an organ.

**intermalle'olar.** Between the malleoli.

**intermam'mary** [ inter- + L. *mamma*, breast ]. Between the breasts.

**intermam'millary** [ inter- + L. *mammilla*, breast, nipple ]. Between the breasts; between the nipples; denoting a line drawn between the two nipples.

**intermarriage** (in'ter-măr'ij). 1. Marriage of relatives. 2. Marriage of persons of different races or cultures.

**intermaxil'la.** *Os incisivum.*

**intermax'illary.** Between the maxillae, or upper jaw bones.

**intermediary** (in'ter-me'dĭ-ĕr-ĭ) [ L. *intermedius*, lying between, fr. *medius*, middle ]. Occurring between.

**intermediate** (in'ter-me'dĭ-āt). 1. Between two extremes; interposed; intervening. 2. A substance, formed in the course of chemical reactions, which then proceeds to participate rapidly in further reactions, so that at any given moment it is present in minute concentrations only. Such substances, when appearing in the course of the reactions involved in metabolism, are metabolic intermediates. 3. In dentistry, a cement base. 4. Intermedius.

**interme'din.** Melanocyte-stimulating *hormone.*

**intermediolateral** (in-ter-me'dĭ-o-lat'er-al). Intermediate, and to one side, not central.

**intermedius** (in-ter-me'dĭ-us) [ L. ] [ NA ]. Intermediate (4); an element or organ between right and left (or lateral and medial) structures.

**intermem'branous.** Between membranes.

**intermeningeal** (in'ter-mē-nin'je-al). Between the meninges.

**intermen'strual.** Between two consecutive menstrual periods.

**intermet'acar'pal.** Between the metacarpal bones.

**intermetameric** (in'ter-met'ah-mēr'ik) Between two metameres; denoting especially the intervertebral disks.

**intermet'atar'sal.** Between the metatarsal bones.

**intermet'atar'seum.** *Os* intermetatarseum.

**intermission** (in-ter-mish'un) [ L. *intermissio,* fr. *intermitto,* to leave off, intermit, fr. *mitto,* to send ]. 1. A temporary cessation of symptoms or of any action. 2. An interval between two paroxysms of a disease such as malaria.

**intermit'.** To cease for a time.

**intermit'tence, intermit'tency.** 1. A condition marked by intermissions or interruptions in the course of a disease or other process or state or in any continued action; denoting especially a loss of one or more pulse beats. 2. The complete cessation of symptoms between two periods of activity of a disease.

**intermit'tent.** Marked by intervals of complete quietude between two periods of activity.

**intermus'cular.** Between the muscles.

**intern** (in'tern or in-tern') [ F. *interne,* inside ]. An advanced student or recent graduate who assists in the medical or surgical care of hospital patients and who resides within the institution.

**inter'nal** [ L. *internus* ]. Interior; away from the surface; often incorrectly used to mean medial.

**inter'naliza'tion.** Adopting as one's own the standards and values of another person or society.

**interna'rial.** Between the nares or nostrils.

**interna'sal.** Internarial.

**International System of Units.** Abbreviated SI (from the French equivalent, Système International). The name was adopted at the 11th General Conference on Weights and Measures of the International Organization for Standardization (ISO) to cover both the coherent units (basic, supplementary, and derived units) and the decimal multi-

ples and submultiples of these units formed by use of the prefixes proposed for general international scientific and technological use. SI proposes seven basic units, meter (m), kilogram (kg), second (s), ampere (A), kelvin (K), candela (cd), mole (mol), for the basic quantities, length, mass, time, electric current, temperature, luminous intensity, and amount of substance. Supplementary units proposed are radian (rad) for plane angle, and steradian (sr) for solid angle. Derived units (such as force, power, frequency) are stated in terms of the basic units, *e.g.,* velocity is in meters per second (m s$^{-1}$). Multiples (prefixes) in descending order are tera- (T, $10^{12}$), giga- (G, $10^9$), mega- (M, $10^6$), kilo- (k, $10^3$), hecto- (h, $10^2$), deca- (da, $10^1$), deci- (d, $10^{-1}$), centi- (c, $10^{-2}$), milli- (m, $10^{-3}$), micro- ($\mu$, $10^{-6}$), nano- (n, $10^{-9}$), pico- (p, $10^{-12}$), femto- (f, $10^{-15}$), atto- (a, $10^{-18}$). Those involving a multiple of $10^3$ are recommended. Compounds of these are not recommended (*e.g.,* m$\mu$ for n).

**interneuromeric** (in'ter-nu-ro-mĕr'ik). Between the neuromeres.

**interneurons** (in'ter-nu'ronz). Combinations or groups of neurons between sensory and motor neurons which govern coordinated activity.

**inter'nist.** A physician trained in internal medicine, as distinguished from a surgeon, obstetrician, etc.

**interno'dal.** Between two nodes; relating to an internode.

**in'ternode.** Internodal *segment.*

**internuclear** (in-ter-nu'kle-ar). Between nerve cell groups in the brain or retina.

**internuncial** (in-ter-nun'sĭ-al) [ L. *inter-nuntius* (or *-nuncius*), a messenger between two parties, fr. *inter,* between, + *nuncius,* a messenger ]. 1. Indicating a neuron functionally interposed between two or more other neurons. 2. Acting as a medium of communication between two organs.

**inter'nus** [ L. ] [ NA ]. Internal.

**interocclusal** (in'ter-ŏ-klu'sal). Between the occlusal surfaces of opposing teeth.

**interoceptive** (in'ter-o-sep'tiv) [ inter- + L. *capio,* to take ]. Relating to the sensory nerve cells innervating the viscera (thoracic, abdominal and pelvic organs, and the cardiovascular system), their sensory end organs, or the information they convey to the spinal cord and the brain.

**interoceptor** (in'ter-o-sep'tor) [ inter- + L. *capio,* to take ]. One of the various forms of small sensory end organs (receptors) situated within the walls of the respiratory and gastrointestinal tracts or in other viscera.

**interol'ivary.** Between the left and right inferior olive of the medulla oblongata.

**interor'bital.** Between the orbits.

**interos'seal.** Interosseous.

**interossei** (in-ter-os'e-i). Plural of interosseus.

**interosseous** (in-ter-os'e-us) [ inter- + L. *os,* bone ]. Lying between or connecting bones; denoting certain muscles and ligaments.

**interosseus,** pl. **interossei** (in'ter-os'e-us, -os'e-i). See under musculus.

**interpal'pebral.** Between the eyelids.

**interparietal** (in'ter-pă-ri'e-tal) [ inter- + L. *paries,* wall ]. Between the walls of a part, or between the parietal bones.

**interparoxysmal** (in'ter-păr'ok-siz'mal). Occurring between successive paroxysms of a disease.

**interpedic'ulate.** Between vertebral pedicles.

**interpedunc'ular.** Between any two peduncles.

**interper'sonal.** Pertaining to relations and social exchanges between persons.

**interphalangeal** (in'ter-fă-lan'je-al). Between two phalanges; denoting the finger or toe joints.

**interphase** (in'ter-fāz). The stage between two successive divisions of a cell nucleus; the stage in which the biochemical and physiologic functions of the cell are performed. Replication of chromatin occurs at this phase.

**interphyletic** (in-ter-fi-let'ik) [ inter- + G. *phylē,* tribe ]. Denoting the transitional forms between two kinds of cells during the course of metaplasia.

**in'terplant.** The material transferred from donor to host in interplanting.

**interplant'ing.** In experimental embryology, the transferring of a primordial cell mass from one embryo to an indifferent environment in another embryo, as in chorioallantoic grafts or intraocular transplants.

**inter'preta'tion.** 1. In psychoanalysis, the characteristic therapeutic intervention of the analyst. 2. In clinical psychology, drawing inferences and formulating the meaning in terms of the psychological dynamics inherent in an individual's responses to psychological tests.

**interpositum** (in'ter-poz'ĭ-tum) [ L. *inter-pono,* pp. *-positus,* to place between ]. See under velum.

**interpu'bic.** Between the two pubic bones.

**interpu'pillary.** Between the pupils; *e.g.,* i. distance.

**interra'dial.** Situated between radii or rays.

**interre'nal.** Between the two kidneys.

**interrenalopathy** (in'ter-re'nal-op'ă-thĭ). Obsolete term for disorder of adrenal gland function.

**interrenotropic** (in-ter-re'no-trop'ik). Obsolete synonym for adrenotropic or adrenocorticotropic.

**interscap'ular.** Between the scapulae.

**interscap'ulum.** The part of the back between the shoulders, or that between the scapulae.

**intersciatic** (in-ter-si-at'ik). Interischiadic.

**intersectio,** pl. **intersectio'nes** (in'ter-sek'shĭ-o) [ L. ] [ NA ]. Intersection; the site of crossing of two structures.
  **i. tendinea** [ NA ], tendinous intersection; a tendinous band or partition running across a muscle.

**intersegmen'tal.** Between two segments, such as metameres or myotomes.

**intersep'tal.** Lying between two septa.

**intersep'toval'vular.** Between the embryonic septum primum and septum spurium.

**intersep'tum** [ L. SEPT- ]. The diaphragm.

**intersex'es.** Individuals exhibiting intersexuality.

**intersex'ual.** Relating to or characterized by intersexuality.

**intersexuality** (in'ter-seks'u-al'ĭ-tĭ). The condition of having both male and female characteristics; being intermediate between the sexes.

**in'terspace.** Any space between two similar objects, such as a costal i. or interval between two ribs.
  **diner'ic i.,** the surface separating two liquid phases.

**interspi'nal.** Between two spines, such as the spinous processes of the vertebrae; interspinous.

**interspina'lis.** See under musculus.

**interspi'nous.** Interspinal.

**interstice,** pl. **interstices** (in-ter'stĭs) [ L. *interstitium,* fr. *sisto,* to stand. STA- ]. A small area, space, or hole in the substance of an organ or tissue.

**interstitial** (in-ter-stish'al). Relating to spaces or interstices in any structure.

**interstitium** (in-ter-stish'um) [ L. ] [ NA ]. Interstice.

**intersystole** (in'ter-sis'to-le). Intersystolic period; the a-c interval (see under interval); the period intervening between the systole of the atrium and that of the ventricle of the heart.

**intertar'sal.** Between the tarsal bones.

**interthal'amic.** Between the thalami.

**intertransversa'lis.** Intertransversarius; see under musculus.

**in'tertrans'verse.** Between the transverse processes of the vertebrae.

**intertriginous** (in'ter-trij'ĭ-nus). Characterized by or related to intertrigo.

**intertrigo** (in-ter-tri'go) [ L. a galling of the skin, fr. *inter,* between, + *tero,* to rub ]. Dermatitis occurring between two folds of the skin, as between the buttocks, between the scrotum and the thigh, etc.

**intertrochanteric** (in'ter-tro-kan-tĕr'ik). Between the two trochanters of the femur.

**intertu'bular.** Between or among tubules.

**interureteral** (in'ter-u-re'ter-al). Between the two ureters.

**interurete'ric.** Interureteral.

**in'terval** [ L. *inter-vallum,* space between breastworks in a camp, an interval, fr. *vallum,* a rampart, wall ]. A time or space between two periods or objects; a break in a current or the course of a disease; a period of rest between two of activity.
  **a-c i., atriocarot'id i., auriculocarot'id i.,** the intersystolic period; the time between the beginning of the atrial and that of the carotid waves in a tracing of the jugular pulse.
  **A-H i.,** the time from initial rapid deflection of A wave to the initial rapid deflection of the His bundle (H) potential; it approximates the conduction time through the A-V node (normally 50 to 120 msec.).
  **A-N i.,** the time between onset of the atrial deflection and the nodal potential (normally 40 to 100 msec.).
  **A-V i.,** the time from the beginning of atrial systole to the beginning of ventricular systole as measured from pressure pulses or cardiac volumne curves in animals, or from the electrocardiogram in man.
  **BH i.,** the time of His bundle deflection (normally 15 to 20 msec.).
  **c-a i., cardioarte'rial i.,** the time between the apex beat of the heart and the radial pulse beat.
  **coupling i.,** the i., usually expressed in hundredths of a second, between a normal sinus beat and the ensuing premature beat.
  **focal i.,** the distance between anterior and posterior focal points of the eye.
  **H-V i.,** the time from the initial deflection of the His bundle (H) potential and the onset of ventricular activity (normally 35 to 45 msec.).
  **interectopic i.,** the distance between consecutive ectopic complexes in the electrocardiogram.
  **i'somet'ric i.,** presphygmic i.
  **lucid i.,** in psychoses or delirium, the rational period appearing in the course of the mental disorder.
  **P-A i.,** the time from onset of P wave to the initial rapid deflection of the A wave in the His bundle electrogram (normally 25 to 45 msec.); it represents the intra-atrial conduction time.
  **passive i.,** the period of rest of the heart.
  **P-J i.,** the time elapsing from the beginning of the P wave to the end of the QRS complex (J for junction between QRS and S-T segment) in the electrocardiogram.
  **postsphyg'mic i.,** postsphygmic period; period of isometric relaxation; the interval in the cardiac cycle following the sphygmic period, *i.e.,* from the closure of the semilunar valves to the opening of the atrioventricular valves.
  **P-P i.,** the distance between consecutive P waves in the electrocardiogram.
  **P-Q i., P-R i.**
  **P-R i.,** P-Q i.; in the electrocardiogram, the time elapsing between the beginning of the P wave and the beginning of the QRS complex; it corresponds to the a-c interval of the venous pulse and is normally 0.12 to 0.20 sec.
  **presphyg'mic i.,** presphygmic period; isometric period or i.; the brief period at the beginning of the ventricular systole during which the pressure is rising before the semilunar valves open.
  **Q-R i.,** the time elapsing from the onset of the QRS complex to the peak of the R wave; measures the time of onset of the intrinsicoid deflection.
  **Q-RB i.,** the time between the onset of the Q wave of the ECG complex and the right bundle-branch potential (normally 15 to 20 msec.).
  **QRS i.,** the duration of the QRS complex in the electrocardiogram.
  **Q-S₂ i.,** electromechanical *systole.*
  **Q-T i.,** in the electrocardiogram, the time elapsing from the beginning of the QRS complex to the end of the T wave. It represents the total duration of electrical activity of the ventricles.
  **R-R i.,** the time elapsing between two consecutive QRS complexes in the electrocardiogram.
  **sphyg'mic i.,** ejection or sphygmic period; the period in the cardiac cycle when the semilunar valves are open and blood is being ejected from the ventricles into the arterial system.
  **Sturm's i.,** the distance between the anterior and posterior focal lines in the astigmatic eye.
  **systolic time i.'s,** see electromechanical *systole;* left ventricular ejection *time;* preejection *period.*

**intervas'cular.** Between blood or lymph vessels.

**interven'tion** A generic term designating what the psychiatrist or psychotherapist does *vis-à-vis* the patient. Psychiatric i.'s include such things as prescribing drugs, instituting commitment proceedings, etc.; psychotherapeutic i.'s include such things as questions, interpretations, etc.

**crisis i.,** a brief psychotherapeutic technique aimed at intervening at the time of an acute life crisis and limited in aim to helping resolve the crisis.

**interventric'ular.** Between the ventricles.

**interver'tebral.** Between two vertebrae.

**intervil'lous.** Between or among villi.

**intes'tinal.** Relating to the intestine.

**intestine** (in-tes'tin) [ L. *intestinum* ]. The digestive tube passing from the stomach to the anus. It is divided primarily into the **small i.** (intestinum tenue) and the **large i.** (intestinum crassum); the small i. is further divided arbitrarily into duodenum, jejunum, and ileum; the large i. is divided into cecum and appendix, ascending, transverse, descending, and sigmoid colons, and rectum. The duodenum is separated from the stomach by the pylorus or pyloric valve, and the ileum is separated from the cecum by the ileocecal valve.

**intes'tinotox'in.** Enterotoxin.

**intesti'num,** pl. **intesti'na,** gen. **intestino'rum** [ L. *intestinus*, internal, ntr. as noun, the entrails, fr. *intus*, within ] 1 [ NA ]. Intestine. 2 [ neuter of *intestinus* ]. Inward; inner.

**i. ce'cum,** blind gut; see cecum.

**i. crassum** [ L. *crassus*, thick ] [ NA ], the large intestine, the portion of the digestive tube extending from the ileocecal valve to the anus, it comprises the cecum, colon, sigmoid colon, and rectum.

**i. il'eum,** twisted intestine; see ileum.

**i. jeju'num,** empty intestine; see jejunum.

**i. rectum,** straight intestine; see rectum.

**i. tenue** [ NA ], small intestine; the portion of the digestive tube between the stomach and the cecum or beginning of the large intestine; it consists of three portions: duodenum, jejunum, and ileum.

**i. tenue mesenteria'le,** the freely movable portion of the small intestine supplied with a mesentery, comprising the jejunum and ileum.

**intima** (in'tĭ-mah) [ L. fem. of *intimus*, inmost ]. 1 [ NA ]. Innermost. 2. The *tunica* intima.

**in'timal.** Relating to the intima or inner coat of a vessel.

**intimitis** (in'tĭ-mi'tis) [ intima + suffix -*itis*, inflammation ]. Inflammation of an intima; endoangiitis (endoarteritis, endophlebitis).

**proliferative i.,** eruption characterized by dusky erythema and small ulcers due to proliferative changes in capillary bed.

**in'toe.** Foot posture (positioning) in which toes are directed toward midline (opposite side) during gait.

**intol'erance.** Abnormal metabolism, excretion, or other disposition of a given substance; term often used to indicate impaired disposal of dietary constituents.

**hereditary fructose i.,** a metabolic error due to deficiency of hepatic fructose 1-phosphate aldolase, the second enzyme in the specific fructose pathway; vomiting and hypoglycemia follow ingestion of fructose; prolonged fructose ingestion in young children results in their failure to thrive and in jaundice, hepatomegaly, albuminuria, aminoaciduria, and sometimes cachexia and death; autosomal recessive inheritance in most families.

**lactose i.,** characterized by abdominal cramps and diarrhea after consumption of food containing lactose, for example, milk or ice cream; believed to reflect a deficiency of intestinal lactase; may appear first in young adults who have previously tolerated milk well as infants.

**intorsion** (in-tor'shun) [ L. *in-torqueo*, pp. *tortus*, to twist. TORS- ]. Adtorsion; conclination; the real or apparent turning of one or both eyes around an anteroposterior axis, so that the upward extension of the vertical meridian of reference rotates nasally from the true vertical.

**intor'tor.** Medial rotator; a muscle that turns a part medialward; see also invertor (for the foot).

**intoxation** (in-tok-sa'shun) [ see intoxication ]. Poisoning, especially by the toxic products of bacteria or poisonous animals, other than alcohol.

**intoxicant** (in-tok'sĭ-kant). 1. Having the power to intoxicate. 2. An intoxicating agent, such as alcohol.

**intoxication** (in-tok'sĭ-ka'shun) [ L. *in*, in, + G. *toxicon*, poison. TOX- ]. Inebriation. 1. Poisoning. 2. Acute alcoholism; drunkenness.

**acid i.,** poisoning by acid products (β-oxybutyric acid, diacetic acid, or acetone), formed in the organism as a result of faulty metabolism, or by acids introduced from without; it is marked by epigastric pain, headache, loss of appetite, constipation, restlessness, odor of acetone in the breath, followed by air hunger, coma, and collapse.

**alkaline i.,** alkalosis.

**anaphylactic i.,** i. following an anaphylactic reaction.

**citrate i.,** a toxic condition that may develop during massive replacement therapy with transfused blood that contains citrate as an anticoagulant; the citrate combines with calcium ions and may result in tetany.

**intestinal i.,** autointoxication.

**men'strual i.,** a condition marked by various morbid symptoms (dermatoses, headache, vomiting, convulsions, one or more) occurring at each menstrual period.

**premenstrual i.,** a condition that sometimes precedes the menstrual period, marked by emotional irritability, breast engorgement, abdominal distention, pelvic congestion, edema, backache, headache, depression, and other symptoms.

**septic i.,** septicemia.

**water i.,** severe overhydration resulting, through diuresis, in salt depletion with salivation, nausea and vomiting, restlessness, weakness, ataxia, tremors, and sometimes convulsions and death.

**intra-** (in'trah-) [ L. within ]. A prefix meaning within. See also endo-.

**intra-abdom'inal.** Within the abdomen.

**intra-acinous** (in-trah-as'ĭ-nus). Within an acinus.

**intra-adenoi'dal.** Within the adenoids.

**intra-arte'rial.** Within an artery or the arteries.

**intra-artic'ular** [ intra- + L. *articulus*, joint ]. Within the cavity of a joint.

**intra-atom'ic.** Referring to situations and events within the atom.

**intra-a'trial.** Within one or both of the atria of the heart.

**intra-aural** (in'trah-aw'ral) [ intra- + L. *auris*, ear ]. Within the ear.

**intra-auric'ular.** 1. Within an auricle (*e.g.,* of the ear). 2. Obsolete synonym for intra-atrial.

**intrabronchial** (in-trah-brong'kĭ-al). Endobronchial; within the bronchi or bronchial tubes.

**intrabuc'cal** [ intra- + L. *bucca*, cheek ]. 1. Within the mouth. 2. Within the substance of the cheek.

**intracanalic'ular.** Within a canaliculus or canaliculi.

**intracap'sular.** Within a capsule, especially the capsule of a joint.

**intracar'diac** [ intra- + G. *kardia*, heart ]. Endocardiac; intracordial; within one of the chambers of the heart.

**intracar'pal.** Within the carpus; among the carpal bones.

**intracartilaginous** (in'trah-kar-tĭ-laj'ĭ-nus). Endochondral; within a cartilage or cartilaginous tissue.

**intracatheter** (in'tra-kath'e-ter). A plastic tube, inserted into a vein, for infusion, injection, or venous pressure monitoring.

**intracelial** (in'trah-se'lĭ-al) [ intra- + G. *koilia*, cavity ]. Endoceliac; within any of the body cavities, especially within one of the ventricles of the brain.

**intracel'lular.** Within a cell or cells.

**in'tracerebel'lar.** Within the cerebellum.

**intracerebral** (in'trah-sĕr'ĕ-bral). Within the cerebrum.

**intracervical** (in'trah-ser'vĭ-kal). Endocervical (1).

**intracisternal** (in'trah-sis-ter'nal). Within one of the subarachnoid cisternae; usually refers to the introduction of a cannula into the cisterna cerebellomedullaris for aspiration of cerebrospinal fluid or the injection of air into the ventricles of the brain.

**intracol'ic.** Within the colon.

**intracor'dial** [ intra- + L. *cor*, heart ]. Intracardiac.

**intracor'onal.** Within the crown portion of a tooth.

**intracorporeal** (in'trah-kor-po're-al) [ intra- + L. *corpus*, body ]. 1. Within the body. 2. Within any structure anatomically styled a corpus.

**intracorpuscular** (in'trah-kor-pus'ku-lar). Within a corpuscle, especially a red blood corpuscle.

**intracos'tal.** On the inner surface of the ribs; denoting an internal intercostal muscle.

**intracra'nial.** Within the skull.

**intrac'table** [ L. *in-tractabilis*, fr. *in-* neg. + *tracto*, to draw, haul ]. Obstinate; refractory; resistant to treatment; difficult to control.

**intracutaneous** (in'trah-ku-ta'ne-us) [ intra- + L. *cutis*, skin ]. Intradermal; within the substance of the skin.

**intracys'tic.** Within a cyst or the urinary bladder.

**in'trad.** Toward the inner part.

**intrader'mal, intrader'mic** [ intra- + G. *derma*, skin ]. Intracutaneous.

**in'traduct.** Within the duct or ducts of a gland.

**intradu'ral.** Within or enclosed by the dura mater.

**intraepider'mal.** Within the epidermis.

**intraepiphysial** (in'trah-ep-ĭ-fiz'ĭ-al). Within the epiphysis of a long bone.

**intraepithelial** (in'trah-ep-ĭ-the'lĭ-al). Within or among the epithelial cells.

**intrafaradization** (in'trah-făr'ă-dĭ-za'shun). The application of a faradic current to the inner surface of a cavity or hollow organ.

**intrafascicular** (in'trah-fă-sik'u-lar). Within the fasciculi of a tissue or structure.

**intrafebrile** (in-trah-fe'bril, in-trah-feb'ril). During the febrile stage of a disease.

**intrafi'lar** [ intra- + L. *filum*, thread ]. Lying within the meshes of a network.

**intrafu'sal.** Applied to structures within the muscle spindle.

**intragal'vaniza'tion.** The application of a galvanic current to the interior of a cavity or hollow organ.

**intragas'tric.** Within the stomach.

**intragemmal** (in'trah-jem'al) [ intra- + L. *gemma*, bud ]. Within any budlike or bulblike body; denoting especially a nerve termination within an end bulb or taste bud.

**intraglan'dular.** Within a gland or glandular tissue.

**intraglob'ular.** Within a globule in any sense. Specifically, intracorpuscular; within a red blood corpuscle.

**intragyral** (in'trah-ji'ral). Within a gyrus or convolution of the brain.

**intrahepat'ic.** Within the liver.

**intrahyoid** (in-trah-hi'oyd). Within the hyoid bone; denoting certain accessory thryoid glands that lie in the hollow or within the substance of the hyoid bone.

**intralaryngeal** (in'trah-lă-rin'je-al). Within the larynx.

**intraligamen'tous.** Within a ligament, especially the broad ligament of the uterus.

**intralo'bar.** Within a lobe of any organ or other structure.

**intralob'ular.** Within a lobule.

**intraloc'ular.** Within the loculi of any structure or part.

**intralu'minal.** Intratubal.

**intramedullary** (in'trah-med'u-lĕr-ĭ). Within (1) the bone marrow; (2) the spinal cord; (3) the medulla oblongata.

**intramem'branous.** 1. Within, or between the layers of, a membrane. 2. Denoting a method of bone formation, as distinguished from endochondral bone formation.

**intrameningeal** (in'trah-mĕ-nin'je-al). Within or enclosed by the meninges of the brain or spinal cord.

**intramolec'ular.** Referring to situations and events within a molecule.

**intramu'ral.** Within the substance of the wall of any cavity or hollow organ.

**intramus'cular.** Within the substance of a muscle.

**intramyocardial** (in'trah-mi'o-kar'dĭ-al). Within the myocardium.

**intramyometrial** (in'trah-mi'o-me'trĭ-al). Within the muscular coat of the uterus.

**intrana'sal.** Within the nasal cavity.

**intrana'tal** [ intra- + L. *natalis*, relating to birth ]. During or at the time of birth.

**intraneural** (in-trah-nu'ral) [ intra- + G. *neuron*, nerve ]. Within a nerve.

**intranuclear** (in'trah-nu'kle-ar). Within the nucleus of a cell.

**intraocular** (in'trah-ok'u-lar). Within the eyeball.

**intraoral** (in'trah-o'ral) [ intra- + L. *os*, mouth ]. Within the mouth.

**intraor'bital.** Within the orbit.

**intraosseous** (in-trah-os'se-us) [ intra- + L. *os*, bone ]. Within bone.

**intraos'teal** Endosteal; intraosseous.

**intraova'rian.** Within the ovary.

**intrao'vular.** Within the ovum.

**intraparietal** (in-trah-pă-ri'e-tal). 1. Intramural. 2. Denoting the intraparietal sulcus.

**intrapar'tum** [ intra- + L. *partus*, childbirth. PARI- ]. During labor and delivery or childbirth.

**intrapel'vic.** Within the pelvis.

**intrapericardiac, intrapericardial** (in'trah-pĕr'ĭ-kar'dĭ-ak, -kar'dĭ-al). Endopericardiac; within the pericardial cavity.

**intraperitoneal** (in'trah-pĕr'ĭ-to-ne'al). Within the peritoneal cavity.

**intraper'sonal.** Intrapsychic.

**intrapi'al.** Within the pia mater.

**intrapleural** (in-trah-plu'ral). Within the pleura or the pleural cavity.

**intrapon'tine.** Within the pons of the brainstem.

**intraprostat'ic.** Within the prostate gland.

**in'traprotoplas'mic.** Within the protoplasm of a cell.

**intrapsychic** (in-trah-sĭ-kik). Intrapersonal; denoting the psychological dynamics which occur inside the mind without reference to the individual's exchanges with other persons or events.

**intrapul'monary.** Within the lungs.

**intrapyretic** (in'trah-pi-ret'ik) [ intra- + L. *pyretos*, fever ]. Intrafebrile.

**intrarec'tal.** Within the rectum.

**intrare'nal** [ intra- + L. *ren*, kidney ]. Within the kidney.

**intraret'inal.** Within the retina.

**intrarrhachidian, intrarachidian,** (in'trah-ră-kid'ĭ-an) [ intra- + G. *rachis*, spine ]. Intraspinal.

**intrascro'tal.** Within the scrotum.

**intraspi'nal.** Within the vertebral canal or spinal cord.

**in'trasplen'ic.** Within the spleen.

**intrastro'mal.** Within the stroma or foundation substance of any organ or part.

**intrasynovial** (in-trah-sĭ-no'vĭ-al). Within the synovial sac of a joint or a synovial tendon sheath.

**intratar'sal.** Within the tarsus; among the tarsal bones.

**intrathe'cal.** Within a sheath; ensheathed.

**intrathoracic** (in'trah-tho-ras'ik). Within the cavity of the chest.

**intraton'sillar.** Within the substance of a tonsil.

**intratu'bal.** Within any tube.

**intratu'bular.** Within any tubule.

**intratympanic** (in'trah-tim-pan'ik). Within the middle ear or tympanic cavity.

**intrauterine** (in'trah-u'ter-in). Within the uterus.

**intravasation** (in-trav'ă-sa'shun) [ intra- + L. *vas*, vessel ]. Entrance of foreign matter into blood vessel.

**intravas'cular.** Within the blood vessels or lymphatics.

**in'travena'tion.** Entrance of foreign matter into vein.

**intrave'nous.** Endovenous; within a vein or veins.

**intraventric'ular.** Within a ventricle of the brain or heart.

**intraves'ical.** Within the bladder, especially the urinary bladder.

**intra vi'tam** [ L. *vita*, life ]. During life.

**intravitelline** (in'tra-vi-tel'in, -ēn). Within the vitellus or yolk.

**intravit'reous.** Within the vitreous humor.

**intrin'sic** [ L. *intrinsecus*, on the inside ]. 1. Inherent; belonging entirely to a part 2. In anatomy, denoting those muscles of the limbs whose origin and insertion are both in the same limb, distinguished from the extrinsic muscles which have their origin in some part of the trunk outside of the pelvic or shoulder girdle; applied also to the ciliary muscle as distinguished from the recti and other orbital muscles which are on the eyeball.

**intro-** [ L. *intro*, into ]. A prefix meaning in or into.

**introdu'cer** [ L. *intro-duco*, to lead into, introduce ]. Intubator; an instrument or stylet for the introduction of an endotracheal tube.

**introflection, introflexion** (in'tro-flek'shun) [ intro- + L. *flecto*, pp. *flectus*, to bend ]. A bending inward.

**introgas'tric** [ intro- + G. *gastēr*, belly, stomach ]. Leading or passed into the stomach.

**intro'itus** [ L. entrance, fr. *intro-eo*, to go into ] [ NA ]. The entrance into a canal or hollow organ, as the vagina.

**introjection** (in-tro-jek'shun) [ intro- + L. *jacere*, to throw ]. A psychological defense mechanism involving appropriation of an external happening and its assimilation by the personality, making it a part of the self.

**intromission** (in-tro-mish'un) [ intro- + L. *mitto*, to send ]. Insertion.

**intromit'tent.** Conveying or sending into a body or cavity.

**introspec'tion** [ intro- + L. *spicere*, to look ]. Looking inward; self-scrutinizing; contemplating one's own mental processes.

**introspec'tive.** Relating to introspection.

**introsusception** (in-tro-sus-sep'shun). Intussusception.

**introversion** (in-tro-ver'shun) [ intro- + L. *verto*, pp. *versus*, to turn ]. 1. The turning of one part within another; invagination. 2. A trait of preoccupation with oneself, in contrast to extraversion.

**introvert** (in'tro-vert). 1. An anatomical structure, such as the intestine, which is turned into itself; an intussusception. 2. One who tends to be introspective and self-centered and who takes small interest in the affairs of others as contrasted with an extrovert.

**introvert** (in-tro-vert'). To invaginate; to pass one part within another.

**intubate** (in'tu-bāt) [ L. *in*, in, + *tuba*, tube ]. 1. To insert a tube into any part. 2. Specifically, to perform intubation of the larynx and trachea.

**intubation** (in-tu-ba'shun). 1. The insertion of a tube into any canal or other part. 2. Specifically, O'Dwyer's method; Bouchut's method; the passage of a specially constructed tube between the vocal cords to relieve stenosis due to the formation of a diphtheritic membrane, to edema, or to cicatricial contraction. 3. Passage of oro- or nasotracheal tube for anesthesia or control of pulmonary ventilation.

**altercursive i.,** diversion of secretion intermittently to the exterior from its normal destination, *e.g.,* of the bile from the intestine.

**aqueductal i.,** insertion of a tube within the aqueduct of Sylvius.

**blind nasotracheal i.,** passage of the endotracheal tube through the nose and into the larynx without the use of a laryngoscope; a procedure used in instances of abnormal anatomy.

**endotracheal i.,** intratracheal i.; passage of a tube into the trachea for maintenance of the airway during anesthesia, or in a patient with an imperilled airway from any cause.

**intratracheal i.,** endotracheal i.

**nasotra'cheal i.,** insertion of a tube through the nose into the trachea; alternative to orotracheal i. in some circumstances.

**orotra'cheal i.,** insertion of a tube through the mouth into the trachea for the relief of respiratory obstruction or for maintenance of the airway during anesthesia or in artificial respiration.

**prolonged nasotracheal i.,** long-term artificial ventilation in infants and very young children for whom tracheostomy is not altogether satisfactory.

**in'tubator.** Introducer.

**intumesce** (in-tu-mes') [ L. *in-tumesco*, to swell up, fr. *tumeo*, to swell ]. To swell up; to enlarge.

**intumescence** (in'tu-mes'ens). 1. Intumescentia (*q. v.*); a swelling or enlargement. 2. The process of enlarging or swelling.

**tympanic i.,** *intumescentia* tympanica.

**intumescent** (in-tu-mes'ent). Enlarging; swelling; becoming enlarged or swollen.

**intumescentia** (in-tu-mes-sen'shĭ-ah) [ Mod. L. ] [ NA ]. Intumescence; an anatomical swelling, enlargement, or prominence.

**i. cervica'lis** [ NA ], cervical enlargement of the spinal cord; a spindle-shaped swelling of the spinal cord extending from the fourth cervical to the first segment, with maximum thickness opposite the fifth or sixth cervical vertebra.

**i. gangliofor'mis,** *ganglion* geniculi.

**i. lumba'lis** [ NA ], lumbar enlargement of the spinal cord; a spindle-shaped swelling of the cord beginning at the level of the tenth thoracic vertebra and tapering into the conus medullaris, with maximum thickness opposite the last thoracic vertebra.

**i. tympan'ica,** tympanic intumescence; a swelling, not ganglionic, on the tympanic branch of the glossopharyngeus nerve; it is regarded as possibly similar to the carotid glomus.

**intussusception** (in'tus-sus-sep'shun) [ L. *intus*, within, + *sus-cipio*, to take up, fr. *sub* + *capio*, to take. CAP- ]. 1. The taking up or receiving of one part within another. 2. Especially the infolding of one segment of the intestine within another. See also invagination.

**colic i.,** the ensheathing of one portion of the colon into another.

**double-barrelled i.,** a second i. occurring which involves the bowel above the first. The first i. is followed by contraction of the bowel wall around it. The solid mass so formed is enveloped by the proximal portion of the bowel and is thus the cause of the second i.

**il'eal i.,** a form in which one portion of the ileum is ensheathed in another portion of the same division of the bowel.

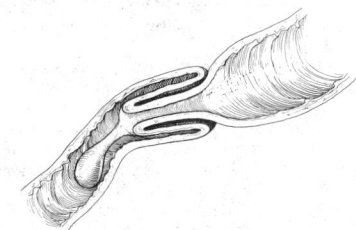

**Ileoileal Intussusception with Pedunculated Tumor**

**ileoce'cal i.,** a form in which the lower segment of the ileum passes through the valve of the colon into the cecum.

**ileocol'ic i.,** a form in which the lower portion of the ileum with the valve of the cecum passes into the ascending colon.

**jeju'nogas'tric i.,** a rare complication following gastrojejunostomy in which the afferent or the efferent loop of bowel is invaginated into the stomach. It is probably due to reverse peristalsis set up in the bowel by some irritable focus.

**ret'rograde i.,** the invagination of a lower segment of the bowel into one just above.

**intussusceptive** (in'tus-sus-sep'tiv). Relating to or characterized by intussusception.

**intussusceptum** (in'tus-sus-sep'tum). The inner segment in an intussusception; that part of the bowel which is received within the other part.

**intussuscipiens** (in'tus-sus-sip'ĭ-enz) [ L. *intus*, within, + *suscipiens*, pr. p. of *suscipio*, to take up ]. The portion of the bowel, in intussusception, which receives the other portion.

**in'ula.** Elecampane.

**in'ulase.** Inulinase.

**in'ulin** (USP, BP). Dahlin; alant starch; alantin; a fructose polysaccharide from the rhizome of *Inula helenium* or *elecampane*, and other plants; a hygroscopic powder. Used by intravenous injection to determine the rate of glomerular filtration (*cf.* i. clearance). Also used in bread for diabetics.

**in'ulinase** (EC 3.2.1.8). Inulase; enzyme acting upon $\beta$-1,2-fructan links in inulin, releasing fructose.

**in′ulol.** Alantol.

**inunction** (in-ungk′shun) [ L. *inunctio,* an anointing, fr. *inunguo,* pp. -*unctus,* to smear on ]. Anointing; the administration of a drug in ointment form applied with rubbing, with the purpose of causing absorption of the active ingredient.

**inustion** (in-us′chun) [ L. *in-uro,* pp. -*ustus,* to burn in, burn ]. The application of the actual cautery.

**in u′tero** [ L. ]. Within the womb; not yet born.

**invaccina′tion.** Accidental inoculation of some disease, *e.g.,* syphilis, during vaccination.

**in vacuo** (in-vak′u-o) [ L. ]. In a vacuum, *i.e.,* under reduced pressure.

**invaginate** (in-vaj′ĭ-nāt) [ L. *in,* in, + *vagina,* a sheath ]. To ensheathe; introvert; insert one part within another part of the same thing.

**invagination** (in-vaj′ĭ-na′shun). 1. Indigitation; the process of invaginating, or of passing one part within another part of the same thing. 2. The state of being invaginated.

**invag′inator.** An instrument for pushing inward any tissue.

**in′valid** [ L. *in*- neg. + *validus,* strong ]. 1. Weak; sick. 2. A sickly person suffering from a disabling but not necessarily completely incapacitating disease.

**in′validism.** The condition of being an invalid.

**inva′sin.** See hyaluronidases.

**inva′sion** [ L. *invasio,* fr. *in-vado,* pp. -*vasus,* to go into, attack ]. 1. The beginning or incursion of a disease. 2. Local spread of a malignant neoplasm by infiltration or destruction of adjacent tissue.

**in′ventory.** A detailed, often descriptive, list of items.

**personality i.,** a psychological test for evaluation of habitual modes of behavior, thinking, and feeling relevant to one's peer group. For specific psychological tests, see subentries under test.

**invermina′tion** [ L. *in,* in, + *vermis* (*vermin*-), worm ]. Helminthiasis.

**inversion** (in-ver′shun) [ L. *inverto,* pp. -*versus,* to turn upside down, to turn about ]. 1. A turning inward, upside down, or in any direction contrary to the existing one. 2. The conversion of a disaccharide or polysaccharide by hydrolysis into a monosaccharide; specifically, the hydrolysis of sucrose to glucose and fructose; so called because of the change in optical activity. 3. A rarely used term for homosexuality. 4. Heat-induced transition of silica, in which the quartz tridymite or cristobalite changes its physical properties as to thermal expansion.

**i. of chromosomes,** see under chromosome.

**i. of the uterus,** a turning of the uterus inside out, usually following childbirth.

**visceral i.,** *situs* inversus.

**in′vert** [ see inversion ]. 1. In chemistry, subjected to inversion, *e.g.,* invert sugar. 2. A rarely used term for a homosexual.

**in′vertase.** β-Fructofuranosidase.

**Invertebrata** (in-ver′te-bra′tah). A general category of the kingdom Animalia (multicellular animals) including those phyla whose members lack a notochord; *i.e.,* all animals except vertebrates in the phylum Chordata.

**invertebrate** (in-ver′te-brāt). 1. Not possessed of a spinal, or vertebral, column. 2. Any animal except the craniate members of the phylum Chordata.

**in′vertin.** β-Fructofuranosidase.

**invert′or** [ see inversion ]. A muscle that inverts or causes inversion or turns a part, such as the foot, inward.

**in′vertose.** Invert *sugar.*

**invest′ing.** 1. In dentistry, covering or enveloping wholly or in part an object such as a denture, tooth, wax form, crown, etc., with a refractory investment material before curing, soldering, or casting. 2. In psychoanalysis, charging an object with psychic energy or cathexis; cathecting an object.

**vacuum i.,** the i. of a pattern within a vacuum.

**invest′ment.** 1. The process of investing, in general. 2. In dentistry, any material used in investing. 3. In psychoanalysis, the psychic charge or cathexis invested in an object.

**refractory i.,** an i. material which can withstand the high temperatures used in soldering or casting.

**invet′erate** [ L. *in-vetero,* pp. -*atus,* to render old, fr. *vetus,* old ]. Chronic; long seated; firmly established; said of a disease or of confirmed habits.

**inviscation** (in-vis-ka′shun) [ L. *in,* in, on, + *viscum,* bird-lime. VISC- ]. 1. Smearing with mucilaginous matter. 2. The mixing of the food, during mastication, with the buccal secretions.

**in vitro** (in ve′tro) [ L. in glass ]. In the test tube; referring to chemical reactions, fermentation, etc., occurring therein, *e.g.,* in cell-free extracts.

**in vivo** (in-ve′vo) [ L. in the living being ]. In the living body; referring to chemical processes occurring within cells, etc., as distinguished from those occurring in cell-free extracts (*in vitro*).

**involucre** (in′vo-lu-ker). Involucrum.

**involucrum,** pl. **involu′cra** (in′vo-lu′krum) [ L. a wrapper, fr. *in-volvo,* to roll up ]. Involucre. 1. An enveloping membrane, *e.g.,* a sheath or sac. 2. The sheath of new bone that forms around a sequestrum.

**invol′untary** [ L. *in*- neg. + *voluntarius,* willing, fr. *volo,* to wish ]. 1. Independent of the will; not volitional. 2. Contrary to the will.

**involution** (in′vo-lu′shun) [ L. *in-volvo,* pp. -*volutus,* to roll up ]. Catagenesis. 1. The return of an enlarged organ, as the puerperal uterus, to normal size. 2. The turning inward of the edges of a part. 3. In psychiatry, the mental decline associated with middle life.

**senile i.,** the retrogression of vital organs and processes incident to aging.

**i. of the u′terus,** the process of reduction of the uterus to its normal nonpregnant size and state following childbirth.

**involu′tional.** Relating to involution.

**iobenzam′ic acid** (USAN). OSBIL; N-(3-amino-2,4,6-tri-iodobenzoyl)-N-phenyl-β-alanine; radiographic contrast medium.

**iocetamic acid** (i′o-se-tam′ik) (USAN). CHOLEBRINE; N-acetyl-N-(3-amino-2,4,6-triiodophenyl)-2-methyl-β-alanine; a radiopaque contrast medium.

**iodamide** (i-o′dă-mīd) (USAN). UROMICO; α,5-diaceta-mide-2,4,6-triiodo-*m*-toluic acid; a radiopaque contrast medium.

**Iodamoeba** (i-od-ă-me′bah) [ iodine + ameba ]. A protozoan genus in the class Rhizopoda, order Amoebida.

**I. bütschlii,** a parasitic amoeba in the large intestine of man; trophozoites are usually 9 to 14 μ in diameter (ranging from 5 to 20 μ), have clear, blunt pseudopodia that form slowly, contain bacteria and debris in vacuoles, and are rarely observed in feces; the cysts are usually 8 to 10 μ in diameter (ranging from 5 to 14 μ), are uninucleate and somewhat irregular in shape, have a thick wall, usually contain a large compact mass of glycogen that stains deeply with a solution of iodine, and contain small deeply staining bodies that resemble granules of volutin; cysts are the forms ordinarily observed in fecal specimens; clinically recognizable amebiasis caused by this organism is rare, but probably occurs, with symptoms resembling those of chronic disease caused by *Entamoeba histolytica;* this amoeba is also found in other primates and is the commonest amoeba of pigs.

**i′odate.** A salt of iodic acid.

**iod′ic.** 1. Relating to, or caused by, iodine or an iodide. 2. Indicating a compound of iodine in its pentavalent state (see i. acid).

**i. acid,** $HIO_3$; crystalline powder, soluble in water; used as an astringent, caustic, disinfectant, deodorant, and intestinal antiseptic.

**i′odide.** The negative ion of iodine, $I^-$.

**i. peroxidase,** iodotyrosine deiodase; iodinase; an oxido-reductase (EC 1.11.1.8) catalyzing reactions between iodine and water to yield iodide and $H_2O_2$; also catalyzes iodination and deiodination of tyrosine compounds.

**iodimetry** (i′o-dim′e-trī) [ iodine + G. *metron,* measure ]. The determination of the amount of iodine in any compound, or the amount consumed in a reaction, as by an unsaturated compound. See also iodometry.

**iodinase.** Iodide peroxidase.

**io′dinate.** To treat or combine with iodine.

**iodine** (i'o-dĭn, i'o-dēn) [ G. *iōdēs*, violet-like, fr. *ion*, a violet, + *eidos*, form ] (USP, BP). Iodum; a nonmetallic chemical element, symbol I, atomic no. 53, atomic weight 126.91. One of the micronutrients or "trace elements," *i.e.*, one essential to life in trace quantities. Used in the manufacture of i. compounds, as a catalyst, and as an important reagent in analytical chemistry. Used medically as an antiseptic, internally in thyroid disease, and as an antidote for alkaloidal poisons.

   **i. number,** i. value; an indication of the quantity of unsaturated fatty acids present in a fat; it represents the number of grams of i. absorbed by each 100 gm. of fat; see also *hydrogen* number.

   **protein-bound i.,** thyroid hormone in its circulating form, consisting of one or more of the iodothyronines bound to one or more of the serum proteins.

   **radioactive i.,** unstable isotopes of $^{127}I$ which give off particulate or electromagnetic radiations to reach a stable or ground state. Usually refers to $^{131}I$, $^{125}I$, $^{132}I$, or $^{123}I$ used as tracers in biology and medicine.

**iodine-123.** $^{123}I$; a radioisotope of iodine with a pure gamma emission and a physical half-life of 13.1 hours; used for studies of thyroid metabolism.

**iodine-125.** $^{125}I$; radioactive iodine isotope; decays by K-capture with a half-life of 60 days; used as a tracer in thyroid studies and as therapy in hyperthyroidism.

**iodine-127.** $^{127}I$; stable, nonradioactive iodine; it is the most abundant iodide isotope found in nature.

**iodine-131.** $^{131}I$; radioactive iodine isotope; beta emitter with a half-life of 8.05 days; used as a tracer in thyroid studies and as therapy in hyperthyroidism and thyroid cancer.

**iodine-132.** $^{132}I$; a gamma-emitting radioisotope of iodine with a physical half-life of 2.4 hours, usually obtained from a tellurium-132 radionuclide generator; used in studies of thyroid metabolism, especially repeat uptakes after short periods of time.

**α-iodine.** Term applied by Kendall to the supposed active principle of the thyroid secretion, now called thyroxine.

**iodine-fast.** Denoting hyperthyroidism unresponsive to iodine therapy, which ultimately develops in most cases so treated.

**iod'inin.** 1,6-Phenazinediol 5,10-dioxide; a deep purple pigment with a copper-like sheen, isolated from *Chromobacterium iodinum*. Antibacterial agent active against *Streptococcus hemolyticus* and *Staphylococcus aureus*, but only slightly active against Gram-negative bacteria.

**iodinophil, iodinophile** (i-o-din'o-fil, -fīl) [ iodine + G. *philos*, fond ]. 1. Staining readily with iodine. 2. Any histologic element that stains readily with iodine.

**iodinoph'ilous.** Iodinophil (1).

**iodip'amide.** BILIGRAFIN; 3,3'-(adipoyldiimino)bis-[ 2,4,6-triiodobenzoic acid ]; a radiographic contrast medium for biliary system. It is also contained in iodipamide meglumine (USP).

   **i. sodium** (USP), radiopaque contrast medium for injection.

**i'odism.** Poisoning by iodine, a condition marked by severe coryza, an acneform eruption, weakness, salivation, and a foul breath, caused by the continuous administration of iodine or one of the iodides.

**i'odize.** To treat or impregnate with iodine.

**iodized oil** (NF). LIPIODOL; an iodine addition product of vegetable oils, containing not less than 38 per cent and not more than 42 per cent of organically combined iodine; a radiopaque medium used in hysterosalpingography.

**iodoacetamide.** $ICH_2—CONH_2$; a chemical reacting readily with sulfhydryl groups and therefore a strong inhibitor of many enzymes.

**io'doace'tic acid.** $ICH_2—COOH$; the sodium salt (sodium iodoacetate) is used to prevent lactic acid production in experiments on striated muscle, presumably by reacting with —SH groups in phosphoglyceraldehyde dehydrogenase.

**iodoalphion'ic acid.** PRIODAX; β-(4-hydroxy-3,5-diiodophenyl)-β-phenylpropionic acid; radiographic contrast medium.

**iodocasein** (i-o-do-ka'sēn). A compound of iodine with casein, in which the iodine is attached to tyrosine molecules; possesses thyroxine activity.

**io'dochlor'hydrox'yquin.** VIOFORM; clioquinol (BP); 5-chloro-7-iodo-8-quinolinol; 5-chloro-8-hydroxy-7-iodoquinoline; iodochlorhydroxyquinoline; used topically as a local anti-infective and in a wide range of dermatoses, intravaginally in *Trichomonas vaginalis* vaginitis, and internally for the treatment of mild or asymptomatic intestinal amebiasis.

**i'odochlor'ol.** Chloriodized oil.

**io'doder'ma.** An eruption of follicular papules and pustules, or a granulomatous lesion, caused by iodine toxicity.

**io'doform.** Triiodomethane; $CHI_3$; a topical antiseptic.

**io'doglob'ulin.** Thyroglobulin.

**io'dogorgo'ic acid.** 3,5-Diiodotyrosine; a precursor of thyroxine.

**io'dogor'gonine.** An iodinated protein first extracted from gorgonian corals; hydrolysis of it yields iodogorgoic acid.

**io'dohip'purate sodium** (BP). HIPPURAN; sodium *o*-iodohippurate; a radiopaque compound used intravenously, orally, or for retrograde urography. When tagged with iodine-131 it is used to measure renal function externally in radioisotopic renography.

**io'dometh'amate sodium.** Iodoxyl (BP); disodium 1-methyl-3,5-diiodo-4-pyridone-2,6-dicarboxylate; disodium 1-methyl-3,5-diiodochelidamate; an organic iodine radiopaque compound used in intravenous urography or retrograde pyelography.

**iodometry** (i'o-dom'e-trī) [ iodine + G. *metron*, measure ]. Analytical techniques involving titrations in which iodine is either formed or consumed, the sudden appearance or disappearance of iodine marking the end point. See also iodimetry.

**io'dopano'ic acid.** Iopanoic acid.

**io'dophen'dylate.** Iophendylate.

**iodophilia** (i-o'do-fil'ĭ-ah) [ iodine + G. *phileō*, to love ]. An affinity for iodine, as manifested by some leukocytes in certain conditions; when treated with a solution of iodine and potassium iodide, normal polymorphonuclear leukocytes are stained a fairly bright yellow; in certain pathologic conditions (such as toxemia, infectious disease, pronounced anemia, and so on), the polymorphonuclear leukocytes are frequently stained diffusely brown or yellow-brown; the reaction may be *intracellular* (as described), or it may occur *extracellularly*, affecting the particles in the immediate vicinity of the leukocytes.

**iodophor** (i-o'do-fōr) [ iodine + G. *phora*, a carrying ]. A combination of iodine with a surfactant carrier, usually polyvinylpyrrolidone. Preparations such as Betadine and Ioprep contain 1 per cent "available" iodine, which is slowly released to become effect against microorganisms. Used as skin disinfectants, particularly for surgical scrubs.

**iodophthalein** (i-o'do-thal'ēn, -fthal'e-in). Tetraiodophenolphthalein; the disodium salt has been used as an indicator in x-ray examination of the gallbladder.

**io'dopro'teins.** Proteins containing iodine which is bound to tyrosine groups; *e.g.*, thyroglobulin, iodocasein, etc.

**iodop'sin.** Visual violet; a visual pigment found in the cones of the retina.

**io'dopy'racet.** DIODRAST; diodone; diethanolamine acetate; 3,5-diiodo-4-pyridone-*N*-acetate; a radiopaque medium used intravenously in urography; also used to determine the renal plasma flow and the renal tubular excretory mass.

**i'odother'apy.** Treatment with iodine.

**io'dothy'ronines.** A group of iodinated amino acids with a diphenyl ether ring system in the side chain; thyroxine is the longest and best known of this group.

**io'doty'rosine.** An iodinated tyrosine; *e.g.*, monoiodotyrosine and diiodotyrosine.

   **i. deiodase,** iodide peroxidase.

**iodox'yl** (BP). Iodomethamate sodium.

**iodu'ria.** Urinary excretion of iodine.

**ioglycam'ic acid** (USAN). BILIVISTAN; 3,3'-(diglycoloyldiimino)bis(2,4,6-triiodobenzoic acid); radiographic contrast medium for biliary system.

**iometer** (i-om'e-ter) [ ion + G. *metron,* measure ]. A chamber for measuring the percentage of ionization.

**i'on** [ G. *iōn,* going ]. An atom or group of atoms carrying a charge of electricity by virtue of having gained or lost one or more valence electrons, usually constituting one of the parts of an electrolyte. The i.'s charged with negative electricity, which travel toward a positive pole (anode), are called anions; those charged with positive electricity, which travel toward a negative pole (cathode), are called cations. I's may exist in solid, liquid, or gaseous environments, although those in liquid (electrolytes) are the most common and familiar.

**aquo-i.,** see *aquo-ion.*

**dipolar i.'s,** i.'s possessing both a negative charge and a positive charge, each localized at a different point in the molecule which thus has both positive and negative "poles"; zwitterions. The amino acids are the most notable dipolar i.'s, containing the positively charged $NH_3$ group and the negatively charged $COO^-$ group.

**gram i.,** the weight in grams of an ion that is equal to the sum of the atomic weights of the atoms making up the ion.

**Ionescu.** See Jonnesco.

**ion exchange.** The process whereby a small ion, constituting part of a salt or acid or base with an immobilized solid polymeric ion, exchanges position with another small ion of like charge in a surrounding liquid (aqueous) medium. See also ion exchanger, anion exchange, cation exchange.

**ion exchanger.** A polymer containing numerous charged groups (*e.g.,* $-SO_3^-$, $-CO_2^-$, $-NR_3^+$) to which mobile ions of opposite charge are attached. If a solution containing other ions of similar charge is passed through the polymer, the new ion may replace (or exchange for) the old; salt water, passing over the appropriate ion exchanger, may exchange $Na^+$ for $H^+$, and $Cl^-$ for $OH^-$, and be thus desalted. Ion exchangers may have differing "preferences" for various otherwise similar ions so that they can be used to effect a chromatographic separation (*e.g.,* $Na^+$ from $K^+$); they have been applied notably to the separation of the rare earth elements in this manner. See also cation exchanger and anion exchanger.

**ion'ic.** Relating to an ion or ions.

**i. strength,** symbolized as $\Gamma/2$ and set equal to $\Sigma 1/2 c_i z_i^2$, where $c_i$ equals the concentration and $z_i$ the charge of each ion present in solution. A number of biochemically important events, *e.g.,* protein solubility and rate of enzyme action, vary with the i. strength of a solution.

**io'nium** [ G. *iōn,* going ]. Thorium-230.

**i'oniza'tion.** 1. Dissociation into ions, occurring when an electrolyte is dissolved in water. 2. Iontophoresis (2).

**i'onize.** To separate into ions; to dissociate atoms or molecules into electrically charged atoms or radicals.

**i'onogram.** Electropherogram.

**i'onone.** A cyclic ketone with an odor of violets; the $\alpha$ and $\beta$ varieties differ in the location of the double bond (the $\beta$ form is given here); provitamins A and vitamin A have ionone configuration in the ring portion; $\alpha$-carotene contains one $\alpha$- and one $\beta$-ionone; $\beta$-carotene, two $\beta$-ionones; and $\gamma$-carotene, one $\beta$-ionone. See carotenoids.

$\beta$-Ionone

**i'onopher'ogram.** Electropherogram.

**ionophose** (i-on'o-fōz, i'on-o-fōz) [ G. *ion,* violet, + *phōs,* light ]. A purple phose.

**iontophoresis** (i-on'to-fo-re'sis) [ ion + G. *phorēsis,* a being borne ]. 1. Term suggested (but not commonly used) to denote movement in an electric field of relatively small ions as distinguished from the movement of large molecules or particles (electrophoresis). 2. Iontotherapy; ionization (2); ionic medication; the introduction into the tissues, by means of an electric current, of the ions of a chosen medicament.

**ion'tophoret'ic.** Relating to iontophoresis.

**iontoquantimeter** (i-on'to-kwon-tim'e-ter) [ ion + L. *quantus,* how much, + G. *metron,* measure ]. A device for determining the quantity of x-rays by measuring the resulting ionization.

**iontotherapy** (i-on'to-thĕr'ă-pī). Iontophoresis (2).

**i'opano'ic acid** (USP, BP). Iodopanoic acid; 3-amino-$\alpha$-ethyl-2,4,6-triiodohydrocinnamic acid; a creamy, organic, radiopaque iodine compound, insoluble in water. Used as a contrast medium in cholecystography.

**i'ophen'dylate** (USP, BP). Iodophendylate; ethyl iodophenylundecylate; a mixture of isomers of ethyl iodophenylundecylate, an absorbable iodized fatty acid of low viscosity. Used for roentgenography of the spinal cord, biliary tree, sinuses, and body cavities.

**iophenox'ic acid.** TERIDAX; $\alpha$-ethyl-3-hydroxy-2,4,6-triiodohydrocinnamic acid; radiographic contrast medium.

**i'opho'bia** [ G. *ios,* poison, + *phobos,* fear ]. Fear of poisons.

**iotacism** (i-o'tă-sizm) [ G. *iōta,* the letter i ]. A speech defect marked by the frequent substitution of an ē sound (that of the Greek iota) for other vowels.

**iothal'amate sodium** (USP). Sodium salt of iothalamic acid; used as a radiopaque medium.

**iothalamic acid** (i'o-thă-lam'ik) (BP, USAN). 5-Acetamido-2,4,6-triiodo-*N*-methylisophthalamic acid; x-ray contrast medium.

**iothiouracil sodium** (i'o-thi'o-u'ră-sil). ITRUMIL sodium; sodium salt of 5-iodo-2-thiouracil; an organic iodine derivative of thiouracil with the thyroid-involuting action of iodine and capable of inhibiting thyroxine production.

**I.P., i.p.** Abbreviation for intraperitoneal, or intraperitoneally.

**ipecac** (ip'e-kak) (USP). Ipecacuanha.

**powdered i.** (USP), used in the preparation of ipecac syrup.

**wild i.,** *Apocynum androsaemifolium.*

**ipecacuanha** (ip-e-kak-u-an'ah) [ native Brazilian word ] (BP). Ipecac; the dried root of *Uragoga (Cephaelis) ipecacuanha* (family Rubiaceae), a shrub of Brazil and other parts of South America; contains emetine, cephaeline, emetamine, ipecacuanhic acid, psychotrine, and methylpsychotrine; has expectorant, emetic, and antidysenteric properties.

**de-emetinized i.,** i. from which the emetic principle has been extracted; has been used as an antidysenteric agent.

**prepared i.** (BP), a fine powder to contain 2 per cent of the total alkaloids of i., calculated as emetine.

**i'podate sodium** (USP). BILOPTIN; ORAGRAFIN sodium; sodium 3-[ (dimethylaminomethylene)amino ]-2,4,6-triiodohydracinnamate; a radiopaque medium.

**ipomea** (i-po-me'ah) [ G. *ips (ip-)*, a worm, + *homoios,* like ]. Orizaba jalap root; Mexican scammony root; the dried root of *Ipomoea orizabensis* (family Convolvulaceae). See also ipomea resin.

**Ipomoea** (i'po-me'ah) [ L. ipomea, *q. v.* ]. A plant genus of the family Convolvulaceae.

**I. rubrocoerulea** var. **praecox,** ololiuqui (*q. v.*); morning glory; the seeds contain lysergic acid amide, isolysergic acide amide, chanoclavine, elymoclavine, and other ergot (indole) alkaloids. Ingestion of the seeds produces hallucinatory and euphoric effects.

**I. versicolor,** *I. tricolor; I. violacea;* pearly gates; the seeds contain hallucinogenic ergot (indole) alkaloids.

**IPPB.** Abbreviation for intermittent positive pressure breathing.

**iproclozide.** SURSUM; *p*-(chlorophenoxy)acetic acid 2-isopropylhydrazide; monoamine oxidase inhibitor.

**iproni'azid phosphate.** MARSILID; 1-isonicotinoyl-2-isopropylhydrazine; an antituberculous and antidepressant agent similar to isoniazid, but more toxic and rarely used. It inhibits monoamine oxidase.

**ipronidazole** (i'pro-ni'dă-zōl) USAN). IPROPRAN; isopropyl-1-methyl-5-nitroimidazole; an antiprotozoal agent.

**iprover'atril.** Verapamil.

**ipsation, ipsism** (ip-sa'shun, ip'sizm) [ L. *ipse,* self (intensive pronoun) ]. Masturbation.

**ipsilat′eral** [ L. *ipse*, same, + *latus* (*later*-), side ]. On the same side; denoting especially motor or sensory disorders occurring on the same side as the causative brain lesion.

**IPSP.** Abbreviation for inhibitory postsynaptic *potential*.

**IPTG.** Abbreviation for isopropylthiogalactoside.

**IQ.** Abbreviation for intelligence *quotient.*

**Ir.** Chemical symbol of the element iridium.

**IRI.** Abbreviation for immunoreactive *insulin.*

**irid-.** See irido-.

**iridal** (i′rĭ-dal, ĭr′ĭ-dal). Relating to the iris; iridic; iridial; iridian.

**iridauxesis** (ĭr-id-awk-se′sis) [ irido- + G. *auxēsis*, enlargement ]. Thickening of the iris following plastic iritis.

**iridectome** (ĭr-ĭ-dek′tōm) [ irido- + G. *tomē*, a cutting ]. A slender scissors used in performing iridectomy.

**iridectomesodialysis** (ĭr-ĭ-dek-to-mes′o-di-al′ĭ-sis) [ irido- + G. *ektomē*, excision, + *mesos*, middle, + *dialysis*, loosening ]. Formation of an artificial pupil by combined excision of iris at its periphery and separation of the adhesions around its inner margin.

**ir′idec′tomize.** To perform an iridectomy.

**iridectomy** (ĭr′ĭ-dek′to-mĭ) [ irido- + G. *ektomē*, excision ]. Excision of a portion of the iris.

   **buttonhole i.,** peripheral i.

   **optical i.,** an i. performed for the purpose of improving the vision by making an artificial pupil, in cases of central opacity of the cornea or lens, keratoconus, etc.

   **peripheral i.,** stenopeic i.; buttonhole i.; in narrow angle glaucoma, the surgical removal of a minute portion of iris at its root; in intracapsular extraction of cataract, removal of one or more minute sections near the peripheral border, leaving the pupillary margin intact.

   **preparatory i.,** one done as a preparatory measure to a cataract operation.

   **stenopeic i.,** peripheral i.

   **therapeutic i.,** one performed for the prevention or cure of disease (for example, glaucoma) in the eye.

**iridectropium** (ĭr′ĭ-dek-tro′pĭ-um) [ irido- + G. *ektropion*, everted eyelid ]. Eversion of part of the iris.

**iridemia** (ĭr′ĭ-de′mĭ-ah) [ irido- + G. *haima*, blood ]. Bleeding from the iris.

**iridencleisis** (ĭr′ĭ-den-kli′sis) [ irido- + G. *enkleiō*, to shut in. CLID- ]. The incarceration of a portion of the iris in a wound of the cornea, either accidentally or as an operative measure in glaucoma to effect filtration.

**iridentropium** (ĭr′ĭ-den-tro′pĭ-um) [ irido- + G. *entropia*, a turning toward ]. Inversion of part of the iris.

**irideremia** (ĭr′id-er-e′mĭ′ah, i′rĭd-) [ irido- + G. *erēmia*, absence ]. A condition wherein the iris is extremely rudimentary, so that it seems to be absent; less correctly termed aniridia.

**irides** (ĭr′ĭ-dēz) [ G. ]. Plural of iris.

**iridescent** (ĭr-ĭ-des′ent) [ G. *iris*, rainbow ]. Presenting a changeable metallic luster like mother of pearl or the plumage of certain birds; nacreous.

**iridesis** (i-rĭd′e-sis) [ irido- + G. *desis*, a binding together ]. Iridodesis; ligature of a portion of the iris brought out through an incision in the cornea.

**irid′ial, irid′ian, irid′ic.** Iridal.

**ir′idin.** 1. Irigenin 7-glucoside; from orris root, *Iris florentina.* 2. Irisin; a resinoid from blue flag, *Iris versicolor;* used as a cholagogue and cathartic.

**irid′ium.** A white, silvery metallic element, symbol Ir, atomic no. 77, atomic weight 192.2.

**iridization** (ĭr′ĭ-dĭ-za′shun, i′rĭ-). An obsolete term denoting the halo appearance surrounding a light observed by sufferers from glaucoma.

**irido-, irid-** (ĭr′ĭ-do-, i′rĭ-do-) [ G. *iris* (*irid*-), rainbow. IRIS ]. Combining forms relating to the iris.

**iridoavulsion** (ĭr′ĭ-do-ă-vul′shun). Avulsion, or tearing away, of the iris.

**iridocapsulitis** (ĭr′ĭ-do-kap-su-li′tis). Iritis with accompanying inflammation of the capsule of the crystalline lens.

**iridocele** (ĭr′ĭ-do-sēl) [ irido- + G. *kēlē*, hernia ]. Myiocephalon; protrusion of a portion of the iris through a corneal defect.

**iridochoroiditis** (ĭr-ĭ-do-ko-roy-di′tis). Inflammation of both iris and choroid.

**iridocoloboma** (ĭr′ĭ-do-kol′o-bo′mah) [ irido- + G. *kolobōma*, coloboma ]. A coloboma, or congenital defect of the iris.

**ir′idoconstric′tor.** Causing contraction of the pupil; denoting especially the circular muscular fibers of the iris.

**ir′idocor′neal.** Relating to the iris and the cornea.

**iridocyclectomy** (ĭr′ĭ-do-si-klek′to-mĭ) [ irido- + G. *kyklos*, circle (ciliary body), + *ektomē*, excision ]. Removal of the iris and ciliary body for excision of tumor.

**iridocyclitis** (ĭr′id-o-si-kli′tis) [ irido- + G. *kyklos*, circle (ciliary body), + suffix - *itis*, inflammation ]. Inflammation of both iris and ciliary body.

**iridocyclochoroiditis** (ĭr′ĭ-do-si′klo-ko-royd-i′tis). Inflammation of the iris, involving the ciliary body and the choroid.

**iridocystectomy** (ĭr′ĭ-do-sis-tek′to-mĭ) [ irido- + G. *kystis*, bladder (capsule), + *ektomē*, excision ]. An operation for making an artificial pupil when posterior synechiae follow extracapsular extraction of cataract; the border of the iris and a portion of the capsule of the lens are drawn out through an incision in the cornea and cut off.

**iridodesis** (ĭr′ĭ-dod′e-sis). Iridesis.

**iridodiagnosis** (ĭr′ĭ-do-di-ag-no′sis). Diagnosis of systemic affections through observation of changes in form and color of the iris.

**iridodialysis** (ĭr′ĭ-do-di-al′ĭ-sis) [ irido- + G. *dialysis*, loosening ]. A colobomatous defect of the iris due to its separation from its ciliary attachment.

**iridodilator** (ĭr′ĭ-do-di-la′tor). Causing dilation of the pupil, applied to the radiating muscular fibers of the iris.

**iridodonesis** (ĭr′ĭ-do-do-ne′sis) [ irido- + G. *doneō*, to shake to and fro ]. Agitated motion of the iris.

**iridokinesis, iridokinesia** (ĭr′ĭ-do-kĭ-ne′sis, -kĭ-ne′zĭ-ah) [ irido- + G. *kinēsis*, movement ]. The movement of the iris in contracting and dilating the pupil.

**ir′idokinet′ic.** Relating to the movements of the iris.

**iridomalacia** (ĭr′ĭ-do-mă-la′shĭ-ah) [ irido- + G. *malakia*, softness ]. Degenerative softening of the iris.

**iridomesodialysis** (ĭr′ĭ-do-mes′o-di-al′ĭ-sis) [ irido- + G. *mesos*, middle, + *dialysis*, loosening ]. Separation of adhesions around the inner margin of the iris.

**ir′idomo′tor.** Iridokinetic.

**iridoncosis** (ĭr′ĭ-dong-ko′sis) [ irido- + G. *onkos*, mass, + suffix - *ōsis*, condition ]. Thickening of the iris.

**iridoncus** (ĭr′ĭ-dong′kus) [ irido- + G. *onkos*, mass ]. A tumefaction of the iris.

**ir′idoparal′ysis.** Iridoplegia.

**ir′idop′athy.** Condition of pathologic lesions in the iris.

**iridoperiphakitis** (ĭr′ĭ-do-pĕr′ĭ-fă-ki′tis) [ irido- + G. *peri*, around, + *phakos*, lentil (lens) ]. Inflammation of the iris and the anterior portion of the capsule of the lens.

**iridoplegia** (ĭr′ĭ-do-ple′jĭ-ah) [ irido- + G. *plēgē*, stroke ]. Paralysis of the sphincter of the iris.

   **accommodation i.,** absence of pupillary contraction during efforts at accommodation.

   **complete i.,** immobilization of the iris.

   **reflex i.,** absence of the pupillary light reflex, as in the Argyll Robertson pupil.

   **sympathetic i.,** i. due to the paralysis of the sympathetically innervated dilator pupillae muscle.

**iridoptosis** (ĭr′ĭ-dop-to′sis) [ irido- + G. *ptosis*, a falling ]. Prolapse of the iris.

**iridorrhexis** (ĭr′ĭ-do-rek′sis) [ irido- + G. *rhēxis*, rupture ]. Tearing the iris from its peripheral attachment in order to increase the breadth of a coloboma.

**iridoschisis** ĭr′ĭ-dos-kĭ-sis) [ irido- + G. *schisma*, cleft. SCHI- ]. Separation of the anterior layer of the iris from the posterior layer; ruptured anterior fibers float in the aqueous.

**iridosclerotomy** (ĭr′ĭ-do-skle-rot′o-mĭ) [ irido- + sclera, *q.v.*, + G. *tomē*, incision ]. An incision involving both sclera and iris.

**iridosteresis** (ĭr′ĭ-do-ste-re′sis) [ irido- + G. *sterēsis*, a loss ]. Loss or absence of all or part of the iris.

**iridotasis** (ĭr'ĭ-dot'ă-sis) [ irido- + G. *tasis*, a stretching. TEN- ]. Borthen's operation; stretching the iris and incarcerating it in the limbal incision; a substitute for iridenclisis in glaucoma.

**iridotomy** (ĭr'ĭ-dot'o-mĭ) [ irido- + G. *tomē*, incision ]. Corotomy; transverse division of some of the fibers of the iris, forming an artificial pupil.

**irigen'in.** A trihydroxy, trimethoxy isoflavone, from iris; component of iridin.

**i'rin.** A lipid-soluble acid found in the human iris and ciliary body and in the irides of other mammals; causes mictic spasm; assayed by its spasmogenic effect on many smooth muscles, notably the hamster colon.

**I'ris** [ G. the plant iris ]. 1. A genus of plants of the family Iridaceae. 2. Orris; the rhizome of *Iris florentina, I. Germanica,* or *I. pallida;* used in the manufacture of various toilet articles. See iridin.

   **I. versicolor,** blue flag; flag lily; occasionally used as a cathartic.

**i'ris,** pl. **ir'ides** [ G. rainbow. The iris of the eye. IRIS ] [ NA ]. The anterior division of the vascular tunic of the eye, a disklike diaphragm, perforated in the center (the pupil), attached marginally to the ciliary body; it is composed of stroma and a double layer of pigmented retinal epithelium from which are derived the sphincter and dilator muscles of the pupil.

   **i. bombé** (e-rĕs'bawn-ba') [ Fr. bulging ], a condition occurring in posterior annular synechia, in which an increase of fluid in the posterior chamber causes a forward bulging of the nonadherent portion of the i.

   **trem'ulous i.,** iridodonesis.

**i'risin.** Iridin (2).

**i'risop'sia** [ G. *iris,* rainbow, + *opsis,* appearance ]. The appearance of rainbow colors about objects.

**irit'ic.** Relating to iritis.

**iritides** (i-rit'ĭ-dēz). Alternate plural of iritis.

**iritis** (i-ri'tis). Inflammation of the iris.

   **i. blenorrhagique à rechutes,** i. recidivans staphylococco-allergica; i. with recurrent hypopyon.

   **i. catamenia'lis,** i. recurring at the menstrual periods.

   **follicular i.,** chronic i. with glassy nodules situated deep down between the anterior and posterior layers of the iris.

   **plastic i.,** i. with a fibrinous exudation.

   **quiet i.,** i. without inflammatory signs such as redness or edema of the cornea.

   **i. recidivans staphylococco-allergica,** i. blenorrhagique à rechutes.

   **serous i.,** inflammation of iris, with serous exudate in anterior chamber.

   **spongy i.,** i. with a fibrinous coagulum in the anterior chamber of the eye.

   **sympathetic i.,** i. consecutive to a similar condition in the other eye.

**irit'omy.** Iridotomy.

**iron** (i'ern, i'run) [ A.S. *iren* ]. Ferrum; a metallic element, symbol Fe, atomic no. 26, atomic weight 55.85. It occurs in the heme of hemoglobin, myoglobin, transferrin, ferritin, and iron-containing porphyrins, and is an essential component of enzymes such as catalase, peroxidase, and the various cytochromes. Iron salts are used in the treatment of iron deficiency anemia. For individual salts not listed below, see subentries under ferric and ferrous.

   **albuminized i.,** i. albuminate; a compound of i. oxide and albumin; rendered soluble by the presence of sodium citrate; occurs as reddish brown, lustrous granules, odorless or nearly so. Used in anemia.

   **i. alum,** ferric ammonium sulfate.

   **i.-dextran complex,** IMFERON; a colloidal solution of ferric hydroxide in complex with partially hydrolyzed dextran. Used in the treatment of iron deficiency anemias by intramuscular injection.

   **i. dextrin,** a complex of dextrin with ferric hydroxide; used intravenously in the treatment of iron deficiency.

   **i. index,** see under index.

   **peptonized i.,** peptonate of i.; a compound of i. oxide and peptone, rendered soluble by the presence of sodium citrate; used in the treatment of iron deficiency anemia.

   **i. protoporphyrin,** a protoporphyrin to which an i. atom is complexed, the most important example being heme.

   **i. pyri'tes,** native sulfide of i.

   **i. sorbitex** (USAN), JECTOFER; i. sorbitol; a complex of iron, sorbitol, and citric acid in stable solution for intramuscular administration in the treatment of iron deficiency anemia in patients who are unable to take sufficient amounts of iron by the oral route.

   **i. sorbitol** (BP), i. sorbitex.

   **i. sulfate,** ferrous sulfate.

**iron-55.** $^{55}$Fe; radioactive i. isotope; positron emitter with half-life of 2.94 years; used (less often than Fe$^{59}$) as tracer in study of i. metabolism.

**iron-59.** $^{59}$Fe; radioactive i. isotope; beta emitter with half-life of 45.1 days; used as tracer in study of i. metabolism.

**i'rone.** A cyclic ketone responsible for the odor of orris root and of violets; occurs as $\alpha$-, $\beta$-, and $\gamma$-irone; used in perfumery.

**irot'omy.** Iridotomy.

**irradiate** (ĭr-ra'dĭ-āt) [ see irradiation ]. To apply radiation from a source to a structure or organism.

**irradiation** (ĭr-ra'dĭ-a'shun) [ L. *ir-radio* (*in-r*), pp. -*radiatus,* to beam forth. RADI- ]. 1. The apparent enlargement of a bright object seen against a dark background. 2. Subjection to the action of rays (*e.g.,* heat, light, radium) for diagnostic or therapeutic purposes. 3. Sub-jection of a substance (*e.g.,* ergosterol) to the action of certain rays (*e.g.,* ultraviolet) in order to impart to it, or to increase its already existing, therapeutic efficiency. 4. The spread of nervous effects (impulses) from one area in the brain or cord, or from a tract, to another tract. See also radiation.

**irrational** (ĭr-rash'un-al) [ L. *irrationalis,* without reason ]. Not rational. 1. Unreasonable (contrary to reason) or unreasoning (not exercising reason). 2. Mentally disordered.

**ir'redu'cible.** Not reducible; incapable of being made smaller; in chemistry, incapable of being made simpler, or of being replaced or hydrogenated or reduced in positive charge.

**irrespirable** (ĭr-rē-spi'ră-bl). 1. Incapable of being breathed; unfit for respiration; denoting a poisonous gas or one containing oxygen in insufficient amount. 2. An aerosol composed of particles with aerodynamic size larger than 10 $\mu$.

**ir'responsibil'ity.** The state of not being responsible.

   **criminal i.,** the state, usually attributed to mental defect or disease, that renders a person not responsbile for his criminal conduct.

**irresuscitable** (ĭr're-sus'ĭ-tă-bl). Incapable of being revived.

**irreversible** (ĭr're-ver'sĭ-bl) [ L. *in-* (*ir-*) neg. + *re-verto,* pp. -*versus,* to turn back. VERT- ]. Permanent.

**irrigate** (ĭr'ĭ-gāt) [ L. *ir-rigo,* pp. -*atus,* to irrigate, fr. *in,* on, + *rigo,* to water ]. To wash out a cavity or wound with water or a medicated fluid.

**irrigation** (ĭr-ĭ-ga'shun) [ see irrigate ]. The washing out of a cavity or wounded surface with a stream of fluid.

**ir'rigator.** An appliance used in irrigation, consisting of a reservoir with a flexible outlet tube.

**ir'ritabil'ity** [ L. *irritabilitas,* fr. *irrito,* pp. -*atus,* to excite ]. The property inherent in protoplasm of reacting to a stimulus.

   **electric i.,** the response of a nerve or muscle to the passage of a current of electricity; in cases of degeneration in nerve or muscle this i. is altered or lost; see modal, qualitative, and quantitative *alteration.*

   **myotatic i.,** the ability of a muscle to contract in response to the stimulus produced by a sudden stretching.

**ir'ritable.** 1. Excitable; capable of reacting to a stimulus. 2. Tending to react immoderately to a stimulus.

**ir'ritant.** 1. Irritating; causing irritation. 2. Any agent with this action.

   **primary i.,** a substance that causes inflammation, particularly of the skin, on first contact or exposure.

**irrita'tion** [ L. *irritatio* ]. 1. Extreme reaction of the tissues to an injury; incipient inflammation. 2. The normal response of nerve or muscle to a stimulus. 3. The evocation of a normal or exaggerated reaction in the tissues by the application of a stimulus.

**ir'rita'tive.** Causing irritation.

**irrumation** (ĭr'ru-ma'shun) [ L. *irrumo*, pp. -*atus*, to give suck ]. Fellatio.

**irrup'tion** (ĭr-rup'shun) [ L. *irruptio*, fr. *irrumpo*, to break in ]. The act or process of breaking through to a surface.

**irrup'tive.** Relating to or characterized by irruption.

**IRV.** Abbreviation for inspiratory reserve *volume*.

**Irvine,** A. Ray, Jr., American ophthalmologist, *1917. See I.'s *syndrome*.

**isauxesis** (i'sawk-ze'sis) [ G. *isos*, even, + *auxēsis*, increase ]. Growth of parts at the same rate as growth of the whole.

**ischemia** (is-ke'mĭ-ah) [ G. *ischō*, to keep back, + *haima*, blood ]. Hypoemia; local anemia due to mechanical obstruction (mainly arterial narrowing) to the blood supply.

    **myocar'dial i.,** inadequate circulation of blood to the myocardium, usually as a result of coronary artery disease; see *angina* pectoris; myocardial *infarction*.

    **postural i.,** the reduced blood pressure and flow induced in a part, *e.g.*, the leg or foot, by raising it above the heart level; used to reduce bleeding during surgical operations on the extremities.

    **i. ret'inae,** diminished blood supply in the retina due to failure of the arterial circulation; it may occur as a result of (1) arterial embolism or spasm, (2) poisoning, as by quinine, or (3) exsanguination from recurring profuse hemorrhages, *e.g.*, in parturition, gastric and duodenal ulcers, and pulmonary tuberculosis; bilateral transitory or permanent blindness may occasionally result from nonfunctioning of the rods and cones.

**ischemic** (is-ke'mik). Relating to or affected by ischemia.

**ischesis** (is-ke'sis) [ G. *ischō*, to hold back ]. Suppression of any discharge, especially of a normal one.

**ischia** (is'kĭ-ah). Plural of ischium.

**ischiadic** (is-kĭ-ad'ik). Ischial.

**ischiadicus** [ L. ] [ NA ]. Ischial or sciatic.

**ischial** (is'kĭ-al). Relating to the hip.

**ischialgia** (is-kĭ-al'jĭ-ah) [ G. *ischion*, hip, + *algos*, pain ]. 1. Ischiodynia; ischioneuralgia; coxalgia; pain in the hip. 2. Sciatica.

**ischiatic** (is-kĭ-at'ik). Ischial.

**ischiatitis** (is-kĭ-ă-ti'tis). Inflammation of the sciatic nerve.

**ischidrosis** (is-ki-dro'sis) [ G. *ischō*, to hold back, + *hidrōsis*, perspiration ]. Anhidrosis; suppression of the perspiration.

**ischio-** (is'kĭ-o) [ G. *ischion*, hip-joint, haunch (ischium) ]. Combining form relating to the ischium.

**ischioanal** (is-kĭ-o-a'nal). Relating to the ischium and the anus.

**ischiobulbar** (is-kĭ-o-bul'bar). Relating to the ischium and the bulb of the urethra.

**ischiocapsular** (is-kĭ-o-kap'su-lar). Relating to the ischium and the capsule of the hip joint; denoting that part of the capsule which is attached to the ischium.

**ischiocavernosus** (is'kĭ-o-kav-er-no'sus). See under musculus.

**ischiocavernous** (is-kĭ-o-kav'er-nus). Relating to the ischium and the corpus cavernosum.

**ischiocele** (is'kĭ-o-sēl) [ ischio- + G. *kēlē*, hernia ]. Sciatic *hernia*.

**ischiococcygeal** (is-kĭ-o-kok-sij'e-al). Relating to the ischium and the coccyx.

**ischiococcygeus** (is-kĭ-o-kok-sij'e-us). See under musculus.

**ischiodynia** (is-kĭ-o-din'ĭ-ah) [ ischio- + G. *odynē*, pain ]. Ischialgia.

**ischiofemoral** (is-kĭ-o-fem'o-ral). Relating to the ischium, or hip bone, and the femur, or thigh bone.

**ischiofibular** (is-kĭ-o-fib'u-lar). Relating to or connecting the ischium and the fibula.

**ischiohebotomy** (is-kĭ-o-he-bot'o-mĭ) [ ischio- + G. *hēbē*, pubes, + *tomē*, incision ]. Division of the ischiopubic ramus and the ascending ramus of the pubes.

**ischiomelus** (is-kĭ-om'e-lus) [ ischio- + G. *melos*, limb ]. Unequal conjoined twins in which the parasite, often only an arm or a leg, arises from the pelvic region of the autosite.

**ischioneuralgia** (is-kĭ-o-nu-ral'jĭ-ah). Ischialgia.

---

**ischionitis** (is'kĭ-o-ni'tis). Inflammation of the ischium.

**ischiopagus** (is'kĭ-op'ă-gus) [ ischio- + G. *pagos*, fixed ]. Conjoined twins united in their ischial region.

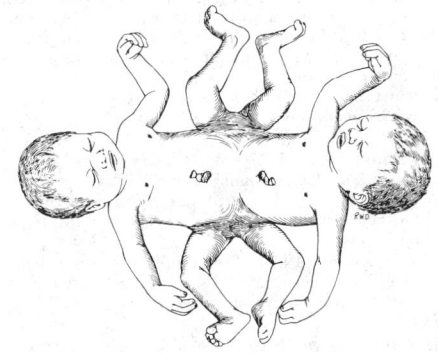

**Ischiopagus**

**ischioperineal** (is-kĭ-o-pĕr-ĭ-ne'al). Relating to the ischium and the perineum.

**ischiopubic** (is'kĭ-o-pu'bik). Relating to both ischium and pubis.

**ischiopubiotomy** (is'kĭ-o-pu-bĭ-ot'o-mĭ) [ ischio- + L. *pubes* + G. *tomē*, incision ]. Ischiohebotomy.

**ischiorectal** (is'kĭ-o-rek'tal). Relating to the ischium and the rectum.

**ischiosacral** (is'kĭ-o-sa'kral). Relating to the ischium and the sacrum.

**ischiothoracopagus** (is'kĭ-o-tho'ră-kop'ă-gus). Iliothoracopagus.

**ischiotibial** (is'kĭ-o-tib'ĭ-al). Relating to or connecting the ischium and the tibia.

**ischiovaginal** (is-kĭ-o-vaj'ĭ-nal). Relating to the ischium and the vagina.

**ischiovertebral** (is-kĭ-o-ver'te-bral). Relating to the ischium and the vertebral column.

**ischium,** gen. **ischii,** pl. **ischia** (is'kĭ-um) [ Mod. L. fr. G. *ischion*, hip ] [ NA ]. *Os* ischii.

**ischochymia** (is-ko-ki'mĭ-ah) [ G. *ischō*, to keep back, + *chymos*, juice ]. Retention of food in the stomach in cases of dilation of that organ.

**ischogalactic** (is'ko-gă-lak'tik) [ G. *ischō*, to keep back, + *gala* (*galakt*-), milk ]. Antigalactic; lactifuge. 1. Causing a suppression of the breast milk. 2. An agent that arrests the secretion of milk.

**ischomenia** (is-ko-me'nĭ-ah) [ G. *ischō*, to keep back, + *mēn*, month. MEN- ]. Suppression of the menses.

**ischuretic** (is-ku-ret'ik). 1. Relating to or relieving ischuria. 2. An agent that relieves retention or suppression of urine.

**ischuria** (is-ku'rĭ-ah) [ G. *ischō*, to keep back, + *ouron*, urine ]. Retention or suppression of urine.

**i'sethi'onate.** 1. A salt or ester of isethionic acid. 2. USAN-approved contraction for 2-hydroxyethanesulfonate, $HOCH_2CH_2SO_3^-$.

**i'sethion'ic acid.** 2-Hydroxyethanesulfonic acid; $HO—CH_2—CH_2—SO_3H$; a colorless, viscous liquid, miscible with water and alcohols. Forms crystalline salts with organic acids.

**Ishihara** (ish-e-har'ah), Shinobu, Japanese ophthalmologist, *1879. See I.'s *test*.

**isinglass** (i'zing-glas) [ Old Ger. *huysenblas*, sturgeon's bladder ]. Ichthyocolla.

**island** (i'land) [ A.S. *igland* ]. Insula; in anatomy, any isolated part, separated from the surrounding tissues by a groove, or marked by difference in structure; see also insula.

    **blood i.,** b. islet; an aggregation of splanchnic mesodermal cells in the embryonic yolk-sac having the potentiality of forming vascular endothelium and primitive blood cells.

**i.'s of Calleja,** dense clusters of very small nerve cells (granule cells) characteristic of the olfactory tubercle at the base of the forebrain.

**Langerhans' i.'s,** Langerhans' islets; pancreatic i.'s or islets; cellular masses varying from a few to hundreds of cells lying in the interstitial tissue of the pancreas; they are composed of different cell types which comprise the endocrine portion of the pancreas, and are the source of insulin and glucagon.

**pancreatic i.'s,** Langerhans' i.'s.

**i. of Reil,** insula (1).

**islet** (i'let). Small island.

**i.'s of Langerhans,** Langerhans' *islands.*

**pancreatic i.'s,** Langerhans' *islands.*

**principal i.'s,** separate globular aggregates made up mostly of endocrine pancreatic tissue; present in some fishes and snakes.

**iso-** [ G. *isos,* equal ]. 1. Prefix meaning equal, like. 2. Extensively used in chemistry to indicate "isomer of" (isomerism), *e.g.,* isocyanate *versus* cyanate; isocitrate *versus* citrate.

**isoadrenocorticism** (i'so-ă-dre'no-kor'tĭ-sizm). Normal state of secretion of the cells of the adrenal cortex. Obsolete usage.

**isoagglutination** (i'so-ăglu-tĭ-na'shun) [ iso- + L. *ad,* to, + *gluten,* glue ]. Isohemagglutination; agglutination of red blood cells as a result of the reaction between an isoagglutinin and specific antigen in or on the cells.

**isoagglutinin** (i'so-ă-glu'tĭ-nin). Isohemagglutinin; an isoantibody that causes agglutination of cells; see also isoantibody.

**i'soagglutin'ogen** [ iso- + agglutinogen, *q.v.* ]. An isoantigen that induces agglutination of the cells to which it is attached upon exposure to its specific isoantibody; see also isoantigen.

**i'soallox'azine.** The tautomeric form of alloxazine, differing from it in the position of a hydrogen atom and a double bond; the ring system is that contained in the various flavins, including riboflavin, *q.v.*

**i. mononucleotide,** term applied by some to cozymase, the coenzyme of Warburg's "old" yellow enzyme; now called riboflavin 5'-phosphate, or flavin mononucleotide.

**isoam'inile.** PERACON; 4-(dimethylamino)-2-isopropyl-2-phenylvaleronitrile; antitussive agent.

**i'soam'ylase.** A hydrolase (EC 3.2.1.68) that cleaves 1,6-α-glucosidic branch linkages in glycogen, amylopectin, and their β-limit dextrins; part of the complex known as debranching enzyme or debranching factor. Pullulanase, amylo-1,6-glucosidase, and exo-1,6-glucosidase have similar activities.

**i'soamylhy'drocupreine.** A topical anesthetic and dental antiseptic.

**isoanaphylaxis** (i'so-an'ă-fi-lak'sis). Anaphylaxis produced in an animal as a result of the injection of serum from another animal of the same species.

**i'soandros'terone.** Epiandrosterone.

**isoantibody** (i'so-an'tĭ-bod-ĭ). [ G. *isos,* equal ]. An antibody that occurs only in some individuals of a species, and reacts specifically with the corresponding isoantigen; the latter does not occur naturally in the cells of the same individual who has the antibody. For specific i.'s of blood groups, see appendix 2, Blood Groups.

**isoantigen** (i'so-an'tĭ-jen). An antigenic substance that occurs only in some individuals of a species, such as the blood group antigens of man. For specific i.'s of blood groups, see appendix 2, Blood Groups.

**isobar** (i'so-bar) [ iso- + G. *baros,* weight ]. 1. A term applied to one of two or more nuclides having the same total number of protons plus neutrons, but with different distribution; *i.e.,* argon-40 with 18 protons and 22 neutrons, potassium-40 with 19 protons and 21 neutrons, and calcium-40 with 20 protons and 20 neutrons. The product of a β-disintegration is an i. of its parent. Nuclear isomers are a special kind of i.; each member of the pair has the same atomic number as well as the same atomic weight. 2. The line connecting points of equal barometric pressure.

**isobaric** (i'so-băr'ik). Having equal weights or pressures.

**isobor'nyl thiocy'anoac'etate, technical.** C₁₃H₁₉NO₂S; pediculicide.

**i'sobu'caine hydrochloride.** 2-(Isobutylamino)-2-methyl-1-propanol benzoate hydrochloride; a local anesthetic used in dentistry.

**isobuteine** (i'so-bu'te-in). A sulfur-containing compound in urine; HOOC—CH(CH₃)—CH₂—S—CH₂—CH-(NH₂)—COOH.

**i'sobu'tyl nitrite.** A liquid present in commercial amyl nitrite, with similar antispasmodic and vasodilator properties.

**i'sobutyr'ic acid.** See butyric acid.

**isobu'zole.** STABINOL; N-(5-isobutyl-1,3,4-thiadiazol-2-yl)-p-methoxybenzenesulfonamide; oral hypoglycemic agent for treatment of diabetes mellitus.

**i'socarbox'azid** (NF, BP). MARPLAN; 1-benzyl-2-(5-methyl-3-isoxazolylcarbonyl)hydrazine; a monoamine oxidase inhibitor used in the treatment of depressive disorders.

**i'socel'lular** [ iso- + L. *cellula,* dim. of *cella,* a storeroom ]. Composed of cells of equal size or of similar character.

**i'socholes'terol.** Lanosterol.

**isochoric** (i'so-ko'rik) [ iso- + G. *chōra,* space ]. Isovolumic.

**isochromatic** (i-so-kro-mat'ik) [ iso- + G. *chrōma,* color ]. 1. Of uniform color; isochroous. 2. Denoting two objects of the same color.

**isochromatophil, isochromatophile** (i'so-kro-mat'o-fil, or fil) [ iso- + G. *chrōma,* color, + *philos,* fond ]. Having an equal affinity for the same dye; said of two or more cells or tissues.

**i'sochro'mosome.** A chromosomal aberration that arises as a result of transverse rather than longitudinal division of the centromere during meiosis; two daughter chromosomes are formed each lacking one chromosome arm but with the other doubled. See fig. under chromosome.

**isochronia** (i'so-kro'nĭ-ah) [ iso- + G. *chronos,* time ]. 1. The state of having the same chronaxie. 2. Agreement, with respect to time, rate, or frequency, between processes.

**isochronous** (i-sok'ro-nus). Occurring during the same time.

**isochroous** (i-sok'ro-us). Isochromatic (1).

**i'socit'rase.** Isocitrate lyase.

**i'socit'ratase.** Isocitrate lyase.

**i'socit'rate dehy'drogenase.** Isocitric acid dehydrogenase; one of two enzymes (EC 1.1.1.41 and .42) that catalyze the conversion of isocitric acid to α-ketoglutaric (2-oxoglutaric) acid, one of the reactions of the tricarboxylic acid cycle. They require either NADP or NAD, respectively.

**i'socit'rate ly'ase** (EC 4.1.3.1). Isocitratase; isocitritase; isocitrase; an enzyme that catalyzes the aldol condensation of glyoxylic acid and succinic acid, forming *threo*-Dₛ-isocitric acid.

**i'socit'ric acid.** Intermediate in the tricarboxylic acid cycle; HOOC—CH₂—CH(COOH)—CH(OH)—COOH.

**i. acid dehydrogenase,** isocitrate dehydrogenase.

**i'socit'ritase.** Isocitrate lyase.

**i'soco'ria** [ iso- + G. *korē,* pupil ]. Equality in the size of the two pupils.

**isocortex** (i'so-kor'teks). Vogt's term for the larger part of the mammalian cerebral cortex, distinguished from the allocortex by being composed of a larger number of nerve cell layers; also called neocortex; homotypic cortex; neopallium. See also *cortex* cerebri.

**i'socy'anate.** The radical —N=C=O, from isocyanic acid.

**i'socy'anide.** A compound whose molecule contains the grouping —NC. Organic i.'s are called isonitriles.

**isocyclic compound** (i'so-si'klik, -sik'lik). See under compound.

**i'socytol'ysin.** A cytolysin that reacts with the cells of certain other animals of the same species, but not with the cells of the individual that formed the i.

**isodactylism** (i'so-dak'tĭ-lizm) [ iso- + G. *daktylos,* finger ]. A condition in which the fingers or toes are approximately of equal length.

**i'sodul'cit.** Rhamnose.

**i′sodynam′ic** [ iso- + G. *dynamis*, force ]. Of equal force or strength; relating to foods or other materials that liberate the same amount of energy on combustion.

**isodynamogenic** (i′so-di′nă-mo-jen′ik, -di-nam′o-) [ iso- + G. *dynamis*, force, + suffix -*gen*, producing ]. 1. Isoenergetic. 2. Producing equal nerve force.

**i′soelec′tric.** Isopotential; of equal electrical potential.

**isoenergetic** (i′so-en-er-jet′ik). Isodynamogenic; exerting equal force; equally active.

**i′soen′zyme.** Isozyme.

**isoerythrolysis** (i′so-ĕ-rith-rol′ĭ-sis). Destruction of erythrocytes by isoantibodies.

   **neonatal i.,** (1) i. in the newborn animal; (2) hemolytic icterus of the newborn.

**isoeth′arine** (USAN). DILABRON; α-(1-isopropylaminopropyl)protocatechuyl alcohol; bronchodilator for treatment of bronchial asthma.

**isoflu′rane** (USAN). FORANE; 2,2,2-trifluoro-1-chloroethyl difluoromethyl ether; a nonflammable, nonexplosive, halogenated ether with potent anesthetic action; an isomer of enflurane devoid of the latter's central nervous system side effects.

**isoflurophate** (i′so-flu′ro-fāt) (USP). FLOROPRYL; diisopropyl fluorophosphate (DFP); diisopropylphosphorofluoridate; [ (CH₃)₂CH—O ]P(O)F; a potent cholinergic agent that acts by irreversible inhibition of cholinesterase. Used in ophthalmology in the treatment of glaucoma and strabismus, reducing intraocular pressure and breaking up peripheral synechias.

**isogamete** (i-so-gam′ēt) [ iso- + G. *gametēs* or *gametē*, husband or wife ]. 1. One of two or more similar cells by the conjugation or fusion of which, with subsequent division, reproduction occurs. 2. A gamete of the same size as the gamete with which it unites.

**isogamy** (i-sog′ă-mĭ) [ iso- + G. *gamos*, marriage ]. Conjugation between two equal gametes, or two individual cells alike in all respects.

**isogeneic** (i′so-jĕ-ne′ik). Isogenic; relating to a group of individuals or strain of animals genetically alike with respect to specified gene pairs; see also isologous.

**isogenesis** (i-so-jen′ĕ-sis) [ iso- + G. *genesis*, production ]. Identity of morphologic development.

**i′sogen′ic.** Isogeneic.

**i′sogen′tiobi′ose.** Isomaltose.

**i′soglu′tamine.** H₂NCO—CH(NH₂)CH₂CH₂COOH; glutamic acid amide.

**isognathous** (i-sog′na-thus) [ iso- + G. *gnathos*, jaw ]. Having jaws of approximately the same width.

**i′sograft** [ iso- + graft ]. Syngeneic graft or homograft; isogeneic graft or homograft; isologous or isoplastic graft; a piece of tissue or organ transplanted from one member of an identical twin pair to another, or between syngeneic animals which are isogeneic with respect to histocompatibility genes.

**isohemagglutination** (i′so-he′mă-glu′tĭ-na′shun) [ iso- + G. *haima*, blood, + L. *ad*, to, + *gluten*, glue ]. Isoagglutination.

**isohemagglutinin** (i′so-he′mă-glu′tĭ-nin). Isoagglutinin.

**i′sohemol′ysin.** An isolysin that reacts with red blood cells.

**isohemolysis** (i′so-he-mol′ĭ-sis) [ iso- + G. *haima*, blood, + *lysis*, dissolution ]. Isolysis; dissolution of red blood cells as a result of the reaction between an isolysin and specific antigen in or on the cells; the isolysin is frequently termed isohemolysin.

**i′sohy′dric.** Said of two substances possessing the same pH.

**isohydruria** [ iso- + hydruria, *q.v.* ]. Fixation of the pH of the urine without the usual variation.

**isohypercytosis** (i′so-hi-per-si-to′sis) [ iso- + G. *hyper*, above, + *kytos*, cell ]. A condition in which the number of leukocytes in the circulating blood is increased, but the relative proportions of the various types (especially the granulocytes) are within the usual range.

**isohypocytosis** (i′so-hi-po-si-to′sis) [ iso- + G. *hypo*, below, + *kytos*, cell ]. A condition in which there is an abnormally small number of leukocytes in the circulating blood, but the relative proportions of the various types (especially the granulocytes) are within the usual range.

**isoiconia** (i-so-i-ko′nĭ-ah) [ iso- + G. *eikōn*, image, + suffix -*ia*, condition ]. Equality of the two retinal images.

**isoiconic** (i-so-i-kon′ik). Marked by or relating to isoiconia.

**i′soim′muniza′tion.** The development of a significant titer of specific antibody as a result of antigenic stimulation with material contained on or in the red blood cells of another individual of the same species; for example, i. is likely to occur when an Rh-negative person is treated with a transfusion of Rh-positive blood from another human being, or an Rh-negative woman has a pregnancy in which the fetus inherits Rh-positive red blood cells (see also erythroblastosis fetalis).

**i′solate** [ It. *isolare;* Mediev. L. *insulo*, pp. -*atus*, to insulate, fr. L. *insula*, island ]. 1. To separate; to set apart by oneself. 2. To free from chemical contaminants. 3. In psychoanalysis, to separate experiences or memories from the affects pertaining to them. 4. That which is isolated.

   **mating i.,** see under mating.

**isola′tion.** The act of isolating, or the condition of being isolated; see isolate.

**isolecithal** (i′so-les′ĭ-thal). Denoting an ovum in which there is a moderate amount of uniformly distributed yolk.

**isoleucine** (i-so-lu′sēn). α-Amino-β-methylvaleric acid; CH₃CH₂CH(CH₃)CH(NH₂)COOH; an amino acid found in almost all proteins; an isomer of leucine and, like it, a dietary essential.

**[8-isoleucine]oxytocin.** Mesotocin.

**isoleukoagglutinin** (i′so-lu′ko-ă-glu′tĭ-nin). Naturally occurring, abnormal antibody in the blood of some persons with certain conditions, capable of agglutinating human polymorphonuclear leukocytes.

**isologous** (i-sol′o-gus) [ iso- + G. *logos*, ratio ]. Isoplastic; syngeneic; syngenic (1); relating to tissue transplant between identical twins or between syngeneic individuals, isogeneic with respect to histocompatibility genes.

**isolysin** (i-sol′ĭ-sin). An antibody that combines with, sensitizes, and results in complement-fixation and dissolution of cells that contain the specific isoantigen; i.'s occur in the blood of some members of a species and they react with the cells of that species, but not with the cells of the individual (or the same type) in which the i.'s are naturally formed.

**isolysis** (i-sol′ĭ-sis) [ iso- + G. *lysis*, dissolution ]. Lysis or dissolution of cells as a result of the reaction between an isolysin and specific antigen in or on the cells. See also isohemolysis, a frequent form of i.

**i′solyt′ic.** Pertaining to, characterized by, or causing isolysis.

**isomal′tase.** Oligo-1,6-glucosidase.

**i′somal′tose.** A disaccharide in which two glucose molecules are attached by an α-1,6 link, rather than an α-1,4 link as in maltose.

**isomastigote** (i-so-mas′tĭ-gōt) [ iso- + G. *mastix*, whip ]. Denoting a protozoan having two or four flagella of equal length at one extremity.

**i′somer** [ iso- + G. *meros*, part ]. One of two or more substances displaying isomerism.

**isom′erase.** A class of enzymes (EC class 5) catalyzing the conversion of a substance to an isomeric form; *e.g.*, glucosephosphate isomerase (EC 5.3.1.9).

**isomeric** (i′so-mĕr′ik). Isomerous; relating to or characterized by isomerism.

**isom′erism** The existence of a chemical compound in two or more forms which are identical with respect to percentage composition but differ as to the position of the atoms within the molecule, and also in physical and chemical properties.

   **geometric i.,** a form of i. displayed by unsaturated or ring compounds where free rotation about a carbon bond is restricted; the i. of a *cis-* or *trans-*compound is an example.

   **optical i.,** stereoisomerism involving the arrangement of substituents about an asymmetric carbon atom or atoms so that there is a difference in the behavior of the various isomers with regard to the extent of their rotation of the plane of polarized light.

   **stereochemical i.,** stereoisomerism.

**structural i.,** i. involving the same atoms in different associations; *e.g.,* the amyl alcohols; leucine and isoleucine; glucose and fructose.

**isom′eriza′tion.** A process in which one isomer is formed from another, as in the action of isomerases.

**isom′erous.** Isomeric.

**isometh′adone.** ISOADANONE; 6-(dimethylamino)-5-methyl-4,4-diphenyl-3-hexanone; analgesic with narcotic properties.

**isometheptene hydrochloride.** OCTIN hydrochloride; 2-methylamino-6-methyl-5-heptane hydrochloride; an unsaturated aliphatic sympathomimetic amine with antispasmodic and vasoconstrictor actions. Used in spastic conditions of the urinary and gastrointestinal tracts and in migraine headaches. Also available as isometheptene mucate.

**isomet′ric** [ iso- + G. *metron,* measure ]. 1. Of equal dimensions. 2. In physiology, opposed to isotonic; refers to the type of muscular contraction that occurs when the ends of the muscle are fixed so that activity is evidenced by increase in tension without change in length; see also isovolumic.

**isometro′pia** [ iso- + G. *metron,* measure, + *ōps (ōp-),* eye ]. Equality in kind and degree of refraction in the two eyes.

**isomor′phic.** Isomorphous.

**isomor′phism** [ iso- + G. *morphē,* shape ]. Similarity of form between two or more organisms or between parts of the body.

**isomor′phous.** Having the same form or shape; morphologically equal.

**isomyl′amine hydrochloride** (USAN). NEURYLAN; 2-(diethylamino)ethyl 1-isopentylcyclohexanecarboxylate hydrochloride; a smooth muscle relaxant.

**isonaph′thol.** β-Naphthol.

**isoni′azid** (USP, BP). Isonicotinic acid hydrazide; $C_6H_7N_3O$; a compound effective in the treatment of tuberculosis.

**i′sonicotin′ic acid.** 4-Carboxypyridine; 4-pyridinecarboxylic acid.
  **i. acid hydrazide,** isoniazid.

**isoni′triles.** Organic isocyanides.

**isonormocytosis** (i-so-nor′mo-si-to′sis) [ iso- + L. *norma,* rule, + G. *kytos,* cell, + suffix *-osis,* condition ]. Normonormocytosis; dinormocytosis; a condition in which the actual number and the relative proportions of the various types of leukocytes in the circulating blood are within normal range.

**isooctylhydrocu′preine.** VUZINE; hydrocupreine 6-methylheptyl ether; antiseptic.

**i′so-osmot′ic.** Isosmotic.

**isop′athy** [ iso- + G. *pathos,* suffering ]. The treatment of disease by means of the causal agent or a product of the same disease; also the treatment of a diseased organ by an extract of a similar organ from a healthy animal. See also homeopathy.

**isopelletierine** (i-so-pel-et′ēr-ēn). An alkaloid derived from *Punica granatum* (family Punicaceae); it has the same composition and anthelmintic properties as pelletierine, but is optically inactive.

**isopentylhydrocu′preine.** EUCUPIN; hydrocupreine isopentyl ether; topical antiseptic with anesthetic properties.

**isophagy** (i-sof′ă-jĭ) [ iso- + G. *phagein,* to eat ]. Autolysis.

**isophane insulin.** See under insulin.

**isophoria** (i′so-fo′rĭ-ah) [ iso- + G. *phora,* movement ]. A condition in which there is no change of muscular imbalance with changes of direction of gaze.

**isopia** (i-so-pī′-ah) [ iso- + G. *ōps (ōp-),* eye ]. Equality in all respects of the two eyes, and of vision.

**isoplassonts** (i-so-plas′onts) [ iso- + G. *plassō,* to form ]. Like-formed entities having certain features in common.

**i′soplas′tic.** Isologous.

**i′sopleth.** A line on a Cartesian nomogram consisting of all points that represent a particular value of a variable; *e.g.,* an isobar is an i. for a particular pressure.

**i′sopoten′tial.** Isoelectric.

**isoprecipitin** (i-so-pre-sip′ĭ-tin) [ iso- + precipitin ]. An antibody that combines with and precipitates soluble antigenic material in the plasma or serum, or in an extract of the cells, from another member, but not all members, of the same species.

**isopren′aline hydrochloride.** Isoproterenol hydrochloride.

**isopren′aline sulphate** (BP). Isoproterenol sulfate.

**i′soprene.** 2-Methylbutadiene; $CH_2=CH—C(CH_3)=CH_2$; an unsaturated C-5 hydrocarbon with a branched chain, which in the plant kingdom is used as the basis for the formation of polymers called the isoprenoids; this includes terpenes, carotenoids, and related pigments, and rubber. The fat-soluble vitamins either are isoprenoid or have isoprenoid side chains; steroids are synthesized *via* isoprenoid intermediates.

**i′sopre′noids.** Compounds whose carbon skeletons consist in whole or in large part of isoprene units joined end to end; notably, carotene, lycopene, and vitamin A. Vitamins K and E and the coenzymes Q have isoprenoid side chains.

**isoprometh′azine.** ISOPHENERGAN; 10-(2-dimethylamino-1-methylethyl)-phenothiazine; antihistaminic.

**i′sopro′pamide iodide** (NF). DARBID; (3-carbamoyl-3,3-diphenylpropyl) diisopropylmethylammonium iodide; a quaternary ammonium compound with anticholinergic activity having peripheral effects similar to those of atropine; antispasmodic and antisecretory agent.

**i′sopro′panol.** Isopropyl alcohol.

**isopropyl alcohol** i′so-pro′pil) (NF, BP). Isopropanol; dimethylcarbinol; $(CH_3)_2CHOH$; an isomer of propyl alcohol and a homologue of ethyl alcohol, similar in its properties, when used externally, to the latter, but more toxic when taken internally. Used as an ingredient of various cosmetics and of medicinal preparations for external use. The NF also lists isopropyl rubbing alcohol, which contains 68 to 72 per cent of isopropyl alcohol (by volume) in water, and is used as a rubefacient.

**i′sopro′pylarter′enol hydrochloride.** Isoproterenol hydrochloride.

**isopropylene vinyl ether.** PROPETHYLENE; $CH_2C(CH_3)-OCHCH_2$; a colorless volatile liquid the vapor of which produces inhalation anesthesia; flammable.

**isopropyl myristate** (NF). ESTERGEL; used in topical medicinal preparations to promote absorption through the skin.

**i′sopro′pylthi′ogalac′toside.** An artificial galactoside capable of inducing β-galactosidase in *Escherichia coli* without being split as are the natural substrates, such as lactose; abbreviated IPTG.

**i′soproter′enol hydrochloride** (USP). ISUPREL; ALUDRINE; isopropylarterenol hydrochloride; isoprenaline hydrochloride; 3,4-dihydroxy-α-[ (isopropylamino)methyl ]-benzyl alcohol hydrochloride; a sympathomimetic β-receptor stimulant possessing the inhibitory properties and the cardiac excitatory, but not the vasoconstrictor, actions of epinephrine. Chemically it differs from epinephrine in having an isopropyl group replacing the methyl group attached to the nitrogen atom. Used in the treatment of bronchial asthma and heart block, including Adams-Stokes attacks.

**i′soproter′enol sulfate.** Isoprenaline sulphate (BP); used for inhalation as an aerosol in the treatment of acute asthmatic attacks and chronic pulmonary emphysema.

**isopter** (i-sop′ter) [ iso- + G. *optēr,* observer. OPS- ]. A curve of equal retinal sensitivity in the visual field designated by a fraction, the numerator being the diameter of the white test object, and the denominator, the testing distance.

**i′sopy′rocalcif′erol.** Thermal decomposition product of calciferol; a stereoisomer of pyrocalciferol and ergosterol.

**isoquin′oline.** Ring structure characteristic of the group of opium alkaloids represented by papaverine.

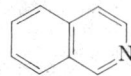

**Isoquinoline**

**isoriboflavin** (i'so-ri'bo-fla-vin). A riboflavin antimetabolite. Differs from riboflavin in that the methyl groups on the isoalloxazine nucleus are in the 5,6 positions rather than the 6,7.

**isorrhea** (i-so-re'ah) [ iso- + G. *rhoia*, a flow ]. Equality of intake and output of water; water equilibrium.

**i'sosen'sitize.** Autosensitize.

**i'sosex'ual.** 1. Relating to the existence of characteristics or feelings of both sexes in one person. 2. Descriptive of somatic characteristics possessed by, or of processes occurring within, an individual that are consonant with the sex of that individual.

**isosmotic** (i'sos-mot'ik). Having the same total osmotic pressure or osmolality as another fluid (ordinarily intracellular fluid); such a fluid is not isotonic if it includes solutes that freely permeate cell membranes.

**i'sosor'bide dinitrate** (USP). ISORDIL; 1,4:3,6-dianhydro-D-glucitol dinitrate; a coronary vasodilator; large doses may produce headache, flushing of the face, palpitation, fainting, and methemoglobinemia.

**Isospora** (i-sos'po-rah) [ iso- + G. *sporos*, seed ]. A genus of coccidia, with species chiefly in mammals; the ripe oocysts contain two sporocysts, each of which contains four sporozoites.

    **I. bel'li,** a relatively rare species occurring in the small intestine of man, commonest in the tropics but probably worldwide; most infections are subclinical, but sometimes may cause mucous diarrhea.

    **I. bigem'ina,** occurs in the small intestine of the dog, cat, fox, mink and possibly other carnivores; the most pathogenic coccidium in dogs and cats, causing enteritis and diarrhea; the oocysts are usually sporulated when passed in the feces; the oocysts are indistinguishable from those of *I. hominis* and *Toxoplasma gondii,* so considerable question remains as to the status of these parasites.

    **I. ca'nis,** a species of worldwide distribution that is mildly pathogenic in dogs and is not infective in cats.

    **I. fe'lis,** found in the small intestine and sometimes the cecum and colon of cats, lions, and other felids; it is only slightly, if at all, pathogenic in cats and is not infective in dogs.

    **I. hom'inis,** a rare species described only from man and capable of causing a mucous diarrhea with anorexia, nausea, and abdominal pain; it is very similar to *I. bigemina* and may prove to be the same species.

    **I. rivol'ta,** occurs in the small intestine of dogs, cats, dingos, and probably other wild carnivores; pathogenic capabilities are about the same as those of *I. bigemina.*

    **I. su'is,** affects the small intestine of the pig, producing mild diarrhea.

**isostere** (i'so-stēr) [ iso- + G. *stereos*, solid ]. One of two or of several atoms or molecules having the same electron arrangement, hence similar properties; *e.g.*, $N_2$ and CO.

**isosthenuria** (i-sos'the-nu'rĭ-ah, i'so-sthe-nu'rĭ-ah) [ iso- + G. *sthenos*, strength, + *ouron*, urine ]. A state in chronic renal disease in which the kidney cannot form urine with a higher or a lower specific gravity than that of protein-free plasma. The specific gravity of the urine becomes fixed around 1.010, irrespective of the fluid intake.

**isosuccinic acid** (i'so-suk-sin'ik). Methylmalonic acid.

**isosulfamer'azine.** PALLIDIN; *N'*-(5-methyl-2-pyrimidinyl)sulfanilamide; antimicrobial agent.

**i'sother'apy.** Treatment of a disease by means of its active causal agent, as in the preventive inoculations against rabies or in the use of bacterial vaccines.

**i'sother'mal** [ iso- + G. *thermē*, heat ]. Having the same temperature.

**i'sothiocy'anate.** The radical of isothiocyanic acid, —N=C=S.

**isothipendyl.** THERUHISTIN; 10-(2-dimethylamino-2-methylethyl)-10*H*-pyrido[ 3,2-*b* ][ 1,4 ]benzothiazine; antihistaminic agent.

**i'soto'cin.** Ichthyotocin.

**i'sotone.** One of several nuclides having the same number of neutrons in their nuclei; *e.g.*, $^{39}_{19}$K, $^{40}_{20}$Ca, $^{56}_{26}$Fe, and $^{58}_{28}$Ni are i.'s.

**isotonia** (i'so-to'nĭ-ah) [ iso- + G. *tonos*, tension ]. Tonic equality; a condition in which tension or osmotic pressure in two substances or solutions is the same.

**i'soton'ic.** 1. Relating to isotonicity or isotonia. 2. Having equal tension; denoting solutions possessing the same osmotic pressure; more specifically, limited to solutions in which cells neither swell nor shrink. Thus, a solution that is isosmotic with intracellular fluid will not be i. if it includes solute, such as urea, that freely permeates cell membranes. 3. Denoting the condition of contraction of a muscle when one end is attached to a light weight which is lifted when the muscle shortens; opposed to isometric.

**isotonicity** (i-so-to-nis'ĭ-tĭ). 1. The quality of possessing and maintaining a uniform tone or tension. 2. The property of a solution in being isotonic.

**isotope** (i'so-tōp) [ iso- + G. *topos*, part, place ]. A term applied to either of two or more nuclides that are chemically identical yet differ in mass number, since their nuclei contain different numbers of neutrons. Individual i.'s are named with the inclusion of their mass number, as carbon-12. This may be symbolized by way of the chemical symbol of the element with the mass number as a superscript either to right or left, as $C^{12}$ or $^{12}C$, the latter being the international official usage. The atomic number (nuclear protons) appears at lower left, *e.g.*, $_6$C.

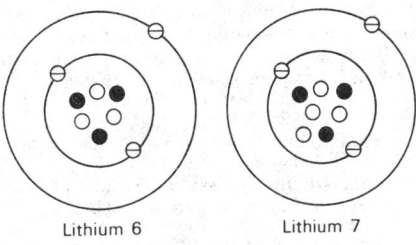

Lithium 6      Lithium 7

**Isotopes of Lithium**
Proton, ●; neutron, ○; electron, ⊖

    **radioactive i.,** an i. with a nuclear composition that is unstable; nuclei of such an i. decompose spontaneously by emission of a nuclear electron (β-particle) or helium nucleus (α-ray) and radiation (γ-rays), thus achieving a stable nuclear composition. Radioactive i.'s are widely used as tracers.

    **stable i.,** a nonradioactive nuclide; an i. of an element that shows no tendency to undergo radioactive breakdown.

**i'sotop'ic.** Of identical chemical composition but differing in some physical property, such as atomic weight.

**i'sotox'in.** A toxin in the blood or tissues of an animal, manifesting no effect on that animal, but toxic to others of the same species.

**i'sotrans'plant.** Isograft.

**i'sotrans'planta'tion.** The act of transferring an isograft.

**i'sotrop'ic, isot'ropous** [ iso- + G. *tropē*, a turn ]. Equal in refracting power.

**isovaleric acid** (i'so-vă-lēr'ik, -lēr'ik). 3-Methylbutyric acid; $(CH_3)_2CHCH_2COOH$.

**isovalericacidemia** (i'so-vă-lēr'ik-as'ĭ-de'mĭ-ah). A disorder of leucine metabolism characterized by the excessive production of isovaleric acid upon protein ingestion or during infectious episodes; severe metabolic acidosis results from the large quantities of acid formed and may cause death; autosomal recessive inheritance.

**i'soval'thine.** $(CH_3)_2CHCH(COOH)—S—CH_2CH-(NH_2)-COOH$; a sulfur-containing compound found in urine.

**i'sovol'ume.** At the same or equal volume; see also isovolumic.

**i'sovolumet'ric.** Isovolumic.

**i'sovolu'mic.** Isovolumetric; isochoric; occurring without an associated alteration in volume; as when, in early ventricular systole, the muscle fibers initially increase their tension without shortening so that ventricular volume remains unaltered. See also isometric.

**isox'suprine hydrochloride** (NF). VASODILAN; 1-(*p*-hydroxyphenyl)-2-[ (1'-methyl-2'-phenoxy)ethylamino ]-1-propanol hydrochloride; a sympathomimetic amine with potent inhibitory effects on vascular, uterine and other smooth muscles; used as a vasodilator in various vascular diseases and as a uterine relaxant.

**i'sozyme.** Isoenzyme; one of a group of enzymes that are very similar in catalytic properties, but may be differentiated by variations in physical properties, such as isoelectric point or electrophoretic mobility. The best known case is lactate dehydrogenase, a tetramer composed of varying amounts of $\alpha$ and $\beta$ subunits (*i.e.*, $4\alpha$; $3\alpha$ plus $1\beta$; $2\alpha$ plus $2\beta$; $1\alpha$ plus $3\beta$; and $4\beta$).

**Israel,** James A., German surgeon, 1848–1926. See I.'s *stain.*

**issue** (ish'u) [ Fr. a going out ]. 1. A suppurating sore, acting as a counterirritant, maintained by the presence of a foreign body in the tissues; it was formerly regarded as a means of escape for peccant humors. 2. A point in question or a matter of dispute.

　**nature-nurture i.,** a controversy concerning the relative importance of heredity (nature) and environment (nurture) in various aspects of individual development, such as intelligence.

**isthmectomy** (is-mek'to-mī) [ G. *isthmos,* isthmus, + *ek-tomē,* excision ]. Median *strumectomy.*

**isthmian** (is'mī-an). Relating to an anatomical isthmus.

**isthmoparalysis** (is'mo-pă-ral'ĭ-sis) [ G. *isthmos,* isthmus, + paralysis ]. Isthmoplegia; faucial paralysis; paralysis of the velum pendulum palati and the muscles forming the anterior pillars of the fauces.

**isthmoplegia** (is'mo-ple'jĭ-ah) [ G. *isthmos,* isthmus, + *plēgē,* stroke ]. Isthmoparalysis.

**isthmus,** pl. **isth'muses, isth'mi** (is'mus) [ G. *isthmos* ] [ NA ]. 1. A constriction connecting two larger parts of an organ or other anatomical structure. 2. A narrow passage connecting two larger cavities. 3. The narrowest portion of the brainstem at the junction between midbrain and hindbrain.

　**i. of aorta,** i. aortae

　**i. aor'tae** [ NA ], isthmus of the aorta; a slight constriction of the aorta immediately distal to the left subclavian artery at the point of attachment of the ductus arteriosus.

　**i. of auditory tube,** i. tubae auditivae.

　**i. of cartilage of ear,** i. cartilaginis auris.

　**i. cartilag'inis au'ris** [ NA ], i. of the cartilage of the ear; a narrow bridge connecting the cartilage of the external acoustic meatus and the lamina tragica with the main portion of the cartilage of the auricle.

　**i. of cingular gyrus,** i. gyri cinguli.

　**i. of external acoustic meatus,** i. meatus acustici externi.

　**i. of fauces,** i. faucium.

　**i. faucium** [ NA ], i. of the fauces; the constricted and short space which establishes the connection between the cavity of the mouth and the oral part of the pharynx.

　**i. glan'dulae thyroid'eae** [ NA ], i. of the thyroid; the central part of the thyroid gland joining the two lateral lobes.

　**Guyon's i.,** i. uteri.

　**i. gy'ri cin'guli** [ NA ], i. of the cingular gyrus; i. of the gyrus fornicatus or limbic lobe; the narrowing of the gyrus cinguli, at its transition with the hippocampal gyrus behind and below the splenium of the corpus callosum, caused by the anterior extension of the conjoined parieto-occipital and calcarine sulci.

　**i. of gyrus fornicatus,** i. gyri cinguli.

　**i. of His,** i. rhombencephali.

　**Krönig's i.,** the narrow straplike portion of the resonant field which extends over the shoulder, connecting the larger areas of resonance over the pulmonary apex in front and behind.

　**i. of limbic lobe,** i. gyri cinguli.

　**i. mea'tus acus'tici exter'ni,** i. of the external acoustic meatus; the narrowest portion of this canal near its deep termination.

　**pharyngeal i.,** i. pharyngonasalis.

　**i. pharyngonasa'lis,** pharyngeal i.; the aperture between the nasal cavity and the nasal portion of the pharynx, corresponding to the choanae.

　**i. pros'tatae** [ NA ], i. of the prostate; the narrow middle part of the prostate anterior to the urethra.

　**i. of prostate,** i. prostatae.

　**i. rhombenceph'ali** [ NA ], rhombencephalic i.; i. of His; (1) a constriction in the embryonic neural tube delineating the mesencephalon from the rhombencephalon; (2) the anterior portion of the rhombencephalon connecting with the mesencephalon.

　**rhombencephalic i.,** i. rhombencephali.

　**i. of thyroid,** i. glandulae thyroideae.

　**i. tu'bae auditi'vae** [ NA ], i. of the auditory (Eustachian) tube; the narrowest portion of the auditory tube at the junction of the cartilaginous and bony portions.

　**i. tu'bae uteri'nae** [ NA ], i. of the uterine tube; the narrow portion of the uterine tube adjoining the uterus.

　**i. u'teri** [ NA ], i. of the uterus; Guyon's i.; ostium uteri internum; os uteri internum; orificium internum uteri; an elongated constriction at the junction of the body and cervix of the uterus.

　**i. of uterine tube,** i. tubae uterinae.

　**i. of uterus,** i. uteri.

　**Vieussens' i.,** *limbus* fossae ovalis.

**itaconic acid** (it'ă-kon'ik). $CH_2 = C(COOH)CH_2COOH$; the decarboxylation product of *cis*-aconitic acid.

**Itard** (e-tar'), Jean M. G., Paris otologist, 1774–1838. See I.-Cholewa *sign.*

**itch** [ A.S. *gikkan* ]. 1. A peculiar irritating sensation in the skin that arouses the desire to scratch. 2. Common name for scabies. 3. Pruritus.

　**azo i.,** itching that occurs among workers in azo dyes.

　**baker's i.,** an eruption on the hands and arms of bakers due to an allergic reaction to flour or other substances handled.

　**barber's i.,** *tinea* sycosis.

　**bath i.,** bath *pruritus.*

　**coolie i.,** cutaneous *ancylostomiasis.*

　**co'pra i.,** a dermatitis occurring in workers in copra mills, caused by the presence of a mite, *Tyrophagus putrescentiae.*

　**Cuban i.,** alastrim.

　**dhobie i.,** *tinea* cruris.

　**frost i.,** *dermatitis* hiemalis.

　**grain i.,** an eruption occasionally noted in farmers and grain handlers, caused by the action of the mite *Pediculoides ventricosus.*

　**grocer's i.,** a vesicular dermatitis seen in grocers and bakers from handling sugar or flour; caused by a mite of the genus *Glycophagus.*

　**ground i.,** cutaneous *ancylostomiasis.*

　**jock i.,** *tinea* cruris.

　**kabure i.,** *schistosomiasis* japonicum.

　**lumberman's i.,** *dermatitis* hiemalis.

　**mad i.,** Aujeszky's *disease.*

　**Malabar i.,** *tinea* imbricata.

　**Norway i.,** Norwegian *scabies.*

　**poultryman's i.,** eruption due to infestation with the mite, *Dermanyssus gallinae.*

　**prairie i.,** pruritus of varied origin, affecting farm laborers.

　**psoroptic i.,** psoroptic *mange.*

　**Saint Ignatius' i.,** pellagra.

　**sarcoptic i.,** sarcoptic *mange.*

　**seven-year i.,** scabies.

　**straw i., straw-bed i.,** dermatitis pediculoides ventricosus; an urticarial eruption caused by the grain itch mite, *Pediculoides ventricosus,* which infests the straw of mattresses.

　**summer i.,** *pruritus* aestivalis.

　**swamp i.,** cutaneous *ancylostomiasis.*

　**swimmer's i.,** (1) cutaneous *ancylostomiasis;* (2) schistosome *dermatitis.*

　**toe i.,** cutaneous *ancylostomiasis.*

　**warehouseman's i.,** eczema of the hands from handling irritating substances.

　**washerwoman's i.,** an eczematous eruption of the hands and arms of washerwomen, dishwashers, and others whose hands are constantly immersed in water.

　**water i.,** (1) cutaneous *ancylostomiasis;* (2) schistosome *dermatitis.*

**winter i.,** *dermatitis* hiemalis.

**itch'ing.** Pruritus; an uncomfortable sensation of irritation of the skin or mucous membranes which causes scratching or rubbing of the affected parts.

**-ite** [ G. *-ites,* fem. *-itis* ]. 1. A suffix denoting "of the nature of," "resembling," the thing to the name of which it is added. 2. In chemistry, denoting a salt of an acid that has the termination -ous. 3. In comparative anatomy, denoting an essential portion of the part to the name of which it is attached. See also -ites.

**i'ter** [ L. *iter*(*itiner-*), a way, road ]. A passage leading from one anatomical part to another.

    **i. a ter'tio ad quar' tum ventric'ulum** [ L. way from the third to the fourth ventricle ], *aqueductus* cerebri.

    **i. chor'dae ante'rius,** Huguier's canal; Civinini's canal; a canal in the Glaserian or petrotympanic fissure, near its posterior edge, through which the chorda tympani nerve issues from the skull.

    **i. chor'dae poste'rius,** *canaliculus* chordae tympani.

    **i. dentis, den'tium,** the route or routes by which one or more teeth erupt.

**i'teral.** Relating to an iter.

**-ites** (i'tēz) [ G. *ites,* m., or *-ites,* n. ]. An adjectival suffix to nouns, corresponding to Latin *-alis, -ale,* or *-inus, -inum,* or English -y, -like, or the hyphenated nouns. The adjective so formed is used without the qualified noun; thus ascites is the short form of *ho askites hydrōps,* abdominal dropsy. The feminine form, *-itis* (agreeing with *nosos,* disease), is so often associated with inflammatory disease, that it has acquired in most cases the significance of inflammation. Tympanites is *ho tympanites oidēma,* the drumlike swelling or tumor, but tympanitis is *hē tympanitis nosos,* the tympanic disease or inflammation of the tympanum, or drum of the ear. See also -ite.

**ithykyphosis, ithycyphosis** (ith'ī-ki-(si)-fo'sis) [ G. *ithys,* straight, + *kyphos,* a hump ]. Pure kyphosis without lateral displacement of the spine.

**ithylordo'sis** (ith'ī-lor-do'sis) [ G. *ithys,* straight, + *lordō-sis,* a forward curvature of the spine, fr. *lordos,* bent backward (opp. of *kyphos,* humped ]. A pure lordosis without lateral curvature of the spine.

**-itis** (i'tis) [ G. fem of *-ites* ]. See -ites.

**Ito,** M. See I.'s *nevus.*

**ITP.** 1. Abbreviation for idiopathic thrombocytopenic purpura. 2. Abbreviation for inosine 5'-triphosphate.

**itramin tosylate.** CARDISAN; 2-aminoethyl nitrate *p*-toluenesulfonate; vasodilator.

**ITyr.** Symbol for monoiodotyrosine.

**IU.** Abbreviation for international *unit.*

**IUB.** Abbreviation for International Union of Biochemistry.

**IUCD.** Abbreviation for intrauterine contraceptive *device.*

**IUD.** Abbreviation for intrauterine *device.*

**IUPAC.** Abbreviation for International Union of Pure and Applied Chemistry.

**I.V., i.v.** Abbreviation for intravenous, or intravenously.

**Ivemark,** Biörn I. See I's syndrome.

**i'vory** [ L. ebur ]. A term applied to the tusks of the elephant, walrus, narwhal, hippopotamus, and warthog, and to all of the teeth of the sperm whale; the material is dentine, which is the inner layer of the tooth derived from the mesoderm. In all of these animals, as well as in several others, the hard enamel layer fails to develop, or develops incompletely, leaving the softer dentin core exposed.

**Ivy loop wiring.** See under wiring.

**Iwanoff's cysts.** See under cyst.

**Ixodes** (ik-so'dēz) [ G. *ixōdes,* sticky, like bird-lime, fr. *ixos,* mistletoe, + *eidos,* form ]. A genus of hard ticks (family Ixodidae), many species of which are parasitic on man and animals; severe reactions frequently follow their bites; they are characterized by an anal groove surrounding the anus anteriorly, absence of eyes and festoons, and marked sexual dimorphism; about 40 species have been described from North America.

    **I. bicor'nis,** a tick found in Mexico whose bite causes fever and extreme malaise.

    **I. cookei,** a tick that is a vector of Powassan virus in Canada.

    **I. holocyc'lus,** a tick of Australia that infests the kangaroo and transmits a paralytic disease to young cattle.

    **I. pacif'icus,** California black-legged tick; a common tick of deer and cattle in California; it may also bite man, sometimes causing severe reactions.

    **I. persulca'tus,** a tick that is a reservoir and vector for Russian spring-summer encephalitis, and is associated with the taiga forest of the USSR and the Kemerovo virus in Western Siberia.

    **I. pilo'sus,** paralysis tick; a tick that infests sheep in South Africa and causes paralysis.

    **I. rici'nus,** castor bean tick; a tick that infests cattle, sheep, and wild animals, and transmits the virus of louping ill, the piroplasm *Babesia bovis,* Central European tick-borne encephalitis virus, Tribec virus, and possibly Japanese B encephalitis virus.

    **I. scapula'ris,** black-legged tick; shoulder tick; found on animals in southern and eastern United States and also capable of inflicting a painful bite to man.

    **I. spinipal'pis,** a tick parasitic on wild rodents in British Columbia and the vector of Powassan virus in mice of the genus *Peromyscus.*

**ixodiasis** (ik'so-di'ā-sis). 1. Skin lesions caused by the bites of certain ticks; in some cases the tick burrows under the skin, causing more or less severe irritation, but in most cases an urticarioid eruption is the only result. 2. Any disease, such as Rocky Mountain fever, that is transmitted through the agency of ticks.

**ixod'ic.** Relating to or caused by ticks.

**ixodid** (iks'o-did). Common name for members of the family Ixodidae.

**Ixod'idae** [ G. *ixōdes,* sticky ]. A family of ticks (order Acarina, suborder Ixodides), the so-called "hard" ticks, because of their rigid body form, presence of a dorsal shield, with an anteriorly projecting capitulum. It includes the genera *Ixodes, Hyalomma, Amblyomma, Boophilus, Margaropus, Dermacentor, Haemaphysalis,* and *Rhipicephalus.* Species in these genera occasionally attack man, a few habitually so; they are concerned with the transmission of many important human and animal diseases and with the causation of tick paralysis. Among the most important diseases transmitted are Rocky Mountain spotted fever, Siberian tick typhus, Boutonneuse fever, epidemic typhus, Queensland tick typhus, Q fever, anaplasmosis, and other rickettsial diseases. *I.* transmit Group B arboviruses (Russian spring-summer encephalitis, Central European tick-borne encephalitis, Omsk hemorrhagic fever, Kyasanur Forest disease, Powassan, Negeishi encephalitis, and possibly Langat), ungrouped viruses (Colorado tick fever, Kemerovo, Tribec, louping ill, Crimean hemorrhagic fever, and Uzbekistan hemorrhagic fever), and possibly other viruses (Japanese B encephalitis, West Nile, Quaranfil, equinine encephalomyelitis, and lymphocytic choriomeningitis). In addition, ixodid ticks transmit tularemia, piroplasma (*e.g.,* canine babesiosis, East Coast fever), hepatozoonosis canis, and tick paralysis.

**Ixodoidea** (iks-o-do-id'e-ah) [ G. *ixōdes,* sticky ]. Superfamily of the order Acarina that includes the families Ixodidae and Argasidae.

**ixomyelitis** (iks-o-mi-ĕ-li'tis) [ G. *ixys,* small of the back ]. Inflammation of the lumbar spinal cord.

# J

**J.** Symbols for (1) joul; (2) Joule's *equivalent;* (3) flux (4).

**jaagziekte, jagiekte** (yahg-ze-ek'te) [ Dutch, *drive sickness* ]. Pulmonary *adenomatosis* of sheep; a South African name for a chronic progressive pneumonia in sheep; it is similar to maedi in Iceland and chronic progressive pneumonia in the United States.

**Jaboulay** (zhă-boo-la'), Mathieu, French surgeon, 1860–1913. See J.'s *amputation, method, operation, pyloroplasty.*

**jack.** The male of the ass family, *Equus asinus.*

**jack'et.** A fixed bandage applied around the body in order to immobilize the spine.

   **Minerva j.,** a plaster of Paris body cast for fracture of spine.

   **Sayre's j.,** a plaster of Paris j., applied while the patient is suspended by the head and axillae.

   **strait j.,** see strait jacket.

**jack'screw.** A threaded device used in appliances for the separation of approximated teeth or jaws.

**Jackson,** Chevalier Q., American otolaryngologist, 1865–1958. See J.'s *sign.*

**Jackson,** Jabez N., American surgeon, 1868–1935. See J.'s *membrane, veil.*

**Jackson,** John Hughlings, English neurologist, 1835–1911. See J.'s *epilepsy, law, rule, sign, syndrome.*

**Jacob,** Arthur, Irish ophthalmologist, 1790–1874. See J.'s *ulcer.*

**Jacob** (zha-kōb'), Francois, French molecular biologist, \*1920. Nobel laureate, 1965, with André Lwoff and Jacques Monod, for their contributions to the understanding of the regulation of gene activity in ontogeny.

**Jacobaeus** (yah-ko-ba'ūs), Hans C., Swedish physician, 1879–1937. See J. *operation.*

**Jacobson,** Ludwig L., Danish anatomist, 1783–1843. See J.'s *anastomosis, canal, cartilage, nerve, organ, plexus, reflex.*

**Jacquart** (zhă-kar'), Henri, French physician, \*1881. See J.'s *angle.*

**Jacquemet** (zhak-ĕ-ma'), Marcel, French anatomist, 1872–1908. See J.'s *recess.*

**Jacquemier** (zhak-me-a'), Jean M., Paris obstetrician, 1806–1879. See J.'s *sign.*

**Jacquemin's test.** See under test.

**Jacques' plexus.** See under plexus.

**jactatio** (jak-ta'shĭ-o) [ L. ]. Jactitation.

**jactitation** (jak'tĭ-ta'shun) [ L. *jactatio,* a tossing, fr. *jacto,* pp. *-atus,* to throw. JAC- ]. Extreme restlessness or tossing about from side to side.

**Jadassohn,** Josef, Breslau dermatologist, 1863–1936. See Borst-J. type intraepidermal *epithelioma,* J.-Pellizzari *anetoderma,* J.-Lewandowsky *syndrome.*

**Jaeger von Jastthal,** (ya'ger) Edward, Vienna ophthalmologist, 1818–1884. See J.'s *test types.*

**Jaffe,** Henry L., U. S. pathologist, \*1896. See J.-Lichtenstein disease.

**Jaffe** (ya'feh), Max, German biochemist, 1841–1911. See J.'s *test.*

**Jahnke's syndrome.** See under syndrome.

**Jakob,** Alfons, German neuropsychiatrist, 1884–1931. See Creutzfeldt-J. *disease.*

**Jaksch** (yaksh), Rudolf von, Austrian physician, 1855–1947. See J.'s *anemia, disease.*

**jal'ap** [ *Jalapa* or *Xalapa,* a Mexican city whence the drug was exported ]. The tuberous root of *Exogonium purga* or *Ipomoea purga* (family Convolvulaceae); used as cathartic.

   **j. resin,** see under resin.

   **wild j.,** man-root; wild scammony; the root of *Ipomoea pandurata.*

**jal'apin.** A resinous glycoside derived from jalap and other convolvulaceous plants.

**James,** William, American psychologist, 1842–1910. See J.-Lange *theory.*

**Janet** (zhan-a'), Pierre M. F., French neurologist, 1859–1947. See J.'s *test.*

**Janeway,** Edward G., American physician, 1841–1911. See J. *lesion.*

**jan'iceps** [ L. *Janus,* an ancient Italic diety having two faces, + *caput,* head ]. Conjoined twins having their two heads fused together, with the faces looking in opposite directions. See also craniopagus, and syncephalus.

   **j. asym'metrus,** iniops; syncephalus asymmetros; a j. with one very small and imperfectly developed face.

   **j. parasit'icus,** a j. in which one of the twins is small and incompletely formed (the parasite) and attached to the more fully formed twin (the autosite).

**Jansen,** Albert, German otologist, 1859–1933. See J.'s *operation.*

**Jansky,** Jan, Prague physician, 1873–1921. See J.-Bielschowsky *disease,* J.'s *classification.*

**Janus green B.** Diethylsafraninazodimethylaniline chloride, $C_{30}H_{31}N_6Cl$; a basic dye used in histology and to stain mitochondria supravitally.

**Jaquet's erythema infantum.** See under erythema.

**jar.** 1. To jolt or shake. 2. A jolting or shaking.

   **heel j.,** the patient standing on tiptoe feels pain on suddenly bringing the heels to the ground: (1) in the spine in the case of Pott's disease; (2) in one lumbar region in case of renal calculus.

**jar'gon** [ Fr. gibberish ]. 1. Language peculiar to a specific field, *e.g.,* laboratory jargon. 2. Paraphasia.

**Jarisch** (yah'rish), Adolf, Austrian dermatologist, 1850–1902. See J.-Herxheimer *reaction.*

**Jarjavay** (zhar-zha-va'), Jean F., French physician, 1815–1868. See J.'s *ligaments.*

**Jarvis,** William C., U. S. laryngologist, 1855–1895. See J.'s *snare.*

**jasmine** (jaz'min, jas'mĭn). Gelsemium.

**Jatropha** (jat'ro-fah) [ G. *iatros,* physician, + *trophē,* nourishment ]. A genus of plants of the family Euphorbiaceae; a poisonous plant found in E. Africa and W. Indies.

   **J. curcas, J. glandulif'era,** Barbados nut; physic-nut; the seed furnishes a purgative oil similar to croton oil.

   **J. u'rens,** a species of South America; the macerated fresh leaves are used as a rubefacient and stimulating poultice; the seeds furnish a purgative oil. The plant bears leaves with stinging hairs that cause itching and faintness.

**jaundice** (jawn'dis) [ Fr. *jaune,* yellow ]. Icterus; a yellowish staining of the integument, sclerae, and deeper tissues and the excretions with bile pigments.

   **acholuric j.,** j. with excessive amounts of unconjugated bilirubin in the circulatory blood and without bile pigments in the blood.

   **black j.,** (1) *icterus* neonatorum; (2) *icterus* melas.

   **Budd's j.,** an obsolete term for acute yellow *atrophy* of the liver.

   **catarrhal j.,** obsolete term for viral *hepatitis* type A.

   **cholestatic j.,** j. produced by inspissated bile or bile plugs in small biliary passages in the liver.

   **chronic acholu'ric j.,** hereditary *spherocytosis.*

   **chronic familial j.,** hereditary *spherocytosis.*

   **congenital hemolytic j.,** hereditary *spherocytosis.*

   **familial nonhemolytic j.,** j. without evidence of liver damage, biliary obstruction, or hemolysis; thought to be due to an inborn error of metabolism in which the excretion of bilirubin by the liver is defective; also called constitutional hepatic dysfunction; benign familial icterus; Gilbert's disease; Hebra's disease (2).

   **hemapheic j.,** urobilin j.

   **hematogenous j.,** hemolytic j.

   **hemohepatogenous j.,** hemolytic j.

   **hemolytic j.,** hematogenous, hemohepatogenous, or toxemic j.; j. resulting from excessive amounts of hemoglobin released by any process (toxic, congenital, or immune) causing hemolysis of erythrocytes.

   **hepatocellular j.,** j. resulting from diffuse injury or inflammation or failure of function of the liver cells.

**hepatogenous j.,** j. resulting from disease of the liver, as distinguished from that supposedly due to blood changes.

**homol'ogous serum j.,** obsolete term for viral *hepatitis* type B.

**infectious j.,** (1) Weil's *disease;* (2) sometimes used in referring to infectious (viral) *hepatitis.*

**latent j.,** increased circulation of bile pigments before clinical j. is apparent.

**leptospiral j.,** in man and animals, j. associated with infection by various species of the genus *Leptospira.*

**malignant j.,** *icterus* gravis.

**malignant j. of dogs,** canine *babesiosis.*

**mechanical j.,** obstructive j.

**j. of the newborn,** *icterus* neonatorum.

**nonobstructive j.,** any j. in which the main biliary passages are not obstructed, *e.g.,* hemolytic j. or j. due to hepatitis.

**nuclear j.,** kernicterus.

**obstructive j.,** mechanical j.; j. resulting from obstruction to the flow of bile into the duodenum, whether intra- or extrahepatic.

**occult j.,** the presence of bile pigments in the blood in amounts inadequate to produce clinical j.

**painless j.,** j. caused by hemolysis or disease of the hepatic parenchyma and occasionally by obstruction at the head of the pancreas or impaction of a stone in the common duct; this condition is not associated with abdominal pain.

**physiologic j.,** physiologic *icterus.*

**regurgitation j.,** j. due to biliary obstruction, the bile pigment having been secreted by the hepatic cells and then reabsorbed into the blood stream.

**retention j.,** j. due to insufficiency of the liver in secreting bile pigment, or to an excess of bile pigment production; the bile pigment does not pass through the liver cells and the van den Bergh test is indirect.

**spherocytic j.,** hemolytic j. associated with spherocytosis.

**toxemic j.,** hemolytic j.

**urobilin j.,** hemapheic j.; any form of nonobstructive j. associated with the appearance of urobilin in the urine.

**jaundice root.** Hydrastis.

**jaw** [ A.S. *ceōwan,* to chew ]. 1. One of the two bony structures, in which the teeth are set, forming the framework of the mouth. 2. Common name for either the maxillae or the mandible.

**crackling j.,** chronic subluxation with clicking on motion.

**drop j.,** paralytic *rabies.*

**Hapsburg j. and lip,** prognathism and pouting lower lip, characteristic of the Hispano-Austrian imperial dynasty.

**India rubber j.,** a pathologic condition in which the osseous tissue of the j. is destroyed and replaced by malignant neoplastic tissue.

**lock-j.,** trismus.

**lower j.,** mandibula.

**lumpy j.,** actinomycosis.

**parrot j.,** a condition caused by protrusion of incisor teeth.

**phossy j.** [ *phosphorus* ], phosphonecrosis; necrosis of the osseous tissue of the j., as a result of poisoning with phosphorus, occurring especially in persons who work with the element.

**upper j.,** maxilla.

**Jaworski** (yah-vor'ske), Walery, Polish physician, 1849–1924. See J.'s *bodies.*

**Jeanselme** (zhaṅ-selm'), A. Edouard, French dermatologist, 1858–1935. See J.'s *nodules.*

**jecorin** (jek'or-in) [ L. *jecur,* liver ]. A nondescript cluco-phospholipid. $C_{105}H_{186}N_5SP_3O_{46}$, first isolated from liver and then identified also in the blood, spleen, muscles, brain, and certain other tissues. Probably not a single substance; soybean j. is a mixture of cephalin(s), galactomonoaraban, and inorganic salts.

**jec'ur,** gen. **jec'oris** [ L. ]. The liver.

**j. adiposum,** fatty metamorphosis of the liver.

**Jeghers,** Harold J., U. S. physician, *1904. See Peutz-J. syndrome.

**jejun-.** See jejuno-.

**jeju'nal.** Relating to the jejunum.

**jejunectomy** (jĕ-ju-nek'to-mĭ) [ jejunum + G. *ektomē,* excision ]. Exsection of all or a part of the jejunum.

**jejunitis** (jĕ-ju-ni'tis). Inflammation of the jejunum.

**jejuno-, jejun-** (jĕ-ju'no-, jej'oo-no, je'ju'no-, je-ju'no-) [ L. *jejunus,* empty. JEJ- ]. Combining forms relating to the jejunum.

**jeju'nocolos'tomy** [ jejuno- + colon + G. *stoma,* mouth ]. Establishment of a communication between the jejunum and the colon.

**jejunoileal** (jĕ-ju'no-il'e-al). Relating to the jejunum and the ileum.

**jejunoileitis** (jĕ-ju'no-il-e-i'tis). Inflammation of jejunum and ileum.

**jejunoileostomy** (jĕ-ju'no-il-e-os'to-mĭ) [ jejuno- + ileum + G. *stoma,* mouth ]. Establishment of a communication between the jejunum and a noncontinuous part of the ileum.

**jejunojejunostomy** (jĕ-ju'no-jĕ-ju-nos'to-mĭ) [ jejuno- + jejuno- + G. *stoma,* mouth ]. A junction between two portions of jejunum.

**jejunoplasty** (jĕ-ju'no-plas-tĭ) [ jejuno- + G. *plastos,* molded ]. A corrective surgical procedure on the jejunum.

**jejunostomy** (jĕ'ju-nos'to-mĭ) [ jejuno- + G. *stoma,* mouth ]. The operative establishment of a fissure through the wall of the abdomen into the jejunum.

**jejunotomy** (jĕ'ju-not'o-mĭ) [ jejuno- + G. *tomē,* incision ]. Incision into the jejunum.

**jejunum** (jĕ-ju'num) [ L. *jejunus,* empty. JEJ- ] [ NA ]. The portion of small intestine, about 8 feet in length, between the duodenum and the ileum.

**Jelks,** John L., U. S. surgeon, *1870. See J.'s *operation.*

**Jellinek** (yel'e-nek), Stefan, Vienna physician, *1871. See J.'s *sign.*

**jel'ly** [ L. *gelo,* to freeze ]. A semisolid, tremulous compound, containing usually some form of gelatin in solution.

**cardiac j.,** term introduced by Davis for the gelatinous, noncellular material between the endothelial lining and the myocardial layer of the heart in very young embryos. Later in development it serves as a substratum for cardiac mesenchyme.

**interlaminar j.,** term introduced by Patten for the gelatinous material between ectoderm and entoderm that serves as the substrate on which mesenchymal cells migrate.

**Wharton's j.,** the mucous connective tissue of the umbilical cord.

**Jendrassik** (yen-drah'shik), Ernö, Hungarian physician, 1858–1936. See J.'s *maneuver.*

**Jenner,** H. D., Canadian physician, *1907. See J.-Kay *unit.*

**Jenner,** Louis, English physician, 1866–1904. See J.'s *stain.*

**Jenner,** Sir William, English physician, 1815–1898. See J.'s *emphysema.*

**Jensen** (yen'sen), Carl O., Danish veterinary surgeon and pathologist, 1864–1934. See J.'s *sarcoma.*

**Jensen** (yen'sen), Edmund Z., Danish ophthalmologist, 1861–1950. See J.'s *disease.*

**jerboa** (jer-bo'ah) [ Ar. *yarbū* ]. A member of the family Dipodidae, small rodents with 10 genera (including the species *Jaculus jaculus,* the desert jumping rat) that inhabit arid areas of Africa and Asia; their hindlimbs are about four times the length of the forelimbs and their auditory bullae are often greatly expanded.

**jerk.** 1. A sudden pull. 2. A sharp muscular contraction following a tap on the muscle or its tendon; muscular or tendon reflex; deep reflex.

**ankle j.,** Achilles *reflex.*

**chin j.,** jaw j.

**crossed j.,** a muscular contraction on one side following a tap on muscle or tendon on the other side.

**crossed adductor knee j.,** crossed j. of adductor femoris muscles.

**crossed knee j.,** crossed j. of patellar tendon.

**elbow j.,** triceps *reflex.*

**jaw j.,** jaw reflex; chin j. or reflex; masseter or mandibular reflex; a spasmodic contraction of the temporal muscles following a downward tap on the loosely hanging mandible.

**knee j.,** patellar *reflex.*

**supinator j.,** brachioradial *reflex.*

**jerks** (pl.). Chorea or any form of tic.

**Jervell,** A. See J. and Lange-Nielsen *syndrome.*

**jervine** (jer'vēn, -vin). Viridine; an alkaloid, $C_{27}H_{39}NO_3$, derived from veratrum or hellebore.

**jes'samine** [ Pers. *yāsmin* ]. Gelsemium.

**Jesuit's bark.** Cinchona.

**jig'ger.** Common name for *Tunga penetrans.*

**Jim'son weed.** Stramonium.

**jird.** A rodent of the genus *Meriones;* distinct from the gerbil, with which it is frequently confused.

**Jk blood group.** See Kidd blood group, appendix 2.

**JNA.** Abbreviation for *Jena Nomina Anatomica,* 1935. See *Nomina Anatomica.*

**Jobert de Lamballe** (zhō-bair'dë-lahñ-bal'), Antoine J., Paris surgeon, 1799–1867. See J. de L.'s *fossa, operation, suture.*

**Joest** (yëst), Ernst, Dresden veterinary pathologist, 1873–1926. See J. *bodies.*

**Joffroy** (zhof-rwah'), Alexis, Paris physician, 1844–1908. See J.'s *reflex, sign.*

**Johne** (yo'neh), H. Albert, German physician, 1839–1910. Gave his name to johnin. See J.'s *bacillus, disease, stain.*

**johnin** (yo'nin) [ A. *Johne* ]. A product analogous to tuberculin but made from the causative organism of Johne's disease grown in a broth medium containing timothy hay bacillus (*Mycobacterium phlei*). It is used as an allergen to provoke reactions in infected animals—a diagnostic agent.

**Johnson,** F. B. See Dublin-J. *syndrome.*

**Johnson,** Frank C., American pediatrician, 1894–1934. See Stevens-J. *syndrome.*

**Johnson,** Harry B. See J.'s *method.*

# JOINT

**joint** [ L. *junctura;* fr. *jungo,* pp. *junctus,* to join. JUNC- ]. Articulatio.

**acromioclavicular j.,** *articulatio* acromioclavicularis.

**ankle j.,** *articulatio* talocruralis.

**antebrachiocarpal j.,** *articulatio* antebrachiocarpea.

**anterior intraoccipital j.,** *synchondrosis* intraoccipitalis anterior.

**arthro'dial j.,** *articulatio* plana.

**atlantooccipital j.,** *articulatio* atlantooccipitalis.

**ball-and-socket j.,** *articulatio* spheroidea.

**biax'ial j.,** one in which there are two principal axes of movement situated at right angles to each other; saddle j.'s are biaxial.

**biloc'ular j.,** one in which the intraarticular disk is complete, dividing the j. into two distinct cavities.

**Budin's obstetrical j.,** *synchondrosis* intraoccipitalis posterior.

**calcaneocuboid j.,** *articulatio* calcaneocuboidea.

**capitular j.,** *articulatio* capitis costae.

**carpal j.'s,** *articulationes* intercarpeae.

**carpometacarpal j.'s,** *articulationes* carpometacarpeae.

**carpometacarpal j. of thumb,** *articulatio* carpometacarpea pollicis.

**cartilag'inous j.,** *junctura* cartilaginea.

**centrodistal j.,** *articulatio* centrodistalis.

**Charcot's j.,** tabetic osteoarthropathy; j. enlargement with osteoarthritis due to trophic disturbances in patients with tabes dorsalis.

**Chopart's j.,** *articulatio* tarsi transversa.

**Clutton's j.'s,** symmetrical arthrosis in cases of congenital syphilis.

**coccyge'al j.,** *junctura* sacrococcygea.

**coch'lear j.,** a variety of hinge j. in which the elevation and depression, respectively, on the opposing articular

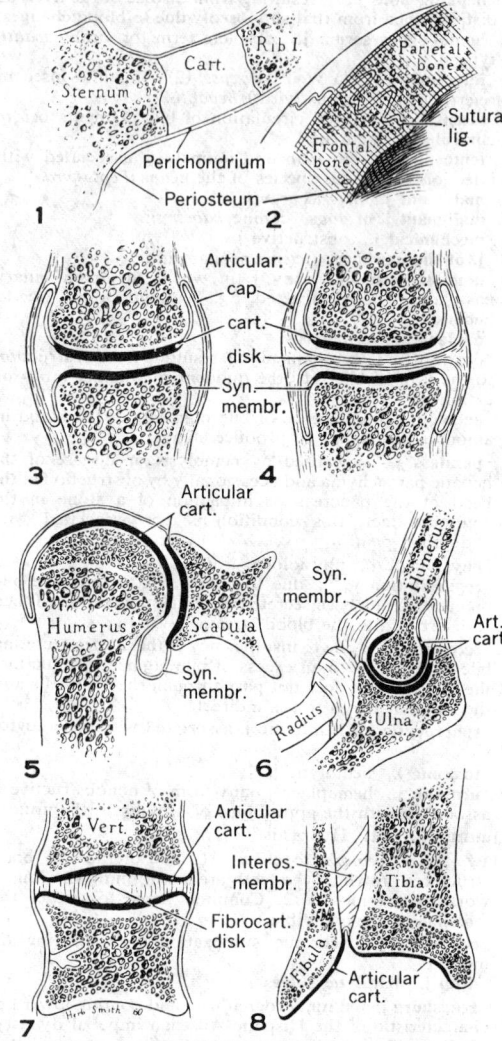

**Types of Joint**

*1,* Cartilaginous, synchondrosis; *2,* fibrous, suture; *3,* synovial, simple; *4,* synovial, with articular disk; *5,* synovial, spheroid (ball and socket); *6,* synovial, ginglymus (hinge); *7,* cartilaginous, symphysis; *8,* fibrous, syndesmosis.

surfaces form part of a spiral, flexion being then accompanied by a certain amount of lateral deviation.

**coffin j.,** the distal interphalangeal articulation of the horse. It is a compound synovial j. between the middle and distal phalanges and also with the distal sesamoid or navicular bone on the caudal side; navicular j.

**compound j.,** one formed of three or more bones.

**condylar j.,** *articulatio* condylaris.

**con'dyloid j.,** *articulatio* condylaris.

**costochon'dral j.'s,** the junctions between the lateral end of each costal cartilage and the sternal end of the corresponding rib.

**cos'totransverse j.'s,** *articulatio* costotransversaria.

**costover'tebral j.'s,** *articulationes* costovertebrales.

**cot'yloid j.,** *articulatio* spheroidea.

**cri'coaryte'noid j.,** *articulatio* cricoarytenoidea.

**cricothy'roid j.,** *articulatio* cricothyroidea.

**Cruveilhier's j.,** *articulatio* atlantoaxialis mediana.

**cubital j.,** *articulatio* cubiti.

**cuboideonavic'ular j.,** a fibrous j. between adjacent parts of the cuboid and navicular bones; occasionally a synovial cavity is found here as an extension of the cuneonavicular j.

**cu'neocu'boid j.,** the synovial articulation between the lateral surface of the lateral cuneiform and the anterior two-thirds of the medial surface of the cuboid.

**cu'neometatar'sal j.'s,** *articulationes* tarsometatarseae.

**cu'neonavic'ular j.,** *articulatio* cuneonavicularis.

**diarthrodial j.,** *junctura* synovialis.

**digital j.'s,** *articulationes* interphalangeae.

**dry j.,** a j. affected with atrophic desiccating changes.

**j.'s of ear bones,** *articulationes* ossiculorum auditis.

**elbow j.,** *articulatio* cubiti.

**ellipsoid'al j.,** *articulatio* ellipsoidea.

**enarthro'dial j.,** *articulatio* spheroidea.

**false j.,** pseudarthrosis.

**femoropatellar j.,** (1) the articulation of the facets on the articular surface of the patella with corresponding surfaces on the femoral condyles; (2) in domestic animals, the *articulatio* femoropatellaris.

**femorotibial j.,** *articulatio* femorotibialis.

**fibrous j.,** *junctura* fibrosa.

**flail j.,** a j. with loss of function caused by loss of the power to stabilize the j. in any plane within its normal range of motion.

**free inferior limb j.'s,** *juncturae* membri inferioris liberi.

**free superior limb j.'s,** *juncturae* membri superioris liberi.

**gin'glymoid j.,** ginglymus.

**gliding j.,** *articulatio* plana.

**gompholic j.,** gomphosis.

**j. of head of rib,** *articulatio* capitis costae.

**hemophilic j.,** hemarthrosis.

**hinge j.,** ginglymus.

**hip j.,** *articulatio* coxae.

**hu'mera'dial j.,** *articulatio* cubiti.

**hu'meroulnar j.,** *articulatio* humeroulnaris.

**hysterical j.,** articular or arthral neuromimesis; a simulation of j. disease, with symptoms of pain, possibly swelling, and impairment of motion; of emotional origin, not dependent upon actual lesion.

**immovable j.,** *junctura* fibrosa.

**incudomalle'olar j.,** *articulatio* incudomallearis.

**incu'dostape'dial j.,** *articulatio* incudostapedia.

**inferior limb girdle j.'s,** *juncturae* cinguli membri inferioris.

**interarticular j.'s,** *juncturae* zygapophyseales.

**intercarp'al j.'s** *articulationes* intercarpeae.

**interchon'dral j.'s,** *articulationes* interchondrales.

**intercu'neiform j.'s,** the articulations between contiguous surfaces of the cuneiform bones.

**intermetacar'pal j.'s,** *articulationes* intermetacarpeae.

**intermetatar'sal j.'s,** *articulationes* intermetatarseae.

**interphalan'geal j.'s,** *articulationes* interphalangeae.

**intersternebral j.'s,** *synchondroses* intersternebrales.

**intertars'al j.'s,** *articulationes* intertarseae.

**intrachondral j.,** *articulatio* intrachondralis.

**jaw j.,** *articulatio* temporomandibularis.

**knee j.,** *articulatio* genus.

**lateral atlantoaxial j.,** *articulatio* atlantoaxialis lateralis.

**lateral atlantoepistrophic j.,** *articulatio* atlantoaxialis lateralis.

**Lisfranc's j.'s,** *articulationes* tarsometatarseae.

**lumbosacral j.,** *junctura* lumbosacralis.

**mandib'ular j.,** *articulatio* temporomandibularis.

**manubriosternal j.,** *synchondrosis* manubriosternalis.

**manubriosternal synovial j.,** *articulatio* synovialis manubriosternalis.

**median atlantoaxial j.,** *articulatio* atlantoaxialis mediana.

**metacar'pophalan'geal j.'s,** *articulationes* metacarpophalangeae.

**metatarsophalan'geal j.'s,** *articulationes* metatarsophalangeae.

**j. mice,** small, fibrous or cartilaginous loose bodies (*q. v.,* under body) in the synovial cavity of a joint.

**middle atlantoepistrophic j.,** *articulatio* atlantoaxialis mediana.

**middle carpal j.,** *articulatio* mediocarpea.

**midtarsal j.,** *articulatio* tarsi transversa.

**mortise j.,** *articulatio* talocruralis.

**movable j.,** *junctura* synovialis or *junctura* cartilaginea.

**multiax'ial j.,** one in which movement occurs in a number of axes; see *articulatio* spheroidea.

**neu'rocent'ral j.,** neurocentral *synchondrosis.*

**peg-and-socket j.,** gomphosis.

**petrooccipital j.,** *synchondrosis* petrooccipitalis.

**phalan'geal j.'s,** *articulationes* interphalangeae.

**pi'sotrique'tral j.,** *articulatio* ossis pisiformis.

**pivot j.,** *articulatio* trochoidea.

**plane j.,** *articulatio* plana.

**polyax'ial j.,** multiaxial j.

**radiocar'pal j.,** *articulatio* radiocarpea.

**radioulnar j., inferior,** *articulatio* radioulnaris distalis.

**radioulnar j., superior,** *articulatio* radioulnaris proximalis.

**ro'tary j., ro'tatory j.,** *articulatio* trochoidea.

**sacrococcyg'eal j.,** *junctura* sacrococcygea.

**sacroiliac j.,** *articulatio* sacroiliaca.

**saddle j.,** *articulatio* sellaris.

**schindyletic j.,** schindylesis.

**screw j.,** cochlear j.

**shoulder j.,** *articulatio* humeri.

**simple j.,** *articulatio* simplex.

**socket j.,** *articulatio* spheroidea.

**spheroid j.,** *articulatio* spheroidea.

**spiral j.,** cochlear j.

**sternal j.'s,** *synchondroses* sternales.

**sternoclavic'ular j.,** *articulatio* sternoclavicularis.

**sternocos'tal j.'s,** *articulationes* sternocostales.

**stifle j.,** the femorotibial articulation in the hind leg of the horse and other quadrupeds; it corresponds to the knee in man.

**subtalar j.,** *articulatio* subtalaris.

**superior limb girdle j.'s,** *juncturae* cinguli membri superioris.

**suture j.,** sutura (2).

**synarthro'dial j.,** *junctura* fibrosa.

**synchondrodial j.,** synchondrosis.

**syndesmodial j., syndesmotic j.,** syndesmosis.

**synovial j.,** *junctura* synovialis.

**talocalcaneal j.,** (1) anterior: *articulatio* talocalcaneonavicularis; (2) posterior: *articulatio* subtalaris; (3) in veterinary anatomy, *articulatio* talocalcanea.

**talocalcaneocentral j.,** *articulatio* talocalcaneocentralis.

**talocalca'neonavic'ular j.,** *articulatio* talocalcaneonavicularis.

**tarsal j.'s,** *articulationes* intertarseae.

**tarsocrural j.,** *articulatio* tarsocruralis.

**tarsometatar'sal j.'s,** *articulationes* tarsometatarseae.

**temporomandibular j.,** *articulatio* temporomandibularis.

**thigh j.,** *articulatio* coxae.

**tibiofib'ular j., inferior,** *syndesmosis* tibiofibularis.

**tibiofib'ular j., superior,** *articulatio* tibiofibularis.

**transverse tarsal j.,** *articulatio* tarsi transversa.

**trochoid j.,** *articulatio* trochoidea.

**uniax'ial j.,** one in which movement is around one axis only.

**uniloc'ular j.,** one in which an intraarticular disk is incomplete or absent, the j. having but a single cavity.

**wedge-and-groove j. or suture,** schindylesis.

**wrist j.,** *articulatio* radiocarpea.

**xiphister'nal j.,** *synchondrosis* xiphosternalis.

**zygapophysial j.'s,** *juncturae* zygapophyseales.

---

**Jolles** (yol'läs), Adolf, Austrian chemist, \*1863. See J.'s *test.*

**Jolly** (yol'le), Friedrich, German neurologist, 1844–1904. See J.'s *reaction.*

**Jolly** (zhŏ-le'), Justin, French histologist, 1870–1953. See Howell-J. *bodies,* J. *bodies.*

**Jones,** Henry Bence. See Bence Jones.

**Jonnesco (Ionesco)** (yon-nes'k̄ ), Thomas, Bucharest surgeon, 1860–1926. See J.'s *fossa.*

**Jonston,** Johns, Scottish physician in Poland, 1603–1675. See J.'s *alopecia, area.*

**Jorissenne** (zhor-is-sen'), Gustav, Belgian physician, \*1846. See J.'s *sign.*

**Joule,** James P., English physicist, 1818–1889. See *joule,* J.'s *equivalent.*

**joule** (jool, jowl) [J. P. *Joule*]. Symbol, J; a unit of energy; the heat generated, or energy expended, by an ampere flowing against an ohm for 1 second; equal to $10^7$ ergs, and to a newton-meter. The joule is an approved multiple of the SI fundamental unit of energy, the erg, and is intended to replace the calorie (= 4.184 J).

**juccuya** (ŭ-koo'yah). Cutaneous *leishmaniasis.*

**ju'gal** [ L. *jugalis,* yoked together, fr. *jugum,* a yoke. JUN- ]. 1. Connecting; yoked. 2. Relating to the zygomatic bone.

**juga'le.** Jugal point; a craniometric point at the union of the temporal and frontal processes of the zygomatic bone. See fig. under craniometric *point.*

**ju'glans,** gen. **juglan'dis** [ L. a walnut, fr. *Jovis* (*Jupiter*) + *glans* (*gland*-), acorn ]. Butternut; the root bark of *Juglans cinerea* (family Juglandaceae), a forest tree of eastern North America; has laxative properties.

**ju'gomax'illary.** Relating to the zygomatic bone and the maxilla.

**jugular** (jug'u-lar, ju'gu-lar) [ L. *jugulum,* throat ]. 1. Relating to the throat or neck. 2. Relating to the j. veins. 3. A j. vein.

**ju'gulum** [ L. collarbone, yoke. JUNC- ] [ NA ]. Neck or throat.

**ju'gum,** pl. **ju'ga** [ L. a yoke. JUNC- ]. 1 [ NA ]. A ridge or furrow connecting two points. 2. A type of forceps.

   **j. alveola're,** pl. **ju'ga alveola'ria,** [ NA ], alveolar yoke; one of the eminences on the outer surface of the alveolar process of the maxilla or mandible, formed by the roots of the incisor teeth.

   **j. penis,** a forceps used for temporary compression of the penis.

   **j. sphenoida'le** [ NA ], a plane surface on the sphenoid bone, in front of the sella turcica, connecting the two lesser wings, and forming part of the anterior cranial fossa.

**juice** (joos) [ L. *jus,* broth ]. 1. The tissue fluid of a plant or animal. 2. A digestive secretion. See also *succus.*

   **appetite j.,** gastric j. secreted upon the sight or smell of food and at the time of eating, influenced by the attractiveness of the food and delight in the food ingested; a conditioned reflex.

   **cancer j.,** turbid, white to yellow-white or gray-white fluid (chiefly plasma) that may be expressed from certain forms of malignant neoplastic tissue, and is likely to contain neoplastic cells and debris; formed especially in relatively large, degenerating, partly necrotic foci of rapidly growing neoplastic tissue.

   **gastric j.,** succus gastricus; the digestive fluid secreted by the glands of the stomach; it is a thin, colorless liquid of acid reaction, containing mainly hydrochloric acid, rennet, the precursor of the proteolytic enzyme (pepsin), and an "intrinsic factor," a mucoprotein, plus mucus.

   **intestinal j.,** succus entericus; an alkaline straw-colored fluid secreted by the crypts of Lieberkühn and the simple follicles. Its enzymes (peptidases, saccharases, nucleases, lecithinase, phosphatase, lipase) complete the hydrolysis of carbohydrates to glucose, fructose, and galactose, and the hydrolysis of protein and lipids. It also contains enterokinase (enteropeptidase), which converts the trypsinogen of the pancreatic j. into trypsin.

   **leper j.,** slightly turbid or almost clear fluid (chiefly plasma) that oozes from a leprous nodule (when the latter is pricked or compressed) and is likely to contain *Mycobacterium leprae,* such material is useful for bacteriologic diagnosis of a lesion presumed to be leprosy.

   **pancreatic j.,** succus pancreaticus; the external secretion of the pancreas; a clear, alkaline fluid containing several enzymes: α-amylase, nucleases, trypsinogen, chymotrypsinogen, and steapsin.

**jumps** [ pl. ]. 1. Nervous twitching; jerks; chorea. 2. *Delirium* tremens.

**junction** (jungk'shun). Junctura (2).

   **amelodental j., amelodentinal j.,** dentinoenamel j.

   **amnioembryonic j.,** the line of amniotic attachment to the periphery of the embryonic disk.

   **anorectal j.,** the site of transition from rectum to anus.

   **cementodentinal j.,** dentinocemental j.; the surface at which the cementum and dentin of the root of a tooth are joined.

   **choled'ochoduode'nal j.,** that part of the duodenal wall traversed by the ductus choledochus, ductus pancreaticus, and ampulla.

   **dentinocemental j.,** cementodentinal j.

   **dentinoenamel j.,** amelodental j.; amelodentinal j.; the surface at which the enamel and the dentin of the crown of a tooth are joined.

   **electrotonic j.,** gap j.; see also synapse.

   **esophagogastric j.,** the line at the cardiac orifice of the stomach where there is a transition from the stratified squamous epithelium of the esophagus to the simple columnar epithelium of the stomach.

   **gap j.,** nexus; electrotonic j. or synapse; an intercellular j. formerly considered to be a tight, membrane-to-membrane j. (zonula occludens) but now shown to have a 20 Å gap between apposed cell membranes. The gap is not blank but contains subunits in the form of polygonal lattices. It occurs in epithelia, between certain nerve cells, and in smooth and cardiac muscle. It is believed to mediate electrotonic coupling which allows ionic currents to pass from one cell to another. See also synapse.

   **intercellular j.'s,** specializations of the cellular margins which contribute to the adhesion or allow for communication between cells; they include the macula adherens (desmosome), zonula adherens, zonula occludens, and nexus (gap junction).

   **j. of lips,** *commissura* labiorum.

   **mucocutaneous j.,** the site of transition from epidermis to the epithelium of a mucous membrane.

   **muscle-tendon j.,** muscle-tendon *attachment.*

   **myoneural j.,** neuromuscular j.; the synaptic connection of the axon of the motor neuron with a muscle fiber; see motor *endplate.*

   **neuroectodermal j.,** neurosomatic j.; the margin of the embryonic neural plate separating it from the embryonic ectoderm; cells from this region form the neural crest.

   **neuromuscular j.,** myoneural j.

   **neurosomatic j.,** neuroectodermal j.

   **sclerocorneal j.,** *limbus* corneae.

   **squamocolumnar j.,** see squamocolumnar.

   **S-T j.,** J *point.*

   **tympanostape'dial j.,** *syndesmosis* tympanostapedia.

**junctura,** pl. **junctu'rae** (jungk-tu'rah) [ L. a joining ] [ NA ]. 1. Articulation; joint. See fig. under joint. 2. Juncture; junction; the point, line, or surface of union of two parts, mainly bones or cartilages.

   **j. cartilagin'ea** [ NA ], cartilaginous joint; a joint in which the apposed bony surfaces are united by cartilage. They are divided into *synchondroses* and *symphyses.* In the former the cartilage connecting the apposed surfaces is, as a rule, ultimately converted to bone, as between the epiphyses and diaphyses of long bones; exceptions are the sternal synchondroses and the cartilaginous union of the first rib and the manubrium of the sternum. In symphyses the bones are connected by a flat disk of fibrocartilage which remains unossified throughout life, *e.g.,* the intervertebral disk and the symphysis pubis.

   **juncturae cing'uli mem'bri inferio'ris** [ NA ], joints of the inferior limb girdle; the joints which unite the sacrum and the two hip bones to form the pelvic girdle; these are the sacroiliac joints, the pubic symphysis, the sacrotuberal and sacrospinal ligaments, and the obturator membrane.

   **juncturae cing'uli mem'bri superio'ris** [ NA ], joints of the superior limb girdle; the joints uniting the scapulae and clavicles to each other and the latter to the sternum forming the superior limb girdle; these are the acromioclavicular and the sternoclavicular joints.

   **j. fibro'sa** [ NA ], fibrous joint; immovable joint (actually slightly movable); a union of two bones by fibrous tissue such that there is no joint cavity and little motion possible. The types of fibrous joints are (a) sutura, (b) syndesmosis, and (c) gomphosis.

   **j. lumbosacra'lis** [ NA ], lumbosacral joint; the articulation of the fifth lumbar vertebra with the sacrum.

   **juncturae mem'bri inferio'ris li'beri** [ NA ], joints of the free inferior limb; the joints uniting the bones of the free inferior limb to one another and to the pelvic girdle; they are the hip joint, knee joint, tibiofibular joints, and joints of the foot.

   **juncturae mem'bri superio'ris li'beri** [ NA ], joints of the free superior limb; the joints uniting the bones of the free superior limb to one another and to the superior limb girlde; they are the shoulder joint, elbow joint, radioulnar joints, and joints of the hand.

**juncturae os'sium** [ NA, NAV ], alternative official NA and NAV name for articulationes; see articulatio.

**j. sacrococcyge'a** [ NA ], sacrococcygeal junction; sacrococcygeal joint; the articulation of the coccyx with the sacrum.

**j. synovia'lis** [ NA ], synovial joint; diarthrosis; movable joint; a joint in which (a) the opposing bony surfaces are covered with a layer of hyaline cartilage or fibrocartilage, (b) there is a joint cavity containing synovial fluid, lined with synovial membrane and reinforced by a fibrous capsule and ligaments, and (c) there is more or less free movement possible.

**juncturae ten'dinum,** *conexus* intertendineus.

**juncturae zygapophysea'les** [ NA ], zygapophysial joints; interarticular joints; the synovial joints between zygapophyses or articular processes of the vertebrae.

**juncture** (jungk'chur). Junctura (2).

**Jung** (yoong), Carl Gustav, Swiss psychiatrist and psychologist, 1875–1961. See Jungian *psychoanalysis.*

**Jung** (yoong), Karl G., Swiss anatomist, 1793–1864. See J.'s *muscle.*

**Jüngling** (yüng'ling), Adolph O., German surgeon, 1884–1944. See J.'s *disease.*

**ju'niper** [ L. the juniper-tree ]. Juniper berries; the dried ripe fruit of *Juniperus communis* (family Pinaceae).

**j. berry oil,** a volatile oil distilled from the fruit of *Juniperus communis;* diuretic.

**j. tar,** cade oil; the empyreumatic volatile oil obtained from the woody portion of *Juniperus oxycedrus;* used externally for skin diseases.

**Junod** (zhü-no'), Victor T., Paris physician, 1809–1881. See J.'s *boot.*

**jurispru'dence.** The science of law, its principles and concepts.

**dental j.,** forensic *dentistry.*

**medical j.,** forensic *medicine.*

**jury-mast.** An upright bar, of which the lower extremity is fixed in a plaster of Paris jacket or spinal support, and the upper recurving extremity carries a sling in which the chin and occiput rest; used as a support to the head in cases of Pott's disease of the cervical vertebrae.

**justo major.** See *pelvis* justo major.

**justo minor.** See *pelvis* justo minor.

**juxtaglomerular** (juks'tah-glo-měr'u-lar). Close to or adjoining a renal glomerulus.

**jux'tallocor'tex.** Voght's collective term for several regions of the cerebral cortex which occupy an intermediate position between the isocortex and the allocortex; see also *cortex* cerebri.

**juxtaposition** (juks-tah-po-zish'un) [ L. *juxta,* near to, + *positio,* a placing, fr. *pono,* pp. *positus,* to place ]. A position side by side; apposition; contiguity.

# K

**κ.** Tenth letter of the Greek alphabet, kappa, *q.v.*

**K.** 1. Chemical symbol for the element potassium (kalium). 2. Abbreviation for phylloquinone (or phylloquinone K). 3. Abbreviation for vitamin K₁ (20).

**K.** Symbol for dissociation constant. Thus, $K_a$ is the symbol for the dissociation constant of an acid; $K_b$, of a base; $K_i$, of an enzyme-inhibitor complex; $K_m$, of the Michaelis-Menten constant; $K_w$, of water. For definitions see under constant.

**°K.** Abbreviation for degrees Kelvin (absolute).

**k.** Symbol for rate or velocity constant; see under constant.

**K and k blood groups.** See Kell blood group, appendix 2.

**Ka.** Abbreviation for kathode or kathodal.

**kabure** (kah-boo'ra). Schistosomiasis japonicum.

**Kaes,** Theodor, German neurologist, 1852–1913. See K.'s *line.*

**kafindo.** Onyalai.

**Kahler,** Otto, Vienna physician, 1849–1893. See K.'s *disease.*

**Kahn,** Reuben L., U.S. bacteriologist, *1887. See K. *test.*

**Kahn and Falta sign.** See under sign.

**kainophobia** (ki'no-fo-bi'ah) [ G. *kainos*, new, + *phobos*, fear ]. Kainotophobia; neophobia; morbid fear of change or of anything new or unfamiliar.

**Kaiserling** (ki'zer-ling), Karl, German pathologist, 1869–1942. See K.'s *method.*

**kak-, kako-** [ G. *kakos*, bad ]. Combining form meaning bad or ill. For words beginning thus and not found here, see cac-, caco-.

**kakerga'sia.** Cacergasia.

**kakesthe'sia.** Cacesthesia.

**kakke** (kak'ka) [ Jap. ]. Beriberi.

**kakos'mia.** Cacosmia.

**kakosto'mia.** Cacostomia.

**kakothen'ics.** Cacogenics.

**kakot'rophy.** Cacotrophy.

**kal-, kali-** [ L. *kalium*, potassium ]. Combining forms relating to potassium. Sometimes the combining form *kalio-* is used (but improperly).

**kala azar** (kah'lah-ah-zahr') [ Hind. *kala*, black, + *azar*, poison ]. Visceral *leishmaniasis.*

**kalafun'gin** (USAN). An antibiotic substance produced by *Streptomyces tanashiensis* var. *kala;* an antifungal agent.

**ka'li** [ see kalium ]. Potassium.

**kalim'eter.** Alkalimeter.

**ka'liope'nia** [ Mod. L. *kalium*, potassium, + G. *penia*, poverty ]. Insufficiency of potassium in the body.

**ka'liope'nic.** Relating to kaliopenia.

**Kalischer,** Siegfried, German physician, *1862. See Sturge-K.-Weber *syndrome.*

**ka'lium** [ Mod. L. fr. Ar. *quali*, potash ]. Potassium.

**kaliuresis** (ka'li-u-re'sis). Kaluresis.

**ka'liuret'ic.** Kaluretic.

**kallak'** [ Eskimo word meaning skin disease ]. A peculiar pustular dermatitis observed among the Eskimos.

**kal'lidin.** See bradykinin.

**kallikrein** (kal'i-kre'in) (EC 3.4.4.21). A blood enzyme that converts kallidinogens into kallidins.

**Kallmann,** Franz Josef, U. S. medical geneticist and psychiatrist, 1897–1965. See K.'s *syndrome.*

**kaluresis** (kal'u-re'sis) [ Mod. L. *kalium*, potassium, + G. *ouresis*, urination ]. Kaliuresis; the increased urinary excretion of potassium.

**kal'uret'ic.** Kaliuretic; relating to, causing, or characterized by kaluresis.

**kama'la, kamee'la.** The hairs and glands from the capsules of *Mallotus philippinensis* (family Euphorbiaceae), a small evergreen tree of India, Africa, and Australia. Occurs in the form of a reddish granular powder; used as an anthelmintic (ascaris and threadworms) and as a dyestuff.

**kan'amy'cin sulfate** (USP). KANTREX; an antibiotic substance derived from strains of *Streptomyces kanamyceticus.* It is a thermostable, water-soluble, polybasic substance consisting of two amino sugars glycosidally linked to deoxystreptamine. The antibacterial activity *in vitro* is nearly identical with that of neomycin. It is active against many aerobic Gram-positive and Gram-negative bacteria (*Aerobacter, Escherichia coli, Proteus, Klebsiella, Neisseria, Shigella and Salmonella*). Excessive doses and prolonged administration may result in irreversible damage to the auditory portion of the eighth cranial nerve. Disturbances of equilibrium may also occur.

**Kanner,** Leo, Austrian psychiatrist in U. S., *1894. See K.'s *syndrome.*

**kanyemba.** Chiufa.

**kaolin** (ka'o-lin) [ Ch. *kao lin*, High Ridge, name of a locality in China where the substance is found in abundance ] (NF). Fuller's earth; white bole; porcelain clay; terra alba; aluminum silicate; powdered and freed from gritty particles by elutriation. Used as a demulcent and adsorbent.

  **heavy k.** (BP), a native hydrated aluminum silicate freed from most of its impurities by elutriation and dried. Used to prepare k. poultice.

  **light k.** (BP), same properties as heavy k.; an adsorbent and demulcent.

**ka'olino'sis.** Pneumonoconiosis caused by the inhalation of clay dust.

**Kaposi** (kap-o'she), Moritz K., Vienna dermatologist, 1837–1902. See K.'s *dermatosis,* varicelliform *eruption, sarcoma.*

**kappa** (kap'ah). Greek letter (κ), symbol for 10th carbon atom.

**Karell** (kah'rel), Philip J., Russian physician, 1806–1886. See K. *diet.*

**Kartagener** (kar'tah-ga'ner), Manes, Swiss physician, *1897. See K.'s *syndrome.*

**Karwinskia humboldtiana.** Coyotillo; a woody shrub or small tree (family Rhamnaceae) that grows in Mexico and parts of the southwest United States; the fruit (an ovoid drupe) and probably other parts of the plant contain a toxic principle that produces a paralysis in man and animals; see buckthorn *polyneuropathy.*

**karyo-** (kar'i-o-) [ G. *karyon*, nut, nucleus ]. Caryo-; combining forms denoting nucleus.

**karyochrome** (kar'i-o-krōm) [ karyo- + G. *chroma,* color ]. A nerve cell body having little or no Nissl substance visible but a nucleus which stains intensely.

**karyoclasis** (kar-i-ok'lă-sis) [ karyo- + G. *klasis,* a breaking ]. Karyorrhexis.

**karyocyte** (kar'i-o-sit) [ karyo- + G. *kytos,* cell ]. A young, immature normoblast.

**karyogamic** (kar'i-o-gam'ik). Relating to or marked by karyogamy.

**karyogamy** (kar'i-og'ă-mi) [ karyo- + G. *gamos,* marriage ]. Fusion of the nuclei of two cells, as occurs in fertilization or true conjugation.

**karyogenesis** (kar-i-o-jen'ē-sis) [ karyo- + G. *genesis,* production ]. Formation of the nucleus of a cell.

**karyogenic** (kar-i-o-jen'ik). Relating to karyogenesis; forming the nucleus.

**karyogonad** (kar-i-o-go'nad) [ karyo- + G. *gone,* generation, descent ]. Micronucleus (2).

**karyogram** (kar'i-o-gram). Karyotype.

**karyokinesis** (kar'i-o-ki-ne'sis) [ karyo- + G. *kinesis,* movement ]. Mitosis.

**kar'yokinet'ic.** Mitotic.

**karyolymph** (kar'i-o-limf) [ karyo- + L. *lympha,* clear water ]. Nuclear sap; the fluid substance contained in the meshes of the linin network of the nucleus.

**karyolysis** (kar'i-ol'i-sis) [ karyo- + G. *lysis,* dissolution ]. Apparent destruction of the nucleus of a cell by swelling and the loss of affinity of its chromatin for basic dyes.

**karyolytic** (kar'i-o-lit'ik). Relating to karyolysis.

**karyomicrosome** (kăr-ĭ-o-mi′kro-sōm) [ karyo- + G. *mikros*, small, + *soma*, body ]. Nucleomicrosome; one of the minute particles or granules making up the substance of the cell nucleus.

**karyomitosis** (kăr′ĭ-o-mi-to′sis). Mitosis.

**kar′yomitot′ic.** Mitotic.;

**karyomorphism** (kăr′ĭ-o-mor′fizm) [ karyo- + G. *morphe*, form ]. 1. Development of the nucleus of a cell. 2. Denoting the nuclear shapes of the cells, especially of the leukocytes.

**karyon** (kăr′ĭ-on) [ G. *karyon*, a nut, kernel ]. Nucleus (1).

**karyophage** (kăr′ĭ-o-fāj) [ karyo- + G. *phagein*, to devour ]. An intracellular protozoan parasite.

**karyoplasm** (kăr′ĭ-o-plazm). Rarely used synonym for nucleoplasm.

**karyoplasmolysis** (kăr′ĭ-o-plaz-mol′ĭ-sis). Achromatolysis.

**karyoplastin** (kăr′ĭ-o-plas′tin). Obsolete term for the achromatic nuclear substance from which it was believed that mitotic spindle fibers arise.

**karyopyknosis** (kăr′ĭ-o-pik-no′sis) [ karyo- + G. *pyknos*, thick, crowded, + suffix *-osis*, condition ]. Cytologic characteristics of the superficial or cornified cells of stratified squamous epithelium in which there is shrinkage of the nuclei and condensation of the chromatin into structureless masses.

**karyorrhexis** (kăr-ĭ-o-rek′sis) [ karyo- + G. *rhexis*, rupture ]. Karyoclasia; fragmentation of the nucleus whereby its chromatin is distributed irregularly throughout the cytoplasm; a stage of necrosis usually followed by karyolysis.

**karyosome** (kăr′ĭ-o-sōm) [ karyo- + G. *sōma*, body ]. A mass of chromatin often found in the interphase cell nucleus representing a more condensed zone of chromatin filaments. Also called chromocenter, chromatin nucleolus, false nucleolus.

**karyostasis** (kăr′ĭ-os′tă-sis) [ karyo- + G. *stasis*, a standing still ]. Interphase.

**karyotheca** (kăr-ĭ-o-the′kah) [ karyo- + G. *thēkē*, box, sheath ]. Nuclear *envelope*.

**karyotype** (kăr′ĭ-o-tip). The chromosome characteristics of an individual or of a cell line, usually presented as a systematized array of metaphase chromosomes from a photomicrograph of a single cell nucleus arranged in pairs in descending order of size and according to the position of the centromere.

**kar′yotyp′ing.** Chromosome analysis.

**karyozoic** (kăr′ĭ-o-zo′ik) [ karyo- + G. *zōon*, animal ]. Denoting a protozoan parasite inhabiting the cell nucleus of its host.

**Kasabach,** Haig H. See K.-Merritt *syndrome.*

**kasai′.** A form of anemia occurring in natives of the Belgian Congo, with associated edema of subcutaneous tissues, depigmented regions in the skin, and various gastrointestinal disturbances; thought to result from deficiencies in nutrition. Termed also Belgian Congo anemia.

**Kashin,** N. I., Russian orthopaedist, 1825–1872. See K.-Bek *disease.*

**kata-** (kat′ah-) [ G. *kata*, down ]. Alternative spelling for cata-, combining form meaning down. For many words beginning with kata- and not found here, see also cata-.;

**kat′achro′masis.** Obsolete term for telophase.

**katathermometer** (kat′ah-ther-mom′e-ter). Psychrometer.

**kathisophobia** (kath′ĭ-so-fo′bĭ-ah) [ G. *kathisis*, a sitting, + *phobos*, fear ]. Morbid fear of sitting down.

**kath′odal, kath′ode.** Abbreviated Ka; obsolete alternative spelling for cathodal, cathode.

**Kathrein′s test.** See under test.

**kat′ion.** Cation.

**Katz,** Bernard, English neurophysiologist, *1911. Nobel laureate, 1970, with Ulf von Euler and Julius Axelrod for their work on humoral transmitter substances and mechanisms at nerve terminals. See Goldman-Hodgkin-K. *equation.*

**kat′zenjam′mer** [ Ger. *Katzenjammer*, headache on morrow of carousal ]. Hangover.

**Kaufmann′s stain for capsules.** See under stain.

**kava** (kah′vah) [ Hawaiian name ]. 1. Methysticum. 2. Yaqona.

**kavaine** (kah-vah-ēn). Methysticine; an alkaloid from the kava root.

**Kay,** Herbert D., English biochemist, *1893. See Jenner-K. *unit.*

**Kayser** (ki′ser), Bernhard, German physician, 1869–1954. See K.-Fleischer *ring.*

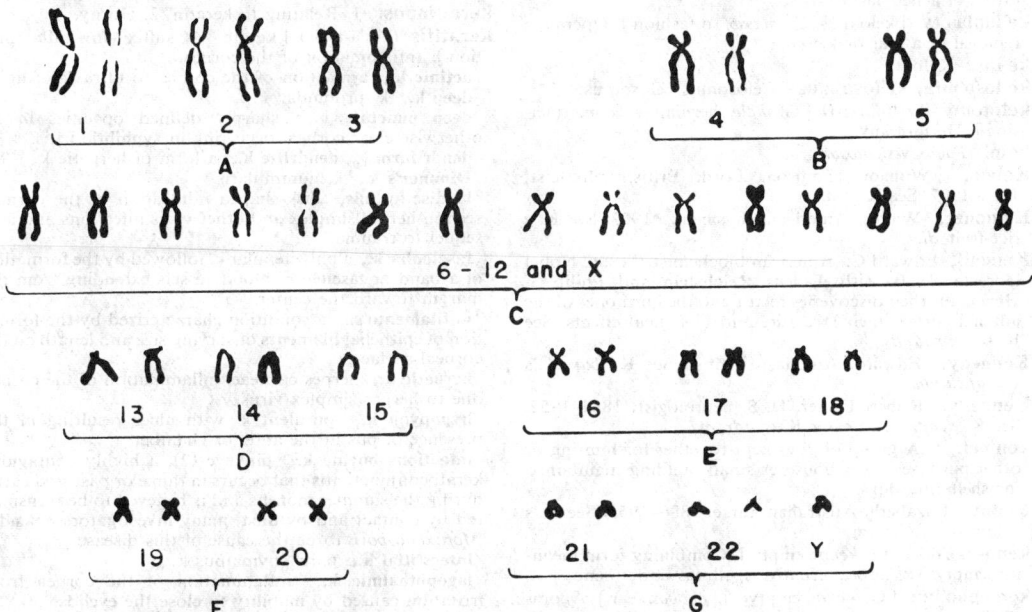

**Karyotype of Normal Male (Human)**
Chromosomes are numbered by pairs, and letters indicate groups of similar morphology. (Courtesy of Dr. H. O. Goodman.)

**Keating-Hart,** Walter V., French physician, 1870–1922. See K.-H. *method.*

**ked.** The sheep ked, *Melophagus ovinus.*

**keel** (kēl). Paratyphoid or salmonellosis of ducklings.

**Keeley,** Leslie E., U. S. physician, 1832–1900. See K. *cure.*

**Keen,** William W., Philadelphia surgeon, 1837–1932. See K.'s *operation, sign.*

**Kehr,** Hans, German surgeon, 1862–1916. See K.'s *incision, sign.*

**keirospasm** (ki'ro-spazm) [ G. *keirō,* to shear ]. Shaving cramp.

**Keith,** Sir Arthur, London anatomist, 1866–1955. See K.'s *bundle,* K. and Flack *node,* K.'s *node.*

**kelectome** (ke'lek-tōm) [ G. *kēlē,* tumor, + *ektomē,* excision ]. An instrument used, like the harpoon, to remove a specimen of tumor substance for examination.

**ke'lis** [ G. *kēlis,* a stain, spot, blemish ]. 1. Morphea; a term sometimes used for localized or circumscribed forms of scleroderma. 2. Keloid.

**Kell blood group.** See appendix 2, Blood Groups.

**Kellie,** George, Scottish anatomist, 18th century. See Monro-K. *doctrine.*

**Kelling,** Georg, German physician, *1866. See K.'s *test.*

**Kelly,** Howard A., American gynecologist, 1858–1943. See K.'s *operation,* rectal *speculum.*

**ke'loid** [ G. *kēlē,* a tumor (or *kēlis,* a spot), + *eidos,* appearance ]. A nodular, frequently lobulated, unusually firm, movable, nonencapsulated, generally linear mass of hyperplastic scar tissue, consisting of relatively large and fairly parallel bands of densely collagenous material separated by irregular bands of cellular fibrous tissue; k.'s occur in the dermis and adjacent subcutaneous tissue, usually after a traumatic injury or a burn, more common in non-Caucasians, and frequently recur in the site after surgical removal.

  **acne k.,** a chronic eruption of fibrous papules which develop at the site of follicular lesions, usually on the back of the neck at the hairline. Also called dermatitis papillaris capilliti; folliculitis keloidalis; sycosis framboesiformis; sycosis nuchae necrotisans.

  **Addison's k.,** morphea.

**ke'loido'sis.** Multiple keloids.

**kelo'ma.** Keloid, especially one that has the gross configuration of a neoplasm.

**ke'loplas'ty** [ keloid + G. *plassō,* to fashion ]. Operative removal of a scar or keloid.

**ke'los.** Keloid.

**ke'loso'mia, ke'loso'mus.** Celosomia, celosomus.

**kelotomy** (ke-lot'o-mī) [ G. *kēlē,* hernia, + *tomē,* incision ]. Herniotomy.

**kelp.** *Fucus vesiculosus.*

**Kelvin,** William Thomson, Lord, British physicist, 1824–1907. See K. *scale.*

**Kempner,** Walter, American physician, *1903. See K.'s rice-fruit *diet.*

**Kendall,** Edward C., American biochemist, *1886. Nobel laureate, 1950, with Tadeus Reichstein and Philip S. Hench, for their discoveries relating to the hormones of the adrenal cortex, their structure and biological effects. See K.'s *compounds.*

**Kennedy,** Edward, American dentist. See K. *bar,* K.'s *classification.*

**Kennedy,** Robert Foster, U. S. neurologist, 1884–1952. See K. *syndrome,* Foster K. *syndrome.*

**ken'nel.** 1. A group of dogs kept together for hunting or other purposes. 2. A house or small building maintained for sheltering dogs.

**Kenny,** Elizabeth, Australian nurse, 1886–1952. See K.'s *treatment.*

**keno-** (ke'no-) [ G. *kenos,* empty ]. Combining form meaning empty; see also alternative spellings under ceno-.

**ken'opho'bia** [ G. *kenos,* empty, + *phobos,* fear ]. Agoraphobia.

**kenotoxin** (ken-o-tok'sin) [ G. *kenos,* empty, exhausted, + *toxicon,* poison ]. Cenotoxin; the "toxin of fatigue"; a hypothetical substance thought to be formed in tissues (especially muscle) as the result of prolonged activity, and presumed to cause (1) the signs and symptoms of fatigue and (2) sleep.

**Kent,** Albert F. Stanley, English physiologist, 1863–1958. See K.'s *bundle,* K.-His *bundle.*

**keph'alin.** Cephalin.

**keph'rine hydrochloride.** Adrenalone.

**Kerandel** (ker-an-del'), Jean F., French physician, *1873. See K.'s *symptom.*

**keraphyllocele** (kĕr-ă-fil'o-sēl) [ G. *keras,* horn, + *phyllon,* leaf, + *kēlē,* hernia, tumor ]. A horn tumor on the internal face of the wall of a horse's foot.

**ker'asin.** Cerasin; a cerebroside found in brain tissue associated with phrenosin and sphingomyelin; it contains lignoceric acid as its characteristic fatty acid; sphingosine and galactose are the other hydrolysis products.

**kerat-.** See kerato-.

**keratectasia** (kĕr-ă-tek-ta'zī-ah) [ kerato- + G. *ektasis,* extrusion. CERAT- ]. Protrusion of the cornea due to pathological weakening of corneal tissue.

**keratec'tomy** [ kerato- + G. *ektomē,* excision ]. Excision of a portion of the cornea.

**keratein** (kĕr'ă-te-in). The reduction product of keratin, in which the disulfide links are reduced to SH groups, the individual peptide chains separated. Differs from keratin, too, in being easily digested.

**keratiasis** (kĕr'ă-ti'ă-sis). Cutaneous warty growths.

**kerat'ic** [ G. *keras* (*kerat-*), horn ]. Horny.

**ker'atin.** Ceratin; a scleroprotein or albuminoid present largely in cuticular structures such as hair, nails, horns, etc.; it contains a relatively large amount of sulfur (human hair is 14 per cent cystine). It is insoluble in the gastric juices and is sometimes used for coating enteric pills that are intended to be dissolved only in the intestine.

**α-keratin.** Keratin in a folded configuration (as in normal hair).

**β-keratin.** Keratin in its extended configuration (as in stretched hair).

**ker'atinases.** Hydrolases (EC 3.4.99.11 and .12) catalyzing the hydrolysis of keratin.

**ker'atiniza'tion.** Cornification; keratin formation or development of horny layer; may also apply to premature formation of keratin.

**ker'atinized.** Cornified; having become horny.

**kerat'inous.** 1. Relating to keratin. 2. Horny.

**keratitis** (kĕr'ă-ti'tis) [ kerato- + suffix -*itis,* inflammation ]. Inflammation of the cornea.

  **actinic k.,** a reaction of the cornea to ultraviolet light.

  **deep k.,** k. profunda.

  **deep punctate k.,** sharply defined opacities in an otherwise clear cornea, occurring in syphilitic iritis.

  **dendriform k., dendritic k.,** a form of herpetic k.

  **Dimmer's k.,** k. nummularis.

  **k. discifor'mis,** disk-shaped infiltration of the cornea, seen in herpes simplex and other virus infections and as a sequel to trauma.

  **fascicular k.,** a phlyctenular k. followed by the formation of a band or fascicle of blood vessels extending from the margin toward the center.

  **k. filamento'sa,** a condition characterized by the formation of epithelial filaments of varying size and length on the corneal surface.

  **herpetic k.,** herpes corneae; inflammation of the cornea due to herpes simplex virus.

  **hypopyon k.,** purulent k. with ulcer resulting in the presence of pus in the anterior chamber.

  **infectious bovine k.,** pinkeye (2); a highly contagious keratoconjunctivitis that occurs in range or pastured cattle during the summer months and is believed to be transmitted by contact and by dust; many investigators consider *Moraxella bovis* to be the cause of this disease.

  **interstitial k.,** parenchymatous k.

  **lagophthalmic k.,** inflammation of the cornea from irritation caused by inability to close the eyelids.

  **marginal k.,** phlyctenular conjunctivitis occurring at the sclerocorneal junction.

  **mycotic k.,** an infection of the cornea of the eye, following trauma or treatment of other corneal lesions with steroid or antibiotic drugs, caused by saprophytic fungi including species of *Aspergillus, Cephalosporium, Curvularia, Fusarium,* and *Penicillium.*

**necrogranulomatous k.,** k. characterized by the formation of necrotizing granulomas; an occasional complication of rheumatoid arthritis or Wegener's granulomatosis.

**neuroparalytic k.,** ulceration of the cornea occurring with trigeminal paralysis.

**k. nummula′ris,** Dimmer's k.; coin-shaped or round, discrete, grayish areas 0.5 to 1.5 mm. in diameter scattered throughout the various layers of the cornea.

**parenchymatous k.,** interstitial k.; a chronic inflammation, with cellular infiltration of the middle and posterior layers of the cornea.

**phlyctenular k.,** scrofulous k.; an inflammation of the corneal conjunctiva with the formation of small red nodules of lymphoid tissue (phlyctenulae) near the limbus.

**k. profun′da,** deep k.; a deep-seated inflammation of the cornea, accompanied with more or less opacity, of benign course; probably an allergic reaction to a chronic infection.

**punctate k., k. puncta′ta,** keratic *precipitates;* see also deep punctate k. and superficial punctate k.

**k. pustulifor′mis profun′da,** k. characterized by circumscribed infiltration of a yellowish color in the deep layers of the cornea without any lesion of the epithelium, accompanied by hypopyon and iritis and a positive serologic reaction.

**reaper's k.,** traumatic k. due to a wound by a spicule of rye or other grain inflicted while harvesting.

**sclerosing k.,** inflammation of the cornea complicating scleritis; characterized by opacification of corneal stroma.

**scrofulous k.,** phlyctenular k.

**serpiginous k.,** a severe, creeping, central, suppurative ulcer usually due to pneumococci; also called ulcus serpens corneae; serpent ulcer of cornea; pneumococcus ulcer.

**superficial punctate k.,** epithelial punctate k. associated with viral conjunctivitis; occasionally may follow exposure to ultraviolet light.

**trachomatous k.,** vascular k. at upper limbus, resulting in pannus.

**vascular k.,** superficial infiltration of the cornea and roughness of the epithelial layer accompanied by a development of blood vessels between Bowman's membrane and the epithelial layer; when pronounced it gives rise to pannus.

**vasculonebulous k.,** rarely used synonym for pannus.

**vesicular k.,** inflammation or degeneration of the cornea with the formation of numerous small vesicles on the surface.

**xerotic k.,** keratomalacia.

**kerato-, kerat-** (kĕr′ă-to-) [ G. *keras,* horn. CERAT- ]. Combining forms denoting (1) the cornea, or (2) horny tissue or cells. For some terms not listed here, see also cerato-.

**keratoacanthoma** (kĕr′ă-to-ak′an-tho′mah). Molluscum pseudocarcinomatosum; molluscum sebaceum; a rapidly growing tumor which may be umbilicated, usually occurring on exposed areas of the skin. Microscopically, the nodule is composed of well differentiated squamous epithelium with a central keratin mass that opens on the skin surface. The lesion invades the dermis, but remains localized and resolves spontaneously if untreated.

**keratoangioma** (kĕr′ă-to-an′jī-o-mah). Angiokeratoma.

**keratoatrophoderma** (kĕr′ă-to-at′ro-fo-der′mah) [ kerato- + G. *atrophia,* atrophy, + *derma,* skin ]. Porokeratosis.

**keratocele** (kĕr′ă-to-sēl) [ kerato- + G. *kēlē,* hernia ]. Hernia of Descemet's membrane through a defect in the outer layer of the cornea.

**keratocentesis** (kĕr′ă-to-sen-te′sis) [ kerato- + G. *kentēsis,* puncture ]. Obsolete term for paracentesis of the cornea.

**keratochromatosis** (kĕr′ă-to-kro-mă-to′sis) [ kerato- + G. *chroma,* color, + suffix *-osis,* condition ]. Discoloration of the cornea.

**keratochromomycosis** (kĕr′ă-to-kro-mo-mi-ko′sis) [ kerato- + G. *chrōma,* color, + *mykēs,* fungus, + suffix *-osis,* condition ]. Corneal ulcer caused by the fungus *Phialophora verrucosa.*

**keratoconjunctivitis** (kĕr′ă-to-kon-jungk′tĭ-vi′tis). Inflammation of the conjunctiva at the border of the cornea.

**epidemic k.,** virus k.; rapidly developing follicular conjunctivitis with marked inflammatory symptoms but a scanty exudate. Corneal subepithelial infiltrations appear 7 to 10 days after the inflammation begins. Caused by adenovirus, usually type 8 and less commonly type 7.

**flash k.,** acute k. caused by intense ultraviolet irradiation, *e.g.,* by exposure of the eyes to a mercury arc lamp.

**k. sicca,** k. associated with lacrimal deficiency; see also Sjögren's *syndrome.*

**superior limbic k.,** a distinct entity, the essential of which is inflammatory edema of the central area of the superior limbus with upward extension, usually bilateral and distinguished by spontaneous sudden resolution or recurrence.

**virus k.,** epidemic k.

**keratoconometer** (kĕr′ă-to-ko-nom′e-ter) [ kerato- + G. *kōnos,* cone, + *metron,* measure ]. An instrument for measuring the degree of keratoconus.

**keratoconus** (kĕr′ă-to-ko′nus) [ kerato- + G. *kōnos,* cone ]. Conical cornea; a conical protrusion of the center of the cornea due to noninflammatory thinning of the stroma; usually bilateral. See also Fleischer's *ring;* Munson's *sign.*

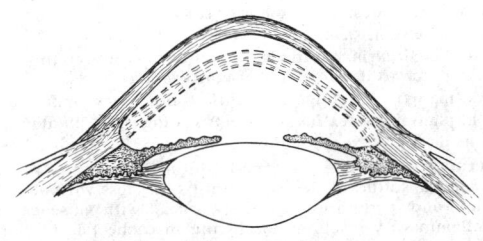

Keratoconus

**keratocricoid.** (kĕr′ă-to-kri′koyd). Ceratocricoid.

**keratoderma** (kĕr′ă-to-der′mah) [ kerato- + G. *derma,* skin ]. 1. Any horny superficial growth. 2. A more or less generalized thickening of the horny layer of the epidermis.

**k. blennorrhag′ica,** *keratosis* blennorrhagica.

**k. eccen′trica,** porokeratosis.

**lymphedematous k.,** mossy *foot.*

**k. palma′ris et planta′ris,** k. symmetrica; the occurrence of symmetrical diffuse or patchy patches of hypertrophy of the horny layer of the epidermis on the palms and soles; an inherited ectodermal dysplasia of considerable variety and of either autosomal dominant or recessive genes.

**k. planta′re sulca′tum,** cracked heel; hyperkeratosis and fissure formation on the soles.

**k. symmet′rica,** k. palmaris et plantaris.

**ker′atodermati′tis** [ kerato- + G. *derma,* skin, + suffix *-itis,* inflammation ]. Inflammation with proliferation of the horny layer of the skin.

**keratoectasia** (kĕr′ă-to-ek-ta′zĭ-ah). Keratectasia.

**ker′atogen′esis** [ kerato- + G. *genesis,* production ]. The production or origin of horny cells or tissue.

**ker′atogenet′ic.** Relating to keratogenesis.

**keratogenous** (kĕr′ă-toj′ĕ-nus). Causing a growth of cells that produce keratin and result in the formation of horny tissue, such as fingernails, scales, feathers, and so on.

**ker′atoglo′bus** [ kerato- + L. *globus,* ball ]. Anterior *megalophthalmus.*

**ker′atoglos′sus.** *Musculus* chondroglossus.

**keratohelcosis** (kĕr′ă-to-hel-ko′sis) [ kerato- + G. *helkōsis,* ulceration ]. Rarely used term meaning ulceration of the cornea.

**ker′atohe′mia** [ kerato- + G. *haima,* blood ]. A disklike collection of blood in the cornea.

**ker′atohy′al.** Ceratohyal.

**keratohyalin** (kĕr′ă-to-hi′ă-lin) [ kerato- + hyalin, *q.v.* ]. The substance in the granules of the stratum granulosum of the epidermis.

**ker′atoid** [ kerato- + G. *eidos,* resemblance ]. Horny; corneous; resembling corneal tissue.

**keratoiritis** (kĕr′ă-to-i-ri′tis) [ kerato- + G. *iris,* iris, + suffix *-itis,* inflammation ]. Inflammation of both cornea and iris.

**hypopyon k.,** suppurative inflammation of the cornea and iris complicated with hypopyon.

**keratoleptynsis** (kĕr′ă-to-lep-tin′sis) [ kerato- + G. *leptynsis,* a making thin. LEP- ]. 1. Gutter dystrophy of the cornea; see under dystrophy. 2. An operation for removing the surface of the cornea and replacement by bulbar conjunctiva for cosmetic reasons.

**keratoleukoma** (kĕr′ă-to-lu-ko′mah) [ kerato- + G. *leukos,* white, + suffix -*ōma,* growth ]. A white corneal opacity.

**keratolysis** (kĕr′ă-tol′ĭ-sis) [ kerato- + G. *lysis,* loosening ]. 1. Separation or loosening of the horny layer of the epidermis. 2. Deciduous skin; specifically, a disease characterized by a shedding of the epidermis recurring at more or less regular intervals.

**k. exfoliati′va,** erythema exfoliativa; erythroderma exfoliativa; a separation of stratum corneum in leaflike flakes on the palms and soles; the cause is unknown.

**k. neonato′rum,** *dermatitis* exfoliativa infantum.

**ker′atolyt′ic.** Relating to keratolysis; desquamative.

**keratoma** (kĕr′ă-to′mah) [ kerato- + G. suffix -*oma,* tumor ]. 1. Callosity. 2. A horny tumor.

**k. diffu′sum,** *ichthyosis* vulgaris.

**k. heredita′ria mu′tilans,** spontaneous amputation of digits due to development of constricting bands.

**k. malig′num,** congenital ichthyosiform *erythroderma.*

**k. planta′re sulca′tum,** *keratosis* palmaris et plantaris.

**senile k.,** *keratosis* senilis.

**keratomalacia** (kĕr′ă-to-mă-la′shĭ-ah) [ kerato- + G. *malakia,* softness ]. Xerotic keratitis; dryness with ulceration and perforation of the cornea, with absence of inflammatory reactions, occurring in cachectic children; results from severe vitamin A deficiency or debilitating disease.

**ker′atome.** Keratotome.

**keratom′eter** [ kerato- + G. *metron,* measure ]. Ophthalmometer; an instrument for measuring the anterior curvature of the corneal surface through observation of the reflective images.

**keratom′etry.** Ophthalmometry; measurement of the degrees of corneal curvature in the principal meridians.

**keratomileusis** (kĕr′ah-to-mi-lu′sis) [ coined by José I. Barraquer, Bogota, who developed the technique, from G. *keras*(*kerat-*), horn, cornea, + *smileusis,* carving ]. Corneal shaping; the shaving off of a sliver of stroma from the underside of a lamellar piece of cornea in order to modify the refractive power of the cornea. A lathe is used to tool the cornea before it is replaced on the eye.

**keratomycosis** (kĕr′ă-to-mi-ko′sis). Disease of the cornea due to the presence of a fungous growth.

**keratonosis** (kĕr′ă-to-no′sis) [ kerato- + G. suffix -*osis,* condition ]. Any abnormal noninflammatory, usually hypertrophic, affection of the horny layer of the skin.

**keratopachyderma** (ker′ă-to-pak-ĭ-der′mah) [ kerato- + G. *pachys,* thick, + *derma,* skin ]. A syndrome of congenital deafness with development of hyperkeratosis of the skin of the palms, soles, elbows, and knees in childhood, and with bandlike constructions of the fingers; autosomal dominant inheritance.

**keratopathy** (kĕr′ă-top′ă-thĭ) [ kerato- + G. *pathos,* suffering, disease ]. A noninflammatory dystrophy of the cornea, as distinguished from keratitis.

**band-shaped k.,** a horizontal, gray, interpalpebral opacity of the cornea, slowly progressing from the limbus; it occurs in hypercalcemia, chronic iridocyclitis, and Still's disease.

**bullous k.,** the formation of large subepithelial bullae in corneal edema, resulting in intense pain when their rupture exposes corneal nerves; it occurs in Fuch's epithelial dystrophy and in advanced stages of glaucoma and iridocyclitis.

**climatic k.,** a bilateral symmetrical corneal dystrophy caused by prolonged exposure to extremes of heat or cold; nodular opacities are limited to the interpalpebral area and vision is only mildly affected.

**discrete colliquative k.,** a softening at the corneal limbus, which perforates outward; seen in young children whose diet consists chiefly of maize.

**striate k.,** edema of the corneal stroma, showing radial tracts; caused by aqueous humor percolating through a damaged endothelium.

**ker′atoplasty** [ kerato- + G. *plassō,* to form ]. Trephining of the cornea; corneal grafting; the removal of a portion of the cornea containing an opacity and the insertion in its place of a piece of the same size and shape removed from elsewhere.

**lamellar k.,** tectonic k. in which only a partial thickness of the donor cornea is used.

**optic k.,** transplantation of transparent corneal tissue to replace a leukoma or scar that obstructs vision.

**tecton′ic k.,** grafting of corneal material on a part where it has been lost, without attempt to restore the transparency.

**ker′atoprosthe′sis** [ kerato- + G. *prosthesis,* addition ]. Replacement of central area of opacified cornea by acrylic plastic.

**keratorhexis, keratorrhexis** (kĕr′ă-to-rek′sis) [ kerato- + G. *rhexis,* a bursting ]. Rupture of the cornea, due to trauma or perforating ulcer.

**keratoscleritis** (kĕr′ă-to-skle-ri′tis). Inflammation of both cornea and sclera.

**ker′atoscope** [ kerato- + G. *skopeō,* to examine ]. Placido's disk; an instrument marked with lines or circles by means of which the corneal reflex can be observed.

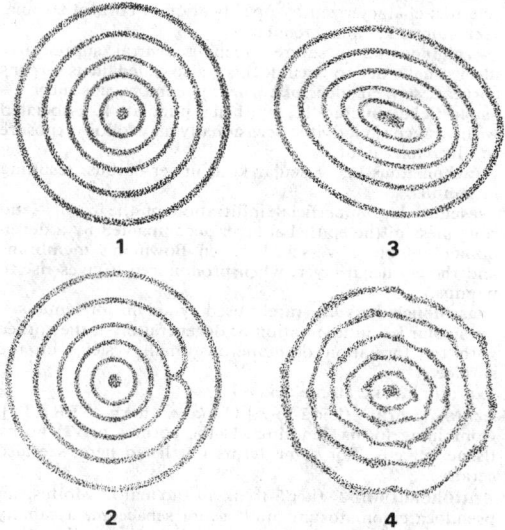

**1**      **3**

**2**      **4**

**Reflections from the Cornea as Seen through a Keratoscope**

*1,* Normal; *2,* foreign body in cornea; *3,* regular astigmatism; *4,* irregular astigmatism.

**keratoscopy** (kĕr′ă-tos′ko-pĭ) [ kerato- + G. *skopeō,* to examine ]. 1. Examination of the reflections from the anterior surface of the cornea in order to determine the character and amount of corneal astigmatism. 2. A term first applied by Cuignet to his method of retinoscopy.

**keratose** (kĕr′ă-tōs). Horny; relating to or marked by keratosis.

**keratosis** (kĕr′ă-to′sis) [ kerato- + G. suffix -*osis,* condition ]. Any lesion on the epidermis marked by the presence of circumscribed overgrowths of the horny layer.

**actinic k.,** k. senilis.

**arsenical k.,** multiple keratoses, most commonly of the palms and soles but also of the fingers and proximal portions of the extremities, resulting from long-term arsenic intoxication; arsenical keratoses may become malignant.

**k. blennorrhag′ica,** keratoderma blennorrhagica; pustules and crusts associated with Reiter's disease; at one time incorrectly believed to be due to gonorrhea.

**k. diffu'sa feta'lis,** *ichthyosis* vulgaris.

**k. follicula'ris,** Darier's or White's disease; k. vegetans; a familial eruption in which keratotic papules develop progressively from childhood, originating from both follicles and intrafollicular epidermis.

**k. follicula'ris contagio'sa,** Brooke's disease (2); a rare condition simulating k. follicularis.

**k. labia'lis,** thickening of stratum corneum on the lips.

**k. ni'gricans,** *acanthosis* nigricans.

**k. obtu'rans,** laminated epithelial plug; an accretion of epithelia in the external auditory canal.

**k. palma'ris et planta'ris,** ichthyosis palmaris et plantaris; keratoma plantare sulcatum; tylosis palmaris et plantaris; a congenital symmetrical k. of the palms and soles.

**k. punctata,** a condition of unknown origin characterized by development of punctate hyperkeratotic lesions on the palms and soles.

**k. ru'bra figura'ta,** *erythrokeratoderma* variabilis.

**seborrheic k., k. seborrhe'ica,** seborrheic wart or verruca; superficial, benign, verrucous lesions consisting of proliferating epidermal cells, especially of basal type, enclosing horn cysts. They usually occur after the third decade, and may be few or numerous.

**senile k., k. seni'lis,** a dyskeratotic (premalignant) warty lesion occurring on the sun-exposed skin of face or hands in aged, light-skinned persons; also called actinic or solar k.; senile keratoma or wart; acanthosis verrucosa; verruca senilis; verruca plana senilis.

**solar k., k. senilis.**

**k. vegetans, k. follicularis.**

**ker'atosul'fate.** A sulfated mucopolysaccharide containing D-galactose in place of the usual uronic acid; found in cartilage, bone, connective tissue, and the cornea.

**ker'atotome.** Keratome; a knife used for incising the cornea.

**keratotomy** (kĕr'ă-tot'o-mĭ) [ kerato- + G. *tomē*, incision ]. Incision through the cornea.

**delimiting k.,** Gifford's operation; incision in the cornea along the margin of an advancing ulcer.

**keraunoneurosis** (kĕ-raw'no-nu-ro'sis) [ G. *keraunos,* thunderbolt, + neurosis ]. A neurosis excited by a stroke of lightning or resulting from fright caused by a thunder storm.

**keraunophobia** (kĕ-raw''no-fo'bĭ-ah) [ G. *keraunos,* thunderbolt, + *phobos,* fear ]. Morbid fear of thunder and lightning.

**Kerckring** (Kerckringius), Theodor, Dutch anatomist, 1640–1693. See K.'s *center, folds, ossicle, valves.*

**ke'rion** [ G. *kērion,* honeycomb; a skin disease, fr. *kēros,* beeswax ]. A granulomatous secondarily infected lesion complicating fungal infection of the hair.

**Celsus' k.,** *tinea* kerion.

**Kerley,** Peter J., English radiologist, *1900. See B *lines* of K.

**kernicterus** (kärn-ik'ter-us) [ Ger. *kern,* kernel (nucleus), + *ikterus,* jaundice ]. Nuclear jaundice; a grave form of icterus neonatorum in which a yellow pigment and degenerative lesions are found in the lenticular nucleus, subthalamus, Ammon's horn, and other areas of intracranial gray matter.

**Kernig,** Vladimir, Russian physician, 1840–1917. See K.'s *sign.*

**Kernohan,** J. W., U. S. pathologist, *1897. See K.'s *notch.*

**keroid** (kĕr'oyd) [ G. *keroeidēs,* horn-like ]. Keratoid; horny.

**kerosene** (kĕr'o-sēn). A mixture of petroleum hydrocarbons, chiefly of the methane series; the fifth fraction in the distillation of petroleum. K. is used as fuel for lamps and stoves; as a degreaser and cleaner; and in insecticides. Contact on human skin can lead to irritation and infection; inhalation may cause headache, drowsiness, coma; swallowing causes irritation, vomiting, and diarrhea. Vomiting should not be induced, as aspiration of vomitus causes pneumonitis.

**kerotherapy** (ke-ro-thĕr'ă-pĭ) [ G. *kēros,* wax, + *therapeia,* treatment ]. Treatment of burns and denuded surfaces with wax or paraffin preparations.

**Kerr,** Harry Hyland, U. S. surgeon, *1881. See Parker-K. *suture.*

**ke'tal.** $R_2C(OR')_2$; a hydrated ketone in which both hydroxyl groups are esterified with alcohols.

**ket'amine hydrochloride** (NF). KETALAR; KETAJECT; DL-2-(o-chlorophenyl)-2-(methylamino)cyclohexanone hydrochloride; a parenterally administered anesthetic characterized by catatonia, profound analgesia, increased sympathetic activity, and little relaxation of skeletal muscles; side effects include sialorrhea and occasional pronounced dysphoria, especially in adults.

**ke'tene.** $CH_2=C=O$; a very reactive acetylating agent, used in chemical synthesis.

**kethox'al** (USAN). 3-Ethoxy-1,1-dihydroxy-2-butanone; an antiviral agent.

**ke'to-.** Combining form used with reference to any compound containing a ketone group.

**ke'to acid.** An acid with the general formula R—CO—COOH.

**3-ketoacid-CoA transferase.** Acetoacetyl-succinic thiophorase; enzyme (EC 2.8.3.5) catalyzing the conversion of acetoacetyl-CoA and succinate into succinyl-CoA and acetoacetate. Malonyl-CoA can substitute for succinyl-CoA and other 3-oxo acids for the acetoacetate.

**ketoacidosis** (ke'to-as'ĭ-do'sis). Acidosis, *e.g.,* diabetic acidosis, caused by the enhanced production of ketone bodies.

**ketoaciduria** (ke'to-as'ĭ-du'rĭ-ah). Excretion of urine having an elevated content of ketonic acids.

**branched chain k.,** maple syrup urine *disease.*

**β-ke'toac'yl-ACP reductase.** 3-Oxoacyl-ACP reductase.

**β-ketoacyl-ACP synthetase.** 3-Oxoacyl-ACP synthase.

**3-ketoacyl-CoA thiolase.** Acetyl-CoA acyltransferase.

**ketobem'idone.** CYMIDON; 1-[ 4-(*m*-hydroxyphenyl)-1-methyl-4-piperidyl ]-1-propanone; analgesic with narcotic properties.

**α-ke'todecarbox'ylase.** Formerly the enzyme system converting pyruvate (a 2-oxoacid) to acetyl-CoA and $CO_2$, with reduction of $NAD^+$ to NADH and the participation of lipoamide and thiamin pyrophosphate. Now known to involve at least three enzymes in succession, pyruvate dehydrogenase, lipoate acetyltransferase, and lipoamide dehydrogenase.

**ketogenesis** (ke-to-jen'e-sis). Production of acetone or other ketones.

**α-ke'toglutar'ic dehydrogenase.** 2-Oxoglutarate dehydrogenase.

**ke'tohep'tose.** A seven-carbon sugar possessing a ketone group; a heptulose.

**2-ke'tohex'ose.** Fructose.

**β-ketohydrogenase** (ke'to-hi'dro-jen-ās). 3-Hydroxyacyl-CoA dehydrogenase.

**ke'tohydrox'yes'trin.** Estrone.

**ke'tol.** An α-ketol has a carbonyl (CO) group adjacent (α) to an alcoholic (OH) group in the chain.

**ke'tole.** Indole.

**k. group,** carbons 1 and 2 of a 2-ketose (HOCH$_2$CO—); transfer of this group (transketolation) from D-xylulose 5'-phosphate to C-1 of aldoses is of importance in various metabolic pathways involving carbohydrates; *e.g.,* in photosynthesis and in the Dickens shunt. The two-carbon unit is transferred as α,β-dihydroxyethyl thiamin pyrophosphate.

**ketolytic** (ke-to-lit'ik). Causing the dissolution of ketone or acetone substances, referring usually to oxidation products of glucose and allied substances.

**ke'tone.** A substance with the group —CO— linking two carbon atoms; there are a number of k.'s, the most important in medicine and the simplest in chemistry being dimethylketone, or acetone.

**k. alcohol,** a compound containing a carbonyl or ketone group (—CO—) as well as a hydroxyl group; *e.g.,* dihydroxyacetone, $HOCH_2$—CO—$CH_2OH$.

**k. body,** acetone body; one of a group of ketones, including acetoacetic acid, its reduction product, β-hydroxybutyric acid, and its decarboxylation product, acetone; high in tissues and body fluids in ketosis.

**ketone-aldehyde mutase.** Lactoyl-glutathione lyase.

**ketonemia** (ke-to-ne′mĭ-ah) [ ketone + G. *haima,* blood ]. The presence of recognizable concentrations of ketone bodies in the plasma.

**keto′nic.** Pertaining to, or possessing the characteristics of, a ketone.

**ke′toniza′tion.** Conversion into a ketone.

**ketonuria** (ke-to-nu′rĭ-ah). Enhanced urinary excretion of ketone bodies.

**ke′topanto′ic acid.** Oxidized precursor of pantoic acid, intermediate on the synthetic pathway between α-ketoiso-valeric acid and pantothenic acid.

**ke′topen′tose.** A five-carbon sugar in which carbons 2,3 or 4 make up part of a carbonyl group; *e.g.,* ribulose.

**ketophenylbu′tazone.** CHEBUTAN; 4-(3-oxobutyl)-1,2-di-phenyl-3,5-pyrazolidinedione; antirheumatic agent.

**β-ketoreductase.** 3-Hydroxyacyl-CoA dehydrogenase.

**ke′tose.** A carbohydrate containing the characterizing group of the ketones (—CO—); the most important is the ketohexose, fructose.

**ketose-1-phosphate aldolase.** Fructose bisphosphate aldolase.

**ketose reductase** (EC 1.1.1.140). D-Sorbitol-6-phosphate dehydrogenase; sorbitol dehydrogenase; an oxidoreductase that interconverts sorbitol and fructose, with NAD as hydrogen acceptor (or donor). See also aldose reductase.

**ketosis** (ke-to′sis) [ ketone + suffix *-osis,* condition ]. A condition characterized by the enhanced production of ketone bodies, as in diabetes mellitus.

  **bovine k.,** a common metabolic disease of cows which appears as a rule within a few weeks after parturition; it is characterized by hypoglycemia, k., ketonuria, loss of appetite, lethargy, loss of milk production, and rapid emaciation.

**17-ke′toster′oids.** Nominally, any steroid with a ketone group on C-17; commonly used to designate urinary $C_{19}$ steroidal metabolites of androgenic and adrenocortical hormones that possess this structural feature.

**α-ketosuccinamic acid** (ke′to-suk′sĭ-nam′ik). $NH_2CO$—$CH_2CO$—COOH; the transamination product of asparagine.

**β-ke′tothi′olase.** Acetyl-CoA acyltransferase.

**Key,** Ernst A.H., Swedish physician, 1832–1901. See K.-Retzius *corpuscles, foramen, sheath.*

**key′way.** The female portion of a precision attachment.

**kg.** Abbreviation for kilogram.

**khat.** The tender fresh parts of *Catha edulis* (*q. v.*).

**khellin** (kel′in) [ Ar. *khella* ]. Dimethoxymethylfurano-chromone; the active principle in extracts of *Ammi visnaga,* an umbelliferous plant growing in the Near East. Used in angina pectoris and asthma.

**KHN.** Abbreviation for Knoop hardness *number.*

**Khorana** (kho-rah′na), Har Gobind, U. S. biochemist born in India, *1922. Nobel laureate, 1968, with Robert W. Holley and Marshall W. Nirenberg, for their interpretation of the genetic code and its function in protein synthesis.

**kick.** A brisk mechanical stimulus.

  **atrial k.,** the vigorous atrial contraction, usually producing an A wave in the apex impulse and an audible fourth heart sound, that improves filling and performance of the stressed ventricle; commonly evoked by aortic stenosis or ischemic heart disease.

  **idioventricular k.,** the increased contractility of the initially contracting ventricular fibers which, by stretching the later contracting fibers, increases their force of contraction.

**kid.** 1. A young goat. 2. The act of giving birth to a k. 3. The meat of a young goat.

**Kidd blood group.** See appendix 2, Blood Groups.

**kidney** (kid′nĭ) [ A.S. *cwith,* womb, belly, + *neere,* kidney ]. One of the two organs (L. *ren,* G. *nephros*) that excrete the urine. The k.'s are bean-shaped organs, about 11 cm. long, 5 cm. wide, and 3 cm. thick lying on either side of the spinal column, posterior to the peritoneum, about opposite the twelfth thoracic and first three lumbar vertebrae.

  **am′yloid k.,** Rokitansky's k.; waxy k.; one in which deposition of amyloid (*i.e.,* amyloidosis) has occurred,

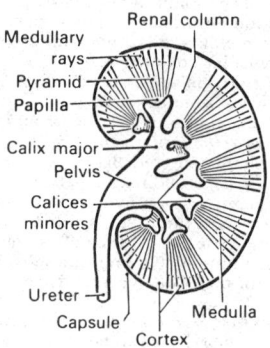

**Kidney**

Diagram of macroscopic structure, as seen on longitudinal section. (From Grant, J. C. B., and Basmajian, J. V.: *Grant's Method of Anatomy,* Ed. 8, The Williams & Wilkins Co., Baltimore, 1971.)

usually in association with some chronic illness such as tuberculosis, osteomyelitis, or other chronic suppurative inflammation. Such k.'s are moderately enlarged and manifest a waxy appearance, grossly; the amyloid is deposited between the endothelium and the basement membrane in the glomerular loops and in the arterioles, apparently beginning as foci of thickening of the basement membranes.

  **Armanni-Ebstein k.,** Armanni-Ebstein change; glycogen vacuolization of the loops of Henle, seen in diabetics before the introduction of insulin.

  **arterio′losclerot′ic k.,** one in which there is sclerosis of the arterioles, *i.e.,* arteriolar nephrosclerosis. Such k.'s tend to be pale red-brown or relatively gray, moderately reduced in size, and firmer than normal organs; the capsular surfaces are evenly, fairly uniformly, finely granular, and may also contain the relatively deep scars resulting from sclerosis of arteries (see arteriosclerotic k.). Most of the arterioles are thickened and hyalinized, thereby resulting in varying degrees of narrowing of the lumens, ischemia, and fibrosis in the interstitial tissue; the scarring eventually leads to fairly uniform contraction of interstitial tissue throughout the organ (especially in the cortex), and groups of dilated tubules bulging outward among the shallow scars lead to the development of the finely granular surface.

  **arteriosclerot′ic k.,** one in which there is sclerosis of arterial vessels that are larger than arterioles. Such k.'s are usually not significantly reduced in size, but are likely to be paler than usual; the capsular surface may be marked by a few, possibly several, conical, relatively deep V-shaped scars that result from fibrosis (and subsequent contraction) of the region supplied by the affected vessel. See also arteriolosclerotic k.

  **artificial k.,** hemodialyzer.

  **cake k.,** a single, unilateral or pelvic k. arising from fusion of bilateral metanephric blastemas.

  **cicatric′ial k.,** the irregularly contracted and deformed k. that results from the scars of chronic pyelonephritis; an obsolete term.

  **cirrhot′ic k.,** a diffusely, fairly evenly scarred k. such as that resulting from sclerosis of arterioles or chronic glomerulonephritis; an obsolete term.

  **contracted k.,** a diffusely scarred k. in which the relatively large amount of abnormal fibrous tissue leads to a moderate or great reduction in the size of the organ, as in arteriolar nephrosclerosis and chronic glomerulonephritis.

  **crush k.,** acute oliguric renal failure following crushing injuries of muscle, first reported in victims of bombing who were trapped inside buildings. The k.'s show the changes of hypoxic nephrosis but the pigment casts in renal tubules contain myoglobin.

  **cyanot′ic k.,** one in which there is an advanced degree of passive congestion.

**cystic k.,** a general term used to indicate a k. that contains one or more cysts, including polycystic disease, solitary cyst, multiple simple cysts, retention cysts (associated with arteriolar nephrosclerosis or pyelonephritis), perinephric cysts (resulting from extravasation of urine), and so on.

**fatty k.,** one in which there is fatty metamorphosis of the parenchymal cells, especially fatty degeneration.

**flea-bitten k.,** the k. seen at autopsy in some cases of bacterial endocarditis, the appearance being caused by diffuse petechial hemorrhages resulting from multiple minute emboli.

**floating k.,** wandering k.; the abnormally mobile k. in nephroptosia.

**fused k.,** horseshoe k.

**Goldblatt k.,** a k. whose arterial blood supply has been compromised, as a consequence of which arterial hypertension develops.

**granular k.,** one in which fairly uniform, diffusely and evenly situated foci of scarring of the interstitial tissue of the cortex (and sometimes scarring of glomeruli), and the associated slight degree of bulging of groups of dilated tubules, leads to the development of a minutely bosselated surface. Such k.'s are observed in patients with arteriolar nephrosclerosis or chronic glomerulonephritis.

**head k.,** pronephros (1).

**hind k.,** metanephros.

**horseshoe k.,** union of the lower or occasionally the upper extremities of the two k.'s by a band of tissue extending across the vertebral column.

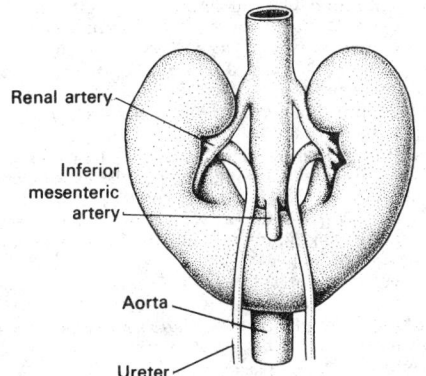

**Horseshoe Kidney**
(From Langman, J.: *Medical Embryology*, Ed. 2, The Williams & Wilkins Co., Baltimore, 1969.)

**larda'ceous k.,** obsolete term for amyloid k.

**large red k.,** enlarged congested k. with increased red appearance seen in acute nephritis; an obsolete term.

**large white k.,** a colloquial, general or nonspecific (and obsolete) term for enlargement and pallor of the k., as observed in certain instances of chronic nonsuppurative interstitial nephritis, amyloidosis, chronic lipoid nephrosis, or nephrosis associated with various infectious diseases or caused by toxic chemical compounds, and so on.

**medullary sponge k.,** cystic disease of the renal pyramids associated with calculus formation and hematuria. Medullary sponge k. differs from cystic disease of the renal medulla (*q.v.* under disease) in that renal failure does not usually develop.

**movable k.,** floating k.

**pal'pable k.,** a slight degree of nephroptosia.

**pelvic k.,** k. that has departed from its usual position, displaced into the pelvis.

**polycys'tic k.,** more properly termed polycystic disease of the k.'s; the condition is characterized by numerous cysts (of varying sizes) scattered diffusely throughout the k.'s, sometimes resulting in organs that tend to resemble grapelike clusters of cysts. The disease is congenital, may be transmitted by either parent, and probably represents the result of a dominant gene. It is thought by some that early generations of nephrons of the metanephros, which

usually become atrophied and disappear, for some unknown reason continue to grow and form cysts.

**pulpy k.,** see enterotoxemia.

**Rokitansky's k.,** amyloid k.

**sclerotic k.,** diffusely, fairly evenly scarred k., such as those observed most frequently in instances of arteriolar nephrosclerosis and chronic glomerulonephritis.

**small red k.,** a contracted k. seen in chronic renal disease.

**surgical k.,** a suppurative form of pyelonephritis.

**wandering k.,** floating k.

**waxy k.,** amyloid k.

**Kieffer's stain.** See under stain.

**Kiel graft.** See under graft.

**Kien** (kēn), Alphonse M. J., German physician, 19th century. See Kussmaul-K. *respiration.*

**Kienböck** (keen'bēk), Robert, Austrian roentgenologist, 1871–1953. See K.'s *atrophy, disease, dislocation, unit.*

**Kiernan,** Francis, English physician, 1800–1874. See K.'s *space.*

**Kiesselbach** (ke'sel-bahkh), Wilhelm, German laryngologist, 1839–1902. See K.'s *area.*

**Kilian,** Hermann F., German gynecologist, 1800–1863. See K.'s *line, pelvis.*

**Killian,** Gustav, German laryngologist, 1860–1921. See K.'s *bundle, operation.*

**kilo-** (kil'o-) [ G. *chilioi,* one thousand ]. A prefix used in the metric system to signify one thousand (10³).

**kilocalorie** (kil'o-kal'o-rī). Large *calorie.*

**kilocycle** (kil'o-si'kl). A thousand cycles; abbreviated kc.

**kil'ogram.** Abbreviated kg; the SI unit of mass; 1000 gm., or 1 cubic decimeter of water; equivalent to 15,432.35 gr., or about 2.205 lb. avoirdupois, or 2.68 lb. troy.

**kil'ogram-meter.** The energy exerted, or work done, when a mass of 1 kg. is raised a height of 1 meter.

**kiloroentgen** (kil-o-rent'gen). Term used to denote an exposure of 1000 roentgens.

**kil'ovolt.** A thousand volts; abbreviated kv.

**kilovolt'meter.** An instrument designed to measure electromotive force (EMF) in kilovolts.

**kilurane** (kil'u-rān). A unit of radioactivity equivalent to 1000 uranium units.

**Kimmelstiel** (kim'el-steel), Paul, German pathologist in the United States, 1900–1970. See K.-Wilson *disease, syndrome.*

**kin-, kine-** [ G. *kinēsis,* movement. CIN- ]. Prefix denoting movement. Words with this same derivation but pertaining specifically to motion picture procedures (*e.g.,* cineradiography) are usually spelled cine-.

**kinanesthesia** (kin-an-es-the'zī-ah) [ G. *kinēsis,* motion, + *an-* priv. + *aisthēsis,* sensation ]. A disturbance of deep sensibility in which there is inability to perceive either direction or extent of movement, the result being ataxia.

**kinase** (ki'nās). Activator. 1. An enzyme catalyzing the conversion of a proenzyme to an active enzyme, *e.g.,* enterokinase (which is an obsolescent term for enteropeptidase). 2. An enzyme catalyzing the transfer of phosphate groups to form triphosphates (ATP). For individual k.'s, see specific name.

**kinematics** (kin'e-mat'iks) [ G. *kinēmatica,* things that move ]. Cinematics; in physiology, the science that deals with movements of the parts of the body.

**kin'emom'eter** [ G. *kinēsis,* movement, + *metron,* measure ]. An electromagnetic device, similar in principle to the velocity ballistocardiograph, used to measure the contraction and relaxation elicited in a tendon reflex.

**kinephantom** (kin'e-fan'tom). False interpretation of seen movement.

**kin'eplastics.** See cineplastic *amputation.*

**kinesalgia** (kin'e-sal'jī-ah) [ G. *kinēsis,* motion, + *algos,* pain ]. Kinesialgia; pain caused by muscular movement.

**kin'escope** [ G. *kinēsis,* motion, + *skopeō,* to examine ]. 1. An instrument for determing the refraction of the eyes; the subject observes the apparent "with" or "against" movement of the test object through a stenopeic slit moved across the front of the eye. 2. An instrument for recording television.

**kinesi-, kinesio-, kineso-** [ G. *kinēsis,* motion ]. Combining forms relating to motion.

**kinesia** (kĭ-ne'zĭ-ah, kĭ-ne'sĭ-ah) [ G. *kinēsis,* movement ]. Motion *sickness.*

**kinesialgia.** Kinesalgia.

**kinesiatrics** (kĭ-ne'sĭ-at'riks) [ G. *kinēsis,* movement, + *iatrikos,* relating to medicine ]. Kinesitherapy.

**kinesics** (kĭ-ne'siks). The study of nonverbal, bodily motion in communication.

**kin'esim'eter** [ G. *kinēsis,* movement, + *metron,* measure ]. Kinesiometer; an instrument for measuring the extent of a movement.

**kinesiodic** (kĭ-ne'sĭ-od'ik) [ G. *kinēsis,* motion, + *hodos,* way ]. Kinesodic; relating to the paths by which motor impulses travel.

**kinesiology** (kĭ-ne'sĭ-ol'o-jĭ) [ G. *kinēsis,* movement, + *-logia* ]. The science or the study of movement, and the active and passive structures involved.

**kinesiometer** (kĭ-ne'sĭ-om'e-ter). Kinesimeter.

**kinesioneurosis** (kĭ-ne'sĭ-o-nu-ro'sis) [ G. *kinēsis,* movement ]. A neurosis, or functional nervous disease, marked by tics, spasms, or other motor disorders.

**kin'esip'athist.** A nonmedical person who treats disease by movements of various kinds.

**kinesipathy** (kin'e-sip'ă-thĭ) [ G. *kinēsis,* movement, + *pathos,* suffering ]. 1. An affection marked by motor disturbances. 2. Kinesitherapy.

**kinesis** (kĭ-ne'sis) [ G. ]. Motion; as a suffix, used to denote movement or activation.

**kinesitherapy** (kĭ-ne-sĭ-thěr'ă-pĭ). Kinesipathy (2); kinesiatrics; treatment by means of a movement regimen; see subentries under movement.

**kinesodic** (kin'e-sod'ik). Kinesiodic.

**kinesophobia** (kĭ-ne'so-fo'bĭ-ah) [ G. *kinēsis,* movement, + *phobos,* fear ]. Morbid fear of movement.

**kinesthesia** (kin'es-the'zĭ-ah) [ G. *kinēsis,* motion, + *aisthēsis,* sensation ]. 1. The sense perception of movement; the muscular sense. 2. An illusion of moving in space.

**kinesthesiometer** (kin'es-the'sĭ-om'e-ter) [ kinesthesia, *q.v.,* + G. *metron,* measure ]. An instrument for determining the degree of muscular sensation.

**kin'esthet'ic.** Relating to kinesthesia.

**kinetic** (kĭ-net'ik) [ G. *kinētikos.* CIN- ]. 1. Relating to motion or movement. 2. A hypothetical substance that is presumed to stimulate ameboid movement in leukocytes.

**kinetics** (kĭ-net'iks). The study of motion, acceleration, or rate of change.

    **chemical k.,** the study of the velocities of chemical reactions.

**kinetin** (kĭ-ne'tin). 6-Furfuryladenine; a plant growth factor.

**kineto-** (kĭ-ne'to-) [ G. *kinētos,* moving, movable ]. Combining form relating to motion.

**kinetocardiogram** (kĭ-ne'to-kar'dĭ-o-gram). Graphic recording of the vibrations of the chest wall produced by cardiac activity.

**kinetocardiograph** (kĭ-ne'to-kar'dĭ-o-graf). A device for recording precordial impulses due to cardiac movement; the absolute displacement of a point on the chest wall is recorded relative to a fixed reference point above the recumbent patient.

**kinetochore** (kĭ-ne'to-kōr) [ kineto- + G. *chōra,* space ]. Centromere.

**kinetogenic** (kĭ-ne'to-jen'ik). Causing or producing motion.

**kinetographic** (kĭ-ne'to-graf'ik). Motorgraphic; relating to kinetography.

**kinetography** (kin'e-tog'ră-fĭ) [ kineto- + G. *graphō,* to write ]. The art of recording graphically movements of any sort.

**kinetoplasm** (kĭ-ne'to-plazm) [ kineto- + G. *plasma,* a thing formed ]. Kinoplasm. 1. The most contractile part of a cell. 2. The cytoplasm of the droplet which covers the sperm head during maturation.

**kinetoplast** (kĭ-ne'to-plast) [ kineto- + G. *plastos,* formed ]. An intensely staining, DNA+, rod-shaped structure found in parasitic flagellates near the base of the

flagellum, often at right angles to the nucleus. Electron micrographs show it to be the part of a single giant mitochondrion filling most of the cytoplasm of amastigote flagellates, the k. portion being visible by light microscopy. It divides independently, along with the basal body, prior to nuclear division. The term formerly included parabasal body and blepharoplast in a locomotory apparatus. See also parabasal *body.*

**kinetoscope** (kĭ-ne'to-skōp) [ kineto- + G. *skopeō,* to examine ]. An apparatus for taking serial photographs to record movement.

**kinetosome** (kĭ-ne'to-sōm) [ kineto- + G. *sōma,* body ]. A rod-shaped or spherical structure that is posterior to the basal granule of a flagellum, is bounded by a double membrane and group of microfibrils (or a single coiled one), and contains DNA. It is the stainable portion of a single mitochondrion running the length of the body.

**King,** Earl J., Canadian biochemist, *1901. See K. *unit,* K.-Armstrong *unit.*

**Kingsley splint.** See under splint.

**ki'nin.** One of a number of widely differing substances having pronounced and dramatic physiological effects. Some k.'s (*e.g.,* kinetin) are plant growth regulators; others (*e.g.,* the polypeptides kallidin, bradykinin) cause contraction of smooth muscle and hypertension, and have become important considerations in pathophysiological processes such as inflammation and shock.

**kink.** An angulation, bend, or twist.

    **Lane's k.,** Lane's *band.*

**kino** (ke'no) [ E. Ind. ]. The inspissated juice of *Pterocarpus marsupium* (family Leguminosae), a forest tree of India and Ceylon. Occurs in the form of dark red, shining, brittle masses of an astringent taste, slightly soluble in water.

**kino-** (kin'o-) [ G. *kineō,* to move ]. Combining form relating to movement.

**kinocentrum** (kin'o-sen'trum) [ kino- + G. *kentron,* center ]. Cytocentrum.

**kinocilium** (ki'no-sil'ĭ-um) [ kino- + cilium, *q.v.* ]. A cilium, usually motile, having nine peripheral double microtubules and two single central ones.

**kin'ohapt** [ kino- + G. *haptein,* to touch ]. An esthesiometer for applying several stimuli to the skin at different distances and frequencies.

**kinomere** (kin'o-mēr) [ kino- + G. *meros,* part ]. Centromere.

**kin'omom'eter** [ kino- + G. *metron,* measure ]. An instrument for measuring degree of motion.

**kin'oplasm.** Kinetoplasm.

**ki'noplasmic.** Relating to kinoplasm (kinetoplasm).

**kinotoxin** (kin'o-tok'sin). Fatigue *toxin.*

**ki'on** [ G. *kiōn,* pillar, the uvula ]. Obsolete term for uvula.

**kion-, kiono-** [ G. *kiōn,* uvula ]. Obsolete combining forms relating to the uvula; for words so beginning, see uvul-, uvulo-.

**Kirk,** Norman Thomas, U. S. Army surgeon, 1888–1960. See K.'s *amputation.*

**Kirkland,** Olin. See K. *knife.*

**Kirschner,** Martin, Greifswald surgeon, 1879–1942. See K.'s *apparatus, wire.*

**Kisch** (kish), Bruno, German physiologist, 1890–1966. See K.'s *reflex.*

**kit.** The young of foxes, mink, and some other wild animals.

**kit'asamy'cin** (USAN). Leucomycin.

**Kitasato** (kit-ă-sah'to), Shibasaburo, Japanese bacteriologist, 1852–1931. See K.'s *bacillus, filter.*

**Kittel,** M., German physician, 19th century. See K.'s *method.*

**Kittrich,** Miroslav. See K.'s *method.*

**Kjeldahl** (kyel'dahl), Johan G. C., Danish chemist, 1849–1900. See K. *apparatus, method,* macro-K. *method,* micro-K. *method.*

**Kjelland** (kyāl'ahnd), Christian, Norwegian obstetrician, *1871. See K.'s *forceps.*

**Klapp,** Rudolph, Berlin surgeon, 1873–1949. See K.'s suction *cup,* K.'s *method.*

**Klebs,** Edwin, German physician, 1834–1913. Gave his name to *Klebsiella*. See K-Loeffler *bacillus*.

**Klebsiella** (kleb-sĭ-el'ah) [ E. *Klebs* ]. A genus of aerobic, facultatively anaerobic, nonmotile, nonsporeforming bacteria (family Enterobacteriaceae) containing Gram-negative, encapsulated rods which occur singly, in pairs, or in short chains. These organisms produce acetylmethylcarbinol and lysine decarboxylase or ornithine decarboxylase. They do not usually liquefy gelatin. Citrate and glucose are ordinarily used as sole carbon sources. These organisms may or may not be pathogenic. They occur in the respiratory, intestinal, or urogenital tracts of man as well as in soil, water, and grain. The type species is *K. pneumoniae*.

**K. ozae'nae,** Abel's bacillus; a species which occurs in cases of ozena and other chronic diseases of the respiratory tract.

**K. pneumo'niae,** Friedländer's bacillus; a species which occurs in soil and water, on grain, and in the intestinal tract of man and other animals. It also occurs in association with several pathological conditions, urinary tract infections, sputum, feces, and metritis in mares. Capsular types 1, 2, and 3 of this organism may be causative agents in pneumonia. Organisms previously identified as nonmotile strains of *Aerobacter aerogenes* are now placed in this species. It is the type species of *K.*

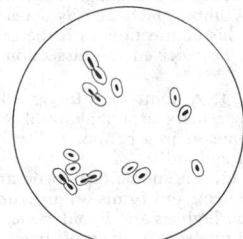

*Klebsiella pneumoniae*

Cells stained to show capsules (original magnification, ×2400).

**K. rhinosclero'matis,** a species found in cases of rhinoscleroma.

**Klein,** Edward E., Hungarian histologist, 1844–1925. See K.'s *muscle*.

**Klein's stain.** See under stain.

**kleptolagnia** (klep'to-lag'nĭ-ah) [ G. *kleptō*, to steal, + *lagneia*, lust, coition ]. Erotic feelings induced by stealing.

**kleptomania** (klep'to-ma'nĭ-ah) [ G. *kleptō*, to steal, + *mania*, insanity ]. A morbid tendency to steal without needing the thing taken.

**klep'toma'niac.** A person exhibiting kleptomania.

**kleptophobia** (klep'to-fo'bĭ-ah) [ G. *kleptō*, to steal, + *phobos*, fear ]. Morbid fear of stealing or of becoming a thief.

**Klinefelter,** Harry F., Jr., American physician, *1912. See K.'s *syndrome*.

**Klippel,** Maurice, French neurologist, 1858–1942. See K.'s *disease*, K.-Feil *syndrome*, K.-Trenaunay-Weber *syndrome*.

**klis'eom'eter.** Cliseometer.

**Kluge** (kloo'gĕ), Karl A. F., German obstetrician, 1782–1844. See K.'s *sign*.

**Klumpke** (kloomp'keh), Augusta Déjérine-K., French neurologist, 1859–1927. See K.'s *paralysis*, K.-Déjérine *syndrome*.

**Klüver,** Heinrich. See K.-Bucy *syndrome*.

**Knapp,** Herman J., New York ophthalmologist, 1832–1911. See K.'s *forceps, streaks, striae*.

**Knaus** (nows), Hermann, German gynecologist, *1892. See K.'s *reaction*, rule of Ogino-K.

**knee** (ne) [ A.S. *cneōw* ]. 1. Genu. 2. See *articulatio* genus (joint of the knee). 3. Any recurved structure resembling a semiflexed knee; see genu (3), and geniculum. 4. In veterinary anatomy, the *articulatio* femorotibialis.

**back-k.,** *genu* recurvatum.

**Brodie's k.,** Brodie's disease (1); chronic hypertrophic synovitis of the k.

**broken k.,** any injury of the k. in the horse, varying in severity from a superficial wound to a fractured bone, and due to violence, usually a fall.

**capped k.,** swelling of the bursa of the extensor metacarpi magnus muscle in cattle, usually caused by injury to the carpus in getting up and down on hard floors; *Brucella abortus* has been isolated from many of these cases.

**housemaid's k.,** prepatellar bursitis; inflammation and swelling of the bursa anterior to the patella, due to traumatism in those who are much on their k.'s.

**locked k.,** a condition in which the k. is prevented from full motion by an internal derangement; may be caused by a malfunctioning cartilage or an osteochondral body within the joint.

**kneecap.** Patella.

**knee-sprung.** Denoting a horse having knees more or less flexed in consequence of traction of the tendons at the back of the leg.

**Knemidokoptes** (ne'mĭ-do-kop'tēz) [ G. *knēmē*, leg, + *coptō*, to cut ]. A genus of microscopic, burrowing sarcoptid mites.

**K. lae'vis var. gal'linae,** the depluming mite that causes irritation at the base of feathers of fowls, particularly of the wings and tail, resulting in feather loss.

**K. mu'tans,** the scaly leg mite that burrows under the scales of the legs of fowls and cage birds, causing thickening, deformity, and crusting.

**K. pi'lae,** causes mange of caged parakeets in the United States.

**knife** (nif). A cutting instrument used in surgery and dissection.

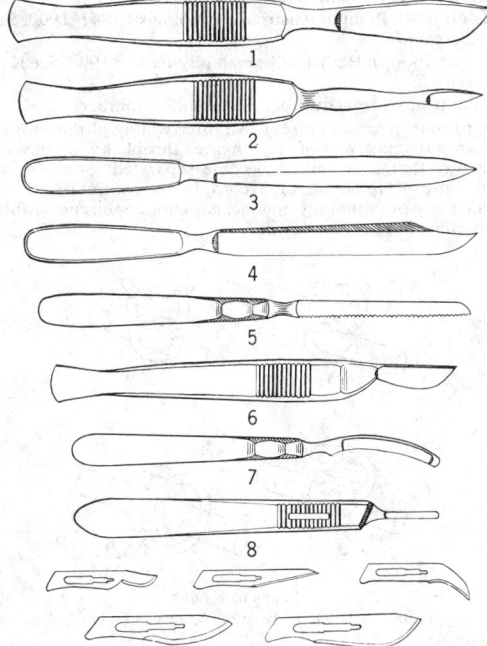

**Types of Knife**

*1*, General operating knife; *2*, tenotome knife; *3*, double-blade amputating knife; *4*, single-blade Liston amputating knife; *5*, Little's operating knife; *6*, Mayo operating knife; *7*, bistoury; *8*, Bard-Parker handle with various blades.

**Beer's k.,** a triangular k. with a sharp point and one sharp edge, formerly used for incision for cataract.

**Brock's k.,** an instrument used in the operation of mitral valvotomy.

**cautery k.,** a k. that sears while cutting, to prevent bleeding.

**fistula k.,** fistulatome.

**Goldman-Fox knives,** a set of knives used in periodontal surgery.

**Graefe's k.,** a narrow-bladed k. used in making a section of the cornea.

**hernia k.,** herniotome; a slender bladed k., with short cutting edge, for dividing the constricting tissues at the mouth of the hernial sac.

**Kirkland k.,** a heart-shaped k. used in gingival surgery.

**lenticular k.,** a scraper resembling a sharp spoon.

**Liston's knives,** long-bladed knives of various sizes used in amputations.

**Merrifield k.,** a long, narrow, triangularly shaped k. used in gingival surgery.

**Thiersch's k.,** a broad, hollow-ground k. for cutting sections of skin in Thiersch's method.

**valvotomy k.,** a k. for performing the operation of mitral valvotomy.

**knismogenic** (nis'mo-jen'ik) [ G. *knismos*, tickling, + suffix -*gen*, production ]. Causing a tickling sensation.

**knismolagnia** (nis'mo-lag'nĭ-ah) [ G. *knismos*, tickling, + *lagneia*, lust ]. Sexual gratification from the act of tickling.

**knitting** (nit'ing). Nonmedical term denoting the process of union of the fragments of a broken bone.

**knob** (nob). A protuberance; a mass; a nodule.

**Englemann's basal k.'s,** obsolete eponym for blepharoplast.

**knock** (nok). 1. Colloquialism for a blow, especially a blow to the head. 2. A sound simulating that of a blow or rap.

**pericardial k.,** an early diastolic sound analogous to the normal third heart sound, but occurring somewhat earlier, due to rapid ventricular filling being abruptly halted by the restricting pericardium.

**knock-knee.** *Genu* valgum.

**Knoll** (nōl), Philipp, Austrian physiologist, 1841–1900. See K.'s *glands.*

**Knoop** (noop), Hedwig, German physician, *1908. See K.'s *theory.*

**Knoop hardness number.** See under number.

**knot** (not) [ A.S. *cnotta* ]. 1. An intertwining of the ends of two cords, tapes, or other elongated flexible bodies in such a way that they cannot become separated; or a similar twining or infolding of a cord in its continuity. 2. In anatomy or pathology, a node, ganglion, or circumscribed swelling suggestive of a k.

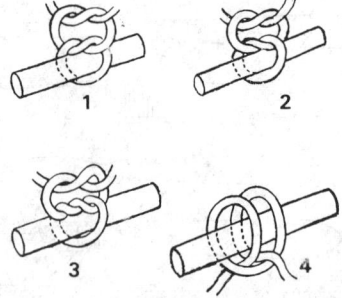

**Types of Knot**

*1*, Granny knot; *2*, square knot; *3*, surgeon's knot; *4*, clove hitch.

**double k.,** (1) one like the square k., in which, after the single k. is made, the ends are turned back and tied again in the same way; (2) friction k.

**false k.'s** (of umbilical cord), local increases in length or varicosity of the umbilical vein, causing markedly apparent twisting of the cord.

**friction k.,** one in which the ends of the cord are passed twice around each other before being pulled taut.

**granny k.,** a double k. in which the two stretches of cord do not pass together under the loop but are separated by it.

**Hensen's knot,** primitive *node.*

**Hubrecht's protochordal k.,** primitive *node.*

**net k.,** karyosome.

**primitive k.,** primitive *node.*

**protochordal k.,** primitive *node.*

**reef k.,** square k.

**square k.,** reef k.; a double k. in which the two stretches of cord pass under the loop in contact with each other.

**Staffordshire k.,** Tait's k.

**stay k.,** two ligatures are passed around an artery side by side and a single k. is tied in each, then the two ends on each side are treated as one and tied together to complete the double k.

**surgeon's k.,** a friction k. made double by recrossing the ends and tying a simple k. over the first.

**syncytial k.,** syncytial bud or sprout; a localized aggregation of syncytiotrophoblastic nuclei in the villi of the placenta during early pregnancy.

**Tait's k.,** a double ligature is passed through the substance of the pedicle of an ovarian tumor; the loop is then reversed over the end of the pedicle and placed between the two free ends of the ligature which are tied over it.

**true k.** (of umbilical cord), actual intertwining of a segment of umbilical cord; circulation is usually not obstructed.

**vital k.,** *noeud* vital.

**Knox,** Robert, Scottish anatomist, 1791–1862. Professor of anatomy at Edinburgh; famed as a teacher but most remembered for his connection with the crimes of Burke and Hare, since he received for dissection the bodies of their victims.

**knuckle** (nuk'l). 1. A joint of a finger when the fist is closed, especially a metacarpophalangeal joint. 2. A kink or loop of intestine, as in a hernia. 3. The knee joint of a pig or calf, used as food.

**cervical aortic k.,** an anomalous aortic arch. The aorta extends into the neck and forms an anteroposterior arch, which may be as high as the hyoid bone. The common carotid artery of one side is given off from the summit of the arch; the common carotid of the other side arises from the more proximal part of the aorta. The pulsating arch may be mistaken for an aneurysm, but the radial pulses are equal.

**knuckling** (nuk'ling). Talipes in the horse, caused by a contraction of the posterior fetlock tendons.

**Kobelt,** George L., German physician, 1804–1857. See K.'s *cyst, tubules.*

**Kober test.** See under test.

**Köbner,** H., German dermatologist, 1838–1904. See K.'s *phenomenon.*

**Koch** (kōkh), Robert, German bacteriologist, 1843–1910. Nobel laureate, 1905, for his investigations and discoveries in relation to tuberculosis. See K.'s *bacilli,* K.-Weeks *bacillus,* K.-Weeks *conjunctivitis,* K.'s *law, lymph, phenomenon, postulates,* K.-Ehrlich *stain,* K.'s old *tuberculin.*

**Koch** (kōkh), Walter, German surgeon, *1880. See K.'s *node.*

**Koch's blue bodies.** See under body.

**Kocher** (ko'kher), E. Theodor, Swiss surgeon, 1841–1917. Nobel laureate, 1909, for his work on the physiology, pathology, and surgery of the thyroid. See K.'s *forceps, incision, operation, sign.*

**Kocks,** Joseph, German surgeon, 1846–1916. See K.'s *operation.*

**Koeberlé** (kë-ber-la'), Eugene, French surgeon, 1828–1915. See K.'s *forceps.*

**Koenig** (kë'nig), Franz, German surgeon, 1832–1910. See K.'s *operation, syndrome.*

**Koerte** (kër'teh), Werner, German surgeon, 1853–1937. See K.-Ballance *operation.*

**Koettstorfer number.** See under number.

**Kogoj,** F. See spongiform *pustule* of K.

**Köhler** (kë'ler), Alban, German roentgenologist, 1874–1947. See K.'s *disease.*

**Köhler,** August, German microscopist, 1866–1948. See K. *illumination.*

**Kohlrausch** (kōl'rowsh), Otto L. B., German physician, 1811–1854. See K.'s *muscle, valves.*

**Kohn,** Hans N., German pathologist, *1866. See K.'s *pores.*

**Kohnstamm** (kōn'stahm), Oskar, German physician, 1871–1917. See K.'s *phenomenon.*

**koilonychia** (koy-lo-nik'ĭ-ah) [ G. *koilos,* hollow, + *onyx* (*onych*-), nail ]. Spoon nail; a malformation of the nails in which the outer surface is concave.

**koilosternia** (koy'lo-ster'nĭ-ah) [ G. *koilos,* hollow, + *sternon,* chest (sternum) ]. *Pectus* excavatum.

**Kojewnikoff (Kozhevnikov),** Aleksei Y., Russian neurologist, 1836–1902. See K.'s *epilepsy.*

**ko'jic acid.** 5-Hydroxy-6-(hydroxymethyl)-4-pyrone; a product of glucose catabolism in some molds.

**koktigen** (kok'tĭ-jen) [ L. *coctus,* pp. of *coquo,* to cook, + suffix *-gen,* producing ]. An antigen for active immunization, prepared by means of heating a suspension of the bacteria in physiologic salt solution, for 30 minutes at 100°C.

**kola** (ko'lah). Cola; the dried cotyledons of *Cola nitida* or other species of *Cola* (family Sterculiaceae). Contains caffeine, theobromine, and a soluble principle, colatin. Used as a cardiac and central nervous system stimulant.

**Kölliker** (kĕl'ik-er), Rudolph A. von, Swiss histologist, 1817–1905. See K.'s dental *crest, glands, layer, reticulum.*

**Kolmer,** John A., American pathologist, *1886. See K. *test.*

**kolp-.** For words beginning thus, see colp-.

**kolyone** (ko'lĭ-ōn). Chalone.

**kolypep'tic.** Colypeptic.

**kolytic** (ko-lit'ik) [ G. *kolyō,* to hinder ]. Denoting an inhibitory action.

**Kondo'leon,** Emmanuel, Athenian surgeon, 1879–1939. See K. *operation.*

**ko'niocor'tex** [ G. *konis,* dust, + L. *cortex,* bark ]. Regions of the cerebal cortex characterized by a particularly well developed inner granular layer (layer 4); this type of cerebral cortex is represented by the primary sensory areas 17 of the visual cortex, areas 1 to 3 of the somatic sensory cortex, and area 41 of the auditory cortex; see also *cortex* cerebri.

**ko'niol'ogy.** Coniology.

**kophe'mia** [ G. *kōphan,* to become stupid, + *phēmē,* word ]. Word *deafness.*

**kopopho'bia** [ G. *kopos,* fatigue, + *phobos,* fear ]. Morbid fear of fatigue.

**Koplik,** Henry, New York physician, 1858–1927. See K.'s *spots,* K.'s *stigma* of degeneration.

**kopr-, kopro-.** For words beginning thus, see copr-, copro-.

**Korányi** (kor-ahn'ye), Baron F. von, Hungarian physician, 1828–1913. See K.'s *method.*

**Korff's fibers.** See under fiber.

**Kornberg,** Arthur, U. S. biochemist, *1918. Nobel laureate, 1959, with Severo Ochoa for their discovery of the mechanisms in the biological synthesis of ribonucleic acid and deoxyribonucleic acid.

**Kornzweig,** A. L. See Bassen-K. *syndrome.*

**koro.** A mental state occurring in Macassars, natives of the Celebes and other parts of the East, in which the subject experiences a sensation that his penis is shriveling or is being drawn into the abdomen.

**koro'nion.** Coronion.

**Korot'koff,** Nikolai S., Russian physician, 1874–1920. See K.'s *sounds, test.*

**Korsakoff** (kor-sah'kawf), Sergei S., Russian neurologist, 1853–1900. See Wernicke-K. *encephalopathy,* K.'s *psychosis, syndrome.*

**ko'sin.** A mixture of α- and β-kosins, obtained from the flowers of *Hagenia abyssinica;* a vermifuge. See also brayera.

**ko'sotox'in.** $C_{26}H_{34}O_{10}$; from the female inflorescence of *Hagenia abyssinica;* a constituent of brayera.

**Kossel,** Albrecht, German biochemist, 1853–1927. Nobel laureate, 1910, for work on the chemistry of the cell and nucleus.

**koumiss** (koo'mis). Kumyss.

**kousso** (koo'so). Brayera.

**Koyanagi,** Yosizo, Japanese ophthalmologist, 20th century. See Vogt-K. *syndrome.*

**Kr.** Chemical symbol of the element krypton.

**Krabbe,** Knud H., Danish neurologist, 1885–1961. See K.'s *disease,* Christensen-K. *disease,* K.'s *syndrome.*

**krait** (krīt). *Bungaris fasciatus;* a very poisonous snake of northern India. Its bite is not associated with local pain, discoloration, or edema but rather with generalized anesthetic and paralytic effects. The neurotoxic symptoms are similar to those induced by cobra venom.

**kra-kra.** Craw-craw.

**Kramer,** John G. H., Austrian physician, 18th century. Gave his name to *Krameria.*

**krame'ria** [ J. G. H. *Kramer* ]. Rhatany; the dried root of *Krameria triandra,* or *K. argentea* (family Leguminosae), shrubs of Peru and of other parts of South America. Formerly used as an astringent.

**Kraske** (krahs'keh), Paul, German surgeon, 1851–1930. See K.'s *operation.*

**kraurosis vulvae** (kraw-ro'sis vul've) [ G. *krauros,* dry, brittle ]. Breisky's disease; leukokraurosis; atrophy and shrinkage of the skin of the vagina and vulva, often accompanied by a chronic inflammatory reaction in the deeper tissues.

**Kraus' reaction.** See under reaction.

**Krause** (krow'zeh), Fedor, German surgeon, 1857–1937. See K.'s *graft, method, operation.*

**Krause** (krow'zeh), Karl F. T., German anatomist, 1797–1868. See K.'s *glands,* median puboprostatic *ligament, muscle, valve.*

**Krause** (krow'zeh), Wilhelm J. F., German anatomist, 1833–1910. See K.'s *bone,* end *bulbs,* respiratory *bundle, membrane.*

**Krauss test.** See under test.

**Krebs,** Sir Hans Adolph, German biochemist in England, *1900. Nobel laureate, 1953, with Fritz A. Lipmann, for his discovery of the citric acid cycle. See K. *cycles,* K.-Henseleit *cycle,* K.-Ringer *solution.*

**Kretschmann,** Friederich, German otologist, 1858–1934. See K.'s *space.*

**Kreysig** (kri'zig), Friedrich L., German physician, 1770–1839. See Heim-K. *sign,* K.'s *sign.*

**Kristeller,** Samuel, German gynecologist, 1820–1900. See K. *technique.*

**Krogh** (krōg), August, Danish physiologist, 1874–1949. Nobel laureate, 1920, for work on the anatomy and physiology of capillaries.

**Kromayer** (kro-mi'er), Ernst L. F., German dermatologist, 1862–1933. See K.'s *lamp.*

**Krompecher** (krōm'pekh-er), Edmund, Budapest pathologist, 1870–1926. See K.'s *tumor.*

**Kronecker** (krōn'ek-er) Karl H., Silesian physiologist, 1839–1914. See K.'s *solution.*

**Krönig** (krö'nig), Georg, Berlin physician, 1856–1911. See K.'s *area, field, isthmus, steps.*

**Krönlein** (krön'lin), Rudolf U., Zurich surgeon, 1847–1910. See K.'s *hernia, operation.*

**Krueger instrument stop.** See under instrument.

**Kru'kenberg,** Adolph, German anatomist, 1816–1877. See K.'s *vein.*

**Kru'kenberg,** Friedrich, German pathologist, 1871–1946. See K.'s *spindle, tumor.*

**Kruse,** Walther, German bacteriologist, 1864–1943. See K.'s *brush,* Shiga-K. *bacillus.*

**krymo-, kryo-** [ G. *krymos, kryos,* cold ]. For words beginning thus, see crymo- and cryo-.

**Kryptok** (krip'tok) [ G. *kryptos,* concealed ]. A bifocal lens made of a flint glass inset fused into a crown glass blank.

**krypton** (krip'ton) [ G. *kryptos,* concealed ]. One of the inert gases, present in small amount in the atmosphere; symbol Kr, atomic no. 36, atomic weight 83.80.

**17-KS.** Abbreviation for 17-ketosteroids.

**kubisagari, kubisagaru** (koo-bĭ-sah-gah'rĭ, koo-bĭ-sah-gah'roo) [ Jap. *kubi,* head, neck, + *sagaru,* to hang down ]. Epidemic *vertigo.*

**Kufs,** H., German psychiatrist, 1871–1955. See K.'s *disease.*

**Kugelberg,** E. See K.-Welander *disease,* Wohlfart-K.-Welander *disease.*

**Kühne** (kü'neh), Heinrich, German histologist. See K.'s *methylene* blue.

**Kühne** (kü'neh), Willy (Wilhelm F.), German physiologist and histologist, 1837–1900. See K.'s *fiber, phenomenon, plate, spindle.*

**Kuhnt** (koont), Hermann, German ophthalmologist, 1850–1925. See K.-Junius *degeneration, disease,* K.'s *spaces.*

**Kulchitsky,** Nicholas, Russian histologist, 1856–1925. See K. *cells.*

**Külz** (külts), Rudolph E., German physician, 1845–1895. See K.'s *cylinders.*

**Kümmell** (küm'el), Hermann, Hamburg surgeon, 1852–1937. See K.'s *disease, spondylitis,* K.-Verneuil *disease.*

**ku'myss** [ Tartar word ]. Koumyss; kumiss; a fermented drink made from mare's milk and sometimes from cow's or ass's milk; a spirituous liquor distilled from it.

**Küntscher nail.** See under nail.

**Kupffer** (koop'fer), Karl W., German anatomist, 1829–1902. See K.'s *cells.*

**kur'chi bark.** Conessi.

**kur'chicine hydrochloride.** An alkaloid obtained from kurchi bark (conessi); has been used in the treatment of amebic dysentery.

**Kurloff** (koor'lawf), Mikhail G., Russian physician, \*1859. See K.'s *bodies.*

**Kürsteiner,** W. See K.'s *canals.*

**kuru** (koo'roo). A progressive, fatal encephalopathy endemic to certain Melanesian tribes in the highlands of New Guinea, and probably of viral origin; it resembles Creutzfeldt-Jakob disease.

**Kurzrok-Ratner test.** See under test.

**Küss** (küs), Emil, Strasburg physiologist, 1815–1871. See K.'s *experiments.*

**Kussmaul** (koos'mowl), Adolph, German physician, 1822–1902. See K.'s *aphasia, coma, disease,* K-Landry *paralysis,* K.'s paradoxical *pulse,* K.'s *respiration,* K.-Kien *respiration,* K.'s *sign,* K.'s *symptom.*

**Küstner,** Heinz, German gynecologist, \*1897. See Prausnitz-K. *reaction,* reversed Prausnitz-K. *reaction.*

**Küstner** (küst'ner), Otto E., German gynecologist, 1849–1931. See K.'s *sign,* Prausnitz-K. *antibody.*

**kv.** Abbreviation for kilovolt.

**Kveim,** Morton A., Norwegian physician, \*1892. See K. *test,* Nickerson-K. *test.*

**kwashiorkor** (kwah-shĭ-or'kor) [ African ]. Infantile pellagra; malignant malnutrition; a disease seen in African natives, particularly children 1 to 3 years old; due to dietary deficiency, particularly of protein; characterized by anemia, edema, pot belly, depigmentation of the skin, loss or change in hair color, marked hypoalbuminemia, and bulky stools containing undigested food. Fatty changes in the cells of the liver, atrophy of the acinar cells of the pancreas, and hyalinization of the renal glomeruli are found postmortem. The term is thought by some to mean "red boy"; by others, "displaced child."

**kyanop'sia.** Cyanopsia.

**kyllo'sis** [ G. *kyllōsis,* a crippling ]. Obsolete term for talipes.

**ky'matism** [ G. *kyma,* wave ]. Myokymia.

**kymboceph'aly.** Cymbocephaly.

**kymogram** (ki'mo-gram). The graphic curve made by a kymograph.

**kymograph** (ki'mo-graf) [ G. *kyma,* wave, + *graphō,* to record ]. An instrument for recording wavelike motions, or modulation; especially for recording variations in blood pressure. It consists of a drum usually revolved by clockwork and covered with smoked paper upon which the curve is inscribed by a stylet or other writing point.

**kymog'raphy.** Use of the kymograph.

**kymoscope** (ki'mo-skōp) [ G. *kyma,* wave, + *skopeō,* to regard ]. An apparatus for measuring the pulse waves, or the variation in blood pressure.

**kynoceph'alus.** Cynocephalus.

**kynurenic acid** (kin'u-re'nik, -ren'ik). 4-Hydroxyquinaldic acid; a product of the metabolism of tryptophan, which appears in human urine probably only in states of marked pyridoxine deficiency.

**kynureninase** (EC 3.7.1.3). A liver enzyme catalyzing the hydrolysis of the kynurenine side chain, with the formation of anthranilic acid and alanine, a reaction in tryptophan catabolism.

**kynurenine** (ki-nu'rĕ-nin, -nēn). 3-Anthraniloylalanine; a product of the metabolism of tryptophan, excreted in the urine in small amounts.

**kynurenine formamidase.** Formamidase.

**kynurenine 3-hydroxylase.** Kynurenine 3-monooxygenase.

**kynurenine 3-monooxygenase** (EC 1.14.13.9). Kynurenine 3-hydroxylase; an enzyme catalyzing addition of 3-OH to L-kynurenine, with the aid of NADPH and $O_2$.

**kyphos** (ki'fos) [ G. ]. A hump.

**ky'phoscolio'sis.** Kyphosis combined with scoliosis; severe, congestive heart failure is not infrequently a complication; it is present in over 1 per cent of cases of cor pulmonale.

**kyphosis** (ki-fo'sis) [ G. *kyphōsis,* hump-back, fr. *kyphos,* bent, hump-backed ]. Cyphosis; Pott's curvature; an abnormal curvature of the spine, with convexity backward.

**kyphot'ic.** Cyphotic; relating to or suffering from kyphosis.

**ky'photone** [ G. *kyphos,* hump, + *tonos,* brace ]. A brace for use in tuberculosis of the spine.

**Kyrle,** J. See K.'s *disease.*

**kyrtorrhachic** (ker-to-rak'ik) [ G. *kyrtos,* curved, + *rhachis,* spine ]. Having a curved lumbar spine with the concavity backward.

**kysth-** [ G. *kysthos,* vagina ]. Obsolete combining form denoting vagina; see colpo-, vagin-.

**kyto-** [ G. *kytos,* a hollow (cell) ]. For words so beginning see cyto-.

# L

**λ.** The 11th letter of the Greek alphabet, lambda, *q. v.*

**L.** 1. Abbreviation for left, *e.g.,* left eye. 2. Symbol for inductance (in henries).

**L, L$_+$, L$_o$, L$_r$.** A series of symbols derived from the Latin *limes* (*i.e.,* boundary or limit), as used in the assay of certain bacterial exotoxins, especially that of *Corynebacterium diphtheriae;* also written L+, Lo, and Lr. See under dose.

***l-.*** A prefix, printed as a lower case italicized letter, indicating a chemical compound to be levorotatory. Opposed to *d-.*

**L-.** A prefix, printed as a small capital letter, indicating a chemical compound to be structurally (sterically) related to L-glyceraldehyde. Opposed to D-.

**La.** Chemical symbol for the element lanthanum.

**lab** [ Ger. ]. A rennet ferment coagulating milk.

**Laband,** Peter F., U. S. dentist, *1900. See L.'s *syndrome.*

**Labbé,** Ernest M., French physician 1870–1939. See L.'s neurociculatory *syndrome.*

**Labbé** (lă-ba'), Leon, French surgeon, 1832–1916. See L.'s *triangle, vein.*

**la belle indifference** [ Fr. ]. A naive, inappropriate lack of emotion or concern for the implications of one's disability, typically seen in persons with conversion hysteria.

**la′bia.** Plural of labium.

**la′bial** [ L. *labium,* lip ]. 1. Relating to the lips or any labium. 2. Toward a lip. 3. One of the letters formed by means of the lips.

**la′bialism.** A form of stammering in which there is confusion in the use of the labial consonants.

**la′bially.** Toward the lips.

**labile** (la′bĭl, la′bil) [ L. *labilis,* liable to slip, fr. *labor,* pp. *lapsus,* to slip ]. 1. Unstable or unsteady; not fixed; characterized by adaptability to alteration or modification, *i.e.,* relatively easily changed, as in cleavage of a molecule or molecular rearrangement in a compound or complex chemical material. 2. Denoting an electrode that is kept moving over the surface during the passage of an electric current. 3. In psychology or psychiatry, denoting free and uncontrolled expression of the emotions; emotionally unstable.

**heat-l.,** destroyed or altered by heat.

**labil′ity.** Instability; relatively easily altered or modified, as complement is destroyed when serum is heated at 56°C.

**labim′eter.** Labidometer.

**labio-** (la′bĭ-o-) [ L. *labium,* lip ]. Combining form relating to the lips.

**labiocervical** (la′bĭ-o-ser′vĭ-kal) [ labio- + L. *cervix,* neck ]. Relating to a lip and a neck; specifically, to the labial or buccal surface of the neck of a tooth.

**labiochorea** (la-bĭ-o-ko-re′ah) [ labio- + G. *choreia,* dance ]. A chronic spasm of the lips interfering more or less with speech.

**la′bioclina′tion.** Positionally inclined more toward lips than is normal; said of a tooth.

**labiodental** (la-bĭ-o-den′tal) [ labio- + L. *dens,* tooth ]. Relating to the lips and the teeth; denoting certain letters the sound of which is formed by both lips and teeth.

**labiogingival** (la′bĭ-o-jin′jĭ-val). Relating to the point of junction of the labial border and the gingival line on the distal or mesial surface of an incisor tooth.

**labioglossolaryngeal** (la′bĭ-o-glos′o-lă-rin′je-al) [ labio- + G. *glōssa,* tongue, + *larynx* ]. Relating to the lips, tongue, and larynx; describing bulbar paralysis in which these parts are involved.

**labioglossopharyngeal** (la′bĭ-o-glos′o-fă-rin′je-al) [ labio- + G. *glōssa,* tongue, + *pharynx* ]. Relating to the lips, tongue, and pharynx; describing bulbar paralysis involving these parts.

**la′biograph** [ labio- + G. *graphō,* to record ]. An instrument for recording the movements of the lips in speaking.

**la′biomen′tal** [ labio- + L. *mentum,* chin ]. Relating to the lower lip and the chin.

**labiomycosis** (la′bĭ-o-mi-ko′sis) [ labio- + G. *mykēs,* fungus, + suffix *-osis,* condition ]. Any disease of the lips due to the presence of a fungus.

**la′biona′sal.** Relating to the upper lip and the nose, or to both lips and the nose; denoting a letter which is both labial and nasal in the production of its sound.

**labiopalatine** (la′bĭ-o-pal′ă-tin). Relating to the lips and the palate.

**la′bioplace′ment.** Positioning (*e.g.,* of a tooth) more toward the lips than normal.

**labioplasty** (la′bĭ-o-plas-tĭ) [ labio- + G. *plassō,* to form ]. Chiloplasty.

**la′bioscro′tal.** Relating to the labium majus and the scrotum.

**labiotenaculum** (la′bĭ-o-te-nak′u-lum). A tenaculum for holding any lip, especially of the os uteri, during an operation.

**la′biover′sion.** Malposition of an anterior tooth axially inclined in a direction toward the lips.

**lab′itome** [ G. *labis,* pincers, + *tomē,* an incision ]. Cutting forceps; a forceps with sharp blades.

**la′bium,** gen. **la′bii,** pl. **la′bia** [ L. ] [ NA ]. 1. A lip. 2. Any lip-shaped structure.

   **l. anterius** [ NA ], anterior lip of the uterus; it projects into the vagina anterior to the ostium of the uterus.

   **l. externum cristae iliacae** [ NA ], external lip of the iliac crest; it gives attachment above to the external oblique and latissimus dorsi muscles and below to the tensor fasciae latae and fascia lata.

   **l. infe′rius o′ris** [ NA ], the lower lip.

   **l. internum cristae iliacae** [ NA ], internal lip of the iliac crest; it gives attachment to parts of the transversus abdominis, quadratus lumborum, and erector spinae muscles.

   **l. laterale lineae asperae femoris** [ NA ], lateral lip of the linea aspera of the femur; it gives attachment to the short head of the biceps femoris and to the lateral intermuscular septum.

   **l. lim′bi tympan′icum** [ NA ], tympanic lip; lower, long, periosteal extension of the limbus laminae spiralis osseae.

   **l. lim′bi vestibula′re** [ NA ], vestibular lip; spiral crest; crista spiralis; lamina dentata; upper, short, periosteal extension of the limbus laminae spiralis osseae which provides the central attachment for the tectorial membrane.

   **l. majus puden′di,** pl. **labia majo′ra** [ NA ], large pudendal lip; one of two rounded folds of integument forming the lateral boundaries of the rima pudendi.

   **l. mediale lineae asperae femoris** [ NA ], medial lip of the linea aspera; the vastus lateralis originates in part from this lip.

   **l. minus puden′di,** pl. **labia mino′ra** [ NA ], small pudendal lip; nympha; one of two narrow longitudinal folds of mucous membrane enclosed in the cleft within the labia majora; posteriorly they gradually merge into the labia majora and join to form the fourchette, or frenulum labiorum pudendi; anteriorly each l. divides into two portions which unite with those of the opposite side in front of the glans clitoridis to form the prepuce.

   **l. o′ris** [ NA ], one of the lips bounding the cavity of the mouth. See also lip (1).

   **l. posterius** [ NA ], posterior lip of the uterus; it bounds the uterine ostium posteriorly and is slightly longer than the anterior lip.

   **l. supe′rius o′ris** [ NA ], the upper lip.

   **l. ure′thrae,** one of the two lateral margins of the ostium urethrae externum.

   **labia u′teri,** l. anterius and l. posterius.

   **l. voca′le,** pl. **labia voca′lia,** *plica* vocalis.

**la′bor** [ L. toil, suffering ]. Delivery; childbirth; the process of expulsion of a fetus from the uterus at the normal termination of pregnancy.

   **dry l.,** xerotocia; l. after spontaneous loss of practically all of the amniotic fluid.

**first stage of l.,** the period of dilation of the os uteri.

**fourth stage of l.,** the period of l. after the birth of the baby during which the membranes and placenta are extruded.

**missed l.,** the occurrence of a few l. pains at the normal term followed by their cessation and the retention of the fetus for an indefinite period. The fetus is usually dead in these circumstances, or it may be extrauterine, *e.g.,* in the abdominal cavity.

**placental stage of l.,** third stage of l.

**precipitate l.,** l. ending in rapid expulsion of the fetus.

**premature l.,** onset of labor before the 37th completed week of pregnancy dated from the last normal menstrual period.

**second stage of l.,** that stage of expulsive effort, beginning with the complete dilation of the cervix and ending with delivery of the infant.

**third stage of l.,** the placental stage, beginning with the delivery of the baby and ending with more or less complete expulsion of the placenta.

**lab'orator'ian.** One who works in a laboratory; in the medical and allied health professions, one who examines or performs tests (or supervises such procedures) with various types of chemical and biologic materials, chiefly as an aid in the diagnosis, treatment, and control of disease, or as a basis for health and sanitation practices.

**laboratory** (lab'o-ră-to-rī) [ Mediev. L. *laboratorium,* a workplace, fr. L. *laboro,* pp. *-atus,* to labor ]. A room or group of rooms, or even a building, that is equipped with apparatus and reagents, and frequently with various types of animals, for the performance of tests and experiments in physics, chemistry, and biology (especially physiology), the preparation of reagents and therapeutic chemical materials, and so on.

**orbital space l.,** a capsule or vehicle designed and equipped for the performance of tests and experiments while in orbit in a space environment.

**personal growth l.,** a sensitivity training l. in which the primary emphasis is on each participant's potentialities for creativity, empathy, and leadership; in such a l. many modalities of experience and expression are utilized. See also sensitivity training *group.*

**labra** (la'brah) [ L. ]. Plural of labrum.

**lab'rocyte.** Mast *cell.*

**la'brum,** pl. **la'bra** [ L. ] [ NA ]. 1. A lip. 2. A lip-shaped structure.

**l. acetabula're** [ NA ], acetabular lip; circumferential cartilage; a fibrocartilaginous rim attached to the margin of the acetabulum of the os coxae.

**l. glenoida'le** [ NA ], glenoidal lip; articular margin; circumferential cartilage; a ring of fibrocartilage of fibrous connective tissue, attached to the margin of the glenoidal cavity of the scapula to increase its depth.

**labyrinth** (lab'ĭ-rinth). 1. Labyrinthus. 2. A group of upright test tubes terminating below in a base of communicating, alternately U -shaped and ∩ -shaped tubes, used for isolating motile from nonmotile organisms in culture, or a motile from a less motile organism (as the typhoid from the colon bacillus), the former traveling faster and farther through the tubes than the latter.

**bony l.,** *labyrinthus* osseus.

**ethmoid'al l.,** *labyrinthus* ethmoidalis.

**Ludwig's l.,** *pars* convoluta lobuli corticalis renis.

**membranous l.,** *labyrinthus* membranaceus.

**os'seous l.,** *labyrinthus* osseus.

**renal l.,** *pars* convoluta lobuli corticalis renis.

**Santorini's l.,** *plexus* venosus prostaticus.

**labyrinthectomy** (lab-ĭ-rin-thek'to-mī) [ labyrinth + G. *ektomē,* excision ]. Excision of the labyrinth.

**labyrinthine** (lab-ĭ-rin'thin). Relating to any labyrinth.

**labyrinthitis** (lab'ĭ-rin-thi'tis). Inflammation of a labyrinth, especially of the internal ear, sometimes accompanied by vertigo; see also *otitis* interna.

**labyrinthotomy** (lab-ĭ-rin-thot'o-mī) [ labyrinth + G. *tomē,* incision ]. Incision into the labyrinth.

**labyrinthus** (lab'ĭ-rin'thus) [ L. fr. G. *labyrinthos,* labyrinth. LABYR- ] [ NA ]. Labyrinth; a term applied to several anatomical structures with numerous intercommunicating cells or canals. 1. The internal or inner ear, composed of the semicircular ducts, vestibule, and cochlea.

2. Any group of communicating cavities, as in each lateral mass of the ethmoid bone, labyrinthus ethmoidalis. 3. *Pars* convoluta lobuli corticalis renis.

**l. ethmoida'lis** [ NA ], ethmoidal labyrinth; lateral mass of the ethmoid bone; a mass of air cells with thin bony walls forming part of the lateral wall of the nasal cavity; the cells are arranged in three groups, anterior, middle, and posterior, and are closed laterally by the orbital plate which forms part of the wall of the orbit.

**l. membrana'ceus** [ NA ], membranous labyrinth; an arrangement of communicating membranous sacs, filled with endolymph and surrounded by perilymph, lying within the cavity of the osseous labyrinth; its chief divisions are: sacculus, utriculus, cochlear duct, and semicircular ducts.

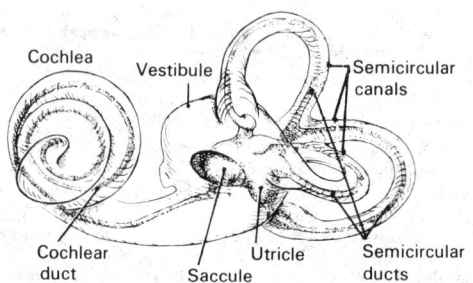

Cochlea    Vestibule    Semicircular canals

Cochlear duct    Saccule    Utricle    Semicircular ducts

**Labyrinthus Membranaceus (Membranous Labyrinth)**

Left membranous labyrinth shown lying within the osseous labyrinth (labyrinthus osseus) of the otic capsule (lateral view).

**l. os'seus** [ NA ], osseous labyrinth; bony labyrinth; a series of cavities (cochlea, vestibule, and semicircular canals) in the petrous portion of the temporal bone which lodge the membranous labyrinth.

**lac,** gen. **lactis** [ L. milk ] [ NA ]. 1. Milk. 2. Any whitish, milky looking liquid.

**l. sul'furis,** precipitated sulfur.

**l. vacci'num,** cow's milk.

**lac'ca.** Shellac.

**lac'case.** Monophenol monooxygenase.

**lacerable** (las'er-ă-bl) [ L. *lacero,* pp. *-atus,* to tear to pieces, fr. *lacer,* mangled ]. Capable of being, or liable to be, torn.

**lacerated** (las'er-a-ted). Torn; rent; having a ragged edge.

**laceration** (las-er-a'shun). 1. A tear or torn wound. 2. The process or act of tearing the tissues.

**brain l.,** a pathologic entity characterized by gross tearing of neural tissue; clinical manifestations depend on the area and extent of tissue involved.

**scalp l.,** traumatic loss of continuity of dermis; may extend into or through subcutaneous tissue and galea aponeurotica.

**lacertus** (lă-ser'tus) [ L. ]. 1. The muscular part of the arm. 2 [ NA ]. Any muscular or fibrous band.

**l. cordis,** one of the trabeculae carneae.

**l. fibro'sus,** *aponeurosis* musculi bicipitis brachii.

**l. of lateral rectus muscle,** l. musculi recti lateralis.

**l. medius,** *ligamentum* longitudinale anterius.

**l. musculi recti latera'lis** [ NA ], l. of the lateral rectus muscle; lateral check ligament; an expansion of the fascia of the lateral rectus to the orbital tubercle of the zygomatic bone.

**lac'erus** [ L. ] [ NA ]. Lacerated.

**lachrymal** (lak'rĭ-mal). Lacrimal.

**lacinia,** pl. **laciniae** (lă-sin-ĭ-ah), [ L. fringe ]. Fimbria.

**lacin'iae tu'bae,** *fimbriae* tubae.

**lacrima,** pl. **lac'rimae** (lak'rĭ-mah) [ L. ] [ NA ]. A tear.

**lacrimal** (lak'rĭ-mal) [ L. *lacrima,* a tear ]. Relating to the tears, their secretion, and the organs concerned therewith.

**lacrimation** (lak'rĭ-ma'shun) [ L. *lacrimatio* ]. The secretion of tears, especially in excess.

**lacrimator** (lak'rĭ-ma-tor) [ L. *lacrima,* tear ]. An agent (such as tear gas) that irritates the eyes and produces tears.

**lacrimatory** (lak'rĭ-mă-to-rĭ). Causing lacrimation.

**lacrimotome** (lak'rĭ-mo-tōm). A fine-bladed knife for use in lacrimotomy.

**lacrimotomy** (lak'rĭ-mot'o-mĭ) [ L. *lacrima*, tear, + G. *tomē*, incision ]. The operation of incising the lacrimal duct or sac.

**lact-, lacti-** [ L. *lac, lactis*, milk ]. Combining form denoting milk.

**lactacidemia** (lak-tas-ĭ-de'mĭ-ah). Lacticacidemia.

**lactagogue** (lak'tă-gog) [ lact- + G. *agōgos*, leading ]. Galactagogue.

**lac'talbu'min.** The albumin fraction of milk. Two proteins are present, termed α-lactalbumin and β-lactalbumin. The former (minor 1.) alters an enzyme in milk so that it becomes capable of synthesizing lactose.

**lac'tam, lac'tim.** Abbreviations of "lactoneamine" and "lactoneimine," and applied to the tautomeric forms —NH—CO— and —N=C(OH)—, respectively, in many purines, pyrimidines, and other substances. The latter form accounts for the acidic properties of uric acid, in particular.

**lac'tase.** β-Galactosidase.

**lac'tate.** 1. A salt or ester of lactic acid. 2. To produce milk in the mammary glands.

**lactate dehydrogenase.** LDH; lactic acid dehydrogenase; name for four enzymes: lactate dehydrogenase (cytochrome) (EC 1.1.2.3); lactate dehydrogenase (EC 1.1.1.27); D-lactate dehydrogenase (cytochrome) (EC 1.1.2.4); and D-lactate dehydrogenase (EC 1.1.1.28). The first of each pair transfers H to ferricytochrome *c* (EC 1.1.2.3 is cytochrome *b₂*), the second to NAD⁺, in catalyzing the oxidation of lactate to pyruvate.

**excess l.,** the increase in 1. concentration beyond that which would be expected from the increase in pyruvate concentration; the increase in 1. concentration resulting from a change in redox potential. It is used as an index of anaerobic carbohydrate metabolism.

**lactate 2-monooxygenase** (EC 1.13.12.4). (L)-Lactate oxidase; (L)-lactic acid oxidase; lactic acid oxidative decarboxylase; an oxidoreductase (flavoprotein) catalyzing oxidation (with O₂) of L-lactate to acetate + CO₂ + H₂O.

**(L)-lactate oxidase.** Lactate 2-monooxygenase.

**lactation** (lak-ta'shun) [ L. *lactatio*, suckle ]. 1. The production of milk. 2. The period following childbirth during which milk is formed in the breasts.

**lacta'tional.** Relating to lactation.

**lacteal** (lak'te-al). 1. Relating to or resembling milk; milky. 2. Chyle vessel; a lymphatic vessel that conveys chyle from the intestine.

**central l.,** the blindly ending lymphatic capillary in the center of an intestinal villus.

**lactenin** (lak'tĕ-nin). An antibacterial agent active against streptococci isolated from cow's milk.

**lactescent** (lak-tes'ent). Resembling milk; milky.

**lactic** (lak'tik). [ L. *lac (lact-)*, milk ]. Relating to milk.

**lactic acid** (USP, BP). CH₃—CHOH—COOH; 2-hydroxypropionic acid; a syrupy, odorless, and colorless liquid obtained by the action of the lactic acid bacillus on milk or milk sugar. A caustic in concentrated form. Used internally to prevent gastrointestinal fermentation; a culture of the bacillus, or milk containing it, is usually given in place of the acid.

**L-lactic acid.** Sarcolactic acid; a dextrorotatory form of lactic acid sometimes excreted in the urine after severe muscular exercise.

**lactic acid dehydrogenase.** Lactate dehydrogenase.

**lacticacidemia** (lak'tik-as'ĭ-de'mĭ-ah) [ lactic acid + G. *haima*, blood ]. The presence of dextrorotatory lactic acid in the circulating blood.

**(L)-lactic acid oxidase.** Lactate 2-monooxygenase.

**lactic acid oxidative decarboxylase.** Lactate 2-monooxygenase.

**lactiferous** (lak-tif'er-us) [ lacti- + L. *fero*, to bear ]. Lactigerous; yielding milk.

**lactifugal** (lak-tif'u-gal). Lactifuge (1).

**lactifuge** (lak'tĭ-fūj) [ lacti- + L. *fugo*, to drive away ]. 1. Lactifugal; galactophygous; causing the arrest of the

secretion of milk. 2. An agent that arrests the secretion of milk.

**lactigenous** (lak-tij'en-us) [ lacti- + suffix -*gen*, producing ]. Producing milk.

**lactigerous** (lak-tij'er-us) [ lacti- + L. *gero*, to carry ]. Lactiferous.

**lac'tim.** See lactam.

**lac'timor'bus** [ lacti- + L. *morbus*, disease ]. Milk *sickness*.

**lac'tinated.** Prepared with or containing milk sugar.

**lacto-** [ L. *lac, lactis*, milk ]. Combining form denoting milk.

**Lactobacillaceae** (lak'to-băs'ĭ-la'se-e). A family of anaerobic to facultatively anaerobic, ordinarily nonmotile bacteria (order Eubacteriales) containing straight or curved, Gram-positive rods which usually occur singly or in chains; motile cells are peritrichous. These organisms have complex organic nutritional requirements; they produce lactic acid from carbohydrates. They are found in fermenting animal and plant products where carbohydrates are available; they are also found in the mouth, vagina, and intestinal tracts of various warm-blooded animals including man. Only a few species are pathogenic. The type genus is *Lactobacillus*.

**lac'tobacil'lic acid.** 2-Hexycyclopropanedecanoic acid; a major constituent of the lipids of lactobacilli; notable for the presence of a cyclopropane ring in the molecule.

**Lactobacillus** (lak-to-bă-sil'us) [ lacto- + bacillus, *q.v.* ]. A genus of microaerophilic or anaerobic, nonsporeforming, ordinarily nonmotile bacteria (family Lactobacillaceae) containing Gram-positive rods which vary from long and slender cells to short coccobacilli. Chains are commonly produced, especially in the later part of the logarithmic phase of growth. Motile cells are peritrichous. These organisms become Gram-negative with increasing age and acidity. There is no branching, clubbing, or bifid formation of the cells. These organisms possess complex nutritional requirements for growth. Their metabolism is fermentative even though growth generally occurs in the presence of air; some of these organisms are strict anaerobes in isolation. They ferment glucose, and at least half of the end product is lactic acid. They are found in dairy products and effluents to grain and meat products, water, sewage, beer, wine, fruits and fruit juices, pickled vegetables, and in sour dough and mash. Some organisms are parasitic in the mouth, intestinal tract, and vagina of many warm-blooded animals, including man. Rarely are these organisms pathogenic. The type species is *L. delbruecki.*

**L. acidoph'ilus,** a species found in the feces of milk-fed infants and also in the feces of older persons on a high milk-, lactose-, or dextrin-containing diet.

**L. bi'fidus,** *Bifidobacterium bifidum.*

**L. bifidus** subsp. **pennsylvanicus,** a bacterium present in human colostrum and milk, in the milk of other mammals, and in the feces of breast-fed infants; associated with a growth factor belonging to a group of N-containing polysaccharides with a high hexosamine content and known as bifidus factor.

**L. brevis,** a species widely distributed in nature, especially in plant and animal products; it is also found in the mouth and intestinal tract of humans and rats.

**L. buch'neri,** a species widely distributed in fermenting substances.

**L. bulgar'icus.** a species used in the production of yogurt.

**L. ca'sei,** a species found in milk and cheese.

**L. catenafor'me,** *Catenabacterium catenaforme;* an anaerobic species found in the intestines and pulmonary cavities of humans.

**L. caucas'icus,** a name applied to an organism which is unrecognizable from its description and for which no cultures exist. Formerly regarded as the type species of *L.* (see *L. delbrueckii*).

**L. cellobio'sus,** a species found in the mouth of man.

**L. coprophi'lus,** a species found in cow dung.

**L. corynifor'mis,** a species found primarily in silage but also in cow dung and dairybarn air.

**L. curva'tus,** a species found in cow dung, dairybarn air, silage, milk, and in a case of endocarditis.

**L. delbrueck'ii,** a species found in fermenting vegetables and grain mashes. It is the type species of the genus *L.*

**L. desidio'sus,** a species found in kefir grains.

**L. fermen'ti,** *L. fermentum.*

**L. fermentum,** *L. fermenti;* a species found widely distributed in nature, especially in fermenting plant and animal products.

**L. fructivorans,** a species isolated from spoiled mayonnaise and salad dressings.

**L. helvet'icus,** a species found in sour milk and Swiss cheese.

**L. heterohiochi,** a species found in spoiled sake.

**L. hilgardii,** a species isolated from California table wines.

**L. homohiochi,** a species found in spoiled sake.

**L. jensenii,** a species isolated from human sources such as vaginal discharge and blood clot.

**L. lactis,** a species found in milk and cheese; not pathogenic.

**L. leichman'nii,** a species found in dairy and plant products.

**L. pastoria'nus,** a species found in sour beer and distillery yeast.

**L. planta'rum,** a species found in dairy products and environments, fermenting plants, silage, sauerkraut, pickled vegetables, spoiled tomato products, sour dough, cow dung, and the human mouth, intestinal tract, and stools.

**L. saliva'rius,** a species found in the mouth and intestinal tract of the hamster, the mouth of man, and the intestinal tract of the hen.

**L. thermoph'ilus,** a thermophilic species so far found only in pasteurized milk.

**L. tricho'des,** a species found in wines containing 20 per cent ethanol and in lees in California, Australia, France, and Spain. In California this organism is commonly referred to as the hair bacillus, cottony bacillus, cottony mold, or Fresno mold.

**L. virides'cens,** a species found in discolored cured meat products such as sausage and bologna.

**lactobutyrometer** (lak'to-bu-tĭ-rom'e-ter) [ lacto- + G. *boutyron,* butter, + *metron,* measure ]. A form of lactocrit.

**lactocele** (lak'to-sēl) [ lacto- + G. *kēlē,* tumor ]. Galactocele.

**lac'tochrome.** Lactoflavin.

**lac'tocrit** [ lacto- + G. *krinō,* to separate ]. An instrument for use in the estimation of the amount of butterfat in milk.

**lac'todensim'eter** [ lacto- + L. *densus,* thick, + G. *metron,* measure ]. A form of galactometer.

**lac'tofla'vin.** 1. Flavin in milk. 2. Riboflavin.

**lactogen** (lak'to-jen) [ lacto- + suffix *-gen,* producing ]. An agent that stimulates milk production or secretion.

**human placental l.,** abbreviated HPL; chorionic "growth hormone-prolactin"; purified placental protein; placenta protein; placental growth hormone; a protein hormone of placental origin; its biological activity weakly mimics that of human pituitary growth hormone and prolactin.

**lactogenesis** (lak-to-jen'e-sis) [ lacto- + G. *genesis,* production ]. Milk production.

**lactogen'ic.** Pertaining to lactogenesis.

**lactoglob'ulin.** Milk globulin; the form of globulin present in milk.

**lactom'eter** [ lacto- + G. *metron,* measure ]. Galactometer.

**lac'tonase.** Gluconolactonase.

**lac'tone.** An organic anhydride formed from a hydroxyacid by the loss of water between the —OH and —COOH groups.

**lac'toperox'idase.** A peroxidase obtained from milk.

*p*-**lactophenetide** LACTOPHENIN; lactyl-*p*-phenetidin; analgesic with antipyretic properties.

**lac'tophos'phate.** A compound of lactic and phosphoric acids.

**lactoprotein** (lak'to-pro'te-in -tēn). Any protein normally present in milk; lactalbumin, lactoglobulin, etc.

**lactorrhea** (lak-to-re'ah) [ lacto- + G. *rhoia,* a flow ]. Galactorrhea.

**lac'toscope** [ lacto- + G. *skopeō,* to view ]. Galactoscope.

**lac'tose** (USP, BP). Milk sugar; saccharum lactis; 4-(β-D-galactosido)-D-glucose; a disaccharide present in mammalian milk and obtained from cow's milk; occurs as α- and β-lactose. Used in modified milk preparations, in food for infants and convalescents, and in pharmaceutical preparations; large doses act as an osmotic diuretic and as a laxative.

**lactosuria** (lak'to-su'rĭ-ah) [ lacto- + G. *ouron,* urine ]. The excretion of lactose (milk sugar) in the urine; a common finding during pregnancy and lactation, and in the newborn, especially premature babies; l. may be associated with anorexia, vomiting and diarrhea.

**lac'tother'apy.** Galactotherapy.

**lac'totro'phin.** Prolactin.

**lactovegetarian** (lak'to-vej-ĕ-ta'rĭ-an). One who lives on a mixed diet of milk and milk products, eggs, and vegetables, but eschews meat.

**lactoyl-glutathione lyase** (lak'to-il-glu-tah-thi'ŏn). Glyoxalase I; aldoketomutase; ketone-aldehyde mutase; methylglyoxalase; a lyase (EC 4.4.1.5) cleaving lactoyl-glutathione to glutathione and methylglyoxal.

**lactucarium** (lak'tu-ka'rĭ-um) [ L. *lactuca,* lettuce ]. Lettuce-opium; the dried milk-juice of *Lactuca virosa* (family Compositae), the wild lettuce of southern and western Europe; contains hyoscyamine, lactucerol, and caoutchouc; has been used as a sedative.

**lacuna,** pl. **lacu'nae** (lă-ku'nah) [ L. a pit, dim. of *lacus,* a hollow, a lake ]. 1 [ NA ]. A small space, cavity, or depression. 2. A gap or defect. 3. An abnormal space between the strata or between the cellular elements of the epidermis. 4. Corneal *space.*

**Blessig's l.,** Blessig's *groove.*

**cartilage l.,** a cavity, within the matrix of cartilage, occupied by a chondrocyte.

**l. cer'ebri,** a small circumscribed loss of brain tissue surrounding one of the small arteries; rupture of the vessel is apt to occur into the cavity so produced.

**Howship's lacunae,** resorption lacunae; tiny depressions, pits or irregular grooves in bone that is being resorbed by osteoclasts.

**intervil'lous l.,** one of the blood spaces in the placenta into which the chorionic villi project.

**lacunae latera'les** [ NA ], parasinoidal sinuses; lateral lakes; lateral expansions of the sinus sagittalis superior of the dura mater, often increasing in width with advancing age until in the very old they may extend 2 cm. lateral to the midline; the endothelium-lined lumen of the l. is usually reduced to a spongelike labyrinth by numerous arachnoid granulations and dural trabeculae.

**l. magna,** a recess on the roof of the fossa navicularis of the penis, formed by a fold of mucous membrane, called Guérin's fold, or the valve of the navicular fossa.

**Morgagni's l.,** l. urethralis.

**l. musculo'rum** [ NA ], the lateral compartment beneath the inguinal (Poupart's) ligament, for the passage of the iliopsoas muscle and femoral nerve; it is separated by the iliopectineal arch from the l. vasorum.

**os'seous l.,** a cavity in bony tissue occupied by an osteocyte.

**l. pharyn'gis,** a depression near the pharyngeal opening of the auditory (Eustachian) tube.

**resorption lacunae,** Howship's lacunae.

**trophoblastic l.,** one of the spaces in the early syncytio-trophoblastic layer of the chorion before the formation of villi. In human embryos maternal blood enters these spaces by the 10th day. With the differentiation of the chorionic villi they become intervillous spaces, sometimes called intervillous lacunae.

**l. urethra'lis,** pl. **lacunae urethrales** [ NA ], urethral l.; Morgagni's l.; one of a number of little recesses in the mucous membrane of the pars spongiosa urethrae into which empty the ducts of the urethral glands.

**l. vaso'rum** [ NA ], vascular compartment; the medial compartment beneath the inguinal ligament, for the passage to the femoral vessels; it is separated from the l. musculorum by the iliopectineal arch.

**lacu'nar.** 1. Relating to a lacuna. 2. Denoting a hiatus or temporary lack of manifestation in a symptom.

**lacunule** (lă-ku'nūl) [ Mod. L. *lacunula,* dim. of L. *lacuna* ]. A very small lacuna.

**la′cus,** pl. **la′cus** [ L. lake ]. A small collection of fluid.

**l. lacrima′lis** [ NA ], lacrimal lake; the small cistern-like area of the conjunctiva at the medial angle of the eye, in which the tears collect after bathing the anterior surface of the eyeball and the conjunctival sac.

**l. semina′lis,** the vault of the vagina after insemination.

**Ladd-Franklin theory.** See under theory.

**Ladendorff** (lah′den-dorf), August, German physician, 19th century. See L.'s *test.*

**La′din,** Louis J., New York obstetrician, \*1862. See L.'s *sign.*

**Lae′laps echidni′nus.** The spiny rat mite, a common worldwide ectoparasite of the wild Norway rat; occasionally found on the house mouse, cotton rat, and other rodents, but rarely on laboratory animals. It is the natural vector of *Hepatozoon muris* and can transmit the agent of tularemia experimentally. Junin virus has been isolated from this species in South America.

**Laënnec,** René T. H., French physician, 1781–1826. See L.'s *cirrhosis, pearls, thrombus.*

**laev-.** For words so beginning see lev-.

**laevulose** (BP). D-Fructose.

**Lafora,** Gonzalo Rodriguez, Spanish neurologist, \*1887. See L. *body,* L.'s *disease.*

**lag.** To move or progress more slowly than normal; to fall behind.

**anaphase l.,** slow movement or no movement of chromosomes during anaphase; results in said chromosomes not being included in one of the daughter cells.

**lagena,** pl. **lage′nae** (lă-je′nah) [ L. flask ]. One of the three parts of the membranous labyrinth of the inner ear of lower vertebrates. In mammals it becomes the cochlea.

**lag′ging.** Retarded or diminished movement of the affected side of the chest in pulmonary tuberculosis.

**lagneia** (lag-na′ah) [ G. ]. 1. Lust. 2. Coition.

**l. furor,** extreme sex urge.

**lagne′sis, lagno′sis** [ G. *lagneia,* lust ]. 1. Nymphomania. 2. Satyriasis.

**lagophthalmia, lagophthalmos** (lag′of-thal′mĭ-ah, lag′-of-thal′mos) [ G. *lagōs,* hare, + *ophthalmos,* eye ]. Hare's eye; failure of the upper eyelid to move down when the patient is asked to close his eye; a defect due to a scar or to involvement of the facial nerve, or occurring as a sequel to ptosis operation.

**Lagrange** (lă-grahn̈zh′), Pierre F., French ophthalmologist, 1857–1928. See L.'s *operation.*

**Lahey,** Frank H., U. S. surgeon, 1880–1935. See L. *forceps.*

**lake** (lāk) [ A.S. *lacu,* fr. L. *lacus,* lake ]. 1. Lacus; a small collection of fluid. 2. To cause blood plasma to become red as a result of the release of hemoglobin from the erythrocytes, as when the latter are suspended in water.

**capillary l.,** the total mass of blood contained in capillary vessels.

**lac′rimal l.,** *lacus* lacrimalis.

**lateral l.'s,** *lacunae* laterales.

**sem′inal l.,** *lacus* seminalis.

**subchorial l.,** subchorial *space.*

**venous l.'s,** thin-walled collections of blood, resembling blood blisters, found commonly in the ears and less often on the lips and on the face and neck of elderly persons.

**Laki-Lorand factor.** See under factor.

**la′ky.** Pertaining to the transparent, bright red appearance of blood serum or plasma, developing as a result of hemoglobin being released from destroyed red blood cells.

**laliatry** (lă-li′ă-trī) [ G. *lalia,* speech, chatter, + *iatria,* cure ]. The study and treatment of speech disorders.

**laliophobia** (lal′ĭ-o-fo′bĭ-ah) [ G. *lalia,* speech, + *phobos,* fear ]. Lalophobia; morbid fear of speaking or stuttering.

**lallation** (lal-la′shun) [ L. *lallo,* pp. -*atus,* to sing lullaby ]. Poor articulation, especially defective enunciation of words containing the letter *l;* see also lambdacism.

**Lallemand** (Lal-mahn̈), Claude F., French surgeon, 1790–1853. See L.'s *bodies,* Trousseau-L. *bodies.*

**lal′ling** [ G. *laleō,* to chatter ]. A form of stammering in which the speech is almost unintelligible.

**lalochezia** (lal′o-ke′zĭ-ah) [ G. *lalia,* speech, + *chezo,* to relieve oneself ]. Emotional discharge gained by uttering indecent or filthy words.

**lalognosis** (lal′og-no′sis) [ G. *lalia,* speech, + *gnosis,* knowledge ]. Understanding of speech.

**laloneurosis** (lal′o-nu-ro′sis) [ G. *laleō,* to chatter, + neurosis ]. A neurosis marked by incoherence or other form of speech defect.

**lal′opathol′ogy.** 1. Lalopathy. 2. The science concerned with speech disorders.

**lalopathy** (lal-op′ă-thī) [ G. *lalia,* speech, + *pathos,* suffering ]. Any form of speech defect.

**lalopho′bia.** Laliophobia.

**laloplegia** (lal′o-ple′jĭ-ah) [ G. *lalia,* speech, + *plēgē,* a stroke ]. Paralysis of the muscles concerned in the mechanism of speech.

**lalorrhea** (lal′o-re′ah) [ G. *lalia,* speech, + *rhoia,* flow ]. Excessive flow of words.

**Lalouette** (lă-loo-et′), Pierre, Paris physician, 1711–1742. See L.'s *pyramid.*

**Lamarck,** Jean-Baptiste P. A., French botanist, zoologist and biological philosopher, 1744–1829. See Lamarckian *theory.*

**lamb.** 1. A young sheep. 2. The act of giving birth to a l. 3. The meat of a l.

**hot house l.'s,** l.'s produced out of season and marketed at 8 to 10 weeks of age during the winter months.

**lambda** (lam′dah) [ The 11th letter of the Greek alphabet, λ, Λ ]. 1. The craniometric point at the junction of the sagittal and lambdoid sutures; see fig. under craniometric *point.* 2. The lower case Greek letter, λ, is used as a symbol for wavelength, Ostwald's solubility *coefficient,* and radioactive *constant;* it is also sometimes used (though not a preferred usage) as a symbol for microliter (μl).

**lambdacism** (lam′dah-sizm) [ G. *lambda,* the letter L ]. 1. Mispronunciation or disarticulation of the letter *l.* 2. Substitution of the letter *l* for the letter *r.* See lallation.

**lamb′doid** [ lambda + G. *eidos,* resemblance ]. Resembling the Greek letter lambda.

**Lambert,** Edward H., U. S. physician, \*1915. See L.-Eaton *syndrome.*

**Lambert,** Johann H., German physicist and mathematician, 1728–1777. Gave his name to lambert.

**lam′bert** [ J.H. *Lambert* ]. A unit of brightness; the brightness of a perfectly diffusing surface emitting or reflecting a total luminous flux of 1 lumen per sq. cm. of surface.

**Lam′blia intestina′lis.** Old term for *Giardia lamblia.*

**lambliasis** (lam-bli′ă-sis). Giardiasis.

**lambo lambo.** *Myositis* purulenta tropica.

**Lambotte** (lahm̈-but′), Albin, Belgian surgeon, 1856–1912. See L.'s *method.*

**lamella,** pl. **lamel′lae** (lă-mel′ah) [ L. dim. of *lamina,* plate, leaf ]. 1. A thin sheet or layer such as occurs in compact bone. 2. Disk; a preparation in the form of a medicated gelatin disk, used as a means of making local applications to the conjunctiva in place of solutions.

**annulate lamellae,** several pairs of parallel, smooth membranes, each pair containing regularly spaced pores resembling those of the nuclear envelope; they occur in germ cells, embryonic cells, and neoplastic cells.

**articular l.,** the compact layer of bone on its articular surface that is firmly attached to the overlying articular cartilage.

**l. of bone,** a concentric, circumferential, or intersititial l.

**circumferential l.,** a bony l. that encircles the outer or inner surface of a bone.

**concen′tric l.,** Haversian l.; one of the tubular layers of bone surrounding the central canal in an osteon.

**elastic l.,** a thin sheet or membrane composed of elastic fibers; not the same as elastic *membrane* (*q.v.*), which usually refers to a condensed mass of fibers, as in an elastic membrane of an artery, whereas an elastic l. may be a looser elastic layer such as found in a vein or the respiratory tract.

**enamel l.,** an organic defect in enamel; a thin, leaflike structure that extends from the enamel surface toward the dentinoenamel junction.

**glandulopreputial l.,** a layer of embryonic epithelial tissue that gives rise to the prepuce.

**ground l.,** interstitial l.

**Haversian l.,** concentric l.

**interme′diate l.,** interstitial l.

**interstitial l.,** intermediate l.; ground l.; one of the lamellae of partially resorbed osteons occurring between newer, complete osteons.

**triangular l.,** *tela* choroidea ventriculi tertii.

**vit′reous l.,** *lamina* basalis choroideae.

**lamellae** (la-mel′e). Plural of lamella.

**lamellar** (lam′ĕ-lar, lă-mel′ar). 1. Lamellate; lamellated; scaly; arranged in thin plates or scales. 2. Relating to lamellae.

**lam′ellate, lam′ellated.** Lamellar (1).

**La Mer,** Victor K. See L. *generator.*

---

# LAMINA

**lamina,** pl. **lam′inae** (lam′ĭ-nah) [ L ] [ NA ]. A thin plate or flat layer.

**l. affix′a** [ NA ], that part of the ependymal medial wall of the lateral ventricle of the embryonic brain that in later development becomes adherent to the superior surface of the thalamus and thus comes to form the floor of the pars centralis of the lateral ventricle; it covers the thalamostriate and choroidal veins.

**alar l. of neural tube,** l. alaris.

**l. ala′ris** [ NA ], alar l. or alar plate of the neural tube; wing plate; the dorsal division of the lateral walls of the neural tube in the embryo (see also l. basalis); the l. alaris gives rise to neurons relaying afferent impulses to higher centers; in the adult such neurons compose the sensory nuclei of the spinal cord and brainstem.

**laminae al′bae cerebel′li** [ NA ], laminae medullares cerebelli; layers of white substance seen on section of the cerebellum.

**l. anterior vagina musculi recti abdominis** [ NA ], anterior layer of the rectus abdominis sheath; the portion of the sheath of the rectus abdominis muscle that lies anterior to the muscle.

**l. ar′cus ver′tebrae** [ NA ], l. of the vertebral arch; neurapophysis; the flattened posterior portion of the vertebral arch from which the spinous process extends.

**basal l.,** basement l.

**basal l. of choroid,** l. basalis choroideae.

**basal l. of neural tube,** l. basalis.

**l. basa′lis** [ NA ], basal l. or basal plate of the neural tube; the ventral division of the lateral walls of the neural tube in the embryo (see also l. alaris). The basal l. contains neuroblasts giving rise to somatic and visceral motor neurons.

**l. basa′lis choroideae** [ NA ], basal layer of the choroid; l. vitrea; vitreous membrane (3); Bruch's membrane; Henle's membrane; the transparent, nearly structureless inner layer of the choroid in contact with the pigmented layer of the retina.

**l. basa′lis cor′poris cilia′ris** [ NA ], basal layer of the ciliary body; the inner layer of the ciliary body, continuous with the basal layer of the choroid.

**basement l.,** basal l.; boundary membrane; the filamentous, ultramicroscopic layer, 500 to 800 Å thick, that occurs at the base of epithelial cells and around muscle and nerve fibers and other microscopic elements; it is a subdivision of the basement membrane (*q.v.,* under membrane) of light microscopists.

**basilar l.,** l. basilaris cochleae.

**l. basila′ris coch′leae** [ NA ], basilar l.; basilar membrane; membrana basilaris; the membrane extending from the osseous spiral l. to the basilar crest of the cochlea; it forms the greater part of the floor of the cochlear duct and supports the organ of Corti.

**l. cartilag′inis cricoi′deae** [ NA ], l. of cricoid cartilage; a quadrate plate forming the posterior part of the cricoid cartilage. It resembles the shield of a signet ring, the arch of the cricoid representing the remainder of the ring.

**l. cartilag′inis latera′lis** [ NA ], lateral cartilaginous layer; official alternative term for l. lateralis.

**l. cartilag′inis media′lis** [ NA ], medial cartilaginous layer; official alternative term for l. medialis.

**l. cartilag′inis thyroi′deae** [ NA ], l. of the thyroid cartilage; one of the paired (dextra et sinistra) quadrilateral plates of the thyroid cartilage that are joined anteriorly and form an open angle posteriorly.

**l. choriocapilla′ris,** l. choroidocapillaris.

**l. choroid′ea,** l. epithelialis.

**l. choroid′ea epithelia′lis,** l. epithelialis.

**l. choroidocapilla′ris** [ NA ], l. choriocapillaris; membrana choriocapillaris; choriocapillary layer; Ruysch's membrane; the internal layer of the choroidea of the eye, composed of a very close capillary network.

**l. cine′rea,** l. terminalis cerebri.

**l. cribro′sa ossis ethmoidalis** [ NA ], cribrum; cribriform plate of the ethmoid bone; a horizontal l. from which are suspended the labyrinth, on either side and the l. perpendicularis in the center; it fits into the ethmoidal notch of the frontal bone and supports the olfactory lobes of the cerebrum, being pierced with numerous openings for the passage of the olfactory nerves.

**l. cribro′sa scle′rae,** perforated layer of the sclera; the portion of the sclera through which pass the fibers of the optic nerve.

**l. of cricoid cartilage,** l. cartilaginis cricoideae.

**l. densa,** the basement membrane of the renal glomerulus; it intervenes between the pedicles of the visceral capsule cells and the endothelium of the glomerular capillaries.

**dental l.,** dental *ledge.*

**l. denta′ta,** *labium* limbi vestibulare.

**dent′oging′ival l.,** dental *ledge.*

**l. dextra cartilaginis thyroidea** [ NA ], right plate of the thyroid cartilage; the thin plate of cartilage forming the right half of the thyroid cartilage.

**l. dura,** the hard layer lining the dental alveoli.

**elastic laminae of arteries,** elastic layers of arteries; (1) external: the fenestrated layer of elastic connective tissue lying immediately outside the smooth muscle of the tunica media; (2) internal: a fenestrated layer of elastic tissue of the tunica intima.

**l. elas′tica ante′rior,** l. limitans anterior corneae.

**l. elas′tica poste′rior,** l. limitans posterior corneae.

**episcleral l.,** l. episcleralis.

**l. episclera′lis** [ NA ], episcleral l.; the layer of loose connective tissue on the external surface of the sclera.

**epithelial l.,** l. epithelialis.

**l. epithelia′lis** [ NA ], epithelial l.; epithelial choroid layer; l. choroidea; l. choroidea epithelialis; the layer of modified ependymal cells that forms the inner layer of the tela choroidea, facing the ventricle.

**l. exter′na cra′nii** [ NA ], the outer table of the skull; the outer compact layer of the cranial bones.

**l. fibrocartilagin′ea interpu′bica,** *discus* interpubicus.

**l. fusca sclerae** [ NA ], brown layer; a thin layer of loose, pigmented connective tissue on the inner surface of the sclera, connecting it with the choroid.

**hepatic laminae,** the plates of liver cells that radiate from the center of the liver lobule.

**l. horizonta′lis os′sis palati′ni** [ NA ], the horizontal plate of the palate bone that forms the posterior part of the bony palate.

**l. inter′na cra′nii** [ NA ], inner table of the skull; the inner compact layer of the cranial bones.

**labiogingival l.,** a band of ectodermal epithelial cells growing into the mesenchyme of the embryonic jaws between the developing lip and the growing gingival elevation; it later opens to form the labiogingival groove.

**lateral medullary l. of corpus striatum,** l. medullaris lateralis corporis striati.

**l. latera′lis** [ NA ], l. cartilaginis lateralis [ NA ]; lateral layer; lateral cartilaginous layer; the narrow lateral portion of the cartilaginous part of the auditory tube.

**l. latera′lis and l. media′lis, proces′sus pterygoid′ei** [ NA ], the lateral and medial pterygoid plates; two bony plates extending downward from the point of union of the body and greater wing of the sphenoid bone on either side.

**l. of lens,** one of a series of concentric layers composed of the lens fibers that make up the substance of the lens.

**l. limitans anterior corneae** [ NA ], anterior limiting layer of the cornea; l. elastica anterior; anterior elastic layer; Bowman's membrane; a thin basement membrane lying between the outer layer of stratified epithelium and the substantia propria of the cornea.

**l. limitans posterior corneae** [ NA ], posterior limiting layer of the cornea; l. elastica posterior; posterior elastic layer; entocornea; Duddell's membrane; Descemet's membrane; vitreous membrane (1); a thin basement membrane between the substantia propria and the endothelial layer of the cornea.

**medial medullary l. of corpus striatum,** l. medullaris medialis corporis striati.

**l. media′lis** [ NA ], l. cartilaginis medialis [ NA ]; medial layer; medial cartilaginous layer; the broad medial portion of the cartilaginous part of the auditory tube.

**laminae medullares cerebelli,** laminae albae cerebelli.

**l. medulla′ris latera′lis cor′poris stria′ti** [ NA ], lateral medullary l. of the corpus striatum; a thin, sharply defined layer of fibers separating the putamen from the globus pallidus.

**l. medulla′ris media′lis cor′poris stria′ti** [ NA ], medial medullary l. of the corpus striatum; a fiber layer separating the medial and lateral segments of the globus pallidus.

**laminae medulla′res thal′ami** [ NA ], medullary layers of thalamus; layers of myelinated fibers appearing on transverse sections of the thalamus, the l. medullaris externa marking the ventral border of the thalamus and delimiting it from the subthalamus and nucleus reticularis thalami, the l. medullaris interna interposed between the mediodorsal and ventral nuclei of the thalamus; the internal medullary l. encloses the intralaminar nuclei (nuclei centromedianus, paracentralis, and centralis lateralis).

**l. membrana′cea** [ NA ], membranous layer; the connective tissue membrane that, with the l. lateralis, completes the lateral and inferior walls of the cartilaginous part of the auditory tube.

**l. modi′oli** [ NA ], plate of the modiolus; a bony plate, the continuation of the modiolus and of the septum between the convolutions of the spiral canal of the cochlea extending upward toward the cupola, forming with the hamulus the helicotrema.

**l. muscula′ris muco′sae** [ NA ], muscular layer of the mucosa; the thin layer of smooth muscle found in most parts of the digestive tube located outside the l. propria mucosae and adjacent to the tela submucosa.

**orbital l. of ethmoid bone,** l. orbitalis ossis ethmoidalis.

**l. orbita′lis ossis ethmoida′lis** [ NA ], orbital l. of ethmoid bone; l. papyracea; paper or papyraceous plate; a thin plate of bone that forms a part of the medial wall of the orbit and bounds the ethmoidal labyrinth laterally.

**osseous spiral l.,** l. spiralis ossea.

**l. papyra′cea,** l. orbitalis ossis ethmoidalis.

**l. parietalis** [ NA ], parietal layer; (1) the outer part of the serous pericardium supported by the fibrous pericardium; (2) the outer part of the tunica vaginalis testis supported by the internal spermatic fascia.

**periclaustral l.,** *capsula* externa.

**l. perpendicula′ris** [ NA ], perpendicular or vertical plate of the ethmoid bone; pars perpendicularis; a thin plate of bone, projecting above the horizontal plate to form the crista galli and depending from it between the two labyrinths.

**l. perpendicula′ris ossis palatini** [ NA ], perpendicular plate of the palate bone; pars perpendicularis; the part that extends vertically in the lateral wall of the nasal cavity.

**l. posterior vaginae musculi recti abdominis** [ NA ], posterior layer of the rectus abdominis sheath; the portion of the sheath of the rectus abdominis muscle that lies posterior to the muscle, its free inferior margin forms the arcuate line.

**l. pretrachea′lis** [ NA ], pretracheal layer; pretracheal fascia; middle cervical fascia; Porter's fascia; the layer of fascia investing the infrahyoid muscles and contributing to the formation of the carotid sheath.

**l. prevertebralis** [ NA ], prevertebral layer; prevertebral fascia; the part of the cervical fascia which covers the bodies of the cervical vertebrae and the muscles attaching to them and to the anterior parts of their transverse processes.

**primary dental l.,** dental *ledge*.

**l. profunda** [ NA ], deep layer; (1) the deep part of the temporal fascia attaching to the medial surface of the zygomatic arch; (2) the deeper fibers of the levator muscle of the superior eyelid which are inserted into the superior tarsal plate.

**l. propria mucosae** [ NA ], the layer of connective tissue underlying the epithelium of a mucous membrane.

**pterygoid laminae,** see l. lateralis and medialis processus pterygoidei.

**l. quadrigem′ina,** l. tecti mesencephali.

**retic′ular l.,** a major component of the basement membrane of the light microscopists; it consists largely of reticular fibers and ground substances.

**rostral l.,** l. rostralis.

**l. rostra′lis,** rostral l. or layer; teniola corporis callosi; a whitish line appearing on perfectly median section of the brain as a thin bridge connecting the rostrum of the corpus callosum with the lamina terminalis; contrary to its appearance, the l. rostralis contains no commissural fibers; instead, it corresponds to the line along which the pia mater reflects from the medial surface of one hemisphere to that of the other.

**l. sep′ti pellu′cidi** [ NA ], l. of the septum pellucidum; one of the two thin layers of the septum pellucidum, often separated from each other by a space, the cavum septi pellucidi.

**l. of septum pellucidum,** l. septi pellucidi.

**l. sinistra cartilaginis thyroidea** [ NA ], left plate of the thyroid cartilage; the thin plate of the thyroid cartilage forming the left half of the thyroid cartilage.

**l. spira′lis os′sea** [ NA ], osseous spiral l.; spiral plate; a double plate of bone winding spirally around the modiolus dividing the spiral canal of the cochlea incompletely into two, scala tympani and scala vestibuli; between the two plates of this l. the fibers of the cochlear nerve reach the spiral organ (of Corti).

**l. spira′lis secunda′ria** [ NA ], secondary spiral plate; a ridge on the outer wall of the first turn of the cochlea opposite the spiral l.

**l. superficialis** [ NA ], superficial layer; (1) the superficial part of the temporal fascia attaching to the lateral surface of the zygomatic arch; (2) the part of the cervical fascia investing the sternocleidomastoid and trapezius and completely encircling the neck; (3) the superficial fibers of the levator muscle of the superior eyelid which are inserted into the skin of the superior eyelid.

**l. suprachoroid′ea** [ NA ], suprachoroid layer; a layer of loose, pigmented connective tissue on the outer surface of the choroid, resembling and attached to the l. fusca sclerae.

**l. su′praneuropor′ica,** that part of the choroid membrane of the third ventricle that forms the roof of the foramen of Monro.

**l. tec′ti mesenceph′ali** [ NA ], tectum mesencephali [ NA ]; quadrigeminal plate; lamina quadrigemina; the roofplate of the midbrain formed by the corpora quadrigemina (a pair of superior and a pair of inferior colliculi).

**l. termina′lis cer′ebri** [ NA ], terminal plate; velum terminale; l. cinerea; a thin plate passing upward from the optic chiasm and forming the anterior wall of the third ventricle.

**l. of thyroid cartilage,** l. cartilaginis thyroideae.

**l. tra′gi** [ NA ], l. of the tragus; a longitudinal curved plate of cartilage, the beginning of the cartilaginous portion of the external acoustic meatus.

**l. of tragus,** l. tragi.

**l. vasculo′sa choroideae** [ NA ], vascular layer of the choroid coat of the eye; Haller's vascular tissue; vascular layer; the outer portion of the choroid containing the largest blood vessels.

**l. of vertebral arch,** l. arcus vertebrae.

**l. visceralis** [ NA ], visceral layer; (1) epicardium; the inner part of the serous pericardium applied directly on the heart; (2) the inner part of the tunica vaginalis testis applied directly to the testis and epididymis.

**l. vit′rea,** l. basalis choroideae.

---

**lam′inagram.** A film taken by a laminagraph.

**lam′inagraph.** Technique whereby tissues above and below the level of a suspected lesion are blurred out to emphasize a specific area.

**laminagraphy** (lam′ĭ-nag′ră-fĭ) [ lamina + G. *graphē,* a writing ]. Sectional roentgenography; tomography.

**lam′inar.** 1. Laminated; arranged in plates or laminae. 2. Relating to any lamina.

**laminar'in.** An algal polysaccharide, made up chiefly of $\beta$-D-glucose residues, obtained from *Laminaria* species (family Laminariaceae). Variable proportions of the glucose chains contain at the potential reducing end a molecule of mannitol that can be sulfated; see l. sulfate.
 **l. sulfate,** l. sulfated to varying degrees; two sulfate groups per glucose unit results in maximum stability and anticoagulant activity similar to that of heparin; l. with fewer sulfate groups has only antilipemic activity.

**lam'inated.** Laminar (1).

**lamination** (lam'ĭ-na'shun). 1. An arrangement in the form of plates or laminae. 2. Embryotomy by removing the head in slices.

**laminectomy** (lam'ĭ-nek'to-mĭ) [ L. *lamina*, layer, + G. *ektomē*, excision ]. Rachiotomy (1); excision of a vertebral lamina; commonly used to denote removal of the posterior arch.

**laminitis** (lam'ĭ-ni'tis). 1. Inflammation of any lamina. 2. Founder; an inflammation of the sensitive lamina to which the hoof of the horse is attached. It may affect only one or all four feet. The front feet are most commonly involved. The condition is very painful. Overfeeding with grain is a common precipitating cause.

**laminotomy** (lam'ĭ-not'o-mĭ) [ L. *lamina*, layer, + G. *tomē*, incision ]. Division of one or more vertebral laminae.

**lamp.** Illuminating device; source of light. See also light.
 **annealing l.,** an alcohol l. with a soot-free flame used to drive off the protective $NH_3$ gas coating from the surface of cohesive gold foil.
 **Eldridge-Green l.,** a lantern used in testing recognition of colored signals. It displays a single light with color filters in rotating disks that can be modified so as to simulate all conditions of weather and atmosphere.
 **Kromayer's l.,** a U-shaped quartz l. of mercury vapor, giving out actinic rays, used in the treatment of skin diseases.
 **mignon l.,** a small electric l. used in cystoscope.
 **slit-l.,** see slitlamp.
 **spirit-l.,** a l., used mainly for heating in laboratory work, in which alcohol is burned.
 **ultraviolet l.,** one that emits rays in the ultraviolet band of the spectrum; see also ultraviolet.
 **uviol l.,** an electric l. with uviol glass, furnishing especially the violet rays, used in phototherapy.

**Lamy,** M. See Maroteaux-L. *syndrome.*

**lamziekte** (lahm'zĕk-teh) [ D. *lam*, lame, + *ziekte*, sickness ]. Botulism.

**lana,** gen. and pl. **lan'ae** (lan'ah) [ L. ]. Wool.

**lanadigenin.** Digoxigenin.

**lanat'osides A, B, C.** Digilanides A, B, and C; the cardioactive precursor glycosides obtained from *Digitalis lanata*. Removal of the acetyl group yields desacetyllanatosides A, B, and C (purpurea glycosides A, B, and C, respectively); removal of the glucose from lanatosides A, B, and C yields acetyl digitoxin, acetylgitoxin, and acetyldigoxin, respectively; removal of glucose and the acetyl group yields digitoxin, gitoxin, and digoxin, respectively. Lanatoside C is official in the NF. See also purpurea glycosides.

**lanat'oside D.** A glycoside from the leaves of *Digitalis lanata*, yielding the genin diginatigenin (12-hydroxygitoxigenin; 16-hydroxydigoxigenin).

**lance** (lans) [ L. *lancea*, a slender spear ]. 1. To incise a part, as an abscess or boil. 2. A lancet.
 **Mauriceau's l.,** a knife with sharp point, used in embryotomy.

**Lancefield,** Rebecca C., New York bacteriologist, *1895. See L. *classification.*

**lancet** (lan'set) [ Fr. *lancette* ]. A surgical knife with a short, wide, sharp-pointed, two-edged blade.
 **gum l.,** a l. used for incising the gum over the crown of an erupting tooth.
 **spring l.,** one the blade of which is set in the handle with a spring.
 **thumb l.,** a l. with short flat blade which folds back, when closed, between two plates of the handle.

**Lancet coefficient.** See under coefficient.

**lancinating** (lan'sĭ-na'ting) [ L. *lancino*, pp. -*atus*, to tear ]. Denoting a sharp cutting or tearing pain.

**Lancisi** (lahn-che'ze), Giovanni M., Italian physician, 1654–1720. See L.'s *striae.*

**Lancisi's sign.** See under sign.

**Landolfi's sign.** See under sign.

**Landolt,** Edmund, Paris oculist, 1846–1926. See L.'s *bodies.*

**Landouzy** (lahn-doo-ze'), Louis, T. J., Paris physician, 1845–1917. See L.-Déjérine *dystrophy*, L.-Grasset *law.*

**Landry** (lahn-dre'), Jean B. O., French physician, 1826–1865. See Kussmaul-L. *paralysis*, L.'s *paralysis.*

**Landschutz tumor.** See under tumor.

**Landsteiner** (lahnd'sti-ner), Karl, Austrian-U. S. pathologist, 1868–1943. Nobel laureate, 1930, for his discovery of human blood groups. See Donath-L. *phenomenon*, L.-Donath *test*, Donath-L. cold *autoantibody.*

**Landström** (lahnd'strĕm), John, Swedish surgeon, 1869–1910. See L.'s *muscle.*

**Landzert** (lahnt'sairt). T., German anatomist, 19th century. See L.'s *fossa*, Grüber-L. *fossa.*

**Lane,** Sir W. Arbuthnot, English surgeon, 1856–1943. See L.'s *band*, L.-Lannelongue *operation*, L.'s *plates*, L.'s *disease.*

**Lang,** Basil T., English ophthalmologist, 1880–1928. See Frost-L. *operation.*

**Lange** (lahng'eh), Carl F. A., German biochemist, *1883. See L.'s *solution*, *test.*

**Lange,** Carl G., Danish psychologist, 1834–1900. See James-L. *theory.*

**Langenbeck** (lahng'en-bek), Bernhard R. K. von, German surgeon, 1810–1887. See L.'s *amputation*, *incision*, *triangle.*

**Langendorff** (lahng'en-dorf), Oscar, German physiologist, 1853–1908. See L.'s *method.*

**Lange-Nielsen,** F. See Jervell and L.-N. *syndrome.*

**Langer,** Carl R., von, Vienna anatomist, 1819–1887. See L.'s *arch, lines, muscle.*

**Langerhans** (lahng'er-hahns), Paul, German anatomist, 1847–1888. See L.'s *cells, granule, islands, islets.*

**Langhans** (lahng'hahns), Theodor, German pathologist, 1839–1915. See L.'s *cells*, giant *cells, layer, stria.*

**Langley,** John N., English physiologist, 1852–1925. See L.'s *granules, test.*

**Langmuir,** Irving, U. S. chemist, 1881–1957. See L. *trough.*

**language** (lang'wij). [ L. *lingua* ]. Any means or form, vocal or other, of expression or communication.
 **body l.,** (1) communication by means of bodily signs, *e.g.*, through the symptoms of hysterical conversion; (2) the expression of thoughts and feelings by means of nonverbal bodily movements, *e.g.*, gestures.

**laniary** (lan'ĭ-ĕr-ĭ) [ L. *laniarius*, to tear to pieces ]. Adapted for tearing; in anatomy, sometimes applied to canine teeth, as l. teeth.

**Lannelongue** (lan-ĕ-loṅg'), Odilon M., French surgeon and pathologist, 1840–1911. See L.'s *foramina, ligament*, Lane-L. *operation.*

**lan'olin** [ L. *lana*, wool, + *oleum*, oil ]. (USP). Hydrous wool fat (BP); adeps lanae hydrosus; the purified, fatlike substance from the wool of sheep, *Ovis aries* (family Bovidae); it contains not less than 25 per cent and not more than 30 per cent of water; used as a water-adsorbable ointment base. See also wool fat.
 **anhydrous l.** (USP), wool fat (BP); l. that contains not more than 0.25 per cent of water; used as a water-adsorbable ointment base.

**lanos'terol.** Isocholesterol; 5α-lanosta-8,24-diene-3β-ol; a sterol present in wool fat. For structure of lanostane, see steroids.

**Lanterman,** A. J., U. S. anatomist in Strasbourg, 19th century. See L.'s *incisures*, Schmidt-L. *clefts, incisures*, L.'s *segments.*

**lan'thanides.** The rare earth elements; see lanthanum.

**lan'thanum** [ G. *lanthanō*, to lie hid ]. A metallic element, symbol La, atomic no. 57, atomic weight 138.92; first of the rare earth elements, which are therefore referred to as lanthanides.

**lanthi'onine.** HOOC—CHNH$_2$—CH$_2$—S—CH$_2$—CHNH$_2$—COOH; *bis*(2-amino-2-carboxyethyl)sulfide; an amino acid resembling cystine but with only one sulfur atom in the molecule rather than two; obtained from wool.

**lanuginous** (lă-nu'jĭ-nus). Covered with lanugo.

**lanugo** (lă-nu'go) [ L. down, woolliness, from *lana*, wool ] [ NA ]. lanugo hair; fine, soft, unmedullated fetal or embryonic hair with minute shafts and large papillae; it appears toward the end of the third month of gestation.

**Lanz** (lahnts), Otto, Amsterdam surgeon, 1865–1935. See L.'s *line*.

**lapac'tic** [ G. *lapaktikos*, fr. *lapassō*, to empty ]. Purgative; laxative.

**laparectomy** (lap'ă-rek'to-mĭ) [ laparo- + G. *ektomē*, excision ]. Excision of strips or gores in the abdominal wall and suture of the edges of the wound, in cases of abnormal laxity of the abdominal muscles.

**laparo-** [ G. *lapara*, flank, loins ]. Combining form denoting the loins or, less properly, the abdomen in general.

**laparocele** (lap'ă-ro-sēl) [ laparo- + G. *kēlē*, hernia ]. Abdominal *hernia*.

**laparocholecystotomy** (lap'ă-ro-ko'le-sis-tot'o-mĭ). Cholecystotomy.

**laparocolectomy** (lap'ă-ro-ko-lek'to-mĭ). Colectomy.

**laparocolostomy** (lap'ă-ro-ko-los'to-mĭ) [ laparo- + G. *kolon*, colon, + G. *stoma*, mouth ]. Formation of an artificial anus, by opening into the colon from the side.

**laparocolotomy** (lap'ă-ro-ko-lot'o-mĭ). Colotomy.

**laparocystectomy** (lap'ă-ro-sis-tek'to-mĭ) [ laparo- + G. *kystis*, cyst, + *ektomē*, excision ]. Removal of an ovarian or other cystic tumor through an incision in the abdominal wall.

**laparocystidotomy** (lap'ă-ro-sis-tĭ-dot'o-mĭ). Laparocystotomy.

**laparocystotomy** (lap'ă-ro-sis-tot'o-mĭ) [ laparo- + G. *kystis*, cyst, + *tomē*, incision ]. 1. Evacuation of the contents of an ovarian or other cystic tumor through an incision in the abdominal wall. 2. Suprapubic *cystotomy*.

**laparoenterostomy** (lap'ă-ro-en-ter-os'to-mĭ) [ laparo- + G. *enteron*, intestine, + *stoma*, mouth ]. Formation of an artificial anus in the loin.

**laparoenterotomy** (lap'ă-ro-en-ter-ot'o-mĭ) [ laparo- + G. *enteron*, intestine, + *tomē*, incision ]. 1. Opening into the intestine through an incision in the loin. 2. Celioenterotomy.

**laparogastroscopy** (lap'ă-ro-gas-tros'ko-pĭ) [ laparo- + G. *gastēr*, stomach, + *skopeō*, to view ]. Inspection of interior of stomach after a gastrotomy.

**laparogastrostomy** (lap'ă-ro-gas-tros'to-mĭ) [ laparo- + G. *gastēr*, stomach, + *stoma*, mouth ]. Celiogastrostomy.

**laparogastrotomy** (lap'ă-ro-gas-trot'o-mĭ) [ laparo- + G. *gastēr*, stomach, + *tomē*, incision ]. Celiogastrotomy.

**laparohepatotomy** (lap'ă-ro-hep'ă-tot'o-mĭ) [ laparo- + G. *hēpar*, liver, + *tomē*, incision ]. Incision into the liver from the side.

**laparohysterectomy** (lap'ă-ro-his-ter-ek'to-mĭ). Abdominal *hysterectomy*.

**laparohystero-oophorectomy** (lap'ă-ro-his'ter-o-o-of'o-rek'to-mĭ) [ laparo- + G. *hystera*, uterus, + oophorectomy ]. Removal of the uterus and ovaries through an incision in the abdominal wall.

**laparohysteropexy** (lap'ă-ro-his'ter-o-pek'sĭ) [ laparo- + G. *hystera*, uterus, + *pēxis*, fixation ]. Abdominal *hysteropexy*.

**lap'arohys'terosal'pingo-o'ophorec'tomy.** Removal of uterus and adnexa (tubes and ovaries) through an abdominal incision.

**laparohysterotomy** (lap'ă-ro-his-ter-ot'o-mĭ) [ laparo- + G. *hystera*, uterus, + *tomē*, incision ]. Abdominal *hysterotomy*.

**laparomyomectomy** (lap'ă-ro-mi'o-mek'to-mĭ). Abdominal *myomectomy*.

**laparomyomotomy** (lap'ă-ro-mi'o-mot'o-mĭ). Celiomyomotomy.

**laparomyositis** (lap'ă-ro-mi'o-si'tis) [ laparo- + G. *mys*, muscle, + suffix *-itis*, inflammation ]. Inflammation of the lateral abdominal muscles.

**laparonephrectomy** (lap'ă-ro-ne-frek'to-mĭ) [ laparo- + G. *nephros*, kidney, + *ektomē*, excision ]. Removal of the kidney through an incision in the loin.

**laparorrhaphy** (lap'ă-ror'ă-fĭ). Celiorrhaphy.

**laparosalpingectomy** (lap'ă-ro-sal'pin-jek'to-mĭ). Abdominal *salpingectomy*.

**laparosalpingo-oophorectomy** (lap'ă-ro-sal'ping-go-o-of'o-rek'to-mĭ). Abdominal salpingo-oophorectomy; removal of the Fallopian tube and ovary through an abdominal incision.

**laparosalpingotomy** (lap'ă-ro-sal'ping-got'o-mĭ). Abdominal *salpingotomy*.

**laparoscope** (lap'ă-ro-skōp) [ laparo- + G. *skopeō*, to view ]. Peritoneoscope.

**laparoscopy** (lap-ă-ros'ko-pĭ). Peritoneoscopy.

**laparosplenectomy** (lap'ă-ro-sple-nek'to-mĭ) [ laparo- + G. *splēn*, spleen, + *ektomē*, excision ]. Removal of the spleen through an incision in the abdominal wall.

**laparosplenotomy** (lap'ă-ro-sple-not'o-mĭ) [ laparo- + G. *splēn*, spleen, + *tomē*, incision ]. Incision through the abdominal wall into the spleen.

**laparot'omize.** To subject to laparotomy.

**laparotomy** (lap'ă-rot'o-mĭ) [ laparo- + G. *tomē*, incision ]. 1. Incision into the loin. 2. Celiotomy.

**laparotrachelotomy** (lap'ă-ro-trak'ē-lot'o-mĭ) [ laparo- + G. *trachēlos*, neck, + *tomē*, incision ]. A low cervical cesarean section.

**laparotyphlotomy** (lap'ă-ro-tif-lot'o-mĭ) [ laparo- + G. *typhlon*, cecum, + *tomē*, incision ]. Typhlotomy through a lateral abdominal incision.

**laparouterotomy** (lap'ă-ro-u'ter-ot'o-mĭ) [ laparo- + uterus + G. *tomē*, incision ]. Abdominal *hysterotomy*.

**Lapham,** Maxwell, E., American obstetrician, *1899. See Friedman-L. *test*.

**lapinization** (lap'ĭ-nĭ-za'shun) [ Fr. *lapin*, rabbit ]. Serial passage of a vaccine in rabbits.

**lapinized** (lap'ĭ-nizd) [ Fr. *lapin*, rabbit ]. Applied to viruses which have been adapted to developing in rabbits by serial transfers in this species. In many instances viruses lose virulence for other species of animals and thus may be used as vaccines.

**Lapicque's law.** See under law.

**la'pis** [ L. ]. A stone.

   **l. divi'nus,** aluminated copper.

   **l. imperia'lis,** silver nitrate, toughened.

**Laplace,** Ernest, Philadelphia surgeon, 1861–1924. See L.'s *forceps*.

**Laplace** (la-plahs), Pierre S. de, French mathemetician, 1749–1827. See L.'s *law*.

**lap'pa** [ L. a burr ]. Burdock; beggars' buttons; the dried root of *Arctium lappa* (family Compositae), a herb of the north temperate zone. Formerly used as an alterative.

**lar'bish.** A form of creeping eruption observed in Senegal.

**lard** [ L. *lardum* ]. Adeps; the rendered fat of swine, particularly of the fat masses found in the abdominal cavity.

   **leaf l.,** that rendered from the firm fat mass found around the kidneys.

   **l. oil,** a fixed oil expressed from l.; used for pharmaceutical purposes.

**lar'icin.** Coniferin.

**lark'spur.** *Delphinium ajacis.*

**Laron type dwarfism.** See under dwarfism.

**Laroyenne** (lar-wah-yen'), Lucien, French surgeon, *1876. See L.'s *operation*.

**Larrey** (lă-ra'), Dominique J., French surgeon, 1766–1842. See L.'s *amputation, cleft,* L.-Weil *disease,* L.'s *ligation*.

**Larsen,** Loren J., U. S. orthopedic surgeon, *1914. See L.'s *syndrome*.

**Larsson,** T. See Sjögren-L. *syndrome*.

**larva,** pl. **larvae** (lar'vah, lar've) [ L. a mask. LARV- ]. 1. The wormlike form of an insect or helminth upon issuing from the egg; a grub, maggot, or caterpillar. 2. The young of fishes or amphibians which often differ in appearance from the adult.

   **filariform l.,** infective strongyliform third-stage l. of the hookworm, *Ascaris,* and other nematodes with penetrating larvae or with larvae that migrate through the body to reach the intestine.

**l. migrans,** see *larva migrans.*

**larvaceous** (lar-va′shus). Larvate.

**lar′val.** 1. Relating to larvae. 2. Larvate.

**lar′va mi′grans.** Larval worms, typically nematodes, that wander for a period in the host tissues but do not develop to the adult stage. This usually occurs in abnormal hosts that inhibit normal development of the parasite.

   **cutaneous l. migrans,** creeping eruption or myiasis; dermatitis linearis migrans; myiasis linearis; an advancing serpiginous or netlike tunneling in the skin, with marked pruritus, caused by wandering hookworm larvae not adapted to intestinal maturation in man; widely distributed in eastern and southern coastal United States and other tropical and subtropical coastal areas. Various hookworms of dogs and cats have been implicated, chiefly *Ancylostoma braziliensis* in the United States, but also *Ancylostoma caninum* of dogs and the European dog hookworm *Uncinaria stenocephala* and cattle hookworm *Bunostomum phlebotomum. Strongyloides* species of animal origin may also contribute to human cutaneous l. migrans, but *A. braziliense* and *A. caninum* are chiefly responsible.

   **spiruroid l. migrans,** extraintestinal migration by nematode larvae of the order Spiruroidea, not adapted to maturation in the human intestine; caused chiefly by species of *Gnathostoma* (*G. spinigerum* and *G. hispidum*) in Japan and Thailand, following ingestion of uncooked fish infected with encapsulated third-stage infective larvae. It may also be possible to become infected from ingestion of infected copepods (the first intermediate host) in contaminated drinking water. The anteriorly spined larvae produce serpiginous tunnels in the skin or may cause subcutaneous or pulmonary abscess, or may invade the eye or brain.

   **visceral l. migrans,** a disease, chiefly of children, caused by ingestion of infective ova of *Toxocara canis* (common intestinal ascarid nematode of dogs), or less commonly by other ascarid nematodes not adapted to man. The larvae hatch in the intestine, penetrate the gut wall, and wander in the viscera, chiefly the liver, for periods of up to 18 or 24 months, producing a sustained high eosinophilia. The condition may be asymptomatic or may be marked by hepatomegaly (with granulomatous lesions caused by encapsulated larvae on the enlarged liver), pulmonary infiltration, fever, cough, and hyperglobulinemia.

**lar′vate, lar′vated** [L. *larva,* mask]. Masked or concealed; applied to a disease with undeveloped, absent, or atypical symptoms.

**larvicide** (lar′vĭ-sīd) [larva + L. *caedo,* to kill]. 1. Destructive to larvae—grubs, caterpillars, etc. 2. An agent that kills larvae.

**larvip′arous** [larva + L. *pario,* to bear]. Larvae-bearing; denoting passage of larvae, rather than eggs, from the body of the female, as in certain nematodes and insects.

**larviphagic** (lar′vĭ-fa′jik) [larva + G. *phagein,* to eat]. Consuming larvae; certain l. fish are used in mosquito control.

**laryng-.** See laryngo-.

**laryngeal** (lă-rin′je-al). Relating in any way to the larynx.

**laryngectomy** (lăr′in-jek′to-mĭ) [laryngo- + G. *ektomē,* excision]. Excision of the larynx.

**laryngemphraxis** (lăr′in-jem-frak′sis) [G. *emphraxis,* a stoppage]. Laryngeal obstruction from any cause.

**larynges** (lă′rin′jēz) [L.]. Plural of larynx.

**laryn′geus** [L.] [NA]. Laryngeal.

**laryngismus** (lăr-in-jiz′mus) [L. fr. G. *larynx,* + suffix *-ismos, -ism*]. A spasmodic narrowing or closure of the rima glottidis.

   **l. paralyt′icus,** "roaring" in horses.

   **l. strid′ulus** [L. *stridulus,* noisy], spasmus glottidis; a spasmodic closure of the glottis, lasting a few seconds, followed by a noisy inspiration; *cf. laryngitis* stridulosa.

**laryngitic** (lăr-in-jit′ik). Relating to or caused by laryngitis.

**laryngitis** (lăr-in-ji′tis) [laryngo- + G. suffix *-itis,* inflammation]. Inflammation of the mucous membrane of the larynx.

   **croupous l.,** inflammation of the larynx associated with respiratory infection and croupy or noisy breathing.

**mem′branous l.,** a form in which there is a pseudomembranous exudate on the vocal cords.

   **l. stridulo′sa,** spasmodic l.; catarrhal inflammation of the larynx in children, accompanied by night attacks of spasmodic closure of the glottis, causing inspiratory stridor.

**laryngo-, laryng-** (lă-ring′go-) [G. *larynx, q.v.*]. Combining forms relating to the larynx.

**laryngocele** (lă-ring′go-sēl) [laryngo- + G. *kēle,* hernia]. An air sac communicating with the larynx through the ventricle, often bulging outward into the tissue of the neck, especially during coughing.

**laryngofissure** (lă-ring′go-fish′ur). Laryngotomy; thyrofissure; thyroidotomy; thyrotomy; thyrochondrotomy; operative opening into the larynx, generally through the midline, commonly done for the excision of early carcinoma or the correction of laryngostenosis.

**laryngograph** (lă-ring′go-graf) [laryngo- + G. *graphō,* to write]. An instrument for making a tracing of the movements of the larynx.

**laryngology** (lăr-ing-gol′o-jĭ) [laryngo- + G. *logos,* study]. The branch of medical science that has to do with the larynx; the specialty of diseases of the larynx.

**laryngomalacia** (lă-ring′go-mă-la′shĭ-ah) [laryngo- + G. *malakia,* a softness]. *Chondromalacia* of larynx.

**laryngoparalysis** (lă-ring′go-pă-ral′ĭ-sis). Paralysis of the laryngeal muscles.

**laryngopathy** (lăr′ing-gop′ă-thĭ) [laryngo- + G. *pathos,* suffering]. Any disease of the larynx.

**laryngophantom** (lă-ring′go-fan′tum) [laryngo- + G. *phantasma,* image. PHAN- ]. A model of the larynx for use in the study of the anatomy or for practice in laryngoscopy.

**laryngopharyngeal** (lă-ring′go-fă-rin′je-al). Relating to both larynx and pharynx or to the laryngopharynx.

**laryngopharyngectomy** (lă-ring′go-făr′in-jek′to-mĭ). Resection or excision of both larynx and pharynx.

**laryngopharyngeus** (lă-ring′go-făr′in-je′us) [L.]. *Musculus* constrictor pharyngeus inferior.

**laryngopharyngitis** (lă-ring′go-făr′in-ji′tis). Inflammation of the larynx and pharynx.

**laryngopharynx** (lă-ring′go-făr′ingks). *Pars laryngea pharyngis.*

**laryngophony** (lăr′ing-gof′o-nĭ) [laryngo- + G. *phōnē,* voice]. The voice sounds heard in auscultation of the larynx.

**laryngophthisis** (lă-ring′go-thi′sis) [laryngo- + G. *phthisis,* a wasting]. Tuberculosis of the larynx.

**laryngoplasty** (lă-ring′go-plas-tĭ) [laryngo- + G. *plassō,* to form]. Reparative or plastic surgery of the larynx.

**laryngoplegia** (lă-ring′go-ple′jĭ-ah) [laryngo- + G. *plēgē,* stroke]. Laryngoparalysis.

**laryngoptosis** (lă-ring′go-to′sis) [laryngo- + G. *ptōsis,* a falling]. An abnormally low position of the larynx at birth, which may be congenital or acquired; does not impair the health of the neonate. Some degree of l. occurs with aging.

**laryngorhinology** (lă-ring′go-ri-nol′o-jĭ) [laryngo- + G. *rhis,* nose, + *logos,* study]. The branch of medical science that has to do with affections of the larynx and of the nose.

**laryngoscope** (lă-ring′go-skōp) [laryngo- + G. *skopeō,* to inspect]. Any of several types of hollow tubes, equipped with electrical lighting, used in examining or operating upon the interior of the larynx through the mouth.

**laryngoscopic** (lă-ring′go-skop′ik). Relating to laryngoscopy.

**laryngoscopist** (lăr′ing-gos′ko-pist). A person skilled in the use of the laryngoscope.

**laryngoscopy** (lăr′ing-gos′ko-pĭ). Inspection of the larynx by means of the laryngoscope.

   **suspension l.,** support of the laryngoscope by leverage from the anterior chest wall or other supportive structure to provide maximum exposure of the pharyngeal cavity and larynx.

**laryngospasm** (lă-ring′go-spazm). Glottidospasm; spasmodic closure of the glottic aperture.

**laryngostenosis** (lă-ring′go-stĕ-no′sis) [laryngo- + G. *stenōsis,* a narrowing]. Stricture or narrowing of the lumen of the larynx.

**laryngostomy** (lăr'ing-gos'to-mĭ) [ laryngo- + G. *stoma*, mouth ]. The establishment of a permanent opening from the neck into the larynx.

**laryngostroboscope** (lă-ring'go-stro'bo-skōp, -strob'o-skōp). Stroboscopic apparatus for observing the motion of the vocal cords during phonation.

**laryngotome** (lă-ring'go-tōm). An instrument for use in laryngotomy.

**dilating l.,** an instrument with almond-shaped extremity, in which is concealed a knife, used for the intralaryngeal division of strictures and cicatricial bands.

**laryngotomy** (lăr-ing-got'o-mĭ) [ laryngo- + G. *tomē*, incision ]. Laryngofissure.

**inferior l.,** cricothyrotomy.

**median l.,** see laryngofissure.

**superior l.,** incision through the thyrohyoid membrane.

**laryngotracheal** (lă-ring'go-tra'ke-al). Relating to both larynx and trachea.

**laryngotracheitis** (lă-ring'go-tra-ke-i'tis). Inflammation of both larynx and trachea.

**avian infectious l.,** a severe, specific, infectious disease of chickens and other birds, caused by a virus; manifested by severe hemorrhagic inflammation of the trachea and upper air passages.

**laryngotracheobronchitis** (lă-ring'go-tra'ke-o-bron-ki'-tis). An acute respiratory disease involving the larynx, trachea, and bronchi, occurring mostly in children under 4 years of age; it is characterized by high fever, severe toxemia, laryngeal obstruction and, sometimes, bronchial or bronchiolar obstruction: croup.

**laryngotracheotomy** (lă-ring'go-tra-ke-ot'o-mĭ) [ laryngo- + trachea, *q.v.*, + G. *tomē*, incision ]. An incision through the cricoid cartilage and the upper tracheal rings.

**laryngoxerosis** (lar-ing'go-ze-ro'sis) [ laryngo- + G. *xērōsis*, a drying up ]. An abnormal dryness of the laryngeal mucous membrane.

**larynx,** pl. **larynges** (lăr'ingks, lă-rin'jēz) [ Mod. L. fr. G. ] [ NA ]. The organ of voice production the part of the respiratory tract between the pharynx and the trachea; it consists of a framework of cartilages and elastic membranes housing the vocal folds and the muscles which control the position and tension of these elements.

**lascivia** (lă-siv'ĭ-ah) [ L. lewdness ]. Satyriasis; nymphomania.

**Lasègue** (lă-seg'), Ernest C., Paris physician, 1816–1883. See L.'s *disease, sign, syndrome.*

**laser** (la'zer) [ acronym coined from *light amplification by stimulated emission of radiation* ]. Optical maser; a device that produces a beam of coherent (nonspreading) monochromatic visible light. High energies are concentrated into a narrow beam and laser treatment of a retina can be completed with so brief a flash that damaging heat in surrounding areas is precluded. Lasers using ruby, argon, krypton, neodymium, and helium-neon are available.

**Lash,** Abraham Fae, U. S. obstetrician-gynecologist, *1898. See L.'s *operation.*

**lash.** An eyelash.

**Las'iohe'lea.** A genus of small, bloodsucking gnats.

**las'situde** [ L. *lassitudo*, fr. *lassus;* weary ]. A sense of weariness.

**latah** (lah'tah) [ Malay, ticklish ]. A nervous affection of the natives of the Malay Peninsula and Archipelago, characterized by an exaggerated physical response to suggestion, the subjects involuntarily uttering cries or executing movements in response to command or in imitation of what they hear or see in others.

**Latarjet** (la-tar-ja'), André, French anatomist, *1877. See L.'s *nerve, vein.*

**latebra** (lat'e-brah) [ L. hiding place ]. A flask-shaped region in large-yolked eggs extending from the animal pole to a dilated terminal portion near the center of the yolk; it contains the main bulk of the white yolk.

**latency** (la'ten-sĭ). 1. The state of being latent. 2. In conditioning, the period of apparent inactivity between the time the stimulus is presented and the moment a response occurs.

**la'tent** [ L. *lateo*, pres. p. *latens* (*-ent-*), to lie hid ]. Not manifest, but potentially discernible.

**laterad** (lat'er-ad) [ L. *latus*, side, + *ad*, to ]. Toward the side.

**lat'eral** [ L. *lateralis*, lateral, fr. *latus*, side ]. 1. On the side. 2. Farther from the median or midsagittal plane. 3. In dentistry, a position either right or left of the midsagittal plane.

**latera'lis** [ L. ] [ NA ]. Lateral.

**lateral'ity.** The state of being toward or on one or other side; or of having a side; specifically, right or left dominance of the cerebral cortex.

**crossed l.,** right dominance of some members, *e.g.*, arm or leg, and left dominance of other members.

**lateriflex'ion, lateriflec'tion.** Lateroflexion.

**latero-** [ L. *lateralis*, lateral, fr. *latus*, side ]. Combining form meaning lateral, to one side, or relating to a side.

**lat'eroabdom'inal.** Relating to the sides of the abdomen, to the loins or flanks.

**laterodeviation** (lat'er-o-de-vĭ-a'shun) [ latero- + L. *devio*, to turn aside, fr. *via*, a way ]. A bending or a displacement to one side.

**lateroduction** (lat'er-o-duk'shun) [ latero- + L. *duco*, pp. *ductus*, to lead ]. A drawing to one side; denoting a movement of a limb or of the eyeball.

**lateroflexion, lateroflection** (lat'er-o-flek'shun) [ latero- + L. *flecto*, pp. *flexus*, to bend ]. A bending or curvature to one side.

**lateroposition** (lat'er-o-po-zish'un). A shift to one side.

**lateropulsion** (lat'er-o-pul'shun) [ latero- + L. *pello*, pp. *pulsus*, to push, drive ]. An involuntary sidewise movement occurring in certain nervous affections.

**laterotorsion** (lat'er-o-tor'shun) [ latero- + L. *torsio*, a twisting ]. A twisting to one side; denoting the turning of the eyeball around its anteroposterior axis.

**lateroversion** (lat'er-o-ver'shun) [ latero- + L. *verto*, pp. *versus*, to turn ]. A turning to one side or the other, denoting especially a malposition of the uterus.

**lathe.** A motor-driven machine with a rotating shaft that can be fitted with various types of cutting instruments, grinding stones and polishing wheels; used in finishing and polishing dental appliances.

**lathyrism** (lath'ĭ-rizm) [ L. *lathyrus*, vetch ]. Githagism; lupinosis. 1. A disease occurring in Abyssinia, Algeria, and India, characterized by various nervous manifestations, tremors, spastic paraplegia, and parasthesias; prevalent in districts where vetches, khasari (*Lathyrus sativus*) and allied species, form the main food. Some, however, regard lathyrism as due to vitamin A deficiency. 2. Poisoning of horses from eating certain varieties of peas, particularly *Lathyrus sativus*, a plant introduced into Europe from India. It is manifested by paralytic symptoms. In experimental l., rats fed a diet rich in sweet-pea meal show skeletal deformities and dissecting aneurysms.

**lathyrogen** (lath'ĭ-ro-jen). An agent or drug, occurring naturally or used experimentally, that induces lathyrism.

**latis'simus** [ L. superlative of *latus*, broad ] [ NA ]. Broadest; a term applied to certain broad flat muscles.

**Latrodec'tus** [ L. *latro*, servant, robber, + G. *dēktēs*, a biter ]. A genus of relatively small spiders, the widow spiders, capable of inflicting highly poisonous, neurotoxic, antagonizing bites; they are responsible, along with *Loxosceles* (the brown spider), for most of the severe reactions from spider envenomation. Medically important species are known from Australia, North and South America, South Africa, and New Zealand. Some venomous species, in addition to *L. mactans*, are *L. bishopi* (the red-legged widow spider), *L. euracaviensis, L. geometricus*, and *L. tredecimguttatus.*

**L. mac'tans,** the black widow spider, a venomous, jet-black spider found in protected dark places; it is especially common in the southern United States; the full grown female (slightly more than 1 cm. long) has a brilliant red dumbbell- or hourglass-shaped mark on the ventral aspect of the abdomen, and her bite may be extremely painful, producing a syndrome mimicking an acute abdominal crisis; some deaths, though rare, have been reported, particularly in small children; the male spider lacks the hourglass mark and is not venomous.

**LATS.** Abbreviation for long-acting thyroid *stimulator.*

**lat'tice.** A regular arrangement of units into an array such that a plane passing through two units of a particular type or in a particular interrelationship will pass through an indefinite number of such units; the atom arrangement in a crystal is an example of such a l.

**latu'mici'din.** Abikoviromycin.

**la'tus** [ L. ]. Broad.

**la'tus,** gen. **lat'eris,** pl. **lat'era** [ L. ] [ NA ]. The side, the flank; the side of the body between the pelvis and the ribs.

**Latzko's cesarean section.** See under section.

**laudable** (law'dă-bl) [ L. *laudabilis,* praiseworthy ]. A term formerly used to describe pus, under the notion that suppuration in a wound favored healing.

**lau'danine.** An isoquinoline alkaloid derived from the mother liquor or morphine, $C_{20}H_{25}NO_4$; it causes tetanoid convulsions, with action similar to that of strychnine.

**laudanosine** (law'dă-no-sēn). An isoquinoline alkaloid obtained from the mother liquor of morphine, $C_{21}H_{27}NO_4$; it causes tetanic convulsions.

**laudanum** (law'dă-num) [ G. *lēdanon,* a resinous gum ]. 1. A tincture containing opium.

**laudex'ium methyl sulfate.** Compound 20; LAUDOLISSIN; LAUDISSINE; 2,2'-decamethylenebis[ 1,2,3,4-tetrahydro-6,7-dimethoxy-2-methyl-1-veratrylisoquinolinium methyl sulfate ]; a muscle relaxant similar in action to *d*-tubocurarine.

**laugh.** See risus.

**Laugier** (lo-zhe-a'), Stanislas, Paris surgeon, 1799–1872. See L.'s *hernia, sign.*

**Laumonier** (lo-mün-e-a'), Jean B., French surgeon, 1749–1818. See L.'s *ganglion.*

**Launois,** Pierre E., French physician, 1856–1914. See L.-Cléret *syndrome.*

**Laurence,** John Zachariah, British ophthalmologist, 1829–1870. See L.-Biedl *syndrome,* L.-Moon-Biedl *syndrome.*

**Laurer's canal.** See under canal.

**lau'ric acid.** Dodecanoic acid; $CH_3(CH_2)_{10}COOH$; a fatty acid occurring in spermaceti, in milk, and in laurel, coconut, and palm oils.

**Lauth,** Charles, English chemist, 1836–1913. See L.'s *violet.*

**Lauth,** Ernst A., Strasbourg physician, 1803–1837. See L.'s *canal.*

**Lauth** (lowth), Thomas, German anatomist and surgeon, 1758–1826. See L.'s *ligament.*

**lavage** (lă-vahzh') [ Fr. from L. *lavo,* to wash ]. The washing out of a hollow organ, as the stomach or lower bowel, by copious injections and rejections of water.

**Lavdovsky,** Michail D., Russian histologist, 1846–1902. See L.'s *nucleoid.*

**lav'ender** [ Mediev. L. *lavandula,* fr. L. *lavo,* to wash; because used in washing ]. Lavandula; the dried flowers of *Lavandula officinalis* (family Labiatae), a shrub of southern Europe. Used as a perfume.

**l. oil** (NF), a volatile oil obtained by distillation from the tops of *Lavendula officinalis;* used as a flavoring and in perfumery.

**laven'dulin.** An antibiotic substance obtained from *Actinomyces lavendulae.*

**Laveran** (lav-er-an'), C. L. Alphonse, French protozoologist, 1845–1922. Gave his name to *Laverania.* Nobel laureate, 1907, for his work on the role played by protozoa in causing disease. See L.'s *disease.*

**Laverania** [ C. *Laveran* ]. An old name for a genus of blood-inhabiting protozoa; the name is no longer valid. See *Plasmodium* and *Haemoproteus.*

**L. mala'riae,** a distinctive generic and specific name for *Plasmodium falciparum,* as suggested by some zoologists who think that the crescentic gametocytes should be the basis for classifying the causal agent of falciparum malaria in a separate genus.

**laveur** (lah-vur') [ Fr. ]. An instrument for irrigation or lavage.

**Lavoisier** (la-vwah'zya), Antoine L., great French chemist, 1743–1794. He discovered that oxygen, which he named, had a function in combustion and that a strict analogy

occurred between combustion and respiration. He was guillotined by the French revolutionists.

---

# LAW

---

**law** [ A.S. *lagu* ]. A principle or rule; a formula expressing a fact or number of facts common to a group of processes or actions.

**Allen's l.,** the more carbohydrate that is taken by a diabetic the less is utilized.

**all or none l.,** Bowditch's l.

**Ambard's l.'s,** (1) with the urinary urea concentration constant, the output of urea varies directly as the square of the concentration of the blood urea; (2) with the blood urea concentration constant, the output of urea varies inversely as the square root of its urinary concentration.

**Ångström's l.,** a substance absorbs light of the same kind, *i.e.,* of the same wavelength, as it emits when luminous.

**Arndt's l.,** weak stimuli excite physiologic activity, moderately strong ones favor it, strong ones retard it, and very strong ones arrest it.

**l.'s of association,** principles formulated by Aristotle to account for the functional relationships between ideas; the l. of contiguity (association) proved most useful to experimental psychologists, culminating in modern studies of respondent conditioning.

**Arrhenius' l.,** only those solutions that have high osmotic pressures are electrically conductive.

**l. of average localization,** visceral pain is most accurately localized in the least mobile viscera, and conversely.

**Avogadro's l., hypothesis, or postulate,** equal volumes of gases contain equal numbers of molecules, the conditions of pressure and temperature being the same.

**Baruch's l.,** the effect of any hydriatic procedure is in direct proportion to the difference between the temperature of the water and that of the skin; when the temperature of the water is above or below that of the skin the effect is stimulating; when the two temperatures are the same the effect is sedative.

**Baumès' l.,** Colles' l.

**Beer's l.,** the intensity of a color or of a light ray is inversely proportional to the depth of liquid through which it is transmitted; it is concluded that the absorption is dependent upon the number of molecules in the path of the ray.

**Behring's l.,** parenteral administration of serum from an immunized person provides a relative, passive immunity to that disease (*i.e.,* prevents it, or favorably modifies its course) in a previously susceptible person.

**Bell's l.,** Bell-Magendie l.; Magendie l.; the ventral spinal roots are motor, the dorsal are sensory.

**Bernoulli's l.,** Bernoulli's principle; Bernoulli's theorem; the velocity of flow of a gas or fluid through a tube is inversely related to its pressure against the side of the tube; *i.e.,* velocity is greatest and pressure lowest at a point of constriction.

**Berthollet's l.,** salts in solution will always react with each other so as to form a less soluble salt, if possible.

**Bladgen's l.,** the depression of the freezing point of dilute solutions is proportional to the amount of the dissolved substance.

**l. of biogenesis, biogenetic l.,** recapitulation *theory.*

**Bowditch's l.,** all or none l.; any stimulus, however feeble, which will excite a cardiac contraction will produce as powerful a contraction as the strongest stimulus; "minimal stimuli cause maximal pulsations."

**Boyle's l.,** Mariotte's l.; the volume of a given quantity of gas varies inversely as the pressure upon it.

**Broadbent's l.,** lesions of the upper segment of the motor tract cause less marked paralysis of the muscles that habitually produce bilateral movements than of those that more commonly act independently of the opposite side.

**Bunsen-Roscoe l.,** reciprocity l.; Roscoe-Brunsen l.; in two photochemical reactions, *e.g.,* the darkening of a photographic plate or film, if the product of the intensity of illumination and the time of exposure are equal, the quantities of chemical material undergoing change will be equal. The retina for short periods of exposure obeys this l.

**Charles' l.,** Gay-Lussac's l.; all gases expand equally on heating, namely, $1/273$ of their volume at 0°C. for every degree Centigrade.

**Colles' l.,** the mother of a syphilitic infant, though she herself has never had any symptoms of the disease, is immune.

**Colles-Baumès l.,** Colles' l.

**l. of constant numbers in ovulation,** the number of ova discharged at each ovulation is nearly constant for any given species.

**l. of contiguity,** when two ideas or events have once occurred in close association they are likely to so occur again, the subsequent occurrence of one tending to elicit the other; this l. figures prominently in modern theories of conditioning and learning.

**l. of contraction,** Pflüger's l.

**Coppet's l.,** solutions having the same freezing point have equal concentrations of dissolved substances.

**Courvoisier's l.,** states that enlargement of the gallbladder with jaundice is likely to result from carcinoma of the head of the pancreas and not from a stone in the common duct, because then the gallbladder is usually scarred from infection and does not distend.

**Cushing's l.,** Cushing's *phenomenon.*

**Dale-Feldberg l.,** an identical chemical transmitter is liberated at all the functional terminals of a single neuron.

**Dalton's l.,** l. of partial pressures; each gas in a mixture of gases exerts a pressure proportionately to the percentage of the gas and quite independently of the presence of the other gases present.

**Dalton-Henry l.,** in dissolving a mixture of gases a fluid will absorb as much of each gas in the mixture as if that were the only gas dissolved.

**Dastre-Morat l.,** dilation of splanchnic blood vessels is associated with constriction of cutaneous vessels, and *vice versa.*

**l. of definite proportions,** Proust's l.; the relative weights of the several elements forming a chemical compound are invariable.

**l. of denervation,** when a structure is denervated, its irritability to certain chemical agents is increased; *e.g.,* the greater sensitivity of the pupil to acetylcholine after section and degeneration of the 3rd nerve, and of the nictitating membrane to adrenaline after excision of the superior cervical ganglion.

**Descartes' l.,** see l. of refraction.

**Donders' l.,** the rotation of the eyeball is determined by the distance of the object from the median plane and the line of the horizon.

**Draper's l.,** states that a chemical change is produced in a photochemical substance only by those rays that are absorbed by that substance.

**Du Bois-Reymond l.,** l. of excitation.

**Dulong-Petit l.,** the heat capacity of the atoms of all simple solid bodies is the same.

**Einthoven's l.,** Einthoven's equation; in the electrocardiogram the potential of any wave or complex in lead II is equal to the sum of the potentials of leads I and III.

**Elliott's l.,** adrenaline acts upon those structures innervated by sympathetic nerve fibers.

**l. of excitation,** Du Bois-Reymond l.; a motor nerve responds, not to the absolute value, but to the alteration of value from moment to moment, of the electric current; *i.e.,* rate of change of intensity of the current is a factor in determining its effectiveness.

**Faraday's l.'s,** (1) the amount of an electrolyte decomposed by an electric current is proportional to the amount of the current; (2) when the same current is passed through several electrolytes, the amounts of the different substances decomposed are proportional to their chemical equivalents.

**Farr's l.,** states that the curve of cases of an epidemic rises rapidly at first, then climbs slowly to a peak from whence the fall is steeper than the previous rise.

**Fechner-Weber l.,** Weber-Fechner l.

**Ferry-Porter l.,** the critical fusion is directly proportional to the logarithm of the light intensity.

**Flatau's l.,** a l. concerning the excentric position of the long spinal tracts; the greater the distance the nerve fibers run lengthwise in the cord, the more they tend toward its periphery.

**Freund's l.,** ovarian tumors, while intrapelvic, lie behind the uterus, but when they grow out of the pelvis, they lie above and in front of the uterus.

**Galton's l.,** l. of regression; with respect to characteristics exhibiting continuous variation, offspring generally tend to resemble their parents; the offspring of parents of extreme types tend to regress toward the mean of the population.

**Gay-Lussac's l.,** Charles' l.

**Gerhardt-Semon l.,** after injury to the recurrent laryngeal nerve the affected vocal cord is paralyzed in a position of adduction.

**Godélier's l.,** tuberculosis of the peritoneum is always associated with tuberculosis of the pleura on one or both sides.

**Graham's l.,** the relative rapidity of diffusion of two gases varies inversely as the square root of the densities.

**Grasset's l.,** Landouzy-Grasset l.

**l. of gravitation,** Newton's l.

**Guldberg-Waage l.,** l. of mass action.

**Haeckel's l.,** recapitulation *theory.*

**Halsted's l.,** transplanted tissue will grow only if there is a lack of that tissue in the host.

**Hamburger's l.,** albumins and phosphates pass from red corpuscles to serum and chlorides pass from serum to cells when blood is acid; reverse occurs when blood is alkaline.

**l. of the heart,** Starling's l.; the energy liberated by the heart when it contracts is a function of the length of its muscle fibers at the end of diastole.

**Hecker's l.,** in every successive childbirth the weight of the child is usually greater than that of its predecessor by from 150 to 200 gm.

**Heidenhain's l.,** glandular secretion is always accompanied by an alteration in the structure of the gland.

**Hellin's l.,** twins occur once in 89 births, triplets once in $89^2$, and quadruplets once in $89^3$.

**Henry's l.,** the amount of gas that can be dissolved in a given quantity of water varies with the pressure; by doubling the pressure twice as much gas passes into solution.

**Hilton's l.,** the nerve supplying a joint supplies also the muscles which move the joint and the skin covering the articular insertion of those muscles.

**Hofacker-Sadler l.'s,** l.'s alledged to be operative in regard to sex determination: (1) when the woman is younger than the man the ratio of male to female births is 113:100; (2) when the woman is older, the ratio is 88.2:100; (3) when the parents are of the same age the ratio is 93.5:100.

**Hooke's l.,** states that the stress applied to stretch or compress a body is proportional to the strain, or change in length thus produced, so long as the limit of elasticity of the body is not exceeded.

**l. of independent assortment,** Mendel's second l.

**l. of initial value,** Wilder's l. of initial value.

**l. of intestine,** myenteric *reflex.*

**l. of inverse square,** intensity of radiation is inversely proportional to the square of the distance.

**l. of isochronism,** a nerve and the muscle which it innervates have the same chronaxie values.

**i'sodynam'ic l.,** for energy purposes, the different foodstuffs may replace one another in accordance with their caloric values when burned in a calorimeter.

**Jackson's l.,** loss of mental functions due to disease retraces in reverse order its evolutionary development.

**Koch's l.,** to establish the specificity of a pathogenic microorganism, it must be present in all cases of the disease, inoculations of its pure cultures must produce the same disease in animals (when it is transmitted to such), and from these it must be again obtained and be propagated in pure cultures.

**Landouzy-Grasset l.,** in lesions of one hemisphere, the patient's head is turned to the side of the affected muscles if there is spasticity, to that of the cerebral lesion if there is paralysis.

**Lapicque's l.,** the chronaxie is inversely proportional to the diameter of an axon.

**Laplace's l.,** the relationship between transmural pressure difference ($\Delta P$), wall tension ($T$), and radius of curvature ($R$) in a concave surface; for a sphere: $\Delta P = 2 T/R$; for a cylinder: $\Delta P = T/R$.

**Le Chatelier's l.,** if external factors such as temperature and pressure disturb a system in equilibrium, adjustment occurs in such a way that the effect of the disturbing factors is reduced to a minimum.

**Leopold's l.,** in anterior insertion of the placenta, the Fallopian tubes project backward; in posterior insertion, they are directed forward.

**Levret's l.,** in cases of placenta previa the insertion of the cord is marginal.

**Lipschutz l. of puberty,** the onset of pubertal changes in the gonad is not determined by changes within the gonad itself, but by maturation of the soma.

**Listing's l.,** when the eye leaves one object and fixes another, it revolves about an axis perpendicular to a plane cutting both the former and the present lines of vision.

**Louis' l.,** (1) pulmonary tuberculosis usually begins in the left lung; (2) every form of tuberculosis is accompanied by pulmonary localization.

**Magendie's l.,** Bell's l.

**Marey's l.,** the pulse rate varies inversely as the blood pressure, *i.e.*, it is slow when the pressure is high; it is an expression of baroreceptor reflex influences on heart rate.

**Marfan's l.,** the healing of localized tuberculosis (*e.g.*, tuberculous cervical lymphadenitis) protects against subsequent development of pulmonary tuberculosis.

**Mariotte's l.,** Boyle's l.

**l. of mass action,** mass l.; Guldberg-Waage l.; the velocity of a chemical reaction is proportional to the active masses (molar concentrations) of the reacting substances.

**Meltzer's l.,** l. of contrary innervation; "all living functions are continually controlled by two opposite forces: augmentation or action on the one hand, and inhibition on the other."

**Mendel's l.'s,** *first l.:* There are factors which affect development; these factors retain their individuality from generation to generation, do not become contaminated when mixed in a hybrid, and become sorted out from one another when the gametes are formed. *Second l.:* Different factors are assorted independently when the gametes are formed. (This law must be modified by the restriction that linked genes do not assort independently.)

**Mendeléeff's l.,** periodic l.; the properties of an element are a periodical function of its atomic weight; that is to say, the elements being arranged in the order of their atomic weights, every element in the series will be related in respect to its properties to the eighth in order before or after it.

**l. of the minimum,** growth and development of plants and animals are determined by the availability of that essential nutrient which is present in the smallest amount.

**Müller's l. of specific nerve energies,** each type of sensory nerve ending, however stimulated, electrically, mechanically, etc., gives rise to its own specific sensation; moreover, each type of sensation depends not upon any special character of the different nerves but upon the part of the brain in which their fibers terminate.

**l. of multiple proportions,** when more than one compound is formed by the chemical union of two elements and the weight of one of the elements is considered as remaining constant, that of the other element varies in the different compounds as a simple multiple of the amount in the lowest of the series.

**l. of multiple variants,** where there is any deviation from the normal in the bones of the hand or foot, the variation is always multiple, involving more than one bone.

**Neumann's l.,** in compounds of analogous chemical constitution, the molecular heat, or the product of the specific heat by the atomic weight, is always the same.

**Newland's l.,** see Mendeléeff's l.

**Newton's l.,** l. of universal gravitation; the attractive force between any two bodies is proportional to the product of their masses, and inversely proportional to the square of the distance between their centers.

**Nysten's l.,** rigor mortis affects first the muscles of the head and spreads toward the feet.

**Ohm's l.,** in an electric current passing through a wire the intensity of the current, in amperes, equals the electromotive force, in volts, divided by the resistance, in ohms. Let $C$ = current in amperes, $E$ = electromotive force in volts, and $R$ = resistance in ohms: then $C = (E/R)$; $E = (C \times R)$; $R = (E/C)$.

**Pascal's l.,** fluids at rest transmit pressure equally in every direction.

**periodic l.,** Mendeléeff's l.

**Pflüger's l.'s,** (1) l. of polar excitation; (2) l. of contraction; the results of the stimulation of an isolated nerve of a frog by opening and closing currents of different intensities and different directions are formulated as follows: CCC > ACC > AOC > COC.

**Poiseuille's l.,** the quantity of fluid flowing from a narrow tube (one comparable in size to the small arteries) is directly proportional to the pressure gradient, the viscosity coefficient, and the fourth power of the diameter of the tube; the mean lineal velocity of the current is proportional to the cross-sectional area of the tube, the pressure gradient, and the viscosity coefficient.

**l. of polar excitation,** Pflüger's l. (1); a given segment of a nerve is irritated by the development of catelectrotonus and the disappearance of anelectrotonus, but the reverse does not hold; *i.e.*, excitation occurs at the cathode when the circuit is closed and at the anode when it is opened.

**Profeta's l.,** the subject of congenital syphilis is immune against the acquired disease.

**Proust's l.,** l. of definite proportions.

**Raoult's l.,** the vapor pressure of a solution is that of the pure solvent multiplied by the mole fraction of the solvent in the solution.

**l. of recapitulation,** recapitulation *theory.*

**l. of reciprocal proportions,** Walton's l.; the relative weights in which two substances form a chemical union singly with a third are the same as, or simple multiples of, those in which they unite with each other.

**l. of referred pain,** pain arises only from irritation of nerves which are sensitive to those stimuli that produce pain when applied to the surface of the body.

**l. of refraction,** for two given media, the sine of the angle of incidence bears a constant relation to the sine of the angle of refraction; also called Snell's l. or Descartes' l.

**l. of regression,** Galton's l.

**Ricco's l.,** for small images, light intensity $\times$ area = constant for the threshold.

**Ritter's l.,** a nerve is stimulated at both the opening and the closing of an electrical current. See l. of polar excitation.

**Roscoe-Bunsen l.,** Bunsen-Roscoe l.

**Rosenbach's l.,** (1) in affections of the nerve trunks or nerve centers, paralysis of the flexor muscles appears later than that of the extensors; (2) in cases of abnormal stimulation of organs with rhythmical functional periodicity, there is often a grouping of the individual acts with corresponding lengthening of the pauses, in such a way that the proportion of total rest and activity remains nearly the same.

**Rubner's l.'s of growth,** (1) the l. of constant energy consumption: the rapidity of growth is proportional to the intensity of the metabolic processes; (2) the l. of the constant growth quotient: in most young mammals 24 per cent of the entire food energy, or calories, is utilized for growth, in man only 5 per cent is utilized.

**second l. of thermodynamics,** the entropy of the universe moves toward a maximum; similarly, the entropy of any isolated microcosm (*e.g.*, a chemical reaction) proceeds spontaneously only in that direction that yields an increase in entropy (*q.v.*). Entropy is maximal at equilibrium. To quote G. N. Lewis: Every process that occurs spontaneously is capable of doing work; to reverse any such process requires the expenditure of work from the outside.

**l. of segregation,** the Mendelian theory of inheritance according to which, in each generation, the ratio of (a) pure dominants, (b) dominants producing descendants in the proportion of three dominants to one recessive, and (c) pure recessives is as 1:2:1.

**Semon's l.,** a l. stating that injury to the recurrent laryngeal nerve results in paralysis of the abductor muscle of the larynx (cricoarytenoid posticus) before paralysis of the adductor muscles.

**Sherrington's l.,** every dorsal spinal nerve root supplies a special territory of the skin (dermatome), which is, however, invaded above and below by fibers from the adjacent spinal segments.

**l. of similars,** see *similia similibus curantur.*

**Snell's l.,** see l. of refraction.

**Spallanzani's l.,** the younger the individual the greater is the regenerative power of its cells.

**Starling's l.,** l. of the heart.

**Stokes's l.,** a muscle lying above an inflamed mucous or serous membrane is frequently the seat of paralysis.

**Tait's l.,** an exploratory laparotomy should be performed in every case of obscure pelvic or abdominal disease that threatens health or life.

**Thoma's l.'s,** the development of blood vessels is governed by dynamic forces acting on their walls as follows: an increase in velocity of blood flow causes dilation of the lumen; an increase in lateral pressure on the vessel wall causes it to thicken; an increase in end-pressure causes the formation of new capillaries.

**Toynbee's l.,** in brain disease due to otitis media, the lateral sinus and cerebellum are involved in case of mastoiditis, the cerebrum in case of inflammation of the tympanic attic.

**van der Kolk's l.,** in a mixed nerve the sensory fibers are distributed to the parts moved by the muscles controlled by the motor fibers.

**van't Hoff's l.,** (1) in stereochemistry, all optically active substances have one or more multivalent atoms united to four different atoms or radicals so as to form in space an unsymmetrical arrangement; (2) the osmotic pressure exerted by any substance in very dilute solution is the same that it would exert if present as gas in the same volume as that of the solution; or, at constant temperature the osmotic pressure of dilute solutions is proportional to the concentration (number of molecules) of the dissolved substance; (3) the velocity of chemical reactions increases between two- and three-fold for each 10°C. rise in temperature.

**Virchow's l.,** there is no special or distinctive neoplastic cell, inasmuch as the component cells of neoplasms originate from preexisting forms.

**Wallerian l.,** after section of the posterior root of a spinal nerve between the root ganglion and the spinal cord, the central portion degenerates; after division of the anterior root, the peripheral portion degenerates; the trophic center of the posterior root is therefore the ganglion, that of the anterior root the spinal cord.

**Walton's l.,** l. of reciprocal proportions.

**Weber's l.,** Weber-Fechner law.

**Weber-Fechner l.,** Fechner-Weber l.; Weber's l.; the intensity of a sensation varies by a series of equal increments (arithmetically) as the strength of the stimulus is increased geometrically; if a series of stimuli is applied and so adjusted in strength that each stimulus causes a just perceptible change in intensity of the sensation, then the strength of each stimulus differs from the preceding one by a constant fraction; thus, if a just perceptible change in a visual sensation is produced by the addition of 1 candle to an original illumination of 100 candles, 10 candles will be required to produce any change in sensation when the original illumination was one of 1000 candles.

**Weigert's l.,** overproduction theory; the loss or destruction of a part or element in the organic world is likely to result in compensatory replacement and overproduction of tissue during the process of regeneration or repair (or both), as in the formation of callus when a fractured bone heals.

**Wilder's l. of initial value,** the direction of response of a body function to any agent depends to a large degree on the initial level of that function.

**Williston's l.,** as the vertebrate scale is ascended, the number of bones in the skull is reduced.

**Wolff's l.,** every change in the form and the function of a bone, or in its function alone, is followed by certain definite changes in its internal architecture and secondary alterations in its external conformation.

---

**Lawford's syndrome.** See under syndrome.

**lawren'cium.** Element number 103; symbol Lw; created and identified at Lawrence Radiation Laboratory, Univer-

sity of California, named in honor of Ernest O. Lawrence, Nobel prize winner who invented the cyclotron.

**laxation** (laks-a′shun) [ see laxative ]. Bowel movement, with or without laxatives.

**laxative** (laks′ă-tiv) [ L. *laxativus,* fr. *laxo,* pp. *-atus,* to slacken, relax ]. 1. Aperient; mildly cathartic; having the action of loosening the bowels. 2. A mild cathartic; a remedy that moves the bowels slightly without pain or violent action.

**laxa′tor tym′pani** [ Mod. L. ]. One of two supposed muscles, probably ligaments of the malleus.

---

# LAYER

---

**layer** (la′er). Stratum; lamina; a sheet of some substance lying upon another, distinguished therefrom by a difference in texture or color or simply not continuous with it.

**aleuron l.,** cells that form the outermost layer of plant endosperm. They are removed with the pericarp during milling.

**ameloblastic l.,** enamel l.; the internal l. of the enamel organ.

**anterior elastic l.,** *lamina* limitans anterior corneae.

**anterior limiting l. of cornea,** *lamina* limitans anterior corneae.

**anterior l. of rectus abdominis sheath,** *lamina* anterior vagina musculi recti abdominis.

**bacillary l.,** l. of rods and cones.

**basal l.,** *stratum* basale.

**basal cell l.,** *stratum* basale epidermidis.

**basal l. of choroid,** *lamina* basalis choroideae.

**blastodermic l.'s,** the primordial cell l.'s on the yolk surface of a telolecithal egg; in earliest stages protoderm, later differentiating into ectoderm, entoderm, and mesoderm.

**cambium l.,** the inner osteogenic l. of the periosteum.

**l.'s of cerebellar cortex,** see *cortex* cerebelli.

**l.'s of cerebral cortex,** see *cortex* cerebri.

**cerebral l. of retina,** *stratum* cerebrale retinae.

**Chievitz' l.,** in the developing retina of an embryo, a transitory zone between the inner and outer neuroblastic l.'s that is devoid of nuclei.

**choriocapillary l.,** *lamina* choroidocapillaris.

**circular l.'s of muscular tunics,** see entries under *stratum* circulare tunicae muscularis.

**circular l. of tympanic membrane,** *stratum* circulare membranae tympani.

**claustral l.,** the l. of gray matter between the external capsule and the white matter of the insula or extreme capsule.

**clear l. of epidermis,** *stratum* lucidum.

**columnar l.,** *stratum* basale epidermidis.

**conjunctival l. of bulb,** *tunica* conjunctiva bulbi.

**conjunctival l. of eyelids,** *tunica* conjunctiva palpebrarum.

**corneal l. of epidermis,** *stratum* corneum epidermidis.

**cornified l. of nail,** *stratum* corneum unguis.

**cutaneous l. of tympanic membrane,** *stratum* cutaneum membranae tympani.

**deep l.,** *lamina* profunda.

**elastic l.'s of arteries,** elastic *laminae* of arteries.

**elastic l.'s of cornea,** see *lamina* limitans anterior corneae and *lamina* limitans posterior corneae.

**enamel l.,** ameloblastic l.

**ependymal l.,** ependymal zone; an inner epithelial l. of cells bordering the lumen of the embryonic neural tube, formed during the latter's stratification, and persisting in modified form throughout life.

**epithelial l.'s,** see epithelium.

**epithelial choroid l.,** *lamina* epithelialis.

**epitrichial l.,** the superficial flattened-cell l. of the epidermis of a young embryo before the definitive stratification has developed.

**fibrous l.,** the outer dense connective tissue l. of the periosteum.

**fillet l.,** *stratum* lemnisci.

**fusiform l.,** multiform l.; spindle-celled l.; l. 6 of the cerebral cortex; see *cortex* cerebri.

**ganglionic l. of cerebellar cortex,** *stratum* gangliosum cerebelli.

**ganglionic l. of cerebral cortex,** l. 5 of the cerebral cortex; see *cortex* cerebri.

**ganglionic l. of optic nerve,** *stratum* ganglionare nervi optici.

**ganglionic l. of retina,** *stratum* ganglionare retinae.

**germ l.,** one of the three primordial cell l.'s (ectoderm, entoderm, mesoderm) established in an embryo during gastrulation and the immediately following stages.

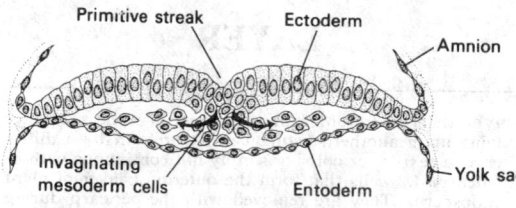

**Embryonic Germ Layers**

Transverse section through the region of the primitive streak of a 16-day presomite human embryo. (From Langman, J.: *Medical Embryology*, Ed. 2, The Williams & Wilkins Co., 1969.)

**germinative l.,** *stratum* germinativum.

**germinative l. of nail,** *stratum* germinativum unguis.

**glomerular l. of olfactory bulb,** a l. composed of spherical bodies, called glomeruli, formed by the synapses of mitral cells with the olfactory nerve fibers derived from the cells of the olfactory epithelium.

**granular l. of cerebellar cortex,** *stratum* granulosum cerebelli.

**granular l.'s of cerebral cortex,** the outer granular l. (l. 2) and inner granular l. (l. 4); see *cortex* cerebri.

**granular l. of epidermis,** *stratum* granulosum epidermidis.

**granular l.'s of retina,** nuclear l.'s of the retina; two l.'s, outer and inner granular l., densely packed with small cell bodies of, respectively, the rod and cone cells, and the bipolar cells of the retina; the outer molecular l. intervenes between the two granular l.'s. The outer granular l., together with the l. of rods and cones, corresponds to the current NA term, stratum neuroepitheliale retinae; the inner granular l. to the stratum ganglionare retinae.

**granular l. of a vesicular ovarian follicle,** *stratum* granulosum folliculi ovarici vesiculosi.

**gray l. of superior colliculus,** *stratum* griseum colliculi superioris.

**half-value l.,** (1) an indicator of penetrability of an x-ray beam; (2) the thickness of a particular material required to decrease the intensity of the beam to one-half.

**Henle's l.,** the outer l. cells of the inner root sheath of the hair follicle.

**Henle's fiber l.,** the l. of inner cone fibers in the central area of the retina.

**Henle's nervous l.,** entoretina.

**horny l. of epidermis,** *stratum* corneum epidermidis.

**horny l. of nail,** *stratum* corneum unguis.

**Huxley's l.,** Huxley's membrane or sheath; the cells of the inner root sheath of the hair follicle.

**infragranular l.,** the cellular band deep to the inner granular l. of the human cerebral cortex which differentiates into the ganglionic l. and multiform l. by the sixth fetal month.

**Kölliker's l.,** the l. of connective tissue in the iris.

**Langhans' l.,** the cytotrophoblast.

**lateral l.,** *lamina* lateralis.

**lateral cartilaginous l.,** *lamina* lateralis.

**latticed l.,** a cortical cell l. in the hippocampus.

**limiting l.'s of cornea,** see *lamina* limitans anterior corneae, and *lamina* limitans posterior corneae.

**longitudinal l.'s of muscular tunics,** see entries under *stratum* longitudinale tunicae muscularis.

**Malpighian l.,** *stratum* germinativum.

**mantle l.,** mantle zone; the nuclear zone of the developing neural tube between the outer (marginal) l. and the inner (ependymal) l.

**marginal l.,** marginal zone; the outer, nonnuclear l. of the embryonic neural tube. Into its fibrous network grow the longitudinal nerve fibers which eventually become the white matter of the cord and brain stem.

**medial l.,** *lamina* medialis.

**medial cartilaginous l.,** *lamina* medialis.

**medullary l.'s of thalamus,** *laminae* medullares thalami.

**membranous l.,** *lamina* membranacea.

**Meynert's l.,** pyramidal cell l.; l. 3 of the cerebral cortex; see *cortex* cerebri.

**molecular l.,** *stratum* moleculare.

**molecular l. of cerebellar cortex,** *stratum* moleculare cerebelli.

**molecular l. of cerebral cortex,** see *cortex* cerebri.

**molecular l.'s of olfactory bulb,** the l.'s, composed mainly of nerve fibers, on the outer and inner sides of the l. of mitral cells of the bulb.

**molecular l. of retina,** *stratum* moleculare retinae.

**monomolecular l.,** a l. or film one molecule thick.

**mucosal l. of tympanic membrane,** *stratum* mucosum membranae tympani.

**multiform l.,** fusiform l.; l. 6 of the cerebral cortex; see *cortex* cerebri.

**neural l. of retina,** *stratum* cerebrale retinae.

**neuroepithelial l. of retina,** *stratum* neuroepitheliale retinae.

**Nitabuch's l.,** Nitabuch's *membrane*.

**nuclear l.'s of retina,** granular l.'s of the retina.

**odontoblastic l.,** a l. of connective tissue cells at the periphery of the dental pulp of the tooth.

**Oehl's l.,** *stratum* lucidum.

**Ollier's l.,** inner or osteogenetic l. of the periosteum.

**optic l.,** *stratum* opticum.

**orbital l. of ethmoid bone,** *lamina* orbitalis ossis ethmoidalis.

**osteogenetic l.,** the inner bone-forming l. of the periosteum.

**palisade l.,** *stratum* basale epidermidis.

**papillary l.,** *stratum* papillare corii.

**parietal l.,** *lamina* parietalis.

**pigmented l. of ciliary body,** *stratum* pigmenti corporis ciliaris.

**pigmented l. of iris,** *stratum* pigmenti iridis.

**pigmented l. of retina,** *stratum* pigmenti retinae.

**plasma l.,** still l.

**plexiform l.,** *stratum* moleculare.

**plexiform l. of cerebral cortex,** molecular l. of cerebral cortex; see *cortex* cerebri.

**plexiform l. of retina,** *stratum* moleculare retinae.

**polymorphous l.,** fusiform (multiform) l. of the cerebral cortex; see *cortex* cerebri.

**posterior elastic l.,** *lamina* limitans posterior corneae.

**posterior limiting l. of cornea,** *lamina* limitans posterior corneae.

**posterior l. of rectus abdominis sheath,** *lamina* posterior vaginae musculi recti abdominis.

**pretracheal l.,** *lamina* pretrachealis.

**prevertebral l.,** *lamina* prevertebralis.

**prickle cell l.,** *stratum* spinosum epidermidis.

**Purkinje's l.,** *stratum* gangliosum cerebelli.

**pyramidal cell l.,** Meynert's l.; l. 3 of the cerebral cortex; see *cortex* cerebri.

**radiate l. of tympanic membrane,** *stratum* radiatum membranae tympani.

**Rauber's l.,** the thinned out trophoblastic membrane over the embryonic disk in developing carnivores and ungulates.

**reticular l. of corium,** *stratum* reticulare corii.

**l.'s of retina,** see retina.

**l. of rods and cones,** bacillary l.; the l. of the retina next to the pigment l. and containing the visual receptors; see retina, layer 2; see also granular l.'s of the retina, and *stratum* neuroepitheliale retinae.

**rostral l.,** *lamina* rostralis.

**Sattler's elastic l.,** the middle l. of the choroid.

**l.'s of skin,** see epidermis and corium.

**sluggish l.,** still l.

**somatic l.,** the external l. of the lateral mesoderm of the embryo, lying adjacent to the ectoderm and together with it constituting the somatopleure.

**spindle-celled l.,** the fusiform l. of the cerebral cortex; see *cortex* cerebri.

**spinous l.,** *stratum* spinosum epidermidis.

**splanchnic l.,** the internal l. of the lateral mesoderm, lying adjacent to the entoderm and together with it forming the splanchnopleure.

**still l.,** sluggish l.; plasma l.; Poiseuille's space; the l. of the blood stream, in the capillary vessels, next to the wall of the vessel; here the current is slow and the white blood cells are seen rolling lazily along the side of the tube, the center of the stream running rapidly and carrying with it the red blood cells.

**subendothelial l.,** the thin l. of connective tissue lying between the endothelium and elastic lamina in the intima of blood vessels.

**subpapillary l.,** the vascular l. of the corium.

**superficial l.,** *lamina* superficialis.

**suprachoroid l.,** *lamina* suprachoroidea.

**Tomes' granular l.,** a thin l. of dentin adjacent to the cementum, appearing granular in ground sections; the granules are small uncalcified spaces.

**vascular l. of choroid coat of eye,** *lamina* vasculosa choroideae.

**visceral l.,** *lamina* visceralis.

**Waldeyer's zonal l.,** *fasciculus* dorsolateralis.

**zonular l.,** *stratum* zonale.

---

**lazaret, lazaretto** (laz'ă-ret, -ret'o) [ It. *lazzaretto,* fr. *lazzaro,* a leper ]. 1. A leper hospital. 2. A hospital for the treatment of contagious diseases; a pest house. 3. A place of detention for persons in quarantine.

**LBF.** Abbreviation for *Lactobacillus bulgaricus* factor (pantetheine, *q.v.*).

**L.D.** Abbreviation for light *difference.*

**LD.** Abbreviation for a lethal dose of a chemical or biologic preparation (*e.g.,* a bacterial exotoxin or a suspension of bacteria), varying in relation to the type of animal and route of administration. See also dose.

**LD$_{50}$.** Abbreviation for the median lethal dose, one that is fatal to 50 per cent of the test animals.

**LDH.** Abbreviation for lactate dehydrogenase.

**Le.** Abbreviation for Lewis blood group; see in appendix 2.

**L.E.** 1. Abbreviation for left eye. 2. Abbreviation for *lupus* erythematosus.

**leaching** (le'ching) [ A.S. *leccan,* to wet ]. Lixiviation.

**lead** (lĕd). Plumbum; a metallic element, symbol Pb, atomic no. 82, atomic weight 207.21, of metallic luster and bluish gray color; it occurs in nature as an oxide or one of the salts, but chiefly as the sulfide, or galena.

**l. acetate,** sugar of l.; has been used as an astringent in diarrhea, and in aqueous solution as a wet dressing in certain dermatoses.

**black l.,** graphite.

**l. car′bonate,** white l.; a heavy white powder, insoluble in water. Occasionally used to relieve irritation in dermatitis. It is used largely in the manufacture of paint and in the arts and is thus productive of l. poisoning.

**l. monoxide,** l. oxide; l. oxide yellow; massicot; litharge; has been used as an ingredient in external applications such as l. plaster.

**l. oxide,** l. monoxide.

**red l.,** l. tetroxide.

**red oxide of l.,** l. tetroxide.

**sugar of l.,** l. acetate.

**l. sulfide,** PbS; galena; the native form in which l. is chiefly found.

**tetraethyl l.,** see under tetraethyl.

**l. tetroxide,** red l.; red oxide of l.; a bright orange-red powder that turns black when heated; used in ointments and plasters.

**white l.,** l. carbonate.

**lead-206.** $^{206}$Pb; the stable l. isotope that ends the uranium-238 radioactive series.

**lead-207.** $^{207}$Pb; the stable l. isotope that ends the uranium-235 radioactive series.

**lead-208** $^{208}$Pb; the stable l. isotope that ends the thorium-232 radioactive series.

**lead** (lĕd). One of the records taken by means of the electrocardiograph.

**bipolar l.,** a record obtained with two electrodes placed on different regions of the body, each electrode contributing significantly to the record, *e.g.* a standard limb l.

**CB l.,** a chest l. with the indifferent electrode placed upon the subject's back.

**CF l.,** a chest l. with the indifferent electrode placed on the subject's left leg.

**chest l.'s.,** precordial l.'s; semidirect l.'s; those in which the exploring electrode is on the chest overlying the heart or its vicinity.

**CL l.,** a chest l. with the indifferent electrode placed on the subject's left arm.

**CR l.,** a chest l. with the indifferent electrode placed on the subject's right arm.

**direct l.,** in electrocardiography, a l. recorded with the exploring electrode placed directly on the surface of the exposed heart.

**esophageal l.,** a record obtained with the exploring electrode lying within the lumen of the esophagus; of particular value in obtaining sizable atrial deflections and therefore helpful in the recognition of arrhythmias.

**indirect l.'s,** standard l.'s.

**intracardiac l.,** the record obtained when the exploring electrode is placed within one of the heart's chambers, usually by means of cardiac catheterization.

**limb l.,** one of the three standard l.'s or one of the unipolar limb l.'s (aVR, aVL, aVF).

**precordial l.'s,** chest l.'s.

**semidirect l.'s,** chest l.'s.

**standard l.,** indirect l.; one of the three original bipolar limb l.'s of the clinical electrocardiogram, designated I, II and III: l. I records the potential difference between the right and left arms; l. II the difference between right arm and left leg; and l. III the difference between left arm and left leg.

**unipolar l.'s,** those in which the exploring electrode is on the chest in the vicinity of the heart or on one of the limbs, while the other or indifferent electrode is the central terminal.

**V l.,** a chest l. with the central terminal as the indifferent electrode.

**learn′ing** A generic term for the relatively permanent change in behavior that occurs as a result of practice. A number of theories to explain l. exist, none of which is acceptable to all psychologists or educators. See also conditioning.

**incidental l.,** passive l.; l. without a direct attempt.

**latent l.,** that l. which is not evident to the observer at the time it occurs, but which is inferred from later performance in which l. is more rapid than would be expected without the earlier experience.

**passive l.,** incidental l.

**rote l.,** the l. of arbitrary relationships, usually by repetition of the l. procedure, without an understanding of the relationships.

**Le Bel-van't Hoff rule.** See under rule.

**Leber** (la'ber) Theodor, German ophthalmologist, 1840–1917. See *amaurosis* congenita of L., L.'s hereditary optic *atrophy,* L.'s *disease, plexus,* L.'s idiopathic stellate *retinopathy.*

**Le Chatelier's law.** See under law.

**lecithal** (les′ĭ-thal) [ G. *lekithos,* egg yolk ]. Having a yolk or pertaining to the yolk of any egg; used especially as a suffix.

**lecithin** (les′ĭ-thin) [ G. *lekithos,* egg yolk ]. Traditional term for 1,2-diacyl-*sn*-glycero-3-phosphorylcholines, or 3-*sn*-phosphatidylcholines (*sn* = stereospecifically numbered), phospholipids that, on hydrolysis, yield two fatty acid molecules and a molecule each of glycerophosphoric acid and choline. There are several varieties of l.; in some, both fatty acids are saturated, others contain only unsaturated acids, *e.g.,* oleic, linoleic, or arachidonic; in others again, one fatty acid is saturated, the other unsaturated. The l.'s are yellowish or brown waxy substances, readily miscible in water, in which they appear under the microscope as irregular elongated particles known as "myelin forms." They are found in nervous tissue, especially in the myelin sheaths, in egg yolk and, generally, as essential constituents of animal and vegetable cells.

**l. acyltransferase,** an enzyme (EC 2.3.1.43) that transfers an acyl residue from a lecithin to cholesterol, forming a 1-acylglycerophosphocholine (a lysolecithin) and a cholesterol ester.

**lec'ithinase.** Phospholipase.
**l. A,** phospholipase A₂.
**l. B,** lysophospholipase.
**l. C,** phospholipase C.
**l. D,** phospholipase D.

**lecithoblast** (les'ĭ-tho-blast) [ G. *lekithos,* egg yolk, + *blastos,* germ ]. One of the cells proliferating to form the yolk-sac entoderm.

**lec'ithopro'tein.** A conjugated protein, with lecithin as the prosthetic group.

**lectin** (lek'tin). A protein of plant (usually seed) or animal source that effects agglutination, precipitation, or other phenomena resembling the action of specific antibody but which is not an antibody in the strict sense in that it was not evoked by an antigenic stimulus; includes plant agglutinins (phytoagglutinins, phytohemagglutinins), plant precipitins, and perhaps certain animal proteins.

**Lederberg** (lā'der-burg), Joshua, U. S. biochemist *1925. Nobel laureate, 1958, with George W. Beadle and Edward L. Tatum, for discoveries concerning genetic recombination and the organization of the genetic material of bacteria.

**Led'erer,** Max, American pathologist, 1885–1952. See L.'s *anemia.*

**ledge.** Shelf; lamina.
**dental l.,** a band of ectodermal cells growing from the epithelium of the embryonic jaws into the underlying mesenchyme. Local buds from the ledge give rise to the primordia of the enamel organs of the teeth. Also called enamel l.; dental shelf; dental lamina; dentogingival lamina.
**enamel l.,** dental l.

**Leduc** (lě-dük'), Stéphane A. N., French physicist, 1853–1939. See L. *current.*

**Lee,** Robert, English physician, 1793–1877. See L.'s *ganglion.*

**leech** [ A.S. *laece,* a physician; a leech, because of its therapeutic use ]. 1. A bloodsucking aquatic annelid worm (genus *Hirudo,* class Hirudinea) formerly used in medicine for local abstraction of blood; for various l. species, see *Hirudo.* 2. To treat medically by applying leeches. 3. A person who gives such treatment.

**Leede** (la'deh), C., German physician, *1882. See Rumpel-L. *sign, test.*

**Leeuwenhoek** (la'wen-hök), Antonj van, Dutch microscopist, 1632–1723. See L.'s *canals.*

**Lee-White method.** See under method.

**Lefèvre,** 38 Paul. See Papillon-L. *syndrome.*

**Le Fort** (lě-for'), Léon C., Paris surgeon, 1829–1893. See L.'s *amputation, fracture.*

**left'handed.** Denoting a person who uses the left hand for writing and other operations for which the right hand is commonly used.

**leg.** The segment of the inferior limb between the knee and the ankle; commonly used to mean the entire inferior limb.
**l. of antihelix,** *crus* anthelicis.
**badger l.,** a condition in which the l.'s are not of equal length.
**bandy-l.,** *genu* varum.
**Barbados l.,** elephantiasis.
**bayonet l.,** incomplete backward dislocation of the bones of the l. with ankylosis of the knee.
**bird-l.,** nonmedical term for atrophy of l. muscles.
**black-l.,** see blackleg.
**boomerang l.,** platycnemia with sharp and curved anterior edge of the tibia.
**bow-l.,** bowleg; see *genu* varum.
**cross l.'s,** scissor l.'s.
**elephant l.,** elephantiasis.
**jimmy l.'s,** restless legs *syndrome.*
**jitter l.'s,** restless legs *syndrome.*
**milk l.,** *phlegmasia* alba dolens.

**restless l.'s,** restless legs *syndrome.*
**rider's l.,** a strain of the adductor muscles of the thigh.
**saber-legged,** denoting a horse in which the angle of the hock is very acute, the feet extending forward under the body.
**scaly l.,** a thickened, encrusted condition of the legs of fowls caused by the mite, *Knemidokoptes mutans.*
**scissor l.'s,** cross l.'s; extreme adduction of both femurs, following hip disease, the two l.'s crossing each other as the person walks.
**tennis l.,** a traumatic lesion of the calf; a rupture of the medial gastrocnemius at the musculotendinous junction.
**trench l.,** trench *shin.*
**white l.,** *phlegmasia* alba dolens.
**x-l.'s,** scissor l.'s.

**Legal** (la'gahl), Emmo, German physician, 1859–1922. See L.'s *test.*

**Legendre** (le-zhahn'dr), Gaston L. J., French physician, *1887. See L.'s *sign.*

**Legg,** Arthur T., Boston surgeon, 1874–1939. See L.'s *disease,* L.-Calvé-Perthes *disease,* L.-Perthes *disease,* L.'s *operation.*

**leghemoglobin** (leg'he-mo-glo'bin). Legoglobin.

**-legia** [ L. *legere,* to read ]. A suffix, of Latin origin, that properly relates to reading and should be distinguished from the Greek derivatives, - *lexis* and - *lexy,* which signify speech.

**legoglobin** (leg'o-glo'bin). Leghemoglobin; a red pigment in the root nodules of legumes, apparently necessary for nitrogen fixation.

**legumin** (lě-gu'min, leg'u-min). A protein contained in peas, beans, and other legumes; it resembles casein and is called vegetable casein.

**leguminivorous** (lě-gu'mĭ-niv'o-rus). Feeding on beans, peas, and other legumes.

**Lehmann,** Orla, Swedish physician. See Börjeson-Forssman-L. *syndrome.*

**Leichtenstern** (līkh'ten-stairn), Otto, German physician, 1845–1900. See L.'s *phenomenon, sign.*

**Leidy,** Joseph, American anatomist and naturalist, 1823–1891. Professor of anatomy at the University of Pennsylvania; he demonstrated the presence of *Trichina spiralis* in swine; described the bacterial flora of the intestine and successfully transplanted malignant tumors.

**Leiner** (li'ner), Karl, Austrian pediatrician, 1871–1930. See L.'s *disease.*

**leio-** (li'o-) [ G. *leios,* smooth ]. Combining form meaning smooth.

**leioder'mia** (li'o-der'mĭ-ah) [ leio- + G. *derma,* skin ]. Smooth, glossy skin.

**leiomyofibroma** (li-o-mi'o-fi-bro'ma). Fibroleiomyoma.

**leiomyoma** (li'o-mi-o'mah) [ leio- + G. *mys,* muscle, + suffix -*oma,* tumor ]. A benign neoplasm derived from smooth (nonstriated) muscle.
**l. cutis,** cutaneous eruption of small painful nodules composed of smooth muscle fibers.
**parasitic l.,** parasitic fibroid; a uterine l. which has become detached from the uterus and adherent to another peritoneal surface from which it derives a blood supply.
**vascular l.,** angioleiomyoma; angiomyofibroma; angiomyoma; telangiectatic fibromyoma; a markedly vascular l., apparently arising from the smooth muscle of blood vessels.
**Zenker's l.,** leiomyosarcoma.

**leiomyomatosis** (li-o-mi'o-mă-to'sis). The state of having multiple leiomyomas throughout the body.

**leiomyosarcoma** (li'o-mi'o-sar-ko'mah) [ leio- + myosarcoma, *q.v.* ]. Zenker's leiomyoma; a malignant neoplasm derived from smooth (nonstriated) muscle.

**leiotrichous** (li-ot'rĭ-kus) [ leio- + G. *thrix,* hair ]. Having straight hair.

**leipo-.** For words so beginning see lipo-.

**Leipzig yellow.** *Chrome* yellow.

**Leishman** (lēsh'man), Sir William B., British surgeon, 1865–1926. Gave his name to *Leishmania.* See L.'s chrome cells, L.-Donovan *body,* L.'s *stain.*

**Leishmania** (lēsh-man'ĭ-ah) [ W. B. *Leishman* ]. A genus of digenetic, asexual, protozoan flagellates (family

Trypanosomatidae) that occur as amastigotes (rounded or ovoid, intracellular, nonflagellated forms) in the macrophages of vertebrate hosts and as promastigotes (elongate, tapered, flagellated, leptomonad forms) in invertebrate hosts and in cultures. The three species are indistinguishable morphologically, but may be separated serologically and on the basis *of their sand fly host, geographic occurrence, and clinical manifestations.

**L. brazilien'sis,** also known as *L. tropica* var. *americana* and *L. tropica* var. *braziliensis;* the causal agent of American or New World mucocutaneous leishmaniasis, endemic in southern Mexico and Central and South America, except for the equatorial region of Chile; clinical or serological variants, such as *L. mexicana, L. peruana, L. guyanensis,* and *L. pifanoi,* have been described, but clear-cut species delineation remains to be satisfactorily established, as the parasites are morphologically indistinguishable; *L. braziliensis* is transmitted by various species of *Lutzomyia* or *Phlebotomus* (sand flies); dogs and possibly other animals serve as reservoir hosts.

**L. cani'num,** described as the *L.* found in dogs with leishmaniasis, especially in Mediterranean countries and in association with children who had visceral leishmaniasis, but now considered a form of *L. donovani* called *L. donovani infantum.*

**L. chaga'si,** a species of *L.* found in South America, chiefly in Brazil, producing visceral leishmaniasis; its taxonomic status is still uncertain.

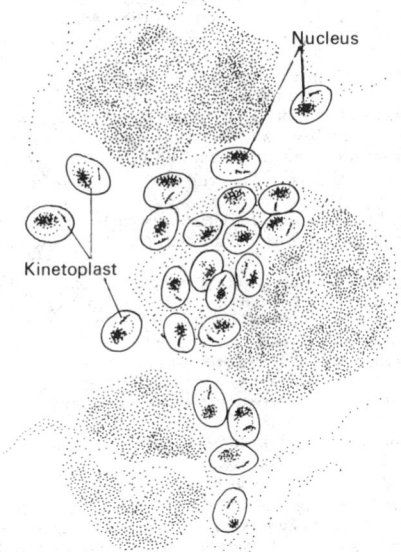

*Leishmania donovani*

Leishmanial forms of parasite in bone marrow smear (×2000). (From Najarian, H. H.: *Textbook of Medical Parasitology,* The Williams & Wilkins Co., Baltimore, 1967.)

**L. donova'ni,** known in the Mediterranian region as *L. donovani* var. *infantum* or *L. infantum;* the causal agent of visceral leishmaniasis, endemic in Mediterranean and adjacent countries, the Middle East, south central USSR, India, China, Kenya, Ethiopia, Sudan, and in parts of South America such as Brazil, Argentina, Colombia, and Venezuela; it is transmitted by various species of *Phlebotomus* (sand flies), such as *P. chinensis, P. argentipes, P. major, P. longipalpis, P. intermedius, P. longicuspis, P. perniciosus, P. orientalis,* each of which is an important vector in a specific endemic area of human infection; dogs and other carnivores serve as reservoir hosts (rodents and small carnivores, but not dogs, in the Sudan; no animal reservoir known in India); The intracellular amastigote form, formerly called the Leishman-Donovan body, multiplies chiefly in macrophages and produces a disease of various

parts of the reticuloendothelial system, causing severe hepatosplenomegaly, which usually is fatal if untreated.

**L. furunculo'sa,** former name for *L. tropica.*

**L. guyanen'sis,** a form of *L.* that transmits a forest form of New World cutaneous leishmaniasis in French Guiana called pian bois.

**L. infan'tum,** a strain of *L.* that causes visceral leishmaniasis in children in the Mediterranean countries; first thought to be different from *L. donovani* on the basis of slightly larger size, more uniform growth in cultures, and apparently greater resistance to antimony compounds, but now considered to be *L. donovani* or (*L. donovani* var. *infantum*).

**L. mexica'na,** a species described from Mexico, Guatemala, and British Honduras; agent of a form of New World cutaneous leishmaniasis called chiclero's ulcer, associated with chicle gum and mahogany forest workers in the Yucatan, Oaxaca in southern Mexico, Petén in Guatemala, and forested regions of Guatemala.

**L. perua'na,** species of *L.* found infecting man in the high Andean valleys of Peru and Bolivia; cause of the distinct form of New World cutaneous leishmaniasis called uta.

**L. pifa'noi,** name proposed for the etiological agent of leishmaniasis tegumentaria diffusa, *q. v.*

**L. trop'ica,** formerly known as *Herpetomonas tropica* and *H. furunculosis;* the causal agent of cutaneous leishmaniasis; formerly endemic throughout the Mediterranean basin, Middle East, parts of southern USSR and elsewhere in Asia, and also reported from West Africa; it is transmitted by *Phlebotomus papatasii* and related species of sand flies; small rodents, the Chinese hamster (*Cricetulus griseus*), and various ground squirrels serve as reservoir hosts.

**leishmaniasis** (lēsh'mă-ni'ă-sis). Infection with a species of *Leishmania.* There are three forms of the disease: (1) visceral l. (kala azar); (2) cutaneous l. (Old World l.); and (3) mucocutaneous l. (American l.). The three forms of the disease, although clinically quite distinct, and each having a definite geographical distribution, are caused by *Leishmania* species which are morphologically identical and which are transmitted by various species of sandfly of the genus *Phlebotomus* or *Lutzomyia.*

**American l., l. americana,** mucocutaneous l.

**anergic l.,** l. tegumentaria diffusa.

**canine l.,** a disease of dogs in the Mediterranean region, Brazil, China and other countries caused by species of *Leishmania* and transmitted by sand flies of the genus *Phlebotomus; L. donovani* causes a visceral form of the disease, while infection with *L. tropica* is manifested by skin lesions; the infections are transmissible to man.

**cutaneous l.,** Old World l.; Oriental or tropical boil, sore, or ulcer; infection with leptomonads (promastigotes) of *Leishmania tropica* inoculated into the skin by the bite of an infected sand fly, *Phlebotomus* (commonly *P. papatasi*). It is endemic in parts of Asia Minor, northern Africa, and India, and is known by innumerable names, each indicating its locality: Aleppo, Bagdad, Delhi, Godovnik, Jericho, Natal boil; Annam, Jeddah, Malabar, Penjdeh, Syrian, Turkestan ulcer; Biskra button; etc. The ulcer begins as a papule that enlarges to a nodule and then breaks down into an ulcer. Two distinctive clinical and epidemiological diseases are recognized in the Soviet Union: a rural, zoonotic, moist, acute form caused by *L. tropica major,* with a reservoir host, the large gerbil, *Rhombomys opimus;* and an urban, anthroponotic, dry, chronic form caused by *L. tropica minor,* without a reservoir host.

**infantile l.,** visceral l. in infants.

**mucocutaneous l.,** New World l.; American l., nasopharyngeal l.; a grave disease caused by *Leishmania braziliensis,* endemic in southern Mexico and Central and South America, except for the equatorial region of Chile. The organism does not invade the viscera, and the disease is limited to the skin and mucous membranes, the lesions resembling the sores of cutaneous l. caused by *Leishmania tropica.* The chancrous sores heal after a time, but some months or years later fungating and eroding forms of ulceration may appear on the tongue and buccal or nasal mucosa in typical cases of espundia (*q. v.*). Many variants of the disease exist, marked by differences in distribution, vector, epidemiology, and pathology, which suggest that it may in fact be caused by as many as eight or nine closely related etiological agents.

na'spharynge'al l., mucocutaneous l.

New World l., mucocutaneous l.

Old World l., cutaneous l.

pseudolepromatous l., l. tegumentaria diffusa.

l. tegumenta'ria diffu'sa, pseudolepromatous l.; anergic l.; a diffuse or disseminated form of cutaneous l. reported recently from widely scattered areas with diverse epidemiological characteristics. The form described from Venezuela was attributed to *Leishmania pifanoi*, but may prove to be a host immunological failure rather than a distinct etiological agent. Nonetheless, the condition is chronic, very difficult to cure, and gives some evidence for specific characteristics based on animal experimentation in Venezuela.

vis'ceral l., kala azar; tropical splenomegaly; Dumdum fever; burdwan fever; cachectic fever; Assam fever; a chronic, disease, highly fatal when untreated, occurring in India, Assam, China, USSR, Kenya, Sudan, and various parts of South America, chiefly Brazil. Caused by the hemoflagellate *Leishmania donovani*, transmitted by the bite of an appropriate vector species of sand fly (*Phlebotomus*). The organisms grow and multiply in macrophages, eventually causing them to burst, and the liberated amastigore parasites then invade other endothelial and parenchymal macrophages, chiefly large mononuclear cells derived from the reticuloendothelial tissues; the bone marrow usually becomes involved, with crowding out of erythroid and myeloid elements, causing leukopenia and anemia. Splenomegaly and hepatomegaly are characteristic, along with enlargement of lymph nodes, fever, fatigue, malaise, and secondary infections.

**leishmaniosis** (lēsh'man-ī-o'sis). Leishmaniasis.

**leishmanoid** (lēsh'mă-noyd). A condition resembling leishmaniasis.

dermal l., post-kala azar dermal l.

post-kala azar dermal l., this condition, first described in India and most characteristic of kala azar in that country, is a chronic, granulomatous, nonulcerating hypopigmented nodular cutaneous outbreak that may appear 6 months to 5 years after spontaneous or drug cure of visceral leishmaniasis (kala azar); 5 to 10 per cent of persons with Indian kala azar are said to develop this condition. It usually follows a progressive, chronic, clinical course and is highly resistant to antimony therapy.

**Leloir** (lěl-wahr), Henri C., French dermatologist, 1855–1896. See L.'s *disease*.

**lema** (le'mah) [ G. *lēmē*, a humor, gum, rheum ]. Secretions from a Meibomian gland, collected at the inner canthus.

**Lembert** (lahn-bair'), Antoine, Paris surgeon, 1802–1851. See L.'s *suture*, Czerny-L. *suture*.

**lememia** (le-me'mī-ah) [ G. *loimos*, plague, + *haima*, blood ]. Pesticemia. 1. The presence of plague bacilli in the peripheral blood stream, with or without grave constitutional symptoms. 2. Septicemic *plague*.

**le'mic** [ G. *loimos*, plague ]. Relating to the plague or any epidemic disease.

**lem'moblast** [ G. *lemma*, husk, + *blastos*, germ ]. In an embryo a cell of neural crest origin capable of forming a cell of the neurolemma sheath.

**lemmocyte** (lem'o-sit) [ G. *lemma*, husk, + *kytos*, cell ]. One of the cells of the neurolemma.

**lemniscus**, pl. **lemnis'ci** (lem-nis'kus) [ L. from G. *lēmniskos*, ribbon or fillet ] [ NA ]. Fillet (1); a bundle of nerve fibers ascending from sensory nuclei in the spinal cord and rhombencephalon to the thalamus.

acoustic l., l. lateralis.

auditory l., l. lateralis.

l. latera'lis [ NA ], acoustic l.; auditory l.; auditory tract; lateral fillet; a bundle of ascending fibers that originate from the cochlear nuclei of the rhombencephalon, enter the corpus trapezoideum, a transverse fiber stratum in which about half their number decussate, and from here turn rostralward along the lateral side of the spinothalamic tract; upon entering the midbrain the lateral lemniscus arches dorsally and enters the inferior colliculus in which all of its fibers terminate. The auditory conduction pathway is transsynaptically extended from here by the brachium of the inferior colliculus to the medial geniculate body of the thalamus, from which in turn the auditory radiation leads to the auditory cortex. Intercalated in the trapezoid body and along the ascending trajectory of the

lemniscus are several cell groups in which part of the fibers synapse and which in turn contribute fibers to the lemniscus: superior olive, nucleus of the trapezoid body, and nuclei of the lateral lemniscus.

l. media'lis [ NA ], medial fillet; ribbon of Reil; Reil's band (2); a band of white fibers taking origin from the gracile and cuneate nuclei and crossing to the opposite side in the lower part of the medulla; thence it passes upward through the center of the medulla oblongata, close to the median raphe; on entering the pons it spreads out laterally to form a flat band ascending over the dorsal border of the pontine nuclei; in the mesencephalon it passes over the dorsal border of the substantia nigra and is displaced laterally by the red nucleus; passing medial to the medial geniculate body, the bundle enters and terminates in the nucleus ventralis posterior of the thalamus. Throughout their course, the fibers of the medial lemniscus retain a somatotopic order such that those originating from the nucleus gracilis and representing the lower extremity lie lateral to those originating in the nucleus cuneatus and representing the arm. The medial lemniscus conveys somatic-sensory information involved in tactile discrimination (two-point discrimination) and proprioceptive awareness.

l. spina'lis [ NA ], *tractus* spinothalamicus.

trigeminal l., l. trigeminalis.

l. trigemina'lis [ NA ], trigeminal l.; collective term denoting the fibers ascending from the sensory nucleus of the trigeminus; one such fiber system originates from the main sensory nucleus, largely decussates, and joins the medial l. with which it enters the nucleus ventralis posterior thalami, terminating in the mediodorsal region of that nucleus; a second, parallel, fiber group follows an ascending course through central parts of the mesencephalic tegmentum ("dorsal trigeminal l."). The l. trigeminalis conveys tactile, pain, and temperature impulses from the skin of the face, the mucous membranes of the nasal and oral cavities, and the eye, as well as proprioceptive information from the facial and masticatory muscles.

**lem'on** [ L. *limon* ]. The fruit of *Citrus limon* (family Rutaceae).

dried l. peel (BP), the dried outer part of the pericarp of the ripe or nearly ripe fruit of *Citrus limon;* used chiefly as a flavor.

l. grass oil, Indian oil of verbena; a volatile oil distilled from the herb *Cymbopogon* (*Andropogon*) *citratus* (family Gramineae), a grass of Ceylon and India; a source of citral, and used in perfumery.

l. juice, the freshly expressed juice of the ripe l., the fruit of *Citrus limon*. Used as a preventive and curative agent in scurvy, and as a refrigerant diuretic in fever, in the form of lemonade.

l. oil (USP), a volatile oil expressed from fresh l. peel; used chiefly in flavoring.

l. yellow, *chrome* yellow.

**Lemuroidea** (lem'u-roy'de-ah) [ L. *lemures*, ghosts, + *eidos*, resemblance ]. A family of primates (lemurs) characterized by long tails, slender bodies, and long limbs; they are agile, restless, and sociable, and eat plants, berries, and animals. The six genera and 16 species are confined to Madagascar and the Comoro Islands.

**length.** Linear distance between two points.

crown-heel l., the total l. or standing height of an embryo or fetus.

crown-rump l., abbreviated CR or CRL; a measurement from the skull vertex to the midpoint between the apices of the buttocks (breech) of an embryo or fetus; permits approximation of embryonic or fetal age.

**Lenhossék**, Michael v., Hungarian anatomist, 1863–1937. See L.'s *processes*.

**lenitive** (len'ī-tiv) [ L. *lenio*, pp. *lenitus*, to soften, fr. *lenis*, mild ]. 1. Soothing; relieving discomfort or pain. 2. A demulcent; an agent that soothes or relieves irritation.

**Lenoir** (lěn-wahr'), Camille A. H., French anatomist, *1867. See L.'s *facet*.

**lens** (lenz) [ L. a lentil. LEN- ]. 1. A piece of glass, quartz, or other transparent substance with one or both surfaces curved, either concave or convex; used for acting upon the rays of light in the way of convergence or divergence. 2 [ NA ]. A transparent biconvex cellular body lying between the iris and the vitreous, one of the refracting media of the eye; it consists of a soft outer part (cortical substance) with a denser central part (nucleus). The anterior surface has a cuboidal epithelium, and at the equator the cells elongate to become lens fibers. The lens is surrounded by a fine membrane (capsule).

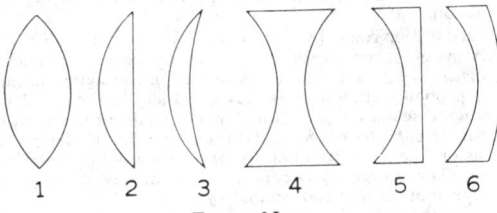

**Types of Lens**

*1*, Biconvex; *2*, planoconvex; *3*, concavoconvex, converging meniscus; *4*, biconcave; *5*, planoconcave; *6*, convexoconcave, diverging meniscus.

**achromatic l.,** a double l., made of two kinds of glass with different dispersive qualities, so selected that one practically neutralizes the light dispersion of the other, without interfering with refraction.

**aplanatic l.,** a l. designed to correct spherical aberration and coma.

**apochromatic l.,** a compound l. designed to correct both spherical and chromatic aberrations.

**aspheric l.,** see aspheric.

**biconcave l.,** double concave l.; concavoconcave l.; a l. that is concave on two opposing surfaces.

**biconvex l.,** double convex l.; convexoconvex l.; a l. with both surfaces convex.

**bifocal l.,** a l. used in cases of presbyopia, in which one portion is suited for distant vision, the other for reading and near work in general; the reading addition may be cemented to the l. (see paster) or fused to the front surface (see kryptok) or ground in one-piece form (see ultex). Other bifocal l.'s are the flat-top Franklin type, or blended invisible.

**cataract l.,** any l. prescribed for aphakia.

**compound l.,** an optical system of two or more lenses.

**concave l.,** a diverging minus power lens; see fig. under refraction.

**concavoconcave l.,** biconcave l.

**concavoconvex l.,** a converging meniscus l. that is concave on one surface and convex on the opposite surface.

**contact l.,** a molded plastic l. that fits over the cornea in direct contact with the sclera or cornea; used to correct refractive errors. A soft, supple, hydrophilic type is advantageous for use in children, aphakia, and conical cornea, and allows healing of penetrating small corneal wounds that are in good apposition. Also available is a silicone type that is easily sterilized and permeable to oxygen and carbon dioxide.

**convex l.,** plus l.; a converging l.; see fig. under refraction.

**convexoconcave l.,** a minus power l. having one surface convex and the opposite surface concave, with the latter having the greater curvature.

**convexoconvex l.,** biconvex l.

**corneal l.,** contact l. of plastic without scleral portions.

**crystalline l.,** l. (2).

**cylindrical l.,** a l. one or both surfaces of which have the curve of a cylinder, either concave (minus) or convex (plus); a cylindric l. refracts the rays of light in only one of its principal meridians; it is used in eyeglasses to correct astigmatism.

**decentered l.,** a l. so mounted that the visual axis does not pass through the axis of the l.

**double concave l.,** biconcave l.

**double convex l.,** biconvex l.

**eye l.,** ocular l.; the upper of the two planoconvex l.'s of Huygens' ocular.

**field l.,** the lower of the two planoconvex l.'s of Huygens' ocular.

**Fresnel l.,** a l. with a surface consisting of a concentric series of zones that duplicate the power of a strong l. or prism but with considerably less thickness.

**immersion l.,** an objective (for a microscope) constructed in such a manner that the lower l. may be moved downward into direct contact with a fluid which is placed on the glass slide being examined; by means of using a fluid with a refractive index closely similar to that of glass, the loss of light is minimized.

**meniscus l.,** a l. having a spherical concave curve on one side and a spherical convex curve on the other. See also relevant subentries under meniscus.

**minus l.,** a concave l.

**ocular l.,** eye l.

**periscopic l.,** a lens with 1.25 D base curve.

**photochromic l.,** a light-sensitive eyeglass that automatically darkens in sunlight and clears in reduced light; two densities are available, transmitting, in full sun, 45 per cent and 20 per cent of the light, respectively.

**planoconcave l.,** a l. that is flat on one side and concave on the other.

**planoconvex l.,** one that is flat on one side and concave on the other.

**plus l.,** a convex l.

**safety l.,** a l. that meets government specifications of impact *resistance* (*q.v.*); the increased impact resistance required for safety lenses is obtained by tempering, an ion-exchange process, or using laminated or plastic lenses, although plastic lenses may warp or scratch.

**slab-off l.,** a l. with a 1 1/2-diopter to 5-diopter base-up inferiorly, produced by grinding a prismatic slab of glass from the lower part of the l.; used in anisomyopia to equalize image displacement when reading.

**spherical l.,** a l. in which all refracting surfaces are spherical.

**spher′ocylin′drical l.,** spherocylinder; a combined spherical and cylindrical l., one surface being spherical, the other cylindrical.

**toric l.,** a spherocylindrical curved l. corresponding in shape to the surface of a torus.

**trial l.'s.,** a series of cylindrical and spherical l.'s used in testing vision.

**trifocal l.,** a l. with segments of three focal powers: distant, intermediate, and near.

**lensometer** (len-zom′e-ter) [ lens + G. *metron*, measure ]. Vertometer; an optical instrument that determines accurately the vertex refractive power, cylinder axis, optical center, and prismatic addition when present in ophthalmic lenses.

**lenticonus** (len′tĭ-ko′nus) [ lens + L. *conus*, cone ]. A conical projection of the anterior or posterior surface of the crystalline lens of the eye, occurring as a developmental anomaly.

**lenticula** (len-tik′u-lah) [ L. dim. of *lens*. LEN- ]. 1. *Nucleus* lentiformis. 2. Lentigo.

**lentic′ular** [ L. *lenticula*, a lentil ]. 1. Relating to or resembling a lens of any kind. 2. Of the shape of a lentil.

**lentic′ulo-op′tic.** Relating to the lentiform nucleus and the optic tract; specifically refers to branches of the middle cerebral artery supplying these structures.

**lentic′ulopap′ular.** Indicating an eruption with dome-shaped or lens-shaped papules.

**lentic′ulostri′ate.** Relating to the nucleus lentiformis and the nucleus caudatus; specifically refers to branches of the middle cerebral artery supplying these gray masses.

**lentic′ulothalam′ic.** Pertaining to the lentiform (lenticular) nucleus and the thalamus.

**lenticulus,** pl. **lenticuli** (len-tik′u-lus) [ L. dim. of *lens, lentis*, a little lens ]. Prosthetophakia; an intraocular lens of inert plastic placed in anterior chamber or behind iris, or clipped to iris after cataract extraction.

**len′tiform.** Lens-shaped; lenticular.

**lentigines** (len-tij′ĭ-nēz) [ L. ]. Plural of lentigo.

**lentiginosis** (len-tij′ĭ-no′sis). Multiple lentigines.

**lentiglo′bus** [ lens + L. *globus*, sphere ]. A rare congenital anomaly showing a prominent spheroid elevation on the posterior surface of the lens.

**lentigo,** pl. **lentigines** (len-ti′go, len-tij′ĭ-nēz) [ L. fr. *lens* (*lent*-), a lentil ]. Lenticula (2); a brown macule resembling a freckle except that the border is usually regular, and microscopic proliferation of rete ridges is present. Scattered solitary nevus cells are seen in the basal cell layer. See also junction *nevus.*

**malig'nant l.,** *melanosis* circumscripta precancerosa.

**senile l.,** liver spot; a variably pigmented l. occurring on exposed skin of older Caucasians.

**lentigomelanosis** (len-ti'go-mel'ă-no'sis). Malignant lesions originating in lentigines.

**lentogenic** (len'to-jen'ik) [ L. *lentus,* sluggish, inactive, + G. suffix *-gen,* producing ]. Denoting the virulence of a virus capable of inducing lethal infection in embryonic hosts after a long incubation period and an inapparent infection in immature and adult hosts; the term is used in characterizing Newcastle disease virus, particularly, strains used as vaccines administered in water or as sprays.

**leontiasis** (le'on-ti'ă-sis) [ G. *leōn* (*leont-*), lion ]. Leonine facies; the appearance of the face of patients with advanced lepromatous leprosy; there are ridges and furrows on the forehead and cheeks.

**l. ossea,** Virchow's disease (2); an overgrowth of the bones of the face, and sometimes of the cranium, causing a general enlargement of all the features.

**leopard's bane.** Arnica.

**Leopold,** Christian G., German physician, 1846–1911. See L.'s *law.*

**lep'er** [ G. *lepra.* LEP- ]. A person who has leprosy.

**lepidic** (lĕ-pid'ik) [ G. *lepis* (*lepid-*), scale, rind. LEP- ]. Relating to scales or a scaly covering layer.

**lep'idine.** 4-Methylquinoline; an oily liquid obtained from cinchonine.

**lepidoma** (lep'ĭ-do'mah) [ G. *lepis,* scale, rind, + suffix *-oma,* tumor ]. Obsolete term for a neoplasm derived from one of the lepidic tissues.

**Lepidoptera** (lep'ĭ-dop'ter-ah) [ G. *lepis,* scale, + *pteron,* wing ]. An order of insects, including the moths and butterflies, characterized by wings covered with delicate scales.

**lepidosis** (lep'ĭ-do'sis) [ G. *lepis,* scale, rind, + suffix *-osis,* condition ]. Any scaly or desquamating eruption.

**lepothrix** (lep'o-thriks) [ G. *lepos,* rind, husk, + *thrix,* hair ]. *Trichomycosis* axillaris.

**lepra** (lep'rah) [ G. leprosy. LEP- ]. 1. Leprosy. 2. Psoriasis.

**l. alba,** macular leprosy with depigmented spots.

**l. alphos,** psoriasis.

**l. anaesthet'ica,** anesthetic *leprosy.*

**l. ar'abum,** tuberculoid *leprosy.*

**l. cuta'nea,** tuberculoid *leprosy.*

**l. graeco'rum,** original name used by Galen (A.D. 150) to designate leprosy.

**l. maculo'sa,** macular *leprosy.*

**l. mu'tilans,** articular *leprosy.*

**l. nervo'rum, l. nervo'sa,** anesthetic *leprosy.*

**l. orienta'lis,** elephantiasis.

**l. tubercula'tum,** tuberculoid *leprosy.*

**Willan's l.,** *psoriasis* circinata.

**leprechaunism** (lep're-kawn-izm) [ Irish *leprechaun,* elf ]. Donohue's disease; a congenital disorder characterized by extreme growth retardation and emaciation, with grotesque elfin facies and large, low-set ears; autosomal recessive inheritance.

**lep'rid** [ G. *lepra,* leprosy, + suffix *-id* (1), *q.v.* ]. Early cutaneous lesion of leprosy.

**leprologist** (lĕ-prol'o-jist). A student of leprosy.

**leprology** (lĕ-prol'o-jĭ) [ G. *lepra,* leprosy, + *logos,* study ]. The science and study of leprosy.

**leproma** (lĕ-pro'mah) [ G. *lepros,* scaly, + suffix *-oma,* tumor ]. A fairly well circumscribed, discrete focus of granulomatous inflammation caused by *Mycobacterium leprae;* the tumorous lesion consists chiefly of an accumulation of large mononuclear phagocytic cells in which the cytoplasm seems finely vacuolated (*i.e.,* foam cells); the foamlike character of the macrophages is related to the engulfing of numerous acid-fast organisms.

**lepro'matous.** Pertaining to, or characterized by, the features of a leproma.

**lep'romin.** An extract of infected tissue used in skin tests of resistance to leprosy; see also l. *reaction.*

**leprosarium** (lep'ro-sār'ĭ-um). A hospital especially designed for the care of those suffering from leprosy, especially those who need expert care.

**lep'rose.** Leprous.

**leprosery** (lep'ro-sĕr-ĭ). A leper home or colony.

**lep'rostat'ic.** 1. Inhibiting to the growth of the bacillus of leprosy (*Mycobacterium leprae*). 2. An agent having this action.

**leprosy** (lep'ro-sĭ) [ G. *lepra,* from *lepros,* scaly. LEP- ]. 1. A name given in Biblical times to various cutaneous diseases, especially those of a chronic or contagious nature; it probably embraced psoriasis and leukoderma. 2. Hansen's disease; chronic granulomatous infection caused by the *Mycobacterium leprae* (Hansen's bacillus). Elephantiasis or true leprosy caused by *M. leprae* was first described by Galen. Leprosy occurs in two relatively stable types: lepromatous and tuberculoid, *q.v.*

**anesthetic l.,** a form affecting the nerves chiefly, marked by hyperesthesia succeeded by anesthesia, by paralysis, ulceration, and various trophic disturbances, terminating in gangrene and mutilation. Also called Danielssen's disease; Danielssen-Boeck disease; dry or trophoneurotic l.; lepra anaesthetica, nervorum, or nervosa.

**artic'ular l.,** lepra mutilans; mutilating l.; a late stage of anesthetic l.

**Astu'rian l.,** pellagra.

**black l.,** see macular l.

**cuta'neous l.,** tuberculoid l.

**dry l.,** anesthetic l.

**dysmorphic l.,** a malignant form which is very unstable; it is frequently positive for lepra bacilli, but the lepromin test is negative. Cutaneous lesions are flat bands or plaques.

**erythe'ma nodo'sum l.,** abbreviated ENL; an acute type of lepromatous reaction with generalized systemic involvement and tender lesions of the face, thighs, and arms.

**Italian l.,** pellagra.

**lepromatous l.,** the malignant form with nodular cutaneous lesions which are infiltrated and have ill-defined borders. The lesions are bacteriologically positive, but the lepromin test is negative.

**Lombardy l.,** pellagra.

**Lucio's l.,** Lucio's l. phenomenon; an acute form of lepromatous leprosy presenting irregularly shaped, intensely erythematous, tender plaques, especially of the legs, with tendency to ulceration and scarring.

**mac'ular l.,** lepra maculosa; anesthetic l. marked by the presence of spots on the skin, either pigmented (black l.) or lighter than normal (white l.).

**Mal'abar l.,** elephantiasis.

**mouse l., murine l.,** rat l.

**nod'ular l.,** tuberculoid l.

**rat l.,** mouse or murine l.; a form of l. occurring in rats, caused by *Mycobacterium lepraemurium;* it appears in two forms, glandular and musculocutaneous. It is slowly but progressively fatal.

**smooth l.,** macular l.

**trophoneurotic l.,** anesthetic l.

**tuberculoid l.,** cutaneous or nodular l.; lepra arabum, cutaneum, or tuberculatum; a benign, stable and resistant form of the disease in which the lepromin reaction is strongly positive and in which the lesions are erythematous, infiltrated plaques with clear-cut edges.

**white l.,** see macular l.

**leprot'ic.** Leprous.

**leprous** (lep'rus). Relating to or suffering from leprosy.

**-lepsis, -lepsy** [ G. *lēpsis,* seizure. LAB- ]. Combining forms denoting seizure.

**leptan'dra** [ G. *leptos,* slender (LEP-), + *anēr*(*andr*-), man (stamen) ]. The rhizome and roots of *Veronica* (*Leptandra*) *virginica* (family Scrophulariaceae); Culver's root; Culver's physic; black-root; a herb of eastern North America; cholagogue cathartic.

**lep'to-** [ G. *leptos,* slender, delicate, weak. LEP- ]. A combining form meaning light, slender, thin, or frail.

**leptocephalous** (lep'to-sef'ă-lus) [ lepto- + G. *kephalē,* head ]. Having an abnormally small head.

**leptocephalus** (lep'to-sef'ă-lus) [ lepto- + G. *kephalē,* head ]. An individual having an abnormally small head.

**leptochroa** (lep'to-kro'ah) [ lepto- + G. *chrōa*, skin ]. Abnormally delicate skin.

**leptochromatic** (lep-to-kro-mat'ik). Having a very fine chromatin network.

**leptocyte** (lep'to-sit) [ lepto- + G. *kytos*, cell ]. A "target" or "Mexican hat" cell, *i.e.*, an unusually thin or flattened red blood cell in which there is (1) a central, rounded area of pigmented material, (2) a middle, clear zone that contains no pigment, and (3) an outer, pigmented rim at the edge of the cell. L.'s are thought to be erythrocytes in which the cellular envelope or membrane is unusually large in proportion to its contents.

**lep'tocyto'sis.** The presence of leptocytes in the circulating blood, as in (1) thalassemia, (2) some instances of jaundice—even in the absence of anemia, (3) occasional examples of hepatic disease—in the absence of jaundice, and (4) some patients who have had the spleen removed.

**leptodactylous** (lep'to-dak'ti-lus) [ lepto- + G. *daktylos*, finger ]. Having slender fingers.

**lep'toder'mic** [ lepto- + G. *derma*, skin ]. Thin-skinned.

**leptomeningeal** (lep'to-mĕ-nin'je-al). Pertaining to the leptomeninges.

**leptomeninges** (lep-to-mĕ-nin'jēz) [ lepto- + G. *mēninx*, pl. *mēninges*, membrane ]. Piarachnoid; pia-arachnoid; meninx tenuis; collective term denoting the soft membranes enveloping brain and spinal cord: pia mater and arachnoidea mater, as distinguished from dura mater, the pachymeninx.

**leptomeningitis** (lep'to-men-in-ji'tis). Arachnoiditis (*q.v.*); pia-arachnitis; inflammation of leptomeninges.

  **basilar l.,** basiarachnitis; basiarachnoiditis; inflammation of the arachnoid at the base of the brain; often found in chronic meningitis of tuberculous, luetic, or mycotic origin.

**leptomeningopathy** (lep'to-men-in-gop'ă-thī). Rarely used term meaning disease of the leptomeninges.

**lep'tomen'inx.** Singular of leptomeninges.

**leptomere** (lep'to-mēr) [ lepto- + G. *meros*, part ]. A very minute particle of living matter; Asclepiades believed the body was composed of an aggregation of vast numbers of l.'s.

**leptomonad** (lep'to-mo'nad, lep-tom'o-nad). 1. Common name for a member of the genus *Leptomonas*. 2. See promastigote.

**Leptomonas** (lep'to-mo'nas, lep-tom'o-nus) [ lepto- + G. *monas*, unit ]. A genus of asexual, monogenetic, parasitic flagellates (family Trypanosomatidae) commonly found in the hindgut of insects.

**leptonema** (lep'to-ne'mah) [ lepto- + G. *nēma*, thread ]. Leptotene.

**leptopel'lic** [ lepto- + G. *pellis*, a bowl (the pelvis) ]. Having an abnormally narrow pelvis.

**leptophonia** (lep'to-fo'nī-ah) [ lepto- + G. *phōnē*, sound, voice ]. Weakness of voice.

**lep'tophon'ic.** Weak-voiced.

**lep'topo'dia** [ lepto- + G. *pous*, foot ]. The state of having slender feet.

**leptoprosope** (lep'to-pro-sōp). A person with leptoprosopia.

**leptoprosopia** (lep'to-pro-so'pī-ah) [ lepto- + G. *prosōpon*, face ]. Narrowness of the face.

**leptoprosopic** (lep'to-pro-so'pik). Having a thin, narrow face.

**leptorrhine** (lep'to-rin) [ lepto- + G. *rhis*, nose ]. Having a thin nose. Applied to a skull with a nasal index below 47 (Frankfort agreement) or 48 (Broca).

**lep'toscope.** An apparatus for measuring cell membranes.

**lep'tosomat'ic** [ lepto- + G. *sōma*, body ]. Leptosomic; having a slender, light, or thin body.

**lep'tosome.** A leptosomatic person.

**lep'to·o'mic.** Leptosomatic.

**Leptospira** (lep'to-spi'rah) [ lepto- + G. *speira*, a coil ]. A genus of aerobic bacteria (order Spirochaetales) containing thin, tightly coiled organisms 6 to 20 μm length. They possess an axial filament, and one or both ends may be bent into a semicircular hook. They stain with difficulty except with Giemsa's stain or silver impregnation. The type species is *L. icterohaemorrhagiae* (however, an effort is underway to make *L. interrogans* the type species of this genus).

  **L. biflexa,** a species found in fresh water; includes the saprophytic leptospires. The organisms in this species are currently regarded as forming a complex with the species *L. interrogans.*

  **L. canic'ola,** a species that causes canicola fever and Stuttgart disease.

  **L. icterohaemorrha'giae,** a species originally found in cases of infectious jaundice (Weil's disease) in man; this species includes the parasitic leptospires. The organisms in this species are currently regarded as forming a complex within the species *L. interrogans. L. icterohaemorrhagiae* is the type species of *Leptospira* (however, an effort is being made to make *L. interrogans* the type species).

  **L. icteroi'des,** a species of organisms morphologically resembling *L. icterohaemorrhagiae*, but somewhat shorter, found in certain cases of yellow fever in America, although not in Africa, and at one time thought to be the cause of that disease.

  **L. inter'rogans,** a species containing parasitic organisms (those formerly placed in *L. icterohaemorrhagiae*) and saprophytic organisms (those formerly placed in *L. biflexa*). This species contains more than a hundred named serotypes. Although *L. icterohaemorrhagiae* is presently the type species of *Leptospira*, an effort is under way to make *L. interrogans* the type species; all leptospires would then belong to a single species, *L. interrogans.*

**lep'tospire.** Common name for any organism belonging to the genus *Leptospira.*

**leptospirosis** (lep-to-spi-ro'sis). Infection with some species of *Leptospira;* see also canicola *fever;* swineherd's *disease;* Weil's *disease.*

**leptospiruria** (lep'to-spi-ru'rī-ah). The presence of organisms of the genus *Leptospira* in the urine, as a result of leptospiras in the renal tubules.

**leptotene** (lep'to-tēn) [ lepto- + G. *tainia*, band, tape ]. Leptonema; early stage of prophase in meiosis in which the chromosomes contract and become visible as long filaments well separated from each other.

**leptothricosis** (lep'to-thrī-ko'sis). An obsolete term for any disease caused by a species of the genus *Leptothrix*. The generic name is no longer valid, and organisms formerly called *Leptothrix* would now probably be classified as actinomycetes, *Nocardia*, or *Corynebacteria.*

  **l. conjuncti'vae.** Parinaud's *conjunctivitis.*

**Leptotrichia** (lep-to-trik'ī-ah) [ lepto- + G. *thrix*, hair ]. A genus of anaerobic, nonmotile bacteria containing Gram-negative, straight or slightly curved rods, 5 to 15 μm in length, with one or both ends rounded, often pointed. Granules are distributed evenly along the long axis, and one or more large granules may localize near the end of the cell. Branched or clubbed forms do not occur. Two or more cells join together and form septate filaments of varying length; in older cultures filaments up to 200 μm may form and twist around each other; large, coccoid bodies may be found within a filament as a cell lyses. Carbon dioxide is essential for optimal growth. Lactic acid is produced from glucose. These organisms occur in the oral cavity of man. The type species is *L. buccalis.*

  **L. bucca'lis,** a species found in the human mouth. It is the type species of the genus *L.*

**lerema** (lĕ-re'mah). Leresis.

**leresis** (lĕ-re'sis) [ G. *lērēsis*, silly talk ]. Lerema; mental weakness marked by garrulity, especially of the aged.

**Leri** (luh-re'), André, French orthopaedic surgeon, 1875–1930. See L.'s *pleonosteosis, sign,* L.-Weill *syndrome.*

**Leriche** (lĕ-rēsh), René, French surgeon, 1879–1955. See L.'s *operation, syndrome.*

**Lermoyez** (ler-moy'āz), Marcel, French otolaryngologist, 1858–1929. See L.'s *syndrome.*

**Leroy,** Jules G. See L.'s *disease.*

**lesbian** (lez'bī-an). 1. One who practices lesbianism; a female homosexual. 2. Pertaining to or practicing lesbianism.

**lesbianism** (lez'bī-an-izm) [ G. *lesbios*, relating to the island of Lesbos ]. Homosexual practices between women. Also called lesbian love; amor lesbicus; female homosexuality; sapphism; tribadism.

**Lesch,** M., U. S. pediatrician, *1939. See L.-Nyhan *syndrome.*

**Leser,** Edmund, German surgeon, 1828–1916. See L.-Trélat *sign.*

**lesion** (le'zhun) [ L. *laedo,* pp. *laesus,* to injure ]. 1. A wound or injury. 2. A more or less circumscribed pathologic change in the tissues. 3. One of the individual points or patches of a multifocal disease.

**Baehr-Lohlein l.,** Lohlein-Baehr l.

**benign lymphoepithelial l.,** adenolymphoma; benign tumor-like masses of lymphoid tissue in the parotid gland, containing scattered small, mainly solid islands of epithelial cells. Sometimes called lymphoepithelioma, but not to be confused with malignant lymphoepitheliomas that arise in the tonsils.

**Bracht-Wachter l.,** a focal collection of lymphocytes and mononuclear cells within the myocardium in bacterial endocarditis.

**caviar l.,** a dilated vein or varicule existing in the venous collecting system under the tongue.

**coin l.'s of lungs,** term given to solitary round, circumscribed shadows found in the lungs in routine x-ray examinations; the subjects at the time are apparently healthy. The l.'s are for the most part tuberculous, but in a fair proportion are carcinomatous; others are cysts, infarcts, or vascular anomalies.

**Councilman's l.,** Councilman *body.*

**Duret's l.,** a cerebral hemorrhage in the neighborhood of the fourth ventricle.

**Ghon's primary l.,** Ghon's *tubercle.*

**gross l.,** one plainly visible to the naked eye.

**Janeway l.,** a small erythematous or hemorrhagic l. seen in some cases of bacterial endocarditis, usually on the palm or sole.

**Lohlein-Baehr l.,** focal embolic glomerulonephritis occurring in bacterial endocarditis.

**precancerous l.,** a noncancerous l. associated with an unusually high incidence of cancer at that site; for example, keratosis senilis.

**ring-wall l.,** a small ring hemorrhage in the brain that stimulates proliferation of a glial ring.

**supranuclear l.,** injury to cerebral (corticonuclear) fibers between the cerebral cortex and brainstem or spinal motor nerve nucleus; it produces an upper motor neuron l.

**wire-loop l.,** thickening of the basement membrane, with fibrinoid staining, of scattered peripheral capillaries in renal glomeruli; characteristic of renal involvement in systemic lupus erythematosus; the appearance of an affected capillary wall resembles a loop used in microbiology.

**Lesser's triangle.** See under triangle.

**Less'haft,** Pyotr F., Russian physician, 1839–1909. See L.'s *triangle.*

**le'thal** [ L. *letalis;* fr. *letum,* death ]. Fatal; mortal; causing death.

**lethal'ity.** Mortality.

**lethargy** (leth'ar-ji) [ G. *lēthargis,* drowsiness ]. A state of deep and prolonged unconsciousness, resembling profound slumber, from which the person can be aroused but into which he immediately relapses. See also consciousness.

**induced l.,** hypnosis.

**le'the** [ G. *lēthē,* forgetfulness ]. Loss of memory; amnesia.

**le'theral** [ G. *lēthē,* forgetfulness ]. Pertaining to amnesia.

**Letterer,** Erich, German pathologist, *1895. See L.-Siwe *disease.*

**Leu.** Symbol for leucine radical.

**leuc-, leuco-** [ G. *leukos,* white ]. For terms beginning thus and not found here, see leuk-, leuko-.

**leucin** (lu'sin). Leukin.

**leucine** (lu'sin). $(CH_3)_2CHCH_2CH(NH_2)COOH$; α-amino-γ-methylvaleric acid; one of the amino acids of proteins; an essential amino acid.

**leucine aminopeptidase.** Aminopeptidase (cytosol).

**[4-leucine] oxytocin.** A synthetic analogue of oxytocin that enhances urinary volume and the renal excretion of sodium, potassium, and chloride ions; it can also reverse the enhanced reabsorption of free water and the antidiuresis produced by arginine vasopressin.

**leucinosis** (lu'si-no'sis). A condition in which there is an abnormally large proportion of leucine in the tissues and body fluids.

**leucinuria** (lu'si-nu'ri-ah). The excretion of leucine in the urine.

**leucism** (lu'sizm) [ G. *leukos,* white ]. A form of incomplete albinism in which nystagmus is absent and the irides are blue.

**leucitis** (lu-si'tis). Scleritis.

**Leucocytozoon** (lu'ko-si'to-zo'on) [ G. *leukos,* white, + *kytos,* cell, + *zōon,* animal ]. *Leukocytozoon;* a genus of sporozoan parasites (family Plasmodiidae, suborder Haemosporina) that attack the immature red blood cells of birds, and are capable of causing acute outbreaks of disease, particularly in turkeys and ducks; vectors are *Simulium* and *Culicoides.*

**L. marchouxi,** a species of unknown pathogenicity, but fairly common in wild doves and pigeons.

**L. sabraze'si,** a cause of leucocytozoonosis of chickens, particularly in Indochina, Malaya, India, Sumatra, and Java.

**L. simon'di,** causes disease in domestic and wild ducks, geese, and related waterfowl in northern United States and Canada; it is severely pathogenic, especially in young birds.

**L. smith'i,** causes disease in domestic turkeys.

**leucocytozoonosis.** Leukocytozoonosis; infection of ducks, turkeys, chickens, pigeons and doves with species of *Leucocytozoon.* The disease is most acute and damaging in young turkeys and ducks, and characterized by enlargement of the spleen and liver, anemia, listlessness, weakness and frequently death.

**leucohar'mine.** Harmine.

**leucoline.** Quinoline.

**leucomycin.** Kitasamycin; antibiotic substance produced by *Streptomyces kitasatoensis;* antimicrobial agent.

**Leuconostoc** (lu-kō-nos'tok) [ G. *leukos,* white, + *nostoc,* a genus of algae (a word coined by Paracelsus) ]. A genus of microaerophilic to facultatively anaerobic bacteria (family Lactobacillaceae) containing Gram-positive, spherical cells which may, under certain conditions, lengthen and become pointed and even form rods. Lactic and acetic acids are produced by these organisms. They are found in plant juices and in milk. The type species is *L. mesen'eroides.*

**L. citrovorum,** a species found in milk and dairy products; growth of these organisms is stimulated by a hemopoietic factor resembling folic acid.

**L. mesenteroi'des,** a species found in fermenting vegetables and other plant materials and in prepared meat products; it is an active slime (dextran) producer, the dextran commonly used as a plasma expander. It is the type species of the genus *L.*

**leucopterin** (lu-kop'ter-in) [ G. *leukos,* white, + *pteron,* a wing ]. 2-Amino-4,6,7-trihydroxypteridine.

**leucovorin** (lu'ko-vo'rin). Folinic acid.

**l. calcium,** calcium folinate; the calcium salt of leucovorin (*i.e.,* folinic acid); for pharmacologic uses, see folinic acid.

**Leudet** (lĕ-da'), Théodor E., French physician, 1825–1887. See L.'s *tinnitus.*

**leuk-.** See leuko-.

**leukanemia** (lu'kă-ne'mi-ah) [leukemia + anemia]. A term (suggested by von Leube) for a rapidly progressive disorder in which the circulating blood manifested changes that closely resembled those of pernicious anemia and myelocytic leukemia (in combination); some observers think that such changes could result from a maturation defect in the precursor of the cells of the erythroid and myeloid series. L. seems to be a rarity; in most instances where pernicious anemia and leukemia are said to be associated, the patient probably has (1) true leukemia, with advanced anemia, or (2) pernicious anemia, with a leukemoid reaction.

**leukapheresis** (lu'kă-fĕ-re'sis) [leuko- + G. *aphairesis,* a withdrawal ]. A procedure, analogous to plasmapheresis, in which leukocytes are removed from the withdrawn blood and the remainder is retransfused into the donor.

**leukasmus** (lu-kaz'mus) [ G. *leukasmos,* a growing white ]. Vitiligo.

**leukemia** (lu-ke'mĭ-ah) [ leuko- + G. *haima*, blood ]. Progressive proliferation of abnormal leukocytes found in hemopoietic tissues, other organs, and usually in the blood in increased numbers. L. is classified by the dominant cell type, and by duration from onset to death. This occurs in *acute l.* within a few months in most cases, and is associated with symptoms that suggest acute infection, with severe anemia, hemorrhages, and slight enlargement of lymph nodes or the spleen. The duration of *chronic l.* exceeds one year, with a gradual onset of symptoms of anemia or marked enlargement of spleen, liver, or lymph nodes.

**acute promyelocytic l.,** l. presenting as a severe bleeding disorder, with infiltration of the bone marrow by abnormal promyelocytes and myelocytes, a low plasma fibrinogen, and defective coagulation.

**aleukemic l.,** subleukemic l.

**aleukocythemic l.,** aleukemic l.

**basophilic l.,** mast cell l.; basophilocytic l.; a form of myelocytic l. in which there are unusually great numbers of basophilic granulocytes in the tissues and circulating blood; in some instances, the immature and mature basophilic forms may represent from 40 to 80 per cent of the total numbers of white blood cells.

**l. cutis,** lymphoderma perniciosa; yellow-brown, red, blue-red, or purple, sometimes nodular lesions associated with diffuse infiltrations or massive accumulations of leukemic cells in the skin; the involvement may be diffuse and generalized, *i.e.,* so-called universal l. cutis, or it may be localized, in which instance the skin of the face is the site of predilection.

**embryonal l.,** stem cell l.

**eosinophilic l., eosinophilocytic l.,** a form of myelocytic l. in which there are conspicuous numbers of eosinophilic granulocytes in the tissues and circulating blood, or in which such cells are predominant; in chronic disease of this type, the total white blood cell count may be as high as 200,000 to 250,000 per cu. mm., with as many as 80 or 90 per cent being eosinophils, chiefly adult forms.

**l. of fowls,** avian *leukosis.*

**granulocytic l.,** myelocytic, myeloid, or myelogenous l.; a form of l. characterized by (1) an uncontrolled proliferation of myelopoietic cells in the bone marrow and in extramedullary sites, and (2) the presence of large numbers of immature and mature granulocytic forms in various tissues (and organs) and in the circulating blood; the total count may range from 1000 (aleukemic variety) to several hundred thousand per cu. mm. The predominant cell is usually of the neutrophilic series, but, in a few instances, eosinophilic or basophilic granulocytes, or even megakaryocytes, may represent the chief form. Early in granulocytic l., the circulating blood may contain excessive numbers of all of the granulocytic forms.

**hairy cell l.,** l. possibly of reticulum cells having numerous fine projections from the cell surface.

**high cell count l.,** a general descriptive term sometimes used to emphasize the occurrence of a greatly increased number of leukocytes in various forms of l., as contrasted with leukemic disease in which the white blood cell count is within normal range or only slightly increased (*i.e.,* aleukemic or subleukemic l.). The term is likely to be used especially in instances where aleukemic or subleukemic l. becomes transformed and the classic findings of l. are observed.

**histiocytic l.,** acute monocytic l.

**hypocytic l.,** subleukemic l.

**leukemic l.,** a redundant term sometimes used to emphasize the occurrence of abundant numbers of leukemic cells in the circulating blood; this classic form of l. is usually termed simply *leukemia.* See also aleukemic l. and subleukemic l.

**leukopenic l.,** a form of lymphocytic, myelocytic, or monocytic l. in which the total number of white blood cells in the circulating blood is in the normal range, or may be diminished to various levels that are significantly less than normal. See also aleukemic and subleukemic l.

**li'enomyelog'enous l.,** splenomyelogenous l.

**lymphatic l.,** lymphocytic l.

**lymphoblastic l.,** acute lymphocytic l. in which the abnormal cells are chiefly (or almost totally) blast forms of the lymphocytic series, or in which unusually large numbers of the immature forms occur in association with adult lymphocytes.

**lymphocytic l.,** lymphoid l.; lymphatic l.; a variety of l. characterized by (1) an uncontrolled proliferation and conspicuous enlargement of lymphoid tissue in various sites (*e.g.,* lymph nodes, spleen, bone marrow, lungs, and so on), and (2) the occurrence of increased numbers of cells of the lymphocytic series in the circulating blood and in various tissues and organs. In chronic disease, the cells are adult lymphocytes, whereas conspicuous numbers of lymphoblasts are observed in the more acute syndromes.

**lymphoid l.,** lymphocytic l.

**lymphosarcoma cell l., lymphosarcomatous l.,** undesirable synonyms for lymphocytic l.

**Mallory l.,** old term for myelocytic l. that is thought to result from chronic poisoning with tar or benzol.

**mast cell l.,** basophilic l.

**mature cell l.,** chronic granulocytic l.

**med'ullary l.,** old term for myelocytic l.

**megakaryocytic l.,** an unusual form of myelopoietic disease that is characterized by (1) a seemingly uncontrolled proliferation of megakaryocytes in the bone marrow, and sometimes by (2) the presence of a considerable number of megakaryocytes in the circulating blood. When bone marrow is examined at various intervals in some instances of chronic myelocytic l., the proliferation of megakaryocytes is more prominent than that of the granulocytes; at such times, the circulating blood may contain megakaryocytes or fragments of megakaryocytic nuclei and cytoplasm, or both, amounting to as much as 5 or 6 per cent of the total number of leukocytes.

**mi'cromyeloblas'tic l.,** a form of myelocytic l. in which relatively large proportions of micromyeloblasts are found in the circulating blood and in bone marrow and other tissues.

**mixed l., mixed cell l.,** terms infrequently used as designations for myelocytic l., thereby emphasizing the occurrence of different types of cells in the myeloid series (*i.e.,* neutrophilic, eosinophilic, and basophilic granulocytes), in contrast to the comparatively monotonous pattern observed in lymphocytic and monocytic l.

**monocyt'ic l.,** a form of l. characterized by large numbers of cells that can be definitely identified as monocytes, in addition to larger, apparently related cells formed from the uncontrolled proliferation of the reticuloendothelial tissue. L. in which these two types of cells seem to "overrun" the usual sites of the reticuloendothelial system, and occur in conspicuous numbers in the circulating blood, is frequently referred to as the Schilling type of monocytic l., or sometimes as true monocytic l. The disease runs an acute or subacute course in older persons, and is characterized by swelling of gums, oral ulceration, bleeding in skin or mucous membranes, secondary infection, and splenomegaly.

**myeloblas'tic l.,** a form of myelocytic l. in which there are large numbers of myeloblasts in various tissues (and organs) and in the circulating blood; the immature forms may amount to 30 to 60 per cent (or even a greater proportion) of the increased total number of white blood cells. Used as a synonym for acute granulocytic l., although myeloblastic l. may be a terminal event in the course of chronic granulocytic l.

**myelocyt'ic l.,** granulocytic l.

**myelogen'ic l., myelog'enous l.,** granulocytic l.

**myeloid l.,** granulocytic l.

**myelomonocyt'ic l.,** Naegeli type of monocytic l.; a variant of granulocytic l. with monocytosis in the peripheral blood.

**Naegeli type of monocytic l.,** myelomonocytic l.

**neutrophilic l.,** an unusual form of chronic granulocytic l. in which the greatly increased number of leukocytes in the circulating blood are mature polymorphonuclear neutrophils, with virtually no young or immature granulocytes being observed.

**plasma cell l.,** an unusual disease characterized by leukocytosis and other signs and symptoms that are suggestive of l., in association with (1) diffuse infiltrations and aggregates of plasma cells in the spleen, liver, bone marrow, and lymph nodes, and (2) the presence of considerable numbers of plasma cells in the circulating blood; the total number of leukocytes in the latter may range from normal levels to 80,000 or 90,000 per cu. mm., and 5 to 90 per cent may be plasma cells. Multiple myelomas are observed in some examples of plasma cell l., but discrete nodules are not formed in bone. Although there are other clinicopathologic differences in the two conditions, they may be phases of the same basic process.

**polymorphocyt′ic l.,** granulocytic l., especially any variety in which the predominant cells are mature, segmented granulocytes.

**Rieder cell l.,** a special form of acute granulocytic l. in which the affected tissues and the circulating blood contain relatively large numbers of atypical myeloblasts (*i.e.,* Rieder cells) that have (1) the usual, faintly granular, immature type of cytoplasm, and (2) a bizarre, comparatively mature nucleus with several wide and deep indentations (suggestive of lobulation).

**Schilling type of monocytic l.,** see monocytic l.

**splenic l.,** a form of l. in which there is an unusually great degree of enlargement of the spleen, as observed frequently in chronic granulocytic l.

**splenomed′ullary l.,** splenomyelogenous l.

**splenomyelog′enous l.,** splenomedullary l.; granulocytic l. associated with conspicuous enlargement of the spleen.

**stem cell l.,** embryonal l.; a form of l. in which the abnormal cells are thought to be the precursors of lymphoblasts, myeloblasts, or monoblasts.

**subleukemic l.,** aleukemic l.; a form of l. in which the characteristic cells are observed in the circulating blood (1) fairly constantly in relatively small numbers, *i.e.,* the total white blood cell count is likely to be less than 10,000 or 12,000 per cu. mm., or (2) irregularly or sporadically in similarly small numbers, or possibly slightly greater proportions.

**symptomat′ic l.,** see temporary l.

**temporary l.,** an undesirable term sometimes used with reference to an unusual degree of leukocytosis, which is not a leukemic condition; also termed symptomatic l.

**leukemic** (lu-ke′mik). Pertaining to, or having the characteristics of, any form of leukemia.

**leukemid** (lu-kem′id) [ leuko- + G. *haima,* blood, + suffix *id* (1), *q.v.* ]. Any nonspecific type of cutaneous lesion that (1) is frequently associated with leukemia (as a feature of the syndrome), but (2) is not a localized accumulation of leukemic cells, and (3) may be observed in other conditions. Petechiae, vesicles, wheals, bullae, hematomas, pustules, papules, and the lesions of exfoliative dermatitis and herpes zoster are examples of l.'s.

**leukemogen** (lu-ke′mo-jen). Any compound, substance, or matter (*e.g.,* benzol, ionizing radiation, and so on) that is known to be (or seems to be) a causal factor in the occurrence of leukemia.

**leukemogenesis** (lu-ke′mo-jen′ē-sis) [ leukemia + G. *genesis,* production ]. The causation (or induction), development, and progression of a leukemic disease.

**leukemogenic** (lu-ke′mo-jen′ik). Pertaining to the causation, induction, and development of leukemia; manifesting the ability to cause leukemia.

**leukemoid** (lu-ke′moyd) [ leukemia + G. *eidos,* resemblance ]. Resembling leukemia in various signs and symptoms, especially with reference to changes in the circulating blood. See also *leukemoid reaction.*

**leukemoid reaction.** A moderate, advanced, or sometimes extreme degree of leukocytosis in the circulating blood, closely similar or possibly identical to that occurring in various forms of leukemia, but not the result of leukemic disease; usually, there is a disproportionate increase in the number of forms (including immature stages) in one series of leukocytes, and various examples of myelocytic, lymphocytic, monocytic, or plasmocytic l. r. may be also indistinguishable from leukocytosis that is associated with certain forms of leukemia. L. r.'s are sometimes observed as a feature of: (1) infectious disease caused by certain bacteria and other biologic agents, *e.g.,* tuberculosis, diphtheria, chickenpox, and others; (2) intoxication of various types, *e.g.,* eclampsia, serious burns, mustard gas poisoning, and others; (3) malignant neoplasms, *e.g.,* carcinoma of the colon or lung, or kidney, and others; (4) acute hemorrhage or hemolysis.

**lymphocytic l. r.,** leukocytosis of varying degrees, with adult lymphocytes and immature forms amounting to 40 per cent (or more) of the total number of white blood cells in the circulating blood; may be observed in association with pertussis, infectious mononucleosis, gonorrhea, chickenpox, and sarcoidosis.

**monocytic l. r.,** leukocytosis of varying degrees, *e.g.,* 30,000 to 40,000 per cu. mm., with adult monocytes and immature forms amounting to 30 per cent (or more) of the total number of white blood cells in the circulating blood; may be observed in association with tuberculosis, especially the first infection, miliary type.

**myelocytic l. r.,** leukocytosis of at least moderate degrees, *e.g.,* 50,000 or more per cu. mm., with a few immature forms, *e.g.,* 1 or 2 per cent myelocytes, but chiefly mature polymorphonuclear leukocytes in the circulating blood; may be observed in association with tuberculosis, chronic osteomyelitis, various types of empyema, malaria, pneumococcal pneumonia, meningococcal meningitis, Hodgkin's disease, and metastases of carcinoma in the bone marrow.

**plasmocytic l. r.,** the presence of unusual numbers of plasma cells, *i.e.,* plasmocytosis, in the bone marrow; may be observed in association with sarcoidosis, rheumatoid arthritis, cirrhosis, Hodgkin's disease, and certain of the socalled collagen diseases.

**leukethiope** (lu-ke′-thĭ-ōp) [ leuko- + *Aithiops,* an Ethiopian ]. Leukoethiope; an albino of the Negro race.

**leukin.** Leucin; endolysin; a thermostable, bactericidal substance extracted from leukocytes.

**leuko-, leuk-** (lu′ko-) [ G. *leukos,* white ]. Combining forms meaning white. For some words beginning thus, see those beginning with leuc- and leuco-.

**leukoagglutinin** (lu′ko-ă-glu′tĭ-nin). An antibody that agglutinates white blood cells.

**leukobilin** (lu′ko-bil′in) [ leuko- L. *bilis,* bile ]. An older term designating the relatively clear, almost colorless, viscid fluid that occurs in the gallbladder or the intestines, or both, as a result of obstruction of the bile ducts in various sites; l., or so-called white bile, is actually the secretion of the mucous membrane, without the usual color resulting from bile pigments.

**leukoblast** (lu′ko-blast) [ leuko- + G. *blastos,* germ ]. An immature white blood cell that is transitional between the lymphoidocyte (or the myeloblast of Naegeli and Downey) and the promyelocyte; the cytoplasm is polychromatophilic or slightly acidophilic and, as compared with the lymphoidocyte, the nuclear network of chromatin is thicker and the nucleoli less distinct.

**granular l.,** promyelocyte.

**leukoblastosis** (lu′ko-blas-to′sis). A general term for the abnormal proliferation of leukocytes, especially that occurring in myelocytic and lymphocytic leukemia.

**leukochloroma** (lu′ko-klo-ro′mah) [ leuko- + G. *chlorōs,* green, + suffix *-oma,* tumor ]. See myelocytomatosis.

**leukocidin** (lu-kos′ĭ-din, lu′ko-si′din) [ leukocyte + L. *caedo,* to kill ]. A heat-labile substance that is elaborated by many strains of *Staphylococcus aureus, Streptococcus pyogenes,* and pneumococci and manifests a destructive action on leukocytes, with or without lysis of the cells.

**leukoco′ria.** Leukokoria.

**leu′kocytac′tic.** Leukocytotactic.

**leukocy′tal.** Leukocytic.

**leu′kocytax′ia.** Leukocytotaxia.

**leu′kocytax′is.** Leukocytotaxia.

**leukocyte** (lu′ko-sit) [ leuko- + G. *kytos,* cell ]. Any one of the white blood cells. They are formed in the myelopoietic, lymphoid, and reticular portions of the reticuloendothelial system in various parts of the body, and are normally present in those sites and in the circulating blood (rarely in other tissues). Under various abnormal conditions, the total numbers or proportions, or both, may be characteristically increased, decreased, or not altered, and they may be present in other tissues and organs. L.'s represent three lines of development from primitive elements, *i.e.,* the myeloid, lymphoid, and monocytic series. On the basis of features observed with various methods of staining with polychromatic dyes (*e.g.,* Wright's stain, and others), cells of the myeloid series are frequently termed granular l.'s, or granulocytes; cells of the lymphoid and monocytic series also have granules in the cytoplasm but, owing to their tiny, inconspicuous size and different properties (frequently not clearly visualized with routine methods), lymphocytes and monocytes are sometimes termed nongranular or agranular l.'s. The granulocytes, or cells of the myeloid series, are commonly known as polymorphonuclear l.'s (also polynuclear or multinuclear l.'s), inasmuch as the mature nucleus is divided into two to five rounded or ovoid lobes that are connected with thin strands or small bands of chromatin. The granulocytes consist of three distinct types, *i.e.*, neutrophils, eosinophils, and basophils, named on the basis of the staining reactions of the cytoplasmic granules. Lymphocytes occur as two, somewhat arbitrary, normal varieties, *i.e.*, small and large lymphocytes; the former represent the ordinary forms and are conspicuously more numerous in the circulating blood and normal lymphoid tissue; the large forms may be found in normal circulating blood, but are more easily observed in lymphoid tissue. The small lymphocytes have nuclei that are deeply or densely stained (the chromatin is coarse and bulky) and almost fill the cells, with only a slight rim of cytoplasm around the nuclei; the large lymphocytes have nuclei that are approximately the same size as, or only slightly larger than, those of the small forms, but there is a broader, easily visualized band of cytoplasm around the nuclei. Monocytes are usually larger than the other l.'s, and are characterized by a relatively abundant, slightly opaque, gray or "muddy" blue cytoplasm that contains myriads of extremely fine granules (somewhat resembling tiny particles of dust). The nuclei of monocytes are usually large and centrally placed and, even when eccentrically located, are completely surrounded by at least a small band of cytoplasm. They are usually indented, reniform, or shaped similarly to a horseshoe, but are sometimes rounded or ovoid.

**acidophilic l.,** eosinophilic l.

**agranular l.,** nongranular l.

**alpha l.,** one that is lysed during the coagulation of blood.

**basophil'ic l.,** basophil; basocyte; basophilocyte; mast l.; a polymorphonuclear l. characterized by many large, coarse, metachromatic granules that are dark purple or blue-black when treated with Wright's or similar stains. The granules usually fill the cytoplasm and may almost mask the nucleus; on the other hand, they are soluble in water and are frequently dissolved during the staining and washing of the blood film. Basophils are unique in that they usually do not occur in increased numbers as the result of acute infectious disease, and their phagocytic qualities are probably not significant. Heparin is formed by basophils, and this substance is effective in preventing coagulation of blood.

**beta l.,** any l. that is not lysed during the coagulation of blood.

**cystinotic l.,** a l. having an enhanced content of cystine; found in patients with disorders characterized by the storage of cystine; within the l., the cystine, largely in noncrystalline form, is associated with dense lysosomal particles.

**endothe'lial l.,** old term for a monocyte, a type of l. thought to be derived from reticuloendothelial tissue; see also monocyte, under leukocyte (above). Sometimes also termed endotheliocyte.

**eosinophil'ic l.,** eosinophil; eosinocyte; acidocyte; acidophilic l.; oxyphilic l.; oxyphil (2); a polymorphonuclear l. characterized by many, large or prominent, refractile, cytoplasmic granules that are fairly uniform in size and bright yellow-red or orange when treated with Wright's or similar stains; the nuclei are usually larger than those of neutrophils, do not stain as deeply, and characteristically have two lobes (a third lobe is sometimes interposed on the connecting strand of chromatin).

**filament polymorphonuclear l.,** any mature polymorphonuclear l., especially a neutrophilic l., in which the lobes of the nucleus are interconnected with a thin strand or filament of chromatin.

**granular l.,** granulocyte; any one of the polymorphonuclear l.'s especially a neutrophilic l. See also basophilic and eosinophilic l.

**heterophil l.,** a type of l. that includes neutrophils of man and equivalent cells of other species.

**hy'aline l.,** old term for a monocyte, and for a mononuclear macrophage in various lesions.

**motile l.,** any l. that manifests active ameboid movement, especially a mature granulocytic l. (eosinophils are less motile than neutrophils or basophils); monocytes manifest a slow, but persistent, wavelike movement.

**neutrophil'ic l.,** neutrophilic granulocyte; the most frequent of the polymorphonuclear l.'s, and also the most active phagocyte among the various types of white blood cells; when treated with Wright's stain (or similar preparations), the fairly abundant cytoplasm is faintly pink, and numerous tiny, slightly refractile, relatively bright pink or violet-pink, diffusely scattered granules are recognizable in the cytoplasm; the deeply stained blue or purple-blue nucleus is sharply distinguished from the cytoplasm and is distinctly lobated, with thin strands of chromatin connecting the three to five lobes.

**nonfilament polymorphonuclear l.,** a neutrophil, basophil, or eosinophil that is not completely matured, *i.e.*, the lobes of the nuclei remain connected with bands of chromatin, in contrast to the thin strands observed in mature cells.

**nongranular l.,** agranular l.; a general, nonspecific term frequently used with reference to lymphocytes, monocytes, and plasma cells; although the cytoplasm of a lymphocyte or monocyte contains tiny granules, it is "nongranular" in comparison with that of a neutrophil, basophil, or eosinophil. See also l.

**nonmotile l.,** a term sometimes used with reference to lymphocytes, monocytes, and plasma cells; although such forms actually have some degree of motility, they are "nonmotile" in comparison with the actively ameboid, neutrophilic, basophilic, and eosinophilic l.'s.

**oxyphilic l.,** eosinophilic l.

**polymorphonuclear l.,** common term for granulocyte or granulocytic l.; polynuclear l.; multinuclear l.; the term includes basophilic, eosinophilic, and neutrophilic l.'s, but is usually used especially with reference to the neutrophilic l.'s.

**segmented l.,** any mature polymorphonuclear l., especially a neutrophilic l.

**transitional l.,** old term for a monocyte.

**Türk's l.,** Türk *cell.*

**leukocythemia** (lu-ko-si-the′mĭ-ah) [ leukocyte + G. *haima*, blood ]. An undesirable term for leukemia.

**leukocytic** (lu′ko-sit′ik). Leukocytal; pertaining to or characterized by leukocytes.

**leukocytoblast** (lu-ko-si′to-blast) [ leukocyte + G. *blastos*, germ ]. A nonspecific term for any immature cell from which a leukocyte develops, including lymphoblast, myeloblast, and the like.

**leukocytogenesis** (lu′ko-si′to-jen′e-sis) [ leukocyte + G. *genesis*, production ]. The formation and development of leukocytes.

**leukocytoid** (lu′ko-si-toyd) [ leukocyte + G. *eidos*, resemblance ]. Resembling a leukocyte.

**leu′kocytol′ysin.** Any substance (including lytic antibody) that causes dissolution of leukocytes.

**leukocytolysis** (lu′ko-si-tol′ĭ-sis) [ leukocyte + G. *lysis*, dissolution ]. Dissolution or lysis of leukocytes.

**leukocytolytic** (lu′ko-si-to-lit′ik). Pertaining to, causing, or manifesting leukocytolysis.

**leukocytoma** (lu′ko-si-to′mah) [ leukocyte + G. suffix *-oma*, tumor ]. A fairly well circumscribed, nodular, dense accumulation of leukocytes.

**leukocytometer** (lu′ko-si-tom′e-ter) [ leukocyte + G. *metron*, measure ]. A standarized glass slide that is suitably ruled for counting the leukocytes in a measured volume of accurately diluted blood (or other specimens).

**leukocytopenia** (lu′ko-si-to-pe′nĭ-ah). Leukopenia.

**leukocytoplania** (lu′ko-si-to-pla′nĭ-ah) [ leukocyte + G. *planē*, a wandering ]. The movement of leukocytes from the lumens of blood vessels, through serous membranes, or in the tissues.

**leukocytopoiesis** (lu′ko-si-to-poy-e′sis) [ leukocyte + G. *poiēsis*, a making ]. The formation and development of various types of white blood cells.

**leukocytosis** (lu-ko-si-to′sis) [ leukocyte + G. suffix *-osis*, condition ]. An abnormally large number of leukocytes, as observed in acute infections. A white blood cell count of 10,000 or more per cu. mm. usually indicates l. Most examples of l. represent a disproportionate increase in the number of cells in the neutrophilic series, and the term is frequently used synonymously with the designation neutrophilia. L. of 15,000 to 25,000 per cu. mm. is frequently observed in various pathologic conditions, and values as high as 40,000 are not unusual. Occasionally, as in some examples of leukemoid reactions, white blood cell counts may range up to 100,000 per cu. mm.

**absolute l.,** an actual increase in the total number of leukocytes in the circulating blood, as distinguished from a relative increase (such as that observed in dehydration).

**ag'onal l.,** terminal l.

**basophilic l.,** basocytosis; the presence of an abnormally large number of basophilic granulocytes in the blood.

**digestive l.,** l. occurring normally after ingestion of food.

**distribution l.,** an abnormally large proportion of one or more types of leukocytes.

**emotional l.,** an abnormally high white blood cell count that is thought to be related only to an emotional disturbance.

**eosinophilic l.,** eosinophilia; a form of relative leukocytosis in which the greatest proportionate increase is in the eosinophils.

**lymphocytic l.,** lymphocytosis.

**monocytic l.,** monocytosis.

**neutrophilic l.,** neutrophilia; see also l. above.

**l. of the newborn,** an apparently "physiologic" l. usually observed in newborn infants; the white blood cell counts are usually greater than 10,000 per cu. mm., and sometimes range to 45,000 per cu. mm., resulting chiefly from increased numbers of neutrophils (especially single and bilobed forms). On the third or fourth day of life, the count generally decreases rapidly, and then fluctuates for several days; beginning about the fourth week of life, a relative lymphocytosis is observed, and this normally continues for a few years.

**physiologic l.,** any form of l. that is associated with apparently normal situations, i.e., one that is not directly related to a pathologic condition. For example, the total number of white blood cells may be temporarily increased during a single day, or from day to day, as well as in the newborn period, during childhood, after strenuous exercise, during attacks of paroxysmal tachycardia, and in association with various other situations.

**relative l.,** an increased proportion of one or more types of leukocytes in the circulating blood, without an actual increase in the total number of white blood cells. For example, a relative l. of all types may be observed in dehydration, a relative lymphocytic l. is normal in childhood, a relative eosinophilic l. is frequently associated with certain parasitologic diseases, and so on.

**terminal l.,** agonal l.; one that occurs in a person just prior to death, especially in one who has a "slow death."

**leukocytotactic** (lu'ko-si-to-tak'tik). Leukocytactic; leukotactic; pertaining to, characterized by, or causing leukocytotaxia.

**leukocytotaxia** (lu-ko-si-to-tak'si-ah) [ leukocyte + G. taxis, arrangement ]. Leukocytaxia; leukotaxia. 1. The active ameboid movement of leukocytes, especially the neutrophilic granulocytes, either toward (**positive l.**) or away from (**negative l.**) certain microorganisms as well as various substances frequently formed in inflamed tissue. 2. The property of attracting or repelling leukocytes.

**leukocytotoxin** (lu'ko-si-to-tok'sin) [ leukocyte + G. toxikon, poison ]. Any substance that causes degeneration and necrosis of leukocytes, including leukolysin and leukocidin.

**Leukocytozoon** (lu-ko-si'to-zo'on). Leucocytozoon.

**leukocytozo'ono'sis.** Leucocytozoonosis.

**leukocyturia** (lu'ko-si-tu'ri-ah) [ leukocyte + G. ouron, urine ]. The presence of leukocytes in urine that is recently voided or collected by means of a catheter.

**leukoderm** (lu'ko-derm) [ leuko- + G. derma, skin ]. A member of one of the white races.

**leukoderma** (lu-ko-der'mah). Leukopathia; achromoderma; hypomelanosis; an absence of pigment, partial or total, in the skin.

**acquired l.,** vitiligo.

**l. acquisi'tum centrifu'gum,** circumnevic vitiligo; Sutton's nevus or disease; halo nevus; a usually benign melanotic nevus in which a central brown mole is surrounded by a uniformly depigmented zone.

**congen'ital l.,** albinism.

**syphilitic l.,** collar or necklace of Venus; melanoleukoderma colli; a fading of the roseola of secondary syphilis, leaving reticulated depigmented and hyperpigmented areas located chiefly on the sides of the neck.

**leukodermatous** (lu'ko-der'mă-tus). Relating to or resembling leukoderma.

**leukodont** (lu'ko-dont). A person having leukodontia.

**leukodontia** (lu'ko-don'shi-ah) [ leuko- + G. odous, tooth ]. The condition of having white teeth.

**leu'kodystro'phia.** Leukodystrophy.

**l. cer'ebri progres'siva,** generic term for the familial leukodystrophies or cerebral scleroses, including the diseases of Krabbe, Scholz, Pelizaeus-Merzbacher and others.

**leukodystrophy** (lu'ko-dis'tro-fi) [ leuko- + G. dys, bad, + trophe, nourishment ]. Leukodystrophia; leukoencephalopathy; sclerosis of the white matter; degeneration of the white matter of the brain characterized by demyelination and glial reaction, probably related to defects of lipid metabolism.

**globoid cell l.,** diffuse infantile familial sclerosis.

**metachromatic l.,** sulfatide lipidosis; sulfatidosis; a metabolic disorder characterized by myelin loss, accumulation of metachromatic lipids (galactosphingosulfatides) in white matter of central and peripheral nervous systems, a marked excess of sulfatide in white matter and in urine, progressive paralysis and dementia; autosomal recessive inheritance. See also Greenfield's disease; Scholz' disease.

**leukoencephalitis** (lu'ko-en-sef-ă-li'tis). Encephalitis restricted to the white matter.

**subacute sclerosing l.,** van Bogaert's encephalitis; thought to be a form of inclusion body encephalitis, q.v.

**leukoencephalopathy** (lu'ko-en-sef'ă-lop'ă-thi) [ leuko- + G. enkephalos, brain, + pathos, suffering ]. Leukodystrophy.

**progressive multifocal l.,** a rare, subacute, afebrile disease characterized by areas of demyelinization surrounded by markedly altered neuroglia, including inclusion bodies in glial cells; it occurs usually in individuals with leukemia, lymphoma, or other debilitating diseases, or in those who have been receiving immunosuppressive treatment.

**leukoerythroblastosis** (lu'ko-ĕ-rith'ro-blas-to'sis). The preferred term for myelophthisic, myelopathic, osteosclerotic, or "leukoerythroblastic" anemia, i.e., any anemic condition resulting from space-occupying lesions in the bone marrow. The circulating blood contains (1) several immature cells of the granulocytic series, and also (2) nucleated red blood cells, frequently in numbers that are disproportionately large in relation to the degree of anemia. Inasmuch as the latter may be only slight (or occasionally not recognizable), l. seems to be a more appropriate term for the condition.

**leukoethiope** (lu'ko-e'thi-ōp). Leukethiope.

**leu'kokerato'sis.** Rarely used term for leukoplakia.

**congenital l., oral,** familial white folded dysplasia.

**leukoko'ria** [ leuko- + G. kore, pupil ]. Leukocoria; reflection from a white mass within the eye giving the appearance of a white pupil.

**leukokraurosis** (lu'ko-kraw-ro'sis). Kraurosis vulvae.

**leukolymphosarcoma** (lu'ko-lim'fo-sar-ko'mah). Leukosarcoma.

**leukol'ysin.** Leukocytolysin.

**leukol'ysis.** Leukocytolysis.

**leukolyt'ic.** Leukocytolytic.

**leukoma** (lu-ko'mah) [ G. whiteness, a white spot in the eye, fr. leukos, white ]. 1. Albugo; a dense, opaque, white opacity of the cornea. 2. Old, undesirable term for lymphoma.

**adhe'rent l.,** anterior synechia causing a dense, white cicatrix of the cornea.

**leukomatous** (lu-ko'mă-tus). Pertaining to, characterized by, or afflicted with leukoma.

**leu'kometh'ylene blue.** The reduced and colorless form of methylene blue.

**leukomyelopathy** (lu'ko-mi'ĕ-lop'ă-thi) [ leuko- + G. myelos, marrow, + pathos, suffering ]. Any system disease involving the white substance or conducting tracts of the spinal cord.

**leukon** (lu'kon). Analogous to the erythron of red blood cells; pertains to all types of leukocytes in the circulating blood, as well as the cells and leukopoietic tissues from which they originate.

**leukonecrosis** (lu'ko-ně-kro'sis) [ leuko- + G. *nekrōsis,* deadness ]. White *gangrene.*

**leukonuclein** (lu-ko-nu'kle-in). An acidic nucleoprotein probably formed from nucleohiston that is present in white blood cells and blood platelets; l. seems to augment the coagulation of blood.

**leukonychia** (lu-ko-nik'ĭ-ah) [ leuko- + G. *onyx (onych-),* nail ]. Leukopathia unguis; achromia unguium; canities unguium; the occurrence of white spots or patches under the nails, due to the presence of air bubbles between the nail and its bed. The decoloration may be total or in the form of lines (striate l.) or dots (punctate l.).

**leukopathia, leukopathy** (lu'ko-path'ĭ-ah, lu-kop'ă-thĭ) [ leuko- + G. *pathos,* disease ]. Leukoderma.
   **acquired l.,** vitiligo.
   **congenital l.,** albinism.
   **l. unguis,** leukonychia.

**leukopedesis** (lu-ko-pe-de'sis) [ leuko- + G. *pēdēsis,* a leaping ]. The movement of white blood cells (especially polymorphonuclear leukocytes) through the walls of capillaries and into the tissues.

**leukopenia** (lu'ko-pe'nĭ-ah) [ leuko(cyte) + G. *penia,* poverty ]. Leukocytopenia; the antithesis of leukocytosis; any situation in which the total number of leukocytes in the circulating blood is less than normal, the lower limit of which is generally regarded as 5000 per cu. mm.
   **basophilic l.,** basocytopenia; a decrease in the number of basophilic granulocytes normally present in the circulating blood (difficult to evaluate, owing to the small and variable number normally present).
   **eosinophilic l.,** a decrease in the number of eosinophilic granulocytes normally present in the circulating blood.
   **lymphocytic l.,** lymphopenia.
   **monocytic l.,** monocytopenia.
   **neutrophilic l.,** neutropenia.

**leukope'nic.** Pertaining to leukopenia.

**leukophlegmasia** (lu-ko-fleg-ma'zĭ-ah) [ leuko- + phlegmasia, *q. v.* ]. Lymphatic *edema.*
   **l. do'lens,** *phlegmasia alba dolens.*

**leukoplakia** (lu'ko-pla'kĭ-ah) [ leuko- + G. *plax,* plate ]. A disturbance of keratinization of mucous membrane, variously present as small opalescent patches or as extensive leathery plaques; occasionally ulcerated. Histologically it may exhibit the features of dyskeratosis: disturbance in the orderly maturation of stratified squamous epithelium and nuclear enlargement; it is then regarded as precancerous. Also called smoker's patches or smoker's tongue; tylosis linguae, psoriasis buccalis; psoriasis linguae; ichthyosis linguae.
   **l. vulvae,** leukoplakic vulvitis; an atrophic thickening and keratinization of the vulvar epithelium, often associated with papillary hypertrophy; the name comes from the white patchy appearance of the lesion.

**leukopoiesis** (lu-ko-poy-e'sis) [ leuko- + G. *poiēsis,* a making ]. The formation and development of the various types of white blood cells.

**leukopoietic** (lu-ko-poy-et'ik). Pertaining to or characterized by leukopoiesis, as manifested by portions of the bone marrow and reticuloendothelial and lymphoid tissues, which form (respectively) the granulocytes, monocytes, and lymphocytes.

**leukoprotease** (lu-ko-pro'te-ās). A proteolytic enzyme, formed in an area of inflammation, which causes liquefaction of dead tissue; it is a product of the polynuclear leukocytes.

**leukopsin** (lu-kop'sin) [ leuko- + G. *opsis,* vision ]. Visual white; the exhausted or decolorized rhodopsin.

**leukoriboflavin** (lu'ko-ri'bo-fla'vin). The colorless nonfluorescing dihydro compound formed by the reduction of riboflavin.

**leukorrhagia** (lu-ko-ra'jĭ-ah) [ leuko- + G. *rhēgnymi,* to burst forth ]. Leukorrhea.

**leukorrhea** (lu-ko-re'ah) [ leuko- + G. *rhoia, flow* ]. Blennorrhea; a discharge from the vagina of a white or yellowish, more or less viscid fluid, containing mucus and pus cells.
   **menstrual l.,** an intermittent l. recurring at or just before each menstrual period.

**leukorrheal** (lu-ko-re'al). Relating to or characterized by leukorrhea.

**leukosarcoma** (lu'ko-sar-ko'mah). Sternberg's l.; leukolymphosarcoma; a variant of malignant lymphoma in which abnormal, immature forms of the lymphocytic series are found in large numbers in the circulating blood of a person with lymphosarcoma involving the lymph nodes and various other tissues and organs: leukemia developing in a person with lymphosarcoma.

**leukosarcomatosis** (lu'ko-sar-ko-mă-to'sis). A condition characterized by numerous, widespread nodules or masses of lymphosarcoma, and the presence of similar cells in the circulating blood. See also leukosarcoma.

**leukoscope** (lu'ko-skōp) [ leuko- + G. *skopeō,* to view ]. A device for testing color vision by the mixture of colors to produce white.

**leukosis** (lu-ko'sis). Abnormal proliferation of one or more of the leukopoietic tissues; the term includes myelosis, certain forms of reticuloendotheliosis, and lymphadenosis.
   **avian l.,** fowl l.; a group of conditions (*e.g.,* lymphoid l., erythroid l., myeloid l.) that occur chiefly in chickens and are characterized by an abnormal proliferation of myelopoietic, erythropoietic, or lymphoid tissues; the etiologic agents are a group of closely related leukoviruses and the conditions are transmissable; see also avian leukosis-sarcoma *complex.*
   **fowl l.,** avian l.
   **lymphoid l.,** a form in which there is a conspicuous degree of proliferation of lymphoid tissue in the lymph nodes and various other sites.
   **myeloblas'tic l.,** a form characterized by an unusual proliferation of myelopoietic tissue (chiefly in the bone marrow, but also in other sites), with the formation of abnormally large numbers of myeloblasts.
   **myelocyt'ic l.,** a condition that is similar to myeloblastic l., except that the predominant cells are slightly more mature, *i.e.,* myelocytes.

**leukotac'tic.** Leukocytotactic.

**leukotax'ia.** Leukocytotaxia.

**leukotax'ine.** A cell-free nitrogenous material prepared from injured, acutely degenerating tissue and from inflammatory exudates.

**leukotax'is.** Leukocytotaxia.

**leukothrombin** (lu-ko-throm'bin). A substance that is derived from leukocytes, is found in the circulating blood, and (in combination with thrombokinase) forms thrombin.

**leukotic** (lu-kot'ik). Pertaining to, characterized by, or manifesting leukosis.

**leu'kotome.** An instrument for performing leukotomy.

**leukotomy** (lu-kot'o-mĭ) [ leuko- + G. *tomē,* a cutting ]. The operation of cutting the white matter of the frontal lobe of the brain.
   **prefrontal l.,** prefrontal *lobotomy.*
   **transor'bital l.,** transorbital *lobotomy.*

**leukotox'in.** Leukocytotoxin.

**leukotrichia** (lu-ko-trik'ĭ-ah) [ leuko- + G. *thrix,* hair ]. Whiteness of the hair.
   **l. annula'ris,** ringed *hair.*

**leukotrichous** (lu-kot'rĭ-kus). Having white hair.

**Levaditi** (la-vah-de'te), Constantin, Roumanian bacteriologist in Paris, 1874–1928. See L. *method.*

**levallorphan tartrate** (lev'al-or'fan) (BP). LORFAN; 1-*N*-allyl-3-hydroxymorphinan tartrate; the *N*-allyl analogue of levorphanol, antagonistic to the actions of narcotic analgesics. Used in the treatment of respiratory depression due to overdosage of narcotics.

**lev'an.** Fructosan, *i.e.,* polyfructose.

**lev'ansu'crase.** Enzyme catalyzing conversion of sucrose into polyfructose (a levan) and free glucose.

**lev'arter'enol bitartrate** (USP). LEVOPHED bitartrate; noradrenaline acid tartrate (BP); L-norepinephrine or L-noradrenaline bitartrate; $(-)$-$\alpha$-(aminomethyl)-3,4-

dihydroxybenzyl alcohol tartrate; for actions and uses, see norepinephrine.

**leva'tor** [ L. a lifter, fr. *levo*, pp. *-atus*, to lift, fr. *levis*, light ]. 1. A surgical instrument for prying up the depressed part in a fracture of the skull. 2 [ NA ]. One of several muscles whose action is to raise the part into which it is inserted.

**level.** Any rank, position, or status in a graded scale of values.

**l. of aspiration,** in clinical psychology, the degree or quality of performance which an individual desires to attain or feels he can achieve.

**Leventhal,** Michael L., U. S. physician, *1901. See Stein-L. *syndrome.*

**lever** (lev'er, le'ver) [ F. *lever*, to lift ]. An instrument used to lift or pry.

**dental l.,** elevator (2).

**leverage** (le'ver-ij). The actual lift or elevating direction of an instrument called a lever or elevator.

**Lévi,** L., French endocrinologist, 1868–1933. See Lorain-L. *dwarfism, infantilism, syndrome.*

**Levin,** Abraham L., U. S. physician, 1880–1940. See L. *tube.*

**Levine,** S. A. See Lown-Ganong-L. *syndrome.*

**Levinea** (lĕ-vin'e-ah) [ M. *Levine* ]. A genus of bacteria (family Enterobacteriaceae) containing Gram-negative motile rods which are peritrichous. Citrate is utilized by these organisms as a sole source of carbon. They are indole- and methyl red-positive, and nitrates are reduced to nitrites. Arginine dihydrolase and ornithine decarboxylase are produced by these organisms, but acetylmethylcarbinol, oxidase, phenylalanine deaminase, and lysine decarboxylase are not produced. They ferment glucose. They are found in human urine samples and may be pathogenic, causing urinary infections. The type species is *L. amalonatica.*

**L. amalonatica,** a species of bacteria found primarily in human feces; occurs as a usual inhabitant of the intestinal tract. It is the type species of the genus *L.*

**L. malonatica,** a species found in human feces, urine, nose, throat, and sputum.

**Levinthal-Cole-Lillie bodies.** See under body.

**lev'ita'tion** [ L. *levitas*, lightness ]. Support of patient on a cushion of air.

**levo-** (le'vo-) [ L. *laevus*, left ]. A prefix denoting left, toward or on the left side.

**le'vocar'dia** [ levo- + G. *kardia*, heart ]. Situs inversus of the other viscera but with the heart normally situated on the left; congenital cardiac lesions are commonly associated.

**le'vocar'diogram.** That part of the bicardiogram, or normal curve, that is the effect of the left ventricle.

**levoclination** (le'vo-klī-na'shun) [ levo- + L. *clino*, pp. *-atus*, to bend ]. Levotorsion (2).

**le'vodo'pa** (USP). *l*-Dopa.

**levoduction** (le-vo-duk'shun) [ levo- + L. *duco*, pp. *ductus*, to lead ]. A rotation of one or both eyes to the left.

**le'voform.** Relating to a substance that rotates the plane of polarized light to the left.

**le'voglu'cose.** Fructose.

**le'vogram.** Electrocardiographic record in experimental animal supposedly representing spread of impulse through the left ventricle, alone.

**levogyrate** (le-vo-ji'rāt) [ levo- + L. *gyro*, to turn in a circle ]. Levorotatory.

**levogyrous** (le'vo-ji'rus). Levorotatory.

**levonordefrin** (le'vo-nor-def'rin). α-(1-Aminoethyl)-3,4-dihydroxybenzyl alcohol; used as a nasal decongestant and as a vasoconstrictor given with infiltration anesthetics.

**levophacetoperane** LIDEPRAN; α-phenyl-2-piperidinemethanol acetate; antidepressant with anorexigenic properties.

**le'vopropox'yphene nap'sylate** (NF). NOVRAD; LETUSIN; CONTRATUSS; α-4-(dimethylamino)-3-methyl-1,2-diphenyl-2-butanol propionate 2-naphthalenesulfonate; an antitussive.

**levorotation** (le-vo-ro-ta'shun) [ levo- + L. *rotare*, to turn ]. 1. Rotation to the left (counterclockwise); see levorotatory. 2. Sinistrotorsion.

**le'voro'tatory.** Turning the plane of polarized light to the left or, more properly, counterclockwise; applied, for instance, to a property of fruit sugar (levulose) as distinguished from grape sugar (glucose or dextrose). As a chemical prefix, usually abbreviated *l-*.

**levorph'anol tartrate** (NF, BP). LEVORPHAN tartrate; LEVO-DROMORAN tartrate; L-3-hydroxy-*N*-methylmorphinan tartrate dihydrate; analgesic similar in action to morphine but more potent and less likely to cause constipation.

**levotorsion** (le'vo-tor'shun) [ levo- + L. *torsio*, a twisting ]. 1. Sinistrotorsion. 2. Levoclination; extorsion of left eye or intorsion of right eye.

**levoversion** (le'vo-ver'zhun) [ levo- + L. *verto*, pp. *versus*, to turn ]. 1. A turning (version) toward the left. 2. In ophthalmology, binocular conjugate movement to the left.

**Levret** (lĕ-vra'), André, French obstetrician, 1703–1780. See L.'s *forceps, law,* Mauriceau-L. *maneuver.*

**lev'ulan.** Fructosan.

**levulic acid.** Levulinic acid.

**lev'ulin.** Fructosan.

**lev'ulinate.** A salt or ester of levulinic acid.

**lev'ulin'ic acid.** Levulic acid; 4-oxovaleric acid; $CH_3COCH_2CH_2COOH$, formed by the action of hot, strong acids on hexoses. See also δ-aminolevulinic acid.

**lev'ulosan.** Fructosan.

**lev'ulose.** D-Fructose.

**levulosemia** (lev'u-lo-se'mī-ah). The presence of fructose (levulose) in the circulating blood.

**levulosuria** (lev'u-lo-su'rī-ah). The excretion of fructose (levulose) in the urine.

**Lévy,** Gabrielle, French neurologist, 1886–1935. See Roussy-L. *disease, syndrome.*

**Lewandowsky,** Felix, 1879–1921. See Jadassohn-L. *syndrome.*

**Lewis,** W. Lee, Chicago chemist, 1898–1943. Inventor of lewisite.

**Lewis,** Sir Thomas, English physician, 1881–1945. See H *factor* of L.

**Lewis blood group.** See appendix 2, Blood Groups.

**Lewis phenomenon.** See under phenomenon.

**lewisite** (lu'ĭ-sīt). Dichloro(2-chlorovinyl)arsine; β-chlorovinyldichloroarsine; $C_2H_2AsCl_3$; a war gas. It is a vesicant, a lung irritant like mustard gas, a systemic poison entering the circulation through the lungs or skin, and a mitotic poison arresting mitosis in the metaphase. Dimercaprol is the antidote.

**Lewy bodies.** See under body.

**-lexis, -lexy** [ G. *-lex-* fr. *legein, lexai,* to speak ]. A suffix, of Greek origin, that properly relates to speech, although often confused with *-legis,* of Latin origin (see -legia), and thus erroneously employed to relate to reading.

**Leyden** (li'den), Ernst V. von, Berlin physician, 1832–1910. Gave his name to *Leydenia.* See L.'s *ataxia, crystals, disease,* L.-Möbius *dystrophy,* L.'s *neuritis.*

**Leyde'nia gemmip'ara** [ E. V. von *Leyden* ]. A presumed protozoan parasite formerly postulated to be present in the ascitic fluid of certain patients with carcinoma.

**Leydig** (li'dig), Franz von, German anatomist, 1821–1908. See L.'s *cells, duct.*

**leydigarche** (li'dig-ar'ke) [ Leydig (see Leydig cells), + G. *arche,* beginning ]. An obsolete term for the beginning of gonadal function in the male, or male puberty.

**Lf, L_f.** See under dose.

**LH.** Abbreviation for luteinizing *hormone.*

**Lhermitte's sign.** See under sign.

**LH-RF.** Abbreviation for luteinizing hormone-releasing *factor.*

**Li.** Chemical symbol of the element lithium.

**Lian's point.** See under point.

**li'ber** [ L. ] [ NA ]. Free; unattached.

**liberomotor** (lib'er-o-mo'tor) [ L. *liber,* free, + *motor,* mover ]. Relating to voluntary movements.

**libidinization** (lī-bid'ĭ-nī-za'shun). Erotization.

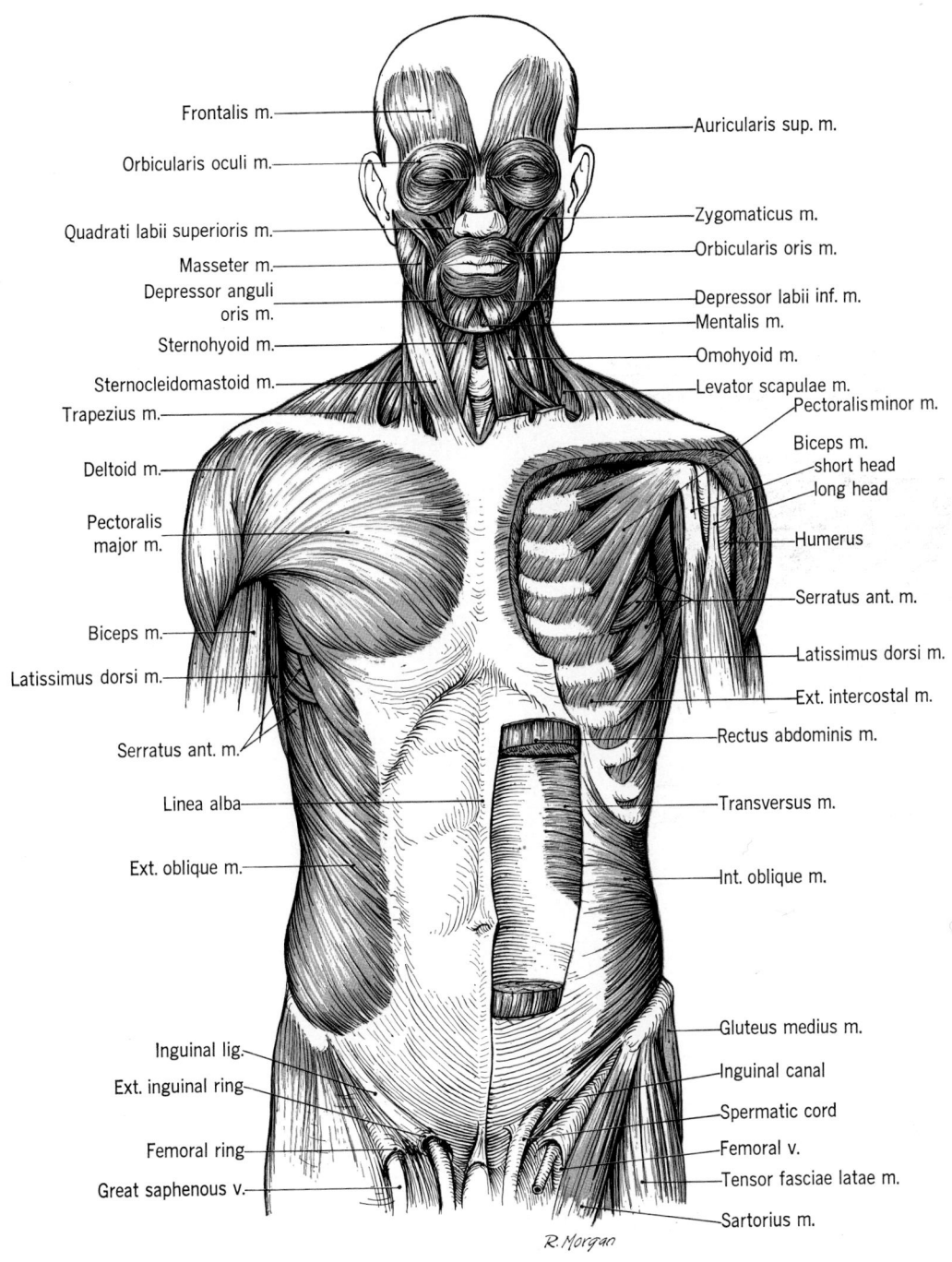

Frontalis m.

Orbicularis oculi m.

Quadrati labii superioris m.

Masseter m.

Depressor anguli oris m.

Sternohyoid m.

Sternocleidomastoid m.

Trapezius m.

Deltoid m.

Pectoralis major m.

Biceps m.

Latissimus dorsi m.

Serratus ant. m.

Linea alba

Ext. oblique m.

Inguinal lig.

Ext. inguinal ring

Femoral ring

Great saphenous v.

Auricularis sup. m.

Zygomaticus m.

Orbicularis oris m.

Depressor labii inf. m.

Mentalis m.

Omohyoid m.

Levator scapulae m.

Pectoralis minor m.

Biceps m.
short head
long head

Humerus

Serratus ant. m.

Latissimus dorsi m.

Ext. intercostal m.

Rectus abdominis m.

Transversus m.

Int. oblique m.

Gluteus medius m.

Inguinal canal

Spermatic cord

Femoral v.

Tensor fasciae latae m.

Sartorius m.

R. Morgan

**PLATE 1**

Muscles of Head, Neck, and Torso, Anterior View

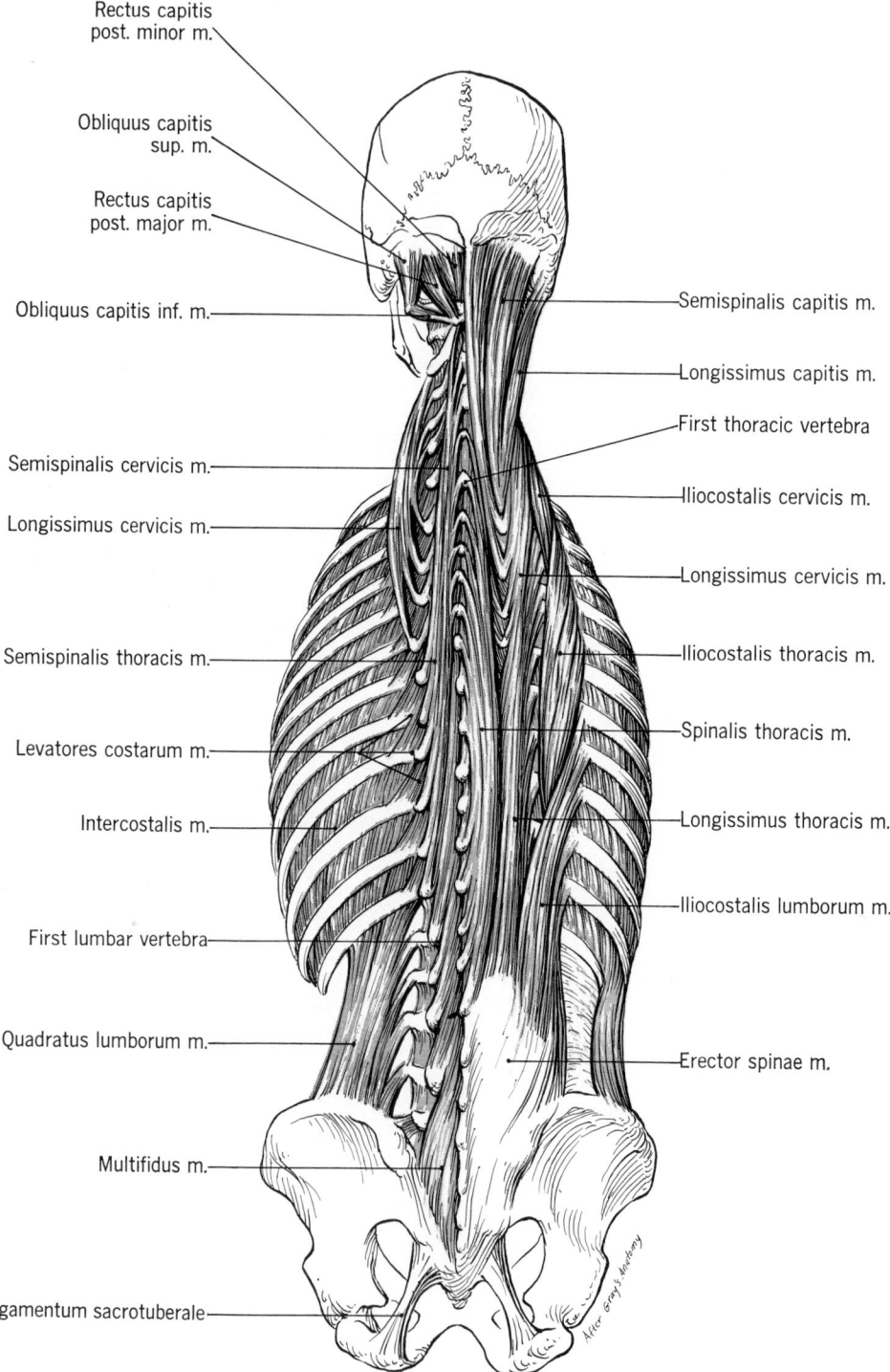

Rectus capitis post. minor m.

Obliquus capitis sup. m.

Rectus capitis post. major m.

Obliquus capitis inf. m.

Semispinalis cervicis m.

Longissimus cervicis m.

Semispinalis thoracis m.

Levatores costarum m.

Intercostalis m.

First lumbar vertebra

Quadratus lumborum m.

Multifidus m.

Ligamentum sacrotuberale

Semispinalis capitis m.

Longissimus capitis m.

First thoracic vertebra

Iliocostalis cervicis m.

Longissimus cervicis m.

Iliocostalis thoracis m.

Spinalis thoracis m.

Longissimus thoracis m.

Iliocostalis lumborum m.

Erector spinae m.

PLATE 2

Muscles of Back, Deep Dissection

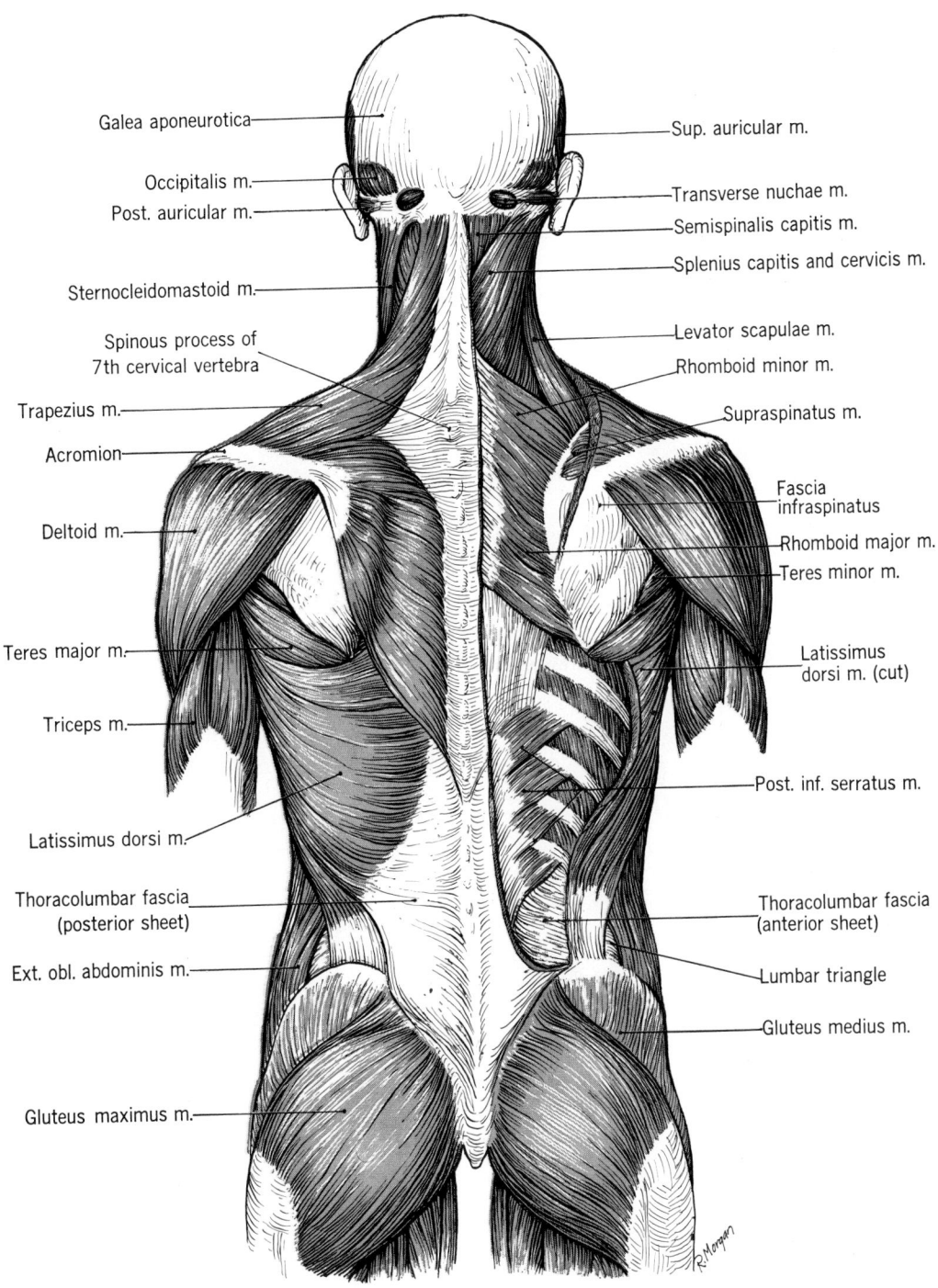

Galea aponeurotica

Occipitalis m.

Post. auricular m.

Sternocleidomastoid m.

Spinous process of
7th cervical vertebra

Trapezius m.

Acromion

Deltoid m.

Teres major m.

Triceps m.

Latissimus dorsi m.

Thoracolumbar fascia
(posterior sheet)

Ext. obl. abdominis m.

Gluteus maximus m.

Sup. auricular m.

Transverse nuchae m.

Semispinalis capitis m.

Splenius capitis and cervicis m.

Levator scapulae m.

Rhomboid minor m.

Supraspinatus m.

Fascia
infraspinatus

Rhomboid major m.

Teres minor m.

Latissimus
dorsi m. (cut)

Post. inf. serratus m.

Thoracolumbar fascia
(anterior sheet)

Lumbar triangle

Gluteus medius m.

R. Morgan

PLATE 3
Muscles of Trunk, Posterior View

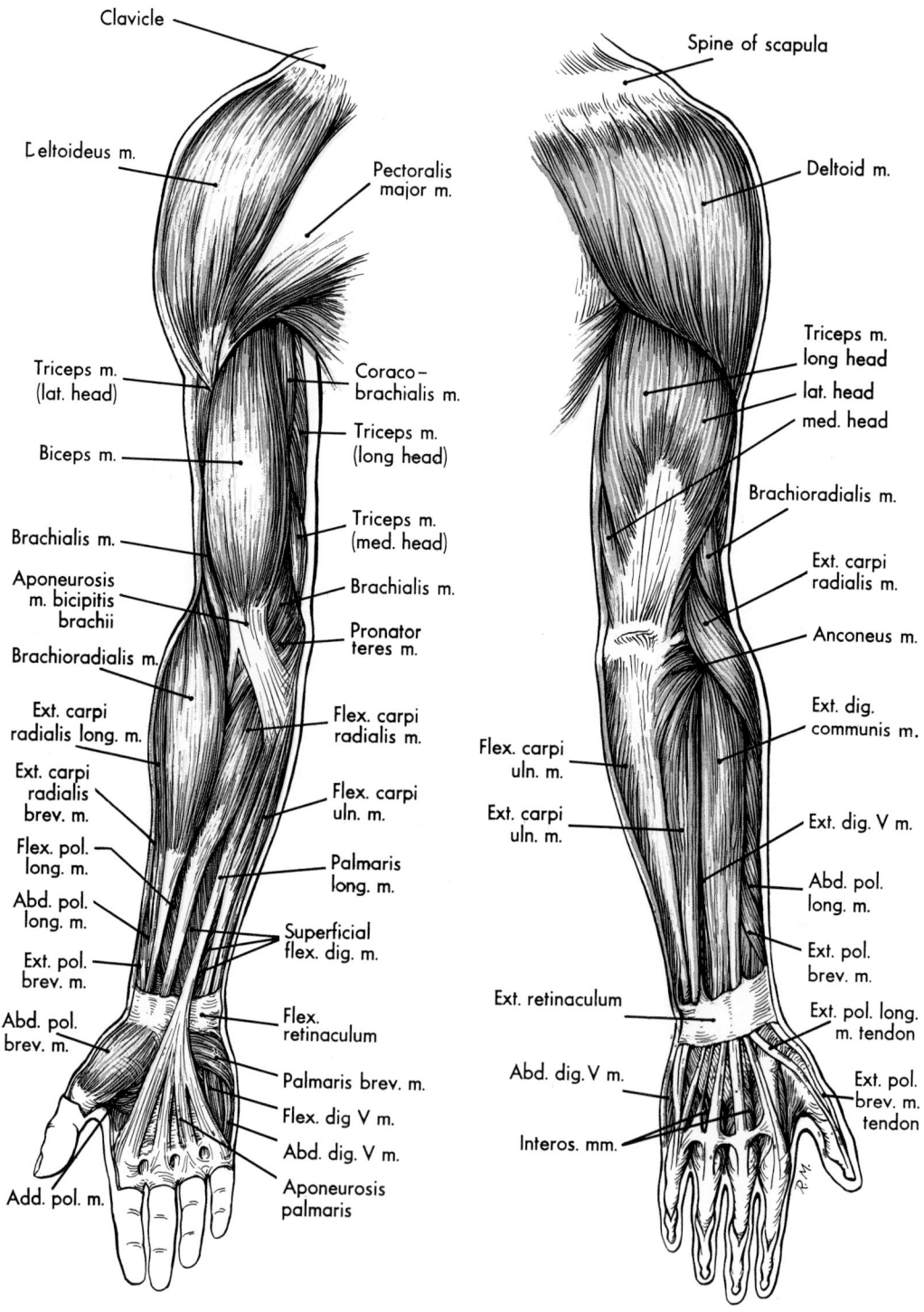

Clavicle

Deltoideus m.

Pectoralis
major m.

Triceps m.
(lat. head)

Coraco-
brachialis m.

Triceps m.
(long head)

Biceps m.

Brachialis m.

Triceps m.
(med. head)

Aponeurosis
m. bicipitis
brachii

Brachialis m.

Pronator
teres m.

Brachioradialis m.

Ext. carpi
radialis long. m.

Flex. carpi
radialis m.

Ext. carpi
radialis
brev. m.

Flex. carpi
uln. m.

Flex. pol.
long. m.

Palmaris
long. m.

Abd. pol.
long. m.

Ext. pol.
brev. m.

Superficial
flex. dig. m.

Abd. pol.
brev. m.

Flex.
retinaculum

Palmaris brev. m.

Flex. dig V m.

Abd. dig. V m.

Add. pol. m.

Aponeurosis
palmaris

Spine of scapula

Deltoid m.

Triceps m.
long head
lat. head
med. head

Brachioradialis m.

Ext. carpi
radialis m.

Anconeus m.

Ext. dig.
communis m.

Flex. carpi
uln. m.

Ext. carpi
uln. m.

Ext. dig. V m.

Abd. pol.
long. m.

Ext. pol.
brev. m.

Ext. retinaculum

Ext. pol. long.
m. tendon

Abd. dig. V m.

Ext. pol.
brev. m.
tendon

Interos. mm.

PLATE 4
Superficial Muscles of Right Upper Limb

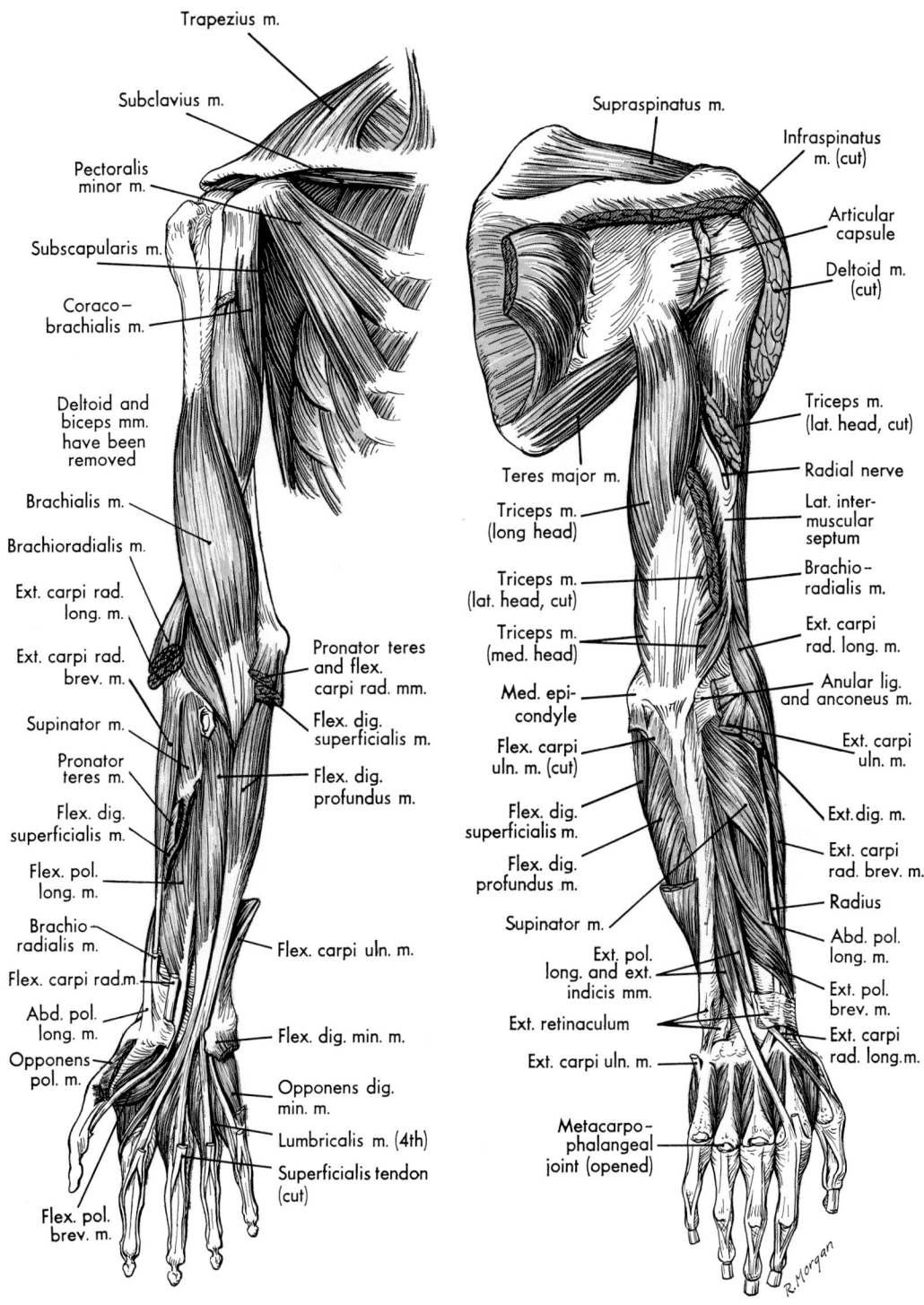

Trapezius m.

Subclavius m.

Pectoralis
minor m.

Subscapularis m.

Coraco-
brachialis m.

Deltoid and
biceps mm.
have been
removed

Brachialis m.

Brachioradialis m.

Ext. carpi rad.
long. m.

Ext. carpi rad.
brev. m.

Supinator m.

Pronator
teres m.

Flex. dig.
superficialis m.

Flex. pol.
long. m.

Brachio-
radialis m.

Flex. carpi rad.m.

Abd. pol.
long. m.

Opponens
pol. m.

Flex. pol.
brev. m.

Pronator teres
and flex.
carpi rad. mm.

Flex. dig.
superficialis m.

Flex. dig.
profundus m.

Flex. carpi uln. m.

Flex. dig. min. m.

Opponens dig.
min. m.

Lumbricalis m. (4th)

Superficialis tendon
(cut)

Supraspinatus m.

Infraspinatus
m. (cut)

Articular
capsule

Deltoid m.
(cut)

Triceps m.
(lat. head, cut)

Radial nerve

Lat. inter-
muscular
septum

Brachio-
radialis m.

Ext. carpi
rad. long. m.

Anular lig.
and anconeus m.

Ext. carpi
uln. m.

Ext.dig. m.

Ext. carpi
rad. brev. m.

Radius

Abd. pol.
long. m.

Ext. pol.
brev. m.

Ext. carpi
rad. long.m.

Teres major m.

Triceps m.
(long head)

Triceps m.
(lat. head, cut)

Triceps m.
(med. head)

Med. epi-
condyle

Flex. carpi
uln. m. (cut)

Flex. dig.
superficialis m.

Flex. dig.
profundus m.

Supinator m.

Ext. pol.
long. and ext.
indicis mm.

Ext. retinaculum

Ext. carpi uln. m.

Metacarpo-
phalangeal
joint (opened)

R. Morgan

## PLATE 5
Muscles of Right Upper Limb, Deep Dissection

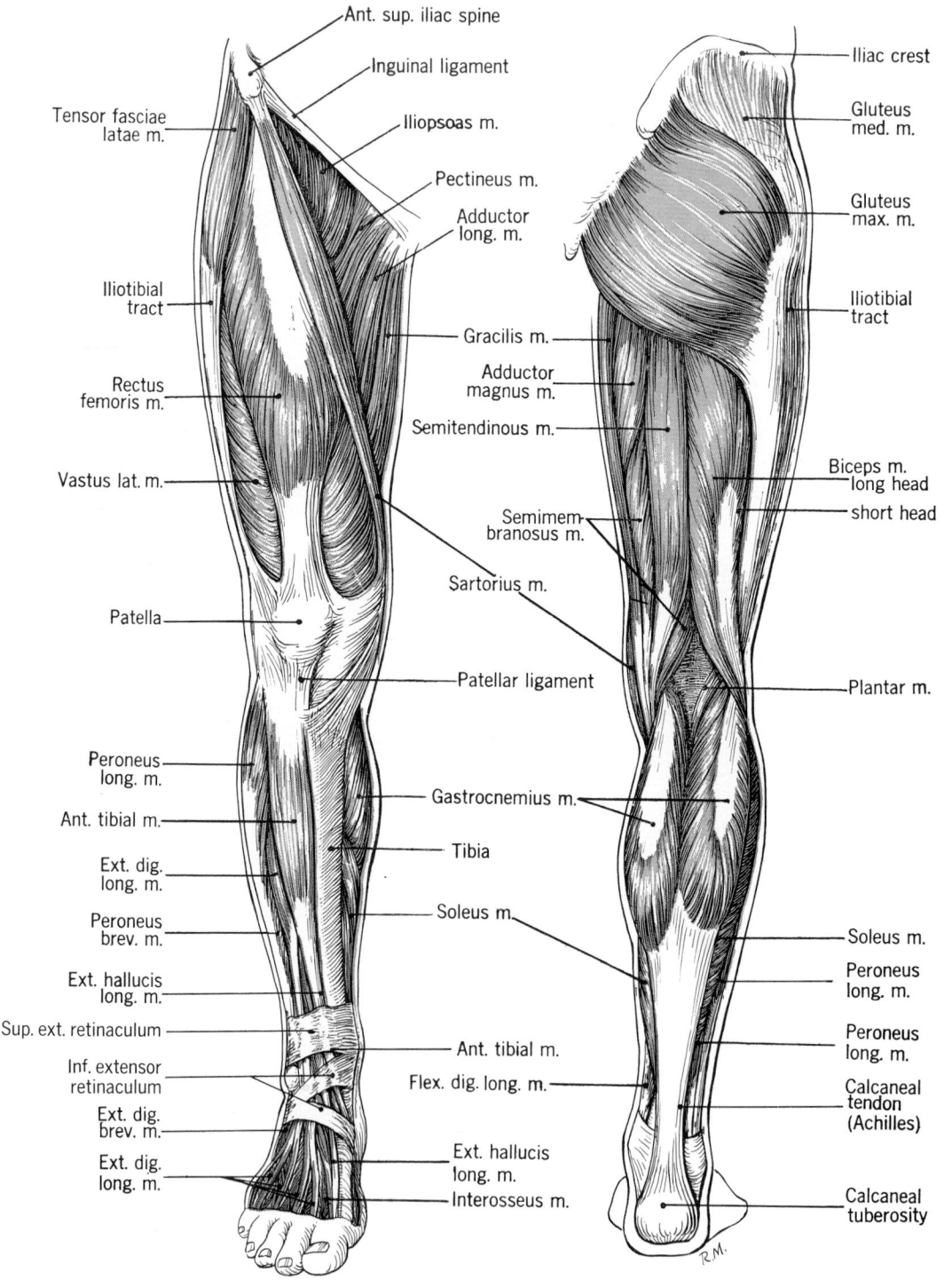

Ant. sup. iliac spine

Inguinal ligament

Iliopsoas m.

Pectineus m.

Adductor long. m.

Tensor fasciae latae m.

Iliotibial tract

Rectus femoris m.

Vastus lat. m.

Patella

Gracilis m.

Adductor magnus m.

Semitendinous m.

Semimem branosus m.

Sartorius m.

Patellar ligament

Iliac crest

Gluteus med. m.

Gluteus max. m.

Iliotibial tract

Biceps m. long head

short head

Plantar m.

Peroneus long. m.

Ant. tibial m.

Ext. dig. long. m.

Peroneus brev. m.

Ext. hallucis long. m.

Sup. ext. retinaculum

Inf. extensor retinaculum

Ext. dig. brev. m.

Ext. dig. long. m.

Gastrocnemius m.

Tibia

Soleus m.

Ant. tibial m.

Flex. dig. long. m.

Ext. hallucis long. m.

Interosseus m.

Soleus m.

Peroneus long. m.

Peroneus long. m.

Calcaneal tendon (Achilles)

Calcaneal tuberosity

R.M.

## PLATE 6
Superficial Muscles of Right Lower Limb

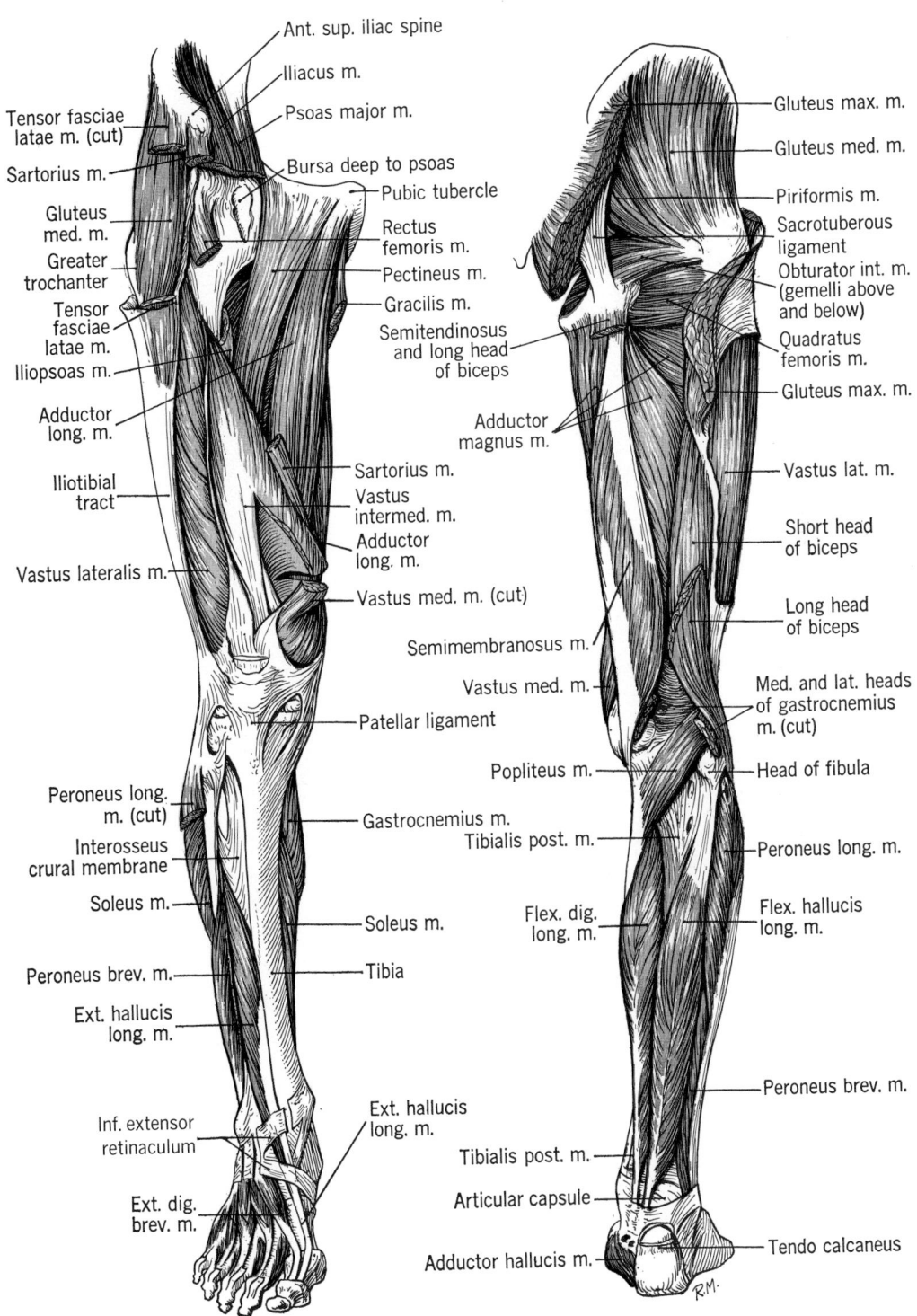

Ant. sup. iliac spine
Iliacus m.
Psoas major m.
Tensor fasciae latae m. (cut)
Sartorius m.
Bursa deep to psoas
Pubic tubercle
Gluteus med. m.
Rectus femoris m.
Greater trochanter
Pectineus m.
Tensor fasciae latae m.
Gracilis m.
Iliopsoas m.
Semitendinosus and long head of biceps
Adductor long. m.
Iliotibial tract
Sartorius m.
Vastus intermed. m.
Adductor long. m.
Vastus lateralis m.
Vastus med. m. (cut)
Semimembranosus m.
Patellar ligament
Peroneus long. m. (cut)
Interosseus crural membrane
Gastrocnemius m.
Soleus m.
Soleus m.
Peroneus brev. m.
Tibia
Ext. hallucis long. m.
Inf. extensor retinaculum
Ext. hallucis long. m.
Ext. dig. brev. m.

Gluteus max. m.
Gluteus med. m.
Piriformis m.
Sacrotuberous ligament
Obturator int. m. (gemelli above and below)
Quadratus femoris m.
Gluteus max. m.
Adductor magnus m.
Vastus lat. m.
Short head of biceps
Long head of biceps
Vastus med. m.
Med. and lat. heads of gastrocnemius m. (cut)
Popliteus m.
Head of fibula
Tibialis post. m.
Peroneus long. m.
Flex. dig. long. m.
Flex. hallucis long. m.
Peroneus brev. m.
Tibialis post. m.
Articular capsule
Adductor hallucis m.
Tendo calcaneus

R.M.

### PLATE 7
Muscles of Right Lower Limb, Deep Dissection

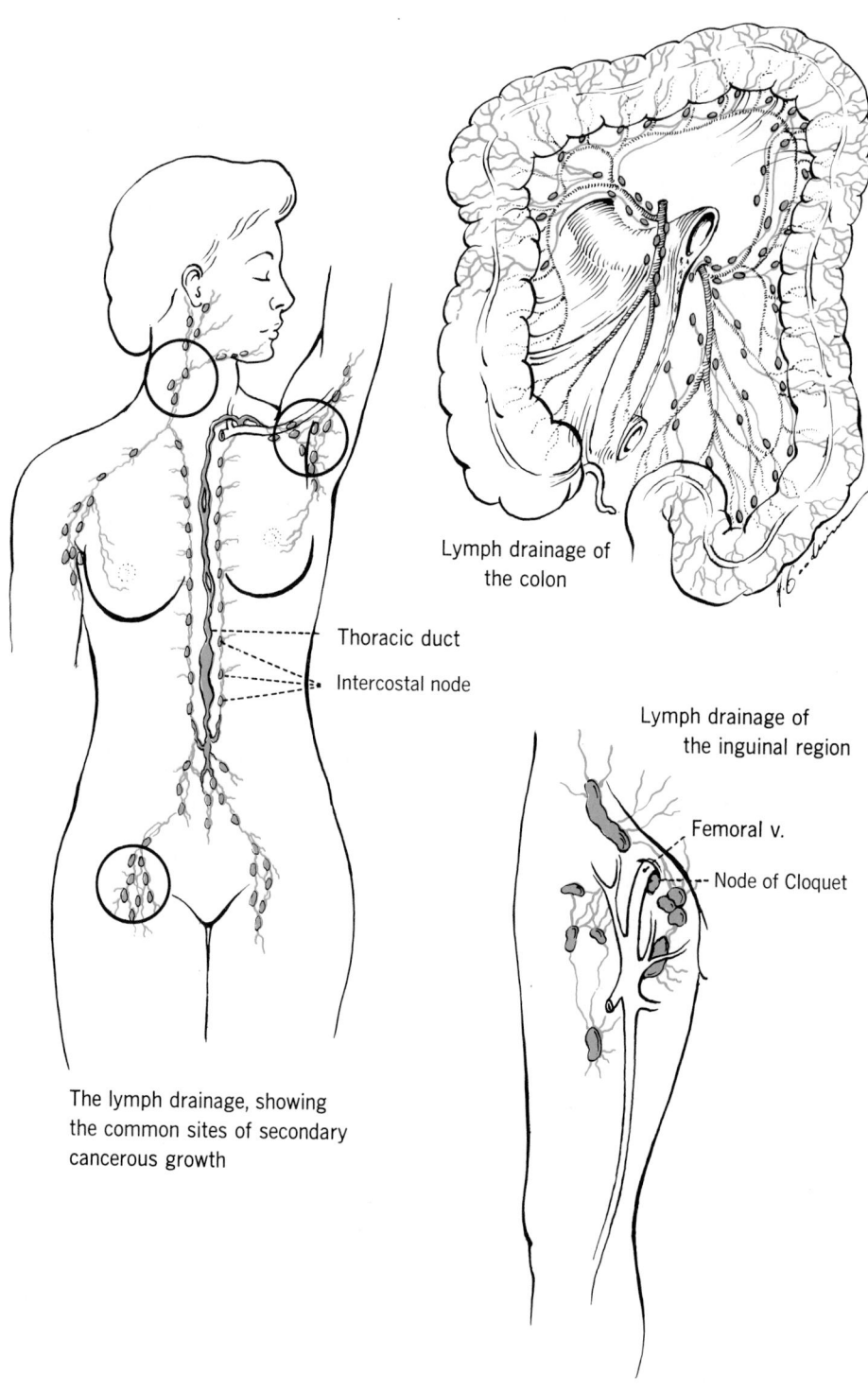

Lymph drainage of
the colon

Thoracic duct

Intercostal node

Lymph drainage of
the inguinal region

Femoral v.

Node of Cloquet

The lymph drainage, showing
the common sites of secondary
cancerous growth

PLATE 8
Lymphatic System

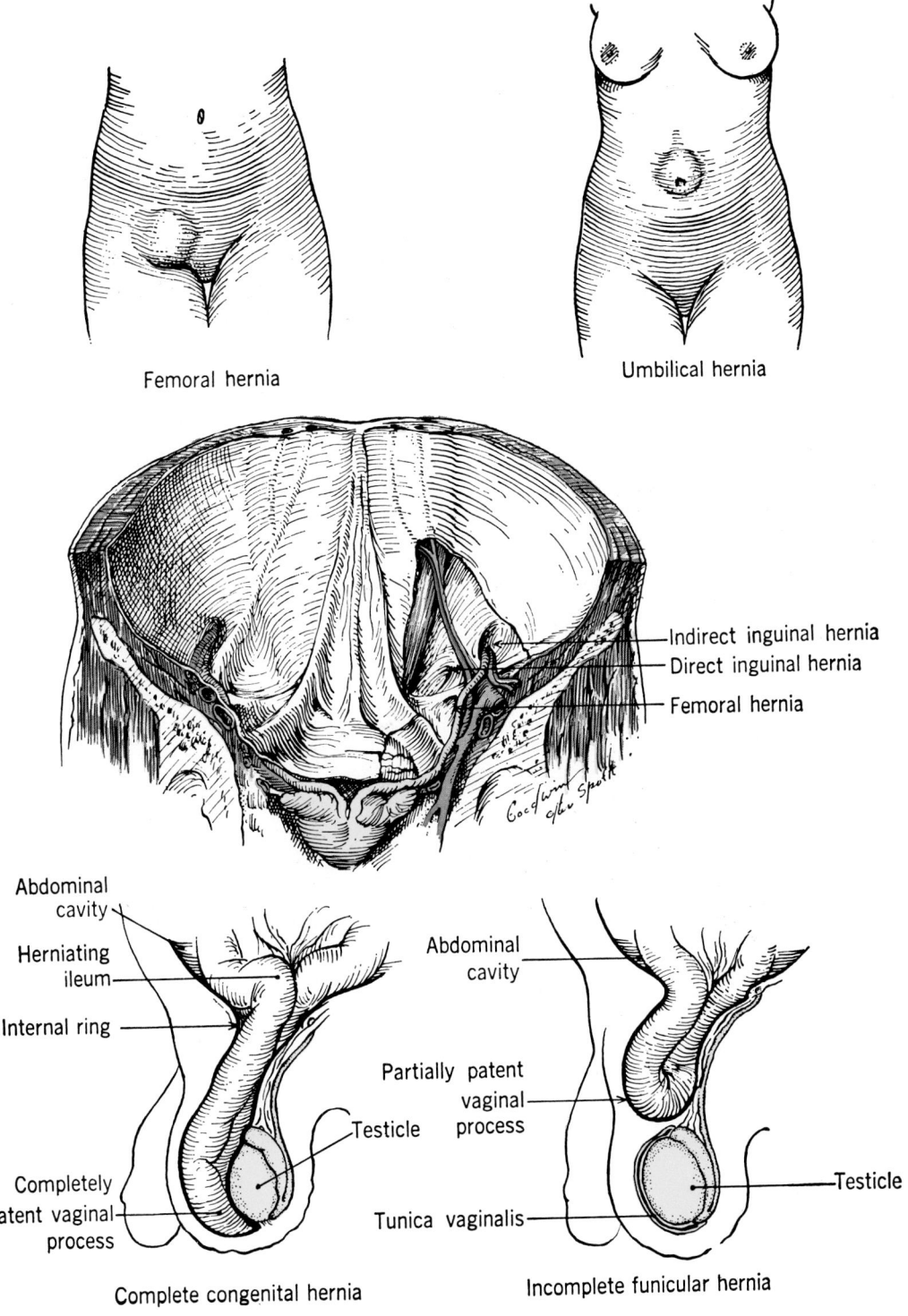

Femoral hernia

Umbilical hernia

Indirect inguinal hernia
Direct inguinal hernia
Femoral hernia

Abdominal cavity

Herniating ileum

Internal ring

Completely patent vaginal process

Testicle

Abdominal cavity

Partially patent vaginal process

Tunica vaginalis

Testicle

Complete congenital hernia

Incomplete funicular hernia

PLATE 9

Hernia of Anterior Abdominal Wall

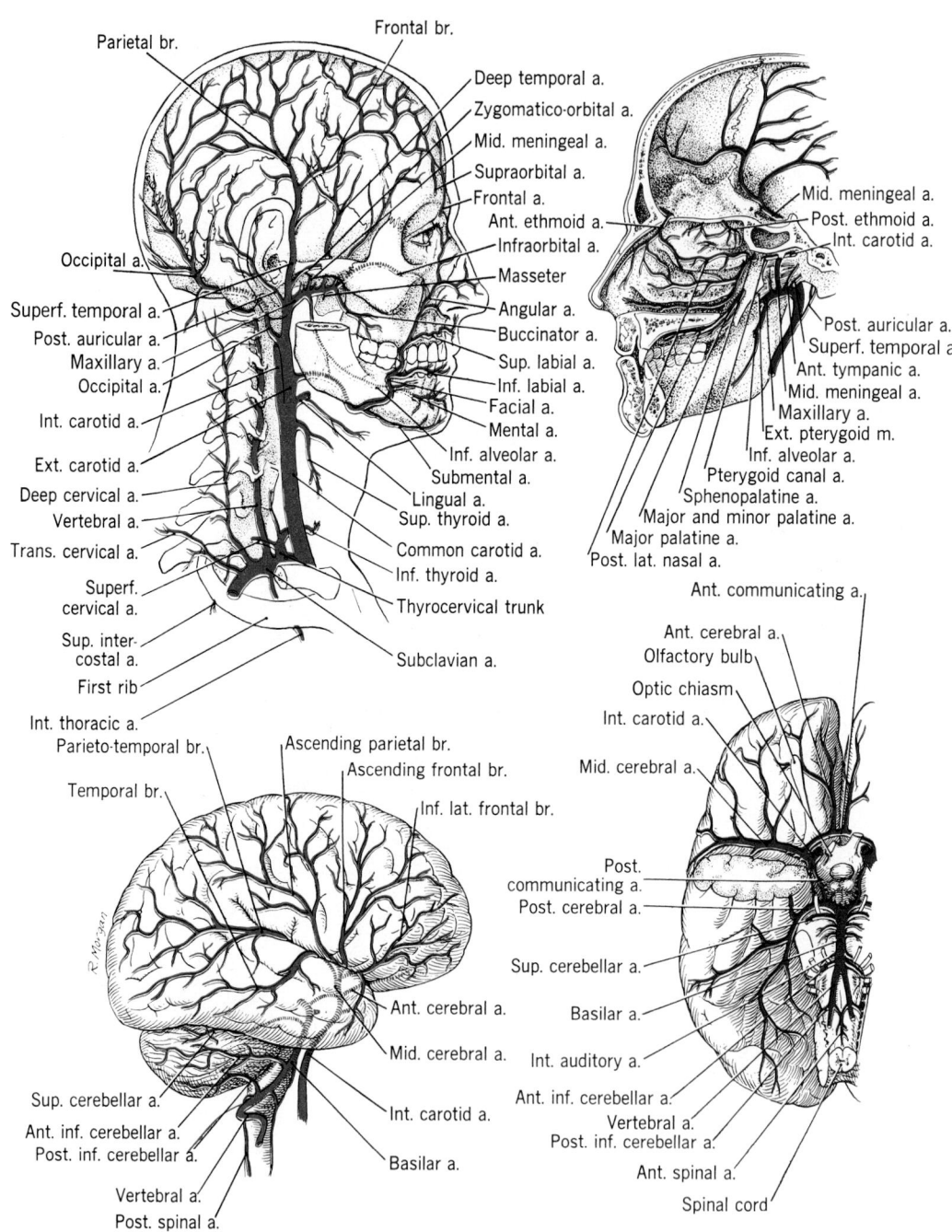

**PLATE 10**
Arteries of Head and Brain

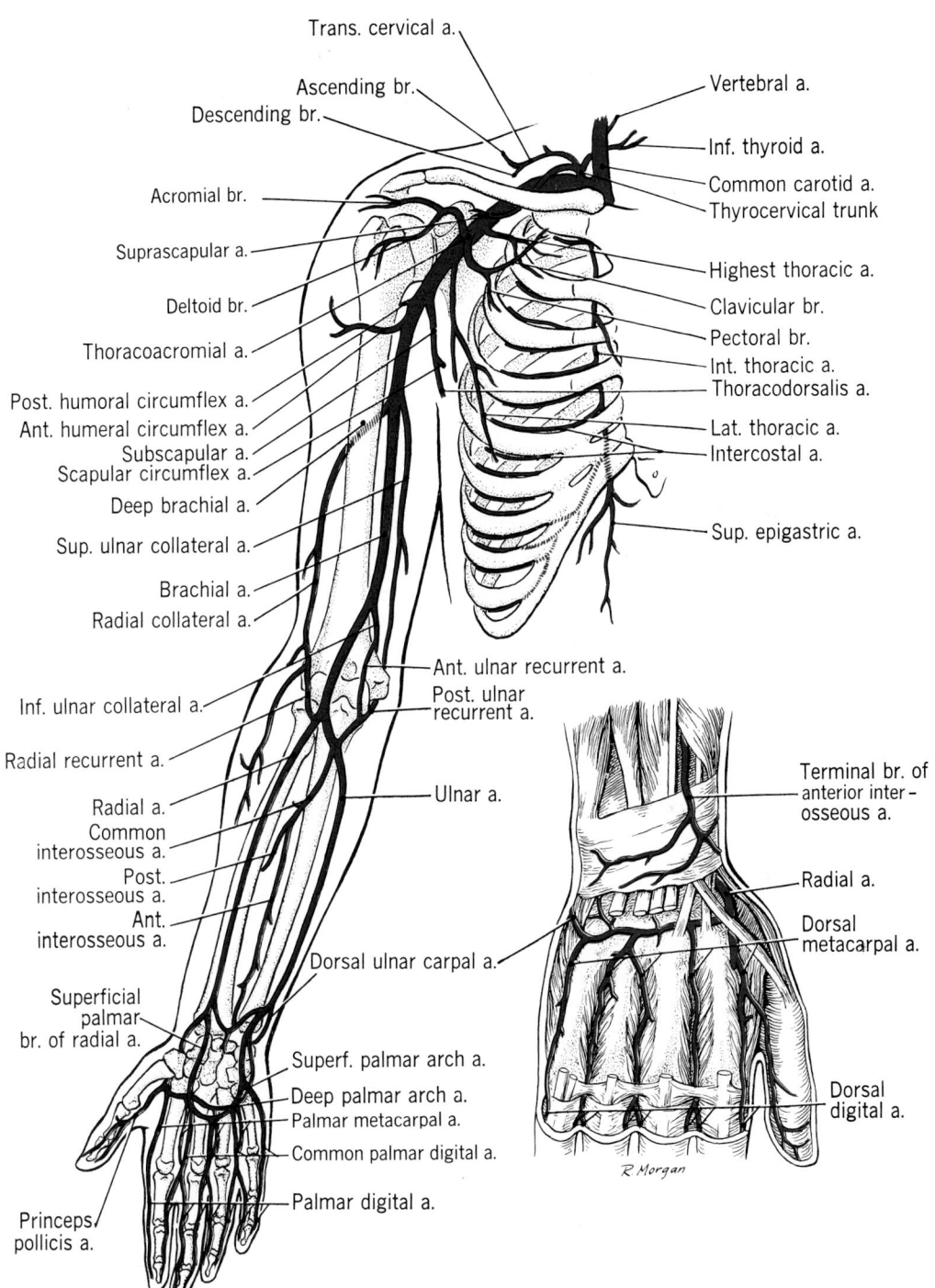

Trans. cervical a.
Ascending br.
Descending br.
Acromial br.
Suprascapular a.
Deltoid br.
Thoracoacromial a.
Post. humoral circumflex a.
Ant. humeral circumflex a.
Subscapular a.
Scapular circumflex a.
Deep brachial a.
Sup. ulnar collateral a.
Brachial a.
Radial collateral a.

Vertebral a.
Inf. thyroid a.
Common carotid a.
Thyrocervical trunk
Highest thoracic a.
Clavicular br.
Pectoral br.
Int. thoracic a.
Thoracodorsalis a.
Lat. thoracic a.
Intercostal a.
Sup. epigastric a.

Inf. ulnar collateral a.
Radial recurrent a.

Ant. ulnar recurrent a.
Post. ulnar recurrent a.

Radial a.
Common interosseous a.
Post. interosseous a.
Ant. interosseous a.

Ulnar a.

Terminal br. of anterior inter-osseous a.
Radial a.
Dorsal metacarpal a.

Superficial palmar br. of radial a.

Dorsal ulnar carpal a.

Superf. palmar arch a.
Deep palmar arch a.
Palmar metacarpal a.
Common palmar digital a.
Palmar digital a.

Dorsal digital a.

Princeps pollicis a.

R. Morgan

PLATE 11
Arteries of Upper Limb and Chest

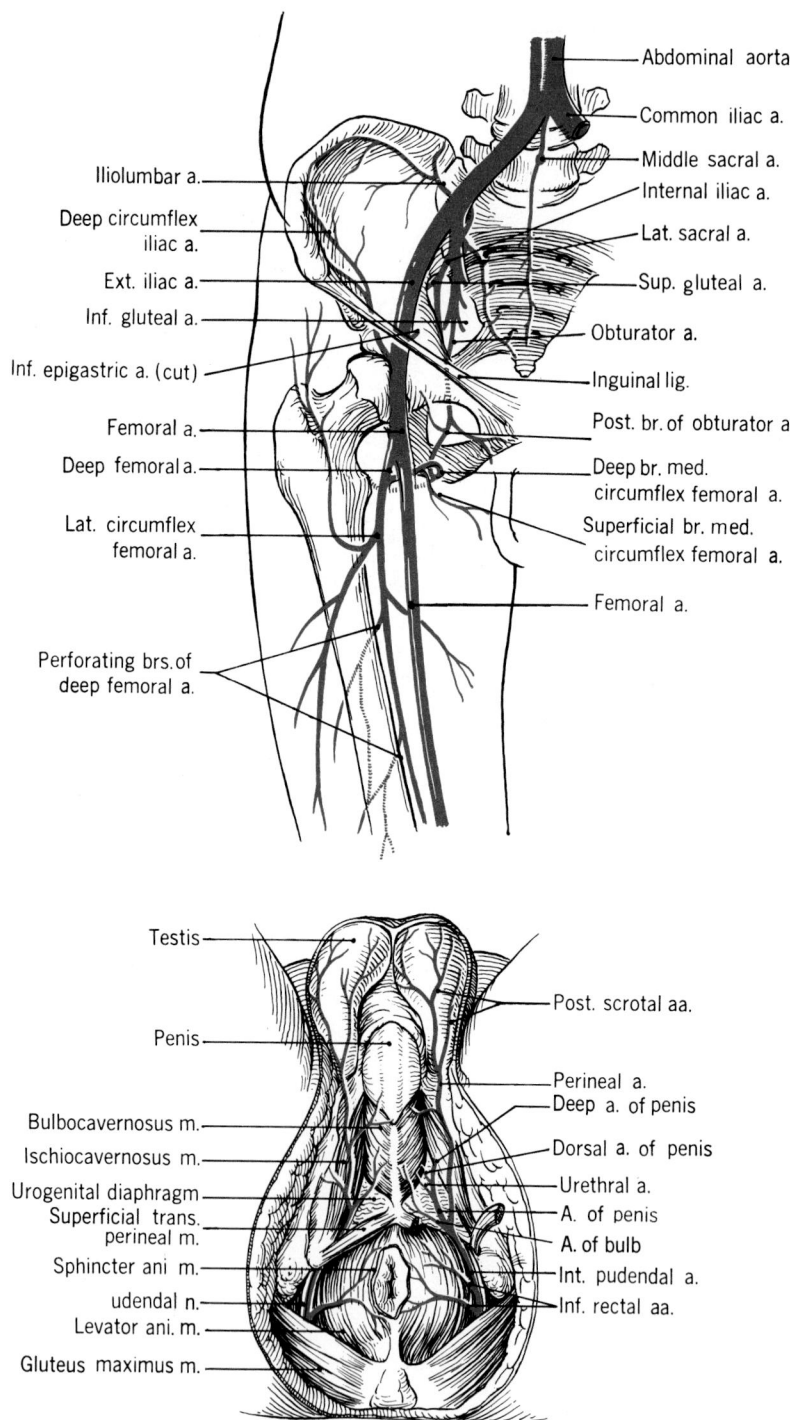

**PLATE 12**

Arteries of Thigh and Perineum

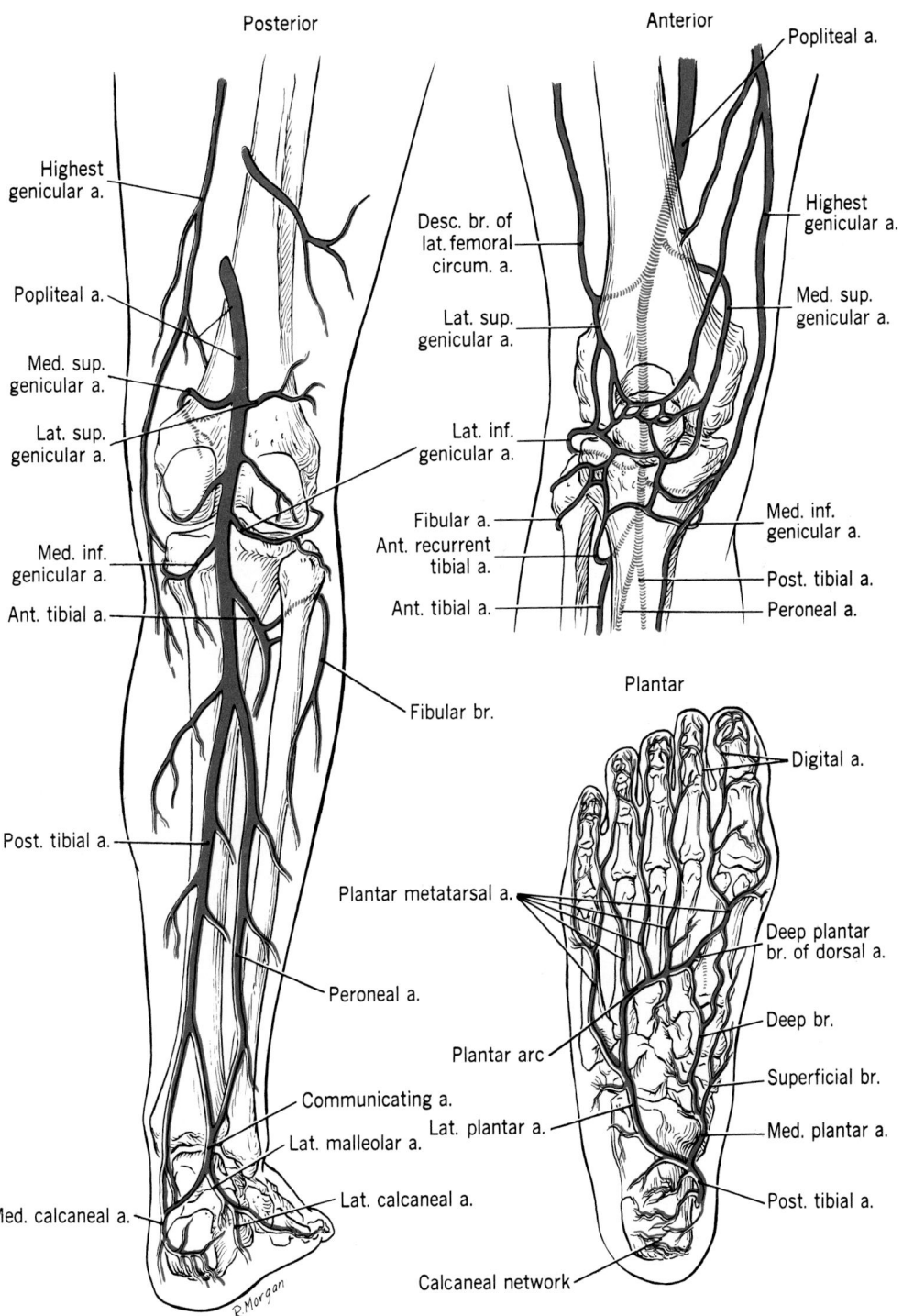

**PLATE 13**

Arteries of Right Lower Extremity in Relation to Bones

PLATES 14, 15, and 16

# MATURATION OF HUMAN BLOOD CELLS

## A PHOTOGRAPHIC PRESENTATION OF HEMATOPOIESIS (X1200)
By John J. Butler, M.D., Lynn C. Wall, and H. L. Gibson

## EXPLANATORY NOTES

The cells pictured are those normally found in blood and bone marrow. They are presented as they appear when stained with Wright's stain except for the reticulocyte, which was stained with brilliant cresyl blue. The arrangement of the chart is designed to show that the transitions between blood cell types are gradual rather than abrupt. The terminology and suggested origins of cells are according to Marcel Bessis.[1]

All of the cell types of the erythrocyte and granulocyte series, which are derived from the hemocytoblast, are found in bone marrow; normally only the more mature forms are found in the peripheral blood.

Thrombocytes, or "platelets," as they are more commonly called, are distributed throughout peripheral blood as well as bone marrow and are considered to be the end product of megakaryocytes, which normally appear only in bone marrow.

The *red arrow* is used to direct attention to the fact that the transition between the hemocytoblast and megakaryoblast shown in the chart has not been accepted by some authorities.

Monocytes, lymphocytes, and plasmocytes—set apart in the chart by *red lines*—in addition to being found in blood or bone marrow, are also found in reticuloendothelial tissue.

To permit easy following of the transitions from the granulocyte series to the erythrocyte series, a certain amount of duplication of the illustrations can be observed.

### REFERENCE

1. BESSIS, M.: *Cytology of Blood and Blood Forming Organs*, Grune & Stratton, Inc., New York, 1956.

### ABOUT THE AUTHORS

Dr. John J. Butler was formerly Director of Medical Education, St. Mary's Hospital, Rochester, New York; formerly Director of Medical Education, St. Michael's Hospital, Newark, New Jersey, and Associate Professor of Medicine, New Jersey School of Medicine, Jersey City.

Mr. Lynn C. Wall and Mr. H. L. Gibson added their expertness as Technical Editors with the Eastman Kodak Co.

### ACKNOWLEDGMENT

The chart and explanatory notes are reproduced through the courtesy of Eastman Kodak Company, Rochester, New York.

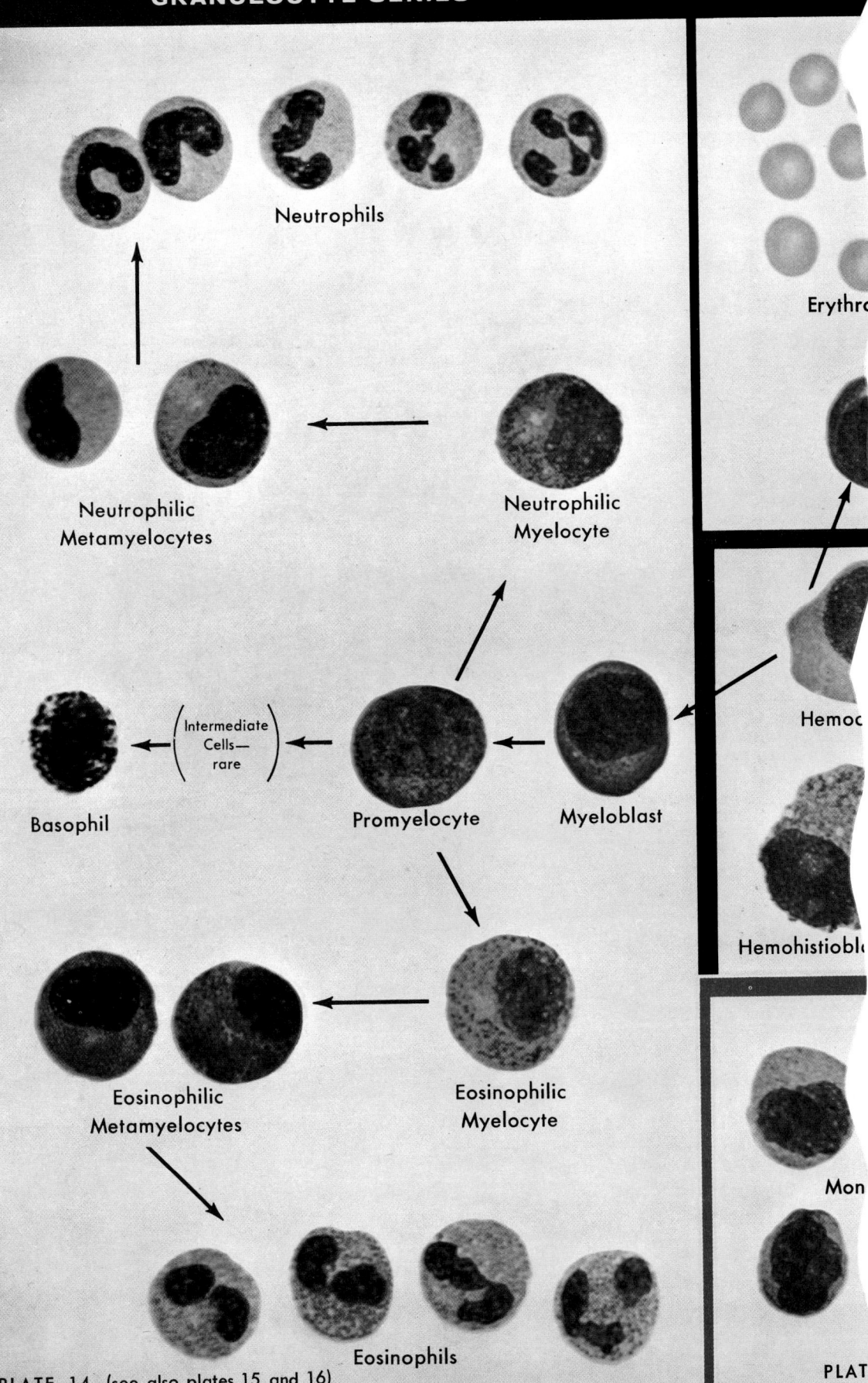

Neutrophils

Neutrophilic
Metamyelocytes

Neutrophilic
Myelocyte

Erythro

Basophil

(Intermediate
Cells—
rare)

Promyelocyte

Myeloblast

Hemoc

Hemohistiobl

Eosinophilic
Metamyelocytes

Eosinophilic
Myelocyte

Mon

Eosinophils

PLATE 14 (see also plates 15 and 16)

PLAT

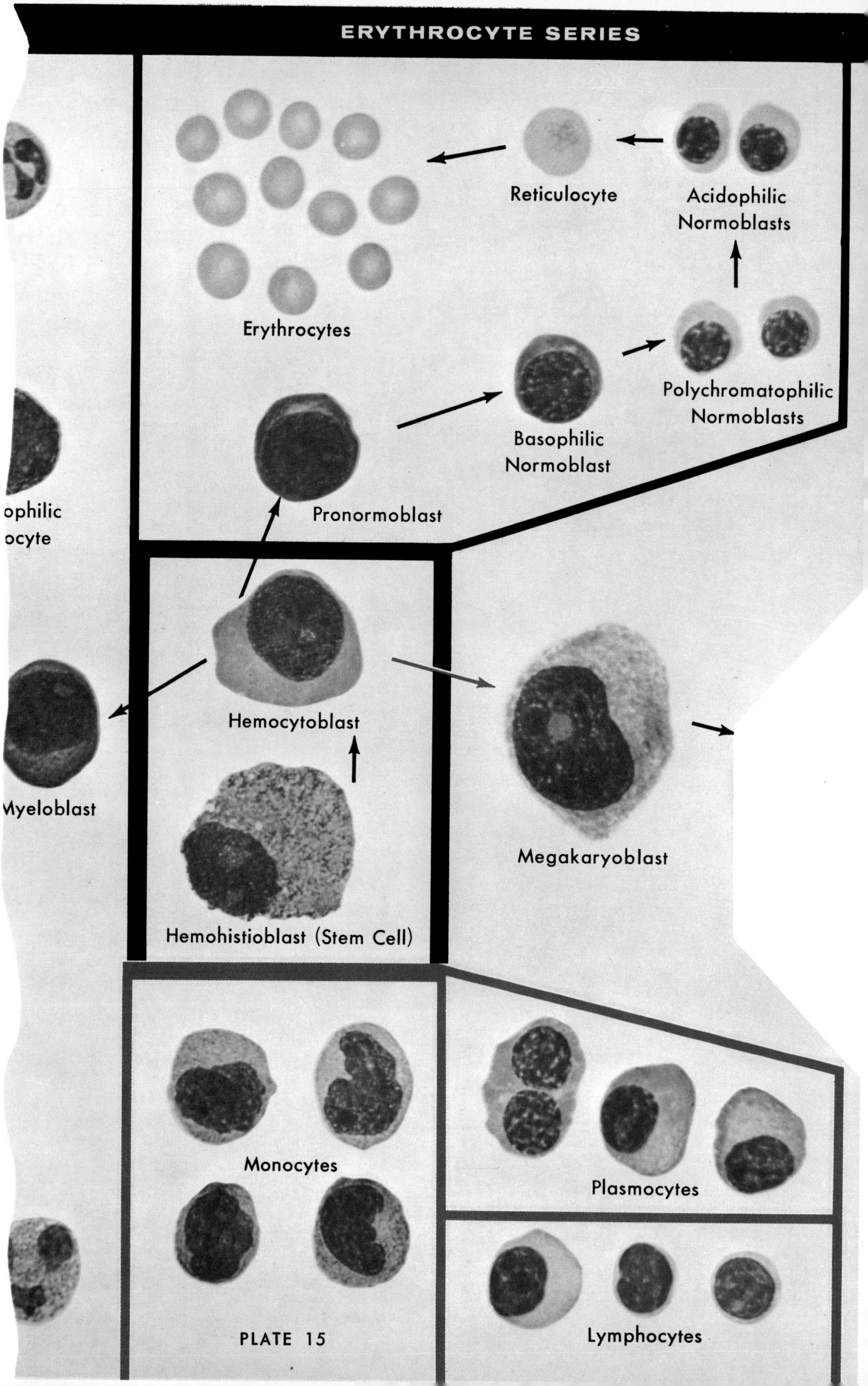

# ERYTHROCYTE SERIES

Erythrocytes

Reticulocyte

Acidophilic Normoblasts

Polychromatophilic Normoblasts

Basophilic Normoblast

Pronormoblast

ophilic ocyte

Myeloblast

Hemocytoblast

Hemohistioblast (Stem Cell)

Megakaryoblast

Monocytes

Plasmocytes

Lymphocytes

PLATE 15

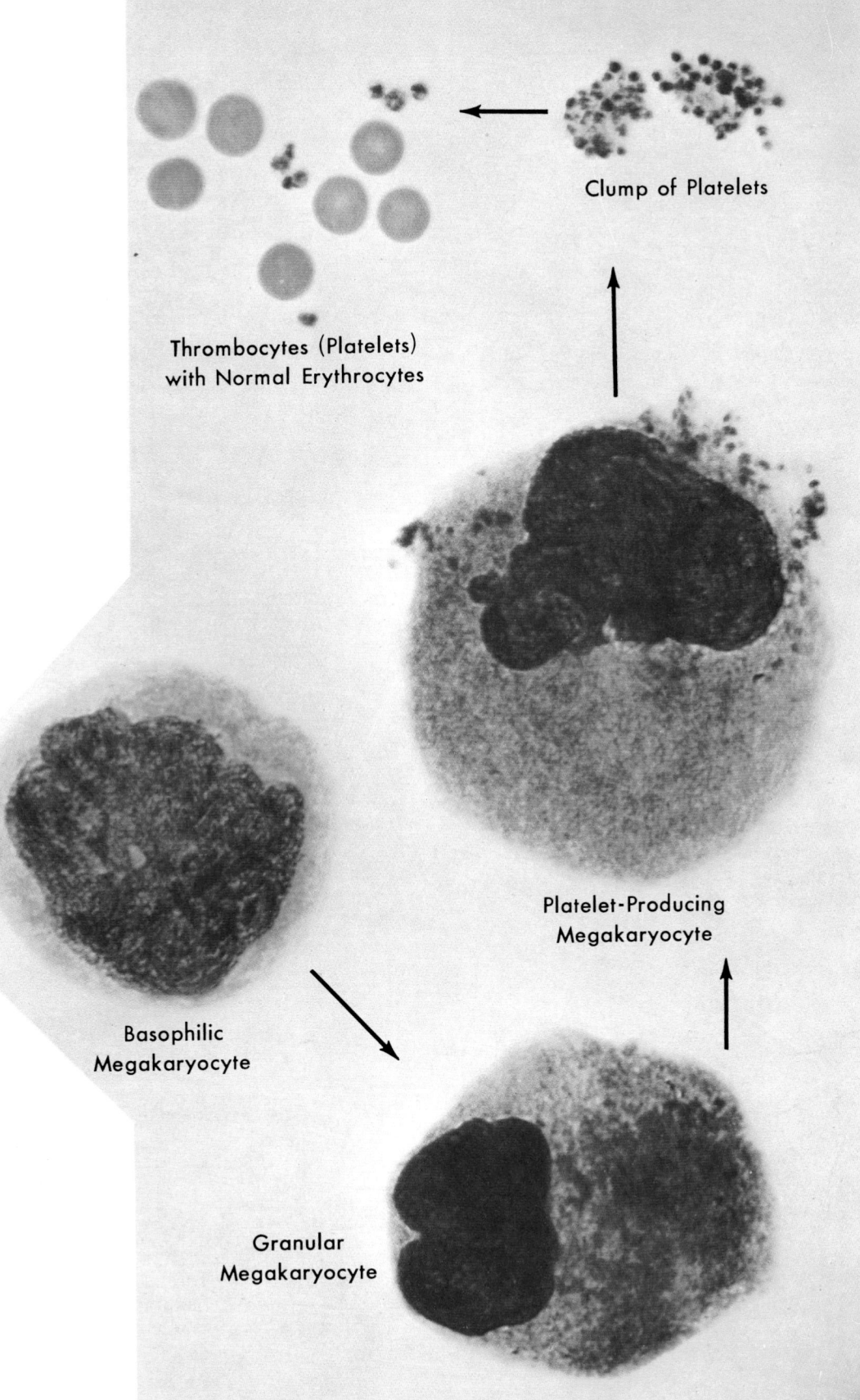

Thrombocytes (Platelets)
with Normal Erythrocytes

Clump of Platelets

Platelet-Producing
Megakaryocyte

Basophilic
Megakaryocyte

Granular
Megakaryocyte

PLATE 16

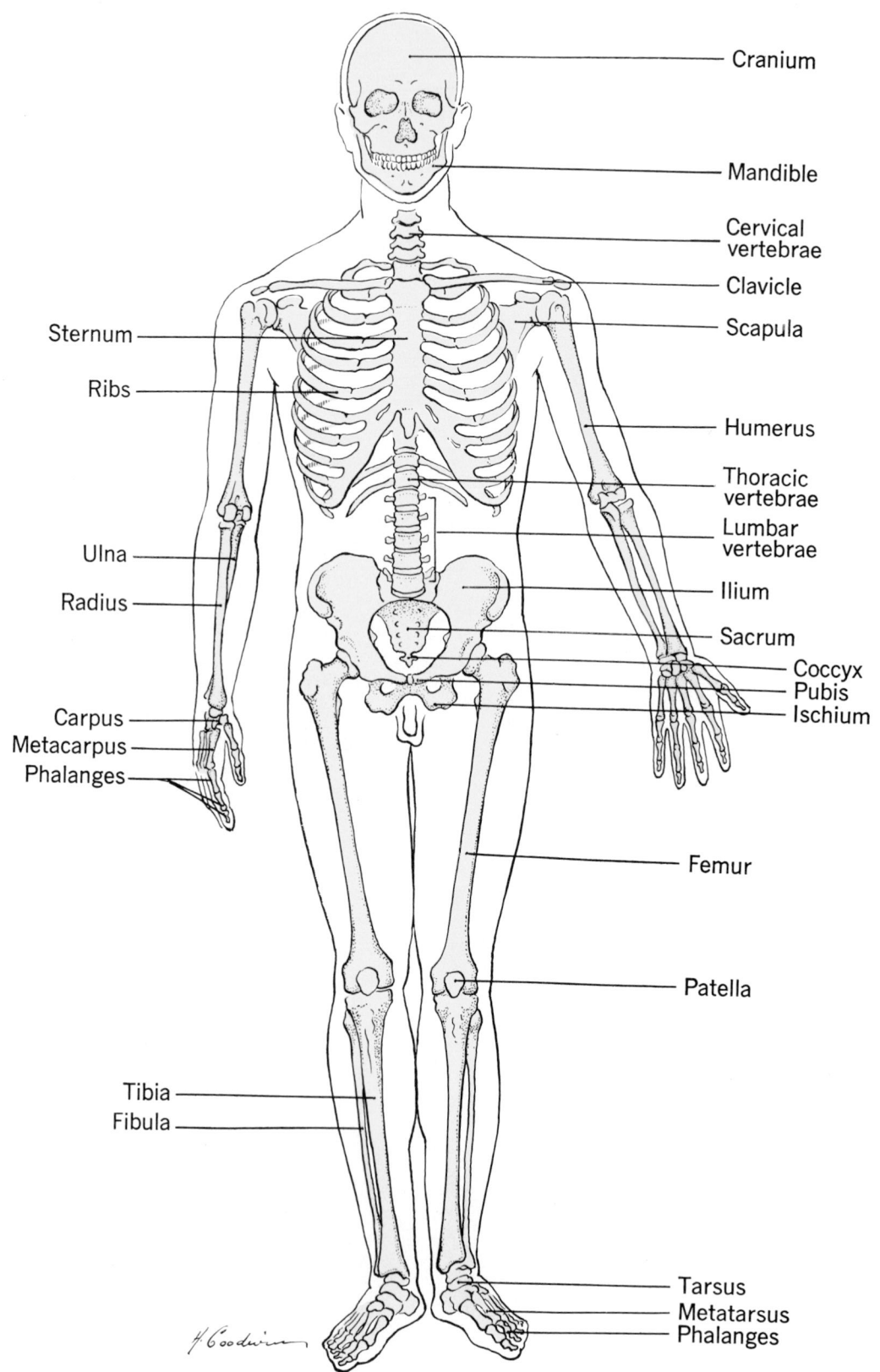

Cranium

Mandible

Cervical vertebrae

Clavicle

Scapula

Sternum

Ribs

Humerus

Thoracic vertebrae

Lumbar vertebrae

Ulna

Radius

Ilium

Sacrum

Coccyx
Pubis
Ischium

Carpus
Metacarpus
Phalanges

Femur

Patella

Tibia
Fibula

Tarsus
Metatarsus
Phalanges

**PLATE 17**

Human Skeleton, Anterior View

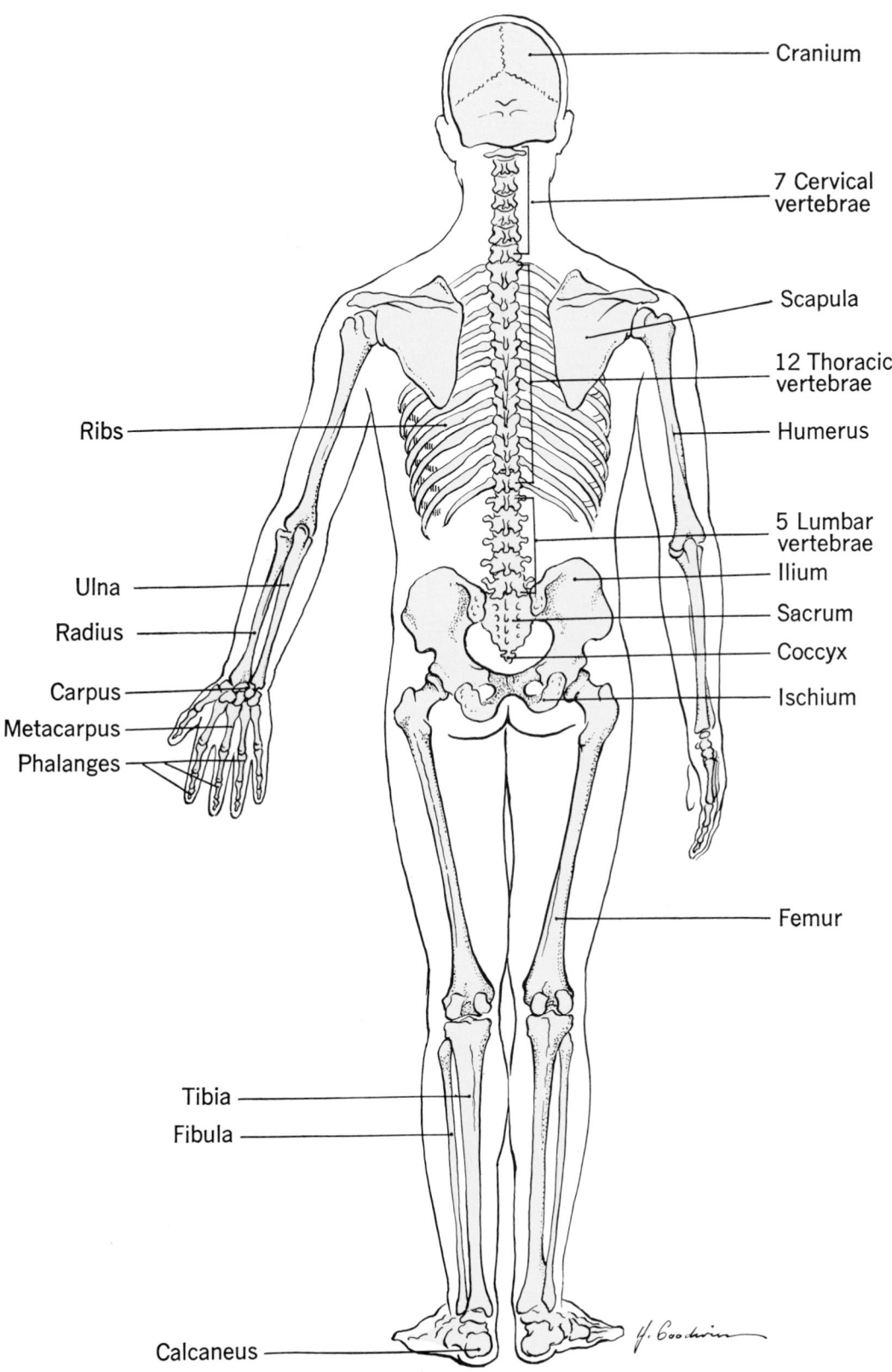

Cranium

7 Cervical
vertebrae

Scapula

12 Thoracic
vertebrae

Humerus

Ribs

5 Lumbar
vertebrae

Ilium

Ulna

Sacrum

Radius

Coccyx

Carpus

Ischium

Metacarpus

Phalanges

Femur

Tibia

Fibula

Calcaneus

**PLATE 18**

Human Skeleton, Posterior View

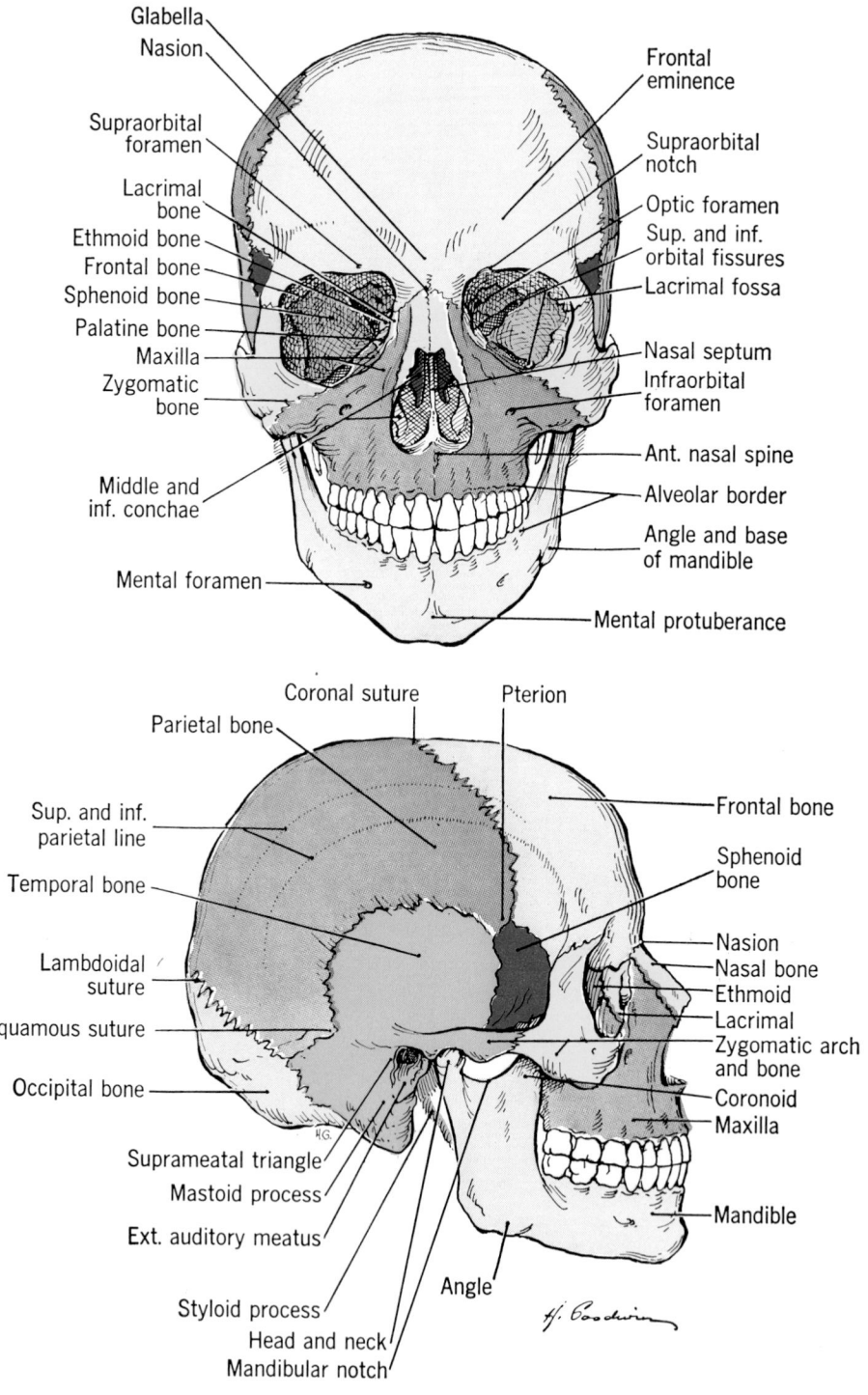

**PLATE 19**

Norma of Skull, Anterior and Lateral Views

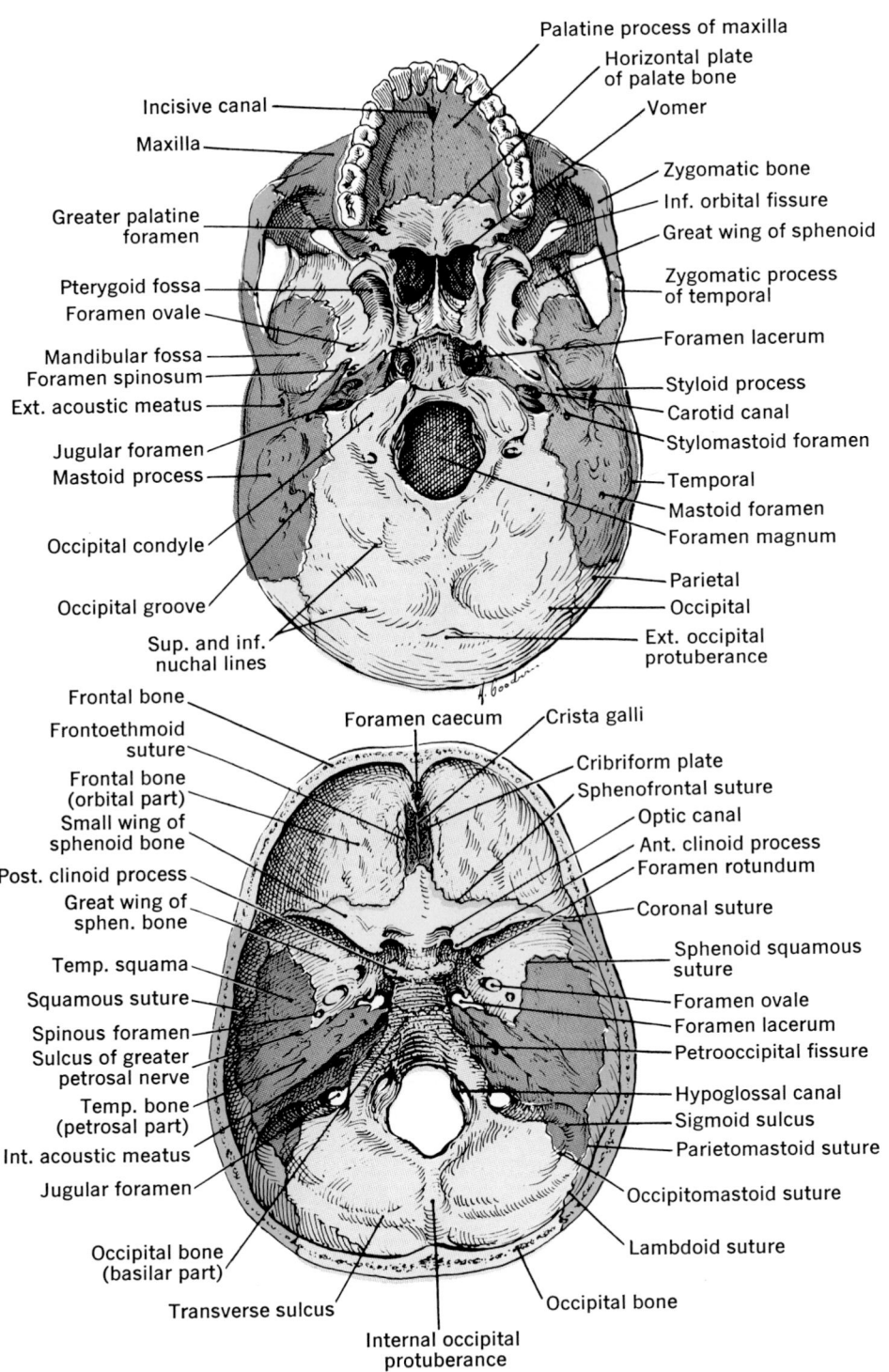

Palatine process of maxilla
Horizontal plate of palate bone
Vomer
Incisive canal
Maxilla
Zygomatic bone
Inf. orbital fissure
Great wing of sphenoid
Greater palatine foramen
Zygomatic process of temporal
Pterygoid fossa
Foramen ovale
Foramen lacerum
Mandibular fossa
Foramen spinosum
Styloid process
Ext. acoustic meatus
Carotid canal
Stylomastoid foramen
Jugular foramen
Mastoid process
Temporal
Mastoid foramen
Foramen magnum
Occipital condyle
Parietal
Occipital
Occipital groove
Ext. occipital protuberance
Sup. and inf. nuchal lines

Frontal bone
Frontoethmoid suture
Foramen caecum
Crista galli
Frontal bone (orbital part)
Cribriform plate
Sphenofrontal suture
Small wing of sphenoid bone
Optic canal
Post. clinoid process
Ant. clinoid process
Foramen rotundum
Great wing of sphen. bone
Coronal suture
Temp. squama
Sphenoid squamous suture
Squamous suture
Foramen ovale
Spinous foramen
Foramen lacerum
Sulcus of greater petrosal nerve
Petrooccipital fissure
Temp. bone (petrosal part)
Hypoglossal canal
Int. acoustic meatus
Sigmoid sulcus
Parietomastoid suture
Jugular foramen
Occipitomastoid suture
Occipital bone (basilar part)
Lambdoid suture
Transverse sulcus
Occipital bone
Internal occipital protuberance

**PLATE 20**

Base of Skull, External and Internal Views

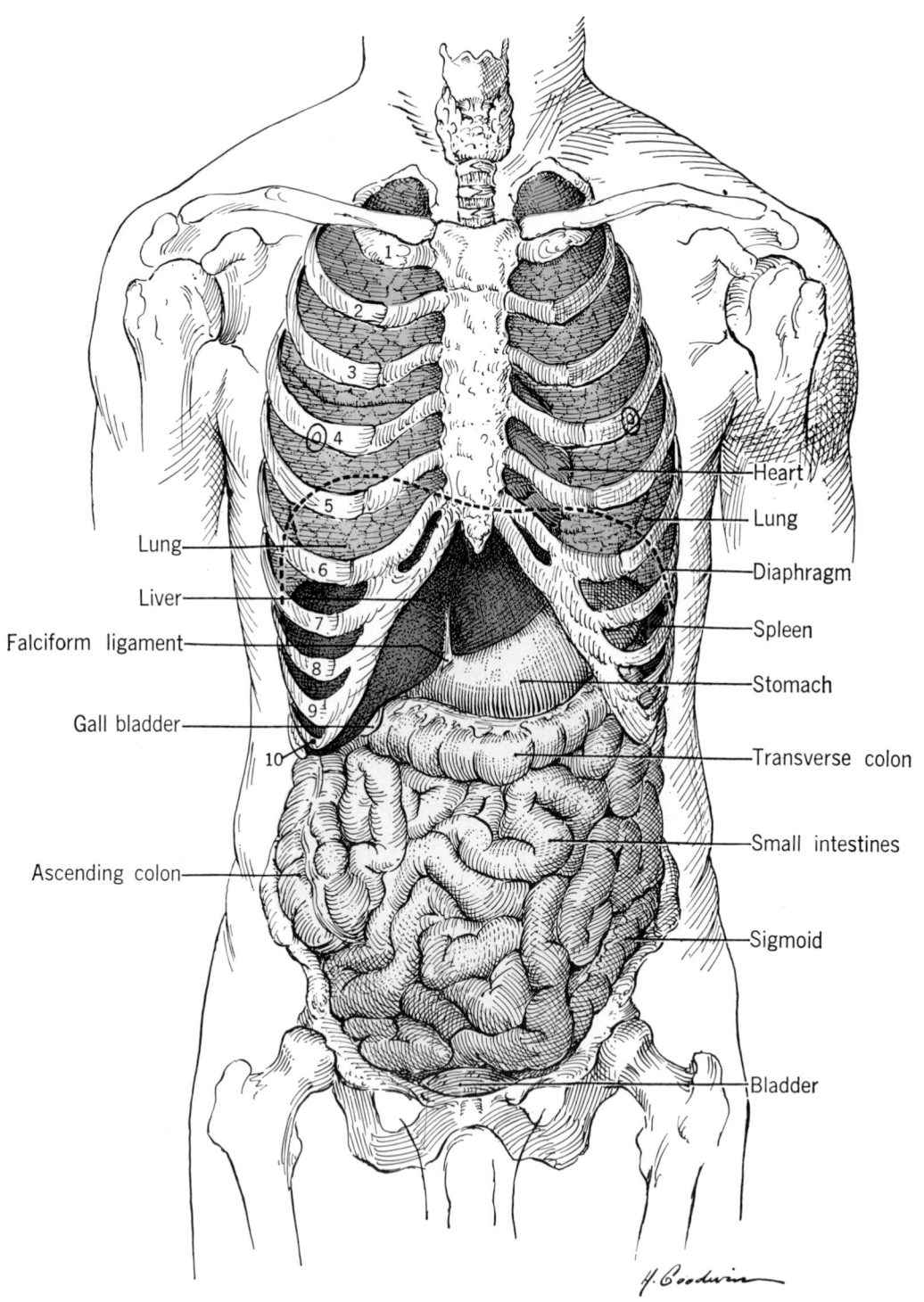

**PLATE 21**
Abdominal and Thoracic Viscera, Anterior View (After Pernkopf)

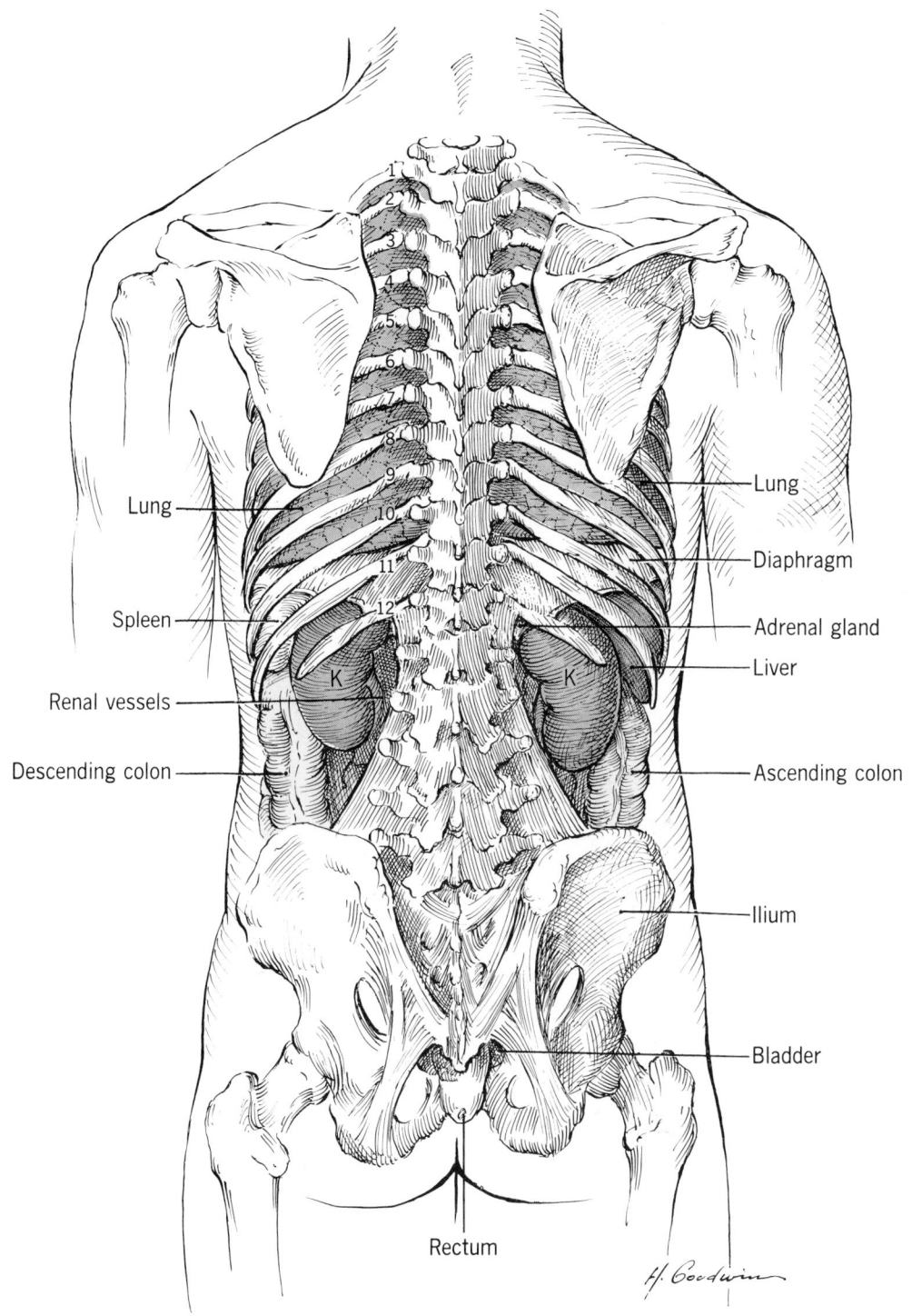

**PLATE 22**

Abdominal and Thoracic Viscera, Posterior View (After Pernkopf)

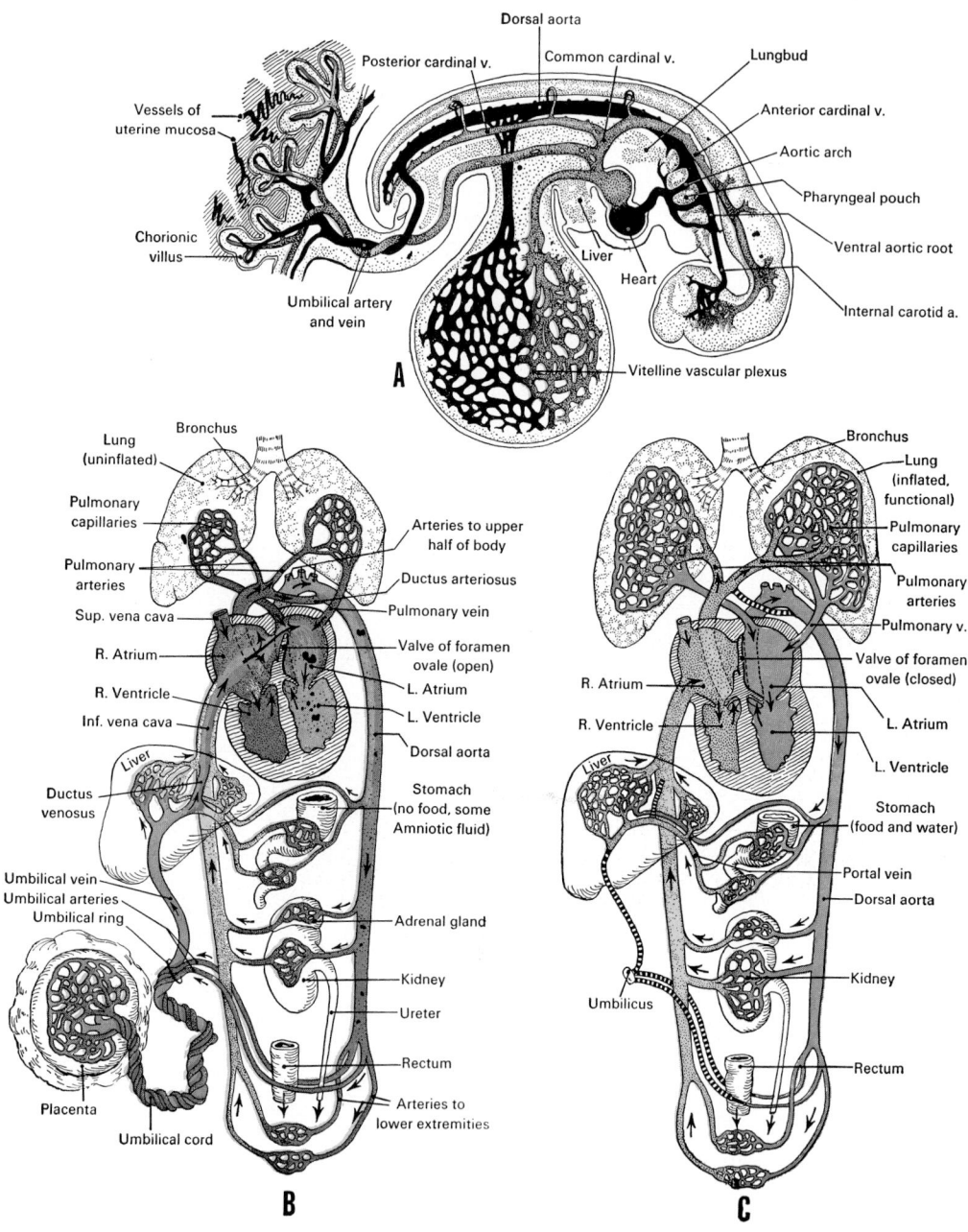

PLATE 23

Circulation

*A*, plan of early embryonic circulation; *B*, plan of fetal circulation at term; *C*, plan of the postnatal circulation. (After Patten, B. M.: *Foundations of Embryology*, Ed. 2, McGraw-Hill, Inc., New York, 1964.)

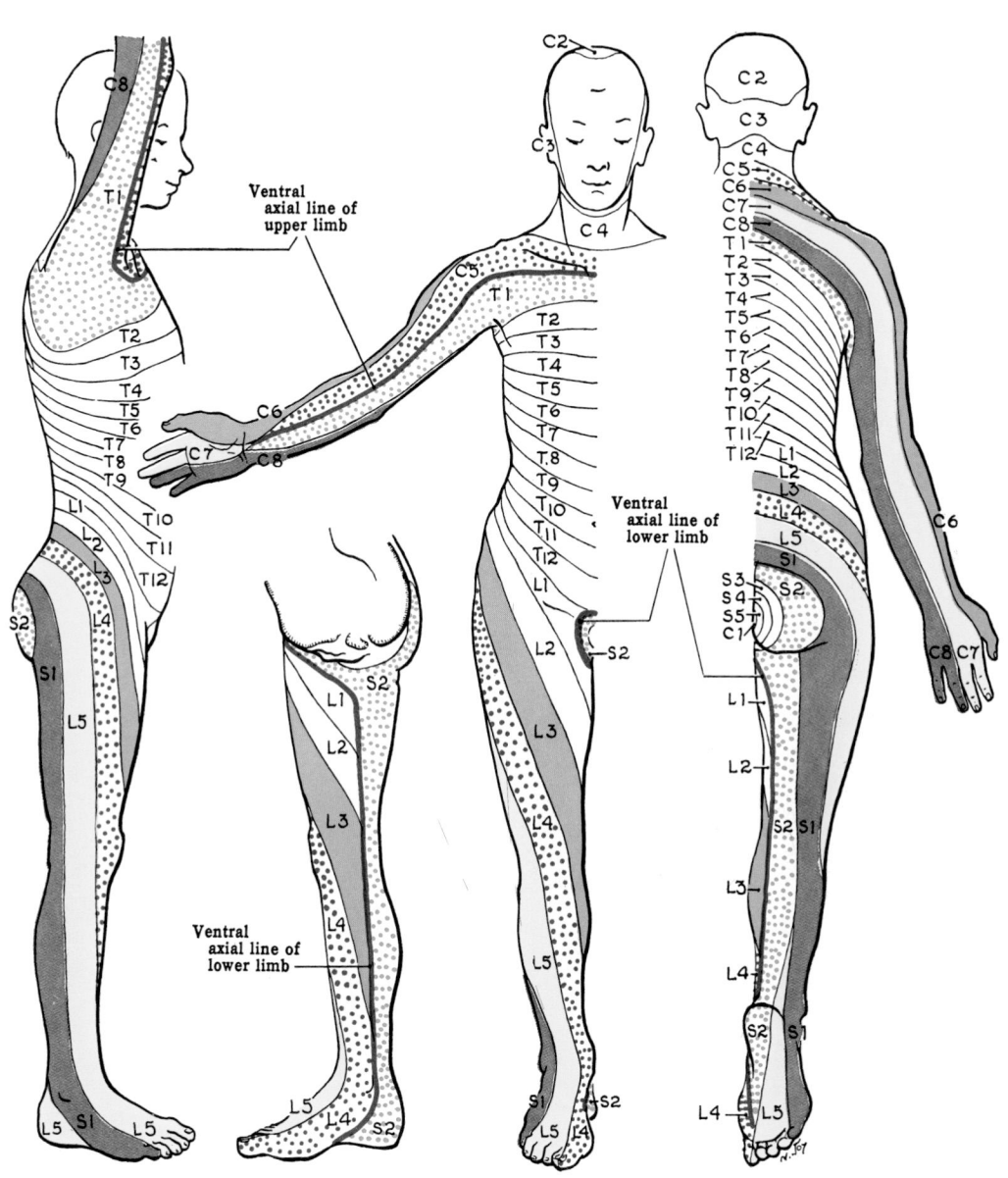

PLATE 24

Dermatomes of the Upper and Lower Limbs

(From Grant, J. C. B.: *An Atlas of Anatomy*, Ed. 5.
The Williams & Wilkins Company, 1962.)

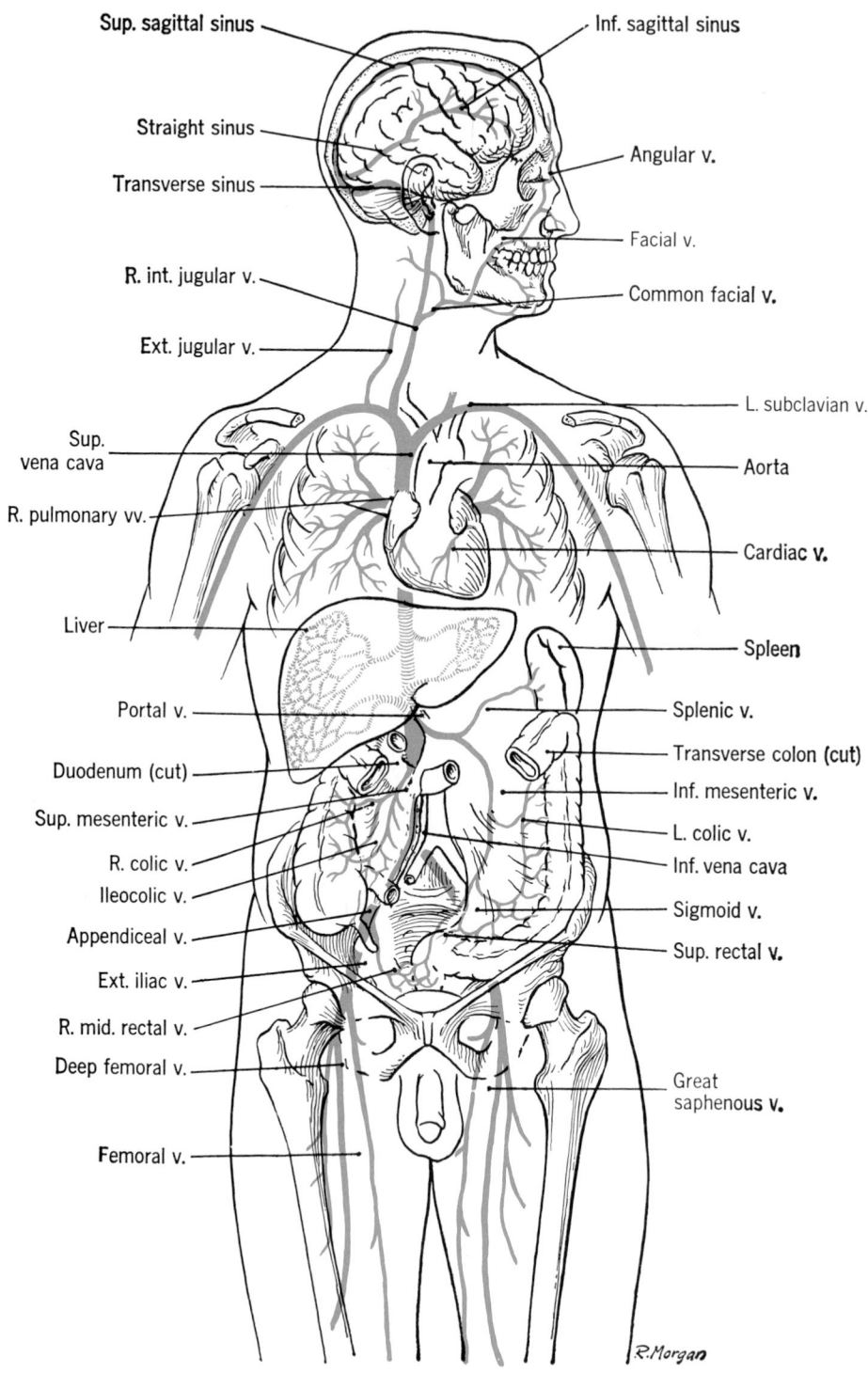

Sup. sagittal sinus — Inf. sagittal sinus

Straight sinus — Angular v.

Transverse sinus — Facial v.

R. int. jugular v. — Common facial v.

Ext. jugular v.

L. subclavian v.

Sup. vena cava — Aorta

R. pulmonary vv. — Cardiac v.

Liver — Spleen

Portal v. — Splenic v.

Duodenum (cut) — Transverse colon (cut)

Sup. mesenteric v. — Inf. mesenteric v.

R. colic v. — L. colic v.

Ileocolic v. — Inf. vena cava

Appendiceal v. — Sigmoid v.

Ext. iliac v. — Sup. rectal v.

R. mid. rectal v.

Deep femoral v. — Great saphenous v.

Femoral v.

R. Morgan

**PLATE 25**
Veins, Anterior View, Viscera Exposed

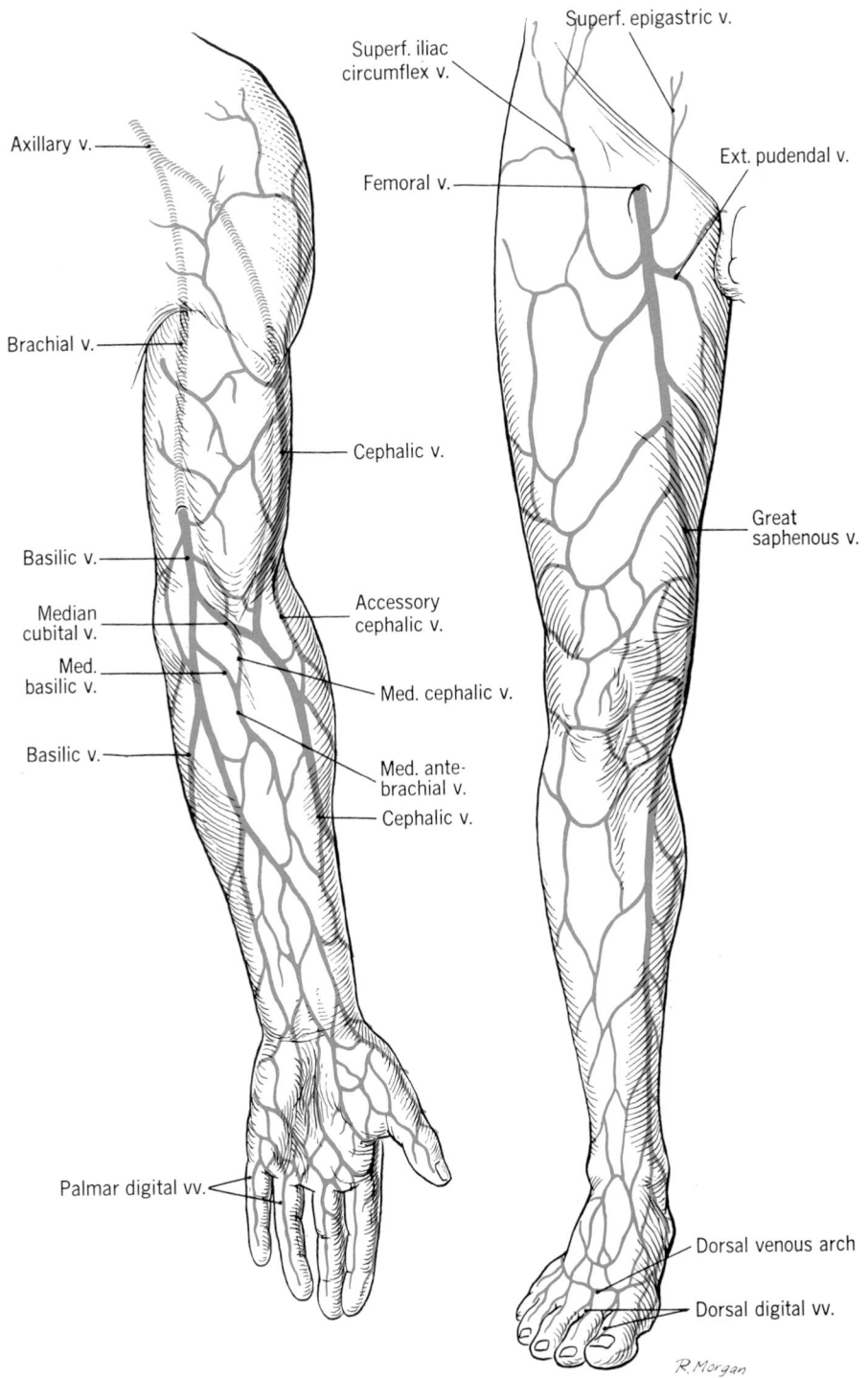

Superf. iliac circumflex v.

Superf. epigastric v.

Axillary v.

Femoral v.

Ext. pudendal v.

Brachial v.

Cephalic v.

Basilic v.

Great saphenous v.

Median cubital v.

Accessory cephalic v.

Med. basilic v.

Med. cephalic v.

Basilic v.

Med. ante-brachial v.

Cephalic v.

Palmar digital vv.

Dorsal venous arch

Dorsal digital vv.

R. Morgan

**PLATE 26**
Veins of Limbs

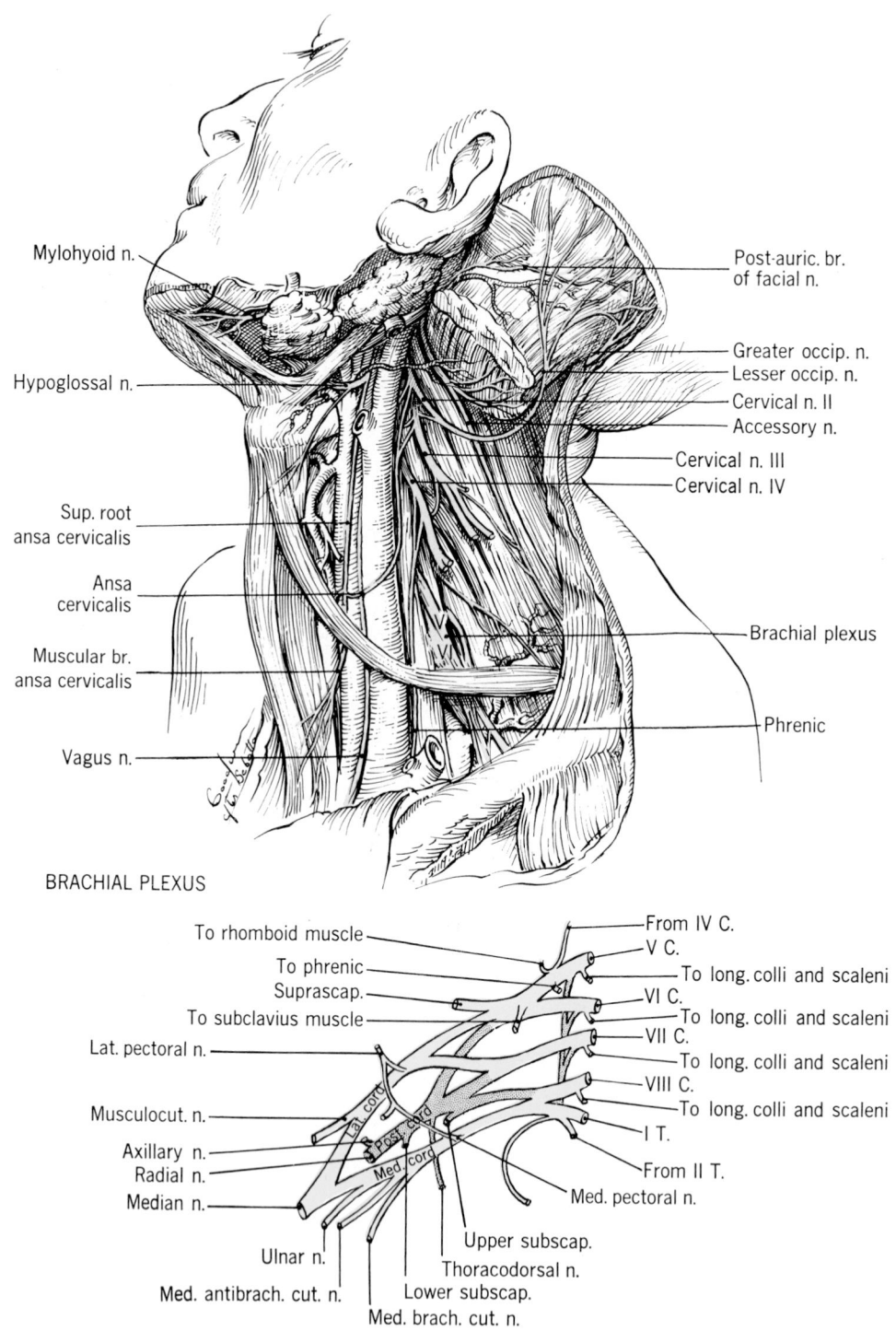

BRACHIAL PLEXUS

**PLATE 27**
Nerves of Neck and Axilla

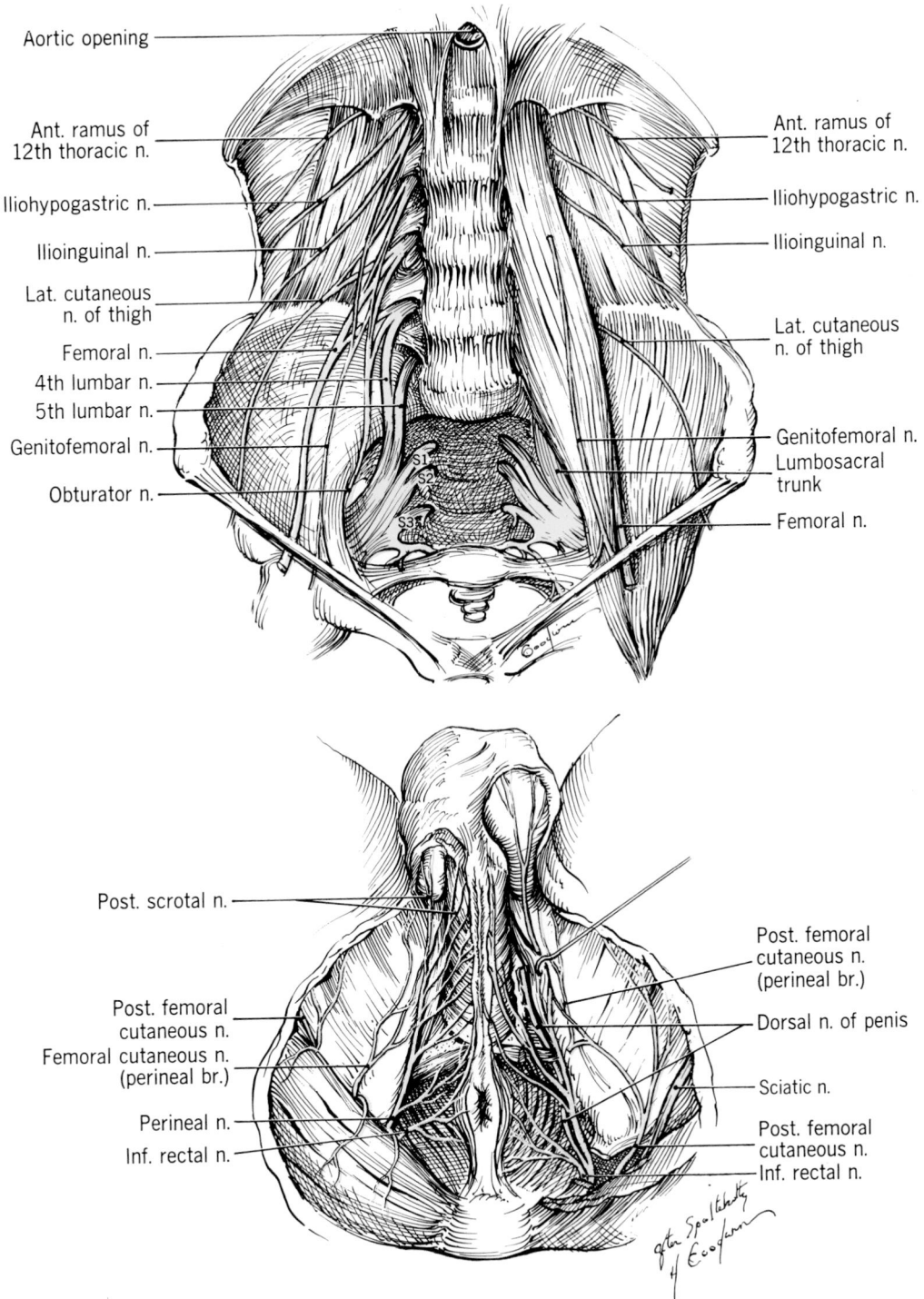

Aortic opening

Ant. ramus of
12th thoracic n.

Iliohypogastric n.

Ilioinguinal n.

Lat. cutaneous
n. of thigh

Femoral n.

4th lumbar n.

5th lumbar n.

Genitofemoral n.

Obturator n.

Ant. ramus of
12th thoracic n.

Iliohypogastric n.

Ilioinguinal n.

Lat. cutaneous
n. of thigh

Genitofemoral n.
Lumbosacral
trunk

Femoral n.

Post. scrotal n.

Post. femoral
cutaneous n.

Femoral cutaneous n.
(perineal br.)

Perineal n.

Inf. rectal n.

Post. femoral
cutaneous n.
(perineal br.)

Dorsal n. of penis

Sciatic n.

Post. femoral
cutaneous n.

Inf. rectal n.

**PLATE 28**
Nerves of Lumbar and Sacral Plexuses

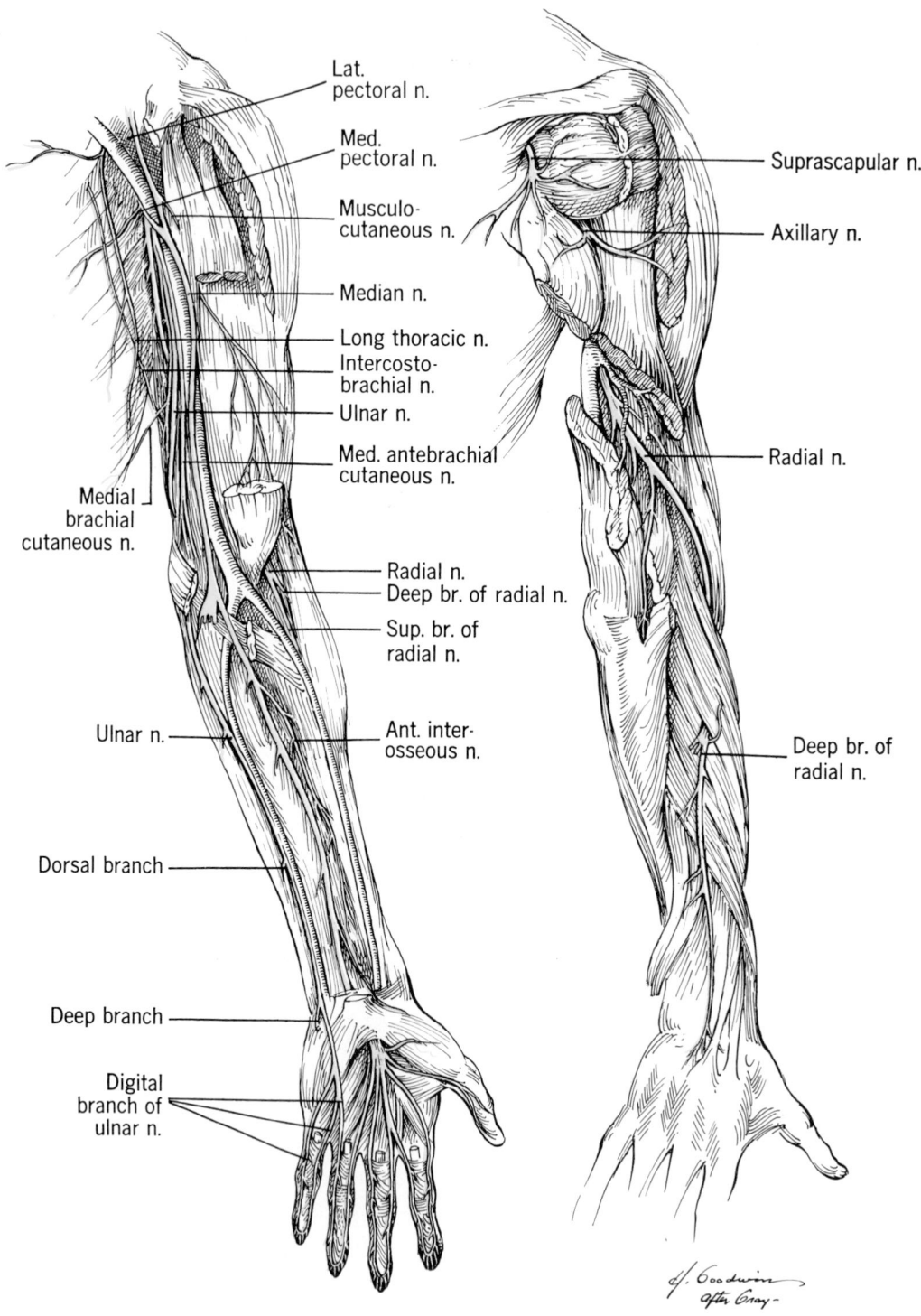

Lat. pectoral n.

Med. pectoral n.

Musculo-cutaneous n.

Median n.

Long thoracic n.

Intercosto-brachial n.

Ulnar n.

Med. antebrachial cutaneous n.

Medial brachial cutaneous n.

Radial n.
Deep br. of radial n.

Sup. br. of radial n.

Ulnar n.

Ant. inter-osseous n.

Dorsal branch

Deep branch

Digital branch of ulnar n.

Suprascapular n.

Axillary n.

Radial n.

Deep br. of radial n.

PLATE 29

Nerves of Superior Limb

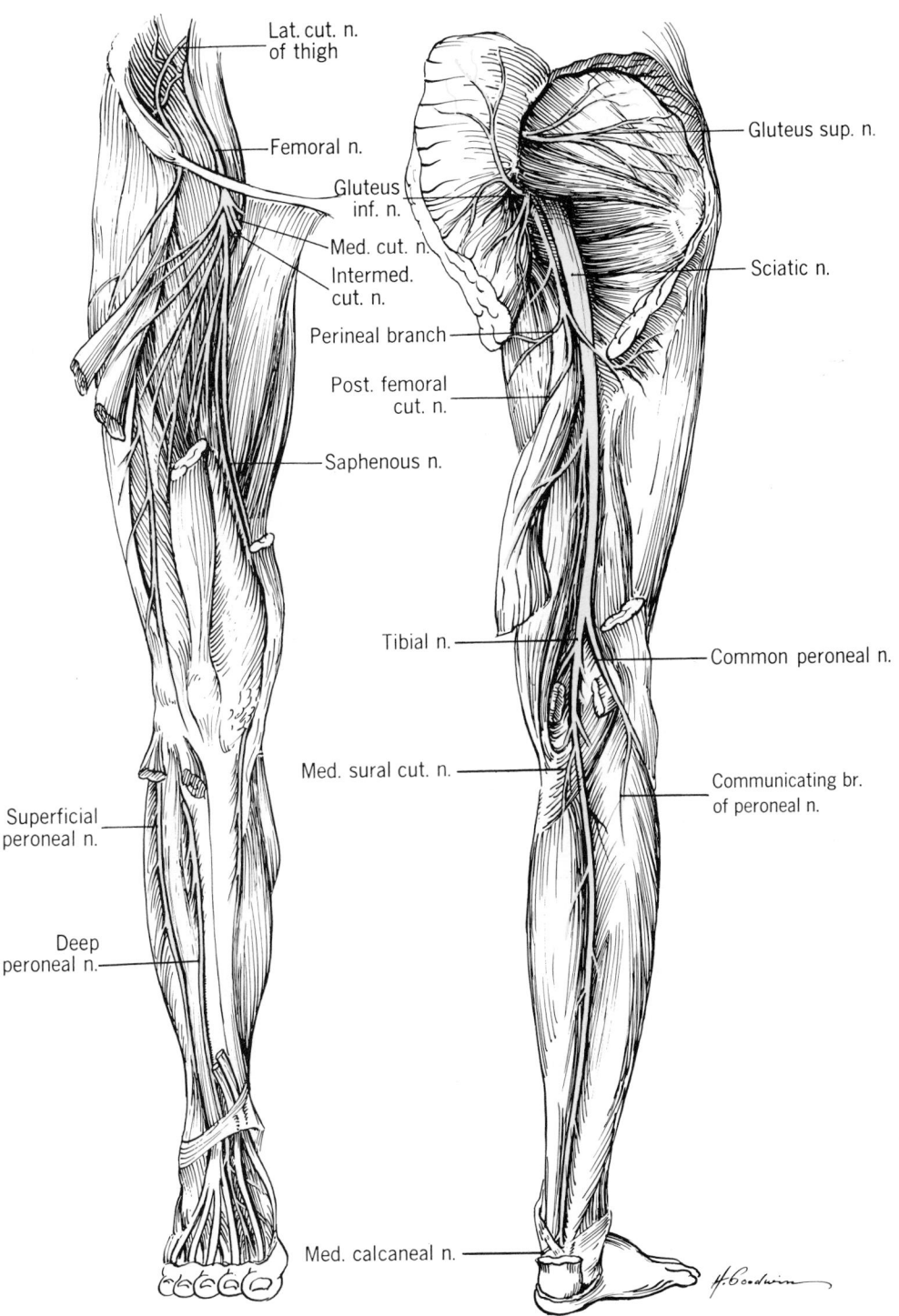

Lat. cut. n. of thigh

Femoral n.

Gluteus inf. n.

Med. cut. n.

Intermed. cut. n.

Perineal branch

Post. femoral cut. n.

Saphenous n.

Tibial n.

Med. sural cut. n.

Superficial peroneal n.

Deep peroneal n.

Med. calcaneal n.

Gluteus sup. n.

Sciatic n.

Common peroneal n.

Communicating br. of peroneal n.

H. Goodwin

**PLATE 30**

Nerves of Inferior Limb

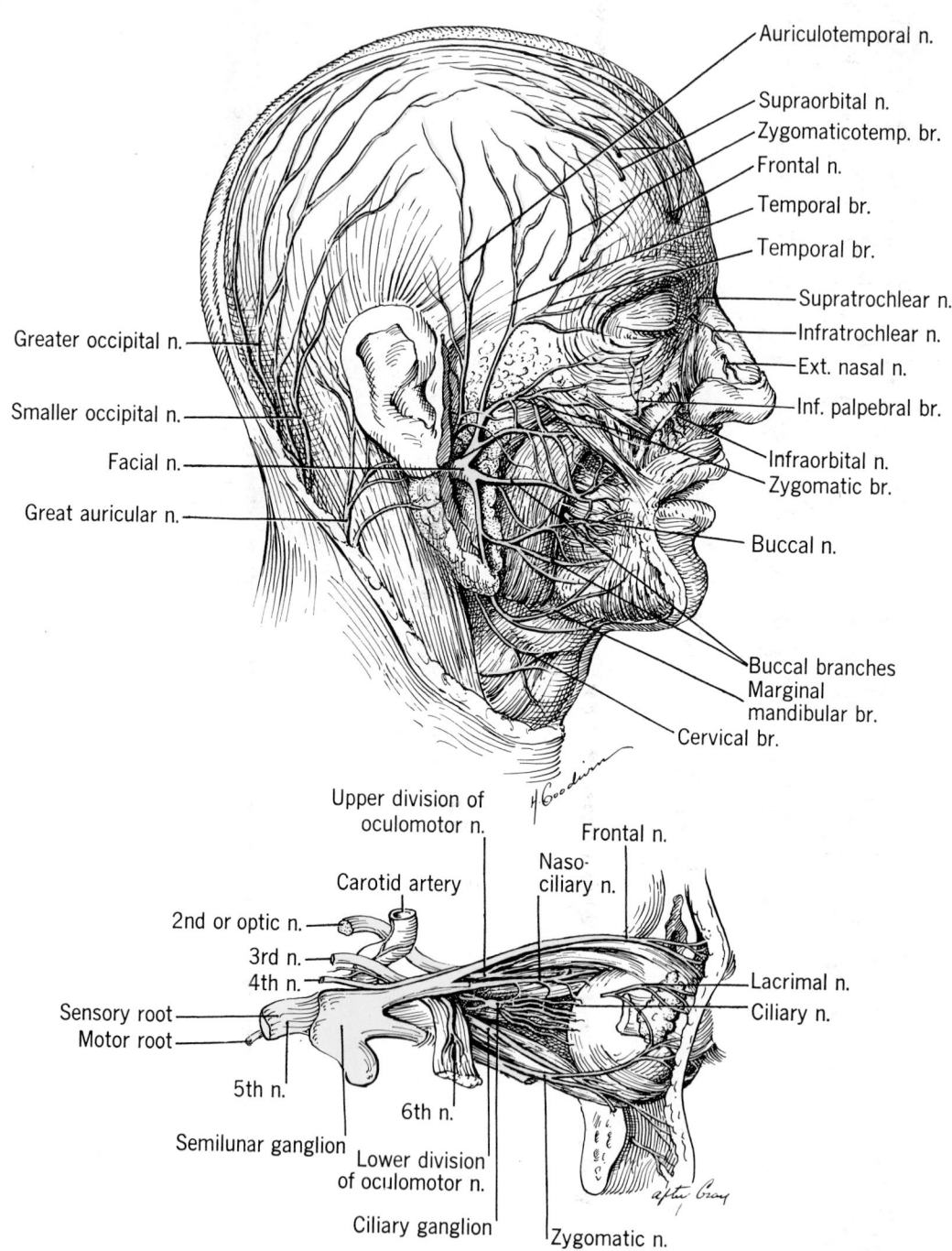

Auriculotemporal n.

Supraorbital n.
Zygomaticotemp. br.
Frontal n.
Temporal br.
Temporal br.

Supratrochlear n.
Infratrochlear n.
Ext. nasal n.
Inf. palpebral br.

Infraorbital n.
Zygomatic br.

Buccal n.

Greater occipital n.

Smaller occipital n.

Facial n.

Great auricular n.

Buccal branches
Marginal
mandibular br.
Cervical br.

Upper division of
oculomotor n.

Frontal n.

Naso-
ciliary n.

Carotid artery

2nd or optic n.

3rd n.
4th n.

Lacrimal n.
Ciliary n.

Sensory root
Motor root

5th n.

6th n.

Semilunar ganglion

Lower division
of oculomotor n.

Ciliary ganglion

Zygomatic n.

PLATE 31

Nerves of Head and Orbit

**libidinous** (lĭ-bid'ĭ-nus) [ L. *libidinosus*, fr. *libido* (*libidin-*), pleasure, desire, fr. *libet*, it pleases ]. Lascivious; erotic; invested with or arousing sexual desire or energy.

**libido** (lĭ-be'do, lĭ-bi'do) [ L. lust ]. 1. Conscious or unconscious sexual desire. 2. Creative energy; *élan vital;* any passionate interest or form of life force. 3. In Jungian psychology, synonymous with psychic *energy* (*q.v.*).

**object l.,** l. invested in the object, in contradistinction to that invested in the ego.

**Libman,** Emanuel, New York physician, 1872–1946. See L.-Sacks *endocarditis, syndrome.*

**Liborius' method.** See under method.

**lice.** Plural of louse.

**lichen** (li'ken) [ G. *leichēn*, lichen; a lichen-like eruption ]. A discrete flat papule or an aggregate of papules giving a patterned configuration resembling lichens growing on rocks.

**l. acumina'tus,** l. planus.

**l. a'grius,** Celsus' papules; acute papular eczema of severe type.

**l. al'bus,** chronic lichenoid dermatitis with depigmentation.

**l. annula'ris,** *granuloma* annulare.

**l. hemorrhag'icus,** a papular eruption due to hemorrhage into the hair follicles.

**l. infan'tum,** *miliaria* rubra.

**l. iris,** ringworm with concentric rings of erythematous papules.

**l. myxedemato'sus,** scleromyxedema; papular mucinosis; a lichenoid eruption of papules or plaques of mucinous edema of the skin in the absence of endocrine disease.

**l. nitidus,** Pinkus' disease; groups of small whitish or pinkish papules; lesions, which are flat-topped, may form linear groups. May involve male genitalia.

**l. nu'chae,** 1. simplex of the neck, usually in women.

**l. obtu'sus,** a form in which the papules are large and rounded instead of flattened.

**l. planopila'ris,** l. planus follicularis.

**l. planus,** l. acuminatus; l. ruber planus; Wilson's l.; eruption of flat-topped, shiny, violaceous papules on flexor surfaces, male genitalia, and buccal mucosa; may form linear groups; individual lesions may be angular or umbilicated; hypertrophic lesions may form on legs.

**l. planus annula'ris,** a form in which the papules are grouped in ring figures.

**l. pla'nus follicula'ris,** l. planopilaris; l. planus of the hair follicles, usually of the scalp.

**l. planus hypertrophicus,** l. planus verrucosus; l. ruber verrucosus; verrucoid or warty lesions occurring on legs and thighs in association with l. planus elsewhere.

**l. planus, oral (erosive),** an oral disease characterized by raw, reddened, painful mucosal lesions with more typical evidences of lichen planus surrounding the eroded areas.

**l. planus, oral (nonerosive),** an oral disease characterized clinically by lesions appearing as a network of fine or thick, violaceous, interlacing lines (Wickham's striae) forming a wide variety of patterns on the oral mucosa.

**l. planus verruco'sus,** l. planus hypertrophicus.

**l. ruber,** an old term originally used to refer to what is presently called l. planus.

**l. ruber moniliformis,** a rare dermatosis consisting of small reddish papules arranged in narrow beaded bands and covering large areas of the body.

**l. ruber planus,** l. planus.

**l. ruber verrucosus,** l. planus hypertrophicus.

**l. sclero'sus et atro'phicus,** Hallopeau's disease (3); an eruption consisting of white atrophic papules; the lesions may be discrete or confluent, and may contain a central depression or a black keratotic plug; often associated with kraurosis vulvae.

**l. scrofulosorum,** papular *tuberculid.*

**l. sim'plex,** Vidal's disease; a small, intensely pruritic, lichenified area in the skin.

**l. spinulosus,** eruption of conical papules which have an adherent scaly surface. Cause is unknown; may be related to l. planus.

**l. stria'tus,** a self-limited papular eruption occurring primarily in children; the lesions are arranged in linear groups and occur on one of the extremities.

**l. strophulo'sus,** *miliaria* rubra.

**l. syphilit'icus,** follicular *syphilid.*

**tropical l., l. tropicus,** *miliaria* rubra.

**l. urticatus,** prurigo infantilis; papular urticaria; urticaria papulosa; a type of papular urticaria occurring in children. Lesions are papules, or small papules and vesicles.

**l. variega'tus** maculopapular *erythroderma.*

**Wilson's l.,** l. planus.

**lichenification** (li'ken-if-ĭ-ka'shun) [ lichen + L. *facio*, to make ]. Lichenization; leathery induration and thickening of the skin due to a chronic inflammation caused by scratching or long-continued irritation.

**licheniformin** (li'ken-ĭ-for'min). One of three antibiotic peptids, A, B, and C, obtained from *Bacillus licheniformis*, moderately active against the tubercle bacillus.

**lichenin** (li'ken-in). Moss starch; a variety of starch obtained from Iceland moss. Used as a demulcent.

**licheniza'tion** (li'ken-ĭ-za'shun). Lichenification.

**lichenoid** (li'ken-oyd). 1. Resembling lichen. 2. Accentuation of normal skin markings observed in cases of chronic eczema.

**Lichtheim** (likht'hīm), Ludwig, German physician, 1845–1928. See Déjerine-L. *phenomenon*, L.'s *sign.*

**licorice** (lik'o-ris). Glycyrrhiza.

**lid** [ A.S. *hlid* ]. Eyelid.

**granular l.'s,** trachoma (1).

**Liddel-Sherrington reflex.** See under reflex.

**lidocaine hydrochloride** (li'do-kān) (USP). XYLOCAINE hydrochloride; lignocaine hydrochloride; diethylamino-2,6-acetoxylidide hydrochloride; a local anesthetic similar in action to procaine hydrochloride but more potent, and possessing pronounced antiarrhythmic and anticonvulsant properties.

**lidofla'zine** (USAN). CLINIUM; 4-[ 4,4-bis(*p*-fluorophenyl)butyl ]-1-piperazineaceto-2',6'-xylidide; coronary vasodilator.

**lie.** The relation which the long axis of the fetus bears to that of the mother.

**longitudinal l.,** that relationship in which the long axis of the fetus is longitudinal and roughly parallel to the long axis of the mother. The presenting part may be either the head or the breech.

**oblique l.,** that relationship in which the fetal axis crosses the maternal axis at an angle (other than a right angle).

**transverse l.,** that relationship in which the long axis of the fetus is transverse or at right angles to that of the mother.

**Lieberkühn** (le'ber-kün), Johann N., German anatomist, 1711–1756. See L.'s *crypts, follicles, glands.*

**lieberkühn** (le'ber-kün) [ J. N. *Lieberkühn* ]. A concave reflector around the objective of a microscope, for the purpose of directing a concentrated beam of light on the material being examined.

**Liebermann** (le'ber-mahn), Leo von S., Hungarian physician, 1852–1926. See Burchard-L. *reaction, test.*

**Liebermeister** (le'ber-mīs-ter), Carl von, German physician, 1833–1901. See L.'s *rule.*

**Liebig** (le'big), Baron Justus von, German chemist, 1803–1873. See L.'s *theory.*

**lie detector.** Polygraph (2).

**li'en** [ L. ] [ NA ]. Spleen.

**l. accesso'rius** [ NA ], accessory spleen; l. succenturiatus; splenculus; splenule; spleneolus; spleniculus; splenunculus; splenulus; lienculus; one of the small globular masses of splenic tissue occasionally found in the neighborhood of the spleen, in one of the peritoneal folds or elsewhere.

**l. mobilis,** floating *spleen.*

**l. succenturia'tus,** l. accessorius.

**lien-, lieno-** (li'en, li'ĕ-no-, li-e'no-) [ L. *lien*, spleen ]. Combining form relating to the spleen. Most terms beginning thus are obsolete or obsolescent, the preferred combining forms being splen- and spleno-.

**lienal** (li'ĕ-nal). Splenic.

**lienculus** (li-en'ku-lus) [ Mod. L. dim. of L. *lien*, spleen ]. *Lien* accessorius.

**lienectomy** (li'ĕ-nek'to-mĭ). Obsolete term for splenectomy.

**lienitis** (li'ĕ-ni'tis). Obsolete term for splenitis.

**lienography** (li'ĕ-nog'rǎ-fĭ). Splenography.

**lienomedullary** (li'ě-no-med'u-lěr-ĭ) [lieno- + G. *medulla,* marrow]. Splenomyelogenous.

**lienomyelogenous** (li'ě-no-mi-ě-loj'ě-nus). Splenomyelogenous.

**lienopancreatic** (li'ě-no-pan'kre-at'ik). Splenopancreatic.

**lienopathy** (li'ě-nop'ǎ-thĭ). Obsolete term for splenopathy.

**li'enore'nal** [lieno- + L. *ren,* kidney]. Splenonephric; splenorenal; relating to the spleen and the kidney.

**lienotoxin** (li'ě-no-tok'sin). [L. *lien,* spleen]. Splenotoxin.

**lienteric** (li-en-těr'ik). Relating to, or marked by, lientery.

**lientery** (li'en-těr-ĭ) [G. *leienteria,* fr. *leios,* smooth, + *enteron,* intestine]. The passage of undigested food in the stools.

**lienunculus** (li'ě-nun'ku-lus) [Mod. L. dim. of L. *lien,* spleen]. *Lien* accessorius.

**Liesegang** (le'seg-ahng), Ralph E., German chemist, 1869–1947. See L. *rings.*

**Lieutaud** (le-ě-to'), Joseph, French physician, 1703–1780. See L.'s *body, triangle, trigone, uvula.*

**life** [A.S. *lif*]. Vitality; the essential condition of being alive; or existence of animals and plants; the state of existence characterized by active metabolism.

**postnatal l.,** that stretch of l. after birth; in man, usually divided into periods: neonatal, infancy, childhood, adolescence, and adulthood.

**prenatal l.,** that stretch of l. between conception and birth; in man, usually divided into embryonic and fetal periods.

**sexual l.,** vita sexualis; in psychiatry and psychoanalysis, the specifically erotic or sexual interests, fantasies, inclinations, and conduct of the patient.

**vegetative l.,** the simple metabolic and reproductive activity of man or animals, apart from the exercise of conscious mental or psychic processes.

**life-span.** 1. The duration of existence of an individual. 2. The normal or average duration of existence of a given species; see also longevity.

# LIGAMENT

**ligament** (lig'ă-ment) [L. *ligamentum,* a band, bandage. LIG-]. 1. A band or sheet of fibrous tissue connecting two or more bones, cartilages, or other structures, or serving as support for fasciae or muscles. See also table of ligamenta. 2. A fold of peritoneum supporting any of the abdominal viscera. 3. Any structure resembling a l. though not performing the function of such. 4. The cordlike remains of a fetal artery or other structure that has lost its original lumen.

**accessory l.'s,** l.'s about a joint that are in addition to the articular capsule. They may lie within, or on the outside of the latter.

**accessory plantar l.'s,** *ligamenta* plantaria.

**accessory volar l.'s,** *ligamenta* palmaria.

**acro'mioclavic'ular l.,** *ligamentum* acromioclaviculare.

**a'lar l.'s,** (1) *ligamenta* alaria; (2) *plicae* alares.

**alveolodental l.,** periodontium.

**an'nular l.,** orbicular l.; one of a number of l.'s encircling various parts; the principal annular l.'s are those of the stapes, digitorum manus, digitorum pedis, radius, trachea. See under *ligamentum* anulare.

**anococcygeal l.,** *ligamentum* anococcygeum.

**anterior costotransverse l.,** *ligamentum* costotransversarium superius.

**anterior l. of head of fibula,** *ligamentum* capitis fibulae anterius.

**anterior l. of malleus,** *ligamentum* mallei anterius.

**anterior sac'rosciat'ic l.,** *ligamentum* sacrospinale.

**anterior talofibular l.,** *ligamentum* talofibulare anterius.

**anterior talotib'ial l.,** *ligamentum* deltoideum.

**anterior tibiofibular l.,** *ligamentum* tibiofibularis anterius.

**apical l. of the dens,** *ligamentum* apicis dentis.

**Arantius' l.,** *ligamentum* venosum.

**arcuate popliteal l.,** *ligamentum* popliteum arcuatum.

**arcuate pubic l.,** *ligamentum* arcuatum pubis.

**arterial l.,** *ligamentum* arteriosum.

**l.'s of auditory ossicles,** *ligamenta* ossiculorum auditus.

**auric'ular l.'s,** *ligamenta* auricularia.

**axis l. of malleus,** *ligamentum* mallei laterale.

**Bardinet's l.,** the posterior band of the ulnar collateral l. of the elbow.

**Barkow's l.,** the l.'s on the anterior and posterior aspects of the elbow joint.

**Bellini's l.,** a fasciculus of the articular capsule l. of the hip extending to the great trochanter.

**Berry's l.,** the lateral l.'s of the thyroid gland.

**Bertin's l.,** *ligamentum* iliofemorale.

**Bichat's l.,** the lower fasciculus of the posterior sacroiliac l.

**bi'furcated l.,** *ligamentum* bifurcatum.

**Bigelow's l.,** *ligamentum* iliofemorale.

**Botallo's l.,** *ligamentum* arteriosum.

**Bourgery's l.,** *ligamentum* popliteum obliquum.

**broad l. of the uterus,** *ligamentum* latum uteri.

**Brodie's l.,** transverse humeral l.

**Burns' l.,** *cornu* superius (2).

**calca'neocu'boid l.,** *ligamentum* calcaneocuboideum.

**calcaneofib'ular l.,** *ligamentum* calcaneofibulare.

**calca'neonavic'ular l.,** *ligamentum* calcaneonaviculare.

**calcaneotib'ial l.,** see *ligamentum* deltoideum.

**Caldani's l.,** *ligamentum* coracoclaviculare.

**Campbell's l.,** suspensory l. of axilla.

**Camper's l.,** *fascia* diaphragmatic urogenitalis inferior.

**capsular l.,** thickened portions of the fibrous membrane of an articular capsule.

**cardinal l.,** one of several fibrous bands running through the base of the broad l. of the uterus beside the vessels and nerves.

**carot'icocli'noid l.,** connects the anterior to the middle clinoid process of the sphenoid bone.

**carpometacarpal l.'s.** *ligamenta* carpometacarpea.

**caudal l.,** *retinaculum* caudale.

**cemental l.,** periodontium.

**cervical l. of the uterus,** Mackenrodt's l.; ligamentum transversalis colli; a fibrous band attached to the uterine cervix and the vault of the lateral fornix of the vagina; continuous with the tissue ensheathing the pelvic vessels.

**check l.'s of eyeball, medial and lateral,** expansions of the sheaths of the medial and lateral rectus muscles of the eyeball which are attached, respectively, to the lacrimal bone and to the orbital (Whitnall's) eminence of the zygomatic bone. They serve to prevent overaction of these muscles.

**check l.'s of odontoid,** *ligamenta* alaria.

**chon'droxiph'oid l.,** *ligamentum* costoxiphoideum.

**cil'iary l.,** *musculus* ciliaris.

**Civinini's l.,** *ligamentum* pterygospinale.

**Clado's l.,** a mesenteric fold running from the broad l. on the right side to the appendix.

**collateral l.'s,** *ligamenta* collateralia.

**Colles' l.,** *ligamentum* reflexum.

**conjugate l.,** ligamentum conjugale; a l. in some mammals which is the homologue of the intraarticular l. present in the joints between the heads of the ribs and the vertebrae.

**conoid l.,** *ligamentum* conoideum.

**Cooper's l.'s,** (1) *ligamenta* suspensoria mammae; (2) *ligamentum* pectineale; (3) *chorda* obliqua.

**cor'acoacro'mial l.,** *ligamentum* coracoacromiale.

**coracoclavic'ular l.,** *ligamentum* coracoclaviculare.

**coracohu'meral l.,** *ligamentum* coracohumerale.

**cornic'ulopharyn'geal l.,** ligamentum jugale; cricosantorinian l.; an elastic band connecting the tip of the corniculate (Santorini's) cartilage and the lamina of the cricoid cartilage, which is attached also to the wall of the pharynx.

**coronary l. of the knee,** portions of the articular capsule of the knee joint which connect the circumference of a semilunar cartilage with the margins of the condyles of the tibia.

**coronary l. of the liver,** *ligamentum* coronarium hepatis.

**costoclavic'ular l.,** *ligamentum* costoclaviculare.

**costocolic l.,** *ligamentum* phrenicocolicum.

**cos'totrans'verse l.,** *ligamentum* costotransversarium.

**costoxiphoid l.,** *ligamentum* costoxiphoideum.

**cotyloid l.,** *labrum* acetabulare.

**cricopharyn′geal l.,** *ligamentum* cricopharyngeum.

**cricosantorin′ian l.,** corniculopharyngeal l.

**cricothy′roid l.,** *ligamentum* cricothyroideum.

**cricotra′cheal l.,** *ligamentum* cricotracheale.

**crucial l.,** (1) *retinaculum* musculorum extensorum; (2) *ligamentum* cruciatum genus; (3) *ligamentum* cruciforme atlantis; (4) *pars* cruciformis vaginae fibrosae.

   **cruciate l. of the atlas,** *ligamentum* cruciforme atlantis.

   **cruciate l.'s of the knee,** *ligamenta* cruciata genus.

   **cruciate l. of the leg,** *retinaculum* musculorum extensorum inferius.

**cru′ciform l.,** *ligamentum* cruciforme atlantis.

**Cruveilhier's l.'s,** the glenoid or plantar l.'s of the metatarsophalangeal articulations.

**cuboideonavic′ular l.,** *ligamentum* cuboideonaviculare.

**cuneocu′boid l.,** *ligamentum* cuneocuboideum.

**cu′neonavic′ular l.'s,** *ligamenta* cuneonavicularia.

**cystoduode′nal l.,** a peritoneal fold that sometimes passes from the gallbladder to the first part of the duodenum.

**deep dorsal sacrococcygeal l.,** *ligamentum* sacrococcygeum dorsale profundum.

**deep transverse metacarpal l.,** *ligamentum* metacarpeum transversum profundum.

**deep transverse metatarsal l.,** *ligamentum* metatarseum transversum profundum.

**deltoid l.,** *ligamentum* deltoideum.

**Denonvilliers' l.,** *ligamentum* puboprostaticum.

**dental l.,** the part of the peridental membrane that surrounds the neck of a tooth.

**dentic′ulate l.,** *ligamentum* denticulatum.

**Denucé's l.,** *ligamentum* quadratum.

**diaphragmatic l. of the mesonephros,** that segment of the urogenital ridge which extends from the mesonephros to the diaphragm.

**dorsal carpal l.,** *retinaculum* extensorum manus.

**dorsal carpometacarpal l.'s,** *ligamenta* carpometacarpea dorsalia.

**dorsal radiocarpal l.,** *ligamentum* radiocarpeum dorsale.

**dorsal sacroiliac l.'s,** *ligamenta* sacroiliaca dorsalia.

**l. of epidid′ymis,** *ligamentum* epididymidis.

**epihyal l.,** *ligamentum* stylohyoideum.

**external collateral l. of the wrist,** *ligamentum* collaterale carpi radiale.

**extracapsular l.'s,** *ligamenta* extracapsularia.

**falciform l.,** *processus* falciformis.

**falciform l. of liver,** *ligamentum* falciforme hepatis.

**Fallopian l.,** *ligamentum* inguinale.

**Ferrein's l.,** *ligamentum* laterale articulationis temporomandibularis.

**fibular collateral l.,** *ligamentum* collaterale fibulare.

**Flood's l.,** a band of the ligamentum coracohumerale, attached to the lower part of the lesser tuberosity of the humerus.

**fundiform l. of foot,** Retzius' l.

**fundiform l. of penis,** *ligamentum* fundiforme penis.

**gastrocolic l.,** *ligamentum* gastrocolicum.

**gastrodiaphragmatic l.,** *ligamentum* gastrophrenicum.

**gastrolienal l.,** *ligamentum* gastrolienale.

**gastrophren′ic l.,** *ligamentum* gastrophrenicum.

**gastrosplen′ic l.,** *ligamentum* gastrolienale.

**genital l.,** an embryonic mesenchymatous band providing support for the internal genitalia.

**genitoinguinal l.,** *ligamentum* genitoinguinale.

**Gerdy's l.,** suspensory l. of axilla.

**Gillette's suspensory l.,** *tendo* cricoesophageus.

**Gimbernat's l.,** *ligamentum* lacunare.

**gingivoden′tal l.,** periodontium.

**glenohu′meral l.'s,** *ligamenta* glenohumeralia.

**glenoid l.,** (1) *labrum* glenoidale; (2) Cruveilhier's l., on the plantar surface of each metatarsophalangeal articulation.

**glossoepiglottic l.,** an elastic ligamentous band passing from the base of the tongue to the epiglottis in the middle glossoepiglottic fold.

**Günz' l.,** a portion of the superficial layer of the obturator membrane.

**hammock l.,** the part of the periodontal l. below the growing end of the root of the tooth.

**l. of head of femur,** *ligamentum* capitis femoris.

**l.'s of head of fibula,** *ligamenta* capitis fibulae.

**Helmholtz' axis l.,** a l. forming the axis about which the malleus rotates; it consists of two portions extending from the anterior and the posterior border, respectively, of the tympanic notch to the malleus.

**Hensing's l.,** the left superior colic l.; a small serous horizontal or oblique fold sometimes found extending between the upper end of the descending colon and the abdominal wall.

**hepatoco′lic l.,** *ligamentum* hepatocolicum.

**hepatoduode′nal l.,** *ligamentum* hepatoduodenale.

**hepatoesophageal l.,** *ligamentum* hepatoesophageum.

**hepatogas′tric l.,** *ligamentum* hepatogastricum.

**hepatore′nal l.,** *ligamentum* hepatorenale.

**Hesselbach's l.,** *ligamentum* interfoveolare.

**Hey's l.,** *cornu* superius (2).

**Holl's l.,** l. joining the corpora cavernosa clitoridis in front of the urinary meatus.

**Hueck's l.,** *ligamentum* pectinatum anguli iridocornealis.

**Humphry's l.,** *ligamentum* meniscofemorale posterius.

**Hunter's l.,** *ligamentum* teres uteri.

**hyoepiglottic l.,** *ligamentum* hyoepiglotticum.

**hypsiloid l.,** *ligamentum* iliofemorale.

**iliofemoral l.,** *ligamentum* iliofemorale.

**iliolumbar l.,** *ligamentum* iliolumbale.

**iliopectineal l.,** *arcus* iliopectineus.

**il′iotrochanter′ic l.,** the lateral strong band of the Y-shaped iliofemoral l.; it is attached below to the tubercle at the upper part of the intertrochanteric line.

**l. of the incus,** *ligamentum* incudis.

**inferior pubic l.,** *ligamentum* arcuatum pubis.

**inferior transverse scapular l.,** *ligamentum* transversum scapulae inferius.

**infundibulo-ovarian l.,** *fimbria* ovarica.

**infundibulopelvic l.,** *ligamentum* suspensorium ovarii.

**in′guinal l.,** *ligamentum* inguinale.

**in′guinal l. of the kidney,** the segment of the mesonephros extending to the inguinal region.

**intercapital l.,** *ligamentum* intercapitale.

**intercar′pal l.'s,** *ligamenta* intercarpea.

**interchon′dral l.'s,** the articular capsules of the synovial joints located at the point of contact of costal cartilages 5, 6, 7, 8, 9, and 10 with adjacent costal cartilages.

**interclavic′ular l.,** *ligamentum* interclaviculare.

**intercli′noid l.,** a band of dura mater connecting the anterior and posterior clinoid processes of the sphenoid bone.

**intercor′nual l.,** *ligamentum* sacrococcygeum laterale.

**intercos′tal l.'s,** *membranae* intercostalia.

**intercu′neiform l.'s,** *ligamenta* intercuneiformia.

**interfo′veo′lar l.,** *ligamentum* interfoveolare.

**in′termetacarp′al l.'s,** *ligamenta* metacarpea.

**intermetatars′al l.'s,** *ligamenta* metatarsea.

**internal collateral l. of the wrist,** *ligamentum* collaterale carpi ulnare.

**interos′seous cu′neometatar′sal l.'s,** *ligamenta* cuneometatarsea interossea.

**interosseous sac′roil′iac l.'s,** *ligamenta* sacroiliaca interossea.

**interosseous talocalcanean l.,** *ligamentum* talocalcaneum interosseum.

**interspinous l.'s,** *ligamentum* interspinale.

**intertransverse l.,** *ligamentum* intertransversarium.

**intraartic′ular l.,** *ligamentum* capitis costae intraarticulare.

**intracapsular l.'s,** *ligamenta* intracapsularia.

**ischiocap′sular l.,** *ligamentum* ischiofemorale.

**ischiofem′oral l.,** *ligamentum* ischiofemorale.

**Jarjavay's l.'s,** uterosacral l.'s.

**jugal l.,** corniculopharyngeal l.

**Krause's l.,** *ligamentum* transversum perinei.

**lacin′iate l.,** *retinaculum* musculorum flexorum.

**lacu′nar l.,** *ligamentum* lacunare.

**Lannelongue's l.'s,** *ligamenta* sternopericardiaca.

**lateral l. of ankle,** consists of the ligamentum calcaneofibulare, ligamentum talofibulare anterius, and ligamentum talofibulare posterius.

**lateral arcuate l.,** *ligamentum* arcuatum laterale.

**lateral l.'s of the bladder,** condensations of fibroareolar tissue which pass one from each side of the bladder to blend with the pelvic fascia; smooth muscle is usually present in this tissue and is referred to as the musculus rectovesicalis.

**lateral collateral l.'s,** *ligamenta* collateralia.

**lateral costotransverse l.,** *ligamentum* costotransversarium laterale.

**lateral l. of elbow,** *ligamentum* collaterale radiale.

**lateral l. of knee,** *ligamentum* collaterale fibulare.

**lateral malleolar l.,** see *ligamentum* tibiofibulare anterius; *ligamentum* tibiofibulare posterius.

**lateral l. of malleus,** *ligamentum* mallei laterale.

**lateral palpebral l.,** *ligamentum* palpebrale laterale.

**lateral puboprostatic l.,** *ligamentum* puboprostaticum laterale.

**lateral sacrococcygeal l.,** *ligamentum* sacrococcygeum laterale.

**lateral talocalcanean l.,** *ligamentum* talocalcaneum laterale.

**lateral tarsal l.,** *ligamentum* palpebrale laterale.

**lateral l. of temporomandibular joint,** ligamentum laterale articulationis temporomandibularis.

**lateral l. of wrist,** *ligamentum* collaterale carpi radiale.

**Lauth's l.,** *ligamentum* transversum atlantis.

**left triangular l.,** *ligamentum* triangulare sinistrum hepatis.

**l. of left vena cava,** *ligamentum* venae cavae sinistrae.

**lienophrenic l.,** *ligamentum* phrenicolienale.

**Lisfranc's l.'s,** *ligamenta* cuneometatarsea interossea.

**Lockwood's l.,** suspensory l. of the eyeball.

**long plantar l.,** *ligamentum* plantare longum.

**longitudinal l.,** *ligamentum* longitudinale.

**lumbocos'tal l.,** *ligamentum* lumbocostale.

**Luschka's l.,** *ligamentum* sternopericardiacum.

**Mackenrodt's l.,** cervical l. of the uterus.

**l.'s of the malleus,** see *ligamentum* mallei anterius, laterale, and superius.

**Mauchart's l.'s,** check l.'s of the eyeball.

**Meckel's l.,** Meckel's *band.*

**medial l.,** *ligamentum* deltoideum.

**medial arcuate l.,** *ligamentum* arcuatum mediale.

**medial calcaneocuboid l.,** *ligamentum* bifurcatum.

**medial collateral l.,** *ligamentum* collaterale tibiale.

**medial l. of elbow,** *ligamentum* collaterale ulnare.

**medial l. of knee,** *ligamentum* collaterale tibiale.

**medial palpebral l.,** *ligamentum* palpebrale mediale.

**medial puboprostatic l.,** *ligamentum* puboprostaticum mediale.

**medial talocalcaneum l.,** *ligamentum* talocalcaneum mediale.

**medial tarsal l.,** *ligamentum* palpebrale mediale.

**medial umbilical l.,** *ligamentum* umbilicale mediale.

**medial l. of wrist,** *ligamentum* collaterale carpi ulnare.

**median arcuate l.,** *ligamentum* arcuatum medianum.

**median thyrohyoid l.,** *ligamentum* thyrohyoideum medianum.

**meniscofemoral l.,** *ligamentum* meniscofemorale.

**metacarpal l.'s,** *ligamenta* metacarpea.

**metatarsal l.'s.,** *ligamenta* metatarsea.

**middle costotransverse l.,** *ligamentum* costotransversarium.

**middle umbilical l.,** *ligamentum* umbilicale medianum.

**nu'chal l.,** *ligamentum* nuchae.

**oblique popliteal l.,** *ligamentum* popliteum obliquum.

**occip'itoaxial l.'s,** l.'s connecting the axis with the occipital bone, ligamenta alaria and ligamentum apicis dentis.

**odon'toid l.,** *ligamenta* alaria.

**orbicular l. of the radius,** *ligamentum* anulare radii.

**ova'rian l.,** *ligamentum* ovarii proprium.

**palmar l.'s,** *ligamenta* palmaria.

**palmar carpometacarpal l.'s,** *ligamenta* carpometacarpea palmaria.

**palmar radiocarpal l.,** *ligamentum* radiocarpeum palmare.

**palmar ul'nocar'pal l.,** *ligamentum* ulnocarpeum palmare.

**patel'lar l.,** *ligamentum* patellae.

**pectinate l. of the iris,** *ligamentum* pectinatum anguli iridocornealis.

**pectine'al l.,** *ligamentum* pectineale.

**periodontal l.,** connective tissue attaching the tooth to the alveolar bone; it consists of collagenous bundles between which are loose connective tissue, blood vessels, lymph vessels, and nerves; also called periodontal or peridental membrane; gingivodental l.; alveolodental l.; cemental l.; alveolar periosteum; periodontium (1).

**Petit's l.,** *plica* rectouterina.

**phrenicoco'lic l.,** *ligamentum* phrenicocolicum.

**phrenicosplen'ic l.,** *ligamentum* phrenicolienale.

**phrenogastric l.,** *ligamentum* gastrophrenicum.

**phrenosplenic l.,** *ligamentum* phrenicolienale.

**pisohamate l.,** *ligamentum* pisohamatum.

**pisometacar'pal l.,** *ligamentum* pisometacarpeum.

**pisounciform l.,** *ligamentum* pisohamatum.

**pi'soun'cinate l.,** *ligamentum* pisohamatum.

**plantar l.'s,** *ligamenta* plantaria.

**plantar calcaneocuboid l.,** *ligamentum* calcaneocuboideum plantare.

**plantar calcaneonavicular l.,** *ligamentum* calcaneonaviculare plantare.

**posterior costotransverse l.,** *ligamentum* costotransversarium laterale.

**posterior cricoarytenoid l.,** *ligamentum* cricoarytenoideum posterius.

**posterior l. of head of fibula,** *ligamentum* capitis fibulae posterius.

**posterior l. of knee,** *ligamentum* popliteum arcuatum.

**posterior sac'roil'iac l.'s,** *ligamenta* sacroiliaca dorsalia.

**posterior sac'rosciat'ic l.,** *ligamentum* sacrotuberale.

**posterior talofibular l.,** *ligamentum* talofibulare posterius.

**posterior talotib'ial l.,** *ligamentum* deltoideum.

**posterior tibiofibular l.,** *ligamentum* tibiofibularis posterius.

**Poupart's l.,** *ligamentum* inguinale.

**proper l. of ovary,** *ligamentum* ovarii proprium.

**pter'ygomandib'ular l.,** *raphe* pterygomandibularis.

**pterygospinal l.,** *ligamentum* pterygospinale.

**pterygospi'nous l.,** *ligamentum* pterygospinale.

**pubocap'sular l.,** *ligamentum* pubofemorale.

**pubofem'oral l.,** *ligamentum* pubofemorale.

**puboprostatic l.,** *ligamentum* puboprostaticum.

**puboves'ical l.,** *ligamentum* pubovesicale.

**pulmonary l.,** *ligamentum* pulmonale.

**quadrate l.,** *ligamentum* quadratum.

**radial collateral l.,** *ligamentum* collaterale radiale.

**radial collateral l. of wrist,** *ligamentum* collaterale carpi radiale.

**radiate l. of rib,** *ligamentum* capitis costae radiatum.

**radiate l. of wrist,** *ligamentum* carpi radiatum.

**reflex l.,** *ligamentum* reflexum.

**Retzius' l.,** fundiform l. of the foot; the deep attachment of the inferior extensor retinaculum in the sinus tarsi; it acts as a sling for the extensor tendons of the toes.

**rhomboid l.,** *ligamentum* costoclaviculare.

**right triangular l.,** *ligamentum* triangulare dextrum hepatis.

**ring l.,** *zona* orbicularis.

**round l. of the femur,** *ligamentum* teres femoris.

**round l. of the liver,** *ligamentum* teres hepatis.

**round l. of the uterus,** *ligamentum* teres uteri.

**sacrospi'nous l.,** *ligamentum* sacrospinale.

**sacrotu'berous l.,** *ligamentum* sacrotuberale.

**Sappey's l.,** the posterior thickened portion of the capsule of the temporomandibular articulation.

**sheath l.'s,** *vagina* fibrosa.

**Simonart's l.'s,** amniotic *bands.*

**Soemmering's l.,** suspensory l. of the lacrimal gland.

**sphenomandib'ular l.,** *ligamentum* sphenomandibulare.

**spinoglenoid l.,** *ligamentum* transversum scapulae inferius.

**spiral l. of the coch'lea,** *ligamentum* spirale cochleae.

**spring l.,** *ligamentum* calcaneonaviculare plantare.

**Stanley's cervical l.'s,** fibers of the capsule of the hip joint reflected onto the neck of the femur.

**stellate l.,** *ligamentum* capitis costae radiatum.

**sternoclavic'ular l.,** *ligamentum* sternoclaviculare.

**sternocos'tal l.,** *ligamentum* sternocostale.

**sternopericar'dial l.,** *ligamentum* sternopericardiacum.

**stylohy'oid l.,** *ligamentum* stylohyoideum.

**stylomandib'ular l.,** *ligamentum* stylomandibulare.

**stylomaxillary l.,** *ligamentum* stylomandibulare.

**superficial dorsal sacrococcygeal l.,** *ligamentum* sacrococcygeum dorsale superficiale.

**superficial transverse metacarpal l.,** *ligamentum* metacarpeum transversum superficiale.

**superficial transverse metatarsal l.,** *ligamentum* metatarseum transversum superficiale.

**superior costotransverse l.,** *ligamentum* costotransversarium superius.

**superior l. of malleus,** *ligamentum* mallei superius.

**superior pubic l.,** *ligamentum* pubicum superius.

**superior transverse scapular l.,** *ligamentum* transversum scapulae superius.

**suprascap′ular l.,** *ligamentum* transversum scapulae superius.

**supraspi′nous l.,** *ligamentum* supraspinale.

**suspensory l. of the axilla,** Gerdy's l.; the continuation of clavipectoral fascia downward to attach to the axillary fascia; it maintains the characteristic hollow of the armpit.

**suspensory l.'s of the breast,** *ligamenta* suspensoria mammae.

**suspensory l. of the clitoris,** *ligamentum* suspensorium clitoridis.

**suspensory l.'s of Cooper,** *ligamenta* suspensoria mammae.

**suspensory l. of crystalline lens,** *zonula* ciliaris.

**suspensory l. of the eyeball,** l. of Lockwood; a thickening of the inferior part of the bulbar sheath which supports the eye within the orbit; it extends between the lateral and medial orbital margins and includes the medial and lateral cheek l.'s.

**suspensory l. of the gonad,** mesentery of the embryonic gonad, derived from the urogenital ridge.

**suspensory l. of the ovary,** *ligamentum* suspensorium ovarii.

**suspensory l. of the penis,** *ligamentum* suspensorium penis.

**suspensory l. of the testis,** the cranial atrophic portion of the urogenital ridge attached to the cranial pole of the intra-abdominal embryonic testis.

**suspensory l. of the thyroid gland,** one of several fibrous bands which pass from the sheath of the thyroid gland to the thyroid and cricoid cartilages.

**sutu′ral l.,** a delicate membrane binding the bones at the cranial sutures.

**synovial l.,** one of the large synovial folds in a joint.

**talocalca′nean l.,** *ligamentum* talocalcaneum.

**talonavic′ular l.,** *ligamentum* talonaviculare.

**tarsal l.'s,** *ligamenta* tarsi.

**tarsometatarsal l.'s,** *ligamenta* tarsometatarsae.

**temporomandib′ular l.,** *ligamentum* laterale articulationis temporomandibularis.

**Teutleben's l.'s,** *ligamentum* pulmonale.

**thyroepiglot′tic l., thyroepiglottid′ean l.,** *ligamentum* thyroepiglotticum.

**thyrohy′oid l.,** *ligamentum* thyrohyoideum.

**tibial collateral l.,** *ligamentum* collaterale tibiale.

**tibiofib′ular l.,** *ligamentum* tibiofibularis.

**tibionavic′ular l.,** see *ligamentum* deltoideum.

**transverse l. of acetab′ulum,** *ligamentum* transversum acetabuli.

**transverse l. of the atlas,** *ligamentum* cruciforme atlantis.

**transverse carpal l.,** *retinaculum* flexorum.

**transverse crural l.,** *retinaculum* musculorum extensorum superius.

**transverse humeral l.,** Brodie's l.; a fibrous band running more or less obliquely from the greater to the lesser tuberosity of the humerus, bridging over the bicipital groove.

**transverse l. of the knee,** *ligamentum* transversum genus.

**transverse l. of the leg,** *retinaculum* musculorum extensorum superius.

**transverse metacar′pal l.,** *ligamentum* metacarpeum transversum profundum.

**transverse metatarsal l.,** *ligamentum* metatarseum transversum profundum.

**transverse l. of pelvis,** *ligamentum* transversum perinei.

**transverse l. of perineum,** *ligamentum* transversum perinei.

**transverse tibiofibular l.,** the distal continuation of the interosseous membrane forming a strong l. that unites the distal end of the tibia and fibula; it lies deep to the posterior tibiofibular l.

**trapezoid l.,** *ligamentum* trapezoideum.

**Treitz′ l.,** *musculus* suspensorius duodeni.

**triangular l.,** *fascia* diaphragmatis urogenitalis inferior; see also *membrana* perinei.

**triangular l.'s of the liver,** *ligamentum* triangulare dextrum hepatis and *ligamentum* triangulare sinistrum hepatis.

**ulnar collateral l.,** *ligamentum* collaterale ulnare.

**ulnar collateral l. of wrist,** *ligamentum* collaterale carpi ulnare.

**urachal l.,** *plica* umbilicalis mediana.

**uterosacral l.,** *plica* rectouterina.

**Valsalva′s l.'s,** *ligamenta* auricularia.

**venous l.,** *ligamentum* venosum.

**ventral sacrococcygeal l.,** *ligamentum* sacrococcygeum ventrale.

**ventral sacroiliac l.'s,** *ligamenta* sacroiliaca ventralia.

**ventric′ular l.,** *ligamentum* vestibulare.

**verte′bropel′vic l.'s,** *ligamenta* iliolumbale, sacrospinale, and sacrotuberale.

**Vesalius′ l.,** *ligamentum* inguinale.

**vesicoumbil′ical l.,** one of the ligaments between the urinary bladder and the umbilicus; the median vesicoumbilical l. is the urachal l.

**vesicouterine l.,** ureterovesical fold; a peritoneal fold extending from the uterus to the posterior portion of the bladder.

**vestib′ular l.,** *ligamentum* vestibulare.

**vocal l.,** *ligamentum* vocale.

**volar carpal l.,** *retinaculum* flexorum.

**Weitbrecht's l.,** *chorda* obliqua.

**Winslow's l.,** *ligamentum* popliteum obliquum.

**Wrisberg's l.,** *ligamentum* meniscofemorale posterius.

**Y-shaped l.,** *ligamentum* iliofemorale.

**yellow l.,** *ligamentum* flavum.

**Zaglas′ l.,** a short thick fibrous band extending from the posterior superior spine of the ilium to the second transverse tubercle of the sacrum.

**Zinn's l.,** *anulus* tendineus communis.

---

**lig′amen′ta** (lig′ă-men′tah) [ L. ]. Plural of ligamentum.

**ligamentopexis** (lig′ă-men-to-pek′sis) [ ligament + G. *pēxis*, fixation ]. Alexander-Adams operation of shortening the round ligaments of the uterus.

**ligamentopexy** (lig′ă-men-to-pek′sĭ). Ligamentopexis.

**ligamentous** (lig′ă-men′tus). Relating to or of the form or structure of a ligament.

---

# LIGAMENTUM

**ligamentum,** pl. **ligamen′ta** (lig′ă-men′tum) [ L. a band, tie, fr. *ligo*, to bind. LIG- ] [ NA ]. Ligament.

**l. acro′mioclavicula′re** [ NA ], acromioclavicular ligament; a fibrous band extending from the acromion of the scapula to the clavicle.

**ligamenta alaria** [ NA ], alar ligaments; odontoid or check ligaments; one of two short stout bands between the side of the dens of the axis and the tubercle on the medial aspect of the occipital condyle.

**l. anococcy′geum** [ NA ], anococcygeal ligament; anococcygeal (Symington's) body; a musculofibrous band that passes between the anus and the coccyx.

**l. anula′re,** annular *ligament*.

**l. anula′re bulbi,** l. pectinatum anguli iridocornealis.

**ligamenta anula′ria digitorum,** *pars* anularis vaginae fibrosae.

**l. anula′re ra′dii** [ NA ], annular ligament of the radius; the ligament that holds the head of the radius in the radial notch of the ulna.

**l. anula′re stapedis** [ NA ], annular ligament of the stapes; a ring of elastic fibers that attaches the base of the stapes to the margin of the fenestra vestibuli.

**ligamenta anula′ria trachea′lia** [ NA ], annular ligaments of the trachea; the fibrous membranes that connect adjacent tracheal cartilages.

**l. ap′icis dentis** [ NA ], apical ligament of the dens; a ligament that extends from the apex of the dens of the axis to the anterior margin of the foramen magnum.

**l. arcua′tum latera′le** [ NA ], lateral arcuate ligament; lateral lumbocostal arch; arcus lumbocostalis lateralis; one of Haller's arches; a thickening of the fascia of the quadratus lumborum muscle between the transverse process of the 1st lumbar vertebra and the 12th rib on either side that gives attachment to a portion of the diaphragm.

**l. arcua′tum media′le** [ NA ], medial arcuate ligament; medial lumbocostal arch; arcus lumbocostalis medialis; one of Haller's arches; a tendinous thickening of the psoas fascia that extends from the body of the first lumbar vertebra to its transverse process on either side. A portion of the diaphragm arises from it.

**l. arcua′tum media′num** [ NA ], median arcuate ligament; a tendinous connection between the crura of the diaphragm that arches in front on the aorta.

**l. arcua′tum pubis** [ NA ], arcuate pubic ligament; inferior pubic ligament; the ligament that arches across the inferior aspect of the pubic symphysis.

**l. arterio′sum** [ NA ], arterial ligament; the remains of the ductus arteriosus.

**ligamen′ta auricula′ria** [ NA ], auricular ligaments; ligaments of Valsalva; the ligaments that attach the auricle to the side of the head; they are three in number, l. **auriculare** anterius; l. **auriculare** posterius, and l. **auriculare** superius.

**ligamen′ta ba′sium,** ligamenta metacarpea; ligamenta metatarsea.

**l. bifurca′tum** [ NA ], bifurcated ligament; a strong ligament that passes distally from the upper margin of the calcaneus, dividing into two portions, the l. calcaneocuboideum and the l. calcaneonaviculare.

**l. calca′neocuboi′deum** [ NA ], calcaneocuboid ligament; the lateral part of the l. bifurcatum.

**l. calca′neocuboi′deum plantare** [ NA ], plantar calcaneocuboid ligament; a strong band that passes forward and medially from the distal end of the calcaneus to the cuboid bone.

**l. calcaneofibula′re** [ NA ], calcaneofibular ligament; the middle of the three fascicles that reinforce the lateral side of the ankle joint, the remaining two being the anterior and posterior talofibular ligaments.

**l. calca′neonavicula′re** [ NA ], calcaneonavicular ligament; the medial part of the l. bifurcatum.

**l. calcaneonavicula′re planta′re** [ NA ], plantar calcaneonavicular ligament; inferior calcaneonavicular ligament; "spring" ligament; a dense fibroelastic ligament that extends from the sustentaculum tali to the plantar surface of the navicular bone. It supports the head of the talus.

**l. calca′neotibia′le,** l. deltoideum (pars tibiocalcanea).

**l. capitis costae intraarticula′re** [ NA ], intraarticular ligament of the costal head; transverse fibers extending within the capsule from the ridge between the two facets on the head of the rib to the intervertebral disk.

**l. capitis costae radia′tum** [ NA ], radiate, stellate, or anterior costovertebral ligament connecting the head of each rib to the bodies of the two vertebrae with which it articulates.

**l. capitis femoris** [ NA ], ligament of the head of the femur; l. teres femoris; a flattened ligament that passes from the fovea in the head of the femur to the borders of the acetabular notch; an artery often passes to the head of the femur with the ligament.

**ligamen′ta capituli fib′ulae** [ NA ], ligaments of the head of the fibula; ligaments anterior and posterior to the superior tibiofibular articulation; they are l. **capitis fibulae anterius** and l. **capitis fibulae posterius,** respectively.

**ligamen′ta capitulo′rum transversa,** l. metacarpeum transversum profundum; l. metatarseum transversum profundum.

**l. capsula′re,** capsular *ligament.*

**l. carpi dorsale,** *retinaculum* extensorum manus.

**l. carpi radia′tum** [ NA ], radiate ligament of the wrist; the ligament that extends from the capitate bone to the scaphoid, lunate, and triquetrum on the palmar side of the wrist.

**l. carpi transversum,** *retinaculum* flexorum.

**l. carpi volare,** *retinaculum* flexorum.

**ligamen′ta carpometacarpe′a** [ NA ], carpometacarpal ligaments, uniting the metacarpal and carpal bones; they are of two sets, dorsal (ligamenta carpometacarpea dorsalia) and palmar (ligamenta carpometacarpea palmaria).

**ligamenta car′pometacarpe′a dorsalia** [ NA ], dorsal carpometacarpal ligaments; fibrous bands that connect the distal row of carpal bones with the metacarpals on their dorsal aspects.

**l. car′pometacarpe′a palma′ria** [ NA ], palmar carpometacarpal ligaments; fibrous bands that connect the palmar surfaces of the carpal and metacarpal bones.

**l. cauda′le,** *retinaculum* caudale.

**l. centra′le,** *filum* terminale.

**l. ceratocricoid′eum,** one of three ligaments (anterius, posterius, and laterale) reinforcing the capsule of the cricothyroid articulation on either side.

**l. collatera′le carpi radia′le** [ NA ], radial collateral ligament of the wrist; external collateral ligament of the wrist; the ligament that extends distally from the styloid process of the radius to the carpal bones.

**l. collatera′le carpi ulna′re** [ NA ], ulnar collateral ligament of the wrist; internal collateral ligament of the wrist; a ligament that passes from the styloid process of the ulna to the pisiform and triquetrum.

**l. collatera′le fibula′re** [ NA ], fibular collateral ligament; the cordlike ligament that passes from the lateral epicondyle of the femur to the head of the fibula.

**l. collatera′le radia′le** [ NA ], radial collateral ligament; lateral ligament of the elbow; medial ligament of the elbow; the ligament that connects the lateral epicondyle of the humerus with the annular ligament and neck of the radius.

**l. collatera′le tibia′le** [ NA ], tibial collateral ligament; medial collateral ligament; the broad fibrous band that crosses the medial side of the knee joint from femur to tibia. It is fused with the medial meniscus.

**l. collatera′le ulna′re** [ NA ], ulnar collateral ligament; the radiating fibrous band that strengthens the medial side of the elbow joint.

**ligamen′ta collatera′lia** [ NA ], medial and lateral collateral ligaments of the metacarpophalangeal (or metatarsophalangeal) and interphalangeal articulations.

**l. colli costae,** l. costotransversarium.

**l. conjuga′le,** conjugate *ligament.*

**l. conoɪd′eum** [ NA ], conoid ligament; the rounded band that connects the conoid tubercle of the clavicle with the coracoid process of the scapula.

**l. coracoacromia′le** [ NA ], coracoacromial ligament; the heavy arched fibrous band that passes between the coracoid process and the acromion above the shoulder joint.

**l. cor′acoclavicula′re** [ NA ], coracoclavicular ligament; Caldani's ligament; the strong ligament that unites the clavicle to the coracoid process; it is subdivided into the l. conoideum and the l. trapezoideum.

**l. coracohumera′le** [ NA ], coracohumeral ligament; the ligament that passes from the base of the coracoid process to the anatomical neck of the humerus close to the greater tubercle.

**l. corniculopharynge′um,** corniculopharyngeal *ligament.*

**l. corona′rium hep′atis** [ NA ], coronary ligament of the liver; peritoneal reflections from the liver to the diaphragm at the margins of the bare area of the liver.

**l. costoclavicula′re** [ NA ], costoclavicular ligament; rhomboid ligament; the ligament that connects the first rib and the clavicle near its sternal end.

**l. costotransversa′rium** [ NA ], costotransverse ligament; l. colli costae; the ligament that connects the dorsal aspect of the neck of a rib to the ventral aspect of the corresponding transverse process.

**l. costotransversa′rium ante′rius,** l. costotransversarium superius.

**l. cos′totransversa′rium laterale** [ NA ], lateral costotransverse ligament; posterior costotransverse ligament; the short quadrangular ligament that passes across behind the costotransverse joint from the tip of the transverse process to the posterior surface of the neck of the rib.

**l. costotransversa′rium poste′rius,** l. costotransversarium laterale.

l. cos'totransversa'rium superius [ NA ], superior costotransverse ligament; anterior costotransverse ligament; the fibrous band that extends upward from the neck of a rib to the transverse process of the next higher vertebra.

l. costoxiphoid'eum [ NA ], costoxiphoid ligament; chondroxiphoid ligament; the ligament that connects the xiphoid process to the seventh, and often to the sixth, costal cartilages.

l. cotyloid'eum, labrum acetabulare.

l. cricoarytenoid'eum posterius [ NA ], posterior cricoarytenoid ligament; the ligament that passes downward from the posterior border of the arytenoid cartilage to the lamina of the cricoid cartilage.

l. cricopharynge'um [ NA ], cricopharyngeal ligament; the lower part of the corniculopharyngeal ligament attached to the lamina of the cricoid cartilage.

l. cricothyroid'eum [ NA ], cricothyroid ligament; the strong band that connects the cricoid and thyroid cartilages in the midline anteriorly. Its upper edge continues into the plica vocalis as the l. vocale.

l. cricotrachea'le [ NA ], cricotracheal ligament; a fibrous band connecting the cricoid cartilage with the first ring of the trachea.

ligamenta crucia'ta digito'rum, pars cruciformis vaginae fibrosae.

ligamenta crucia'ta genus [ NA ], cruciate ligaments of the knee; these consist l. cruciatum anterius and l. cruciatum posterius which pass from the intercondylar area of the tibia to the intercondylar fossa of the femur.

l. crucia'tum atlan'tis, l. cruciforme atlantis.

l. crucia'tum cruris, retinaculum musculorum extensorum inferius.

l. crucia'tum ter'tium genus, l. meniscofemorale.

l. cruciforme atlantis [ NA ], cruciform ligament of atlas; the strong ligament that lies posterior to the dens of the axis; it consists of a transverse part (l. transversum atlantis) and longitudinal fibers (fasciculi longitudinales).

l. cuboid'eonavicula're [ NA ], cuboideonavicular ligament; one of two ligaments, l. cuboideonaviculare dorsale and l. cuboideonaviculare plantare, which unite the cuboid and navicular bones of the tarsus.

l. cu'neocuboid'eum [ NA ], cuneocuboid ligament; one of three ligaments, l. cuneocuboideum dorsale, l. cuneocuboideum interosseum, and l. cuneocuboideum plantare, which unite the cuneiform and cuboid bones of the tarsus.

ligamenta cuneometatar'sea interossea [ NA ], interosseous cuneometatarsal ligaments; Lisfranc's ligaments; ligaments that pass from the cuneiform bones to the metatarsals, the one from the first cuneiform to the second metatarsal being the strongest.

ligamenta cuneonavicula'ria [ NA ], cuneonavicular ligaments; fibrous bands arranged in two sets of ligaments, dorsal (ligamenta cuneonavicularia dorsalia) and plantar (ligamenta cuneonavicularia plantaria), which strengthen the capsule of the cuneonavicular joint.

l. deltoid'eum [ NA ], l. mediale [ NA ]; deltoid ligament; medial ligament; it consists of the following four parts which pass downward from the medial malleolus of the tibia to the tarsal bones: pars tibionavicularis, pars tibiocalcanea, pars tibiotalaris anterior and pars tibiotalaris posterior.

l. denticula'tum [ NA ], denticulate ligament; a dural septum placed in the frontal plane and extending longitudinally along each side of the thoracic and cervical segments of the spinal cord; it is attached to the lateral side of the cord by about 21 segmental, toothlike medial extensions that fuse with the cord's pial coverings; the interval between each two successive denticulate attachments provides the opening through which the corresponding dorsal root passes ventrally to join the ventral root.

l. ductus veno'si, l. venosum.

l. duode'norena'le, a fold of periotoneum occasionally passing from the termination of the hepatoduodenal ligament to the front of the right kidney.

l. epididym'idis [ NA ], ligament of the epididymis; one of two folds of the tunica vaginalis above (l. e. superius) and below (l. e. inferius) the sinus epididymidis supporting the epididymis.

ligamenta extracapsularia [ NA ], extracapsular ligaments; ligaments associated with a synovial joint but separate from and external to its articular capsule.

l. falcifor'me, processus falciformis.

l. falcifor'me hep'atis [ NA ], falciform ligament of the liver; a crescentic fold of peritoneum extending to the surface of the liver from the diaphragm and anterior abdominal wall. The round ligament lies in its free inferior border.

l. flavum [ NA ], yellow ligament; one of the paired ligaments of yellow elastic fibrous tissue, which bind together the laminae of adjoining vertebrae.

l. fundifor'me penis [ NA ], fundiform ligament of penis; a band of elastic fibers that extends from the linea alba above the pubic symphysis splitting to surround the penis before attaching to the fascia of the penis.

l. gastrocol'icum [ NA ], gastrocolic ligament; the portion of the greater omentum that extends between the stomach and the transverse colon.

l. gastroliena'le [ NA ], gastrosplenic ligament; the portion of the greater omentum that lies between the greater curvature of the stomach and the hilus of the spleen.

l. gastrophren'icum [ NA ], gastrophrenic or gastrodiaphragmatic ligament; the portion of the greater omentum that extends from the greater curvature of the stomach to the inferior surface of the diaphragm.

l. genitoinguina'le [ NA ], genitoinguinal ligament; plica gubernatrix; a fold of the mesorchium in the fetus containing the gubernaculum testis.

ligamenta glenohumeralia [ NA ], glenohumeral ligaments; three fibrous bands that reinforce the articular capsule of the shoulder joint. They are attached to the margin of the glenoid cavity of the scapula and to the anatomic neck of the humerus.

l. glenoida'le, labrum glenoidale.

l. hep'atocol'icum [ NA ], hepatocolic ligament; an inconstant extension of the hepatoduodenal ligament to the transverse colon.

l. hep'atoduodena'le [ NA ], hepatoduodenal ligament; the portion of the lesser omentum that connects the liver and duodenum.

l. hepatoesopha'geum, hepatoesophageal ligament; the part of the lesser omentum that extends between the liver and the abdominal portion of the esophagus.

l. hep'atogas'tricum [ NA ], hepatogastric ligament; the part of the lesser omentum that extends between the liver and lesser curvature of the stomach.

l. hepatorena'le [ NA ], hepatorenal ligament; a prolongation of the coronary ligament downward over the right kidney.

l. hyoepiglot'ticum [ NA ], hyoepiglottic ligament; a short elastic band that unites the epiglottis to the upper border of the hyoid bone.

l. hyothy'roid'eum latera'le, l. thyrohyoideum.

l. hyothy'roid'eum me'dium, l. thyrohyoideum medianum.

l. iliofemora'le [ NA ], iliofemoral ligament; Y-shaped ligament of Bigelow; a triangular ligament attached by its apex to the anterior inferior spine of the ilium and rim of the acetabulum, and by its base to the anterior intertrochanteric line of the femur. The strong medial band is attached to the lower part of the intertrochanteric line; the strong lateral part is fixed to the tubercle at the upper part of this line. The bands diverge, forming a Y-like figure with a weak area between.

l. iliolumba'le [ NA ], iliolumbar ligament; the strong ligament that connects the fourth and fifth lumbar vertebrae with the ilium.

l. iliopectinea'le, arcus iliopectineus.

l. in'cudis [ NA ], one of two ligaments of the incus: l. incudis posterius, attaching the short process of the incus to the fossa incudis; and l. incudis superius, a thin ligament running from the body of the incus to the roof of the epitympanic recess.

l. inguina'le [ NA ], inguinal ligament; Vesalius' ligament; Poupart's ligament; crural or femoral arch; Fallopian arch; a fibrous band formed by the inferior border of the aponeurosis of the external oblique that extends from the anterior superior spine of the ilium to the pubic tubercle.

l. intercapita'le [ NAV ], intercapital ligament; formerly referred to as the conjugal ligament; a part of the l. capitis costae intraarticulare; it connects the heads of opposite ribs by passing over the intervertebral fibrocartilage, and thus holds the ribs in their articular sockets; not present in man but well developed in the dog and cat.

**ligamenta intercarpe'a** [ NA ], intercarpal ligaments; three sets of short fibrous bands that bind together the two rows of carpal bones; according to their location they are named **l. intercarpea dorsalia, l. intercarpea interossea,** and **l. intercarpea palmaria.**

**l. interclavicula're** [ NA ], interclavicular ligament; a strong ligament that interconnects the two sternoclavicular joints across the upper border of the manubrium.

**ligamenta intercosta'lia,** *membranae* intercostalia.

**ligamenta intercu'neifor'mia** [ NA ], intercuneiform ligaments; fibrous bands that unite the cuneiform bones; they are arranged in three sets, **l. intercuneiformia dorsalia, l. intercuneiformia interossea,** and **l. intercuneiformia plantaria.**

**l. interfoveola're** [ NA ], interfoveolar ligament; Hesselbach's ligament; fibrous or muscular strands that lie medial to the deep inguinal ring, extending from the lower border of the transversus muscle to the lacunar ligament and pectineal fascia.

**l. interspinale** [ NA ], interspinous ligament; bands of fibrous tissue that connect the spinous processes of adjacent vertebrae.

**l. intertransversarium** [ NA ], intertransverse ligament; one of the ligaments that connect the transverse processes of adjacent vertebrae.

**ligamenta intracapsula'ria** [ NA ], intracapsular ligaments; ligaments located within and separate from the articular capsule of a synovial joint.

**l. is'chiocapsula're,** l. ischiofemorale.

**l. ischiofemora'le** [ NA ], ischiofemoral ligament; ischiocapsular ligament; the thickened part of the capsule of the hip joint that passes from the ischium upward and laterally over the femoral neck; some of its fibers continue into the zona orbicularis.

**l. juga'le,** corniculopharyngeal *ligament.*

**l. lacinia'tum,** *retinaculum* musculorum flexorum.

**l. lacuna're** [ NA ], lacunar ligament; Gimbernat's ligament; a curved fibrous band that passes horizontally backward from the medial end of the inguinal ligament to the pectineal line; it forms the medial boundary of the femoral ring.

**l. latera'le,** l. collaterale.

**l. laterale articulatio'nis tem'poromandibula'ris** [ NA ], lateral ligament of the temporomandibular joint; Ferrein's ligament; the capsular ligament that passes obliquely down and backward across the temporomandibular joint.

**l. la'tum pulmo'nis,** l. pulmonale.

**l. la'tum u'teri** [ NA ], broad ligament of the uterus; the peritoneal fold passing from the lateral margin of the uterus to the wall of the pelvis on either side.

**l. lienorenale** [ NA ], l. phrenicolienale.

**l. longitudin'ale** [ NA ], longitudinal ligament; one of two extensive fibrous bands, the **l. longitudinale anterius** and the **l. longitudinale posterius,** that interconnect the bodies of the vertebrae throughout the length of the spinal column; they attach firmly to the intervertebral disks.

**l. lumbocosta'le** [ NA ], lumbocostal ligament; a strong band that unites the twelfth rib with the tips of the transverse processes of the first and second lumbar vertebrae.

**l. mal'lei anterius** [ NA ], anterior ligament of the malleus; consists of two portions: Meckel's band, passing from the base of the anterior process to the spine of the sphenoid through the petrotympanic fissure; and the anterior ligament of Helmholtz, extending from the anterior aspect of the neck of the malleus to the anterior boundary of the tympanic notch.

**l. mal'lei latera'le** [ NA ], lateral ligament of the malleus; a short fan-shaped ligament converging from the posterior half of the tympanic notch to the neck of the malleus.

**l. mal'lei superius** [ NA ], superior ligament of the malleus; a ligament extending from the head of the malleus to the roof of the epitympanic recess.

**l. malle'oli latera'lis,** see l. tibiofibularis anterius and posterius.

**l. media'le** [ NA ], l. deltoideum.

**l. menis'ci latera'lis,** l. meniscofemorale posterius.

**l. meniscofemora'le** [ NA ], meniscofemoral ligament; one of two bands, the **l. meniscofemorale anterius** and the **l. meniscofemorale posterius,** which extend upward from the posterior part of the lateral meniscus; they pass in front of and behind the posterior cruciate ligament to reach the medial condyle of the femur.

**ligamenta metacarpea** [ NA ], metacarpal ligaments; ligaments of the bases of the metacarpals; these consist of three groups of ligaments (**l. metacarpea dorsalia, l. metacarpea interossea,** and **l. metacarpea palmaria**) which interconnect the bases of the second to fifth metacarpals.

**l. metacarpeum transversum profundum** [ NA ], deep transverse metacarpal ligament; the ligament that interconnects the heads of the second to fifth metacarpals. It lies in the plane of the palmar interosseous fascia.

**l. metacar'peum transversum superficia'le** [ NA ], superficial transverse metacarpal ligament; Gerdy's fibers; a thickening of the superficial fascia in the most distal part of the palm.

**ligamenta metatarsea** [ NA ], metatarsal ligaments; ligaments of the bases of the metatarsals; these consist of three groups of ligaments (**l. metatarsea dorsalia, l. metatarsea interossea,** and **l. metatarsea plantaria**) which unite the bases of the metatarsals to each other.

**l. metatarseum transversum profundum** [ NA ], deep transverse metatarsal ligament; the ligament that interconnects the heads of the metatarsals.

**l. metatarseum transversum superficia'le** [ NA ], superficial transverse metatarsal ligament; l. natatorium; a thickening of the superficial fascia under the heads of the metatarsal bones.

**l. natato'rium,** l. metacarpeum transversum superficiale.

**ligamenta navicula'ricuneifor'mia,** l. cuneonavicularia.

**l. nuchae** [ NA ], nuchal ligament; apparatus ligamentosus colli; a saggital ligamentous band at the back of the neck, formed of thickened supraspinous ligaments; it extends from the external occipital protuberance to the posterior border of the foramen magnum, cranially, to the seventh cervical spinous process, caudally.

**l. orbicula're ra'dii,** l. anulare radii.

**ligamenta ossiculorum auditus** [ NA ], ligaments of the auditory ossicles; the ligaments connecting the ear bones with one another and with the walls of the tympanic cavity.

**l. ova'rii proprium** [ NA ], proper ligament of the ovary; ovarian ligament; a cordlike bundle of fibers passing to the side of the uterus from the lower end of the ovary, between the folds of the broad ligament.

**ligamenta palma'ria** [ NA ], palmar ligaments; accessory volar ligaments; the fibrocartilaginous plates, one located on the anterior aspect of each metacarpophalangeal and interphalangeal joint, that are firmly attached to the bases of the phalanges and articulate with the heads of the next proximal bones.

**l. palpebra'le externum,** l. palpebrale laterale.

**l. palpebra'le latera'le** [ NA ], lateral palpebral ligament; the band that attaches the tarsal plates to the orbital eminence of the zygomatic bone.

**l. palpebra'le media'le** [ NA ], medial palpebral ligament; the fibrous band that attaches the medial ends of the tarsal plates to the maxilla at the medial orbital margin.

**l. patel'lae** [ NA ], patellar ligament; a strong flattened fibrous band passing from the apex and adjoining margins of the patella to the tuberosity of the tibia.

**l. pectina'tum anguli iridocornea'lis** [ NA ], pectinate ligament of the iridocorneal angle; Gerlach's valvula; radiating fibers from the posterior limiting lamina of the cornea that pass across to the iris, forming a meshwork of spaces of the iridocorneal angle.

**l. pectina'tum ir'idis,** l. pectinatum anguli iridocornealis.

**l. pectinea'le** [ NA ], pectineal ligament; Cooper's ligament; a thick, strong fibrous band that passes laterally from the lacunar ligament along the pectineal line of the pubis.

**l. phrenicocol'icum** [ NA ], phrenicocolic ligament; sustenaculum lienis; costocolic ligament; a triangular fold of peritoneum attached to the left flexure of the colon and to the diaphragm, on which rests the inferior pole or extremity of the spleen.

**l. phrenicoliena'le** [ NA ], phrenicosplenic ligament; the portion of the greater omentum which extends from the spleen to the diaphragm.

**l. pisohama'tum** [ NA ], pisohamate ligament; pisounci-nate ligament; a strong fibrous band that extends from the pisiform bone to the hook of the hamate.

**l. pisometacarpe'um** [ NA ], the pisometacarpal liga-ment; a strong fibrous band extending from the pisiform bone to the base of the fifth metacarpal bone. This ligament, together with the pisohamate ligament, forms the insertion of the flexor carpi ulnaris.

**ligamenta planta'ria** [ NA ], plantar ligaments; accessory plantar ligaments; the counterparts in the foot of the ligamenta palmaria, in the hand.

**l. planta're longum** [ NA ], long plantar ligament; a strong ligament that extends from the calcaneus to the cuboid and lateral metatarsals on the plantar aspect of the foot.

**l. poplite'um arcua'tum** [ NA ], arcuate popliteal liga-ment; a broad fibrous band attached above to the lateral condyle of the femur and passing medially and downward in the posterior part of the capsule of the knee joint, arching over the tendon of the popliteus muscle.

**l. poplite'um obli'quum** [ NA ], oblique popliteal liga-ment; a fibrous band that extends across the back of the knee from the insertion of the semimembranosus on the medial condyle of the tibia to the lateral condyle of the femur.

**l. pterygospina'le** [ NA ], pterygospinal ligament; ptery-gospinous ligament; a membranous ligament extending from the spine of the sphenoid to the upper part of the posterior border of the lateral pterygoid lamina.

**l. pu'bicum superius** [ NA ], superior pubic ligament; fibers that pass transversely above the pubic symphysis.

**l. pubocapsula're,** l. pubofemorale.

**l. pubofemora'le** [ NA ], pubofemoral ligament; pubo-capsular ligament; a thickened part of the capsule of the hip joint that extends from the superior ramus of the pubis to the intertrochanteric line of the femur.

**l. puboprostat'icum** [ NA ], puboprostatic ligament, the localized thickening of the superior fascia of the pelvic diaphragm anteriorly that anchors the prostate and neck of the bladder to the pubis on each side. It is composed of medial and lateral parts and usually contains smooth muscle.

**l. puboprostat'icum latera'le,** l. puboprostaticum.

**l. puboprostat'icum media'le,** l. puboprostaticum.

**l. pubovesica'le** [ NA ], pubovesical ligament; in the female the fascial thickening comparable to the l. pubopro-staticum.

**l. pulmona'le** [ NA ], pulmonary ligament; the reflection of pleura from the mediastinum to the lung which continues as a two-layered fold below the root of the lung.

**l. quadratum** [ NA ], quadrate ligament; fibers that pass from the distal margin of the radial notch of the ulna to the neck of the radius.

**l. radia'tum,** l. capitis costae radiatum.

**l. radiocarpe'um dorsa'le** [ NA ], dorsal radiocarpal ligament; the ligament that extends from the distal end of the radius posteriorly to the proximal row of carpals.

**l. radiocarpe'um palmare** [ NA ], palmar radiocarpal ligament; a strong ligament that passes from the distal end of the radius to the proximal row of carpal bones on the anterior surface of the wrist joint.

**l. reflex'um** [ NA ], reflex ligament; Colles' ligament; fascia triangularis abdominis; triangular fascia; a triangu-lar fibrous band extending from the aponeurosis of the external oblique to the pubic tubercle of the opposite side.

**l. sacrococcyge'um dorsale profundum** [ NA ], deep dorsal sacrococcygeal ligament; the continuation of the posterior longitudinal ligament uniting the sacrum and coccyx.

**l. sacrococcygeum dorsale superficiale** [ NA ], superficial dorsal sacrococcygeal ligament; the continuation of the supraspinal ligament from the sacrum to the coccyx.

**l. sacrococcygeum laterale** [ NA ], lateral sacrococcygeal ligament; a ligament that extends from the lateral inferior margin of the sacrum to the transverse process of the first coccygeal vertebra.

**l. sacrococcygeum ventrale** [ NA ], ventral sacrococcyg-eal ligament; the continuation of the anterior longitudinal ligament uniting the sacrum and coccyx.

**l. sacrodura'le,** fibrous filaments running from the middle line of the spinal dura to the posterior ligament of the sacrum.

**ligamenta sacroili'aca dorsalia** [ NA ], dorsal sacroiliac ligaments; heavy fibrous bands that pass from the ilium to the sacrum posterior to the sacroiliac joint; they consist of long and short ligaments.

**ligamenta sacroili'aca interos'sea** [ NA ], interosseous sacroiliac ligaments; short obliquely directed fibrous bands that pass between the sacrum and ilium in the narrow cleft behind the auricular surfaces of these bones.

**ligamenta sacroili'aca ventralia** [ NA ], ventral sacroiliac ligaments; the strong fibrous bands that reinforce the sacroiliac joint anteriorly.

**l. sacroili'acum poste'rius,** l. sacroiliaca dorsalia.

**l. sacrospina'le** [ NA ], sacrospinous ligament; the fibrous band that passes from the ischial spine to the sacrum and coccyx.

**l. sacrospino'sum,** l. sacrospinale.

**l. sacrotubera'le** [ NA ], sacrotuberous ligament; the ligament that passes from the ischial tuberosity to the ilium, sacrum, and coccyx.

**l. sacrotubero'sum,** l. sacrotuberale.

**l. sero'sum,** serous band or ligament; a supporting band, composed chiefly of a fold of peritoneum, attaching certain of the viscera to the abdominal wall or to each other.

**l. sphenomandibula're** [ NA ], sphenomandibular liga-ment; the fibrous band that passes from the spine of the sphenoid bone to the lingula of the mandible.

**l. spira'le coch'leae** [ NA ], spiral ligament of the cochlea; the thickened periosteal lining of the bony cochlea forming the outer wall of the cochlear duct.

**l. ster'noclavicula're** [ NA ], sternoclavicular ligament; one of two ligaments, **l. sternoclaviculare anterius** and **l. sternoclaviculare posterius,** which reinforce the capsule of the sternoclavicular joint.

**l. sternocosta'le** [ NA ], sternocostal ligament; one of the two sets of chondrosternal ligaments connecting the rib cartilages and the sternum; these are **l. sternocostale intraarticulare** and **ligamenta sternocostalia radiata.**

**ligamenta sternoper'icardi'aca** [ NA ], sternopericardial ligaments; Lannelongue's ligaments; fibrous bands that pass from the pericardium to the sternum.

**l. sty'lohyoid'eum** [ NA ], stylohyoid ligament; a fibrous cord that passes from the tip of the styloid process to the lesser cornu of the hyoid bone; it is occasionally ossified.

**l. stylomandibula're** [ NA ], stylomandibular ligament; stylomaxillary ligament; a condensation of the deep cervi-cal fascia extending from the tip of the styloid process of the temporal bone to the posterior border of the angle of the jaw.

**l. supraspina'le** [ NA ], supraspinous ligament; the longitudinal fibrous band attached to the tips of the spinous processes of the vertebrae: in the cervical region it is altered to form the ligamentum nuchae.

**l. suspenso'rium clitor'idis** [ NA ], suspensory ligament of clitoris; a fibrous band that extends from the pubic symphysis to the fascia of the clitoris.

**ligamenta suspenso'ria mam'mae** [ NA ], suspensory ligaments of the breast; suspensory ligaments of Cooper; well developed retinacula cutis that extend from the overlying skin to the fibrous stroma of the mammary gland.

**l. suspenso'rium ova'rii** [ NA ], suspensory ligament of ovary; infundibulopelvic ligament; a band of peritoneum that extends upward from the upper pole of the ovary; it contains the ovarian vessels and ovarian plexus of nerves.

**l. suspenso'rium penis** [ NA ], suspensory ligament of penis; a fibrous band that extends from the pubic symphy-sis to the deep fascia of the penis.

**l. talocalca'neum** [ NA ], talocalcanean ligament; one of several ligaments that unite the talus and calcaneus; these include the **l. talocalcaneum interosseum,** the **l. talocalca-neum laterale,** and the **l. talocalcaneum mediale.**

**l. talofibula're anterius** [ NA ], anterior talofibular ligament; the part of the lateral ligament of the ankle joint that extends from the lateral malleolus to the neck of the talus.

**l. talofibula're posterius** [ NA ], posterior talofibular ligament; the nearly horizontal fibrous band that unites the lateral malleolus with the posterior border of the talus.

**l. talonavicula're** [ NA ], talonavicular ligament; the broad band that passes from the dorsal side of the neck of the talus to the dorsal surface of the navicular bone.

**l. talotibia'le anterius,** see under l. deltoideum.

**l. talotibia'le posterius,** see under l. deltoideum.

**l. tarsa'le externum,** l. palpebrale laterale.

**l. tarsa'le internum,** l. palpebrale mediale.

**ligamenta tarsi** [ NA ], tarsal ligaments; the ligaments that interconnect the tarsal bones; they are grouped into three sets (**ligamenta tarsi dorsalia, ligamenta tarsi interossea,** and **ligamenta tarsi plantaria**), and are individually named according to their attachments.

**ligamenta tarsometatarse'a** [ NA ], tarsometatarsal ligaments; the ligaments that unite tarsal and metatarsal bones; they are arranged in dorsal, interosseous, and plantar sets.

**l. temporomandibula're,** l. laterale articulationis temporomandibularis.

**l. teres fem'oris,** l. capitis femoris.

**l. teres hep'atis** [ NA ], round ligament of the liver, the remains of the umbilical vein.

**l. teres u'teri** [ NA ], round ligament of the uterus; a fibromuscular band that is attached to the uterus on either side in front of and below the opening of the fallopian tube; it passes through the inguinal canal to the labium majus.

**l. tes'tis,** the caudal portion of the embryonic urogenital ridge; the upper third of the gubernaculum testis.

**l. thyroepiglot'ticum** [ NA ], thyroepiglottic ligament; an elastic band that connects the petiole of the epiglottis to the interior of the thyroid cartilage near the superior thyroid notch.

**l. thyrohyoi'deum** [ NA ], l. hyothyroideum laterale; thyrohyoid ligament; a band that extends from the superior cornu of the thyroid cartilage to the tip of the greater cornu of the hyoid bone.

**l. thyrohyoi'deum medianum** [ NA ], l. hyothyroideum medium; median thyrohyoid ligament; the central thickened portion of the thyrohyoid membrane.

**l. tibiofibula're ante'rius** [ NA ], anterior tibiofibular ligament; the ligament that binds the anterior aspect of the tibiofibular syndesmosis.

**l. tibiofibula're me'dium,** *membrana* interossea cruris.

**l. tibiofibula're poste'rius** [ NA ], posterior tibiofibular ligament; the fibrous band that crosses the posterior aspect of the tibiofibular syndesmosis.

**l. tibionavicula're,** see under l. deltoideum.

**ligamenta trachea'lia** [ NA ], ligamenta anularia trachealia.

**l. transversa'lis colli,** cervical *ligament* of the uterus.

**l. transver'sum acetab'uli** [ NA ], transverse ligament of acetabulum; the ligament that passes across the acetabular notch.

**l. transver'sum atlan'tis** [ NA ], see under l. cruciforme atlantis.

**l. transver'sum cruris,** *retinaculum* musculorum extensorum pedis superius.

**l. transver'sum genus** [ NA ], transverse ligament of the knee; a transverse band that passes between the lateral and medial menisci in the anterior part of the knee joint.

**l. transver'sum pelvis,** l. transversum perinei.

**l. transversum perinei** [ NA ], transverse ligament of the perineum; Krause's ligament; the thickened anterior border of the urogenital diaphragm, formed by the fusion of its two fascial layers.

**l. transver'sum scap'ulae infe'rius** [ NA ], inferior transverse scapular ligament; spinoglenoid ligament; an inconstant fibrous band that passes from the lateral border of the spine of the scapula to the posterior margin of the glenoid cavity.

**l. transver'sum scap'ulae supe'rius** [ NA ], superior transverse scapular ligament; suprascapular ligament; the strong fibrous band that bridges the scapular notch.

**l. trapezoid'eum** [ NA ], trapezoid ligament; the part of the coracoclavicular ligament that attaches to the trapezoid line of the clavicle.

**l. triangula're,** *fascia* diaphragmatis urogenitalis inferior.

**l. triangula're dextrum hepatis** [ NA ], right triangular ligament; a triangular fold of peritoneum that passes from the right lobe of the liver to the diaphragm; it is continuous with the coronary ligament.

**l. triangula're sinis'trum hepatis** [ NA ], left triangular ligament; a triangular fold of peritoneum that extends from the left lobe of the liver to the diaphragm.

**l. tuber'culi costae,** l. costotransversarium laterale.

**l. ulnocarpeum palmare** [ NA ], palmar ulnocarpal ligament; the fibrous band that passes from the ulnar styloid process to the carpal bones.

**l. umbilica'le latera'le,** an old name for l. umbilicale mediale.

**l. umbilica'le media'le** [ NA ], medial umbilical ligament; the obliterated umbilical artery that persists as a fibrous cord passing upward alongside the bladder to the umbilicus.

**l. umbilica'le medianum** [ NA ], middle umbilical ligament; contained in the plica umbilicalis mediana; the remnant of the urachus; it persists as a midline fibrous cord between the apex of the bladder and the umbilicus.

**l. ve'nae ca'vae sinis'trae,** ligament of the left vena cava; the obliterated left common cardinal vein.

**l. veno'sum** [ NA ], venous ligament; ligament of Arantius; a thin fibrous cord, lying in the fossa ductus venosi, the remains of the ductus venosus of the fetus.

**l. ventriculare,** l. vestibulare.

**l. vestibula're** [ NA ], vestibular ligament; ventricular ligament; the thin fibrous layer that lies in the ventricular fold of the larynx.

**l. voca'le** [ NA ], vocal ligament; the band that extends on either side from the thyroid cartilage to the vocal process of the arytenoid cartilage; it is the upper border of the conus elasticus of the larynx.

**ligand** (lig'and, li'gand) [ L. *ligo,* to bind ]. An organic molecule attached to a central metal ion by multiple coordination bonds; the porphyrin portion of heme, the corrin nucleus of the $B_{12}$ vitamins, etc., are l.'s.

**li'gase.** Generic term for enzymes (EC class 6) catalyzing the joining of two molecules coupled with the breakdown of a pyrophosphate bond in ATP or a similar compound; l.'s are commonly known as synthetases.

**li'gate** [ L. *ligo,* pp. *-atus,* to bind ]. To apply a ligature; to constrict a blood vessel or the pedicle of a tumor by means of a tightly tied thread or fillet.

**ligation** (li-ga'shun) [ L. *ligatio,* fr. *ligo,* to bind. LIG- ]. The application of a ligature.

**Larrey's l.,** l. of the femoral artery immediately below Poupart's ligament.

**pole l.,** l. at root of an organ to shut off or to diminish blood supply.

**surgical l.,** in dentistry, the surgical exposure of an unerupted tooth so that a metal ligature can be placed around its cervix and fastened to an orthodontic appliance to facilitate eruption.

**tooth l.,** the binding together of teeth with wire for stabilization and immobilization following traumatic injury or during periodontal therapy.

**li'gator.** An instrument used in the ligation of vessels in deep and nearly inaccessible parts.

**ligature** (lig'a-chūr) [ L. *ligatura,* a band or tie, fr. *ligo,* to tie. LIG- ]. 1. A thread, wire, fillet, or the like, tied tightly around a blood vessel, the pedicle of a tumor, or other structure in order to constrict it. 2. Ligation.

**Desault's l.,** l. of the femoral artery in its passage through the adductor muscle, for the cure of popliteal aneurysm.

**elastic l.,** one of india rubber which slowly constricts the part by reason of its contractility.

**occluding l.,** l. to shut off completely the distal blood supply.

**provisional l.,** one applied to an artery in continuity at the beginning of an operation to prevent hemorrhage, but removed when the operation is completed.

**soluble l.,** a l. of catgut or other animal material, which eventually is absorbed or becomes organized.

**Stannius' l.,** a l. placed either around the junction between the sinus venosus and atrium of the frog or turtle heart (first Stannius' l.) or around the atrioventricular junction (second Stannius' l.); demonstrates that the cardiac impulse is conducted from sinus venosus to atria to ventricle, but that successive chambers possess automaticity since each may continue to beat, but the atria now have a slower rate than the sinus venosus and the ventricle either does not contract or beats at a slower rate than the atria.

**suboccluding l.,** l. to diminish blood supply and encourage collateral circulation.

**light** (līt) [ A.S. *leōht* ]. Electromagnetic radiations to which the retina is sensitive and which thus render visible the object whence they proceed. See also subentries under **lamp.**

**arc l.,** arc lamp; a device that produces bright light when an electric current is made to spark continuously across a gap between two incandescent electrodes, usually of carbon.

**cold l.,** (1) l. produced enzymatically by certain luminous insects (the firefly), fungi, protozoa, bacteria, etc., which is accompanied by a negligible production of heat, chemical energy being converted directly into l. energy; see luciferin, luciferase; (2) fluorescent l. as opposed to incandescent l.

**cone of l.,** see under cone.

**Finsen l.,** the violet and ultraviolet rays of the spectrum filtered out of the sunlight by a hollow planoconvex lens filled with an ammoniacal solution of copper sulfate; usually, instead of the filtered sunlight, the carbon electric arc is used, the rays being made parallel by two planoconvex lenses. It was formerly used in the treatment of cutaneous tuberculosis.

**idioretinal l.,** intrinsic l.

**infrared l.,** see infrared.

**intrin'sic l.,** idioretinal l.; a very faint glow seen on looking at the retina in the dark.

**po'larized l.,** l. in which, as a result of reflection or transmission through certain media, the vibrations are all in one plane, transverse to the ray, instead of in all planes.

**reflected l.,** l. directed backward from a mirror.

**refracted l.,** bent rays of l. changed in passage from one transparent medium to another of unequal density; see also refraction.

**Simpson l.,** a lamp emitting ultraviolet rays, produced by an electric arc between two electrodes, one of tungstate of iron and the other of manganese.

**transmitted l.,** l. passed through a transparent medium.

**Wood's l.,** ultraviolet l. formed by filtering l. through Wood's *glass, q.v.*

**light'ening.** The feeling of decreased abdominal distention during the later weeks of pregnancy following the descent of the fetal head into the pelvic inlet.

**Lignac,** G. O. E., Dutch pediatrician. See L.-Fanconi *syndrome.*

**lig'nin** [ L. *lignum,* wood ]. A polymer of coniferyl alcohol accompanying cellulose and present in vegetable fiber and wood cells; source of vanillin (by oxidation of l.).

**lignocaine hydrochloride** (lig'no-kān) (BP). Lidocaine hydrochloride.

**lignoceric acid** (lig'no-sēr'ik, -sēr'ik). Tetracosanoic acid; $CH_3$—$(CH_2)_{22}$—COOH; present in one type of sphingomyelin.

**lig'num,** gen. **lig'ni** [ L. ]. Wood.

**Lilienthal,** Howard, U. S. surgeon, 1861–1946. See L.'s *probe.*

**Lillie,** R. D., U. S. pathologist, *1896. See Levinthal-Cole-L. *bodies,* L.'s allochrome *stain,* azure-eosin *stain.*

**Lilly,** John C., U. S. physiologist, *1915. See Silverman-L. *pneumotachograph.*

**limb** [ A.S. *lim* ]. 1. An extremity; a member; an arm or leg. 2. A segment of any jointed structure.

**ampullary l.'s of semicircular ducts,** *crura* membranacea ampullaria.

**anacrotic l.,** the ascending l. of an arterial pulse tracing.

**anterior l. of internal capsule,** *crus* anterius capsulae internae.

**anterior l. of stapes,** *crus* anterius stapedis.

**l.'s of bony semicircular canals,** *crura* ossea canales semicirculares.

**common l. of membranous semicircular ducts,** *crus* membranaceum commune ductus semicircularis.

**l. of helix,** *crus* helicis.

**lateral l.,** *crus* laterale.

**medial l.,** *crus* mediale.

**pelvic l.,** an inferior l.

**phantom l.,** after amputation of a l. or a portion of it, the patient experiences sensations (sometimes called stump

hallucinations) as though the part were still intact; various types of paresthesias or severe pain may be complained of.

**posterior l. of internal capsule,** *crus* posterius capsulae internae.

**posterior l. of stapes,** *crus* posterius stapedis.

**retrolenticular l. of internal capsule,** *pars* retrolentiformis capsulae internae.

**simple membranous l. of semicircular duct,** *crus* membranaceum simplex ductus semicircularis.

**siren l.,** see sirenomelia.

**sublenticular l. of internal capsule,** *pars* sublentiformis capsulae internae.

**superior l.,** *membrum* superius.

**thoracic l.,** a superior l.

**lim'bic.** Relating to (1) a limbus, or (2) the limbic *system.*

**limbus,** pl. **lim'bi** (lim'bus) [ L. a border ] [ NA ]. The edge, border, or fringe of a part.

**l. alveola'ris,** *arcus* alveolaris.

**l. corneae** [ NA ], corneal margin; sclerocorneal junction; the margin of the cornea overlapped by the sclera.

**l. fos'sae ova'lis** [ NA ], margin of the fossa ovalis; anulus ovalis; Vieussens' anulus or isthmus; a muscular ring surrounding the fossa ovalis in the wall of the right atrium of the heart.

**l. lam'inae spira'lis osseae** [ NA ], the border of the spiral lamina; the thickened periosteum covering the upper plate of the lamina spiralis ossea of the cochlea.

**l. membra'nae tym'pani,** margin of the tympanic membrane attaching to the tympanic sulcus.

**limbi palpebra'les** [ NA ], borders of the eyelids; anterior and posterior margins of the lids.

**l. penicilla'tus,** brush *border.*

**l. stria'tus,** striated *border.*

**Vieussens' l.,** l. fossae ovalis.

**lime** (līm). 1. Fruit of the l. tree, *Citrus medica* (family Rutaceae), the juice of which is used to make an acidulous drink. 2. Calx; calcium oxide; CaO; an alkaline earth occurring in grayish white masses (quicklime). On exposure to the atmosphere it becomes converted into calcium hydrate and calcium carbonate (air-slaked lime). The direct addition of water to calcium oxide produces calcium hydrate (slaked lime).

**chlorinated l.** (BP), bleaching powder; obtained by the action of chlorine on calcium hydroxide; used to prepare surgical chlorinated soda solution and as a disinfectant and deodorant.

**sulfurated l.,** calcium sulfide, crude.

**limen,** gen. **liminis,** pl. **limina** (li'men, lim'ĭ-nah) [ L. ] [ NA ]. Threshold (3); entrance; the external opening of a canal.

**l. in'sulae** [ NA ], threshold of the island of Reil; the band of transition between the anterior portion of the gray matter of the insula and the anterior perforated substance; it is formed by a narrow strip of olfactory cortex along the lateral side of the lateral olfactory stria.

**l. nasi** [ NA ], threshold of the nose; a ridge marking the boundary between the nasal cavity proper and the vestibule.

**limes nul.** See symbol $L_0$, under dose.

**limes tod.** See symbol $L_+$, under dose.

**liminal** (lim'ĭ-nal) [ L. *limen* (*limin-*), a threshold ]. 1. Pertaining to a threshold. 2. Pertaining to a stimulus just strong enough to excite a tissue, *e.g.,* nerve or muscle.

**liminometer** (lim'ĭ-nom'e-ter) [ L. *limen,* threshold, + G. *metron,* measure ]. An instrument for measuring the strength of stimulus which is barely sufficient to produce a reflex response.

**lim'it** [ L. *limes,* boundary ]. Boundary; end.

**l. dextrin, dextrinase, dextrinosis,** see the nouns.

**elastic l.,** the greatest stress to which a material may be subjected and still be capable of returning to its original dimensions when the forces are released.

**proportional l.,** the greatest stress that a material is capable of sustaining without any deviation from proportionality of stress to strain (Hooke's law).

**quantum l.,** the shortest wavelength found in an x-ray spectrum.

**limitaneus** [ L. situated on the borders ] [ NA ]. Pertaining to the borders or margins of a structure or organ.

**limitrophic** (lim'ĭ-trof'ik) [ L. *limes* (*limit*-), limit, + G. *trophē*, nourishment ]. Controlling nutrition; denoting the sympathetic nervous system.

**Limna'tis nilot'ica.** The horse leech; a species of land-leech of Southern Europe and North Africa which may infest the nostrils or gullet and, attaching itself to the mucous membrane, cause hemorrhages and anemia.

**limnemia** (lim-ne'mĭ-ah) [ G. *limnē*, marsh, + *haima*, blood ]. Chronic malaria; malarial cachexia.

**limnemic** (lim-ne'mik). Suffering from malarial cachexia.

**limnology** (lim-nol'o-jĭ) [ G. *limnē*, pool, + *logos*, study ]. Study of the physical, chemical, meteorological, and biological conditions in fresh water; of importance to ecology.

**Limnotrag'us spek'ei** [ G. *limnē*, pool, + *tragos*, a he-goat ]. Former name for *Strepsiceros spekei*.

**li'mon**, gen. **limo'nis** [ L. ]. Lemon.

**lim'onene.** Cinene; cajeputene; caoutchin; *p*-mentha-1,8-diene; a substance present in several oils; one of the constituents of the terpenes.

Limonene

**limophoitas** (li'mo-foy'tas) [ G. *limos*, hunger, + *phoitas*, frenzy ]. Psychosis induced by starvation.

**limophthisis** (li-mof'thĭ-sis) [ G. *limos*, hunger, + *phthisis*, wasting ]. Emaciation from lack of sufficient nourishment.

**limosis** (li-mo'sis) [ G. *limos*, hunger ]. Hunger, especially abnormal or inordinate hunger.

**li'mother'apy** [ G. *limos*, hunger, + therapy ]. Hunger therapy.

**limp'ing.** Walking lame, with a yielding step; see also claudication.

**Linacre** (lin'ak-er) Thomas, English priest and physician, 1460–1524; physician to Henry VIII; founded lectureships in medicine at Cambridge and Oxford; translated Galen's works into Latin correcting the inaccuracies of previous editions.

**lina'ria** [ L. *linum*, flax ]. Toad flax; snap dragon; the plant *Linaria vulgaris* (family Scrophulariaceae). Diuretic and laxative; has been used in hemorrhoids.

**lincomycin** (lin'ko-mi-sin) (USAN). An antibacterial substance, $C_{18}H_{34}N_2O_6S$, produced by *Streptomyces lincolnensis;* active against Gram-positive organisms. Official in the BP as lincomycin hydrochloride.

**linc'ture, linc'tus** [ L. *lingo*, pp. *linctus*, to lick ]. Electuary; confection; originally a medical preparation taken by licking.

**Lind,** James, British naval surgeon, 1716–94. Remembered for his advocacy of lemon juice as a preventive of scurvy and for his graphic account of this disease which he eradicated from the British Navy.

**lin'dane.** GAMMEXANE; 1,2,3,4,5,6-hexachlorocyclohexane; used as scabicide, pediculocide, and insecticide (10 times more toxic for house flies than DDT). Official in the USP and BP as gamma-benzene hexachloride.

**Lindau,** Arvid, Swedish pathologist, *1892. See L.'s *disease, tumor,* von Hippel-L. *disease.*

**Lindbergh,** Charles A., American aviator, *1902. See Carrel-L. *pump.*

**Lindeman's cannula.** See under cannula.

**Lindner,** Karl, Austrian ophthalmologist, 1883–1961. See L.'s *bodies.*

**Lindqvist,** Johan Torsten, Swedish physician, *1906. See Fahraeus-L. *effect.*

# LINE

**line** [ L. *linea,* a linen thread, a string, line, fr. *linum*, flax ]. 1. A mark, strip, or streak; see also linea. 2. A unit of measurement used by histologists in the 19th century; it varied in different countries from $^1/_{10}$ to $^1/_{12}$ of an English inch, but the most widely used unit was the Paris l., *q.v.*

**absorption l.'s,** numerous dark l.'s in the solar spectrum due to absorption by the solar atmosphere, and also by that of the earth; the phenomenon is due to the fact that rays passing from an incandescent body through a cooler medium are absorbed by elements in that medium. These elements would give out the same rays if the medium were itself made incandescent.

**accretion l.'s.,** l.'s seen in microscopic sections of the enamel, marking successive layers of added material.

**alve'olona'sal l.,** a l. connecting the alveolar point and the nasion.

**Amberg's lateral sinus l.,** a l. dividing the angle formed by the anterior edge of the mastoid process and the temporal l.

**anocutaneous l.,** pectinate l.

**ar'cuate l.,** *linea arcuata.*

**ax'illary l.,** *linea axillaris.*

**azygos venous l.,** medial sympathetic l.; a longitudinal venous channel lying dorsilateral to the aorta and medial to the sympathetic trunk in the embryo; the right side forms the azygos vein, the left side forms the hemiazygos vein.

**B l.'s of Kerley,** fine horizontal l.'s a few centimeters above the costophrenic angle in the chest x-ray; seen in patients with pulmonary hypertension secondary to mitral stenosis and thought to be due to distention of interlobular lymphatics with edema fluid.

**Baillarger's l.'s,** Baillarger's bands; two laminae of white fibers that course parallel to the surface of the cerebral cortex and are visible as outer and inner l.'s in sections cut perpendicular to the surface; the l. of Gennari in the calcarine cortex represents the outer of these lines.

**base l.,** a l. corresponding to the base of the skull, passing from the infraorbital ridge to the midline of the occiput, cutting the external auditory meatus.

**basina'sal l.,** a l. connecting the basion and the nasion.

**Beau's l.'s,** the transverse corrugations on the fingernails after typhoid fever and other systemic diseases.

**l. of Bechterew,** band of Bechterew; l. of Kaes; in the fresh brain, a faintly visible white l. on the cerebral cortex, composed of tangential fibers in layer 3, superficial to the much more numerous fibers composing Baillarger's l. in layer 5.

**blood l.,** a l. of descent or ancestry of several generations.

**blue l.,** a bluish discoloration along the dental edges of the gums, seen in chronic lead or bismuth poisoning.

**Bolton-nasion l.,** Bolton *plane.*

**Brödel's bloodless l.,** l. in section of the kidney demarcating the areas of distribution of the anterior and posterior branches of the renal artery.

**Bryant's l.,** the base of Bryant's triangle along which the trochanter moves in fracture of the neck of the femur.

**Burton's l.,** a bluish l. on the free border of the gums, occurring in lead poisoning.

**calcification l.'s of Retzius,** incremental l.'s of rhythmic deposition of successive layers of enamel matrix during development.

**Camper's l.,** the l. running from the inferior border of the ala of the nose to the superior border of the tragus of the ear.

**cell l.,** in tissue culture, the cells growing in the first or later subculture from a primary culture; see also established cell l.

**cement l.,** the refractile boundaries of osteons or interstitial lamellar systems in compact bone.

**cervical l.,** a continuous anatomical irregular curved line marking the cervical end of the crown of a tooth.

**Chamberlain's l.,**  a l. drawn from the posterior margin of the hard palate to the dorsum of the foramen magnum; in basilar impression, the odontoid process rises above this l.

**Chaussier's l.,**  the anteroposterior l. of the corpus callosum as appearing on median section of the brain.

**Clapton's l.,**  a greenish discoloration of the dental margin of the gums in cases of chronic copper poisoning.

**cleavage l.'s,**  when a pin is driven into the skin of the cadaver, the opening made is linear, owing to the special distribution of the subcutaneous fibrous connective tissue bundle. These l.'s, known as Langer's l.'s, take definite directions varying with the region of the body surface.

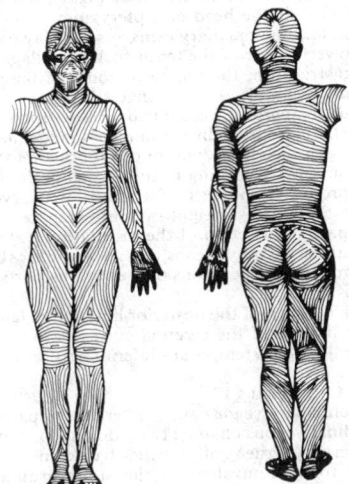

**Cleavage Lines of the Skin**
(After Langer)

**Conradi's l.,**  a l. extending from the base of the ensiform cartilage to the apex beat of the heart, corresponding approximately to the lower edge of the cardiac area.

**Correra's l.,**  a l. between lungs and thoracic cage, seen on x-ray.

**costoclavic'ular l.,**  parasternal l.

**costophrenic septal l.'s,**  B l.'s of Kerley.

**Crampton's l.,**  a l. from the apex of the cartilage of the last rib downward and forward nearly to the crest of the ilium, then forward parallel with it to a little below the anterior superior spine; a guide to the common iliac artery.

**Daubenton's l.,**  the occipital l. passing between the opisthion and the nasion.

**l. of demarcation,**  see under demarcation.

**dentate l.,**  pectinate l.

**developmental l.'s,**  developmental *grooves.*

**Dobie's l.,**  Z l.

**Douglas' l.,**  *linea* arcuata.

**Eberth's l.'s,**  l.'s appearing between the cells of the myocardium when stained with silver nitrate.

**epiphysial l.,**  *linea* epiphysialis.

**established cell l.,**  cells growing in culture after at least 70 subcultures at intervals of 3 days.

**Farre's l.,**  a whitish l. marking the insertion of the mesovarium on the ovary.

**Feiss l.,**  a l. running from the medial malleolus to the plantar aspect of the first metatarsophalangeal joint.

**l. of fixation,**  see under fixation.

**Fleischner l.'s,**  linear shadows on the roentgenogram of the chest, indicating foci of atelectasis.

**Fraunhofer's l.'s,**  a number of the most prominent of the absorption l.'s of the solar spectrum.

**fulcrum l.,**  opening axis; rotational axis; an imaginary l. around which a removable partial denture tends to rotate.

**fulcrum l., retentive,**  (1) an imaginery l. connecting the retentive points of clasp arms on retaining teeth adjacent to mucosa-borne denture bases; (2) an imaginary l. connecting the retentive points of clasp arms, around

which l. the denture tends to rotate when subjected to forces such as the pull of sticky foods.

**fulcrum l., stabilizing,**  an imaginary l. connecting occlusal rests, around which l. the denture tends to rotate under masticatory force.

**l. of Gennari,**  band, stria, or stripe of Gennari; a prominent white line appearing in perpendicular sections of the visual cortex (Brodmann's area 17) at about mid-thickness of the cortical gray matter, corresponding to the particularly well developed outer line of Baillarger of that cortical area, and composed largely of tangentially disposed intracortical association fibers.

**glu'teal l.,**  *linea* glutea.

**Granger's l.,**  in x-ray of skull, a l. produced by the groove of the optic nerve.

**Gubler's l.,**  the level of the superficial origin of the trigeminus on the pons, a lesion below which causes Gubler's paralysis.

**gum l.,**  the position of the margin of the gingiva in relation to the teeth in the dental arch.

**Haller's l.,**  *linea* splendens.

**Hampton l.,**  a radiolucent density indicating mucosal edema, contrasted against the radiopaque barium in benign gastric ulcerations.

**Harris' l.'s,**  transverse l.'s seen under the x-ray near the epiphyses of the long bones.

**Head's l.'s,**  Head's zones; tender l.'s or zones; bands of cutaneous hyperesthesia associated with acute or chronic inflammation of the viscera.

**Hensen's l.,**  H *band.*

**highest nuchal l.,**  *linea* nuchae suprema.

**Hilton's white l.,**  white l. of anal canal.

**Holden's l.,**  an indistinct furrow or wrinkle in the groin, passing outward between the anterior superior spine of the ilium and the great trochanter, indicating the position of the capsule of the hip joint.

**Hudson's l.,**  Hudson-Stähli l.; Stahl's l.; linea corneae senilis; a brown, somewhat wavy horizontal l. across the lower third of the cornea, occasionally seen in the aged and also in association with corneal opacities.

**Hudson-Stähli l.,**  Hudson's l.

**Hunter's l.,**  *linea* alba.

**iliopectin'eal l.,**  *linea* terminalis.

**incremental l.'s,**  Owen's l.'s; the l.'s, perhaps caused by imperfect calcification or other growth phenomena, seen passing through the dentin. When seen in the enamel, they are referred to as l.'s of Retzius.

**inferior nuchal l.,**  *linea* nuchae inferior.

**inferior temporal l.,**  *linea* temporalis inferior.

**infracos'tal l.,**  subcostal l.

**intercondy'lar l.,**  *linea* intercondylaris.

**intermediate l. of iliac crest,**  *linea* intermedia cristae iliacae.

**interspi'nal l.,**  Lanz's l.; a horizontal l. drawn between the two anterior superior spines of the ilia.

**intertrochanter'ic l.,**  *linea* intertrochanterica.

**intertuber'cular l.,**  an imaginary transverse l., drawn at the level of the iliac crests, at a point corresponding to the tubercle about 2 inches behind the anterior superior spine on either side; it divides the umbilical from the hypogastric zones of the abdomen.

**isoelectric l.,**  the base line of the electrocardiogram.

**l. of Kaes,**  l. of Bechterew.

**Kilian's l.,**  a transverse l. marking the promontory of the pelvis.

**Langer's l.'s,**  cleavage l.'s.

**Lanz's l.,**  interspinal l.

**lateral l.,**  see lateral line *system.*

**lateral sympathetic l.,**  thoracolumbar venous l.

**lead l.,**  an irregular dark deposit in the gums found in lead poisoning, particularly in people with poor oral hygiene.

**lip l., high,**  the greatest height to which the lip is raised in normal function or during the act of smiling broadly.

**lip l., low,**  (1) the lowest position of the lower lip during the act of smiling or voluntary retraction; (2) the lowest position of the upper lip at rest.

**M l.,**  M band; mesophragma; a fine l. in the center of the A band in the myofibrils of striated muscle fibers.

**mam'illary l.,**  *linea* mamillaris.

**mam'mary l.,**  a transverse l. drawn between the two

nipples.

**McKees' l.,** a l. drawn from the tip of the cartilage of the eleventh rib to a point an inch and a half to the inner side of the anterior superior spine, then curved downward, forward, and inward to just above the internal abdominal ring; a guide to the common iliac artery.

**medial sympathetic l.,** azygos venous l.

**median l.,** *linea mediana.*

**Mees' l.'s,** Mees' stripes; horizontal white bands of the nails seen in chronic arsenical poisoning, and occasionally in leprosy.

**mercurial l.,** a bluish brown pigmentation seen at the gingival margin and associated with mercury poisoning (mercurial stomatitis).

**Meyer's l.,** a l. through the axis of the big toe and passing the midpoint of the heel in a normal foot.

**midax'illary l.,** a perpendicular l. passing through the center of the axilla.

**midclavic'ular l.,** *linea mamillaris.*

**milk l.,** mammary *ridge.*

**Monro's l.,** Monro-Richter l.

**Monro-Richter l.,** a l. passing from the umbilicus to the left anterior superior spine of the ilium.

**mylohy'oid l.,** *linea mylohyoidea.*

**nasobas'ilar l.,** basinasal l.

**Nélaton's l.,** a l. drawn from the anterior superior spine of the ilium to the tuberosity of the ischium; normally the great trochanter lies in this l., but in cases of iliac dislocation of the hip or fracture of the neck of the femur the trochanter is felt above the l.; called also Roser-Néla-ton l.

**nipple l.,** *linea mamillaris.*

**Obersteiner-Redlich l.,** Obersteiner-Redlich *zone.*

**oblique l.,** *linea obliqua.*

**l. of occlusion,** the alignment of the occluding surfaces of the teeth in the horizontal plane; see also occlusal *plane.*

**Ogston's l.,** a l. drawn from the tubercle of the femur to the intercondyloid notch; a guide to resection of the internal condyle for knock-knee.

**Owen's l.'s,** incremental l.'s.

**paraster'nal l.,** a perpendicular l., nearly continuous with Poupart's l., running midway between the nipple and the outer border of the sternum.

**Paris l.,** a unit of microscopic measurement as used in Kölliker's *Mikroskopische Anatomie;* it was equal to 0.0888138 of an inch.

**pectinate l.,** anocutaneous l.; dentate l.; the l. between the simple columnar epithelium of the rectum and the strati-fied epithelium of the anal canal.

**pectin'eal l.,** *linea pectinea.*

**pleuroesophageal l.,** a l. seen normally in an x-ray of the chest. It has no pathologic significance.

**Poirier's l.,** a l. extending from the nasion to a little above the lambda.

**poplit'eal l.,** *linea musculi solei.*

**Poupart's l.,** a perpendicular l. passing through the center of Poupart's ligament on either side; it marks off the hypochondriac, lumbar, and iliac from the epigastric, umbilical, and hypogastric regions, respectively.

**precentral l.,** a l. on the head, running from the midpoint on the vertex between the glabella and the inion, down-ward and forward; it corresponds to the superior and inferior precentral sulci.

**profile l.,** in roentgenography of the stomach, the thin l. delineating the stomach as seen by means of x-rays when barium is ingested and a thin rubber balloon then swallowed and distended within the stomach. The barium is thus spread and pressed against the gastric mucosa.

**pure l.,** see isogenic *strain.*

**Reid's base l.,** a l. drawn from the lower margin of the orbit to the auricular point (center of the aperture of the external auditory canal) and extending backward to the center of the occipital bone.

**l.'s of Retzius,** see (1) calcification l.'s of Retzius; (2) incremental l.'s.

**Richter-Monro l.,** Monro-Richter l.

**Roser-Nélaton l.,** Nélaton's l.

**sagittal l.,** any anteroposterior l.

**Salter's incremental l.'s,** transverse l.'s sometimes seen in dentin, due to improper calcification.

**Schreger's l.'s,** l.'s seen in enamel in reflected light due to crossing of groups of rods.

**semilunar l.,** *linea semilunaris.*

**Sergent's white l.,** white l.

**Shenton's l.,** a curved l. or arch, formed by the top of the obturator foramen and the inner side of the neck of the femur, seen in a skiagram of the normal joint; it is disturbed in many lesions of the hip joint, such as congenital dislocation.

**Spigelius' l.,** *linea semilunaris.*

**spiral l.,** *linea intertrochanterica.*

**Stahl's l.,** Hudson's l.

**sternal l.,** the midline of the sternum.

**Stocker's l.,** a fine l. of melanotic pigment in the corneal epithelium near the head of a pterygium.

**subcostal l.,** an imaginary transverse l., drawn at the level of the lower border of the tenth costal cartilage; it divides the epigastric from the umbilical zones of the abdomen.

**superior nuchal l.,** *linea nuchae superior.*

**superior temporal l.,** *linea temporalis superior.*

**survey l.,** clasp guideline; Cummer's guideline; (1) the l. indicating the height of contour of a tooth after the cast has been positioned according to the chosen path of insertion; (2) a l. produced on a cast of a tooth by a survey scriber; it marks the greatest height of contour in relation to the chosen path of insertion of the restoration; (3) a l. drawn on a tooth or teeth by means of a surveyor for the purpose of determining the positions of the various parts of a clasp or clasps.

**Sylvian l.,** the l. of the posterior limb of the lateral sulcus (Sylvian fissure) of the cerebral cortex.

**temporal l.,** *linea* temporalis inferior and *linea* temporalis superior.

**tender l.'s,** Head's l.'s.

**thoracolumbar venous l.,** lateral sympathetic l.; a longitudinal venous channel lying dorsilateral to the aorta and lateral to the sympathetic trunk in the embryo; thought to be equivalent to the supracardinal veins in lower mammals.

**Topinard's l.,** a l. running between the glabella and the mental point.

**trapezoid l.,** *linea trapezoidea.*

**Ullmann's l.,** the l. of displacement in spondylolisthesis.

**Veslingius' l.,** *raphe scroti.*

**vibrating l.,** the imaginary l. across the posterior part of the palate, marking the division between the movable and immovable tissues.

**l. of vision,** visual *axis.*

**Wagner's l.,** a narrow, whitish, slightly curved l., representing an area of preliminary calcification, at the junction of the epiphysis and diaphysis of a long bone.

**white l.,** Sergent's white l.; a pale streak appearing in 30 to 60 seconds after scratching the skin and lasting for several minutes, regarded as a sign of diminished arterial tension.

**white l. of anal canal,** Hilton's white l.; a bluish pink, narrow, wavy zone in the mucosa of the anal canal below the pectinate l. at the level of the interval between the subcutaneous part of the external sphincter and the lower border of the internal sphincter.

**Z l.,** one of the cross striations in a muscle fiber which bisects the I band in the myofibrils and occurs at the limits of the sarcomere. Also called Z band or disk; Dobie's l.; Krause's membrane; telophragma; inophragma; Amici's disk; intermediate disk.

**l.'s of Zahn,** striae of Zahn; riblike markings seen by the naked eye on the surface of antemortem thrombi; they consist of a branching framework of platelets and fibrin separating the coagulated blood cells.

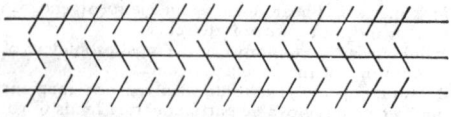

Zöllner's Lines

**Zöllner's l.'s,** figures devised to show the possibility of optical delusions; a common one consists of two parallel l.'s which are met by numerous short lines obliquely placed, the parallel lines then seeming to converge or diverge.

# LINEA

**linea,** gen. and pl. **lin'eae** (lin'e-ah) [ L. ] [ NA ]. A line; a long narrow mark, strip, or streak distinguished, in anatomy, from the adjacent tissues by color, texture, or elevation.

**l. adminic'ulum,** see *adminiculum* lineae albae.

**l. alba** [ NA ], white line; a fibrous band running vertically the entire length of the center of the anterior abdominal wall, receiving the attachments of the oblique and transverse abdominal muscles.

**l. al'bicans,** pl. **lin'eae albican'tes,** *striae* cutis distensae.

**l. arcua'ta** [ NA ], arcuate line; (1) the iliac portion of the terminal line of the pelvis; (2) semicircular line; line of Douglas; a crescentic line, not always clearly defined, which marks the lower limit of the posterior layer of the sheath of the rectus abdominis muscle.

**l. as'pera** [ NA ], rough line; a rough ridge with two pronounced lips running down the posterior surface of the shaft of the femur; the outer lip (labium laterale) is a continuation of the crista glutea, the inner lip (labium mediale) of the linea intertrochanterica; it affords attachment to the vastus medialis, adductor longus, adductor magnus, adductor brevis, the short head of the biceps, and the vastus lateralis muscles.

**lineae atroph'ica,** *striae* cutis distensae.

**l. axilla'ris** [ NA ], axillary line; one of three vertical parallel lines used as guides in physical diagnosis; the anterior passes through the anterior axillary fold, and the posterior through the posterior axillary fold, while the midaxillary line passes through the center of the axillary space.

**l. cor'neae seni'lis,** Hudson's *line.*

**l. epiphysia'lis** [ NA ], epiphysial line; the line of junction of the epiphysis and diaphysis of a long bone where growth in length occurs.

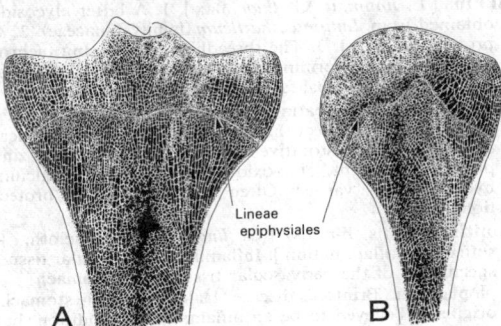

Lineae epiphysiales

A          B

**Lineae Epiphysiales**
Epiphysial lines of (*A*) proximal end of tibia and (*B*) proximal end of humerus.

**l. glute'a** [ NA ], gluteal line; one of three rough curved lines on the outer surface of the ala of the ilium, named **l. glutea anterior** (or middle), **inferior,** and **posterior;** the two areas bounded by these give attachment to the gluteus minimus muscle below and gluteus medius above.

**l. intercondylaris** [ NA ], intercondylar line; a faint transverse ridge separating the floor of the intercondyloid notch from the popliteal surface of the femur; it affords attachment to the posterior portion of the articular capsule of the knee.

**l. interme'dia cristae ili'acae** [ NA ], intermediate line of the iliac crest; the intermediate surface of the crest of the ilium between the outer and inner lips.

**l. intertrochanter'ica** [ NA ], intertrochanteric line; spiral line; a rough line that separates the neck and shaft of the femur anteriorly; it passes downward and medially from the greater trochanter and continues into the medial lip of the linea aspera.

**l. mamilla'ris** [ NA ], l. medioclavicularis [ NA ]; mamillary line; midclavicular line; a perpendicular line passing through the nipple on either side, it corresponds closely to a perpendicular line dropped from the midpoint of the clavicle.

**l. media'na** [ NA ], median line; (1) the center line dividing the central body surface into right and left; (2) the intersection of the midsagittal plane with the maxillary and mandibular dental arches.

**l. media'na ante'rior** [ NA ], anterior median line; anterior midline; a perpendicular line along the anterior midline of the body.

**l. media'na poste'rior** [ NA ], posterior median line; posterior midline; a perpendicular line that passes along the midline of the body posteriorly.

**l. medioclavicula'ris** [ NA ], l. mamillaris.

**l. musculi solei** [ NA ], line for the soleus muscle; soleal line; popliteal line; a ridge which extends obliquely downward and medially across the back of the tibia from the fibular articular facet; it gives origin to the soleus muscle.

**l. mylohyoid'ea** [ NA ], mylohyoid line; internal oblique line; a ridge on the inner surface of the mandible running from the inferior to the mental spine upward and backward to the ramus behind the last molar tooth; it gives attachment to the mylohyoid muscle and superior constrictor of the pharynx.

**l. nigra,** black line; the l. alba in pregnancy, which then becomes pigmented.

**l. nuchae inferior** [ NA ], inferior nuchal line; a ridge that extends laterally from the external occipital crest toward the jugular process of the occipital bone.

**l. nu'chae media'na,** *crista* occipitalis externa.

**l. nuchae superior** [ NA ], superior nuchal line; the ridge that extends laterally from the external occipital protuberance toward the lateral angle of the occipital bone; it gives attachment to the trapezius, sternocleidomastoid, and splenius capitis muscles.

**l. nuchae supre'ma** [ NA ], highest nuchal line; a line above and parallel to the superior nuchal line on the external surface of the occipital bone; it gives attachment to the epicranial aponeurosis and occipitalis muscle.

**l. obli'qua** [ NA ], oblique line; (1) a ridge on the outer surface of the thyroid cartilage that gives attachment to the sternothyroid and thyrohyoid muscles; (2) the line on the external surface of the mandible that extends from the mental tubercle to the ramus and separates the alveolar and basilar parts of the bone.

**l. pectine'a** [ NA ], pectineal line; a ridge running down the posterior surface of the shaft of the femur from the lesser trochanter to which the pectineus muscle attaches.

**l. poplite'a,** l. musculi solei.

**l. scapula'ris** [ NA ], scapular line; a line passing vertically downward from the inferior angle of the scapula.

**l. semicircula'ris,** l. arcuata (2).

**l. semiluna'ris** [ NA ], semilunar line; line of Spigelius; the slight groove in the external abdominal wall parallel to the lateral edge of the rectus sheath.

**l. spira'lis,** l. intertrochanterica.

**l. splendens,** Haller's line; a thickened band of pia mater along the midline of the anterior surface of the spinal cord.

**l. tempora'lis inferior** [ NA ], inferior temporal line; the lower of two curved lines on the parietal bone; it marks the limit of attachment of the temporal muscle.

**l. tempora'lis superior** [ NA ], superior temporal line; the upper of two curved lines on the parietal bone; the temporal fascia is attached to it.

**l. termina'lis** [ NA ], terminal line; iliopectineal line; an oblique ridge on the inner surface of the ilium and continued on the pubis, which forms the lower boundary of the iliac fossa; it separates the true from the false pelvis.

**l. transver'sa** [ NA ], transverse line; one of four ridges that cross the pelvic surface of the sacrum; these mark the positions of the intervertebral disks between the bodies of the five sacral vertebrae in the immature bone.

**l. trapezoi'dea** [ NA ], trapezoid line; the area on the inferior surface of the clavicle near its lateral extremity on which the trapezoid ligament attaches.

**linear** (lin'e-ar). Pertaining to or resembling a line.

**line'breeding.** A practice of successive inbreeding of closely related individuals with the object of concentrating the genetic characteristics of some individual, or group.

**li'ner.** A layer of protective material.

  **asbestos l.,** a layer of asbestos used to line a dental casting ring so that during the heating and expansion of the investment the compression of the l. will free the investment from the restraint of the ring.

**Lineweaver,** H. See L.-Burk *equation.*

**Ling,** Per Henrik, Swedish hygienist, 1776–1839. See L.'s *method.*

**Lingelsheimia** (ling'el-shi'mī-ah) [ W. von *Lingelsheim* ]. *Acinetobacter.*

  **L. anitrata,** *Acinetobacter calcoaceticus.*

**ling'ism.** Ling's *method.*

**lingua,** gen. and pl. **lin'guae** (ling'gwah) [ L. tongue ] [ NA ]. 1. The tongue; a mobile mass of muscular tissue covered with mucous membrane, occupying the cavity of the mouth and forming part of its floor, constituting also by its posterior portion the anterior wall of the pharynx. It bears the organ of taste and assists in mastication, deglutition, and articulation. 2. One of a number of tongue-like anatomical structures.

  **l. cerebel'li,** *lingula* cerebelli.

  **l. dissec'ta,** geographical *tongue.*

  **l. fissura'ta,** fissured tongue; usually a normal variant when fissures are in the midline; severe forms may occur in association with clefts of palate or lip.

  **l. frena'ta,** a tongue with a very short frenum constituting tongue-tie.

  **l. geograph'ica,** geographical *tongue.*

  **l. nigra,** black *tongue.*

  **l. plica'ta,** furrowed *tongue.*

**lingual** (ling'gwal). 1. Glossal; relating to the tongue or any tongue-like part. 2. Next to or toward the tongue. 3. One of the letters, *t, d,* the sound of which is made with the tip of the tongue.

**lingually** (ling'gwal-ī). Toward the tongue.

**Linguatula** (ling-gwat'u-lah) [ L. *linguatulus,* tongued ]. A genus of endoparasitic bloodsucking arthropods (family Linguatulidae) commonly known as tongue worms and also called Pentastomida; once thought to be degenerate Acarina, but now generally considered to be a small but distinctive early offshoot of the Arthropoda. Adult worms are found in lungs or air passages of various hosts (*e.g.,* reptiles, birds, carnivores); young worms are found in a great variety of hosts, including man, but chiefly in animals that are prey.

  **L. rhina'ria,** *L. serrata.*

  **L. serra'ta,** *L. rhinaria;* commonest in Europe, but also found in the United States, South America, and probably elsewhere; the adult is a whitish, soft, flattened, annulated worm equipped with hooks by which it attaches itself to the nasal mucosa of dogs and other canids; the larvae develop in the liver and lymph nodes of rodents, swine, cattle, and sometimes man and other primates.

**linguatuliasis** (ling'gwat'u-li'ā-sis). Linguatulosis; infestation with *Linguatula.*

**Linguatulidae** (ling-gwat'u-lī-de). One of the families of Pentastomida of medical interest, the other being the Porocephalidae. L. have flattened bodies; adults inhabit the nasal cavities of various carnivores, such as the dog and cat, and larval forms are found in tissues of rodents, herbivores, and other animals; both larvae and adults have been reported from man.

**linguatulosis** (ling-gwat'u-lo'sis). Linguatuliasis.

**linguiform** (ling'gwī-form). Tongue-shaped.

**lingula,** pl. **lin'gulae** (ling'gu-lah) [ L. dim. of *lingua,* tongue. LING- ] [ NA ]. 1. A term applied to several tongue-shaped processes. 2. When not qualified, the l. cerebelli.

  **l. cerebel'li** [ NA ], lingula (2); tongue of the cerebellum; a tongue-shaped sequence of flattened cerebellar folia forming the anterior (or superior) extreme of the cerebellar vermis, extending forward on the surface of the velum medullare superius between the two emerging superior cerebellar peduncles.

  **l. mandib'ulae** [ NA ], mandibular tongue; a pointed tongue of bone overlapping the mandibular foramen, giving attachment to the sphenomandibular ligament.

  **l. pulmonis sinistri** [ NA ], lingula of the left lung; a projection from the upper lobe of the left lung which bounds the cardiac notch inferiorly.

  **l. sphenoida'lis** [ NA ], a slender process projecting posteriorly between the body and greater wing of the sphenoid bone, on either side, forming an independent element at birth.

**lingulectomy** (ling'u-lek'to-mī). 1. Glossectomy. 2. Excision of the lingular portion of the left upper lobe of the lung.

**linguo-** (ling'gwo-) [ L. *lingua,* tongue ]. Combining form relating to the tongue.

**linguoclina'tion** (ling'gwo-kli-na'shun). The axial inclination of a tooth when the crown is inclined toward the tongue more than is normal.

**linguoclu'sion** (ling'gwo-klu'zhun). The displacement of a tooth toward the interior of the dental arch, or toward the tongue; see also lingual occlusion.

**linguodistal** (ling-gwo-dis'tal). Relating to the lingual and distal part of the tooth, *e.g.,* the l. cusp. See also distolingual.

**linguogingival** (ling-gwo-jīn'jī-val). 1. Relating to the gingival third of the lingual surface of a tooth. 2. Relating to the angle or point of junction of the lingual border and gingival line on the distal or mesial surface of an incisor tooth.

**linguo-occlusal** (ling'gwo-ŏ-klu'sal). Relating to the line of junction of the lingual and occlusal surfaces of a tooth.

**linguopapillitis** (ling'gwo-pap'ī-li'tis). Small painful ulcers involving the papillae on the tongue margins.

**linguoversion** (ling'gwo-ver'ghun). Malposition of an anterior tooth axially inclined in a direction toward the tongue.

**liniment** (lin'ī-ment) [ L. fr. *lino,* to smear ]. Embrocation; a liquid preparation for external application or application to the gums; they may be clear dispersions, suspensions, or emulsions, and are frequently applied by friction to the skin; used as counterirritants, rubefacients, anodynes, or cleansing agents.

**li'nin** [ L. *linum,* fr. G. *linon,* flax ]. 1. A bitter glycoside obtained from *Linum catharticum* (family Linaceae). 2. A protein in linseed. 3. The threadlike, nonstaining (achromatic) substance forming the network of the cell nucleus, containing in its meshes the nucleoplasm.

**lining** (li'ning). A coating applied to a wall or walls of a tooth cavity to protect the pulp from thermal or chemical irritation by the restorative material. Usually made of zinc phosphate cement, zinc-oxide eugenol cement, calcium hydroxide, or a varnish. Often referred to as pulp protection.

**linitis** (lī-ni'tis, li-ni'tis) [ G. *linon,* flax, linen cloth, + suffix -*itis,* inflammation ]. Inflammation of cellular tissue, specifically of the perivascular tissue of the stomach.

  **l. plas'tica,** Brinton's disease (1); leather-bottle stomach; originally believed to be an inflammatory condition, but now recognized to be due to infiltrating scirrhous carcinoma causing extensive thickening of the wall of the stomach.

**linkage** (lingk'ij). 1. Chemical covalent bond. 2. Association of genes in inheritance, due to the fact that they are in the same chromosome pair. See also cis- and trans-.

  **genetic l.,** see l. (2).

  **medical record l.,** the assemblage of lifetime or long term individual medical histories from vital and medical data derived from multiple sources.

  **sex l.,** a form of inheritance related to sex as a result of the gene concerned being carried on the X chromosome. A man receives all his sex-linked genes from his mother and transmits them to his daughters but not to his sons; a recessive sex-lined character is much more likely to be expressed in the male. See also sex *chromosome;* sex-linked *gene.*

**Linognathus** (lī-nog'nă-thus) [ G. *linon,* flax, thread, + *gnathos,* jaw ]. A genus of sucking lice (order Anoplura, family Linognathidae).

**L. africa'nus,** the African blue louse of sheep and goats.

**L. ovil'lus,** the sheep body louse.

**L. peda'lis,** the foot louse of sheep; occurs on the legs and feet of sheep where there is no wool.

**L. seto'sus,** the sucking louse of the dog and other canids.

**L. stenop'sis,** the sucking louse of goats.

**L. vituli,** the "long-nosed" sucking louse, ox louse, or blue louse of cattle.

**lino'leate.** Salt of linoleic acid.

**linole'ic acid** [ L. *linum,* flax, + *oleum,* oil ]. Octadecadienoic acid; linolic acid; $CH_3(CH_2)_4CH=CHCH_2CH=CH(CH_2)_7COOH$; an unsaturated fatty acid occurring widely in plant glycerides; essential in nutrition.

**linolen'ic acid.** Octadecatrienoic acid; $CH_3(CH_2CH=CH)_3CH_2(CH_2)_6COOH$; an unsaturated fatty acid essential in nutrition.

**lino'lic acid.** Linoleic acid.

**lin'seed** [ G. *linon,* flax ]. Flaxseed; the dried ripe seed of *Linum usitatissimum* (family Linaceae), the fiber of which is used in the manufacture of linen; the chief source is Russia. An infusion is used as a demulcent in catarrhal affections of the respiratory and urogenital tracts, and the ground seeds are used in making poultices.

**l. oil,** flaxseed oil; a fatty oil expressed from the ripe seeds of *Linum usitatissimum;* used in the preparation of lime liniment.

**lint** [ O.E. *lin,* flax ]. A soft, absorbent material used in surgical dressings. It was formerly made by scraping or raveling old linen cloths; now usually in the form of a thick, loosely woven material, sheet l. or patent l.

**lio-.** For words so beginning and not found here, see *leio.*

**li'othy'ronine.** 3,5,3'-Triiodothyronine.

**l. sodium.** See under sodium.

**li'otrix** (USP). THYROLAR; a mixture of liothyronine sodium and levothyroxine sodium; used as a thyroid hormone.

**lip-.** See lipo-.

**lip** [ A.S. *lippa* ]. 1. Labium oris; one of the two muscular folds with an outer mucosa having a stratified squamous epithelial surface layer which bound the mouth anteriorly. 2. Any liplike structure bounding a cavity or groove; see also labium; labrum.

**anterior l. of uterus,** *labium* anterius.

**cleft l.,** harelip; cheiloschisis; chiloschisis; a congenital facial deformity of the l. (usually the upper l.) due to a mesodermal deficiency or failure of fusion in one or more of the embryologic processes that form the upper l.; frequently but not necessarily associated with cleft alveolus and cleft palate.

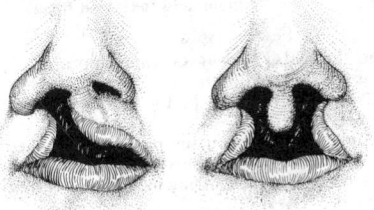

**Cleft Lip**
*Left,* unilateral; *right,* bilateral

**external l. of iliac crest,** *labium* externum cristae iliacae.

**Hapsburg l.,** see Hapsburg *jaw.*

**internal l. of iliac crest,** *labium* internum cristae iliacae.

**large pudendal l.,** *labium* majus pudendi.

**l.'s of linea aspera of femur,** (1) *labium* laterale lineae asperae femoris; (2) *labium* mediale lineae asperae femoris.

**lower l.,** *labium* inferius oris.

**posterior l. of uterus,** *labium* posterius.

**rhombic l.,** the thickened alar plate of the embryonic rhombencephalon.

**small pudendal l.,** *labium* minus pudendi.

**tympanic l.,** *labium* limbi tympanicum.

**upper l.,** *labium* superius oris.

**vestibular l.,** *labium* limbi vestibulare.

**lipacidemia** (lip'-i-de'mi-ah) [ lipo- + G. *haima,* blood ]. The presence of a fatty acid in the circulating blood.

**lipaciduria** (lip'as'i-du'ri-ah) [ lipo- + G. *ouron,* urine ]. The excretion of one or more fatty acids in the urine.

**liparocele** (lip'ä-ro-sel) [ G. *liparos,* fatty, + *kele,* tumor, hernia ]. 1. Old term for a mass of adipose tissue in the scrotum. 2. An omental hernia.

**liparodyspnea** (lip'ä-ro-disp-ne'ah) [ G. *liparos,* fatty, + dyspnea ]. Dyspnea in the grotesquely obese.

**liparomphalus** (lip'ä-rom'fä-lus) [ G. *liparos,* fatty, + *omphalos,* umbilicus ]. A fairly well circumscribed mass of adipose tissue situated in the region of the umbilicus.

**lip'ase.** In general, any fat-splitting or lipolytic enzyme, *e.g.,* triacylglycerol lipase, phospholipase $A_2$, diacylglycerol lipase, all of which cleave a fatty acid residue from the glycerol residue in a neutral fat or a phospholipid.

**pancreatic l.,** triacylglycerol lipase.

**lipectomy** (lip-ek'to-mi) [ lipo- + G. *ektome,* excision ]. Adipectomy; surgical removal of fatty tissue, such as has been proposed in cases of adiposity.

**lipedema** (lip'e-de'mah) [ lipo- + G. *oidema,* swelling ]. Chronic swelling, usually of the lower extremities, particularly in middle-aged women; caused by the widespread, even distribution of subcutaneous fat and fluid.

**lipemia** (lip-e'mi-ah) [ lipid + G. *haima,* blood ]. The presence of an abnormally large amount of lipids in the circulating blood; also known as hyperlipemia; hyperlipidemia; hyperlipoidemia; lipidemia; lipoidemia.

**alimentary l.,** relatively transient l. occurring after the ingestion of foods with a large content of fat.

**diabetic l.,** the development of lactescent plasma upon ingestion of dietary lipids; a rare manifestation of uncontrolled diabetes mellitus; it is caused by defective metabolism of dietary lipids, and abolished by the administration of insulin.

**postprandial l.,** alimentary l.

**l. retina'lis,** a creamy appearance of the retinal blood vessels when the lipoids of the blood are over 5 per cent, also seen in some cases of leukemia or diabetes.

**lip'id** [ G. *lipos,* fat ]. Fat; "fat-soluble," the name denoting substances extracted from animal or vegetable cells by nonpolar or "fat" solvents (ethanol, ether, chloroform, petroleum ether, benzene, etc.). Lipid is an operational term describing a solubility characteristic, not a chemical substance. Included in the heterogeneous collection of materials thus extractable are fatty acids, glycerides and glyceryl ethers, phospholipids, sphingolipids, alcohols and waxes, terpenes, steroids, and "fat-soluble" vitamins. Formerly also called lipide, lipin, lipoid (all of which are now obsolete).

**lipidemia** (lip'i-de'mi-ah). Lipemia.

**lipidosis,** pl. **lipido'ses** (lip'i-do'sis) [ lipid + G. suffix *-osis,* condition ]. Inborn or acquired disorder of lipid metabolism.

**cerebral l.,** cerebral *sphingolipidosis.*

**cerebroside l.,** Gaucher's *disease.*

**ganglioside l.,** gangliosidosis.

**glycolipid l.,** Fabry's *disease.*

**sphingomyelin l.,** Niemann-Pick *disease.*

**sulfatide l.,** metachromatic *leukodystrophy.*

**lip'in.** Lipid.

**Lipmann,** Fritz A., German biochemist in the U. S. *1899. Nobel laureate, 1953, with Sir Hans A. Krebs for the discovery of coenzyme A and its importance for intermediary metabolism.

**lipo-, lip-** (lip'o-) [ G. *lipos,* fat ]. Combining forms relating to fat, or lipid.

**lipo'amide.** See lipoic acid.

**l. dehydrogenase** (EC 1.6.4.3), diaphorase; lipoyl dehydrogenase; an enzyme (a flavoprotein) catalyzing the oxidation of dihydrolipoamide by NAD+ to lipoamide, thus completing the oxidative decarboxylation sequence of pyruvate initiated by pyruvate dehydrogenase (lipoate).

**l. disulfide,** oxidized lipoic acid in amide combination with the ϵ-amino group of a lysine of pyruvic acid dehydrogenase.

**lipoarthritis** (lip'o-ar-thri'tis) [ lipo- + arthritis, *q.v.* ]. Inflammation of the periarticular fatty tissues of the knee.

**lip'oate.** A salt or ester of lipoic acid.

**l. acetyltransferase** (EC 2.3.1.12), thioltransacetylase A; an enzyme (a transferase) catalyzing reaction between acetyldihydrolipoate, the product of the pyruvate dehydrogenase reaction, and CoA to yield acetyl-CoA and dihydrolipoate.

**lipoatrophia** (lip'o-ă-tro'fi-ah) [ L. fr. G. *lipos,* fat, + *a*-priv., + *trophē,* nourishment ]. Atrophy of body fat.

**l. circumscrip'ta,** localized fat atrophy.

**lip'oblast** [ lipo- + G. *blastos,* germ ]. An embryonic fat cell.

**lip'oblasto'ma.** Liposarcoma.

**lipocaic** (lip-o-ka'ik) [ lipo- + G. *kaiō* to burn ]. A pancreatic hormone associated with fat metabolism in the liver. It is lipotropic in action, preventing the accumulating of fat in the liver in depancreatized dogs.

**lipocardiac** (lip'o-kar'di-ak) [ lipo- + G. *kardia,* heart ]. 1. Relating to fatty heart. 2. One suffering from fatty degeneration of the heart.

**lipocatabolic** (lip'o-kat'ă-bol'ik). Relating to the breakdown (catabolism) of fat.

**lipocele** (lip-o-sēl) [ lipo- + G. *kēlē,* tumor ]. Adipocele; the presence of fatty tissue, without intestine, in a hernia sac.

**lipoceratous** (lip'o-sēr'ă-tus). Adipoceratous.

**lipocere** (lip'o-sēr) [ lipo- + L. *cera,* wax ]. Adipocere.

**lipochondrodystrophy** (lip'o-kon'-dro-dis'-tro-fī). Hurler's *syndrome.*

**lipochrome** (lip'o-krōm) [ lipo- + G. *chroma,* color ]. 1. A pigmented lipid, such as lutein or carotene. 2. A term sometimes used to designate the "wear-and-tear" pigments, *i.e.,* lipofuscin, hemofuscin, ceroid, and so on; more precisely, l.'s are yellow pigments that seem to be identical to carotene and xanthophyll (both of which are plant pigments), and they are frequently found in the serum, skin, adrenal cortex, corpus luteum, and arteriosclerotic plaques, as well as in the liver, spleen, and adipose tissue; l.'s do not stain with the ordinary dyes for fat. 3. The pigment produced by certain bacteria.

**lipoclasis** (lī-pok'lă-sis) [ lipo- + G. *klasis,* a breaking ]. Lipolysis.

**lip'oclas'tic.** Lipolytic.

**lip'ocor'ticoid.** A principle of the adrenal cortex that is supposed to influence fat deposition; its existence has not been proved.

**lipocorticotrophic (-tropic)** (lip'o-kor'ti-ko-trof'ik, -trop'ik). Indicating an action of the anterior lobe of the hypophysis that is supposed to increase, through the adrenal cortex, the accumulation of fat in the fat depots. Obsolete.

**lipocrit** (lip'o-krit) [ lipo- + G. *krinō,* to separate ]. An apparatus and procedure for separating and volumetrically analyzing the amount of lipid in blood or other body fluid.

**lipocyte** (lip'o-sīt) [ lipo- + G. *kytos,* cell ]. Fat *cell.*

**lipodermoid** (lip'o-der'moyd) [ lipo- + dermoid ]. A congenital yellowish white, fatty, benign tumor located subconjunctivally.

**lipodieresis** (lip-o-di-ĕr'e-sis) [ lipo- + G. *diairesis,* division ]. Lipolysis.

**lipodystrophia** (lip'o-dis-tro'fi-ah) [ lipo- + G. *dys*-, bad, difficult, + *trophē,* nourishment ]. Lipodystrophy.

**l. intestina'lis,** Whipple's *disease.*

**l. progessi'va superior,** progressive *lipodystrophy.*

**lipodystrophy** (lī-po-dis'tro-fī). Lipodystrophia; defective metabolism of fat.

**congenital total l.,** characterized by almost complete lack of subcutaneous fat, accelerated rate of growth and skeletal development during the first 3 to 4 years of life, muscular hypertrophy, cardiac enlargement, hepatosplenomegaly, hypertrichosis, phebomegaly, renal enlargement, hyperlipemia, and hypermetabolism; probably autosomal recessive inheritance.

**insulin l.,** dystrophic atrophy of subcutaneous tissues in diabetics at the site of frequent injections of insulin.

**intestinal l.,** Whipple's *disease.*

**progressive l.,** lipodystrophia progressiva superior; Barraquer's disease; Simon's disease; a condition characterized by a more or less complete loss of the subcutaneous fat of the upper part of the torso, the arms, neck, and face, sometimes with an increase of fat in the tissues about and below the pelvis.

**lipoferous** (lip-of'er-us). 1. Transporting fat. 2. Sudanophil.

**lipofibroma** (lip'o-fi-bro'mah). A benign neoplasm of fibrous connective tissue, with conspicuous numbers of adipose cells.

**lipofuscin** (lip-o-fus'in). Brown pigment granules representing lipid-containing residues of lysosomal digestion, seen in many tissues; for example, adjacent to the nuclei of myocardial cells.

**lipofuscinosis** (lip'o-fus-ĭ-no'sis). Abnormal storage of any one of a group of fatty pigments.

**ceroid l.,** late juvenile type of cerebral *sphingolipidosis.*

**lipogenesis** (lip'o-jen'ĕ-sis) [ lipo- + G. *genesis,* production ]. The production of fat, either fatty degeneration or fatty infiltration; term also applied to the normal deposition of fat or to the conversion of carbohydrate or protein to fat.

**lipogen'ic.** Adipogenic; adipogenous; lipogenous; relating to lipogenesis; fat-producing.

**lipogenous** (lī-poj'ĕ-nus). Lipogenic.

**lipogranuloma** (lip'o-gran'u-lo'mah). Paraffinoma; oleoma; oleogranuloma; eleoma; oil tumor; a nodule or focus of granulomatous inflammation (usually of the foreign-body type) in association with lipid material deposited in tissues, *e.g.,* after the injection of certain oils, and so on.

**lip'ogran'ulomato'sis.** 1. The presence of lipogranulomas. 2. The local inflammatory reaction to necrosis of adipose tissue.

**lipohe'mia.** Obsolete synonym for lipemia.

**lipo'ic acid.** 6,8-Dithio-*n*-octanoic acid; thioctic acid; protogen; acetate-replacing factor; pyruvate-oxidation factor; factor II; it functions as the amide (lipoamide) in the —S—S— form in the transfer of "active aldehyde," the two-carbon fragment resulting from decarboxylation of pyruvate, from α-hydroxyethyl thiamin pyrophosphate to acetyl-CoA, itself being reduced (to the —SH—SH form) in the process. It is present in yeast and liver extracts.

$$
\begin{array}{cc}
S\!\!-\!\!\!\!-\!\!\!\!-\!\!\!\!-\!\!\!\!-\!\!\!\!-\!\!\!\!-\!\!\!\!-S \\
CH_2\!\!-\!\!CH_2\!\!-\!\!CH\!\!-\!\!(CH_2)_4\!\!-\!\!COOH
\end{array}
$$

**Lipoic acid (oxidized form)**

**lipoid** (lip'oyd) [ lipo- + G. *eidos,* appearance ]. 1. Resembling fat. 2. Lipid.

**anisotrop'ic l.,** a l. in the form of doubly refractive droplets.

**brain l.,** impure cephalin, possessing marked hemostatic action when locally applied.

**isotrop'ic l.,** a l. occurring in the form of singly refractive droplets.

**lipoidemia** (lip'oy-de'mĭ-ah). Lipemia.

**lipoidosis** (lip-oy-do'sis). The presence of anisotropic lipoids in the cells.

**l. corneae,** *arcus* senilis.

**l. cutis et mucosae,** lipid *proteinosis.*

**lipolipoidosis** (lip'o-lip'oy-do'sis). Fatty infiltration, both neutral fats and anisotropic lipoids being present in the cells; see also liposis (2).

**lipolysis** (lī-pol'ĭ-sis) [ lipo- + G. *lysis,* dissolution ]. Lipoclasis; lipodieresis; the splitting up (hydrolysis), or chemical decomposition, of fat.

**lipolytic** (lip'o-lit'ik). Relating to or causing lipolysis.

**lipoma** (lī-po'mah) [ lipo- + G. suffix -*oma,* tumor ]. Adipose tumor; a benign neoplasm of adipose tissue, comprised of mature fat cells.

**l. annula′re colli,** an encircling growth of l. (or coalescent l.'s) in the neck, resulting in a collar-like enlargement.

**l. arbores′cens,** an irregularly shaped l. involving the synovial membrane of a joint, resulting in finger-like or treelike, hyperplastic folds in the villi.

**l. capsula′re,** a well circumscribed mass resulting from a greatly increased amount of adipose tissue adjacent to the breast.

**l. caverno′sum,** telangiectatic l.

**l. du′rum,** old term sometimes used for a subcutaneous l., or even a sebaceous cyst.

**l. fibro′sum,** fibrolipoma.

**infiltrating l.,** liposarcoma.

**lipoblastic l.,** liposarcoma.

**l. ossif′icans,** a l. in which metaplasia occurs and small foci of bone are formed.

**l. petrif′icans,** a l. in which degeneration and necrosis results in a considerable amount of dystrophic calcification.

**l. sarcomato′des, l. sarcomato′sum,** liposarcoma.

**telangiectat′ic l.,** l. cavernosum; a l. that contains several to numerous, relatively large, apparently dilated vascular channels and spaces, in association with capillaries of the usual size.

**lipomatoid** (lī-po′mah-toyd). Resembling a lipoma, frequently said of accumulations of adipose tissue that is not thought to be neoplastic.

**lipomatosis** (lip′o-mă-to′sis). Adiposis.

**l. neurot′ica,** *adiposis* dolorosa.

**lipo′matous.** Pertaining to or manifesting the features of lipoma, or characterized by the presence of a lipoma (or lipomas).

**lipomeningocele** (lip′o-mě-ning′go-sēl) [ lipo- + G. *mēninx,* membrane, + *kēlē,* tumor ]. An intraspinal cauda equinal lipoma associated with a spina bifida.

**li′pome′ria** [ G. *leipō,* leave, leave behind, lack, + *meros,* a part ]. The congenital absence of a limb or other part.

**lip′ometabol′ic.** Relating to lipid metabolism.

**lip′ometab′olism.** Lipid metabolism.

**lipomucopolysaccharidosis** (lip′o-mu′ko-pol-ĭ-sak′ă-rĭ-do′sis). Mucolipidosis I.

**lipomyoma** (lip-o-mi-o′mah) [ Mod. L. fr. G. *lipos,* fat, + *mys (myo-),* muscle, + *-ōma* ]. Probably a form of mesenchymoma.

**liponucleoproteins** (lip′o-nu′kle-o-pro′te-inz, -pro′tēnz). Associations or complexes containing lipids, nucleic acids, and proteins.

**Liponyssus** (lip-o-nis′us) [ lipo- + G. *nyssō,* to prick ]. *Ornithonyssus.*

**lip′opec′tic.** Marked by lipopexia.

**lipopenia** (lip-o-pe′nĭ-ah) [ lipo- + G. *penia,* poverty ]. An abnormally small amount, or a deficiency, of lipids in the body.

**lipopenic** (lip′o-pe′nik). 1. Relating to or characterized by lipopenia. 2. An agent or drug that produces a reduction in the concentration of lipids in the blood.

**lip′opep′tid.** A compound or complex of lipid and amino acids.

**lipopexia** (lip′o-pek′sĭ-ah) [ lipo- + G. *pēxis,* fixation ]. Adipopexia; the accumulation of lipids in the body.

**lipophage** (lip′o-fāj) [ G. *lipos,* fat, + *phagein,* to eat ]. A cell that ingests fat.

**lipophagia** (lip′o-fa′jĭ-ah). Lipophagy.

**l. granulomato′sis,** Whipple's *disease.*

**lipophagic** (lip-o-fa′jik). Relating to lipophagy.

**lipophagy** (lip-of′a-jī) [ lipo- + G. *phagein,* to eat ]. Lipophagy; the ingestion of fat by a lipophage.

**lipophanerosis** (lip′o-fan-er-o′sis) [ lipo- + G. *phaneros,* visible, + suffix *-osis,* condition ]. A change in certain cells whereby previously invisible fat becomes demonstrable as small sudanophilic droplets. See fatty *degeneration.*

**lipophil** (lip′o-fil) [ lipo- + G. *philos,* fond of ]. Capable of dissolving, of being dissolved in, or of absorbing lipids; opposite of hydrophil. All lipids are, by definition, lipophils. See also lipid.

**lipophore** (lip′o-fōr) [ lipo- + G. *phoros,* bearing ]. Xanthophore.

**lip′ophos′phodies′terase I.** Phospholipase C.

**lip′ophos′phodies′terase II.** Phospholipase D.

**lipophrenia** (li′po-fre′nĭ-ah) [ G. *leipō,* to leave behind, lack, + *phrēn,* mind ]. Mental failure.

**lipopolysaccharide** (lip′o-pol′ĭ-sak′ar-id). A compound or complex of lipid and carbohydrate.

**lipoprotein** (lip′o-pro′te-in, -tēn). Complexes or compounds containing lipid and protein.

**l. lipase,** diacylglycerol lipase.

**α-lipoprotein.** A lipoprotein fraction of relatively small molecular weight, rich in phospholipids; found in the $α_1$-globulin fraction of human plasma.

**β-lipoprotein.** A lipoprotein fraction of relatively large molecular weight, rich in cholesterol; found in the β-globulin fraction of human plasma.

**liposarcoma** (lip′o-sar-ko′mah) [ lipo- + *sarx,* flesh, + suffix *-oma,* tumor ]. A malignant neoplasm that may occur in any site in the body, but especially in the retroperitoneal tissues, the thigh, popliteal space, and gluteal region, usually deep in the intermuscular or periarticular planes; histologically, l.'s consist chiefly of immature, anaplastic lipoblasts of varying sizes (including giant forms), with bizarre nuclei and vacuoles of varying sizes in the cytoplasm, usually in association with a rich network of capillaries. L.'s may include foci of fully developed fat cells, as well as relatively undifferentiated, immature mesenchymal tissue; the demonstration of droplets and globules of fat (by means of special stains) is helpful in recognizing the nature of the neoplasm. Termed also lipoblastoma, infiltrating or lipoblastic lipoma; lipoma sarcomatodes; lipoma sarcomatosum; Abernethy's sarcoma.

**liposis** (lī-po′sis) [ lipo- + G. suffix *-osis,* condition ]. 1. Adiposis. 2. Fatty infiltration, neutral fats being present in the cells; see also lipolipoidosis.

**general l.,** obesity.

**lipos′itol.** Inositol.

**lip′osol′uble.** Fat-soluble.

**lipostomy** (li-pos′to-mī) [ G. *leipō,* to lack, + *stoma,* mouth ]. Congenital absence of the mouth.

**lip′othi′amide py′rophos′phate.** Name once given to the coenzymes of the multi-enzyme complex catalyzing the formation of acetyl-CoA from pyruvate and involving lipoamide and diphosphothiamin, on the assumption that the lipoamide and thiamin pyrophosphate are a single compound. See lipoic acid.

**lipothymia** (li′po-thi′mĭ-ah) [ G. *leipō,* to leave, + *thymos,* mind, soul ]. Syncope; fainting.

**li′pothy′mial.** Syncopal.

**lip′otroph′ic.** Relating to lipotrophy.

**lipotrophy** (lī-pot′ro-fī) [ lipo- + G. *trophē,* nourishment ]. The increase of fat in the body.

**lip′otrop′ic.** 1. Pertaining to substances preventing or correcting the fatty liver of choline deficiency (*e.g.,* arsenocholine, or methyl donors for choline synthesis). 2. Relating to lipotropy.

**lipotropy** (lī-pot′ro-pī) [ lipo- + G. *trope,* turning ]. 1. Affinity of basic dyes for fatty tissue. 2. Prevention of accumulation of fat in the liver. 3. Affinity of nonpolar substances for each other; see lyophilic.

**lipovaccine** (lip′o-vak′sēn). A vaccine having a vegetable oil as a menstruum; see adjuvant *vaccine.*

**lipovitellin** (lip′o-vī-tel′in). Vitellin.

**lipoxanthine** (lip′o-zan′thin) [ lipo- + G. *xanthos,* yellow ]. Yellow lipochrome.

**lipox′enous.** Pertaining to lipoxeny.

**lipoxeny** (li-pok′sĕ-nī, lī-pok′sĕ-nī) [ G. *leipō,* to leave, + *xenos,* host ]. Desertion of the host by a parasite when the development of the latter is complete.

**lipox′idase.** Lipoxygenase.

**lipox′ygenase** (EC 1.13.11.12). Lipoxidase; carotene oxidase; an enzyme that catalyzes the oxidation of unsaturated fats with $O_2$ to yield a peroxide of the fat.

**lipoyl dehydrogenase** (lip′o-il). Lipoamide dehydrogenase.

**lip′ping.** The formation of a liplike structure, as at the articular end of a bone in osteoarthritis.

**lippitude, lippitudo** (lip'ĭ-tūd) [ L. fr. *lippus*, blear-eyed ]. Blear *eye*.

**Lipschutz,** A. See L. *law* of puberty.

**Lipschütz** (lip'shuts), Benjamin, Austrian physician, 1878–1931. See L. *cells*, L.'s *ulcer*.

**lipuria** (lĭ-pu'rĭ-ah) [ lipo- + G. *ouron*, urine ]. Adiposuria; the excretion of lipid in the urine.

**lipu'ric.** Pertaining to lipuria.

**liquefacient** (lik'we-fa'shent) [ L. *lique–facio*, pp. *-factus*, pres. p. *-faciens*, to make fluid, fr. *liquo*, to dissolve, melt ]. 1. Making liquid; causing a solid to become liquid. 2. Denoting an agent supposed to cause the resolution of a solid tumor by liquefying its contents; resolvent.

**liquefaction** (lik-we-fak'shun). The act of becoming liquid; change from a solid to a liquid form.

**liquefactive** (lik'we-fak'tiv). Relating to liquefaction; liquefacient.

**liquescent** (lĭ-kwes'ent) [ L. *liquesco*, to become liquid ]. Becoming or tending to become liquid; deliquescent.

**liqueur** (lik-ĕr') [ Fr. ]. A cordial; a spirit containing sugar and aromatics.

**liquid** (lik'wid) [ L. *liquidus* ]. 1. Flowing. 2. An inelastic fluid, like water, that is neither solid nor gaseous.
　**Cotunnius' l.,** perilympha.

**Liquidambar** (lik'wid-am'bar) [ L. *liquidus*, liquid + *ambar*, amber ]. A genus of trees of the witch-hazel family, *Hamamelidaceae*, source of storax.

**liquidus.** The line on a constitution diagram above which temperature all metal is liquid.

**liquor,** gen. **liquo'ris,** pl. **liquo'res** (lik'er, lik'wor) [ L. ]. 1. Any liquid or fluid. 2 [ NA ]. A term used for certain body fluids. 3. The pharmacopeial term for any aqueous solution (not a decoction or infusion) of a nonvolatile substance and for aqueous solutions of gases; see also solution.
　**l. amnii,** amniotic *fluid*.
　**l. cerebrospina'lis** [ NA ], cerebrospinal fluid (CSF); neurolymph; a fluid secreted by the choroid plexuses of the ventricles of the brain, filling the ventricles and the subarachnoid cavities of the brain and spinal cord.
　**l. cotunnii,** perilympha.
　**l. enter'icus,** intestinal secretions.
　**l. follic'uli,** the fluid within the antrum of the ovarian follicle.
　**malt l.,** a beverage brewed from malt, such as beer or ale.
　**Morgagni's l.,** a fluid found post mortem between the epithelium and the fibers of the crystalline lens, resulting from the liquefaction of a semifluid material existing there during life.
　**mother l.,** the saturated solution remaining after a crystallization or precipitation.
　**Scarpa's l.,** endolympha.
　**spir'ituous l.,** a strong alcoholic l. obtained by distillation, such as whiskey.
　**vi'nous l.,** wine.

**liquorice** (lik'o-ris) (BP). Glycyrrhiza.

**liquorrhea** (lik'o-re'ah) [ L. *liquor*, fluid, + *rhoia*, flow ]. The flow of liquid.

**Lisfranc** (lis-frahnk'), Jacques, French surgeon, 1790–1847. See L.'s *amputation, joint, ligament, operation, tubercle.*

**lisp'ing.** Mispronunciation of the sibilants *s* and *z* ; also called sigmatism or parasigmatism.

**Lissauer** (lis'ow-er), Heinrich, German neurologist, 1861–1891. See L.'s *bundle, fasciculus, paresis, tract,* marginal *zone.*

**lissencephalia** (lis'en-sĕ-fa'lĭ-ah) [ G. *lissos*, smooth, + *enkephalos*, brain ]. Agyria.

**lissencephalic** (lis'en-sĕ-fal'ik). Having a brain with few and shallow convolutions; see also agyria.

**lissencephaly** (lis'en-sef'ă-lĭ) [ G. *lissos*, smooth, + *enkephalos*, brain ]. Agyria.

**lissosphincter** (lis'so-sfingk'ter) [ G. *lissos*, smooth, + sphincter, *q.v.* ]. A sphincter of smooth musculature.

**lissothricic** (lis-o-thris'ik) [ G. *lissos*, smooth, + *thrix*, hair ]. Having straight hair.

**Lister,** Joseph (later Lord Lister), English surgeon, 1827–1912. Noted for his establishment of antiseptic methods in surgery and the use of antiseptics in the operating room. Gave his name to *Listerella, Listeria,* listerism. See L.'s *dressing, method, tubercle.*

**Listerella** (lis'ter-el'ah) [ Joseph *Lister* ]. 1. A genus of myxomycetes. 2. In bacteriology, a rejected generic name sometimes cited as a synonym of *Listeria.* The type species is *L. hepatolytica.*

**Listeria** (lis-tēr-ĭ-ah) [ Joseph *Lister* ]. A genus of aerobic to microaerophilic, motile, peritrichous bacteria (family Corynebacteriaceae) containing small, coccoid, Gram-positive rods; these organisms tend to produce chains of three to five cells and, in the rough state, elongated and filamentous forms. Cells 18 to 24 hours old may show a palisade arrangement with a few V or Y forms. They produce acid but no gas from glucose. They are found in the feces of man and other animals, on vegetation, and in silage and are parasitic on poikilothermic and warm-blooded animals, including man. The type species is *L. monocytogenes.*
　**L. denitrificans,** a species found in cooked blood of beef; pathogenic to rats and mice when injected intraperitoneally.
　**L. grayi,** a species found in the feces of chinchillas.
　**L. monocytog'enes,** a species causing meningitis, encephalitis, septicemia, endocarditis, abortion, abscesses, and local purulent lesions; it is often fatal. It is found in healthy ferrets, insects, and the feces of chinchillas, ruminants, and man, as well as in sewage, decaying vegetation, silage, soil, and fertilizer.

**listeriosis** (lis-tēr'ĭ-o'sis). [ fr. organism *Listeria* ]. Listeria meningitis; circling disease (in sheep); a sporadic disease of animals and occasionally man caused by the bacterium, *Listeria monocytogenes.* The infection in sheep and cattle frequently involves the central nervous system, causing various neurologic signs; in monogastric animals and fowl the chief manifestations are septicemia and necrosis of the liver.

**lis'terism.** Lister's *method.*

**Listing,** Johann B., German physicist, 1808–1882. See L.'s reduced *eye*, L.'s *law.*

**Liston,** Robert, London surgeon, 1794–1847. See L.'s *forceps, knives, shears, splint.*

**liter** (le'ter) [ Fr. fr. G. *litra*, a pound ]. A measure of capacity of 1000 cubic centimeters, or 1 cubic decimeter, the equivalent of 1.0567 quarts.

**lith-.** See litho-.

**lithagogue** (lith'ă-gog) [ litho- + G. *agōgos*, a drawing forth ]. 1. Causing the dislodgment or expulsion of calculi, especially urinary calculi. 2. An agent that is credited with causing the partial solution and expulsion of urinary calculi.

**litharge** (lith'arj) [ litho- + G. *argyros*, silver ]. Lead monoxide.

**lithecbole** (lĭ-thek'bo-le) [ litho- + G. *ekbolē*, ejection ]. Ejection of a calculus.

**lithectasy** (lĭ-thek'tă-sĭ) [ litho- + G. *ektasis*, a stretching out ]. The urethral extraction of a vesical calculus after a preliminary dilation of this canal.

**lithectomy** (lĭ-thek'to-mĭ) [ litho- + G. *ektomē*, excision ]. Excision of a calculus; see also lithotomy.

**lithemia** (lĭ-the'mĭ-ah) [ lithic (uric) acid + G. *haima*, blood ]. Uricacidemia.

**lithemic** (lĭ-the'mik). Pertaining to, causing, or manifesting an abnormally large amount of uric acid in the circulating blood.

**lithiasis** (lĭ-thi'ă-sis) [ litho- + G. suffix *-iasis*, condition ]. 1. The so-called uric acid diathesis. 2. The formation of calculi of any kind, especially of biliary or urinary calculi.
　**l. conjuncti'vae,** deposits of cellular degeneration into hard masses in Henle's glands.
　**pancreatic l.,** the formation of stones in the pancreas, usually associated with chronic inflammation and obstruction of the pancreatic ducts.

**lith'ic acid.** Uric acid.

**lithicosis** (lith'ĭ-ko'sis) [ G. *lithikos*, of stone ]. Pneumonoconiosis.

**lith'ium,** gen. **lith'ii** [ Mod. L. fr. G. *lithos*, a stone ]. An element of the alkali metal group, symbol Li, atomic no. 3, atomic weight 6.940. See fig. under isotope.

**l. bromide,** LiBr; a white deliquescent powder, used as a sedative and hypnotic.

**l. carbonate** (USP, BP). Li₂CO₃; used as an antirheumatic and antilithic agent, and in the treatment of hypomanic and manic phases of manic-depressive states.

**l. citrate,** Li₃C₆H₅O₇.4H₂O, used as a diuretic and antirheumatic, and in the treatment of manic psychosis.

**efferves'cent l. citrate,** a preparation containing l. citrate, sodium bicarbonate, tartaric acid, and citric acid; same use as potassium or sodium citrate.

**litho-, lith-** [ G. *lithos*, stone ]. Combining forms relating to a stone or calculus, or to calcification.

**Litho'bius.** A genus of centipedes characterized by 15 pairs of legs. Species common in the United States include *L. multidentatus* and *L. forficatus.*

**lithocenosis** (lith'o-se-no'sis) [ litho- + G. *kenōsis,* an emptying, fr. *kenos,* empty ]. Litholapaxy.

**lith'ocholan'ic acid.** See *cholic*acid.

**lith'ochol'ic acid.** 3α-Hydroxy-5β-cholan-24-oic acid; 3α-hydroxy-5β-cholanic acid (for cholane structure, see steroids); one of the bile acids isolated from human bile. See cholic acid.

**lith'oclast** [ litho- + G. *klastos,* broken ]. A powerful lithotrite.

**lithoclysma** (lith-o-kliz'mah) [ litho- + G. *klysma,* clyster, fr. *klyzō,* to wash away ]. The injection of calculary solvents into the bladder.

**lithoconion** (lith-o-ko'nī-on) [ litho- + G. *konis,* dust ]. A form of lithotrite.

**lithocystotomy** (lith'o-sis-tot'o-mī) [ litho- + G. *kystis,* bladder, + *tomē,* incision ]. Vesical lithotomy.

**lithodialysis** (lith'o-di-al'ī-sis) [ litho- + G. *dialysis,* a breaking up ]. The fragmentation or solution of a calculus.

**lithogenesis, lithogeny** (lith-o-jen'ē-sis, lith-oj'ē-ni) [ litho- + G. *genesis,* production ]. The formation of calculi.

**lithogenous** (lith-oj'e-nus). Calculus-forming.

**lithoid** (lith'oyd) [ litho- + G. *eidos,* resemblance ]. Resembling a calculus or stone.

**lithokelyphopedion, lithokelyphopedium** (lith'o-kel'ī-fo-pe'dī-on, or -um) [ litho- + G. *kelyphos,* husk, shell, + *paidion,* child ]. A lithopedion in which the fetal parts in contact with the surrounding membranes, as well as the membranes, are calcified.

**lithokelyphos** (lith'o-kel'ī-fos) [ litho- + G. *kelyphos,* rind, shell ]. A type of lithopedion in which the fetal membranes alone undergo calcification.

**lith'olabe** [ litho- + G. *lambanein, labein,* to grasp ]. An instrument for holding a bladder calculus during its removal.

**litholapaxy** (li-thol'ă-pak'sĭ) [ litho- + G. *lapaxis,* an emptying out ]. Lithocenosis; the operation of crushing a stone in the bladder and washing out the fragments through a catheter of wide lumen.

**lithology** (li-thol-o-ji) [ litho- + G. *logos,* study ]. The branch of medical science relating to calculi or concretions.

**litholysis** (li-thol'ī-sis) [ litho- + G. *lysis,* dissolution ]. The dissolving of urinary calculi.

**lith'olyte.** An instrument for injecting calculary solvents.

**lithometer** (li-thom'e-ter) [ litho- + G. *metron,* measure ]. An instrument for measuring the size of a vesical calculus.

**lithometra** (lith'o-me'trah) [ litho- + G. *mētra,* womb ]. Calcification of the uterine tissues.

**lithomyl** (lith'o-mil) [ litho- + G. *mylē,* mill ]. An instrument for pulverizing a stone in the bladder.

**lithonephria** (lith-o-nef'rī-ah) [ litho- + G. *nephros,* kidney, + suffix -*ia,* condition ]. Stone in the kidney.

**lithonephritis** (lith'o-ne-fri'tis). Nephritis associated with calculus formation.

**lithonephrotomy** (lith'o-ne-frot'o-mī) [ litho- + G. *nephros,* kidney, + *tomē,* incision ]. Incision into the kidney for the removal of a calculus.

**lithopedion, lithopedium** (lith'o-pe'dī-on, -um) [ Litho- + G. *paidion,* small child ]. A retained fetus, usually extrauterine, which has become calcified.

**lithophone** (lith'o-fōn) [ litho- + G. *phōnē,* sound ]. An instrument that gives a sound when in contact with a stone in the bladder.

**lithoscope** (lith'o-skōp) [ litho- + G. *skopeō,* to view ]. Cystoscope.

**lithosis** (lĭ-tho'sis) [ litho- + G. suffix -*osis,* condition ]. Pneumonoconiosis.

**lithotome** (lith'o-tōm). A knife used in lithotomy.

**lithotomist** (lĭ-thot'o-mist). A person skilled in lithotomy.

**lithotomy** (lĭ-thot'o-mī) [ litho- + G. *tomē,* incision ]. Cutting for stone; a cutting operation for the removal or excision (lithectomy) of a calculus, especially a vesical calculus.

**bilateral l.,** one in which the perineal incision is made transversely across the median raphe.

**high l.,** suprapubic l.

**lateral l.,** one in which the perineum is incised to one side of the median line.

**marian l.** [ L. *mas (mar-),* male ], median l.

**median l.,** an operation in which the perineal incision is made in the line of the median raphe.

**perine'al l.,** any operation for stone in which the bladder is approached by an incision in the perineum.

**prerectal l.,** l. by an incision in midline of perineum anterior to anus.

**suprapu'bic l.,** one in which the bladder is entered by an incision immediately above the symphysis pubis.

**vag'inal l.,** one in which the bladder is entered through an incision in the vagina.

**lithotony** (lĭ-thot'o-ni) [ litho- + G. *tonos,* a stretching ]. Extraction of a stone from the bladder through a small incision which is then dilated instrumentally.

**lith'otre'sis** [ litho- + G. *trēsis,* a boring ]. The boring of holes in a calculus to facilitate its crushing.

**ul'trason'ic l.,** the demolition of calculi by high frequency sound waves; in the experimental stage.

**lithotripsy** (lith'o-trip'sĭ) [ litho- + G. *tripsis,* a rubbing ]. The operation of crushing a stone in the bladder or urethra.

**lith'otrip'tic.** 1. Relating to lithotripsy. 2. An agent that effects the dissolution of a calculus.

**lith'otrip'tor.** Lithotrite.

**lith'otrip'toscope.** An instrument used in lithotriptoscopy.

**lithotriptoscopy** (lith'o-trip-tos'ko-pī) [ litho- + G. *tribō,* to rub, crush, + *skopeō,* to view ]. Crushing of a stone in the bladder under direct vision.

**lith'otrite** [ litho- + G. *tero,* pp. *tritus,* to rub ]. Lithoclast; lithotriptor; an instrument used to crush a stone in the bladder or urethra.

**lithotrity** (lĭ-thot'rĭ-tĭ). The operation of crushing a calculus in the bladder or urethra.

**lithous** (lith'us). Calculous; calculary; relating to a calculus.

**lithuresis** (lith'u-re'sis) [ litho- + G. *ourēsis,* urination ]. The passage of gravel in the urine.

**lith'urete'ria** [ litho- + G. *ourētēr,* ureter ]. Stone in the ureter.

**lithuria** (lĭ-thu'rĭ-ah) [ lithic (acid) + G. *ouron,* urine ]. The excretion of uric acid or urates in large amount in the urine.

**lit'mus** [ a corruption of *lacmus,* fr. Dutch *lakmoes* ]. Lacmus; a blue coloring matter obtained from *Roccella tinctoria* and other species of lichens, the principal component of which is azolitmin; used as an indicator; it is reddened by acids and turned blue again by alkalies.

**Litten,** Moritz, Berlin physician, 1845–1907. See L.'s *phenomenon.*

**lit'ter** [ Fr. *litière;* fr. *lit,* bed ]. 1. A stretcher or portable couch for moving the sick or wounded. 2. Brood (1); a group of animals of the same parents, born at the same time. 3. Sawdust or other dry material used as bedding for poultry or other animals.

**Little,** William J., English surgeon, 1810–1894. See L.'s *disease,* Stromeyer-L. *operation,* L.'s *paralysis.*

**Little's area.** See under area.

**Littré,** Alexis, Paris anatomist, 1658–1726. See L.'s *gland, hernia.*

**littritis** (lit-tri'tis). Inflammation of Littré's glands.

**Litzmann** (lits'mahn), Karl K. T., German gynecologist, 1815–1890. See L.'s *obliquity.*

**live′birth, live birth.** The birth of an infant who shows evidence of life after birth; see also liveborn *infant.*

**livedo** (lī-ve′do) [ L. lividness, fr. *liveo,* to be black and blue ]. A bluish discoloration of the skin, either in limited patches or general.

**l. racemo′sa,** l. reticularis.

**l. reticular′ris,** l. racemosa; dermatopathia pigmentosa reticularis; a purplish network-patterned discoloration of the skin caused by dilation of capillaries and venules due to (1) alteration of a site or (2) changes in underlying larger vessels; rarely appears as a developmental defect.

**l. reticula′ris idiopath′ica,** an extensive and permanent form of l. reticularis; in rare instances associated with central arterial disease.

**l. reticula′ris symptomat′ica,** a discoloration or mottling of the skin due to some demonstrable cause, such as seen in erythema ab igne, in certain tuberculids, or due to the action of cold.

**l. telangiectat′ica,** a permanent mottling of the skin due to an anomaly, probably congenital, of the cutaneous capillaries; a form of l. reticularis.

**livedoid** (liv′e-doyd). Pertaining to or resembling livedo.

**liv′er** [ A.S. *lifer* ]. Hepar; jecur; the largest gland of the body, lying beneath the diaphragm in the right hypochondrium and upper part of the epigastrium; it is of irregular shape and weighs from 3 to 3½ pounds, or about 1/40 the weight of the body. It secretes the bile and is also of great importance in both carbohydrate and protein metabolism.

**brimstone l.,** a bright yellow, bile-stained l., seen in congenital syphilis and acute yellow atrophy.

**cardiac l.,** cardiac *cirrhosis.*

**desiccated l.,** desiccated l. substance; the dried, undefatted powder prepared from mammalian l.'s used as food by man; contains riboflavin, nicotinic acid, and choline. Used in the treatment of macrocytic anemias and as a nutritional supplement.

**frosted l.,** hyaloserositis (*q.v.*) of the liver; also called Zuckergussleber; icing l.; sugar-icing l.; Curschmann's disease.

**gin-drinkers' l.,** alcoholic *cirrhosis.*

**hobnail l.,** Laënnec's cirrhosis (*q.v.*), the contraction of scar tissue and hepatic cellular regeneration causing a nodular appearance of the surface.

**icing l.,** frosted l.

**infantile l.,** obsolete term for biliary cirrhosis of children.

**larda′ceous l.,** waxy l.

**nutmeg l.,** chronic passive congestion of the l., causing accentuation of the lobular pattern with red central and yellow or tan periportal zones.

**sugar-icing l.,** frosted l.

**tropical l.,** chronic congestion of the l. resulting in hypertrophic cirrhosis, with occasionally lardaceous or fatty degeneration, occurring in northerners who have lived for many years in the tropics.

**wandering l.,** hepatoptosia.

**waxy l.,** lardaceous l.; amyloid degeneration of the l.

**liv′etin.** A protein in egg yolk.

**liv′id** [ L. *lividus,* being black and blue ]. Having a black and blue or a leaden or ashy gray color, as in discoloration from a contusion, congestion, or cyanosis.

**lividity** (lī-vid′ĭ-tĭ). The state of being livid.

**li′vor** [ L. a black and blue spot ]. The livid discoloration of the skin on the dependent parts of a corpse.

**lixiviation** (lik-siv′ĭ-a′shun) [ L. *lixivius,* made into lye, fr. *lix,* lye ]. The removal of the soluble constituents of a substance by running water through it; leaching.

**lixivium** (lik-siv′ĭ-um) [ L. ntr. of *lixivius,* made into lye ]. Lye.

**Lloyd's reagent.** See under reagent.

**L.M.** Abbreviation for licentiate in midwifery.

**LNPF.** Abbreviation for lymph node permeability *factor.*

**Lo, L₀.** See under dose.

**load.** A departure from normal body content, as of water, salt, or heat; positive l.'s are quantities in excess of the normal; negative l.'s are quantities in deficit.

**electronic pacemaker l.,** the impedance to the output, the standard l. being 500 ohms resistance ± 1 per cent.

**loading** (lo′ding). Administration of a substance for the purpose of testing metabolic function.

**salt l.,** the administration of 2 gm. of sodium chloride (with a regular diet) three times a day for four days; a diagnostic test in primary aldosteronism, in which the salt loading produces the typical plasma electrolyte pattern.

**Loa loa.** African eye worm; a species of the superfamily Filarioidea that is the causal agent of loiasis. It is indigenous to the western part of equatorial Africa, especially in the region of the Congo River. The adult worms are white or gray-white, cylindroid, and threadlike, the males averaging 25 to 35 by 0.3 to 0.4 mm. (with a curved tail) and the females ranging from 50 to 60 by 0.4 to 0.6 mm.; microfilariae are ensheathed, with nuclei in the tip of the tail and tiny wartlike nodules on the cuticle. The life cycle resembles that of *Wuchereria* species; man is the only known definitive host, and parasites are transmitted by *Chrysops* or tabanid flies. Infective larvae from the latter require 3 years (or more) to mature in man, and the adult forms may persist in man as long as 17 years. The older names include *Strongylus loa, Filaria oculi humani,* and *Dracunculus loa.* See also loiasis.

**lo′bar.** Relating to any lobe.

**lo′bate.** Lobose; lobed; divided into lobes; lobe-shaped; denoting a bacterial colony with a deeply undulate margin.

**lobe** [ G. *lobos,* lobe ]. 1. Lobus. 2. A rounded projecting part, as the l. of the ear; see also lobuli; lobulus. 3. One of the larger divisions of the crown of a tooth, formed from a distinct point of calcification.

**anterior l. of hypophysis,** *lobus* anterior hypophyseos.

**caudate l.,** *lobus* caudatus.

**l.'s of cerebrum,** *lobi* cerebri.

**cuneiform l.,** *lobulus* biventer.

**ear l.,** the lower fleshy part of the auricle, or pinna.

**falciform l.,** *gyrus* cinguli.

**flocculonodular l.,** the small posterior and inferior subdivision of the cerebellar cortex that borders the line of attachment of the choroid roof of the rhomboid fossa, and consists of the left and right flocculus together with the unpaired nodulus (the most posterior of the folia composing the vermis cerebelli). Its major afferent connections come from the vestibular nuclei and directly from the vestibular nerve; it projects largely to the vestibular nuclei, both directly and by way of the nucleus fastigii.

**frontal l.,** *lobus* frontalis cerebri.

**Home's l.,** the enlarged middle l. of the prostate gland.

**inferior l. of lung,** *lobus* inferior pulmonis.

**left l.,** *lobus* sinister.

**left l. of liver,** *lobus* hepatis sinister.

**limbic l.,** as originally defined by Broca: the nearly closed ring of the brain structures surrounding the hilus of the cerebral hemisphere of mammals; it is composed of the gyrus fornicatus (gyrus cinguli and gyrus parahippocampalis), the hippocampus, and the amygdala.

**lingual l.,** cingulum (3).

**lower l. of lung,** *lobus* inferior pulmonis.

**l.'s of mammary gland,** *lobi* glandulae mammariae.

**middle l. of prostate,** *lobus* medius prostatae.

**middle l. of right lung,** *lobus* medius pulmonis dextri.

**occipital l.,** *lobus* occipitalis cerebri.

**parietal l.,** *lobus* parietalis cerebri.

**posterior l. of hypophysis,** *lobus* posterior hypophyseos.

**l. of prostate,** *lobus* prostatae.

**pyramidal l.,** *lobus* pyramidalis.

**quadrate l.,** (1) *lobus* quadratus; (2) *lobulus* quadrangularis; (3) precuneus.

**renal l.,** *lobus* renalis.

**Riedel's l.,** lobus linguiformis; lobus appendicularis; an occasional tongue-like process extending downward from the right l. of the liver lateral to the gallbladder; a similar process may, though rarely, extend from the left lobe.

**right l.,** *lobus* dexter.

**right l. of liver,** *lobus* hepatis dexter.

**Spigelius' l.,** *lobus* caudatus.

**superior l. of lung,** *lobus* superior pulmonis.

**supplemental l.,** in dental anatomy, an extra l.; one that is not included in the typical formation of a tooth.

**temporal l.,** *lobus* temporalis.

**l.'s of thyroid gland,** *lobi* glandulae thyroideae.

**upper l. of lung,** *lobus* superior pulmonis.

**lobec′tomy** [ G. *lobos,* lobe, + *ektomē,* excision ]. Excision of a lobe of any organ or gland.

**lobelia** (lo-be'lĭ-ah). Asthma-weed; wild tobacco; the dried leaves and tops of *Lobelia inflata* (family Lobeliaceae). The fluidextract and the tincture have been used as an expectorant in asthma and chronic bronchitis. Contains several alkaloids: lobeline, lobelamine, lobelanidine, lobelanine, norlobelanine, norlobelanidine, and isolobelanine.

**lobeline** (lo'bĕ-lēn, lob'ē-lēn, -lin). A piperidylacetophenone; an alkaloid of *Lobelia inflata;* it has the same actions as nicotine, but is less potent.

   **l. sulfate,** occurs in yellow friable masses soluble in water. Used in whooping cough and asthma, and has been suggested as a smoking deterrent.

**lo'bi** [ L. ]. Plural of lobus.

**lobitis** (lo-bi'tis). Inflammation of a lobe.

**Lobo,** Jorge, Brazilian physician. See L.'s *disease.*

**lobodontia** (lo'bo-don'shĭ-ah) [ G. *lobos,* lobe, + *odous,* tooth ]. The presence of multiple dental anomalies resulting in teeth resembling those of a carnivore.

**lobomycosis** (lo-bo-mi-ko'sis). Keloidean blastomycosis; Lobo's disease; a chronic infection of the skin resulting in fibrous nodules or keloids that contain budding, thick-walled cells, which are presumably fungi, although the organism has never been definitely cultured and it has not been possible to infect laboratory animals; the presumed causative agent has been variously designated as *Blastomyces loboi, Glenosporella loboi, Glenosporopsis amazonica, Loboa loboi,* or *Paracoccidioides loboi.*

**lobopodium,** pl. **lobopo'dia** (lo'bo-po'dĭ-um) [ G. *lobos,* lobe, + *pous,* foot ]. A thick, lobose pseudopodium.

**lo'bose, lo'bous.** Lobate.

**lobotomy** (lo-bot'o-mī) [ G. *lobos,* lobe, + *tomē,* a cutting ]. 1. Incision into a lobe for any purpose. 2. Division of one or more nerve tracts in a lobe of the cerebrum.

   **prefrontal l.,** prefrontal leukotomy; division of one or more nerve tracts in the prefrontal area of the brain for surgical treatment of pain and emotional disease.

   **transor'bital l.,** transorbital leukotomy; l. by an approach through the roof of the orbit, behind the frontal sinus.

**Lobry de Bruyn-van Ekenstein transformation.** See under transformation.

**Lobstein,** Johann F. G., German pathologist, 1777–1835. See L.'s *ganglion, placenta, syndrome.*

**lobster-claw.** See lobster-claw *deformity.*

**lob'ular.** Relating to a lobule.

**lob'ulate, lob'ulated.** Divided into lobules.

**lobule** (lob'ūl). Lobulus.

   **ansiform l.,** comprises the greater part of the hemisphere of the cerebellum; its superior and inferior surfaces are separated by the horizontal fissure.

   **anterior lunate l.,** *lobulus* semilunaris superior.

   **l. of auricle,** *lobulus* auriculae.

   **biventral l.,** *lobulus* biventer.

   **central l.,** *lobulus* centralis cerebelli.

   **crescentic l.'s of the cerebellum,** *lobulus* semilunaris inferior and *lobulus* semilunaris superior.

   **l.'s of epididymis,** *lobuli* epididymidis.

   **hepatic l.,** *lobulus* hepatis.

   **inferior parietal l.,** *lobulus* parietalis inferior.

   **inferior semilunar l.,** *lobulus* semilunaris inferior.

   **l.'s of mammary gland,** *lobuli* glandulae mammariae.

   **paracentral l.,** *lobulus* paracentralis.

   **portal l. of liver,** a polygonal mass of liver tissue that has as its center a portal canal and at its periphery several venae centrales hepatis. See also liver *acinus.*

   **posterior lunate l.,** *lobulus* semilunaris inferior.

   **pulmonary l.,** a pyramidal mass of lung tissue whose sides are bounded by the incomplete interlobular septa and whose base, which is about an inch in diameter, usually faces the surface of the lung. Some lobules occupy a more central position and are irregular in shape.

   **quadrangular l.,** *lobulus* quadrangularis.

   **quadrate l.,** (1) *lobulus* quadrangularis; (2) precuneus.

   **renal cortical l.,** *lobulus* corticalis renalis.

   **respiratory l.,** a unit of pulmonary tissue that includes a respiratory bronchiole, alveolar ducts, sacs and alveoli.

   **slender l.,** *lobulus* gracilis.

   **superior parietal l.,** *lobulus* parietalis superior.

   **superior semilunar l.,** *lobulus* semilunaris superior.

   **l.'s of testis,** *lobuli* testis.

   **l.'s of thymus,** *lobuli* thymi.

   **l.'s of thyroid gland,** *lobuli* glandula thyroideae.

**lobulet, lobulette** (lob'u-let'). A very small lobule or one of the smaller subdivisions of a lobule.

**lobulus,** gen. and pl. **lob'uli** (lob'u-lus) [ Mod. L. dim. of *lobus,* lobe ] [ NA ]. Lobule; a small lobe or subdivision of a lobe.

   **l. auric'ulae** [ NA ], lobule of the auricle; the lowest part of the auricle; it consists of fat and fibrous tissue not reinforced by the auricular cartilage.

   **l. biven'ter** [ NA ], biventral lobule; cuneiform lobe; l. biventralis; l. cuneiformis; a lobule on the undersurface of each cerebellar hemisphere, divided by a curved sulcus into a lateral and medial portion; it corresponds to the pyramid of the vermis.

   **l. biventra'lis,** l. biventer.

   **l. centra'lis cerebel'li** [ NA ], central lobule; a division of the superior vermis of the cerebellum between the lingula and the monticulus.

   **l. cli'vi,** declive.

   **l. cortica'lis rena'lis** [ NA ], renal cortical lobule; reniculus (1); one of the subdivisions of the kidney, consisting of the pars radiata or medullary ray and the pars convoluta having renal corpuscles and convoluted tubules.

   **l. cul'minis,** culmen.

   **l. cune'iform'is,** l. biventer.

   **lobuli epididym'idis** [ NA ], lobules of the epididymis; coni epididymidis; vascular cones; coni vasculares; Haller's cones; consisting of the coiled portion of the efferent ductules that constitute the head of the epididymis. These join the ductus epididymidis.

   **l. folii,** the part of the superior vermis of the cerebellum lying immediately behind the fissura prima and in front of the l. clivi.

   **l. fusifor'mis,** *gyrus* fusiformis.

   **lobuli glan'dulae mamma'riae** [ NA ], lobules of the mammary gland; subdivisions of the lobes of the mammary gland.

   **lobuli glan'dulae thyroi'deae** [ NA ], lobules of the thyroid gland; the subdivisions of the lobes, consisting of incompletely separated, irregular groups of thyroid follicles (20 to 40 in number) bound together by delicate connective tissue.

   **l. grac'ilis,** slender lobule; the anterior portion of the posterioinferior lobule of the cerebellum, the posterior portion being the l. semilunaris inferior; the two correspond to the tuber of the vermis.

   **l. hep'atis** [ NA ], hepatic lobule; the polygonal histologic unit of the liver consisting of masses of liver cells arranged around a central vein, a terminal branch of one of the hepatic veins; at the periphery are located branches of the portal vein, hepatic artery and bile duct.

   **l. paracentra'lis** [ NA ], paracentral lobule; a division of the medial aspect of the pallium, lying above the sulcus cinguli and bounded by the precentral sulcus in front and the pars marginalis of the sulcus cinguli behind.

   **l. parieta'lis infe'rior** [ NA ], inferior parietal lobule; inferior parietal gyrus; the area of the parietal lobe of the cerebrum lying below the interparietal sulcus; it contains the angular and the supramarginal gyri.

   **l. parieta'lis supe'rior** [ NA ], superior parietal lobule; superior parietal gyrus; the area of the convex surface of the parietal lobe of the cerebrum lying between the longitudinal fissure and the interparietal sulcus behind the posterior central gyrus; it is continuous with the precuneus on the medial aspect of the hemisphere.

   **l. quadrangula'ris** [ NA ], quadrate or quadrangular lobe or lobule; l. quadratus (1); the main portion of the superior part of each hemisphere of the cerebellum, corresponding to the monticulus of the vermis; it is divided into two portions, the anterior and the posterior crescentic lobules, corresponding to the culmen and the declive of the vermis.

   **l. quadra'tus,** (1) l. quadrangularis; (2) precuneus.

   **l. semiluna'ris infe'rior** [ NA ], inferior semilunar lobule; posterior lunate lobule; the part of the superior surface of the cerebellar hemisphere lying behind the fissura prima.

   **l. semiluna'ris supe'rior** [ NA ], superior semilunar lobule; anterior lunate lobule, the part of the superior surface of the cerebellar hemisphere lying in front of the fissura prima, and adjoining the l. culminis.

**lobuli tes'tis** [ NA ], lobules of the testis; the subdivisions of the parenchyma of the testis formed by delicate fibrous septa that pass inward from the tunica albuginea to converge at the mediastinum testis.

**lobuli thy'mi** [ NA ], lobules of the thymus; areas of thymic tissue 0.5 to 2 mm. in diameter with a cortex and medulla.

**lo'bus,** gen. and pl. **lo'bi** [ LL. fr. G. *lobos*] [ NA ]. Lobe; one of the subdivisions of an organ or other part, bounded by fissures, connective tissue septa, or other structural demarcations. See also lobe.

**l. ante'rior hypophys'eos** [ NA ], adenohypophysis [ NA ]; anterior lobe of the hypophysis; l. glandularis of hypophysis; it consists of the pars distalis, pars intermedia, and pars tuberalis (pars infundibularis); see also hypophysis.

**l. appendicula'ris,** Riedel's *lobe.*

**l. az'ygos,** a small accessory lobe, pyramidal in form, sometimes found on the lower part of the inner aspect of the right lung.

**l. cauda'tus** [ NA ], caudate lobe; Spigelius' lobe; a small lobe of the liver situated posteriorly between the sulcus for the vena cava and the fissure for the ligamentum venosum.

**lobi cer'ebri** [ NA ], lobes of the cerebrum; the major divisions of the cerebral hemisphere, including the frontal, parietal, temporal, and occipital lobes.

**l. cli'vi,** the clivus monticuli and the posterior crescentic lobules of the cerebellum considered as one lobe.

**l. dexter,** [ NA ], right lobe; the right subdivision of several glands, *e.g.,* prostate, thyroid, thymus.

**l. falcifor'mis,** *gyrus* cinguli.

**l. fronta'lis cer'ebri** [ NA ], frontal lobe; the portion of each cerebral hemisphere anterior to the fissure of Rolando, or central sulcus.

**lobi glan'dulae mamma'riae** [ NA ], lobes of the mammary gland; the 15 to 20 separate lobes of the mammary gland that comprise the corpus mammae. Each is drained by a single lactiferous duct.

**lobi glan'dulae thyroi'deae** [ NA ], lobes of the thyroid gland; the two major divisions of the gland lying on the right (l. dexter) and left (l. sinistra) side of the trachea and connected by the isthmus. A smaller pyramidal lobe is frequently present as an upward extension from the isthmus.

**l. glandularis of hypophysis,** l. anterior hypophyseos.

**l. hep'atis dexter** [ NA ], right lobe of the liver; the largest lobe of the liver, it is separated from the left lobe above and in front by the falciform ligament and from the caudate and quadrate lobes by the sulcus for the vena cava and the fossa for the gallbladder. It contains two segments, anterior and posterior.

**l. hep'atis sinis'ter** [ NA ], left lobe of the liver; it is separated from the right lobe above and in front by the falciform ligament, and from the quadrate and caudate lobes by the fissure for the ligamentum teres and the fissure for the ligamentum venosum; the distribution of the portal vein, hepatic artery, and bile ducts does not correspond to the gross lobar divisions of the liver. It contains two segments, medial and lateral.

**l. infe'rior pulmo'nis** [ NA ], inferior or lower lobe of the lung; it is located below and behind the oblique fissure and contains five bronchopulmonary segments, superior, medial basal, anterior basal, lateral basal and posterior basal.

**l. linguiformis,** Riedel's *lobe.*

**l. me'dius prosta'tae** [ NA ], middle lobe of prostate; Morgagni's caruncle; the portion of the prostate lying between the urethra and the ejaculatory ducts; indistinct unless hypertrophied.

**l. me'dius pulmo'nis dex'tri** [ NA ], middle lobe of the right lung; it is located anteriorly between the horizontal and oblique fissures and includes lateral and medial bronchopulmonary segments.

**l. occipita'lis cer'ebri** [ NA ], occipital lobe; the posterior, somewhat pyramid-shaped part of each cerebral hemisphere, demarcated by no distinct surface markings from the parietal and temporal lobes on the cerebral convexity, but sharply delineated from the parietal lobe by the deep parietooccipital sulcus on the medial surface.

**l. parieta'lis cer'ebri** [ NA ], parietal lobe; the middle portion of each cerebral hemisphere, separated from the frontal lobe by the central (Rolandic) sulcus, from the temporal lobe by the lateral (Sylvian) sulcus in front and an imaginary line continuing it posteriorly, and from the occipital lobe only partially by the parietooccipital sulcus on its medial aspect.

**l. poste'rior hypophys'eos** [ NA ], neurohypophysis [ NA ]; pars nervosa hypophyseos; the posterior lobe of the hypophysis; see hypophysis.

**l. prosta'tae** [ NA ], lobe of the prostate; one of the lateral lobes (right or left) or the middle lobe or isthmus of the prostate; in the adult the lobes are ill-defined.

**l. pyramida'lis** [ NA ], pyramidal lobe; Morgagni's appendix; an inconstant narrow lobe of the thyroid gland that arises from the upper border of the isthmus and extends upward, sometimes as far as the hyoid bone.

**l. quadra'tus** [ NA ], quadrate lobe (1); a lobe on the inferior surface of the liver located between the fossa for the gallbladder and the fissure for the ligamentum teres.

**l. rena'lis** [ NA ], renal lobe; one of the subdivisions of the kidney, consisting of a renal pyramid and the cortical tissue associated with it.

**l. sinis'ter** [ NA ], left lobe; the left subdivision of several glands, *e.g.,* prostate, thyroid, thymus.

**l. supe'rior pulmo'nis** [ NA ], superior or upper lobe of the lung; on the right it lies above the oblique and horizontal fissures and includes the apical, posterior and anterior bronchopulmonary segments; on the left it lies above the oblique fissure and contains the apicoposterior, anterior, superior lingular and inferior lingular segments.

**l. tempora'lis** [ NA ], temporal lobe; a long lobe, the lowest of the major subdivisions of the cortical mantle, forming the posterior two-thirds of the ventral surface of the cerebral hemisphere, separated from the frontal and parietal lobes above it by the fissure of Sylvius, arbitrarily delineated by an imaginary plane from the occipital lobe with which it is continuous posteriorly. The temporal lobe has a heterogeneous composition: in addition to a large neocortical component consisting of the superior, middle, and inferior temporal gyri and the lateral and medial occipitotemporal gyri, it includes the largely juxtallocortical parahippocampal gyrus with its paleocortical (olfactory) uncus and, beneath the latter, the amygdala.

**lo'cal** [ L. *localis,* fr. *locus,* place ]. Having reference or confined to a limited part; not general or systemic.

**localization** (lo'kal-ĭ-za'shun). 1. Limitation to a definite area. 2. The reference of a sensation to its point of origin. 3. The determination of the location of a morbid process.

**auditory l.,** in sensory psychology, the naming or pointing to positions from which sounds emanate.

**cerebral l.,** the mapping of the cerebral cortex into areas and the correlation of the various areas with cerebral function, or the diagnosis of the situation in the cerebrum of a brain lesion from the signs and symptoms manifested by the patient or from a study of the electroencephalogram.

**germinal l.,** the determination in very young embryos of the presumptive areas for specific organs or structures.

**pneumotaxic l.,** l. on a grid of basal structures in the brain outlined by ventriculography.

**spatial l.,** the reference of a visual sensation to a definite locality in space.

**localized** (lo'kal-izd). Restricted or limited to a definite part.

**lo'calizer.** In ophthalmology: 1. An apparatus for determining the location of a solid particle imbedded in the eyeball. 2. A visual training instrument used to establish correct localization in the treatment of amblyopia or anopsia.

**lo'cator.** An instrument for finding the position of an object.

**Berman-Moorhead l.,** a device for finding fragments of metal in tissue.

**electroacoustic l.,** an instrument for finding foreign body in tissue by sound on contact.

**lochia** (lo'kĭ-ah) [ G. neut. pl. of *lochios,* relating to childbirth, fr. *lochos,* childbirth ]. The discharge from the vagina of mucus, blood, and tissue debris, following childbirth.

**l. alba,** l. purulenta; the later discharge no longer tinged with blood.

**l. cruen'ta,** the earlier discharge stained with blood.

**l. purulen'ta,** l. alba.

**l. rubra,** l. cruenta.

**l. sanguinolen'ta,** thick, dark red vaginal discharge seen a few days after delivery.

**l. sero'sa,** a thin and watery l.

**lochial** (lo'kĭ-al). Relating to the lochia.

**lochiometra** (lo-kĭ-o-me'trah) [ G. *mētra*, womb ]. Distention of the uterus with retained lochia.

**lochiometritis** (lo-kĭ-o-me-tri'tis). Puerperal metritis.

**lochioperitonitis** (lo'kĭ-o-pĕr'ĭ-to-ni'tis). Puerperal peritonitis.

**lochiopyra** (lo-kĭ-op'ĭ-rah) [ lochia + G. *pyr*, fire, fever ]. Puerperal *fever*.

**lochiorrhagia** (lo-kĭ-ŏ-ra'jĭ-ah) [ lochia + G. *rhēgnymi*, to burst forth. RHAG- ]. Lochiorrhea.

**lochiorrhea** (lo-kĭ-ŏ-re'ah) [ lochia + G. *rhoia*, a flow ]. A profuse flow of the lochia.

**lochioschesis** (lo-kĭ-os'kĭ-sis) [ lochia + G. *schesis*, retention ]. Retention of the lochia.

**loci** (lo'si). Plural of locus.

**Locke,** Frank S., British physiologist, 1871–1949. See L.'s *solution*, L.-Ringer *solution*.

**lock'jaw.** Trismus.

**Lockwood,** Charles B., English surgeon, 1858–1914. See L.'s *ligament*.

**loco** (lo'ko) [ Sp. crack-brained ]. Locoweed disease; a disease affecting cattle on the great plains of the western United States, caused by eating the locoweed; it is characterized by paresis, incoordination, dullness, and a tendency to become solitary in habit.

**locoed** (lo'kōd). Poisoned by the loco weed.

**locoism** (lo'ko-izm). Poisoning by loco weed.

**lo'como'tive.** Locomotor.

**locomotor** (lo'ko-mo'tor) [ L. *locus*, place, + L. *moveo*, pp. *motus*, to move ]. Locomotive; locomotory; relating to locomotion, or movement from one place to another.

**locomoto'rial.** Relating to the locomotorium.

**locomoto'rium** [ L. *locus*, place, + *motorius*, moving ]. The locomotor apparatus of the body.

**locomo'tory.** Locomotor.

**locular** (lok'u-lar). Relating to a loculus.

**loc'ulate.** Containing numerous loculi.

**loculation** (lok-u-la'shun). 1. A loculate region in an organ or tissue, or a loculate structure formed between surfaces of organs, mucous or serous membranes, and so on. 2. The process that results in the formation of a loculus or loculi.

**loculus,** pl. **loc'uli** (lok'u-lus) [ L. dim. of *locus*, place ]. A small cavity or chamber.

**lo'cum te'nens** [ L. *locus*, place, + *teneo*, pres. p. *tenens*, to hold ]. A substitute; a physician taking another's practice during the temporary absence or incapacity of the latter.

**locus,** pl. **loci** (lo'kus, lo'si) [ L. ] [ NA ]. A place; usually, a specific site.

**l. ceru'leus** [ NA ], substantia ferruginea [ NA ]; l. cinereus; l. ferrugineus; a shallow depression, of a blue color in the fresh brain, lying laterally in the most anterior portion of the rhomboidal fossa near the cerebral aqueduct; it corresponds to the location, closely under the floor of the ventricle, of a group of about 20,000 melanin-pigmented neuronal cell bodies whose norepinephrine-containing axons have a remarkably wide distribution in the cerebellum as well as in the hypothalamus and cerebral cortex.

**l. cine'reus,** l. ceruleus.

**l. ferrugin'eus,** l. ceruleus.

**l. minor'is resisten'tiae,** a place of less resistance, any part or organ which is more susceptible than the others to the attack of a morbific agent.

**l. ni'ger,** *substantia* nigra.

**l. perfora'tus anti'cus,** *substantia* perforata anterior.

**l. perfora'tus posti'cus,** *substantia* perforata posterior.

**Loeb,** Leo, American pathologist, *1869. See L.'s *deciduoma*.

**Loeffler** (lĕf'ler), Friedrich A. J., German bacteriologist and surgeon, 1852–1915. See L.'s *bacillus*, Klebs-L. *bacillus*, L.'s blood culture *medium*, caustic *solution*, L.'s *stain*, L.'s *methylene* blue.

**Loeffler,** Wilhelm. See Löffler, Wilhelm.

**loeffleria** (lĕf-le'rĭ-ah). A condition in which the Klebs-Loeffler bacillus of diphtheria is present without producing any symptoms.

**Loenen's sign.** See under sign.

**Loeschia** (lĕ'shyah). A genus of the order Gymnamoebidae, designed to include many forms formerly in the genus *Amoeba*, but no longer used.

**Loevit** (lĕ'vit), Moritz, Austrian pathologist, 1851–1918. See L.'s *cells*.

**Loewenthal** (lĕv'en-tahl), Wilhelm, German physician, 1850–1894. See L.'s *bundle, reaction, tract*.

**Loewi,** Otto, German pharmacologist in New York, 1873–1961. Nobel laureate 1936 with Sir Henry H. Dale for investigations on the transmission of nerve impulses by chemical substances.

**Löffler** (lĕf'ler), Wilhelm, Swiss physician, *1887. See L.'s *disease, endocarditis, pneumonia, syndrome*.

**Löffleria.** See loeffleria.

**log-.** See logo-.

**logadi'tis** [ G. *logades*, the whites of the eyes, + suffix -*itis*, inflammation ]. Obsolete term for scleritis.

**logagnosia** (log'ag-no'sĭ-ah) [ logo- + G. *agnosia*, ignorance ]. Aphasia.

**logagraphia** (log-ă-graf'ĭ-ah) [ logo- + G. *a-* priv. + *graphō*, to write ]. Agraphia.

**logamnesia** (log'am-ne'zĭ-ah) [ logo- + G. *amnēsia*, forgetfulness ]. Aphasia.

**Logan's bow.** See under bow.

**logaphasia** (log-ă-fa'zĭ-ah) [ logo- + G. *aphasia*, speechlessness ]. Aphasia of articulation.

**logasthenia** (log'as-the'nĭ-ah) [ logo- + G. *astheneia*, weakness ]. Aphasia.

**loget'ronog'raphy.** A method of printing in which special details are emphasized by purely electronic means in very dense or very thin low contrast area in a manner that allows the desired emphasis to be obtained. Used especially in emphasizing details of x-ray films.

**-logia** [ G. *logos*, discourse, treatise ]. 1. A Greek suffix, expressing in a general way the study of the subject noted in the body of the word, or a treatise on the same; the English equivalent is -logy, or, with the connecting vowel, -ology. A number of words thus formed have been transformed bodily from the Greek, as *osteologia*, osteology; others have been formed on this model, as urology, laryngology, etc. 2 [ G. *legō*, to collect ]. A suffix with the signification of collecting, picking, as in carphologia, picking imaginary bits of straw or lint.

**logo-, log-** [ G. *logos*, word, discourse ]. Combining forms relating to speech, or words.

**logokophosis** (log'o-ko-fo'sis) [ logo- + G. *kophōsis*, deafness ]. Obsolete term for auditory *aphasia*.

**logoneurosis** (log-o-nu-ro'sis) [ logo- + neurosis ]. Any neurosis associated with a speech defect.

**logopathy** (log-op'ă-thĭ) [ logo- + G. *pathos*, suffering ]. Any speech disorder.

**logope'dia.** Logopedics.

**logopedics** (log'o-pe'diks) [ logo- + G. *pais* (*paid-*), child ]. A branch of science dealing with the physiology and pathology of the organs of speech and with the correction of speech defects.

**logoplegia** (log-o-ple'jĭ-ah) [ logo- + G. *plēgē*, stroke ]. Paralysis of the organs of speech.

**logorrhea** (log'o-re'ah) [ logo- + G. *rhoia*, a flow ]. Garrulousness.

**logospasm** (log'o-spazm) [ logo- + G. *spasmos*, spasm ]. 1. Stuttering. 2. Explosive *speech*.

**log'other'apy** [ logo- + G. *therapeia*, cure ]. A form of psychotherapy which places special emphasis on the patient's spiritual life and on the physician as "medical minister."

**log'wood.** Hematoxylon.

**-logy** [ G. *logos*, treatis, discourse ]. See -*logia*.

**Lohlein-Baehr lesion.** See under lesion.

**Lohnstein** (lōn'stin), Theodor, German physician, 1866–1918. See L.'s *saccharimeter*.

**loiasis** (lo-i'ă-sis). Calabar swelling; fugitive swelling; a chronic disease caused by *Loa loa*, with symptoms and signs first occurring approximately 3 to 4 years after a bite by an infected tabanid fly. When the infective larvae mature, the adult worms move about in an irregular course through the connective tissue of the body (as much as 1 cm. per minute), frequently becoming visible beneath the skin and mucous membranes, *e.g.*, in the back, scalp, chest, inner surface of the lip, conjunctiva, and so on. The worms provoke hyperemia and exudation of fluid, but cause no serious damage, and the acute reaction subsides as the parasites move on. The patient is annoyed by the "creeping" in the tissues and intense itching, as well as occasional pain, especially when the swelling is in the region of tendons and joints; most patients manifest an eosinophilia of 10 to 30 or 40 per cent in the circulating blood.

**loim-.** For words beginning thus, see those beginning with lem-.

**loin** (loyn) [ Fr. *longe;* E. *lumbus* ]. Lumbus.

**loliism** (lo'lĭ-izm) [ L. *lolium,* darnel, tares ]. Giddiness, tremor, green vision, dilated pupils, great prostration, and sometimes vomiting—symptoms of poisoning by the seeds of a grass, *Lolium temulentum,* in the form of flour made into bread.

**Lombard voice-reflex test.** See under test.

**lombricine.** A phosphagen (guanidinoethylserylphosphate) found in earthworms.

**lo'mofun'gin** (USAN). An antibiotic from *Streptomyces lomondensis;* possesses antifungal activity.

**lomy'cin.** Griseomycin.

**Long,** Crawford W., American surgeon, 1815–1878. He was the first to use ether as an anesthetic in a surgical operation (1842) but this work was not published until 1849.

**Long,** John H., American physician, 1856–1927. See L.'s *coefficient, formula.*

**longevity** (lon-jev'ĭ-tĭ). Macrobiosis; the duration of a particular life beyond the norm for the species; see also life-span.

**longissimus** (lon-jis'ĭ-mus) [ L. superlative of *longus,* long ] [ NA ]. Longest; see under musculus.

**longitudinal** (lon'jĭ-tu'dĭ-nal) [ L. *longitudo,* length ]. Running lengthwise; in the direction of the long axis of the body or any of its parts.

**longitudina'lis** [ NA ]. Longitudinal.

**longitype** (lon'jĭ-tĭp). Ectomorph.

**Longmire,** William P., Jr., Los Angeles surgeon, *1913. See L.'s *operation.*

**long'sight'edness.** Hyperopia.

**lon'gus** [ L. long ] [ NA ]. Long; see under musculus.

**Looney,** Joseph M., American biochemist, *1896. See Folin-L. *test.*

**loop** [ M.E. *loupe* ]. 1. A curve or complete bend in a cord or other cylindrical body, forming an oval or circular ring. 2. A more or less sharp and more or less complete bend or curve in a nerve or blood vessel or urinary tubule. 3. A wire (usually 3.5 inches long), usually of platinum or nichrome, fixed into a handle (about 10 inches long) at one end and bent into a circle (inside diameter ordinarily about 4 mm.) at the other; the l. is rendered sterile by flaming and is then used to transfer microorganisms.

**Biebl l.,** a portion of the small intestine is brought out to a subcutaneous location and the continuity of the intestine is kept intact. The muscles of the abdominal wall are brought together so that the intestine passes out through one opening through the muscles, passes along under the skin, and enters the abdominal cavity through another opening in the abdominal muscles. Mann prepared two modifications of the Biebl l.

**bulboventricular l.,** the portion of the early somite embryonic cardiac tube which will become the ventricle and bulbus cordis.

**capillary l.'s,** small blood vessels in papillae of corium.

**gamma l.,** the reflex arc consisting of small anterior horn cells, their small gamma fibers to the intrafusal bundle producing its contraction, which stimulates the afferent impulses that pass through the posterior root to the anterior horn cells, inducing a stretch reflex.

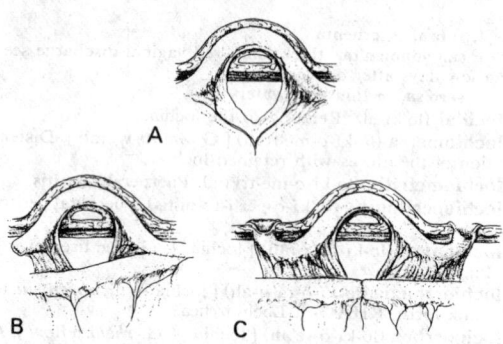

**Biebl Loop (A), and Mann's Modifications of the Biebl Loop (B and C)**

(From Youmans, W. B.: *Nervous and Neurohumoral Regulation of Intestinal Motility, Monographs in the Physiological Sciences,* Interscience Publishers, Inc., New York, 1949. Used with permission.)

**Gerdy's interatrial l.,** a muscular fasciculus in the interatrial septum of the heart, passing backward from the atrioventricular groove.

**Granit's l.,** the efferent gamma axon innervates intrafusal fibers in the muscle spindle and influences the sensory output, forming a reflex l.

**Henle's l.,** nephronic l.

**Hyrtl's l.,** Hyrtl's anastomosis; a communicating l. between the right and left hypoglossal nerves, lying between the geniohyoid and genioglossus muscles or in the substance of the geniohyoid; it is found in about one in ten persons.

**lenticular l.,** *ansa* lenticularis.

**memory l.,** an electronic device for retrieving data that had been displayed upon the oscilloscope at an earlier time; used for reviewing electrical events immediately preceding a specific disturbance.

**Meyer-Archambault l.,** the fibers of the visual radiation which loop around the tip of the temporal horn.

**nephronic l.,** Henle's l.; Henle's ansa; the U-shaped part of the nephron extending from the proximal to the distal

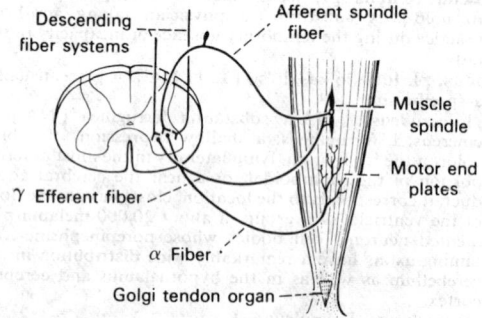

**Schematic Diagram of the Gamma Loop**

Gamma efferent fibers pass to the polar portions of the muscle spindle. Contractions of the intrafusal fibers in the polar parts of the spindle stretch the nuclear bag region and thus cause an efferent impulse to be conducted centrally. The afferent fibers from the spindle synapse upon an alpha motor neuron, whose peripheral processes pass to extrafusal muscle fibers, thus completing the loop. Both alpha and gamma motor neurons can be influenced by descending fiber systems from supraspinal levels. (From Truex, R. C., and Carpenter, M. B.: *Human Neuroanatomy,* Ed. 6, The Williams & Wilkins Co., Baltimore, 1969.)

convoluted tubules and consisting of descending and ascending limbs; see fig. under nephron.

**peduncular l.,** *ansa* peduncularis.

**l.'s of spinal nerves,** *ansae* nervorum spinalium.

**subclavian l.,** *ansa* subclavia.

**vector l.,** an irregularly elliptical curve representing the average direction and magnitude of the heart's action from moment to moment throughout the cardiac cycle. See also vector (2), and vectorcardiogram.

**ventricular l.,** the l. in the conoventricular region of the embryonic heart.

**Vieussens' l.,** *ansa* subclavia.

**Looser,** Emil, Swiss physician, 1877–1936. See L.'s *zones.*

**lop-ear.** A congenital deformity of the external ear, with poor development of helix and anthelix.

**lophodont** (lof'o-dont) [ G. *lophos,* ridge, + *odous,* tooth ]. Having the crowns of the molar teeth formed in transverse or longitudinal crests or ridges; opposed to bunodont.

**Lophoph'ora williamsii.** *Anhalonium lewinii* (family Cactaceae); the botanical origin of peyote, mescal button; it contains over a dozen alkaloids, of which mescaline is the most important; others are pellotine, anhalomine, anhalonidine, anhalamine, anhalinine, anhalidine, and lophophorine.

**lophophorine** (lo-fof'o-rin, rēn). *N*-Methylanhalonine; an alkaloid, $C_{13}H_{17}NO_3$, from *Lophophora williamsii.*

**lophot'richate.** Lophotrichous.

**lophotrichous** (lo-fot'rī-kus) [ G. *lophos,* crest, + *thrix,* hair ]. Lophotrichate; referring to a bacterial cell with two or more flagella at one or both poles.

**lo'premone** (USAN). 5-Oxo-L-propyl-L-histidyl-L-prolinamide; a synthetic thyrotropin-releasing hormone.

**Lorain** (lor-an'), Paul, French physician, 1827–1875. See L.'s *disease;* L.-Lévi *dwarfism, infantilism, syndrome.*

**lora'zepam** (USAN). 7-Chloro-5-(*o*-chlorophenyl)-1,3-dihydro-3-hydroxy-2*H*-1,4-benzodiazepin-2-one; an antianxiety drug.

**lordoscoliosis** (lor'do-sko-lī-o'sis) [ G. *lordos,* bent back, + *skoliōsis,* crookedness, fr. *skolios,* bent, aslant ]. Combined backward and lateral curvature of the spine.

**lordo'sis** [ G. *lordōsis,* a bending backward ]. Hollow back, saddle back; anteroposterior curvature of the spine, generally lumbar with the convexity looking anteriorly.

**lordot'ic.** Pertaining to or marked by lordosis.

**Lorenz,** Adolf, Vienna surgeon, 1854–1946. See L.'s *method, operation, sign.*

**Lorenz,** Konrad, Austrian ethologist working in Germany, *1903. Nobel laureate, 1973, with Karl Ritter von Frisch and Nikolas Tinbergen, for their discoveries concerning organization and elicitation of individual and social behavior patterns.

**lor'etin.** Ferron; 7-iodo-8-hydroxyquinoline-5-sulfonic acid; topical antiseptic and intestinal amebicide.

**Loschmidt's number.** See under number.

**lota tokelau.** *Tinea* imbricata.

**lo'tio** [ L. ]. Lotion.

**lotion** (lo'shun) [ L. *lotio,* a washing, fr. *lavo,* to wash ]. A wash; a class of pharmacopeial preparations that are liquid suspensions or dispersions intended for external application; some consist of finely powdered, insoluble solids held in more or less permanent suspension by suspending agents or surface-active agents, or both; others are oil-in-water emulsions stabilized by surface-active agents.

**Louis** (loo-e'), Antoine, Paris surgeon, 1723–1792. See L.'s *angle.*

**Louis** (loo-e'), Pierre C. A., Paris physician, 1787–1872. See L.'s *law.*

**Louis-Bar,** Denise. See L.-B. *syndrome.*

**loupe** (loop) [ Fr. ]. A magnifying lens.

**binocular l.,** a magnifying device, attached to spectacles or a headband, worn as an aid when performing delicate operations.

**louse** pl. **lice** (lows), [ A.S. *lūs* ]. Common name for *Bovicola, Haematopinus, Linognathus, Pediculus, Trichodectes,* and a variety of biting lice (order Mallaphaga) and sucking lice (order Anoplura). Other important lice are *Felicola subrostrata* (cat l.), *Goniocotes gallinae* (fluff l.), *Goniodes dissimilis* (brown chicken l.), *Haemodipsus ventri-*

*cosus* (rabbit l.), *Lipeurus caponis* (wing l.), *Menacanthus stramineus* (chicken body l.), *Phthirus pubis* (crab or pubic l.), and *Polyplax serratus* (mouse l.).

**biting l.,** chewing l.; feather l.; ectoparasites (order Mallophaga) chiefly found on birds, where they feed on feathers, hair, epidermal debris, and (less commonly) on blood; they possess nipper-like, heavily sclerotized mandibles and a characteristic broad head; many species are host-specific.

**lousiness** (low'zī-nes). Pediculosis.

**Lovén** (lo-vān'), Otto C., Swedish physician, 1835–1904. See L. *reflex.*

**Low,** George C., English physician, 1872–1952. See Castellani-L. *sign.*

**Lowe,** Charles U., U. S. pediatrician, *1921. See L.'s *syndrome,* L.-Terrey-MacLachlan *syndrome.*

**Löwe,** Karl F., German optician, *1874. See L.'s *ring.*

**Löwenberg** (lĕ'ven-berg), Benjamin B., Paris laryngologist, *1836. See L.'s *canal, forceps, scala.*

**Löwenstein,** L. W. See Buschke-L. *tumor.*

**Lower,** Richard, English physician and physiologist, 1631–1691. See L.'s *rings, tubercle.*

**Lown,** Bernard, U. S. cardiologist. See L.-Ganong-Levine *syndrome.*

**loxarthron, loxarthrus** (loks-sar'thron, -thrus) [ G. *loxos,* slanting, + *arthron,* joint ]. Rarely used term for deformity of a joint without dislocation or fracture, such as knock-knee or clubfoot.

**loxia** (lok'sī-ah) [ G. *loxos,* oblique, slanting ]. Torticollis.

**loxophthalmus** (loks'of-thal'mus) [ G. *loxos,* slanting, + *ophthalmos,* eye ]. Obsolete term for strabismus.

**Loxosceles** (loks-os'ē-lēz) [ G. *loxos,* oblique, + *skelos,* leg ]. A genus of venomous spiders, the brown spiders, marked by a fiddle-shaped pattern on the cephalothorax, and found chiefly in South America. They inflict a highly ulcerative, spreading dermal lesion at the site of the bite (see loxoscelism). Important species include *L. laeta,* the Chilean brown spider; *L. reclusus,* the brown spider of North America; and *L. rufipes,* the Peruvian brown spider.

**loxoscelism** (loks-os'ē-lizm). A clinical illness produced by the brown recluse spider, *Loxosceles reclusus,* of North America; characterized by gangrenous slough at the site of the bite, nausea, malaise, fever, hemolysis, and thrombocytopenia.

**loxot'ic** [ G. *loxotēs,* obliquity ]. Slanting; distorted; awry.

**loxotomy** (lok'sot'o-mī) [ G. *loxos,* slanting, + *tomē,* incision ]. Amputation by means of an oblique incision through the soft parts; distinguished from a circular amputation.

**Loxotre'ma ova'tum** [ G. *loxos,* slanting, + *trēma,* a hole; L. *ovatus,* egg-shaped ]. *Metagonimus yokogawai.*

**lozenge** (loz'enj) [ Fr. *losange,* from *losangé,* rhombic ]. Troche.

**L.P.N.** Abbreviation for licensed practical nurse.

**Lr, L_r.** See under dose.

**L.R.C.P.** Abbreviation for Licentiate of the Royal College of Physicians.

**L.R.C.P.E.** Abbreviation for Licentiate of the Royal College of Physicians (Edinburgh).

**L.R.C.P.I.** Abbreviation for Licentiate of the Royal College of Physicians (Ireland).

**L.R.C.S.** Abbreviation for Licentiate of the Royal College of Surgeons.

**L.R.C.S.E.** Abbreviation for Licentiate of the Royal College of Surgeons (Edinburgh).

**L.R.C.S.I.** Abbreviation for Licentiate of the Royal College of Surgeons (Ireland).

**LRF.** Abbreviation for (1) liver residue *factor;* (2) luteinizing hormone-releasing *factor.*

**L.R.F.P.S.** Abbreviation for Licentiate of the Royal Faculty of Physicians and Surgeons, a Scottish institution.

**L.S.A.** Abbreviation for Licentiate of the Society of Apothecaries.

**LSD.** Abbreviation for lysergic acid diethylamide.

**LSH.** Abbreviation for lutein-stimulating *hormone.*

**LTH.** Abbreviation for luteotropic *hormone.*

**Lu.** 1. Chemical symbol of the element lutetium. 2. Abbreviation for Lutheran blood group; see appendix 2.

**Lubarsch** (loo'barsh), Otto, German pathologist, 1860–1933. See L.'s *crystals.*

**Luc,** Henri, French laryngologist, 1855–1925. See L.'s *operation,* Caldwell-L. *operation,* Ogston-L. *operation.*

**lucan'thone hydrochloride** (BP, USAN). NILODIN; MIRACIL; 1,2'-diethylaminoethylamino-4-methylthiaxanthone hydrochloride. Used in the treatment of urinary schistosomiasis (*Schistosoma haematobium*) and intestinal schistosomiasis (*S. mansoni*).

**Lucas,** Richard C., English anatomist and surgeon, 1846–1915. See L.'s *groove.*

**Lucas-Championnière** (lü-kah'shahṅ-pe-on-e-air'), Just M. M., French surgeon, 1843–1913. See L.-C.'s *disease.*

**lucen'somycin.** ETRUSCOMYCIN; antibiotic isolated from cultures of *Streptomyces lucensis;* antifungal agent.

**lucent** (lu'sent) [ L. *lucere,* to shine ]. Bright; clear; translucent.

**Lucibacterium** (lu'si-bak-tēr-ī-um) [ L. *lucere,* to shine, + bacterium ]. A genus of aerobic to facultatively anaerobic, motile, peritrichous bacteria containing Gram-negative rods. Their metabolism is fermentative, and they are usually luminescent. They occur on the surfaces of dead fish and in sea water. The type species is *L. harveyi.*
  **L. harveyi,** *Photobacterium harveyi;* a species of luminescent bacteria found in sea water; it is the type species of the genus *L.*

**lucidification** (lu-sid'ī-fī-ka'shun) [ L. *lucidus,* clear, + *facere,* to make ]. Clarification.

**lucidity** (lu-sid'ī-tī) [ L. *lucidus,* clear ]. Clarity, especially mental clarity.

**lu'cidus** [ L. ] [ NA ]. Lucent.

**lucif'erase.** An enzyme present in certain luminous bacteria, worms, insects, and other organisms, that acts to bring about the oxidation of luciferin. The energy produced in the process is liberated as light, without significant heat ("cold light").

**lucif'erin.** Generic term for the chemical substances present in certain luminous worms, bacteria, insects, and other organisms that when acted upon by an oxidative enzyme, luceriferase, produce a bluish green light.

**lucifugal** (lu-sif'u-gal) [ L. *lux,* light, + *fugio,* to flee from ]. Avoiding light.

**Lucilia** (lu-sil'ī-ah). A genus of blowflies of the family Calliphoridae.
  **L. cae'sar,** a species whose larvae formerly were used in the treatment of septic wounds.
  **L. cuprina,** the most important cause of blowfly strike of sheep in Australia and South Africa.
  **L. illus'tris,** a metallic blue-green blowfly widely distributed in North America; the eggs are deposited chiefly on animal carcasses.
  **L. serica'ta,** *Phaenicia sericata.*

**Lucio,** R. See L.'s *leprosy,* L.'s leprosy *phenomenon.*

**lucipetal** (lu-sip'ī-tal) [ L. *lux,* light, + *peto,* to seek ]. Seeking light.

**lucites** pl. of **luci'tis** (lu-si'tēz) [ L. *lux,* light, + *-itis,* inflammation ]. Diseases in which actinic rays play a major etiologic role.

**Lucké,** Balduin, U. S. pathologist. See L.'s *adenocarcinoma, carcinoma, virus.*

**Lücke** (lük'eh), George A., German surgeon, 1829–1894. See L.'s *test.*

**lucotherapy** (lu'ko-thĕr'ă-pī) [ L. *lux,* light, + G. *therapeia,* therapy ]. Phototherapy.

**lu'dic** [ G. *ludus,* game ]. Unreal; playlike.

**Ludloff** (lood'lawf), Karl, Breslau surgeon, *1864. See L.'s *sign.*

**Ludwig** (lood'vig), Daniel, German anatomist, 1625–1680. See L.'s *angle.*

**Ludwig** (lood'vig), Karl F. W., eminent German anatomist and physiologist, 1816–1895. Famous as a teacher of over 200 eminent scientists and for his unselfish devotion to science, much of his work being published under the names of his pupils or jointly with them. See depressor *nerve* of L., L.'s *ganglion, labyrinth, stromuhr.*

**Luer,** German instrument maker, †1883. See L.'s *syringe.*

**lues** (lu'ēz) [ L. *pestilence* ]. A plague, or pestilence; specifically, syphilis.
  **l. vene'rea,** syphilis.

**luetic** (lu-et'ik). Syphilitic.

**lumba'go** [ L. fr. *lumbus,* loin ]. Pain in mid and lower back; a descriptive term not specifying cause.
  **ische'mic l.,** a lumbar type of intermittent claudication; a vascular form of backache characterized by a painful cramp of the muscles in the lumbar region excited by the exertion of walking or standing and promptly relieved by rest.

**lum'bar** [ L. *lumbus,* a loin ]. Relating to the loins, or the part of the back and sides between the ribs and the pelvis.

**lum'bariza'tion.** Fusion between the transverse processes of the 5th lumbar and the 1st sacral vertebrae.

**lum'bi** [ L. ]. Plural of lumbus.

**lum'boabdom'inal.** Relating to the sides and front of the abdomen.

**lumbocolostomy** (lum'bo-ko-los'to-mī) [ L. *lumbus,* loin, + G. *kolon,* colon, + *stoma,* mouth ]. The formation of an artificial anus by opening into the colon in the left lumbar region.

**lumbocolotomy** (lum'bo-ko-lot'o-mī) [ L. *lumbus,* loin, + G. *kolon,* colon, + *tomē,* incision ]. Incision into the colon in the left lumbar region.

**lumbocostal** (lum'bo-kos'tal) [ L. *lumbus,* loin, + *costa,* rib ]. 1. Relating to the lumbar and the hypochondriac regions. 2. Relating to the lumbar spine and the ribs; denoting a ligament connecting the first lumbar vertebra with the neck of the twelfth rib.

**lumbodynia** (lum'bo-din'ī-ah) [ L. *lumbus,* loin, + *odynē,* pain ]. Obsolete term for lumbago.

**lumboiliac** (lum-bo-il'ī-ak). Lumboinguinal.

**lumboinguinal** (lum'bo-ing'givī-nal) [ L. *lumbus,* loin, + *inguen* (*inguin-*), groin ]. Lumboiliac; relating to the lumbar and the inguinal regions.

**lumboovarian** (lum-bo-o-va'rī-an). Relating to the ovary and the lumbar regions.

**lumbosacral** (lum'bo-sa'kral). Relating to the lumbar vertebrae and the sacrum.

**lumbrical** (lum'brī-kal) [ L. *lumbricus,* earthworm ]. 1. Relating to or resembling an earthworm; vermiform; lumbricoid. 2. *Musculus* lumbricalis.

**lumbrica'lis** [ L. *lumbricus,* an earthworm ]. See *musculus* lumbricalis.

**lumbricide** (lum'brī-sid) [ L. *lumbricus,* worm, + *caedo,* to kill ]. 1. Destructive to lumbricoid (intestinal) worms. 2. An agent that kills such worms.

**lumbricoid** (lum'brī-koyd) [ L. *lumbricus,* earthworm, + G. *eidos,* resemblance ]. 1. Resembling an earthworm; vermiform; denoting a shape like an earthworm. 2. A roundworm parasitic in the human intestine, *Ascaris lumbricoides.*

**lumbricosis** (lum'brī-ko'sis). Infestation with lumbricoids or round intestinal worms.

**lumbricus** (lum'brī-kus) [ L. earthworm ]. 1 [ NA ]. Lumbricoid (1). 2. An intestinal parasitic worm, *Ascaris lumbricoides.*

**lum'bus,** gen. **lum'bi** [ L. ] [ NA ]. Loin; the part of the side and back between the ribs and the pelvis.

**lu'men,** pl. **lu'mina** [ L. light, window ]. 1. The space in the interior of a tubular structure, such as an artery or the intestine. 2. The unit of luminous flux; the luminous flux emitted in a solid angle of 1 steridian by a uniform point source of light having a luminous intensity of 1 candela.
  **residual l.,** residual *cleft.*

**lumichrome** (lu'mik-rōm). 6,7-Dimethylalloxazine; riboflavin minus its ribityl side chain; produced by ultraviolet irradiation in acid solution.

**lumiflavin** (lu'mī-fla'vin). 6,7,9-Trimethylisoalloxazine; a yellow photoderivative of riboflavin, bearing a methyl group in place of the ribityl; produced by ultraviolet irradiation in alkaline solution.

**lu'mina** [ L. ]. One of the plural forms of lumen.

**lu'minal.** Relating to the lumen of a blood vessel or other tubular structure.

**luminescence** (lu'mĭ-nes'ent) [ L. *lumen*, light ]. Emission of light from a body at room temperature.

**luminiferous** (lu'mĭ-nif'er-us) [ L. *lumen*, light, + *fero*, to carry. FER- ]. Producing or conveying light.

**luminophore** (lu'mĭ-no-fōr) [ L. *lumen*, light, + G. *phoros*, bearing ]. An atom or atomic grouping which, when present in an organic compound, increases its ability to luminesce.

**luminous** (lu'mĭ-nus) [ L. *lumen*, light ]. Emitting light, with or without accompanying heat.

**lumirhodopsin** (lu'mĭ-ro-dop'sin). An intermediate between rhodopsin and opsin plus *trans*-retinal during bleaching of rhodopsin by light.

**lumisterol** (lu-mis'ter-ol). Sterol X; $9\beta,10\alpha$-ergosta-5,7,22-trien-3$\beta$-ol (for structure of ergostane, see steroids); an irradiation product of ergosterol which has apparently no antirachitic action. It differs from ergosterol in configuration of methyl group at C-10. See also vitamin $D_1$.

**lumpectomy.** Tylectomy.

**"lumpers."** Those who classify diseases into a few large groups according to similarities, rather than into many small groups because of differences ("splitters").

**lu'nacy** [ L. *luna*, moon ]. 1. Formerly, a form of insanity characterized by alternating lucid and insane periods, believed to be influenced by phases of the moon. 2. Any form of insanity. 3. Insanity as defined variously by law.

**lu'nar** [ L. *luna*, moon ]. 1. Relating to the moon or to a month. 2. Lunate (1); crescentic; crescent-shaped; semilunar; resembling the moon, especially a half moon. 3. Relating to silver (the moon was the symbol of silver in alchemy).

**luna're.** *Os* lunatum.

**lu'nate.** 1. Lunar (2); crescent-shaped. 2. Relating to the lunate bone (os lunatum).

**lu'natic** [ L. *luna*, moon ]. An obsolete term for a mentally ill person.

**lunatomalacia** (lu-na'to-mă-la'shĭ-ah). Kienböck's *disease*.

**luna'tus** [ L. ] [ NA ]. Semilunar; crescent-shaped; having the shape of a half moon.

**lung** [ A.S. *lungen* ]. One of a pair of viscera occupying the cavity of the thorax, the organs of respiration in which aeration of the blood takes place. As a rule, the right l. is slightly larger than the left and is divided into three lobes (an upper, a middle, and a lower or basal), while the left has but two lobes (an upper and a basal). Each l. is irregularly conical in shape, presenting a blunt upper extremity (the apex), a concave base following the curve of the diaphragm, an outer convex surface (facies costalis), an inner or mediastinal surface (facies mediastinalis), a thin and sharp anterior border (margo anterior), and a thick and rounded posterior border (margo posterior).

   **bird-breeder's l.,** bird-fancier's l.; extrinsic allergic alveolitis caused by inhalation of particulate avian emanations; sometimes specified by avian species, *e.g.*, pigeon-breeder's l., budgerigan-breeder's l.

   **bird-fancier's l.,** bird-breeder's l.

   **black l.,** a form of pneumoconiosis common in coal miners; characterized by deposit of carbon particles in the lung.

   **butterfly l.,** hemorrhagic markings appearing on an animal's l. after inoculation with *Leptospira icterohaemorrhagiae.*

   **cardiac l.,** engorged l. due to mitral stenosis or a failing left ventricle.

   **collier's l.,** anthracosis.

   **farmer's l.,** thresher's l.; extrinsic allergic alveolitis caused by inhalation of spores of the mold *Thermopolyspora polyspora* as a result of disturbing moldy hay.

   **fibroid l.,** a l. that is the seat of chronic interstitial pneumonia.

   **fluid l.,** edema of the l.

   **honeycomb l.,** the radiological and gross appearance of the l.'s resulting from diffuse fibrosis and cystic dilation of bronchioles; of unknown cause or a sequel of several diseases, including eosinophilic granuloma and sarcoidosis.

   **iron l.,** Drinker *respirator.*

   **malt-worker's l.,** extrinsic allergic alveolitis caused by

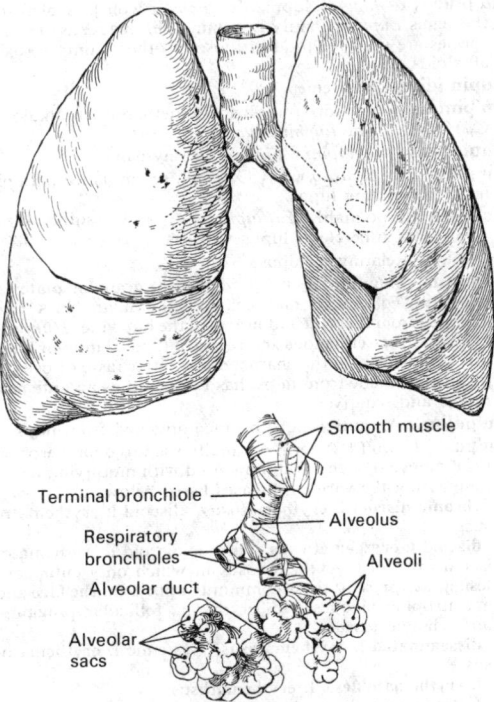

Smooth muscle

Terminal bronchiole

Respiratory bronchioles

Alveolar duct

Alveolar sacs

Alveolus

Alveoli

**Lungs and Terminal Respiratory Units of Bronchial Tree**

inhalation of spores of *Aspergillus clavatus* from contaminated barley during the manufacture of beer.

   **mason's l.,** silicosis occurring in stone masons.

   **miner's l.,** anthracosis.

   **Momsen l.,** a rebreathing bag system equipped with a $CO_2$-absorber and a pressure-relief valve; developed about 1930 for escape from sunken submarines.

   **mushroom-worker's l.,** extrinsic allergic alveolitis caused by inhalation of spores of the mold *Thermopolyspora polyspora* or *Micromonospora vulgaris* from contaminated mushrooms under cultivation.

   **postperfusion l.,** a condition in which small areas of atelectasis with pulmonary arteriovenous shunting develop in patients who have undergone cardiac surgery involving the use of an extracorporeal circulation.

   **quiet l.,** the collapse of a lung during thoracic operations to facilitate surgical procedure by absence of movement.

   **thresher's l.,** farmer's l.

   **trench l.,** a condition marked by paroxysmal attacks of rapid breathing, but without any signs of organic disease.

   **ure'mic l.,** perihilar edema of the l. associated with renal failure and hypertension; the peripheral parts of the l. remain clear.

   **welder's l.,** relatively benign form of pneumoconiosis resulting from deposition of fine metallic particles in the lung; associated with welding.

   **wet l.,** the l. in pulmonary edema.

**lung'motor.** A device similar to the pulmotor, used to pump air or a mixture of air and oxygen into the lungs in cases of asphyxia.

**lung'worms.** Nematodes that inhabit the air passages of animals, chiefly in the family Metastrongylidae (or Protostrongylidae). See *Dictyocaulus, Metastrongylus, Protostrongylus, Muellerius, Aeleurostrongylus,* and *Crenosoma.*

**lunula,** pl. **lu'nulae** (lu'nu-lah) [ L. dim. of *luna*, moon ] [ NA ]. The pale arched area at the proximal portion of the nail plate; the half moon. See fig. under unguis.

   **l. val'vulae semiluna'ris** [ NA ], l. of the semilunar valve; the free border of a semilunar valve at each side of the nodulus valvulae semilunaris or corpora Arantii.

**lu'piform.** Lupoid.

**lu'pine** [ L. *lupinus,* lupine, fr. *lupus,* a wolf ]. A plant of the genus *Lupinus* (family Leguminosae); the seeds of some species are used for fodder; those of others contain toxic alkaloids.

**lupin'idine.** Sparteine.

**lu'pinine.** Octahydroquinolizine-1-methanol; an alkaloid, $C_{10}H_{19}NO$, from *Lupinus luteus.*

**lupino'sis** [ L. *lupinus,* lupine ]. Lathyrism.

**lu'poid** [ L. *lupus, q.v.,* + G. *eidos,* resemblance ]. Lupiform; resembling lupus.

**lupoma** (lu-po'mah) [ L. *lupus, q.v.,* + G. suffix *-oma,* tumor ]. A tubercle of lupus vulgaris.

**lu'pous.** Relating to lupus.

**lu'pulin.** Humulin; a sticky, yellowish, granular material consisting of entire multicellular glandular hairs (trichomes) from the fruit and bracts of the hop vine, *Humulus lupulus;* the essential oils and resins of these glandular hairs are responsible for the characteristic bitter taste of beer or medicinals made from hops; has been used as an antispasmodic and sedative.

**lu'pulon.** An antibiotic substance obtained from hops.

**lu'pus** [ L. wolf ]. A term originally used to depict erosion (as if gnawed) of the skin, now used with modifying terms designating the various diseases listed below.

   **chronic discoid l. erythematosus,** discoid l. erythematosus.

   **discoid l. erythemato'sus,** chronic discoid l. erythematosus; a form of l. erythematosus in which only cutaneous lesions are present; these commonly appear on the face and are atrophic plaques with erythema, follicular plugging, and telangiectasia.

   **disseminated l. erythematosus,** systemic l. erythematosus.

   **l. erythemato'des,** l. erythematosus.

   **l. erythemato'sus,** l. erythematodes; l. superficialis; ulerythema centrifugum; Biett's disease; Cazenave's disease; erythema centrifugum; a systemic illness which may be chronic (characterized by skin lesions alone), subacute (characterized by skin lesions that are more disseminate and present more acute features both clinically and histologically than those seen in the chronic discoid phase), or systemic or disseminated (in which the L.E. cell test may be positive and in which there is almost always involvement of vital structures. See also discoid l. erythematosus and systemic l. erythematosus.

   **l. erythemato'sus profun'dus,** l. erythematosus affecting the deep corium and giving rise to deep-seated, firm, rubbery nodules, usually of the face.

   **l. hypertroph'icus,** l. tumidus; a form of l. vulgaris in which the tubercles are grouped into prominent nodules.

   **l. livido,** persistent cyanotic lesions on the extremities, associated with the cutaneous manifestations of Raynaud's disease.

   **l. lymphat'icus,** *lymphangioma* circumscriptum.

   **l. milia'ris dissemina'tus fa'ciei,** a millet-like papular eruption of the face, associated with a positive anergy to tuberculin and (histopathologically) to tuberculoid structure.

   **l. mu'tilans,** cutaneous tuberculosis with extensive destruction of tissue, *e.g.,* amputation of fingers; or erosion of the skin or cartilage of the nose.

   **l. papillomato'sus,** *tuberculosis* cutis verrucosa.

   **l. per'nio,** sarcoid lesions involving ears and hands. The lesions resemble those of frostbite.

   **l. psori'asis,** a form of l. vulgaris in which there is a formation of scales simulating psoriasis.

   **l. sclero'sus,** a permanent thickening of the skin due to excessive connective tissue formation in l. vulgaris lesions.

   **l. seba'ceus,** l. erythematosus with lesions on the face in butterfly areas.

   **l. serpigino'sus,** a cutaneous tuberculous lesion that spreads peripherally; it heals with scar formation as it spreads.

   **l. superficia'lis,** l. erythematosus.

   **systemic l. erythematosus,** disseminated l. erythematosus; an inflammatory connective tissue disease with variable features, frequently including fever, weakness and fatigability, joint pains or arthritis resembling rheumatoid arthritis, erythematous skin lesions on the face, neck, or upper extremities, lymphadenopathy, pleurisy or pericardi-

tis, glomerular lesions, anemia, hyperglobulinemia, and a positive L.E. cell test.

   **l. tuberculosus,** l. vulgaris.

   **l. tu'midus,** l. hypertrophicus.

   **l. verruco'sus,** *tuberculosis* cutis verrucosa.

   **l. vulga'ris,** tuberculosis cutis luposa; l. tuberculosus; cutaneous tuberculosis with characteristic nodular lesions on the face, particularly about the nose and ears.

   **l. vulga'ris erythematoi'des,** Leloir's disease; a form of cutaneous tuberculosis having a superficial resemblance to l. erythematosus.

   **Willan's l.,** l. vulgaris, especially of the cheek.

**lura** (lu'rah) [ L. the mouth of a bottle ]. The contracted termination of the infundibulum of the brain.

**lu'ral.** Pertaining to the lura.

**Luria,** Salvador, U. S. bacteriologist, *1912. Nobel laureate 1969, with Max Delbrück and Alfred Hershey for their contributions to the understanding of the molecular biology of bacteriophage.

**lu'ridine.** Obsolete term for choline.

**Luschka,** Hubert, German anatomist, 1820–1875. See L.'s *bursa, cartilage, ducts, foramen, gland,* cystic *glands, ligament, sinus, tonsil.*

**lust** [ A.S. pleasure, desire ]. Sexual desire, especially of a very intense or self-indulgent character.

**Lust's sign.** See under sign.

**lu'sus natu'rae** [ L. a sport of nature ]. A monstrosity or conspicuous congenital abnormality.

**lute** (lūt) [ L. *lutum,* mud ]. To seal or fasten with wax or cement.

**luteal** (lu'te-al) [ L. *luteus,* saffron-yellow ]. Relating to the corpus luteum; l. cells, l. hormone, etc.

**lutein** (lu'te-in) [ L. *luteus,* saffron-yellow ]. 1. The yellow pigment in the corpus luteum, in the yolk of eggs, or any lipochrome. 2. Xanthophyll. 3. Dried, powdered corpora lutea of hog, formerly used as progesterone source.

**luteinization** (lu'te-in'ĭ-za'shun). The transformation of the mature ovarian follicle and its theca interna into a corpus luteum after ovulation; the formation of luteal tissue.

**luteinize** (lu'te-ĭ-nīz). To form luteal tissue.

**luteinoma** (lu'te-ĭ-no'mah). Luteoma.

**Lutembacher** (loo'tem-bah-shay), René, French physician, *1884. See L.'s *syndrome.*

**luteogenic** (lu'te-o-jen'ik). Leuteinizing; inducing the production or growth of corpora lutea.

**lu'teohor'mone.** Progesterone.

**lu'teol, lu'teole.** Xanthophyll.

**luteolin** (lu'te-o'lin). 3',4',5,7-Tetrahydroflavone.

**luteol'ysin.** A postulated secretory product of the uterine endometrium that causes degeneration of corpora lutea, either by a direct action or by stimulating luteolytic secretions from the anterior pituitary gland.

**luteolysis** (lu'te-ol'ĭ-sis). The degeneration or destruction of ovarian luteinized tissue.

**luteoma** (lu-te-o'mah). Luteinoma; an ovarian tumor of granulosa or theca cell origin in which luteinization has occurred, producing progesterone effects on the uterine mucosa.

   **pregnancy l.,** a benign lutein cell tumor of the ovary.

**luteosterone** (lu-te-os'ter-ōn). A steroid occurring in corpus luteum. Obscure and obsolete designation.

**luteotropic, luteotrophic** (lu'te-o-trop'ik, -trof'ik). Having a stimulating action on the development and function of the corpus luteum.

**luteotropin, luteotrophin** (lu'te-o-tro'pin, -tro'fin). Luteotropic *hormone.*

**lutetium, lutecium** (lu-te'shĭ-um) [ L. *Lutetia,* Paris ]. Cassiopeium; a rare element, symbol Lu, atomic no. 71, atomic weight 174.99.

**lute'us** [ L. ] [ NA ]. Luteal.

**Lutheran blood group.** See appendix 2, Blood Groups.

**lu'tutrin.** LUTREXIN; water-soluble, protein-like fraction extracted from the corpus luteum of sows' ovaries; it resembles relaxin; it causes uterine relaxation and is used in dysmenorrhea.

**Lutz,** A. See L.-Splendore-Almeida *disease.*

**lux** [ L. light ]. Meter-candle; candle-meter; a unit of light or illumination; the reception of a luminous flux of 1 lumen per sq. meter of surface.

**luxa′tio** [ L. *luxo,* pp. *-atus,* to dislocate ]. Luxation; dislocation.
  **l. erec′ta,** subglenoid dislocation of the head of the humerus; the arm is raised and abducted and cannot be lowered.
  **l. imperfec′ta,** sprain.
  **l. perinea′lis,** a condition in which the head of the femur is dislocated to the perineum.

**luxation** (luks-a′shun) [ L. *luxatio* ]. 1. Dislocation. 2. In dentistry, the partial or complete separation of a tooth from its socket.
  **Malgaigne′s l.,** l. of head of radius beneath the annular ligament.

**Luxol fast blue.** A copper phthalocyanin dye used as a stain for myelin in nerve fibers.

**lux′us** [ L. extravagance, luxury ]. Excess of any sort.

**Luys** (lü-ēs′), Georges, Paris surgeon, *1870. See L.'s *separator.*

**Luys** (lü-ēs′), Jules B., French physician, 1828–1897. See L.'s *body, centre* médian de L., *corpus* luysi, L.'s *nucleus.*

**Lw.** Symbol for lawrencium.

**Lwoff,** André, French molecular biologist, *1902. Nobel laureate, 1965, with Jacques Monod and François Jacob, for their contributions to the understanding of regulation of gene activity in ontogeny.

**ly′ase.** Class name for those enzymes removing groups nonhydrolytically (EC class 4). Prefixes such as "hydro-," "ammonia-," etc., are used to indicate the type of reaction. Decarboxylases are carboxy-lyases. Trivial names for lyases include synthases, decarboxylase, aldolase, dehydratase; *cf.* synthase, synthetase.

**lycanthropy** (li-kan′thro-pĭ) [ G. *lykos,* wolf, + *anthropos,* man ]. The insane delusion that the subject is a wolf, possibly a mental atavism of the werewolf superstition.

**lycoc′tonine.** An alkaloid, $C_{25}H_{41}NO_7$, obtained from *Aconitum lycoctonum,* an exceedingly poisonous species of aconite; also occurs in other species of *Aconitum* and *Delphinium.*

**lycopene** (li′ko-pēn). Red pigment of the tomato that may be considered chemically as the parent substance from which all natural carotenoid pigments are derived. It is an unsaturated hydrocarbon, made up of 8 isoprene units, two of the hydrogenated with 11 conjugated double bonds. See also carotenoids.

**lycopenemia** (li′ko-pe-nĭ′-ah) [ lycopene + G. *haima,* blood ]. A condition in which there is a high concentration of lycopene in the blood, producing carotenoid-like yellowish pigmentation of the skin; found in people who consume excessive amounts of tomatoes or tomato juice.

**Lycoperdon** (li′ko-per′don) [ G. *lykos,* wolf, + *perdesthai,* to break wind ]. Puffball; a genus of fungi (family Lycoperdaceae) some species have been used medicinally; the spores of *L. bovista* ( *L. gemmatum, L. caelatum*) and of *L. pyriforme* may produce a persisting pneumonitis, lycoperdonosis.

**lycoperdonosis** (li′ko-per-don-o′sis). A persisting pneumonitis following inhalation of spores of the puffballs *Lycoperdon pyriforme* and *L. bovista;* nasal inhalation of puffball spores is a folk medicine treatment for epistaxis.

**lycopodium** (li′ko-po′dĭ-um) [ G. *lykos,* wolf, + *pous,* foot ]. Vegetable sulfur; club moss; the spores of *Lycopodium clavatum* (family Lycopodiaceae) and other species of *L.;* a yellow, tasteless, and odorless powder. Used as a dusting powder and in pharmacy to prevent the agglutination of pills in a box.

**lycopus** (li′ko-pus) [ G. *lykos,* wolf, + *pous,* foot ]. Bugleweed; the whole plant *Lycopus virginicus* (family Labiatae), a herb of eastern and central North America; hemostatic and astringent; has been used in diarrhea.
  **L. europae′us,** the bitter bugleweed of Europe. Has been used as astringent and tonic.

**lycorexia** (li′ko-rek′sĭ-ah) [ G. *lykos,* wolf, + *orexis,* appetite ]. Bulimia.

**ly′corine.** Narcissine.

**ly′dimy′cin** (USAN). An antibiotic produced by *Streptomyces lydicus;* possesses antifungal activity.

**lye** (li) [ A.S. *leáh* ]. Lixivium; the liquid obtained by leaching wood ashes; see potassium hydroxide and sodium hydroxide.

**Lyell,** A. See L.'s *disease.*

**ly′gophil′ia** [ G. *lygē,* twilight, + *phileō,* to love ]. Abnormal preference for dark places.

**lying-in.** 1. Confinement; labor; childbirth. 2. Relating to childbirth; obstetrical.

**lymecycline.** MUCOMYCIN; tetracycline-methylene lysine; antimicrobial agent.

**Lymnaea** (lim-ne′ah) [ G. *limnē,* marsh ]. A genus of snails, species of which are invertebrate hosts for the giant liver fluke, *Fasciola gigantica,* and other trematodes.

**lymph-.** See lympho-.

**lymph** (limf) [ L. *lympha,* clear spring water ]. Lympha [ NA ]; a clear, transparent, sometimes faintly yellow and slightly opalescent fluid that is collected from the tissues throughout the body, flows in the lymphatic vessels (through the lymph nodes), and is eventually added to the venous blood circulation. L. consists of a clear liquid portion, varying numbers of white blood cells (chiefly lymphocytes), and a few red blood cells.
  **aplas′tic l.,** 1. containing a relatively large number of leukocytes, but comparatively little fibrinogen; such l. does not form a good clot and manifests only slight tendency to become organized. Termed also corpuscular l.
  **blood l.,** l. exuded from the blood vessels and not derived from the fluid in the tissue spaces.
  **corpus′cular l.,** aplastic l.
  **croupous l.,** a form of inflammatory l. with an unusually large content of fibrinogen; as a result of the fibrin that is formed in relatively dense mats, a pseudomembrane is likely to be produced.
  **euplas′tic l.,** l. that contains relatively few leukocytes, but a comparatively high concentration of fibrinogen; such l. clots fairly well and tends to become organized with fibrous tissue.
  **fibrinous l.,** euplastic l. or croupous l.
  **humanized l.,** vaccine l. derived from vaccinia lesions in the skin of human beings.
  **inflammatory l.,** plastic l.; a faintly yellow, usually coagulable fluid ( *i.e.,* euplastic l.) that collects on the surface of an acutely inflamed membrane or cutaneous wound.
  **intercellular l.,** the fluid in the potential spaces between cells in the various organs and tissues.
  **intravascular l.,** l. within the lymphatic vessels, in contrast to intercellular l. and l. that has exuded from the vessels.
  **Koch's l.,** tuberculin.
  **plastic l.,** inflammatory l.
  **tissue l.,** true l., *i.e.,* l. derived chiefly from fluid in tissue spaces (in contrast to blood l.).
  **vaccine l., vaccinia l.,** that collected from the vesicles of vaccinia infection, and used for active immunization against smallpox.

**lympha** (lim′fah) [ L. ] [ NA ]. Lymph.

**lymphaden** (limb′ā-den) [ lymph- + G. *adēn,* gland ]. Lymph node.

**lymphaden-.** See lymphadeno-.

**lymphadenectasia** (lim-fad′ē-nek-ta′zĭ-ah). Enlargement of a lymph node that results from an increased amount of lymph and acute hyperplasia, in contrast to that occurring in such lesions as malignant lymphoma, granulomatous inflammation, and so on.

**lymphadenectasis** (lim-fad′ē-nek′tă-sis) [ lymphadeno- + G. *ektasis,* a stretching ]. Lymphadenectasia.

**lymphadenectomy** (lim-fad′ē-nek′to-mī) [ lymphadeno- + G. *ektomē,* excision ]. Excision of lymph nodes.

**lymphadenia** (lim′fă-de′nĭ-ah) [ lymphadeno- + G. suffix *-ia,* condition ]. Persistent or chronic hyperplasia of lymph nodes, thereby resulting in hypertrophy (in contrast to lymphadenectasia).
  **l. os′sea,** old term for multiple myeloma.

**lymphadenism** (lim-fad′ē-nizm). 1. Any condition characterized by lymphadenia. 2. The signs and symptoms associated with lymphadenia or lymphadenoma.

**lymphadenitis** (lim'fad-ĕ-ni'tis) [ lymphadeno- + G. suffix -itis, inflammation ]. Inflammation of a lymph node or lymph nodes.

**caseous l.,** a specific disease of sheep, characterized by slowly progressing caseation necrosis of the lymph nodes, particularly those of the thorax. It is caused by a bacterium, *Corynebacterium pseudotuberculosis.*

**nonbacterial regional l.,** cat-scratch *disease.*

**paracaseous l.,** paratuberculous l.

**paratuber'culous l.,** paracaseous l.; chronic inflammation of certain lymph nodes, apparently not specifically tuberculous (*i.e.,* tubercle bacilli are not demonstrable), but associated with proved tuberculous inflammation in another part or organ of the body.

**lymphadeno-, lymphaden-** (lim-fad'ĕ-no-) [ L. *lympha,* spring water (lymph), + G. *adēn,* gland ]. Combining forms relating to the lymph nodes.

**lymphadenography** (lim'fad-ĕ-nog'ră-fī) [ lymphadeno- + G. *graphō,* to write ]. X-ray after 5 cc. of opaque (iodized) oil are injected into center of an enlarged lymph node.

**lymphadenoid** (lim-fad'ĕ-noyd) [ lymphadeno- + G. *eidos,* resemblance ]. Relating to, or resembling, or derived from a lymph node.

**lymphadenoma** (lim-fad'ĕ-no'mah) [ lymphadeno- + G. suffix -oma, tumor ]. 1. An enlarged lymph node. 2. An infrequently used, undesirable term for Hodgkin's disease.

**lymphadenomatosis** (lim-fad'ĕ-no-mă-to'sis). A condition characterized by the presence of several to numerous, enlarged lymph nodes, as in lymphosarcoma, Hodgkin's disease, and the like.

**lymphadenomatous** (lim-fad'ĕ-no'mă-tus). Pertaining to or having the features of lymphadenoma.

**lymphadenopathy** (lim-fad'ĕ-nop'ă-thī) [ lymphadeno- + G. *pathos,* suffering ]. Any disease process affecting a lymph node or lymph nodes.

**dermatopathic l.,** lipomelanic reticulosis; enlargement of lymph nodes, with proliferation of histiocytes and macrophages containing fat or melanin; secondary to various forms of dermatitis, particularly with pruritus or exfoliation.

**lymphadenosis** (lim-fad'ĕ-no'sis) [ lymphadeno- + G. suffix -osis, condition ]. The basic, underlying proliferative process that results in enlargement of lymph nodes, as in lymphocytic leukemia, certain inflammations, and so on.

**benign l.,** infectious *mononucleosis.*

**malignant l.,** malignant lymphoma.

**lymphadenovarix** (lim-fad'ĕ-no-va'riks) [ lymphadeno- + L. *varix, q.v.* ]. Varicose deformity of a lymph node associated with lymphangiectasis.

**lymphagogue** (limf'ă-gog) [ lymph + G. *agōgos,* drawing forth ]. An agent that increases the formation and flow of lymph.

**lymphangeitis** (lim-fan'je-i'tis). Lymphangitis.

**lymphangi-.** See lymphangio-.

**lymphangial** (lim-fan'jī-al). Relating to a lymphatic vessel.

**lymphangiectasis, lymphangiectasia** (lim-fan'jī-ek'tă-sis, -ek-ta'zī-ah) [ lymphangio- + G. *ektasis,* a stretching ]. Lymphectasia; telangiectasia lymphatica; dilation of the lymphatic vessels; the basic process that may result in the formation of a lymphangioma.

**cavernous l.,** *lymphangioma* cavernosum.

**lymphangiectatic** (lim-fan'jī-ek-tat'ik). Relating to or characterized by lymphangiectasis.

**lymphangiectodes** (lim-fan'jī-ek-to'dēz) [ lymphangio- + G. *ektasis,* a stretching, + *eidos,* appearance ]. *Lymphangioma* circumscriptum.

**lymphangiectomy** (lim-fan'jī-ek'to-mī) [ lymphangio- + G. *ektomē,* excision ]. Excision of a lymph channel.

**lymphangiitis** (lim-fan'jī-i'tis). Lymphangitis.

**lymphangio-, lymphangi-** (lim-fan'jī-o-) [ L. *lympha,* lymph, + G. *angeion,* vessel ]. Combining forms relating to the lymphatic vessels.

**lymphangioendothelioma** (lim-fan'jī-o-en'do-the-lī-o'-mah). Lymphendothelioma; a neoplasm consisting of irregular groups or small masses of endothelial cells, as well as congeries of tubate structures that are thought to be derived from lymphatic vessels and are lined with endothelial cells; such neoplasms are similar to a hemangi-oendothelioma, except that blood vessels are conspicuous in the latter.

**lymphangiography** (lim-fan'jī-og'ră-fī) [ lymphangio- + G. *graphō,* to write ]. Visualization of lymph vessels by x-ray following the injection of a contrast medium.

**lymphangiology** (lim-fan'jī-ol'o-jī) [ lymphangio- + G. *logos,* study ]. The branch of medical science that pertains to the lymphatic system.

**lymphangioma** (lim-fan'jī-o'mah) [ lymphangio- + G. suffix -oma, tumor ]. A fairly well circumscribed nodule or mass of lymphatic vessels or channels that vary in size, are frequently greatly dilated, and are lined with normal endothelial cells; lymphoid tissue is usually present in the peripheral portions of the lesions, but may not be observed unless several sections are examined. Similarly to hemangiomas, l.'s are present at birth, or shortly thereafter, and probably represent anomalous development of lymphatic vessels (rather than true neoplasms). L.'s occur most frequently in the neck and axilla, but may also develop in the arm, inguen, mesentery, retroperitoneum, and other sites.

**l. capilla're varico'sum,** l. circumscriptum.

**l. caverno'sum,** cavernous lymphangiectasia; cavernoma lymphaticum; a condition of conspicuous dilation of lymphatic vessels in a fairly circumscribed region, frequently with the formation of cavities or "lakes" filled with lymph.

**l. circumscrip'tum,** l. superficium simplex; l. capillare varicosum; lupus lymphaticus; a congenital nevoid lesion consisting of a circumscribed group of tense lymph vesicles. The surface may be verrucous due to a thickened keratin layer over the vesicles.

**l. cys'ticum,** cystic lymphangiectasia; a condition characterized by a fairly well circumscribed group of several or numerous, cystlike, dilated vessels or spaces lined with endothelium and filled with lymph.

**l. simplex,** simple lymphangiectasia; a circumbscribed region or focus of several to numerous lymphatic vessels that are moderately dilated.

**l. superfic'ium simplex,** l. circumscriptum.

**l. tubero'sum multiplex,** a cutaneous lesion characterized by multiple, slightly red, cystlike nodules (located chiefly on the trunk), resulting from fairly large lymphatic vessels and spaces, and groups of proliferating endothelial cells; the lesion has some gross resemblance to spiradenoma, except for the characteristic location.

**l. xanthelasmoid'eum,** a capillary l. with colloid degeneration of the elastic tissues of the skin, characterized by yellow-brown or gray-brown plaques that may be only slightly raised above the surface of the skin.

**lymphangiomatous** (lim-fan'jī-o'mă-tus). Pertaining to, characterized by, or containing a lymphangioma (or lymphangiomas).

**lymphangion** (lim-fan'jī-on) [ L. *lympha,* lymph, + G. *angeion,* vessel ]. A lymphatic vessel; see vas lymphaticum.

**lymphangiophlebitis** (lim-fan'jī-o-flē-bi'tis). Inflammation of the lymphatic vessels and veins.

**lymphangioplasty** (lim-fan'jī-o-plas'tī) [ lymphangio- + G. *plassō,* to form ]. The formation of artificial lymphatics by the introduction of buried silk threads, with the object of draining the tissues (*e.g.,* of the "brawny arm" in cases of mammary carcinoma) when the lymphatic vessels are obliterated.

**lymphangiosarcoma** (lim-fan'jī-o-sar-ko'mah). A malignant neoplasm derived from vascular tissue, *i.e.,* an angiosarcoma, in which the neoplastic cells originate from the endothelial cells of lymphatic vessels.

**lymphangiotomy** (lim-fan'jī-ot'o-mī) [ lymphangio- + G. *tomē,* incision ]. Incision of lymphatic vessels.

**lymphangitis** (lim'fan-ji'tis) [ lymphangio- + G. suffix -itis, inflammation ]. Inflammation of the lymphatic vessels.

**l. carcinomatosa,** extensive lymphatic permeation by tumor cells, with surrounding fibrosis, producing visible or palpable cords, especially in pleura or skin overlying a carcinoma.

**l. epizootica** (ep-ī-zo-ot'ī-kah), a l. involving the lymph channels of the skin of the legs and chest of the horse.

Lesions are rarely found elsewhere. The causative agent is a yeastlike organism, *Zymonema farciminosum.*

**lymphatic** (lim-fat′ik) [ L. *lymphaticus,* frenzied; Mod. L. use, of or for lymph ]. 1. Pertaining to lymph, a vascular channel that transports lymph, or a lymph node. 2. Sometimes pertaining to a sluggish or phlegmatic characteristic.

    **afferent l.'s,** the l. vessels that enter the nodes.
    **efferent l.'s,** the l. vessels that leave the lymph nodes.

**lymphaticostomy** (lim-fat-ĭ-kos′to-mĭ) [ lymphatic + G. *stoma,* mouth ]. Making an opening into a lymphatic duct.

**lymphat′icus** [ L. ] [ NA ]. Lymphatic.

**lymphatism** (lim′fă-tizm). 1. A condition in which there is an excess in the lymphoid or tonsillar structures. 2. The lymphatic temperament. 3. A condition characterized by sluggishness in the vital processes.

**lymphatitis** (lim-fă-ti′tis) [ lymphatic + G. suffix *-itis,* inflammation ]. Inflammation of the lymphatic vessels or lymph nodes.

**lymphatology** (lim′fă-tol′o-jĭ) [ lymphatic + G. *logos,* study ]. The study of the lymphatic system.

**lymphatolysis** (lim′fă-tol′ĭ-sis) [ lymphatic + G. *lysis,* dissolution ]. Destruction of the lymphatic vessels or lymphoid tissue, or both.

**lymphatolytic** (lim′fă-to-lit′ik). Pertaining to or characterized by lymphatolysis.

**lymphectasia** (lim-fek-ta′zĭ-ah) [ lymph + G. *ektasis,* a stretching ]. Lymphangiectasis.

**lymphedema** (limf′e-de′mah) [ lymph + G. *oidēma,* a swelling ]. Swelling (especially in subcutaneous tissues) as a result of obstruction of lymphatic vessels or lymph nodes and the accumulation of large amounts of lymph in the affected region.

    **congenital l.,** see hereditary l.
    **hereditary l.,** trophedema; permanent pitting edema usually confined to the lower extremities; two types, congenital (Milroy's or Nonne-Milroy disease), or with onset at about the age of puberty (Meige's disease); autosomal dominant inheritance.
    **l. precox,** primary l.
    **primary l.,** a form observed chiefly in young women and girls, characterized by diffuse swelling of the lower extremities.

**lymphemia** (lim-fe′mĭ-ah) [ lymph(ocyte) + G. *haima,* blood ]. The presence of unusually large numbers of lymphocytes or their precursors, or both, in the circulating blood.

**lymphendothelioma** (limf-en′do-the′lĭ-o′mah). Lymphangioendothelioma.

**lymphenteritis** (lim-fen′ter-i′tis) [ lymph + G. *enteron,* intestine, + suffix *-itis,* inflammation ]. Inflammation of the peritoneal covering of the intestine.

**lympherythrocyte** (limf′e-rith′ro-sit). Anerythrocyte.

**lymphization** (lim′fĭ-za′shun). The formation of lymph.

**lymphnoditis** (limf′no-di′tis). Lymphadenitis.

**lympho-, lymph-** (lim′fo-) [ L. *lympha,* lymph ]. Combining forms relating to lymph.

**lymphoadenoma** (lim′fo-ad′ĕ-no′mah). Lymphadenoma.

**lymphoblast** (lim′fo-blast) [ lympho- + G. *blastos,* germ ]. A young, immature cell that matures into a lymphocyte; l.'s are characterized by (1) a more abundant cytoplasm, (2) a nucleus in which the chromatin is finer than that in a lymphocyte (but coarser than that in the myeloblast), and (3) one or two rather prominent nucleoli.

**lymphoblas′tic.** Pertaining to the production of lymphocytes.

**lymphoblastoma** (lim-fo-blas-to′mah) [ lymphoblast + G. suffix *-oma,* tumor ]. A form of malignant lymphoma in which the chief cells are lymphoblasts, the term is sometimes used synonymously with lymphosarcoma.

    **giant follicular l.,** Brill-Symmers disease; follicular lymphoma; a slowly progressive l., frequently limited for a considerable time to a single group of lymph nodes, in which the normal structure is replaced by follicular aggregates of lymphoblasts a millimeter or two in diameter, separated by lymphocytes; giant follicular l. eventually shows widespread involvement of the lymph nodes and spleen and frequent transformation to lymphosarcoma.

**lymphoblastomid** (lim′fo-blas-to′mid) [ lymphoblastoma + suffix *-id* (1), *q. v.* ]. Cutaneous lesion signifying presence of lymphoblastoma.

**lymphoblastosis** (lim-fo-blas-to′sis) [ lymphoblast + G. suffix *-osis,* condition ]. The presence of lymphoblasts in the peripheral blood; sometimes used as a synonym for acute lymphocytic leukemia.

**lymphocele** (lim′fo-sēl) [ lympho- + G. *kēlē,* tumor ]. Lymphocyst; a cystic mass that contains lymph.

**lymphocerastism** (lim-fo-sĕr′as-tizm) [ lympho- + G. *kerastos,* mixed, mingled. CERAS- ]. The process of formation of cells in the lymphocytic series.

**lym′phocine′sia.** Lymphokinesis.

**lymphocyst** (lim′fo-sist) [ lympho- + G. *kystis,* bladder ]. Lymphocele.

**lymphocyte** (lim′fo-sīt) [ lympho- + G. *kytos,* call ]. Lymph cell; lymphoid cell; lympholeukocyte; a white blood cell formed in lymphoid tissue throughout the body, *e.g.,* lymph nodes, spleen, thymus, tonsils, Peyer's patches, and sometimes in bone marrow. L.'s are generally small (7 to 8 μ), but larger forms are frequent (10 to 20 μ); with Wright's (or a similar) stain, the nucleus is deeply colored (purple-blue), and is composed of dense aggregates of chromatin within a sharply defined nuclear membrane; the nucleus is usually round, but may be slightly indented, and is eccentrically situated within a relatively small amount of light blue cytoplasm that ordinarily contains no granules. On the other hand, especially in the larger forms, the cytoplasm may be fairly abundant and includes several, bright red-violet, fine granules; in contrast to granules of the myeloid series of cells, those in l.'s do not yield a positive oxidase or peroxidase reaction. In normal adult persons, l.'s comprise approximately 22 to 28 per cent of the total number of leukocytes in the circulating blood. See color plate 15.

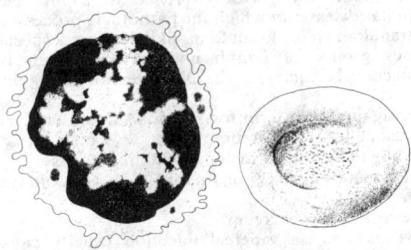

**Human Lymphocyte (*left*)**
With red blood cell, to show comparative sizes

    **B l.,** B cell (2); an immunologically important l. that is not thymus-dependent, is of short life, and resembles the bursa-derived l. of birds in that it is responsible for the production of immunoglobulins and does not play a role in cell-mediated sensitivity (immunity); areas in man and other mammals, analogous to the bursa of Fabricius, have not been identified but it is assumed that they exist. See also T l.

    **Rieder's l.,** an abnormal form of l. that has a greatly indented (or lobed), slightly twisted nucleus; such cells are usually observed in certain examples of chronic lymphocytic leukemia.

    **T l.,** T cell; a thymocyte-derived l. of immunological importance; it is of long life (months to years), is responsible for the delayed-type (cell-mediated) sensitivity, and, in the presence of transforming agents (mitogens), differentiates and divides. See also B l.

    **transformed l.,** see lymphocyte *transformation.*

**lymphocythemia** (lim′fo-si-the′mĭ-ah). Lymphocytosis.

**lymphocytic** (lim′fo-sit′ik). Pertaining to or characterized by lymphocytes.

**lymphocytoblast** (lim-fo-si′to-blast) [ lymphocyte, + G. *blastos,* germ ]. Lymphoblast.

**lymphocytoma** (lim'fo-si-to'mah) [ lymphocyte + G. suffix -oma, tumor ]. A circumscribed nodule or mass of mature lymphocytes, grossly resembling a neoplasm.

**lymphocytopenia** (lim'fo-si-to-pe'nĭ-ah). Lymphopenia.

**lymphocytopoiesis** (lim'fo-si-to-poy-e'sis) [ lymphocyte + G. poiēsis, a making ]. The formation of lymphocytes.

**lymphocytosis** (lim'fo-si-to'sis). Lymphocytic leukocytosis; achroacytosis; lymphocythemia; a form of actual or relative leukocytosis in which there is an increase in the number of lymphocytes.

**Lymphocytozoon** (lim'fo-si-to-zo'on) [ lymphocyte + G. zōon, animal ]. A supposed genus of parasitic ameboid cells found in lymphocytes or uninuclear leukocytes.

    **L. coba'yae,** see Kurloff's *body.*

**lymphoderma** (lim'fo-der'mah) [ lympho- + G. derma, skin ]. A condition resulting from any disease of the cutaneous lymphatic vessels.

    **l. pernicio'sa,** *leukemia cutis.*

**lymphoduct** (lim'fo-dukt) [ lympho- + L. ductus, a leading ]. Lymphatic vessel; *vas* lymphaticum.

**lymphoepithelioma** (lim'fo-ep-ĭ-the-lĭ-o'mah). A poorly differentiated squamous cell carcinoma involving lymphoid tissue in the region of the tonsils and nasopharynx; composed of irregular sheets, or small groups, of neoplastic epithelial cells (squamous or undifferentiated), with a slight to moderate amount of fibrous stroma that contains numerous lymphocytes. L.'s metastasize at an early stage to cervical lymph nodes. Also called Schmincke's tumor.

**lymphogenesis** (lim'fo-gen'ĕ-sis) [ lympho- + G. genesis, production ]. Lymph production.

**lymphogen'ic.** Lymphogenous.

**lymphogenous** (lim-foj'ĕ-nus). 1. Lymphogenic; originating from lymph or the lymphatic system. 2. Producing lymph.

**lymphoglandula** (lim'fo-glan'du'lah). *Nodus* lymphaticus.

**lymphogranuloma** (lim'fo-gran-u-lo'mah). 1. An old, nonspecific term used with reference to a few basically dissimilar diseases in which the pathologic processes result in granulomas or granuloma-like lesions, especially in various groups of lymph nodes (which then become conspicuously enlarged). 2. Old term for Hodgkin's disease.

    **l. benignum,** old term for Boeck's sarcoid (sarcoidosis).

    **l. inguina'le,** l. venereum.

    **l. malignum,** old term for Hodgkin's disease.

    **Schaumann's l.,** old eponym for Boeck's sarcoid (sarcoidosis).

    **venereal l.,** l. venereum.

    **l. vene'reum,** a venereal infection usually caused by *Chlamydia,* and characterized by a transient genital ulcer and inguinal adenopathy in the male; in the female, perirectal nodes are involved and rectal stricture is a common occurrence. Also known by numerous synonyms, including venereal l.; l. inguinale; lymphopathia venereum; inguinal poradenitis; poradenolymphitis; climatic or tropical bubo; Favre-Durand-Nicolas disease; Frei's bubo or disease, Nicolas-Favre disease.

**lymphogranulomatosis** (lim-fo-gran'u-lo-mă-to'sis). Any condition characterized by the occurrence of multiple and widely distributed lymphogranulomas. Note types under lymphogranuloma.

**lymphography** (lim-fog'ră-fi) [ lympho- + graphō, to write ]. The delineation of lymph vessels or nodes by injecting dyes or radiopaque material and taking photographs or x-rays.

**lymphoid** (lim'foyd) [ lympho- + G. eidos, appearance ]. 1. Resembling lymph or lymphatic tissue, or pertaining to the lymphatic system. 2. Adenoid.

**lymphoidectomy** (lim-foy-dek'to-mĭ) [ lymphoid + G. ektomē, excision ]. Excision of lymphoid tissue.

**lymphoidocyte** (lim-foy'do-sīt). A primitive mesenchymal cell believed to be capable of differentiating into all types of lymphoid cells, including lymphocytes, littoral cells, and reticular cells of lymph nodes.

**lymphoidotoxemia** (lim-foy'do-tok-se'mĭ-ah). *Status* lymphaticus.

**lymphokinesis** (lim'fo-kĭ-ne'sis) [ lympho- + G. kinēsis, movement ]. Lymphocinesia. 1. The circulation of lymph

in the lymphatic vessels and through the lymph nodes. 2. The movement of lymph in the semicircular canals of the inner ear.

**lympholeukocyte** (lim'fo-lu'ko-sīt). Lymphocyte.

**lymphology** (lim-fol'o-jĭ) [ lympho- + G. logos, study ]. Lymphangiology.

**lymphoma** (lim-fo'mah) [ lympho- + G. suffix -oma, tumor ]. A general term that includes various, abnormally proliferative, probably neoplastic diseases of the lymphoid tissues, e.g., lymphosarcoma, leukosarcoma, lymphocytic leukemia, Hodgkin's disease, and so on; ordinarily termed malignant l.

    **benign l. of the rectum,** lymphoid polyp; a rectal polyp composed of lymphoid tissue with follicle formation, covered by mucosa.

    **Burkitt's l.,** a malignant l. reported in African children, frequently involving facial bones, ovaries, and abdominal lymph nodes, which are infiltrated by lymphoblasts with scattered, pale macrophages containing nuclear debris. The geographical distribution of Burkitt's l. suggested that it may be transmitted by biting insects and caused by a virus or malarial infection. Occasional cases of l. with similar features have been reported in the United States. See also Epstein-Barr *virus.*

    **follicular l.,** giant follicular *lymphoblastoma.*

**lymphomatoid** (lim-fo'mă-toyd). Resembling a lymphoma.

**lymphomatosis** (lim'fo-mă-to'sis). Any condition characterized by the occurrence of multiple, widely distributed sites of involvement with lymphoma.

    **avian l.,** fowl l.; a group of virus-induced transmissible diseases of chickens and some other birds in which there is lymphoid cell infiltration or formation of lymphomatous tumors in various tissues and organs; the two principal diseases are (1) the avian leukosis-sarcoma virus-induced lymphoid leukosis, involving the bursa fabricii and various visceral organs, and (2) Marek's disease, caused by a herpesvirus and involving primarily the peripheral nerves and gonads and, to a lesser and more variable extent, other visceral organs, skin, muscle, and the eye; the lesion site prompted other names for avian l., such as big liver disease, gray eye, white eye, ocular lymphomatosis, visceral lymphomatosis, neurolymphomatosis gallinarum, fowl paralysis, and range paralysis.

    **fowl l.,** avian l.

    **ocular l.,** see avian l.

    **visceral l.,** see avian l.

**lympho'matous.** Pertaining to or characterized by lymphoma.

**lymphomegaloblast** (lim'fo-meg'ă-lo-blast). A megaloblast that does not contain hemoglobin.

**lymphomonocyte** (lim-fo-mon'o-sīt) [ lympho(cyte) + monocyte ]. A large uninuclear leukocyte.

**lymphomyelocyte** (lim-fo-mi'ĕ-lo-sīt). Myeloblast.

**lymphomyeloma** (lim-fo-mi'ĕ-lo'mah) [ lympho- + G. myelos, marrow, + suffix -oma, tumor ]. A medullary neoplasm that consists of uninuclear, relatively small cells with morphologic features resembling those of lymphocytic forms.

**lymphomyxoma** (lim'fo-mik-so'mah) [ lympho- + G. myxa, mucus, + suffix -oma, tumor ]. A soft nonmalignant neoplasm that contains lymphoid tissue in a matrix of loose, areolar connective tissue.

**lymphonodus,** pl. **lymphono'di** (lim'fo-no'dus) [ lympho- + L. nodus, node ] [ NA ]. *Nodus* lymphaticus.

    **lymphonodi anorecta'les,** anorectal or hemorrhoidal lymph nodes.

    **lymphonodi prelarynge'i,** two or three small lymph nodes in front of the lower portion of the larynx.

    **lymphonodi retropharynge'i,** *nodi* lymphatici retropharyngei.

    **lymphonodi submenta'les,** *nodi* lymphatici submentales.

**lymphopathia** (lim'fo-path'ĭ-ah). Lymphopathy.

    **l. vene'reum,** old term for lymphogranuloma venereum.

**lymphopathy** (lim-fop'ă-thĭ) [ lympho- + G. pathos, suffering ]. Any disease of the lymphatic vessels or lymph nodes.

**lymphopenia** (lim'fo-pe'nĭ-ah) [ lympho- + G. penia, poverty ]. Lymphocytopenia; lymphocytic leukopenia; a reduction, relative or absolute, in the number of lymphocytes in the circulating blood.

**lymphoplasmia** (lim'fo-plaz'mĭ-ah). Absence of hemoglobin in red blood cells.

**lym'phoplas'ty.** Lymphangioplasty.

**lymphopoiesis** (lim-fo-poy-e'sis) [ lympho- + G. *poiēsis,* a making ]. The formation of lymphocytes.

**lymphopoietic** (lim'fo-poy-et'ik). Pertaining to or characterized by lymphopoiesis.

**lymphoreticulosis** (lim'fo-rĕ-tik'u-lo'sis). Proliferation of the reticuloendothelial cells of the lymph glands.

    **benign inoculation l.,** cat-scratch *disease.*

**lymphorrhagia** (lim'fo-ra'jĭ-ah) [ lympho- + G. *rhēgnymi,* to burst forth. RHAG- ]. Lymphorrhea.

**lymphorrhea** (lim'fo-re'ah) [ lympho- + G. *rhoia,* a flow ]. An escape of lymph on the surface from ruptured, torn, or cut lymphatic vessels.

**lymphorrhoid** (lim'fo-royd). A dilation of a lymph channel, resembling hemorrhoid.

**lymphosarcoma** (lim'fo-sar-ko'mah) [ lympho- + G. *sarkōma,* sarcoma ]. A form of malignant lymphoma in which there is neoplastic proliferation of abnormal lymphocytes and immature cells of that series, resulting in the occurrence of multiple enlarged lymph nodes and infiltration of various tissues.

    **l. cutis,** appears on the skin as small to large, dull reddish, smooth papules or nodules; may be primary in the skin or associated with l. of lymphoid tissues; may also appear as an area of lichenification resembling chronic eczema.

**lymphosarcomatosis** (lim'fo-sar-ko'mă-to'sis). A condition characterized by the presence of multiple, widely distributed masses of lymphosarcoma.

**lympho'sis.** Undesirable term for lymphocytic *leukemia.*

**lymphostasis** (lim-fos'tă-sis) [ lympho- + G. *stasis,* a standing still ]. Obstruction of the normal flow of lymph.

**lymphotaxis** (lim'fo-tak'sis) [ lympho- + G. *taxis,* orderly arrangement ]. The exertion of an effect that attracts or repels lymphocytes.

**lymphotrophy** (lim-fot'ro-fī) [ lympho- + G. *trophē,* nourishment ]. Nourishment of the tissues by lymph in parts devoid of blood vessels.

**lymphuria** (lim-fu'rĭ-ah) [ lympho- + G. *ouron,* urine ]. Discharge of lymph in the urine.

**Lynen** (le'nen), Feodor, German biochemist, *1911. Nobel laureate, 1964, with Konrad Bloch, for contributions to the knowledge concerning reactions involved in biosynthesis of cholesterol and fatty acids.

**lynestrenol** (lin-es'tren-ol) (USAN, BP). ORGAMETIL; ORGANMETRIL; ethinylestrenol; 17α-ethynylestr-4-en-17β-ol; 3-desoxynorlutin; ethinylestrenol; a progestational agent, used with mestranol as an oral contraceptive.

**lyo-** (li'o-) [ G. *lyō,* to loosen, dissolve ]. Combining form relating to dissolution. See also lyso-.

**lyoenzymes** (li'o-en'zimz). Extracellular *enzymes.*

**lyolysis** (li-ol'ĭ-sis). See solvolysis.

**Lyon,** B. B. Vincent, American physician, 1880–1953. See Meltzer-L. *test.*

**Lyon,** James A., U. S. physician, 1882–1955. See L. and Horgan *method.*

**Lyon,** Mary F., British geneticist. See L. *hypothesis.*

**lyophil** (li'o-fil). Lyophilic.

**lyophilic** (li'o-fil'ik) [ lyo- + G. *phileō,* to love ]. Lyophil; lyophile; in colloid chemistry, denoting a dispersed phase having a pronounced affinity for the dispersion medium; when the dispersed phase is l., the colloid is usually a reversible one. Compare hydrophilic.

**lyophilization** (li-of'ĭ-lĭ-za'shun). The process of isolating a solid substance from solution by freezing the solution and evaporating the ice under vacuum; freeze-drying.

**lyophobe** (li'o-fōb). Lyophobic.

**lyophobic** (li'o-fo'bik) [ lyo- + G. *phobos,* fear ]. Lyophobe; denoting a dispersed phase having but slight affinity for the dispersion medium; when the dispersed phase is l. the colloid is usually an irreversible one. Compare hydrophobic.

**lyosorption** (li'o-sorp'shun). The adsorption of a liquid on a solid surface.

**lyotropic** (li-o-trop'ik) [ lyo- + G. *tropē,* a turning ]. Lyophilic; readily soluble.

**Lyozo'on atroph'icans** (li-o-zo'on ā-trof'i-kanz). Obsolete term applied to inclusion bodies found in trachoma-like disease (epitheliosis desquamativa) seen in Samoa.

**lypothymia** (li'po-thi'mĭ-ah) [ G. *lypē,* pain, grief, + *thymos,* mind ]. Lypemania; obsolete term for melancholia.

**ly'pressin** (USP). Lysine vasopressin.

**lyra** (li'rah) [ L. and G. lyre ]. A lyre-shaped structure; specifically, the commissura fornicis (lyra davidis, or lyre of David).

    **l. uteri'na,** *plicae* palmatae.

**Lys.** Symbol for lysine or its radicals in peptides.

**lys-.** See lyso-.

**ly'sate.** The material (cellular debris and fluid) produced by lysis.

**lyse** (līz). To break up, to disintegrate, *e.g.,* as applied to cells; to effect lysis.

**lysemia** (li-se'mĭ-ah) [ lyso- + G. *haima,* blood ]. Disintegration or dissolution of red blood cells and the occurrence of hemoglobin in the circulating plasma and in the urine.

**lysergamide.** Lysergic acid amide.

**lysergic acid** (li-sur'jik). D-Lysergic acid; a cleavage product of alkaline hydrolysis of ergot alkaloids; molecular weight 268.3; occurs as shiny crystals, slightly soluble in water.

Lysergic acid

    **l. acid amide,** lysergamide; ergine; a psychotomimetic agent present in *Rivea corymbosa* and *Ipomoea tricolor;* possesses less hallucinogenic potency than l. acid diethylamide.

    **l. acid diethylamide,** LSD; lysergide; peripherally, a serotonin antagonist; 1 to 2 μg. per kg. induces schizophrenic-like states in humans, with hallucinations that are visual rather than auditory; its use may precipitate psychoses. It is occasionally used in the treatment of chronic alcoholism and psychotic disorders.

    **l. acid monoethylamide,** a psychotomimetic agent present in *Rivea corymbosa* and *Ipomoea tricolor;* possesses less hallucinatory potency than l. acid diethylamide.

**lysergide.** Lysergic acid diethylamide.

**lys'idine.** Methylglyoxalidine; 2-methyl-2-imidazoline; has been used in the treatment of the uric acid diathesis and to prevent radiation injury.

**lysimeter** (li-sim'e-ter) [ lyso- + G. *metron,* measure ]. An apparatus for determining the degree of solubility of any substance.

**ly'sin.** 1. A specific complement-fixing antibody that acts destructively on cells and tissues; the various types are designated in accordance with the form of antigen that stimulates the production of the l., *e.g.,* hemolysin, bacteriolysin, and so on. 2. Any substance which causes lysis.

**β-lysin.** A thermostable bactericidal substance present in serum. The designation β was applied in early years to distinguish this substance from thermolabile substances (α -lysins, *i.e.,* antibodies) that mediate the action of complement.

**lysine** (li'sēn). $NH_2(CH_2)_4CH(NH_2)COOH$; an α-amino acid found in many proteins; distinguished by an ε-amino group.

    **l. decarboxylase** (EC 4.1.1.18), an enzyme that catalyzes the decarboxylation of l., with the production of the diamine, cadaverine.

**l. vasopressin,** [ Lys[8] ]vasopressin; lypressin; vasopressin containing lysine in position 8; antidiuretic hormone formed in pigs, hippotami, and peccaries.

**lysinemia** (li′sĭ-ne′mĭ-ah). Increased concentration of lysine in the blood, associated with mental and physical retardation.

**lysin′ogen.** An antigen that stimulates the formation of a specific lysin.

**lysinogenic** (li′sĭ-no-jen′ik). Having the property of a lysinogen.

**lysinuria** (li′sĭ-nu′rĭ-ah). The presence of lysine in the urine.

**lysis** (li′sis) [ G. dissolution or loosening ]. 1. The gradual subsidence of the symptoms of an acute disease, a form of the curative process, distinguished from crisis. 2. The destruction of red blood cells, bacteria, and other antigens, by a specific lysin; according to the form of antigen destroyed, the process is called hemolysis, nephrolysis, bacteriolysis, and so on.

**lyso-, lys-** (li′so-) G. *lysis,* a loosening or dissolution ]. Combining forms relating to lysis, or dissolution.

**ly′soceph′alin.** A lysophosphatidic acid esterified with ethanolamine or serine, *i.e.,* a lysophosphatidyl serine or ethanolamine; analogous to lycolecithin, lysophosphatidyl choline.

**lysogen** (li′so-jen) [ lysin + G. suffix -*gen,* producing ]. 1. Something capable of inducing lysis. 2. A bacterium in the state of lysogeny.

**lysogenesis** (li′so-jen′ĕ-sis). The production of lysins.

**lysogenic** (li′so-jen′ik). 1. Causing or having the power to cause lysis, indicating the action of certain antibodies and chemical substances. 2. Pertaining to bacteria in the state of lysogeny.

**lysogenicity** (li′so-jĕ-nis′ĭ-tĭ). The property of being lysogenic.

**lysogenization** (li′so-jĕ-nĭ-za′shun, li-soj′ĕ-nĭ-za′shun). The process by which a bacterium becomes lysogenic.

**lysogeny** (li-soj′ĕ-nĭ). The phenomenon of a culture of a bacterial strain being capable of inducing, by means of its contained bacteriophage, general lysis in a culture of another bacterial strain without itself undergoing obvious lysis; in such lysogenic cultures probacteriophage is associated with the genome of all the bacteria, rendering the bacteria immune to infection by the free bacteriophage always present in the culture due to constant dissociation, at a slow rate, of probacteriophage and freeing of infectious particles.

**ly′soki′nase.** Term proposed for activator agents, such as streptokinase, urokinase, or staphylokinase, that produce plasmin by indirect or multiple-stage action on plasminogen.

**lysolecithin** (li′so-les′ĭ-thin). A lecithin (phosphatidyl choline) from which one fatty acid residue has been removed by partial hydrolysis, as by phospholipase $A_1$ or $A_2$. L.'s are good detergents, emulsifiers of dietary lipid, and hemolytic agents.

**ly′solec′ithinase.** Lysophospholipase.

**ly′sophos′phatid′ic acid.** A phosphatidic acid in which only one of the hydroxyl groups of the glycerol is esterified. The prefix lyso- derives from the fact that the acids are good detergents and as such can lyse cells (*cf.* lysolecithin, lysocephalin).

**ly′sophos′phati′dyl ser′ine.** Phosphatidyl serine from which one fatty acid residue has been removed from the glycerol moiety; *cf.* lysophosphatidic acid.

**ly′sophos′pholip′ase.** Phospholipase B; lecithinase B, lysolecithinase; a hydrolase (EC 3.1.1.5) removing the single acyl group from a lysolecithin, leaving glycerophosphinicocholine.

**ly′sopine.** $N^2$-(2-Lactyl)lysine; found in, and active in promoting growth of, crown-gall tumors in plants; similar in structure and action to octopine.

**lysosome** (li′so-sōm) [ lyso- + G. *soma,* body ]. Autophagic vacuole; a cytoplasmic, membrane-bound particle, 0.5 $\mu$ or less in diameter, containing hydrolyzing enzymes.
  **definitive l.'s,** secondary l.'s.
  **primary l.'s,** cytoplasmic bodies produced at the Golgi apparatus where hydrolytic enzymes are incorporated; they fuse with phagosomes or pinosomes to become secondary l.'s.
  **secondary l.'s,** definitive l.'s; l.'s in which lysis takes place, owing to the activity of hydrolytic enzymes; they are believed to eventually become residual bodies.

**lysozyme** (li′so-zīm). Muramidase; mucopeptide glycohydrolase; enzyme (EC 3.2.1.17) hydrolyzing 1,4-$\beta$ links between N-acetylmuramic acid and N-acetylglucosamine, and thus destructive to cell walls of certain bacteria; it is present in tears and some other fluids of the body, in egg white, and in some plant tissues.

**lyssa** (lis′ah) [ G. *madness* ]. 1 [ NAV ]. "Worm" (3); a cartilage in the tongue of the dog. 2. Old term for rabies.

**ly′syl.** The univalent radical of lysine.

**lytic** (lit′ik). Pertaining to lysis in either sense.

**lytta** (lit′ah). Old term for rabies.

**lyx′itol.** A pentitol (reduced lyxose) occurring in lyxoflavin.

**lyx′ofla′vin.** A compound similar to riboflavin except that D-lyxitol is present in place of the D-ribitol group; present in small quantity in cardiac muscle.

**lyx′ose.** An aldopentose isomeric with ribose. For structure, see sugars.

**lyx′ulose.** The 2-keto derivative of lyxose.

**lyze** (līz). Lyse.

# M

μ [ mu, 12th letter of the G. alphabet ]. 1. Symbol for micro- (10⁻⁶), micron, micrometer. 2. Symbol for dynamic viscosity.

μμ. Symbol for micromicro- (*i.e.,* pico, p).

**M.** 1. Abbreviation for myopia or myopic. 2. Abbreviation, in prescriptions, for *misce,* mix. 3. Symbol for a blood factor; see MNSs blood group, appendix 2.

**M.** Symbol for moles per liter (also written M or *M*); see molar (4).

**M + Am.** Abbreviation for compound myopic astigmatism.

**m.** Abbreviation for (1) meter; (2) minim; (3) milli-; (4) mass.

***m*-.** Abbreviation, in chemistry, for *meta*-.

**mμ.** Abbreviation for millimicro- (now known as nano-, *q. v.*).

**ma.** Abbreviation for milliampere.

**MAC.** Abbreviation for minimal alveolar (anesthetic) *concentration.*

**Mac-.** For proper names beginning thus, see also Mc-.

**Macaca** (mă-kahk′ah) [ Pg. *macaco,* monkey ]. A large genus of Old World monkeys (family Cercopithecidae that includes the macaque and rhesus monkeys, and the barbary apes; found in Gibraltar, N. Africa, S. Asia, East Indies, Philippines, and Japan. At least 26 different generic names have been applied to macaques. The rhesus macaques, *M. mulatta,* range from altitudes of 10,000 ft. in Kashmir eastward through Assam, Tonkin, and China, to Fukien and Formosa. They live in large troops, are good swimmers, and are noisy and pugnacious. Their gestation period is 5 to 7 mohths, and usually only one young is born; the life-span in captivity is about 30 years.

**macaque** (mă-kahk′) [ Fr. ]. See *Macaca.*

**Macdowel's frenulum.** See under frenulum.

**mace** (mās) [ Mediev. L. *macia,* mace, prob. fr. L. *macir,* fr. G. *maker,* an Indian spice ]. *Myristica fragrans* (family Myristicaceae); the arillode, or husk, surrounding the nutmeg. Used for the same purposes as nutmeg.

**Mace.** Proprietary name for chloracetophenone (the classical lacrimator) in a light petroleum dispersant and a Freon-like propellant.

**MacEod syndrome.** See under syndrome.

**macerate** (mas′er-āt) [ see maceration ]. To soften by steeping or soaking.

**maceration** (mas-er-a′shun) [ L. *macero,* pp. *-atus,* to soften by soaking ]. 1. Softening by the action of a liquid 2. Softening of tissues after death by nonputrefactive (sterile) autolysis; seen especially in the stillborn, with separation of the epidermis by bullae.

**Macewen** (mak-u′en), Sir William, Scottish surgeon, 1848–1924. See M.'s *operation, sign, symptom, triangle.*

**Mach,** Ernst, Austrian scientist, 1838–1916. See M.'s *band,* M. *number.*

**Machado-Guerreiro test.** See under test.

**Mache** (mah′kheh), Heinrich, Vienna physicist, *1876. See M. *unit.*

**machine** (mă-shēn) [ L. *machina,* contrivance ]. Any mechanical apparatus or device.

**anesthesia m.,** equipment used for inhalation anesthesia, including flowmeters, vaporizers, and sources of compressed gases, but not including the anesthetic circuit (*q. v.*) or mechanisms for elimination of carbon dioxide.

**panoramic rotating m.,** an x-ray machine using a reciprocating motion of the tube and extraoral film to produce radiographs of all the teeth and surrounding structures.

**macies** (mă′se-ēz) [ L. leanness ]. Emaciation.

**Macintosh,** Charles, Scottish chemist, 1766–1843. See M. *blockers,* M.'s *sheet.*

**Mackay,** Ralph S. See M.-Marg *tonometer.*

**Mackenrodt** (mahk′en-rot), Alwin K., German gynecologist, 1859–1925. See M.'s *incision, ligaments.*

**Mackenzie,** Sir James, Scottish physician practicing in London, 1853–1925. See M.'s *polygraph.*

**Mackenzie,** Richard J., Scottish surgeon, 1821–1854. See M.'s *amputation.*

**MacLachlan,** E. A. See Lowe-Terrey-M. *syndrome.*

**MacLean,** Charles, British physician, 1788–1824. See M.-Maxwell *disease.*

**Macleod,** John J. R., Scottish physiologist in Canada, 1876–1935. Nobel laureate, 1923, with Frederick G. Banting for their discovery, with Charles H. Best, of insulin.

**Macleod,** Roderick, Scottish physician, 1795–1852. See M.'s *rheumatism.*

**Macleod,** W. M. See M.'s *syndrome.*

**MacNeal,** Ward J., U. S. bacteriologist, 1881–1946. See Novy-M. blood *agar,* M.'s *stain.*

**macr-.** See macro-.

**Macracanthorhynchus** (mak′ră-kan′tho-ringk′us) [ macro- + G. *akantha,* thorn, + *rhynchos,* snout ]. A genus of thorny-headed worms (class Acanthocephala).

**M. hirudina′ceus,** the thorny-headed Acanthocephala of the pig, formerly called *Echinorhynchus gigas* and *Gigantorhynchus hirudinaceus;* it inhabits the intestinal tract and causes nodules proboscis develop at the site of penetration of the spiny proboscis of each worm; it is said to occur occasionally in man.

**macrencephaly, macrencephalia** (mak′ren-sef′ă-lĭ, -sĕ-fa′lĭ-ah) [ macro- + G. *enkephalos,* brain ]. Hypertrophy of the brain; the condition of having a large brain.

**macro-, macr-** (mak′ro-) [ G. *makros,* large ]. Combining form meaning large, long. See also mega-, megalo-.

**mac′roam′ylase.** Descriptive term applied to a form of serum amylase in which the enzyme is present as a complex, joined to a globulin; the molecular weight of the enzyme alone is 50,000, whereas that of the complex probably exceeds 160,000, which explains why renal excretion of the complex is not appreciable.

**macroamylasemia** (mak′ro-am′ĭ-la-se′mĭ-ah) [ macroamylase + G. *haima,* blood ]. A form of hyperamylasemia, in which a portion of serum amylase exists as macroamylase.

**macrobacterium** (mak′ro-bak-tēr′ĭ-um). Megabacterium.

**macrobiosis** (mak′ro-bi-o′sis) [ macro- + G. *bios,* life ]. Longevity.

**macrobiote** (mak′ro-bi′ōt) [ macro- + G. *bios,* life ]. An organism that is long-lived.

**mac′robiot′ic.** 1. Long-lived. 2. Tending to prolong life.

**mac′robiot′ics.** The study of the prolongation of life.

**mac′roblast** [ macro- + G. *blastos,* germ ]. A large erythroblast.

**m. of Naegeli,** pronormoblast; see discussion under erythroblast.

**macroblepharia** (mak′ro-blĕ-făr′ĭ-ah) [ macro- + G. *blepharon,* eyelid, + suffix *-ia,* condition ]. The state of having abnormally large eyelids.

**macrobrachia** (mak-ro-bra′kĭ-ah) [ macro- + G. *brachiōn,* arm ]. Condition of having abnormally large or long arms.

**macrocardia** (mak′ro-kar′dĭ-ah). Cardiomegaly.

**macrocardius** (mak′ro-kar′dĭ-us) [ macro- + G. *kardia,* heart ]. An individual with an abnormally large heart.

**macrocephalic, macrocephalous** (mak′ro-sĕ-fal′ik, -sef′ă-lus) [ macro- + G. *kephalē,* head ]. Relating to or characterized by macrocephaly.

**macrocephalus** (mak′ro-sef′ă-lus). A fetus with an abnormally large head.

**macrocephaly, macrocephalia** (mak′ro-sef′ă-lĭ, -sĕ-fa′lĭ-ah) [ macro- + G. *kephalē,* head ]. The condition of having an abnormally large head; see also dolichocephaly and megacephaly.

**macrocheilia, macrochilia** (mak′ro-ki′lĭ-ah) [ macro- + G. *cheilos,* lip ]. Macrolabia; cavernous lymphangioma of the lip; a condition of permanent swelling of the lip, resulting from the presence of greatly distended lymph spaces.

**macrocheiria, macrochiria** (mak'ro-ki'rĭ-ah) [ macro- + G. *cheir,* hand ]. Cheiromegaly; chiromegaly; megalocheiria; megalochiria; a condition characterized by abnormally large hands.

**macrochemistry** (mak-ro-kem'is-trĭ). The use of chemical tests, the reactions of which (color change, effervescence, etc.) are visible to the naked eye; distinguished from microchemistry.

**macrochilia** (mak'ro-ki'lĭ-ah). Macrocheilia.

**macrochiria** (mak-ro-ki'rĭ-ah). Macrocheiria.

**macrochylomicron** (mak'ro-ki'lo-mi'kron). An unusually large chylomicron.

**macrochylomicronemia** (mak'ro-ki-lo-mi'kro-ne'mĭ-ah). The presence of macrochylomicrons in large numbers in the blood, often associated with hypercholesterolemia, and regarded as a possible factor in the pathogenesis of arteriosclerosis.

**macrocnemia** (mak'ro-ne'mĭ-ah) [ macro- + G. *knēmē,* leg ]. A condition in which there is an enlargement of the shins.

**macrococcus** (mak'ro-kok'us). Megacoccus.

**macrocolon** (mak'ro-ko'lon). A sigmoid colon of unusual length; a variety of megacolon.

**macroconidium,** pl. **macroconidia** (mak'ro-ko-nid'ĭ-um). 1. A conidium, or exospore, of large size. 2. In fungi, the larger of two types of conidia that bear both macroconidia and microconidia.

**macrocornea** (mak'ro-kor'ne-ah). Megalocornea; a cornea of unusual size.

**macrocra'nium.** An enlarged skull, especially the bones containing the brain, as seen in hydrocephalus; the face appears relatively small in comparison.

**macrocryoglobulin** (mak'ro-kri-o-glob'u-lin). A macroglobulin that has the properties of a cryoglobulin.

**macrocryoglobulinemia** (mak'ro-kri-o-glob'u-lin-e'mĭ-ah). The presence of cold-precipitating macroglobulins in the peripheral blood. Such macrocryoglobulins are often called cold hemagglutinins.

**macrocyst** (mak'ro-sist). A cyst of macroscopic proportions.

**mac'rocy'tase.** According to Metchnikoff, a cytase or complement, formed by the large uninuclear leukocytes, which is effective in the destruction of tissue cells, blood cells, etc.

**macrocyte** (mak'ro-sīt) [ macro- + G. *kytos,* a hollow (cell) ]. A large erythrocyte, such as those observed in pernicious anemia.

**macrocythemia** (mak'ro-si-the'mĭ-ah) [ macrocyte + G. *haima,* blood ]. The occurrence of unusually large numbers of macrocytes in the circulating blood; macrocytosis; megalocytosis or megalocythemia.

hyperchromat'ic m., an inexact term frequently used for macrocytes that contain an unusually large amount of hemoglobin, but are actually normochromic; although the total mass of hemoglobin is greater than normal (owing to the large cells), the percentage of hemoglobin in the cells is not greater than normal.

**macrocytosis** (mak'ro-si-to'sis) [ macrocyte + G. suffix *-osis,* condition ]. Macrocythemia.

**macrodactyl'ia, macrodac'tylism, macrodac'tyly.** Megadactyly.

**macrodont** (mak'ro-dont) [ macro- + G. *odous* (*odont-*), tooth ]. Megadont; megalodont. 1. A tooth of abnormally large and frequently distorted proportions, tending to occur bilaterally and often following a genetic pattern. 2. Denoting a skull with a dental index above 44.

**macrodontia, macrodontism** (mak'ro-don'shĭ-ah, -don'-tizm). Megalodontia; megadontism; the state of having abnormally large teeth.

**macroencephalon** (mak'ro-en-sef'ă-lon) [ macro- + G. *enkephalos,* brain ]. Megaloencephalon.

**macroerythroblast** (mak'ro-e-rith'ro-blast). A large erythroblast.

**macroerythrocyte** (mak'ro-e-rith'ro-sīt). Macrocyte.

**macroesthesia** (mak'ro-es-the'zĭ-ah) [ macro- + G. *aisthēsis,* sensation ]. A subjective sensation of large size of all objects touched.

**macrogamete** (mak-ro-gam'ēt) [ macro- + G. *gametē,* wife ]. Megagamete; the female element in anisogamy, or conjugation of unicellular organisms of unequal size; it is the larger of the two cells, more full of reserve material, and but little if at all motile.

**macrogametocyte** (mak'ro-gă-me'to-sit). Macrogamont; the mother cell producing the macrogametes in Protozoa.

**mac'rogam'ont.** Macrogametocyte.

**macrogamy** (mă-krog'ă-mĭ) [ macro- + G. *gamos,* marriage ]. Conjugation of two adult cells or gametes.

**mac'rogas'tria.** Megalogastria.

**mac'rogen'esy** [ macro- + G. *genesis,* origin, production ]. Obsolete synonym for gigantism.

**macrogenitosomia** (mak'ro-jen'ĭ-to-so'mĭ-ah) [ macro- + L. *genitalis,* genital, + G. *sōma,* body ]. Excessive bodily and genital development.

m. pre'cox, Pellizzi's syndrome; an example of precocious puberty in which gonadal maturation and the adolescent growth spurt in bodily height occur in the first decade of life. It is often associated with a pineal tumor; however, there is not general agreement about the location of the causative lesion. It has been noted that lesions in hypothalamic areas known to regulate gonadotrophin secretion are also often present.

m. pre'cox su'prarena'lis, precocious somatic growth and isosexual maturation of secondary sexual characteristics, as the consequence of an adrenocortical tumor.

**macrogingivae** (mak'ro-jin-ji've). Clinical state characterized by generalized enlargement of the gingivae.

**macroglia** (mă-krog'lĭ-ah) [ macro- + G. *glia,* glue ]. Astrocyte.

**macroglobulin** (mak'ro-glob-u-lin). Plasma globulin that has an unusually large molecular weight, *e.g.,* as much as 1,000,000.

**mac'roglob'uline'mia.** The presence of macroglobulins in the circulating blood, as in some patients with multiple myeloma.

Waldenström's m., Waldenström's syndrome; Waldenström's purpura; hyperglobulinemic purpura; m. occurring in elderly persons, especially women; characterized by proliferation of cells resembling lymphocytes or plasma cells in the bone marrow; anemia; increased sedimentation rate; and hyperglobulinemia with a narrow peak in γ-globulin or $β_2$-globulin at about 19 S units. The spleen, liver, or lymph nodes are often enlarged and there is frequently purpura or mucosal bleeding.

**mac'roglos'sia** [ macro- + G. *glōssa,* tongue ]. Megaloglossia; pachyglossia; enlargement of the tongue, due usually to local lymphangiectasia, or to muscular hypertrophy.

**macrognathia.** (mak'rog-nath'ĭ-ah, mak'ro-na'thĭ-ah) [ macro- + G. *gnathos,* jaw, + suffix *-ia,* condition ]. Enlargement or elongation of the jaw.

**macrography** (mă-krog'ră-fĭ) [ macro- + G. *graphō,* to write ]. Writing with very large letters.

**macrogyria** (mak'ro-ji'rĭ-ah) [ macro- + G. *gyros,* circle (gyrus) ]. Convolutions of the cerebral cortex congenitally larger than normal.

**mac'rola'bia** [ macro- + L. *labium,* lip ]. Macrocheilia.

**macroleukoblast** (mak-ro-lu'ko-blast). An unusually large leukoblast.

**mac'rolides.** A class of antibiotics discovered in streptomycetes, characterized by molecules made up of large-ring lactones; *e.g.,* erythromycin.

**mac'roma'nia** [ macro- + G. *mania,* frenzy ]. 1. Megalomania. 2. A delusion that all objects surrounding the subject, or the subject himself or his members, are of immense size.

**macromastia, macromazia** (mak'ro-mas'tĭ-ah, -ma'zĭ-ah) [ macro- + G. *mastos,* breast ]. Abnormally large breasts.

**macromelia** (mak'ro-me'lĭ-ah) [ macro- + G. *melos,* limb ]. Megalomelia; abnormal large size of one or more of the extremities.

**macromelus** (mă-krom'e-lus). An individual with macromelia.

**macromere** (mak'ro-mēr) [ macro- + G. *meros,* part ]. A blastomere of large size (as in amphibia).

**macromerozoite** (mak-ro-me-ro-zoīt). Megamerozoite; a large merozoite.

**mac'rometh'od.** The usual method of chemical examinations, tests, etc. in which ordinary quantities are used; the opposite of micromethod.

**macromolecule** (mak'ro-mol'e-kūl). A molecule of colloidal size, notably proteins, nucleic acids, and polysaccharides.

**mac'romon'ocyte.** An unusually large monocyte.

**macromyeloblast** (mak'ro-mi'ē-lo-blast). An abnormally large myeloblast.

**mac'ronor'moblast.** 1. A large normoblast. 2. A large, incompletely hemoglobiniferous, nucleated red blood cell with a "cart-wheel" nucleus.

**macronormochromoblast** (mak-ro-nor'mo-kro'mo-blast). Macroerythroblast.

**macronucleus** (mak'ro-nu'kle-us). 1. Meganucleus; a nucleus that occupies a relatively large portion of the cell, or the larger nucleus where two (or more) are present in a cell. 2. Trophonucleus; nutrition, somatic, motion, or trophic nucleus; specifically, the larger of the two nuclei in ciliates; it governs the vegetative metabolic functions and has nothing to do with reproduction. See also micronucleus (2).

**macronychia** (mak-ro-nik'ī-ah) [ macro- + G. *onyx,* nail ]. Megalonychosis; abnormal size of the fingernails or toenails.

**mac'ropar'asite.** A parasite, such as a louse or an intestinal worm, that is visible to the naked eye.

**mac'ropathol'ogy.** The phase of pathology that pertains to the gross anatomical changes in disease.

**macropenis** (mak'ro-pe'nis). Macrophallus; megalopenis; megalophallus; an abnormally large penis.

**macrophage** (mak'ro-fāj) [ macro- + G. *phagein,* to eat ]. Macrophagocyte; any large ameboid mononuclear phagocytic cell, regardless of origin; see also phagocyte, and reticuloendothelial *system.*

**macrophagocyte** (mak'ro-fag'o-sīt). Macrophage.

**macrophallus** (mak-ro-fal'lus) [ macro- + G. *phallos,* penis ]. Macropenis.

**macrophthalmia** (mak'rof-thal-mī-ah) [ macro- + G. *ophthalmos,* eye ]. Megalophthalmus.

**macroplasia** (mak-ro-pla'zī-ah) [ macro- + G. *plasis,* molding, formation ]. Obsolete term for gigantism.

**mac'ropo'dia** [ macro- + G. *pous,* foot ]. Megalopodia; pes gigas; the state of having large feet.

**macropolycyte** (mak'ro-pol'ī-sīt) [ macro- + G. *polys,* many, + *kytos,* cell ]. An unusually large polymorphonuclear neutrophilic leukocyte that contains a multisegmented nucleus (*e.g.,* 8, 10, or more lobes); the arrangement of chromatin is less compact than in the normal neutrophil, and the cytoplasmic granules tend to be larger and more acidophilic. Such changes frequently precede significant alterations in the red blood cells, *e.g.,* as in pernicious anemia and certain other forms of anemia.

**macropromyelocyte** (mak'ro-pro-mi'ē-lo-sīt). An unusually large promyelocyte.

**macroprosopia** (mak'ro-pro-so'pī-ah) [ macro- + G. *prosōpon, face* ]. Megaprosopia; a condition in which the face is large, out of proportion to the size of the cranial vault.

**macroprosopous** (mak'ro-pro'so-pus, -pro-so'pus) Megaprosopous; relating to or exhibiting macroprosopia.

**macroprosopus** (mak'ro-pro'so-pus, -pro-so'pus) An individual with macroprosopia.

**macropsia** (mă-krop'sī-ah) [ macro- + G. *opsis,* vision ]. Megalopsia; megalopia; the subjective perception of objects as larger than they are.

**macrorrhinia** (mak'ro-rin'ī-ah) [ macro- + G. *rhis* (*rhin-*), nose ]. Excessive size of the nose, either congenital or pathologic.

**macroscelia** (mak'ro-se'lī-ah) [ macro- + G. *skelos,* leg ]. Abnormally increased length or thickness of the legs.

**macroscopic** (mak'ro-skop'ik). Relating to macroscopy.

**macroscopy** (mă-kros'ko-pī) [ macro- + G. *skopeō,* to view ]. The examination of objects with the naked eye.

**mac'rosig'moid.** Megasigmoid; enlargement or dilation of the sigmoid colon.

**macrosis** (mă-kro'sis) [ G. ]. A lengthening, or an increase in volume generally.

**macrosmatic** (mak'roz-mat'ik) [ macro- + G. *osmē,* smell ]. Denoting an abnormally keen olfactory sense.

**macrosomia** (mak'ro-so'mī-ah) [ macro- + G. *sōma,* body ]. Megasomia; abnormally large size of the body.

**macrosplanchnic** (mak'ro-splangk'nik). Megalosplanchnic.

**mac'rospore** [ macro- + G. *sporos,* seed ]. Megaspore; megalospore; one of the larger spores of certain protozoans, their size being due to their paucity.

**macrostereognosis** (mak'ro-stēr'ī-og-no'sis) [ macro- + G. *stereos,* solid, + *gnōsis,* recognition ]. An error of perception in which objects appear larger than they are.

**macrostomia** (mak'ro-sto-mī-ah) [ macro- + G. *stoma,* mouth ]. Abnormally large size of the mouth.

**mac'rostruc'ture.** Gross structure in contrast to microstructure.

**macrotia** (mak-ro'shī-ah) [ macro- + G. *ous,* ear, + suffix *-ia,* condition ]. Congenital excessive enlargement of the auricle.

**mac'rotome** [ macro- + G. *tomē,* cutting ]. An instrument for making gross anatomical sections.

**macrotys.** Cimicifuga.

**mac'roworld.** A neologism for macrocosm, usually meaning the environment and physical world outside the organism.

**macula,** pl. **mac'ulae** (mak'u-lah) [ L. a spot ]. Spot; macule. 1 [ NA ]. A small spot, perceptibly different in color from the surrounding tissue. 2. A small, discolored patch or spot on the skin, neither elevated above nor depressed below the skin's surface; see also subentries under spot.

**maculae acusticae,** see m. sacculi and m. utriculi.

**m. adherens,** desmosome.

**m. al'bida,** pl. **maculae albidae,** m. lactea; gray-white or white, rounded or irregularly shaped, slightly opaque patches or spots that are sometimes observed post mortem in the epicardium, especially in middle-aged or older persons; they result from fibrous thickening, and sometimes hyalination, of the epicardium. Similar lesions may also occur in the visceral layer of the peritoneum.

**m. atroph'ica,** an atrophic glistening white spot in the skin.

**m. ceru'lea,** blue spot; a bluish stain on the skin caused by the bites of fleas or lice.

**m. commu'nis,** the thickened area in the medial wall of the auditory vesicle that later becomes subdivided to form the maculae of the sacculus and utriculus and the cristae of the ampullae of the semicircular ducts.

**m. cor'neae,** corneal spot; a moderately dense opacity of the cornea.

**m. cribro'sa,** pl. **maculae cribrosae,** [ NA ], one of three areas (inferior, middle, and superior) on the wall of the vestibule of the labyrinth, marked by numerous foramina giving passage to nerve filaments supplying portions of the membranous labyrinth; sometimes a fourth (m. cribrosa quarta) is described, giving passage to the cochlear nerve.

**m. den'sa,** a densely packed collection of special staining cells in the distal tubular epithelium, in direct apposition to the juxtaglomerular cells; they may function as chemoreceptors feeding information to justaglomerular.

**false m.,** an extrafoveal point of fixation.

**m. flava,** a yellowish spot at the anterior extremity of the rima glottidis where the two vocal folds join.

**m. germinati'va,** germinal *spot.*

**m. gonorrho'ica,** Saenger's m.; a spot of brighter red than the surrounding membrane, the congested lips of the duct of Bartholin's gland, sometimes seen in gonorrhea.

**m. lac'tea,** m. albida.

**m. lu'tea,** m. retinae.

**mongolian maculae,** mongolian *spots.*

**m. ret'inae** [ NA ], m. lutea; yellow spot; area centralis; a small, orange-yellow, oval area, 3 by 5 mm., on the inner surface of the retina slightly below and lateral to the optic disk at a point corresponding to the posterior pole of the eyeball, and therefore in the visual axis. At its center is the fovea centralis, which provides the best visual acuity under photopic conditions.

**m. sac'culi** [ NA ], saccular spot; the oval neuroepithelial sensory area in the anterior wall of the saccule. Hair cells of the neuroepithelium support the membrana statoconiorum and have terminal arborizations of vestibular nerve fibers around their bodies.

**Saenger's m.,** m. gonorrhoica.

**m. tendin'ea,** m. albida.

**m. utric'uli** [ NA ], utricular spot; the neuroepithelial sensory area in the inferolateral wall of the utricle. Hair cells of the neuroepithelium support the membrana statoconiorum and have terminal arborizations of vestibular nerve fibers around their bodies.

**macular, maculate** (mak'u-lar, -lāt). Relating to or marked by macules; spotted.

**maculation** (mak'u-la'shun). The formation of macules; the presence of macules.

**macule** (mak'ūl) [ L. *macula,* spot ]. Macula.

**maculocerebral** (mak'u-lo-sěr'ĕ-bral). Relating to the macula lutea and the brain; denoting a type of nervous disease marked by degenerative lesions in both the retina and the brain.

**maculoerythematous** (mak'u-lo-ĕr-ĭ-the'mă-tus). Denoting lesions that are erythematous and macular, covering wide areas.

**maculopapule** (mak'u-lo-pap'ūl). A lesion with a sessile base; a broad lesion that slopes from a papule in the center.

**maculopathy** (mak'u-lop'ă-thi). Macular retinopathy; any pathological condition of the macula lutea.

**cystic m.,** cystic degeneration of the retinal macula; it may occur after cataract extraction or in idiopathic senile macular degeneration.

**familial pseudoinflammatory m.,** familial pseudoinflammatory macular *degeneration.*

**nicotinic acid m.,** m. observed in persons taking 3000 mg. or more of nicotinic acid daily for reduction of serum cholesterol; normal vision returns after this medication is discontinued.

**MacWilliam,** John A., English physician, 1857–1937. See M.'s *test.*

**mad** [ A.S. *gemād* ]. 1. Rabid. 2. Insane. 3. Mentally ill.

**mad'aro'sis** [ G. a falling off of the eyelashes, fr. *madaō,* to fall off (of hair) ]. Loss of the eyebrows or of the eyelashes.

**mad'der** [ A.S. *maedere* ]. Turkey red; the dried and powdered root of *Rubia tinctorum* (family Rubiaceae); it contains several glycosides which upon fermentation give the red dyes, alizarin and purpurin. When m. (or alizarin) is fed to young animals, the calcium in newly deposited bone salt, hydroxyapatite, is stained red.

**Maddox,** Ernest E., English ophthalmologist, 1860–1933. See M. double *prism,* M.'s *rod.*

**Mad'elung,** Otto W., German surgeon, 1846–1926. See M.'s *deformity, disease, neck.*

**madescent** (mă-des'ent) [ L. *madesco,* to become moist ]. Becoming moist; slightly moist.

**madidans** (mad'ĭ-danz) [ L. *madido,* pres. p. -*ans,* to moisten ]. Moist; denoting certain skin lesions.

**Madlener operation.** See under operation.

**mad'ness.** The state of being mad.

**dumb m.,** paralytic *rabies.*

**madra buba.** The primary lesion of yaws.

**Madsen,** Thorvald J. M., *1870. See Arrhenius-M. *theory.*

**Madurella** (mad'u-rel'ah) [ *Madura,* India ]. A genus of the Fungi Imperfecti, including a number of species that may be causal agents of maduromycosis.

**M. myceto'mi,** a species of fungi causing maduromycosis. Synonymous terms include *M. bovoi, M. oswaldoi, M. ramiroi, M. tabarkae, M. tozeuri, M. americana, M. ikedai, M. lackawanna,* and *Glenospora khartiymensis. M. grisea* is a separate species causing maduromycosis.

**maduromycosis** (mad'u-ro-mi-ko'sis). Madura boil; Bouffardi's black mycetoma; Madura foot; fungous foot; a chronic mycotic infection, usually involving the feet (and rarely the hands and other sites), caused by a varied group

of filamentous fungi of several species and genera (*e.g., Allescheria, Aspergillus, Sterigmatocystis, Penicillium, Madurella, Indiella, Glenospora, Monosporium, Cephalosporium,* and *Phialophora*); the disease is characterized by the formation of tumefactions and sinuses, from which serosanguineous or "oily" exudate drains. The exudate contains characteristic granules of variable colors, *e.g.,* yellow, white, orchid, red, brown, or black. One of the principal types of mycetoma, *q. v.*

**maedi** (ma'dē) [ Icelandic, dyspnea ]. A chronic, progressive, contagious pneumonia of sheep caused by a virus with a long incubation period. It is seen primarily in Iceland, but similar diseases have been reported from the Netherlands and (infrequently) from North America; occasionally confused with pulmonary adenomatosis of sheep, but generally believed to be a separate disease.

**ma'fenide** (USP). MARFENIL; SULFAMYLON; 4-homosulfanilamide hydrochloride; $\alpha$-amino-*p*-toluenesulfonamide hydrochloride; a topical antibacterial agent active against anaerobic pathogens.

**m. acetate** (USP), the preferred salt for ointment.

**m. hydrochloride,** the preferred salt for solution.

**Maffucci** (mah-foo'che), Angelo, Italian physician, 1847–1903. See M. *syndrome.*

**mag'aldrate** (USP). RIOPAN; RIPON; a chemical combination of aluminum hydroxide and magnesium hydroxide, used as an antacid.

**Magendie** (mă-zhahn-de'), Franc̣ois, French physiologist, 1783–1855. One of the outstanding experimental physiologists of the 19th century; he demonstrated that the posterior spinal nerve roots transmitted only sensory impulses and confirmed Bell's observation that the anterior roots were purely motor. See M.'s *foramen, law,* M.-Hertwig *sign, syndrome,* M.'s *spaces.*

**mag'enstrasse** [ Ger. *Magen,* stomach, + *Strasse,* road ]. The name sometimes applied to the passageway which food takes after it passes through the cardia, namely along the lesser curvature into the gastroduodenal junction.

**mag'got.** A fly larva; grub.

**cheese m.,** *Philopia casei.*

**wool m.,** the larva of one of several species of blowflies which deposit eggs on sheep, causing myiasis; fleece worm.

**magistral** (maj'is-tral) [ L. *magister,* master ]. Denoting a preparation compounded according to a physician's prescription; opposed to officinal (derived from a druggist's stock).

**Magitot** (mahzh-e-to'). Emile, French oral surgeon and investigator, 1833–1897. Noted especially for his early experimental studies of dental caries. See M.'s *disease.*

**magma** (mag'mah) [ G. a soft mass or salve, fr. *massō,* to knead ]. 1. A soft mass left after extraction of the active principles. 2. A salve or thick paste.

**m. reticula're,** delicate noncellular strands running between the yolk-sac and the outer wall of the blastocyst.

**magna'lium.** A type of alloy of aluminum with a high content of magnesium, lighter in weight, but harder, than aluminum.

**Magnan** (man-yon'), Valentin J. J., Paris psychiatrist, 1835–1916. See M.'s trombone *movement,* M.'s *sign.*

**magnesia** (mag-ne'zhuh) [ see magnesium ]. Magnesium oxide.

**m. and alumina oral suspension** (USP), a mixture of magnesium hydroxide and variable amounts of aluminum oxide; used as an antacid.

**cal'cined m.,** magnesium oxide.

**m. le'vis,** light m.; see magnesium oxide.

**m. magma,** milk of m.

**milk of m.** (USP), mixture of magnesium hydroxide (BP); m. magma; an aqueous suspension of magnesium hydroxide; antacid and laxative.

**m. pondero'sa,** heavy m.; see magnesium oxide.

**magnesium** (mag-ne'zhĭ-um) [ Mod. L. fr. G. *Magnēsia,* a region in Thessaly. MAG- ]. A mineral element, symbol Mg, atomic no. 12, atomic weight 24.32, of silvery luster, oxidizing to the alkaline earth magnesia. It burns with an intense white light, very rich in actinic rays, and is therefore used in photography.

**m. aluminum silicate** (USP), GELUSIL; aluminum magnesium silicate; magnesium aluminosilicate dihydrate; antacid.

**m. ben′zoate,** has been used in gout and rheumatoid arthritis.

**m. car′bonate** (NF, BP), used in gastric and intestinal acidity and as a laxative. The USP recognizes the light and heavy m. carbonate under the same title, but in the BP there are two separate monographs.

**m. chloride** (USP, BP), $MgCl_2 \cdot 6H_2O$; has been used as a laxative.

**m. citrate,** $Mg_3(C_6H_5O_7)_2 \cdot 14H_2O$; laxative.

**m. citrate, effervescent,** m. carbonate, citric acid, sodium bicarbonate, and sugar, moistened with alcohol, passed through a sieve, and dried to a coarse granular powder; used as a laxative.

**m. hydroxide** (NF), $Mg(OH)_2$; antacid and laxative.

**m. lactate,** laxative.

**m. oxide** (USP, BP), magnesia; calcined magnesia; used as an antacid and laxative. The USP recognizes both the light and heavy m. oxide under the same title, but in the BP there are two separate monographs.

**m. perox′ide,** decomposes in water to hydrogen peroxide; used as an ingredient in dentifrices and in antiseptic dusting powder.

**m. phosphate, tribasic,** (NF), tertiary m. phosphate, $Mg_3(PO_4)_2 \cdot 5H_2O$; used as an antacid, but does not produce systemic alkalization; 1 gm. is equivalent in neutralizing power to about 0.46 gm. of sodium bicarbonate.

**m. stearate** (USP, BP), a compound of m. with variable proportions of stearic and palmitic acids; used in the preparation of tablets, as a lubricant, and as an ingredient in some baby powders.

**m. sulfate** (USP, BP), Epsom salt; the active ingredient of most of the natural laxative waters. It is a promptly acting cathartic particularly useful in certain poisonings; also used in the treatment of increased intracranial pressure, eclampsia, and edema. Applied locally it has anti-inflammatory action; when administered intravenously it acts as an anticonvulsant and anesthetic.

**m. sulfate, dried** (BP), exsiccated m. sulfate; dried Epsom salts.

**m. sulfate, effervescent,** effervescent Epsom salt; m. sulfate, sodium bicarbonate, tartaric acid, and citric acid, moistened, passed through a sieve, and dried to a coarse granular powder; purgative.

**m. trisil′icate** (USP, BP), $2MgO \cdot 3SiO_2 \cdot nH_2O$; a compound of m. oxide and silicon dioxide with varying proportions of water; occurs in nature as meerschaum, pararepiolite, and repiolite; gastric antacid.

**mag′net** [ G. *magnes.* MAG- ]. Lodestone; magnetite; native magnetic oxide of iron; a body which has the property of attracting particles of iron, cobalt, nickel, or any of various metallic alloys, and which has magnetic polarity, *i.e.,* when freely suspended, it tends to assume a definite direction between the magnetic poles of the earth. This is a natural m.; an artificial m. is a bar or horseshoe-shaped piece of iron or steel which has been made magnetic by contact with another m. or, as in an electromagnet, by passage of electric current around a metallic (iron) core.

**Haab′s m.,** a very powerful electric m. used for drawing out chips of iron or steel which have become imbedded in the eyeball.

**magnet′ic.** Relating to a magnet; possessing magnetism.

**magnetism** (mag′nĕ-tizm). 1. The property of mutual attraction or repulsion possessed by magnets. 2. The science that has to do with magnets and their properties.

**animal m.,** mesmerism.

**magnetization** (mag′nĕ-tĭ-za′shun). Rendering magnetic.

**magnetoelectricity** (mag-ne′to-e-lek-tris′ĭ-tĭ). Electricity generated by the action of a magnet.

**magnetoencephalogram** (mag-ne′to-en-sef′ă-lo-gram). Abbreviated MEG; a gauss-time record of the magnetic field of the brain.

**magnetoencephalography** (mag-ne′to-en-sef-ă-log′ră-fĭ). The process of recording the brain's magnetic field.

**magnetometer** (mag′ne-tom′e-ter). An instrument for detecting and measuring the magnetic field.

**magneton** (mag′nĕ-ton). A unit of measurement of the magnetic moment of a particle (*e.g.,* atom or subatomic particle).

**Bohr m.,** electron m.; a constant in the equation relating the difference in energies between parallel and antiparallel spin alignments of electrons in a magnetic field; used in electron spin resonance (ESR) spectrometry for detection and estimation of free radicals; it is the net magnetic moment of one unpaired electron.

**electron m.,** Bohr m.

**nuclear m.,** a constant in the equation relating the difference in energies between parallel and antiparallel spin alignments of atomic nuclei in a magnetic field; used in nuclear magnetic resonance (NMR) spectrometry.

**magnetother′apy.** Treatment of disease by the application of a magnet.

**magnification** (mag′nĭ-fĭ-ka′shun) [ L. *magnifico,* pp. *-atus,* to magnify, fr. *magnus,* great, + *facio,* to make ]. 1. The seeming increase in size of an object viewed under the microscope; when noted, this increased size is expressed by a figure preceded by $\times$, indicating the number of times its diameter is enlarged. 2. The increased amplitude of a tracing, as of a muscular contraction, caused by the use of a lever with a long writing arm, *i.e.,* one in which the fulcrum is placed nearer to the muscle than to the writing point.

**mag′nitude.** Size or extent.

**average pulse m.,** the amplitude of pulse averaged throughout its duration; identical with peak amplitude for a square wave or pulse without droop.

**peak m.,** the greatest pulse amplitude.

**magnocellular** (mag′no-sel′u-lar) [ L. *magnus,* large, + cellular ]. Composed of cells of large size.

**magnolia** (mag-nōl′yah) The bark of various species of *Magnolia* (family Magnoliaceae), sweet bay; swamp laurel; beaver tree; shrubs and trees of the eastern coast of North America. Formerly used as a bitter tonic and diaphoretic.

**mag′num** [ L. *magnus,* large ]. *Os* capitatum.

**Magnus,** Rudolph, German physiologist, 1873–1927. See M.'s *sign* (of death).

**mag′nus** [ L. ] [ NA ]. Large; great; denoting a structure of large size.

**Magovern-Cromie prosthesis.** See under prosthesis.

**Maher** (ma′her), J. J. E., New York physician, 1857–1931. See M.'s *disease.*

**Mah′ler,** Richter A., German obstetrician, 19th century. See M.'s *sign.*

**Ma-huang** (mah-hwahng) [ Chinese ]. *Ephedra equisetina.*

**maidenhead** (ma′den-hed). The hymen; virginity.

**maidism** (ma′dizm) [ *Zea mays,* maize ]. Pellagra.

**Maier,** Rudolf, German physician, 1824–1888. See M.'s *sinus.*

**maieusiomania** (mi-u-sĭ-o-ma′nĭ-ah) [ G. *maieusis,* childbirth, + *mania,* frenzy ]. Puerperal *insanity.*

**maieusiophobia** (mi-u-sĭ-o-fo′bĭ-ah) [ G. *maieusis,* childbirth, + *phobos,* fear ]. Extreme dread of childbirth.

**maieutics** (mi-u′tiks) [ G. *maieusis,* childbirth or midwifery, fr. *maia,* mother, midwife ]. Obsolete term for obstetrics.

**maim** (mām). 1. To disable or cripple by an injury. 2. A hurt; injury; trauma.

**Maimonides** or **Moses ben Maimon** (mi-mon′id-ēz), Jewish physician (1135–1208) of the Arabian period; court physician to the Sultan Saladin; he wrote a work on health (*Book of Counsel*) and a tract on poisons.

**main** (man) [ Fr. ]. Hand.

**m. d′accoucheur,** accoucheur's *hand.*

**m. en crochet** (oń krō-sha′), a permanent flexure of the fourth and fifth fingers, resembling the hand of a woman crocheting with three fingers bent to guide the thread.

**m. en griffe,** griffin-claw *hand.*

**m. fourché,** cleft *hand.*

**m. succulente** (sü-kü-lont′), edema of the hand.

**maintainer** (mān-ta′ner). A device utilized to hold or keep teeth in a given position.

**space m.,** space retainer; an orthodontic appliance used to prevent the loss of space or the shifting of teeth following extraction or premature loss of teeth.

**maise oil** (māz) (BP). Corn oil.

**Maissiat** (may-se-ā), Jacques H., Paris anatomist, 1805–1878. See M.'s *band*.

**Majocchi** (mah-yok'ke), Domenico, Italian dermatologist, 1849–1929. See M.'s *disease*.

**ma'jor** [ L. comparative of *magnus*, great ] [ NA ]. Larger or greater in size of two similar structures.

**Makeham's hypothesis.** See under hypothesis.

**Maklakoff,** C., Russian ophthalmologist. See M. applanation *tonometer*.

**mal** (mahl) [ Fr. fr. L. *malum*, an evil ]. A disease or disorder; an evil.

**m. comitial** (kŭ-me-se-al'), epilepsy.

**m. de caderas,** a disease of horses in some South American countries, due to *Trypanosoma equinum*. The disease is manifested by emaciation, remittent fever, weakness (especially of the hind quarters, from which the disease gets its name), and eventually death. The trypanosome has a reservoir in a wild animal, the capybara. Cattle, sheep, and goats are only mildly affected. Man is not involved.

**m. de Cayenne,** elephantiasis.

**m. de la rosa, m. rosso,** pellagra.

**m. de los pintos,** pinta.

**m. de Meleda** (ma-la'dah), endemic symmetrical keratodermia of the extremities occurring on the island of Meleda off the coast of Dalmatia.

**m. de mer,** seasickness.

**m. de San Laz'aro,** elephantiasis.

**grand m.** (grahṅ), generalized *epilepsy*.

**haut m.** (o') [ Fr. high ], generalized *epilepsy*.

**m. morado,** onchocerciasis.

**m. perforant,** perforating ulcer of the foot; see under ulcer.

**m. perforant' palatin** (pă-lă-taṅ'), a perforating ulcer of the roof of the mouth opening into the nasal cavity.

**petit m.** (pĕ-te') [ Fr. small ], see petit mal *epilepsy*.

**mal-** [ L. *malus*, bad. MAL- ]. Combining form meaning ill or bad.

**mala** (ma'lah) [ L. cheek bone ]. 1 [ NA ]. Cheek. 2. *Os zygomaticum*.

**mal'abar nut.** Adhatoda.

**mal'absorp'tion.** Imperfect, inadequate or otherwise disordered gastrointestinal absorption.

**Malacarne** (mah-lah-car'na), Michele V. G., Italian surgeon, 1744–1816. See M.'s *pyramid, space*.

**malachite green** (mal'ă-kīt) [ G. *malachē*, a mallow ]. Tetramethyl-di-*p*-aminotriphenylcarbinol; a dye that has been used as a wound antiseptic and in the treatment of mycotic skin infections.

**malacia** (mă-la'shĭ-ah) [ G. *malakia*, a softness. MALAC- ]. Malacoma; malacosis; mollities; a softening or loss of consistency and contiguity in any of the organs or tissues. Also used as combining form in suffix position.

**metaplastic m.,** *osteitis* fibrosa cystica.

**myeloplastic m.,** *osteogenesis* imperfecta.

**malacic** (mă-la'sik). Malacotic.

**malaco-** [ G. *malakos*, soft; *malakia*, a softness. MALAC- ]. Combining form meaning soft or softening.

**malacoma** (mal'ă-ko'mah) [ malaco- + G. suffix *-oma*, tumor ]. Malacia.

**malacoplakia** (mal'ă-ko-pla'kĭ-ah) [ malaco- + G. *plax*, plate, plaque ]. Malakoplakia; a rare lesion in the mucous of the urinary bladder, more frequently in women; characterized by numerous mottled, yellow and gray, soft plaques and nodules that consist of numerous macrophages and calcospherites (Michaelis-Guttmann bodies). The condition is most likely to occur in malnourished persons, in association with coliform infections, tuberculosis, or sarcoid.

**malacosis** (mal'ă-ko'sis). Malacia.

**malacosteon** (mal'ă-kos'te-on) [ malaco- + G. *osteon*, bone ]. Osteomalacia.

**malacotic** (mal'ă-kot'ik). Pertaining to or characterized by malacia.

**malacotomy** (mal'ă-kot'o-mĭ) [ malaco- + G. *tomē*, incision ]. Incision of soft parts, especially of the abdominal wall.

**malactic** (mă-lak'tik) [ G. *malaktikos*, softening ]. Emollient.

**maladie** (mal'ah-de') [ Fr. ]. Malady.

**m. de Roger** [ Fr. ], Roger's *disease*.

**m. du coit** (mal-ă-de' dü ko-e')[ Fr. disease from coitus ], dourine.

**mal'adjust'ment.** In the mental health professions, an inability to cope with the problems and challenges of everyday living.

**social m.,** m. without manifest psychiatric disorder, as that occasioned by cultural shock or conflict.

**malady** (mal'ă-dĭ) [ Fr. *maladie*, illness ]. Disease; illness; especially a chronic, usually fatal, disease.

**malagma** (mă-lag'mah) [ G. a poultice. MALAC- ]. A cataplasm or emollient.

**malaise** (mă-lāz') [ Fr. discomfort ]. A feeling of general discomfort or uneasiness, an out-of-sorts feeling, often the first indication of an infection or other disease.

**mal'akopla'kia.** Malacoplakia.

**ma'lar.** Relating to the mala, the cheek or cheek bones.

**malaria** (mă-la'rĭ-ah, mă-lăr'ĭ-ah) [ It. *malo* (fem. *mala*), bad, + *aria*, air, referring to the old theory of the miasmatic origin of the disease. MAL- ]. Marsh fever; paludal fever; jungle fever; a disease caused by the presence of a haemosporidian protozoan parasite (*Plasmodium*) of the red blood cells. The disease is transmitted by the bite of an infected femal mosquito of the genus *Anopheles*, which has previously sucked the blood of a person suffering from m. The parasite has a sexual cycle in the body of the mosquito followed by production of sporozoites which collect in the salivary glands (gametogeny and then sporogeny), and an exoerythrocytic schizogenous cycle in the liver cells of the human host, followed by a series of erythrocytic schizogenous cycles repeated at regular intervals; production of gametocytes in other red cells provides the future gametes for another mosquito infection. See also *Plasmodium* species.

**acute m.,** may be intermittent or remittent; a malarial attack or paroxysm consists of a chill accompanied and followed by fever with its attendant general symptoms, and terminates in a sweating stage; the paroxysms, caused by release of merozoites from infected cells, recur every 48 hours in tertian (vivax or ovale) m., every 72 hours in quartan (malariae) m., and at indefinite but frequent intervals, usually about 48 hours, in malignant tertian (falciparum) m.

**autochthonous m.,** disease acquired by mosquito transmission in an area where m. regularly occurs.

**avian m.,** plasmodial infections of domestic and wild birds, transmitted chiefly by culicine mosquitoes.

**benign tertian m.,** vivax m.

**bilious remittent m.,** a form of m. characterized by bilious vomiting, bilious diarrhea, etc.

**chronic m.,** malarial cachexia; develops after frequently repeated attacks of one of the acute forms, usually falciparum m. It is characterized by profound anemia, enlargement of the spleen, emaciation, mental depression, sallow complexion, edema of ankles, feeble digestion, and muscular weakness.

**m. comatosa,** falciparum m. complicated by coma.

**double tertian m.,** see quotidian m.

**falciparum m.,** malignant tertian fever or malaria; aestivoautumnal fever; falciparum fever; caused by *Plasmodium falciparum*, the most pathogenic malarial parasite of man; 48-hour malarial paroxysms of severe form with acute cerebral or renal manifestations in severe cases, chiefly caused by the large number of red blood cells affected and the tendency for infected red cells to become sticky and clump, blocking capillaries.

**imported m.,** m. acquired outside of a given specific area (such as the United States).

**induced m.,** m. acquired by artificial means, such as *via* blood transfusion, common syringes, or malariotherapy.

**intermittent m.,** a malarial fever, usually of the tertian or quartan type, in which there is complete apyrexia, with absence of the other symptoms, in the intervals between the paroxysms.

**introduced m.,** disease acquired by mosquito transmission from an imported case in an area where m. is not a regular occurrence.

**malariae m.,** quartan m.; quartan fever; a malarial fever the paroxysms of which recur every 72 hours, or fourth day, reckoning the day of the paroxysm as the first; due to the schizogeny and invasion of new red blood corpuscles by the sporozoan blood protozoan, *Plasmodium malariae.*

**nonan m.,** a malarial fever the paroxysms of which occur every ninth day, *i.e.,* every eighth day following the preceding paroxysm, the day of each paroxysm being included in the computation.

**ovale m., ovale tertian m.,** m. caused by *Plasmodium ovale.*

**pernicious m.,** falciparum m. in which the symptoms are severe and are complicated by gastroenteric, hemorrhagic, or cerebral disturbances.

**quartan m.,** malariae m.

**quotidian m.,** quotidian fever; m. in which the paroxysms occur daily; it is usually a double tertian, in which there is an infection by two distinct groups of *Plasmodium vivax* parasites sporulating alternately every 48 hours, but may also be an infection by the pernicious form of malarial parasite, *Plasmodium falciparum,* combined with *Plasmodium vivax,* or infection by two distinct *P. falciparum* generations.

**relapsing m.,** renewal of clinical activity at some interval after the primary attack.

**remittent m.,** a malarial fever, usually of the severer falciparum type, in which the temperature falls more or less but not to the normal in the interval between two pronounced paroxysms.

**simian m.,** plasmodial infections of monkeys, as with human m., transmitted chiefly by anopheline mosquitoes. A number of species are recognized, especially in southeast Asia and Africa; among these are species that appear identical with the four human forms and may be derived from them.

**tertian m.,** vivax m.

**vivax m.,** tertian or benign tertian m.; tertian or vivax fever; a malarial fever the paroxysms of which recur every 48 hours or every other day (every third day, reckoning the day of the paroxysm as the first). It is caused by the sporulation and invasion of new red blood corpuscles by the sporozoan protozoan blood parasite, *Plasmodium vivax.*

**malarial** (mă-la′rĭ-al, mă-lăr′ĭ-al). Pertaining to or affected with malaria.

**malariology** (mă-la-rĭ-ol′o-jĭ). A study of malaria in all its relations.

**malariotherapy** (mă-la′rĭ-o-thĕr′ă-pĭ). Treatment of syphilitic and other affections by inoculation with malarial organisms; no longer used.

**malarious** (mă-la′rĭ-us, mă-lăr′ĭ-us). Relating to or characterized by the prevalence of malaria.

**Malassez** (mal-ah-sa′), Louis C., French physiologist, 1842–1910. See M.'s *stain,* M.'s epithelial *rests.*

**Malassezia furfur.** A fungus which causes tinea versicolor (pityriasis versicolor); the proper name for *Microsporon furfur.*

**mal′assimila′tion.** Incomplete or faulty assimilation.

**mal′ate.** A salt or ester of malic acid.

**malate-condensing enzyme.** Malate synthase.

**mal′ate dehydrogenase.** An enzyme that catalyzes, through NAD or NADP, the dehydrogenation of malate to oxaloacetate or its decarboxylation to pyruvate. At least six are known (EC 1.1.1.37–.40, 1.1.1.82–.83); they are distinguished by their products, use of NAD or NADP, and specificity of substrate. Other names include malic acid dehydrogenase; "malic" enzyme; pyruvic-malic carboxylase; malic dehydrogenase.

**mal′ate synthase** (EC 4.1.3.2). Malate-condensing enzyme; glyoxylate transacetase; an enzyme catalyzing the condensation of acetyl-CoA with glyoxylate to form malate.

**malathion** (mal′ă-thi′on, mă-la′thĭ-on). *S*-(1,2-Dicarboxyethyl) *O,O*-dimethyldithiophosphate; an organophosphorous compound used as an insecticide and veterinary ectoparasiticide; considered to be less toxic than parathion.

**malaxation** (mal′ak-sa′shun) [ L. *malaxo,* pp. -*atus,* to soften. MALAC- ]. 1. The formation of ingredients into a

mass for pills and plasters. 2. A kneading process in massage.

**mal′diges′tion.** Imperfect digestion.

**male** (māl) [ L. *masculus,* fr. *mas,* male ]. 1. In zoology, denoting the sex to which those belong that produce spermatozoa; an individual of the male sex. 2. Masculine.

**genetic m.,** (1) an individual with a normal m. karyotype, including one X and one Y chromosome; see fig. under karyotype; (2) an individual whose cell nuclei do not contain Barr sex chromatin bodies, which are normally present in females and absent in m.'s; patients with ambiguous sexual development and those with Turner's syndrome and classed as genetic m.'s or genetic females by absence or presence of Barr bodies even though their sex chromosome complement may be abnormal.

**maleic acid** (mă-le′ik) (BP). The *cis* isomer of fumaric acid; used for preparing maleat salts of antihistaminics and similar drugs.

$$\begin{array}{c} \text{CHCOOH} \\ \| \\ \text{CHCOOH} \end{array}$$

Maleic acid

**malemission** (mal′e-mish′un) [ mal- + L. *e-mitto,* pp. *missus,* to send out ]. Failure of the semen to be ejected from the penis in coitus.

**Malerba** (mahl-er′bah), Pasquale, Italian physician, 1849–1917. See M.'s *test.*

**mal′erup′tion.** Faulty eruption of teeth.

**mal′forma′tion.** Failure of proper or normal development.

**Arnold-Chiari m.,** Arnold-Chiari *deformity.*

**mal′func′tion.** Disordered, inadequate or abnormal function.

**Malgaigne** (mal-gān′yuh), Joseph F., Paris surgeon, 1806–1865. See M.'s *amputation, apparatus, fossa, hernia, hooks, luxation, triangle.*

**Malherbe,** A. See M.'s *disease,* calcifying *epithelioma.*

**malic acid** (mal′ik, ma′lik). Hydroxysuccinic acid; HOOCCH$_2$CHOHCOOH; an acid found in apples and various other tart fruits; an intermediate in the tricarboxylic acid cycle.

**malic acid dehydrogenase.** Malate dehydrogenase.

**malic dehydrogenase.** Malate dehydrogenase.

**"malic" enzyme.** Malate dehydrogenase.

**malignancy** (mă-lig′nan-sĭ). The property or condition of being malignant.

**malignant** (mă-lig′nant) [ L. *maligno,* pres. p. -*ans* (*ant-*), to do anything maliciously. MAL- ]. Resistant to treatment; occurring in severe form, and frequently fatal; tending to become worse and lead to an ingravescent course; in the case of a neoplasm, having the property of uncontrollable growth and dissemination, or recurrence after removal, or both.

**malig′nin.** A presumed intracellular substance that was formerly postulated as the chief factor in certain neoplastic cells being malignant, inasmuch as it manifested a digestive action on normal tissue.

**malinger** (mă-ling′ger) [ Fr. *malingre,* poor, weakly. MAL- ]. To sham; to feign an illness, usually in order to escape work, excite sympathy, or gain compensation.

**malingerer** (mă-ling′ger-er). One who feigns illness.

**malingering** (mă-ling′ger-ing). Feigning illness.

**malinterdigitation** (mal′in-ter-dij′ĭ-ta′shun). Faulty intercuspation of teeth.

**Mall,** Franklin P., American anatomist and embryologist, 1862–1917. See M.'s *formula, ridge,* periportal *space.*

**malleable** (mal′e-ă-bl) [ L. *malleus,* a hammer ]. Capable of being shaped by being beaten or by pressure; a property of certain metals such as gold and silver.

**malleation** (mal′e-a′shun) [ L. *malleus,* a hammer ]. A sort of hammering movement of the hands against the thighs, a form of tic.

**mallebrin.** Aluminum chlorate nonahydrate.

**mallein** (mal'e-in). A product analogous to tuberculin but made from the growth products of the organism of glanders (*Actinobacillus mallei*). It is an allergen used to provoke reactions in animals affected with glanders—a diagnostic agent.

**malleinization** (mal'e-in'ĭ-za'shun). Inoculation with mallein.

**malleoincudal** (mal'e-o-ing'ku-dal). Relating to the malleus and the incus in the tympanum.

**malleolar** (mă-le'o-lar). Relating to one or both malleoli.

**malleolus, pl. malle'oli** (mă-le'o-lus) [ L. dim. of *malleus*, hammer ] [ NA ]. A rounded bony prominence such as those on either side of the ankle joint.
   **m. latera'lis** [ NA ], lateral m.; extramalleolus; external or outer m.; the process at the lateral side of the lower end of the fibula, forming the projection of the lateral part of the ankle.
   **m. media'lis** [ NA ], medial m.; internal or inner m.; the process at the medial side of the lower end of the tibia, forming the projection of the medial side of the ankle.

**Malleomy'ces.** *Pseudomonas.*
   **M. mallei,** *Pseudomonas mallei;* type species of the genus *M.*
   **M. pseudomallei,** *Pseudomonas pseudomallei.*

**malleotomy** (mal'e-ot'o-mĭ) [ malleus + G. *tomē*, incision ]. 1. Division of the malleus. 2. Division of the ligaments holding the malleoli in apposition in order to permit their separation in certain cases of clubfoot.

**malleus, gen. and pl. mallei** (mal'e-us, mal'e-i) [ L. a hammer ] [ NA ]. Hammer; the largest of the three auditory ossicles, resembling a club rather than a hammer; it is regarded as having a head or capit, below which is the neck or collum, and from this diverge the handle or manubrium, and the slender, anterior process; from the base or the manubrium the short lateral process arises. The manubrium and lateral process are firmly attached to the tympanic membrane, and the head articulates with a saddle-shaped surface on the body of the incus.

**Mallophaga** (mă-lof'ă-gah) [ G. *mallos*, wool, + *phagein*, to eat ]. An order of biting lice that cause irritation by feeding on hair, feathers, and skin, and on blood and exudates when present; most species are found on birds, but some are found on common domestic animals.

**Mallory,** Frank B., American pathologist, 1862–1941. See M. *bodies, stains.*

**Mallory,** G. Kenneth, American pathologist, *1926. See M.-Weiss *syndrome.*

**Mallory leukemia.** See under leukemia.

**malnutrition** (mal-nu-trish'un). Faulty nutrition resulting from malassimilation, poor diet, or overeating.
   **malignant m.,** kwashiorkor.

**malocclusion** (mal'o-klu'zhun). 1. Any deviation from a physiologically acceptable contact of opposing dentitions. 2. Any deviation from a normal occlusion.

**malonic acid** (mă-lo'nik, mă-lon'ik). HOOC—CH₂— COOH; a dicarboxylic acid of importance in intermediary metabolism.

**malonic mononitrile.** Cyanoacetic acid.

**mal'onyl.** The radical derived from malonic acid.
   **m. transacylase,** an enzyme (EC 2.3.1.39) transferring malonyl from malonyl-CoA to ACP; a key step in fatty acid synthesis.

**malonylurea** (mal'o-nil-u-re'ah). Barbituric acid.

**mal'oplasty** [ L. *mala*, cheek, + G. *plassō*, to form ]. Genyplasty; plastic surgery of the cheek.

**Malpighi** (mahl-pe'ge), Marcello, Italian anatomist, histrologist, and embryologist, 1628–1694. His many fundamental discoveries in the minute structure of animals and plants entitle him to be called the founder of histology. His observations in embryology were also outstanding. See Malpighian *body, canal, capsule, corpuscle, gland, glomerulus, layer, nodule, pyramid, rete, stigmas, stratum, tuft, tubules, vesicles.*

**malposition** (mal-po-zish'un). Faulty or abnormal position of a part or of the body.

**mal'prac'tice.** Mistreatment of a disease or injury through ignorance, carelessness, or criminal intent.

**malprax'is.** Malpractice.

**mal'presenta'tion.** Faulty presentation of the fetus; presentation of any part other than the occiput.

**mal'rota'tion.** Failure during embryonic development of normal rotation of all or any portion of the intestinal tract.

**malt** (mawlt) [ A.S. *mealt* ]. The seed of barley or other grain, artificially germinated and dried, containing dextrin, maltose, small amounts of glucose, and amylolytic enzymes. Used in the form of an extract as a digestive and flavoring agent.

**maltase** (mawl-tās). α-Glucosidase.
   **acid m.,** exo-1,4-α-glucosidase.

**maltose** (mawl-tōs). Malt sugar; 4-(α-D-glucosido)-D-glucose; a disaccharide formed in the hydrolysis of starch and consisting of two glucose residues bound by a 1,4-α-glycoside link.

**mal'totet'rose.** A saccharide made up of four glucose units in the α-1,4 linkage.

**ma'lum** [ L. an evil ]. A disease.
   **m. artic'ulorum seni'lis,** arthritis in the aged.
   **m. caducum,** epilepsy.
   **m. cordis,** heart disease.
   **m. coxae,** disease of the hip.
   **m. cox'ae seni'le,** senile hip disease; deformity of the head of the femur caused by ischemic damage.
   **m. minus,** petit mal *epilepsy.*
   **m. per'forans pe'dis,** perforating ulcer of the foot; see under ulcer.
   **m. vene'reum,** syphilis.
   **m. vertebra'le suboccipita'le,** Rust's *disease.*

**malunion** (mal-ūn'yun). Incomplete union, or union in a faulty position, after fracture or a wound of the soft parts.

**Maly** (mah'le), Richard L., Austrian physiological chemist, 1839–1894. See M.'s *test.*

**mamanpian** (mă-moń-pe-oń'). Yaw.

**mamelon** (mam'ē-lon) [ Fr. nipple ]. One of the rounded prominences, three in number, on the cutting edge of an incisor tooth when it first pierces the gum.

**mam'elonated** [ Fr. *mamelon*, nipple ]. Having rounded, teatlike elevations; nodulated.

**mam'elonation.** The formation of rounded projections or nodules on bony and other structures.

**mamil-, mamilli-** [ L. *mamilla*, nipple ]. Combining forms relating to the mamillae; for words beginning thus, see also mammil-, mammilli-.

**mamilla, pl. mamil'lae** (mă-mil'ah) [ L. nipple ]. 1 [ NA ]. A small rounded elevation resembling the female breast. 2. *Papilla mammae.*

**mamilla're** [ L. ] [ NA ]. Mamillary.

**mamilla'ria.** See *corpus* mamillare.

**mam'illary.** Relating to or shaped like a nipple.

**mam'illate, mam'illated.** Studded with nipple-like projections.

**mamilla'tion.** 1. A nipple-like projection. 2. The condition of being mamillated.

**mamil'liform** [ L. *mamilla*, nipple, + *forma*, form ]. Nipple-shaped.

**mamma, gen. and pl. mammae** (mam'ah, mam'e) [ L. ] [ NA ]. Breast; mammary gland; the organ of milk secretion; one of two large hemispheric projections situated in the subcutaneous layer over the pectoralis major muscle on either side of the chest; it is rudimentary in the male. See *glandula* mammaria.
   **m. accesso'ria** [ NA ], accessory breast; supernumerary m.; a milk secreting gland located elsewhere than at the normal place on the chest and existing in addition to the two usual mammae.
   **m. errat'ica,** a supernumerary breast aberrantly located, *i.e.,* in some part other than the milk line.
   **m. masculina** [ NA ], male breast; m. virilis; one of the two, usually rudimentary, mammary glands in the male.
   **m. viri'lis,** m. masculina.

**mam'mal.** An animal of the class Mammalia.

**mammalgia** (mă-mal'jĭ-ah) [ L. *mamma*, breast, + G. *algos*, pain ]. Mastodynia.

**Mammalia** (mă-ma'lĭ-ah) [ L. *mamma*, breast ]. The highest class of living organisms; it includes all the vertebrate animals (monotremes, marsupials, and placentals) that suckle their young, possess hair, and (except for the egg-laying monotremes) bring forth living young rather than eggs.

**mam'maplasty.** Mammoplasty.

**mam'mary.** Relating to the breasts.

**mammectomy** (mă-mek'to-mĭ) [ L. *mamma*, breast, + *ektomē*, excision ]. Mastectomy.

**mam'miform** [ L. *mamma*, breast, + *forma*, form ]. Resembling a breast; breast-shaped.

**mammil-, mammilli-** [ L. *mammilla (mamilla)*, nipple ]. Combining forms relating to the mamillae; for words beginning thus, see also mamil-, mamilli-.

**mammillaplasty** (mă-mil'ă-plas-tĭ) [ L. *mammilla*, nipple, + G. *plassō*, to form ]. Theleplasty.

**mammillitis** (mam'ĭ-li'tis) [ L. *mamilla*, nipple, + G. suffix *-itis*, inflammation ]. Thelitis.

**mammitis** (mă-mi'tis) [ L. *mamma*, breast, + G. suffix *-itis*, inflammation ]. Mastitis.

**mammo-** [ L. *mamma*, breast ]. Combining form relating to the breasts.

**mammogens I and II** (mam'o-jen) [ mammo- + G. suffix *-gen*, producing ]. See mammogenic *hormones*.

**mam'mogram.** Roentgenogram of the breast.

**mammography** (mă-mog'ră-fĭ) [ mammo- + G. *graphō*, to write ]. Roentgenographic examination of the breast.

**mam'moplasty** [ mammo- + G. *plassō*, to mold ]. Mammaplasty; an operation for the correction of sagging pendulous breasts or inadequate breasts; it consists of excision of skin and glandular tissue and fixation of the glands in their normal positions.

**mam'mose.** 1. Mammiform. 2. Having large breasts.

**mammotomy** (mă-mot'o-mĭ) [ mammo- + G. *tomē*, incision ]. Mastotomy.

**mammotroph** (mam'o-trof). A cell of the adenohypophysis that produces an effect in the mammary glands.

**mammotrophic** (mam'o-trof'ik) [ mammo- + G. *trophē*, nourishment ]. Mammotropic.

**mammotropic** (mam'o-trop'ik) [ mammo- + G *tropos*, a turning ]. Mammotrophic; having a stimulating effect upon the development, growth, or function of the mammary glands.

**mam'motro'pin, mam'motro'phin.** Obsolete term for prolactin.

**Man.** Symbol for mannose or its radicals in polysaccharides.

**manaca** (man'ă-kah) [ Braz. ]. Vegetable mercury; the dried root of *Brunfelsia hopeana*, or *Francisca uniflora* (family Solanaceae), a plant of Brazil lowlands. Has been used in rheumatism and syphilis.

**Manchester ovoid.** See under ovoid.

**manchette** (män-shet') [ Fr. ]. A circular band formed mainly of microtubules at the caudal pole of the nucleus of a developing spermatozoon.

**manco'na bark.** Erythrophleum.

**man'delate.** A salt or ester of mandelic acid.

**mandel'ic acid.** Phenylglycolic acid; hydroxytoluic acid; $C_6H_5CHOHCOOH$; a urinary antibacterial agent (both bactericidal and bacteriostatic).

**Mandelin's reagent.** See under reagent.

**mandelytropine.** Homatropine.

**mandible** (man'dĭ-bl). Mandibula.

**mandibula,** pl. **mandib'ulae** (man-dib'u-lah) [ L. a jaw, fr. *mando*, pp. *mansus*, to chew ] [ NA ]. Mandible; mandibulum; jaw bone; inferior jaw; a U-shaped bone, forming the lower jaw, articulating by its upturned extremities with the temporal bone on either side.

**mandib'ular.** Relating to the lower jaw.

**mandibulectomy** (man-dib'u-lek'to-mĭ) [ mandibula + G. *ektomē*, excision ]. Excision of the lower jaw.

**mandib'ulofa'cial.** Relating to the mandible and the face.

**mandib'ulo-oc'ulofa'cial.** Relating to the mandible and the orbital part of the face.

**mandibulopharyngeal** (man-dib'u-lo-fă-rin'je-al). Relating to the mandible and the pharynx; denoting a space between the pharynx and the ramus of the mandible, in which are found the internal carotid artery, the internal

jugular vein, and the vagus, glossopharyngeal, accessory, and hypoglossal nerves.

**mandib'ulum.** Mandibula.

**mandragora** (man-drag'o-rah) [ G. *mandragoras* ]. The European mandrake, *Mandragora officinalis*, or *Atropa mandragora* (family Solanaceae), the mandrake of the Bible. Its properties are similar to those of stramonium, hyoscyamus, and belladonna.

**mandrag'orine.** A mydriatic alkaloid from mandragora, similar to atropine and scopolamine.

**man'drake** [ thr. L. fr. G. *mandragoras* ]. 1. Mandragora. 2. Podophyllum.

**man'drel, man'dril** [ G. *mandra*, a stable; the bed in which a ring's stone is set ]. 1. The shaft, spindle, or handle to which a tool is attached and by means of which it is rotated. 2. Mandrin.

**man'drill.** Common name for a species of monkey of the genus *Cynocephalus*, with a short tail and stout, doglike head.

**man'drin** [ Fr. *mandrin*, mandrel ]. Mandrel (2); a stiff wire inserted in the lumen of a soft catheter in order to give it shape and firmness while passing through the urethra.

**maneuver** (mă-nu'ver) [ Fr. *manoeuvre*, fr. L. *manu operari*, to work by hand ]. A planned movement or procedure.

    **Adelmann's m.,** forcible flexion of the extremities to arrest arterial hemorrhage.

    **Bill's m.,** forceps rotation of the head before attempting to bring the head down.

    **Bracht m.,** in a breech presentation, a procedure to extract the head.

    **Brandt-Andrews m.,** the expression of the placenta by grasping the umbilical cord with one hand and placing the other hand on the abdomen, with the fingers over the anterior surface of the uterus at the junction of the lower uterine segment and the corpus uteri.

    **Buzzard's m.,** testing the patellar reflex while the sitting patient makes firm pressure on the floor with the toes.

    **Credé's m.'s,** Credé's *methods*.

    **Giffard's m.,** to flex the aftercoming head, one or two fingers are placed in the baby's mouth while traction is exerted with the other hand upon the shoulders.

    **Hampton m.,** rolling a supine patient on his right and then left side to obtain an air contrast x-ray film of the antrum and duodenum in gastrointestinal fluoroscopy.

    **Hillis m.,** the impression maneuver is pressure on the fundus while a finger in the rectum determines the descent of the head into the pelvis (engagement).

    **Hueter's m.,** in passing a stomach tube one presses the patient's tongue downward and forward with the left forefinger.

    **Jendrassik's m.,** a method of emphasizing the patellar reflex: the subject hooks his hands together by the flexed fingers and pulls against them with all his strength.

    **key-in-lock m.,** DeLee's operation; a method by which obstetrical forceps are used to rotate the fetal head.

    **Leopold's m.'s,** four m.'s employed to determine fetal position: The first m. determines what is in the fundus; the second evaluates the fetal back and small parts; the third palpates the presenting part above the symphysis; the fourth determines the direction and degree of flexion of the head.

    **Mauriceau's m.,** Mauriceau-Levret m.; a method of assisted breech delivery in which the infant's body is astraddle the right forearm, and the middle finger of the right hand is in the fetal mouth to maintain flexion while traction is made upon the shoulders by the other hand.

    **Mauriceau-Levret m.,** Mauriceau's m.

    **McDonald's m.,** measurement of uterus from the upper border of the symphysis to a line tangential to the fundus over the abdomen with a tape to determine the height of the uterus. This figure divided by 3.5 gives the approximate age of the fetus in lunar months.

    **Müller's m.,** (1) pressure is made on the fetal head while a finger in the vagina determines whether the head will enter the pelvis; (2) Müller's *experiment*.

    **Osiander's m.,** Saxtorph m.

    **Pajot's m.,** Saxtorph m.

    **Pinard's m.,** in management of a frank breech, pressure on the popliteal space is made by the index finger while the other three fingers flex the leg while wiping it along the other thigh as the foot is brought down and out.

**Prague m.,** a procedure for extracting the aftercoming head.

**Ritgen's m.,** delivery of a child's head by pressure on the perineum while controlling the speed of delivery by pressure with the other hand on the head.

**Saxtorph m.,** Osiander's m.; Pajot's m.; traction downward on forceps lock with one hand while traction is made with the other hand so that the head is brought down in the axis of the birth canal.

**Scanzoni's m.,** forceps rotation and traction in a spiral course, with reapplication of forceps for delivery.

**Sellick's m.,** pressure applied to the cricoid cartilage, to prevent regurgitation during endotracheal intubation in the anesthetized patient.

**Valsalva m.,** (1) Valsalva experiment; forced expiratory effort with closed nose and mouth to inflate the Eustachian tubes and middle ears; *e.g.,* as used by persons descending from high altitudes; (2) any forced expiratory effort against a closed airway, whether at the nose and mouth or at the glottis, the reverse of Müller's *experiment;* because high intrathoracic pressure impedes venous return to the right atrium, this m. is used to study cardiovascular effects of raised peripheral venous pressure and decreased cardiac filling and cardiac output.

**Wigand m.,** an assisted breech delivery with pressure above the symphysis while the fetus lies astraddle the operator's other arm.

**manganese** (mang'gă-nēz) [ Mod. L. *manganesium, manganum,* an altered form of *magnesium.* MAG- ]. A metallic element resembling, and often associated in ores with iron; symbol Mn, atomic no. 25, atomic weight 54.94. Manganous salts are sometimes used in medicine.

**m. citrate, soluble,** m. and sodium citrate; manganous citrate rendered soluble by means of sodium citrate; said to increase the hematinic effect of iron.

**m. hypophosphite,** manganous hypophosphite; formerly used as a hematinic.

**m. lactate,** pale reddish crystals, soluble in water; has been used in anemia.

**m. sulfate,** manganous sulfate; light pinkish, prismatic crystals, freely soluble in water; used as a preventive against perosis.

**mangan'ic.** Denoting the trivalent cation of manganese, Mn$^{3+}$.

**manganous** (mang'gă-nus). Denoting the divalent cation of manganese, Mn$^{2+}$.

**man'ganum** [ L. ]. Manganese.

**mange** (mānj) [ Fr. *manger,* to eat ]. A cutaneous disease of domestic and wild animals caused by any one of several genera of skin burrowing mites. In man, this condition is called scabies or itch.

**chorioptic m.,** m. caused by mites of the genus *Chorioptes;* in many cases it involves the skin of much of the body.

**demodectic m.,** follicular m.; an infection of the hair follicles and sebaceous glands with *Demodex folliculorum;* it occurs in man and a number of domesticated animals; although it causes a benign disease in most species, this organism can cause severe and extensive dermatitis ("red mange") in dogs.

**ear m.,** otodectic m.

**follicular m.,** demodectic m.

**foot m.,** chorioptic m. affecting only the foot regions.

**notoedric m.,** m. of cats caused by the mite, *Notoedres cati.*

**otodectic m.,** ear m.; disease resulting from heavy infestation with *Otodectes cynotis* in the ears of dogs, cats, foxes, and other carnivores and manifested by head shaking, continual ear scratching, and ear droop; observed in severe cases are torticollis, circling, epileptoid fits with purulent inflammation and discharge of the external ear, and possible perforation of the tympanic membrane. See also otoacariasis.

**psoroptic m.,** psoroptic itch; hair loss or m. caused by infestation with *Psoroptes,* the scale-eating mites.

**red m.,** demodectic m. in dogs.

**sarcop'tic m.,** sarcoptic itch; a cutaneous disease due to the itch mite, *Sarcoptes scabiei.*

**mania** (ma'nĭ-ah) [ G. frenzy ]. An emotional disorder characterized by great psychomotor activity, excitement, a rapid passing of ideas, exaltation, and unstable attention.

**alcoholic m.,** acute excitement due to excessive intake of alcohol; sometimes used synonymously with delirium tremens.

**m. à po'tu,** an acute m. associated with hallucinations, due to chronic alcoholic poisoning; see also alcoholic m. and delirium tremens.

**dancing m.,** see chorea.

**doubting m.,** *folie* du doute.

**epileptic m.,** manic excitement in a person afflicted with epilepsy; often associated with destructive behavior.

**peracute m.,** acute maniacal excitement; see under excitement.

**puer'peral m.,** postpartum *psychosis.*

**religious m.,** m. with display of religious ideas and emotions.

**transitory m.,** manic excitement of short duration.

**unproductive m.,** a behavior exhibiting a lack of spontaneity in speech, and occasional muteness; sometimes observed in manic-depressive psychosis.

**-mania** [ G. frenzy ]. Combining form used in the suffix position, usually referring to an abnormal love for, or morbid impulse toward, some specific object, place, or action (*e.g.,* megalomania, kleptomania).

**maniac** (ma'nĭ-ak). 1. One suffering from mania. 2. An obsolete term for a mentally ill or disturbed person.

**maniacal** (ma-ni'ă-kal). Relating to or characterized by mania; wild; furious.

**manic** (man'ik, ma'nik). Relating to mania; frenzied.

**manic-depressive.** 1. Pertaining to manic-depressive *psychosis* (*q.v.*). 2. One suffering from manic-depressive psychosis.

**man'icy.** Behavior characteristic of the manic phase of manic-depressive psychosis.

**man'ifesta'tion.** In medicine, the display or disclosure of characteristic signs or symptoms of an illness.

**behavioral m.,** a m. characterized by defects in personality structure with minimal anxiety and little or no sense of distress, indicative of a psychiatric disorder; occasionally encephalitis or head injury will produce the clinical picture which is properly diagnosed as chronic brain disorder with behavioral m.'s.

**neurotic m.,** a m. characterized by such defenses as depression, conversion, dissociation, displacement, phobia formation, or repetitive thoughts and acts being utilized to handle anxiety; in contrast to psychotic m.'s, gross distortion or falsification of reality is not exhibited and gross disintegration of the personality is not usually observed.

**psychophysiologic m.,** a m. characterized by the visceral expression of affect, the symptoms due to a chronic and exaggerated state of the physiologic expression of emotion with the feeling repressed; such m.'s are commonly characteristic of psychosomatic disorders.

**psychotic m.,** a m. characterized by a varying degree of personality disintegration and distortion or falsification of reality in various spheres; persons exhibiting such a m. fail in effective relationships to other people or to their work.

**manikin** (man'ĭ-kin) [ dim. of *man* ]. A model, especially one with removable pieces, of the human body or any of its parts; see also phantom (2).

**maniphalanx** (man'ĭ-fa'langks) [ L. *manus,* hand, + *phalanx, q.v.* ]. A phalanx of the hand; a bony segment of a finger; distinguished from pediphalanx.

**manipulation** (mă-nip'u-la'shun) [ Mediev. L. *manipulo,* pp. *-atus,* to lead by the hand, fr. L. *manipulus,* a handful, fr. *manus,* hand, + *pleo,* to fill ]. Any manual operation, as palpation, extracting the fetus in difficult labor, expressing the placenta, etc.

**conjoined m.,** the use of both hands in an obstetric operation, one being on the abdomen, the other in the vagina.

**Mann,** Frank C., American surgeon, 1887–1962. See M.-Bollman *fistula,* M.-Williamson *operation, ulcer.*

**manna** (man'ah) [ L. fr. G. *manna,* fr. Heb. *mān* ]. A saccharine exudation from *Fraxinus ornus,* flowering ash, a tree of the Mediterranean shores. It occurs as **m. cannel-**

lata, a flake m., **m. in lacrimis**, m. in tears or small flakes, and **m. communis** or **m. in sortis**, m. in sorts. Used as a laxative, especially for children.

**Turkish m.**, trehala.

**man′nans.** Mannosans; polysaccharides of mannose, found in various legumes and in the ivory nut.

**man′nerism.** A peculiar or unusual characteristic mode of movement, action, or speech.

**manninositose** (man-ni′no-si′tōz). A compound of mannose and inositol.

**mannite** (man′īt). D-Mannitol; manna sugar.

**man′nitol** (USP, BP). Mannite; the hexahydric alcohol derived by reduction of fructose. Used in renal function testing to measure glomerular filtration, and intravenously as an osmotic diuretic.

**m. hexanitrate**, MAXITATE; nitromannitol; an explosive compound formed by the nitration of m. When diluted with carbohydrate substances (1 part of m. hexanitrate to 9 or more parts of carbohydrate) it is not explosive, and is used as a vasodilator and hypotensive agent; it is slower in action than nitroglycerin.

**Mannkopf**, Emil W., German physician, 1836–1918. See M.'s *sign.*

**man′nohep′tulose.** See D-*manno*-heptulose, under heptulose.

**mannomus′tine.** DEGRANOL; 1-6-bis(2-chloroethyl-amino)-1,6-dideoxy-D-mannitol dihydrochloride; antineoplastic agent.

**man′nosans.** Mannans.

**man′nose.** An aldohexose obtained from various plant sources (*i.e.*, from mannans). For structure, see sugars.

**mannose-1-phosphate guanylyltransferase.** GDP-mannose phosphorylase; a transferase (EC 2.7.7.22) that catalyzes the transfer of GDP to mannose of mannose 1-phosphate.

**man′noside.** A glycoside of mannose.

**man′nosido′sis.** Congenital deficiency of α-mannosidase; associated with mental retardation, kyphosis, enlarged tongue, and vacuolated lymphocytes, with accumulation of mannose in tissues.

**mannuronic acid** (man′u-ron′ik). The uronic acid derived from the oxidation of mannose.

**manometer** (mă-nom′e-ter) [ G. *manos*, thin, scanty, + *metron*, measure ]. An instrument for indicating the pressure of gases or vapor, or the tension of the blood.

**airway pressure m.**, an instrument that reflects the inspiratory pressure required to inflate the lung with a given volume of gas during assisted or controlled respiration.

**aneroid m.**, dial m.; one in which the pressure is indicated by a revolving pointer moved by the diaphragm on a metallic box exhausted of air.

**dial m.**, aneroid m.

**mercurial m.**, one in which the varying pressures are shown by differences of elevation in a column of mercury.

**manomet′ric.** Relating to a manometer.

**manometry** (mă-nom′e-trĭ) [ see manometer ]. Measurement of pressure of gases by means of a manometer.

**manos′copy.** Manometry.

**Manson**, Sir Patrick, London authority on tropical medicine, 1844–1922. Gave his name to *Mansonella* and *Mansonia*. See M.'s *disease, pyosis, schistosomiasis,* eye worm.

**Mansonella** (man′so-nel′ah). Generic term for Ozzard's filarial parasite, *M. ozzardi,* suggested by Faust (1929) in honor of Sir Patrick Manson, who had previously studied the organism and named it *Filaria ozzardi* (1897).

**M. demarquayi**, a filarial parasite that, for several years, was thought to be a distinct species, but is now regarded as a variety of *M. ozzardi.*

**M. ozzar′di**, a filarial parasite occurring in Yucatan, Panama, Colombia, northern Argentina, British and French Guiana, and the islands of St. Vincent and Dominica; the microfilariae are not ensheathed, and there are no nuclei in the pointed tail. The life cycle is similar to that of *Wuchereria bancrofti;* man is the only known definitive host, and the intermediate hosts are the punkies

or biting midges, *Culicoides furens* and possibly *C. paraensis.* See also mansonelliasis.

**M. tucumana**, a filarial parasite that was first thought to be a distinct species, but later proved to be a variety of *M. ozzardi.*

**mansonelliasis** (man′so-něl-i′ă-sis). The condition caused by *Mansonella ozzardi;* infective larvae may be transmitted when biting midges feed on man. After migration, the adult males and females live in the serous cavities (especially the peritoneal cavity) and in the mesenteric and perivisceral adipose tissue. The worms apparently cause little or no permanent damage in the connective tissue, and the human hosts usually manifest no symptoms of disease; occasionally, a saccular dilation of lymphatic vessels or an enlarged lymph node may result.

**Mansonia** (man-so′nī-ah) [ P. *Manson* ]. A genus of brown or black medium-sized mosquitoes (tribe Culicini), often having banded abdomen and legs. Larvae and pupae have modified breathing tubes enabling them to pierce aquatic plants and obtain air in that manner; surface-active larvicides are therefore ineffectual, and control largely depends upon plant-clearing operations. *M.* mosquitoes are distributed worldwide, and in tropical areas are important vectors of *Brugia malayi;* in some areas they also transmit *Wuchereria bancrofti.*

**Mansonoides** (man′so-noy′dēz). A subgenus of *Mansonia.*

**man′tle.** 1. A covering layer. 2. The pallium.

**brain m.**, pallium.

**myoepicardial m.**, the dorsal wall of the primitive pericardium which in the early somite embryo becomes both the epicardium and the myocardium.

**Mantoux** (mahn-too′), Charles, French physician, 1887–1947. See M. *test.*

**manubrium**, pl. **manu′bria** (mă-nu′brĭ-um) [ L. handle. MANI-2 ] [ NA ]. The portion of the sternum or of the malleus that represents the handle.

**m. mal′lei** [ NA ], handle of the malleus; the portion that extends downward, inward, and backward from the neck of the malleus. It is embedded throughout its length in the tympanic membrane.

**m. sterni** [ NA ], episternum; the upper segment of the sternum, a flattened, roughly triangular bone, occasionally fused with the body of the sternum, forming with it a slight angle, the sternal angle.

**manudynamometer** (man′u-di-nă-mom′e-ter) [ L. *manus,* hand, + G. *dynamis,* force, + *metron,* measure ]. In dentistry, a device for measuring the force exerted by the thrust of an instrument.

**manus**, gen. and pl. **manus** (ma′nus) [ L. ] [ NA ]. Hand; the distal portion of the superior limb, comprised of the carpus, metacarpus, and digits.

**m. cava**, a condition of extreme concavity of the palm of the hand.

**m. extensa**, clubhand with deviation backward.

**m. flexa**, clubhand with forward deviation.

**m. plana**, loss of normal arches of the hand; flat hand.

**m. superextensa**, m. extensa.

**m. valga**, clubhand with deviation to the ulnar side.

**m. vara**, clubhand with deviation to the radial side.

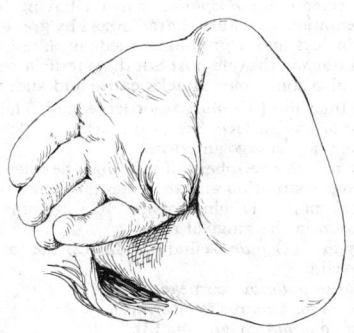

**Manus Vara**
Clubhand with radial deviation.

**manustupration** (man'u-stu-pra'shun) [ L. *manus*, hand, + *stupro*, pp. *stupratus*, to defile ]. Masturbation.

**MAOI.** Abbreviation for monoamine oxidase inhibitor (see under monoamine).

**map'pine.** Bufotenine.

**maransis** (mă-ran'sis). Obsolete term for marasmus.

**marantic** (mă-ran'tik) [ G. *marantikos*, wasting. MARA- ]. Marasmic.

**maraschino** (mar'ă-ske'no) [ Sp. ]. A cordial originally made in Dalmatia from a special sort of cherry growing in that country.

**marasmic** (mă-raz'mik). Marantic; relating to or suffering from marasmus.

**marasmoid** (mă-raz'moyd) [ G. marasmus, *q.v.*, + *eidos*, resemblance ]. Resembling marasmus.

**marasmus** (mă-raz'mus) [ G. *marasmos*, withering. MARA- ]. Athrepsia (1); marantic atrophy; marcor; pedatrophia; cachexia, especially in young children, most commonly due to prolonged dietary deficiency of protein and calories.

**marc** (mark) [ Fr. fr. *marcher*, to trample ]. The residue remaining after percolation of a drug.

**Marcacci** (mar-kah'che), Arturo, Italian physiologist, 1854–1915. See M.'s *muscle*.

**Marchand** (mar-shant'), Felix, German pathologist, 1846–1928. See M.'s *adrenals*, wandering *cell*.

**Marchant** (mar-shahn'), Gérard T. J., French surgeon, 1850–1903. See M.'s *zone*.

**Marchesani** (mar-ka-sah'ne), Oswald, 1900–1952. See M.'s *syndrome*, Weill-M. *syndrome*.

**Marchetti,** Andrew A., U. S. obstetrician and gynecologist, 1901–1970. See Marshall-M. *operation*.

**Marchi** (mar'ke), Vittorio, Italian physician, 1851–1908. See M.'s *fluid, method, reaction, tract*.

**Marchiafava** (mar-ke-ah-fah'vah), Ettore, Italian pathologist, 1847–1935. See M.-Bignami *disease*, M.-Micheli *anemia, syndrome*.

**marcid** (mar'sid) [ L. *marcidus*; fr. *marceo*, to wither ]. Emaciating; tabid; wasting away.

**Marcille** (mar-se'ē), Maurice, 1871–1941. See M.'s *triangle*.

**Marckwald** (mark'valt), Max, German surgeon, 1844–1923. See M.'s *operation*.

**marcor** (mar'kor) [ L. fr. *marceo*, to wither. MARA- ]. Marasmus.

**Marcus Gunn,** Robert. See *Gunn*, Robert Marcus.

**Maréchal** (mar-a-shal'), Louis-Eugène, French physician, 19th century. See M.'s *test*.

**Marek,** Josef, Hungarian scientist. See M.'s *disease*.

**Marey** (mar-a'), Ettienne J., French physiologist, 1830–1904. See M.'s *law*.

**Marfan** (mar-fahn'), Antoine Bernard-Jean, French pediatrician, 1858–1942. See M.'s *disease, law, syndrome*.

**Marg,** Elwin. See Mackay-M. *tonometer*.

**margaric acid** (mar-găr'ik, mar'gă-rik). Heptadecanoic acid; $CH_3(CH_2)_4COOH$; the 17-carbon saturated fatty acid.

**Margaropus** (mar-găr'o-pus). A genus of ixodid ticks closely resembling *Boophilus*, but not having festoons or ornamentations; they are characterized by greatly enlarged posterior legs and a prolonged median plate.

**M. winthemi,** the one-host South American winter horse tick; it also sometimes attacks cattle and sheep.

**margin** (mar'jin) [ L. *margo*, border, edge ]. The boundary or edge of any surface. See also margo.

**anterior m.,** *margo* anterior.

**cavity m.,** the periphery of a filling, the line of junction between a restoration and the external surface of a tooth.

**cervical m.,** (1) gingival m.; (2) termination of a restoration in the gingival area.

**ciliary m.,** (1) *margo* ciliaris iridis; (2) the tarsal border of an eyelid.

**corneal m.,** *limbus* corneae.

**falciform m.,** *margo* falciformis.

**fibular m.,** *margo* lateralis (3).

**free m.,** *margo* liber.

**frontal m.,** *margo* frontalis.

**gingival m.,** that part of the free gingiva that is localized at the labial, buccal, and lingual aspects of the teeth.

**inferior m.,** *margo* inferior.

**inferolateral m.,** *margo* inferior (1).

**inferomedial m.,** *margo* medialis (1).

**interosseous m.,** *margo* interosseus.

**lacrimal m.,** *margo* lacrimalis.

**lambdoid m.,** *margo* lambdoideus.

**lateral m.,** *margo* lateralis.

**mastoid m.,** *margo* mastoideus.

**medial m.,** *margo* medialis.

**mesovarian m.,** *margo* mesovaricus.

**nasal m.,** *margo* nasalis.

**occipital m.,** *margo* occipitalis.

**parietal m.,** *margo* parietalis.

**posterior m.,** *margo* posterior.

**m. of safety,** m. between the therapeutic dose and the lethal dose of a drug.

**squamous m.,** *margo* squamosus.

**superior m.,** *margo* superior.

**superomedial m.,** *margo* superior (1).

**ulnar m.,** *margo* medialis (2).

**zygomatic m.,** *margo* zygomaticus.

**marginal** (mar'jī-nal). Relating to a margin.

**margination** (mar'jī-na'shun). A phenomenon that occurs during the relatively early phases of an inflammation; as a result of dilation of capillaries and slowing of the blood stream, leukocytes tend to occupy the periphery of the cross-sectional lumen and adhere to the endothelial cells that line the vessels.

**m. of placenta,** *placenta* marginata.

**margines** (mar'jī-nēz) [ L. ]. Plural of margo.

**marginoplasty** (mar'jī-no-plas'tī). Plastic or reparative surgery of the tarsal border of an eyelid.

**margo,** gen. **mar'ginis,** pl. **mar'gines** (mar'go) [ L. margin ] [ NA ]. Edge; margin; border.

**m. anterior** [ NA ], anterior margin; anterior border; (1) a ridge on the shaft of the fibula to which is attached the anterior intermuscular septum of the leg; (2) the sharp margin separating the costal and mediastinal surfaces of the lung; (3) the sharp margin between the anterior and inferior surfaces of the pancreas; (4) the ridge on the shaft of the radius extending from the radial tuberosity to the anterior part of the styloid process; (5) the rounded, free, anterior portion of the testis; (6) the subcutaneous ridge of the tibia that extends from the tuberosity to the anterior part of the medial malleolus; (7) the ridge on the body of the ulna that extends from the tuberosity to the anterior part of the styloid process.

**m. cilia'ris i'ridis** [ NA ], ciliary margin of the iris; the peripheral border of the iris attached to the ciliary body.

**m. dexter cordis** [ NA ], right margin of the heart; the border between the sternocostal and diaphragmatic surfaces of the heart; it is fairly well defined in fixed hearts but is rounded and indefinite in the living heart.

**m. falciform'is** [ NA ], falciform margin; the sharply curved, free margin of the saphenous opening in the fascia lata; medially it ends in a superior and an inferior horn.

**m. fibula'ris** [ NA ], fibular margin; an alternate term for m. lateralis (3).

**m. fronta'lis** [ NA ], frontal margin; (1) the margin of the parietal bone that articulates with the frontal bone; (2) the margin of the greater wing of the sphenoid that articulates with the frontal bone.

**m. incisa'lis** [ NA ], incisal margin; incisal, cutting, or shearing edge; the part of an anterior tooth farthest from the apex of the root.

**m. infe'rior** [ NA ], inferior margin or border; (1) m. inferolateralis; inferolateral margin; the irregular, discontinuous margin of the cerebral hemisphere at the junction of the inferior and superolateral surfaces; (2) the sharp border of the liver that separates the diaphragmatic and visceral surfaces; (3) the sharp border of the lung that separates the diaphragmatic surface from the costal and mediastinal surfaces; (4) the border of the pancreas separating the inferior and posterior surfaces; (5) the border of the spleen separating the renal and diaphragmatic surfaces.

**m. inferolatera'lis** [ NA ], inferolateral margin; an alternate term for m. inferior (1).

**m. inferomedia′lis** [ NA ], inferomedial margin; an alternate term for m. medialis (1).

**m. infraorbita′lis** [ NA ], infraorbital margin; the lower border of the entrance to the orbit, formed by the maxilla medially and the zygomatic bone laterally.

**m. interosseus** [ NA ], interosseous margin; interosseous crest; (1) the ridge along the lateral side of the body of the ulna to which is attached the interosseous membrane; (2) the ridge along the medial side of the radius to which is attached the interosseous membrane; (3) the ridge along the medial border of the fibula to which is attached the interosseous membrane; (4) the ridge along the lateral border of the tibia to which is attached the interosseous membrane.

**m. lacrima′lis** [ NA ], lacrimal margin; the margin of the nasal surface of the maxilla that articulates with the lacrimal bone.

**m. lambdoid′eus** [ NA ], lambdoid margin; the margin of occipital squama that articulates with the parietal bones in the lambdoid suture.

**m. latera′lis** [ NA ], lateral margin; (1) the convex lateral border of the kidney; (2) m. radialis; the radial or lateral border of the forearm; (3) m. fibularis; fibular margin; the border of the foot between the small toe and the heel; (4) the ridge on the humerus that extends from the greater tubercle to the lateral epicondyle; (5) the sides of the nail extending from the concealed to the free borders; (6) the border of the scapula extending from the glenoid fossa to the inferior angle.

**m. liber** [ NA ], free margin; (1) the distal border of the nail that overhangs the tip of the digit; (2) the posterior margin of the ovary.

**m. lin′guae** [ NA ], margin of the tongue; the lateral border that separates the dorsum from the inferior surface of the tongue on each side, the two borders meeting anteriorly at the apex.

**m. mastoid′eus** [ NA ], mastoid margin; the margin of the occipital squama that articulates with the mastoid part of the temporal bone.

**m. media′lis** [ NA ], medial margin; (1) m. inferomedialis; inferomedial margin; the irregular border of the cerebral hemisphere at the junction of the inferior and medial surfaces; (2) m. ulnaris; ulnar margin; the ulnar or medial border of the forearm; (3) m. tibialis; tibial border; the border of the foot from the great toe to the heel; (4) the ridge on the humerus that extends from the crest of the lesser tubercle to the medial epicondyle; (5) the concave border of the kidney; (6) the border of the scapula that extends from the superior angle to the inferior angle; (7) the paravertebral border of the suprarenal gland; (8) the rounded border of the tibia that separates the posterior and medial surfaces.

**m. mesovaricus** [ NA ], mesovarian margin; the border of the ovary to which the mesovarium is attached.

**m. nasalis** [ NA ], nasal margin; the border of the frontal bone that articulates with the nasal bones.

**m. occipitalis** [ NA ], occipital margin; (1) the posterior margin of the parietal bone that articulates with the occipital squama; (2) that part of the petrous part of the temporal bone that articulates with the occipital squama.

**m. occul′tus un′guis** [ NA ], occult border of the nail; the proximal border of the nail entirely covered by the nail wall.

**m. palpe′brae**, margin of the eyelid.

**m. parietalis** [ NA ], parietal margin; (1) the margin of the frontal bone that articulates with the parietal bone; (2) the margin of the greater wing of the sphenoid that articulates with the parietal bone; (3) the border of the squamous part of the temporal bone that articulates with the parietal bone.

**m. posterior** [ NA ], posterior margin; (1) the ridge on the posterior aspect of the fibula extending from the head to the medial aspect of the peroneal groove; (2) the ridge on the radius that extends from the tuberosity to the tubercle on the posterior aspect of the distal extremity; (3) the sinous ridge on the posterior aspect of the ulna that extends from near the olecranon to the styloid process; (4) the rounded posterior portion of the testis into which the vessels enter.

**m. posterior partis petrosae ossis temporalis** [ NA ], posterior border of the petrous part of the temporal bone;

the margin of the petrous part of the temporal bone that extends from the apex to the jugular notch, it articulates with the basal and jugular portions of the occipital bone.

**m. pupilla′ris i′ridis** [ NA ], pupillary margin of the iris; the inner border of the iris that forms the edge of the pupil.

**m. radialis** [ NA ], m. lateralis (2).

**m. sagittalis** [ NA ], sagittal border; the medial border of the parietal bone entering into the sagittal suture.

**m. sphenoidalis** [ NA ], sphenoidal border; the part of the border of the squamous part of the temporal bone that articulates with the greater wing of the sphenoid.

**m. squamo′sus** [ NA ], squamous margin; (1) the margin of the greater wing of the sphenoid bone that articulates with the squamous part of the temporal bone; (2) the lateral border of the parietal bone that articulates with the squamous part of the temporal bone.

**m. supe′rior** [ NA ], superior margin; (1) m. superomedialis; the curved margin of the cerebral hemisphere at the junction of the superolateral and medial surfaces; (2) the border of the body of the pancreas that separates the anterior and posterior surfaces; (3) the border of the scapula that extends from the glenoid fossa to the superior angle; (4) the notched border of the spleen that separates the gastric and diaphragmatic surfaces; (5) the border of the suprarenal gland at the superior junction of the anterior and posterior surfaces.

**m. superior partis petrosae ossis temporalis** [ NA ], superior border of the petrous part of the temporal bone; the margin that separates the anterior and posterior surfaces of the petrous part of the temporal bone.

**m. superomedialis** [ NA ], m. superior (1).

**m. supraorbitalis** [ NA ], supraorbital margin; supraorbital arch; the curved superior border of the aditus orbitae.

**m. tibialis** [ NA ], m. medialis (3).

**m. ulnaris** [ NA ], m. medialis (2).

**m. u′teri** [ NA ], border of the uterus; the right or left margin of the uterus along which the broad ligament is attached. The uterine tube and round ligament attach to the uterus at the upper part of the border.

**m. zygomaticus** [ NA ], zygomatic margin; the border of the greater wing of the sphenoid that articulates with the zygomatic bone.

**Marie,** Pierre, Paris neurologist, 1853–1940. See M.'s *ataxia,* M.'s *disease,* Charcot-M.-Tooth *disease,* Bamberger-M. *disease,* M.-Strümpell *disease,* Strümpell-M. *disease,* Brissaud-M. *syndrome,*

**marihuana** (măr′ĭ-wah′nah) [ derivation doubtful; possibly fr. Sp. *Maria-Juana,* Mary-Jane ]. Alternative spellings are mariguana, marijuana; popular name for the dried flowering leaves of *Cannabis sativa,* which are smoked as cigarettes or "reefers." In the United States the term marihuana includes any part of, or any extracts from, the female plant; see also cannabis.

**Marinesco,** Georges, Rumanian neurologist, 1863–1938. See M.'s succulent *hand,* M.-Garland *syndrome,* M.-Sjögren *syndrome.*

**marinobu′fotoxin.** A poison produced by the parotid gland of *Bufo marinus,* a large toad native to South and Central America; used in tropical countries for insect control.

**Marion,** H., French pediatrician. See M.'s *disease.*

**Mariotte** (mar-e-ot′), Edmé, French physicist, 1620–1684. See M.'s *experiment, law,* blind *spot.*

**mariposia** (măr′ĭ-po′zĭ-ah) [ L. *mare,* the sea, + G. *posis,* drinking ]. Thallasoposia; sea water drinking.

**Marjolin** (mar-zhŏ-laň′), Jean N., French physician, 1780–1850. See M.'s *ulcer.*

**marjoram** (mar′jo-ram). Sweet marjoram, leaf marjoram, garden marjoram. The leaves, with and without a small portion of the flowering tops of *Majorana hortensis* (*Origanum majorana*) (family Labiatae), are used as seasoning and medicinally as stimulant, carminative and emmenagogue.

**mark** [ A.S. *mearc* ]. 1. Any spot, line, or other figure on the cutaneous or mucocutaneous surface, visible through difference in color, elevation, or other peculiarity. 2. Infundibulum (8).

**alignment m.,** m.'s made in tracings while the kymograph or other recording apparatus is at rest in order to indicate the time relations between two tracings inscribed one above the other, *e.g.*, jugular and radial pulses.

**dhobie m.,** dhobie mark *dermatitis.*

**port-wine m.,** *nevus* flammeus.

**strawberry m.,** strawberry *nevus.*

**Unna's m.,** nape *nevus.*

**washerman's m.,** dhobie mark *dermatitis.*

**Markee,** Joseph E., American anatomist, 1904–1970. See M. *test.*

**mark′er.** A device used to make a mark or to indicate measurement.

**Amsler's m.,** a caliper compass, used in eye surgery.

**time m.,** an instrument, usually run by clockwork, that marks the time, usually in seconds or fractions of seconds, on a kymograph record in physiologic experiments.

**Marme's reagent.** See under reagent.

**marmorated** (mar′mo-ra′ted) [ L. *marmoratus,* marbled ]. Denoting a streaked appearance of the skin, like marble; see also *cutis* marmorata.

**mar′mot** [ Fr. *marmotte* ]. Woodchuck; groundhog; a hibernating rodent; may serve as reservoir host of plague bacillus; and may harbor ticks which transmit Rocky Mountain spotted fever.

**Maroteaux,** Pierre. See M.-Lamy *syndrome.*

**Marquis' reagent.** See under reagent.

**marrianolic acid** (măr′ĭ-ă-no′lik). 2-Carboxy-1,2,3,4,4a,9,10,10a-octahydro-7-hydroxy-2-methyl-1-phenanthreneacetic acid; a potent estrogen formed by exposure of 16-keto-17$\beta$-estradiol to alkali, with cleavage of the D ring (see steroids).

**marrow** (măr′o) [ A.S. *mearh* ]. 1. The soft, fatty substance filling the medullary cavities and cancellous extremities of the long bones. 2. Any soft gelatinous or fatty material resembling the m. of bone. See also medulla.

**bone m.,** *medulla* ossium.

**red m.,** *medulla* ossium rubra.

**spinal m.,** *medulla* spinalis.

**yellow m.,** *medulla* ossium flava.

**marrubium** (mă-ru′bĭ-um) [ L. hoarhound ]. Hoarhound; horehound; the leaves and tops of *Marrubium vulgare* (family Labiatae), a herb of Europe and Asia; used as an expectorant and diaphoretic, chiefly in domestic medicine in the form of candy.

**Marsh,** Hadleigh, U. S. veterinary pathologist, 1888–1971. See M.'s ovine progressive *pneumonia.*

**Marshall,** Eli K., American pharmacologist, *1889. See M.'s *method.*

**Marshall,** John, English anatomist, 1818–1891. See M.'s vestigial *fold,* oblique *vein.*

**Marshall,** Victor F., U. S. urologist. See M.-Marchetti *operation.*

**Marshall Hall.** See Hall.

**Marshalla′gia marshal′li.** One of the medium stomach worms of the nematode family Trichostrongylidae; it usually is found in the abomasum of sheep, goats, camels, and various wild ruminants.

**marsh′mallow root.** Althea.

**marsupial** (mar-su′ĭ-al) [ L. *marsupium,* a pouch ]. 1. A member of the order of mammals (Marsupalia) which includes kangaroos, wombats, bandicoots, opossums, etc., the female of which has an abdominal pouch for carrying the young; opossums the only marsupials found outside of Australia and the neighboring islands. Of or pertaining to marsupials.

**marsupialization** (mar-su′pĭ-al-ĭ-za′shun) [ L. *marsupium,* pouch ]. An operation for treatment of a cyst; the sac is opened and emptied of its contents, and its edges are stitched to the external incision, which is kept open until the interior incision closes by granulation.

**marsupium** (mar-su′pĭ-um) [ L. pouch ]. Scrotum.

**Martegiani** (mar-tej-ah′ne), Carlo, Italian anatomist, 20th century. See M.'s *area, funnel.*

**martensitic** (mar′ten-sit′ik). In stainless steels, denoting ferromagnetic alloys that can be hardened by heat treatment. They contain chromium as the chief addition to the iron.

**martial** (mar′shal) [ L. *Mars* (*Mart-*), Roman god of war; in old chem., iron ]. Ferruginous; chalybeate; relating to or containing iron.

**Martin,** August E., Berlin gynecologist, 1847–1933. See M.'s *pelvimeter, tube.*

**Martin,** Henry A., American surgeon, 1824–1884. See M.'s *bandage, disease.*

**Martin,** Thomas C., American physician, 1864–1926. See M.'s *speculum.*

**Martinotti,** Giovanni, Italian physician, 1857–1928. See M.'s *cells.*

**martius yellow.** 2,4-Dinitro-$\alpha$-naphthol; an acid dye, $C_{10}H_6N_2O_5$, used as a plasma stain in plant and animal histology, and as a light filter for photomicrography.

**Martorell,** F. See M.'s *syndrome*

**Marx's stain.** See under stain.

**maschaladenitis** (mas′kal-ad′ē-ni′tis) [ G. *maschalē,* axilla, + *adēn,* gland, + suffix *-itis,* inflammation ]. Inflammation of the axillary glands.

**maschale** (mas′kal-e) [ G. ]. Axilla.

**maschalephidrosis** (mas-kal-ef-ĭ-dro′sis) [ G. *maschalē,* axilla, + *ephidrōsis,* perspiration ]. Sweating in the axillae.

**maschaliatria** (mas-kal-e-at′rĭ-ah) [ G. *maschalē,* axilla, + *iatreia,* healing ]. Medication by means of inunction in the axilla, where absorption is prompt.

**maschaloncus** (mas-kal-ong′kus) [ G. *maschalē,* axilla, + *onkos,* mass. ONC-1 ]. A neoplasm in the axilla.

**maschalyperidrosis** (mas′kal-i′per-i-dro′sis) [ G. *maschalē,* axilla, + *hyper,* over, + *hidrōs,* sweat ]. Excessive sweating in the axillae.

**masculine** (mas′ku-lin) [ L. *masculus,* male, fr. *mas,* male ]. Relating to or marked by the characteristics of the male sex.

**masculinity** (mas′ku-lin′ĭ-tĭ). The characteristics of a male.

**masculinization** (mas′ku-lin-ĭ-za′shun) [ L. *masculus,* male ]. The condition marked by the attainment of male characteristics.

**masculinize** (mas′ku-lĭ-nīz). To confer the qualities or characteristics peculiar to the male.

**masculinovoblastoma** (mas′ku-lin-o′vo-blas-to′mah). An ovarian neoplasm that causes varying degrees of masculinization, *e.g.,* male-type distribution of hair, change in voice, hypertrophy of the clitoris, and so on; the neoplasm consists of cords or anastomosing columns of cells with vesicular nuclei and indistinct cytoplasm, and is usually well vascularized. M.'s are thought by some to be derived from rests of adrenal cortical tissue, and they are morphologically similar to certain types of arrhenoblastoma.

**masculi′nus** [ L. ] [ NA ]. Masculine.

**masculonucleus** (mas′ku-lo-nu′kle-us). Arsenoblast.

**maser** (ma′zer) [ an acronym, coined from *microwave amplification by stimulated emission of radiation* ]. A device that produces a beam of monochromatic radiation, characteristically in the microwave region, but also (depending on the materials used) in the infrared and visible light regions. The monochromaticity of the radiation makes it possible to use the steady, unvarying frequency as a highly accurate time measure ("atomic clock"). It can also be used as a very sensitive detector of very weak signals in radio-astronomy, radar, etc.

**optical m.,** laser.

**Masini** (mah-se′ne), Giulio, Italian physician, 1874–1937. See M.'s *sign.*

**mask.** 1. Any of a variety of disease states producing alteration or discoloration of the skin of the face. 2. The expressionless appearance seen in certain diseases; *e.g.,* Parkinsonian facies. 3. A facial bandage. 4. A gauze shield designed to cover the mouth and nose for maintenance of antiseptic conditions. 5. A device for administration of anesthetics and for breathing oxygen.

**BLB m.,** a m. designed for breathing oxygen at high altitudes; devised by Boothby, Lovelace, and Bulbulian.

**ecchymot′ic m.,** traumatic asphyxia; pressure stasis; a dusky discoloration of the head and neck occurring when the trunk has been subjected to sudden and extreme compression.

**Hutchinson's m.,** the sensation in tabes dorsalis as if the face were covered with a m. or with cobwebs.

**luet'ic m.,** a dirty, brownish yellow pigmentation, blotchy in character, resembling that of chloasma, occurring on the forehead, temples, and sometimes cheeks in the subjects of tertiary syphilis.

**Mikulicz' m.,** a wire frame, to which gauze is attached, used as a m. to cover the mouth and nose of the surgeon while operating.

**nonrebreathing m.,** a m., used in inhalation anesthesia, fitted with both an inhalation valve and an exhalation valve so that all exhaled gas is vented to the external atmosphere, thus assuring that the patient will inhale only the anesthetic mixture delivered from the anesthesia machine.

**surgical m.,** a m. of folded gauze used for covering the mouth and nose of the surgeon, nurse, etc. during operations.

**tropical m.,** *chloasma* bronzinum.

**Tuttle's m.,** a wire frame over which gauze is spread, so shaped as to cover the face below the eyes of the surgeon when operating.

**u'terine m.,** *chloasma* uterinum.

**masked** (maskt). Concealed.

**mask'ing.** 1. The "drowning" of a weak sound by a louder one, *e.g.*, the inaudibility of a voice of ordinary intensity in the roar of traffic; for any given intensity, low pitched tones have a greater m. effect than those of a high pitch. In hearing testing, the use of a noise applied to one ear while testing the hearing acuity of the other ear. 2. The hiding of smaller rhythms in the brain wave record by larger and slower ones whose wave form they distort. 3. In dentistry, an opaque covering used to camouflage the metal parts of a prosthesis.

**Maslow,** Abraham H., U. S. psychologist, 1908–1970. See M.'s *hierarchy.*

**Masoch,** Leopold von Sacher-, Austrian novelist, 1836–1895. Gave his name to masochism.

**masochism** (maz'o-kizm, mas'o-kizm) [ L. von Sacher-*Masoch* ]. 1. Algolagnia; a form of perversion in which sexual pleasure is heightened in the person who is beaten and maltreated; the opposite of sadism. 2. A general orientation in life that personal suffering relieves guilt and leads to a reward.

**masochist** (mas'o-kist). The passive party in the practice of masochism.

**masque** (mask) [ Fr. ]. Mask.

   **m. biliaire,** periocular hyperpigmentation seen not infrequently in middle-aged women, probably unrelated to any systemic disease.

**mass** [ L. *massa*, a dough-like mass ]. 1. Massa. 2. In pharmacy, a soft solid preparation containing an active medicinal agent, of such consistency that it can be divided into small pieces and rolled into pills. 3. One of the seven fundamental quantities of the SI system of units; often confused with weight (which see). Its unit is the kilogram (symbol kg), defined as the mass of the international prototype of the kilogram, which is made of platinum-iridium and kept at the International Bureau of Weights and Measures.

   **apperceptive m.,** the already existing knowledge base in a similar or related area with which the new perceptual material is articulated.

   **filar m.,** reticular *substance* (1).

   **inner cell m.,** the group of cells at the embryonic pole of the blastocyst which are concerned in the formation of the body of the embryo.

   **pilular m.,** any soft solid drug m. that is of the proper consistency to be made into pills.

   **tigroid m.'s,** see tigroid.

   **tubular excretory m.,** the m. of functioning excretory tubules of the kidney, determined from the excretion of Diodrast when large doses are used.

**massa,** gen. and pl. **massae** (mas'sah, mas'se) [ L. ] [ NA ]. Mass; a lump or aggregation of coherent material.

   **m. interme'dia,** *adhesio* interthalamica.

   **m. lateralis atlantis** [ NA ], lateral mass of the atlas; the thick lateral part of the atlas on each side that articulates above with the occipital condyle and below with the axis.

**massage** (mă-sahzh') [ Fr. from G. *massō,* to knead ]. A method of manipulation of the body by rubbing, pinching, kneading, tapping, etc.

**cardiac m.,** manual rhythmic compression of the ventricles to maintain the circulation.

**closed chest m.,** external cardiac m.; rhythmic compression of the heart between sternum and spine by depressing the lower sternum backward with heels of hands, the patient lying supine.

**external cardiac m.,** closed chest m.

**gingival m.,** mechanical stimulation of the gingiva by rubbing or pressure.

**nerve-point m.,** gelotripsy.

**open chest m.,** rhythmic manual compression of the ventricles of the heart with the hand inside the thoracic cavity.

**vibratory m.,** seismotherapy; sismotherapy; very rapid tapping of the surface effected by means of an instrument, usually with elastic tip.

**Masselon** (mah-sel-awn'), M. Julián, Paris physician, 1844–1917. See M.'s *spectacles.*

**masseter** (mă-se'ter) [ G. *masētēr,* masticator ]. See *musculus* masseter.

**masseur** (mas-ër') [ Fr. see *massage* ]. 1. A man who massages. 2. An instrument used in mechanical massage.

**masseuse** (mas-ëz'). A woman who massages.

**mas'sicot.** Lead monoxide.

**mas'sother'apy** [ G. *massō,* to knead, + *therapeia,* treatment ]. The therapeutic use of massage.

**mast-.** See masto-.

**mastadenitis** (mast-ad-ĕ-ni'tis) [ masto- + G. *adēn,* gland, + suffix *-itis,* inflammation ]. Mastitis.

**mastadenoma** (mast'ad-ĕ-no'mah) [ masto- + G. *adēn,* gland, + *-ōma* ]. A benign neoplasm (adenoma) of the breast.

**mastalgia** (mas-tal'jĭ-ah) [ masto- + G. *algos,* pain ]. Mastodynia.

**mastatrophy, mastatrophia** (mas-tat'ro-fī, mast'ā-tro'fī-ah) [ masto- + atrophy ]. Atrophy or wasting of the breasts.

**mastauxe** (mast-awk'se) [ masto- + G. *auxē,* increase ]. Hypertrophy of the breast.

**mastectomy** (mas-tek'to-mī) [ masto- + G. *ektomē,* excision ]. Mammectomy; amputation of the breast.

**Master,** Arthur M., American physician, *1895. See M.'s two-step exercise *test.*

**masthelcosis** (mas-thel-ko'sis) [ masto- + G. *helkōsis,* ulceration ]. Ulceration of the breast.

**mastic** (mas'tik) [ G. *mastichē,* the resin of the mastich tree ]. Mastich; mastiche; a resinous exudate from *Pistacia lentiscus* (family Anacardiaceae), a small tree of the Mediterranean shores. Used in chewing gum, as enteric coating, and as temporary filling material in dentistry.

**masti'cate.** To chew; see mastication.

**mastication** (mas'tī-ka'shun) [ L. *mastico,* pp. *-atus,* to chew ]. The process of chewing food in preparation for deglutition and digestion; the act of grinding or comminuting with the teeth.

   **components of m.,** see under component.

**masticatory** (mas'tī-kă-to-rī). Relating to mastication.

**mastica'tus** [ L. ] [ NA ]. Masticated; chewed.

**mastich, mastiche** (mas'te-ke). Mastic.

**Mastigophora** (mas'tī-gof'o-rah) [ G. *mastix* (*mastig-*), a whip, + *phoros,* bearing ]. Flagellates; a superclass of Protozoa which possess one or more flagella for locomotion, and a single vesicular nucleus; *Volvox, Trypanosoma,* and *Euglena* are examples. It consists of two classes: Phytomastigina, to which *Euglena* belongs, contains chlorophyll and in its nutrition is holophytic; the other, Zoomastigina, lacks chromatophores; it includes the parasitic genera *Trypanosoma* and *Leishmania.*

**mastigote** (mas'tī-gōt) [ G. *mastix,* a whip ]. An individual flagellate.

**masti'tis** (mas'ti'tis) [ masto- + G. suffix *-itis,* inflammation ]. Mammitis; mastadenitis; inflammation of the breast.

   **bovine m.,** garget; a disease complex which occurs in acute, gangrenous, chronic, and subclinical forms of inflammation of the bovine udder, and is due to a variety of infectious agents. Animal care, hygiene, and management are important factors in this dairy cow disease of great economic import.

**chronic cystic m.,** fibrocystic *disease* of the breast.

**gargan'tuan m.,** chronic inflammation of the breast with great enlargment of the gland.

**glandular m.,** parenchymatous m.

**interstitial m.,** inflammation of the connective tissue of the mammary gland.

**m. neonator'um,** m. in the newborn.

**ovine m.,** bluebag; an acute inflammation of the sheep udder, usually gangrenous, caused by *Staphylococcus aureus* and *Pasteurella mastidis.*

**parenchy'matous m.,** glandular m.; inflammation of the secreting tissue of the breast.

**phleg'monous m.,** abscess or cellulitis of the breast.

**plasma cell m.,** a condition of the breasts characterized by tumor-like indurated masses containing numerous plasma cells. Though clinically it resembles malignant disease (attachment to skin and enlargement of axillary lymph nodes), it is not neoplastic. Some cases result from mammary duct ectasia, *q. v.*

**puer'peral m.,** m. occurring in the later part of the puerperium; usually a suppurative m.

**retromam'mary m.,** submammary m.

**stagna'tion m.,** caked breast; painful distention of the breast occurring during the latter days of pregnancy and the first days of lactation.

**submam'mary m.,** retromammary m.; paramastitis; inflammation of the tissues lying deep to the mammary gland.

**sup'purative m.,** inflammation of the breast due to infection with pyogenic bacteria.

**masto-, mast-** [ G. *mastos,* breast ]. Combining forms relating to the breast.

**mastoccipital** (mast'ok-sip'ĭ-tal). Masto-occipital.

**mastochondroma** (mas-to-kon-dro'mah) [ masto- + G. *chondros,* cartilage, + suffix -*oma,* tumor ]. A benign cartilaginous neoplasm of the breast.

**mastocyte** (mas'to-sīt). Mast *cell.*

**mastocytogenesis** (mas'to-si'to-jen'ē-sis). The formation and development of mast cells.

**mastocytoma** (mas'to-si-to'mah) [ mastocyte + G. suffix -*oma,* tumor ]. A fairly well circumscribed accumulation or nodular focus of mast cells, grossly resembling a neoplasm.

**mastocytosis** (mas'to-si-to'sis) [ mastocyte + G. suffix -*osis,* condition ]. Urticaria pigmentosa, particularly with mast cell infiltration of viscera as well as skin.

**mastodynia** (mas'to-din'ĭ-ah) [ masto- + G. *odynē,* pain ]. Mastalgia; mazodynia; mammalgia; pain in the breast; see also mammary *neuralgia.*

**mastoid** (mas'toyd) [ masto- + G. *eidos,* resemblance ]. 1. Resembling a mamma; breast-shaped. 2. Relating to the m. process, antrum, cells, etc.

**mastoidal** (mas-toy'dal). Mastoid (2).

**mastoidectomy** (mas'toy-dek'to-mĭ) [ mastoid (process) + G. *ektomē,* excision ]. Hollowing out of the mastoid process by curretting, gouging, drilling, or otherwise removing the bony partitions forming the mastoid cells.

**radical m.,** typanomeatomastoidectomy; an operation to exteriorize and join the mastoid air cells, the middle ear space, and the external meatus, often for extensive cholesteatoma.

**mastoideocentesis** (mas-toyd'e-o-sen-te'sis) [ mastoid + G. *kentēsis,* puncture ]. The operation of drilling or chiseling into the mastoid cells and antrum.

**mastoi'deus** [ L. ] [ NA ]. Mastoid.

**mastoiditis** (mas'toy-di'tis). Inflammation of any part of the mastoid process. See also *otitis* mastoidea.

**Bezold's m.,** primary m.

**sclerosing m.,** a chronic m. in which the trabeculae are greatly thickened, almost or entirely obliterating the cells.

**mastoidotomy** (mas'toy-dot'o-mĭ) [ mastoid (process) + G. *tomē,* cutting ]. Wilde's incision; incision into the subperiosteum or the mastoid process of the temporal bone.

**mastology** (mas-tol'o-jĭ) [ masto- + G. *logos,* study ]. Mazology; the branch of medical science that has to do with the breasts—their anatomy, physiology, pathology, etc.

**mastomenia** (mas'to-me'nĭ-ah) [ masto- + G. *mēn,* month ]. Vicarious menstruation from the mammae.

**mastoncus** (mas-tong'kus) [ masto- + G. *onkos,* mass ]. A tumor or swelling of the breasts.

**masto-occipital** (mas'to-ok-sip'ĭ-tal). Mastoccipital; relating to the mastoid portion of the temporal bone and to the occipital bone, denoting the suture uniting them.

**mastoparietal** (mas'to-pă-ri'ē-tal). Relating to the mastoid portion of the temporal bone and to the parietal bone, denoting the suture uniting them.

**mastopathy** (mas-top'ă-thĭ) [ masto- + G. *pathos,* suffering ]. Mazopathy; any disease of the breasts.

**mastopexy** (mas'to-pek'sĭ) [ masto- + G. *pēxis,* fixation ]. Mazopexy; an operation for correcting an exaggerated sagging of the breasts.

**mastoplasia** (mas-to-pla'zĭ-ah) [ masto- + G. *plasis,* a molding ]. Mazoplasia; enlargement of the breast.

**mastoplasty** (mas'to-plas'tĭ) [ masto- + G. *plassō,* to form ]. Plastic operation on the breast.

**mastoptosis** (mas'top-to'sis, mas'to-to'sis) [ masto- + G. *ptōsis,* a falling ]. Ptosis or sagging of the breast.

**mastorrhagia** (mas'to-ra'jĭ-ah) [ masto- + G. *rhēgnymi,* to burst forth ]. Hemorrhage from a breast.

**mastoscirrhus** (mas-to-skĭr' (sĭr')us). A scirrhous carcinoma of the breast.

**mastosquamous** (mas'to-skwa'mus). Relating to the mastoid and the squamous portions of the temporal bone.

**mastosyrinx** (mas'to-sĭr'ingks) [ masto- + G. *syrinx,* tube ]. Fistula of the breast.

**mastotomy** (mas-tot'o-mĭ) [ masto- + G. *tomē,* incision ]. Mammotomy; incision of the breast.

**mas'turbate** [ L. *masturbari,* pp. *masturbatus* ]. To practice masturbation.

**masturbation** (mas'tur-ba'shun) [ L. *masturbatio* ]. Erotic stimulation of the genital organs usually resulting in orgasm, achieved by manual or other stimulation exclusive of sexual intercourse, in both heterosexual and homosexual relations.

**false m.,** peotillomania.

**Masugi,** M. See M.'s *nephritis.*

**Mat'as,** Rudolph, U. S. surgeon, 1860–1957. See M.'s *operation.*

**maté** (mah-tā') [ Sp. *maté,* a vessel in which the leaves are prepared ]. Paraguay tea; the dried leaves of *Ilex paraguayensis* and other species of *Ilex* (family Aquifoliaceae), shrubs growing in Paraguay and Brazil. They contain caffeine and tannin. Used in South American countries as a beverage and medicinally as a diuretic and diaphoretic, and for the relief of headache.

**ma'ter** [ L. ] [ NA ]. Mother; that which nourishes or forms.

**materia** (mă-tēr'ĭ-ah) [ L. substance-MAT- ]. Substance; matter.

**m. alba** [ L. white matter ], accumulation or aggregation of microorganisms, desquamated epithelial cells, blood cells and food debris loosely adherent to surfaces of plaques, teeth, gingiva or dental appliances.

**m. med'ica** [ L. medical matter ], (1) the branch of medical science that treats of the origin and preparation of drugs, their doses, and their mode of administration; (2) any agent used therapeutically.

**material** (mă-tēr'ĭ-al) [ L. *materialis,* fr. *materia,* substance ]. Elements, parts, or constituents.

**base m.,** any substance from which a denture base may be made, such as shellac, acrylic resin, vulcanite, polystyrene, metal, etc.

**dental m.,** any m. used in dentistry, such as restorative dental m.'s, accessory dental m.'s, and oral dental m.'s.

**impression m.,** any substance or combination of substances used for making a negative reproduction or impression.

**restorative dental m.'s,** m.'s used to replace oral tissues in dentistry; *e.g.,* amalgam, gold alloys, cements, procelain, plastics, and denture m.'s.

**surface-active m.,** surfactant.

**materies morbi** (mă-te'rĭ-ēz mor'bi) [ L. the matter of disease ]. The substance acting as the immediate cause of a disease.

**maternal** (mă-ter′nal) [ L. *maternus,* fr. *mater,* mother ]. Relating to or derived from the mother.

**maternity** (mă-ter′nĭ-tĭ) [ see maternal ]. Motherhood.

**Mathews,** Joseph M., American physician, *1847. See M.'s *speculum.*

**matico** (mat-e′ko) [ Sp. ]. The leaves of *Piper angustifolium* (family Piperaceae), a small tree of Peru and Boliva. Has been used as a local astringent, and internally in the treatment of diarrhea.

**ma′ting.** The pairing of male and female for the purpose of reproduction.

**assortative m.,** m. in which pairing of male and female is not random with respect to one or more specified characters; if mated pairs are alike more often than expected by chance, there is positive assortative m.; if mated pairs are different more often than expected by chance, there is negative assortative m.

**m. isolate,** a population separated from its neighbors by any means (cultural, geographic, etc.) so that all or most m.'s occur within the population group.

**random m.,** panmixis; m. in which the pairing of male and female with respect to one or more characters occurs with the frequency that would be predicted by chance, based on the frequency of the characters in the population.

**mat′rass** [ Fr. *matras* ]. A long-necked glass vessel used for heating dry substances in chemical manipulations.

**mat′rical.** Matricial; relating to any matrix.

**matrica′ria** [ L. *matrix,* womb. MAT- ]. German chamomile; wild chamomile; horse gowan; the flowers of *Matricaria chamomilla* (family *Compositae*). Tonic. Used externally as an infusion in contusions and other inflammation.

**matrices** (ma′trĭ-sēz, mat′rĭ-sēz) [ L. ]. Plural of matrix.

**matricial** (mă-trish′al). Matrical.

**matricide** (mat′rĭ-sĭd) [ L. *mater,* mother, + *caedo,* to kill ]. 1. The killing of one's mother. 2. One who commits such an act.

**matrilineal** [ L. *mater,* mother, + *linea,* line ]. Related to descent through the female line.

**matrix,** pl. **ma′trices** (ma′triks, mat′riks) [ L. womb; female breeding animal. MAT- ]. 1. The womb. 2 [ NA ]. The formative portion of (*a*) a tooth, (*b*) a nail. 3. The intercellular substance of a tissue. 4. A mold in which anything is cast or swaged; a counterdie; a specially shaped instrument, plastic material, or metal strip used for holding and shaping the material used in filling a tooth cavity.

**amalgam m.,** a device used during placement of the amalgam mass within a compound cavity preparation, facilitating proper condensation and contour thereof by providing a confining wall.

**bone m.,** the intercellular substance of bone tissue consisting of collagen fibers, ground substance, and inorganic bone salts.

**cartilage m.,** the intercellular substance of cartilage consisting of fibers and ground substance; **territorial m.** is the more basophilic area around isogenous groups.

**mitochondrial m.,** m. mitochondrialis.

**m. mitochondria′lis,** mitochondrial m.; the finely granular substance occupying the space enclosed by the inner membrane of a mitochondrium.

**nail m.,** m. unguis.

**m. un′guis** [ NA ], nail m.; nailbed; the area of the corium on which the nail rests; it is extremely sensitive and presents numerous longitudinal ridges on its surface. According to some anatomists the nailbed is the portion covered by the body of the nail, the nail m. being only the part on which the root of the nail rests. See fig. under unguis.

**Matson,** D. D., U. S. neurosurgeon, 1913–1969. See M. *operation.*

**mat′ter** [ L. *materies,* substance. MAT- ]. 1. Substance. 2. Pus.

**gray m.,** *substantia grisea.*

**pontine gray m.,** *nuclei pontis.*

**white m.,** *substantia alba.*

**maturate** (mat′u-rate) [ L. *maturo,* pp. -*atus,* to make ripe, fr. *maturus,* ripe ]. To suppurate.

**maturation** (mat′u-ra′shun) [ L. *maturatio,* a ripening, fr. *maturus,* ripe ]. 1. A stage of cell division in the formation of sex cells during which the number of chromosomes in the germ cells is reduced to one-half the number characteristic of the species; see also meiosis; reduction of *chromosomes.* 2. The process of achieving full development or growth. 3. The development changes that lead to maturity.

**mature** (mă-tūr′) [ L. *maturus,* ripe ]. 1. Ripe; fully developed. 2. To ripen; to become fully developed.

**maturity** (mă-tūr′ĭ-tĭ). A state of ripeness or completed growth.

**Mauchart** (mow′khart), Burkhard D., German anatomist, 1696–1751. See M.'s *ligament.*

**Maurer** (mow′rer), Georg, German physician in Sumatra, *1909. See M.'s *dots, clefts.*

**Mauriceau** (mo-re-so′), François, French obstetrician, 1637–1709. See M.'s *lance,* M.'s *maneuver,* M-Levret *maneuver.*

**Mauthner** (mowt′ner), Ludwig, Austrian physician, 1840–1894. See M.'s *cell, fiber, sheath, test.*

**maxilla,** gen. and pl. **maxil′lae** (mak-sil′ah) [ L. jawbone ] [ NA ]. Upper jaw bone; an irregularly shaped bone, supporting the superior teeth and taking part in the formation of the orbit, hard palate, and nasal cavity.

**maxillary** (mak′sĭ-lĕr-ĭ). Relating to the maxilla, or upper jaw.

**maxillitis** (mak′sĭ-li′tis). Inflammation of the maxilla.

**maxil′loden′tal.** Relating to the upper jaw and its associated teeth.

**maxil′lofa′cial.** Pertaining to the jaws and face, particularly with reference to specialized surgery of this region.

**maxil′loju′gal.** Relating to the maxilla and the zygomatic bone.

**maxil′lomandib′ular.** Relating to the upper and lower jaws.

**maxillopalatine** (mak-sil′o-pal′ă-tĭn). Relating to the maxilla and the palatine bone.

**maxillotomy** (mak′sĭ-lot′o-mĭ) [ maxilla + G. *tomē,* incision ]. Surgical sectioning of the maxilla to allow movement of all or a part of the maxilla into the desired portion.

**maxil′lotur′binal.** Relating to the inferior turbinated bone, concha nasalis inferior.

**maximum** (mak′sĭ-mum) [ L. neuter of *maximus,* greatest ]. 1. Fastigium (2). 2. The greatest amount, value, or degree attained or attainable.

**glucose transport m.,** the maximal rate of reabsorption of glucose from the glomerular filtrate; it amounts to approximately 320 mg. per minute in man.

**transport m.,** symbol Tm; tubular m.; the maximal rate of secretion or reabsorption of a substance by the renal tubules.

**tubular m.,** transport m.

**maximus** [ L. ] [ NA ]. In anatomy, greatest.

**Maxwell,** Alice Freeland, San Francisco obstetrician-gynecologist, 1890–1961. See Goldberg-M. *syndrome.*

**Maxwell,** James Clerk, English physicist, 1831–1879. See M.'s *spot.*

**Maxwell,** James L., English physician in Formosa, 19th century. See MacLean-M. *disease.*

**Maxwell,** Patrick W., Dublin ophthalmologist, 1856–1917. See M.'s *ring.*

**May,** R. See M.-Hegglin *anomaly.*

**Maydl** (mi′dl), Karl, Prague surgeon, 1853–1903. See M.'s *hernia, method.*

**Mayer,** Karl, Austrian neurologist, 1862–1932. See M.'s *reflex.*

**Mayer,** Karl, W., German gynecologist, 1795–1868. See M.'s *pessary.*

**mayidism** (ma′id-izm) [ *Zea mays,* maize ]. Pellagra.

**Mayo,** Charles H., American surgeon, 1865–1939. See M.'s *treatment.*

**Mayo,** William J., American surgeon, 1861–1939. See M.'s *operation, vein.*

**Mayo-Robson,** Sir Arthur W., English surgeon, 1853–1933. See M.-R.'s *point, position.*

**Mayou,** Marmaduke Stephen, London ophthalmologist, 1876–1934. See Batten-M. *disease.*

**maza** (ma′zah) [ G. a barley cake, fr. *massō,* to knead ]. Obsolete term for the placenta.

**mazamor'ra.** Name given in Puerto Rico to a dermatitis caused by penetration of the skin by ancylostome larvae.

**maze** [ M.E. *masen*, to confuse ]. A labyrinth; frequently used to study higher functions of the nervous system in rats.

**ma'zindol** (USAN). SANOREX; an isoindole anorexiant that is distinctive in not having the phenethylamine chain common to sympathomimetic amines.

**mazo-.** 1 [ G. *mazos*, breast ]. Combining form relating to the breast; for most terms beginning thus, see masto-. 2 [ G. *maza*, barley cake (placenta) ]. Combining form (rarely used) relating to the placenta.

**mazocacothesis** (ma'zo-kă-koth'e-sis) [ G. *maza*, placenta, + *kakos*, bad, + *thesis*, a placing ]. Placenta previa.

**mazodynia** (ma'zo-din'ĭ-ah). Mastodynia.

**mazology** (ma-zol'o-jĭ). Mastology.

**mazolysis** (ma-zol'ĭ-sis) [ G. *maza*, placenta, + *lysis*, a loosening ]. Detachment of the placenta.

**mazopathy, mazopathia.** 1 [ G. *maza*, a barley cake (placenta), + *pathos*, suffering ]. Any disease of the placenta. 2 [ G. *mazos*, breast ]. Mastopathy.

**mazopexy** (ma'zo-pek'sĭ). Mastopexy.

**mazoplasia** (ma'zo-pla'zĭ-ah). Mastoplasia.

**Mazzoni** (mat-zo'ne), Vittorio, Italian physician, 19th century. See M.'s *corpuscle*, Golgi-M. *corpuscle*.

**M.b.** Abbreviation in prescription writing for L. *misce bene*, mix well.

**Mb, MbCO, MbO₂.** Abbreviations for myoglobin and its combinations with CO and O₂.

**MBC.** Abbreviation for maximum breathing *capacity*.

**M.C.** Abbreviation for (1) *Magister Chirurgiae*, Master of Surgery, (2) Medical Corps.

**mc.** Older abbreviation for millicurie (now mCi).

**McArdle,** B., London pediatrician. See M.'s *disease*, M.-Schmid-Pearson *disease*.

**McArthur,** Louis L., American surgeon, 1858–1934. See M.'s *method*.

**McBurney,** Charles, New York surgeon, 1845–1914. See M.'s *incision, point*.

**McCall,** J. O. See M's *festoon*.

**McCarthy,** Daniel J., U. S. neurologist, 1874–1958. See M.'s *reflexes*.

**McClintock,** Alfred H., Irish physician, 1822–1881. See M.'s *sign*.

**McDonald,** Ellice, U. S. gynecologist, 1876–1955. See M.'s *maneuvers*.

**McGavin method.** See under method.

**McGoon's technique.** See under technique.

**McIndoe,** Archibald H., British surgeon, 1900–1960. See M.'s *operation*.

**McKees' line.** See under line.

**McLean,** Franklin C., U. S. physiologist, *1888. See M.'s *formula*.

**McMurray test.** See under test.

**McPhail test.** See under test.

**McVay,** Chester B., U. S. surgeon, *1911. See M.'s *operation*.

**Md.** Chemical symbol of the element mendelevium.

**M.D.** Abbreviation of *Medicinae Doctor*, Doctor of Medicine.

**M.D.S.** Abbreviation of Master of Dental Surgery.

**M.E.** Abbreviation of Mache Einheit; see Mache *unit*.

**Me.** Abbreviation for the methyl radical, CH₃⁻.

**meal** (mēl). The food consumed at regular intervals or at a specified time.
   Boyden m., a m. consisting of three or four egg yolks, beaten up in milk and seasoned with sugar, port wine, etc., used to test the evacuation time of the gallbladder; 2/3 to 3/4 of the contents will be normally evacuated within 40 minutes.
   test m., toast and tea, or crackers and tea, or gruel or other bland food, given to stimulate gastric secretion before withdrawing gastric contents for analysis.

**mean.** A statistical measurement of central tendency or average derived from adding a set of values and then dividing the sum by the number of values.

**standard error of the m.,** a statistical index of the probability that a given sample m. is representative of the m. of the population from which the sample was drawn.

**measle** (me'zl). 1. The larva (*Cysticercus cellulosae*) of *Taenia solium*, the pork tapeworm. 2. The larva (*Cysticercus bovis*) of *Taenia saginata*, the beef tapeworm.

**measles** (me'zlz) [ D. *maselen* ]. 1. Morbilli; rubeola; an acute exanthematous disease, caused by an RNA virus seemingly related to myxoviruses, and marked by fever and other constitutional disturbances, a catarrhal inflammation of the respiratory mucous membranes, and a generalized maculopapular eruption of a dusky red color, followed by a branny desquamation. The eruption occurs early on the buccal mucous membrane in the form of the so-called Koplik's spots, a fact utilized in the early diagnosis of the disease. The average incubation period is from 10 to 12 days. 2. A disease of swine caused by the presence of *Cysticercus cellulosae*, the m. or larva of *Taenia solium*, the pork tapeworm. 3. A disease of cattle caused by the presence of *Cysticercus bovis*, the m. or larva of *Taenia saginata*, the beef tapeworm of man.
   black m., hemorrhagic m.
   German m., rubella.
   hemorrhag'ic m., a severe form in which the eruption is dark in color due to an effusion of blood into the skin.
   three-day m., rubella.
   tropical m., a disease of uncertain character, somewhat resembling roetheln, occurring in southern China.

**measly** (me'zlĭ). Pertaining to pork or beef infected with the cysticerci of *Taenia solium* or *T. saginata*, respectively.

**meatal** (me-a'tal). Relating to a meatus.

**meato-** [ L. *meatus*, q.v. ]. Combining form relating to a meatus.

**meatomastoidectomy** (me'ă-to-mas-toy-dek'to-mĭ). A modified mastoidectomy to exteriorize mastoid air cells into the external auditory meatus, preserving the tympanic cavity and ossicles.

**meatometer** (me'ă-tom'e-ter) [ meato- + G. *metron*, measure ]. An instrument for measuring the size of a meatus, especially the meatus of the urethra.

**meatoplasty** (me'ă-to-plas-tĭ). Reparative or reconstructive surgery of a meatus or canal, *e.g.*, the external auditory meatus.

**meatorrhaphy** (me'ă-tor'ă-fĭ) [ meato- + G. *rhaphē*, suture ]. Closing by suture the wound made in a previous meatotomy.

**meatoscope** (me-at'o-skōp) [ meato- + G. *skopeō*, to view ]. A form of speculum for examining a meatus, especially the meatus of the urethra.

**meatoscopy** (me-ă-tos'ko-pĭ) [ meato- + G. *skopeō*, to view ]. Inspection, usually instrumental, of any meatus, especially of the meatus of the urethra.
   ure'teral m., inspection, through a cystoscope, of the orifices of the ureters in the wall of the bladder.

**meatotome** (me-at'o-tōm). A knife with short cutting edge for use in meatotomy.

**meatotomy** (me-ă-tot'o-mĭ) [ meato- + G. *tomē*, incision ]. Porotomy; an incision made to enlarge the meatus of the urethra.

**meatus,** pl. **meatus** (me-a'tus) [ L. a going, a passage, fr. *meo*, pp. *meatus*, to go, pass ] [ NA ]. A passage or channel, especially the external opening of a canal.
   m. acus'ticus externus [ NA ], external acoustic or auditory m.; antrum auris; auditory canal; the passage leading inward through the tympanic portion of the temporal bone, from the auricle to the membrana tympani; it consists of an osseous (internal) portion and a fibrocartilaginous (external) portion, the **m. acusticus externus cartilagineus.**
   m. acus'ticus internus [ NA ], internal acoustic or internal auditory m.; a canal running from the internal acoustic pore, through the petrous portion of the temporal bone, ending at the fundus where a thin plate of bone separates it from the vestibule; it gives passage to the facial and vestibulocochlear nerves together with the labyrinthine artery and veins.
   external auditory m., m. acusticus externus.
   fish-mouth m., a red and swollen condition of the orifice of the urethra (urinary m.) in gonorrhea.

**internal auditory m.,** m. acusticus internus.

**m. nasi** [ NA ], the three passages in the nasal cavity formed by the projection of the conchae, the **m. nasi inferior** lies below the inferior concha, the **m. nasi medius** between the middle and inferior conchae, the **m. nasi superior** between the superior and middle conchae.

**m. na′sopharynge′us** [ NA ], nasopharyngeal passage; the posterior part of the nasal cavity from the posterior limits of the conchae to the choanae.

**m. urina′rius,** *ostium* urethrae externum.

**meban′azine.** ACTOMOL; (α-methylbenzyl)hydrazine; antidepressant with inhibitory effect on monoamine oxidase.

**meben′dazole** (USAN). Methyl 5-benzoyl-2-benzimidazolecarbamate; anthelmintic.

**mebev′erine hydrochloride** (USAN). DUSPATALIN; 4-[ ethyl(*p*-methoxy-α-methylphenethyl)amino ]butyl veratrate hydrochloride; intestinal antispasmodic.

**mebhy′droline.** OMERIL; 5-benzyl-1,3,4,5-tetrahydro-2-methyl-2*H*-pyrido[ 4,3-*b* ]indole; antihistaminic agent.

**mebrophenhy′dramine.** BROMADRYL; 2-(*p*-bromo-α-methyl-α-phenyl-benzyloxy)-*N,N*-dimethylethylamine; antihistaminic agent.

**mebu′tamate** (USAN). CAPLA; carbamic acid 2-sec-butyl-2-methyltrimethylene ester; chemically, it differs only slightly from meprobamate, and possesses similar CNS-depressant properties. Used as a centrally acting hypotensive agent.

**mecamylamine hydrochloride** (mek′ă-mil′ă-mēn) (BP). INVERSINE hydrochloride; 3-methylaminoisocamphane hydrochloride; a secondary amine that blocks transmission of impulses at autonomic ganglia (similar to but more effective than hexamethonium); used in the management of severe hypertension.

**mechanical** (me-kan′ĭ-kal) [ G. *meckanikos*, relating to a machine, fr. *mēchanē*, a contrivance, machine ]. 1. Performed by means of some apparatus, not manually. 2. Explaining phenomena in terms of mechanics. 3. Automatic.

**mechan′icorecep′tor.** Mechanoreceptor.

**mechanics** (me-kan′iks) [ see mechanical ]. The science of the action of forces in promoting motion or equilibrium.

**body m.,** the study of the action of muscles in producing motion or posture of the body.

**mechanism** (mek′ă-nizm) [ G. *mēchanē*, a contrivance ]. 1. An arrangement or grouping of the parts of anything that has a definite action. 2. The means by which an effect is obtained.

**association m.,** the cerebral m. whereby the memory of past sensations may be compared or associated with present ones.

**countercurrent multiplication m.,** postulated scheme of production of hypertonic urine by the kidney.

**defense m.,** (1) a psychological means of coping with conflict or anxiety, *e.g.,* conversion, denial, dissociation, rationalization, repression, and sublimation; (2) the psychic structure underlying a coping strategy; (3) immunological m.

**Douglas′ m.,** m. of spontaneous evolution in transverse lie; extreme lateral flexion of the vertebral column with birth of the lateral aspect of thorax before the buttocks.

**Duncan′s m.,** the passage of the placenta from the uterus with the rough side foremost.

**feedback m.,** see feedback *inhibition.*

**gating m.,** occurrence of the maximum refractory period among cardiac conducting cells approximately 2 mm. proximal to the terminal Purkinje fibers in the ventricular muscle, beyond which the refractory period is shortened through a sequence of Purkinje cells, transitional cells, and muscular cells; gating m. may be a cause of ventricular aberration, bidirectional tachycardia, and concealed extrasystoles.

**immunological m.,** defense m. (3); the groups of cells (chiefly lymphocytes and cells of the reticuloendothelial system) that function in establishing active acquired immunity or induced sensitivity.

**ping-pong m.,** a special case of bi-bi reaction (*q.v.,* under reaction), in which an enzyme reacts with one substrate to form a product and a modified enzyme, the latter then reacting with a second substrate to form a second, final

product, and regenerating the original enzyme. Schematically:

$$E + S_1 \rightarrow EM + P_1$$
$$EM + S_2 \rightarrow E + P_2$$
$$\text{Sum: } S_1 + S_2 \rightarrow P_1 + P_2$$

**pressoreceptive m.,** pressoreceptor *system,* especially of the carotid sinuses and aortic arch.

**proprioceptive m.,** the m. of sense of position and movement, by which we are able to adjust our muscular movements to a great degree of accuracy and to maintain our equilibrium.

**Schultze′s m.,** expulsion of the placenta with the fetal surface foremost.

**mechanocardiography** (mek′ă-no-kar-dĭ-og′ră-fĭ). The use of graphic tracings reflecting the mechanical effects of the heart beat, such as the carotid pulse tracing or apexcardiogram.

**mechanocyte** (mek′ă-no-sīt). An *in vitro* tissue culture fibroblast.

**mechanophobia** (mek′ă-no-fo′bĭ-ah) [ G. *mēchanē,* machine, + *phobos,* fear ]. Morbid fear of machinery.

**mechanoreceptor** (mek′ă-no-re-sep′tor). Mechanicoreceptor; a receptor which has the role of responding to mechanical pressures; *e.g.,* receptors in the carotid sinuses, touch receptors in the skin.

**mechanotherapy** (mek′ă-no-thěr′ă-pĭ) [ G. *mēchanē,* machine, + *therapeia,* treatment ]. Treatment of disease by means of apparatus or mechanical appliances of any kind.

**mèche** (māsh) [ Fr. wick ]. A strip of gauze or other material used as a tent or drain.

**mechlorethamine hydrochloride** (mek′lōr-eth′ă-mēn) (USP). MUSTARGEN hydrochloride; mustine hydrochloride; nitrogen mustard (*q.v.*); HN2; 2,2′-dichloro-*N*-methyldiethylamine hydrochloride; methyl-bis(beta-chloroethyl)amine hydrochloride; it is cytotoxic for all cells, but with a special affinity for bone marrow, lymphatic tissues, and rapidly proliferating cells of certain neoplasms. Used for the palliative treatment of Hodgkin′s disease, lymphosarcoma, and certain chronic leukemias.

**mecism** (me′sizm) [ G. *mēkos,* length, + suffix *-ismos,* condition ]. Abnormal elongation of the body or one or more of its parts.

**Mecistocirrus** (me-sis′to-sīr′us) [ G. *mēkistos,* very long, + L. *cirrus,* curl, the protruding male organ of a nematode ]. A monotypic genus of trichostrongylid nematodes forming its own family, Mecistocirrinae, and consisting of a single species, *M. digitatus;* it is not grossly distinguished from *Haemonchus contortus* and has about the same effect on the host. *M.* is distributed chiefly in Asia and is found in cattle, sheep, buffalo, bison, the stomach of pigs, and rarely in man.

**Mecke′s reagent.** See under reagent.

**Meckel,** Johann F., Sr., German anatomist and obstetrician, 1714–1774. See M.′s *band, cavity, ganglion, ligament, space.*

**Meckel,** Johann F., the younger, German comparative anatomist and embryologist, 1781–1833. See M.′s *cartilage, diverticulum, plane.*

**meckelectomy** (mek′el-ek′to-mĭ) [ Meckel′s ganglion + G. *ektomē,* excision ]. Excision of the sphenopalatine, or Meckel′s ganglion.

**meclizine hydrochloride** (mek′lĭ-zēn) (USP). BONAMINE hydrochloride; meclozine hydrochloride; 1-(*p*-chlorobenzhydryl)-4-(*m*-methylbenzyl) piperazine dihydrochloride. Antihistaminic agent useful in the prevention and relief of motion sickness and symptoms caused by vestibular disorders.

**meclofenox′ate.** LUCIDRIL; (*p*-chlorophenoxy)acetic acid 2-(dimethylamino)ethyl ester; analeptic.

**mecloqualone** (mek-lo-kwah′lōn) (USAN). 3-(*o*-Chlorophenyl)-2-methyl-4(3*H*)-quinazolinone; sedative and hypnotic.

**meclox'amine citrate.** MELIDORM; 2-[ ($p$-chloro-$\alpha$-methyl-$\alpha$-phenylbenzyl) oxy ]-$N,N$-dimethylpropylamine citrate; sedative and hypnotic.

**mec'lozine hydrochloride** (BP). Meclizine hydrochloride.

**mecometer** (me-kom'e-ter) [ G. *mēkos*, length, + *metron*, measure ]. An instrument, like calipers with a scale attachment, for ready measurement of the newborn child.

**mec'onate** [ G. *mēkōn*, poppy ]. A salt or ester of meconic acid.

**mecon'ic acid.** 3-Hydroxy-4-oxy-4$H$-pyran-2,6-dicarboxylic acid; obtained from opium; it forms soluble salts (meconates) with many of the alkaloids of opium.

**mec'onin.** Opianyl; $C_{10}H_{10}O_4$; the lactone of meconic acid, found also in *Hydrastis canadensis*; hypnotic.

**meconiorrhea** (me-ko'nĭ-o-re'ah) [ meconium + G. *rhoia*, flow ]. The passage, by the newborn infant, of an abnormally large amount of meconium.

**meconism** (me'ko-nizm) [ G. *mēkōn*, the poppy ]. Opium addiction or poisoning.

**meconium** (me-ko'nĭ-um) [ L. fr. G. *mēkōnion*, dim. of *mēkōn*, poppy ]. 1. The first intestinal discharges of the newborn infant, greenish in color and consisting of epithelial cells, mucus, and bile. 2. Opium.

**Medawar** (med'ah-war). Peter B., English biologist, *1915. Nobel laureate, 1960, with F. Macfarlane Burnet for the discovery of acquired immunological tolerance.

**medazepam** (mĕ-daz'e-pam, mĕ-da'ze-pam) (USAN). NOBRIUM; 7-chloro-2,3-dihydro-1-methyl-5-phenyl-1$H$-benzodiazepine monohydrochloride; an antianxiety agent.

**med'falan.** Medphalan.

**media** (me'dĭ-ah) [ L. fem. of *medius*, middle ]. 1. *Tunica media*. 2. Plural of medium.

**mediad** (me'dĭ-ad). Toward the middle line.

**medial** (me'dĭ-al) [ L. *medialis*, middle ]. Relating to the middle or center; nearer to the median or midsagittal plane.

**medialecithal** (me'dĭ-ă-les'ĭ-thal) [ L. *medialis*, medial, + G. *lekithos*, egg yolk ]. Denoting an egg with a moderate amount of yolk, as in amphibians.

**media'lis** [ L. ] [ NA ]. Medial.

**median** (me'dĭ-an) [ L. *medianus*, middle ]. 1. Central; middle; lying in the midline. 2. The middle value in a set of measurements; like the mean, a measure of central tendency.

**media'num** [ L. ] [ NA ]. Median.

**media'nus** [ L. ] [ NA ]. Median.

**mediastinal** (me'dĭ-as-ti'nal). Relating to the mediastinum.

**mediastinitis** (me'dĭ-as-tī-ni'tis). Inflammation of the cellular tissue of the mediastinum.

**mediastinography** (me'dĭ-as-tī-nog'ră-fī) [ mediastinum + G. *graphō*, to write ]. X-ray of the mediastinum.

   **gaseous m.**, x-ray of mediastinum after injection of air (artificial pneumomediastinum).

**mediastinopericarditis** (me'dĭ-as-ti'no-pĕr'ĭ-kar-di'tis). Inflammation of the pericardium and of the surrounding mediastinal cellular tissue.

**me'diastin'oscope.** Instrument designed by Eric Carlens for inspection of mediastinum through a suprasternal incision.

**mediastinoscopy** (me'dĭ-as-tī-nos'ko-pī) [ mediastinum + G. *skopeō*, to view ]. Exploration of the mediastinum through a suprasternal incision, designed for biopsy of paratracheal lymph nodes.

**mediastinotomy** (me'dĭ-as-tī-not'o-mī) [ mediastinum + G. *tomē*, incision ]. Incision into the mediastinum.

**mediastinum** (me'dĭ-as-ti'num) [ Mod. L. a middle septum, fr. Mediev. L. *mediastinus*, medial, fr. L. *mediastinus*, a lower servant, fr. *medius*, middle ]. 1. A septum between two parts of an organ or a cavity. 2 [ NA ]. Interpulmonary septum; the median partition of the thoracic cavity, covered by the mediastinal pleura and containing all the thoracic viscera and structures except the lungs. It is divided arbitrarily into four parts: the **superior m. (m. superius)** is that part lying above the pericardium; it contains the arch of the aorta and the vessels arising from

it, the brachiocephalic veins, and upper portion of the superior vena cava, the trachea, the esophagus, the thoracic duct, the thymus, and the phrenic, vagus, cardiac, and left recurrent laryngeal nerves. The **middle m. (m. medium)** contains the pericardium and its contents and the phrenic nerves and accompanying vessels. The **anterior m. (m. anterius)** is the narrow space between the pericardium and the sternum containing some lymph nodes and vessels and branches of the internal thoracic artery. The **posterior m. (m. posterius)** lies between the pericardium and the vertebral column, below the level of the fourth thoracic vertebra; it contains the descending aorta, thoracic duct, esophagus, azygos veins, and vagus nerves.

   **m. testis** [ NA ], septum of the testis; corpus Highmori; Highmore's body; a mass of fibrous tissue continuous with the tunica albuginea, projecting into the testis from its posterior border.

**mediate** (me'dĭ-it, -āt) [ L. *mediatus*, fr. *medio*, pp. *-atus*, to divide in the middle ]. 1. Situated between two parts; intermediate. 2. To effect something by means of an intermediary substance (*e.g.*, complement-mediated phagocytosis).

**mediation** (me'dĭ-a'shun). The action of an intermediary substance (mediator).

**mediator** (me'dĭ-a'tor). An intermediary substance or thing.

**medicable** (med'ĭ-kă-bl). Admitting of treatment with hope of cure.

**medical** (med'ĭ-kal) [ L. *medicalis*, fr. *medicus*, physician (see medicus) ]. 1. Relating to medicine or the practice of medicine. 2. Medicinal.

**medic'ament** [ L. *medicamentum*, medicine, *q.v.* ]. A medicine; a medicinal application; a remedy.

**med'icamento'sus** [ L. ]. Relating to a drug; a term characterizing a drug eruption.

**medicate** (med'ĭ-kāt) [ L. *medico*, pp. *-atus*, to heal ]. 1. To treat disease by the giving of drugs. 2. To impregnate with a medicinal substance.

**med'ica'ted.** Impregnated with a medicinal substance.

**medication** (med'ĭ-ka'shun). 1. The act of medicating (see medicate), in either sense. 2. A medicinal substance, or medicament.

   **arrhenic m.**, treatment of disease by means of the organic preparations of arsenic, the cacodylates, and methylarsinates.

   **ionic m.**, iontophoresis (2).

   **preanesthetic m.**, drugs administered prior to an anesthetic to decrease anxiety and to obtain a smoother induction to, maintenance of, and emergency from anesthesia.

**med'ica'tor.** 1. One who gives medicaments for the relief of disease; a term sometimes applied in derision to one who prescribes drugs for every minor ailment. 2. An instrument for use in making therapeutic applications to the deeper parts.

**me'dicephal'ic.** Median cephalic; denoting the communicating vessel between the median and the cephalic veins of the forearm.

**medicinal** (mĕ-dis'ĭ-nal). 1. Relating to medicine having curative properties. 2. Medical.

**medicine** [ L. *medicina*, fr. *medicus*, physician (see medicus) ]. 1. A drug. 2. The art of preventing or curing disease; the science that treats of disease in all its relations. 3. The study and treatment of general diseases or those affecting the internal parts of the body, distinguished from surgery.

   **adolescent m.**, see ephebiatrics.

   **aerospace m.**, see space m.

   **aviation m.**, the study and practice of physiology, pathology, and other branches of m. as they apply to aviation.

   **clinical m.**, the study and practice of m. in relation to the actual patient; the art of m. as distinguished from laboratory science.

   **domestic m.**, treatment of minor ailments by simple remedies in the home by a member of the family; see also folk m.

   **eclectic m.**, (1) a cult of medical practitioners in America, now defunct. They used preparations of indigenous plants which they thought were specific cures when certain signs or symptoms occurred; (2) Greek and Roman physicians, affiliated with no medical sect, who adopted the practice and teachings which they considered best from all past and present systems. Some members of this group were diligent compilers of great medical writings of the past.

**empiric m.,** see empirical *treatment.*

**experimental m.,** the scientific investigation of medical problems by experimentation upon animals or by clinical research.

**federal m.,** state m.

**folk m.,** treatment of ailments in the home by remedies and simple measures based upon experience and knowledge handed on from generation to generation.

**forensic m.,** legal m.; medical jurisprudence; medicolegal science; (1) the relation and application of medical facts to legal problems, as in the presentation of autopsy findings in murder trials; (2) the law in its bearing on the practice of medicine.

**group m.,** the practice of m. by a group of physicians, each of whom as a rule confines himself to some special field; such a group often shares a common suite of consulting rooms, laboratories, x-ray equipment, etc., and is called a clinic.

**internal m.,** the branch of m. dealing with nonsurgical diseases of a constitutional nature in adults.

**legal m.,** forensic m.

**military m.,** the practice of any branch of m. as applied to the special circumstances associated with military operations.

**nuclear m.,** the clinical discipline concerned with the diagnostic, therapeutic, and investigative uses of radionuclides, excluding the therapeutic use of sealed radiation sources.

**patent m.,** a nostrum; a m., usually of secret composition or protected by a patent, and advertised to the public, often with false or extravagant claims.

**physical m.,** the study and treatment of disease mainly by mechanical and other physical methods.

**practice of m.,** the practical application of scientific medical principles, or of the theory of m., to the diagnosis and treatment of disease.

**preventive m.,** the branch of medical science that treats of the prevention of disease.

**proprietary m.,** a medicinal compound the formula and mode of manufacture of which are the property of the maker.

**psychiat'ric m.,** psychiatry.

**psychosomatic m.,** the study and treatment of diseases, disorders, or abnormal states in which psychological processes and reactions are believed to play a prominent role.

**quack m.,** a compound advertised falsely as curative of a certain disease or diseases.

**railway m.,** treatment of injuries resulting from railways, including also the sanitation of cars and of stations, the ocular and physical examination of engineers and other employees, etc.

**rational m.,** scientific m.; rational therapeutics; m. based upon fundamental causes and medical knowledge as opposed to empiric m.

**socialized m.,** state m. (2).

**space m.,** the field of m. that deals with diseases or derangements of body functions of men and animals in space vehicles, removed from a gravitational field, and exposed to the hazards of radiant energy and perhaps other hazards, such as isolation, claustrophobia, mechanical difficulty with alimentation and excretion, rapid decompression, and decomposition.

**spagir'ic m.** [ Early mod. L. *spagiricus,* pertaining to alchemy or chemistry; probably coined by Paracelsus fr. G. *spaō,* to tear open, + *ageirō,* to collect ], term given to the medical system expounded by Paracelsus that stressed the treatment of disease by various types of chemical substances.

**state m.,** (1) public m.; the branch of medical science that deals with statistics, hygiene, the prevention and overcoming of epidemics, etc.; (2) the control of medical practice by an organization of the government, the practitioners being an integral part of the organization from which they draw their pay and to which the public contributes in some form or other.

**static m.,** a system of therapeutics based upon the varying weight of the body in relation to the amount of food taken and the total excretion.

**third party m.,** the intervention between physician and patient of a third party or agency in the patient-physician relationship.

**tropical m.,** the branch of m. that deals with diseases, mainly of parasitic origin, of tropical countries.

**veterinary m.,** medical science as applied to the study of animals in health and disease and to the diagnosis and treatment of the diseases.

**war m.,** military m.

**medico-** (med'ĭ-ko-) [ L. *medicus,* physician ]. Combining form meaning medical.

**medicobiologic, -biological** (med'ĭ-ko-bi-o-loj'ik, -loj'-ĭ-kal). Pertaining to the biologic aspects of medicine.

**medicochirurgical** (med'ĭ-ko-ki-rur'jĭ-kal) [ medico- G. *cheirourgia,* surgery ]. Relating to both medicine and surgery, or to both physicians and surgeons.

**medicolegal** (med'ĭ-ko-le'gal) [ medico- + L. *legalis,* legal ]. Relating to both medicine and the law; see forensic *medicine.*

**medicomechanical** (med'ĭ-ko-me-kan'ĭ-kal). Relating to both medicinal and mechanical measures in therapeutics.

**medicophysical** (med'ĭ-ko-fiz'ĭ-kal). Relating to disease and the condition of the body generally; as m. examination, in which a person is examined in order to determine the presence or absence of disease as well as to note the general physical condition.

**medicopsychology** (med'ĭ-ko-si-kol'o-jĭ). Psychology in its relation to medicine.

**medicus** (med'ĭ-kus) [ L. fr. *medeor,* to heal ]. Physician.

**Medin** (ma'dĕn), Oskar, Swedish physician, 1874–1928. See M.'s *disease,* Heine-M. *disease.*

**medio-, medi-** (me'dĭ-o-, me'dĭ-) [ L. *medius,* middle ]. Combining forms meaning middle, or median.

**mediocarpal** (me'dĭ-o-kar'pal). Mesocarpal; midcarpal; relating to the central part of the carpus; denoting the articulation of the carpal bones with each other.

**medioccipital** (me'dĭ-ok-sip'ĭ-tal). Midoccipital.

**me'diodens** [ medio- + L. *dens,* tooth ]. A supernumerary tooth located between the two maxillary central incisors.

**me'diodor'sal.** Relating to the median plane and the dorsal plane.

**me'diolat'eral.** Relating to the median plane and a side.

**me'dionecro'sis.** Necrosis of a tunica media.

**m. of the aorta,** cystic medial *necrosis.*

**m. aortae idiopathica cystica,** cystic medial *necrosis.*

**me'diotar'sal.** Midtarsal; mesotarsal; relating to the middle of the tarsus; denoting the articulations of the tarsal bones with each other.

**mediotype** (me'dĭ-o-tip). Mesomorph.

**medisect** (me'dĭ-sekt) [ L. *medius,* middle, + *seco,* pp. *sectus,* to cut ]. To incise in the median line.

**medium,** pl. **media** (me'dĭ-um, me'dĭ-ah) [ L. neuter of *medius,* middle ]. 1. A means; anything through which an action is performed. 2. A substance through which impulses or impressions are transmitted. 3. Culture m.; a substance, either solid or liquid, used for the cultivation of microorganisms. 4. The liquid vehicle holding a substance in solution or suspension.

**clearing m.,** one used in histology for making specimens transparent or transparent.

**contrast m.,** any material opaque to the x-rays, such as barium, used in roentgenography to visualize the stomach, intestine, or other organ.

**culture m.,** m. (3).

**dispersion m.,** external *phase.*

**Dorset's egg m.,** a m. for cultivating the tubercle bacillus; it consists of the whites and yolks of four fresh eggs and 25 ml. of a 0.95 per cent sodium chloride solution.

**Eagle's Basal M.,** a solution of various salts containing 13 naturally occurring amino acids, several vitamins, two antibiotics, and phenol red; used as a tissue culture medium

**Eagle's Minimum Essential M.** (abbreviated MEM); similar to Eagle's Basal Medium but with different amounts and a few exclusions (*e.g.*, antibiotics and phenol red); used as a tissue culture medium.

**Endo's m.,** Endo *agar.*

**external m.,** external *phase.*

**Loeffler's blood culture m.,** a culture m. consisting of 3 parts beef blood serum and sheep blood serum and 1 part beef bouillon containing 1 per cent peptone, 1 per cent glucose, and 1/2 per cent sodium chloride.

**mounting m.,** a substance, usually resinous, used for mounting a cover glass on histologic suspensions.

**passive m.,** one that produces no change in the specimens placed in it.

**separating m.,** (1) any coating which serves to prevent one surface from adhering to another; (2) in dentistry, a material usually applied to a cast to facilitate separation from the resin denture base after curing; a coating on impressions to facilitate removal of the cast.

**Simmons' citrate m.,** an agar medium on which Enterobacteriaceae grow through citrate utilization.

**me'dius** [ L. ] [ NA ]. Middle; denoting an anatomical structure that is between two other similar structures or that is midway in position.

**MEDLARS.** Abbreviation for Medical Literature Analysis and Retrieval System, a computerized index system of the U. S. National Library of Medicine.

**MEDLINE** (MEDLARS-on-line). A telephone linkage between a number of medical libraries in the United States and MEDLARS for rapid provision of medical bibliographies.

**medmain.** 2-Methyl-3-ethyl-5-dimethylaminoindole; an experimental serotonin (5-hydroxytryptamine) antagonist.

**medorrhea** (me-dor-re'ah) [ G. *mēdos* (sing.), the bladder, *medea* (pl.), the genitals, + *rhoia*, flow ]. Gleet.

**medphalan** (med'fă-lan). Medfalan; D-phenylalanine mustard; D-sarcolysine; D-3-[ *p*-[ *bis*-(2-chloroethyl)amino ]-phenyl ]-alanine; an antineoplastic agent.

**medrogestone** (med'ro-jis'tŏn)    (USAN).   COLPRONE; 6,17α-dimethyl-4,6-pregnadiene-3,20-dione (for pregnane structure, see steroids); an oral progestin.

**medrox'yproges'terone acetate** (USP). DEPO-PROVERA; PROVERA; 17α-hydroxy-6α-methylprogesterone; a progestational agent that is active orally as well as parenterally, and more potent than progesterone; used, in combination with ethynyl estradiol, as an oral contraceptive.

**medryl'amine.** HISTAPHEN; 2-(*p*-methoxy-α-phenylbenzyloxy-*N,N*-dimethylethylamine; antihistaminic.

**med'rysone**    (USP).   HMS;    11β-hydroxy-6α-methylpregn-4-ene-3,20-dione; a glucocorticoid used topically as an anti-inflammatory agent.

**medulla,** pl. **medul'lae** (me-dul'ah) [ L. marrow, fr. *medius,* middle ] [ NA ]. Any soft marrow-like structure, especially in the center of a part. Specifically, (1) m. ossium, (2) m. spinalis, (3) m. oblongata.

**m. glan'dulae suprarena'lis** [ NA ], m. of the adrenal gland; it is composed principally of anastomosing cords of cells in the core of the gland; the cells display a chromaffin reaction because of the presence of epinephrine and norepinephrine in their granules.

**m. of hair shaft,** the central axis of some hairs, containing air spaces in white hair; the medullary portion is surrounded by the cortex.

**m. no'di lymphat'ici,** [ NA ], m. of a lymph node; the central portion of a node consisting of cordlike masses of lymphocytes separated by lymph sinuses; it reaches the surface of the node at the hilus.

**m. oblonga'ta** [ NA ], myelencephalon; the lowest subdivision of the brainstem, immediately continuous with the spinal cord, extending from the lower border of the decussation of the pyramidal tracts up to the pons; its ventral surface resembles that of the spinal cord except for the bilateral prominence of the inferior olive; the dorsal surface of its upper half forms part of the floor of the fourth ventricle. Motor nuclei of the m. oblongata include the hypoglossal nucleus, the dorsal motor nucleus, and the nucleus ambiguus of the vagus; sensory nuclei include the nuclei of the posterior column (gracilis and cuneatus), the

cochlear and vestibular nuclei, the midportion of the spinal nucleus of the trigeminus, and the nucleus of the solitary tract.

**m. ossium** [ NA ], the bone marrow; the tissue filling the cavities of bones, having a stroma of reticular fibers and cells. It may be yellow (m. ossium flava) because the meshes of the reticular network are filled with fat, or red (m. ossium rubra) because the meshes contain the developmental stages of erythrocytes, granular leukocytes, and megakaryocytes.

**m. ossium flava** [ NA ], yellow bone marrow; see m. ossium.

**m. ossium rubra** [ NA ], red bone marrow; see m. ossium.

**m. renis** [ NA ], medulla of the kidney; the inner, darker portion of the kidney parenchyma consisting of the renal pyramids.

**m. spina'lis** [ NA ], spinal marrow; spinal cord; the elongated cylindrical portion of the cerebrospinal axis, or central nervous system, which is contained in the spinal or vertebral canal.

**medul'ladrenalec'tomy.** Removal of the medullary portion of the adrenal gland.

**medul'lar.** Medullary.

**medullary** (med'uh-lĕr-ĭ, mĕ-dul'ĕr-ĭ, med'u-lĕr-ĭ). Relating to the medulla or marrow.

**med'ullated.** 1. Having a medulla or medullary substance. 2. Myelinated.

**medullation** (med'uh-la'shun, med'u-). 1. Acquiring, or the act of formation of, marrow or medulla. 2. Myelination.

**med'ullec'tomy** [ medulla + G. *ektomē,* excision ]. Excision of any medulla substance.

**medullization** (med'uh-lĭ-za'shun, med'u-). The enlargement of the medullary spaces in rarefying osteitis.

**medullo-** (med'uh-lo-, mĕ-dul'o-, med'u-lo-) [ L. *medulla, q. v.* ]. Combining form meaning medulla.

**medulloarthritis** (med-ul'o-ar-thri'tis). Inflammation of the cancellous articular extremity of a long bone.

**med'ulloblast.** Cells of the neural tube that may develop into nerve cells or neuroglial cells.

**med'ulloblasto'ma.** Neurospongioma; a term used to define a glioma consisting of neoplastic cells that resemble the undifferentiated cells of the primitive medullary tube. M.'s are usually located in the vermis of the cerebellum, frequently extend into the fourth ventricle and adjacent cerebellar tissue, and may be implanted discretely or coalescently on the surfaces of the cerebellum, brainstem, and spinal cord; they comprise approximately 3 per cent of all intracranial neoplasms, are usually found in children, and are approximately twice as frequent in boys as in girls. The neoplastic cells are fairly uniform in size and shape, rounded or ovoid, and have hyperchromatic nuclei that are situated in an inconspicuous, relatively scant cytoplasm; they tend to occur individually, in small and poorly defined groups, or, occasionally, in a pseudorosette pattern.

**med'ullocell.** Myelocyte.

**medulloepithelioma** (med'uh-lo-ep-ĭ-the-lĭ-o'mah). A primitive, rapidly growing glioma thought to originate from the cells of the embryonic medullary canal; although such neoplasms may occur, satisfactory criteria for conclusive identification are lacking, and most observers include them with ependymomas.

**medullomyoblastoma** (med'uh-lo-mi'o-blas-to'mah). A rare histologic variant of medulloblastoma with scattered smooth and striated muscle cells incorporated into the neoplasm.

**Meeh-DuBois formula.** See under formula.

**Mees' lines** or **stripes.** See Mees' *lines.*

**mefenam'ic acid** (BP, USAN). PONSTEL; *N*-(2,3-xylyl)anthranilic acid; analgesic with anti-inflammatory properties.

**mefen'orex hydrochloride** (USAN). ANEXATE; *N*-(3-chloropropyl)-α-methylphenethylamine hydrochloride; a sympathomimetic drug with anorexic activity.

**mefex'amide** (USAN). TIMODYNE; *N*-[ 2- diethylamino)ethyl ]-2-(*p*-methoxyphenoxy)acetamide;   antidepressant.

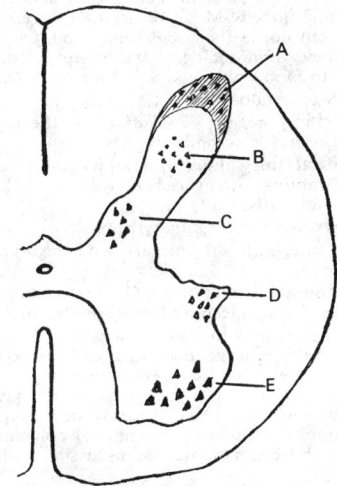

**Main Cell Groups in the Thoracic Region of the
Spinal Cord**

*a*, Substantia gelatinosa of Rolando; *b*, chief sensory nucleus; *c*, dorsal nucleus; *d*, intermediolateral cell column (sympathetic); *e*, ventral horn cells (motor).

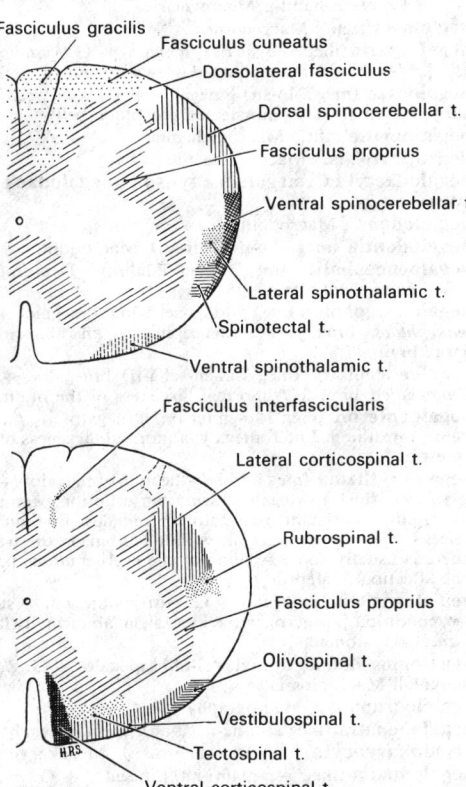

Fasciculus gracilis
Fasciculus cuneatus
Dorsolateral fasciculus
Dorsal spinocerebellar t.
Fasciculus proprius
Ventral spinocerebellar t.
Lateral spinothalamic t.
Spinotectal t.
Ventral spinothalamic t.

Fasciculus interfascicularis
Lateral corticospinal t.
Rubrospinal t.
Fasciculus proprius
Olivospinal t.
Vestibulospinal t.
Tectospinal t.
Ventral corticospinal t.

**Tracts of Brain and Spinal Cord**

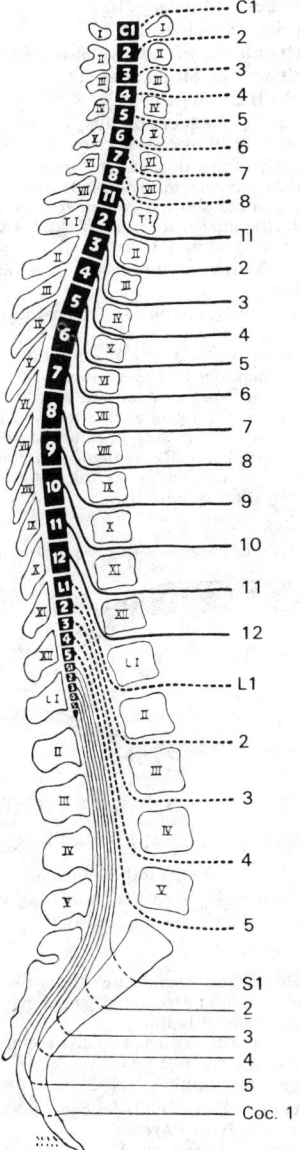

**Segments of Spinal Cord (Medulla Spinalis)**

Diagram of the position of the spinal cord segments with
reference to the bodies and spinous processes of the vertebrae.
Note also the place of origin of the nerve roots from the spinal
cord and their emergence from the corresponding intervertebral foramina (Haymaker and Woodhall). (From Truex, R. C.;
*Strong and Elwyn's Human Neuroanatomy*, Ed. 5, The Williams & Wilkins Co., Baltimore, 1964.)

839

**mega-** (meg'ah-) [ G. *megas*, big ]. 1. Combining form meaning large, oversize; see also macro- and megalo-. 2. A prefix used in the metric system to signify one million ($10^6$).

**meg'abacte'rium.** Macrobacterium; a bacterium of unusually large size.

**meg'ablad'der.** Megalocystis.

**meg'acar'dia.** Cardiomegaly.

**meg'acar'yoblast.** Megakaryoblast.

**meg'acar'yocyte.** Megakaryocyte.

**meg'acepha'lia.** Megacephaly.

**megacephalic, megacephalous** (meg'ah-sĕ-fal'ik, -sef'-ă-lus). Relating to or characterized by megacephaly.

**megacephaly** (meg'ah-sef'ă-lĭ) [ mega- + G. *kephalē*, head ]. Megacephalia; macrocephaly; megalocephaly; megalocephalia; a condition in which the head is abnormally large. Usually applied to an adult skull with a capacity of over 1450 cc., and may be congenital or acquired.

**megacin.** Bacteriocin produced by strains of *Bacillus megaterium*.

**megacoccus** (meg'ah-kok'us). Macrococcus; a coccus of unusually large size.

**megacolon** (meg'ah-ko'lon). A condition of extreme dilation and hypertrophy of the colon.

    **congenital m.,** m. congenitum; Myà's disease; Hirschsprung's disease; congenital dilation and hypertrophy of the colon due to absence or marked reduction in the number of ganglion cells (aganglionosis) of the myenteric plexus of the rectum and a varying but continuous length of gut above the rectum.

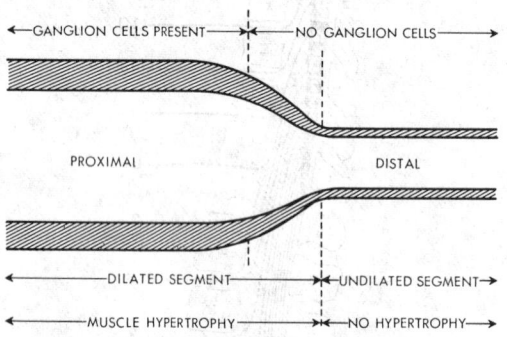

←—GANGLION CELLS PRESENT—→ ←— NO GANGLION CELLS —→

PROXIMAL      DISTAL

←——DILATED SEGMENT——→ ←—UNDILATED SEGMENT—→

←——MUSCLE HYPERTROPHY——→ ←—NO HYPERTROPHY—→

**Congenital Megacolon**

(From Bodian, M., Stephens, F. D., and Ward, B. C. H.: *Lancet 1:* 6, 1949. Used with permission.)

    **idiopathic m.,** m., found in children or adults, without distal obstruction or absence of ganglion cells; the muscle of the dilated colon is thin.

    **toxic m.,** acute nonobstructive dilation of the colon, seen in fulminating ulcerative colitis.

**meg'acycle.** One million cycles.

**megadactyl** (meg'ah-dak'til) [ mega- + G. *daktylos*, finger ]. Denoting large fingers.

**megadactyl'ia, megadac'tylism.** Megadactyly.

**megadactyly** (meg'ah-dak'tĭ-lĭ) [ mega- + G. *daktylos*, digit ]. Megadactylia; megalodactylia; macrodactylia; dactylomegaly; a condition characterized by enlargement of one or more digits (fingers or toes).

**megadolichocolon** (meg'ah-dol'ĭ-ko-ko'lon) [ mega- + G. *dolichos*, long, + *kolon*, colon ]. Excessive length and dilation of colon.

**meg'adont** [ mega- + G. *odous* (*odont-*), tooth ]. Macrodont.

**meg'adon'tism.** Macrodontia.

**megadyne** (meg'ah-dīn). One million dynes.

**megaesophagus** (meg'ah-e-sof'ah-gus). Great enlargement of the lower portion of the esophagus, as seen in patients with chronic cardiospasm.

**megagamete** (meg-ah-gam'ēt). Macrogamete.

**megagnathia** (meg'ah-na'the-ah). Macrognathia.

**megakaryoblast** (meg'ah-kär'ĭ-o-blast). The precursor of a megakaryocyte. See color plate 15.

**megakaryocyte** (meg'ah-kär'ĭ-o-sīt) [ mega- + G. *karyon*, nut (nucleus), + *kytos*, hollow vessel (cell) ]. A large cell (as much as 100 $\mu$ in diameter) with a nucleus that is usually multilobed. M.'s are normally present in bone marrow, but not in the circulating blood. On the basis of morphologic, immunologic, and chemical studies, they give rise to blood platelets. See color plate 16.

**megal-** See megalo-.

**megalac'ria** [ megal- + G. *akros*, at the top or end ]. Obsolete term for acromegaly.

**megalecithal** (meg'ah-les'ĭ-thal) [ mega- + G. *lekithos*, yolk ]. Denoting an egg rich in yolk, as in bony fishes, reptiles, and birds.

**meg'alerythe'ma.** Megaloerythema.

**megalgia** (meg-al'jĭ-ah) [ megal- + G. *algos*, pain ]. Very severe pain.

**megalo-, megal-, -megaly** [ G. *megas* (*megal-*), large ]. Combining forms meaning large; see also macro-, mega-.

**megaloblast** (meg'ă-lo-blast) [ megalo- + G. *blastos*, + germ, sprout ]. A large, nucleated, embryonic type of cell that is a precursor of erythrocytes in an abnormal erythropoietic process observed almost exclusively in pernicious anemia. Its four stages of development are (1) promegaloblast, (2) basophilic m., (3) polychromatic m., and (4) orthochromatic m. See discussion under erythroblast.

    **m. of Sabin,** pronormoblast; see discussion under erythroblast.

**megalocardia** (meg'ă-lo-kar'dĭ-ah) [ megalo- + G. *kardia*, heart ]. Cardiomegaly.

**megalocephaly, megalocephalia** (meg'ă-lo-sef'ă-lĭ, -sĕ-fa'lĭ-ah). Megacephaly.

**megalocheiria, megalochiria** (meg'al-o-ki'rĭ-ah) [ megalo- + G. *cheir*, hand ]. Macrocheiria.

**meg'alocor'nea.** Macrocornea.

**megalocystis** (meg'ă-lo-sis'tis) [ megalo- + G. *kystis*, bladder ]. Megabladder; an enlarged or overdistended bladder.

**megalocyte** (meg'ă-lo-sīt) [ megalo- + G. *kytos*, cell ]. A large (10 to 20 $\mu$) nonnucleated red blood cell.

**meg'alocythe'mia.** Macrocythemia.

**meg'alocyto'sis.** Macrocythemia.

**megalodactyl'ia, megalodac'tylism, megalodac'tyly.** Megadactyly.

**meg'alodont.** Macrodont.

**megalodontia** (meg-al-o-don'shĭ-ah). Macrodontia.

**megaloencephalic** (meg'ă-lo-en'sĕ-fal'ik). Denoting a brain of unusual size.

**megaloencephalon** (meg'ă-lo-en-sef'ă-lon) [ megalo- + G. *enkephalos*, brain ]. Macroencephalon; an abnormally large brain.

**megaloencephaly** (meg'ă-lo-en-sef'ă-lĭ) [ megalo- + G. *enkephalon*, brain ]. Abnormal largeness of the brain.

**megaloenteron** (meg'ă-lo-en'ter-on) [ megalo- + G. *enteron*, intestine ]. Enteromegaly; abnormal largeness of the intestine.

**megaloerythema** (meg'ă-lo-ĕr'ĭ-the'mah) [ megalo- + G. *erythēma*, flush ]. Megalerythema; an eruption beginning as rapidly coalescing rose-colored macules, first on the cheeks, then on the extremities, but seldom on the trunk; there is usually some swelling of the erythematous parts; the affection is afebrile.

**meg'alogas'tria** [ megalo- + G. *gastēr*, stomach, + suffix *-ia*, condition ]. Macrogastria; megastria; abnormally large size of the stomach.

**megaloglossia** (meg'ă-lo-glos'sĭ-ah) [ megalo- + G. *glōssa*, tongue ]. Macroglossia.

**meg'alograph'ia.** Macrography.

**megalohepatia** (meg'al-o-he-pat'ĭ-ah). Hepatomegaly.

**megalokaryocyte** (meg'ă-lo-kär'ĭ-o-sit). Megakaryocyte.

**megalomania** (meg'ă-lo-ma'nĭ-ah) [ megalo- + G. *mania*, frenzy ]. A delusion of grandeur; insanity in which the patient believes himself to be a person of great importance, wealth, or intellect.

**megalomaniac** (meg'ă-lo-ma'nĭ-ak). A person exhibiting megalomania.

**meg'alome'lia.** Macromelia.

**megalonychosis** (meg'al-on-ik-o'sis) [ megalo- + G. *onyx*, nail, + suffix -*osis*, condition ]. Macronychia.

**megalopenis** (meg'ă-lo-pe'nis). Macropenis.

**megalophallus** (meg'ă-lo-fal'us). Macropenis.

**megalophthalmus** (meg'al-of'thal'mus) [ megalo- + G. *ophthalmos*, eye ]. Macrophthalmia; abnormally large eyes occurring as a developmental anomaly.

  **anterior m.,** keratoglobus; m. affecting the anterior segment of the eyeball, with associated changes in the zonular ligament and the lens.

**meg'alo'pia.** Macropsia.

**megalopodia** (meg'ă-lo-po'dĭ-ah) [ megalo- + G. *pous*, foot ]. Macropodia.

**meg'alop'sia.** Macropsia.

**megalosplanchnic** (meg'ă-lo-splangk'nik) [ megalo- + G. *splanchnon*, viscus ]. Macrosplanchnic; having abnormally large viscera.

**meg'alosple'nia.** Splenomegaly.

**megalospore** (meg'al-o-spōr). 1. Macrospore. 2. Megalosporon.

**megalos'poron** [ megalo- + G. *sporos*, seed ]. *Trichophyton megalosporon.*

**megalosyndactyly, megalosyndactylia** (meg'ă-lo-sin-dak'tĭ-lĭ, -dak-til'ĭ-ah) [ megalo- + G. *syn*, together, + *daktylos*, finger ]. A condition of webbed or fused fingers or toes of large size.

**megaloureter** (meg'ă-lo-u-re'ter). Megaureter; a congenitally enlarged ureter without evidence of obstruction or infection.

**megalourethra** (meg'ă-lo-u-re'thrah). Megaurethra; congenital dilation of the urethra.

**megamerozoite** (meg'ah-mĕr'o-zo'ĭt). Macromerozoite.

**meg'anu'cleus.** Macronucleus.

**megaprosopia** (meg'ah-pro-so'pĭ-ah) [ mega- + G. *prosopon*, face ]. Macroprosopia.

**megaprosopous** (meg'ah-pros'o-pus). Macroprosopous.

**megarectum** (meg-ah-rek'tum). Extreme dilation of the rectum.

**megaseme** (meg'ah-sēm) [ mega- + G. *sēma*, sign ]. Denoting an orbital aperture with an index above 89.

**megasigmoid** (meg'ah-sig'moyd). Macrosigmoid.

**meg'aso'mia.** Macrosomia.

**meg'aspore.** Macrospore.

**megastria** (meg-as'trĭ-ah). Megalogastria.

**megathrombocyte** (meg'ă-throm'bo-sīt) [ mega- + G. *thrombos*, clot, + *kytos*, cell ]. A large blood platelet, especially a young one recently released from the bone marrow.

**megaureter** (meg'ah-u-re'ter). Megaloureter.

**megaurethra** (meg'ah-u-re'thrah). Megalourethra.

**meg'avolt.** A unit of electromotive force, equal to one million volts.

**megestrol acetate** (mĕ-jes'trōl) (USAN, BP). NIAGESTINE; 17α-hydroxy-6-methylpregna-4,6-diene-3,20-dione acetate; a synthetic progestin with progestational effects similar to those of progesterone; used in threatened and habitual abortion, endometriosis, and menstrual disorders; claimed to be superior to 19-nor compounds as an antifertility agent because it has less effect on the endometrium and vagina; in combination with ethynyl estradiol, it acts as an oral contraceptive.

**meglumine** (meg'lu-mēn). USAN-approved contraction for *N*-methylglucamine.

  **m. acetrizoate,** VASURIX; a radiographic contrast medium.

  **m. diatrizoate** (USP), CARDIOGRAFIN; GASTROGRAFIN; RENOGRAFIN; methylglucamine diatrizoate; *N*-methylglucamine salt of 3,5-diacetamido-2,4,6-triiodobenzoic acid; a water-soluble organic iodine compound used for excretory urography for contrast visualization of the cardiovascular system, and orally for roentgenography of the gastrointestinal tract.

  **m. iothalamate** (USP, BP), CONRAY; *N*-methylglucamine of 5-acetamido-2,4,6-triiodo-*N*-methylisophthalmic acid (60 per cent solution); a diagnostic radiopaque medium for intravascular use in angiography and urography.

**megohm** (meg'ōm). A unit of electrical resistance, equal to one million ohms.

**megophthalmus** (meg'of-thal'mus). Megalophthalmus.

**megoxycyte** (meg-ok'sĭ-sīt). Megoxyphil.

**megoxyphil, megoxyphile** (meg-oks'ĭ-fil, or fīl) [ mega- + G. *oxys*, acid, + *phileō*, to like ]. An eosinophilic leukocyte, containing coarse granules.

**me'grim.** Migraine.

**Mehlis' gland.** See under gland.

**mehl'nährscha'den** [ Ger. ]. A syndrome seen in young children as a result of severe malnutrition, especially a deficiency of protein and an excess of carbohydrate; it is characterized by hypoproteinemia, edema, enlargement of the liver, and diarrhea: it appears to be closely related to kwashiorkor.

**Meibom** (mi'bōm), Hendrik, German anatomist, 1638–1700. See Meibomian *conjunctivitis, cyst, gland, sty.*

**meibomitis, meibomianitis** (mi'bo-mi'tis, mi-bo'mĭ-ă-ni'-tis). Inflammation of the Meibomian glands.

**Meibo'mius.** See Meibom.

**Meige** (mehzh), Henri, French physician, 1866–1940. See M.'s *disease.*

**Meigs** (megz), Joe V., Boston gynecologist, 1892–1963. See M.'s *syndrome.*

**Meinicke** (mi'nik-eh), Ernst, German physician, 1878–1945. See M. *test.*

**meio-.** For words beginning thus and not found here, see mio-.

**meiosis** (mi-o'sis) [ G. *meiōsis*, a lessening ]. Meiotic division; the special process of cell division that results in the formation of gametes, consisting of two nuclear divisions in rapid succession that result in the formation of four gametocytes each containing half the number of chromosomes found in somatic cells.

**meiotic** (mi-ot'ik). Pertaining to meiosis.

**Meissner** (mīs'ner), Georg, German histologist, 1829–1905. See M.'s *corpuscles, plexus.*

**mel-, melo-.** 1 [ G. *melos*, limb ]. Combining form indicating limb. 2 [ G. *mēlon*, cheek ]. Combining form indicating cheek. 3 [ L. *mel, mellis*, honey; G. *meli, melitos*, honey ]. Combining form relating to honey or sugar. 4 [ G. *mēlon*, sheep ]. Combining form relating to sheep.

**mel.** 1. Honey. 2. Unit of pitch; a pitch of 1000 mels results from a simple tone of frequency 1000 c.p.s., 40 db. above the normal threshold of audibility.

**melag'ra** [ G. *melos*, limb, + *agra*, seizure ]. Rheumatic or myalgic pains in the arms or legs.

**melal'gia** [ G. *melos*, a limb, + *algos*, pain ]. Pain in a limb; specifically, burning pain in the feet extending up the leg and even to the thigh, thickening of the walls of the blood vessels with obliteration of the vascular lumina; thought to be a vitamin deficiency disease.

**melamine formaldehyde.** melamine resin; see under resin.

**melam'pyrin.** Galactitol.

**melan-, melano-** [ G. *melas*, black. MELAN- ]. Combining forms meaning black or extreme darkness of hue.

**melancholia** (mel-an-ko'lĭ-ah) [ melan- + G. *cholē*, bile. See humoral doctrine ]. Melancholy. 1. Tristimania; a mental disorder marked by apathy and indifference to one's surroundings, mental sluggishness, and depression. 2. A symptom occurring in other conditions, marked by depression of spirits and by a sluggish and painful process of thought.

  **acute m.,** simple, functional m., marked by insomnia, emaciation, and a subnormal temperature.

  **m. agitata,** agitated *depression.*

  **m. attoni'ta,** m. stuporosa; in schizophrenia, the catatonic state characterized by immobility and muscular rigidity.

  **chronic m.,** hypochondriacal m.; a form of involutional m. marked by depression, anxiety, restlessness, and more or less hypochondria.

  **climacteric m.,** involutional m.

  **convulsive m.,** depression related to epileptic occurrences.

  **hypochondri'acal m.,** chronic m.

**involutional m.,** climacteric m.; depressive disorder of middle life, commonly associated with the male or female climacteric.

**panphobic m.,** morbid generalized dread.

**paretic m.,** depression which precedes paresis.

**puberty m.,** depression with feelings of inferiority, usually occurring at puberty.

**recurrent m.,** acute or simple m. that shows a tendency to recur after longer or shorter periods of remission.

**sexual m.,** depression with concern about impotence, inadequacy, or venereal disease.

**m. simplex,** acute m.

**m. stuporo'sa,** m. attonita.

**suicidal m.,** depression with impulses to commit suicide.

**melancholiac** (mel-an-ko'li-ak). A person suffering from melancholia.

**melancholy** (mel-an-kol'i). Melancholia.

**melanedema** (mel'an-e-de'mah) [ melan- + G. *oidēma,* swelling ]. Anthracosis.

**melanemia** (mel'ă-ne'mi-ah) [ melan- + G. *haima,* blood ]. The presence of dark brown, almost black, or black granules of insoluble pigment (melanin) in the circulating blood.

**melanephidrosis** (mel'an-ef'i-dro'sis) [ melan- + G. *ephidrōsis,* perspiration ]. Melanidrosis; a form of chromidrosis in which the sweat is nearly black.

**mélangeur** (ma-loṅ-zhër') [ Fr. mixer ]. A glass tube with a bulb at one extremity, used for diluting the blood collected for microscopic examination.

**melanidrosis** (mel'an-i-dro'sis). Melanephidrosis.

**melanif'erous** [ melan- (melanin) + L. *ferro,* to carry ]. Containing melanin or other black pigment.

**mel'anin** [ G. *melas(melan-),* black ]. Dark brown to black polymers of indole 5,6-quinone and/or 5,6-dihydroxyindole 2-carboxylic acid that normally occur in the skin, hair, pigmented coat of the retina, and inconstantly in the medulla and zona reticularis of the adrenal gland. The material may be formed *in vitro* or biologically by oxidation of tyrosine or tryptophan; the usual mechanism is the enzymatic oxidation of tyrosine to 3,4-dihydroxyphenylalanine (dopa) by monophenol monooxygenase, and the further oxidation (probably spontaneous) of this intermediate to melanin.

**artificial m., factitious m.,** melanoid.

**mel'anism.** Unusually marked, diffuse, melanin pigmentation of body hair of mammalian species; see also melanosis.

**melano-** (mel'ă-no-). See melan-.

**melanoameloblastoma** (mel'ă-no-am'e-lo-blas-to'mah). Melanotic neuroectodermal *tumor.*

**mel'anoblast** [ melano- + G. *blastos,* germ, sprout ]. A cell derived from the neural crest; they migrate to various parts of the body during the relatively early phases of embryonic life, and then become mature melanocytes capable of forming melanin. See also melanophore.

**mel'anocarcino'ma.** See melanoma.

**melanochrous** (mel-an-ok'ro-us) [ melano- + G. *chroa,* complexion. CHROM- ]. Having dark complexion; dark-skinned; brunette.

**melanocomous** (mel'an-ok'o-mus) [ melano- + G. *komē,* hair of the head ]. Melanotrichous.

**melanocyte** (mel'ă-no-sīt) [ melano- + G. *kytos,* cell ]. Pigment cell of the skin; melanodendrocyte; a cell located at the dermoepidermal junction having branching processes by means of which melanosomes are transferred to epidermal cells, resulting in pigmentation.

**mel'anocyto'ma.** A variety of benign pigmented nevus on the optic disk.

**mel'anoden'drocyte** [ melano- + G. *dendron,* tree, + *kytos,* a hollow (cell) ]. Melanocyte.

**mel'anoderm** [ melano- + G. *derma,* skin ]. A member of one of the black races.

**mel'anoder'ma** [ melano- + G. *derma,* skin ]. An abnormal darkening of the skin by deposition of excess melanin, or of metallic substances such as silver and iron.

**m. cachectico'rum,** m. of the cachectic; m. occurring in certain chronic diseases, such as malaria and tuberculosis.

**m. chloas'ma,** melasma.

**parasitic m.,** vagabond's disease; vagrant's disease; Greenhow's disease; excoriations and m. caused by scratching the bites of the body louse, *Pediculus corporis.*

**racial m.,** the normally dark skin of Negroes and certain other races.

**m. senile,** melasma universale; cutaneous pigmentation occurring in the aged.

**mel'anoder'mati'tis.** Excessive deposit of melanin in an area of dermatitis.

**mel'anoder'mic.** Relating to or marked by melanoderma.

**melanoepithelioma** (mel'ă-no-ep-i-the'li-o'mah). Melanoma.

**melanogen** (mě-lan'o-jen, mel'ă-no-jen) [ melano- + G. suffix -*gen,* producing ]. A colorless substance that may be converted into melanin; for example, some patients with widespread metastases of melanoma excrete m. in their urine, and melanin is formed when the urine is exposed to air (*i.e.,* oxidized) for a few hours.

**melanogenemia** (mel'ă-no-jě-ne'mi-ah) [ melanogen + G. *haima,* blood ]. The presence of melanin precursors in the blood; may occur in malignant melanoma with metastasis.

**melanogenesis** (mel'ă-no-jen'ě-sis) [ melanin + G. *genesis,* production ]. The formation of melanin by living cells.

**mel'anoglos'sia** [ melano- + G. *glōssa,* tongue ]. Black *tongue.*

**mel'anoid.** A dark pigment that resembles melanin; formed from glucosamines in chitin.

**melanoleukoderma** (mel'ă-no-lu'ko-der'mah) [ melano- + G. *leukos,* white, + *derma,* skin ]. Marbled, or marmorated, skin.

**m. col'li,** syphilitic *leukoderma.*

**melanoma** (mel'ă-no'mah) [ melano- + G. suffix, -*ōma,* tumor ]. Melanotic cancer; melanotic sarcoma; malignant m.; a malignant neoplasm derived from cells that are capable of forming melanin; may occur in the skin of any part of the body, in the eye, or, rarely, in the mucous membranes of the genitalia, anus, oral cavity, or other sites. In the early phases, the lesion is characterized by proliferation of cells at the dermal-epidermal junction, and the neoplastic cells soon invade adjacent tissue extensively. The cells vary in amount and pigmentation of cytoplasm; the nuclei are relatively large and frequently bizarre in shape, with prominent acidophilic nucleoli; mitotic figures tend to be numerous. M.'s frequently metastasize widely, and the regional lymph nodes, liver, lungs, and brain are likely to be involved. Most examples of this neoplasm occur in patients who are more than 30 years of age, and approximately 60 per cent originate in a pigmented mole. For emphasis in distinguishing them from benign pigmented lesions, m.'s are usually termed **malignant m.;** they are also known as melanoblastoma, melanocarcinoma, melanosarcoma, nevocarcinoma, nevomelanoma, melanotic malignant tumor, and so on.

**amelanotic m.,** an anaplastic m. consisting of cells derived from melanoblasts but not forming melanin.

**benign juvenile m.,** spindle cell nevus; epithelioid cell nevus; a benign, slightly pigmented or red superficial small skin tumor; most common in children but also appearing in adults; composed of spindle-shaped, epithelioid, and multinucleated cells with moderately small nuclei.

**Cloudman m.,** a transplantable m. that arose spontaneously in a mouse of DBA strain, and which grows and metastasizes in mice of related strains.

**m. de novo,** a form of malignant m. that seems to originate in a site where there was no preexisting lesion; *e.g.,* a nevus.

**Harding-Passey m.,** a melanin-forming tumor that arose spontaneously in a non-inbred mouse, and that is transplantable to mice of many strains but does not ordinarily metastasize.

**malignant m.,** melanoma.

**malignant lentigo m.,** malignant m. arising from a malignant lentigo; the prognosis is better than for a nevocytic malignant m.

**nevocytic malignant m.,** malignant m. arising from a preexisting pigmented nevus.

**subungual m.,** melanotic *whitlow.*

**melanomatosis** (mel'ă-no'mă-to'sis) [ melanoma + G. suffix -*osis,* condition ]. A condition characterized by numerous, widespread lesions of melanoma.

**melanonychia** (mel'ă-no-nik'ĭ-ah) [ melano- + G. *onyx* (*onych*-), nail ]. Black pigmentation of the nails.

**mel'anop'athy** [ melano- + G. *pathos,* suffering ]. 1. Any disease marked by pigmentation of the skin. 2. Melanoderma; melasma.

**melanophage** (mel'ă-no-fāj, mĕ-lan'o-fāj) [ melano- + G. *phagein,* to eat ]. Melanophore (1).

**melanophora** (mel'ă-nof'o-rah) [ melano- + G. *phora,* a carrying ]. Intermittent discharge of free melanin from conjunctiva; cause is unknown, but this condition appears to be controlled by administration of pituitary extract.

**melanophore** (mel'ă-no-fōr, mĕ-lan'o-fōr) [ melano- + G. *phoros,* bearing ]. 1. Melanophage; in human histology and pathology, a phagocytic cell that contains melanin, but does not form the pigment. See also melanoblast. 2. In general biology, a cell that is capable of forming melanin.

**melanoplakia** (mel'ă-no-pla'kĭ-ah) [ melano- + G. *plax,* plate, plaque ]. The occurrence of pigmented patches on the tongue and buccal mucous membrane.

**mel'anopro'tein.** A protein complex with melanin.

**melanorrhagia** (mel'ă-no-ra'jĭ-ah) [ melano- + G. *rhēgnymi,* to burst forth. RHAG- ]. Melena.

**melanorrhea** (mel'ă-no-re'ah) [ melano- + G. *rhoia,* a flow ]. Melena.

**mel'anosarco'ma.** Melanoma.

**melanoscirrhus** (mel'ă-no-skĭr'us, -sĭr'us) [ melano- + G. *skirrhos,* a hardened tumor ]. A relatively unusual form of melanoma, in which there is an abundant stroma of dense fibrous tissue, *i.e.,* scirrhous melanoma.

**melanosis** (mel'ă-no'sis) [ melano- + G. suffix -*osis,* condition ]. 1. Abnormal, dark brown or brown-black pigmentation of various tissues or organs, as the result of melanins or, in some situations, other substances that resemble melanin to varying degrees. M. of the skin, for example, may occur in sunburn, during pregnancy, as a result of Addison's disease, and so on. 2. Cachexia resulting from widespread metastases of melanoma.

  **m. circumscrip'ta precancero'sa,** a brown or black mottled lesion resembling a lentigo in which there are junctional nests of melanocytes showing nuclear abnormality, usually occurring in older persons and regarded as premalignant or as a malignant melanoma *in situ;* development of a dark papule or nodule indicates an invasion of the dermis; also known as Hutchinson's or melanotic freckle; malignant lentigo; precancerous m. of Dubreuilh.

  **m. coli,** m. of the large intestinal mucosa due to accumulation of pigment of uncertain composition within macrophages in the lamina propria.

  **m. corii degenerativa,** a congenital abnormality in which pigment is deposited in whorls and streaks; vesicles occasionally occur. May be associated with cardiac or neurologic disorders.

  **neurocutaneous m.,** cutaneous giant pigmented nevi associated with m. of the leptomeninges; malignant melanomas may develop in the skin or meninges.

  **oculodermal m.,** Ota's nevus; pigmentation of the conjunctiva and skin around the eye, usually unilateral; seen especially in females of Oriental races.

  **precancerous m. of Dubreuilh,** m. circumscripta precancerosa.

  **Riehl's m.,** a brown pigmentary condition of the exposed portions of the skin of the neck and face, thought to result from materials, such as oil, contacted in various occupations.

**mel'anos'ity.** Darkness of complexion.

**melanosome** (mel'ă-no-sōm) [ melano- + G. *sōma,* body ]. The generally oval pigment granule (0.2 by 0.6 μ) produced by melanocytes.

**mel'anot'ic.** Relating to or characterized by melanosis.

**melanotrichous** (mel'ă-not'rĭ-kus) [ melano- + G. *thrix* (*trich*-), hair ]. Melanocomous; having black hair.

**melanotroph** (mel'ă-no-trof) [ melano- + G. *trophē,* nourishment ]. A cell of the hypophysis that produces melanocyte-stimulating hormone (MSH).

**mel'anous.** Dark-complexioned; brunette.

**melanurenic acid.** Melanurin; a dark pigment sometimes found in the urine.

**melanuria** (mel'ă-nu'rĭ-ah) [ melano- + G. *ouron,* urine ]. The excretion of urine of a dark color, resulting from the presence of melanin or other pigments or from the action of phenol, creosote, resorcin, and other coal tar derivatives.

**melanu'ric.** Pertaining to or characterized by melanuria.

**melan'urin.** Melanurenic acid.

**melar'soprol** (BP). MEL B; 2-*p*-(4,6-diamino-1,3,5-triazine-2-ylamino) phenyl-4-hydroxymethyl-1,3,2-dithioarsolan; used in the treatment of the meningoencephalitic stages of trypanosomiasis; may produce a fatal reactive encephalopathy.

**melasma** (mĕ-laz'mah) [ G. a black color, a black spot. MELAN- ]. Melanoderma chloasma; a patchy or generalized pigmentation of the skin.

  **m. addiso'nii,** obsolete term for Addison's *disease.*

  **m. gravida'rum,** chloasma; pigmentation of the skin in pregnancy.

  **m. suprarena'le,** obsolete term for Addison's *disease.*

  **m. universa'le,** *melanoderma* senile.

**mel'ato'nin.** *N*-Acetyl-5-methoxytryptamine; formed by the mammalian pineal gland. It appears to depress gonadal function in mammals and is known to cause contraction of amphibian melanophores; only preliminary evidence exists about other possible effects.

**melena** (mel-e'nah) [ G. *melaina,* fem. of *melas,* black ]. Melanorrhea; melanorrhagia; the passage of dark colored, tarry stools, due to the presence of blood altered by the intestinal juices.

  **m. neonato'rum,** m. of the newborn, a form occurring in young infants.

  **m. spu'ria,** the passage of blood which has been swallowed, especially that swallowed by nurslings from a fissured nipple.

  **m. vera,** true m. as distinguished from m. spuria.

**melenemesis** (mel-e-nem'e-sis) [ G. *melas,* black, + *emesis,* vomiting ]. The vomiting of dark colored or blackish material; see also black *vomit.*

**Meleney,** F. L., U. S. surgeon, 1889–1963. See M.'s synergistic *gangrene,* M.'s *ulcer.*

**melengestrol acetate** (mel'en-jes'trōl) (USAN). 17α-Acetoxy-6-methyl-16-methylene-4,6-pregnadiene-3,20-dione; a progestational agent.

**melezitose** (mĕ-lez'ĭ-tōs). A trisaccharide occurring in the exudations of various plants; a condensation product of two glucose residues and a fructose residue.

**meli-** [ G. *meli,* honey. MEL-1 ]. Combining form relating to honey or sugar.

**mel'ibi'ase.** α-Galactosidase.

**mel'ibi'ose.** 6-*O*-α-D-Galactopyranosyl-D-glucose; a disaccharide (an isolactose) formed by the hydrolysis of raffinose under the catalytic influence of β-fructofuranosidase.

**melicera, meliceris** (mel-ĭ-se'rah, mel-ĭ-se'ris) [ G. *melikēris,* a tumor, fr. *melikēron,* honeycomb, fr. *meli,* honey, + *kēros,* wax ]. A hygroma or other type of cyst that contains a relatively thick, tenacious, semifluid material.

**melioidosis** (me'lĭ-oy-do'sis) [ G. *melis,* a distemper of asses, + *eidos,* resemblance, + suffix -*osis,* condition ]. Pseudoglanders; an infectious disease of rodents in India and Southeast Asia, which is communicable to man. The characteristic lesion is a small caseous nodule, found generally throughout the body, which breaks down into an abscess; the symptoms vary according to the tracts or organs involved; the pathogenic organism is *Pseudomonas pseudomallei.*

**melis'sa** [ G. a bee ]. Balm; sweet balm; lemon lobelia; sweet Mary; the leaves the tops of *Melissa officinalis* (family Labiatae), a plant of southern Europe; diaphoretic.

**melis'sic acid.** $CH_3(CH_2)_{28}COOH$; a fatty acid present in beeswax.

**melissophobia** (mĕ-lis'o-fo'bĭ-ah) [ G. *melissa,* bee, + *phobos,* fear ]. Morbid fear of bees.

**melis'syl.** Myricyl.

  **m. alcohol,** myricyl alcohol; 1-triacontanol; $CH_3$-$(CH_2)_{29}OH$; an alcohol present in beeswax.

**melitagra** (mel'ĭ-tag'rah) [ G. *meli* (*melit*-), honey, + *agra,* a seizure ]. Eczema with soft, honey-like crusts.

**melitemia** (mel'ĭ-te'mĭ-ah) [ G. *meli* (*melit-*), honey, + *haima*, blood ]. Glycemia.

**meliten'sis.** Brucellosis.

**melitis** (me-li'tis) [ G. *mēlon*, cheek, + *-itis* ]. Inflammation of the cheek.

**melitococcosis** (mel'ĭ-to-kok-o'sis). Brucellosis.

**melitoptyalism** (mel'ĭ-to-ti'ă-lizm) [ G. *meli*, honey, + *ptyalon*, saliva ]. Glycoptyalism.

**mel'itose.** Raffinose; a crystalline dextrorotatory trisaccharide obtained from the manna of the Tasmanian eucalyptus built up of residues of galactose, glucose, and fructose.

**melitra'cen hydrochloride** (USAN). TRAUSABUN; 9,10,dihydro-10,10-dimethyl-9-(3-dimethylaminopropylidene)anthracene hydrochloride; antidepressant.

**melituria** (mel'ĭ-tu'rĭ-ah) [ G. *meli*, honey, + *ouron*, urine ]. Obsolete term for glycosuria.

**Melkersson,** E., Swedish physician. See M.'s *syndrome*.

**melli'tum,** gen. **melli'ti,** pl. **melli'ta** [ L. neut. of *mellitus*, honeyed ]. A pharmaceutical preparation with honey as an excipient.

**melo-** (mel'o-, me'lo-). See mel-.

**mel'ocervicoplas'ty.** Plastic surgery on cheek and neck.

**melo'mania** [ G. *melos*, song + *mania*, frenzy ]. An abnormal fascination with or devotion to music.

**melom'elus** [ G. *melos* + *melos*, limb ]. A malformed fetus with normal and rudimentary accessory limbs.

**me'lonoplas'ty** [ G. *mēlon*, cheek, + *plassō*, to form ]. Meloplasty (1); plastic surgery of the cheek; repair of a defect in the cheek by grafting or the sliding of tissue from a neighboring part.

**Melophagus** (me-lof'ă-gus) [ G. *mēlon*, sheep, + *phagein*, to eat ]. A genus of louse flies (family Hippoboscidae) that includes the ectoparasite of sheep, *M. ovinus;* see also *Hippobosca.*

  **M. ovi'nus,** ked; a wingless, flattened, hairy, leathery parasitic fly found in the wool of sheep and on goats; it is cosmopolitan in sheep, in which it sucks blood and causes much skin irritation.

**mel'oplasty** [ G. *melos*, limb, + *plassō*, to form ]. 1. Melonoplasty. 2. Reparative or plastic surgery of the extremities.

**melorheostosis** (mel'o-re-os-to'sis) [ G. *melos*, limb, + *rheos*, stream, + *osteon*, bone, + *-ōsis* ]. Rheostosis confined to the extremities; also known as osteopathia hyperostotica congenita; osteosis eburnisans monomelica.

**melosal'gia** [ G. *melos*, limb, + *algos*, pain ]. Pain in the lower limbs.

**meloschisis** (me-los'kĭ-sis) [ G. *mēlon*, cheek, + *schisis*, a cleaving ]. A congenital cleft in the cheek.

**melotia** (me-lo'shĭ-ah) [ G. *mēlon*, cheek, + *ous*, ear ]. Congenital displacement of the auricle.

**melphalan** (mel'fă-lan) (BP, USP). ALKERAN; L-phenylalanine mustard; L-sarcolysine; L-3-[ *p-* [ *bis* (2-chloroethyl)-amino ] phenyl ] alanine; a phenylalanine derivative of nitrogen mustard. An alkalylating antineoplastic agent, sometimes used in multiple myeloma; bone marrow depression may occur.

**Meltzer** (melt'ser), Samuel J., American physiologist, 1851–1920. See M.'s *law, reaction,* M.-Auer *test,* M.-Lyon *test.*

**mem'ber** [ L. *membrum* ]. A limb.

  **virile m.,** penis.

**mem'bra** [ L. ] [ NA ]. Limbs; plural of membrum.

---

# MEMBRANA

---

**membrana,** gen, and pl., **membra'nae** (mem-bra'nah) [ L. ] [ NA ]. Membrane; a thin sheet or layer of pliable tissue, serving as a covering or envelope of a part, the lining of a cavity, as a partition or septum, or to connect two structures.

  **m. abdom'inis,** peritoneum.

  **m. adamantin'ea,** *cuticula* dentis.

  **m. adventi'tia,** (1) *tunica* adventitia; (2) *decidua* capsularis.

  **m. atlan'tooccipita'lis anterior** [ NA ], anterior atlantooccipital membrane; the fibrous layer that extends from the anterior arch of the atlas to the anterior margin of the foramen magnum.

  **m. atlan'tooccipita'lis posterior** [ NA ], posterior atlantooccipital membrane; the fibrous membrane that attaches between the posterior arch of the atlas and the posterior margin of the foramen magnum.

  **m. basa'lis duc'tus semicircula'ris** [ NA ], the basal membrane underlying the epithelium of the semicircular duct.

  **m. basila'ris,** *lamina* basilaris cochleae.

  **m. capsula'ris,** the portion of the lens capsule that covers the posterior surface of the lens.

  **m. cap'sulopupilla'ris,** the portion of the m. pupillaris that extends laterally from the pupil to the anterior surface of the lens.

  **m. carno'sa,** *tunica* dartos.

  **m. cer'ebri,** any one of the cerebral meninges.

  **m. chor'iocapilla'ris,** *lamina* choroidocapillaris.

  **m. cordis,** pericardium.

  **m. cortica'lis,** m. vitellina.

  **m. cricothyroid'ea,** *conus* elasticus.

  **m. decid'ua** [ NA ], decidua; Hunter's membrane; caduca; the mucous membrane of the pregnant uterus which has already undergone certain changes, under the influence of the ovulation cycle, to fit it for the implantation and nutrition of the ovum. Named decidua from the fact that it is cast off after labor. See also fig. and subentries under decidua.

  **m. e'boris,** the lining membrane of the pulp cavity of a tooth, consisting of the odontoblastic layer.

  **m. fibroelas'tica laryn'gis** [ NA ], a layer of elastic fibers, taking the place in the larynx of the submucosa.

  **m. fibro'sa** [ NA ], fibrous membrane; fibrous articular capsule; the outer fibrous part of the capsule of a synovial joint which may in places be thickened to form capsular ligaments.

  **m. flac'cida,** *pars* flaccida membranae tympani.

  **m. fus'ca,** the pigment layer between the choroid and the sclera of the eyeball.

  **m. germinati'va,** blastoderm.

  **m. granulo'sa,** *stratum* granulosum folliculi ovarici vesiculosi.

  **m. hyaloid'ea,** m. vitrea.

  **m. hyothyroid'ea,** m. thyrohyoidea.

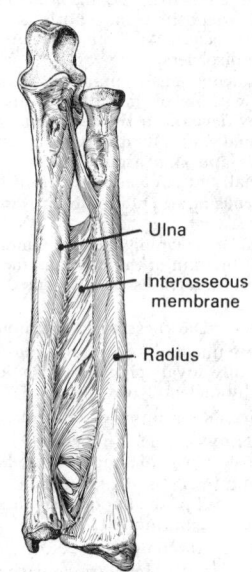

**Interosseous Membrane of the Forearm**

**membranae intercosta'lia** [ NA ], intercostal membranes; the membranous layers between ribs; one, the **m. intercostalia externa,** replaces the external intercostal muscle anteriorly, and a second, the **m. intercostalia interna,** similarly replaces the internal intercostal muscle posteriorly.

**m. interos'sea antebra'chii** [ NA ], interosseous membrane of the forearm; the dense membrane that connects the interosseous margins of the radius and ulna.

**m. interos'sea cru'ris** [ NA ], interosseous membrane of the leg; the dense fibrous layer that connects the interosseous margins of the tibia and fibula.

**m. lim'itans,** limiting *membrane.*

**m. lim'itans gli'ae,** a dense, resilient membrane forming the true capsule of the brain and spinal cord, composed of the processes of astrocytes (macroglia cells) and covered throughout by the pia mater which firmly adheres to it; the two membranes are collectively called the pial-glial membrane.

**m. muco'sa,** *tunica* mucosa.

**m. nic'titans,** *plica* semilunaris conjunctivae (2).

**m. obturato'ria** [ NA ], obturator membrane; the thin membrane of strong interlacing fibers filling the obturator foramen.

**m. perinei** [ NA ], perineal membrane; an alternate term for *fascia* diaphragmatis urogenitalis inferior.

**m. pituito'sa,** *tunica* mucosa nasi.

**m. preforma'ta,** a layer of dentin when it first appears between ameloblasts and odontoblasts.

**m. propria ductus semicircularis** [ NA ], the meshwork of connective tissue fibers between the semicircular duct and the bony semicircular canal; it encloses the perilymph in its spaces.

**m. pupilla'ris** [ NA ], pupillary membrane; Wachendorf's membrane; a thin, vascular membrane, forming the anterior portion of the capsule of the lens and occluding the pupil in fetal life; it normally disappears about the seventh month, but may persist and cause congenital blindness.

**m. quadrangula'ris** [ NA ], quadrangular membrane; the elastic membrane that extends from the ventricular fold of the larynx upward to the aryepiglottic fold; it attaches anteriorly to the epiglottis.

**m. reticula'ris** [ NA ], reticular membrane; the membrane formed by cuticular plates of the cells of the spiral organ of Corti; it appears netlike when viewed from above.

**m. sero'sa,** (1) *tunica* serosa; (2) serosa (2).

**m. seroti'na,** *decidua* basalis.

**m. spira'lis** [ NA ], spiral membrane; alternate term for *paries* tympanicus ductus cochlearis.

**m. stape'dis** [ NA ], membrane of the stapes; the delicate mucosal layer that bridges the space between the crura and base of the stapes.

**m. statoconio'rum** [ NA ], statoconial membrane; otolithic membrane; a gelatinous membrane supported by the hairs of the hair cells of the maculae of the saccule and utriculus of the inner ear; adhering to the surface are numerous crystalline particles called statoconia.

**m. sterni** [ NA ], sternal membrane; interlacing fibers from the anterior costosternal ligaments covering the anterior surface of the sternum.

**m. stria'ta,** *zona* striata.

**m. succin'gens** [ L. *succingere,* to surround ], the pleura.

**m. suprapleura'lis** [ NA ], suprapleural membrane; Sibson's fascia; Sibson's aponeurosis; the thickened portion of endothoracic fascia extending over the cupola of the pleura and reinforcing it; it attaches to the inner border of the first rib and to the transverse process of the seventh cervical vertebra.

**m. synovia'lis** [ NA ], synovial membrane; stratum synoviale; the connective tissue membrane that lines the cavity of a synovial joint and produces the synovial fluid. It does not cover the articular cartilage of the bones.

**m. tecto'ria** [ NA ], tectorial (roof) membrane; apparatus ligamentosus weitbrechti; posterior occipitoaxial ligament; the upper continuation of the anterior part of the posterior longitudinal ligament attached to the upper surface of the basilar portion of the occipital bone and the bodies of the second and third cervical vertebrae.

**m. tectoria ductus cochlea'ris** [ NA ], tectorial membrane of the cochlear duct; a gelatinous membrane that overlies

the spiral organ (Corti) in the inner ear. See fig. under cochlea.

**m. tensa,** *pars* tensa membranae tympani.

**m. thyrohyoidea** [ NA ], m. hyothyroidea; thyrohyoid membrane; a thin, fibrous, membranous sheet filling the gap between the hyoid bone and the thyroid cartilage.

**m. tym'pani** [ NA ], tympanic membrane; membrane of the tympanum; eardrum; drum membrane; drumhead; a thin, tense membrane forming the greater part of the lateral wall of the tympanic cavity and separating it from the external acoustic meatus; it constitutes the boundary between the external and middle ear. It is covered on both surfaces with epithelium, and in the pars tensa has an intermediate layer of outer radial and inner circular collagen fibers.

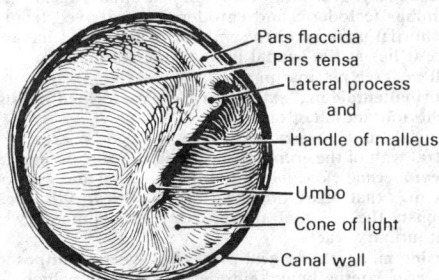

**Right Membrana Tympani**
As seen through an aural speculum

**m. tym'pani secunda'ria** [ NA ], secondary tympanic membrane; Scarpa's membrane; the membrane closing the fenestra cochleae or rotunda.

**m. versic'olor,** tapetum (2).

**m. vestibula'ris** [ NA ], *paries* vestibularis ductus cochlearis.

**m. vibrans,** *pars* tensa membranae tympani.

**m. vitelli'na,** (1) vitelline membrane; ovular membrane; the membrane enveloping the yolk; the thickened cell membrane of large-yolked ova; (2) sometimes used to designate the zona pellucida of a mammalian ovum.

**m. vit'rea** [ NA ], vitreous membrane; m. hyaloidea; hyaloid membrane; membranous thickening of the stroma of the vitreous, forming a capsule of this body.

**membrana'ceous.** Membranous.
**mem'branate.** Of the nature of a membrane.

# MEMBRANE

**membrane** [ L. *membrana,* a skin or membrane that covers parts of the body, fr. *membrum,* a member ]. See membrana.

**accidental m.,** false m.

**allantoid m.,** allantois.

**alveolodental m.,** periodontium.

**anal m.,** the dorsal portion of the embryonic cloacal m. after its division by the urorectal septum.

**anterior atlantooccipital m.,** *membrana* atlantooccipitalis anterior.

**arachnoid m.,** arachnoidea.

**atlantoccip'ital m.,** *membrana* atlantooccipitalis.

**basement m.,** basilemma; a thin layer, from 6 μ thick in the adult trachea to less than 1 μ in other regions, that intervenes between epithelium and connective tissue. With some stains it appears clear and amorphous, but it is argyrophilic with silver stains and positive for stains reacting with protein polysaccharide. With the electron microscope a finely filamentous layer less than 0.01 μ is seen which has also been called a basement m. by some or, more appropriately, a basal lamina, basement lamina, or boundary membrane. In addition to the basal (basement) lamina there is usually present a reticular lamina containing reticular fibers and ground substances.

**basilar m.,** *lamina* basilaris cochleae.

**Bichat's m.,** the inner elastic m. of arteries.

**Bogros' serous m.,** m. between the posterior pole of the eyeball and the intervaginal space (of Tenon).

**boundary m.,** basement *lamina.*

**Bowman's m.,** *lamina* limitans anterior corneae.

**Bruch's m.,** *lamina* basalis choroideae.

**Brunn's m.,** the epithelium of the olfactory region of the nose.

**bucconasal m.,** oronasal m.; a thin, transient epithelial sheet separating the primitive nasal cavity from the stomodeum in the 7-week-old human embryo.

**buccopharyngeal m.,** oral m.; oropharyngeal m.; a bilaminar (ectoderm and entoderm) m. derived from the prochordal plate; after the embryonic head fold has taken place it lies at the caudal limit of the stomodeum.

**cell m.,** see plasma m.

**chorioallantoic m.,** extraembryonic m. formed by fusion of chorion and allantois.

**cloac'al m.,** a transitory m. in the caudal area of the ventral wall of the embryo, separting the entodermal from the ectodermal cloaca; it is divided into anal and genitourinary m.'s that break down during the 8th to 9th week to establish the external opening for the alimentary and genitourinary tracts.

**closing m.'s,** pharyngeal m.'s; thin sheets, composed of ectoderm externally and entoderm internally, which separate the pharyngeal pouches from overlying branchial clefts in the early embryo.

**Corti's m.,** *membrana* tectoria ductus cochlearis.

**cricothy'roid m.,** *conus* elasticus.

**cricotracheal m.,** *ligamentum* cricotracheale.

**cricovocal m.,** *conus* elasticus.

**croupous m.,** false m.

**deciduous m.,** *membrana* decidua.

**Descemet's m.,** *lamina* limitans posterior corneae.

**diphtherit'ic m.,** the false m. forming on the mucous surfaces in diphtheria.

**drum m.,** *membrana* tympani.

**Duddell's m.,** *lamina* limitans posterior corneae.

**dysmenorrhe'al m.,** a m., resembling the decidua, cast off in cases of membranous dysmenorrhea.

**egg m.,** the investing envelope of the ovum; *primary,* produced from ovarian cytoplasm; *secondary,* the product of the ovarian follicle; *tertiary,* secreted by the lining of the oviduct.

**elastic m.,** one formed of elastic connective tissue fibers, present in the trachea, the coats of the arteries, and elsewhere.

**embryonic m.,** fetal m.

**enamel m.,** the internal layer of the enamel organ formed by the enamel cells.

**epipapillary m.,** (1) a congenital m. covering the optic cup; (2) the glial remnants of Bergmeister's *papilla, q.v.*

**exocelomic m.,** Heuser's m.; a layer of cells delaminated from the inner surface of the blastocystic cytotrophoblast and from the envelope of the primary yolk sac during the second week of embryonic life.

**false m.,** pseudomembrane; croupous m.; neohymen; plica (2); a more or less thick, tough fibrinous exudate on the surface of a mucous m. or the skin.

**fen'estrated m.,** elastic lamina, as in elastica interna of arteries.

**fertilization m.,** a viscous m. formed on the inner surface of the vitelline m. from the cytoplasm of the egg cell after entry of the sperm, preventing the entry of additional sperm.

**fetal m.,** embryonic m.; a structure or tissue developed from the fertilized ovum but which does not form part of the embryo proper; one of those structures.

**fibrous m.,** *membrana* fibrosa.

**Fielding's m.,** tapetum (2).

**flaccid m.,** *pars* flaccida membranae tympani.

**germ m.,** germinal m.; blastoderm.

**glassy m.,** (1) the basement m. present between the stratum granulosum and the theca interna of a vesicular ovarian follicle; it becomes very prominent in large atretic

follicles; (2) hyaline m. (2); the basement m. of the hair follicle.

**Henle's m.,** *lamina* basalis choroideae.

**Henle's fenestrated m.,** elastic *lamina.*

**Heuser's m.,** exocelomic m.

**Hunter's m.,** *membrana* decidua.

**hyaline m.,** (1) the thin, clear basement m. beneath certain epithelia; (2) glassy m. (2).

**hy'aloid m.,** *membrana* vitrea.

**hyoglossal m.,** a delicate fibrous m. that extends between the hyoid bone and the tongue.

**intercostal m.'s,** *membranae* intercostalia.

**interosseous m. of forearm,** *membrana* interossea antebrachii.

**interosseous m. of leg,** *membrana* interossea cruris.

**ivory m.,** *membrana* eboris.

**Jackson's m.,** Jackson's veil; a thin vascular m. or veil-like adhesion, covering the anterior surface of the ascending colon from the cecum to the right flexure; it may cause obstruction by kinking of the bowel.

**keratog'enous m.,** *matrix* unguis.

**Krause's m.,** Z *line.*

**limiting m. of neural tube,** the inner and outer aspects of the developing neural tube, formed from foot-plates of the cytoplasmic processes of ependymal cells passing centripetally and centrifugally, respectively.

**limiting m. of retina,** membrana limitans; one of two layers of the retina. The internal limiting m. is formed by the expanded inner ends of Müller's fibers; the outer limiting m. is not a membrane but a row of junctional complexes.

**med'ullary m.,** endosteum.

**mucous m.'s,** see entries under *tunica* mucosa.

**Nasmyth's m.,** *cuticula* dentis.

**nictitating m.,** *plica* semilunaris conjunctivae (2).

**Nitabuch's m.,** Nitabuch's layer or stria; a layer of fibrin between the boundary zone of compact endometrium and the cytotrophoblastic shell in the placenta.

**nuclear m.,** nuclear *envelope.*

**ob'turator m.,** *membrana* obturatoria.

**olfactory m.,** that part of the nasal mucosa having olfactory receptor cells and glands of Bowman.

**oral m.,** buccopharyngeal m.

**oronasal m.,** bucconasal m.

**oropharyngeal m.,** buccopharyngeal m.

**otolithic m.,** *membrana* statoconiorum.

**ovular m.,** *membrana* vitellina.

**Payr's m.,** a fold of peritoneum that crosses over the left flexure of the colon.

**pericardiopleural m.,** pleuropericardial m.

**peridental m.,** periodontium.

**perineal m.,** *membrana* perinei.

**periodontal m.,** periodontium.

**perior'bital m.,** periorbita.

**pharyngeal m.'s,** closing m.'s.

**pial-glial m.,** the dual outer lining of the brain and spinal cord, composed of the membrana limitans gliae and the pia mater.

**pitu'itary m.,** *tunica* mucosa nasi.

**placental m.,** the semipermeable layer of tissue separating the maternal from the fetal blood.

**plasma m.,** the protoplasmic boundary of all cells which controls permeability and may serve other functions through surface specializations; for example, absorption by microvilli and formation of pinocytotic vesicles; also known as cytomembrane; cell membrane; plasmalemma; cytolemma; plasmolemma. See schematic diagram under cell.

**pleuropericardial m.,** pericardiopleural m.; a tissue fold jutting into the embryonic pericardioperitoneal canals; it separates the developing pericardium from the pleural cavity.

**pleuroperitoneal m.,** pleuroperitoneal fold; a tissue fold jutting into the caudal portion of the embryonic pericardioperitoneal canal; it develops into the dorsal portion of the definitive diaphragm.

**posterior atlantooccipital m.,** *membrana* atlantooccipitalis posterior.

**postsynaptic m.,** that part of the plasma m. of a neuron or muscle fiber with which an axon terminal forms a synaptic junction. In many instances, part at least of such a small postsynaptic m. patch shows characteristic morphological modifications such as greater thickness and higher electron-density, believed to correspond to the transmitter-sensitive receptor site of such synapses.

**presynaptic m.,** that part of the plasma m. of an axon terminal that faces the plasma m. of the neuron or muscle fiber with which the axon terminal establishes a synpatic junction. In many synaptic junctions the presynaptic membrane exhibits structural characteristics, such as conical, electron-dense internal protrusions, that distinguish it from the remainder of the axon's plasma m. See also synapse.

**prolig′erous m.,** *cumulus* oophorus.

**prophylac′tic m.,** pyogenic m.

**pu′pillary m.,** *membrana* pupillaris.

**pyogen′ic m.,** prophylactic m.; a layer of pus cells that have not yet autolyzed, lining an abscess cavity.

**quadrangular m.,** *membrana* quadrangularis.

**Reissner's m.,** *paries* vestibularis ductus cochlearis.

**retic′ular m.,** *membrana* reticularis.

**Rivinus' m.,** *pars* flaccida membrane tympani.

**Ruysch's m.,** *lamina* choroidocapillaris.

**Scarpa's m.,** *membrana* tympani secundaria.

**Schneiderian m.,** *tunica* mucosa nasi.

**Schultze's m.,** *regio* olfactoria tunicae mucosae nasi.

**secondary tympanic m.,** *membrana* tympani secundaria.

**semiper′meable m.,** a m. that allows the passage of water and small ions or molecules, but not of large molecules or colloidal matter.

**serous m.,** *tunica* serosa.

**Shrapnell's m.,** *pars* flaccida membranae tympani.

**spiral m.,** *paries* tympanicus ductus cochlearis.

**m. of stapes,** *membrana* stapedis.

**statoconial m.,** *membrana* statoconiorum.

**sternal m.,** *membrana* sterni.

**stri′ated m.,** *zona* striata.

**suprapleural m.,** *membrana* suprapleuralis.

**syno′vial m.,** *membrana* synovialis.

**tecto′rial m.,** *membrana* tectoria.

**tectorial m. of cochlear duct,** *membrana* tectoria ductus cochlearis.

**thy′rohy′oid m.,** *membrana* thyrohyoidea.

**Toldt's m.,** the anterior layer of the renal fascia.

**Tourtual's m.,** *membrana* quadrangularis.

**tympanic m.,** *membrana* tympani.

**m. of tympanum,** *membrana* tympani.

**un′dulating m., un′dulatory m.,** a locomotory organelle of certain flagellate (trypanosome and trichomonad) parasites, consisting of a finlike extension of the limiting m. with the flagellar sheath; wavelike rippling of the undulating m. produces a characteristic movement.

**unit m.,** when seen with the electron microscope, a trilaminar m. about 75 Å thick. It has been suggested that not only the cell but other membranous structures such as endoplasmic reticulum, mitochondria, etc., have unit m.'s.

**urogenital m.,** the ventral portion of the embryonic cloacal m. after its division by the urorectal septum.

**urorect′al m.,** in the embryo, urorectal septum separating the cloaca into urogenital sinus and rectum.

**u′teroepicho′rial m.,** *decidua* parietalis.

**vestib′ular m.,** *paries* vestibularis ductus cochlearis.

**virginal m.,** hymen.

**vitelline m.,** *membrana* vitellina.

**vitreous m.,** (1) *lamina* limitans posterior corneae; (2) *membrana* vitrea; (3) *lamina* basalis choroideae.

**Wachendorf's m.,** *membrana* pupillaris.

**yolk m.,** *zona* pellucida.

**Zinn's m.,** the anterior layer of the iris.

---

**mem′branec′tomy** [ membrane + G. *ektomē*, excision ]. Removal of the inner membrane of a subdural hematoma.

**membranelle** (mem′bră-nel′). A minute membrane formed of fused cilia, found in certain of the Ciliata.

**membra′niform.** Of the appearance or character of a membrane.

**membranocartilaginous** (mem′bră-no-kar-tĭ-laj′ĭ-nus). 1. Partly membranous and partly cartilaginous. 2. Derived from both membrane and cartilage; denoting certain bones.

**membranoid** (mem′bră-noyd). Membraniform.

**membranous** (mem′bră-nus). Relating to or of the form of a membrane.

**mem′broid.** A membranous capsule, resistant to the action of the gastric juice but dissolving in the intestine, used for enclosing medicaments which it is desired to introduce unaltered into the duodenum.

**membrum,** pl. **membra** (mem′brum, mem′brah) [ L. member ] [ NA ]. A limb; a member.

**m. inferius** [ NA ], inferior limb; pelvic limb; lower extremity; the hip, thigh, leg, ankle, and foot.

**m. mulieb′re,** clitoris.

**m. superius** [ NA ], superior limb; thoracic limb; upper extremity; the shoulder, arm, forearm, wrist, and hand.

**m. vir′ile,** the penis.

**mem′ory** [ L. *memoria* ]. 1. A general term for the recollection of that which was once experienced or learned. 2. The psychic function of storing in the subconscious and retrieving an idea or impression that the mind had once been conscious of or had learned.

**affect m.,** the emotional element recurring whenever a significant experience is recalled.

**an′terograde m.,** m. for things after an event such as a brain injury.

**remote m.,** m. for events of long ago as opposed to recent events.

**retrograde m.,** m. for things preceding an event such as a brain injury.

**screen m.,** in psychoanalysis, a consciously tolerable m. that unwittingly serves as a cover for another associated m. which would be emotionally painful if recalled.

**senile m.,** m. for remote events, as characteristically seen in aged persons.

**short term m.,** m. involving intervals less than half a minute in length; abbreviated STM.

**subconscious m.,** information not immediately available for recall.

**mem′otine hydrochloride** (USAN). 3,4-Dihydro-1-[ (*p*-methoxyphenoxy)methyl ]isoquinoline hydrochloride; an antiviral drug.

**menacme** (mĕ-nak′me) [ G. *mēn*, month, + *akmē*, prime. AC- ]. The period of menstrual activity in a woman's life.

**menadiol** (men′ă-di′ol). Vitamin $K_4$.

**m. diacetate,** acetomenaphthone; 2-methyl-1,4-naphthohydroquinone diacetate; menadiol acetylated at both OH's. Used in the preoperative treatment of obstructive jaundice, in hemorrhagic disease of the newborn, and prophylactically to prevent neonatal hemorrhage.

**m. sodium diphosphate,** SYNKAYVITE; vitamin K analogue; tetrasodium 2-methyl-1,4-naphthalenediol-*bis*(dihydrogen phosphate); a dihydro derivative of menadione, with similar vitamin K activity.

**menadione** (men-ă-di′ōn) (NF). Menaphthone; menaquinone (*q.v.*); vitamin $K_3$; 2-methyl-1,4-naphthoquinone; a synthetic preparation at least twice as active as vitamin $K_1$. Used in hemorrhagic diatheses due to low prothrombin content of blood.

**m. reductase,** NAD(P)H dehydrogenase (quinone).

**m. sodium bisulfite** (NF), HYKINONE; menaphthone sodium bisulfite; possesses the same action and used for the same purposes as m. or vitamin K. It differs, however, from m. in being water-soluble.

**menaph′thone.** 1. Menaquinone. 2. Menadione.

**menaquinone** (men′ă-kwĭ-nōn′, -kwin′ōn). Abbreviation, MQ or MK; 2-methyl-1,4-naphthoquinone; root of a group of compounds that are 3-multiprenyl derivatives of menaquinone; specifically applied to the latter (vitamin $K_3$), which is also known as menadione (*q.v.*).

**Menaquinone**

**menaquinone-6.** Menaquinone-K₆ (abbreviated MQ-6 or MK-6 or MK₆); vitamin K₂ or K₂(30); hexaprenyl-menaquinone; prenylmenaquinone-6; 2-methyl-3-hexaprenyl-1,4-naphthoquinone; isolated from putrified fish meal; potency about 60 per cent of that of vitamin $K_1$ (phylloquinone).

**menarche** (mĕ-nar′ke) [ G. *mēn*, month, + *archē*, beginning ]. The establishment of the menstrual function; the time of the first menstrual period or flow.

**Mendel,** Gregor J., Austrian geneticist, 1822–1884. See Mendelian *character, inheritance, ratio*, M.'s *laws*.

**Mendel,** Kurt, German neurologist, 1874–1946. See Bechterew-M. *reflex*, M.'s instep *reflex*.

**Mendeléeff** (also seen Mendeleev) (men-da-la′ef), Dimitri (also seen Dmitri) I., Russian chemist, 1834–1907. Gave his name to mendelevium. See M.'s *law*.

**mendelevium** (men′dĕ-le′vī-um) [ *D. Mendeléeff* ]. Element no. 101, prepared in 1955 by bombardment of einsteinium (element no. 99) with alpha particles. Symbol Md.

**mendelism** (men′del-izm). The hereditary principles derived from Mendel's laws.

**Mendelson,** Curtis L., U. S. physician, *1913. See M.'s *syndrome*.

**menelip′sis.** Menolipsis.

**Ménétrier,** Pierre E., French physician, 1859–1935. 1935. See M.'s *disease, syndrome*.

**Menge** (men′geh), Karl, German gynecologist, 1864–1945. See M.'s *pessary*.

**Menghini needle.** See under needle.

**menhidrosis, menidrosis** (men′hi-dro′sis, -ĭ-dro′sis) [ G. *mēn*, month, + *hidrōsis*, perspiration ]. Monthly sweating, sometimes bloody, from the skin occurring as a form of vicarious menstruation.

**Ménière** (mān-yair′), Prosper, French physician, 1799–1862. See M.'s *disease, syndrome*.

**mening-.** See meningo-.

**meningeal** (mĕ-nin′je-al). Relating to the meninges.

**meningeocortical** (mĕ-nin′jē-o-kor′tĭ-kal). Meningocortical.

**meningeorrhaphy** (mĕ-min′je-or′ă-fĭ) [ G. *mēninx* (*mēning-*), membrane, + *rhaphē*, suture ]. Suture of the cranial or spinal meninges or of any membrane.

**meninges** (mĕ-nin′jēz). Plural of meninx.

**meningioma** (mĕ-nin′jĭ-o′mah) [ mening- + G. suffix *-oma*, tumor ]. A neoplasm that originates in the arachnoidal tissue, usually occurring in adults more than 30 years of age; m.'s comprise approximately 15 per cent of all intracranial neoplasms, and 25 per cent of intraspinal neoplasms. The most frequent form consists of elongated, fusiform cells in whorls and pseudolobules, and psammoma bodies are frequently observed; in addition to this type, *i.e.*, the meningothelial m., one may recognize angiomatous, chondromatous, osteomatous, lipomatous, melanotic, and fibrosarcomatous varieties. M.'s are typically slow in growth, tend to be oval in shape and compressive, rather than invasive, of brain tissue; the commonest locations are along the superior sagittal sinus, along the sphenoid ridge, or in the vicinity of the optic chiasm.

**meningiomatosis** (mĕ-nin′jĭ-o-mă-to′ sis). The presence of multiple meningiomas, sometimes seen in von Recklinghausen's disease.

**meningism** (men′in-jizm). Pseudomeningitis; a condition of irritation of the brain or spinal cord in which the symptoms simulate a meningitis, but in which no actual inflammation of these membranes is present.

**meningitic** (men′in-jit′ik). Relating to or characterized by meningitis.

**meningitis** pl. **meningit′ides** (men-in-ji′tis) [ mening- G. suffix *-itis*, inflammation ]. Inflammation of the membranes of the brain or spinal cord; see also arachnoiditis; leptomeningitis.

  **basilar m.,** m. at the base of the brain, due usually to tuberculosis, syphilis, or any low grade chronic granulomatous process; may result in an internal hydrocephalus.

  **cerebrospinal m.,** meningococcal m.

  **epidemic cerebrospi′nal m.,** meningococcal m.

  **epidural m.,** *pachymeningitis* externa.

  **external m.,** *pachymeningitis* externa.

  **internal m.,** *pachymeningitis* interna.

  **listeria m.,** listeriosis.

  **meningococcal m.,** cerebrospinal m.; cerebrospinal fever; epidemic cerebrospinal m.; an acute infectious disease affecting children and young adults, caused by a special microorganism, the meningococcus (*Neisseria meningitidis*); the symptoms are nasopharyngeal catarrh, headache, vomiting, convulsions, stiffness in the neck (nuchal rigidity), photophobia, constipation, cutaneous hyperesthesia, a purpuric or herpetic eruption, and the presence of Kernig's sign; in cases of recovery, blindness, deafness, and paralysis are frequent sequelae.

  **neoplastic m.,** neoplastic arachnoiditis; infiltration of subarachnoid space by neoplastic cells, typically medulloblastoma or metastatic carcinoma.

  **occlusive m.,** leptomeningitis causing occlusion of the spinal fluid pathways.

  **otitic m.,** infection of the meninges secondary to mastoiditis.

  **serous m.,** acute m. with secondary external hydrocephalus.

  **tuberculous m.,** inflammation of the cerebral leptomeninges marked by the presence of granulomatous inflammation; it is usually confined to the base of the brain (basilar m., Whytt's disease) and is accompanied in children by an accumulation of spinal fluid in the ventricles (acute hydrocephalus).

**meningo-, mening-** (mĕ-ning′go-) [ G. *mēninx*, membrane. MENIN- ]. Combining forms relating to meninges.

**meningocele** (mĕ-ning′go-sēl) [ meningo- + G. *kēlē*, tumor ]. A protrusion of the membranes of the brain or spinal cord through a defect in the skull or spinal column.

  **spurious m.,** traumatic m.; an extracranial accumulation of cerebrospinal fluid, due to meningeal tear.

  **traumatic m.,** spurious m.

**meningococcemia** (mĕ-ning′go-kok-se′mĭ-ah). The presence of meningococci (*Neisseria meningitidis*) in the circulating blood.

**meningococcus** (mĕ-ning′go-kok′us) [ meningo- + G. *kokkos*, berry ]. *Neisseria meningitidis*.

**meningocortical** (mĕ-ning′go-kor′tĭ-kal). Meningeocortical; relating to the meninges and the cortex of the brain.

**meningocyte** (mĕ-ning′go-sīt) [ meningo- + G. *kytos*, cell ]. A mesenchymal epithelial cell of the subarachnoid space; it may become a macrophage.

**meningoencephalitis** (mĕ-ning′go-en-sef′ă-li′tis) [ meningo- + G. *enkephalos*, brain, + suffix *-itis*, inflammation ]. Cerebromeningitis; encephalomeningitis; an inflammation of the brain and its membranes.

  **biundulant m.,** tick-borne *encephalitis*, Central European subtype.

  **eosinophilic m.,** a disease caused by infection with the rat lungworm, *Angiostrongylus cantonensis*, whose larvae, ingested with infected slugs or land snails (or some unidentified transport host), migrate from intestine to the meninges of the brain where the febrile, eosinophilic meningoencephalitis is produced. The disease is usually mild, of short duration, and characterized by fever, eosinophilia, and white blood cells (rarely nematode larvae) in the spinal fluid.

  **mumps m.,** a usually benign nervous system infection arising during the active phase of clinical mumps parotiditis.

  **syphilitic m.,** a secondary or tertiary stage manifestation of syphilis; rarely fatal.

  **trypanosomal m.,** a subacute or chronic inflammatory disease of the brain caused by the pathogenic protozoa, *Trypanosoma gambiense* or *Trypanosoma rhodesiense;* see also gambian *trypanosomiasis*.

**meningoencephalocele** (mĕ-ning′go-en-sef′ă-lo-sēl) [ meningo- + G. *enkephalos*, brain, + *kēlē*, hernia ]. Encephalomeningocele; a protrusion of the meninges and brain through a congenital defect in the cranium, usually in the frontal or occipital region.

**meningoencephalomyelitis** (mĕ-ning′go-en-sef′ă-lo-mi-ĕ-li′tis) [ meningo- + G. *enkephalos*, brain, + *myelos*, marrow, + suffix *-itis*, inflammation ]. Inflammation of the brain and spinal cord together with their membranes.

**meningoencephalopathy** (mĕ-ning′go-en-sef′ă-lop′ă-thĭ) [ meningo- + G. *enkephalos*, brain, + *pathos*, suffering ]. Encephalomeningopathy; disorder affecting the meninges and the brain.

**meningomyelitis** (mĕ-ning′go-mi′ĕ-li′tis) [ meningo- + G. *myelos*, marrow, + suffix - *itis*, inflammation ]. Inflammation of the spinal cord and of its enveloping arachnoid and pia mater, and less commonly also of the dura mater.

**meningomyelocele** (mĕ-ning′go-mi′ĕ-lo-sēl) [ meningo- + G. *myelos*, marrow, + *kēlē*, tumor ]. Myelomeningocele; a protrusion of the membranes and cord through a defect in the vertebral column.

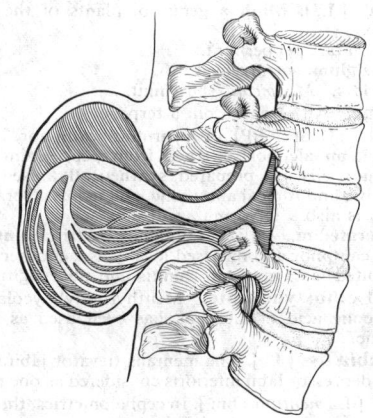

Meningomyelocele

**meningo-osteophlebitis** (mĕ-ning′-go-os-te-o-fle-bi′tis). Inflammation of the veins of the periosteum.

**meningopathy** (men′ing-gop′ă-thĭ) [ meningo- + G. *pathos*, suffering ]. Any disease of the cerebral or spinal meninges.

**meningoradicular** (mĕ-ning′go-ră-dik′u-lar) [ meningo- + L. *radix*, root ]. Relating to the meninges and the cranial or spinal nerve roots.

**meningoradiculitis** (mĕ-ning′go-ră-dik′u-li′tis). Inflammation of the meninges and roots of the nerves.

**meningorrhachidian** (mĕ-ning′go-ră-kid′ĭ-an) [ meningo- + G. *rhachis*, spine ]. Relating to the spinal cord and its membranes.

**meningorrhagia** (mĕ-ning′go-ra′jĭ-ah) [ meningo- + G. *rhēgnymi*, to burst forth ]. Hemorrhage into or beneath the cerebral or spinal meninges.

**meningosis** (men′ing-go′sis) [ meningo- + G. suffix -*ōsis*, condition ]. Membranous union of bones, as in the skull of the newborn.

**meningovascular** (mĕ-ning′go-vas′ku-lar). Concerning the blood vessels in the meninges; or the meninges and blood vessels.

**meninguria** (men′ing-gu′rĭ-ah) [ meningo- + G. *ouron*, urine ]. The passage of membraniform shreds in the urine.

**meninx,** gen. **meningis,** pl. **meninges** (me′ningks, men-′ingks, mĕ-nin′jes, -jēz) [ Mod. L. fr. G. *mēninx*, membrane. MENIN- ] [ NA ]. Any membrane; specifically, one of the membranous coverings of the brain and spinal cord. See also arachnoidea, dura mater, pia mater.
    **m. fibro′sa,** rarely used term for dura mater.
    **m. primiti′va,** the embryonic loose mesenchymatous tissue surrounding the brain and spinal cord; from it the three definitive meninges are derived.
    **m. sero′sa,** arachnoidea.
    **m. ten′uis,** the leptomeninges.
    **m. vasculo′sa,** rarely used term for pia mater.

**meniscectomy** (men′ĭ-sek′to-mĭ) [ G. *mēniskos*, crescent (meniscus) + *ektomē*, excision ]. Excision of a meniscus, usually from the knee joint.

**meniscitis** (men′ĭ-si′tis) [ G. *mēniskos*, crescent (meniscus),

+ suffix -*itis*, inflammation ]. Inflammation of an interarticular cartilage.

**meniscocyte** (mĕ-nis′ko-sīt) [ G. *mēniskos*, a crescent, + *kytos*, a hollow (cell) ]. Sickle *cell*.

**meniscocytosis** (mĕ-nis-ko-si-to′sis) [ meniscocyte + G. suffix -*osis*, condition ]. Sickle cell *anemia*.

**meniscotome** (mĕ-nis′ko-tōm) [ G. *mēniskos*, crescent (meniscus) + *tomē*, incision ]. An instrument used in the removal of a meniscus.

**meniscus,** pl. **menis′ci,** (mĕ-nis′kus) [ G. *mēniskos*, crescent. MEN- ]. 1. Meniscus *lens*. 2 [ NA ]. A crescent-shaped structure.
    **articular m.,** m. articularis.
    **m. articula′ris** [ NA ], articular meniscus; articular crescent; a crescent-shaped intraarticular fibrocartilage found in certain joints.
    **converging m.,** positive m.; a m. in which the convexity exceeds the concavity.
    **diverging m.,** negative m.; a convexoconcave lens in which the concavity has a greater radius than the convexity.
    **lateral m.** m. lateralis.
    **m. latera′lis** [ NA ], lateral m.; external semilunar fibrocartilage, attached to the lateral border of the upper articular surface of the tibia.
    **medial m.,** m. medialis.
    **m. media′lis** [ NA ], medial m.; falciform cartilage; internal semilunar fibrocartilage of the knee joint; attached to the medial border of the upper articular surface of the tibia.
    **negative m.,** diverging m.
    **periscopic m.,** aplanatic *lens*.
    **positive m.,** converging m.
    **tactile m.,** m. tactus.
    **m. tac′tus** [ NA ], tactile m.; tactile disk; Merkel's tactile disk; Merkel's corpuscle; a specialized tactile sensory nerve ending in the skin characterized by a terminal cuplike expansion of the nerve fiber in contact with a single modified epithelial cell.

**Menkes,** John H., U. S. neurologist, *1928. See M.'s *syndrome*.

**meno-** [ G. *mēn*, month. MEN- ]. Combining form denoting relationship to the menses.

**menocelis** (men-o-se′lis) [ meno- + G. *kēlis*, spot ]. A dark macular or petechial eruption sometimes occurring in cases of amenorrhea.

**menoc′tone** (USAN). 2-(8-Cyclohexyloctyl)-3-hydroxy-1,4-naphthoquinone; an antimalarial drug.

**menolip′sis** [ meno- + G. *leipsis*, a failing or lacking ]. Menelipsis; amenorrhea; temporary cessation of menstruation.

**menometrorrhagia** (men′o-me′tro-ra′jĭ-ah) [ meno- + G. *mētra*, uterus, + *rhēgnymi*, to burst forth ]. Irregular or excessive bleeding during menstruation and between menstrual periods; this is a symptom but not an acceptable diagnosis.

**menopausal** (men′o-paw-zal). Associated with or occasioned by the menopause.

**menopause** (men′o-pawz) [ meno- + G. *pausis*, cessation ]. Permanent cessation of the menses; termination of the menstrual life.

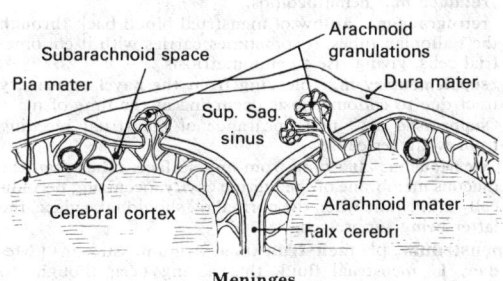

Meninges

Coronal section to show the cerebral meninges in relation to the brain.

**menophania** (men'o-fa'nĭ-ah) [ meno- + G. *phainō*, to show ]. The first sign of the menses at puberty.

**menoplania** (men'o-pla'nĭ-ah) [ meno- + G. *plane*, a wandering ]. Vicarious *menstruation*.

**Men'opon.** A genus of biting lice (family Menoponidae, order Mallophaga) found only on birds; it includes important pests that infect domestic fowl.

    **M. gal'linae,** *M. pallidum;* the shaft louse of poultry; it is light yellow and about 1.7 to 2.0 mm. long, and is found on barnyard fowl, ducks, and pigeons.

    **M. pal'lidum,** *M. gallinae.*

**menorrhagia** (men'o-ra'jĭ-ah) [ meno- + G. *rhēgnymi*, to burst forth ]. Excessively profuse or prolonged menstruation.

**menorrhalgia** (men'o-ral'jĭ-ah) [ meno- + G. *algos*, pain ]. Dysmenorrhea.

**menorrhea** (men'o-re'ah) [ meno- + G. *rhoia*, flow ]. 1. Normal menstruation. 2. Menorrhagia.

**menoschesis** (mĕ-nos'ke-sis, men'o-ske'sis) [ meno- + G. *schesis*, retention ]. Suppression of menstruation.

**men'osep'sis** [ meno- + G. *sēpsis*, putrefaction ]. Blood poisoning due to the absorption of septic material from a retained menstrual discharge.

**menostasis, menostasia** (mĕ-nos'tă-sis, men'o-sta'zĭ-ah) [ meno- + G. *stasis*, a standing ]. Amenorrhea.

**menostaxis** (men-o-stak'sis) [ meno- + G. *staxis*, a dripping ]. Unduly prolonged menstrual flow.

**menothermal** (men'o-ther'mal) [ meno- + G. *thermē*, heat ]. Denoting the menopausal hot flashes.

**men'otro'pins** (USP). PERGONAL; extract of postmenopausal urine containing primarily the follicle-stimulating hormone; see also human menopausal *gonadotropin.*

**menouria** (men-o-u'rĭ-ah) [ meno- + G. *ouron*, urine, + suffix -*ia*, condition ]. Menstruation occurring through the urinary bladder as a result of vesicouterine fistula.

**menoxenia** (men-o-ze'nĭ-ah) [ meno- + G. *xenos*, strange ]. Any abnormality of menstruation.

**menses** (men'sēz) [ L. pl. of *mensis*, month. MEN- ]. A periodic physiologic hemorrhage, occurring at approximately 4-week intervals, and having its source from the uterine mucous membrane. Under normal circumstances, the bleeding is preceded by ovulation and predecidual changes in the endometrium. See also menstrual *cycle.*

**menstrual** (men'stru-al) [ L. *menstrualis* ]. Catamenial; relating to the menses.

**menstruant** (men'stru-ant). Menstruating.

**menstruate** (men'stru-āt) [ L. *menstruo*, pp. -*atus*, to be menstruant. MEN- ]. To perform menstruation; to pass through the catamenial period.

**menstruation** (men-stru-a'shun) [ see menstruate ]. Menorrhea (1); the periodic discharge of a bloody fluid from the uterus.

    **anov'ular m.,** menstrual bleeding without the discharge of an ovum; it occurs in subhuman primates as well as in women. In women an ovum may be found retained within the follicle which later undergoes degeneration or, rarely, may become impregnated and result in an ovarian pregnancy.

    **anovula'tional m.,** anovular m.

    **nonovula'tional m.,** anovular m.

    **retained m.,** hematocolpos.

    **retrograde m.,** a flow of menstrual blood back through the Fallopian tubes; it sometimes carries with it endometrial cells, giving rise to endometriosis.

    **supplementary m.,** bleeding from the navel or urinary tract due to endometriosis occurring at the time of m.

    **suppressed m.,** nonappearance of menstrual bleeding from whatever cause.

    **vicarious m.,** bleeding from any surface, other than the mucous membrane of the uterine cavity, occurring periodically at the time when the normal m. should take place, the latter being suppressed.

**menstruum,** pl. **menstrua** (men'stru-um, -stru-ah) [ Mediev. L. menstrual fluid, this having been thought to possess markedly solvent properties, ntr. of L. *menstruus*, monthly. MEN- ]. A solvent, a fluid containing another substance in solution.

**mensual** (men'su-al, -shu-al) [ L. *mensis*, month ]. Monthly.

**mensuration** (men'su-ra'shun) [ L. *mensuratio*, fr. *mensuro*, to measure ]. Measurement.

**mentag'ra** [ L. tetter on the chin, fr. *mentum*, chin, + G. *agra*, a seizure ]. Sycosis.

**mentagrophyton** (men'tă-gro-fi'ton). *Trichophyton mentagrophytes.*

**men'tal.** 1 [ L. *mens* (*ment*-), mind ]. Relating to the mind. 2 [ L. *mentum*, chin ]. Relating to the chin; genial.

**menta'lis** [ L. ]. See under musculus.

**mental'ity.** The functional condition of the mind; mental activity.

**Menten,** Maud R. See Michaelis-M. *constant, hypothesis.*

**Men'tha** [ L. ]. Mint; a genus of plants of the family Labiatae.

    **M. piperi'ta,** peppermint.

    **M. pule'gium,** pennyroyal.

    **M. vi'ridis,** *M. spicata;* spearmint.

**men'thane.** An essential oil, a terpene.

**men'thol** (USP, BP). Peppermint camphor; *p*-menthan-3-ol; an alcohol obtained from peppermint oil or other mint oils, or prepared synthetically; used as an antipruritic and topical anesthetic, and in nasal sprays and inhalers; is also a flavoring agent.

    **camphorated m.,** a liquid obtained by triturating equal parts of camphor and m. Used locally as a counterirritant and (diluted) as a spray in rhinitis and pharyngitis.

**men'thyl ethox'yac'etate.** Menthyl ethylglycolate; the ethylglycolic acid of menthol; has been used as a local anesthetic.

**men'tolabia'lis** [ L. ]. The mentalis (levator labii inferioris) and depressor labii inferioris considered as one muscle.

**men'ton** [ L. *mentum*, chin ]. In cephalometrics, the lowermost point in the symphysial shadow as seen on a lateral jaw projection.

**men'tum,** gen. **men'ti** [ L. ] [ NA ]. The chin.

**menyan'thes.** Buckbean.

**mep'acrine hydrochloride** (BP). Quinacrine hydrochloride.

**mepar'fynol.** DORMISON; 3-methyl-1-pentyn-3-ol; hypnotic and sedative; weak but nontoxic in sedative doses; it is used as an anticonvulsant in subtoxic doses, but may cause hepatic damage; drug dependence may develop.

**mep'azine ac'etate.** PACATAL acetate; 10-[ (1-methyl-3-piperidyl)methyl ]phenothiazine acetate. A phenothiazine derivative with actions and uses similar to those of chlorpromazine. Used as a tranquilizing drug in neuroses and psychoses and for its calming and antiemetic effects in surgery and obstetrics. Also available as m. hydrochloride.

**mepen'zolate bro'mide** (NF). CANTIL; 1-methyl-3-piperidyl benzilate methylbromide. Anticholinergic drug used for the relief of spasm and hypermotility of the small intestine and colon. It also relaxes the sphincter of Oddi, and suppresses pancreatic and gastric secretion.

**meper'idine hydrochloride** (USP). DEMEROL; ISONIPE-CAINE; DOLANTIN; pethidine hydrochloride; ethyl 1-methyl-4-phenylisonipecotate hydrochloride; a narcotic, analgesic, sedative, and antispasmodic; may produce physical and psychic dependence.

**mephen'esin** (NF). MYANESIN; TOLSEROL; 3-*o*-toloxy-1,2-propanediol; a skeletal muscle relaxant. Also available as m. carbamate (TOLSERAM).

**mephenox'alone.** TREPIDONE; 5-[ (*o*-methoxyphenoxy)methyl ]-2-oxazolidinone; a mild tranquilizer and muscle relaxant.

**mephen'termine** (NF). WYAMINE; *N*-α ,α-trimethylphenethylamine; a sympathomimetic amine.

    **m. sulfate** (USP, BP), WYAMINE sulfate; used topically as a nasal decongestant and systemically for its pressor effects in acute hypotensive states.

**mephenytoin** (mĕ-fen'ĭ-to-in) (NF). PHENANTOIN; MESANTOIN; methion; 5-ethyl-3-methyl-5-phenylhydantoin; an anticonvulsant; it is more potent than diphenylhydantoin but may produce rash, fever, blood dyscrasias, and aplastic anemia; seldom used.

**mephit'ic** [ L. *mephitis*, a noxious exhalation ]. Foul; poisonous; noxious.

**meph'obarb'ital** (NF). MEBARAL; 5-ethyl-1-methyl-5-phenylbarbituric acid; used as a sedative and long-acting hypnotic; and as an anticonvulsant in the management of epilepsy.

**mepicy'cline.** AMBRAVEINE; *N*-{[ 4-(2-hydroxyethyl)-1-piperazinyl ]methyl}tetracycline; antimicrobial agent.

**mepiperphenidol** (mep'ĭ-per-fen'ĭ-dōl). DARSTINE; 1-(3-hydroxy -5- methyl -4- phenylhexyl)-1- methylpiperidinium bromide; an anticholinergic agent.

**mepivacaine hydrochloride** (me-piv'ă-kān) (USP). CARBOCAINE hydrochloride; *dl-N*-methylpipecolic acid; 2,6-dimethylanilide hydrochloride; a potent local anesthetic agent similar in action to lidocaine. It is less toxic than lidocaine and has a longer duration of action; the addition of epinephrine or other vasoconstrictor drug is not necessary. It is used for infiltration, regional nerve block, peridural and caudal anesthesia.

**mepred'nisone** (NF). BETAPAR; 17,21-dihydroxy-16β-methylpregna-1,4-diene-3,11,20-trione; a glucocorticoid for oral use.

**mepro'bamate** (USP, BP). EQUANIL; MEPROSPAN; MEPROTABS; MILTOWN (and many others); 2-methyl-2-*n*-propyl-1,3-propanediol dicarbamate; a skeletal muscle relaxant with action similar to that produced by mephenesin (central interneuronal blockade) but of longer duration. Used in the management of certain disorders associated with abnormal motor activity. Also used as a mild hypnotic in simple insomnia and as an antianxiety agent in the treatment of psychoneuroses and tension states.

**mep'rylcaine hydrochloride.** ORACAINE; 2-methyl-2-(propylamino)-1-propanol benzoate hydrochloride; a local anesthetic used in dentistry.

**mepyramine maleate** (me-pĭr'ă-mēn) (BP). Pyrilamine maleate.

**mepyrapone** (me-pĭr'ă-pōn). Metyrapone.

**mequidox** (mek'wĭ-doks) (USAN). 2-Methyl-2-quinoxalinemethanol 1,4-dioxide; an antibacterial drug.

**-mer.** 1. A suffix attached to a prefix such as mono-, di-, tri-, poly-, etc., to indicate the smallest unit of a repeating structure; see monomer, polymer. 2. Suffix denoting a member of a particular group, as in isomer, enantiomer.

**meralein sodium** (mĕr'a-lēn) (USAN). MERODICEIN; *O*-[ 6-hydroxy-5-(hydroxymercuri) -2,7-diiodo-3-oxo-3*H*-xanthen-9-yl ]benzenesulfonic acid sodium salt; topical antiseptic.

**meralgia** (me-ral'jĭ-ah) [ G. *mēros*, thigh, + *algos*, pain ]. Pain in the thigh.
  **m. paraesthet'ica,** tingling, formication, itching, and other forms of paresthesia in the outer side of the lower part of the thigh in the area of distribution of the external cutaneous branch of the femoral nerve; there may be pain, but the skin is usually hypesthetic to the touch. Also called Bernhardt's disease or syndrome, or Roth-Bernhardt's disease.

**meral'luride.** MERCUHYDRIN; *N*-[ [ 2-methoxy-3-[ (1,2,3,6-tetrahydro- 1,3-dimethyl-2,6-dioxopurin- 7-yl)-mercuri ]propyl ]carbamoyl ]succinamic acid; a mercurial diuretic.

**merbro'min.** MERCUROCHROME; the disodium salt of 2,7-dibrom-4-hydroxymercurifluorescein; an organic mercurial antiseptic compound.

**mercap'tal.** A substance derived from an aldehyde by the replacement of the bivalent oxygen by two thioalkyl groups.

**mercap'tan.** 1. Thioalcohol or thiol; a class of substances in which the oxygen of an alcohol has been replaced by sulfur; they form white compounds with mercuric oxide. 2. In dentistry, a class of elastic impression compounds sometimes referred to as rubber base materials.

**mercap'to-.** A prefix indicating the presence of a thiol group —SH.

**mercaptoacetic acid** (mer-kap'to-ă-se'tik). Thioglycolic acid.

**β -mercaptoethylamine.** Cysteamine.

**mercap'tol, mercap'tole.** A substance derived from a ketone by the replacement of the bivalent oxygen by two thioalkyl groups.

**mercaptom'erin sodium** (USP). THIOMERIN sodium; (γ-carboxymethylmercaptomercuri -β- methoxy) propylcamphoramic acid disodium salt; an effective mercurial diuretic, less toxic to the heart than other mercurial diuretics given by injection.

**mercap'topu'rine** (USP, BP). PURINETHOL; 6-purinethiol; an analogue of hypoxanthine and of adenine; used in the treatment of acute leukemia in children.

**mer'captu'ric acid.** A condensation product of cysteine with compounds such as bromobenzene.

**Mercier** (mer-se-a'), Louis A., French urologist, 1811–1882. See M.'s *bar, barrier, sound, valve.*

**mer'cocre'sols.** A mixture consisting of equal parts by weight of *sec*-amyltricresol and *o*-hydroxyphenylmercuric chloride. Possesses fungicidal, germicidal, and bacteriostatic action.

**mercumat'ilin.** CUMERTILIN; 8-(2'-methoxy-3'-hydroxymercuripropyl) coumarin-3-carboxylic acid (mercumallylic acid) and theophylline; a mercurial diuretic. Also available as m. sodium.

**mercurial** (mer-ku'rĭ-al). 1. Relating to mercury. 2. Any salt of mercury used medicinally.

**mercurialentis** (mer-ku'rĭ-ă-len'tis). A brown discoloration of the anterior capsule of the crystalline lens caused by mercury; early sign of mercurial poisoning.

**mercurialism** (mer-ku'rĭ-ă-lizm). Mercury *poisoning.*

**mercu'rializa'tion.** The being or the bringing under the therapeutic influence of mercury.

**mercu'rialize.** 1. To impregnate with mercury. 2. To bring under the therapeutic influence of mercury.

**p-mercu'riben'zoate.** A commonly used enzyme inhibitor, because of its reaction with sulfhydryl groups. Usually *p*-chloromercuribenzoate or *p*-hydroxymercuribenzoate is used.

**mercu'ric.** Denoting a salt of mercury in which the ion of the metal is bivalent, as in corrosive sublimate, mercuric chloride, $HgCl_2$; the mercurous chloride is calomel, $HgCl$.
  **m. benzoate,** has been used in the treatment of syphilis.
  **m. chloride,** mercury bichloride; mercury perchloride; corrosive mercury chloride; corrosive sublimate; $HgCl_2$; topical antiseptic and disinfectant for inanimate objects.
  **m. chloride, ammoniated,** ammoniated mercury.
  **m. cyanide,** cyanuret of mercury; $Hg(CN)_2$; has been used as antisyphilitic and antiseptic.
  **m. iodide, red,** mercury biniodide; mercury deutoiodide; $HgI_2$; has been used as an antiseptic and as a disinfectant for inanimate objects.
  **m. oleate,** ointment-like preparation used in parasitic skin diseases.
  **m. oxide, red,** red precipitate of $HgO$; has been used externally as an antiseptic in chronic skin diseases and fungus infections.
  **m. oxide, yellow,** yellow precipitate of $HgO$; used externally as an antiseptic in the treatment of inflammatory conditions of the eyelids and the conjunctivae.
  **m. oxycyanide,** $HgOHg(CN)_2$; has been used by injection in the treatment of syphilis.
  **m. salicylate,** mercury subsalicylate; used externally in the treatment of parasitic and fungus skin diseases.
  **m. succinimide,** m. imidosuccinate; has been used as an antisyphilitic agent.
  **m. sulfide, black,** ethiops mineral; $HgS$; occurs as a mineral in California; used commercially as a pigment.
  **m. sulfide, red,** cinnabar; Paris red; vermilion; the ore from which metallic mercury is obtained.

**Mercurio** (mer-koo're-o), Geronimo S., Italian obstetrician, 1550–1595. See M.'s *position.*

**mercurophen** (mur-ku'-ro-fen). Sodium hydroxymercury-*o*-nitrophenolate; a local antiseptic, recommended for the treatment of external diplococcic infections.

**mer'curophyl'line sodium.** MERCUZANTHIN; the sodium salt of β -methoxy-γ -hydroxymercuripropylamide of trimethylcyclopentanedicarboxylic acid, and theophylline. A mercurial diuretic.

**mercurous** (mer-ku'rus, mer'ku-rus). Denoting a salt of mercury in which the ion of the metal is univalent, as in calomel, mercurous chloride, $HgCl$; the mercuric chloride is corrosive sublimate, $HgCl_2$.

**m. acetate,** CH$_3$COOHg; has been used in syphilis and externally in skin diseases.

**m. chloride,** calomel; mild mercury chloride; mercury monochloride; mercury protochloride; mercury subchloride; sweet precipitate; HgCl; has been used as an intestinal antiseptic, laxative and antisyphilitic.

**m. iodide,** yellow mercury iodide; mercury protoiodide; HgI; used externally as ointment in eye diseases; formerly used in syphilis.

**mercury** (mer′ku-rĭ) [ L. *Mercurius,* Mercury, the god of trade, messenger of the gods, in Mediev. L. quicksilver, mercury ]. Quicksilver; hydrargyrum; a heavy, silvery, liquid metal, symbol Hg, atomic no. 80, atomic weight 200.6. Used in thermometers, barometers, manometers, and other scientific instruments. Some of its salts (see under mercurous and mercuric) and organic mercurials are used in medicine as antiseptics, parasiticides, antisyphilitics, and diuretics.

**ammoniated m.,** mercuric chloride, ammoniated; white precipitate; white mercuric precipitate; HgNH$_2$Cl; used in ointment for the treatment of skin diseases.

**vegetable m.,** manaca.

**mere-, mero-** [ G. *mēros,* part ]. Combining forms meaning part; also indicating one of a series of similar parts, as in blastomere or metamere.

**Merendino's technique.** See under technique.

**merergasia** (mer-er-gă′zĭ-ah) [ G. *meros,* part, + *ergasia,* work ]. A mild form of mental incapacity.

**mer′ethox′ylline procaine.** DICURIN procaine; dehydro-2-[ *N*-(3′-hydroxymercuri-2′-methoxyethoxy) -propylcarbamyl ]phenoxyacetic acid (merethoxylline), 2-diethylaminoethyl *p*-aminobenzoate (procaine) and theophylline; a mixture of procaine salt of merethoxylline and anhydrous theophylline; used as a mercurial diuretic.

**meridian** (mĕ-rid′ĭ-an) [ L. *meridianus,* pertaining to midday, on the south side, southern, fr. *meridies,* midday, fr. *medius,* middle, + *dies,* day ]. 1. A line encircling a globular body at right angles to its equator and touching both poles, or the half of such a circle extending from pole to pole. 2. In acupuncture, the lines connecting different anatomical sites.

**m. of cornea,** any line bisecting the cornea through its apex.

**m.'s of eye,** *meridiani* bulbi oculi.

**meridia′ni.** Plural of meridianus.

**meridia′nus,** pl. **meridia′ni** [ L. ] [ NA ]. Meridian.

**meridiani bul′bi oc′uli** [ NA ], lines surrounding the surface of the eyeball passing through both anterior and posterior poles.

**meridional** (mĕ-rid′ĭ-o-nal). Relating to a meridian.

**Mering** (ma′ring), Joseph von, German physician, 1849–1908. Noted for his studies with Minkowski of phlorizin diabetes and pancreatic diabetes.

**merispore** (mĕr′ĭ-spōr) [ G. *meros,* a part, + *sporos,* seed ]. A secondary spore; a spore resulting from the segmentation of another (compound or septate) spore.

**meris′tic** [ G. *meristikos,* suitable for dividing ]. Symmetrical; that which can be divided evenly; denoting bilateral or longitudinal symmetry in the arrangement of parts in one organism.

**Merkel,** Friedrich S., German anatomist and physiologist, 1845–1919. See M.'s *corpuscle,* M.'s tactile *cell,* tactile *disk.*

**Merkel,** Karl L., German anatomist and laryngologist, 1812–1876. See M.'s *filtrum* ventriculi, *fossa, muscle.*

**mero-.** See mere-.

**meroacrania** (mĕr′o-ă-kra′nĭ-ah) [ mero- + G. *a-* priv. + *kranion,* skull ]. Congenital lack of a part of the cranium other than the occipital bone.

**meroanencephaly** (mer′o-an-en-sef′ă-lĭ) [ mero- + G. *an-* priv. + *enkephalos,* brain ]. A type of anencephaly in which the brain and cranium are present in a rudimentary form.

**meroblas′tic** [ mero- + G. *blastos,* germ ]. Denoting a type of cleavage in a markedly telolecithal ovum. See meroblastic *cleavage.*

**merocele** (me′ro-sēl) [ G. *mēros,* thigh, + *kele,* hernia ]. Femoral *hernia.*

**merocrine** (mĕr′o-krin, -krĭn, -krēn) [ mero- + G. *krinō,* to separate ]. See under gland.

**merodiastolic** (mĕr′o-di-ă-stol′ik) [ mero- + diastole, *q.v.* ]. Partially diastolic; relating to a part of the diastole of the heart.

**merogenesis** (mĕr′o-jen′ĕ-sis) [ mero- + G. *genesis,* production ]. Reproduction by segmentation.

**merogenet′ic, merogen′ic.** Relating to merogenesis.

**merogony** (mĕ-rog′o-nĭ) [ mero- + G. *gonē,* generation ]. 1. The incomplete development of an ovum which has been disorganized. 2. A form of asexual multiple fission (schizogony), typical of sporozoan protozoa, in which the nucleus divides several times before the cytoplasm divides; the dividing cell (schizont) breaks up to form daughter cells (merozoites) in this asexual phase of the life cycle.

**meromicrosomia** (mĕr′o-mi′kro-so′mĭ-ah) [ mero- + G. *mikros,* small, + *sōma,* body ]. Abnormal smallness of some portion of the body; local dwarfism.

**mer′omy′osin.** A product of the tryptic digestion of myosin; a subunit of myosin; two types are produced, H-m. and L-m.

**H-m.** [ H for "heavy" ], one of the relatively heavy products of the action of trypsin on myosin; molecular weight about 232,000.

**L-m.** [ L for "light" ], the relatively low molecular weight product of the tryptic digestion of myosin; molecular weight about 96,000.

**meropia** (mĕ-ro′pĭ-ah) [ mero- + G. *ōps,* vision ]. Incomplete blindness.

**merorachischisis, merorrhachischisis** (mĕr′o-răkis′kĭ-sis) [ mero- + G. *rhachis,* spine, + *schisis,* fissure ]. Mesorrhachischisis; rachischis partialis; fissure of a portion of the spinal cord.

**merosmia** (mĕ-roz′mĭ-ah) [ mero- + G. *osmē,* smell ]. A condition analogous to color blindness, in which the perception of certain odors is wanting.

**merosystolic** (mĕr′o-sis-tol′ik) [ mero- + systole, *q.v.* ]. Partially systolic; relating to a portion of the systole of the heart.

**merotomy** (mĕ-rot′o-mĭ) [ mero- + G. *tomē,* incision ]. The procedure of cutting into parts, as the cutting of a cell into separate parts to study their capacity for survival and development.

**merozoite** (mĕr′o-zo′ĭt) [ mero- + G. *zōon,* animal ]. Endodyocyte; schizozoite; zoite; the motile infective stage of sporozoan protozoa that results from schizogony or a similar type of asexual reproduction; *e.g.,* endodyogeny or endopolygeny. M.'s form at the surface of schizonts, blastophores, or invaginations into schizonts, and are responsible for the vast reproductive powers of sporozoan parasites; this is seen in human malaria, where the cyclic production of m.'s produces the typical fever and chill syndrome.

**me′rozy′gote** [ mero- + *zygotos,* yoked ]. In microbial genetics, an organism that, in addition to its own original genome (endogenote), contains a fragment (exogenote) of a genome from another organism; the relatively small size of the exogenote permits a diploid condition for only a limited region of the endogenote.

**merphalan** (mer′fă-lan). Sarcolysine; the racemic mixture of melphalan and medphalan; an antineoplastic agent.

**Merrifield knife.** See under knife.

**Merritt,** Katharine K., U. S. pediatrician, *1886. See Kasabach-M. *syndrome.*

**mersalyl** (mer′să-lil). SALYRGAN; sodium salt of salicyl-(3-hydroxymercuric-2-methoxypropyl) -amide-*o*-acetic acid; a mercurial diuretic.

**m. acid** (BP), a mixture of *o*-carboxymethylsalicyl-(3-hydroxymercuric-2-methoxypropyl)-amide and its anhydrides. Same use as m.

**m. sodium and theophylline,** MERSALYN; SALYRGAN-THEOPHYLLINE; sodium *o*-[ 3-hydroxymercuri-2-methoxypropyl)carbamoyl ]phenoxyacetate and theophylline; similar to m., but more effective.

**Méry** (ma-re′), Jean, Paris anatomist, 1645–1722. See M.'s *glands.*

**Merzbacher** (mairts′bakh-er), Ludwig, German physician in Argentina, *1875. See M.-Pelizaeus *disease.*

**mes-.** See meso-.

**mes′acon′ic acid.** Methylfumaric acid; $CH_3C(COOH)=CHCOOH$.

**mesad** (mes′ad, me′zad) [ G. *mesos*, middle, + L. *ad*, to ]. Passing or extending toward the median plane of the body or of a part.

**mesal** mes′al, me′zal) [ G. *mesos*, middle ]. Rarely used term referring to the median plane of the body or a part.

**mesameboid** (mes-ă-me′boyd) [ mes- + G. *amoibē*, change (ameba), + *eidos*, resemblance ]. Minot′s term for a primitive, "wandering" cell derived from mesoderm, probably a hemocytoblast.

**mesangial** (mes-an′jī-al). Referring to the mesangium.

**mesangium** (mes-an′jī-um) [ mes- + G. *angeion*, vessel ]. A central part of the renal glomerulus between capillaries; mesangial cells are phagocytic and for the most part separated from capillary lumina by endothelial cells.

**mesaortitis** (mes-a-or-ti′tis) [ mes- + aortitis, *q.v.* ]. Inflammation of the middle or muscular coat of the aorta.

**mesareic, mesaraic** (mes′ă-ra′ik) [ G. *mesaraion*, mesentery, fr. *mesos*, middle, + *araia*, flank, belly ]. Mesenteric.

**mesarteritis** (mes-ar-ter-i′tis) [ mes- + arteritis, *q.v.* ]. Inflammation of the middle (muscular) coat of an artery.

**mesaticephalic** (mē-sat′ī-sē-fal′ik) [ G. *mesatos*, midmost, + *kephalē*, head ]. Mesocephalic.

**mesatipellic, mesatipelvic** (mē-sat′ī-pel′ik, -pel′vik) [ G. *mesatos*, midmost, + *pellis*, a bowl (pelvis) ]. Denoting an individual with a pelvic index between 90° and 95°. The superior strait has a round appearance, with the transverse diameter longer than the anteroposterior by 1 cm. or less.

**mesaxon** (mez-ak′son, mes-). The plasma membrane of the neurolemma which is folded in to surround a nerve axon. In electron micrographs the double layer is similar to a mesentery in appearance.

**mescal buttons** (mes′kal). Peyote; see *Lophophora williamsii;* also mescaline.

**mescaline** (mes′kă-lēn). 3,4,5-Trimethoxyphenethylamine; the most active alkaloid present in the buttons of a small cactus, *Lophophora williamsii (q. v.)*. M. produces psychotomimetic effects similar to those produced by LSD: alteration in mood, changes in perception, reveries, visual hallucinations, delusions, depersonalization, mydriasis, hippus, and increases in body temperature and blood pressure. Psychic dependence, tolerance, and cross tolerance to LSD and psilocybin develop.

**mescalism** (mes′kă-lizm). Addiction to mescaline, the main symptom of which is the production of visions of great beauty.

**mesectic** (mē-sek′tik) [ mes- + G. *echō*, to have. ECT- ]. An obsolete term denoting a specimen of blood that has a normal percentage saturation of oxygen at any given pressure.

**mesectoderm** (mes-ek′to-derm) [ mes- + ectoderm, *q.v.* ]. 1. The cells in the area around the dorsal lip of the blastopore where separation of mesoderm and ectoderm is being accomplished. 2. Ectomesenchyme; that part of the mesenchyme derived from ectoderm, especially from the neural crest in the cephalic region in very young embryos.

**mesencephalic** (mes-en′sē-fal′ik, mez-). Relating to the mesencephalon.

**mesencephalitis** (mes′en-sef′ă-li′tis). Inflammation of the midbrain (mesencephalon); sometimes noted in *Listeria* infection of the nervous system.

**mesencephalon** (mes′en-sef′ă-lon) [ mes- + G. *enkephalos*, brain ] [ NA ]. The midbrain; that part of the brainstem that develops from the middle of the three primary cerebral vesicles of the embryo (the caudal of these being the rhombencephalon or hindbrain, the rostral the prosencephalon or forebrain). In the adult, the mesencephalon is characterized gross-anatomically by the unique conformation of its roofplate, the tectum mesencephali or lamina quadrigemina, composed of the bilaterally paired superior and inferior colliculus, and by the massive and likewise paired prominence of the crus cerebri or cerebral peduncle at its ventral surface. On transverse section, the patent central canal of the mesencephalon (the aqueductus cerebri or Sylvian aqueduct) is seen to be surrounded by a prominent ring of gray matter poor in myelinated fibers;

this central (or circumaqueductal) gray substance is ventrally and laterally adjoined by the myelin-rich midbrain tegmentum, dorsally by the quadrigeminal plate. Prominent cell groups of the mesencephalon include the motor nuclei of the trochlear and oculomotor nerves, the red nucleus, and the substantia nigra.

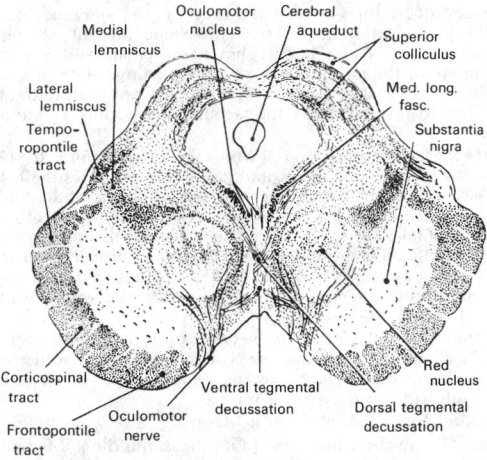

**Mesencephalon**

Cross section, showing some of the more important tracts and gray masses. (From Ranson, S. W., and Clark, S. L.: *Anatomy of the Nervous System*, W. B. Saunders Company, Philadelphia, 1959.)

**mesencephalotomy** (mes′en-sef′ă-lot′o-mī) [ mesencephalon + G. *tomē*, incision ]. 1. The sectioning of any structure in the midbrain, especially of the spinothalamic tracts for the relief of unbearable pain. 2. Mesencephalic spinothalamic *tractotomy*.

**mesenchyma** (mē-seng′kī-mah). Mesenchyme.

**mesenchymal** (mē-seng′kī-mal, mes′eng-ki′mal). Relating to the mesenchyme.

**mesenchyme** (mes′en-kīm) [ mes- + G. *enkyma*, infusion ] [ NA ]. 1. An aggregation of mesenchymal cells. 2. A primordial embryonic tissue consisting of mesenchymal cells, usually stellate in form, supported in a loose, fluid, homogeneous ground substance (see mesenchymal *cell* and interlaminar *jelly*).

    **interzonal m.,** an area of avascular m. between adjacent skeletal elements in the embryo; it denotes the region of future joints.

    **synovial m.,** vascular m. surrounding the interzonal m.; it develops into the synovial membrane of a joint.

**mesenchymoma** (mes-en-ki-mo′mah). A neoplasm in which there is a mixture of mesenchymal derivatives, other than fibrous tissue. A **benign m.** may contain foci of vascular, muscular, adipose, osteoid, osseous, and cartilaginous tissue; such neoplasms are sometimes classed under a compounded name, *e.g.*, angioleiomyolipoma, and the like, but the broader term may be preferred. A similar mixture of two or more types of mesenchymal cells that are malignant (other than fibrous tissue cells) may also occur, and such neoplasms should be termed **malignant m.**

**mesenter′ic.** Relating to the mesentery.

**mesenteriolum** (mes-en-ter-i′o-lum) [ Mod. L. dim. of *mesenterium*, mesentery ]. A small mesentery, as one of an intestinal diverticulum.

    **m. proces′sus vermifor′mis,** mesoappendix.

**mesenteriopexy** (mes′en-těr′ī-o-pek′sī) [ mesentery + G. *pēxis*, fixation ]. Mesopexy; attachment of a torn or incised mesentery.

**mesenteriorrhaphy** (mes-en-těr′ī-or′ă-fī) [ mesentery + G. *rhaphē*, suture ]. Mesorrhaphy; suture of the mesentery.

**mesenteriplication** (mes′en-těr′ī-pli-ka′shun) [ mesentery + L. *plico*, pp. *-atus*, to fold ]. Reducing the redundancy of a mesentery by making one or more tucks in it.

**mesenteritis** (mes'en-ter-i'tis). Inflammation of the mesentery.

**mesenterium** (mes'en-těr'ĭ-um) [ Mod. L. ] [ NA ]. Mesentery.

    **m. dorsale commune,** the mesentery proper as distinguished from the mesocolon, mesorectum, and mesoappendix.

**mesenteron** (mes-en'ter-on) [ mes- + G. *enteron*, intestine ]. 1. Old term for the embryonic midgut. 2. The midportion of the insect alimentary canal and site of digestion; the m. may possess anterior finger-like projections, the gastric ceca, and a tubular anterior midgut, followed posteriorly by the saccular ventriculus, or stomach.

**mesentery** (mes'en-těr-ĭ) [ Mod. L. *mesenterium,* fr. G. *mesenterion,* fr. G. *mesos,* middle, + *enteron,* intestine ]. 1. A double layer of peritoneum attached to the abdominal wall and enclosing in its fold a portion or all of one of the abdominal viscera, conveying to it its vessels and nerves. 2. Specifically, the fan-shaped fold of peritoneum encircling the greater part of the small intestines (jejunum and ileum) and attaching it to the posterior abdominal wall.

**mesh'work.** See network.

    **trabecular m.,** trabecular network; trabecular zone; a m. of collagen fibers at the angle of the anterior chamber of the eye, within which are the endothelium-lined spatia anguli iridocornealis (of Fontana).

**mesiad** (me'zĭ-ad, mes'ĭ-ad). Mesad.

**mesial** (me'zĭ-al, mes'ĭ-al) [ G. *mesos,* middle ]. Median; middle; mesal; toward the middle line or apex of the dental arch.

**mesio-** (me'zĭ-o-, me'sĭ-o-) [ G. *mesos,* middle ]. Combining form (especially in dentistry) meaning mesial, *q. v.*

**mesiobuccal** (me'zĭ-o-buk'al). Relating to the mesial and buccal surfaces of a tooth; denoting especially the angle formed by the junction of these two surfaces.

**mesiobucco-occlusal** (me'zĭ-o-buk'o-ok-lu'sal). A term designating the angle formed by the junction of the mesial, buccal, and occlusal surfaces of a bicuspid or molar tooth.

**me'siobuc'copul'pal.** Relating to the angle denoting the junction of mesial, buccal and pulpal surfaces in a tooth cavity preparation.

**me'siocer'vical.** 1. Relating to the line angle of a cavity preparation at the junction of the mesial and cervical walls. 2. Pertaining to the area of a tooth at the junction of the mesial surface and the cervical region.

**mesioclusion** (me'zĭ-ok-lu'zhun). Mesio-occlusion.

**mesiodens** (me'zĭ-o-denz) [ mesio- + L. *dens,* tooth ]. A supernumerary tooth located in the midline of the anterior maxillae, between the maxillary central incisor teeth.

**me'siodis'tal.** Denoting the plane or diameter of a tooth cutting its mesial and distal surfaces.

**mesiodistocclusal** (me'zĭ-o-dist'o-klu'sal, -zal). Term used in dentistry to denote the three-surface cavity or cavity preparation or restoration (class 2, Black classification) in the premolars (bicuspids) and molars; abbreviated MOD.

**mesiogingival** (me'zĭ-o-jin'jĭ-val). Relating to the angle formed by the junction of the mesial surface with the gingival line of a tooth.

**mesioincisal** (me'zĭ-o-in-si'sal, -zal). Relating to the mesial and incisal surfaces of a tooth; denoting the angle formed by their junction.

**me'siola'bial.** Relating to the mesial and labial surfaces of a tooth; denoting especially the angle formed by their junction.

**mesiolingual** (me'zĭ-o-ling'gwal). Relating to the mesial and lingual surfaces of a tooth; denoting especially the angle formed by their junction.

**mesiolinguo-occlusal** (me'zĭ-o-ling'gwo-o-klu'sal, -zal). Denoting the angle formed by the junction of the mesial, lingual, and occlusal surfaces of a bicuspid or molar tooth.

**mesiolinguopulpal** (me'zĭ-o-ling'gwo-pul-pal). Relating to the angle denoting the junction of the mesial, lingual and pulpal surfaces in a tooth cavity preparation.

**mesion** (me'zĭ-on, mes'ĭ-on). Meson.

**mesio-occlusal** (me'zĭ-o-o-klu'sal, -zal). Denoting the angle formed by the junction of the mesial and occlusal surfaces of a bicuspid or molar tooth.

**mesio-occlusion** (me'zĭ-o-o-klu'zhun). 1. A forward position of a tooth in relation to its opponent in the other jaw. 2. A forward position of the teeth in the lower jaw in relation to those of the upper jaw when the jaws are closed and at rest.

**me'sioplace'ment.** Mesial displacement; malposition of a tooth from its usual position toward the direction of the midline.

**me'siopul'pal.** Pertaining to the inner wall or floor of a cavity preparation on the mesial side of a tooth.

**me'siover'sion.** Malposition of a tooth axially inclined in a direction toward the midline of the dental arch.

**Mesmer,** F. A., Austrian physician, 1733–1815. Gave his name to mesmerism and mesmerize.

**mes'merism** [ F. *Mesmer* ]. Animal magnetism; a system of therapeutics from which were developed hypnotism and therapeutic suggestion.

**mes'merize.** An obsolete term for hypnotize.

**meso-, mes-** (mes'o-, mez'o-, me'zo-, me'so-) [ G. *mesos,* middle ]. Prefix meaning middle, or mean, or used to give an indication of intermediacy. A meson is a particle of intermediate mass between that of a proton and an electron; a meso-compound is optically inactive (intermediate, between the D and L extremes); a mesothorax is the middle segment of the thorax, and so on.

**mesoappendix** (mes'o-ă-pen'diks) [ NA ]. Mesentery of the appendix; mesenteriolum processus vermiformis; the short mesentery of the appendix lying behind the terminal ileum.

**mesoarium** (mes-o-a'rĭ-um). Mesovarium.

**mes'obi'lane.** Mesobilirubinogen; a reduced mesobilirubin with no double bonds between the pyrrole rings and, consequently, colorless. See also bilirubinoids.

**mes'obi'lene.** See bilirubinoids.

**mesobilene-b.** See bilirubinoids.

**mesobilirubin** (mes'o-bil'ĭ-ru'bin). A compound differing from bilirubin only in that the vinyl groups of bilirubin are reduced to ethyl groups. See also bilirubinoids.

**mesobilirubinogen** (mes'o-bil'ĭ-ru-bin'o-jen). Mesobilane.

**mesobiliviolin** (mes'o-bil'ĭ-vi-o'lin). See bilirubinoids.

**mes'oblast** [ meso- + G. *blastos,* germ ]. Mesoderm.

**mes'oblaste'ma** [ meso- + G. *blastēma,* a sprout ]. All the cells collectively which constitute the early undifferentiated mesoderm.

**mes'oblaste'mic.** Relating to or derived from the mesoblastema.

**mes'oblas'tic.** Relating to or derived from the mesoderm.

**mesobronchitis** (mes'o-brong-ki'tis). Inflammation of the middle, or muscular, coat of the bronchi.

**mesocardia** (mes'o-kar'dĭ-ah) [ meso- + G. *kardia,* heart ]. 1. Atypical position of the heart in a central position in the chest, as in early embryonic life. 2. Plural of mesocardium.

**mesocardium,** pl. **mesocar'dia** (mes'o-kar'dĭ-um) [ meso- + G. *kardia,* heart ]. The double layer of splanchnic mesoderm supporting the embryonic heart in the pericardial cavity.

    **dorsal m.,** the part of the m. that is dorsal to the embryonic heart.

    **ventral m.,** the part of the m. that lies ventral to the embryonic cardiac tube. It is transitory in all vertebrates, and in the higher mammals it breaks through as soon as its component layers make contact.

**mes'ocar'pal.** Mediocarpal.

**mesocecal** (mes'o-se'kal). Relating to the mesocecum.

**mesocecum** (mes'o-se'kum) [ meso- + cecum, *q. v.* ]. The mesentery of the cecum, occasionally present.

**mesocephalic** (mes'o-sĕ-fal'ik) [ meso- + G. *kephalē,* head ]. Mesocephalous; mesaticephalic; normocephalic; having a head of medium length; denoting a skull with a cephalic index between 75 and 80 and with a capacity of 1350 to 1450 cc., or an individual with such a skull.

**mes'oceph'alous.** Mesocephalic.

**mes'ocol'ic.** Relating to the mesocolon.

**mesocolon** (mes'o-ko'lon) [ meso- + *kolon,* colon ] [ NA ]. The fold of peritoneum attaching the colon to the posterior abdominal wall; it is variously called ascending (m.

ascendens), transverse (m. transversum), descending (m. descendens), and pelvic or sigmoid (m. sigmoideum), corresponding to the respective divisions of the colon; the ascending and descending portions are usually more or less deficient or absent.

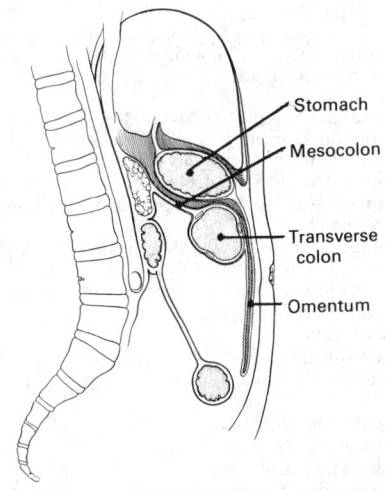

**Mesocolon**

**mesocolopexy** (mes'o-ko'lo-pek'sĭ) [ meso- + G. *kolon*, colon, + *pēxis*, fixation ]. Mesocoloplication; an operation for shortening the mesocolon by making a fold in it and suturing; for the correction of undue mobility and ptosis of the colon.

**mesocoloplication** (mes'o-ko'lo-pli-ka'shun) [ meso- + G. *kolon*, colon, + L. *plico*, pp. *-atus*, to fold ]. Mesocolopexy.

**mes'ocord.** A fold of amnion that sometimes binds a segment of the umbilical cord to the placenta.

**mesocuneiform** (mes-o-ku'ne-ĭ-form). *Os* cuneiforme intermedium.

**mes'oderm** [ meso- + G. *derma*, skin ]. Mesoblast; the middle of the three primary germ layers of the embryo; it gives origin to all connective tissues, all body musculature, blood, cardiovascular and lymphatic systems, most of the urogenital system, and the lining of the pericardial, pleural, and peritoneal cavities.

    **branchial m.,** m. surrounding the primitive stomodeum and pharynx; it becomes the pharyngeal arches.

    **extraembryonic m.,** primary m.; cells or tissues which, though derived from the zygote, are not part of the embryo proper but form the fetal membranes.

    **gastral m.,** m. in lower vertebrates formed by constriction from the roof of the archenteron or yolk sac.

    **intermediate m.,** a continuous band of m. between the segmented paraxial m. medially and the lateral plate m. laterally; from it develops the nephrogenic cord.

    **intraembryonic m.,** secondary m.; m. derived from the primitive streak and lying between the ectoderm and entoderm.

    **lateral m.,** lateral plate m.

    **lateral plate m.,** lateral m.; the peripheral thinned out portion of intraembryonic m. which is continuous with the extraembryonic m. beyond the margins of the embryonic disk; in it develops the intraembryonic celom.

    **paraxial m.,** a thickened mass lying at either side of the midline embryonic notochord; on segmentation, it forms the paired somites.

    **primary m.,** extraembryonic m.

    **prostomial m.,** m. that arises in lower vertebrates by continued proliferation at the lateral lips of the blastopore.

    **secondary m.,** intraembryonic m.

    **somatic m.,** after foundation of the intraembryonic celom, the m. adjacent to the ectoderm in the early embryo.

    **splanchnic m.,** the layer of lateral plate m. adjacent to the entoderm.

    **visceral m.,** the splanchnic m. or the branchial m.

**mes'oder'mic.** Relating to the mesoderm.

**mes'odiastol'ic.** Middiastolic.

**mes'odont** [ meso- + G. *odous*, tooth ]. Having teeth of medium size; denoting a skull with a dental index between 42 and 43.9.

**mes'oduode'nal.** Relating to the mesoduodenum.

**mesoduodenum** (mes'o-du'o-de'num, -du-od'ĕ-nal). The mesentery of the duodenum.

**mesoenteriolum** (mes'o-en-ter-i'o-lum). Mesenteriolum.

**mesoepididymis** (mes-o-ep-ĭ-did'ĭ-mis) [ meso- + epididymis, *q.v.* ]. An occasional fold of the tunica vaginalis binding the epididymis to the testis.

**mes'ogas'ter.** Mesogastrium.

**mes'ogas'tric.** Relating to the mesogastrium.

**mesogastrium** (mes'o-gas'trĭ-um) [ meso- + G. *gastēr*, stomach ] [ NA ]. In the embryo, the mesentery in relation with the dilated portion of the enteric canal which is the future stomach.

**mes'ogen'ic** [ meso- + G. suffix *-gen*, producing ]. Denoting the virulence of a virus capable of inducing lethal infection in embryonic hosts, after a short incubation period, and an inapparent infection in immature and adult hosts; used in characterizing Newcastle disease virus, particularly strains used in parenteral vaccination of chickens.

**mes'ogenita'le.** The embryonic mesentery by which the genital ridge is connected to the mesonephros.

**mesoglia** (mĕ-sog'lĭ-ah) [ meso- + G. *glia*, glue ]. Mesoglial cells; neuroglial cells of mesodermal origin; see also microglia.

**mes'oglio'ma.** Undesirable term for oligodendroglioma.

**mesogluteal** (mes'o-glu'te-al). Relating to the musculus gluteus medius.

**mesoglute'us.** *Musculus* gluteus medius.

**mesognathic** (mes'o-nath'ik, -og-nath'ik). 1. Relating to the mesognathion. 2. Mesognathous.

**mesognathion** (mes'o-na'thĭon, -og-na'thĭ-on, -nath'ĭ-on) [ meso- + G. *gnathos*, jaw ]. The lateral segment of the premaxillary or incisive bone external to the endognathion.

**mesog'nathous.** Having a face with slightly projecting jaw, one with a gnathic index from 98 to 103.

**mesoileum** (mes-o-il'e-um). The mesentery of the ileum.

**mesojejunum** (mes'o-jĕ-ju'num). The mesentery of the jejunum.

**mesolepidoma** (mes'o-lep'ĭ-do'mah) [ meso- + G. *lepis*, rind (LEP-), + suffix *-oma*, tumor ]. A neoplasm derived from the persistent embryonic mesothelium.

    **atypical m.,** carcinoma of one of the urogenital organs or of the serous membranes.

    **typical m.,** adenoma of the urogenital organs or of the serous membranes.

**mesol'obus** [ meso- + L. *lobus*, lobe ]. *Corpus* callosum.

**mesolymphocyte** (mez-o-lim'fo-sit) [ meso- + lymphocyte ]. A mononuclear leukocyte of medium size, probably a lymphocyte, with deeply staining nucleus of large size, but relatively smaller than that in most of the lymphocytes.

**mesomere** (mes'o-mēr) [ meso- + G. *meros*, part ]. 1. A blastomere of a size intermediate between a macromere and a micromere. 2. Archaic term for intermediate mesoderm.

**mesomeric** (mes'o-mĕr'ik). Pertaining to mesomerism.

**mesom'erism.** The displacement of electrons within a molecule in such a way as to create fractional charges on different parts of the molecule.

**mesometritis** (mes'o-me-tri'tis) [ meso- + G. *mētra*, uterus, + suffix *-itis*, inflammation ]. Myometritis.

**mesometrium** (mes'o-me'trĭ-um) [ meso- + G. *mētra*, uterus ] [ NA ]. The broad ligament of the uterus, below the mesosalpinx.

**mes'omorph** [ meso- + G. *morphē*, form ]. Mediotype; a constitutional body type or build (biotype or somatotype) in which tissues that originate from the mesoderm prevail. From the morphological standpoint, there is a balance between trunk and limbs. See also hypermorph, hypomorph, ectomorph, endomorph.

**mes′omorph′ic.** Relating to mesomorphs.

**mes′on** [ G. neuter of *mesos*, middle ]. An elementary particle having a rest mass intermediate in value between the mass of an electron and that of a proton.

**mes′oneph′ric.** Relating to the mesonephros.

**mesonephroma** (mes′o-ne-fro′mah). Mesometanephric carcinoma; Wolffian duct carcinoma; a relatively rare neoplasm of the ovary, thought to originate in mesonephric structures that become misplaced in ovarian tissue during embryonic development; characterized by a tubular pattern, with focal proliferation of epithelial cells; so-called glomeruloid structures are typical, *i.e.*, small convolutions or tufts of tiny tubate formations with capillaries extending into the spaces. M.'s are usually gray-white, sometimes partly encapsulated, with foci of hemorrhage or necrosis, thereby resembling a carcinoma or malignant teratoma of the ovary.

**mesonephros,** pl. **mesonephroi** (mes′o-nef′ros, nef′roy) [ meso- + G. *nephros*, kidney ] [ NA ]. Wolffian body; one of three excretory organs appearing in the evolution of vertebrates. In those forms that have developed a metanephros the m. lies cephalic to it, between it and the regressing pronephros. In young mammalian embryos the m. is well developed and is functional for a time before the establishing of the metanephros which is their definitive kidney. In older embryos the m. undergoes regression as an excretory organ but its duct system is retained in the male as the epididymis and ductus deferens.

**mesoneuritis** (mes′o-nu-ri′tis). Inflammation of a nerve or of its connective tissue without involvement of its sheath.

   **nodular m.,** inflammation of the connective tissue beneath the nerve sheath, with the formation of circumscribed fibrous thickenings.

**meso-ontomorph** (mes-o-on′to-morf) [ meso- + G. *ōn*, being, + *morphē*, form ]. A broad, stocky individual.

**mesopexy** (mes′o-pek-si). Mesenteriopexy.

**mesophil, mesophile** (mes′o-fil, -fil) [ meso- + G. *philos*, fond ]. A microorganism with an optimum temperature between 25°C. and 40°C., but growing within the limits of 10°C. and 45°C.

**mes′ophil′ic.** Pertaining to a mesophil.

**mesophlebitis** (mes′o-flē-bi′tis) [ meso- + phlebitis, *q. v.* ]. Inflammation of the middle coat of a vein.

**mesophragma** (mes-o-frag′mah) [ meso- + G. *phragma*, a fence ]. M *line*.

**mesophryon** (mes-of′ri-on) [ meso- + Gr. *ophrys*, eyebrow ]. Glabella.

**meso′pic** [ meso- + G. *opsis*, vision ]. Pertaining to illumination between the photopic and scotopic ranges.

**mes′opor′phyrin.** Porphyrin compounds resembling the protoporphyrins except that the vinyl side chains of the latter are reduced to ethyl side chains (*e.g.*, mesobilane).

**mesoprosopic** (mes′o-pro-sop′ik, -so′pik) [ meso- + G. *prosōpon*, face ]. Having a face of moderate width, *i.e.*, with a facial index of about 90.

**mesopsyche** (mes-o-si′ke) [ meso- + G. *psychē*, soul ]. Mesencephalon.

**mes′opul′monum** [ meso- + L. *pulmo*, lung ]. The mesentery of the embryonic lung.

**mesorchial** (mes-or′ki-al). Relating to the mesorchium.

**mesorchium** (mes-or′ki-um) [ meso- + G. *orchis*, testis ]. 1 [ NA ]. A fold of tunica vaginalis testis in the fetus supporting the mesonephros and the developing testis. 2. A fold of peritoneum in the adult between the testis and epididymis.

**mes′orec′tum.** The peritoneal investment of the rectum, covering the upper part only.

**mesorid′azine besylate** (NF). SERENTIL; 10-[ 2-(1-methyl-2-piperidyl)ethyl ]-2-(methylsulfinyl)phenothiazone; biotransformation product of thioridazine; an antipsychotic agent.

**mesoropter** (mes′o-rop′ter) [ meso- + G. *horos*, boundary, + *optērios*, concerning sight ]. The normal position of the eyes at rest.

**mesorrhachischisis** (mes′o-ră-kis′ki-sis). Merorrhachischisis.

**mesorrhaphy** (mes-or′ă-fi). Mesenteriorrhaphy.

**mesorrhine** (mes′o-rin) [ meso- + G. *rhis* (*rhin*-), nose ]. Having a nose of moderate width. Denoting a skull with a nasal index from 47 to 51 (Frankfort agreement) or 48 to 53 (Broca).

**mes′osal′pinx** [ meso- + G. *salpinx*, trumpet. SALP- ] [ NA ]. The part of the broad ligament investing the uterine (Fallopian) tube.

**mesoscope** (mes′o-skōp) [ meso- + G. *skopeō*, to view ]. An instrument for viewing objects that are larger than microscopic but cannot be seen distinctly with the naked eye.

**mesoseme** (mes′o-sēm) [ meso- + G. *sēma*, sign ]. Denoting an orbital aperture with an index between 84 and 89; characteristic of the Caucasian race.

**mes′osig′moid.** The mesocolon of the sigmoid colon.

**mesosigmoiditis** (mes-o-sig-moy-di′tis). Inflammation of the mesosigmoid.

**mesosigmoidopexy** (mes-o-sig-moy′do-pek-si). Surgical fixation of the mesosigmoid.

**mes′oso′matous.** Denoting a person of medium height.

**mesosomia** (mes′o-so′mi-ah) [ meso- + G. *sōma*, body ]. Medium height.

**mesostenium** (mes′o-ste′ni-um). Mesentery (2).

**mes′oster′num** [ meso- + G. *sternon*, chest ]. *Corpus sterni.*

**mes′osyph′ilis.** Secondary *syphilis.*

**mes′osystol′ic.** Midsystolic.

**mes′otar′sal.** Mediotarsal.

**mesotendineum** (mes′o-ten-din′e-um) [ NA ]. Mesotendon; the synovial layers that pass from a tendon to the wall of a tendon sheath in certain places where tendons lie within osteofibrous canals.

**mes′oten′don.** Mesotendineum.

**mes′othe′lial.** Relating to the mesothelium.

**mesothelioma** (mes′o-the′li-o′mah) [ mesothelium + G. suffix -*oma*, tumor ]. A rare neoplasm derived from the lining cells of the pleura and peritoneum; m.'s have been reported in asbestosis. They grow as thick sheets covering the viscera, and are composed of spindle cells or fibrous tissue which may enclose glandlike spaces lined by cuboidal cells. The prognosis is bad. Similar tumors have been reported arising in the female genital tract.

   **benign m. of genital tract,** adenomatoid *tumor.*

**mesothelium,** pl. **mesothe′lia** (mes′o-the′li-um) [ meso- + epithelium ] [ NA ]. A single layer of flattened cells forming an epithelium that lines serous cavities, *e.g.*, peritoneum, pleura, pericardium.

**mes′otho′rium.** The first two disintegration products of thorium; mesothorium 1 is $^{228}$Ra, a beta emitter with a half-life of 6.7 years, decaying into mesothorium 2, which is $^{228}$Ac, a beta emitter with a half-life of 6.13 hours, which disintegrates to radiothorium ($^{228}$Th).

**mes′oto′cin.** [ 8-Isoleucine ]oxytocin; a neurohypophysial hormone formed by lungfish and some amphibia; its physiological effects in these animals are unknown.

**mes′otron.** Obsolete synonym for meson (2).

**mes′otrop′ic** [ meso- + G. *tropē*, a turning ]. Turned toward the median plane.

**mesouranic** (mes′o-u-ran′ik) [ meso- + G. *ouranos*, palate ]. Having a palatal index between 110 and 115.

**mesovarium,** pl. **mesova′ria** (mes′o-va′ri-um) [ meso- + L. *ovarium*, ovary ]. [ NA ]. A short peritoneal fold connecting the anterior border of the ovary with the posterior layer of the broad ligament of the uterus.

**Mesozoa** (mes′o-zo′ah) [ meso- + G. *zōon*, animal ]. A large group of the Metazoa with a single external layer of primitive digestive cells, and no internal digestive cavity, thus resembling certain kinds of Protozoa. They are regarded by some observers as intermediate between unicellular and multicellular animals, or possibly a degenerate group.

**mes′senger.** 1. That which carries a message. 2. Having message-carrying properties.

   **first m.,** a hormone that has a transaction with the second m. (cyclic AMP) at or near the cell membrane.

   **second m.,** adenosine 3′:5′-cyclic phosphate.

**messenger RNA.** See under ribonucleic acid.

**mestranol** (mes'tră-nŏl) (USP, BP). 3-Methoxy-19-nor-17α-pregna-1,3,5(10)-trien-20-yn-17-ol; the 3 methyl ether of ethynyl estradiol (for structure of estradiol and parent pregnane, see steroids); an estrogen used in many oral contraceptive preparations.

  **m. plus chlormadinone acetate with m.**, C-QUENS; a sequential orally effective preparation consisting of the estrogen, mestranol, given from the 5th through the 19th days of the menstrual cycle, and the mixture of the progestogen, chlormadinone acetate, given from the 20th to the 24th days.

**mestan'olone.** ANDROSTALONE; 17β-hydroxy-17-methyl-5α-androstan-3-one; androgenic steroid with anabolic properties.

**mesul'phen.** MITIGAL; 2-7-dimethylthianthrene; topical scabicide with antipruritic properties.

**mes'uran'ic.** Mesouranic.

**mes'ylate.** USAN-approved contraction for methanesulfate, $CH_3SO_3^-$.

**Met.** Symbol for methionine or its radicals in peptides.

**meta-** (met'ah-) [ G. after, between, over ]. 1. In medicine and biology, a prefix used to denote the concept of after, subsequent to, behind, or hindmost. 2. A prefix denoting joint action, or sharing. 3. In chemistry a prefix denoting that a compound is formed by two substitutions in the benzene ring arranged unsymmetrically, i.e., linked to the first and third, second and fourth, third and fifth, etc., carbon atoms of the ring. For chemical terms beginning with *meta-*, or its abbreviation, *m-*, and not found here, see under the specific name.

**metabasis** (mĕ-tab'ă-sis) [ G. a passing over, change, fr. *metabainō*, to pass over. BAS- ]. A change of any kind in symptoms or course of a disease.

**met'abi'osis** [ meta- + G. *biōsis*, way of life ]. Dependence of one organism on another for its existence.

**metabol'ic.** Relating to metabolism.

**met'abolim'eter.** An apparatus for measuring the rate of basal metabolism; a modified calorimeter.

**metab'olin.** Metabolite.

**metabolism** (mĕ-tab'o-lizm) [ G. *metabolē*, change. BAL- ]. Tissue change; the sum of the chemical changes whereby the function of nutrition is effected. It consists of anabolism, or those energy-consuming processes that convert small molecules into large (*e.g.*, amino acids to proteins), and catabolism, or those energy-producing processes that convert large molecules into small (*e.g.*, glycogen to pyruvic acid).

  **basal m.**, basal metabolic rate (BMR); heat production of an individual at the lowest level of cell chemistry in the waking state; or the minimal amount of cell activity associated with the continuous organic functions of respiration, circulation, and secretion. It is determined upon the fasting subject (first thing in the morning without breakfast) at complete bodily and mental rest and a room temperature of 20°C.

  **carbohy'drate m.**, the changes that carbohydrates undergo in the tissues: oxidation, breakdown, and synthesis.

  **elec'trolyte m.**, the changes which the various essential minerals, sodium, potassium, calcium, magnesium, etc., undergo in the fluids and tissues of the body.

  **fat m.**, the chemical changes, oxidation, decomposition, and synthesis, that fats undergo in the tissues.

  **protein m.**, the chemical changes, decompositions, and synthesis, that protein undergoes in the tissues.

  **respiratory m.**, the exchange of respiratory gases in the lungs and the oxidation of foodstuffs in the tissues with the production of carbon dioxide and water.

  **water of m.**, see under water.

**metabolite** (mĕ-tab'o-līt). Any product (foodstuff, intermediate, waste product) of metabolism, especially of catabolism.

**metab'oli'zable.** Capable of taking part in metabolic reactions within the organism.

**met'abuteth'amine hydrochloride.** UNACAINE; 2-(isobutylamino)ethanol *m*-aminobenzoate monohydrochloride; a local anesthetic used in dentistry.

**metabutox'ycaine hydrochloride.** PRIMACAINE hydrochloride; 2-butoxy-3-aminobenzoic acid β-diethylamino-

ethyl ester hydrochloride; local anesthetic for dental extraction.

**met'acar'pal.** Relating to the metacarpus.

**metacarpectomy** (met'ah-kar-pek'to-mī) [ metacarpus + G. *ektomē*, excision ]. Excision of one or all of the metacarpals.

**metacarpophalangeal** (met'a-kar'po-fă-lan'je-al). Relating to the metacarpus and the phalanges; denoting the articulations.

**metacarpus**, pl. **metacar'pi** (met'ah-kar'pus) [ meta- + G. *karpos*, wrist ] [ NA ]. The five bones of the hand between the carpus and the phalanges.

**metacasein** (met-ah-ka'se-in). One of the nondescript intermediates in the digestion of casein.

**metacentric** (met'ah-sen'trik). See m. chromosome.

**metacercaria** (met'ah-ser-kăr'ĭ-ah) [ meta- + G. *kerkos*, tail ]. The encysted stage in the life history of a fluke, prior to the final stage of transfer to the definitive host. M. may attach themselves to blades of grass or other vegetation and are then ingested by herbivores, in the case of *Fasciola* and similar forms, or they enter muscles of fish (fish "grubs") in the case of strigeids, or of crayfish in the case of *Paragonimus*, etc.

**metachloral** (met-ah-klo'ral). See *m*-chloral.

**metachloridine** (met'ah-klōr'ĭ-dēn, -din). *N*-(5-Chloro-2-pyrimidyl)metanilamide; an antimalarial agent.

**metachromasia** (met'ah-kro-ma'zĭ-ah) [ meta- + G. *chrōma*, color ]. Metachromatism (2); the condition in which a cell or tissue component takes on a color different from the dye solution with which it is stained.

**metachromatic** (met'ah-kro-mat'ik). Metachromophil; said of cells or dyes which exhibit metachromasia.

**metachromatism** (met'ah-kro'mă-tizm) [ meta- + G. *chrōma*, color ]. 1. Any color change, whether natural or produced by staining fluids. 2. Metachromasia.

**metachromophil, metachromophile** (met-ah-kro'mo-fil, -fīl) [ meta- + G. *chrōma*, color, + *philos*, fond ]. Metachromatic.

**metachrosis** (met'ah-kro'sis) [ meta- + G. *chrōsis*, a coloring ]. A change of color, such as occurs in certain animals, *e.g.*, the chameleon, by expansion and contraction of chromatophores.

**metacone** (met'ah-kōn) [ meta- + G. *kōnos*, cone ]. The distobuccal cusp of an upper molar tooth.

**metaconid** (met-ah-kon'id, -ko'nid) [ meta- + -conid, *q.v.* ]. The mesolingual cusp of a lower molar tooth.

**metaconule** (met-ah-kon'ūl) [ meta- + G. *kōnos*, a cone ]. The distal intermediate cusp of an upper molar tooth.

**met'acre'sol.** *m*-Cresol; one of the three isomeric cresols; a local antiseptic with a higher germicidal power than phenol and less toxic to animal tissues; used in disinfectants and fumigants.

  **m. ac'etate**, *m*-cresyl acetate; *m*-tolyl acetate; a cresol derivative used as a topical antiseptic and fungicide.

**metacryptozoite** (met'ah-krip'to-zo'īt) [ meta- + G. *kryptos*, hidden, + *zōon*, animal ]. The exoerythrocytic stage that develops from merozoites formed by the first, or cryptozoite, generation; the cryptozoite and metacryptozoite generations comprise the primary exoerythrocytic stages of malaria development (prepatent period) prior to infection of the blood.

**metacyesis** (met-ah-si-e'sis) [ meta- + G. *kyesis*, pregnancy ]. Extrauterine pregnancy.

**metadysentery** (met'ă-dis'en-tĕr-ī). An old term for bacillary dysentery, caused by *Bacillus ceylonensis* A. *B. ceylonensis* B. or *B. metadysentericus*.

**metagenesis** (met'ah-jen'ĕ-sis) [ meta- + G. *genesis*, production ]. Alternation of *generation*.

**met'aglob'ulin.** A partially hydrolyzed globulin (nondescript term).

**Metagonimus** (met-ah-gon'ĭ-mus) [ meta- + G. *gonimos*, productive ]. A genus of flukes in the superfamily Heterophyoidea. They encyst on fish and infect various fish-eating animals, including man.

  **M. yokoga'wai**, Yokogawa's fluke; formerly called *Loxotrema ovatum;* an intestinal fluke widely distributed in the Far East and Balkan states; the smallest fluke that infects man, 1 to 2.5 mm. long. It is passed from

*Semisulcospira* snails to cyprinoid fish, then to man and other fish-eating mammals and birds.

**met'agrip'pal.** Postgrippal; occurring as a sequel of grippe or influenza.

**metaicteric** (met-ah-ik'ter-ik) [ meta- + G. *ikterikos*, jaundiced ]. Occurring as a sequel of jaundice.

**metainfective** (met'ah-in-fek'tiv). Occurring subsequent to an infection; denoting specifically a febrile condition that is sometimes observed during convalescence from an infectious disease.

**metakinesia** (met'ah-kī-ne'zī-ah). Metakinesis.

**metakinesis** (met'ah-kī-ne'sis) [ meta- + G. *kinēsis*, movement ]. Moving apart; the separation of the two chromatids of each chromosome and their movement to opposite poles in the anaphase of mitosis.

**met'al** [ L. *metallum*, a mine, a mineral, fr. G. *metallon*, a mine, pit ]. One of the electropositive elements, either amphoteric or basic; usually characterized by properties such as luster, malleability, ductility, the ability to conduct electricity, and the tendency to lose electrons in chemical reaction rather than gaining electrons.

**alkali m.,** one of the members of the family Li, Na, K, Rb, Cs, all of which have highly ionized hydroxides, which are alkalies.

**alkali-earth m.,** see alkaline *earths.*

**Babbitt m.,** an alloy of antimony, copper, and tin; used occasionally in dentistry.

**base m.,** one that is readily oxidized, *e.g.,* iron, copper.

**basic m.,** base m.

**colloidal m.,** a colloidal solution of a m. obtained by passing electric sparks between terminals of the m. through distilled water.

**d'Arcet's m.,** an alloy of lead, bismuth, and tin; used in dentistry.

**earth m.,** one of the third group of the periodic system, aluminum, etc.

**fusible m.,** one with a low melting point.

**light m.,** one with a specific gravity of less than 4.

**noble m.,** one that cannot be oxidized by heat alone, nor readily dissolved by acid, *e.g.,* gold, platinum.

**rare-earth m.,** elements of the third group of the periodic system from atomic numbers 57 to 72.

**respiratory m.,** one present in certain respiratory pigments; iron, manganese, copper, vanadium.

**Rose's m., Rose m.,** an alloy of bismuth 2, lead 1, and tin 1.

**metalbu'min.** A substance found in ovarian cysts and sometimes in the urine. See also pseudomucin and paralbumin.

**metal'dehyde.** A polymer of acetaldehyde.

**metal'lic.** Relating to, composed of, or resembling metal.

**metallo-** (mĕ-tal'o-, met'ă-lo-) [ see metal ]. Combining form relating to metal, or meaning metallic.

**metal'locy'anide.** A compound of cyanogen with a metal forming an ionic radical that combines with a basic element to form a salt; *e.g.,* potassium ferricyanide, $K_3Fe(CN)_6$.

**metal'loen'zyme.** An enzyme containing a metal (ion) as an integral part of its active structure; *e.g.,* cytochromes (Fe; Cu), aldehyde oxidase (Mo), catechol oxidase (Cu), carbonic anhydrase (Zn).

**metal'lofla'vodehy'drogenase.** An oxidizing enzyme, containing one of the flavin nucleotides as coenzyme plus a metal ion that is also necessary to the action; the metal may be iron (as in succinate dehydrogenase), copper (as in urate oxidase), or molybdenum (as in xanthine oxidase).

**met'alloid** [ metallo- + G. *eidos*, resemblance ]. Resembling a metal in at least one amphoteric form; thus silicon, germanium, arsenic, selenium, and even carbon can be considered metalloids, since all in one form or another conduct electricity more easily than true nonmetals (*e.g.,* sulfur and chlorine) will; also called semiconductors.

**metallophilia** (mĕ-tal'o-fil'ĭ-ah) [ metallo- + G. *philos*, fond ]. Affinity for metal salts; *e.g.,* the affinity of the cytoplasm of cells of the reticuloendothelial system for silver carbonate stain and salts of gold and iron.

**metal'lophobia** (mĕ-tal'o-fo'bĭ-ah) [ G. *metallon*, metal, + *phobos*, fear ]. Morbid fear of metal objects.

**metal'lopor'phyrin.** A combination of a porphyrin with a metal, *e.g.,* iron (hematin), magnesium (as in chlorophyll), copper (in hemocyanin), zinc, cobalt, etc.

**metal'lopro'teins.** Proteins with a more or less tightly bound metal ion or ions, hemoglobin being the best known case.

**metalloscopy** met'ă-los'ko-pĭ) [ metallo- + G. *skopeō,* to examine ]. Testing the action of various metals applied to the surface of the body.

**met'allother'apy.** Siderism; treatment of various neuroses by the external application of metal disks to the skin.

**metaluetic** (met'ah-lu-et'ik). Metasyphilitic.

**met'amer** [ meta- + suffix -mer, *q.v.* ]. A substance, thing, or color that is similar to, but ultimately differentiable from, some other substance, thing, or color.

**metamere** (met'ah-mēr) [ meta- + G. *meros,* part ]. One of a series of homologous segments in the body; see also somite.

**metamer'ic.** Relating to or showing metamerism, or occurring in a metamere.

**metam'erism.** 1. A type of body structure exhibiting a series of segments or metameres one behind another. The metameres are serially homologous and in such primitive forms as the annelids are almost alike in structure. In the vertebrates specialized in the cephalic region masks the underlying metamerism, but it is still clearly evident in the serially repeated vertebrae, ribs, and intercostal muscles, and the spinal nerves. In young vertebrate embryos the basic metameric plan of structure is much more clearly evident than it remains in the adult. 2. In chemistry, sometimes (rarely) used as a synonym for isomerism.

**met'amid'ium.** A derivative of phenanthridinium and an aromaric diamidine; a prophylactic and curative agent of promising effectiveness in African trypanosomiasis.

**metamorphopsia** (met'ah-mor-fop'sĭ-ah) [ meta- + G. *morphē,* shape, + *opsis,* vision ]. A condition in which objects appear distorted in various ways.

**metamorphosis** (met'ah-mor'fo-sis, -mor-fo'sis) [ G. transformation; *meta,* beyond, over, + *morphē,* form ]. A change in form, structure, or function.

**complete m.,** the development of the larva into the pupa and adult; the latter is entirely different from the first two forms of the insect.

**fatty m.,** fatty change; the appearance of microscopically visible droplets of fat in the cytoplasm of cells.

**incomplete m.,** the development of a nymph into the imago which in many respects resembles the former.

**retrograde m.,** catabolism (2).

**met'amorphot'ic.** Relating to or marked by metamorphosis.

**metamyelocyte** (met'ah-mi'el-o-sīt) [ meta- + G. *myelos,* marrow, + *kytos,* cell ]. Immature granulocyte; juvenile cell of Schilling; a transitional form of myelocyte with nuclear construction that is intermediate between the mature myelocyte (myelocyte C of Sabin) and the two-lobed granular leukocyte. See color plate 14.

**metamfepyramone hydrochloride.** EFFILONE; 2-(dimethylamino)propiophenone hydrochloride; anorexic agent.

**met'aneph'rine.** 3-*O*-Methylepinephrine; 3-methoxyepinephrine; a catabolite of epinephrine found, together with normetanephrine, in the urine and in some tissues; results from the action of catechol-*O*-methyltransferase on epinephrine. It has no sympathomimetic actions.

**metanephrogenic, metanephrogenous** (met'ah-nef'rojen'ik, -ne-froj'ē-nus) [ meta- + G. *mephros,* kidney, + suffix -*gen,* producing ]. Applied to the more caudal part of the intermediate mesoderm which, under the inductive action of the metanephric diverticulum, has the potency to form metanephric tubules.

**metanephros,** pl. **metanephroi** (met'ah-nef'ros, -roy) [ meta- + G. *nephros,* kidney ]. Hind kidney; the most caudally located of the three excretory organs appearing in the evolution of the vertebrates. It becomes the permanent kidney of mammals. In mammalian embryos it is formed caudal to the mesonephros and develops later, as the mesonephros undergoes regression.

**metaneutrophil, metaneutrophile** (met-ah-nu'tro-fil, -fil) [ meta- + L. *neuter,* neither, + G. *philos,* fond ]. Not staining true with neutral dyes.

**metanil yellow.** An acid dye, $C_{18}H_{14}N_3O_3SNa$, used as a plasma and connective tissue stain.

**met'apep'tone.** One of the nondescript stages in peptone formation.

**met'aphase** [ meta- + G. *phasis*, an appearance ]. The stage of mitosis or meiosis in which the chromosomes become aligned on the equatorial plate of the cell with the centromeres mutually repelling each other. In mitosis and in the second meiotic division the centromeres of each chromosome divide and the two daughter centromeres are directed toward opposite poles of the cell. In the first division of meiosis the centromeres do not divide but the centromeres of each pair of homologous chromosomes become directed toward opposite poles.

**metaphos'phatase.** Endopolyphosphatase.

**met'aphosphor'ic acid.** Glacial phosphoric acid.

**metaphrenia** (met'ah-fre'nĭ-ah) [ meta- + G. *phren*, mind ]. The psychology, orientation, or life style of one whose energies have at least temporarily withdrawn from close interpersonal relationships, such as the family, and are directed to practical, gainful interests, such as business.

**metaphysial, metaphyseal** (met'ah-fiz-ĭ-al). Relating to a metaphysis.

**metaphysis,** pl. **metaphyses** (mĕ-taf'ĭ-sis, -sēz) [ meta- + G. *physis*, growth ]. The growth zone between the epiphysis and diaphysis during development of a bone.

**metaphysitis** (mĕ-taf'ĭ-si'tis). Inflammation of the metaphysis, or line of union of the epiphysis and diaphysis of a long bone.

**metaplasia** (met-ah-pla'zĭ-ah) [ G. *metaplasis*, transformation ]. The abnormal transformation of an adult, fully differentiated tissue of one kind into a differentiated tissue of another kind; m. is an acquired condition, in contrast to heteroplasia (*q. v.*).

   **apocrine m.,** alteration of acinar epithelium of breast tissue to resemble apocrine sweat glands; seen commonly in fibrocystic disease of the breasts.

   **autoparenchy'matous m.,** m. occurring in the parenchymal cells proper to the tissue.

   **intestinal m.,** the transformation of mucosa, particularly in the stomach, into glandular mucosa resembling that of the intestines, although usually lacking villi.

   **myeloid m.,** a syndrome characterized by anemia, enlargement of the spleen, nucleated red blood cells and immature granulocytes in the circulating blood, and conspicuous foci of extramedullary hemopoiesis in the spleen and liver. The condition occurs in some persons who have another disease (*e.g.*, cancer, tuberculosis, leukemia, Hodgkin's disease), and is termed secondary or symptomatic myeloid m.; it also occurs as an apparently primary illness, and is then termed primary or agnogenic myeloid m. or myelofibrosis, or myelosclerosis, because of the presence of an associated fibrosis of the bone marrow of unknown cause. The condition may develop in the course of polycythemia rubra vera. There is a high incidence of development of myeloid leukemia.

   **squamous m.,** the transformation of glandular or mucosal epithelium into stratified squamous epithelium.

   **squamous m. of amnion,** *amnion* nodosum.

**metap'lasis** [ G. a transformation. PLAS- ]. 1. Haeckel's term for the stage of completed growth or development of the individual. 2. Metaplasia.

**metaplasm** (met'ah-plazm) [ meta- + G. *plasma*, something formed ]. Cell *inclusions.*

**met'aplas'tic.** Pertaining to metaplasia or metaplasis.

**met'aplex'us** [ meta- + L. *plexus*, an interweaving ]. The choroid plexus in the fourth ventricle of the brain.

**metapneumonic** (met'ah-nu-mon'ik). Occurring after or as a sequel of pneumonia.

**metapophysis** (met'ă-pof'ĭ-sis) [ meta- + G. *apophysis*, a process ]. *Processus* mammillaris.

**met'apore** [ meta- + G. *poros*, pore ]. *Apertura* ventriculi quarti.

**met'apro'tein.** A derived protein obtained by the action of acids or alkalies; it is soluble in weak acids or alkalies, but insoluble in neutral solutions.

   **acid m.,** acid albumin or albuminate, obtained by the action of acid on protein.

**al'kali m.,** alkali albumin or albuminate, obtained by the action of an alkali on protein.

**met'aproter'enol sulfate** (USAN). Orciprenaline sulphate (BP); ALUPENT; 3,5-dihydroxy-α-[ (isopropylamino)methyl ]benzyl alcohol sulfate; a sympathomimetic bronchodilator used for the treatment of bronchial asthma.

**metapsychology** (met'ah-si-kol'o-jĭ) [ G. *meta,* beyond, transcending, + psychology ]. 1. A systematic attempt to discern and describe what lies beyond the empirical facts and laws of psychology, such as the relations between body and mind, or concerning the place of the mind in the universe. 2. In psychoanalysis, or psychoanalytic m., psychology concerning the fundamental assumptions of the Freudian theory of the mind, which entail five more or less distinct points of view: the dynamic (concerning psychologic forces); the economic (concerning psychologic energy); the structural (concerning psychologic configurations); the genetic (concerning psychologic origins); and the adaptive (concerning psychologic relations with the environment).

**met'apyret'ic** [ meta- + G. *pyretos*, fever ]. Postfebrile.

**met'aram'inol bitartrate** (USP). Metaraminol tartrate (BP); ARAMINE bitartrate; *l*-α-(1-aminoethyl)-*m*-hydroxybenzyl alcohol hydrogen *d*-tartrate; a potent sympathomimetic amine used for the elevation and maintenance of blood pressure in acute hypotensive states and topically as a nasal decongestant.

**metarteriole** (met'ar-tēr'ĭ-ōl) [ meta- + arteriole ]. One of the small peripheral blood vessels between the arterioles and the true capillaries that contain scattered groups of smooth muscle fibers in their walls.

**metarubricyte** (met'ah-ru'brĭ-sīt). Orthochromatic normoblast; see discussion under erythroblast.

   **pernicious anemia type m.,** orthochromatic megaloblast; see discussion under erythroblast.

**metastable** (met'ah-sta'bl) [ meta- + L. *stabilis*, stable ]. 1. Of uncertain stability; in a condition to pass into another phase when slightly disturbed. Water, for example, when cooled below the freezing point may remain liquid but will at once congeal if a piece of ice is added. Gunpowder is metastable. 2. Denoting the excited condition of the nucleus of a radionuclide isomer that reaches a lower energy state by the process of isomeric transition decay without changing its atomic number or weight; for example, $^{99m}_{43}Tc \rightarrow ^{99}_{43}Tc + \gamma$.

**metastasis,** pl. **metastases** (mĕ-tas'tă-sis, -sēz) [ G. a removing, fr. *meta,* in the midst of, + *stasis,* a placing. STA- ]. 1. The shifting of a disease, or its local manifestations, from one part of the body to another, as is seen in mumps when the symptoms referable to the parotid gland subside and the testis becomes affected. 2. In cancer, the appearance of neoplasms in parts of the body remote from the seat of the primary tumor. 3. Transportation of bacteria from one part of the body to another, through the blood streams (**hematogenous m.**) or through lymph channels (**lymphogenous m.**).

   **m. ad nervos,** a reflex nervous disturbance.

   **biochemical m.,** the transportation and induction of abnormal immunochemical specificities in apparently normal organs.

   **calcareous m.,** the deposit of calcareous material in remote tissues in the event of extensive resorption of osseous tissue in caries, malignant neoplasms, and so on.

   **crossed m.,** the passage of any substance from the venous to the arterial circulation without passing through the lungs, as through a persistent ductus arteriosus or foramen ovale.

   **direct m.,** transportation in the direction of the blood or lymph stream.

   **implantation m.,** transportation along a free surface.

   **paradoxical m.,** (1) crossed m.; (2) retrograde m.

   **pulsating metastases,** metastases to bone, usually from hypernephromas, occasionally from thyroid tumors; they may have rather extensive expansile pulsation and a continuous bruit.

   **retrograde m.,** m. occurring in a direction opposed to that of the blood current.

transplantation m., m. from one tissue to another.

**metas′tasize.** To pass into or invade by metastasis.

**met′astat′ic.** Relating to metastasis.

**met′aster′num.** *Processus* xiphoideus.

**metastrongyle** (met-ah-stron′jil). Common name for members of the genus *Metastrongylus.*

**Metastrongylus** (met-ah-stron′jĭ-lus) [ meta- + G. *strongylos,* round ]. A genus of nematode lungworms (family Metastrongylidae, sometimes called Protostrongylidae) and the only genus in its subfamily (Metastrongylinae). The four known species are found only in pigs; transmission is by earthworm intermediate hosts.

**M. a′pri,** a common lungworm of the pig; it occurs in the larger bronchi of wild and domestic pigs, where it is highly pathogenic, causing verminous pneumonia, consolidation of the lungs, emmphysema, loss of condition, and reduced growth; it may also transmit swine influenza and hog cholera.

**M. elonga′tus,** *M. salmi.*

**M. pudendotec′tus,** a common lungworm of the pig, considerably smaller than *M. apri,* and also important in the transmission of swine influenza and hog cholera.

**M. sal′mi,** *M. elongatus;* occurs in the trachea, bronchi, and bronchioles of domestic and wild pigs.

**metasyphilis** (met′ah-sif′ĭ-lis). 1. The constitutional state due to congenital syphilis without local lesions. 2. Parasyphilis.

**met′asyphilit′ic.** Metaluetic. 1. Relating to metasyphilis. 2. Following or occurring as a sequel of syphilis. 3. Parasyphilitic.

**met′atar′sal.** Relating to the metatarsus or to one of the metatarsal bones.

**metatarsalgia** (met′ah-tar-sal′jĭ-ah) [ meta- + G. *algos,* pain ]. Pain in the forepart (metatarsal region) of the foot.

**metatarsectomy** (met′ah-tar-sek′to-mĭ) [ metarsus + G. *ektomē,* excision ]. Excision of the metatarsus.

**metatarsophalangeal** (met′ah-tar′so-fă-lan′je-al). Relating to the metatarsal bones and the phalanges; denoting the articulations between them.

**metatarsus,** pl. **metatar′si** (met′ah-tar′sus) [ meta- + G. *tarsos,* tarsus ]. [ NA ]. The distal portion of the foot between the instep and the toes, having as its skeleton the five long bones (metatarsal bones) articulating posteriorly with the cuboid and cuneiform bones and distally with the phalanges.

**m. adduc′tova′rus,** fixed deformity of the foot in which both adductus and varus vectors contribute to the resultant foot posture.

**m. adduc′tus,** a fixed deformity of the foot in which the forepart of the foot is angled away from the main longitudinal axis of the foot toward the midline; usually congenital in origin.

**m. atav′icus,** abnormal shortness of the first metatarsal bone as compared with the second.

**m. la′tus,** talipes transversoplanus; spread foot; broad foot; deformity caused by sinking down of the transverse arch of the foot.

**m. va′rus,** fixed deformity of the foot in which the forepart of the foot is rotated on the long axis of the foot, so that the plantar surface faces the midline of the body.

**metathalamus** (met′ah-thal′ă-mus) [ meta- + G. *thalamos,* thalamus ] [ NA ]. The most caudal part of the thalamus, composed of the medial and lateral geniculate bodies.

**metathesis** (mĕ-tath′e-sis) [ meta- + G. *thesis,* a placing ]. 1. The transfer of a pathologic product (*e.g.,* a calculus) from one place to another where it causes less inconvenience or injury, when it is not possible or expedient to remove it from the body. 2. Double decomposition, wherein a compound, A-B, reacts with another compound, C-D, to yield A-C + B-D, or A-D + B-C.

**metathrombin** (met-ah-throm′bin). An inactive derivative of fibrin formed during the process of contraction of the coagulum.

**met′atrop′ic** [ meta- + G. *tropē,* a turning ]. Denoting a changing back or reversion to a previous state.

**met′atyp′ical.** Pertaining to tissue that is formed of elements identical to those occurring in that site under normal

conditions, but the various elements are not arranged in the usual, normal pattern.

**metaxalone** (mĕ-tak′să-lōn) (USAN). SKELAXIN; 5-[ (3,5-xylyloxy)methyl ]-2-oxazolidinone; 5-(3,5-dimethylphenoxymethyl)-2-oxazolidinone; a centrally acting skeletal muscle relaxant. It blocks polysynaptic reflexes without affecting monosynaptic reflexes. Side effects (liver damage, hemolytic anemia) occur frequently.

**Metazoa** (met′ah-zo′ah) [ meta- + G. *zōon,* animal ]. A subkingdom of the animal kingdom, including all the multicellular animal organisms in which the cells are differentiated and form tissues; distinguished from the Protozoa, or unicellular animal organisms.

**metazoonosis** (met′ah-zo-o-no′sis) [ meta- + G. *zōon,* animal, + *nosos,* disease ]. A zoonosis that requires both a vertebrate and an invertebrate host for completion of its life cycle; for example, the arborvirus, snail-vectored, and insect-vectored helminth infections of man and other vertebrates.

**metcaraphen** NETRIN; 1-(3′,4′-dimethylphenyl)-1-cyclopentanecarboxylic acid 2-diethylaminoethyl ester; intestinal antispasmodic with anticholinergic properties.

**Metchnikoff,** Elie, Russian biologist in Paris, 1845–1916. Nobel laureate, 1908, with Paul Ehrlich, for their work on immunity. See M.'s *theory.*

**met′encephal′ic.** Relating to the metencephalon.

**metencephalon** (met′en-sef′ă-lon) [ meta- + G. *enkephalos,* brain ] [ NA ]. The anterior of the two major subdivisions of the rhombencephalon (the posterior being the myelencephalon or medulla oblongata), composed of the pons and the cerebellum.

**meteorism** (me′te-or-izm) [ G. *meteōrismos,* a lifting up ]. Tympanites.

**meteoropathy** (me′te-or-op′ă-thĭ) [ G. *meteōra,* things high in the air, + *pathos,* suffering ]. Ill health due to climatic conditions.

**meteorophobia** (me′te-or-o-fo′bĭ-ah). Morbid fear of meteors.

**meteorotropic** (me-te-or-o-trop′ik) [ meteorology, the science of the weather, + G. *tropos,* a turning ]. Denoting diseases affected in their incidence by the weather.

**me′ter** [ Fr. *metre;* G. *metron,* measure ]. A measure of length; the equivalent of 39.37 inches.

**atom m.,** Angstrom *unit.*

**rate m.,** a device that continuously displays the magnitude of events averaged over varying time intervals.

**sight m.,** a device for measuring light, calibrated in footcandles.

**ventilation m.,** a m. used to measure tidal and minute ventilatory volumes.

**Venturi m.,** a device for measuring flow of a fluid in terms of the drop in pressure when the fluid flows into the constriction of a Venturi tube.

**meter-candle.** Lux.

**metergasia** (met′er-ga′zĭ-ah) [ G. *meta,* denoting change, + *ergasia,* work ]. Change of function.

**metestrus, metestrum** (met-es′trus, -trum) [ meta- + estrus, *q. v.* ]. The period between estrus and diestrus in the estrous cycle.

**metfor′min hydrochloride** (BP, USAN). DIABEFAGOS; 1,1-dimethylbiguanide hydrochloride; oral hypoglycemic agent.

**meth-, metho-.** Chemical prefixes usually denoting a methyl or methoxy group.

**meth′acho′line chloride** (NF). MECHOLYL chloride; acetyl-β-methylcholine chloride; Mecholyl chloride; a derivative of acetylcholine; a parasympathomimetic used as a vasodilator in peripheral vascular disease, and for inducing hyperemia in arthritis, its action being brought about locally by iontophoresis. Also available (NF) as m. bromide.

**methacrylate resin** (meth-ak′nĭ-lāt). See under resin.

**methacrylic acid** (meth′ă-kril′ik). Methylacrylic acid; occurs in oil from Roman camomile; used in the manufacture of methacrylate resins and plastics; methyl ester polymerizes easily to a transparent plastic known as LUCITE or PLEXIGLAS.

**methacycline hydrochloride** (meth'ă-si'klēn). (NF, BP). RONDOMYCIN; 6-methylene-5-hydroxytetracycline hydrochloride; an antimicrobial agent.

**meth'adone hydrochloride** (USP, BP). AMIDONE hydrochloride; DOLOPHINE hydrochloride (and others); 6-dimethylamino-4,4-diphenyl-3-heptanone hydrochloride; a synthetic narcotic drug; an orally effective analgesic similar in action to morphine but with slightly greater potency and longer duration; produces psychic and physical dependence, but withdrawal symptoms are relatively mild. Used as a replacement (oral route) for morphine and heroin; also used during withdrawal treatment in morphine and heroin addiction.

**methallatal.** MOSIDAL; 5-ethyl-5-(2-methylallyl)-2-thiobarbituric acid; used in treatment of motion sickness.

**methallenestril** (meth'ă-len-es'tril). VALLESTRIL; α,α-dimethyl- β-ethyl-6-methoxy-2-naphthalene propionic acid; an orally effective, nonsteroid estrogenic compound.

**methallibure** (mĕ-thal'ĭ-būr) (USAN). AIMAX; methyl-6-(1-methylallyl)-2,5-diothiobiurea; an anterior pituitary activator for swine.

**meth'amphet'amine hydrochloride.** METHEDRINE; PERVITIN; methylamphetamine hydrochloride; d-desoxyephedrine hydrochloride; d-N,α-dimethylphenethylamine hydrochloride. A sympathomimetic agent that exerts greater stimulating effects upon the central nervous system than does amphetamine. It depresses the motility of the gastrointestinal tract and allays hunger. M. is widely used by drug abusers via the oral and intravenous ("mainlining") routes; strong psychic dependence may develop.

**methampyrone.** NOVALGIN; (antipyrinylmethylamino)-methanesulfonic acid sodium salt; analgesic and antipyretic agent.

**methandi'enone** (BP). Methandrostenolone.

**methan'driol.** Methylandrostenediol; the methyl derivative of androstenediol, with similar actions and uses.

**methandrostenolone** (meth-an'dro-sten'o-lōn). (NF). DANABOL; NEROBOL; methandienone; 17β-hydroxy-17α-methyl-1,4-androstadiene-3-one (for androstane structure, see steroids); a methylated dehydrotestosterone; an orally effective anabolic steroid that may promote nitrogen retention when combined with an adequate diet; in addition, it can exert typically androgenic effects.

**meth'ane** [ meth(yl) + -ane ]. Marsh gas; $CH_4$; an odorless gas produced by the decomposition of organic matter; it is explosive when mixed with 7 or 8 volumes of air, constituting then the firedamp in coal mines.

**meth'anol.** Methyl alcohol.

**methan'theline bromide** (NF). BANTHINE; β-diethylaminoethyl-9-xanthenecarboxylate methobromide; $C_{21}H_{26}BrNO_3$; a parasympatholytic (anticholinergic) drug used in the management of peptic ulcer.

**meth'aphen'ilene hydrochloride.** N,N-dimethyl-N'-(α-thenyl)-N'-phenylethylenediamine hydrochloride; a histamine-antagonizing agent.

**methapyrilene** (meth'ă-pir'ĭ-lēn). HISTADYL; SEMIKON; THENYLENE; 2-[ (2-dimethylaminoethyl)-2-thenylamino ]-pyridine; a histamine antagonist.
   **m. fumarate** (NF), administered topically on the skin.
   **m. hydrochloride** (NF), the preferred salt for oral or parenteral use.

**methaqualone** (meth-ak'wah-lōn) (NF, BP). QUAALUDE; SOMNAFAC; SOPOR; PAREST; 2-methyl-3-o-tolyl-4(3H)-quinazolinone; a sedative and hypnotic resembling short-acting barbiturates; a drug of abuse, known on the street as "sopors."

**metharbital** (meth-ar'bĭ-tal) (NF). GEMONIL; 5,5-diethyl-1-methylbarbituric acid. An N-methylated derivative of barbital with anticonvulsant properties similar to those of phenobarbital. Used to control various types of epileptic seizures, particularly in young children.

**methargen.** VIACUTAN; 2,2'-dinaphthylmethane-3,3'-disulfonic acid disilver salt; topical antiseptic agent.

**methazol'amide** (USP). NEPTAZANE; N-(4-methyl-2-sulfamoyl-Δ²-1,3,4-thiadiazolin-5-ylidene)acetamide; a carbonic anhydrase inhibitor used in glaucoma, as an adjunct to conventional miotic therapy, and in epilepsy in conjunction with usual antiepileptics.

**MetHb.** Abbreviation for methemoglobin.

**methdil'azine hydrochloride** (NF). TACARYL hydrochloride; 10-(1-methyl-3-pyrrolidylmethyl)phenothiazine hydrochloride; a phenothiazine compound with antihistaminic activity; used in the treatment of various dermatoses to relieve pruritus.

**methemalbumin** (met'hēm-al-bu'min, -hem-al'bu-min) An abnormal compound formed in the blood as a result of heme combining with plasma albumin; found in some patients with black water fever or paroxysmal nocturnal hemoglobinuria. The presence of m. in plasma has been decribed as a means of differentiating severe (hemorrhagic) from mild (edematous) pancreatitis. It also has been described in other acute abdominal conditions such as strangulation obstruction and mesenteric artery occlusion. Formerly termed pseudomethomoglobin.

**methemoglobin** (met-he-mo-glo'bin). MetHb; a transformation product of oxyhemoglobin because of the oxidation of the normal $Fe^{2+}$ to $Fe^{3+}$; found in sanguineous effusions and in the circulating blood after poisoning with acetanilid, potassium chlorate, and other substances; it contains oxygen in firm union with ferric iron, thus being chemically different from oxygenated hemoglobin (oxyhemoglobin). Also called ferrihemoglobin.
   **m. reductase,** a flavoenzyme catalyzing the recuction of m. to hemoglobin in the red cell; absent in familial methemoglobinemia.

**methemoglobinemia** (met-he-mo-glo-bin-e'mĭ-ah or meth-e-mo-) [ methemoglobin + G. *haima*, blood ]. The presence of methemoglobin in the circulating blood.
   **acquired m.,** enterogenous m.; secondary m.; m. caused by various chemical agents, such as nitrites.
   **congenital m.,** primary or hereditary m.; congenital methemoglobic c.; (1) m. due to formation of any one of a group of abnormal hemoglobins collectively known as hemoglobin M (*q.v.*); slate-gray cyanosis occurs in early infancy, without pulmonary or cardiac disease, and is resistant to ascorbic acid or methylene blue therapy; autosomal dominant inheritance; (2) m. due to deficiency of DPNH-diaphorase, the enzyme responsible for reduction of intraerythrocyte methemoglobin; cyanosis is improved by ascorbic acid or methylene blue; autosomal recessive inheritance.
   **enterogenous m.,** acquired m.
   **primary m.,** congenital m.
   **secondary m.,** acquired m.

**methemoglobinuria** (met-he-mo-glo-bin-u'rĭ-ah, meth-e-mo-) [ methemoglobin + G. *ouron*, urine ]. The presence of methemoglobin in the urine.

**methen'amine** (NF). FORMIN; UROTROPIN; hexamine; hexamethylenamine; hexamethylenetetramine; ammonioformaldehyde; $C_6H_{12}N_4$; a condensation product obtained by the action of ammonia upon formaldehyde.
   **m. anhydromethylene citrate,** CITRAMIN; FORMANOL; hexamethylenetetramine anhydromethylene citrate; a urinary antiseptic.
   **m. camphorate,** AMPHOTROPIN; hexamethylenetetramine camphorate; used in cystitis, pyelitis, and nephritis.
   **m. hippurate** (USAN), HIPPRAMINE; HIPREX; hexamethylenetetramine hippurate; used as urinary antiseptic.
   **m. man'delate** (USP), $C_{14}H_{20}N_4O_3$; a urinary anti-infective.
   **m. salicylate,** UROTROPIN salicylate; SALIFORMIN; hexamethylenetetramine salicylate; uric acid solvent and urinary antiseptic.
   **m. sulfosalicylate,** SULFHEXET; hexamethylenetetramine sulfosalicylate; a urinary antiseptic.
   **m. tetraiodide,** SIOMINE; hexamethylenetetramine tetraiodide; $(CH_2)_6N_4I_4$; used to produce effects of iodides; it is decomposed into m. and iodide in the intestine.

**meth'ene.** Methylene.

**methen'olone acetate** (USAN). PRIMONABOL; 17β-hydroxy-1β-methyl-5α-andros-1-en-3-one 17-acetate; anabolic agent.

**methicil'lin sodium** (BP, USAN). Sodium methicillin (USP); DIMOCILLIN-RT; STAPHCILLIN; sodium 2,6-dimethoxyphenylpenicillin monohydrate; a semisynthetic penicillin salt for parenteral administration; restriction of its use to infections caused by penicillin G-resistant staphylococci is recommended. It is less effective than penicillin G in infections caused by hemolytic streptococci, pneumococci, gonococci, and penicillin G-sensitive staphylococci.

**methim′azole** (USP). 1-Methylimidazole-2-thiol; an antithyroid drug similar in action to propylthiouracil.

**methi′odal sodium.** See under sodium.

**methi′onine.** CH₃S—CH₂CH₂CHNH₂—COOH; L-methionine; 4-methylthio-L-2-aminobutyric acid; an amino acid essential in the diet; the most important natural source of "active methyl" groups in the body, hence usually involved in methylations *in vivo.* See also DL-methionine.

   **active m.,** S-adenosylmethionine.

   **m. adenosyltransferase** (EC 2.5.1.6, formerly 2.4.2.13), methionine-activating enzyme; an enzyme catalyzing the condensation of methionine and ATP, forming S-adenosylmethionine ("active methionine").

   **m. sulfoxime,** a toxic derivative of m. formed when proteins containing it are treated with nitrogen chloride (a compound sometimes used in the bleaching of flour) to give —SO(NH)CH₃ in place of —SCH₃.

**DL-methionine.** A lipotropic agent useful as an adjunct in the treatment of liver diseases; in severe forms of liver diseases large doses exaggerate the toxemia.

**methisazone** (me-this′ă-zōn) (USP). MARBORAN; 1-methylindole-2,3-dione 3-thiosemicarbazone; antiviral agent.

**methitural** (meth′ĭ-tu′ral). NERAVAL; 5-1-methylbutyl)-5-[ 2-(methylthio)ethyl ]-2-thiobarbituric acid sodium salt; a nonvalatile general anesthetic for intravenous use, similar to thiopental but with less potency and more rapid emergence. Used in emergency and minor surgery, for induction and basal anesthesia. It may cause respiratory and circulatory depression at levels providing adequate muscular relaxation.

**methix′ene hydrochloride** (USAN). TREMOQUIL; 1-methyl-3-(thioxanthen-9-ylmethyl)piperidine hydrochloride; intestinal antispasmodic with anticholinergic properties.

**metho-.** See meth-.

**meth′ocar′bamol** (NF). ROBAXIN; 2-hydroxy-3-o-methoxyphenoxypropyl carbamate. Chemically related to mephenesin carbamate, it is slower in onset of action but of longer duration. Used as a centrally acting skeletal muscle relaxant which may be administered intravenously, intramuscularly or orally.

---

# METHOD

**meth′od** [ G. *methodos;* fr. *meta,* after, + *hodos,* way ]. The mode or manner or sequence of events of performing an operation, making a test, etc.

   **Abbott's m. of treatment of scoliosis,** use of a series of plaster jackets applied after partial correction of the curvature by external force.

   **Achard-Castaigne m.,** methylene blue *test.*

   **activated sludge m.,** a m. of sewage disposal in which the sewage is treated with 15 per cent bacterially active, liquid sludge. In the presence of an ample supply of oxygen, the colloidal material of the sewage is coagulated and undergoes sedimentation.

   **Ahlfeld's m.,** (1) a m. for determining the duration of pregnancy by measuring the length of the fetal ovoid and calculating the age of the fetus from Haas's rule. The length of the fetal ovoid is measured by means of a pelvimeter one arm of which passes through the abdominal wall upon the fundus of the uterus; the other arm is inserted into the vagina and impinges upon the presenting part; (2) hand disinfection with hot water and alcohol.

   **air dent m.,** a m. of grinding teeth by the application of abrasives impelled by compressed air; see also airbrasive.

   **Altmann-Gersh m.,** the m. of rapidly freezing a tissue and dehydrating it in a vacuum.

   **Anel's m.,** ligation of an artery immediately above (on the proximal side of) an aneurysm.

   **Antyllus′ m.,** ligature of the artery above and below an aneurysm, followed by incision into and emptying of the sac.

   **Aristote′lian m.,** a m. of study that stresses the relation between a general category and a particular object.

   **auxanographic m.,** diffusion m. for the study of bacterial enzymes; agar is mixed with the material (such as starch or milk) which is to serve as an indicator of the enzyme action and is inoculated and plated; if the bacteria produce enzymes digesting the admixed material, there will be a zone of clearing in the medium about each colony.

   **Baer's m.,** injection of sterilized oil into an ankylosed joint, after the adhesions have been broken up, to prevent their reformation.

   **Bandi's m.,** an obsolete m. for the identification of *Vibrio cholerae,* based on observing agglutinated vibrios in feces incubated for 3 hours in peptone water that contains varied concentrations of specific antiserum.

   **Bang's m. for eliminating tuberculosis from dairy herds,** an early m. that involved segregation of diseased cows, removal of calves from the infected environment immediately after birth, and feeding them with tuberculosis-free milk; eventually the tuberculous animals are slaughtered.

   **Bang's m. for microestimation of blood constituents,** (1) an obsolete m. for determining the quantities of urea, glucose, albumin, and certain other constituents of blood by testing with only a few drops of blood collected on blotting paper; (2) an obsolete m. for analyzing glucose in urine, based on adding an aliquot of the specimen to an excess of boiling alkaline solution of copper thiocyanate, and then titrating the excess reagent with a volumetric solution of hydroxylamine sulfate.

   **Bangerter's m.,** pleoptics.

   **Baréty's m.,** a modified extension m. for the treatment of hip disease and fracture of the thigh.

   **Barraquer's m.,** zonulolysis.

   **Beck's m.,** gastrostomy in which a permanent opening into the stomach is made by means of a tube made from the greater curvature of the stomach.

   **Bergonié m.,** general faradization for the reduction of fat.

   **Bethea's m.,** a m. for the detection of unilateral impairment of expansion of the pulmonary apices. The examiner, standing behind the patient, places the tips of his fingers on the upper surfaces of corresponding ribs high up in the axillae; unilateral impairment of expansion is indicated by the lessened respiratory movement of the rib on the affected side.

   **Beuttner's m.,** an obsolete m. of partial extirpation of the adnexa, with preservation of a portion of the ovaries, and transverse cuneiform excision of the fundus of the uterus.

   **Bielschowsky's m.,** a m. of treating tissues with silver nitrate to demonstrate reticular fibers in histology.

   **Bier's m.,** (1) intravenous regional *anesthesia;* (2) Bier's hyperemia; constriction hyperemia; treatment of various surgical conditions by artificial hyperemia induced by suction or by constriction of the proximal portion of the limb.

   **Bobroff's m.,** treatment of cyst of the liver by incision and removal of the lining membrane, followed by suture of the incision and closure of the abdomen without lavage or drainage.

   **Born m. of wax plate reconstruction,** the making of three-dimensional models of structures from serial sections; it depends on the building up of a series of wax plates, cut out to scaled enlargements of the individual sections involved in the region to be reconstructed.

   **Bouchut's m.,** intubation of the larynx, first suggested by Bouchut, but not adopted because of the imperfection of the tubes used; revived independently by O'Dwyer.

   **Braquehaye's m.,** closure of a vesicovaginal fistula by invagination, after denudation, of the vaginal mucous membrane.

   **Brasdor's m.,** treatment of aneurysm by ligation of the artery immediately below (on the distal side of) the tumor.

   **Buist's m.,** a m. for the resuscitation of an infant born asphyxiated; the child is simply transferred from one hand of the obstetrician to the other alternately, being held supine on one hand, prone on the other, thus causing alternate inspiration and expiration.

   **Callahan's m.,** chloropercha m.

   **Carpue's m.,** Indian m.

   **Charters′ m.,** a method of toothbrushing utilizing a restricted circular motion with the bristles inclined coronally at a 45 degree angle.

**Chayes' m.,** a m. of replacing lost teeth, devised by Chayes in the early part of the 20th century; a mechanical device for the fixation and stabilization of the dental prosthesis allows "movement in function" of the abutment teeth.

**Chervin's m.,** a gymnastic m. of treating stuttering.

**chloropercha m.,** a m. of filling the root canals of teeth by dissolving gutta-percha cones in a chloroform-rosin medium within the root canal. Also called Callahan's m. or Johnson's m.

**Ciacco's m.,** a m. for demonstrating complex insoluble intracellular lipids; using fixation in a formalin-dichromate solution, paraffin embedding, staining with Sudan III or IV, examination in aqueous mountant.

**closed circuit m.,** a m. for measuring oxygen consumption in which the subject rebreathes an initial quantity of oxygen through a carbon dioxide absorber and the decrease in the volume of oxygen being rebreathed is noted.

**closed plaster m.,** a m. of treating war wounds in which, after débridement, the limb is encased completely in a close-fitting plaster of Paris bandage. The cast is left intact for an indefinite period. This method was used extensively by Trueta in the Spanish Civil War.

**confrontation m.,** a m. of perimetry; the examiner compares the visual fields of the patient with his own by facing the patient who has one eye covered and the other fixed upon the corresponding (confronting) eye of the examiner. The examiner then holds his finger midway between the patient and himself and moves it slowly in different directions until the patient fails to see it. In each instance the finger is moved again toward the original position until it is just seen by the subject.

**cooled-knife m.,** the cutting of frozen sections with a knife cooled to a few degrees below the freezing point.

**copper-sulfate m.,** a m. for the determination of specific gravity of blood or plasma; a series of small bottles is set up containing solutions of copper sulfate graded in specific gravity by increments of 0.004; a drop of blood or plasma is delivered from the tip of a medicine dropper into each of several bottles within the expected range of the blood or plasma sample. The specific gravity of the copper sulfate solution in which the drop of blood or plasma remains suspended indefinitely indicates the specific gravity of the sample.

**correlational m.,** a m., most often used in clinical and other applied areas of psychology, to study the relationship which exists between one characteristic and another in an individual.

**Credé's m.'s,** Credé's maneuvers; (1) instillation of one drop of a 2 per cent solution of silver nitrate into each eye of the newborn infant, to prevent ophthalmia neonatorum; (2) resting the hand on the fundus uteri from the moment of the expulsion of the fetus, and gently rubbing in case of hemorrhage or failing contraction; then, when the afterbirth is loosened it is expelled by firm compression or squeezing of the fundus by the hand; (3) use of manual pressure on bladder, particularly a paralyzed bladder, to express urine.

**cross-sectional m.,** in developmental psychology, the study of the life span involving comparison of groups of individuals at different age levels, as contrasted with the longitudinal m. (*q. v.*).

**Cuignet's m.,** retinoscopy.

**Dick m.,** Dick *test.*

**Dieffenbach's m.,** a plastic operation for covering a defect by sliding a flap with broad pedicle.

**diffusion m.,** auxanographic m.

**direct m.,** in dentistry, a term usually applied to inlay technic in which the wax pattern is made directly in the prepared cavity in the tooth.

**disk sensitivity m.,** a procedure for testing the relative effectiveness of various antibiotics; small disks of paper (or other suitable material) are impregnated with known, appropriate amounts of antibiotic, and then placed on the surface of semisolid medium that has been previously inoculated with the organism being tested. After suitable periods of incubation at 37°C., the lack of growth in zones about the various disks indicates the relative effectiveness of the antibiotic.

**double antibody m.,** double antibody *precipitation.*

**Edman m.,** see phenylisothiocyanate.

**Eggleston m.,** rapid digitalization by means of large doses of digitalis leaf or tincture frequently repeated.

**Eicken's m.,** facilitation of hypopharyngoscopy by means of forward traction on the cricoid cartilage by a laryngeal probe.

**Emerson m.,** a m. of artificial respiration, with the subject prone. The hips are alternately raised (inspiration) and lowered (expiration). When the hips are raised the diaphragm descends, the spine being hyperextended. This m. is now outmoded and has been replaced by direct or indirect mouth-to-mouth resuscitation.

**Emmet's m.,** an operative procedure for the repair of lacerated perineum.

**epidermic m.,** the application of remedies to the surface of the skin in order to obtain their constitutional effects.

**experimental m.,** in experimental psychology, contol of environmental, physiological, or attitudinal factors to observe dependent changes in aspects of experience and behavior.

**flash m.,** sterilization of milk by raising it rapidly to a temperature of 178°F. and, after holding it there for a short time, reducing it rapidly to 40°F.

**flotation m.,** any of several procedures for concentrating various types of helminthic eggs, as a means of more reliable results when eggs are difficult to find in direct examination. The flotation m.'s are based on the principle that most helminthic eggs float on the surface of a liquid that has a sufficiently high specific gravity, *e.g.*, approximately 1.180; thus, a small amount of test feces may be thoroughly mixed with approximately 10 parts of saturated solution of common table salt, and protozoan cysts and helminthic eggs tend to float on the surface, from which they may be collected on a coverslip. In addition to this **simple flotation m.,** one may also use a **zinc sulfate flotation centrifugation m.:** the fecal specimen is suspended in tap water and strained through wet gauze (to remove coarse particles); the filtrate is centrifugated at top speed for 45 to 60 seconds, and the sediment is resuspended in tap water; after three or four washings and centrifugations, the sediment is finally suspended in 33 per cent solution of zinc sulfate and centrifugated at top speed for 45 to 60 seconds; a bacteriologic loop may be used to skim the surface layer, which contains the cysts and eggs.

**Frenkel's m.,** treatment of the ataxia of tabes dorsalis by means of systematic exercises.

**Gärtner's m.,** a m. of measuring venous pressure, based upon Gärtner's vein phenomenon; with the patient sitting erect a vein is selected on the back of the hand which is held horizontal a little below the level of the right atrium, and then slowly raised; when the vein is observed to collapse, the distance between its level and that of the atrium is measured with a millimeter rule; this distance gives the venous pressure in millimeters of blood. The vein itself is thus used as a manometer communicating with the right atrium.

**Gatch m.,** a m. of hyperextension of the spine in compression fracture; head of patient is at foot of bed, with knee gatch under spine.

**Gerota's m.,** injection of the lymphatics with a dye that is soluble in chloroform or ether but not in water; alkanin, red sulfide of mercury, and Prussian blue are said to be suitable for this purpose.

**Golgi's m.,** a m. of staining nerve cells and their processes, nerve fibers, and the neuroglia cells: (*a*) rapid m. (for embryonic specimens): place in Golgi's osmiobichromate solution, wash in distilled water, and dip in a 75 per cent solution of silver nitrate; (*b*) mixed m.: place in Müller's fluid for 4 or 5 days, then in Golgi's osmiobichromate solution for 24 hours, and finally in a 75 per cent solution of silver nitrate; (*c*) slow m.: harden in Müller's fluid for 5 or 6 weeks, then stain with (1) a 0.5 per cent solution of silver nitrate, and (2) a 0.75 per cent solution of silver nitrate soaking indefinitely in the latter.

**Gram's m.,** Gram *stain.*

**Gräupner's m.,** a test of the sufficiency of the heart muscle. If a normal subject takes a measured amount of exercise, the pulse rate rises, and after it has begun to fall the systolic blood pressure begins to rise, reaching its maximum a few minutes after the pulse rate; in the case of a weakened heart the blood pressure reaction is delayed and diminished in amount; in seriously weakened hearts there is no rise, but rather a fall in blood pressure.

**Gruber's m.**, a modification of the Politzer m. in which the patient does not swallow, but says "hoc" at the instant of compression of the bag.

**Guyon's m.**, treatment of ingrowing toenail by the excision of a wedge-shaped piece from the side of the great toe.

**Hamilton's m.**, sponge *graft.*

**Hammerschlag's m.**, a hydrometric m. of determining the specific gravity of the blood by allowing a drop of blood to fall into each of a series of tubes containing mixtures of chloroform and benzene of known graded specific gravities; the specific gravity of that mixture in which the drop remains exactly suspended, neither rising nor falling, corresponds to the specific gravity of the blood sample.

**Hegar's m.**, treatment of sciatica by stretching the nerve trunk, the thigh being forcibly flexed on the abdomen while the knee is maintained in extension.

**Hilton's m.**, division of the nerves supplying the part, for the relief of pain in ulcers.

**Hirschberg's m.**, a m. of measuring the amount of deviation of a strabismic eye, by observing the reflection of a light fixated by the straight eye on the cornea of the deviating eye.

**Howe's silver precipitation m.**, ammoniacal silver nitrate is carefully applied to carious dentin; silver is precipitated by light and reducing agents such as eugenol, formaldehyde solution 10 per cent and hydroquinone, will stain tooth structure, therefore use is limited to posterior teeth only.

**Hung's m.**, Wilson's m.; a simple flotation m. for detecting helminth eggs in the feces. A sample of feces is mixed with saline and a watch glass filled to the brim with the mixture; when a glass slide is placed in contact with the surface of the fluid the eggs float to the surface and adhere to the undersurface of the slide.

**immunofluorescence m.'s**, any m. in which a fluorescent-labeled antibody is used to detect the presence or determine the location of the corresponding antigen. See fluorescein isothiocyanate.

**impedance m.**, a m. for localizing brain structures by measuring impedance of electric current.

**Indian m.**, Carpue's m.; rhinoplasty by means of a skin flap taken from the forehead; ancient technique used in India where noses were often cut off as a punishment.

**indirect m. for making inlays**, indirect technique; a method whereby the inlay is constructed entirely on a model made from an impression of the prepared tooth or teeth in the mouth.

**indophe′nol m.**, a m. of determining quantitatively the amount of vitamin C in plant and animal tissue based on the rapid reduction of a standardized indophenol solution to a colorless compound by vitamin C in acid solution.

**introspective m.**, in the branch of psychology called functionalism, the systematic study of mental phenomena by contemplating the processes in one's own conscious experiences.

**Italian m.**, Tagliacotian *operation.*

**Jaboulay's m.**, suture of arteries by splitting up the cut ends a short distance and then suturing the flaps together, applying intima to intima; called also the broad marginal confrontation m.

**Johnson's m.**, chloropercha m.

**Kaiserling's m.**, a m. of preserving histologic and pathologic specimens without altering the color; the specimens are immersed in a solution of potassium nitrate 10, potassium acetate 30, formalin 750, distilled water to make 1000.

**Keating-Hart's m.**, fulguration in the treatment of external cancer or of the field of operation after the removal of a malignant growth.

**Kittel's m.**, dispersion of the uratic deposits in gouty joints by massage and manipulation.

**Kittrich's m.**, a cytodiagnostic m. for detecting amniotic discharge by staining a fresh vaginal smear with 0.05 per cent Nile blue sulfate, whereby any fetal epidermal cells will be stained orange to red and all other cells stained blue.

**Kjeldahl m.**, a m. for determining the amount of nitrogen in an organic substance by digesting it with concentrated sulfuric acid in the presence of appropriate catalysts and distilling and determining the ammonia from the ammonium sulfate thus formed.

**Klapp's m.**, treatment of scoliosis by a series of systematic crawling movements whereby the spine is bent laterally and made more flexible.

**Korányi's m.**, a m. of percussion, usually auscultatory percussion; a finger of the examiner's left hand is held vertically against the chest wall while percussion is made by the finger of the right hand tapping its second phalanx.

**Krause's m.**, Krause's graft; skin grafting by means of large strips the entire thickness of the skin but without any of the subcutaneous fat; an application of Wolfe's m. to general surgery.

**Lambotte's m.**, treatment of fractures of the extremities by means of an apparatus, called a *fixateur,* which consists of an extensible steel frame fastened to the bone by pegs inserted above and below the seat of fracture. The apparatus maintains the spatial relationship of the pegs.

**Langendorff's m.**, perfusion of the isolated mammalian heart by carrying fluid under pressure into the sectioned aorta, and thus into the coronary system.

**Lee-White m.**, coagulation time of venous blood is determined in tubes of standard bore at body temperature.

**Levaditi m.**, the use of Cajal's nerve fibril stain for the staining of *Treponema pallidum* in sections; thus impregnated with silver they appear black.

**Liborius' m.**, a m. for culturing anaerobic bacteria; a stab culture is made in the appropriate agar medium, then more of the same medium is liquefied and poured into the test tube on top of the stab culture, effectually sealing it from the air.

**Ling's m.**, lingism; gymnastic exercises (as in Swedish movements) without the use of apparatus.

**Lister's m.**, antiseptic surgery, first advocated by Lister in an article published in 1867. The operation was performed under a cloud of diluted carbolic acid spray, the instruments were dipped in a carbolic solution before use, and the wound was dressed with a thick layer of carbolized gauze. From this was developed the present practice of aseptic surgery.

**longitudinal m.**, in developmental psychology, the study of the life span of one individual involving comparisons of different age levels, as contrasted with cross-sectional m. (*q. v.*).

**Lorenz' m.**, manual, nonbloody reduction of congenital dislocation of the hip, the head of the femur being retained in place by a plaster of Paris splint.

**Lyon and Horgan m.**, the division and ligation of both superior and both inferior thyroid arteries, thereby decreasing the amount of blood entering the gland and cutting off all stimuli from the sympathetic nervous system; an obsolete m. for the relief of angina pectoris and congestive heart failure.

**macro-Kjeldahl m.**, a procedure for analyzing the content of nitrogenous compounds in urine, serum, or other specimens; the test material is treated with a digestion mixture (copper sulfate and sulfuric acid), heated thoroughly, and then alkalinized with a solution of sodium hydroxide; ammonia is then distilled from the mixture, trapped in a boric acid-indicator solution, and titrated with standard hydrochloric or sulfuric acid. The macro-Kjeldahl method, so termed in order to distinguish it from the micromodification, is usually used for determining relatively greater amounts of nitrogen, *e.g.,* 20 to 100 mg.; see also micro-Kjeldahl m.

**Marchi's m.**, hardening the specimen for 8 to 10 days in Müller's fluid, followed by immersion for from 1 to 3 weeks in the same with the addition of $\frac{1}{2}$ part of a 1 per cent solution of osmic acid; fat and degenerating nerve fibers stain black.

**Marshall's m.**, a quantitative procedure for estimating free and conjugated sulfanilamide in body fluids.

**Maydl's m.**, insertion of the ureters into the rectum in cases of exstrophy of the bladder.

**McArthur's m.**, anteroclysis by means of a catheter introduced into the bile duct, in toxic cases following operation on the gallbladder.

**McGavin m.**, filigree *implantation.*

**micro-Astrup m.**, an interpolation technique for acid-base measurement, based on pH and the use of the Siggaard-Andersen nomogram to determine the base deficit as an expression of metabolic acidosis and the arterial $PCO_2$ as an expression of respiratory acidosis or alkalosis.

**micro-Kjeldahl m.,** a modified Kjeldahl procedure designed for the analysis of nitrogenous compounds in relatively small quantities, *e.g.,* specimens in which the total content of nitrogen is in the range of 1 to a few mg. See also macro-Kjeldahl m.

**Momburg's m.,** production of artifical anemia of the pelvis and lower extremities by compression of the abdominal aorta by means of elastic tubing encircling the abdomen midway between the border of the ribs and the iliac crests.

**Moore's m.,** treatment of aneurysm by the introduction of silver or zinc wire into the sac to induce fibrin deposition.

**Müller's m.,** (1) resection of the sclera for detachment of the retina; (2) the obstetrician with one hand passed through the cervix holds the fetal head in flexion, while with the other hand on the abdomen he endeavors to force the head into the brim of the pelvis, thus getting an idea of the possible amount of molding of the head.

**Murphy's m.,** (1) treatment of peritonitis, after operation, by drainage from the lower part of the abdomen or the pelvis (this being favored by the Fowler position), and by continuous irrigation of the lower bowel with physiologic saline solution, the irrigation being made so slowly (Murphy drip) as to secure the absorption of the fluid; (2) arterial suture by invagination of the ends of the vessel over a removable cylinder in two pieces.

**Nakanishi's m.,** a m. for vital staining of bacteria; a slide is treated with hot methylene blue solution until it acquires a sky-blue color, and then a drop of an emulsion of the bacteria is put on the cover glass and the latter is laid on the slide; by this means the bacteria are stained differentially, some parts more intensely than others.

**Needles' split cast m.,** split cast m.

**Nikiforoff's m.,** the fixing of blood films by immersion for 5 to 15 minutes in absolute alcohol, a mixture of equal parts of alcohol and ether, or pure ether.

**Ochsner's m.,** treatment of appendicitis, when operation is not advisable, by peristaltic rest secured by abstention from the use of cathartics and of food by the mouth, by gastric lavage for the relief of nausea and meteorism, and by rectal irrigation (but not large enemas).

**O'Dwyer's m.,** (1) intubation of the larynx; (2) treatment of simple ulcers of the vocal cords by the insertion of a tube coated with alum and gelatin.

**Ollier's m.,** see Thiersch's m.

**Olshausen's m.,** treatment of congenital umbilical hernia by separation of the skin around the sac, removal of Wharton's jelly, reduction of the hernia *en masse* without opening the sac, and suture of the skin.

**open circuit m.,** a m. for measuring oxygen consumption and carbon dioxide production by collecting the expired gas over a known period of time and measuring its volume and composition.

**Orsi-Grocco m.,** palpatory percussion of the heart.

**Pachon's m.,** cardiography, the patient lying on the left side.

**Pappenheim's m.,** a m. for differentiation between the tubercle bacillus and the smegma bacillus; the preparation is stained with hot carbol-fuchsin solution, and then treated with an alcoholic solution of rosolic acid and methylene blue to which glycerin is added; tubercle bacilli are stained bright red, but smegma bacilli are decolorized.

**Paracel'sian m.,** the use of chemical agents only in the treatment of disease.

**parallax m.,** localization of a foreign body by observation of the shadow upon the fluoroscopic screen while the tube is moving at determined distances from the body.

**Pavlov m.,** the m. of studying conditioned reflex activity by the observation of a motor indicator, such as the salivary or electroencephalogram response.

**Perthes' m.,** continuous aspiration of a pleuritic exudate, the drainage tube passing into an airtight receiving vessel which is connected with water power exhaust.

**Politzer m.,** inflation of the Eustachian tube and tympanum by forcing air into the nasal cavity at the instant the patient swallows.

**Porges m.,** a m. of destroying the capsule of bacteria by heating with $N/4$ hydrochloric acid and neutralizing with NaOH.

**Pratt's m.,** orificial *surgery.*

**Purmann's m.,** treatment of aneurysm by extirpation of the sac.

**Quick's m.,** Quick's *test.*

**Rehfuss m.,** fractional m. of test meal examination; a fine tube with fenestrated metal tip is left in the stomach after an Ewald test meal, and small quantities (6 or 8 cc.) of the stomach contents are removed at 15-minute intervals and examined.

**Reverdin's m.,** Thiersch's m.

**Ribera's m.,** production of artificial anemia of the lower extremities by means of compression by an elastic spica the circular turn of which is made around the waist.

**Rideal-Walker m.,** see Rideal-Walker *coefficient.*

**Roux's m.,** division of the inferior maxilla in the median line, to facilitate the operation of ablation of the tongue.

**Scarpa's m.,** cure of aneurysm by ligation of the artery at some distance above the sac.

**Schäfer's m.,** an obsolete m. of resuscitation in cases of drowning or asphyxia; the patient is laid face downward and natural breathing is imitated by gentle intermittent pressure over the lower part of the thorax at the rate of about 15 times a minute.

**Schede's m.,** Schede's clot; supplying the defect in bone, after removal of a sequestrum or scraping away carious material, by allowing the cavity to fill with blood which may become organized.

**Schick m.,** Schick *test.*

**Schlösser's m.,** injection of alcohol into the foramina of exit of the branches of the fifth nerve, for the relief of trigeminal neuralgia.

**Schmidt-Thannhauser m.,** used for the fractionation of nucleic acid, based upon the fact that ribonucleic acid but not deoxyribonucleic acid is hydrolyzed to nucleotides by alkali. Treatment may be carried out at room temperature, the ribonucleic acid being completely hydrolyzed in $\pm 2$ hours in 0.75 N NaOH; usually 18 hours and 0.3 N NaOH are used.

**Schwartz' m.,** treatment of varicose veins by multiple ligatures and sometimes excision of large varices.

**Shaffer-Hartman m.,** an obsolete m. for the quantitative determination of glucose in biological fluids; Benedict's quantitative reagent is added to urine or blood after removal of the proteins, and the mixture boiled in alkaline solution; sulfuric acid is added, and iodate in the reagent reacts with iodide, causing the liberation of free iodine that oxidizes the reduced copper; the remaining free iodine is titrated with thiosulfate, using starch solution to indicate the end point.

**Sippy's m.,** treatment of gastric ulcer by neutralizing the free acid of the gastric juice, with a view to prevent further corrosive action.

**socio-experiential m.,** a m. used in the study of an individual's subjective states without the intervention of the experimenter.

**Somogyi-Shaffer-Hartman m.,** Shaffer-Hartman m.

**split cast m.,** Needles' split cast m.; (1) a procedure for placing indexed casts on an articulator to facilitate their removal and replacement on the instrument; (2) the procedure of checking the ability of an articulator to receive or be adjusted to a maxillomandibular relation record.

**Stas-Otto m.,** a m. of extraction of alkaloids from plants and animal bodies; the substance is digested in alcohol and tartaric acid, then the fatty and resinous matters are precipitated with water, the fluid is treated with an alkali, and the alkaloids are extracted with ether or chloroform.

**Stroganoff's m.,** treatment of eclampsia by morphine, chloral hydrate, and shielding the patient from all external sources of irritation, and rapid delivery.

**Thane's m.,** a m. for indicating the position of the central sulcus (of Rolando) of the brain; the upper end of the sulcus corresponds to the midpoint of a line drawn from the glabella to the inion.

**Theden's m.,** treatment of aneurysms or of large sanguineous effusions by compression of the entire limb by means of a roller bandage.

**Thiersch's m.,** Thiersch's graft; dermoepidermic graft; Reverdin's m.; Ollier's graft or m.; skin grafting with films of epidermis with a portion of the dermis, shaved off in strips and applied to the surface after shaving down the granulations; the m. was published in 1874 but had been previously recommended by Ollier of Lyons in 1872.

**thi'ochrome m.,** a m. for the determination of thiamin based upon the production of thiochrome when the vitamin is oxidized by alkaline ferricyanide to yield the fluorescent compound, thiochrome.

**Uhlenhuth's m.,** (1) precipitin test for human blood by means of an immune serum obtained from rabbits or horses which have received repeated injections of human blood; (2) a m. of the examination of tuberculous sputum by the addition of antiformin.

**ultropaque m.,** ultropak m.; a rapid m. for examining thick (1 to 3 mm.) sections of fresh tissue with the ultramicroscope, making use of an objective built in an illuminator so that the light is reflected down upon the tissue.

**van Ermengen's m.,** a m. for staining flagella; the cover-slip preparation is immersed for an hour in a mixture of glacial acetic acid, osmic acid, and tannic acid solutions, washed in water and then alcohol, immersed for two seconds in 0.5 per cent silver nitrate solution, transferred to a solution of gallic and tannic acids and fused potassium acetate in water, and finally returned to the silver solution and then washed in water.

**Wardrop's m.,** treatment of aneurysm by ligation of the artery at some distance beyond the sac, leaving one or more branches of the artery between the sac and the ligature.

**Westergren m.,** a procedure for estimating the sedimentation rate of red blood cells in fluid blood; 4.5 ml. of venous blood are mixed with 0.5 ml. of 3.8 per cent aqueous solution of sodium citrate, and a special, standard pipet (2-mm. bore, 300 mm. long, graduated at 1-mm. intervals from zero to 200) is filled to the zero mark and placed in an upright position in a special rack. The fall of the red blood cells, in millimeters, is observed in 1 hour; the normal rate for men is zero to 15 mm. (average, 4 mm.), and for women zero to 20 mm. (average, 5mm.).

**Wheeler m.,** a surgical procedure for correction of cicatricial ectropion.

**Wij's m.,** a m. for determining the iodine value of a fat using iodine chloride.

**Willems' m.,** treatment of wounded joints by active mobilization.

**Wilms' m.,** perineal prostatectomy through a lateral incision.

**Wilson's m.,** Hung's m.

**Wolfe's m.,** treatment of ectropion by incision and the insertion of a large graft, the entire thickness of the skin but without any subcutaneous fat.

**Yasuda's m.,** a m. for determining the iodine number using pyridine sulfate dibromide.

---

**meth'odism.** Solidism.

**meth'odist.** A follower of methodism.

**meth'ohex'ital sodium** (USP). BREVITAL sodium; methohexitone; sodium α-dl-methyl-5-allyl-5-(1-methyl-2-pentynyl) barbiturate; an ultrashort-acting barbiturate used intravenously for induction and for general anesthesia of short duration. It is compatible with the skeletal muscle relaxants, and has the advantage that the recovery period is short.

**methohex'itone** (BP). Methohexital sodium.

**methoin** (meth'o-in) (BP). Mephenytoin.

**metho'nium compounds.** Agents that block impulses in ganglia, e.g., hexamethonium, and are used in arterial hypertension.

**methophen'azine.** FRENOLON; 3,4,5-trimethoxybenzoic acid 2-{4-[ 3-(2-chlorophenothiazin-10-yl)propyl ]-1-piperazinyl}ethyl ester; antipsychotic agent.

**methopho'line** (USAN). VERSIDYNE; 1-(p-chlorophenethyl)-1,2,3,4-tetrahydro-6,7-dimethoxy-2-methylisoquinoline; analgesic.

**methop'terin.** 10-Methylfolic acid; 10-methylpteroylglutamic acid; a folic acid antagonist.

**methomania** (meth-o-ma'nĭ-ah) [ G. methe, strong drink, + mania, frenzy ]. A pathological craving for intoxicants.

**methorphinan** (meth-or'fĭ-nan). 3-Hydroxy-N-methylmorphinan; C$_{17}$H$_{23}$NOHBr; see dextromethorphan and levorphanol.

**meth'oser'pidine** (BP). DECASERPYL; 10-methoxydeserpidine; used in the treatment of hypertension.

**meth'otrex'ate** (USP, BP). Amethopterin; 4-amino-10-methylfolic acid; a folic acid antagonist used parenterally for leukemia and other neoplastic diseases.

**methotrimeprazine** (meth'o-tri-mep'ră-zēn) (NF). LEVOPROM; SINOGAN-DEBIL; NIRVAN; 10-[ 3-(dimethylamino)-2-methylpropyl ]-2-methoxyphenothiazine; a phenothiazine analgesic, nearly as potent as morphine but producing less respiratory depression and no addiction.

**methox'amine hydrochloride** (USP). VASOXYL hydrochloride; α-(1-aminoethyl)-2,5-dimethoxybenzyl alcohol; β-hydroxy-β-(2,5-dimethoxyphenyl) isopropylamine hydrochloride; a sympathomimetic amine.

**methoxsalen** (mĕ-thok'să-len) (USP). MELOXINE; OXSORALEN; δ-lactone of 3-(6-hydroxy-7-methoxybenzofuranyl) acrylic acid. A methoxypsoralen derivative; increases melanin production in the skin when exposed to ultraviolet light. Used orally and topically in the treatment of idiopathic vitiligo; also used as a suntan accelerator and sun protectant.

**methoxy-.** Chemical prefix denoting addition of a methoxyl group (CH$_3$O—).

**methox'yflu'rane** (NF, BP). PENTHRANE; 2,2-dichloro-1,1-difluoroethyl methyl ether; a potent, nonflammable, nonexplosive, inhalation anesthetic; low vapor pressure makes induction of anesthesia slow; very high lipid solubility may prolong recovery; adverse side effects may include high output renal failure.

**methox'yl.** The group —OCH$_3$.

**methox'yphen'amine hydrochloride** (NF). ORTHOXINE; β-(o-methoxyphenyl)isopropylmethylamine hydrochloride; a sympathomimetic amine with a predominant bronchodilator action.

**methoxypro'mazine maleate.** MOPAZINE; 10-(3-dimethylaminopropyl)-2-methoxyphenothiazine maleate; antipsychotic agent.

**meth'scopol'amine bromide** (NF). PAMINE bromide; LESCOPINE bromide; epoxytropine tropate methylbromide; a parasympatholytic drug similar to atropine, but more selective; a gastrointestinal antispasmodic used in the management of peptic ulcers, gastritis, intestinal hypermotility and hyperhidrosis.

**meth'scopol'amine nitrate.** SKOPOLATE nitrate; epoxytropine tropate methyl nitrate; has the same action and uses as m. bromide.

**methsuximide** (meth-suk'sĭ-mid) (NF). CELONTIN; N,2-dimethyl-2-phenylsuccinimide; an antiepileptic effective against petit mal and psychomotor epilepsy. Psychic disturbances and liver, kidney and bone marrow damage may occur.

**methyclothiazide** (meth'ĭ-klo-thi'ă-zīd) (NF). ENDURON; 6-chloro-3-(chloromethyl)-3,4-dihydro-2-methyl-2H-1,2,4-benzothiadiazine-7-sulfonamide-1,1-dioxide; an orally effective diuretic and antihypertensive agent of the thiazide group, used in the treatment of edema associated with congestive heart failure, renal disease, hepatic cirrhosis, and premenstrual tension, and in steroid therapy.

**methyl** (meth'il) [ G. methy, wine, + hylē, wood ]. The radical, —CH$_3$.

**active m.,** a m. group attached to a quaternary ammonium ion or a tertiary sulfonium ion which can take part in transmethylation reactions; m. groups in choline and in S-adenosylmethionine are examples.

**m. alcohol** (NF), wood alcohol; methanol; carbinol; wood naphtha; wood spirit; pyroxylic spirit; pyroligneous spirit; CH$_3$OH; a flammable, toxic, mobile liquid, used as an industrial solvent, antifreeze, and in chemical manufacture. Ingestion may result in severe acidosis, visual impairment, and other effects on the central nervous system.

**m. aldehyde,** formaldehyde.

**angular m.,** a m. group attached to carbon 10 (between rings A and B) or to carbon 13 (between rings C and D) of the steroid nucleus.

**m. blue,** an acid triphenylmethane dye, $C_{37}H_{27}N_3O_9S_2$-$Na_2$, used as a plasma and collagen stain for demonstrating Negri bodies.

**m. cysteine hydrochloride,** ACDRILE; mucolytic agent.

**m. donors,** compounds that, in living tissue, are capable of supplying m. groups for transfer to other compounds; quaternary ammonium compounds, such as choline, and tertiary sulfonium compounds, such as *S*-adenosylmethionine, are the chief naturally occurring m. donors; other substances that may act as donors when introduced into tissue, as dimethylthetin, are also known.

**m. ether,** dimethyl ether; $CH_3OCH_3$; a weak inhalation anesthetic with convulsant properties.

**m. green,** a basic triphenylmethane dye, $C_{26}H_{33}N_3Cl_2$, used as a chromatin stain and, in combination with pyronin, for differential staining of ribonucleic acid (red) and deoxyribonucleic acid (green).

**m. hydroxybenzoate** (BP), methylparaben.

**m. isobutyl ketone** (NF), 4-methyl-2-pentanone, an alcohol denaturant; in high concentrations it has narcotic action; in relatively low concentrations it may be irritating to the eyes and mucous membranes.

**m. methacrylate,** a thermoplastic; the main material used for denture bases.

**m. nicotinate,** MIDALGAN; nicotinic acid methyl ester; used as rubefacient.

**m. orange,** sodium salt of helianthine; *p*-(*p*-dimethylaminophenyl)azobenzenesulfonic acid; used as a pH indicator, red at 3.1, yellow at 4.4.

**m. red** (USP), *p*-dimethylaminoazobenzene-*o*-carboxylic acid; a pH indicator at pH 4.4, red; 6.2, yellow; used for estimation of urin pH.

**m. salicylate** (USP, BP), betula oil; sweet birch oil; teaberry oil; methyl ester of salicylic acid; oil of wintergreen; produced synthetically or distilled from *Gaultheria procumbens* or from *Betula lenta.* The distilled variety was called oleum gaultheria and oleum betulae. Used externally and internally for the treatment of various forms of rheumatism. See also gaultheria oil.

**m. violet 6B,** pentamethylbenzyl-*p*-rosaniline hydrochloride; used as indicator, 0.1 per cent solution; at pH 0.1 yellow, 1.5 blue, 3.2 violet.

**m. yellow,** *butter* yellow.

**methylamphetamine hydrochloride** (BP). Methamphetamine hydrochloride.

**meth'ylate.** 1. To mix with methyl alcohol. 2. To introduce a methyl group. 3. A compound of a metal ion with methyl alcohol.

**meth'ylated.** Mixed or compounded with methyl alcohol.

**methyla'tion.** The addition of methyl groups.

**methylatropine bromide** (meth'il-at'ro-pēn, -pin). TROPIN; atropine methylbromide; a cycloplegic.

**meth'ylbenzetho'nium chloride** (NF). DIAPARENE chloride; benzyldimethyl {2-[2-(*p*-1,1,3,3-tetramethylbutyl-cresoxy)ethoxy]-ethyl} ammonium chloride. A quaternary ammonium compound having a surface action like other cationic detergents; generally germicidal and bacteriostatic. Used to rinse infant diapers and bed linen in the prevention of ammonia dermatitis.

**meth'ylben'zol.** Toluene.

**meth'ylcel'lulose** (USP). CELLOTHYL; METHOCEL; methylcellulose 450 (BP); a methyl ether of cellulose; forms a colorless liquid when dissolved in water, alcohol, or ether. Used to increase bulk of intestinal contents and thus to relieve constipation, or of the gastric contents to reduce appetite in obesity; also used dissolved in water as a spray to cover burned areas.

3 (or 20)-**meth'ylcholan'threne.** A highly carcinogenic hydrocarbon that can be formed chemically from deoxycholic or cholic acids, or from cholesterol. The choice between 3- or 20- for the methyl group depends upon whether hydrocarbon (inner) or steroid (outer) numbering is chosen. In the latter case, the formal relationship to the cholic acids and cholesterol is clear.

**methyl 2-cyanoacrylate** (si'ă-no-ak'rĭ-lāt). Methyl α-cyanoacrylate; 2-cyanoacrylic acid methyl ester; a rapidly polymerizing substance used experimentally for hemostasis.

**methylcysteine synthase.** Cystathionine β-synthase.

**meth'yldo'pa** (USP, BP). ALDOMET; (L)-3-(3,4-dihydroxyphenyl)-2-methylalanine; an orally effective hypotensive agent related to the catecholamines; used in the treatment of primary hypertension. It produces fewer untoward reactions than do other hypotensive drugs, but tolerance may develop and reversible hepatic toxicity has been observed.

**meth'yldo'pate hydrochloride** (USP). ALDOMET ester; (L)-3-(3,4-dihydroxyphenyl)-2-methylalanine ethyl ester hydrochloride; same action and uses as methyldopa.

**meth'ylene.** The radical, —$CH_2$—.

**m. bichloride,** dichloromethane.

**m. blue** (USP, BP), 3,7-bis(dimethylamino)phenazathionium chloride; tetramethylthionine chloride; a basic dye used in histology and microbiology; also used as an antidote for methemoglobinemia.

Kuhne's **m. blue,** m. blue 1.5, absolute alcohol 10. 5 per cent phenol solution 100.

Loeffler's **m. blue,** a stain for bacteria; add 30 cc. of alcohol containing 0.3 gm. m. blue to 100 cc. of a 0.01 per cent solution of potassium hydroxide.

new **m. blue,** a basic thiazin dye, $C_{18}H_{22}N_3SCl$, used for supravital staining of reticulocytes in blood smears.

**m. white,** leukomethylene blue.

**methylenophil, methylenophile** (meth'ĭ-lēn'o-fil, -fīl) [ methylene + G. *philos*, fond ]. Methylenophilic; staining readily with methylene blue; denoting certain cells and histologic structures.

**methylenophil'ic, methylenoph'ilous.** Methylenophil.

**methylergometrine maleate** (meth'il-er'go-met'rēn mal'e-āt) (BP). Methylergonovine maleate.

**methylergonovine maleate** (meth'il-er'go-no'vēn mal'e-āt). METHERGINE maleate; methylergometrine maleate; *d*-lysergic acid-*dl*-hydroxybutylamide-2-maleate. A partially synthesized derivative of lysergic acid with oxytocic action, used to prevent or treat postpartum uterine atony and hemorrhage.

**methylglu'camine.** Meglumine.

**m. diatrizoate,** meglumine diatrizoate.

**m. iodipamide** (USP), INTRABILIX; bis-*N*-methylglucamine salt of *N,N*-adipyl-bis-(3-amino-2,4,6-triiodobenzoic acid); a water-soluble organic iodine compound used for intravenous cholangiography and cholecystography.

**meth'ylglyox'al.** Pyruvaldehyde; pyruvic aldehyde; $Ch_3$—$CO_3$—CHO.

**m. bisguanylhydrazone,** 1,1'-[(methylethenediylidene)-dinitro]diguanidine; antineoplastic agent.

**meth'ylglyox'alase.** Lactoyl-glutathione lyase.

*n*-**methylgrana'tonine.** Pseudopelletierine; $C_9H_{15}$-$NO2H_2O$; an alkaloid from the bark of the root of *Punica granatum,* pomegranate; see also granatum.

**methylhexaneamine** (meth'il-hek-sān'ă-mēn, -min). FORTHANE; 4-methyl-2-hexylamine; a volatile sympathetic amine base. Used as an inhalant to constrict the nasal mucosa.

**meth'ylki'nase.** Methyltransferase.

**methylmalon'ic aciduria.** Excretion of excessive amounts of methylmalonic acid in urine due to deficiency of activity of methylmalonyl-CoA mutase. Two types occur: (1) a congenital metabolic error resulting in severe ketoacidosis developing shortly after birth; urine also contains long chain ketones; (2) an acquired type, developing in vitamin $B_{12}$ deficiency.

**meth'ylmercap'tan.** Methanethiol; $CH_3SH$.

3 (or 20)-Methylcholanthrene

**methylnortestos'terone** Normethandrone.

**meth'ylol.** Hydroxymethyl; the monovalent radical, —CH₂OH.

**meth'ylose.** A sugar in which the carbon atom farthest from the carbonyl group is a methyl (CH₃); an ω-deoxysugar.

**meth'ylpar'aben** (USP). NIPAGIN; methyl hydroxybenzoate (BP); methyl *p*-hydroxybenzoate; an antifungal preservative.

**meth'ylpen'tose.** A hexose (a 6-deoxyhexose) in which carbon-6 is part of a methyl group; *e.g.,* rhamnose and fucose.

**meth'ylphen'idate hydrochloride** (USP). RITALIN hydrochloride; methyl α-phenyl-2-piperidineacetate hydrochloride; a central nervous system stimulant used to produce mild cortical stimulation in various types of depressions; commonly used in the treatment of hyperkinetic or hyperactive children.

**meth'ylprednis'olone** (NF, BP). MEDROL; 6-α-methylprednisolone. Has greater anti-inflammatory potency and produces less sodium and water retention than prednisolone. Suitable for oral administration.

    **m. acetate** (USP), DEPO-MEDROL; MEDROL acetate; VERIDERM; 6-methylprednisolone-21-acetate. Has the same actions and uses as m. Aqueous suspensions are suitable for intrasynovial and soft tissue injection.

    **sodium m. succinate** (USP), SOLU-MEDROL; sodium 6-methylprednisolone-21-succinate. It has the same metabolic and anti-inflammatory actions as the parent compound, m. Because of its solubility it can be administered in small volumes.

**methyl-*n*-propyl ether.** METOPRYL; CH₃O(CH₂)CH₃; an effective inhalation anesthetic; disadvantages include flammability, cardiovascular depression, and vagal stimulation.

**meth'ylpyrocatechin** (meth'il-pi-ro-kat'e-kin). Guaiacol.

**meth'ylresor'cinol.** Orcinol.

**methylrosaniline chloride** (meth'il-ro-zan'ĭ-lēn, -lin) (USP). Gentian violet (USP); crystal violet (BP); C₂₅H₃₀N₃Cl; hexamethyl-*p*-rosaniline chloride; a histological and bacterial stain; has been used in the treatment of burns, wounds, and infections of the skin and mucous membranes, and internally for pinworms and certain fluke infestations.

**meth'ylsul'fonal.** Sulfonethylmethane.

**meth'yltestos'terone** (USP, BP). METANDREN; a methyl derivative of testosterone, with the same actions and uses, except that it is active when given orally or sublingually.

**methylthioadenosine.** Thiomethyladenosine; adenosine carrying an —SCH₃ group in place of OH at position 5′; the —SCH₃ group is transferred to α-aminobutyric acid to form methionine in some bacteria.

**methylthiouracil** (meth'il-thi-o-u'ră-sil) (NF, BP). 6-Methyl-2-thiouracil; antithyroid compound with the same action as thiouracil but a smaller dose is required.

**8-methyltocol** (meth'il-to'kol). δ-Tocopherol.

**meth'yltrans'ferase** (EC 2.1.1.). Transmethylase; methylkinase; any enzyme transferring methyl groups from one compound to another.

**methyprylon** (meth'ĭ-pri'lon) (NF). Methyprylone (BP); NOLUDAR; 3,3-diethyl-2,4-dioxo-5-methylpiperidine; a sedative and hypnotic.

**methysergide maleate** (meth'ĭ-ser'jĭd) (USP). SANSERT; N-[ 1-(hydroxymethyl)propyl ]-1-methyl -D-lysergamide bimaleate; a serotonin antagonist, weakly adrenolytic, chemically related to methylergonovine. Used in the prophylactic treatment of vascular headache (migraine). Untoward effects are common.

**methys'ticine.** Kavaine.

**methysticum** (mĕ-this'tĭ-kum). Kava or kava-kava, the root of *Piper methysticum* (family Piperaceae), a plant of the Pacific islands, used by the natives as an intoxicant. Has been used in diarrhea and in inflammatory affection of the urogenital tract.

**MetMb.** Abbreviation for metmyoglobin.

**metmyoglobin** (met'mi'o-glo-bin). Myoglobin in which the ferrous ion of the heme prosthetic group is oxidized to ferric ion.

**metoclo'pramide hydrochloride** (USAN). PASPERTIN; 4-amino-5-chloro-*N*-[ 2-(diethylamino)-ethyl ]-*o*-anisamide hydrochloride; antiemetic agent.

**meto'lazone** (USAN). ZAROXOLYN; 7-chloro-1,2,3,4-tetrahydro-2-methyl-4-oxo-3-*o*- tolyl-6-quinazolinesulfonamide; a diuretic with antihypertensive activity.

**metonymy** (mĕ-ton'o-mī) [ meta- + G. *ōnyma,* name ]. Imprecise or circumscribed labeling of objects or events, said to be characteristic of the language disturbance of schizophrenics; *e.g.,* the patient speaks of having had a "menu" rather than a "meal."

**metopagus** (mĕ-top'ă-gus) [ G. *metōpon,* forehead, + *pagos,* something fixed ]. Conjoined twins united at the forehead.

**meto'pic** [ G. *metōpon,* forehead ]. Relating to the forehead or anterior portion of the cranium.

**metopion** (mĕto'pī-on) [ G. *metōpon,* forehead ]. A craniometric point midway between the frontal eminences.

**met'opism** [ G. *metōpon,* forehead ]. The persistence of the frontal suture in the adult.

**metopodyn'ia** [ G. *metōpon,* forehead, + *odynē,* pain ]. Frontal headache.

**met'opon hydrochlo'ride.** Methyl DILAUDID; methyldihydromorphinone hydrochloride; a derivative of morphine and with the same pharmacologic action, but has double the analgesic potency and is free from emetic action; its efficacy by oral administration is relatively high.

**metopoplasty** (met'o-po-plas'tĭ, mĕ-top'o-plas'tĭ) [ G. *metōpon,* forehead, + *plassō,* to form ]. Reparative surgery of the skin or bone of the forehead.

**metoposcopy** (met'o-pos'ko-pī) [ G. *metōpon,* forehead, + *skopeō,* to view ]. The study of physiognomy.

**metopyrone.** Metyrapone.

**Metorchis** (met-or'kis) [ G. *meta,* behind, + *orchis,* testicle ]. A genus of opisthorchid fish-borne flukes parasitic in the gallbladder of fish-eating mammals and birds; it is especially common in north temperate regions.

    **M. conjunc'tus,** a species that occurs in cats and dogs, and has occasionally been found in man.

**metoser'pate** (USAN). PACITRAN; methyl 11,17α,18α-trimethoxy-3β,20α-yohimban-16β-carboxylate monohydrochloride; a sedative for veterinary use.

**metox'enous** [ G. *meta,* beyond, + *xenos,* host ]. Denoting a parasite with two cycles of existence passed on different hosts.

**metox'eny** [ G. *meta,* beyond, + *xenos,* host ]. 1. Heterecism. 2. Change of host by a parasite.

**metra-, metr-** [ G. *mētra,* uterus ]. Combining forms denoting the uterus.

**metra** (me'trah) [ G. uterus. MAT- ]. Uterus.

**metralgia** (me-tral'jĭ-ah) [ metra- + G. *algos,* pain ]. Hysteralgia.

**metramania** (mĕ-tra-ma'nĭ-ah) [ metra- + G. *mania,* frenzy ]. Hysteromania; a generic term for certain psychoendocrine disturbances caused by uterine disease.

**metrane'mia** [ metra- + G. *an-* priv. + *haima,* blood ]. Local anemia of the uterus.

**metranoicter** (me-tran-oyk'ter) [ metra- + G. *anoigō,* to open ]. An instrument by which dilation of the os uteri is effected by means of two to four blades or branches passed into the os and then separated.

**me'tratome** [ metra- + G. *tomē,* incision ]. Hysterotome.

**metrat'omy.** Hysterotomy.

**metrato'nia** [ metra- + G. *a-* priv. + *tonos,* tension ]. Atony of the uterine walls after childbirth.

**metratrophy, metratrophia** (me-trat'ro-fī, me-trătro'fī-ah) [ metra- atrophy ]. Uterine atrophy.

**metrauxe** (me-trawk'se) [ metra- + G. *auxē,* increase ]. Hypertrophy of the uterus.

**metrectasia** (me'trek-ta'zĭ-ah) [ metra- + G. *ektasis,* extension ]. Dilation of the uterus.

**metrectomy** (me-trek'to-mī) [ metra- + G. *ektomē,* excision ]. Obsolete term for hysterectomy.

**metrecto'pia, metrec'topy** [ metra- + G. *ektopos,* out of place ]. Displacement of the uterus.

**metreurynter** (me'tru-rin'ter) [ metra- + G. *eurynō,* to dilate ]. Hystereurynter.

**metreurysis** (me-tru'rĭ-sis) [ metra- + G. *eurynō*, to dilate ]. Hystereurysis.

**me'tria** [ G. *mētra*, uterus ]. Pelvic cellulitis or other inflammatory affection in the puerperal period.

**met'ric** [ G. *metrikos*, fr. *metron*, measure ]. Quantitative; relating to measurement. See metric *system*.

**metriocephalic** (met'rĭ-o-se-fal'ik) [ G. *metrios*, moderate, fr. *metron*, measure, + *kephalē*, head ]. Having a well proportioned head as regards height; denoting a skull with an index between 72 and 77. Similar to orthocephalic.

**metri'tis** [ G. *mētra*, uterus, + suffix *-itis*, inflammation ]. Hysteritis; uteritis; inflammation of the uterus.

**metrizo'ate sodium** (USAN). ISOPAQUE; 3-acetamido-5-(*N*-methylacetamido)-2,4,6-triiodobenzoic acid sodium salt; radiographic contrast medium.

**metro-** (me'tro-, met'ro-) [ G. *metra*, uterus. MAT- ]. Combining form relating to the uterus. See also hystero-, utero-.

**metrocele** (me'tro-sēl) [ metro- + G. *kēlē*, hernia ]. Hysterocele.

**metroclyst** (me'tro-klist) [ metro- + G. *klystēr*, a washing out ]. A uterine irrigator.

**metrocolpocele** (me-tro-kol'po-sēl) [ metro- + G. *kolpos*, bosom (vagina), + *kēlē*, hernia ]. Prolapse of the uterus.

**metrocystosis** (me'tro-sis-to'sis) [ metro- + G. *kystis*, cyst, + suffix *-osis*, condition ]. The formation of uterine cysts.

**metrocyte** (me'tro-sīt) [ G. *mētēr*, mother, + *kytos*, a hollow (cell) ]. A mother *cell*.

**metrodynamometer** (me'tro-di'nă-mom'e-ter) [ metro- + G. *dynamis*, power, + *metron*, measure ]. An instrument for measuring the force of uterine contractions.

**me'trodyn'ia** [ metro- G. *odynē*, pain ]. Hysteralgia.

**me'trofibro'ma.** A fibroma of the uterus.

**metrography** (me-trog'ră-fī) [ metro- + G. *graphō*, to write ]. Hysterography.

**metrolymphangitis** (me'tro-lim-fan-ji'tis) [ metro- + lymphangitis, *q.v.* ]. An inflammation of the uterine lymphatics.

**metromalacia** (me'tro-mă-la'shĭ-ah) [ metro- + G. *malakia*, softness ]. Pathologic softening of the uterine tissues.

**me'tromalaco'ma, me'tromalaco'sis.** Metromalacia.

**met'roma'nia** [ G. *metron*, measure, + *mania*, frenzy ]. Mania for incessant writing of verses.

**metronidazole** (met'ro-nid'ă-zōl) (USP, BP). FLAGYL; 2-methyl-5-nitroimidazole-1-ethanol; an orally effective trichomonicide used in the treatment of infections caused by *Trichomonas vaginalis*. The incidence of untoward reactions is low.

**metronoscope** (mē-tron-'o-skōp) [ G. *metron*, measure, + *skopeō*, to view ]. A tachistoscopic apparatus that exposes for timed intervals short selections of printed matter for reading; used in testing and developing reading speed.

**metroparalysis** (me'tro-pă-ral'ĭ-sis) [ metro- + paralysis, *q.v.* ]. Flaccidity or paralysis of the uterine muscle during or immediately after childbirth.

**metropath'ia** [ L. ]. Metropathy.

   **m. hemorrhag'ica,** abnormal, excessive, often continuous uterine bleeding due to persistence and exaggeration of the follicular phase of the menstrual cycle. The endometrium is the seat of glandular hyperplasia with cyst formation (see Swiss cheese *endometrium*).

**me'tropath'ic.** Relating to or caused by uterine disease.

**metropathy** (me-trop'ă-thī) [ metro- + G. *pathos*, suffering ]. Any disease of the uterus.

**metroperitonitis** (me'tro-pĕr'ĭ-to-ni'tis) [ metro- + peritonitis, *q.v.* ]. Perimetritis; inflammation of the uterus involving the peritoneal covering.

**metrophlebitis** (me'tro-flĕ-bi'tis) [ metro- + G. *phleps*, vein, + suffix *-itis*, inflammation ]. Inflammation of the uterine veins usually following childbirth.

**me'troplasty.** Uteroplasty.

**metroptosis, metroptosia** (me'trop-to'sis, -to'sĭ-ah) [ metro- + G. *ptōsis*, a falling ]. Hysteroptosis; falling or prolapse of the uterus.

**metrorrhagia** (me'tro-ra'jĭ-ah) [ metro- + G. *rhēgnymi*, to burst forth. RHAG- ]. Irregular, acyclic bleeding from the uterus, particularly between periods.

   **m. myopath'ica.** postpartum hemorrhage due to flaccidity of the uterine muscle.

**metrorrhea** (me'tro-re'ah) [ metro- + G. *rhoia*, a flow ]. A discharge of mucus or pus from the uterus.

**metrorrhexis** (me'tro-rek'sis) [ metro- + G. *rhēxis*, rupture ]. Hysterorrhexis.

**metrorthosis** (met'ror-tho'sis) [ metro- + G. *orthōsis*, a making straight ]. The correction of a displacement of the uterus.

**metrosalpingitis** (me-tro-sal-pin-ji'tis) [ metro- + G. *salpinx*, trumpet (oviduct), + suffix *-itis*, inflammation ]. Inflammation of the uterus and of one or both Fallopian tubes.

**metrosalpingography** (me-tro-sal-pin-gog'raf-ī) [ metro- + G. *salpinx*, tube, + *graphō*, to write ]. Hysterosalpingography.

**metroscirrhus** (me'tro-skĭr'us, -sĭr'us) [ metro- + G. *skirrhos*, a hard tumor ]. A scirrhous cancer of the uterus with a predominance of connective tissue.

**metroscope** (me'tro-skōp) [ metro- + G. *skōpeō*, to view ]. Hysteroscope.

**metrostaxis** (me'tro-stak'sis) [ metro- + G. *staxis*, a dripping ]. A dripping of blood from the uterine mucous membrane; a small but continuous uterine hemorrhage.

**metrostenosis** (me'tro-stē-no'sis) [ metro- + G. *stenosis*, a narrowing ]. A narrowing of the uterine cavity.

**me'trotome.** Hysterotome.

**metrotomy** (me-trot'o-mĭ) [ metro- + G. *tomē*, incision ]. Hysterotomy.

**metrourethrotome** (met'ro-u-re'thro-tōm) [ G. *metron*, measure, + *ourēthra*, urethra, + *tomos*, cutting ]. A form of urethrotome with which, by means of a screw attachment, the exact extent of division of the urethra can be regulated.

**metryperesthesia** (me-tri'per-es-the'sĭ-ah) [ G. *metra*, uterus, + *hyper*, overmuch, + *aisthēsis*, sensation ]. Extreme sensitiveness or hyperesthesia of the uterus.

**metryperkinesis, metryperkinesia** (me-tri'per-kĭ-ne'sis, -kĭ-ne'zĭ-ah) [ G. *mētra*, uterus, + *hyper*, overmuch, + *kinēsis*, movement ]. Excessive labor pains.

**metrypertrophia** (me-tri'per-tro'fĭ-ah) [ G. *mētra*, uterus, + *hyper*, overmuch, + *trophē*, nourishment ]. Hypertrophy of the uterus.

**M. et sig.** Abbreviation for L. *misce et signa*, mix and write, or label.

**metyrapone** (mĕ-tĭr'ă-pōn) (USP, BP). METROPIONE; METOPIRONE; mepyrapone; metopyrone; 2-methyl-1,2-di-3-pyridyl-1-propanone; an inhibitor of adrenocortical steroid C-11β hydroxylation; administered orally or intravenously to determine the ability of the pituitary gland to increase its secretion of corticotropin. Because 11-deoxycortico-steroids, a consequence of metyrapone administration, only weakly inhibit pituitary corticotropin secretion, the normal pituitary gland will appreciably increase its output of this hormone.

**meturedepa** (USAN). TURLOC; [ bis(2,2-dimethyl-1-aziridinyl)phosphinyl ]carbamic acid ethyl ester; antineoplastic agent.

**Mev.** The symbol for 1 million electron-volts, or $10^6$ ev.

**meval'dic acid.** $CHO—CH_2—C(CH_3)(OH)—CH_2—COOH$; 3-hydroxy-3-methylglutaraldehydic acid; see mevalonic acid.

**mev'alon'ic acid.** $HOCH_2—CH_2—C(CH_3)(OH)—CH_2—COOH$; a dihydroxy acid; precursor of squalene and steroids.

**mexenone.** UVISTAT; 2-hydroxy-4-methoxy-4'-methylbenzophenone; sun-screening agent.

**Meyenburg,** H. von. See M.'s *complex, disease,* M.-Altherr-Uehlinger *syndrome.*

**Meyer,** Adolf, American psychiatrist, 1866–1950. See M.-Archambault *loop.*

**Meyer,** Edmund V., Berlin laryngologist, 1864–1931. See M.'s *cartilages.*

**Meyer,** Georg H., German anatomist, 1815–1892. See M.'s *disease, line, sinus.*

**Meyer,** Hans H., German pharmacologist, 1853–1939. See M.-Overton *theory* of narcosis.

**Meyer,** Willy, American surgeon, 1854–1932. See M.'s *reagent.*

**Meyerhof,** Otto F., German biochemist, 1884–1951. Nobel laureate, 1922, with A. V. Hill, for the discovery of the fixed relationship between the consumption of oxygen and the metabolism of lactic acid in muscle. See Embden-M. *pathway,* Embden-M.-Parnas *pathway.*

**Meyer-Schwickerath,** Gerd. See M.-S. and Weyers *syndrome.*

**Meynert** (mi'nert), Theodor H., Vienna neurologist, 1833–1892. See M.'s *bundle, cells, commissure, fasciculus, layer.*

**Meynet** (ma-na'), Paul C. H., French physician, 1831–1892. See M.'s *nodosities.*

**meze'reon, meze'reum** [ Ar. *māzariyūn,* camellia ]. The bark of *Daphne mezereum* (family Thymelaeaceae); wild pepper; spurge olive. Formerly used in the treatment of rheumatism, syphilis and indolent skin ulcers.

**Mg.** Chemical symbol of the element magnesium.

**mg.** Abbreviation for milligram.

**mho** (mo) [ *ohm* reversed ]. The unit of electrical conductivity; the conductivity of a body having the resistance of one ohm.

**mianserin hydrochloride** (me-an'ser-in) (USAN). 1,2,3,4,10,14b-Hexahydro-2-methyldibenzo[ *c,f* ] pyrazino- [ 1,2-α ]azepine monohydrochloride; an antihistaminic with antiserotonin activity.

**miasm, miasma** (mi'azm, mi-az'mah) [ G. *miasma,* stain ]. Noxious effluvia or emanations, formerly regarded as the cause of malaria and of various epidemic diseases.

**mi'asmat'ic.** Relating to or caused by miasma.

**miasmology** (mi'az-mol'o-ji) [ G. *miasma,* miasm, + *logos,* study ]. The science that deals with air pollutants and aerosols in general, and especially in relation to human health.

**Mibelli** (me-bel'e), Vittorio, Italian dermatologist, 1860–1910. See M.'s *angiokeratoma, disease.*

**mica** (mi'kah) [ L. ]. A crumb or small morsel.
m. pa'nis, breadcrumb.

**mice.** See mouse; *Mus.*
joint m., see under joint.

**micel'lar.** Having the properties of an assemblage of micelles, *i.e.,* of a gel.

**micelle** (mi-sel', mi-sel') [ L. *micella,* small morsel, dim. of *mica,* morsel, grain ]. A term created by Nägeli (1817–1891) for elongated, sub(light)microscopic particles detected by hydrogels, of supramolecular character and crystalline structure. More recently defined as one of two classes of colloidal particle, consisting of many molecules, the other class being single macromolecules light- or submicroscopic in size. A m. is thus a structural unit of the disperse phase in a gel, a unit whose repetition in three dimensions constitutes the micellar structure of the gel. The term is frequently misused to denote the individual particles in free suspension or solution, or the unit structure of a crystal.

**Michaelis,** L., U. S. chemist, 1875–1949. See M.-Gutmann *body,* M.-Menten *constant, hypothesis.*

**Micheli** (me-ka'le), Ferdinando, Italian physician, 1872–1936. See Marchiafava-M. *anemia,* Marchiafava-M. *syndrome.*

**micon'azole nitrate** (USAN). 1-[ 2,4-Dichloro-β- [ (2,4-dichlorobenzyl)oxy ]phenethyl ]imidazole mononitrate; an antifungal agent.

**micr-.** See micro-.

**micracoustic** (mi'kră-koo'stik) [ micro- + G. *akoustikos,* relating to hearing, fr. *akouō,* to hear ]. Microcoustic. 1. Relating to faint sounds. 2. Magnifying very faint sounds so as to make them audible.

**mi'crencepha'lia.** Micrencephaly.

**micrencephalon** (mi-kren-sef'ă-lon) [ micro- + G. *enkephalos,* brain ]. Microencephalon. 1. The cerebellum. 2. Rarely used term meaning an abnormally small brain.

**mi'crenceph'alous.** Having a small brain.

**micrencephaly** (mi'kren-sef'ă-lī) [ micro- + G. *enkephalos,* brain ]. Micrencephalia; microencephaly; abnormal smallness of the brain.

**micro-** (mi'kro-) [ G. *mikros,* small ]. A prefix denoting smallness. (1) When prefixed to a term denoting a unit of any kind, it denotes the one-millionth of such unit; (2) applied to words denoting chemical examination, methods, etc., it means that minimal quantities of the substance to be examined are used—a drop or two, for example, in place of one or more cubic centimeters; (3) a combining form meaning microscopic.

**microabscess** (mi'kro-ab'ses). A very small circumscribed collection of leukocytes in solid tissues.
**Munro's m.,** Munro's abscess; a microscopic collection of leukocytes found in the stratum corneum at the granular layer in psoriasis.
**Pautrier's m.,** Pautrier's abscess; a microscopic lesion in the epidermis, seen in mycosis fungoides; it is composed of the same type of cells as those that form the infiltrate in the corium.

**microaerobion** (mi'kro-a-er-o'bī-on). A microaerophilic microorganism.

**microaerophil, microaerophile** (mi-kro-a'er-o-fil, -fil) [ micro- + G. *aēr,* air, + *philos,* fond ]. 1. An aerobic bacterium that requires oxygen, but less than is present in the air, and grows best under modified atmospheric conditions. 2. Microaerophilic; microaerophilous; relating to such an organism.

**microaerophilic** (mi-kro-a'er-o-fil'ik). Microaerophil (2).

**microaerophilous** (mi-kro-a'er-of'ī-lus). Microaerophil (2).

**microaerosol** (mi'kro-a'er-o-sol). A suspension in air of particles that are submicronic or, more frequently, from 1 to 10 μ in diameter.

**microaerotonometer** (mi'kro-a'er-o-to-nom'e-ter) [ micro- + aerotonometer, *q.v.* ]. An instrument for measuring volume of gases in blood.

**microanalysis** (mi'kro-ă-nal'ī-sis). Special analytic techniques involving unusually small samples.

**microanatomist** (mi'kro-ă-nat'o-mist). Histologist.

**microanatomy** (mi'kro-ă-nat'o-mī). Histology.

**microaneurysm** (mi'kro-an'u-rizm). Focal dilation of retinal capillaries in diabetics, or arteriolocapillary junctions in many organs in thrombotic thrombocytopenic purpura.

**microangiography** (mi'kro-an' jī-og'ră-fī). The radiography of the finer vessels of an organ after the injection of a contrast medium and enlarging the resulting radiogram.

**microangiopathy** (mi'kro-an-jī-op'ă-thī). Capillaropathy.
**thrombotic m.,** thrombosis within small blood vessels, as in thrombotic thrombocytopenic *purpura, q. v.*

**microangioscopy** (mi'kro-an'jī-os'ko-pī). Capillarioscopy.

**microarteriography** (mi'kro-ar-tēr-ī-og'ră-fī). Microangiography.

**mi'crobal'ance.** A balance designed for use in weighing unusually small samples of materials.

**microbe** (mi'krōb) [ Fr. fr. G. *mikros,* small, + *bios,* life ]. A very minute organism; originated by Sédillot in France in 1878, the word was offered as an alternative to the many terms then in use for the large variety of microorganisms; modern usage has retained the originally intended broad meaning, both microscopic and ultramicroscopic organisms (including spirochetes, bacteria, rickettsiae, and viruses) being included within its scope. These organisms form a biologically distinctive group, all having a procaryotic genetic mechanism.

**micro'bial.** Microbic; microbiotic (2); relating to a microbe or microbes.

**mi'crobialler'gic.** Allergic to microbial agents; denoting an allergic reaction caused by sensitivity to specific microbial agents (bacteria) or bacterial protein.

**micro'bic.** Microbial.

**microbicidal** (mi-kro'bi-si'dal). Destructive to microbes; microbicide.

**microbicide** (mi-kro'bī-sid) [ microbe + L. *caedo,* to kill ]. 1. Microbicidal. 2. An agent destructive to microbes; a germicide; an antiseptic.

**micro'bid** [ micro- + G. *bios,* life, + *eidés,* resembling; see -id ]. Cutaneous allergic response to superficial bacterial infection.

**microbiologic** (mi-kro-bi-o-loj'ik). Relating to microbiology.

**mi'crobiol'ogist.** One who pursues the science of microbiology.

**microbiology** (mi'kro-bi-ol'o-jī) [ Fr. *microbiologie* ]. The science dealing with microbes (microscopic and ultramicroscopic organisms).

**micro'bion.** Obsolete term for microbe.

**microbiot'ic.** 1. Short-lived. 2. Microbial.

**mi'crobism.** Infection with microbes.

   **latent m.,** the presence of pathogenic microorganisms in the body, which give rise to no symptoms; the condition of a bacilli carrier.

**mi'croblast** [ micro- + G. *blastos,* sprout, germ ]. A small, nucleated, red blood cell.

**microblepharia** (mi'kro-blĕ-făr'ĭ-ah) [ micro- + G. *blepharon,* eyelid, + suffix *-ia,* condition ]. Microblepharism; microblepharon; a rare developmental anomaly characterized by eyelids of abnormally short vertical dimension.

**microbleph'arism, microbleph'aron.** Microblepharia.

**mi'crobody.** Peroxisome.

**microbrachia** (mi-kro-bra'kĭ-ah) [ micro- + G. *brachiōn,* arm ]. Abnormal smallness of the arms.

**microbrachius** (mi-kro-bra'kĭ-us). A malformed individual with rudimentary arms.

**microbren'ner** [ micro- + Ger. *Brenner,* burner ]. An electric cautery with needle point.

**microcar'dia** [ micro- + G. *kardia,* heart ]. Abnormally small size of the heart.

**microcar'dius.** An individual with an abnormally small heart.

**microcen'trum** [ micro- + G. *kentron,* center ]. Cytocentrum.

**microcepha'lia.** Microcephaly.

**microcephalic** (mi'kro-sĕ-fal'ik). Microcephalous; having a small head; denoting a skull with a capacity below 1350 cc., or an individual having such a skull.

**microceph'alism.** Microcephaly.

**microceph'alous.** Microcephalic.

**microcephalus** (mi'kro-sef'ă-lus). 1. One with an abnormally small head. 2. An individual with rudimentary or imperfectly developed head.

**microcephaly** (mi'kro-sef'ă-lī) [ micro- + G. *kephalē,* head ]. Microcephalia; microcephalism; abnormal smallness of the head; see microcephalic.

   **encephaloclastic m.,** complex growth disturbances in the brain as a result of regressive changes in fetal life.

   **schizencephalic m.,** dysgenic process resulting in focal cerebral defects.

**microcheilia, microchilia** (mi-kro-ki'lĭ-ah) [ micro- + G. *cheilos,* lip ]. Smallness of the lips.

**microcheiria, microchiria** (mi'kro-ki'rĭ-ah) [ micro- + G. *cheir,* hand ]. Smallness of the hands.

**michrochemical** (mi'kro-kem'ĭ-kal). Relating to microchemistry.

**microchemistry** (mi'kro-kem'is-trī) 1. The chemistry of microscopic objects. 2. Microscopic observation of chemical reactions.

**microchi'lia.** Microcheilia.

**microchi'ria.** Microcheiria.

**microcinematography** (mi'kro-sin-e-mă-tog'ră-fī) [ micro- + G. *kinēma,* movement, + *graphō,* to write ]. The application of moving pictures taken through magnifying lenses to the study of an organ or system in motion; *e.g.,* the circulation in living embryos.

**mi'crocir'cula'tion.** Circulation in the smallest vessels, namely arterioles, capillaries, and venules.

**microclyster** (mi'kro-klis'ter) [ micro- + G. *klystēr,* enema, fr. *klyzō,* to wash out ]. A very small rectal injection; *e.g.,* a teaspoonful or two of glycerin.

**Micrococcaceae** (mi-kro-kok-a'se-e). A family of bacteria (order Eubacteriales) containing Gram-positive spherical cells which occur singly or in pairs, tetrads, packets, irregular masses, or even chains. Rarely are these organisms motile. Free living, saprophytic, parasitic, and pathogenic species occur. The type genus is *Micrococcus.*

**micrococcin** (mi-kro-kok'sin). Micrococcin P.; an antibiotic obtained from a strain of *Micrococcus* resembling *M. varians;* it has some antituberculous activity.

**Micrococcus** (mi'kro-kok-us) [ micro- + G. *kokkos,* berry ]. A genus of bacteria (family Micrococcaceae) containing Gram-positive, spherical cells that occur in irregular masses, never in packets. Some species are motile or produce motile mutants. These organisms are saprophytic, facultatively parasitic or parasitic but are not truly pathogenic. The type species is *M. luteus.* It is the type genus of the family Micrococcaceae.

   **M. can'didus,** a species found in skin secretions, milk, and dairy products.

   **M. conglomera'tus,** a species found in infections, milk, dairy products, dairy utensils, and water.

   **M. cryoph'ilus,** a species found in frozen meat products.

   **M. flavus,** a species found in skin gland secretions, milk, dairy products, and dairy utensils.

   **M. lu'teus,** a saprophytic species found in milk and dairy products and on dust particles. It is the type species of the genus *M.*

   **M. morrhua,** a species found in sea-water brine, sea salt, and salt lakes; also found in association with a red discoloration of salted fish.

   **M. ure'ae,** a species found in stale urine or in soil containing urine.

   **M. varians,** a species found in body secretions, dairy products, dairy utensils, dust, and fresh and salt water.

**microcolon** (mi'kro-ko'lon). A small colon.

**microcoria** (mi'kro-ko'rĭ-ah) [ micro- + G. *korē,* pupil ]. Congenital contraction of the pupil (miosis).

**microcornea** (mi'kro-kor'ne-ah). A condition in which the cornea is thinner and flatter than normal.

**microcoulomb** (mi-kro-koo'lom). An electrical microunit of quantity, the one-millionth of a coulomb.

**microcoustic** (mi-kro-koo'stik). Micracoustic.

**microcrys'talline.** Occurring in minute crystals.

**microcurie** (mi'kro-ku're). A measure of radium emanation, one-millionth of a curie; $3.7 \times 10^4$ disintegrations per second; abbreviated $\mu$Ci.

**microcyst** (mi'kro-sist). A tiny cyst, frequently of such dimensions that a magnifying lens or microscope is required for observation.

**microcy'tase.** According to Metchnikoff, a cytase or complement that is formed by the multinuclear leukocytes and is capable of destroying bacteria.

**microcyte** (mi'kro-sīt) [ micro- + G. *kytos,* cell ]. Microerythrocyte; a small (5 $\mu$ or less) non-nucleated red blood cell.

**microcythemia** (mi'kro-si-the'mĭ-ah) [ microcyte + G. *haima,* blood ]. Microcytosis; the presence of many microcytes in the circulating blood.

**microcyto'sis.** [ microcyte + G. suffix *-osis,* condition ]. Microcythemia.

**microdactylia** (mi'kro-dak-til'ĭ-ah). Microdactyly.

**microdactylous** (mi'kro-dak'tĭ-lus). Relating to or characterized by microdactyly.

**microdactyly** (mi'kro-dak'tĭ-lī) [ micro- + G. *dactylos,* finger, toe ]. Smallness or shortness of the fingers or toes.

**mi'crodeter'mina'tion.** See micro- (2).

**microdissection** (mi'kro-dī-sek'shun). Dissection of tissues under a microscope or magnifying glass, usually done by teasing the tissues apart by means of needles.

**mi'crodont** [ micro- + G. *odous* (*odont-*), tooth ]. Having small teeth; denoting a skull with a dental index below 41.9.

**microdontia** (mi'kro-don'shĭ'ah) [ micro- + G. *odous,* tooth ]. Microdontism; a condition in which a single tooth, or pairs of teeth, or the whole dentition may be disproportionately smaller than body build. See also microdont.

**microdon'tism.** Microdontia.

**microdose** (mi'kro-dōs). A very small dose.

**mi'crodrep'anocyto'sis** [ microcytosis + drepanocytosis ]. A chronic hemolytic anemia resulting from interaction of the genes for sickle cell anemia and thalassemia.

**microelectrode** (mi'kro-e-lek'trōd). An electrode of very fine caliber consisting usually of a fine wire or a glass tube of capillary diameter (10 $\mu$ to 1 mm.) drawn to a fine point and filled with saline or a metal such as gallium or indium (while melted). Used in physiologic experiments to stimulate or to record action currents from a very small area of tissue.

**mi'croenceph'alon.** Micrencephalon.

**mi'croenceph'aly.** Micrencephaly.

**microerythrocyte** (mi'kro-ĕ-rith'ro-sīt). Microcyte.

**mi'croes'tima'tion.** See micro- (2).

**mi'croevolu'tion.** The evolution of bacteria and other microorganisms through mutations.

**mi'crofar'ad.** A microunit of electrical capacity, the millionth part of a farad.

**microfilaremia** (mi'kro-fil-ă-re'mĭ-ah). Infection of the blood with microfilariae.

**microfilaria,** pl. **microfila'riae** (mi'kro-fĭ-lăr'ĭ-ah). Term for embryos of all forms of filarial nematodes in the superfamily Filarioidea (*q.v.*); see also *Filaria*. This term has sometimes been used as a genus name; *e.g., Microfilaria bancrofti, Microfilaria diurna, Microfilaria malaya*.

**microgamete** (mi-kro-gam'ēt) [ micro- + G. *gametēs*, husband ]. The male element in anisogamy, or conjugation of cells of unequal size; it is the smaller of the two cells and actively motile.

**microgametocyte** (mi-kro-gam'e-to-sīt). Microgamont; the mother cell producing the microgametes, or male elements of sexual reproduction in Protozoa.

**microgam'ont.** Microgametocyte.

**microgamy** (mi-krog'ă-mī) [ micro- + G. *gamos*, marriage ]. Conjugation between two young cells, the recent product of sporulation or some other form of reproduction.

**microgas'tria** [ micro- + G. *gastēr*, stomach ]. Smallness of the stomach.

**microgenia** (mi'kro-je'nĭ-ah) [ micro- + G. *geneion*, chin ]. Abnormal smallness of the chin.

**microgenitalism** (mi-kro-jen'ĭ-tal-izm). Abnormal smallness of the external genital organs.

**microglia** (mi-krog'lĭ-ah) [ micro- + G. *glia*, glue ]. Microglia or microglial cells; Hortega cells; small neuroglial cells of mesodermal origin which may become phagocytic, hence are considered elements of the reticuloendothelial system.

**microgliacyte** (mi-kro-gli'ă-sīt) [ micro- + G. *glia*, glue, + *kytos*, cell ]. A cell, especially an embryonic cell, of the microglia.

**microglioma** (mi-krog'lĭ-o'mah) [ microglia + G. suffix *-oma*, tumor ]. An intracranial neoplasm of microglial cell origin that is structurally similar to reticulum cell sarcoma.

**microgliosis** (mi-krog'lĭ-0'sis) [ microglia + G. suffix *-osis*, condition ]. Presence of microglia in nervous tissue secondary to injury.

**microglos'sia** [ micro- + G. *glōssa*, tongue ]. Smallness of the tongue.

**micrognathia** (mi'kro-na'thĭ-ah, mi-krog-nath'ĭ-ah) [ micro- + G. *gnathos*, jaw ]. Smallness of the jaws, especially of the underjaw.

    **m. with peromelia,** Hanhart's syndrome; hypoplasia of the mandible with malformed and missing teeth, birdlike face, severe deformities of the hands and forearms and sometimes of feet and legs; probably due to a recessive gene.

**microgonioscope** (mi'kro-go'nĭ-o-skōp) [ micro- + G. *gōnia*, angle, + *skopeō*, to examine ]. An instrument for measuring minute angles, used in the study of glaucoma.

**mi'crogram.** The millionth part of a gram, equivalent to about ¹⁄₆₈₀₀₀ grain. Symbol, $\mu$g.

**mi'crograph** [ micro- + G. *graphō*, to write ]. 1. An instrument that magnifies the microscopic movements of a diaphragm by means of light interference and records them on a moving photographic film; it may be used for recording various pulse curves, sound waves, and any

forms of motion that may be communicated through the air to a diaphragm. 2. Photomicrograph.

**micrography** (mi-krog'ră-fī) [ micro- + G. *graphō*, to write ]. 1. Writing with very minute letters, sometimes observed in psychoses and in paralysis agitans. 2. A description of microscopic objects; a treatise on histology.

**microgyria** (mi-kro-ji'rĭ-ah) [ micro- + G. *gyros*, convolution ]. Abnormal narrowness of the cerebral convolutions.

**microhepatia** (mi-kro-hep-ah'tĭ-ah) [ micro- + G. *hepar* (*hepat*-), liver ]. Abnormal smallness of the liver.

**microhm** (mi'krōm). Micro-ohm; a microunit of electrical resistance; the millionth of an ohm.

**mi'croincin'era'tion.** Spodography; combustion, in a furnace, of organic constituents in a tissue section, so that the remaining mineral ash can be examined microscopically.

**microincision** (mi-kro-in-sizh'un). Micropuncture; destruction of cellular organelles by ruby laser beam.

**mi'croinva'sion.** Invasion of tissue immediately adjacent to a carcinoma in situ, the earliest stage of malignant neoplastic invasion.

**mi'crokymat'other'apy** [ micro- + G. *kyma*, a wave, + *therapeia*, treatment ]. Microwave therapy; treatment with high frequency radiations, 3,000,000,000 cycles (3000 megacycles) per second, at a wavelength of 10 cm.

**mi'crolens.** A small, thin corneal contact lens with single curve, diameter 9.5 mm., and thickness 0.15 to 0.30 mm.

**microlentia** (mi'kro-len'shĭ-ah). Spherophakia.

**microleukoblast** (mi-kro-lu'ko-blast). Micromyeloblast; myeloblast.

**microliter** (mi'kro-le-ter). The millionth part of a liter, about ¹⁄₇₀ drop. Symbol, $\mu$l.

**mi'crolith** [ micro- + G. *lithos*, stone ]. A minute calculus, usually multiple, constituting a coarse sand called gravel.

**microlithiasis** (mi-kro-lĭ-thi'ă-sis). The formation, presence, or discharge of minute concretions, or gravel.

    **pulmonary alveolar m.,** microscopic granules of calcium or bone disseminated throughout the lungs.

**micrology** (mi-krol'o-jī) [ micro- + G. *logos*, study ]. The science of microscopic objects, of which histology is a branch.

**micromania** (mi'kro-ma'nĭ-ah) [ micro- + G. *mania*, frenzy ]. A delusion of self-depreciation, or that one's own body is of minute size.

**mi'cromanip'ulation.** Dissection, teasing, stimulation, etc., under the microscope, of minute structures, *e.g.,* tissue cells or unicellular organisms.

**mi'cromanip'ulator.** An instrument used in micromanipulation, whereby microdissection, microinjection, and other maneuvers are performed, usually with the aid of a microscope.

**microma'zia** [ micro- + G. *mazos*, breast ]. Condition in which the breasts are rudimentary and functionless.

**micromegaly** (mi'kro-meg'ă-lī) [ micro- + G. *megas*, large ]. Progeria.

**micromelia** (mi'kro-me'lĭ-ah) [ micro- + G. *melos*, limb ]. The condition of having disproportionately short or small limbs; see also achondroplasia.

**microm'elus.** A malformed individual with rudimentary limbs.

**micromere** (mi'kro-mēr) [ micro- + G. *meros*, a part ]. A blastomere of small size.

**micromerozoite** (mi'kro-mĕr'o-zo'īt). A small merozoite.

**mi'crome'ter.** Micron; millionth part of a meter; symbol, $\mu$(disfavored) or $\mu$m.

**microm'eter** [ micro- + G. *metron*, measure ]. A device for measuring various types of objects in an accurate and precise manner; in medicine and biology, the term is usually used with reference to a glass slide or lens that is accurately marked for measuring microscopic forms.

    **caliper m.,** a gauge with a calibrated m. screw for the measurement of thin objects such as microscope cover glasses and slides.

    **filar m.,** an ocular micrometer with a line moved by a ruled drum such that a movement of the line of 0.005 mm. or less may be made in relation to fixed parallel lines.

**ocular m.,** a glass disk that fits in a microscope eyepiece and that has a ruled scale; when calibrated with a slide m., direct measurements of a microscopic object can be made.

**slide m.,** a scale made on a microscope slide with lines ruled in divisions, usually, of 0.01 mm.

**mi'crometh'od.** See micro- (2).

**microm'etry.** Measurement of objects with some type of micrometer and a microscope.

**mi'cromi'cro-.** A prefix (symbol $\mu\mu$) sometimes used to signify one-trillionth ($10^{-12}$); preferred term is now pico-, *q. v.*

**mi'cromi'crogram.** Picogram, $10^{-12}$ gram; abbreviated $\mu\mu g$ (or pg).

**micromicron** (mi-kro-mi'kron). The millionth of a micron, or a meter $\times 10^{-12}$; expressed by the Greek letters $\mu\mu$. Preferred term is now picometer (pm).

**mi'cromo'lar.** Denoting a concentration of $10^{-6}$ mol per liter ($10^{-6}$ M or 1 $\mu$M).

**micromole** (mi'kro-mōl). One millionth of a mole; abbreviated $\mu$mole.

**micromo'toscope** [ micro- + L. *motus,* motion, + G. *skopeō,* to view ]. A cinematoscope for representing the movements of amebas and other motile microscopic objects.

**micromyces** (mi'kro-mi'sēz) [ micro- + G. *mykēs,* fungus ]. A microscopic fungus; bacterium.

**micromyelia** (mi'kro-mi-e'lī-ah) [ micro- + G. *myelos,* marrow ]. Abnormal smallness or shortness of the spinal cord.

**micromyeloblast** (mi-kro-mi'el-o-blast). A small myeloblast, often the predominating cell in myeloblastic leukemia.

**micromyelolymphocyte** (mi'kro-mi'el-o-lim'fo-sīt) [ micro- + G. *myelos,* marrow, + L. *lympha,* clear water (lymph), + G. *kytos,* cell ]. Myeloblast.

**mi'cron.** Micrometer (preferred by many workers); the millionth of a meter; symbol, $\mu$.

**microneedle** (mi'kro-nee'dl). A small glass needle used in micrurgical manipulation.

**mi'croneme** [ micro- + G. *nema,* thread ]. Toxoneme (so called because first described from *Toxoplasma*); sarconeme; a small, osmiophilic, cordlike twisted organelle found in the anterior region of many sporozoans, and one of the characteristics that helps to define the subphylum Apicomplexa.

**micronew'ton.** One-millionth of a newton.

**micron'ic.** Of the size of 1 micron.

**micronod'ular** [ G. *mikros,* small ]. Characterized by the presence of minute nodules; denoting a somewhat coarser appearance than that of a granular tissue or substance.

**micronucleus** (mi-kro-nu'kle-us). 1. A small nucleus in a large cell, or the smaller nuclei in cells that have two or more such structures. 2. Specifically, the smaller of the two nuclei in ciliates dividing mitotically; it contains the specific inheritable material; also called germ, gonad, gametic, or reproductive nucleus; and karyogonad.

**micronu'trients.** Essential food factors required in only small quantities by the body; *i.e.,* vitamins, trace minerals.

**micronychia** (mi'kro-nik'ī-ah) [ micro- + G. *onyx,* nail ]. Abnormal smallness of nails.

**micro-ohm.** Microhm.

**microorganism** (mi'kro-or'gan-izm). A microscopic organism (plant or animal).

**micropar'asite.** A parasitic microorganism.

**micropathol'ogy** [ micro- + G. *pathos,* suffering, + *logos,* study ]. 1. Morbid histology; the microscopic study of changes in tissues and cells associated with disease. 2. Microbiology (bacteriology, virology, mycology, and so on) in relation to disease.

**micrope'nis.** Microphallus; abnormally small penis.

**microperox'isomes.** Small *peroxisomes, q. v.*

**microphage** (mi'kro-fāj) [ micro- + phag(ocyte) ]. Microphagocyte; a polymorphonuclear leukocyte that is phagocytic. See also phagocyte.

**microphag'ocyte.** Microphage.

**mi'cropha'kia** [ micro- + G. *phakos,* lens ]. Spherophakia.

**microphallus** (mi-kro-fal'us). Micropenis.

**micropho'bia** [ micro- + G. *phobos,* fear ]. Fear of small objects, bacteria, or parasites.

**mi'crophone** [ micro- + G. *phōnē,* sound ]. An instrument for magnifying sounds.

**micropho'nia, microph'ony** [ micro- + G. *phōnē,* voice ]. Weakness of voice.

**micropho'noscope.** A stethoscope with a diaphragm attachment for magnifying the sound.

**micropho'tograph.** A minute photograph of any object; to be distinguished from photomicrograph, which is a photograph of a microscopic object.

**microphthalmia, microphthalmos** (mi'krof-thal'mī-ah, -thal'mos) [ micro- + G. *ophthalmos,* eye ]. Nanophthalmia; nanophthalmos; the presence of one or both eyeballs of abnormally small size.

**microphthalmus** (mi'krof-thal'mus). Nanophthalmus; an individual with microphthalmia.

**micropipette, micropipet** (mi'kro-pī-pet', -pi-pet'). A pipette designed for the measurement of very small volumes.

**mi'cropla'nia** [ micro- + L. *planus,* flat ]. Decreased horizontal diameter of erythrocytes.

**microplasia** (mi+kro-pla'zī-ah) [ micro- + G. *plasis,* a shaping, forming ]. Dwarfism; stunted growth.

**microplethysmography** (mi'kro-pleth'iz-mog'ră-fī) [ micro- + plethysmography, *q. v.* ]. The technique of measuring minute changes in the volume of a part as a result of blood flow into or out of it.

**micropo'dia** [ micro- + G. *pous,* foot ]. The state of having small feet.

**mi'cropore** [ micro- + G. *poros,* pore ]. An organelle formed by the pellicle of all stages of sporozoan protozoa of the subphylum Apicomplexa; it is also found in developmental stages that may lack the inner pellicle layer. The m. is composed of two concentric rings (in transverse section), the inner of which corresponds with an invagination of the outer pellicle membrane. M.'s thus far observed seem to serve as feeding organelles; their role in nonfeeding developmental forms is unknown. This organelle was first called a micropyle, then an ultracytostome.

**micropromyelocyte** (mi-kro-pro-mi'el-o-sīt). A cell derived from a promyelocyte.

**microprosopus** (mi'kro-pro'so-pus, -pro-so'pus) [ micro- + G. *prosōpon,* face. OPO- ]. An individual with abnormally small or imperfectly developed face.

**microp'sia** [ micro- + G. *opsis,* sight ]. The subjective perception of objects as smaller than they actually are.

**mi'cropuncture.** Microincision.

**micropus** (mi'kro-pus, mi-kro'pus) [ micro- + G. *pous,* foot ]. A person with very small feet.

**micropyle** (mi'kro-pīl) [ micro- + G. *pylē,* gate ]. 1. A minute opening believed to exist in the investing membrane of certain ova as a point of entrance for the spermatozoon. 2. Former name for micropore.

**mi'croradiog'raphy.** Making radiograms that can be enlarged.

**microrefractometer** (mi'kro-re-frak-tom'e-ter). A refractometer used in the study of blood cells.

**microres'pirom'eter.** An apparatus for measuring the utilization of oxygen by small particles of isolated tissues or cells or particles of cells.

**microscope** (mi'kro-skōp) [ micro- + G. *skopeō,* to view ]. An instrument that gives an enlarged image of an object or substance that is minute or not visible with the naked eye; usually the term denotes a compound m. (see fig.); for low magnifications the term simple m., or magnifying glass, is used.

**binocular m.,** a m. having two eyepieces; it may be a compound m. or a stereoscopic m.

**color-contrast m.,** Rheinberg m.; a variety of m. in which the condenser stop is of one color and the annulus is a complement of it so that unstained objects are observed in one color on a field of the other.

**comparator m.,** a device constructed with one or more m.'s having micrometer eyepieces used to measure dimensional changes during setting or temperature changes.

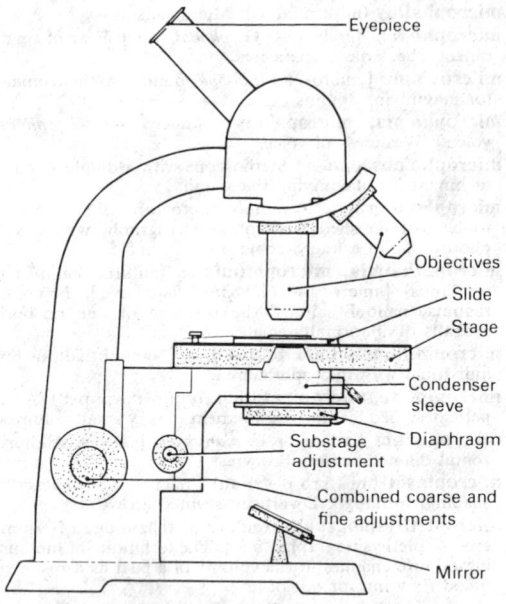

Eyepiece

Objectives

Slide

Stage

Condenser sleeve

Substage adjustment

Diaphragm

Combined coarse and fine adjustments

Mirror

**A Compound Light Microscope**
Diagram showing principal parts

**compound m.,** one consisting of two or more lenses.

**corneal m.,** biomicroscope.

**darkfield m.,** a m. that has a special condenser and objective with a diaphragm or stop such that light is scattered from the object observed with the result that the object appears bright on a dark background.

**electron m.,** a visual and photographic m. in which electron beams with wavelengths thousands of times shorter than visible light are utilized in place of light, thereby allowing much greater magnification; in this technique, the electrons are transmitted through a very thin section of an embedded, dehydrated specimen maintained in a vacuum.

**fluorescent m.,** see fluorescence *microscopy.*

**flying spot m.,** a m. in which a moving spot of light is imaged in the object plane, the energy transmitted by the specimen being detected with a photoelectric cell; the light source may be a cathode ray tube, a scanning disk or drum, or an oscillating mirror.

**Greenough m.,** stereoscopic m.

**infrared m.,** a m. that is equipped with infrared transmitting optics and that measures the infrared absorption of minute samples with the aid of photoelectric cells; images may be observed with image converters or television.

**interference m.,** a specially constructed m. in which the entering light is split into two beams which pass through the specimen and are recombined in the image plane where interference effects make transparent (invisible) refractile object details become visible as intensity differences. This instrument permits measurements of light retardation, index of refraction, and thickness and mass of specimen, and is useful in the examination of living or unstained cells.

**laser m.,** a m. in which a laser beam is focused on a microscopic field, causing it to vaporize; the emitted radiation is analyzed by means of a microspectrophotometer; at a low intensity the laser is employed as the light source in an interference m.

**opaque m.,** epimicroscope.

**operating m.,** surgical m.

**phase m.,** a specially constructed m. which employs a special condenser and objective containing a phase-shifting ring whereby small differences in index of refraction are made visible as intensity or contrast differences in the image. This instrument is particularly useful for examining structural details in transparent specimens such as living or unstained cells and tissues.

**polarizing m.,** a m. equipped with a polarizer and analyzer; formerly the polars were made of calcite prisms, but more recently Polaroid film has been used. The conventional polarizing m. is useful only for the study of birefringence and linear dichroism.

**Rheinberg m.,** color-contrast m.

**scanning electron m.,** a m. in which the object is examined point by point directly by an electron beam, and an image is formed on a television screen; with this method an unembedded specimen is viewed by reflected and secondary electrons, thus giving the surface image a three-dimensional quality.

**simple m., single m.,** one that consists of a single magnifying lens; a magnifying glass.

**slitlamp m.,** biomicroscope.

**stereoscopic m.,** Greenough m.; a m. having double eyepieces and objectives and thus independent light paths, giving a three-dimensional image.

**stroboscopic m.,** a m. which has a light source that flashes at a constant rate so that an analysis of the motility of an object may be made; it may be used for high speed or low speed (time-lapse) cinephotomicrography.

**surgical m.,** operating m.; a binocular m. used in delicate eye and ear surgery; in the standing type of m., a motorized zoom system (see zoom) operated by hand or foot controls provides an adjustable working distance; in headborne models, interchangeable oculars provide the magnification needed.

**television m.,** a m. in which the image is observed by a television camera which produces a television display; it is used for quantitative studies, display to a large audience, or examinations in ultraviolet and infrared regions of the spectrum.

**ultra-m.,** see ultramicroscope.

**ultrasonic m.,** one that has lenses designed to use acoustic energy so that the ultrasonic wavelengths may be utilized; by means of transducers the information is translated to a form that may be visualized or recorded.

**ultraviolet m.,** a m. having optics of quartz and fluorite which allow transmission of light waves shorter than those of the visible spectrum, *i.e.,* below 400 mμ (manometers); the image is made visible by photography, fluorescence of special glasses, or television. In a scanning instrument the receptor is a multiplier phototube.

**x-ray m.,** one in which images are obtained by using x-rays as an energy source; these are recorded on a very fine-grained film, or the image is enlarged by projection. If film is used it may be examined with the light m. at fairly high magnifications.

**microscop'ic, microscop'ical.** 1. Of minute size; visible only with the aid of the microscope. 2. Relating to a microscope.

**microscopy** (mi-kros'ko-pī). Investigation of minute objects by means of a microscope.

**fluorescence m.,** a procedure based on the fact that fluorescent materials emit visible light when they are irradiated with invisible ultraviolet rays; some materials manifest this property naturally, whereas others may be treated with fluorescent solutions (somewhat analogous to staining). When the absorption of the specimen is in the relatively long ultraviolet range, a filter that transmits these radiations is used, and a yellow filter is placed on or in the ocular; the field is then dark, and any yellow or red fluorescence becomes visible.

**immunofluorescence m.,** see immunofluorescence.

**mi'crosec'ond.** One millionth of a second; $10^{-6}$ second.

**microseme** (mi'kro-sēm) [ micro- + G. *sēma,* sign ]. Denoting a skull with an orbital index below 84.

**mi'crosides.** Fatty acid esters of trehalose and mannose isolated from diphtheria bacilli.

**microsmatic** (mi'kroz-mat'ik) [ micro- + G. *osmē,* sense of smell ]. Having the sense of smell poorly developed.

**mi'crosome** [ micro- + G. *sōma,* body ]. One of the small spherical vesicles derived from the endoplasmic reticulum after disruption of cells by centrifugation.

**microsomia** (mi'-kro-so'mī-ah) [ micro- + G. *sōma,* body ]. Dwarfism; smallness of body.

**microspectrophotometry** (mi'kro-spek'tro-fo'tom'ē-trī). A technique for characterizing and quantitating minute cellular constituents by their absorption spectra.

**microspectroscope** (mi'kro-spek'tro-skōp). An instrument for observing the spectrum of microscopic objects.

**microspherocytosis** (mi'kro-sfe-ro-si-to'sis). A condition of the blood seen in hemolytic icterus in which small spherocytes are predominant. The red blood cells are smaller and more globular than normal.

**microsphygmy** (mi'kro-sfig'mī) [ micro- + G. *sphygmos*, pulse ]. Microsphyxia; smallness of the pulse.

**microsphyxia** (mi'kro-sfik'sī-ah) [ micro- + G. *sphyxis*, pulse ]. Microsphygmy.

**microsplanchnic** (mi'kro-splangk'nik) [ micro- + G. *splanchna*, viscera ]. Referring to smallness of the abdominal viscera.

**microsplenia** (mi-kro-sple'nī-ah). Abnormal smallness of the spleen.

**micros'porid** [ micro- + suffix -id, *q.v.* ]. Cutaneous allergic response to infection with one of the species of *Microsporum*.

**Microspo'rida**. An order of the protozoan subphylum Cnidospora (or Microspora) characterized by minute spores with a single long coiled tubular filament enclosing the infective cell or sporoplasm. They are typically parasites of invertebrates and lower vertebrates, although fish and higher vertebrates (including man) have been infected. This order includes parasites of mammals, such as *Nosema cuniculi* (rabbits, rats, dogs, man), *Nosema muris* (laboratory mice), and *Thelohania apodemi* (rodents).

**Micros'poron.** *Microsporum.*

**mi'crosporo'sis.** Skin eruption caused by one of the species of *Microsporum*; ringworm of the skin.

   **m. cap'itis,** *tinea* tonsurans.

**Microsporum** (mi'kros'po-rum, mi'kro-spo'rum) [ micro- + G. *sporos*, seed ]. *Microsporon*; a genus of pathogenic fungi causing dermatophytosis and tinea; in appropriate culture media, characteristic macroconidia and microconidia are seen.

   **M. audoui'nii,** an anthrophilic species that causes epidemic tinea tonsurans in children.

   **M. ca'nis,** a zoophilic species that causes sporadic tinea tonsurans in children.

   **M. cook'ei,** a geophilic species that has been isolated from various animals (none of which had recognizable lesions) and soil.

   **M. distor'tum,** a zoophilic species that causes infection in man (tinea tonsurans) and animals.

   **M. ferrugin'eum,** an anthropophilic species that causes tinea tonsurans, primarily in the Far East and middle Europe.

   **M. furfur,** *Malassezia furfur.*

   **M. na'num,** a geophilic species that has been isolated from man, hogs, and soil.

**Microsporum** M. na'num, a geophilic species that has been isolated from man, hogs, and soil.

**microsteth'ophone** [ micro- + G. *stethos*, chest, + *phōnē*, sound ]. A form of amplifying stethoscope.

**microsteth'oscope.** A form of magnifying stethoscope.

**microsto'mia** [ micro- + G. *stoma*, mouth ]. Smallness of the oral aperature.

**microsur'gery.** Surgical procedures performed under the magnification of a special surgical microscope. See also microincision and micromanipulation.

**microsyringe** (mi'kro-sī-rinj', -sīr'inj). A hypodermic syringe having a micrometer screw attached to the piston, whereby accurately measured minute quantities of fluid may be injected.

**microthe'lia** [ micro- + G. *thēlē*, nipple ]. Smallness of the nipples.

**microtia** (mi-kro'shī-ah) [ micro- + G. *ous,* ear, + suffix *-ia*, condition ]. Smallness of the auricle or pinna of the ear.

**mi'crotome.** An instrument for making sections for examination under the microscope.

**microtomy** (mi-krot'o-mī) [ micro- + G. *tomē,* incision ]. Section-cutting; the making of thin sections of tissues for examination under the microscope.

**microtonometer** (mi'kro-to-nom'e-ter) [ micro- + G. *tonos,* tone, + *metron,* measure ]. A small tonometer invented by Krogh, originally intended for animals but later adapted to man, for determining the tensions of

oxygen and carbon dioxide in arterial blood. It provides the means of bringing a small bubble of air into gaseous equilibrium with a sample of blood obtained by arterial puncture.

**Microtrombid'ium wichman'ni.** A mite or harvest bug of New Guinea. It is parasitic on human skin, causing severe itching.

**mi'crotro'pia** [ micro- + G. *trope,* a turn, turning ]. A strabismus of less than 5 degrees; it is characterized by lessened acuity and eccentric fixation of the involved eye, which shows a slight central scotoma and harmonious anomalous retinal correspondence.

**mi'crotu'bule.** A cylindrical cytoplasmic element 100 to 270 Å in diameter and variable in length; m.'s increase in number during mitosis and occur widely in plant and animal cells, where they may be related to cell motility.

   **subpellicular m.,** subpellicular fibril; m. of certain protozoa found in several stages of sporozoan life cycles; in sporozoites and merozoites of the coccidia, these m.'s are distributed in a regular subpellicular pattern, from anterior to posterior regions, each originating at the polar ring and extending to the nucleus.

**micro'tus** [ micro- + G. *ous,* ear ]. An individual with microtia.

**Micro'tus** [ micro- + G. *ous,* ear ]. A genus of voles that may transmit ratbite fever.

**microvil'lus,** pl. **microvil'li.** One of the minute projections of cell membranes greatly increasing surface area. Microvilli form the striated or brush borders of certain cells.

**mi'crovolt.** One millionth of a volt; $10^{-6}$ volt.

**mi'crowaves.** Microelectric waves; that portion of the radio wave spectrum of shortest wavelength, including the region with wavelengths of 1 mm. to 30 cm. (1000 to 300,000 megacycles per second); used in radar.

**mi'croweld'ing.** A method of fastening or joining stainless steel sutures or such sutures to needles.

**microxyphil** (mi-krok'sī-fil) [ micro- + G. *oxys,* acid, + *philos,* fond ]. A multinuclear oxyphil leukocyte.

**microzoon** (mi'kro-zo'on) [ micro- + G. *zōon,* animal ]. A microscopic form of the animal kingdom; a protozoon.

**micrurgical** (mi-krer'jī-kal) [ micro- + G. *ergon,* work ]. Relating to the manipulation of minute structures under the microscope. See also micromanipulation, microsurgery, and microdissection.

**miction** (mik'shun). Micturition.

**micturate** (mik'tu-rāt) [ see micturition ]. Urinate.

**micturition** (mik-tu-rish'un) [ L. *micturio,* to desire to make water ]. 1. Urination. 2. The desire to urinate or frequency of urination.

**M.I.D.** Abbreviation for minimal infecting *dose.*

**mid-** [ A.S. *mid, midd* ]. Combining form meaning middle.

**mid'body.** A group of granules formed in the equatorial part of the spindle during anaphase of mitosis.

**mid'brain.** Mesencephalon.

**mid'carpal.** Mediocarpal.

**midgracile** (mid-gras'il). Denoting an occasional fissure dividing the gracile lobe of the cerebellum into two parts.

**mid'gut.** 1. The central portion of the digestive tube; the small intestine. 2. The portion of the embryonic gut tract between the foregut and the hindgut.

**midmenstrual** (mid'men'stru-al). Denoting the period about midway between two menstrual periods.

**midoccipital** (mid'ok-sip'ĭ-tal). Relating to the central portion of the occiput; medioccipital.

**mid'pain.** Intermenstrual *pain.*

**mid'plane.** Pelvic plane of least dimensions; see under plane.

**midriff** [ A.S. *mid,* middle, + *hrif,* belly ]. Diaphragma (2).

**mid'section.** A cut or section through the middle of an organ.

**mid'sternum.** *Corpus* sterni.

**mid'tarsal.** Mediotarsal.

**mid'wife** (mid'wif) [ A.S. *mid,* with, + *wif,* wife ]. A woman who attends women in confinement; see also accoucheuse.

**midwifery** (mid'wĭf'rĭ). The practice and art of assisting women in childbirth.

**Miescher** (me'sher), Johann F., Swiss pathologist, 1811–1887. See M.'s *tubes*.

**migraine** (mi'grān, mī-grān') [ through O. Fr. fr. G. *hēmikrania*, pain on one side of the head, fr. *hēmi-*, half, + *kranion*, skull ]. Sick, bilious, blind, or vascular headache; hemicrania; megrim; a symptom complex occurring periodically and characterized by pain in the head, usually unilateral, vertigo, nausea and vomiting, photophobia, and scintillating appearances of light. Classified as classic m., common m., cluster headache, hemiplegic or ophthalmoplegic m., and lower half hemiplegic m.

**abdominal m.,** paroxysmal abdominal pain without apparent cause; probably due to epilepsy; responds to anticonvulsant drugs but not to ergotamine tartrate.

**classic m.,** headache with visual or other prodromes.

**common m.,** sick headache without prodromes.

**ful'gurating m.,** m. coming on abruptly and with violence.

**Harris' m.,** periodic migrainous *neuralgia*.

**hemiplegic m.,** a form associated with transient hemiplegia.

**ophthal'mic m.,** a form accompanied by marked disturbances of vision.

**ophthalmoplegic m.,** a form associated with paralysis of the eye muscles.

**mi'grate** [ L. *migro*, pp. *-atus*, to move from place to place ]. To wander; to pass from one part to another in an organ or in the body; said of certain diseases or symptoms.

**migration** (mi-gra'shun) [ L. *migratio* (see migrate) ]. 1. Passing from place to place, said of certain morbid processes or symptoms. 2. Diapedesis.

**epithelial m.,** apical shift of epithelial attachment, exposing more of the tooth crown.

**m. of ovum,** the transperitoneal passage of an ovum from the ovarian follicle into the uterine tube (oviduct).

**tooth m.,** the naturally occurring movement of a tooth.

**Migula** (me'goo-lah), Walter, German naturalist, \*1863. His early (1900) classification of bacteria was based chiefly on morphologic resemblance.

**Mikity,** V. G. See Wilson-M. *syndrome*.

**Mikulicz** (mik'oo-lich), Johannes von M.-Radecki, Polish surgeon in Breslau, 1850–1905. See M.-Vladimiroff *amputation*, M.'s *aphthae, cells, clamp, disease, drain, mask, operation*, Heineke-M. *pyloroplasty*, M.'s *pad, syndrome*; Sjögren-M. *syndrome*.

**Miles,** William E., British surgeon, 1869–1947. See M.'s *operation, resection*.

**mil'foil.** *Achillea*.

**mil'ia.** Plural of milium.

**Milian,** Gaston, French dermatologist, 1871–1945. See M.'s *disease, erythema*.

**miliaria** (mil'ĭ-ăr'ĭ-ah) [ L. *miliarius*, relating to millet, fr. *milium*, millet ]. An eruption of minute vesicles and papules due to retention of fluid at the mouths of the sweat follicles.

**m. alba,** m. with vesicles containing a milky fluid.

**apocrine m.,** Fox-Fordyce *disease*.

**m. crystalli'na,** sudamina; a noninflammatory form of m. in which the vesicles are filled with clear fluid.

**m. papulo'sa,** m. rubra.

**m. profunda,** m. rubra.

**pus'tular m.,** m. tropicalis; an eruption of pustules that occurs usually in very hot weather and mostly on the flexor aspects of the limbs, the groins, and the axillae. The lesions are situated at the orifices of sweat glands.

**m. ru'bra,** an eruption of papules and vesicles at the mouths of the sweat follicles, accompanied by redness and inflammatory reaction of the skin. Also called strophulus, lichen infantum, lichen strophulosus, tropical lichen, m. papulosa, m. profunda, m. vesiculosa, and known by many lay terms such as gum, heat, tooth, summer, or wildfire rash, or prickly heat.

**m. tropicalis,** pustular m.

**m. vesiculo'sa,** m. rubra.

**miliary** (mil'ĭ-ĕr-ĭ, mil'yă-rĭ) [ see miliaria ]. 1. Resembling a millet seed in size (about 2 mm.). 2. Marked by the presence of nodules of millet seed size on any surface.

**milieu** (mēl-yü) [ Fr. *mi*, fr. L. *medius*, middle, + *leiu*, fr. L. *locus*, place ]. 1. Surroundings; environment. 2. In psychiatry, the social setting of the mental patient, *e.g.*, the hospital.

**m. intérieur, m. interne,** the internal environment; the fluids bathing the tissue cells of multicellular animals.

**mil'ium,** pl. **mil'ia** [ L. millet ]. A small subepidermal keratin cyst, usually multiple, therefore commonly referred to in the plural; also known as pearly or sebaceous tubercle; tuberculum sebaceum.

**colloid milia,** actinic *elastosis*.

**milk** [ A.S. *meolc* ]. 1. A white liquid, containing proteins, sugar, and lipids, secreted by the mammary glands, designed for the nourishment of the young. 2. Any whitish, milky fluid; *e.g.*, the juice of the cocoanut or a suspension of various metallic oxides. 3. A pharmacopeial preparation that is a suspension of insoluble drugs in a water medium; distinguished from gels mainly in that the suspended particles of m. are larger; formerly called magma.

**acidoph'ilus m.,** m. inoculated with a culture of *Bacillus acidophilus*.

**m. of bismuth,** see under bismuth.

**bud'deized m.,** see Budde *process*.

**certified m.,** raw m.; cow's m. that has not more than the maximal permissible limit of 10,000 bacteria per ml. at any time prior to delivery to the consumer, and that must be cooled to 50°F. or less and maintained at that temperature until delivery.

**certified pasteurized m.,** cow's m.; the maximum permissible limit for bacteria should not be more than 10,000 bacteria per ml. before pasteurization and not more than 500 bacteria per ml. after pasteurization; it must be cooled to 45°F. or less and maintained at that temperature until delivery.

**condensed m.,** a thick liquid prepared by the partial evaporation of cow's m., with or without the addition of sugar.

**crop m.,** pigeon's m.

**fortified vitamin D m.,** m. produced through direct addition of vitamin D; standardized at 400 units (USP) per quart.

**irradiated vitamin D m.,** cow's m. exposed in a thin film to ultraviolet light and standardized to contain 400 units (USP) of vitamin D per quart.

**lactobac'illary m.,** m. inoculated with a culture of *Bacillus acidophilus, B. bulgaricus*, or other lactic acid-forming microorganism.

**m. of magnesia,** see under magnesia.

**metab'olized vitamin D m.,** yeast m.; m. produced by feeding irradiated yeast to cows; standardized to contain not less than 400 units (USP) per quart.

**modified m.,** cow's m. altered, by increasing the fat and reducing the amount of protein, to resemble in composition human m.

**perhy'drase m.,** m. treated by the addition of hydrogen peroxide. See Budde *process*.

**pigeon's m.,** crop m.; a secretion formed by glands in the mucosa of the pigeon's crop with which the young are fed; it is increased under the influence of prolactin.

**skim m., skimmed m.,** the aqueous (noncream) part of m. from which casein is isolated.

**m. of sulfur,** precipitated sulfur.

**u'terine m.,** a whitish fluid secretion between the villi of the placenta; pabulum of the uterus. It nourishes the implanting ovum.

**vitamin D m.,** cow's m. to which vitamin D has been added, to contain 400 USP units of vitamin D per quart.

**witch's m.,** hexenmilch; a secretion of colostrum-like m. sometimes occurring in the glands of newborn infants of either sex 3 to 4 days after birth and lasting a week or two; due to endocrine stimulation from the mother before birth.

**milk'ing.** Stripping; running the finger along a compressible tube, such as the urethra, with the object of expressing its contents.

**Milkman,** Louis A., U. S. roentgenologist, 1895–1951. See M.'s *syndrome*.

**milk'pox.** Alastrim.

**Millard** (me-lar'), Auguste L. J., Paris physician, 1830–1915. See M.-Gubler *syndrome*.

**Miller,** Thomas G., American physician, *1886. See M.-Abbott *tube.*

**Milles' syndrome.** See under syndrome.

**milli-** [ L. *mille,* one thousand ]. A prefix used in the metric system to signify one thousandth ($10^{-3}$).

**mil'liam'pere.** One thousandth of an ampere; abbreviated ma.

**mil'libar.** One-thousandth of a bar; standard atmospheric pressure is 1013 millibars.

**millicurie** (mil'ĭ-ku're). A unit of radioactivity equivalent to 3.7 × $10^7$ disintegrations per second; abbreviated mCi.

**milliequivalent** (mil'ĭ-e-kwiv'ă-lent). Abbreviated mEq or meq; $10^{-3}$ equivalent; $10^{-3}$ mole divided by valence.

**milligram.** One thousandth of a gram. Abbreviated mg.
  **m. hour,** milligramage; a unit of exposure in radium therapy, *i.e.,* the application of 1 mg. of radium during 1 hr.

**milligramage** (mil'ĭ-gram-āj). *Milligram* hour.

**mil'lilam'bert.** One thousandth of a lambert; a unit of brightness equal to 0.929 lumen per square foot (roughly, 1 equivalent footcandle).

**milliliter** (mil'ĭ-le'ter). One thousandth of a liter, or 1 cubic centimeter; about 15 minims. Abbreviated ml.

**mil'lime'ter.** One thousandth of a meter, roughly $1/25$ inch. Abbreviated mm.

**millimicro-.** A prefix sometimes used to signify one billionth ($10^{-9}$); equivalent of nano-, which is the preferred usage.

**millimicron** (mil'ĭ-mi'kron). One thousandth of a micron; abbreviated mμ. Equivalent of nanometer, which is the preferred usage.

**millimole** (mil'ĭ-mōl). One thousandth of a gram-molecule. Abbreviated mmole.

**mil'ling-in.** The procedure of refining the occlusion of teeth by the use of abrasives between their occluding surfaces while the dentures are rubbed together in the mouth or on the articulator; see also selective *grinding* and milled-in *paths.*

**mil'linor'mal.** One thousandth of the normal, denoting the strength of a solution; see normal (3).

**milliosmole** (mil'ĭ-oz'mōl). A term for expressing the osmotic pressure exerted by a certain concentration of an ion in a solution; the milligrams of ion per liter divided by the atomic weight of the ion indicates the number of m.'s. In instances of univalent ions, 1 m. is equal to 1 milliequivalent, but 1 m. is equal to 2 milliequivalents of a bivalent ion.

**millipede** (mil'lĭ-pēd) [ milli- + L. *pes, pedis,* foot ]. A venomous nonpredaceous arthropod of the order Diplopoda, characterized by two pairs of legs per leg-bearing segment. The venom is purely defensive, oozed or squirted from pores along the body, producing irritation to the skin or severe inflammation if it reaches the eyes.

**mil'lisec'ond.** One thousandth of a second; abbreviated msec.

**mil'livolt.** One thousandth of a volt; abbreviated mv.

**Millon** (me-yoñ'), Auguste N. E., French chemist, 1812–1867. See M.'s *reaction, reagent,* M.-Nasse *test.*

**Mills,** Charles K., U. S. neurologist, 1845–1931. See M.'s *disease.*

**milphae** (mil'fe) [ G. *milphai* (pl. only) ]. Milphosis; loss of eyelashes or eyebrows or both.

**milphosis** (mil-fo'sis) [ G. *milphōsis* ]. Milphae.

**Milroy,** William F., American physician, 1855–1942. See M.'s *disease.*

**milt.** The sperm and seminal fluid of fish.

**Milton,** John L., English dermatologist, 1820–1898. See M.'s *disease.*

**mimesis** (mĭ-me'sis, mi-me'sis) [ G. *mimēsis,* imitation, fr. *mimeomai,* to mimic ]. 1. Hysterical simulation of organic disease. 2. The symptomatic imitation of one organic disease by another.

**mimet'ic** [ G. *mimētikos,* imitative ]. Relating to mimesis; simulating.

**mimic** (mim'ik) [ G. *mimikos,* imitating, fr. *mimos,* a mimic ]. Imitative; simulating; mimetic.

**mimmation** (mĭ-ma'shun) [ Ar. *mim,* the letter m ]. A form of stammering in which the m-sound is given to various letters.

**mimo'sis** [ G. *mimos,* mimic ]. Mimesis.

**mind** [ A.S. *gemynd* ]. 1. The psyche; the organ or seat of consciousness, remembering, reasoning, and willing. 2. The organized totality of all mental processes and psychic activities, with emphasis on the relatedness of the phenomena.

**mind-reading.** Telepathy.

**mineral** (min'er-al) [ L. *mineralis,* pertaining to mines, fr. *mino,* to mine ]. Any homogeneous inorganic material found in the earth's crust.
  **m. oil** (USP, BP), white m. oil; heavy liquid petrolatum; liquid paraffin; liquid petroleum; a mixture of liquid hydrocarbons obtained from petroleum.
  **m. oil, light** (NF), light liquid paraffin, light liquid petrolatum; light white m. oil; a mixture of liquid hydrocarbons obtained from petroleum; used as a vehicle.

**mineral'ocoid.** Mineralocorticoid.

**mineralocorticoid** (min'er-al-o-kor'tĭ-koyd). One of the steroid principles of the adrenal cortex that influences salt (sodium and potassium) metabolism.

**min'im** [ L. *minimus,* least ]. 1. A fluid measure, one sixtieth of a fluidrachm; in the case of water about one drop. 2. Smallest; least; the smallest of several similar structures.

**minimus** [ L. ] [ NA ]. Smallest.

**min'ocy'cline hydrochloride** (USP). MINOCIN; an antibacterial drug.

**minor** [ L. ] [ NA ]. Smaller; lesser; denoting the smaller of two similar structures.

**Minot,** George R., U. S. physician, 1885–1950. Nobel laureate, 1934, with George H. Whipple and William P. Murphy, for their discoveries concerning liver therapy in cases of anemia.

**mint** [ G. *mintha* ]. Mentha.

**mio-** [ G. *meiōn,* less. MIO- ]. Combining form meaning less.

**miocardia** (mi'o-kar'dĭ-ah) [ mio- + G. *kardia,* heart ]. Systole.

**miodidymus** (mi-o-did'ĭ-mus) [ mio- + G. *didymos,* twin ]. Miodymus; unequal conjoined twins with the smaller head fused to the larger in the occipital region.

**miodymus** (mi-od'ĭ-mus). Miodidymus.

**miolecithal** (mi'o-les'ĭ-thal) [ mio- + G. *lekithos,* egg yolk ]. Denoting an egg with little yolk which is uniformly dispersed throughout the egg.

**mionectic** (mi'o-nek'tik) [ mio- + G. *echō,* to have ]. An obsolete term denoting less than the normal; used especially with reference to blood that has an abnormally low percentage of saturation with oxygen at a certain pressure.

**miopragia** (mi-o-pra'jĭ-ah) [ mio- + G. *prassō,* to do ]. Diminished functional activity in a part.

**miopus** (mi-o'pus) [ mio- + G. *ōps,* eye ]. Unequal conjoined twins with heads united in such a manner that one face is rudimentary.

**mio'sis** [ G. *meiosis,* a lessening ]. 1. The period of decline of a disease in which the intensity of the symptoms begins to diminish. 2. Contraction of the pupil. 3. Sometimes incorrectly used as an alternative spelling for meiosis, *q.v.*
  **paralytic m.,** contraction of the pupil due to paralysis of the radiating muscular fibers.
  **spastic m.,** m. due to spasmodic contraction of the circular muscular fibers.

**miosphygmia** (mi'o-sfig'mĭ-ah) [ mio- + G. *sphygmos,* pulse ]. A situation in which pulse beats are fewer than heart beats.

**miot'ic.** 1. Relating to or characterized by miosis. 2. An agent that causes the pupil to contract.

**miracidium,** pl. **miracid'ia** (mi'rä-sid'ĭ-um) [ G. *meirakidion,* boy ]. The ciliated first-stage larva of a trematode that emerges from the egg and must penetrate into the tissues of an appropriate intermediate host snail if it is to continue its life cycle. This is followed by development into a mother sporocyst, followed by production of a number of offspring of successive larval generations. See also sporocyst (1).

**Mirchamp's sign.** See under sign.

**mire** (mēr) [ L. *miror*, pp. -*atus*, to wonder at ]. One of the test objects in the ophthalmometer, by means of the images of which the amount of astigmatism is calculated.

**mires'trol.** A substance obtained from the tuberous roots of *Pueraria mirifica.* As active an estrogen as estradiol when injected, and more potent than diethylstilbestrol when given by mouth.

**mir'ror** [ Fr. *miroir*, fr. L. *miror*, to wonder at ]. A polished surface reflecting the rays of light from objects in front of it.

**head m.,** a circular concave m. attached to a head band, used to project a beam of light into a cavity, such as the nose or larynx, for purposes of examination and permitting binocular vision.

**mouth m.,** a small m. on a handle used to facilitate visualization in the examination of the teeth.

**van Helmont's m.,** *centrum* tendineum.

**mirror-writing.** Retrography; writing backward, from right to left, the letters appearing like ordinary writing seen in a mirror.

**miryach'it.** A nervous affection observed in Siberia; similar to palmus, latah, or the jumper disease of Maine.

**misan'dria** [ G. *miseō,* to hate, + *anēr, andros,* male ]. Fear of men.

**misanthropy** (mis-an'thro-pī) [ G. *miseō,* to hate, + *anthrōpos,* man ]. Aversion to people; hatred of mankind.

**miscarriage** (mis-kăr'ij) Spontaneous expulsion of the products of pregnancy before the middle of the second trimester.

**miscarry** (mis-kăr'ī). To have a miscarriage.

**misce** (mis'e) [ L. imperative of *misceo,* to mix ]. In prescription writing the direction given to the pharmacist to mix the ingredients; it is usually abbreviated to *M.*

**miscegenation** (mis'ē-jĕ-na'shun) [ L. *misceo,* to mix, + *genus,* descent, race ]. Marriage or interbreeding of individuals of different races.

**miscible** (mis'ĭ-bl) [ L. *misceo,* to mix ]. Capable of being mixed and remaining so after the mixing process ceases.

**mis'diagno'sis.** Wrong or mistaken diagnosis.

**miserere mei** (me-sa-ra'ra ma'e) [ L. have pity on me ]. An old term for volvulus or ileus.

**miserotia** (mis'ē-ro'shĭ-ah) [ G. *miseō,* to hate, + *eros,* physical love ]. The dislike of physical love.

**misocainia** (mis-o-ki'nī-ah) [ G. *miseō,* to hate, + *kainos,* new ]. Misoneism.

**misogamy** (mī-sog'ă-mī) [ G. *miseō,* to hate, + *gamos,* marriage ]. Aversion to marriage.

**misogyny** (mī-soj'ē-nī) [ G. *miseō,* to hate, + *gynē,* woman ]. Aversion to or hatred of women.

**misologia** (mis'o-lo'jī-ah) [ G. *miseō,* to hate, + *logos,* reasoning, discussion ]. Aversion to talking or to mental activity.

**misoneism** (mis-o-ne'izm) [ G. *miseō,* to hate, + *neos,* new ]. Misocainia; dislike of and disinclination to accept new ideas; extreme conservatism.

**misope'dia, misop'edy** [ G. *miseō,* to hate, + *pais* (*paid-*), child ]. Aversion to or hatred of children.

**mist.** Abbreviation of *mistura,* mixture.

**mistletoe** (mis'l-tō). See viscum.

**mistu'ra,** gen. and plural **misturae** [ L. see MIST- ]. Mixture.

**Mitchell,** Silas Weir, American neurologist, poet, and novelist, 1829–1914. See M.'s *disease, treatment.*

**mite** [ A.S. ]. A minute arthropod of the order Acarina, which includes a vast assemblage of parasitic and (primarily) free-living organisms. Most are still undescribed, and only a relatively small number are of medical or veterinary importance (1) as vectors or intermediate hosts of pathogenic agents, (2) by directly causing dermatitis or tissue damage, or (3) by causing blood or tissue fluid loss. The six-legged larvae of trombiculid m.'s are parasitic of man and many mammals and birds, and are important as vectors of scrub typhus and other rickettsial agents. Some important m.'s are *Demodex folliculorum* (follicular or mange m.), *Dermonyssus gallinae* (chicken m.), *Ornithonyssus bursa* (tropical fowl m.), *Ornithonyssus sylviarum* (northern fowl m.), *Pediculoides ventricosus* (grain itch m.),

*Sarcoptes scabei* (itch m.), and *Trombicula akamushi* (vector of scrub typhus).

**chigger m.,** see *Trombicula.*

**mitel'la** [ L. dim. of *mitra,* a bandage, band ]. A sling for the arm.

**mith'ramy'cin** (USP). MITHRACIN; an antibiotic produced by *Streptomyces argillaceus* and *S. tanashiensis;* possesses antineoplastic activity.

**mithridatism** (mith'rī-da'tizm, mith-rid'ă-tizm) [ *Mithridates,* King of Pontus (132–63 B.C.), who is said to have acquired immunity to poison by this means, and to have succeeded so well that he failed later in an attempt at suicide ]. Immunity against the action of a poison produced by small and gradually increasing doses of the same.

**miticidal** (mi'tĭ-si'dal). Destructive to mites.

**miticide** (mi'tĭ-sīd) [ mite + L. *caedo,* to kill ]. An agent destructive to mites.

**mit'igate** [ L. *mitigo,* pp. -*atus,* to make mild or gentle, fr. *mitis,* mild, + *ago,* to do, make ]. To make weaker or milder; sometimes erroneously used for militate.

**mi'tis** [ L. ]. Mild.

**mitochondria** (mit'o-kon'drī-ah, mi'to-). Plural of mitochondrion.

**mitochondrial** (mit'o-kon'drī-al, mi'to-). Relating to mitochondria.

**mitochondrion,** pl. **mitochondria** (mit'o-kon'drī-on, mi'to-) [ G. *mitos,* thread, + *chondros,* granule, grits ]. An organelle of the cell cytoplasm consisting of two sets of membranes, a smooth continuous outer coat and an inner membrane arranged in tubules or more often in folds that form platelike double membranes called cristae; mitochondria are the principal energy source of the cell and contain the cytochrome enzymes of terminal electron transport and the enzymes of the citric acid cycle, fatty acid oxidation and oxidative phosphorylation.

**m. of hemoflagellates,** the "mother m.," from which smaller mitochondria appear to arise.

**mi'tocro'min** (USAN). Antibiotic produced by *Streptomyces viridochromogenes;* possesses antineoplastic activity.

**mitogen** (mi'to-jen) [ mitosis + G. suffix -*gen,* producing ]. Transforming agent; a substance that stimulates mitosis and lymphocyte transformation (*q.v.*); m.'s include not only the substances associated with lectins, but also substances from streptococci (associated with streptolysin S) and from strains of α-toxin-producing staphylococci.

**mitogenesis** (mit-o-jen'e-sis) [ mitosis + G. *genesis,* origin ]. The process of induction of mitosis in a cell.

**mitogenetic** (mi'to-jĕ-net'ik). Pertaining to the factor or factors causing cell mitosis.

**mi'tomal'cin** (USAN). Antibiotic produced by *Streptomyces malayensis;* possesses antineoplastic activity.

**mitomycin.** Antibiotic produced by *Streptomyces caespitosus;* antineoplastic.

**mi'toplasm** [ G. *mitos,* thread, + *plasma,* thing formed ]. Chromatin.

**mitosis,** pl. **mitoses** (mi-to'sis, -sēz) [ G. *mitos,* threat ]. Karyokinesis; mitotic division; indirect nuclear division; the usual process of cell reproduction consisting of a sequence of modifications of the nucleus (prophase, prometaphase, metaphase, anaphase, telophase) that result in the formation of two daughter cells with exactly the same chromosome and deoxyribonucleic acid (DNA) content as that of the original cell. See also mitotic *cycle.*

**asymmet'rical m.,** a form of m. in which the chromosomes are unequal in number in the two daughter nuclei, in consequence either of irregular distribution or of a reduction of chromosomes in one nucleus.

**het'erotype m.,** a variety of m. in which the halved chromosomes are united at their ends forming ring figures.

**multipo'lar m.,** a pathologic form in which the spindle has three or more poles resulting in the formation of a corresponding number of nuclei.

**somat'ic m.,** the ordinary process of m. as it occurs in the somatic or body cells, characterized by the formation of a definite number of chromosomes, varying according to the species; in the human subject this number is 46. See fig. under karyotype.

**mi'totane** (USP). LYSODREN; 1,1-dichloro-2-(*o*-chlorophenyl)-2-(*p*-chlorophenyl)ethane; an antineoplastic agent.

**mitot′ic.** Relating to or marked by mitosis.

**mi′tra** [ L. ] [ NA ]. Mitral (2).

**mi′tral** [ L. *mitra*, a coif or turban ]. 1. Relating to the mitral or bicuspid valve. 2. Shaped like a bishop's miter; denoting a structure resembling the shape of a headband or turban.

**mi′traliza′tion.** Straightening of the left heart border in the chest x-ray due to increased prominence of the left atrial appendage and/or the pulmonary salient.

**Mitsuda,** K. See M. *reaction.*

**Mittelschmerz** (mit′el-schmĕrts) [ Ger. middle pain ]. Abdominal pain occurring at the time of ovulation, resulting from irritation of the peritoneum by bleeding from the ovulation site.

**mix′ing.** The mingling or blending of particles or components, especially of different kinds.

   **phenotypic m.,** the condition in which bacteriophage particles released from a bacterium with a mixed infection have components from both the infecting phages.

**mix′ture** [ L. *mixtura* or *mistura* ]. 1. A mutual incorporation of two or more substances, without chemical union, the physical characteristics of each of the components being retained. A **mechanical m.** is a m. of particles or masses distinguishable as such under the microscope or in other ways, a **physical m.** is a more intimate m. of molecules as obtains in the case of gases and many solutions. 2. In chemistry, a mingling together of two or more substances without the occurrence of a reaction by which they would lose their individual properties; *i.e.,* without permanent gain or loss of electrons. 3. In pharmacy, a preparation, consisting of a liquid holding an insoluble medicinal substance in suspension by means of acacia, sugar, or some other viscid material.

   **A.C.E. m.,** a m. of 1 part alcohol, 2 parts chloroform, and 3 parts diethyl ether; once popular as an inhalation anesthetic.

   **binary m.,** a m. of two substances.

   **Bordeaux m.,** a plant fungicidal m., comprising copper sulfate (5 parts) and calcium oxide (5 parts) in water (400 parts) freshly mixed; the CaO is added to the $CuSO_4$ solution.

   **Carrel's m.,** paraffin melting at 52°C., 18; paraffin melting at 20°C., 6; beeswax, 2; castor oil, 1. Used to keep grafts in place on an ulcerated surface.

   **explosive m.,** a m., particularly an anesthetic m., capable of extremely rapid or almost instantaneous combustion, and with an expansive force that is destructive.

   **extemporaneous m.,** one prepared at the time ordered, according to the directions of a prescription, as distinguished from a stock preparation.

**Miyagawa** (me′yă-gah-wah) Yoneji, Japanese bacteriologist, *1885. See M. *bodies.*

**Miyagawanella** (me′yă-gah′wă-nel′ah) [ Y. *Miyagawa* ]. Formerly considered a genus of Chlamydiaceae, but now synonymous with *Chlamydia.*

**MK.** Abbreviation for menaquinone.

**MK-6, MK₆.** Abbreviations for menaquinone-6.

**ml.** Abbreviation for milliliter.

**M.L.D., m.l.d.** Abbreviation for minimal lethal dose. Frequently also written as MLD, and sometimes mld. See under dose.

**M.L.D.₅₀, m.l.d.₅₀.** Frequently also written as $MLD_{50}$, and sometimes mld₅₀. See under dose.

**mm.** Abbreviation for millimeter.

**Mn.** Chemical symbol for the element manganese.

**M'Naghten,** Daniel, British criminal, tried in March, 1843. See M. *rule* (on criminal responsibility).

**mneme** (ne′me) [ G. *mnēmē,* memory ]. 1. A word used by Richard Semon to denote the ability to remember which he believed all living cells possessed. 2. The enduring quality in the mind that accounts for the facts of memory; the engram of a specific experience. 3. The fact that an organism is enduringly modified by stimulation.

**mnemenic, mnemic** (ne-men′ik, ne′mik). Relating to memory.

**mnemism** (ne′mizm) [ G. *mnēmē,* memory ]. Mnemic hypothesis.

**mnemonics** (ne-mon′iks) [ G. *mnēmonikos,* mnemonic, pertaining to memory ]. The art of improving the memory; a system for aiding the memory.

**mnemotechne, mnemotechnics** (ne-mo-tek′ne, ne-mo-tek′nics) [ G. *mnēmē,* memory, + *technē,* art ]. Mnemonics.

**MNSs blood group.** See appendix 2, Blood Groups.

**M.O.** Abbreviation for Medical Officer.

**Mo.** Chemical symbol of the element molybdenum.

**mobilization** (mo′bī-lī-za′shun) [ see mobilize ]. 1. Making movable; restoring the power of motion in a joint. 2. The act of mobilizing; starting a hitherto quiescent process on a round of physiologic activity.

   **stapes m.,** an operation to remobilize the footplate of the stapes to relieve conductive hearing impairment caused by its immobilization through otosclerosis or middle ear disease.

**mobilize** (mo′bī-līz) [ Fr. *mobiliser,* to liberate, make ready, fr. L. *mobilis,* movable ]. To liberate material stored in the body; to excite quiescent material, such as glycogen, to physiologic activity.

**Mobitz,** Woldemar, German cardiologist, *1889. See M. types A-V *block.*

**Möbius** (mё′be-oos), Paul J., German physician, 1853–1907. See Leyden-M. *dystrophy,* M.'s *disease, sign, syndrome.*

**MOD.** Abbreviation for mesiodistocclusal.

**modality** (mo-dal′ĭ-tĭ) [ Mediev. L. *modalitas,* fr. L. *modus,* a mode ]. 1. Any form of electrical or physiomedical therapeutics. 2. Various forms of sensation, *e.g.,* touch, vision, etc.

**mode** [ L. *modus,* a measure, quantity ]. In a set of measurements, that value which appears most frequently.

**mod′el.** 1. A representation of something, usually idealized and modified to make it conceptually easier to understand; *e.g.,* a physical representation, such as a scale m. of an anatomical structure, or a mathematical representation of the functioning of a system. 2. Something to be imitated. 3. In dentistry, a cast.

   **articulating m.,** articulating *cast.*

   **Bingham m.,** a m. representing the flow behavior of a Bingham plastic, in the idealized case.

   **computer m.,** computer simulation; a mathematical representation of the functioning of a system, presented in the form of a computer program.

   **study m.,** diagnostic *cast.*

**modifica′tion.** A nonhereditary change in an organism; *e.g.,* one that is acquired from its own activity or environment.

   **behavior m.,** the systematic use of principles of conditioning and learning to teach simple skills (*e.g.,* reading or spelling) or to alter undesirable behavior.

**modiolus,** pl. **modi′oli** (mo′di′o-lus) [ L., the nave of a wheel ] [ NA ]. Columella cochleae; the central cone-shaped core of spongy bone about which turns the spiral canal of the cochlea. 2. Modiolus labii; a point near the corner of the mouth where several muscles of facial expression converge.

**modulation** (mod′u-la′shun) [ L. *modulari,* to measure off properly ]. 1. The functional and morphologic fluctuation of cells in response to changing environmental conditions. 2. Systematic variation in a characteristic (*e.g.,* frequency, amplitude) of a sustained oscillation to code additional information.

   **m. transfer function,** in depicting radionuclide distribution, the efficiency, at a given spatial frequency, of transferring the m. of the object that of the image; it is a more complete expression of spatial resolution and is used to evaluate imaging systems and their compenents; abbreviated MTF.

**Moeller** (mё′ler), Alfred, German bacteriologist, *1868. See M.'s *bacillus, stain.*

**Moeller** (mё′ler), Julius O. L., German surgeon, 1819–1887. See M.'s *glossitis.*

**mofebu′tazone.** MOBUZON; 4-butyl-1-phenyl-3,5-pyrazolidinedione; anti-inflammatory agent used for treatment of arthritis.

**mogiarthria** (moj-ĭ-ar'thrĭ-ah) [ G. *mogis*, with difficulty, + *arthroun*, to articulate ]. Speech defect due to muscular incoordination.

**mogigraphia** (moj-ĭ-graf'ĭ-ah) [ G. *mogis*, with difficulty, + *graphē*, writing ]. Writer's *cramp*.

**mogilalia** (moj-ĭ-la'lĭ-ah) [ G. *mogis*, with difficulty, + *lalia*, speech ]. Molilalia; stuttering stammering, or any speech defect.

**mogiphonia** (moj-ĭ-fo'nĭ-ah) [ G. *mogis*, with difficulty, + *phōnē*, voice ]. Laryngeal spasm occurring in public speakers as a result of overuse of the voice.

**mogitocia** (moj-ĭ-to'sĭ-ah) [ G. *mogis*, with difficulty, + *tokos*, childbirth ]. Dystocia; difficult labor.

**Mohrenheim** (mo'ren-hīm), Joseph J. F. von, Austrian surgeon, †1799. See M.'s *fossa*, *space*.

**Mohs,** Frederick E., U. S. surgeon *1910. See M.'s chemo-surgery *technique*.

**Mohs,** Friedrich, German mineralogist, 1773–1839. See M. *scale*.

**moiety** (moy'ĭ-te) [ M.E. *moite*, a half ]. Originally a half, now (loosely) one of two or more parts into which something is divided.

**mol.** Abbreviation for mole.

**mola** [ L. ] [ NA ]. A structure having the shape or function of a millstone.

**mo'lal.** Denoting one mole of solute dissolved in 1000 gm. of solvent; to be distinguished from molar. Molal solutions provide a definite ratio of solute to solvent molecules.

**molal'ity.** The concentration of a solution expressed in mols per kilogram of pure solvent.

**mo'lar.** 1 [ L. *molaris*, relating to a mill ]. Grinding. 2. A molar tooth; a grinder; see *dens* molaris. 3 [ L. *moles*, mass ]. Massive; relating to a mass; not molecular. 4. Denoting a concentration of 1 gram-molecular weight (1 mol) of solute per liter of solution, the common unit of concentration in chemistry; abbreviated M. 5. Adjective indicating a specific quantity, *e.g.*, molar volume (volume of 1 mol). 6. Relating to or associated with hydatidiform mole, *e.g.*, molar pregnancy.

   **first m.,** sixth permanent tooth or fourth deciduous tooth in the maxilla and mandible on either side of the midsagittal plane of the head following the arch form.

   **first permanent m.,** first m.

   **Moon's m.'s,** small dome-shaped first m. teeth occurring in hereditary syphilis.

   **mulberry m.,** a primary or permanent tooth with a nonanatomical depression in its surface caused by hypoplasia of enamel.

   **second m.,** seventh permanent or fifth deciduous tooth in the maxilla and mandible on either side of the midsagittal plane of the head following the arch form.

   **sixth-year m.,** the first permanent m. tooth.

   **third m.,** eighth permanent tooth in the maxilla and mandible on either side of the midsagittal plane of the head following the arch form.

   **twelfth-year m.,** the permanent second m. tooth.

**molar'iform** [ molar (tooth) + L. *forma*, form ]. Having the form of a molar tooth.

**molarity** (mo-lăr'ĭ-tĭ). The concentration of a solution expressed in mols per liter of solution.

**mold,** Mould. 1. A multicellular fungous growth. 2. A shaped receptacle into which wax is pressed or fluid plaster is poured in making a cast. 3. To shape a mass of plastic material according to a definite pattern. 4. To change in shape; denoting especially the adaptation of the fetal head to the pelvic canal. 5. The term used to specify the shape of an artificial tooth (or teeth).

**mold'ing.** Shaping by means of a mold.

   **border m.,** tissue m.; tissue-trimming; muscle-trimming; the shaping of an impression material by the manipulation or action of the tissues adjacent to the borders of an impression.

   **compression m.,** (1) the act of pressing or squeezing together to form a shape in a mold; (2) the adaptation of a plastic material to the negative form of a split mold by pressure; see also injection m.

   **injection m.,** the adaptation of a plastic material to the negative form of a closed mold by forcing the material into

the mold through appropriate gateways. See also compression m.

   **tissue m.,** border m.

**mole.** 1 [ A.S. *māēl* (L. *macula*), a spot ]. *Nevus* pigmentosus. 2 [ L. *moles*, mass ]. An intrauterine mass formed by the degeneration of the partly developed products of conception. 3 (abbreviated mol.). Gram molecule; the unit of "amount" of substance; one of the seven base units in the SI system of units. The mole is defined as that amount of substance that contains as many "elementary entities" as there are atoms in 0.0120 kg. of carbon-12. "Elementary entities" may be atoms, molecules, ions, or any describable entity or defined mixture of entities. In practical terms, the mole is $6.0225 \times 10^{23}$ "elementary entities." See also Avogadro's *number*.

   **blood m.,** fleshy m.

   **Breus m.,** an aborted ovum in which the fetal surface of the placenta presents numerous hematomata, there is an absence of blood vessels in the chorion, and the ovum is much smaller than it should be according to the duration of the pregnancy.

   **car'neous m.,** fleshy m.

   **cystic m.,** hydatidiform m.

   **false m.,** an intrauterine polypus.

   **fleshy m.,** (1) a shapeless fetal mass; (2) a shapeless mass of the secundines retained after abortion.

   **grape m.,** hydatidiform m.

   **hairy m.,** *nevus* pilosus.

   **hydat'id m., hydatid'iform m.,** cystic m.; grape m.; vesicular m.; a vesicular or polycystic mass resulting from the proliferation of the trophoblast, with hydropic degeneration and avascularity of the chorionic villi.

   **maternal m.,** fleshy m. (2).

   **spider m.,** arterial *spider*.

   **stone m.,** uterine calculus; wombstone; a fleshy m. which has undergone calcareous degeneration.

   **true m.,** fleshy m. (1).

   **vesic'ular m.,** hydatidiform m.

**molecular** (mo-lek'u-lar). Relating to molecules.

**molecule** (mol'e-kūl) [ Mod. L. *molecula*, dim. of L. *moles*, mass ]. The smallest possible quantity of a di-, tri-, or polyatomic substance that retains the chemical properties of the substance. A molecule of $H_2SO_4$ contains two atoms of H, one of S, and four of O.

**Moliaceae** (mol'ĭ-a'se-e). A family of Fungi Imperfecti in the order Moniliales, which includes *Sporotrichum schenckii*, causative agent of sporotrichosis.

**molilalia** (mol'ĭ-la'lĭ-ah) [ G. *molis*, with difficulty (a later form of *mogis*), + *lalia*, talking ]. Mogilalia.

**molimen,** pl. **molim'ina** (mo-li'men, mo'li-men) [ L. an endeavor ]. An effort; the laborious performance of a normal function.

   **m. climacte'reium virile,** a condition resembling neurasthenia, occurring in men of 45 to 55 years of age; may be psychosomatic or due to alteration in testicular androgen secretion.

   **menstrual molimina,** the unpleasant symptoms, feeling of weight in the pelvis, nervous and circulatory disturbances, etc., experienced during the menstrual period.

**molin'done hydrochloride** (USAN). 3-Ethyl-6,7-dihydro-2-methyl-5-(morpholinomethyl)indol-4(5*H*)-one monohydrochloride; a sedative with antianxiety activity.

**Mol'isch,** Hans, Vienna chemist, 1856–1937. See M.'s *test*.

**Moll,** Jacob A., Dutch oculist, 1832–1914. See M.'s *gland*.

**mollis** [ L. ] [ NA ]. Mollities.

**mollities** (mol-ish'ĭ-ēz) [ L. *mollis*, soft. MOLL- ]. 1. Characterized by a soft consistency. 2. Malacia (1).

   **m. os'sium,** osteomalacia.

**Mollusca** (mol-us'kah) [ L. *mollusca*, a nut with a thin shell, fr. *mollis*, soft ]. A phylum of the subkingdom Metazoa with soft, unsegmented bodies, consisting of an anterior head, a dorsal visceral mass and a ventral foot. Most forms are enclosed in a protective calcareous shell. M. includes the classes Gastropoda (snails, whelks, slugs), Pelecypoda (oysters, clams, mussels), Cephalopoda (squids, octopuses), Amphineura (chitons), Scaphopoda (tooth shells), and a recently discovered class of primitive metameric mollusks, Monoplacophora.

**molluscous** (mol-us'kus). Relating to or resembling molluscum.

**molluscum** (mol-us'kum) [ L. *molluscus*, soft. MOLL- ]. A disease marked by the occurrence of soft, rounded tumors of the skin.

    **m. contagiosum,** m. sessile; m. verrucosum; m. epitheliale; condyloma subcutaneum; an infectious disease of the skin, caused by a virus, characterized by the appearance of few to numerous small pearly umbilicated papular epithelial lesions which contain numerous inclusion bodies known as m. bodies.

    **m. epithelia'le,** m. contagiosum.

    **m. fibrosum,** neurofibromatosis.

    **m. fibrosum gravida'rum,** *fibroma* molluscum gravidarum.

    **m. pen'dulum,** *fibroma* pendulum.

    **m. pseu'docar'cinomato'sum,** keratoacanthoma.

    **m. seba'ceum,** keratoacanthoma.

    **m. sessi'le,** m. contagiosum.

    **m. verruco'sum,** m. contagiosum.

**Moloney,** P. J. See M. *test.*

**Moloy,** Howard C., American obstetrician, 1903–1953. See Caldwell-M. *classification.*

**molt** [ L. *muto*, to change ]. Moult; to cast off feathers, hair, or cuticle; to undergo ecdysis; see also desquamate.

**mol wt.** Abbreviation for molecular *weight.*

**molybdate** (mo-lib'dāt). A salt of molybdic acid.

**molybden'ic.** Molybdenous; relating to molybdenum.

**molyb'denize.** To impregnate with a salt of molybdic acid, such as ammonium molybdate; denoting a method of demonstrating nerve fibrils.

**molyb'denous.** Molybdenic.

**molybdenum** (mo-lib'dĕ-num) [ G. *molybdaina*, a piece of lead; a metal, prob. galena, fr. *molybdos*, lead ]. A silvery white metallic element, symbol Mo, atomic no. 42, atomic weight 95.95.

**molybdenum-99.** $^{99}$Mo; a reactor-produced radioisotope of molybdenum with a half-life of 68.3 hours; used in the manufacture of radionuclide generators for the production of technetium-99m.

**molyb'dic.** Denoting molybdenum in the 6+ state, as in $MoO_3$.

    **m. acid,** $MoO_3 \cdot H_2O$; a yellowish crystalline acid, forming salts called molybdates.

**molyb'dous.** Denoting molybdenum in the 4+ state, as in $MoO_2$.

**molysmophobia** (mō-liz'mo-fo'bī-ah) [ G. *molysma*, filth, infection, + *phobos*, fear ]. Mysophobia; a morbid fear of infection.

**Momburg,** Fritz A., German surgeon, 1870–1939. See M.'s *method.*

**mom'ism.** Excessive or overbearing mothering, especially as attributed to American cultural stereotypes.

**Momsen,** Charles B., Sr., U. S. naval officer, 1896–1967. See M. *lung.*

**mon-.** See mono-.

**monad** (mo'nad, mon'ad) [ G. *monas*, the number one, unity ]. 1. A univalent element. 2. A unicellular organism. 3. Specifically, a flagellate. 4. The single chromosome derived from a tetrad after the first and second maturation divisions.

**Monadida** (mon-ad'ī-dah). Monadina; an order of Zoomastigophora, embracing cells, often ameboid in form, provided with one or more flagella at one end.

**mon'adin.** Monad.

**Monadina** (mon'ă-di'nah). Monadida.

**Monakow** (mo-nah'kov), Constantin von, Swiss histologist, 1853–1930. See M.'s *bundle, nucleus, syndrome, tract.*

**monam'ide.** Monoamide.

**monam'ine.** Monoamine.

**monam'inu'ria.** Monoaminuria.

**monarda** (mon-ar'dah). The leaves of *Monarda punctata* (family Labiatae), American horsemint, a labiate plant of the United States east of the Mississippi; the main commercial source of natural thymol; used as a carminative in colic.

**monarthric** (mon-ar'thrik). Monarticular.

**mon'arthri'tis.** Arthritis of a single joint.

**mon'artic'ular.** Uniarticular; monarthric; relating to a single joint.

**Mo'nas** [ G. single, a unit ]. 1. A genus of flagellates of the order Monadida. 2. A monad.

**monas'ter** [ mono- + G. *astēr*, star ]. The single star figure in mitosis.

**mon'atheto'sis.** Athetosis affecting one hand or foot.

**mon'atom'ic.** 1. Relating to or containing a single atom. 2. Univalent.

**monauchenos** (mon-aw'kĕ-nus) [ mono- + G. *auchēn*, neck ]. Single-necked; see *dicephalus* monauchenos.

**monaural** (mon-aw'ral) [ mono- + L. *auris*, ear ]. Pertaining to one ear.

**monaxon'ic** [ mono- + G. *axōn*, axle ]. 1. Having but one axis, being therefore elongated and slender. 2. Having one axon.

**Mönckeberg** (mĕn'ka-bairg), Johann G., German pathologist, 1877–1925. See M.'s *arteriosclerosis, calcification, degeneration.*

**Mondeville** (mon-de-ve'yuh), Henri de, 1260–1320. French anatomist and surgeon, professor at Montpellier and author of surgical text; he was among the first to advocate cleanliness in surgery.

**Mondino.** See Mundinus.

**Mondonesi** (mon-do-na'zi), Filippo, Italian physician. See M.'s *reflex.*

**Mondor,** Henri, French surgeon, 1885–1962. See M.'s *disease.*

**mo'ner** [ G. *monērēs*, solitary, fr. *monos*, alone ]. Obsolete designation for a non-nucleated mass of protoplasm.

**Monera** (mo-ne'rah) [ pl. of Mod. L. *moneron*, fr. G. *monērēs*, solitary ]. A name given by Haeckel to protozoan organisms having no defined nucleus.

**mon'esthet'ic** [ mono- + G. *aisthēsis*, sense perception ]. Relating to a single sense or sensation.

**monestrous** (mon-es'trus). Having but one estrous cycle in a mating season.

**mon'etite.** $2CaOP_2O_5H_2O$; a naturally occurring calcium phosphate.

**Mon'gol.** An individual of the Mongolian race.

**mon'gol.** An individual with mongolism.

    **translocation m.,** a patient in whom mongolism is due to translocation of a major portion of chromosome 21 to another chromosome, and who also has two normal no. 21 chromosomes; he is thus effectively trisomic for chromosome 21 but has a chromosome count of 46; see also Down's *syndrome.*

**mongo'lian.** 1. Mongoloid. 2. Relating to a member of the Mongolian race.

**mon'golism** (so called because the facial appearance resembles that of a Mongol). Down's *syndrome.*

**mon'goloid.** Mongolian (1); relating to or characterized by mongolism.

**Monie'zia expan'sa.** The broad tapeworm (family Anoplocephalidae) of sheep; also reported from calves. It is the most common tapeworm of sheep, occurring in the small intestine and reaching a length of 12 to 15 feet; infections are usually benign. Cysticercoids develop in soil-dwelling mites commonly ingested with grass by herbivores.

**mon'ilated.** Moniliform.

**monilethrix** (mo-nil'ĕ-thriks) [ L. *monile*, necklace, + G. *thrix*, hair ]. Beaded or moniliform hair; a condition in which the hairs are brittle and show a series of constrictions, giving the appearance of a string of fusiform beads; a developmental ectodermal defect, probably due to underlying metabolic disorder.

**Monilia** (mo-nil'ĭ-ah) [ L. *monile*, necklace ]. Generic term for a large group of molds or fungi that are commonly known as fruit molds; a few closely related pathogenic organisms formerly classified in this genus are now properly termed *Candida.*

    **M. al'bicans,** *Candida albicans.*

    **M. psilo'sis,** a species formerly thought by some observers to be the pathogenic organism in sprue; probably synonymous with *Candida albicans.*

**monil'ial.** Precisely, pertaining to fungi of the genus *Monilia*, but, in medicine, frequently used with reference to the genus *Candida*.

**moniliasis** (mo'nĭ-li'ă-sis). Moniliosis; infection with any species of *Monilia*; it includes thrush and certain dermatomycoses and bronchomycoses.

**monil'iform** [ L. *monile*, necklace, + *forma*, appearance ]. Monilated; beaded.

**Moniliformis** (mo-nil'ĭ-for'mis). A genus of the class (or phylum) Acanthocephala, the thorny-headed worms.

  **M. du'bius,** the common spiny-headed worm of house rats, transmitted by infected cockroaches, *Periplaneta americana;* a few infections in man have been reported.

  **M. monilifor'mis,** normally found in rodents but not usually a parasite of man.

**moniliid** (mo-nil'e-id). Minute macular or papular lesions occurring as an allergic reaction to monilial infection. *Candida albicans* cannot be recovered from the m.

**moniliosis** (mo-nil'ĭ-o'sis). Moniliasis.

**mon'ism** [ G. *monos*, single ]. A metaphysical system in which all of reality is conceived as a unified whole.

**monis'tic.** Pertaining to monism.

**mon'itor.** A device that records specified data for a given series of events, operations, or circumstances.

  **cardiac m.,** an electronic m. which, when connected to the patient, signals each heart beat with a flashing light, an electrocardiographic curve, or an audible signal.

**Moniz** (mo-nesh'), Antonio Egas, Portuguese neurosurgeon, 1874–1955. Nobel laureate, 1949, with Walter R. Hess, for the discovery of the therapeutic value of leukotomy in certain psychoses.

**monkey-paw.** A contracture of the hand resulting from median nerve palsy; the thumb cannot be opposed to the tips of the fingers.

**monks'hood.** See aconite.

**mono-, mon-** [ G. *monos*, single ]. Prefix denoting the participation or involvement of a single element or part; see also uni-.

**mon'oam'ide.** A molecule containing one amide group.

**mon'oam'ine.** A molecule containing one amine group.

  **m. oxidase,** amine oxidase (flavin-containing).

  **m. oxidase inhibitors,** abbreviated MAOI; hydrazine (—NHNH₂) and hydrazide (—CONHNH₂) derivatives, such as isocarboxazid, that inhibit several enzymes, and raise the brain norepinephrine and 5-hydroxytryptamine levels; used as antidepressant and hypotensive agents.

**monoaminuria** (mon'o-am'in-u'rĭ-ah). The excretion of any monoamine in the urine.

**monobac'illary.** Relating to or caused by one species of bacillus, denoting an infection.

**monobacte'rial.** Associated with one species only of bacteria, said of an infection.

**monoba'sic.** Denoting an acid with only one replaceable hydrogen atom, or only one replaced hydrogen atom.

**monoben'zone** (NF). BENOQUIN; *p*-benzyloxyphenol; a melanin-pigment inhibiting agent; used topically for the treatment of hyperpigmentation caused by formation of melanin.

**mon'oblast** [ mono- + G. *blastos*, germ ]. An immature cell that develops into a monocyte.

**mon'oblep'sia** [ mono- + G. *blepsis*, sight ]. A condition in which vision is better with one eye than with two.

**monobrachius** (mon'o-bra'kĭ-us) [ mono- + G. *brachiōn*, arm ]. An individual with but one arm.

**mon'obro'mated.** Monobrominated; denoting a chemical compound with one atom of bromine per molecule.

**monocar'dian.** Having a heart with a single atrium and ventricle.

**monoceph'alus.** Syncephalus.

**monochlorphen'amide.** SOLURAN; 4-chloro-*m*-benzenedisulfonamide; diuretic.

**monochord** (mon'o-kord). An instrument used in hearing tests.

  **Schultze's m.,** a device formed of a metal wire tightly stretched and provided with an appliance for shortening the length of its vibrating portion, when rubbed or plucked; used to determine the upper tone limit of hearing.

**monochorea** (mon-o-ko-re'ah). Chorea affecting the head alone or only one extremity.

**monochorial** (mon'o-ko'ri-al). Monochorionic.

**monochorionic** (mon'o-ko-rĭ-on'ik). Monochorial; relating to or having a single chorion; denoting monovular twins.

**monochroic** (mon-o-kro'ik). Monochromatic.

**monochromasia** (mon'o-kro-ma'zĭ-ah). Monochromatism.

**monochromatic** (mon'o-kro-mat'ik). 1. Monochroic; monochromic; having but one color. 2. Indicating a pure spectral color of a single wavelength. 3. Relating to or characterized by monochromatism.

**monochromatism** (mon'o-kro'mă-tizm) [ mono- + G. *chrōma*, color ]. 1. The state of having or exhibiting only one color. 2. Achromatopsia.

**monochromatophil, monochromatophile** (mon'o-kro-mat'o-fil, -fil) [ mono- + G. *chrōma*, color, + *philos*, fond ]. 1. Taking only one stain. 2. A cell or any histologic element staining with only one kind of dye.

**monochro'mic.** Monochromatic.

**monochro'mophil, monochro'mophile.** Monochromatophil.

**monoclinic** (mon'o-klin'ik) [ mono- + G. *klinein*, to incline ]. Relating to crystals with a single oblique inclination.

**monocra'nius** [ mono- + G. *kranion*, cranium ]. Syncephalus.

**monocrotaline** (mon'o-cro'tă-lin). Crotaline; an alkaloid in the seeds, leaves and stems of *Crotalaria spectabilis* (family Leguminosae), a plant poisonous to livestock and poultry in the southern United States.

**monocrotic** (mon'o-krot'ik) [ mono- + G. *krotos*, a beat ]. Denoting a pulse the curve of which presents no notch in the downward line.

**monocrotism** (mon-ok'ro-tizm) [ mono- + G. *krotos*, a beat ]. The state in which the pulse is monocrotic.

**monocular** (mon-ok'u-lar) [ mono- + L. *oculus*, eye ]. Relating to, affecting, or visible by, one eye only.

**monoculus** (mon-ok'u-lus) [ L. a one-eyed man, a hybrid word fr. G. *monos*, single, + L. *oculus*, eye ]. 1. Cyclops. 2. A bandage applied to one eye only.

**monocyte** (mon'o-sīt) [ mono- + G. *kytos*, cell ]. A relatively large mononuclear leukocyte (16 to 22 μ) in diameter. M.'s normally constitute 3 to 7 per cent of the leukocytes of the circulating blood; in addition, they are normally found in lymph nodes, spleen, bone marrow, and loose connective tissue. When treated with the usual dyes, m.'s manifest an abundant, pale blue or blue-gray cytoplasm that contains numerous, fine, dustlike, red-blue granules, and vacuoles are frequently present; the nucleus is usually indented, or slightly folded, and has a stringy chromatin structure that seems more condensed where the delicate strands are in contact. See also monocytoid *cell*, endothelial *leukocyte*, and color plate 15.

**monocytopenia** (mon'o-si-to-pe'nĭ-ah) [ mono- + G. *kytos*, cell, + *penia*, poverty ]. Monocytic leukopenia; monopenia; diminution in the number of monocytes in the circulating blood.

**monocytosis** (mon'o-si-to'sis). Monocytic leukocytosis; an abnormal increase in the number of monocytes in the circulating blood.

  **avian m.,** bluecomb *disease* of chickens.

**Monod** (mo-no'), Jacques, French molecular biologist, \*1910. Nobel laureate, 1965, with François Jacob and André Lwoff, for their contributions to the understanding of the regulation of gene activity in ontogeny.

**monodactyly, monodactylism** (mon'o-dak'-tĭ-lĭ, -dak'-tĭ-lizm) [ mono- + G. *daktylos*, digit ]. The presence of a single finger on the hand, or a single toe on the foot.

**mon'odermo'ma** [ mono- + G. *derma*, skin, + suffix -*ōma*, tumor ]. A neoplasm composed of tissues from a single germinal layer.

**monodiplopia** (mon'o-dĭ-plo'pĭ-ah). Monocular *diplopia*.

**mon'odisperse.** Of relatively uniform size; said of aerosol suspensions with size variation of less than ± 20 per cent.

**mon'oethanol'amine** (NF). 2-Aminoethanol; a surfactant; the oleate is used as a sclerosing agent in the treatment of varicose veins.

**monofactorial** (mon'o-fak-to'rĭ-al). Pertaining to a single factor.

**monogamet'ic.** Homogametic.

**monog'amy** [ mono- + G. *gamos*, marriage ]. The marriage (human) or mating (animal) system in which each partner has but one mate.

**monogenesis** (mon-o-jen'ĕ-sis) [ mono- + G. *genesis*, origin, production ]. 1. The production of similar organisms in each generation; see metagenesis. 2. The production of young by a single parent as in nonsexual generation and parthenogenesis. 3. The process of parasitizing a single host, in which the life cycle of the parasite is passed; *e.g.*, *Boophilus annulatus*, the one-host cattle tick, or trematodes of the order Monogenea.

**monogenet'ic.** Monoxenous; relating to monogenesis.

**monogenous** (mŏ-noj'ĕ-nus). Asexually produced, as by fission, gemmation, or sporulation.

**monogerminal** (mon'o-jer'mĭ-nal). Unigerminal.

**mon'ograph** [ mono- + G. *graphē*, a writing ]. A treatise on a particular subject or class of subjects.

**monohy'brid.** The offspring of parents that differ in one character.

**monohy'drated.** Containing or united with a single molecule of water per molecule of substance.

**monohy'dric.** Having but one hydrogen atom in the molecule.

**monoideism** (mon-o-i-de'izm) [ mono- + G. *idea*, form, idea ]. A harping on one idea; a slight degree of monomania.

**mon'oinfec'tion.** Simple infection with a single variety of microorganism.

**monoiodotyrosine** (mon'o-i-o'do-ti'ro-sēn). Symbol ITyr; tyrosine with one ring H replaced by I; one of the iodinated amino acids present in thyroid hydrolysates.

**monoisonitrosoacetone** (mon'o-i'so-ni-tro-so-as'e-tōn). A cholinesterase reactivator that can penetrate the blood-brain barrier readily and cause significant reactivation of phosphorylated acetylcholinesterase in the central nervous system; used to protect human beings and animals against otherwise lethal poisoning with organophosphorous anticholinesterase agents.

**mon'olay'ers.** Films, one molecule thick, formed on water by certain substances, such as proteins and fatty acids, characterized by molecules containing some atom groupings that are soluble in water and other atom groupings that are insoluble in water.

**monolocular** (mon'o-lok'u-lar) [ mono- + L. *loculus*, a small place ]. Unicameral; having one cavity, as in a fat cell.

**monolu'pine.** Anagyrine.

**mon'oma'nia** [ mono- + G. *mania*, frenzy ]. Monopsychosis; an obsession or abnormally extreme enthusiasm for a single idea or subject; a psychosis marked by the limitation of the symptoms more or less strictly to a certain group, as the delusion in paranoia.

**monomaniac** (mon'o-ma'nĭ-ak). 1. One exhibiting monomania. 2. Characterized by or relating to monomania.

**monomas'tigote.** A mastigote having but one flagellum.

**monomel'ic** [ mono- + G. *melos*, limb ]. Relating to one limb.

**mon'omer** [ mono- + suffix -mer, *q.v.* ]. 1. The molecular unit that, by repetition, constitutes a large structure or polymer. Thus, ethylene, $CH_2=CH_2$, is the monomer of polyethylene . . . $CH_2CH_2CH_2CH_2$ . . . or $H(CH_2)_nH$; adenylic acid is the monomer of poly(adenylic acid). 2. The protein structural unit of a virion capsid; see virion.

**monomeric** (mon'o-mĕr'ik) [ mono- + G. *meros*, part ]. 1. Consisting of a single part. 2. In genetics, relating to a hereditary disease or characteristic controlled by genes at a single locus. 3. Consisting of monomers.

**monometal'lic.** Containing but one atom of a metal in the molecule.

**monomicro'bic.** Denoting a monoinfection, or an infection due to the presence of a single species of microbe, whether bacterium or protozoon.

**monomolecular** (mon'o-mo-lek'u-lar). Referring to a single molecule.

**monomor'phic** [ mono- + G. *morphē*, shape ]. Of one shape; unchangeable in shape.

**monomphalus** (mon-om'fă-lus) [ mono- + G. *omphalos*, umbilicus ]. Omphalopagus.

**monomyoplegia** (mon'o-mi'o-ple'jĭ-ah) [ mono- + G. *mys*, muscle, + *plēgē*, a stroke ]. Paralysis limited to one muscle.

**monomyositis** (mon-o-mi-o-si'tis). Inflammation of a single muscle.

**mononeural, mononeuric** (mon'o-nu'ral, -nu'rik). 1. Having only one neuron. 2. Supplied by a single nerve.

**mononeuralgia** (mon'o-nu-ral'jĭ-ah). Pain along the course of one nerve.

**mononeuritis** (mon'o-nu-ri'tis). Inflammation of a single nerve.

m. **mul'tiplex**, inflammation of several nerves in unrelated portions of the body.

**mononeuropathy** (mon'o-nu-rop'ă-thĭ). Disease involving a single nerve.

m. **multiplex**, involvement of several individual nerves.

**mononoea** (mon'o-ne'ah) [ mono- + G. *noēsis*, idea ]. Fixation of the mind on one subject.

**mononuclear** (mon'o-nu'kle-ar). Uninuclear.

**mononucleosis** (mon'o-nu'kle-o'sis). The presence of abnormally large numbers of mononuclear leukocytes in the circulating blood, especially with reference to forms that are not normal.

**infectious m.**, benign lymphadenosis; glandular fever; an acute, febrile illness that is probably caused by a virus, but the causal agent has not been clearly identified; characterized by fever, sore throat, enlargement of lymph nodes and spleen, and leukopenia that changes to lymphocytosis during the second week; the circulating blood usually contains abnormal, large lymphocytes that have a resemblance to monocytes, and there is heterophil antibody that may be completely adsorbed on beef erythrocytes, but not on guinea pig kidney antigen. Collections of the characteristic abnormal lymphocytes may be present not only in the lymph nodes and spleen, but in various other sites, *e.g.*, the meninges, brain, myocardium, and so on.

**mon'onu'cleotide.** Nucleotide.

**monooxygenases** (mon'o-ok'sĭ-jĕ-na-sez). Oxidoreductases that induce the incorporation of one atom of oxygen from $O_2$ into the substance being oxidized. M.'s are classified in EC sub-subgroups 1.13.12 and 1.14.13 – .99; see, for example, monophenol monooxygenase.

**monoparesis** (mon'o-pă-re'sis, -păr'e-sis). Paresis affecting a single extremity or part of an extremity.

**monoparesthesia** (mon'o-păr-es-the'zĭ-ah). Paresthesia affecting a single region only.

**monopath'ic.** Relating to a single disease or to a disease affecting a single part.

**monop'athy** [ mono- + G. *pathos*, suffering ]. 1. A single uncomplicated disease. 2. A local disease affecting only one organ or part.

**monope'nia.** Monocytopenia.

**monophagism** (mo-nof'ă-jizm) [ mono- + G. *phagein*, to eat ]. Habitual eating of but one kind of food or but one meal a day.

**monophasia** (mon'o-fa'zĭ-ah) [ mono- + G. *phasis*, speech ]. Inability to speak other than a single word or sentence.

**monophasic** (mon-o-fa'zik). 1. Marked by monophasia. 2. Characterized by only one phase. 3. Pertaining to a psychiatric disorder with one phase, as opposed to a diphasic disorder like manic-depressive psychosis.

**monophenol monooxygenase** (EC 1.14.18.1). *o*-Diphenol oxidase; *p*-diphenol oxidase; phenol oxidase; tyrosinase; catechol oxidase; cresolase; polyphenol oxidase; phenolase; laccase; urushiol oxidase; a copper-containing oxidoreductase that catalyzes the oxidation of *o*-diphenols to *o*-quinones, utilizing $O_2$; also catalyzes the oxidation of monophenols such as tyrosine to dihydroxyphenylalanine (dopa), a precursor of melanin and epinephrine (catecholamines).

**monopho'bia** [ mono- + G. *phobos*, fear ]. Morbid fear of solitude or of being left alone.

**monophtalmus** (mon'of-thal'mus) [ mono- + G. *ophthalmos*, eye ]. Cyclops.

**monophyletic** (mon'o-fi-let'ik) [ mono- + G. *phylē*, tribe ]. 1. Having a single source of origin; derived from one line of descent; opposed to polyphyletic. 2. In hematology, relating to polyphyletism.

**monophyletism** (mon-o-fi'lĕ-tizm) [ mono- + G. *phylē*, tribe ]. Monophyletic theory; in hematology, the theory that all the blood cells are derived from one common stem cell or histioblast.

**monophyodont** (mon'o-fi'o-dont) [ mono- + G. *phyō*, to grow, + *odous* (*odont*-), tooth ]. Having one set of teeth only; without deciduous dentition; compare diphyodont and polyphyodont.

**mon'oplasmat'ic** [ mono- + G. *plasma*, thing formed ]. Formed of but one tissue.

**mon'oplast** [ mono- + G. *plastos*, formed ]. A unicellular organism that retains the same structure or form throughout its existence.

**monoplas'tic.** Undergoing no change in structure, relating to a monoplast.

**monoplegia** (mon'o-ple'ji-ah) [ mono- + G. *plēgē*, a stroke ]. Paralysis of one limb.

  **m. masticato'ria,** unilateral paralysis of the muscles of mastication (masseter, temporal, pterygoid).

**monoploid** (mon'o-ployd). Haploid.

**monopo'dia** [ mono- + G. *pous*, foot ]. A malformation in which there is only one foot externally recognizable.

**mon'ops** [ mono- + G. *ōps*, eye ]. Cyclops.

**monopsychosis** (mon-o-si-ko'sis). Monomania.

**monoptychial** (mon'o-tik'ī-al) [ mono- + G. *ptychē*, fold ]. Arranged in a single but folded layer, as the cells in the epithelium of the gallbladder or certain glands.

**mon'opus** [ mono- + G. *pous*, foot ]. See *sympus* monopus.

**monorchia** (mon-or'kī-ah). Monorchism.

**monorchid** (mon-or'kid). 1. Monorchidic. 2. Monorchis.

**monorchidic** (mon-or-kid'ik). 1. Having but one testis. 2. Having apparently but one testis, the other being undescended.

**monorchidism** (mon-or'kī-dizm). Monorchism.

**monorchis** (mon-or'kis) [ mono- + G. *orchis*, testis ]. A person with monorchidism.

**monorchism** (mon-or-kizm) [ mono- + G. *orchis*, testis ]. Monorchidism; a condition in which but one testis is apparent, the other being absent or undescended.

**monorecidive** (mon'o-res'ī-dēv') [ mono- + L. *recidivus*, relapsing ]. A late or tertiary manifestation of syphilis which takes the form of an ulcerated papule located at the site of the original chancre. Such a lesion is called a monorecidive lesion. See also *chancre* redux.

**monorhinic** (mon'o-rin'ik) [ mono- + G. *rhis* (*rhin*-), nose ]. Single-nosed; used to characterize conjoined twins in which cephalic fusion has left only a single nose evident.

**monosaccharide** (mon-o-sak'ă-rīd). A carbohydrate that cannot form any simpler sugar by simple hydrolysis. The pentoses and hexoses are m.'s.

**monoscelous** (mon'o-sel'us, -skel'us) [ mono- + G. *skelos*, leg ]. Having only one leg.

**monoscenism** (mon'o-se'nizm) [ mono- + G. *skēnē*, tent (stage drop) ]. Morbid concentration on some past experience.

**mon'ose.** Monosaccharide.

**mon'osome** [ mono- + chromosome ]. Accessory *chromosome.*

**monosomia** (mon'o-so'mī-ah) [ mono- + G. *sōma*, body ]. A state in which, in conjoined twins, the trunks are completely merged although the heads remain separate.

**monoso'mic.** Relating to monosomy.

**monoso'mous.** Characterized by or pertaining to monosomia.

**monosomy** (mon'o-so'mī) [ see monosome ]. State of an individual or cell that has lost one member of a pair of homologous chromosomes; in man the state of a cell with 45 chromosomes, exclusive of balanced translocations.

**mon'ospasm.** Spasm affecting only one muscle or group of muscles, or a single extremity.

**mon'ospermy** [ mono- + G. *sperma*, seed ]. Fertilization through the entrance of only one spermatozoon into the egg.

**Monospo'rium apiosper'mum.** The imperfect stage of the fungus *Allescheria boydii*, *q. v.*

**Monostoma** (mo-nos'to-mah) [ mono- + G. *stoma*, mouth ]. Archaic name for a genus of flukes, or trematodes, based on the presence of a single sucker.

  **M. lentis,** a species reported from the crystalline lens of the human eye.

**monostotic** (mon'os-tot'ik) [ mono- + G. *osteon*, bone ]. Involving only one bone.

**monostra'tal** [ mono- + L. *stratum*, layer ]. Composed of a single layer.

**monosub'stituted.** In chemistry, denoting an element or radical, only one atom of which is found in each molecule of a substitution compound.

**mon'osymptomat'ic.** Denoting a disease or morbid condition manifested by only one marked symptom.

**monosynaptic** (mon'o-sĭ-nap'tik). Referring to direct neural connections (those not involving an intermediary neuron); *e.g.*, the direct connection between primary sensory nerve cells and motor neurons characterizing the monosynaptic reflex arc.

**monosyphilide** (mo-no-sif'ī-lēd). Marked by the occurrence of a single syphilitic lesion.

**monoter'penes.** Hydrocarbons or their derivatives formed by the condensation of two isoprene units, and containing, therefore, 10 carbon atoms; *e.g.*, camphor.

**monother'mia** [ mono- + G. *thermē*, heat ]. Evenness of bodily temperature; absence of an evening rise in fever.

**monothi'oglyc'erol** (NF). α-Monothioglycerol; thioglycerol; used to promote wound healing.

**monotocous** (mo-not'o-kus) [ mono- + G. *tokos*, birth ]. Producing a single offspring at a birth.

**Monotremata** (mon'o-tre'mă-tah) [ mono- + G. *trēma*, a hole ]. Monotremes; an order of egg-laying mammals that have a cloaca or common chamber which receives digestive, urinary, and reproductive products; only Australia has such forms: the duck-billed platypus (*Ornithorhynchus*) and the echidna (*Tachyglossus*).

**monotreme** (mon'o-trēm). A member of the order Monotremata.

**Monotricha** (mo-not'rī-kah) [ mono- + G. *thrix*, hair ]. A group of protozoans having a single flagellum.

**monotrichate** (mon-o-trik'āt). Monotrichous.

**monotrichous** (mo-not'rī-kus). Monotrichate; uniflagellate; denoting a microorganism possessing a single flagellum or cilium.

**monova'lence.** Univalence; a valence of one; the state of being monovalent.

**monova'lent.** 1. Univalent; having the combining power of an atom of hydrogen; denoting a valence of one. 2. Pertaining to a monovalent (specific) *antiserum.*

**monox'enous** [ mono- + G. *xenos*, stranger ]. Monogenetic.

**monox'ide.** Any oxide having only one atom of oxygen (*e.g.*, carbon monoxide, CO).

**monozygotic** (mon'o-zi-got'ik) [ mono- + G. *zygōtos*, yoked ]. Denoting twins derived from a single fertilized ovum; see under twin.

**Monro,** Alexander, Scottish anatomist and surgeon, 1697–1767. See *bursa* of M.

**Monro,** Alexander, Jr., Scottish anatomist, 1733–1817. See M.'s *doctrine*, M.-Kellie *doctrine*, M.'s *foramen*, M.'s *line*, M.-Richter *line*, Richter-M. *line*, M.'s *sulcus*.

**mons,** gen. **montis,** pl. **montes** (monz, mon'tis, mon'tēz) [ L. a mountain ] [ NA ]. An anatomical prominence or slight elevation above the general level of the surface.

  **m. pu'bis** [ NA ], pubic mound; m. veneris; the prominence caused by a pad of fatty tissue over the symphysis pubis in the female.

  **m. ure'teris,** a pinkish prominence on the wall of the bladder marking each ureteral orifice.

  **m. ven'eris** [ L. *Venus* ], m. pubis.

**Monson,** G. S. See M. *curve,* anti-Monson *curve.*

**mon′ster** [ L. *monstrum,* an evil omen, a prodigy, a wonder, fr. *moneo,* to advise, warn ]. Term frequently appearing in the older literature to designate a grossly malformed fetus.

   **compound m.,** one in which there are parts, more or less imperfectly developed, of more than one individual.

   **double m.,** conjoined *twins.*

   **Gila m.** (he′lah) [ *Gila,* a river in Arizona ], a large poisonous lizard, *Heloderma suspectum* and *H. horridum,* of New Mexico, Arizona, and northern Mexico.

   **parasitic m.,** the smaller and less well developed of unequal conjoined twins attached as a "parasite" on the more nearly normal twin.

   **triplet m.,** a compound m., containing parts of three individuals.

   **twin m.,** conjoined *twins.*

**Monteggia** (mon-ted′jah), Giovanni B., Italian surgeon, 1762–1815. See M.'s *fracture.*

**Montgomery,** William F., Irish physician, 1797–1859. See M.'s *follicle, gland, tubercle.*

**monticulus,** pl. **montic′uli** (mon-tik′u-lus) [ L. dim. of *mons,* mountain ]. 1 [ NA ]. Any slight rounded projection above a surface. 2. The central portion of the superior vermis forming a projection on the surface of the cerebellum; its anterior and most prominent portion is called the culmen, its posterior sloping portion, the declive.

**mood.** The emotional state of an individual.

**mood swing.** Oscillation of a person's emotional feeling tone between periods of euphoria and depression.

**Moon,** Henry, English surgeon, 19th century. See M.'s *molars.*

**Moon,** Robert C., American ophthalmologist, 1844–1914. See Laurence-M.-Biedl *syndrome.*

**Moore,** Charles H., English surgeon, 1821–1870. See M.'s *method.*

**Moore,** Edward M., U. S. surgeon, 1814–1902. See M.'s *fracture.*

**Moore,** Robert Foster, British ophthalmologist, 1878–1963. See M.'s lightning *streaks.*

**Mooren,** Albert, German oculist, 1828–1899. See M.'s *ulcer.*

**Mooser bodies.** See under body.

**Morand** (mor′ahn′), Sauveur F., Paris surgeon, 1697–1773. See M.'s *foot, spur.*

**Morax,** Victor, Paris ophthalmologist, 1866–1935. See M.-Axenfeld *conjunctivitis, diplobacillus.*

**Moraxel′la** (V. *Morax*) A genus of obligately aerobic, nonmotile bacteria containing Gram-negative coccoids or short rods which usually occur in pairs. They do not produce acid from carbohydrates. They are oxidase-positive and penicillin-sensitive. These organisms are parasitic on the mucous membranes of man and other mammals. The type species is *M. lacunata.*

   **M. bovis,** a species isolated from ophthalmia (pink eye) of cattle.

   **M. kingae,** a species found in the throat, nose, blood, a bone lesion, and a joint; pathogenicity is uncertain, and it is uncertain whether this organism belongs to the genus *M.*

   **M. lacunata,** a species causing conjunctivitis in man. It is the type species of the genus *M.*

   **M. nonliquefa′ciens,** a species found in the respiratory tract of man, especially in the nose; usually not pathogenic, but occasionally causes sinusitis.

   **M. osloen′sis,** a species found in the genitourinary tract, blood, spinal and chest fluids, and nose; rarely found in the respiratory tract. Usually not pathogenic, although some strains have been isolated from serious pathological conditions in man.

   **M. phenylpyrouvica,** *M. phenylpyruvica.*

   **M. phenylpyru′vica,** *M. phenylpyrouvica; M. polymorpha;* a species found in the genitourinary tract, blood, cerebrospinal fluid, and in pus from various lesions; pathogenicity unknown.

   **M. polymor′pha,** *M. phenylpyruvica.*

**mor′bid** [ L. *morbidus,* ill, fr. *morbus,* disease ]. 1. Diseased or pathologic. 2. In psychology, abnormal or deviant.

**morbid′ity.** 1. A diseased state. 2. The ratio of sick to well in a community; morbility; see also morbidity *rate.*

**morbif′ic** [ L. *morbus,* disease, + *facio,* to make ]. Pathogenic.

**morbigenous** (mor-bij′ĕ-nus) [ L. *morbus,* disease, + G. suffix *-gen,* producing ]. Pathogenic.

**morbil′ity.** Morbidity.

**morbil′li** [ Mediev. L. *morbillus,* dim. of L. *morbus,* disease. MORB- ]. Measles.

**morbil′liform** [ see morbilli ]. Resembling measles.

**morbilous** (mor-bil′us) [ see morbilli ]. Relating to measles.

**mor′bus** [ L. disease. MORB- ]. Disease. For varieties of morbus, see under disease.

   **m. virgin′eus,** chlorosis.

**morcel** (mor-sel′) [ Fr. *morceler,* to subdivide ]. To remove piecemeal.

**morcellation** (mor′sĕ-la′shun) [ Fr. *morceler,* to subdivide ]. Taking away by bits; a mode of removal of a tumor or hypertrophied tissue by nipping or crushing off little bits at a time.

**morcellement** (mor-sel-mon′) [ Fr. ]. Morcellation.

**mor′dant** [ L. *mordeo,* to bite ]. 1. A substance capable of combining with a dye and the material to be dyed, thereby increasing the affinity or binding of the dye. Alum is commonly used as a m. to promote staining with hematoxylin. 2. To treat with a m.

**Morel,** Benoît A., French psychiatrist, 1809–1873. See M.'s *ear,* Stewart-M. *syndrome.*

**Morelli,** Italian physician, †1918. See M.'s *test.*

**Morgagni** (mor-gahn′ye), Giovanni B., Italian anatomist and pathologist, 1682–1771. See M.'s *appendix, cartilage, caruncle, cataract, columns, concha, crypts, cyst, disease, foramen, fossa, fovea, frenulum, frenum, globules, humor, hydatid, lacuna, liquor, nodule, prolapse, retinaculum, sinus, spheres, syndrome,* M.-Adams-Stokes *syndrome,* M.'s *valve, ventricle.*

**Morgan,** Harry de R., British physician, 1863–1931. See M.'s *bacillus.*

**Morgan,** Thomas Hunt, American geneticist, 1866–1945. Nobel laureate, 1933, for his work on chromosomes and genes in heredity.

**morgue** (morg) [ Fr. ]. Mortuary. 1. A building where unidentified dead are kept pending identification before burial. 2. A building or room in a hospital where the dead are kept pending autopsy, burial, or cremation.

**moria** (mo′rĭ-ah) [ G. *mōria,* folly, fr. *mōros,* stupid, dull ]. 1. Foolishness; dullness of comprehension; hebetude. 2. A mental state marked by frivolity, joviality, an inveterate tendency to jest, and inability to take anything seriously.

**moribund** (mor′ĭ-bund) [ L. *moribundus,* dying, fr. *morior,* to die ]. Dying; at the point of death.

**mor′in.** A yellow dye, $C_{15}H_{10}O_7$, obtained from Cuba wood or yellow Brazil wood; it is used as a fluorochrome for detection of certain metals.

**mor′ioplasty** [ G. *morion,* piece, + *plassō,* to form ]. Plastic surgery for restoring parts lost by injury or disease.

**Morison,** James R., British surgeon, 1853–1939. See Drummond-M. *operation, pouch* of M.

**Mörner,** K. A.,H., Swedish chemist, 1855–1917. See M.'s *test.*

**morn′ing glo′ry.** 1. *Ipomoea rubrocoerulea.* 2. *Rivea corymbosa.*

**Moro,** Ernst, German physician, 1874–1951. See M.'s *reflex.*

**mo′ron** [ G. *mōros,* stupid ]. An obsolete term for a subclass of mental retardation (*q.v.*).

**morox′ydine.** VIRONIL; 4-morpholinecarboximidoylguanidine; antiviral agent.

**morph-.** See morpho-.

**morphazin′amide hydrochloride.** PIAZOLIN; morinamide hydrochloride; *N*-(morpholinomethyl)pyrazinecarboxamide hydrochloride; antituberculous agent.

**morphe′a** (mor-fe′ah) [ G. *morphē,* form, figure. MORPH- ]. Circumscribed scleroderma; Addison's keloid; a cutaneous lesion or lesions characterized by indurated plaques of thickened dermal fibrous tissue, of a whitish or yellowish white color surrounded by a pinkish or purplish halo.

**m. acroter'ica,** m. confined chiefly to the extremities.

**m. alba,** a form of m. in which there is little pigmentation.

**m. gutta'ta,** white spot disease; small discrete, white, waxy, indurated lesions due to localized degenerative changes in the fibrous tissue.

**m. herpetifor'mis,** m. distributed along the course of distribution of a nerve, as in herpes zoster.

**m. linea'ris,** m. in which lesions are arranged in bands.

**m. pigmentosa,** localized scleroderma in which there is pigmentation.

**morpheme** (mor'fēn) [ morph- + G. *phēmē,* voice ]. The smallest linguistic unit with a meaning.

**morphine** (mor'fēn, mor-fēn') [ L. *Morpheus,* the god of dreams or of sleep. MORPH- ]. Morphium; morphia; $C_{17}H_{19}NO_3$; the major phenanthrene alkaloid of opium; contains 9 to 14 per cent of anhydrous morphine. It produces a combination of depression and excitation in the central nervous system and some peripheral tissues; predominance of either central stimulation or depression depends upon the species and dose; repeated administration leads to the development of tolerance, physical dependence, and (if abused) psychic dependence. It is a reliable, effective analgesic for almost every type of pain; also produces sedation and allays anxiety.

**m. hydrochloride** (BP), occurs as white acicular or cubical crystals of bitter taste, soluble in about 25 parts of water.

**m. sulfate** (USP), m. sulphate (BP); feathery, silky crystals or a white crystalline powder of bitter taste; when exposed to the air it gradually loses water of crystallization; a narcotic analgesic.

**morphinism** (mor'fĭ-nizm). Morphine habit; the habitual use of morphine.

**morphinization** (mor'fĭ-nĭ-za'shun). Bringing under the influence of morphine.

**morphinomania** (mor'fĭ-no-ma'nĭ-ah). Morphiomania; pathological and psychological craving for morphine, or the pathological and abnormal psychological conditions resulting from excessive use of morphine.

**morphiomania** (mor'fĭ-o-ma'nĭ-ah). Morphinomania.

**morpho-, morph-** [ G. *morphē,* form, shape. MORPH- ]. Combining forms relating to form, shape, or structure.

**morphocytology** (mor'fo-si-tol'o-jĭ) [ morpho- + G. *kytos,* cell, + *logos,* study ]. The science or study dealing with the morphologic features (*i.e.,* size, shape, structure, and visible contents) of cells, as distinguished from chemical reactions and function, and from histology.

**morphogenesis** (mor'fo-jen'ĕ-sis) [ morpho- + G. *genesis,* production ]. The differentiation of cells and tissues in the early embryo which results in establishing the form and structure of the various organs and parts of the body.

**morphogenetic** (mor'fo-jĕ-net'ik). Relating to morphogenesis.

**morphography** (mor-fog'ră-fĭ) [ morpho- + G. *graphē,* a writing ]. The study of or a treatise on the form and structure of animals and plants.

**mor'pholine salicylate.** RETARCYL; 1,4-tetrahydrooxazine orthoxybenzoate; antirheumatic agent.

**morphologic** (mor-fo-loj'ik). Relating to morphology.

**morphology** (mor-fol'o-jĭ) [ morpho- + G. *logos,* study ]. The science which treats of the configuration or the structure of animals and plants.

**morphometry** (mor-fom'e-trĭ) [ morpho- + G. *metron,* measure ]. The measurement of the different parts entering into the configuration of bodies.

**morphon** (mor'fon) [ G. *morphē,* form ]. Any one of the individual structures entering into the formation of an organism; a morphologic element, such as a cell.

**morphosis** (mor-fo'sis) [ G. formation, act of forming ]. Mode of development of a part.

**mor'phosyn'thesis** [ morpho- + synthesis, *q.v.* ]. An awareness of space and of body schema represented in the parietal lobes of the cerebral cortex.

**morphotype** (mor'fo-tip) [ morpho- + G. *typos,* stamp, model ]. A group (infrasubspecific) of bacterial strains distinguishable from other strains of the same species on

the basis of morphological characters which may or may not be associated with a change in serological state.

**Morquio** (mor-ke'o), Louis, Montevideo physician, 1867–1935. See M.'s *disease,* Brailsford-M. *disease,* M.-Ullrich *disease,* M.'s *syndrome.*

**morrhuate** (mor'ru-āt) [ fr. *Gadus morrhua,* cod ]. Salts of fatty acids derived from cod liver oil.

**Morris,** John McL., U. S. surgeon, *1914. See M.'s *syndrome.*

**mors** [ L. ]. Death.

**m. thy'mica,** sudden death in children, usually the result of infection; formerly attributed to an enlarged thymus. See also crib *death;* sudden death *syndrome.*

**mor'sal** [ L. *morsus,* a biting, fr. *mordeo,* pp. *morsus,* to bite ]. Denoting the masticatory, grinding, or occlusal surface of a tooth.

**mor'sulus** [ Mod. L. dim. of L. *morsus,* a bite ]. Troche.

**mor'sus** [ L. a bite ]. A bite.

**mor'tal** [ L. *mortalis,* fr. *mors,* death ]. 1. Fatal; destructive to life. 2. Destined to die.

**mortality** (mor-tal'ĭ-tĭ) [ L. *mortalitus,* fr. *mors* (*mort-*), death ]. 1. The state of being mortal. 2. Statistically, death rate; the ratio of the number of deaths to a given population in a given situation; see also mortality *rate* and fatality *rate.*

**mor'tar** [ L. *mortarium* ]. A vessel with rounded interior in which crude drugs and other substances are crushed or bruised by means of a pestle.

**Mortierel'la.** A genus of saprophytic fungi belonging to the class Phycomycetes (Zygomycetes) and the family Mucoraceae; they are commonly found in nature and may cause phycomycosis in man.

**mortif'erous** [ L. *mortiferus,* fr. *mors* (*mort-*), death, + *fero,* to bear ]. Fatal; lethal; causing death.

**mortification** (mor'tĭ-fĭ-ka'shun) [ L. *mors* (*mort-*), death, + *facio,* to make ]. Gangrene.

**Mortimer's disease.** See under disease.

**mortinatal'ity** [ L. *mors* (*mort-*), death, + *natalis,* relating to birth ]. Natimortality.

**Morton,** Dudley J., U.S. orthopaedist, 1884–1960. See M.'s *syndrome.*

**Morton,** Samuel G., U. S. physician, 1799–1851. See M.'s *plane.*

**Morton,** Thomas G., American physician, 1835–1903. See M.'s *neuralgia.*

**Morton,** William J., American neurologist, 1846–1920. See M.'s *current.*

**mortuary** (mor'tu-ĕr-ĭ) [ L. *mortuus,* dead, part. adj. fr. *morior,* pp. *mortuus,* to die ]. 1. Relating to death or to burial. 2. Morgue.

**morula** (mor'u-lah) [ Mod. L. dim. of L. *morus,* mulberry ]. The mass of blastomeres resulting from the early cleavage divisions of the zygote. In ova with little yolk the m. is a spheroidal mass of cells taking its name from its resemblance to a mulberry. In forms with considerable yolk the configuration of the m. stage is greatly modified. See fig. under cleavage.

**morulation** (mor'u-la'shun). The formation of the morula.

**moruloid** (mor'u-loyd). Resembling a morula.

**Morvan** (mor-van'), Augustin M., French physician, 1819–1897. See M.'s *chorea, disease.*

**mosaic** (mo-za'ik) [ Mod. L. *mosaicus, musaicus,* pertaining to the Muses, artistic ]. 1. Tessellated; inlaid; resembling inlaid work. 2. The juxtaposition in an organism of genetically different tissues, resulting from somatic mutation (gene mosaicism), an anomaly of chromosome division resulting in two or more types of cells containing different numbers of chromosomes (chromosome mosaicism) or chimerism (see chimera).

**mosaicism** (mo-zā'ĭ-sizm). Condition of being mosaic; see mosaic (2).

**erythrocyte m.,** compound serologic types in twin cattle or sheep due to the fusion of the placental vessels of the twins. It is thought that each twin possesses hematopoietic tissue derived in part from its own embryonic cells and in part from the embryonic cell of its twin. The red cells are therefore of two antigenic types, the blood giving a double hemolytic reaction; that is, some red cells are hemolzed by one type of antibody, some by another. See also freemartin.

**Moschowitz,** E., U. S. physician, 1879–1964. See M.'s *disease.*

**moschus** (mos'kus) [ G. *moschos,* musk ]. Musk.

**Mosher,** Harrison P., American surgeon, *1867. See M. *drain.*

**Mosler,** Karl F., German physician, 1831–1911. See M.'s *diabetes.*

**mosquito,** pl. **mosqui'toes** (mus-ke'to) [ Sp. dim. of *mosca,* fly, fr. L. *musca,* a fly ]. A blood-sucking dipterous insect of the family Culicidae; see *Aedes, Anopheles, Culex,* and *Stegomyia,* the genera containing most of the species instrumental in the transmission of various protozoa and other animal forms of disease-producing parasites.

**moss** [ A.S. *meōs* ]. 1. A delicate, low growing, cryptogamous plant of the class Musci. 2. Popularly, any one of a number of lichens and seaweeds.

    **Ceylon m.,** a source of agar-agar.

    **club m.,** lycopodium.

    **Cor'sican m.,** helminthochorton.

    **Iceland m.,** cetraria.

    **Irish m.,** chondrus (2).

    **mus'keag m.,** sphagnum m.

    **pearl m.,** chondrus (2).

    **sphag'num m.,** muskeag m.; peat m.; a highly absorbent m. used as a substitute for absorbent cotton or gauze in surgical dressing and sanitary napkins.

    **m. starch,** lichenin.

**Moss,** Gerald, New York physician, *1931. See M. *tube.*

**Moss,** Melvin L., U. S. oral pathologist, *1923. See Gorlin-Chaudhry-M. *syndrome.*

**Mosso,** Angelo, Italian physiologist, 1846–1910. See M.'s *ergograph, sphygmomanometer.*

**Moszkowicz** (mos'ko-viks), Ludwig, Austrian surgeon, 1873–1945. See M.'s *test.*

**Motais** (mō-teh'), Ernst, French ophthalmologist, 1845–1913. See M.'s *operation.*

**mote** (mōt) [ A.S. *mot* ]. A small particle; a speck.

    **blood m.'s,** hemoconia.

**mother** (muth'er) [ A.S. *mōdor* ]. 1. The female parent. 2. Any cell or other structure from which other similar bodies are formed.

    **m. of vinegar,** see under vinegar.

**motile** (mo'til) [ see motion ]. 1. Having the power of spontaneous movement. 2. Denoting the type of mental imagery in which the person learns and recalls most readily that which he has felt, as contrasted with audile and visile. 3. A person having such mental imagery.

**motil'ity.** The power of spontaneous movement.

**motion** (mo'shun) [ L. *motio,* movement, fr. *moveo,* pp. *motus,* to move. MOV- ]. 1. Movement; change of place or position. 2. Specifically, a movement of the bowels; defecation. 3. The matter discharged from the rectum; a stool.

**motivation** [ ML. *motivus,* moving ]. In psychology, the aggregate of all the individual motives and drives operative in an individual at any given moment which influence will and cause behavior. The individual motives and drives can be operating in concert or antagonistic to one another. See also drive, motive, and their subentries.

    **personal m.,** an individual's predispositions and expectations that give meaning and direction to personality functioning.

**mo'tive** [ L. *moveo,* to move, to set in motion ]. 1. Learned drive; a predisposition, need, or specific state of tension within an individual which arouses, maintains, and directs behavior toward a goal. 2. The reason attributed to or given by an individual for a behavioral act.

    **achievement m.,** a chronic need to succeed in the face of recognizable obstacles; its strength is usually diagnosed from recurring themes in stories told by the individual while taking a thematic apperception test or from other assessment instruments used by clinical psychologists.

    **mastery m.,** the need to be assertive, to stand out in a crowd, to be dominant.

**motofacient** (mo-to-fa'shi-ent) [ L. *motus,* motion, + *facio,* to make ]. Causing motion; denoting the second phase of muscular activity in which actual movement is produced.

**motoneuron** (mo'to-nu'ron). Motor *neuron.*

**mo'tor** [ L. a mover, fr. *movere,* to move ]. That which imparts movement. Applied to living organisms, the term refers to: 1 [ NA ]. In anatomy and physiology, those neural structures which by the impulses generated and transmitted by them cause muscle fibers or pigment cells to contract, or glands to secrete; see also motor *cortex;* motor *endplate;* motor *neuron.* 2. In psychology, the organism's overt reaction to a stimulus (motor response).

    **m. oc'uli,** *nervus* oculomotorius.

    **plastic m.,** an artificial point of attachment, on an amputation stump, to which is fastened the cord or extensor by which movement is transmitted to an artificial limb, in cinematization.

**mo'torgraph'ic.** Kinetographic.

**moto'rial.** Relating to motion, to a motor nerve or the motor nucleus.

**moto'rius** [ L. moving ]. Motor *nerve.*

**motormeter** (mo'tor-me'ter). A device for determining the amount, force, and rapidity of movement.

**mottling** (mot'ling) [ E. *motley,* variegated in color ]. Macular lesions of varying shades or colors.

**moulage** (moo-lazh') [ F. a molding ]. A reproduction in wax of a skin lesion, tumor, or other pathologic state.

**mould.** Mold.

**moult.** Molt.

**mound'ing.** Myoedema.

**mount.** 1. To prepare for microscopic examination. 2. To climb on for purposes of copulation.

**mount'ing.** In dentistry, the laboratory procedure of attaching the maxillary and/or mandibular cast to an articulator.

    **split cast m.,** (1) a cast with key grooves on its base, mounted on an articulator for the purpose of easy removal and accurate replacement; split remounting metal plates may be used instead of grooves in casts; (2) a means for testing the accuracy of articulator adjustment.

**mourn.** 1. To express grief or sorrow as a result of loss. 2. In psychoanalysis, mourning is the frequently unexpressed process of responding to loss of a cathectic object. In contrast to malancholia, it usually does not involve loss of self-esteem.

**mouse.** A small rodent belonging to the genus *Mus.*

    **NZB mice,** an inbred strain of mice developed in New Zealand which, when adult, exhibit autoimmune hemolytic anemia and renal disease.

**mouth** [ A.S. *mūth* ]. 1. Os (1); stoma (2); expanded upper portion of the digestive tract, containing the tongue and the teeth; it is bounded by the lips anteriorly, the cheeks laterally, the arch of the palate above (roof of the m.), below by muscular tissue (floor of the m.), and passes posteriorly into the pharynx through the isthmus of the fauces. 2. Os (2) or ostium; orifice; the opening, usually the external opening, of a cavity or canal.

    **denture sore m.,** inflammation of the oral mucosa caused by ill fitting dentures, allergic response to the denture base, Candida infection, or a combination of the three.

    **parrot m.,** a condition of the horse in which the upper jaw is relatively longer than the lower, resulting in elongation of the upper incisors.

    **sore m.,** see soremouth.

    **tapir m.,** protrusion of the lips due to weakness of the oral muscle in certain forms of juvenile muscular dystrophy.

    **trench m.,** Vincent's *disease.*

    **m. of the womb,** *ostium* uteri.

**mouth stick.** A prosthesis which is held by the teeth and utilized by handicapped persons to perform such actions as typing, painting, and lifting small objects.

**mouth'wash.** Collutorium.

**move'ment** [ L. *moveo,* pp. *motus,* to move ]. 1. The act of changing position, of passing from one place to another; said of the entire body or of one or more of its numbers or parts. 2. A discharge of feces from the rectum.

    **active m.,** m. effected by the organism itself, unaided by external influences.

    **adversive m.,** a rotation of the eyes, head, or trunk about the long axis of the body.

**after-m.,** Kohnstamm's *phenomenon.*

**ame'boid m.,** the m. characteristic of leukocytes and protozoan organisms of the class Rhizopodea. See also streaming m.

**assistive m.,** in massage, a m. which the partially paralyzed muscle of the patient would be unable to perform unaided but which is effected with the graduated assistance of the operator.

**associated m.,** involuntary m. in a limb corresponding to one voluntarily executed in its fellow.

**Bennett m.,** the bodily lateral m. or lateral shift of the mandible resulting from the m.'s of the condyles along the lateral inclines of the mandibular fossae in lateral jaw m.'s.

**border m.'s,** any extreme compass of mandibular m. limited by bone, ligaments, or soft tissues. Usually applied to horizontal manidibular m.'s.

**border tissue m.'s** the action of the muscles and other tissues adjacent to the borders of a denture.

**Brownian m.,** erratic, nondirectional, zigzag m. observed in certain colloidal solutions (when viewed with an ultramicroscope), and in suspensions of light particulate matter, *e.g.,* bacterial cells (when viewed with a microscope); the m. results from the jostling or bumping of the larger particles by the molecules in the suspending medium, which are therefore in continuous motion.

**Brownian-Zsigmondy m.,** Brownian m.

**chore'ic m.,** an involuntary spasmodic twitching or jerking in groups of muscles not associated in the production of definite purposeful m.'s.

**ciliary m.,** the thythmic, sweeping m. of the cilia of epithelial cells or protozoan organisms of the class Ciliata or the sculling m. of flagella, effected possibly by the alternate contraction and relaxation of contractile threads (myoids) on one side of the cilium or flagellum.

**circus m.,** circus rhythm; "a term applied to a contraction or excitation wave traveling continuously in circular fashion around a ring of muscle or through the wall of the heart" (Lewis).

**conjugate m. of the eyes,** m. of the two eyes in the same direction; see also version (4).

**decomposition of m.,** a manifestation of cerebellar disease in which a muscular movement is not carried out smoothly but in a series of separate motions.

**disjugate m. of the eyes,** m. of the two eyes in opposite directions, as in convergence or divergence.

**fetal m.,** the m. characteristic of the fetus in utero; usually commences between the 12th and 16th weeks of pregnancy.

**hinge m.,** an opening or closing m. of the mandible on the hinge axis.

**intermediary m.'s,** in dentistry, all m.'s between the extremes of mandibular excursions.

**jaw m.'s,** mandibular m.'s.

**lateral m.,** in dentistry, denotes m. of the mandible to the side.

**Magnan's trombone m.,** an involuntary forward and back m. of the tongue when it is drawn out of the mouth.

**mandibular m.,** (1) m.'s of the lower jaw; (2) all changes in position of which the mandible is capable.

**mandibular m.'s, free,** (1) any mandibular m.'s made without tooth interference; (2) any uninhibited m.'s of the mandible.

**mandibular m.'s, functional,** all natural, proper, or characteristic m.'s of the mandible made during speech, mastication, yawning, swallowing, and other associated m.'s.

**mass m.,** mass *peristalsis.*

**molec'ular m.,** Brownian m.

**morphogenetic m.,** the streaming of cells in the early embryo to form tissues or organs.

**muscular m.,** m. caused by the contraction of the protoplasm of the muscle cell.

**neurobiotactic m.,** the streaming of nerve cells toward the area from which they receive the most stimuli.

**opening m.,** in dentistry, m. of the mandible executed during jaw separation.

**passive m.,** allokinesis (1); m. imparted to an organism or any of its parts by external agency; m. of any joint effected by the hand of another person, or by mechanical means, without participation of the subject himself.

**pendular m.,** a to-and-fro m. of the intestine, without any propelling or peristaltic action, whereby the contents are churned and thoroughly mixed with the intestinal ferments.

**protoplas'mic m.,** m. produced by the inherent power of contraction and relaxation of protoplasm; such m.'s are of three kinds: muscular, streaming, and ciliary.

**rapid eye m.'s,** symmetrical quick m.'s occurring many times during a single night's sleep, in clusters for 5 to 60 minutes; scanning m.'s associated with dreaming. Abbreviated REM.

**reflex m.,** allokinesis (2); an involuntary m. resulting from a sensory stimulus.

**resistive m.,** in massage, a m. made by the patient against the efforts of the operator, or one forced by the operator against the resistance of the patient.

**saccadic m.,** (1) a quick jump of the eyes from one fixation point to another as in reading; (2) the rapid return m. of a jerky nystagmus, as in labyrinthine and optokinetic nystagmus.

**streaming m.,** the form of m. characteristic of the protoplasm of leukocytes, amebae, and other unicellular organisms; it consists in the massing of the protoplasm at some point where surface pressure is least and its extrusion in the form of a pseudopod; the protoplasm may return to the body of the cell, resulting in the retraction of the pseudopod, or the entire mass may flow into the latter and thereby result in locomotion of the cell.

**Swedish m.,** Swedish gymnastics; a form of kinesitherapy in which certain systemztized m.'s of the body and limbs are regulated by resistance made by an attendant.

**translatory m.,** the motion of the body at any instant when all points within the body are moving at the same velocity and in the same direction.

**vermicular m.,** peristalsis.

**Zsigmondy's m.'s,** Brownian m.'s.

**moxa** (mok'sah) [ Jap. *moe kusa,* burning herb ]. 1. A cone or cylinder of cotton wool or other combustible material, placed on the skin and ignited in order to produce counterirritation. 2. A button-shaped iron, heated in the fire or electrically, and applied as a cautery; actual cautery; galvanic m.

**moxibustion** (mok'sī-bus'chun) [ moxa + (com)-bustion ]. The production of counterirritation by means of a moxa.

**MPD.** Abbreviation for maximal permissible *dose.*

**MQ.** Abbreviation for menaquinone.

**MQ-6, MQ₆.** Abbreviation for menaquinone-6.

**M.R.C.P.** Abbreviation for Member of the Royal College of Physicians.

**M.R.C.P.E.** Abbreviation for Member of the Royal College of Physicians (Edinburgh).

**M.R.C.P.I.** Abbreviation for Member of the Royal College of Physicians (Ireland).

**M.R.C.S.** Abbreviation for Member of the Royal College of Surgeons.

**M.R.C.S.E.** Abbreviation for Member of the Royal College of Surgeons (Edinburgh).

**M.R.C.S.I.** Abbreviation for Member of the Royal College of Surgeons (Ireland).

**M.R.C.V.S.** Abbreviation for Member of the Royal College of Veterinary Surgeons.

**MRD, m.r.d.** Abbreviation for minimal reacting *dose.*

**mRNA.** Abbreviation for messenger RNA; see under ribonucleic acid.

**msec.** Abbreviation for millisecond.

**MSH.** Abbreviation for melanocyte-stimulating *hormone.*

**MTF.** Abbreviation for *modulation* transfer function.

**mu** [ G. ]. The twelfth letter of the Greek alphabet. $\mu$, *q.v.*

**m.u.** 1. Abbreviation for mouse *unit.* 2. Abbreviation for Mache *unit.*

**mu'avine.** An alkaloid from muavi bark, obtained from an African tree of the genus *Erythrophloeum*; it is similar in its properties to erythrophleine.

**mu'case.** Mucinase.

**Much** (mookh), Hans C. R., German physician, 1880–1932. See M.'s *bacillus,* M.'s *reaction,* M.-Holzmann *reaction,* M.-Weiss *stain.*

**Mucha,** V., Austrian dermatologist, 1877–1919. See M.-Habermann *disease.*

**muci-** (mu'sī-) [ L. *mucus, q. v.* ]. Combining form for mucus, mucous, or mucin. See also muco-.

**mucic acid** (mu'sik). Galactaric acid; the aric acid derived from *d*-galactose; noteworthy for optical inactivity, because of *meso* configuration, and for being the least soluble of the aric acids.

**mu'cicar'mine.** A mucin stain containing aluminum chloride 0.5, carmine 1, distilled water 2, heated for 2 min. and then diluted with 100 ml. of 50 per cent alcohol.

**mucid** (mu'sid). Mucilaginous; slimy.

**mucif'erous.** Muciparous.

**mucification** (mu'sī-fī-ka'shun) [ L. *mucus* + *facio,* to make ]. A change produced in the vaginal mucosa of spayed experimental animals following stimulation with estrogen, characterized by the formation of tall columnar cells secreting mucus.

**mu'ciform.** Resembling mucus.

**mucigenous** (mu-sij'ĕ-nus). Muciparous.

**mucihematein** (mu'sī-he'mă-te-in). A staining fluid consisting of aluminum chloride 0.1, hematin 0.2, glycerin 40, water 60.

**mucilage** (mu'sī-lij) [ L. *mucilago* ]. A pharmacopeial preparation consisting of a solution in water of the mucilaginous principles of vegetable substances. Used as a soothing application to the mucous membranes and in the preparation of official and extemporaneous mixtures.

**mucilaginous** (mu-sī-laj'ĭ-nus). 1. Resembling mucilage; viscid; sticky. 2. Muciparous.

**mu'cin.** Secretions containing mucopolysaccharides, as those from the goblet cells of the intestine, the submaxillary glands, and other mucous glandular cells. M. is also present in the ground substance of connective tissue, especially during development when it is known as mucous connective tissue. M. is soluble in alkaline water and precipitated by acetic acid.

    **gastric m.,** prepared from mucosa of hog's stomach by pepsin-hydrochloric acid digestion and precipitation of the supernatant fluid with 60 per cent alcohol; a white or yellowish powder which forms a viscous opalescent fluid with water. Used in peptic ulcer for its protective and lubricating action.

**mu'cinase.** Mucase; mucopolysaccharidase; hyaluronidase, spreading factor. Specifically applied to hyaluronate lyase, hyaluronoglucosidase, and hyaluronoglucuronidase (the hyaluronidases, *q. v.*), but more loosely to any enzyme, such as lysozyme and neuraminidase, that hydrolyzes mucopolysaccharide substances (mucins).

**mucinemia** (mu'sī-ne'mī-ah) [ mucin + G. *haima,* blood ]. Myxemia; the presence of mucin in the circulating blood.

**mucinogen** (mu'sin'o-jen) [ mucin + G. suffix *-gen,* producing ]. A protein-carbohydrate compound (glycoprotein) that forms mucin through the imbibition of water.

**mu'cinoid.** 1. Mucoid. 2. Resembling mucin.

**mucinolytic** (mu'sī-no-lit'ik). Possessing the property of bringing about the hydrolysis of mucin, as by a mucinase.

**mucinosis** (mu'sī-no'sis) [ mucin + G. suffix *-osis,* condition ]. A condition in which mucin is present in the skin in excessive amounts.

    **follicular m.,** a relatively unusual, benign eruption of discrete lesions on the face or scalp in which there are cystic mucinous changes in the pilosebaceous units in the involved area.

    **papular m.,** *lichen* myxedematosus.

**mu'cinous.** Relating to or containing mucin.

**mucinuria** (mu'sī-nu'rĭ-ah) [ mucin + G. *ouron,* urine ]. The presence of mucin in the urine.

**mucip'arous** [ mucin + L. *pario,* to bring forth, bear ]. Muciferous; mucigenous; mucilaginous (2); producing mucus.

**mucitis** (mu-si'tis). Inflammation of a mucous membrane.

**Muckle,** T. J. See M.-Wells *syndrome.*

**muco-** (mu'ko-) [ L. *mucus, q. v.* ]. Combining form for mucus, mucous, or mucosa (mucous membrane). See also muci-.

**mucocele** (mu'ko-sēl) [ muco- + G. *kēlē,* tumor, hernia ]. 1. A cyst or cystlike structure that contains mucus. 2. A

mucous polypus. 3. A retention cyst of the lacrimal sac. 4. A cystic disease of the paranasal sinuses producing erosion of the surrounding bone.

**mucoclasis** (mu-kok'lă-sis) [ muco- + G. *klasis,* a breaking off ]. Denudation of any mucous surface.

**mucocolitis** (mu-ko-ko-li'tis). Mucous *colitis.*

**mucocolpos** (mu'ko-kol'pos) [ muco- + G. *kolpos,* vagina ]. Mucus in the vagina.

**mu'cocuta'neous.** Cutaneomucosal; relating to mucous membrane and skin; denoting the line of junction of the two at the nasal, oral, vaginal, and anal orifices.

**mucoenteritis** (mu'ko-en-ter-i'tis). 1. Inflammation of the intestinal mucous membrane. 2. Mucomembranous *enteritis.*

**mucoepidermoid** (mu'ko-ep-ĭ-der'moyd). Denoting a mixture of mucus-secreting and epithelial cells; see also m. *carcinoma.*

**mu'coglob'ulin.** A glycoprotein or mucoprotein in which the protein component is a globulin.

**mu'coid** [ mucus + G. *eidos,* appearance ]. 1. Mucin, mucoprotein, or mucopolysaccharide. 2. Muciform or mucinous.

**mucoitin sulfuric acids** (mu-ko'ī-tin). Obsolete term for sulfated mucopolysaccharides (chondroitin sulfates, dermatan sulfate, keratosulfate, heparin, heparan sulfate).

**mucolipidosis,** pl. **mucolipidoses** (mu'ko-lip'ī-do'sis, -sēz). Any of a group of metabolic storage diseases characterized by visceral storage of acid mucopolysaccharides and glycolipids, but without excess mucopolysaccharides in the urine; autosomal recessive inheritance.

    **m. I,** lipomucopolysaccharidosis; m. with mild Hurler-like symptoms, mild dysostosis multiplex, and moderate mental retardation.

    **m. II,** I-cell or inclusion cell disease; Leroy's disease; m. with severe Hurler-like symptoms, dyostosis multiplex, mental retardation, and abnormal coarse inclusions in fibroblasts.

    **m. III,** pseudopolydystrophy; m. with mild Hurler-like symptoms, restricted joint mobility, short stature, mild mental retardation, and dysplastic skeletal changes.

**mucolysis** (mu-kol'ī-sis) [ muco- + G. *lysis,* dissolution ]. The solution, digestion, or liquefaction of mucus.

**mucolyt'ic.** Capable of dissolving, digesting, or liquefying mucus.

**mucomembranous** (mu'ko-mem'bră-nus). Relating to a mucous membrane.

**mu'copep'tide.** Peptide found in combination with polysaccharides containing muramic or sialic acids; see also mucoprotein.

    **m. glucohydrolase,** lysozyme.

**muc'operios'teal.** Relating to mucoperiosteum.

**mucoperiosteum** (mu'ko-pĕr-ī-os'te-um). Mucous membrane and periosteum so intimately united as to form practically a single membrane, as that covering the hard palate.

**mu'copolysac'charidase.** Mucinase.

**mu'copolysac'charide.** A complex of protein and polysaccharide; a general term, usually implying that the polysaccharide component is a major part of the complex, in contradistinction to mucoprotein. M.'s include the blood group substances.

**mucopolysaccharidosis** (mu'ko-pol-ī-sak'ă-rī-do'sis). Term embracing a group of diseases that have in common a disorder in metabolism of mucopolysaccharides, as evidenced by excretion of various mucopolysaccharides in urine; the mucopolysaccharides comprise much of the ground substance of connective tissue, and these diseases include various defects of bone, cartilage, and connective tissue.

    **type I m.,** Hurler's *syndrome.*

    **type IS m.,** Scheie's *syndrome.*

    **type II m.,** Hunter's *syndrome.*

    **type III m.,** Sanfilippo *syndrome.*

    **type IV m.,** Morquio *syndrome.*

    **type V m.,** former designation for Scheie's *syndrome.*

    **type VI m.,** Maroteaux-Lamy *syndrome.*

    **type VII m.,** m. due to β-glucuronidase deficiency.

**mucopolysacchariduria** (mu'ko-pol-ī-sak'ă-rī-du'rī-ah). The excretion of mucopolysaccharides in the urine.

**mu'copro'tein.** A protein-polysaccharide complex; a general term, usually implying that the protein component is the major part of the complex, in contradistinction to mucopolysaccharide. M.'s include the α₁- and α₂-globulins of serum (and others). Sometimes called glycoproteins.

**mu'copu'rulent.** Pertaining to an exudate that is chiefly purulent (pus), but containing relatively conspicuous proportions of mucous material.

**mucopus** (mu'ko-pus'). Mycopus; a mucopurulent discharge; a mixture of mucous material and pus.

**Mu'cor.** A genus of saprophytic fungi belonging to the class Phycomycetes (Zygomycetes) and the family Mucoraceae; they may cause phycomycosis in man.

**mu'cor** [ L. mold, fr. *muceo*, to be moldy ]. A common name for several species of molds frequently found on dead and decaying vegetable matter, bread, and the like.

**Mucoraceae** (mu'kor-a'se-e) [ L. *mucor*, mold ]. A family of fungi in the class Phycomycetes, which includes terrestrial, aquatic, and sometimes parasitic organisms; the family M. includes the genera *Mucor, Absidia, Rhizopus,* and *Mortierella*. Although the various species of the four genera are ordinarily saprophytic, free-living forms, some of them cause phycomycosis in man.

**mu'corin.** A protein present in certain mucors or molds.

**mucormycosis** (mu'kor-mī-ko'tis). A general term that includes conditions occasionally caused by, or associated with, various species in the family Mucoraceae, *e.g., Absidia, Mortierella,* and *Rhizopus.*

**mucosa** (mu-ko'sah) [ L. fem. of *mucosus*, mucous ]. See *tunica mucosa.*

  **alveolar m.,** the mucous membrane apical to the attached gingiva.

  **gingival m.,** that portion of the oral mucous membrane that covers the alveolar process of the jaws and surrounds the necks of the teeth. Gingival m. is demarcated from lining m. on the facial aspect by a clearly defined line which marks the mucogingival junction. On the palatal surface, the gingiva blends imperceptibly with the palatal m.

  **olfactory m.,** *regio* olfactoria tunicae mucosae nasi.

  **respiratory m.,** *regio* respiratoria tunicae mucosae nasi.

**muco'sal.** Relating to the mucosa or mucous membrane.

**mucosanguineous, mucosanguinolent** (mu'ko-sang-gwin'e-us, -o-lent) [ muco- + L. *sanguis*, blood ]. Pertaining to an exudate or other fluid material that has a relatively high content of blood and mucus.

**mucoserous** (mu'ko-se'rus). Pertaining to an exudate or secretion that consists of both mucus and serum or a watery component.

**mu'cosin.** Name given a disaccharide obtained by hydrolysis of hyaluronic acid.

**mucositis** (mu'ko-si'tis). An obsolete term meaning inflammation of a mucous membrane surface.

**mucostatic** (mu'ko-stat'ik) [ muco- + G. *stasis*, a standing ]. 1. Denoting the normal, relaxed condition of mucosal tissues covering the jaws. 2. Arresting the secretion of mucus.

**muco'sus** [ L. ] [ NA ]. Mucous.

**mucous** (mu'kus) [ L. *mucosus*, mucous, fr. *mucus* ]. Relating to mucus or a m. membrane.

**mucoviscidosis** (mu'ko-vis'ī-do'sis). Viscidosis.

**mucro,** pl. **mucro'nes** (mu'kro) [ L. point, sword ]. A term applied to the pointed extremity of a structure.

  **m. cordis,** *apex* cordis.

  **m. sterni,** *processus* xiphoideus.

**mu'cronate** [ L. *mucronatus*, pointed ]. Relating to or resembling a sword; ensiform; xiphoid.

**mucu'na** [ a native Brazilian name ]. The hairs adherent to the pods of the cowhage, *Mucuna pruriens*, and the Florida bean, *M. urens;* anthelmintic.

**mucus** (mu'kus) [ L. ] [ NA ]. The clear, viscid secretion of the mucous membranes, consisting of mucin, epithelial cells, leukocytes, and various inorganic salts suspended in water.

**Mueller electronic tonometer.** See under tonometer.

**Muelle'rius capilla'ris.** One of the commonest hair lungworms (subfamily Protostrongylinae) of sheep, goats, and deer. It is smaller than *Dictyocaulus*, inhabits the smaller bronchi and lung parenchyma, and is relatively nonpathogenic to its host.

**muffle** (muf'l). A refractory core wound with resistant wire for electrical heating; or similar core for gas, etc.

**muhin'yo.** Native name of a continued fever prevalent in Uganda, probably brucellosis.

**muira puama** (moo-e'rah poo-ah'mah) [ Native Brazilian, wooden strength ]. The wood of *Liriosma ovata* (family Oleaceae), a tree of Brazil; antidysenteric and aphrodisiac.

**Mulder,** Johannes, Dutch anatomist, 1769–1810. See M.'s *angle.*

**Mules,** Philip H., English ophthalmologist, 1843–1905. See M.'s *operation.*

**muliebria** (mu'lī-e'brī-ah) [ L. neut pl. of *muliebris*, relating to *mulier*, a woman ]. The female genital organs.

**muliebrity** (mu-lī-eb'rī-tī) [ L. *mulier*, a woman ]. 1. The state of being a woman. 2. The normal or abnormal assumption of female characteristics.

**mull** [ Hindu, *malmal, mulmul* ]. 1. A soft thin cotton cloth, a kind of muslin. 2. Mulla.

**mulla** (mul'lah). Mull (2); an ointment or cerate, consisting of the medicinal agent in a base of a mixture of suet and lard with the occasional addition of wax or lead plaster, spread on mull, or soft muslin. These preparations are no longer official.

**Müller** (mü'ler), Friedrich von, German physician, 1858–1941. See M.'s *sign, steatoma.*

**Müller** (mü'ler), Heinrich, German anatomist, 1820–1864. See M.'s radial *cell*, M.'s *fibers, muscle, trigone.*

**Muller,** Herman J., U. S. geneticist, 1890–1967. Nobel laureate, 1946, for the discovery of the production of mutations by means of x-ray irradiation.

**Müller** (mü'ler), Hermann F., German histologist, 1866–1898. See formol-M. *fluid*, M.'s *fluid.*

**Müller** (mü'ler), Johannes P., German anatomist, physiologist, and pathologist, 1801–1858. See M.'s (or Müllerian) *canal, capsule, duct, experiment, law, tubercle.*

**Müller,** P. See M.'s *maneuver.*

**Müller,** Paul H., Swiss chemist, *1899. Nobel laureate, 1948, for his discovery of DDT as a contact insecticide.

**Müller,** W. See Geiger-M. *counter, tube.*

**Müller's method.** See under method.

**Mülle'rian.** Relating to Müller, usually Johannes, as in Müllerian ducts.

**multan'gular.** Having many angles.

**multi-** [ L. *multus*, much, many ]. Prefix denoting many, properly joined only to words of Latin derivation; the equivalent in words of Greek origin is *poly-.*

**mul'tiartic'ular** [ multi- + L. *articulus*, joint ]. Relating to or involving many joints; polyarthric.

**multicap'sular.** Having numerous capsules.

**multicel'lular.** Composed of many cells.

**Multiceps** (mul'ti-seps) [ multi- + L. *caput*, head ]. A genus of taeniid tapeworms in which the larval forms occur in the form of a coenurus (multiple scoleces invaginated within a single cyst).

  **M. mul'ticeps,** the mature form occurs in the intestines of dogs, the coenurus in the brains of herbivorous animals, especially sheep; the cyst is often called *Coenurus cerebralis.*

  **M. seria'lis,** mature form found in the intestine of dogs, the coenurus in the subcutaneous tissues of rabbits.

**multicus'pid.** A multicuspidate tooth.

**multicus'pidate.** 1. Having more than two cusps. 2. A tooth with three or more cusps or projections on the crown; a multicuspid; a molar tooth.

**multifamilial** (mul-tī-fă-mil'ī-al). Denoting a familial disease that attacks the children in several successive generations.

**multifeta'tion.** Superfetation.

**mul'tifid** [ L. *multifidus*, fr. *multus*, much, + *findo*, to cleave. FIS- ]. Divided into many clefts or segments.

**multif'idus** [ L. ]. 1 [ NA ]. Multifid. 2. See *musculus* multifidus.

**multifocal** (mul-tī-fo'kăl). Relating to or arising from many foci.

**mul'tiform.** Polymorphic (1).

**multiglan'dular.** Pluriglandular.

**multigrav'ida** [ multi- + L. *gravida*, pregnant ]. A pregnant woman who has been pregnant two or more times previously.

**multi-infection** (mul-tī-in-fek'shun). Mixed infection with two or more varieties of microorganisms developing simultaneously.

**multilo'bar, multilo'bate, multilobed** (mul-tī-lōbd'). Having several lobes.

**multilob'ular.** Having many lobules.

**multiloc'ular.** Many-celled; having many compartments or loculi.

**multimammae** (mul-tī-mam'e) [ multi- + L. *mamma*, breast ]. Polymastia.

**multino'dal.** Having many nodes.

**multinod'ular, multinod'ulate.** Having many nodules.

**multinu'clear.** Having two or more nuclei.

**multinu'cleated.** Multinuclear.

**multinucleo'sis.** Polynucleosis.

**multip'ara** [ multi- + L. *pario*, to bring forth, to bear ]. A woman who has given birth at least two times to an infant or infant, whether alive or dead, weighing 500 gm. or more or having an estimated length of gestation of at least 20 weeks.
  **grand m.,** a m. who has given birth seven or more times.

**multipar'ity.** The condition of being a multipara.

**multip'arous.** Relating to a multipara.

**multipartial** (mul'ti-par'shal). Polyvalent, with respect to an antiserum.

**multiple** (mul'tī-pl) [ L. *multiplex*, fr. *multus*, many, + *plico*, pp. -*atus*, to fold. PLIC- ]. Manifold; repeated several times; occurring in several parts at the same time, as m. arthritis, m. neuritis.

**multipo'lar.** Having more than two poles; denoting a nerve cell in which the branches project from several points.

**multiroot'ed.** Having more than two roots.

**multirota'tion.** Mutarotation.

**multisynaptic** (mul'tī-sī-nap'tik). Polysynaptic.

**multiva'lence.** The state of being multivalent.

**multiva'lent.** [ multi- + L. *valentia*, power ]. 1. In chemistry, having a combining power of more than one atom of hydrogen. 2. Efficacious in more than one direction. 3. See polyvalent (2).

**mum'mifica'tion** [ mummy + L. *facio*, to make ]. 1. Dry gangrene. 2. The shrivelling of a dead and retained fetus. 3. In dentistry, preservation of dead pulp tissue by means of antiseptics and other chemical agents.

**mumps** [ dialectic Eng. *mump*, a lump or bump ]. Epidemic *parotiditis*.
  **metastat'ic m.,** m. complicated by participation of the testis or the mamma.

**mu mu** [ G. letter μ ]. The millionth part of a micron; used chiefly as a measurement of the length of light rays; micromicron; usually written μμ.

**Munchausen** (münch'how-zen), Baron Karl F. H. von, German author of fabulous stories, 1720–1797. See M. *syndrome*.

**Mundinus,** or **Mondino d'Luzzi,** Italian anatomist, *circa* 1280. Professor of anatomy at Bologna; wrote a human anatomy, *Anatomia*, which was the standard anatomical text for over a century; taught anatomy by dissection for which his text was used as a guide. He was the most renowned anatomist before Vesalius.

**Munro,** John C., American surgeon, 1858–1910. See M.'s *point*.

**Munro's abscess, microabscess.** See under microabscess.

**Munsell,** Hazel E., American chemist, *1891. See Sherman-M. *unit*.

**Münzer,** E. See *tract* of M. and Wiener.

**mu'ral** [ L. *muralis;* fr. *murus*, wall ]. Relating to the wall of any cavity.

**muramic acid** (mu-ram'ik). 2-Amino-3-*O*-(D-1-carboxyethyl)-2-deoxy-D-glucose; glucosamine and lactate in ether linkage between the 3 and 2 positions, respectively; a constituent of the mureins in bacterial cell walls.

**muram'idase.** Lysozyme.

**mureins** (mu're-inz). Peptidoglycans composing the sacculus or cell casing of bacteria, consisting of linear polysaccharides of alternating *N*-acetylglucosamine and *N*-acetylmuramic acid units, to the lactate side chains of which are linked oligopeptides; independent chains are cross-linked in three dimensions *via* the peptides or the 6-OH groups (the latter may be linked *via* phosphate to a teichoic acid).

**Muret** (mü-ra'), Paul-Louis, French physician, *1878. See Quénu-M. *sign*.

**murexide** (mu-rek'sīd, -sid). The ammonium salt of purpuric acid, formerly used as a dye, but superseded by the aniline colors.

**murex'ine.** Urocanylcholine; β-(4-imidazolyl)acrylcholine; present in the hypobranchial body of *Murex trunculus* and other species of mollusk. It has powerful nicotinic and curariform actions.

**mu'riate** [ L. *muria*, brine ]. The former term for chloride.

**muriat'ic** [ L. *muriaticus*, pickled in brine, fr. *muria*, brine ]. Hydrochloric; relating to brine.
  **m. acid,** hydrochloric acid.

**Muridae** (mu'rī-de) [ L. *mus*(*mur-*), a mouse ]. The largest family of Rodentia embracing the Old World mice and rats; it is the largest family of mammals.

**murine** (mu'rīn, -rin, -rēn) [ L. *murinus*, relating to mice, fr. *mus*(*mur-*), a mouse ]. Relating to animals of the family Muridae.

**Murless,** B. C., South African obstetrician. See M. head *extractor*.

**mur'mur** [ L. ]. Susurrus; a soft sound, like that made by a somewhat forcible expiration with the mouth open, heard on auscultation of the heart, lungs, or blood vessels. Also used of a variety of other-than-soft sounds, which may be loud, harsh, frictional, etc. Many organic cardiac m.'s are loud and harsh; pericardial m.'s are friction rubs.
  **accidental m.,** an evanescent cardiac m. not due to valvular lesion.
  **anemic m.,** a nonvalvular m. heard on auscultation of the heart and large blood vessels in cases of profound anemia.
  **aortic m.,** one produced at the aortic orifice, either obstructive or regurgitant.
  **arterial m.,** a m. heard on auscultating an artery.
  **at'riosystol'ic m.,** presystolic m.
  **Austin Flint m.,** Flint's m.
  **bellows m.,** a blowing m.; bruit de soufflet.
  **brain m.** (1) Fischer's cerebral m.; a systolic m., sometimes heard in patients with rickets, with the stethoscope applied to the anterior fontanelle or the temporal region; (2) sounds produced by intracranial aneurysms or arterial venous aneurysms in congenital dysplastic angiomatosis.
  **Cabot-Locke m.,** an early diastolic m., like that of aortic insufficiency, heard best at the left lower sternal border in severe anemia.
  **cardiac m.,** a m. produced within the heart, at one of its orifices.
  **car'diopul'monary m.,** an innocent extracardiac m., synchronous with the heart's beat but disappearing when the breath is held, believed due to movement of air in a segment of lung compressed by the contracting heart.
  **car'diorespi'ratory m.,** cardiopulmonary m.
  **Carey Coombs m.,** Coombs m.; a blubbering apical middiastolic m. occurring in the acute stage of rheumatic mitral valvulitis and disappearing as the valvulitis subsides.
  **Cole-Cecil m.,** the diastolic m. of aortic insufficiency when well or predominantly heard in the left axilla.
  **continuous m.,** one that is heard without interruption throughout systole and into diastole.
  **Coombs m.,** Carey Coombs m.
  **crescendo m.,** a m. that increases in intensity and suddenly ceases; the presystolic m. of mitral stenosis.
  **Cruveilhier-Baumgarten m.,** a venous m. heard over collateral veins, connecting portal and caval venous systems, on the abdominal wall.

**diamond-shaped m.,** a crescendo-decrescendo m., from the shape of the frequency intensity curve of the phonocardiogram.

**diastolic m.,** one heard during diastole.

**Duroziez' m.,** see Duroziez' *symptom.*

**dynamic m.,** a heart m. due to anemia or to any cause other than a valvular lesion.

**early diastolic m.,** one that begins with the second heart sound, as the m. of aortic insufficiency.

**ejection m.,** a diamond-shaped systolic m. ending before the second heart sound and produced by the ejection of blood into aorta or pulmonary artery.

**endocardial m.,** one arising, from any cause, within the heart.

**exocardial m.,** a pericardial friction m.

**extracar'diac m.,** a m. heard over the precordium but originating from structures other than the heart; the term includes pericardial friction rubs and cardiopulmonary m.'s.

**Fischer's cerebral m.,** brain m. (1).

**Flint's m.,** a diastolic m., similar to that of mitral stenosis, heard at the cardiac apex in some cases of free aortic insufficiency; it is thought to be caused by the turbulent regurgitating stream from the aorta mixing into the stream simultaneously entering from the left ventricle through the mitral valve, and perhaps by the posterior movement of the anterior leaflet of the mitral valve in that turbulence.

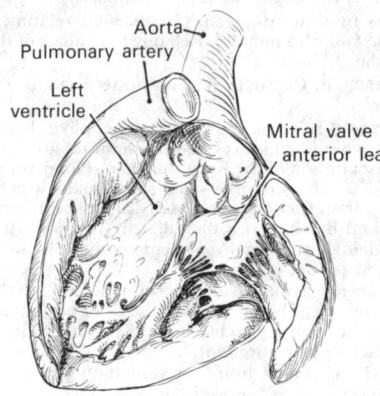

**Flint's Murmur**
Mechanism of production

**Fräntzel's m.,** m. of mitral stenosis when louder at its beginning and end than in its midportion.

**functional m.,** inorganic m.; a cardiac m. not associated with a heart lesion.

**Gibson m.,** the typical continuous "machinery-like" m. of patent ductus arteriosus.

**Graham Steell's m.,** an early diastolic m. of pulmonic insufficiency secondary to pulmonary hypertension, as in mitral stenosis.

**hemic m.,** a cardiac or vascular m. heard in anemic persons who have no valvular lesion, probably due to the increased blood velocity that characterizes anemia.

**Hodgkin-Key m.,** a musical diastolic m. associated with retroversion of an aortic cusp.

**holosystol'ic m.,** pansystolic m.

**hour-glass m.,** one in which there are two areas of maximum loudness decreasing to a point midway between the two.

**innocent m.,** one that is not caused by or indicative of organic heart disease.

**inorganic m.,** functional m.

**late apical systolic m.,** a m. ordinarily considered benign, or even extracardiac, with a possible relationship to pericardial disease; it often represents mitral insufficiency, often localized and of moderate severity but with propensity for developing pacterial endocarditis; it is frequently associated with systolic *click, q.v.*

**late diastolic m.,** presystolic m.

**machinery m.,** the long "continuous" rumbling m. of patent ductus arteriosus.

**mid-diastolic m.,** one beginning after the A-V valves have opened in diastole, *i.e.,* an appreciable time after the second heart sound, as the m. of mitral stenosis.

**mill wheel m.,** water wheel m.; churning cardiac m. produced by air embolism to the heart.

**mitral m.,** one produced at the mitral valve, either obstructive or regurgitant.

**muscular m.,** the sound produced by contracting muscular tissue.

**musical m.,** a cardiac m. having a musical character.

**nun's m.,** venous *hum.*

**obstructive m.,** one caused by narrowing of one of the valvular orifices.

**organic m.,** one caused by an organic lesion.

**pansystolic m.,** holosystolic m.; one occupying the entire systolic interval, from first to second sound.

**pericardial m.,** a friction sound, synchronous with the heart movements, heard in certain cases of pericarditis.

**pleuropericardial m.,** a pleural friction sound over the pericardial region, synchronous with the heart's action, and simulating a pericardial m.

**presystolic m.,** atriosystolic m.; late diastolic m.; one heard at the end of ventricular diastole (during atrial systole), usually due to obstruction at one of the atrioventricular orifices.

**pul'monary m., pulmon'ic m.,** a m. produced at the pulmonary orifice of the heart, either obstructive or regurgitant.

**regur'gitant m.,** one due to leakage or backward flow at one of the valvular orifices of the heart.

**respiratory m.,** vesicular *respiration.*

**Roger's m.,** bruit de Roger; loud pansystolic m. maximal at left sternal border, caused by small ventricular septal defect.

**sea gull m.,** a musical m. erroneously supposed to imitate the sea gull's cry.

**seesaw m.,** to-and-fro m.

**Steell's m.,** Graham Steell's m.

**sten'osal m.,** an arterial m. due to narrowing of the vessel from pressure or organic change.

**Still's m.,** an innocent musical m. resembling the noise produced by a twanging string.

**systol'ic m.,** a m. heard during ventricular systole.

**to-and-fro m.,** see-saw m.; m.'s heard in both systole and diastole of the heart, as in aortic stenosis and insufficiency.

**tricus'pid m.,** a m. produced at the tricuspid orifice, either obstructive or regurgitant.

**vascular m.,** one originating in a blood vessel.

**venous m.,** one heard over a vein.

**vesicular m.,** vesicular *respiration.*

**water wheel m.,** mill wheel m.

**Murphy,** John B., American surgeon, 1857–1916. See M.'s *button, drip, method,* kidney *punch.*

**Murphy,** William P., Boston physician, *1892. Nobel laureate, 1934, with George H. Whipple and George R. Minot, for their discoveries concerning liver therapy in cases of anemia.

**murrina** (moor-re'nah) [ Fr. *morine;* Sp. *morriña,* cattle plague, prob. fr. L. *morior,* to die ]. A disease of horses, mules, camels, and dogs (cattle seem to be immune) caused by the presence in the blood of *Trypanosoma evansi.* It is marked by emaciation, weakness, anemia, edema, ecchymotic conjunctivitis, fever, and more or less pronounced paralysis of the hind legs; in Panama, it affects chiefly horses. It is widely distributed mechanically by tabanid flies but not cyclically by tsetse flies. As a disease in camels, it is called el debab in Algeria, mbori in Sudan, and guifar in Chad. See also derrengadera, and surra.

**Mus** [ L. *mus* (*mur*-), a mouse. MUSCU- ]. A genus of the family Muridae that includes about 16 species of mice; domesticated strains are numerous and genetically well defined, the most popular being the albino and piebald strains. The gestation period of the mouse is 18 to 21 days, the litter size is 3 to 14 in number, and the stage of maturity to breed can be attained in 35 days. Although not native to the Western Hemisphere, species of *Mus* are found throughout this hemisphere, as well as the rest of the world. Only characteristics of dentition and jaws separate *Mus* from *Rattus* (the rat).

**Musca,** pl. **mus'cae** (mus'kah, mus'e, mus'ke) [ L. fly ]. A genus of diptera or flies.

**M. domes'tica,** the common housefly; an abundant member of the insect order Diptera, universally associated with humans, particularly under unsanitary conditions; it breeds in filth and organic waste, and is involved in the mechanical transfer of numerous pathogens.

**M. vomito'ria,** blowfly or flesh fly.

**muscae volitantes** (mus'se or mus'ke vol-ĭ-tan'tēs) [ L. pl. of *musca,* fly; pres. p. pl. of *volito,* to fly to and fro, fr. *volo,* to fly ]. Opplotentes; an appearance as of moving spots before the eyes.

**muscarine** (mus'kă-rēn, -rin). The cholinergic substance present in *Amanita muscaria* (fly agaric mushroom) and other mushrooms (*Inocybe* species); the quaternary trimethylammonium salt of 2-methyl-3-hydroxy-5-(aminomethyl)tetrahydrofuran; pharmacologic effects resemble those of acetylcholine and postganglionic parasympathetic stimulation (cardiac inhibition, vasodilation, salivation, lacrimation, bronchoconstriction, gastrointestinal stimulation). See also muscarinic.

**muscarin'ic.** 1. Having a muscarine-like action, *i.e.,* producing effects that resemble postganglionic parasympathetic stimulation. 2. An agent that stimulates the postganglionic parasympathetic receptor. See also muscarine, and nicotinic.

**mus'carinism.** Mycetism.

**muscegenetic** (mus'e-jen-et'ik). Muscegenic; producing muscae volitantes.

**muscegenic** (mus'e-jen'ik). Muscegenetic.

**Mus'ci** [ L. pl. of *muscus,* moss ]. The class of plants that includes the mosses.

**muscicide** (mus'sĭ-sid) [ L. *musca,* fly, + *caedo,* to kill ]. An agent destructive to flies.

**Muscidae** (mus'ĭ-de) [ L. *musca,* fly ]. A family of flies (order Diptera) including the houseflies (*Musca*) and stable flies (*Stomoxys*).

---

# MUSCLE

---

**muscle** (mus'el) [ L. *musculus*]. Microscopically, m. consists predominantly of contractile cells and may be classified as skeletal m., cardiac m., or smooth m. (*q.v.*). The latter is lacking in transverse striations characteristic of the other varieties. For reference to gross anatomical muscles, see musculus and color plates 1 to 7.

**m.'s of abdomen,** *musculi* abdominis.

**abductor m. of great toe,** *musculus* abductor hallucis.

**abductor m. of little finger,** *musculus* abductor digiti minimi manus.

**abductor m. of little toe,** *musculus* abductor digiti minimi pedis.

**adductor m. of great toe,** *musculus* adductor hallucis.

**adductor m. of thumb,** *musculus* adductor pollicis.

**Aeby's m.,** *musculus* cutaneomucosus.

**Albinus' m.,** (1) *musculus* risorius; (2) *musculus* scalenus minimus.

**anconeus m.,** *musculus* anconeus.

**antagonistic m.'s,** those having an opposite function, the contraction of one neutralizing that of the other.

**anterior auricular m.,** *musculus* auricularis anterior.

**anterior cervical intertransverse m.'s,** *musculi* intertransversarii anteriores cervicis.

**anterior scalene m.,** *musculus* scalenus anterior.

**anterior serratus m.,** *musculus* serratus anterior.

**anterior straight m. of head,** *musculus* rectus capitis anterior.

**anterior tibial m.,** *musculus* tibialis anterior.

**antigravity m.'s,** the m.'s that maintain the posture characteristic of a given animal species. In most mammals they are the extensor m.'s.

**m. of antitragus,** *musculus* antitragicus.

**appendicular m.,** one of the skeletal m.'s of the limbs.

**articular m.,** *musculus* articularis.

**articular m. of elbow,** *musculus* articularis cubiti.

**articular m. of knee** *musculus* articularis genus.

**axial m.,** one of the skeletal m.'s of the trunk or head.

**Bell's m.,** a band of muscular fibers, forming a slight fold in the wall of the bladder, running from the uvula to the opening of the ureter on either side, bounding the trigonum.

**biceps m. of arm,** *musculus* biceps brachii.

**biceps m. of thigh,** *musculus* biceps femoris.

**bipennate m.,** *musculus* bipennatus.

**Bochdalek's m.,** *musculus* triticeoglossus.

**Bovero's m.,** *musculus* cutaneomucosus.

**Bowman's m.,** *musculus* ciliaris.

**brachial m.,** *musculus* brachialis.

**brachiocephalic m.,** *musculus* brachiocephalicus.

**brachioradial m.,** *musculus* brachioradialis.

**Braune's m.,** *musculus* puborectalis.

**broadest m. of back,** *musculus* latissimus dorsi.

**bronchoesophageal m.,** *musculus* bronchoesophageus.

**Brücke's m.,** Crampton's m.; the part of the ciliary m. formed by the meridional fibers.

**cardiac m.,** the muscle of the heart; myocardium; it consists of anastomosing, transversely striated m. fibers formed of cells united at intercalated disks; nuclei are centrally located and the longitudinally arranged myofibrils have considerable sarcoplasm around them; connective tissue is limited to reticular and fine collagenous fibers.

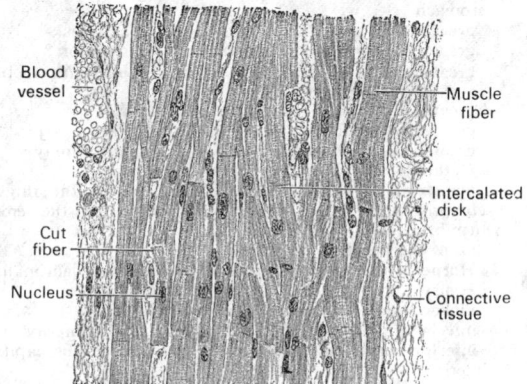

Cardiac Muscle

(From Copenhaver, W. M.: *Bailey's Textbook of Histology,* Ed. 15, The Williams & Wilkins Co., Baltimore, 1964.)

**Casser's perforated m.,** the coracobrachialis through which the musculocutaneous nerve frequently passes.

**cervical interspinal m.,** *musculus* interspinalis cervicis.

**cervical rotator m.'s,** *musculi* rotatores cervicis.

**cheek m.,** *musculus* buccinator.

**ciliary m.,** *musculus* ciliaris.

**m.'s of coccyx,** *musculi* coccygei.

**Coiter's m.,** *musculus* corrugator supercilii.

**coracobrachial m.,** *musculus* coracobrachialis.

**corrugator m.,** *musculus* corrugator supercilii.

**cowl m.,** *musculus* trapezius.

**Crampton's m.,** Brücke's m.

**cremaster m.,** *musculus* cremaster.

**cricothyroid m.,** *musculus* cricothyroideus.

**cutaneomucous m.,** *musculus* cutaneomucosus.

**cutaneous m.,** *musculus* cutaneus.

**dartos m.,** *tunica* dartos.

**deep transverse m. of perineum,** *musculus* transversus perinei profundus.

**deltoid m.,** *musculus* deltoideus.

**depressor m. of epiglottis,** *musculus* thyroepiglotticus.

**depressor m. of eyebrow,** *musculus* depressor supercilii.

**depressor m. of lower lip,** *musculus* depressor labii inferioris.

**depressor m. of septum,** *musculus* depressor septi.

**digas'tric m.,** (1) a m. with two fleshy bellies separated by a fibrous insertion; (2) *musculus* digastricus.

**dilator m.,** (1) *musculus* dilator; (2) *musculus* dilator pupillae.

**dorsal m.'s,** *musculi* dorsi.

**dorsal sacrococcygeal m.,** *musculus* sacrococcygeus dorsalis.

**Dupré's m.,** *musculus* articularis genu.

**Duverney's m.,** *pars* lacrimalis musculi orbicularis oculi.

**elevator m. of prostate,** *musculus* levator prostatae.

**elevator m. of thyroid,** *musculus* levator glandulae thyroideae.

**elevator m. of upper lip,** *musculus* levator labii superioris.

**elevator m. of upper lip and wing of nose,** *musculus* levator labii superioris alaeque nasi.

**epicranial m.,** *musculus* epicranius.

**erector m.'s of the hairs,** *musculi* arrectores pilorum.

**erector m. of spine,** *musculus* erector spinae.

**external pterygoid m.,** *musculus* pterygoideus lateralis.

**external sphincter m. of anus,** *musculus* sphincter ani externus.

**m.'s of the eyball,** *musculi* bulbi.

**femoral m.,** *musculus* vastus intermedius.

**fixator m.,** a m. that acts as a stabilizer of one part of the body during movement of another part.

**fu'siform m.,** *musculus* fusiformis.

**Gantzner's m.,** a group of m. fibers, which, although normally connecting the superficial and deep m.'s of the hand, appears as an entirely separate bundle.

**Gavard's m.,** oblique fibers in the muscular coat of the stomach.

**great adductor m.,** *musculus* adductor magnus.

**greater pectoral m.,** *musculus* pectoralis major.

**greater posterior straight m. of head,** *musculus* rectus capitis posterior major.

**greater psoas m.,** *musculus* psoas major.

**greater rhomboid m.,** *musculus* rhomboideus major.

**greater zygomatic m.,** *musculus* zygomaticus major.

**Guthrie's m.,** *musculus* sphincter urethrae.

**hamstring m.'s,** the m.'s at the back of the thigh, comprising the biceps, the semitendinosus, and the semimembranosus.

**m. of the heart,** cardiac m.

**Horner's m.,** *musculus* orbicularis oculi pars lacrimalis.

**Houston's m.,** *compressor* venae dorsalis penis.

**iliococcygeal m.,** *musculus* iliococcygeus.

**inferior lingual m.,** *musculus* longitudinalis inferior.

**inferior oblique m. of head,** *musculus* obliquus capitis inferior.

**iliopsoas m.,** *musculus* iliopsoas.

**inferior posterior serratus m.,** *musculus* serratus posterior inferior.

**inferior straight m.,** *musculus* rectus inferior.

**inferior tarsal m.,** *musculus* tarsalis inferior.

**infrahyoid m.'s,** *musculi* infrahyoidei.

**innermost intercostal m.,** *musculus* intercostalis intimus.

**intermediate great m.,** *musculus* vastus intermedius.

**internal pterygoid m.,** *musculus* pterygoideus medialis.

**internal sphincter m. of anus,** *musculus* sphincter ani internus.

**interspinal m.'s,** *musculi* interspinales.

**intertransverse m.'s,** *musculi* intertransversarii.

**involuntary m.'s,** m.'s not under control of the will; except in the case of the heart, they are smooth (nonstriated) m.'s.

**Jung's m.,** *musculus* pyramidalis auriculae.

**Klein's m.,** *musculus* cutaneomucosus.

**Kohlrausch's m.,** the longitudinal m.'s of the rectal wall.

**Krause's m.,** *musculus* cutaneomucosus.

**Landström's m.,** microscopic m. fibers in the fascia behind and about the eyeball, attached anteriorly to the lids and anterior orbital fascia; its action is to draw the eyeball forward and the lids backward, resisting the pull of the four orbital m.'s.

**Langer's m.,** axillary *arch.*

**large m. of helix,** *musculus* helicis major.

**m.'s of larynx,** *musculi* laryngis.

**lateral cricoarytenoid m.,** *musculus* cricoarytenoideus lateralis.

**lateral great m.,** *musculus* vastus lateralis.

**lateral lumbar intertransverse m.'s,** *musculi* intertransversarii laterales lumborum.

**lateral pterygoid m.,** *musculus* pterygoideus lateralis.

**lateral straight m.,** *musculus* rectus lateralis.

**lateral straight m. of the head,** *musculus* rectus capitis lateralis.

**lesser rhomboid m.,** *musculus* rhomboideus minor.

**lesser zygomatic m.,** *musculus* zygomaticus minor.

**long abductor m. of thumb,** *musculus* abductor pollicis longus.

**long adductor m.,** *musculus* adductor longus.

**long extensor m. of digits,** *musculus* extensor digitorum longus.

**long extensor m. of great toe,** *musculus* extensor hallucis longus.

**long extensor m. of thumb,** *musculus* extensor pollicis longus.

**long palmar m.,** *musculus* palmaris longus.

**long peroneal m.,** *musculus* peroneus longus.

**lumbar interspinal m.,** *musculus* interspinalis lumborum.

**lumbar quadrate muscle,** *musculus* quadratus lumborum.

**lumbar rotator m.'s,** *musculi* rotatores lumborum.

**Marcacci's m.,** a sheet of smooth m. fibers underlying the areola and nipple of the mammary gland.

**m.'s of mastication,** see *musculus* masseter, temporalis, pterygoideus lateralis, and pterygoideus medialis.

**medial great m.,** *musculus* vastus medialis.

**medial lumbar intertransverse m.'s,** *musculi* intertransversarii mediales lumborum.

**medial pterygoid m.,** *musculus* pterygoideus medialis.

**medial scalene m.,** *musculus* scalenus medius.

**medial straight m.,** *musculus* rectus medialis.

**Merkel's m.,** *musculus* ceratocricoideus.

**mucocutaneous m.,** *musculus* cutaneomucosus.

**Müller's m.,** (1) *musculus* orbitalis; (2) Rouget's m.; circular fibers of the musculus ciliaris; (3) *musculus* tarsalis superior.

**Myerholtz' m.,** radial smooth m. fibers beneath the areola of the nipple.

**nasal m.,** *musculus* nasalis.

**m.'s of neck,** *musculi* colli.

**m. of notch of helix,** *musculus* incisurae helicis.

**oblique arytenoid m.,** *musculus* arytenoideus obliquus.

**oblique m. of auricle,** *musculus* obliquus auriculae.

**occipitofrontal m.,** *musculus* occipitofrontalis.

**ocular m.'s,** see appropriate entries under *musculus* rectus and *musculus* obliquus.

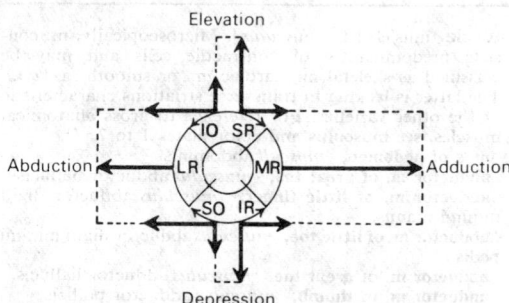

**Ocular Muscles**

Diagram showing actions. Length of arrow denotes relative contribution to movement in the indicated direction. *IO,* inferior oblique; *SO,* superior oblique; *LR,* lateral rectus; *SR,* superior rectus; *MR,* medial rectus; *IR,* inferior rectus. (After Marquez.)

**Oehl's m.'s,** strands of m. fibers in the chordae tendineae of the left atrioventricular valve.

**opposer m. of little finger,** *musculus* opponens digiti minimi.

**opposer m. of thumb,** *musculus* opponens pollicis.

**orbicular m.,** *musculus* orbicularis.

**orbicular m. of eye,** *musculus* orbicularis oculi.

**orbicular m. of mouth,** *musculus* orbicularis oris.

**orbital m.,** *musculus* orbitalis.

**palatoglossus m.,** *musculus* palatoglossus.

**palatopharyngeal m.,** *musculus* palatopharyngeus.

**pal'atouvula'ris m.,** *musculus* uvulae.

**panniculus carnosus m.,** (1) a sheet of m., lying beneath the skin, by which the skin can be made to shiver; it is especially well developed in the horse; often called the flyshaker; (2) in man, platysma.

**papillary m.,** *musculus* papillaris.

**pectinate m.,** *musculus* pectinatus.

**pectineal m.,** *musculus* pectineus.

**pennate m.,** see *musculus* bipennatus and *musculus* unipennatus.

**perineal m.'s,** *musculi* perinei.

**piriform m.,** *musculus* piriformis.

**plantar m.,** *musculus* plantaris.

**plantar quadrate m.,** *musculus* quadratus plantae.

**pleuroesophageal m.,** *musculus* pleuroesophageus.

**popliteal m.,** *musculus* popliteus.

**posterior auricular m.,** *musculus* auricularis posterior.

**posterior cervical intertransverse m.'s,** *musculi* intertransversarii posteriores cervicis.

**posterior cricoarytenoid m.,** *musculus* cricoarytenoideus posterior.

**posterior scalene m.,** *musculus* scalenus posterior.

**posterior tibial m.,** *musculus* tibialis posterior.

**Pozzi's m.,** *musculus* extensor digitorum brevis manus.

**procerus m.,** *musculus* procerus.

**pubococcygeal m.,** *musculus* pubococcygeus.

**puboprostatic m.,** *musculus* puboprostaticus.

**puborectal m.,** *musculus* puborectalis.

**pubovaginal m.,** *musculus* pubovaginalis.

**pubovesical m.,** *musculus* pubovesicalis.

**pyramidal m.,** *musculus* pyramidalis.

**pyramidal m. of auricle,** *musculus* pyramidalis auriculae.

**quadrate m. of loins,** *musculus* quadratus lumborum.

**quadrate pronator m.,** *musculus* pronator quadratus.

**quadrate m. of sole,** *musculus* quadratus plantae.

**quadrate m. of thigh,** *musculus* quadratus femoris.

**quadrate m. of upper lip,** *musculus* quadratus labii superioris.

**quadriceps m. of thigh,** *musculus* quadriceps femoris.

**radial flexor m. of wrist,** *musculus* flexor capri radialis.

**rectococcygeal m.,** *musculus* rectococcygeus.

**rectourethral m.,** *musculus* rectourethralis.

**rectovesical m.,** *musculus* rectovesicalis.

**Reisseissen's m.'s,** microscopic smooth m. fibers in the smallest bronchial tubes.

**rider's m.'s,** the adductor m.'s of the thigh, which come into play especially in horseback riding.

**Riolan's m.,** (1) marginal fibers of the palpebral part of the musculus oculi; (2) *musculus* cremaster.

**risorius m.,** *musculus* risorius.

**round pronator m.,** *musculus* pronator teres.

**rotator m.'s,** *musculi* rotatores.

**Rouget's m.,** Müller's m. (2).

**Ruysch's m.,** the muscular tissue of the fundus uteri.

**salpingopharyngeal m.,** *musculus* salpingopharyngeus.

**Santorini's m.,** (1) *musculus* risorius; (2) *musculus* incisurae helicis; (3) an incomplete band of nonstriated muscular fibers beneath the contrictor urethrae.

**scalp m.,** *musculus* epicranius.

**Sebileau's m.,** deep fibers of the dartos tunic which pass into the scrotal septum.

**second tibial m.,** *musculus* tibialis secundus.

**semimembranosus m.,** *musculus* semimembranosus.

**semispinal m.,** *musculus* semispinalis.

**semispinal m. of head,** *musculus* semispinalis capitis.

**semispinal m. of neck,** *musculus* semispinalis cervicis.

**semispinal m. of thorax,** *musculus* semispinalis thoracis.

**semitendinous m., semitendinosus m.,** *musculus* semitendinosus.

**shawl m.,** *musculus* trapezius.

**short abductor m. of thumb,** *musculus* abductor pollicis brevis.

**short adductor m.,** *musculus* adductor brevis.

**short extensor m. of thumb,** *musculus* extensor pollicis brevis.

**short flexor m. of little finger,** *musculus* flexor digiti minimi brevis manus.

**short flexor m. of little toe,** *musculus* flexor digiti minimi brevis pedis.

**short palmar m.,** *musculus* palmaris brevis.

**short peroneal m.,** *musculus* peroneus brevis.

**Sibson's m.,** *musculus* scalenus minimus.

**skeletal m.,** *musculus* skeleti (*q.v.*); a skeletal m. is one consisting of elongated, multinucleated, transversely striated skeletal muscle fibers (see under fiber), together with connective tissues, blood vessels, and nerves. Individual m. fibers are surrounded by fine reticular and collagen fibers, the endomysium; bundles (fascicles) of m. fibers are surrounded by irregular connective tissue called the perimysium. The entire m. is surrounded, except at the m. tendon junction, by a dense connective tissue, the epimysium.

**smaller m. of helix,** *musculus* helicis minor.

**smaller pectoral m.,** *musculus* pectoralis minor.

**smaller posterior straight m. of the head,** *musculus* rectus capitis posterior minor.

**smaller psoas m.,** *musculus* psoas minor.

**smallest scalene m.,** *musculus* scalenus minimus.

**smooth m.,** unstriated m.; involuntary m.; one of the m.'s of the internal organs, blood vessels, hair follicles, etc. The contractile elements of smooth m. are elongated, usually spindle-shaped cells with centrally located nuclei. They may vary in length from 20 to 200 $\mu$, or may be even longer in the pregnant uterus. Although transverse striations are lacking, fine myofibrils occur. The smooth m. fibers are bound together into sheets or bundles by reticular fibers, and frequently elastic fiber nets are also abundant.

**smooth m. of the ciliary body,** *musculus* ciliaris.

**Soemmering's m.,** *musculus* levator glandulae thyroideae.

**sphincter m.,** *musculus* sphincter.

**sphincter m. of common bile duct,** *musculus* sphincter ductus choledochi.

**sphincter m. of pancreatic duct,** *musculus* sphincter ductus pancreatici.

**sphincter m. of the pupil,** *musculus* sphincter pupillae.

**sphincter m. of pylorus,** *musculus* sphincter pylori.

**sphincter m. of urethra,** *musculus* sphincter urethrae.

**sphincter m. of urinary bladder,** *musculus* sphincter vesicae.

**spinal m.,** *musculus* spinalis.

**spinal m. of head,** *musculus* spinalis capitis.

**spinal m. of the neck,** *musculus* spinalis cervicis.

**spinal m. of thorax,** *musculus* spinalis thoracis.

**spindle-shaped m.,** *musculus* fusiformis.

**splenius m. of the head,** *musculus* splenius capitis.

**stapedius m.,** *musculus* stapedius.

**sternal m.,** *musculus* sternalis.

**sternochondroscapular m.,** *musculus* sternochondroscapularis.

**sternoclavicular m.,** *musculus* sternoclavicularis.

**sternocleidomastoid m.,** *musculus* sternocleidomastoideus.

**sternohyoid m.,** *musculus* sternohyoideus

**sternothyroid m.,** *musculus* sternothyroideus.

**straight m. of abdomen,** *musculus* rectus abdominis.

**straight m. of thigh,** *musculus* rectus femoris.

**strap m.'s,** *musculi* infrahyoidei.

**striated m.,** skeletal or cardiac m. in which cross striations occur in the fibers; sometimes the term striated m. is used as a synonym for skeletal m.

**styloglossus m.,** *musculus* styloglossus.

**stylohyoid m.,** *musculus* stylohyoideus.

**stylopharyngeal m.,** *musculus* stylopharyngeus.

**subanconeus m.,** *musculus* articularis cubiti.

**subclavian m.,** *musculus* subclavius.

**subcostal m.,** *musculus* subcostalis.

**subcrural m.,** *musculus* articularis genus.

**subquadricipital m.,** *musculus* articularis genus.

**subscapular m.,** *musculus* subscapularis.

**superficial lingual m.,** *musculus* longitudinalis superior.

**superficial transverse m. of perineum,** *musculus* transversus perinei superficialis.

**superior auricular m.,** *musculus* auricularis superior.

**superior oblique m. of head,** *musculus* obliquus capitis superior.

**superior posterior serratus m.,** *musculus* serratus posterior superior.

**superior straight m.,** *musculus* rectus superior.

**superior tarsal m.,** *musculus* tarsalis superior.

**supinator m.,** *musculus* supinator.

**supraclavicular m.,** *musculus* supraclavicularis.

**suprahyoid m.'s,** *musculi* suprahyoidei.

**supraspinous m.,** *musculus* supraspinatus.

**suspensory m. of duodenum,** *musculus* suspensorius duodeni.

**synergis'tic m.'s,** m.'s having a similar and mutually helpful function or action.

**tailor's m.,** *musculus* sartorius.

**temporal m.,** *musculus* temporalis.

**temporoparietal m.,** *musculus* temporoparietalis.

**tensor m. of fascia lata,** *musculus* tensor fasciae latae.

**tensor tarsi m.,** *musculus* orbicularis oculi pars lacrimalis.

**tensor m. of the tympanic membrane,** *musculus* tensor tympani.

**tensor m. of velum palatini,** *musculus* tensor veli palatini.

**teres major m.,** *musculus* teres major.

**teres minor m.,** *musculus* teres minor.

**Theile's m.,** *musculus* transversus perinei superficialis.

**third peroneal m.,** *musculus* peroneus tertius.

**thoracic interspinal m.,** *musculus* interspinalis thoracis.

**thoracic intertransverse m.'s,** *musculi* intertransversarii thoracis.

**thoracic rotator m.'s,** *musculi* rotatores thoracis.

**m.'s of thorax,** *musculi* thoracis.

**thyroarytenoid m.,** *musculus* thyroarytenoideus.

**thyroepiglottic m., thyroepiglottidean m.,** *musculus* thyroepiglotticus.

**thyrohyoid m.,** *musculus* thyrohyoideus.

**Tod's m.,** *musculus* obliquus auriculae.

**m.'s of tongue,** *musculi* linguae.

**Toynbee's m.,** *musculus* tensor tympani.

**tracheloclavicular m.,** *musculus* tracheloclavicularis.

**m. of tragus,** *musculus* tragicus.

**transverse m. of the abdomen,** *musculus* transversus abdominis.

**transverse arytenoid m.,** *musculus* arytenoideus transversus.

**transverse m. of auricle,** *musculus* transversus auriculae.

**transverse m. of the chin,** *musculus* transversus menti.

**transverse m. of the nape,** *musculus* transversus nuchae.

**transverse m. of thorax,** *musculus* transversus thoracis.

**transverse m. of the tongue,** *musculus* transversus linguae.

**trapezius m.,** *musculus* trapezius.

**Treitz' m.,** *musculus* suspensorius duodeni.

**triceps m. of the arm,** *musculus* triceps brachii.

**triceps m. of the calf,** *musculus* triceps surae.

**ulnar flexor m. of wrist,** *musculus* flexor carpi ulnaris.

**unipennate m.,** *musculus* unipennatus.

**unstriated m., unstriped m.,** smooth m.

**Valsalva's m.,** *musculus* tragicus.

**ventral sacrococcygeal m.,** *musculus* sacrococcygeus ventralis.

**vertical m. of the tongue,** *musculus* verticalis linguae.

**vestigial m.,** an imperfect structure in man corresponding to a functioning m. in the lower animals.

**vocal m.,** *musculus* vocalis.

**voluntary m.,** one whose action is under the control of the will; all the striated m.'s, except the heart, are voluntary m.'s.

**Wilson's m.,** (1) *musculus* sphincter urethrae; (2) certain fibers of the levator ani.

**wrinkler m. of eyebrow,** *musculus* corrugator supercilii.

---

**mus'cle-bound.** Said of one whose individual muscles are large or overdeveloped but whose muscles function poorly together for concerted action. Though muscles are strong, they are dyssynergic.

**mus'cle-trim'ming.** Border *molding.*

**mus'cone.** Muskone.

**muscular** (mus'ku-lar). Relating to a muscle or the muscles.

**muscula'ris** [ Mod. L. muscular ]. The muscular coat of a hollow organ or tubular structure.

**m. muco'sae,** *lamina* muscularis mucosae.

**muscularity** (mus'ku-lăr'ĭ-tĭ). The state or condition of having well developed muscles.

**mus'cularize.** To change into muscle substance, as the partial conversion of cicatricial tissue after the healing of a wound of muscle.

**mus'culature.** The arrangement of the muscles in a part or in the body as a whole.

**mus'culin.** A globulin in muscle, coagulable by slight heat (87°C., 116.6°F.).

**mus'culoap'oneurot'ic.** Relating to muscular tissue and an aponeurosis of origin or insertion.

**musculocutaneous** (mus'ku-lo-ku-ta'ne-us). Relating to both muscle and skin; denoting certain nerves that give off sensory fibers to the skin and motor fibers to the underlying muscles.

**mus'culomem'branous.** Relating to both muscular tissue and membrane; denoting certain muscles, such as the occipitofrontalis, that are largely membranous.

**mus'culophren'ic.** Relating to the muscular portion of the diaphragm; denoting an artery supplying this part.

**mus'culoskel'etal.** Relating to muscles and to the skeleton, as, for example, the m. system.

**mus'culospi'ral.** Denoting the musculospiral nerve; see *nervus* radialis.

**mus'culoten'dinous.** Relating to both muscular and tendinous tissues.

**mus'culotrop'ic.** Affecting, acting upon, or attracted to muscular tissue.

---

# MUSCULUS

---

**musculus,** gen. and pl. **musculi** (mus'ku-lus, mus'ku-li) [ L. a little mouse, a muscle, fr. *mus* (*mur*-), a mouse. MUSCU- ] [ NA ]. Muscle; one of the contractile organs of the body by which movements of the various organs and parts are effected. The typical muscle is a mass of muscle fibers (venter or belly), attached at each extremity, by means of a tendon, to a bone or other structure; the more proximal or more fixed attachment is called the *origin,* the more distal or more movable attachment is the *insertion;* the narrowing part of the belly which is attached to the tendon of origin is called the caput or head. See color plates 1 to 7. For histologic descriptions, see muscle, and relevant subentries under muscle.

**musculi abdom'inis** [ NA ], muscles of the abdomen; muscles forming the wall of the abdomen including rectus abdominis, external and internal oblique muscles, transversus abdominis, and quadratus abdominis.

**m. abductor digiti minimi manus** [ NA ], abductor of the little finger; m. abductor digiti quinti; *origin,* pisiform bone and pisohamate ligaments; *insertion,* medial side of base of proximal phalanx of the little finger; *nerve supply,* ulnar; *action,* abducts and flexes little finger.

**m. abductor digiti minimi pedis** [ NA ], abductor of the little toe; m. abductor digiti quinti; *origin,* lateral and medial processes of calcaneus; *insertion,* lateral side of proximal phalanx of fifth toe; *nerve supply,* lateral plantar nerve, *action,* abducts and flexes little toe.

**m. abduc'tor hallu'cis** [ NA ], abductor of great toe; *origin,* medial process of tuber calcanei, flexor retinaculum, and plantar aponeurosis; *insertion,* medial side of proximal phalanx of great toe; *nerve supply,* medial plantar; *action,* abducts great toe.

**m. abduc'tor pol'licis brevis** [ NA ], short abductor of thumb; m. abductor pollicis; *origin,* ridge of trapezium and flexor retinaculum; *insertion,* lateral side of proximal phalanx of thumb; *nerve supply,* median; *action,* abducts thumb.

**m. abduc'tor pol'licis longus** [ NA ], long abductor of thumb; *origin,* interosseous membrane and posterior surfaces of radius and ulna; *insertion,* lateral side of base of first metacarpal bone; *nerve supply,* radial; *action,* abducts and assists in extending thumb.

**m. accelera'tor uri'nae,** m. bulbospongiosus.

**m. accessorius gluteus minimus,** m. scansorius.

**m. adduc'tor brevis** [ NA ], short adductor muscle; *origin,* superior ramus of pubis; *insertion,* upper third of medial lip of linea aspera; *nerve supply,* obturator; *action,* adducts thigh.

**m. adduc'tor hallu'cis** [ NA ], adductor of great toe; *origin*, by two heads, the caput transversum from the capsules of the lateral four metatarsophalangeal joints and the caput obliquum from the lateral cuneiform and bases of the third and fourth metatarsal bones; *insertion*, lateral side of base of proximal phalanx of great toe; *nerve supply*, lateral plantar; *action*, adducts great toe.

**m. adduc'tor longus** [ NA ], long adductor muscle; *origin*, symphysis and crest of pubis; *insertion*, middle third of medial lip of linea aspera; *nerve supply*, obturator; *action*, adducts thigh.

**m. adduc'tor magnus** [ NA ], great adductor muscle; *origin*, ischial tuberosity and ischiopubic ramus; *insertion*, linea aspera and adductor tubercle of femur; *nerve supply*, obturator and sciatic; *action*, adducts and extends thigh.

**m. adduc'tor min'imus**, a small flat muscle constituting the upper portion of the adductor magnus, *inserted* into space above linea aspera.

**m. adduc'tor pol'licis** [ NA ], adductor of the thumb; *origin*, by two heads, the caput transversum from the shaft of the third metacarpal and the caput obliquum from the front of the base of the second metacarpal, the trapezoid and capitate bones; *insertion*, medial side of base of proximal phalanx of thumb; *nerve supply*, ulnar; *action*, adducts thumb.

**m. ancone'us** [ NA ], anconeus muscle; m. anconeus quartus; *origin*, back of lateral condyle of humerus; *insertion*, olecranon process and posterior surface of ulna; *nerve supply*, radial; *action*, extends forearm and abducts ulna in pronation of wrist.

**m. antitrag'icus** [ NA ], muscle of the antitragus; a band of transverse muscular fibers on the outer surface of the antitragus, arising from the border of the intertragic notch and inserted into the anthelix and cauda helicis.

**musculi arrecto'res pilo'rum** [ NA ], erector muscles of the hairs; bundles of smooth muscle fibers, attached to the deep part of the hair follicles, passing outward alongside the sebaceous glands to the papillary layer of the corium; they act to pull the hairs erect.

**m. articula'ris** [ NA ], articular muscle; a muscle that inserts directly onto the capsule of a joint, acting to retract the capsule in certain movements.

**m. articula'ris cu'biti** [ NA ], articular muscle of the elbow; subanconeus muscle; the name applied to a small slip of the medial head of the triceps that inserts into the capsule of the elbow joint.

**m. articula'ris genus** [ NA ], articular muscle of the knee; m. subcrureus; *origin*, lower fourth of anterior surface of shaft of femur; *insertion*, capsule of knee joint; *nerve supply*, femoral; *action*, retracts suprapatellar bursa.

**m. aryepiglot'ticus** [ NA ], the fibers of the oblique arytenoid muscle that extend from the summit of the arytenoid cartilage to the side of the epiglottis; *action*, constricts the laryngeal aperture.

**m. arytenoid'eus obli'quus** [ NA ], oblique arytenoid muscle; *origin*, muscular process of arytenoid cartilage; *insertion*, summit of arytenoid cartilage of opposite side and the aryepiglottic fold as far as the epiglottis; *nerve supply*, recurrent laryngeal; *action*, narrows rima glottidis.

**m. arytenoid'eus transver'sus** [ NA ], transverse arytenoid muscle; a band of muscular fibers passing between the two arytenoid cartilages posteriorly; *nerve supply*, recurrent laryngeal; *action*, narrows the rima glottidis.

**m. aryvoca'lis**, a number of the deeper fibers of the vocalis muscle attached directly to the outer side of the true vocal cord.

**m. attol'lens au'rem** or **auric'ulam**, m. auricularis superior.

**m. a'ttrahens au'rem** or **auric'ulam**, m. auricularis anterior.

**m. auricula'ris ante'rior** [ NA ], anterior auricular muscle; m. attrahens aurem or auriculam; *origin*, galea aponeurotica; *insertion*, cartilage of auricle; *action*, draws pinna of ear upward and forward; *nerve supply*, facial. Considered by some to be the anterior part of the m. temporoparietalis.

**m. auricula'ris posterior** [ NA ], posterior auricular muscle; m. retrahens aurem or auriculam; *origin*, mastoid process; *insertion*, posterior portion of root of auricle; *action*, draws back the pinna; *nerve supply*, facial.

**m. auricula'ris superior** [ NA ], superior auricular muscle; m. attollens aurem or auriculam; attollens aurem, auriculam; *origin*, galea aponeurotica; *insertion*, cartilage of auricle; *action*, draws pinna of ear upward and backward; *nerve supply*, facial. Considered by some to be the posterior part of the m. temporoparietalis.

**m. az'ygos u'vulae,** m. uvulae.

**m. biceps bra'chii** [ NA ], biceps muscle of arm; *origin*, long head (caput longum) from supraglenoidal tuberosity of scapula, short head (caput breve) from coracoid process; *insertion*, tuberosity of radius; *nerve supply*, musculocutaneous; *action*, flexes and supinates forearm.

**m. biceps fem'oris** [ NA ], biceps muscle of thigh; *origin*, long head (caput longum) from tuberosity of ischium, short head (caput breve) from lower half of lateral lip of linea aspera; *insertion*, head of fibula; *nerve supply*, long head, tibial, short head, peroneal; *action*, flexes knee and rotates leg laterally.

**m. biceps flexor cruris,** m. biceps femoris.

**m. bipenna'tus** [ NA ], bipennate muscle; a muscle with a central tendon toward which the fibers converge on either side like the barbs of a feather.

**m. biven'ter mandib'ulae,** m. digastricus.

**m. brachia'lis** [ NA ], brachial muscle; *origin*, lower two-thirds of anterior surface of humerus; *insertion*, coronoid process of ulna; *nerve supply*, musculocutaneous and (usually) radial; *action*, flexes forearm.

**m. brachiocephal'icus** [ NAV ], brachiocephalic muscle; in animals, a compound muscle passing from the brachium or humerus to the head and the dorsal cervical raphe; the clavicular insection or clavicle subdivides the muscle.

**m. brachioradia'lis** [ NA ], brachioradial muscle; m. supinator longus; *origin*, lateral supracondylar ridge of humerus; *insertion*, front of base of styloid process of radius; *nerve supply*, radial; *action*, flexes forearm and assists slightly in supination.

**m. bronchoesophage'us** [ NA ], bronchoesophageal muscle; muscular fascicles, arising from the wall of the left bronchus, which reinforce the musculature of the esophagus.

**m. buccina'tor** [ NA ], *origin*, posterior portion of alveolar portion of maxilla and mandible and pterygomandibular ligament or raphe; *insertion*, orbicularis oris at angle of mouth; *action*, flattens cheek, retracts angle of mouth; *nerve supply*, facial.

**m. buccopharynge'us,** see m. constrictor pharyngis superior.

**musculi bul'bi** [ NA ], muscles of the eyeball; the muscles within the orbit including the four rectus muscles; two oblique muscles, and the levator of the superior eyelid.

**m. bulbocaverno'sus,** m. bulbospongiosus.

**m. bulbospongiosus** [ NA ], m. ejaculator seminis; m. bulbocavernosus; m. ejaculator or accelerator urinae; m. sphincter vaginae; In the male: *origin*, the inferior fascia of the urogenital diaphragm, fascia on the dorsum of the bulb of the penis; *insertion*, central tendon of the perineum and the median raphe on the free surface of the bulb; *action*, constricts bulbous urethra. In the female: *origin*, the dorsum of the clitoris, the corpus cavernosum, and the inferior fascia of the urogenital diaphragm; *insertion*, central tendon of the perineum; *nerve supply*, pudendal; *action*, acts as a weak sphincter of the vagina.

**m. caninus,** m. levator anguli oris.

**musculi cap'itis** [ NA ], muscles of the head; the muscles of expression, of mastication, and the suboccipital muscles in general.

**m. cephalopharynge'us,** m. constrictor pharyngis superior.

**m. ceratocricoid'eus** [ NA ], a fasciculus from the m. cricoarytenoideus posterior inserted into the inferior cornu of the thyroid cartilage.

**m. ceratopharynge'us,** see m. constrictor pharyngis medius.

**m. cervica'lis ascen'dens,** m. iliocostalis cervicis.

**m. chondroglos'sus** [ NA ], ceratoglossus; keratoglossus; muscular fibers occasionally separated from the hyoglossus, but usually forming part of it.

**m. chondropharynge'us,** see m. constrictor pharyngis medius.

**m. cilia'ris** [ NA ], ciliary muscle; Bowman's muscle; the smooth muscle of the ciliary body; it consists of circular fibers (fibrae circulares, or Müller's muscle) and radiating fibers (fibrae meridionales, or Brücke's muscle); *action*, it changes the shape of the lens in the process of accommodation. See fig. under eye.

**m. clei'doepitro'chlea'ris**, the anterior portion of the deltoid, arising from the clavicle.

**m. cleidomastoid'eus**, the portion of the sternocleidomastoid muscle passing between the clavicle and the mastoid process.

**m. cleidooccipita'lis**, the portion of the sternocleidomastoid muscle between the clavicle and the superior curved line of the occipital bone.

**musculi coccygei** [ NA ], muscles of the coccyx; the muscles of the coccyx considered as a group, including the m. coccygeus and the inconstant m. sacrococcygeus ventralis and dorsalis.

**m. coccyge'us** [ NA ], coccygeal muscle; m. ischiococcygeus; *origin*, spine of ischium and sacrospinous ligament; *insertion*, sides of lower part of sacrum and upper part of coccyx; *nerve supply*, 3d and 4th sacral; *action*, assists in raising and supporting pelvic floor.

**musculi col'li** [ NA ], muscles of the neck; the anterolateral muscles of the neck including the platysma, sternocleidomastoid, suprahyoid muscles, infrahyoid muscles, longus colli and scalene muscles.

**m. compres'sor naris**, see m. nasalis.

**m. compres'sor ure'thrae**, m. sphincter urethrae.

**m. constric'tor pharyn'gis infe'rior** [ NA ], m. laryngopharyngeus; *origin*, outer surfaces of thyroid and cricoid cartilages, as the **pars thyropharyngea** and the **pars cricopharyngea**; *insertion*, pharyngeal raphe in the posterior portion of wall of pharynx; *nerve supply*, pharyngeal plexus; *action*, narrows lower part of pharynx in swallowing.

**m. constric'tor pharyn'gis me'dius** [ NA ], *origin*, stylohyoid ligament, lesser cornu of the hyoid bone (**pars chondropharyngeus**) and greater cornu of the hyoid bone (**pars ceratopharyngeus**); *insertion*, pharyngeal raphe in the posterior wall of the pharynx; *nerve supply*, pharyngeal plexus; *action*, narrows pharynx in the act of swallowing.

**m. constric'tor pharyn'gis supe'rior** [ NA ], m. cephalopharyngeus; *origin*, medial pterygoid plate (**pars pterygopharyngea**), pterygomandibular raphe (**pars buccopharyngea**), mylohyoid line of mandible (**pars mylopharyngea**), and the mucous membrane of the floor of the mouth and the side of the tongue (**pars glossopharyngea**); *insertion*, pharyngeal raphe in the posterior wall of the pharynx; *nerve supply*, pharyngeal plexus; *action*, narrows pharynx.

**m. constric'tor ure'thrae**, m. sphincter urethrae.

**m. coracobrachia'lis** [ NA ], *origin*, coracoid process of scapula; *insertion*, middle of medial border of humerus; *nerve supply*, musculocutaneous; *action*, adducts and flexes the arm.

**m. corruga'tor cutis ani**, smooth muscle fibers radiating from the anal opening superficial to the external sphincter.

**m. corruga'tor supercil'ii** [ NA ], Coiter's muscle; corrugator muscle; wrinkler muscle of eyebrow; *origin*, from orbital portion of m. orbicularis oculi and nasal prominence; *insertion*, skin of eyebrow; *action*, draws medial end of eyebrow downward and wrinkles forehead vertically; *nerve supply*, facial.

**m. cremas'ter** [ NA ], cremaster muscle; Riolan's muscle (2); *origin*, from m. obliquus internus and inguinal ligament; *insertion*, cremasteric fascia and pubic tubercle; *action*, raises testicle; *nerve supply*, genitofemoral; in the male the muscle envelops the spermatic cord and testis, in the female the round ligament of the uterus.

**m. cricoarytenoid'eus latera'lis** [ NA ], lateral cricoarytenoid muscle; *origin*, upper margin of arch of cricoid cartilage; *insertion*, muscular process of arytenoid; *nerve supply*, recurrent laryngeal; *action*, narrows rima glottidis.

**m. cricoarytenoid'eus posterior** [ NA ], posterior cricoarytenoid muscle; *origin*, depression on posterior surface of lamina of cricoid; *insertion*, muscular process of arytenoid; *nerve supply*, recurrent laryngeal; *action*, widens rima glottidis.

**m. cricopharynge'us**, see m. constrictor pharyngis inferior.

**m. cricothyroid'eus** [ NA ], cricothyroid muscle; *origin*, anterior surface of arch of cricoid; *insertion*, **pars recta**,

anterior or straight part, passes upward to ala of thyroid, **pars obliqua**, posterior or oblique part, passes more outward to inferior cornu of thyroid; *nerve supply*, superior laryngeal; *action*, makes vocal folds tense.

**m. cuta'neomuco'sus**, cutaneomucous or mucocutaneous muscle; a labial muscle formed by sagittal fibers running from the skin to the mucous membrane. Also called compressor muscle of the lips; Aeby's, Bovero's, Klein's, or Krause's muscle; "sucking muscle."

**m. cuta'neus** [ NA ], cutaneous muscle; a muscle that lies in the subcutaneous tissue and attaches to the skin; it may or may not have a bony attachment. The muscles of expression are the chief examples of cutaneous muscles in the human.

**m. deltoid'eus** [ NA ], deltoid muscle; *origin*, lateral third of clavicle, lateral border of acromion process, lower border of spine of scapula; *insertion*, lateral side of shaft of humerus a little above its middle; *nerve supply*, axillary from 5th and 6th cervical through brachial plexus; *action*, abduction, flexion, extension, and rotation of arm.

**m. depressor an'guli oris** [ NA ], m. triangularis; *origin*, lower border of lower jaw anteriorly; *insertion*, blends with other muscles in lower lip near angle of mouth; *action*, pulls down corners of mouth; *nerve supply*, facial.

**m. depressor la'bii inferioris** [ NA ], depressor of the lower lip; m. quadratus labii inferioris; *origin*, anterior portion of lower border of mandible; *insertion*, m. orbicularis oris and skin of lower lip; *action*, depresses lower lip; *nerve supply*, facial.

**m. depressor septi** [ NA ], depressor of the septum; a vertical fasciculus from the m. orbicularis oris passing upward along the median line of the upper lip, and inserted into the cartilaginous septum of nose.

**m. depressor supercilii** [ NA ], depressor of the eyebrow; fibers of the orbital part of the m. orbicularis oculi which insert in the eyebrow.

**m. detru'sor uri'nae**, the external longitudinal layer of the muscular coat of the bladder.

**m. diaphrag'ma**, see diaphragma.

**m. digas'tricus** [ NA ], digastric muscle; two-bellied muscle; m. biventer mandibulae; consists of two bellies united by a central tendon which is connected to the body of the hyoid bone; *origin*, by posterior belly (venter posterior) from digastric groove medial to the mastoid process; *insertion*, by anterior belly (venter anterior) into lower border of mandible near symphysis; *action*, elevates the hyoid when mandible is fixed; depresses the mandible when hyoid is fixed; *nerve supply*, posterior belly from facial, anterior belly by mylohyoid from third division of trigeminal.

**m. dilatator**, m. dilator.

**m. dila'tor**, m. dilatator; dilator muscle; a muscle which opens an orifice or dilates the lumen of an organ; it is the dilating or opening component of a pylorus (the other component is the m. sphincter).

**m. dila'tor i'ridis**, m. dilator pupillae.

**m. dila'tor na'ris**, see m. nasalis.

**m. dila'tor pupil'lae** [ NA ], m. dilator iridis; dilator muscle; the radial muscular fibers extending from the sphincter pupillae to the ciliary margin; some anatomists regard them as elastic, not muscular, in man.

**m. dila'tor pylo'ri gastroduodena'lis**, the longitudinal muscular fibers that open the gastroduodenal junction.

**m. dila'tor pylo'ri ilea'lis**, the longitudinal muscular fibers that open the ileal orifice at the level of the cecocolic junction.

**musculi dor'si** [ NA ], dorsal muscles; the muscles of the back in general, including those attaching the shoulder girdle to the trunk posteriorly, the posterior serratus muscles, and the erector spinae.

**m. ejacula'tor sem'inis**, m. bulbospongiosus.

**m. epicra'nius** [ NA ], epicranial muscle; scalp muscle; composed of the galea aponeurotica and the muscles inserting into it, *i.e.*, the m. occipitofrontalis and m. temporoparietalis.

**m. epitroch'leoancone'us**, an occasional muscle *arising* from the back of the medial condyle of the humerus, and *inserted* into the medial side of the olecranon process.

**m. erec'tor clitor'idis**, m. ischiocavernosus.

**m. erec'tor penis**, m. ischiocavernosus.

**m. erec'tor spi'nae** [ NA ], erector muscle of the spine; sacrospinalis; *origin*, from sacrum, ilium, and spines of lumbar vertebrae; it divides into three columns, the *iliocostalis, longissimus*, and *spinalis*, which insert into ribs and vertebrae with additional muscle slips joining the columns at successively higher levels; *action*, extends spinal column; *nerve supply*, posterior branches of spinal nerves.

**m. exten'sor brevis digito'rum**, m. extensor digitorum brevis.

**m. exten'sor brevis pol'licis**, m. extensor pollicis brevis.

**m. exten'sor carpi radia'lis brevis** [ NA ], *origin*, lateral epicondyle of humerus; *insertion*, base of third metacarpal bone; *nerve supply*, radial; *action*, extends and abducts wrist radialward.

**m. exten'sor carpi radia'lis longus** [ NA ], *origin*, lateral supracondylar ridge of humerus; *insertion*, back of base of second metacarpal bone; *nerve supply*, radial; *action*, extends and abducts wrist radialward.

**m. exten'sor carpi ulna'ris** [ NA ], *origin*, lateral epicondyle of humerus (caput humerale) and oblique line and posterior border of ulna (caput ulnare); *insertion*, base of fifth metacarpal bone; *nerve supply*, radial (posterior interosseous); *action*, extends and abducts wrist ulnarward.

**m. exten'sor coccy'gis**, m. sacrococcygeus dorsalis.

**m. exten'sor dig'iti minimi** [ NA ], m. extensor digiti quinti proprius; *origin*, lateral epicondyle of humerus; *insertion*, dorsum of proximal phalanx of little finger; *nerve supply*, radial (posterior interosseous); *action*, extends little finger.

**m. exten'sor digito'rum** [ NA ], *origin*, lateral epicondyle of humerus; *insertion*, by four tendons into the base of the proximal and middle and base of the distal phalanges; *nerve supply*, radial (posterior interosseous); *action*, extends fingers.

**m. exten'sor digito'rum brevis** [ NA ], *origin*, dorsal surface of calcaneus; *insertion*, by four tendons fusing with those of the extensor digitorum longus, and by a slip attached independently to the base of the proximal phalanx of the great toe; *nerve supply*, deep peroneal; *action*, extends toes.

**m. exten'sor digitorum brevis manus**, a short extensor muscle of the fingers of rare occurrence, and comparable to the short extensor of the toes.

**m. exten'sor digito'rum commu'nis**, m. extensor digitorum.

**m. exten'sor digito'rum longus** [ NA ], long extensor of the digits; *origin*, lateral condyle of tibia, upper two-thirds of anterior margin of fibula; *insertion*, by four tendons to the dorsal surfaces of the bases of the proximal, middle, and distal phalanges of the 2d to 5th toes; *nerve supply*, deep branch of peroneal; *action*, extends the four lateral toes.

**m. exten'sor hallu'cis brevis** [ NA ], the medial belly of m. extensor digitorum brevis, the tendon of which is inserted into the base of the proximal phalanx of the great toe.

**m. exten'sor hallu'cis longus** [ NA ], long extensor of the great toe; *origin*, lateral surface of tibia and interosseous membrane; *insertion*, base of distal phalanx of great toe; *action*, extends the great toe; *nerve supply*, anterior tibial.

**m. exten'sor in'dicis** [ NA ], m. extensor indicis proprius; *origin*, dorsal surface of ulna; *insertion*, dorsum of proximal phalanx of index finger; *nerve supply*, radial; *action*, assists in extending the forefinger.

**m. exten'sor longus digitorum**, m. extensor digitorum longus.

**m. exten'sor longus pol'licis**, m. extensor pollicis longus.

**m. exten'sor min'imi dig'iti**, m. extensor digiti minimi.

**m. exten'sor ossis metacar'pi pol'licis**, m. abductor pollicis longus.

**m. exten'sor pol'licis brevis** [ NA ], short extensor of the thumb; *origin*, dorsal surface of radius; *insertion*, base of proximal phalanx of thumb; *nerve supply*, radial; *action*, extends and abducts the thumb.

**m. exten'sor pol'licis longus** [ NA ], long extensor of the thumb; *origin*, posterior surface of ulna; *insertion*, base of distal phalanx of thumb; *nerve supply*, radial; *action*, extends distal phalanx of thumb.

**m. fibula'ris brev'is** [ NA ], m. peroneus brevis.

**m. fibula'ris long'us** [ NA ], m. peroneus longus.

**m. fibula'ris ter'tius** [ NA ], m. peroneus tertius.

**m. flexor accesso'rius** [ NA ], m. quadratus plantae.

**m. flexor brevis digito'rum**, m. flexor digitorum brevis.

**m. flexor brevis hallu'cis**, m. flexor hallucis brevis.

**m. flexor brevis min'imi dig'iti**, m. flexor digiti minimi.

**m. flexor carpi radia'lis** [ NA ], radial flexor of the wrist; *origin*, medial condyle of humerus; *insertion*, anterior surface of bases of 2d and 3d metacarpal bones; *nerve supply*, median; *action*, flexes and abducts wrist radialward.

**m. flexor carpi ulna'ris** [ NA ], ulnar flexor of the wrist; *origin*, humeral head (caput humerale) from medial condyle of humerus, ulnar head (caput ulnare) from olecranon and upper three-fifths of posterior border of ulna; *insertion*, pisiform bone; *nerve supply*, ulnar; *action*, flexes and abducts wrist ulnarward.

**m. flex'or dig'iti min'imi brev'is ma'nus** [ NA ], *origin*, hamulus of hamate bone; *insertion*, medial side of proximal phalanx of little finger; *nerve supply*, ulnar; *action*, flexes proximal phalanx of little finger.

**m. flex'or dig'iti min'imi brev'is pe'dis** [ NA ], *origin*, base of metatarsal bone of the little toe and sheath of m. peroneus longus; *insertion*, lateral surface of base of proximal phalanx of little toe; *nerve supply*, lateral plantar; *action*, flexes the proximal phalanx of the little toe.

**m. flexor digito'rum brevis** [ NA ], *origin*, medial tubercle of calcaneus and central portion of plantar fascia; *insertion*, middle phalanges of four lateral toes by tendons perforated by those of the flexor longus; *nerve supply*, medial plantar; *action*, flexes lateral four toes.

**m. flexor digito'rum longus** [ NA ], *origin*, middle third of posterior surface of tibia; *insertion*, by four tendons, perforating those of the flexor brevis, into bases of distal phalanges of four lateral toes; *nerve supply*, tibial nerve; *action*, flexes 2d to 5th toes.

**m. flexor digito'rum profun'dus** [ NA ], *origin*, anterior surface of upper third of ulna; *insertion*, by four tendons, piercing those of the superficialis, into base of distal phalanx of each finger; *nerve supply*, ulnar and median (anterior interosseous muscle); *action*, flexes distal phalanges of fingers.

**m. flexor digito'rum superficialis** [ NA ], *origin*, humero-ulnar head (caput humeroulnare) from the medial epicondyle of the humerus, the medial border of the coronoid process, and a tendinous arch between these points, radial head (caput radiale) from the oblique line and middle third of the lateral border of the radius; *insertion*, by four split tendons, passing to either side of the profundus tendons, into sides of middle phalanx of each finger; *nerve supply*, median; *action*, flexes middle phalanges of the fingers.

**m. flexor hallu'cis brevis** [ NA ], *origin*, medial surface of cuboid and middle and lateral cuneiform bones; *insertion*, by two tendons, embracing that of the flexor longus hallucis, into the sides of the base of the proximal phalanx of the great toe; *nerve supply*, medial and lateral plantar; *action*, flexes great toe.

**m. flexor hallu'cis longus** [ NA ], *origin*, lower two-thirds of posterior surface of fibula; *insertion*, base of distal phalanx of great toe; *nerve supply*, medial plantar; *action*, flexes great toe.

**m. flexor longus digito'rum**, m. flexor digitorum longus.

**m. flexor longus hallu'cis**, m. flexor hallucis longus.

**m. flexor longus pol'licis**, m. flexor pollicis longus.

**m. flexor pol'licis brevis** [ NA ], *origin*, superficial portion from flexor retinaculum of wrist, deep portion from ulnar side of first metacarpal bone; *insertion*, base of proximal phalanx of thumb; *nerve supply*, median and ulnar; *action*, flexes proximal phalanx of thumb.

**m. flexor pol'licis longus** [ NA ], *origin*, anterior surface of middle third of radius; *insertion*, distal phalanx of thumb; *nerve supply*, median palmar interosseous); *action*, flexes distal phalanx of thumb.

**m. flexor profun'dus digito'rum**, m. flexor digitorum profundus.

**m. flexor subli'mis digito'rum**, m. flexor digitorum superficialis.

**m. fronta'lis**, see m. occipitofrontalis.

**m. fusifor'mis** [ NA ], fusiform muscle; spindle-shaped muscle; one that has a fleshy belly, tapering at either extremity.

**m. gastrocne'mius** [ NA ], *origin*, by two heads (caput laterale and caput mediale) from the lateral and medial condyles of the femur; *insertion*, with soleus by tendo calcaneus (achillis) into lower half of posterior surface of calcaneus; *nerve supply,* tibial; *action,* plantar flexion of foot.

**m. gemel'lus inferior** [ NA ], *origin,* tuberosity of ischium; *insertion,* tendon of m. obturator internus; *nerve supply* and *action* rotates thigh laterally.

**m. gemel'lus superior** [ NA ], *origin,* ischial spine and margin of lesser sciatic notch; *insertion,* tendon of m. obturator internus; *nerve supply* and *action* rotates thigh laterally.

**m. genioglos'sus** [ NA ], m. geniohyoglossus; one of the paired lingual muscles; *origin,* mental spine of the mandible; *insertion,* lingual fascia beneath the mucous membrane and epiglottis; *nerve supply,* hypoglossal; *action,* depresses and protrudes the tongue.

**m. geniohyoid'eus** [ NA ], geniohyoid; *origin,* mental spine of mandible; *insertion,* body of hyoid bone; *action,* draws hyoid forward, or depresses jaw when hyoid is fixed; *nerve supply,* fibers from 1st and 2d cervical accompanying hypoglossal.

**m. glossopalati'nus,** m. palatoglossus.

**m. glossopharynge'us,** see m. constrictor pharyngis superior.

**m. glute'us maximus** [ NA ], *origin,* ilium behind posterior gluteal line, posterior surface of sacrum and coccyx, and sacrotuberous ligament; *insertion,* iliotibial band of fascia lata and gluteal ridge of femur; *nerve supply,* inferior gluteal; *action,* extends thigh.

**m. glute'us medius** [ NA ], *origin,* ilium between anterior and posterior gluteal lines; *insertion,* lateral surface of great trochanter; *nerve supply,* superior gluteal; *action,* abducts and rotates thigh.

**m. glute'us minimus** [ NA ], *origin,* ilium between anterior and inferior gluteal lines; *insertion,* great trochanter of femur; *nerve supply,* superior gluteal; *action,* abducts thigh.

**m. glu'teus quar'tus,** m. scansorius.

**m. grac'ilis** [ NA ], *origin,* ramus of pubis near symphysis; *insertion,* shaft of tibia below medial tuberosity; *nerve supply,* obturator; *action,* adducts thigh, flexes knee, rotates leg medially.

**m. hel'icis major** [ NA ], large muscle of the helix; a narrow band of muscular fibers on the anterior border of the helix arising from the spine and inserted at the point where the helix becomes transverse.

**m. hel'icis minor** [ NA ], smaller muscle of the helix; a band of oblique fibers covering the crus helicis.

**m. hyoglos'sus** [ NA ], *origin,* body and greater horn of hyoid bone; *insertion,* side of the tongue; *nerve supply,* hypoglossal; *action,* retracts and pulls down side of tongue.

**m. hypopharynge'us,** see m. constrictor pharyngis medius.

**m. ili'acus** [ NA ], *origin,* iliac fossa; *insertion,* tendon of psoas, anterior surface of lesser trochanter, and capsule of hip joint; *nerve supply,* lumbar plexus; *action,* flexes thigh and rotates it medially.

**m. ili'acus minor,** the fibers of the iliacus arising from the anterior inferior iliac spine and inserted into the iliofemoral ligament; they are sometimes distinctly separate from the rest of the muscle.

**m. iliocapsula'ris,** m. iliacus minor.

**m. il'iococcyge'us** [ NA ], iliococcygeal muscle; the posterior part of the levator ani arising from the tendinous arch of the levator ani muscle and inserting on the anococcygeal ligament and coccyx.

**m. iliocosta'lis** [ NA ], the lateral division of the erector spinae, having three subdivisions: m. iliocostalis lumborum, m. iliocostalis thoracis, and m. iliocostalis cervicis.

**m. iliocosta'lis cervi'cis** [ NA ], m. cervicalis ascendens; *origin,* angles of upper six ribs; *insertion,* transverse processes of middle cervical vertebrae; *action,* extends, abducts, and rotates cervical vertebrae; *nerve supply,* posterior divisions of upper thoracic nerves.

**m. iliocosta'lis dorsi,** m. iliocostalis thoracis.

**m. iliocosta'lis lumbo'rum** [ NA ], m. sacrolumbalis; *origin,* with erector spinae; *insertion,* the angles of lower six ribs; *action,* extends, abducts, and rotates lumbar vertebrae; *nerve supply,* dorsal branches of thoracic and lumbar.

**m. iliocosta'lis thoracis** [ NA ], m. iliocostalis dorsi; *origin,* medial side of angles of lower six ribs; *insertion,* angles of upper six ribs; *action,* extends, abducts, and

rotates thoracic vertebrae; *nerve supply,* dorsal branches of thoracic nerves.

**m. iliopso'as** [ NA ], iliopsoas muscle; a compound muscle, consisting of the m. iliacus and m. psoas major.

**m. incisi'vus la'bii inferior'is,** inferior incisive bundle of origin of m. orbicularis oris.

**m. incisi'vus la'bii superior'is,** superior incisive bundle of origin of m. orbicularis oris.

**m. incisu'rae hel'icis** [ NA ], muscle of the notch of the helix; Santorini's muscle; m. intertragicus.

**m. infracosta'lis,** pl. **infracosta'les,** m. subcostalis.

**musculi infrahyoi'dei** [ NA ], infrahyoid muscles; strap muscles; the small, flat muscles inferior to the hyoid bone including the sternohyoideus, omohyoideus, sternothyroideus, thyrohyoideus and levator glandulae thyroideae.

**m. infraspina'tus** [ NA ], *origin,* infraspinous fossa of scapula; *insertion,* middle facet of great tubercle of humerus; *nerve supply,* suprascapular from 5th to 6th cervical; *action,* extends arm and rotates it laterally.

**m. intercosta'lis externus,** pl. **intercosta'les externi** [ NA ], each arises from lower border of one rib and passes obliquely downward and forward to be inserted into the upper border of rib below; *action,* contract during inspiration, also maintain tension in the intercostal spaces to resist mediolateral movement; *nerve supply,* intercostal.

**m. intercosta'lis internus,** pl. **intercosta'les interni** [ NA ], each arises from lower border of rib and passes obliquely downward and backward to be inserted into upper border of rib below; *action,* contract during expiration, also maintain tension in the intercostal spaces to resist mediolateral movement; *nerve supply,* intercostal.

**m. intercosta'lis intimus** pl. **intercosta'les intimi** [ NA ], innermost intercostal; a layer parallel to the internal intercostal muscle but separated from it by the intercostal vessels and nerves.

**m. interos'seus dorsa'lis manus,** pl. **interos'sei dorsa'les** [ NA ], four in number; *origin,* sides of adjacent metacarpal bones; *insertion,* proximal phalanges and extensor expansion, 1st on radial side of index, 2d on radial side of middle finger, 3d on ulnar side of middle finger, 4th on ulnar side of ring finger; *nerve supply,* ulnar; *action,* abducts index, abducts or adducts middle finger, abducts ring finger.

**m. interos'seus dorsa'lis pedis,** pl. **interos'sei dorsa'les** [ NA ], four muscles; *origin,* from sides of adjacent metatarsal bones; *insertion,* 1st into medial, 2d to lateral side of proximal phalanx of 2d toe, 3d and 4th into lateral side of proximal phalanx of 3d and 4th toes; *nerve supply,* lateral plantar; *action,* 1st adducts 2d toe; 2d, 3d, and 4th abduct 2d, 3d, and 4th toes.

**m. interos'seus palma'ris,** pl. **interos'sei palma'res** [ NA ], m. interosseus volaris; three in number; *origin,* 1st from ulnar side of 2d metacarpal, 2d and 3d from radial sides of 4th and 5th metacarpals; *insertion,* 1st into ulnar side of index, 2d and 3d into radial sides of ring and little fingers; *nerve supply,* ulnar; *action,* adducts fingers toward axis of middle finger.

**m. interos'seus planta'ris,** pl. **interos'sei planta'res** [ NA ], three muscles; *origin,* the medial side of the 3d, 4th, and 5th metatarsal bones; *insertion,* corresponding side of proximal phalanx of the same toes; *nerve supply,* lateral plantar; *action,* adducts three lateral toes.

**m. interos'seus vola'ris,** m. interosseus palmaris.

**musculi interspina'les** [ NA ], interspinal muscles; the paired muscles between spinous processes of adjacent vertebrae; subdivided into cervical, thoracic, and lumbar muscles.

**m. interspina'lis cervi'cis** [ NA ], cervical interspinal muscle; *origin,* tubercle of spinous process of cervical vertebra; *insertion,* tubercle of spinous process of next superior vertebra; *nerve supply,* dorsal branches of cervical nerves; *action,* extends the neck.

**m. interspina'lis lumbo'rum** [ NA ], lumbar interspinal muscles; *origin,* superior margin of lumbar spinous process; *insertion,* inferior margin of next superior spinous process; *nerve supply,* dorsal branches of lumbar nerves; *action,* extends lumbar vertebrae.

**m. interspina'lis thora'cis** [ NA ], thoracic interspinal muscle; often poorly developed or absent muscles between spinous process of thoracic vertebrae; *nerve supply,* dorsal branches of thoracic nerves; *action,* extends thoracic vertebrae.

**musculi intertransversa'rii** [ NA ], intertransverse muscles; the paired muscles between transverse processes of adjacent vertebrae; there are anterior and posterior muscles in the cervical region; lateral and medial muscles in the lumbar region; and single muscles in the thoracic region.

**musculi intertransversa'rii anterio'res cervi'cis** [ NA ], anterior cervical intertransverse muscles; *origin,* anterior tubercle of cervical transverse process; *insertion,* anterior tubercle of next superior transverse process; *nerve supply,* ventral branch of cervical nerves; *action,* abducts cervical vertebrae.

**musculi intertransversa'rii latera'les lumbo'rum** [ NA ], lateral lumbar intertransverse muscles; *origin,* transverse processes of lumbar vertebrae; *insertion,* next superior transverse process; *nerve supply,* ventral branches of lumbar nerves; *action,* abducts lumbar vertebrae.

**musculi intertransversa'rii media'les lumbo'rum** [ NA ], medial lumbar intertransverse muscles; *origin,* accessory and mamillary processes of lumbar vertebrae; *insertion,* corresponding processes of next superior vertebra; *nerve supply,* dorsal branches of lumbar nerves; *action,* abducts lumbar vertebrae.

**musculi intertransversa'rii posterio'res cervi'cis** [ NA ], posterior cervical intertransverse muscles; *origin,* pars lateralis, posterior tubercle of cervical transverse process; pars medialis; transverse process; *insertion,* corresponding parts of next superior transverse process; *nerve supply,* pars lateralis; ventral branches of cervical nerves; pars medialis, dorsal branches of cervical nerves; *action,* abducts cervical vertebrae.

**musculi intertransversa'rii thora'cis** [ NA ], thoracic intertransverse muscles; *origin,* transverse processes of thoracic vertebrae; *insertion,* next superior transverse process; *nerve supply,* dorsal branches of thoracic nerves; *action,* abducts thoracic vertebrae.

**m. ischiocaverno'sus** [ NA ], m. erector penis (or clitoridis); *origin,* ramus of ischium; *insertion,* corpus cavernosum penis (or clitoridis); *nerve supply,* perineal; *action,* maintains the penis, or clitoris, erect.

**m. ischiococcyge'us,** m. coccygeus.

**m. keratopharynge'us,** see m. constrictor pharyngis medius.

**musculi laryn'gis** [ NA ], muscles of the larynx; the intrinsic muscles that regulate the length, position and tension of the vocal cords and adjust the size of the openings between the aryepiglottic folds, the ventricular folds and the vocal folds.

**m. laryngopharynge'us,** m. constrictor pharyngis inferior.

**m. latis'simus dorsi** [ NA ], broadest muscle of the back; *origin,* spinous processes of lower 5 or 6 thoracic and the lumbar vertebrae, median ridge of sacrum, and outer lip of iliac crest; *insertion,* with teres major into posterior lip of bicipital groove of humerus; *action,* adducts arm, rotates it medially, and extends it; *nerve supply,* thoracodorsal from brachial plexus.

**m. leva'tor alae nasi,** alar insertion of m. levator labii superioris alaeque nasi.

**m. leva'tor an'guli oris** [ NA ], m. caninus; *origin,* canine fossa of maxilla; *insertion,* orbicularis oris and skin at angle of mouth; *action,* raises angle of mouth; *nerve supply,* facial.

**m. leva'tor an'guli scap'ulae,** m. levator scapulae.

**m. leva'tor ani** [ NA ], formed by m. puborectalis, m. levator prostatae (m. pubovaginalis), m. pubococcygeus, and m. iliococcygeus; *origin,* back of pubis, tendinous arch of the levator ani, and spine of ischium; *insertion,* anococcygeal ligament, sides of the lower part of the sacrum and of coccyx; *nerve supply,* 4th sacral; *action,* draws the anus upward in defecation; supports the pelvic viscera.

**m. leva'tor costae,** pl. **levato'res costa'rum** [ NA ], the musculi levatores costarum breves arise from the transverse processes of last cervical and eleven thoracic vertebrae and are *inserted* into ribs next below, between angle and tubercle; the musculi levatores costarum longi are *inserted* into the second rib below their origin; *action,* raise ribs; *nerve supply,* intercostal.

**m. leva'tor glan'dulae thyroid'eae** [ NA ], elevator of the thyroid gland; a fasciculus occasionally passing from the thyrohyoid muscle to the isthmus of the thyroid gland.

**m. leva'tor la'bii inferio'ris,** m. mentalis.

**m. leva'tor la'bii superio'ris** [ NA ], elevator of the upper lip; caput infraorbitale quadrati labii superioris; *origin,* maxilla below infraorbital foramen; *insertion,* orbicularis oris of upper lip; *action,* elevates upper lip; *nerve supply,* facial.

**m. leva'tor la'bii superio'ris alae'que na'si** [ NA ], elevator of the upper lip and wing of the nose; caput angulare quadrati labii superioris; *origin,* root of nasal process of maxilla; *insertion,* ala of nose and m. orbicularis oris of upper lip; *action,* elevates upper lip and wing of nose; *nerve supply,* facial.

**m. leva'tor pala'ti,** m. levator veli palatini.

**m. leva'tor palpe'brae superio'ris** [ NA ], *origin,* orbital surface of the lesser wing of the sphenoid, above and anterior to the optic canal; *insertion,* skin of eyelid, tarsal plate, and orbital walls, by medial and lateral expansions of the aponeurosis of insertion; *nerve supply,* oculomotor; *action,* raises the upper eyelid.

**m. levator prostatae** [ NA ], elevator of the prostate; in the male, the most medial fibers of the levator ani muscle that extend from the pubis into the fascia of the prostate.

**m. leva'tor scap'ulae** [ NA ], m. levator anguli scapulae; *origin* from posterior tubercles of transverse processes of four upper cervical vertebrae; *insertion* into superior angle of scapula; *action,* raises the scapula; *nerve supply,* dorsal nerve of scapula from brachial plexus.

**m. leva'tor ve'li palati'ni** [ NA ], m. levator palati; *origin,* apex of petrous portion of temporal bone and lower part of cartilaginous auditory (Eustachian) tube; *insertion,* aponeurosis of soft palate; *nerve supply,* pharyngeal plexus; *action,* raises soft palate.

**musculi lin'guae** [ NA ], muscles of the tongue; the extrinsic muscles include the genioglossus, hyoglossus, chondroglossus, styloglossus and glossopalatinus; the intrinsic muscles are the vertical, transverse and the superior and inferior longitudinal.

**m. longis'simus** [ NA ], the intermediate division of the erector spinae muscle having three subdivisions, m. longissimus capitis, m. longissimus cervicis, and m. longissimus thoracis.

**m. longis'simus cap'itis** [ NA ], m. trachelomastoideus; m. transversalis capitis; m. complexus minor; *origin,* from transverse processes of upper thoracic and transverse and articular processes of lower and middle cervical vertebrae; *insertion* into mastoid process; *action,* keeps head erect, draws it backward or to one side; *nerve supply,* dorsal branches of cervical.

**m. longis'simus cervi'cis** [ NA ], m. transversalis cervicis or colli; *origin,* transverse processes of upper thoracic vertebrae; *insertion,* transverse processes of middle and upper cervical vertebrae; *action,* extends cervical vertebrae *nerve supply,* dorsal branches of lower cervical and upper thoracic.

**m. longis'simus dor'si,** m. longissimus thoracis.

**m. longis'simus thoracis** [ NA ], m. longissimus dorsi; *origin* with iliocostalis and from transverse processes of lower thoracic vertebrae; *insertion,* by lateral slips into most or all of the ribs between angles and tubercles and into tips of transverse processes of upper lumbar vertebrae, and by medial slips into accessory processes of upper lumbar and transverse processes of thoracic vertebrae; *action,* extends vertebral column; *nerve supply,* thoracic and lumbar.

**m. longitudina'lis inferior** [ NA ], inferior lingual; an intrinsic muscle of the tongue, cylindrical in shape, occupying the under part on either side.

**m. longitudina'lis superior** [ NA ], superficial lingual; an intrinsic muscle of the tongue, running from base to tip on the dorsum just beneath the mucous membrane.

**m. longus cap'itis** [ NA ], m. rectus capitis anticus major; *origin,* anterior tubercles of transverse processes of 3d to 6th cervical vertebrae; *insertion,* basilar process of occipital bone; *action,* twists or bends neck forward; *nerve supply,* cervical plexus.

**m. longus colli** [ NA ], *medial portion* arises from the bodies of the 3d thoracic to the 5th cervical vertebrae and is inserted into the bodies of the 2d to 4th cervical vertebrae; *superolateral portion* arises from the anterior tubercles of the transverse processes of the 3d to 5th cervical vertebrae and is inserted into the anterior tubercle of the atlas; the *inferolateral portion* arises from the bodies of the 1st to 3d thoracic vertebrae and is inserted into the anterior tubercles of the transverse processes of the 5th and 6th cervical vertebrae; *action*, twists and bends neck forward; *nerve supply*, ventral branches of cervical.

**m. lumbrica'lis manus**, pl. **lumbrica'les ma'nus** [ NA ], four in number; *origin*, the two lateral, from the radial side of the tendons of the flexor digitorum profundus going to the index and middle fingers, the two medial, from the adjacent sides of the 2d and 3d, and 3d and 4th tendons; *insertion*, radial side of extensor tendon on dorsum of each of the four fingers; *nerve supply*, the two radial by the median, the two ulnar by the ulnar; *action*, flexes the proximal and extends the middle and distal phalanges.

**m. lumbrica'lis pedis**, pl. **lumbrica'les pedis** [ NA ], four muscles; *origin*, 1st from tibial side of tendon to 2d toe of flexor digitorum longus, 2d, 3d, and 4th from adjacent sides of all four tendons of this m.; *insertion*, tibial side of extensor tendon on dorsum of each of the four lateral toes; *nerve supply*, lateral and medial plantar; *action*, flex the proximal and extend the middle and distal phalanges.

**m. masse'ter** [ NA ], *origin*, pars superficialis, inferior border of the anterior two-thirds of the zygomatic arch; pars profunda, inferior border and medial surface of the zygomatic arch; *insertion*, lateral surface of ramus and coronoid process of the mandible; *action*, closes jaw; *nerve supply*, masseteric from third division of trigeminal.

**m. menta'lis** [ NA ], m. levator labii inferioris; *origin*, incisor fossa of mandible; *insertion*, skin of chin; *action*, raises and wrinkles skin of chin and pushes up lower lip; *nerve supply*, facial.

**m. multif'idus** [ NA ], m. multifidus spinae; *origin*, from the sacrum, sacroiliac ligament, mammillary processes of the lumbar vertebrae, transverse processes of thoracic vertebrae, and articular processes of last four cervical vertebrae; *insertion* into the spinous processes of all the vertebrae up to and including the axis; *action*, rotates vertebral column; *nerve supply*, dorsal branches of spinal.

**m. multifidus spinae**, m. multifidus.

**m. mylohyoid'eus** [ NA ], *origin*, mylohyoid line of mandible; *insertion*, upper border of hyoid bone and raphe separating muscle from its fellow; *action*, elevates floor of mouth and the tongue, depresses jaw when hyoid is fixed; *nerve supply*, mylohyoid from third division of trigeminal.

**m. mylopharynge'us**, see m. constrictor pharyngis superior.

**m. nasa'lis** [ NA ], nasal muscle; consists of the pars transversa, arising from the maxilla on each side and passing across the bridge of the nose, and the pars alaris, arising from the maxilla and attaching to the ala of the nose. The pars alaris dilates the nostrils. *Nerve supply*, facial.

**m. obli'quus auric'ulae** [ NA ], oblique muscle of the auricle; a thin band of oblique muscular fibers extending from the upper part of the eminence of the concha to the convexity of the helix, running across the groove corresponding to the crus anthelicis inferior.

**m. obli'quus cap'itis inferior** [ NA ], inferior oblique muscle of the head; *origin*, spinous process of axis; *insertion*, transverse process of the atlas; *action*, rotates head; *nerve supply*, suboccipital.

**m. obli'quus cap'itis superior** [ NA ], superior oblique muscle of the head; *origin*, transverse process of atlas; *insertion*, outer third of inferior curved line of occipital bone; *action*, rotates head; *nerve supply*, suboccipital.

**m. obli'quus externus abdom'inis** [ NA ], *origin*, 5th to 12th ribs; *insertion*, anterior half of lateral lip of iliac crest, inguinal ligament, and anterior layer of the sheath of the rectus; *action*, diminishes capacity of abdomen, draws thorax downward; *nerve supply*, lower thoracic.

**m. obli'quus inferior** [ NA ], *origin*, orbital plate of maxilla lateral to the lacrimal groove; *insertion*, sclera between the superior and lateral recti; *nerve supply*, oculomotor; *action*, laterally rotates the eyeball on its anteroposterior axis; directs pupil of eye upward and outward.

**m. obli'quus inter'nus abdom'inis** [ NA ], *origin*, iliac fascia deep to lateral part of inguinal ligament, anterior half of crest of ilium, and lumbar fascia; *insertion*, 10th to 12th ribs and sheath of rectus; some of the fibers from inguinal ligament terminate in the falx inguinalis; *action*,

diminishes capacity of abdomen, bends thorax forward; *nerve supply*, lower thoracic.

**m. obli'quus superior** [ NA ], *origin*, above the medial margin of the optic canal; *insertion*, by a tendon passing through the trochlea, or pulley, and then reflected backward, downward, and laterally to the sclera between the superior and lateral recti; *nerve supply*, trochlear nerve; *action*, laterally rotates eyeball on its anteroposterior axis; directs pupil of eye downward and outward.

**m. obtura'torius externus** [ NA ], *origin*, lower half of margin of obturator foramen and adjacent part of external surface of obturator membrane; *insertion*, trochanteric fossa of femur trochanter; *nerve supply*, obturator; *action*, rotates thigh laterally.

**m. obtura'torius internus** [ NA ], *origin*, pelvic surface of obturator membrane and margin of obturator foramen; *insertion*, medial surface of great trochanter; *nerve supply*, sacral plexus; *action*, rotates thigh laterally.

**m. occipita'lis**, see m. occipitofrontalis.

**m. occipitofronta'lis**, [ NA ], occipitofrontal muscle; it is a part of m. epicranius; the occipital belly (venter occipitalis) arises from the occipital bone and inserts into the galea aponeurotica; the frontal belly (venter frontalis) arises from the galea and inserts into the skin of the eyebrow and nose; *action*, to move the scalp; *nerve supply*, facial.

**m. omohyoid'eus** [ NA ], formed of two bellies attached to intermediate tendon; *origin*, by inferior belly from upper border of scapula between superior angle and notch; *insertion*, by superior belly into hyoid bone; *action*, depresses hyoid; *nerve supply*, upper cervical through ansa cervicalis.

**m. opponens digiti minimi** [ NA ], opposer of the little finger; *origin*, hamulus of the hamate bone and flexor retinaculum; *insertion*, shaft of 5th metacarpal; *nerve supply*, ulnar; *action*, draws ulnar side of hand toward center of palm.

**m. oppo'nens dig'iti quin'ti**, m. opponens digiti minimi.

**m. oppo'nens min'imi dig'iti**, m. opponens digiti minimi.

**m. oppo'nens pol'licis** [ NA ], opposer of the thumb; *origin*, ridge of trapezium and flexor retinaculum; *insertion*, anterior surface of 1st metacarpal bone; *nerve supply*, median; *action*, opposes thumb to other fingers.

**m. orbicula'ris** [ NA ], orbicular muscle; a sphincter-like sheet of muscle that encircles an orifice such as the mouth or the palpebral fissures.

**m. orbicula'ris oc'uli** [ NA ], orbicular muscle of eye; m. orbicularis palpebrarum; consists of three portions: (*a*) **pars orbitalis**, or external portion, arises from frontal process of maxilla and nasal process of frontal bone, encircles aperture of orbit, and is inserted near origin; (*b*) **pars palpebralis**, or internal portion, arises from medial palpebral ligament, passes through each eyelid, and is inserted into lateral palpebral raphe; (*c*) **pars lacrimalis**, tensor tarsi or Horner's muscle, arises from posterior lacrimal crest and passes across lacrimal sac to join palpebral portion; *action*, closes eye, wrinkles forehead vertically; *nerve supply*, facial.

**m. orbicula'ris o'ris** [ NA ], orbicular muscle of mouth; m. sphincter oris; *origin*, by nasolabial band from septum of the nose, by superior incisive bundle from incisor fossa of maxilla, by inferior incisive bundle from lower jaw each side of symphysis; *insertion*, fibers surround mouth between skin and mucous membrane of lips and cheeks, and are blended with other muscles; *action*, closes lips; *nerve supply*, facial.

**m. orbicula'ris palpebra'rum**, m. orbicularis oculi.

**m. orbita'lis** [ NA ], orbital muscle; Müller's muscle; a rudimentary nonstriated muscle, crossing the infraorbital groove and sphenomaxillary fissure, intimately united with the periosteum of the orbit.

**m. orbitopalpebra'lis**, m. levator palpebrae superioris.

**musculi ossiculo'rum audi'tus** [ NA ], the m. stapedius and m. tensor tympani.

**m. palatoglos'sus** [ NA ], palatoglossus muscle; m. glossopalatinus; forms anterior pillar of fauces; *origin*, oral surface of soft palate; *insertion*, side of tongue; *nerve supply*, pharyngeal plexus; *action*, raises back of tongue and narrows fauces.

**m. palatopharyngeus** [ NA ], palatopharyngeal muscle; m. pharyngopalatinus; forms the posterior pillar of the fauces; *origin*, soft palate; *insertion*, posterior border of

m. **sacrococcyge'us posterior,** m. sacrococcygeus dorsalis.

m. **sacrococcyge'us ventralis** [ NA ], ventral sacrococcygeal muscle; an inconstant muscle on the pelvic surfaces of the sacrum and coccyx, the remains of a portion of the caudal musculature of lower animals.

m. **sacrolumba'lis,** m. iliocostalis lumborum.

m. **sacrospina'lis,** m. erector spinae.

m. **salpingopharynge'us** [ NA ], salpingopharyngeal muscle; *origin,* medial lamina of cartilaginous part of auditory tube; *insertion,* muscular layer of pharynx in association with m. palatopharyngeus; *nerve supply,* pharyngeal plexus; *action,* assists in elevating pharynx and opening auditory tube during swallowing.

m. **sarto'rius** [ NA ], tailor's muscle; *origin,* anterior superior spine of ilium; *insertion,* medial border of tuberosity of tibia; *nerve supply,* femoral; *action,* flexes thigh and leg, rotates leg medially and thigh laterally.

m. **scale'nus anterior** [ NA ], anterior scalene muscle; m. scalenus anticus; *origin,* anterior tubercles of transverse processes of 3d to 6th cervical vertebrae; *insertion,* scalene tubercle of 1st rib; *action,* raises 1st rib; *nerve supply,* cervical plexus.

m. **scalenus anticus,** m. scalenus anterior.

m. **scale'nus me'dius** [ NA ], medial scalene muscle; *origin,* costotransverse lamellae of transverse processes of 2nd to 6th cervical vertebrae; *insertion,* 1st rib posterior to subclavian artery; *action,* raises 1st rib; *nerve supply,* cervical plexus.

m. **scale'nus min'imus** [ NA ], smallest scalene muscle; an occasional independent muscular fasciculus between the scalenus anterior and medius, and having the same action and innervation as they.

m. **scale'nus posterior** [ NA ], m. scalenus posticus; posterior scalene muscle; *origin,* posterior tubercles of transverse processes of 4th to 6th cervical vertebrae; *insertion,* lateral surface of 2d rib; *action,* elevates 2d rib; *nerve supply,* cervical and brachial plexuses.

m. **scalenus posticus,** m. scalenus posterior.

m. **scanso'rius,** m. accessorius gluteus minimus; m. gluteus quartus; anterior fibers of the gluteus minimus (according to some anatomists the piriformis) which are sometimes distinct from the main portion of the muscle.

m. **semimembrano'sus** [ NA ], semimembranosus muscle; *origin,* tuberosity of ischium; *insertion,* medial condyle of tibia and by membrane to tibial collateral ligament of knee joint, popliteal fascia, and lateral condyle of femur; *nerve supply,* tibial; *action,* flexes leg and rotates it medially and makes capsular ligament of knee joint tense.

m. **semispina'lis** [ NA ], semispinal muscle; the superficial part of the transverospinal muscle; comprised of m. semispinalis capitis, m. semispinalis cervicis, and m. semispinalis thoracis.

m. **semispina'lis cap'itis** [ NA ], semispinal muscle of the head; m. complexus; *origin,* transverse processes of five or six upper thoracic and articular processes of four lower cervical vertebrae; *insertion,* occipital bone between superior and inferior nuchal lines; *action,* rotates head and draws it backward; *nerve supply,* dorsal branches of cervical.

m. **semispina'lis cervi'cis** [ NA ], semispinal muscle of the neck; m. semispinalis colli, continuous with m. semispinalis thoracis; *origin,* transverse processes of 2d to 5th thoracic vertebrae; *insertion,* spinous processes of axis and 3d to 5th cervical vertebrae; *action,* extends cervical spine; *nerve supply, dorsal* branches of cervical and thoracic.

m. **semispina'lis colli,** m. semispinalis cervicis.

m. **semispina'lis dorsi,** m. semispinalis thoracis.

m. **semispina'lis thoracis** [ NA ], semispinal muscle of the thorax; *origin,* transverse processes of 5th to 11th thoracic vertebrae; *insertion,* spinous processes of first four thoracic and 5th and 7th cervical vertebrae; *action,* extends vertebral column; *nerve supply,* dorsal branches of cervical and thoracic.

m. **semitendino'sus** [ NA ], semitendinous muscle; semitendinosus muscle; *origin,* ischial tuberosity; *insertion,* medial surface of upper fourth of shaft of tibia; *nerve supply,* tibial; *action,* extends thigh, flexes leg and rotates it medially.

m. **serra'tus anterior** [ NA ], anterior serratus muscle; m. serratus magnus; costoscapularis; *origin,* from center of lateral aspect of first 8 to 9 ribs; *insertion,* superior and inferior angles and intervening medial margin of scapula; *action,* rotates scapula and pulls it forward, elevates ribs; *nerve supply,* long thoracic from brachial plexus.

m. **serra'tus magnus,** m. serratus anterior.

m. **serra'tus posterior inferior** [ NA ], inferior posterior serratus muscle; *origin,* with latissimus dorsi, from spinous processes of two lower thoracic and two upper lumbar vertebrae; *insertion,* into lower borders of last four ribs; *action,* draws lower ribs backward and downward; *nerve supply,* 9th to 12th intercostal.

m. **serra'tus posterior superior** [ NA ], superior posterior serratus muscle; *origin,* from spinous processes of two lower cervical and two upper thoracic vertebrae; *insertion,* into lateral side of angles of 2d to 5th ribs; *nerve supply,* 1st to 4th intercostals.

m. **skel'eti** [ NA ], skeletal muscle; a striated muscle connected at either or both extremities with the bony framework of the body; it may be an appendicular or an axial muscle. For histologic description, see skeletal *muscle.*

m. **sol'eus** [ NA ], soleus muscle; *origin,* posterior surface of head and upper third of shaft of fibula, oblique line and middle third of medial margin of tibia, and a tendinous arch passing between tibia and fibula over the popliteal vessels; *insertion,* with gastrocnemius by tendo calcaneus (Achillis) into tuberosity of calcaneus; *nerve supply,* tibial; *action,* plantar flexion of foot.

m. **sphenosal'pingostaphyli'nus,** m. tensor veli palatini.

m. **sphincter** [ NA ], sphincter muscle; a muscle that encircles a duct, tube or orifice in such a way that its contraction constricts the lumen or orifice. It is the closing component of a pylorus (the outer component is the m. dilator).

m. **sphincter ampullae hepatopancreat'icae** [ NA ], Glisson's sphincter; Oddi's sphincter; the smooth muscle sphincter of the hepatopancreatic ampulla.

m. **sphincter ani externus** [ NA ], external sphincter muscle of the anus; a fusiform ring of striated muscular fibers surrounding the anus, attached posteriorly to the coccyx and anteriorly to the central tendon of the perineum; it is subdivided into a **pars subcutanea, pars superficialis,** and **pars profunda.**

m. **sphincter ani internus** [ NA ], internal sphincter muscle of the anus; a smooth muscle ring, formed by an increase of the circular fibers of the rectum, situated at the upper end of the anal canal.

m. **sphincter duc'tus choledo'chi** [ NA ], choledochal sphincter; Boyden's sphincter; sphincter muscle of the common bile duct; smooth muscle sphincter at the terminal end of the common bile duct.

m. **sphincter duc'tus pancrea'tici,** sphincter muscle of the pancreatic duct; smooth muscle sphincter of the main pancreatic duct within the duodenal papilla.

m. **sphincter oris,** m. orbicularis oris.

m. **sphincter pupil'lae** [ NA ], sphincter muscle of the pupil; a ring of smooth muscle fibers surrounding the pupillary border of the iris.

m. **sphincter pylo'ri** [ NA ], sphincter muscle of the pylorus; pyloric sphincter; a thickening of the circular layer of the gastric musculature encircling the gastroduodenal junction.

m. **sphincter ure'thrae** [ NA ], m. compressor urethrae; m. constrictor urethrae; m. sphincter urethrae membranaceae; sphincter muscle of the urethra; Wilson's muscle; *origin,* ramus of pubis; *insertion,* with fellow in median raphe behind and in front of urethra; *nerve supply,* pudendal; *action,* constricts membranous urethra.

m. **sphincter urethrae membranaceae,** m. sphincter urethrae.

m. **sphincter vagi'nae,** m. bulbospongiosus.

m. **sphincter vesi'cae,** sphincter muscle of the urinary bladder; anulus urethralis; traditionally recognized as a vesical sphincter made up of a thickening of the middle muscular layer of the bladder around the urethral opening; although no anular sphincter exists, a sphincteric action is attributed to the bundle of muscles in the region of the neck (of the urinary bladder).

m. **spina'lis** [ NA ], spinal muscle; the medial component of the erector spinae muscle; it is comprised of m. spinalis capitis, m. spinalis cervicis, and m. spinalis thoracis.

**m. spina'lis cap'itis** [ NA ], biventer cervicis; spinal muscle of head; an inconstant extension of spinalis cervicis to the occipital bone, sometimes fusing with semispinalis capitis.

**m. spina'lis cervi'cis** [ NA ], spinal muscle of the neck; m. spinalis colli; inconstant or rudimentary; *origin*, spinous processes of 6th and 7th cervical; *insertion*, spinous processes of axis and 3d cervical vertebra; *action*, extends cervical spine; *nerve supply*, dorsal branches of cervical.

**m. spina'lis colli**, m. spinalis cervicis.

**m. spina'lis dorsi**, m. spinalis thoracis.

**m. spina'lis thoracis** [ NA ], m. spinalis dorsi; spinal muscle of the thorax; *origin*, spinous processes of upper lumbar and two lower thoracic vertebrae; *insertion*, spinous processes of middle and upper thoracic vertebrae; *action*, supports and extends vertebral column; *nerve supply*, dorsal branches of thoracic and upper lumbar.

**m. sple'nius cap'itis** [ NA ], splenius muscle of the head; *origin*, from spinous processes of last four cervical and first three thoracic vertebrae; *insertion*, into outer half of superior nuchal line of occipital and mastoid process; *action*, rotates head, the two together draw head backward; *nerve supply*, dorsal branches 2d to 8th cervical.

**m. sple'nius cervi'cis** [ NA ], splenius muscle of the neck; m. splenius colli; *origin*, from spinous processes of 3d to 5th (or 4th to 6th) cervical vertebrae; *insertion*, posterior tubercles of transverse processes of 1st and 2d (sometimes 3d) cervical vertebrae; *action*, rotates neck, both together extend neck; *nerve supply*, dorsal branches of upper cervical.

**m. sple'nius colli**, m. splenius cervicis.

**m. stape'dius** [ NA ], stapedius; stapedius muscle; *origin*, internal walls of pyramidal eminence in tympanic cavity; *insertion*, neck of the stapes; *action*, draws head of stapes backward; *nerve supply*, facial.

**m. sterna'lis** [ NA ], sternal muscle; an inconstant muscle, running parallel to the sternum across the costosternal origin of the pectoralis major, and usually connected with the sternocleidomastoid and rectus muscles and the pectoralis major.

**m. sternochon'droscapula'ris**, sternochondroscapular muscle; an occasional muscle arising from the manubrium sterni and first costal cartilage and passing outward and backward to be inserted into the upper border of the scapula.

**m. sternoclavicula'ris**, sternoclavicular muscle; an occasional muscle, a slip from the subclavius muscle, passing from the upper part of the sternum to the clavicle beneath the pectoralis major.

**m. ster'noclei'domastoid'eus** [ NA ], sternocleidomastoid muscle; *origin*, by two heads from anterior surface of manubrium sterni and sternal end of clavicle; *insertion*, mastoid process and lateral half of superior nuchal line of occipital bone; *action*, turns head obliquely to opposite side; when acting together, flex the neck and extend the head; *nerve supply*, accessory.

**m. sternofascia'lis**, an occasional muscular slip arising from the manubrium sterni and inserted into the fascia of the neck.

**m. sternohyoid'eus** [ NA ], sternohyoid muscle; *origin*, posterior surface of manubrium sterni and 1st costal cartilage; *insertion*, body of hyoid bone; *action*, depresses hyoid bone; *nerve supply*, upper cervical through ansa cervicalis.

**m. sternothyroid'eus** [ NA ], sternothyroid muscle; *origin*, posterior surface of manubrium sterni and 1st or 2d costal cartilage; *insertion*, oblique line of thyroid cartilage; *action*, depresses larynx; *nerve supply*, upper cervical through the ansa hypoglossi.

**m. styloauricula'ris**, styloauricular muscle; an occasional small muscle extending from the root of the styloid process to the cartilage of the meatus of the ear.

**m. styloglos'sus** [ NA ], styloglossus muscle; *origin*, lower end of styloid process; *insertion*, side and under surface of tongue; *nerve supply*, hypoglossal; *action*, retracts tongue.

**m. stylohyoid'eus** [ NA ], stylohyoid muscle; *origin*, styloid process of temporal bone; *insertion*, hyoid bone by two slips on either side of central tendon of digastric; *action*, elevates hyoid bone; *nerve supply*, facial.

**m. stylolarynge'us**, that part of the stylopharyngeus which is inserted into the thyroid cartilage.

**m. stylopharynge'us** [ NA ], stylopharyngeal muscle; *origin*, root of styloid process; *insertion*, thyroid cartilage and wall of pharynx; *nerve supply*, glossopharyngeal; *action*, elevates pharynx and larynx.

**m. subcla'vius** [ NA ], subclavian muscle; *origin*, 1st costal cartilage; *insertion*, inferior surface of acromial end of clavicle; *action*, fixes clavicle or elevates 1st rib; *nerve supply*, subclavian from brachial plexus.

**m. subcosta'lis**, pl. **subcosta'les** [ NA ], subcostal muscle; m. infracostalis; one of a number of inconstant muscles having the same direction as the intercostales interni, but passing deep to one or more ribs.

**m. subcuta'neus colli**, platysma.

**m. subscapula'ris** [ NA ], subscapular muscle; *origin*, subscapular fossa; *insertion*, lesser tuberosity of humerus; *nerve supply*, upper and lower subscapular from 5th and 6th cervical; *action*, rotates arm medially.

**m. supina'tor** [ NA ], supinator muscle; m. supinator radii brevis; *origin*, lateral epicondyle of humerus and supinator ridge of ulna; *insertion*, anterior and lateral surface of radius; *nerve supply*, radial (posterior interosseous); *action*, supinates the forearm.

**m. supina'tor longus**, m. brachioradialis.

**m. supraclavicula'ris**, supraclavicular muscle; an anomalous muscular slip running from the upper edge of the manubrium sterni outward to about the middle of the upper surface of the clavicle.

**musculi suprahyoi'dei** [ NA ], suprahyoid muscles; the group of muscles attached to the upper part of the hyoid bone including the digastricus, stylohyoideus, mylohyoideus, and geniohyoideus.

**m. supraspina'lis**, one of a number of muscular bands passing between the tips of the spinous processes of the cervical vertebrae.

**m. supraspina'tus** [ NA ], supraspinous muscle; *origin*, supraspinous fossa of scapula; *insertion*, great tuberosity of humerus; *nerve supply*, suprascapular from 5th and 6th cervical; *action*, abducts arm.

**m. suspenso'rius duode'ni** [ NA ], suspensory muscle of the duodenum; muscle of Treitz; ligament of Treitz; a broad flat band of smooth muscle and fibrous tissue attached to the right crus of the diaphragm and to the duodenum at its junction with the jejunum.

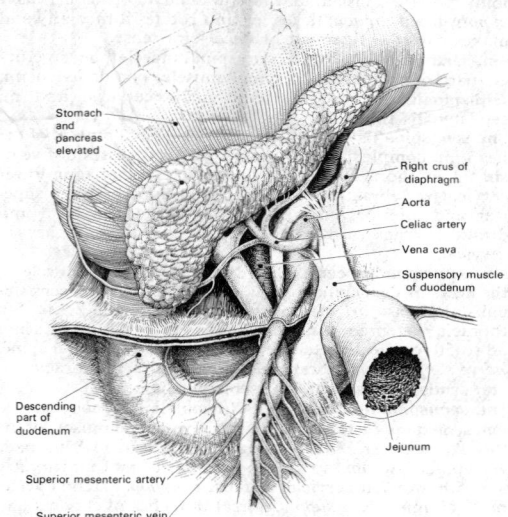

Stomach and pancreas elevated

Right crus of diaphragm

Aorta

Celiac artery

Vena cava

Suspensory muscle of duodenum

Descending part of duodenum

Jejunum

Superior mesenteric artery

Superior mesenteric vein

**Suspensory Muscle of Duodenum (Ligament or Muscle of Treitz)**

**m. tarsalis inferior** [ NA ], inferior tarsal muscle; poorly developed smooth muscle in the lower eyelid that acts to widen the palpebral fissure.

m. **tarsalis superior** [ NA ], superior tarsal muscle; a well defined layer of smooth muscle that extends from the aponeurosis of the m. levator palpebrae superioris to the superior tarsus; it is innervated by sympathetic nerves and acts to hold the upper lid in an elevated position.

m. **tempora'lis** [ NA ], temporal muscle; *origin*, temporal fossa; *insertion*, anterior border of ramus and apex of coronoid process of mandible; *action*, closes jaw; *nerve supply*, deep temporal branches of third division of trigeminal.

m. **temporoparieta'lis** [ NA ], temporoparietal muscle; the part of m. epicranius that arises from the lateral part of the galea aponeurotica and inserts in the cartilage of the auricle. See also m. auricularis anterior and m. auricularis superior.

m. **tensor fasciae latae** [ NA ], tensor muscle of the fascia lata; m. tensor fasciae femoris; *origin*, anterior superior spine and adjacent lateral surface of the ilium; *insertion*, iliotibial band of fascia lata; *nerve supply*, superior gluteal; *action*, tenses fascia lata; flexes, abducts and medially rotates thigh.

m. **tensor pala'ti**, m. tensor veli palatini.

m. **tensor tarsi**, m. orbicularis oculi pars lacrimalis.

m. **tensor tym'pani** [ NA ], tensor muscle of the tympanic membrane; *origin*, the cartilaginous part of the auditory (Eustachian) tube and the walls of its canal just above the bony portion of the auditory tube; *insertion*, handle of the malleus; *nerve supply*, branches of trigeminal through the otic ganglion; *action*, draws the handle of the malleus medialward and tenses the tympanic membrane.

m. **tensor veli palati'ni** [ NA ], tensor muscle of the velum palatini; m. tensor palati; m. sphenosalpingo-staphylinus; dilator tubae; *origin*, scaphoid fossa of sphenoid, and wall of cartilaginous auditory (Eustachian) tube; *insertion*, posterior border of hard palate and aponeurosis of soft palate; *nerve supply*, branches of trigeminal nerve through the otic ganglion; *action*, tenses the soft palate; opens auditory tube.

m. **teres major** [ NA ], teres major muscle; *origin*, inferior angle and lower third of border of scapula; *insertion*, medial border of intertubercular groove of humerus; *nerve supply*, lower subscapular from 5th and 6th cervical; *action*, adducts and extends arm and rotates it medially.

m. **teres minor** [ NA ], teres minor muscle; *origin*, upper two-thirds of the lateral border of scapula; *insertion*, lower facet of great tuberosity of humerus; *nerve supply*, axillary from 5th and 6th cervical; *action*, adducts arm and rotates it laterally.

m. **tetragonus**, platysma.

**musculi thora'cis** [ NA ], muscles of the thorax; the muscles attaching to the rib cage including the pectoral muscles, serratus anterior, subclavius, levator muscles, intercostal muscles, transverse thoracic muscle, subcostal muscles and diaphragm.

m. **thyroarytenoid'eus** [ NA ], thyroarytenoid muscle; m. thyroarytenoideus externus; *origin*, inner surface of thyroid cartilage; *insertion*, muscular process and outer surface of arytenoid; *nerve supply*, recurrent laryngeal; *action*, shortens vocal cords.

m. **thyroarytenoid'eus externus**, m. thyroarytenoideus.

m. **thyroarytenoid'eus internus**, m. vocalis.

m. **thyroepiglot'ticus** [ NA ], thyroepiglottic or thyroepiglottidean muscle; depressor muscle of the epiglottis; *origin*, inner surface of thyroid cartilage in common with m. thyroarytenoideus; *insertion*, aryepiglottic fold and margin of epiglottis; *nerve supply*, recurrent laryngeal; *action*, depresses base of epiglottis.

m. **thyrohyoid'eus** [ NA ], thyrohyoid muscle; apparently a continuation of the sternothyroid; *origin*, oblique line of thyroid cartilage; *insertion*, body of hyoid bone; *action*, approximates hyoid bone to the larynx; *nerve supply*, upper cervical passing with hypoglossal.

m. **thyropharynge'us**, see m. constrictor pharyngis inferior pars thyropharyngea.

m. **tibia'lis anterior** [ NA ], anterior tibial muscle; m. tibialis anticus; *origin*, upper two-thirds of lateral surface of tibia, interosseous membrane, and intermuscular septum; *insertion*, medial cuneiform and base of first metatarsal; *nerve supply*, deep peroneal; *action*, dorsal flexion and inversion of foot.

m. **tibia'lis gra'cilis**, m. plantaris.

m. **tibia'lis posterior** [ NA ], posterior tibial muscle; m. tibialis posticus; *origin*, soleal line and posterior surface of tibia, the head and shaft of the fibula between the medial crest and interosseous border, and the posterior surface of interosseous membrane; *insertion*, navicular, three cuneiform, cuboid, and 2nd, 3rd, and 4th metatarsal bones; *nerve supply*, tibial; *action*, produces plantar flexion and inversion of foot.

m. **tibia'lis secun'dus**, second tibial muscle; an inconstant muscle, of small size, arising from the back of the tibia and inserted into the articular capsule of the ankle joint.

m. **tibiofascia'lis anterior** or **anti'cus**, separate fibers of the tibialis anterior inserted into the fascia of the dorsum of the foot.

m. **trachea'lis** [ NA ], the band of smooth muscular fibers in the fibrous membrane connecting posteriorly the ends of the tracheal rings.

m. **tracheloclavicula'ris**, tracheloclavicular muscle; an anomalous muscle occasionally arising from the cervical vertebrae and inserted into the lateral end of the clavicle.

m. **trachelomastoid'eus**, m. longissimus capitis.

m. **trag'icus** [ NA ], muscle of the tragus; a band of vertical muscular fibers on the outer surface of the tragus of the ear.

m. **transversa'lis abdom'inis**, m. transversus abdominis.

m. **transversa'lis cap'itis**, m. longissimus capitis.

m. **transversa'lis cervi'cis** or **colli**, m. longissimus cervicis.

m. **transversa'lis nasi**, see m. nasalis pars transversa.

m. **transversospina'lis** [ NA ], the group of muscles that originate from transverse processes of vertebrae and pass to spinous processes of higher vertebrae; they act as rotators and include the semispinalis (capitis, cervicis, thoracis), multifidus, and rotatores (cervicis, thoracis, lumborum).

m. **transver'sus abdom'inis** [ NA ], transverse muscle of the abdomen; m. transversalis abdominis; *origin*, 7th to 12th costal cartilages, lumbar fascia, iliac crest, and inguinal (Poupart's) ligament; *insertion*, xiphoid cartilage and linea alba and, through falx inguinalis, pubic tubercle and pecten; *action*, compresses abdominal contents; *nerve supply*, lower thoracic.

m. **transver'sus auric'ulae** [ NA ], transverse muscle of the auricle; a band of sparse muscular fibers on the cranial surface of the auricle, extending from the eminence of the concha to the eminence of the scapha.

m. **transver'sus linguae** [ NA ], transverse muscle of the tongue; an intrinsic muscle of the tongue, the fibers of which arise from the septum and radiate to the dorsum and sides.

m. **transver'sus menti** [ NA ], transverse muscle of the chin; inconstant fibers of the m. depresser anguli oris which continue into the neck and cross to the opposite side inferior to the chin.

m. **transver'sus nuchae** [ NA ], transverse muscle of the nape; an occasional muscle passing between the tendons of the trapezius and sternocleidomastoid, possibly a fasciculus of the auricularis posterior.

m. **transver'sus perine'i profun'dus** [ NA ], deep transverse muscle of the perineum; *origin*, ramus of ischium; *insertion*, with its fellow in a median raphe; *nerve supply*, pudendal; *action*, assists sphincter urethrae.

m. **transver'sus perine'i superficia'lis** [ NA ], superficial transverse muscle of the perineum; an inconstant muscle; *origin*, ramus of ischium; *insertion*, central tendon of perineum; *nerve supply*, pudendal; *action*, draws back and fixes the central tendon of the perineum.

m. **transver'sus thora'cis** [ NA ], transverse muscle of thorax; triangularis sterni; *origin*, dorsal surface of xiphoid cartilage and lower portion of dorsal surface of body of sternum; *insertion*, 2nd to 6th costal cartilages; *action*, narrows chest; *nerve supply*, intercostal.

m. **trape'zius** [ NA ], trapezius muscle; *origin*, medial third of superior nuchal line of the occipital bone, external occipital protuberance, ligamentum nuchae, spinous processes of 7th cervical and the thoracic vertebrae and corresponding supraspinous ligaments; *insertion*, lateral third of posterior surface of clavicle, medial side of acromion, and upper border of the spine of the scapula;

*action*, draws head to one side or backward, rotates scapula; *nerve supply*, accessory and cervical plexus.

**m. triangularis,** m. depressor anguli oris.

**m. triangula′ris la′bii inferior′is,** m. depressor anguli oris.

**m. triangula′ris la′bii superior′is,** m. levator anguli oris.

**m. triangula′ris sterni,** m. transversus thoracis.

**m. triceps brachii** [ NA ], triceps muscle of the arm; *origin*, long or scapular head (caput longum) lateral border of scapula below glenoid fossa, lateral head (caput laterale) lateral and posterior surface of humerus below greater tubercle, medial head (caput mediale) posterior surface of humerus below radial groove; *insertion*, olecranon of ulna; *nerve supply*, radial; *action*, extends forearm.

**m. triceps surae** [ NA ], triceps of the calf, the gastrocnemius and soleus considered as one muscle.

**m. triti′ceoglos′sus,** Bochdalek's muscle; an occasional thin band of muscular fibers passing between the root of the tongue and the cartilago triticea.

**m. unipenna′tus** [ NA ], unipennate muscle; a muscle with a lateral tendon to which the fibers are attached obliquely, like one half of a feather.

**m. u′vulae** [ NA ], muscle of the uvula; azygos uvulae; *origin*, posterior nasal spine; *insertion*, forms chief bulk of the uvula; *nerve supply*, pharyngeal plexus; *action*, raises the uvula.

**m. vastus exter′nus,** m. vastus lateralis.

**m. vastus interme′dius** [ NA ], intermediate great muscle; crureus; *origin*, upper three-fourths of anterior surface of shaft of femur; *insertion*, tibial tuberosity by way of common tendon of quadriceps femoris and ligamentum patellae; *action*, extends leg; *nerve supply*, femoral.

**m. vastus inter′nus,** m. vastus medialis.

**m. vastus latera′lis** [ NA ], lateral great muscle; m. vastus externus; *origin*, lateral lip of linea aspera as far as great trochanter; *insertion*, tibial tuberosity by way of common tendon of quadriceps femoris and ligamentum patellae; *action*, extends leg; *nerve supply*, femoral.

**m. vastus media′lis** [ NA ], medial great muscle; m. vastus internus; *origin*, medial lip of linea aspera; *insertion*, tibial tuberosity by way of common tendon of quadriceps femoris and ligamentum patellae; *action*, extends leg; *nerve supply*, femoral.

**m. ventricula′ris,** fibers of the thyroarytenoid which pass into the false vocal cord.

**m. vertica′lis linguae** [ NA ], vertical muscle of the tongue; an intrinsic muscle of the tongue, consisting of fibers that pass from the aponeurosis of the dorsum to the aponeurosis of the inferior surface.

**m. voca′lis** [ NA ], vocal muscle; m. thyroarytenoideus internus; *origin*, depression between the two laminae of thyroid cartilage; *insertion*, vocal process of arytenoid; *nerve supply*, recurrent laryngeal; *action*, shortens and relaxes vocal cords.

**m. zygomat′icus,** m. zygomaticus major.

**m. zygomat′icus major** [ NA ], greater zygomatic muscle; m. zygomaticus; *origin*, zygomatic bone anterior to temporozygomatic suture; *insertion*, muscles at angle of mouth; *action*, draws upper lip upward and laterally; *nerve supply*, facial.

**m. zygomat′icus minor** [ NA ], lesser zygomatic muscle; caput zygomaticum quadrati labii superioris; *origin*, zygomatic bone posterior to zygomaticomaxillary suture; *insertion*, orbicularis oris of upper lip; *action*, draws upper lip upward and outward; *nerve supply*, facial.

---

**musenna** (mu-sen′ah). The bark of *Albizzia anthelmintica* (family Leguminoseae), a tree of Abyssinia; teniafuge.

**mush′bite.** A maxillomandibular record made by introducing a mass of soft wax into the patient's mouth and instructing the patient to bite into it to the desired degree; not a generally accepted procedure.

**mu′sicother′apy.** Melodiotherapy; treatment of mental disorders by means of music.

**musk.** Moschus; the dried secretion from the preputial follicles of *Moschus moschiferus* (family Moschidae), the musk deer, a native of Tibet and central Asia; contains muskone, an odorous agent used in perfumery.

**mus′kone.** Muscone; 3-methylcyclopentadecanone; a 15-carbon cyclic ketone, resembling civetone; the odoriferous component of musk.

**Musset** (mü-sa′), L. C. Alfred de, French poet, 1810–1857; first person in whom M.'s sign was studied. See M.'s *sign*.

**mussitation** (mus′ĭ-ta′shun) [ L. *mussito*, to murmur constantly, fr. *musso*, pp. *-atus*, to mutter ]. Movements of the lips as if speaking, but without sound; observed in delirium and in semicoma.

**Mussy.** See Guéneau de Mussy.

**must** [ L. *mustum*, new wine, ntr. of *mustus*, fresh, sc. *vinum*, wine ]. Unfermented juice of the grape or other fruits.

**mus′tard** [ O. Fr. *moustarde*, fr. L. *mustum*, must ]. The dried ripe seeds of *Brassica alba* (family Cruciferae), white m. and black m.; see *Sinapis*.

**black m.,** the dried ripe seed of *Brassica* (*Sinapis*) *nigra* or of *B. juncea;* it is the source of allyl isothiocyanate; contains sinigrin (potassium myronate); myrosin; sinapine sulfocyanate; erucic, behenic, and synapolic acids; and fixed oil; prompt emetic, rubefacient, and condiment.

**m. chlorohydrin,** hemisulfur m.

**m. gas,** di(2-chloroethyl) sulfide; dichlorodiethyl sulfide; yperite; vesicating gas; $S(CH_2CH_2Cl)_2$. It was introduced as a poison gas in World War I; contact with the skin causes vesication and sloughing, and inhalation may result in bronchopneumonia. It is the progenitor of the so-called nitrogen m.'s (*q.v.*) used in cancer chemotherapy.

**hemisulfur m.,** mustard chlorohydrin; 2-(2-chloroethylthio)ethanol; antineoplastic agent.

**nitrogen m.'s,** compounds of the general formula $R—N(CH_2CH_2Cl)$; the prototype is HN2, nitrogen mustard, in which R is $CH_3$. Also some have been used therapeutically for their destructive action upon lymphoid tissue in lymphosarcoma, leukemia, Hodgkin's disease, and certain other cancers. See also mechlorethamine hydrochloride.

**m. oils,** term applied to organic isothiocyanates (*e.g.,* benzyl mustard oil) in general, but more specifically to allyl isothiocyanate, *q.v.* They are metabolically convertible to thiocyanates and may thus lead to goiter.

**m. oil, expressed,** the fixed oil expressed from the seeds of *Brassica alba* and *B. nigra;* it contains the glycerides of oleic, arachidic, and other fatty acids; used as salad oil and in the manufacture of oleomargarine.

**m. oil, volatile,** allyl isothiocyanate.

**uracil m.,** see under uracil.

**white m.,** the ripe seeds of *Brassica* (*Sinapsis*) *alba;* less pungent than black m., but with the same constituents and uses.

**mus′tine hydrochloride** (BP). Mechlorethamine hydrochloride.

**mu′tacism.** Mytacism.

**mutagen** (mu′tă-jen) [ L. *muto*, to change, + G. suffix *-gen*, producing ]. Mutagenic agent; any agent that causes the production of a mutation, *e.g.,* radioactive substances, x-rays, or certain chemical substances.

**chemical m.,** any chemical substance that causes mutation, *e.g.,* acridines, alkylating agents, base analogues, nitrous acid, etc.

**frame-shift m.,** a m. such as an acridine derivative that causes a reading frame-shift mutation, *q.v.*

**mu′tagen′esis.** The production of a mutation.

**mu′tagen′ic.** Having the power to cause mutations.

**mu′tant.** An individual possessing one or more genes that have undergone mutation.

**amber m.,** a fanciful term for one of the several known nonsense *triplets*.

**ochre m.,** a term for one of the several known nonsense *triplets*.

**mu′taro′tase.** Aldose mutarotase.

**mu′tarota′tion.** The process of changing specific rotation; a solution of D-glucose, for example, recrystallized from its solution in acetic acid and freshly dissolved in water, gives a rotation of $[\alpha]_D^{20} = +112.2°$, but when recrystallized from a boiling aqueous solution it shows an initial rotation of $[\alpha]_D^{20} = +18.7°$; either solution upon standing slowly changes its specific rotation to a value of $[\alpha]_D^{20} = +52.7°$.

**mu'tase.** Any enzyme that catalyze the apparent migration of groups within one molecule; sometimes the transfer is from one molecule to another, as for phosphoglucomutase and phosphoglyceromutase (both are phosphotransferases). True mutases include, *e.g.*, phosphoglycerate phosphomutase.

**mutation** (mu-ta'shun) [ L. *muto*, pp. *-atus*, to change ]. 1. A change in the character of a gene that is perpetuated in subsequent divisions of the cell in which it occurs; a change in the sequence of base pairs in the chromosomal DNA molecule. 2. De Vries' term for the sudden production of a species, as distinguished from variation.

   **frame-shift m.,** reading frame-shift m.

   **induced m.,** a m. caused by the application of an external stimulus, *e.g.*, irradiation to the germ cells.

   **mis'sense m.** [ L. *mitto*, to send away ], a m. in which a base-pair substitution results in a condon that causes insertion of a different amino acid into the growing polypeptide chain, giving rise to an altered protein.

   **natural m.,** a m. occurring spontaneously, and not due to an artificial external stimulus; see induced m.

   **nonsense m.,** a m. in which a base-pair substitution results in a codon that cannot be "translated," causing cessation of growth of the polypeptide chain.

   **point m.,** a m. that involves a single nucleotide; it may consist of loss of a nucleotide, substitution of one nucleotide for another, or the insertion of an additional nucleotide.

   **reading frame-shift m.,** frame-shift m.; a m. that results from a nucleotide insertion into, or deletion from, the normal DNA sequence; because the exact sequence in which nucleotides occur (not specific nucleotides) is the determining factor in the formation of triplets (codons), the inserted or deleted nucleotide results in a shift from the normal in each group of three nucleotides subsequent to the insertion or deletion.

   **somat'ic m.,** a m. occurring in the general body cells (as opposed to the germ cells).

   **suppressor m.,** a second m. which occurs at a site on the chromosome different from that of the first m., and which cancels the effect of the first.

   **transition m.,** a point m. involving substitution of one base pair for another, *i.e.*, replacement of one purine for another and of one pyrimidine for another pyrimidine without change in the purine-pyrimidine orientation.

   **transversion m.,** a point m. involving base substitution in which the orientation of purine and pyrimidine is reversed, in contradistinction to transition m.

**mute** [ L. *mutus* ]. 1. Dumb. 2. A person who has not the faculty of speech.

**mutilation** (mu'tĭ-la'shun) [ L. *mutilatio*, fr. *mutilo*, pp. *-atus*, to maim ]. 1. Maiming; the removal or destruction of any conspicuous or essential part of the body. 2. The condition of being mutilated; the loss of an important part.

**mu'tism** [ L. *mutus*, mute ]. Dumbness; speechlessness. 1. The state of being silent. 2. Organic or functional absence of the faculty of speech.

   **akinet'ic m.,** a syndrome characterized by m., loss of voluntary and emotional movement, and apparent loss of emotional feeling; related to lesions of the upper brain stem.

**mu'ton.** In genetics, the smallest unit of a chromosome in which alteration can be effective in causing a mutation.

**mutualism** (mu'tu-al-izm). Symbiosis.

**mutualist** (mu'tu-al-ist) [ L. *mutuus*, in return, mutual ]. Symbion.

**muzzle** (muz'l). The snout of an animal; the prominent nose and mouth.

**mv.** Abbreviation of millivolt.

**MVV.** Abbreviation for maximum voluntary *ventilation*.

**MW.** Abbreviation for molecular *weight*.

**my.** Abbreviation of myopia.

**Myà** (me-ah'), Giuseppe, Italian physician, 1857–1911. See M.'s *disease*.

**myalgia** (mi-al'jĭ-ah) [ G. *mys*, muscle, + *algos*, pain ]. Myodynia; myosalgia; muscular pain.

   **epidemic m.,** epidemic *pleurodynia*.

   **m. ther'mica,** heat *cramps*.

**my'asthe'nia** [ G. *mys*, muscle, + *astheneia*, weakness ]. Muscular weakness.

   **m. angiosclerot'ica,** intermittent *claudication*.

   **m. cordis,** amyocardia.

   **m. gravis,** Goldflam disease; Hoppe-Goldflam disease; asthenic bulbar or bulbospinal paralysis; a chronic progressive muscular weakness, beginning usually in the face and throat, unaccompanied by atrophy; due to a defect in myoneural conduction.

**my'asthen'ic.** Relating to myasthenia.

**myatonia, myatony** (mi-at-o'nĭ-ah, mi-at'o-nĭ) [ G. *mys*, muscle, + *a* priv. + *tonos*, tone ]. Amyotonia; abnormal extensibility of a muscle.

   **m. congenita,** *amyotonia* congenita.

**myatrophy** (mi-at'ro-fĭ). Myoatrophy.

**my'carose.** 2,6-Dideoxy-3-*C*-methyl*ribo*hexose; a methylated dideoxy sugar found as part of the spiramycins, carbomycins, and erythromycins. The 3-*O*-methyl derivative is called cladinose.

**mycelia** (mi-se'lĭ-ah). Plural of mycelium.

**myce'lian.** Pertaining to mycelium.

**mycelioid** (mi-se'lĭ-oyd) [ mycelium + G. *eidos*, resemblance ]. Resembling a mycelium.

**mycelium,** pl. **myce'lia** (mi-se'lĭ-um) [ G. *mykēs*, fungus, + *hēlos*, nail, wart, excrescence on animal or plant ]. The mat or complex group of protoplasmic units, or the entangled mass of tubelike or filamentous structures, *i.e.*, hyphae, that represents the "body" of plant forms classified as Eumycetes (including Phycomycetes, Ascomycetes, Fungi Imperfecti, and Basidiomycetes).

   **aerial m.,** the portion of m. that grows upward or outward from the surface of the substrate, and from which propagative spores develop in or on characteristic structures that are distinctive for various generic groups.

   **coenocytic m.,** nonseptate m.

   **nonseptate m.,** coenocytic m.; one in which there are no septa, or "cross-walls," in the hyphae; inasmuch as the latter are not divided into numerous individual cells, the multinucleated protoplasm may flow throughout the tubelike structures.

   **reproductive m.,** an aerial m. from which various types of reproductive spores develop.

   **septate m.,** one in which septa, or "cross-walls," divide the hyphae into numerous uninucleated or multinucleated cells.

   **substrate m.,** the network of hyphae growing within a solid medium.

   **vegetative m.,** the portion of m. that grows downward or inward, thereby penetrating the substrate and providing the means by which nutriments are absorbed.

**mycet-, myceto-** [ G. *mykēs*, fungus ]. Combining forms relating to fungus. See also myco-.

**my'cete** [ G. *mykēs*, fungus ]. A fungus.

**mycethemia** (mi'se-the'mĭ-ah) [ G. *mykēs*, fungus, + *haima*, blood ]. Mycohemia; the presence of some form of fungus in the circulating blood.

**mycetism, mycetis'mus** (mi'se-tizm, -tiz'mus) [ G. *mykēs*, fungus ]. Mushroom poisoning; muscarinism.

   **m. cholifor'mis,** due to a poisonous principle in *Amanita phalloides;* the symptoms are severe abdominal pains, vomiting, diarrhea with the passage of blood and mucus, and collapse.

   **m. nervo'sa,** caused by muscarine present in *Amanita muscaria;* the symptoms are mainly those resembling the stimulation of cholinergic nerve endings, *e.g.*, cardiac slowing, salivation, lacrimation, sweating, vomiting, diarrhea, and cardiovascular collapse; atropine is used as an antidote.

**mycetogenetic, mycetogenic** (mi-se'to-jĕ-net'ik, -jen'ik, mi'se-to-) [ G. *mykēs*, fungus, + *gennētos*, begotten ]. Mycetogenous; caused by fungi.

**mycetogenous** (mi'se-toj'ĕ-nus). Mycetogenetic.

**myceto'ma.** 1. A chronic infection usually involving the feet (and rarely the hands and other sites), and characterized by the formation of tumefactions and multiple draining sinuses. The exudate contains granules of variable colors, *e.g.*, yellow, white, red, brown, or black. M. is caused by two principal groups of microorganisms: (1) actinomycetes, including *Nocardia madurae, Streptomyces* *somaliensis, Streptomyces (Nocardia) pelletieri, N. brasiliensis,* and *N. asteroides;* and (2) true fungi, including *Madurella mycetomi, M. grisea, Phialophora jeanselmei, Allescheria boydii,* and *Cephalosporium* species. Actinomycotic m. is caused by actinomycetes; maduromycosis is caused by true fungi. 2. Any tumor produced by filamentous fungi.

**Bouffardi's black m.,** maduromycosis.

**Bouffardi's white m.,** a form common in India and found occasionally in Somaliland; caused by the organism *Streptomyces (Indiella) somaliensis.* In this variety, the muscles, tendons, and bones of the foot are destroyed by the disease process. Numerous draining sinuses discharge yellowish grains, clustered like fish roe.

**Brumpt's white m.,** due to *Allescheria boydii* (formerly called *Monosporium apiospermum* or *Indiella manson)* occurs in India; small, white, hard granules are discharged through the draining sinuses.

**Carter's black m.,** caused by *Madurella mycetomi.* Prevalent in Italy, parts of Africa, and India. The grains are dark brown or black.

**Nicolle's white m.,** caused by a species of aspergillus. Relatively large granules, about the size of a pea, are produced. Infection occurs from barley grain.

**Raynier's white m.,** caused by *Indiella reynieri.*

**Vincent's white m.,** caused by *Nocardia madurae* (formerly called *Actinomyces madurae* or *Discomyces madurae*); a form occurring in North Africa, India, the Argentine, and Cuba.

**Mycetozoa** (mi-se'to-zo'ah) [ G. *mykēs (mykēt-),* fungus, + *zōon,* animal ]. Microscopic animal forms, frequently known as slime animals, that consist of an irregular, semifluid mass of multinucleated, ameboid protoplasm; although grouped as a subclass in the Rhizopoda (Sarcodina), some of the mycetozoan forms closely resemble certain species of pseudomycetes and are sometimes classified as members of Myxomycetes, *i.e.,* the slime molds.

**my'cid** [ G. *mykēs,* fungus, + -id, *q.v.* ]. An allergic reaction to a distant focus of mycotic infection.

**myco-** (mi'ko-) [ G. *mykēs,* fungus ]. Combining form relating to fungus.

**my'cobac'idin.** Actithiazic acid; 4-oxo-2-thiazolidinehexanoic acid; an antibiotic produced by *Streptomyces virginiae* and other species of *Streptomyces.* Highly active against mycobacteria.

**my'cobacte'ria** Organisms belonging to the genus *Mycobacterium.*

**group I m.,** photochromogens; m. that produce a bright yellow color when grown in the presence of light. Organisms placed in this group appear to belong to the species *Mycobacterium kansasii.*

**group II m.,** scotochromogens; m. that produce a yellow pigment even when grown in the dark; when grown in the light, the pigment is orange. These organisms behave as do saprophytes in man and are nonpathogenic to laboratory animals.

**group III m.,** nonchromogens; m. that are either colorless or that slowly produce a light yellow pigment when grown in the presence of light. Organisms placed in this group belong to the species *Mycobacterium intracellulare.*

**group IV m.,** m. that grow rapidly and that do not produce pigment. Organisms placed in this group belong to such species as *Mycobacterium ulcerans* and *M. marinum.*

**Mycobacteriaceae** (mi'ko-bak-tēr'ī-a'se-e). A family of aerobic bacteria (order Actinomycetales) containing Gram-positive, spherical to rod-shaped cells. Branching does not occur under ordinary cultural conditions. They may or may not be acid-fast. They occur in soil and dairy products and as parasites on man and other animals. The type genus is *Mycobacterium.*

**mycobacteriosis** (mi'ko-bak-tēr'ī-o'sis). Infection with mycobacteria.

**Mycobacterium** (mi'ko-bak-tēr'ī-um) [ myco- + bacterium ]. A genus of aerobic, nonmotile bacteria (family Mycobacteriaceae) containing Gram-positive, acid-fast, slender, straight or slightly curved rods; slender filaments occasionally occur, but branched forms rarely are produced. Parasitic and saprophytic species occur. The type

species is *M. tuberculosis.* It is the type genus of the family Mycobacteriaceae.

**M. absces'sus,** a species orginally found in a traumatic infection of the human knee.

**M. avium,** a species causing tuberculosis in fowl and other birds.

**M. balnei,** a later, subjective synonym of *M. marinum.*

**M. bovis,** *M. tuberculosis* subsp. *bovis;* bovine tubercle bacillus; a species which is the primary cause of tuberculosis in cattle; transmissible to man and other animals, causing tuberculosis.

**M. fortu'itum,** a saprophytic species found in soil and in infections of humans, cattle, and cold-blooded animals.

**M. intracellula're,** Battey bacillus; a species found in lung lesions and sputum of man; may cause bone and tendon-sheath lesions in rabbits; some strains are pathogenic for mice.

**M. johnei,** *M. paratuberculosis;* a species causing Johne's disease, a chronic diarrhea in cattle.

**M. kansasii,** a species causing a tuberculosis-like pulmonary disease; also found to cause infections (and usually lesions) in spinal fluid, spleen, liver, pancreas, testes, hip joint, knee joint, finger, wrist, and lymph nodes.

**M. leprae,** Hansen's bacillus; leprosy bacillus; an obligately parasitic species of man which causes leprous lesions; confined largely to the skin, testes, and peripheral nerves.

**M. lepraemu'rium,** a species which causes an endemic disease of rats; the disease occurs chiefly in the skin and lymph nodes, causing induration, alopecia, and eventually ulceration.

**M. maria'num,** a subjective synonym of *M. scrofulaceum.*

**M. mari'num,** a species causing spontaneous tuberculosis in salt water fish; it also occurs in other cold-blooded animals, in some swimming pools, irrigation canals and ditches, and ocean beaches. *M. balnei* is a later, subjective synonym of *M. marinum.*

**M. micro'ti,** a species causing generalized tuberculosis in voles; transmissible to guinea pigs, rabbits, and calves, causing localized infections.

**M. par'atuberculo'sis.** *M. johnei.*

**M. phle'i,** timothy hay bacillus; Moeller's grass bacillus; a species found in soil and dust and on plants.

**M. platypoeci'lus,** a species found in skin ulcers, liver, spleen, gills, and kidneys of diseased platyfish.

**M. scrofula'ceum,** a species frequently associated with cervical adenitis in children; also found in a skin lesion of a leprosy patient. A subjective synonym is *M. marianum.*

**M. smeg'matis,** a saprophytic species of bacteria found in smegma from the genitalia of man and many of the lower animals; it is also found in soil, dust, and water.

**M. thamno'pheos,** a species found as a parasite in the garter snake and other cold-blooded vertebrates; experimentally it causes tuberculosis in snakes, frogs, lizards, and fish; it is not pathogenic for guinea pigs, rabbits, or fowl.

**M. tuberculo'sis,** Koch's bacillus; tubercle bacillus; a species which causes tuberculosis in man. It is the type species of the genus *M.*

**M. tuberculo'sis** subsp. **bovis,** *M. bovis.*

**M. ulcerans,** a species causing skin ulcers in man; transmissible to rats and mice.

**M. xenopei,** *M. xenopi.*

**M. xenopi,** *M. xenopei;* a species found in a skin lesion of a cold-blooded animal, *Xenopus laevis.*

**mycobactin** (mi'ko-bak'tin). A complex lipid factor reported to be required for the growth of *Mycobacterium tuberculosis* in human plasma; appears to be identical with the lipid factor extracted from *M. phlei* and essential for the growth of *M. johnei.*

**mycocide** (mi'ko-sīd) [ myco- + L. *caedo,* to kill ]. Fungicide.

**My'coder'ma** [ myco- + G. *derma,* skin ]. 1. An obsolete term for a genus of *Schizomycetes,* to which belongs the mother of vinegar. 2. A genus of yeast.

**my'coder'mati'tis.** Mycodermomycosis.

**my'coder'momyco'sis.** Mycodermatitis; a cutaneous mycotic infection.

**mycogastritis** (mi-ko-gas-tri'tis) [ myco- + G. *gastēr,* stomach, + suffix *-itis,* inflammation ]. Inflammation of the stomach due to the presence of a fungus, not a bacterium.

**mycohe′mia.** Mycethemia.

**mycol′ic acid.** Mykol; an acid alcohol, containing free hydroxyl groups, found in certain bacteria; this waxy substance appears to be primarily responsible for the acid-fastness of the bacteria which contain it.

**mycologist** (mi-kol′o-jist). A student of fungi and of the diseases caused by them

**mycology** (mi-kol′o-jĭ) [ myco- + G. *logos*, study ]. Science in relation to fungi: their classification, edibility, cultivation, etc.

**mycomycin.** 3,5,7,8-Tridecatetraene-10,12-diynoic acid; a fatty acid produced by an actinomycete, notable for the presence of acetylenic bonds in the molecule.

**mycomyringitis** (mi′ko-mĭr-in-ji′tis) [ myco- + Mod. L. *myringa*, drum-membrane, + G. suffix *-itis*, inflammation ]. Myringomycosis; inflammation of the membrana tympani caused by the presence of *Aspergillus* or other fungus.

**mycophylaxin** (mi′ko-fi-lak′sin) [ myco- + G. *phylaxis*, protection ]. A biologic substance that is thought to provide some degree of protection against infection and its complications, by means of destructive effects on the causal bacterium or fungus.

**Mycoplasma.** (mi′ko-plaz-mah) [ myco- + G. *plasma*, something formed (plasm) ]. *Asterococcus;* a genus of aerobic to facultatively anaerobic bacteria (family Mycoplasmataceae) containing Gram-negative cells which do not possess a true cell wall. They do not revert to bacteria containing cell walls or cell wall fragments. The cells are bounded by a three-layered membrane. The minimal reproductive units of these organisms are 0.2 to 0.3 μm in diameter. The cells are pleomorphic, and in liquid media appear as coccoid bodies, rings, or filaments. Colonies usually consist of a central core, growing down into the medium, surrounded by superficial peripheral growth. They require sterol for growth. They also require enrichment with serum or ascitic fluid. These organisms are found in humans and other animals and are parasitic to pathogenic. The type species is *M. mycoides.*

**M. agalactiae,** a species causing contagious agalactia of sheep and goats, a common disease in the Mediterranean region.

**M. ana′tis,** a species found in ducks.

**M. argini′ni,** a species found in sheep, goats, and tissue cultures.

**M. arthrit′idis,** a species found in various infected lesions of rats.

**M. bovigenita′lium,** a species found in the lower genital tract of cattle.

**M. bovirhi′nis,** a species found in the bovine respiratory tract.

**M. bucca′le,** *M. orale 2;* a species which is an infrequent parasitic inhabitant of the human oropharynx; it is the predominant mycoplasma in the oropharynx of nonhuman primates.

**M. canis,** a species found in the genital tract and throat of dogs.

**M. conjuncti′vae** subsp. **ovis,** a subspecies associated with pinkeye of sheep.

**M. dispar,** a species found in pneumonic lungs of calves.

**M. edwardii,** a species found in the respiratory tract and occasionally in the genital tract of dogs.

**M. fau′cium,** *M. orale 3;* a species which is a rare member of the normal flora of the human oropharynx; it is occasionally found in the oropharynx of nonhuman primates.

**M. feliminu′tum,** a species found in cats.

**M. fe′lis,** a species found in cats.

**M. fermen′tans,** a species found in ulcerative genital lesions associated with fusiform bacilli and spirilla and also on the apparently normal genital mucosa of humans.

**M. gallina′rum,** a species found in the normal and diseased upper respiratory tracts of fowl.

**M. gallisep′ticum,** a species associated with a chronic respiratory disease of fowl.

**M. gatea,** a species found in cats.

**M. granula′rum,** *Acholeplasma granularum.*

**M. hominis,** a species found in the genital tract and anal canal of humans; also found in the blood of a patient with puerperal speticemia and in pus of a bronchopleural fistula.

**M. hyorhinis,** a species found in the nasal cavity of swine; causes a generalized infection in swine involving the serous membranes of the thoracic and abdominal cavities. The relationship of this organism to atrophic rhinitis is not clear.

**M. hyosyno′viae,** a species found in the joints and respiratory tracts of swine.

**M. hypopneumo′niae,** a species believed to be the cause of mycoplasma pneumonia of pigs.

**M. iners,** a species occurring as a commensal in poultry.

**M. laidlawii,** *Acholeplasma laidlawii.*

**M. maculo′sum,** a species found in the vagina and throat of dogs.

**M. meleagridis,** a species found in turkeys.

**M. mycoi′des,** a species containing two subspecies: *M. mycoides* subsp. *mycoides,* the type subspecies, and *M. mycoides* subsp. *capri.* The former causes pleuropneumonia in cattle; the latter causes pleuropneumonia in goats. It is the type species of the genus *M.*

**M. neuroly′ticum,** a species found in normal and diseased mice; causes "rolling disease."

**M. ora′le 1,** *M. pharyngis.*

**M. ora′le 2,** *M. buccale.*

**M. orale 3,** *M. faucium.*

**M. pharyn′gis,** *M. orale* 1; a species occurring as a commensal in the human oropharynx.

**M. pneumo′niae,** Eaton agent; a species causing primary atypical pneumonia in man.

**M. pulmo′nis,** a species found in the normal and diseased lungs of rats.

**M. saliva′rium,** a species found in human saliva.

**M. spumans,** a species found in the vagina and semen of dogs.

**M. suida′niae,** a species found in the lungs of swine.

**M. syno′viae,** a species found in the hock joint of a fowl; causes synovitis in chickens.

**T-mycoplasma** [ T = tiny ], *Ureaplasma.*

**Mycoplasmatales** (mi′ko-plaz′mă-ta′lēz). An order of Gram-negative bacteria containing cells which are bounded by a three-layered membrane but which do not possess a true cell wall. The minimal reproductive units are 0.2 to 0.3 μm in diameter. Pathogenic and saprophytic species occur. These organisms possess a peculiar mode of reproduction characterized by the breaking up of branched filaments into coccoid, filterable elementary bodies. The order includes the so-called pleuropneumonia-like *organisms* (PPLO), *q.v.*

**mycoprecipitin** (mi′ko-pre-sip′ĭ-tin). A substance causing a precipitation from fungus cultures.

**my′copro′tein.** Protein of fungi or of bacteria.

**mycopus** (mi′ko-pus′). Mucopus.

**my′cose.** Trehalose.

**mycosis** (mi-ko′sis) [ myco- + G. suffix *-osis*, condition ]. Any disease caused by the presence of fungi.

   **m. cu′tis chron′ica,** a chronic dermatomycosis; a chronic skin disease caused by the presence of a fungus.

   **m. favo′sa,** favus.

   **m. framboesioi′des,** yaws.

   **m. fungoi′des,** a chronic progressive reticulosis of the dermis with a proliferation of abnormal cellular elements, a liquefaction necrosis and invasion of the epidermis with the formation of clear spaces containing mononuclear cells (Pautrier's abscesses). Initially, the disease simulates an inflammatory reaction such as eczema or nonspecific exfoliative dermatitis; this premycotic phase is followed in some cases by the development of indurated lesions and tumors of the skin. Also called Alibert's disease; fibroma fungoides; granulosarcoid; granulosarcoma; granuloma sarcomatodes.

   **Gilchrist's m.,** North American *blastomycosis.*

   **m. intestina′lis,** gastroenteric form of anthrax, the symptoms of which are those of gastroenteritis followed by toxemia and general depression.

   **m. leptoth′rica,** obsolete and incorrect usage for pharyngitis caused by the presence of *Leptothrix buccalis.* The organism cited is now known to be a bacterium and not a fungus (see *L. buccalis*); furthermore, there is no evidence that it is a true pathogen capable of producing pharyngitis.

**mycostat'ic.** Fungistatic.

**mycos'terols.** Sterols obtained from fungi.

**mycot'ic.** Relating to a mycosis.

**my'cotoxina'tion, my'cotox'iniza'tion.** Preventive or curative inoculation with any bacterial toxin.

**mydaleine** (mi-da'le-ēn) [ G. *mydaleos*, moldy, fr. *mydos*, dampness ]. A poisonous ptomaine formed in putrefying liver and other viscera; it acts specifically upon the heart, causing arrest of its action in diastole.

**mydatox'in** [ G. *mydos*, dampness, decay, + *toxikon*, poison ]. A ptomaine from putrefying viscera and flesh.

**mydriasis** (mid-ri'ă-sis) [ G. ]. Dilation of the pupil.

    **alternating m.,** m. alternately affecting each eye; due to a disorder of the central nervous system. Also called bounding, leaping, or springing m.

    **bounding m.,** alternating m.

    **paralytic m.,** pupillary dilation due to paralysis of the sphincter pupillae induced by anticholinergic drugs given topically or systemically, or resulting from lesions of midbrain or oculomotor nerve, contusion of eyeball, or glaucoma.

    **spasmodic m.,** spastic m.

    **spastic m.,** spasmodic m., spastic contraction of the dilator pupillae from sympathomimetic drugs applied topically or resulting from irritation of the synpathetic pathway.

**mydriatic** (mid'ri-at'ik). 1. Causing mydriasis or dilation of the pupil. 2. An agent that dilates the pupil.

**myectomy** (mi-ek'to-mi) [ G. *mys*, muscle, + *ektomē*, excision ]. Exsection of a portion of a muscle.

**myectopy, myectopia** (mi-ek'to-pi, mi'-ek-to'pi-ah) [ G. *mys*, muscle, + *ektopos*, out of place ]. Dislocation of a muscle.

**myel-, myelo-** [ G. *myelos*, medulla, marrow. Combining form denoting relationship to (1) the bone marrow, (2) the spinal cord and medulla oblongata, or (3) the myelin sheath of nerve fibers.

**myelalgia** (mi-el-al'ji-ah) [ myel- + G. *algos*, pain ]. Pain in the spinal cord or its membranes.

**myelapoplexy** (mi'el-ap'o-plek'si) [ myel- + G. *apoplēxia*, apoplexy ]. Hematomyelia.

**myelatelia** (mi'el-ă-te'li-ah) [ myel- + G. *ateleia*, incompleteness, fr. *a*- priv. + *telos*, end, fulfilment ]. A developmental defect of the spinal cord.

**myelauxe** (mi-el-awk'se) [ myel- + G. *auxē*, increase ]. Hypertrophy of the spinal cord.

**myele'mia** [ myel- + G. *haima*, blood ]. Myelocytosis.

**myelencephalon** (mi'el-en-sef'ă-lon) [ myel- + G. *enkephalos*, brain ] [ NA ]. *Medulla* oblongata.

**myel'ic.** Relating to (1) the spinal cord, or (2) bone marrow.

**my'elin.** 1. The lipoproteinaceous material enveloping the axon of myelinated nerve fibers, composed of regularly alternating layers of lipids (cholesterol, phospholipids, sphingolipids, phosphatides) and protein; see also myelin *sheath*. 2. Droplets of lipid formed during autolysis and postmortem decompostion.

**my'elinated.** Medullated (2); having a myelin sheath.

**myelination** (mi'ĕ-li-na'shun). Myelinization; myelinogenesis; medullation (2) the acquisition, development, or formation of a myelin sheath around a nerve fiber.

**myelinic** (mi'ĕ-lin'ik). Relating to myelin.

**my'eliniza'tion.** Myelination.

**myelinoclasis** (mi'ĕ-li-nok'lă-sis) [ myelin + G. *klasis*, a breaking ]. Destruction of myelin; see also demyelination, dysmyelination.

**myelinogenesis** (mi'ĕ-lin-o-jen'ĕ-sis) [ myelin + G. *genesis*, production ]. Myelination.

**myelinolysis** (mi'ĕ-li-nol'i-sis) [ myelin + G. *lysis*, dissolution ]. Dissolution of the myelin sheaths of nerve fibers.

    **central pontine m.,** localized loss of myelin within the midbase of the pons; related to malnutrition and often to alcoholism.

**myelitic** (mi'ĕ-lit'ik). Relating to or affected by myelitis.

**myelitis** (mi'ĕ-li'tis) [ myel- + G. suffix -*itis*, inflammation ]. Inflammation (1) of the spinal cord (also called notomyelitis), or (2) of the bone marrow.

    **acute transverse m.,** acute softening of the spinal cord; an acute inflammation, limited in longitudinal extent, involving the entire thickness of the spinal cord.

    **apoplec'tiform m.,** Hayem's disease; inflammation involving chiefly the gray matter of the spinal cord, in which paralysis occurs with suddenness.

    **ascending m.,** progressive inflammation involving successively higher areas of the spinal cord.

    **bulbar m.,** inflammation of the medulla oblongata.

    **concussion m.,** traumatic myelopathy.

    **Foix-Alajouanine m.,** subacute necrotizing m.

    **funicular m.,** (1) inflammation involving any of the columns of the spinal cord; (2) subacute combined *degeneration* of the spinal cord.

    **subacute necrotizing m.,** Foix-Alajouanine m.; angiodysgenetic myelomalacia; a disorder of the lower spinal cord resulting in progressive paraplegia.

    **systemic m.,** inflammation confined to special tracts of the spinal cord.

    **transverse m.,** inflammation involving the entire thickness of the spinal cord, but of limited longitudinal extent.

**myelo-** (mi'ĕ-lo-). See myel-.

**myeloarchitectonics** (mi'ĕ-lo-ar'ki-tek-ton'iks). The pattern of myelinated nerve fibers in the brain, as distinguished from cytoarchitectonics.

**my'eloblast** [ myelo- + G. *blastos*, germ ]. Lymphomyelocyte; an immature cell (10 to 18 μ in diameter) in the granulocytic series, occurring normally in bone marrow, but not in the circulating blood (except in certain diseases). When stained with the usual dyes, the cytoplasm is light blue, nongranular, and variable in amount, sometimes being only a thin rim around the nucleus; the latter is deep purple-blue with finely divided, punctate, thread-like chromatin that is somewhat condensed at the periphery. A few light blue nucleoli are usually present in the nucleus, and these generally disappear as the m. matures into a promyelocyte and then a myelocyte. M.'s ordinarily yield a negative reaction with peroxidase. See color plate 14.

**my'eloblaste'mia** [ myeloblast + G. *haima*, blood ]. The presence of myeloblasts in the circulating blood.

**my'eloblasto'ma** [ myeloblast + G. suffix -*oma*, tumor ]. A nodular focus or fairly well circumscribed accumulation of myeloblasts, as sometimes observed in acute myeloblastic leukemia and chlorosis.

**my'eloblasto'sis.** The presence of unusually large numbers of myeloblasts in the circulating blood, or tissues, or both (as in acute leukemia).

    **avian m.,** fowl m.; an expression of disease caused by the avian leukosis-sarcoma virus; characterized by progressive anemia, enormous numbers of myeloblasts in the blood, weakness, and death.

    **fowl m.,** avian m.

**myelocele** (mi'ĕ-lo-sēl) [ myelo- + G. *kēle*, hernia ]. Protrusion of the spinal cord in spina bifida. 2 [ G. *myelos*, marrow, + *koilia*, a hollow ]. The central canal of the spinal cord.

**myelocyst** (mi'ĕ-lo-sist) [ myelo- + G. *kystis*, bladder ]. Any cyst (usually lined with columnar or cuboidal cells) that develops from a rudimentary medullary canal in the central nervous system.

**my'elocyst'ic.** Pertaining to or characterized by the presence of a myelocyst.

**myelocystocele** (mi'ĕ-lo-sis'to-sēl) [ myelo- + G. *kystis*, bladder, + *kēlē*, tumor ]. Spina bifida containing spinal cord substance.

**myelocystomeningocele** (mi'ĕ-lo-sis'to-mē-ning'go-sēl) [ myelo- + G. *kystis*, bladder, + *mēninx* (*mēning*-), membrane, + *kēlē*, hernia ]. Spina bifida with protrusion of spinal cord matter and meninges.

**myelocyte** (mi'ĕ-lo-sīt) [ myelo- + G. *kytos*, cell ]. 1. A young cell of the granulocytic series, occurring normally in bone marrow, but not in circulating blood (except in certain diseases). When stained with the usual dyes, the cytoplasm is distinctly basophilic and relatively more abundant than in myeloblasts or promyelocytes, even though m.'s are smaller cells; numerous cytoplasmic granules (*i.e.,* neutrophilic, eosinophilic, or basophilic) are present in the more mature forms of m.'s, and the first two types are peroxidase-positive. The nuclear chromatin is coarser than that observed in myeloblasts, but it is relatively faintly stained and lacks a well defined membrane; the nucleus is fairly regular in contour (*i.e.,* not indented), and seems to be "buried" beneath the numerous cytoplasmic granules. See color plate 14. 2. A nerve cell of the gray matter of the brain or spinal cord.

m. A, the youngest form of m., characterized by only a few (not more than ten) cytoplasmic granules, which are most reliably demonstrated by means of staining with neutral red. The mitochondria are numerous, and resemble those of the myeloblast.

m. B, the intermediate form of m., characterized by approximately 30 to 100 (or more) cytoplasmic granules scattered among the mitochondria; the latter are less numerous than in m.'s of the A stage, and they are frequently displaced toward the periphery of the cell.

m. C, the most mature of the m.'s characterized by numerous cytoplasmic granules that are recognizable as neutrophilic, eosinophilic, and basophilic; with neutral red these are stained, respectively, red, bright yellow, and deep maroon; C m.'s are frequently larger than earlier forms. If the nucleus is indented, the m. is maturing into a metamyelocyte.

**myelocythemia** (mi'ĕ-lo-si-the'mĭ-ah) [ myelocyte + G. *haima,* blood ]. The presence of myelocytes in the circulating blood, especially in persistently large numbers (as in myelocytic leukemia).

**myelocytic** (mi'ĕ-lo-sit'ik). Pertaining to or characterized by myelocytes.

**myelocytoma** (mi'ĕ-lo-si-to'mah) [ myelocyte + G. suffix *-oma,* tumor ]. A nodular focus or fairly well circumscribed, relatively dense accumulation of myelocytes, as in certain tissues of persons with myelocytic leukemia.

**myelocytomatosis** (mi'ĕ-lo-si'to-mă-to'sis). 1. A form of tumor involving chiefly the myelocytes. 2. A rare leukosis of fowl marked by the presence of white tumors composed of myeloid cells, located principally along the sternum and in the liver.

**myelocytosis** (mi'ĕ-lo-si-to'sis) [ myelocyte + G. suffix *-osis,* condition ]. The occurrence of abnormally large numbers of myelocytes in the circulating blood, or tissues, or both.

**myelodiastasis** (mi'ĕ-lo-di-as'tă-sis) [ myelo- + G. *diastasis,* separation ]. Softening and destruction of the spinal cord.

**myelodysplasia** (mi'ĕ-lo-dis-pla'zĭ-ah) [ myelo- + G. *dys-,* difficult, + *plasis,* a molding ]. 1. An abnormality in development of the spinal cord. 2. Inappropriate term for spina bifida occulta.

**my'elofibro'sis.** Myelosclerosis; centrosclerosis; ostemyelofibrotic syndrome; fibrosis of the bone marrow, especially generalized, associated with myeloid metaplasia of the spleen and other organs, leukoerythroblastic anemia, and thrombocytopenia, although the bone marrow often contains many megakaryocytes.

**myelogenesis** (mi'ĕ-lo-jen'ĕ-sis). The development of bone marrow.

**myelogenetic, myelogenic** (mi'ĕ-lo-jen-et'ik, -jen'ik) 1. Relating to myelogenesis. 2. Myelogenous; produced by or orginating in the bone marrow.

**myelogenous** (mi'ĕ-loj'ĕ-nus). Myelogenetic (2).

**myelogone, myelogonium** (mi'ĕ-lo-gōn, -go'nĭ-um) [ myelo- + G. *gonē,* seed ]. 1. Myeloblast. 2. An immature white blood cell (of the myeloid series) that is characterized by (1) a relatively large, fairly deeply stained, finely reticulated nucleus that contains palely stained nucleoli, and (2) a scant amount of rimlike, nongranular, moderately basophilic cytoplasm. M.'s are difficult to distinguish from lymphoblasts and monoblasts, unless one evaluates them in relation to the more mature forms usually associated with the younger cells.

**myelography** (mi'ĕ-log'ră-fi) [ myelo- + G. *graphē,* a drawing ]. Visualization or photography of the spinal cord after the injection of a radiopaque substance into the spinal arachnoid space.

**myeloic** (mi'ĕ-lo'ik). Pertaining to the tissue and precursor cells from which neutrophils, eosinophils, and basophils are derived.

**myeloid** (mi'ĕ-loyd). 1. Pertaining to, derived from, or manifesting certain features of the bone marrow. 2. Sometimes used with reference to the spinal cord. 3. Pertaining to certain characteristics of myelocytic forms, but not necessarily implying origin in the bone marrow.

**my'eloido'sis.** General hyperplasia of myeloid tissue.

**myeloleukemia** (mi'ĕ-lo-lu-ke'mĭ-ah). A form of leukemia in which the abnormal cells are derived from myelopoietic tissue. See leukemia and subentries.

**my'elolipo'ma.** A misnomer for certain nodular foci that are not neoplasms, but probably represent accumulations of cells derived from localized proliferation of reticuloendothelial tissue in the blood sinuses of the adrenal glands. Grossly, the nodules may seem to be adipose tissue, but they actually are foci of bone marrow; in one type, there is a predominance of fat, with only slight numbers of myeloid elements and relatively large numbers of erythropoietic cells; in the second type, there is a predominance of myeloid elements, with relatively few erythroid cells. True lipomas rarely originate in such nodules, which are apparently not clinically significant.

**myelolymphocyte** (mi'ĕ-lo-lim'fo-sīt). An abnormal form of the lymphocytic series in the bone marrow, and presumed to be formed in that tissue.

**my'elol'ysis.** The breaking down of myelin.

**myeloma** (mi'ĕ-lo'mah) [ myelo- + G. suffix *-oma,* tumor ]. A tumor composed of cells derived from hemopoietic tissues of the bone marrow.

endothelial m., Ewing's *tumor.*

giant cell m., giant cell *tumor* of bone.

multiple m., Kahler's disease; myelomatosis; myelomatosis multiplex; myeloma multiplex; an unusual disease that occurs more frequently in men than in women, and is ordinarily regarded as a malignant neoplasm that originates in bone marrow and involves chiefly the skeleton. The clinical features are attributable to the sites of involvement and to abnormalities in formation of plasma protein. the disease if characterized by numerous diffuse foci or nodular accumulations of abnormal plasma cells in bone marrow of various bones, especially the skull, and occasionally in extraskeletal sites. The myeloma cells produce abnormal proteins in the serum and urine; those formed in any one example of multiple m. are different from all other m. proteins, as well as different from normal serum proteins; the most frequent abnormalities in the metabolism of protein are (1) the occurrence of Bence Jones proteinuria, (2) a great increase in γ-globulin in the plasma, (3) the occasional formation of cryo-globulin, and (4) a form of primary amyloidosis. The Bence Jones protein is not a derivative of abnormal serum protein, but seems to be formed *de novo* from amino acid precursors. See also plasma cell m.

m. multiplex, multiple m.

plasma cell m., a term sometimes used for either of two conditions: (1) multiple m.; (2) plasmacytoma of bone, which is usually a solitary lesion and not associated with the occurrence of Bence Jones protein or other disturbances in the metabolism of protein (as observed in multiple m.). Some observers emphasize that the solitary lesion probably represents an early phase of classic multiple m., or an example of the latter in which only one focus is recognized.

**my'elomala'cia** [ myelo- + G. *malakia,* a softness ]. Softening of the spinal cord.

angiodysgenetic m., subacute necrotizing *myelitis.*

**my'elomato'sis.** A disease characterized by the occurrence of myelomas in various sites.

multiple m., multiple *myeloma.*

m. multiplex, multiple *myeloma.*

**myelomenia** (mi'ĕ-lo-me'nĭ-ah) [ myelo- + G. *mēniaia,* menses, fr. *mēn,* month ]. Spinal hemorrhage occurring as a form of vicarious menstruation.

**myelomeningocele** (mi'ĕ-lo-mĕ-ning'go-sēl) [ myelo- + G. *mēninx,* membrane, + *kēlē,* hernia ]. Spina bifida with protrusion of both the cord and its membranes.

**my'elomere** [ myelo- + G. *meros*, part ]. A neuromere of the spinal cord.

**myelomonocyte** (mi'ĕ-lo-mon'o-sit). Myelocyte (1).

**my'elon** [ G. *myelon*, later ntr. form of *myelos*, marrow ]. Obsolete term for medulla spinalis (spinal cord).

**myeloneuritis** (mi'ĕ-lo-nu-ri'tis). Neuromyelitis.

**myelon'ic.** Relating to the spinal cord.

**my'eloparal'ysis.** Spinal *paralysis*.

**my'elopath'ic.** Relating to myelopathy.

**my'elop'athy** [ myelo- + G. *pathos*, suffering ]. 1. Disturbance or disease of the spinal cord. 2. A disease of the myelopoietic tissues.

    **compressive m.,** destruction of spinal cord tissue caused by pressure from neoplasms, hematomas, or other masses.

    **diabetic m.,** degenerative changes in spinal cord tissue noted in some patients with diabetes mellitus.

    **radiation m.,** damage to the spinal cord from excessive exposure to x-rays.

**my'eloperox'idase.** Verdoperoxidase.

**my'elop'etal** [ myelo- + L. *peto*, to seek ]. Proceeding in a direction toward the spinal cord; said of different nerve impulses.

**myelophthisic** (mi'ĕ-lo-tiz'ik, -thiz'ik). Relating to or suffering from myelophthisis.

**myelophthisis** (mi'ĕ-lof'thĭ-sis, mi'ĕ-lo-ti'sis, -te'sis) [ myelo- + G. *phthisis*, a wasting away ]. 1. Wasting or atrophy of the spinal cord as in tabes dorsalis. 2. Panmyelophthisis; replacement of hemopoietic tissue in the bone marrow by abnormal tissue, usually fibrous tissue or malignant tumors which are most commonly metastatic carcinomas.

**my'eloplaque.** Myeloplax.

**my'eloplast** [ myelo- + G. *plastos*, formed ]. Any of the leukocytic series of cells in the bone marrow, especially young forms.

**my'eloplax** [ myelo- + G. *plax*, a flat stone, plaque ]. Myeloplaque; old terms for any multinucleated giant cell occurring in bone marrow.

    **Robin's m.'s,** an old eponym for osteoclasts.

**myeloplegia** (mi'ĕ-lo-ple'jĭ-ah) [ myelo- + G. *plēgē*, a stroke ]. Spinal *paralysis*.

**myelopoiesis** (mi'ĕ-lo-poy-e'sis) [ myelo- + G. *poiēsis*, a making ]. The formation of the tissue elements of bone marrow, or any of the types of blood cells derived from bone marrow, or both processes.

**my'elopoiet'ic.** Relating to myelopoiesis.

**my'eloprolif'erative.** Pertaining to or characterized by unusual proliferation of myelopoietic tissue.

**my'eloradic'uli'tis** [ myelo- + L. *radicula*, root, + G. suffix -*itis*, inflammation ]. Inflammation of the spinal cord and nerve roots.

**my'eloradic'ulodyspla'sia** [ myelo- + L. *radicula*, root, + dysplasia ]. Congenital maldevelopment of the spinal cord and spinal nerve roots.

**myeloradiculopathy** (mi'ĕ-lo-rǎ-dik'u-lop'ǎ-thĭ) [ myelo- + L. *radicula*, root, + G. *pathos*, disease ]. Radiculomyelopathy; disease involving the spinal cord and nerve roots.

**my'eloradic'ulopolyneuroni'tis.** Guillain-Barré *syndrome*.

**myelorrhagia** (mi'ĕ-lo-ra'jĭ-ah) [ myelo- + G. *rhēgnymi*, to burst forth ]. Hematomyelia.

**myelorrhaphy** (mi'ĕ-lor'ǎ-fĭ) [ myelo- + G. *rhaphē*, a seam ]. Suture of a wound of the spinal cord.

**my'elosarco'ma** [ myelo- + G. *sarx*, flesh, + suffix -*ōma*, tumor ]. A malignant neoplasm derived from bone marrow or one of its cellular elements.

**my'elosarco'mato'sis.** Widespread myelosarcomas.

**myeloschisis** (mi'ĕ-los'kĭ-sis) [ myelo- + G. *schisis*, a cleaving ]. A cleft spinal cord as a result of the failure of the neural folds to close as is normally the case in the formation of the neural tube; inevitably spina bifida is a sequel.

**myelosclerosis** (mi'ĕ-lo-skle-ro'sis) [ myelo- + G. *sklērō-sis*, induration ]. Myelofibrosis.

**my'elo'sis.** 1. A condition characterized by abnormal proliferation of tissue or cellular elements of bone marrow, *e.g.*, multiple myeloma, myelocytic leukemia, erythroblas-

temia, myelocytosis, and the like. 2. A condition in which there is abnormal proliferation of medullary tissue in the spinal cord, as in a glioma.

    **aleukemic m.,** subleukemic m.; m. with a normal or subnormal leukocyte count.

    **chronic nonleukemic m.,** a condition in which there is abnormal proliferation of leukopoietic tissue that results in immature white blood cells in the circulating blood, but the total count is within the normal range.

    **erythremic m.,** a neoplastic process involving the erythropoietic tissue; characterized by anemia, irregular fever, splenomegaly, hepatomegaly, hemorrhagic disorders, and numerous erythroblasts in all stages of maturation (with disproportionately large numbers of less mature forms) in the circulating blood. Postmortem studies reveal primitive erythroblasts and reticuloendothelial cells, not only in hemopoietic organs, but also in the kidneys, adrenal glands and other sites. Acute and chronic forms are recognized; the former is also called Di Guglielmo's disease and acute erythremia; in the latter, there is less prominence of the immature cells.

    **funicular m.,** subacute combined *degeneration* of the spinal cord.

    **leukemic m.,** (1) myelocytic or (2) myeloblastic *leukemia*.

    **leukopenic m.,** aleukemic *leukemia*.

    **subleukemic m.,** aleukemic m.

**myelospongium** (mi'ĕ-lo-spun'jĭ-um) [ myelo- + G. *spongos*, sponge ]. The fibrocellular meshwork in the spinal cord of the embryo, from which the neuroglia is developed.

**my'elosyph'ilis.** Syphilis of the spinal cord.

**my'elosyringo'sis.** Syringomyelia.

**myelotome** (mi'ĕ-lo-tōm) [ myelo- + G. *tomos*, cutting ]. An instrument used in making serial sections of the spinal cord.

**my'elot'omy** [ myelo- + G. *tomē*, incision ]. Incision of the spinal cord.

    **Bischof's m.,** longitudinal incision of the spinal cord through lateral column for spasticity.

    **commissural m.,** midline m.

    **midline m.,** commissural m., commissurotomy (2); section of the midline transverse fibers of the spinal cord.

**myelotoxic** (mi'ĕ-lo-tok'sik). 1. Inhibitory, depressant, or destructive to one or more of the components of bone marrow. 2. Pertaining to, derived from, or manifesting the features of diseased bone marrow.

**myenteric** (mi'en-tĕr'ik). Relating to the myenteron.

**myen'teron** [ G. *mys*, muscle, + *enteron*, intestine ]. The muscular coat, or muscularis, of the intestine.

**Myerholtz' muscle.** See under muscle.

**myesthesia** (mi-es-the'zĭ-ah) [ G. *mys*, muscle, + *aisthēsis*, sensation ]. Kinesthetic sense; muscular sense; mesoblastic sensibility; deep sensibility; myoesthesia; the sensation felt in muscle when contracting.

**myiasis** (mi-i'ǎ-sis) [ G. *myia*, a fly. MYI- ]. Strike; any infection due to the invasion of the tissues or cavities of the body by the larvae of dipterous insects.

    **aural m.,** invasion of the external, middle, or inner ear by larvae of dipterous insects.

    **creeping m.,** cutaneous *larva migrans*.

    **intestinal m.,** larvae in the gastrointestinal tract. There are some twenty species of dipterous insects whose larvae may inhabit the human intestine, including those of the domestic fly, cheese mite, and *Fannia canicularis*, a fly resembling the housefly.

    **m. linea'ris,** cutaneous *larva migrans*.

    **nasal m.,** fly larva invasion of the nasal passages, due most commonly in America to primary screwworms, the larvae of *Callitroga hominivorax*, which develop in the nasal or aural cavity.

    **ocular m.,** ophthalmomyiasis; invasion of the conjunctival sac or eyeball by larvae of flies, *e.g.*, *Hypoderma bovis*, *H. lineata*, *Sarcophaga*, or *Gastrophilus intestinalis*.

    **m. oestruo'sa,** m. due to a species of the *Oestridae*, the gadflies or botflies.

    **subcuta'neous m.,** invasion of the subcutaneous tissues by the larvae of dipterous insects.

    **wound m., traumatic m.,** the infestation of a surface wound or other open lesion by fly larvae.

**myiocephalon, myiocephalum** (mi-i-o-sef'a-lon, or -lum) [ G. *myia*, fly, + *kephalē*, head. MYI- ]. Iridocele.

**myiodesopsia** (mi-i-o-des-op'sī-ah) [ G. *myiōdēs*, like flies (MYI-), + *opsis*, vision ]. Myodesopsia; myopsis; the condition in which muscae volitantes are seen.

**myiosis** (mi-i-o'sis). Myiasis.

**myitis** (mi-i'tis) [ G. *mys*, muscle, + *-itis* ]. Myositis.

**my'kol.** Mycolic acid.

**myl'abris** [ G. a cockroach found in mills and bakehouses, fr. *mylē*, mill ]. The dried beetle, *Mylabris phalerata;* a vesicant, like cantharis.

**mylohyoid** (mi'lo-hi'oyd) [ G. *mylē*, a mill, in pl. *mylai*, molar teeth. MYL- ]. Relating to the molar teeth, or posterior portion of the lower jaw, and to the hyoid bone; denoting various structures; see under nerve, muscle, region, and sulcus.

**mylohyoideus** (mi-lo-hi-o-id'e-us). *Musculus* mylohyoideus.

**myo-** (mi'o-) [ G. *mys*, muscle. MUSCU- ]. Combining form relating to muscle.

**myoalbumin** (mi'o-al-bu'min). Albumin in muscle tissue, possibly the same as serum albumin.

**myoarchitectonic** (mi'o-ar'kī-tek-ton'ik) [ myo- + G. *architektonikos*, relating to construction ]. Relating to the structural arrangement of muscle or of fibers in general.

**myoatrophy** (mi-o-at'ro-fī). Myatrophy; muscular atrophy.

**my'oblast** [ myo- + G. *blastos*, germ ]. Sarcogenic cell; sarcoblast; a primitive muscle cell with the potentiality of developing into a muscle fiber.

**myoblas'tic.** Relating to a myoblast or to the mode of formation of muscle cells.

**myoblastoma** (mi'o-blas-to'mah) [ myo- + G. *blastos*, germ, + suffix *-oma*, tumor ]. A tumor of immature muscle cells; *e.g.*, embryonal rhabdomyosarcoma.

    **granular cell m.,** Granular cell *tumor.*

**myobra'dia** [ myo- + G. *bradys*, slow ]. Sluggish reaction of muscle following stimulation.

**myocar'dial.** Relating to the myocardium.

**myocardiograph** (mi'o-kar'dī-o-graf) [ myo- + G. *kardia*, heart, + *graphō*, to record ]. An instrument composed of a tambour with recording lever attachment, by means of which a tracing is made of the movements of the heart muscle.

**myocardiopathy** (mi'o-kar-dī-op'ă-thī) [ myocardium + G. *pathos*, suffering ]. Cardiomyopathy; disease of the myocardium.

    **primary m.,** myocardial disease of unknown cause.

**myocardiorraphy** (mi'o-kar-dī-or'ă-fī) [ myocardium + G. *raphē*, suture ]. Suture of wounds of the myocardium.

**myocardi'tis.** Inflammation of the muscular walls of the heart.

    **acute isolated m.,** Fiedler's m.; an acute interstitial m. of unknown cause, the endocardium and pericardium being unaffected.

    **Fiedler's m.,** acute isolated m.

    **fragmentation m.,** fragmentation of the myocardium; see under myocardium.

    **in'durative m.,** chronic m. leading to hardening of the muscular wall of the heart.

**myocardium,** pl. **myocar'dia** (mi'o-kar'dī-um) [ myo- + G. *kardia*, heart ] [ NA ]. The middle layer of the heart, consisting of cardiac *muscle* (*q. v.*).

    **fragmentation of the m.,** a transverse rupture of the muscular fibers of the heart, especially those of the papillary muscles.

**myocardo'sis.** 1. A condition marked by symptomatic signs of cardiac trouble without any discoverable pathologic lesion. 2. Any degenerative condition of the heart muscle except myofibrosis.

**myocele** (mi'o-sēl). 1 [ myo- + G. *kēlē*, hernia ]. Protrusion of muscle substance through a rent in its sheath. 2 [ myo- + G. *koilia*, a cavity ]. Somite cavity; the small cavity that appears in somites.

**myocelialgia** (mi'o-se-lī-al'jī-ah) [ myo- + G. *koilia*, the belly, + *algos*, pain ]. Pain in the abdominal muscles.

**myocelitis** (mi-o-se-li'tis) [ myo- + G. *koilia*, belly, + suffix *-itis*, inflammation ]. Inflammation of the abdominal muscles.

**myocellulitis** (mi-o-sel-u-li'tis) [ myo- + Mod. L. *cellularis*, cellular (tissue), + G. suffix *-itis*, inflammation ]. Inflammation of muscle and cellular tissue.

**myocerosis** (mi'o-se-ro'sis) [ myo- + G. *kēros*, wax ]. Waxy degeneration of the muscles.

**myochrome** (mi'o-krōm). Cytochrome *c.*

**myochronoscope** (mi'o-kron'o-skōp) [ myo- + G. *chronos*, time, + *skopeō*, to examine ]. An instrument for timing a muscular impulse, for determining the interval between the application of the stimulus and the muscular movement in response.

**myocinesimeter** (mi'o-sin-e-sim'ī-ter). Myokinesimeter.

**myoclonia** (mi'o-klo'nī-ah) [ myo- + G. *klonos*, a tumult ]. Any disorder characterized by myoclonus.

    **fi'brillary m.,** the twitching of a limited part or group of fibers of a muscle.

    **infectious m.,** chorea.

**myoclon'ic.** Showing myoclonus.

**myoclonus** (mi-ok'lo-nus, mi'o-klo'nus) [ myo- + G. *klonus*, tumult ]. Clonic spasm or twitching of a muscle or group of muscles.

    **m. multiplex,** a disorder marked by rapid contractions occurring simultaneously or consecutively in various unrelated muscles. Also called Friedreich's disease; polyclonia; polymyoclonus; paramyoclonus.

    **noctur'nal m.,** frequently repeated muscular jerks occurring at the moment of dropping off to sleep. Similar jerks that awaken a sleeper occur occasionally in all normal persons.

    **palatal m.,** rhythmic contractions of the soft palate, the facial muscles and the diaphragm, related to lesions of the olivocerebellar pathways.

**myocolpitis** (mi-o-kol-pi'tis) [ myo- + G. *kolpos*, bosom (vagina), suffix *-itis*, inflammation ]. Inflammation of the muscular tissue of the vagina.

**myocom'ma,** pl. **myocom'mata** [ myo- + G. *komma*, a coin or the stamp of a coin ]. Myoseptum; the connective tissue septum separating adjacent myotomes.

**myocrismus** (mi'o-kris'mus) [ myo- + G. *krizō*, to squeak ]. A creaking sound sometimes heard on ausculatation of a contracting muscle.

**my'ocyte** [ myo- + G. *kytos*, cell ]. A muscle cell.

    **Anitschkow m.,** cardiac *histiocyte.*

**myocytoma** (mi'o-si-to'mah). A benign neoplasm derived from muscle, usually nonstriated type.

**my'odegenera'tion.** Muscular degeneration.

**myode'mia** [ myo- + G. *dēmos*, tallow ]. Fatty degeneration of muscle.

**myodesop'sia.** Myiodesopsia.

**myodiastasis** (mi'o-di-as'tă-sis) [ myo- + G. *diastasis*, separation ]. Separation of muscle.

**myodiopter** (mi'o-di-op'ter). The contractile power of the ciliary muscle required to raise the refractive power of the lens by 1 diopter.

**myodynamia** (mi'o-di-na'mī-ah) [ myo- + G. *dynamis*, power ]. Muscular strength.

**my'odynam'ics.** Dynamics of muscular action.

**myodynamometer** (mi'o-di'nă-mom'e-ter) [ myo- + G. *dynamis*, force, + *metron*, measure ]. An instrument for determining the muscular strength.

**myodynia** (mi'o-din'ī-ah) [ myo- + G. *odynē*, pain ]. Myalgia.

**myodystony** (mi-o-dis'to-nī) [ myo- + G. prefix *dys-*, difficult, + *tonos*, tone, tension ]. A condition of slow relaxation, interrupted by a succession of slight contractions, following electrical stimulation of a muscle.

**myodystrophia** (mi'o-dis-tro'fī-ah). Muscular *dystrophy.*

    **m. feta'lis,** *arthrogryposis* multiplex congenita.

**myodystrophy** (mi-o-dis'tro-fī) [ myo- + G. prefix *dys-*, difficult, poor, + *trophē*, nourishment ]. Muscular *dystrophy.*

**myoedema** (mi'o-e-de'mah) [ myo- + G. *oidēma*, swelling ]. A localized contraction of a degenerating muscle, occurring at the point of a sharp blow; the response is independent of the nerve supply. Also called idiomuscular contraction; mounding; myoidema.

**my'oelas'tic.** Pertaining to closely associated smooth muscle fibers and elastic connective tissue.

**myoelec'tric.** Relating to the electrical properties of muscle.

**myoendocarditis** (mi-o-en-do-kar-di'tis) [ myo- + G. *endon*, within, + *kardia*, heart, + suffix *-itis*, inflammation ]. Inflammation of the muscular wall and lining membrane of the heart.

**my'oepithe'lial.** Relating to myoepithelium.

**my'oepithelio'ma** [ myo- + epithelium, *q.v.*, + G. suffix *-ōma*, tumor ]. Nodular *hidradenoma*.

**myoepithelium** (mi'o-ep-ĭ-the'lĭ-um) [ myo- + epithelium, *q.v.* ]. Spindle-shaped cells arranged longitudinally or obliquely around sweat glands and the secretory alveoli of the mammary gland. Stellate myoepithelial cells occur around lacrimal and some salivary gland secretory units. The myoepithelial cells are contractile and resemble smooth muscle cells.

**myoesthesis, myoesthesia** (mi'o-es-the'sis, -the'zĭ-ah). Myesthesia.

**myofascitis** (mi'o-fă-si'tis) [ myo- + fascitis ]. *Myositis* fibrosa.

**myofi'bril** [ myo- + Mod. L. *fibrilla*, fibril ]. Myofibrilla; muscular fibril; one of the fine longitudinal fibrils occurring in a skeletal, cardiac, or smooth muscle fiber. In striated muscle the fibril is made up of ultramicroscopic thick and thin myofilaments.

**myofibrilla**, pl. **myofibril'lae** (mi'o-fi-bril'ah). Myofibril.

**myofibro'ma.** A benign neoplasm that consists chiefly of fibrous connective tissue, with variable numbers of muscle cells forming portions of the neoplasm.

**myofibro'sis.** Chronic myositis with diffuse hyperplasia of the interstitial connective tissue pressing upon and causing atrophy of the muscular tissue.
  **m. cordis,** m. of the heart walls.

**my'ofibrosi'tis.** Inflammation of the perimysium.

**myofil'aments.** The ultramicroscopic threads making up myofibrils in striated muscle. Thick ones contain myosin and thin ones actin.

**my'ofunc'tional.** Relating to function of muscles.

**myogen** (mi'o-jen) [ myo- + G. suffix *-gen*, producing ]. Myosinogen; the proteins extracted from muscle with cold water, largely the enzymes promoting glycolysis. From the residue, alkaline 0.6 M KC1 extracts actin and myosin as actomyosin; myosin is separable into two meromyosins by proteinase treatment.

**myogenesis** (mi'o-jen'ĕ-sis) [ myo- + G. *genesis*, origin ]. The formation of muscle cells or fibers.

**myogenet'ic, myogen'ic.** 1. Originating in or starting from muscle. 2. Relating to the origin of muscle cells or fibers.

**myogenous** (mi-oj'en-us). Myogenetic.

**myoglo'bin.** Myohemoglobin; the oxygen-transporting protein of muscle, resembling blood hemoglobin in function, but containing only one heme as part of the molecule (rather than the four of hemoglobin), and with a molecular weight but one-quarter that of hemoglobin.

**my'oglobinu'ria.** The excretion of myoglobin in the urine, as in certain instances of crush syndrome, advanced or protracted ischemia of muscle, and so on. The condition may be paroxysmal.

**myoglob'ulin.** Globulin present in muscle tissue.

**myoglobulinemia** (mi'o-glob'u-lin-e'mĭ-ah). The presence of myoglobulin in the blood.
  **idiopathic paroxysmal m.,** inborn deficiency of muscle phosphorylase causing muscle pains and myoglobinuria after exercise; may lead to acute renal failure.

**myoglobulinuria** (mi'o-glob'u-lin-u'rĭ-ah). The excretion of myoglobulin in the urine.
  **paralytic m.,** *azoturia* of horses.

**myognathus** (mi-og'nă-thus) [ myo- + G. *gnathos*, jaw ]. An unequal conjoined twin in which the rudimentary head of the parasite is attached to the lower jaw of the autosite by muscle and skin only.

**my'ogram** [ myo- + G. *gramma*, a drawing ]. Muscle curve; the tracing made by a myograph.

**my'ograph** [ myo- + G. *graphō*, to write ]. A recording instrument by which tracings are made of muscular contractions.
  **palate m.,** palatograph.

**myograph'ic.** Relating to a myogram, or the record of a myograph.

**myography** (mi-og'ră-fĭ). 1. The recording of muscular movements by the myograph. 2. Descriptive myology; a description of or treatise on the muscles.

**my'ohem'atin.** Cytochrome *c*.

**myohemoglobin** (mi'o-he'mo-glo-bin). Myoglobin.

**my'oid** [ myo- + G. *eidos*, appearance ]. 1. Resembling muscle. 2. One of the fine, contractile, threadlike masses of protoplasm found in certain epithelial cells in the simpler forms of animals. 3. A contractile part of retinal cones in certain fish and amphibia.

**myoidema** (mi-oy-de'mah) [ myo- + G. *oidēma*, swelling ]. Myoedema.

**my'oidism.** The condition of myoedema.

**my'oino'sitol.** See under inositol.

**myoischemia** (mi'o-is-ke'mĭ-ah) [ myo- + ischemia, *q.v.* ]. A condition of localized deficiency or absence of blood supply in muscular tissue.

**myokero'sis.** Myocerosis.

**my'oki'nase.** Adenylate kinase.

**myokinesimeter** (mi'o-kin-ĕ-sim'ĕ-ter) [ myo- + G. *kinesis*, movement, + *metron*, measure ]. Myocinesimeter; a device for registering the exact time and extent of contraction of the larger muscles of the lower extremity in response to electric stimulation.

**myokymia** (mi'o-ki'mĭ-ah) [ myo- + G. *kyma*, wave ]. A benign condition, often familial, characterized by an irregular twitching of most of the muscles.
  **hereditary m.,** a syndrome consisting of m., hypoglycemia, and disturbed thyroid function.

**myolem'ma.** Sarcolemma.

**myolipo'ma.** A benign neoplasm that consists chiefly of fat cells (adipose tissue), with variable numbers of muscle cells forming portions of the neoplasm.

**myologia** (mi'o-lo'jĭ-ah) [ NA ]. Myology.

**myol'ogist.** One learned in the knowledge of muscles.

**myology** (mi-ol'o-jĭ) [ myo- + G. *logos*, study ]. The branch of science that deals with the muscles and their accessory parts, tendons, aponeuroses, bursae, and fasciae.
  **descriptive m.,** myography (2).

**myolysis** (mi-ol'ĭ-sis) [ myo- + G. *lysis*, dissolution ]. Dissolution or liquefaction of muscular tissue, frequently preceded by degenerative changes such as infiltration of fat, atrophy, fatty degeneration, hydropic degeneration, and so on.
  **cardiotox'ic m.,** cardiomalacia occurring in fever and various systemic infections.

**myoma** (mi-o'mah) [ myo- + G. suffix *-oma*, tumor ]. A benign neoplasm of muscular tissue; usually of smooth (nonstriated) type, *i.e.*, leiomyoma; that derived from striated muscle is termed rhabdomyoma.
  **m. levicellula're** [ L. *levis*, smooth ], leiomyoma.
  **m. prae'vium,** a muscular tumor obstructing the delivery of the child.
  **m. sarcomato'des,** a m. that seems to develop at an unusually rapid rate, eventually becoming malignant, *i.e.*, myosarcoma.
  **m. striocellula're** [ L. *stria*, a furrow ], rhabdomyoma.
  **m. telangiecto'des,** angiomyoma.

**myomalacia** (mi'o-mă-la'shĭ-ah) [ myo- + G. *malakia*, softness ]. Pathologic softening of muscular tissue.
  **m. cordis,** cardiomalacia.
  **Zenker's m. cordis,** softening of cardiac muscle, as the result of degenerative changes in the myocardium.

**myo'matous.** Pertaining to or characterized by the features of a myoma.

**myomectomy** (mi'o-mek'to-mĭ) [ myoma + G. *ektomē*, excision ]. Operative removal of a myoma, specifically of a uterine myoma.
  **abdominal m.,** celiomyomectomy; laparomyomectomy; removal of a myoma of the uterus through an abdominal incision.
  **vaginal m.,** colpomyomectomy; removal of a myoma of the uterus through the vagina.

**myomelanosis** (mi'o-mel'ă-no'sis) [ myo- + G. *melanōsis*, becoming black ]. Abnormal dark pigmentation of muscular tissue. See also melanosis.

**myomere** (mi'o-mēr) [ myo- + G. *meros*, a part ]. The muscular segment within a metamere.

**myom'eter** [ myo- + G. *metron*, measure ]. An instrument for measuring the extent of a muscular contraction.

**myometri'tis** [ myo- + G. *mētra*, uterus, + suffix *-itis*, inflammation ]. Inflammation of the muscular wall of the uterus.

**myometrium** (mi'o-me'trĭ-um) [ myo- + G. *mētra*, uterus ] [ NA ]. The muscular wall of the uterus.

**myomitochondrion**, pl. **myomitochondria** (mi'o-mi'-to-kon'dre-on). Sarcosome (2); a mitochondrion of a muscle fiber.

**myomotomy** (mi'o-mot'o-mĭ) [ myoma + G. *tomē*, incision ]. Incision into a myoma.

**myon** [ G. *mys*, muscle ]. An individual muscle.

**my'onecro'sis.** Necrosis of muscle.

**myoneme** (mi'o-nēm) [ myo- + G. *nēma*, thread ]. 1. A muscle fibril. 2. One of the contractile fibrils of certain protozoans; thought to function in an analogous fashion to metazoan muscle fibers.

**myoneural** (mi-o-nu'ral) [ myo- + G. *neuron*, nerve ]. Relating to both muscle and nerve; denoting specifically the synapse of the motor neuron with striated muscle fibers: myoneural junction or motor endplate. See also neuromuscular.

**myoneuralgia** (mi'o-nu-ral'jĭ-ah) [ myo- + G. *neuron*, nerve, + *algos*, pain ]. Myalgia.

 **postural m.,** muscle pain associated with cramped position, stress of standing with improper posture, etc.

**myoneurasthenia** (mi'o-nu-ras-the'nĭ-ah). The condition of muscular weakness associated with neurasthenia.

**myoneuroma** (mi'o-nu-ro'mah) [ myo- + *neuron*, nerve, + G. suffix *-oma*, tumor ]. A tumefaction consisting chiefly of abnormally proliferating Schwann cells, with variable numbers of muscle cells forming portions of the mass. M.'s are probably malformations, rather than true neoplasms.

**myon'osus** [ myo- + G. *nosos*, disease ]. Myopathy; any disease of muscular tissue.

**myonymy** (mi-on'ĭ-mĭ) [ myo- + G. *onyma* or *onoma*, name ]. Nomenclature of the muscles.

**myopachynsis** (mi-o-pă-kin'sis) [ myo- + G. *pachynsis*, a thickening ]. Muscular hypertrophy.

**myopal'mus** [ myo- + G. *palmos*, a quivering ]. Muscle twitching.

**myoparal'ysis.** Muscular paralysis.

**myoparesis** (mi'o-pă-re'sis, -păr'e-sis). Slight muscular paralysis.

**myopath'ic.** 1. Relating to disease of the muscles. 2. One suffering from disease of a muscle, especially the heart muscle or myocardium.

**myop'athy** [ myo- + G. *pathos*, suffering ]. Any abnormal condition or disease of the muscular tissues; commonly designates a disorder involving skeletal muscle.

 **carcinomatous m.,** Lambert-Eaton *syndrome*.

 **centronuclear m.,** myotubular m.; generalized muscle weakness and atrophy beginning in childhood, slowly progressive; on biopsy of skeletal muscle, the nuclei of most muscle fibers are seen to be located near the center of the fiber (the normal position for a 10-week embryo) rather than at the periphery of the fiber; familial incidence.

 **distal m.,** m. affecting predominantly the distal portions of the limbs; onset is usually after age 40, with weakness and wasting of small muscles of the hands; autosomal dominant inheritance.

 **mitochondrial m.,** weakness and hypotonia of muscles, primarily those of the neck, shoulder, and pelvic girdles, with onset in infancy or childhood; on biopsy, giant, bizarre mitochondria are seen located between muscle fibrils just beneath the sarcolemma.

 **myotubular m.,** centronuclear m.

 **nemaline m.** rod m.; congenital, nonprogressive muscle weakness that is most evident in the proximal muscles; named after the characteristic nemaline (threadlike) rods seen in the muscle cells composed of Z-band material.

 **ocular m.,** a specific type of progressive muscular dystrophy that begins with the gradual onset of ptosis and sequential involvement of the other extraocular muscles.

 **rod m.,** nemaline m.

 **thyrotoxic m.,** extreme muscular weakness in severe thyrotoxicosis affecting muscles of limbs and trunk as well as those used in speech and swallowing.

**myope** (mi'ōp). A nearsighted person; one suffering from myopia.

**myopericarditis** (mi-o-pĕr-ĭ-kar-di'tis) [ myo- + pericarditis ]. Inflammation of the muscular wall of the heart and of the enveloping pericardium.

**myoperitonitis** (mi'o-pĕr'ĭ-to-ni'tis). Inflammation of the parietal peritoneum with myositis of the abdominal wall.

**myophage** (mi'o-fāj) [ myo- + G. *phagein*, to eat ]. A phagocyte that ingests muscle cells or portions of such cells.

**my'ophone** [ myo- + G. *phōnē*, sound ]. An instrument to enable one to hear the murmur of muscular contractions.

**myopia** (mi-o'pĭ-ah) [ G. fr. *myo*, to shut, + *ōps*, eye ]. Shortsightedness; nearsightedness; a condition in which, in consequence of an error in refraction or of elongation of the globe of the eye, parallel rays are focused in front of the retina.

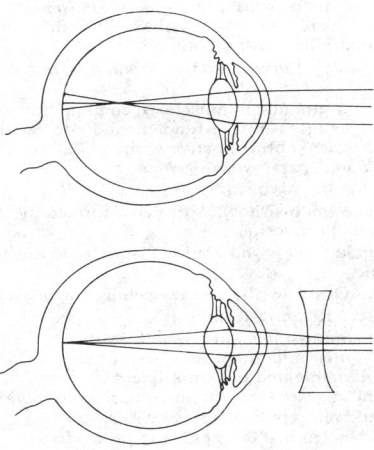

**Myopia**
 *Top*, diagram showing the course of parallel rays in unaided myopia; *bottom*, after correction by the concave lens indicated.

 **axial m.,** m. due to elongation of the globe of the eye.

 **chromic m.,** a form of color blindness in which colors can be recognized in objects near the eye, but cannot be distinguished at long distances.

 **curvature m.,** m. due to refractive errors consequent upon excessive corneal curvature.

 **index m.,** m. due to error of refraction consequent upon a variation in the index of refraction of the media of the eye.

 **pathologic m.,** progressive m. marked by fundus changes, posterior staphyloma, and subnormal corrected acuity.

 **prodromal m.,** second *sight*.

 **senile lenticular m.,** second *sight*.

**myopic** (mi-op'ik, -o'pik). Relating to or suffering from myopia.

**my'oplasm** [ myo- + G. *plasma*, a thing formed ]. The contractile portion of the muscle cell, as distinguished from the sarcoplasm.

**myoplas'tic.** Relating to the plastic surgery of the muscles, or to the use of muscular tissue in supplying defects.

**myoplasty** (mi'o-plas'tĭ) [ myo- + G. *plassō*, to form ]. Plastic surgery of muscular tissue.

**myopo'lar.** Relating to muscular polarity, or to the portion of muscle between two electrodes.

**my'opro'tein.** Protein occurring in muscle.

**myoproteose** (mi'o-pro'te-ōs). A protein in muscle plasma.

**myop'sis.** Myiodesopsia.

**myorhythmia** (mi'o-rith'mĭ-ah) [ myo- + G. *rhythmos,* rhythm ]. A form of hyperkinesia in which the tremor rate (2 to 4 per second) is irregular and slower than in alternating tremor, with greater frequency and higher voltage of the associated spike potentials in the electromyogram.

**myorrhaphy** (mi-or'ă-fĭ) [ myo- + G. *raphē,* seam ]. Suture of a wound in a muscle.

**myorrhexis** (mi'o-rek'sis) [ myo- + G. *rhēxis,* a rupture ]. Tearing of a muscle.

**myosalgia** (mi-o-sal'jĭ-ah). Myalgia.

**myosalpingitis** (mi'o-sal-pin-ji'tis) [ myosalpinx + G. suffix -*itis,* inflammation ]. Inflammation of the muscular tissue of the uterine tube.

**myosalpinx** (mi'o-sal'pingks) [ myo- + salpinx, *q.v.* ]. The muscular tunic of the uterine tube.

**myosarcoma** (mi'o-sar-ko'mah). A general term for a malignant neoplasm derived from muscular tissue, *i.e.,* leiomyosarcoma (from smooth or nonstriated muscle) and rhabdomyosarcoma (from striated muscle).

**myosclerosis** (mi'o-skle-ro'sis). Chronic myositis with hyperplasia of the interstitial connective tissue.

**myoseism** (mi'o-sīzm) [ myo- + G. *seismos,* a shaking, shock, fr. *seiō,* fut. *seisō,* to shake ]. Nonrhythmic spasmodic muscular contractions.

**myosep'tum** [ myo- + L. *saeptum,* a barrier ]. Myocomma.

**my'osin.** A globulin in muscle. In combination with actin, it forms actomyosin, the fundamental contractile unit of muscle (the myofibril), active with ATP.

    **Fürth's m.,** paramyosinogen.

**myosin'ogen.** Myogen.

**myosinose** (mi'o-sī-nōs). A proteose formed by the partial hydrolysis of myosin.

**myosinuria** (mi'o-sī-nu'rĭ-ah). The excretion of myosin in the urine.

**myo'sis.** Obsolete alternative spelling for miosis (2).

**myosit'ic.** Relating to myositis.

**myositis** (mi-o-si'tis) [ myo- + G. suffix -*itis,* inflammation ]. Myitis; inflammation of a muscle.

    **acute disseminated m.,** multiple m.

    **cervical m.,** see posttraumatic neck *syndrome.*

    **epidemic m.,** epidemic *pleurodynia.*

    **m. epidem'ica acu'ta,** epidemic *pleurodynia.*

    **m. fibro'sa,** myofascitis; interstitial m.; Froriep's induration; induration of a muscle through an interstitial growth of fibrous tissue.

    **infectious m.,** inflammation of the voluntary muscles, marked by swelling and pain, affecting usually the shoulders and arms, though almost the entire body may be involved.

    **interstitial m.,** m. fibrosa.

    **multiple m.,** acute disseminated m.; pseudotrichiniasis; pseudotrichinosis; dermatomyositis (*q.v.*); the occurrence of multiple foci of acute inflammation in the muscular tissue and overlying skin in various parts of the body, accompanied with fever and other signs of systemic infection.

    **m. ossif'icans,** ossification or deposit of bone in muscle.

    **m. ossif'icans circumscrip'ta,** local deposit of bone in a muscle, usually following prolonged trauma; *e.g.,* riders' bone.

    **m. ossif'icans progressi'va,** a rare disease, beginning in early life, characterized by progressive ossification of the muscles; it is not strictly a m., but a noninflammatory ossification.

    **m. purulen'ta trop'ica,** tropical myositis or pyomyositis; lambo lambo; bungpagga; a disease observed in Samoa and also in tropical Africa, marked by rheumatoid pains in the extremities, fever of a remittent or intermittent type, and abscesses in the muscles in various parts of the body. Death may result from pyemia. The causative organisms are *Staphylococcus aureus* and *Streptococcus pyogenes,* but the disease is usually associated with parasitic infections.

    **tropical m.,** m. purulenta tropica.

**my'ospasm, myospas'mus.** Spasmodic muscular contraction.

    **cervical m.,** see posttraumatic neck *syndrome.*

**myosthenometer** (mi'o-sthĕ-nom'e-ter) [ myo- + G. *sthenos,* strength, + *metron,* measure ]. An instrument for measuring the power of muscle groups.

**myostroma** (mi'o-stro'mah) [ myo- + G. *strōma,* mattres ]. The supporting connective tissue or framework of muscular tissue.

**myostro'min.** A protein found in muscle stroma.

**myosu'ria.** Myosinuria.

**myotac'tic** [ myo- + L. *tactus,* a touching ]. Relating to the muscular sense.

**myotasis** (mi-ot'ă-sis) [ myo- + G. *tasis,* a stretching ]. Stretching of a muscle.

**myotat'ic.** Relating to myotasis.

**myotenositis** (mi'o-ten'o-si'tis) [ myo- + G. *tenōn,* tendon, + suffix -*itis,* inflammation ]. Inflammation of a muscle with its tendon.

**myotenotomy** (mi'o-tĕ-not'o-mĭ) [ myo- + G. *tenōn,* tendon, + *tomē,* incision ]. Tenontomyotomy; tenomyotomy; cutting through the principal tendon of a muscle, with division of the muscle itself in whole or in part.

**myother'mic** [ myo- + G. *thermē,* heat ]. Relating to the increased temperature in muscular tissue resulting from its contraction.

**my'otome** [ myo- + G. *tomos,* a cut. TOM- ]. 1. A knife for dividing muscle. 2. Muscle plate; in embryos, that part of the somite that gives rise to skeletal muscle. 3. All muscles derived from one somite and innervated by one segmental spinal nerve. 4. In primitive vertebrates, the muscular part of a metamere.

**myotomy** (mi-ot'o-mĭ) [ myo- + G. *tomē,* excision ]. 1. Anatomy of the muscles; dissection of the muscles. 2. Surgical division of a muscle.

**my'otone.** Myotony.

**myoto'nia** [ myo- + G. *tonos,* tension, stretching. TEN- ]. Delayed relaxation of a muscle after an initial contraction.

    **m. acquis'ita,** Talma's disease; acquired m. following injury or disease.

    **m. atroph'ica,** myotonic *dystrophy.*

    **m. congen'ita,** Thomsen's disease; a hereditary disease marked by momentary tonic spasms occurring when a voluntary movement is attempted.

    **m. dystroph'ica,** myotonic *dystrophy.*

    **m. neonato'rum,** neonatal *tetany.*

**myoton'ic.** Pertaining to or exhibiting myotonia.

**myotonoid** (mi-ot'o-noyd) [ myo- + G. *tonos,* tone, tension, + *eidos,* resemblance ]. Denoting a muscular reaction, naturally or electrically excited, characterized by a slow (lazy) contraction and, especially, relaxation.

**myot'onus** [ myo- + G. *tonos,* tension, stretching ]. A tonic spasm or temporary rigidity of a muscle or group of muscles.

**myot'ony** [ myo- + G. *tonos,* tension ]. Myotone; muscular tonus or tension.

**myot'rophy** [ myo- + G. *trophē,* nourishment ]. Nutrition of muscular tissue.

**my'otube.** A skeletal muscle fiber during a developmental stage; a few myofibrils occur at the periphery and the central core is occupied by nuclei and sarcoplasm so that the fiber has a tubular appearance; it was formerly called a myotubule; however, the electron microscope shows smaller tubular elements.

**my'otu'bule.** Former term for myotube.

**myriachit** (mir-yah'chit) [ Kalmuk? ]. An affection similar to latah, observed in Siberia.

**myrica** (mĭr'ĭ-kah). Bayberry bark; the bark of *Myrica cerifera* (family Myricaceae); used in diarrhea and icterus and externally in sore throat.

**myricin** (mĭr'ĭ-sin). Myricyl palmitate, chief constituent of beeswax; white, almost odorless solid.

**myricyl** (mĭr'ĭ-sil). Melissyl; $CH_3(CH_2)_{29}$—; an alkyl radical occurring in the long chain esters of beeswax.

    **m. alcohol,** melissyl alcohol.

**myring-.** See myringo-.

**myringa** (mĭ-ring'gah) [ Mod. L. drum membrane ]. *Membrana* tympani.

**myringectomy** (mĭr-in-jek'to-mĭ) [ myring- + G. *ektomē,* excision ]. Excision of the tympanic membrane.

**myringitis** (mĭr-in-ji'tis) [ myring- + G. suffix *-itis*, inflammation ]. Tympanitis; inflammation of the tympanic membrane.

**m. bulbo'sa,** myringodermatitis.

**myringo-, myring-** (mĭ-ring'go-) [ Mod. L. *myringa, q. v.* ]. Combining forms relating to the membrana tympani.

**myringodectomy** (mĭ-ring'go-dek'to-mĭ). Myringectomy.

**myringodermatitis** (mĭ-ring'go-der-mă-ti'tis) [ myringo- + dermatitis ]. Myringitis bulbosa; inflammation of the meatal or outer surface of the drum membrane and the adjoining skin of the external auditory canal.

**myringomycosis** (mĭ-ring'go-mi-ko'sis). Mycomyringitis.

**myringoplasty** (mĭ-ring'go-plas'tĭ) [ myringo- + G. *plassō*, to form ]. Operative repair of a damaged tympanic membrane.

**myringostapediopexy** (mĭ-ring'go-sta-pe'dĭ-o-pek'sĭ) [ *myringo-* + L. *stapes*, stirrup (stapes), + G. *pēxis*, fixation ]. A technique of tympanoplasty in which the drum membrane or grafted drum membrane is brought into functional connection with the stapes.

**myringotome** (mĭ-ring'go-tōm) [ myringo- + G. *tomē*, excision ]. A knife used for paracentesis of the tympanic membrane.

**myringotomy** (mĭr-ing-got'o-mĭ) [ myringo- + G. *tomē*, excision ]. Paracentesis tympani; tympanotomy; incision of the tympanic membrane; paracentesis of the drum membrane.

**myrinx** (mi'ringks, mĭr'ringks) [ Mod. L. *myringa, q. v.* ]. *Membrana* tympani.

**myristica** (mĭ-ris'ti-kah) [ G. *myrizō*, to anoint, fr. *myron*, an unguent ]. Nutmeg.

**m. oil** (NF), nutmeg oil.

**myris'tic acid.** Tetradecanoic acid; $CH_3$—$(CH_2)_{12}$—COOH; a saturated fatty acid present as an acylglycerol in milk, vegetable fats, and cod liver oil.

**myris'ticin.** A constituent of nutmeg thought to be responsible, at least in part, for the bizarre central nervous system symptoms produced by the ingestion of large amounts of nutmeg.

**myristin** (mĭ-ris'tin). An acylglycerol of myristic acid occurring in nutmeg oil and other oils.

**myristoleic acid** (mĭ-ris'to-le'ik). 9-Tetradecenoic acid; a 14-carbon unsaturated fatty acid with a double bond between carbons 9 and 10.

**myrmecia** (mĭr-me'shĭ-ah) [ G. *murmex*, ant ]. Verruca simplex with epidermal cells containing inclusion bodies; the wart has the configuration of an ant hill.

**myro'sinase.** Thioglucosidase.

**myrrh** (mur) [ G. *myrrha* ]. A gum resin from *Commiphora molmol* and *C. phora abyssinica* (family Burseraceae) and other species of *C.,* a shrub of Arabia and Eastern Africa; used as an astringent, tonic, and stimulant, and locally for diseases of the oral cavity and in mouthwashes.

**myrtillin** (mur'til-lin). A galactoside present in leaves of the blueberry, *Vaccinium myrtillus* (family Ericaceae); lowers blood sugar and may cause hepatic injury.

**myrtle** (mur'tl) [ L. *myrtus*, the myrtle tree ]. The leaves of *Myrtus communis* (family Myrtaceae); used as an astringent in vesical and bronchial catarrhs.

**myrtol** (mur'tol). A distillate of the essential oil of myrtle; consists of eucalyptol and *d*-pinine; has been used in bronchitis, cystitis, and menorrhagia.

**mysophilia** (mi'so-fil'ĭ-ah) [ G. *mysos*, defilement, + *philos*, fond ]. A sexual interest in excretions.

**mysophobia** (mi-so-fo'bĭ-ah) [ G. *mysos*, defilement, + *phobos*, fear ]. A morbid fear of dirt or defilement from touching familiar objects.

**mytacism** (mi'tă-sizm) [ G. *my*, the letter μ ]. Mutacism; a form of stammering in which the letter *m* is frequently substituted for other consonants.

**mytatrienediol.** MANVENE; 3-methoxy-16-methyl-1,3,5(10)-estratriene-16β,17β-diol; an estrogen with hypolipemic properties.

**myurous** (mi-u'rus) [ G. *mys*, mouse, + *ouros*, tail ]. Gradually decreasing, as a mouse's tail, in thickness; rarely used term denoting certain symptoms in process of cessation, and also the heart beat in certain cases in which it grows feebler and feebler for a while and then strengthens.

**myx-.** See myxo-.

**myxadenitis** (miks'ad-e-ni'tis) [ myx- + G. *adēn*, gland, + suffix *-itis*, inflammation ]. Inflammation of the mucous glands.

**m. labia'lis,** *cheilitis* glandularis.

**myxadenoma** (miks-ad-e-no'mah). A benign neoplasm derived from glandular epithelial tissue, *i.e.,* an adenoma, in which the loose connective tissue of the stroma has a resemblance to relatively primitive mesenchymal tissue.

**myxangitis** (miks-an-ji'tis) [ myx- + G. *angeion*, vessel, + suffix *-itis*, inflammation ]. Inflammation of the ducts of the mucous glands.

**myxasthenia** (miks-as-the'nĭ-ah) [ myx- + G. *astheneia*, weakness ]. Faulty secretion of mucus.

**myxedema** (miks'e-de'mah) [ myx- + G. *oidema*, swelling ]. Gull's disease; hypothyroidism characterized by a relatively hard edema of subcutaneous tissue, dryness and loss of hair, subnormal temperature, hoarseness, muscle weakness, and slow return of a muscle after a tendon jerk to the neutral position; caused by removal or loss of functioning thyroid tissue.

**circumscribed m.,** pretibial m.; nodules and plaques of mucoid edema of the skin, usually in the pretibial region, occurring in some patients with hyperthyroidism.

**congenital m.,** cretinism.

**infantile m.,** m. beginning during infancy in consequence of some acquired injury of the thyroid gland or of the presence of cretinism.

**operative m.,** *cachexia* strumipriva.

**pituitary m.,** m. resulting from inadequate secretion of the thyrotropic hormone; commonly occurs in association with inadequate secretion of other anterior pituitary hormones.

**pretibial m.,** circumscribed m.

**myxedem'atoid.** Resembling myxedema.

**myxedem'atous.** Relating to myxedema.

**myxemia** (mik-se'mĭ-ah) [ myx- + G. *haima*, blood ]. Mucinemia.

**myxo-, myx-** (mik'so-) [ G. *myxa*, mucus ]. Combining forms relating to mucus.

**myxochondrofibrosarcoma** (mik'so-kon'dro-fi'-bro-sar-ko'ma) [ myxo- + G. *chondros*, cartilage, + L. *fibra*, fiber, + G. *sarx*, flesh, + suffix *-ōma*, tumor ]. A malignant neoplasm derived from fibrous connective tissue, *i.e.,* a fibrosarcoma, in which there are intimately associated foci of cartilaginous and myxomatous tissue.

**myxochondroma** (mik'so-kon-dro'mah) [ myxo- + G. *chondros*, cartilage, + suffix *-oma*, tumor ]. Myxoma enchondromatosum; a benign neoplasm of cartilaginous tissue, *i.e.,* a chondroma, in which the stroma has a resemblance to relatively primitive mesenchymal tissue.

**Myxococcid'ium stegomy'iae.** A protozoon once found in the body of the mosquito, *Stegomyia calopus,* that had fed on the blood of a patient with yellow fever; the organism was then postulated, incorrectly, to be the causal agent of yellow fever.

**myxocystoma** (mik'so-sis-to'mah) [ myxo- + G. *kystis,* bladder, + suffix *-ōma,* tumor ]. Myxoid cystoma; any benign cystic neoplasm in which the cysts are lined with epithelium and contain a relatively viscid mucoid material.

**myxocyte** (miks'o-sīt) [ myxo- + G. *kytos,* cell ]. One of the stellate or polyhedral cells present in mucous tissue.

**myxoder'mia** [ myxo- + G. *derma,* skin ]. Edematous softening of the skin.

**myxofibro'ma** [ myxo- + L. *fibra,* fiber, + G. suffix *-ōma,* tumor ]. Fibroma myxomatodes; myxoma fibrosum; a benign neoplasm of fibrous connective tissue in which focal or diffuse degenerative changes result in portions that resemble primitive mesenchymal tissue.

**myxofibrosarcoma** (mik'so-fi'bro-sar-ko'mah) [ myxo- + L. *fibra,* fiber, + G. *sarx,* flesh, + suffix *-ōma,* tumor ]. A malignant neoplasm of fibrous connective tissue, *i.e.,* fibrosarcoma, in which (1) focal or diffuse degenerative changes or (2) growth of less differentiated anaplastic cells results in portions that resemble primitive mesenchymal tissue.

**myxoglobulosis** (mik'so-glob-u-lo'sis) [ myxo- + L. *globulus,* globule, + G. suffix *-osis,* condition ]. The presence of mucous cysts in the appendix.

**myx'oid** [ myxo- + G. *eidos*, resemblance ]. Mucoid; resembling mucus.

**myxoidedema** (mik'soyd-e-de'mah). A severe coryza.

**myxoinoma** (mik'so-ĭ-no'mah) [ myxo- + G. *is*(*in*-), fiber, + suffix -*ōma*, tumor ]. Obsolete term for myxofibroma.

**myx'olip'ofi'brosarco'ma.** An undesirable term for malignant *mesenchymoma*, indicating the multiple differentiated cell types present.

**myxolipo'ma** [ myxo- + G. *lipos*, fat, + suffix -*ōma*, tumor ]. Lipoma myxomatodes; myxoma lipomatosum; a benign neoplasm of adipose tissue, *i.e.*, lipoma, in which focal or diffuse degenerative changes result in portions that resemble mucoid mesenchymal tissue.

**myxoma** (mik-so'mah) [ myxo- + G. suffix -*ōma*, tumor ]. A neoplasm derived from connective tissue, consisting chiefly of polyhedral and stellate cells that are loosely embedded in a soft, mucoid matrix, thereby resembling primitive mesenchymal tissue.

  **atrial m.,** a primary cardiac neoplasm arising most commonly in the left atrium; it may resemble an organized mural thrombus, and the symptoms may include cardiac murmurs that change with alteration of body position.

  **m. enchondromato'sum,** myxochondroma.

  **m. fibro'sum,** myxofibroma.

  **m. lipomato'sum,** myxolipoma.

  **m. sarcomato'sum,** myxosarcoma.

**myxomatosis** (mik'so-mă-to'sis). 1. A fatal disease of rabbits marked by edema and swelling of the mucous membranes and the development of myxomatous growths of mucous membranes and skin; due to a virus. 2. Myxomatous degeneration. 3. Multiple myxomas.

  **infectious m.,** a highly contagious and almost invariably fatal disease of domesticated rabbits and European hares, caused by a virus, and characterized by gelatinous tumors in all parts of the body. The disease is transmitted by mosquitoes. It has been used successfully to reduce the wild hare population of certain areas of Australia.

**myxo'matous.** 1. Pertaining to or characterized by the features of a myxoma. 2. Said of tissue that resembles primitive mesenchymal tissue.

**myxomycetes** (mik'so-mi-se'tēz) [ myxo- + G. *mykēs*, fungus ]. The slime molds or slime fungi; saprophytic fungi that occur on rotting vegetation.

**myxoneuroma** (mik'so-nu-ro'mah) [ myxo- + G. *neuron*, nerve, + suffix -*ōma*, tumor ]. 1. A tumefaction resulting from abnormal proliferation of Schwann cells, in which focal or diffuse degenerative changes result in portions that resemble primitive mesenchymal tissue. 2. Obsolete term for a neurilemoma, meningioma, or glioma in which the stroma is myxomatous in nature.

**myxopapilloma** (mik'so-pap-ĭ-lo'mah) [ myxo- + L. *papilla*, a nipple, + G. suffix -*ōma*, tumor ]. A benign neoplasm of epithelial tissue, *i.e.*, papilloma, in which the stroma resembles primitive mesenchymal tissue.

**myxopoiesis** (mik'so-poy-e'sis) [ myxo- + G. *poiēsis*, a making ]. Mucus production.

**myxorrhea** (mik'so-re'ah) [ myxo- + G. *rhoia*, a flow ]. Blennorrhea.

  **m. gas'trica,** gastromyxorrhea.

**myxosarco'ma** [ myxo- + G. *sarx*, flesh, + suffix -*ōma*, tumor ]. Myxoma sarcomatosum; a malignant neoplasm derived from connective tissue elements, *i.e.*, sarcoma; characterized by immature, relatively undifferentiated, and primitive cells that are polyhedral or stellate in shape, and contain bizarre, hyperchromatic nuclei; the anaplastic cells grow rapidly and invade extensively, resulting in tissue that resembles primitive mesenchyme in its gross features.

**myx'ospore** [ myxo- + G. *sporos*, seed ]. One of a number of spores occurring embedded in a gelatinous mass, noted in certain fungi and protozoan organisms.

**Myxosporidia** (mik'so-spo-rid'ĭ-ah). An order of Cnidosporidia with pansporoblastic reproduction, the spores having polar capsules containing threads; a number of the members of this order are parasitic in metazoan organisms, both vertebrate and invertebrate.

**myx'ovirus.** See under virus.

**myze'sis** [ G. *myzeō*, to suck ]. Sucking.

# N

ν. Greek nu; symbol for kinematic *viscosity*.

**N.** 1. Chemical symbol of the element nitrogen. 2. Designation for an inherited blood factor; see MNSs blood group, in appendix 2.

N. Chemical abbreviation for normal concentration; see normal (3).

**n.** Abbreviation for (1) nasal; (2) nano-.

**N.A.** Abbreviation for numerical *aperture*.

**NA.** Abbreviation for *Nomina Anatomica*.

**Na.** Chemical symbol for the element sodium (natrium).

**Naboth** (nah'bōt), Martin, Leipzig anatomist and physician, 1675–1721. See Nabothian *cyst, follicle, gland*.

**nacreous** (na'kre-us) [ Fr. *nacre*, mother-of-pearl ]. Iridescent; lustrous; like mother-of-pearl.

**N.A.D.** Abbreviation for (1) no appreciable disease; (2) nothing abnormal detected (British usage).

**NAD.** Abbreviation for nicotinamide adenine dinucleotide.

**NAD+.** Abbreviation for nicotinamide adenine dinucleotide (oxidized form).

**NADH.** Abbreviation for nicotinamide adenine dinucleotide (reduced form).

**NADH dehydrogenase** (EC 1.6.99.3). Cytochrome *c* reductase; an iron-containing flavoprotein oxidizing NADH to NAD+.

**NADH dehydrogenase (quinone).** Enzyme (EC 1.6.99.5) oxidizing NADH with quinones (*e.g.*, menaquinone) as acceptors.

**NADH-hydroxylamine reductase** (EC 1.6.6.11). Enzyme reducing hydroxylamine to ammonia with NADH as hydrogen donor.

**nadide** (USAN). ENZOPRIDE; 3-carbamoyl-1-β-D-ribofuranosylpyridinium hydroxide; a narcotic antagonist.

**Nadi reaction.** See under reaction.

**NAD nucleosidase** (EC 3.2.2.5). See nucleosidases.

**NADP.** Abbreviation for nicotinamide adenine dinucleotide phosphate.

**NADP+.** Abbreviation for nicotinamide adenine dinucleotide phosphate (oxidized form).

**NADPH.** Abbreviation for nicotinamide adenine dinucleotide phosphate (reduced form).

**NADPH dehydrogenase** (EC 1.6.99.1). "Old yellow enzyme"; Warburg's "old yellow enzyme"; a flavoprotein (FMN) oxidizing NADPH to NADP+.

**NADPH dehydrogenase (quinone)** (EC 1.6.99.6). A flavoprotein similar to NADH dehydrogenase (quinone), but oxidizing NADPH.

**NAD(P)H dehydrogenase (quinone)** (EC 1.6.99.2). Menadione reductase; quinone reductase; phylloquinone reductase; DT-diaphorase; a flavoprotein oxidizing NADH or NADPH to NAD+ or NADP+ with quinones (*e.g.*, menadione) as hydrogen acceptors.

**NAD(P) nucleosidase** (EC 3.2.2.6). See nucleosidases.

**Naegeli,** Otto, Swiss physician, 1871–1938. See N. type of monocytic *leukemia*.

**naepaine hydrochloride** (ne'pān). AMYLSINE hydrochloride; 2-amylaminoethyl-*p*-aminobenzoate hydrochloride; a local (topical) anesthetic.

**nafcillin** (naf'sil'in). 6-(2-Ethoxy-1-naphthamido)penicillin; a semisynthetic penicillin derived from 6-aminopenicillanic acid; resistant to penicillinase, and effective against *Staphylococcus aureus*.

**n. sodium** (USP), UNIPEN; a penicillinase-resistant penicillin.

**Naff'ziger,** Howard C., San Francisco surgeon, 1884–1961. See N. *operation, syndrome*.

**nafiverine.** NAFTIDAN; 1,4-piperazinediethanol bis(α-methyl-1-naphthaleneacetate; intestinal antispasmodic.

**naf'ronyl oxalate** (USAN). DUSODRIL; 2-(diethylamino)-ethyl tetrahydro-α-(1-naphthylmethyl)-2-furanpropionate oxalate; a vasodilator drug.

**naf'talos** (USAN). MARETIN; *N*-hydroxynaphthalimide diethyl phosphate; veterinary anthelmintic.

**nagana** (nah-gah'nah). An acute or chronic disease of cattle, dogs, pigs, horses, sheep, goats, and many wild animals in tropical and South Africa; it is marked by fever, anemia, and cachexia, varying in severity with the strain and the host. The name is a collective term for infections with *Trypanosoma brucei, T. congolense*, and *T. vivax*.

**nagarse.** A proteinase elaborated by *Bacillus subtilis*.

**Nagel** (nah'gel), Willibald, A., German ophthalmologist and physiologist, 1870–1911. See N.'s *photometer, test*.

**Nägele** (na'gel-e), Franz K., German obstetrician, 1777–1851. See N.'s *obliquity, pelvis, rule*.

**Nageotte** (naj-ot'), Jean, French histologist, 1866–1948. See N. *cells*.

**nail** [ A.S. *naegel* ]. 1. Unguis. 2. A slender rod of metal, bone, or other solid substance, used sometimes in surgery to fasten together the divided extremities of a broken bone.

   **egg shell n.,** a thinning of the n. with separation from the matrix and upcurving at the anterior border.

   **Hippocratic n.'s,** the coarse, curved n.'s capping the Hippocratic fingers.

   **ingrown n.,** ingrowing toenail; acronyx; onychocryptosis; onyxis; unguis aductus; unguis incarnatus; a toenail, one edge of which is overgrown by the nailfold, producing a pyogenic granuloma; due to faulty trimming of the toenails or pressure from a tight shoe.

   **Küntscher n.,** a n. used for internal fixation of a fracture.

   **parrot-beak n.,** a markedly curved fingernail.

   **racket n.,** broad, flat thumbnail of unknown origin.

   **reedy n.,** one marked by longitudinal ridges and furrows.

   **Smith-Petersen n.,** a flanged n. for pinning a fracture of the neck of the femur.

   **spoon n.,** koilonychia.

**nailbed.** *matrix* unguis.

**nail'ing.** Act of holding ends of fractured bone with a nail.

**Naja** (nah'jah) [ Hind. *nāg*, a snake ]. A genus of highly venomous serpents (family Elapidae), the cobras.

**Nakanishi** (nah-kah-nish'e), K., Japanese physician. See N.'s *method*.

**nal'buphine hydrochloride** (USAN). 17-(Cyclobutylmethyl)-4,5α-apoxymorphinan-3,6α,14-triol hydrochloride; narcotic antagonist with analgesic activity.

**nal'idix'ic acid** (NF). NEGGRAM; 1-ethyl-1,4-dihydro-7-methyl-4-oxo-1,8-naphthyridine-3-carboxylic acid; an orally effective antibacterial agent used in the treatment of genitourinary tract infections; effective against *Escherichia coli* and several species of *Proteus*. A high degree of resistance can rapidly develop.

**nalorphine** (nal'or-fēn, nal-or'fēn). NALLINE; *N*-allylnormorphine; $C_{19}H_{21}NO_3$; antagonizes most of the depressant and stimulatory effects of morphine and related narcotic analgesics. Precipitates severe withdrawal symptoms in morphine addicts. Used in the diagnosis of suspected morphine addiction and to counteract the respiratory depression produced by morphine and related compounds. Available as n. hydrobromide (BP) and n. hydrochloride.

**nalox'one hydrochloride** (USP). NARCAN; 1-*N*-allyl-7,8-dihydro-14-hydroxymorphinone hydrochloride; a potent antagonist of all narcotics, including pentazocine; unique because of absence of pharmacological action when administered without narcotics.

**nan'drolone.** 17β-Hydroxy-4-estrene-3-one (for estrene structure, see steroids); a semisynthetic, parenterally administered, anabolic steroid that may promote nitrogen retention when combined with an adequate diet; in addition, it can exert typically androgenic effects.

   **n. decanoate** (NF, BP), DECA-DURABOLIN; an anabolic androgen.

   **n. phenpropionate** (NF), DURABOLIN; n. phenylpropionate; a moderately long-acting synthetic anabolic androgen; used in preparing patients for surgery and for patients recovering from surgery, burns, fracture, infection, and trauma.

   **n. phenylpropionate** (BP), n. phenpropionate.

**nan'ism** [ G. *nanos*; L. *nanus*, dwarf ]. Dwarfism.

   **Paltauf's n.,** lymphatic *infantilism*.

**pituitary n.,** pituitary *dwarfism.*

**symptomatic n.,** n. associated with delayed and deficient ossification, dentition, and sexual development; an obscure and obsolete phrase that could refer to n. arising from various causes.

**nano-** (nan-o-, na'no-) [ G. *nānos,* dwarf ]. 1. Combining form relating to dwarfism (nanism). 2. A prefix used in the metric system to signify one-billionth ($10^{-9}$) of any unit; equivalent of millimicro-.

**nanocephalia** (nan'o-sĕ-fa'lĭ-ah). Nanocephaly.

**nanocephalous, nanocephalic** (nan'o-sef'ă-lus, -se-fal'ik). Having a very small head.

**nanoceph'alus.** An individual with nanocephaly.

**nanocephaly** (nan'o-sef'ă-lĭ) [ nano- + G. *kephale,* head ]. Nanocephalia; a condition in which the head is very small or imperfectly developed.

**nanocormia** (nan'o-kor'mĭ-ah) [ nano- + G. *kormos,* trunk ]. Extreme smallness of the body compared with the head and extremities.

**nanocor'mus.** An individual with nanocormia.

**na'nogram.** A billionth of a gram; $10^{-9}$ gram.

**nan'oid** [ nano- + G. *eidos,* resemblance ]. 1. Dwarfish. 2. A pygmy.

**nanome'lia** [ nano- + G. *melos,* limb ]. Extreme smallness of the extremities.

**nanomelous** (nă-nom'e-lus). Having very small extremities.

**nanomelus** (nă-nom'e-lus). A fetus with disproportionately small or undeveloped extremities.

**nanom'eter.** One billionth of a meter, $10^{-9}$ meter; abbreviated nm.

**nanophthalmia, nanophthalmos** (nan'of-thal'mĭ-ah, -mos) [ nano- + G. *ophthalmos,* eye ]. Microphthalmia.

**nan'ophthal'mus.** Microphthalmus.

**Nano'phyetes salmin'cola.** *Troglotrema salmincola;* a digenetic fish-borne fluke (family Nanophyetidae) of dogs and other fish-eating mammals. Dogs ingesting fish (especially salmon or other members of the trout family) infected with the metacercariae of this fluke may, in turn, acquire from them *Neorickettsia helmintheca,* the agent of salmon poisoning.

**nanoso'ma, nanoso'mia** [ nano- + G. *sōma,* body ]. Dwarfism.

**n. essentia'lis,** physiologic dwarfism; see physiologic *dwarf.*

**n. infan'tilis,** obsolete term for pituitary *infantilism.*

**nanoso'mus.** A dwarf.

**na'nous.** Dwarfish.

**nanukayami** (nah-noo-kah-yah'mĭ). Seven-day fever of Japan. Like autumn fever, it occurs in the fall, but is caused by *Leptospira hebdomadis.*

**na'nus** [ L.; G. *nanos* ]. 1. A dwarf. 2. A pigmy.

**NAP.** Abbreviation for *Nomina Anatomica Parisiensia.*

**na'palm.** A gasoline gel incendiary agent, prepared by adding naphthenate and palmitate to gasoline.

**nape.** Nucha.

**nap'elline.** An alkaloid (or a mixture of several compounds) from the root of *Aconitum napellus,* possibly identical with aconine.

**na'pex.** The area of the scalp just below the occipital protuberence.

**naphaz'oline hydrochloride** (USP). PRIVINE hydrochloride; naphthazoline hydrochloride; 2-(1-naphthylmethyl)-2-imidazoline hydrochloride; a sympathomimetic amine; used as a topical vasoconstrictor. Naphazoline nitrate, with same uses, is also available (BP).

**naphtha** (naf'thah) [ G. See NAPH- ]. Petroleum benzin. **wood n.,** methyl alcohol.

**naphthalene** (naf'thă-lēn). Tar camphor; naphthalin; a hydrocarbon obtained from coal tar; used for many purposes in industry and is also used in some moth repellents. It is carcinogenic, causing bladder tumors in industrial workers, and is toxic.

**naphthalin** (naf'thă-lin). Naphthalene.

**naphthanthracene** (naf-than'thră-sēn). Benzanthrene.

**naphthaz'oline** (BP). Naphazoline.

**naphthol** (naf'thol). A phenol of naphthalene; $C_{10}H_7OH.$

**n. yellow S,** an acid dye, $C_{10}H_4N_2O_8SNa_2,$ used as a stain for microspectrophotometry of basic proteins.

**α-naphthol.** 1-Naphthol; 1-hydroxynaphthalene; used in microscopy.

**β-naphthol.** Betanaphthol; isonaphthol; 2-naphthol; 2-hydroxynaphthalene; a phenol occurring in coal tar and also prepared from naphthalene. Formerly used as an intestinal antiseptic, and externally for scabies, eczema, and other skin diseases.

**naph'tholate.** A compound of naphthol in which the hydrogen in the hydroxyl radical is substituted by a base.

**naphthoquinone** (naf'tho-kwin'ōn). A quinone derivative of naphthalene; either 1,4-naphthoquinone, derivatives of which have vitamin K activity (see menaquinone), or 1,2-naphthoquinone; reducible to naphthohydroquinone.

$$\text{O} \quad \underset{-2H}{\overset{+2H}{\rightleftharpoons}} \quad \text{OH}$$

1, 4-Naphthoquinone

**naphthyl** (naf'thil). The radical of naphthalene, $C_{10}H_7.$

**α-naph'thylthiourea'a.** ANTU; 1-(1-naphthyl)-2-thiourea; a derivative of thiourea; a highly toxic antithyroid agent, especially to small mammals, causing pulmonary edema, fatty degeneration of the liver, and low body temperature. Used as a rat poison.

**Napier's aldehyde test.** See under test.

**naprapathy** (nă-prap'ă-thĭ) [ Bohemian *napravit,* to correct, + G. *pathos,* suffering ]. A system of therapeutic manipulation based on the theory that morbid symptoms are dependent upon strained or contracted ligaments in the spine, thorax, or pelvis.

**nap'sylate.** USAN-approved contraction for 2-naphthalenesulfonate.

**Narath,** Albert, Utrecht surgeon, 1864–1924. See N.'s *operation.*

**narceine** (nar'se-ēn). An alkaloid of opium; $C_{23}H_{27}NO_8.$ Ethylnarceine is a narcotic, analgesic, and antitussive.

**narcism** (nar'sizm). Narcissism.

**narcissine** (nar-sis'ēn). Lycorine; amarylline; belamarine; an alkaloid prepared from the bulb of the daffodil, *Narcissus pseudonarcissus.* Emetic and cathartic.

**narcissism** (nar-sis'izm, nar'sĭ-sizm) [ G. *Narkissos,* the son of a river god who conceived a consuming passion for the reflection of himself which he saw in a fountain ]. 1. Self-love; autosexualism; autophilia; sexual attraction toward one's own person. 2. A state in which the individual regards everything in relation to himself and not to other persons or things.

**primary n.,** in psychoanalysis, the original psychic energy embodied or invested in the ego.

**secondary n.,** in psychoanalysis, the psychic energy, once attached to external objects, now withdrawn from those objects and reinvested in the ego.

**narco-** (nar'ko-) [ G. *narkoun,* to benumb, deaden ]. Combining form relating to stupor or narcosis.

**narcoanal'ysis.** Narcosynthesis; psychotherapeutic treatment under light anesthesia, originally used in acute combat cases during World War II. See also narcotherapy.

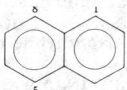

**Naphthalene**

**narcohypnia** (nar-ko-hip′nĭ-ah) [ narco- + G. *hypnos*, sleep ]. A general numbness sometimes experienced at the moment of waking.

**narcohypnosis** (nar-ko-hip-no′sis) [ narco- + G. *hypnos*, sleep ]. Stupor or deep sleep induced by hypnosis.

**nar′colepsy** [ narco- + G. *lēpsis*, seizure ]. Sleep epilepsy; paroxysmal sleep; hypnolepsy; Friedmann's disease; Gélineau's syndrome; a sudden uncontrollable disposition to sleep occurring at irregular intervals, with or without obvious predisposing or exciting cause, usually involving an abnormality in sleep-stage sequencing.

**narcomania** (nar′ko-ma′nĭ-ah) [ narco- + G. *mania*, frenzy ]. 1. A craving for narcotics. 2. Insanity resulting from narcotic addiction.

**narcomaniac** (nar′ko-ma′nĭ-ak). A subject of narcomania.

**narcosis** (nar-ko′sis) [ G. a benumbing, fr. *narkoō*, to benumb, fr. *narkē*, numbness ]. General and nonspecific reversible depression of neuronal excitability, produced by a number of physical and chemical agents, usually resulting in stupor rather than in anesthesia. The use of the term narcosis as a synonym for anesthesia is obsolescent.

nitrogen n., (1) n. produced by nitrogenous materials such as occurs in certain forms of uremia and hepatic coma; (2) the stuporous condition characterized by loss of judgment and skill attributed to an increased pressure of nitrogen as occurs with divers breathing air during underwater operations; commonly referred to as "rapture of the deep."

**narcosyn′thesis.** Narcoanalysis.

**narcother′apy.** Psychotherapy conducted with the patient under the influence of a sedative or narcotic drug, such as Pentothal sodium.

**narcot′ic** [ G. *narkōtikos*, benumbing ]. 1. Nonspecifically, any substance producing stupor associated with analgesia. 2. Specifically, a drug derived from opium or opium-like compounds, with potent analgesic effects associated with significant alteration of mood and behavior, and with the potential for dependence and tolerance following repeated administration. 3. Capable of inducing a state of stuporous analgesia.

*dl*-**nar′cotine.** Gnoscopine.

*l*-α-**nar′cotine.** Noscapine.

**nar′cotism.** 1. Stupor induced by a narcotic drug. 2. Addiction to narcotics.

**nar′cotize.** To bring under the influence of a narcotic.

**na′ris,** gen. sing. **narium,** pl. **nares** [ L. ] [ NA ]. Nostril; the anterior opening, on either side of the nasal cavity.
anterior n., n.
posterior n., choana.

**nasal** (na′zal) [ L. *nasus*, nose ]. Rhinal; relating to the nose.

**nascent** (nas′ent, na′sent) [ L. *nascor*, pres. p. *nascens*, to be born ]. 1. Beginning; being born or produced. 2. Denoting the state of a chemical element at the moment it is set free from one of its compounds.

**Nas′ik vi′brio.** See under vibrio.

**nasioiniac** (na′zĭ-o-in′ĭ-ak). Relating to the nasion and the inion; denoting the distance in a straight line between the frontonasal suture and the external occipital protuberance.

**nasion** (na′zĭ-on) [ L. *nasus*, nose ]. A point on the skull corresponding to the middle of the nasofrontal suture. See fig. under craniometric *points*.

**Nas′myth,** Alexander, London dentist, †1847. See N.'s *cuticle, membrane*.

**naso-** (na′zo-) [ L. *nasus*, nose ]. Combining form relating to the nose.

**nasoantral** (na′zo-an′tral). Relating to the nose and the maxillary sinus.

**nasociliary** (na′zo-sil′ĭ-ĕr-ĭ). See *nervus* nasociliaris.

**nasofrontal** (na′zo-frun′tal). Relating to the nose and the forehead, or to the nasal cavity and the frontal sinuses.

**nasolabial** (na′zo-la-bī′al) [ naso- + G. *labium*, lip ]. Relating to the nose and the upper lip.

**nasolacrimal** (na′zo-lak′rĭ-mal). Relating to the nasal and the lacrimal bones, or to the nasal cavity and the lacrimal ducts.

**naso-oral** (na′zo-o′ral). Relating to the nose and the mouth.

**nasopalatine** (na′zo-pal′ă-tīn, -tin). Relating to the nose and the palate.

**nasopharyngeal** (na′zo-fă-rin′je-al). Rhinopharyngeal; relating to the nose or the nasal cavity and the pharynx or to the rhinopharynx or nasopharynx.

**nasopharyngitis** (na′zo-făr-in-ji′tis). Rhinopharyngitis.

**nasopharyngoscope** (na′zo-fă-ring′go-skōp). Telescopic instrument, electrically lighted, for examination of the nasal passages and the nasopharynx.

**nasopharynx** (na′zo-făr′ingks). *Pars* nasalis pharyngis.

**nasorostral** (na′zo-ros′tral). Relating to the nasal cavity and the rostrum of the sphenoid bone.

**nasoscope** (na′zo-skōp). Rhinoscope.

**nasosinusitis** (na′zo-si-nus-i′tis). Inflammation of the nasal cavities and of the accessory sinuses.

**na′sus** [ L. ] [ NA ]. The nose. 1. *Nasus externus*. 2. The portion of the respiratory pathway above the hard palate; it includes both the nasus externus and the cavum nasi.
n. exter′nus [ NA ], external nose; the visible portion of the nose which forms a prominent feature of the face; it consists of a root, dorsum and apex from above downward and is perforated inferiorly by the two nostrils separated by the septum.

**na′tal.** 1 [ L. *natalis*, fr. *nascor*, pp. *natus*, to be born ]. Relating to birth. 2 [ L. *nates*, buttocks ]. Relating to the buttocks or nates.

**natal′ity** [ see natal ]. The birth rate; the ratio of births to the general population.

**nates** (na′tēz) [ L. pl. of *natis* ] [ NA ]. The buttocks; the prominence formed by the gluteal muscles on either side.

**natimortality** (na′tĭ-mor-tal′ĭ-tĭ) [ L. *natus*, birth ]. Mortinatality; the perinatal death rate; the proportion of fetal and neonatal deaths to the general natality.

**National Formulary.** An official compendium issued by the American Pharmaceutical Association for the purpose of providing standards and specifications which can be used to evaluate the quality of pharmaceuticals and therapeutic agents; abbreviated NF.

**Nativelle** (nat-e-vel′), Adolphe, French pharmacist, 19th century. See N.'s *digitalin*.

**natremia, natriemia** (na-tre′mĭ-ah, na′trī-e′mĭ-ah) [ natrium, *q.v.*, sodium, + G. *haima*, blood ]. The presence of sodium in the blood.

**na′trium** [ Ar. *natrūm*, fr. G. *nitron*, carbonate of soda. NITR- ]. Sodium.

**natriuresis** (na′trī-u-re′sis) [ natrium, *q.v.*, + G. *ouron*, urine ]. Urinary excretion of sodium; commonly designates enhanced sodium excretion, which may occur in certain diseases or as a result of the administration of diuretic drugs.

**na′triuret′ic.** 1. Pertaining to or characterized by natriuresis. 2. A chemical compound that may be used as a means of retarding the tubular reabsorption of sodium ions from glomerular filtrate, thereby resulting in greater amounts of that ion in the urine.

**na′tron.** A native hydrous sodium carbonate.

**na′turopath.** One who practises naturopathy exclusively.

**na′turopath′ic.** Relating to or by means of naturopathy.

**na′turop′athy** [ see PATH- ]. A system of therapeutics in which neither surgical nor medicinal agents are used, dependence being placed only on natural (nonmedicinal) forces.

**na′tus** [ L. ] [ NA ]. Natal.

**Nauheim treatment** (now′hīm) [ *Nauheim*, Germany ]. See under treatment.

**naupathia** (naw-path′ĭ-ah) [ G. *naus*, ship, + *pathos*, suffering ]. Seasickness.

**nausea** (naw′ze-ah, naw′zhah) [ L. fr. G. *nausia*, seasickness, fr. *naus*, ship ]. Sickness at the stomach; an inclination to vomit.
epidemic n., epidemic *vomiting*.
n. gravida′rum [ L. gen. pl. of *gravida*, a pregnant woman ], the morning sickness of pregnant women.

**nauseant** (naw′ze-ant). 1. Nauseating; causing nausea. 2. An agent that causes nausea.

**nauseate** (naw′ze-āt). To make sick at the stomach.

**nauseated** (naw′ze-a′ted). Affected with nausea.

**nauseous** (naw'ze-us, naw'shus). Causing nausea.

**na'vel** [ A.S. *nafela* ]. Umbilicus.

**navicula** (nă-vik'u-lah) [ L. dim of *navis,* ship ]. A small boat-shaped structure.

**navicular** (nă-vik'u-lar) [ L. *navicularis,* relating to shipping ]. Boat-shaped; scaphoid.

**naviculararthritis** (nă-vik'u-lar-thri'tis) [ navicular + arthritis ]. Navicular *disease.*

**Nb.** Chemical symbol of the element niobium.

**Nd.** Chemical symbol of the element neodymium.

**Ne.** Chemical symbol of the element neon.

**nealbarbitone** (ne'al-bar'bĭ-tōn) (BP). NEVENTAL; CENSEDAL; 5-allyl-5-neopentylbarbituric acid; sedative and hypnotic.

**near'sight'edness.** Myopia.

**nearthrosis** (ne-ar-thro'sis) [ G. *neos,* new, + *arthrōsis,* a jointing ]. Pseudarthrosis.

**nebramy'cin** (USAN). A complex of substances produced by *Streptomyces tenebrarius;* antibacterial.

**nebula,** pl. **neb'ulae** (neb'u-lah) [ L. fog, cloud, mist. NEB- ]. 1. A faint, foglike opacity of the cornea. 2. A class of oily preparations, intended for application by atomization; see spray.

**nebularine** (neb'u-lăr'in). Ribosylpurine; purine ribonucleoside; a slightly toxic nucleoside isolated from the mushroom *Agaricus nebularis.*

**nebulization** (neb'u-lĭ-za'shun) [ L. *nebula,* mist ]. Spraying; vaporization.

**nebulize** (neb'u-līz) [ L. *nebula,* mist ]. To break up a liquid into a fine spray or vapor; to vaporize.

**neb'uli'zer.** An atomizer; a vaporizer; an apparatus for throwing a liquid in the form of a fine spray or vapor.

**jet n.,** an atomizer that uses the gas stream to break the liquid into small particles.

**spinning disk n.,** a n. in which water is broken up into small particles as it is thrown from a spinning disk by centrifugal force.

**ultrasonic n.,** a humidifier using high-frequency electric power to energize a transducer that vibrates 1,350,000 times per second and breaks water up into particles of 0.5 to 3 $\mu$ in size in its nebulizing chamber; used in inhalation therapy.

**Necator** (ne-ka'tor) [ L. a murderer ]. A genus of nematode hookworms (family Ancylostomatidae, subfamily Necatorine) distinguished by two chitinous cutting plates in the buccal cavity and fused male copulatory spicules.

**N. america'nus,** the so-called New World hookworm, although also prevalent in the tropics of Central and South Africa, southern Asia, and Polynesia; the filariform larvae enter the venules of the dermis and subcutaneous tissues, and pass to the heart and lungs, where they migrate upward in the bronchi and trachea and then downward in the alimentary tract; the larvae mature in the jejunum, and the adults live in the small intestine, causing abdominal discomfort, diarrhea (usually with melena), and cramps; anorexia, loss of weight, and hypochromic microcytic anemia may occur in advanced disease; see also ancylostomiasis and fig. under *Ancylostoma duodenale.*

**N. suil'lus,** a species found in the small intestine of pigs.

**necatoriasis** (ne-ka'to-ri'ă-sis). Disease caused by *Necator;* see also ancylostomiasis.

**Necheles' tube.** See under tube.

**neck** [ A.S. *hnecca* ]. Cervix; collum; trachelos. 1. The part between the shoulders or thorax and the head. 2. In anatomy, any constricted portion having a fancied resemblance to the n. of an animal. 3. The germinative portion of an adult tapeworm which develops the segments or proglottids; the region of cestode segmentation behind the scolex.

**anatomical n. of the humerus,** *collum* anatomicum humeri.

**back of the n.,** nucha.

**buffalo n.,** combination of moderate kyphosis with thick heavy fat pad on the n., seen especially in persons with Cushing's disease or syndrome.

**bull n.,** heavy, thick n., caused by hypertrophied muscles or enlarged cervical lymph nodes.

**dental n.,** *collum* dentis.

**n. of femur,** *collum* femoris.

**n. of gallbladder,** *collum* vesicae felleae.

**n. of glans penis,** *collum* glandis penis.

**limber n.,** botulism.

**Madelung's n.,** Madelung's disease confined to the n.

**n. of malleux,** *collum* mallei.

**nape of the n.,** nucha; scruff.

**pit of the n.,** *incisura* jugularis (3).

**n. of radius,** *collum* radii.

**n. of rib,** *collum* costae.

**n. of scapula,** *collum* scapulae.

**scruff of the n.,** nucha; nape.

**stiff n.,** torticollis.

**surgical n. of the humerus,** *collum* chirurgicum humeri.

**n. of talus,** *collum* tali.

**n. of a tooth,** *collum* dentis.

**n. of uterus,** *cervix* uteri.

**webbed n.,** the broad n. due to lateral folds of skin extending from the clavicle to the head; occurs in Turner's syndrome.

**n. of the womb,** *cervix* uteri.

**wry n.,** torticollis.

**neck'lace.** Term used to describe a skin rash that encircles the neck.

**Casal's n.,** a dermatitis partly or completely encircling the lower part of the neck in pellagra.

**n. of Venus,** syphilitic *leukoderma.*

**necr-.** See necro-.

**necrectomy** (nĕ-krek'to-mĭ) [ necr- + G. *ektomē,* excision ]. Necronectomy; operative removal of any necrosed tissue.

**necre'mia** [ G. *nekros,* dead, + *haima,* blood ]. Obsolete designation for a condition characterized by death of a large proportion of the red blood cells.

**necro-, necr-** (nek'ro-) [ G. *nekros,* corpse ]. Combining forms relating to death or to necrosis.

**necrobacillosis** (nek'ro-bă'sĭ-lo'sis). Coagulation necrosis caused by the action of *Sphaerophorus necrophorus* and other anaerobic microorganisms.

**nec'robio'sis** [ necro- + G. *bios,* life ]. 1. The physiologic or normal death of cells or tissues as a result of changes associated with development, aging, or use ("wear-and-tear" degeneration). 2. Necrosis of a small area of tissue.

**n. lipoid'ica,** or **n. lipoid'ica diabetico'rum,** a condition, not necessarily associated with diabetes, in which atrophic, shiny lesions, one or more, develop on the legs. The histopathologic picture shows necrobiosis in the cutis. Also (less correctly) termed dermatitis atrophicans lipoides diabetica.

**nec'robiot'ic.** Pertaining to or characterized by necrobiosis.

**necrocytosis** (nek'ro-si-to'sis) [ necro- + G. *kytos,* cell, + suffix -*osis,* condition ]. A process that results in, or a condition that is characterized by, the abnormal or pathologic death of cells.

**necrogenic** (nek'ro-jen'ik) [ necro- + G. *genesis,* origin ]. Relating to, living in, or having origin in dead matter.

**necrogenous** (nĕ-kroj'en-us). Necrogenic.

**necrogranulomatous** (nek'ro-gran-u-lo'mah-tus). Having the characteristics of a granuloma with central necrosis. See, *e.g.,* necrogranulomatous *keratitis.*

**necrologist** (nĕ-krol'o-jist). A student of, or one expert in, the interpretation of mortality statistics.

**necrology** (nĕ-krol'o-jĭ) [ necro- + G. *logos,* study ]. The science of the collection, classification, and interpretation of mortality statistics.

**necrolysis** (nĕ-krol'ĭ-sis) [ necro- + G. *lysis,* loosening ]. Necrosis and loosening of tissue.

**toxic epidermal n.,** abbreviated TEN; epidermolysis necroticans combustiformis; erythema necroticans combustiformis; Lyell's disease; scalded skin syndrome; a syndrome in which a large portion of the skin becomes intensely erythematous and peels off in the manner of a second-degree burn, often simultaneous with the formation of flaccid bullae; several causes have been assigned, including drug sensitivity; prognosis is grave, except where early steroid therapy is instituted.

**nec′roma′nia** [ necro- + G. *mania,* frenzy ]. 1. A morbid tendency to dwell with longing on death. 2. A morbid attraction to dead bodies.

**necrometer** (nĕ-krom′e-ter) [ necro- + G. *metron,* measure ]. An instrument for measuring a dead body or any of its parts or organs.

**necronectomy** (nek′ro-nek′to-mī). Necrectomy.

**nec′ropar′asite.** Saprophyte.

**necropathy** (nĕ-krop′ă-thī) [ necro- + G. *pathos,* disease ]. A tendency to tissue death or gangrene.

**necrophagous** (nĕ-krof′ă-gus) [ necro- + G. *phagein,* to eat ]. 1. Living on carrion. 2. Necrophilous.

**necrophilia** (nek′ro-fil′ī-ah) [ necro- + G. *phileō,* to love ]. Necrophilism. 1. A morbid fondness for being in the presence of dead bodies. 2. The impulse to sexual contact, or the act of such contact, with the dead body, usually of males with female corpses.

**necrophilism** (nĕ-krof′ī-lizm). Necrophilia.

**necrophilous** (nĕ-krof′ī-lus) [ necro- + G. *philos,* fond ]. Having a preference for dead tissue; denoting certain bacteria.

**nec′ropho′bia** [ necro- + G. *phobos,* fear ]. Morbid fear of corpses.

**necropneumonia** (nek-ro-nu-mo′nī-ah) [ necro- + pneumonia ]. Gangrene of the lungs; any of several forms of pneumonia associated with necrosis or death of lung tissue.

**nec′ropsy** [ necro- + G. *opsis,* view ]. Autopsy.

**nec′rosad′ism** [ necro- + sadism, *q. v.* ]. Sexual gratification derived by mutilating corpses.

**necros′copy** [ necro- + G. *skopeō,* to examine ]. Autopsy.

**necrose** (nĕ-krōz′). 1. To cause necrosis. 2. To become the site of necrosis.

**nec′rosin.** A term suggested by Menkin as the name for an active principle isolated from exudates of acute inflammation, causing necrosis of cells.

**necrosis** (ne-kro′sis) [ G. *nekrōsis,* death, fr. *nekroō,* to make dead ]. The pathologic death of one or more cells, or of a portion of tissue or organ, resulting from irreversible damage; the most frequent visible alterations are nuclear: (1) pyknosis, *i.e.,* shrunken and abnormally dark basophilic staining; (2) karyolysis, *i.e.,* swollen and abnormally pale basophilic staining; or (3) karyorrhexis, *i.e.,* rupture and fragmentation of the nucleus. After such changes, the outlines of individual cells are indistinct, and affected cells may become merged, sometimes forming a focus of coarsely granular, amorphous, or hyaline material. The changes vary in degree and extent of involvement in different situations.

**aseptic n.,** n. occurring in the absence of infection.

**Balser's n.,** pancreatitis with areas of fat n., associated occasionally with fat n. in the omentum and mesentery.

**caseation n.,** caseous n.

**ca′seous n.,** caseation n.; caseous degeneration; n. characteristic of certain inflammations, *e.g.,* tuberculosis, histoplasmosis, and others; represents n. with loss of separate structures of the various cellular and histologic elements; the affected tissue manifests the friable, crumbly consistency and dull, opaque quality observed in cheese.

**central n.,** that involving the deeper or inner portions of a tissue, or an organ or its units; for example, central n. of the liver is that occurring in the cells adjacent to the central veins.

**coagulation n.,** a type of n. in which the affected cells or tissue are converted into a dry, dull, fairly homogeneous eosinophilic mass without nuclear staining, as a result of the coagulation of protein (such as that occurring in an infarct); microscopically, the necrotic process involves chiefly the cells, and remnants of histologic elements (*e.g.,* elastin, collagen, muscle fibers, and so on) may be recognizable, as well as "ghosts" of cells and portions of cell membranes. True coagulation n. may be caused by heat, formaldehyde, phenol, mercuric chloride, and other agents that instantly destroy the vital processes of the tissue, including the enzymes that would continue to alter the devitalized cellular substance.

**colliq′uative n.,** liquefactive n.

**cystic medial n.,** medionecrosis of the aorta; medionecrosis aortae idiopathica cystica; mucoid medial degeneration; loss of elastic and muscle fibers in the aortic media, with accumulation of mucopolysaccharide, sometimes in cyst-like spaces between the fibers. Cystic medial n. is a disease of unknown cause, which may be inherited (in Marfan's syndrome) and which predisposes to dissecting aneurysms.

**epiphysial aseptic n.,** aseptic n. of bony epiphyses, probably due to ischemia. It may affect the upper end of the femur (Perthes, Legg's, or Legg-Calvé-Perthes disease, osteochondritis deformans juvenilis, coxa plana, pseudocoxalgia); the tibial tubercle (Osgood-Schlatter disease); the tarsal navicular bone or the patella (Kohler's disease); the second metatarsal head (Freiberg's disease); vertebral bodies (Scheuermann's disease); the capitellum of the humerus (Panner's disease).

**fat n.,** steatonecrosis; the death of adipose tissue, characterized by the formation of small (1 to 4 mm.), dull, chalky, gray or white foci; these represent small quantities of calcium soaps formed in the affected tissue when fat is hydrolyzed into glycerol and fatty acids.

**fibrinoid n.,** n. in which the necrotic tissue has some staining reactions resembling fibrin and becomes deeply eosinophilic, homogenous, and refractile.

**focal n.,** the occurrence of numerous, relatively small or tiny, fairly well circumscribed, usually spheroidal portions of tissue that manifests coagulative, caseous, or gummatous n.; focal n. is frequently observed only in histologic sections, but the foci may be as large as 1 to 3 mm. and macroscopically visible. Arbitrarily, foci larger than that are usually not termed focal n. The small foci are characteristically associated with agents that are hematogenously disseminated.

**ischemic n.,** n. caused by hypoxia resulting from local deprivation of blood supply; see also infarction.

**laminar cortical n.,** the breaking down of a definite cell layer in the cerebral cortex, encountered typically after temporary cardiac arrest or perinatal hypoxia.

**liquefactive n.,** colliquative n.; a type of n. characterized by a fairly well circumscribed, microscopically or macroscopically visible lesion that consists of the dull, opaque or turbid, gray-white to yellow-gray, soft or boggy, partly or completely fluid remains of tissue that became necrotic and was digested by enzymes, especially proteolytic enzymes liberated from disintegrating leukocytes. Liquefactive n. is classically observed in abscesses, and frequently in infarcts of the brain.

**mummification n.,** dry *gangrene.*

**n. progre′diens,** progressive sloughing.

**progressive emphysem′atous n.,** gas *gangrene.*

**renal papillary n.,** necrotizing papillitis; n. of renal papillae, occurring in acute pyelonephritis, especially in diabetics, or in analgesic nephropathy. Renal failure may result.

**simple n.,** a stage of coagulation n.; the occurrence of a coarsely granular or hyaline change in the cytoplasm, and the lack of a recognizable nucleus, with the general configuration of the dead cells being relatively unchanged.

**subcutaneous fat n. of newborn,** *sclerema* neonatorum.

**suppurative n.,** liquefactive n. with pus formation.

**total n.,** (1) complete n. of the cytologic and histologic elements in a portion of tissue, as in caseous n., or (2) death of an entire organ or part.

**n. ustilagin′ea,** gangrene caused by the long-continued use of ergot.

**Zenker's n.,** Zenker's *degeneration.*

**zonal n.,** n. predominantly affecting or limited to an anatomical zone, especially parts of the hepatic lobules defined according to proximity to either the portal tracts or central (hepatic) veins.

**nec′rosper′mia** [ necro- + G. *sperma,* seed ]. A condition in which there are dead or immobile spermatozoa in the semen.

**necros′teon, necrosteo′sis** [ necro- + G. *osteon,* bone ]. Gangrene of bone.

**necrot′ic.** Pertaining to or affected by necrosis.

**nec′rotize.** To cause necrosis.

**necrot′omy** [ necro- + G. *tomē,* cutting ]. 1. Dissection. 2. Operation for the removal of a sequestrum or necrosed portion of bone.

**osteoplas′tic n.,** operation to remove bone sequestrum through a window of bone hinged on one side, which is then replaced.

**necrozo'osperm'ia** [ necro- + G. *zōon*, animal, + *sperma*, seed ]. Obsolete synonym for necrospermia.

**needle** (ne'dl). 1. A slender, usually sharp-pointed, instrument used for puncturing the tissues, for guiding the thread or wire in suturing, or for passing a ligature around an artery. 2. To separate the tissues by means of one or two n.'s, in the dissection of small parts. 3. To perform discission of a cataract by means of a n. or very slender knife.

   **an'eurysm n., artery n.,** a blunt-pointed, curved n., set in a handle, with the eye at the point, used for passing a ligature beneath and around an artery.

   **aspirating n.,** a hollow n. used for withdrawing fluid from a cavity, an aspirator tube being attached to one end, the other being thrust into the cavity.

   **atraumatic n.,** an eyeless surgical n. with the thread fastened by adhesive means.

   **cataract n.,** a form of n. or very slender knife used in the removal or the discission of a cataract.

   **couching n.,** see couching.

   **Deschamps' n.,** a n. with a long shaft for passing sutures in the deep tissues.

   **Emmet's n.,** a strong n. with the eye in the point, having a wide curve, and set in a handle.

   **exploring n.,** a stout n. with a longitudinal groove, which is thrust into a tumor or cavity in order to determine whether or not fluid is present, the latter escaping externally along the groove.

   **Fischer's n.,** an instrument used in the operation for artificial pneumothorax.

   **Francke's n.,** a small lancet-shaped n., operated by a spring, used to evacuate a small effusion of blood.

   **Frazier's n.,** a n. for draining lateral ventricles of brain.

   **Gillmore n.,** a device for obtaining the setting time of dental cement.

   **Hagedorn n.,** a curved surgical n. flattened on the sides.

   **hypodermic n.,** a hollow n. similar to, but smaller than an aspirating n., attached to a syringe; used for injecting liquids beneath the skin or for withdrawing fluid for examination from an abscess or cyst.

   **knife n.,** a very narrow, needle-pointed knife used in the operation of discission of a cataract.

   **lumbar puncture n.,** a n. for entering the spinal canal or cisterna magna, having a bore of at least 1 mm. and being 40 mm. long; it is provided with a stylet.

   **Menghini n.,** a biopsy n. for liver tissue.

   **Salah's sternal puncture n.,** a wide-bore n. for obtaining samples of red marrow from the sternum.

   **spatula n.,** a minute n. used by eye surgeons for splitting the sclera.

   **stop-n.,** a surgical n., with the eye at the tip, the shank of which has a projecting shelf to arrest the n. when it has passed the desired distance through the tissues.

   **Vicat n.,** a device for obtaining the setting time of plaster and other materials.

   **Vim-Silverman n.,** a n. with a stylet and removable, double-pronged, tweezer-like cutters for obtaining a core of tissue for biopsy, especially of liver or kidney.

**needle-holder.** Needle-carrier; needle forceps; instrument used for grasping a needle when passing sutures in a cavity or other part not easily reached by the fingers.

**Needles,** J. W., U. S. dentist. See N.'s split cast *method*.

**need'ling.** 1. Discission of a soft or of a secondary cataract. 2. Treatment of an aneurysm by the insertion of a fine needle far enough to reach the opposite wall, the intima of which is then scratched so as to roughen it and induce coagulation.

**Neelsen** (näl'sen), Friedrich K. A., German pathologist, 1854–1894. See Ziehl-N. *method*.

**neencephalon** (ne-en-sef'ă-lon) [ G. *neos*, new, + *enkephalos*, brain ]. Neoencephalon; Edinger's term for the higher levels of the central nervous system superimposed upon the metameric or propriospinal system (paleencephalon).

**Neftel,** William B., U. S. neurologist, 1830–1906. See N.'s *disease*.

**nega'tion.** Denial.

**nega'tive G.** Gravity in a foot-to-head direction in flying, or in standing on one's head; the reverse of positive G.

**nega'tive S.** See flotation *constant*.

**neg'ativism.** A tendency to do the opposite of what one is requested to do, or to stubbornly resist for no apparent reason.

**neg'atrons.** Electrons; so called to emphasize their negative charge in contradistinction to the positive charge carried by the otherwise similar positron.

**Negri** (na'gre), Adelchi, Italian physician, 1876–1912. See N. *bodies*, N. *corpuscles*.

**Negro's phenomenon.** See under phenomenon.

**Neill-Mooser reaction.** See under reaction.

**Neisser** (ni'ser), Albert L. S., Breslau physician, 1855 –1916. Gave his name to *Neisseria*. See N.'s *coccus*.

**Neisser** (ni'ser), Ernst, German physician, *1863. See N.-Doering *phenomenon*.

**Neisser** (ni'ser), Albert L. S., Breslau physician, 1855– 1916. Gave his name to *Neisseria*. See N.'s *coccus*.

**Neisseria** (ni-se'rĭ-ah) [ A. *Neisser* ]. A genus of aerobic to facultatively anaerobic bacteria (family Neisseriaceae) containing Gram-negative cocci which occur in pairs with the adjacent sides flattened. These organisms are parasites of animals so far as known. The type species is *N. gonorrhoeae*.

   **N. catarrha'lis,** *Branhamella catarrhalis*.

   **N. ca'viae,** a species found in the pharyngeal region of guinea pigs and perhaps of other animals.

   **N. flava,** a species found in the mucous membranes of the human respiratory tract.

   **N. flaves'cens,** a species found in cerebrospinal fluid in cases of meningitis; probably occurs in the mucous membranes of the human respiratory tract.

   **N. gonorrhoe'ae,** gonococcus; Neisser's coccus; a species which causes gonorrhea and other infections in man. It is the type species of the genus *N*.

   **N. haemolysans,** a species found in the mucous membranes of the human respiratory tract.

   **N. meningitidis,** meningococcus; Weichselbaum's coccus; a species found in the nasopharynx of man but not in other animals; causes epidemic cerebrospinal fever (meningitis).

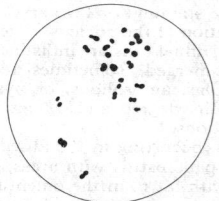

*Neisseria meningitidis*
(Original magnification, × 2400)

   **N. sicca,** a species found in the mucous membranes of the human respiratory tract.

   **N. subfla'va,** a species found in the mucous membranes of the human respiratory tract; easily confused with *N. meningitidis*.

**Nélaton** (na-lă-toń'), Auguste, French surgeon, 1807– 1873. See N.'s *catheter, dislocation, fibers, line,* Roser-N. *line,* N.'s *sphincter, tumor*.

**Nelson,** Don H., U. S. internist, *1925. See N. *syndrome, tumor*.

**nem** [ Ger. *Nahrung, Einheit, Milch*, nourishment, unit, milk ]. The caloric value of 1 gram of mother's milk of a definite composition; it is a unit of comparison of food values, equivalent to about $2/3$ calorie; 1 calorie equals $1\frac{1}{2}$ nem.

**nema-, nemat-, nemato-** (nem'ah-, ne'mah-) [ G. *nēma*, thread ]. Combining forms meaning thread, threadlike.

**nemathelminth** (nem-ah-thel'minth). A member of the phylum Nemathelminthes.

**Nemathelminthes** (nem-ah-thel-min'thēz) [ nemat- + G. *helmins, helminthos,* worm ]. Aschelminthes.

**nematocide** (ne-mat'o-sīd) [ nematode + L. *caedo*, to kill ]. 1. Destructive to nematode worms. 2. An agent that kills nematodes.

**nematocyst** (nem'ă-to-sist) [ nemato- + G. kystis, bladder ]. Cnida; cnidocyst; a stinging cell of coelenterates consisting of a poison sac and a coiled barbed sting capable of being ejected and penetrating the skin of an animal on contact; of considerable consequence in large jelly fish and in the Portuguese "man-of-war," whose large numbers of these stinging cells can cause great pain and even death.

**Nematoda** (nem'ă-to'dah) [ nemat- + G. *eidos*, form ]. A class in the phylum Aschelminthes, including the species that are parasitic in man and the far greater number of nonparasitic species. For practical purposes, the parasitic nematodes may be regarded in two groups, based on their habitat in the human body: (1) the intestinal roundworms—e.g., the genera *Ascaris, Trichuris, Ancylostoma, Necator, Strongyloides, Enterobius,* and *Trichinella;* (2) the filarial roundworms of the blood, lymphatic tissues, and viscera—e.g., the genera *Wuchereria, Mansonella, Acanthocheilonema, Loa, Onchocerca,* and *Dracunculus.*

**nematode** (nem'ă-tōd). A common name for any parasitic worm of the class Nematoda.

**Ne'matodirel'la longis'simespicula'ta.** One of the thread-necked trichostrongyle nematodes in the small intestine of sheep, goats, reindeer, moose, musk ox, and pronghorn.

**Nematodirus** (nem'ă-to'dī-rus). The thread-necked or thin-necked trichostrongyles; a genus of slender, relatively long nematodes (family Trichostrongylidae) occurring in herbivorous animals, usually in the small intestine. Generally, they are not believed to be highly pathogenic except in poorly fed animals in which heavy infections occur.

    **N. abnorma'lis,** occurs in sheep, goats, camels, and mule deer; very common in the United States.

    **N. filicol'lis,** occurs worldwide in sheep, goats, oxen, and various wild ruminants.

    **N. helvetia'nus,** occurs in cattle, sheep, goats, and camels in Europe, Asia, and the Americas.

    **N. lanceola'tus,** occurs in sheep and pronghorns in the Americas.

    **N. lepo'ris,** occurs in the duodenum of domestic rabbits and wild cottontail rabbits in North America.

    **N. spathi'ger,** the commonest species, widespread and abundant, found in the small intestines of sheep, cattle, camels, and other ruminants.

**nem'atodo'sis.** Infection with nematode parasites.

**nem'atoid.** Relating to the nematodes.

**nem'atol'ogist.** A scientist trained and experienced in nematology.

**nematology** (nem'ă-tol'o-jī) [ nemadode + G. *logos,* study ]. The science dealing with nematoid worms in all their relations.

**nematospermia** (nem'ă-to-sper'mĭ-ah) [ G. *mēma (nēmat-),* thread, + *sperma,* seed ]. Spermatozoa with an elongated tail, such as in man; opposed to spherospermia.

**neo-** [ G. *neos,* new ]. Prefix meaning new or recent.

**neoantigen** (ne'o-an'tĭ-jen). New specific antigen which appears in a cell after infection by oncogenic virus, such as the T antigen which follows infection with SV40.

**neoarsphen'amine.** NEOSALVARSAN; consists chiefly of sodium 3,3'-diamino-4,4'-dihydroxyarsenobenzene methanal sulfoxylate; an antisyphilitic.

**neoarthro'sis.** Pseudarthrosis.

**Neoas'caris vitulo'rum.** The large roundworm occurring in the small intestine of cattle, water buffalo, and (rarely) sheep. Although uncommon in the United States, it is a serious cattle parasite in many other areas. Experimental infection has been produced in rodents and man.

**ne'obi'ogen'esis** [ neo- + G. *bios,* life, + *genesis,* origin ]. The theory that life can originate from nonliving matter.

**neoblas'tic** [ neo- + G. *blastos,* germ, offspring ]. Developing in or characteristic of new tissue.

**neocerebellum** (ne-o-sĕr-e-bel'um). The lateral lobe or hemisphere of the cerebellum which developed latest in the phylogeny of vertebrates, and is particularly prominent in mammals; the term distinguishes this subdivision of the cerebellum from the paleocerebellum.

**neochymotrypsinogen** (ne'o-ki'mo-trip-sin'o-jen). An intermediate in the conversion of chymotrypsin to α-chymotrypsin by one of two alternate routes (the other route involving π-chymotrypsin as intermediate) by chymotrypsin cleavage.

**neocinchophen** (ne'o-sin'ko-fen). The ethyl ester of 6-methyl-2-phenylquinolin-4-carboxylic acid; same action and uses as cinchophen, but appears to be less toxic.

**neocinet'ic.** Neokinetic.

**neocortex** (ne'o-kor'teks). Isocortex.

**neocystostomy** (ne'o-sis-tos'to-mĭ) [ neo- + G. *kystis,* bladder, + *stoma,* mouth ]. An operation in which the ureter or a segment of the ileum is inserted into the bladder.

    **ureteral n.,** when the ureter is severed and in part destroyed and end-to-end anastomosis is not feasible, the upper segment of the ureter is inserted into the bladder.

    **ure'teroil'eal n.,** restoration of the continuity of the urinary tract by anastomosing the upper segment of a partially destroyed ureter to a segment of ileum the lower end of which is inserted into the bladder; resorted to when a ureter is severed and cannot be sutured end to end.

**neocytosis** (ne-o-si-to'sis) [ neo- + G. *kytos,* cell, + suffix *-osis,* condition ]. Skeocytosis; presence of immature cells in the peripheral blood; see also *shift* to the left.

**neodymium** (ne'o-dim'ĭ-um) [ neo- didymium, *q.v.* ]. One of the rare earth elements; symbol Nd, atomic no. 60, atomic weight 144.27.

**neoencephalon** (ne-o-en-sef'ă-lon). Neencephalon.

**neofe'tal.** Relating to the neofetus.

**neofe'tus.** The intrauterine organism in the transition period between embryo and fetus.

**neoforma'tion.** 1. The formation of neoplasia, or a neoplasm. 2. Sometimes used to indicate the process of regeneration, or a regenerated tissue or part.

**neogala** (ne-og'ă-lah) [ neo- + G. *gala,* milk ]. The first milk formed in the breasts after childbirth.

**neogenesis** (ne'o-jen'ĕ-sis) [ neo- + G. *genesis,* origin ]. Regeneration; new formation.

**neogenet'ic.** Pertaining to or characterized by neogenesis.

**neohy'men** [ neo- + G. *hymēn,* membrane ]. False *membrane.*

**neokinetic** (ne'o-kĭ-net'ik) [ neo- + G. *kinētikos,* relating to movement ]. Neocinetic; denoting one of the divisions of the motor system, the function of which is the transmission of isolated synergic movements of voluntary origin; it represents a more highly specialized form of movement than the paleokinetic function.

**neolal'lism** [ neo- + G. *laleō,* to chatter ]. The use of neologisms in speech.

**neologism** (ne-ol'o-jizm) [ neo- + G. *logos,* word ]. 1. A new word or phrase, or an old word used in a new sense. 2. A form of lalopathy in which the patient coins new and meaningless words.

**neomem'brane.** False *membrane.*

**neomorph, neomorphism** (ne'o-morf, ne'o-mor'fizm) [ neo- + G. *morphē,* form ]. A new formation; a structure found in higher organisms, no, or only slight, traces of which exist in lower orders.

**neomy'cin sulfate** (USP, BP). The sulfate of an antibacterial substance produced by the growth of *Streptomyces fradiae,* active against a variety of Gram-positive and Gram-negative bacteria.

**ne'on** [ G. *neos,* new ]. An inert gaseous element in the atmosphere, separated from argon by Ramsay in 1898; symbol Ne, atomic no. 10, atomic weight 20.183.

**neona'tal** [ neo- + L. *natalis,* relating to birth ]. Newborn; relating to the period immediately succeeding birth and continuing through the first month of life.

**neonate** (ne'o-nāt) [ L. *neonatus,* newborn ]. A newborn or neonatal infant; see also neonatal.

**ne'onatol'ogy** [ neo- + L. *natus,* pp. born, + G. *logos,* theory ]. The study of disorders of the newborn.

**neonatus** (ne'o-na'tus) [ L. newborn ]. Neonate.

**neonic'otine.** Anabasine.

**neopal'lium.** Isocortex.

**neopathy** (ne-op'ă-thī) [ neo- + G. *pathos,* disease ]. A new lesion or pathologic process.

**neophilism** (ne-of'ĭ-lizm) [ neo- + G. *phileō*, to love ]. Morbid fascination or love for novelty, especially new persons or places.

**neopho'bia** [ neo- + G. *phobos*, fear ]. Morbid aversion to or dread of novelty or the unknown.

**neophen'ylal'anine.** Dimethylphenylalanine.

**neophrenia** (ne'o-fre'nĭ-ah) [ neo- + G. *phrēn*, mind ]. Any major mental disorder (psychosis) occurring in childhood; similar disorders in adolescents were once called hebephrenia, and in old age, presbyophrenia.

**neoplasia** (ne'o-pla'zĭ-ah) [ neo- + G. *plasis*, a molding ]. The pathologic process that results in the formation and growth of a tumor, *i.e.*, a neoplasm, *q.v.*

**ne'oplasm** [ neo- + G. *plasma*, thing formed ]. New growth; an abnormal tissue that grows by cellular proliferation more rapidly than normal and continues to grow after the stimuli that initiated the new growth cease. N.'s show partial or complete lack of structural organization and functional coordination with the normal tissue; they usually form a distinct mass of tissue. The term tumor, which literally means "swelling " (of various types), is frequently used synonymously with the word neoplasm. The behavior of n.'s may be either benign (see benign *tumor*) or malignant (see cancer).

**histoid n.,** one characterized by a cytohistologic pattern that closely resembles the tissue from which the neoplastic cells are derived.

**neoplas'tic.** Pertaining to or characterized by neoplasia, or containing a neoplasm.

**neopyrithi'amin.** (ne'o-pĭr'ĭ-thi'ă-min). A thiamin antimetabolite, differing from thiamin in that the thiazole ring of the thiamin molecule is replaced by a pyridine ring.

**neoret'inene B.** 11-*cis*-Retinol; see under retinol.

**Neorickett'sia helmin'theca.** A rickettsia-like organism that is the agent of salmon poisoning; it is transmitted by the metacercariae of *Nanophyes salmincola*.

**neostigmine bromide** (ne-o-stig'min) (USP, BP). PROSTIGMIN; $C_{12}H_{19}BrN_2O_2$; a synthetic compound, closely similar in action to physostigmine (eserine; a reversible cholinesterase inhibitor, used in the treatment of myasthenia gravis, postoperative distention, urinary retention, overdose of tubocurarine, and as a pregnancy test. Neostigmine methylsulfate (USP, BP) is also available for parenteral administration.

**neostomy** (ne-os'to-mĭ) [ neo- + G. *stoma*, mouth ]. Surgical construction of a new or artificial opening.

**neostriatum** (ne-o-stri-a'tum). The caudate nucleus and putamen considered as one and distinguished from the globus pallidus (paleostriatum).

**neostrophingic** (ne'o-stro-fin'jik) [ neo- + G. *strophē*, a turning, + E. hinge ]. A "new turning," describing surgical mobilization of the mitral valve by extension of the arcuate line in valve closure a little past the normal limits at both ends, thus rehinging the septal leaflet and making it more flexible.

**neoteny** (ne-ot'ĕ-nĭ) [ neo- + G. *tenō*, to stretch ]. Prolongation of the larval state, as in the Mexican tiger salamander or axolotl, or in certain termite castes held in the larval stage as future replacements of the queen; *cf.* pedogenesis.

**neothal'amus.** The portion of the thalamus projecting to the neocortex.

**neoty'rosine.** Dimethyltyrosine; a tyrosine antimetabolite.

**neovi'tamin A.** One of the *cis-trans* isomers of vitamin A; obsolete.

**nepen'thic** [ G. *nēpenthēs*, free from sorrow ]. Inducing peace or forgetfulness; a tranquilizer.

**nephelometer** (nef'e-lom'e-ter) [ G. *nephelē*, cloud, + *metron*, measure ]. NEB-. An instrument for estimating the number of particles (*e.g.*, bacteria and the like) in a suspension, by matching its opacity with that of one of a series of standardizing tubes that contain precipitates of barium sulfate (or other insoluble salt) of varying density.

**nephelometry** (nef'e-lom'e-trĭ). The semiquantitative estimation of the concentration of particles in a suspension (*e.g.*, bacterial cells in an antigenic preparation), by

means of comparing it with the standard suspensions in a nephelometer.

**nephelopia** (nef'e-lo'pĭ-ah) [ G. *nephelē*, cloud, + *ōps*, eye ]. Dimness of vision due to cataract or cloudiness of the cornea.

**nephr-.** See nephro-.

**nephradenoma** (nef'rad-ĕ-no'mah) [ nephr- + adenoma ]. Adenoma of the kidney.

**nephralgia** (ne-fral'jĭ-ah) [ nephr- + G. *algos*, pain ]. Pain in the kidney.

**nephral'gic.** Relating to nephralgia.

**nephrapostasis** (nef'ră-pos'tă-sis) [ nephr- + G. *apostasis*, abscess ]. Abscess of the kidney; pyonephrosis.

**nephrasthenia** (nef-ras-the'nĭ-ah) [ nephr- + G. *asthenia*, weakness ]. A mild nephrosis; a condition of imperfect functioning of the kidney, giving rise to slight urinary signs, but without actual disease of the renal tubules.

**nephrato'nia, nephrat'ony** [ nephr- + G. *a-* priv. + *tonos*, tension ]. Diminished functional activity of the kidneys.

**nephrectasia, nephrectasy** (nef'rek-ta'zĭ-ah, ne-frek'tă-sis) [ nephr- + G. *ektasis*, a stretching ]. Dilation of the pelvis of the kidney.

**nephrec'tomize.** To perform nephrectomy upon.

**nephrectomy** (ne-frek'to-mĭ) [ nephr- + G. *ektomē*, excision ]. The operation of removing a kidney.

**abdominal n.,** removal of the kidney through an anterior incision, involving a double incision of the peritoneum.

**paraperitoneal n.,** n. performed by an incision in the side below the ribs, the kidney being reached by a blunt dissection behind the peritoneum.

**nephredema** (nef're-de'mah) [ nephr- + G. *oidēma*, swelling ]. Edema caused by renal disease; rarely, edema of the kidney.

**nephrelcosis** (nef'rel-ko'sis) [ nephr- + G. *helkōsis*, ulceration ]. Ulceration of the mucous membrane of the pelvis or calices of the kidney.

**nephremorrhagia** (nef'rem-o-raj'ĭ-ah) [ nephr- + hemorrhage, *q.v.* ]. Hemorrhage from or into the kidney.

**nephric** (nef'rik). Renal; relating to the kidney.

**nephridium, pl. nephrid'ia** (ne-frid'ĭ-um) [ G. *nephridios*, relating to the kidney ]. One of the paired, segmentally arranged excretory tubules of invertebrates such as the annelids.

**nephrit'ic.** Relating to or suffering from nephritis.

**nephritides** (nef-frit'ĭ-dēz). Plural of nephritis.

**nephritis, pl. nephritides** (ne-fri'tis) [ nephr- + G. suffix *-itis*, inflammation ]. Inflammation of the kidneys.

**acute n.,** acute *glomerulonephritis.*

**acute interstit'ial n.,** an acute inflammation of the interstitial tissues of the kidney, with less obvious involvement of the glomeruli and tubules, which may occur during an acute infection.

**analgesic n.,** analgesic nephropathy; chronic interstitial n. with renal papillary necrosis, occurring in patients with a long history of excessive consumption of analgesics, especially those containing phenacetin.

**anti-basement membrane n.,** glomerulonephritis produced by autologous or heterologous antibodies to kidney, the kidney, the latter known as anti-kidney serum n., *e.g.*, Masugi's n.

**anti-kidney serum n.,** experimental glomerulonephritis produced by injection of antiserum to kidney, *e.g.*, Masugi's n.

**chronic n.,** chronic *glomerulonephritis.*

**Ellis types 1 and 2 n.,** Ellis types 1 and 2 *glomerulonephritis.*

**embolic n.,** focal embolic *glomerulonephritis.*

**focal n.,** focal *glomerulonephritis.*

**glomer'ular n.,** glomerulonephritis.

**n. gravidarum,** n. developing in pregnancy.

**hemorrhagic n.,** acute glomerulonephritis accompanied by hematuria.

**hereditary n.,** familial renal disease progressing to chronic renal failure, especially in males; associated with nerve deafness.

**immune complex n.,** an immune complex disease (*q.v.*) resulting from glomerular deposits, as in membranous glomerulonephritis.

**interstit'ial n.,** a form in which the interstitial connective tissue is chiefly affected.

**lupus n.,** diffuse glomerulonephritis occurring in some patients with systemic lupus erythematosus; characterized by hematuria and a progressive course culminating in renal failure, often without hypertension. The term is sometimes also applied to the nephrotic syndrome in patients with systemic lupus.

**Masugi's n.,** glomerulonephritis produced by injecting into rats a rabbit antiserum prepared against rat kidney tissue suspensions.

**parenchy'matous n.,** inflammation of the stroma of the kidneys; the chronic form constitutes what has been called the large white *kidney.*

**salt-losing n.,** Thorn's syndrome; a rare disorder resulting from renal tubular damage of unknown etiology; it mimics adrenocortical insufficiency in that abnormal renal loss of sodium chloride occurs, accompanied by azotemia, acidosis, dehydration, and vascular collapse. Responds to replacement of sodium chloride, but not to mineralocorticoid therapy.

**scarlati'nal n.,** acute glomerulonephritis occurring as a complication of scarlet fever.

**serum n.,** induced glomerulonephritis; glomerulonephritis occurring in serum sickness or in animals injected with foreign serum protein.

**subacute n.,** subacute *glomerulonephritis.*

**sup'purative n.,** a focal n. with abscess formation in the kidney.

**syphilit'ic n.,** a rare complication of the secondary stage of syphilis. The kidney shows tubular degeneration and spirochetes are present in the tubules.

**transfusion n.,** the renal tubular damage resulting from the transfusion of incompatible blood. The hemoglobin of the hemolyzed red cells is deposited as casts in the renal tubules whose walls are damaged in a manner the nature of which is not clearly understood. Blockage of the tubules by the insoluble hemoglobin is also a factor in the uremic state which frequently results.

**trench n.,** war n.; glomerulonephritis occurring in soldiers subjected to cold and wet in muddy trenches.

**tuberculous n.,** n., mainly of the interstitial type, due to the tubercle bacillus.

**uranium n.,** an experimental n. produced by the administration of uranium nitrate.

**war n.,** trench n.

**nephro-, nephr-** (nef'ro-) [ G. *nephros,* kidney ]. Combining forms relating to the kidney.

**neph'roblasto'ma.** Wilms' *tumor.*

**nephrocalcinosis** (nef'ro-kal-sĭ-no'sis) [ nephro- + calcinosis ]. A form of renal lithiasis that is characterized by diffusely scattered foci of calcification in the kidneys; the deposits of calcium phosphate, calcium oxalate monohydrate, and similar compounds are usually demonstrable radiologically.

**nephrocapsectomy** (nef'ro-kap-sek'to-mĭ) [ nephro- + L. *capsula,* a small box, + G. *ektomē,* excision ]. Edebohl's operation; decortication, or decapsulation, of the kidney, in order to provide a more abundant blood supply and thereby increase the functional activity of the organ in cases of chronic nephritis.

**neph'rocar'diac** [ nephro- + G. *kardia,* heart ]. Cardiorenal.

**nephrocele** (nef'ro-sēl). 1 [ nephro- + G. *kēlē,* hernia ]. Hernial displacement of a kidney. 2 [ nephro- + G. *koilōma,* a hollow (celom) ]. Nephrotomic cavity; nephrocelom; in lower vertebrates the developmental cavity connecting the myocele with the celom. kidney.

**nephrocelom** (nef'ro-se'lom) [ nephro- + G. *koilōma,* a hollow (celom) ]. Nephrocele (2).

**nephrocolic, nephrocolica** (nef'ro-kol'ik, -kol'ĭ-kah). Renal *colic.*

**nephrocystanastomosis** (nef'ro-sist'an-as-to-mo'sis) [ nephro- + G. *kystis,* bladder, + *anastomōsis,* an outlet ]. The establishment of an artificial connection between the kidney and the bladder, in case of permanent obstruction of the ureter.

**nephrocystitis** (nef-ro-sis-ti'tis) [ nephro- + G. *kystis,* bladder, + suffix *-itis,* inflammation ]. Inflammation of both kidney and bladder.

**nephrocystosis** (nef'ro-sis-to'sis) [ nephro- + G. *kystis,* cyst, + suffix *-osis,* condition ]. The formation of renal cysts.

**nephroerysipelas** (nef'ro-ĕr'ĭ-sip'e-las). Acute interstitial nephritis occurring with erysipelas.

**neph'rogenet'ic, neph'rogen'ic** [ nephro- + G. *genēsis,* origin ]. Giving rise to kidney tissue.

**nephrogenous** (nef-roj'ē-nus). Arising from kidney tissue.

**neph'rogram.** Roentgenogram of the kidney after the intravenous injection of a radiopaque substance.

**nephrography** (ne-frog'rä-fĭ) [ nephro- + G. *graphō,* to write ]. Radiography of the kidney.

**neph'rohydro'sis.** Hydronephrosis.

**neph'roid.** (nef'royd) [ nephro- + G. *eidos,* resemblance ]. Reniform; kidney-shaped; resembling a kidney.

**neph'rolith** [ nephro- + G. *lithos,* stone ]. Renal *calculus.*

**nephrolithiasis** (nef'ro-lĭ-thi'ă-sis). The presence of renal calculi.

**nephrolithotomy** (nef'ro-lĭ-thot'o-mĭ) [ nephro- + G. *lithos,* stone, + *tomē,* incision ]. Incision into the kidney for the removal of a renal calculus.

**nephrology** (ne-frol'o-jĭ) [ nephro- + G. *logos,* study ]. The branch of medical science that deals especially with the kidneys.

**nephrolysin** (ne-frol'ĭ-sin). An antibody that causes destruction of the cells of the kidneys, formed in response to the injection of an emulsion of renal substance; it is specific for the species from which the antigen was prepared.

**nephrolysis** (ne-frol'ĭ-sis) [ nephro- + G. *lysis,* dissolution ]. 1. Freeing of the kidney from adhesions of inflammatory origin, with preservation of the capsule. 2. Destruction of renal cells as a result of the effects of a nephrolysin.

**nephrolyt'ic.** Pertaining to, characterized by, or causing nephrolysis.

**nephroma** (ne-fro'mah) [ nephro- + G. suffix *-oma,* tumor ]. A tumor arising from renal tissue.

**mesoblastic n.,** Wilms' *tumor.*

**nephromalacia** (nef'ro-mă-la'shĭ-ah) [ nephro- + G. *malakia,* softness ]. Softening of the kidneys.

**nephromegaly** (nef-ro-meg'ă-lĭ) [ nephro- + G. *megas,* great ]. Extreme hypertrophy of one or both kidneys.

**nephromere** (nef'ro-mēr) [ nephro- + G. *meros,* a part ]. That portion of the intermediate mesoderm that gives rise to segmented kidney tubules.

**neph'ron** [ G. *nephros,* kidney ]. The functional unit of the kidney, consisting of the renal corpuscle, the proximal convoluted tubule, the nephronic loop, and the distal convoluted tubule.

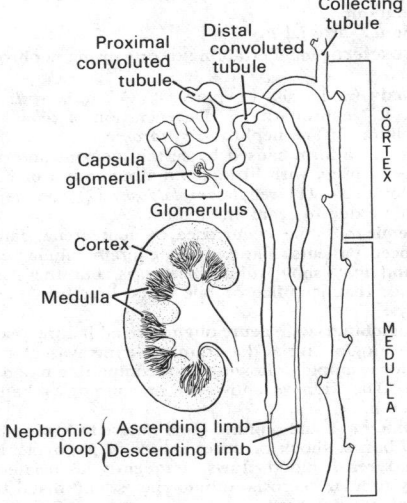

**Diagram of the Nephron**

**nephroncus** (nef-rong'kus) [ nephro- + G. *onkos*, tumor ]. Renal neoplasmal tumor.

**nephropathy** (nef'rop'ă-thī) [ nephro- + G. *pathos*, suffering ]. Any disease of the kidney.

**analgesic n.**, analgesic *nephritis*.

**hypokalemic n.**, vacuolar nephrosis; vacuolation of the epithelial cytoplasm of renal convoluted tubules in patients seriously depleted of potassium by any cause; the vacuoles do not contain fat or glycogen; concentrating ability is impaired.

**nephropexy** (nef'ro-pek'sī) [ nephro- + G. *pēxis*, fixation ]. The operative fixation of a floating kidney.

**nephrophthisis** (nef-rof'thī-sis, -tĭ-sis) [ nephro- + G. *phthisis*, a wasting ]. 1. Suppurative nephritis with wasting of the substance of the organ. 2. Tuberculosis of the kidney.

**familial juvenile n.**, cystic *disease* of renal medulla, autosomal recessive type.

**nephroptosis, nephroptosia** (nef'rop'to'sis, -to'sī-ah) [ nephro- + G. *ptōsis*, a falling ]. A downward displacement or falling of the kidney.

**nephropyelitis** (nef'ro-pi-ĕ-li'tis). Pyelonephritis.

**neph'ropy'eloplas'ty** [ nephro- + G. *pyelos*, trough (pelvis), + *plassō*, to form ]. A plastic procedure on kidney pelvis.

**nephropyosis** (nef'ro-pi-o'sis) [ nephro- + G. *pyōsis*, suppuration ]. Suppuration of the kidney.

**nephrorrhagia** (nef'ro-ra'jī-ah) [ nephro- + G. *rhēgnymi*, to break forth ]. Nephrhemorrhagia.

**nephrorrhaphy** (nef-ror'ă-fī) [ nephro- + G. *raphē*, a suture ]. Nephropexy by suturing the kidney in place.

**nephrosclerosis** (nef'ro-skle-ro'sis) [ nephro- + G. *sklērosis*, hardening ]. Induration of the kidney from overgrowth and contraction of the interstitial connective tissue.

**arterial n.**, arterionephrosclerosis; senile n.; patchy atrophic scarring of the kidney due to gradual narrowing of the lumens of large branches of the renal artery, occurring in old or hypertensive persons and occasionally causing hypertension.

**arteriolar n.**, arteriolonephrosclerosis; benign n.; Gull-Sutton disease; renal scarring due to arteriolar sclerosis resulting from longstanding hypertension. The kidneys are finely granular and mildly or moderately contracted. There is hyaline thickening of the walls of afferent glomerular arterioles and hyaline scarring of scattered glomeruli. Chronic renal failure develops infrequently.

**benign n.**, arteriolar n.

**malignant n.**, the renal changes in malignant hypertension; subcapsular petechiae are seen, and necrosis in the walls of scattered afferent glomerular arterioles. The urine contains red blood cells and casts, and uremia is a common termination.

**senile n.**, arterial n.

**neph'rosclerot'ic.** Pertaining to or causing nephrosclerosis.

**nephrosis** (ne-fro'sis) [ nephro- + G. suffix *-osis*, condition ]. 1. Nephropathy. 2. Degeneration of renal tubular epithelium. 3. The nephrotic *syndrome*.

**acute n.**, a form caused by certain poisons and marked by scanty urine with little or no albuminuria or edema.

**amyloid n.**, (1) renal *amyloidosis;* (2) the nephrotic syndrome due to renal amyloidosis.

**cholemic n.**, the occurrence of acute renal failure in jaundiced patients. The kidneys contain tubular casts of bile and may show tubular necrosis, but there is little evidence that jaundice or bile casts directly damage the kidneys.

**hemoglobinuric n.**, acute oliguric renal failure associated with hemoglobinuria, due to massive intravascular hemolysis, for example, following an incompatible blood transfusion. The kidneys show the morphologic changes of hypoxic n.

**hypoxic n.**, acute oliguric renal failure following hemorrhage, burns, shock or other causes of hypovolemia and reduced renal blood flows; frequently associated with patchy tubular necrosis, tubulorrhexis, and distal tubular casts of hemoglobin.

**lipoid n.**, n., occurring most frequently in children marked by edema and albuminuria and an increase in cholesterol in the blood, but otherwise with fairly good renal function. The tubular epithelium is vacuolated by cholesterol droplets, but the glomeruli show only minimal changes. The foot processes of the glomerular epithelial cells are fused. This change is probably secondary to the proteinuria. The cause of the increased glomerular permeability to plasma protein is unknown.

**lower nephron n.**, in which the distal parts of the renal tubules are chiefly affected.

**osmotic n.**, swelling of renal tubular epithelium associated with glomerular filtration of sugars. The swelling is due to formation of cytoplasmic vesicles by pinocytosis, and is reversible, probably with no dysfunction, when produced by glucose or mannitol. Large doses of sucrose intravenously have been reported to produce renal failure in animals.

**toxic n.**, acute oliguric renal failure due to chemical poisons, for example, mercuric chloride; septicemia, or bacterial toxemia; frequently associated with extensive necrosis of proximal convoluted tubules.

**vacuolar n.**, hypokalemic *nephropathy*.

**nephrospasia, nephrospasis** (nef-ro-spa'sī-ah, nef-ros'pă-sis) [ nephro- + G. *spasis*, a pulling. SPA- ]. Floating kidney in which the organ is attached only by the blood vessels entering at the hilus.

**nephros'toma, neph'rostome** [ nephro- + G. *stoma*, mouth ]. One of the ciliated funnel-shaped openings by which pronephric and some primitive mesonephric tubules communicate with the celom.

**nephrostomy** (ne-fros'to-mī) [ nephro- + G. *stoma*, mouth ]. The establishment of an opening between the pelvis of the kidney and the external surface of the body.

**nephrot'ic.** Relating to, caused by, or similar to nephrosis.

**neph'rotome** [ nephro- + G. *tomē*, a cutting. TOM- ]. The intermediate mesoderm, sometimes so designated because it gives rise to nephric primordia.

**nephrotomic** (nef'ro-tom'ik). Relating to the nephrotome.

**neph'rotom'ogram.** Sectional x-rays of the kidney.

**neph'rotomog'raphy.** X-ray examination of the kidney by tomography.

**nephrotomy** (ne-frot'o-mī) [ nephro- + G. *tomē*, incision ]. Incision into the substance of the kidney.

**nephrotox'ic.** Pertaining to nephrotoxin; poisonous to the cells of the kidney; nephrolytic.

**nephrotox'in.** A cytotoxin that is specific for cells of the kidney.

**nephrotresis** (nef'ro-tre'sis) [ nephro- + G. *trēsis*, a boring ]. The establishment of a permanent opening into the kidney from the loin for the purpose of giving exit to the renal excretion.

**nephrotroph'ic.** Renotrophic.

**nephrotrop'ic.** Renotrophic.

**neph'rotuberculo'sis.** Tuberculosis of the kidney; renal tuberculosis.

**nephroty'phoid.** Acute nephritis, or symptoms suggesting it (lumbar pain, albuminuria, edema, etc.), caused by the typhoid bacilli or their toxin in a case of typhoid fever.

**nephroty'phus.** Acute hemorrhagic nephritis occurring as a complicating lesion in typhus fever.

**nephroureterectomy** (nef'ro-u-re'ter-ek'to-mī) [ nephro- + ureter + G. *ektomē*, excision ]. Surgical removal of a kidney and its ureter.

**neph'roure'terocystec'tomy** [ nephro- + ureter, + G. *kystis*, bladder, + *ektomē*, excision ]. Removal of kidney, ureter, and part of bladder.

**nepiology** (nep-ĭ-ol'o-jī) [ G. *nepios* (adj.), infant, + *logos*, study ]. The branch of pediatrics dealing with young infants.

**neptunium** (nep-tu'nī-um) [ planet, *Neptune* ]. A transuranian radioactive element; symbol Np, atomic no. 93; parent element of the n. radioactive series (not found in nature).

**nequinate** (nĕ-kwin'āt) (USAN). STATYL; methyl 7-(benzyloxy) -6- butyl-1, 4- dihydro-4-oxo-3-quinolinecarboxylate; a coccidiostat for poultry.

**Néri's sign.** See under sign.

**nerian'tin.** A glucoside from *Nerium oleander* (family Apocynaceae), oleander.

**neriin** (ne'rĭ-in). A glucoside from the leaves and bark of the oleander; belongs to digitalis group of glucosides.

**neriine** (ne'rĭ-ēn). Conessine.

**Nernst,** Walther, Berlin physicist, 1864–1941. See N.'s *equation, theory.*

**neroli oil** (nĕr'o-lĭ, nēr-). Orange flower oil; see under orange.

# NERVE

**nerve** [ L. nervus. NERV- ]. Nervus. 1. For gross anatomical definition and reference to NA nomenclature for nerves, see nervus; see also color plates 27 to 31 for gross relationships of n.'s. 2. Microscopically, a n. is a bundle composed of one or more fascicles of myelinated or unmyelinated n. fibers, or more often mixtures of both, together with accompanying connective tissue and blood vessels. The connective tissue within the fascicle and around the neurolemma of individual n. fibers is called endoneurium; that forming a sheath around each fascicle, perineurium; and that around the entire n. and between fascicles, epineurium.

**abducent n.,** *nervus* abducens.

**accelerator n.'s,** the slender n.'s establishing the sympathetic innervation of the heart. Originating from the ganglion cells of the superior, middle, and inferior cervical ganglion of the sympathetic trunk, hence unmyelinated, the efferent fibers of the accelerator n.'s upon stimulation increase the heart rate.

**accessory n.,** *nervus* accessorius.

**accessory phrenic n.'s,** *nervi* phrenici accessorii.

**acoustic n.,** *nervus* vestibulocochlearis.

**af'ferent n.,** centripetal or esodic n.; a n. conveying impulses from the periphery to the central nervous system.

**Andersch's n.,** *nervus* tympanicus.

**anococcygeal n.'s,** *nervi* anococcygei.

**anterior ampullar n.,** *nervus* ampullaris anterior.

**anterior antebrachial n.,** *nervus* interosseus anterior.

**anterior auricular n.'s,** *nervi* auriculares anteriores.

**anterior crural n.,** *nervus* femoralis.

**anterior ethmoidal n.,** *nervus* ethmoidalis anterior.

**anterior interosseous n.,** *nervus* interosseus anterior.

**anterior labial n.'s,** *nervi* labiales anteriores.

**anterior scrotal n.'s,** *nervi* scrotales anteriores.

**anterior supraclavicular n.,** *nervus* supraclavicularis medialis.

**anterior thoracic n.,** *nervus* pectoralis.

**anterior tibial n.,** *nervus* peroneus profundus.

**aortic n.,** depressor n. of Ludwig; Cyon's n.; Ludwig's n.; a branch of the vagus which ends in the aortic arch and base of the heart; composed entirely of afferent fibers; its stimulation elicits a brainstem reflex which causes slowing of the heart, dilation of the peripheral vessels, and a fall in blood pressure.

**Arnold's n.,** *ramus* auricularis vagi.

**articular n.,** *nervus* articularis.

**auditory n.,** see *nervus* vestibulocochlearis.

**augmentor n.'s,** accelerator n.'s, called augmentor because their action is to increase the force as well as the rate of the heart beat.

**auriculotemporal n.,** *nervus* auriculotemporalis.

**autonomic n.,** a bundle of nerve fibers belonging or relating to the autonomic nervous system.

**axillary n.,** *nervus* axillaris.

**baroreceptor n.,** pressoreceptor n.

**Bell's respiratory n.,** *nervus* thoracicus longus.

**bigem'inal n.,** *nervus* bigeminus.

**Bock's n.,** *ramus* pharyngeus.

**buccal n.,** *nervus* buccalis.

**buc'cinator n.,** *nervus* buccalis.

**caroticotympanic n.,** *nervus* caroticotympanicus.

**cavernous n.'s of clitoris,** *nervi* cavernosi clitoridis.

**cavernous n.'s of penis,** *nervi* cavernosi penis.

**centrif'ugal n.,** efferent n.

**centrip'etal n.,** afferent n.

**cervical n.'s,** *nervi* cervicales.

**chorda tym'pani n.,** *chorda* tympani.

**circumflex n.,** *nervus* axillaris.

**coccygeal n.,** *nervus* coccygeus.

**cochlear n.,** see *nervus* vestibulocochlearis.

**common fibular n.,** *nervus* peroneus communis.

**common palmar digital n.'s,** *nervi* digitales palmares communes.

**common peroneal n.,** *nervus* peroneus fibularis communis.

**common plantar digital n.'s,** *nervi* digitales plantares communes.

**cranial n.'s,** *nervi* craniales.

**cubital n.,** *nervus* ulnaris.

**cutaneous n.,** *nervus* cutaneus.

**cutaneous cervical n.,** *nervus* transversus colli.

**Cyon's n.,** aortic n.

**dead n.,** misnomer for a dead pulp of a tooth.

**deep fibular n.,** *nervus* peroneus profundus.

**deep peroneal n.,** *nervus* peroneus fibularis profundus.

**deep petrosal n.,** *nervus* petrosus profundus.

**deep temporal n.'s,** *nervi* temporales profundi.

**dental n.,** (1) layman's term for a dental pulp; (2) see entries under *nervus* alveolaris.

**depressor n. of Ludwig,** aortic n.

**dorsal n. of clitoris,** *nervus* dorsalis clitoridis.

**dorsal digital n.'s,** *nervi* digitales dorsales.

**dorsal digital n.'s of the foot,** *nervi* digitales dorsales pedis.

**dorsal interosseous n.,** *nervus* interosseus posterior.

**dorsal lateral cutaneous n.,** *nervus* cutaneus dorsalis lateralis.

**dorsal medial cutaneous n.,** *nervus* cutaneus dorsalis medialis.

**dorsal n. of penis,** *nervus* dorsalis penis.

**dorsal n. of scapula,** *nervus* dorsalis scapulae.

**dorsal n.'s of the toes,** *nervi* digitales dorsales pedis.

**ef'ferent n.,** centrifugal or exodic n.; a n. conveying impulses from the central nervous system to the periphery.

**eighth cranial n.,** *nervus* vestibulocochlearis.

**eleventh cranial n.,** *nervus* accessorius.

**esod'ic n.,** afferent n.

**excitor n.,** a n. conducting impulses that stimulate to increased function.

**excitore'flex n.,** a visceral n. the special function of which is to cause reflex action.

**exod'ic n.,** efferent n.

**n. of external acoustic meatus,** *nervus* meatus acustici externi.

**external carotid n.'s,** *nervi* carotici externi.

**external respiratory n. of Bell,** *nervus* thoracicus longus.

**external saphenous n.,** *nervus* suralis.

**facial n.,** *nervus* facialis.

**femoral n.,** *nervus* femoralis.

**fifth cranial n.,** *nervus* trigeminus.

**first cranial n.,** see *nervi* olfactorii.

**fourth n.,** *nervus* trochlearis.

**fourth lumbar n.,** furcal n.

**frontal n.,** *nervus* frontalis.

**furcal n.,** *nervus* furcalis; the fourth lumbar nerve, the ventral branch of which is forked to enter into the formation of both lumbar and sacral plexuses.

**Galen's n.,** Galen's *anastomosis.*

**gan'gliated n.,** a sympathetic n.

**Gaskell's n.'s,** rarely used eponym for the accelerator n.'s of the heart.

**genitocru'ral n.,** *nervus* genitofemoralis.

**genitofemoral n.,** *nervus* genitofemoralis.

**glossopharyngeal n.,** *nervus* glossopharyngeus.

**great auricular n.,** *nervus* auricularis magnus.

**great sciatic n.,** *nervus* ischiadicus.

**greater occipital n.,** *nervus* occipitalis major.

**greater palatine n.,** *nervus* palatinus major.

**greater petrosal n.,** *nervus* petrosus major.

**greater splanchnic n.,** *nervus* splanchnicus major.

**greater superficial petrosal n.,** *nervus* petrosus major.

**hemorrhoid'al n.'s,** *plexus* rectalis superior; *plexus* rectalis medii; *nervi* rectales inferiores.

**Hering's sinus n.,** *ramus* sinus carotici nervi glossopharyngei.

**hypogastric n.,** *nervus* hypogastricus.

**hypoglossal n.,** *nervus* hypoglossus.

**iliohypogastric n.,** *nervus* iliohypogastricus.
**ilioinguinal n.,** *nervus* ilioinguinalis.
**inferior alveolar n.,** *nervus* alveolaris inferior.
**inferior cervical cardiac n.,** *nervus* cardiacus cervicalis inferior.
**inferior cluneal n.'s,** *nervi* clunium inferiores.
**inferior dental n.,** *nervus* alveolaris inferior.
**inferior gluteal n.,** *nervus* gluteus inferior.
**inferior hemorrhoidal n.'s,** *nervi* rectales inferiores.
**inferior laryngeal n.,** *nervus* laryngeus inferior.
**inferior maxillary n.,** *nervus* mandibularis.
**inferior rectal n.'s,** *nervi* rectales inferiores.
**inferior vesical n.'s,** several small n.'s passing from the pudendal plexus to the bladder.
**infraorbital n.,** *nervus* infraorbitalis.
**infratrochlear n.,** *nervus* infratrochlearis.
**inhib'itory n.,** a n. conveying impulses that diminish functional activity in a part.
**intercostal n.'s,** *nervi* intercostales.
**intercostobrachial n.'s,** *nervi* intercostobrachiales.
**intercostohu'meral n.'s,** *nervi* intercostobrachiales.
**intermediary n.,** *nervus* intermedius.
**intermediate n.,** *nervus* intermedius.
**intermediate dorsal cutaneous n.,** *nervus* cutaneus dorsalis intermedius.
**intermediate supraclavicular n.,** *nervus* supraclavicularis intermedius.
**internal carotid n.,** *nervus* caroticus internus.
**internal saphenous n.,** *nervus* saphenus.
**interosseous n. of leg,** *nervus* interosseus cruris.
**Jacobson's n.,** *nervus* tympanicus.
**jugular n.,** *nervus* jugularis.
**lacrimal n.,** *nervus* lacrimalis.
**Latarjet's n.,** *plexus* hypogastricus superior.
**lateral ampullar n.,** *nervus* ampullaris lateralis.
**lateral cutaneous n. of forearm,** *nervus* cutaneus antebrachii lateralis.
**lateral cutaneous n. of thigh,** *nervus* cutaneus femoris lateralis.
**lateral plantar n.,** *nervus* plantaris lateralis.
**lateral popliteal n.,** *nervus* peroneus fibularis communis.
**lateral supraclavicular n.,** *nervus* supraclavicularis lateralis.
**lateral sural cutaneous n.,** *nervus* cutaneus surae lateralis.
**lesser occipital n.,** *nervus* occipitalis minor.
**lesser palatine n.'s,** *nervi* palatini minores.
**lesser splanchnic n.,** *nervus* splanchnicus minor.
**lesser superficial petrosal n.,** *nervus* petrosus minor.
**lingual n.,** *nervus* lingualis.
**long buccal n.,** *nervus* buccalis.
**long ciliary n.,** *nervus* ciliaris longus.
**long saphenous n.,** *nervus* saphenus.
**long subscapular n.,** *nervus* thoracodorsalis.
**long thoracic n.,** *nervus* thoracicus longus.
**lower lateral cutaneous n. of arm,** *nervus* cutaneus brachii lateralis inferior.
**lowest splanchnic n.,** *nervus* splanchnicus imus.
**Ludwig's n.,** aortic n.
**lumbar n.'s,** *nervi* lumbales.
**lumbar splanchnic n.'s,** *nervi* splanchnici lumbales.
**lumboin'guinal n.,** femoral branch of genitofemoral n.; see *nervus* genitofemoralis.
**mandibular n.,** *nervus* mandibularis.
**masseteric n.,** *nervus* massetericus.
**masticator n.,** *radix* motoria nervi trigemini.
**medial cutaneous n. of arm,** *nervus* cutaneus brachii medialis.
**medial cutaneous n. of forearm,** *nervus* cutaneus antebrachii medialis.
**medial cutaneous n. of leg,** *nervus* cutaneus surae medialis.
**medial plantar n.,** *nervus* plantaris medialis.
**medial popliteal n.,** *nervus* tibialis.
**medial supraclavicular n.,** *nervus* supraclavicularis medialis.
**median n.,** *nervus* medianus.
**mental n.,** *nervus* mentalis.
**middle cervical cardiac n.,** *nervus* cardiacus cervicalis medius.
**middle cluneal n.'s,** *nervi* clunium medii.

**middle meningeal n.,** *ramus* meningeus medius nervi maxillaris.
**middle supraclavicular n.,** *nervus* supraclavicularis intermedius.
**mixed n.,** a n. containing both afferent and efferent fibers.
**motor n.,** motorius; an efferent n. conveying an impulse that excites muscular contraction.
**motor n. of face,** *nervus* facialis.
**musculocutaneous n.,** *nervus* musculocutaneus.
**musculocuta'neous n. of leg,** *nervus* peroneus superficialis.
**musculospiral n.,** *nervus* radialis.
**mylohyoid n.,** *nervus* mylohyoideus.
**nasal n.,** *nervus* nasociliaris.
**nasociliary n.,** *nervus* nasociliaris.
**nasopalatine n.,** *nervus* nasopalatinus.
**ninth cranial n.,** *nervus* glossopharyngeus; under the old nomenclature, which counted but nine cranial n.'s, the ninth was what is now the twelfth (hypoglossal).
**obturator n.,** *nervus* obturatorius.
**oculomotor n.,** *nervus* oculomotorius.
**olfactory n.,** see *nervi* olfactorii.
**ophthalmic n.,** *nervus* ophthalmicus.
**optic n.,** *nervus* opticus.
**orbital n.,** *nervus* zygomaticus.
**parasympathetic n.'s,** one of the n.'s of the parasympathetic nervous system.
**pathetic n.,** *nervus* trochlearis.
**pectoral n.,** *nervus* pectoralis.
**pelvic splanchnic n.'s,** *nervi* splanchnici pelvini.
**perineal n.'s,** *nervi* perineales.
**peroneal communicating n.,** *ramus* communicans peroneus.
**phrenic n.,** *nervus* phrenicus.
**pneumogas'tric n.,** *nervus* vagus.
**popliteal communicating n.,** *nervus* cutaneus surae medialis.
**posterior ampullar n.,** *nervus* ampullaris posterior.
**posterior antebrachial n.,** *nervus* interosseus posterior.
**posterior auricular n.,** *nervus* auricularis posterior.
**posterior cutaneous n. of arm,** *nervus* cutaneus brachii posterior.
**posterior cutaneous n. of forearm,** *nervus* cutaneus antebrachii posterior.
**posterior ethmoidal n.,** *nervus* ethmoidalis posterior.
**posterior femoral cutaneous n.,** *nervus* cutaneus femoris posterior.
**posterior interosseous n.,** *nervus* interosseus posterior.
**posterior labial n.'s,** *nervi* labiales posteriores.
**posterior scapular n.,** *nervus* dorsalis scapulae.
**posterior scrotal n.'s,** *nervi* scrotales posteriores.
**posterior supraclavicular n.,** *nervus* supraclavicularis lateralis.
**posterior thoracic n.,** *nervus* thoracicus longus.
**presacral n.,** *plexus* hypogastrica superior.
**pressor n.,** an afferent n., stimulation of which excites a reflex vasoconstriction, thereby raising the blood pressure.
**pressorecep'tor n.,** baroreceptor n.; a n. composed of afferent fibers the endings of which are sensitive to increases in mechanical pressure; the term specifically refers to sensory n.'s innervating the walls of hollow organs.
**proper palmar digital n.'s,** *nervi* digitales palmares proprii.
**proper plantar digital n.'s,** *nervi* digitales plantares proprii.
**pterygoid n.,** *nervus* pterygoideus.
**n. of pterygoid canal,** *nervus* canalis pterygoidei.
**pterygopalatine n.'s,** *nervi* pterygopalatini.
**pudendal n.,** *nervus* pudendus.
**pudic n.,** *nervus* pudendus.
**radial n.,** *nervus* radialis.
**recurrent n.,** *nervus* laryngeus recurrens.
**recurrent laryngeal n.,** *nervus* laryngeus recurrens.
**recurrent meningeal n.,** *ramus* meningeus medius nervi maxillaris.
**n. to the rhomboid,** *nervus* dorsalis scapulae.
**saccular n.,** *nervus* saccularis.
**sacral n.'s,** *nervi* sacrales.
**sacral splanchnic n.'s,** *nervi* splanchnici sacrales.
**saphenous n.,** *nervus* saphenus.

**sciatic n.,** *nervus* ischiadicus.

**second cranial n.,** *nervus* opticus.

**secre'tory n.,** a n. conveying impulses that excite functional activity in a gland.

**sensory n.,** an afferent n. conveying impulses that are processed by the central nervous system so as to become part of the organism's perception of self and its environment.

**seventh cranial n.,** nervus facialis; under the old nomenclature, which counted but nine cranial n.'s, the seventh included what are now called the seventh and the eighth (facial and vestibulocochlear or octavus).

**short ciliary n.,** *nervus* ciliaris brevis.

**short saphenous n.,** *nervus* suralis.

**sinus n. of Hering,** *ramus* sinus carotici nervi glossopharyngei.

**sinuvertebral n.,** *ramus* meningeus nervi spinalis.

**sixth cranial n.,** *nervus* abducens.

**small deep petrosal n.,** *nervus* caroticotympanicus.

**small sciatic n.,** *nervus* cutaneus femoris posterior.

**smallest splanchnic n.,** *nervus* splanchnicus imus.

**n. of smell,** see *nervi* olfactorii.

**somat'ic n.,** one of the n.'s of sensation or motion, as distinguished from the trophic and secretory n.'s.

**space n.,** one of the branches of the auditory n. distributed to the semicircular canals.

**spinal n.'s,** *nervi* spinales.

**spinal accessory n.,** *nervus* accessorius.

**splanchnic n.,** one of the n.'s supplying the viscera; see entries under *nervus* splanchnicus.

**n. to stapedius muscle,** *nervus* stapedius.

**subclavian n.,** *nervus* subclavius.

**subcostal n.,** *nervus* subcostalis.

**sublingual n.,** *nervus* sublingualis.

**suboccipital n.,** *nervus* suboccipitalis.

**subscapular n.,** *nervus* subscapularis.

**superficial cervical n.,** *nervus* transversus colli.

**superficial fibular n.,** *nervus* peroneus superficialis.

**superficial peroneal n.,** *nervus* peroneus superficialis.

**superior alveolar n.'s,** *nervi* alveolares superiores.

**superior cervical cardiac n.,** *nervus* cardiacus cervicalis superior.

**superior cluneal n.'s,** *nervi* clunium superiores.

**superior dental n.'s,** *nervi* alveolares superiores.

**superior gluteal n.,** *nervus* gluteus superior.

**superior laryngeal n.,** *nervus* laryngeus superior.

**superior maxillary n.,** *nervus* maxillaris.

**supraorbital n.,** *nervus* supraorbitalis.

**suprascapular n.,** *nervus* suprascapularis.

**supratrochlear n.,** *nervus* supratrochlearis.

**sural n.,** *nervus* suralis.

**sympathetic n.,** one of the n.'s of the sympathetic nervous system.

**temporomandibular n.,** *nervus* zygomaticus.

**n. of tensor veli palatini muscle,** *nervus* tensoris veli palatini.

**tenth cranial n.,** *nervus* vagus.

**tento'rial n.,** *ramus* tentorii.

**terminal n.'s,** *nervi* terminales.

**third cranial n.,** *nervus* oculomotorius.

**third occipital n.,** *nervus* occipitalis te.tius.

**third sacral n.,** *nervus* bigeminus.

**thoracic n.'s,** *nervi* thoracici.

**thoracic cardiac n.'s,** *nervi* cardiaci thoracici.

**thoracodorsal n.,** *nervus* thoracodorsalis.

**tibial n.,** *nervus* tibialis.

**tibial communicating n.,** *nervus* cutaneus surae medialis.

**Tiedemann's n.,** a n. accompanying the central artery of the retina in the optic n.

**transverse nerve of neck,** *nervus* transversus colli.

**trifacial n.,** *nervus* trigeminus.

**trigeminal n.,** *nervus* trigeminus.

**trochlear n.,** *nervus* trochlearis.

**twelfth cranial n.,** *nervus* hypoglossus.

**tympanic n.,** *nervus* tympanicus.

**ulnar n.,** *nervus* ulnaris.

**upper lateral cutaneous n. of arm,** *nervus* cutaneus brachii lateralis superior.

**utricular n.,** *nervus* utricularis.

**utriculoampullar n.,** *nervus* utriculoampullaris.

**vaginal n.'s,** *nervi* vaginales.

**vagus n.,** *nervus* vagus.

**Valentin's n.,** connects the sphenopalatine ganglion with the sixth n.

**vascular n.,** *nervus* vascularis.

**vasomo'tor n.,** a motor n. effecting dilation (vasodilator n.) or contraction (vasoconstrictor n.) of the blood vessels.

**vertebral n.,** *nervus* vertebralis.

**vestibular n.,** see *nervus* vestibulocochlearis.

**vestibulocochlear n.,** *nervus* vestibulocochlearis.

**Vidian n.,** *nervus* canalis pterygoidei.

**volar interosseous n.,** *nervus* interosseus anterior.

**Wrisberg's n.,** (1) *nervus* cutaneus brachii medialis; (2) *nervus* intermedius.

**zygomatic n.,** *nervus* zygomaticus.

---

**ner'vi** [ L. ] [ NA ]. Plural of nervus.

**nervimotil'ity.** Neurimotility; capability of movement in response to a nervous stimulus.

**nervimo'tion.** Movement in response to a nervous stimulus.

**nervimo'tor.** Neurimotor; relating to a motor nerve.

**ner'vine.** 1. Acting therapeutically, especially as a sedative, upon the nervous system. 2. An agent that increases nerve force and lessens irritability.

**ner'vone.** A cerebroside containing nervonic acid.

**nervon'ic acid.** A 24-carbon straight-chain fatty acid unsaturated between C-15 and C-16.

**ner'vosism** [ L. *nervosus* ]. 1. Neurasthenia (1). 2. Hypothetical dependence of psychiatric conditions upon alterations of nerve force.

**nervous** (ner'vus) [ L. *nervosus* ]. 1. Relating to a nerve or the nerves. 2. Easily excited or agitated; suffering from instability.

**ner'vousness.** A condition of unrest and of irritability.

---

# NERVUS

---

**ner'vus,** gen. and pl. **ner'vi** [ L. NERV- ] [ NA ]. Nerve; a whitish cord, made up of nerve fibers arranged in bundles (fascicles) held together by a connective tissue sheath. Stimuli are transmitted from the central nervous system to the periphery or the reverse through the fibers. Nerve branches are given in the definition of the major nerve; many are also listed and defined under ramus. See also nerve (for histological description), and color plates 27 to 31.

**n. abdu'cens** [ NA ], abducent nerve; 6th cranial nerve; a small motor nerve supplying the lateral rectus muscle of the eye; its origin is in the dorsal part of the tegmentum of the pons just below the surface of the rhomboidal fossa, and it emerges from the brain in the fissure between the medulla oblongata and the posterior border of the pons; in its intracranial trajectory, the longest of all cranial nerves, it passes along the cavernous sinus and enters the orbit through the superior orbital fissure.

**n. acesso'rius** [ NA ], accessorius willisii; accessory nerve; spinal accessory nerve; 11th cranial nerve; arises by two sets of roots, cranial and spinal; the former emerge from the side of the medulla and unite to form the internal ramus; the latter emerge from the ventrolateral part of the spinal cord from the first five cervical segments and unite to form the external ramus; the internal ramus joins the vagus in the jugular foramen supplying the muscles of the pharynx, soft palate and larynx; the external ramus supplies the sternocleidomastoid and trapezius muscles.

**n. acu'sticus,** n. vestibulocochlearis.

**n. alveolaris inferior** [ NA ], inferior alveolar nerve; inferior dental nerve; one of the terminal branches of the mandibular, it enters the mandibular canal to be distributed to the lower teeth, periosteum, and gingiva of the mandible; a branch, the mental nerve, passes through the mental foramen to supply the skin of the lower lip and chin.

**nervi alveolares superiores** [ NA ], superior alveolar nerves; superior dental nerves; three branches (posterior, middle, and anterior) of the maxillary nerve that enter the maxilla to supply the upper teeth and gingiva.

**n. ampulla'ris ante'rior** [ NA ], anterior ampullar nerve; a branch of the utriculoampullar nerve that supplies the crista ampullaris of the anterior semicircular duct.

**n. ampulla'ris latera'lis** [ NA ], lateral ampullar nerve; a branch of the utriculoampullar nerve that supplies the crista ampullaris of the lateral semicircular duct.

**n. ampulla'ris poste'rior** [ NA ], posterior ampullar nerve; a branch of the vestibular part of the eighth nerve that supplies the crista ampullaris of the posterior semicircular duct.

**nervi anococcygei** [ NA ], anococcygeal nerves; several small nerves arising from the coccygeal plexus, supplying the skin over the coccyx.

**n. antebra'chii ante'rior** [ NA ], official alternative term for n. interosseus anterior.

**n. antebra'chii poste'rior** [ NA ], official alternative term for n. interosseus posterior.

**n. articula'ris** [ NA ], articular nerve; a branch of a nerve supplying a joint.

**nervi auricula'res anterio'res** [ NA ], anterior auricular nerves; branches of the auriculotemporal nerve that supply the tragus and upper part of the auricle.

**n. auricula'ris magnus** [ NA ], great auricular nerve; arises from the 2d and 3d cervical, supplies the skin of part of the ear, adjacent portion of the scalp, cheek, and angle of the jaw.

**n. auricula'ris poste'rior** [ NA ], posterior auricular nerve; the first extracranial branch of the facial nerve; it passes behind the ear, supplying the auricularis posterior and intrinsic muscles of the auricle and, through its occipital branch, innervating the occipital belly of the occipitofrontal muscle.

**n. auric'ulotempora'lis** [ NA ], auriculotemporal nerve; a branch of the mandibular, usually by two roots embracing the middle meningeal artery; it passes backward beneath the lateral pterygoid muscle, between the sphenomandibular ligament and the neck of the mandible, and through the parotid gland, terminating in the skin of the temple and scalp; it sends branches to the external acoustic meatus, tympanic membrane, parotid gland and auricle as well as a communicating branch to the facial nerve.

**n. axilla'ris** [ NA ], axillary nerve; circumflex nerve; arises from the posterior cord of the brachial plexus in the axilla, passes downward and laterally with the posterior circumflex artery, and winds round the surgical neck of the humerus supplying the deltoid and teres minor muscles.

**n. bigem'inus** [ L. twin ], bigeminal nerve; the third sacral nerve, the ventral division of which divides to enter into the formation of both sacral and pudendal plexuses.

**n. buccalis** [ NA ], buccal nerve; buccinator nerve; long buccal nerve; a sensory branch of the mandibular division of the trigeminal nerve; it passes downward and forward on the buccinator muscle to supply the buccal mucous membrane and skin of the cheek near the angle of the mouth.

**n. canal'is pterygoi'dei** [ NA ], radix facialis [ NA ]; facial root; nerve of the pterygoid canal; Vidian nerve; the nerve constituting the motor and sympathetic roots of the pterygopalatine ganglion; it is formed in the foramen lacerum by the union of the greater petrosal and the deep petrosal nerves, and runs through the pterygoid canal to the pterygopalatine fossa.

**n. cardiacus cervica'lis inferior** [ NA ], inferior cervical cardiac nerve; a nerve passing from the cervicothoracic ganglion of the sympathetic, to the cardiac plexus.

**n. cardiacus cervica'lis medius** [ NA ], middle cervical cardiac nerve; a bundle of fibers running downward, from the middle cervical ganglion of the sympathetic, along the subclavian artery (on the left) or the brachiocephalic (on the right side) to join the cardiac plexus.

**n. cardiacus cervica'lis superior** [ NA ], superior cervical cardiac nerve; a nerve which arises from the lower part of the superior cervical ganglion of the sympathetic, and passes down to form, with branches of the vagus, the cardiac plexus.

**nervi cardiaci thoracici** [ NA ], thoracic cardiac nerves; branches from the second to fifth segments of the thoracic

sympathetic trunk that passes forward to enter the cardiac plexus.

**nervi carotici externi** [ NA ], external carotid nerves; a number of sympathetic nerve fibers extending upward from the superior cervical ganglion along the external carotid artery, forming the external carotid plexus.

**n. carot'icotympan'icus,** pl. **nervi carot'icotympan'ici** [ NA ], carotico tympanic nerve; small deep petrosal nerve; one of two sympathetic branches from the internal carotid plexus to the tympanic plexus.

**n. caroticus internus** [ NA ], internal carotid nerve; a sympathetic nerve extending upward from the superior cervical ganglion along the internal carotid artery, forming the internal carotid plexus.

**nervi caverno'si clitor'idis** [ NA ], cavernous nerves or plexus of the clitoris; they correspond to the nervi cavernosi penis in the male.

**nervi caverno'si pe'nis** [ NA ], cavernous nerves or plexus of the penis; two nerves, major and minor, derived from the inferior hypogastric plexus supplying sympathetic and parasympathetic fibers to the corpus cavernosum.

**nervi cervica'les** [ NA ], cervical nerves whose nuclei of origin are situated in the cervical spinal cord.

**n. cervica'lis superficia'lis,** n. transversus colli.

**n. cilia'ris brev'is** pl. **nervi cilia'res brev'es** [ NA ], short ciliary nerve; one of a number of branches of the ciliary ganglion, supplying the ciliary muscles, iris, and tunics of the eyeball.

**n. cilia'ris longus,** pl. **nervi cilia'res lon'gi** [ NA ], long ciliary nerve; one of two or three branches of the nasociliary nerve, supplying the ciliary muscles, iris, and cornea.

**nervi clunium inferiores** [ NA ], inferior cluneal nerves, branches of the posterior femoral cutaneous nerve supplying the skin of the lower half of the gluteal region.

**nervi clunium medii** [ NA ], middle cluneal nerves; terminal branches of the dorsal rami of the sacral nerves, supplying the skin of the mid-gluteal region.

**nervi cluninum superiores** [ NA ], superior cluneal nerves; terminal branches of the dorsal rami of the lumbar nerves, supplying the skin of the upper half of the gluteal region.

**n. coccygeus** [ NA ], coccygeal nerve; a small nerve, the lowest of the spinal nerves, entering into the formation of the coccygeal plexus.

**n. cochlea'ris,** see n. vestibulocochlearis.

**nervi crania'les** [ NA ], cranial nerves; those nerves that emerge from, or enter, the brain, in contrast to the spinal nerves. The twelve paired cranial nerves are the olfactory, optic, oculomotor, trochlear, trigeminal, abducens, facial, vestibulocochlear, glossopharyngeal, vagal, accessory, and hypoglossal. The first two of these, although traditionally included among the cranial nerves, histologically are not true nerves but control brain tracts.

**n. cuta'neus** [ NA ], cutaneous nerve; a mixed nerve supplying a region of the skin, including its blood vessels, smooth muscle and glands.

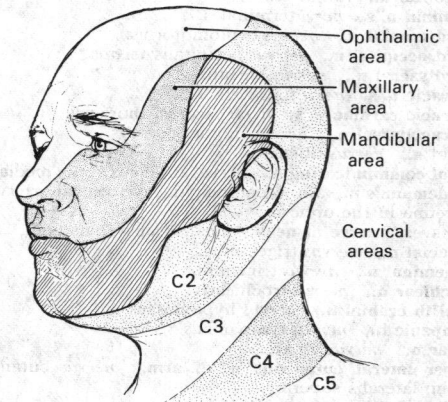

**Cutaneous Nerve Supply of the Face**

**n. cutaneus antebrachii lateralis** [ NA ], lateral cutaneous nerve of the forearm; terminal cutaneous branch of the musculocutaneous nerve; it supplies the skin of the radial side of the forearm.

**n. cutaneus antebrachii medialis** [ NA ], medial cutaneous nerve of the forearm; arises from the medial fasciculus of the brachial plexus, passes downward in company with the brachial artery and then the basilic vein, and supplies the skin of the flexor and ulnar surfaces of the forearm.

**n. cutaneus antebrachii posterior** [ NA ], posterior cutaneous nerve of the forearm; distal lower lateral cutaneous branch of the radial, supplying the skin of the dorsal surface of the forearm.

**n. cutaneus brachii lateralis inferior** [ NA ], lower lateral cutaneous nerve of the arm; a branch of the radial nerve supplying the skin of the lower lateral aspect of the arm. It frequently is a branch of the posterior antebrachial nerve.

**n. cutaneus brachii lateralis superior** [ NA ], upper lateral cutaneous nerve of the arm; a branch of the axillary supplying the skin over the lower portion of the deltoid and for a distance below its insertion.

**n. cutaneus brachii medialis** [ NA ], medial cutaneous nerve of the arm; lesser internal cutaneous nerve; nerve of Wrisberg (1); arises from the medial fasciculus of the brachial plexus, unites in the axilla with the second intercostal nerve, and supplies the skin of the medial side of the arm.

**n. cutaneus brachii posterior** [ NA ], posterior cutaneous nerve of the arm; upper lateral cutaneous branch of the radial nerve; a branch of the radial supplying the skin of the posterior surface of the arm.

**n. cutaneus dorsalis intermedius** [ NA ], intermediate dorsal cutaneous nerve; the lateral terminal branch of the superficial peroneal nerve, supplying the dorsum of the foot and dorsal nerves to the toes.

**n. cutaneus dorsalis lateralis** [ NA ], dorsal lateral cutaneous nerve; the continuation of the sural nerve in the foot, supplying the lateral margin and dorsum.

**n. cutaneus dorsalis medialis** [ NA ], dorsal medial cutaneous nerve; the medial terminal branch of the superficial peroneal nerve, supplying the dorsum of the foot and dorsal nerves to the toes.

**n. cutaneus femoris lateralis** [ NA ], lateral cutaneous nerve of the thigh; arises from the second and third lumbar nerves, supplies the skin of the anterolateral and lateral surfaces of the thigh.

**n. cutaneus femoris posterior** [ NA ], posterior femoral cutaneous nerve; small sciatic nerve; arises from the first three sacral nerves, supplies the skin of the posterior surface of the thigh and of the popliteal region. It gives off a perineal branch that passes to the scrotum or labia majora.

**n. cutaneus surae lateralis** [ NA ], lateral sural cutaneous nerve; it arises from the common peroneal in the popliteal space and is distributed to the skin of the inferolateral surface of the calf.

**n. cutaneus surae medialis** [ NA ], medial cutaneous nerve of the leg; tibial or popliteal communicating nerve; arises from the tibial in the popliteal space, passes down the calf between the two heads of the gastrocnemius and unites in the middle of the leg with the communicating branch of the common peroneal to form the sural nerve, distributed to the skin of the distal and lateral surfaces of the leg and ankle.

**nervi digitales dorsales** [ NA ], dorsal digital nerves; nerves of the hand supplying the skin of the dorsal surface of the fingers.

**nervi digitales dorsales pedis** [ NA ], dorsal digital nerves of the foot; dorsal nerves of the toes; nerves of the foot supplying the skin of the proximal and middle phalanges.

**nervi digita'les palma'res commu'nes** [ NA ], common palmar digital nerves; four nerves in the palm that send branches (nervi digitales palmares proprii) to adjacent sides of two digits; three are branches of the median, one is from the ulnar.

**nervi digita'les palma'res pro'prii** [ NA ], proper palmar digital nerves; ten palmar nerves of the digits of the hand derived from common palmar digital nerves; each nerve supplies a palmar quadrant of a digit and a part of the dorsal surface of the distal phalanx.

**nervi digita'les planta'res commu'nes** [ NA ], common plantar digital nerves; these include three nerves derived from the medial plantar and one from the lateral plantar that supply the skin of the ball of the foot and terminate as proper plantar digital nerves to the side of each toe.

**nervi digita'les planta'res pro'prii** [ NA ], proper plantar digital nerves; the ten nerves derived from the common plantar digital nerves; each nerve supplies a plantar quadrant of a toe and part of the dorsal surface of the distal phalanx.

**n. dorsalis clitoridis** [ NA ], dorsal nerve of the clitoris; the deep terminal branch of the pudendal, supplying especially the glans clitoridis.

**n. dorsalis penis** [ NA ], dorsal nerve of the penis; the deep terminal branch of the pudendal running along the dorsum of the penis, supplying the skin of the penis, the prepuce, and the glans.

**n. dorsalis scapulae** [ NA ], dorsal nerve of the scapula; posterior scapular nerve; nerve to the rhomboids; arises from the fifth to seventh cervical nerves and passes downward to supply the levator scapulae and the rhomboideus major and minor muscles.

**nervi erigentes** [ L. *erigens*, erecting ] [ NA ], *nervi* splanchnici pelvini.

**n. ethmoidalis anterior** [ NA ], anterior ethmoidal nerve; a branch of the nasociliary nerve.

**n. ethmoidalis posterior** [ NA ], posterior ethmoidal nerve; a branch of the nasociliary nerve.

**n. facia'lis** [ NA ], facial nerve; seventh cranial nerve; the motor nerve of the face; its origin is in the tegmentum of the lower portion of the pons, and it emerges from the brain at the posterior border of the pons; it leaves the cranial cavity through the internal acoustic meatus where it is joined by the n. intermedius, traverses the facial canal in the petrous portion of the temporal bone, and makes its exit through the stylomastoid foramen; it passes through the parotid gland and reaches the facial muscles through various branches.

**n. femoralis** [ NA ], femoral nerve; anterior crural nerve; arises from the second, third, and fourth lumbar nerves in the substance of the psoas muscle and enters the thigh lateral to the femoral vessels; it supplies muscles and skin of the anterior region of the thigh.

**n. fibularis communis** [ NA ], n. peroneus communis.

**n. fibularis profundus** [ NA ], n. peroneus profundus.

**n. fibularis superficialis** [ NA ], n. peroneus superficialis.

**n. frontalis** [ NA ], frontal nerve; a branch of the ophthalmic which divides within the orbit into the supratrochlear and the supraorbital nerves.

**n. furca'lis** [ L. ], furcal *nerve.*

**n. genitofemora'lis** [ NA ], genitofemoral nerve; genitocrural nerve; arises from the first and second lumbar nerves, passes distad along the anterior surface of psoas major muscle and divides into genital and femoral branches.

**n. glossopharyn'geus** [ NA ], glossopharyngeal nerve; ninth cranial nerve; it emerges from the rostral end of the medulla and passes through the jugular foramen to supply sensation to the pharynx and posterior third of the tongue; it also carries motor fibers to the stylopharyngeus muscle and the parasympathetic fibers to the otic ganglion.

**n. gluteus inferior** [ NA ], inferior gluteal nerve; arises from the fifth lumbar and first and second sacral, and supplies the gluteus maximus muscle.

**n. gluteus superior** [ NA ], superior gluteal nerve; arises from the fourth and fifth lumbar and first sacral nerves, and supplies the gluteus medius and minimus and tensor fasciae latae muscles.

**n. hemorrhoida'lis,** see *plexus* rectalis superior; *plexus* rectales medii; *plexus* rectales inferiores; *nervi* rectales inferiores.

**n. hypogastricus** [ NA ], hypogastric nerve; one of the two nerve trunks (right and left) which lead from the superior hypogastric plexus into the pelvis to join the inferior hypogastric plexuses.

**n. hypoglos'sus** [ NA ], hypoglossal nerve; twelfth cranial nerve; arises from an oblong nucleus in the medulla and emerges by several roots between the pyramid and the olive; it passes through the hypoglossal canal, then courses downward and forward to supply all the intrinsic muscles of the tongue.

**n. iliohypogastricus** [ NA ], iliohypogastric nerve; arises from the first lumbar nerve; it supplies the abdominal muscles and the skin of the lower part of the anterior abdominal wall.

**n. ilioinguinalis** [ NA ], ilioinguinal nerve; arises from the first lumbar, passes through the superficial inguinal ring to supply the skin of the upper medial thigh and scrotum or labia majora.

**n. impar,** *filum* terminale.

**n. infraorbita'lis** [ NA ], infraorbital nerve; the continuation of the maxillary nerve after it has entered the orbit, traversing the infraorbital canal to reach the face; it supplies the upper incisors, canine and premolars, the upper gums, the inferior eyelid and conjunctiva, part of the nose and the superior lip.

**n. infratrochlea'ris** [ NA ], infratrochlear nerve; a branch of the nasociliary running beneath the pulley of the superior oblique muscle to the front of the orbit, and supplying the skin of the eyelids and root of the nose.

**nervi intercosta'les** [ NA ], intercostal nerves; ventral branches of the thoracic nerves.

**nervi intercostobrachia'les** [ NA ], intercostobrachial nerves; branches of the second and third intercostal nerves which pass to the skin of the medial side of the arm.

**n. interme'dius** [ NA ], intermediary or intermediate nerve; nerve of Wrisberg (2); pars intermedia (3); portio intermedia; a root of the facial nerve containing sensory fibers whose cell bodies are located in the geniculate ganglion and autonomic fibers whose cell bodies are located in the superior salivatory nucleus.

**n. interos'seus ante'rior** [ NA ], n. antebrachii anterior [ NA ]; anterior interosseous or antebrachial nerve; volar interosseous nerve; a branch of the median supplying the flexor pollicis longus, part of flexor digitorum profundus and the pronator quadratus muscles.

**n. interosseus cruris** [ NA ], interosseous nerve of the leg; a nerve given off from one of the muscular branches of the tibial which passes down over the posterior surface of the interosseous membrane supplying it and the two bones of the leg.

**n. interos'seus dorsa'lis,** n. interosseous posterior.

**n. interos'seus poste'rior** [ NA ], n. antebrachii posterior [ NA ]; n. interosseus dorsalis; posterior interosseous or antebrachial nerve; dorsal interosseous nerve; the deep terminal branch of the radial nerve, supplying the supinator and all the extensor muscles in the forearm.

**n. ischiadicus** [ NA ], sciatic nerve; great sciatic nerve; arises from the sacral plexus, passes through the greater sciatic foramen and down the thigh, at about the middle of which it divides into the common peroneal and tibial nerves.

**n. jugularis** [ NA ], jugular nerve; a communicating branch between the superior cervical ganglion of the sympathetic and the inferior ganglion of the vagus and the inferior ganglion of the glossopharyngeal.

**nervi labiales anteriores** [ NA ], anterior labial nerves; branches of the ilioinguinal nerve distributed to the labia majora.

**nervi labiales posteriores** [ NA ], posterior labial nerves; terminal branches of the perineal nerve, supplying the skin of the posterior portion of the labia and the vestibule of the vagina, corresponding to the posterior scrotal nerve in the male.

**n. lacrimalis** [ NA ], lacrimal nerve; a branch of the ophthalmic, supplying the upper eyelid, conjunctiva, and lacrimal gland.

**n. laryngeus inferior** [ NA ], inferior laryngeal nerve; terminal branch of the recurrent laryngeal; it supplies all laryngeal muscles except the cricothyroid and the mucosa inferior to the vocal folds.

**n. laryngeus recurrens** [ NA ], recurrent laryngeal nerve; recurrent nerve; a branch of the vagus curving upward, on the right side round the root of the subclavian artery, on the left side round the arch of the aorta, then passing up behind the common carotid artery and between the trachea and the esophagus to the larynx; it supplies cardiac, tracheal and esophageal branches terminating as the inferior laryngeal nerve.

**n. laryngeus superior** [ NA ], superior laryngeal nerve; a branch of the vagus at the inferior ganglion; at the thyroid cartilage it divides into two branches, the internal laryngeal nerve supplies the mucous membrane of the larynx superior to the vocal folds, and the external laryngeal nerve supplies the inferior pharyngeal constrictor and the cricothyroid muscle.

**n. lingualis** [ NA ], lingual nerve; one of the branches of the mandibular, passing medial to the lateral pterygoid muscle, between the medial pterygoid and the mandible, and beneath the mucous membrane of the floor of the mouth to the side of the tongue over the anterior two-thirds of which it is distributed: it supplies also the mucous membrane of the floor of the mouth.

**nervi lumbales** [ NA ], lumbar nerves; five nerves on each side, emerging from the lumbar portion of the spinal cord; the first four nerves enter into the formation of the lumbar plexus, the fourth and fifth into that of the sacral plexus.

**n. mandibularis** [ NA ], mandibular nerve; the third division of the trigeminal nerve formed by the union of sensory fibers from the trigeminal (Gasserian) ganglion and the motor root in the foramen ovale, through which the nerve emerges; its branches are: meningeal, masseteric, deep temporal, lateral and medial pterygoid, buccal, auriculotemporal, lingual, and inferior alveolar.

**n. massetericus** [ NA ], masseteric nerve; a muscular branch of the mandibular nerve passing to the medial surface of the masseter muscle which it supplies.

**n. maxillaris** [ NA ], maxillary nerve; the second division of the trigeminal, passing from the trigeminal (Gasserian) ganglion through the foramen rotundum into the pterygopalatine fossa, where it gives off the pterygopalatine nerve and continues forward to give off the zygomatic nerve and enter the orbit, where it is named the infraorbital.

**n. meatus acustici externi** [ NA ], nerve of the external acoustic meatus; a branch of the auriculotemporal nerve supplying the lining of the external acoustic meatus.

**n. medianus** [ NA ], median nerve; formed by the union of medial and lateral roots from the medial and lateral cords of the brachial plexus, respectively; it supplies muscular branches in the anterior region of the forearm and muscular and cutaneous branches in the hand.

**n. mentalis** [ NA ], mental nerve; a branch of the inferior alveolar, arising in the mandibular canal and passing through the mental foramen to the chin and lower lip.

**n. musculocutaneus** [ NA ], musculocutaneous nerve; arises from lateral cord of the brachial plexus, passes through the coracobrachialis muscle, and then downward between the brachialis and biceps, supplying these three muscles and being prolonged as the lateral cutaneous nerve of the forearm.

**n. mylohyoideus** [ NA ], mylohyoid nerve; a small branch of the inferior alveolar given off just before the nerve enters the mandibular foramen, distributed to the anterior belly of the digastric and to the mylohyoid muscle.

**n. nasocilia'ris** [ NA ], nasociliary nerve; nasal nerve; a branch of the ophthalmic in the superior orbital fissure, passing through the orbit, entering the cranial cavity through the anterior ethmoidal foramen, and then the nasal cavity, through the nasal fissure; its branches are the long root of the ciliary ganglion, the long ciliary nerves, the infratrochlear, and nasal branches, supplying the mucous membrane of nose, the skin of the tip of the nose, and the conjunctiva.

**n. nasopalatinus** [ NA ], nasopalatine nerve; a branch from the pterygopalatine ganglion, passing through the sphenopalatine foramen, down the nasal septum, and through the incisive foramen to supply the mucous membrane of the hard palate.

**nervi nervo'rum** [ L. nerves of nerves ], nerves distributed to the sheaths of nerve trunks.

**n. obturatorius** [ NA ], obturator nerve; arises from the second, third, and fourth lumbar nerves in the psoas muscle, crosses the brim of the pelvis, and enters the thigh through the obturator canal; it supplies muscles and skin on the medial side of the thigh.

**n. occipitalis major** [ NA ], greater occipital nerve; medial branch of the dorsal ramus of the second cervical nerve; sends branches to the semispinalis capitis and multifidus cervicis, but is mainly cutaneous, supplying the back part of the scalp.

**n. occipitalis minor** [ NA ], lesser occipital nerve; arises from the second and third cervical nerves; supplies the skin of the posterior surface of the pinna and the adjacent portion of the scalp.

**n. occipitalis tertius** [ NA ], third occipital nerve; medial branch of the dorsal ramus of the third cervical nerve; this is usually joined with the greater occipital, but may exist as an independent nerve supplying cutaneous branches to the scalp and nucha.

**n. octa'vus** [ NA ], n. vestibulocochlearis.

**n. oculomoto'rius** [ NA ], oculomotor nerve; third cranial nerve; supplies all the extrinsic muscles of the eye, except the lateral rectus and superior oblique, it also supplies the levator palpebrae superioris, the ciliary muscle, and the sphincter pupillae; its origin is in the midbrain below the cerebral aqueduct, it emerges from the brain in the interpeduncular fossa, pierces the dura mater to the side of the posterior clinoid process, passes through the cavernous sinus and enters the orbit through the superior orbital fissure.

**nervi olfacto'rii** [ NA ], olfactory nerve; first cranial nerve; nerve of smell; collective term denoting the numerous olfactory filaments: slender fascicles each composed of the thin, unmyelinated axons of 8 to 12 of the bipolar olfactory receptor cells in the olfactory portion of the nasal mucosa. The olfactory filaments pass through the cribriform plate of the ethmoid bone and enter the olfactory bulb, where they terminate in synaptic contact with mitral cells, tufted cells, and granule cells. See also *tractus* olfactorius.

**n. ophthalmicus** [ NA ], ophthalmic nerve; the ophthalmic branch of the trigeminal; passes forward from the trigeminal ganglion in the lateral wall of the cavernous sinus, entering the orbit through the superior orbital fissure; through its branches, frontal, lacrimal, and nasociliary, it supplies sensation to the orbit and its contents, the anterior part of the nasal cavity, and the skin of the nose and forehead.

**n. op'ticus** [ NA ], optic nerve; second cranial nerve; taking origin from the retina, passes out of the orbit through the optic canal to the chiasm, where part of the fibers cross to the opposite side and pass through the optic tract to the geniculate bodies and superior colliculus. See fig. under *tractus* opticus.

**n. palati'nus major** [ NA ], greater palatine nerve; a branch of the pterygopalatine ganglion that passes downward through the greater palatine canal to supply the mucosa and glands of the hard palate, and the anterior part of the soft palate.

**nervi palati'ni mino'res** [ NA ], lesser palatine nerves; usually two, these nerves emerge through the lesser palatine foramina and supply the mucosa and glands of the soft palate and uvula. They are branches of the pterygopalatine ganglion and contain fibers of the maxillary and facial nerves.

**n. pectora'lis** [ NA ], pectoral nerve; anterior thoracic nerve; one of two nerves, medial and lateral, that arise from the medial and lateral cords of the brachial plexus, respectively, and pass to the pectoral muscles.

**nervi perineales** [ NA ], perineal nerves; the superficial terminal branches of the pudendal nerve, supplying most of the muscles of the perineum as well as the skin of that region.

**n. perone'us commu'nis** [ NA ], n. fibularis communis [ NA ]; common peroneal or fibular nerve; lateral popliteal nerve; one of the terminal divisions of the sciatic, passing through the lateral portion of the popliteal space to opposite the head of the fibula where it divides into the superficial and deep peroneal nerves.

**n. perone'us profun'dus** [ NA ], n. fibularis profundus [ NA ]; deep peroneal or fibular nerve; anterior tibial nerve; one of the terminal branches of the common peroneal nerve, passing into the anterior compartment of the leg it supplies the tibialis anterior, extensor hallucis longus, extensor digitorum longus, and peroneus tertius muscles, and also the skin of the great toe and medial surface of the second toe.

**n. perone'us superficia'lis** [ NA ], n. fibularis superficialis [ NA ]; superficial peroneal or fibular nerve; musculocutaneous nerve of the leg; a branch of the common peroneal which passes downward in front of the fibula to supply the

long and short peroneal muscles and terminate in the skin of the dorsum of the foot and toes.

**n. petrosus major** [ NA ], greater petrosal nerve; greater superficial petrosal nerve; the parasympathetic root of the pterygopalatine ganglion; a branch from the knee of the facial nerve running through the canal and groove on the anterior surface of the petrous part of the temporal bone to the foramen lacerum and the pterygoid canal to reach the pterygopalatine ganglion.

**n. petrosus minor** [ NA ], lesser petrosal nerve; lesser superficial petrosal nerve; the parasympathetic root of the otic ganglion, derived from the tympanic plexus; it leaves the tympanic cavity through the canal for the lesser petrosal nerve and passes within the cranium to the sphenopetrosal fissure, or to the foramen ovale, or to a small foramen near it through which it reaches the otic ganglion.

**n. petrosus profundus** [ NA ], deep petrosal nerve; great deep petrosal branch of the carotid plexus; the sympathetic part of the nerve of the pterygoid canal; it arises from the internal carotid plexus and joins the greater petrosal at the entrance of the pterygoid canal.

**n. pharyngeus,** *ramus* pharyngeus.

**n. phren'icus** [ NA ], phrenic nerve; arises from the cervical plexus, chiefly from the fourth nerve, passes downward in front of the scalenus anterior and enters the thorax between the subclavian artery and vein behind the sternoclavicular articulation; it then passes in front of the root of the lung to the diaphragm; it is mainly the motor nerve of the diaphragm but sends sensory fibers to the pericardium (ramus pericardiacus), and branches (rami phrenicoabdominales) that communicate with branches from the celiac plexus.

**nervi phren'ici accesso'rii** [ NA ], accessory phrenic nerves; accessory nerve strands that arise from the fifth cervical nerve, often as branches of the nerve to the subclavius, passing downward to join the phrenic nerve.

**n. plantaris lateralis** [ NA ], lateral plantar nerve; one of the two terminal branches of the tibial nerve; it courses along the lateral side of the sole, dividing into superficial and deep branches. It supplies the skin of the lateral aspect of the sole and the lateral one and one-half toes, it innervates the intrinsic muscles of the plantar part of the foot with the exception of the abductor hallucis and the flexor digitorum brevis.

**n. plantaris medialis** [ NA ], medial plantar nerve; one of the two terminal branches of the tibial nerve; it courses along the medial aspect of the sole to supply the abductor hallucis and flexor digitorum brevis and, by way of common and proper digital branches, to innervate the skin of the medial part of the foot and medial three and one-half toes.

**n. presacra'lis** [ NA ], official alternative name for *plexus* hypogastricus superior.

**n. pterygoideus** [ NA ], pterygoid nerve; one of two motor branches, lateral and medial, of the mandibular, supplying the lateral and medial pterygoid muscles.

**nervi pter'ygopalati'ni** [ NA ], pterygopalatine nerves; nervi sphenopalatini; two short branches, given off by the maxillary in the pterygopalatine fossa, which constitute the short (sensory) roots of the pterygopalatine (Meckel's) ganglion.

**n. puden'dus** [ NA ], pudendal nerve; pudic nerve; plexus pudendus nervosus; formed by fibers from the second, third, and fourth sacral nerves; it passes through the greater sciatic foramen and accompanies the internal pudendal artery, terminating as the dorsal nerve of the penis or of the clitoris.

**n. radialis** [ NA ], radial nerve; musculospiral nerve; arises from the posterior cord of the brachial plexus; it curves round the posterior surface of the humerus and passes down to the cubital fossa where it divides into its two terminal branches, the superficial ramus and the deep ramus; it supplies muscular and cutaneous branches to the dorsal aspect of the arm and forearm.

**nervi rectales inferiores** [ NA ], inferior rectal nerves; inferior hemorrhoidal nerves; several branches of the pudendal nerve that pass to the sphincter ani externus and the skin of the anal region.

**n. saccula'ris** [ NA ], saccular nerve; a branch of the vestibular nerve going to the macula sacculi.

**nervi sacrales** [ NA ], sacral nerves; five nerves issuing from the sacral foramina on either side; three enter into the formation of the sacral plexus, and three into that of the pudendal plexus, the third sacral going to both plexuses.

**n. saphenus** [ NA ], saphenous nerve; long or internal saphenous nerve; a branch of the femoral, extending from the femoral triangle to the foot, becoming cutaneous on the medial side of the knee; it supplies sensation to the skin of the leg and foot, by way of infrapatellar and medial crural cutaneous branches.

**nervi scrotales anteriores** [ NA ], anterior scrotal nerves; branches of the ilioinguinal nerve; distributed to the skin of the root of the penis, and the anterior surface of the scrotum.

**nervi scrotales posteriores** [ NA ], posterior scrotal nerves; several terminal branches of the perineal nerve supplying the skin of the posterior portion of the scrotum, corresponding to the posterior labial nerve in the female.

**n. spermat'icus exter'nus,** *ramus* genitalis.

**nervi sphenopalati'ni,** nervi pterygopalatini.

**nervi spina'les** [ NA ], spinal nerves; the nerves emerging from the spinal cord; there are 31 pairs, each attached to the cord by two roots, anterior and posterior, or ventral and dorsal; the latter is provided with a circumscribed enlargement, the spinal ganglion; the two roots unite in the intervertebral foramen, and the nerve almost immediately divides again into ventral and dorsal rami, or anterior and posterior primary divisions, the former supplying the foreparts of the body and the limbs, the latter the muscles and skin of the back.

**n. splanchnicus imus** [ NA ], lowest splanchnic nerve; smallest splanchnic nerve; a nerve containing the sympathetic fibers for the renal plexus, usually contained in the lesser splanchnic nerve, but occasionally existing as an independent nerve.

**nervi splanchnici lumbales** [ NA ], lumbar splanchnic nerves; branches from the lumbar sympathetic trunks that pass anteriorly to join the celiac, intermesenteric, aortic, and superior hypogastric plexuses.

**n. splanchnicus major** [ NA ], greater splanchnic nerve; arises from the fifth or sixth to the ninth or tenth thoracic sympathetic ganglia and passes downward along the bodies of the thoracic vertebrae, to join the celiac plexus.

**n. splanchnicus minor** [ NA ], lesser splanchnic nerve; arises from the last two thoracic sympathetic ganglia and passes to the aorticorenal ganglion.

**nervi splanch'nici pelvi'ni** [ NA ], nervi erigentes [ NA ]; pelvic splanchnic nerves; branches from the second, third, and fourth sacral nerves that join the inferior hypogastric plexus; they carry parasympathetic and sensory fibers.

**nervi splanchnici sacra'les** [ NA ], sacral splanchnic nerves; branches from the sacral sympathetic trunk that pass to the inferior hypogastric plexus.

**n. stapedius** [ NA ], nerve to the stapedius muscle; a branch of the facial arising in the facial canal and innervating the stapedius muscle.

**n. statoacus'ticus,** n. vestibulocochlearis.

**n. subclavius** [ NA ], subclavian nerve; a branch from the superior trunk of the brachial plexus supplying the subclavius muscle.

**n. subcostalis** [ NA ], subcostal nerve; the ventral ramus of the twelfth thoracic nerve; it courses below the last rib, supplies parts of the abdominal muscles and gives off cutaneous branches to the skin of the lower abdominal wall and to the gluteal region.

**n. sublingualis** [ NA ], sublingual nerve; a branch of the lingual to the sublingual gland and mucous membrane of the floor of the mouth.

**n. suboccipita'lis** [ NA ], suboccipital nerve; dorsal ramus of the first cervical nerve, passing through the suboccipital triangle and sending branches to the rectus capitis posterior major and minor, obliquus capitis superior and inferior, rectus capitis lateralis, and semispinalis capitis.

**n. subscapula'ris** [ NA ], subscapular nerve; a branch of the posterior cord of the brachial plexus, supplying the subscapularis muscle.

**n. supraclavicularis intermedius** [ NA ], middle supraclavicular nerve; intermediate supraclavicular nerve; one of several nerves arising from the cervical plexus which pass

down across the clavicle to supply the skin, in the infraclavicular region.

**n. supraclavicularis lateralis** [ NA ], lateral supraclavicular nerve; posterior supraclavicular nerve; one of several branches of the cervical plexus which descend to the skin over the acromion and deltoid region.

**n. supraclavicularis medialis** [ NA ], medial supraclavicular nerve; anterior supraclavicular nerve; one of several nerves arising from the cervical plexus which supply the skin over the upper medial part of the thorax.

**n. supraorbita'lis** [ NA ], supraorbital nerve; a branch of the frontal leaving the orbit through the supraorbital foramen or notch and dividing into branches distributed to the forehead and scalp, upper eyelid, and frontal sinus.

**n. suprascapula'ris** [ NA ], suprascapular nerve; arises from the fifth and sixth cervical, passes downward parallel to the cords of the brachial plexus, then through the suprascapular foramen, supplying the supraspinatus and infraspinatus muscles, and also sending branches to the shoulder joint.

**n. supratrochlea'ris** [ NA ], supratrochlear nerve; a branch of the frontal supplying the medial part of the upper eyelid, the central part of the skin of the forehead, and the root of the nose.

**n. suralis** [ NA ], sural nerve; short or external saphenous nerve; formed by the union of the medial sural cutaneous from the tibial and the peroneal communicating branch of the common peroneal, about the middle of the calf; thence it accompanies the small saphenous vein around the lateral malleolus to the dorsum of the foot.

**nervi tempora'les profun'di** [ NA ], deep temporal nerves; two branches, anterior and posterior, from the mandibular nerve, supplying the temporal muscles.

**n. tensoris tympani** [ NA ], nerve of the tensor tympani muscle; a muscular branch of the otic ganglion supplying the tensor tympani muscle.

**n. tensoris veli palatini** [ NA ], nerve of the tensor veli palatini muscle; a muscular branch of the otic ganglion, supplying the tensor veli palatini muscle.

**n. tentorii,** *ramus* tentorii.

**nervi termina'les** [ NA ], terminal nerves; delicate plexiform nerve strands passing parallel and medial to the olfactory tracts, distributing peripherally with the olfactory nerves and passing centrally into the anterior perforated substance. They are considered to have an autonomic function but the exact nature of this is unknown.

**nervi thoracici** [ NA ], thoracic nerves; twelve nerves on each side, mixed motor and sensory, supplying the muscles and skin of the thoracic and abdominal walls.

**n. thoracicus longus** [ NA ], long thoracic nerve; posterior thoracic; external respiratory nerve of Bell; arises from the fifth, sixth, and seventh cervical nerves, descends the neck behind the brachial plexus, and is distributed to the serratus anterior muscle.

**n. thoracodorsa'lis** [ NA ], thoracodorsal nerve; long subscapular nerve; arises from the posterior cord of the brachial plexus; it contains fibers from sixth, seventh, and eighth cervical nerves and supplies the latissimus dorsi muscle.

**n. tibia'lis** [ NA ], tibial nerve; medial popliteal nerve; one of the two major divisions of the sciatic nerve, it courses down the back of the leg to terminate as the medial and lateral plantar nerves in the foot. It supplies the hamstring muscles, the muscles of the back of the leg and the plantar aspect of the foot, as well as the skin on the back of the leg and sole of the foot.

**n. transversus colli** [ NA ], transverse nerve of the neck; superficial cervical nerve; cutaneous cervical nerve; a branch of the cervical plexus that supplies the skin over the anterior triangle of the neck.

**n. trigem'inus** [ NA ], trigeminal nerve; trifacial nerve; fifth cranial nerve; the chief sensory nerve of the face and the motor nerve of the muscles of mastication; its nuclei are in the mesencephalon and in the pons extending down into the cervical portion of the spinal cord; it emerges by two roots, sensory and motor, from the lateral portion of the surface of the pons, and enters a cavity of the dura mater, cavum trigeminale (of Meckel), at the apex of the petrous portion of the temporal bone, where the sensory root expands to form the trigeminal (Gasserian) ganglion; from there the three divisions (ophthalmic, maxillary, and mandibular) branch forth.

**n. trochlea′ris** [ NA ], trochlear nerve; fourth nerve; pathetic nerve; supplies the superior oblique muscle of the eye; its origin is in the midbrain below the cerebral aqueduct, its fibers decussate in the superior medullary velum, and it emerges from the brain at the side of the frenulum and enters the orbit through the superior orbital fissure.

**n. tympanicus** [ NA ], tympanic nerve; Jacobson's nerve; a nerve from the inferior ganglion of the glossopharyngeal, passing to the tympanic cavity, forming there the tympanic plexus which supplies the mucous membrane of the tympanic cavity mastoid cells, and auditory tube; parasympathetic fibers also pass through the tympanic nerve to the otic ganglion to supply the parotid gland.

**n. ulnaris** [ NA ], ulnar nerve; arises through the medial cord of the brachial plexus from the eighth cervical and first thoracic nerves, passes down the arm, through the interval between the olecranon and the medial condyle of the humerus, and down the ulnar side of the forearm to the hand; it gives off numerous muscular and cutaneous branches in the forearm and supplies intrinsic muscles of the hand and the skin of the medial side of the hand.

**n. utricula′ris** [ NA ], utricular nerve; a branch of the utriculoampullar nerve, supplying the macula of the utricle.

**n. utric′uloampulla′ris** [ NA ], utriculoampullar nerve; a division of the vestibular part of the eighth nerve; it gives off branches to the macula of the utricle (n. utricularis) and to the cristae of the ampullae of the anterior and lateral semicircular ducts (n. ampullaris anterior, n. ampullaris lateralis).

**nervi vaginales** [ NA ], vaginal nerves; several nerves passing from the uterovaginal plexus to the vagina.

**n. va′gus** [ NA ], vagus nerve; pneumogastric nerve; tenth cranial nerve; arises by numerous small roots from the side of the medulla oblongata, between the glossopharyngeal above and the accessory below; it leaves the cranial cavity by the jugular foramen and passes down to supply the larynx, lungs, heart, esophagus, stomach, and most of the abdominal viscera; it is a mixed nerve.

**n. vascula′ris** [ NA ], vascular nerve; a small nerve filament that supplies the wall of a blood vessel.

**n. vertebra′lis** [ NA ], vertebral nerve; a branch from the cervicothoracic ganglion that ascends along the vertebral artery to the level of the axis or atlas, giving branches to the cervical nerves and meninges.

**n. vestibula′ris,** see n. vestibulocochlearis.

**n. vestibulocochlea′ris** [ NA ], n. octavus [ NA ]; vestibulocochlear nerve; eighth cranial nerve; acoustic nerve; n. acusticus; n. statoacusticus; a composite sensory nerve innervating the receptor cells of the membranous labyrinth. The nerve consists of two major, anatomically and functionally distinct components: (1) The **radix superior** [ NA ], also called radix vestibularis [ NA ]; pars vestibularis nervi octavi [ NA ]; nervus vestibularis; vestibular nerve; superior or vestibular root or part of the vestibulocochlear nerve. It is made up of the centrally directed axonal processes of the bipolar sensory neurons which compose the ganglion vestibulare (Scarpa's ganglion, located in the vestibulum of the bony labyrinth) and which, with their peripheral processes innervate the neuroepithelial receptor cells (hair cells) of the vestibular organ (organ of equilibrium): macula utriculi, macula sacculi, and cristae ampullares. From the vestibular ganglion in the vestibulum of the bony labyrinth the radix superior gains access to the cranial cavity by passing in fascicles through the vestibular areas and the foramen singulare at the bottom of the bony internal auditory meatus; continuing medially it enters the brainstem in the lateral extreme of the pontomedullary groove (cerebellopontine angle); passing dorsomedially between the corpus restiforme and the tractus spinalis nervi trigemini it distributes its fibers to the nuclei vestibulares and to the flocculus, nodulus, and nucleus fastigii of the cerebellum. (2) The **radix inferior** [ NA ], also called radix cochlearis [ NA ], pars cochlearis nervi octavi [ NA ], nervus cochlearis; cochlear nerve; auditory nerve; inferior or cochlear root or part of the vestibulocochlear nerve. It is made up of the central processes of the bipolar neurons which compose the ganglion spirale cochleae (Corti's ganglion) in the canalis spiralis modioli of the bony cochlea; the peripheral processes of these neurons innervate the four rows of neuroepithelial receptor cells (hair cells) of the organum spirale (Corti's organ, organ of hearing). The radix inferior enters the cranial cavity by passing in fascicles through the tractus spiralis foraminosus at the bottom of the internal auditory meatus; it enters the brainstem through the pontomedullary groove, closely adhering to the caudoventral aspect of the radix superior, and distributes its fibers to the ventral and dorsal cochlear nuclei in the floor of the lateral recess of the fourth ventricle.

**n. zygomat′icus** [ NA ], zygomatic nerve; orbital or temporomalar nerve; a branch of the maxillary in the inferior orbital fissure through which it passes. It divides into a ramus zygomaticotemporalis and a ramus zygomaticofacialis, which supply the skin of the temporal and zygomatic regions.

---

**nesidiectomy** (ne-sid′ĭ-ek′to-mĭ) [ G. *nēsidion,* islet, dim. of *nēsos,* island, + *ektomē,* excision ]. Excision of islet tissue of the pancreas.

**nesidioblast** (ne-sid′ĭ-o-blast) [ G. *nēsidion,* dim. of *nēsos,* island, + *blastos,* germ ]. A pancreatic islet-forming cell.

**nesidioblastoma** (ne-sid′ĭ-o-blas′to′mah) [ G. *nēsidion,* dim. of *nēsos,* island, + blastoma ]. Islet cell *adenoma.*

**nesid′ioblasto′sis.** Hyperplasia of the cells of the islets of Langerhans.

**Nessler,** A., German chemist, 1827–1905. See N.'s *reagent.*

**nesslerize** (nes′ler-īz). To treat with Nessler's reagent; used in the determination of urea nitrogen in the blood and in the urine.

**nest** [ A.S. ]. A group or collection of similar objects; see also nidus.

**Brunn's n.'s,** glandlike invaginations of surface transitional epithelium in the mucosa of the lower urinary tract.

**cell n.'s,** a small focus or accumulation of one type of cell that is different from the other cells in the tissue.

**egg n.,** one of the clumps of cells resulting from the breaking up of the egg tubes, and later developing into a primary ovarian follicle.

**epithe′lial n.'s,** epithelial pearls; onion bodies; multiple, discrete, rounded or ovoid, compact, whorled aggregates or small masses of neoplastic epidermoid tissue, frequently formed as a characteristic part of the growth of well differentiated squamous cell carcinomas; the n.'s may vary from 40 to 50 to 100 or 150 $\mu$ in diameter (sometimes larger), and consist of several, moderately compressed, centrally located, polygonal cells that are bounded by irregular laminations of deeply acidophilic keratin and flattened epithelial cells with pyknotic nuclei.

**nes′tia, nes′tis** [ G. *nēstis,* fasting ]. Abstinence from food.

**nestiatria** (nes-tĭ-at′rĭ-ah) [ G. *nēstis,* fasting, + *iatreia,* medical treatment ]. Hunger *therapy.*

**nestiostomy** (nes-tĭ-os′to-mĭ) [ G. *nēstis,* jejunum, + *stoma,* mouth. NEST- ]. Jejunostomy.

**nes′tis.** Nestia.

**nes′tither′apy.** Hunger *therapy.*

**net.** Network; reticulum.

**Chiari's n.,** abnormal fibrous or lacelike strands in the right atrium, extending from the margins of the coronary or caval valves and attaching to the atrial wall along the line of the crista terminalis. They result when the resorption of septum spurium (*q. v.*) is markedly less than normal.

**chromidial n.,** a reticulum of basophilic-staining material in the cytoplasm of certain cells.

**Netherton,** Earl W., U. S. dermatologist. See N.'s *syndrome.*

**Netterhynchus armillatus.** *Armillifer armillatus.*

**nettle** (net′l) [ A.S. *netele* ]. Urtica.

**Nettleship,** Edward, English dermatologist, 1845–1913. See N.'s *disease.*

**net′work.** 1. A structure bearing a resemblance to a woven fabric; rete; reticulum. See also net. 2. The persons in a patient's environment, especially as significant for the course of the illness.

**acromial n.,** *rete* acromiale.

**articular n. of elbow,** *rete* articulare cubiti.

**articular n. of knee,** *rete* articulare genus.

**chromatin n.,** the appearance of basophilic material after fixation in the nuclei of many cells; see also chromatin.

**dorsal carpal n.,** *rete* carpi dorsale.

**dorsal venous n. of hand,** *rete* venosum dorsale manus.

**n. of heel,** *rete* calcaneum.

**linin n.,** see linin (3).

**patellar n.,** *rete* patellae.

**peritar'sal n.,** the lymphatic vessels along the margin of the eyelid.

**Purkinje's n.,** the n. formed by Purkinje's fibers beneath the endocardium.

**subpap'illary n.,** the capillary blood vessels in the deeper layers of the skin.

**trabecular n.,** trabecular *meshwork.*

**Neubauer** (noy'bow-er), Johann E., German anatomist, 1742–1777. See N.'s *artery.*

**Neufeld** (noy'feld), Fred, German bacteriologist, *1869. See N. *reaction,* capsular *swelling.*

**Neumann** (noy'mahn), Ernst F. C., German histologist, anatomist, and pathologist, 1834–1918. See N.'s *cells, sheath,* Rouget-N. *sheath.*

**Neumann** (noy'mahn), Franz E., German physicist, 1798–1895. See N.'s *law.*

**Neumann** (noy'mahn), Isidor, Vienna dermatologist, 1832–1906. See N.'s *disease.*

**neur-, neuri-** (nūr-, nu'rī-) [ G. *neuron,* nerve. NERV- ]. Combining form denoting nerve.

**neuradynamia** (nūr'ă-di-na'mĭ-ah) [ neur- + G. *a-*priv. + *dynamis,* force ]. Neurasthenia.

**neuragmia** (nūr-ag'mĭ-ah) [ neur- + G. *agmos,* fracture ]. The rupture or tearing asunder of a nerve.

**neural** (nūr'al) [ G. *neuron,* nerve. NERV- ]. Relating to any structure that is composed of nerve cells or their processes, or that on further development will give rise to nerve cells.

**neuralgia** (nūr-al'jī-ah) [ neur- + G. *algos,* pain ]. Nerve pain; facial ague; pain of a severe, throbbing, or stabbing character in the course or distribution of a nerve.

**degenerative n.,** n. caused by degenerative changes in the nerve or its central origin.

**epilep'tiform n.,** trigeminal n.

**facial n.,** trigeminal n.

**n. facia'lis vera,** geniculate n.

**Fothergill's n.,** trigeminal n.

**genic'ulate n.,** n. facialis vera; Hunt's n.; geniculate otalgia; a severe paroxysmal lancinating pain deep in the ear, on the anterior wall of the external meatus, and on a small area just in front of the pinna.

**hallu'cinatory n.,** reminiscent n.; an impression of local pain persisting after an attack of n. has ceased.

**Hunt's n.,** geniculate n.

**idiopath'ic n.,** nerve pain not due to any apparent lesion of the nerve itself.

**intercos'tal n.,** pain in the chest wall due to neuralgia of one or more of the intercostal nerves.

**mam'mary n.,** mastodynia; intercostal n. of the branches of the upper dorsal nerves of one side.

**Morton's n.,** neuralgia of an interdigital nerve, usually the anastomotic branch between the medial and lateral plantar nerves.

**occipital n.,** see posttraumatic neck *syndrome.*

**periodic migrainous n.,** Harris' migraine; recurrent facial pain and headache, more common in men than in women.

**red n.,** erythromelalgia.

**reminis'cent n.,** hallucinatory n.

**sciatic n.,** sciatica.

**stump n.,** pain referred to the absent part, caused by pressure on neuromas in an amputation stump.

**suboccipital n.,** see posttraumatic neck *syndrome.*

**supraorbital n.,** n. of the supraorbital nerve.

**symptomatic n.,** n. occurring as a symptom of some local or systemic disease not involving primarily the nerve structures.

**trifacial n.,** trigeminal n.

**trigeminal n.,** severe, paroxysmal bursts of pain in one or more branches of the trigeminal nerve; often induced by touching trigger areas in or about the mouth. Also called

trifacial, facial, epileptiform, or Fothergill's n.; tic douloureaux; prosopalgia; prosoponeuralgia; trismus dolorificus.

**neural'gic.** Relating to, resembling, or of the character of, neuralgia.

**neural'giform.** Resembling or of the character of neuralgia.

**neuramebimeter** (nūr'am-e-bim'e-ter) [ neur- + G. *amoibē,* exchange, return, answer, + *metron,* measure ]. An instrument for measuring the rapidity of response of a nerve to any stimulus.

**neuraminic acid** (nūr'ă-min'ik). 5-Amino-3,5-dideoxy-D-*glycero*-D-*galacto*-nonulosonic acid; an aldol condensation product of mannosamine and pyruvic acid, linking the C-1 of the former to the C-3 of the latter. The *N*- and *O*-acyl derivatives of n. are known as sialic acids and are constituents of gangliosides and of the polysaccharide components of muco- and glycoproteins from many tissues, secretions, and species.

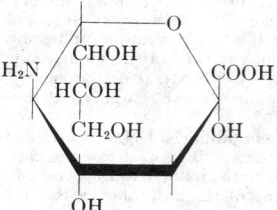

Neuraminic acid

**neuramin'idase.** Sialidase; an enzyme (EC 3.2.1.18) that cleaves terminal acylneuraminic residues from oligosaccharides, glycoproteins, or glycolipids; it is present as a surface antigen in myxoviruses.

$\alpha_2$-**neuraminoglycoprotein.** C1-esterase inhibitor (see under esterase).

**neuranagenesis** (nūr'an-ă-jen'e-sis) [ neur- + G. *ana,* up, again, + *genesis,* generation ]. Regeneration of a nerve.

**neurapophysis** (nūr'ă-pof'ĭ-sis) [ neur- + G. *apophysis,* offshoot ]. *Lamina* arcus vertebrae.

**neurapraxia** (nūr'ă-prak'sĭ-ah) [ neur- + apraxia, *q.v.* ]. Injury to nerve resulting in paralysis but unattended by degeneration and followed by rapid and complete recovery of function.

**neurarchy** (nūr'ar-kī) [ neur- + G. *archē,* dominion ]. The dominant action of the nervous system over the physical processes of the body.

**neurasthenia** (nūr'as-the'nĭ-ah) [ neur- + G. *astheneia,* weakness ]. 1. Nervosism (1); nervous exhaustion; an ill-defined condition, commonly following depression, characterized by vague functional fatigue. 2. Considered by some as a stage in the recovery from a schizophrenic episode in which the patient appears apathetic or unable to reengage with his pre-illness responsibilities and relationships.

**angiopath'ic n., angioparalyt'ic n.,** pulsating n.; a form of mild n. in which the chief complaint is of a universal throbbing or sense of pulsation throughout the body.

**gastric n.,** a condition marked by gastric atony and distention, dyspepsia, and mild neurasthenic symptoms.

**n. gravis,** a condition of extreme and lasting n.

**n. precox,** primary n.; a form of nervous exhaustion appearing in the adolescent period.

**pulsating n.,** angiopathic n.

**sexual n.,** a form in which sexual erethism, weakness, or perversion is a marked symptom.

**traumatic n.,** posttraumatic *syndrome.*

**tropical n.,** n. occurring in Europeans resident in the tropics marked by headache, insomnia, failure of concentration, loss of memory, and general disinterestedness in life.

**neurastheniac** (nūr-as-the'nī-ak). One suffering from neurasthenia.

**neurasthenic** (nūr'as-then'ik). 1. Relating to, or suffering from neurasthenia. 2. One suffering from neurasthenia; a neurastheniac.

**n. helmet,** a feeling of pressure over the entire cranium in certain cases of neurasthenia.

**neuratrophy** (nūr-at'ro-fĭ) [ neur- + G. *atrophia,* atrophy ]. Obsolete term, meaning atrophy or defective nutrition of the nerves or central nervous system.

**neuraxis** (nūr-ak'sis). The axial, unpaired part of the central nervous system: spinal cord, rhombencephalon, mesencephalon, and diencephalon, in contrast to the paired cerebral hemisphere or telencephalon.

**neuraxon, neuraxone** (nūr'ak'son, -sōn) [ neur- + G. *axōn,* axis ]. Axon.

**neurectasis, neurectasia, neurectasy** (nūr-ek'tă-sis, -ek-ta'zĭ-ah, -ek'tă-sĭ) [ neur- + G. *ektasis,* extension ]. Nerve-stretching; neurotension; neurotony; the operation of stretching a nerve or nerve trunk.

**neurectomy** (nu-rek'to-mĭ) [ neur- + G. *ektomē,* excision ]. Neuroectomy; excision of a segment of a nerve.

**presacral n.,** presacral sympathectomy; Cotte's operation; removal of the presacral plexus to relieve severe dysmenorrhea.

**retrogasserian n.,** trigeminal *rhizotomy.*

**neurectopia, neurectopy** (nūr'ek-to'pĭ-ah, -ek'to-pĭ) [ neur- + G. *ektopos,* fr. *ek,* out of, + *topos,* place ]. 1. Dislocation of a nerve trunk. 2. A condition in which a nerve follows an anomalous course.

**neurenteric** (nūr'en-tĕr'ik) [ neur- + G. *enteron,* intestine ]. Relating, in the embryo, to both the neural tube and the enteric canal; see neurenteric *canal.*

**neur'epithe'lium.** Neuroepithelium.

**neurergic** (nūr'er'jik) [ neur- + G. *ergon,* work ]. Relating to the activity of a nerve.

**neurexeresis** (nūr'ek-sĕr'e-sis) [ neur- + G. *exairesis,* a taking out, fr. *haireō,* to grasp, take ]. Tearing out or evulsion of a nerve.

**neuri-** (nu'rĭ-). See neur-.

**neuriatria, neuriatry** (nu-rĭ-at'rĭ-ah, nu-rĭ-at'rĭ) [ neur- + G. *iatreia,* medical treatment ]. Treatment of nervous diseases.

**neuricity** (nu-ris'ĭ-tĭ). Nervous energy; the property inherent in nervous matter.

**neu'ridine.** A ptomaine, spermine.

**neurilemma** (nu'rĭ-lem'ah). Neurolemma.

**neurilemoma** (nu'rĭ-lĕ-mo'mah) [ neurilemma + G. suffix *-oma,* tumor ]. Neurinoma; neuroschwannoma; schwannoma (2); Schwann's tumor (2); a benign, encapsulated neoplasm in which the fundamental component is structurally identical to the syncytium of Schwann; the neoplastic cells proliferate within the endoneurium, and the perineurium forms the capsule. The neoplasm may originate from a peripheral or sympathetic nerve, or from various cranial nerves, particularly the eighth nerve; when the nerve is small, it is usually found (if at all) in the capsule of the neoplasm; if the nerve is large, the n. may develop within the sheath of the nerve, the fibers of which may then spread over the surface of the capsule as the neoplasm enlarges. Microscopically, n.'s are composed of combinations of two types of tissue, *i.e.,* Antoni types A and B (see below); either of the two types may be predominant in various examples of n.'s. See also neurofibroma.

**acoustic n.,** acoustic *neurinoma.*

**Antoni type A n.,** relatively solid or firm neoplastic tissue that consists of Schwann cells arranged in twisting bundles and associated with delicate reticulin fibers. The nuclei of the Schwann cells are frequently grouped in parallel rows (*i.e.,* so-called palisades), and the nuclei and fibers sometimes form exaggerated tactile corpuscles, termed Verocay bodies.

**Antoni type B n.,** relatively soft neoplastic tissue that consists of Schwann cells in a haphazard or nondescript type of arrangement among reticulin fibers and tiny cystlike foci; fat-laden macrophages may be observed in some of the larger neoplasms.

**neuril'ity.** The property of conducting stimuli, inherent in nerves.

**neurimotility** (nu'rĭ-mo-til'ĭ-tĭ). Nervimotility.

**neurimo'tor.** Nervimotor.

**neu'rine.** $CH_2=CH-N^+(CH_3)_3OH^-$; trimethylvinylammonium hydroxide; a toxic amine; a product of decomposing animal matter (dehydration of choline); also a poisonous constituent of mushrooms.

**neurino'ma.** Neurilemoma.

**acoustic n.,** a benign neoplasm of the intracranial segment of the eighth cranial nerve, producing cerebellar, lower crainial nerve, and brainstem signs and symptoms; also known as acoustic neurilemoma, neuroma, or schwannoma; cerebellopontine angle tumor; eighth nerve tumor.

**neurit, neurite** (nu'rit, nu'rĭt) [ G. *neuritēs,* of a nerve ]. Axon.

**neuritic** (nu-rit'ik). Relating to neuritis.

**neuritis,** pl. **neuritides** (nu-ri'tis, nu-rit'ĭ-dēz) [ neuri- + G. suffix *-itis,* inflammation ]. Inflammation of a nerve, marked by neuralgia, hyperesthesia, anesthesia, or parasthesia, paralysis, muscular atrophy in the region supplied by the affected nerve, and by abolition of the reflexes.

**adventitial n.,** inflammation of the sheath of a nerve; see also perineuritis.

**ascending n.,** inflammation progressing upward along a nerve trunk in a direction away from the periphery.

**axial n.,** parenchymatous n.

**central n.,** parenchymatous n.

**descending n.,** inflammation progressing downward along a nerve trunk in a direction toward the periphery.

**Eichhorst's n.,** interstitial n.

**endemic n.,** beriberi; see also nutritional *polyneuropathy.*

**Fallopian n.,** facial *palsy.*

**interstitial n.,** Eichhorst's n.; inflammation of the connective tissue framework of a nerve.

**intraocular n.,** inflammation of the retinal portion of the optic nerve.

**Leyden's n.,** fatty degeneration of the fibers of the affected nerve.

**multiple n.,** polyneuritis.

**occipital n.,** see posttraumatic neck *syndrome.*

**optic n.,** neuropapillitis; inflammation of the optic nerve; see also *neuromyelitis* optica.

**parenchymatous n.,** axial n.; central n.; inflammation of the nervous substance proper, the axons, and myelin.

**retrobulbar n.,** inflammation of the orbital portion of the optic nerve; noted in certain intoxications.

**sciatic n.,** inflammation of the sciatic nerve, causing sciatica.

**segmental n.,** inflammation occurring at several points along the course of a nerve; see also segmental *neuropathy.*

**suboccipital n.,** see posttraumatic neck *syndrome.*

**toxic n.,** n. due to the action of alcohol, lead, arsenic, or some other poison.

**traumatic n.,** inflammation of a nerve following an injury.

**neuro-** (nu'ro-) [ G. *neuron,* nerve. NERV- ]. Combining form denoting nerve or relating to the nervous system.

**neuroallergy** (nu'ro-al'er-jĭ). An allergic reaction in nervous tissue.

**neu'roanas'tomo'sis.** Surgical formation of a junction between nerves.

**neuroanatomy** (nu'ro-an-at'o-mĭ). The anatomy of the nervous system.

**neuroarthropathy** (nu'ro-ar-throp'ă-thĭ) [ neuro- + G. *arthron,* joint, + *pathos,* suffering, disease ]. A trophoneurosis affecting one or more joints.

**neurobiotaxis** (nu-ro-bi-o-tak'sis) [ neuro- + G. *bios,* life, + *taxis,* arrangement ]. The tendency of the nerve cells to move toward the area from which they receive the most stimuli.

**neu'roblast** [ neuro- + G. *blastos,* germ ]. An embryonic nerve cell.

**neuroblasto'ma.** A malignant neoplasm characterized by immature, only slightly differentiated nerve cells of embryonic type, *i.e.,* neuroblasts, which are histogenetically intermediate between (1) medulloblasts and neurocytes of the central nervous system, or (2) migrant cells from the neural crest and neurocytes of the peripheral nervous system. The typical cells are relatively small forms (10 to 15 $\mu$ in diameter) with disproportionately large, darkly staining, vesicular nuclei and scant, palely acidophilic cytoplasm; they are arranged in sheets, irregular clumps, and cordlike groups, and also occur individually and in pseudorosettes (with nuclei arranged peripherally about the centrally directed cytoplasmic processes). Ordinarily, the stroma is sparse, and foci of necrosis and hemorrhage are not unusual. Cellular differentiation to neurons is sometimes seen. N.'s occur more frequently in infants and children (more than 50 per cent in the first two years of life, and an additional 20 to 25 per cent prior to the age of ten years), and those observed in adult patients tend to be less malignant; maturation to ganglioneuroma after a period of years has been reported. The most frequent primary sites for n. are in the mediastinal and retroperitoneal regions (approximately 30 per cent associated with the adrenal glands), and widespread metastases to the liver, lungs, lymph nodes, cranial cavity and skeleton are very common.

   **olfactory n.,** olfactory neuroepithelioma; olfactory esthesioneurocytoma; a rare benign or slowly growing malignant tumor of primitive nerve cells, usually arising in the olfactory area of the nasal cavity.

   **n. sympathet'icum embryona'le,** sympathoblastoma.

**neurocar'diac** [ neuro- + G. *kardia,* heart ]. 1. Relating to the nerve supply of the heart. 2. Relating to a cardiac neurosis.

**neurocele** (nu'ro-sēl) [ neuro- + G. *koilos,* hollow ]. Rarely used collective term for the central cavity of the cerebrospinal axis; the combined ventricles of the brain and central canal of the spinal cord.

**neu'rochem'istry.** The chemistry of nerve material, metabolism, and function.

**neurochitin** (nu-ro-ki'tin) [ neuro- + G. *chitōn,* tunic ]. Neurokeratin.

**neurochoroiditis** (nu-ro-ko'roy-di'tis). Inflammation of the choroid coat of the eye and the optic nerve.

**neurochorioretinitis** (nu-ro-ko'rī-o-ret-in-i'tis). Inflammation of the choroid coat of the eye, the retina, and the optic nerve.

**neurocladism** (nu-rok'lă-dizm) [ neuro- + G. *klados,* a young branch ]. Odogenesis; the outgrowth of axons from the central stump to bridge the gap in a cut nerve.

**neuroclonic** (nu'ro-klon'ik) [ neuro- + G. *klonos,* a tunnel (clonus). Affected by, or pertaining to, rhythmical spasms caused by irritation of the nervous system.

**neurocranium** (nu'ro-kra'nī-um) [ neuro- + G. *kranion,* skull ]. The part of the skull enclosing the brain, as distinguished from the bones of the face.

   **cartilaginous n.,** in the embryo, that part of the base of the skull first laid down in cartilage and then ossified.

   **membranous n.,** the vault of the embryonic skull which is ossified in membrane.

**neurocristopathy** (nu'ro-kris-top'ă-thī) [ neuro- + L. *crista,* crest, + G. *pathos,* suffering ]. Maldevelopment or neoplasia of tissues of neural crest origin.

**neurocyte** (nu'ro-sīt) [ neuro- + G. *kytos,* cell ]. Neuron.

**neurocytolysis** (nu'ro-si-tol'ĭ-sis) [ neuro- + G. *kytos,* cell, + *lysis,* dissolution ]. Destruction of neurons.

**neurocytoma** (nu-ro-si-to'mah) [ neuro- + G. *kytos,* cell, + suffix -*oma,* tumor ]. Ganglioneuroma.

**neu'roden'drite.** Dendrite (1).

**neu'roden'dron.** Dendrite (1).

**neurodermatitis** (nu'ro-der'mă-ti'tis) [ neuro- + G. *derma,* skin, + suffix -*itis,* inflammation ]. Neurodermatosis; a chronic lichenified skin lesion, localized or disseminated; a term loosely applied to atopic dermatitis or lichen simplex chronicus.

**neu'rodermato'sis.** Neurodermatitis.

**neurodynamic** (nu'ro-di-nam'ik) [ neuro- + G. *dynamis,* force ]. Pertaining to nervous energy.

**neurodynia** (nu'ro-din'ĭ-ah) [ neuro- + G. *odynē,* pain ]. Neuralgia.

**neuroectoderm** (nu'ro-ek'to-derm). That central region of the early embryo's ectoderm which in further development forms the brain and spinal cord, and also gives rise to the nerve cells and neurolemma or Schwann cells of the peripheral nervous system.

**neu'roectoder'mal.** Relating to the neuroectoderm.

**neuroectomy** (nu'ro-ek'to-me). Neurectomy.

**neu'roenceph'alomyelop'athy.** Disease of the brain, spinal cord, and nerves.

**neu'roen'docrine.** 1. Pertaining to the anatomical and functional relationships between the nervous system and the endocrine apparatus. 2. Descriptive of cells that release a hormone into the circulating blood in response to a neural stimulus. Such cells may compose a peripheral endocrine gland, *e.g.,* the insulin-secreting beta cells of the islets of Langerhans in the pancreas and the adrenaline-secreting chromaffin cells of the adrenal medulla; others are neurons in the brain, *e.g.,* the neurons of the supraoptic nucleus that release antidiuretic hormone from their axon terminals in the posterior lobe of the hypophysis.

**neu'roen'docrinol'ogy.** The knowledge or study of the anatomical and functional relationships between the nervous system and the endocrine apparatus.

**neu'roepithe'lial.** Relating to the neuroepithelium.

**neuroepithelioma** (nu'ro-ep-ĭ-the'lĭ-o-mah). A relatively rare type of glioma (usually of the retina) that consists of bands or irregular columns, and occasional rosettes or looplike groups, of cuboidal or columnar ectodermal cells in a trabecular stroma of cellular fibrous tissue. The neoplastic cells resemble primitive forms that develop into specialized sensory epithelium (such as that in the organ of Corti) or the cerebrospinal axis. Histologically, the n. is similar to the medulloepithelioma.

   **olfactory n.,** olfactory *neuroblastoma.*

**neuroepithelium** (nu'ro-ep-ĭ-the'lĭ-um) [ NA ]. Neuroepithelial cells; epithelial cells specialized for the reception of external stimuli. Most neuroepithelial cells, notably the hair cells of the inner ear and the receptor cells of the taste buds, are not true neurons but transducer cells that stand in synaptic contact with the peripheral endings of sensory ganglion cells. The neuroepithelial receptor cells of the olfactory epithelium, by contrast, are true peripheral neurons whose extremely thin, unmyelinated axons compose the olfactory filaments that enter the olfactory bulb of the cerebral hemisphere. The NA also applies the term to the rods and cones of the retina.

   **n. cris'tae ampulla'ris** [ NA ], n. of the ampullary crest; the specialized sensory hair cells in the ampullary crest of the ampulla of each semicircular duct.

   **n. mac'ulae** [ NA ], n. of the macula; the specialized sensory hair cells of the epithelium of the macula sacculi and macula utriculi.

**neurofi'bril.** A filamentous structure seen with the light microscope in the nerve cell's body, dendrites, axon, and sometimes synaptic endings. N.'s are aggregations of much finer ultramicroscopic elements, the microfilaments and microtubules. The original notion according to which the n.'s are the essential conducting elements of the neural impulse has been disproved; their functional significance remains to be established.

**neurofi'brillar.** Relating to neurofibrils.

**neurofibroma** (nu'ro-fi-bro'mah). Fibroma molluscum (1); Schwann's tumor (1); schwannoma (1); a moderately firm, benign, nonencapsulated tumor resulting from proliferation of Schwann cells in a disorderly pattern that includes portions of nerve fibers; in neurofibromatosis (*q.v.*), n.'s may be solitary but are more often multiple.

   **multiple n.'s,** neurofibromatosis.

   **plexiform n.,** a type of n. in which the proliferation of Schwann cells occurs from the inner aspect of the nerve sheath, thereby resulting in an irregularly thickened, distorted, tortuous structure; in some instances, the process extends along the course of the nerve and may eventually involve the spinal roots and the spinal cord. See also plexiform *neuroma.*

**neurofibromatosis** (nu'ro-fi-bro'mă-to'sis). von Recklinghausen's disease; neuromatosis; molluscum fibrosum; multiple neurofibromas; small, discrete, pigmented skin lesions (café-au-lait spots, pigmented nevi) that develop in infancy or early childhood, followed by development of multiple subcutaneous neurofibromas that may slowly increase in number and size over many years; neurofibromas may develop on nerve trunks anywhere; compression of the spinal cord by a neurofibroma arising from a spinal nerve root is not uncommon; malignant change (sarcoma, schwannoma) is an infrequent complication; the disease is sometimes associated with acoustic neurinomas or other intracranial neoplasms. Autosomal dominant inheritance with marked clinical variability.

**abortive n.,** incomplete n.

**incomplete n.,** abortive n.; multiple neurofibromas with minimal manifestations, perhaps limited to café-au-lait spots or pigmented nevi of skin; individuals with minimal lesions may have offspring with severe involvement.

**neurogangliitis** (nu′ro-gang-gli-i′tis). Obsolete term for inflammation of a nerve ganglion.

**neuroganglion.** Ganglion (1).

**neurogas′tric.** Relating to the innervation of the stomach.

**neurogenesis** (nu′ro-jen′e-sis) [ neuro- + G. *genesis*, production ]. The formation of the nervous system.

**neurogen′ic, neurogenet′ic.** 1. Originating in, or starting from, or caused by, the nervous system or nerve impulses. 2. Relating to neurogenesis.

**neurogenous** (nu-roj′ē-nus). Neurogenic (1).

**neuroglia** (nu-rog′lī-ah) [ neuro- + G. *glia*, glue ]. Glia; Kölliker's reticulum; non-neuronal cellular elements of the central and peripheral nervous system; formerly believed to be merely supporting cells but now thought to have important metabolic functions, since they are invariably interposed between neurons and the blood vessels supplying the nervous system. In central nervous tissue they include oligodendroglia cells, astrocytes, ependymal cells, and microglia cells. The satellite cells of ganglia and the neurolemmal or Schwann cells around peripheral nerve fibers can be interpreted as the oligodendroglia cells of the peripheral nervous system.

**neurogliacyte** (nu-rog′lī-ah-sīt) [ neuro- + G. *glia*, glue, + *kytos*, cell ]. A neuroglia cell; see neuroglia.

**neurog′lial, neurog′liar.** Relating to neuroglia.

**neurog′liomato′sis.** The occurrence of neoplastic growth of neuroglial cells in the brain or spinal cord; the term is used especially with reference to a relatively large neoplasm or to multiple foci.

**neu′rogram** [ neuro- + G. *gramma*, something written ]. The imprint on the brain substance left behind after every mental experience, *i.e.*, the engram or physical register of the mental experience, stimulation of which retrieves and reproduces the original experience, thereby producing memory.

**neurohe′mal** [ neuro- + hemal, relating to blood vessels ]. Descriptive of structures containing neurosecretory neurons, whose axons form no synapses with other neurons and whose axonal endings are modified to permit storage and release into the circulation of neurosecretory material.

**neurohistol′ogy.** The microscopic anatomy of the nervous system.

**neu′rohor′mone.** A hormone liberated by nerve impulses; formed by neurosecretory cells.

**neu′rohu′mor.** The active chemical substance (*e.g.*, epinephrine and norepinephrine) liberated at nerve endings with exciting effect on adjacent structures.

**neurohypophysial** (nu′ro-hi-po-fiz′ī-al). Relating to the neurohypophysis.

**neurohypophysis** (nu′ro-hi-pof′ī-sis) [ neuro- + hypophysis, *q.v.* ] [ NA ]. Official alternative term for *lobus* posterior hypophyseos (posterior lobe of the hypophysis); see also hypophysis.

**neuroid** (nu′royd) [ neuro- + G. *eidos*, resemblance ]. 1. Resembling a nerve; nervelike. 2. Neurapophysis.

**neuroinduction** (nu-ro-in-duk′shun). Suggestion.

**neurokeratin** (nu′ro-kĕr′ă-tin) [ neuro- + G. *keras*, horn ]. Neurochitin. 1. The proteinaceous network that remains of the myelin sheath of axons following fixation and the removal of the fatty material; the reticular appearance is probably a fixation artifact. 2. The insoluble protein matter of brain remaining after extraction with solvents following proteolytic digestion; it differs in composition from other keratins.

**neurokyme** (nu′ro-kīm) [ neuro- + G. *kyma*, wave ]. Neurorrheuma; nervous energy.

**neurolapine** (nu′ro-lap′ēn) [ neuro- + Fr. *lapin*, rabbit ]. Neurovirus in the rabbit.

**neurolemma** (nu′ro-lem′ah) [ neuro- + G. *lemma*, husk, LEP- ]. Neurilemma; sheath of Schwann; a cell that enfolds one or more axons of the peripheral nervous system; in myelinated fibers its plasma membrane forms the lamellae of myelin.

**neu′rolep′sy** [ neuro- + G. *lepsis*, seizure ]. State characterized by hypnosis and blockade of vegetative reflexes.

**neu′rolept.** Neuroleptic *agent*.

**neuroleptanesthesia** (nu′ro-lept-an′es-the′zī-ah). A technique of general anesthesia based upon intravenous administration of neuroleptic drugs, together with inhalation of a weak anesthetic such as nitrous oxide, with or without curare or curare-like drugs.

**neurolep′tic.** 1. A neuroleptic *agent*. 2. Denoting a condition similar to that produced by such an agent.

**neurol′ogist.** One versed in the science of neurology; a specialist in the treatment of nervous diseases.

**neurology** (nu-rol′o-jī) [ neuro- + G. *logos*, study ]. The branch of medical science that has to do with the nervous system and its disorders.

**neurolymph** (nu′ro-limf) [ neuro- + L. *lympha*, clear water ]. *Liquor* cerebrospinalis.

**neurolymphomatosis** (nu′ro-lim-fo-mă-to′sis). Lymphoblastic invasion of a nerve.

**n. gallina′rum,** see avian *lymphomatosis*.

**neurolysin** (nu-rol′ī-sin). An antibody causing destruction of ganglion and cortical cells, obtained by the injection of brain substance.

**neurolysis** (nu-rol′ī-sis) [ neuro- + G. *lysis*, dissolution ]. 1. Destruction of nerve tissue. 2. Freeing of a nerve from inflammatory adhesions.

**neurolyt′ic.** Relating to neurolysis.

**neuroma** (nu′ro′mah) [ neuro- + G. suffix -*oma*, tumor ]. An old, general term for any neoplasm derived from cells of the nervous system; on the basis of newer knowledge pertaining to the cytologic and histologic characteristics, such neoplasms are now classified in more specific categories, *e.g.*, ganglioneuroma, neurilemoma, pseudoneuroma, and others.

**acoustic n.,** acoustic *neurinoma*.

**amputation n.,** traumatic n.

**n. cu′tis,** neurofibroma of the skin.

**false n.,** traumatic n.

**fibrillary n.,** plexiform n.

**plexiform n.,** fibrillary n.; a tumefaction that consists of irregular bands and whorls of nerve fibers (myelinated or not myelinated) in a stroma of cellular fibrous tissue; the lesion probably represents an anomaly, rather than a neoplasm. See also plexiform *neurofibroma*.

**n. telangiecto′des,** a neurofibroma with a conspicuous number of blood vessels, some of which have unusually large lumens (in proportion to the thickness of the walls).

**traumatic n.,** amputation or false n.; pseudoneuroma; the proliferative mass of Schwann cells and neurites that may develop at the proximal end of a severed or injured nerve; a traumatic n. is not a neoplasm.

**Verneuil's n.,** a nodular enlargement of the cutaneous nerves.

**n. verum,** ganglioneuroma.

**neuromalacia** (nu′ro-mă-la′shī-ah) [ neuro- + G. *malakia*, softness ]. Pathologic softening of nervous tissue.

**neu′romast.** See lateral line sense *organ*.

**neuromatosis** (nu′ro-mă-to′sis). Neurofibromatosis.

**neuromelanin** (nu′ro-mel′ă-nin). A modified form of melanin pigment normally found in certain neurons of the nervous system, especially in the substantia nigra and locus ceruleus.

**neuromelitococcosis** (nu′ro-mel′ī-to-kok-o′sis). An old term for Malta fever (brucellosis) with pronounced nervous (cerebral) complications.

**neuromere** (nu′ro-mēr) [ neuro- + G. *meros*, part ]. Rhombomere; neural segment; that part of the neural tube within a metamere.

**neuromime′sis** [ neuro- + G. *mimēsis*, imitation ]. Hysterical or neurotic simulation of disease.

**neu′romimet′ic.** Relating to the action of a drug that mimics the response of an effector organ to nerve impulses.

**neuromus′cular.** Referring to the relationship between nerve and muscle, in particular to the motor innervation of skeletal muscles and its pathology (*e.g.*, neuromuscular disorders). See also myoneural.

**neu'romyasthe'nia** [ neuro- + G. *mys,* muscle, + *a*- priv. + *sthenos,* strength ]. Muscular weakness, usually of emotional origin.

**epidemic n.,** Akureyri or Iceland disease; benign or epidemic myalgic encephalomyelitis; an epidemic disease often with insidious onset and characterized by stiffness of the neck and back, headache, diarrhea, fever, and localized muscular weakness; it is restricted almost exclusively to adults, affecting women more than men; first described in Iceland (Akureyri) but outbreaks have occurred in various parts of the world, including England and the United States; etiology is not known, deaths have been rare, and histological descriptions therefore not available.

**neuromyelitis** (nu'ro-mi-el-i'tis) [ neuro- + G. *myelos,* marrow, + suffix -*itis,* inflammation ]. Myeloneuritis; neuritis combined with spinal cord inflammation.

**n. op'tica,** Devic's disease; a demyelinating disorder associated with transverse myelopathy and optic neuritis.

**neu'romyop'athy** [ neuro- + G. *mys,* muscle, + pathos, disease ]. A disorder of muscle, anatomical or physiological, that directly reflects a disease or disorder of nerve supplying the muscle.

**neuromyositis** (nu'ro-mio-o-si'tis) [ neuro- + G. *mys,* muscle, + suffix -*itis,* inflammation ]. Neuritis with inflammation of the muscles with which the affected nerve or nerves are in relation.

**neuron** (nu'ron) [ G. *neuron,* a nerve. NERV- ]. 1. Neurone; nerve cell; neurocyte; the morphologic and functional unit of the nervous system, consisting of the nerve cell body, the dendrites, and the axon. 2. Obsolete synonym for axon.

**autonomic motor n.,** see motor n.

**bipolar n.,** a n. that has two processes arising from opposite poles of the cell body.

**gamma motor n.'s,** see gamma motor *system.*

**ganglionic motor n.,** see motor n.

**intercalary n.,** internuncial n.

**internuncial n.,** intercalary n.; a n. interposed between and connecting two other n.'s.

**lower motor n.,** a term used in clinical neurology to indicate the motor n., as opposed to the "upper motor n.'s" of the motor cortex that contribute to the pyramidal or corticospinal tract; see also motor n.

**motor n.,** a nerve cell in the spinal cord, rhombencephalon, or mesencephalon characterized by having an axon that leaves the central nervous system to establish a functional connection with an effector (muscle or glandular) tissue. Somatic motor n.'s directly synapse with striated muscle fibers by motor endplates; visceral or autonomic motor n.'s (preganglionic motor n.'s), by contrast, innervate smooth muscle fibers or glands only by the intermediary of a second, peripheral, n. (postganglionic or ganglionic motor n.) located in an autonomic ganglion. See also motor *endplate* and *systema* nervosum autonomicum.

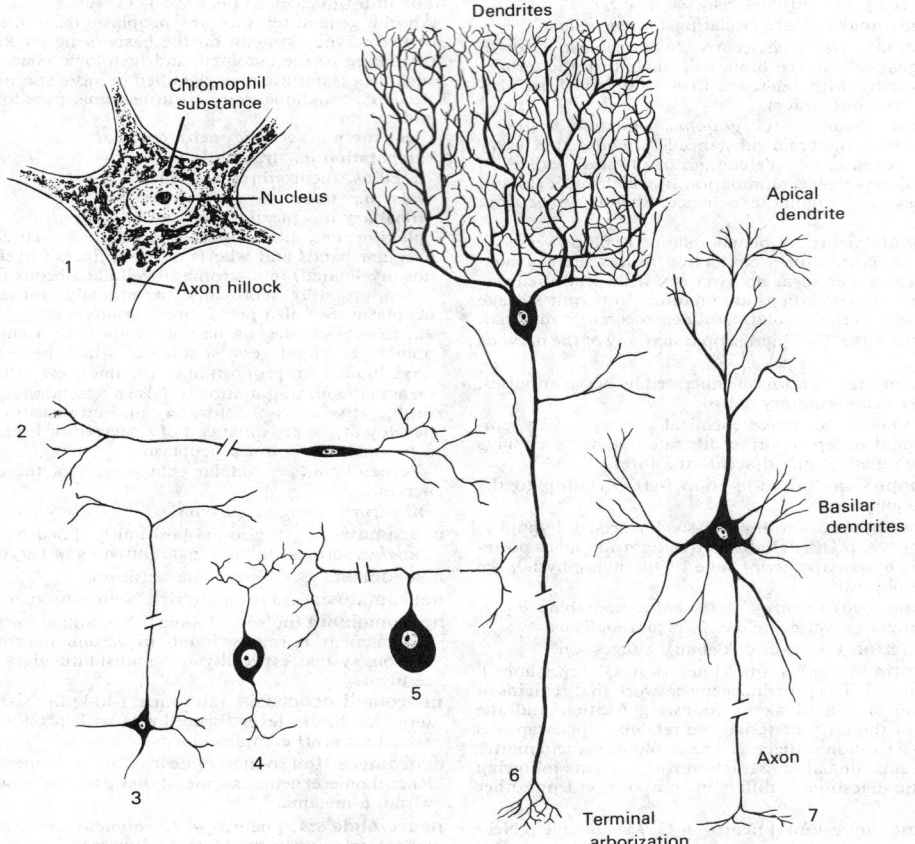

Dendrites

Chromophil substance

Nucleus

Axon hillock

Apical dendrite

Basilar dendrites

Axon

Terminal arborization

**Some Types of Neuron**

*1,* Typical nerve cell body showing internal structure; *2,* horizontal cell (of Cajal) from cerebral cortex; *3,* cell of Martinotti; *4,* bipolar cell; *5,* unipolar cell (posterior root ganglion; *6,* Purkinje cell; *7,* pyramidal cell of motor area of cerebral cortex. Sheaths are not shown.

**multipolar n.,** a n. with several processes, usually an axon and three or more dendrites.

**postganglionic motor n.,** see motor n.

**preganglionic motor n.,** see motor n.

**pseudounipolar n.,** unipolar n.

**somatic motor n.,** see motor n.

**unipolar n.,** pseudounipolar n.: pseudounipolar or unipolar cell; a n. the cell body of which emits a single, axonal process that resulted from the fusion of two polar processes during development; at a variable distance from the cell body the process divides into a peripheral axon branch extending outward as a peripheral afferent (sensory) nerve fiber, and a central axon branch that enters into synaptic contact with n.'s in the spinal cord or brainstem. With the single known exception of the n.'s composing the mesencephalic nucleus of the trigeminus, unipolar n.'s are the exclusive neural elements of the sensory ganglia. The lack of dendritic processes of these primary sensory n.'s is only apparent: the dendritic pole of the unipolar n. is represented by the unmyelinated terminal ramifications of the peripheral axon branch.

**upper motor n.'s,** clinical term indicating those n.'s of the motor cortex that contribute to the formation of the pyramidal or corticospinal and corticobulbar tracts, as against the "lower motor n.'s" innervating the skeletal muscles. Although not motor n.'s in the strict sense, these cortical n.'s became colloquially classified as motor n.'s because of the severe disorders of movement resulting from destruction of the motor cortex or the pyramidal tract. See also motor n., and motor *cortex.*

**visceral motor n.,** see motor n.

**neuronal** (nu′ro-nal, nu-ro′nal). Pertaining to a neuron.

**neu′rone.** Neuron.

**neuronephric** (nu′ro-nef′rik) [ neuro- + G. *nephros,* kidney ]. Relating to the nerve supply of the kidney.

**neuronevus** (nu′ro-ne′vus). Intradermal *nevus.*

**neuronitis** (nu-ron-i′tis). Degenerative inflammation of nerve cells.

**neuronophage** (nu-ron′o-fāj) [ neuron + G. *phagein,* to eat ]. A phagocyte that ingests neuronal elements; see microglia.

**neuronophagia, neuronophagy** (nu-ron′o-fa′jĭ-ah, nu′-ro-nof′a-jĭ) [ neuron + G. *phagein,* to eat ]. Phagocytosis of nerve cells.

**neuronyxis** (nu′ro-nik′sis) [ neuro- + G. *nyxis,* pricking ]. Acupuncture of a nerve.

**neuro-ophthalmology** (nu′ro-of-thal-mol′o-jĭ). Neurophthalmology; that branch of medical science pertaining to the visual representation in the central nervous system.

**neu′ropapilli′tis.** Optic *neuritis.*

**neuroparal′ysis.** Paralysis resulting from disease of the nerve supplying the affected part.

**neu′ropath.** One who suffers from or is predisposed to some disease of the nervous system.

**neuropath′ic.** Relating in any way to neuropathy.

**neuropathogen′esis** [ neuro- + G. *pathos,* suffering, + *genesis,* origin ]. The origin or causation of a disease of the nervous system.

**neuropathol′ogy.** Pathology of the nervous system.

**neuropathy** (nu′rop′ă-thĭ) [ neuro- + G. *pathos,* suffering ]. 1. A classical term for any disorder affecting any segment of the nervous system. 2. In contemporary usage, a disease involving the cranial or spinal nerves.

**asymmetric motor n.,** n. in which the loss of function is more marked in the extremities of one side of the body.

**diabet′ic n.,** a combined sensory and motor n., typically symmetric and segmental, and involving, as well, autonomic fibers; seen frequently in older diabetic persons.

**diphtheritic n.,** a rapidly developing peripheral n. caused by a toxin elaborated by *Corynebacterium diphtheriae.*

**entrapment n.,** a region of traumatic neuritis in which the nerve is maintained in an irritated state by external pressure created by encroachment or impingement from a nearby anatomical configuration; *e.g.,* pressure on the median nerve by swollen tendons and their sheaths in the carpal tunnel lead to the carpal tunnel syndrome.

**familial amyloid n.,** a disorder found largely in the Portuguese, beginning in the third decade of life, with paresis, amyotrophy, trophic alterations, and sensory changes; autosomal dominant inheritance.

**hereditary sensory radicular n.,** n. characterized by the occurrence of severe, relapsing foot ulcerations of neuropathic origin, destruction of terminal digits of feet and hands, and a loss of sensation; autosomal dominant inheritance.

**isoniazid n.,** an axonal form of n. seen in some patients treated with isoniazid.

**lead n.,** a progressive, often symmetric, segmental peripheral n. seen in chronic lead intoxication; characterized by wrist-drop.

**leprous n.,** a slowly developing granulomatous n. caused by *Mycobacterium leprae* and commonly seen in leprosy.

**segmental n.,** demyelination of scattered segments of peripheral nerves, with relating sparing of axons; noted in diabetes, arsenic poisoning, lead poisoning, diphtheria, and leprosy.

**symmetric distal n.,** n. in which the motor weakness is equal on the two sides of the body.

**vitamin $B_{12}$ n.,** subacute combined *degeneration* of the spinal cord.

**neuropharmacology** (nu′ro-far′mă-kol′o-jĭ). The study of drugs that exert effects on neuronal tissue.

**neurophilic** (nu-ro-fil′ik) [ neuro- + G. *philos,* fond ]. Neurotrophic.

**neuropho′nia** [ neuro- + G. *phōnē,* voice ]. A spasm or tic of the muscles of phonation causing involuntary sounds or cries.

**neur′ophthalmol′ogy.** Neuro-ophthalmology.

**neurophysine** (nu′ro-fiz′ēn). A protein found in the hypothalamus and pars nervosa; on bioassay it has exhibited the properties of oxytocin and vasopressin, and is postulated to participate in the transport and storage of neurohypophysial hormones.

**neurophysiology** (nu′ro-fiz-ĭ-ol′o-jĭ). Physiology of the nervous system.

**neuropil, neuropile** (nu′ro-pil, -pīl) [ neuro- + G. *pilos,* felt ]. The complex, feltlike net of axonal, dendritic, and glial arborizations that forms the bulk of the central nervous system's gray matter, and in which the nerve cell bodies lie embedded.

**neu′roplasm.** The protoplasm of a nerve cell.

**neuroplasty** (nu′ro-plas′tĭ) [ neuro- + G. *plassō,* to form ]. Plastic surgery of the nerves.

**neuroplegic** (nu′ro-ple′jik) [ neuro- + G. *plēgē,* a stroke ]. Pertaining to paralysis due to nervous system disease.

**neuropodia** (nu′ro-po′dĭ-ah) [ pl. of *neuropodium* or *neuropodion,* fr. neuro- + G. *podion,* little foot ]. Axon *terminals.*

**neuropore** (nu′ro-pōr) [ neuro- + G. *poros,* pore ]. An opening in the embryo leading from the central canal of the neural tube to the exterior.

**neuropsychiatry** (nu′ro-si-ki′ă-trĭ). The specialty dealing with both organic and functional diseases of the nervous system.

**neuropsycholog′ic, neuropsycholog′ical.** Pertaining to neuropsychology.

**neuropsychology** (nu′ro-si-kol′o-jĭ). A subspecialty of clinical psychology concerned with the study of the relationships between the brain and behavior, including the diagnosis of brain pathology from the results of psychological tests and assessment techniques.

**neuropsychopath′ic.** Relating to neuropsychopathy.

**neuropsychopathy** (nu-ro-si-kop′ă-thĭ). An emotional illness of neurologic and/or functional origin.

**neuropsychopharmacology** (nu′ro-si′ko-far-mă-kol′o-jĭ). Psychopharmacology.

**neuropsychosis** (nu-ro-si-ko′sis). Obsolete term for what is now called psychosis.

**neurora′diol′ogy.** X-ray studies of the central nervous system.

**neurorecidive** (nu′ro-res′ĭ-dēv) [ neuro- + L. *recidivus,* recurring ]. Neurorelapse.

**neurorecurrence** (nu′ro-re-kur′ens). Neurorelapse.

**neurorelapse** (nu′ro-re-laps′). Neurorecurrence; neurorecidive; the recurrence of neurological symptoms upon initiation of antisyphilitic therapy.

**neuroretinitis** (nu′ro-ret-ĭ-ni′tis). Inflammation of the retina and of the optic nerve.

**neurorrhaphy** (nu-ror'ă-fĭ) [ neuro- + G. *rhaphē*, suture ]. Joining together, usually by suture, of the two parts of a divided nerve.

**neurorrheuma** (nu-ro-ru'mah) [ neuro- + G. *rheuma*, current ]. Neurokyme.

**neurosarcocleisis** (nu-ro-sar-ko-kli'sis) [ neuro- + G. *sarx*, flesh, + *kleisis*, closure ]. An operation for the relief of neuralgia, which consists in resection of one of the walls of the osseous canal traversed by the nerve and the transportation of the latter into the soft tissues.

**neurosarco'ma.** An old, general term for a malignant neoplasm derived from cells of the nervous system.

**neuroschwannoma** (nu'ro-shwah-no'mah). Neurilemoma.

**neurosciences** (nu'ro-si'en-sez). The scientific disciplines concerned with the development, structure, function, chemistry, pharmacology, and pathology of the nervous system.

**neu'rosecre'tion.** The release of a secretory substance from the axon terminals of certain nerve cells in the brain into the circulating blood. The secretory product may be a true hormone, *e.g.*, the antidiuretic hormone released from the axon terminals of the neurons composing the supraoptic nucleus of the hypothalamus; in the case of the so-called releasing-factor neurons of the hypothalamus the cell product is not a systemic hormone in its own right but elicits the release of trophic hormones by the anterior lobe of the hypophysis, substances that in turn stimulate peripheral endocrine glands to release their systemically active hormones.

**neurosecretory** (nu'ro-se'kre-tor-ĭ, -se'kre'to-rĭ). Relating to neurosecretion.

**neurosis,** pl. **neuroses** (nu-ro'sis, -sēz) [ neuro- + G. suffix -*osis*, condition ]. A psychological or behavioral disorder in which anxiety is the primary characteristic. Defense mechanisms or any of the phobias are the adjustive techniques which an individual learns in order to cope with this underlying anxiety. In contrast to the psychoses, persons with a n. do not exhibit gross distortion of reality or disorganization of personality. 2. A functional nervous disease, or one which is dependent upon no evident lesion. 3. A peculiar state of tension or irritability of the nervous system; any form of nervousness.

**accident n.,** traumatic n.

**anxiety n.,** chronic abnormal distress and worry to the point of panic, associated with overaction of the sympathetic nervous system.

**association n.,** one in which association of ideas causes mental repetition of an experience.

**battle n.,** war n.

**cardiac n.,** cardioneurosis; anxiety concerning the state of the heart, as a result of palpitation, chest pain, or other symptom not due to heart disease. See also neurocirculatory *asthenia*.

**character n.,** a subclass of personality disorders.

**compensation n.,** the development of symptoms of n. believed to be motivated by the desire for, and hope of, monetary gain.

**compulsive n.,** obsessive-compulsive n.

**conversion hysteria n.,** conversion *hysteria*.

**expectation n.,** a condition in which anticipation of an event produces neurotic symptoms.

**experimental n.,** a behavior disorder produced experimentally, as when an organism is required to make a discrimination of extreme difficulty and "breaks down" in the process.

**fatigue n.,** neurasthenia or psychasthenia.

**military n.,** war n.

**noogenic n.,** in existential psychiatry, the neurotic symptomatology resulting from existential frustration.

**obsessive-compulsive n.,** compulsive n.; a disorder characterized by the persistent and repetitive intrusion of unwanted thoughts, urges, or actions that the individual is unable to prevent. The compulsive thoughts may consist of single words, ideas, or ruminations often perceived by the sufferer as nonsensical; the repetitive urges or actions vary from simple movements to complex rituals. Anxiety and distress is the underlying emotion or drive state, and the ritualistic behavior is a learned method of reducing the anxiety.

**occupation** or **professional n.,** occupation or professional spasm; local chorea; a functional disorder of a group of muscles used chiefly in one's occupation, marked by the occurrence of spasm, paresis, or incoordination on attempt to repeat the habitual movements. See also subentries under cramp.

**Oedipal n.,** continuation of the Oedipus *complex* (*q. v.*) into adulthood.

**pension n.;** a type of compensation n., motivated by the desire for premature retirement on pension.

**postconcussion n.,** neurosis following cerebral concussion; a type of traumatic n.; see also neuropsychologic *disorder.*

**posttraumatic n.,** traumatic n.

**sexual n.,** a mental disorder of the sexual function, *e.g.,* impotence.

**n. tarda,** neurotic patterns developing in older people, related to organic cerebral lesions.

**torsion n.,** *dysbasia* lordotica progressiva.

**transference n.,** in psychoanalysis, the phenomenon of the patient's developing a strong emotional relationship with the analyst, symbolizing an emotional relationship with a family figure; analysis of this n. comprises an important part of psychoanalytic treatment.

**traumatic n.,** any functional nervous disorder following an accident or injury.

**war n.,** battle n.; military n.; a stress condition or mental disorder induced by conditions existing in warfare; see also shell-shock.

**neu'rospasm.** Muscular spasm or twitching caused by a disordered nerve supply.

**neurosplanchnic** (nu'ro-splangk'nik) [ neuro- + G. *splanchnon,* a viscus ]. Neurovisceral.

**neurospongioma** (nu-ro-spon-jĭ-o'mah). Medulloblastoma.

**neurospongium** (nu'ro-spon'jĭ-um, -spun'jĭ-um) [ neuro- + G. *spongion,* small sponge ]. 1. Obsolete term for the plexus of neurofibrils within nerve cells. 2. Obsolete designation for the reticular layer of the retina.

**Neurospora** (nūr-os'por-ah) [ neuro- + G. *spora,* seed ]. Pink bread mold; a genus of fungi of the class Ascomycetes, grown in cultures and used in researches in genetics and in cellular biochemistry.

**neurosthenia** (nu-ro-sthe'nĭ-ah) [ neuro- + G. *sthenos,* force ]. A condition in which the nerves respond with abnormal force or rapidity to slight stimuli.

**neurosur'geon.** A surgeon specializing in operations on the nervous system.

**neurosur'gery.** Surgery of the nervous system.

**neurosu'ture.** Neurorrhaphy.

**neurosyphilis** (nu-ro-sif'ĭ-lis). Nervous system manifestations of syphilis, including tabes dorsalis, general paresis, meningovascular syphilis.

**neurotabes** (nu'ro-ta'bēz) [ neuro- + L. *tabes,* a wasting away ]. Déjérine's n.; polyneuritis with ataxic symptoms.

**Déjérine's peripheral n.,** neurotabes.

**neurotendinous** (nu'ro-ten'dĭ-nus). Relating to both nerves and tendons.

**neurotension** (nu'to-ten'shun). Neurectasia.

**neurothele** (nu'ro-thēl) [ neuro- + G. *thēlē,* nipple ]. Nerve *papilla.*

**neurotherapeutics, neurotherapy** (nu'ro-thĕr-ă-pu'tiks, -thĕr'ă-pĭ). The treatment of nervous disorders.

**neurothlipsis, neurothlipsia** (nu'ro-thlip'sis, -sĭ-ah) [ neuro- + G. *thlipsis,* pressure ]. Pressure on one or more nerves.

**neurotic** (nu-rot'ik). 1. Relating to or suffering from a neurosis. 2. One who suffers from a neurosis, or functional nervous disorder.

**neuroticism** (nu-rot'ĭ-sizm). The condition or psychological trait of being neurotic.

**neurotization** (nu'ro-tĭ-za'shun). The acquiring of nervous substance; the regeneration of a nerve.

**neu'rotize.** To provide with nerve substance.

**neurotmesis** (nu'rot-me'sis) [ neuro- + G. *tmēsis,* a cutting, TOM- ]. The condition in which there is complete division of a nerve.

**neurotology** (nu'ro-tol'o-ji) [ neuro- + G. *ous (ot-)*, ear, + *logos*, study ]. The science dealing with labyrinthine affections and with the brain lesions complicating disease of the ear.

**neu'rotome** [ neuro- + G. *tomē*, a cutting ]. A very slender knife or needle, used for teasing apart nerve fibers in microdissection.

**neurotomy** (nu-rot'o-mi) [ neuro- + G. *tomē*, a cutting ]. Operative division of a nerve.

**retrogasserian n.,** trigeminal *rhizotomy.*

**neurotonic** (nu'ro-ton'ik). 1. Relating to neurotony. 2. Strengthening or stimulating impaired nervous action. 3. An agent that improves the tone or force of the nervous system.

**neurotony** (nu-rot'o-ni) [ neuro- + G. *tonos*, tension ]. Neurectasia.

**neurotox'ic.** Poisonous to nervous substance.

**neurotox'in.** Neurolysin.

**neurotransmission** (nu'ro-trans-mish'un) Neurohumoral *transmission.*

**neurotransmitter** (nu'ro-trans-mit'er) [ neuro- + L. *transmitto*, to send across ]. Any specific chemical agent released by a presynaptic cell, upon excitation, that crosses the synapse to stimulate or inhibit the postsynaptic cell.

**neurotrauma** (nu-ro-traw'mah) [ neuro- + G. *trauma*, injury ]. 1. Trauma of the nervous system. 2. Neurotrosis; trauma or wounding of a nerve.

**neurotrip'sy** [ neuro- + G. *tripsis*, a rubbing ]. The operative crushing of a nerve.

**neurotrophic** (nu'ro-trof'ik). Relating to neurotrophy.

**neurotrophy** (nu-rot'ro-fi) [ neuro- + G. *trophē*, nourishment ]. Nutrition and metabolism of tissues under nervous influence.

**neurotropic** (nu'ro-trop'ik). Relating to neurotropy; having an affinity for the nervous system.

**neurotropy, neurotropism** (nu-rot'ro-pi, -pizm) [ neuro- + G. *trope*, a turning ]. 1. Affinity of basic dyes for nervous tissue. 2. The attraction of certain pathogenic microorganisms, poisons, and nutritive substances toward the nerve centers.

**neurotrosis** (nu'ro-tro'sis) [ neuro- + G. *trōsis*, a wounding ]. Neurotrauma (2).

**neurotubule** (nu'ro-tu-būl). One of the microtubules, 100 to 200 Å in diameter, occurring in the cell body, dendrites, axon, and in some synaptic endings of neurons.

**neurovaccine** (nu'ro-vak'sēn). A fixed or standardized vaccine virus of definite strength, obtained by continued passage through the brain of rabbits.

**neu'rovarico'sis, neu'rovaricos'ity** [ neuro- + L. *varix*, varicosis ]. A condition marked by multiple swellings along the course of a nerve.

**neurovas'cular.** Relating to both nervous and vascular systems; relating to the nerves supplying the walls of the blood vessels, the vasomotor nerves.

**neuroveg'etative.** Neurovisceral.

**neurovi'rus.** Vaccine virus modified by means of passage into and growth in nervous tissue.

**neurovisceral** (nu-ro-vis'er-al) [ neuro- + L. *viscera*, the internal organs ]. Neurovegetative; neurosplanchnic; referring to the innervation of the internal organs by the autonomic nervous system.

**neurula,** pl. **neu'rulae** (nu'ruh-lah) [ neur- + L. dim. suffix *-ulus* ]. The stage in embryonic development in which the formation of the neural plate and its closure to form the neural tube are prominent processes.

**neurulation** (nu'ruh-la'shun) [ see neurula ]. The processes involved in the formation of the neurula stage.

**Neusser** (noy'ser), Edmund von, Austrian physician, 1852–1912. See N.'s *granules.*

**neutral** (nu'tral) [ L. *neutralis*, fr. *neuter*, neither ]. 1. Exhibiting no positive properties; indifferent. 2. In chemistry, neither acid nor alkaline.

**n. red,** toluylene red; aminodimethylaminotoluaminozine hydrochloride; used (1) as indicator: pH 6.8, red; 8.0, yellow; (2) as a vital dye to stain granules and vacuoles in living cells; (3) in testing the secretion of acid by the stomach, it being given with a test meal.

**neu'traliza'tion.** 1. The conversion of the entire amount of an acid or a base into a salt by the addition of an exactly sufficient quantity of a base or of an acid, respectively. 2. The change in reaction of a solution from acid or alkaline to neutral by the addition of just a sufficient amount of an alkaline or of an acid substance, respectively. 3. The rendering ineffective of any action, process, or potential.

**neu'tralize.** 1. To render ineffective. 2. To effect neutralization.

**neutretto** (nu-tret'o) [ neutron + It. dim. suffix *-etto* ]. A supposed nuclear particle intermediate in mass between the neutrino and the neutron.

**neutrino** (nu-tre'no) [ neutron + It. dim. suffix *-ino* ]. A subatomic particle having zero rest mass and no charge; traveling always at the speed of light and interacting with matter only very rarely.

**neutro-, neutr-** (nu'tro-) [ L. *neutralis*, fr. *neuter*, neither ]. Combining forms meaning neutral.

**neutroclusion** (nu'tro-klu'zhun) [ neutro- + occlusion ]. Normal *occlusion.*

**neutrocyte** (nu'tro-sit) [ neutro- + G. *kytos*, cell ]. Neutrophil.

**neutrocytopenia** (nu'tro-si-to-pe'ni-ah) [ neutrocyte + G. *penia*, poverty ]. Neutropenia.

**neutrocytosis** (nu'tro-si-to'sis). Neutrophilia.

**neutron** [ L. *neuter*, neither ]. Electrically neutral particle in the nucleus of the atom with a mass practically that of a proton; in isolation, it breaks down to a proton and an electron with a half-life of about 12 minutes. See fig. under atom.

**epither'mal n.,** a n. having an energy in the range immediately above the thermal range, *i.e.*, having an energy between a few hundredths and approximately 100 ev.

**neutropenia** (nu-tro-pe'ni-ah) [ neutrophil + G. *penia*, poverty ]. Neutrophilic leukopenia; neutrocytopenia; the presence of abnormally small numbers of neutrophils in the circulating blood.

**cyclic n.,** periodic n.

**periodic n.,** cyclic n.; n. recurring at regular intervals (14 to 45 days), in association with various types of infectious diseases, *e.g.*, stomatitis, cutaneous ulcers, furuncles, arthritis, and others.

**neutrophil, neutrophile** (nu'tro-fil, -fil) [ neutro- + G. *philos*, fond ]. Neutrocyte. 1. A mature white blood cell in the granulocytic series, formed by myelopoietic tissue of the bone marrow (sometimes also in extramedullary sites), and released into the circulating blood, where they normally represent from 54 to 65 per cent of the total number of leukocytes. When stained with the usual Romanowsky type of dyes, n.'s are characterized by: (1) a nucleus that is dark purple-blue, lobated (three to five distinct lobes joined by thin strands of chromatin), and has a rather coarse network of fairly dense chromatin; (2) a cytoplasm that is faintly pink (sharply contrasted with the nucleus) and contains numerous, fine or tiny, pink or violet-pink granules, *i.e.*, not acidophilic or basophilic (as in eosinophils or basophils). The precursors of n.'s, in order of increasing maturity, are (1) myeloblasts, (2) myelocytes, and (3) metamyelocytes or "juvenile" forms, including the "stabkernige" or staff cells, which are also known as stabs or band forms. Although the terms neutrophilic leukocytes and neutrophilic granulocytes include younger cells in which neutrophilic granules are recognized, the two expressions are frequently used as synonyms for n.'s, which are mature forms unless otherwise indicated by a modifying term, such as immature n. See also leukocyte, leukocytosis, and their subentries. 2. The term n. is also used with reference to any cells or tissues that manifest no special affinity for acid or basic dyes, *i.e.*, the cytoplasm stains approximately equally with either type of dye. See color plate 14.

**band n.,** stab *cell.*

**hypersegmented n.,** an aged and degenerated n. in which there may be 6 to 10 lobes in the nucleus.

**immature n.,** a young n.; the term is usually used with reference to stab n.'s (or other "juvenile" n.'s), neutrophilic granulocytes in which the nucleus is indented but not distinctly segmented.

**juvenile n.,** a metamyelocyte; any cell of the granulocytic series in which the neutrophilic granules are recognizable and the nucleus is indented (the first phase of segmentation).

**mature n.,** segmented n.

**segmented n.,** mature n.; a fully matured n. that has at least 2 (and as many as 5) distinct lobes in the nucleus and manifests active ameboid motion.

**stab n.,** stab *cell*.

**neutrophil'ia.** Neutrocytosis; neutrophilic leukocytosis; also frequently used synonymously with leukocytosis, inasmuch as the latter is generally the result of an increased number of meutrophilic granulocytes in the circulating blood (or in the tissues, or both). N. is usually *absolute*, that is, there is an increase in the total number of leukocytes as well as an increased percentage of neutrophils. In some instances, n. may be *relative*, that is, there is an increased percentage of neutrophils, but the total number of all types of leukocytes may be within the normal range.

**neutrophil'ic.** 1. Pertaining to or characterized by neutrophils, as an exudate in which the predominant cells are n. granulocytes. 2. Characterized by a lack of affinity for acid or basic dyes, *i.e.*, staining approximately equally with either type.

**neutrophilopenia** (nu'tro-fil'-o-pe'nĭ-ah) [ neutrophil + G. *penia*, poverty ]. Neutropenia.

**neutroph'ilous.** Neutrophilic (2).

**neutrotaxis** (nu-tro-tak'sis) [ neutrophil + G. *taxis*, arrangement ]. A phenomenon in which neutrophilic leukocytes are stimulated by a substance in such a manner that (1) they are attracted and move toward it—*positive n.*, or (2) they are repelled and move away from it—*negative n.*; in some instances, there is no effect, and this condition is sometimes termed *indifferent n.*

**ne'vi** [ L. ]. Plural of nevus.

**ne'vocarcino'ma** [ nevus + carcinoma ]. A malignant melonoma that is presumed to have originated in a nevus.

**ne'void** [ L. *naevus*, mole (nevus), + G. *eidos*, resemblance ]. Resembling a nevus.

**ne'volipo'ma** [ nevus + lipoma ]. Nevus lipomatodes; nevus mollusciformis; unsatisfactory terms for a lesion that is basically a nevus, with a stroma of fibrous and adipose elements.

**ne'vose, ne'vous.** Marked with nevi; nevoid.

**nevoxanthoendothelioma** (ne'vo-zan'tho-en-do-the-le-o'-mah) [ nevus + G. *xanthos*, yellow, + endothelioma ]. Juvenile xanthogranuloma; a lesion usually found in young children. Lesions are reddish papules, and may be single or multiple.

**ne'vus,** pl. **ne'vi** [ L. *naevus*, mole, birthmark ]. 1. Birthmark; a circumscribed malformation of the skin, especially if colored by hyperpigmentation or increased vascularity; it may be predominantly epidermal, adnexal, melanocytic, or mesodermal, or a compound overgrowth of these tissues. 2. A benign localized overgrowth of melanocytes arising in the skin early in life.

**n. ane'micus,** a functional developmental defect characterized by pale, round or oval, flat lesions, indistinguishable from surrounding normal skin on diascopy.

**n. angiecto'des,** n. vascularis.

**n. angiomato'des,** a diffuse angiomatous formation in the subcutaneous connective tissue.

**n. arachnoi'deus,** arterial *spider*.

**n. ara'neus,** arterial *spider*.

**blue n.,** a dark blue or blue-black n. covered by smooth skin, formed by melanin-pigmented spindle cells in the lower dermis; of mesodermal origin.

**blue rubber-bleb nevi,** a syndrome characterized by erectile, easily compressible, thin-walled hemangiomatous nodules, widely distributed in the skin and in the alimentary canal, and sometimes in other tissues. Lesions in the gut may perforate or cause hemorrhage and the patient may be anemic from continual bleeding.

**capillary n.,** capillary hemangioma of the skin.

**n. caverno'sus,** cavernous *hemangioma*.

**comedo n.,** n. comedonicus.

**n. comedon'icus,** comedo n.; n. follicularis keratosus; congenital linear keratinous cystic invaginations of the

epidermis, with failure of development of normal pilosebaceous follicles.

**compound n.,** a n. in which there are abnormalities of dermal structures, such as the pilosebaceous, in addition to proliferation of melanocytes.

**epidermic-dermic n.,** junction n.

**epithelioid cell n.,** benign juvenile *melanoma*.

**n. flam'meus,** port-wine mark or stain; a large n. vascularis having a purplish color; it is usually found on the head and neck and persists throughout life.

**n. follicula'ris kerato'sus,** n. comedonicus.

**halo n.,** *leukoderma* acquisitum centrifugum.

**intradermal n.,** neuronevus; a n., in which nests of melanocytes are found in the dermis but not at the epidermal-dermal junction. Benign pigmented nevi become intradermal when they cease to grow in adult life.

**Ito's n.,** pigmentation of skin innervated by lateral branches of the supraclavicular nerve and the lateral cutaneous nerve of the arm.

**junction n.,** epidermic-dermic n.; consists of nests of n. cells in the basal cell zone—at junction of the epidermis and dermis; appears as a slightly raised flat, nonhairy pigmented (dark brown or black) tumor about the size of a pea.

**n. lipomato'des, n. lipomato'sus,** nevolipoma.

**n. lupus,** *angioma* serpiginosum.

**n. lymphat'icus,** cutaneous lymphangioma.

**n. molluscifor'mis,** nevolipoma.

**nape n.,** so-called Unna's mark; a pale, vascular birthmark found on the nape of the neck in 25 to 50 per cent of normal persons.

**Ota's n.,** oculodermal *melanosis*.

**n. papillomato'sus,** a prominent wartlike mole.

**paving-stone n.,** shagreen *skin*.

**n. pigm'ento'sus,** mole (1); a congenital pigmented lesion of varying size, raised or level with the skin.

**n. pilo'sus,** hairy mole; a mole covered with a more or less abundant growth of hair.

**n. sanguin'eus,** n. vascularis.

**n. seba'ceus,** congenital sebaceous gland hyperplasia; a n. or hamartoma composed of mature sebaceous glands.

**spider n.,** arterial *spider*.

**n. spillus** [ G. *spilos*, stain ], a flat mole.

**spindle cell n.,** benign juvenile *melanoma*.

**n. spongio'sus albus muco'sae,** white sponge n. of the mucosa; a congenital white spongy lesion of the mucous membranes (buccal, rectal, and vaginal).

**strawberry n.,** strawberry birthmark or mark; a small n. vascularis resembling a strawberry in size, shape, and color; it usually disappears spontaneously in early childhood.

**Sutton's n.,** *leukoderma* acquisitum centrifugum.

**systematized n.,** a developmental dysplasia of the skin; extensive, patterned, and usually unilateral.

**n. u'nius lat'eris,** a congenital linear n. limited to one side of the body.

**n. vascula'ris, n. vasculo'sus,** capillary or superficial angioma; n. angiectodes or sanguineus; a congenital red discoloration of the skin, of irregular size and boundaries, caused by an overgrowth of the cutaneous capillaries; most of these capillary hemangiomas (*q. v.*) regress spontaneously; strawberry n. and n. flammeus are types of n. vascularis.

**n. veno'sus,** one formed of a patch of dilated venules.

**woolly-hair n.,** allotrichia circumscripta; a circumscribed congenital kinking or woolliness of scalp hair; it appears during infancy (or as late as age 19) in a previously normal hair site and enlarges for a period of 2 to 3 years.

**new'born.** 1. Neonate; a baby that has recently been born. 2. Neonatal (*q. v.*); indicating an infant recently born.

**Newcastle disease.** See under disease.

**New Hampshire rule.** See under rule.

**Newland's law.** See under law.

**Newton,** Sir Isaac, English physicist, 1642–1727. See Newtonian *aberration, constant* (of gravitation), *flow, viscosity*; N.'s *disk, law*.

**new'ton.** [ I. *Newton* ]. Derived unit of force in the SI system, expressed as meters-kilograms per second squared (m kg s$^{-2}$).

**newton-meter.** A unit of the mks system (see mks *unit*); energy expended, or work done, by a force of 1 newton acting through a distance of 1 meter; equal to a joule ($10^7$ ergs).

**nexus,** pl. **nexus** (nek'sus) [ L. interconnection ]. Gap *junction.*

**Nezelof,** C., French pathologist, *1922. See N. *syndrome,* N. type of thymic *alymphoplasia.*

**NF.** Abbreviation for *National Formulary.*

**ng.** Abbreviation for nanogram.

**NGF.** Abbreviation for nerve growth *factor.*

**N.H.S.** Initials of National Health Service (England).

**NH$_2$-terminal.** Amino-terminal.

**Ni.** Chemical symbol of the element nickel.

**ni'acin** (NF). Nicotinic acid.

**ni'acinam'ide** (USP, BP). Nicotinamide.

**nial'amide** (BP). NIAMID; *N*-benzyl-*β*-(isonicotinoylhydrazine) propionamide; a monoamine oxidase inhibitor used in the treatment of depressive disorders.

**niche** (nitch, nēsh) [ Fr. ]. An eroded or ulcerated area which is detected by contrast radiography; *e.g.,* an x-ray with barium in the stomach or duodenum. See also Haudek's n.

   **enamel n.,** enamel *crypt.*

   **Haudek's n.,** an apparent projection from the wall of the stomach sometimes seen in roentgenograms of gastric ulcer, due actually to the filling of the cavity of the ulcer with bismuth.

**nickel** (nik'l) [ abbrev. fr. Ger. *kupfer-nickel,* name of copper-colored ore from which nickel was first obtained; *nickel,* the Ger. word for a dwarfish imp ]. A metallic element, symbol Ni, atomic no. 28, atomic weight 58.71, closely resembling cobalt and often associated with it.

   **Raney n.,** see under Raney.

**Nickerson-Kveim test.** See under test.

**nick'ing.** Localized constrictions in retinal blood vessels.

   **A-V n.,** arteriovenous n.; constriction of retinal vein where it is crossed by an artery.

**Nicklès** (ne-klĕs'), François J. J., French chemist, 1821–1869. See N.'s *test.*

**niclo'samide** (NF, BP). CESTOCID; FENASAL; YOMESAN; *N*-(2'-chloro-4'-nitrophenyl)-5-chlorosalicylamide; an effective, relatively nontoxic teniacide.

**nicofu'ranose.** VASPERDIL; fructose 1,3,4,6-tetranicolinate; peripheral vasodilator.

**Nicol,** William, Edinburgh physicist, 1768–1851. See N. *prism.*

**Nicolaier** (ne-ko-li'er), Arthur, German physician, *1862. See N.'s *bacillus.*

**Nicolas** (ne'kŭ-lah), J., French physician. See Favre-Durand-N. *disease,* N.-Favre *disease.*

**Nicolle** (nĭ-kul'), Charles J. H., French microbiologist, 1866–1936. Nobel laureate, 1928, for his work on typhus. See N.'s white *mycetoma,* N.'s *stain.*

**nicotin'amide** (BP). Nicotinic acid amide; niacinamide (for structure, see nicotinamide adenine dinucleotide); biologically active amide of nicotinic acid, used in the prevention and treatment of pellagra.

**nicotinamide adenine dinucleotide.** NAD; formerly known as diphosphopyridine nucleotide (DPN), coenzyme I; cozymase; codehydrogenase I. It consists of ribosylnicotinamide 5'-phosphate (NMN) and adenosine 5'-phosphate (AMP) linked by pyrophosphate formation between the two phosphate groups. Attached as a prosthetic group to a protein, it serves as a respiratory enzyme (hydrogen acceptor and donor) through alternate oxidation and reduction (NAD$^+$⇌NADH). The large number of enzymes acting upon or with NAD (or NADP) in this manner are listed in EC subgroup 1.6. Definitions of those enzymes named in terms of NAD or NADP are alphabetized under these abbreviations.

**nicotinamide adenine dinucleotide phosphate.** NADP; formerly known as triphosphopyridine nucleotide (TPN) and coenzyme II; a coenzyme of many oxidases (dehydrogenases), in which the reaction NADP$^+$ + 2H ⇌ NADPH + H$^+$ takes place. The third phosphoric group

**Oxidized NAD (NAD$^+$)**
*Arrow* indicates location of the third phosphoric group in NADP.

**Reduced NAD (NADH) (Nicotinamide moiety)**
* Denotes that remainder of NADH formula is identical with that shown for NAD$^+$.

esterifies the 2'-hydroxyl of the adenosine moiety of NAD. See also entries under NADP.

**nicotin'amide mononucleotide.** A condensation product of nicotinamide and ribose 5-phosphate, linking the N of nicotinamide to the (*β*) C-1 of the ribose; in NAD, ring is linked by the 5'-P to the 5'-P of AMP.

**nic'otinate.** Ester of nicotinic acid. Some n.'s are used in ointments as rubefacients.

**nicotine** (nik'o-tēn). 1-Methyl-2-(3-pyridyl)pyrrolidine; a poisonous volatile alkaloid, derived from tobacco and responsible for many of the effects of tobacco; an important tool in physiologic and pharmacologic investigation. It first stimulates (small doses) then depresses (large doses) at autonomic ganglia and myoneural junctions. Also used as an insecticide and fumigant. It forms salts with most acids. See also nicotinic.

**Nicotine**

**nic'otinehy'droxam'ic acid methi'odide.** An effective cholinesterase reactivator, with actions that are most marked at the skeletal neuromuscular junction; antidotal effects are less striking at autonomic effector sites, and insignificant in the central nervous system.

**nicotin'ic.** Nicotine-like; relating to the stimulating action of acetylcholine and other nicotinic agents on autonomic ganglia, adrenal medulla, and the motor end-plate of striated muscle. See also nicotine, and muscarinic.

   **n. acid** (BP), niacin; 3-carboxypyridine; pyridine-3-carboxylic acid; anti-black tongue factor; anti-pellagra factor; P-P (pellagra-preventing) factor; part of the vitamin B complex. It is used in the prevention and treatment of pellagra, as a vasodilator, and as a cholesterol-lowering agent.

**n. acid amide,** nicotinamide.

**n. alcohol,** nicotinyl alcohol.

**nicotin'omimet'ic.** Mimicking the action of nicotine.

**nicotinuric acid** (nik'o-tī-nu'rik). Nicotinic acid combined with glycine in amide linkage.

**nic'otin'yl alcohol** (USAN). RONIACOL; RONICOL; nicotinic alcohol; 3-pyridinemethanol; same action and use as nicotinyl tartrate.

**nic'otin'yl tartrate.** RONIACOL tartrate; 3-pyridinemethanol tartrate; a relatively weak peripheral vasodilator related to nicotinic acid; used in peripheral vascular disorders such as Raynaud's disease, acrocyanosis, and chilblains.

**nicoumalone** (nī-koo-mă-lōn) (BP). Acenocoumarin.

**nictation** (nik-ta'shun). Nictitation.

**nictitate** (nik'tī-tāt) [ see nictitation ]. To wink.

**nictitation** (nik-tī-ta'shun) [ L. *nicto,* pp. *-atus,* to wink, fr. *nico,* to beckon ]. Winking.

**ni'dal.** Relating to a nidus, or nest; focal.

**nidation** (ni-da'shun) [ L. *nidus,* nest ]. The embedding of the early embryo in the uterine mucosa.

**ni'dus,** pl. **ni'di** [ L. nest ]. 1. A nest. 2. The nucleus or central point of origin of a nerve. 3. A focus or point of lodgment and development of a pathogenic organism.

**n. a'vis** [ L. bird's nest ], a deep depression on each side of the inferior surface of the cerebellum, between the uvula and the biventral lobe, in which the tonsil rests.

**n. hirun'dinis** [ L. swallow's nest ], n. avis.

**Niemann** (ne'mahn), Albert, German physician, 1880–1921. See N.-Pick *cell, disease.*

**Niewenglowski** (nya-ven-glov'ske), Gaston H., Paris scientist, 19th century. See N. *rays.*

**nifen'azone.** NICOPYRON; *N*-antipyrinylnicotinamide; analgesic and antipyretic.

**nifu'ratel** (USAN). POLMIROR; 5-[ (methylthio)methyl ]-3-[ (5-nitrofurfurylidene)amino ]-2-oxazolidinone; trichomonacide.

**nifu'rimide** (USAN). *dl*-4-Methyl-1-[ (5-nitrofurfurylidene)amino ]-2-imidazolidinone; an antibacterial drug.

**nifuroxime** (ni'fu-rok'sēm, -sim) (NF). MICOFUR; *anti*-5-nitro-2-furaldoxime; a furan derivative, principally effective against *Candida albicans.*

**nifurprazine.** FURENAZIN; 3-amino-6-[ 2-(5-nitro-2-furyl)-vinyl ]pyridazine; topical antibacterial agent.

**ni'ger** [ L. ] [ NA ]. Black.

**nigerose** (ni'jē-rōs). A disaccharide obtained among the hydrolysis of amylopectins, consisting of two glucose residues bound in a 1–3 linkage; 3-*O*-α-D-glucopyranosyl-D-glucose.

**night'guard.** A device used to stabilize the teeth and reduce the traumatic effects of bruxism.

**Nightingale,** Florence, English nurse, 1820–1910. During the Crimean War (1854) with a staff of nurses she established a hospital for the treatment of the sick and wounded. Later, she founded a training school for nurses at St. Thomas's Hospital, London; is looked upon as the founder of modern nursing.

**night'mare** [ *A.S. nyht,* night, + *mara,* a demon ]. Aneirodynia gravis; a terrifying dream in which one is unable to cry for help or to escape from a seemingly impending evil.

**night'shade.** Any of a number of plants of the genus *Solanum,* and of some other genera of the family Solanaceae.

**deadly n.,** belladonna.

**night-terrors.** Pavor nocturnus; a disorder allied to nightmare, occurring in children. The child awakes screaming with fright, the alarm persisting for a time during a state of semiconsciousness.

**ni'gra** [ L. fr. *niger,* black ]. In neuroanatomy, the *substantia* nigra.

**ni'gricans** [ L. fr. *niger,* black ]. Blackish.

**nigrities** (ni-grish'ī-ēz) [ L. blackness, fr. *niger,* black ]. Black pigmentation.

**n. lin'guae,** black *tongue.*

**nigrosin, nigrosine** (ni'gro-sin, -sēn). A variable mixture of blue-black aniline dyes; used as a histologic stain for nervous tissue and as a background stain for studying unstained bacteria.

**Nigros'pora.** A genus of rapidly growing fungi that produces shiny, black conidia in cultures; considered to be a common contaminant.

**nigrostriatal** (ni'gro-stri-a'tal). Referring to the efferent connection of the substantia nigra (*q.v.*) with the striatum.

**NIH.** Abbreviation for National Institutes of Health, of the U. S. Public Health Service.

**nihilism** (ni'ī-lizm, ni'hī-lizm) [ L. *nihil,* nothing ]. 1. In psychiatry, the delusion of the nonexistence of everything especially of the self or part of the self. 2. Engagement in acts which are totally destructive to one's own purposes and those of one's group.

**therapeutic n.,** a disbelief in the efficacy or value of therapy (*e.g.,* of drugs, psychotherapy, etc.).

**niketh'amide** (BP). CORAMINE; *N,N-* diethylpyridine-3-carboxamide; *N,N*-diethylnicotinamide; it acts mainly on the central nervous system, as a respiratory and cardiovascular stimulant.

**Nikiforoff** (ne-ke-for'awf), Mikhail, Russian dermatologist, *1858. See N.'s *method.*

**Nikol'sky,** Pyotr V., Russian dermatologist, *1855. See N.'s *sign.*

**Nile blue A.** A basic oxazin dye, $C_{20}H_{20}N_3OCl$, used as a fat and vital stain; as an indicator, it changes from blue to purplish red at pH 10 to 11.

**nim'azone** (USAN). 3-(*p*-Chlorophenyl)-4-imino-2-oxo-1-imidazolidineacetonitrile; an anti-inflammatory drug.

**ninhydrin.** 1,2,3-Indantrione hydrate; triketohydrindene hydrate; reacts with free amino acids to yield $CO_2$, $NH_3$, and an aldehyde, the $NH_3$ produced yielding a colored product (diketohydrindylidene-diketohydrinamine, a bi-indane derivative). The reaction is widely used for the colorimetric quantitation of amino acids.

**niobium** (ni-o'bī-um) [ G. *Niobē,* daughter of Tantalus, after whom the element tantalum was named ]. A rare metallic element, symbol Nb, atomic no. 41, atomic weight 92.91, usually found with tantalum; it was formerly called columbium (Cb).

**niphablepsia** (nif-ă-blep'sĭ-ah) [ G. *nipha,* snow, + *ablepsia,* blindness ]. Snow *blindness.*

**niphotyphlosis** (nif-o-ti-flo'sis) [ G. *nipha,* snow, + *typhlōsis,* blindness. TYPH- ]. Severe snow blindness.

**nipple** (nip'l) [ dim. of A.S. *neb,* beak, nose (?) ]. *Papilla* mammae.

**Nirenberg** (nir'en-berg), Marshall W., U. S. biochemist, *1922. Nobel laureate, with Har Gobind Khorana and Robert W. Holley, for their interpretation of the genetic code and its function in protein synthesis.

**niridazole** (ni-rid'ă-zōl) (USAN). AMBILHAR; 1-(5-nitro-2-thiozolyl)-2-imidazolidinone; used for the treatment of schistosomiasis, amebiasis, and dracontiasis.

**Nisbet,** William, English physician, 1759–1822. See N.'s *chancre.*

**ni'sin.** An antibiotic agent isolated from cultures of *Streptococcus lactis* which is active against streptococcal infections in mice and against the tubercle bacillus, staphylococci, pneumococci, and several other bacteria *in vitro.*

**Nissen,** Rudolf, Swiss surgeon, *1896. See N.'s *operation.*

**Nissl** (nis'l), Franz, Heidelberg neurologist, 1860–1919. See N. *bodies, degeneration, granules, stain, substance.*

**nit** [ A.S. *knitu* ]. 1. The ovum of a louse; it is found attached to the hair or clothing of the patient by a layer of chitin. 2. A unit of luminance; a luminous intensity of 1 candela per sq. meter of orthogonally projected surface.

**Nitabuch,** Raissa, German physician, 19th century. See N.'s *layer, membrane, stria.*

**ni'ter** [ G. *nitron,* soda, formerly not distinguished from potash. NITR- ]. Potassium nitrate.

**cubic n.,** sodium nitrate.

**ni'ton.** Radon.

**ni'trate.** A salt of nitric acid.

**nitra′zepam** (BP, USAN). MOGADAN; MOGADON; 1,3-di-hydro-7-nitro-5-phenyl-2$H$-1,4-benzodiazepin-2-one; hypnotic and sedative.

**nitric acid** (ni′trik) (NF). $HNO_3$; used as a local caustic.
  **fuming n. acid,** contains about 91 per cent nitric acid; used as a caustic. The fumes are dangerous.

**nitric oxide reductase.** See nitrogenase.

**ni′trida′tion.** Formation of nitrides; formation of nitrogen compounds through the action of ammonia (analogous to oxidation).

**ni′tride.** A compound of nitrogen and one other element; e.g., magnesium nitride, $Mg_3N_2$.

**ni′trifica′tion.** 1. The bacterial conversion of nitrogenous matter into nitrates. 2. The treatment of a material with nitric acid.

**ni′trile.** An alkyl cyanide; named for the acid formed in hydrolysis; thus $CH_3$—CN is methyl cyanide but acetonitrile.

**ni′trilo-.** Prefix indicating the presence of a cyanide group, —C≡N.

**ni′trilomalon′ic acid.** Cyanoacetic acid.

**ni′trimuriat′ic acid.** Nitrohydrochloric acid.

**ni′trite.** A salt of nitrous acid.

**nitritocobalamin** (ni′trī-to-ko-bal′ă-min). Vitamin $B_{12c}$; resembles cyanocobalamin (vitamin $B_{12}$) except that the cyanide group is replaced by a nitrite ($NO_2$) group. See also vitamin $B_{12}$.

**nitritu′ria.** The presence of nitrites in urine, as a result of the action of *Escherichia coli, Proteus vulgaris,* and other microorganisms that may reduce nitrates.

**ni′tro-.** Prefix denoting the group —$NO_2$.

**nitroben′zene, nitroben′zol.** $C_6H_5NO_2$; used in the manufacture of aniline dyes.

**nitrocel′lulose.** Pyroxylin.

**nitrochlor′oform.** Chloropicrin.

**nitrofu′rans.** Antimicrobials (e.g., nitrofurazone) effective against Gram-positive and Gram-negative organisms.

**nitrofurantoin** (ni′tro-fu-ran′to-in) (USP, BP). FURADANTIN; $N$-(5-nitro-2-furfurylidene)-1-aminohydantoin. A urinary antibacterial agent with a wide range of activity against both Gram-positive and Gram-negative organisms. The USP lists n. sodium, for injection.

**nitrofu′razone** (NF). Furacin; 5-nitro-2-furaldehyde semicarbazone; a topical bacteriostatic and bactericidal agent.

**nitrogen** (ni′tro-jen) [ L. *nitrum,* niter, + suffix -*gen,* to produce ]. 1. A gaseous element, symbol N, atomic no. 7, atomic weight 14.007; it forms about 77 parts by weight of the atmosphere. Also called azote, which is the root of azo. 2 (USP). $N_2$; contains not less than 99.0 per cent, by volume, of $N_2$; used as a diluent for medicinal gases, and for air replacement in pharmaceutical preparations.
  **n. balance,** the difference between total n. ingested and the total n. excreted by an organism; in an adult, presumably not growing, this should be zero at a given intake or above; during growth, as in children, the balance is positive, that is, more is taken in than is excreted; in starvation, malnutrition, certain febril diseases, and injuries, the balance may become negative (sometimes referred to as imbal∗nce).
  **blood urea n.,** abbreviated BUN; urea is the most prevalent of nonprotein nitrogenous compounds in blood; whole blood normally contains 10 to 15 mg. of urea per 100 ml. See also urea n.
  **n. cycle,** see under cycle.
  **n. equivalent,** the nitrogen content of protein, used in calculating the protein breakdown in the body from the niotrogen excreted in the urine, 1 gm. of nitrogen being equal to 6.25 gm. of protein catabolized.
  **filtrate n.,** nonprotein n.; *i.e.,* the n. in various compounds that normally pass through the glomerular filtration, or through a filter in the laboratory (after proteins are precipitated).
  **n. group,** five trivalent or quinquivalent elements: nitrogen, phosphorus, arsenic, antimony, and bismuth; their hydrogen compounds are basic; their oxyacids vary from monobasic to tetrabasic.
  **heavy n.,** nitrogen-15.

  **n. lag,** the length of time after the ingestion of a given protein before an amount of n. equal to that in this protein has been excreted in the urine.
  **n. monoxide,** nitrous oxide.
  **n. mustards,** see under mustard.
  **nonprotein n.,** the n. content of other than protein bodies— of urea for example; about one half the nonprotein n. in the blood is contained in the urea molecule. Abbreviated NPN.
  **n. partition,** n. distribution; the determination of the distribution of n. in the urine among the various constituents.
  **n. pentoxide,** $N_2O_5$; nitric acid anhydride. It forms nitric acid when dissolved in water.
  **rest n.,** nonprotein n.
  **undetermined n.,** the n. of blood, urine, etc., other than urea, uric acid, amino acids, etc., that can be directly estimated; in blood it amounts to about 25 mg. per 100 ml.
  **urea n.,** the portion of n. in a biological sample, such as blood or urine, that derives from its content of urea. See also blood urea n.
  **urinary n.,** the n. excreted as urea, amino acids, uric acid, etc., in the urine; each gram of urinary n. indicates the breakdown in the body of 6.25 gm. of protein. See also n. equivalent.

**nitrogen-13** ($^{13}$N). A cyclotron-produced, positron-emitting radioisotope of nitrogen with a physical half-life of 10 minutes; used in protein metabolism studies.

**nitrogen-14** ($^{14}$N). The common nitrogen isotope, making up 99.635 per cent of natural nitrogen.

**nitrogen-15** ($^{15}$N). Heavy nitrogen; the less common stable nitrogen isotope, making up 0.365 per cent of natural nitrogen.

**nitrogenase** (ni′tro-jĕ-nās). General term used to describe enzyme systems that catalyze the reduction of molecular nitrogen to ammonia in nitrogen-fixing bacteria. Specifically applied to nitric oxide reductase (EC 1.7.99.2), which catalyzes the reaction between $N_2$ and NO, a first step in the process.

**nitrogenous** (ni-troj′ĕ-nus). Relating to or containing nitrogen.

**nitroglycerin** (ni′tro-glis′er-in). Glonoin; glyceryl trinitrate; trinitroglycerin; $C_3H_5(NO_3)_3$; a yellowish oily fluid formed by the action of sulfuric and nitric acids on glycerin. It is explosive. Used as a vasodilator, especially in angina pectoris. Official (USP) as tablets.

**nitrohy′drochlo′ric acid.** Aqua regia (so called because it can dissolve the noble metals); nitrimuriatic acid; contains nitric acid 18, hydrochloric acid 82 volumes. A fuming, corrosive, yellowish liquid, used as a local caustic. Caution!

**nitroman′nitol.** Mannitol hexanitrate.

**nitromer′sol** (NF). METAPHEN; the anhydride of 4-nitro-3-hydroxymercuriorthocresol; a synthetic organic mercurial compound, used as an antiseptic for skin and mucous membranes.

**nitrom′eter** [ nitrogen + G. *metron,* measure ]. A device for collecting and measuring the nitrogen set free in a chemical reaction.

**ni′tron.** 1,4-Diphenyl-3,5-*end*-anilodihydrotriazole; used as a reagent for the determination of nitric acid, for it is one of the few substances to form an insoluble nitrate.

**$N$-$o$-nitrophenylsulfenyl.** Nps; a radical easily attached to $NH_2$ groups, used in peptide synthesis and protein chemistry.

**nitroprus′side.** Sodium nitroprusside; $Na_2Fe(CN)_5NO$.

**nitroso-.** Nitrosyl; prefix denoting a compound containing the univalent atom group, —N=O.

**$p$-nitrosulf′athi′azole.** Nisulfazole; $p$-nitro-$N$-2-thiazolylbenzenesulfonamide; a sulfonamide, administered rectally and used only in the treatment of ulcerative colitis.

**ni′trosyl.** A univalent radical or atom group, —N=O, forming the nitroso compounds; prefix, nitroso.

**ni′trous.** Denoting a nitrogen compound containing one less atom than the nitric compounds; one in which the nitrogen is present in its trivalent state.
  **n. acid,** $HNO_2$.
  **n. ether,** ethyl nitrite; spirit of ethyl nitrite; $C_2H_5NO_2$; sedative, diuretic, and diaphoretic.

**n. oxide** (USP, BP), dinitrogen monoxide; nitrogen monoxide; laughing gas; $N_2O$; a nonflammable, nonexplosive gas that will support combustion. It is widely used as a rapidly acting, rapidly reversible, nondepressant, and nontoxic inhalation analgesic to supplement other anesthetics and analgesics; its anesthetic potency alone is inadequate to provide surgical anesthesia.

**nitroxanthic acid** (ni'tro-zan'thik). Picric acid.

**nitrox'oline.** ENTEROCOL; 5-nitro-8-quinolinol; antibacterial agent.

**nitrox'yl.** HNO.

**ni'tryl.** The radical $—NO_2$ of the nitro compounds.

**njovera** [ Native ]. A disease of children in Southern Rhodesia; a nonvenereal disease indistinguishable from syphilis and due to an organism, so far as is known, identical with *Treponema pallidum.* The disease is probably the same as bejel.

**N.K.** Initials of *Nomenklatur Kommission,* Committee on Nomenclature of the German Anatomical Society, appointed to revise or supplement the BNA (1895).

**nm.** Abbreviation for nanometer.

**NMN.** Abbreviation for nicotinamide mononucleotide.

**NMR.** Abbreviation for nuclear magnetic *resonance.*

**No.** Chemical symbol of the element nobelium.

**no.** Abbreviation for number (*q.v.*).

**nobelium** (no-bel'ĭ-um) [ *Nobel* Institute ]. Element with atomic no. 102, symbol No, prepared in 1957 by bombardment of curium (element no. 96) with carbon nuclei at the Nobel Institute for Physics in Stockholm. Hence the name.

**Noble's position.** See under position.

**Noble-Collip procedure.** See under procedure.

**Nocard** (nō-kar'), Edmund I. E., French veterinarian, 1850–1903. Gave his name to *Nocardia.* See Preisz-N. *bacillus.*

**nocar'damin.** $C_{27}H_{48}N_6O_9$; a crystalline antibiotic obtained from *Nocardia;* active against the tubercle bacillus.

**Nocardia** (no-kar'dĭ-ah) [ E. *Nocard* ]. A genus of aerobic, nonmotile bacteria (family Actinomycetaceae) containing occasionally weakly acid-fast slender rods or filaments, frequently swollen and occasionally branched, forming a mycelium. Conidia are not produced by these organisms. They are mainly saprophytic, but they may produce disease in man and other animals. The type species is *N. farcinica.*

**N. africana,** a species found in a case of mycetoma of a foot in South Africa.

**N. asteroides,** a species found in conditions resembling pulmonary tuberculosis; also found in a cerebral abscess in man.

**N. blackwellii,** a species found in the hock joint of a foal.

**N. caprae,** a species found in lesions of goats.

**N. ca'viae,** *N. otitidis-caviarum.*

**N. cuniculi,** a species found in rabbits.

**N. farcinica,** a species associated with a disease in cattle resembling chronic tuberculosis; transmissible to guinea pigs, cattle, and sheep but not to rabbits, dogs, horses, or monkeys. It is the type species of the genus *N.*

**N. fordii,** a species found in a human spleen in a case of acholuric jaundice.

**N. gibsonii,** *Streptomyces gibsonii.*

**N. leishmanii,** a species found in a fatal case of lung disease and pericarditis in man.

**N. lutea,** a species found in a case of actinomycosis of the lacrimal gland.

**N. madu'rae,** a species which causes some cases of Madura foot.

**N. minutis'sima,** *Microsporum minutissimum.*

**N. otitidis-caviarum,** *N. caviae;* a species found in infected middle ears of guinea pigs in Sumatra.

**N. pelletieri,** a species found in a case of crimson-grained mycetoma in Nigeria.

**N. polychromogenes,** a species found in the blood of a horse, and in soil.

**N. pretoriana,** a species found in a case of mycetoma of the chest wall of a South African native.

**N. pulmonalis,** a species found in bovine infections.

**N. rangoonensis,** a species found in a case of human pulmonary streptotrichosis.

**N. transvalensis,** a species found in a case of mycetoma of the foot in South Africa.

**nocardiosis** (no-kar'dĭ-o'sis). Any of the several pathological entities which may follow infection with microorganisms of the genus *Nocardia.*

**granulo'matous n.,** a form characterized by emaciation, abdominal distention, and the replacement of lymphoid tissue in lymph nodes and spleen by granulomatous tissue.

**Nocht,** Bernhard A. E., German hygienist, 1857–1927. See N.'s *stain.*

**noci-** (no'sĭ-) [ L. *noceo,* to injure, hurt ]. Combining form relating to hurt, pain, or injury.

**nociassociation** (no-sĭ-as-so-sĭ-a'shun) [ noci- + association ]. The discharge of nervous energy, in the form of shock or exhaustion, following overstimulation of the nociceptors by trauma, surgical operation, or chronic disease.

**nociceptive** (no-sĭ-sep'tiv) [ see nociceptor ]. Capable of appreciation or transmission of pain.

**nociceptor** (no'sĭ-sep'tor) [ noci- + L. *capio,* to take ]. A peripheral nerve organ or mechanism for the appreciation and transmission of painful or injurious stimuli.

**nocifensor** (no'sĭ-fen'sor) [ noci- + L. *fendo* (only in compounds), to strike, ward off ]. Denoting processes or mechanisms that act to protect the body from injury. Specifically, a system of nerves in the skin and mucous membranes that react to adjacent injury by vasodilation.

**no'ci-in'fluence.** Injurious or harmful influence.

**nociperception** (no'sĭ-per-sep'shun) [ noci- + perception ]. The appreciation of injurious influences, referring to nerve centers.

**noct-** (nokt-) [ L. *nox,* night ]. Combining form meaning night, nocturnal; see also nycto-.

**noctalbuminuria** (nok'tal-bu'mĭ-nu'rĭ-ah). Nyctalbuminuria.

**noctambulation** (nok-tam'bu-la'shun). Somnambulism.

**noctam'bulism.** Somnambulism.

**nocturia** (nok-tu'rĭ-a) [ noct- + G. *ouron,* urine ]. Urinating at night, often because of increased nocturnal secretion of urine.

**noctur'nal** [ L. *nocturnus,* of the night ]. Pertaining to the hours of darkness; the opposite of diurnal (1).

**no'dal.** Relating to any node.

**node** [ L. *nodus,* a knot ]. 1. A knob; nodosity; a circumscribed swelling. 2. A circumscribed mass of differentiated tissue; see nodus. 3. A knuckle, or finger joint.

**anterior mediastinal lymph n.'s,** *nodi* lymphatici mediastinales anteriores.

**anterior tibial lymph n.,** *nodus* lymphaticus tibialis anterior.

**apical lymph n.'s,** *nodi* lymphatici apicales.

**Aschoff and Tawara's n.,** *nodus* atrioventricularis.

**a'trioventric'ular n.,** *nodus* atrioventricularis.

**A-V n.,** *nodus* atrioventricularis.

**axillary lymph n.'s,** *nodi* lymphatici axillares.

**Babès' n.'s,** collections of lymphocytes in the central nervous system found in rabies.

**bronchopulmonary lymph n.,** *nodus* lymphaticus bronchopulmonalis.

**buccal lymph n.'s,** *nodi* lymphatici buccales.

**celiac lymph n.'s,** *nodi* lymphatici celiaci.

**central lymph n.'s,** *nodi* lymphatici centrales.

**n. of Cloquet,** Rosenmuller's node or gland; one of the deep inguinal lymph n.'s located in or adjacent to the femoral canal; sometimes mistaken for a femoral hernia when enlarged.

**common iliac lymph n.'s,** *nodi* lymphatici iliaci communes.

**coronary n.,** the uppermost part of the A-V n.

**cubital lymph n.'s,** *nodi* lymphatici cubitales.

**deep cervical lymph n.'s,** *nodi* lymphatici cervicales profundae.

**deep inguinal lymph n.'s,** *nodi* lymphatici inguinales profundi.

**diaphragmatic n.'s,** *nodi* lymphatici phrenici.

**Dürck's n.'s,** a small cell infiltration of the perivascular lymphatic tissue, throughout the brain, cord, and meninges, occurring in human trypanosomiasis.

**epigastric lymph n.'s,** *nodi* lymphatici epigastrici.

external iliac lymph n.'s, *nodi* lymphatici iliaci externi.

**Féréol's n.'s,** ephemeral cutaneous nodules in acute articular rheumatism.

**epitroch'lear n.'s,** nodi lymphatici cubitales; see under nodus.

**Flack's n.,** *nodus* sinuatrialis.

**gastroduodenal lymph n.'s,** *nodi* lymphatici pylorici.

**Haygarth's n.'s,** Haygarth's nodosities; exostoses from the margins of the articular surfaces and from the periosteum and bone in the neighborhood of the joints of the fingers, leading to ankylosis and associated with lateral deflection of the fingers toward the ulnar side; they occur in arthritis deformans.

**Heberden's n.'s,** Heberden's nodosities; Rosenbach's disease (1); hard nodules (exostoses) about the size of a pea or smaller, found on the terminal phalanges of the fingers in osteoarthritis; they are enlargements of the tubercles at the articular extremities of the distal phalanges.

**hemal n.,** hemolymph n.; hemal, hemolymph, or vascular gland; a lymphoid structure in which the blood sinuses are present in place of lymph sinuses; hemal n.'s occur in ruminants and some other mammals, but their presence in man is questioned.

**hemolymph n.,** hemal n.

**Hensen's n.,** primitive n.

**hepatic lymph n.'s,** *nodi* lymphatici hepatici.

**ileocolic lymph n.'s,** *nodi* lymphatici ileocolici.

**inferior mesenteric lymph n.'s,** *nodi* lymphatici mesenterici inferiores.

**intercostal lymph n.'s,** *nodi* lymphatici intercostalis.

**internal iliac lymph n.'s,** *nodi* lymphatici iliaci interni.

**jugulodigas'tric n.,** *nodus* lymphaticus jugulodigastricus.

**jugulo-omohyoid lymph n.,** *nodus* lymphaticus jugulo-omohyoideus.

**Keith's n.,** *nodus* sinuatrialis.

**Keith and Flack n.,** *nodus* sinuatrialis.

**Koch's n.,** *nodus* sinuatrialis.

**lateral lymph n.'s,** *nodi* lymphatici laterales.

**left colic lymph n.'s,** *nodi* lymphatici colici sinistri.

**left gastric lymph n.'s,** *nodi* lymphatici gastrici sinistri.

**left gastroepiploic lymph n.'s,** *nodi* lymphatici gastroepiploici sinistri.

**lingual lymph n.'s,** *nodi* lymphatici linguales.

**lumbar lymph n.'s,** *nodi* lymphatici lumbales.

**lymph n.,** *nodus* lymphaticus.

**lymph n.'s of elbow,** *nodi* lymphatici cubitales.

**mandibular lymph n.'s,** *nodi* lymphatici mandibulares.

**middle colic lymph n.'s,** *nodi* lymphatici colici medii.

**milkers' n.'s,** paravaccinia.

**occipital lymph n.'s,** *nodi* lymphatici occipitales.

**Osler n.,** a tender cutaneous lesion characteristic of subacute bacterial endocarditis; small, raised, and discolored, these n.'s usually appear in the pads of fingers or toes.

**pancreaticosplenic lymph n.'s,** *nodi* lymphatici pancreaticolienales.

**parasternal lymph n.'s,** *nodi* lymphatici parasternales.

**paratracheal n.,** lymph n. found on each side of the trachea.

**parotid lymph n.'s,** *nodi* lymphatici parotidei.

**pectoral lymph n.'s,** *nodi* lymphatici pectorales.

**phrenic lymph n.'s,** *nodi* lymphatici phrenici.

**popliteal lymph n.'s,** *nodi* lymphatici poplitei.

**posterior mediastinal lymph n.'s,** *nodi* lymphatici mediastinales posteriores.

**pretracheal n.,** lymph n. located anteriorly to the trachea.

**primitive n.,** primitive knot; Hensen's n. or knot; Hubrecht's protochordal knot; a local thickening of the blastoderm at the cephalic end of the primitive streak of the embryo.

**pulmonary lymph n.'s,** *nodi* lymphatici pulmonales.

**pyloric lymph n.'s,** *nodi* lymphatici pylorici.

**Ranvier's n.,** a short interval in the myelin sheath of a nerve fiber, occurring between each two successive segments of the myelin sheath; at the n., the axon is invested only by short, finger-like cytoplasmic processes of the two neighboring Schwann cells or, in the central nervous system, oligodendroglia cells. See also myelin *sheath.*

**retroauricular lymph n.'s,** *nodi* lymphatici retroauriculares.

**retropharyngeal lymph n.'s,** *nodi* lymphatici retropharyngei.

**right colic lymph n.'s,** *nodi* lymphatici colici dextri.

**right gastric lymph n.'s,** *nodi* lymphatici gastrici dextri.

**right gastroepiploic lymph n.'s,** *nodi* lymphatici gastroepiploici dextri.

**Rosenmüller's n.,** n. of Cloquet.

**n. of Rouviere,** lateral retropharyngeal n. of the nodi lymphatici retropharyngei.

**S-A n.,** *nodus* sinuatrialis.

**sacral lymph n.'s,** *nodi* lymphatici sacrales.

**signal n.,** Virchow's n.; jugular gland; a firm supraclavicular lymph n., especially on the left side, sufficiently enlarged that it is palpable from the cutaneous surface; such a lymph n. is so termed because it may be the first recognized, *presumptive* evidence of a malignant neoplasm in one of the viscera. A signal n. that is *known* to contain a metastasis from a malignant neoplasm is sometimes designated by an old eponym, Troisier's ganglion or Troisier's n.

**singer's n.'s,** singer's nodules; vocal nodules; trachoma of the vocal bands; teacher's nodes; chorditis nodosa or tuberosa; small, circumscribed, beadlike enlargements on the vocal cords, caused by overuse or abuse of the voice in singing, especially high notes.

**sinoa'trial n.,** *nodus* sinuatrialis.

**sinus n.,** *nodus* sinuatrialis.

**subdigastric n.,** *nodus* lymphaticus jugulodigastricus.

**submandibular lymph n.'s,** *nodi* lymphatici submandibulares.

**submental lymph n.'s,** *nodi* lymphatici submentales.

**subscapular lymph n.'s,** *nodi* lymphatici subscapulares.

**superficial cervical lymph n.'s,** *nodi* lymphatici cervicales superficiales.

**superior gastric lymph n.'s,** *nodi* lymphatici gastrici sinistri.

**superficial inguinal lymph n.'s,** *nodi* lymphatici inguinales superficiales.

**superior mesenteric lymph nodes,** *nodi* lymphatici mesenterici superiores.

**supraclavicular n.,** a lymph n. situated at a level just above the clavicle.

**Tawara's n.,** *nodus* atrioventricularis.

**teachers' n.'s,** singer's n.'s.

**tracheal lymph n.'s,** *nodi* lymphatici tracheales.

**tracheobronchial lymph n.'s,** *nodi* lymphatici tracheobronchiales.

**Troisier's n.,** see signal n.

**Virchow's n.,** signal n.

**vital n.,** *noeud* vital.

**no'di** [ L. ]. Plural of nodus.

**no'dose** [ L. *nodosus* ]. Having nodes or knotlike swellings.

**nodos'itas** [ L. fr. *nodos,* a knot ]. Nodosity.

**n. crin'ium** [ L. gen. pl. of *crinis,* hair ], trichorrhexis nodosa.

**nodos'ity** [ L. *nodositas* ]. 1. A node; a knoblike or knotty swelling. 2. The condition of being nodose.

**Haygarth's n.'s,** Haygarth's *nodes.*

**Heberden's n.'s,** Heberden's *nodes.*

**Meynet's n.'s.** small, movable, subcutaneous connective tissue nodules, formed at times in the neighborhood of the affected joints in acute articular rheumatism.

**no'dous, nod'ular, nod'ulate, nod'ula'ted.** Nodose.

**nod'ula'tion.** The formation or the presence of nodules.

**nodule** (nod'ūl) [ L. *nodulus,* dim. of *nodus,* knot ]. A small node; see also nodulus.

**aggregated n.'s,** *folliculi* lymphatici aggregati.

**Albini's n.'s,** minute fibrous n.'s on the margins of the mitral and tricuspid valves of the heart, sometimes present in the newborn. They were described previously by Cruveilhier.

**apple jelly n.'s,** descriptive term for the papular lesions of lupus vulgaris, as they appear on diascopy.

**Arantius' n.,** *nodulus* valvulae semilunaris.

**Aschoff n.'s,** Aschoff *bodies.*

**Bianchi's n.,** *nodulus* valvulae semilunaris.

**Bohn's n.'s,** Epstein's *pearls.*

**Caplan's n.'s,** see Caplan's *syndrome.*

**cold n.,** clinical jargon for a thyroid n. with a much lower uptake of radioactive iodine than the surrounding parenchyma; about one in four solitary cold n.'s prove to be malignant.

**cutaneous n.,** see dermatofibroma.

**enamel n.,** odontoma; circumscribed mass of enamel substance.

**Gamna-Gandy n.'s,** Gamna-Gandy *bodies.*

**Hoboken's n.'s,** Hoboken's gemmules; gross dilations on the outer surface of the umbilical arteries.

**hot n.,** clinical jargon for a thyroid n. with a much higher uptake of radioactive iodine than the surrounding parenchyma; hot n.'s are benign.

**Jeanselme's n.'s,** Steiner's tumors; juxta-articular n.'s; a form of tertiary yaws that is characterized by the occurrence of n.'s on the arms and legs, situated usually near the joints.

**juxta-articular n.'s,** Jeanselme's n.'s.

**lymph n.,** *folliculus* lymphaticus.

**Malpighian n.,** *folliculus* lymphaticus lienalis.

**milkers' n.'s,** paravaccinia.

**Morgagni's n.,** *nodulus* valvulae semilunaris.

**Paterson's n.'s,** molluscum *corpuscles.*

**pulp n.,** pulp *stone.*

**rheumatoid n.'s,** subcutaneous n.'s, occurring most commonly over bony prominences, in some patients with rheumatoid arthritis. Microscopically, the n.'s are foci of fibrinoid necrosis, surrounded by a palisade of fibroblasts.

**Schmorl's n.,** prolapse of the nucleus pulposus into the spongiosa of a vertebra.

**secondary n.,** the lighter-staining center of a lymphatic n.; it might be either a reaction center consisting largely of macrophages, or a germinal center of lymphocytes, many undergoing mitosis.

**siderotic n.'s,** Gamna-Gandy *bodies.*

**singer's n.'s, vocal n.'s,** singer's *nodes.*

**solitary n.'s of intestine,** *folliculi* lymphatici solitarii.

**nodulous** (nod'u-lus). Nodose.

**nodulus,** pl. **noduli** (nod'u-lus, -li) [ L. dim. of *nodus*, knot ]. 1 [ NA ]. Nodule; a small node. 2 [ NA ]. The posterior extremity of the inferior vermis of the cerebellum, forming with the velum medullare posterius the central portion of the flocculonodular lobe.

**n. carot'icus,** *glomus* caroticum.

**n. lymphat'icus,** *folliculus* lymphaticus.

**n. val'vulae semiluna'ris,** pl. **nod'uli valvula'rum semiluna'rium** [ NA ], corpus arantii; Arantius', Morgagni's, or Bianchi's nodule; a nodule at the center of the free border of each semilunar valve at the beginning of the pulmonary artery and aorta.

# NODUS

**no'dus,** pl. **no'di** [ L. a knot ] [ NA ]. Node; in anatomy, a circumscribed mass of tissue.

**n. atrioventricula'ris** [ NA ], atrioventricular node; A-V node; node of Aschoff and Tawara; a small node of specialized muscle fibers located near the ostium of the coronary sinus; it gives rise to the atrioventricular bundle of the conduction system of the heart.

**n. lymphat'icus** [ NA ], lymph node; lymphonodus; one of numerous round, oval, or bean-shaped bodies located along the course of lymphatic vessels. They vary greatly in size (1 to 25 mm. in diameter) and usually present a depressed area, the hilus, on one side through which blood vessels enter and efferent lymphatic vessels emerge. The structure consists of a fibrous capsule and internal trabeculae supporting lymphoid tissue and lymph sinuses. The lymphoid tissue is arranged in follicles in the cortex and cords in the medulla of a node. Afferent vessels enter a node at many points of its periphery.

**nodi lymphatici apicales** [ NA ], apical lymph nodes; the group of lymph nodes located at the apex of the axillary fossa which receive lymphatic drainage from the other groups of axillary nodes.

**nodi lymphat'ici axilla'res** [ NA ], axillary lymph nodes; they are numerous and consist of several groups, apical, central, lateral, pectoral, and subscapular, which receive the lymphatic drainage from the upper limb, shoulder

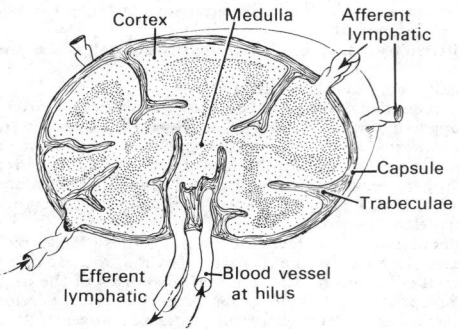

**Nodus Lymphaticus (Cross Section)**

girdle and mammary gland; they drain into the subclavian trunk.

**n. lymphat'icus bronchopulmona'lis** [ NA ], bronchopulmonary lymph node; one of the lymph nodes in the hilus of the lung that receives lymph from the pulmonary nodes.

**nodi lymphatici bucca'les** [ NA ], buccal lymph nodes; small nodes along the course of the facial artery that drain the eyelids, conjunctiva, nose and cheek, sending efferent vessels to the submandibular nodes.

**nodi lymphat'ici celi'aci** [ NA ], celiac lymph nodes; nodes located along the celiac trunk; they drain lymph from the stomach, duodenum, pancreas, spleen and biliary tract.

**nodi lymphatici centrales** [ NA ], central lymph nodes; nodes located around the midportion of the axillary artery, they receive afferent vessels from the lateral, subscapular and pectoral nodes and send efferent vessels to the apical nodes.

**nodi lymphat'ici cervica'les profun'dae** [ NA ], deep cervical lymph nodes; the chain of nodes located along the great vessels from the base of the skull to the root of the neck; they are usually subdivided into upper and lower groups by the omohyoid muscle. They receive the lymphatic drainage of the head and neck and terminate in the jugular lymphatic trunk on each side.

**nodi lymphat'ici cervica'les superficia'les** [ NA ], superficial cervical lymph nodes; nodes located along the external jugular vein as it crosses the sternocleidomastoid muscle; they drain the auricle and lower part of the parotid region and send efferent vessels to the deep cervical nodes.

**nodi lymphat'ici col'ici dex'tri** [ NA ], right colic lymph nodes; located along the right colic artery, these nodes drain the upper part of the ascending colon.

**nodi lymphat'ici col'ici me'dii** [ NA ], middle colic lymph nodes; nodes along the middle colic artery and its branches that drain the right colic flexure and most of the transverse colon.

**nodi lymphat'ici col'ici sinis'tri** [ NA ], left colic lymph nodes; small nodes along the left colic artery and its branches that drain the left flexure and upper part of the descending colon. Efferent vessels pass to the inferior mesenteric nodes.

**nodi lymphat'ici cubita'les** [ NA ], cubital lymph nodes; lymph nodes of the elbow; epitrochlear nodes; one or two small superficial nodes lying along the basilic vein above the medial epicondyle; they receive afferents from the ulnar side of the forearm and hand and send efferents to the lateral axillary nodes.

**nodi lymphat'ici epigas'trici** [ NA ], epigastric lymph nodes; three or four nodes placed along the inferior epigastric vessels; they receive afferents from the lower abdominal wall and empty into the external iliac nodes.

**nodi lymphat'ici gas'trici dex'tri** [ NA ], right gastric lymph nodes; small nodes along the course of the right gastric artery that drain part of the lesser curvature of the stomach.

**nodi lymphat'ici gas'trici sinis'tri** [ NA ], left gastric lymph nodes; superior gastric lymph nodes; nodes located along the left gastric artery and its branches; they are divided into paracardial, upper and lower groups.

**nodi lymphatici gastroepiploici dextri** [ NA ], right gastroepiploic lymph nodes; inferior gastric lymph nodes; nodes located in the greater omentum along the right gastroepiploic artery that drain part of the greater curvature of the stomach and the greater omentum.

**nodi lymphatici gastroepiploici sinistri** [ NA ], left gastroepiploic lymph nodes; nodes located in the greater omentum along the left gastroepiploic artery that drain part of the greater curvature of the stomach and greater omentum.

**nodi lymphat'ici hepat'ici** [ NA ], hepatic lymph nodes; located along the hepatic artery as far as the porta hepatis, these nodes drain the liver, gall bladder, stomach, duodenum and pancreas and send efferents to the celiac nodes.

**nodi lymphatici ileocolici** [ NA ], ileocolic lymph nodes; nodes along the ileocolic artery and its branches that drain the terminal ileum, cecum, vermiform appendix, and lower part of the ascending colon.

**nodi lymphatici iliaci communes** [ NA ], common iliac lymph nodes; nodes located in association with the common iliac artery that receive afferent vessels from the external and internal iliac lymph nodes and send efferent vessels to the lumbar nodes.

**nodi lymphatici iliaci externi** [ NA ], external iliac lymph nodes; nodes located along the external iliac artery that receive afferent vessels from the inguinal nodes, lower abdominal wall, and pelvic viscera and send efferent vessels to the common iliac nodes.

**nodi lymphat'ici ili'aci inter'ni** [ NA ], internal iliac lymph nodes; nodes that lie along the internal iliac artery and its branches; they receive lymph from the pelvic viscera, the gluteal region, and the deep parts of the perineum, and send efferent vessels to the common iliac nodes.

**nodi lymphat'ici inguina'les profun'di** [ NA ], deep inguinal lymph nodes; several small nodes deep to the fascia lata and medial to the femoral vein; they receive lymph from the deep structures of the lower limb, from the glans penis and from superficial inguinal nodes. Efferents pass to the external iliac nodes.

**nodi lymphat'ici inguina'les superficia'les** [ NA ], superficial inguinal lymph nodes; a group of twelve to twenty nodes that lie in the subcutaneous tissue below the inguinal ligament and along the terminal part of the great saphenous vein. They drain the skin of the lower abdominal wall, perineum, buttock, external genitalia and lower limb.

**nodi lymphat'ici intercosta'les** [ NA ], intercostal lymph nodes; one or two small nodes located posteriorly in each intercostal space; they receive lymph from the parietal pleura, intercostal space, and posterior body wall. The nodes in the upper spaces empty into the thoracic duct; the nodes in the lower spaces form a descending intercostal trunk that opens into the cisterna chyli.

**n. lymphat'icus ju'gulodigas'tricus** [ NA ], jugulodigastric or subdigastric lymph node; a prominent node in the upper deep cervical chain lying between the digastric muscle and the internal jugular vein; it receives lymphatic drainage from the tongue and palatine tonsil.

**n. lymphat'icus ju'gulo-omohyoid'eus** [ NA ], jugulo-omohyoid lymph node; a node of the lower deep cervical group that lies just above the intermediate tendon of the omohyoid muscle; its afferent vessels drain the tongue and submental nodes and it sends efferent vessels to the lower deep cervical nodes.

**nodi lymphatici laterales** [ NA ], lateral lymph nodes; the most laterally located group of the axillary nodes; they receive lymph drainage from the entire free superior limb and send efferent vessels to the central lymph nodes.

**nodi lymphat'ici lingua'les** [ NA ], lingual lymph nodes; two or three small nodes that lie along the hyoglossus in the course of the lymphatic vessels draining the tongue.

**nodi lymphat'ici lumba'les** [ NA ], lumbar lymph nodes; nodes located along the aorta as right and left lateral aortic, preaortic and retroaortic groups; they receive lymph from the common iliac nodes and from the territory corresponding to that supplied by the paired branches of the aorta plus the inferior mesenteric artery; they drain by paired lumbar trunks into the cisterna chyli.

**nodi lymphat'ici mandibula'res** [ NA ], mandibular lymph nodes; small nodes along the facial artery as it crosses the mandible.

**nodi lymphat'ici mediastina'les anterio'res** [ NA ], anterior mediastinal lymph nodes; located in the superior mediastinum in relation to the great vessels, these nodes receive lymph from the thymus, pericardium and sternal nodes; their efferent vessels join those of the tracheal nodes to form the bronchomediastinal trunks.

**nodi lymphat'ici mediastina'les posterio'res** [ NA ], posterior mediastinal lymph nodes; nodes located along the thoracic aorta; they receive vessels from the esophagus, diaphragm, liver and pericardium and send efferents to the thoracic duct and inferior tracheobronchial nodes.

**nodi lymphat'ici mesenter'ici inferio'res** [ NA ], inferior mesenteric lymph nodes; nodes located along the inferior mesenteric artery and its branches that drain the upper part of the rectum, the sigmoid colon and descending colon.

**nodi lymphat'ici mesenter'ici superio'res** [ NA ], superior mesenteric lymph nodes; the numerous nodes located in the mesentery along the superior mesenteric artery and its branches to the jejunum and ileum, from which they receive lymph.

**nodi lymphat'ici occipita'les** [ NA ], occipital lymph nodes; one or two small nodes along the occipital vessels close to the trapezius muscle that receive afferents from the posterior scalp and drain into the deep cervical nodes.

**nodi lymphat'ici pancreaticoliena'les** [ NA ], pancreaticosplenic lymph nodes; nodes lying along the course of the splenic artery that receive lymph from the stomach, spleen, and pancreas and send efferent vessels to the celiac nodes.

**nodi lymphat'ici par'asterna'les** [ NA ], parasternal lymph nodes; a number of small nodes that lie along the course of the internal thoracic vessels. Lymph enters these nodes from the anterior intercostal spaces, pericardium, diaphragm, liver and mammary gland. The efferent vessels pass upward to join the bronchomediastinal trunk of the same side.

**nodi lymphat'ici parotide'i** [ NA ], parotid lymph nodes; two groups of small nodes are present; superficial nodes on the surface of the parotid receive vessels from the auricle, scalp, eyelids, and cheek and drain into deep parotid and deep cervical nodes; deep nodes receive lymph from the external acoustic meatus, middle ear, auditory tube, soft palate and nasal cavity and drain into deep cervical nodes.

**nodi lymphatici pectorales** [ NA ], pectoral lymph nodes; nodes located along the inferior margin of the pectoralis major muscle; they receive afferent vessels from the mammary gland and anterior thoracic wall and send efferent vessels to the central and apical nodes in the axilla.

**nodi lymphat'ici phren'ici** [ NA ], phrenic lymph nodes; diaphragmatic nodes; three groups of small nodes, anterior, middle, and posterior, on the upper surface of the diaphragm; they receive afferents from the liver, diaphragm, intercostal spaces and send efferents to parasternal and posterior mediastinal nodes.

**nodi lymphat'ici poplite'i** [ NA ], popliteal lymph nodes; six or seven small nodes located in the popliteal fossa along the popliteal vessels and termination of the small saphenous vein. They receive lymph from the skin of the back of the leg, the deep structures of the leg, and the knee joint, and send efferents principally to the deep inguinal nodes.

**nodi lymphat'ici pulmona'les** [ NA ], pulmonary lymph nodes; small nodes that occur along the bronchi within the lung; they receive the drainage from localized areas of the lung and send efferents to bronchopulmonary nodes.

**nodi lymphat'ici pylo'rici** [ NA ], pyloric or gastroduodenal lymph nodes; nodes located on the head of the pancreas below the duodenum and along the right gastroepiploic artery; they drain the stomach and duodenum.

**nodi lymphat'ici re'troauricula'res** [ NA ], retroauricular lymph nodes; two or three nodes that lie posterior to the mastoid process; they receive afferent lymphatic vessels from the scalp and auricle and send efferent vessels to the deep cervical nodes.

**nodi lymphat'ici re'tropharyng'ei** [ NA ], retropharyngeal lymph nodes; lymphonodi retropharyngei; they lie behind the lateral border of the nasopharynx on the prevertebral fascia, receiving afferent vessels from the auditory tube, nasopharynx, atlantooccipital and atlantoaxial joints, and drain into lower nodes of the deep cervical group.

**nodi lymphat'ici sacra'les** [ NA ], sacral lymph nodes; nodes in the concavity of the sacrum that drain the rectum and posterior pelvic wall.

**nodi lymphat'ici submandibula'res** [ NA ], submandibular lymph nodes; four or five nodes that lie between the mandible and the submandibular gland; they receive vessels from the face below the eye and from the tongue and drain into the deep cervical nodes, particularly the jugulodigastric node.

**nodi lymphat'ici submenta'les** [ NA ], submental lymph nodes; lymphonodi submentales; small nodes that lie superficial to the mylohyoid muscle; they receive afferents from the lower lip, chin, and the tip of the tongue, and send efferents to the deep cervical nodes.

**nodi lymphatici subscapulares** [ NA ], subscapular lymph nodes; nodes of the axillary region located along the subscapular artery and its branches; they receive afferent vessels from the dorsal surface of the thorax and scapular region and send efferent vessels to the central and apical nodes.

**n. lymphat'icus tibia'lis ante'rior** [ NA ], anterior tibial lymph node; a small, inconstant node in front of the interosseous membrane along the upper part of the anterior tibial vessels.

**nodi lymphat'ici trachea'les** [ NA ], tracheal lymph nodes; nodes along the sides of the trachea that drain the trachea and esophagus and empty into the bronchomediastinal trunk.

**nodi lymphat'ici tracheobronchia'les** [ NA ], tracheobronchial lymph node; ten or twelve lymph nodes situated near the bifurcation of the trachea; they are arranged in superior and inferior groups (nodi lymphatici tracheobronchiales superiores and inferiores).

**n. sinuatria'lis** [ NA ], sinoatrial node; atrionector; S-A node; Koch's node; Keith's node; Keith and Flack's node; sinus node; the mass of specialized cardiac muscle fibers that normally acts as the "pacemaker" of the cardiac conduction system. It lies under the epicardium at the upper end of the sulcus terminalis.

---

**noematic** (no-e-mat'ik) [ G. *noēma* (*noēmat-*), perception, a thought ]. Noetic; relating to the mental processes.

**noesis** (no-e'sis) [ G. *noēsis*, thought, intelligence ]. Cognition, especially through direct and self-evident knowledge.

**noetic** (no-et'ik). Noematic.

**noeud vital** (nü ve-tal') [ Fr. ]. Vital node or knot; a circumscript region in the lower part of the medulla oblongata, near the apex of the calamus scriptorius, interpreted by Flourens (1858) as a nerve center controlling respiration.

**Nogu'chi,** Hideyo, Japanese bacteriologist in New York, 1876–1928. Gave his name to *Noguchia.*

**Nogu'chia** [ H. *Noguchi* ]. A genus of aerobic to facultatively anaerobic, motile, peritrichous bacteria (family Brucellaceae) containing small, slender, Gram-negative encapsulated rods. These organisms are present in the conjunctiva of man and other animals affected by a follicular type of disease. The type species is *N. granulosis.*

**N. cunic'uli,** a species which causes conjunctival folliculosis in rabbits.

**N. granulo'sis,** a species regarded by some as a cause of trachoma in man; it produces a granular conjunctivitis in monkeys and apes. It is the type species of the genus *N.*

**N. sim'iae,** a species which causes conjunctival folliculosis in monkeys (*Macacus rhesus*).

**noise** (noyz). Unwanted additions to a signal not arising at its source; *e.g.,* the 60-cycle frequency wave in an electrocardiogram.

**no'li me tan'gere** [ L. "touch me not," fr. *John 20: 17*]. Obsolete term for rodent *ulcer.*

**no'ma** [ G. *nomē*, a spreading (sore) ]. A gangrenous stomatitis, usually beginning in the mucous membrane of the corner of the mouth or cheek, and then progressing fairly rapidly to involve the entire thickness of the lips or cheek (or both), with conspicuous necrosis and complete sloughing of tissue; usually observed in poorly nourished children and debilitated adults, especially in lower socioeconomic groups, and frequently preceded by another disease, *e.g.,* kala azar, dysentery, and scarlet fever. A similar process (n.

pudendi, n. vulvae) may also involve the labia majora. Several organisms are usually found in the necrotic material, but fusiform bacilli, *Borrelia* organisms, staphylococci, and anaerobic streptococci are most frequently observed. Also known as stomatonecrosis; stomatonoma; corrosive ulcer; cancrum oris; water canker or cancer.

**nomen** [ L. ] [ NA ]. Name.

**Nom'ina Anatom'ica.** A revision of the BNA system of anatomical terminology which was started in 1950 in Oxford, adopted by the Sixth International Congress of Anatomists meeting in Paris in July 1955, and modified by the Seventh International Congress in New York in 1960, by the Eight International Congress in Weisbaden in 1965, and by the Ninth International Congress in Leningrad in 1970. It was prepared by the International Anatomical Nomenclature Committee. The terms are indicated in this dictionary by the sign [ NA ].

**no'mogen'esis** [ G. *nomos,* law, + *genesis,* origin ]. A theory that evolution proceeds by predetermined law and cannot be modified by environment or chance events.

**nom'ogram** [ G. *nomos,* law, + *gramma,* something written ]. Nomograph; a series of scales arranged so that calculations can be performed graphically.

**blood volume n.,** predicts blood volume on the basis of the individual's weight and height.

**Cartesian n.,** a n. based on rectangular coordinates, representing two variables, on which a family of isopleths is superimposed for each of the additional variables involved.

**d'Ocagne n.,** an alignment chart consisting of an arrangement of three or more graduated lines (straight or curved), each constituting a scale of values of a variable, constructed so that any straight line crossing these scales connects the simultaneously compatible values; from values for any two variables, the values of all other variables can be determined.

**Radford n.,** predicts necessary tidal volume for artificial respiration on the basis of respiratory rate, body weight, and sex; correction factors are supplied for activity, fever, altitude, metabolic acidosis, and alterations in dead space.

**Siggaard-Andersen n.,** predicts acid-base composition of blood by slope and position of a buffer line constructed when $PCO_2$ on a logarithmic scale is plotted against pH.

**nom'ograph** ]G. *nomos,* law, + *graphō,* to write ]. Nomogram.

**nom'othet'ic** [ G. *nomos,* law, + *thesis,* a placing ]. Denoting the discovery of general laws pertaining to the behavior of groups of individuals as groups, as opposed to idiographic.

**nom'otop'ic** [ G. *nomos,* law, custom, + *topos,* place ]. Relating to, or occurring at, the usual or normal place.

**no'nan** [ L. *nonus,* ninth ]. Occurring on the ninth day; see nonan *malaria.*

**n-nonanoic acid.** Pelargonic acid.

**Nonbursata** (non-bur-sah'tah) [ L. *non,* not, + Mediev. L. *bursa,* purse ]. A nontaxonomic division of Nematoda embracing those in which the bursa copulatrix in the male is only a skin fold containing no fleshy ribs, as seen in *Trichuris.*

**nonca'riogen'ic.** Not caries-producing.

**nonchromogen** (non-kro'mo-jen). See group III *mycobacteria.*

**non compos mentis** [ L. *non,* not, + *compos,* participating, competent, + *mens,* gen. *mentis,* mind ]. Not of sound mind; mentally incapable of managing one's affairs.

**nonconduc'tor.** Anything that does not transmit electrical current, or heat, as the case may be.

**nondisjunc'tion.** Failure of the pairs of chromosomes to separate at the miotic stage of karyokinesis, with the result that both chromosomes are carried to one daughter cell and none to the other.

**non'elec'trolyte.** A substance with molecules which do not, in solution, dissociate to ions, and, therefore, do not carry an electric current.

**nonigravida** (no'nĭ-grav'ĭ-dah, non'ĭ-) [ L. *nonus,* ninth, + *gravida,* pregnant ]. A woman pregnant for the ninth time.

**non'inva'sive.** Descriptive of diagnostic procedures which do not involve the insertion of needles, cannulas, or other devices that require penetration of the skin.

**nonipara** (no-nip'ă-rah, non-ip'ă-rah) [ L. *nonus*, ninth, + *pario*, to bear ]. A woman who has borne nine children.

**nonmed'ullated.** Unmyelinated.

**nonmyelinated** (non-mi'ĕ-li-na'ted). Unmyelinated.

**Nonne** (non'eh), Max, German physician, 1861–1959. See N.-Milroy *disease*.

**non-neoplas'tic, non'neoplas'tic.** Not neoplastic.

**non-nucleated.** Having no nucleus.

**non'occlu'sion.** Failure of a tooth to contact an opponent.

**non'ose** [ L. *nonus*, ninth ]. $C_9H_{18}O_9$; any sugar with nine carbon atoms. Neuraminic acid is the aldonic acid of a nonulose.

**nonparous** (non-păr'us). Nulliparous.

**nonproprietary name** (non-pro-pri'ĕ-tĕr-ī). A short, public name of a chemical, which may be a drug, that is not subject to trademark (proprietary) rights; often mistakenly called generic name, *q.v.*

**non'rota'tion.** Lack of rotation to a normal position.

**n. of intestine,** lack of developmental turning, resulting in small intestine being on the right of the abdomen and colon on the left.

**nonsecre'tor.** An individual whose saliva does not contain antigens of the ABO blood group; see also secretor.

**non'union.** Failure of healing of a fractured bone.

**no'nus** [ L. ninth ]. The ninth cranial nerve of the old nomenclature, now called the twelfth or hypoglossal nerve.

**nonva'lent.** Having no valency because entering into union with no other element; denoting, in chemistry, an element such as argon.

**nonvi'able.** Incapable of independent existence; often denoting a prematurely born fetus; also denoting a microorganism incapable of metabolic or reproductive activity.

**Noonan's syndrome.** See under syndrome.

**noprylsulf'amide.** SOLUCIN; 1-phenyl-3-*p*-sulfamoylanilino-1,3-propanedisulfonic acid disodium salt; antibacterial agent.

**nor-.** 1. Chemical prefix denoting (a) elimination of one methylene group from a chain, the highest permissible locant being used; (b) contraction of a (steroid) ring by one $CH_2$ unit, the locant being the capital letter identifying the ring. Elimination of two methylene groups is denoted by the prefix dinor-; three groups, by trinor-, etc. 2. Chemical prefix denoting "normal" (*i.e.*, unbranched chain of carbon atoms) in aliphatic compounds, as opposed to branched, *e.g.*, leucine, norleucine.

**noradren'aline.** *l*-Noradrenaline; see *l*-norepinephrine.

**n. acid tartrate** (BP), levarterenol bitartrate.

**norbol'ethone** (USAN). GENABOL; *dl*-13-ethyl-17-hydroxy-18,19-dinor-17α-pregn-4-en-3-one; anabolic steroid.

**norbor'nane.** Norcamphane; bicyclo[ 2.2.1 ]heptane; parent of camphor and related to many essential oils (*e.g.*, camphene, the boracols, citronella).

Norbornane

**norcam'phane.** Norbornane.

**nordef'rin hydrochloride.** COBEFRIN hydrochloride; *dl*-α-(1-aminoethyl)-3,4-dihydroxybenzyl alcohol hydrochloride; a sympathomimetic and vasoconstrictor.

*l*-**norepinephrine** (nor'ep-ī-nef'rin). LEVOPHED; *l*-Noradrenaline; *l*-arterenol; levarterenol; *l*-α-(aminomethyl)-3,4-dihydroxybenzyl alcohol; a catecholamine hormone. The natural form is D, although the L form has some activity. The base is considered to be the postganglionic adrenergic mediator. It is present in the adrenal medulla and in adult animals of most species in much smaller amounts than epinephrine. It may be present in pheochromocytoma. It possesses the excitatory actions of epinephrine, but has minimal inhibitory effects. It has feeble effects on bronchial smooth muscle and metabolic processes, and differs from epinephrine in its cardiovascular action, chiefly vasoconstriction, exerting little effect upon the cardiac output. Listed in the USP as levarterenol bitartrate, *q.v.*

**nor'ethan'drolone** (NF, BP). NILEVAR; 17α-ethyl-19-nortestosterone; 17α-ethyl-17-hydroxy-19-nor-androst-4-en-3-one. A mildly androgenic steroid similar chemically and pharmacologically to testosterone. Used principally to stimulate protein anabolism.

**noreth'indrone** (USP). NORLUTIN; norethisterone (BP); 19-norethisterone; 19-nor-17α-ethinyltestosterone; 17α-ethynl-17β-hydroxy-4-estren-3-one (for structure of testerone and estrane, see steroids); a potent orally effective progestational agent with some estrogenic and androgenic activity. Therapeutically, it is used as a substitute for progesterone and, in combination with an estrogen, as an oral contraceptive.

**n. acetate** (USP), NORLUTATE; norethisterone acetate; 17-hydroxy-19-nor-17α-pregn-4-en-20-yn-3-one acetate; an orally active progestin with some estrogenic and androgenic activity; used to treat endometriosis and, with an estrogen, as an oral contraceptive.

**n. with mestranol,** ORTHO-NOVUM; a mixture of a progestational and an estrogenic agent orally effective in preventing conception when taken from the 5th through the 24th day of the cycle.

**nor'ethis'terone** (BP). Norethindrone.

**norethynodrel** (nor'ĕ-thin'o-drel) (BP, USAN). An orally active progestin with some estrogenic activity; used as a progestational agent and, in combination with mestranol, as an oral contraceptive.

**n. with mestranol,** ENOVID; an oral contraceptive preparation; also used to treat dysfunctional uterine bleeding, dysmenorrhea, and endometriosis, and to postpone menstruation for medical reasons.

**norflurane** (nor-flŭr'ăn) (USAN). 1,1,1,2-Tetrafluoroethane; an inhalation anesthetic.

**norleucine** (nor-lu'sin). α-Amino-*n*-caproic acid; 2-aminohexanoic acid. A synthetic amino acid, isomeric to leucine and isoleucine, but not found in proteins; $CH_3(CH_2)_3CHNH_2COOH$.

**norma,** pl. **nor'mae** (nor'mah) [ L. a carpenter's square ] [ NA ]. A line or pattern defining the contour of a part; extended to denote the outline of a surface, referring especially to the various aspects of the cranium. See color plates 19 and 20.

**n. anterior,** n. frontalis.

**n. basila'ris,** n. ventralis; n. inferior; basis cranii externa; the outline of the inferior aspect of the skull.

**n. facia'lis,** n. frontalis.

**n. fronta'lis,** the outline of the skull viewed from in front.

**n. inferior,** n. basilaris.

**n. latera'lis,** n. temporalis.

**n. occipita'lis,** the outline of the skull viewed from behind.

**n. posterior,** n. occipitalis.

**n. sagitta'lis,** the outline of a sagittal section through the skull.

**n. superior,** n. verticalis.

**n. tempora'lis,** the profile of the skull; the outline of the skull viewed from either side.

**n. ventra'lis,** n. basilaris.

**n. vertica'lis,** the outline of the superior surface of the skull, or of a vertical section.

**nor'mal** [ L. *normalis*, according to pattern ]. 1. Typical; usual; healthy; according to the rule or standard. 2. In bacteriology, nonimmune; untreated; denoting an animal, or the serum or substance contained therein of an animal, that has not been experimentally immunized against any microorganism or its products. 3. Symbol N; denoting a solution containing 1 equivalent of replaceable hydrogen or hydroxyl per liter; the molarity of $H^+$ or $OH^-$ in a strong acid or base; thus 1 M HCl is 1 N, but 1 M $H_2SO_4$ is 2 N. 4. In psychiatry and psychology, denoting a state of effective function which is satisfactory to both the individual and his social milieu.

**normal'ity.** The state of being normal.

**nor'maliza'tion.** The making normal or according to the standard; the reducing or strengthening of a solution to make it normal; adjusting one curve to another by multiplication of the points of the one by some arbitrary factor.

**nor'malize.** To make normal or of the proper strength or standard.

**normetanephrine** (nor-met'ah-nef'rin). 3-*O*-Methylnorepinephrine; 3-*O*-methylnoradrenaline; 3-*O*-methylarterenol; α-(aminomethyl)vanillyl alcohol; a catabolite of norepinephrine found, together with metanephrine, in the urine and some tissues; results from the action of catechol-*O*-methyltransferase on norepinephrine. It has no sympathomimetic actions.

**normeth'adone.** TICARDA; 6-dimethylamino-4,4-diphenyl-3-hexanone; antitussive with narcotic properties.

**normeth'androne.** Methylnortestosterone; 17β-hydroxy-17-methylestr-4-en-3-one; progestational agent.

**normo-** [ L. *normalis*, normal, according to pattern ]. Combining form meaning normal, usual.

**normobaric** (nor'mo-băr'ik) [ normo- + G. *baros*, weight ]. Denoting a barometric pressure equivalent to sea level pressure.

**nor'moblast** [ normo- + G. *blastos*, sprout, germ ]. A nucleated red blood cell, the immediate precursor of a normal erythrocyte in man. Its four stages of development are (1) pronormoblast, (2) basophilic n.; (3) polychromatic n.; and (4) orthochromatic n. See discussion under erythroblast.

  **acidophilic n.,** orthochromatic n.; see discussion under erythroblast.

**normocapnia** (nor'mo-kap'nĭ-ah) [ normo- + G. *kapnos*, vapor ]. A state in which the arterial carbon dioxide pressure is normal, about 40 mm. Hg; see also eucapnia.

**normocephalic** (nor'mo-sĭ-fal'ik) [ normo- + G. *kephalē*, head ]. Mesocephalic (1).

**normochromia** (nor-mo-kro'mĭ-ah) [ normo- + G. *chrōma*, color ]. Normal color; referring to blood in which the amount of hemoglobin in the red blood cells is normal.

**normochro'mic.** Being normal in color; referring especially to red blood cells that possess the normal quantity of hemoglobin.

**normocyte** (nor'mo-sīt) [ normo- + G. *kytos*, cell ]. Normoerythrocyte; a non-nucleated erythrocyte of normal size (averaging 7.5 μ); a normal, healthy red blood cell.

**normocyto'sis.** A normal state of the blood with regard to its component formed elements.

**normoerythrocyte** (nor'mo-ĕ-rith'ro-sīt). Normocyte.

**normogenesis** (nor'no-jen'ĕ-sis) [ normo- + G. *genesis*, origin ]. A developmental process that approximates that which is the average for the majority of individuals in a species.

**normoglycemic** (nor-mo-gli-se'mik). Denoting a normal blood concentration of glucose.

**normokale'mia, normokalie'mia.** A normal level of potassium in the blood.

**nor'monor'mocyto'sis.** Isonormocytosis.

**normo-orthocytosis** (nor'mo-or'tho-si-to'sis) [ normo- + G. *orthos*, correct, + *kytos*, cell, + *-ōsis* ]. A condition of the blood in which the total number of white blood cells is increased, but the relative proportion of the different varieties is normal.

**normoplasia** (nor-mo-pla'zĭ-ah) [ normo- + G. *plasis*, a forming ]. A specific differentiation characteristic of a cell within normal limits.

**normoske'ocyto'sis** [ normo- + G. *skaios*, left, + *kytos*, cell, + *-ōsis* ]. A condition of the blood in which the white blood cells are normal in number, but there is a shift to the left. See also shift.

**normosthenuria** (nor-mo-sthē-nu'rĭ-ah) [ normo- + G. *sthenos*, strength, + *ouron*, urine ]. The excretion of normal urine in normal amount.

**normoten'sive.** Normotonic (2); indicating a normal arterial blood pressure.

**normother'mia** [ normo- + G. *thermē*, heat ]. Environmental temperature that does not cause increased or depressed activity of body cells (Herrmann).

**normoton'ic.** 1. Eutonic; relating to or characterized by normal muscular tone. 2. Normotensive. 3. A person possessing normal muscular tonus.

**normoto'pia** [ normo- + G. *topos*, place ]. The state of being in the normal place.

**normotop'ic.** Relating to normotopia; in the right place.

**normovolemia** (nor-mo-vol-e'mĭ-ah) [ normo- + volume, *q.v.,* + G. *haima*, blood ]. Normal blood with regard to volume; *i.e.,* neither oligohemia nor polyhemia.

**normoxia** (nor-mok'sĭ-ah) [ normo- + oxygen ]. A state in which the partial pressure of oxygen in the inspired gas is equal to that of air at sea level, about 150 mm. Hg.

**norophthalmic acid** (nor'of-thal'mik). *N*ˢ-[ 1-(Carboxymethylcarbamoyl)ethyl ]glutamine; a tripeptide, an analogue of glutathione (cysteine replaced by alanine), found in the lens of the eye.

**norpipanone.** HEXALGON; 4,4-diphenyl-6-(1-piperidyl)-3-hexanone; analgesic agent.

**Norrie,** Gordon, Danish ophthalmologist. See N.'s *disease.*

**Norris,** Richard, English physiologist, 1831–1916. See N.'s *corpuscles.*

**norsteroids** (nor'stěr'oydz). Steroids in which an angular methyl group is missing; most commonly, it is the group between the A and B rings (C-19).

**nortriptyline hydrochloride** (nor-trip'tĭ-lēn) (NF, BP), AVENTYL hydrochloride; 10,11-dihydro-*N*-methyl-5*H*-dibenzol[ a,d ]cycloheptene-Δ⁵,γ-propylamine hydrochloride; antidepressant with mild tranquilizing properties.

**norvaline** (nor-val'ēn, -va'lēn). α-Aminovaleric acid; $CH_3(CH_2)_2CHNH_2COOH$; the straight chain analogue of valine; not found in proteins.

**noscapine** (nos'kă-pēn) (NF, BP). Opianine; *l*-α-narcotine; 2-methyl-8-methoxy-6,7-methylenedioxy-1-(6,7-dimethoxy-3-phthalidyl)-1,2,3,4-tetrahydroisoquinoline. An isoquinoline alkaloid occurring in opium to the extend of 6 per cent. Has papaverine-like action on smooth muscle. It suppresses the cough reflex and is used as an antitussive. It appears to be without addiction liability.

**nose** (nōz) [ A.S. *nosu* ]. Nasus.

  **brandy n.,** rhinophyma.

  **cleft n.,** a n. with a furrow where the bridge is normally present; due to failure of complete convergence of the paired primordia.

  **copper n.,** rhinophyma.

  **dog n.,** goundou.

  **external n.,** *nasus externus.*

  **hammer n.,** rhinophyma.

  **potato n.,** a nasal deformity resulting from an overdevelopment of the lateral cartilages.

  **rum n.,** rhinophyma.

  **saddle n.,** a n. with markedly depressed bridge, seen in congenital syphilis or after injury from trauma or operation.

  **toper's n.,** rhinophyma.

**nose'bleed.** Epistaxis.

**Nose'ma** [ G. *nosēma*, plague, fr. *noséo*, to be sick, fr. *nosos*, disease ]. A genus of the order Microsporida (phylum Protozoa), including certain species, *e.g., N. apis, N. bombycis,* and others, that are pathogenic for certain invertebrates.

**nosencephalus** (nos'en-sef'ă-lus) [ G. *nosos*, disease, + *enkephalos*, brain ]. Obsolete term for anencephalus.

**nose'piece.** A microscope attachment, consisting of several objectives surrounding a central pivot.

**nosetiology** (nōs'e-tĭ-ol'o-jĭ) [ G. *nosos*, disease, + *aitia*, cause, + *logos*, study ]. Study of the causes of disease.

**noso-** (nos'o-, no'so-) [ G. *nosos*, disease ]. Combining form relating to disease.

**nosochthonography** (nos'ok-tho-nog'ră-fĭ) [ noso- + G. *chthōn*, the earth, + *graphē*, a description ]. Geomedicine.

**nosocomial** (nos'o-ko'mĭ-al) [ G. *nosokomeion*, hospital ]. 1. Relating to a hospital. 2. Denoting a new disorder (unrelated to the patient's primary condition) associated with being treated in a hospital.

**nosocomion, nosocomium** (nos-o-ko'mĭ-on, or -um) [ G. *nosokomeian*, hospital, fr. *nosos*, disease, + *komeō*, to take care of ]. A hospital.

**nos'ode** [ noso- + G. *eidos*, appearance ]. An agent administered in minute doses in the treatment of the disease which, in larger amount, it causes; an isopathic term, signifying a bacterine or bacterial vaccine.

**nosogenesis, nosogeny** (nos'o-jen'ĕ-sis, nos-oj'ĕ-nĭ) [ noso- + G. *genesis*, production ]. Pathogenesis.

**nosogenic** (nos-o-jen'ik). Pathogenic.

**nosogeography** (nos'o-je-og'ră-fĭ). Geomedicine.

**nosog'rapher.** A writer on diseases.

**nos'ograph'ic.** Relating to nosography, or the description of diseases.

**nosography** (no-sog'ră-fĭ) [ noso- + G. *graphē*, description ]. A treatise on pathology or the practice of medicine.

**nosologic** (nos-o-loj'ik). Relating to nosology.

**nosology** (no-sol'o-jĭ) [ noso- + G. *logos*, study ]. The classification of diseases.

**psychiatric n.,** psychonosology.

**nos'oma'nia** [ noso- + G. *mania*, insanity ]. An unfounded, morbid belief that one is suffering from some special disease.

**nosometry** (no-som'e-trĭ) [ noso- + G. *metron*, measure ]. The measurement of morbidity or of the sickness rate in the several occupations and social conditions; see also pathometry.

**nosomycosis** (nos'o-mi-ko'sis) [ noso- + G. *mykēs*, fungus ]. Any disease caused by a fungus.

**nosonomy** (no-son'o-mĭ) [ noso- + G. *nomos*, law ]. Nosology.

**nos'opar'asite.** 1. A microparasite found in association with a certain disease and modifying its course, but not the actual cause of the morbid process. 2. A pathogenic parasite attacking only diseased tissues, *e.g.*, one of a number of protozoans which excite dysenteric symptoms only when a catarrhal or other nonspecific form of colitis is present.

**nosophilia** (nos'o-fil'ĭ-ah) [ noso- + G. *phileō*, to love ]. A morbid desire to be sick.

**nosophobia** (nos'o-fo'bĭ-ah) [ noso- + G. *phobos*, fear ]. Pathophobia; an inordinate dread and fear of disease.

**nosophyte** (nos'o-fīt) [ noso- + G. *phyton*, plant ]. A pathogenic microorganism of the plant kingdom.

**nosopoietic** (nos'o-poy-et'ik) [ noso- + G. *poiēsis*, a making ]. Pathogenic.

**Nosopsyllus** (nos'o-sil'us) [ noso- + G. *psylla*, flea ]. A genus of flea commonly found on rodents.

**N. fascia'tus,** the northern rat flea that infrequently transmits the plague bacillus to man.

**nos'otaxy** [ noso- + G. *taxis*, arrangement ]. Nosology.

**nos'otox'ic.** Relating to a nosotoxin or to nosotoxicosis.

**nos'otoxico'sis** [ noso- + G. *toxicon*, poison ]. A morbid state caused by a nosotoxin.

**nos'otox'in.** Any toxin associated with a disease.

**nosotrophy** (nos-ot'ro-fĭ) [ noso- + G. *trophē*, nourishment ]. Care of the sick.

**nos'otrop'ic** [ noso- + G. *tropē*, a turning ]. Directed against the pathologic changes or symptoms of a disease; opposed to etiotropic.

**nostalgia** (nos-tal'jĭ-ah) [ G. *nostos*, a return (home), + *algos*, pain ]. Homesickness; philopatridomania; the longing to return home or to familiar surroundings.

**nostoma'nia** [ G. *nostos*, return, homecoming, + *mania*, frenzy ]. An obsessive or abnormal interest in nostalgia, especially as an extreme manifestation of homesickness.

**nos'tril.** Naris.

**flare of the n.'s,** *alae* nasi.

**nostrum** [ L. neuter of *noster*, our, "our own remedy" ]. A quack medicine; a therapeutic agent, secret or patented, offered to the general public as a specific remedy for any disease or class of diseases.

**no'tal** [ G. *nōtos*, the back ]. Relating to the back.

**notalgia** (no-tal'jĭ-ah) [ G. *nōtos*, the back, + *algos*, pain ]. Obsolete term for dorsalgia.

**notancephalia** (no'tan-sĕ-fa'lĭ-ah) [ G. *nōtos*, back, + *an*-priv. + *kephalē*, head ]. A fetal malformation characterized by a deficiency in the occipital region of the skull.

**notanencephalia** (no'tan-en'sĕ-fāl'ĭ-ah) [ G. *nōtos*, back, + *an*-priv. + *enkephalos*, brain ]. A malformation marked by defective development or absence of the cerebellum.

**nota'tin.** Glucose oxidase.

# NOTCH

**notch.** Emargination; incisura; an indentation at the edge of any structure.

**acetab'ular n.,** *incisura* acetabuli.

**angular n.,** *incisura* angularis.

**anterior n. of cerebellum,** *incisura* cerebelli anterior.

**anterior n. of ear,** *incisura* anterior auris.

**aor'tic n.,** the slight n. in the sphygmographic tracing caused by the rebound at the closure of the aortic valves.

**n. of apex of heart,** *incisura* apicis cordis.

**auric'ular n.,** (1) *incisura* anterior auris; (2) *incisura* terminalis auris.

**cardiac n.,** *incisura* cardiaca.

**n. in cartilage of external acoustic meatus,** *incisura* cartilaginis meatus acustici externi.

**cerebellar n.,** *incisura* cerebelli.

**clavicular n.,** *incisura* clavicularis.

**costal n.,** *incisura* costalis.

**cot'yloid n.,** *incisura* acetabuli.

**craniofacial n.,** a defect in the osseous partition between the orbital and nasal cavities.

**dicrotic n.,** the n. in a pulse tracing which precedes the second or dicrotic wave.

**digastric n.,** *incisura* mastoidea.

**ethmoid'al n.,** *incisura* ethmoidalis.

**fibular n.,** *incisura* fibularis.

**frontal n.,** *incisura* frontalis.

**greater sciatic n.,** *incisura* ischiadica major.

**hamular n.,** pterygomaxillary n.

**Hutchinson's crescentic n.,** the semilunar n. on the incisal edge of the upper middle incisors in Hutchinson's teeth, seen also occasionally in the upper lateral incisors, the lower incisors, and rarely the cuspids.

**iliosciatic n.,** *incisura* ischiadica major.

**inferior thyroid n.,** *incisura* thyroidea inferior.

**interarytenoid n.,** *incisura* interarytenoidea.

**interclavic'ular n.,** *incisura* jugularis (3).

**intercon'dyloid n.,** *fossa* intercondylaris.

**intertragic n.,** *incisura* intertragica.

**intervertebral n.,** *incisura* vertebralis.

**ischiat'ic n.,** *incisura* ischiadica.

**jugular n.,** *incisura* jugularis.

**Kernohan's n.,** an abnormal indentation of intracranial tissue compressed against the incisura of the tentorium.

**lacrimal n.,** *incisura* lacrimalis.

**lesser sciatic n.,** *incisura* ischiadica minor.

**mandib'ular n.,** *incisura* mandibulae.

**marsupial n.,** *incisura* cerebelli posterior.

**mastoid n.,** *incisura* mastoidea.

**nasal n.,** *incisura* nasalis.

**pancreatic n.,** *incisura* pancreatis.

**pari'etal n.,** *incisura* parietalis.

**parot'id n.,** the space between the ramus of the mandible and the mastoid process of the temporal bone.

**poplit'eal n.,** *area* intercondylaris posterior.

**posterior n. of cerebellum,** *incisura* cerebelli posterior.

**preoccipital n.,** *incisura* preoccipitalis.

**presternal n.,** *incisura* jugularis (3).

**pter'ygoid n.,** *incisura* pterygoidea.

**pterygomaxillary n.,** hamular n.; the n. or fissure between the tuberosity of the maxilla and the hamulus of the pterygoid process of the sphenoid bone.

**radial n.,** *incisura* radialis.

**Rivinus' n.,** *incisura* tympanica.

**n. for round ligament of liver,** *incisura* ligamenti teretis hepatis.

**sacrosciatic n.,** the n. of the pelvic outlet on either side, formed by the ischium in front, the sacrum behind, and the ilium above; in life it is converted into a foramen by the sacrospinous ligaments.

**scapular n.,** *incisura* scapulae.

**semilunar n.,** (1) *incisura* cerebelli anterior; (2) *incisura* trochlearis.

**sigmoid n.,** *incisura* mandibulae.

**sphenopal'atine n.,** *incisura* sphenopalatina.

sternal n., *incisura* jugularis (3).
superior thyroid n., *incisura* thyroidea superior.
supraor'bital n., *incisura* supraorbitalis.
suprascapular n., *incisura* scapulae.
suprasternal n., *incisura* jugularis (3).
n. of tentorium, *incisura* tentorii.
terminal n., *incisura* terminalis auris.
trochlear n., *incisura* trochlearis.
tympanic n., *incisura* tympanica.
ulnar n., *incisura* ulnaris.
umbil'ical n., *incisura* ligamenti teretis.
vertebral n., *incisura* vertebralis.

---

**notched.** Indented; emarginate.

**notencephalocele** (no-ten-sef'al-o-sēl) [ G. *nōtos*, back, + *enkephalos*, brain, + *kēlē*, hernia ]. A malformation in the occipital portion of the cranium with protrusion of brain substance.

**no'tenceph'alus.** A fetus with notencephalocele.

**Nothnagel** (nōt'nah-gel), Carl W. H., Vienna physician, 1841–1905. See N.'s *syndrome, test.*

**notochord** (no'to-kord) [ G. *nōtos*, back, + *chordē*, cord, string ]. 1. In primitive vertebrates, the primary axial supporting structure of the body; an important organizer for determining the final form of the nervous system and related structures. 2. In embryos, the axial fibrocellular cord about which the vertebral primordia develop. Vestiges of it persist in the adult as the nucleii pulposi of the intervertebral disks. Also called chorda dorsalis; chorda vertebralis; head process.

**notochordal** (no-to-kor'dal). Relating to the notochord.

**Notoedres cati** (no'to-ed'rēz ka'ti). Sarcoptic mange mite of cats; also called *Sarcoptes scabei minor.*

**notomelus** (no-tom'ě-lus) [ G. *nōtos*, back, + *melos*, limb ]. A malformed individual with one or more accessory limbs attached to the back.

**notomyelitis** (no-to-mi-el-i'tis) [ G. *nōtos*, back, + *myelos*, marrow, + *-itis* ]. Myelitis; inflammation of the spinal cord.

**noumenal** (noo'men-al) [ G. *nooumenos*, perceived; pres. p. pass. of *noeō*, to perceive, think ]. Intellectually, not sensuously, intuitional; relating to the object of pure thought divorced from all concepts of time or space.

**nous** (noos or nows) [ G. mind, reason ]. A word originally used by Anaxagoras by which he meant an all-knowing all-pervading spirit or force; in later Greek philosophy it came to mean simply mind, reason, or intellect.

**novobi'ocin.** CARDELMYCIN; ALBAMYCIN; streptonivicin; an antibacterial substance produced by fermentation from cultures of *Streptomyces niveus* or *S. spheroides*, effective against penicillin-resistant *Staphylococcus* and *Proteus.* Also available (BP) as n. calcium and n. sodium.

**Novy,** Frederick G., American bacteriologist, 1864–1957. See N.-MacNeal *agar.*

**noxa** (nok'sah) [ L. injury, fr. *noceo*, to injure ]. Anything that exerts a harmful influence, such as trauma, poison, etc.

**noxious** (nok'shus) [ L. *noxius*, injurious, fr. *noceo*, to injure ]. Injurious.

**noxythi'olin.** NOXYFLEX; 1-(hydroxymethyl)-3-methyl-2-thiourea; antibacterial and antifungal agent.

**Np.** Chemical symbol of the element neptunium.

**NPH insulin.** See under insulin.

**NPN.** Abbreviation for nonprotein *nitrogen.*

**Nps.** Abbreviation for *N-o*-nitrophenylsulfenyl.

**N-terminal.** Amino-terminal.

**nu.** Thirteenth letter of the Greek alphabet, *ν.* Symbol for kinematic *viscosity.*

**nubecula** (nu-bek'u-lah) [ L. dim. of *nubes*, cloud ]. A faint cloud or cloudiness.

**nubile** (nu'bil) [ L. *nubilis*, fr. *nubo*, pp. *nuptus*, to marry ]. Fit for marriage; sexually mature; said of a young woman at puberty.

**nubil'ity.** The state of being nubile.

**nucha** (nu'kah) [ Fr. *nuque* ] [ NA ]. The nape of the neck; the back of the neck.

**nuchal** (nu'kal). Relating to the nucha.

**Nuck,** Anton, Dutch anatomist, 1650–1692. See N.'s *canal, diverticulum, hydrocele.*

**nucl-.** See nucleo-.

**nuclear** (nu'kle-ar). Relating to a nucleus.

**nuclease** (nū'kle-ās) General term for enzymes that catalyze the hydrolysis of nucleic acid into nucleotides or oligonucleotides by cleaving phosphodiester linkages (see ribonucleases, deoxyribonucleases, guanyloribonuclease, spleen endonuclease, nucleate endonuclease, exonuclease, endonuclease).
azotobacter n., nucleate *endonuclease.*
micrococcal n., spleen *endonuclease.*
mung bean n., nucleate *endonuclease.*

**nucleated** (nu'kle-a'ted). Provided with a nucleus, a characteristic of all true cells.

**nucleate endonuclease.** See under endonuclease.

**nuclei** (nu'kle-i). Plural of nucleus.

**nucleic acid** (nu-kle'ik). A family of substances of large molecular weight, found in chromosomes, nucleoli, mitochondria, and cytoplasm of all cells, and in viruses. In combination with proteins they are called nucleoproteins. On hydrolysis they yield purines, pyrimidines, phosphoric acid, and a pentose, either D-ribose or D-deoxyribose. From the last, the nucleic acids derive their more specific names, ribonucleic acid and deoxyribonucleic acid. Nucleic acids are linear (*i.e.*, unbranched) polymers of nucleotides in which the 5' phosphate of each one is esterified with the 3' hydroxyl of the preceding nucleotide.
n. acid base, purine base; see under purine.
infectious n. acid, nucleic acid that is capable of effecting transfection (*q.v.*).

**nucleiform** (nu'kle-ĭ-form). Shaped like or having the appearance of a nucleus.

**nucleinase** (nu'kle-in-ās). Obsolete term for nuclease.

**nucleinic base.** Obsolete term for purine.

**nucleo-, nucl-** (nu'kle-o-) [ L. *nucleus, q.v.* NUC- ]. Combining forms for nucleus or nuclear.

**nucleocapsid** (nu'kle-o-kap'sid). See virion.

**nucleochylema** (nu-kle-o-ki-le'mah) [ nucleo- + G. *chylos*, juice ]. Karyolymph.

**nucleochyme** (nu'kle-o-kīm). Karyolymph.

**nucleofugal** (nu'kle-of'u-gal) [ nucleo- + L. *fugio*, to flee ]. 1. Moving within the cell body in a direction away from the nucleus. 2. Moving in a direction away from a nerve nucleus; said of nerve transmission.

**nucleohistone** (nu'kle-o-his'tōn). A complex of histone and deoxyribonucleic acid, the form in which the latter is usually found in cells; n. may be viewed as a salt between the basic protein and the nucleic acid.

**nucleoid** (nu'kle-oyd) [ nucleo- + G. *eidos*, resemblance ]. 1. Nucleiform. 2. A nuclear inclusion body. 3. The genome of microorganisms (microbes); see also nucleus; virion.
Lavdovsky's n., astrosphere.

**nucle'olar.** Relating to a nucleolus.

**nucle'oli.** Plural of nucleolus.

**nucle'oliform.** Resembling a nucleolus.

**nucleoloid** (nu-kle'o-loyd) [ nucleolus + G. *eidos*, resemblance ]. Nucleoliform.

**nucleolonema** (nu-kle'o-lo-ne'mah) [ nucleolus + G. *nema*, thread ]. The irregular network or rows of fine granules of ribonucleoprotein composing the greater part of nucleolus as seen in the electron microscope.

**nucleolus, pl. nucle'oli** (nu-kle'o-lus) [ L. dim of *nucleus*, a nut, kernel ]. 1 [ NA ]. A small spherical mass of basophilic material within the substance of the nucleus of a cell; it is usually single, but there may be from two to five nucleoli. It is composed of an apparently structureless pars amorpha and the nucleolonema. 2. A more or less central body in the vesicular nucleus of certain protozoa in which an endosome is lacking but one or more Feulgen-positive (DNA +) nucleoli are present; characteristic of Sporozoa, certain flagellates, opalinids, dinoflagellates, and radiolarians among the Protozoa. The chromatin material is distributed throughout the nucleus rather than peripherally, as in the endosome type of nucleus. Formerly called plasmosome and endosome, *q.v.*
chromatin n., karyosome.
false n., karyosome.

**nu′cleomi′crosome.** Karyomicrosome.

**nu′cleon.** One of the subatomic particles of the atomic nucleus; *i.e.*, either a proton or a neutron.

**nucleopetal** (nu′kle-op′ĕ-tal) [ nucleo- + L. *peto*, to seek ]. 1. Moving in the cell body in a direction toward the nucleus. 2. Moving in a direction toward a nerve nucleus; said of a nervous impulse.

**Nucleophaga** (nu-kle-of′ă-gah) [ nucleo- + G. *phagein*, to eat ]. A sporozoan parasite of amebae, which destroys the nucleus of its host; the parasite is thought to be a microsporidia.

**nucleophil, nucleophile** (nu′kle-o-fil, -fīl) [ nucleo- + G. *philos*, fond ]. 1. The electron donor in a chemical reaction in which a pair of electrons is picked up by an electrophil. 2. Nucleophilic; relating to a nucleophil.

**nu′cleophil′ic.** Nucleophil (2).

**nu′cleophos′phatase.** Nucleotidase.

**nucleoplasm** (nu′kle-o-plazm). Karyoplasm; the protoplasm, or colloid portion of the nucleus of a cell, including the karyolymph.

**nu′cleopro′tein.** A nondescript complex of protein and nucleic acid; chromosomes and viruses are largely n. in nature. See nucleohistone.

**nucleoreticulum** (nu′kle-o-re-tik′u-lum) [ nucleo- + L. *reticulum*, dim. of *rete*, net ]. The intranuclear network of chromatin or linin.

**nucleorrhexis** (nu′kle-o-rek′sis) [ nucleo- + G. *rhēxis*, rupture ]. Fragmentation of a cell nucleus.

**nu′cleosi′dases.** Enzymes that catalyze the hydrolysis of nucleosides, releasing the purine or pyrimidine base, including nucleosidase (EC 3.2.2.1), inosine (EC 3.2.2.2), uridine n. (EC 3.2.2.3), AMP n. (EC 3.2.2.4), NAD n. (EC 3.2.2.5), and NAD(P) n. (EC 3.2.2.6).

**nu′cleoside.** A compound of a sugar (notably ribose or deoxyribose) with a purine or pyrimidine base by way of an *N*-glycosyl link. (See adenosine, cytidine, guanosine, uridine, thymidine, also deoxyadenosine, etc.)

**n. deaminase,** see deaminase.

**n. diphosphates,** the 5′-pyrophosphoric acid esters of nucleosides; *i.e.*, nucleosides in which the H of one of the ribose hydroxyls (usually the 5′) is replaced by a pyrophosphoric radical; *e.g.*, adenosine diphosphate (ADP). Distinguished from bisphosphates which have two orthophosphate groups on two different C—O groups of the sugar.

**n. diphosphate kinase,** enzyme (a phosphotransferase) catalyzing transfer of one phosphate group from ATP to a nucleoside diphosphate to yield a nucleoside triphosphate.

**n. diphosphate sugars,** n. diphosphates linked through the 5′-diphosphate group with a simple or complex carbohydrates, *e.g.*, GDP-mannose, UDP-glucose (UDPG), dTDP-glucosamine.

**n. diphosphokinase,** n. diphosphate kinase.

**n. phosphate,** a nucleotide, *e.g.*, AMP.

**n. phosphorylases,** enzymes that catalyze the phosphorolysis of a n. forming the free purine or pyrimidine plus ribose (or deoxyribose) 1-phosphate; purine n. p. (EC 2.4.2.1), uridine p. (EC 2.4.2.3), thymidine p. (EC 2.4.2.4).

**n. triphosphate,** a n. in which the H of one of the ribose hydroxyls (usually the 5′) is replaced by a triphosphate group, —PO(OH)—O—PO(OH)—O—PO(OH)$_2$; *e.g.*, adenosine triphosphate, ATP.

**nu′cleospin′dle.** The fusiform body in mitosis.

**nucleoti′dase.** A phosphohydrolase (EC 3.1.3.31) releasing nucleosides and phosphate from nucleotides. See also nucleotidases.

**nu′cleoti′dases.** Enzymes that catalyze the hydrolysis of nucleotides into phosphoric acid and nucleosides. Specificities are indicated by prefixes: 5′-nucleotidase (EC 3.1.3.5) acts on nucleoside 5′-phosphates; 3′-nucleotidase (EC 3.1.3.6) on 3′-phosphates; phosphoadenylate 3′-nucleotidase (EC 3.1.3.7) on adenosine 3′,5′-bisphosphate (releasing the 3′ phosphate group).

**nu′cleotide.** Mononucleotide; originally a combination of a nucleic acid purine or pyrimidine, one sugar (usually ribose or deoxyribose), and a phosphate group; by extension, any compound containing a heterocyclic compound bound to a phosphorylated sugar by an *N*-glycosyl link, as

adenosine phosphate and flavin mononucleotide. For the individual nucleotides, see specific names (*e.g.*, adenylic acid or adenine ribonucleotide).

**n. pair,** see under pair.

**nucleotidyltransferase** (nu′kle-o-ti′dil-trans′fer-ās) (EC class 2.7.7). Enzymes (transferases) transferring nucleotide residues (nucleotidyls) from nucleoside di- or triphosphates into dimer or polymer forms. Some n.'s bear specific names (*e.g.*, adenylyltransferases), or trivial names indicating the linkage hydrolyzed in the synthesis (pyrophosphorylases, phosphorylases), or names of the material synthesized (RNA or DNA polymerase).

**nu′cleotox′in.** A toxin acting upon the cell nuclei.

# NUCLEUS

**nucleus,** pl. **nu′clei** (nu′kle-us) [ L. a little nut, the kernel, stone of fruits, the inside of a thing, dim. of *nux*, nut ]. 1. In cytology, typically a rounded or oval mass of protoplasm within the cytoplasm of a plant or animal cell. It is surrounded by a nuclear envelope, which encloses chromatin, linin, one or more nucleoli, and karyolymph, and undergoes mitosis during cell division; see fig. under cell. 2. By extension, because of similar function, the genome of microorganisms (microbes) that is relatively simple in structure, lacks a nuclear membrane, and does not undergo mitosis during replication. 3 [ NA ]. In neuroanatomy, a group of nerve cells in the brain or spinal cord that can be demarcated more or less sharply from neighboring groups on the basis of either differences in cell type or the presence of a surrounding zone of nerve fibers or cell-poor neuropil. 4. Any substance—foreign body, mucus, crystal, etc-.—around which a urinary or other calculus is formed. 5. The central portion of an atom (composed of protons and neutrons) where most of the mass and all of the positive charge are concentrated.

**abdu′cens n.,** n. nervi abducentis.

**n. of abducent nerve,** n. nervi abducentis.

**n. abducen′tis,** n. nervi abducentis.

**accessory cuneate n.,** n. cuneatus accessorius.

**accessory olivary nuclei,** see n. olivaris accessorius dorsalis and n. olivaris accessorius medialis.

**n. accum′bens sep′ti,** the region of fusion between the caput nuclei caudati and the putamen, covered on the ventral side by the olfactory tubercle. The name ("a nucleus leaning against the septum") refers to a medial, hook-shaped expansion of this anteroventral region of the striatum which curves under the bottom of the frontal horn of the lateral ventricle and ascends for some distance into the ventral half of the septal region.

**n. acu′sticus,** see n. nervi vestibulocochlearis.

**n. a′lae cine′reae,** n. dorsalis nervi vagi.

**almond n.,** *corpus* amygdaloideum.

**ambiguous n.,** n. ambiguus.

**n. ambig′uus** [ NA ], ambiguous n.; a very slender, longitudinal column of motor neurons in the ventrolateral region of the medulla oblongata; its efferent fibers leave with the vagus and glossopharyngeal nerve and innervate the striated muscle fibers of the pharynx (including the musculus levator veli palatini) and the vocal cord muscles of the larynx.

**n. amyg′dalae,** *corpus* amygdaloideum.

**amyg′daloid n.,** *corpus* amygdaloideum.

**anterior nuclei of thalamus,** nuclei anteriores thalami.

**nuclei anterio′res thal′ami** [ NA ], anterior nuclei of the thalamus; three groups of nerve cells together forming the tuberculum anterius thalami: the relatively large anteroventral n., the anteromedial n., and the small (but large-celled) anterodorsal n. The nuclei receive the mamillothalamic tract from the mamillary body, and additional afferents by way of the fornix; they project collectively to the cortex of the cingulate and parahippocampal gyrus.

**n. anterodorsa′lis** [ NA ], anterodorsal thalamic n.; see nuclei anteriores thalami.

**n. anteromedia′lis** [ NA ], anteromedial thalamic n.; see nuclei anteriores thalami.

**n. anteroventra'lis** [ NA ], anteroventral thalamic n.; see nuclei anteriores thalami.

**arcuate nuclei,** nuclei arcuati.

**arcuate n.,** n. arcuatus.

**nuclei arcua'ti** [ NA ], arcuate nuclei; a variable assembly of small cell groups, probably outlying components of the pontine nuclei, on the ventral and medial aspects of the pyramid in the medulla oblongata.

**n. arcua'tus,** arcuate n.; (1) the n. semilunaris of Flechsig; a component of the n. ventralis posterior thalami; (2) posterior periventricular n.; a cell group in the hypothalamus, located in the lowest part of the infundibulum adjacent to the median eminence.

**atomic n.,** see nucleus (5).

**auditory n.,** see n. nervi vestibulocochlearis.

**n. basa'lis of Ganser,** a large group of large cells in the substantia innominata, ventral to the lentiform n.

**Bechterew's n.,** (1) n. vestibularis superior; see nuclei vestibulares; (2) n. centralis tegmenti superior; see nuclei raphes.

**Blumenau's n.,** the lateral cuneate n. of the medulla oblongata.

**branchiomotor nuclei,** special visceral efferent (or motor) nuclei; collective term for those motoneuronal nuclei of the brainstem (n. ambiguus, facial motor n., motor n. of the trigeminus) that develop from the branchiomotor column of the embryo and innervate striated muscle fibers developed from the mesenchyme of the branchial arches (muscles of mastication, facial musculature, pharynx and vocal cord muscles).

**Burdach's n.,** n. cuneatus.

**caudate n.,** n. caudatus.

**n. cauda'tus** [ NA ], caudate n.; caudatum; an elongated curved mass of gray matter, consisting of an anterior thick portion, the caput or head, which projects into the anterior horn of the lateral ventricle, a portion extending along the floor of the body of the lateral ventricle as the corpus, and an elongated curved thin portion, the cauda or tail, which curves downward and backward in the temporal lobes to the wall of the descending horn.

**n. centra'lis latera'lis thal'ami,** the most lateral of the intralaminar nuclei of the thalamus.

**n. centra'lis tegmen'ti supe'rior,** Bechterew's n. (2); see nuclei raphes.

**centromedian n.,** n. centromedianus.

**n. centromedia'nus** [ NA ], centromedian n.; centrum medianum; centre médian of Luys; a large, lentil-shaped cell group, the largest and most caudal of the intralaminar nuclei, located in the lamina medullaris interna of the thalamus between the mediodorsal n. and ventrobasal n.; so called by Luys because of its prominent appearance on frontal sections midway between anterior and posterior pole of the human thalamus. The n. receives numerous fibers from the internal segment of the globus pallidus by way of the fasciculus thalamicus of the ansa lenticularis, as well as from area 4 of the motor cortex; its major efferent connection is with the putamen.

**Clarke's n.,** n. thoracicus.

**cochlear nuclei,** nuclei cochleares.

**nuclei cochlea'res** [ NA ], cochlear nuclei; nuclei nervi cochlearis; the n. cochlearis dorsalis and n. cochlearis ventralis, located on the dorsal and lateral surface of the inferior cerebellar peduncle, in the floor of the lateral recess of the rhomboid fossa. They receive the incoming fibers of the cochlear part of the vestibulocochlear nerve and are the major source of origin of the lateral lemniscus or central auditory pathway.

**n. collic'uli inferio'ris** [ NA ], the nerve cell groups composing the colliculus inferior.

**convergence n. of Perlia,** Perlia's n.

**n. cor'poris genicula'ti media'lis** [ NA ], n. of the medial geniculate body; the nerve cell groups composing the medial geniculate body (corpus geniculatum mediale).

**nuclei cor'poris mamilla'ris** [ NA ], the cell groups composing the corpus mamillare (mamillary body): a single, large-celled lateral n. and a larger, bipartite medial n.

**n. cor'poris trapezoi'dei,** n. of the trapezoid body; this cell group is renamed n. ventralis corporis trapezoidei in the latest NA.

**nuclei of cranial nerves,** nuclei nervorum cranialium.

**cuneate n.,** n. cuneatus.

**n. cunea'tus** [ NA ], cuneate n.; n. of Burdach; n. funiculi cuneati; the larger, middle one of the three nuclei of the posterior column (dorsal column or dorsal funiculus) of the spinal cord. Located near the dorsal surface of the medulla oblongata at and below the level of the obex, the n. receives posterior root fibers corresponding to the sensory innervation of the upper extremity (arm and hand) of the same side. Togerher with its medial companion n., the n. gracilis, it is the major source of origin of the medial lemniscus.

**n. cunea'tus accesso'rius** [ NA ], accessory cuneate n.; lateral or external cuneate n.; Monakow's n.; a cell group lateral to the n. cuneatus which receives posterior-root fibers corresponding to the proprioceptive innervation of the arm and hand. It projects to the cerebellum by way of the cuneocerebellar tract, and can be considered the upper-extremity equivalent of Clarke's column, or n. thoracicus of the spinal cord.

**n. of Darkschewitsch (Darkschevich),** an ovoid cell group in the central gray substance rostral to the oculomotor nucleus, receiving fibers from the vestibular nuclei by way of the medial longitudinal fasciculus, and itself projecting caudally, by way of that fiber bundle, to the oculomotor, abducens, and trochlear nuclei.

**deep cerebellar nuclei,** collective term for the nuclei dentatus, globosus, emboliformis, and tecti or fastigii of the cerebellum.

**Deiters' n.,** n. vestibularis lateralis; see nuclei vestibulares.

**dentate n. of cerebellum,** n. dentatus cerebelli.

**n. denta'tus cerebel'li** [ NA ], dentate n. of the cerebellum; dentatum; corpus dentatum; the most lateral and largest of the deep cerebellar nuclei; it receives the axons of the Purkinje cells of the neocerebellum; together with the more medially located nuclei globosus and emboliformis it is the major source of fibers composing the massive superior cerebellar peduncle or brachium conjunctivum.

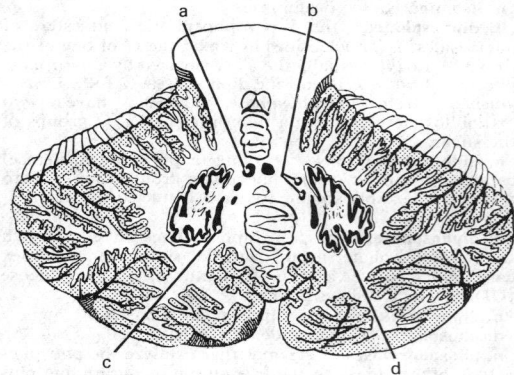

**Cerebellar Nuclei**

*a*, Nucleus fastigii; *b*, nucleus globosus; *c*, nucleus emboliformis; *d*, nucleus dentatus.

**descending n. of the trigeminus,** n. tractus spinalis nervi trigemini.

**diploid n.,** a n. containing the diploid or normal double complement of chromosomes.

**dorsal n.,** n. thoracicus.

**dorsal accessory olivary n.,** n. olivaris accessorius dorsalis.

**dorsal motor n. of vagus,** n. dorsalis nervi vagi.

**dorsal n. of vagus,** n. dorsalis nervi vagi.

**n. dorsa'lis,** n. thoracicus.

**n. dorsa'lis cor'poris trapezoi'dei** [ NA ], oliva superior; superior olive; superior olivary n.; a circumscript, bipartite cell group located ventrolaterally in the lower pontine tegmentum, immediately dorsal to the trapezoid body; the n. receives fibers from both the ipsilateral and contralateral cochlear nuclei, and contributes fibers to the lateral (auditory) lemniscus of both sides. It is believed to be prominently involved in the function of spatial localization of sound.

**n. dorsa'lis ner'vi va'gi** [ NA ], dorsal n. of the vagus; dorsal motor n. of the vagus; n. alae cinereae; the visceral motor n. located in the vagal trigone (ala cinerea) of the floor of the fourth ventricle. It gives rise to the parasympathetic fibers of the vagus nerve innervating the heart muscle and the smooth musculature and glands of the respiratory and intestinal tracts.

**dorsomedial n.,** n. medialis thalami.

**dorsomedial hypothalamic n.,** n. dorsomedialis hypothalami.

**n. dorsomedia'lis hypothal'ami** [ NA ], dorsomedial hypothalamic n.; an oval cluster of cells located dorsal to the ventromedial hypothalamic n.

**droplet nuclei,** dried residue of droplets, *e.g.,* from sneezing and coughing, that carry airborne infection.

**Edinger-Westphal n.,** a small group of preganglionic parasympathetic motor neurons at the rostral pole of the oculomotor n. of the midbrain; the axons of these motor neurons leave the brain with the oculomotor nerve and synapse on the cells of the ciliary ganglion which in turn innervate the sphincter muscle of the pupil and ciliary muscle. Destruction of this n. or its efferent fibers causes maximal paralytic dilation of the pupil.

**emboliform n.,** n. emboliformis.

**n. embolifor'mis** [ NA ], emboliform n.; embolus (2); a small elongated mass of gray matter in the central white substance of the cerebellum just internal to the hilus of the dentate n.

**external cuneate n.,** n. cuneatus accessorius.

**facial motor n.,** n. nervi facialis.

**n. facia'lis,** n. nervi facialis.

**n. fascic'uli gra'cilis,** n. gracilis.

**n. fastig'ii** [ NA ], n. tecti; roof n.; fastigatum; the most medial of the deep cerebellar nuclei, lying medial to the n. interpositus, near the midline, in the white matter underneath the vermis of the cerebellar cortex. It receives the axons of Purkinje cells in the vermis, especially the latter's caudal part, and also receives fibers from the vestibular nerve and vestibular nuclei. Its major projection is to the vestibular nuclei and medullary reticular formation.

**n. fibro'sus lin'guae,** *septum* linguae.

**n. filifor'mis,** n. paraventricularis.

**n. funic'uli cunea'ti,** n. cuneatus.

**n. funic'uli gra'cilis,** n. gracilis.

**gamet'ic n.,** micronucleus (2).

**n. gelatino'sus,** n. pulposus.

**germ n.,** micronucleus (2).

**n. globo'sus** [ NA ], spherical n.; a group of two or three small masses of gray substance in the white central core of the cerebellum, to the inner side of and a little ventral to the n. emboliformis.

**n. of Goll,** n. gracilis.

**gonad n.,** micronucleus (2).

**n. gra'cilis** [ NA ], n. fasciculi gracilis; n. funiculi gracilis; n. of Goll; the medial one of the three nuclei of the dorsal column, the remaining two being the n. cuneatus and the n. cuneatus accessorius. The n. gracilis corresponds to a slight prominence of the dorsal surface of the medulla oblongata, the clava. It receives dorsal-root fibers corresponding to the sensory innervation of the leg, and projects, by way of the medial lemniscus, to the n. ventralis posterior of the thalamus.

**gustatory n.,** see n. tractus solitarii.

**n. haben'ulae** [ NA ], habenular n.; ganglion habenulae; the gray matter of the habenula, composed of a small-celled medial and a larger-celled lateral habenular n.; both nuclei receive fibers from basal forebrain regions (septum, n. basalis, lateral preoptic n.); the lateral habenular n. receives an additional projection from the medial segment of the globus pallidus. Both nuclei project by way of the fasciculus retroflexus to the n. interpeduncularis and a medial zone of the midbrain tegmentum.

**habenular n.,** n. habenulae.

**hypoglossal n.,** n. nervi hypoglossi.

**n. of hypoglossal nerve,** n. nervi hypoglossi.

**inferior olivary n.,** n. olivaris.

**inferior salivary n.,** n. salivatorius inferior.

**inferior vestibular n.,** n. vestibularis inferior; see nuclei vestibulares.

**intercalated n.,** n. intercalatus.

**n. intercala'tus** [ NA ], intercalated n.; n. of Staderini, a small collection of nerve cells in the medulla oblongata lying lateral to the hypoglossal n.

**intermediolateral n.,** n. intermediolateralis.

**n. intermediolatera'lis,** intermediolateral n.; intermediolateral cell column; the cell column that forms the lateral horn of the spinal cord's gray matter. Extending from the first thoracic through the second lumbar segment, the column contains the autonomic motor neurons that give rise to the preganglionic fibers of the sympathetic system.

**intermediomedial n.,** n. intermediomedialis.

**n. intermediomedia'lis,** intermediomedial n.; a small group of scattered visceral motor neurons immediately ventral to the n. thoracicus or column of Clarke in the thoracic and upper two lumbar segments of the spinal cord; like the larger n. intermediolateralis it gives rise to preganglionic fibers of the sympathetic nervous system.

**interpeduncular n.,** n. interpeduncularis.

**n. interpeduncula'ris** [ NA ], interpeduncular n. or ganglion; Gudden's ganglion; intercrural ganglion; ganglion isthmi; a median, unpaired, ovoid cell group at the base of the midbrain tegmentum between the left and right cerebral peduncles; it receives the fasciculus retroflexus from the habenula, and projects to the raphe region (nuclei raphes) and central gray substance of the midbrain.

**n. interpos'itus,** collective term denoting the nuclei globosus and emboliformis of the cerebellum.

**interstitial n. of Cajal,** n. interstitialis.

**n. interstitia'lis** [ NA ], interstitial n. of Cajal; a group of widely spaced, medium-sized neurons in the dorsomedial region of the upper mesencephalic tegmentum, immediately lateral to the n. of Darkschewitsch; together with the latter, the n. interstitialis is closely associated with the fasciculus longitudinalis medialis, via which it receives fibers from the vestibular nuclei and projects caudally to the oculomotor n. and cervical segments of the spinal cord. It is believed to be involved in the integration of head and eye movements.

**intralaminar nuclei of thalamus,** nuclei intralaminares thalami.

**nuclei intralamina'res thal'ami** [ NA ], intralaminar nuclei of the thalamus; collective term denoting several cell groups embedded in the internal medullary lamina of the thalamus; n. centralis lateralis, n. paracentralis, and farthest caudally, the large n. centromedianus. The first two of these receive afferents from the cerebral cortex, brainstem, reticular formation, cerebellum, and spinal cord, and project more or less diffusely to large regions of the frontal and parietal cortex. See also n. centromedianus.

**Klein-Gumprecht shadow nuclei,** shadow nuclei in degenerating lymphoidocytes and macrolymphocytes in leukemia.

**lateral cuneate n.,** n. cuneatus accessorius.

**n. of lateral lemniscus,** n. lemnisci lateralis.

**lateral n. of medulla oblongata,** n. lateralis medullae oblongatae.

**lateral reticular n.,** n. lateralis medullae oblongatae.

**lateral n. of thalamus,** n. lateralis thalami.

**lateral tuberal nuclei,** nuclei tuberales.

**lateral vestibular n.,** n. vestibularis lateralis; see nuclei vestibulares.

**n. latera'lis medul'lae oblonga'tae** [ NA ], lateral n. of medulla oblongata; lateral reticular n.; a group of cells in the medulla oblongata, located between the inferior olive and the descending trigeminal n., receiving fibers from the spinal cord and motor cortex and projecting to the cerebellum.

**n. latera'lis thal'ami** [ NA ], lateral n. of the thalamus; the largest of the major subdivisions of the thalamus; the composite n. lateralis includes, from before backward, the n. lateralis anterior or dorsalis, n. lateralis intermedius, n. lateralis posterior, and pulvinar. Together, these cell groups form most of the free dorsal surface of the posterior half of the thalamus. The n. lateralis projects to a very large region of parietal, occipitoparietal, and temporal cortex. Its afferent connections are largely obscure, but the n. lateralis posterior and pulvinar are known to receive a projection from the superior colliculus.

**n. lemnis'ci latera'lis** [ NA ], n. of the lateral lemniscus; a substantial cell mass embedded in the anterior stretch of the lateral lemniscus, immediately below the latter's entry into the inferior colliculus; the n. represents a synaptic way-station for part of the fibers of the lateral lemniscus.

**n. of lens,**  n. lentis.

**lenticular n.,**  n. lentiformis.

**lentiform n.,**  n. lentiformis.

**n. lentifor'mis**  [ NA ], lentiform n.; lenticular n.; the large, cone-shaped mass of gray matter forming the central core of the cerebral hemisphere. The convex base of the cone, oriented laterally and rostrally, is formed by the putamen which together with the caudate nucleus composes the small-celled striatum. The apical part of the lentiform n., oriented medially and caudally, consists of the large-celled globus pallidus or pallidum. The lentiform n. is placed ventral and lateral to the thalamus and caudate n., from which it is separated by the internal capsule. Together with the caudate n. it composes the corpus striatum.

**n. len'tis**  [ NA ], n. of the lens; the core or inner dense portion of the lens of the eye.

**n. of Luys,**  n. subthalamicus.

**main sensory n. of the trigeminus,**  n. sensorius principalis nervi trigemini.

**masticatory n., n. masticato'rius,**  n. motorius nervi trigemini.

**medial accessory olivary n.,**  n. olivaris accessorius medialis.

**n. of medial geniculate body,**  n. corporis geniculati medialis.

**medial n. of thalamus,**  n. medialis thalami.

**medial central n. of thalamus,**  n. medialis centralis thalami.

**medial vestibular n.,**  n. vestibularis medialis; see nuclei vestibulares.

**n. media'lis centra'lis thal'ami**  [ NA ], medial central n. of the thalamus; a small cell group in the massa intermedia of the thalamus, occupying the midline region of the internal medullary lamina, between the left and the right n. paracentralis.

**n. media'lis thal'ami**  [ NA ], medial n. of the thalamus; mediodorsal or dorsomedial n.; a large, composite cell group in the dorsomedial region of the thalamus projecting to the entire extent of the frontal cortex anterior to the motor cortex (area 4) and premotor cortex (area 6). The afferent connections of the n. medialis are incompletely known; they include afferents from the olfactory cortex and amygdala.

**mediodorsal n.,**  n. medialis thalami.

**mesencephalic n. of the trigeminus,**  n. tractus mesencephali nervi trigemini.

**Monakow's n.,**  n. cuneatus accessorius.

**motor nuclei,**  nuclei originis.

**motor n. of facial nerve,**  n. nervi facialis.

**motor n. of trigeminus,**  n. motorius nervi trigemini.

**n. moto'rius nervi trigem'ini**  [ NA ], masticatory n.; n. masticatorius; motor n. of the trigeminus; a group of motor neurons innervating the muscles of mastication (masseter, temporalis, internal and external pterygoid muscles) and the musculi tensor tympani and tensor veli palatini. The n. lies in the upper pontine tegmentum medial to the main sensory n. of the trigeminus; its outgoing fibers form the portio minor of the trigeminal nerve.

**n. ner'vi abducen'tis**  [ NA ], n. of the abducent (sixth cranial) nerve; n. abducentis; abducens n.; a group of motor neurons in the lower part of the pons, innervating the lateral rectus muscle of the eye.

**nuclei ner'vi cochlea'ris,**  nuclei cochleares.

**nuclei nervo'rum crania'lium**  [ NA ], nuclei of the cranial nerves; groups of nerve cells associated with the cranial nerves either as motor nuclei (nuclei originis) or sensory nuclei (nuclei terminationis).

**n. ner'vi facia'lis**  [ NA ], facial motor n.; motor n. of the facial nerve; n. facialis; a group of motor neurons located in the ventrolateral region of the lower pontine tegmentum and innervating the facial muscles, the stapedius muscle in the middle ear, the posterior limb of the musculus digastricus, and the stylohyoid muscle.

**n. ner'vi hypoglos'si**  [ NA ], n. of the hypoglossal nerve; hypoglossal n.; the motor n. innervating the musculature of the tongue; it is located in the medulla oblongata near the midline, immediately beneath the floor of the inferior recess of the rhomboid fossa.

**n. ner'vi oculomoto'rii**  [ NA ], n. of the oculomotor nerve; oculomotor n.; the composite group of motor neurons innervating all of the external eye muscles except the nusculus rectus lateralis and musculus obliquus superior, and including the musculus levator palpebrae superioris. The most rostral component of the n. is the preganglionic parasympathetic n. of Edinger-Westphal which innervates the musculi sphincter pupillae and ciliaris. The oculomotor n. lies in the rostral half of the midbrain, near the midline in the most ventral part of the central gray substance.

**n. ner'vi trochlea'ris**  [ NA ], n. of the trochlear nerve; trochlear n.; a group of motor neurons innervating the superior oblique muscle of the contralateral eye. The n. lies in the caudal half of the midbrain, behind the oculomotor n., in the most ventral part of the central gray substance, near the midline.

**nuclei ner'vi vestib'ulocochlea'ris**  [ NA ], the combined cochlear and vestibular nuclei in the brain stem that receive the incoming fibers of the eighth cranial nerve; see nuclei cochleares and nuclei vestibulares.

**n. ni'ger,**  *substantia* nigra.

**nutrition n.,**  macronucleus (2).

**oculomotor n.,**  n. nervi oculomotorii.

**n. oliva'ris**  [ NA ], inferior olivary n.; a large aggregate of small, densely packed nerve cells arranged in a strongly folded lamina that is shaped like a purse with the opening or hilus directed medially. It corresponds in position to the oliva, or olive, a marked ovoid elevation of the ventral surface of the medulla oblongata lateral to the pyramidal tract. It projects to all parts of the contralateral half of the cerebellar cortex by way of the olivocerebellar tract, and is believed to be the major source of cerebellar climbing fibers. Its afferent connections are imperfectly understood; they include afferents from the spinal cord and probably motor cortex, but its major input appears to be conveyed by the central tegmental tract originating at rostral levels of the brainstem.

**n. oliva'ris accesso'rius dorsa'lis**  [ NA ], dorsal accessory olivary n.; a detached part of the n. olivaris dorsal to the latter's main body.

**n. oliva'ris accesso'rius media'lis**  [ NA ], medial accessory olivary n.; n. pyramidalis (obs.); a detached part of the n. olivaris placed medial to the latter's main body, against the lateral side of the medial lemniscus and pyramidal tract.

**nuclei of origin,**  nuclei originis.

**nuclei ori'ginis**  [ NA ], nuclei of origin; motor nuclei; collections of motor neurons (forming a continuous column in the cord, discontinuous in the medulla and pons) giving origin to the spinal and cranial motor nerves.

**Pander's n.,**  a disk-shaped accumulation of white yolk immediately below the blastoderm in an avian egg.

**paracentral n. of thalamus,**  n. paracentralis thalami.

**n. paracentra'lis thal'ami,**  paracentral n. of the thalamus; one of the intralaminar nuclei of the thalamus, placed medial to the n. centralis lateralis.

**paraventricular n.,**  n. paraventricularis.

**n. paraventricula'ris**  [ NA ], paraventricular n.; n. filiformis; a triangular group of large neurons in the periventricular zone of the anterior half of the hypothalamus. The cells of the n. are very similar to those of the supraoptic n.; the axons of about 20 per cent of their number join in the formation of the supraopticohypophysial tract and must therefore be functionally associated with the posterior lobe of the hypophysis.

**Perlia's n.,**  Spitzka's n.; convergence n. of Perlia; a small cell group located between the oculomotor nuclei of the left and right side. Since it is placed between the groups of motor neurons innervating, respectively, the left and right medial rectus muscles, the n. is traditionally considered to represent an integrating mechanism for ocular convergence.

**pontine nuclei,**  nuclei pontis.

**nuclei pon'tis**  [ NA ], pontine nuclei; pontine gray matter; the very large mass of gray matter filling the ventral part of the metencephalon, or pons. The pontine nuclei are of fairly homogeneous architecture; they project to the cortex of the contralateral cerebellar hemisphere by way of the large middle cerebellar peduncle, or brachium pontis. Their main afferents come from the entire extent of the cerebral neocortex by way of the longitudinal pontine bundles. Thus, the pontine nuclei form a major way-station in the impulse conduction from the cerebral cortex to the cerebellum.

**n. poste′rior hypothal′ami** [ NA ], posterior hypothalamic n.; a large, periventricular hypothalamic n. located dorsal to the mamillary body, continuous with the central gray substance of the mesencephalon.

**posterior hypothalamic n.,** n. posterior hypothalami.

**posterior periventricular n.,** n. arcuatus (2).

**prerubral n.,** the gray matter of field H₂; see *fields* of Forel.

**n. pulpo′sus** [ L. fleshy ] [ NA ], n. gelatinosus; the soft fibrocartilage central portion of the intervertebral disk; it is regarded as a derivative of the notochord.

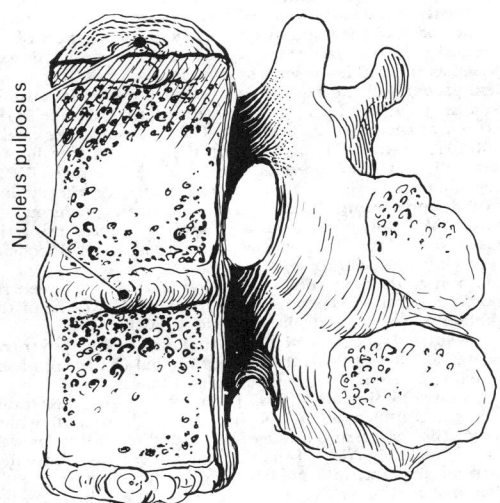

**Nucleus Pulposus**

**n. pyramida′lis,** obsolete term for n. olivaris accessorius medialis.

**raphe nuclei,** nuclei raphes.

**nuclei raph′es,** raphe nuclei; collective term denoting a variety of unpaired nerve cell groups in and along the median plane of the mesencephalic tegmentum: the n. centralis tegmenti superior of Bechterew, and the n. raphis dorsalis, n. raphis ventralis, and n. raphis anterior. The last three of these include neurons characterized by containing the indolamine transmitter agent serotonin; their serotonin-carrying axons extend rostrally to the hypothalamus, septum, hippocampus, and cingulate gyrus.

**red n.,** n. ruber.

**reduction n.,** a n. that degenerates in the cell during the changes incident to fertilization.

**reproductive n.,** micronucleus (2).

**reticular nuclei of the brainstem,** the vaguely delineated cell groups composing the gray matter of the reticular formation of the rhombencephalon and mesencephalon. In general, large-celled territories occupy the medial two-thirds of the reticular formation: n. gigantocellularis medullae oblongatae, nuclei tegmenti pontis caudalis and oralis. See also *formatio* reticularis.

**reticular n. of thalamus,** n. reticularis thalami.

**n. reticula′ris thal′ami** [ NA ], reticular n. of the thalamus; a sheet of fairly large neurons covering the lateral and ventral sides and the anterior pole of the thalamus; its reticular appearance is caused by the numerous fascicles of the thalamic peduncles which traverse the n. The n. receives numerous fibers from the cerebral cortex and projects fibers caudalward into the thalamus.

**Roller′s n.,** (1) lateral n. of the accessory nerve; (2) a small bulbar n. lying immediately anterior to the hypoglossal n., believed to be an accessory hypoglossal n.

**roof n.,** n. fastigii.

**n. ru′ber** [ NA ], red n.; a large, well defined, somewhat elongated cell mass, of reddish-gray hue in the fresh brain, located in the rostral part of the mesencephalic tegmentum. The n. receives a massive projection from the contralateral half of the cerebellum by way of the superior cerebellar peduncle, and an additional projection from the ipsilateral motor cortex. Its efferent connections are with the contralateral half of the rhombencephalic reticular formation and spinal cord by way of the rubrobulbar and rubrospinal tracts.

**n. salivato′rius infe′rior** [ NA ], inferior salivary n.; a group of preganglionic parasympathetic motor neurons located in the reticular formation of the medulla oblongata dorsal to the n. ambiguus; its axons leave the brain with the glossopharyngeal nerve and govern secretion from the parotid gland by the intermediary of the ganglion oticum.

**n. salivato′rius supe′rior** [ NA ], superior salivary n.; a group of preganglionic parasympathetic motor neurons situated rostrally and laterally to the inferior salivary n.; it governs secretion of the lacrimal, sublingual, and submaxillary glands by way of the facial nerve and the sphenopalatine and submandibular ganglia.

**Schwalbe′s n.,** n. vestibularis medialis; see nuclei vestibulares.

**secondary sensory nuclei,** nuclei terminationis.

**segmentation n.,** the compound n. in the impregnated ovum, formed by the conjugation of the nuclei of the germ cell and of the sperm cell, or the female and the male pronucleus.

**n. semiluna′ris of Flechsig,** n. arcuatus (1).

**n. senso′rius principa′lis ner′vi trigem′ini** [ NA ], n. sensorius superior nervi trigemini; the main sensory n. of the trigeminal nerve.

**n. senso′rius supe′rior ner′vi trigem′ini,** n. sensorius principalis nervi trigemini.

**shadow n.,** a n. that has lost its pigment and staining properties.

**sole nuclei,** an accumulation of skeletal muscle fiber nuclei at the myoneural junction.

**n. of solitary tract,** n. tractus solitarii.

**somatic n.,** macronucleus (2).

**somatic motor nuclei,** collective term indicating the motor nuclei innervating the tongue masculature (n. nervi hypoglossi) and the external eye muscles (n. nervi abducentis, n. nervi trochlearis, and n. nervi oculomotorii).

**special visceral efferent (or motor) nuclei,** branchiomotor nuclei.

**sperm n.,** the head of the spermatozoon, become spheroidal, after it has entered the ovum.

**spherical n.,** n. globosus.

**spinal n. of accessory nerve,** n. spinalis nervi accessorii.

**spinal n. of the trigeminus,** n. tractus spinalis nervi trigemini.

**n. spina′lis ner′vi accesso′rii** [ NA ], spinal n. of the accessory nerve; a slender column of motor neurons extending longitudinally through the central part of the ventral horn of the upper four segments of the spinal cord, giving origin to the pars spinalis of the accessory nerve.

**Spitzka′s n.,** Perlia′s n.

**Staderini′s n.,** n. intercalatus.

**Stilling′s n.,** n. thoracicus.

**subthalamic n.,** n. subthalamicus.

**n. subthalam′icus** [ NA ], subthalamic n.; n. or body of Luys; corpus luysi; a circumscript n., shaped like a biconvex lens, located in the ventral part of the subthalamus on the dorsal surface of the cerebral peduncle, immediately rostral to the substantia nigra. The n. receives a massive projection from the lateral segment of the globus pallidus, and itself projects to both pallidal segments, as well as to the mesencephalic tegmentum.

**superior olivary n.,** n. dorsalis corporis trapezoidei.

**superior salivary n.,** n. salivatorius superior.

**superior vestibular n.,** n. vestibularis superior; see nuclei vestibulares.

**supraoptic n.,** n. supraopticus hypothalami.

**n. supraop′ticus hypothal′ami** [ NA ], supraoptic n.; a large-celled n. in the hypothalamus located over the lateral border of the optic tract; it gives rise to the supraopticohypophysial tract which passes to the posterior lobe of the hypophysis. It is a neurosecretory n.; its neurons produce a hormone, the antidiuretic hormone, which is released into the general circulation from their axon terminals in the posterior lobe of the hypophysis.

**n. tec'ti,** n. fastigii.

**nuclei tegmen'ti** [ NA ], tegmental nuclei of Gudden; two small, round cell groups in the caudal part of the midbrain, associated with the mamillary body by way of the mamillary peduncle and mamillotegmental tract.

**terminal nuclei,** nuclei terminationis.

**nuclei termina'les,** nuclei terminationis.

**nuclei terminatio'nis** [ NA ], nuclei terminales; terminal nuclei; secondary sensory nuclei; collective term indicating those nerve cell groups in the rhombencephalon and spinal cord in which the afferent fibers of the spinal and cranial nerves terminate.

**thoracic n.,** n. thoracicus.

**n. thorac'icus** [ NA ], thoracic n.; dorsal n.; n. dorsalis; Clarke's n. or column; Stilling's n. or column; a column of large neurons located in the base of the posterior gray column of the spinal cord, extending from the first thoracic through the second lumbar segment; it gives rise to the dorsal spinocerebellar tract of the same side.

**n. trac'tus mesenceph'ali ner'vi trigem'ini** [ NA ], mesencephalic n. of the trigeminus; a long, narrow plate of unipolar neurons extending throughout the length of the midbrain, in and along the lateral angle of the central gray substance. The n. is the single known instance of primary sensory neurons enclosed in the central nervous system instead of in a peripheral sensory ganglion. Its peripheral axonal processes go out with the trigeminal nerve and terminate in the muscles of mastication, probably also in the external eye muscles.

**n. trac'tus solita'rii** [ NA ], n. of the solitary tract; a slender cell column extending sagittally through the dorsal part of the medulla oblongata, closely beneath the floor of the rhomboid fossa, immediately lateral to the sulcus limitans. It is the visceral sensory (visceral afferent) n. of the brainstem, receiving the afferent fibers of the vagus, glossopharyngeal, and facial nerves by way of the tractus solitarius. The caudal two-thirds of the n. process impulses originating in the pharynx, larynx, intestinal and respiratory tracts, and heart and large blood vessels (examples: the aortic and sinus nerves); its upper one-third receives impulses from the taste buds and is also known as the gustatory n.

**n. trac'tus spina'lis ner'vi trigem'ini** [ NA ], descending n. of the trigeminus; spinal n. of the trigeminus; the long sensory n. extending from the caudal border of the main sensory n. of the trigeminus down through the lateral region of the rhombencephalon into the upper three segments of the spinal cord's dorsal horn. The n. receives the fibers of the sensory root (portio major) of the trigeminus which descend along its lateral border as the tractus spinalis (or tractus descendens) nervi trigemini.

**n. of trapezoid body,** n. ventralis corporis trapezoidei.

**trochlear n.,** n. nervi trochlearis.

**n. of trochlear nerve,** n. nervi trochlearis.

**trophic n.,** macronucleus (2).

**tuberal nuclei,** nuclei tuberales.

**nuclei tubera'les** [ NA ], tuberal nuclei; lateral tuberal nuclei; two or three small, encapsulated, round or ovoid clusters of cells in the lateral hypothalamic area along the surface of the tuber cinereum; their connections and functional significance are unknown.

**ventral n. of the thalamus,** n. ventralis thalami.

**ventral anterior n. of thalamus,** n. ventralis anterior thalami.

**ventral intermediate n. of thalamus,** n. ventralis intermedius thalami.

**ventral lateral n. of thalamus,** n. ventralis intermedius thalami.

**ventral posterior n. of thalamus,** n. ventralis posterior thalami.

**ventral posterolateral n. of thalamus,** n. ventralis posterolateralis thalami.

**ventral posteromedial n. of thalamus,** n. ventralis posteromedialis thalami.

**n. ventra'lis ante'rior thal'ami,** ventral anterior n. of the thalamus (abbreviated VA); the most rostral of the subdivisions of the ventral n., receiving projections from the globus pallidus and projecting to the motor cortex.

**n. ventra'lis cor'poris trapezoi'dei** [ NA ], n. of the trapezoid body; a cell group embedded among the fibers of the trapezoid body, the major decussation of the central auditory pathway, in the lower pons. The n. receives fibers from the contralateral cochlear nuclei and itself contributes fibers to the ascending auditory system or lateral lemniscus.

**n. ventra'lis interme'dius thal'ami** [ NA ], n. ventralis lateralis (abbreviated VL); ventral intermediate or ventral lateral n. of the thalamus; the composite middle third of the ventral n. receiving partially overlapping projections from the contralateral half of the cerebellum (by way of the superior cerebellar peduncle) and the ipsilateral globus pallidus; the n. projects to the motor cortex.

**n. ventra'lis latera'lis,** n. ventralis intermedius thalami.

**n. ventra'lis poste'rior interme'dius thal'ami,** ventral posterior intermediate (VPI) n. of the thalamus; see n. ventralis posterior thalami.

**n. ventra'lis poste'rior thal'ami,** ventrobasal n.; ventral posterior n. of the thalamus; the large posterior part of the ventral n. of the thalamus receiving the somatic sensory lemnisci (medial lemniscus, spinothalamic tract, trigeminal lemniscus) and the ascending gustatory (taste) lemniscus, and projecting in turn by way of the internal capsule to the cortex of the postcentral gyrus. The n. is somatotopically subdivided into (1) a n. ventralis posterolateralis (n. ventralis posterior lateralis, commonly abbreviated VPL) representing the leg; (2) a n. ventralis posterior intermedius (VPI) representing the arm; (3) a n. ventralis posteromedialis (n. ventralis posterior medialis, VPM) representing the face; and (4) a n. arcuatus (semilunar n. of Flechsig) receiving the gustatory lemniscus.

**n. ventra'lis posterolatera'lis thal'ami** [ NA ], ventral posterolateral or ventral posterior lateral (VPL) n. of the thalamus; see n. ventralis posterior thalami.

**n. ventra'lis posteromedia'lis thal'ami** [ NA ], ventral posteromedial or ventral posterior medial (VPM) n. of the thalamus; see n. ventralis posterior thalami.

**n. ventra'lis thal'ami** [ NA ], ventral n. of the thalamus; a large, complex cell mass the external border of which forms the ventral and much of the lateral boundary, as well as the rostral border, of the thalamus; it can be subdivided into an anterior, intermediate, and posterior part.

**ventrobasal n.,** n. ventralis posterior thalami.

**ventromedial n. of hypothalamus,** n. ventromedialis hypothalami.

**n. ventromedia'lis hypothal'ami** [ NA ], ventromedial n. of the hypothalamus; a circumscript ovoid group of small neurons in the medial zone of the tuberal region of the hypothalamus. Bilateral destruction of this n. in the rat leads to severe obesity. It receives numerous fibers from the amygdala via the stria terminalis; its efferent connections are obscure.

**vestibular nuclei,** nuclei vestibulares.

**nuclei vestibula'res** [ NA ], vestibular nuclei; a group of four nuclei, the n. vestibularis lateralis (Deiters' n.), n. vestibularis medialis (Schwalbe's n.), n. vestibularis superior (Bechterew's n.), and n. vestibularis inferior, located in the lateral region of the hindbrain closely beneath the floor of the rhomboid fossa. They receive the incoming fibers of the vestibular nerve, are reciprocally connected with the n. fastigii and flocculonodular lobe of the cerebellum, and project by way of the medial longitudinal fasciculus to the abducens, trochlear, and oculomotor nuclei and to the ventral horn of the spinal cord, on both left and right side. The n. vestibularis lateralis in addition projects to the ipsilateral ventral horn of the spinal cord by the vestibulospinal tract.

---

**nuclide** (nu'klīd). A particular (atomic) nuclear species with defined characteristics and properties. See also isotope.

**Nuel** (nü-el'), Jean P., Belgian ophthalmologist and otologist, 1847–1920. See N.'s *space.*

**Nuhn** (noon), Anton, Heidelberg anatomist, 1814–1889. See N.'s *gland.*

**nulligravida** (nul'ĭ-grav'ĭ-dah) [ L. *nullus,* none, + *gravida,* pregnant ]. A woman who has never conceived.

**nullipara** (nul-ip'ă-rah) [ L. *nullus,* none, + *pario,* to bear ]. A woman who has never borne any children.

**nullipar'ity.** The condition of having borne no children.

**nullip'arous.** Never having borne children.

**nullisomic** (nul'ĭ-so'mik) [ L. *nullus*, none, + G. *sōma*, body ]. Lacking both members of a single pair of chromosomes.

**num'ber.** The place of any unit in a series; abbreviated No.

   **atomic n.**, charge n.; the n. of negatively charged electrons in an uncharged atom, or the number of protons in its nucleus; it indicates the position of the element in the periodic system.

   **Avogadro's n.**, the n. of molecules in one gram-molecular weight of any compound; defined as the number of atoms in 0.012 kg. of pure carbon-12; it equals $6.02 \times 10^{23}$.

   **Brinell hardness n.**, a n. related to the size of the permanent impression made by a ball indenter of specified size (usually 10 mm. in diameter) pressed into the surface of the material under a specified load,

$$ \text{BHN} = \cfrac{P}{\cfrac{\pi D}{2} \left( D - \sqrt{D^2 - d^2} \right)} $$

where $P$ = applied load in kg., $D$ = diameter of the ball in mm. and $d$ = diameter of the impression in mm.

   **charge n.**, atomic n.

   **dibucaine n.**, see under dibucaine.

   **electronic n.**, the n. of electrons in the outermost orbit (valence shell) of an element.

   **Hehner n.**, the weight of the nonvolatile fatty acids yielded by 5 gm. of a saponified fat or oil.

   **hydrogen n.**, see under hydrogen.

   **iodine n.**, see under iodine.

   **Knoop hardness n.**, a n. obtained by dividing the load in kg. applied to pyramid-shaped diamond of specific size divided by the projected area of the impression: KHN = $L/A$, where $A$ = the projected area of the impression in sq. mm., and $L$ = the load in kg. This is used for measurements of hardness of any materials, especially very hard and brittle substances such as tooth dentin and enamel.

   **Koettstorfer n.**, saponification number; see under saponification.

   **Loschmidt's n.**, the n. of molecules in 1 ml. of gas at 0°C. and 1 atmosphere of presssure; Avogadro's n. divided by 22,400.

   **Mach n.** (mock), a n. representing the ratio between the speed of an object moving through a fluid medium, such as air, and the speed of sound in the same medium.

   **mass n.**, the mass of the atom of a particular isotope relative to hydrogen-1 (or to 1/12 the mass of carbon-12); generally very close to the whole number represented by the sum of the protons and neutrons in the atomic nucleus of the isotope; indicated in the name or symbol of the isotope, thus: oxygen-16 or $^{16}$O; not to be confused with the atomic weight of an element, which may include a number of isotopes in natural proportion.

   **Polenské n.**, the n. of ml. of 0.1 N KOH required to neutralize the nonvolatile fatty acids obtained from 5 gm. of a saponified fat or oil.

   **Reichert-Meissl n.**, volatile fatty acid n.; an index of the volatile acid content of a fat; the n. of ml. of 0.1 N KOH required to neutralize the soluble volatile fatty acids in 5 gm. of fat. that has been saponified, acidified to liberate the fatty acids, and then steam-distilled.

   **saponification n.**, see under saponification.

   **thi'ocyan'ogen n.**, see under thiocyanogen.

   **transport n.**, the fraction of the total current carried through a solution by a particular type of ion present in that solution.

   **wave n.**, the n. of waves (of any wave form such as light or sound) per unit length.

**numb'ness.** A peculiar sensation due to combined anesthesia and paresthesia.

   **waking n.**, night palsy; a temporary n. and paresis of the extremities experienced on waking or after lying down for a long period.

**num'miform.** Nummular.

**nummular** (num'u-lar) [ L. *nummus*, coin ]. Nummiform. 1. Discoid or coin-shaped; denoting the thick mucous sputum in certain respiratory diseases. 2. Arranged like stacks of coins, denoting the association of the red blood corpuscles with flat surfaces apposed, forming rouleaux.

**nummulation** (num'u-la'shun). The formation of nummular masses.

**Nunn's gorged corpuscles.** See under corpuscles.

**nunnation** (nun-a'shun) [ Ar. *nūn*, the letter n. ]. A form of stammering in which the *n* sound is given to other consonants.

**nurse** [ O. Fr. *nourice*, fr. L. *nutrix*, wet-nurse, nurse, fr. *nutrio*, to sucke, to tend ]. 1. To suckle; to give suck to an infant. 2. To perform all the necessary offices in the care of the sick. 3. A woman who has the care of an infant or young child. 4. One who has the care of a sick person, performing all the necessary offices in relation to the toilet, giving of food and medicine, etc., under the direction of a physician.

   **n. anesthetist,** a person who, after completing basic educational requirements as a nurse, is additionally trained for 1 to 2 years in the administration of anesthetics, in order to function thereafter as an anesthetist under the direction of a physician.

   **charge n.**, a n. in charge of a hospital ward.

   **community n., district n.**, a visiting n. whose field of action is limited to a certain district.

   **dry n.**, a child's n. who does not suckle the infant.

   **general duty n.**, one who does not specialize in any form of group nursing, but who is available for any duty of her profession.

   **graduate n.**, one who has been graduated from a recognized training school.

   **head n.**, (1) supervisor; a graduate n. at the head of the nursing staff in a hospital; called "sister" in Great Britain; (2) charge n.

   **health n.**, a community n., charged with the duty of instructing the families to which she is sent in general hygiene and the prevention of disease.

   **hospital n.**, one on duty in the wards of a hospital; see general duty, group, and special nursing.

   **monthly n.**, one attending confinement cases, engaged usually for a period of four weeks.

   **practical n.**, one who has had experience in the care of the sick and has received more or less instruction from the physicians with whom she has worked, but who is not a graduate of a training school.

   **private duty n.**, one who is not a member of the hospital staff, but is called upon to take special care of an individual patient.

   **probationer n.**, a young woman in a training school who is not yet accepted as a student but is under observation as to her fitness for nursing duty.

   **public health n.**, a graduate n. working under the direction of a public health official, who acts as the connecting link between that official and the lay public, and whose duties in relation to the community and the health office are similar on a large scale to the more restricted duties of the school n.

   **registered n.**, a graduate n. who has satisfied the state authorities regarding her qualifications and is entitled to affix the initials R.N. to her name.

   **school n.**, a graduate n. who examines the children in one or more schools, reporting any serious or infectious disease or eye or ear defect among the pupils to the school physician, and carrying out his directions in the care of defectives and in relation to the hygiene of the school and of the pupils' homes.

   **scrub n.**, one who has scrubbed arms and hands, donned sterile gloves and, usually, a sterile gown, and passes instruments to the operating surgeon.

   **sick n.**, see n. (4).

   **special n.**, (1) one who specializes in the care of patients suffering from diseases of a particular class, such as surgical cases, tuberculosis, children's diseases, etc.; (2) private n.

   **student n.**, an undergraduate member of a hospital training school.

   **theatre n.** in Great Britain the chief assistant to the theatre (operating room) sister.

   **trained n.**, same as graduate n.

**visiting n.,** one who has charge of several sick persons, visiting each every day and performing the necessary offices.

**wet n.,** a woman who suckles a child not her own.

**nurs'ing.** Feeding an infant at the breast; tending and taking care of a child; caring for the mentally or physically ill or infirm; in general, performing the duties of a nurse in any sense.

**divisional n.,** group n.

**general duty n.,** the work of a hospital nurse who is not in charge of one (special n. (1)) or more (group n.) patients, or of one suffering from a disease of a particular group (special n. (2)), but is available for any duty of her profession.

**group n.,** a development of special n. (1) in which one nurse has the care of two or more patients in the same neighborhood.

**industrial n.,** caring for the sick or injured in large industrial plants; the work of one or more whole time nurses, assisting the medical officer of the plant.

**n. home,** a convalescent home or small private hospital.

**special n.,** (1) service rendered by a nurse to one patient only; (2) service restricted to the n. of those suffering from maladies of a particular class, such as surgical, pediatric, psychiatric, obstetrical, etc.

**Nussbaum** (noos'bowm), Johann N. von, German surgeon, 1829–1890. See N.'s *bracelet.*

**Nussbaum** (noos'bowm), Moritz, German histologist, 1850–1915. See N.'s *experiment.*

**nutation** (nu-ta'shun) [ L. *annuere*, to nod ]. The act of nodding, especially involuntary nodding.

**nut'gall.** Galla; gall (3); oak apple; an excrescence on the oak, *Quercus infectoria* (family Fagaceae) and other species of *Quercus*, caused by the deposit of the ova of a fly, *Cynips gallae tinctorae.* An astringent and styptic, by virtue of the tannin it contains.

**nut'meg.** Myristica; the dried ripe seed of *Myristica fragrans* (family Myristicaceae), ), deprived of its seed coat and arillode; an aromatic stimulant, carminative, condiment, and source of volatile and expressed nutmeg oils; it is consumed for its bizarre central nervous system effects; see also myristicin.

**n. oil,** myristica oil; the volatile oil distilled from the dried kernels of the ripe seeds of *Myristica fragrans;* used as a flavoring agent and a carminative; in large quantities, may produce narcosis and delirium.

**n. oil, expressed,** n. butter; oil of mace; fixed oil expressed from *Myristica fragrans;* rubefacient.

**n. oil, volatile,** see n. oil.

**nutricius** [ L. ] [ NA ]. Nourishing; nutritious.

**nutrient** (nu'tri-ent) [ L. *nutriens*, fr. *nutrio*, to nourish ]. An item of food; may be essential or nonessential.

**nu'trilites** [ L. *nutrio*, to suckle, nourish ]. Essential nutritional factors.

**nutrition** (nu-trish'un) [ L. *nutritio*, fr. *nutrio*, to nourish ]. 1. A function of living plants and animals, consisting in the taking in and assimilation through chemical changes (metabolism) of material whereby tissue is built up and energy liberated; its successive stages are known as digestion, absorption, assimilation, and excretion; in highly organized animals digestion is preceded by mastication and deglutition, and excretion is effected by expiration, perspiration, urination, and defecation. 2. The study of the food and drink requirements of human beings or animals for maintenance, growth, activity, reproduction, and lactation.

**nutriture** [ L. *nutritura*, a nursing, fr. *nutrio*, to suckle, nourish ]. State or condition of the nutrition of the body; state of the body with regard to nourishment.

**Nuttall,** George H. F., American biologist, 1862–1937. See N.'s *stain.*

**Nuttal'lia** [ G. H. F. *Nuttall* ]. Former name for *Babesia.*

**nux vom'ica** [ Mod. L. emetic nut, fr. L. *nux,* nut, + *vomo,* to vomit ] (BP). Strychnos seed; poison nut; Quaker button; the seed of *Strychnos nux-vomica* (family Logeniaceae), a tree of tropical Asia; it contains two alkaloids, strychnine and brucine; has been used as a bitter tonic and central nervous system stimulant.

**nyct-.** See nycto-.

**nyctalbuminuria** (nik-tal-bu-min-u'ri-ah) [ nyct- + albumin + G. *ouron,* urine ]. Noctalbuminuria; a form of cyclic albuminuria, occurring at night.

**nyctalgia** (nik-tal'ji-ah) [ nyct- + G. *algos,* pain ]. Night pain; denoting especially the osteocopic pains of syphilis occurring at night.

**nyctalopia** (nik'ta-lo'pi-ah) [ nyct- + G. *alaos,* obscure, + *ōps,* eye ]. Night blindness; nocturnal amblyopia; inability to see as well as persons with normal sight at night or in a dim light.

**n. with congenital myopia,** a condition evident in the first year of life and characterized by low visual acuity, strabismus, or nystagmus; x-linked recessive inheritance.

**nycterine** (nik'ter-in, nik'ter-in) [ G. *nykterinos* ]. 1. By night. 2. Dark; obscure.

**nycterohemeral** (nik-ter-o-he'mer-al) [ G. *nykteros,* by night, nightly (NOCT-), + *hēmera,* day ]. Both daily and nightly.

**nycto-, nyct-** (nik'to-) [ G. *nyx,* night. NOCT- ]. Combining forms for night, nocturnal.

**nyctophilia** (nik-to-fil'i-ah) [ nycto- + G. *philos,* fond ]. Scotophilia; preference for the night or darkness.

**nyctophobia** (nik'to-fo'bi-ah) [ nycto- + G. *phobos,* fear ]. Scotophobia; morbid fear of night or of the dark.

**Nyctotherus** (nik-to-the'rus) [ G. *nyktothēras,* one who hunts by night, fr. *thēraō,* to hunt, fr. *thēr,* wild beast ]. A genus of Ciliophora one species of which, *N. faba,* has been reported, though rarely, from the human intestine; it is generally found in amphibia.

**nyctotyphlosis** (nik'to-tif-lo'sis) [ nycto- + G. *typhlōsis,* blindness, fr. *typhlos,* blind ]. Nyctalopia.

**nyctu'ria.** Nocturia.

**Nyhan,** W. L. See Lesch-N. *syndrome.*

**nylidrin hydrochloride** (ni'li-drin, nil-) (NF). ARLIDIN hydrochloride; 1-(p-hydroxyphenyl)-2-(1-methyl-3-phenylpropylamino) propanol hydrochloride; a sympathomimetic similar to isoproterenol; produces vasodilation of arterioles of skeletal muscles and increases muscle blood flow. Used in the treatment of peripheral vascular diseases.

**nymph** (nimf) [ G. *nymphē,* maiden, NYMPH- ]. The earliest stage in the development of certain insects (*e.g.,* the locusts) immediately after hatching. It resembles the adult in many respects, but shows certain important differences. It grows without any intermediate stage into the imago or adult form.

**nympha,** pl. **nym'phae** (nim'fah) [ Mod. L. fr. G. *nymphē,* a bride. NYMPH- ]. One of the labia minora.

**nymphal** (nim'fal). 1. Pertaining to a nymph. 2. Pertaining to the nymphae (labia minora).

**nymphectomy** (nim-fek'to-mi) [ nympha + G. *ektomē,* excision ]. Surgical removal of the hypertrophied nymphae.

**nymphitis** (nim-fi'tis) [ nympha + G. suffix *-itis,* inflammation ]. Inflammation of the nymphae.

**nympho-, nymph-** (nim'fo-, nimf-) [ L. *nympha, q.v.* NYMPH- ]. Combining forms relating to the nymphae (labia minora).

**nym'phola'bial.** Relating to the nymphae, or labia minora, and the labia majora; denoting a furrow between the two labia on each side.

**nympholepsy** (nim'fo-lep'si) [ nympho- + G. *lēpsis,* a seizure. LAB- ]. Ecstasy; transport; especially one of an erotic nature.

**nym'phoma'nia** [ nympho- + G. *mania,* frenzy ]. Andromania; estromania; extreme eroticism, or sexual desire, in women.

**nym'phoma'niac.** A woman exhibiting nymphomania.

**nym'phomani'acal.** Pertaining to, or exhibiting, nymphomania.

**nymphoncus** (nim-fongk'us) [ nympho- + G. *onkos,* tumor ]. A swelling or hypertrophy of one or both labia minora.

**nymphotomy** (nim-fot'o-mi) [ nympho- + G. *tomē,* incision ]. An incision into the nymphae, or the clitoris.

**nystagmic** (nis-tag'mik). Relating to or suffering from nystagmus.

**nystag'miform.** Nystagmoid.

**nystag′mogram.** The tracing produced by nystagmography.

**nystag′mograph.** An apparatus for indicating graphically the movements of the eyeball in nystagmus; the receiving tambour is placed on the upper lid of the closed eye, the oscillations being recorded by means of a registering apparatus similar to that of the cardiograph

**nystagmography** (nis′tag-mog′rǎ-fi). The technique of documenting nystagmus via amplifiers and a pen recorder.

**electro-n.,** see electronystagmography.

**photoelectric n.,** a more recent technique based on photosensor oculography; it provides a greater electric potential than electro-oculography and portable apparatus.

**nystagmoid** (nis-tag′moyd) [ nystagmus + G. *eidos*, resemblance ]. Nystagmiform; resembling nystagmus.

**nystagmus** (nis-tag′mus) [ G. *nystagmos*, a nodding, fr. *nystazō*, to be sleepy, nod ]. Rhythmical oscillation of the eyeballs, either horizontal, rotary, or vertical.

**n. against the rule,** miner's n. excited when the eyes are directed downward.

**ataxic n.,** dissociated n.

**aural n.,** labyrinthine n.

**caloric n.,** see Bárány's *sign.*

**central n.,** reflex from stimulation arising in the central nervous system.

**Cheyne's n.,** a n. with a rhythm like that of Cheyne-Stokes respiration.

**congenital n.,** (1) congenitally predetermined n. caused by lesions sustained in utero or at the time of birth; (2) inherited n., usually sex-linked, without associated neurologic lesions and nonprogressive; (3) the n. associated with albinism, achromatopsia, and hypoplasia of the macula.

**dissociated n.,** incongruent n.; ataxic n.; in internuclear ophthalmoplegia, when abduction is attempted, the eye with the paralyzed medial rectus shows only a fine n., while the other eye has a course, slow, jerky n. with rapid component in the direction of lateral gaze.

**end-position n.,** a jerky, physiologic n. occurring in a normal individual when attempts are made to fixate a point at the limits of the field of fixation.

**fixation n.,** opticokinetic n.

**incongruent n.,** dissociated n.

**jerk n.,** n. in which the oscillations are faster in one direction than in the other, so that the combined cycle has a characteristic jerky rhythm.

**labyrinthine n.,** aural n.; a mixed horizontal and rotary n. in presence of labyrinthine manifestations, *e.g.,* vertigo.

**latent n.,** jerk n. that is brought out by covering one eye.

**lateral n.,** a form in which the eyes oscillate from side to side.

**miner's n.,** n. occurring in coal miners who wield the pick while lying on the side in a constrained position; when not constantly present it can be elicited by turning the eyes upward.

**ocular n.,** a continuous wandering or searching movement of the eye.

**opticokinetic n., optokinetic n.,** n. brought on by visual stimuli; also called fixation or railroad n.

**pal′atal n.,** a clonic spasm of the levator palati muscle, causing an audible click.

**pendular n.,** n. characterized by oscillations that, in some positions of gaze, are approximately equal in rate for the two directions.

**railroad n.,** opticokinetic n.

**n. retractorius,** irregular jerks of the eye backward into the orbit when the patient attempts to look in one or the other direction.

**ro′tatory n.,** a slight movement of the eyes around the visual axis.

**see-saw n.,** a disjunctive vertical pendular n.; said to be ocular in origin.

**vertical n.,** an up-and-down oscillation of the eyes.

**vestib′ular n.,** n. occurring as a reflex of disease of the ear; when due to otic irritation the more rapid eye movement is toward the side of the affected ear; when due to paralysis of one vestibular nerve it is toward the sound side; see Bárány's *sign.*

**voluntary n.,** a special case of pendular n. in which the subject can at will cause his eyes to make extremely fine and rapid horizontal oscillations (500 to 600 per minute).

**nystatin** (nis′tǎ-tin) (USP, BP). Mycostatin; an antibiotic substance isolated from cultures of *Streptomyces noursei.* Effective in the treatment of all forms of moniliasis, particularly monilial infections of the intestine, skin, and mucous membranes.

**Nysten's law.** See under law.

**nyxis** (nik′sis) [ G. ]. A pricking; puncture; paracentesis.

# O

**O.** 1. Chemical symbol of the element oxygen. 2. In formulas for electrical reactions, abbreviation for opening. 3. Abbreviation for *oculus*, eye. 4. Abbreviation for *octarius*, pint. 5. Symbol for a blood group in the ABO system. See ABO blood group, appendix 2. 6. An abbreviation derived from *ohne Hauch* (*i.e.*, without a film), used as a designation for (*a*) antigens that occur in the bacterial cell—in contrast to those in the flagella, or (*b*) specific antibodies for such somatic antigens, or (*c*) the agglutinative reaction between somatic antigen and its antibody. 7. Symbol for orotidine.

**o-.** In chemistry, abbreviation for *ortho-*.

**oak.** Quercus.

**oari-, oario-** (o'ā-rī-, o-ăr'ī-o-) [ G. *ōarion*, a small egg, dim. of *ōon*, egg ]. Rarely used combining forms denoting ovary; for most such words, see ovario-, oophoro-.

**oarialgia** (o'a-rī-al'jī-ah) [ oari- + G. *algos*, pain ]. Ovarialgia.

**oaric** (o-ăr'ik). Ovarian.

**oariotomy** (o-ăr'ī-ot'o-mī). Ovariotomy.

**oaritis** (o-ăr-i'tis). Oophoritis.

**oarium** (o-ăr'ī-um) [ G. *ōarion*, a small egg ]. Ovary.

**oath** (ōth). A solemn affirmation or attestation. See Hippocratic Oath, under Hippocrates, and the Veterinarian's Oath, under veterinarian.

**obcecation** (ob'se-ka'shun) [ L. *ob-*, near, + *caecitas*, blindness, fr. *caecus*, blind ]. Partial blindness.

**obdormition** (ob-dor-mish'un) [ L. *ob-dormio*, pp. -*itus*, to sleep ]. Numbness of an extremity, due to pressure on the sensory nerve.

**O'Beirne** (o-burn'), James, Irish surgeon, 1786–1862. See O.'s *sphincter*.

**obe'liac.** Relating to the obelion.

**obe'liad.** Toward the obelion.

**obelion** (ŏ-be'lĭ-on) [ G. *obelos*, a spit ]. A craniometric point on the sagittal suture between the parietal foramina near the lambdoid suture. See fig. under craniometric *point*.

**Ober,** Frank R., U. S. surgeon, *1881. See O.'s *operation*.

**Obermayer,** Friedrich, Vienna physician, 1861–1925. See O.'s *test*.

**Obermeier,** Otto H. F., German physician, 1843–1873. See O.'s *spirillum*.

**Obersteiner,** H., Austrian neurologist, 1847–1922. See O.-Redlich *line, zone*.

**obese** (o-bēs') [ L. *obesus*, fat, partic. adj., fr. *ob-edo*, pp. -*esus*, to eat away, devour ]. Extremely fat or corpulent.

**obe'sity** [ see obese ]. Fatness; corpulence; general adiposity; an abnormal increase of fat in the subcutaneous connective tissues.

**hypothalamic o.,** o. caused by disease of the hypothalamus.

**morbid o.,** o. sufficient to prevent normal activity; in extreme cases (Pickwickian syndrome) respiratory failure is brought on by slight exertion or by assuming a horizontal position.

**simple o.,** ordinary o.; o. resulting when caloric intake exceeds energy expenditure.

**o'bex** [ L. barrier ] [ NA ]. The point on the midline of the dorsal surface of the medulla oblongata that marks the caudal angle of the rhomboid fossa or fourth ventricle. It corresponds to a small, transverse medullary fold overhanging the calamus scriptorius.

**obfuscation** (ob-fus-ka'shun) [ L. *ob-fusco*, pp. -*atus*, to darken, fr. *fuscus*, dark, tawny ]. 1. A rendering dark or obscure. 2. Confusion. 3. Obscurantism.

**ob'ject.** 1. Anything to which thought or action is directed. 2. In psychoanalysis, that through which an instinct can achieve its aim. 3. Also in psychoanalysis, often used synonymously with aim.

**good o.,** in psychoanalysis, the good or supporting aspects of an important person in the patient's life, especially of a parent or parent-surrogate.

**sex o.,** a person toward whom another is sexually attracted.

**test o.,** an o. having very fine surface markings, mounted on a slide, used to determine the defining power of the o. lens of a microscope.

**objec'tive** [ L. *ob-jicio*, pp.-*jectus*, to throw before, fr. *jacio* ]. 1. The lens or lenses in the lower end of a microscope, by means of which the rays coming from the object examined are brought to a focus. See fig. under microscope. 2. Viewing events or phenomena as they exist in the external world, impersonally or in an unprejudiced way; open to observation by oneself and by others; the opposite of subjective.

**achromatic o.,** an o. that is corrected for two colors chromatically, and one color spherically.

**apochromatic o.,** an o. in which chromatic aberration is corrected for three colors and spherical abberation is corrected for two.

**immersion o.,** a high power o. used with a drop of oil between the lens and the specimen on the slide. Similar lenses are available for use with water as the immersing liquid.

**obligate** (ob'lĭ-gāt) [ L. *ob-ligo*, pp. -*atus*, to bind to ]. Without an alternative pathway; see obligate *parasite*.

**oblique** (ob-lēk') [ L. *obliquus* ]. Slanting; deviation from the perpendicular or the horizontal.

**obliquity** (ob-lik'wĭ-tī). Asynclitism.

**Litzmann o.,** posterior asynclitism; inclination of the fetal head so that the biparietal diameter is oblique in relation to the plane of the pelvic brim, the posterior parietal bone presenting to the parturient canal.

**Nägele o.,** anterior asynclitism; inclination of the fetal head in cases of flat pelvis, so that the biparietal diameter is oblique in relation to the plane of the brim, the anterior parietal bone presenting to the parturient canal.

**obliquus** (ob-li'kwus) [ L. slanting, oblique ] [ NA ]. Denoting a structure having an oblique course or direction; a name given, with further qualification, to several muscles; see under musculus.

**obliteration** (ob-lit'er-a'shun) [ L. *oblittero*, to blot out ]. Blotting out, especially by filling of a natural space or lumen by fibrosis or inflammation.

**oblivis'cence** [ L. *oblivio*, to forget ]. Forgetfulness.

**oblongata** (ob-long-gah'tah) [ L. fem. of *oblongatus*, from *oblongus*, rather long ]. *Medulla* oblongata.

**obmutescence** (ob-mu-tes'ens) [ L. *ob-mutesco*, to become dumb, fr. *mutus*, dumb ]. Dumbness; loss of the voice or of the power of speech.

**obnubilation** (ob-nu-bil-a'shun) [ L. *ob-nubilo*, pp. -*atus*, to overcloud, befog, fr. *nubes*, a cloud ]. A beclouded mental state.

**obscurantism** (ob-skūr'an-tizm). Obfuscation (3); a deliberate attempt to keep others from understanding.

**obser'ver** [ L. *observo*, to watch ]. One who perceives, notices, or watches.

**nonparticipant o.,** an investigator who studies a group of subjects engaged in certain activities (*e.g.*, group psychotherapy) but does not directly participate in these activities; presumably, he is able to study them more objectively.

**participant o.,** an investigator who, while studying the activities of a group of subjects (*e.g.*, in group psychotherapy), also participates in their activities; presumably, he is thus able to gain more detailed, relevant information.

**obsession** (ob-sesh'un) [ L. *obsideo*, pp. -*sessus*, to besiege, fr. *sedeo*, to sit ]. A condition, usually associated with anxiety and dread, in which one idea constantly fills the mind despite one's efforts to ignore or dislodge it.

**impulsive o.,** an o. accompanied by action, sometimes becoming a mania (*q. v.*).

**inhibitory o.,** an o. involving an impediment to action, usually representing a phobia (*q. v.*).

**obses'sive-compul'sive.** Having a tendency to perform certain repetitive acts or ritualistic behavior to relieve anxiety; see also obsessive-compulsive *neurosis* and obsessive-compulsive *personality*.

**obsolescence** (ob'so-les'ens) [ L. *obsolescere*, to grow out of use ]. Falling into disuse; denoting the abolition of a function.

**obstet'ric, obstet'rical.** Relating to obstetrics.

**obstetrician** (ob'stĕ-trish'un) [ see obstetrics ]. One who is skilled in the medical care of a woman during pregnancy and childbirth.

**obstet'rics** [ L. *obstetrix*, a midwife, fr. *ob-sto*, to stand before, denoting the position formerly taken by the midwife ]. The branch of medicine that has to do with the care of the pregnant woman during pregnancy, parturition, and the puerperium.

**obstipation** (ob'stĭ-pa'shun) [ L. *ob*, against, + *stipo*, pp. -*atus*, to crowd ]. Intestinal obstruction; severe constipation.

**obstruction** (ob-struk'shun) [ L. *obstructio* ]. Blockage or clogging, *e.g.*, by occlusion or stenosis.
 **closed-loop o.**, o. of a segment of intestine by rotation on a fixed point (see volvulus); frequently causes impairment of circulation from and to the affected segment bowel, resulting in strangulation and gangrene; the segment of intestine contained in the hernia may also become a closed-loop o. when compression occurs at the neck of the sac.
 **uteropelvic o.**, a blocking or stenosis at the junction of the renal pelvis and ureter, usually resulting in stasis, hydronephrosis, and calyceal clubbing.

**obstruent** (ob'stru-ent) [ L. *ob-struo*,pp. -*structus*, to build against, obstruct ]. 1. Obstructing; blocking advance. 2. An agent that obstructs or prevents a normal discharge, especially a discharge from the bowels.

**obtund'** [ L. *ob-tundo*, pp. -*tusus*, to beat against, blunt ]. To dull or blunt, especially to blunt sensation or deaden pain.

**obtun'dent.** 1. Dulling; making less acute. 2. An agent that blunts sensibility or deadens pain.

**obturation** (ob'tu-ra'shun) [ see obturator ]. A stopping up or obstructing; occlusion.

**ob'turator** [ L. *obturo*, pp. -*atus*, to occlude or stop up ]. 1. Any structure that occludes an opening. 2. Denoting a large opening in the lower part of the hip bone, the obturator foramen, the occluding membrane of the same, or any of several parts in relation to this foramen. 3. A prosthesis used to close a congenital or acquired opening in the palate.

**obtuse** (ob-tūs') [ see obtund ]. 1. Dull in intellect; of slow understanding. 2. Blunt; not acute.

**obtusion** (ob-tu'zhun). 1. Dullness of sensibility. 2. Dulling or deadening sensibility.

**occipital** (ok-sip'ĭ-tal). Relating to the occiput.

**occipital'lis** [ L. ]. The posterior belly of the scalp muscle; see *musculus* epicranius.

**occipitalization** (ok'sip'ĭ-tal-ĭ-za'shun). Bony ankylosis between the atlas and occipital bone.

**occipito-** (ok-sip'ĭ-to-) [ L. *occiput, q.v.* ]. Combining form for occiput, occipital.

**occipitoatloid** (ok-sip'ĭ-to-at'loyd). Relating to the occipital bone and the atlas; denoting the articulation between the two bones.

**occipitoaxial, occipitoaxoid** (ok-sip'ĭ-to-aks'ĭ-al, -ak'-soyd). Relating to the occipital bone and the axis, or epistropheus.

**occipitobregmatic** (ok-sip'ĭ-to-breg-mat'ik). Relating to the occiput and the bregma; denoting a measurement in craniometry.

**occip'itofa'cial.** Relating to the occiput and the face.

**occip'itofron'tal.** 1. Relating to the occiput and the forehead. 2. Relating to the occipital and frontal lobe of the cerebral cortex.

**occip'itofronta'lis** [ L. ]. See under musculus.

**occip'itomas'toid.** Relating to the occipital bone and the mastoid process.

**occip'itomen'tal.** Relating to the occiput and the chin.

**occipitoparietal** (ok-sip'ĭ-to-pă-ri'e-tal). Relating to the occipital and the parietal bones.

**occip'itotem'poral.** Relating to the occiput and the temple, or the occipital and the temporal bones.

**occip'itothalam'ic.** Relating to the nerve fibers leading from the occipital lobe of the cerebral cortex to the thalamus.

**occiput,** gen. **occip'itis** (ok'sĭ-put) [ L. See CAP-1 ] [ NA ]. The back of the head.

**occlude** (o-klūd) [ see occlusion ]. To close or bring together.

**occlu'der.** In dentistry, a name given to some articulators.

**occlusal** (o-klu'zal). 1. Pertaining to occlusion or closure. 2. In dentistry, pertaining to the contacting surfaces of opposing occlusal units (teeth or occlusion rims), or the masticating surfaces of the posterior teeth.

**occlusion** (o-klu'zhun) [ L. *oc-cludo*, pp. -*clusus*, to shut up, fr. *ob*, against, + *claudo*, to close. CLAUS- ]. 1. The act of closing or the state of being closed. 2. In chemistry, the absorption of a gas by a metal or the inclusion of one substance within another (as in a gelatinous precipitate). 3. Any contact between the incising or masticating surfaces of the upper and lower teeth. 4. The relationship between the occlusal surfaces of the maxillary and mandibular teeth when they are in contact.
 **abnormal o.**, an arrangement of the teeth which is not considered to be within the normal range of variation.
 **afunctional o.**, a malocclusion which does not permit normal function of the dentition.
 **anterior o.**, (1) mesio-occlusion; (2) the o. of anterior teeth.
 **balanced o.**, balanced bite; balanced articulation; the simultaneous contacting of the upper and lower teeth on the right and left and in the anterior and posterior occlusal areas in centric and eccentric positions within the functional range. It is thought of primarily in the mouth, but may be arranged and observed on articulators. This o. is developed to prevent a tipping or rotating of the denture bases in relation to the supporting structures.
 **buccal o.**, malposition of a tooth toward the cheek; also the occlusion as seen from the buccal side of the teeth.
 **centric o.**, centric contact; (1) the relation of opposing occlusal surfaces which provides the maximum planned contact and/or intercuspation; (2) the o. of the teeth when the mandible is in centric relation to the maxillae.
 **components of o.**, see under component.
 **coronary o.**, blockage of a coronary vessel usually by thrombosis and usually leading to infarction of the myocardium.
 **curve of o.**, see under curve.
 **distal o.**, (1) distocclusion; (2) a tooth occluding in a position distal to normal.
 **eccentric o.**, any o. other than centric.
 **edge-to-edge o.**, edge-to-edge bite; end-to-end bite or o.; an o. in which the anterior teeth of both jaws meet along their incisal edges when the teeth are in centric o.
 **end-to-end o.**, edge-to-edge o.
 **functional o.**, (1) any tooth contacts made within the functional range of the opposing teeth surfaces; (2) o. which occurs during function.
 **gliding o.**, dental *articulation*.
 **hyperfunctional o.**, occlusal stress of tooth or teeth exceeding normal physiologic demands.
 **labial o.**, malposition of a tooth in a labial direction; also the o. as seen from the labial side of the arches.
 **lateral o.**, malposition of a tooth or an entire dental arch in a direction away from the midline.
 **lingual o.**, (1) linguoclusion; (2) the interdigitation of the teeth as seen from the internal or lingual aspect.
 **mechanically balanced o.**, a balanced o. without reference to phsyiologic considerations, as on an articulator.
 **mesenteric artery o.**, obstruction of arterial flow in the mesenteric circulation by an embolus or thrombus; usually refers to o. of the superior mesenteric artery, although atherosclerotic narrowing may involve all three major splanchnic branches (celiac, superior, and inferior mesenteric).
 **mesial o.**, an o. in which the mandibular teeth articulate with the maxillary teeth in a position anterior to normal; a mesioclusion; an angle class III malocclusion.
 **neutral o.**, an arrangement of teeth such that the maxillary and mandibular first permanent molars are in normal anteroposterior relation; neutroclusion; an angle class I malocclusion.

**normal o.,** that arrangement of teeth and their supporting structure which is usually found in health and which approaches an ideal or standard arrangement.

**pathogenic o.,** an occlusal relationship capable of producing pathologic changes in the supporting tissues.

**physiologic o.,** o. in harmony with functions of the masticatory system.

**physiologically balanced o.,** a balanced o. that is in harmony with the temperomandibular joints and the neuromuscular system.

**plane of o.,** occlusal *plane.*

**posterior o.,** the most effective contact of the molar and bicuspid teeth of both jaws which allows for all the natural movements of the jaws essential to normal mastication and closure.

**postnormal o.,** an o. in which the mandibular teeth articulate with the maxillary teeth in a position posterior to normal; a distoclusion; an angle class II malocclusion.

**protrusive o.,** that which results when the mandible is protruded forward from centric position.

**retrusive o.,** a biting relationship in which the mandible is more distally placed than is considered normal; an angle class II malocclusion; a distoclusion.

**spherical form of o.,** an arrangement of teeth which places their occlusal surfaces on the surface of an imaginary sphere (usually 8 inches in diameter) with its center above the level of the teeth. See also Monson *curve.*

**torsive o.,** torsoclusion.

**traumatic o.,** traumatogenic o.

**traumatogenic o.,** traumatic o.; a malocclusion capable of producing injury to the teeth and/or associated structures.

**working o.,** working *contacts.*

**occlu'sive.** Serving to close; denoting a bandage or dressing that closes a wound and protects it from the air.

**oc'clusom'eter.** Gnathodynamometer.

**occult** (ŏ-kult', ok'ult) [ L. *oc-culo,* pp. *-cultus,* to cover, hide, fr. *ob-* + *celo,* to hide ]. 1. Hidden; concealed. 2. Denoting a concealed hemorrhage, the blood being so changed as not to be readily recognized. See occult *blood.*

**occultus** [ L. ] [ NA ]. Occult.

**octavus** [ L. ] [ NA ]. The eighth, specifically the vestibulocochlear nerve.

**occupa'tion.** Any activity in which one engages; especially, one regularly engaged in for pay, as one's job.

**prescribed o.,** in occupational therapy, an activity which has been prescribed by the physician for a particular patient.

**occupa'tional.** Relating to occupation.

**Oceanospirillum** (o'shen-o-spi-ril'um) [ L. *oceanus,* ocean, + *spirillum,* coil ]. A genus of motile, nonsporeforming, aerobic bacteria (family Spirillaceae) containing Gram-negative, rigid, helical cells which are 0.3 to 1.2 μm in diameter. Motile cells contain bipolar fascicles of flagella. There is no growth anaerobically with nitrate. These organisms are chemoorganotrophic and possess a strictly respiratory metabolism; they neither oxidize nor ferment carbohydrates. These organisms are found in marine environments. There are at present five species in this genus, of which the type species is *O. linum.*

**ocellus,** pl. **ocell'i** (o-sel'us) [ L. dim. of *oculus,* eye ]. 1. Eyespot (2); the simple eye found in many invertebrates. 2. Facet of the compound eye of an insect.

**ochlesis** (ok-le'sis) [ G. *ochlēsis,* disturbance, fr. *ochlos,* a crowd ]. A disorder occasioned or aggravated by overcrowding.

**Ochoa,** Severo, Spanish biochemist in the United States, *1905. Nobel laureate, 1959, with Arthur Kornberg, for their discovery of the mechanisms in the biological synthesis of ribonucleic acid and deoxyribonucleic acid.

**ochrodermatosis** (o'kro-der-mă-to'sis) [ G. *ōchros,* pale yellow, sallow, + *derma,* skin, + suffix *-osis,* condition ]. Yellow disease (2); a bright yellow or saffron coloration of the skin sometimes observed in Europeans living in tropical countries, especially India; it disappears on change of residence to the hills.

**ochrodermia** (o'kro-der'mĭ-ah) [ G. *ōchros,* pale yellow, + *derma,* skin ]. Yellow discoloration of skin.

**ochrometer** (o-krom'e-ter) [ G. *ōchros,* pale yellow, + *metron,* measure ]. An instrument for determining the capillary blood pressure; one of two adjacent fingers is compressed by a rubber balloon until blanching of the skin occurs, when the force necessary to accomplish this color change is read in millimeters of mercury.

**ochronosis** (o-kron-o'sis) [ G. *ōchros,* pale yellow, + *nosos,* disease ]. A pathologic condition observed in certain patients with alkaptonuria, characterized by pigmentation of the cartilages and sometimes other tissues, such as muscle, epithelial cells, and connective tissue; it may affect also the sclera, mucous membrane of the lips, and skin of the ears, face, and hands; the urine may be dark-colored and pigmented casts may be found in it. The pigmentation is thought to result from a substance similar to melanin, produced by the action of tyrosinase on tyrosine and phenylalanine.

**exogenous o.,** darkening of the cornea and of the skin of the face and hands from prolonged exposure to phenol or resinol.

**ocular o.,** symmetrical pigmentary deposits in the corneal periphery and a diffuse scleral and episcleral pigmentation in the region of the rectus muscles.

**ochronotic** (o-kron-ot'ik). Relating to or characterized by ochronosis.

**Ochsner** (oks'ner), Albert J., Chicago surgeon, 1858–1925. See O.'s *method.*

**oc'rylate** (USAN). Octyl-2-cyanoacrylate; a tissue adhesive for surgery.

**oct-, octa-, octi-, octo-** [ G. *oktō,* L. *octo,* eight ]. Combining forms meaning eight.

**octad** (ok'tad) [ L. *octo,* eight ]. 1. Octavalent. 2. An octavalent element or radical.

**oc'tameth'yl py'rophosphor'amide.** OMPA; an anticholinesterase that is used as a plant insecticide; also occasionally used in myasthenia gravis.

**octamylamine.** OCTISAMYL; *N*-isopentyl-1,5-dimethylhexylamine; intestinal antispasmodic with anticholinergic properties.

**octan** (ok'tan) [ L. *octo,* eight ]. Applied to fever, the paroxysms of which recur every eighth day, the day of each paroxysm being included in the count.

**octapep'tide.** A peptide made up of eight amino acid residues. The posterior pituitary hormones, oxytocin and vasopressin, are o.'s.

**oc'taploid.** See polyploid.

**oc'taploidy.** See polyploidy.

**octa'rius** [ L. *octo,* eight ]. The eighth of a gallon; a pint; abbreviation, O.

**octavalent** (ok'tah-va'lent, ok-tav'ă-lent) [ octa- + L. *valeo,* to have power ]. Denoting a chemical element or radical having a combining power or valency of eight; an octad.

**octigravida** (ok'tĭ-grav'ĭ-dah) [ octi- + L. *gravida,* pregnant woman ]. A woman pregnant for the eighth time.

**octipara** (ok-tip'ă-rah) [ octi- + L. *pario,* to bear ]. A woman who has borne eight children.

**octo-, octi-.** See oct-.

**Octomitidae** (ok-to-mit'ĭ-de) [ octo- + G. *mitos,* thread ]. A family in the class Mastigophora of the Protozoa; includes flagellated organisms with six to eight flagella arranged in pairs and a body that is bilaterally symmetric. *Giardia mesnili* (*G. lamblia*), a parasite in the human intestine, is in this family.

**Octom'itus hom'inis.** A species of tiny flagellated protozoan organisms sometimes occurring as a parasite in the human intestine; probably a commensal, although some observers regard it as a causal agent of diarrhea.

**octopamine hydrochloride.** NORDEN; norsynephrine hydrochloride; α-(aminomethyl)-*p*-hydroxybenzyl alcohol; sympathomimetic amine.

**oc'topine.** *N*-1-(2-Lactyl)arginine; a substituted arginine found in octopus muscle, crown-gall tumors of plants, and elsewhere.

**oc'tose.** A sugar, containing eight carbon atoms, prepared in the laboratory but not occurring in nature; an octulosonic acid forms part of the repeating unit of the polysaccharides of the complex lipopolysaccharides of the *Enterobacteriaceae* constituting the characteristic somatic

O antigens; it is a condensation product of arabinose and phosphoenolpyruvate analogous to neuraminic acid.

**octoxynol** (NF). Polyethylene glycol mono[ *p*-(1,1,3,3-tetramethylbutyl)phenyl ]ether; a surfactant.

**oc'tyl gal'late** (BP). Octyl 3,4,5-trihydroxybenzoate; an antioxidant.

**oc'tylphenox'y polyethox'yeth'anol.** Mono-*p*-isooctyl phenyl ether of polyethylene glycol; a surface-active (wetting) agent.

**ocular** (ok'u-lar) [ L. *oculus*, eye ]. 1. Relating to the eye; visual; ophthalmic. 2. The eyepiece of a microscope, the lens or lenses at the upper end of a microscope, by means of which the image focused by the objective is viewed. See fig. under microscope.

   **compensating o.,** one that compensates and corrects for the effects of chromatic aberration in the objective.

   **Huygens' o.,** the compound o. of a microscope, composed of two planoconvex lenses so arranged that the plane side of each is uppermost.

   **Ramsden's o.,** an eyepiece of a microscope, consisting of two planoconvex lenses with convexities turned to each other.

   **wide field o.,** one that gives a larger than usual field of view and a high eyepoint.

**oc'ularist** [ L. *oculus*, eye ]. One skilled in the design, fabrication, and fitting of artificial eyes and the making of prostheses associated with the appearance or function of the eyes.

**oculen'tum,** pl. **oculen'ta** [ Mod. L. fr. L. *oculus*, eye ]. Ophthalmic *ointment*.

**oculi** (ok'u-li) [ L. ]. Plural of oculus.

**oculist** (ok'u-list) [ L. *oculus*, eye ]. Ophthalmologist.

**oculo-** (ok'u-lo-) [ L. *oculus*, eye ]. Combining form meaning eye, ocular.

**oculoauriculovertebral** (ok'u-lo-aw-rik'u-lo-ver'te-bral). Relating to the eyes, the ears, and the vertebrae.

**oculocardiac** (ok'u-lo-kar'dī-ak). Relating to the eyes and the heart.

**oculocerebrorenal** (ok'u-lo-sĕr'e-bro-re'nal). Relating to the eyes, the brain, and the kidneys.

**oculocutaneous** (ok'u-lo-ku-ta'ne-us). Relating to the eyes and the skin.

**oculodentodigital** (ok'u-lo-den'to-dij'ī-tal). Relating to the eyes, the teeth, and the fingers.

**oc'uloder'mal.** Relating to the eyes and the skin.

**oculofacial** (ok-u-lo-fa'shal). Relating to the eyes and the face.

**oculography** (ok'u-log'ră-fī) [ oculo- + G. *graphē*, a writing ]. A method of recording eye position and eye movements.

   **electro-o.,** see electro-oculography.

   **photosensor o.,** with eyes in primary position exposed to red light, photocells that are directed to the nasal and temporal limbus of the corneas respectively record the difference in potential occasioned by eye movements, the resulting oculogram being similar to that of the electro-oculogram.

**oculogyria** (ok-u-lo-ji'rī-ah) [ oculo- + G. *gyros*, circle ]. The limits of rotation of the eyeballs.

**oculogyric** (ok-u-lo-ji'rik). Referring to rotation of the eyeballs; characterized by oculogyria.

**oculomandibulodyscephaly** (ok'u-lo-man-dib'u-lo-dissef'ă-lī). *Dyscephalia* mandibulo-oculofacialis.

**oc'ulomo'tor** [ L. *oculomotorius*, fr. oculo- + L. *motorius*, moving ]. 1. Relating to or causing movements of the eyeball. 2. Pertaining to the o. nerve.

**oc'ulomoto'rius** [ L. ]. *Nervus* oculomotorius.

**oc'ulomyco'sis.** Ophthalmomycosis.

**oc'ulona'sal** [ oculo- + L. *nasus*, nose ]. Relating to the eyes and the nose.

**oculopathy** (ok'u-lop'ă-thī). Ophthalmopathy.

**oc'ulopu'pillary.** Pertaining to the pupil of the eye.

**oculoreaction** (ok'u-lo-re-ak'shun). Ophthalmoreaction.

**oc'ulover'tebral.** Relating to the eyes and vertebrae.

**oc'ulozygomat'ic.** Relating to the orbit or its margin and the zygomatic bone.

**oc'ulus,** gen. and pl. **oc'uli** [ L. ] [ NA ]. Eye; the organ of vision, consisting of the eyeball and the optic nerve. See fig. under eye.

**O.D.** 1. Abbreviation for *oculus dexter* [ L. ], right eye. 2. Abbreviation for Doctor of Optometry.

**od** [ G. *hodos*, way ]. A force assumed to be exerted upon the nervous system by magnets.

**odaxesmus** (o'dak-sez'mus) [ G. *odaxēsmos*, an irritation, fr. *odax* (adv.), by biting. ]. A biting sensation; a form of paresthesia.

**odaxetic** (o'dak-set'ik) [ G. *odaxēsmos*, an irritation ]. 1. Causing formication or itching. 2. A substance or agent that causes this.

**Oddi,** Ruggero, Italian physician, 19th century. See *sphincter* of O.

**odditis** (od-i'tis). Inflammation of the junction of the duodenum and common bile duct at the sphincter of Oddi.

**-odes** (o'dēz) [ G. *eidos*, form, resemblance. OID- ]. A suffix meaning: having the form of; like; resembling.

**odogenesis** (o-do-jen'e-sis) [ G. *hodos*, path, + *genesis*, source ]. Neurocladism.

**odont-, odonto-** [ G. *odous* (*odont-*), tooth ]. Combining forms, properly in words formed from Greek roots, denoting a tooth or teeth.

**odontagra** (o'don-tag'rah) [ odonto- + G. *agra*, seizure ]. Obsolescent term for toothache thought to be gouty origin.

**odontalgia** (o'don-tal'jī-ah) [ odont- + G. *algos*, pain ]. Toothache.

**odontal'gic.** Relating to or marked by odontalgia.

**odontatrophy, odontatrophia** (o'don-tat'ro-fī, o-don'-tă-tro'fī-ah) [ odont- + atrophy ]. Imperfect formation of the teeth.

**odontectomy** (o'don-tek'to-mī) [ odont- + G. *ektomē*, excision ]. The removal of teeth by the reflection of a mucoperiosteal flap and excision of bone from around the root or roots before the application of force to effect the tooth removal.

**odon'terism** [ odont- + G. *erismos*, quarrel ]. Chattering of the teeth.

**odontexesis** (o-don'tek-se'sis) [ odont- + G. *xesis*, a scraping ]. The act of scaling teeth (see scaling).

**odonti'asis.** Teething.

**odon'tinoid.** 1. Resembling dentin. 2. A small excrescence from a tooth, most common on the root or neck. 3. Toothlike.

**odonti'tis.** Pulpitis.

**odonto-.** See odont-.

**odontoameloblastosarcoma** (o-don'to-am'ĕ-lo-blas'to-sar-ko'mah). Ameloblastic sarcoma; probably a misnomer, applied to ameloblastic fibromas with a poorly differentiated connective tissue component. The clinical course appears to be benign.

**odon'toblast** [ odonto- + G. *blastos*, sprout, germ ]. One of a layer of columnar cells, lining the pulp cavity of a tooth; odontoblastic processes extend into the dentinal tubules.

**odon'toblasto'ma** [ odontoblast + G. suffix *-oma*, tumor ]. 1. A tumor composed of neoplastic epithelial and mesenchymal cells that may differentiate into cells able to produce calcified tooth substances. 2. A odontoma in its early formative stage.

**odontobothrion** (o-don-to-both'rī-on) [ odonto- + G. *bothrion*, a little pit ]. *Alveolus* dentalis.

**odontocele** (o-don'to-sēl) [ odonto- + G. *kēlē*, tumor ]. Alveolodental *cyst*.

**odontochirurgical** (o-don-to-ki-rur'jī-kal) [ odonto- + G. *cheirurgia*, surgery ]. Relating to dental surgery.

**odon'toclast** [ odonto- + G. *klastos*, broken ]. One of the cells believed to produce absorption of the roots of the milk teeth.

**odontodynia** (o-don'to-din'ī-ah) [ odonto- + G. *odynē*, pain ]. Toothache.

**odontodysplasia** (o-don'to-dis-pla-zī'ah) [ odonto- + dysplasia, *q.v.* ]. *Odontogenesis* imperfecta.

**odontogenesis** (o-don'to-jen'ĕ-sis) [ odonto- + G. *genesis*, production ]. Odontogeny; odontosis; the process of development of the teeth.

**o. imperfec'ta,** odontodysplasia; dysgenesis of the enamel, dentin, and pulp of primary or secondary teeth.

**odontogeny** (o-don-toj'ē-nĭ). Odontogenesis.

**odon'toid** [ odont- + G. *eidos,* resemblance ]. 1. Shaped like a tooth. 2. Relating to the dens or o. process of the second cervical vertebra.

**odontol'ogy** [ odonto- + G. *logos,* study ]. Dentistry.
  **forensic o.,** forensic *dentistry.*

**odontolox'ia, odontol'oxy** [ odonto- + G. *loxos,* slanting ]. Odontoparallaxis.

**odontolysis** (o-don-tol'ĭ-sis) [ odonto- + G. *lysis,* dissolution ]. Erosion of the teeth; see erosion (3).

**odontoma** (o'don-to'mah) [ odonto- + G. suffix *-oma,* tumor ]. 1. A tumor of odontogenic origin. 2. A tumor composed of differentiated cells of the tooth germ that lay down tooth substance in an abnormal pattern.
  **ameloblastic o.,** ameloblastodontoma; a form of soft o. in which ameloblasts comprise a conspicuous part of the hamartoma; may be confused histologically with ameloblastomas that have a relatively loose, edematous stroma.
  **radicular o.,** an o. positioned on or near the root of a tooth.

**odontoneuralgia** (o-don'to-nūr-al'jĭ-ah). Facial neuralgia caused by a carious tooth.

**odontonomy** (o'don-ton'o-mĭ) [ odonto- + G. *onoma,* name ]. Dental nomenclature.

**odon'tonosol'ogy** [ odonto- + G. *nosos,* disease, + *logos,* study ]. Odontology; dentistry.

**odontoparallaxis** (o-don'to-păr-ă-lak'sis) [ odonto- + G. *parallaxis,* alternation ]. Odontoloxia; irregularity of the teeth.

**odontopathy** (o'don-top'ă-thĭ) [ odonto- + G. *pathos,* suffering ]. Any disease of the teeth or of their sockets.

**odontopho'bia** [ odonto- + G. *phobos,* fear ]. Morbid fear of teeth.

**odon'toplast** [ odonto- + G. *plassō,* to form ]. Odontoblast.

**odontoprisis** (o'don-top'rĭ-sis) [ odonto- + G. *prisis,* a sawing, a grinding ]. Grinding together of the teeth.

**odontoptosis** (o-don-top-to'sis, o-don-to-to'sis) [ odonto- + G. *ptosis,* a falling ]. Drooping downward of an upper tooth due to the loss of its lower antagonist(s).

**odontorrhagia** (o-don-to-ra'jĭ-ah) [ odonto- + G. *rhēgnymi,* to burst forth ]. Profuse bleeding from the socket after the extraction of a tooth.

**odon'tortho'sis** [ odonto- + G. *orthos,* straight ]. Obsolete term for orthodontics.

**odontoschism** (o-don'to-skizm, -sizm) [ odonto- + G. *schisma,* a cleft ]. Fissure of a tooth.

**odont'oscope.** An optical device, similar to a closed circuit television system, that projects the oral cavity onto a screen for multiple viewing.

**odontoscopy** (o'don-tos'ko-pĭ) [ odonto- + G. *skopeō,* to view ]. 1. Examination of the oral cavity by means of the odontoscope. 2. An examination of the markings in prints of the cutting edges of the teeth; used, like fingerprints, as a method of personal identification.

**odonto'sis.** Odontogenesis.

**odontosmegma** (o-don'to-smeg'mah) [ odonto- + G. *smegma,* unguent ]. Anything (powder, paste, or wash) used in cleaning the teeth.

**odontother'apy.** Treatment of diseases of the teeth.

**odontotomy** (o-don-tot'o-mĭ) [ odonto- + G. *tomē,* incision ]. Cutting into the crown of a tooth.
  **prophylactic o.,** a preventive operation in which imperfectly formed developmental grooves, pits, and fissures are opened up by means of a bur and filled in order to obviate future decay.

**o'dor** [ L. ]. Scent; an emanation from any substance that stimulates the olfactory cells in the organ of smell.

**o'dorant.** Odoriferous.

**odoratism** (o-dor'ă-tizm) [ fr. *Lathyrus odoratus,* sweet pea ]. See lathyrism and osteolathyrism.

**odorif'erous** [ odor + L. *fero,* to bear ]. Odorant; odorous; having a scent, perfume, or odor.

**odorimeter** (o'dor-im'e-ter). Instrument for performing odorimetry.

**odorimetry** (o'dor-im'e-trī) [ odor + G. *metron,* measure ]. The determination of the comparative power of different substances in exciting olfactory sensations.

**odor'iphore** [ odor + G. *phoros,* bearing ]. A group or radical that imparts odor to a compound of which it is a part; osmophore.

**odorivection** (o'dor-ĭ-vek'shun) [ odor + L. *vector,* a carrier ]. Conveying or bearing an odor, as on the air.

**odorography** (o'dor-og'ră-fĭ) [ odor + G. *graphē,* a description ]. Description of odors.

**o'dorous.** Odoriferous.

**O'Dwyer,** Joseph P., New York physician, 1841–1898. See O'D.'s *method, tube.*

**odyn-, odyno-** [ G. *odyne,* pain ]. Combining forms meaning pain.

**odynacusis** (o-din'ă-koo'sis) [ odyn- + G. *akouō,* to hear ]. Hypersensitiveness of the organ of hearing, so that noises cause actual pain.

**odynometer** (o'dĭ-nom'e-ter) [ odyno- + G. *metron,* measure ]. Algesiometer.

**odynophagia** (o-din'o-fa'jĭ-ah) [ odyno- + G. *phagein,* to eat ]. Dysphagia.

**odynophobia** (o-din'o-fo'bĭ-ah) [ odyno- + G. *phobos,* fear ]. Algophobia.

**odynopoeia** (od-in-o-pe'ĭ-ah) [ odyno- + G. *poieō,* to make ]. The bringing on or strengthening of labor pains.

**oe-.** For words so beginning and not found here, see e-.

**Oedipal** (ed'ĭ-pal). Relating to Oedipus, *q. v.*

**oedipism** (ed'ĭ-pizm) [ *Oedipus, q. v.* ]. 1. Self-infliction of injury to the eyes, usually an attempt at evulsion. 2. Manifestation of Oedipus complex.

**Oedipus** (ed'ĭ-pus). King of Thebes, who unwittingly killed his father and married his mother. Upon learning the truth of these events, he killed his mother and also tore out his own eyes because they had betrayed him in not revealing the truth. See oedipism, O. *complex,* Oedipal *neurosis, period.*

**Oehl,** Eusebio, Italian anatomist, 1827–1903. See O.'s *layer, muscles.*

**Oehler** (ē'ler), Johannes, German physician, *1879. See O.'s *symptom.*

**oenanthol** (e-nan'thol). $CH_3(CH_2)_5CHO$; heptyl aldehyde; heptanal.

**Oersted,** Hans-Christian, Danish physicist, 1777–1851. Gave his name to oersted.

**oersted** (ur'sted) [ H. C. *Oersted* ]. Symbol H; unit of magnetic field intensity; the magnetic field intensity that exerts a force of 1 dyne on unit magnetic pole.

**oesophagostomiasis** (e-sof'a-go-sto-mi'ă-sis) [ G. *oisophagos,* gullet (esophagus), + *stoma,* mouth, + suffix *-iasis,* condition ]. Nodular *disease.*

**Oesophagostomum** (e-sof'ă-gos'to-mum) [ G. *oisophagos,* gullet (esophagus), + *stoma,* mouth ]. A genus of strongyle nematodes (subfamily Oesophagostominae) that encyst in the intestinal wall of herbivores and primates, causing nodular disease. Larvae appear to stimulate host reaction in the intestinal wall, forming nodules in which they complete their development (unless the host is immune); they then leave the nodule and feed as adults in the lumen of the large intestine.
  **O. apios'tomum,** a species that encysts under the submucosa of the intestine of man, and occasionally causes dysentery, as reported in Northern Nigeria and central Africa; also a common parasite of monkeys and apes.
  **O. brevicau'dum,** occurs in the cecum and colon of pigs in North America and India.
  **O. brump'ti,** a species described from African monkeys and reported occasionally in man.
  **O. columbia'num,** occurs in sheep, goats, and wild African antelopes; except when present in large numbers, it does not appear to greatly affect the health of the host.
  **O. denta'tum,** affects the colon of swine; the lesions are similar to those in sheep.
  **O. georgia'num,** occurs in the cecum and colon of pigs in the United States.

**O. quadrispinula'tum,** occurs in the cecum and colon of pigs in the Americas, Europe, and southeast Asia.

**O. radia'tum,** occurs worldwide in cattle and water buffalo; the lesions are similar to those of sheep.

**O. stephanos'tomum,** occurs in chimpanzees, monkeys and gorillas in Africa, but also reported from man and monkeys in Brazil.

**O. venulo'sum,** occurs worldwide in the cecum and colon of cattle, sheep, goats, deer, and many other ruminants.

**oestrids** (est'ridz) [ see *Oestrus* ]. Common name for botflies of the family Oestridae, such as *Oestrus*.

**Oestrus** (es'trus) [ G. *oistros,* gadfly ]. A genus of tissue-invading myiasis flies, the head botflies in the family Oestridae.

**O. o'vis,** a grayish brown, robust, hairy, bee-like botfly, imported from Europe, now a serious pest in parts of the United States; larvae are deposited by the adult fly in the nostrils of the sheep, and inch-long larvae develop in the paranasal sinuses, causing considerable mucous discharge and distress in old or weak sheep.

**official** (ŏ-fish'al) [ L. *officialis,* fr. *officium,* a favor, service, fr. *opus,* work, + *facio,* to do ]. Authoritative; denoting a drug or a chemical or pharmaceutical preparation recognized as standard in the Pharmacopeia (*q.v.*); see also officinal.

**officinal** (ŏ-fis'ĭ-nal) [ L. *officina,* shop ]. Denoting a chemical or pharmaceutical preparation kept in stock, as distinguished from one prepared extemporaneously according to a physician's prescription, or a magistral preparation. An officinal preparation is often, though not necessarily, official.

**-ogen.** Often mistakenly construed as a combining form, whereas, actually, the "o" is the final letter of a preceding combining form. See -gen.

**Ogino,** Kyusaka, Japanese physician, 20th century. See *rule* of O.-Knaus.

**Ogston,** Alexander, Scottish surgeon, 1844–1929. See O.'s *line,* O.-Luc *operation,* O.'s *operation.*

**Oguchi,** Chita, Japanese ophthalmologist, 1875–1945. See O.'s *disease.*

**O'Hara,** Michael, Jr., U. S. surgeon, 1869–1926. See O'H. *forceps.*

**Ohm** (ōm), Georg S., German physicist, 1787–1854. Gave his name to ohm. See O.'s *law.*

**Ohm** (ōm), Reinhard, German physician, *1875. See O.'s *instrument.*

**ohm** (ōm) [ G. S. *Ohm* ]. The practical unit of electrical resistance. The international o. is the resistance of a column of mercury at 0°C., 106.3 cm. long, with a constant cross-sectional area (1 sq. mm.), having a mass of 14.4521 gm.; roughly, the resistance of a copper wire 50 m. long and 1 mm. in diameter; the resistance of any conductor allowing 1 ampere of current to pass under the electromotive force (EMF) of 1 volt.

**ohmammeter** (ōm'am'e-ter). A combined ohmmeter and ammeter.

**ohm'meter.** An instrument for determining the resistance, in ohms, of a conductor.

**ohne Hauch** [ Ger. without breath ]. A term used to designate the nonspreading growth of nonflagellated bacteria on agar media; also applied to somatic agglutination. See also O *antigen.*

**oi-.** For words so beginning and not found here, see e-.

**-oid** [ G. *eidos,* form, resemblance. OID- ]. A suffix denoting resemblance to the thing indicated by the preceding element of the compound; joined properly to words formed from Greek roots; equivalent to -form.

**oidia** (o-id'ĭah). Plural of *Oidium.*

**oidiomycetes** (o-id'ĭ-o-mi-se'tes) [ oidium + G. *mykēs,* fungus ]. The common name for a group of fungi in which segmentation of the hyphae results in the formation of rectangular arthrospores (a type of thallospore) that are frequently termed oidia (singular, oidium).

**oidiomycetic** (o-id-ĭ-o-mi-se'tik). Pertaining to or characterized by oidiomycetes.

**oidiomycosis** (o-id'ĭ-o-mi-ko'sis) [ *oidium* + G. *mykes,* fungus, + suffix *-osis,* condition ]. A general term formerly used with reference to certain mycotic diseases thought to be caused by species of *Oidium,* but now classified more specifically in other genera, *e.g., Candida albicans, Blastomyces dermatitidis, Trichophyton schoenleini.*

**oidiomycotic** (o-id'ĭ-om-i-kot'ik). Pertaining to oidiomycosis.

**oidium,** pl. **oidia** (o-id'ĭ-um, o-id'ĭ-ah) [ Mod. L. dim. of G. *ōon,* egg ]. A free, thin-walled hyphal cell derived either by fragmentation of a somatic hypha into component cells or from an oidiophore; such a free o. is frequently called an arthrospore.

**Oidium** (o-id'ĭ-um) [ Mod. L. dim. of G. *ōon,* egg ]. An obsolete generic name for fungi having the features of the oidiomycetes, *q.v.*

**O. al'bicans,** an obsolete name for *Candida albicans.*

**O. lactis,** obsolete name for *Geotrichum candidum.*

**O. schönlein'ii,** obsolete name for *Trichophyton schoenleini.*

**O. ton'surans,** obsolete name for *Trichophyton tonsurans.*

**O. tropica'le,** obsolete name for *Candida tropicalis.*

**oikomania** (oy'ko-ma'nĭ-ah). Ecomania.

**oil** [ L. *oleum;* G. *elaion,* originally olive oil ]. A liquid of fatty consistence and unctuous feel, insoluble in water, soluble or not in alcohol, freely soluble in ether, and inflammable. O.'s are variously classified into animal, vegetable, and mineral o.'s according to their source (the mineral o.'s are probably of remote animal and vegetable origin); into fixed or fatty and volatile or ethereal or essential o.'s, the former being permanent, leaving a stain on an absorbent surface, the latter evaporating when exposed to the air and being capable of distillation; and into drying and nondrying (fatty) o.'s, the former becoming gradually thicker when exposed to the air and finally drying to a varnish, the latter not drying but liable to become rancid on exposure. The volatile o.'s are of vegetable origin; the fatty o.'s are of both animal and vegetable origin. Volatile o.'s are prepared by distillation, distillation with steam, expression, or extraction; fixed o.'s are obtained by expression or extraction. Many of the o.'s, both fixed and volatile, are used in medicine. For individual o.'s, see the specific names.

**essential o.'s,** plant products, usually somewhat volatile, giving the odors and tastes characteristic of the particular plant, thus possessing the essence, *e.g.,* citral, pinene, geraniol, camphor, menthane, terpenes. See also volatile o.

**ethereal o.** volatile o.

**fatty o.,** fixed o.; an o. which cannot be distilled; it is chemically a glyceride of a fatty acid; by substitution of the glycerine by an alkaline base it is converted into a soap; the consistence varies with the temperature, some being liquid (o.'s proper), others semisolid (fats), and others solid (tallows) at ordinary temperatures; but o.'s are congealed by cold and the solids are liquified by heat; the fatty o.'s are of both animal and vegetable origin.

**fixed o.,** fatty o.

**volatile, essential,** or **ethereal o.,** a substance of oily consistence and feel, derived from a plant and containing the principles to which the odor and taste of the plant are due; it is capable of distillation. Many volatile o.'s, identical with or closely resembling the natural o.'s, can be made synthetically. Volatile o.'s are used in medicine as stimulants, stomachics, correctives, carminatives, and for purposes of flavoring.

**oint'ment** [ O. Fr. *oignement;* L. *unguo,* pp. *unctus,* to smear ]. Salve; unguent; a semisolid preparation usually containing medicinal substances and intended for external application. O. bases used as vehicle fall into four general classes: Hydrocarbon bases (oleaginous o. bases) keep medicaments in prolonged contact with the skin, act as occlusive dressings, and are used chiefly for emollient effects. Absorption bases either permit the incorporation of aqueous solutions with the formation of a water-in-oil emulsion or are water-in-oil emulsions that permit the incorporation of additional quantities of aqueous solutions; such bases permit better absorption of some medicaments and are useful as emollients. Water-removable bases (creams) are oil-in-water emulsions containing petrolatum, anhydrous lanolin, or waxes; they may be washed from the skin with water, and are thus more acceptable for cosmetic reasons; they favor absorption of serous discharges in dermatological conditions. Water-soluble bases (greaseless ointment bases) contain only water-soluble substances.

**eye o.,** ophthalmic o.

**ophthalmic o.,** eye o.; oculentum; a special o. for application to the eye. Special precautions must be taken in the preparation of an ophthalmic o.; the finished o. must be free from particles and must be nonirritating to the eye.

**ol.** Abbreviation of L. *oleum*, oil.

**-ol.** A suffix denoting that a substance is an alcohol or a phenol.

**OLA.** Abbreviation for occipitolevoanterior; see under position.

**olamine** (ol'ă-mēn). USAN-approved contraction for ethanolamine.

**oleaginous** (o-le-aj'ĭ-nus) [ L. *oleagineus*, pertaining to *olea*, the olive tree ]. Oily; greasy.

**oleander** (o'le-an'der). The bark and leaves of *Nerium oleander* (family Apocynaceae), a shrub of the eastern Mediterranean; a diuretic and heart tonic.

**oleandomycin phosphate** (o'le-an'do-mi'sin). LANDOMYCIN phosphate; an antibiotic substance produced by species of *Streptomyces antibioticus*. It is effective against staphylococci, streptococci, and pneumococci and some Gram-negative bacteria and is used in the treatment of staphyloccic infections, especially those refractory to erythromycin, penicillin, streptomycin, and the tetracyclines.

**oleate** (o'le-āt). 1. A salt of oleic acid. 2. A pharmacopeial preparation consisting of a combination or solution of an alkaloid or metallic base in oleic acid. Used as an inunction.

**olecranarthritis** (o-lek'ran-ar-thri'tis) [ olecranon + G. *arthron*, joint, + *-itis* ]. Obsolete term for inflammation of the elbow joint.

**olecranarthrocace** (o-lek'ran-ar-throk'a-se) [ olecranon + G. *arthron*, joint + *kakos*, bad ]. Obsolete term for tuberculosis of the elbow joint.

**olecranarthropathy** (o-lek'ran-ar-throp'ă-thĭ) [ olecranon + G. *arthron*, joint, + *pathos*, suffering ]. Any disease of the elbow; an obsolete usage.

**olecranon** (o-lek'rā-non, o-le-kra'non) [ G. the head or point of the elbow, fr. *ōlenē*, ulna, + *kranion*, skull, head ] [ NA ]. Tip of the elbow; the prominent curved proximal extremity of the ulna, the upper and posterior surface of which gives attachment to the tendon of the triceps muscle, the anterior surface entering into the formation of the trochlear notch; called also o. process.

**o'lefin.** Any one of a group of hydrocarbons possessing one or more double bonds in the carbon chain. The simplest is ethylene.

**ole'ic** [ L. *oleum*, oil ]. Relating to oil.

**o. acid** (USP, BP), octadecenoic acid; an organic acid prepared from fats; used in the preparation of oleates and lotions.

**olein** (o'le-in). Trioleoyl glycerol; triolein; glyceryl ester of oleic acid, found in fats and oils.

**olenitis** (o'len-i'tis) [ G. *ōlenē*, elbow, + suffix *-itis*, inflammation ]. Obsolete term for inflammation of the elbow.

**oleo-** (o'le-o-) [ L. *oleum*, oil ]. Combining form relating to oil; see also eleo-.

**oleochrysotherapy** (o'le-o-kris'o-thĕr'ă-pĭ) [ oleo- + G. *chrysos*, gold, + *therapeia*, therapy ]. Treatment with gold in a fat or oil vehicle.

**oleogo'menol.** Gomenol.

**oleo'ma.** Lipogranuloma.

**oleometer** (o'le-om'e-ter) [ oleo- + G. *metron*, measure ]. An instrument like a hydrometer for determining the specific gravity of oils.

**oleopal'mitate.** A double salt of oleic and palmitic acids.

**oleoresin** (o'le-o-rez'in). 1. A compound of an essential oil and resin, present in certain plants. 2. A pharmaceutical preparation; see subentries under aspidium, capsicum, and ginger.

**oleosaccharum,** pl. **oleosacchara** (o-le-o-sak'ar-um) [ oleo- + G. *saccharon*, sugar ]. Oil sugar; a class of preparations made by the trituration of a volatile oil (anise, fennel, lemon, etc.) with sugar. Used as a diluent or corrigent of powerful or bad tasting drugs in powder form.

**oleostearate** (o'le-o-ste'ă-rāt). A double salt of oleic and stearic acids.

**oleosus** (o-le-o'sus) [ L. fr. *oleum*, oil ]. Greasy; relating to defects of the sebaceous apparatus.

**oleotherapy** (o'le-o-thĕr'ă-pĭ) [ oleo- + G. *therapeia*, therapy ]. Eleotherapy; treatment of disease by oil given internally or applied externally.

**oleothorax** (o'le-o-tho'raks) [ oleo- + thorax ]. Eleothorax; the introduction of mineral oil or a mixture of gomenol and olive oil into the pleural cavity, either with or without artificial pneumothorax, to make compression of the lung in pulmonary tuberculosis, for the relief of pyothorax, or to meet other indications.

**o'leovi'tamin.** A solution of a vitamin in an edible oil.

**o. A and D** (NF), a solution of vitamins A and D in fish liver oil or in an edible vegetable oil.

**oleum,** gen. **o'lei,** pl. **o'lea** (o'le-um) [ L. ]. Oil.

**oleyl alcohol** (o-le'il). A mixture of aliphatic alcohols consisting chiefly of $CH_3(CH_2)_7CH=CH(CH_2)_7CH_2OH$. Used as an emulsifying aid and in the preparation of cold cream; found in fish oils.

**olfactie, olfacty** (ol-fak'tĭ) [ see olfaction ]. The unit of smell; the threshold of olfactory stimulation, or the point where the smell is just received in the olfactometer.

**olfaction** (ol-fak'shun) [ L. *ol- facio*, pp. *-factus*, to smell ]. Osmesis. 1. Smell (2); the sense of smell. 2. The act of smelling.

**olfactology** (ol'fak-tol'o-jĭ) [ olfaction *(q.v.)* + G. *logos*, study ]. Study of the sense of smell.

**ol'factom'eter** [ L. *olfactus*, smell, + G. *metron*, measure ]. A device for estimating the keenness of the sense of smell.

**ol'factom'etry.** Determination of the degree of sensibility of the olfactory organ.

**olfactophobia** (ol-fak'to-fo'bĭ-ah) [ L. *olfactus*, smell, + G. *phobos*, fear ]. Morbid fear of odors.

**olfac'tory** [ see olfaction ]. Relating to the sense of smell.

**olfactus** [ L. ] [ NA ]. Olfactory.

**olfacty** (ol-fak'tĭ). Olfactie.

**olib'anum** [ Ar. *al*, the, + *lubān*, frankincense ]. Oriental frankincense; thus; thuris; a gum resin from several trees of the genus *Boswellia* (family Burseraceae); has been used as a stimulant expectorant in bronchitis, for fumigations, and as incense.

**olig-.** See oligo-.

**oligamnios** (ol'ĭ-gam'nĭ-os). Oligoamnios.

**oligemia** (ol-ĭ-ge'mĭ-ah) [ oligo- + G. *haima*, blood ]. Olighemia; oligohemia; hypovolemia; a deficiency in the amount of blood in the body.

**olige'mic.** Pertaining to or marked by oligemia.

**olighe'mia.** Oligemia.

**olighidria, oligidria** (ol'ig-hid'rĭ-ah, -id'rĭ-ah) [ oligo- + G. *hidrōs*, sweat ]. Scanty perspiration.

**oligo-, olig-** (ol'ĭ-go-) [ G. *oligos*, few ]. 1. Combining form meaning "a few" or "a little." 2. In chemistry, used in contrast to "poly-" in describing polymers; *e.g.*, oligosaccharide.

**oligoamnios** (ol'ĭ-go-am'nĭ-os) [ oligo- + amnion ]. Oligohydramnios; oligamnios; deficiency in the amount of the amniotic fluid.

**oligobiop'sy.** Needle *biopsy*.

**oligocar'dia** (ol'ĭ-go- + G. *kardia*, heart ]. Bradycardia.

**oligocholia** (ol'ĭ-go-ko'lĭ-ah) [ oligo- + G. *cholē*, bile ]. A deficient secretion of bile.

**oligochromemia** (ol-ĭ-go-kro-me'mĭ-ah) [ oligo- + G. *chrōma*, color, + *haima*, blood ]. A deficiency in the total amount of hemoglobin in all of the red blood cells.

**oligochylia** (ol'ĭ-go-ki'lĭ-ah) [ oligo- + G. *chylos*, juice ]. Hypochylia; a deficiency of the gastric juice.

**oligochymia** (ol'ĭ-go-ki'mĭ-ah) [ oligo- + G. *chymos*, juice ]. A deficiency of chyme.

**oligocystic** (ol'ĭ-go-sis'tik) [ oligo- + G. *kystis*, bladder, cyst ]. Consisting of only a few cysts, as occasionally observed in certain examples of hydatidiform mole and other lesions that ordinarily have numerous cysts.

**oligocythemia** (ol'ĭ-go-si-the'mĭ-ah) [ oligo- + G. *kytos*, a cell, + *haima*, blood ]. Globular anemia; a deficiency in the total quantity of red blood cells in the body.

**ol'igodac'tyly, oligodactyl'ia** [ oligo- + G. *daktylos*, finger or toe ]. The presence of fewer than five digits on one or more extremities.

**oligoden'dria.** Oligodendroglia.

**oligodendroblast** (ol'ĭ-go-den'dro-blast). A primitive glial cell that is the normal precursor cell of the oligodendrocyte.

**oligodendroblastoma** (ol'ĭ-go-den'dro-blas-to'mah). A rare neoplasm of oligodendroblast origin and more rapid in growth than the oligodendroglioma.

**oligodendrocyte** (ol'ĭ-go-den'dro-sīt). A cell of the oligodendroglia.

**oligodendroglia** (ol'ĭ-go-den-drog'lĭ-ah) [ oligo- + G. *dendron*, tree, + *glia*, glue ]. Oligodendria; one of the three types of glia cells (the other two being macroglia or astrocytes, and microglia) that, together with nerve cells, compose the tissue of the central nervous system. Oligodendroglia cells are characterized by having a variable number of veil-like or sheetlike processes which, wrapped each around an individual axon, form the myelin sheath of nerve fibers in the central nervous system (*cf.* Schwann cells in the peripheral nervous system); they accordingly are more numerous in white matter than in gray matter.

**oligodendroglioma** (ol'ĭ-go-den-dro-gli-o'mah). A relatively rare, moderately well differentiated, relatively slowly growing glioma that occurs most frequently in the cerebrum of adult persons. The neoplasm is grossly homogeneous, fairly well circumscribed, moderately firm, and somewhat gritty in consistency. Interstitial calcification is sufficiently dense to be detected by x-rays of the skull. Microscopically, an o. is characterized by numerous, small, round or ovoid oligodendroglial cells with small, deeply stained nuclei (rarely observed in mitosis), and palely stained, indistinct cytoplasm; the neoplastic cells are rather uniformly distributed in a sparse, fibrillary stroma.

**ol'igodip'sia** [ oligo- + G. *dipsa*, thirst ]. Abnormal absence of thirst; see also hypodipsia.

**oligodontia** (ol'ĭ-go-don'shĭ-ah) [ oligo- + G. *odous*, tooth ]. 1. The condition of having less than a full complement of teeth. 2. Hypodontia.

**oligodynamic** (ol'ĭ-go-di-nam'ik) [ oligo- + G. *dynamis*, power ]. Active in very small quantity; denoting, for example, the germicidal effect of an exceedingly dilute solution (such as one to one hundred million) of copper in distilled water.

**oligoerythrocythemia** (ol'ĭ-go-ĕ-rith'ro-si-the'mĭ-ah) [ oligo- + erythrocyte + G. *haima*, blood ]. Erythropenia.

**oligogalactia** (ol'ĭ-go-gă-lak'tĭ-ah, -shĭ-ah) [ oligo- + G. *gala*, milk ]. A deficiency in the secretion of milk.

**oligogenics** (ol'ĭ-go-jen'iks) [ oligo- + G. *genea*, offspring ]. Birth control.

**oligoglucan-branching glycosyltransferase.** 1,4-α-Glucan 6-α-glucosyltransferase.

**oligo-1,6-glucosidase** (EC 3.2.1.10). Limit dextrinase; isomaltase; a glucanohydrolase cleaving α-1,6 links in isomaltose and dextrins produced from starch and glycogen by α-amylase.

**oligohe'mia** [ oligo- + G. *haima*, blood ]. Oligemia.

**oligohydramnios** (ol'ĭ-go-hi-dram'nĭ-os) [ oligo- + G. *hydōr*, water, + amnion ]. Oligoamnios.

**oligohydruria** (ol'ĭ-go-hi-dru'rĭ-ah) [ oligo- + G. *hydōr*, water, + *ouron*, urine ]. Excretion of small quantities of urine as seen in dehydration.

**oligolecithal** (ol'ĭ-go-les'ĭ-thal) [ oligo- + G. *lekithos*, yolk ]. Having but little yolk; denoting an egg in which there is only a little scattered deutoplasm.

**oligoleukocythemia** (ol'ĭ-go-lu'ko-si-the'mĭ-ah) [ oligo- + leukocyte + G. *haima*, blood ]. Leukopenia.

**oligoma'nia** [ oligo- + G. *mania*, insanity ]. Obsolete term for monomania.

**oligomenorrhea** (ol'ĭ-go-men-o-re'ah) [ oligo- + menorrhea, *q.v.* ]. Scanty menstruation.

**oligomor'phic** [ oligo- + G. *morphē*, form ]. Presenting few changes of form; not polymorphic.

**ol'igonatal'ity.** Low birth rate; one that is below normal.

**oligonephronic** (ol'ĭ-go-nef-ron'ik). Characterized by a reduced number of nephrons.

**ol'igonu'cleotide.** A compound made up of the condensation of a small number of nucleotides.

**ol'igopep'sia.** Hypopepsia.

**oligophosphatu'ria** [ oligo- + phosphate + G. *ouron*, urine ]. Hypophosphaturia.

**oligoplas'mia.** Deficiency in the amount of blood plasma.

**oligoplas'tic** [ oligo- + G. *plassō*, to form ]. Deficient in reparative power.

**oligopnea** (ol'ĭ-gop-ne'ah, ol'ĭ-gop'ne-ah) [ oligo- + G. *pnoē*, breath ]. Infrequent respiration.

**oligopo'sia, oligop'osy** [ oligo- + G. *posis*, drink ]. The drinking of little fluid; the absence of thirst.

**oligoptyalism** (ol'ĭ-go-ti'ă-lizm) [ oligo- + G. *ptyalon*, saliva ]. Oligosialia; a scanty secretion of saliva.

**oligor'ia** [ G. *oligōria*, negligence, slight esteem, fr. *oligos*, little, + *ōra*, care, regard ]. An abnormal indifference toward or dislike of persons or things.

**ol'igosac'charide.** A compound made up of the condensation of a small number of monosaccharide units.

**oligosialia** (ol'ĭ-go-si-a'lĭ-ah) [ oligo- + G. *sialon*, saliva ]. Oligoptyalism.

**oligosper'matism, oligosper'mia** [ oligo- + G. *sperma*, seed ]. A subnormal concentration of spermatozoa in the penile ejaculate.

**ol'igosymptomat'ic.** Having few or minor symptoms.

**oligosynaptic** (ol'ĭ-go-sĭ-nap'tik). Paucisynaptic; referring to neural conduction pathways that are interrupted by only a few synaptic junctions, *i.e.*, made up of a sequence of only few nerve cells, in contrast to polysynaptic pathways.

**ol'igothy'mia** [ oligo- + -thymia, *q.v.* ]. Poverty or loss of affect.

**oligotrichia** (ol'ĭ-go-trik'ĭ-ah). Hypotrichosis.

**oligotrichosis** (ol'ĭ-go-trĭ-ko'sis). Hypotrichosis.

**oligotro'phia, oligot'rophy** [ oligo- + G. *trophē*, nourishment ]. Deficient nutrition.

**oligozoospermatism, oligozoospermia** (ol'ĭ-go-zo'o-sper'mă-tizm, -sper'mĭ-ah) [ oligo- + G. *zōon*, animal, + *sperma*, seed ]. Oligospermatism.

**oligure'sia, oligure'sis** [ oligo- + G. *ourēsis*, urination ]. Oliguria.

**oliguria** (ol'ĭ-gu'rĭ-ah) [ oligo- + G. *ouron*, urine ]. Oliguresia; scanty urination.

**olisthe** (o-lis'the) [ G. *olisthēma*, a slipping ]. A slipping, especially of two opposing joint surfaces; an incomplete luxation.

**oliva,** pl. **oli'vae** (o-li'vah) [ L. ] [ NA ]. Olive (1); inferior olive; olivary eminence; olivary body; corpus olivare; a smooth, oval prominence of the ventrolateral surface of the medulla oblongata corresponding to the nucleus olivaris.
  **o. infe'rior,** the oliva.
  **o. supe'rior,** *nucleus* dorsalis corporis trapezoidei.

**ol'ivary.** 1. Relating to the oliva. 2. Relating to or shaped like an olive.

**olive** (ol'iv) [ L. *oliva* ]. 1. Oliva. 2. The o. tree or its fruit, a member of the genus *Olea* (family Oleaceae).
  **inferior o.,** oliva.
  **superior o.,** *nucleus* dorsalis corporis trapezoidei.

**olive oil** (USP, BP). The expressed oil of the fruit of *Olea europaea;* used as a cholagogue, laxative, and emollient, and in the preparation of liniments.

**Oliver,** William S., English physician, 1836–1908. See O.'s *sign,* O.-Cardarelli *sign.*

**olivifugal** (ol'ĭ-vif'u-gal) [ oliva + L. *fugio*, to flee ]. In a direction away from the olive.

**olivipetal** (ol'ĭ-vip'ĕ-tal) [ oliva + L. *peto*, to seek ]. In a direction toward the olive.

**olivocochlear** (ol'ĭ-vo-kok'le-ar). See olivocochlear *bundle.*

**ol'ivopon'tocerebel'lar.** Relating to the olivary nucleus, the basis pontis, and the cerebellum.

**Ollier** (ʊl-e-a') Léopold L. X. E., French surgeon, 1830–1900. See O.'s *disease, graft, layer, method, theory.*

**-ology.** See -logia.

**ololiuqui** (o'lo-lyu'ke). A hallucinogen used in ceremonies by the Aztec Indians in Mexico; see also *Rivea corymbosa* and *Ipomoea rubrocoerulea.*

**olophonia** (ol'o-fo'nĭ-ah) [ G. *oloos,* destroyed, lost, + *phōnē,* voice ]. Impaired speech due to an anatomical defect in the vocal organs.

**OLP.** Abbreviation of occipitolevoposterior.

**Olshausen** (ols'how-zen), Robert von, Berlin obstetrician, 1835–1915. See O.'s *method, operation.*

**Olszewski,** J. See Steele-Richardson-O. *syndrome.*

**-oma** [ G. *-ōma* ]. A suffix, properly added only to words derived from Greek roots, meaning a tumor or neoplasm.

**omacephalus** (o'mă-sef'ă-lus) [ G. *ōmos,* shoulder, + a-priv. + *kephalē,* head ]. A malformed fetus with a very imperfectly developed head or none at all, and without upper extremities.

**omag'ra** [ G. *ōmos,* shoulder, + *agra,* a seizure ]. Obsolete term for gouty inflammation of the shoulder joint.

**omalgia** (o-mal'jĭ-ah) [ G. *ōmos,* shoulder, + *algos,* pain ]. Omodynia; pain in the shoulder joint or in the deltoid muscle.

**omarthritis** (o-mar-thri'tis) [ G. *ōmos,* shoulder, + *arthritis* ]. Obsolete term for inflammation of the shoulder joint.

**omasitis** (o'mă-si'tis). Inflammation of the omasum.

**omasum** (o-ma'sum) [ L. bullock's tripe ]. Psalterium (2); third stomach division of a ruminant.

**ombrophobia** (om-bro-fo'bĭ-ah) [ G. *ombros,* a rain storm, + *phobos,* fear ]. A morbid fear of rain.

**omega melancholium** (o'meg-ah mel-an-kol'ĭ-um) [ G. *ōmega,* the last letter of the Greek alphabet, *ōmega,* "great o"; L. and G. *melancholia,* fr. *melas* (*melan-*), black, + *cholē,* bile ]. A wrinkle of the shape of the lower case Greek omega (ω) between the eyebrows; assumed to indicate a state of melancholy.

**omen'tal.** Relating to the omentum.

**omentec'tomy** [ omentum + G. *ektomē,* excision ]. Epiploectomy; omentumectomy; resection or excision of the omentum.

**omenti'tis.** Epiploitis.

**omento-, oment-** [ L. *omentum, q.v.* ]. Combining forms relating to the omentum. See also epiplo-.

**omen'tofixa'tion.** Omentopexy.

**omen'topexy** [ omento- + G. *pēxis,* fixation ]. Epiplopexy; omentofixation. 1. Suture of the great omentum to the abdominal wall to induce collateral portal circulation. 2. Suture of the omentum to another organ to increase arterial circulation. See also omentoplasty.

**omen'toplasty** [ omento- + G. *plassō,* to form, manipulate ]. Epiploplasty; surgical disposition of the great omentum to cover or fill a defect, augment arterial or portal venous circulation, absorb effusions, or increase lymphatic drainage; see also omentopexy.

**omentorrhaphy** (o-men-tor'ă-fĭ) [ omento- + G. *rhaphē,* suture ]. Epiplorrhaphy; suture of an opening in the omentum.

**omen'tovol'vulus.** Twisting of the omentum.

**omen'tulum** [ Mod. L. dim. of *omentum* ]. Omentum minus.

**omen'tum,** pl. **omen'ta** [ L. the membrane that encloses the bowels. OMENT- ] [ NA ]. A fold of peritoneum passing from the stomach to another abdominal organ.

  **gastrocolic o.,** o. majus.

  **gastrohepat'ic o.,** o. minus.

  **gastrosplen'ic o.,** *ligamentum* gastrolienale.

  **greater o.,** o. majus.

  **lesser o.,** o. minus.

  **o. majus** [ NA ], greater or gastrocolic o.; epiploon; caul (2); velum (3); a fold passing from the greater curvature of the stomach to the transverse colon, hanging like an apron in front of the intestines.

  **o. minus** [ NA ], lesser or gastrohepatic o.; a peritoneal fold passing from the margins of the porta hepatis and the bottom of the fossa ductus venosi to the lesser curvature of the stomach and to the upper border of the duodenum for a distance of about an inch beyond the gastroduodenal pylorus.

**omentumectomy** (o-men'tum-ek'to-mĭ). Omentectomy.

**omnip'otence of thought.** A childish thought process whereby instantaneous realization of fantasies and wishes is expected.

**omniv'orous** [ L. *omnis,* all, + *voro,* to eat ]. Living on food of all kinds, upon both animal and vegetable food.

**omo-** [ G. *ōmos,* shoulder ]. Combining form indicating relationship to the shoulder.

**o'moclavic'ular.** Relating to the shoulder and the clavicle; denoting an anomalous muscle attached to the coracoid process or upper edge of the scapula and to the clavicle.

**omodynia** (o'mo-din'ĭ-ah) [ omo- + G. *odynē,* pain ]. Omalgia.

**omohy'oid.** *Musculus* omohyoideus.

**omophagia** (o'mo-fa'jĭ-ah) [ G. *ōmos,* raw, + *phagein,* to eat ]. The eating of raw food, especially of raw flesh.

**omothy'roid.** Denoting a band of muscular fibers passing between the superior cornu of the thyroid cartilage and the omohyoid muscle.

**OMP.** Abbreviation for *orotidylic* acid or orotidylate.

**omphal-, omphalo-** (om'fal-, om'fă-lo-) [ G. *omphalos,* navel (umbilicus) ]. Combining form denoting relationship to the umbilicus.

**omphalectomy** (om'fă-lek'to-my) [ omphal- + G. *ektomē,* excision ]. Excision of the umbilicus or of a neoplasm connected with it.

**omphalelcosis** (om'fal-el-ko'sis) [ omphal- + G. *helkōsis,* ulceration ]. Ulceration at the umbilicus.

**omphal'ic** [ G. *omphalos,* umbilicus ]. Umbilical.

**omphalitis** (om'fă-li'tis). Inflammation of the umbilicus and surrounding parts.

**omphalo-.** See omphal-.

**omphaloangiopagus** (om'fă-lo-an'jĭ-op'ă-gus) [ omphalo- + G. *angeion,* vessel, + *pagos,* something fixed ]. Unequal conjoined twins in which the parasite derives its blood supply from the placenta of the autosite.

**omphalocele** (om'fă-lo-sēl) [ omphalo- + G. *kēlē,* hernia ]. Exomphalos; congenital eventration at the umbilicus.

**omphalochorion** (om'fă-lo-ko'rĭ-on). Yolk-sac chorion; a chorion supplied by the omphalomesenteric blood vessels.

**om'phaloenter'ic.** Relating to the umbilicus and the intestine.

**om'phalomesenter'ic.** Relating to the umbilicus and the mesentery or intestine.

**omphalopagus** (om'fă-lop'ă-gus) [ omphalo- + G. *pagos,* something fixed ]. Monomphalus; conjoined twins united at their umbilical regions.

**omphalophlebitis** (om'fă-lo-flē-bi'tis) [ omphalo- + G. *phleps,* vein, + suffix *-itis,* inflammation ]. Inflammation of the umbilical veins.

**omphalopleure** (om'fă-lo-ploor) [ omphalo- + G. *pleura,* rib, side ]. The primitive yolk sac wall in the marsupials, composed of layers of ectoderm and entoderm.

**omphalorrhagia** (om'fă-lo-ra'jĭ-ah) [ omphalo- + G. *rhēgnymi,* to burst forth ]. Bleeding from the umbilicus.

**omphalorrhea** (om'fă-lo-re'ah) [ omphalo- + G. *rhoia,* flow ]. A serous discharge from the umbilicus.

**omphalorrhexis** (om'fă-lo-rek'sis) [ omphalo- + G. *rhēxis,* rupture ]. Rupture of the umbilical cord during childbirth.

**omphalos** (om'fă-los) [ G. navel ]. [ NA ]. Umbilicus.

**omphalosite** (om'fă-lo-sit) [ omphalo- + G. *sitos,* food ]. The parasitic member of unequal monochorial twins which derives its blood supply from the placenta of the autosite. It is not capable of independent existence after birth and separation from the placenta.

**omphalospinous** (om'fă-lo-spi'nus). Relating to the umbilicus and the anterior superior spine of the ilium; denoting a line connecting these two parts on which is situated McBurney's point.

**omphalotomy** (om'fă-lot'o-mĭ) [ omphalo- + G. *tomē,* incision ]. Cutting of the umbilical cord at birth.

**om'phalotrip'sy** [ omphalo- + G. *tripsis,* a rubbing ]. Crushing, instead of cutting, the umbilical cord after childbirth.

**omphalovesical** (om'fă-lo-ves'ĭ-kal). Vesicoumbilical.

**omphalus** (om'fă-lus) [ G. *omphalos,* navel ]. Umbilicus.

**o'nanism** [ *Onan*, son of Judah, who practiced it. Genesis 38:9 ]. 1. Coitus interruptus; withdrawal by the male before the completion of the sexual act, in order to prevent insemination and fecundation of the ovum. 2. Incorrectly used by some as synonymous with masturbation.

**o'nanist.** One who practices onanism.

**Onanoff** (aw-nah-nawf'), Jacques, Paris physician, *1859. See O.'s *reflex, sign*.

**oncho-.** For words beginning thus, and not found here, see onco-.

**Onchocerca** (ong'ko-ser'kah) [ G. *onkos*, a barb (ONC-2), + *kerkos*, tail ]. *Oncocerca;* elongated filariform nematodes (family Onchocercidae) that inhabit the connective tissue of their hosts, usually within firm nodules in which these parasites are coiled and entangled.

**O. cervica'lis,** common in the ligamentum nuchae of horses, mules, and asses, where it has been suspected of playing a role in fistulous withers and poll evil.

**O. gibso'ni,** a species that infests cattle, buffalo, and sheep in Australia, Southeast Asia, India, and Egypt.

**O. liena'lis,** inhabits the connective tissue around the ligamentum nuchae, tibiofemoral ligament, spleen capsule, and other sites in cattle and buffalo; although widely distributed, it is not common in the United States.

**O. vol'vulus,** the blinding nodular worm; a species that causes onchocerciasis in man in parts of Central America and central and west Africa.

**onchocerciasis** (ong'ko-ser-si'ă-sis). Oncocerciasis; onchocercosis; coast erysipelas; volvulosis; blinding disease; mal morado; infection with *Onchocerca* (especially *O. volvulus*), marked by nodular swellings forming a fibrous cyst enveloping the coiled parasites. Microfilariae move freely out of the nodule and escape into the intercellular lymph in the dermis. Ocular complications may develop, with blindness frequently occurring in advanced cases, probably as a result of the sensitization of the cornea to the microfilariae.

**ocular o.,** ocular complications, such as keratitis, iridocyclitis, or retrobulbar neuritis, caused by the microfilariae of *Onchocerca volvulus*.

**onchocercid** (ong'ko-ser'kid). Common name for members of the family Onchocercidae.

**Onchocercidae** (ong'ko-ser'kĭ-de). A family of nematode parasites (superfamily Filarioidea) that includes the genus *Onchocerca*.

**onchocercosis** (ong-ko-ser-ko'sis). Onchocerciasis.

**onco-** (ong'ko-) [ G. *onkos*, bulk, mass. ONC- 1 ]. Combining form meaning a tumor or some relation to a tumor, or to bulk, volume.

**Oncocer'ca.** *Onchocerca*.

**oncocerci'asis.** Onchocerciasis.

**oncocyte** (ong'ko-sit) [ onco- + G. *kytos*, cell ]. A large, granular, acidophilic tumor cell containing numerous mitochondria; a neoplastic oxyphil cell.

**on'cocyto'ma.** Oxyphil cell *adenoma*.

**oncogenesis** (ong'ko-jen'ĕ-sis) [ onco- + G. *genesis*, production ]. Origin and growth of a neoplasm.

**oncogen'ic.** Oncogenous.

**oncogenous** (ong'koj'ĕ-nus). Causing, inducing, or being suitable for the formation and development of a neoplasm.

**oncograph** (ong'ko-graf) [ onco- + G. *graphē*, a record ]. A recording oncometer, or the recording portion of an oncometer.

**oncography** (ong'kog'ră-fĭ). Graphic representation, by means of a special apparatus, of the size and configuration of an organ.

**oncoides** (ong-koy'dēz) (onco- + G. *eidos*, resemblance ]. Turgidity; turgor; intumescence.

**oncology** (ong-kol'o-jĭ) [ onco- + G. *logos*, study ]. The study or science dealing with the physical, chemical, and biologic properties and features of neoplasms, and including causation and pathogenesis.

**oncolysis** (ong-kol'ĭ-sis) [ onco- + G. *lysis*, dissolution ]. The destruction of a neoplasm; sometimes used with reference to the reduction of any swelling or mass.

**oncolytic** (ong'ko-lit'ik). Pertaining to, characterized by, or causing oncolysis.

**onco'ma** [ G. *onkos*, mass, + suffix *-oma*, tumor ]. Obsolescent term for neoplasm or tumor.

**oncometer** (ong-kom'e-ter) [ onco- + G. *metron*, measure ]. An instrument for measuring the size and configuration of the kidneys and other organs. 2. The measuring, as distinguished from the recording part of the oncograph.

**oncomet'ric.** Relating to oncometry.

**oncom'etry.** Measurement of the size of an organ.

**oncor'navi'ruses.** RNA tumor *viruses*.

**oncosis** (ong-ko'sis) [ G. *onkōsis*, swelling, fr. *onkos*, bulk, mass. ONC-1 ]. A condition characterized by the formation of one or more neoplasms or tumors.

**oncosphere** (ong'-ko-sfēr) [ onco- + G. *sphaira*, sphere ]. Hexacanth.

**on'cother'apy.** Treatment of tumors.

**oncot'ic.** Relating to or caused by edema or any swelling (oncosis).

**oncotomy** (ong-kot'o-mĭ) [ onco- + G. *tomē*, incision ]. Incision of an abscess, cyst, or other tumor.

**oncotropic** (ong'ko-trop'ik) [ onco- + G. *tropē*, a turning ]. Tumoraffin; manifesting a special affinity for neoplasms or neoplastic cells; denoting a drug, radiant energy, or other force acting especially on new growths.

**one-carbon-fragment.** The name given to the formyl group or to the active methyl group that takes part in transformylation or transmethylation reactions; by means of these reactions a single carbon atom is added to a compound being biosynthesized, adding a methyl group as in thymidine formation, adding a hydroxymethyl group as in serine biosynthesis, or closing a ring as in purine formation. Tetrahydrofolate and *S*-adenosylmethionine are the transfer agents of the one-carbon units.

**oneiric** (o-ni'rik) [ G. *oneiros*, dream ]. 1. Pertaining to dreams. 2. Pertaining to the clinical state of oneirophrenia.

**oneirism** (ō-ni'rizm) [ G. *oneiros*, dream ]. A waking dream state.

**oneirocritical** (on-i-ro-krit'ĭ-kl) [ G. *oneiros*, dream, + *kritikōs*, skilled in judgment ]. Pertaining to the logic of dreams.

**oneirodynia** (on-i-ro-din'ĭ-ah) [ G. *oneiros*, dream, + *odynē*, pain ]. An unpleasant or painful dream.

**o. acti'va,** somnambulism.

**o. gra'vis,** nightmare.

**oneirogmus** (o'ni-rog'mus) [ G. *oneirōgmos*, an effusion of semen during sleep ]. Wet dream; nocturnal emission of semen related to erotic dreams.

**oneirol'ogy** [ G. *oneiros*, dream, + *logos*, study ]. The study of dreams.

**oneirophrenia** (o-ni'ro-fre'nĭ-ah) [ G. *oneiros*, dream, + *phrēn*, mind ]. A state in which hallucinations occur, caused by such conditions as prolonged deprivation of sleep, sensory isolation, and a variety of drugs.

**oneiroscopy** (o-ni-ros'ko-pĭ) [ G. *oneiros*, dream, + *skopeō*, to examine ]. Dream analysis; diagnosis of a person's mental state by a study of his dreams.

**o'nioma'nia** [ G. *ōnios*, for sale, + *mania*, insanity ]. The morbidly exaggerated need or urge to buy beyond the realistic needs of the individual.

**oni'ric.** Oneiric.

**-onium.** A suffix indicating a positively charged compound ion, as ammonium ($NH_4^+$), phosphonium ($PH_4^+$), carbonium ($\rightarrow C^+$).

**onium compounds.** See under compound.

**onko-.** For words beginning thus, see oncho- and onco-.

**onlay.** A metal (usually gold) cast restoration of the occlusal surface of a posterior or the lingual surface of an anterior tooth the entire surface of which is in dentin, leaving no side walls. Retention in the anterior tooth is by pins and in the posterior by pins and/or boxes in retentive grooves in the buccal and lingual walls.

**onomatology** (on'o-mă-tol'o-jĭ) [ G. *onoma* (*onomat-*), name, + *logos*, study ]. Terminology; nomenclature; the science of naming objects; the vocabulary of a science.

**onomatomania** (on'o-mat'o-ma'nĭ-ah) [ G. *onomo*, name, + *mania*, frenzy ]. An abnormal impulse to dwell upon certain words and their supposed significance, or to frantically try to recall a particular word.

**onomatophobia** (on'o-mat'o-fo'bī-ah) [ G. *onomo*, name, + *phobos*, fear ]. Abnormal dread of certain words or names because of their supposed significance.

**onomatopoiesis** (on'o-mat'o-poy-ee'sis) [ G. *onoma*, name, + *poiēsis*, making ]. The making of a name or word, especially to express or imitate a natural sound (*e.g.*, hiss, crash, boom). In psychiatry, the tendency to make new words of this type is said to characterize some persons with schizophrenia; see also neologism.

**ontogenesis** (on'to-jen'ē-sis). Ontogeny.

**ontogenet'ic.** Relating to ontogeny.

**ontogeny** (on-toj'ē-nī) [ G. *ōn*, being, + *genesis*, origin. ONT- ]. Ontogenesis; the development of the individual, as distinguished from phylogenesis, or the evolutionary development of the species.

**onyalai** (on'ī-al'ā). Chilopa; akembe; kafindo; an acute disease affecting natives of Central Africa, characterized by bloody vesicles of the mouth and other mucous surfaces, hematuria, and melena. Defective nutrition may be the cause.

**onych-.** See onycho-.

**onychalgia** (on'ī-kal'jī-ah) [ onycho- + G. *algos*, pain ]. Pain in the nails.

**onychatrophia, onychatrophy** (on'ī-kă-tro'fī-ah, on-ik-at'ro-fī) [ onycho- + G. *atrophia*, atrophy ]. Atrophy of the nails.

**onychauxis** (on-ī-kawk'sis) [ onycho- + G. *auxē*, increase ]. Marked overgrowth of fingernails or toenails.

**onychectomy** (on'ī-kek'to-mī) [ onycho- + G. *ectomē*, excision ]. The ablation of a toenail or fingernail.

**onychia** (o-nik'ī-ah) [ onycho- + G. suffix -*ia*, condition ]. Onychitis; onyxitis; inflammation of the matrix of the nail.
  **o. latera'lis,** paronychia.
  **o. malig'na,** Wardrop's disease; acute o. occurring spontaneously in debilitated patients, or in response to slight trauma.
  **o. periungua'lis,** paronychia.
  **o. sic'ca,** a condition characterized by brittle nails.

**onychitis** (on-ī-ki'tis). Onychia.

**onycho-, onych-** (on'ī-ko-) [ G. *onyx*, nail ]. Combining forms meaning nail.

**onychocryptosis** (on'ī-ko-krip-to'sis) [ onycho- + G. *kryptō*, to conceal ]. Ingrown *nail*.

**onychodystrophy** (on'ī-ko-dis'tro-fī) [ onycho- + G. prefix *dys*-, bad, + *trophē*, nourishment ]. Dystrophic changes in nails occurring as a congenital defect or due to any illness or injury that may cause a malformed nail.

**onychograph** (on'ī-ko-graf) [ onycho- + G. *graphō*, to write ]. An instrument for recording the capillary blood pressure as shown by the circulation under the nail.

**onychogrypho'sis.** Onychogryposis.

**onychogryposis** (on-ī-ko-gri-po'sis) [ onycho- + G. *grypōsis*, a curvature ]. Onychogryphosis; gryposis unguium; enlargement with increased curvature of the fingernails or toenails.

**onychoid** (on'ī-koyd) [ onycho- + G. *eidos*, resemblance ]. Resembling in structure or form a fingernail.

**onychology** (on'ī-kol'o-jī) [ onycho- + G. *logos*, treatise ]. Study of the nails.

**onycholysis** (on'ī-kol'ī-sis) [ onycho- + G. *lysis*, loosening ]. Loosening of the nails, beginning at the free border, and usually incomplete.

**onychoma** (on-ī-ko'mah) [ onycho- + G. suffix -*ōma*, tumor ]. A tumor arising from the nail bed.

**onychomadesis** (on'ī-ko-mă-de'sis) [ onycho- + G. *madēsis*, a growing bald, fr. *madaō*, to be moist, (of hair) fall off ]. Complete shedding of the nails usually associated with a systemic illness.

**onychomalacia** (on'ī-ko-mă-la'shī-ah) [ onycho- + G. *malakia*, softness ]. Abnormal softness of the nails.

**onychomycosis** (on'ī-ko-mi-ko'sis) [ onycho- + G. *mykes*, fungus, + suffix -*ōsis*, condition ]. ringworm of the nails; tinea unguium; a fungus infection of the nails, causing thickening, roughness, and splitting; it may be caused by species of *Microsporum* or *Trichophyton*.
  **o. favo'sa,** favus involving the nails.

**onychonosus** (on-ī-kon'o-sus) [ onycho- + G. *nosos*, disease ]. Onychopathy.

**onychopathic** (on-ī-ko-path'ik). Relating to or suffering from any disease of the nails.

**onychopathology** (on'ī-ko-pă-thol'o-jī). Study of diseases of the nails.

**onychopathy** (on'ī-kop'ă-thī) [ onycho- + G. *pathos*, suffering ]. Onychonosus; onychosis; any disease of the nails.

**onychophage** (on'ī-ko-fāj) [ see onychophagy ]. Onycophagist; one who bites the fingernails.

**onychophagia** (on-ī-ko-fa'jī-ah). Onycophagy.

**onychophagist** (on-ī-kof'ă-jist). Onychophage.

**onychophagy** (on-ī-kof'ă-jī) [ onycho- + G. *phagein*, to eat ]. Nailbiting.

**onychophosis** (on'ī-ko-fo'sis). A growth of horny epithelium in the nailbed.

**onychophyma** (on'ī-ko-fi'mah) [ onycho- + G. *phyma*, growth ]. Swelling or hypertrophy of the nails.

**onychoptosis** (on'ī-kop-to'sis) [ onycho- + G. *ptōsis*, a falling ]. Falling off of the nails.

**onychorrhexis** (on'ī-ko-rek'sis) [ onycho- + G. *rhēxis*, a breaking ]. Abnormal brittleness of the nails with splitting of the free edge.

**onychosis** (on-ī-ko'sis). Onychopathy.

**onychostroma** (on'ī-ko-stro'mah) [ onycho- + G. *strōma*, bedding ]. *Matrix* unguis.

**onychotillomania** (on'ī-kot'ī-lo-ma'nī-ah) [ onycho- + G. *tillein*, to pluck, + *mania*, insanity ]. A tendency to pick at the nails.

**onychotomy** (on'ī-kot'o-mī) [ onycho- + G. *tomē*, cutting ]. Incision into a toenail or fingernail.

**onychotrophy** (on-ī-kot'ro-fī) [ onycho- + G. *trophē*, nourishment ]. Nutrition of the nails.

**onyx** (on'iks) [ G. nail ]. 1. Unguis. 2. A collection of pus in the anterior chamber of the eye, resembling a fingernail; see also hypopyon.

**onyx'is.** Ingrown *nail*.

**onyxitis** (on-iks-i'tis). Onychia.

**oo-** (o'o-) [ G. *ōon*, egg. OO- ]. Combining form denoting egg, ovary. See also ovi- and ovo-.

**o'oblast** [ G. *ōon*, egg, + *blastos*, germ ]. A primordial cell from which the ovum is developed.

**oocyesis** (o-o-si-e'sis) [ G. *ōon*, egg, + *kyēsis*, pregnancy ]. Ovarian *pregnancy*.

**o'ocyst** [ G. *ōon*, egg, + *kystis*, bladder ]. The encysted form of the fertilized macrogamete, or zygote, in which sporogonic multiplication occurs, resulting in the formation of sporozoites, infectious agents for the next stage of the sporozoan life cycle.

**oocytase** (o-o-si'tās). A cytase acting destructively upon the ovarian cells.

**oocyte** (o'o-sīt) [ G. *ōon*, egg, + *kytos*, a hollow (cell) ]. The immature ovum.
  **primary o.,** an o. during its growth phase and prior to completion of the first maturation division.
  **secondary o.,** an o. in which the first meiotic division is completed. The second meiotic division usually stops short of completion unless fertilization occurs.

**oocytin** (o-o-si'tin). Substance that causes the formation of fertilization membranes in ova.

**oogenesis** (o-o-jen'ē-sis) [ G. *ōon*, egg, + *genesis*, origin ]. The process of formation and development of the ovum.

**oogenetic, oogenic, oogenous** (o'o-jě-net'ik, o-o-jen'ik, o-oj'ē-nus). Producing ova.

**oogonium,** pl. **oogonia** (o'o-go'nī-um) [ G. *ōon*, egg, + *gonē*, generation ]. 1. The primitive egg mother cell, from which the oocytes are developed. 2. In fungi, the female gametangium bearing one or more eggs.

**ookinesis, ookinesia** (o'o-kī-ne'sis, -zī-ah) [ G. *ōon*, egg, + *kinēsis*, movement ]. The chromosomal movements of the egg during maturation and fertilization.

**ookinete** (o'o-kī-nēt, -ki'nēt) [ G. *ōon*, egg, + *kinētos*, motile ]. The motile zygote of the malarial organism that penetrates the mosquito stomach to form an oocyst under the outer gut lining; the contents of the oocyst subsequently divide to produce numerous sporozoites.

**oolemma** (o-o-lem'ah) [ G. *ōon*, egg, + *lemma*, sheath ].

The plasma membrane of the oocyte.

**oophagia, oophagy** (o-o-fa'jĭ-ah, o-of'a-jĭ) [ G. *ōon*, egg, + *phagein*, to eat ]. The habitual eating of eggs; subsisting largely on eggs.

**oophor-, oophoro-** [ Mod. L. *oophoron*, ovary, fr. G. *ōophoros*, egg-bearing, fr. *ōon*, egg, + *phoros*, bearing. OO- ]. Combining forms denoting the ovary; for such words not found here, see also ovari-, ovario-.

**oophoralgia** (o-of'or-al'jĭ-ah) [ oophor- + G. *algos*, pain ]. Ovarialgia.

**oophorectomy** (o-of'or-ek'to-mĭ) [ G. *ōon*, egg, + *phoros*, bearing, + *ectomē*, excision ]. Ovariectomy.

**oophoritis** (o-of-or-i'tis) [ G. *ōon*, egg, + *phoros*, a bearing, + -*itis* ]. Ovaritis; oaritis; oothecitis; inflammation of an ovary.

**oophoro-.** See oophor-.

**oophorocystectomy** (o-of'or-o-sis-tek'to-me). Excision of an ovarian cyst.

**oophorocystosis** (o-of'or-o-sis-to'sis). Oothecocystosis; ovarian cyst formation.

**oophorohysterectomy** (o-of'or-o-his'ter-ek'to-mĭ). Ovariohysterectomy.

**oophoroma** (o-of-or-o'mah). Ovarioncus; oothecoma; an ovarian tumor.

**oophoromalacia** (o-of'or-o-mă-la'shĭ-ah) [ oophoro- + G. *malakia*, softness ]. Oothecomalacia; softening of ovary.

**oophoroma'nia** (o-of'or-o-ma'nĭ-ah). Oothecomania; mental disorder associated with ovarian disease.

**oophoron** (o-of'or-on) [ Mod. L. ovary, fr. G. *ōon*, egg, + *phoros*, bearing ]. Ovary.

**oophoropathy** (o-of-or-op'ă-thĭ). Ovariopathy.

**oophoropeliopexy** (o-of'or-o-pel'ĭ-o-pek'sĭ) [ oophoro- + G. *pellis*, pelvis, + *pēxis*, fixation ]. Oophororrhaphy.

**oophoropexy** (o-of'or-o-pek'sĭ) [ oophoro- + G. *pēxis*, fixation ]. Oothecopexy; surgical fixation or suspension of ovary.

**oophoroplasty** (o-of'or-o-plas'tĭ). Plastic operation upon an ovary.

**oophororrhaphy** (o-of-o-ror'ă-fĭ) [ oophoro- + G. *rhaphē*, suture ]. Oothecorrhaphy; oophoropeliopexy; suspension of ovary by attachment to pelvic wall.

**oophorosalpingectomy** (o-of'or-o-sal-pin-jek'to-mĭ). Ovariosalpingectomy.

**oophorosalpingitis** (o-of'or-o-sal-pin-ji'tis) [ oophoro- + salpingitis, *q.v.* ]. Ovariosalpingitis.

**oophorostomy** (o-of-or-os'to-mĭ) [ oophoro- + G. *stoma*, mouth ]. Ovariostomy.

**oophorotomy** (o-of-or-ot'o-mĭ) [ oophoro- + G. *tomē*, incision ]. Ovariotomy.

**oophorrhagia** (o-of-or-rā'jĭ-ah) [ oophoro- + G. *rhēgnymi*, to burst forth ]. Ovarian hemorrhage.

**ooplasm** (o'o-plazm) [ G. *ōon*, egg, + *plasma*, a thing formed ]. The protoplasmic portion of the ovum.

**o'opor'phyrin.** Protoporphyrin; the coloring matter in the brown egg shell.

**oosperm** (o'o-sperm) [ G. *ōon*, egg, + *sperma*, seed ]. The fertilized ovum.

**Oospora** (o-os'po-rah) [ G. *ōon*, egg, + *sporos*, seed ]. An obsolete generic name used synonymously either with the actinomycetes or with the group of fungi formerly designated as *Oidium*. Because oospores are not involved, the obsolete terms are improper and should not be used.

    **O. cani'na,** *Mycoderma caniunum*, a species causing favus in dogs which is sometimes transmitted to man, producing lesions resembling ordinary ringworm.

**oosporangium** (o'o-spo-ran'jĭ-um) [ oospore + G. *angeion*, vessel. ANGI- ]. A sac containing oospores.

**oospore** (o'o-spōr) [ see *Oospora* ]. A thick-walled fungus spore which develops from a female gamete either through fertilization or parthenogenesis.

**oosporosis** (o'os-po-ro'sis). Infection with a species of *Oospora*, usually *O. canina*.

**oothec-, ootheco-** [ Mod. L. *ootheca*, *q.v.* ]. Obsolescent combining forms denoting the ovary; for most such words, see oophor-, and ovari-.

**ootheca** (o-oth-e'kah) [ Mod. L. fr. G. *ōon*, egg, + *thēkē*, box, case ]. Ovary.

**oothecalgia** (o-oth-e-kal'jĭ-ah) [ ootheca + G. *algos*, pain ]. Ovarialgia.

**oothecectomy** (o-oth-e-sek'to-mĭ) [ ootheca + G. *ektomē*, excision ]. Ovariectomy.

**oothecitis** (o-oth-e-si'tis) [ ootheca + G. suffix -*itis*, inflammation ]. Oophoritis.

**oothecocele** (o-oth-e'co-sēL) [ ootheca + G. *kēlē*, hernia ]. Ovariocele.

**oothecocentesis** (o-oth-e'ko-sen-te'sis) [ ootheca + G. *kentēsis*, puncture ]. Ovariocentesis.

**oothecocyesis** (o-oth-e'ko-si-e'sis) [ ootheca + G. *kyēsis*, pregnancy ]. Ovarian *pregnancy*.

**oothecocystosis** (o-oth-e'ko-sis-to'sis) [ ootheca + G. *kystis*, cyst ]. Oophorocystosis.

**oothecohysterectomy** (o-oth-e'ko-his-ter-ek'to-mĭ) [ ootheca + G. *hystera*, uterus, + *ektomē*, excision ]. Ovariohysterectomy.

**oothecoma** (o-oth-e-ko'mah) [ ootheca + G. suffix -*oma*, tumor ]. Oophoroma.

**oothecomalacia** (o-oth-e'ko-mă-la'shĭ-ah) [ ootheca + G. *malakia*, softness ]. Oophoromalacia.

**oothecomania** (o-oth-e'ko-ma'nĭ-ah). Oophoromania.

**oothecopathy** (o-oth-e-kop'ath-ĭ) [ ootheca + G. *pathos*, suffering ]. Ovariopathy.

**oothecopexy** (o-oth-e'ko-pek-sĭ) [ ootheca + G. *pēxis*, fixation ]. Oophoropexy.

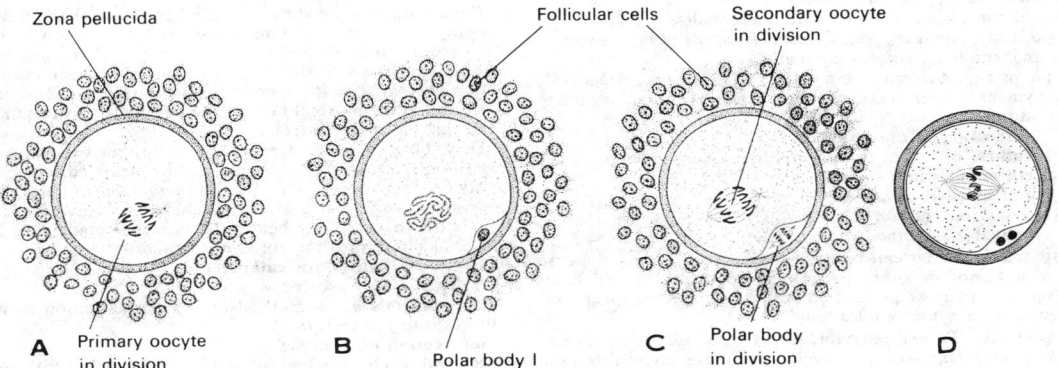

Zona pellucida    Follicular cells    Secondary oocyte in division

A   Primary oocyte in division     B    Polar body I     C   Polar body in division     D

**Maturation of the Oocyte**

*A*, primary oocyte showing first miotic division; *B*, secondary oocyte and first polar body; *C*, secondary oocyte showing second miotic division immediately after ovulation; *D*, completion of secondary miotic division with production of second polar body immediately after fertilization. (From Langman, J.: *Medical Embryology*, Ed. 2, The Williams & Wilkins Co., Baltimore, 1969.

**oothecorrhaphy** (o-oth-e-kor'af-ĭ) [ ootheca + G. *rhaphē*, suture ]. Oophororrhaphy.

**oothecorrhexis** (o-oth-e-ko-rek'sis) [ ootheca + G. *rhēxis*, rupture ]. Ovariorrhexis.

**oothecosalpingectomy** (o-oth-e'ko-sal-pin-jek'to-mĭ) [ ootheca + G. *salpinx* (*salping*), trumpet (oviduct), + *ektomē*, excision ]. Ovariosalpingectomy.

**oothecosalpingitis** (o-oth-e'co-sal-pin-ji'tis) [ ootheca + salpingitis ]. Ovariosalpingitis.

**oothecostomy** (o-oth-e-kos'to-mĭ) [ ootheca + G. *stoma*, mouth ]. Ovariostomy.

**oothecotomy** (o-oth-e-kot'o-mĭ) [ ootheca + G. *tomē*, incision ]. Ovariotomy.

**o'otid** [ G. *ōotidion*, a diminutive egg; see -id (2) ]. The nearly mature ovum after the first maturation has been completed and the second initiated. In most higher mammals the second maturation division is not completed unless fertilization occurs.

**ootype** (o'o-tip) [ G. *ōon*, egg, + *typos*, stamp, print ]. The central portion of the ovarian complex of trematodes in which fertilization takes place and the vitellarian or eggshell materials are coated over the egg; this occurs in a rapid, stamping-mill sequence, after which eggs pass into the uterus for tanning of the shell, storage, and passage toward the genital pore.

**opac'ifica'tion** [ L. *opacus*, shady ]. 1. The process of making opaque. 2. The formation of opacities.

**opacity** (o-pas'ĭ-tĭ) [ L. *opacitas, shadiness* ]. 1. A lack of transparency; an opaque or nontransparent area. 2. Mental dullness.

**snowball o.**, a spherical, white body seen in the vitreous in asteroid hyalosis.

**opalescent** (o-pal-es'ent) [ Fr. fr. L. *opalus*, opal ]. Resembling an opal in the display of various colors; denoting certain bacterial cultures.

**opal'gia** [ G. *ōps* (*ōp-*), eye, face, + *algos*, pain ]. Opsialgia; pain about the eye.

**Opalski**, Adam, Polish physician, 1897–1963. See O. *cell*.

**opaque** (o-pāk') [ Fr. fr. L. *opacus*, shady ]. Impervious to light; not translucent or only slightly so.

**opeidoscope** (op-i'do-skōp) [ G. *ops* (*op-*), a voice, + *eidos*, appearance, + *skopeō*, to view ]. An apparatus by which the vibrations of a diaphragm, started by the voice, move a mirror by which a ray of light is reflected on a screen.

**o'pen** [ A.S. ]. 1. Exposed to the air; said of a wound. 2. A term applied to females of most animal species indicating that they are not pregnant; a market term.

**o'pening.** Aperture; see also fossa, ostium, and orifice.

**bite o.** vertical dimension increase; see under dimension.

**cardiac o.**, *ostium* cardiacum.

**ileocecal o.**, *ostium* ileocecale.

**o. of inferior vena cava**, *ostium* venae cavae inferioris.

**pharyngeal o. of auditory tube**, *ostium* pharyngeus tubae auditivae.

**piriform o.**, *apertura* piriformis.

**pulmonary o.**, *ostium* trunci pulmonalis.

**o.'s of pulmonary veins**, *ostia* venarum pulmonalium.

**saphenous o.**, *hiatus* saphenus.

**o. of superior vena cava**, *ostium* venae cavae superioris.

**tympanic o. of auditory tube**, *ostium* tympanicum tubae auditivae.

**ureteral o.**, *ostium* ureteris.

**urethral o.'s**, see *ostium* urethrae externum and *ostium* urethrae internum.

**o. of uterus**, *ostium* uteri.

**vaginal o.**, *ostium* vaginae.

**vertical o.**, vertical *dimension*.

**op'erable.** That can be operated upon; denoting the case of a tumor or other pathologic condition in which an operation can be performed with a reasonable expectation of cure or symptomatic relief.

**op'erant.** Target behavior; target response; in conditioning, any behavior or specific response chosen by the experimenter; its frequency is intended to increase or decrease by the judicious pairing with it of a reinforcer when it occurs.

**op'erate** [ L. *operor*, pp. -*atus*, to work, fr. *opus*, work ]. 1. To cause a movement of the bowels; said of a laxative or cathartic remedy. 2. To work upon the body by the hands or by means of cutting or other instruments for the purpose of correcting a deformity, removing a tumor or a limb, etc.

---

# OPERATION

**op'era'tion.** 1. Any surgical procedure. 2. The act, manner, or process of functioning.

**Abbé-Estlander o.**, the transfer of a full-thickness flap from one lip of the oral cavity to fill a defect in the other lip, using an arterial pedicle to insure survival of the graft.

**Adams' o. for ectropion**, excision of a wedge from the lateral margin of the eyelid in order to shorten it.

**Albee's o.**, an o. for producing ankylosis of the hip; the upper surface of the head of the femur is sliced off and the corresponding point of the edge of the acetabulum is squared, so that the two freshened bony surfaces may rest in contact.

**Albert's o.**, exsection of the articular ends of the tibia and femur to obtain ankylosis of the knee.

**Alexander-Adams o.**, shortening of the round ligaments of the uterus.

**Ammon's o.**, (1) blepharoplasty by transplantation from the cheek; (2) dacryocystotomy.

**Anagnostakis' o.**, Hotz-Anagnostakis o.

**Annandale's o.**, (1) exsection of the internal condyle of the femur for knock knee; (2) fixation by sutures of a loose cartilage in the knee joint.

**Arlt's o.**, transplantation of the eyelashes back from the edge of the lid in trichiasis.

**Babcock's o.**, extirpation of the varicosed saphenous vein by introducing an olive-tipped sound, and fastening the vein to it, and then drawing the latter out.

**Badal's o.**, laceration of the infratrochlear nerve for the relief of pain in glaucoma.

**Baldy's o.**, Webster's o.; an o. for retrodisplacement of the uterus, consisting in bringing the round ligaments through the perforated broad ligaments and attaching them to each other and to the back of the uterus; no longer due because of high incidence of intestinal obstruction.

**Ball's o.**, division of the sensory nerve trunks supplying the anus, for relief of pruritus ani.

**Bassini's o.**, an o. for the radical cure of hernia; after reduction of the hernia, the sac is twisted, ligated, and cut off, obliterating the canal; then a new canal is made by uniting the edges of the rectus and internal oblique muscles and joining them to the transversalis fascia and Poupart's ligament, placing on this the cord, and covering the latter by the external oblique.

**Baudelocque's o.**, an incision through the posterior cul-de-sac of the vagina for the removal of the ovum, in extrauterine pregnancy.

**Beck I o.**, a procedure, designed to increase the blood supply to the myocardium, consisting in abrasion of the epicardium and lining of the parietal pericardium, application of an irritant to these surfaces, partial occlusion of the coronary sinus at its opening into the right atrium, and grafting of mediastinal fat and the parietal pericardium to the surface of the heart.

**Beck II o.**, a two-stage procedure designed to improve the blood supply to the myocardium by placing a vein graft between the aorta and the coronary sinus; later the coronary sinus is partially occluded to increase the pressure therein and thereby induce retrograde flow of arterial blood into the coronary capillaries.

**Beer's o.**, flap o. for cataract.

**Belfield's o.**, vasostomy.

**Bergenhem's o.**, a method for the implantation of the ureter into the rectum.

**bifurcation o.**, Lorenz' o.

**Billroth's o.'s** o.'s for cancer of the stomach; I, excision of the pylorus with end-to-end anastomosis of stomach and duodenum; II, resection of the pylorus with the greater part of the lesser curvature of the stomach, closure of the cut ends of the duodenum and stomach, followed by a posterior gastrojejunostomy.

**Bischoff's o.,** total removal of the gravid uterus by the abdominal route.

**Blalock-Hanlon o.,** the creation of a large atrial septal defect as a palliative procedure for complete transposition of the great arteries.

**Blalock-Taussig o.,** an o. for congenital malformations of the heart, *e.g.,* stenosis at the pulmonary orifice and a septal defect with cyanosis, in which an abnormally small volume of blood passes through the pulmonary circuit; blood from the systemic circulation is directed to the lungs by anastomosing the innominate, right or left subclavian or a carotid artery to the pulmonary artery.

**Blaskovics' o.,** resection of the musculus levator palpebrae superioris for remedying blepharoptosis.

**bloodless o.,** one performed with loss of little or no blood.

**Bonnet's o.,** enucleation of the eyeball.

**Borthen's o.,** iridotasis.

**Bouilly's o.,** excision of a part of the mucous membrane of the cervix uteri, leaving a portion at each side to avoid the production of atresia.

**Bowman's o.,** (1) double-needle o. for dilaceration of a cataract, two lance-pointed needles being introduced through opposite sides of the cornea, the points meeting in the center of the lens and then being separated by moving the handles toward each other; (2) slitting the canaliculus for the relief of stenosis, to evacuate an abscess of the lacrimal sac, etc.

**Bozeman's o.,** hysterocystocleisis; an o. for uterovaginal fistula, the cervix uteri being attached to the bladder and opening into its cavity.

**Brailey's o.,** stretching of the supratrochlear nerve for the relief of pain in glaucoma; a modification of Badal's o.

**Brauer's o.,** cardiolysis.

**Bricker o.,** utilizes an isolated segment of ileum to conduct urine from ureters to skin surface.

**Brock o.,** transventricular valvotomy for relief of pulmonic stenosis.

**Brunschwig's o.,** (1) pancreatoduodenectomy; (2) total pelvic *exenteration.*

**Burow's o.,** (1) a flap o. for closing a defect in the lip; (2) blepharoplasty in which triangles of skin adjacent to sides of prepared sliding flap are excised to facilitate mobility.

**Caldwell-Luc o.,** radical exenteration of the contents of the maxillary antrum through an opening made in the supradental (canine) fossa above the second molar tooth.

**capital o.,** an o. of such magnitude or involving vital organs to such an extent that it is *per se* dangerous to life.

**Caslick's o.,** an o. for the correction of faulty conformation of the vulva of the mare, a frequent cause of low grade vaginitis and infertility. It consists of surgical closure of the dorsal portion of the vulva.

**Celsus' o.,** (1) circular amputation by a single sweep of the knife; (2) lithotomy performed by cutting directly upon the stone pressed into the perineum by two fingers in the rectum.

**cesarean o.,** see cesarean *section* and cesarean *hysterectomy.*

**Codivilla's o.,** surrounding the line of pseudoarthrosis with osteoperiosteal grafts taken from the tibia.

**concrete o.'s,** in the psychology of Piaget, a stage of development in thinking, occurring approximately between 7 and 11 years of age, during which a child becomes capable of reasoning about concrete situations.

**Cotte's o.,** presacral neurectomy.

**Cotting's o.,** cutting off the flesh at each side of the toe in cases of ingrowing toenail.

**Critchett's o.,** removal of the anterior portion of the eyeball.

**Dana's o.,** posterior *rhizotomy.*

**Dandy o.,** (1) third *ventriculostomy;* (2) suboccipital trigeminal *rhizotomy.*

**Daviel's o.,** extracapsular cataract extraction.

**decompression o.'s,** see decompression.

**de Grandmont's o.,** an o. for the correction of ptosis of the eyelid.

**DeLee's o.,** key-in-lock *maneuver.*

**Drummond-Morison o.,** omentopexy for ascites; an obsolete procedure.

**Dudley's o.,** (1) an obsolete procedure for the relief of retrodisplacement, consisting of shortening the round ligaments by fastening them to an oval denuded area on the

anterior uterine wall; (2) splitting the cervix uteri for the relief of obstructive dysmenorrhea.

**Dührssen's o.,** vaginal fixation of the uterus.

**Dupuy-Dutemps o.,** a modification of the Toti operation for stenosis of the lacrimal duct.

**Edebohls' o.,** nephrocapsectomy.

**Elliot's o.,** trephining of the eyeball, at the corneoscleral margin, to relieve tension in glaucoma.

**Emmet's o.,** trachelorrhaphy.

**equil'ibrating o.,** tenotomy of the healthy antagonist of a paralyzed eye muscle.

**Esser's o.,** epithelial *inlay.*

**Estes o.,** an o. for sterility in which a portion of an ovary is implanted on one uterine cornua.

**Estlander's o.,** resection of a part of one or more ribs and excision of the affected pleura in chronic empyema.

**exploratory o.,** one made in order to ascertain the condition present.

**Farabeuf's o.,** ischiohebotomy.

**fenestra'tion o.,** a surgical procedure producing an opening from the external auditory canal to the membranous labyrinth, used to improve hearing in the conduction type of hearing impairment.

**Finney's o.,** a form of gastroduodenostomy in which a large opening is formed, insuring free emptying from the stomach.

**Finsterer's o.,** Hofmeister's o.

**flap o.,** (1) flap *amputation;* (2) in dental surgery, an o. in which a portion of the mucoperiosteal tissues are surgically detached from the underlying bone or impacted tooth for better access and visibility in exploring the area covered by the tissue; **modified flap o.'s** allow for variation in the design, direction, and number of incisions in creating a mucoperiosteal flap. See also subentries under flap.

**Foley's o.,** Y-plasty procedure for ureteropelvic junction stricture.

**formal o.'s,** in the psychology of Piaget, a stage of development in thinking, occurring approximately between 11 and 15 years of age, during which a child becomes capable of reasoning about abstract situations; reasoning at this stage is comparable to that of normal adults but less sophisticated.

**Fothergill's o.,** Manchester o.

**Frazier-Spiller o.,** a subtemporal trigeminal *rhizotomy.*

**Fredet-Ramstedt o.,** pyloromyotomy.

**Freund's o.,** (1) total abdominal hysterectomy for uterine cancer; (2) chondrotomy to relieve Freund's anomaly.

**Freyer's o.,** suprapubic excision of the prostate gland.

**Frommel's o.,** shortening of the uterosacral ligaments by the abdominal route, for retrodeviation.

**Frost-Lang o.,** insertion of a gold ball after the enucleation of the eyeball, then union of the superior and inferior recti muscles by a suture including the overlying conjunctiva.

**Fukala's o.,** removal of the lens for the relief of very pronounced myopia.

**Galbiati's o.,** bilateral pelvitomy or ischiopubiotomy, through the rami forming the obturator foramina, with symphyseotomy.

**Gifford's o.,** delimiting *keratotomy.*

**Gigli's o.,** pubiotomy.

**Gill bone-block o.,** the insertion of a wedge of bone taken from the os calcis, to restrict plantar flexion in cases of drop foot or of pes equinus, due to overaction of the calf muscles.

**Gilliam's o.,** an o. for retroversion of uterus by suturing round ligaments to abdominal wall fascia.

**Gillies' o.,** (1) correction of ectropion by epithelial outlay, the skin of the eyelid being made thereby; (2) a technique for reducing fractures of the zygoma and the zygomatic arch through an incision in the temporal region above the hairline.

**Gonin o.,** closure of a laceration in the retina through cauterization, in the treatment of detachment of the retina.

**Graefe's o.,** removal of cataract by a limbal incision with capsulotomy and iridectomy.

**Gritti's o.,** Gritti's *amputation.*

**Halsted's o.'s,** (1) an o. for the radical cure of inguinal hernia; (2) amputation of the breast for carcinoma with removal of the pectoralis major and minor and lymphatic structures of the axilla.

**Haynes' o.,** drainage of the cisterna magna in the treatment of acute suppurative meningitis.

**Heaney's o.,** technique for vaginal hysterectomy.

**Heile o.,** a subarachnoid ureterostomy.

**Heine's o.,** cyclodialysis.

**Heisrath's o.,** an o. for trachoma, consisting of excision of the tarsal folds.

**Heller o.,** esophagomyotomy.

**Herbert's o.,** an o. for obtaining a filtering cicatrix in glaucoma by cutting and displacing, without removing, a wedge-shaped scleral flap.

**Hey's o.,** Hey's *amputation.*

**Hibbs' o.,** ankylosis of the spine in Pott's disease; the spinous processes and laminae are denuded of periosteum, the processes are "green-stick" fractured at the bases and turned down so that their tips rest against the broken bases of the processes below; then a sliver of bone is raised from the lower edge of each lamina and turned down so as to unite with the lamina below; finally the periosteum and split supraspinous ligaments are reunited over the spine.

**Hoffa's o.,** hollowing out the acetabulum and reduction of the head of the femur after severing the muscles inserted into the upper portion of the bone, in cases of congenital dislocation of the hip.

**Hofmeister's o.,** Finsterer's o.; partial gastrectomy with closure of a portion of the lesser curvature and retrocolic anastomosis of remainder to jejunum.

**Horsley's o.,** subpial resection of an area of cortex for the relief of athetoid and convulsive movements of an upper extremity.

**Hotz-Anagnostakis o.,** an o. for the correction of entropion and trichiasis of cicatricial origin.

**Huggins' o.,** orchidectomy for cancer of prostate.

**Hunter's o.,** ligation of the artery on the proximal side and at some distance from the sac, for the cure of aneurysm.

**Indian o.,** a plastic o. for restoration of the nose by means of a flap taken from the forehead.

**interval o.,** an o. performed during a period of quiescence or of intermission, as in appendicitis after an acute attack has passed away, but when a recurrence may be expected.

**Italian o.,** Tagliacotian o.

**Jaboulay's o.,** interpelviabdominal *amputation.*

**Jacobaeus o.,** pleurolysis; locating pleural adhesions by the aid of an endoscope and then dividing them with the electric cautery.

**Jansen's o.,** an o. for frontal sinus disease, the lower wall and lower portion of the anterior wall being removed and the mucous membrane curetted away.

**Jelks' o.,** an o. for rectal stricture, especially one of perirectal origin; an anteroposterior incision is made on each side of the anus, through which the fibrous tissue surrounding the rectum is incised.

**Jobert de Lamballe's o.,** closure of a vesicovaginal fissure by autoplasty.

**Kazanjian's o.,** surgical extension of the vestibular sulcus of edentulous ridges to increase their height and to improve denture retention; see also ridge *extension.*

**Keen's o.,** removal of sections of the posterior branches of the spinal nerves to the affected muscles, and of the spinal accessory nerve, as a cure for torticollis.

**Kelly's o.,** (1) correction of retroversion of the uterus by plication of uterosacral ligaments; (2) correction of urinary stress incontinence by vaginally placing sutures beneath the bladder neck.

**Killian's o.,** an o. for frontal sinus disease; a skin incision is made from the inner third of the edge of the orbit to the root of the nose, the periosteal incision being a little higher up; the entire anterior wall is removed and the mucous membrane is curetted away; the ethmoid cells are scraped out through an opening in the nasal process of the maxillary bone, and the upper wall of the orbit is removed as well.

**Kocher's o.,** resection of the wrist by means of an incision on the ulnar side of the dorsum.

**Kocks' o.,** shortening of the base of the broad ligament, through the vagina, for prolapse or retroversion of the uterus.

**Koenig's o.,** shelving o.; in congenital dislocation of the hip, reduction of the dislocation and formation of a lip to the upper edge of the acetabulum by an osteoperiosteal strip cut from the surface of the ilium.

**Koerte-Ballance o.,** operative anastomosis of the facial and hypoglossal nerves for the relief of facial paralysis.

**Kondoleon o.,** excision of strips of subcutaneous connective tissue for the relief of elephantiasis.

**Kraske's o.,** removal of the coccyx and excision of the left wing of the sacrum in order to afford approach for resection of the rectum for cancer or stenosis.

**Krause's o.,** extradural o. for the removal of the Gasserian ganglion in trigeminal neuralgia.

**Krönlein's o.,** resection of the anterior portion of the lateral wall of the orbit.

**Lagrange's o.,** a combined iridectomy and sclerectomy performed in glaucoma for the purpose of forming a filtering cicatrix.

**Lane-Lannelongue o.,** a decompression o. consisting in removal segments of bone from the roof of the skull.

**Laroyenne's o.,** puncture of Douglas' cul-de-sac to evacuate the pus and to secure drainage in cases of pelvic suppuration.

**Lash's o.,** removal of a wedge of the internal cervical os with suturing of the internal os into a tighter canal structure.

**Legg's o.,** transplantation of the tensor fascia into the femur in cases of weakness of the gluteus medius muscle.

**Leriche's o.,** periarterial *sympathectomy.*

**Lisfranc's o.,** Lisfranc's *amputation.*

**Longmire's o.,** intrahepatic cholangiojejunostomy with partial hepatectomy for biliary obstruction.

**Lorenz' o.,** a bifurcation o. for congenital dislocation of the hips; an oblique osteotomy of the upper femur with placement of the distal end in the acetabulum.

**Luc's o.,** Caldwell-Luc o.

**Macewen's o.,** supracondyloid osteotomy of the femur for knock-knee.

**Madlener o.,** tubal sterilization by clamp and tie.

**magnet o.,** the drawing out of a fragment of iron or steel from the eyeball by means of a powerful electromagnet.

**major o.,** an o. of great extent or involving vital organs, thereby exposing the patient directly to danger of death.

**Manchester o.** [ *Manchester*, England ], Fothergill's o.; a vaginal o. for prolapse uteri consisting of cervical amputation and parametrial fixation (cardinal ligaments) anterior to the uterus.

**Mann-Williamson o.,** an o. performed on experimental animals (dogs) in research on peptic ulcer, the duodenum with its alkaline secretions being transplanted into the ileum and the cut end of the jejunum anastomosed to the pylorus. The animals develop ulcers in the jejunum which receives directly the gastric juice.

**marcellation o.,** vaginal hysterectomy in which the uterus is removed by lateral halves after being split.

**Marckwald's o.,** an o. for stenosis of the external os uteri, consisting in the excision of two wedge-shaped pieces from opposite sides of the portio vaginalis, and suturing the edges of the defects.

**Marshall-Marchetti o.,** an o. for stress incontinence, performed retropubically.

**Matas' o.,** aneurysmoplasty.

**Matson o.,** a subarachnoid ureterostomy.

**Mayo's o.,** an o. for the radical cure of umbilical hernia; the neck of the sac is exposed by two elliptical incisions, the gut is returned to the abdomen, the sac and adherent omentum are cut away, and the walls of the opening are overlapped with mattress sutures.

**McIndoe's o.,** colpopoiesis.

**McVay's o.,** repair of inguinal and femoral hernias by suture of the aponeurosis of the transversus abdominis muscle and its associated fasciae to the pectineal ligament (of Cooper).

**mika o.** [ Australian native term ], the establishment of a permanent fistula in the bulbous portions of the urethra in order to render the man incapable of procreating; said to be a practice among certain Australian tribes.

**Mikulicz' o.,** (1) exsection of the sternocleidomastoid muscles in torticollis; (2) excision of bowel in two stages, first, exteriorizing the diseased area, suturing efferent and afferent limbs together, and closing the abdomen around them, after which the diseased part is excised; second, at a later time, cutting the spur with an enterotome and closing the stoma extraperitoneally.

**Mikulicz-Vladimiroff o.,** Mikulicz-Vladimiroff *amputation.*

**Miles' o.,** one-stage abdominoperineal radical o. for carcinoma of the rectum.

**minor o.,** an o. of slight extent and not in itself dangerous to life.

**Motais' o.,** transplantation of the middle third of the tendon of the superior rectus muscle of the eyeball into the upper lid, between the tarsus and skin, to supplement the action of the levator muscle in ptosis.

**Mules' o.,** evisceration of the eyeball followed by the insertion within the sclera of a hollow ball of glass, gold, or some other nonirritating material, to give support to an artificial eye.

**Naffziger o.,** orbital decompression for severe malignant exophthalmos by removal of the lateral and superior orbital walls.

**Narath's o.,** omentopexy for ascites; an obsolete procedure.

**Nissen's o.,** fundoplication.

**Ober's o.,** fasciotomy.

**Ogston's o.,** (1) separation of the internal condyle of the femur, followed by forcible straightening of the limb, for the correction of knock knee; (2) treatment of flatfoot by removal of the adjacent articular surfaces of the talus and navicular bone in order to effect ankylosis between them.

**Ogston-Luc o.,** an o. for frontal sinus disease; skin incision from inner third of edge of orbit toward root of nose or outward; the periosteum is pushed upward and outward, and the sinus is opened on outer side of median line; then wide opening is made by curetting nasofrontal duct, interior of sinus, and anterior ethmoid cells.

**Olshausen's o.,** an o. to correct retroversion of the uterus; the uterus is suspended by suturing the midportion of the round ligament of the uterus to the anterior rectus sheath.

**Ord's o.,** an o. for overcoming fresh adhesions in the joints.

**Paci's o.,** an o. for congenital dislocation of hip.

**Panas' o.,** connecting the upper eyelid with the occipitofrontalis muscle, for the relief of congenital ptosis.

**Pancoast's o.,** division of the trigeminal nerve at the foramen ovale.

**Phelps' o.,** division of all the soft parts on the inner border of the foot, including the ligaments and tendons, followed by forcible correction, in the treatment of talipes varus.

**Physick's o.,** iridectomy with the formation of a circular opening.

**plastic o.,** reparative o.; one undertaken to restore lost parts or lost functions.

**Pólya's o.,** Pólya gastrectomy; partial gastrectomy with retrocolic anastomosis of the full width of stomach to jejunum.

**Pomeroy's o.,** excision of a ligated portion of the Fallopian tubes.

**Poncet's o.,** (1) lengthening of the tendo Achillis for talipes equinus; (2) perineal urethrostomy; (3) perineotomy; perineal cystotomy in prostatic disease.

**Porro o.,** cesarean *hysterectomy.*

**Pott's o.,** Potts' anastomosis; direct side-to-side anastomosis between aorta and pulmonary artery as a palliative procedure in Fallot's tetralogy.

**Putti-Platt o.,** a procedure for recurrent dislocation of shoulder joint.

**radical o.,** a thorough o. intended to cure the abnormal condition and prevent its recurrence.

**radical o. for hernia,** an o. by which the hernia is reduced, and the canal through which the gut descended is obliterated.

**Ramstedt o.,** Fredet-Ramstedt o.

**Récamier's o.,** curettage of the uterus.

**Reed's o.,** ligature in sections of the plexus of veins in tubo-ovarian varicocele.

**Ridell's o.,** removal of the entire anterior and inferior walls of the frontal sinus, for chronic inflammation of that cavity.

**Roux-en-Y o.,** the distal end of the divided jejunum is anastomosed to the stomach and the proximal end is implanted into the side of the jejunum, about three inches below the first anastomosis.

**Ruotte's o.,** venoperitoneostomy.

**Saemisch's o.,** incision of the cornea to evacuate pus.

**Saenger's o.,** cesarean section followed by careful closure of the uterine wound by three tiers of sutures.

**Salzer's o.,** excision of the mandibular division of the trigeminal nerve.

**Schauta-Amreich vaginal o.,** an extensive extirpation of the uterus and the adnexa, using the vaginal approach facilitated by the Schuchardt paravaginal incision (see Schuchardt's o.).

**Schroeder's o.,** excision of diseased endocervical mucosa.

**Schuchardt's o.,** paravaginal rectal displacement incision; a surgical technique of making the upper vagina accessible for fistula closure or radical surgery per vaginam.

**Schwartze o.,** an o. for mastoiditis; an incision is made from the temporal line to the apex of the mastoid process, parallel to and 1/4 inch behind the attachment of the pinna; then the mastoid antrum is cautiously opened and free drainage is established for the escape of pus.

**Schwartze-Stacke o.,** a mastoid o. combining the main features of the Schwartze and the Stacke o.'s.

**scleral buckling o.,** an o. performed in retinal detachment to indent the sclerochoroidal wall.

**seton o.,** an o. for advanced glaucoma; passage of a suture or seton into the anterior chamber to act as a wick.

**shelving o.,** Koenig's o.

**Shirodkar o.,** purse-string suturing of an incompetent cervical os with a nonabsorbent suture material; a cerclage procedure.

**Siebold's o.,** pubiotomy.

**Sigault's o.,** symphysiotomy.

**Simon's o.,** (1) colpocleisis; (2) repair of a ruptured perineum by suturing first the vaginal mucous membrane and then the cutaneous surface.

**Smith's o., Smith-Indian o.,** a surgical technique for removal of cataract within the capsule.

**Smith-Robinson o.,** interbody fusion through an anterior cervical approach.

**Spinelli o.,** an o. splitting the anterior wall of the prolapsed uterus and reversing the organ preliminary to reposition.

**Stacke o.,** the pinna and cartilaginous auditory canal are separated from their attachments and turned forward; the outer wall of the attic is now removed and the external wall of the antrum, so that tympanum, aditus, and antrum make but one cavity, thus giving free exit to pus in mastoiditis.

**stapes mobilization o.,** fracture of tissue immobilizing the stapes to restore hearing, especially used in patients with otosclerosis.

**Stoffel's o.,** division of certain motor nerves for the relief of spastic paralysis.

**Stoltz' o.,** pubiotomy.

**Stookey-Scarff o.,** third *ventriculostomy.*

**Stromeyer-Little o.,** an o. for abscess of the liver, the pus being found by a cannula and the abscess being then opened by the knife running along the cannula as a guide.

**Sturmdorf's o.,** conical removal of the endocervix.

**subcutaneous o.,** an o., as for the division of a tendon, performed without incising the skin other than by a minute opening made by the entering knife.

**Syme's o.,** (1) Syme's *amputation;* (2) excision of the tongue; (3) external urethrotomy.

**Tagliacotian o.,** Italian o.; a plastic o. in which the skin flap is taken from a distant part; especially rhinoplasty, in which the new nose is fashioned from the forearm which is bound firmly to the face until the flap is solidly united in its new position.

**Tait's o.,** a form of perineoplasty.

**talc o.,** poudrage; pericardial poudrage; application of magnesium silicate powder to the epicardium, designed to create a sterile granulomatous pericarditis and thus promote pericardial anastomoses with the coronary circulation.

**Talma's o.,** omentopexy for ascites; an obsolete procedure.

**Tansini's o.,** (1) an o. for the removal of a cyst of the liver; (2) amputation of the breast with removal of all the skin covering it, the loss being compensated for by a generous flap taken from the back.

**TeLinde o.,** modified radical *hysterectomy.*

**Terrillon's o.,** removal of hydatids by gradual constriction with an elastic ligature.

**Torek o.,** (1) an o. for the removal of a carcinoma of the thoracic portion of the esophagus; (2) an o. for bringing down an undescended testicle.

**Toti's o.,** dacryocystorrhinostomy.

**Trendelenburg's o.,** (1) ligation of the saphena magna for the cure of varicose veins; (2) excision of varicose veins; (3) synchondroseotomy; (4) pulmonary embolectomy.

**Urban's o.,** extended radical mastectomy, including *en bloc* resection of internal mammary lymph nodes, part of the sternum, and costal cartilages, in continuity with the origin of the greater pectoral muscle.

**Verhoeff's o.,** sclerotomy combined with electrolytic punctures for detachment of the retina.

**Vermale's o.,** a double-flap transfixion amputation.

**Vidal's o.,** subcutaneous ligature of the veins for the cure of varicocele.

**Wagner's o.,** osteoplastic resection of the skull.

**Waters' o.,** an extraperitoneal cesarean section.

**Webster's o.,** Baldy's o.

**Weir's o.,** appendicostomy.

**Wertheim's o.,** a radical o. for carcinoma of the uterus in which as much as possible of the vagina is excised and there is wide lymph node excision.

**Wheelhouse's o.,** external *urethrotomy.*

**Whipple's o.,** pancreatoduodenectomy.

**Whitehead's o.,** excision of hemorrhoids by two circular incisions above and below involved veins, allowing normal mucosa to be pulled down and sutured to anal skin.

**Williams' o.,** colpopoiesis.

**Wilms' o.,** resection of the ribs anteriorly and posteriorly so that the chest may be flattened and the lungs compressed by the sinking in of the chest wall; it is resorted to in certain cases of pulmonary tuberculosis.

**Wölfler's o.,** anterior *gastroenterostomy.*

**Wyeth's o.,** bloodless amputation of the hip, hemorrhage being controlled by a strong elastic tube held in place by long needles transfixing the tissues above the joint.

**Wylie's o.,** intra-abdominal shortening of the round ligaments; each ligament is folded on itself and held by sutures, the opposing surfaces being freshened.

**Ziegler's o.,** a V-shaped iridotomy for the formation of an artificial pupil.

---

**op'era'tive.** 1. Relating to, or effected by means of an operation. 2. Active; effective.

**op'era'tor.** In genetics, operator *gene.*

**opercular** (o-per'ku-lar). Relating to an operculum.

**oper'culated.** Provided with a lid (operculum); denoting the eggs of certain parasitic worms such as the trematodes (except the schistosomes) and the broad fish tapeworm.

**operculitis** (o-per'ku-li'tis) [ operculum + G. suffix -*itis*, inflammation ]. Pericoronitis.

**oper'culum,** gen. **oper'culi,** pl. **oper'cula** (o-per'ku-lum) [ L. cover or lid, fr. *operio*, pp. *opertus*, to cover ]. 1. Anything resembling a lid or cover. 2 [ NA ]. Specifically, in anatomy the portions of the frontal (o. frontale), parietal (o. frontoparietale), and temporal (o. temporale), lobes bordering the lateral sulcus and covering the insula. 3. A bit of mucus sealing the endocervical canal of the uterus after conception has taken place. 4. In parasitology, the lid or caplike cover of a trematode egg. 5. The attached flap in tear of retinal detachment. 6. The mucosal flap partially or completely covering an unerupted tooth.

**occip'ital o.,** a portion of the occipital lobe of the brain cut off by the ape fissure, rarely present in man.

**trophoblastic o.,** the mushroom-shaped plug of fibrin that fills the aperture in the endometrium made by the implanting ovum.

**op'eron.** A genetic functional unit that controls production of messenger RNA; it consists of an operator gene and two or more structural genes located in sequence in the cis position on one chromosome. See fig. under protein.

**ophiasis** (o-fi'ä-sis) [ G. fr. *ophis*, snake ]. A form of alopecia areata in which the loss of hair occurs in bands partially or completely encircling the head.

**Ophidia** (o-fid'i-ah) [ G. *ophidion*, dim. of *ophis*, a serpent ]. The snakes, a suborder of the class *Reptilia.*

**ophidiasis** (o'fi-di'ä-sis) [ G. *ophidion*, dim. of *ophis*, a serpent ]. Ophidism; poisoning by a snake.

**ophid'ic.** Relating to snakes.

**ophidin** (o'fi-din). A β-alanyl 2-methylhistidine dipeptide found in snake muscle. See also anserine.

**ophidiophobia** (o-fid-i-o-fo'bi-ah) [ G. *ophidion*, a small snake, + *phobos*, fear ]. A morbid fear of snakes.

**ophidism** (o'fid-izm). Ophidiasis.

**ophioxylin** (o'fi-ok'si-lin). An amaroid from *Rauwolfia Serpentina* (family Apocynaceae), or dogbane; oxytocic, antiperiodic, and anthelmintic.

**ophritis** (of-ri'tis) [ G. *ophrys*, eyebrow, + suffix -*itis*, inflammation ]. Ophryitis; dermatitis in the region of the eyebrows.

**ophryitis** (of-re-i'tis). Ophritis.

**oph'ryon** [ G. *ophrys*, eyebrow ]. The point on the midline of the forehead just above the glabella (1). See fig. under craniometric *point.*

**Ophryoscolecidae** (of're-o-sko-les'i-de) [ G. *ophrys*, eyebrow, + *scolex*, *q.v.* ]. A family of ciliate protozoa occurring in the rumen and reticulum of ruminant animals and characterized by having cilia arranged in spiral membranelles around the mouth (adoral) and in some genera also in a dorsal (metoral) position. The most important genera are *Entodinium, Diplodinium, Epidinium* and *Ophryoscolex.* They are thought to contribute to ruminant nutrition by converting cellulose in plant material ingested by the ruminant into readily digestible animal protein of their own bodies.

**ophryosis** (of-re-o'sis) [ G. *ophrys*, eyebrow, + suffix -*osis*, condition ]. Spasmodic twitching of the upper portion of the orbicularis palpebrarum muscle causing a wrinkling of the eyebrow.

**ophthalm-.** See ophthalmo-.

**ophthalmacrosis** (of-thal-mä-kro'sis) [ ophthalmo- + G. *makros*, large ]. Enlargement of the eye.

**oph'thalmag'ra** [ ophthalmo- + G. *agra*, seizure ]. Gouty inflammation of the eye or any of its parts.

**ophthalmalgia** (of'thal-mal'ji-ah) [ ophthalmo- + G. *algos*, pain ]. Ophthalmodynia; pain in the eyeball.

**ophthalmatrophia, ophthalmatrophy** (of-thal'mä-tro'fi-ah, of'thal-mat'ro-fi). Atrophy of the eyeball.

**ophthalmectomy** (of'thal-mek'to-mi) [ ophthalmo- + G. *ektomē*, excision ]. Enucleation of the eyeball.

**ophthalmedema** (of-thal'me-de'mah) [ ophthalmo- + G. *oidema*, swelling ]. Edema of the orbit, conjunctiva, and eyelids.

**ophthalmia** (of-thal'mi-ah) [ G. ]. 1. Severe, often purulent, conjunctivitis. 2. Inflammation of the deeper structures of the eye.

**catarrhal o.,** mucous o.; a mild form of conjunctivitis with mucopurulent secretion.

**caterpillar-hair o.,** o. nodosa.

**o. eczematosa,** phlyctenosis; superficial vascularization of the conjunctiva and sclera with scattered yellow phlyctenules at the limbus and in the cornea.

**Egyptian o.,** trachoma.

**electric o.,** conjunctivitis caused by the irritation from actinic light in electric welding.

**gonorrheal o.,** blennorrhea conjunctivalis; acute purulent conjunctivitis excited by the presence of the gonococcus.

**granular o.,** trachoma (1).

**metastatic o.,** (1) sympathetic o; (2) choroiditis in pyemia.

**migratory o.,** sympathetic o.

**mucous o.,** catarrhal o.

**o. neonato'rum,** blennorrhea neonatorum; gonococcal conjunctivitis in the newborn.

**neuroparalytic o.,** corneal inflammation or ulceration following lesion of the ophthalmic branch of the trigeminal nerve.

**o. nodo'sa,** caterpillar-hair o.; pseudotuberculous o.; the presence of nodular swellings on the conjunctiva, due to penetration of ocular tissues by the hairs of caterpillars.

**periodic o.,** moon blindness; an acute iridocyclitis of horses, involving one or both eyes; it subsides only to recur at intervals of varying length and usually ends in blindness; the cause is uncertain but some have associated it with *Leptospira;* it does not appear to be contagious.

**phlycten'ular o.,** phlyctenular *conjunctivitis.*

**pseu'dotuber'culous o.,** o. nodosa.

**pu'rulent o.,** purulent conjunctivitis, usually of gonorrheal origin.

**scrof'ulous o.,** phlyctenular *conjunctivitis.*

**spring o.,** vernal *conjunctivitis.*

**sympathet'ic o.,** a serous or plastic uveitis caused by a perforating wound of the uvea followed by a similar severe reaction in the other eye that may eventuate to bilateral blindness. Also called migratory, transferred, or metastatic o.

**transferred o.,** sympathetic o.

**ophthal'mic** [ G. *ophthalmikos* ]. Ocular; relating to the eye.

**ophthal'mic acid.** A tripeptide occurring in calf lens, similar to glutathione but differing in the replacement of cysteine by α-amino-*n*-butyric acid (*i.e.,* in the replacement of —SH by —CH₃). Compare norophthalmic acid. O. acid is a potent inhibitor of glyoxalase.

**ophthalmicus** [ L. ] [ NA ]. Ophthalmic.

**ophthalmit'ic.** Relating to inflammation of the eye.

**ophthalmitis** (of-thal-mi'tis). Ophthalmia.

**ophthalmo-, ophthalm-** (of-thal'mo-) [ G. *ophthalmos,* eye. OPH- ]. Combining forms denoting relationship to the eye.

**ophthalmoblennorrhea** (of-thal'mo-blen-or-ē'ah) [ ophthalmo- + G. *blenna,* mucus, + *rhoia,* flow ]. Purulent, usually gonorrheal, ophthalmia.

**ophthal'mocarcino'ma.** Carcinoma of the eye.

**ophthalmocele** (of-thal'mo-sēl) [ ophthalmo- + G. *kēlē,* hernia ]. Rarely used term meaning exophthalmos.

**ophthalmocentesis** (of-thal'mo-sen-te'sis) [ ophthalmo- + G. *kentēsis,* puncture ]. Surgical puncture of the eye.

**ophthalmodesmitis** (of-thal'mo-dez-mi'tis) [ ophthalmo- + G. *desmos,* band, + suffix -*itis,* inflammation ]. Ophthalmic tenonitis; inflammation of the tendons or fibrous structure of the eye.

**ophthal'modiagno'sis.** Diagnosis of an infectious disease by means of the ophthalmoreaction.

**ophthalmodiaphanoscope** (of-thal'mo-di'ah-fan'o-skōp) [ ophthalmo- + diaphanoscope, *q.v.* ]. An instrument for viewing the interior of the eye by transmitted light.

**ophthalmodiastimeter** (of-thal'mo-di-ă-stim'e-ter) [ ophthalmo- + G. *diastasis,* separation, + *metron,* measure ]. A device for adjusting the lenses of spectacles and eyeglasses so that their optical centers correspond to the visual axes of the eyes.

**ophthalmodonesis** (of-thal'mo-do-ne'sis) [ ophthalmo- + G. *doneō,* to agitate ]. Trembling motion of the eyes.

**ophthal'modynamom'eter** [ ophthalmo- + G. *dynamis,* power, + *metron,* measure ]. 1. An instrument for determining the power of convergence of the eyes as regards the near point of vision. 2. An instrument that measures the blood pressure in the retinal vessels.

**Bailliart's o.,** an instrument that measures the apparent diastolic and systolic blood pressure of the central retinal artery; of value in diagnosing occlusion of the proximal carotid system and in assessing the effect of ligation of the carotid artery.

**optical-corneal pressure o.,** an o. in which the head of the slitlamp applanation tonometer is replaced by a —60 D fundus lens; graded pressure is delivered against the cornea while the observer views the slitlamp image of the central retinal artery through this lens.

**suction o.,** an o. with a suction disk which provides increased ocular pressure during ophthalmoscopic observation of the retinal artery.

**ophthal'modynamom'etry** [ ophthalmo- + G. *dynamis,* power, + *metron,* measure ]. 1. The process of measuring the degree of power of the extraocular muscles. 2. The measurement of blood pressure in the retinal vessels by means of an ophthalmodynamometer.

**ophthalmodynia** (of-thal'mo-din'ĭ-ah) [ ophthalmo- + G. *odynē,* pain ]. Ophthalmalgia.

**ophthalmo-eikonometer** (of-thal'mo-i'ko-nom'e-ter) [ ophthalmo- + G. *eikon,* image, + *metron,* measure ].

Ophthalmoiconometer; an instrument for measuring aniseikonia.

**ophthal'mofun'doscope** [ ophthalmo- + L. *fundus,* bottom, + G. *skopeō,* to view ]. Obsolete term for ophthalmoscope.

**ophthal'mogram.** The record made by an ophthalmograph, or the similar record made by electro-oculography.

**ophthal'mograph.** An instrument that records eye movements during reading by photographing a mark on the cornea or making a tracing of light reflexes.

**ophthalmography** (of'thal-mog'ră-fĭ) [ ophthalmo- + G. *graphē,* a description ]. 1. Use of the ophthalmograph. 2. A treatise on or description of the eyes.

**ophthalmoiconometer** (of-thal-mo-i'ko-nom'e-ter). Ophthalmo-eikonometer.

**ophthalmoleukoscope** (of-thal'mo-lu'ko-skōp) [ ophthalmo- + G. *leukos,* white, + *skopeō,* to examine ]. A polarizing instrument, used in examining for color blindness, in which the controlled color intensities produce a white mixture.

**ophthal'molith** [ ophthalmo- + G. *lithos,* stone ]. Dacryolith.

**ophthalmol'ogist.** One skilled in ophthalmology; an oculist; a specialist in diseases and refractive errors of the eye.

**ophthalmology** (of'thal-mol'o-jĭ) [ ophthalmo- + G. *logos,* study ]. The branch of medical science that has to do with the eye, its diseases and refractive errors.

**ophthalmomalacia** (of-thal'mo-mă-la'shĭ-ah) [ ophthalmo- + G. *malakia,* softness ]. Abnormal softening of the eyeball.

**ophthalmomelanosis** (of-thal'mo-mel'ă-no'sis). Melanotic discoloration of the conjunctiva and adjoining tissues.

**ophthalmometer** (of'thal-mom'e-ter) [ ophthalmo- + G. *metron,* measure ]. Keratometer.

**oph'thalmom'etry.** Keratometry.

**ophthalmomycosis** (of-thal-mo-mi-ko'sis) [ ophthalmo- + G. *mykēs,* fungus, + suffix -*osis,* condition ]. Oculomycosis; any disease of the eye or its appendages caused by the growth of a fungus.

**ophthalmomyiasis** (of-thal'mo-mi-i'ă-sis). Ocular *myiasis.*

**ophthalmomyitis** (of-thal-mo-mi-i'tis) [ ophthalmo- + G. *mys,* muscle, + suffix -*itis,* inflammation ]. Ophthalmomyositis; inflammation of the extrinsic muscles of the eye.

**ophthalmomyositis** (of-thal-mo-mi-o-si'tis). Ophthalmomyitis.

**ophthalmomyotomy** (of-thal'mo-mi-ot'o-mĭ) [ ophthalmo- + G. *mys,* muscle, + *tomē,* incision ]. Division of any of the extrinsic eye muscles.

**ophthalmoneuritis** (of-thal'mo-nu-ri'tis). Inflammation of the optic nerve.

**ophthal'moparal'ysis.** Ophthalmoplegia.

**ophthalmopathy** (of'thal-mop'ă-thĭ) [ ophthalmo- + G. *pathos,* suffering ]. Oculopathy; any disease of the eyes.

**endocrine o.,** exophthalmos caused by orbital mesenchymitis associated with hyperthyroidism.

**external o.,** any disease of the conjunctiva, cornea, or adnexa of the eye.

**internal o.,** any disease of the retina, lens, or other internal structures of the eyeball.

**ophthalmophacometer** (of-thal'mo-fa-kom'e-ter) [ ophthalmo- + G. *phakos,* lentil (lens), + *metron,* measure ]. An instrument for measuring the refractive power of the crystalline lens of the eye, using the Purkinje images.

**ophthalmophantom** (of-thal'mo-fan'tom). A model of the eye used for demonstration or for practicing surgery.

**ophthalmophlebotomy** (of-thal'mo-flē-bot'o-mĭ) [ ophthalmo- + G. *phleps,* vein, + *tomē,* incision ]. Incision of a conjunctival vein to relieve congestion.

**ophthalmophthisis** (oph-thal-mof'thĭ-sis) [ ophthalmo- + G. *phthisis,* a wasting. PHTH- ]. 1. Ophthalmomalacia. 2. *Phthisis* bulbi.

**ophthal'moplasty** [ ophthalmo- + G. *plassō,* to form ]. Reparative or plastic surgery of the eye.

**ophthalmoplegia** (of-thal'mo-ple'jĭ-ah) [ ophthalmo- + G. *plēgē,* stroke ]. Paralysis of one or more of the motor nerves of the eye.

**exophthal'mic o.,** protrusion of the eyeballs; o. due to orbital edema, stretching and paresis of the ocular muscles, incidental to certain thyroid disorders.

**o. exter'na,** Ballet's disease; paralysis affecting one or more of the nerves supplying the extrinsic eye muscles.

**fascic'ular o.,** o. due to a lesion in the pons.

**infectious o.,** transient or permanent nuclear paralysis of eye muscles, including the intraocular muscles, in encephalitis lethargica.

**o. inter'na,** paralysis affecting only the branches of the third nerve supplying the iris and ciliary muscle.

**o. internuclearis,** disordered movement of the extraocular muscles due to injury of the coordinating pathways in the brain stem.

**nu'clear o.,** o. due to a lesion of the nuclei of origin of the motor nerves of the eye.

**orbital o.,** o. due to some lesion within the orbit.

**Parinaud's o.,** paralysis of conjugate vertical movement upward; less often, downward.

**o. partia'lis,** incomplete o.; o. involving only one or two of the extrinsic or intrinsic ocular muscles.

**o. progressi'va,** Graefe's disease; progressive upper bulbar palsy, due to degeneration of the nuclei of the motor nerves of the eye.

**o. tota'lis,** paralysis of all the motor nerves of the eye, those supplying both the extrinsic and the intrinsic muscles.

**ophthalmople'gic.** 1. Relating to or marked by ophthalmoplegia. 2. An agent causing paralysis of the eye muscles, especially of the intrinsic muscles; a cycloplegic.

**ophthalmoptosis, ophthalmoptosia** (of-thal-mop-to'sis, -to'sĭ-ah) [ ophthalmo- + G. *ptōsis,* a falling ]. Obsolete term for exophthalmos.

**ophthalmopyorrhea** (of-thal'mo-pi-o-re'ah) [ ophthalmo- + G. *pyon,* pus, + *rhoia,* flow ]. Ophthalmorrhea.

**ophthalmoreaction** (of-thal'mo-re-ak'shun). Oculoreaction; an evanescent mild inflammatory reaction of the conjunctiva excited by the instillation of an antigen (allergen) in a sensitive (allergic) individual.

**ophthalmorrhagia** (of-thal-mo-ra'jĭ-ah) [ ophthalmo- + G. *rhēgnymi,* to burst forth ]. Hemorrhage from the eye.

**ophthalmorrhea** (of-thal-mo-re'ah) [ ophthalmo- + G. *rhoia,* flow ]. Ophthalmopyorrhea; a mucous or purulent discharge from the eye.

**ophthalmorrhexis** (of-thal-mo-rek'sis) [ ophthalmo- + G. *rhēxis,* rupture ]. Rupture of the eyeball.

**ophthal'moscope** [ ophthalmo- + G. *skopeō,* to examine ]. Funduscope; ophthalmofundoscope; an instrument

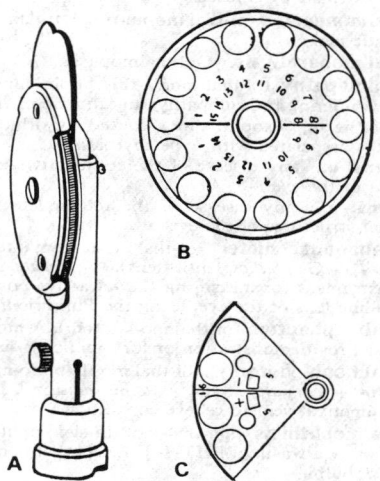

**Ophthalmoscope**
Self-lit electric monocular type. *A,* head, containing illuminating system and refraction disks; *B,* principle refraction disk with plus and minus lenses; *C,* supplementary lenses of stronger power.

for use in examination of the interior of the eye.

**binocular o.,** stereo-ophthalmoscope; one that uses a directed beam from an electric lamp and two adjustable oculars instead of the battery of lenses used in the monocular o.; a stereoscopic view of the fundus is obtainable by the use of apparatus separately designed for direct or indirect ophthalmoscopy.

**luminous o.,** one consisting of a prism which directs the light from an electric lamp contained in the instrument; in the head of the instrument is a battery of lenses which may be rotated in front of the peephole in monocular instruments.

**reflecting o.,** one consisting of a concave mirror with a hole in the center; the mirror serves to illuminate, by the reflection of a light beside the patient, the ocular media and the fundus of the eye, which the examiner observes through the central hole.

**oph'thalmos'copy.** Examination of the fundus of the eye by means of the ophthalmoscope.

**direct o.,** examination of the eye at close range, the image seen being an erect one.

**indirect o.,** examination of the fundus at nearly arm's length by means of the interposition of a convex lens, the image being an inverted one.

**medical o.,** ophthalmoscopic examination of the eye as an aid in diagnosis.

**metric o.,** o. as an aid to the determination of refractive errors of the eye.

**ophthalmostasis, ophthalmostasia** (of'thal-mos'tă-sis, of-thal-mo-sta'sĭ-ah) [ ophthalmo- + G. *stasis,* standing ]. Holding the eyeball immovable by means of the ophthalmostat.

**ophthalmostat** (of-thal'mo-stat). An instrument for holding the eyeball in order to prevent involuntary movements during an operation.

**ophthalmosteresis** (of-thal'mo-ste-re'sis) [ ophthalmo- + G. *stereō,* to deprive ]. Absence of an eye.

**ophthal'mothermom'eter.** A thermometer for determining the temperature of the eye.

**ophthal'motonom'eter.** Tonometer (2).

**ophthal'motonom'etry.** Tonometry (2).

**ophthal'motox'in.** A specific cytotoxin obtained by means of injections of emulsions of the ciliary body.

**ophthalmotrope** (of-thal'mo-trōp) [ ophthalmo- + G. *tropos,* a turning ]. A model of the two eyes, to each of which are attached weighted cords pulling in the direction of the six extrinsic eye muscles. Used to demonstrate the action of the ocular muscles singly or in various combinations.

**ophthal'movas'cular.** Relating to the blood vessels of the eye.

**ophthalmoxerosis** (of-thal-mo-ze-ro'sis). Xerophthalmia.

**ophthalmoxysis** (of-thal'mo-zi'sis, of'thal-mok'sĭ-sis) [ ophthalmo- + G. *xyō,* to scrape ]. Operation of lightly scraping the conjunctiva.

**ophthalmoxyster** (of-thal-mo-zis'ter, of-thal-moks-is'ter) [ ophthalmo- + *xystēr,* a scraper, fr. *xyō,* to scrape ]. A conjunctival curette, or instrument for lightly scraping the conjunctiva.

**ophthalmus** (of-thal'mus) [ L. fr. G. *ophthalmos* ]. The eye; oculus.

**-opia** [ G. *ōps,* eye ]. Suffix meaning vision.

**o'pianine.** Noscapine.

**o'pianyl.** Meconin.

**opiate** (o'pĭ-āt). Any preparation or derivative of opium.

**opioid** (o'pĭ-oyd). Designating synthetic narcotics that resemble opiates in action but are not derived from opium.

**opiomania** (o-pĭ'o-ma-nĭ-ah). Opium *addiction.*

**opiophagism, opiophagy** (o-pĭ-of'a-jizm, o-pĭ-of'a-jĭ) [ G. *opion,* opium, + *phagein,* to eat ]. Opium-eating; see opium *addiction.*

**opip'ramol hydrochloride** (USAN). ENSIDON; 4-[ 3-(5 *H*-dibenz[ *b,f* ]azepin-5-yl)propyl ]-1-piperazineethanol dihydrochloride; antidepressant agent.

**opisthenar** (o-pis'the-nar) [ G. back of the hand, from *opisthen,* behind, + *thenar,* palm of the hand ]. Dorsum of the hand.

**opisthiobasial** (o-pis'thĭ-o-ba'sĭ-al). Relating to both opisthion and basion; denoting a line connecting the two, or the distance between them.

**opisthion** (o-pis'thĭ-on) [ G. *opisthios*, posterior ]. The middle point on the posterior margin of the foramen magnum, opposite the basion.

**opisthionasial** (o-pis'thĭ-o-na'zĭ-al). Relating to the opisthion and the nasion; denoting the distance between the two points.

**opistho-** (op'is-tho-, o'pis'tho-) [ G. *opisthen*, at the rear, behind ]. Combining form meaning backward, behind, dorsal.

**opisthocheilia, opisthochilia** (op'is-tho-ki'lĭ-ah) [ opistho- + G. *cheilos*, lip ]. Recession of the lips.

**opisthomastigote** (o-pis'tho-mas'tĭ-gōt) [ opistho- + G. *mastix*, whip ]. Term now used instead of herpetomonad for the stage of development of certain insect and plant parasitizing flagellates to avoid confusion between the stage and the genus *Herpetomonas*. In this stage the flagellum arises from the kinetoplast located behind the nucleus and emerges from the anterior end of the organism. An undulating membrane is absent.

**opisthoporeia** (o-pis'tho-po-ri'ah, -re'ah) [ opistho- + G. *poreia*, a walking, fr. *poreuō*, to go, walk ]. Involuntary walking backward; frequently connected with parkinsonism.

**opisthorchiasis** (op'is-thor-ki'ă-sis). Infection with the Asiatic liver fluke, *Opisthorchis viverrini*, or other opisthorchiids.

**opisthorchiid** (op'is-thor'ke-id). Common name for members of the family Opisthorchiidae.

**Opisthorchiidae** (op'is-thor-ke'ĭ-de). A family of trematodes that includes the genera *Opisthorchis* and *Clonorchis*.

**Opisthorchis** (op-is-thor'kis) [ opistho- + G. *orchis*, testis ]. Genus of digenetic trematodes (family Opisthorchiidae) found in the bile ducts or gallbladder of fish-eating mammals, birds, and fish.

  O. felin'eus, the cat liver fluke; an inhabitant of the bile ducts and gallbladder, frequently found as a parasite of man in eastern Europe, Siberia, India, Japan, and southeast Asia; adults are lancet-shaped, thin, relatively transparent, and hermaphroditic; sizes range from 7 to 12 by 2 to 3 mm.; ingested eggs hatch in *Bithynia* snails, cercariae encyst on various species of fish, and man acquires the infection by ingesting raw or inadequately cooked fish; the parasites sometimes cause no evidence of disease, but cholangitis, biliary cirrhosis, and chronic pancreatitis may occur.

  O. sinen'sis endemic in Japan, Korea, most of China, and southeast Asia; adults are flattened or spatulate, transparent, flabby, hermaphroditic, and 1 to 2.5 by 0.3 to 0.6 cm.; ingested eggs hatch in suitable snails (*e.g., Bulinus* and *Parafossalurus* species), cercariae encyst on fish, and man acquires infection by ingesting inadequately cooked fish; the parasites sometimes cause no evidence of disease, but cholangitis, periportal fibrosis of the liver (sometimes cirrhosis), and various nervous symptoms may occur; see also *Clonorchis sinensis*.

  O. viverri'ni, a species closely related to O. *felineus*, very common in man in Thailand; causes opisthorchiasis.

**opisthotic** (op-is-tho'tik) [ opistho- + G. *ous* (*ōt-*), ear ]. Behind the ear.

**opisthotonic** (op'is-thot'o-nik, o-pis'tho-ton'ik). Relating to or characterized by opisthotonos.

**opisthotonoid** (op'is-thot'o-noyd). Resembling opisthotonos.

**opisthotonos, opisthotonus** (op'is-thot'o-nus) [ opistho- + G. *tonos*, tension, stretching ]. Tetanus dorsalis; tetanus posticus; a tetanic spasm in which the spine and extremities are bent with convexity forward, the body resting on the head and the heels.

**opium** (o'pĭ-um) [ L. fr. G. *opion*, poppy-juice ] (USP, BP). Gum opium; succus thebaicus; meconium (2); the air-dried, milky exudation obtained by incising the unripe capsules of *Papaver somniferum* or its variety *P. album* (family Papaveraceae). It contains some 20 alkaloids, including morphine, 9 to 16 per cent; noscapine, 4 to 8 per cent; codeine, 0.8 to 2.5 per cent; papaverine, 0.5 to 2.5 per cent; thebaine, 0.5 to 2 per cent. It is used as an analgesic,

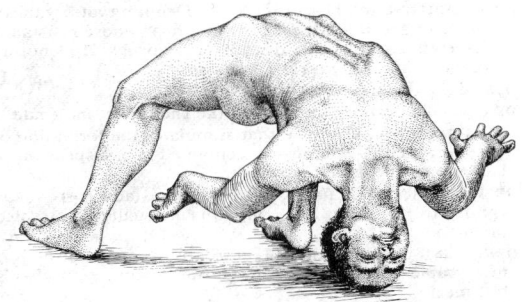

Opisthotonos

hypnotic, and diaphoretic, in diarrhea and spasmodic conditions.

  Boston o., pudding o.; o. so diluted after importation as barely to meet the official requirements.

  denarcotized o., deodorized o.

  deodorized o., denarcotized o.; powdered o. treated with purified petroleum benzine which removes certain nauseating and odorous constituents.

  granulated o., o. dried and reduced to a coarse powder; it contains 10 to 10.5 per cent anhydrous morphine.

  powdered o. (USP, BP), dried and finely powdered o. containing 10 per cent of morphine.

  pudding o., Boston o.

**opiumism** (o'pĭ-um-izm). Opium *addiction*.

**opo-**. 1 [ G. *opos*, juice. OPIO- ]. A prefix to pharmacological terms meaning juice. 2 [ G. *ōps*, face, eye. OPO- ]. Combining form relating to the face or eye.

**op'obal'samum** [ G. *opobalsamon*, the juice of the balsam tree, fr. *opos*, juice, + *balsamon* ]. *Balm* of Gilead.

**opocephalus** (op'o-sef'ă-lus) [ G. *ōps*, eye, face, + *kephalē*, head ]. A fetus without mouth or nose, with a rudimentary jaw and single eye, or two eyes very close together.

**opodidymus** (op'o-did'ĭ-mus) [ G. *ōps*, eye, face, + *didymos*, twin ]. Conjoined twins with a single body, but with two heads, fused behind but partly separated in the facial region.

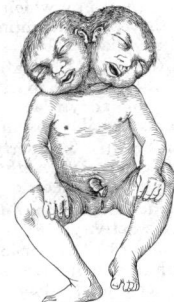

Opodidymus

**Oppenheim,** Hermann, Berlin neurologist, 1858–1919. See O.'s *disease, gait, reflex, syndrome*, Ziehen-O. *disease*.

**Oppenheimer,** Isaac, New York physician, 1855–1928. See O. *treatment*.

**oppilation** (op'ĭ-la'shun) [ L. *oppilatio*, fr. *op-pilo* (*obp-*), pp. *-atus*, to stop up, fr. *pilo*, to ram down ]. Constipation; obstipation.

**op'pila'tive.** Obstructive to any secretion.

**opploten'tes** [ G. *opsis*, vision, + *plōtos*, floating ]. *Muscae* volitantes.

**oppo'nens** [ L. *op-pono* (*obp-*), pres. p. *-ens*, to place against, oppose ]. A name given to several adductor muscles of the fingers or toes, by the action of which these digits are opposed to the others.

**opportunistic** (op'or-tu-nis'tik). 1. Denoting an organism capable of causing disease only in a host whose resistance is lowered, *e.g.*, by other diseases or by drugs. 2. Denoting a disease caused by an o. organism.

**opsialgia** (op'sĭ-al'jĭ-ah). Opalgia.

**op'sin.** The protein portion of the rhodopsin molecule.

**opsin'ogen.** A substance that stimulates the formation of opsonin, such as the antigen contained in a suspension of bacteria used for immunization.

**opsitocia** (op'sĭ-to'sĭ-ah) [ G. *opsi*, late (adv.), + *tokos*, childbirth ]. Labor following an unusually protracted pregnancy.

**opsiuria** (op'-sĭ-u'rĭ-ah) [ G. *opsi*, late, + *ouron*, urine ]. A more rapid excretion of urine during fasting than after a full meal.

**opsoclonus** (op'so-klo'nus) [ G. *ōps*, *ōpos*, eye, + *klonos*, confused motion ]. Rapid, irregular, nonrhythmic movements of the eye in horizontal and vertical directions.

**op'sogen.** Opsinogen.

**opsoma'nia** [ G. *opson*, seasoning, + *mania*, frenzy ]. A longing for a particular article of diet, or for highly seasoned food.

**opson'ic.** Relating to opsonins or to their utilization.

**op'sonin** [ G. *opsonion*, provisions. OPSO- ]. Antibody that combines with specific antigen and sensitizes it in such a manner that it is more readily engulfed by phagocytes. Certain o. is present in normal serum, and is effective against various microorganisms, whereas other types of o. are formed only in response to suitable stimulation by a specific antigen (either during a disease, or as a result of artificial immunization).

  **common o.,** normal o.

  **immune o.,** specific o.

  **normal o.,** that normally present in the blood, *i.e.*, without stimulation by a known, specific antigen; it is relatively thermolabile and reacts with various organisms.

  **specific o.,** that formed in response to stimulation by a specific antigen, either as a result of an attack of a disease, or injections with a suitably prepared suspension of the specific microorganism. Specific o. is more heat-stable than normal o., and reacts only with microorganisms that contain the specific antigens that stimulated formation of the antibody.

  **thermolabile o.,** normal o.

**op'sonist.** One who uses opsonic technique.

**opsoniza'tion.** The process by which bacteria are altered in such a manner that they are more readily and more efficiently engulfed by phagocytes.

**opsonocytophagic** (op'son-o-si'to-fa'jik) [ opsonin + G. *kytos*, a hollow (cell), + *phagein*, to eat ]. Pertaining to the increased efficiency of phagocytic activity of the leukocytes in blood that contains specific opsonin.

**opsonology** (op-son-ol'o-jĭ). Formerly an area of study dealing with opsonins, especially with methods of demonstrating and analyzing their effects.

**opsonom'etry.** The determination of the opsonic index or the opsonocytophagic activity.

**opsonophilia** (op-son-o-fil'ĭ-ah) [ opsonin + G. *phileō*, to love ]. The condition in which bacteria readily unite with opsonins, thereby sensitizing them for more effective phagocytosis.

**opsonophilic** (op-son-o-fil'ik). Pertaining to, characterized by, or resulting in opsonophilia.

**op'sonother'apy.** Opsonic *therapy*.

**optesthesia** (op'tes-the'zĭ-ah) [ G. *optikos*, optical, + *aisthēsis*, sensation ]. Visual sensibility to light stimuli.

**op'tic.** Optical.

**optical** (op'tĭ-kal) [ G. *optikos* ]. Relating to the eye, vision, or optics.

**optician** (op-tish'an). One who practices opticianry.

**opticianry** (op-tish'an-rĭ). The professional practice of filling prescriptions for ophthalmic lenses, dispensing spectacles, and making and fitting contact lenses.

**optico-, opt-.** See opto-.

**opticociliary** (op'tĭ-ko-sil'ĭ-ĕr-ĭ). Relating to the optic and ciliary nerves.

**opticokinetic** (op'tĭ-ko-kĭ-net'ik). Optokinetic.

**opticon** (op'tĭ-kon). A portable electronic device that enables a totally blind person to visualize objects.

**op'ticopu'pillary.** Relating to the optic nerve and the pupil.

**op'tics** [ G. *optikos*, fr. *ōps*, eye. OPO- ]. The science that treats of the properties of light, its refraction and absorption, and of the refracting media of the eye in that relation.

  **fiber o.,** the conduction of light from a source through a bundle of glass or plastic fibers; in wide use for illumination of endoscopic systems. See also fiberscope.

**optimism** (op'tĭ-mizm) [ L. *optimus*, best ]. The habit of looking on the best side of everything, of believing that there is good in everything.

  **therapeutic o.,** a belief in the efficacy of drugs and other therapeutic agents in the treatment of diseases; opposed to therapeutic pessimism.

**op'timum** [ L. ntr. sing. of *optimus*, best ]. The best or most suitable, denoting, for example, the dose of a remedy, the temperature for bacterial cultures, etc.

**opto-, optico-** [ G. *optikos*, optical, from *ōps*, eye. OPO- ]. Combining forms meaning optical.

**op'togram** [ opto- + G. *gramma*, a picture ]. The image formed by the decoloration of the visual purple in an excised eye.

**optokinet'ic** [ opto- + G. *kinēsis*, movement ]. Opticokinetic; pertaining to the occurrence of nystagmus-like twitchings or movements of the eye when the subject looks at moving objects.

**optome'ninx** [ opto- + G. *mēninx*, membrane ]. Retina.

**optom'eter** [ opto- + G. *metron*, measure ]. An instrument for determining the refraction of the eye.

  **objective o.,** refractometer.

**optom'etrist.** One who practices optometry.

**optom'etry.** 1. The profession concerned with the examination of the eyes and related structures to determine the presence of vision problems, eye disease, or other abnormalities, and of the prescription and adaptation of lenses and other optical aids or the use of visual training for maximum visual efficiency. 2. The use of an optometer.

**optomyometer** (op-to-mi-om'e-ter) [ opto- + G. *mys*, muscle, + *metron*, measure ]. An instrument for determining the relative power of the extrinsic muscles of the eye.

**op'totypes** [ opto- + G. *typos*, type ]. Test letters; see *test type*.

**ora** (o'rah) [ L. ]. Plural of L. *os*, the mouth.

**ora,** pl. **orae** (o'rah, o're) [ L. ] [ NA ]. An edge or a margin.

  **o. serra'ta** [ NA ]. the serrated extremity of the pars optica retinae; it is a little behind the ciliary body, marking the limits of the percipient portion of the membrane.

**o'rad** [ L. *os*, mouth, + *ad*, to ]. Toward the mouth.

**o'ral** [ L. *os* (*or-*), mouth ]. 1. Relating to the mouth. 2. Rostral or cephalad; toward the anterior (snout) end of an organism; the opposite of caudal.

**orale** (o-ra'lĭ) [ Mod. L. punctum *orale*, oral point, fr. L. *os* (*or-*), mouth ]. A point at the lingual side of the alveolar termination of the premaxillary suture.

**oral'ity.** Referring to the psychic organization derived from, and characteristic of, the oral period of psychosexual development.

**oralogy** (o-ral'o-jĭ) [ Mod. L. *oralis*, relating to the mouth, + G. *logos*, study ]. 1. The practice of dental and oral hygiene in its relation to the general health. 2. Stomatology.

**Oram,** S. See Holt-O. *syndrome*.

**orange** (or'enj) [ O.F. *orenge*, fr. Ar. *nâranj*, the initial *n* being absorbed in Fr. article *une* ]. 1. The fruit of the orange tree, *Citrus aurantium* (family Rutaceae). 2. A color between yellow and red in the spectrum; for individual orange dyes see specific name.

  **bitter o. peel,** the dried rind of the unripe but fully grown fruit; a flavoring agent.

  **bitter o. peel, dried** (BP), the dried outer part of the pericarp of the ripe, or nearly ripe, fruit; it contains not less than 2.5 per cent v/w of volatile oil.

  **bitter o. peel, fresh,** the outer part of the pericarp of the ripe, or nearly ripe, fruit; used to prepare the tincture and the syrup.

**bitter o. peel oil,** a volatile oil obtained by expression from the fresh peel of the bitter o.

**o. flower oil** (NF), neroli oil; a volatile oil distilled from the fresh flowers of *Citrus aurantium;* used as a flavoring and in perfume.

**o. oil** (USP), sweet o. oil; a volatile oil obtained by expression from the fresh peel of the ripe fruit of *Citrus sinensis;* flavoring agent.

**sweet o. oil,** o. oil.

**o. wood,** a soft wood used in dentistry for the placement of bridges, crowns, etc., by biting pressure. It is also used as a burnishing point in the polishing of root surfaces.

**orange G.** An acid azo dye, $C_{16}H_{10}N_2O_7S_2Na_2$, used as a cytoplasmic stain in histologic techniques.

**Orbeli,** Leon A., Russian scientist, 1882–1958. See O. *effect.*

**orbicular** (or-bik'u-lar) [ L. *orbiculus,* a small disk, dim. of *orbis,* circle ]. Annular; circular.

**orbicula're** [ L. fr. *orbiculus,* a small disk ]. Orbicular *bone.*

**orbicula'ris** [ L. fr. *orbiculus,* a small disk ]. 1 [ NA ]. Circular; denoting a circular or disk-shaped structure. 2. *Musculus* orbicularis.

**orbic'ulus cilia'ris** [ Mod. L. ] [ NA ]. Ciliary disk; anulus ciliaris; pars plana; the darkly pigmented posterior zone of the ciliary body continuous with the retina at the ora serrata.

**or'bit.** Orbita.

**orbita,** gen. **or'bitae** (or'bĭ-tah, -te) [ L. a wheel-track, fr. *orbis,* circle ] [ NA ]. Orbit; orbital cavity; eye socket; the bony cavity containing the eyeball and its adnexa; it is formed of parts of seven bones: the frontal, maxillary, sphenoid, lacrimal, zygomatic, ethmoid, and palatine bones.

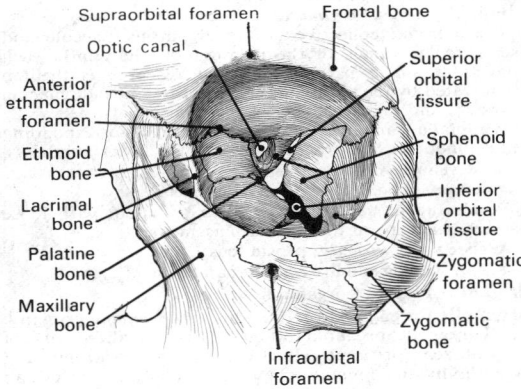

Supraorbital foramen — Frontal bone
Optic canal
Anterior ethmoidal foramen
Ethmoid bone
Lacrimal bone
Palatine bone
Maxillary bone
Infraorbital foramen
Superior orbital fissure
Sphenoid bone
Inferior orbital fissure
Zygomatic foramen
Zygomatic bone

**The Orbit**

**or'bital.** Relating to the orbits.

**orbita'le** [ L. of an orbit ]. In cephalometrics, the lowermost point in the lower margin of the bony orbit that may be felt under the skin.

**orbitography** (or'bĭ-tog'ră-fĭ) [ L. *orbita,* orbit, + G. *graphō,* to write ]. A diagnostic technique for radiographic evaluation in suspected blow-out fracture of the orbit, using a water-soluble iodinated compound injected over the orbital floor.

**or'bitona'sal.** Relating to the orbit and the nose or nasal cavity.

**orbitonometer** (or'bĭ-to-nom'e-ter) [ L. *orbita,* orbit, + G. *metron,* measure ]. An instrument for measurement of the resistance offered to pressing the eyeball backwards into its socket.

**orbitonom'etry.** Measurement by means of the orbitonometer.

**orbitopagus** (or'bĭ-top'ă-gus) [ L. *orbita,* orbit, + G. *pagos,* something fixed ]. Teratoma orbitae; unequal conjoined twins in which the parasitic fetus, usually very imperfectly developed, is attached at an orbit of the autosite.

**orbitosphenoid** (or'bi-to-sfe'noyd). Relating to the orbit and the sphenoid bone.

**orbitot'omy** [ L. *orbita,* orbit, + *tomas,* cut ]. Surgical incision into the orbit.

**orcein** (or'se-in). A mixture of reddish brown pigments obtained by the oxidation of orcinol in the presence of ammonia. The alcoholic solution, of a purple color, is used as a stain in histology and microparasitology, specifically, as a stain for elastic fibers and chromosomes.

**orchectomy** (or-kek'to-mĭ). Orchiectomy.

**orchella** (or-kel'ah). Archil.

**orcheo-.** For words beginning thus, see orchio-.

**orchi-, orchid-, orchio-** (or'ki-, or'kĭ-o-) [ G. *orchis,* testis. ORCH- ]. Combining forms denoting relationship to the testes.

**orchialgia** (or-kĭ-al'jĭ-ah) [ orchi- + G. *algos,* pain ]. Pain in the testis; didymalgia; orchidynia; orchioneuralgia; orchidalgia.

**orchiatrophy** (or-kĭ-at'ro-fĭ). Atrophy or shrinking of the testis.

**orchiauxe** (or-kĭ-awk'se) [ orchi- + G. *auxē,* increase ]. Obsolete term meaning enlargement of the testis.

**orchichorea** (or-kĭ-ko-re'ah) [ orchi- + G. *choreia,* a dance ]. Involuntary rising and falling movements of the testis.

**orchidalgia** (or-kĭ-dal'jĭ-ah). Orchialgia.

**orchidectomy** (or-kĭ-dek'to-mĭ). Orchiectomy.

**orchidic** (or-kid'ik). Relating to the testis.

**orchiditis** (or'kĭ-di'tis). Orchitis.

**orchido-** (or'kĭ-do-). See orchi-; for words beginning thus and not found here, see those beginning with orchio-.

**orchidoptosis** (or'kĭ-dop-to'sis) [ orchido- + G. *ptosis,* a falling ]. Ptosis of the male genitals.

**orchidorraphy** (or-kĭ-dor'ă-fĭ). Orchiopexy.

**orchiectomy** (or-kĭ-ek'to-mĭ) [ orchi- + G. *ektomē,* excision ]. Castration; orchidectomy; orchectomy; removal of one or both testes.

**orchiencephaloma** (or'kĭ-en-sef-al-o'ma) [ orchi- + G. *enkephalos,* brain, + suffix *-oma,* tumor ]. A general, nonspecific term for a relatively soft or encephaloid neoplasm of the testes.

**orchiepididymitis** (or'kĭ-ep'ĭ-did'ĭ-mi'tis) [ orchi- + epididymis, + G. suffix *-itis,* inflammation ]. Inflammation of the testis and epididymis.

**orchil** (or'kil). Archil.

**orchilytic** (or'kĭ-lit'ik) [ orchi- + G. *lytikos,* causing dissolution ]. Destructive to the testis.

**orchio-.** See orchi-.

**orchiocatabasis** (or'kĭ-o-kă-tab'ă-sis) [ orchio- + G. *katabasis,* a descent ]. Obsolete term meaning descent of the testis.

**orchiocele** (or'kĭ-o-sēl) [ orchio- + G. *kēlē,* hernia tumor ]. 1. A tumor of the testis. 2. A testis retained in the inguinal canal.

**orchiococcus** (or'kĭ-o-kok'us) [ orchio- + G. *kokkos,* berry (coccus) ]. An old term for any Gram-negative diplococcus that resembles the gonococcus but is more easily cultivated on ordinary media; it is sometimes found in vaginal secretions. Such bacteria are now classified as species of *Neisseria,* along with *N. gonorrhoeae.*

**orchiodynia** (or'kĭ-o-din'ĭ-ah) [ orchi- + G. *odynē,* pain ]. Orchialgia.

**orchiomyeloma** (or'kĭ-o-mi-ĕ-lo'mah) [ orchio- + G. *myelos,* marrow, + suffix *-oma,* tumor ]. Orchiencephaloma.

**orchioncus** (or-kĭ-ong'kus) [ orchio- + G. *onkos,* bulk, mass ]. A neoplasm of the testis.

**orchioneuralgia** (or'kĭ-o-nu-ral'jĭ-ah) [ orchio- + G. *neuron,* nerve, + *algos,* pain ]. Orchialgia.

**orchiopathy** (or-kĭ-op'ă-thĭ) [ orchio- + G. *pathos,* suffering ]. Disease of a testis.

**orchiopexy** (or'kĭ-o-pek'sĭ) [ orchio- + G. *pēxis,* fixation ]. Orchiorrhaphy; orchidorrhaphy; surgical treatment of an undescended testicle by freeing it and attaching it to the thigh.

**orchioplasty** (or'kī-o-plas-tī) [ orchio- + G. *plassō*, to form ]. Plastic surgery of the testis.

**orchiorrhaphy** (or-kī-or'ă-fī) [ orchio- + G. *rhaphē*, a suture ]. Orchiopexy.

**orchioscheocele** (or'kī-os'ke-o-sēl) [ orchi- + G. *osche*, scrotum, + *kēlē*, tumor, hernia ]. A tumefaction or mass involving the testis in association with a scrotal hernia.

**orchioscirrhus** (or-kī-o-skīr', sīr'us) [ orchio- + G. *skirrhos*, a hardened swelling or tumor ]. An unusually firm neoplasm or sclerosis of the testis.

**or'chiother'apy.** Treatment with testicular extracts.

**orchiotomy** (or-kī-ot'o-mī) [ orchio- + G. *tome*, incision ]. Orchotomy; incision into a testis.

**orchis** pl. **orchises** (or'kis, or'kī-sēz) [ G. testis, an orchid. ORCH- ]. The testis.

**orchit'ic.** Relating to orchitis.

**orchitis** (or-ki'tis) [ orchi- + G. suffix *-itis*, inflammation ]. Orchiditis; inflammation of the testis.

  **o. parotid'ea,** o. associated with mumps.

  **traumat'ic o.,** simple inflammation of the testis caused by mechanical injury.

  **o. variolo'sa,** o. complicating smallpox.

**orchotomy** (or-kot'o-mī). Orchiotomy.

**or'cin.** Orcinol.

**or'cinol.** Orcin; methylresorcinol; 3,5-dihydroxytoluene; obtained from certain lichens, species of *Roccella*. Used as an external antiseptic in various skin diseases, and in chemistry as a reagent for pentoses.

**orcipren'aline sulphate** (BP). Metaproterenol sulfate.

**Ord,** William M., London surgeon, 1834–1902. See O.'s *operation.*

**Ord.** Symbol for orotidine.

**ORD.** Abbreviation for optical rotatory *dispersion.*

**ordeal bark** (or'de-al). Erythrophleum.

**ordeal bean.** Physostigma.

**or'der** [ L. *ordo*, regular arrangement ]. In biological classification, the division just below the class (or subclass) and above the family.

  **pecking o.,** the establishment of a graded dominance in members of a group by the use of aggression.

**or'derly.** A male attendant in a hospital ward.

**orectic** (o-rek'tik). Pertaining to or characterized by orexia.

**orex'ia** (o-rek'sī-ah) [ G. *orexis*, appetite ]. 1. The affective and conative aspects of an act, in contrast to the cognitive aspect. 2. Appetite.

**orexigenic** (o-rek'sī-jen'ik). Appetite-stimulating.

**orf.** Contagious *ecthyma.*

**or'gan** [ G. *organon*, a tool, organ. ERG- ]. Any part of the body exercising a specific function, as of respiration, secretion, digestion, etc.; see also organum.

  **accessory o.'s,** supernumerary o.'s.

  **accessory o.'s of the eye,** *organa* oculi accessoria.

  **an'nulospiral o.,** annulospiral *ending.*

  **Bidder's o.,** a small structure adjacent to the ovary in certain toads; it resembles ovarian tissue and can substitute for the ovaries after ovariectomy.

  **Chievitz' o.,** a transient embryonic ectodermal outgrowth associated with the developing parotid gland; it usually disappears completely.

  **Corti's o.,** *organum* spirale.

  **enamel o.,** a circumscribed mass of ectodermal cells budded off from the dental lamina. It becomes cup-shaped and develops on its internal face the ameloblast layer of cells which produce the enamel cap of a developing tooth.

  **end o.,** the special structure containing the terminal of a nerve fiber in peripheral tissue such as muscle, tissue, skin, mucous membrane, or glands; see also subentries under ending.

  **floating o.,** wandering o.

  **flower-spray o. of Ruffini,** flower-spray *ending.*

  **genital o.'s.** *organa* genitalia.

  **Golgi tendon o.,** neurotendinous o. or spindle; a proprioceptive sensory nerve ending embedded among the fibers of a tendon, often near the musculotendinous junction; it is compressed and activated by any increase of the tendon's tension, whether caused by active contraction or passive stretch of the corresponding muscle.

  **gustatory o.,** *organum* gustus.

  **o. of hearing,** *organum* vestibulocochleare.

  **intromittent o.,** penis.

  **Jacobson's o.,** *organum* vomeronasale.

  **lateral line sense o.,** neuromast o.; a structure in fish consisting of a long groove or canal extending along each side of the trunk and tail and branching in the head region; the groove or tube is lined with neuroepithelial cells, some of which are in groups known as neuromasts; its function appears to be the detection of vibrations of low frequency.

  **neuromast o.,** lateral line sense o.

  **neurotendinous o.,** Golgi tendon o.

  **olfactory o.,** *organum* olfactus.

  **ptotic o.,** wandering o.

  **Rosenmüller's o.,** epoophoron and paroophoron.

  **sense o.'s,** *organa* sensuum.

  **o. of smell,** *organum* olfactus.

  **spiral o.,** *organum* spirale.

  **subcommissural o.,** a microscopic organ, made up of columnar ciliated ependymal cells facing the lumen of the cerebral aqueduct, located beneath the posterior commissure of the brain.

  **supernumerary o.'s,** accessory o.'s; o.'s exceeding the normal number, which may arise from multiple foci of organization in an organ-formative field originally greater in extent than that of the definitive main o. Supernumerary o.'s are aberrant but frequently are not a cause of disease, although illness may persist if they are left in the body after therapeutic removal of the main o.

  **target o.,** target (3); a tissue or o. upon which a hormone exerts its action; the target o. may be an endocrine gland (*e.g.,* the adrenal cortex is a target o. for ACTH), a nonendocrine gland (*e.g.,* the prostate is a target o. for androgens), or a type of tissue (*e.g.,* axillary and pubic hair follicles are target tissues for androgens).

  **taste o.,** *organum* gustus.

  **o. of touch,** *organum* tactus.

  **uropoietic o.'s,** *organa* uropoetica.

  **vestibular o.,** collective term for the utricle, saccule, and semicircular canals of the membranous labyrinth, each having a single patch of ciliated receptor epithelium innervated by the vestibular nerve: macula sacculi, macula utriculi, and cristae of the semicircular canals.

  **vestigial o.,** an imperfect structure in man corresponding to a functioning structure or o. in the lower animals.

  **o. of vision,** *organum* visus.

  **vomeronasal o.,** *organum* vomeronasale.

  **wandering o.,** floating or ptotic o.; an o. with loose attachments, permitting its displacement.

  **Weber's o.,** *utriculus* prostaticus.

  **o.'s of Zuckerkandl,** *corpora* paraaortica.

**or'gana.** Plural of organum.

**organelle** (or'gă-nel) [ Mod. L. dim. of G. *organon*, organ ]. Cell organelle; organoid (3); one of the specialized parts of a protozoan or tissue cell serving for the performance of some individual function; these subcellular units include all types of mitochondria, the Golgi apparatus, cell center and centrioles, granular and agranular cytoplasmic reticulum, lysosomes, plasma membrane, and certain fibrils, as well as plastids of plant cells.

  **paired o.'s,** rhoptries.

**organ'ic** [ G. *organikos* ]. 1. Relating to an organ. 2. Relating to an animal or vegetable organism. 3. Organized; structural.

**organicism** (or-gan'ī-sizm). A theory which attributes all diseases, in particular, all mental disorders, to organic lesions.

**organ'icist.** One who believes in, or subscribes to the views of, organicism.

**organism** (or'gă-nizm). Any living individual, whether plant or animal, considered as a whole.

  **pleuropneumonia-like o.'s,** (PPLO), the original name given to a group of bacteria which did not possess cell walls. These o.'s isolated from animals, man, soil, and sewage are now assigned to the order Mycoplasmatales (*q.v.*). *Mycoplasma pneumoniae* is the cause of primary atypical pneumonia of man.

**or'ganiza'tion.** 1. An arrangement of distinct but mutually dependent parts. 2. The conversion of coagulated blood, exudate, or dead tissue into fibrous tissue.

**pregenital o.,** in psychoanalysis, the o. or arrangement of the libido in the stages prior to that of genital primacy.

**or'ganize.** To provide with, or to assume, a structure.

**or'ganizer.** Spemann's term originally applied to a group of cells on the dorsal lip of the blastopore which induces differentiation of cells in the embryo, controlling the growth and development of adjacent parts. The term is now generally applied to any group of cells having such a controlling influence. The effects are brought about through the action of a chemical of a steroid nature called the evocator.

    **nucle'olar o.,** nucleolar zone; the chromosome region that is active in nucleolus formation.

    **primary o.,** the o. situated on the dorsal lip of the blastopore.

**organo-** (or'gă-no-) [ G. *organon*, organ. ERG- ]. Combining form meaning organ, or organic.

**organoferric** (or'gă-no-fĕr'ik). Relating to an organic compound containing an iron atom within the molecule.

**organogel** (or-gan'o-jel). Same as a hydrogel, with an organic liquid instead of water as the dispersion means.

**organogenesis** (or'gă-no-jen'ĕ-sis) [ organo- + G. *genesis*, origin ]. The formation of organs during development.

**organogenetic, organogenic** (or'gă-no-jĕ-net'ik, -jen'ik). Relating to organogenesis.

**organogeny** (or-gan-oj'ĕ-nĭ). Organogenesis.

**or'ganog'raphy** [ organo- + G. *graphē*, a writing ]. A treatise on, or description of, the organs of the body.

**organoid** (or'gă-noyd) [ organo- + G. *eidos*, resemblance ]. 1. Resembling in superficial appearance or in structure any of the organs or glands of the body. 2. Composed of glandular or organic elements, and not of a single tissue; pertaining to certain neoplasms (*e.g.*, an adenoma) that contain cytologic and histologic elements arranged in a pattern that closely resembles or is virtually identical to a normal organ; see also histoid. 3. Organelle.

**organoleptic** (or'gă-no-lep'tik) [ organo- + G. *lēptikos*, disposed to accept. LAB- ]. 1. Stimulating any of the organs of sensation. 2. Susceptible to a sensory stimulus.

**organology** (or'gă-nol'o-jĭ) [ organo- + G. *logos*, study ]. The branch of science that deals with the anatomy, physiology, development, and functions of the various organs.

**organoma** (or'gă-no'mah) [ organo- + G. suffix *-oma*, tumor ]. A neoplasm that contains cytologic and histologic elements in such an arrangement that specific types of tissue, *e.g.*, thyroid glands, intestinal mucosa, ovarian stroma and follicles, and the like, may be identified in various parts; see also teratoma and dermoid *cyst.*

**or'ganomeg'aly.** Visceromegaly.

**organ'omercu'rial.** Any organic mercurial compound; *e.g.*, merbromin and thiomersol.

**or'ganometal'lic.** Denoting an organic compound containing one or more metallic atoms in its structure.

**organon,** pl. **organa** (or'gă-non, or'gă-nah) [ G. organ. ERG- ]. Organum.

**organonomy** (or'gă-non'o-mĭ) [ organo- + G. *nomos*, law ]. The body of laws regulating the life processes of organized beings.

**organonymy** (or'gă-non'ĭ-mĭ) [ organo- + G. *onyma*, name ]. The nomenclature of the organs of the body, as distinguished from toponymy.

**organopathy** (or'gă-nop'ă-thĭ) [ organo- + G. *pathos*, suffering ]. Any disease especially affecting one of the organs of the body.

**organopexy, organopexia** (or'gă-no-pek'sĭ, -pek'sĭ-ah) [ organo- + G. *pēxis*, fixation ]. The fixation by suture or otherwise of a floating or ptotic organ.

**organoscopy** (or'gă-nos'ko-pĭ) [ organo- + G. *skopeō*, to view ]. Visualization of abdominal contents by endoscope inserted through abdominal wall.

**organ'osol.** Same as hydrosol, with an organic liquid instead of water as the dispersion means.

**or'ganotax'is** [ organo- + G. *taxis*, orderly arrangement ]. Tendency to migrate to a certain organ selectively.

**or'ganother'apy.** Treatment of disease by preparations made from endocrine organs. Now that the chemical

nature of many hormones is known, synthetic preparations are frequently used instead of an extract of the gland.

**organotrophic** (or'gă-no-trof'ik) [ organo- + G. *trophē*, nourishment ]. Pertaining to the nourishment of an organ.

**organotrop'ic.** Pertaining to or characterized by organotropism.

**organotropism** (or-gă-not'ro-pizm) [ organo- + G. *tropē*, a turning ]. Organotropy; the special affinity of particular drugs, pathogens, or other agents for particular organs or their component parts; *cf.* parasitotropism.

**organotropy** (or'gă-not'ro-pĭ). Organotropism.

**organ-specific.** Denoting or pertaining to a serum produced by the injection of the cells of a certain organ or tissue that, when injected into another animal, destroys the cells of the corresponding organ.

**organum,** pl. **organa** (or'gă-num, or'gă-nah) [ L. organ. ERG- ]. [ NA ]. An organ.

    **o. auditus,** o. vestibulocochleare.

    **or'gana genita'lia** [ NA ], the genital organs; the reproductive organs. The organa genitalia feminina (female genital organs), include the ovaries, uterus, uterine tubes, vagina, clitoris, and vulva. The organa genitalia masculina (male genital organs) include the testes, penis, seminal vesicles, and prostate.

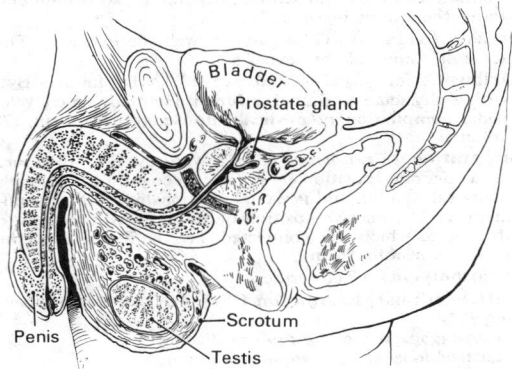

**Male Genital Organs**

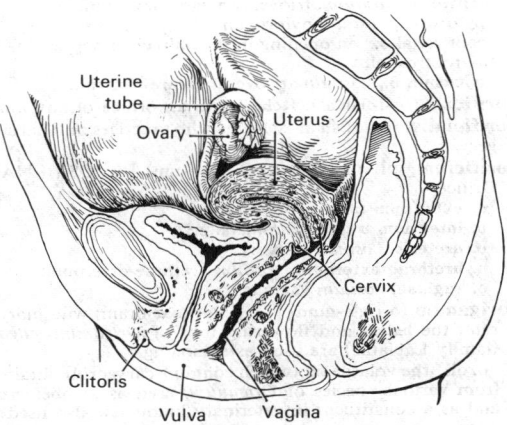

**Female Genital Organs**

    **o. gus'tus** [ NA ], gustatory organ; organ of taste; located in the papillae of the mucous membrane of the tongue, chiefly in the vallate papillae.

    **or'gana oc'uli acceso'ria** [ NA ], the accessory organs of the eye, consisting of the eyelids, lacrimal apparatus, and extrinsic muscles of the eyeball.

    **o. olfac'tus** [ NA ], olfactory organ; organ of smell; the olfactory region in the superior portion of the nasal cavity.

**organa sen'suum** [ NA ], sense organs; the organs of special sense, including the eye, ear, olfactory organ, taste organs, and the accessory structures associated with these organs.

**o. spira'le** [ NA ], spiral organ; Corti's organ; acoustic papilla; a prominent ridge of highly specialized epithelium in the floor of the ductus cochlearis overlying the membrana basilaris, containing four rows of hair cells, or cells of Corti (the ciliated auditory receptor cells innervated by the cochlear nerve) supported by various columnar cells: the pillars of Corti, cells of Hensen, and cells of Claudius. The o. spirale is partly overhung by an awning-like shelf, the membrana tectoria, the free marginal zone of which is covered by a gelatinous substance in which the cilia of the hair cells are embedded.

**o. tac'tus,** organ of touch; any one of the sensory end organs.

**organa uropoet'ica** [ NA ], uropoietic organs; organs concerned in the excretion of urine.

**o. vestibulocochlea're** [ NA ], organ of hearing, including the external, middle, and internal ear.

**o. visus** [ NA ], the organ of vision; the eye and its adnexa.

**o. vomeronasa'le** [ NA ], Jacobson's organ; a fine horizontal canal, ending in a blind pouch, in the mucous membrane of the nasal septum, beginning just behind and above the ductus incisivus.

**orgasm** (or'gazm) [ G. *orgaō,* to swell, be excited ]. The acme or climax of the sexual act.

**Oribasius** (or-ĭ-ba'sĭ-us), *ca.* 325–403 A.D., famous Byzantine physician to Emperor Julian. He made an encyclopedic compilation of medical knowledge comprising 70 volumes.

**orientation** [ Fr. *orienter,* to set toward the East, therefore in a definite position ]. 1. The recognition of one's temporal, spatial, and personal relationships and environment. 2. The relative position of an atom with respect to the one to which it is connected, *i.e.,* the direction of the bond connecting them.

**orientomycin.** Cycloserine.

**orifice** (or'ĭ-fis) [ L. *orificium.* OS- ]. Any aperture or opening.

**esophagogastric o.,** *ostium* cardiacum.

**gastroduodenal o.,** *ostium* pyloricum.

**golf-hole ure'teral o.,** a retracted funnel-shaped condition of the ureteral o. in the wall of the bladder, due often to tuberculosis or a secondary sclerosis of the ureter.

**mitral o.,** *ostium* atrioventriculare sinistrum.

**pyloric o.,** *ostium* pyloricum.

**root canal o.,** an opening in the pulp chamber leading to the root canal.

**tricuspid o.,** *ostium* atrioventriculare dextrum.

**orificial** (or-ĭ-fish'al). Relating to an orifice of any kind.

**orificialist** (or-ĭ-fish'al-ist). One who practices orificial surgery.

**orificium,** pl. **orificia** (or-ĭ-fish'ĭ-um) [ L. OS ] [ NA ]. Orifice.

**o. exter'num u'teri,** *ostium* uteri.

**o. inter'num u'teri,** *isthmus* uteri.

**o. ureteris,** *ostium* ureteris.

**o. urethrae externum,** *ostium* urethrae externum.

**o. vaginae,** *ostium* vaginae.

**origanum** (o-rig'ă-num) [ L. ]. Pot marjoram; wild marjoram; the leaves and flowering tops of *Origanum vulgare* (family Labiatae) are used as seasoning.

**o. oil,** the volatile oil (which contains carvacrol) obtained from various species of *Origanum;* used as a rubefacient and as a constituent in veterinary liniments; also used in microscopic techniques.

**origin** (or'ĭ-jin) [ L. *origo,* source, beginning, fr. *orior,* to rise ]. 1. The less movable of the two points of attachment of a muscle, that which is attached to the more fixed part of the skeleton. 2. The starting point of a cranial or spinal nerve. The former have two o.'s: the **ental, deep,** or **real o.,** the cell group in the brain or medulla, whence the fibers of the nerve begin, and the **ectal, superficial,** or **apparent o.,** the point where the nerve emerges from the brain.

**origo** [ L. ] [ NA ]. Origin.

**orizaba jalap root.** Ipomea.

**Orla-Jensen** (yen'sen), Sigurd, Danish physiologic chemist, *1870. See O.-J.'s classification of bacteria, under *Bacterium.*

**Ormond,** J. K. See O.'s *disease.*

**Orn.** Symbol for ornithine or its radical.

**or'nate** [ L. *ornatus,* decorated ]. In ixodid ticks, describing the patterning (gray or white markings on a dark background) of the scutum.

**or'nithine.** $NH_2(CH_2)_3CHNH_2COOH$; the amino acid formed when arginine is hydrolyzed by arginase; not a constituent of proteins, but an important intermediate in the urea cycle.

**o. acetyltransferase,** glutamate acetyltransferase.

**o. cycle,** see under cycle.

**o. decarboxylase** (EC 4.1.1.17), a bacterial enzyme catalyzing the decarboxylation of ornithine to putrescine.

**o. transcarbamoylase (carbamoyltransferase)** (EC 2.1.3.3), enzyme catalyzing formation of citrulline from ornithine and carbamoyl phosphate.

**Ornithodoros** (or'nĭ-thod'o-rus) [ G. *ornis* (*ornith-*), bird, + *doros,* a leather bag ]. A genus of soft ticks (family Argasidae) several species of which are vectors of pathogens of various relapsing fevers. They are characterized by a capitulum hidden below the hood and by disks and mamillae of the integument that are continuous from dorsal to ventral surfaces in a variety of patterns.

**O. coria'ceus,** pajaroello; common in the mountainous coastal areas of California; adults readily attack deer, cattle, and man, and have an irritating, painful bite.

**O. herm'si,** a rodent parasite and vector of relapsing fever spirochetes, such as *Borrelia hermsii,* in the western United States and Canada.

**O. lahoren'sis,** possibly a transmitter of *Borrelia persica,* the agent of Persian relapsing fever.

**O. maroca'nas,** probably the vector of *Borrelia hispanica,* the agent of Spanish relapsing fever.

**O. mouba'ta complex,** a group of four species in Africa; the taxonomy and ecology of this complex is of great significance because its members are vectors of relapsing fever spirochetes. Members of the complex include *O. moubata* (various hosts), *O. compactus* (tortoises), *O. apertus* (porcupines), and *O. porcinus* (warthogs); a domestic subspecies of *O. porcinus,* in turn, forms three strains that feed chiefly on man, fowl, and swine.

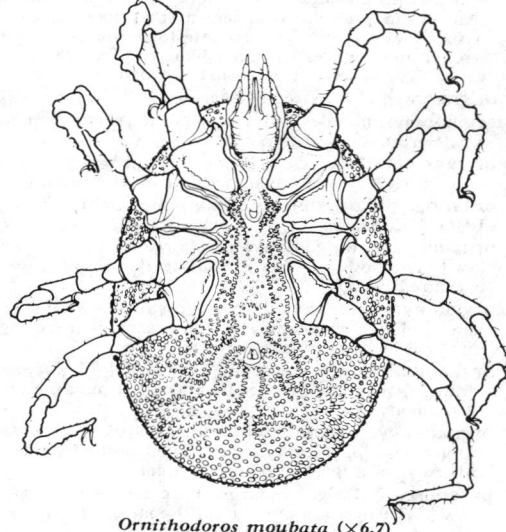

*Ornithodoros moubata* (×6.7)

(From Najarian, H. H.: *Textbook of Medical Parasitology,* The Williams & Wilkins Co., Baltimore, 1967.)

**O. pappil'ipes,** "Persian bug," found in Russia and the Near East; transmits *Spirochaeta persica,* the pathogen in Iran of relapsing fever.

**O. ru'dis,** an important vector of relapsing fever spirochetes in Central and South America; possibly another·complex similar to *O. moubata* complex.

**O. par'keri,** a tick of the western United States and vector of *Borrelia parkeri.*

**O. savi'gni,** a species transmitting *Borrelia kochii,* an agent of relapsing fever of East Africa, Southern Egypt, Abyssinia, and Southwestern Asia.

**O. talajé,** found in Mexico and in Central and South America, where it feeds on wild rodents, domestic animals and man; it delivers a painful, irritating bite and is a vector of relapsing fever.

**O. tholoza'ni,** a species transmitting *Borrelia persica,* the agent of Persian relapsing fever.

**O. turica'ta,** a tick that readily attacks animals and man in the southern portion of the United States and Mexico; it is a vector of *Borrelia turicatae,* an agent of relapsing fever; the bite is painful and irritating.

**O. venezuelen'sis,** the vector of *Borrelia venezuelensis,* the cause of the relapsing fever of Colombia and Venezuela and other mountainous parts of South America.

**O. verruco'sus,** vector of *Borrelia caucasica, q. v.*

**Ornithonyssus** (or'nĭ-thon'ĭ-sus) [ G. *ornis* (*ornith-*), bird, + *nyssus,* to prick ]. A genus of mites; formerly called *Liponyssus.*

**O. baco'ti,** the tropical rat mite, a possible vector of murine typhus.

**O. bur'sa,** the tropical fowl mite.

**O. sylvia'rum,** the northern fowl mite.

**ornitho'sis** [ G. *ornis* (*ornith-*), bird, + suffix *-osis,* condition ]. Parrot disease (2); a disease in nonpsittacine birds caused by *Chlamydia psittaci.* It occurs in domestic fowls, ducks, pigeons, turkeys, and many wild birds. It is contracted by man by contact with these birds; generally, but not always, o. in man is milder than psittacosis.

**ornithu'ric acid.** $N^2,N^5$-Dibenzoylornithine; condensation product formed by birds after ingestion of benzoic acid, and excreted in urine; analogous to hippuric acid formation in mammals.

**Oro.** Symbol for orotic acid or orotate.

**oro-.** 1 [ L. *os, oris,* mouth. OS- ]. Combining form relating to the mouth. 2 [ L. *orrhos,* whey, serum. ORO- ]. Alternative spelling for orrho-; For some terms beginning with oro- or orrho-, see also sero-.

**orodiagnosis** (or-o-di-ag-no'sis). Obsolete term for serodiagnosis.

**orodigitofacial** (o'ro-dij'ĭ-to-fa'shal). Relating to the mouth, fingers, and face.

**orofa'cial.** Relating to the mouth and face.

**orolingual** (o'ro-ling'gwal). Relating to the mouth and the tongue.

**or'omeningi'tis.** Serositis.

**o'rona'sal.** Relating to the mouth and the nose.

**oropharynx** (o'ro-făr'ingks). [ L. *os* (*or-*), mouth ]. *pars oralis pharyngis.*

**or'orrhe'a.** Orrhorrhea.

**orosomucoid** (or'o-so-mu'koyd). An $\alpha_1$-globulin in plasma, 40 per cent carbohydrate.

**orotate.** A salt or ester of orotic acid.

**o. phosphoribosyltransferase** (EC 2.4.2.10), orotidylic acid phosphorylase; a phosphoribosyltransferase synthesizing orotidylate from orotate and 5-phosphoribose 1-diphosphate (PPRibP).

**orot'ic acid.** 6-Carboxyuracil; uracil 6-carboxylic acid; an important intermediate in the formation of the pyrimidine nucleotides.

**orot'ic acidu'ria** [ orotic acid + G. *ouron,* urine ]. A disorder of pyrimidine metabolism characterized by megaloblastic anemia, leukopenia, retarded growth, and urinary excretion of orotic acid; recessive inheritance.

**orot'idine.** Symbol, Ord; 1-ribosylorotate; orotic acid ribonucleoside; uridine-6-carboxylic acid.

**orotidylic acid** (o-rot'ĭ-dil'ik). OMP; orotidine 5'-phosphate; orotidine phosphoric acid.

**o. acid phosphorylase,** orotate phosphoribosyltransferase.

**orphen'adrine citrate** (NF, BP). NORFLEX; same action and use as orphenadrine hydrochloride.

**orphen'adrine hydrochloride** (BP). DISIPAL; *N,N*-dimethyl-2(*o*-methyl-α-phenylbenzoyloxy)ethylamine hydrochloride; the *o*-methyl analogue of diphenhydramine hydrochloride. It reduces spasm of voluntary muscles, probably by action on the cerebral motor areas. Used in the symptomatic treatment of paralysis agitans and drug-induced parkinsonism.

**orrho-, oro-** (or'o-) [ G. *orrhos, oros,* whey, serum. ORO- ]. Combining forms meaning serum; for words beginning thus and not found here, see sero-.

**orrhomeningitis** (or-o-men-in-ji'tis). Serositis.

**orrhorrhea** (or-o-re'ah) [ orrho- + G. *rhoia,* a flow ]. Any condition in which an abnormally large amount of a thin, watery, clear, colorless or faintly straw-colored fluid oozes or flows from various structures, *e.g.,* nasal membranes, urethra.

**or'ris.** *Iris.*

**orseillin.** A red disazo acid dye, $C_{24}H_{18}N_4O_7S_2Na_2$, used as a fungal and bacterial stain.

**Orsi,** Francesco, Italian physician, 1828–1890. See O.-Grocco *method.*

**Orth** (ort), Johannes J., German pathologist, 1847–1923. See O.'s *fluid, stain.*

**orthergasia** (orth'er-ga'zi-ah) [ G. *orthos,* straight, correct, + *ergasia,* work ]. Normal intellectual and emotional adjustment.

**orthe'sis.** Orthosis.

**orthet'ics.** Orthotics.

**ortho-** [ Gr. *orthos,* correct, straight ]. 1. A prefix meaning straight, normal, or in proper order. 2. Specifically, in chemistry, denoting that a compound has two substitutions on adjacent carbon atoms in a benzene ring. It is abbreviated *o-.* See also *meta-* and *para-,* indicating separated by one and separated by two (carbon atoms), respectively.

**orthoacid** (or'tho-as'id). An acid in which the number of hydroxyl groups equals the valence of the acid-forming element; *e.g.,* C(OH)$_4$, which may be termed orthocarbonic acid. When there is no such acid, the one that most nearly approaches this condition is sometimes called an o.; *e.g.,* PO(OH)$_3$, which is orthophosphoric acid; CH$_3$— C(OCH$_3$)$_3$, trimethyl orthoacetate; C(OCH$_3$)$_4$, tetramethyl orthocarbonate.

**orthoarteriotony** (or'tho-ar-te-rĭ-ot'o-nĭ) [ ortho- + G. *artēria,* artery, + *tonos,* tension ]. Normal blood pressure.

**orthobio'sis** [ ortho- + G. *biōsis,* life ]. Correct living, both hygienically and morally.

**orthocaine** (or'tho-kān). ORTHOFORM; the methyl ester of 3-amino-4-hydroxybenzoic acid; a surface anesthetic agent used (usually as a dusting powder) for burns, ulcers, etc.

**orthocephalic** (or'tho-sē-fal'ik) [ ortho- + G. *kephalē* head ]. Having a well proportioned head as regards height. Denoting a skull with a vertical index between 70 and 75. Similar to metriocephalic.

**orthoceph'alous.** Orthocephalic.

**orthochorea** (or'tho-ko-re'ah). A form of chorea in which the spasms occur only or chiefly when the patient is in the erect posture.

**orthochromatic** (or'tho-kro-mat'ic) [ ortho- + G. *chrōma,* color ]. Euchromatic; orthochromophil; denoting any tissue or cell that stains the color of the dye used, *i.e.,* the same color as the dye solution with which it is stained (as opposed to metachromatic).

**orthochromophil, orthochromophile** (or-tho-kro'mo-fil, or fil) [ ortho- + G. *chrōma,* color, + *philos,* fond ]. Orthochromatic.

**orthocrasia** (or-tho-kra'zi-ah) [ ortho- + G. *krasis,* a mixing, temperament. CRAS- ]. A condition in which there is a normal reaction to drugs, ingested proteins, etc.; distinguished from idiosyncrasy and eucrasia.

**orthocytosis** (or-tho-si-to'sis) [ ortho- + G. *kytos,* cell, + suffix *-osis,* condition ]. A condition in which all of the cellular elements in circulating blood are mature forms, irrespective of the proportions of various types and total numbers.

**orthodigita** (or-tho-dij'ĭ-tah) [ ortho- + L. *digitus,* finger or toe ]. Correction of malformations of fingers or toes.

**or'thodont** [ ortho- + G. *odous*, tooth ]. A person having normal teeth.

**orthodontia** (or-tho-don'shǐah). Orthodontics.

**or'thodont'ics** [ ortho- + G. *odous*, tooth ]. Orthodontia; that branch of dentistry concerned with the correction and prevention of irregularities and malocclusion of the teeth.

  **surgical o.,** the correction of occlusal abnormalities by the surgical repositioning of segments of the mandible or maxillae containing one to several teeth; or the bodily repositioning of entire jaws to improve function and esthetics.

**or'thodont'ist.** A dental specialist who practices orthodontics.

**orthodro'mic** [ ortho- + G. *dromos*, course ]. Denoting the propagation of an impulse along an axon in the normal direction.

**orthogenesis** (or-tho-jen'ē-sis) [ ortho- + G. *genesis*, origin ]. The doctrine that evolution is definitely governed by intrinsic factors, and occurs in definite directions.

**orthogenic** (or-tho-jen'ik). Relating to orthogenesis.

**orthogenics** (or-tho-jen'iks). The science dealing with the study and treatment of mental and physical defects that obstruct or retard normal development.

**orthognathic, orthognathous** (or'tho-nath'ik, or-thog'nă-thus) [ ortho- + G. *gnathos*, jaw ]. Having a face without projecting jaw, one with a gnathic index below 98.

**or'thograde** [ ortho- + L. *gradior*, pp. *gressus*, to walk ]. Walking or standing erect; denoting the posture of man; opposed to pronograde.

**orthokeratology** (or'tho-kĕr-ă-tol'o-jǐ) [ ortho- + G. *keras*, horn (cornea), + *logos*, science ]. A method of improving unaided vision by molding the cornea with contact lenses.

**or'thokinet'ics** [ ortho- + G. *kinētikos*, movable, fr. *kineō*, to move ]. A method advocated for the treatment of hypertrophic osteoarthritis in which an attempt is made to change muscular action from one group of muscles to another set of muscles in order to protect the diseased joint.

**orthome'lic** [ ortho- + G. *melos*, limb ]. Correcting malformations of arms or legs.

**orthom'eter** [ ortho- + G. *metron*, measure ]. An instrument for determining the degree of protrusion or retraction of the eyeballs.

**orthomolecular** (or-tho-mo-lek'u-lar). Designating the normal chemical constituents of the body, including substances formed endogenously and those acquired through the diet.

**orthopae'dic, orthope'dic.** Relating to orthopaedics.

**orthopaedics, orthopedics** (or-tho-pe'diks) [ ortho- + G. *pais* (*paid*-), child ]. The medical specialty concerned with the preservation, restoration, and development of form and function of the extremities, spine, and associated structures by medical, surgical, and physical methods.

  **dental o.,** orthodontics.

**orthopae'dist, orthope'dist.** One who practices orthopaedics.

**or'thopan'tograph.** A panoramic radiographic device that permits visualization of the entire dentition, alveolar bone, and other contiguous structures on a single extraoral film.

**orthope'dics.** Orthopaedics.

**orthopercussion** (or'tho-per-kush'un). Very light percussion of the chest, made in a sagittal direction (*i.e.,* anteroposteriorly, and not perpendicularly to the wall of the chest) by one finger striking the knuckle of the pleximeter finger bent at a right angle, the impact being transmitted through the two phalanges (middle and distal) to the tip of the finger resting in an intercostal space. It is used to determine the size of the heart, the faint percussion sound disappearing when the heart is reached even though that may be overlapped by a layer of the lung. Called also Goldscheider's method.

**orthophoria** (or'tho-fo'rǐ-ah) [ ortho- + G. *phora*, motion ]. Absence of heterophoria; the condition of binocular fixation in which the lines of sight meet at a distant or near point of reference in the absence of a fusion stimulus.

  **asthen'ic o.,** o. with low relative convergence.

**orthopho'ric.** Pertaining to orthophoria.

**orthophos'phate.** Any form (salt or ester) of orthophosphoric acid.

  **inorganic o.,** symbol, $P_i$; any ion or salt form of $H_3PO_4$; for example, $H_2PO_4^-$, $HPO_4=$, or $PO_4$.

**orthophrenia** (or'tho-fre'nǐ-ah) [ ortho- + G. *phrēn*, mind ]. 1. Soundness of mind. 2. A condition of normal interpersonal relationships.

**orthopnea** (or-thop-ne'ah, or-thop'ne-ah) [ ortho- + G. *pnoē*, a breathing ]. Discomfort on breathing in any but the erect sitting or standing position.

**orthopneic** (or'thop-ne'ik). Relating to or suffering from orthopnea.

**orthopraxia, orthopraxy** (or-tho-prak'sǐ-ah, -prak'sǐ) [ ortho- + G. *praxis*, a doing, making ]. Obsolete terms for orthopaedics.

**orthoprosthesis** (or'tho-pros'the-sis, -pros-the'sis). An appliance used in the management of prosthetic problems related to alignment of teeth.

**orthopsychiatry** (or-tho-si-ki'ă-trǐ). The science relating to the study and treatment of disorders of behavior, especially in children.

**Orthoptera** (or-thop'ter-ah) [ ortho- + G. *pteron*, a wing ]. An order of the Insecta to which belong the locusts and grasshoppers.

**orthop'tic.** Relating to orthoptics.

**orthop'tics** [ ortho- + G. *optikos*, relating to sight ]. The study and treatment of defective binocular vision, of defects in the action of the ocular muscles, or of faulty visual habits.

**orthop'tist.** One skilled in orthoptics.

**orthoscope** (or'tho-skōp) [ ortho- + G. *skopeō*, to view ]. 1. An instrument by means of which one is able to draw the various normas of the skull. 2. An instrument by which water is held in contact with the eye, thereby eliminating corneal refraction.

**orthoscop'ic.** 1. Relating to the orthoscope. 2. Having normal vision. 3. Denoting an object correctly observed by the eye.

**orthoscopy** (or-thos'ko-pǐ). Examination of the eye with the orthoscope.

**ortho'sis** [ G. *orthōsis*, a making straight ]. Orthesis; the correction of maladjustments.

**orthostat'ic.** Relating to or caused by the erect posture.

**orthostatism** (or'tho-stat'izm) [ ortho- + G. *statos*, standing ]. The upright position.

**orthostereoscope** (or'tho-stěr'ǐ-o-skōp). An instrument for stereoscopic x-ray.

**or'thosympathet'ic.** Referring to the sympathetic component of the autonomic nervous system, as distinguished from parasympathetic; see *systema* nervosum autonomicum.

**or'thotast** [ ortho- + G. *tassō*, to arrange ]. An instrument for the gradual straightening of an abnormally curved bone.

**orthothanasia** (orth-o-thă-na'zǐ-ah) [ ortho- + G. *thanatos*, death ]. 1. The art and science of normal or natural death and dying. 2. A term sometimes used to denote the deliberate stopping of artificial or heroic means of maintaining life.

**orthot'ics.** Orthetics; the science that deals with the making and fitting of orthopaedic appliances.

**or'thotist.** A maker and fitter of orthopaedic appliances.

**orthot'onos, orthot'onus** [ ortho- + G. *tonos*, tension ]. A form of tetanic spasm in which the neck, limbs, and body are held fixed in a straight line.

**orthotop'ic** [ ortho- + G. *topos*, place ]. In the normal or usual position.

**orthotrop'ic** [ ortho- + G. *tropē*, a turn ]. Extending or growing in a straight, especially a vertical, direction.

**or'thovolt'age.** Median voltage of 250 kv.

**O.S.** Abbreviation for oculus sinister [ L. ], left eye.

**Os.** Chemical symbol of the element osmium.

**os,** gen. **o'ris,** pl. **o'ra** [ L. mouth. OS- ]. 1 [ NA ]. The mouth. 2. Term applied sometimes to an opening into a hollow organ or canal, especially one with thick or fleshy edges.

incompetent cervical o., a defect in the muscular ring at the internal o. allowing premature dilation of the cervix.

**Scanzoni's second o.,** pathologic retraction *ring*.

**o. u'teri exter'num,** *ostium* uteri.

**o. u'teri inter'num,** *isthmus* uteri.

# OS

**os,** gen. **os'sis,** pl. **os'sa** [ L. bone. OS- ] [ NA ]. Bone; a portion of osseous tissue of definite shape and size, forming a part of the animal skeleton; in man there are 200 distinct ossa in the skeleton, not including the ossicula auditus of the tympanic cavity or the ossa sesamoidea other than the two patellae. A bone consists of a dense outer layer of compact substance or cortical substance covered by the periosteum, and an inner loose, spongy substance; the central portion of a long bone is filled with marrow. Bones of the human skeleton are illustrated in color plates 17 and 18. For histological definition, see bone.

**o. acromia'le,** an acromion that is joined to the scapular spine by fibrous rather than by bony union.

**o. breve** [ NA ], short bone; as opposed to a long bone, one whose dimensions are approximately equal. It consists of a layer of cortical substance enclosing spongy substance and marrow.

**o. calcis** [ NA ], calcaneus.

**o. capita'tum** [ NA ], capitate (2); capitate bone; o. magnum; the largest of the carpal bones; located in the distal row.

**ossa carpi** [ NA ], carpal bones; see carpus (2) and the individual bones o. scaphoideum, o. lunatum, o. triquetrum, o. pisiforme, o. trapezium, o. trapezoideum, o. capitatum, o. hamatum.

**o. centra'le** [ NA ], central bone; a small bone occasionally found on the dorsal aspect of the wrist between the scaphoid, capitate, and trapezoid; it is developed as an independent cartilage in early fetal life but usually becomes fused with the scaphoid; it occurs normally in most monkeys.

**o. centra'le tarsi,** o. naviculare.

**o. clitoris,** a small bone located in the clitoris of many carnivorous mammals. It is homologous with the o. penis of the male.

**o. coccygis** [ NA ], coccygeal bone; coccyx; tail bone; the small bone at the end of the vertebral column in man, formed by the fusion of four rudimentary vertebrae. It articulates above with the sacrum.

**o. compeda'le** [ NAV ], the proximal or first phalanx of ungulates.

**o. cordis,** each of two irregular, three-pronged bones which are found in the right and left fibrous trigones of the heart of the ox and deer. The greatest dimension of the larger bones may attain a length of 6 cm. in the ox.

**o. corona'le** [ NAV ], the second or middle phalanx of ungulates.

**o. costa'le** [ NA ], the bony part of a rib.

**o. cox'ae,** (1) [ NA ], coxal bone; hip bone; innominate bone; haunch bone; a large flat bone formed by the fusion of the ilium, ischium, and pubis (in the adult), constituting the lateral half of the pelvis; it articulates with its fellow anteriorly, with sacrum posteriorly and with the femur laterally; (2) huckle *bone* (1).

**ossa cranii** [ NA ], cranial bones; bones of the cerebral cranium; the bones surrounding the brain; they are the paired parietal and temporal and the unpaired occipital, frontal sphenoid and ethmoid.

**o. cuboi'deum** [ NA ], cuboid bone; a bone of the distal row of the tarsus, articulating with the calcaneus, lateral cuneiform, navicular (occasionally), and fourth and fifth metatarsal bones.

**o. cuneiforme intermedium** [ NA ], intermediate, middle or second cuneiform bone; a bone of the distal row of the tarsus, articulates with the medial and lateral cuneiform, navicular, and second metatarsal bones.

**o. cuneiforme laterale** [ NA ], lateral cuneiform, third cuneiform, or wedge bone; a bone of the distal row of the tarsus, articulates with the intermediate cuneiform, cuboid, navicular, and second, third, and fourth metatarsal bones.

**o. cuneiforme mediale** [ NA ], medial cuneiform, first cuneiform, or wedge bone; the largest of the three cuneiform bones, the medial bone of the distal row of the tarsus, articulating with the intermediate cuneiform, navicular, and first and second metatarsal bones.

**ossa digito'rum manus** [ NA ], bones of the digits of the hand; the phalanges and sesamoid bones of the fingers; see also phalanx (1).

**ossa digito'rum pedis** [ NA ], bones of the digits of the foot; the phalanges and sesamoid bones of the toes; see also phalanx (1).

**o. ethmoida'le** [ NA ], ethmoid bone; an irregularly shaped bone lying between the orbital plates of the frontal and anterior to the sphenoid bone; it consists of two lateral masses of thin plates enclosing air cells, attached above to a perforated horizontal lamina, the cribriform plate, from which descends a median vertical or perpendicular plate in the interval between the two lateral masses; the bone articulates with the sphenoid, frontal, maxillary, lacrimal, palatine bones and the inferior nasal concha, and the vomer, and enters into the formation of the anterior cranial fossa, the orbits, and the nasal cavity.

**ossa faciei** [ NA ], facial bones; bones of the visceral cranium; the bones surrounding the mouth and nose and contributing to the orbits; they are the paired maxilla, zygomatic, nasal, lacrimal, palatine, and inferior nasal concha; and the unpaired vomer, mandible, and hyoid.

**o. fronta'le** [ NA ], frontal bone; the large single bone forming the forehead and the upper margin and roof of the orbit on either side; it articulates with the parietal, nasal, ethmoid, maxillary, and zygomatic bones, and with the lesser wings of the sphenoid.

**o. hamatum** [ NA ], hamate bone; hooked bone; unciform bone; the bone on the medial (ulnar) side of the distal row of the carpus; it articulates with the fourth and fifth metacarpal, triquetral, lunate, and capitate.

**o. hyoi'deum,** (1) [ NA ], hyoid bone; lingual or tongue bone; a U-shaped bone lying between the mandible and the larynx, suspended from the styloid processes by slender stylohyoid ligaments; (2) see *apparatus* hyoideus.

**o. ilium** [ NA ], ilium [ NA ]; iliac or flank bone; the broad, flaring portion of the hip bone, distinct at birth but later becoming fused with the ischium and pubis; it consists of a body, which joins the pubis and ischium to form the acetabulum and a broad thin portion, called the ala or wing.

**o. incae,** o. interparietale.

**o. incisi'vum** [ NA ], incisive bone; intermaxillary bone; premaxilla; premaxillary bone; Kölliker's dental crest; the anterior and inner portion of the maxilla, which in the fetus and sometimes in the adult is a separate bone; the incisive suture runs from the incisive canal between the lateral incisor and the canine tooth. According to Albrecht, this is further divided by a suture between the two incisor teeth on each side into two bones, the endognathion and the mesagnathion.

**o. intermaxilla're,** o. incisivum.

**os intermedium,** o. lunatum.

**o. intermetatar'seum,** a supernumerary bone at the base of the first metatarsal, or between the first and second metatarsal bones, usually fused with one or other or with the medial cuneiform bone.

**o. interparieta'le** [ NA ], interparietal bone; incarial bone; o. incae; the upper part of the squama of the occipital bone, developed in membrane instead of in cartilage as is the rest of the occipital, and occasionally (especially in ancient Peruvian skulls) existing as a separate bone, separated from the remainder of the occipital by the sutura mendosa.

**o. ischii** [ NA ], ischium [ NA ]; ischial bone; the lower and posterior part of the hip bone, distinct at birth but later becoming fused with the ilium and pubis. It consists of a body, where it joins the ilium and superior ramus of the pubis to form the acetabulum, and a ramus joining the inferior ramus of the pubis.

**o. japon'icum,** a bipartite or tripartite zygomatic bone, found with greater frequency in the Japanese than in other races.

**o. lacrima'le** [ NA ], lacrimal bone; o. unguis an irregularly rectangular thin plate, forming part of the medial wall of the orbit behind the frontal process of the maxilla; it articulates with the inferior nasal concha, ethmoid, frontal, and maxillary bones.

**o. lon'gum** [ NA ], long bone; pipe bone; one of the elongated bones of the extremities, consisting of a tubular shaft (diaphysis) and two extremities (epiphyses) usually wider than the shaft. The shaft is composed of compact bone surrounding a central medullary cavity.

**o. lunatum** [ NA ], lunate bone; semilunar bone; o. intermedium; one of the proximal row in the carpus between the scaphoid and triquetral; it articulates with the radius, scaphoid, triquetral, hamate, and capitate.

**o. magnum,** o. capitatum.

**o. mala're,** o. zygomaticum.

**ossa membri inferioris** [ NA ], bones of the inferior limb; these include the inferior limb girdle (hip bone) and the skeleton of the free inferior limb (femur, tibia, fibula, patella, tarsus, metatarsus, and bones of the toes).

**ossa membri superioris** [ NA ], bones of the superior limb; these include the superior limb girdle (scapula and clavicle) and the skeleton of the free superior limb (humerus, radius, ulna, wrist bones, metacarpus, and bones of the fingers).

**o. metacarpa'le,** pl. **ossa metacarpalia** [ NA ], one of the metacarpal bones, five long bones forming the skeleton of the metacarpus or palm they are numbered I-V, beginning with the bone on the radial or thumb side, and articulate with the bones of the distal row of the carpus and with the five proximal phalanges.

**o. metatarsa'le,** pl. **ossa metatarsalia** [ NA ], one of the metatarsal bones; the five long bones forming the skeleton of the anterior portion of the foot, articulating posteriorly with the three cuneiform and the cuboid bones, anteriorly with the five proximal phalanges.

**o. multan'gulum majus,** o. trapezium.

**o. multan'gulum minus,** o. trapezoideum.

**o. nasa'le** [ NA ], nasal bone; an elongated rectangular bone which, with its fellow, forms the bridge of the nose; it articulates with the frontal bone superiorly, the ethmoid and the frontal process of the maxilla posteriorly, and its fellow medially.

**o. navicula're** [ NA ], navicular bone; o. centrale tarsi; central bone of the ankle; a bone of the tarsus on the medial side of the foot articulating with the head of the talus, the three cuneiform bones, and occasionally the cuboid.

**o. navicula're manus,** o. scaphoideum.

**o. occipita'le** [ NA ], occipital bone; a bone at the lower and posterior part of the skull, consisting of three parts (basilar, condylar, and squamous), enclosing a large oval hole, the foramen magnum; it articulates with the parietal and temporal bones on either side, the sphenoid anteriorly, and the atlas below.

**o. odontoi'deum,** the dens of the axis when anomalously not fused with the body of this bone.

**o. orbiculare,** *processus* lenticularis incudis.

**o. palati'num** [ NA ], palatine bone; an irregularly shaped bone posterior to the maxilla, which enters into the formation of the nasal cavity, the orbit, and the hard palate; it articulates with the maxilla, inferior nasal concha, sphenoid, and ethmoid bones, the vomer and its fellow of the opposite side.

**o. parieta'le** [ NA ], parietal bone; a flat, curved bone of irregular quadrangular shape, at either side of the vault of the cranium; it articulates, with its fellow medially, with the frontal anteriorly, the occipital posteriorly, and the temporal and sphenoid inferiorly.

**o. pe'nis** [ NAV ], baculum; penis bone; a bone of variable size and shape, located in the glans penis or glans clitoris of all animals, except man, ungulates, elephants, whales, and a few others; it is particularly well developed in carnivora, and in the dog it may reach a length of more than 10 cm.; its size and shape is often a characteristic of a species.

**o. pisifor'me** [ NA ], pisiform bone; lentiform bone; a small bone resembling a pea in size and shape, in the first row of the carpus, lying on the anterior surface of the distal end of the triquetral with which alone it articulates; it gives insertion to the tendon of the flexor carpi ulnaris muscle.

**o. planum** [ NA ], flat bone; a type of bone characterized by its thin, flattened shape, such as the scapula or certain of the cranial bones.

**o. pneumat'icum** [ NA ], pneumatic bone; hollow bone; one that is hollow or contains many air cells, such as the mastoid process of the temporal bone.

**o. premaxilla're,** o. incisivum.

**o. pterygoid'eum,** *processus* pterygoideus.

**o. pubis** [ NA ], pubic bone; pubes; the anteroinferior portion of the hip bone, distinct at birth but later becoming fused with the ilium and ischium; it is composed of a body which articulates with its fellow at the symphysis pubis, and two rami; the superior ramus enters into the formation of the acetabulum, the inferior ramus fuses with the ramus of the ischium.

**o. pyramida'le,** o. triquetrum.

**o. rostra'le** [ NAV ], a thick, roughly four-sided bone located in the snout of the hog.

**o. sacrum** [ NA ], sacrum; sacred bone (so called because it was believed to escape disintegration and to serve as the basis for the resurrected body); the segment of the vertebral column forming part of the pelvis; a broad, slightly curved, spade-shaped bone, thick above, thinner below, closing in the pelvic girdle posteriorly. It is formed by the fusion of five originally separate sacral vertebrae; it articulates with the last lumbar vertebra, the coccyx, and the hip bone on either side.

**o. scaphoi'deum** [ NA ], scaphoid bone; navicular bone of the hand; the largest bone of the proximal row of the carpus on the radial or thumb side, articulating with the radius, lunate, capitate, trapezium, and trapezoid.

**o. sesamoi'deum,** pl. **ossa sesamoi'dea** [ NA ], sesamoid bone; a bone formed in a tendon where it passes over a joint.

**o. sphenoida'le** [ NA ], sphenoid bone; a bone of most irregular shape occupying the base of the skull; it is described as consisting of a central portion, or body, and six processes: two greater wings, two lesser wings and two pterygoid processes; it articulates with the occipital, frontal, ethmoid, and vomer, and with the paired temporal, parietal, zygomatic, palatine and sphenoidal concha bones.

**o. subtibia'le,** an inconstant bone found very rarely in the distal articular end of the tibia.

**o. suprasterna'le,** pl. **ossa suprasternalia** [ NA ], suprasternal bone; episternal bone; Breschet's bones; one of the small ossicles occasionally found in the ligaments of the sternoclavicular articulation.

**ossa sutura'rum** [ NA ], sutural, epactal, or Wormian bones; Andernach's ossicles; small irregular bones found along the sutures of the cranium, particularly related to the parietal bone.

**o. syl'vii,** *processus* lenticularis incudis.

**ossa tarsi** [ NA ], tarsal bones see tarsus.

**o. tempora'le** [ NA ], temporal bone; a large irregular bone situated in the base and side of the skull; it consists of three parts, squamous, tympanic and petrous, which are distinct at birth; the petrous part contains the vestibulocochlear organ; the bone articulates with the sphenoid, parietal, occipital, and zygomatic bones, and by a synovial joint with the mandible.

**o. tibia'le posterius** or **posti'cum,** a sesamoid bone in the tendon of the tibialis posterior muscle, occasionally fused with the tuberosity of the navicular.

**o. trape'zium** [ NA ], trapezium bone; o. multangulum majus; greater multangular bone; a bone in the distal row of the carpus; it articulates with the 1st and 2nd metacarpals, scaphoid, and trapezoid bones.

**o. trapezoi'deum** [ NA ], trapezoid bone; lesser multangular bone; o. multangulum minus; a bone in the distal row of the carpus; it articulates with the second metacarpal, trapezium, capitate, and scaphoid.

**o. triangula're,** (1). o. trigonum; (2) o. triquetrum.

**o. tribasila're,** the single bone resulting from the fusion in infancy of the occipital and temporal bones at the base of the cranial cavity.

**o. trigo'num** [ NA ], triangular bone; an independent ossicle sometimes present in the tarsus; usually it forms part of the talus, constituting the posterior process.

**o. triquetrum** [ NA ], triquetral bone; cubital bone; three-cornered bone; cuneiform or pyramidal bone; a bone on the medial side of the proximal row of the carpus, articulating with the lunate, pisiform, and hamate.

**o. unguis,** o. lacrimale.

**o. vesalea'num,** Vasalius' bones; the tuberosity of the fifth metatarsal bone sometimes existing as a separate bone.

**o. zygomaticum** [ NA ], zygomatic bone; yoke bone; jugal bone; malar bone; cheek bone; mala; zygoma (1); a quadrilateral bone which forms the prominence of the cheek; it articulates with the frontal, sphenoid, temporal, and maxillary bone.

---

**osazone** (o'să-zōn). Dihydrazone; the compound formed by certain sugars (*e.g.,* glucose, galactose, fructose) with excess hydrazines, possessing two hydrazones on carbons 1 and 2 instead of only one at C-1, as in the ordinary hydrazone. O.'s are used in characterizing and in identifying certain sugars, *e.g.,* as in the phenylhydrazine test for glucose.

**osce'do** [ L. ]. 1. Aphthae. 2. Yawning.

**osche-, oscheo-** [ G. *oschē,* scrotum ]. Combining forms denoting the scrotum.

**oscheal** (os'ke-al). Scrotal.

**oscheitis** (os-ke-i'tis) [ osche- + G. suffix *-itis,* inflammation ]. Oschitis; inflammation of the scrotum.

**oschelephantiasis** (osk'el-ĕ-fan-ti'ă-sis) [ osche- + elephantiasis ]. An enlargement or elephantiasis of the scrotum.

**oscheocele** (os'ke-o-sēl) [ oscheo- + G. *kēlē,* hernia, tumor ]. 1. Scrotal *hernia.* 2. Oscheoncus.

**oscheohydrocele** (os-ke-o-hi'dro-sēl) [ oscheo- + G. *hydōr,* water, + *kēlē,* tumor ]. Scrotal hydrocele.

**oscheolith** (os'ke-o-lith) [ oscheo- + G. *lithos,* stone ]. A mass of concretions in the sebaceous glands of the scrotum.

**oscheoma** (os-ke-o'mah). Oscheoncus.

**oscheoncus** (os-ke-ong'kus) [ osche- + G. *onkos,* mass, bulk ]. Oscheoma; oscheocele (2); a tumor of the scrotum.

**oscheoplasty** (os'ke-o-plas-tĭ) [ oscheo- + *plassō,* to form ]. Scrotoplasty.

**oschitis** (os-ki'tis). Oscheitis.

**oscillation** (os'ĭ-la'shun) [ L. *oscillatio,* fr. *oscillo,* to swing ]. 1. A to-and-fro movement. 2. A stage in the vascular changes in inflammation in which the accumulation of leukocytes in the small vessels arrests the passage of blood and there is simply a to-and-fro movement at each cardiac contraction.

**os'cillator.** An apparatus somewhat like a vibrator, used to give a form of mechanical massage.

**oscillograph** (os'ĭ-lo-graf). An instrument that records oscillations, usually electrical.

**cathode ray o.,** an o. that permits amplification of electrical oscillations and allows for multichannel leads to record electrical change simultaneously from many areas.

**oscillography** (os'ĭ-log'ră-fĭ). Study of the records made by an oscillograph.

**oscillometer** (os'ĭ-lom'e-ter) [ L. *oscillo,* to swing, + G. *metron,* measure ]. An apparatus for measuring oscillations of any kind, especially those of the blood stream in sphygmometry; see also sphygmo-oscillometer.

**oscillometric** (os'ĭ-lo-mat'rik). Relating to the oscillometer or the records made by its use.

**oscillom'etry.** Use of the oscillometer.

**oscillopsia** (os'ĭ-lop'sĭ-ah) [ L. *oscillo,* to swing, + G. *opsis,* vision ]. The subjective sensation of oscillation of objects viewed.

**oscilloscope** (os'ĭ-lo-skōp). Oscillograph.

**oscine** (os'sēn). Scopoline.

**oscitate** (os'ĭ-tāt) [ L. *oscito,* fr. *os,* mouth, + *cieo,* to put in motion ]. To yawn; to gape.

**oscitation** (os'ĭ-ta'shun) [ L. *oscitatio;* see oscitate ]. Yawning; gaping.

**osculum,** pl. **os'cula** (os'ku-lum) [ L. dim.of *os,* mouth ]. A pore or minute opening.

**-ose.** 1. In chemistry, a termination usually indicating a carbohydrate. 2 [ L. *-osus* ]. Suffix appended to some Latin roots, with significance of the commoner *-ous.*

**Osgood,** Robert B., American orthopedic surgeon, *1873. See O.-Schlatter *disease.*

**Osiander,** Friederick Benjamin, German professor of midwifery, 1759–1825. See O.'s *maneuver.*

**-osis** [ G. ]. A suffix, properly added only to words formed from Greek roots, meaning a process, condition, or state, usually abnormal or diseased; denoting primarily any production or increase, physiologic or pathologic (leukocytosis, tuberculosis); and secondarily an invasion, and increase within the organism, of parasites (coccidiosis); in the latter sense, it is similar to and often interchangeable with -iasis, as seen in trichinosis, trichiniasis.

**Osler,** Sir William, Canadian-American physician, 1849–1919. See O.'s *disease, node, sign,* Rendu-O.-Weber *disease, syndrome.*

**os'mate.** A salt of osmic acid.

**osmatic** (oz-mat'ik) [ G. *osmē,* smell ]. Relating to olfaction, or the sense of smell.

**osmesis** (oz-me'sis) [ G. *osmēsis,* smelling ]. Olfaction.

**os'mic acid.** Osmium tetroxide; $OsO_4$; a volatile caustic; a strong oxidizing agent; colorless crystals, poorly soluble in water, but soluble in organic solvents; the aqueous solution is a fat stain and tissue fixative for electron microscopy.

**osmicate** (oz'mĭ-kāt). To stain with osmic acid.

**os'mica'tion, os'mifica'tion.** The fixation of tissue with an osmic acid solution.

**osmics** (oz'miks) [ G. *osmē,* smell ]. The science of olfaction.

**osmidrosis** (oz'mĭ-dro'sis) [ G. *osmē,* smell, + *hidrōs,* sweat ]. Bromidrosis.

**osmiophilic** (oz'mĭ-o-fil'ik) [ osmium + G. *phileō,* to love ]. Readily stained with osmic acid.

**osmiophobic** (oz'mĭ-o-fo'bik) [ osmium + G. *phobos,* fear ]. Not readily stained with osmic acid.

**osmium** (oz'mĭ-um) [ G. *osmē,* smell, because of the strong odor of the tetroxide ]. A metallic element of the platinum group, symbol Os, atomic no. 76, atomic weight 190.2.

**o. tetroxide,** osmic acid.

**osmo-.** 1 [ G. *osmos,* impulsion ]. Combining form relating to osmosis. 2 [ G. *osmē,* smell ]. Combining form relating to smell or odors.

**osmocep'tor.** Osmoreceptor.

**osmodysphoria** (oz'mo-dis-fo'rĭ-ah) [ G. *osmē,* smell, + *dys-,* bad, + *phora,* a carrying ]. An abnormal dislike of certain odors.

**osmogen** (os'mo-jen) [ osmo(sis) + G. suffix *-gen,* producing ]. A substance from which an enzyme may be formed.

**os'mol.** The molecular weight of a solute, in grams, divided by the number of ions or particles into which it dissociates in solution.

**osmolagnia** (oz'mo-lag'nĭ-ah). Osphresiolagnia.

**os'molal'ity.** Osmotic concentration, defined as the number of osmols ($\Phi n$mols, where $\Phi$ is the osmotic coefficient, and $n$ is the number of particles or ions formed upon dissociation of a solute in solution; *e.g.,* $n = 2$ for sodium chloride and $n = 1$ for glucose) of a solute per kg. of solvent (water). Thus o. is given by $\Phi nc$, where $c$ is the molal concentration of solute. The o. of a given solution is numerically equal to the molality of an ideal solution of a nonelectrolyte having the same freezing point. It is approximated by the quotient of the freezing point depression of an aqueous solution below that of water ($\Delta$°C.) and the molal freezing point depression for water (*ca.* 1.86°C. per mol of undissociated solute per kg. of water); *i.e.,* o. = $\Delta / 1.86$.

**osmo'lar.** Osmotic.

**osmolarity** (os'mo-lăr'ĭ-tĭ). The osmotic concentration of a solution expressed as osmols of solute per liter of solution.

**osmology** (oz-mol'o-jĭ). 1. Osphresiology; the study of odors, their production, and their effects. 2. The study of osmosis.

**osmom'eter.** An instrument for measuring osmosis.

**osmophil, osmophilic** (os'mo-fil, -fil'ik) [ osmo(sis) + G. *phileō,* to love ]. Flourishing in a medium of high osmotic pressure.

**osmophobia** (oz'mo-fo'bĭ-ah) [ G. *osmē,* smell, + phobia ]. Osphresiophobia.

**osmophore** (oz'mo-fōr). Odoriphore.

**os'morecep'tor.** Osmoceptor. 1 [ G. *osmos*, impulsion ]. A receptor in the central nervous system (probably the hypothalamus) that responds to changes in the osmotic pressure of the blood. 2 [ G. *osmē*, smell ]. A receptor that receives olfactory stimuli.

**os'moreg'ulatory.** Influencing the degree and rapidity of osmosis.

**os'mose.** To subject to osmosis; to diffuse by osmosis.

**osmo'sis** [ G. *ōsmos*, a thrusting, an impulsion ]. The phenomenon of the passage of certain fluids and solutions through a membrane or other porous substance. The rapidity of the passage of two fluids separated by a membrane is not always equal, particularly when the two fluids represent solutions of different solutes or of different concentrations where the membrane is semipermeable, *i.e.*, permeable to molecules of solvent but not to those of the solute; the phenomenon of the more rapid passage is called endosmosis, that of the slower passage is called exosmosis; these terms also, and more commonly, indicate the direction, endosmosis being the passage of the fluid from without into a vessel, exosmosis being the reverse of this: the two terms are now largely outmoded and have been replaced by simply o., which represents the net passage of fluid from the less concentrated to the more concentrated side of the membrane.

**osmos'ity.** The measure of the osmotic pressure of a solution given numerically by the molarity (or, loosely, by the millimolarity) of a sodium chloride solution having the same osmotic pressure; approximated by the quotient Δ/3.64. See also osmolality.

**os'mother'apy** [ osmosis + therapy ]. Dehydration by means of injections of hypertonic solutions of sodium chloride, dextrose, urea or mannitol; or orally glycerine, 1 to 1.5 gm. per kg., isosorbide 1.5 to 2 gm. per kg., or glycine, 25 gm. per 250 ml. of water.

**osmot'ic.** Relating to osmosis.

**osphresio-** (os-fre'zĭ-o-) [ G. *osphresis*, smell ]. Combining form relating to odors or the sense of smell.

**osphresiolagnia** (os-fre'zĭ-o-lag'nĭ-ah) [ osphresio- + G. *lagneia*, lust ]. Sexual excitement produced by odors.

**osphresiologic** (os-fre-zĭ-o-loj'ik). Relating to osphresiology.

**osphresiology** (os-fre'zĭ-ol'o-jĭ) [ osphresio- + G. *logos*, study ]. Osmology (1).

**osphresiophilia** (os-fre'zĭ-o-fil'ĭ-ah) [ osphresio- + G. *phileō*, to love ]. Unusual interest in odors.

**osphresiophobia** (os-fre'zĭ-o-fo'bĭ-ah) [ osphresio- + G. *phobos*, fear ]. Osmophobia; olfactophobia; morbid fear of certain odors.

**osphre'sis** [ G. *osphrēsis*, smell ]. Olfaction.

**osphret'ic.** Olfactory.

**osphyalgia** (os-fĭ-al'jĭ-ah) [ G. *osphys*, loin, + *algos*, pain ]. Obsolete term for lumbago.

**os'phyarthro'sis** [ G. *osphys*, loin, + arthrosis ]. Obsolete term for inflammation of the hip.

**osphyitis** (os-fĭ-i'tis) [ G. *osphys*, loin, + -*itis* ]. Obsolete term for lumbago.

**osphyomyelitis** (os'fĭ-o-mi'ĕ-li'tis) [ G. *osphys*, loin, + *myelos*, marrow, + -*itis* ]. Obsolete term meaning inflammation of the spinal cord in the lumbar region.

**ossa** (os'ah) [ L. ]. Plural of L. *os*, bone.

**ossein, osseine** (os'e-in) [ L. *os*, bone ]. Collagen.

**os'selet** [ L. dim. of *os*, bone ]. A periostitis of the anterior margin of the third metacarpal bone or first phalanx near the fetlock and a cause of lameness in horses, particularly young race horses in training. There is first a painful, soft swelling and later exostosis.

**osseo-** (os'se-o-) [ L. *osseus*, bony. OS- ]. Combining form meaning bony. For other combining forms relating to bone, see osse-, osteo-.

**osseoalbu'moid.** Osteoalbuminoid; ostealbumoid; a protein derived from ossein.

**osseocartilaginous** (os-e-o-kar-tĭ-laj'ĭ-nus). Osteochondrous; relating to, or composed of, both bone and cartilage.

**osseomu'cin.** The ground substance of bony tissue.

**osseomucoid** (os-e-o-mu'koyd). A mucoid derived from ossein.

**osseous** (os'e-us) [ L. *osseus* ]. Bony.

**ossi-** (os'ĭ-) [ G. *os*, bone. OS- ]. Combining form denoting bone. For words beginning thus and not found here, see oste- and osteo-.

**ossicle** (os'ĭ-kl) [ L. *ossiculum*, dim. of *os*, bone ]. Ossiculum.
  **Andernach's o.'s,** *ossa* suturarum.
  **au'ditory o.,** *ossiculum* auditus.
  **Bertin's o.'s,** *conchae* sphenoidales.
  **epac'tal o.,** *os* suturae.
  **Kerckring's o.,** Kerckring's *center*.

**ossicula** (ŏ-sik'u-lah) [ L. ]. Plural of ossiculum.

**ossicular** (ŏ-sik'u-lar). Pertaining to an ossicle.

**ossiculectomy** (os-ik'u-lek'to-mĭ) [ L. *ossiculum*, ossicle, + G. *ektomē*, excision ]. Removal of the ossicles of the middle ear.

**ossiculot'omy** [ L. *ossiculum*, ossicle, + G. *tomē*, incision ]. Division of one of the processes of the ossicles of the middle ear, or of a fibrous band causing ankylosis between any two ossicles.

**ossiculum, pl. ossicula** (ŏ-sik'u-lum, -lah) [ L. dim. of *os*, bone ] [ NA ]. Ossicle; bonelet; a small bone; specifically, one of the bones of the tympanic cavity or middle ear.
  **o. audi'tus** [ NA ], auditory ossicle; ear bone; one of the small bones of the middle ear; malleus, incus, or stapes; they are articulated to form a chain for the transmission of sound from the tympanic membrane to the oval window.

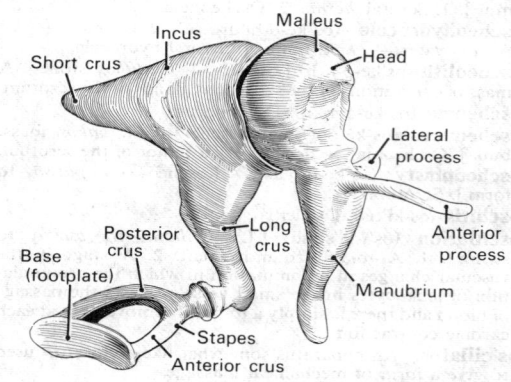

**Ossicula Auditus**

**ossicula mentalia,** small nodules of bone that appear at the symphysis menti shortly before birth and fuse with the mandible after birth.

**ossiferous** (ŏ-sif'er-us) [ ossi- + L. *fero*, to bear ]. Osseous; containing bone.

**ossif'ic.** Relating to a change into or formation of bone.

**ossification** (os'ĭ-fĭ-ka'shun) [ L. *ossificatio*, fr. *os*, bone, + *facio*, to make ]. 1. The formation of bone. 2. A change into bone.
  **endochondral o.,** the formation of osseous tissue within cartilage; the process by which bones grow in length. In long bones endochondral o. is seen at the epiphysial cartilage plate by formation of bone trabeculae on a framework of unresorbed cartilage, by the action of osteoblasts.
  **intramembranous o.,** membranous o.
  **membranous o.,** intramembranous o.; the development of osseous tissue within connective tissue such as that of the skull.
  **metaplas'tic o.,** the formation of irregular foci of bone (sometimes including bits of bone marrow) in various soft structures, such as the muscles, lungs, brain, and other sites where osseous tissue is abnormal.

**ossifluence** (ŏ-sif'lu-ens). Obsolescent term for osteolysis.

**os'siform** [ ossi- + L. *forma*, form ]. Osteoid.

**ossify** (os'ĭ-fi) [ ossi- + L. *facio*, to make ]. To form bone or change into bone.

**ost-, oste-.** See osteo-.

**ostal'gia.** Ostealgia.

**osteal** (os'te-al) [ G. *osteon*, bone ]. Osseous; bony.

**ostealbumoid** (os-te-al-bu'moyd). Osseoalbumoid.

**ostealgia** (os-te-al'jĭ-ah) [ osteo- + G. *algos*, pain ]. Osteo-dynia; ostalgia; osteocope; pain in a bone.

**osteal'gic.** Relating to or marked by bone pain.

**osteanabrosis** (os'te-an-ă-bro'sis) [ osteo- + G. *anabrōsis*, an eating up ]. Atrophy of bone.

**osteanagenesis** (os'te-an'ă-jen'ē-sis). Osteoanagenesis.

**osteanaphysis** (os'te-ă-naf'ĭ-sis) [ osteo- + G. *anaphysis*, a growing again ]. Osteoanagenesis.

**ostearthritis** (os'te-ar-thri'tis). Osteoarthritis.

**ostearthrotomy** (os'te-ar-throt'o-mĭ). Osteoarthrotomy.

**ostectomy** (os-tek'to-mĭ) [ osteo- + G. *ektomē*, excision ]. Osteectomy; osteoectomy; surgical removal of a segment of bone or an entire bone.

**ostectopy** (os-tek'to-pĭ) [ osteo- + G. *ek*, out of, + *topos*, place ]. Osteectopia; displacement of a bone.

**osteectomy** (os'te-ek'to-mĭ). Ostectomy.

**osteectopia** (os'te-ek-to'pĭ-ah). Ostectopy.

**ostein, osteine** (os'te-in). Ossein.

**osteitic** (os-te-it'ik). Ostitic; relating to or affected by oste-itis.

**osteitis** (os-te-i'tis) [ osteo- + G. suffix *-itis*, inflamma-tion ]. Ostitis; inflammation of bone.

    **alveolar o.,** alveoalgia.

    **o. carno'sa,** o. fungosa.

    **caseous o.,** tuberculous caries in bone.

    **central o.,** osteomyelitis; endosteitis.

    **o. conden'sans generalisa'ta,** obsolete term for osteope-trosis.

    **condensing o.,** sclerosing o.

    **cortical o.,** periostitis with involvement of the superficial layer of bone.

    **o. defor'mans,** Paget's disease (1).

    **o. fibro'sa cir'cumscrip'ta,** Albright's *disease.*

    **o. fibro'sa cys'tica,** increased osteoclastic resorption of calcified bone with replacement by fibrous tissue, due to primary hyperparathyroidism or other causes of the rapid mobilization of mineral salts. Also known as Recklinghau-sen's disease of bone; metaplastic malacia; o. fibrosa generalisata; osteodystrophia fibrosa; hemorrhagic osteo-myelitis; parathyroid osteosis.

    **o. fibro'sa disseminat'a,** Albright's *disease.*

    **o. fibro'sa gen'eralisat'a,** o. fibrosa cystica.

    **formative o.,** sclerosing o.

    **o. fungo'sa,** o. carnosa; chronic o. with dilated Haversian canals filled with a vascular granulation tissue.

    **hematog'enous o.,** any o. caused by infection carried in the blood stream.

    **localized o. fibro'sa,** Albright's *disease.*

    **multifocal o. fibro'sa,** polyostotic fibrous *dysplasia.*

    **o. ossif'icans,** condensing or rarefying o.; chronic o. accompanied by absorption of ostein and widening of the intraosteal spaces, the whole bone becoming more or less cancellated.

    **Pagetoid o.,** o. fibrosa cystica with marked deformity of the bones.

    **renal o. fibrosa,** renal *rickets.*

    **sarco'matous o.,** myelomatosis.

    **scleros'ing o.,** condensing or formative o.; Garré's disease; fusiform thickening of long bones of unknown cause; the disease has been considered a form of chronic nonsuppurative osteomyelitis.

    **o. tuberculo'sa mul'tiplex cys'tica,** Jüngling's disease; an o. of tuberculous origin, marked by numerous small cavities in the osseous substance.

**ostembryon** (os-tem'brĭ-on) [ osteo- + G. *embryon*, em-bryo ]. Archaic for lithopedion.

**oste'mia** [ osteo- + G. *haima*, blood ]. Congestion or hyperemia of a bone.

**ostempyesis** (os-tem-pi-e'sis) [ osteo- + G. *empyēsis*, sup-puration ]. Suppuration in bone.

**osteo-, ost-, osteo-** [ G. *osteon*, bone. OS- ]. Combining forms relating to bone.

**os'teoalbu'minoid.** Osseoalbumoid.

**osteoanagenesis** (os'te-o-an-ă-jen'ē-sis) [ osteo- + G. *ana,* again, + *genesis*, generation ]. Osteanagenesis; osteanaph-ysis; reproduction of bone.

**osteoanesthesia** (os'te-o-an'es-the'zĭ-ah). Loss of sensa-tion in bone.

**osteoarthritis** (os-te-o-ar-thri'tis). Degenerative joint *dis-ease.*

    **endemic o. defor'mans,** a disease observed in a province of Russia, in which a very large proportion of the inhabitants suffered from softening of the articular ends of the bones, thickening of the joints, crepitus, and partial ankylosis.

    **hyperplas'tic o.,** pulmonary *osteoarthropathy.*

**osteoarthropathy** (os'te-o-ar-throp'ă-thĭ) [ osteo- + G. *arthron*, joint, + *pathos*, suffering ]. A trophic disorder affecting bones and joints with periosteal and articular proliferation and severe pain, related to clubbing of the fingers; often found in association with disease of the lungs, pleura, or mediastinum.

    **hypertroph'ic pul'monary o.,** Marie-Bamberger disease or syndrome; Marie's disease; pneumogenic or pulmonary o.; expansion of the distal ends, or the entire shafts, of the long bones, sometimes with erosions of the articular cartilages and thickening and villous proliferation of the synovial membranes, and frequently clubbing of fingers. The affection occurs in chronic pulmonary disease, in heart disease, and occasionally in other acute and chronic disorders.

    **idiopathic hypertrophic o.,** primary o., not secondary to pulmonary or other progressive lesions, which may occur alone (acropathy) or as part of the syndrome of pachyder-moperiostosis.

    **pneumogenic a.,** hypertrophic pulmonary o.

    **pulmonary o.,** hypertrophic pulmonary o.

    **tabetic o.,** Charcot's *joint.*

**osteoarthrotomy** (os'te-o-ar-throt'o-mĭ) [ osteo- + G. *ar-thron*, joint, + *tomē*, incision ]. Ostearthrotomy; surgical removal of the articular end of a bone.

**os'teoblast** [ osteo- + G. *blastos*, germ ]. Osteoplast; a bone-forming cell derived from mesenchyme; it forms the osseous matrix in which it becomes enclosed as an osteocyte.

**osteoblas'tic.** Relating to the osteoblasts.

**os'teoblasto'ma.** Giant osteoid osteoma; an uncommon benign tumor of osteoblasts with areas of osteoid and calcified tissue, occurring most frequently in the spine of a young person.

**osteocampsia** (os'te-o-kamp'sĭ-ah) [ osteo- + G. *kampsis,* a bending ]. Curvature of a bone, as in rickets or osteomalacia.

**osteocar'cino'ma.** An undesirable, nonspecific term for (1) a metastasis of carcinoma in a bone, or (2) a carcinoma that contains foci of osseous tissue (as a result of metaplasia).

**osteocartilaginous** (os-te-o-kar-tĭ-laj'ĭ-nus). Osseocarti-laginous.

**osteocele** (os'te-o-sēl) [ osteo- + G. *kēlē*, tumor ]. A scro-tal tumefaction or mass that contains portions of osseous tissue.

**osteochondritis** (os-te-o-kon-dri'tis) [ osteo- + G. *chon-dros,* cartilage, + suffix -*itis,* inflammation ]. Inflammation of a bone with its cartilage.

    **o. defor'mans juveni'lis,** epiphysial aseptic *necrosis* (*q. v.*) of the upper end of the femur.

    **o. defor'mans juveni'lis dorsi,** epiphysial aseptic *necrosis* (*q. v.*) of vertebral bodies.

    **o. dissecans,** osteochrondrosis dissecans; osteochondrol-ysis; complete or incomplete separation of a portion of joint cartilage and underlying bone.

**os'teochon'drodystro'phia defor'mans.** Osteochondro-dystrophy.

**osteochondrodystrophy** (os'te-o-kon'dro-dis'tro-fĭ). Term for a group of disorders of bone and cartilage that includes the Morquio *syndrome* (*q. v.*) and similar condi-tions.

**os'teochondrol'ysis.** *Osteochondritis* dissecans.

**osteochondroma** (os-te-o-kon-dro'mah) [ osteo- + G. *chondros*, cartilage, + suffix -*oma*, tumor ]. Solitary osteocartilaginous exostosis; a benign cartilaginous neoplasm that consists of a pedicle of normal bone (protruding from the cortex) covered with a rim of proliferating cartilage cells. O.'s may originate from any bone that is preformed in cartilage, but they are most frequent near the ends of long bones, usually in patients who are 10 to 25 years of age. The lesions are frequently not noticed, unless they are traumatized or of large size; sometimes they are multiple.

**osteochondromatosis** (os-te-o-kon-dro-mă-to'-sis). Hereditary multiple *exostoses*.

**osteochondrosarcoma** (os'te-o-kon'dro-sar-ko'-ma) [ osteo- + G. *chondros*, cartilage, + *sarx*, flesh, + suffix -*oma*, tumor ]. Chondrosarcoma arising in bone. Sarcomas in bone containing foci of neoplastic cartilage as well as bone are classified as osteogenic sarcomas.

**osteochondrosis** (os-te-o-kon-dro'sis) [ osteo- + G. *chondros*, cartilage, + suffix -*osis*, condition ]. Any of a group of disorders of one or more ossification centers in children, characterized by degeneration or aseptic necrosis followed by recalcification; includes the various forms of epiphysial aseptic necrosis, *q. v.*

**o. dissecans,** *osteochondritis* dissecans.

**osteochondrous** (os'te-o-kon'drus) [ osteo- + G. *chondros*, cartilage ]. Osseocartilaginous.

**osteoclasia, osteoclasis** (os'te-o-kla'zĭ-ah, os'te-ok'lă-sis) [ osteo- + G. *klasis*, fracture ]. 1. Osteoclasty; intentional fracture of a misshapen bone in order to correct deformity. 2. Osteolysis.

**os'teoclast** [ osteo- + G. *klastos*, broken ]. 1. Osteophage; a large multinucleated cell with abundant acidophilic cytoplasm, functioning in the absorption and removal of osseous tissue; once termed Robin's myeloplax. 2. An instrument used to break a misshapen bone to correct the deformity.

**osteoclas'tic.** Pertaining to osteoclasts, especially with reference to their activity in the absorption and removal of osseous tissue.

**osteoclasto'ma.** Giant cell *tumor* of bone.

**os'teoclasty.** Osteoclasia (1).

**osteocope** (os'te-o-kōp) [ G. *osteokopos*, bone-breaking, bone-racking ]. Severe pain in the bones; specifically the night pains of syphilis.

**osteocop'ic.** Relating to severe bone pain.

**osteocra'nium** [ osteo- + G. *kranion*, skull ]. The cranium of the fetus after ossification of the membranous cranium has advanced so far as to give it firmness.

**osteocystoma** (os'te-o-sis-to'mah). Solitary bone *cyst*.

**osteocyte** (os'te-o-sīt) [ osteo- + G. *kytos*, cell ]. Bone cell; osseous cell; a cell of osseous tissue which occupies a lacuna and has processes which extend into canaliculi.

**osteoden'tin** [ osteo- + L. *dens*, tooth ]. Calcified deposit that is neither bone nor dentin in structure but is something in between.

**osteodermatopoikilosis** (os'te-o-der'mă-to-poy'kĭ-lo-sis) [ osteo- + G. *derma*, skin, + *poikilos*, dappled, + suffix -*osis*, condition ]. Osteopoikilosis with skin lesions, most commonly small fibrous nodules on the posterior aspects of the thighs and buttocks.

**osteoder'matous.** Pertaining to or characterized by osteodermia.

**osteodermia** (os-te-o-der'mĭ-ah) [ osteo- + G. *derma*, skin ]. *osteosis* cutis.

**osteodesmosis** (os'te-o-dez-mo'sis) [ osteo- + G. *desmos*, a band (tendon), + suffix -*osis*, condition ]. The transformation of tendon into bony tissue.

**osteodiastasis** (os'te-o-di-as'tă-sis) [ osteo- + G. *diastasis*, a separation ]. Separation of two adjacent bones, as of the cranium.

**osteodyn'ia** [ osteo- + G. *odynē*, pain ]. Ostealgia.

**osteodystrophia** (os-te-o-dis-tro'fĭ-ah). Osteodystrophy.

**o. fibro'sa,** *osteitis* fibrosa cystica.

**osteodystrophy** (os-te-o-dis'trof-ĭ) [ osteo- + G. *dys*, difficult, imperfect, + *trophē*, nourishment ]. Defective formation of bone.

**renal o.,** generalized bone changes resembling osteomalacia and rickets or osteitis fibrosa, occurring in children or adults with chronic renal failure.

**osteoectasia** (os'te-o-ek-ta'sĭ-ah) [ osteo- + G. *ektasis*, a stretching ]. Hyperphosphatasia.

**osteoectomy** (os-te-o-ek'to-mĭ). Ostectomy.

**osteoepiphysis** (os'te-o-e-pif'ĭ-sis). An epiphysis of a bone.

**os'teofibro'ma.** A benign lesion of bone, probably not a true neoplasm, consisting chiefly of fairly dense, moderately cellular, fibrous connective tissue in which there are small foci of osteogenesis. Most examples of this condition, especially in the maxilla and mandible, probably represent foci of fibrous dysplasia. A few examples of fibrous lesions with foci of osteogenesis, especially in vertebral bodies, may be neoplasms.

**osteogen** (os'te-o-jen) [ osteo- + G. suffix -*gen*, producing ]. The substance forming the inner layer of the periosteum from which new bone is formed.

**osteogenesis** (os'te-o-jen'ĕ-sis) [ osteo- + G. *genesis*, production ]. Osteosis (2); ostosis (2); the formation of bone.

**o. imperfec'ta,** fragilitas ossium; brittle bones; myeloplastic malacia; Durante's disease; a condition of abnormal fragility and plasticity of bone, with recurring fractures on minimal trauma, deformity of long bones, usually bluish color of sclerae, and, in many cases, the development of otosclerosis. There is extreme variation in severity and clinical findings; the terms *o. imperfecta congenita* and *o. imperfecta tarda* are used to indicate more severe and less severe cases, respectively. Inheritance is autosomal dominant in most families, but a rare autosomal recessive type also exists.

**o. imperfec'ta cys'tica,** cystic formation in growing bone.

**osteogen'ic, osteogenet'ic.** Relating to osteogenesis.

**osteogenous** (os-te-oj'ĕ-nus). Osteogenic.

**osteogeny** (os-te-oj'ĕ-nĭ). Osteogenesis.

**osteography** (os'te-og'ră-fĭ) [ osteo- + G. *graphē*, a writing ]. A treatise on or description of the bones.

**osteohalisteresis** (os'te-o-hal-is-ter-e'sis) [ osteo- + G. *hals*, salt, + *sterēsis*, privation ]. Softening of the bones through absorption or insufficient supply of the mineral portion.

**osteohypertrophy** (os'te-o-hi-per'tro-fĭ) [ osteo- + G. prefix *hyper-*, over, + *trophē*, nourishment ]. A condition characterized by overgrowth of bones.

**osteoid** (os'te-oyd) [ osteo- + G. *eidos*, resemblance ]. 1. Relating to or resembling bone. 2. Osseous tissue prior to calcification.

**osteoino'ma.** Obsolete term for osteofibroma.

**osteolathyrism** (os'te-o-lath'ĭ-rizm) [ osteo- + lathyrism, *q. v.* ]. An experimental disease in rats that are fed the seeds of certain species of *Lathyrus* (e.g., *L. odoratus*, sweet pea), or such nitriles as aminoacetonitrile or β-aminopropionitrile; the chief pathologic changes occur in connective tissue structures, as follows: (1) fibroblastic, chondroblastic, and osteoblastic proliferative changes in the periosteum; (2) degeneration, necrosis, and atypical proliferation of epiphysial cartilages; (3) an increase in adipose tissue of the bone marrow; (4) sometimes proliferation of synovial membranes; and (5) relatively large foci of extensive destruction of elastic fibers in the aorta, especially in the thoracic aorta.

**osteolipochondroma** (os'te-o-lip'o-kon-dro'mah) [ osteo- + G. *lipos*, fat, + *chondros*, cartilage, + suffix -*oma*, tumor ]. A benign neoplasm of cartilaginous tissue, in which metaplasia occurs and foci of adipose cells and osseous tissue are formed.

**osteolo'gia** [ L. ] [ NA ]. Osteology.

**osteol'ogist.** A person versed in osteology.

**osteology** (os'te-ol'o-jĭ) [ osteo- + G. *logos*, study ]. The anatomy of the bones; the science that treats of the bones and their structure.

**osteolysis** (os'te-ol'ĭ-sis) [ osteo- + G. *lysis*, dissolution ]. Osteoclasia (2); softening, absorption, and destruction of bony tissue.

**osteolyt'ic.** Pertaining to, characterized by, or causing osteolysis.

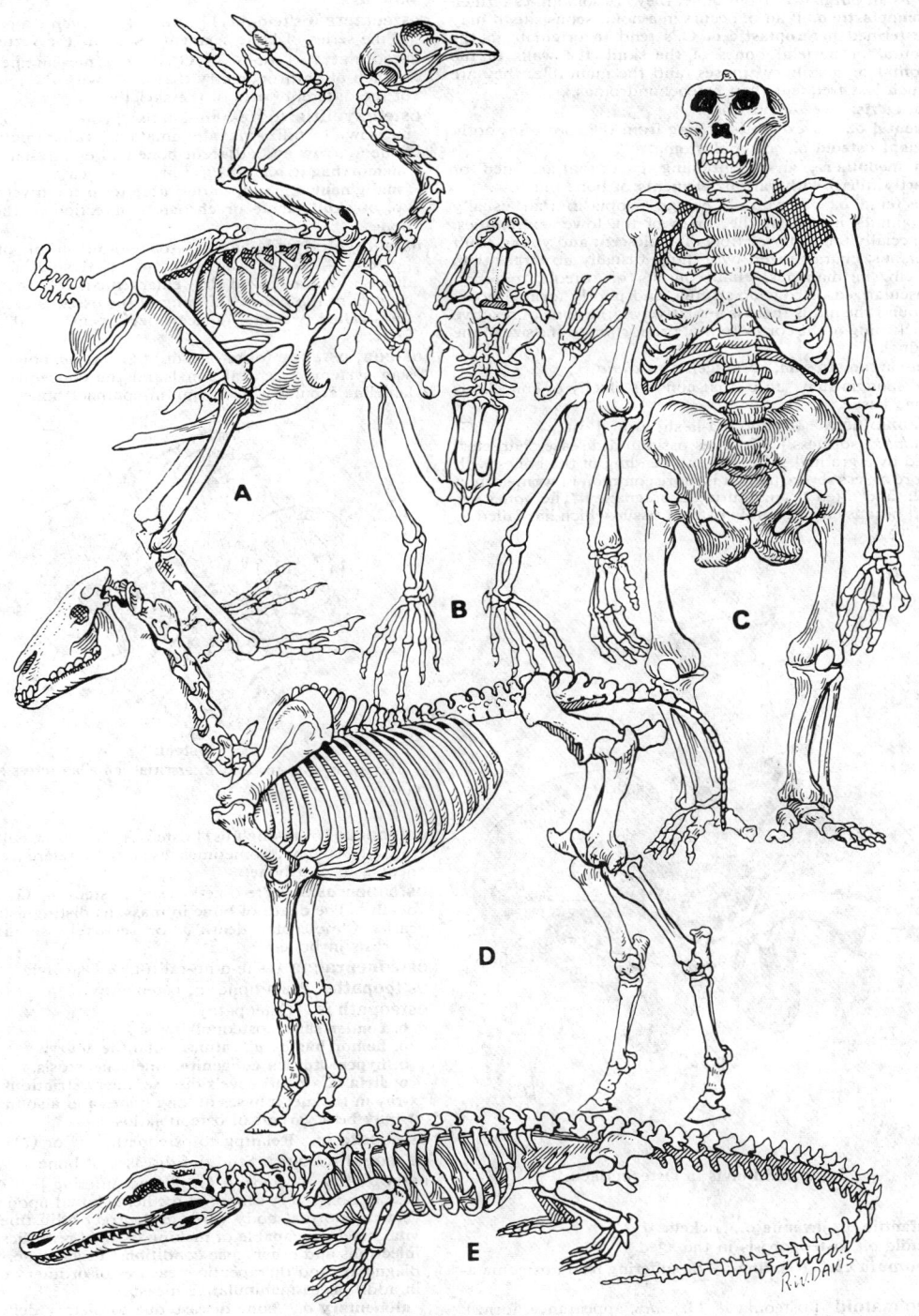

**Comparative Osteology**

*A*, Domestic fowl; *B*, frog; *C*, gorilla; *D*, horse; *E*, alligator

**osteo'ma** [ osteo- + G. suffix -*oma*, tumor ]. A benign neoplasm consisting of osteoblastic connective tissue that forms osteoid tissue and new bone, which may become fairly compact. When such neoplasms occur within bone, or as an outgrowth from bone, they are sometimes termed **homoplastic o.**; if an o. occurs in a nonosseous site, it may be termed **heteroplastic o.** O.'s tend to originate in the frontal or parietal bones of the skull, the walls of the frontal or maxillary sinuses, and the mandible; they are much less frequent than osteochondromas.

    **o. cu'tis,** see *osteosis* cutis.

    **dental o.,** an exostosis arising from the root of a tooth.

    **giant osteoid o.,** osteoblastoma.

    **o. medulla're,** an o. containing spaces that are filled (or partly filled) with various elements of bone marrow.

    **os'teoid o.,** a painful, benign neoplasm that usually originates in one of the bones of the lower extremities, especially the femur or tibia of adolescent and young adult persons; characterized by a nidus (usually no larger than 1 cm. in diameter) that consists of osteoid material, vascularized osteogenic stroma, and poorly formed bone; around the nidus there is a relatively large zone of reactive thickening of the cortex (out of proportion to the size of the nidus).

    **o. sarcomato'sum,** osteogenic *sarcoma*.

    **o. spongio'sum,** an o. that consists chiefly of concellous bone tissue.

**osteomalacia** (os'te-o-mă-la'shĭ-ah) [ osteo- + G. *malakia*, softness ]. Mollities ossium; a disease characterized by a gradual softening and bending of the bones with more or less severe pain; it is more common in women than men and often begins during a pregnancy. The bones are soft because they contain osteoid tissue which has failed to calcify.

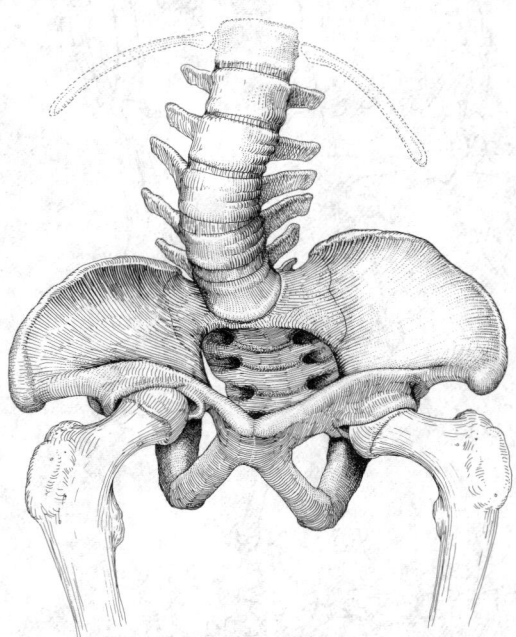

**Spine and Pelvis in Osteomalacia**

    **infantile o., juvenile o.,** rickets.

    **senile o.,** osteoporosis in the aged.

**osteomala'cic.** Relating to, or suffering from, osteomalacia.

**osteo'matoid** [ osteoma + G. *eidos*, appearance, form ]. An abnormal nodule or small mass of overgrowth of bone, usually occurring bilaterally and symmetrically, in juxtaepiphysial regions, especially in long bones of the lower extremities. The lesions are not actually neoplasms, but represent anomalous developments in which there are outpouchings of the cortex (in contrast to a growth superimposed on the cortex). O.'s are more properly termed exostoses (bulging outward) or enostoses (bulging inward).

**osteomere** (os'te-o-mēr) [ osteo- + G. *meros*, a part ]. One of the series of bone segments, such as the vertebrae.

**osteom'etry** [ osteo- + G. *metron*, measurement ]. The branch of anthropometry that deals with the relative size of the different parts of the skeleton.

**osteomyelitis** (os-te-o-mi-ĕ-li'tis) [ osteo- + G. *myelos*, marrow, + suffix -*itis*, inflammation ]. Inflammation of the bone marrow and adjacent bone and epiphysial cartilage.

    **hemorrhag'ic o.,** *osteitis* fibrosa cystica.

    **malig'nant o.,** old, undesirable term for myelomatosis.

    **o. of skull (acute or chronic),** infection of the cranial bones.

**osteomyelodysplasia** (os'te-o-mi'ĕ-lo-dis-pla'-zĭ-ah) [ osteo- + G. *myelos*, marrow, + dysplasia, *q.v.* ]. A disease characterized by enlargement of the marrow cavities of the bones, thinning of the osseous tissue, large, thin-walled vascular spaces, leukopenia, and irregular fever.

**osteon, osteone** (os'te-on, -ōn) [ G. *osteon*, bone ]. Haversian system; a central canal and the concentric osseous lamellae around it occurring in compact bone.

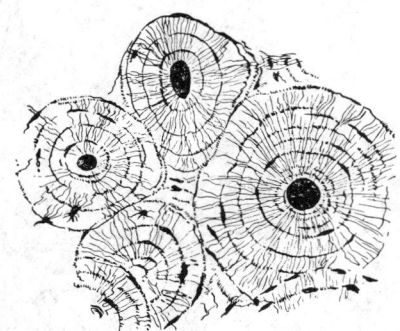

**Osteon**
Haversian systems and interstitial lamellae (cross section) of bone.

**osteoncus** (os'te-ong'kus) [ osteo- + G. *onkos*, bulk (swelling) ]. Osteoma; sometimes used with reference to any neoplasm of a bone.

**osteonecrosis** (os'te-o-ne-kro'sis) [ osteo- + G. *nekrōsis*, death ]. The death of bone in mass, as distinguished from caries ("molecular death"), or relatively small foci of necrosis in bone.

**osteoneuralgia** (os'te-o-nu-ral'jĭ-ah). Ostealgia.

**os'teopath.** Practitioner of osteopathy.

**osteopath'ia.** Osteopathy.

    **o. conden'sans,** osteopoikilosis.

    **o. hemorrhagica infantum,** infantile *scurvy*.

    **o. hyperostot'ica congenita,** melorheostosis.

    **o. stria'ta,** Voorhoeve's disease; linear striations seen by x-ray in the metaphyses of long bones and also flat bones; it may be a variant of osteopoikilosis.

**osteopath'ic.** Relating to osteopathy (1) or (2).

**os'teopathol'ogy.** Study of diseases of bone.

**osteop'athy** [ osteo- + G. *pathos*, suffering ]. 1. Any disease of bone. 2. A school of medicine based upon the idea that the normal body when in "correct adjustment" is a vital machine capable of making its own remedies against infections and other toxic conditions. Practitioners use the diagnostic and therapeutic measures of ordinary medicine in addition to manipulative measures.

    **alimentary o.,** bone disease due to dietary deficiency.

    **dissem'inated condensing o.,** obsolete term for osteopetrosis.

**osteope'dion** [ osteo- + G. *paidion*, dim. of *pais*, a child ]. Archaic for lithopedion.

**osteope′nia** [ osteo- + G. *penia*, poverty ]. 1. Decreased calcification or density of bone; a descriptive term applicable to all skeletal systems in which such a condition is noted; carries no implication about causality. 2. Reduced bone mass due to inadequate osteoid synthesis.

**osteoperiostitis** (os′te-o-pĕr′ĭ-os-ti′tis). Inflammation of the periosteum and of the underlying bone.

**osteopetrosis** (os-te-o-pe-tro′sis) [ osteo- + G. *petra*, stone, + suffix -*osis*, condition ]. Albers-Schönberg disease; marble bones; marble bone disease; inherited excessive formation of dense trabecular bone and calcified cartilage, especially in long bones, leading to obliteration of marrow spaces and to anemia.

   **o. ac′ro-osteoly′tica,** pyknodysostosis.

   **o. gallina′rum,** a virus-induced bone tumor of chickens.

**osteopetrot′ic.** Relating to osteopetrosis.

**osteophage** (os′te-o-fāj) [ osteo- + G. *phagein*, to eat ]. Osteoclast (1).

**osteophagia** (os′te-o-fa′jī-ah) [ osteo- + G. *phagein*, to eat ]. Eating of bones; perverted appetite seen in cattle suffering from mineral (phosphorus or calcium) deficiency.

**osteophlebitis** (os′te-o-flĕ-bi′tis) [ osteo- + G. *phleps*, vein, + suffix -*itis*, inflammation ]. Inflammation of the veins of a bone.

**osteophone** (os′te-o-fōn) [ osteo- + G. *phōnē*, voice ]. An appliance similar to the audiphone for helping the deaf to hear.

**osteophony** (os′te-of′o-nī). Bone *conduction*.

**osteophore** (os′te-o-fōr) [ osteo- + G. *phoros*, bearing ]. A bone-crushing forceps with strong blades and teeth. See fig. under forceps.

**osteophy′ma** [ osteo- + G. *phyma*, tumor ]. Osteophyte.

**osteophyte** (os′te-o-fit) [ osteo- + G. *phyton*, plant ]. Osteophyma; a bony outgrowth.

**osteoplaque** (os′te-o-plak) [ osteo- + Fr. *plaque*, plate ]. Any osseous layer.

**os′teoplast** [ osteo- + G. *plassō*, to form ]. Osteoblast.

**osteoplas′tic.** 1. Relating to osteogenesis; osteogenic. 2. Relating to osteoplasty.

**os′teoplasty** [ osteo- + G. *plassō*, to form ]. Bone grafting; reparative or plastic surgery of the bones.

**osteopoikilosis** (os′te-o-poy′kī-lo′sis) [ osteo- + G. *poikilos*, dappled, + suffix -*osis*, condition ]. Osteopathia condensans; an inherited condition of mottled or spotted bones, caused by widespread small foci of compact bone in the substantia spongiosa; see also *osteopathia striata.*

**osteoporosis** (os′te-o-po-ro′sis) [ osteo- + G. *poros*, pore, + suffix -*osis*, condition ]. Reduction in the quantity of bone or atrophy of skeletal tissue; it occurs in postmenopausal women and elderly men, resulting in bone trabeculae that are scanty, thin, and without osteoelastic resorption.

**osteoporot′ic.** Pertaining to, Characterized by, or causing a porous condition of the bones.

**osteopsathyrosis** (os′te-op-sath-i-ro′sis) [ osteo- + G. *psathyros*, friable ]. Old term for *osteogenesis* imperfecta.

**os′teora′dionecro′sis.** Necrosis of bone produced by ionizing radiation; may occur as a complication of radiotherapy of cancer.

**osteorrhagia** (os′te-o-ra′jī-ah) [ osteo- + G. *rhēgnymi*, to burst forth ]. Bleeding from bone.

**osteorrhaphy** (os-te-or′ă-fī) [ osteo- + G. *rhaphē*, suture ]. Osteosuture; wiring together the fragments of a broken bone.

**os′teosarco′ma.** Osteogenic *sarcoma.*

**osteosclerosis** (os′te-o-skle-ro′sis) [ osteo- + G. *sklērōsis*, hardness ]. Abnormal hardening or eburnation of bone.

   **o. congen′ita,** achondroplasia.

   **o. fra′gilis generalisa′ta,** obsolete term for osteopetrosis.

**osteosclerotic** (os′te-o-skle-rot′ik). Relating to, due to, or marked by hardening of bone substance.

**osteoscope** (os′te-o-skōp) [ osteo- + G. *skopeō*, to view ]. An apparatus enclosing certain bones of standard density and thickness, used for testing an x-ray machine.

**osteosis** (os′te-o′sis) [ osteo- + G. suffix -*osis*, condition ]. 1. Ostosis (1); a morbid process in bone. 2. Osteogenesis.

   **o. cu′tis,** dermostosis; osteodermia; bone formed in the skin by osseous metaplasia of calcium deposits; also called osteoma cutis, although not neoplastic.

   **parathy′roid o.,** *osteitis* fibrosa cystica.

   **renal fibrocys′tic o.,** renal *rickets.*

**osteospongioma** (os′te-o-spon′jī-o′mah) [ osteo- + G. *spongos*, sponge, + suffix -*oma*, tumor ]. A general, nonspecific term for a neoplasm in bone that results in thinning and fragmentation (thus, in softening) of the cortex.

**osteosteatoma** (os′te-o-ste′ă-to′mah) [ osteo- + G. *stear*, suet, fat, + suffix -*oma*, tumor ]. A benign mass, usually a lipoma or sebaceous cyst, in which small foci of bony elements are present.

**osteostixis** (os′te-o-stik′sis) [ osteo- + G. *stixis*, a pricking ]. Trephining or simple puncture of a bone.

**osteosuture** (os-te-o-su′chur). Osteorrhaphy.

**osteosynthesis** (os-te-o-sin′the-sis). Bringing the ends of a fractured bone into close apposition.

**osteotabes** (os′te-o-ta′bēz) [ osteo- + L. *tabes*, wasting ]. Atrophy of the bone marrow.

**osteotelangiectasia** (os′te-o-tĕ-lan′jī-ek-ta′zī-ah) [ osteo- + G. *telos*, end, + *angeion*, vessel, + *ektasis*, extension ]. An undesirable term for a sarcoma of bone in which there are numerous, relatively large vascular channels and capillaries.

**os′teothrombo′sis.** Thrombosis in one or more of the veins of a bone.

**os′teotome** [ osteo- + G. *tomē*, incision ]. A chisel for use in cutting bone.

**osteotomoclasia, osteotomoclasis** (os-te-ot′o-mo-kla′-zī-ah, os-te-ot′o-mok′lă-sis) [ osteo- + G. *tomē*, incision, + *klasis*, fracture ]. An operation for the straightening of a pathologically curved bone, by partial division with the osteotome followed by forcible bending of the remaining portion of the bone.

**osteot′omy** [ osteo- + G. *tomē*, incision ]. Osteoectomy; cutting a bone, usually by means of a saw or chisel, for the removal of a sequestrum, the correction of knock-knee or other deformity, or for any purpose whatever. O. for the correction of knock-knee or other deformity may be cuneiform, *i.e.,* the removal of a wedge from the convex side of the curve; or linear, cutting through the shaft or articular extremity of the bone by a straight incision.

**osteotribe** (os′te-o-trib) [ osteo- + G. *tribō*, to bruise, to grind down ]. An instrument for crushing off bits of necrosed or carious bone.

**osteotrite** (os′te-o-trīt) [ osteo- + L. *tritus*, a grinding, a wearing off ]. An instrument with conical or olive-shaped tip having a cutting surface, resembling a dental burr, used for the removal of carious bone.

**osteotrophy** (os′te-ot′ro-fī) [ osteo- + G. *trophē*, nourishment ]. Nutrition of osseous tissue.

**osteotylus** (os′te-ot′ī-lus) [ osteo- + G. *tylos*, callus ]. The callus ensheathing the ends of a broken bone.

**os′teotympan′ic** [ osteo- + G. *tympanon*, drum ]. Otocranial.

**Ostertagia** (os′ter-ta′jī-ah) [ R. von *Ostertag* ]. A genus of small, slender, bloodsucking trichostrongyle nematodes found in the abomasum (rarely in the small intestine) of sheep, goats, cattle, and other ruminants; commonly called the medium stomach worm or the brown stomach worm (since they are usually brown when fresh). The larvae penetrate the stomach mucosa, giving rise to small nodules; heavy infections do much damage.

   **O. biso′nis,** occurs in the abomasum of bison, cattle, and deer.

   **O. circumcinc′ta,** occurs worldwide in the abomasum of sheep, goats, camels, and wild ruminants; it is the most economically important species found in sheep.

   **O. lyra′ta,** occurs in the abomasum of cattle and wild ruminants.

   **O. occidenta′lis,** occurs in the abomasum of sheep, goats, pronghorn, mule deer, and other ruminants.

   **O. orlof′fi,** occurs in the abomasum of sheep, cattle, mule deer, and Barbary sheep in North America and the USSR.

   **O. osterta′gi,** occurs in the abomasum of cattle, sheep, and many wild ruminants; chiefly a cattle parasite (sheep being resistant), and one of the most important ones in many areas.

**O. trifurca'ta,** occurs in the abomasum of sheep and goats, and reported from many wild ruminants.

**osthexia** (os-theks'ĭ-ah) [ G. *osteon*, bone, + *hexis*, state or habit of body, fr. *echō*, fut. *hexō*, to have ]. Obsolescent term for ossification in tissue sites that do not normally develop into bone.

**ostia** (os'tĭ-ah) [ L. ]. Plural of ostium.

**os'tial.** Relating to any orifice, or ostium.

**osti'tic.** Osteitic.

**osti'tis.** Osteitis.

**ostium,** pl. **os'tia** (os'tĭ-um) [ L. door, entrance, mouth. OS- ] [ NA ]. A small opening, especially one of entrance into a hollow organ or canal.

**o. abdomina'le** or **o. abdomina'le tu'bae uteri'na** [ NA ], the fimbriated or ovarian extremity of an oviduct.

**o. aortae** [ NA ], aortic o.; o. arteriosum (2); the opening from the left ventricle into the ascending aorta; it is guarded by the aortic valve.

**o. appendicis vermiformis** [ NA ], the opening of the vermiform appendix into the lumen of the cecum.

**o. arterio'sum,** (1) o. trunci pulmonalis; (2) o. aortae.

**ostia atrioventricula'ria dex'trum et sinis'trum** [ NA ], atrioventricular openings; the two openings, right (tricuspid orifice) and left (mitral orifice), which lead from the atria into the ventricles of the heart.

**o. cardi'acum** [ NA ], cardiac opening; esophagogastric orifice; the trumpet-shaped opening of the esophagus into the stomach.

**o. ileoceca'le** [ NA ], ileocecal opening; the opening of the terminal ileum into the large intestine at the transition between the cecum and the ascending colon.

**o. inter'num,** o. uterinum tubae.

**o. pharynge'um tubae auditi'vae** [ NA ], pharyngeal opening of the auditory (Eustachian) tube, in the upper part of the nasopharynx about half an inch behind the posterior extremity of the inferior concha on each side.

**o. primum,** a brief designation for interatrial *foramen primum*.

**o. pyloricum** [ NA ], pyloric orifice; gastroduodenal orifice; the opening between the stomach and the superior part of the duodenum.

**o. secundum,** a brief designation for interatrial *foramen secundum*.

**o. trunci pulmona'lis** [ NA ], pulmonary opening; o. arteriosum (1); the opening of the pulmonary trunk from the right ventricle, guarded by the pulmonary valve.

**o. tympan'icum tu'bae auditi'vae** [ NA ], tympanic opening of the auditory (Eustachian) tube, in the anterior part of the tympanic cavity below the canal for the tensor tympani muscle.

**o. ure'teris** [ NA ], orificium ureteris; the o. of the ureter in the bladder, situated one at each upper and outer angle of the trigone, the lower angle being occupied by the internal orifice of the urethra.

**o. ure'thrae exter'num** [ NA ], external urethral opening; meatus urinarius; orificium urethrae externum; (1) the slitlike opening of the urethra in the glans penis; (2) the external orifice of the urethra (in the female) in the vestibule, usually upon a slight elevation, the papilla urethrae.

**o. ure'thrae inter'num** [ NA ], the internal opening or orifice of the urethra, at the anterior and inferior angle of the trigone, the upper and outer angles being occupied by the orifices of the ureters.

**o. uteri** [ NA ], o. of the uterus; o. uteri externum; os uteri externum; orificium externum uteri; the mouth of the womb; the vaginal opening of the uterus.

**o. uteri externum,** o. uteri.

**o. uteri internum,** *isthmus* uteri.

**o. uteri'num tubae** [ NA ], o. internum; the uterine opening of the oviduct.

**o. vagi'nae** [ NA ], the vaginal opening; orificium vaginae; the narrowest portion of the canal, in the floor of the vestibule posterior to the urethral orifice.

**o. ve'nae ca'vae inferio'ris** [ NA ], opening of the inferior vena cava; the orifice through which the inferior vena cava opens into the right atrium.

**o. ve'nae ca'vae superio'ris** [ NA ], opening of the superior vena cava; the point of entry of the superior vena cava into the right atrium.

**ostia vena'rum pulmona'lium** [ NA ], openings of the pulmonary veins; the orifices of the pulmonary veins, usually two on each side, in the wall of the left atrium.

**o. venosum,** o. atrioventriculare sinistrum et dextrum.

**os'tomate** [ L. *ostium*, mouth ]. One who has an ostomy.

**os'tomy** [ L. *ostium*, mouth ]. An artificial stoma or opening into the gastrointestinal canal.

**osto'sis.** 1. Osteosis (1). 2. Osteogenesis.

**ostraceous** (os-tra'shus) [ Ostraeacea, group including the oysters ]. Resembling oyster shells; denoting the heaping up of scales seen in psoriasis.

**os'treotox'ism** [ G. *ostreon*, oyster, + *toxikon*, poison ]. Poisoning from eating infected or contaminated oysters.

**Ostwald's solubility coefficient.** See under *coefficient*.

**OT.** Abbreviation for Koch's old *tuberculin*.

**ot-** (ōt-) [ G. *ous*, ear. OT- ]. Combining form relating to the ear.

**Ota,** M. T. See O.'s nevus.

**otalgia** (o-tal'jĭ-ah) [ ot- + G. *algos*, pain ]. Earache.

**genic'ulate o.,** geniculate *neuralgia*.

**reflex o.,** pain referred to the ear from disease in another part, most commonly laryngeal, tonsillar or nasopharyngeal.

**otal'gic.** 1. Relating to otalgia, or earache. 2. A remedy for earache.

**othematoma** (o-the-mă-to'mah) [ ot- + G. *haima*, blood, + suffix -*oma*, tumor ]. Hematoma auris; insane ear; a purplish, rounded, hard swelling of the external ear, resulting from an effusion of blood between the cartilage and perichondrium; it may be caused by an inadvertent trauma in the insane.

**othemorrhagia** (o-them-o-raj'ĭ-ah) [ ot- + G. *haima*, blood, + *rhēgnymi*, to burst forth ]. Bleeding from the ear.

**other-directed.** Pertaining to a person readily influenced by the attitudes of others.

**otiatria, otiatrics** (o-tī-at'rĭ-ah, -ĭ-at'riks) [ or- + G. *iatreia*, treatment ]. The treatment of diseases of the ear.

**o'tic** [ G. *otikos*, fr. *ous*, ear ]. Relating to the ear.

**oticus** [ L. ] [ NA ]. Otic.

**otit'ic.** Relating to otitis.

**otitis** (o-ti'tis) [ ot- + G. suffix -*itis*, inflammation ]. Inflammation of the ear.

**aviation o.,** *aerotitis* media.

**o. desquamati'va,** o. externa with a copious brawny desquamation.

**o. diphtherit'ica,** diphtheritic inflammation of the external auditory meatus.

**o. externa,** inflammation of the external auditory canal.

**o. externa circumscrip'ta,** o. furunculosa; furunculosis of the external auditory canal.

**o. externa diffu'sa,** inflammation of the entire extent of the external auditory meatus.

**o. externa hemorrhag'ica,** inflammation, marked by the presence of one or more vesicles filled with blood on the wall of the bony portion of the external auditory canal.

**o. furunculo'sa,** o. externa circumscripta.

**o. interna,** labyrinthitis.

**o. in'tima,** o. interna.

**o. labyrin'thica,** o. interna.

**o. mastoid'ea,** mastoiditis; inflammation of the mastoid antrum and cells.

**o. media,** inflammation of the middle ear, or tympanum.

**o. media catarrha'lis,** serous o.

**o. media purulen'ta,** o. media suppurativa.

**o. media suppurati'va,** suppurative inflammation of the middle ear.

**o. mycot'ica,** a fungous growth in the external auditory meatus, usually of *Aspergillus niger*.

**parasitic o.,** otoacariasis.

**serous o.,** o. media catarrhalis; inflammation of middle ear mucosa, often accompanied by accumulation of fluid, secondary to Eustachian tube abstraction.

**oto-** (o'to-) [ G. -*ous*, ear. OT- ]. Combining forms relating to the ear.

**otoacariasis** (o'to-ak'ă-ri'ă-sis) [ oto- + acariasis ]. Parasitic otitis; an infection in the auditory canal of cats, dogs, foxes, and other animals caused by auricular mites, chiefly *Otodectes cynotis*. The mites swarm in the ears and cause considerable discomfort and tenderness; in extreme cases, they cause symptoms such as loss of appetite, wasting, and fits. See also otodectic *mange*.

**otoantritis** (o-to-an-tri'tis). Inflammation of the mastoid antrum.

**otobiosis** (o-to-bi-o'sis). Presence of larvae and the characteristic spiny nymphs of *Otobius megnini* in the external auditory canal of cattle, horses, cats, dogs, deer, coyotes, and other domestic and wild animals; they may remain in the ear for several months before dropping out to pupate and mature. Several records of human infection are known.

**Oto'bius.** A genus of argasid ticks similar to *Ornithodoros* but characterized by a granulated integument, a hypostome that is vestigial in the adult but well developed in the spiny nymphs, and the absence of eyes and hood. Two species are recognized, *O. lagophilus* and *O. megnini*.

    **O. lagoph'ilus,** the face tick of rabbits.

    **O. megni'ni,** the spinose ear tick that causes otobiosis in horses, cattle, sheep, dogs, and some wild animals; it occurs in the southwestern parts of the United States, where it is an important pest, and is also distributed worldwide.

**otocephalus** (o'to-sef'ă-lus). An individual with otocephaly.

**otocephaly** (o'to-sef'ă-li) [ oto- + G. *kephalē*, head ]. A malformation characterized by markedly defective development of the lower jaw (micrognathia or agnathia) and the union or close approach of the ears (synotia) on the front of the neck.

**otocerebritis** (o-to-sĕr-e-bri'tis). Otoencephalitis.

**otocleisis** (o-to-kli'sis) [ oto- + G. *kleisis*, closure ]. 1. Closure of the Eustachian tube. 2. Closure, by a new growth or accumulation of cerumen, of the external auditory meatus.

**otoco'nia.** Plural of otoconium.

**otoco'nium,** pl. **otoco'nia.** Statoconium; see statoconia.

**otocra'nial.** Relating to the otocranium.

**otocranium** (o'to-kra'nĭ-um) [ oto- + G. *kranion*, cranium ]. The bony case of the internal and middle ear, consisting of the petrous portion of the temporal bone.

**otocyst** (o'to-sist) [ oto- + G. *kystis*, a bladder ]. 1. The embryonic auditory vesicle. 2. An organ, analogous to the utricle of mammals, possessed by certain invertebrates. It contains small calcareous grains, or grains of sand.

**Otodec'tes.** A genus of ear mites (family Psoroptidae) consisting of a single species, *O. cynotis*.

    **O. cynot'is,** the cause of otodectic mange in dogs, cats, and other carnivores; the entire lifespan of this mite is spent in the ears (rarely on the body) of the host, where it feeds on epidermal debris; it can be found in the encrusted material scraped from infected ears.

**otodyn'ia** [ oto- + G. *odynē*, pain ]. Earache.

**otoencephalitis** (o'to-en-sef-ă-li'tis) [ oto- + G. *enkephalos*, brain, + suffix *-itis*, inflammation ]. Otocerebritis; inflammation of the brain by extension of the process from the middle ear and mastoid cells.

**otoganglion** (o'to-gang'glĭ-on). Ganglion oticum.

**otogenic, otogenous** (o'to-jen'ik, o-toj'ĕ-nus) [ oto- + G. suffix *-gen*, producing ]. Of otic origin; originating within the ear, especially from inflammation of the ear.

**otography** (o-tog'ră-fī) [ oto- + G. *graphē*, a writing ]. A treatise on, or a description of the ear.

**otolaryngol'ogist** (o'to-lăr-in-gol'o-jist). A physician who specializes in otolaryngology.

**otolaryngology** (o'to-lăr'ing-gol'o-jī) [ oto- + G. *larynx*, + *logos*, study ]. The combined specialties of diseases of the ear and larynx, often including upper respiratory tract and many diseases of the head and neck, tracheobronchial tree, and esophagus.

**otolith, otolite** (o'to-lith, o'to-līt) [ oto- + G. *lithos*, stone ]. 1. Statoconium; see statoconia. 2. Otosteon (2).

**otologic** (o'to-loj'ik). Relating to otology.

**otol'ogist.** Aurist; one versed in otology; a specialist in diseases of the ear.

**otology** (o-tol'o-jī) [ oto- + G. *logos*, study ]. The branch of medical science that embraces the study, diagnosis, and treatment of diseases of the ear and related structures.

**otomassage** (o'to-mă-sahzh). Systematic and regular movement imparted to the tympanic membrane and ossicles, by means of sound waves, rapid jets of air in the external auditory meatus, or vibratory tapping of the drum membrane.

**otometry** (o'tom-ĕ-trī) [ oto- + G. *metron*, measure ]. The technology of hearing aid prescription based on measurement of sound pressure levels required to attain comfortable loudness sensation in speech frequency range.

**otomu'cormyco'sis.** Mucormycosis of the ear.

**otomyces** (o-to-mi'sēz) [ oto- + G. *mykēs*, fungus ]. Any fungus growing in the external auditory meatus.

**otomycosis** (o'to-mi-ko'sis) [ oto- + G. *mykēs*, fungus ]. An infection due to the presence of a fungus in the external auditory canal.

**otoneuralgia** o'to-nu-ral'jī-ah) [ oto- + G. *neuron*, nerve, + *algos*, pain ]. Earache of neuralgic origin, not caused by inflammation.

**otopalatodigital** (o'to-pal'ă-to-dij'ĭ-tal). Relating to the ears, palate, and fingers.

**otop'athy** [ oto- + G. *pathos*, suffering ]. Any disease of the ear.

**otopharyngeal** (o'to-fă-rin'je-al). Relating to the middle ear and the pharynx.

**o'toplasty** [ oto- + G. *plassō*, to form ]. Reparative or plastic surgery of the auricle of the ear.

**otopolypus** (o'to-pol'ĭ-pus) [ oto- + L. *polypus*, polyp ]. A polyp in the external auditory meatus, usually arising from the middle ear.

**otopyorrhea** (o-to-pi-o-re'ah) [ oto- + G. *pyon*, pus, + *rhoia*, a flow ]. Chronic otitis media with perforation of the drum membrane and a purulent discharge.

**otorhinolaryngology** (o'to-ri'no-lăr'ing-gol'o-jī) [ oto- + G. *rhis*, nose, + *larynx*, larynx, + *logos*, study ]. The combined specialties of diseases of the ear, nose, and larynx. See also otolaryngology.

**otorhinology** (o'to-ri-nol'o-jī) [ oto- + G. *rhis*, nose, + *logos*, study ]. Study of disease of the ear and nose.

**otorrhagia** (o-to-ra'jī-ah) [ oto- + G. *rhēgnymi*, to burst forth ]. Bleeding from the ear.

**otorrhea** (o-to-re'ah) [ oto- + G. *rhoia*, flow ]. A discharge from the ear.

    **cerebrospinal fluid o.,** discharge of cerebrospinal fluid through the external auditory meatus.

**otosalpinx** (o'to-sal'pingks) [ oto- + G. *salpinx*, trumpet ]. Tuba auditiva.

**otosclerosis** (o'to-skle-ro'sis) [ oto- + G. *sklērosis*, hardening ]. A new formation of spongy bone about the stapes and fenestra vestibuli (ovalis), resulting in progressively increasing deafness, without signs of disease in the Eustachian tube or tympanic membrane; see also Bezold's *triad*.

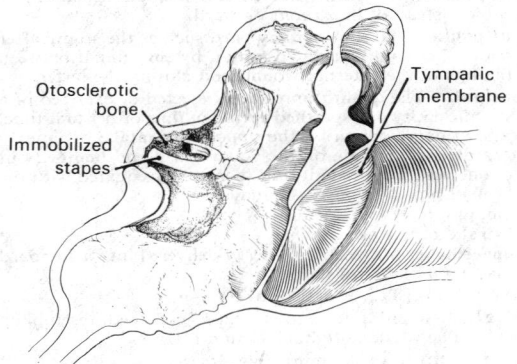

Otosclerotic bone

Tympanic membrane

Immobilized stapes

**Otosclerosis**

**otoscope** (o'to-skōp) [ oto- + G. *skopeō*, to view ]. An instrument for examining the drum membrane or auscultating the ear. In England, generally called auriscope.

**Siegle's o.**, an ear speculum with a bulb attachment by which the air pressure can be varied, thus imparting movement to the membrana tympani, if intact, while under inspection.

**Toynbee's o.**, a rubber tube with an earpiece at each end, by means of which the otologist can listen to the sounds in the patient's ear during politzerization; called also Toynbee's diagnostic tube.

**otoscopy** (o-tos'ko-pī) [ oto- + G. *skopeō*, to view ]. Inspection of the ear, especially of the drum membrane.

**ostosteal** (o-tos'te-al) [ oto- + G. *osteon*, bone ]. Relating to the ossicles of the ear.

**otosteon** (o-tos'te-on) [ oto- + G. *osteon*, bone ]. 1. One of the ossicles of the ear. 2. A concretion in the ear, larger than a statoconium.

**otot'omy** [ oto- + G. *tomē*, incision ]. Anatomy of the ear; dissection of the ear.

**ototoxic** (o'to-tok'sik) [ oto- + G. *toxikon*, poison ]. Having a toxic action upon the ear.

**ototoxici'ty.** The property of being ototoxic.

**Ott,** Isaac, American physiologist, 1847–1916. See O.'s *test.*

**Otto,** Adolph W., German surgeon, 1786–1845. See O.'s *disease*, O. *pelvis.*

**O.U.** Abbreviation for oculus uterque [ L. ], each eye; both eyes.

**ouabain** (wah'bah-in) (USP). G-strophanthin; acocantherin; $C_{29}H_{44}O_{12}8H_2O$; a glycoside from ouabaio, obtained from the wood of *Acocanthera ouabaio* or from the seeds of *Strophanthus gratus;* an African arrow poison. Its action is qualitatively identical to that of strophanthus and the digitalis glycosides. Used for rapid digitalization.

**Ouchterlony,** O. See O.'s *test.*

**Ouidin,** Paul, French roentgenologist, 1851–1923. See O. *current.*

**oul-.** For words beginning thus, see ul-.

**ounce** [ L. *unica*, the twelfth part (of a pound or foot) hence also inch ]. Abbreviation oz.; a weight containing 480 gr., or $1/12$ pound troy and apothecaries' weight, or $437^{1}/_2$ gr., $1/16$ pound avoirdupois; the apothecary o. (used in the USP) contains 8 drams, and is equivalent to 31.10349 gm. The avoirdupois o. is equivalent to 28.35 gm.

**-ous.** A suffix denoting that the element to the name of which it is attached is in one of its lower valencies, *e.g.,* phosphorous acid, $H_3PO_3$.

**out'lay.** A graft applied on the exterior of a bone.

**epithelial o.,** a procedure similar to epithelial inlay in which the edges of the cavity are not tightly closed, but have intervals of nonapproximation through which the new epithelium grows out around the margins of the wound.

**out'let.** An exit or opening of a passageway.

**pelvic o.,** *apertura pelvis inferior.*

**out'patient.** A patient treated in a hospital dispensary or clinic instead of in a room or ward.

**out'pocket.** To shut out any part, such as the stump after removal of a pudunculated tumor, by engaging it between the lips of the external wound and closing the latter.

**out'put.** The quantity produced, ejected or excreted of a specific entity in a specified period of time or per unit time, *e.g.,* urinary sodium o.; the opposite of intake or input.

**cardiac o.,** minute o.; the volume of blood pumped out of one ventricle per unit time, commonly equated with the flow of blood through the lungs.

**minute o.,** cardiac o.

**stroke o.,** stroke *volume.*

**pacemaker o.,** electrical energy delivered into a standard load (500 ohms resistance).

**ova** (o'vah) [ L. ]. Plural of ovum.

**o'val.** 1. Relating to an ovum. 2. Egg-shaped; resembling in outline the longitudinal section of an egg.

**ovalbumin** (o'val-bu'min). Egg *albumin.*

**o'valocyte** [ L. *ovalis*, oval, + G. *kytos*, cell ]. Elliptocyte.

**o'valocyto'sis.** Elliptocytosis.

**ovarialgia** (o-văr'ī-al'jī-ah) [ ovario- + G. *algos*, pain ]. Oarialgia; oothecalgia; ovarian pain.

**ovarian** (o-văr'ī-an). Relating to the ovary.

**ovariectomy** (o-văr'ī-ek'to-mī) [ ovario- + G. *ektomē*, excision ]. Oothecectomy; oophorectomy; ovariosteresis; excision of ovaries.

**ovario-, ovari-** (o-văr'ī-o-) [ L. *ovarium*, ovary. OV- ]. Combining forms denoting ovary; for such words not found here, see also oophor-, oophoro-.

**ovariocele** (o-văr'ī-o-sēl) [ ovario- + G. *kēlē*, hernia ]. Oothecocele; hernia of an ovary.

**ovariocentesis** (o-văr'ī-o-sen-te'sis) [ ovario- + G. *kentēsis*, puncture ]. Oothecocentesis; puncture of an ovary or an ovarian cyst.

**ovariocyesis** (o-văr'ī-o-si-e'sis) [ ovario- + G. *kyēsis*, pregnancy ]. Ovarian *pregnancy.*

**ovariodysneuria** (o-văr'ī-o-dis-nu'rī-ah) [ ovario- + G. *dys-*, bad, + *neuron*, nerve ]. Ovarian pain or neuralgia.

**ovariogenic** (o-văr'ī-o-jen'ik) [ ovario- + G. suffix *-gen*, producing ]. Originating in the ovary.

**ovariohysterectomy** (o-văr'ī-o-his'ter-ek'to-mī) [ ovario- + G. *hystera*, uterus, + *ektomē*, excision ]. Oophorohysterectomy; oothecohysterectomy; removal of ovaries and uterus.

**ovariolytic** (o-văr'ī-o-lit'ik) [ ovario- + G. *lysis*, dissolution ]. Destructive to the ovary.

**ovarioncus** (o-văr'ī-ong'kus) [ ovario- + G. *onkos*, tumor ]. Oophoroma.

**ovariopathy** (o-văr'ī-op'ă-thī) [ ovario- + G. *pathos*, suffering ]. Oophoropathy; oothecopathy; any disease of the ovary.

**ovariorrhexis** (o-văr'ī-o-rek'sis) [ ovario- + G. *rhēxis*, rupture ]. Oothecorrhexis; rupture of an ovary.

**ovariosalpingectomy** (o-văr'ī-o-sal-pin-jek'to-mī) [ ovario- + salpingectomy ]. Oophorosalpingectomy; oothecosalpingectomy; operative removal of an ovary and the corresponding oviduct.

**ovariosalpingitis** (o-văr'ī-o-sal-pin-ji'tis) [ ovario- + salpingitis ]. Oophorosalpingitis; oothecosalpingitis; inflammation of ovary and oviduct.

**ovariosteresis** (o-văr'ī-o-ste-re'sis) [ ovario- + G. *sterēsis*, deprivation, loss ]. Ovariectomy.

**ovarios'tomy** [ ovario- + G. *stoma*, mouth ]. Oothecostomy; oophorostomy; establishment of a temporary fistula for drainage of a cyst of the ovary.

**ovar'iotes'tis.** Obsolete synonym for ovotestis.

**ovariot'omist.** Historically, one who is skilled in the operation for removing the ovaries.

**ovariot'omy** [ ovario- + G. *tomē*, incision ]. Oariotomy; oothecotomy; oophorotomy; an incision in an ovary, *e.g.,* a biopsy or a wedge excision.

**normal o.,** historically, removal of an apparently healthy ovary.

**ovaritis** (o'vă-ri'tis). Oophoritis.

**ovarium,** pl. **ovaria** (o-văr'ī-um, -ah) [ Mod. L. fr. *ovum*, egg. OV- ] [ NA ]. Ovary.

**o. biparti'tum,** an ovary separated into two parts.

**o. disjunc'tum,** an ovary more or less completely divided into two parts.

**o. gyra'tum,** an ovary showing curved or irregular grooves or furrows.

**o. loba'tum,** an ovary marked off by deep furrows into two or more parts or lobes.

**o. masculi'num,** *appendix* testis.

**ovarius** [ NA ]. Ovarian; relating to the ovary.

**ovary** (o'vă-rī) [ Mod. L. *ovarium*, fr. *ovum*, egg. OV- ]. Ovarium; oarium; ootheca; oophoron; one of the paired reproductive glands in the female, containing the ova or germ cells. Its stroma is a vascular connective tissue containing numbers of ovarian follicles enclosing the ova; surrounding this is a more condensed layer of stroma called the tunica albuginea.

**mulberry o.,** term applied to the type of o. produced by the administration of anterior pituitary extracts to immature rats; such o.'s contain many follicles in various stages of development; on their surface, many corpora lutea are

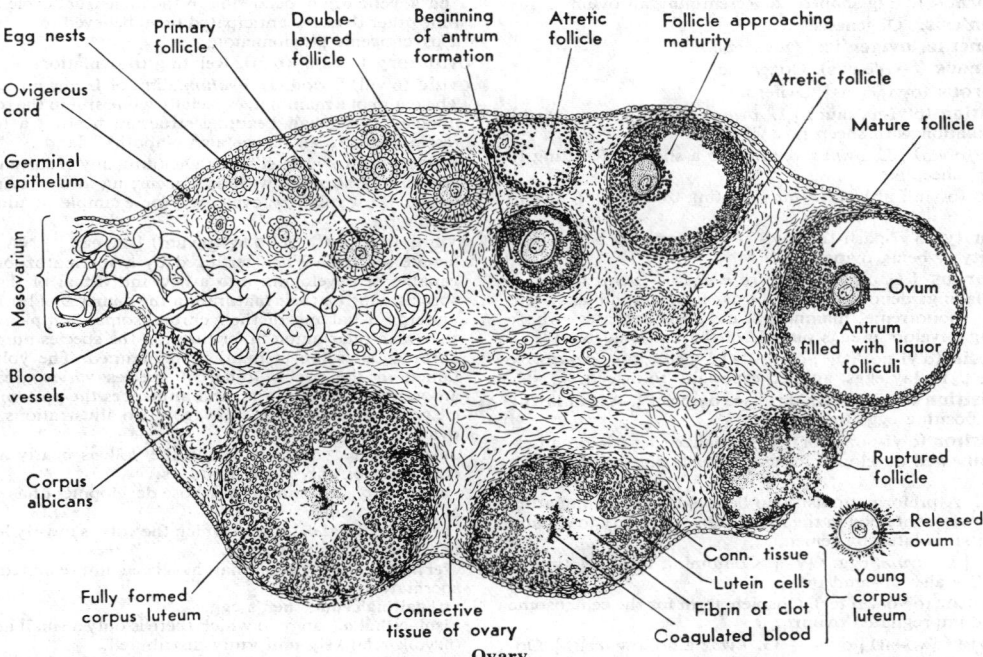

Egg nests
Ovigerous cord
Germinal epithelum
Mesovarium
Blood vessels
Corpus albicans
Fully formed corpus luteum

Primary follicle
Double-layered follicle
Beginning of antrum formation
Atretic follicle
Follicle approaching maturity
Atretic follicle
Mature follicle
Ovum
Antrum filled with liquor folliculi
Ruptured follicle
Released ovum
Young corpus luteum
Conn. tissue
Lutein cells
Fibrin of clot
Coagulated blood
Connective tissue of ovary

**Ovary**

Schematic diagram showing sequence of events in origin, growth, and rupture of ovarian follicle and formation and retrogression of corpus luteum. Follow clockwise around ovary, starting at mesovarium. (From Patten, B. M.: *Human Embryology*, Ed. 3, McGraw-Hill Book Co., New York, 1968. Used with permission.)

prominently evident and thus the gland somewhat resembles a mulberry.

**polycystic o.,** enlarged cystic o.'s, pearl white in color, with thickened tunica albuginea, characteristic of the Stein-Leventhal syndrome. Clinical features are abnormal menses, obesity, and evidence of masculinization, such as hirsutism and clitoromegaly.

**third o.,** an accessory o.

**o'verbite.** Vertical *overlap*.

**overclo'sure.** Occlusal vertical dimension decrease; see under dimension.

**o'vercompensa'tion.** 1. An exaggeration of personal capacity to overcome a real or imagined inferiority. 2. The process in which a psychologic deficiency inspires exaggerated correction.

**overden'ture.** Overlay *denture*.

**overdeter'mina'tion.** In psychoanalysis, a term indicating the multiple causation of a single behavioral or emotional reaction, mental symptom, or dream.

**overerup'tion** (o'ver-e-rup'shun). The occlusal projection of a tooth beyond the line of occlusion.

**overexten'sion.** Extension of a limb or any of its segments beyond what is normal.

**o'vergrowth.** Hypertrophy; hyperplasia.

**o'verhang.** An excess of dental filling material beyond the cavity margin or normal tooth contour.

**overhydra'tion.** Hyperhydration.

**o'verjet, o'verjut.** Horizontal *overlap*.

**o'verlap.** 1. A surgical procedure in which one layer of tissue is sutured above or under another to gain additional strength. 2. An extension or projection of one tissue over another.

**horizontal o.,** horizontal overjet or overjut; the projection of the upper anterior and/or posterior teeth beyond their antagonists in a horizontal direction.

**vertical o.,** overbite; (1) the extention of the upper teeth over the lower teeth in a vertical direction when the opposing posterior teeth are in contact in centric occlusion; (2) the distance that teeth lap over their antagonists vertically; this term is used especially for the distance that

the upper incisal edges drop below the lower ones, but may also be used to describe the vertical relations of opposing cusps; (3) the relationship of the maxillary incisors to the mandibular incisors when the incisal edges pass each other in centric occlusion.

**o'verlay.** An addition to an already existing condition.

**emotional o.,** the emotional component of an organic disability.

**overlearn'ing.** In the psychology of memory, continuation of practice beyond the point where one is able to perform according to specified criterion. Typically, retention is longer after o. as compared with retention after practice only to the point of performance meeting the specified criterion.

**overresponse** (o'ver-rĕ-spons'). An abnormally strong reaction to a stimulus.

**overriding** (o'ver-ri'ding). 1. The slipping of the lower fragment of a broken long bone up alongside the proximal portion. 2. Descriptive of a fetal head which is palpable above the symphysis because of cephalopelvic disproportion.

**o'vertoe.** Condition in which the great toe overlies the adjacent toes.

**Overton,** E. See Meyer-O. *theory* of narcosis.

**o'vertone.** Any of the tones, other that the lowest or fundamental tone, of which a sound is composed.

**psychic o.,** the mental associations related to any stimulus.

**overventila'tion.** Hyperventilation.

**ovi-** (o'vĭ-) [ L. *ovum*, egg. OV- ]. Combining form relating to egg. See also ovo- and oo-.

**ovicap'sule.** Archaic term for ovarian follicle.

**ovicidal** (o'vĭ-si'dal) [ ovi- + L. *caedo*, to kill ]. Causing death of the ovum.

**ovidu'cal.** Oviductal.

**oviduct** (o'vĭ-dukt) [ ovi- + L. *ductus*, a leading, fr. *duco*, pp. *ductus*, to lead ]. *Tuba uterina*.

**oviduc'tal.** Oviducal; relating to a uterine tube.

**ovif'erous** [ ovi- + L. *fero*, to carry ]. Carrying or containing ova.

**o'viform.** 1. Egg-shaped. 2. Resembling an ovum.

**ovigen'esis.** Oogenesis.

**ovigenet'ic, ovigen'ic.** Oogenetic.

**ovigenous** (o-vij'ĕ-nus). Oogenetic.

**ovigerous** (o-vij'er-us). Oviferous.

**ovination** (o'vī-na'shun) [ L. *ovinus*, relating to a sheep ]. Inoculation with sheep pox virus.

**ovine** (o'vīn) [ L. *ovinus*, relating to a sheep ]. Relating to sheep; sheeplike.

**ovinia** (o-vin'ī-ah) [ L. *ovinus*, relating to a sheep ]. Sheeppox.

**oviparity** (o'vī-păr'ī-tī) [ ovi- + L. *pario*, to bear ]. The quality of being oviparous.

**ovip'arous** [ L. *oviparus*, fr. *ovum*, egg, + *pario*, to bear ]. Egg-laying; denoting those birds, fish, amphibians, reptiles, monotreme mammals, and invertebrates whose young develop in eggs outside of the maternal body.

**oviposit** (o'vī-poz'it) [ ovi- + L. *pono*, pp. *positus*, to place ]. To lay eggs; applied especially to insects.

**oviposition** (o'vī-po-zish'un) [ see oviposit ]. Act of laying or depositing eggs by insects.

**ovipositor** (o'vī-poz'ī-tor). A specialized female organ especially well developed in insects for laying or depositing eggs.

**o'vist.** A preformationist who believed that the miniature body was contained in the female sex cell, ready to expand when stimulated by semen.

**o'vo-** [ L. *ovum*, egg. OV- ]. Combining form relating to egg. See also oo- and ovi-.

**ovocenter** (o'vo-sen'ter). Obsolete term for the centrosome of the impregnated ovum.

**ovocyte** (o'vo-sīt) [ ovo- + G. *kytos*, a hollow (cell) ]. Oocyte.

**ovofla'vin.** A flavin found in eggs.

**ovogen'esis.** Oogenesis.

**ovoglob'ulin.** Egg globulin.

**ovogo'nium** [ ovo- + G. *gonē*, generation ]. Oogonium.

**ovoid** (o'voyd) [ ovo- + G. *eidos*, resemblance ]. Oviform; egg-shaped.

   **fetal o.,** the form of the fetus *in utero*. Its length is about one-half of the length of the fetus.

   **Manchester o.,** an egg-shaped radium applicator for placement in the lateral vaginal fornices.

**ovolarviparous** (o'vo-lar-vip'ă-rus) [ ovo- + L. *larva*, a mask, + *pario*, to bear ]. Denoting certain nematodes and other invertebrates in which the eggs are hatched within the female, and the larvae developed or protected within the uterus until the correct time for their emergence.

**ovomu'cin.** A glycoprotein in egg.

**ovomucoid** (o'vo-mu'koyd). Mucoprotein obtained from egg white.

**ovoplasm** (o'vo-plazm). The protoplasm of an unfertilized egg.

**ovopro'togen.** Lipoic acid (protogen A).

**ovose'rum.** An egg albumin antiserum specific for albumin of eggs of the same species as that from which the antigen was obtained.

**ovotestis** (o'vo-tes'tis). A gonad in which both testicular and ovarian components are present; a form of hermaphroditism.

**o'vover'din.** A chromoprotein with a carotenoid prosthetic group found in lobster eggs.

**o'vovitel'lin** [ ovo- + L. *vitellus*, yolk ]. Vitellin.

**ovoviviparous** (o'vo-vi-vip'ă-rus) [ ovo- + L. *viviparus*, bringing forth alive, fr. *vivus*, alive, + *pario*, to bear ]. Denoting those fish, amphibians, and reptiles that produce eggs which hatch within the body of the parent and then are born alive.

**ovular** (o'vu-lar). Relating to an ovule.

**ovulation** (o'vu-la'shun). The release of an ovum from the ovarian follicle.

   **amen'strual o.,** o. in the absence of menstruation, as is believed to occur sometimes in women. Conceptually obscure.

   **anes'trous o.,** discharge of ova occurring in animals without estrus.

   **paracyclic o.,** o. occurring in the menstrual cycle at any time other than the anticipated time; believed to be usually a psychogenic phenomenon.

**ovulatory** (o'vu-lă-to-rī). Relating to ovulation.

**ovule** (o'vūl) [ Mod. L. *ovulum*, dim. of L. *ovum*, egg ]. 1. The ovum of a mammal, especially while still in the ovarian follicle. 2. A small beadlike structure bearing a fancied resemblance to an o.; see also Naboth's glands.

**ovulocyclic** (o'vu-lo-si'klik). Denoting any recurrent phenomenon associated with and occurring at a certain time within the ovulatory cycle, as, for example, ovulocyclic porphyria.

**ovum,** gen. **ovi,** pl. **ova** (o'vum) [ L. egg ] [ NA ]. The female sex cell. When fertilized by a spermatozoon, it is capable of developing into a new individual of the same species. During their maturation the gametes of both sexes undergo a halving of their chromosomal complement so that with their union in fertilization the species number of chromosomes (46 in man) is maintained. The yolk contained in the ova of different species varies greatly in amount and distribution, and influences the pattern of the cleavage division. See cleavage; also illustrations under ovary, ovarian *follicle.*

   **alec'ithal o.,** an o. in which the yolk is nearly absent, consisting of only a few particles.

   **blighted o.,** a fertilized o. whose development has ceased at an early stage.

   **centrolec'ithal o.,** one in which the yolk is mostly located near the center of the egg.

   **fertilized o.,** the o. that has been impregnated by a spermatozoon.

   **o. gallina'ceum,** hen's egg.

   **isolecithal o.,** an o. in which there is only a small amount of yolk relatively uniformly distributed.

   **Peter's o.,** an o. having a presumptive fertilization age of about 13 days. For many years it was one of very few young human embryos recovered in good condition, and its study furnished many facts regarding early embryonic changes. Many younger human embryos have since been recovered. As in the case of the Peter's o., the noteworthy ones are likely to be known to embryologists under the name of the investigator recovering and describing them, as in the outstanding Hertig-Rock series of young embryos.

   **primitive o.,** ooblast.

   **telolec'ithal o.,** on o. in which there is a large amount of yolk massed at the vegetative pole, as in the eggs of birds and reptiles.

**Owen,** Richard, English anatomist, 1804–1892. See O.'s *lines;* interglobular *space* of O.

**Owren,** Paul A., Norwegian physician, 20th century. See O.'s *disease.*

**oxa-.** Term inserted in names of organic compounds to signify presence or addition of oxygen atom(s). See also oxo-, oxy-.

**oxacid** (oks-as'id) An acid containing oxygen as well as hydrogen atoms; oxyacid.

   **inorganic o.,** an inorganic acid containing one or more oxygen atoms in the molecule; *e.g.,* $H_2SO_4$, $HNO_3$.

   **organic o.,** one containing carboxyl, COOH, plus an oxo (*e.g.,* keto) or hydroxy group.

**oxacil'lin sodium** (USP). PROSTAPHLIN; RESISTOPEN; 5-methyl-3-phenyl-4-isoxazolylpenicillin sodium; used in the oral therapy of penicillin-resistant staphylococcal infections.

**ox'alate.** A salt of oxalic acid.

**oxale'mia** [ oxalate + G. *haima*, blood ]. The presence of an abnormally large amount of oxalates in the blood.

**oxal'ic acid.** An acid, HOOC—COOH, found in many plants and vegetables, particularly in buckwheat (family Polygoniaceae) and *Oxalis* (family Oxalidaceae); used as a hemostatic in veterinary medicine, but toxic when ingested by man; also used in the removal of ink and other stains, and as a general reducing agent.

**oxaloacetate transacetase** (ok'să-lo-as'e-tāt trans-as'e-tās). *Citrate* synthase.

**ox'aloace'tic acid.** Ketosuccinic acid; $HOOC-COCH_2-COOH$; a ketodicarboxylic acid; an important intermediate in the tricarboxylic acid cycle; the product formed when aspartic acid acts as amine donor in transamination reactions.

**oxalo′sis.** Widespread deposition of calcium oxalate crystals in the kidneys, bones, arterial media and myocardium; urinary excretion of oxalate is increased. May be an acquired disorder, as in oxalate poisoning, or represent one aspect of a heritable disorder, primary hyperoxaluria and o.

**oxalosuccinic acid** (ok′să-lo-suk-sin′ik). HOOC—CO—CH(COOH)—CH₂—COOH; the product of the dehydrogenation of isocitric acid under the catalytic influence of isocitrate dehydrogenase; an intermediate of the tricarboxylic acid cycle.

**ox″alosuccin′ic carbox′ylase.** Isocitrate dehydrogenase.

**oxaluria** (ok′să-lu′rĭ-ah) [ oxalate + G. *ouron*, urine ]. The excretion of an abnormally large amount of oxalates, especially calcium oxalate, in the urine.

**oxalu′ric acid.** NH₂CONHCOCOOH, derived from uric acid or parabanic acid; the ureide of oxalic acid.

**ox′alyl.** The radical —CO—CO— (from oxalic acid).

**oxalylurea** (ok′să-lil-u-re′ah). Parabanic acid; the cyclic (end-to-end) amide anhydride of oxaluric acid; an oxidation product of uric acid.

**oxam′ide.** The diamide of oxalic acid, NH₂CO—CONH₂.

**oxammo′nium.** Hydroxylamine.

**oxan′amide.** QUIACTIN; 2-ethyl-3-propylglycidamide; a mild sedative used primarily in the management of anxiety and tension associated with psychoneurotic disorders.

**oxan′drolone** (NF). ANAVAR; 17β-hydroxy-17α-methyl-2-oxa-5α-androstan-3-one (C-2 replaced by O in the androstane nucleus; for structure of androstane, see steroids). A synthetic orally effective anabolic steroidal lactone, used to promote growth in children and nitrogen retention in patients of all ages; however, effective doses may produce virilization and other untoward effects associated with androgenic hormones.

**oxaphenamide.** DRIBAZIL; 4′-hydroxysalicylanilide; choleretic agent.

**oxapropa′nium iodide.** DILVASENE; (1,3-dioxolan-4-ylmethyl)trimethylammonium iodide; parasympathomimetic drug.

**oxazepam** (ok-sa′zĕ-pam). (NF). SERAX; 7-chloro-1,3-dihydro-3-hydroxy-5-phenyl-2H-1,4-benzodiazepin-2-one; a benzodiazepine chemically and pharmacologically related to chlordiazepoxide and diazepam; an antianxiety agent used in the treatment of anxiety tension and various psychoneurotic disorders.

**ox′azin.** Oxyiminodiphenylimine; C₁₂H₁₀ON₂; parent substance of a series of biological dyes; *e.g.*, gallocyanin, brilliant cresyl blue.

**ox′azole.** The fundamental ring system, C₃H₃ON.

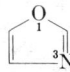

1,3-Oxazole

**oxeladin.** PECTAMON; 2-ethyl-2-phenylbutyric acid 2-(2-diethylaminoethoxy)ethyl ester; antitussive agent.

**ox′idant.** The substance that is reduced and that therefore, oxidizes the other component of an oxidation-reduction system.

**oxidase** (ok′sĭ-dās). Classically, one of a group of enzymes now termed oxidoreductases (EC class 1) that bring about oxidation by the addition of oxygen to a metabolite or by the removal of hydrogen or of one or more electrons. Those removing hydrogen are now termed dehydrogenases. The term oxidase is now used for those cases in which O₂ acts as an acceptor (of H or of electrons); peroxidase (EC class 1.11) is the term used where H₂O₂ acts as acceptor. For individual o.'s, see the specific names.

 **direct o.,** originally, an o. catalyzing the transfer of O₂ directly to other bodies; now termed oxygenase (EC class 1.13).

 **indirect o.,** originally, one that acts by reducing a

peroxide; now termed peroxidase (EC class 1.11).

**oxida′sis.** Oxidation by an oxidase.

**oxidation** (ok′sĭ-da′shun). Combination with oxygen; or increasing the valence of an atom or ion by the loss from it of hydrogen or of one or more electrons thus rendering it more electropositive, as when iron is changed from the ferrous (2+) to the ferric (3+) state (+ = electropositive charge, the loss of an electron).

 **beta-o.,** o. of the β-carbon (carbon 3) of a fatty acid, forming the β-keto acid analogue; of importance in fatty acid catabolism.

 **omega-o.,** oxidation at the carbon atom farthest removed (ω-carbon) from the carboxyl group (carbon 1).

**oxida′tion-reduc′tion.** Any chemical oxidation or reduction reaction, which must, *in toto*, comprise both oxidation and reduction. Often abbreviated redox. The basis for calling all oxidative enzymes (see oxidase) oxidoreductases.

**oxida′tive.** Having the power to oxidize; referring to a process involving oxidation.

**oxide** (ok′sĭd). A compound of oxygen with another element or a radical (*e.g.*, mercuric oxide, HgO; ethylene oxide).

 **acid o.,** an acid anhydride; an oxide of an electronegative element or radical; it can combine with water to form an acid, *e.g.*, P₂O₅ (phosphorus pentoxide) + 3 H₂O → 2 H₃PO₄ (phosphoric acid).

 **basic o.,** a base anhydride; an oxide of an electropositive element or radical; it can combine with water to form a base; *e.g.*, CaO (calcium oxide) + H₂O → Ca(OH)₂ (calcium hydroxide).

 **indifferent o.,** neutral o.

 **neutral o.,** one that is neither an acid nor a base, *e.g.*, water (hydrogen oxide), H₂O.

**oxidization** (ok′sĭ-dĭ-za′shun). Oxidation.

**ox′idize.** To combine or cause an element or radical to combine with oxygen or to lose electrons.

**ox′idoreduc′tase.** An enzyme (EC class 1) catalyzing an oxidation-reduction reaction. Trivial names for o.'s include dehydrogenase, reductase, oxidase (where O₂ is the H acceptor), oxygenase (where O₂ is incorporated into the substrate), peroxidase (H₂O₂ is the acceptor; catalase is an exception), hydroxylase (coupled oxidation of two donors). See also oxidase.

**oxido′sis.** Rarely used synonym for acidosis.

**ox′igram.** A continuous record of the oxygen saturation of the blood.

**oxime** (ok′sim). A compound resulting from the action of hydroxylamine, NH₂OH, on a ketone or an aldehyde to yield the group =N—OH attached to the former carbonyl carbon atom.

**oxim′eter.** An instrument for determining photoelectrically the oxygen saturation of a sample of blood in a translucent part, such as the pinna of the ear. It consists of an electric light bulb and a photoelectric cell placed, respectively, at the front and back of the pinna; red light rays are transmitted by oxyhemoglobin, but only slightly by reduced hemoglobin.

**oxim′etry.** Measurement with an oximeter of the oxygen saturation of hemoglobin in a sample of blood.

**oxo-.** Prefix denoting addition of oxygen (*e.g.*, oxotestosterone); often used in place of keto- in systematic nomenclature; see also oxa-, hydroxy-, oxy-.

**3-oxoacyl-ACP reductase.** β-Ketoacyl-ACP reductase; an enzyme (EC 1.1.1.100) reducing acetoacetyl-ACP to hydroxybutyryl-ACP, with NADPH as hydrogen donor; part of the synthesis of fatty acids involving ACP.

**3-oxoacyl-ACP synthase.** β-Ketoacyl-ACP synthetase; acyl-malonyl-ACP synthase; enzyme (EC 2.3.1.41) condensing malonyl-ACP and acetyl-ACP to acetoacetyl-ACP + ACP + CO₂, and similar reactions, steps in fatty acid synthesis.

**oxoges′tone phenpropionate** (USAN). 20-β-Hydroxy-19-norpregn-4-en-2-one hydrocinnamate; a progestational agent.

**2-oxoglutarate dehydrogenase** (EC 1.2.4.2). α-Ketoglutaric dehydrogenase; an enzyme or enzyme group that catalyzes the oxidative decarboxylation of 2-ketoglutaric acid to succinyl hydrolipoate; requires thiamin pyrophosphate. The succinyl group is later transferred to CoA; the reduced lipoate is oxidized by $NAD^+$.

**oxolamine citrate.** OXORMIN; 5-(2-diethylaminoethyl)-3-phenyl-1,2,4-oxadiazole citrate; used for treatment of bronchopulmonary infections.

**oxo'nium ion.** Hydronium ion.

**ox'ophenar'sine hydrochloride** (USP, BP). MAPHARSEN; 3-amino-4-hydroxyphenylarsineoxide hydrochloride; an antisyphilitic and antitrypanosomal agent.

**17-oxosteroid** (ok'so-stĕr'oyd). 17-Ketosteroid.

**oxpren'olol hydrochloride** (USAN). TRASICOR; (+)-1-[ *o*- (Allyloxy)phenoxy ]-3-(isopropylamino)-2-propanol hydrochloride; a $\beta$-receptor blocking agent with coronary vasodilator activity.

**ox'triphyl'line** (NF). CHOLEDYL; choline theophyllinate; a true salt of theophylline. It has mild diuretic, myocardial stimulating vasodilator, and bronchodilator actions, with the same uses as theophylline, but better absorbed and less irritating.

**oxy-** (ok'sĭ-) [ G. *oxys*, keen. OX- ]. Combining form meaning (1) sharp, pointed (oxycephaly); (2) acid (oxydesis); (3) acute (oxyesthesia); (4) shrill (oxyphonia) (5) quick (incorrectly used for ocy-, from G. *ōkys*, swift, as in oxytocia); (6) in chemistry, denoting the presence of oxygen in the substance whose name follows, either added or substituted, *e.g.*, oxybiotin. See also oxo-, hydroxy-.

**oxyacanthine** (ok'sĭ-ā-kan'thēn). Berbine; vinetine; an alkaloid, $C_{37}H_{40}N_2O_6$, from *Berberis vulgaris* (family Berberidaceae), isomeric with berbamine. It causes paralysis of the cerebrospinal centers.

**oxyacid** (ok'sĭ-as'id). Oxacid.

**oxyacoia, oxyakoia** (ok'sĭ-ā-koy'ah) [ G. *oxys*, acute, + *akoē*, hearing ]. Increased sensitiveness to noises, occurring in facial paralysis, especially when the stapedius muscle is paralyzed.

**oxyaphia** (ok'sĭ-a'fī-ah) [ G. *oxys*, acute, + *haphē*, touch ]. Hyperaphia.

**oxybarbit'urates.** Hypnotics of the barbiturate group in which the atom attached at the carbon-2 position is oxygen.

**oxyben'zone** (USP). 2-Hydroxy-4-methoxybenzophenone; an ultraviolet screen for use in skin ointments and lotions.

**oxybi'otin.** An analogue and antimetabolite of biotin, in which the heterocyclic sulfur atom is replaced by oxygen.

**oxyblep'sia** [ G. *oxys*, acute, + *blepō*, to see ]. Oxyopia.

**oxybu'tynin chloride** (USAN). TROPAX; $\alpha$-phenylcyclohexaneglycolic acid 4-(diethylamino)-2-butynyl ester hydrochloride; intestinal antispasmodic.

**oxybutyria** (ok'sĭ-bu-tĭr'ĭ-ah). The presence of oxybutyric acid in the blood, or its excretion in the urine.

**ox'ycalorim'eter.** A calorimeter measuring energy content of substances in terms of oxygen consumed.

**oxycel'lulose.** Cellulose that has been oxidized by $NO_2$ or other oxidizing agents to the point where all or most of the glucose residues have been converted to glucuronic acid residues; used as an adsorbent in chromatography or other absorption processes. See also oxidized *cellulose*.

**oxycepha'lia.** Oxycephaly.

**oxycephal'ic, oxyceph'alous.** Relating to or characterized by oxycephaly.

**oxycephaly** (ok'sĭ-sef'ă-lĭ) [ G. *oxys*, pointed, + *kephalē*, head ]. Oxycephalia; acrocephaly; hypsicephaly; turricephaly; tower skull; a type of craniosynostosis in which there is premature closure of the lambdoid and coronal sutures, resulting in an abnormally high, peaked, or conically shaped skull.

**oxychlo'ride.** A compound of oxygen with a metallic chloride; *e.g.*, a chlorate or perchlorate.

**oxychromatic** (ok'sĭ-kro-mat'ik) [ G. *oxys*, sour, acid, + *chrōma*, color ]. Acidophilic.

**oxychromatin** (ok'sĭ-kro'mă-tin). Oxyphil chromatin; chromatin which stains with acid dyes, as in interphase nuclei.

**oxyco'done** (USAN). PERCODAN; 14-hydroxydihydrocodeinone; narcotic analgesic.

**11-oxycor'ticoids.** Cortical steroids bearing an alcohol or ketonic group on carbon-11, *e.g.*, cortisone and cortisol.

**ox'ydase.** Oxidase.

**oxydesis** (ok'sĭ-de'sis) [ G. *oxys*, sour, acid, + *desis*, a binding together ]. The acid-binding power of the blood indicated by the amount of a centinormal solution of HCl that can be added to a given quantity of oxalated blood without causing agglutination of the red blood cells.

**oxydet'ic.** Pertaining to oxydesis.

**oxyesthesia** (ok'sĭ-es-the'zĭ-ah) [ G. *oxys*, acute, + *aisthēsis*, sensation ]. Hyperesthesia.

**oxygen** (ok'sĭ-jen). 1. A gaseous element, symbol O, atomic no. 8, atomic weight 15.999+ on basis of $^{13}C = 12.0000$; the most abundant and widely distributed of all the chemical elements in the earth's crust. It combines with most of the other elements to form oxides, and is essential to animal and plant life. 2 (USP, BP). A medicinal gas that contains not less than 99.0 per cent, by volume, of $O_2$.

   **heavy o.,** oxygen-18.

   **high pressure o.,** hyperbaric o.

   **hyperbaric o.,** high pressure o.; o. at a pressure greater than 1 atmosphere. See also hyperbaric *oxygenation*.

   **singlet o.,** an excited or higher energy form of o.; characterized by the spin of a pair of electrons in opposite directions, whereas electron spin is unidirectional in normal molecular o. Because of its great reactivity, singlet o. is a probable intermediate in most photo-oxidation reactions. Although it exists for no more than 0.1 sec. it may react with atmospheric pollutants to foster smog formation and may have harmful biological effects.

**oxygen-15.** $^{15}O$; a cyclotron-produced, positron-emitting radioisotope of oxygen with a physical half-life of 2 minutes; used in studies of respiratory function.

**oxygen-16.** $^{16}O$; the common o. isotope, making up 99.759 per cent of natural o.; previously the standard nuclide for the mass numbers on the physical scale, its mass number

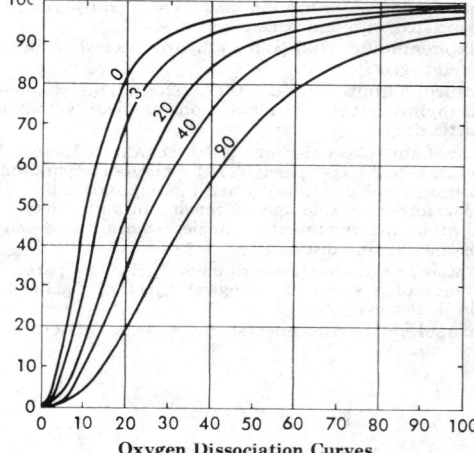

**Oxygen Dissociation Curves**

Hemoglobin exposed to 0, 3, 20, 40, and 90 mm. $CO_2$ pressures. *Ordinates*, per cent saturation with oxygen; *abscissae*, oxygen pressures. (After Barcroft.)

being arbitrarily set equal to 16.000000. The standard is now $^{12}C$, set equal to 12.000000.

**oxygen-17.** $^{17}O$; the rarest of the stable o. isotopes, making up 0.037 per cent of natural o.

**oxygen-18.** $^{18}O$; a stable o. isotope making up 0.204 per cent of natural o.

**oxygenase** (ok'sĭ-jĕ-nās). Direct oxidase; one of a group of enzymes catalyzing direct incorporation of $O_2$ into the substrates (EC class 1.13), *e.g.*, tryptophan 2,3-dioxygenase (tryptophan pyrrolase) catalyzing reaction between $O_2$ and tryptophan to form formylkynurenine.

**oxygenate** (ok'sĭ-jĕ-nāt). To accomplish oxygenation.

**oxygenation** (ok'sĭ-jĕ-na'shun) Addition of oxygen to any chemical or physical system.

   **apneic o.,** diffusion *respiration*.

hyperbaric o., an increased amount of oxygen in organs and tissues resulting from the administration of oxygen in a compression chamber at an ambient pressure greater than 1 atmosphere.

**oxygen'ic.** Pertaining to or containing oxygen.

**ox'ygenize.** Oxidize.

**oxygeusia** (ok'sĭ-gu'sĭ-ah) [ G. oxys, acute, + geusis, taste ]. Hypergeusia.

**ox'yhematopor'phyrin.** A derivative of hematoporphyrin sometimes found in the urine; it is distinguished from urohematoporphyrin on the basis of a red color reaction; cf. urorosein, urorubin.

**ox'yheme.** Hematin.

**ox'yhemochro'mogen.** Hematin.

**oxyhemoglo'bin.** Hemoglobin in combination with oxygen. It is the form of hemoglobin present in arterial blood, and is scarlet or bright red when dissolved in water. Termed also oxygenated hemoglobin; see also hemoglobin.

**oxyhy'drogen.** A mixture of oxygen and hydrogen the combustion of which produces a brilliant white light when the flame is directed against a piece of lime.

**oxyiodide** (ok'sĭ-i'o-dīd). A compound of oxygen with a metallic iodide, e.g., an iodate or periodate.

**oxykrin'in.** Secretin.

**oxyla'lia** [ G. oxys, swift, + lalia, speech ]. Abnormally rapid speaking.

**oxymes'terone.** ORANABOL; 4,17β-dihydroxy-17-methylandrost-4-en-3-one; anabolic steroid.

**oxymetazoline hydrochloride** (ok'sĭ-met'ă-zo-len) (USP). AFRIN; 6-tert-butyl-3-(2-imidazolin-2-ylmethyl)-2,4-dimethylphenol hydrochloride; a vasoconstrictor used topically to reduce swelling and congestion of the nasal mucosa.

**oxymeth'olone** (NF). ADROYD; ANADROL; 17β-hydroxy-2-(hydroxymethylene)-17-methyl-5α-androstan-3-one (for structure of androstane, see steroids); a semisynthetic, orally effective, anabolic steroid that may promote nitrogen retention when combined with an adequate diet; however, effective doses may produce virilization and other untoward effects associated with androgenic hormones.

**oxymethurea.** METHURAL; 1,3-bis(hydroxymethyl)urea; topical antiseptic.

**oxymor'phone hydrochloride** (NF). NUMORPHAN; 14-hydroxydihydromorphinone hydrochloride; a semisynthetic narcotic analgesic closely related chemically to hydromorphone. Its actions are similar to those of morphine, but more potent.

**oxymy'oglo'bin.** Myoglobin in its oxygenated form, analogous in structure to oxyhemoglobin.

**oxyner'vone.** Hydroxynervone.

**α-oxynervonic acid.** Hydroxynervonic acid.

**oxyneu'rine.** Betaine.

**oxyntic** (ok-sin'tik) [ G. oxynō, to sharpen, make sour, acid. OX- ]. Acid-forming, as are the parietal cells of gastric glands.

**oxyo'pia** [ G. oxys, acute, + ōps, eye ]. Oxyblepsia; extreme acuteness of vision.

**oxyo'sis.** Obsolete synonym for acidosis.

**oxyosmia** (ok-sĭ-oz'mĭ-ah) [ G. oxys, acute + osmē, sense of smell ]. Hyperosmia.

**oxyosphresia** (ok'sĭ-os-fre'zĭ-ah) [ G. oxys, acute, + osphrēsis, smell ]. Hyperosmia.

**oxypathia** (ok-sĭ-path'ĭ-ah) [ G. oxys, acute, + pathos, suffering ]. Hyperpathia.

**oxyper'tine** (USAN). EQUIPERTINE; 5,6-dimethoxy-2-methyl-3-[ 2-(4-phenyl-1-piperazinyl)ethyl ]indole; an antianxiety agent. Also available as the hydrochloride (INTEGRIN).

**oxyphenbutazone** (ok'sĭ-fen-bu'tă-zōn) (NF, BP). TANDEARIL; 1-(p-hydroxyphenyl)-2-phenyl-4-butyl-3,5-pyrazolidine-dione monohydrate; an orally effective analgesic and anti-inflammatory agent used (usually in short courses) for rheumatoid arthritis and gout.

**oxyphencyclimine hydrochloride** (ok'sĭ-fen-si'klĭ-mēn) (NF, BP). DARICON; the hydrochloride of 1,4,5,6-tetrahydro-1-methylpyrimidin-2-ylmethyl-α-cyclohexyl-α-hydro-xy-α-phenylacetate; an anticholinergic agent used as a smooth muscle antispasmodic.

**oxyphenisatin acetate** (ok'sĭ-fē-ni'să-tin) (USAN). ISACEN; acetphenolisatin; 3,3-bis-(p-acetoxyphenyl)oxindole; cathartic with pharmacologic properties resembling those of phenolphthalein, except that it is not absorbed from the gastrointestinal tract.

**oxyphenonium bromide** (ok'sĭ-fē-no'mĭ-um). ANTRENYL bromide; diethyl(2-hydroxyethyl)methylammonium bromide α-phenyl-α-cyclohexylglycolate. A quaternary ammonium compound with anticholinergic action. Used for the adjunctive management of peptic ulcer and other conditions of the gastrointestinal tract associated with hyperacidity and hypermotility.

**oxyphil, oxyphile** (ok'sĭ-fil, -īl) [ G. oxys, sour, acid, + philos, fond ]. 1. Oxyphyl cell. 2. Eosinophilic leukocyte. 3. Oxyphilic.

**oxyphil'ic.** Oxyphil (3); having an affinity for acid dyes; denoting certain cell or tissue elements.

**oxypho'nia** [ G. oxys, sharp, + phōnē, voice ]. Shrillness or high pitch of the voice.

**ox'ypolygel'atin.** A modified gelatin used as a plasma extender in transfusions. Abbreviated OPG.

**oxypu'rine.** A purine containing oxygen as part of the molecule; e.g., guanine, xanthine, uric acid.

**oxyrhine** (ok'sĭ-rīn) [ G. oxys, sharp, + rhis (rhin-), noxe ]. Having a sharp-pointed nose.

**oxyrygmia** (ok-sĭ-rig'mĭ-ah) [ G. oxys, acid, + erygmos, eructation ]. Acid eructation.

**ox'ysalt.** A salt formed from an oxyacid.

**Oxyspirura mansoni** (ok'-se-spi-roo'rah man-so'ne). Manson's eye worm; a widely distributed spirurid nematode parasite found under the nictitating membrane in the eye of turkeys, chickens, peafowl, quail, and grouse. The larvae develop to the infective stage in cockroaches.

**ox'yspore** [ G. oxys, sharp, + sporos, seed ]. Sporozoite.

**oxytalan** (ok-sit'ă-lan) [ G. oxys, acid, + talas, suffering, resisting; coined term probably intended to mean "resistant to acid hydrolysis" ]. A type of connective tissue fiber histochemically distinct from collagen or elastic fibers described in the periodontal membrane and gingivae.

**oxytet'racy'cline.** (USP, NF). TERRAMYCIN; oxytetracycline dihydrate (BP); the dihydrate of 4-dimecenecarboxamide. An antibiotic produced by the actinomycete, Streptomyces rimosus, present in the soil. It is active against a large number of pathogenic microorganisms, including bacteria, rickettsiae, spirochetes, and some viruses. Has also been used with some success in amebic dysentery and typhoid fever. o. hydrochloride (USP, BP) and o. calcium (NF) are also available, with the same uses.

**oxythi'amin.** A molecule similar to that of thiamin but with a hydroxyl group replacing the amino group on the pyrimidine ring; a thiamin antagonist capable of inducing symptoms of thiamin deficiency on administration; increases thiamin excretion.

**oxytocia** (ok'sĭ-to'sĭ-ah) [ G. oxys, swift, + tokos, childbirth ]. Rapid parturition.

**oxytocic** (ok'sĭ-to'sik). 1. Hastening childbirth. 2. An agent that promotes the rapidity of labor.

**oxyto'cin.** PITOCIN; α-hypophamine; a nonapeptide hormone of the neurohypophysis, differing from human vasopressin in having leucine at position 8 and isoleucine at position 3. It causes myometrial contractions at term and promotes milk release during lactation, and is used for the induction or stimulation of labor, in the management of postpartum hemorrhage and atony, and to relieve painful breast engorgement. Listed in USP and BP as o. injection.

**oxyto'cinase.** The enzyme that inactivates oxytocin.

**oxyuriasis** (ok-sĭ-u-ri'ă-sis). Oxyurosis; disease manifestations from infection with pinworms (oxyurids).

**oxyuricide** (ok'sĭ-u'rĭ-sīd) [ oxyurid + L. caedo, to kill ]. 1. Destructive to pinworms. 2. An agent that destroys pinworms.

**oxyurid** (ok'sĭ-u'rid) [ see Oxyuris]. Common name for members of the family Oxyuridae.

**Oxyuridae.** A family of parasitic nematodes found in the intestine of many animals. It includes the genera Aspicula-

*ris, Enterobius, Oxyuris, Passalurus,* and *Syphacia.*

**Oxyuris** (ok'sĭ-u'ris) [ G. *oxys,* sharp, + *oura,* tail ]. A genus of nematodes commonly called pinworms, although the pinworm of man is the closely related form, *Enterobius vermicularis.*

O. e'qui, horse pinworm; a common parasite of horses in all parts of the world; it inhabits the large intestine.

**ox'yuro'sis.** Oxyuriasis.

**oz.** Abbreviation for ounce.

**oze'na** [ G. *ozaina,* a fetid polypus, fr. *ozō,* to smell ]. A disease characterized by intranasal crusting, atrophy, and fetid odor.

**o'zenous.** Relating to ozena.

**ozoce'rite.** Ozokerite.

**ozochrotia** (o-zo-kro'shĭ-ah) [ G. *ozō,* to smell, + *chroa,* skin. CHROM- ]. Bromidrosis.

**ozokerite** (o-zo-kēr'ĭt). Ozocerite; mineral wax; mineral tallow; a mixture of paraffinic and cycloparaffinic hydrocarbons occurring in nature; it has a higher melting point than synthetic paraffin, and is used as a substitute for beeswax.

purified o., ceresin.

**ozonator** (o'zo-na'tor). An apparatus for generating ozone and diffusing it in the atmosphere of a room.

**ozone** (o'zōn) [ G. *ozō,* to smell. OZ- ]. O₃; air containing a perceptible amount of $O_3$ has an odor suggesting chlorine or $SO_2$. It is formed by an electric discharge or by the slow combustion of phosphorus; a powerful oxidizing agent.

**o'zonide.** A compound of ozone with an unsaturated organic compound.

**o'zonize.** To saturate or impregnate with ozone.

**ozonolysis** (o'zo-nol'ĭ-sis) [ ozone + G. *lysis,* dissolution ]. The splitting of a double bond in a hydrocarbon chain upon treatment with ozone, with the formation of two aldehydes; used to determine the structure of the unsaturated fatty acids.

**ozonom'eter.** A modified form of ozonoscope, in which by a series of test papers the amount of ozone in the atmosphere may be estimated.

**ozonophore** (o-zo'no-fōr) [ ozone + *phoros,* bearing ]. 1. A red blood cell, or erythrocyte. 2. A protoplasmic granule.

**ozonoscope** (o-zo'no-skōp). Filter paper saturated with starch and potassium iodide or with litmus and potassium iodide; it turns blue in the presence of ozone.

**ozostomia** (o'zo-sto'mĭ-ah) [ G. *ozō,* to smell, + *stoma,* mouth ]. Halitosis; bad breath; a foul odor from the mouth.

# P

**P.** 1. Chemical symbol for the element phosphorus. 2.Abbreviation for Pharmacopeia. 3. Symbol for phosphoric residue in nucleic acid terminology. 4. Followed by a subscript, it refers to the plasma concentration of the substance indicated by the subscript. 5. Blood group designation; see P blood group, appendix 2, Blood Groups. 6. Symbol for pressure or partial *pressure*, frequently with subscripts indicating location and chemical species.

**P$_i$.** Symbol for inorganic *orthophosphate*.

**P$_1$.** Abbreviation for parental *generation*.

**P$_{700}$.** That pigment in chloroplasts bleached by light of wavelengths about 700 nm.

**P$_{870}$.** The pigment in bacterial chromatophores bleached by light of wavelengths about 870 nm.

**p.** Abbreviation for (1) pupil, (2) optic papilla, (3) phosphoric ester or phosphate in polynucleotide symbolism, (4) pico- (10$^{-12}$).

**p-.** Abbreviation for *para-* (3).

**Pa.** 1. Chemical symbol of the element protactinium. 2. Abbreviation for pascal.

**Paas** (pahs), H. R., German physician. See P.'s *disease.*

**PABA.** Abbreviation for *p*-aminobenzoic acid.

**pab'lum.** A precooked infant food, a mixture of wheat, oat, and corn meals, wheat embryo, alfalfa leaves, brewers' yeast, iron, and sodium chloride.

**pab'ular.** Relating to pabulum, or food.

**pabulin** (pab'u-lin) [ L. *pabulum,* food ]. The products of digestion in the blood just after the digestion of food.

**pabulum** (pab'u-lum) [ L. ]. Food; nutriment; aliment.

**Pacchioni** (pak-e-o'ne), Antonio, Italian anatomist, 1665–1726. See Pacchionian *bodies, depressions, foramen, glands, granulations.*

**pace.** A gait of horses in which the fore and hind legs of the same side act together.

**pace'follower.** Any cell in excitable tissue that responds to stimuli from a pacemaker.

**pace'maker.** 1. Any rhythmic center controlling the heart's activity; normally, the sinus node. See also the various types of pulse *generators.* 2. In chemistry, the substance whose rate of reaction sets the pace for a series of chain reactions; the rate-limiting reaction; a "bottleneck."

   **artificial p.,** any device that substitutes for the normal cardiac p. and controls the rhythm of the heart. The device may be implanted in the chest, with electrodes attached to the external cardiac surface, or passed through the venous circulation into the right side of the heart (pervenous p.).

   **demand p.,** a form of artificial p. usually implanted into cardiac tissue; because its output of electrical stimuli can be inhibited by endogenous cardiac electrical activity, this type of p. reduces the risk that a serious arrhythmia will develop as a result of the collective impact of stimuli originating from the p. and from the heart itself.

   **ectopic p.,** any p. other than the sinus node.

   **electric cardiac p.,** an electric device that can substitute for the normal cardiac p., controlling the heart's rhythm by a series of artificial electric discharges.

   **external p.,** an artificial cardiac p. whose electrodes for delivering rhythmical electrical stimuli to the heart are placed externally on the chest wall.

   **fixed-rate p.,** an artificial p. that emits electrical stimuli at a constant frequency; usually implanted into cardiac tissue, where it maintains heart rate at a constant, predetermined value.

   **shifting p.,** wandering p.

   **wandering p.,** shifting p.; a disturbance of the normal cardiac rhythm in which the site of the controlling p. shifts from beat to beat, usually between the sinus and A-V nodes.

**pachismus** (pă-kiz'mus). Pachynis.

**pachometer** (pă-kom'e-ter). Pachymeter.

**Pachon** (pa-shawn'), Michel V., French physiologist, 1867–1938. See P.'s *method, test.*

**pachy-** (pak'ĭ-) [ G. *pachys,* thick ]. Prefix to words formed from Greek roots, signifying thick.

**pachyacria** (pak'ĭ-ak'rĭ-ah) [ pachy- + G. *akron,* tip ]. Obsolete synonym for (1) hypertrophic pulmonary osteoarthropathy, and (2) acromegaly.

**pachyblepharon** (pak'ĭ-blef'ă-ron) [ pachy- + G. *blepharon,* eyelid ]. Tylosis ciliaris; thickening of the tarsal border of the eyelid.

**pachycephalic, pachycephalous** (pak'ĭ-sĕ-fal'ik, -sef'ă-lus). Relating to or marked by pachycephaly.

**pachycephaly, pachycephalia** (pak'ĭ-sef'ă-lĭ, -sĕ-fa'lĭ-ah) [ pachy- + G. *kephalē,* head ]. Abnormal thickness of the skull.

**pachycheilia, pachychilia** (pak-ĭ-ki'lĭ-ah) [ pachy- + G. *cheilos,* lip ]. Swelling or abnormal thickness of the lips.

**pachycholia** (pak'ĭ-ko'lĭ-ah) [ pachy- + G. *cholē,* bile ]. Inspissation of the bile.

**pachychromatic** (pak'ĭ-kro-mat'ik). Having a coarse chromatin reticulum.

**pachychymia** (pak'ĭ-ki'mĭ-ah) [ pachy- + G. *chymos,* juice ]. Inspissation of the chyme.

**pachycolpismus** (pak'ĭ-kol-piz'mus) [ pachy- + G. *kolpos,* bosom, vagina ]. Pachyvaginitis.

**pachydactylia** (pak'ĭ-dak-til'ĭ-ah). Pachydactyly.

**pachydactylous** (pak'ĭ-dak'tĭ-lus). Relating to or characterized by pachydactyly.

**pachydactyly** (pak'ĭ-dak'tĭ-lĭ) [ pachy- + G. *daktylos,* finger or toe ]. Enlargement of the fingers or toes, especially extremities.

**pachyderma** (pak'ĭ-der'mah) [ pachy- + G. *derma,* skin ]. Abnormally thick skin; see also elephantiasis.

   **p. laryn'gis,** a circumscribed connective tissue hyperplasia at the posterior commissure of the larynx.

   **p. lymphangiectat'ica,** elephantiasis due to lymph stasis.

   **p. ora'lis,** familial white folded *dysplasia.*

   **p. verruco'sa,** chronic elephantiasis due to lymph stasis.

   **p. vesicae,** elephantiasis with nodules comprised of lymph vesicles on skin surface.

**pachydermatocele** (pak'ĭ-der-mat'o-sēl) [ pachy- + G. *derma,* skin, + *kēlē,* tumor ]. 1. *Cutis* laxa. 2. A huge neurofibroma.

**pachydermatosis** (pak'ĭ-der-mă-to'sis). Pachyderma.

**pachydermatous** (pak'ĭ-der'mă-tus). Relating to pachyderma.

**pachydermia** (pak'ĭ-der'mĭ-ah). Pachyderma.

**pachydermic** (pak'ĭ-der'mik). Pachydermatous.

**pachydermoperiostosis** (pak-ĭ-der'mo-per'ĭ-os-to'sis) [ pachy- + G. *derma,* skin, + periostosis ]. A syndrome characterized by clubbing of the digits, periosteal new bone formation especially over the distal ends of the long bones, coarsening of the facial features with thickening, furrowing and oiliness of the skin of the face and forehead; there is seborrheic hyperplasia with wide-open sebaceous pores filled with plugs of sebum. About half of patients have affected relatives, often with minor or incomplete forms of the syndrome; probably of autosomal dominant inheritance.

**pachyglossia** (pak-ĭ-glos'ĭ-ah) [ pachy- + G. *glōssa,* tongue ]. Macroglossia.

**pachygnathous** (pak-ig'nath-us) [ pachy- + G. *gnathos,* jaw ]. Characterized by a large or thick jaw.

**pachygyria** (pak-ĭ-ji'rĭ-ah) [ pachy- + G. *gyros,* circle ]. Unusually thick convolutions of the cerebral cortex, related to defective development.

**pachyhymenia** (pak'ĭ-hi-me'nĭ-ah) [ pachy- + G. *hymān,* membrane ]. Pachymenia.

**pachyhymenic** (pak'ĭ-hi-men'ik). Pachymenic.

**pachyleptomeningitis** (pak'ĭ-lep'to-men-in-ji'tis) [ G. *pachys,* thick, + *leptos,* thin (LEP-), + *mēninx* (*mēning-*), membrane, + *-itis* ]. Inflammation of all the membranes of the brain or spinal cord.

**pachylosis** (pak-ĭ-lo'sis) [ G. *pachylos,* rather coarse ]. A condition of roughness, dryness and thickening of the skin, usually on the lower extremities.

**pachymenia** (pak′ī-me′nī-ah) [ pachy- + G. *hymēn*, a membrane ]. Pachyhymenia; thickening of the skin or contiguous membranes.

**pachymenic** (pak′ī-men′ik). Pachyhymenic; marked by or relating to pachymenia.

**pachymeningitis** (pak-ī-men-in-ji′tis) [ pachy- + G. *mēninx*, membrane, + suffix -*itis*, inflammation ]. Perimeningitis; inflammation of the dura mater.

  **p. externa,** external meningitis; epidural meningitis; inflammation of the outer surface of the dura mater.

  **hemorrhagic p.,** subdural *hemorrhage.*

  **hypertrophic cervical p.,** a fibrotic and inflammatory thickening of spinal pachymeninges, particularly in the cervical region, resulting in spinal nerve radiculopathy; believed to be of syphilitic etiology.

  **p. interna,** internal meningitis; inflammation of the inner surface of the dura mater.

  **pyogenic p.,** suppurative inflammation of the dura, often spreading from a neighboring osteomyelitis.

**pach′ymeningop′athy** [ pachy- + G. *mēninx* (*mēning-*), membrane, + *pathos*, disease ]. Disease of the dura mater.

**pachymeninx** (pak′ī-me′ningks) [ pachy- + G. *mēninx*, membrane ]. The dura mater.

**pachymeter** (pă-kim′e-ter) [ pachy- + G. *metron*, measure ]. An instrument for measuring the thickness of any object, especially of thin objects such as a plate of bone or a membrane.

  **optical p.,** a special split ocular substituted for the eyepiece of a slitlamp; it measures corneal thickness by alignment of its anterior and posterior surfaces.

**pachynema** (pak′ī-ne′mah) [ pachy- + G. *nēma*, thread ]. Pachytene.

**pachynsis** (pă-kin′sis) [ G. a thickening ]. Any pathologic thickening.

**pachyntic** (pă-kin′tic). Relating to pachynsis.

**pachyonychia** (pak′ī-o-nik′ī-ah) [ pachy- + G. *onyx*, nail ]. Abnormal thickness of the fingernails or toenails.

  **p. congen′ita,** Jadassohn-Lewandowsky syndrome; a congenital deformity characterized by an abnormal thickness and elevation of nail plates with palmar and plantar hyperkeratosis; the tongue is whitish and glazed due to papillary atrophy.

**pachyotia** (pak-ī-o′shī-ah) [ pachy- + G. *ous*, ear ]. Thickness and coarseness of the auricles of the ears.

**pach′yperiosti′tis** [ pachy- + periostitis ]. Proliferative thickening of the periosteum caused by inflammation.

**pachyperitonitis** (pak′ī-pĕr′ī-to-ni′tis) [ pachy- + peritonitis ]. Productive peritonitis; inflammation of the peritoneum with thickening of the membrane.

**pachypleuritis** (pak-ī-plu-ri′tis) [ pachy- + pleura + -*itis*, ]. Productive pleurisy; inflammation of the pleura with thickening of the membrane.

**pachypodous** (pă-kip′o-dus) [ pachy- + G. *pous*, foot ]. Having large thick feet.

**pach′ysalpingi′tis.** Chronic parenchymatous salpingitis.

**pachysalpingo-oothecitis** (pak-e-sal′pin-go-o-o-the-si′tis) [ pachy- + G. *salpinx*, trumpet, + Mod. L. *ootheca*, ovary, + -*itis* ]. Pachysalpingo-ovaritis.

**pachysalpingo-ovaritis** (pak-e-sal′pin-go-o-var-i′tis) [ pachy- + salpinx + Mod. L. *ovarium*, ovary, + G. -*itis* ]. Pachysalpingo-oothecitis; chronic parenchymatous inflammation of the ovary and Fallopian tube.

**pachysomia** (pak-ī-so′mī-ah) [ pachy- + G. *sōma*, body ]. Pathologic thickening of the soft parts of the body, notably in acromegaly.

**pachytene** (pak′ī-tēn) [ pachy- + G. *tainia*, band, tape ]. Pachynema; the stage of prophase in meiosis in which pairing of homologous chromosomes is complete and the paired homologues may twine about each other as they continue to shorten; longitudinal cleavage occurs in each chromosome to form two sister chromatids so that each homologous chromosome pair becomes a set of four intertwined chromatids called a bivalent.

**pachyvaginalitis** (pak′ī-vaj′ī-nal-i′tis) [ pachy- + Mod. L. (tunica) *vaginalis*, + G. suffix -*itis*, inflammation ]. Chronic inflammation with thickening of the tunica vaginalis testis.

**pachyvaginitis** (pak′ī-vaj′ī-ni′tis) [ pachy- + vagina + G. suffix -*itis*, inflammation ]. Chronic colpitis with thickening and induration of the vaginal walls.

  **p. cys′tica,** *colpohyperplasia* cystica.

**Paci,** Agostino, Italian surgeon. See P.'s *operation.*

**Pacini** (pah-che′ne), Filippo, Italian anatomist, 1812–1883. See Pacinian *corpuscle,* Vater-P. *corpuscle.*

**pacinitis** (pă-sin (chin)-i′tis). Inflammation of the Pacinian corpuscles.

**pack.** 1. To fill or stuff; to tampon. 2. To enwrap; to envelop the body in a wet sheet or blanket. 3. The process of enveloping one in a wet sheet or blanket, or the material so used. 4. In dentistry, to apply a dressing or covering to a surgical site. 5. In dentistry, a surgical dressing or cement used to cover a wound.

  **cold p.,** a p. in a sheet wrung out of cold water.

  **dry p.,** a p. enveloping one in dry, warmed blankets in order to induce profuse perspiration.

  **hot p.,** a p. in a sheet wrung out of hot water.

  **wet p.,** the usual form of p. in a sheet wrung out of hot or cold water.

**pack′er** 1. An instrument for use in tamponing the vagina or other cavity. 2. Plugger.

**pack′ing.** 1. Tamponing; filling a natural cavity or a wound with cotton-wool, gauze, or other material. 2. The material used for packing. 3. The application of a wet pack. 4. The act of filling a mold.

  **denture p.,** filling and compressing a denture base material into a mold in a flask.

**pad.** A bundle of soft material forming a cushion, used in making pressure on a part, in relieving pressure, or in filling a depression so that dressings may fit snugly.

  **abdominal p.,** large dressing for absorption of drainage after laparotomy.

  **dinner p.,** a p. of moderate thickness placed over the pit of the stomach before the application of a plaster jacket; after the plaster has set the p. is removed, leaving space for varying conditions of abdominal distention.

  **fat p.,** see *fat-pad.*

  **knuckle p.'s,** congenital condition in which thick p.'s of skin appear over the proximal phalangeal joints.

  **Mikulicz' p.,** a p. made from several layers of gauze folded into a rectangular shape; used as a sponge, for packing off the viscera in abdominal operations, and in other ways.

  **Passavant's p.,** Passavant's *cushion.*

  **periarterial p.,** see juxtaglomerular *body.*

  **retromolar p.,** pear-shaped area; a cushioned mass of tissue, frequently pear-shaped, located on the alveolar process of the mandible behind the area of the last natural molar tooth.

  **sucking p., suctorial p.,** *corpus* adiposum buccae.

**P.ae.** Abbreviation in prescription writing for L. *partes aequales,* equal parts.

**Paecilomyces** (pe-sil-o-mi′sēz). A genus of saprophytic imperfect fungi whose conidia-bearing hyphae superficially resemble the *penicillus* of *Penicillium;* isolated as contaminants of skin and sputum.

**paed-.** For words so beginning see under ped-.

**Pagenstecher** (pah′gen-stek-er), Alexander, German ophthalmologist, 1828–1879. See P.'s *circle, thread.*

**Paget** (paj′et), Sir James, English surgeon, 1814–1899. See P.'s *abscess, cells, disease,* Pagetoid *osteitis.*

**pagophagia** (pa′go-fa-jī-ah) [ G. *pagos,* frost, + *phagein,* to eat ]. The ingestion of ice; sometimes associated with iron deficiency anemia.

**-pagus** [ G. *pagos,* something fixed, fr. *pēgnymi,* to fasten together. PAG- ]. A termination denoting conjoined twins, the first element of the word denoting the point of attachment; *cf.* -didymus.

**PAH.** Abbreviation for *p*-aminohippuric acid.

**paidol′ogy.** Pedology.

**paidonyx** (pa′do-niks) [ G. *pais,* child, + *onyx,* nail ]. Rudimentary nail.

**pain** [ L. *poena,* a fine, a penalty ]. 1. Suffering, either physical or mental; an impression on the sensory nerves causing distress or, when extreme, agony. 2. One of the uterine contractions occurring in childbirth.

  **after-p.'s,** see afterpains.

**bearing-down p.,** a uterine contraction accompanied with straining and tenesmus; usually appearing in the second stage of labor.

**dream p.,** hypnalgia.

**expulsive p.'s,** effective labor p.'s; those associated with contraction of the uterine muscle.

**false p.'s,** ineffective uterine contractions, preceding and sometimes resembling true labor, but distinguishable from it by the lack of progressive effacement and dilation of the cervix.

**girdle p.,** a painful sensation encircling the body like a belt, occurring in tabes dorsalis or other spinal cord disease.

**growing p.'s,** aching p.'s, frequently felt at night, in the limbs of growing children; attributed variously to growth, rheumatic state, faulty posture, fatigue, or ill-defined psychic causes.

**heterotopic p.,** referred p.

**homotopic p.,** p. felt at the point of injury.

**hunger p.,** cramp in the epigastrium associated with hunger.

**intermenstrual p.,** mittelschmerz.

**labor p.'s,** parodynia; rhythmical uterine contractions which under normal conditions increase in quality, frequency, and duration, culminating in vaginal delivery of the infant.

**middle p.,** Mittelschmerz.

**mind p.,** psychalgia.

**nerve p.,** neuralgia.

**organic p.,** pain caused by an organic lesion.

**phantom limb p.,** see phantom *limb.*

**psychogenic p.,** mental or imaginary p.; p. without demonstrable organic lesion.

**referred p.,** heterotopic p.; telalgia; p. perceived as coming from a situation remote from its actual origin. An example of such a referred visceral p. is the arm, elbow, or wrist p. felt in angina pectoris, or the p. above the clavicle in diaphragmatic pleurisy.

**rest p.,** p. occurring usually in the extremities during rest in the sitting or lying position.

**soul p.,** psychalgia.

**tracheal p.,** trachealgia.

**paint.** A solution or suspension of one or more medicaments applied to the skin with a brush or large applicator. Usually used in treatment of widespread eruptions.

**carbol-fuchsin p.,** Castellani's p.; one containing boric acid, phenol, resorcinol, fuchsin, acetone and alcohol in water, *q.s.* Used in the treatment of superficial mycotic infections.

**Castellani's p.,** carbol-fuschin p.

**pair.** Two objects considered together because of similarity, for a common purpose, or because of some attracting force between them.

**base p.,** nucleotide p.; the complex of two heterocyclic nucleic acid bases, one a pyrimidine and the other a purine, brought about by hydrogen bonding between the 1 and 6 positions of the purine and the 3 and 4 positions of the pyrimidine; base pairing is the essential element in the structure of DNA proposed by Watson and Crick in 1953; usually guanine is paired with cytosine (G.C), and adenine with thymine (A.T) or uracil (A.U).

**conjugate acid-base p.,** in protonic solvents (*e.g.,* $H_2O$, $NH_3$, acetic acid), two molecular species differing only in the presence or absence of a hydrogen ion; as, carbonic acid/bicarbonate ion or ammonium ion/ammonia; the basis of buffer action (most buffers comprise a conjugate acid-base pair).

**nucleotide p.,** base p.

**pajaroello** (pah-har-wa′o). *Ornithodoros coriaceus.*

**Pajot** (pă-zho′), Charles, Paris obstetrician, 1816–1896. See P.'s *hook, maneuver.*

**Palade,** George, Romanian-born electron microscopist, *1912. Nobel laureate, 1974, with Albert Claude and Christian deDuve, for their discoveries concerning the structural and functional organization of the cell. See P. *granule.*

**palatal** (pal′ă-tal). Palatine; relating to the palate or the palate bone.

**pal′ate** [ L. *palatum,* palate ]. Palatum.

**bony p.,** *palatum* osseum.

**Byzantine arch p.,** incomplete fusion of the palatal process with the nasal spine.

**cleft p.,** palatum fissum; palatoschisis; uranoschisis; a congenital fissure in the median line of the p., often associated with cleft lip.

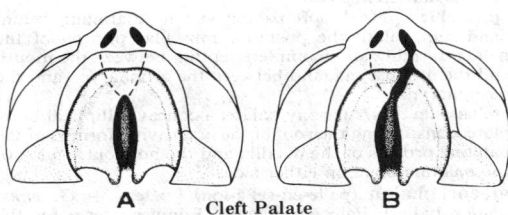

**Cleft Palate**

*A,* isolated cleft palate; *B.* cleft palate combined with unilateral anterior cleft. (From Langman, J.: *Medical Embryology,* Ed. 2, The Williams & Wilkins Co., Baltimore. 1969.)

**falling p.,** uvuloptosis.

**Gothic p.,** an abnormally highly arched p.

**hard p.,** *palatum* durum.

**pen′dulous p.,** soft p.; uvula.

**primary p.,** primitive p.; in the early embryo, the mesodermal shelf separating anteriorly the oral cavity below from the primitive nasal cavities above.

**primitive p.,** primary p.

**secondary p.,** the posterior portion of the embryonic p. which gives rise to the hard p. behind the incisive canal and the soft p.

**soft p.,** *palatum* molle.

**palat′iform.** Palate-shaped; resembling the palate.

**palatine** (pal′ă-tin). Palatal.

**palatitis** (pal′ă-ti′tis). Uranisconitis; inflammation of the palate.

**palato-** [ L. *palatum,* palate ]. Combining form meaning palate.

**pal′atoglos′sal.** Relating to the palate and the tongue, or to the palatoglossus muscle.

**palatoglos′sus.** *Musculus* palatoglossus.

**palatognathous** (pal′ă-tog′nă-thus) [ palato- + G. *gnathos,* jaw ]. Having a cleft palate.

**pal′atogram.** A registration of tongue action against the palate made by placing soft wax on a baseplate.

**pal′atograph** [ palato- G. *graphō,* to record ]. Palate myograph; palatomyograph; an instrument used in recording the movements of the soft palate in speaking and during respiration.

**pal′atomax′illary.** Relating to the palate and the maxilla.

**palatomy′ograph** [ G. *mys,* muscle, + *graphō,* to record ]. Palatograph.

**palatona′sal.** Relating to the palate and the nasal cavity.

**palatopharyngeal** (pal′ă-to-fă-rin′je-al). Relating to palate and pharynx.

**pal′atopharynge′us** [ L. ]. *Musculus* palatopharyngeus.

**palatopharyngorrhaphy** (pal′ă-to-făr′ing-or′ă-phī) [ palato- + pharynx + G. *raphē,* suture ]. Staphylopharyngorrhaphy.

**pal′atoplasty** [ palato- + G. *plassō,* to form ]. Staphyloplasty; uraniscoplasty; uranoplasty; plastic surgery of the palate.

**palatoplegia** (pal′ă-to-ple′jī-ah) [ palato- + G. *plēgē,* stroke ]. Staphyloplegia; paralysis of the muscles of the soft palate.

**palatorrhaphy** (pal′ă-tor′ă-fī) [ palato- + G. *rhaphē,* suture ]. Uraniscorrhaphy; uranorrhaphy; staphylorrhaphy; suture of a cleft palate.

**pal′atosalpinge′us** [ L. ]. *Musculus* palatosalpingeus.

**palatoschisis** (pal-ă-tos′kĭ-sis) [ palato- + G. *schisis,* fissure ]. Cleft *palate.*

**palatum,** pl. **pala′ti** (pă-la′tum) [ L. ] [ NA ]. Palate; uraniscus; the roof of the mouth; the bony and muscular partition between the oral and nasal cavities; popularly the uvula.

**p. durum** [ NA ], hard palate; the anterior part of the palate, consisting of the bony palate covered above by the mucous membrane of the floor of the nose and below by the mucoperiosteum of the roof of the mouth which contains the palatine vessels, nerves, and mucous glands.

**p. fissum,** cleft *palate.*

**p. mol′le** [ NA ], soft palate; velum palatinum; velum pendulum palati; the posterior muscular portion of the palate, forming an incomplete septum between the mouth and the oropharynx, and between the oropharynx and the nasopharynx.

**p. osseum** [ NA ], bony palate; a concave elliptical bony plate, constituting the roof of the oral cavity, formed of the palatine process of the maxilla and the horizontal plate of the palatine bone on either side.

**paleencephalon** (pa′le-en-sef′ă-lon) [ paleo- + G. *enke-phalos,* brain ]. Paleoencephalon; Edinger's term for the metameric nervous *system.*

**paleo-, pale-** (pa′le-o-, pal′e-o-) [ G. *palaios,* old, ancient ]. Combining forms meaning old or primitive (primary, early).

**paleocerebellum** (pa′le-o-sĕr′e-bel′um). The phylogenetically older part of the cerebellum represented by the flocculonodular lobe, as distinguished from middle parts of the vermis and cerebellar hemisphere.

**paleocortex** (pa′le-o-kor′teks). The phylogenetically oldest part of the cortical mantle of the cerebral hemisphere represented by the olfactory cortex; the archicortex of the hippocampus is often included in the term; see also *cortex cerebri.*

**paleoencephalon** (pa′le-o-en-sef′ă-lon). Paleencephalon.

**paleogenesis** (pa′le-o-jen′e-sis) [ paleo- + G. *genesis,* origin ]. The hereditary transmission of peculiarities of organization, in absolute latency for periods of indefinite length; invoked by Hutchinson in explanation of certain human disease—the dappled skin of leukoderma colli, for example, a similar marking occurring normally in the deer and horse; the condition in both animals and man being an inheritance from some infinitely remote common ancestor.

**pa′leogenet′ic.** Relating to paleogenesis.

**paleokinetic** (pa′le-o-kĭ-net′ik) [ paleo- + G. *kinētikos,* relating to movement ]. Denoting the primitive motor mechanisms underlying muscular reflexes and automatic, stereotyped movements.

**paleopathology** (pa-le-o-pă-thol′o-jĭ) [ paleo- + pathology ]. The science of disease in prehistoric terms as revealed in bones, mummies, and archaeologic artifacts as well as statues, drawings, carvings, paintings on stone, amulets, and other objects.

**paleostriatal** (pa′le-o-stri-a′tal). Relating to the paleostriatum.

**paleostriatum** (pal-e-o-stri-a′tum) [ paleo- + L. *striatum, q. v.* ]. Term denoting the pallidum (globus pallidus), and expressing the hypothetical notion that this component of the corpus striatum developed earlier in evolution than did the "neostriatum" or striatum (caudate nucleus and putamen).

**paleothalamus** (pa′le-o-thal′ă-mus). The intralaminar nuclei, believed to be the components of the thalamus to develop earliest in evolution.

**Palfyn (Palfin),** Jean, Ghent surgeon and anatomist, 1650–1730. See P.'s *sinus.*

**palikinesia, palicinesia** (pal-ĭ-kĭ-ne′zĭ-ah, -sĭ-ne′zĭ-ah) [ G. *palin,* again, + *kinēsis,* movement ]. Involuntary repetition of movements.

**palilalia** (pal-ĭ-la′lĭ-ah) [ G. *palin,* again, + *lalia,* a form of speech ]. Paliphrasia.

**pal′inal** [ G. *palin,* backward ]. Moving backward.

**palindromia** (pal-in-dro′mĭ-ah) [ G. a running back, fr. *palin,* back, + *dromos,* a running ]. A relapse or recurrence of a disease.

**palindrom′ic.** Relapsing; recurring.

**palingenesis** (pal′in-jen′ĕ-sis) [ G. *palin,* again, + *genesis,* production ]. The appearance during embryonic development of structural features characteristic of phylogenetically ancestral types.

**palinopsia** (pal′ĭ-nop′sĭ-ah) [ G. *palin,* again, + *opsis,* vision ]. Abnormal recurring visual imagery noted by old persons having other visual disorders.

**paliphrasia** (pal-ĭ-fra′zĭ-ah) [ G. *palin,* again, + *phrasis,* speech ]. Palilalia; involuntary repetition of words or sentences in talking.

**palirrhea** (pal′ĭ-re′ah) [ G. *palirrhoia,* a flowing back ]. 1. The return of a discharge after its cessation. 2. Regurgitation.

**pal′isade** [ Fr. *palissade,* fr. L. *palus,* a pale, stake ]. A row of stakes; in pathology, a row of elongated nuclei.

**palla′dium** [ fr. the asteroid, Pallas ]. A metallic element resembling platinum, symbol Pd, atomic no. 46, atomic weight 106.4.

**pallanesthesia** (pal′an-es-the′zĭ-ah) [ G. *pallō,* to quiver, + *anaisthēsia,* insensibility ]. Apallesthesia; absence of pallesthesia.

**pallescense** (pal-es′ens) [ L. *palesco,* to become pale, fr. *palleo,* to be pale ]. Pallor.

**pallesthesia** (pal′es-the′zĭ-ah) [ G. *pallō,* to quiver, + *aisthesis,* sensation ]. The appreciation of vibration—a form of pressure sense; it is most acute when the vibrating tuning fork is applied over a bony prominence. Also called pallesthetic bone; vibratory sensibility.

**pal′lesthet′ic.** Pertaining to pallesthesia.

**pal′lial.** Relating to the pallium.

**palliate** (pal′ĭ-āt) [ L. *palliatus* (adj.), dressed in a *pallium,* cloaked ]. To mitigate; to reduce the severity of; to relieve slightly.

**pal′liative.** Mitigating; reducing the severity of; denoting a method of treatment of a disease or of its symptoms.

**pal′lidal.** Relating to the pallidum.

**pallidectomy** (pal′ĭ-dek′to-mĭ) [ pallidum + G. *ektomē,* excision ]. Excision or destruction of the globus pallidus, usually by stereotaxy; prefix may indicate the method used, *e.g.,* chemopallidectomy (destruction by a chemical agent), cryopallidectomy (destruction by cold).

**pallidoamygdalotomy** (pal′ĭ-do-ă-mig′dă-lot′o-mĭ). Production of lesions in the globus pallidus and amygdaloid nuclei.

**pallidoansotomy** (pal′id-o-an-sot′o-mĭ). Production of lesions in the globus pallidus and ansa lenticularis.

**pallidotomy** (pal′ĭ-dot′o-mĭ) [ pallidum + G. *tomē,* incision ]. Surgical section of nerve fibers coming from the globus pallidus; done to produce changes in pathologic involuntary movements in man.

**pal′lidum** [ L. *pallidus,* pale ]. *Globus* pallidus.

**pallium** (pal′ĭ-um) [ L. cloak ] [ NA ]. Mantle; brain mantle; the cerebral cortex with the subjacent white substance.

**pal′lor** [ L. ]. Paleness, as of the skin.

cachectic p., achromasia (1).

**palm** (pahm) [ L. *palma.* PALM-1 ]. Palma; palma manus; vola manus; the flat of the hand; the flexor or anterior surface of the hand, exclusive of the thumb and fingers; the opposite of the dorsum.

liver p., erythema of the thenar and hypothenar eminences.

**palma,** pl. **pal′mae** (pal′mah) [ L. ] [ NA ]. Palm.

**p. ma′nus** [ NA ], palm of the hand; see palm.

**palmar** (pahl′mar) [ L. *palmaris,* fr. *palma* ]. Referring to the palm of the hand; volar.

**palma′ris** [ L. ] [ NA ].Palmar.

**pal′mature** [ L. *palma,* palm ]. Adhesion or webbing of the fingers.

**pal′mellin.** A red coloring matter formed by an alga, *Palmella cruenta.*

**Palmer,** Walter L. See P. acid test for peptic ulcer, under test.

**palmic** (pal′mik). Beating; throbbing; relating to a palmus.

**pal′mital′dehyde.** $CH_3(CH_2)_{14}CHO$; the 16-carbon aldehyde corresponding to palmitic acid; a constituent of plasmalogens.

**pal′mitate.** A salt of palmitic acid.

**palmit′ic acid.** Hexadecanoic acid; a saturated fatty acid, $C_{16}H_{32}O_2$; occurring in palm oil and other fats.

**pal′mitin.** Tripalmitin; the triglyceride of palmitic acid, occurring in palm oil.

**palmitoleic acid** (pal'mĭ-to-le'ik). An unsaturated 16-carbon acid; one of the common constituents of the glycerides of human adipose tissue.

**palmityl alcohol** (pal'mĭ-til). Cetyl alcohol.

**palmodic** (pal'mod'ik). Relating to palmus (1).

**palmoscopy** (pal-mos'ko-pī) [ G. *palmos*, pulsation, + *skopeō*, to examine ]. Examination of the cardiac pulsation.

**pal'mus**, pl. **pal'mi** [ G. *palmos*, pulsation, quivering ]. 1. Facial *tic*. 2. Rhythmical fibrillary contractions in a muscle. 3. The heart beat.

**palpable** (pal'pă-bl) [ see palpation ]. 1. Perceptible to touch; that can be palpated. 2. Evident; plain.

**pal'pate**. To examine by feeling and pressing with the palms of the hands and the fingers.

**palpa'tion** [ L. *palpatio*, fr. *palpo*, pp. -*atus*, to touch, stroke. PALP- ]. 1. Examination by means of the hands, to outline the organs or tumors of the abdomen, to determine the degree of resistance of various parts, to feel the heart beat, the vibrations in the chest, etc. 2. Touching; feeling or perceiving by the sense of touch.

  **light-touch p.**, a method of determining the outlines of the thoracic and abdominal organs by lightly palpating the surface with the tip of a finger.

**pal'patopercus'sion**. Examination by means of combined palpation and percussion.

**palpe'bra**, pl. **palpe'brae**, gen. pl. **palpebra'rum** [ L. ] [ NA ]. Eyelid; one of the two movable folds of skin (upper and lower eyelids) lined with conjunctiva in front of the eyeball.

  **p. III** [ NAV ], alternate term for *plica* semilunaris conjunctivae (2).

  **p. inferior** [ NA ], lower eyelid.

  **p. superior** [ NA ], upper eyelid.

  **p. ter'tia**, *plica* semilunaris conjunctivae (2).

**pal'pebral**. Relating to an eyelid or the eyelids.

**palpebra'lis** [ L. ]. *Musculus* levator palpebrae superioris.

**pal'pebrate** [ L. *palpebra*, eyelid ]. 1. Having eyelids. 2. To wink.

**palpebration** (pal'pe-bra'shun) [ L. *palpebratio* ]. Winking.

**palpebritis** (pal'pe-bri'tis) [ L. *palpebra*, eyelid, + G. suffix -*itis*, inflammation ]. Obsolete term for blepharitis.

**palpitatio cordis**. Palpitation of the heart.

**palpitation** (pal-pĭ-ta'shun) [ L. *palpitatio*, fr. *palpito*, pp. -*atus*, to throb. PALP- ]. Forcible pulsation of the heart, perceptible to the patient, usually with an increase in frequency, with or without irregularity in rhythm.

**palsy** (pawl'zī) [ a corruption thru O. Fr. fr. L. and G. *paralysis* ]. Paralysis (q.v.); often used to connote partial paralysis, or paresis.

  **Bell's p.**, facial p.

  **birth p.**, obstetrical paralysis; paralysis, hemiplegia or diplegia, due to cerebral hemorrhage occurring at birth or to anoxic injury of the fetal brain *in utero*.

  **brachial birth p.**, paralysis of the arm due to injury received at birth; there are three types, the whole arm type, the upper arm (Erb's) type, and the forearm (Klumpke) type.

  **bulbar p.**, progressive bulbar *paralysis*.

  **cerebral p.**, defect of motor power and coordination related to damage of the brain.

  **craft p.**, an occupational neurosis, such as writer's cramp.

  **creeping p.**, progressive muscular *atrophy*.

  **crutch p.**, paralysis of the arm caused by the pressure of the crosspiece of a crutch.

  **diver's p.**, see bends.

  **Erb's p.**, Duchenne-Erb or Erb's paralysis; a type of brachial birth p. in which there is paralysis of the muscles of the upper arm (deltoid, biceps, anterior brachial, and long supinator muscles) due to a lesion of the brachial plexus or of the roots of the fifth and sixth cervical nerves.

  **facial p.**, Bell's p.; facial paralysis; Fallopian neuritis; facioplegia; prosopoplegia; a unilateral paralysis of the facial muscles supplied by the seventh nerve.

  **Féréol-Graux p.**, paralysis, of nuclear origin, of the external rectus muscle of one eye and the internal rectus of the other.

  **lead p.**, lead paralysis; paralysis of the extensor muscles of the wrist causing wrist-drop; occurs in lead poisoning.

  **night p.**, waking *numbness*.

  **posticus p.**, paralysis of the cricoarytenoideus posticus muscle, resulting in the vocal cord being held in or near the midline.

  **pressure p.**, paralysis due to pressure on a nerve trunk or on the spinal cord.

  **progressive supranuclear p.**, a heterogeneous degeneration involving the brainstem, basal ganglia, and cerebellum, with nuchal dystonia and dementia.

  **scrivener p.**, writer's *cramp*.

  **shaking p.**, **trembling p.**, parkinsonism (1).

  **wasting p.**, progressive muscular *atrophy*.

**Paltauf** (pahl'towf), Arnold, German physician, 1860–1893. See P.'s *infantilism, nanism*.

**Paltauf** (pahl'towf), Richard, Vienna pathologist, 1858–1924. See P.'s modification of Gram's stain, under *stain*, P.-Sternberg *disease*.

**pal'udal** [ L. *palus*, marsh ]. 1. Marshy. 2. Malarial.

**paludism** (pal'u-dizm) [ L. *palus*, marsh ]. Malaria.

**pam'abrom**. PAMPRIN; 8-bromotheophylline compound with 2-amino-2-methyl-1-propanol; diuretic.

**pam'aquine**. PLASMOCHIN; an antimalarial agent, active against avian malaria and against the gametocytes of all malarial forms in man; it is more toxic than chloroquine or primaquine and has been replaced by primaquine.

**pam'oate**. USAN-approved contraction for 4,4'-methylenebis[ 3-hydroxy-2-naphthoate).

**pampin'iform** [ L. *pampinus*, a tendril, + *forma*, form ]. Having the shape of a tendril; denoting a vinelike structure.

**pampiniformis** [ L. ] [ NA ]. Pampiniform.

**pampinocele** (pam-pin'o-sēl) [ L. *pampinus*, tendril, + G. *kēlē*, tumor ]. Varicocele.

**pan-** [ G. *pas*, all. PAN- ]. Prefix to words derived from Greek roots, implying all, entire.

**panacea** (pan-ă-se'ah) [ G. *panakeia*, universal remedy (fr. Panacea, Aesculapius' daughter) ]. A cure-all; a remedy claimed to be curative of all diseases.

**panagglutinable** (pan-ă-glu'tĭ-nă-bl). Agglutinable with all types of human serum; denoting erythrocytes having this property.

**panagglu'tinins**. Agglutinins that react with all human erythrocytes.

**Panama bark**. Quillaja.

**panangiitis** (pan'an-jī-i'tis) [ pan- + angiitis ]. Inflammation involving all the coats of a blood vessel.

**pan'arteri'tis** [ pan- + L. *arteria*, artery, + G. suffix -*itis*, inflammation ]. An inflammatory disorder of the arteries characterized by involvement of all structural layers of the vessels.

**panarthri'tis**. 1. Inflammation involving all the tissues of a joint. 2. Inflammation of all the joints of the body.

**Panas** (pă-nah'), Photinos, Paris ophthalmologist, 1832–1903. See P.'s *operation*.

**panatrophy** (pan-at'ro-fī). 1. Atrophy of all the parts of a structure. 2. General atrophy of the body.

**panblas'tic** [ pan- + G. *blastos*, germ ]. Relating to all the primary germ layers.

**pancardi'tis**. Inflammation of all the structures of the heart, including endocardium, myocardium, and epicardium.

**panchrest** (pan'krest) [ pan- + G. *chrēstos*, useful ]. Panacea.

**Pancoast**, H. K., American roentgenologist, 1875–1939. See P. *syndrome, tumor*.

**Pancoast**, Joseph, U. S. surgeon, 1805–1882. See P.'s *operation, suture*.

**pancolectomy** (pan'ko-lek'to-mī). Extirpation of the entire colon.

**pancreas**, pl. **pancreata** (pan'kre-as, pan'kre-a'tah) [ G. *pankreas*, the sweetbread, fr. *pas* (*pan*), all, + *kreas*, flesh. PAN- ] [ NA ]. An elongated lobulated gland, devoid of capsule, extending from the concavity of the duodenum to the spleen; it consists of a flattened head (caput) within the duodenal cavity, an elongated three-sided body (corpus) extending transversely across the abdomen, and a tail (cauda) in contact with the spleen. The gland secretes the pancreatic juice, discharged into the intestine, and internal secretions, insulin and glucagon. See fig. on p. 1020.

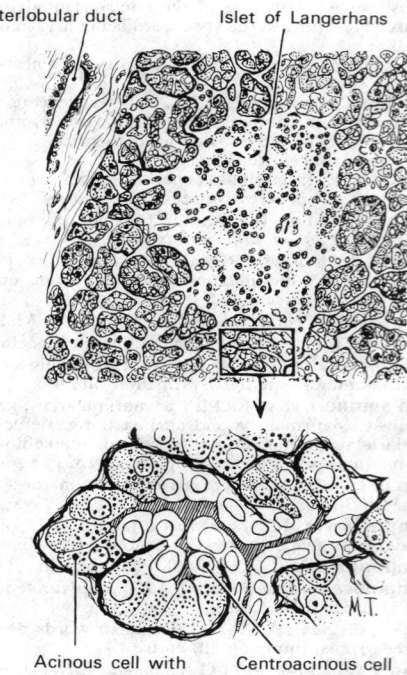

Interlobular duct          Islet of Langerhans

Acinous cell with          Centroacinous cell
zymogen granules

**Pancreas (Cross Section)**

**p. accesso′rium** [ NA ], a detached portion of pancreatic tissue sometimes found in the wall of the stomach or of the duodenum.

**annular p.,** a ring of p. encircling the duodenum.

**Aselli's p.,** see *nodi* lymphatici mesenterici.

**p. divisum** bifid or divided p.; a congenital failure of the embryonic primordia to unite completely.

**dorsal p.,** that portion of the pancreatic primordium of the embryo that arises as a dorsal bud from the foregut entoderm.

**lesser p.,** *processus* uncinatus pancreatis.

**p. minus,** *processus* uncinatus pancreatis.

**small p.,** *processus* uncinatus pancreatis.

**tail of p.,** *cauda* pancreatis.

**uncinate** or **unciform p.,** *processus* uncinatus pancreatis.

**ventral p.,** that portion of the primordium of the pancreas that arises, together with the hepatic diverticulum, as a ventral bud from the foregut entoderm.

**Willis' p.,** *processus* uncinatus pancreatis.

**Winslow's p.,** *processus* uncinatus pancreatis.

**pancreat-** [ G. *pankreas,* pancreas. PAN- ]. Combining form relating to the pancreas.

**pancreatalgia** (pan′kre-ă-tal′jĭ-ah) [ pancreat- + G. *algos,* pain ]. Pain arising from the pancreas or felt in or near the region of the pancreas.

**pancreatectomy** (pan′kre-ă-tek′to-mĭ) [ pancreat- + G. *ektomē,* excision ]. Pancreectomy; excision of the pancreas.

**pancreatemphraxis** (pan′kre-at-em-frak′sis) [ pancreat- + G. *emphraxis,* a stoppage ]. Obstruction in the pancreatic duct, causing swelling of the gland.

**pancreathelcosis** (pan′kre-ath-el-ko′sis) [ pancreat- + G. *helkōsis,* ulceration ]. Suppurative inflammation or abscess of the pancreas.

**pancreatic** (pan-kre-at′ik). Relating to the pancreas.

**pancreatico-** (pan′kre-at′ĭ-ko-). Combining form relating to the pancreas; for most terms beginning thus, see pancreato-.

**pancreaticoduodenal** (pan-kre-at′ĭ-ko-du′o-de′nal, -du-od′ĕ-nal). Relating to the pancreas and the duodenum.

**pancreatin** (pan′kre-ă-tin) (NF, BP). A mixture of the enzymes from the pancreas of the ox or hog, occurring in the form of a cream-colored powder. Used internally as a digestive, and also as a peptonizing agent in preparing predigested foods; it contains the proteolytic trypsin, the amylolytic amylopsin, and the lipolytic steapsin.

**pancreatitis** (pan′kre-ă-ti′tis). Inflammation of the pancreas.

**acute hemorrhagic p.,** an acute inflammation of the pancreas accompanied by the formation of necrotic areas and frequently, though not invariably, hemorrhages into the substance of the gland. Clinically, it is marked by sudden severe abdominal pain, nausea, fever, and leukocytosis. Areas of fat necrosis are present on the surface of the pancreas and in the omentum due to the action of the escaped pancreatic enzyme (trypsin and lipase).

**pancreato-** (pan′kre-ă-to-, pan-kre-at′o-) [ G. *pankreas,* pancreas. PAN- ]. Combining form relating to the pancreas.

**pancreatocholecystostomy** (pan-kre-at′o-ko-le-sis-tos′-to-mĭ, pan′kre-ă-to-). A surgical anastomosis between a pancreatic cyst or fistula and the gallbladder.

**pancreatoduodenectomy** (pan-kre-at′o-du-o-dĕ-nek′to-mĭ, pan′kre-ă-to-). Brunschwig's operation (1); Whipple's operation; excision of all or part of the pancreas together with the duodenum.

**pancreatoduodenostomy** (pan-kre-at′o-du-o-de-nos′to-mĭ, pan′kre-ă-to-). Surgical anastomosis of a pancreatic duct, cyst, or fistula to the duodenum.

**pancreatogastrostomy** (pan-kre-at′o-gas-tros′to-mĭ, pan′kre-ă-to-). Surgical anastomosis of a pancreatic cyst or fistula to the stomach.

**pancreatogenic** (pan′kre-ă-to-jen′ik). Pancreatogenous.

**pancreatogenous** (pan′kre-ă-toj′e-nus). Pancreatogenic; of pancreatic origin; formed in the pancreas.

**pancreatog′raphy** (pan′kre-ă-tog′ră-fĭ) [ pancreato- + G. *graphō,* to write ]. Visualization of the pancreas on x-ray films, after injection of radiopaque material into the duct.

**pancreatojejunostomy** (pan-kre-at′o-jĕ-ju-nos′to-mĭ, pan′kre-ă-to-). Surgical anastomosis of a pancreatic duct, cyst, or fistula to the jejunum.

**pancreatolith** (pan-kre-at′o-lith) [ pancreato- + G. *lithos,* stone ]. Pancreolith; pancreatic calculus; a pancreatic concretion.

**pancreatolithectomy** (pan-kre-at′o-lĭ-thek′to-mĭ, pan′-kre-ă-to-) [ pancreato- + G. *lithos,* stone, + *ektomē,* excision ]. Pancreatolithotomy.

**pancreatolithiasis** (pan-kre-at′o-lĭ-thi′ă-sis, pan′kre-ă-to-). Stones in the pancreas, usually found in the pancreatic duct system.

**pancreatolithotomy** (pan-kre-at′o-lĭ-thot′o-mĭ, pan′kre-ă-to-) [ pancreato- + G. *lithos,* stone, + *tomē,* incision ]. Pancreolithotomy; pancreatolithectomy; incision of the pancreas for the removal of concretion.

**pancreatolysis** (pan′kre-ă-tol′ĭ-sis) [ pancreato- + G. *lysis,* dissolution ]. Destruction of the substance of the pancreas.

**pancreatolytic** (pan′kre-ă-to-lit′ik). Relating to pancreatolysis.

**pancreatomegaly** (pan′kre-ă-to-meg′ă-lĭ) [ pancreato- + G. *megas,* great ]. Abnormal enlargement of the pancreas.

**pancreatomy** (pan′kre-at′o-mĭ). Pancreatotomy.

**pancreatopathy** (pan′kre-ă-top′ă-thĭ) [ pancreato- + G. *pathos,* suffering ]. Pancreopathy; any disease of the pancreas.

**pancreatopep′tidase E.** Elastase.

**pancreatotomy** (pan′kre-ă-tot′o-mĭ) [ pancreato- + G. *tomē,* incision ]. Pancreatomy; incision of the pancreas for the removal of a new growth, evacuation of a calculus, etc.

**pancreatropic** (pan-kre-ă-trop′ik) [ pancreat- + G. *tropi-kas,* relating to a turning ]. Exerting an action on the pancreas.

**pancreectomy** (pan′kre-ek′to-mĭ). Pancreatectomy.

**pan′crelip′ase** (NF). COTAZYM; a concentrate of pancreatic enzymes standardized for lipase content; a lipolytic used for substitution therapy.

**pancreo-** (pan′kre-o-). See pancreato-.

**pan′creopriv′ic** [ pancreo- + L. *privus*, deprived of ]. Without a pancreas.

**pan′creozy′min.** A hormone, found in intestinal mucosa, that stimulates the secretion of pancreatic enzymes.

**pancuro′nium bromide** (USAN). PAVULON; 2β,16β-dipiperidino-5α-androstane-3α,17β-diol diacetate dimethobromide; a nondepolarizing steroidal neuromuscular blocking agent resembling curare but without the potential of curare for ganglionic blockade, histamine release, or hypotension.

**pancytopenia** (pan-si-to-pe′nĭ-ah) [ pan- + G. *kytos*, cell, + *penia*, poverty ]. Pronounced reduction in the number of erythrocytes, all types of white blood cells, and the blood platelets in the circulating blood.
  **congenital p.,** Fanconi's *anemia.*
  **Fanconi's p.,** Fanconi's *anemia.*

**pandemic** (pan-dem′ik) [ pan- + G. *dēmos*, the people ]. Denoting a disease affecting or attacking the population of an extensive region; extensively epidemic.

**pan′demic′ity.** The state or condition of being pandemic.

**Pander,** Heinrich C. von, German anatomist and embryologist, 1794–1865. See P.'s *nucleus.*

**pandiculation** (pan-dik′u-la′shun) [ L. *pandiculor*, to stretch oneself, fr. *pando*, to spread out ]. The act of stretching, as when awaking.

**Pandy,** Kalman, Hungarian neurologist, *1868. See P.'s *test, reaction.*

**panencephalitis** (pan′en-sef-ă-li′tis). A diffuse encephalitis of the central nervous sytem involving both the white and gray matter.
  **nodular p.,** Pette-Döring disease; probably a form of subacute sclerosing p., *q. v.*
  **subacute sclerosing p.,** a diffuse encephalitis seemingly the same as inclusion body *encephalitis, q. v.*

**panendoscope** (pan-en′do-skōp) [ pan- + G. *endon*, within, + *skopeō*, to view ]. A cystoscope that permits visualization of the entire interior of the bladder.

**panesthesia** (pan-es-the′zĭ-ah) [ pan- + G. *aisthēsis*, sensation ]. The sum of all the sensations experienced by a person at one time; see also cenesthesia.

**Paneth** (pah′nāt), Josef, German physician, 1857–1890. See P.'s granular *cells.*

**pang.** A sudden sharp, brief pain.
  **breast p.,** *angina pectoris.*

**pangenesis** (pan-jen′ĕ-sis) [ pan- + G. *genesis*, production ]. The theory of Darwin that every separate part of the organism reproduces itself in the progeny, each ovule and spermatozoon containing a particle or germ thrown off from each separate unit in the parent organism.

**pangenetic** (pan′jĕ-net′ik). Panmeristic; relating to pangenesis.

**pan′globinope′nia.** A hypothetical hereditary inhibition of hemoglobin synthesis involving all hemoglobin polypeptide chains, distinct from thalassemia.

**panglossia** (pan-glos′ĭ-ah) [ pan- + G. *glōssa*, tongue ]. Garrulity.

**pan′hidro′sis.** Panidrosis.

**pan′hydrom′eter** [ pan- + G. *hydōr*, water, + *metron*, measure ]. A hydrometer for use in determining the specific gravity of any liquid.

**panhygrous** (pan-hy′grus) [ pan- + G. *hygros*, damp ]. Universally moist.

**panhyperemia** (pan-hi-per-e′mĭ-ah) [ pan- + G. *hyper*, over, + *haima*, blood ]. Universal congestion or hyperemia; plethora.

**panhypopituitarism** (pan′hi-po-pĭ-tu′ĭ-tă-rizm). A state in which the secretion of all anterior pituitary hormones is inadequate or absent; caused by a variety of disorders that result in destruction of substantially all of the anterior pituitary gland.

**pan′ic** [ fr. G. god *Pan*, who was presumed to inspire terror ]. A violent and unreasoning anxiety and fear.
  **homosexual p.,** an acute, severe attack of anxiety based on unconscious conflicts regarding homosexuality.

**panic′ulus** [ L. dim. of *pannus*, cloth ] [ NA ]. Panniculus; a sheet or layer of tissue.
  **p. adipo′sus** [ NA ], the superficial fascia which contains more or less fatty deposit in its areolar substance.

**p. carno′sus,** the skeletal muscle layer in the superficial fascia represented in man by the platysma muscle; it is much more extensive in lower mammals.

**panidrosis** (pan′ĭ-dro′sis) [ pan- + G. *hidros*, sweat ]. Panhidrosis; sweating of entire surface of body.

**pan′immu′nity.** A general immunity to all infectious diseases.

**pa′nis** [ L. ]. Bread.

**panleukope′nia.** Feline infectious enteritis; distemper (2); feline agranulocytosis; cat plague; cat fever; a highly contagious and fatal disease of cats, particularly young cats, caused by a virus. It is manifested by severe leukopenia, prostration, fever, and diarrhea; its course is 5 to 7 days.

**pan′meris′tic** [ pan- + G. *meros*, part ]. Pangenetic.

**pan′mix′is** [ pan- + G. *mixis*, intercourse ]. Random *mating.*

**panmyelophthisis** (pan-mi′ĕ-lof′thĭ-sis). Myelophthisis (2).

**panmyelosis** (pan-mi′ĕ-lo′sis) [ pan- + G. *myelos*, marrow, + suffix *-osis*, condition ]. Myeloid metaplasia with abnormal immature blood cells in the spleen and liver, associated with myelofibrosis.

**Panner,** H. J. See P.'s *disease.*

**panneuritis** (pan-nu-ri′tis). Rarely used term meaning extreme polyneuritis.
  **p. endem′ica,** beriberi.

**panniculitis** (pă-nik′u-li′tis) [ panniculus + G. suffix *-itis*, inflammation ]. Inflammation of the panniculus adiposus of the abdominal wall.
  **nodular nonsup′purative p.,** Weber-Christian disease; a condition marked by recurring attacks of fever and the formation of tender subcutaneous nodules; necrotic areas infiltrated by lipid macrophages are present in subcutaneous fat; the cause is unknown.

**panniculus,** pl. **pannic′uli** (pă-nik′u-lus) [ L. dim. of *pannus*, cloth ]. Paniculus.

**pan′nus,** pl. **pan′ni** [ L. cloth ]. A membrane of granulation tissue covering a normal surface, particularly the articular cartilages in rheumatoid arthritis and the cornea in trachoma; see also corneal p.
  **corneal p.,** p. covering the upper half of, or sometimes the entire, cornea; a frequent complication of trachoma. It occurs in three forms: p. crassus (thick), in which the blood vessels are many and the opacity very dense; p. siccus (dry), p. with dry, glossy surface; p. tenuis (thin), in which the blood vessels are few and the opacity slight.

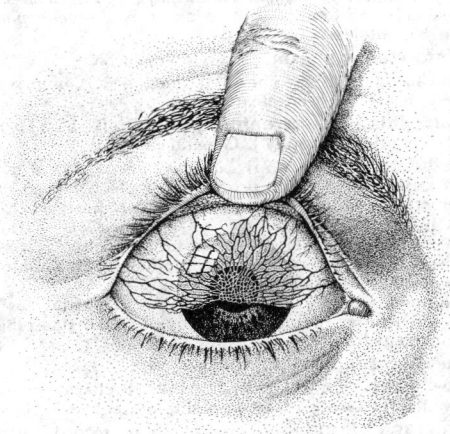

**Pannus**

**phlycten′ular p.,** p. occurring in phlyctenular conjunctivitis.

**panod′ic** [ pan- + G. *hodos*, way ]. Panthotic; pollodic; denoting a wide and extreme diffusion of a nerve impulse.

**pan'opho'bia.** A state of general apprehension, or fear of everything; pantophobia; panphobia.

**panophthalmia, panophthalmitis** (pan'of-thal'mĭ-ah, -of'thal-mi'tis) [ pan- + G. *ophthalmos*, eye ]. Inflammation of the eyeball in all its parts.

**panop'tic** [ pan- + G. *optikos*, relating to vision ]. All-revealing, denoting the effect of multiple or differential staining; see under stain.

**panotitis** (pan'o-ti'tis) [ pan- + G. *ous*, ear, + suffix *-itis*, inflammation ]. General inflammation of all parts of the ear; specifically, a disease described by Politzer which begins as an otitis interna, the inflammation subsequently extending to the middle ear and neighboring structures.

**panphobia** (pan-fo'bĭ-ah) [ pan- + G. *phobos*, fear ]. Panophobia.

**panplegia** (pan-ple'jĭ-ah) [ pan- + G. *plēgē*, stroke ]. Paralysis of the four extremities.

**Pansch,** Adolf, German anatomist, 1841–1887. See P.'s *fissure.*

**pan'sclero'sis.** Universal sclerosis of an organ or part.

**pansinuitis** (pan-sin-u-i'tis). Pansinusitis.

**pansinusitis** (pan-si-nus-i'tis). Pansinuitis; inflammation of all the accessory sinuses of the nose on one or both sides.

**panspermia, panspermatism** (pan-sper'mĭ-ah, pan-sper'mă-tizm) [ pan- + G. *sperma*, seed ]. The hypothetical doctrine of the omnipresence of minute forms and spores of animal and vegetable life, thus accounting for apparent spontaneous generation.

**pan'spo'roblast** [ pan- + G. *sporos*, seed, + *blastos*, germ ]. The reproductive area in the myxosporidia containing both vegetative and germinal nuclei.

**pan'sporoblas'tic.** Referring to a pansporoblast.

**pansystolic** (pan'sis-tol'ik). Holosystolic; lasting throughout systole, extending from first to second heart sound.

**pant** [ Fr. *panteler*, to gasp ]. To breathe rapidly and shallowly.

**pant-.** See panto-.

**pantalgia** (pan-tal'jĭ-ah) [ pant- + G. *algos*, pain ]. Pain involving the entire body.

**pantachromatic** (pant'ak'ro-mat'ik). Completely achromatic.

**pantam'ides.** A class of antibacterial substances derived from pantothenic acid.

**pantamor'phia** [ pant- + G. *a-* priv. + *morphē*, shape ]. Shapelessness; general or over-all malformation.

**pantamor'phic.** Relating to or characterized by pantamorphia.

**pantanencephaly, pantanencephalia** (pan-tan'en-sef'ă-lĭ, -sē-fa'lĭ-ah) [ pant- + G. *an-* priv. + *enkephalos*, brain ]. Complete anencephaly.

**pant'ankylobleph'aron.** Ankyloblepharon.

**pantaphobia** (pan'tă-fo'bĭ-ah) [ pant- + G. *a-* priv. + *phobos*, fear ]. Absolute fearlessness.

**pantatrophia, pantatrophy** (pan-tă-tro'fĭ-ah, pan-tat'-ro-fi) [ pant- + atrophy ]. General atrophy.

**pantetheine** (pan'te-the'in) *Lactobacillus bulgaricus* factor (LBF); the condensation product of pantothenic acid and aminoethanethiol, *N*-pantothenyl-2-aminoethanethiol, HOCH₂—C(CH₃)₂—CHOH—CO—NH—CH₂—CH₂—CO—NH—CH₂—CH₂—SH; an intermediate in biosynthesis of CoA via 4'-phosphopantetheine (phosphate on the terminal —CH₂O group) and ATP.

$\quad$**p. kinase** (EC 2.7.1.34), an enzyme that catalyzes the phosphorylation of pantetheine by ATP to pantetheine 4'-phosphate.

**panthodic** (pan-thod'ik). Panodic.

**panto-, pant-** [ G. *pas*, all. PAN- ]. Prefixes to words derived from Greek roots, implying all, entire.

**pan'tograph** [ panto- + G. *graphō*, to record ]. 1. An instrument for reproducing drawings by a system of levers whereby a recording pencil is made to follow the movements of a stylet passing along the lines of the original. 2. An instrument for reproducing graphically the outlines of the chest. 3. In dentistry, an instrument used to record mandibular border movements that may be transferred to make equivalent settings on an articulator.

**pantoic acid.** HOCH₂—C(CH₃)₂—CHOH—COOH, the β-alanine amide of which is pantothenic acid, a constituent of CoA.

**pantomor'phia** [ panto- + G. *morphē*, shape ]. 1. The condition of an organism, as an amoeba, that is capable of assuming all shapes. 2. Perfect shapeliness or symmetry.

**pantomor'phic.** Capable of assuming all shapes.

**pantonine.** An amino acid identified in *Escherichia coli,* which may be an intermediate in the biosynthesis of pantothenic acid by that organism, containing NH₂ in place of the α-OH group of pantothenic acid.

**pantopho'bia.** Panophobia.

**pantoscopic** (pan'to-skop'ik) [ panto- + G. *skopeō*, to view ]. Fit for observing objects at all distances; denoting bifocal lenses.

**pantothen'ate.** A derivative of pantothenic acid.

$\quad$**p. synthetase** (EC 6.3.2.1), pantoate activating enzyme; converts pantoate and β-alanine to pantothenate with cleavage of ATP to AMP and PPᵢ.

**pantothen'ic acid.** *N*-(2,4-dihydroxy-3,3-dimethylbutyryl)-3-aminopropionic acid; the β-alanine amide of pantoic acid; HOCH₂—C(CH₃)₂—CHOH—CO—NH—CH₂—CH₂—COOH. A growth substance widely distributed in plant and animal tissues; part of the vitamin B₂ complex formerly called filtrate factor Y; part of coenzyme A. It is essential for growth of yeast and certain bacteria; deficiency in diet causes a dermatitis in chicks and rats and achromotrichia in the latter.

**pantothen'yl.** The acyl radical of pantothenic acid, present in pantotheine and CoA.

**pantoyl** (pan'to-il). The acyl radical of pantoic acid present in pantothenic acid and CoA.

**pantoyltaurine** (pan'to-il-taw'rin, -rēn). A pantothenic acid antimetabolite, analogous to that vitamin in structure except that taurine replaces β-alanine in the molecule.

**Panum's area.** See under area.

**Panzerherz** [ Ger. ]. Armored *heart.*

**panzootic** (pan-zo-ot'ik) [ pan- + (epi)zootic ]. Pandemic in relation to any of the lower animals.

**pap.** A food of soft consistence, like that of breadcrumbs soaked in milk or water.

**papain** (pap-a'in). Papayotin; caricin; a proteolytic enzyme (EC 3.4.22.2) obtained from papaya latex; used as a protein digestant and as a meat tenderizer.

**Papanicolaou** (pah-pah-nik'o-low), George N., Greek U. S. physician, anatomist, and cytologist, 1883–1962. See P. *examination, smear, stain.*

**Papaver** (pă-pa'ver, pă-pav'er) [ L. poppy ]. A genus of plants, one species of which, *P. somniferum* (family Papaveraceae), furnishes opium.

**papaveraldine** (pă-pav'er-al-din). Xanthaline.

**papav'erine.** A benzylisoquinoline alkaloid of opium. It is not a narcotic but it has mild analgesic action; does not evoke tolerance and has no addiction liability. It is a powerful spasmolytic. Also available as p. hydrochloride (NF, BP).

**papaw** (pă-paw'). See papaya.

**papaya** (pă-pi'yah, pă-pa'yah) [ Sp. ]. Carica; the fruit of the papaw (pawpaw), *Carica papaya* (family Caricaceae), a tree of tropical America. It possesses a proteolytic action and is the source of papain.

**papayotin** (pap-a'yo-tin). Papain.

**pa'per** [ L. *papyrus;* G. *papyros,* a kind of rush, from which writing paper was made ]. Charta. 1. A square of p. folded over so as to form an envelope containing a dose of any medicinal powder. 2. A piece of blotting p. or filter p. impregnated with a medicinal solution and dried; when burned the fumes are inhaled in the treatment of asthma and other respiratory affections. 3. Test p.

$\quad$**absorption p.,** fat-free filter p., used in fat and resin determinations.

$\quad$**alkanin p.,** Boettger's test p.; anchusin p.; filter p. dipped in a 3 per cent alcoholic solution of alkanin and dried; alkalies turn it blue or green, acids red.

$\quad$**anchusin p.,** alkanin p.

$\quad$**articulating p.,** occluding p.

azolitmin p., filter p., dipped in a solution of azolitmin and dried; used as an indicator, acids turning the purplish red to bright red, and alkalis turning it blue.

biuret p., strips of filter p. immersed in biuret reagent and allowed to dry.

Congo red p., p. impregnated with Congo red; used as a pH indicator, changing from blue-violet at 3.0 to red at 5.0.

filter p., an unsized p. used in pharmacy and chemistry for filtering solutions; many varieties are used for paper chromatography.

litmus p., blotting p. stained with litmus; used to test the reaction of urine and other fluids, being turned red if the fluid is acid.

occluding p., articulating p.; an inked p. or ribbon interposed between natural or artificial teeth to determine cusp contact when the teeth are in centric occlusion.

test p., a piece of filter p. impregnated with a solution of litmus or other test agent and dried; used as a test of the reaction of a fluid.

# PAPILLA

papilla, pl. papillae (pă-pil'ah, pă-pil'e) [ L. a nipple, dim. of *papula*, a pimple ]. [ NA ]. Any small nipple-like process.

acoustic p., *organum* spirale.

Bergmeister's p., in the embryonic eye a small mass of glial fibers and nuclei forming a transitory conical investment of the hyaloid artery at its emergence into the vitreous chamber. Vestiges of it may persist as a prepapillary membrane.

bile p., p. duodeni major.

p. of breast, p. mammae.

circumvallate p., p. vallata.

clavate papillae, papillae fungiformes.

conic papillae, papillae conicae.

papillae con'icae [ NA ], conic papillae; numerous projections on the dorsum of the tongue, scattered among the filiform papillae and similar to them, but shorter.

papillae co'rii [ NA ], papillae of the corium; papillae dermis; dermal papillae; the superficial projections of the corium or dermis that interdigitate with recesses in the overlying epidermis. They contain vascular loops and specialized nerve endings, and are arranged in ridgelike lines best developed in the hand and foot.

papillae of corium, papillae corii.

dentinal p., p. dentis.

p. den'tis [ NA ], dentinal p.; a projection of the mesenchymal tissue of the developing jaw into the cup of the enamel organ. Its outer layer becomes specialized columnar cells, the odontoblasts, that form the dentin of the tooth.

dermal papillae, papillae corii.

papillae dermis [ NA ], papillae corii.

p. duodeni major [ NA ], major duodenal p.; Santorini's major caruncle; point of opening of the common bile duct and pancreatic duct into the duodenum; it is located posteriorly in the descending part of the duodenum.

p. duodeni minor [ NA ], minor duodenal p.; Santorini's minor caruncle; the site of the opening of the accessory pancreatic duct into the duodenum, located anterior to and slightly superior to the major p.

filiform papillae, papillae filiformes.

papillae filifor'mes [ NA ], filiform papillae; numerous elongated conical projections on the dorsum of the tongue.

papillae folia'tae [ NA ], foliate papillae; numerous projections arranged in several transverse folds upon the lateral margins of the tongue just in front of the palatoglossus muscle.

foliate papillae, papillae foliatae.

fungiform papillae, papillae fungiformes.

papillae fungifor'mes [ NA ], fungiform or clavate papillae; numerous minute elevations on the dorsum of the tongue, of a fancied mushroom shape, the tip being broader than the base. The epithelium of many of these papillae have taste buds.

hair p., p. pili.

ileal p., *valva* ileocecalis.

p. inci'siva [ NA ], incisive p.; palatine p.; a slight elevation at the anterior extremity of the raphe of the palate.

incisive p., p. incisiva.

interdental p., interproximal p.; the gingiva that fills the interproximal space between two adjacent teeth.

interproximal p., interdental p.

lacrimal p., p. lacrimalis.

p. lacrimalis [ NA ], lacrimal p.; a slight projection from the margin of each eyelid near the medial commisure, in the center of which is the punctum lacrimale or opening of the lacrimal duct.

lenticular p., p. lenticularis; one of the projections on the dorsum of the tongue, similar to, but less elevated than, the fungiform papillae.

lingual p., (1) p. lingualis; (2) the lingual portion of gingiva filling interproximal space between adjacent teeth. In molar and premolar areas, there may be separate lingual and buccal papillae.

p. lingua'lis, pl. papillae lingua'les [ NA ], lingual p. (1); one of numerous variously shaped projections of the mucous membrane of the dorsum of the tongue.

major duodenal p., p. duodeni major.

p. mam'mae [ NA ], p. of the breast; nipple; mamilla (2); teat; thele; thelium; a wartlike projection at the apex of the mamma, on the surface of which the lactiferous ducts open; it is surrounded by a circular pigmented area, the areola.

minor duodenal p., p. duodeni minor.

nerve p., neurothele; one of the papillae in the skin containing a tactile corpuscle or other form of end organ.

p. nervi optici, *discus* nervi optici.

optic p., *discus* nervi optici.

palatine p., p. incisiva.

parotid p., p. parotidea.

p. parotidea [ NA ], parotid p.; the projection at the opening of the parotid duct into the vestibule of the mouth opposite the neck of the upper second molar tooth.

p. pili [ NA ], hair p.; a knoblike indentation of the bottom of the hair follicle, upon which the hair bulb fits like a cap; it is derived from the corium and contains vascular loops for the nourishment of the hair root.

renal p., p. renalis.

p. rena'lis, pl. papillae rena'les [ NA ], renal p.; the apex of a renal pyramid which projects into a minor calyx; some 10 to 25 openings of papillary ducts occur on its tip, forming the area cribrosa.

tactile p., one of the papillae of the skin containing a tactile cell or corpuscle.

urethral p., p. urethralis; the slight projection in the vestibule of the vagina marking the urethral orifice

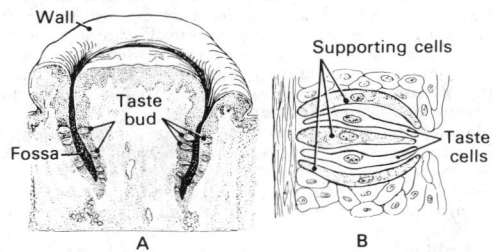

**Papilla Vallata**

*A*, microscopic section of papilla vallata of tongue; *B*, structure of taste bud.

p. valla'ta, pl. papillae valla'tae [ NA ], vallate p.; circumvallate p.; one of eight or ten projections from the dorsum of the tongue forming a row anterior to and parallel with the sulcus terminalis; each p. is surrounded by a circular trench (fossa) having a slightly raised outer wall (vallum); on the sides of the vallate p. and the opposed margin of the vallum are numerous taste buds.

vallate p., p. vallata.

vascular papillae, dermal papillae containing vascular loops.

---

**pap'illary.** Relating to, resembling, or provided with papillae.

**papillate** (pap'ĭ-lāt). Papillary.

**papillectomy** (pap'ĭ-lek'to-mĭ) [ papilla + G. *ektomē*, excision ]. Surgical removal of any papilla.

**papilledema** (pă-pil'e-de'mah) [ papilla + edema ]. Choked disk; edema of the optic disk; may be due to raised intracranial pressure, or part of a diffuse retinal edema, as in malignant hypertension.

**papilliferous** (pap'ĭ-lif'er-us) [ papilla + L. *fero*, to bear ]. Provided with papillae.

**papil'liform.** Resembling or shaped like a papilla.

**papillitis** (pap'ĭ-li'tis) [ papilla + G. suffix -*itis*, inflammation ]. Inflammation of the optic disk or renal papilla.
  **necrotizing p.,** see renal papillary *necrosis.*

**papillo-, papill-** [ L. *papilla, q.v.* ]. Combining forms for papilla, papillary.

**papilloadenocystoma** (pă-pil'o-ad'e-no-sis-to'mah). A benign epithelial neoplasm characterized by glands or gland-like structures, formation of cysts, and finger-like projections of neoplastic cells covering a core of fibrous connective tissue.

**papillocarcinoma** (pă-pil'o-kar-sĭ-no'mah) [ papilla + G. *karkinōma*, cancer ]. 1. A papilloma that has become malignant. 2. A carcinoma that is characterized by papillary, finger-like projections of neoplastic cells in association with cores of fibrous stroma as a supporting structure.

**papilloma** (pap'ĭ-lo'mah) [ papilla + G. suffix -*oma*, tumor ]. A circumscribed benign epithelial tumor projecting from the surrounding surface; more precisely, a benign epithelial neoplasm consisting of villous or arborescent outgrowths of fibrovascular stroma covered by neoplastic cells.
  **p. acumina'tum,** *condyloma* acuminatum.
  **p. canalic'ulum,** a papillomatous benign tumor arising within the duct of a gland.
  **canine oral p.,** warts affecting mucous membranes of young dogs, caused by a papovirus approximately 40 to 50 mμ in diameter.
  **p. diffusum,** widespread occurrence of p.'s.
  **duct p.,** intraductal p.
  **p. durum,** a hard p.; a wart, corn or cutaneous horn.
  **fibroepithelial p.,** skin *tag.*
  **hard p.,** p. durum.
  **Hopmann's p.,** Hopmann's polyp; a papillomatous overgrowth of the nasal mucous membrane.
  **infectious p. of cattle,** cattle warts; single or multiple rough nodules on the skin and mucous membranes caused by a virus; in young cattle, which are most susceptible, they are most numerous on the head, neck and shoulders; in cows they usually affect the udder and teats.
  **p. inguina'le trop'icum,** a cutaneous eruption, occurring in Colombia, characterized by numerous slender pink vegetations in the inguinal region.
  **intracys'tic p.,** one growing within a cystic adenoma, filling the cavity with a mass of branching epithelia processes.
  **intraductal p.,** duct p.; a small, often impalpable, benign p. arising in a lactiferous duct and frequently causing bleeding from the nipple.
  **p. mol'le,** soft p.
  **p. neuropath'icum** or **neurot'icum,** a papillomatous eruption or growth following the course of a nerve.
  **rabbit p.,** see Shope p.
  **rabbit oral p.,** a virus disease of rabbits characterized by nodules located usually on the lower surface of the tongue, but never on the skin as in Shope p.
  **Shope p.,** a common, virus-induced, wart of the wild cottontail rabbit of North America.
  **soft p.,** p. molle; (1) a p. with but a thin layer of horny epithelium; (2) any small soft growth, *e.g.,* a soft mole or nevus.
  **transitional cell p.,** a benign papillary tumor of transitional epithelium; in the urinary tract it is called transi-

tional cell *carcinoma* (*q.v.*), grade 1, because of the likelihood of its recurrence.
  **p. vene'reum,** *condyloma* acuminatum.
  **villous p.,** a p. composed of slender, finger-like excrescences occurring in the bladder or large intestines, from the duroid plexus of the lateral cerebral ventricle, or within the mammary gland.
  **zymotic p.,** yaws.

**papillomatosis** (pap'ĭ-lo-mă-to'sis). 1. The development of numerous papillomas. 2. Papillary projections of the epidermis forming a microscopically undulating surface.

**papillo'matous.** Relating to a papilloma.

**Papillon,** M. M. See P.-Lefèvre *syndrome.*

**Papillon-Léage.** See P.-L. and Psaume *syndrome.*

**papilloretinitis** (pap'ĭ-lo-ret'ĭ-ni'tis). Retinopapillitis; papillitis with extension of the inflammation to neighboring parts of the retina.

**papillula,** pl. **papil'lulae** (pă-pil'u-lah) [ Mod. L. dim. of L. *papilla* ]. 1. A small papilla. 2. Nipple.

**Papin** (pă-pań'), Denis, French physicist, 1647–1714. See P.'s *digester.*

**papovavirus** (pă-po'vah-vi'rus). See under virus.

**Pappenheim** (pah'pen-hīm), Artur, German physician, 1870–1916. See P.'s *stain,* Unna-P. *stain.*

**pap'pose, pap'pous** [ G. *pappos,* down ]. Downy.

**pap'pus** [ G. *pappos,* down ]. The first downy growth of beard.

**PAPS.** Abbreviation for adenosine 3'-phosphate 5'-phosphosulfate.

**papula,** pl. **pap'ulae** (pap'u-lah) [ L. ]. Papule.

**pap'ular.** Relating to papules.

**papula'tion.** The formation of papules.

**papule** (pap'ūl) [ L. *papula,* pimple ]. A small, circumscribed, solid elevation on the skin.
  **Celsus' p.'s,** *lichen* agrius.
  **follicular p.,** a papular lesion arising about a hair follicle; not specific for any condition.
  **moist p., mucous p.,** *condyloma* latum.
  **split p.'s,** p.'s at commissures of mouth seen in some cases of secondary syphilis.

**papulif'erous** [ papule + L. *fero,* to bear ]. Having papules.

**papulo-, papul-** [ L. *papula,* papule ]. Combining forms for papule.

**papuloerythematous** (pap'u-lo-ĕr'ĭ-them'ă-tus). Denoting an eruption of papules on an erythematous surface.

**pap'ulopus'tular.** Denoting an eruption composed of papules and pustules.

**pap'ulopus'tule.** A papule surmounted by a pustule.

**papulo'sis.** The occurrence of numerous widespread papules.
  **malignant atrophic p.,** Degos' syndrome; a fatal cutaneovisceral syndrome, characterized by pathognomonic umbilicated porcelain-white papules with elevated telangiectatic annular borders, followed by the development of intestinal ulcers which perforate, causing peritonitis.

**papulosquamous** (pap'u-lo-skwa'mus) [ papulo- + L. *squamosus,* scaly (squamous) ]. Denoting an eruption composed of both papules and scales.

**pap'ulovesic'ular.** Denoting an eruption composed of papules and vesicles.

**papyraceous** (pap'ĭ-ra'shus) [ L. *papyraceus,* made of *papyrus* ]. Like parchment or paper.

**papyraceus** [ L. ] [ NA ]. Papyraceous.

**Paquelin** (pak-lań'), Claude A., Paris physician, 1836–1905. See P.'s *cautery.*

**par** [ L. equal ]. A pair; specifically a pair of cranial nerves, *e.g.,* **p. nonum,** ninth pair, glossopharyngeal, **p. vagum,** the vagus or tenth pair.

**para-** (păr'ah-, păr'ă-) [ G. alongside of, near ]. A prefix denoting (1) a departure from the normal; (2) an involvement of two like parts, a pair as the two lower extremities; (3) a compound formed by two substitutions in the benzene ring arranged symmetrically, *i.e.,* linked to opposite carbon atoms in the ring. In chemical terms it is usually abbreviated *p-*, and those beginning thus but not listed here are alphabetized under the specific name.

**para** (păr'ah) [ L. *pario*, to bring forth. PARI- ]. A woman who has given birth to an infant or infants; see parity.

**para I.** Primipara.

**para II.** Secundipara.

**para III.** Tertipara.

**para IV.** Quadripara.

**para V.** Quintipara.

**para VI.** Sextipara.

**para-ac'tinomyco'sis.** Pseudactinomycosis.

**para-appendicitis.** Periappendicitis.

**paraballism** (păr'ăbal'izm) [ para- + G. *ballismos*, jumping about ]. Severe jerking movements of both legs.

**parabanic acid.** Oxalylurea.

**parabio'sis** [ para- + G. *biōsis*, life ]. 1. The fusion of whole eggs or embryos, as occurs in conjoined twins. 2. Temporary loss of nerve conductivity. 3. Surgical joining of the vascular systems of two individuals.

**parabiot'ic.** Relating to, or characterized by, parabiosis.

**parablasto'ma.** A neoplasm formed of structures of parablastic origin.

**parablep'sia** [ para- + G. *blepsis*, sight ]. Perverted vision, as in visual illusions or hallucination.

**parabu'lia** [ para- + G. *boulē*, will ]. Perversion of volition or will; one impulse is checked and replaced by another.

**paracanthoma** (păr'ak-an-tho'mah) [ para- + G. *akantha*, a thorn, + suffix -*oma*, tumor ]. A neoplasm arising from abnormal hyperplasia of the prickle cell layer of the skin.

**paracanthosis** (păr'ak-an-tho'sis). 1. The development of paracanthomas. 2. A division of tumors that includes the cutaneous epitheliomas.

**paracar'mine.** A staining fluid consisting of a solution of calcium chloride and carminic acid in 75 per cent alcohol.

**paracasein** (păr'ah-ka'se-in). The compound produced by the action of rennin upon Kcasein (which liberates a glycoprotein), and that precipitates with calcium ion as the insoluble curd.

**Paracel'sus** or Aureolus Theophrastus Bombastus von Hohenheim. A Swiss physician, 1493–1541; professor of medicine at Basel (Basle). His teachings were a strange mixture of conceit, showmanship, senseless bombast, mysticism, astrology, and sound medical wisdom; he contributed to pharmacy, pharmacology, and therapeutics. See also Paracelsian *method.*

**paracenesthesia** (păr'ah-se'nes-the'zĭ-ah) [ para- + G. *koinos*, common, + *aisthestai*, to perceive ]. Deterioration in one's sense of bodily well-being, *i.e.*, of the normal functioning of its organs.

**paracentesis** (păr'ah-sen-te'sis) [ G. *parakentēsis*, a tapping for dropsy, fr. *para*, beside, + *kentēsis*, puncture ]. Tapping (2); the passage into a cavity of a trocar and cannula or other hollow instrument for the purpose of removing fluid. The operation is variously designated, according to the cavity punctured.

  **p. abdom'inis,** p. of the abdomen; also called abdominocentesis, celiocentesis, celioparacentesis, peritoneocentesis.

  **p. cap'itis,** cephalocentesis.

  **p. cordis,** cardiocentesis.

  **p. cor'neae,** p. of the cornea; tapping of the anterior chamber of the eye.

  **p. ovarii,** needle exploration of the ovary for a cyst.

  **p. pericar'dii,** pericardiocentesis.

  **p. pulmo'nis,** pneumonocentesis.

  **p. thora'cis,** thoracentesis.

  **p. tym'pani,** myringotomy.

  **p. vesi'cae,** p. of the bladder.

**paracentet'ic.** Relating to paracentesis.

**paracen'tral.** Close to or alongside the center or some structure designated "central."

**paraceph'alus** [ para- + G. *kephalē*, head ]. A rarely used term denoting an omphalosite with a conspicuously malformed head which is usually rudimentary.

**paracet'amol** (BP). Acetaminophen.

**parachlorophenol** (păr'ah-klo'ro-fe'nol) (USP). *p-*Chlorophenol; used in dentistry as a local anti-infective. Also available as camphorated p. (USP).

**paracholera** (păr-ah-kol'er-ah). A disease clinically resembling Asiatic cholera but due to a vibrio specifically different from *Vibrio cholerae* (Koch).

**parachordal** (păr'ah-kor'dal) [ para- + G. *chordē*, cord ]. Alongside the anterior portion of the notochord in the embryo; designating the cartilaginous bars on either side which enter into the formation of the base of the skull.

**parachroia** (păr-ah-kroy'ah) [ para- + G. *chroia*, color ]. 1. Parachroma (1). 2. Obsolete term for dichromatism.

**parachroma** (păr'ah-kro'mah) [ para- + G. *chrōma*, color ]. 1. Parachromatosis; abnormal coloration of the skin. 2. Obsolete term for dichromatism.

**parachromatism** (păr'ah-kro'mă-tizm). Dichromatism.

**parachromatopsia** (păr'ah-kro'mă-top'sĭ-ah) [ para- + G. *chrōma*, color, + *opsis*, vision ]. Dichromatism.

**parachromatosis** (păr'ah-kro-mă-to'sis). Parachroma (1).

**parachymosin** (păr'ah-ki'mo-sin). An enzyme resembling chymosin (rennin).

**paracine'sia, paracine'sis.** Parakinesia, parakinesis.

**paracmasis** (păr-ak'mă-sis). Paracme.

**paracmastic** (păr'ak-mas'tik). Relating to the paracme; declining; past the prime; denoting the stage of subsidence of a fever, or the stage of senescence or physical decline.

**paracme** (păr-ak'me) [ G. the point at which the prime is past; fr. *para*, beyond, + *akmē*, highest point, prime ]. 1. The stage of subsidence of a fever. 2. The period of life beyond the prime; the decline or stage of involution of the organism.

**Par'acoccid'ioid'es brazilien'sis.** The pathogen of South American blastomycosis.

**paracoli'tis.** Inflammation of the peritoneal coat of the colon.

**paracolpi'tis** [ para- + G. *kolpos*, vagina, + suffix -*itis*, inflammation ]. Inflammation of the cellular tissues surrounding the vagina.

**paracol'pium** [ para- + G. *kolpos*, vagina ]. The tissues alongside the vagina.

**paracone** (păr'ah-kōn) [ para- + G. *kōnos*, cone ]. The mesiobuccal cusp of an upper molar tooth.

**par'acon'id.** The mesiobuccal cusp of a lower molar tooth.

**paracor'tex.** Deep cortex; tertiary cortex; thymus-dependent zone; the area of a lymph node between the subcapsular cortex and the medullary cords; it contains mostly the long-lived lymphocytes derived from the thymus.

**paracou'sis.** Paracusis.

**paracu'sia.** Paracusis.

**paracusis** (păr'ă-koo'sis) [ para- + G. *akousis*, hearing ]. Paracusia; paracousis. 1. Impaired hearing. 2. Auditory illusion or hallucination.

  **false p.,** Willis' p.; the apparent increase in auditory acuity of a deaf person to conversation in noisy surroundings due to his companion unconsciously raising his voice.

  **p. loci,** loss or diminution of the power of determining the direction of sound.

  **Willis' p.,** false p.

**paracyesis** (păr'ah-si-e'sis) [ para- + G. *kyēsis*, pregnancy ]. Extrauterine *pregnancy.*

**paracys'tic** [ para- + G. *kystis*, bladder ]. Alongside or near the bladder.

**paracystitis** (păr'ah-sis-ti'tis) [ para- + G. *kystis*, bladder, + suffix -*itis*, inflammation ]. Inflammation of the connective tissue and other structures about the urinary bladder.

**paracys'tium** [ para- + G. *kystis*, bladder ]. The tissues adjacent to the urinary bladder.

**paracy'tic** [ para- + G. *kytos*, cell ]. 1. Relating to cells other than those normal to the part where they are found. 2. Between or among, but independent of, cells.

**paradenitis** (păr'ad'ĕ-ni'tis) [ para- + G. *adēn*, gland, + suffix -*itis*, inflammation ]. Inflammation of the tissues adjacent to a gland.

**paraden'tal.** Periodontal.

**paraden'tium.** Periodontium.

**paradidymal** (păr'ah-did'ĭ-mal). 1. Relating to the paradidymis. 2. Alongside the testis.

**paradidymis,** pl. **paradidymides** (păr'ah-did'ĭ-mis, -dĭ-dim'ĭ-dēz) [ para- + G. *didymos*, twin, in pl. *didymoi*, testes ] [ NA ]. Parepididymis; a small body sometimes attached to the front of the lower part of the spermatic cord above the head of the epididymis; the remmants of tubules of the mesonephros.

**paradip'sia** [ para- + G. *dipsa*, thirst ]. Perverted appetite for fluids ingested without relation to bodily need.

**paradonto'sis.** Periodontosis.

**paradox** (păr'ă-doks) [ G. *paradoxos*, incredible, beyond belief, fr. *doxa*, belief ]. That which is apparently, though not actually, inconsistent with or opposed to the known facts in any case.

    **Weber's p.**, if a muscle is loaded beyond its power to contract it may elongate.

**para-equilibrium** (păr'ah-e'kwĭ-lib'rĭ-um). Vertigo, often associated with nausea, nystagmus, and muscular weakness, due to irritation of the vestibular apparatus of the ear.

**paraesthesia** (păr-es-the'zĭ-ah). Paresthesia.

**paraffin** (păr'ă-fin) [ L. *parum*, little, + *affinis*, neighboring, akin, so called because of its slight tendency to chemical reaction ]. 1. One of the methane series of acyclic hydrocarbons. 2. Hard p.

    **chlor'inated p.**, CHLORCOSANE; used as a solvent for dichloramine-T.

    **hard p.** (BP), p. (2); a purified mixture of solid hydrocarbons derived from petroleum.

    **liquid p.** (BP), mineral oil.

    **white soft p.** (BP), white petrolatum.

    **yellow soft p.** (BP), petrolatum.

**paraffinoma** (păr'ă-fĭ-no'mah) A tumefaction, usually a granuloma, caused by the prosthetic or therapeutic injection of paraffin into the tissues. The term is sometimes used with reference to similar lesions resulting from the injection of any oil, wax, or the like. See lipogranuloma.

**parafibrin'ogen.** A substance obtained in association with the precipitation of fibrinogen by means of sodium chloride.

**paraflagel'la.** Plural of paraflagellum

**paraflagellate** (păr'ah-flaj'ĕ-lāt). 1. Having one or more paraflagella. 2. Paramastigote.

**paraflagellum**, pl. **paraflagel'la** (păr'ah-flă-jel'um). A minute accessory flagellum sometimes present in addition to the oridinary flagellum of certain protozoans.

**parafollic'ular.** Associated with a follicle.

**paraformaldehyde** (par'ah-for-mal'de-hīd). Trioxymethylene; a polymer of formaldehyde; used as a disinfectant fumigant and topically in the treatment of various skin disorders.

**parafuchsin** (par-ah-fook'sin). Pararosanilin.

**paragammacism** (păr'ah-gam'ă-sizm) [ para- + G. *gamma*, the letter g ]. Faulty pronunciation of the sounds of g and k, or their substitution by other letters. See also gammacism.

**paragang'lia.** Plural of paraganglion.

**paraganglio'ma.** Chromaffin tumor; a neoplasm usually derived from the chromaffin tissue of a paraganglion or the medulla of the adrenal gland; when such a neoplasm produces hormone, it is usually termed pheochromocytoma.

    **nonchromaffin p.**, chemodectoma.

**paraganglion**, pl. **paraganglia** (păr'ah-gang'glĭ-on, -glĭ-ah). [ NA ]. Chromaffin body; a small, roundish body containing chromaffin cells; a number of such bodies may be found retroperitoneally near the aorta and in organs such as the kidney, liver, heart, and gonads.

**paragene** (păr'ah-jēn [ para- + gene ]. Replicating unit, other than a nucleus gene, that contains nucleoprotein and is involved in various aspects of metabolism in organisms; extrachromosomal hereditary determinants. Also called plasmid.

**paragen'ital.** Alongside the gonads.

**parageusia** (păr-ah-gu'sĭ-ah, -ju'sĭ-ah) [ para- + G. *geusis*, taste ]. Disordered or perverted sense of taste.

**parageu'sic.** Relating to parageusia.

**paraglob'ulin.** A globulin present in the blood plasma, lymph, and fluid exudates, precipitated by ammonium or magnesium sulfate.

**paraglobulinu'ria** [ paraglobulin + G. *ouron*, urine ]. The excretion of serum globulin in the urine.

**paragnathus** (păr'ag-nath'us) [ para- + G. *gnathos*, jaw ]. 1. An individual with an accessory lower jaw. 2. A parasitic fetus attached to the jaw of the autosite.

**paragnomen** (păr'ag-no'men) [ para- + G. *gnōmēn*, acc. case of *gnōmē*, judgment ]. An unexpected reaction.

**paragomphosis** (păr'ah-gom-fo'sis) [ para- + G. *gomphoō*, to nail or bolt, fr. *gomphos*, a bolt ]. Impaction of the head of the child in a narrowed parturient canal.

**paragonimiasis** (păr'ah-gon'ĭ-mi'ă-sis). Pulmonary distomiasis; endemic hemoptysis; parasitic hemoptysis; infection with a worm of the genus *Paragonimus*, especially *P. westermani*.

**Paragonimus** (păr'ah-gon'ĭ-mus) [ para- + G. *gonimos*, with generative power ]. A genus of trematode lung flukes that are parasitic in man and a wide variety of mammals that feed upon crustacea carrying the metacercariae.

    **P. kellicot'ti**, prevalent in certain wild animals, and occurs in dogs, in the Great Lakes region of the United States; it is morphologically similar to *P. westermani*.

    **P. rin'geri**, a species once thought to be distinct, but now regarded as *P. westermani*.

    **P. westerman'i**, Bronchial fluke; lung fluke; causes paragonimiasis and is found chiefly in Japan, Korea, Formosa, China, Philippines, and Thailand. Adult worms are ovoid, red-brown, 8 to 12 by 4 to 6 mm., and 3 mm. thick. Eggs are coughed up in sputum or swallowed and passed in the feces; miracidia invade *Melania* snails and the stumpy-tailed cercaria crawl into muscles and viscera of crayfish or crabs. Man acquires infection by ingesting raw or inadequately cooked crustacea, and the metacercariae then excyst in the duodenum, invade the wall of the gut, and migrate through the serous membranes and diaphragm into the lungs; the developing parasites cause an intense inflammatory reaction and eventually form fibrous-walled nodules that usually contain a pair of adult worms, exudate, eggs, and the remains of red blood cells; the fibroparasitic nodules may become contiguous and form multiloculated cystlike structures. In some instances, the flukes involve the brain, liver, peritoneum, intestine, or skin. Formerly termed *Distoma westermani, D. ringeri*, and *P. ringeri*.

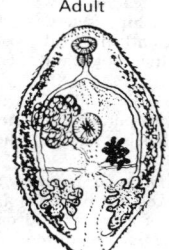
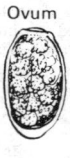

Adult      Ovum

*Paragonimus westermani*
Modified after Jeffrey, H. C., and Leach, R. M.: *Atlas of Medical Helminthology and Protozoology*, Churchill Livingstone, Edinburgh, 1966.)

**paragonorrheal** (păr'ah-gon-o-re'al). Indirectly related to or consequent upon gonorrhea.

**paragram'matism.** Paraphasia.

**paragranulo'ma.** A cellular infiltrate with some features of a granuloma, especially with a relatively good prognosis.

    **Hodgkin's p.**, an indolent form of Hodgkin's disease, in which a few lymph nodes are enlarged by an infiltrate replacing the normal structure, composed of reticulum cells with pole-staining nuclei, occurring as scattered single cells separated by lymphocytes. After a variable interval, up to many years, the condition transforms into a more rapidly progressive and widespread lymphoma, usually the ordinary type of Hodgkin's disease.

**paragraphia** (păr-ah-graf'ĭ-ah) [ para- + G. *graphō*, to write ]. 1. Loss of the power of writing from dictation, although the words are heard and comprehended. 2. Writing one word when another is intended.

**parahem'atin.** A ferriporphyrin linked to two moles of a nitrogenous base; now termed (base) ferriporphyrins.

**parahemophilia** (păr'ah-he'mo-fil'ĭ-ah). A hemorrhagic tendency, due to deficiency in factor V.

**parahepat'ic.** Adjacent to the liver.

**parahidro'sis.** Paridrosis.

**parahormone** (păr'ah-hor'mōn). A substance, product of ordinary metabolism, not produced for a specific purpose, that acts like a hormone in modifying the activity of some distant organ; a familiar example is the action of carbon dioxide on the control of breathing.

**parahypno'sis.** (păr'ah-hip-no'sis) Disordered sleep, such as nightmare or somnambulism.

**parahypophysis** (păr'ah-hi-pof'ĭ-sis). A small mass of pituitary tissue, or tissue resembling in structure the anterior lobe of the hypophysis, occasionally found in the dura mater lining of the sella turcica.

**parakeratosis** (păr'ah-kĕr'ă-to'sis) [ para- + keratosis, *q.v.* ]. The retention of nuclei in the cells of the stratum corneum of the epidermis. This is observed in many scaly dermatoses such as psoriasis and exfoliative dermatitis.

   **p. ostra'cea,** p. scutularis.

   **porcine p.,** a skin disease of young pigs characterized by a hard, scaly, proliferation of the surface layers of the skin. The extremities are commonly affected first, but it may involve the entire body. It is thought to be due to a deficiency of fatty acids occasioned by an excessive demand because of the great growth rate of this species in early life. Zinc salts appear to influence this disease favorably.

   **p. psoriasifor'mis,** an eruption marked by the presence of thick scales resembling those of psoriasis.

   **p. scutula'ris,** p. ostracea; a disease of the scalp marked by the formation of crusts that envelop the hairs.

   **p. variega'ta,** parapsoriasis.

**parakinesia, parakinesis** (păr'ah-kĭ-ne'zĭ-ah, -kĭ-ne'sis) [ para- + G. *kinēsis*, movement ]. Any motor abnormality.

**parala'lia** [ para- + G. *lalia*, talking ]. Any speech defect; especially one in which one letter is habitually substituted for another.

   **p. litera'lis,** stammering.

**paralambdacism** (păr'ah-lam'dă-sizm) [ para- + G. *lambda*, letter l ]. Mispronunciation of the letter l, or the substitution of some other letter for it. See also lambdacism.

**paralbu'min.** An albuminous substance, a mixture of metalbumin and serum albumin, found in the fluid of ovarian cysts and in ascites.

**paraldehyde** (păr-al'de-hīd) (USP, BP). Paracetaldehyde; a polymer, $(CH_3CHO)_3$, of acetaldehyde; a safe, potent hypnotic and sedative suitable for oral, rectal, intravenous, and intramuscular administration; its offensive odor limits its use.

**paraleprosis** (păr-ah-lĕ-pro'sis). The presence of certain trophic or nerve changes suggesting an attenuated form of leprosy in regions where the disease has long prevailed.

**paralepsy** (par-ah-lep'sĭ) [ G. para- + *lepsis*, seizure ]. 1. A temporary attack of mental inertia and hopelessness. 2. A sudden alteration in mood or emotional tension.

**paralexia** (păr'ah-lek'sĭ-ah) [ para- + G. *lexis*, speech ]. Misapprehension of written or printed words, other meaningless words being substituted for them in reading.

**paralgesia** (păr'al-je'zĭ-ah) [ para- + G. *algēsis*, the sense of pain ]. Painful paresthesia; any disorder or abnormality of the sense of pain.

**paral'gia** [ para- + G. *algos*, pain ]. Abnormal or unusual pain.

**paral'inin.** Karyolymph.

**parallac'tic.** Relating to a parallax.

**parallagma** (păr'ă-lag'mah) [ G. ]. Displacement or over-riding of the ends of a broken bone.

**parallax** (păr'ă-laks) [ G. alternately, fr. *par-allassō*, to make alternate, fr. *allos*, other ]. 1. The apparent displacement of an object by a change in the position from which it is viewed. 2. See phi *phenomenon.*

   **binoc'ular p.,** stereoscopic p.; the difference in the angles formed by the lines of sight to two objects situated at

different distances from the eyes. This angular difference is a factor in the visual perception of depth.

   **heteron'ymous p.,** the apparent movement of an object toward the closed eye; noted in exophoria.

   **homon'ymous p.,** the apparent movement of an object toward the open eye when one is closed; noted in esophoria.

   **stereoscopic p.,** binocular p.

   **vertical p.,** the relative vertical displacement of the image when each eye is closed in turn; see in vertical diplopia, or heterophoria.

**parallelism** (păr'ă-lel-izm) [ para- + G. *allēlōn*, of one another (gen. pl.), fr, *allos*, other ]. 1. The state of being structurally parallel. 2. In psychology, the doctrine that for every conscious process there is a corresponding or parallel organic process, without asserting a causal interrelation between the two parallel systems.

**parallelometer** (păr'ă-lel-om'e-ter). 1. An instrument for measuring or accomplishing parallelism. 2. An apparatus used for paralleling the attachments and abutments for fixed or removable partial dentures.

**parallergic** (păr'ă-ler'jik). Denoting an allergic state in which the body becomes predisposed to nonspecific stimuli following original sensitization with a specific allergen.

**paralogia** (păr'ă-lo'jĭ-ah) [ G. *paralogia*, a fallacy, fr. *para*, beside, + *logos*, reason ]. Paralogism; paralogy; false reasoning, involving self-deception.

   **thematic p.,** false reasoning in relation chiefly to one theme or subject, upon which the mind dwells insistently.

**paralogism** (pă-ral'o-jizm). Paralogia.

**paralogy** (pă-ral'o-jĭ). Paralogia.

**paral'ysin.** Agglutinin.

**paralysis,** pl. **paralyses** (pă-ral'ĭ-sis, -sēz) [ G. fr. para- + *lysis*, a loosening. LY- ]. 1. Palsy (*q.v.*); loss of power of voluntary movement in a muscle through injury or disease of its nerve supply. 2. Anesthesia; loss of sensation in a part. 3. Loss of any function, as of secretion or of mental action.

   **acute ascending p.,** Landry's p.; Kussmaul-Landry p.; a p. of rapid course beginning in the legs and involving progressively the trunk, arms, and neck, ending sometimes in death in from one to three weeks.

   **acute atroph'ic p.,** acute anterior *poliomyelitis.*

   **acute infectious p.,** acute anterior *poliomyelitis.*

   **p. agitans,** parkinsonism (1).

   **anterior spinal p.,** anterior *poliomyelitis.*

   **ascending p.,** p. that advances progressively from the periphery toward the nerve center, or from the lower toward the upper portions of the body.

   **asthe'nic bulbar,** or **bulbospi'nal p.,** *myasthenia* gravis.

   **atrophic spinal p.,** anterior *poliomyelitis.*

   **Brown-Séquard's p.,** (1) a reflex flaccid paraplegia occurring in the course of some affections of the urinary tract; (2) Brown-Séquard's *syndrome.*

   **bulbar p.,** progressive bulbar p.

   **central p.,** p. due to a lesion in the brain or spinal cord.

   **Chastek p.,** a disease of foxes and mink caused by feeding raw fish of certain types which contain an enzyme destructive of thiamin; the thiamin deficiency causes loss of appetite, emaciation, and finally paralysis and death.

   **compression p.,** p. due to compression of a nerve, usually of the arm, due to prolonged pressure, *e.g.*, during sleep, or from the pressure of a crutch.

   **conjugate p.,** p. of one or more of the external muscles of the eye, resulting in loss of conjugate movement of the eyes.

   **crossed p.,** alternate *hemiplegia.*

   **crutch p.,** a form of compression p.

   **decu'bitus p.,** a form of compression p. due to pressure on a limb during sleep.

   **diphtherit'ic p.,** postdiphtheritic p.

   **diver's p.,** caisson *disease.*

   **Duchenne's p.,** childhood muscular *dystrophy.*

   **Duchenne-Erb p.,** Erb's *palsy.*

   **epidem'ic p.,** acute anterior *poliomyelitis.*

   **Erb's p.,** Erb's *palsy.*

   **Erb's spinal p.,** chronic myelitis of syphilitic origin.

   **essential p. of children,** acute anterior *poliomyelitis.*

   **facial p.,** facial *palsy.*

   **famil'ial periodic p.,** see periodic p.

**faucial p.,** isthmoparalysis.

**fowl p.,** see avian *lymphomatosis.*

**general p. of the insane,** paresis (2).

**ginger p.,** jake p.

**global p.,** p. of both whole sides of the body; survival is usually of short duration.

**gloss′ola′biolaryn′geal p., gloss′ola′biopharyn′geal p.,** progressive bulbar p.

**Gubler's p.,** alternate *hemiplegia.*

**hyperkalemic periodic p.,** adynamia episodica hereditaria; a form of periodic p. (*q.v.*) in which the serum potassium level is elevated during attacks; onset occurs in infancy, attacks are frequent but relatively mild, myotonia is often present; autosomal dominant inheritance.

**hypokalemic periodic p.,** a form of period p. (*q.v.*) in which the serum potassium level is low during attacks; onset usually occurs between the ages of 7 and 21 years; attacks may be precipitated by exposure to cold, high carbohydrate meal, or alcohol, may last hours to days, and may cause respiratory p.; autosomal dominant inheritance with reduced penetrance in females.

**immunological p.,** lack of specific antibody production after exposure to large doses of the antigen; immunological p. disappears when the antigen is eliminated.

**infantile p.,** acute anterior *poliomyelitis.*

**infantile spinal p.,** acute anterior *poliomyelitis.*

**infectious bulbar p.,** Aujeszky's *disease.*

**jake p.,** ginger p.; neuropathy produced by drinking synthetic Jamaica ginger (popular name "jake") containing triorthocresylphosphate.

**Klumpke's p.,** Klumpke-Déjérine syndrome; atrophic p. of the forearm and small muscles of the hand together with paralysis of the cervical sympathetic, due often to injury at birth.

**Kussmaul-Landry p.,** acute ascending p.

**labial p.,** progressive bulbar p.

**Landry's p.,** acute ascending p.

**lead p.,** lead *palsy.*

**Little's p.,** acute anterior *poliomyelitis.*

**mimetic p.,** p. of the facial muscles.

**mixed p.,** combined motor and sensory p.

**morning p.,** infantile p. in which the stage of fever is slight or absent, a child being put to bed well and waking up paralyzed.

**motor p.,** loss of the power of muscular contraction.

**musculospi′ral p.,** p. of the muscles of the forearm due to injury of the radial (musculospiral) nerve.

**myogen′ic p.,** acute anterior *poliomyelitis.*

**normokalemic periodic p.,** sodium-responsive periodic p.; a form of periodic p. (*q.v.*) in which the serum potassium level is within normal limits during attacks; onset usually occurs between the ages of 2 and 5 years; there is often severe quadriplegia, usually improved by the administration of sodium salts; autosomal dominant inheritance.

**obstetrical p.,** birth *palsy.*

**ocular p.,** complete p. of extraocular and intraocular muscles.

**parturient p.,** milk *fever* (2).

**periodic p.,** term for a group of diseases characterized by recurring episodes of muscular weakness or flaccid p. without loss of consciousness, speech, or sensation; attacks begin when the patient is at rest, and there is apparent good health between attacks. See hyperkalemic periodic p., hypokalemic periodic p., and normokalemic periodic p.

**postdiphtherit′ic p.,** diphtheritic p.; p. affecting the uvula most frequently, but also any other muscle, due to toxic neuritis; it comes on, as a rule, in the second or third week following the beginning of the attack of diphtheria.

**posti′cus p.,** p. of the posterior cricothyroid muscles.

**Pott's p.,** Pott's *paraplegia.*

**progressive bulbar p.,** bulbar p. or palsy; labial p.; glossolabiolaryngeal p.; glossolabiopharyngeal p.; Duchenne's disease; Erb's disease; a progressive atrophy and p. of the muscles of the tongue, lips, palate, pharynx, and larynx, occurring in later life and due to atrophic degeneration of the neurons innervating these muscles.

**pseudobul′bar p.,** p. of the lips and tongue, simulating progressive bulbar p., due to cerebral lesions, involving the upper motor neurons bilaterally. There is difficulty in speech and swallowing, with emotional instability. Some-

times referred to as "laughing sickness," because spasmodic, mirthless laughter is a common symptom.

**pseudohypertroph′ic muscular p.,** childhood muscular *dystrophy.*

**range p.,** see avian *lymphomatosis.*

**Remak's p.,** lead *palsy.*

**sensory p.,** loss of sensation; anesthesia.

**sleep p.,** sleep dissociation; a condition in which upon waking in the morning the person is aware of his surroundings but is unable to move.

**sodium-responsive periodic p.,** normokalemic periodic p.

**spastic spinal p.,** spastic *diplegia.*

**spinal p.,** myeloparalysis; myeloplegia; rachioplegia; loss of motor power due to a lesion of the spinal cord.

**supranuclear p.,** p. due to lesions above the primary motor neurons.

**tick p.,** an ascending p. caused, mainly in children, by sustained bites of ticks of the genera *Dermacentor* and *Ixodes,* which are found in the western United States, British Columbia, and other regions; it also occurs in dogs, calves, and sheep.

**Todd's p.,** temporary p. that occurs in the limb or limbs involved in the Jacksonian convulsions of epilepsy after the fit is over; it lasts ordinarily not longer than a few days.

**Todd's postepileptic p.,** Todd's p.

**p. vacil′lans,** chorea.

**vasomotor p.,** vasoparesis.

**wasting p.,** progressive muscular *atrophy.*

**Zenker's p.,** paresthesia and p. in the area of the external popliteal nerve.

**paralyssa** (păr′ă-lis′ah) [ paralysis + G. *lyssa,* madness (rabies) ]. Trinidad disease; a paralytic form of rabies occurring in Trinidad and Brazil, caused by the bite of the vampire bat (*Desmodus*).

**paralytic** (păr′ă-lit′ik) 1. Relating to paralysis. 2. A person suffering from paralysis.

**paralyzant** (pă-ral′ī-zant). 1. Causing paralysis. 2. Any agent, such as curare, that causes paralysis.

**paralyze** (păr′ă-līz). To produce paralysis in.

**paralyzer** (păr′ă-li′zer). 1. Anything causing paralysis. 2. Any substance inhibiting a chemical reaction (inhibitor).

**paramagnet′ic.** Having the property of paramagnetism.

**paramag′netism.** The property of being magnetic, as shown by assuming a position parallel with the lines of force between the two poles of a magnet.

**paramastigote** (păr′ah-mas′tĭ-gōt) [ para- + G. *mastix,* whip ]. A mastigote having two flagella, one long and one short.

**paramastitis** (păr-ah-mas-ti′tis) [ para- + G. *mastos,* breast, + suffix -*itis,* inflammation ]. Submammary *mastitis.*

**paramas′toid.** Near the mastoid process.

**parame′cin.** Name used for a substance or substances liberated by some strains of *Paramecium aurelia* or by symbiotes present in cultures of them and poisonous to other strains of *Paramecia.*

**Paramecium** (păr′ah-me′shĭ-um, -sī-um) [ G. *paramēkēs,* rather long, fr. *mēkos,* length ]. A genus of ciliates, the members of which are of rather elongated form and some of large size even visible to the naked eye.

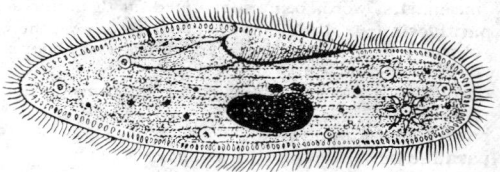

*Paramecium* (×140)

**parame′dian.** Near the middle line.

**paramed′ical.** Related to the medical profession in an adjunctive capacity, *e.g.,* denoting allied fields such as nursing, physical therapy, speech therapy, etc.

**parame′nia** [ para- + G. *mēn,* month ]. Any disorder or irregularity of menstruation.

**parame'sial.** Paramedian.

**paramesonephric** (păr'ah-mes-o-nef'rik). Close to or alongside the embryonic mesonephros.

**parameter** (pă-ram'e-ter) [ para- + G. *metron*, measure ]. One of many ways of measuring or describing an object or evaluating a subject. Examples are: (a) In a mathematical expression, an arbitrary constant which can possess different values, each value defining other expressions, and can determine the specific form but not the general nature of the expression; *e.g.*, in the equation $y = a + bx$, $a$ and $b$ are parameters. (b) In statistics, a term used to define a characteristic of a population, in contrast to a sample from that population; *e.g.*, the mean and standard deviation of a total population. (c) In psychoanalysis, any tactic, other than interpretation, used by the analyst to further the patient's progress.

**paramethadione** (păr'ah-meth'ă-di'ōn) (USP, BP). PARADIONE; 3,5-dimethyl-5-ethyloxazolidine-2,4-dione; used in petit mal epilepsy.

**parameth'asone.** 6α-Fluoro-11β,17α,21-trihydroxy-16α-methyl-1,4-pregnadiene-3,20-dione (see steroids). A semisynthetic steroid (a derivative of prednisolone, hence of pregnane), with anti-inflammatory effects and toxicity similar to those of cortisol (see also cortisone). Not useful in treatment of adrenal insufficiency because it causes little sodium retention.
  **p. acetate** (NF), MONOCORTIN; acetic ester of p. at C-21; a glucocorticoid useful in the treatment of rheumatoid arthritis and other collagen diseases, allergic conditions, and certain hematologic disorders.

**paramet'ric.** Relating to the parametrium, or structures immediately adjacent to the uterus.

**parametrismus** (păr'ah-me-triz'mus) [ parametrium + G. *trismos*, a creaking ]. Painful spasm of the muscular fibers in the broad ligaments.

**parametrit'ic.** Relating to parametritis.

**parametritis** (păr-ah-me-tri'tis) [ parametrium + G. suffix -*itis*, inflammation ]. Pelvic cellulitis; inflammation of the cellular tissue adjacent to the uterus.

**parametrium,** pl. **parame'tria** (păr'ah-me'trĭ-um) [ para- + G. *mētra*, uterus ] [ NA ]. The connective tissue of the pelvic floor extending from the fibrous subserous coat of the supracervical portion of the uterus laterally between the layers of the broad ligament.

**paramim'ia** [ para- + G. *mimia*, imitation ]. The use of gestures unsuited to the words which they accompany.

**paramnesia** (păr-am-ne'zĭ-ah) [ para- + G. *amnēsia*, forgetfulness ]. False recollection, events being recalled which have never occurred.

**Paramoeba** (păr-ă-me'bah). *Craigia.*

**paramo'lar.** A supernumerary tooth lying between, lingual, or buccal to the maxillary or mandibular molars.

**par'amorph.** An individual in which a structural change has been induced by environmental influences without any corresponding genetic change.

**paramor'phan.** Dihydromorphine hydrochloride.

**paramor'phia** [ para- + G. *morphē*, shape ]. Any abnormality in form or structure.

**paramor'phic.** Relating to a paramorph.

**paramor'phine.** Thebaine.

**Paramphistomum** (păr'am-fis'to-mum) [ para- + G. *amphistomos*, having a double mouth, fr. *amphi*, two-sided, + *stoma*, mouth ]. Rumen fluke; a genus of digenetic trematodes parasitic in the rumen or paunch of cattle. Species described in cattle include *P. microbothrioides, P. cervi,* and *P. liorchis.*

**paramu'cin.** A glycoprotein found in ovarian and certain other cysts, insoluble in water like mucin, but unlike mucin precipitated by tannin.

**paramu'sia.** Loss of the ability to read or to render music correctly.

**paramyloidosis** (pă-ram'ĭ-loy-do'sis). A variety of amyloid deposit seen in lymph nodes in some chronic nonspecific inflammations and in primary localized amyloidosis; histologic reactions are the same as in amyloidosis.

**paramyoclonus** (păr'ah-mi-ok'lo-nus) [ para- + G. *mys*, muscle, + *klonos*, a tumult ]. *Myoclonus* multiplex.

**paramyosinogen** (păr'ah-mi-o-sin'o-jen). v. Fürth's myosin; a coagulable globulin, constituting about 20 per cent of the protein of muscle plasma.

**paramyotonia** (păr'ah-mi-o-to'nĭ-ah). An atypical form of myotonia.
  **atax'ic p.,** a disorder characterized by a tonic muscular spasm on attempted movement, associated with slight paresis and ataxia.
  **congenital p., p. congenita,** Eulenburg's disease; a nonprogressive disease characterized by myotonia induced by exposure of muscles to cold; there are episodes of intermittent flaccid paralysis, but no atrophy or hypertrophy of muscles; autosomal dominant inheritance.
  **symptomatic p.,** a temporary rigidity of the muscles when first attempting to walk.

**paramyotonus** (păr'ah-mi-ot'o-nus). Paramyotonia.

**paramyxovirus** (păr'ah-mik'so-vi'rus). See under virus.

**paranalgesia** (păr-an'al-je'zĭ-ah) [ para- + analgesia, *q.v.* ]. Analgesia of the lower half of the body.

**parana'sal.** Alongside the nose.

**paraneph'ric.** 1. Relating to the paranephros. 2. In the region of the kidney.

**paranephros,** pl. **paranephroi** (păr'ah-nef'ros, -nef'roy) [ para- + G. *nephros*, kidney ]. *Glandula* suprarenalis.

**paranesthesia** (păr'an-es-the'zĭ-ah) [ para- + anesthesia, *q.v.* ]. Anesthesia of the lower half of the body.

**paraneu'ral** [ para- + G. *neuron*, nerve ]. Near or alongside a nerve.

**parangi** (pă-rang'ge, pă-ran'je). A disease similar to yaws, occurring in Ceylon.

**paranoia** (păr'ă-noy'ah) [ G. derangement, madness, fr. para- + *noeō*, to think ]. A severe but rare mental disorder marked by the presence of systematized delusions, often of a persecutory character, in an otherwise intact personality. When symptoms are relatively mild and mental illness is not present, the condition is called paranoid *personality* (*q.v.*).
  **acute hallucinatory p.,** a form in which there are interjected periods of hallucinations in addition to the systematized delusions.
  **litigious p.,** p. querulans.
  **p. origina'ria,** a form occurring in children.
  **p. querulans,** litigious p.; a morbid state characterized by discontent and the disposition to complain of imaginary slights.

**paranoiac** (păr'ah-noy'ak). 1. Relating to or affected with paranoia. 2. A person suffering from paranoia.

**paranoid** (păr'ah-noyd). Resembling paranoia.

**paranoidism** (păr'ah-noy-dizm). The paranoiac character; the condition of one suffering from paranoia.

**parano'mia** [ para- + G. *onoma*, name ]. A form of aphasia in which objects are called by the wrong names.

**paranuclear** (par-ah-nu'kle-ar). 1. Paranucleate. 2. Outside of, but near the nucleus.

**paranucleate** (păr'ah-nu'kle-āt). Relating to or having a paranucleus.

**paranucleolus** (păr'ah-nu-kle'o-lus). See sex *chromatin.*

**paranucleus** (păr'ah-nu'kle-us). An accessory nucleus, or small mass of chromatin lying outside of, though near, the nucleus.

**paraomphalic** (păr'ah-om-fal'ik) [ para- + G. *omphalos*, umbilicus ]. Paraumbilical.

**par'aop'erative.** Relating to the accessories of an operation, the preparation of the patient, asepsis, selection and care of the instruments, etc.

**paraovarian** (păr'ah-o-văr'ĭ-an). Parovarian (2); beside or in the neighborhood of the ovary.

**paraox'on.** MINTACOL; BAYER E 600; diethyl-4-nitrophenyl phosphate; an organophosphorous cholinesterase inhibitor used in insecticides. Parathion is converted in the liver to p.

**parapancreatic** (par'ah-pan-kre-at'ik). Near or alongside of the pancreas.

**paraparesis** (păr'ah-păr'e-sis) [ para- + paresis, *q.v.* ]. A slight degree of paralysis, affecting the lower extremities.

**paraparetic** (păr'ah-pă-ret'ik). 1. Relating to paraparesis. 2. A person with paraparesis.

**parapedesis** (păr'ah-pe-de'sis) [ para- + G. *pedēsis*, a bending, deflection ]. Excretion or secretion through an abnormal channel.

**parapep'tone.** Syntonin; acid albumin; albuminoids resulting from the incomplete proteolysis of albumin, intermediate between that and peptone; obtained by arresting the artificial digestion of a protein by neutralizing the previously acid pepsin solution.

**paraperitoneal** (păr'ah-pĕr'ĭ-to-ne'al). Outside of or alongside the peritoneum.

**parapestis** (păr-ah-pes'tis) [ para- + G. *pestis*, plague ]. Ambulant *plague*.

**paraphasia** (păr'ah-fa'zĭ-ah) [ para- + G. *phasis*, speech ]. Paraphrasia; paragrammatism; pseudagrammatism; jargon (2); a form of aphasia in which the patient has lost the power of speaking correctly. He substitutes one word for another, and jumbles his words and sentences in such a way as to make his speech unintelligible.

**thematic p.,** incoherent speech that wanders from the theme or subject under discussion.

**parapha'sic.** Relating to paraphasia.

**paraphemia** (păr'ah-fe'mĭ-ah) [ para- + G. *phēmē*, speech ]. A form of aphasia in which the patient constantly uses the wrong words.

**paraphia** (pă-ra'fĭ-ah) [ para- + G. *haphē*, touch ]. Parapsia; pseudaphia; pseudesthesia (1); any disorder of the sense of touch.

**paraphil'ia** [ para- + G. *philos*, fond ]. Sexual practices that are socially prohibited; see also sexual *perversion*.

**paraphimosis** (păr'ah-fi-mo'sis) [ para- + G. phimosis ]. 1. Constriction of the glans penis by a foreskin, with narrow orifice, which has been retracted behind the corona and cannot be drawn forward. 2. A retraction of the lid behind a protruding eyeball.

**parapho'nia** [ para- + G. *phōnē*, voice ]. Any disorder of the voice, especially a change in its tone.

**paraphora** (pă-raf'o-rah) [ G. a going aside, derangement. PHER- ]. Slight emotional disturbance.

**paraphrasia** (păr'ah-fra'zĭ-ah) [ para- + G. *phrasis*, speech ]. Paraphasia.

**paraphronia** (păr'ah-fro'nĭ-ah) [ G. *paraphrōn*, deranged, + *-ia*, condition ]. Decreased mentality accompanied by character change.

**paraphysial, paraphyseal** (păr'ah-fiz'ĭ-al). Pertaining to the paraphysis.

**paraphysis,** pl. **paraphyses** (pă-raf'ĭ-sis, -sēz) [ G. an offshoot. PHYS- ]. A median organ developing from the roofplate of the diencephalon in certain lower vertebrates.

**parapineal** (păr-ah-pin'e-al). Beside the pineal; denoting the visual or photoreceptive portion of the pineal body present, if not functioning, in certain lizards.

**par'aplasm** [ para- + G. *plasma*, a thing formed ]. 1. Hyaloplasm. 2. Malformed material.

**paraplas'tic.** Relating to paraplasm.

**paraplec'tic** [ G. *paraplēktikos*, paralyzed ]. Paraplegic.

**paraplegia** (păr-ah-ple'jĭ-ah) [ G. a stroke on one side, hemiplegia, fr. *para*, beside, + *plēgē*, a stroke. PLES- ]. Paralysis of both lower extremities and, generally, the lower trunk.

**ataxic p.,** progressive ataxia and paresis of the leg muscles due to sclerosis of the lateral and posterior funiculi of the spinal cord.

**congenital spastic p.,** infantile spastic p.; a spastic paralysis of the lower extremities occurring in the infant, due to meningeal hemorrhage following injury at birth; a form of obstetric paralysis or birth palsy.

**p. doloro'sa,** painful p.; paralysis of the lower extremities in which the affected parts, in spite of loss of motion and sensation, are the seat of excruciating pain; it occurs in certain cases of cancer of the spinal cord.

**p. in extension,** fixation of the paralyzed legs in extension, due to release of the antigravity mechanism.

**infantile spastic p.,** congenital spastic p.

**p. in flexion,** the fixation of the paralyzed legs in a flexed posture; usually in transection of the spinal cord.

**Pott's p.,** paralysis of the lower part of the body and the extremities, due to pressure on the spinal cord in Pott's disease of the spine.

**senile p.,** (1) simple weakness of the lower extremities, without atrophy or changes in the reflexes, occurring in the aged; (2) an acute p. due to hemorrhage or thrombosis of the spinal arteries; (3) a slowly developing paralysis of the lower, eventually of the upper, extremities, with involvement of the sphincters, due to softening of the anterior cornua of the spinal cord in the aged.

**spastic p.,** tetanoid p.; paresis of the lower extremities with increased irritability and spasmodic contraction of the muscles.

**superior p.,** paralysis of both arms.

**tetanoid p.,** spastic p.

**paraple'gic.** Relating to or suffering from paraplegia.

**parapoplexy** (păr-ap'o-plek'sĭ). Pseudoapoplexy.

**parapraxia** (păr'ah-prak'sĭ-ah) [ para- + G. *praxis*, a doing ]. A condition analogous to paraphasia and paragraphia in which there is a defective performance of purposive acts, *e.g.,* slips of the tongue, or mislaying of objects.

**paraprocti'tis** [ para- + G. *prōktos*, anus, + suffix *-itis*, inflammation ]. Inflammation of the cellular tissue surrounding the rectum.

**paraproctium,** pl. **paraproc'tia** (păr'ah-prok'shĭ-um, -tĭ-um) [ para- + G. *prōktos*, anus ]. The cellular tissue surrounding the rectum.

**paraprostatitis** (păr'ah-pros-tă-ti'tis) [ para- + L. *prostata*, prostate, + suffix *-itis*, inflammation ]. Extraprostatitis; inflammation of the tissue around the prostate gland.

**parapro'tein.** An abnormal plasma protein, such as macroglobulin, cryoglobulin, and myeloma protein.

**par'aproteine'mia.** The presence of abnormal proteins in the blood.

**parapsia** (pă-rap'sĭ-ah) [ para- + G. *hapsis*, touch ]. Paraphia.

**parapsoriasis** (păr-ah-so-ri'ă-sis). Parakeratosis variegata; xanthoerythrodermia perstans; a chronic dermatosis of unknown origin; it may appear as small or large scaling papules or in plaques.

**p. en plaque,** a benign form of parapsoriasis.

**p. lichenoi'des,** *poikiloderma* atrophicans vasculare.

**p. lichenoi'des et variolifor'mis acu'ta,** *pityriasis* lichenoides et varioliformis acuta.

**p. variolifor'mis,** *pityriasis* lichenoides et varioliformis acuta.

**parapsychology** (păr'ah-si-kol'o-jĭ). The study of extrasensory perception, such as thought transference (telepathy) and clairvoyance.

**parapsychosis** (păr'ah-si-ko'sis). A transitory psychotic episode.

**paraquat.** 1,1'-Dimethyl-4,4'-dipyridilium; a weedkiller that produces delayed toxic effects on the liver, kidneys, and lungs when ingested; progressive interstitial pneumonia with proliferation of alveolar lining cells may develop.

**pararec'tal.** Near the rectum or rectus muscle.

**parareflexia** (păr'ah-re-flek'sĭ-ah). A condition characterized by abnormal reflexes.

**pararhotacism** (păr'ah-ro'tă-sizm) [ para- + G. *rho*, the letter r ]. Mispronunciation of the letter *r*. See also rhotacism.

**pararosan'ilin.** Parafuchsin; C.I. Basic Red 9; a tri(aminophenyl)methane hydrochloride; an important red biologic stain.

**pararrhyth'mia.** A cardiac dysrhythmia in which two independent rhythms coexist, but not as a result of A-V block; p. thus includes parasystole and A-V dissociation (2), but not complete A-V block.

**parar'thria** [ para- + G. *arthron*, joint ]. A faulty mode of articulating.

**Parasaccharomyces** (păr'ah-sak'ă-ro-mi'sēz) [ para- + G. *sakcharon*, sugar, + *mykēs*, fungus ]. An obsolete generic name proposed in 1909 for a fungus isolated from ulcerations and later from nails and the respiratory tract. Species have been isolated from the intestine of persons with a spruelike disease; however, the fungus is not believed to be the causative agent. Probably identical with *Monilia* and *Candida*.

**parasa'cral.** Alongside the sacrum.

**parasalpingitis** (păr-ah-sal-pin-ji'tis) [ para- + salpinx, *q. v.,* + suffix *-itis*, inflammation ]. Inflammation of the tissues surrounding the Fallopian tube or the Eustachian tube.

**Paras′caris equo′rum.** *Ascaris equorum;* a large heavy-bodied ascarid nematode extremely common in the small intestine of horses and other equids. Larvae may develop in man or mice, but do not reach the adult stage.

**parasecre′tion.** Obsolete term for abnormal secretion.

**par′asexual′ity.** Abnormal or perverted sexuality.

**parasigmatism** (păr′ah-sig′mă-tizm) [ para- + G. *sigma,* the letter s ]. Sigmatism; lisping; mispronunciation of the letter *s.*

**parasinoidal** (păr′ah-si-noy′dal). Near a sinus in any sense, but particularly a cerebral sinus.

**parasite** (păr′ah-sīt) [ G. *parasitos,* a guest, fr. *para,* beside, + *sitos,* food ]. 1. An organism that lives on or in another and draws its nourishment therefrom. 2. In the case of a fetal inclusion or conjoined twins, the more or less incomplete twin that derives its support from the more nearly normal one called the autosite.

    **autistic p.,** autochthonous p.; a p. descended from the tissues of the host.

    **autochthonous p.,** autistic p.

    **commensal p.,** see commensal.

    **facultative p.,** an organism that may lead an independent existence or live as a parasite; opposed to obligate p.

    **incidental p.,** one that normally lives on another than its present host.

    **in′quiline p.,** see inquiline.

    **malignant tertian p.,** *Plasmodium falciparum.*

    **obligate p.,** one that cannot lead an independent nonparasitic existence; opposed to facutative p.

    **quartan p.,** *Plasmodium malariae.*

    **specific p.,** one that habitually lives on its present host.

    **temporary p.,** an organism accidentally ingested that survives briefly in the intestine.

    **tertian p.,** *Plasmodium vivax.*

**parasitemia** (păr′ah-si-te′mĭ-ah). The presence of parasites in the circulating blood; the term is used especially with reference to malarial and other protozoan forms, and microfilariae.

**parasit′ic.** 1. Relating to or of the nature of a parasite. 2. Denoting microorganisms that normally grow only in or on the living body.

**parasit′icide** [ parasite + L. *caedo,* to kill ]. 1. Destructive to parasites. 2. An agent that destroys parasites.

**parasitism** (păr′ah-sī-tizm). The process of parasitic infestation (usually restricted to external p.) or infection (usually restricted to internal p.) by which a parasite exists on or in a host organism.

    **multiple p.,** a condition in which parasites of different species parasitize a single host; in contrast to superparasitism (excessive parasitization by the same species).

**par′asitize.** To invade as a parasite.

**parasitocenose** (păr′ah-si′to-se-nōz) [ parasite + G. *koinos,* common, together ]. Parasite-host ecosystem; complex of all parasite species and individuals associated with a specific host.

**parasitogenic** (păr′ah-si′to-jen′ik) [ parasite + G. suffix -*gen,* producing ]. 1. Caused by certain parasites. 2. Favoring parasitism.

**parasitol′ogist.** One who is learned in the science of parasitology.

**parasitology** (păr′ah-si-tol′o-jī) [ parasite + G. *logos,* study ]. The branch of zoology and of medicine that treats of parasitism in all its relations.

**parasitome** (păr′ah-si-tōm) [ parasite + suffix -*ome* (fr. G. -*ōma*), group, mass ]. All individuals of all developmental stages of a single parasite species in one host.

**parasitophobia** (păr′ah-si-to-fo′bĭ-ah) [ parasite + G. *phobos,* fear ]. Morbid fear of parasites.

**parasitosis** (păr′ah-si-to′sis). Infestation with parasites.

**parasitotropic** (păr′ah-si-to-trop′ik). Pertaining to or characterized by parasitotropism.

**parasitotropism** (păr′ah-si-tot′ ro-pizm) [ parasite + G. *tropē,* a turning ]. Parasitotropy; the special affinity of particular drugs or other agents for parasites rather than for their hosts, including microparasites that infect a larger parasite; *cf.* organotropism.

**parasitotropy** (păr′ah-si-tot′ro-pī). Parasitotropism.

**paraspadia, paraspadias** (păr′ah-spa′dĭ-ah, -dĭ-us) [ G. *para-spaō,* to draw aside. SPA- ]. A condition in which there is a lateral opening into the urethra.

**paraster′nal.** Alongside the sternum.

**parastru′ma** [ para- + L. *struma, q.v.* ]. A goitrous tumefaction resulting from enlargement of a parathyroid gland.

**par′asympathet′ic.** Pertaining to a division of the autonomic nervous system; see *systema* nervosum autonomicum.

**parasympathet′icus** [ L. ] [ NA ]. Parasympathetic.

**parasym′patholyt′ic.** Parasympathoparalytic.

**parasympathomimetic** (păr′ah-sim′pă-tho-mĭ-met′ik) [ para- + G. *sympatheia,* sympathy, + *mimētikos,* imitative ]. Relating to drugs or chemicals having an action resembling that caused by stimulation of parasympathetic nervous system. See also cholinomimetic.

**parasym′pathoparalyt′ic.** Parasympatholytic; relating to an agent that annuls or antagonizes the effects of the parasympathetic nervous system, *e.g.,* atropine.

**parasympathotonia** (păr′ah-sim′pă-tho-to′nĭ-ah). Vagotonia.

**parasynanche** (păr′ah-sĭ-nang′ke) [ para- + cynanche, *q.v.* ]. Rheumatic inflammation of the muscles of the throat, or any angina, especially parotitis.

**parasynapsis** (păr′ah-si-nap′sis) [ para- + G. *synapsis,* a connection, junction ]. Union of chromosomes side to side in the process of "reduction."

**parasynovitis** (păr′ah-si-no-vi′tis) [ para- + synovitis ]. Inflammation of the tissues immediately adjacent to a joint.

**parasyphilis** (păr′ah-sif′ĭ-lis). Parasyphilosis; quaternary syphilis; any affection indirectly due to syphilis.

**parasyphilit′ic.** Denoting certain diseases supposed to be indirectly due to syphilis, though presenting none of the recognized anatomicopathologic lesions of that infection; *e.g.,* tabes dorsalis, general paralysis, paresis (2).

**parasyphilo′sis.** Parasyphilis.

**parasystole** (păr′ah-sis′to-le) [ para- + G. *systolē,* a contracting ]. A second automatic rhythm existing simultaneously with normal sinus rhythm, the parasystolic center being protected from the sinus impulses so that its rhythm is undisturbed.

**paratax′ia.** Parataxis.

**paratax′ic.** Pertaining to parataxis.

**paratax′is** [ para- + G. *taxis,* orderly arrangement ]. Parataxia; the psychological state or repository of attitudes, ideas, and experiences accumulated during personality development that are not effectively assimilated or integrated into the growing mass and residue of the other attitudes, ideas, and experiences of an individual's personality.

**paraten′on** [ para- + G. *tenōn,* tendon ]. The material, fatty or synovial, between a tendon and its sheath.

**parater′minal.** Near or alongside any terminus.

**parathi′on.** An organic phosphate insecticide, highly poisonous to animals and man. Great care must be used in applying it in the presence of livestock. It is an irreversible inhibitor of cholinesterases.

**parathor′mone.** Parathyroid *hormone.*

**parathymia** (păr′ah-thi′mĭ-ah) [ para- + G. *thymos,* soul, mind, THYM- ]. Misdirection of the emotional faculties; disordered mood.

**parathy′roid.** 1. Adjacent to the thyroid gland. 2. *Glandula* parathyroidea.

**parathyroidectomy** (păr′ah-thi′roy-dek′to-mī) [ parathyroid + G. *ektomē,* excision ]. Excision of the parathyroid glands.

**parathyrotropic, parathyrotrophic** (păr′ah-thi′ro-trop′ik, -trof′ik) [ parathyroid + G. *tropē,* a turning; *trophē,* nourishment ]. Influencing the growth or activity of the parathyroid glands.

**paratrichosis** (păr′ah-trī-ko′sis) [ para- + G. *trichōsis,* making or being hairy, fr. *thrix* ( *trich-* ), hair ]. Any disorder in the growth of the hair, with particular reference to quantity.

**paratrip'sis** [ G. friction, fr. *para*, beside, + *tripsis*, rubbing ]. 1. Chafing. 2. Obsolete term for retardation of catabolism or tissue waste.

**paratrip'tic.** Causing or caused by chafing.

**paratrophic** (păr'ah-trof'ik) [ para- + G. *trophē*, nourishment ]. Deriving sustenance from living organic material; parasitic; see also metatrophic, prototrophic.

**paratuber'culo'sis.** 1. A condition marked by symptoms of tuberculosis, in which the presence of the tubercle bacillus cannot be demonstrated; 2. Tuberculid; a scrofulous eruption; an inflammatory lesion of the skin due to the action of tuberculous toxin in the blood.

**paratuber'culous.** Relating to paratuberculosis.

**paratyphlitis** (păr'ah-ti-fli'tis) [ para- + G. *typhlon*, cecum, + suffix -*itis*, inflammation ]. Inflammation of the connective tissue adjacent to the cecum.

**paratyphoid** (păr'ah-ti'foyd). Resembling in some respects, yet not the same as, typhoid.

**paratypic, paratypical** (păr'ah-tip'ik, -tip'ĭ-kal) [ para- + G. *typos*, type ]. Deviating more or less from a type.

**paraumbilical** (păr'ah-um-bil'ĭ-kal). Paraomphalic; near the umbilicus.

**paraurethral** (păr'ah-u-re'thral). Alongside the urethra.

**paravaccinia** (par'ah-vak-sin'ĭ-ah) [ para- + vaccinia, *q.v.* ]. Milkers' nodules or nodes; pseudocowpox; an infection caused by a pox virus transmitted from cow udders to the fingers of milkers, producing nodules and lymphangitis, and occasionally widespread papular or papulovesicular eruption; human infection is transferable to uninfected cows. See also paravaccinia virus.

**paravaginal** (păr'ah-vaj'ĭ-nal). Alongside the vagina.

**paravaginitis** (păr'ah-vaj'ĭ-ni'tis). Inflammation of the cellular tissue alongside the vagina.

**paraval'vular.** Alongside or in the vicinity of a valve.

**paravenous** (păr'ah-ve'nus). Beside a vein.

**paraver'tebral.** Alongside a vertebra or the vertebral column.

**paraves'ical.** Paracystic; alongside the bladder.

**paraxanthine** (păr-ah-zan'thin). A xanthine base, $C_7H_8N_4O_2$, that is a urinary metabolite of ingested xanthines and that may be formed in excess in cases of gout.

**paraxial** (păr-ak'sĭ-al). By the side of the axis of any body or part.

**paraxon** (păr-ak'son) [ para- + G. *axōn*, axis ]. A collateral branch of an axon.

**parazoon** (păr-ah-zo'on) [ para- + G. *zōon*, animal ]. An animal parasite.

**parben'dazole** (USAN). Methyl 5-butyl-2-benzimidazolecarbamate; anthelmintic.

**parch'ment crack'ling.** The sensation as of the crackling of stiff paper or parchment, noted on palpation of the skull in cases of craniotabes.

**Paré** (par-a'), Ambroïse, French surgeon, 1510–1590. The most influential surgeon of his time and said to be the originator of modern surgery. See P.'s *suture*.

**parectasis, parectasia** (păr'ek'tă-sis, -ek-ta'zĭ-ah) [ G. *parektasis*, extrusion, fr. *para*, beside, + *ektasis*, extension ]. Extreme distention of a cavity or other part.

**parectropia** (păr-ek-tro'pĭ-ah) [ G. *par-ektropē*, a turning aside ]. Apraxia.

**paregor'ic** [ G. *parēgorkos*, soothing ] (USP). An antiperistaltic containing powdered opium, anise oil, benzoic acid, camphor, glycerin, and diluted alcohol.

**pareira** (pă-ra'ĭ-rah) [ Pg. *parreira*, vine trained against a wall ]. Pareira brava, the root of *Chondodendron tomentosum* and other species of *Chondodendron* (family Menispermaceae), a vine of tropical America; one of the chief sources of *d*-tubocurarine. It has diuretic and urinary antiseptic properties.

**parelectronomic** (păr'e-lek'tro-nom'ik) [ para- + G. *ēlektron*, amber (electricity), + *nomos*, law ]. Not subject to the laws of electricity, *i.e.*, not excited by an electric stimulus.

**parencephalia** (păr'en-sĕ-fa'lĭ-ah) [ para- + G. *enkephalos*, brain ]. A condition of imperfect cerebral development.

**parencephalitis** (păr'en-sef'ă-li'tis) [ parencephalon + G. suffix -*itis*, inflammation ]. Inflammation of the cerebellum.

**parencephalocele** (păr-en-sef'ă-lo-sēl) [ parencephalon + G. *kēle*, hernia ]. Protrusion of the cerebellum through a defect in the cranium.

**parenceph'alous.** Relating to parencephalia or to a parencephalus.

**parencephalus** (păr'en-sef'ă-lus) [ para- + G. *enkephalos*, brain ]. A fetus with imperfect cerebral development.

**parenchyma** (pă-reng'kĭ-mah) [ G. anything poured in beside, fr. *parencheō*, to pour in beside. CHY- ]. 1 [ NA ]. The distinguishing or specific cells of a gland or organ, contained in and supported by the connective tissue framework, or stroma. 2. The endoplasm of a protozoan cell.

**p. testis** [ NA ], the parenchyma of the testis, consisting of the seminiferous tubules located within the lobules.

**parenchymal** (pă-reng'kĭ-mal). Parenchymatous.

**parenchymatitis** (pă-reng'kĭ-mă-ti'tis). Inflammation of the parenchyma or differentiated substance of a gland or organ.

**parenchymatous** (păr'eng-kim'ă-tus). Relating to the parenchyma; parenchymal.

**paren'teral** [ para- + G. *enteron*, intestine ]. By some other means than through the intestinal canal, referring particularly to the introduction of nutritive material into veins and subcutaneous tissues.

**parepicele** (păr-ep'ĭ-sēl) [ para- + G. *epi*, upon, + *koilia*, a hollow ]. The lateral recess of the fourth ventricle of the brain.

**parepididymis** (păr'ep'ĭ-did'ĭ-mis). Paradidymis.

**parepithymia** (păr'ep-ĭ-thi'mĭ-ah) [ para- + G. *epithymia*, desire ]. Morbid longing; perverted desire or craving.

**parerethisis** (păr'ĕ-re'thĭ-sis) [ para- + G. *erethizō*, to excite ]. Perverted excitement.

**parergasia** (păr'er-ga'zĭ-ah) [ para- + G. *ergasia*, work ]. Schizophrenia.

**paresis** (pă-re'sis, par'e-sis) [ G. a letting go, slackening, paralysis, fr. *pariēmi*, to let go ]. 1. Partial or incomplete paralysis. 2. Dementia paralytica; general paralysis of the insane; a disease of the brain, syphilitic in origin, marked by progressive dementia, tremor, speech disturbances, and increasing muscular weakness; in a large proportion of cases there is a preliminary stage of irritability often followed by exaltation and delusions of grandeur.

**Lissauer's p.,** a disease characterized by physical and mental deterioration, seizures, hemiplegia, and aphasia.

**parturient p.,** milk *fever (2)*.

**paresthesia** (păr-es-the'zĭ-ah) [ para- + G. *aisthēsis*, sensation ]. Paraesthesia; an abnormal spontaneous sensation, such as of burning, pricking, tickling, or tingling.

**Berger's p.,** p. of the legs in young patients, especially at the beginning of a movement.

**paresthet'ic.** Relating to or marked by paresthesia.

**parethox'ycaine hydrochloride.** INTRACAINE hydrochloride; *p*-ethoxybenzoic acid 2-diethylaminoethyl ester; local anesthetic.

**paret'ic.** Relating to or suffering from paresis.

**pareunia** (păr-u'nĭ-ah) [ G. *pareunos*, lying beside, fr. *para*, beside, + *eunē*, a bed ]. Sexual intercourse.

**pargyline hydrochloride** (par'jĭ-lēn) (NF). EUTONYL; *N*-methyl-*N*-(2-propynyl)-benzylamine hydrochloride; a nonhydrazine monoamine oxidase inhibitor; an antihypertensive agent. Concurrent use of certain drugs that affect the central nervous system, and the liberal use of alcohol and cheese should be avoided.

**parhor'mone.** Parahormone.

**paridrosis** (păr'ĭ-dro'sis) [ para- + G. *hidrōsis*, sweating ]. Parahidrosis; any derangement of perspiration.

**paries**, gen. **pari'etis,** pl. **pari'etes** (păr'ĭ-ēz, pa'rĭ-ēz) [ L. wall. PARIE- ] [ NA ]. A wall, as of the chest, abdomen, or any hollow organ.

**p. anterior vaginae** [ NA ], the anterior wall of the vagina; it is somewhat shorter than the posterior wall and at its upper end is penetrated by the cervix uteri.

**p. anterior ventriculi** [ NA ], the anterior wall or surface of the stomach.

p. **caroticus cavi tym'pani** [ NA ], carotid, or anterior, wall of the middle ear; it contains the opening of the auditory (Eustachian) tube.

p. **exter'nus duc'tus cochlea'ris** [ NA ], external wall of the cochlear duct; the wall that faces the outer side of the cochlea.

p. **infe'rior or'bitae** [ NA ], inferior wall, or floor, of the orbit; it is the shortest of the four walls of the orbit and slopes upward from the orbital margin. The maxilla and orbital process of the palatine bone comprise it.

p. **jugula'ris cavi tym'pani** [ NA ], jugular wall of the middle ear; fundus tympani; inferior wall, or floor, of the tympanic cavity; a thin plate of bone separating the tympanic cavity from the jugular fossa.

p. **labyrinthicus cavi tym'pani** [ NA ], labyrinthic, or medial, wall of the middle ear; a bony layer separating the middle from the internal ear or labyrinth, it contains the fenestra vestibuli (ovalis) and the fenestra cochleae (rotunda).

p. **latera'lis or'bitae** [ NA ], lateral wall of the orbit; a triangular wall formed by the zygomatic bone, the greater wing of the sphenoid and a small part of the frontal bone. Posteriorly it is bounded by the superior and inferior orbital fissures.

p. **mastoid'eus cavi tym'pani** [ NA ], mastoid, or posterior, wall of the middle ear, containing the opening into the mastoid antrum.

p. **me'dialis or'bitae** [ NA ], medial wall of the orbit; the thin, rectangular wall formed by the orbital plate of the ethmoid, lacrimal, frontal and a small part of the sphenoid bones. The fossa for the lacrimal sac lies at its anterior limit.

p. **membrana'ceus cavi tym'pani** [ NA ], membranous, or lateral, wall of the middle ear, formed mainly by the membrana tympani.

p. **membrana'ceus tracheae** [ NA ], membranous wall of the trachea; the part of the tracheal wall posteriorly that is not reinforced by tracheal cartilages.

p. **posterior vaginae** [ NA ], the posterior wall of the vagina.

p. **posterior ventriculi** [ NA ], the posterior wall of the stomach; that part of the gastric wall that faces the omental bursa.

p. **supe'rior or'bitae** [ NA ], superior wall, or roof, of the orbit; formed by the orbital plate of the frontal bone and the lesser wing of the sphenoid bone, the optic canal opens at its posterior limit. An indentation, the fossa for the lacrimal gland, is located in the anterolateral part of the roof.

p. **tegmenta'lis tym'pani** [ NA ], tegmental wall of the middle ear; the superior wall, or roof, of the tympanic cavity, formed by the tegmen tympani of the temporal bone.

p. **tympan'icus duc'tus cochlea'ris** [ NA ], tympanic wall of the cochlear duct; membrana spiralis [ NA ]; spiral membrane; the wall that separates the cochlear duct from the scala tympani; it consists of the osseous spiral lamina and the basilar membrane.

p. **vestibula'ris ductus cochlea'ris** [ NA ], vestibular wall of the cochlear duct; membrana vestibularis; vestibular membrane; Reissner's membrane; the membrane separating the ductus cochlearis from the scala vestibuli. It consists of squamous epithelial cells with microvilli toward the ductus, a basement membrane, and a thin layer of connective tissue toward the scala. See fig. under cochlea.

**parietal** (pă-ri'e-tal). Relating to the wall of any cavity.

**parietes** (pă-ri'e-tēz) [ L. ]. Plural of paries.

**parieto-** (pă-ri'e-to-) [ L. paries, wall. PARIE- ]. Combining form meaning parietal; denoting relationship to any wall or to any paries.

**pari'etofron'tal.** Relating to the parietal and the frontal bones or the parts of the cerebral cortex corresponding thereto.

**parietography** (pă-ri'e-tog'ră-fi) [ parieto- + G. graphē, a writing ]. A combination of pneumoperitoneum and air study of the stomach.

**pari'etomas'toid.** Relating to the parietal bone and the mastoid portion of the temporal bone.

**parietooccipital** (pă-ri'e-to-ok-sip'i-tal). Relating to the parietal and occipital bones or to the parts of the cerebral cortex corresponding thereto.

**pari'etosphe'noid.** Relating to the parietal and the sphenoid bones.

**parietosplanchnic** (pă-ri'e-to-splangk'nik). Parietovisceral.

**parietosquamosal** (pă-ri'e-to-skwa-mo'sal). Relating to the parietal bone and the squamous portion of the temporal bone.

**pari'etotem'poral.** Relating to the parietal and the temporal bones.

**parietovisceral** (pă-ri'e-to-vis'er-al). Parietosplanchnic; relating to the wall of a cavity and to the contained viscera.

**Parinaud** (par-e-no'), Henri, Paris ophthalmologist, 1844–1905. See P.'s *conjunctivitis, ophthalmoplegia, syndrome.*

**pa'ri pas'su** [ L. ]. At the same rate or proportion.

**Paris green.** Cupric acetoarsenite; an insecticide (for Colorado beetle) and a pigment.

**Paris yellow.** *Chrome* yellow.

**parity** (păr'i-ti) [ L. pario, to bear. PARI- ]. The state of having given birth to an infant or infants, alive or dead, weighing at least 500 gm. or having an estimated length of gestation of at least 20 weeks; a multiple birth is considered as a single parous experience.

**Park,** Henry, Liverpool surgeon, 1744–1831. See P.'s *aneurysm.*

**Park,** William H., American bacteriologist, 1863–1939. See P.-Williams *bacillus, fixative.*

**Parker,** Edward Mason, U. S. surgeon, 1860–1941. See P.-Kerr *suture.*

**Parker,** George H., U. S. zoologist, 1864–1955. See P.'s *fluid.*

**Parker,** Willard, New York surgeon, 1800–1884. See P.'s *incision.*

**Parkinson,** James, English physician, 1755–1824. See P.'s *disease, facies.*

**Parkinson,** Sir John, English physician, *1885. See Wolff-P.-White *syndrome.*

**parkinso'nian.** 1. Relating to parkinsonism. 2. A sufferer from parkinsonism (1).

**parkinsonism** (par'kin-son-izm). 1. Paralysis agitans; Parkinson's disease; shaking palsy; spasmus agitans; a neurological syndrome usually resulting from arteriosclerotic changes in the basal ganglia and characterized by rhythmical muscular tremors, rigidity of movement, festination, droopy posture, and masklike facies. 2. A syndrome similar to p. appearing as a side effect of certain antipsychotic drugs.

**parmelin.** Atranorin.

**paroa'rium.** Paroophoron.

**paroccipital** (păr'ok-sip'i-tal) [ para- + occipital ]. Near or beside the occipital bone or the occiput.

**par'odonti'tis.** Periodontitis.

**parodontium** (par-o-don'shi-um) [ para- + G. odous, tooth ]. The tissues that surround, support and are attached to the teeth; includes the periodontium, gingivae, cementum, and alveolar bone.

**parodynia** (păr-o-din'i-ah) [ L. pario, to bear, + G. odynē, pain ]. Labor *pains.*

p. **perver'sa,** cross *birth.*

**parole** (pa-rōl'). In psychiatry, term for conditional release of a formally committed patient from a mental hospital prior to formal discharge, so that the patient may be returned to the hospital if necessary without fresh legal action.

**par'olfac'tory.** Associated with or related to the olfactory system.

**parolivary** (păr-ol'i-ver-i) [ para- + L. oliva, olive ]. By the side of or near the oliva.

**paromomycin sulfate** (păr'o-mo-mi'sin) (NF, BP). HUMATIN; a broad spectrum antibiotic produced by *Streptomyces rimosus* forma *paromomycinus;* used in the treatment of bacterial enteritis and amebiasis, and for preoperative suppression of intestinal bacteria.

**paromphalocele** (păr-om′fă-lo-sēl) [ para- + G. *omphalos*, umbilicus, + *kēlē*, tumor, hernia ]. 1. A tumor near the umbilicus. 2. A hernia through a defect in the abdominal wall near the umbilicus.

**Paro′na**, Francesco, Italian surgeon, 19th century. See P.'s *space*.

**paroneiria, paroniria** (păr-o-ni′rī-ah) [ para- + G. *oneiros*, dream ]. Disagreeable or terrifying dreams.

**p. salax**, restlessness in sleep, with lascivious dreams and nocturnal emissions.

**paronychia** (păr-o-nik′ī-ah) [ para- + G. *onyx*, nail ]. Onychia lateralis; onychia periungualis; inflammation of the nail fold with separation of the skin from the proximal portion of the nail; may be due to bacteria or fungi.

**paronychial** (păr-o-nik′ī-al). Relating to paronychia.

**paroophoritis** (păr′o-of′o-ri′tis) [ paroophoron + G. suffix *-itis*, inflammation ]. Inflammation of tissues adjacent to the ovaries.

**paroophoron** (păr′o-of′o-ron) [ para- + oophoron (*q.v.*), ovary ] [ NA ]. Parovarium; paroarium; organ of Rosen-müller; a few scattered rudimentary tubules in the broad ligament between the epoophoron and the uterus; remnants of the tubules and glomeruli of the lower part of the Wolffian body.

**parophthalmia** (păr′of-thal′mī-ah) [ para- + G. *ophthalmos*, eye ]. Inflammation of the tissues around the eye.

**parophthalmoncus** (păr-of′thal-mong′kus) [ para- + G. *ophthalmos*, eye, + *onkos*, mass, swelling ]. A neoplasm or other type of discrete mass near the eye.

**parop′sis** [ para- + G. *opsis*, vision ]. 1. Any disorder of vision. 2. False vision impression observed in the hemianoptic field.

**parorchidium** (păr-or-kid′ī-um) [ para- + G. *orchis*, testis ]. Ectopic *testis*.

**parorchis** (păr-or′kis) [ para- + G. *orchis*, testis ]. The epididymis.

**parorexia** (păr′o-rek′sī-ah) [ para- + G. *orexis*, appetite ]. Perverted appetite.

**parosmia** (păr-oz′mĭ-ah) [ para- + G. *osmē*, the sense of smell ]. Parosphresia; any disorder of the sense of smell, especially the subjective perception of odors that do not exist.

**parosphresia** (păr′os-fre′zĭ-ah) [ para- + G. *osphrēsis*, smell ]. Parosmia.

**paros′teal**. Relating to the tissues immediately adjacent to the periosteum of a bone.

**parosteitis** (păr-os-te-i′tis) [ para- + G. *osteon*, bone, + suffix *-itis*, inflammation ]. Parostitis; inflammation of the tissues immediately adjacent to a bone.

**parosteo′sis, parosto′sis** [ para- + G. *osteon*, bone, + suffix *-osis*, condition ]. 1. The development of bone in an unusual location, as in the skin. 2. Abnormal or defective ossification.

**parosti′tis**. Parosteitis.

**parotic** (pă-rot′ik) [ para- + G. *ous*, ear ]. Near or beside the ear.

**parotid** (pă-rot′id) [ G. *parōtis* (*parōtid-*), the gland beside the ear, fr. *para*, beside, + *ous* (*ōt-*), ear. OT- ]. Situated near the ear; denoting several structures in this neighborhood. Usually refers to the p. salivary gland.

**parotidectomy** (pă-rot′ĭ-dek′to-mī) [ parotid + G. *ektomē*, excision ]. Surgical removal of the parotid gland.

**parotiditis** (pă-rot′ĭ-di′tis). Parotitis; inflammation of the parotid gland.

**epidemic p.**, mumps; an acute viral infectious and contagious disease caused by a paramyxovirus characterized by inflammation and swelling of the parotid gland, sometimes of other salivary glands, and occasionally by inflammation of the testis, ovary, pancreas, or meninges.

**postoperative p.**, an acute inflammation of the parotid gland occurring in the postoperative period, especially in debilitated or dehydrated patients; frequently results in abscess formation and rapidly spreading cellulitis that may become fatal.

**parotidoauricularis** (pă-rot′ĭ-do-aw-rik-u-la′ris). 1. An occasional band of muscle fibers passing from the surface of the parotid gland to the auricle. 2. Relating to the parotid gland and the external ear.

**par′otin**. A proteinaceous substances, obtained from bovine parotid glands, that is said to have hormonal activity; in animals, p. causes hypocalcemia, has effects on mesenchyman tissues, produces first leukopenia and then leukocytosis, and promotes calcification of dentin.

**S-p.**, a parotin-like substance obtained from the submaxillary glands of various animals.

**saliva p. A**, a parotin-like substance obtained from human saliva.

**parotis** [ L. ] [ NA ]. Parotid.

**paroti′tis**. Parotiditis.

**parous** (păr′us) [ L. *pario*, to bear ]. Pertaining to parity; having given birth to an infant or infants.

**parova′rian**. 1. Relating to the paroophoron. 2. Paraovarian.

**parovariot′omy** [ parovarium + G. *tomē*, incision ]. Incision into or removal of a tumor of the parovarium.

**parovari′tis**. Inflammation of the parovarium.

**parova′rium** [ para- + L. *ovarium*, ovary ]. Paroophoron.

**parox′ypro′pione**. PROFENONE; *p*-hydroxypropiophenone; an inhibitor of pituitary gonadotropic hormone.

**paroxysm** (păr′ok-sizm) [ G. *paroxysmos*, fr. *paroxynō*, to sharpen, irritate, fr. *oxys*, sharp. OX- ]. 1. A sharp spasm or convulsion. 2. A sudden onset of a symptom or disease, especially one with recurrent manifestations such as the chills and rigor of malaria.

**paroxysmal** (păr′ok-siz′mal). Relating to or occurring in paroxysms.

**parricide** (păr′ĭ-sīd) [ L. *parricidium*, killing of close kin ]. 1. The killing of one's parent (either patricide or matricide). 2. A person who commits such an act.

**Parrot** (pă-ro′), Joseph M. J., French physician, 1829–1883. See P.'s *disease, ulcer*.

**Parry**, Caleb H., English physician, 1755–1822. See P.'s *disease*.

# PARS

**pars**, pl. **par′tes** [ L. *pars* (*part-*) a part ] [ NA ]. A part; a portion.

**p. abdominalis** [ NA ], abdominal part; (1) see *musculus* pectoralis major; (2) the part of the esophagus inferior to the diaphragm; (3) the part of the ureter between the renal pelvis and the brim of the pelvis.

**p. ala′ris** [ NA ], alar part; see *musculus* nasalis.

**p. alveola′ris mandib′ulae** [ NA ], alveolar part of the mandible; the portion of the body of the mandible that surrounds and supports the lower teeth.

**p. amorpha**, the dense central area in some nucleoli; see also p. granulosa.

**p. ante′rior** [ NA ], anterior part; (1) the part of the diaphragmatic surface of the liver deep to the costal arches and xiphoid process; (2) the anterior part of the anterior commissure of the brain.

**p. anula′ris vagi′nae fibro′sae** [ NA ], anulus of the fibrous sheath; ligamentum anularis digitorum; one of the two circular fibrous bands of the fibrous sheaths of the fingers and toes attached to the shaft of the proximal and middle phlanges.

**p. ascen′dens** [ NA ], ascending part; see duodenum.

**p. basa′lis arte′riae pulmona′lis** [ NA ], basal part of the pulmonary artery; see arteria pulmonalis dextra and arteria pulmonalis sinistra.

**p. basila′ris os′sis occipita′lis** [ NA ], basal part of the occipital bone; the part of the bone that lies anterior to the foramen magnum and joins with the body of the sphenoid bone.

**p. basila′ris pon′tis**, p. ventralis pontis.

**p. buccopharyn′gea** [ NA ], buccopharyngeal part; see *musculus* constrictor pharyngis superior.

**p. cardi′aca ventric′uli** [ NA ], cardiac part of the stomach; the area of the stomach close to the cardiac opening which contains the cardiac glands.

**p. cartilagin′ea sep′ti na′si**, *cartilago* septi nasi.

**p. cartilagin′ea tu′bae auditi′vae** [ NA ], cartilaginous part of the auditory tube; that portion of the auditory tube that is supported by cartilage; it continues anteromedially from the osseous part to open into the nasopharynx.

**p. cavernosa,** p. spongiosa.

**p. ce′ca ret′inae,** the embryological anterior part of the retina that gives rise to the p. ciliaris retinae and p. iridica retinae.

**p. centra′lis ventric′uli latera′lis** [ NA ], cella media; body of the lateral ventricle of the brain, extending from the interventricular foramen (of Monro) to the splenium of the corpus callosum.

**p. ceratopharyn′gea** [ NA ], ceratopharyngeal part; see *musculus* constrictor pharyngis medius.

**p. cervica′lis esoph′agi** [ NA ], cervical part of the esophagus; the part of the esophagus located in the neck.

**p. cervica′lis medul′lae spina′lis** [ NA ], cervical part of the spinal cord; the upper part of the spinal cord giving rise to the cervical spinal nerves.

**p. chondropharyngea** [ NA ], chondropharyngeal part; see *musculus* constrictor pharyngis medius.

**p. cilia′ris ret′inae** [ NA ], ciliary part of the retina; the part of the retina covering the ciliary body posteriorly. See fig. under retina.

**p. clavicula′ris** [ NA ], clavicular part; see *musculus* pectoralis major.

**p. cochlea′ris ner′vi octa′vi** [ NA ], cochlear part of the eighth nerve; see *nervus* vestibulocochlearis.

**p. convolu′ta lo′buli cortica′lis re′nis** [ NA ], convoluted part of the kidney lobule; labyrinthus (3); renal labyrinth; Ludwig's labyrinth; it consists of proximal and distal convoluted tubules and the associated renal corpuscles supplied by branches of the interlobular arteries.

**partes corporis humani** [ NA ], parts of the human body; the head, neck, trunk, and limbs.

**p. costa′lis diaphragma′tis** [ NA ], costal part of the diaphragm; the part of the diaphragm that arises from the inner aspect of the lower six costal cartilages and the lower four ribs and inserts on the anterolateral part of the central tendon.

**p. cricopharyn′gea** [ NA ], cricopharyngeal part; see *musculus* constrictor pharyngis inferior.

**p. cruciformis vaginae fibrosae** [ NA ], cruciform part of the fibrous sheath; ligamenta cruciata digitorum; the fibers of the fibrous sheath of the fingers and toes which form X-shaped patterns over the region of the interphalangeal joints.

**p. cupula′ris** [ NA ], cupular or cupulate part; the dome-shaped, highest portion of the epitympanic recess.

**p. cys′tica,** the smaller caudal division of the primitive embryonic hepatic bud; it gives origin to the gallbladder and cystic duct.

**p. descen′dens** [ NA ], descending part; see duodenum.

**p. dex′tra** [ NA ], right part; the part of the diaphragmatic surface of the liver deep to the bodies of the lower ribs on the right side.

**p. dista′lis lo′bi anterio′ris hypophys′eos** [ NA ], distal part of the anterior lobe of the hypophysis; it consists of anastomosing cords or clumps of cells (chromophil and chromophobe cells of varying kinds) separated by a profuse network of sinusoidal capillaries and a minimal amount of stroma. See also hypophysis.

**p. dorsa′lis pon′tis** [ NA ], dorsal part of the pons; tegmentum of the pons; the part of the pons bounded at the sides by the middle cerebellar peduncles and anteriorly by the p. ventralis pontis; it is continuous with the tegmentum of the mesencephalon and contains long tracts such as the medial and lateral lemnisci, cranial nerve nuclei, and reticular formation.

**p. feta′lis placen′tae** [ NA ], placenta fetalis; fetal placenta; the chorionic portion of the placenta, containing the fetal blood vessels, from which the funis arises; specifically, in man it is developed from the chorion frondosum.

**p. flac′cida membranae tympani** [ NA ], Shrapnell's membrane; Rivinus' membrane; flaccid part of the tympanic membrane; see fig. under *membrana* tympani.

**p. fronta′lis corpo′ris callo′si,** *forceps* minor.

**partes genitales femininae externae** [ NA ], parts of the female genitalia; the female pudendum and clitoris.

**partes genitales masculinae externae** [ NA ], parts of the male external genitalia; the penis and scrotum.

**p. glossopharyngea** [ NA ], glossopharyngeal part; see *musculus* constrictor pharyngis superior.

**p. granulosa,** the granular part of the nucleolonema which surrounds the p. amorpha of the nucleolus.

**p. hepat′ica,** the larger cranial division of the primitive embryonic hepatic bud; it gives rise to the liver proper.

**p. horizonta′lis,** horizontal part; see duodenum.

**p. inferior** [ NA ], inferior part; (1) see duodenum; (2) the vein draining the inferior lingular bronchopulmonary segment; (3) the part of the vestibular ganglion which receives fibers from the macula of the saccule and the ampulla of the posterior semicircular duct.

**p. inflex′a,** one of the two posterior reflections **(p. i. lateralis, p. i. medialis)** of the wall of a horse's hoof; see bar.

**p. infraclavicula′ris plex′us brachia′lis** [ NA ], infraclavicular part of the brachial plexus; the part that extends from the level of the clavicle downward into the axilla. It includes the cords of the plexus and their branches.

**p. infraloba′ris** [ NA ], infralobar part; the vein draining the posterior segment of the right lung that emerges inferior to the superior lobe; tributary to the posterior branch of the right superior pulmonary vein.

**p. infrasegmentalis** [ NA ], p. intersegmentalis [ NA ]; infrasegmental or intersegmental part; a vein receiving blood from adjacent bronchopulmonary segments; it emerges from the inferior margin of a segment to become a tributary of a branch of a pulmonary vein.

**p. infundibula′ris lo′bi anterio′ris hypophys′eos** [ NA ], infundibular part of the anterior lobe; formerly called the p. tuberalis; the upward extension of the anterior lobe that wraps around the infundibular stalk. The cells as seen with the light microscope are slightly basophilic but nongranular. See also hypophysis.

**p. in′tercartilagin′ea rimae glottidis** [ NA ], intercartilaginous part of glottic opening; the opening between the vocal processes of the arytenoid cartilages.

**p. interme′dia,** intermediate part; (1) [ NA ], the part of the anterior lobe of the hypophysis between the pars distalis and the posterior lobe; it usually contains follicles of variable size with colloid material; chromophobe and basophil cells may also be present, the latter sometimes migrating into the posterior lobe; (2) *commissura* bulborum; (3) *nervus* intermedius.

**p. intermembrana′cea ri′mae glot′tidis** [ NA ], intermembranous part of glottic opening; the portion of the opening anterior to the vocal processes of the arytenoid cartilages bounded by the vocal ligaments.

**p. intersegmentalis** [ NA ], official alternate term for p. infrasegmentalis.

**p. intraloba′ris** [ NA ], intralobar part; the vein draining the apical and posterior segments of the right lung; tributary to the posterior branch of the right superior pulmonary vein.

**p. intrasegmenta′lis** [ NA ], intrasegmental part; a vein emerging from the bronchopulmonary segment it drains; a tributary to a branch of a pulmonary vein.

**p. irid′ica ret′inae** [ NA ], iridial part of the retina; two layers of pigmented cells, derived from the primitive optic cup, that cover the posterior surface of the iris. See fig. under retina.

**p. labialis** [ NA ], labial part; the major part of the obicularis oris muscle within the body of the lips.

**p. lacrima′lis mus′culi orbicula′ris oc′uli,** see *musculus* orbicularis oculi.

**p. laryngea pharyngis** [ NA ], laryngeal part of the pharynx; hypopharynx; laryngopharynx; the part of the pharynx lying below the aperture of the larynx and behind the larynx; it extends from the vestibule of the larynx to the esophagus at the level of the inferior border of the cricoid cartilage.

**p. latera′lis** [ NA ], lateral part; (1) see *arcus* pedis longitudinalis; (2) the lateral mass of the sacrum formed by the fused costal elements; (3) exoccipital bone; the part of the occipital bone that lies on either side of the foramen magnum; (4) see *musculi* intertransversarii posteriores cervicis; (5) the vein draining the lateral bronchopulmonary segment of the middle lobe of the right lung.

**p. lumba'lis diaphragma'tis** [ NA ], lumbar part of the diaphragm; vertebral part of diaphragm; the portion of the diaphragm that arises from the upper lumbar vertebrae and from the medial and lateral arcuate ligaments. See *crus* dextrum, *crus* sinistrum, *ligamentum* arcuatum.

**p. lumba'lis medul'lae spina'lis** [ NA ], lumbar part of the spinal cord; that part of the cord from which the five pairs of lumbar nerves originate.

**p. marginalis** [ NA ], marginal part; the part of the orbicularis oris muscle located in the margin of the lips, *i.e.*, the red area.

**p. mastoid'ea**, mastoid part; the portion of the petrous part of the temporal bone bearing the mastoid process.

**p. medialis** [ NA ], medial part; (1) see *arcus* pedis longitudinalis; (2) see musculi intertransversarii posteriores cervicis; (3) the vein draining the medial bronchopulmonary segment of the middle lobe of the right lung.

**p. mediastinalis** [ NA ], mediastinal part; the part of the medial surface of a lung in contact with the mediastinum.

**p. membrana'cea septi atrio'rum,** *septum* atrioventriculare.

**p. membrana'cea septi interventricula'ris** [ NA ], membranous septum (2); the membranous portion of the interventricular septum of the heart.

**p. membrana'cea septi nasi** [ NA ], the membranous part of the nasal septum; the small portion of the nasal septum anterior to the portion supported by the cartilage of the nasal septum.

**p. membrana'cea urethrae masculinae** [ NA ], membranous part of the male urethra; the portion of the male urethra, about 1 cm. in length, extending from the prostate to the beginning of the urethra in the corpus spongiosum just beyond the bulb.

**p. mobilis septi nasi** [ NA ], the anterior movable part of the nasal septum formed by the medial crus of the greater alar cartilage on each side.

**p. muscula'ris sep'ti interventricula'ris cor'dis** [ NA ], the muscular portion of the interventricular septum of the heart.

**p. mylopharyngea** [ NA ], mylopharyngeal part; see *musculus* constrictor pharyngis superior.

**p. nasa'lis ossis frontalis** [ NA ], nasal portion of the frontal bone which lies between the two orbital parts anteriorly and forms part of the roof of the nasal cavity.

**p. nasa'lis pharyngis** [ NA ], nasal part of the pharynx; pharyngonasal cavity; epipharynx; rhinopharynx; nasopharynx; the part of the pharynx that lies above the soft palate; anteriorly it opens into the nasal cavity.

**p. nervo'sa hypophys'eos,** *lobus* posterior hypophyseos.

**p. obliqua,** [ NA ], oblique part; see *musculus* cricothyroideus.

**p. occipita'lis corpo'ris callo'si,** *forceps* major.

**p. opercula'ris,** the posterior one of the three small cortical convolutions together forming the frontal operculum, the other two being the p. orbitalis and p. triangularis.

**p. op'tica ret'inae** [ NA ], *stratum* cerebrale retinae.

**p. oralis pharyngis** [ NA ], oral part of the pharynx; oropharynx; the portion of the pharynx that lies posterior to the mouth; it is continuous above with the nasopharynx and below with the laryngopharynx.

**p. orbita'lis,** orbital part; (1) [ NA ], the portion of the frontal bone that contributes to the formation of the orbits; (2) [ NA ], see *musculus* orbicularis oculi; (3) [ NA ], see *glandula* lacrimalis; (4) the anterior one of three small cortical convolutions that together form the frontal operculum.

**p. os'sea septi nasi** [ NA ], bony part of the nasal septum; the major portion of the nasal septum supported by the ossea septi nasi, *q. v.*

**p. os'sea tu'bae auditi'vae** [ NA ], bony part of the auditory tube; the portion of the auditory tube that passes from the tympanic cavity anteromedially through the semicanalis tubae auditivae.

**p. palpebralis** [ NA ], palpebral part; (1) see *musculus* orbicularis oculi; (2) see *glandula* lacrimalis.

**p. parasympath'ica systema'tis nervo'si autonom'ici** [ NA ], parasympathetic part of the autonomic nervous system; see parasympathetic nervous *system* and *systema* nervosum autonomicum.

**p. pelvi'na,** (1) [ NA ], pelvic part; the part of the ureter between the brim of the pelvis and the urinary bladder; (2) the upper pelvic portion of the embryologic urogenital sinus.

**p. perpendicula'ris,** (1) *lamina* perpendicularis ossis palatini; (2) *lamina* perpendicularis.

**p. petro'sa ossis temporalis** [ NA ], petrous bone; petrous portion of the temporal bone; pyramid; the part of the temporal bone that contains the structures of the inner ear.

**p. phal'lica,** the lower portion of the urogenital sinus, related to the base of the genital or phallic tubercle.

**p. pharyn'gea hypophys'eos** [ NA ], pharyngeal hypophysis; residual tissue derived from the hypophysial diverticulum which lies in the lamina propria of the lining of the nasopharynx; its cells and their arrangement are identical with those of the pars distalis.

**p. plana,** *orbiculus* ciliaris.

**p. poste'rior** [ NA ], posterior part; (1) that portion of the diaphragmatic surface of the liver that includes the bare area and the caudate lobe; (2) the posterior portion of the anterior commissure of the brain.

**p. profunda** [ NA ], deep part; (1) see *musculus* masseter; (2) see *glandula* parotis; (3) see *musculus* sphincter ani externus.

**p. prostat'ica urethrae** [ NA ], the prostatic part of the male urethra; about 2.5 cm. in length, that traverses the prostate.

**p. pterygopharyngea** [ NA ], pterygopharyngeal part; see *musculus* constrictor pharyngis superior.

**p. pylo'rica ventric'uli** [ NA ], pyloric part of the stomach; that portion of the stomach between the angular notch and the pylorus; its mucosa contains pyloric glands.

**p. quadrata** [ NA ], quadrate part; the part of the medial segment of the liver which includes the quadrate lobe.

**p. radia'ta lo'buli cortica'lis re'nis** [ NA ], medullary ray; Ferrein's pyramid; processus ferreini; the center of the renal lobule, which has the shape of a small, steep pyramid, consisting of straight tubular parts. These may be either ascending or descending limbs of the nephronic loop or collecting tubules.

**p. recta** [ NA ], straight part; see *musculus* cricothyroideus.

**p. retrolentifor'mis cap'sulae inter'nae** [ NA ], retrolenticular limb of the internal capsule; that portion of the capsule that passes caudate to the lentiform nucleus and contains among other fiber systems the larger part of the optic or geniculocalcarine radiation.

**p. sella'ris,** *sella* turcica.

**p. spongio'sa ure'thrae masculi'nae** [ NA ], spongiose part of the male urethra; spongy urethra; penile urethra; the portion of the male urethra, about 15 cm. in length, which traverses the corpus spongiosum.

**p. squamo'sa os'sis tempora'lis** [ NA ], squama temporalis; the squamous portion of the temporal bone.

**p. sterna'lis diaphragma'tis** [ NA ], sternal part of the diaphragm; the small slip on each side that arises from the inner surface of the xiphoid process and inserts on the central tendon.

**p. sternocostalis** [ NA ], sternocostal part; see *musculus* pectoralis major.

**p. subcutanea** [ NA ], subcutaneous part; see *musculus* sphincter ani externus.

**p. sublentifor'mis cap'sulae inter'nae** [ NA ], sublenticular limb of the internal capsule; the part of the internal capsule that passes below the caudal third of the lentiform nucleus, and contains the auditory radiation as well as that part of the optic radiation that represents the upper part of the contralateral half of the binocular visual field.

**p. superficialis** [ NA ], superficial part; (1) see *musculus* masseter; (2) see *glandula* parotis; (3) see *musculus* sphincter ani externus.

**p. superior** [ NA ], superior part; (1) see duodenum; (2) the convex superior portion of the diaphragmatic surface of the liver; (3) the vein that drains the superior lingular bronchopulmonary segment; (4) the part of the vestibular ganglion that receives fibers from the macula of the utricle and the ampullae of the anterior and lateral semicircular ducts.

**p. supraclavicula'ris plex'us brachia'lis** [ NA ], supraclavicular part of the brachial plexus, including the roots, trunks and divisions. This part of the plexus gives rise to the dorsal scapular, long thoracic, suprascapular and subclavian nerves.

**p. sympath'ica systema'tis nervo'si autonom'ici** [ NA ], sympathetic part of the autonomic nervous system; see sympathetic nervous *system* and *systema* nervosum autonomicum.

**p. tec'ta duode'ni,** hidden portion of the duodenum; part of duodenum covered by the root of the transverse mesocolon, the coalescence of the ascending mesocolon, and the root of the mesentery.

**p. tec'ta pancreatis,** hidden portion of the pancreas; part of pancreas covered by the root of the transverse mesocolon, the coalescence of the ascending mesocolon, and the root of the mesentery.

**p. tec'ta rena'lis,** hidden portion of the kidney; part of kidney covered by the root of the transverse mesocolon.

**p. tec'ta uretera'lis,** hidden portion of the right ureter; part of right ureter covered (crossed) by the root of the mesentery, and of the left ureter covered (crossed) by the root of the sigmoid mesocolon.

**p. tensa membranae tympani** [ NA ], tense part of the tympanic membrane; the greater portion of the membrana tympani which is tense and firm, contrasting with the small triangular pars flaccida. See fig. under *membrana* tympani.

**p. thorac'ica esoph'agi** [ NA ], thoracic part of the esophagus; the part of the esophagus between the thoracic inlet and the diaphragm.

**p. thorac'ica medul'lae spina'lis** [ NA ], thoracic part of the spinal cord; the portion of the cord that gives rise to the twelve paired thoracic spinal nerves.

**p. thyropharynge'a** [ NA ], thyropharyngeal part; see *musculus* constrictor pharyngis inferior.

**p. tibiocalcanea** [ NA ], tibiocalcaneal part; the part of the medial ligament that extends from the medial malleolus to the sustentaculum tali of the calcaneus.

**p. tibionavicularis** [ NA ], tibionavicular part; the part of the medial ligament that extends from the medial malleolus to the navicular bone.

**p. tibiotalaris anterior** [ NA ], anterior tibiotalar part; the part of the medial ligament that extends from the medial malleolus to the neck of the talus.

**p. tibiotalaris posterior** [ NA ], posterior tibiotalar part; the part of the medial ligament that extends from the medial malleolus to the posterior process of the talus.

**p. transversa** [ NA ], transverse part; (1) see *musculus* nasalis; (2) the long unbranched part of the left branch of the portal vein.

**p. triangula'ris,** the middle one of three small convolutions which together compose the frontal operculum of the cerebral cortex, the other two being the p. orbitalis and p. opercularis.

**p. tuberalis of hypophysis,** p. infundibularis lobi anterioris hypophyseos.

**p. tympan'ica ossis temporalis** [ NA ], the tympanic portion of the temporal bone, forming the greater part of the wall of the external acoustic meatus.

**p. umbilicalis** [ NA ], umbilical part; the highly branched part of the left branch of the portal vein; the round and venous ligaments attach to this part.

**p. uterina** [ NA ], uterine part; (1) the part of the uterine tube located within the wall of the uterus; (2) maternal placenta; placenta uterina; the part of the placenta derived from the uterine tissue; see also placenta.

**p. ventra'lis pon'tis** [ NA ], p. basilaris pontis; basilar or ventral part of the pons; the large ventral part of the pons occupied by the nuclei pontis, traversed lengthwise by the longitudinal pontine bundles composed of corticopontine, corticobulbar, and corticospinal fibers, and transversally by bundles of the pontocerebellar fibers converging laterally to form the middle cerebellar peduncle or brachium pontis.

**p. vertebralis** [ NA ], vertebral part; the part of the medial surface of the lung in contact with the vertebral bodies.

**p. vestibula'ris ner'vi octa'vi** [ NA ], vestibular part of the eighth nerve; see *nervus* vestibulocochlearis.

---

**pars'ley.** A garden herb of the genus *Petroselinum* (family Umbelliferae), the root of which has been used as an emmenagogue.

**p. camphor,** apiol.

**pars-planitis.** A clinical syndrome consisting of peripheral nodular inflammation of the retina and/or pars plana, massive exudation into the overlying vitreous base, and edema of the posterior pole. There are two types, massive exudative and diffuse inflammatory.

**part.** See pars.

**abdominal p.,** *pars* abdominalis.

**alar p.,** *pars* alaris.

**alveolar p. of mandible,** *pars* alveolaris mandibulae.

**anterior p.,** *pars* anterior.

**anterior movable p. of nasal septum,** *pars* mobilis septi nasi.

**anterior p. of pons,** *pars* basilaris pontis.

**anterior tibiotalar p.,** *pars* tibiotalaris anterior.

**ascending p.,** *pars* ascendens; see duodenum.

**basal p. of occipital bone,** *pars* basilaris ossis occipitalis.

**basal p. of pulmonary artery,** *pars* basalis arteriae pulmonalis.

**basilar p. of pons,** *pars* ventralis pontis.

**bony p. of auditory tube,** *pars* ossea tubae auditivae.

**bony p. of nasal septum,** *pars* ossea septi nasi.

**buccopharyngeal p.,** *pars* buccopharyngea; see *musculus* constrictor pharyngis superior.

**cardiac p. of stomach,** *pars* cardiaca ventriculi.

**cartilaginous p. of auditory tube,** *pars* cartilaginea tubae auditivae.

**ceratopharyngeal p.,** *pars* ceratopharyngea; see *musculus* constrictor pharyngis medius.

**cervical p. of esophagus,** *pars* cervicalis esophagi.

**cervical p. of spinal cord,** *pars* cervicalis medullae spinalis.

**chondropharyngeal p.,** *pars* chondropharyngea; see *musculus* constrictor pharyngis medius.

**ciliary p. of the retina,** *pars* ciliaris retinae.

**clavicular p.,** *pars* clavicularis.

**convoluted p. of kidney lobule,** *pars* convoluta lobuli corticalis renis.

**costal p. of diaphragm,** *pars* costalis diaphragmatis.

**cricopharyngeal p.,** *pars* cricopharyngea; see *musculus* constrictor pharyngis inferior.

**cruciform p. of the fibrous sheath,** *pars* cruciformis vaginae fibrosae.

**cupular p., cupulate p.,** *pars* cupularis.

**deep p.,** *pars* profunda; see *musculus* masseter; *glandula* parotis; *musculus* sphincter ani externus.

**descending p.,** *pars* descendens.

**distal p. of anterior lobe of hypophysis,** *pars* distalis lobi anterioris hypophyseos.

**dorsal p. of pons,** *pars* dorsalis pontis.

**p.'s of the female external genitalia,** *partes* genitales femininae externae.

**flaccid p. of tympanic membrane,** *pars* flaccida membranae tympani.

**glossopharyngeal p.,** *pars* glossopharyngea; see *musculus* constrictor pharyngis superior.

**p.'s of the human body,** *partes* corporis humani.

**inferior p.,** *pars* inferior.

**infraclavicular p. of brachial plexus,** *pars* infraclavicularis plexus brachialis.

**infralobar p.,** *pars* infralobaris.

**infrasegmental p.,** *pars* infrasegmentalis.

**infundibular p. of anterior lobe of hypophysis,** *pars* infundibularis lobi anterioris hypophyseos.

**intercartilaginous p. of glottic opening,** *pars* intercartilaginea rimae glottidis.

**intermediate p.,** *pars* intermedia.

**intermembranous p. of glottic opening,** *pars* intermembranacea rimae glottidis.

**intralobar p.,** *pars* intralobaris.

**intrasegmental p.,** *pars* intrasegmentalis.

**iridial p. of retina,** *pars* iridica retinae.

**labial p.,** *pars* labialis.

**laryngeal p. of pharynx,** *pars* laryngea pharyngis.

**lateral p.,** *pars* lateralis.

**lumbar p. of diaphragm,** *pars* lumbalis diaphragmatis.

**lumbar p. of spinal cord,** *pars* lumbalis medullae spinalis.

**p.'s of the male external genitalia,** *partes* genitales masculinae externae.

**marginal p.,** *pars* marginalis.

**mastoid p.,** *pars* mastoidea.

**medial p.,** *pars* medialis.

**mediastinal p.,** *pars* mediastinalis.

**membranous p.'s,** see subentries under *pars* membranaceae.

**mylopharyngeal p.,** *pars* mylopharyngea; see *musculus* constrictor pharyngis superior.

**nasal p. of pharynx,** *pars* nasalis pharyngis.

**oblique p.,** *pars* obliqua; see *musculus* cricothyroideus.

**optic p. of retina,** *stratum* cerebrale retinae.

**oral p. of pharynx,** *pars* oralis pharyngis.

**orbital p.,** *pars* orbitalis.

**palpebral p.,** *pars* palpebralis; see *musculus* orbicularis oculi; see *glandula* lacrimalis.

**parasympathetic p. of autonomic nervous system,** *pars* parasympathica systematis nervosi autonomici.

**pelvic p.,** *pars* pelvina.

**posterior p.,** *pars* posterior.

**posterior tibiotalar p.,** *pars* tibiotalaris posterior.

**pterygopharyngeal p.,** *pars* pterygopharyngea; see *musculus* constrictor pharyngis superior.

**pyloric p. of stomach,** *pars* pylorica ventriculi.

**quadrate p.,** *pars* quadrata.

**right p.,** *pars* dextra.

**soft p.'s,** the nonbony and noncartilaginous tissues of the body.

**spongiose p. of the male urethra,** *pars* spongiosa urethrae masculinae.

**sternal p. of diaphragm,** *pars* sternalis diaphragmatis.

**sternocostal p.,** *pars* sternocostalis; see *musculus* pectoralis major.

**straight p.,** *pars* recta; see *musculus* cricothyroideus.

**subcutaneous p.,** *pars* subcutanea; see *musculus* sphincter ani externus.

**superficial p.,** *pars* superficialis; see *musculus* masseter; *glandula* parotis; *musculus* sphincter ani externus.

**superior p.,** *pars* superior.

**supraclavicular p. of brachial plexus,** *pars* supraclavicularis plexus brachialis.

**sympathetic p. of autonomic nervous system,** *pars* sympathica systematis nervosi autonomici.

**tense p. of the tympanic membrane,** *pars* tensa membranae tympani.

**thoracic p. of esophagus,** *pars* thoracica esophagi.

**thoracic p. of spinal cord,** *pars* thoracica medullae spinalis.

**thyropharyngeal p.,** *pars* thyropharyngea; see *musculus* constrictor pharyngis inferior.

**tibiocalcaneal p.,** *pars* tibiocalcanea.

**tibionavicular p.,** *pars* tibionavicularis.

**transverse p.,** *pars* transversa.

**umbilical p.,** *pars* umbilicalis.

**uterine p.,** *pars* uterina.

**ventral p. of the pons,** *pars* ventralis pontis.

**vertebral p.,** *pars* vertebralis.

**partes.** Plural of pars.

**parthenogen'esis** [ G. a *parthenos*, virgin, + *genesis*, product ]. Apogamia; apomixia; a form of nonsexual reproduction, or agamogenesis, in which the female reproduces its kind without fecundation by the male.

**parthenology** (par-then-ol'o-jī) [ G. *parthenos*, virgin, + *logos*, study ]. The branch of gynecology which deals with the genital apparatus of the virgin.

**parthenopho'bia** [ G. *parthenos*, virgin, + *phobos*, fear ]. Morbid fear of girls.

**particle** (par'tĭ-kl) [ L. *particula*, dim. of *pars*, part ]. A very small piece or portion of anything.

**alpha p.,** a p. consisting of two neutrons and two protons (the nucleus of the helium atom) emitted by the atoms of such radioactive nuclides as $^{238}$U, $^{232}$Th, $^{226}$Ra, etc.

Alpha Particle

**beta p.,** an electron, either positively (positron) or negatively (negatron) charged, emitted during beta decay of a radionuclide.

**chromatin p.'s,** fine bluish dots thought to represent remnants of the nucleus, occasionally seen in stained erythrocytes.

**Dane's p.'s,** the larger spherical forms of hepatitis-associated antigens.

**elementary p.,** 1. Blood *platelet.* 2. One of the units occurring on the matrical surface of mitochondrial cristae; the head of the p., which measures about 90 Å, attaches to the membrane of the crista by a stalk 50 Å in length; the p.'s may be concerned with the electron transport system.

**kappa p.'s,** inheritable cytoplasmic symbionts, once thought to be p.'s mainly or exclusively of DNA, occurring in some strains of *Paramecium;* capable of producing something that is lethal to other strains.

**Zimmermann's elementary p.,** platelet.

**partic'ulate.** Relating to or occurring in the form of fine particles.

**partic'ulates.** Formed elements, discrete bodies, as contrasted with the surrounding liquid or semiliquid material, *e.g.,* granules or mitochondria in cells.

**partigen** (par'tĭ-jen). Partial antigen; a term coined by Hans Much to denote a constituent of a natural antigen, the latter being regarded as a mixture of partial antigens.

**parturient** (par-tu'rĭ-ent) [ L. *parturio*, to be in labor. PARI- ]. Relating to or being in the process of parturition or childbirth.

**parturifacient** (par-tu-rĭ-fa'shent) [ L. *parturio*, to be in labor, + *facio*, to make ]. Oxytocic. 1. Inducing or accelerating labor. 2. An agent that induces or accelerates labor.

**parturiometer** (par-tu'rĭ-om'e-ter) [ L. *parturitio*, parturition, + G. *metron*, measure ]. A device for determining the force of the uterine contractions in childbirth.

**parturition** (par-tu-rish'un) [ L. *parturitio*, fr. *parturio*, to be in labor. PARI- ]. Childbirth; labor; giving birth to a child.

**double p.,** split p.; a phenomenon characterized by two successive p.'s, in which fully grown newborn are delivered at each p., and in which the two p.'s are separated by an interval in time that is appreciable, but definitely shorter than the normal term of pregnancy; observed to occur in women and various animals; may represent superfetation, superfecundation, or an embryonic diapause.

**split p.,** double p.

**par'tus** [ L. *partus* (noun), fr. *pario*, to bear ]. Parturition.

**p. agrippi'nus,** breech *delivery.*

**p. caesa'rius,** delivery by cesarean section.

**p. prepara'tor,** preparer for parturition; denoting any remedy or therapeutic measure designed to render an approaching labor safer or easier.

**p. seroti'nus,** delayed labor.

**p. siccus,** a dry labor; one in which the amniotic fluid is scanty or flows away prematurely before the onset of labor.

**parulis,** pl. **parulides** (pă-ru'lis, pă-ru'lĭ-dēz) [ G. *paroulis,* gumboil, fr. *para,* beside, + *oulon,* gum. UL- ]. Gingival abscess.

**parumbilical** (păr'um-bil'ĭ-kal). Paraumbilical.

**parvicellular** (par'vĭ-sel'u-lar) [ L. *parvus,* small, + Mod. L. *cellularis,* cellular ]. Relating to or composed of cells of small size.

**Parvobacteriaceae** (par'vo-bak-te'rĭ-a'se-e). Brucellaceae.

**par'voline.** A ptomaine, $C_9H_{13}N$, from decaying fish.

**parvule** (par'vūl) [ L. *parvulus,* very small, fr. *parvus,* small ]. A pillule; pellet; granule; a minute pill.

**par'vus** [ L. ] [ NA ]. Small.

**PAS.** Abbreviation for (1) *p*-aminosalicylic acid (also abbreviated PASA), and (2) periodic acid-Schiff (*q. v.* under stain).

**Pascal,** Blaise, French scientist, 1623–1662. See P.'s *law.*

**pas'cal.** Abbreviated Pa; a derived unit of pressure in the SI system, expressed in newtons per square meter.

**Pascheff's conjunctivitis.** See under conjunctivitis.

**Paschen** (pah'shen), Enrique, German physician, 1860–1936. See P. *bodies.*

**pasini'azide.** DIPASIC; isoniazid 4-aminosalicylate; antituberculostatic agent.

**paspalism** (pas'pal-izm) [ G. *paspalos*, a kind of millet, fr. *pas*, all, + *palē*, meal ]. Poisoning by seeds of a species of grass, *Paspalum scrobiculatum*.

**pas'sage** [ Mediev. L. *passo*, to pass ]. 1. The act of passing. 2. A discharge, as from the bowels or of urine. 3. The inoculation of a series of animals with the same strain of a pathogenic micro-organism whereby the virulence usually is increased, but is sometimes diminished. 4. A channel, duct, pore, or opening.

**Passal'urus ambig'uus.** Rabbit pinworm; an oxyurid nematode found abundantly in the cecum and large intestine of rabbits.

**Passavant** (pah'sah-fahnt), Philippas G., German physician, 1815–1893. See P.'s *cushion*, P.'s *bar, pad, ridge*.

**Passey,** R. D. See Harding-P. *melanoma*.

**passiflora** (pas'ĭ-flo'rah) [ L. *passio*, passion, + *flos* (*flor-*), flower ]. Passion-flower; *Passiflora incarnata* (family *Passifloraceae*); a climbing herb of the southern United States. The dried flowering and fruiting top has been used in neuralgia, dysmenorrhea, and insomnia, and as an application to hemorrhoids and for burns.

**passion** (pash'un) [ L. *passio*, fr. *patior*, pp. *passus*, to suffer ]. 1. Intense emotion. 2. Obsolete term for suffering or pain.

**passional** (pash'un-al). Relating to any of the passions; emotional.

**passive** (pas'iv) [ L. *passivus*, fr. *patior*, to endure ]. Not active; submissive.

**passivism** (pas'ĭ-vizm) [ see passive ]. 1. An attitude of submission. 2. A form of sexual perversion in which the subject, usually the male, is submissive to the will of the partner, either male or female, in sexual practices. See also pathic.

**passiv'ity.** 1. The condition of a metal having formed a protective oxide coating. Rustless metals and aluminum become passive in air. 2. In dentistry, the quality or condition of inactivity or rest assumed by the teeth, tissues, and denture when a removable partial denture is in place but not under masticatory pressure.

**pas'ta,** gen. and pl. **pas'tae** [ L. ]. Paste.

**paste** (pāst) [ L. *pasta* ]. A soft semisolid of firmer consistence than pap, but soft enough to flow slowly and not to retain its shape. Two classes of p.'s are recognized by the USP: one is prepared from hydrogels such as hydrated pectin; the other class consists of stiff, thick ointments which do not melt at body temperature, and are more absorptive and less greasy than ointments.

   **dermatologic p.,** a class of preparations consisting of starch, dextrin, sulfur, calcium carbonate or zinc oxide made into a p. with glycerin, soft soap, petrolatum, or some fat, with which is incorporated some medicinal substance.

   **desensitizing p.,** an ointment, usually caustic, coagulating or cytotoxic, formulated to be applied to the cervix of a tooth for the purpose of obtunding pain from sensitive, exposed cementum or dentin.

   **devitalizing p.,** a p. which when applied to the dentin or to an exposed pulp will destroy it. The principal ingredient of such a p. is arsenic trioxide or paraformaldehyde.

**pas'ter.** The segment forming the part for near vision in two-piece bifocal lenses.

**pas'tern** [ O. Fr. *pasturon*, pasture; because the shackle of a horse out at pasture is attached to this part of the leg ]. The part of the leg of a horse and similar animals that lies between the fetlock joint and the hoof.

**Pasteur** (pahs-tër'), Louis, eminent French chemist and bacteriologist, 1822–1895. His first important contribution was the splitting of racemic acid ($C_4H_6O_6$), an optically inactive form of tartaric acid, into the *d*- and *l*-forms; this laid the foundation of stoichochemistry. His greatest work was in the field of bacteriology and immunology which started from his investigations into fermentative processes; he showed that all fermentative action was brought to an end by heating to a temperature of 60°C. and furnished evidence which disproved the prevailing theory of spontaneous generation; conquered the diseases of silk worms which threatened to bankrupt the silk industry in France. Later, turning his attention to the diseases of animals and of man, he discovered the bacteria of septic infection (*Staphylococcus pyogenes* and *Streptococcus pyogenes*). Discovering by accident that the virulence of bacteria may undergo attenuation, he originated the method of immunization based on this principle and produced vaccines against anthrax and hydrophobia. See P.'s *effect*, P.-Chamberland *filter*, P.'s *theory, vaccine*.

**Pasteurella** (pas-tur-el'ah) [ L. *Pasteur* ]. A genus of aerobic to facultatively anaerobic, nonmotile bacteria (family Brucellaceae) containing small, Gram-negative, ellipsoidal to elongated rods which, with special methods, show bipolar staining. These organisms are parasites of man and other animals, including birds. The type species is *P. multocida*.

   **P. anatipestifer,** a species associated with a disease of ducklings.

   **P. haemolytica,** a species found in cases of penumonia in sheep and cattle.

   **P. multocida,** a species which causes chicken cholera and hemorrhagic septicemia in warm-blooded animals. It is the type species of the genus *P*.

   **P. novicida,** a species pathogenic for white mice, guinea pigs, and hamsters; it produces lesions in experimental animals similar to those found in cases of tularemia. It is not known to infect man.

   **P. pestis,** *Yersinia pestis*.

   **P. pfaffii,** a species found in an epidemic of septicemia in canaries where it caused a necrotic enteritis; pathogenic for canaries, sparrows, pigeons, white mice, guinea pigs, and rabbits; not pathogenic for chickens.

   **P. pseudotuberculo'sis,** *Yersinia pseudotuberculosis*.

   **P. septicaemiae,** a species which causes fatal septicemia in young geese.

   **P. tularen'sis,** *Francisella tularensis*.

**pasteurellosis** (pas'tur-ĕ-lo'sis). Infection with bacteria of the group *Pasteurella*, including hemorrhagic septicemia, plague, tularemia, and pseudotuberculosis.

**pasteurization** (pas'tur-ĭ-za'shun) [ L. *Pasteur* ]. The heating of milk, wines, fruit juices, etc., for about 30 minutes at 68°C. (154.4°F.) whereby the living bacteria are destroyed, but the flavor or bouquet is preserved; the spores are unaffected, but are kept from developing by immediately cooling the liquid to 10°C. (50°F.) or lower. See also sterilization.

**pasteurize** (pas'tur-īz). To treat milk or other liquids after the manner described under pasteurization.

**pas'teuri'zer.** An apparatus used in the pasteurization of fluids.

**Pastia,** C., Roumanian physician. See P.'s *sign*.

**pastil, pastille** (pas'til, pas-tēl') [ Fr. *pastille*; L. *pastillus*, a roll (of bread), dim. of *panis*, bread ]. 1. A small mass of benzoin and other aromatic substances to be burned for fumigation. 2. A troche.

   **Sabouraud's p.'s,** disks of barium platinocyanide in a mixture of acetate of starch and collodion, which undergo a color change when exposed to the x-rays, the degree of change indicating, like Holzknecht's chromoradiometer, the strength of the rays.

**past-pointing.** A test of the integrity of the vestibular apparatus of the ear; the person, seated in a revolving chair, is rotated to the right ten rounds, the eyes being closed, then his right index finger, with arm horizontal, is brought to touch the tip of the examiner's finger; now he raises his arm vertically and is told to touch the examiner's finger again on bringing the arm once more to the horizontal; if the vestibular apparatus is normal, the finger will be brought down several inches to the right of the examiner's finger because he then has the sensation of rotation to the left. The reverse is true of rotation to the left. This test is also used in connection with caloric stimulation.

**patagium,** pl. **pata'gia** (pă-ta'jĭ-um) [ L. a gold edging on a woman's gown ]. A winglike membrane.

   **cer'vical p.,** *pterygium* colli.

**Patau,** Klaus, U. S. geneticist. See P.'s *syndrome*.

**patch.** 1. A small circumscribed area differing in color or structure from the surrounding surface. 2. See patch *test*.

   **butterfly p.,** butterfly (2).

   **cotton wool p.'s,** areas of exudate seen in hypertensive retinopathy.

**herald p.,** the initial manifestation of .tyriasis rosea, consisting of a large, solitary lesion, pre ding sometimes by several days or weeks the general e uption.

   **Hutchinson's p.,** salmon p.

   **moth p.,** chloasma.

   **mucous p.,** an oval to round, yellow-gray to white, maturated lesion or lesions occurring on the mucous membranes; usually seen in secondary syphilis.

   **opaline p.,** a mucous p. of silver-gray appearance.

   **Peyer's p.'s,** *folliculi* lymphatici aggregati.

   **salmon p.,** Hutchinson's p.; interstitial or parenchymatous keratitis giving rise to neovascularization of the cornea.

   **smoker's p.'s,** leukoplakia.

   **soldier's p.'s,** milk *spots* (1).

**patefaction** (pa-te-fak'shun) [ L. *pate-facio,* pp. *-factus,* to make lie open, fr. *pateo,* to lie open ]. A laying open.

**Patein** (pat-an'), G., French physician, 1857–1928. See P.'s *albumin.*

**patel'la,** gen. and pl. **patellae** [ L. a small plate, the kneecap, dim. of *patina,* a shallow disk, fr. *pateo,* to lie open ] [ NA ]. Kneecap; the large sesamoid bone, in the combined tendon of the extensors of the leg, covering the anterior surface of the knee.

   **floating p.,** a p. riding high on effusion of the knee.

   **slipping p.,** spontaneous or easily provoked dislocation of the p.

**patel'lar.** Relating to the patella.

**patellectomy** (pat'e-lek'to-mi) [ patella + G. *ektome,* excision ]. Excision of the patella.

**patel'liform.** Of the shape of the patella.

**patellometer** (pat'e-lom'e-ter) [ patella + G. *metron,* measure ]. Instrument for measuring the patellar reflex.

**patency** (pa'ten-si). The state of being freely open or patulous.

   **probe p.** (of foramen ovale), a term introduced by Patten to cover incomplete fibrous adhesion of an adequate valvula foraminis ovalis in the postnatal closure of the foramen ovale.

**pa'tent** [ L. *patens,* pres. p. of *pateo,* to lie open ]. Open; expanded.

**Pat'erson,** Robert, Scottish physician, 1814–1889. See P.'s *corpuscles, nodules.*

**Paterson-Kelly syndrome.** See under syndrome.

**path-, patho-, -pathy** [ G. *pathos,* suffering, disease. PATH- ]. Combining forms meaning disease.

**path** [ A.S. *paeth* ]. A road or way; the course taken by an electric current or by nervous impulses. See also pathway.

   **condyle p.,** the p. traveled by the mandibular condyle in the temporomandibular joint during the various mandibular movements.

   **condyle p., lateral,** the p. of the condyle in the glenoid fossa when a lateral mandibular movement is made.

   **generated occlusal p.,** a registration of the p.'s of movement of the occlusal surfaces of mandibular teeth on a plastic or abrasive surface attached to the maxillary arch; see also functional chew-in *record.*

   **incisal p.,** incisal *guidance.*

   **p. of insertion,** see under insertion.

   **milled-in p.'s,** milled-in curves; (1) contours carved by various mandibular movements into the occluding surface of an occlusion rim, by teeth or studs placed in the opposing occlusion rim; the curves or contours may be carved into wax, modeling plastic, or plaster of Paris; (2) occlusal curves developed by masticatory or gliding movements of occlusion rims which are composed of materials including abrasives; see also functional chew-in *record.*

   **occlusal p.,** (1) a gliding occlusal contact; (2) the p. of movement of an occlusal surface.

**pathema** (pa-the'mah) [ G. *pathema,* suffering. PATH- ]. Any disease or morbid condition.

**pathematology** (pa-the'ma-tol'o-ji) [ G. *pathema,* (*pathemat-*), suffering, + *logos,* study ]. Pathology, especially mental pathology.

**pathergasia** (path'er-ga'zi-ah) [ G. *pathos,* disease, + *ergasia,* work ]. A physiologic or anatomical defect that limits normal emotional adjustment.

**pathergy** (path'er-ji) [ G. *pathos,* disease, + *ergon,* work ]. A term suggested to include reactions of all kinds resulting from a state of altered activity, both allergic (immune) and nonallergic.

**pathetic** (pa-thet'ik) [ G. *pathetikos,* relating to the feelings ]. 1. Denoting that which arouses sorrow or pity. 2. Denoting the fourth cranial nerve (pathetic nerve, or nervus patheticus), the *nervus* trochlearis, *q.v.*

**path'etism** [ G. *pathetos,* subject to suffering ]. Mesmerism; hypnotism.

**path'etist.** A mesmerizer; a hypnotist.

**path'finder.** A filiform bougie for introduction through a narrow stricture end to serve as a guide for the passage of a larger sound or catheter.

**pathic** (path'ik) [ G. *pathikos,* remaining passive ]. A person who assumes the passive role in any abnormal sexual act. See also passivism.

**patho-.** See path-.

**pathoamine** (path-o-am'en). A ptomaine.

**path'oanat'omy.** Pathologic *anatomy.*

**path'obiol'ogy.** Pathology.

**path'oclis'is** [ patho- + G. *klisis,* bending, proneness ]. A specific tendency to sensitivity to special toxins; a tendency for toxins to attack certain organs.

**pathocrin'ia** [ patho- + G. *krinein,* to separate ]. Obsolete term meaning disorder of the glands of internal secretion.

**pathocure** (path'o-kūr). The disappearance of a neurosis upon the outbreak of an organic disease.

**pathodixia** (path'o-dik'si-ah) [ patho- + G. *deiknunai,* to show ]. A morbid desire to exhibit one's injured or diseased part.

**pathodontia** (path-o-don'shi-ah) [ patho- + G. *odous,* tooth ]. The science dealing with diseases of the teeth.

**pathofor'mic** [ patho- + L. *formo,* to form ]. Relating to the beginning of disease; denoting especially certain symptoms occurring in the transition period between a normal and a diseased state.

**pathogen** (path'o-jen) [ patho- + suffix *-gen,* to produce ]. Any virus, microorganism, or other substance causing disease.

   **opportunistic p.,** an organism that is capable of causing disease only when the host's resistance is lowered, *e.g.,* by other diseases or drugs.

**pathogenesis** (path'o-jen'e-sis) [ patho- + G. *genesis,* production ]. The mode of origin or development of any disease or morbid process.

   **drug p.,** the production of morbid symptoms by drugs.

**pathogen'ic, pathogenet'ic.** Morbific; morbigenous; nosopoietic; causing disease.

**pathogenicity** (path'o-je-nis'i-ti). The condition of being pathogenic or of causing disease.

**pathogeny** (pa-thoj'e-ni). Pathogenesis.

**pathognomonic** (pa-thog'no-mon'ik) [ see pathognomy ]. Pathognostic; characteristic or indicative of a disease; denoting especially one or more typical symptoms.

**pathognomy** (pa-thog'no-mi) [ patho- + G. *gnome,* a mark, a sign. Diagnosis by means of a study of the typical symptoms of a disease, or of the subjective sensations of the patient.

**pathognostic** (path-og-nos'tik) [ patho- + G. *gnostikos,* pertaining to knowledge ]. Pathognomonic.

**pathog'raphy** [ patho- + G. *graphe,* a description ]. A treatise on or description of disease; a treatise on pathology.

**pathole'sia** [ path- + G. *lesis,* choice, will ]. Any impairment or abnormality of the will.

**pathologic** (path-o-log'ik). Pertaining to pathology; morbid; diseased; resulting from disease.

**pathol'ogist.** A physician who is specially trained and experienced in anatomical, experimental, clinical pathology. P.'s are doctors of medicine who practice chiefly in the laboratory, serving as consultants to their clinical colleagues (especially with reference to histologic diagnoses on tissue removed for biopsy, and the selection of diagnostic tests and interpretation of laboratory results), performing postmortem studies, and designing and participating in research of various types (case studies, experimental, and so on).

**pathology** (pă-thol'o-jĭ) [ patho- + G. *logos*, study, treatise ]. The medical science, and specialty practice, that deals with all aspects of disease, but with special reference to the essential nature, the causes, and development of abnormal conditions, as well as the structural and functional changes that result from the disease processes. Although there are disciplines known as animal p. and plant p., the term is ordinarily construed to mean *human* p. when used without a modifier.

    **anatomical p.**, the subspecialty of p. that pertains to the gross and microscopic study of organs and tissues removed for biopsy or during postmortem examination, and also the interpretation of the results of such study. Termed also pathologic or morbid anatomy.

    **animal p.**, the science or study dealing with diseases of animal.

    **cellular p.**, (1) the interpretation of diseases in terms of cellular alterations, the ways in which cells fail to maintain homeostasis; (2) sometimes used as a synonym for cytopathology.

    **clinical p.**, (1) in a strict sense, any part of the medical practice of p. (including anatomic p. or pathologic anatomy) as it pertains to the care of patients; (2) the subspecialty in p. that deals with the theoretical and technical aspects (*i.e.*, the methods or procedures) of chemistry, bacteriology, virology, mycology, parasitology, immunology, hematology, biophysics, and so on, as they pertain to the diagnosis of disease and the care of patients, as well as the prevention of disease and welfare of the community.

    **comparative p.**, the p. of diseases of animals, especially in relation to human p.

    **dental p.**, oral p.

    **functional p.**, that pertaining to abnormalities in function of a tissue, organ, or part, with or without associated changes in structure.

    **geographic p.**, the study of disease in its relation to climate and to the various parts of the earth's surface.

    **humoral p.**, the thesis that disorders in the fluids of the body, especially the blood, are the basic factors in disease.

    **medical p.**, that pertaining to various diseases not suitable for treatment by means of surgery.

    **molecular p.**, the study of biochemical and biophysical cellular mechanisms which are the basic factors in disease.

    **oral p.**, dental p.; the branch of dentistry concerned with the gross and microscopic nature of diseases of the teeth, jaws and tissues lining the mouth.

    **plant p.**, the science or study dealing with diseases of plants, especially the higher forms.

    **surgical p.**, a field in anatomical p., dealing with examination of tissues removed from living patients for the purpose of diagnosis of disease and guidance in the care of patients.

    **vegetable p.**, plant p.

**pathom'eter** [ patho- + G. *metron*, measure ]. A device for recording the varying incidence of the exanthemas and other infectious diseases, endemic or epidemic in a certain locality.

**pathomet'ric.** Relating to pathometry.

**pathometry** (pă-thom'e-trĭ) [ patho- + G. *metron*, measure ]. 1. Determination of the proportionate number of individuals affected with a certain disease at a given time, and of the conditions leading to an increase or decrease in this number. 2. The measurement of illness and of incapacity resulting from trauma, as regards both the individual affections and the sum total of disability, in the several occupations and social conditions; see also nosometry.

**pathomimesis** (path'o-mĭ-me'sis) [ patho- + G. *mimēsis*, imitation ]. Pathomimicry; mimicry of disease, whether intentional or unconscious.

**pathomimicry** (path-o-mim'ĭ-krĭ). Pathomimesis.

**pathomiosis** (path'o-mi-o'sis) [ patho- + G. *meiōsis*, a lessening ]. The attitude of a patient which leads him to minimize his disease.

**pathomor'phism.** Abnormal morphology.

**pathoneurosis** (path'o-nu-ro'sis). A neurotic preoccupation with real illness.

**pathono'mia, pathon'omy** [ patho- + G. *nomos*, law ]. The science of the laws of morbid changes.

**pathopho'bia** [ patho- + G. *phobos*, fear ]. A morbid fear of disease.

**path'ophysiol'ogy.** Derangement of function seen in disease; alteration in function as distinguished from structural defects.

**pathopoiesis** (path'o-poy-e'sis). [ patho- + G. *poiēsis*, making ]. The mode of production of disease.

**pathopsychology** (path-o-si-kol'o-jĭ) [ patho- + psychology, *q. v.* ]. The study of deviations from normal psychological processes.

**patho'sis** [ patho- + suffix -*osis*, condition ]. A state of disease; a diseased condition; a finding, *e.g.*, periapical p., pulmonary p., etc.

**pathotropism** (path-ot'ro-pizm) [ patho- + G. *tropos*, a turning ]. Attraction of drugs toward diseased structures.

**path'way.** 1. A collection of axons establishing a conduction route for nerve impulses from one group of nerve cells to another group or to an effector organ composed of muscle or gland cells. 2. Any sequence of chemical reactions leading from one compound to another; if taking place in living tissue, usually referred to as a **biochemical p.**

    **Embden-Meyerhof p.**, the anaerobic glycolytic p. by which glucose (most notably in muscle) is converted to lactic acid.

    **Embden-Meyerhof-Parnas p.**, Embden-Meyerhof p.

**patient** (pa'shent) [ L. *patiens*, pres. p. of *patior*, to suffer ]. One who is suffering from any disease and is under treatment for it; not to be confused with "case," *q. v.*

    **target p.**, in psychoanalytic group therapy, the p. being analyzed in turn by another member p.

**pat'ricide** [ L. *pater*, father, + *caedō*, to kill ]. 1. The killing of one's father. 2. A person who commits such an act.

**Patrick,** Hugh T., Chicago neurologist, 1860–1938. See P.'s *test.*

**patrilineal** (pat'rĭ-lin'e-al) [ L. *pater*, father, + *linea*, line ]. Related to descent through the male line.

**pat'ten** [ Fr. *patin*, a clog ]. A support placed under one shoe to equalize the length of the two legs, when one is shorter than the other, or when one is artificially lengthened by a brace or splint.

**pat'tern.** 1. A design. 2. In dentistry, a form used in making a mold, as for an inlay or partial denture framework.

    **action p.**, according to Crile's theory, a complicated set of tracks or grooves (figuratively speaking), partly congenital and partly acquired, for the conduction of stimuli and impulses in the brain, in virtue of which a certain stimulus is apt to be followed by a certain action, the action induced by the stimulus varying in each individual according to the action p. in his brain.

    **juvenile p.**, precordial T-wave inversion in the electrocardiogram, resembling that seen in normal children; it occurs as a normal variant in some adults, especially Negroes.

    **occlusal p.**, occlusal *form.*

    **wax p.**, a wax form of shape which, when invested and burned out or otherwise eliminated, will produce a mold in which a casting may be made.

**patulin** (pat'u-lin). Clavacin; clavatin; claviformin; a hydroxy furopyranone; a bacteriostatic and bactericidal principle isolated from at least four kinds of mold: *Aspergillus clavatus, Penicillium claviforme, P. patulum,* and *P. expansum.*

**patulous** (pat'u-lus) [ L. *patulus*, fr. *pateo*, to lie open ]. Patent; lying freely open.

**paucisynaptic** (paw'sĭ-sĭ-nap'tik) [ L. *paucus*, few, + synapse, *q. v.* ]. Oligosynaptic.

**Paul,** Gustav, Vienna physician, 1859–1935. See P.'s *reaction, test.*

**Paul** of Aegina, Greek eclectic surgeon, 625–690 A.D. An assiduous compiler of the works of his predecessors; wrote an *Epitome* of medicine in seven volumes in which lithotomy, trephining, surgery of the eye, tonsillectomy, and amputation of the breast were described.

**Pauli's principle.** See under principle.

**Pauling,** Linus C., American chemist, *1901. See P.-Corey *helix,* P.'s *theory.*

**paulocardia** (paw-lo-kar'dī-ah) [ G. *paula,* a pause, fr. *pauō,* to cease, + *kardia,* heart ]. 1. A sensation that the heart has stopped beating. 2. A condition in which the period of rest in the cardiac cycle is unduly prolonged.

**Pauly reaction.** See under reaction.

**paunch** (pawnch). Rumen, or largest compartment of the stomach of the cow or other ruminant.

**pause** (pawz) [ G. *pausis,* cessation ]. Temporary stop.

**compensatory p.,** the p. following an extrasystole, when the p. is long enough to compensate for the prematurity of the extrasystole; the short cycle ending with the extrasystole plus the p. following the extrasystole together equal two of the regular cycles.

**postextrasystolic p.,** the somewhat prolonged cycle immediately following an extrasystole.

**preautomat'ic p.,** a temporary p. in cardiac activity before an automatic pacemaker escapes (see escape).

**sinus p.,** a spontaneous interruption in the regular sinus rhythm, the p. lasting for a period that is not an exact multiple of the sinus cycle; sinus arrest; sinus standstill.

**Pautrier** (po-tre-a'), Lucien M. A., French physician, 1876–1959. P.'s *abscess, microabscess.*

**Pauzat** (po-zǎ'), Jean E., French physician, 19th century. See P.'s *disease.*

**pave'ment** [ L. *pavimentum,* a floor, pavement, fr. *pavio,* to beat, ram down ]. Any structure resembling a p. or a tiled floor.

**pa'vex.** An apparatus for producing passive vascular exercise in peripheral circulatory disorders by means of alternate positive and negative pressure.

**Pavlov** (pahv'lawf), Ivan P., Russian physiologist, 1849–1936. Nobel prize-winner 1904; noted for his investigations of the digestive glands; originated the method of sham feeding; discovered conditioned reflexes. See P. *method, pouch, reflex, stomach.*

**pa'vor** [ L. ]. Fear; terror.

**p. noctur'nus,** *night-terrors.*

**Pavy,** Frederick W., English physician, 1829–1911. See P.'s *disease, reagent.*

**Pawlik** (pahv'lik), Karel, Prague obstetrician, 1849–1914. See P.'s *grip.*

**paw'paw.** See papaya.

**Paxton,** F. V., English physician. See P.'s *disease.*

**Payr** (pīr), Erwin, German surgeon, 1871–1946. See P.'s *clamp, membrane, sign.*

**PB.** Symbol for barometric *pressure.*

**Pb.** Chemical symbol for the element lead (plumbum).

**PBI.** Abbreviation for protein-bound *iodine.*

**PCMB** (*pCMB*). Abbreviation for *p*-chloromercuribenzoic acid (now replaced by ClHgBzOH).

**Pco₂** or **pCO₂.** Symbol for partial pressure (tension) of carbon dioxide; see partial *pressure.*

**P-congenitale.** The P-wave pattern in the electrocardiogram seen in some cases of congenital heart disease, consisting of tall peaked P waves in leads I, II, aVF, and aVL, with predominant positivity of diphasic waves in V1-2. See also Spannungs-P.

**Pd.** Chemical symbol for the element palladium.

**p.d.** Abbreviation of prism *diopter.*

**P-dex'trocardia'le.** An electrocardiographic syndrome characteristic of overloading of the right atrium, often erroneously called P-pulmonale (*q.v.*) because the syndrome can result from any overloading of the right atrium (*e.g.,* tricuspid stenosis) and independently of cor pulmonale.

**peach kernel oil.** See persic oil.

**Péan** (pa-oṅ'), Jules, Paris surgeon, 1830–1898. See P.'s *forceps.*

**peanut oil** (USP). Arachis oil; oil extracted from the kernels of one or more cultivated varieties of *Arachis hypogaea* (family *Leguminosae*); used as a solvent for intramuscular injections.

**pearl.** 1. A concretion formed around a grain of sand or other foreign body within the shell of certain mollusks. 2. A small hollow sphere of thin glass containing amyl nitrite

or other fluid for inhalation; the p. is crushed in a handkerchief and its contents are inhaled. 3. One of a number of small tough masses of mucus occurring in the sputum in asthma.

**Elschnig p.'s,** remnants of partially absorbed lens following surgical capsulotomy or injury to the capsule.

**enamel p.,** enameloma.

**epithe'lial p.'s,** epithelial *nests.*

**Epstein's p.'s,** Bonn's nodules; Epstein's cysts; multiple, small, white, epithelial inclusion cysts found in the midline of the palate in most newborn infants; probably developmental in origin.

**gouty p.,** a concretion of sodium urate on the cartilage of the ear, occurring in the gouty.

**keratin p.,** squamous p.

**Laënnec's p.'s,** small, round, translucent, tenacious bodies in the sputum of some persons with asthma; when floated in water, they become unfurled and are then recognizable as Curschmann's spirals.

**squamous p.,** keratin p.; a focus of central keratinization within concentric layers of abnormal squamous cells; seen in squamous cell carcinoma.

**pearl-ash.** Impure potassium carbonate.

**Pearson,** Carl M. See McArdle-Schmid-P. *disease.*

**peb'bles.** Lenses for eyeglasses cut from colorless rock crystal, or quartz.

**peccant** (pek'ant) [ L. *peccans* (-*ant-*), pres. p. of *pecco,* to sin ]. Morbid; unhealthy; producing disease.

**peccatiphobia** (pek'kah-tī-fo'bī-ah) [ L. *pecco,* to sin, + G. *phobos,* fear ]. Morbid fear of sinning.

**pecilo-.** See poikilo–.

**pecilocin.** VARIOTIN; *N*-(8'-hydroxy-6'-methyl-*trans-trans-cis*-dodeca-2',4',6'-trienoyl)-2-pyrrolidone; antifungal agent.

**Pecquet** (pek-a'), Jean, French anatomist, 1622–1674. See P.'s *cistern, duct, receptaculum, reservoir.*

**pec'tase.** An enzyme, present in fruits, that converts pectin to pectic acid; used in the clarification of fruit juices.

**pec'ten** [ L. comb ] 1 [ NA ]. A structure with comblike processes or projections. 2. The middle third of the anal canal.

**p. ossis pubis** [ NA ], p. pubis; pectineal line of the pubis; the continuation on the superior ramus pubis of the terminal line, forming a sharp ridge.

**p. sclerae,** a pleated membrane that extends from the optic disk into the vitreous body in birds.

**pectenitis** (pek-ten-i'tis) [ L. *pecten,* a comb, + -*itis* ]. Inflammation of the sphincter ani.

**pecteno'sis.** Exaggerated enlargement of the pecten band.

**pectic** (pek'tik) [ G. *pēktos,* stiff, curdled ]. Relating to any of the pectic substances or materials; see pectin.

**p. acid,** galacturonic acid.

**pectin** (pek'tin) (NF). Broad, generic term for what are now called pectic substances or pectic materials; a gelatinous substance extracted from fruits, where it is presumed to exist as protopectin (pectose), that is largely responsible for the gelling of fruit juices. P. consists largely of long chains of galacturonic acid units. The commercial p.'s are sometimes called pectinic acid. Used in the preparation of jams, jellies, and similar food products; therapeutically, to control diarrhea, usually in conjunction with other agents; has also been used as a plasma expander.

**pec'tinase.** Polygalacturonase.

**pec'tinate.** Combed; comb-shaped.

**pectineal** (pek-tin'e-al). Ridged; relating to the os pubis or to any comblike structure.

**pectine'us** [ L. ]. 1. Pectineal. 2. See *musculus* pectineus.

**pectin'ic acids.** See pectin.

**pectin'iform.** Pectinate.

**pectization** (pek-tī-za'shun) [ G. *pēktikos,* curdling ]. In colloidal chemistry, the same as coagulation.

**pec'toral** [ L. *pectoralis;* fr. *pectus,* breast bone ]. Relating to the chest.

**pectoralgia** (pek'to-ral'jī-ah) [ L. *pectus* (*pector-*), chest, + G. *algos,* pain ]. Pain in the chest.

**pectoriloquy** (pek-to-ril'o-kwī) [ L. *pectus,* chest, + *loquor,* to speak ]. Pectorophony; transmission of the voice sound through the pulmonary structures, so that it is audible on auscultation of the chest; it indicates either solidification of the pulmonary structures or the presence of a large cavity.

   **aphonic p.,** Baccelli's *sign.*

   **whispered p.,** the transmission of the whisper in the same way as that of the voice in ordinary p.

**pectorophony** (pek′to-rof′o-nĭ) [ L. *pectus,* chest, + G. *phōnē,* voice ]. Pectoriloquy.

**pec′tose.** Protopectin; see pectin.

**pectous** (pek′tus). 1. Relating to or consisting of pectin or pectose. 2. Denoting a firm, coagulated condition sometimes assumed by a gel, which is permanent in that the substance cannot be made to reassume the gel form.

**pectus,** gen. **pec′toris,** pl. **pec′tora** (pek′tus) [ L. ] [ NA ]. The thorax; the chest; especially the anterior wall, the breast.

   **p. carina′tum** [ L. *carina,* keel ], pigeon breast; chicken breast; keeled chest; flattening of the chest on either side with forward projection of the sternum, like the keel of a boat.

   **p. excava′tum,** a hollow at the lower part of the chest caused by a backward displacement of the xiphoid cartilage. Also called pectus recurvatum; funnel breast or chest; foveated chest; chonechondrosternon; koilosternia.

   **p. recurva′tum,** p. excavatum.

**ped-, pedi-, pedo-.** 1 [ G. *pais,* child. PAED-, PED- ]. Combining forms meaning child. 2 [ L. *pes,* foot. PES- ]. Combining forms relating to feet.

**ped′al** [ L. *pedalis,* fr. *pes* (*ped*-), a foot ]. Relating to the feet, or to any structure called pes.

**peda′lis** [ L. ] [ NA ]. Pedal.

**pedarthrocace** (ped′ar-throk′ă-se) [ G. *pais* (*paid*-), child, + *arthron,* joint, + *kakos,* bad ]. Joint disease in children.

**pedatro′phia, pedat′rophy** [ G. *pais* (*paid*-), child, + atrophy ]. Marasmus.

**ped′erast.** A person given to pederasty.

**pederasty** (ped′er′as′tĭ) [ G. *paiderastia;* fr. *pais* (*paid*-), boy, + *eraō,* to long for ]. Coitus per anum, or anal intercourse, especially when practiced on boys.

**Pedersen's speculum.** See under speculum.

**pedesis** (pe-de′sis) [ G. *pedēsis,* a leaping, fr. *pēdaō,* fut. -*ēsō,* to leap ]. Brownian *movements.*

**pedial′gia.** Pedionalgia.

**pediatric** (pe-dĭ-at′rik) [ G. *pais* (*paid*-), child, + *iatrikos,* relating to medicine ]. Relating to the study and treatment of children in health and disease.

**pediatrician** (pe-dĭ-ă-trish′an). Pediatrist; a medical practitioner who specializes in the diseases of children.

**pediatrics** (pe′dĭ-at′riks) [ G. *pais* (*paid*-), child, + *iatreia,* medical treatment ]. Pediatry; the branch of medical science that treats of children in their hygienic, physiologic, and pathologic relations; the specialty of the diseases of children.

**pediatrist** (pe-dĭ-at′rist). Pediatrician.

**pediatry** (pe′dĭ-at′rĭ, pe-dĭ′ă-trĭ). Pediatrics.

**pedicel** (ped′ĭ-sel) [ Mod. L. *pedicellus,* dim. of L. *pes,* foot ]. Foot process; footplate (2); the secondary process of a podocyte which helps form the visceral capsule of a renal corpuscle.

**ped′icellate, ped′icellated.** Pedunculate.

**pedicellation** (ped-ĭ-sel-la′shun). Formation of a pedicle or peduncle.

**pedicle** (ped′ĭ-kl) [ L. *pediculus,* dim. of *pes,* foot. PES- ]. 1. Pediculus (1). 2. Peduncle (2). 3. A tubed stalk by means of which a skin graft made at a distant site is later moved to a desired position.

   **p. of arch of a vertebra,** *pediculus* arcus vertebrae.

   **Filatov-Gillies tubed p.,** the long edges of the graft are sewn together, leaving both ends attached to induce a blood supply parallel to the long axis of the flap, and to prevent any granulation or scar tissue formation on its deep surface.

**pedicterus** (pe-dik′ter-us) [ G. *pais* (*paid*-), child, + *ikteros,* jaundice ]. *Icterus* neonatorum.

**pedicular** (pĕ-dik′u-lar). Relating to pediculi, or lice.

**pedic′ulate.** Pedunculate.

**pedicula′tion** [ L. *pediculus,* louse ]. Pediculosis; infestation with lice.

**pediculi** (pĕ-dik′u-li) [ L. ]. Plural of pediculus.

**pediculicide** (pĕ-dik′u-lĭ-sĭd) [ L. *pediculus,* louse, + *caedo,* to kill ]. An agent used to destroy lice.

**Pediculoi′des ventrico′sus** [ Mod. L. fr. L. *pediculus,* louse, + *venter,* belly ]. The grain itch mite; a mite infesting straw or grain and causative of straw itch or grain itch.

**pediculopho′bia** [ L. *pediculus,* louse, + G. *phobos,* fear ]. Morbid fear of infestation with lice.

**pediculosis** (pĕ-dik′u-lo′sis) [ L. *pediculus,* louse, + G. suffix -*osis,* condition ]. Lousiness; phthiriasis; the state of being infested with pediculi or lice.

   **p. cap′itis,** the presence of lice on the hair of the head.

   **p. cor′poris,** p. vestimenti; the presence of body lice. See also parasitic *melanoderma.*

   **p. palpebra′rum,** the presence of lice in the eyelashes.

   **p. pu′bis,** the presence of pubic lice.

   **p. vestimen′ti, p. vestimento′rum,** p. corporis.

**pedic′ulous.** Infested with pediculi; lousy.

**Pediculus** (pĕ-dik′u-lus) [ L. ]. A genus of lice of the family Pediculidae; animal parasites that live in the hair (*P. capitis, P. pubis*) or clothing (*P. corporis*) and feed on the body.

   **P. huma′nus,** the species of louse infecting man.

   **P. humanus** var. **capitis,** the head louse of man.

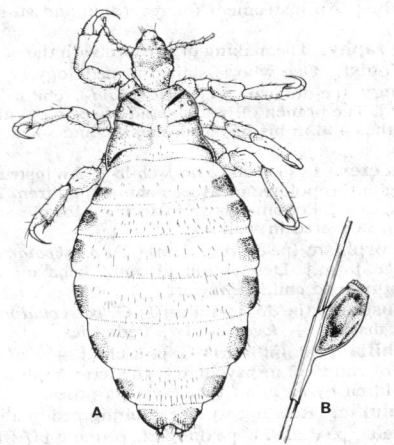

***Pediculus humanus* var. *capitis***

*A,* the female head louse (×20); *B,* egg or nit (×15), attached to hair. (From Najarian, H. H.: *Textbook of Medical Parasitology,* The Williams & Wilkins Co., Baltimore, 1967.)

   **P. humanus** var. **corporis,** sometimes termed *P. vestimenti* or *P. corporis;* the body louse or clothes louse, which lives in the clothing and feeds on the body.

   **P. pu′bis,** *Phthirus pubis.*

   **P. vestimen′ti,** *P. humanus* var. *corporis.*

**pediculus,** pl. **pedic′uli** (pĕ-dik′u-lus) [ L. pedicle. PES- ] 1 [ NA ]. Pedicle (1); a constricted portion or stalk. 2. A louse; see *Pediculus.*

   **p. arcus vertebrae** [ NA ], pedicle of the arch of a vertebra; the constricted portion of the arch on either side extending from the body to the lamina.

**pedicure** (ped′ĭ-kūr) [ L. *pes* (*ped*-), foot, + *cura,* treatment ]. 1. Obsolete term for podiatrist. 2. Care and treatment of the feet.

**pediluvium** (ped′ĭ-lu′vĭ-um) [ L. *pes* (*ped*-), foot, + *luo,* to wash ]. A foot bath.

**pedionalgia** (ped′ĭ-o-nal′jĭ-ah) [ G. *pedion,* a plain, sole of the foot, + *algos,* pain ]. Metatarsalgia; pedialgia; pedioneuralgia; pain in the sole of the foot.

**ped′ioneural′gia.** Pedionalgia.

**ped′iopho′bia** [ G. *paidion,* a little child, + *phobos,* fear ]. Morbid fear aroused by the sight of a child or of a doll.

**pediphalanx** (ped′ĭ-fa′langks) [ L. *pes* (*ped-*), foot, + phalanx ]. A phalanx of the foot, distinguished from maniphalanx.

**pedo-** (pe′do-, ped′o-). See ped-.

**pedobaromacrometer** (pe′do-băr′o-mă-krom′e-ter) [ G. *pais* (*paid-*), child, + *baros*, weight, + *makros*, length, + *metron*, measure ]. A form of scales for weighing a baby and at the same time measuring its length.

**pedobarometer** (pe′do-bă-rom′e-ter) [ G. *pais* (*paid-*), child, + *baros*, weight, + *metron*, measure ]. Scales for weighing a baby.

**pedodontia** (pe′do-don′shĭ-ah). Pedodontics.

**pedodontics** (pe′do-don′tiks) [ G. *pais*, child, + *odous*, tooth ]. Pedodontia; dental care and treatment of children.

**pe′dodon′tist.** A dentist who practices pedodontics.

**pedodynamometer** (ped′o-di-nă-mom′e-tur) [ L. *pes* (*ped-*), foot, + G. *dynamis*, force, + G. *metron*, measure ]. An instrument for measuring the strength of the leg muscles.

**pedogenesis** (pe′do-jen′ĕ-sis) [ G. *pais* (*paid-*), child, + *genesis*, origin ]. Permanent larval stage with sexual development, as in certain gall midges (genus *Miastor*); *cf.* neoteny.

**ped′ogram.** A record made by the pedograph.

**pedograph** (ped′o-graf) [ L. *pes* (ped-), foot, + G. *graphō*, to write ]. An instrument for recording and studying the gait.

**pedog′raphy.** The making of a record with the pedograph.

**pedol′ogist.** One who is skilled in pedology.

**pedology** (pe-dol′o-jĭ) [ G. *pais* (*paid-*), child, + *logos*, study ]. The branch of biology and of sociology that deals with the child in his physical, mental, and social development.

**pedom′eter.** 1 [ G. *pais* (*paid-*), child ].. An instrument for taking anthropologic measurements of children. 2 [ L. *pes* (*ped-*), foot ]. Podometer; an instrument for measuring the distance covered in walking.

**pedomorphism** (pe′do-mor′fizm) [ G. *pais* (*paid*), child, + *morphē*, form ]. Description of adult behavior in terms appropriate to child behavior.

**pedonosology** (pe′do-no-sol′o-jĭ) [ G. *pais* (*paid-*), child, + *nosos*, disease, + *logos*, study ]. Pediatrics.

**pedophilia** (pe′do-fil′ĭ-ah) [ G. *pais*, child, + *philos*, fond ]. Love of children; in psychiatry, the term implies the love of children by an adult for sexual purposes.

**pe′dophil′ic.** Relating to or exhibiting pedophilia.

**peduncle** (pĕ-dung′kl, pe′dung-kl, ped′ung-kl) [ Mod. L. *pedunculus*, dim. of *pes*, foot ]. 1. Pedunculus. 2. Pedicle (2); a constricted portion, stalk, or stem forming the attachment of a nonsessile tumor.

   **cerebral p.,** see *pedunculus* cerebri and *crus* cerebri.
   **p. of corpus callosum,** *gyrus* subcallosus.
   **inferior cerebellar p.,** *pedunculus* cerebellaris inferior.
   **inferior thalamic p.,** *pedunculus* thalami inferior.
   **lateral thalamic p.,** *pedunculus* thalami lateralis.
   **p. of mamillary body,** *pedunculus* corporis mamillaris.
   **middle cerebellar p.,** *pedunculus* cerebellaris medius.
   **olfactory p.,** in man and other primates, this term is synonymous with olfactory tract (see *tractus* olfactorius).
   **superior cerebellar p.,** *pedunculus* cerebellaris superior.
   **ventral thalamic p.,** *pedunculus* thalami ventralis.

**peduncular** (pĕ-dung′ku-lar). Relating to a peduncle.

**pedun′culate, pedun′culated.** Pedicellate; pediculate; stalked; having a peduncle; not sessile.

**pedunculotomy** (pĕ-dung′ku-lot′o-mĭ) [ peduncle + G. *tomē*, incision ]. 1. A total or partial section of a cerebral peduncle. 2. A mesencephalic pyramidal *tractotomy.*

**pedun′culus,** pl. **pedun′culi** (pĕ-dung′ku-lus) [ Mod. L. dim. of *pes*, foot. PES- ] [ NA ]. Peduncle (1); a stalk or stem; in neuroanatomy, term loosely applied to a variety of stalklike connecting structures in the brain, composed either exclusively of white matter (*e.g.*, p. cerebellaris) or of white and gray matter (*e.g.*, p. cerebri).
   **p. cerebella′ris infe′rior** [ NA ], inferior cerebellar peduncle; corpus restiforme; restiform body; a large bundle of nerve fibers extending up under the lateral recess of the rhomboid fossa, then curving steeply dorsalward into the cerebellum. It is made up of the dorsal spinocerebellar tract

and the cerebellar afferents originating in the ipsilateral nucleus cuneatus accessorius, vestibular nuclei, and lateral reticular nucleus, and in the contralateral inferior olive. The vestibulocerebellar fibers are placed medially in the p. and are often separately identified as the juxtarestiform body. The inferior cerebellar p. also contains fibers from the nucleus fastigii of the cerebellum to the vestibular nuclei and medullary reticular formation.
   **p. cerebella′ris me′dius** [ NA ], middle cerebellar peduncle; brachium pontis; the largest of three paired cerebellar peduncles, composed entirely of fibers that originate in the nuclei pontis, cross the midline in the pars basilaris pontis, and emerge on the opposite side as a massive bundle arching dorsally along the lateral side of the pontine tegmentum into the cerebellum; it is distributed chiefly to the cortex of the cerebellar hemisphere.
   **p. cerebella′ris supe′rior** [ NA ], superior cerebellar peduncle; brachium conjunctivum cerebelli; a large bundle of nerve fibers that originates from the nuclei dentatus and interpositus and emerges from the cerebellum in the rostral direction, along the lateral wall of the superior recess of the fourth ventricle. The bundle submerges from the dorsal surface of the brainstem into the mesencephalic tegmentum, where all of its fibers cross in the massive decussatio brachii conjunctivi. A large part of the bundle terminates in the red nucleus; the remainder continues rostrally to the nuclei ventralis lateralis, ventralis anterior, and centralis lateralis of the thalamus.
   **p. cer′ebri** [ NA ], cerebral peduncle; originally denoting either of the two halves of the midbrain (a relatively narrow "neck" connecting the forebrain to the hindbrain), this term later came to refer to the crus cerebri together with the midbrain tegmentum, and is now even used occasionally to indicate the crus cerebri (basis pedunculi): the massive bundle of corticofugal fibers on either side at the ventral surface of the midbrain.
   **p. cor′poris callo′si** [ NA ], *gyrus* subcallosus.
   **p. cor′poris mamilla′ris** [ NA ], peduncle of the mamillary body; fasciculus pedunculomamillaris; a fascicle of nerve fibers passing to the mamillary body along the ventral surface of the midbrain; it consists of fibers that originate from the tegmental nuclei of Gudden.
   **p. of the pineal body,** see habenula (2).
   **p. thal′ami infe′rior** [ NA ], inferior thalamic peduncle; a large fiber bundle emerging from the anterior part of the thalamus in the ventral direction, in part joining the medial fibers of the internal capsule, in other part curving laterally around the medial margin of the capsule into the substantia innominata. Many of its fibers establish a reciprocal connection of the mediodorsal nucleus of the thalamus with the orbital gyri of the frontal lobe, but numerous other fibers constitute a conduction system from the amygdala and olfactory cortex to the mediodorsal nucleus. See also *ansa* peduncularis.
   **p. thal′ami latera′lis,** lateral thalamic peduncle; the massive group of fibers that emerges from the laterodorsal side of the thalamus to join the corona radiata; it reciprocally connects the lateral nucleus and the geniculate bodies of the thalamus with the corresponding regions of the cerebral cortex.
   **p. thal′ami ventra′lis,** ventral thalamic peduncle; the massive system of fiber bundles emerging through the ventral, lateral, and anterior borders of the thalamus to join the internal capsule; it contains the fibers reciprocally connecting the ventral thalamic nuclei with the precentral and postcentral gyri of the cerebral cortex.

**peel′ing** [ M.E. *pelen* ]. A stripping off or loss of skin, as in sunburn, postscarlatinal peeling, or toxic epidermal necrolysis.

**pee′nash** [ East Indian ]. Rhinitis caused by insect larvae in the nasal passages.

**PEEP.** Abbreviation for positive end-expiratory *pressure.*

**peg′anine.** Vasicine.

**peg.** A cylindrical projection.
   **rete p.'s,** rete *ridges.*

**pe′jorism** [ L. *pejor*, worse ]. A pessimistic attitude.

**Pel** (peel), Pieter K., Dutch physician 1852–1919. See P.'s crises, P.-Ebstein *disease,* P.-Ebstein *symptom.*

**pelade** (pĕ-lad′, -lahd′) [ Fr. *peler*, to remove the hair from a hide ]. Alopecia.

**pelage** (pel'ij) [ Fr. ]. The hairy covering of the body of animals; *e.g.*, the fur or coat.

**pel'argon'ic acid.** *n*-Nonanoic acid, $CH_3(CH_2)_7COOH$.

**pel'argon'idin.** A flavone derivative of the aglycon of the glycoside pelargonin, one of the plant pigments known as anthocyanins.

**Pelger,** Karel, Amsterdam physician, 1885–1931. See P.-Huët nuclear *anomaly.*

**pelidno'ma** [ G. *pelidnos*, livid, + suffix *-oma*, tumor ]. Pelioma; a circumscribed livid patch on the skin.

**pelio'ma.** Pelidnoma.

**peliosis** (pe'lĭ-o'sis, pel'ĭ-o'sis) [ G. *peliōsis*, a livid spot, livor ]. Purpura.

  **p. hepatis,** the presence in hepatic lobules of multiple microscopic pools of blood which may become lined by endothelium, or organized; a rare condition that may result from congestion of the liver with necrosis.

**Pelizaeus** (pa-le-zi'us), Friedrich, German neurologist, \*1850. See Merzbacher-P. *disease.*

**pellagra** (pĕ-lag'rah, pĕ-la'grah) [ It. *pelle*, skin, + *agro*, rough ]. Erythema endemicum; Asturion, Italian, or Lombardy leprosy; elephantiasis italica; st. Ignatius' itch; maidism; mal de la rosa; psychoneurosis maidica; an affection characterized by gastrointestinal disturbances, erythema followed by desquamation, and nervous and mental disorders. It may occur because of a poor diet, alcoholism, or some other disease upsetting nutrition. Its main cause is a deficiency of niacin, which may be made up to some extent by dietary tryptophan. It is most common in maize-eating persons, perhaps because of toxic material as well as low tryptophan and niacin in the diet.
  **infantile p.,** kwashiorkor.
  **secondary p.,** p. resulting from any morbid condition which upsets nutrition by increasing the requirement or reducing the available supply of vitamins. The treatment is that of p. plus attending to the underlying disease.
  **p. sine p.,** p. without characteristic erythema or dermatitis.

**pellag'roid.** Resembling pellagra.

**pellag'rous.** Relating to or suffering from pellagra.

**pel'lant** [ L. *pello*, to drive ]. Depurative; causing the removal of "peccant humors."

**Pellegrini** (pel-a-gre'ne), Augusto, Italian surgeon, 19th century. See P.'s *disease.*

**pellet** (pel'et) [ Fr. *pelote;* L. *pila*, a ball ]. 1. A pilule, granule, or minute pill. 2. A small, rod-shaped or ovoid dosage form that is sterile and is composed essentially of pure steroid hormones in compressed form, intended for subcutaneous implantation in body tissues; p.'s serve as a depot providing for the slow release of the hormone over an extended period of time.

**Pelletier** (pel-et-e-a'), Pierre J., French chemist, 1788–1842. Gave his name to pelletierine.

**pelletierine** (pel'e-tēr-ēn, -in) [ P. *Pelletier* ]. Punicine; β-(2-piperidyl)propionaldehyde; a volatile liquid alkaloid; one of four alkaloids from pomegranate bark (pelletierine, isopelletierine, methylisopelletierine, and pseudopelletierine). Has been used as a teniacide in the form of tannates.

**pellicle** (pel'ĭ-kl) [ L. *pellicula*, dim of *pellis*, skin ]. 1. Literally and nonspecifically, a thin skin. 2. A film or scum on the surface of a liquid. 3. Cell boundary of sporozoites and merozoites of the protozoan subphylum Apicomplexa (Sporozoa), consisting of an outer unit membrane and an inner layer of two unit membranes.
  **brown p.,** a brownish to black coating that forms near the gingival portion of teeth as a result of improper brushing.

**pellicular, pelliculous** (pĕ-lik'u-lar, -lus). Relating to a pellicle.

**pellis** [ L. ] [ NA ]. Cutis.

**Pellizzari,** C. See Jadassohn-P. *anetoderma.*

**Pellizzi,** G. B. See P.'s *syndrome.*

**pellote** (pa-yo'ta) [ Aztec, *peyotl* ]. Peyote.

**pel'lotine.** *N*-Methylanhalonidine; an alkaloid from *Lophophora williamsii,* a Mexican cactus. The hydrochloride has been used as a hypnotic and in maniacal excitement.

**pellucid** (pel-lu'sid) [ L. *pellucidus* ]. Translucent; allowing the passage of light.

**pellu'cidus** [ L. ] [ NA ]. Pellucid.

**pelma** (pel'mah) [ G. ]. The sole of the foot; planta.

**pelmat'ic** [ G. *pelma*, sole ]. Relating to the sole of the foot.

**pelmat'ogram** [ G. *pelma* (*pelmat-*), sole of the foot, + *gramma,* a picture ]. An imprint of the sole of the foot, made by resting the inked foot on a sheet of paper, or by pressing the greased foot on a plaster of Paris paste.

**pelohemia** (pe'lo-he'mĭ-ah) [ G. *pēlos,* mud, wine-lees, + *haima,* blood ]. Obsolete term for inspissation of the blood.

**pelop'athy** [ G. *pēlos,* mud, + *pathos,* suffering ]. Pelotherapy.

**pe'lother'apy** [ G. *pēlos,* mud, + *therapeia,* treatment ]. Treatment of disease by means of mud baths.

**pelt.** The hide of animals on which the hair, fur, or wool is left.

**pel'ta** [ L. a shield ]. A crescentic, silver-staining, membranous organelle located anteriorly near the base of the flagella in certain flagellate protozoa related to *Trichomonas.*

**pelta'tion** [ L. *pelta,* a light shield ]. The prophylactic influence of inoculation with an antitoxic serum or with a vaccine.

**pelvi-, pelvio-, pelvo-** [ L. *pelvis,* basin (pelvis). PELV- ]. Combining forms relating to the pelvis.

**pel'vic** Relating to a pelvis.
  **p. direction,** the curved line denoting the direction of the axis of the canal of the pelvis.

**pelvicephalography** (pel'vĭ-sef'ă-log'ră-fĭ) [ pelvi- + G. *kephalē,* head, + *graphō,* to write ]. Pelvocephalography; roentgenographic mensuration of the birth canal and of the fetal head.

**pelvicephalometry** (pel'vĭ-sef'ă-lom'ē-trĭ) [ pelvi- + G. *kephalē,* head, + *metron,* measure ]. Measurement of the pelvic diameters in relation to those of the fetal head.

**pelvicliseometer** (pel'vĭ-kliz-e-om'e-ter) [ pelvi- + G. *klisis,* inclination, + *metron,* measure ]. An instrument for measuring the degree of inclination of the pelvis.

**pelvifixa'tion.** Surgical attachment of a floating pelvic organ to the wall of the cavity.

**pel'vigraph** [ pelvi- + G. *graphō,* to write ]. An instrument whereby the contour and dimensions of the pelvis may be drawn to scale.

**pelvilithotomy** (pel'vĭ-lĭ-thot'o-mĭ) [ pelvi- + G. *lithos,* stone, + *tomē,* incision ]. Pyelolithotomy; pelviolithotomy; nephrolithotomy; operative removal of a calculus from the pelvis of the kidney.

**pelvim'eter.** An instrument shaped like calipers for measuring the diameters of the pelvis.
  **Budin's p.,** an instrument fashioned like a large pair of calipers for measuring the diameters of the female pelvis.
  **Martin's p.,** an instrument for measuring certain diameters of the female pelvis; its arms are like those of a large calipers, but reversed.

**pelvimetry** (pel-vim'e-trĭ) [ pelvi- + G. *metron,* measure ]. Measurement of the diameters of the pelvis.
  **manual p.,** estimation of the length of the diameters of the pelvis by the spread of the fingers in the vagina.
  **stereoscopic p.,** roentgenographic mensuration of the pelvis by stereoscopy; two x-ray films are shot under the same conditions except the x-ray tube distance, for which correction is made for distortion.

**pelviolithotomy** (pel'vĭ-o-lĭ-thot'o-mĭ). Pelvilithotomy.

**pelvioperitonitis** pel'vĭ-o-pĕr-ĭ-to-ni'tis). Pelvic *peritonitis.*

**pel'vioplasty** [ pelvio- + G. *plassō,* to form ]. Symphysiotomy or pubiotomy for enlargement of the pelvic outlet.

**pelvioscopy** (pel'vĭ-os'ko-pĭ) [ pelvio- + G. *skopeō,* to view ]. Examination of the pelvis to determine its diameters or for any other purpose.

**pelviotomy** (pel'vĭ-ot'o-mĭ) [ pelvio- + G. *tomē,* incision ]. 1. Symphysiotomy or pubiotomy. 2. An incision into the pelvis of the kidney for the removal of a calculus or for any other purpose.

**pelviperitonitis** (pel-vĭ-pĕr-ĭ-to-ni'tis). Pelvic *peritonitis.*

# PELVIS

**pelvis,** pl. **pelves** (pel′vis, pel′vēz) [ L. basin. PELV- ]. 1
[ NA ]. The massive cup-shaped ring of bone, with its
ligaments, at the lower end of the trunk, formed of the os
coxae (the pubic bone, ilium, and ischium) on either side
and in front, and the sacrum, and coccyx posteriorly. 2.
Any basin-like or cup-shaped cavity, as the p. of the
kidney.

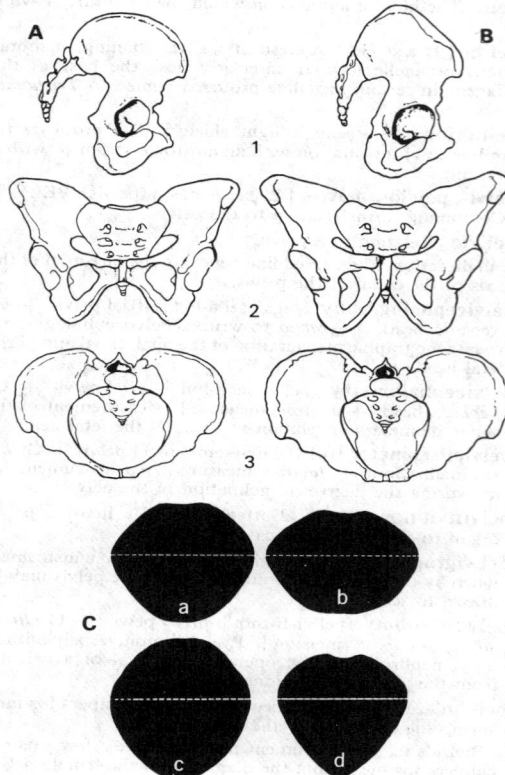

**Pelvis**

*A,* female; *B,* male; *1,* lateral view; *2,* front view; *3,* inlet
view; *C,* types of female pelvis: *a,* gynecoid; *b,* platypelloid;
*c,* anthropoid; *d,* android. (From Fitzpatrick, E., and Eastman, N. J.: *Zabriskie's Obstetrics for Nurses,* J. B. Lippincott Co., Philadelphia, 1960.)

**p. aequabil′iter justo minor,** p. justo minor.

**an′droid p.,** male type (funnel p.).

**an′thropoid p.,** apelike p.; long anteroposterior diameter
and narrow transverse diameter.

**assimila′tion p.,** a deformity in which the transverse
processes of the last lumbar vertebra are fused with the
sacrum, or the last sacral with the first coccygeal body.

**beaked p.,** osteomalacic p.

**brachypellic p.,** transverse oval p.; one in which the
transverse diameter is more than 1 cm. longer but less than
3 cm. longer than the anteroposterior diameter.

**caoutchouc p.,** India rubber p.; rubber p.; a p. in a case
of osteomalacia in which the bones are still soft.

**Chrobak p.,** one deformed in consequence of hip joint
disease.

**contracted p.,** a p. with less than normal measurements
in any diameter.

**cordate p., cor′diform p.,** heart-shaped p.; one with
sacrum projecting forward between the ilia, giving to the
brim a heart shape.

**Deventer's p.,** a p. with shortened anteroposterior
diameter.

**dol′ichopellic p.,** longitudinal oval p.; one in which the
anteroposterior diameter is longer than the transverse.

**dwarf p.,** p. nana; a very small p., in which the several
bones are united by cartilage as in the infant.

**false p.,** p. major.

**flat p.,** p. plana; one in which the anteroposterior
diameter is uniformly contracted, the sacrum being dislocated forward between the iliac bones.

**frozen p.,** hardened p.; a condition in which the true p.
is indurated throughout, especially by carcinoma.

**funnel-shaped p.,** one in which the pelvic inlet dimensions
are normal, but the outlet is contracted in the transverse
or in both transverse and anteroposterior diameters.

**p. of the gallbladder.** Hartmann's *pouch.*

**gyn′ecoid p.,** normal female type.

**hardened p.,** frozen p.

**India rubber p.,** caoutchouc p.

**inverted p.,** split p. with separation at pubis.

**p. justo major,** a symmetrical p. with greater than normal
measurements in all diameters.

**p. justo minor,** one of female type, but with all its
diameters smaller than normal.

**juvenile p.,** a p. justo minor in which the bones are
slender.

**Kilian's p.,** osteomalacic p.

**kyphoscoliot′ic p.,** a p. with marked anteroposterior
curvature of the spine combined with lateral spinal
curvature, usually due to severe rickets.

**kyphot′ic p.,** p. with marked anteroposterior curvature of
spine combined with lateral spinal curvature, usually due
to severe rickets.

**large p.,** p. major.

**lordot′ic p.,** a deformed p. associated with lordosis.

**p. major** [ NA ], large p.; false p.; the expanded portion
of the p. above the brim.

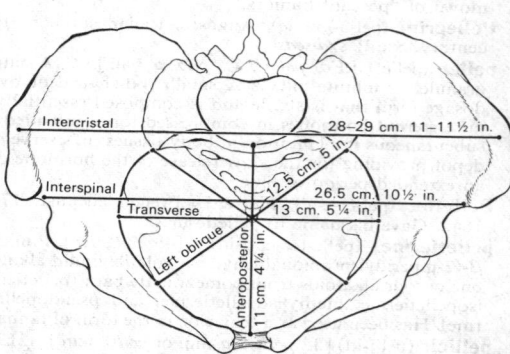

**Diameters of Pelvis Major and Pelvic Brim**

**malacos′teon p.,** osteomalacic or rachitic p.

**masculine p.,** (1) a p. justo minor in which the bones are
large and heavy; (2) a slight degree of funnel-shaped p. in
the woman, in which the shape approximates that of the
male p.

**mesat′ipellic p.,** round p.; one in which the anteroposterior and transverse diameters are equal or the transverse
diameter is not more than 1 cm. longer than the anteroposterior.

**p. minor** [ NA ], small p.; true p.; the cavity of the p.
below the brim or superior aperture.

**Nägele's p.,** an obliquely contracted or unilateral
synostotic p., marked by arrest of development of one
lateral half of the sacrum, usually ankylosis of the
sacroiliac joint on that side, rotation of the sacrum toward
the same side, and deviation of the symphysis pubis to the
opposite side.

**p. obtec'ta,** a form of kyphotic p. in which the angular curvature is low down and extreme so that the spinal column projects horizontally across the inlet of the p.

**osteomalacic p.,** Kilian's p.; p triradiata; beaked p.; rostrate p.; acanthopelvis; acanthopelyx; pelvic deformity in osteomalacia; the pressure of the trunk on the sacrum and lateral pressure of the femoral heads produce a pelvic aperture that is three-cornered or has the shape of a heart or cloverleaf, while the pubic bone becomes beak-shaped. **Otto p.,** Otto's *disease.*

**p. plana,** flat p.

**platypel'lic p.,** flat oval p., in which the transverse diameter is more than 3 cm. longer than the anteroposterior.

**platypel'loid p.,** simple flat p.

**Prague p.,** spondylolisthetic p.

**pseudo-osteomala'cic p.,** an extreme degree of rachitic p., resembling the puerperal osteomalacic p., in which the pelvic canal is obstructed by a forward projection of the sacrum, and an approximation of the acetabula.

**rachit'ic p.,** a contracted and deformed p., most commonly a flat p., occurring from rachitic softening of the bones in early life.

**renal p.,** p. renalis.

**p. rena'lis** [ NA ], renal p.; a flattened funnel-shaped expansion of the upper end of the ureter receiving the calices, the apex being continuous with the ureter.

**ren'iform p.,** a modified cordate p., with a long transverse diameter, giving the brim a kidney shape.

**Robert's p.,** one which is narrowed transversely in consequence of the almost entire absence of the alae of the sacrum.

**Rokitansky''s p.,** spondylolisthetic p.

**rostrate p.,** osteomalacic p.

**rubber p.,** caoutchouc p.

**scoliot'ic p.,** a deformed p. associated with lateral curvature of the spine.

**small p.,** p. minor.

**spider p.,** narrow calices of renal p.

**p. spino'sa** projection of pubis into p.

**split p.,** one in which the symphysis pubis is absent, the pelvic bones being separated by quite an interval; it is usually associated with exstrophy of the bladder.

**spon'dylolisthet'ic p.,** Prague p.; Rokitansky's p.; one whose brim is more or less occluded by a dislocation forward of the body of the lower lumbar vertebra.

**p. spu'ria,** p. major.

**p. triradia'ta,** osteomalacic p.

**true p.,** p. minor.

**p. vera,** p. minor.

---

**pelvisa'cral.** Relating to both the pelvis, or hip bones, and the sacrum.

**pelviscope** (pel'vĭ-skōp) [ pelvi- + G. *skopeō, to view* ]. An instrument for examining the interior of the pelvis.

**pelvitherm** (pel'vĭ-therm) [ pelvi- + G. *thermē,* heat ]. An instrument for applying heat to the pelvic organ.

**pelvit'omy.** Pelviotomy.

**pelviureterography** (pel-vĭ-u-re-ter-og'rā-fĭ). Pyelography.

**pelvo-.** See pelvi-.

**pel'vocephalog'raphy.** Pelvicephalography.

**pelvos'copy.** Pelvioscopy.

**pel'vospondyli'tis ossif'icans** [ L. *pelvis,* basin, + G. *spondylos,* vertebra, + *-itis;* L. *os,* bone, + *facere,* to make ]. Deposit of bony substance between the vertebrae of the sacrum.

**pelyco-, pelyc-** (pel'ĭ-ko-) [ G. *pelyx,* bowl (pelvis). PELV- ]. Rarely used combining forms relating to the pelvis; see also pelvi-, pelvo-.

**pelycology** (pel'ĭ-kol'o-jĭ). The study of the pelvis in all its relations, especially the female pelvis in its relation to pregnancy and childbirth.

**pem'oline** (USAN). DELTAMINE; 2-imino-5-phenyl-4-oxazolidinone; psychostimulant.

**pemphigoid** (pem'fĭ-goyd) [ G. *pemphix,* blister, + *eidos,* resemblance ]. 1. Resembling pemphigus. 2. A disease resembling pemphigus but histologically nonacantholytic and generally benign.

**benign mucosal p.,** cicatricial p.; ocular pemphigus; a chronic disease that produces adhesions and progressive cicatrization and shrinkage of the conjunctivae and nonacantholytic vesicles, and also produces denuded areas of oral mucosa.

**bullous p.,** a chronic, generally benign disease of old age and early childhood; it is characterized by tense nonacantholytic bullae in which serum antibodies are localized to the epidermal basement membrane, causing detachment of the entire epidermis.

**cicatrical p.,** benign mucosal p.

**pemphigus** (pem'fĭ-gus) [ G. *pemphix,* a blister ]. A general term used to designate the chronic bullous diseases, p. foliaceus, p. erythematosus, or p. vegetans; also used with a modifying adjective to designate a variety of blistering skin diseases.

**p. acu'tus,** bullous fever; a pyogenic infection due to local trauma; it responds to antibiotic therapy; if untreated, the condition may become extensive and the patient seriously ill.

**p. contagio'sus,** Manson's pyosis; a superficial pyogenic infection.

**p. croupo'sus,** p. diphtheriticus; the formation of a false membrane on the raw surface left after rupture of the bullae.

**p. diphtherit'icus,** p. crouposus.

**p. erythemato'sus,** Senear-Usher disease or syndrome; an eruption involving the scalp, face, and trunk; the lesions are scaling erythematous macules and blebs, combining the clinical features of both lupus erythematosus and p. vulgaris; the bullae are subcorneal; some authorities believe this to be a variant of p. foliaceus.

**familial benign chronic p.,** Hailey and Hailey disease; recurrent eruption of vesicles and bullae that become scaling and crusted lesions with vesicular borders, predominantly of the neck, groin, and axillary regions; irregular autosomal dominant inheritance.

**p. folia'ceus,** a generally chronic form of p. in which extensive exfoliative dermatitis, with no perceptible blistering, may be present in addition to the bullae; crusted superficial epidermal lesions are usually present at the site of ruptured bullae.

**p. gangreno'sus,** (1) *dermatitis* gangrenosa infantum; (2) bullous *impetigo* of the newborn.

**p. hyster'icus,** an eruption of bullae occurring as a manifestation of conversion hysteria.

**p. lepro'sus,** an eruption of bullae, occurring sometimes in the course of anesthetic leprosy.

**p. neonato'rum,** *dermatitis* exfoliativa neonatorum.

**ocular p.,** benign mucosal *pemphigoid.*

**p. veg'etans,** (1) Neumann's disease; a form of p. vulgaris in which vegetations develop on the eroded surfaces left by ruptured bullae; new bullae continue to form; (2) Hallopeau's disease (2); a chronic benign vegetating form of pemphigus, with lesions commonly in the axillae and perineum; spontaneous remissions and occasionally permanent healing occur.

**p. vulga'ris,** a serious systemic illness in which the previously fatal outcome has been modified by active and persistent treatment; this disease is characterized by an eruption of flaccid acantholytic suprabasal vesicles over the entire body, with erosions on the mucous membranes; the condition results from the action of autoimmune antibodies that localize to interepithelial sites, causing separation of desmosomal attachments, and responds to systemic steroid therapy.

**pem'pidine.** PEROLYSEN; secondary amine of the mecamylamine group, effective as a ganglionic blocking agent. Also available as p. tartrate (BP), with the same uses.

**pen'cil** [ L. *penicillum,* a paint-brush. PENI- ]. 1. A roll of material in the form of a cylinder. 2. A stick, especially of caustic substances, pointed like a p. for local application. 3. All the rays of light focused at a given point.

**Pendred's syndrome.** See under syndrome.

**penec'tomy** [ L. *penis,* + G. *ektomē,* excision ]. Surgical removal of penis.

**pen'etrance** [ see penetration ]. The frequency, usually expressed as a percentage, with which a mutant gene produces its characteristic effect in those individuals possessing it; p. may be specified at the level of clinical disease or at the level of laboratory recognition of a susceptible genotype.

**pen'etrate.** To pierce; to pass into the deeper tissues or into a cavity.

**penetration** (pen'ē-tra'shun) [ L. *penetratio*, fr. *penetro*, pp. *-atus*, to enter ]. 1. Piercing; entering. 2. Mental acumen. 3. In optics, focal *depth*.

**penetrom'eter.** Radiosclerometer; a device for measuring the penetrating power of the x-rays from any given tube, and thus determining the degree of hardness of the tube.

**-penia** [ G. *penia*, poverty ]. Combining form used in the suffix position to denote deficiency.

**pe'nial.** Penile.

**pe'niapho'bia** [ G. *penia*, poverty, + *phobos*, fear ]. Morbid fear of poverty.

**penici'din.** An antibiotic obtained from several species of penicillin. Active against both Gram-positive and Gram-negative bacteria.

**penicil'lamine.** 1. A degradation product of penicillin; β,β-dimethylcysteine. 2 (USP, BP). Chelating agent used in the treatment of lead poisoning and hepatolenticular degeneration; also available as p. hydrochloride (BP).

**penicil'lanate.** A salt of penicillanic acid.

**penicillan'ic acid.** A penicillin (a penicillinic acid) without the characterizing R group (that is, with H— replacing RCONH— in the structure of penicillins, *q. v.*).

**penicil'late.** 1. Pertaining to a penicillus. 2. Having a tuftlike structure.

**penicil'lic acid.** An antibiotic produced by *Penicillium puberulum*, a mold found on maize, and from *P. cyclopium*. Active against Gram-positive and Gram-negative bacteria but toxic to animal tissues.

Penicillic acid

**penicillin** (pen'ĭ-sil'in) [ L. *penicillus*, a hair-pencil. PENI- ]. 1. Originally, an antibiotic substance obtained from cultures of the molds *Penicillium notatum* or *P. chrysogenum*. 2. One of a family of natural or synthetic variants of penicillinic acid. They are mainly bacteriostatic in action, but are also slightly bactericidal. They are especially active against Gram-positive organisms, and show a particularly low toxic action on animal tissue. A filtrate of a culture of *P. notatum* contains several penicillin compounds designated F, G, X, and K (or, according to the British nomenclature, I, II, III, and IV, respectively), and dihydropenicillin. Penicillin G (benzylpenicillin) is the compound in most common use. It comprises over 85 per cent of the penicillin salts (sodium, potassium, aluminum, and procaine). Penicillin K (*n*-heptylpenicillin) is less stable than penicillin G; penicillin F (2-pentenylpenicillin) and dihydropenicillin, though as stable and as effective as penicillin G, are produced by the mold in very small amounts. Penicillins are effective when administered orally, intramuscularly, intravenously, subcutaneously, or by inhalation as an aerosol or a dust. The dose varies with the infection and the mode of administration, from 100,000 to 500,000 units at intervals of 3 to 6 hours.

Penicillin

**p. I,** p. F.
**p. II,** p. G.
**p. III,** p. X.
**p. IV,** p. K.

**allylmercaptomethylpenicillin,** p. O.

**aluminum p.,** the trivalent aluminum salt of an antibiotic substance or substances produced by the growth of the molds *Penicillium notatum* or *P. chrysogenum*. Used for oral or sublingual administration.

α-**aminobenzylpenicillin,** ampicillin.

**amorphous p.,** the calcium, potassium, or sodium salt of the antimicrobial acid produced by the growth of *Penicillium notatum* or related organisms under appropriate conditions.

**amylpenicillin sodium,** see under amylpenicillin.

**p. B.,** glucose oxidase.

**benz'athine p. G** (USP, BP), BICILLIN; PERMAPEN; benzylpenicillin compound with *N,N*-dibenzylethylenediamine (2:1); a relatively insoluble preparation that may remain in the body for 1 to 2 weeks.

**benzathine phenoxymethyl p.** (NF), p. for oral use.

**benzylpenicillin** (BP), p. G.

**buffered crystalline p. G,** crystalline potassium p. G or crystalline sodium p. G buffered with not less than 4 per cent and not more than 5 per cent of sodium citrate.

**chlor'oprocaine p. O,** DEPO-CER-O-CILLIN chloroprocaine; a crystalline salt of 2-chloroprocaine and p. O, insoluble in water. The level of the antibiotic in the blood persists for 24 hours. Its antibacterial activity is similar to that of p. O and G.

**dihydropenicillin F,** *n*-amylpenicillin; p. dihydro-F; R = $CH_3CH_2CH_2CH_2CH_2$—; a natural p. in which the hydrocarbon group is *n*-amyl. See also amylpenicillin sodium.

**2,6-dimethoxyphenylpenicillin sodium,** methicillin sodium.

**L-ephenamine p. G.,** the salt of p. G with the antiallergic base *N*-methyl-1,2-diphenyl-2-hydroxyethylamine.

**6-(2-ethoxy-1-naphthamido)penicillin,** nafcillin.

**p. F** (or **I**), 2-pentenylpenicillin; R = $CH_3CH_2CH=CHCH_2$—; see also the main entry.

**p. G** (or **II**), benzylpenicillin; R = $C_6H_5CH_2$—; see also the main entry.

*n*-**heptylpenicillin,** p. K.

**hydrabamine p. G.,** COMPOCILLIN; a dipenicillin compound, a mixture of p. G salts consisting chiefly of the salt of the diacidic base *N,N*-bis-(dehydroabietyl) ethylenediamine.

**hydrabamine phenoxymethylpenicillin** (NF), COMPOCILLIN-V; preparation and uses analogous to those of hydrabamine p. G.

*p*-**hydroxybenzylpenicillin,** p. X.

**p. K** (or **IV**), *n*-heptylpenicillin; R = $CH_3(CH_2)_6$—; see also the main entry.

**5-methyl-3-*o*-chlorophenyl-4-isoxazolylpenicillin sodium,** cloxacillin sodium.

**5-methyl-3-phenyl-4-isoxazolylpenicillin sodium,** oxacillin sodium.

**p. N,** cephalosporin N.

**p. O,** allylmercaptomethylpenicillin; R = $CH_2=CH$—$CH_2$—$S$—$CH_2$—; produced by growing the mold in a medium containing allylmercaptomethylacetic acid.

**2-pentenylpenicillin,** p. F.

α-**phenoxyethylpenicillin potassium,** phenethicillin potassium.

**p. phenoxymethyl** (USP), p. V.

α-**phenoxypropylpenicillin potassium,** propicillin.

**potassium p. G** (USP), potassium benzylpenicillin; contains 85 to 90 per cent of p. G.

**potassium p. O,** potassium salt of allylmercaptomethylpenicillin (p. O); a distinctly hypoallergenic p.

**p. potassium phenoxymethyl** (USP), p. V for oral administration.

**procaine p. G** (USP), procaine p. (BP); procaine benzylpenicillin; the procaine salt of p. G; has a more prolonged action than p. G.

**sodium p. G** (NF), sodium benzylpenicillin; the sodium salt of p. G; contains not less than 85 per cent of p. G.

**sodium p. O,** the sodium salt of allylmercaptomethylpenicillin; it is less likely to cause sensitivity or allergic reactions than p. G.

**p. V,** p. phenoxymethyl (USP); phenoxymethylpenicillin (BP); R = $C_6H_5$ $OCH_2$—; obtained from *Penicillium chrysogenum* Q 176; a crystalline, nonhydroscopic acid, very stable even in high humidity; it resists destruction by gastric juice.

**p. X** (or **III**),  *p*-hydroxybenzylpenicillin; R = $HOC_6H_4CH_2$—; one of the early natural p.'s studied clinically and shown to be inferior to benzylpenicillin.

**penicil'linase.** 1. An enzyme (EC 3.5.2.6) that brings about the hydrolysis of penicillin to penicilloic acid; found in most staphylococcus strains that are naturally resistant to penicillin. 2 (NF). NEUTRAPEN; a purified enzyme preparation obtained from cultures of a strain of *Bacillus cereus;* used in the treatment of slowly developing or delayed penicillin reactions.

**penicil'linate.** A salt of a penicillinic acid (*i.e.,* of a penicillin).

**penicillin'ic acid.** 1. Penicillins. 2. Penicillin (*q.v.*) with H— replacing R—.

**penicilliosis** (pen-ĭ-sil-ĭ-o'sis). Any disease caused by a species of *Penicillium.*

**Penicillium** (pen'ĭ-sil'ĭ-um) [ L. *penicillus,* paint-brush ]. A saprophytic mold, a genus of the Fungi of the class Ascomycetes, order Aspergillales; yields several antibiotic substances.

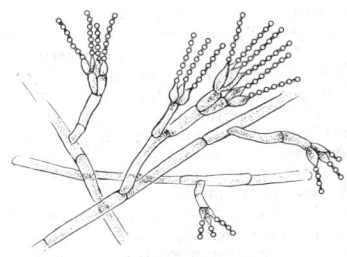

**Penicillium**

**P. aurantio-virens,** produces the antibiotic puberulic acid.

**P. claviforme,** produces the antibiotic, patulin.

**P. chrysogenum,** yields penicillin.

**P. citrinum,** yields citrinin.

**P. cyclopium,** yields penicillic acid.

**P. expansum,** produces patulin.

**P. glaucum,** the common mildew.

**P. notatum,** from which penicillin and notatin are derived.

**P. patulum,** produces patulin.

**P. puberulum,** yields penicillic acid and puberulic acid.

**penicilloic acid** (pen'ĭ-sĭ-lo'ik). Alkali and bacterial degradation product of a penicillin, resulting from hydrolysis of the 1,7 bond.

**penicilloyl polylysine** (pen'ĭ-sil'o-il). CILLIGEN; a preparation of polylysine and a penicillenic acid; used intradermally in the diagnosis of penicillin sensitivity; sensitive persons may react with systemic manifestations, including generalized cutaneous eruptions.

**penicillus,** pl. **penicil'li** (pen'ĭ-sil'us) [ L. a painter's brush ] [ NA ]. One of the tufts formed by the repeated subdivision of the minute arterial twigs in the spleen.

**penile** (pe'nil). Penial; relating to the penis.

**penil'lic acids.** Acid degradation products of penicillins, produced by cleavage of the 1,7 bond, forming penicilloic acid, and formation of a bond between the exocyclic carbon and N-1 with elimination of $H_2O$ from those two and the exocyclic NH.

**pen'in.** 6-Aminopenicillanic acid ($NH_2$ replaces RCONH— in penicillin, *q.v.*); an intermediate in the synthesis of penicillins.

**pe'nis** [ L. tail. PENI- ] [ NA ]. Coles; membrum virile; phallus; priapius; intromittent organ; the organ of copulation in the male; it is formed of three columns of erectile tissue, two arranged laterally on the dorsum (corpora cavernosa p.) and one median below (corpus spongiosum); the urethra traverses the latter; the extremity (glans p.) is formed by an expansion of the corpus spongiosum, and is more or less completely covered by a free fold of skin (preputium).

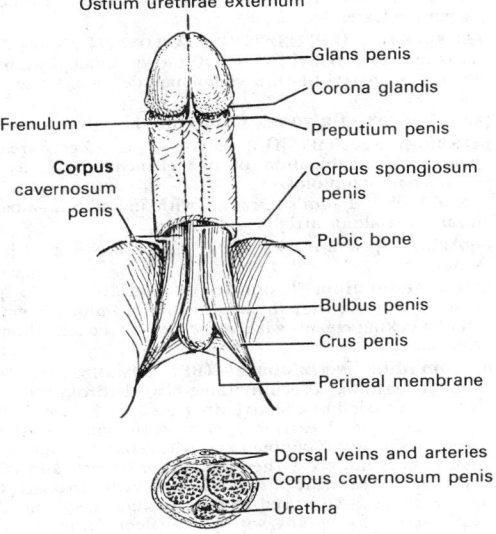

**Penis**

*Top*, skin and subcutaneous tissue removed in part to show structure of root of penis; *bottom*, transverse section of penis.

**bifid p.,** diphallus.

**p. capti'vus,** a rare accident during coitus, in which the p. is firmly held by spasmodic contraction of the vaginal and perineal musculature, preventing its withdrawal.

**clubbed p.,** a deformity of the p. when erect, consisting in a more or less marked curve to one or the other side or toward the scrotum.

**double p.,** diphallus.

**p. femin'eus,** clitoris.

**p. luna'tus,** chordee.

**p. mulie'bris,** clitoris.

**p. palma'tus,** a p. more or less completely enclosed by the scrotum.

**webbed p.,** one whose undersurface is joined to the front of the scotum by a fold of skin.

**penischisis** (pe-nis'kĭ-sis) [ L. *penis* + G. *schisis,* fissure ]. A fissure of the penis resulting in an abnormal opening into the urethra, either above (epispadia), below (hypospadia), or to one side (paraspadia).

**peni'tis.** Phallitis; priapitis; inflammation of the penis.

**pen'nate** [ L. *pennatus,* fr. *penna,* feather ]. Penniform; feathered; resembling a feather.

**pen'niform** [ L. *penna,* feather, + *forma,* form ]. Pennate.

**pen'nyroy'al.** A name in folk medicine given to *Mentha pulegium an aromatic p.*), or to *Hedeoma pulegeoides* (American p.) (family Labiatae); aromatic stimulant formerly used as an emmenagogue.

**pe'noscro'tal.** Relating to both penis and scrotum.

**Penrose,** Charles B., American gynecologist, 1862–1925. See P. *drain.*

**penta-, pent-** (pen'tah-) [ G. *pente,* five ]. Combining forms meaning five.

**pentaba'sic** [ penta- + G. *basis,* base ]. Denoting an acid having five replaceable hydrogen atoms.

**pen'tad** [ G. *pentas,* the number five ]. 1. A collection of five things in some way related. 2. In chemistry, a quinquevalent element.

**pentadactyl, pentadactyle** (pen-tah-dak'til) [ penta- + G. *daktylos,* finger ]. Having five fingers or toes on each hand or foot.

**pentaerythritol** (pen'tah-e-rith'ri-tol). $C(CH_2OH)_4$.

**diluted p. tetranitrate** (NF). PERITRATE; it is diluted with an inert ingredient, such as lactose, since the undiluted compound may explode upon percussion. It possesses vasodilator action similar to that of other slow acting organic nitrates.

**pentagas'trin** (BP, USAN). PEPTAVLON; *N*-[ *N*-[ *N*-[ *N*-(*N*-tert-* butoxycarbonyl-*β*- alanyl)-L-tryptophanyl ]-L-methionyl ]-L-aspartyl ]-L-phenylalaninamide; a gastric acid stimulator.

**pentahydrox'yfla'vone.** Quercetin, the aglycon of rutin.

**pentalogy** (pen'tal'o-jī) [ penta- + G. *logos,* treatise, word ]. A combination of five elements, such as five concurrent symptoms.

   **p. of Fallot,** Fallot's tetralogy with, in addition, a patent foramen ovale or atrial septal defect.

**pentamer** (pen'tă-mer) [ penta- + G. *meros,* part ]. See virion.

**pen'tametho'nium bromide** or **iodide.** C-5; pentamethylene-*bis*[ trimethylammonium bromide ]; a ganglionic blocking agent with same use as hexamethonium chloride.

**pentam'idine isethi'onate** (BP). LOMIDINE; *p,p'*-(pentamethylenedioxy)dibenzamidine-bis(*β*-hydroxyethanesulfonate); a toxic but effective drug used in the prophylaxis and treatment of early stages of both types of African sleeping sickness (Gambian and Rhodesian trypanosomiasis). It does not cross the blood-brain barrier, and is not effective in treatment of the advanced (neurological) stage of the disease. Also used to treat leishmaniasis that does not respond to therapy with pentavalent antimonials.

**pentapip'eride fumarate.** LYSPAFEN; 2-methyl-2-phenylvaleric acid 1-methyl-4-piperidyl ester fumarate; intestinal antispasmodic.

**pentaquine** (pen'tah-kwīn). 8-(5-Iso-propylamino)-6-methoxyquinoline; an antimalarial agent closely related chemically to pamaquine but less toxic and more effective. It is administered with quinine, the two drugs acting synergically. Active against *P. Plasmodium vivax* infections.

**Pentastoma** (pen-tas'to-mah) [ penta- + G. *stoma,* mouth ]. Older name for a genus of Pentastomida or tongue worms, now called *Linguatula;* the highly specialized arthropods formerly thought to be degenerate mites.

   **P. denticula'tum,** formerly called *Porocephalus denticulatus;* the larva of *Linguatula rhinaria,* which is sometimes parasitic in the nose of man and other mammals; adults are found in lungs of reptiles.

**pentastomiasis** (pen'tah-sto-mi'ă-sis). Infection of herbivorous animals, swine, and man with the larval form of Pentastomida. The lesions occur principally in the lymph nodes of the digestive tract, where they often resemble those of tuberculosis.

**Pentastomida** (pen'tah-stom'ĭ-dah) [ see *Pentastoma* ]. The tongue worms; a group of parasitic wormlike animals considered to form a distinct class within the phylum Arthropoda; they are strongly modified by parasitism to form elongate, pseudosegmented, wormlike organisms with two pairs of anterior, hollow, fanglike hooks. This group includes two genera reported from man, *Linguatula* and *Porocephalus,* both placed in the order Porocephalida.

**pentatomic** (pent'ă-tom'ik) [ penta- + atomic ]. 1. Denoting a chemical element, five atoms of which occur in the molecule. 2. Denoting a chemical compound having five replaceable hydrogen atoms.

**Pen'tatrichom'onas** [ penta- + *Trichomonas* ]. A genus of parasitic protozoan flagellates, formerly part of the genus Trichomonas but now separated as a distinct genus by the presence of five anterior flagella and a granular parabasal body; see *Trichomonas.*

   **P. hom'inis,** formerly *Trichomonas hominis;* lives as a commensal in the colon on man and other primates, dogs, cats, oxen, and various rodents.

**pentavalent** (pen-tav'ă-lent, pen'tah-va'lent) [ penta- + L. *valeo,* to have power ]. Quinquevalent; having a combining power equal to five atoms of hydrogen.

**pentazocine** (pen-ta'zo-sēn) (NF). TALWIN; 1,2,3,4,-5,6-hexahydro-6,11-dimethyl-3- (3-methyl-2-butenyl) -2,6-methano-3-benzazocin-8-ol; a benzomorphan analgesic which is a promising alternative to morphine. It has minimum addiction liability; is unsatisfactory in preventing the abstinence syndrome; and is a weak narcotic antagonist. Requires parenteral administration.

**pentdyopent** (pent-di-o-pent') [ G. *pente,* 5, + *dyo,* 2, + *pente,* 5, (5-2-5), indicating the spectroscopic localization by a line with its maximum at 525 micromicrons ]. A decomposition product of the blood pigment, found in the urine in a number of diseases and toxic disorders; when there is doubt as to which organ is diseased, the absence of pentdyopent from the urine is regarded as negating a hepatic disorder.

**pen'tene.** Amylene.

**pentetate trisodium calcium** (pen'tĕ-tāt) (USAN). Calcium trisodium salt of diethylenetriaminepentaacetic acid, *q. v.,* for uses.

**pentethylcy'clanone hydrochloride.** EXOPAN; 2-(1-cyclopenten-1-yl)-2-(2-morpholinoethyl)cyclopentanone hydrochloride; antitussive.

**pen'thanil.** Diethylenetriaminepentaacetic acid.

**penthienate bromide** (pen-thi'e-nāt). MONODRAL bromide; 2-diethylaminoethyl-*α*-cyclopentyl-2-thiopheneglycolate methylbromide; an anticholinergic agent with atropine-like effects; used as an adjunct in the treatment of peptic ulcers and to relieve pylorospasm and spastic colon.

**pen'tobar'bital** (NF). NEMBUTAL; pentobarbitone; 5-(ethyl-5-methylbutyl)barbituric acid; a sedative and short-acting hypnotic, used for preoperative medication.

**pentobar'bitone** (BP). Pentobarbital.

**pentolinium tartrate** (pen'to-lin'ĭ-um) (NF, BP). ANSOLYSEN tartrate; pentamethylene-1,1'-bis-(1-methylpyrrolidinium bitartrate; a quaternary ammonium compound with potent ganglionic blocking action; used in the management of severe and malignant hypertension and peripheral vasospastic diseases.

**pen'tosan.** An oligosaccharide of a pentose.

**pen'tose.** A monosaccharide containing five carbon atoms in the molecule (*e.g.,* arabinose, lyxose, ribose, and xylose).

   **p. nucleotide,** a nucleotide having a p. as the sugar component.

**pen'tose nucle'ic acid.** Older term for ribonucleic acid.

**pentosu'ria.** The excretion of one or more pentoses in the urine.

   **alimentary p.,** the urinary excretion of L -arabinose and L-xylose, as the result of the excessive ingestion of fruits containing these pentoses.

   **essential p.,** primary p.; a benign heritable disorder in which the urinary output of L-xylose is 1 to 4 gm. per 24 hours; occurs principally in Jewish people; believed to reflect defective oxidation of glucuronic acid.

   **primary p.,** essential p.

**pentox'ide.** [ G. *pente,* five ]. An oxide containing five oxygen atoms; *e.g.,* phosphorus p., $P_2O_5$.

**pentulose** (pen'tu-lōs). A ketopentose; *e.g.,* ribulose.

**pen'tylenetet'razol.** LEPTAZOL; METRAZOL; $C_6H_{10}N_4$; a powerful stimulant to the central nervous system; used to cause generalized convulsion in the shock treatment of emotional states and as a respiratory stimulant.

**peotillomania** (pe'o-til-o-ma'nĭ-ah) [ G. *peos,* penis, + *tillō,* to pull out (of hair), + *mania,* frenzy ]. False masturbation; pseudomasturbation; a nervous tic consisting in constant pulling of the penis.

**peotomy** (pe-ot'o-mī) [ G. *peos,* penis, + *tomē,* cutting ]. Amputation of the penis.

**pe'po** [ G. *pepōn,* a gourd or melon ]. Pumpkin seed; the dried seed of *Cucurbita pepo* (family Cucurbitaceae); teniacide.

**Pepper,** William, Jr., American physician, 1874–1947. See P. *syndrome.*

**pep'permint** (USP). The dried leaves and flowering tops of *Mentha piperita* (family Labiatae); carminative and antiemetic.

   **p. camphor,** menthol.

   **p. oil** (USP, BP), the volatile oil distilled with steam from the fresh, overground parts of the flowering plant of *Mentha piperita,* rectified by distillation and neither partially nor wholly dementholized; a flavor.

**pep'sase.** Peptic.

**pep'sic.** Peptic.

**pep'sin** [ G. *pepsis,* digestion. PEP- ]. Pepsin A.

   **p. A** (EC 3.4.23.1), formerly pepsin; a digestive enzyme (protease) of the gastric juice, formed from pepsinogen; it

hydrolyzes peptide bonds, preferably adjacent to phenylalanine and leucine residues, thus reducing proteins to smaller molecules (peptones).
**p. B** (EC 3.4.23.2), similar to p. A; formed from pepsinogen B.
**p. C** (EC 3.4.23.3), similar to p. A.
**pep'sinate.** To mix pepsin with.
**pepsinif'erous.** Producing pepsin.
**pepsinogen** (pep-sin'o-jen) [ pepsin + G. suffix -*gen*, producing ]. A proenzyme formed and secreted by the chief cells of the gastric mucosa; the acidity of the gastric juice and pepsin itself remove 42 amino acid residues from p. to form active pepsin.
**pepsinogenous** (pep-sin-oj'ĕ-nus). Producing pepsin.
**pepsinu'ria** [ pepsin + G. *ouron*, urine ]. Excretion of pepsin in the urine.
**pepsiten'sin.** A hypertensive peptide produced by the action of pepsin upon the angiotensinogen fraction of blood plasma. Similar in action and composition to angiotensin.
**pep'tic** [ G. *peptikos*, fr. *peptō*, to digest. PEP- ]. Relating to the stomach, to gastric digestion, or to pepsin.
**pep'tidase.** An enzyme capable of hydrolyzing one of the peptide links of a peptide. Carboxypeptidases, aminopeptidases, etc., are p.'s (EC Class 3.4, peptide hydrolases).
**pep'tide.** A compound of two or more amino acids in which the carboxyl group of one is united with the amino group of the other, with the elimination of a molecule of water, thus forming a peptide bond, —CO—NH—.
  **adrenocorticotropic p.,** a p. with ACTH activity isolated from pituitary extracts.
  **p. bond,** see under bond.
  **heteromeric p.,** a p. which, on hydrolysis, yields substances other than amino acids in addition to amino acids; *e.g.,* pteroylglutamic acid.
  **phenylthiocarbamoyl p.,** PTC p., formed by combination of phenylisothiocyanate and an α-amino group of a peptide.
  **PTC p.,** abbreviation for phenylthiocarbamoyl p.
  **S p.,** see S *protein.*
  **sigma p.,** a p. with one end bonded to a point within the chain, usually by means of the disulfide group of a cystine residue, so that only one end of the p. is free; so called since the p. chain has then the rough shape of the Greek letter sigma.
  **p. synthetase** (EC sub-subclass 6.3.2), any enzyme that catalyzes the synthesis of peptide bonds.
**pep'tidogly'cans.** Glycans to which are attached short polypeptides.
**peptidoid** (pep'tĭ-doyd). A condensation product of two amino acids involving at least one condensing group other than the α-carboxyl or α-amino groups; glutathione is one natural example.
**peptidolytic** (pep'tĭ-do-lit'ik) [ peptide + G. *lytikos*, solvent ]. Causing the cleavage or digestion of peptides.
**peptization** (pep'tĭ-za'shun). In colloid chemistry, an increase in the degree of dispersion, tending toward a uniform distribution of the dispersed phase; the formation of a sol from a gel.
**pep'tize.** In colloidal chemistry, to transform a gel into a sol, as when dry gelatine is "dissolved" or dispersed in water.
**Peptococcaceae** (pep'to-kok-a'ce-e). A family of nonmotile, nonsporeforming, anaerobic bacteria (order Eubacteriales) containing Gram-positive (staining may be equivocal) cocci, 0.5 to 1.6 μm in diameter, which occur singly, in pairs, tetrads, and irregular masses but not in three-dimensional, cubic packets. These organisms are chemoorganotrophic and have complex nutritional requirements. Carbohydrates may or may not be fermented by these organisms which produce gas, principally $CO_2$ and usually $H_{27}$ from amino acids, or carbohydrates, or both. They are found in the mouth and intestinal and respiratory tracts of man and other animals; they are frequently found in the normal and pathological human female urogenital tracts. The type genus is *Peptococcus.*
**Peptococcus** (pep'to-kok'us) [ G. *peptō*, to digest, + *kokkos,* berry ]. A genus of nonmotile, anaerobic, chemoorganotrophic bacteria (family Peptococcaceae) containing

Gram-positive, spherical cells that occur singly, in pairs, tetrads, or irregular masses, rarely in short chains. They are frequently found in association with pathological conditions. The type species is *P. niger.*
  **P. activus,** a species found in cases of puerperal septicemia and in the female genital tract.
  **P. aerogenes,** a species found primarily on human mucous surfaces; also found in cases of puerperal fever, in the female genital tract, and in the tonsils and nose.
  **P. anaerobius,** a species found in appendices, the female genital tract, in cases of cystitis and draining sinus, and in tidal bay mud.
  **P. asaccharolyticus,** a species found in the human large intestine, buccal cavity, pleura, uterus, and vagina.
  **P. constellatus,** a species found in tonsils, purulent pleurisy, appendix, the nose, throat, and gums, and infrequently on the skin and in the vagina.
  **P. niger,** a species found once, in the urine of an aged woman; type species of the genus *P.*
**peptocrinine** (pep-to-krin'ēn). An extract of the intestinal mucosa resembling secretin.
**peptogenic, peptogenous** (pep'to-jen'ik, pep-toj'ĕ-nus). 1. Producing peptones. 2. Promoting digestion.
**peptolysis** (pep-tol'ĭ-sis). The hydrolysis of peptones.
**peptolyt'ic.** 1. Pertaining to peptolysis. 2. Denoting an enzyme or other agent that hydrolyses peptones.
**pep'tonate.** A compound of peptone, acting as an acid, with a base.
**pep'tone.** A descriptive term applied to intermediate polypeptide products formed in partial hydrolysis of proteins. In general, p.'s are soluble in water, diffusible, and not coagulable by heat. Used in bacterial culture media.
  **Hoechst's p.,** silk p.
  **silk p.,** a preparation of p. derived from silk. Used for the identification of peptolytic enzymes that induce changes in its optical activity or the precipitation of tyrosin.
**peptone'mia** [ peptone + G. *haima,* blood ]. The presence of peptones in the circulating blood.
**pepton'ic.** Relating to or containing peptone.
**pep'toniza'tion.** The conversion, by enzymic action, of native protein, as for example curdled milk, into the soluble peptone.
**pep'tonize.** To convert native protein into peptone.
**pep'tonoid.** A substance supposed to resemble peptone.
**peptonu'ria** [ peptone + G. *ouron,* urine ]. The excretion of peptones in the urine.
**Peptostreptococcus** (pep'to-strep'to-kok-us) [ G. *peptō,* to digest, + *streptos,* curved, + *kokkus,* berry ]. A genus of nonmotile, anaerobic, chemoorganotrophic bacteria (family Peptococcaceae) containing spherical to ovoid, Gram-positive cells which occur in pairs and short or long chains. These organisms are found in normal and pathological female genital tracts and blood in puerperal fever, in respiratory and intestinal tracts of normal humans and other animals, in the oral cavity, and in pyogenic infections, putrefactive war wounds, and appendicitis; they may be pathogenic. The type species is *P. anaerobius.*
  **P. anaero'bius,** a species found in the mouth, intestinal and respiratory tracts, and cavities, especially the vagina, of man and other animals; it may be pathogenic. It is the type species of the genus *P.*
  **P. evolutus,** a species found in the human respiratory tract, mouth, and vagina.
  **P. foetidus,** a species found in abscesses, blood, intestinal tracts, vaginas, and mouths of humans and other animals; it is sometimes fatal.
  **P. interme'dius,** a species found in human respiratory and digestive tracts, oral cavity, and vagina. It has been isolated from various pathological conditions.
  **P. lanceola'tus,** a species found in the human mouth, vagina, and intestinal tract. It has been isolated from putrid diarrhoea, dental infection, vulvovaginitis, and arthritic and other abscesses.
  **P. magnus,** a species found in putrefying butcher's meat and in a case of appendicitis.
  **P. mi'cros,** a species found in natural cavities of man and other animals. It has been isolated from various pathological conditions.

**P. morbillorum,** a species found in the nose, throat, eyes, ears, mucous secretions, and blood in cases of measles; being irrelevant, however, to the etiology of measles; probably present normally, developing as a secondary invader.

**P. paleopneumoniae,** a species found in the baccal pharyngeal cavity and the upper respiratory tract of man.

**P. parvulus,** a species isolated from the mouth and the respiratory tract.

**P. plagarumbelli,** a species commonly found in septic war wounds.

**P. productus,** a species found in natural cavities of man, especially the respiratory.

**P. putridus,** a species found in the human mouth and intestinal tract but especially in the human vagina.

**pep′totox′in.** 1. A toxic substance obtained from peptone. 2. A poisonous product formed at a certain stage in the digestion of protein and disappearing at a later stage.

**peptozyme** (pep′to-zīm) [ G. *peptō*, to digest, + *zymē*, leaven. ZE- ]. A substance, supposed to be derived from certain tissues used in the preparation of peptone, which has the property of preventing the coagulation of the blood.

**per-** [ L. through, throughout, extremely ]. 1. A prefix meaning through; carrying an idea of intensity (super). 2. In chemistry, denoting either (a) more or most, with respect to the amount of a given element (usually oxygen) or radical contained in a compound, or (b) the degree of substitution for hydrogen (as in peroxides, peroxy acids, *e.g.*, hydrogen peroxide, peroxyformic acid).

**peracephalus** (per-ă-sef′ă-lus) [ per- + G. *a-* priv. + *kephalē*, head ]. An omphalosite lacking head and arms and with a defective thorax. Typically the body consists of little more than pelvis and legs.

**peracetate** (per-as′e-tāt). Salt or ester of peracetic acid.

**perace′tic acid.** Peroxyacetic acid; acetyl hydroperoxide; a peroxide of acetic acid, $CH_3—CO—O—OH$.

**peracid** (per-as′id). Peroxy acid; an acid containing a peroxide group (—O—OH) as for instance peracetic acid.

**per a′num** [ L. ]. By or through the anus.

**perarticulation** (per′ar-tik′u-la′shun) [ per- + L. *articulatio*, joint ]. *Junctura* synovialis.

**peratodynia** (pĕr′ă-to-din′ī-ah) [ G. *peratos*, on the opposite side, + *odynē*, pain ]. Cardialgia.

**perax′illary.** Through the axilla.

**per′azine.** TAXILAN; 10-[ 3-(4-methyl-1-piperazinyl)propyl ]phenothiazine; antipsychotic agent.

**perbo′ric acid.** Pyroboric *acid.*

**percen′tile.** The rank position of an individual in a serial array of data, stated in terms of what percentage of the group he equals or exceeds.

**percept** (per′sept) [ L. *perceptum*, a thing perceived ]. 1. That which is perceived; the complete mental image, formed by the process of perception, of an object present in space. 2. In clinical psychology, a single unit of perceptual report, such as one of the responses to an inkblot in the Rorschach test.

**perception** (per-sep′shun). Awareness; consciousness; esthesia; the mental process of becoming aware of or recognizing an object. The process is primarily cognitive rather than affective or conative, although all three aspects are manifested.

**after-p.,** see afterperception.

**depth p.,** the ability to judge depth or distance in space by vision.

**extrasensory p.,** ESP; p. by means other than through the ordinary senses; *e.g.*, telepathy (mind reading or thought transference), clairvoyance, and precognition are forms of extrasensory p.

**facial p.,** the p. of objects through sensation in the skin of the face; supposedly present in the blind.

**percep′tive.** Relating to or having the power of perception.

**perceptiv′ity.** The power of perception.

**percepto′rium.** Sensorium (2).

**perchlo′ric acid.** $HClO_4$; the highest in oxygen content of the series of chlorine acids.

**perchlo′ride.** A chloride containing the highest possible amount of chlorine.

**percolation** (per′ko-la′shun) [ L. *percolatio*, fr. per- + *colare*, to strain ]. 1. Filtration. 2. Extraction of the soluble portion of a solid mixture by passing a solvent liquid through it. 3. Passage of saliva or other fluids into the interface between tooth structure and restoration; sometimes induced by thermal changes.

**per′cola′tor.** A funnel-shaped vessel used for the process of percolation in pharmacy.

**Percomorphi** (per-ko-mor′fi) [ G. *perkē*, perch, + *morphē*, form ]. An order of fishes resembling in some anatomical features the perches, the oil from the livers of which is rich in vitamins A and D.

**percomorph oil.** A liver oil from fish of the order Percomorphi, standardized to contain not less than 60,000 units of vitamin A (USP) and 8500 units of vitamin D (USP) per gram.

**per contiguum** (per kon-tig′u-um) [ per- + L. *contiguus*, touching, fr. *tango*, to touch ]. In contiguity; touching; denoting the mode of spread of an inflammation or other morbid process that passes into an adjacent contiguous structure.

**per continuum** (per kon-tin′u-um) [ per- + L. *continuus*, holding together, continuous, fr. *teneo*, to hold ]. In continuity; continuous; denoting the mode of spread of an inflammation or other morbid process from one part to another through continuous tissue.

**percuss** (per-kuss′) [ see percussion ]. To perform percussion.

**percussion** (per-kush′un) [ L. *percussio*, fr. *per-cutio*, pp. *-cussus*, to beat, fr. *quatio*, to shake, beat ]. 1. A diagnostic procedure designed to determine the density of a part by means of tapping the surface with the finger or a plessor. 2. A form of massage, consisting of repeated blows or taps of varying force.

**auscul′tatory p.,** auscultation of the chest or other part at the same time that p. is made.

**bimanual p.,** immediate p. in which the finger of one hand taps the other hand.

**clavicular p.,** p., usually direct, along the entire clavicle to demonstrate dullness—particularly in apical pulmonary tuberculosis.

**deep p.,** heavy p. to obtain information about deeply situated organs or structures.

**direct p.,** immediate p.

**finger p.,** p. in which a finger of one hand is used as a plessimeter and one of the other hand as a plessor.

**immediate p.,** the striking of the part under examination directly with the finger or a plessor, without the intervention of another finger or plessimeter.

**mediate p.,** p. effected by the intervention of a finger or a thin plate of ivory or other substance (plessimeter) between the striking finger or hammer and the part percussed.

**palpatory p.,** finger p. in which the attention is fixed upon the resistance of the tissues under the finger as well as upon the sound elicited.

**p. sound,** see under sound.

**threshold p.,** p. effected by means of a glass rod as a plessimeter, the rod being inclined to the wall of the chest or abdomen and touching it only by one extremity.

**percussor** (per-kus′sor). A hammer used for making percussion; a plessor.

**percutaneous** (per′ku-ta′ne-us). Through unbroken skin, as in absorption by inunction.

**pereirine** (per-a′e-rēn). An alkaloid derived from the bark of *Geissospermum loeve* (family Apocynaceae), a tree of Brazil; the bark is used in Brazil as an antipyretic.

**perencephaly** (pe-ren-sef′a-lī) [ G. *pēra*, a purse, a wallet, + *enkephalos*, brain ]. A condition marked by one or more cerebral cysts.

**Perez,** Bernard, French physician, 1836–1903. See P. *reflex.*

**Perez,** George V., Teneriffe (Canary Islands) physician, †1920. See P.'s *sign.*

**perfec′tionism.** A tendency to set rigid high standards of performance for oneself.

**perfla′tion** [ L. *per-flo*, pp, *-flatus*, to blow through. FLAT- ]. Blowing air into or through a cavity or canal in order to force apart its walls or to expel any contained pus or other material.

**perfla′von.** LADFLAVON; 1,2,3,4-tetrahydro-1,3-dimethyl-2,6-dioxopurine-7-acetic acid compound with 7-[ 2-(dimethylamino)-ethoxy ]flavone; antianginal drug.

**per′forans** [ L. perforating ]. A term applied to several muscles and nerves which, in their course, perforate other structures.

**per′forated** [ L. *perforatus*, fr. *per-foro*, pp. *-atus*, to bore through ]. Pierced with one or more holes.

**perforation** (per′fo-ra′shun) [ see perforated ]. An abnormal opening in a hollow organ or viscus.
  **Bezold's p.,** p. on the inner surface of the mastoid portion of the temporal bone.

**per′forator.** An instrument for perforation of the head in craniotomy.

**perforato′rium.** A rod or fibrous cone located between the acrosome and the anterior pole of the nucleus in the spermatozoa of toads and birds; there does not seem to be a corresponding formed structure in the subacrosomal space of mammalian spermatozoa.

**perfora′tus** [ L. ] [ NA ]. Perforated; denoting a structure pierced by another.

**perfor′mic acid.** H—CO—O—OH; peroxyformic acid; an organic peracid used in cleaving disulfide links in peptides, by oxidizing cystine to cysteic acid.

**perfrigeration** (per-frij′er-a′shun) [ L. *per-frigero*, pp. *-atus*, to make cold, fr. *frigus*, cold ]. A minor degree of frostbite.

**perfusate** (per′fu-zāt) [ see perfusion ]. A liquid, solution, or colloidal suspension that has been passed (1) over a special surface, *e.g.,* a column of baffles or a charged plate, or (2) through an appropriate structure, *e.g.,* a semipermeable membrane or porcelain filter or a tissue or organ.

**perfusion** (per-fu′zhun) [ L. *perfusio*, fr. per- + *fusio*, a pouring, fr. *fundo*, pp. *fusus*, to pour ]. Artificial passage of fluid through blood vessels.
  **regional p.,** p. of part of the body, especially a limb, and particularly with chemotherapeutic agents for treatment of a malignant tumor, primary recurrent or metastatic.

**perhex′iline maleate** (USAN). PEXID; 2-(2,2-dicyclohexylethyl)piperidine maleate; a coronary vasodilating drug.

**perhydrocyclopenta[ *a* ]phenanthrene. Tetracyclic ste**-roid nucleus; see under steroid.

**perhydrocyclopentenophenanthrene.** Misnomer for perhydrocyclopenta[ *a* ]phenanthrene.

**peri-** (per′ĭ-) [ G. around ]. A prefix carrying the idea of around, about.

**periacinal, periacinous** (pĕr-ĭ-as′ĭ-nal, -ĭ-nus). Surrounding an acinus.

**periadenitis** (pĕr-ĭ-ad-ē-ni′tis) [ peri- + G. *adēn*, gland, + *-itis* ]. Inflammation of the tissues surrounding a gland.
  **p. muco′sa necrot′ica recur′rens,** Mikulicz' aphthae; Sutton's disease; a severe form of recurrent aphthous stomatitis, with large lesions, regional adenopathy, and healing with scar formation.

**perianal** (pĕr-ĭ-a′nal). Circumanal.

**periangiocholitis** (pĕr-ĭ-an′jĭ-o-ko-li′tis) [ peri- + G. *angeion*, vessel, + *cholē*, bile, + *-itis* ]. Pericholangitis.

**periangitis** (pĕr-ĭ-an-ji′tis) [ peri- + G. *angeion*, a vessel, + *-itis* ]. Perivasculitis; inflammation of the adventitia of a blood vessel or of the tissues surrounding it or a lymphatic vessel; including periarteritis, periphlebitis, and perilymphangitis.

**periaortic** (pĕr′ĭ-a-or′tik). Surrounding or adjacent to the aorta.

**periaortitis** (pĕr-ĭ-a-or-ti′tis). Inflammation of the adventitia of the aorta and of the tissues surrounding it.

**periapex** (pĕr′ĭ-a′peks) [ peri- L. *apex*, tip ]. The periapical structures, particularly periodontal membrane and adjacent bone.

**periapical** (pĕr-ĭ-ap′ĭ-kal). 1. At or around the apex of a root of a tooth. 2. Denoting the periapex.

**periappendicitis** (pĕr′ĭ-ă-pen-dĭ-si′tis). Para-appendicitis; inflammation of the tissue surrounding the vermiform appendix.

**p. decidua′lis,** the presence of decidual cells in the peritoneum of the vermiform appendix in cases of right tubal pregnancy with adhesions between the Fallopian tube and the appendix.

**periappendicular** (pĕr′ĭ-ă-pen-dik′u-lar). Surrounding an appendix, especially the vermiform appendix.

**periarterial** (pĕr′ĭ-ar-tēr′ĭ-al). Surrounding an artery.

**periarteritis** (pĕr-ĭ-ar-ter-i′tis). Inflammation of the outer coat, or adventitia, of an artery.
  **p. nodo′sa,** *polyarteritis* nodosa.

**periarthric** (pĕr′ĭ-ar′thrik). Circumarticular.

**periarthritis** (pĕr-ĭ-ar-thri′tis) [ peri- + arthritis ]. Inflammation of the parts surrounding a joint.
  **scapulohumeral p.,** subdeltoid or subacromial bursitis; Duplay's disease; periarthrosis humeroscapularis; p. with calcification of the subacromial bursa, frequently bilateral.

**periarthro′sis humeroscapula′ris.** Scapulohumeral *periarthritis*.

**periarticular** (pĕr′ĭ-ar-tik′u-lar). Circumarticular.

**periatrial** (pĕr′ĭ-a′trĭ-al). Surrounding the atrium of the heart.

**periauricular** (pĕr′ĭ-aw-rik′u-lar). 1. Periatrial. 2. Perionchal. 3. Around the external ear.

**periaxial** (pĕr′ĭ-ak′sĭ-al). Surrounding an axis.

**periaxillary** (pĕr′ĭ-ak′sĭ-lĕr-ĭ). Circumaxillary.

**periaxonal** (pĕr′ĭ-ak′so-nal) [ peri- + G. *axōn*, axis ]. Surrounding the axon of a nerve.

**per′iblast** [ peri- + G. *blastos*, germ ]. A specialized region of yolk surface immediately peripheral to the blastoderm in telolecithal eggs.

**periblep′sis** [ peri- + G. *blepsis*, looking ]. The staring expression of an insane person.

**peribronchial** (pĕr-ĭ-brong′kĭ-al). Surrounding a bronchus or the bronchi.

**peribronchiolar** (pĕr-ĭ-brong′kĭ-o′lar). Surrounding the bronchioles.

**peribronchiolitis** (pĕr-ĭ-brong′kĭ-o-li′tis). Inflammation of the tissues surrounding the bronchioles.

**peribronchitis** (pĕr-ĭ-brong-ki′tis). Inflammation of the tissues surrounding the bronchi or bronchial tubes.

**per′ibuc′cal.** Surrounding the cheek.

**peribul′bar.** Surrounding any bulb, especially the eyeball or the bulb of the urethra.

**peribur′sal.** Surrounding a bursa.

**pericanalicular** (pĕr′ĭ-kan′ă-lik′u-lar). Surrounding a canaliculus.

**pericardectomy** (per-ĭ-kar-dek′to-mĭ). Pericardiectomy.

**pericar′diac, pericar′dial.** 1. Surrounding the heart. 2. Relating to the pericardium.

**pericar′dicente′sis.** Pericardiocentesis.

**pericardiectomy** (pĕr-ĭ-kar-dĭ-ek′to-mĭ) [ pericardium + G. *ektomē*, excision ]. Pericardectomy; excision of a portion of the pericardium. Done for constrictive pericarditis.

**pericardiocentesis** (pĕr-ĭ-kar′dĭ-o-sen-te′sis) [ peri- + G. *kardia*, heart, + *kentesis*, puncture ]. Pericardicentesis; paracentesis pericardii; paracentesis of the pericardium; surgical puncture of the pericardium.

**pericar′dioperitone′al.** Relating to the pericardial and peritoneal cavities.

**pericar′diophren′ic** [ pericardium + G. *phrēn*, diaphragm ]. Relating to the pericardium and the diaphragm.

**pericar′diopleur′al.** Relating to the pericardial and pleural cavities.

**pericardiorrhaphy** (pĕr′ĭ-kar-dĭ-or′ă-fĭ) [ pericardium + G. *rhaphē*, suture ]. Suture of a wound of the pericardium.

**pericardiostomy** (pĕr′ĭ-kar-dĭ-os′to-mĭ) [ pericardium + G. *stoma*, mouth ]. Making a more or less permanent opening into the pericardium.

**pericardiotomy** (pĕr′ĭ-kar-dĭ-ot′o-mĭ) [ pericardium + G. *tomē*, incision ]. Pericardotomy; incision into the pericardium.

**pericardit′ic.** Relating to pericarditis.

**pericardi′tis.** Inflammation of the pericardium.
  **adhesive p.,** adherent pericardium; p. with adhesions between the two pericardial layers, between the pericar-

dium and heart, or between the pericardium and neighboring structures.

**p. calculo'sa,** p. marked by calcific deposits in the pericardium.

**p. callo'sa,** chronic p. with no characteristic symptoms other than signs of obstructed return of venous blood to the heart.

**chronic constrictive p.,** tuberculous or other infection of the pericardium, with thickening of the membrane and constriction of the cardiac chambers. The condition is marked clinically by small pulse volume, enlargement of the liver, engorgement of the veins of the neck, and sometimes edema. Syncope may occur during effort. The condition is treated by surgical removal (decortication, pericardiectomy) of the thickened pericardium.

**fibrinous p.,** acute p. with fibrinous exudate; also known as cor hirsutum, tomentosum, or villosum; hairy heart; p. sicca or villosa, shaggy pericardium; trichocardia.

**internal adhesive p.,** concretio *cordis.*

**p. oblit'erans,** inflammation of the pericardium leading to adhesion of the two layers, obliterating the sac; see also adhesive p.

**rheumatic p.,** fibrinous p. occurring in acute rheumatic fever.

**p. sic'ca,** fibrinous p.

**uremic p.,** fibrinous p. seen in chronic renal failure.

**p. villo'sa,** fibrinous p.

**pericardium,** pl. **pericar'dia** (pĕr-ĭ-kar'dĭ-um) [ L. fr. G. *pericardion,* the membrane around the heart. CARD- ]. Capsula cordis; membrana cordis; the fibroserous membrane, consisting of mesothelium and submesothelial connective tissue, covering the heart and beginning of the great vessels; it is a closed sac having two layers—that immediately surrounding the heart, the visceral layer, or epicardium, and the outer parietal layer, forming the sac, composed of strong fibrous tissue (p. fibrosum) lined with serous membrane (p. serosum). The phrenic nerve divides the pericardium into an antephrenic and a retrophrenic portion; the pulmonary hilus divides both portions into a suprahilar, a hilar, and an infrahilar portion of the pericardium.

**adherent p.,** adhesive *pericarditis.*

**bread-and-butter p.,** the visceral and parietal surfaces of the p. resemble those of two pieces of buttered bread that have been pressed together and then pulled apart.

**p. fibro'sum** [ NA ], see p.

**p. sero'sum** [ NA ], see p.

**shaggy p.,** fibrinous *pericarditis.*

**pericardot'omy.** Pericardiotomy.

**pericecal** (pĕr'ĭ-se'kal). Perityphlic; surrounding the cecum.

**pericecitis** (pĕr-ĭ-se-si'tis). Periappendicitis.

**pericel'lular.** Pericytial; surrounding a cell.

**pericemental** (pĕr'ĭ-se-men'tal). Periodontal.

**pericementitis** (pĕr'ĭ-se-men-ti'tis). An inflammatory reaction of the periodontium, and its adjacent structures, which may be caused by trauma or infection; see also periodontitis.

**apical p.,** inflammation of the tissues surrounding the apex of the tooth.

**chronic septic apical p.,** a longstanding inflammation of the apex of a tooth.

**pericen'tral.** Surrounding the center.

**perichareia** (pĕr'ĭ-kă-ri'ah) [ G. excessive joy, fr. *chairō,* to rejoice ]. Delirious rejoicing.

**pericholangitis** (pĕr-ĭ-ko-lan-ji'tis) [ peri- + G. *cholē,* bile, + *angeion,* vessel, + -*itis* ]. Periangiocholitis; inflammation of the tissues around the bile ducts.

**perichondral, perichondrial** (pĕr'ĭ-kon'dral, -kon'drĭ-al). Relating to the perichondrium.

**perichondritis** (pĕr-ĭ-kon-dri'tis). Inflammation of the perichondrium.

**relapsing p.,** Meyenburg's disease; Meyenberg-Altherr-Uehlinger syndrome; generalized chondromalacia; a generalized disease of connective tissue characterized by p. and resulting deformation of cartilages of ears, nose, larynx, or trachea.

**perichondrium** (pĕr-ĭ-kon'drĭ-um) [ peri- + G. *chondros,* cartilage ] [ NA ]. The dense, irregular connective tissue membrane around cartilage.

**perichord** (pĕr'ĭ-kord). Sheath of the notochord.

**perichordal** (pĕr-ĭ-kor'dal). Relating to the perichord.

**perichoroidal** (pĕr-ĭ-ko-roy'dal). Surrounding the choroid coat of the eye.

**perichrome** (pĕr'ĭ-krōm) [ peri- + G. *chrōma,* a color ]. Denoting a nerve cell in which the chromophil substance, or stainable material, is scattered throughout the cytoplasm.

**pericolic** (pĕr'ĭ-kol'ik). Surrounding or encircling the colon.

**pericolitis** (pĕr'ĭ-ko-li'tis). Serocolitis; inflammation of the connective tissue or peritoneum surrounding the colon.

**p. dextra,** p. involving the ascending colon.

**p. sinistra,** perisigmoiditis.

**perico'loni'tis.** Pericolitis.

**pericolpi'tis** [ peri- + G. *kolpos,* bosom (vagina), + suffix -*itis,* inflammation ]. Perivaginitis.

**periconchal** (pĕr'ĭ-kong'kal). Surrounding the concha of the auricle.

**pericor'neal.** Surrounding the cornea; perikeratic.

**per'icor'onal.** Around the crown of a tooth.

**pericoronitis** (pĕr-ĭ-kor-o-ni'tis) [ peri- + L. *corona,* crown, + G. suffix -*itis,* inflammation ]. Operculitis; inflammation around the crown of a tooth, usually of an incompletely erupted mandibular third molar; could also occur on any upper or lower molar during eruption.

**pericra'nial.** Relating to the pericranium; surrounding the skull.

**pericrani'tis.** Inflammation of the pericranium.

**pericranium** (pĕr'ĭ-kra'nĭ-um) [ peri- + G. *kranion,* skull ] [ NA ]. Periosteum of the skull.

**pericy'azine.** NEULACTIL; 10-[ 3-(4-hydroxypiperidino)-propyl ]phenothiazine-2-carbonitrile; antipsychotic agent.

**pericystic** (pĕr'ĭ-sis'tik) [ peri- + G. *kystis,* bladder ]. 1. Surrounding the urinary bladder. 2. Surrounding the gallbladder. 3. Surrounding a cyst.

**pericystitis** (pĕr-ĭ-sis-ti'tis). Inflammation of the tissues surrounding a bladder, especially the urinary bladder.

**pericystium** (pĕr'ĭ-sis'tĭ-um) [ peri- + G. *kystis,* bladder, cyst ]. 1. The tissues surrounding the urinary bladder or gallbladder. 2. A vascular investment of a cystic tumor.

**per'icyte** [ peri- + G. *kytos,* cell ]. Perithelial cell; pericapillary cell; adventitial cell; one of the slender connective tissue cells in close relationship to the outside of the capillary wall.

**capillary p.'s,** Rouget's *cells.*

**pericytial** (pĕr'ĭ-sish'ĭ-al, -sit'ĭ-al). Pericellular.

**peridec'tomy** [ peri- + G. *ektomē,* excision ]. Peritectomy.

**per'idens** [ peri- + L. *dens,* tooth ]. A supernumerary tooth erupting on the outer aspect of the dental arches.

**periden'tal.** Periodontal.

**peridenti'tis.** Periodontitis.

**peridentium** (pĕr'ĭ-den'tĭ-um). Periodontium.

**per'iderm, perider'ma** [ peri- + G. *derma,* skin ]. Epitrichium; the outermost layer of the epidermis of the embryo and fetus up to the sixth month of intrauterine life; desquamated epitrichial cells are a considerable component of the vernix caseosa.

**perider'mal, perider'mic.** Relating to the periderm.

**peridesmic** (pĕr'ĭ-dez'mik). 1. Periligamentous; surrounding a ligament. 2. Relating to the peridesmium.

**peridesmitis** (pĕr'ĭ-dez-mi'tis) [ peri- + G. *desmos,* band, + suffix -*itis,* inflammation ]. Inflammation of the connective tissue surrounding a ligament.

**peridesmium** (pĕr'ĭ-dez'mĭ-um) [ peri- + G. *desmion (desmos),* band ]. The connective tissue membrane surrounding a ligament.

**peridiastole** (pĕr-ĭ-di-as'to-le). Prediastole.

**peridiastol'ic.** Prediastolic.

**perididymis** (pĕr'ĭ-did'ĭ-mis) [ G. *didymos,* twin, pl. *didymoi,* testes ]. *Tunica albuginea testis.*

**perididymitis** (pĕr-ĭ-did-ĭ-mi'tis). Inflammation of the perididymis.

**perid'ium** [ G. *peridion*, dim. of *pera*, leather pouch ]. A specialized hyphal structure forming an outer wall around the ascus of Ascomycetes.

**per'idiverticuli'tis.** Inflammation of the tissues around an intestinal diverticulum.

**peridu'odeni'tis.** Inflammation around the duodenum.

**peridu'ral.** Epidural.

**periencephalitis** (pĕr'ĭ-en-sef'ă-li'tis) [ peri- + G. *enkephalos*, brain ]. Inflammation of the cerebral membranes, particularly leptomeningitis or inflammation of the pia mater.

**periendothelioma** (pĕr-ĭ-en-do-the-lĭ-o'mah). Perithelioma.

**perienter'ic.** Surrounding the intestine.

**perienteritis** (pĕr-ĭ-en-ter-i'tis). Seroenteritis; inflammation of the peritoneal coat of the intestine.

**perien'teron** [ peri- + G. *enteron*, intestine ]. Archaic term for perivisceral *cavity*.

**periependymal** (pĕr'ĭ-e-pen'dĭ-mal). Surrounding the ependyma.

**periesophageal** (pĕr'ĭ-e-sof'ă-je'al). Surrounding the esophagus.

**periesophagitis** (pĕr-ĭ-e-sof'ă-ji'tis). Inflammation of the tissues surrounding the esophagus.

**perifo'cal.** Surrounding a focus; denoting the tissues or the blood that they contain in the vicinity of an infective focus.

**perifollic'ular.** Surrounding a hair follicle; term usually used to describe the histopathologic appearance of the infiltrate surrounding a hair follicle.

**perifolliculitis** (pĕr'ĭ-fo-lik-u-li'tis). The presence of an inflammatory infiltrate surrounding hair follicles. Frequently occurs in conjunction with folliculitis.

   **p. absce'dens et suffo'diens,** dissecting cellulitis; a chronic dissecting folliculitis of the scalp.

   **superficial pustular p.,** Bockhart's *impetigo.*

**periganglionic** (pĕr'ĭ-gang-glĭ-on'ik). Surrounding a ganglion, especially a nerve ganglion.

**perigas'tric** [ peri- + G. *gaster*, belly, stomach ]. Surrounding the stomach.

**perigastri'tis.** Inflammation of the peritoneal coat of the stomach.

**perigemmal** (pĕr'ĭ-jem'al) [ peri- + L. *gemma*, bud ]. Circumgemmal.

**periglandulitis** (pĕr-ĭ-glan-du-li'tis). Inflammation of the tissues surrounding a gland.

**periglot'tic** [ peri- + G. *glōssa* or *glōtta*, tongue ]. Around the tongue, especially around the base of the tongue and the epiglottis, or around the glottis (laryngis), the rima glottidis.

**periglot'tis** [ G. *periglottis*, covering of the tongue ]. The mucous membrane of the tongue.

**perihepat'ic** [ peri- + G. *hēpar*, liver ]. Surrounding the liver.

**perihepatitis** (pĕr-ĭ-hep-ă-ti'tis) [ peri- + G. *hēpar*, liver, + *-itis* ]. Hepatic capsulitis; hepatitis externa; inflammation of the serous, or peritoneal, covering of the liver.

**periher'nial.** Surrounding a hernia.

**peri-implantoclasia** (per'ĭ-im-plan'to-kla'zĭ-ah) [ peri- + L. *im*, in, + *planto*, to plant, + G. suffix *klasis*, breaking up ]. In dentistry, a general term implying disease of the supporting bone involving an implant; the disease may be exfoliative, resorptive, traumatic, or ulcerative in nature.

**perije'juni'tis.** Inflammation around the jejunum.

**perikaryon,** pl. **perika'rya** (pĕr-ĭ-kăr'ĭ-on) [ peri- + G. *karyon*, kernel ]. 1. The cytoplasm; periplast; protoplasm surrounding the nucleus. 2. The body of the odontoblast, excluding tubules. 3. The cell body of the nerve cell, as distinguished from its axon and dendrites.

**perikerat'ic** [ peri- + G. *keras*, horn ]. Pericorneal.

**perikymata,** sing. **perikyma** (pĕr'ĭ-ki'mă-tah, -ki'mah) [ peri- + G. *kyma*, wave ]. The transverse ridges and grooves on the surface of tooth enamel.

**perilabyrinthitis** (pĕr'ĭ-lab'ĭ-rin-thi'tis). Inflammation of the parts about the labyrinth.

**perilaryngeal** (pĕr'ĭ-lă-rin'je-al). Surrounding the larynx.

**perilaryngitis** (pĕr'ĭ-lăr-in-ji'tis). Inflammation of the tissues around the larynx.

**perilentic'ular.** Surrounding the lens of the eye.

**periligamen'tous.** Peridesmic.

**per'ilymph.** Perilympha.

**perilympha** (pĕr'ĭ-lim'fah) [ peri- + L. *lympha*, a clear fluid (lymph) ] [ NA ]. Perilymph; Cotunnius' liquid; liquor cotunnii; the fluid contained within the osseus labyrinth, surrounding and protecting the membranous labyrinth.

**perilymphangial** (pĕr'ĭ-lim-fan'jĭ-al). Surrounding a lymphatic vessel.

**perilymphangitis** (pĕr-ĭ-lim-fan-ji'tis). Inflammation of the tissues surrounding a lymphatic vessel.

**perilymphatic** (pĕr'ĭ-lim-fat'ik). 1. Surrounding a lymphatic structure (node or vessel); relating to lymph. 2. The spaces and tissues surrounding the membranous labyrinth of the inner ear.

**perimasti'tis** [ peri- + G. *mastos*, breast ]. Inflammation of the connective tissue around the breast.

**perimeningitis** (pĕr-ĭ-men-in-ji'tis). Pachymeningitis.

**perim'eter** [ G. *perimetros*, circumference, fr. *peri*, around, + *metron*, measure ]. 1. A circumference, edge, or border. 2. An instrument for delimiting the field of vision and measuring the degree of strabismus.

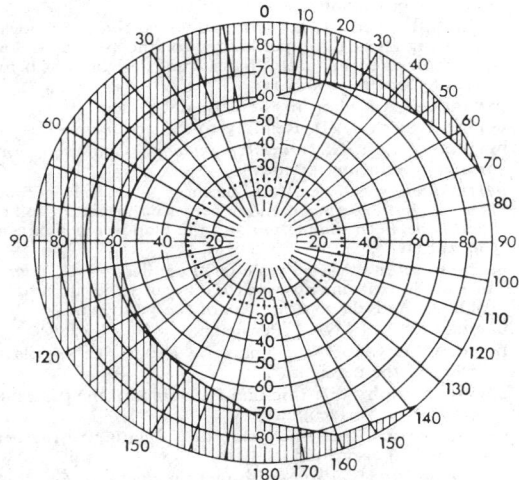

**Perimeter Chart of Right Eye**
The unshaded area is sensitive to light

   **arc p.,** a p. consisting of a semicircular frame at the center of which the patient looks while a white object is moving along the arc, the exact point where it becomes visible or invisible being noted and recorded on a chart.

   **Goldmann p.,** a projection p. that adds further precision by controlling the surrounding illumination.

   **projection p.,** one that uses as target a spot of light that can be regulated rapidly as to size, brightness, and color, and moves silently at any desired speed.

**perimet'ric.** 1 [ G. *peri*, around, + *mētra*, uterus ]. Surrounding the uterus; relating to the perimetrium. 2 [ G. *perimetros*, circumference ]. Relating to the circumference of any part or area. 3. Relating to perimetry.

**perimetrit'ic.** Relating to or marked by perimetritis.

**perimetritis** (pĕr'ĭ-me-tri'tis) [ perimetrium + G. suffix *-itis*, inflammation ]. Metroperitonitis.

**perimetrium,** pl. **perimetria** (pĕr'ĭ-me'trĭ-um, -me'trĭ-ah) [ peri- + G. *mētra*, uterus ] [ NA ]. Tunica serosa uteri [ NA ]; the serous (peritoneal) coat of the uterus.

**perim'etry** [ G. *perimetros*, circumference ]. The determination of the limits of the visual field.

   **flicker p.,** a technique of p. using the criterion of critical fusion frequency (*q. v.* under frequency).

   **kinetic p.,** mapping of the visual field by using a moving test object.

**quantitative p.,** a plotting of the visual field in isopters of equal retinal perceptiveness.

**static p.,** exploration of the visual field by using test objects at fixed positions and gradually increasing luminance to the threshold of visibility.

**perimyelis** (pĕr'ĭ-mi'ĕ-lis) [ peri- + G. *myelos,* marrow ]. Endosteum.

**perimyelitis** (pĕr'ĭ-mi'ĕ-li'tis). Endosteitis.

**perimyoendocarditis** (pĕr-ĭ-mi'o-en-do-kar-di'tis). Endoperimyocarditis.

**perimyositis** (pĕr-ĭ-mi-o-si'tis). Inflammation of the loose cellular tissue surrounding a muscle.

**perimysial** (pĕr'ĭ-mis'ĭ-al, -miz'ĭ-al). Relating to the perimysium; surrounding a muscle.

**perimysiitis, perimysitis** (pĕr'ĭ-mis'ĭ-i'tis, -mī-si'tis). 1. Inflammation of the perimysium. 2. Perimyositis.

**perimysium,** pl. **perimysia** (pĕr'ĭ-mis'ĭ-um, -miz'ĭ-um, -ĭ-ah) [ peri- + G. *mys,* muscle ] [ NA ]. The fibrous sheath enveloping each of the primary bundles of skeletal muscle fibers.

**p. externum,** epimysium.

**p. internum,** in the older literature, a term referring to the connective tissue around secondary and tertiary fascicles and individual fibers and also to the supporting framework of the myocardium.

**perina'tal** [ peri- + L. *natus,* pp. of *nascor,* to be born ]. Occurring during, or pertaining to, the periods before, during, or after the time of birth. Time designations before and after birth are arbitrary.

**per'inate.** An infant in the perinatal period.

**perineal** (pĕr'ĭ-ne'al). Relating to the perineum.

**perineo-** [ L. fr. G. *perineon, perinaion* ]. Combining form meaning perineum, perineal.

**perineocele** (pĕr-ĭ-ne'o-sēl) [ perineo- + G. *kēlē,* hernia ]. A hernia in the perineal region, between the rectum and the vagina, between the rectum and the bladder, or alongside the rectum.

**perineometer** (pĕr'ĭ-ne-om'e-ter) [ perineo- + G. *metron,* measure ]. Instrument used to measure the strength of voluntary muscle contractions of the perineum.

**perineon** [ L. ] [ NA ]. Perineum.

**perineoplasty** (pĕr'ĭ-ne'o-plas'tĭ). Reparative or plastic surgery of the perineum.

**perineorrhaphy** (pĕr'ĭ-ne-or'ă-fĭ). Suture of the perineum, performed in perineoplasty.

**perineoscrotal** (pĕr-ĭ-ne'o-skro'tal). Relating to the perineum and the scrotum.

**perineostomy** (pĕr'ĭ-ne-os'to-mĭ) [ perineo- + G. *stoma,* mouth ]. Urethrostomy through the perineum.

**perineosynthesis** (pĕr-ĭ-ne'o-sin'thĕ-sis). Perineoplasty in a case of extensive laceration of the perineum.

**perineotomy** (pĕr'ĭ-ne-ot'o-mĭ). Incision into the perineum as in external urethrotomy, lithotomy, etc., or to facilitate childbirth. See also episiotomy.

**perineovaginal** (pĕr-ĭ-ne'o-vaj'ĭ-nal). Relating to the perineum and the vagina.

**perinephrial** (pĕr'ĭ-nef'rĭ-al). Relating to the perinephrium.

**perinephric** (pĕr'ĭ-nef'rik). Perirenal; surrounding the kidney in whole or part.

**perinephritis** (pĕr'ĭ-ne-fri'tis). Inflammation of perinephric tissue.

**perinephrium,** pl. **perinephria** (pĕr'ĭ-nef'rĭ-um, -nef'-rĭ-ah) [ peri- + G. *nephros,* kidney ]. The connective tissue and fat surrounding the kidney.

**perineum,** pl. **perinea** (pĕr'ĭ-ne'um, -ne'ah) [ L. fr. G. *perineon, perinaion* ]. 1 [ NA ]. The area between the thighs extending from the coccyx to the pubis and lying below the pelvic diaphragm. 2. The external surface of the central tendon of the perineum, lying between the vulva and the anus in the female and the scrotum and the anus in the male.

**watering-pot p.,** a p. riddled with fistulas resulting from urethral stricture.

**perineural** (pĕr'ĭ-nu'ral) [ peri- + G. *neuron,* nerve ]. Surrounding a nerve.

**perineurial** (pĕr'ĭ-nu'rĭ-al). Relating to the perineurium.

**perineuritis** (pĕr-ĭ-nu-ri'tis). Inflammation of the perineurium. See also adventitial *neuritis.*

**perineurium,** pl. **perineuria** [ L. fr. peri- + G. *neuron,* nerve ]. The connective tissue sheath surrounding a fascicle of nerve fibers in a peripheral nerve; it consists of concentric layers of closely united flattened cells which alternate with layers of fine collagenous fibers having a predominantly longitudinal direction.

**perinuclear** (pĕr-ĭ-nu'kle-ar). Surrounding a nucleus.

**perioc'ular.** Circumocular.

**period** (pĕr'ĭ-od) [ G. *periodos,* a way round, a cycle, fr. *peri,* around, + *hodos,* way ]. 1. A certain duration or division of time. 2. One of the stages of a disease, *e.g.,* p. of incubation, p. of convalescence. See also entries under stage and phase.

**absolute refractory p.,** the p. following excitation when no response is possible regardless of the intensity of the stimulus.

**amphibolic p.,** amphibolic *stage.*

**critical p.,** (1) in the first hours after birth, the p. of maximum imprintability; the period before and after which imprinting is difficult or impossible; (2) in animals, a p. when socialization is possible.

**eclipse p.,** eclipse phase; phage eclipse; the period of time between infection by (or induction of) bacteriophage, or other virus, and the appearance of mature virus within the cell.

**effective refractory p.,** the p. during which impulses may appear but are too weak to be conducted.

**ejection p.,** sphygmic *interval.*

**induction p.,** the interval between an initial injection of antigen and the appearance of demonstrable antibodies in the blood.

**intersystolic p.,** a-c *interval.*

**intrapartum p.,** in obstetrics, the p. from the onset of labor to the end of the third stage of labor.

**isoelectric p.,** the p. occurring in the electrocardiogram between the end of the S wave and the beginning of the T wave during which electrical forces are acting in directions such as to neutralize each other so that there is no difference in potential under the two electrodes.

**isometric p.,** presphygmic *interval.*

**isometric p. of cardiac cycle,** that p. in which, though the cardiac muscle is excited and the pressure in the ventricles rises, the muscle fibers do not shorten; it extends from the closure of the atrioventricular valves to the opening of the semilunar valves.

**latency p.,** latency *phase.*

**latent p.,** (1) the p. elapsing between the application of a stimulus and the obvious response, *e.g.,* contraction of a muscle; (2) the p. of incubation of an infectious disease before the appearance of the prodromal symptoms.

**missed p.,** the failure of menstruation to occur in any month at the expected time.

**mitotic p.'s,** see mitotic *cycle.*

**monthly p.,** menses.

**Oedipal p.,** Oedipal *phase.*

**postsphygmic p.,** postsphygmic *interval.*

**presphygmic p.,** presphygmic *interval.*

**preejection p.,** the interval between onset of QRS complex and cardiac ejection; electromechanical systole minus ejection time.

**puerperal p.,** the p. elapsing between the termination of labor and the return of the generative tract to its normal condition; the 6 weeks following the completion of labor.

**pulse p.,** the reciprocal of the repetition rate, *e.g.,* the interval between leading edges of successive pulses.

**refractory p.,** the p. following effective stimulation, during which excitable tissue such as heart muscle and nerve fails to respond to a stimulus of threshold intensity (*i.e.,* excitability is depressed).

**refractory p. of electronic pacemaker,** the time required to restore full sensitivity after detecting cardiac activity or delivering a pacing impulse.

**relative refractory p.,** the p. between the effective refractory p. and the end of the refractory p.; fibers then respond only to high intensity stimuli and the impulses conduct more slowly than normally.

**safe p.,** the p. in the menstrual cycle when conception is least likely to occur, namely, about 10 days before or after the onset of menstruation, since ovulation occurs about midway between two menstrual p.'s.

**silent p.,** the cessation of electrical responses from the contracting muscle during the experimental elicitation of a tendon jerk.

**sphygmic p.,** sphygmic *interval.*

**total refractory p.,** the absolute refractory p. plus the relative refractory p.

**vulnerable p. (of heart),** a brief time during the cardiac cycle when stimuli are particularly likely to induce repetitive activity like fibrillation which persists after the stimulus has ceased; for the ventricle, it occurs during the latter part of systole, during the relative refractory period coincident with the inscription of the T wave of the electrocardiogram.

**Wenckebach p.,** a sequence of cardiac cycles in the electrocardiogram ending in a dropped beat due to A-V block, the preceding cycles showing progressively lengthening P-R intervals. The P-R interval following the dropped beat is again shortened.

**periodate** (per-i'o-dāt). A salt of periodic acid.

**periodic** (pēr-ĭ-od'ik). Recurring at regular intervals; denoting a disease with regularly recurring exacerbations or paroxysms.

**periodic acid** (per-i'o-dik). HIO₄, but existing in solution usually in hydrated form.

**periodicity** (pēr'ĭ-o-dis'ĭ-tĭ). The tendency to recurrence at regular intervals.

**periodontal** (pēr'ĭ-o-don'tal) [ peri- + G. *odous,* tooth ]. Pericemental; peridental; around a tooth.

**periodontia** (pēr-ĭ-o-don'shĭ-ah). 1. Plural of periodontium. 2. Periodontics.

**periodontics** (pēr'ĭ-o-don'tiks) [ peri- + G. *odous,* tooth ]. Periodontia; the branch of dentistry concerned with the study of the normal tissues and the treatment of abnormal conditions of the tissues immediately about the teeth.

**per'iodon'tist.** A dentist who specializes in periodontics.

**periodontitis** (pēr'ĭ-o-don-ti'tis) [ periodontium + G. suffix *-itis,* inflammation ]. Rigg's disease; stomatitis ulcerosa chronica; a disease of the periodontium, evidence by inflammation of the gingivae, resorption of the alveolar bone, degeneration of the periodontal membrane (ligament), migration of the epithelia attachment apically, and formation of periodontal pockets.

**chronic p.,** a slowly progressive inflammatory disease that extends from the marginal gingiva to destroy alveolar bone and periodontal membrane; usually accompanied by pathologic deepening of the gingival sulcus to form a periodontal pocket.

**p. complex,** resorption of the alveolar process in a vertical nature with pockets of uneven depth on adjacent teeth with traumatic occlusion as a factor.

**p. simplex,** resorption of the alveolar process in a horizontal fashion with pockets of even depth on adjacent teeth; traumatic occlusion is not a factor.

**sup'purative p.,** pyorrhea alveolaris; inflammatory disease of periodontium, accompanied by purulent exudate.

**periodontium,** pl. **periodontia** (pēr'ĭ-o-don'shĭ-um, -shĭ-ah) [ L. fr. peri- + G. *odous,* tooth ] [ NA ]. Periodontal, alveolodental, or peridental membrane; alveolodental, gingivodental, or cemental ligament; peridentium; periosteum; tapetum alveoli; the connective tissue attaching the tooth to the alveolar bone. See also parodontium.

**periodontoclasia** (pēr'ĭ-o-don'to-kla'zĭ-ah) [ periodontium + *klasis,* breaking ]. Periodontolysis; destruction of periodontal tissues, gingiva, pericementum, alveolar bone, and cementum.

**per'iodontol'ysis** [ periodontium + G. *lysis,* dissolution ]. Periodontoclasia.

**periodontosis** (pēr'ĭ-o-don-to'sis) [ periodontium + G. suffix *-osis,* condition ]. A noninflammatory degenerative disease of the attachment apparatus characterized by looseness and migration of teeth.

**periomphalic** (pēr'ĭ-om-fal'ik) [ peri- + G. *omphalos,* umbilicus ]. Periumbilical; around or near the umbilicus.

**perionychia** (pēr-ĭ-o-nik'ĭ-ah). Perionyxis; inflammation of the perionychium.

**perionychium,** pl. **perionychia** (pēr-ĭ-o-nik'ĭ-um, -nik'-ĭ-ah) [ peri- + G. *onyx,* nail ]. Eponychium (2).

**perionyx** pĕr'ĭ-on'iks [ peri- + G. *onyx,* nail ] [ NA ]. A remnant of the eponychium remaining in the narrow fold overlapping the proximal part of the lunula.

**perionyxis** (pĕr'ĭ-o-nik'sis). Perionychia.

**perioophoritis** (pĕr'ĭ-o-of'o-ri'tis) [ peri- + G. *oophoron,* ovary, + suffix *-itis,* inflammation ]. Perioothecitis; periovaritis; inflammation of the peritoneal covering of the ovary.

**perioophorosalpingitis** (pĕr'ĭ-o-of'o-ro-sal'pin-ji'tis) [ peri- + G. *oophoron,* ovary, + salpingitis ]. Perioothecosalpingitis; perisalpingo-ovaritis; inflammation of the peritoneum and other tissues around the ovary and oviduct.

**perioothecitis** (pĕr'ĭ-o'o-the-si'tis) [ peri- + Mod. L. *ootheca,* ovary, + G. suffix *-itis,* inflammation ]. Perioophoritis.

**perioothecosalpingitis** (pĕr-ĭ-o-ō-the'ko-sal-pin-ji'tis) [ G. *peri,* around, + Mod. L. *ootheca,* ovary, + salpingitis ]. Perioophorosalpingitis.

**per'iophthal'mic** [ peri- + G. *ophthalmos,* eye ]. Circumocular.

**periophthalmitis** (pĕr'ĭ-of'thal-mi'tis). Inflammation of the periophthalmic tissues.

**periople** (pĕr'ĭ-ōpl) [ G. *peri,* around, + *hoplon,* implement, shield ]. Corium limbi; a region of the pododerm; the thin, hard, relatively impervious, outer layer of the horn wall of the hoof of an animal. See fig. under hoof.

**per'iop'lic.** Pertaining to the periople.

**perio'ral.** Around the mouth.

**perior'bit.** Periorbita.

**periorbita** (pĕr-ĭ-or'bĭ-tah) [ peri- + L. *orbita,* orbit ] [ NA ]. Periorbit; orbital fascia; the periosteum of the orbit of the eye.

**perior'bital.** 1. Relating to the periorbita. 2. Circumorbital.

**periorchitis** (pĕr-ĭ-or-ki'tis) [ peri- + G. *orchis,* testis, + suffix *-itis,* inflammation ]. Inflammation of the tunica vaginalis testis.

**p. hemorrha'gica,** chronic hematocele of the tunica vaginalis testis.

**per'iost.** Periosteum.

**perios'teal.** Relating to the periosteum.

**periosteitis** (per-ĭ-os-te-i'tis). Periostitis.

**periosteo-** (pĕr'ĭ-os'te-o-) [ Mod. L. *periosteum,* q. v. ]. Combining form for periosteum, periosteal.

**periosteoma** (pĕr'ĭ-os'te-o'mah). Periostoma; periosteophyte; a neoplasm derived from the periosteum.

**periosteomedullitis** (pĕr-ĭ-os'te-o-mĕ-duh-li'tis) [ periosteo- + L. *medulla,* marrow, + G. suffix *-itis,* inflammation ]. Periosteomyelitis.

**periosteomyelitis** (pĕr-ĭ-os'te-o-mi-ĕ-li'tis) [ periosteo- + G. *myelos,* marrow, + suffix *-itis,* inflammation ]. Osteomyelitis; periosteomedullitis; inflammation of the entire bone, with the periosteum and marrow.

**periosteophyte** (pĕr'ĭ-os'te-o-fīt) [ periosteo- + G. *phyton,* growth ]. Periosteoma.

**periosteosis** (pĕr'ĭ-os'te-o'sis). Periostosis; the formation of a periosteoma.

**periosteotome** (pĕr'ĭ-os'te-o-tōm). Periostotome; a strong scapel-shaped knife, for cutting the periosteum.

**periosteotomy** (pĕr'ĭ-os-te-ot'o-mī) [ periosteo- + G. *tomē,* incision ]. Periostotomy; the operation of cutting through the periosteum to the bone.

**perios'teous.** Periosteal.

**periosteum,** pl. **periostea** (pĕr'ĭ-os'te-um, -te-ah) [ Mod. L. fr. G. *periosteon,* ntr. of adj. *periosteos,* round the bones, fr. *peri,* around, + *osteon,* bone ] [ NA ]. The thick fibrous membrane covering the entire surface of a bone except its articular cartilage. In young bones it consists of two layers: an inner which is osteogenic, forming new bone tissue, and an outer connective tissue layer conveying the blood vessels and nerves supplying the bone. In older bones the osteogenic layer is reduced. See also perichondral *bone.*

**alveolar p., p. alveola're,** periodontium.

**p. cra'nii,** pericranium.

**periostitis** (pĕr'ĭ-os-ti'tis). Periosteitis; inflammation of the periosteum.

**albuminous p.,** periosteal *ganglion.*

**alveolar p.,** alveolitis.

**dental p.,** inflammation of periodontal ligament.

**orbital p.,** inflammation of periorbital soft tissues.

**periosto'ma.** Periosteoma.

**periosto'sis,** pl. **periosto'ses.** Periosteosis.

**periostosteitis** (pĕr-ĭ-os'tos-te-i'tis) [ periosteum + G. *osteon*, bone, + suffix *-itis*, inflammation ]. Inflammation of a bone with involvement of the periosteum.

**perios'totome.** Periosteotome.

**periostot'omy.** Periosteotomy.

**periotic** (pĕr'ĭ-o'tik, -ot'ik) [ peri- + G. *ous*, ear ]. Surrounding the internal ear; referring to the petromastoid portion of the temporal bone, or the spaces and tissues in the bony labyrinth that surround the membranous labyrinth.

**periovaritis** (pĕr'ĭ-o'vă-ri'tis). Perioophoritis.

**periovular** (pĕr'ĭ-o'vu-lar). Surrounding the ovum.

**peripachymeningitis** (pĕr'ĭ-pak'ĭ-men'in-ji'tis) [ peri- + pachymeninx (dura mater) + G. suffix *-itis*, inflammation ]. Inflammation of the parietal layer of the dura mater.

**peripancreatitis** (pĕr-ĭ-pan-kre-ă-ti'tis). Inflammation of the peritoneal coat of the pancreas.

**peripap'illary.** Surrounding a papilla.

**peripatetic** (pĕr'ĭ-pă-tet'ik) [ G. *peripatēsis*, a walking about ]. Walking around; sometimes used to describe a patient with "walking" typhoid.

**peripe'nial.** Surrounding the penis.

**periphacitis** (pĕr-ĭ-fă-si'tis) [ peri- + G. *phakos*, lentil (lens), + suffix *-itis*, inflammation ]. Periphakitis; presumed inflammation of the capsule of the crystalline lens of the eye.

**periphaki'tis.** Periphacitis.

**peripharyngeal** (pĕr'ĭ-fă-rin'je-al). Surrounding the pharynx.

**peripherad** (pĕ-rif'er-ad) [ G. *periphereia*, periphery (PHER-), + L. *ad*, to ]. In a direction toward the periphery.

**periph'eral.** Relating to or situated at the periphery.

**peripheraphose** (per-if'er-ă-fōz) [ G. *periphereia*, periphery, + *a-* priv. + *phōs*, light ]. Peripherophose; the subjective sensation of a dark spot or patch, the cause residing in the eye itself or the optic nerve.

**peripheria** [ L. ] [ NA ]. Periphery.

**periph'erocen'tral.** Relating to both the periphery and the center of the body or any part.

**peripherophose** (per-if'er-o-fōz). Peripheraphose.

**periphery** (per'if'er-ĭ) [ G. *periphereia*, fr. *peri*, around, + *pherō*, to carry. PHER- ]. 1. The part of a body away from the center, the outer part or surface. 2. Denture *border*.

**periphlebitic** (pĕr'ĭ-flĕ-bit'ik). Relating to periphlebitis.

**periphlebitis** (pĕr-ĭ-flĕ-bi'tis) [ peri- + G. *phleps*, vein, + suffix *-itis*, inflammation ]. Inflammation of the outer coat of a vein or of the tissues surrounding it.

**per'iplast** [ peri- + G. *plastos*, formed ]. An obsolete term that referred variously to the cytoplasm of a cell, to the centrosphere, or to the stroma of an organ.

**perip'loca** [ G. *peri-plokē*, a winding around, fr. *plekō*, to twine, plait ]. The bark and stems of *periploca graeca* (family Asclepiadaceae), climbing dogbane; silk vine; a plant of Southern Europe; has been used as a cardiac tonic.

**perip'locin.** Glucoperiplocymarin; periplocoside; a cardiotonic glycoside from periploca.

**peripo'lar.** Surrounding the pole or poles of any body, or any electric or magnetic poles.

**peripolesis** (per-ĭ-po-le'sis) [ peri- + G. *poleomai*, to wander ]. Penetration of migrating cells between fixed tissue cells that are normally in close contact.

**per'ipori'tis** [ peri- + G. *poros*, pore, + suffix *-itis*, inflammation ]. Miliary papules and papulovesicles with staphylococcic infection; most frequently on the face and in infants.

**peripor'tal.** Peripylic; surrounding the portal vein.

**periproctic** (pĕr'ĭ-prok'tik) [ peri- + G. *prōktos*, anus ]. Circumanal.

**periproctitis** (pĕr'ĭ-prok-ti'tis). Perirectitis; inflammation of the areolar tissue about the rectum.

**periprostat'ic.** Surrounding the prostate.

**periprostatitis** (pĕr-ĭ-pros-tă-ti'tis). Inflammation of the tissues surrounding the prostate.

**peripylephlebitis** (pĕr-ĭ-pi'le-flĕ-bi'tis) [ peri- + G. *pylē*, gate, + *phleps*, vein, + *-itis* ]. Inflammation of the tissues around the portal vein.

**peripy'lic** [ peri- + G. *pylē*, portal, gate ]. Periportal.

**peripyloric** (pĕr'ĭ-pi-lor'ik, -pī-lor'ik). Surrounding the pylorus.

**perirectal** (pĕr'ĭ-rek'tal). Surrounding the rectum.

**perirectitis** (pĕr'ĭ-rek-ti'tis). Periproctitis.

**perirenal** (pĕr'ĭ-re'nal [ peri- + L. *ren*, kidney ]. Perinephric.

**perirhinal** (pĕr'ĭ-ri'nal) [ peri- + G. *rhis*, nose ]. Around the nose or nasal cavity.

**perisalpingitis** (pĕr-ĭ-sal-pin-ji'tis) [ peri- + G. *salpinx*, trumpet, + suffix *-itis*, inflammation ]. Inflammation of the peritoneum covering the Fallopian tube.

**perisalpingo-ovaritis** (pĕr'ĭ-sal-ping'go-o-vă-ri'tis) [ peri- + G. *salpinx*, trumpet, + ovary + G. suffix *-itis*, inflammation ]. Perioophorosalpingitis.

**perisalpinx** (pĕr'ĭ-sal'pingks) [ peri- + G. *salpinx* (*salping-*), trumpet ]. The peritoneal covering of the uterine tube.

**periscopic** (pĕr'ĭ-skop'ik) [ peri- + G. *skopeō*, to view ]. Denoting that which gives the ability to see objects to one side as well as in the direct axis of vision.

**perisigmoiditis** (pĕr-ĭ-sig-moy-di'tis). Pericolitis sinistra; inflammation of the connective tissues surrounding the sigmoid flexure, giving rise to symptoms, referable to the left iliac fossa, similar to those of perityphlitis in the right iliac fossa.

**perisinuous** (pĕr'ĭ-sin'u-us). Surrounding a sinus, especially a sinus of the dura mater.

**perispermatitis** (pĕr'ĭ-sper-mă-ti'tis). Inflammation of the tissues around the spermatic cord.

**p. sero'sa,** hydrocele of the spermatic cord.

**perisplanchnic** (pĕr'ĭ-splangk'nik) [ peri- + G. *splanchna*, viscera ]. Perivisceral; surrounding any viscus or viscera.

**perisplanchnitis** (pĕr'ĭ-splangk-ni'tis) [ peri- + G. *splanchna*, viscera, + suffix *-itis*, inflammation ]. Inflammation surrounding any viscus or viscera.

**perisplen'ic.** Around the spleen.

**perisplenitis** (per-ĭ-sple-ni'tis). Inflammation of the peritoneum covering the spleen.

**perispondyl'ic** [ peri- + G. *spondylos*, vertebra ]. Perivertebral.

**perispondylitis** (pĕr-ĭ-spon-dī-li'tis) [ peri- + G. *spondylos*, vertebra, + suffix *-itis*, inflammation ]. Inflammation of the tissues about a vertebra.

**perissodactyl, perissodactylous** (pĕ-ris'o-dak'til, -dak'-tĭ-lus) [ G. *perissos*, odd, + *dactylos*, finger or toe ]. Imparidigitate.

**peristalsis** (pĕr'ĭ-stal'sis) [ peri- + G. *stalsis*, constriction. STAL- ]. The vermiform movement of the intestine or other tubular structure; a wave of alternate circular contraction and relaxation of the tube by which the contents are propelled onward.

**mass p.,** mass movement; forcible peristaltic movements of short duration, occurring only three or four times a day, which move the contents of the large intestine from one division to the next, as from the ascending to the transverse colon.

**reversed p.,** antiperistalsis; a wave of contraction in a direction the reverse of normal, by which the contents of the tube are forced backward.

**peristal'tic.** Relating to peristalsis.

**peristal'tin.** A water-soluble glycoside, possible constituent of cascara sagrada; laxative.

**peristaphylitis** (pĕr'ĭ-staf-ĭ-li'tis) [ peri- + G. *staphylē*, uvula, + *-itis* ]. Inflammation of the soft palate and parts about the uvula.

**peristasis** (pĕ-ris'tă-sis) [ peri- + G. *stasis*, a standing still ]. Peristatic hyperemia; phases of inactivity of vasoconstriction in inflammation.

**peristole** (pĕ-ris'to-le) [ peri- + G. *stellō*, to contract. STAL- ]. The tonic activity of the walls of the stomach whereby the organ contracts about its contents; contrasting with the peristaltic waves passing from the cardia toward the pylorus (peristalsis).

**peristolic** (pĕr'ĭ-stol'ik). Relating to peristole.

**peristoma** (pĕ-ris'to-mah, per'ĭ-sto'mah). Peristome.

**peristomal, peristomatous** (pĕr'ĭ-sto'mal, -sto'mă-tus). Perioral.

**peristome** (pĕr'ĭ-sto'm) [ peri- + G. *stoma*, mouth ]. Peristoma; a groove leading from the cytostome in ciliates and certain other forms of protozoa.

**per'iston.** A plasma substitute consisting of fractionated polyvinyl pyrrolidone; mean molecular weight, 50,000.

**peristrumitis** (pĕr-ĭ-stru-mi'tis) [ peri- + L. *struma*, goiter ]. Perithyroiditis.

**peristrumous** (pĕr'ĭ-stru'mus) [ peri- + L. *struma*, goiter ]. Situated about or near a goiter.

**perisynovial** (pĕr'ĭ-sĭ-no'vĭ-al). Around a synovial membrane.

**perisystole** (pĕr-ĭ-sis'to-le). Presystole.

**perisystol'ic.** Presystolic.

**peritectomy** (pĕr'ĭ-tek'to-mĭ) [ peri- + G. *ektomē*, excision ]. Peridectomy; peritomy; the removal of a paracorneal strip of the conjunctiva for the relief of pannus.

**peritendineum**, pl. **peritendinea** (pĕr-ĭ-ten-din'e-um, -e-ah) [ L. fr. peri- + G. *tenōn*, tendon ] [ NA ]. One of the fibrous sheaths surrounding the primary bundles of fibers in a tendon.

**peritendinitis** (pĕr'ĭ-ten-dĭ-ni'tis). Peritenonitis; inflammation of the sheath of a tendon.

  **p. calcarea,** a lime or calcium (chalky) deposit around a tendon.

  **p. sero'sa,** ganglion (2).

**peritenon** (pĕr'-ĭ-ten-on) [ peri- + G. *tenōn*, tendon ]. *Vagina tendinis.*

**peritenontitis** (pĕr-ĭ-ten-on-ti'tis). Peritendinitis.

**perithecium**, pl. **perithecia** (per-ĭ-thē'sĭ-um) [ peri- + G. *thēkē*, flask ]. Among certain fungi, a flask-shaped hollow structure that contains the asci; a flask-shaped ascocarp.

**perithelioma** (pĕr'ĭ-the-lĭ-o'mah). A neoplasm thought to be derived from the perithelial cells of the vascular adventitial tissues.

**perithelium**, pl. **perithelia** (pĕr'ĭ-the'lĭ-um, -lĭ-ah) [ peri- + G. *thēlē*, nipple ]. The connective tissue that surrounds smaller vessels and capillaries.

  **Eberth''s p.,** an incomplete layer of connective tissue cells encasing the blood capillaries.

**perithoracic** (pĕr-ĭ-tho-ras'ik). Surrounding or encircling the thorax.

**perithyroiditis** (pĕr-ĭ-thi-roy-di'tis). Peristrumitis; inflammation of the capsule or tissues surrounding the thyroid gland.

**perit'omist.** One who performs circumcision.

**perit'omize.** To perform peritomy upon.

**peritomy** (pe-rit'o-mĭ) [ G. *peritomē*, fr. *peri*, around, + *tomē*, incision ]. 1. Peritectomy. 2. Circumcision.

**peritoneal** (pĕr'ĭ-to-ne'al). Relating to the peritoneum.

**peritonealgia** (pĕr-ĭ-to-ne-al'jĭ-ah) [ peritoneum + G. *algos*, pain ]. Pain in the peritoneum.

**peritoneo-** (pĕr'ĭ-to-ne'o-) [ L. *peritoneum, q.v.* ]. Combining form relating to the peritoneum.

**peritoneocentesis** (pĕr'ĭ-to-ne'o-sen-te'sis) [ peritoneum + G. *kentēsis*, puncture ]. Paracentesis of the abdomen.

**peritoneoclysis** (pĕr'ĭ-to-ne-ok'lĭ-sis) [ peritoneum, + G. *klysis*, a washing out ]. Irrigation of the abdominal cavity.

**peritoneopathy** (pĕr'ĭ-to-ne-op'ă-thĭ) [ peritoneum, + *pathos*, suffering ]. Inflammation or other disease of the peritoneum.

**peritoneopericardial** (pĕr'ĭ-to-ne'o-pĕr'ĭ-kar'dĭ-al). Relating to the peritoneum and the pericardium.

**peritoneopexy** (pĕr'ĭ-to-ne'o-pek-sĭ) [ peritoneum + G. *pēxis*, fixation ]. A suspension or fixation of the peritoneum.

**peritoneoplasty** (pĕr'ĭ-to-ne'o-plas-tĭ) [ peritoneum + G. *plassō*, to form ]. Loosening adhesions and covering the raw surfaces with peritoneum to prevent reformation.

**peritoneoscope** (pĕr'ĭ-to-ne'o-skōp) [ peritoneum + G. *skopeō*, to view ]. Laparoscope; an endoscope for examining the peritoneal cavity.

**peritoneoscopy** (pĕr'ĭ-to-ne-os'ko-pĭ). Abdominoscopy; celioscopy; laparoscopy; ventroscopy; examination of the contents of the peritoneum through an electrically lighted tubular instrument passed through the abdominal wall.

**peritoneotomy** (pĕr'ĭ-to-ne-ot'o-mĭ) [ peritoneum + G. *tomē*, incision ]. Incision of the peritoneum.

**peritoneum**, pl. **peritonea** (pĕr'ĭ-to-ne'um, -ne'ah) [ Mod. L. fr. G. *peritonaion*, fr. *periteino*, to stretch over. TEN- ] [ NA ]. The serous sac consisting of mesothelium and a thin layer of irregular connective tissue, that lines the abdominal cavity and covers most of the viscera contained therein. It forms two sacs, the peritoneal (or greater) sac and the omental bursa (lesser sac) connected by the foramen epiploicum (of Winslow).

  **p. parieta'le** [ NA ], the layer of p. lining the abdominal walls.

  **p. viscera'le** [ NA ], the layer of p. investing the abdominal organs.

**peritonism** (pĕr'ĭ-to-nizm). 1. A symptom complex marked by vomiting, pain, and shock, in inflammation of any of the abdominal viscera in which the peritoneum is involved. 2. Pseudoperitonitis; a neurosis in which the symptoms simulate those of peritonitis.

**peritonitis** (pĕr'ĭ-to-ni'tis). Inflammation of the peritoneum.

  **adhesive p.,** a form in which a fibrinous exudate occurs, matting together the intestines and various other organs.

  **benign paroxysmal p.,** familial paroxysmal *polyserositis.*

  **bile p.,** inflammation of the peritoneum caused by the escape of bile into the free peritoneal cavity.

  **chemical p.,** p. due to the escape of bile, contents of the gastrointestinal tract, or pancreatic juice into the peritoneal cavity; shock and peritoneal exudation due to chemical injury may precede any associated infection.

  **chyle p.,** due to free chyle in the peritoneal cavity.

  **circumscribed p.,** localized p.

  **p. defor'mans,** a chronic p. in which thickening of the membrane and contracting adhesions cause shortening of the mesentery and kinking and retraction of the intestines.

  **diaphragmat'ic p.,** p. affecting mainly the peritoneal surface of the diaphragm.

  **diffuse p.,** general p.

  **p. encap'sulans,** a localized fibrous or adhesive p. remaining after a generalized p. has nearly disappeared; it is marked by pain, constipation, and a palpable tumor.

  **fibrocaseous p.,** p. characterized by caseation and fibrosis, usually caused by the tubercle bacillus.

  **gas p.,** inflammation of the peritoneum accompanied by an intraperitoneal accumulation of gas.

  **general p.,** p. diffused throughout the peritoneal cavity.

  **localized p.,** p. confined to a circumscribed region of the peritoneal cavity.

  **meco'nium p.,** p. caused by intestinal perforation in the fetus during or shortly after birth, usually associated with congenital obstruction.

  **pelvic p.,** pelviperitonitis; inflammation, more or less strictly localized, of the peritoneum surrounding the uterus and Fallopian tubes; usually gonorrheal, tuberculous, or septic.

  **periodic p.,** periodic *abdominalgia.*

  **tuberculous p.,** p. caused by the tubercle bacillus.

**peritonize** (pĕr'ĭ-to-nīz). To cover with peritoneum, referring usually to the procedure in an operation for the anastomosis of the stomach or intestine.

**peritonsillar** (pĕr'ĭ-ton'sĭ-lar). Around a tonsil or the tonsils.

**peritonsillitis** (pĕr'ĭ-ton'sĭ-li'tis). Inflammation of the connective tissue above and behind the tonsil.

**peritracheal** (pĕr-ĭ-tra'ke-al). About the trachea.

**peritrichal** (pĕ-rit'rĭ-kal). Peritrichous (2).

**peritrichate** (pĕ-rit'rĭ-kat, pĕr'ĭ-trik'āt). Peritrichous (2).

**peritrichic** (pĕr'ĭ-trik'ik). Peritrichous (2).

**Peritrichida** (pĕr'ĭ-trik'ĭ-dah) [ peri- + G. *thrix*, hair ]. An order of Ciliata of cylindrical shape with the cilia usually limited to the zone surrounding the mouth opening.

**peritrichous** (pĕ-rit'rĭ-kus) [ peri- + G. *thrix*, hair ]. 1. Relating to cilia or other appendicular organs projecting from the periphery of a cell. 2. Peritrichal; peritrichate; peritrichic; having flagella uniformly distributed over a cell; used especially with reference to bacteria.

**peritrochanter'ic** (pĕr-ĭ-tro-kan-tĕr'ik). Around a trochanter.

**perituber'culo'sis.** Paratuberculosis.

**perityphlic** (pĕr'ĭ-tif'lik) [ peri- + G. *typhlon*, cecum ]. Pericecal.

**perityphlitis** (pĕr'ĭ-tif-li'tis). Obsolete term for periappendicitis.

**periumbilical** (pĕr'ĭ-um-bil'ĭ-kal). Periomphalic.

**periungual** (pĕr'ĭ-ung'gwal) [ peri- + L. *unguis*, nail ]. Surrounding a nail; involving the nail folds.

**periureteral, periureteric** (pĕr'ĭ-u-re'ter-al, -u're-tĕr'ik). Surrounding one or both ureters.

**periureteritis** (pĕr-ĭ-u-re'ter-i'tis) [ peri- + ureter + suffix -*itis*, inflammation ]. Inflammation of the tissues about a ureter.

   **p. plastica,** idiopathic retroperitoneal *fibrosis*.

**periurethral** (pĕr'ĭ-u-re'thral). Surrounding the urethra.

**periurethritis** (pĕr'ĭ-u-re-thri'tis) [ peri- + urethra + suffix -*itis*, inflammation ]. Inflammation of the parts about the urethra.

**periuterine** (pĕr'ĭ-u'ter-in). Perimetric (1).

**periuvular** (pĕr'ĭ-u'vu-lar). Around the uvula.

**perivaginitis** (pĕr'ĭ-vaj'ĭ-ni'tis). Pericolpitis; inflammation of the connective tissue around the vagina.

**perivascular** (pĕr'ĭ-vas'ku-lar) [ peri- + L. *vasculum*, vessel ]. Surrounding a blood or lymph vessel.

**perivasculitis** (pĕr'ĭ-vas-ku-li'tis). Periangitis.

**perive'nous.** Surrounding a vein.

**periver'tebral.** Perispondylic; around a vertebra or vertebrae.

**perives'ical** [ peri- + L. *vesica*, bladder ]. Pericystic.

**perivisceral** (pĕr-ĭvis'er-al). Perisplanchnic.

**perivisceritis** (pĕr-ĭ-vis-er-i'tis) [ peri- + L. *viscere* + G. -*itis* ]. Inflammation surrounding any viscus or viscera.

**perivitel'line** [ peri- + L. *vitellus*, yolk ]. Surrounding the vitellus or yolk.

**periwinkle** (pĕr'ĭ-wing'kl). *Vinca rosea.*

**per'kinism** [ E. *Perkins* ]. A form of quackery in which disease is purported to be treated by applying metals with magnetic and magic properties.

**Perkins,** E., British ophthalmologist. See P. *tonometer.*

**Perkins,** Elisha, New England physician, 1741–1799. Gave his name to perkinism.

**per'lapine** (USAN). 6-(4-Methyl-1-piperazinyl)morphanthridine; a hypnotic drug.

**perlèche** (per-lesh') [ Fr. *per*, intensive, + *lécher*, to lick ]. Commissural cheilitis (1).

**Perlia** (per'le-ah), Richard, German ophthalmologist, 19th century. See P.'s *nucleus*, convergence *nucleus* of P.

**perlingual** (per-ling'gwal) [ L. *per*, through, + *lingua*, tongue ]. Through or by way of the tongue; a method of medication.

**Perls** (perlz), Max, German pathologist, 1843–1881. See P.'s *test*.

**perlsucht** (perl'zukht) [ Ger. *perle*, pearl, + *sucht*, disease ]. Pearl *disease*.

**per'manens** [ L. ] [ NA ]. Permanent; in anatomy, denoting a structure which persists as opposed to a deciduous structure.

**permanganate** (per-mang'gă-nāt). A salt of permanganic acid.

**permangan'ic acid.** An acid, $HMnO_4$, derived from manganese, forming permanganates with bases; see also *potassium* permanganate.

**permeability** (per'me-ă-bil'ĭ-tĭ). The property of being permeable.

**permeable** (per'me-ă-bl) [ L. *permeabilis* (see permeation) ]. Pervious; permitting the passage of liquids.

**permeant** (per'me-ant) [ L. *permeabilis* (see permeation) ]. Able to pass through a particular semipermeable membrane.

**permease** (per'me-ās). The enzyme-like name attached to the property, in bacteria, of concentrating carbohydrates and their glycosides.

**permeation** (per-me-a'shun) [ L. *per-meo*, pp. -*meatus*, to pass through ]. The extension of a malignant neoplasm by proliferation of the cells continuously along the blood vessels or lymphatics.

**perniciosiform** (per-nish'ĭ-o'sĭ-form). Apparently pernicious; denoting a condition or disease that appears to be, but is not actually, pernicious or malignant.

**pernicious** (per-nish'us) [ L. *perniciosus*, destructive, fr. *pernicies*, destruction, fr. *per*, through, + *nex* (*nec*-), slaughter ]. Destructive; harmful; denoting a disease of severe character and usually fatal without specific treatment.

**pernio'sis.** [ L. *pernio*, chilblain, + G. suffix, -*osis*, condition ]. Chilblain.

**pe'ro-** [ G. *pēros*, maimed ]. Combining form meaning maimed or malformed.

**perobrachius** (pe-ro-bra'kĭ-us) [ pero- + G. *brachiōn*, arm ]. An individual with congenitally defective hands and forearms.

**perocephalus** (pe-ro-sef'ă-lus) [ pero- + G. *kephalē*, head ]. An individual with congenitally defective face and head.

**perochirus** (pe-ro-ki'rus) [ pero- + G. *cheir*, hand ]. An individual with congenitally defective hands.

**pe'rocor'mus** [ pero- + G. *kormos*, trunk ]. Perosomus.

**perodactylia** (pe'ro-dak-til'ĭ-ah). Perodactyly.

**perodactylus** (pe-ro-dak'tĭ-lus). An individual with perodactyly.

**perodactyly** (pe'ro-dak'tĭ-lĭ) [ pero- + G. *daktylos*, finger or toe ]. Perodactylia; a congenital condition characterized by deformed fingers or toes.

**perogen** (per'o-jen). A preparation of sodium perborate that when mixed with the accompanying catalyzer, liberates 10 per cent of the oxygen in the salt.

**peromelia** (pe-ro-me'lĭ-ah) [ pero- + G. *melos*, limb ]. Peromely; severe congenital malformations of extremities, including absence of hand or foot.

**peromelus** (pĕ-rom'e-lus). An individual with peromelia.

**perom'ely.** Peromelia.

**perone** (per-o'ne) [ G. *peronē*, brooch, the small bone of the arm or leg, the fibula, fr. *peirō*, to pierce ]. Fibula.

**peroneal** (pĕr-o-ne'al) [ L. *peroneus*, fr. G. *peronē*, fibula ]. Relating to the fibula, to the lateral side of the leg, or to the muscles there present.

**peroneotibial** (pĕr'o-ne'o-tib'ĭ-al). Tibiofibular; relating to the fibula and the tibia.

**perone'us** [ L. ] [ NA ]. Peroneal.

**per'onine.** Benzylmorphine hydrochloride; a narcotic analgesic related to morphine.

**peropus** (pe'ro-pus) [ pero- + G. *pous*, foot ]. A person with congenitally defective feet.

**peroral** (per-o'ral) [ L. *per*, through, + *os* (*or*-), mouth ]. Through the mouth; *e.g.*, the p. administration of a drug.

**per os** [ L. ]. By or through the mouth.

**perosis** (pe-ro'sis) [ pero- + G. suffix -*osis*, condition ]. A nutritional disease of young birds (*e.g.*, chicks and turkeys) characterized by shortening and thickening of the limb bones and a deformity known as "slipped tendon." Manganese, biotin, and choline are preventives; overcrowding, confinement, and wire floors without roosts are predisposing factors.

**perosomus** (pe-ro-so'mus) [ pero- + G. *sōma*, body ]. Perocormus; an individual with congenitally defective body.

**perosplanchnia** (pe'ro-splank'nĭ-ah) [ pero- + G. *splanchnon*, viscus ]. Congenital malformation of the viscera.

**perosseous** (per-os'e-us) [ L. *per*, through, + *os*, bone ]. Through bone.

**perot'ic.** Affected with perosis.

**peroxi-.** See peroxy-.

**perox'idases** (EC subclass 1.11.1). Hydrogen peroxide reducing oxidoreductases; enzymes in animal and plant tissues that catalyze the dehydrogenation (oxidation) of various substances in the presence of hydrogen peroxide, which acts as hydrogen acceptor, being converted to water in the process. If the oxidized substance is iodide, yielding iodine, the enzyme may be termed iodide peroxidase (EC 1.11.1.8) and be involved in the iodination of tyrosine (as tyrosine iodinase or thyroid peroxidase).

**perox'ide.** That oxide of any series that contains the greatest number of oxygen atoms; applied most correctly to compounds containing an —O—O— link, as in hydrogen peroxide (H—O—O—H).

**perox'isome** [ peroxide + G. *sōma*, body ]. Microbody; an organelle which, in most subhuman mammals, has an electron-dense core or nucleoid containing urate oxidase; other oxidative enzymes also occur.

**peroxy-.** Prefix denoting the presence of an extra O atom, as in peroxides, peroxy acids (*e.g.*, hydrogen peroxide, peroxyformic acid).

**peroxyace'tic acid.** Peracetic acid.

**peroxyace'tyl nitrate.** Major pollutant responsible for eye and nose irritation in smog.

**peroxyfor'mic acid.** Performic acid.

**perox'yl.** H—O—O; one of the free radicals presumed formed as a result of the bombardment of tissue by high energy radiation. Compare superoxide.

**perpendicula'ris** [ L. ] [ NA ]. Perpendicular; denoting a structure or part of a structure that forms a right angle.

**perphen'azine** (NF, BP). TRILAFON; 2-chloro-10-{3-[ 4-(2-hydroxyethyl)piperazinyl ]propyl} phenothiazine; a phenothiazine compound similar in chemical structure, pharmacologic actions, and uses to prochlorperazine but more potent; an antipsychotic agent and antiemetic.

**per pri'mam, per pri'mam intentio'nem** [ L. ]. By first intention; denoting a manner of healing of a wound. See under intention.

**per rec'tum** [ L. ]. By or through the rectum.

**persalt** (per'sawlt'). In chemistry, any salt that contains the greatest possible amount of the acid radical.

**per sal'tum** [ L. ]. At a leap; at one bound; not gradually or through different stages.

**per secun'dam, per secun'dam intentio'nem** [ L. ]. By second intention; denoting a manner of healing of a wound. See under intention.

**perseveration** (per-sev-er-a'shun). [ L. *persevero*, to persist ]. 1. The constant repetition of a meaningless word or phrase. 2. The duration of a mental impression, measured by the rapidity with which one impression follows another as determined by the revolving of a two-colored disk. 3. In clinical psychology, the repetition of a previously appropriate or correct response, even though the repeated response has since become inappropriate or incorrect.

**per'sic oil** (NF). The fixed oil expressed from the kernels of varieties of *Prunus armeniaca* (apricot kernel oil) or *Prunus persica* (peach kernel oil). Used as a vehicle.

**persim'mon.** Diospyros.

**per'sio.** Cudbear.

**persis'tence** [ L. *persisto*, to abide, stand firm ]. Obstinate continuation of characteristic behavior, or of existence in spite of opposition or adverse environmental conditions.

 **microbial p.,** the phenomenon of survival, in high concentration of an antimicrobial substance, of microbes that seem not to be resistant variants (mutants) since their progeny are fully susceptible.

**persis'ter.** That which, or one who, is capable of *persistence, q.v.*

 **bacterial p.'s,** bacteria that exhibit the phenomenon of microbial *persistence, q.v.*

**persona** (per-so'nah) [ L. *per*, through, + *sonare*, to sound: from the small megaphone in ancient dramatic masks, to aid in projecting the actor's voice ]. In Jungian psychology, the outer character, as opposed to anima (inner personality); the assumed personality used to mask the true one.

**per'sonal'ity.** 1. The unique self; the organized system of attitudes and behavioral predispositions by which one impresses and establishes relationships with others. 2. An individual with a particular p. pattern.

 **allotropic p.,** see allotropic (2).

 **authoritarian p.,** a cluster of p. traits reflecting a desire for security and order, *e.g.*, rigidity, highly conventional outlook, unquestioning obedience, scapegoating, and a desire for structured lines of authority.

**basic p.,** see basic personality *type.*

**compulsive p.,** one characterized by rigidity, extreme inhibition, and excessive concern with conformity and adherence to standards of conscience either for himself or others.

**cyclothymic p.,** a p. disorder in which a person experiences regularly alternating periods of elation and depression, usually not related to external circumstances.

**dual p.,** a mental disturbance in which a person assumes alternately two different identities without either p. being consciously aware of the other; see also double *consciousness.*

**histrionic p.,** hysterical p.

**hysterical p.,** histrionic p.; a condition in which a person, typically immature, dependent, self-centered, and often vain, exhibits unstable, overreactive, and excitable behavior intended to gain attention even though he may not be aware of this intent; this condition does not include the extreme forms of hysteria.

**inadequate p.,** a p. disorder, characterized by ineptness and emotional and physical instability, which renders the individual unable to cope with the normal vicissitudes of life.

**multiple p.,** a particular schizophrenic or dissociative reaction in which two or more distinct conscious p.'s alternately prevail in the same person, without either p. being aware of the other.

**paranoid p.,** a p. disorder characterized by hypersensitivity, rigidity, unwarranted suspicion, jealousy, and a tendency to blame others and ascribe evil motives to them; though neither a neurosis or psychosis, it interferes with the individual's ability to maintain interpersonal relationships.

**passive-aggressive p.,** a p. disorder in which aggressive feelings are manifested in passive ways, especially through mild obstructionism and stubbornness.

**psychopathic p.,** psychopath.

**schizoid p.,** a disorder with characteristics similar to those of schizophrenia but in milder form, *e.g.*, pathological shyness, oversensitivity, and seclusiveness to the point of avoiding close or competitive relationships; autistic thinking without loss of reality recognition is common in this condition.

**shut-in p.,** a person who responds inadequately to contacts with other people.

**split p.,** nontechnical term for schizophrenia; now rarely used.

**syntonic p.,** a stable p., one characterized by even temperament.

**person-years.** The number of people in a population multiplied by their life expectancy.

**perspiration** (per 'spī-ra'shun) [ L. *per-spiro*, pp. *-atus*, to breathe everywhere ]. 1. Sweating; diaphoresis; the excretion of fluid by the sweat glands of the skin. 2. All fluid loss through normal skin, whether by sweat gland secretion or by diffusion through other skin structures. 3. Sweat; the fluid excreted by the sweat glands; it consists of water containing sodium chloride and phosphate, urea, ammonia, ethereal sulfates, creatinine, fats, and other waste products; the average daily quantity is estimated at about 1500 gm. (3.3 lb.). See also subentries under sweat.

**insensible p.,** p. that evaporates before it is perceived as fluid on the skin. The term sometimes includes evaporation from the lungs.

**sensible p.,** the p. excreted in large quantity, or when there is much humidity in the atmosphere, so that it appears as moisture on the skin.

**perstillation** (per-stī-la'shun) [ L. *per*, through, + *stillo*, to trickle, distil ]. See pervaporation.

**persuasion** (per-swa'zhun). The act of influencing the mind of another, by authority, argument, or reason; an important element in most types of psychotherapy.

**persul'fate.** Salt of a persulfuric acid.

**persul'fide.** 1. That one of a series of sulfides that contains more atoms of sulfur than any other; a polysulfide. Compare perthio. 2. The sulfur analogue of a peroxide.

**persulfu'ric acid.** Peroxymonosulfuric acid, $H_2SO_5$; Caro's acid or peroxydisulfuric acid.

**per tertiam intentionem** per ter'shĭ-am in-ten-shĭ-o'-nem). By third intention; denoting a manner of healing of a wound. See under intention.

**Perthes** (pair'tās), Georg C., German surgeon, 1869–1927. See P.'s *disease,* Calvé-P. *disease,* Legg-Calvé-P. *disease,* Legg-P. *disease,* P.'s *incision, method, test.*

**perthio-** (per-thī'o-). Prefix denoting substitution of sulfur for every oxygen in a compound (*e.g.,* perthiocarbonic acid, $H_2CS_3$).

**Pertik,** Otto, Hungarian pathologist, 1852–1913. See P.'s *diverticulum.*

**per tu'bam** [ L. ]. Through a tube.

**pertussis** (per-tus'is) [ L. *per,* very (intensive), + *tussis,* cough ]. Whooping cough; an acute infectious disease caused by *Bordetella pertussis,* and marked by recurrent attacks to spasmodic coughing continued until the breath is exhausted, then ending with a deep noisy inspiration; the lesion, other than those caused by the violent cough, is a catarrh of the respiratory passages.

**pertussoid** (per-tus'oyd) [ pertussis + G. *eidos,* resemblance ]. A cough, often influenzal, resembling whooping cough in its general features.

**Peru'vian bark.** Cinchona.

**pervap'ora'tion** [ L. *per,* through, + *vapor,* steam ]. The heating of a liquid within a dialyzing bag suspended over a hot plate, evaporation taking place rapidly through the membrane; any colloids in solution remain within the bag while crystalloids diffuse out and crystallize on the outer surface of the bag (perstillation).

**perversion** (per-ver'zhun, -shun) [ L. *perversio,* fr. *per-verto,* pp. *-versus,* to turn about ]. A deviation from a societal norm, especially concerning sexual interests or behavior.

    **polymorphous p.,** (1) in psychoanalytic theory, a child's variegated sexual activity and interests; (2) in general, the manifold p.'s shown by an adult.

    **sexual p.,** sexual deviation; paraphilia; sexual practice considered medically abnormal, morally wrong, or legally prohibited.

**per'vert.** One who practices perversions.

**per vi'as natura'les** [ L. ]. Through the natural passages; denoting, for example, the birth of a child in the natural way and not by cesarean section; or the passage at stool of a foreign body that has been swallowed, instead of its removal by an abdominal section.

**pervigilium** (per'vĭ-jil'ĭ-um) [ L. a watching all night ]. Wakefulness; mild insomnia.

**per'vious** [ L. *pervius,* fr. *per,* through, + *vis,* a way ]. Permeable; capable of giving passage to anything, such as heat, moisture, light, etc.

**pes,** gen. **pe'dis,** pl. **pe'des** [ L. ]. 1 [ NA ]. The foot. 2. Any footlike or basal structure or part. 3. See p. pedunculi. 4. Talipes or clubfoot; in this sense always qualified by a word expressing the form of clubfoot, *e.g.,* p. cavus, p. planus; see talipes.

    **p. abductus.** *talipes* valgus.

    **p. adductus,** *talipes* varus.

    **p. anseri'nus,** (1) *plexus* parotideus; (2) the tendinous expansions of the sartorius, gracilis, and semitendinosus muscles at the medial border of the tuberosity of the tibia.

    **p. ca'vus,** *talipes* cavus.

    **p. equi'noval'gus,** *talipes* equinovalgus.

    **p. equi'nova'rus,** *talipes* equinovarus.

    **p. febric'itans,** elephantiasis.

    **p. gi'gas,** macropodia.

    **p. hippocam'pi** [ NA ], foot of the hippocampus; digitationes hippocampi; the anterior thickened extremity of the hippocampus.

    **p. pedun'culi,** *crus* cerebri.

    **p. pla'nus,** *talipes* planus.

    **p. prona'tus,** *talipes* valgus.

    **p. valgus,** *talipes* valgus.

    **p. va'rus,** *talipes* varus.

**pessary** (pes'ă-rĭ) [ L. *pessarium, fr.* G. *pessos,* an oval stone used in certain games ]. 1. An appliance of varied form, introduced into the vagina to support the uterus or to correct any displacement. 2. A medicated vaginal suppository.

    **diaphragm p.,** a ring with the opening covered with some material such as Neoprene, providing a platform to

support uterus, bladder or rectum, or to prevent conception.

    **Dumontpallier's p.,** Mayer's p.; an elastic ring p.

    **Gariel's p.,** a hollow rubber p. which can be inflated, made in the form of (1) a ring or (2) a pear.

    **Hodge's p.,** a double-curve oblong p. employed for the correction of retrodeviations of the uterus.

    **Mayer's p.,** Dumontpallier's p.

    **Menge's p.,** a ring p. with a central horizontal bar into which a detachable handle is inserted.

    **ring p.,** a ring of rubber, plastic, or metal in which the cervix rests; designed to support the uterus and to correct prolapse of that organ.

**pes'simism** [ L. *pessimus,* worst, irreg. superl. of *malus,* bad ]. A tendency to look on the dark side of life.

    **therapeutic p.,** a disbelief in the curative virtues of remedies in general and especially of drugs.

**pessulum, pessum** (pes'u-lum, pes'um) [ L. a pessary (both forms), fr. G. *pessos.* See pessary ]. Pessary.

**pes'sus** [ G. *pessos,* a pessary ]. Pessary (2).

**pest** [ L. *pestis* ]. Plague (2).

    **fowl p.,** fowl *plague.*

    **swine p.,** hog *cholera.*

**pesticemia** (pes-tĭ-se'mĭ-ah) [ L. *pestis,* plague, + G. *haima,* blood ]. Lememia.

**pes'ticide.** A very general term signifying an agent that destroys fungi, insects, rodents, or any other pest.

**pes'tilence** [ L. *pestilentia* ]. 1. The plague. 2. An epidemic of any infectious disease.

**pestilential** (pes-tĭ-len'shal). Pestiferous; relating to, or tending to produce, a pestilence.

**pes'tis** [ L. ]. Plague (2).

    **p. am'bulans,** ambulant *plague.*

    **p. ful'minans,** bubonic *plague.*

    **p. ma'jor,** bubonic *plague.*

    **p. mi'nor,** ambulant *plague.*

    **p. sid'erans,** septicemic *plague.*

    **p. variolo'sa,** smallpox.

**pestle** (pes'l) [ L. *pistillum,* fr. *pinso,* or *piso,* to pound ]. An instrument in the shape of a rod with one rounded and weighted extremity, used for bruising, breaking, and triturating substances in a mortar.

**petechiae,** sing. **petechia** (pe-te'kĭ-e, pe-te'kĭ-ah, pe-tek'-) [ Mod. L. form of It. *peteechie* ]. Minute hemorrhagic spots, of pinpoint to pinhead size, in the skin.

**petechial** (pe-te'kĭ-al, pe-tek'ĭ-al). Relating to or accompanied or characterized by petechiae.

**petechiasis** (pe-tĕ-ki'ă-sis). Formation of petechiae or purpura.

**Peters,** A. See P.'s *anomaly.*

**Peters,** Hubert, Vienna obstetrician, 1859–1934. See P.'s *ovum.*

**Petersen,** C. F., Kiel surgeon, 1845–1908. See P.'s *bag.*

**peth'idine hydrochloride** (BP). Meperidine hydrochloride.

**pet'iolate, pet'iolated** [ L. *petiolus,* petiole ]. Stalked or pedunculate.

**petiole** (pet'ĭ-ōl). Petiolus.

**pet'ioled.** Petiolate.

**peti'olus** [ L. dim. of *pes* (foot), the stalk of a fruit. PES- ]. Petiole; a stem or pedicle.

    **p. epiglot'tidis** [ NA ], the lower end or pedicle of the cartilage of the epiglottis, attached to the superior notch of the thyroid cartilage.

**Petit,** Alexis T., French physician, 1791–1820. See Dulong-P. *law.*

**Petit** (pet-e'), Antoine, French surgeon and anatomist, 1718–1794. See P.'s *ligaments.*

**Petit** (pet-e'), Francois P. du, French surgeon and anatomist, 1664–1741. See P.'s *canal, sinus.*

**Petit** (pet-e'), Jean L., Paris surgeon, 1674–1750. See P.'s *hernia, herniotomy, triangle.*

**Petit** (pet-e'), Paul, French anatomist, *1889. See P.'s *aponeurosis.*

**petit mal** (pĕ-te'mal). See under epilepsy.

**petr-.** See petro-.

**Petri** (pa'tre), Julius, German bacteriologist, 1852–1921. See P. *dish.*

**petrichloral** (pet'rĭ-klo'ral). PERICLOR; pentaerythritol chloral; a derivative of chloral. Used as a hypnotic and sedative, particularly for elderly persons.

**petrifaction** (pet'rĭ-fak'shun) [ L. *petra,* rock + *facio,* to make ]. Fossilization; calcification; conversion into stone.

**pétrissage** (pa-tre-sazh') [ Fr. kneading ]. A manipulation in massage, consisting in a kneading of the muscles.

**petro-, petr-** (pet'ro-) [ L. *petra,* rock; G. *petros,* stone ]. Combining forms for (1) stone, stony; (2) petrous, petrosal.

**petroccipital** (pet'rok-sip'ĭ-tal). Petrooccipital.

**pet'rola'tum** (NF). Yellow soft paraffin (BP); amber p.; petroleum jelly; paraffin jelly; a yellowish mixture of the softer members of the paraffin or methane series of hydrocarbons, obtained from petroleum as an intermediate product in its distillation. Used as a soothing application to burns and abrasions of the skin, and as a base for ointments.

    **hy'drophilic p.** (USP), composed of cholesterol 30 gm., stearyl alcohol 30 gm., white wax 80 gm., white p. 860 gm., to make 1000 gm.

    **light liquid p.** (NF), light *mineral oil.*

    **liquid p.,** (1) mineral oil.

    **white p.** (USP), white soft paraffin (BP); of the same composition as p. except that care is taken in its preparation to keep it colorless. Used for the same purposes as p.

**petroleum** (pĕ-tro'le-um) [ L. *petra,* rock, + *oleum,* oil ]. Rock oil; coal oil; mineral oil; a mixture of liquid hydrocarbons found in the earth in various parts of the world; its source is uncertain but it is believed to be derived from fossilized animal and plant remains; the p. of the United States is from rocks of the Devonian period, the Russian p. from tertiary formations. Besides its use for lighting and heating purposes p. is the source of petrolatum.

    **p. benzin,** p. ether; benzin; benzine; purified benzin; naphtha; purified, low boiling fractions distilled from p. consisting of hydrocarbons, chiefly of the methane series. Highly flammable; its vapors, when mixed with air and ignited, may explode; used as a solvent.

    **p. ether,** p. benzin.

**pet'romas'toid.** Relating to the petrous and the mastoid portions of the temporal bone, which are usually united at birth, forming the p. portion.

**petrooccipital** (pet'ro-ok-sip'ĭ-tal). Denoting the cranial suture between the occipital bone and the petrous portion of the temporal.

**pet'ropharynge'us.** See under musculus.

**petrosa,** pl. **petrosae** (pĕ-tro'sah, -se) [ L. fr. *petra,* rock ]. The petrous portion of the temporal bone.

**petro'sal.** Relating to the petrosa.

**pet'rosal'pingostaphyli'nus** [ petrosa + G. *salpinx,* trumpet, + *staphylē,* uvula ]. *Musculus* levator veli palatini.

**petrositis** (pet'ro-si'tis). Petrousitis; an inflammation involving the petrous portion of the temporal bone and its air cells.

**petro'somas'toid.** Petromastoid.

**petrosphenoid** (pet'ro-sfe'noyd). Relating to the petrous portion of the temporal bone and to the sphenoid bone.

**petrosquamosal, petrosquamous** (pet'ro-skwa-mo'sal, -skwa'mus). Relating to the petrous and the squamous portions of the temporal bone.

**pet'rostaphyli'nus** [ G. *petra,* stone, + *staphylē,* uvula ]. *Musculus* levator veli palatini.

**petro'sus** [ L. ] [ NA ]. Petrosal.

**petrous** (pet'rus, pe'trus) [ L. *petrosus,* fr. *petra,* a rock ]. 1. Of stony hardness. 2. Petrosal.

**petrousitis** (pet'rus-i'tis). Petrositis.

**Pette,** H., German physician. See P.-Döring *disease.*

**Pettit** (pet-e'), Auguste, French physician, 19th century. See Bachman and P. *test.*

**Peutz,** J. L. A. See P.-Jeghers *syndrome.*

**pexin** (pek'sin). Rennin.

**pexinogen** (pek'sin'o-jen). Renninogen.

**pexis** (pek'sis) [ G. *pēxis,* fixation. PAG- ]. The fixation of substances in the tissues.

**-pexy** [ G. *pēxis,* fixation ]. Suffix meaning fixation, usually surgical.

**Peyer** (pi'er), Johann K., Swiss anatomist, 1653–1712. See P.'s *glands, patches.*

**peyote, peyotl** (pa-yo'te, pa-yo'tl) [ Sp. ] (also called pellote; mescal buttons). See mescaline and *Lophophora williamsii.*

**Peyronie** (pa-ron-e'), Francois de la, French surgeon, 1678–1747. See P.'s *disease.*

**Peyrot** (pa-ro'), Jean J., Paris surgeon, 1843–1918. See P.'s *thorax.*

**Pezzer** (pez-a'), O. de, French physician, 19th century. See P. *catheter.*

**Pfannenstiel** (pfahn'en-stel), Johann, German gynecologist, 1862–1909. See P.'s *incision.*

**Pfaundler,** Meinhard von, German physician, 1872–1947. See P.-Hurler *syndrome.*

**Pfeiffer** (pfi'fer), Emil, German physician, 1846–1921. See P.'s *disease.*

**Pfeiffer** (pfi'fer), Richard F., German physician, *1858. Gave his name to *Pfeifferella.* See P.'s blood *agar, bacillus, phenomenon.*

**Pfeifferella** (pfi-fer-el'lah) [ R. F. J. *Pfeiffer* ]. An obsolete genus of bacteria, the type species of which, *P. mallei,* formerly was placed in the genus *Actinobacillus* and presently is placed in the genus *Pseudomonas.*

**Pflü'ger,** Eduard F. W., German physiologist, 1829–1910. See P.'s *laws, tubules.*

**Pfuhl** (pfool), Eduard, German physician, 1852–1905. See P.'s *sign.*

**pg.** Abbreviation for picogram.

**PGR.** Abbreviation for psychogalvanic *response.*

**Ph.** Symbol for the phenyl radical, $C_6H_5$—.

**pH.** Symbol for the logarithm of the reciprocal of the H ion concentration. A solution with pH 7.00 is neutral, one with a pH of more than 7.0 is alkaline, one with a pH lower than 7.00 is acid.

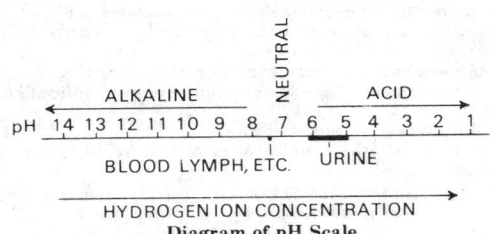

**Diagram of pH Scale**

**optimum pH,** the pH at which an enzymatic or any other reaction or process is most effective.

**PHA.** Abbreviation for phytohemagglutinin.

**phacitis** (fă-si'tis) [ G. *phakos,* lentil (lens), + suffix *-itis,* inflammation ]. Phakitis; presumed inflammation of the crystalline lens of the eye.

**phaco-** (fak'o-) [ G. *phakos,* lentil (lens), anything shaped like a lentil ]. Combining form usually meaning lens-shaped, or relating to a lens; also denotes "mother-spot," as in phacomatosis, *q. v.*

**phacoanaphylaxis** (fak'o-an'-ă-fi-lak'sis). Anaphylaxis or hypersensitiveness to protein of the crystalline lens.

**phacocele** (fak'o-sēl) [ phaco- + G. *kēlē,* hernia ]. Hernia of the crystalline lens of the eye, as when extruded through a rupture of the sclera beneath the conjunctiva.

**phacocyst** (fak'o-sist) [ phaco- + G. *kystis,* bladder ]. *Capsula* lentis.

**phacocystectomy** (fak'o-sis-tek'to-mĭ) [ phaco- + G. *kystis,* bladder, + *ektomē,* excision ]. Surgical removal of a portion of the capsule of the crystalline lens.

**phacoemulsification** (fak'o-e-mul-sĭ-fi-ka'shun). A method of emulsifying and aspirating a cataract with the use of a low frequency ultrasonic needle.

**phacoerysis** (fak″o-er′ĭ-sis) [ phaco- + G. *erysis*, pulling, drawing off ]. Extraction of the crystalline lens by means of a suction cup called the erysiphake.

**phacoid** (fak′oyd) [ phaco- + G. *eidos*, resemblance ]. Of lentil shape.

**phacolysis** (fă-kol′ĭ-sis) [ phaco- + G. *lysis*, dissolution ]. Operative breaking down and removal of the crystalline lens.

**phacolyt′ic.** Characterized by or referring to phacolysis.

**phacoma** (fă-ko′mah) [ phaco- + G. suffix *-oma*, tumor ]. A hamartoma found in phacomatosis, *q.v.*

**phacomalacia** (fak′o-mă-la′shĭ-ah) [ phaco- + G. *malakia*, softness ]. Softening of the crystalline lens, as may occur in hypermature cataract.

**phacomatosis** (fak′o-mă-to′sis) [ Van der Hoeve's coinage fr. G. *phakos*, mother-spot ]. A generic term for a group of hereditary diseases characterized by hamartomas involving multiple tissues; *e.g.*, Lindau's disease, neurofibromatosis, Sturge-Weber syndrome, tuberous sclerosis.

**phacometachoresis** (fak′o-met-ă-ko-re′sis) [ phaco- + G. *metachōrēsis*, change of place ]. Obsolete term for luxation or subluxation of lens.

**phacometer** (fă-kom′e-ter) [ phaco- + G. *metron*, measure ]. Obsolete synonym for lensometer.

**phacoscope** (fak′o-skōp) [ phaco- + G. *skopeō*, to view ]. An instrument in the form of a dark chamber for observing the changes in the crystalline lens during accommodation.

**Phaeni′cia serica′ta,** A common blowfly of the dipteran family Calliphoridae found in the northern United States and in Canada.

**-phage, -phagia, -phagy** [ G. *phagein*, to eat. PHAG- ]. Combining forms, used in the suffix position, meaning eating or devouring.

**phage** (fāj). Bacteriophage.

β **p.,** β *corynebacteriophage.*

**defective p.,** defective *bacteriophage.*

**p. eclipse,** see eclipse *period.*

**p. lambda,** *coliphage* λ.

**T p.,** T *coliphage.*

**T-even p.,** see T *coliphage.*

**phagedena** (faj-e-de′nah) [ G. *phagedaina*, a canker ]. An ulcer that rapidly spreads peripherally, destroying the tissues as it increases in size.

**p. gangrenosa,** severe gangrene with sloughing.

**p. nosocomialis,** gangrene arising in a hospital from cross infection.

**sloughing p.,** decubitus *ulcer.*

**p. trop′ica,** the tropical ulcer of Old World cutaneous leishmaniasis.

**phagedenic** (faj-e-den′ik). Relating to or having the characteristics of phagedena.

**phago-** (fag′o-) [ G. *phagein*, to eat. PHAG- ]. Combining form, used in the prefix position, meaning eating or devouring.

**phagocyte** (fag′o-sīt) [ phago- + G. *kytos*, cell ]. Carrier cell; scavenger cell; a cell possessing the property of ingesting bacteria, foreign particles, and other cells. P.'s are divided into two general classes; *microphages,* polymorphonuclear leukocytes which ingest chiefly bacteria; and *macrophages,* mononucleated cells (histiocytes and monocytes) which are largely scavengers, ingesting dead tissue and degenerated cells.

**educated p.,** a p. which, following an infection, has acquired the ability to withstand the poison of a further infection of the same kind.

**phagocytic** (fag′o-sit′ik). Relating to phagocytes or phagocytosis.

**phagocy′tin.** A very labile bactericidal substance that may be isolated from polymorphonuclear leukocytes.

**phagocytize** (fag′o-si-tīz). Phagocytose.

**phagocytoblast** (fag′o-si′to-blast) [ phagocyte + G. *blastos,* germ ]. A primitive cell developing into a phagocyte.

**phagocytolysis** (fag′o-si-tol′ĭ-sis) [ phagocyte + G. *lysis,* dissolution ]. 1. Phagolysis; destruction of phagocytes, or leukocytes, occurring in the process of blood coagulation or as the result of the introduction of certain antagonistic foreign substances into the body. 2. A spontaneous

breaking down of the phagocytes, preliminary (according to Metchnikoff) to the liberation of cytase, or complement.

**phagocytolytic** (fag′o-si-to-lit′ik). Relating to phagocytolysis; phagolytic.

**phagocytose** (fag′o-si-tōz). Phagocytize; to englobe and destroy bacteria and other foreign substances; denoting the action of the phagocytic cells.

**phagocytosis** (fag′o-si-to′sis) [ phagocyte + G. suffix *-osis,* condition ]. The process of ingestion and digestion by cells; the substances ingested are other cells, bacteria, bits of necrosed tissue, foreign particles, etc.

**induced p.,** p. occurring when bacteria subjected to the action of blood serum are brought in contact with leukocytes.

**spontaneous p.,** p. occurring when a culture of bacteria is brought in contact with washed leukocytes in an indifferent medium, such as a physiologic salt solution.

**phagodynamometer** (fag′o-di′nă-mom′e-ter) [ phago- + G. *dynamis,* force, + *metron,* measure ]. A device for measuring the force required to chew various foods.

**phagokaryosis** (fag′o-kăr-ĭ-o′sis) [ phago- + G. *karyon,* kernel (nucleus), + suffix *-osis,* condition ]. An assumed phagocytic action of the cell nucleus.

**phagol′ysis.** Phagocytolysis.

**phagolyt′ic.** Phagocytolytic.

**phagomania** (fag′o-ma′nĭ-ah) [ phago- + G. *mania,* frenzy ]. Bulimia; morbid desire to eat.

**phagophobia** (fag′o-fo′bĭ-ah) [ phago- + G. *phobos,* fear ]. Morbid fear of eating.

**phagosome** (fag′o-sōm) [ phago- + G. *soma,* body ]. A vacuole containing bacteria or other ingested particles; lysosomes become fused with it.

**phagotype** (fag′o-tīp) [ phago- + G. *typos,* type ]. In microbiology, a subdivision of a species distinguished from other strains therein by sensitivity to a certain bacteriophage or set of bacteriophages.

**phak-, phako-.** For words so beginning and not listed here, see phac-.

**phaki′tis.** Phacitis.

**phak′omato′sis.** Phacomatosis.

**phako′ma.** Phacoma.

**phalacrosis** (fal′ă-kro′sis) [ G. *phalakrōsis,* fr. *phalos,* shining, white, fr. *phaō,* to shine ]. Obsolete term for alopecia.

**phalangeal** (fă-lan′je-al). Relating to a phalanx.

**phalangectomy** (fal-an-jek′to-mī). Excision of one or more of the phalanges of hand or foot.

**phalanges** (fă-lan′jēz) [ L. ] [ NA ]. Plural of phalanx.

**phalangette** (fal-an-jet′) [ Fr. dim. of *phalange,* phalanx ]. The distal or ungual phalanx.

**drop p.,** falling of the distal phalanx of a finger, and inability to extend it, when the hand is prone, due to an overstretching or rupture of the extensor tendons of the finger near their insertion into the base of the affected segment.

**phalanx,** gen. **phalan′gis,** pl. **phalan′ges** (fa′langks, fă-langks′) [ L. fr. G. *phalanx* (*-ang-*), line of soldiers, bone between two joints of the fingers and toes ]. 1 [ NA ]. One of the long bones of the fingers or toes, 14 in number for each hand or foot, two for the thumb or great toe, and three each for the other four digits; they are designated as proximal, middle, and distal, beginning from the metacarpus. The distal p. is sometimes called the **ungual p.** because of the flattened tuberosity, at its termination which supports the nail. 2. One of a number of cuticular plates, arranged in several rows, on the surface of the spiral organ (of Corti); they are the heads of the outer row of pillar cells and of phalangeal cells, and between them are the free ends of the hair cells.

**tufted p.,** one of the terminal phalanges of the fingers in acromegaly; it has an expanded extremity, and in shape somewhat resembles a sheaf of wheat.

**ungual p.,** the distal p. of each of the fingers and toes.

**phall-, phalli-.** See phallo-.

**phallalgia** (fal-al′jĭ-ah) [ phall- + G. *algos,* pain ]. Phallodynia.

**phallectomy** (fal-ek′to-mī) [ phall- + G. *ektomē,* excision ]. Amputation of the penis.

**phallic** (fal'ik) [ G. *phallos*, penis ]. 1. Relating to the penis. 2. In psychoanalysis, relating to the penis especially during the phases of infantile psychosexuality; see also phallic *phase*.

**phallicism** (fal'ĭ-sizm). Phallism; phallic worship; worship of the male genital.

**phalliform** (fal'ĭ-form). Phalloid.

**phal'lism.** Phallicism.

**phallitis** (fal-i'tis). Penitis.

**phallo-, phall-, phalli-** (fal'o-) [ G. *phallos*, penis ]. Combining forms relating to the penis.

**phallocampsis** (fal'o-kamp'sis) [ phallo- + G. *kampsis*, a bending ]. Any curvature of the erect penis; see also chordee.

**phallocrypsis** (fal'o-krip'sis) [ phallo- + G. *krypsis*, concealment ]. Dislocation and retraction of the penis.

**phallodynia** (fal'o-din'ĭ-ah) [ phallo- + G. *odynē*, pain ]. Phallalgia; pain in the penis.

**phalloid** (fal'oyd) [ phallo- + G. *eidos*, resemblance ]. Resembling in shape a penis.

**phalloidine** (fă-loy'din, -dēn). A cyclic peptide produced by the poisonous mushroom, *Amanita phalloides*.

**phalloncus** (fal-ong'kus) [ phallo- + G. *onkos*, mass ]. A tumor or swelling of the penis.

**phalloplasty** (fal'o-plas-tī) [ phallo- + G. *plassō*, to form ]. Reparative or plastic surgery of the penis.

**phallorrhagia** (fal-o-ra'je-ah) [ phallo- + G. *rhēgnymi*, to burst forth ]. Hemorrhage of the penis.

**phallorrhea** (fal-o-re'ah) [ phallo- + G. *rhoia*, flow ]. Discharge from the penis.

**phallus,** pl. **phalli** (fal'us, fal'i) [ L.; G. *phallos* ]. Penis.

**phanero-** (fan'er-o-) [ G. *phaneros*, visible. PHAN- ]. Combining form meaning visible, manifest.

**phanerogenic** (fan-er-o-jen'ic) [ phanero- + G. *genesis*, origin ]. Denoting a disease the etiology of which is manifest; opposed to cryptogenic.

**phaneromania** (fan'er-o-ma'nĭ-ah) [ phanero- + G. *mania*, frenzy ]. Constant preoccupation with some external part, as plucking the beard, pulling the lobe of the ear, picking at a pimple, etc.

**phaneroscope** (fan'er-o-skōp) [ phanero- + G. *skopeō*, to view ]. A lens used to concentrate the light from a lamp upon the skin, to facilitate examination of lesions of the skin and subcutaneous tissues.

**phanerosis** (fan-er-o'sis) [ phanero- + G. suffix -*osis*, condition ]. The act or process of becoming visible.

**fatty p.,** presumed unmasking of previously invisible fat in the cytoplasm of cells; marked fatty metamorphosis is associated with an absolute increase in the fat content of cells, so that the occurrence of p. is doubted.

**phanerozoite** (fan'er-o-zo'it) [ phanero- + G. *zōon*, animal ]. An exoerythrocytic tissue stage of malaria infection other than the primary exoerythrocytic stages (cryptozoite and metacryptozoite generations); consists chiefly of reinfection of the liver by merozoites produced by a blood infection (not found in falciparum malaria).

**phanquone** (fan'kwōn). ENTOBEX; 4,7-phenanthroline-5,6-dione; amebicide.

**phantasia** (fan-ta'zĭ-ah) [ G. appearance. PHAN- ]. Fantasy.

**phantasm** (fan'tazm) [ G. *phantasma*, an appearance. PHAN- ]. Phantom (1); the mental imagery produced by fantasy.

**phantasmagoria** (fan-taz'mă-go'rĭ-ah). A fantastic sequence of haphazardly associative imagery.

**phantasmatomoria** (fan-taz'mă-to-mo'rĭ-ah) [ G. *phantasma*, an appearance, + *mōria*, folly ]. Dementia with childish fantasies.

**phantasmol'ogy** [ G. *phantasma*, an appearance, + *logos*, study ]. The study of spiritualistic manifestations and of apparitions.

**phantasmoscopia, phantasmoscopy** (fan-taz'mo-sko'pĭ-ah, fan-taz-mos'ko-pī) [ G. *phantasma*, an appearance, + *skopeō*, to view ]. The form of delusion consisting of the seeing of phantoms.

**phantom** (fan'tom) [ G. *phantasma*, an appearance. PHAN- ]. 1. Phantasm. 2. A model, especially a transparent one, of the human body or any of its parts; see also manikin.

**Schultze's p.,** a model of a female pelvis used in demonstrating the mechanism of childbirth and the application of forceps.

**phan'tomize.** In psychiatry, to create a phantom.

**phar'macal.** Pharmaceutical.

**pharmaceutic, pharmaceutical** (far-mă-su'tik, far-mă-su'tĭ-kal) [ G. *pharmakeutikos*, relating to drugs ]. Relating to pharmacy or to pharmaceutics.

**pharmaceutics** (far'mă-su'tiks). 1. Pharmacy. 2. The science of pharmaceutical systems, *i.e.*, preparations, dosage forms, etc.

**pharmaceutist** (far-mă-su'tist). Pharmacist.

**pharmacist** (far'mă-sist) [ G. *pharmakon*, a drug ]. A druggist; a pharmaceutist; an apothecary; one who prepares and dispenses drugs and has knowledge concerning their properties.

**pharmaco-** (far'mă-ko-) [ G. *pharmakon*, drug, medicine ]. Combining form relating to drugs.

**phar'macochem'istry.** Pharmaceutical *chemistry*.

**phar'macodiagno'sis.** Use of drugs in diagnosis.

**phar'macodynam'ic.** Relating to drug action.

**pharmacodynamics** (far'mă-ko-di-nam'iks) [ pharmaco- + G. *dynamis*, force ]. The study of the actions of drugs on the living organism.

**phar'macoen'docrinol'ogy.** The pharmacology of endocrine function.

**phar'macogenet'ics.** The study of genetically determined variations in responses to drugs in man or in laboratory organisms.

**pharmacog'nosist.** One skilled in pharmacognosy.

**pharmacognosy** (far'mă-kog'no-sī) [ pharmaco- + G. *gnōsis*, knowledge ]. A branch of pharmacology that deals with the physical characteristics and botanical sources of crude drugs.

**pharmacography** (far'mă-kog'ră-fī) [ pharmaco- + G. *graphē*, description ]. A treatise on or description of drugs.

**phar'macokinet'ics** [ pharmaco- + G. *kinēsis*, movement ]. Movements of drugs within biological systems, as affected by uptake, distribution, elimination, and biotransformation.

**pharmacol'ogist.** One who specializes in pharmacology.

**pharmacology** (far'mă-kol'o-jī) [ pharmaco- + G. *logos*, study ]. The science that deals with drugs, their sources, appearance, chemistry, actions, and uses.

**biochemical p.,** a branch of p. that deals with the biochemical mechanisms responsible for the actions of drugs.

**marine p.,** a branch of p. that deals with pharmacologically active substances present in aquatic plants and animals; its objective is to find and develop new therapeutic agents.

**phar''macoma'nia** [ pharmaco- + G. *mania*, frenzy ]. A morbid impulse to take drugs.

**pharmacopedics, pharmacopedia** (far'mă-ko-pe'diks, -pe'dĭ-ah) [ pharmaco- + G. *paideia*, instruction, fr. *pais* (*paid*-), a child ]. The teaching of pharmacy and pharmacodynamics.

**Pharmacopeia, Pharmacopoeia** (far'mă-ko-pe'ah) [ G. *pharmakopoiia*, fr. *pharmakon*, a medicine, + *poieo*, to make ]. A work containing monographs of therapeutic agents, standards for their strength and purity, and directions for making preparations. The various national pharmacopeias are referred to by abbreviations, of which the following are the most frequently encountered: *U.S.P.*, the Pharmacopeia of the United States of America (United States Pharmacopeia); *B.P.*, British Pharmacopoeia; *Codex medicamentarius*, the French Pharmacopeia; *I.C. Add.* (or *B.A.*), the Indian and Colonial Addendum to the B.P.; *I.P.*, International Pharmacopeia; *P. Austr.*, the Austrian Pharmacopeia; *P.G.*, the German Pharmacopeia (D.A.B.); *P. Helv.*, the Swiss Pharmacopeia. The first edition of the U.S.P. was compiled in 1820; it has since been revised every ten years, and recently every five years, by the United States Pharmacopeial Convention, composed of physicians, scientists, and pharmacists. The work was made a legal standard by the terms of the National Food and Drugs Act in January, 1907.

**pharmacopeial** (far'mă-ko-pe'al). Relating to the Pharmacopeia; denoting a drug in the list of the Pharmacopeia; see also official.

**phar'macophil'ia** [ pharmaco- + G. *phileō*, to love ]. A morbid fondness for taking drugs.

**pharmacophobia** (far'mă-ko-fo'bī-ah) [ pharmaco- + G. *phobos*, fear ]. Morbid fear of taking drugs.

**pharmacopsychosis** (far'mă-ko-si-ko'sis) [ pharmaco- + psychosis ]. Drug *addiction*.

**phar'macother'apy** [ pharmaco- + G. *therapeia*, therapy ]. Treatment of disease by means of drugs; see also chemotherapy.

**pharmacy** (far'mă-sī) [ G. *pharmakon*, drug ]. 1. The act of preparing and dispensing drugs. 2. A drugstore.

**Pharm. D.** Abbreviation for Doctor of Pharmacy.

**pharyng-.** See pharyngo-.

**pharyngalgia** (făr'ing-gal'jī-ah) [ pharyng- + G. *algos*, pain ]. Pharyngodynia; pain in the pharynx.

**pharyngeal** (fă-rin'je-al) [ Mod. L. *pharyngeus* ]. Relating to the pharynx.

**pharyngectomy** (făr'in-jek'to-mī) [ pharyng- + G. *ektomē*, excision ]. Excision of a part of the pharynx.

**pharyngemphraxis** (făr'in-jem-frak'sis) [ pharyng- + G. *emphraxis*, a stoppage ]. Pharyngeal obstruction.

**pharynges** (fă-rin'jēz). Plural of pharynx.

**pharyngeus** (făr'in-je'us) [ Mod. L. ]. Pharyngeal.

**pharyngismus** (făr'in-jiz'mus). Pharyngospasm; spasm of the muscles of the pharynx.

**pharyngitic** (făr'in-jit'ik). Relating to pharyngitis.

**pharyngitis** (făr'in-ji'tis) [ pharyng- + G. suffix *-itis*, inflammation ]. Inflammation of the mucous membrane and underlying parts of the pharynx.

    **atroph'ic p.**, p. sicca; chronic p. accompanied by more or less atrophy of the mucous glands and absence of their secretion.

    **croupous p.**, p. associated with an exudate resembling a membrane.

    **follic'ular p.**, granular p.

    **gan'grenous p.**, putrid sore throat; gangrenous inflammation of the pharyngeal mucous membrane.

    **glandular p.**, granular p.

    **granular p.**, follicular or glandular p.; a form of p. in which the lymphoid follicles are enlarged, studding the mucous membrane as minute nodules or granules.

    **p. herpet'ica**, p. characterized by vesicular eruption or shallow ulcers.

    **p. hypertroph'ica latera'lis**, a form of chronic p. in which the glazed central portion is bounded on either side by a band of red, thickened mucous membrane.

    **membranous p.**, inflammation accompanied by a fibrinous exudate, forming a nondiphtheritic false membrane.

    **p. sicca**, atrophic p.

    **p. ulcero'sa**, Vincent's *disease*.

**pharyngo-, pharyng-** (fă-ring'go-) [ Mod. L. fr. G. *pharynx, q.v.* ]. Combining forms relating to the pharynx.

**pharyngocele** (fă-ring'go-sēl) [ pharyngo- + G. *kēlē*, hernia ]. A diverticulum from the pharynx.

**pharyn'gocerato'sis.** Pharyngokeratosis.

**pharyngodynia** (fă-ring'go-din'ī-ah) [ pharyngo- + G. *odynē*, pain ]. Pharyngalgia.

**pharyngoepiglottic, pharyngoepiglottidean** (fă-ring'go-ep'ī-glot'ik, -glō-tid'e-an). Relating to the pharynx and the epiglottis.

**pharyngoesophageal** (fă-ring'go-e-sof'ă-je'al). Relating to the pharynx and the esophagus.

**pharyngoesophagoplasty** (fă-ring'go-e-sof'ă-go-plas'tī). Any plastic procedure on pharynx and esophagus.

**pharyn'goglos'sal.** Relating to the pharynx and the tongue.

**pharyngoglos'sus.** *Musculus* glossopharyngeus.

**pharyngokeratosis** (fă-ring'go-kĕr-ă-to'sis) [ pharyngo- + G. *keras* (*kerat-*), horn ]. A thickening of the lining of the lymphoid follicles of the pharynx, with the formation of a tough, firmly adherent, pseudomembranous exudate.

**pharyngolaryngeal** (fă-ring'go-lă-rin'je-al). Relating to both the pharynx and the larynx.

**pharyngolaryngitis** (fă-ring'go-lăr'in-ji'tis). Inflammation of both the pharynx and the larynx.

**pharyngolith** (fă-ring'go-lith) [ pharyngo- + G. *lithos*, stone ]. Pharyngeal calculus; a concretion in the pharynx.

**pharyngology** (făr'ing-gol'o-jī) [ pharyngo- + G. *logos*, study ]. The medical science concerned with the study, diagnosis, and treatment of the pharynx.

**pharyn'gomax'illary.** Relating to the pharynx and the maxilla.

**pharyngomycosis** (fă-ring'go-mi-ko'sis) [ pharyngo- + G. *mykēs*, a fungus ]. Invasion of the mucous membrane of the pharynx by fungi.

**pharyn'gona'sal.** Relating to the pharynx and the nasal cavity.

**pharyngo-oral** (fă-ring'go-o'ral) [ pharyngo- + L. *os* (*or-*), mouth ]. Relating to the pharynx and the mouth.

**pharyngopalatine** (fă-ring'go-pal'a-tīn). Relating to the pharynx and the palate.

**pharyng'opalati'nus** [ L. ]. *Musculus* palatopharyngeus.

**pharyngopathy, pharyngopathia** (făr'ing-gop'ă-thī, fă-ring'go-path'ī-ah) [ pharyngo- + G. *pathos*, suffering ]. Any disease of the pharynx.

**pharyngoperistole** (fă-ring'go-pĕ-ris'to-le) [ pharyngo- + G. *peristolē*, a drawing out ]. Narrowing of the lumen of the pharynx.

**pharyngoplasty** (fă-ring'go-plas'tī) [ pharyngo- + G. *plassō*, to form ]. Plastic surgery of the pharynx.

**pharyngoplegia** (fă-ring'go-ple'jī-ah) [ pharyngo- + G. *plēgē*, stroke ]. Paralysis of the wall of the pharynx.

**pharyngorhinitis** (făring'go-ri-ni'tis). Inflammation of the rhinopharynx, or of the mucous membrane of the pharynx and the nasal fossae.

**pharyngorhinoscopy** (fă-ring'go-ri-nos'ko-pī) [ pharyngo- + G. *rhis*, nose, + *skopeō*, to view ]. Inspection of the rhinopharynx and posterior nares by means of the rhinoscopic mirror.

**pharyngoscleroma** (fă-ring'go-skle-ro'mah) [ pharyngo- + G. *sklērōma*, an induration ]. A scleroma, or indurated patch, in the mucous membrane of the pharynx.

**pharyngoscope** (fă-ring'go-sko'p) [ pharyngo- + G. *skopeō*, to view ]. An instrument like a laryngoscope, used for inspection of the mucous membrane of the pharynx.

**pharyngoscopy** (făr'in-gos'ko'pī) [ pharyngo- + G. *skopeō*, to view ]. Inspection and examination of the pharynx.

**pharyngospasm** (făring'go-spazm). Pharyngismus.

**pharyn'gostaphyli'nus** [ L. fr. pharyngo- + G. *staphylē*, uvula ]. *Musculus* palatopharyngeus.

**pharyngostenosis** (fă-ring'go-stĕ-no'sis) [ pharyngo- + G. *stenōsis*, a narrowing ]. Stricture of the pharynx.

**pharyngotomy** (făr'ing-got'o-mī) [ pharyngo- + G. *tomē*, incision ]. Any cutting operation upon the pharynx either from without or from within.

**pharyngotonsillitis** (fă-ring'go-ton'sī-li'tis) [ pharyngo- + tonsillitis ]. Inflammation of the pharynx and tonsils.

**pharyngotyphoid** (fă-ring'go-ti'foyd). Typhoid fever in which angina is prominent among the initial symptoms.

**pharyngoxerosis** (fă-ring'go-ze-ro'sis) [ pharyngo- + G. *xe-⅜rīsis*, a drying up ]. Dryness of the pharyngeal mucous membrane.

**pharynx**, gen. **pharyngis**, pl. **pharynges** (făr'ingks, fă-rin'jis, fă-rin'jēz) [ Mod. L. fr. G. *pharynx* (*pharyng-*), the throat, the joint opening of the gullet and windpipe ] [ NA ]. The upper expanded portion of the digestive tube, between the esophagus below and the mouth and nasal cavities above and in front.

    **laryngeal p.**, *pars* laryngea pharyngis.

    **nasal p.**, *pars* nasalis pharyngis.

    **oral p.**, *pars* oralis pharyngis.

**phase** (fāz) [ G. *phasis*, an appearance. PHAN- ]. 1. One of the stages in which a thing appears during its course of change or development. 2. A homogeneous, physically distinct, and separable portion of a heterogeneous system; *e.g.*, oil, gum, and water are three p.'s of an emulsion. 3. The time relationship between two or more events. 4. A particular part of a recurring time-pattern or wave-form. See also stage, and period, and their subentries.

**anal p.,** in psychoanalytic personality theory, the stage of psychosexual development occurring when a child is between 1 and 3 years; during this period his activities, interests, and concerns are centered around his anal zone.

**apophylac'tic p.,** negative p. or p. of diminished blood resistance following the injection in vaccine therapy.

**aqueous p.,** the water portion of a system consisting of two liquid p.'s, one mainly water, the other a liquid immiscible with water (*e.g.*, benzene, ether).

**continuous p.,** external p.

**dispersed p.,** the particles contained in a colloid solution or dispersion.

**dispersion p.,** external p.

**eclipse p.,** eclipse *period*.

**external p.,** the dispersion or external medium or fluid in which a disperse is suspended.

**genital p.,** in psychoanalytic personality theory, the final stage of psychosexual development; it occurs during puberty. In this stage the individual's psychosexual development is so organized that sexual gratification can be achieved from genital-to-genital contact and the capacity exists for a mature, affectionate relationship with an individual of the opposite sex.

**in p.,** moving in the same direction at the same time; a possible characteristic of two simultaneous oscillations of similar frequency.

**internal p.,** dispersed p.; the particles contained in a colloid solution.

**lag p.,** A brief period in the course of a bacterial culture, especially at the beginning, during which the growth is very slow or scarcely appreciable.

**latency p.,** latency period; in psychoanalytic personality theory, the period of psychosexual development in children extending from about age 5 to the beginning of adolescence at age 12; the apparent cessation of sexual preoccupation during this period stems from a strong, aggressive blockade of libidinal and sexual impulses in an effort to avoid Oedipal relationships. During this p., boys and girls are inclined to choose friends and join groups of their own sex.

**logarithmic p.,** a period in the course of a bacterial culture in which maximal multiplication is occurring by geometrical progression; thus if the logarithms of their numbers are plotted against the time they will form a straight upward line.

**luteal p.,** that portion of the menstrual cycle extending from the time of formation of the corpus luteum to the time when menstrual flow begins; usually 14 days in length.

**meiotic p.,** reduction p.; the stage of nuclear changes in the sexual cells during which reduction of the chromosomes takes place; it embraces the cell generations of spermatocytes and oocytes.

**negative p.,** the period during which the opsonic index is lowered following the injection of a vaccine.

**Oedipal p.,** Oedipal period; in psychoanalysis, a stage in the psychosexual development of the child, characterized by erotic attachment to the parent of the opposite sex, repressed because of fear of the parent of the same sex; usually occurring between the ages of 3 and 6 years.

**oral p.,** in psychoanalytic personality theory, the earliest stage in psychosexual development; it lasts through the first 18 months of life. During this period the oral zone is the center of the infant's needs, expression, gratification, and pleasurable erotic experiences; it has a strong influence on the organization and development of the child's psyche.

**out of p.,** not in p., moving in opposite directions at the same time; 180° out of p.; a possible characteristic of two simultaneous oscillations of similar frequency.

**phallic p.,** in psychoanalytic personality theory, the stage in psychosexual development occurring when a child is between 2 and 6 years of age; during this period, interest, curiosity, and pleasurable experiences are centered around the penis in boys and the clitoris in girls.

**positive p.,** the period following the negative p., during which the opsonic index rises.

**postmeiotic p.,** postreduction p.; the stage following that of reduction of the chromosomes in the sexual cells, representing the mature forms of these cells, ending with the conjugation of the nuclei in the impregnated ovum.

**postreduc'tion p.,** postmeiotic p.

**pregenital p.,** in psychoanalysis, the psychosexual development p.'s preceding the genital p.

**premeiotic p.,** prereduction p.; the stage of nuclear changes in the sexual cells before the reduction of the chromosomes, embracing the cell generations up to that of the spermatogonia and oogonia.

**pre-Oedipal p.,** in psychoanalysis, the p.'s of psychosexual development preceding the Oedipal p.

**prereduc'tion p.,** premeiotic p.

**reduction p.,** meiotic p.

**short luteal p.,** a period of 10 days or less between ovulation and the onset of menses; it is frequently associated with infertility.

**stationary p.,** the period in the course of a bacterial culture during which the multiplication of the organisms becomes gradually less and finally ceases.

**supernormal recovery p.,** a brief period during the recovery of cardiac muscle following excitation when the muscle is abnormally excitable; corresponds to the U wave in the electrocardiogram.

**synap'tic p.,** synapsis.

**phaseolin** (fă-se'o-lin). An antifungal substance from *Phaseolus vulgaris* (family Leguminoseae), the French bean.

**Phasmidia** (faz'mid'ĭ-ah) [ G. *phasma*, appearance. PHAN- ]. A subclass of the class Nematoda in which phasmids (caudal sensory organs) are present. This group includes most of the common nematodes of man and domestic animals. See also Aphasmidia.

**phasmopho'bia** [ G. *phasma*, apparition, + *phobos*, fear ]. Morbid fear of ghosts.

**phatnorrhagia** (fat'no-ra'jĭ-ah) [ G. *phatnē*, manger (alveolus), + G. *rhēgnymi*, to burst forth ]. Alveolar hemorrhage.

**Ph.D.** Abbreviation for Doctor of Philosophy.

**Phe.** Symbol for phenylalanine or its radical.

**pheasant's-eye.** The herb *Adonis vernalis*.

**Phelps,** Abel M., U. S. surgeon, 1851–1902. See P.'s *operation*.

**phen-, pheno-** [ fr. G. *phainō*, to appear, show forth. PHAN- ]. Combining form denoting: (1) appearance; (2) derivation from benzene.

**phenacaine hydrochloride** (fen'ă-kān) (NF). HOLOCAINE hydrochloride; bis-(*p*-ethoxyphenyl)-acetamidine hydrochloride; potent local surface anesthetic used in ophthalmology.

**phenacemide** (fĕ-nas'e-mīd) (NF). PHENURONE; phenylacetylurea; an anticonvulsant with a slight sedative action; used in the treatment of epilepsy. It has serious side effects.

**phenacetin** (fĕ-nas'e-tin) (BP). Acetophenetidin; *p*-acetaminophenetide; *p*-acetphenetidine; $C_2H_5O-C_6H_4-NHCOCH_3$; analgesic and antipyretic.

**phenaceturic acid** (fĕ-nas'e-tu'rik). Phenylaceturic acid; $C_6H_5-CH_2-CO-NH-CH_2-COOH$; end product of the metabolism of phenylated fatty acids with even numbers of carbon atoms; *cf.* hippuric acid.

**phenac'ridane chloride.** ACRIZANE chloride; 9-[ *p*-(hexoloxy)phenyl ]-10-methylacridinium chloride; topical antiseptic.

**phenactropinium chloride** (fĕ-nak'tro-pin'ĭ-um). TROPHENIUM; 8-phenacylhomatropinium chloride; a ganglionic blocking agent.

**phenadoxone hydrochloride** (fen'ă-dok'sōn). HEPTONE; heptazone hydrochloride; 6-morpholino-4,4-diphenylheptan-3-one hydrochloride; a narcotic that is a congener of methadone but less potent.

**phenaglycodol** (fen'ă-gli'ko-dol). ULTRAN; 2-*p*-chlorophenyl-3-methyl-2,3-butanediol; a mild central nervous system depressant similar in action to meprobamate. It is used in the treatment of anxiety and simple neuroses.

**phenakistoscope** (fen'ă-kis'to-skōp) [ G. *phenakistēs*, deceiver, + *skopeō*, to view ]. An instrument consisting of a slotted disk with figures arranged around the center through which the figures are viewed in motion by means of a mirror; see also zoetrope.

**phenam'ine.** Phenocoll.

**phenanthrene** (fĕ-nan'thrĕn). $C_{14}H_{10}$; a compound isomeric with anthracene, derived from coal tar; used as a basis for the synthesis of various dyes and drugs.

**Phenanthrene**

**p. nucleus,** term given incorrectly to the steroid nucleus (cyclopenta[ *a* ]phenanthrene).

**phenarsenamine** (fen-ar-sen-am'ēn). Arsphenamine.

**phenar'sone sulfox'ylate.** ALDARSONE; sodium 3-amino-4-hydroxyphenylarsonate-*N*-methanolsulfoxylate; a pentavalent arsenical; used in trichomonal vaginitis and in neurosyphilis; administered as an insufflation of the powder (with kaolin) for trichomonas vaginitis, and in solution in distilled water intravenously in neurosyphilis.

**phe'nate.** Carbolate; a salt of phenic acid.

**phenazocine** (fĕ-naz'o-sēn). PRIMADOL; 2'-hydroxy-5,9-dimethyl-2-phenethyl-6,7-benzomorphan; a potent analgesic when given intramuscularly or intravenously, less effective orally. It may have cumulative effects in man; produces respiratory depression, constipation, and psychic and physical dependence.

**phenaz'oline hydrochloride.** Antazoline hydrochloride.

**phenazopyridine hydrochloride** (fĕ-naz'o-pīr'ĭ-dēn, -din) (NF). PYRIDACIL; AZODYNE; MALLOPHENE; PYRIDIUM; 2,6-diamino-3-(phenylazo)pyridine hydrochloride; urinary antiseptic and anesthetic.

**phenben'zamine.** ANTERGAN; *N*-benzyl-*N'*,*N'*-dimethyl-*N*-phenylethylenediamine; antihistaminic.

**phenbu'tamide.** DIAPEROS; 1-butyl-3-(phenylsulfonyl)-urea; oral hypoglycemic agent.

**phencarbamide** (fen-kar-bam'id) (USAN). TRIPHENAMIL; ESCORPAL; diphenylthioacetic acid *S*-(2-diethylaminoethyl) ester; an anticholinergic agent used as an antispasmodic (urinary and lower gastrointestinal tract).

**phency'clidine hydrochloride** (USAN). SERNYL; 1-(1-phenylcyclohexyl)piperidine hydrochloride; a dissociative anesthetic for parenteral administration.

**phen'dimet'razine tartrate.** PLEGINE; (*d*-3,4-dimethyl-2-phenylmorpholine)-bitartrate; an anorexic agent useful in the management of simple obesity. The side effects are similar to those produced by amphetamine (insomnia and palpitation).

**phenelzine sulfate** (fen'el-zēn) (BP). NARDIL; a monoamine inhibitor used as an antidepressant.

**phenes'terine.** FENESTRIN; { *p*-[ bis(2-chloroethyl)amino ]phenyl}acetic acid cholesterol ester; antineoplastic agent.

**phenet'amine.** LICARAN; 2-(α-cyclohexylbenzyl)-*N*,*N*,*N'*,*N'*-tetraethyl-1,3-propanediamine; intestinal antispasmodic.

**phenethar'bital.** PYRICTAL; 5,5-diethyl-1-phenylbarbituric acid; anticonvulsant with antipyretic properties.

**phenethicillin potassium** (fĕ-neth'ĭ-sil'in) (NF, BP). CHEMIPEN; DARCIL; MAXIPEN; SYNCILLIN; α-phenoxyethylpenicillin potassium; a penicillin preparation that is stable in gastric acid and is rapidly but only partially absorbed from the gastrointestinal tract.

**phenetidin** (fĕ-net'ĭ-din). 4-Aminophenetole; a substance formed in the course of manufacture of acetophenetidin; used in dyes.

**phenetidinuria** (fĕ-net'ĭ-dĭ-nu'rĭ-ah). The presence of phenetidin in the urine.

**phenetsal.** SALOPHEN; acetaminosalol; salicylic acid ester of acetyl-*p*-aminophenol; analgesic, antipyretic, and intestinal antiseptic.

**pheneturide** (fĕ-net'u-rīd). Phenylethylacetylurea; (2-phenylbutyryl)urea; an antiepileptic similar in action to phenacemide; used (mainly in Europe) for psychomotor epilepsy. It may produce personality changes, aplastic anemia, and liver damage.

**phenfor'min hydrochloride** (USP, BP). DBI; 1-phenyl-biguanide monohydrochloride; an oral hypoglycemic agent used mainly in conjunction with insulin or sulfonyl-urea oral hypoglycemic agents in the management of diabetic patients; it will not produce hypoglycemia in normal human subjects.

**phenglutarimide hydrochloride** (fen'glu-tăr'ĭ-mīd). ATURBAN; the hydrochloride of α-2-diethylaminoethyl-α-phenylglutarimide; an antihistaminic agent used to decrease or prevent motion sickness, and to control Ménière's disease and vomiting. It should not be used in pregnancy. Its anticholinergic action may make it useful in the treatment of the Parkinsonian syndrome.

**phengophobia** (feng''go-fo'bĭ-ah) [ G. *phengos,* daylight, + *phobos,* fear ]. Morbid fear of the daylight.

**phe'nic acid.** Phenol.

**phenicar'bazide.** KYROGENIN; 1-phenylsemicarbazide; antipyretic agent.

**phenin'damine tartrate** (NF, BP). THEPHORIN tartrate; 2-methyl-9-phenyltetrahydro-1-pyridindene tartrate; an antihistaminic.

**phenindione** (fĕ-nin'di-ōn) (NF, BP). DANILONE; phenylindanedione; 2-phenyl-1,3-indanedione: a synthetic anticoagulant with action and uses similar to those of bishydroxycoumarin.

**pheniramine maleate** (fĕ-nīr'ă-mēn, -min). TRIMETON maleate; prophenpyridamine maleate; 1-phenyl-1-(2-pyridyl)-3-dimethylaminopropane maleate; an antihistaminic agent.

**pheni'sonone.** DAPANONE; 3',4'-dihydro-2-isopropyl-aminopropiophenone; bronchodilator.

**phenmetrazine hydrochloride** (fen-met'ră-zēn) (NF, BP). PRELUDIN; 2-phenyl-3-methyltetrahydro-1,4-oxazine hydrochloride; a secondary amine related pharmacologically to amphetamine, exerting an appetite-depressant effect; used in the management of simple obesity.

**pheno-.** See phen-.

**phenobarbital** (fe-no-bar'bĭ-tal) (USP). LUMINAL; phenobarbitone; phenylethylmalonylurea; phenylethylbarbituric acid; $CO(NHCO)_2C(C_2H_5)(C_6H_5)$; slightly soluble in water; sedative and hypnotic.

    **p. sodium** (USP), LUMINAL sodium; phenobarbitone sodium (BP); sodium phenylethylbarbiturate; the monosodium salt of p., a white powder, very soluble in water; used for the same purpose as p.

**phe'nobar'bitone** (BP). Phenobarbital.

**phen'obuti'odil.** VESIPAQUE; 2-(2,4,6-triiodophenoxy)-butyric acid; radiographic contrast medium for cholecystography.

**phe'nocoll.** PHENAMINE; 2-amino-*p*-acetophenetidide; glycocoll-*p*-phenetidide; has been used as analgesic, antipyretic, diaphoretic.

    **p. hydrochloride,** aminoacetophenetidin hydrochloride; has been used in neuralgia and, combined with piperazine, in rheumatoid arthritis.

**phenocopy** (fe'no-kop'ĭ) [ G. *phainō,* to appear, + *copy* ]. 1. An individual with clinical or laboratory characteristics that would ordinarily assign him to a specific phenotype with respect to genetic abnormality, but whose characteristics are of environmental rather than genetic etiology. 2. A condition of environmental etiology that mimics a condition usually of genetic etiology.

**phe'nodin.** Hematin.

**phe'nol** (USP, BP). Phenyl alcohol; phenic acid; carbolic acid; $C_6H_5OH$; occurs in the form of colorless crystals, liquefied by the addition of 10 per cent of water; antiseptic and disinfectant; locally escharotic in concentrated form and anesthetic in 3 to 4 per cent solutions; internally a powerful escharotic poison (olive oil recommended as an antidote).

    **camphorated p.,** camphorated carbolic acid; consists of p., camphor, and liquid petrolatum. Used as a local anesthetic and for the relief of toothache.

    **liquefied p.** (USP, BP), liquefied carbolic acid; p. liquefied by the addition of 10 per cent of water.

    **p. oxidase,** monophenol monooxygenase.

    **p. red,** phenolsulfonphthalein.

**phe'nolase.** Monophenol monooxygenase.

**phe'nolated.** Phenicated; carbolated; impregnated or mixed with phenol.

**phenolemia** (fe-nol-e'mĭ-ah) [ phenol + G. *haima*, blood ]. The presence of phenols in the blood.

**phenology** (fĕ-nol'o-jĭ) [ G. *phainō*, to appear, + *logos*, study ]. The study of the biological rhythms of plants and animals, particularly those rhythms showing seasonal variation.

**phenolphthalein** (fe'nol-thal'e-in, -thal'e-in) (NF, BP). Obtained by the action of phenol on phthalic anhydride; used as a hydrogen ion indicator; also used as a laxative.

**phe'nolphthal'ol.** EGMOL; *o*-[ bis(*p*-hydroxyphenyl)-methyl ]benzyl alcohol; cathartic.

**phenolsulfonphthalein** (fe'nol-sulf'-ōn-thal'e-in, -'thal'-e-in) (BP). Phenol red; occurs as a bright to dark red crystalline powder. It is used as an indicator, being yellow at pH 6.8 and red at pH 8.4; also used by parenteral injection as a test for renal function.

**phenoltetrachlorophthalein sodium** (fe'nol-tet-rah-klo'ro-thal'e-in, -thal'e-in). A synthetic dye formerly used as a liver function test and as a hypodermic purgative.

**phenoltetraiodophthalein sodium** (fe-nol-tet-rah-i'o-do-thal'e-in, -thal'e-in). Phentetiothalein sodium.

**phenoluria** (fe-nol-u'rĭ-ah). The excretion of phenols in the urine.

**phenomenology** (fe-nom'e-nol'o-jĭ) [ phenomenon, *q.v.*, + G. *logos*, study ]. 1. The systematic description and classification of phenomena without attempt at explanation or interpretation. 2. The study of human experiences, irrespective of objective-subjective distinctions. See also existential *psychology*.

---

# PHENOMENON

---

**phenomenon,** pl. **phenom'ena** (fe-nom'e-non) [ G. *phainomenon*, ntr. pres. p. pass. of *phainō*, to cause to appear. PHAN- ]. 1. A symptom; an occurrence of any sort, whether ordinary or extraordinary, in relation to a disease. 2. Any unusual fact or occurrence.

**adhesion p.,** immune adherence p.; erythrocyte adherence p.; red cell adherence p.; a p. recognized in a variety of forms since the early years of the 20th century and manifested by the adherence of antigen-antibody-complement complex to "indicator cells" (microorganisms, platelets, leukocytes, or erythrocytes), the reaction being sensitive and specific for the antigen and antibody in the complex and requiring only the first four components of complement. When the antigen is a microorganism, adherence can be determined microscopically; when the antigen-antibody-complement complex is soluble, adherence causes agglutination of the indicator cells; when the antigen is on the surface of a cell (*e.g.*, leukocyte), the "target cell"-antibody-complement complex forms a rosette around the indicator cell.

**aqueous influx p.,** Ascher's aqueous influx p.; the filling of the laminary vein, which normally carries blood and aqueous, with aqueous when the junction of the aqueous vein and the recipient vein is partially occluded by pressure of a glass rod; indicates higher pressure within the aqueous vein than within the recipient vein.

**Arias-Stella p.,** Arias-Stella *effect*.

**arm p.,** Pool's p. (2).

**Arthus p.,** a form of allergic inflammatory reaction observed in rabbits that become progressively more sensitive to an antigen (*e.g.*, horse serum) administered as a series of subcutaneous injections spaced at intervals of several days; the fifth or sixth dose is likely to result in a persistent swelling and firm indurated region that eventually becomes necrotic; the reaction is not confined to the region adjacent to the sites of previous injections, but is frequently observed at any site where the critical injection is made. A similar response may be observed when a cutaneous dose of antigen is administered to a rabbit sensitized 3 to 5 weeks previously by means of a series of 2 or 3 weekly intravenous doses of the same antigen. The reaction is caused by the inflammation that results from the deposition of antigen-antibody complexes in tissue spaces and in blood vessel walls, most of the damage seemingly being due to the polymorphonuclear leukocytes that phagocytize the deposits. The p., as described by Arthus, seems to be peculiar to rabbits, but similar reactions are observed in guinea pigs, rats, and dogs, as well as in man, under appropriate conditions.

**Ascher's aqueous influx p.,** aqueous influx p.

**Aschner's p.,** oculocardiac *reflex*.

**Ashley's p.,** oculocardiac *reflex*.

**Ashman's p.,** aberrant ventricular conduction of a beat ending a short cycle that is preceded by a longer cycle during atrial fibrillation.

**Aubert's p.,** a bright perpendicular line appears to incline to one side when the observer turns the head to the opposite side in a dark room.

**autoscopic p.,** the encountering of an image of oneself, the image being an illusion, a hallucination, or a vivid fantasy.

**Babinski's p.,** Babinski's *sign* (1).

**Becker's p.,** pulsation in the retinal arteries in exophthalmic goiter.

**Bell's p.,** a patient with peripheral facial paralysis cannot close the eyelids of the affected side without at the same time moving the eyeball upward and outward.

**Bordet's p.,** the basis of a test for identifying the species of animal from which an unknown protein is derived. See under test.

**Bordet-Gengou p.,** the p. of complement fixation, observed during a historically important experiment dealing with the unity of alexin (complement), that has proved of great practical value; when alexin (complement)-containing serum is added to a mixture of bacteria and specific antibody, the alexin is removed (fixed) and is not available to lyse subsequently added erythrocytes sensitized with specific antibody. The observations were later extended by Gengou (see Gengou p.).

**breakoff p., breakaway p.,** the occurrence, during high-altitude flight, of a sensation of being totally detached from the earth and one's fellow man.

**Browning's p.,** *therapia* sterilisans divergens.

**cer'vicolum'bar p.,** a sense of weakness in the lower extremities on movement of the neck when a lesion is present in the upper portion of the spinal cord; or sensations referrrd to the neck when a lesion exists in the lower portion of the cord.

**cogwheel p.,** Negro's p.; a sudden brief halt in usually smooth respiration or other motor activity.

**constancy p.,** in perception, the tendency for brightness, color, size, or shape to remain relatively perceptually constant despite changes in any conditions of observation, *e.g.*, light or position.

**crossed phrenic p.,** hemisection of the cord above the exit of the phrenic nerve paralyzes the ipsilateral half of the diaphragm; if the contralateral phrenic nerve is then sectioned or blocked, contractions on the ipsilateral side are resumed.

**Cushing's p.,** Cushing's law; rise in systemic blood pressure as a result of increased intracranial tension.

**Danysz p.,** reduction of the neutralizing effect of an antitoxin when toxin is mixed with it in divided portions, rather than adding the same total quantity of toxin in one step.

**Debré p.,** in measles, the failure of the rash to develop at the site of immune serum injection.

**declamping p.,** declamping shock; shock or hypotension following release of clamps from a large portion of the vascular bed, as from the aorta; apparently caused by transient pooling of blood in a previously ischemic area.

**déjà entendu p.** (de-zhah'oṅ-toṅ-dü') [ Fr. heard before ], the feeling a person has that something he has just heard has been heard by him at some other time.

**déjà vécu p.** (da-zhah va-kü), a feeling that a new experience has happened before.

**déjà vu p.** (da-zhah-vü') [ Fr. already seen ], the mental impression of having seen something which has been seen before. Every normal person has had this experience, but in certain emotional or organic disorders it may occur frequently or may be continuous.

**Déjérine's hand p.,** Déjérine's reflex; clonic contractions of the flexors of the hand (wrist) on tapping the dorsum of the hand or the volar side of the forearm near the wrist; it occurs in normal persons but is exaggerated in pyramidal tract lesions.

**Déjérine-Lichtheim p.,** Lichtheim's *sign.*

**Denys-Leclef p.,** enhanced phagocytosis by leukocytes of microorganisms in the presence of immune serum.

**d'Herelle p.,** Twort-d'Herelle p.

**diaphragm p.,** Litten's p.; phrenic p.; phrenic wave; a lowering of the line of retraction on the side of the chest (marking the insertion of the diaphragm) during inspiration, and elevation of the same during expiration; it is absent in cases of distention of the pleural sac; see also paradoxical diaphragm p.

**dip p.,** complete disappearance of ventricular excitability followed by progressive recovery within a few microseconds at the end of excitation; the muscle as a whole repolarizes somewhat inhomogeneously, so that this period is one of special sensitivity to exogenous or endogenous stimuli and reentry.

**Donath-Landsteiner p.,** the hemolysis which results in a sample of blood of a subject of paroxysmal hemoglobinuria when it is cooled to around 5°C. and then warmed again.

**Doppler p.,** Doppler *effect.*

**Duckworth's p.,** respiratory arrest before cardiac arrest as a result of intracranial disease.

**Ehret's p.,** a sudden throb felt by the finger on the brachial artery, as the pressure in the cuff falls during a blood pressure estimation; said to indicate fairly accurately the diastolic pressure.

**Ehrlich's p.,** the difference between the amount of diphtheria toxin that will exactly neutralize one unit of antitoxin and that which, added to one unit of antitoxin, will leave one lethal dose free is greater than one lethal dose of toxin; in other words, it is necessary to add more than one lethal dose of toxin to a neutral mixture of toxin and antitoxin to make the mixture lethal. This is the basis of the L₊ dose.

**elec′tromagnet′okinet′ic p.,** the migration of electrically neutral particles in a magnetic field traversed by an electric current.

**Erben's p.,** (1) in a case of neurasthenia, if the patient squats or stands bent far over, several slow heart beats occur; (2) the local temperature of the knee on the painful side is reduced in sciatica; (3) pain in sciatica is increased by hyperflexion of the sound leg.

**erythrocyte adherence p.,** adhesion p.

**escape p.,** after initial constrictions, the failure of the pupil of an eye with retrobulbar neuritis to constrict as the eyes are repeatedly stimulated alternately.

**facia′lis p.,** light rubbing of the skin or a tap on the zygoma causes a quick contraction of the lip and ala nasi; sometimes percussion above the zygoma causes contraction of the lip only; observed in tetany and sometimes in exophthalmic goiter.

**finger p.,** Gordon's sign; a sign of organic hemiplegia; the patient's arm resting with the elbow on a table, the examiner grasps the wrist and makes pressure with his thumb on the radial side of the pisiform bone; if the hemiplegia is organic, some or all of the patient's fingers become extended and spread out in a fanlike form.

**foot p.,** ankle *clonus.*

**Förster's p.,** a limitation of the primary normal visual field; an object brought gradually from without toward the fixed point is seen sooner than normal, whereas the preception of one moved from the center toward the periphery is lost sooner than normal; the visual field is therefore greater in the first case than in the second, which is the reverse of the normal; the p. occurs in neurasthenia.

**Friedreich's p.,** the tympanitic percussion sound over a pulmonary cavity is slightly raised in pitch on deep inspiration.

**Galassi's pupillary p.,** orbicularis pupillary *reflex.*

**Gallavardin's p.,** dissociation between the noisy and musical elements of the murmur of aortic stenosis, the musical element being better heard at the left sternal border and at the cardiac apex while the noisy element is better heard at the aortic area.

**Gärtner's vein p.,** fullness of the veins of the arm and hand below heart level and collapse at a certain variable distance above.

**generalized Shwartzman p.,** Sanarelli p.; Sanarelli-Shwartzman p.; when both the preparative injection of endotoxin-containing filtrate and the provocative injection are given intravenously 24 hours apart, the animal usually dies within 24 hours after the second inoculation; the characteristic lesions in the rabbit include widespread hemorrhages and bilateral cortical necrosis of the kidney; the p. is associated with a marked fall in the number of circulating leukocytes and platelets.

**Gengou p.,** an extension of the Bordet-Gengou p.; Gengou's experiments showed that noncellular antigens, when mixed with specific antibody, also fix alexin (complement).

**gestalt p.,** see gestalt.

**Goldblatt p.,** Goldblatt's hypertension; arterial hypertension resulting from partial occlusion of a renal artery.

**Grasset's p.,** Grasset-Gaussel p.; in organic paralysis of the lower extremity, the patient, lying on his back, can raise either limb separately, but not both together.

**Grasset-Gaussel p.,** Grasset's p.

**Gunn p.,** jaw-winking *syndrome.*

**Hamburger's p.,** *chloride* shift.

**Hapke's p.,** an abnormally prominent presentation of the parietal bone of the head of the first of twins, lying deep in the pelvis.

**Hata's p.,** contrary effect; exacerbation of an infectious disease when, in chemotherapy, a small dose is given of a remedy which is but little parasitotropic, such as methylene blue.

**hip p.,** Joffroy's *reflex.*

**hip-flexion p.,** when a hemiplegic attempts to raise himself from a lying posture he first flexes the hip on the paralyzed side, and the same movement takes place when he lies down again.

**Hochsinger's p.,** pressure to the inner side of the biceps muscle causes closure of the fist in tetany.

**Hoeppli p.,** an eosinophilic hyaline fringe that occasionally surrounds schistosome eggs entrapped in granulomas or pseudotubercles, probably a complex of egg antigen and host globulin.

**Hoffmann's p.,** excessive irritability of the sensory nerves to electrical or mechanical stimuli in tetany.

**Houssay p.,** see Houssay *animal.*

**Hunt's paradoxical p.,** in dystonia musculorum deformans, if an attempt is made at plantar flexion of the foot when the foot is in dorsal spasm the only response is an increase of the extensor, or dorsal, spasm; if, however, the patient is told to extend the foot which is already in a state of strong dorsal flexion there will be a sudden movement of plantar flexion; the same p., *mutatis mutandis,* is observed when there is a condition of strong plantar flexion.

**hunting p.,** hunting *reaction.*

**immune adherence p.,** adhesion p.

**jaw-winking p.,** see jaw-winking *syndrome.*

**knee p.,** patellar *reflex.*

**Köbner's p.,** isomorphic response; an isomorphic reaction seen in response to trauma in psoriasis, lichen planus, and verruca plana juvenilis.

**Koch's p.,** rise of temperature and increase of the local lesion, in a tuberculous subject, following an injection of tuberculin.

**Kohnstamm's p.,** aftermovement; a slow, involuntary elevation of the arm after strong pressure against a firm object.

**Kühne's p.,** when a constant current is passed through a muscle, an undulation is seen to pass from the positive to the negative pole.

**L.E. p.,** the formation of L.E. cells in bone marrow or blood on adding serum from patients with disseminated lupus erythematosus.

**leg p.,** Pool's p. (1).

**Leichtenstern's p.,** Leichtenstern's *sign.*

**Lewis p.,** hydrophagocytosis.

**Litten's p.,** diaphragm p.

**Lucio's leprosy p.,** Lucio's *leprosy.*

**Marcus Gunn p.,** jaw-winking *syndrome.*

**Negro's p.,** cogwheel p.

**Neisser-Doering p.,** the lack of hemolytic action in human serum due to the presence of an antihemolytic substance capable of neutralizing the hemolysin normally present; the p. is rare, but has been observed especially in cases of arteriosclerosis and cirrhotic kidney.

**orbicula′ris p.,** unilateral constriction of the pupil when an effort is made to close eyelids forcibly held apart.

**paradoxical diaphragm p.,** in pyopneumothorax, hydropneumothorax, and some cases of injury, the diaphragm on the affected side rises during inspiration and falls during expiration.

**paradoxical pupillary p.,** paradoxical pupillary *reflex*.

**perone′al p.,** tapping the peroneal nerve below the head of the fibula causes dorsal flexion and abduction of the foot.

**Pfeiffer's p.,** the alteration and complete disintegration of cholera vibrios when introduced into the peritoneal cavity of an immunized guinea pig, or into that of a normal one if immune serum is injected at the same time; extended to include bacteriolysis in general. The animal is immunized by means of intraperitoneal injections of a culture of the pathogenic bacteria, in gradually increasing doses, until many times the fatal dose is borne; if now a minute quantity of this animal's serum is injected into another animal, the latter is rendered immune against the same bacteria.

**phi p.,** parallax test; an illusion of movement, as seen in motion pictures and certain electric signs, which occurs by means of successive visual impressions at intervals of $1/15$ to $1/20$ seconds. When an occluder is passed from one eye to the other while a small distant light is observed, the light seems to move with the occluder in exophoria, but in an opposite direction in esophoria.

**phrenic p.,** diaphragm p.

**Pool's p.,** (1) leg p.; Pool-Schlesinger sign; Schlesinger's sign; in tetany, spasm both of the extensor muscles of the knee and of the calf muscles when the extended leg is flexed at the hip; (2) arm p.; in tetany, contraction of the arm muscles, resembling that from stimulation of the ulnar nerve, following stretching of the brachial plexus by elevating the arm above the head with the forearm extended.

**psi p.,** a p. that includes both psychokinesis and extrasensory perception.

**Purkinje's p.,** Purkinje shift; if the spectrum is viewed in bright light (cone vision) the region of maximal brightness is in the yellow; when the illumination of the spectrum is reduced and the eye dark-adapted (rod vision), the region of maximal brightness will be found to have shifted toward the blue end of the spectrum, the blues becoming brighter.

**quellung p.,** Neufeld capsular *swelling*.

**radial p.,** dorsal flexion of the hand occurring involuntarily with palmar flexion of the fingers.

**Raynaud's p.,** spasm of the digital arteries with blanching and numbness of the fingers occurring secondary to another disease.

**rebound p.,** Stewart-Holmes *sign*.

**reclotting p.,** thixotropy.

**red cell adherence p.,** adhesion p.

**reentry p.,** see reentry.

**release p.,** the increased tonus and hyperirritability of muscle-stretch reflexes which occur following damage of the upper portions of the extrapyramidal system.

**Ritter-Rollet p.,** on equal electrical stimulation of motor nerve trunks, the flexor and abductor muscle groups react more readily than the extensors and adductors.

**R-on-T p.,** a premature ventricular (QRS) complex in the electrocardiogram interrupting the T wave of the preceding beat.

**Rust's p.,** in cancer or caries of the upper cervical vertebrae the patient will always support the head by the hands when changing from the recumbent to the sitting posture or the reverse.

**Sanarelli p.,** generalized Shwartzman p.

**Sanarelli-Shwartzman p.,** generalized Shwartzman p.

**Schellong-Strisower p.,** a reduction of the systolic blood pressure, accompanied sometimes by vertigo, on rising from the horizontal to the erect posture.

**Schiff-Sherrington p.,** when the cord is transected in the midthoracic region or a little lower, the stretch and other postural reflexes of the upper extremity become exaggerated; if the transection is made in the sacral cord a similar effect is observed in the lower limbs. The effect is regarded as a release p., *i.e.*, release from an inhibitory influence

normally exerted by the spinal segments below the transection.

**Schramm's p.,** a gaping sphincter vesicae through which a cystoscopic view can be obtained of part or all of the posterior urethra; interpreted by Schramm as a sign of paralysis of the muscles of the pelvic floor from disease or injury of the spinal cord.

**Schüller's p.,** in cases of functional hemiplegia the patient usually turns to the sound side in walking, but to the affected side in case of an organic lesion.

**Schultz-Charlton p.,** Schultz-Charlton *reaction*.

**Sherrington p.,** after the muscles of the leg have been deprived of their motor innervation by sectioning the ventral roots containing fibers for the sciatic nerve, and allowing time for the degeneration of the fibers to occur, stimulation of the sciatic nerve causes slow contraction of the muscles.

**shot-silk p.,** shot-silk *reflex*.

**Shwartzman p.,** Shwartzman reaction; a rabbit is so prepared by the intradermal injection of a small quantity of a suspension or of a filtrate of a culture of *Salmonella typhi*, or certain other Gram-negative bacteria, that it will develop a hemorrhagic and necrotic lesion at the site of this preparatory inoculation following the intravenous injection, after a latent period (usually 24 hours); the active material which prepares the animal is "endotoxin," a complex macromolecular phospholipid-polysaccharide which forms an integral part of the cell wall of the Gram-negative bacteria; substances capable of provoking the reaction in the prepared animals include not only those capable of preparing the animal but also other substances which are incapable of serving as preparative materials such as starch and agar, animal serums, and antigen-antibody precipitates.

**Soret's p.,** in a solution kept in a long, upright tube at room temperature, the upper part, being the warmer, is also the more concentrated.

**staircase p.,** treppe.

**steal p.,** see steal.

**Strassman's p.,** in the third stage of labor, failure of placental detachment is recognized by transmission of pressure from the fundus uteri to the umbilical vein which becomes engorged.

**Strümpell's p.,** dorsal flexion of the great toe, sometimes of the entire foot, in a paralyzed limb when the extremity is drawn up against the body, flexing both knee and hip.

**symbiotic fermentation p.,** "two organisms, neither of which alone produces gas fermentation in certain carbohydrates, may do so when living in symbiosis or when artifically mixed" (Castellani).

**Theobald Smith's p.,** observed in guinea pigs which had survived use for diphtheria antitoxin standardization, the animals having been rendered highly susceptible to subsequent inoculation of horse serum.

**tib′ial p.,** Strümpell's p.

**toe p.,** Babinski's *sign* (1).

**tongue p.,** Schultze's *sign*.

**Twort p.,** Twort-d'Herelle p.

**Twort-d'Herelle p.,** Twort p.; d.'Herelle p.; bacteriophagia; lysis of bacteria by bacteriophage. Discovered by Twort in 1916 in cultures of staphylococci on agar media, and observed in 1917 by d'Herelle following his discovery of the "lytic substance" (bacteriophage) in the stool of a dysentery (*Shigella dysenteriae*) patient.

**Tyndall p.,** the visibility of floating particles in gases or liquids when illuminated by a ray of sunlight and viewed at right angles to the illuminating ray.

**Van Allen phenomena,** belts of intense cosmic radiation surrounding the earth at very high altitudes, exceeding 600 miles. First reported by Dr. James A. Van Allen, State University of Iowa, from measurements obtained from the two Explorer satellites in 1958.

**Wenckebach p.,** progressive lengthening of A-V conduction time (P-R interval) until a beat is dropped; following the dropped beat the P-R interval is again shortened.

**Westphal's p.,** Westphal's *sign*.

**Westphal-Piltz p.,** (1) tonic *pupil*; (2) spasm of orbicularis oculi and pupillary muscles.

**Wever-Bray p.,** the action potentials in the acoustic nerve that correspond to auditory stimuli reaching the cochlea.

**phenoper'idine.** LEALGIN; 1-(3-hydroxy-3-phenylpropyl)-4-phenylisonipecotic acid ethyl ester; analgesic.

**phe'nothi'azine.** Thiodiphenylamine; dibenzothiazine; a compound widely used for the treatment of intestinal nematodes in animals. Without central nervous system depressant activity itself, it serves as the parent compound for synthesis of a large number of antipsychotic compounds, including promethazine, chlorpromazine, mepazine, prochlorperazine.

**Phenothiazine**

**phenotype** (fe'no-tip) [ G. *phainō,* to display, show forth, + *typos,* model. TYP- ]. In genetics, a category or group to which an individual may be assigned on the basis of one or more characteristics observable clinically or by laboratory means that reflect genetic variation or gene-environment interaction. A p. may include more than one genotype. For examples, see ABO blood group, appendix 2.

**phen'otyp'ic.** Relating to phenotype.

**phenox'yben'zamine hydrochloride** (NF, BP). DIBENZYLINE; (2-chloroethyl)-*N*-(1-methyl-2-phenoxyethyl) benzylamine hydrochloride; a potent adrenergic (α-receptor) blocking agent of the β-haloalkylamines; selectively blocks the excitatory response of smooth muscle and exocrine glands to epinephrine; used in the treatment of peripheral vascular diseases.

**2-phenoxyeth'anol.** PHENOXETOL; 1-hydroxy-2-phenoxyethane; an antibacterial agent used in the topical treatment of wound infections; it is active against Gram-negative bacteria that are resistant to most other antiseptics.

**phenoxymethylpenicillin** (USP, BP). Penicillin V.

**phenozygous** (fe-noz'ĭ-gus) [ G. *phainō,* to show, + *zygon,* yoke ]. Having a narrow cranium as compared with the width of the face, so that when the skull is viewed from above, the zygomatic arches are visible.

**phenpen'termine tartrate.** MODATROP; α,α,β-trimethylphenethylamine; anorexigenic agent.

**phenpro'bamate.** GAMAQUIL; carbamic acid 3-phenylpropyl ester; skeletal muscle relaxant with antianxiety action.

**phenprocoumon** (fen-pro-koo'mon) (NF). LIQUAMAR; 3-(1'-phenylpropyl)-4-hydroxycoumarin; a long-acting, orally effective anticoagulant.

**phenpro'pionate.** USAN-approved contraction for 3-phenylpropionate.

**phensux'imide** (NF). MILONTIN; *N*-methyl-2-phenylsuccinimide; an anticonvulsant drug used in the treatment of petit mal epilepsy; less effective than trimethadione but apparently free from serious side effects.

**phen'tanyl.** Fentanyl citrate.

**phen'termine** (USAN). IONAMIN; α,α-dimethylphenethylamine; a sympathomimetic used as an appetite depressant; may cause palpitation and insomnia. Also available as the hydrochloride.

**phentetiothalein sodium** (fen-tet-i'o-thal'e-in). Phenoltetraiodophthalein sodium; used as a test of hepatic function and to aid in the x-ray examination of the gallbladder.

**phentol'amine hydrochloride** (NF). REGITINE hydrochloride; 2-(*N-p*-tolyl-*N-m*-hydroxyphenylaminomethyl)-imidazoline hydrochloride; an adrenergic (α-receptor) blocking agent.

**phentol'amine mesylate** (USP). REGITINE methanesulfonate; phentolamine methanesulfonate (BP); same actions as phentolamine hydrochloride, for intravenous use only.

**phenyl** (fen'il). The univalent radical, $C_6H_5$—, of phenol.

**p. aminosalicylate** (USAN), *p*-aminosalicylic acid phenyl ester; an antituberculous drug.

**p. salicylate,** SALOL; the salicylic ester of phenol; the phenylic ester of salicylic acid; intestinal analgesic and antipyretic; has been used in the treatment of rheumatism, diarrhea, and pharyngitis, as an enteric coating for tablets, and in ointments for sunburn prevention.

**phen'ylace'tic acid.** $C_6H_5CH_2COOH$; an abnormal product of phenylalanine catabolism, appearing in the urine in phenylpyruvic oligophrenia.

**phen'ylacetur'ic acid.** Phenaceturic acid.

**phen'ylac'etylure'a.** Phenacemide.

**phen'ylacrylic acid** (fen'il-ă-kril'ik). Cinnamic acid.

**phenylalaninase** (fen'il-al'ă-nin-ās). Phenylalanine 4-monooxygenase.

**phen'ylal'anine.** 2-Amino-3-phenylpropionic acid; one of the common amino acids in proteins; $C_6H_5CH_2$—$CH(NH_2)$—COOH.

**phenylalanine 4-hydroxylase.** Phenylalanine 4-monooxygenase.

**phenylalanine 4-monooxygenase.** Phenylalaninase; phenylalanine 4-hydroxylase; an enzyme (EC 1.14.16.1) that catalyzes the oxidation of phenylalanine to tyrosine with O₂ and tetrahydrobiopterin, the latter forming the dihydro derivative, which is reduced by NADPH and a reductase to the active form. The hereditary failure to produce this enzyme causes phenylketonuria.

**phenylalanyl chain** (fen'il-al'ă-nil). See under chain.

**phenyl'amine.** Aniline.

**phen'ylbu'tazone** (USP, BP). 1,2-Diphenyl-4-butyl-3,5-pyrazolidinedione; a pyrazolone derivative; an analgesic, antipyretic, anti-inflammatory, and uricosuric agent; used especially in painful musculoskeletal disorders.

**1-phenylcyclohexylamine** (fen'il-si-klo-hek-sil'ă-men). Parent compound of a number of parenteral dissociative anesthetics, including cyclohexamine, phencyclidine, and ketamine.

**1-Phenylcyclohexylamine**

**phen'ylenedi'amine hydrochloride.** A light reddish crystalline powder; used in the manufacture of dyes and as a reagent.

**phen'yleph'rine hydrochloride** (USP, BP). NEOSYNEPHRINE hydrochloride; (—)-*m*-hydroxy-α-[ (methylamino)-methyl ]benzyl alcohol hydrochloride; a sympathomimetic amine; a powerful vasoconstrictor, used as a nasal decongestant and mydriatic.

**phen'yleth'yl alcohol** (NF). Phenethyl alcohol; 2-phenylethanol; benzyl carbinol; $C_6H_5CH_2CH_2OH$. Natural constituent of some volatile oils (rose, geranium, and neroli). Used as an antibacterial agent in ophthalmic solutions.

**phen'yleth'ylbarbitu'ric acid.** Phenobarbital.

**phen'yleth'yl carbamate.** Phenylurethan.

**phen'ylglycol'ic acid.** Mandelic acid.

**phen'ylhy'drazine.** Hydrazinobenzene; $C_6H_5NHNH_2$; a colorless liquid, the hydrochloride of which is used as a reagent for the detection of sugars, aldehydes, and ketones.

**phenylindanedione** (fen'il-in'dān-di-ōn). Phenindione.

**phenylisothiocyanate** (fen'il-i'so-thi'o-si'ă-nāt). $C_6H_5$—N=C=S, a reagent that condenses with the free *N*-terminal amino group of a peptide chain to form a phenylthiohydantoin in the Edman method of determining the nature of *N*-terminal amino acids. Abbreviated PhNCS.

**phenylketonuria** (fen'il-ke'to-nu'rī-ah) [ phenyl + ketone, + g. *ouron,* urine ]. Common abbreviation, PKU; Følling's disease; congenital deficiency of phenylalanine hydroxylase causing inadequate formation of tyrosine, elevation of serum phenylalanine, urinary excretion of phenylpyruvic acid, and accumulation of phenylalanine and its metabolites that produce brain damage resulting in severe mental retardation, often with seizures, other neurologic abnormalities such as retarded myelination, and deficient melanin formation that predisposes to eczema; autosomal recessive inheritance; brain damage can be prevented by a low phenylalanine diet.

**phenyllactic acid** (fen'il-lak'tik). $C_6H_5CH_2CHOHCOOH$; a product of phenylalanine catabolism, prominently appearing in the urine in phenylketonuria.

**phen'ylmercu'ric acetate** (NF). NYLMERATE; SCUTL; RIOGEN; TAG fungicide; PMA; PMAC; acetoxyphenylmercury; a bacteriostatic preservative, fungicide, and herbicide (especially for crabgrass).

**phen'ylmercu'ric nitrate** (NF, BP). MERPHENYL nitrate (basic); basic phenylmercuric nitrate; a mixture of phenylmercuric nitrate and phenylmercuric hydroxide; antiseptic; used for the prophylactic disinfection of the intact skin or of minor wounds.

**phen'ylmeth'yl acetone.** Acetophenone.

**phen'ylpropanol'amine hydrochloride** (NF). PROPADRINE hydrochloride; α-(1-aminoethyl)-benzyl alcohol; a sympathomimetic amine, used as a nasal decongestant and bronchodilator.

**1,4-bis-2-(5-phenyloxazolyl)-benzene.** POPOP; a scintillation agent, used in radioisotope measurement.

**phen'ylpro'pylmethyl'amine hydrochloride.** VONEDRINE hydrochloride; a sympathomimetic drug; used as a nasal decongestant.

**phenylsulfonic acid** (fen-il-sul-fon'ik). Benzenesulfonic acid, $C_6H_5SO_3H$.

**phen'ylthi'ocar'bamide.** Phenylthiourea.

**phenylthiocarbamoyl peptide.** See under peptide.

**phenylthiohydantoin** (fen'il-thi-o-hi-dan'to-in). PTH; the compound formed from an amino acid in the Edman method of protein degradation.

**phenylthiourea** (fen'il-thi-o-u-re'ah). Phenylthiocarbamide; a substance that tastes bitter to some persons but is tasteless to others. The ability to taste this substance is inherited and is dependent upon a single gene pair. "Tasters" are either homozygous or heterozygous for the dominant allele. Phenylthiourea contains the N—C=S group upon which the taste peculiarity apparently depends, for goitrogenic or antithyroid substances, e.g., thiourea and thiouracil, which also contain this group, possess the same property with respect to taste.

**phenyltolox'amine.** BRISTAMIN; N,N-dimethyl-2-(α-phenyl-o-tolyloxy)-ethylamine; antihistaminic.

**phen'yltrimeth'ylammo'nium.** PTMA; a highly selective stimulant of the motor end-plates of skeletal muscle.

**phenylurethan** (fen'il-u're-than). Phenylurethane; phenylethyl carbamate; ethyl carbanilate; has been used as antipyretic, analgesic, and antirheumatic.

**phenyramidol hydrochloride** (fen'i-ram'i-dol) (USAN). ANALEXIN; α-(2-pryidylaminomethyl)benzyl alcohol hydrochloride; a moderately effective analgesic comparable in potency to aspirin, and a muscle relaxant. It has no anti-inflammatory action.

**phen'ytoin sodium** (BP). See diphenylhydantoin.

**pheo-** (fe'o-). 1. Prefix denoting same substituents on a phorbin or phorbide (porphyrin) residue as are present in chlorophyll, excluding any ester residues and Mg. 2 [ G. *phaios*, dusky ]. Combining form meaning dusky, gray, or dun.

**pheochrome** (fe'o-krōm) [ G. *phaios*, dusky, + *chrōma*, color ]. 1. Chromaffin. 2. Staining darkly with chromic salts.

**pheochromoblast** (fe-o-kro'mo-blast) [ G. *phaios*, dusky, + *chrōma*, color, + *blastos*, sprout, offspring ]. A primitive chromaffin cell which, with sympathetoblasts, enters into the formation of the adrenal gland.

**pheochromoblastoma** (fe'o-kro-mo-blas-to'mah). Pheochromocytoma.

**pheochromocyte** (fe'o-kro'mo-sīt) [ pheochrome + G. *kytos*, cell ]. A chromaffin cell of a sympathetic paraganglion, medulla of an adrenal gland, or of a pheochromocytoma.

**pheochromocytoma** (fe-o-kro-mo-si-to'mah). A functional chromaffinoma, derived from cells in the adrenal medullary tissue and characterized by the secretion of catecholamines, resulting in hypertension which may be paroxysmal and associated with attacks of palpitation, headache, nausea, dyspnea, anxiety, pallor, and profuse

sweating. P.'s are nearly always benign. See also paraganglioma.

**pheophor'bide.** A chlorophyllide; what remains of a chlorophyll molecule when the magnesium atom and the phytyl group have been removed, the latter by chlorophyllase; see pheophytin.

**pheophor'bin.** A chlorophyllide; what remains of chlorophyll molecule when the magnesium atom has been removed and the phytyl and methyl esters hydrolyzed to the free acids.

**pheophy'tin.** A chlorophyllide; the porphyrin derivative remaining when the magnesium ion of a chlorophyll is removed (by dilute acid).

**pher'omones** [ G. *pherein*, to carry, + *horman*, to excite, stimulate ]. Substances secreted to the outside by an individual, and perceived by a second individual of the same species, thereby producing a change in the sexual or social behavior of that individual. P.'s represent one type of ectohormone.

**phethenylate sodium** (fe-then'ī-lāt). 5-Phenyl-5-(2-thienyl)-hydantoin; $C_{13}H_{10}N_2O_2S$; An anticonvulsant effective in the management of grand mal, petit mal, and psychomotor epilepsy, but withdrawn from the market because of toxicity.

**Ph.G.** 1. Abbreviation for *Pharmacopoeia germanica;* German Pharmacopoeia. 2. Abbreviation for Graduate in Pharmacy.

**phi'al** [ G. *phialē*, a drinking-bowl ]. Vial.

**Phialophora verrucosa** (fi'ă-lof'o-rah věr'u-ko'sah) [ G. *phialē*, a bowl, + *phoreō*, to carry; L. *verrucosus*, warty, fr. *verruca*, a wart ]. A genus of fungi causative of chromoblastomycosis.

**-phil, -phile, -philic, -philia** [ G. *philos*, fond, loving; *phileō*, to love ]. Combining forms, used in the suffix position, to denote affinity for, or craving for. See also philo-.

**philiater** (fil-i'a-tur) [ G. *philos*, fond, + *iatreia*, practice of medicine ]. One interested in the study of medicine.

**Philinus** of Cos, Greek physician, c. 250 B.C. Outstanding figure of the school of empirics.

**Philip,** Robert W., Scottish physician, 1857–1939. See P.'s *glands.*

**Phillippe** (fil-ēp'), Claudien, French anatomist, 1866–1903. See P.'s *triangle.*

**Phillips' catheter.** See under catheter.

**Phillipson's reflex.** See under reflex.

**philo-** (fil'o-) [ G. *philos*, fond, loving; *phileō*, to love ]. Combining form, used in the prefix position, to denote affinity or craving for.

**philomimesia** (fil'o-mī-me'sī-ah) [ philo- + G. *mimēsis*, imitation ]. Morbid impulse to imitate or mimic.

**philoneism** (fil'o-ne'izm) [ philo- + G. *neos*, new ]. An extreme love of novelty.

**phil'opatridoma'nia** [ G. *phileō*, to love, + *patris*, fatherland, + *mania*, frenzy ]. Nostalgia.

**Philop'ia ca'sei.** Cheese maggot; may cause intestinal myiasis.

**philoprogenitive** (fil'o-pro-jen'ī-tĭv) [ philo- + L. *progenies*, offspring, progeny ]. 1. Procreative, producing offspring. 2. In psychiatry, pedophilic; manifesting an erotic or abnormal love for children.

**philtrum,** pl. **philtra** (fil'trum, -trah) [ L. from G. *philtron*, a love-charm, depression on upper lip, fr. *phileo*, to love ]. 1. A philter or love potion. 2 [ NA ]. The infranasal depression; the groove in the midline of the upper lip.

**phimosis,** pl. **phimoses** (fi-mo'sis, -sēz) [ G. a muzzling, fr. *phimos*, a muzzle ]. Narrowness of the opening of the prepuce, preventing its being drawn back over the glans.

    **p. vagina'lis,** narrowness of the vagina.

**phimot'ic.** Pertaining to phimosis.

**phleb-.** See phlebo-.

**phlebalgia** (flē-bal'jī-ah) [ phlebo- + G. *algos*, pain ]. Pain originating in a vein.

**phlebarteriectasia** (fleb'ar-tēr'ī-ek-ta'zī-ah) [ phlebo- + G. *arteria*, artery, + *ektasis*, a stretching ]. General dilation of the blood vessels.

**phlebectasia** (fleb'ek-ta'zĭ-ah) [ phlebo- + G. *ektasis*, a stretching ]. Dilation of the veins; varicosity.

**phlebectomy** (flĕ-bek'to-mĭ) [ phlebo- + G. *ektomē*, excision ]. Venectomy; excision of a segment of a vein, performed sometimes for the cure of varicose veins; see also strip (2).

**phlebectopia, phlebectopy** (fleb'ek-to'pĭ-ah, flĕ-bek'to-pĭ) [ phlebo- + G. *ektopos*, out of place ]. Dislocation or abnormal course of a vein.

**phlebemphraxis** (fleb'em-frak'sis) [ phlebo- + G. *emphraxis*, a stoppage ]. Venous thrombosis.

**phlebeurysm** (fleb'u-rizm) [ phlebo- + G. *eurys*, wide ]. Pathologic dilation (varix) of a vein.

**phlebismus** (flĕ-biz'mus) [ phlebo- + G. suffix -*ismos*, condition ]. Venous congestion and phlebectasia.

**phlebit'ic.** Relating to inflammation of a vein.

**phlebitis** (flĕ-bi'tis) [ phlebo- + G. suffix -*itis*, inflammation ]. Inflammation of a vein.
  **adhesive p.,** a form of p. in which the walls adhere, leading to obliteration of the vessel.
  **p. nodula'ris necroti'sans,** p. in which tuberculous nodules are formed in the skin. The lesions spread peripherally and undergo central necrosis.
  **puer'peral p.,** *phlegmasia* alba dolens.
  **sinus p.,** inflammation of a cerebral sinus.

**phlebo-, phleb-** (fleb'o-) [ G. *phleps*, vein ]. Combining forms denoting vein.

**phlebocholosis** (fleb-o-ko-lo'sis) [ phlebo- + G. *cholos*, maimed ]. Disease of a vein.

**phleboclysis** (flĕ-bok'lĭ-sis) [ phlebo- + G. *klysis*, a washing out ]. The intravenous injection of an isotonic solution of dextrose or other substances in quantity.
  **drip p.,** venoclysis; intravenous injection of a liquid drop by drop, by the drip method.

**phlebodynamics** (fleb'o-di-nam-iks) [ phlebo- + G. *dynamis*, force ]. Laws and principles governing blood pressures and flow within the venous circulation.

**phleb'ogram** [ phlebo- + G. *gramma*, something written ]. Venogram (2); a tracing of the jugular venous pulse.

**phleb'ograph** [ phlebo- + G. *graphō*, to write ]. A venous sphygmograph; an instrument for making a tracing of the venous pulse.

**phlebography** (flĕ-bog'rä-fĭ) [ phlebo- + G. *graphē*, a writing ]. 1. A treatise on or a description of the veins. 2. The recording of the venous pulse. 3. Roentgenography of the veins; see also venography.

**phleb'oid** [ phlebo- + G. *eidos*, resemblance ]. 1. Resembling a vein. 2. Relating to a vein or veins; venous. 3. Containing many veins.

**phleb'olite.** Phlebolith.

**phlebolith** (fleb'o-lith) [ phlebo- + G. *lithos*, stone ]. Vein stone; a concretion in a vein resulting from the calcification of an old thrombus.

**phlebolithiasis** (fleb'o-lĭ-thi'ă-sis). The formation of phleboliths.

**phlebology** (flĕ-bol'o-jĭ) [ phlebo- + G. *logos*, study ]. The branch of medical science that treats of the anatomy and diseases of the veins.

**phlebomanometer** (fleb'o-mă-nom'e-ter). A manometer for measuring venous blood pressure.

**phlebometritis** (fleb'o-me-tri'tis) [ phlebo- + G. *metra*, uterus, + suffix -*itis*, inflammation ]. Inflammation of the uterine veins.

**phlebomyomatosis** (fleb'o-mi-o-mă-to'sis) [ phlebo- + myoma, *q.v.,* + suffix -*osis*, condition ]. Thickening of the walls of a vein by an overgrowth of muscular fibers arranged irregularly, intersecting each other without any definite relation to the axis of the vessel.

**phlebophlebostomy** (fleb'o-flĕ-bos'to-mĭ). Venovenostomy.

**phlebophthalmotomy** (fleb-of-thal-mot'o-mĭ) [ phlebo- + G. *ophthalmos*, eye, + *tomē*, incision ]. Ophthalmophlebotomy.

**phleboplasty** (fleb'o-plas'tĭ) [ phlebo- + G. *plassō*, to fashion ]. Repair of a defect or wound of a vein.

**phleborrhagia** (fleb-o-ra'je-ah) [ phlebo- + G. *rhēgnymi*, to burst forth ]. Venous hemorrhage; bleeding from a vein.

**phleborrhaphy** (flĕ-bor'ă-fĭ) [ phlebo- + G. *rhaphē*, seam ]. Venisuture; suture of a vein.

**phleborrhexis** (fleb'o-rek'sis) [ phlebo- + G. *rhēxis*, rupture ]. Rupture of a vein.

**phlebosclerosis** (fleb'o-skle-ro'sis) [ phlebo- + G. *sklērōsis*, hardening ]. Fibrous hardening of the walls of the veins.

**phlebostasis** (flĕ-bos'tä-sis) [ phlebo- + G. *stasis*, a standing still ]. Venostasis. 1. Abnormally slow motion of blood in veins, usually with venous distention. 2. Treatment of congestive heart failure by compressing proximal veins of the extremities with tourniquets ("bloodless phlebotomy").

**phlebostenosis** (fleb'o-stĕ-no'sis) [ phlebo- + G. *stenōsis*, a narrowing ]. Narrowing of the lumen of a vein from any cause.

**phlebostrep'sis** [ phlebo- + G. *strepsis*, a twisting ]. Twisting the cut or torn end of a vein to arrest hemorrhage.

**phleb'othrombo'sis** [ phlebo- + G. *thrombōsis*, *q.v.* ]. Thrombosis, or clotting, in a vein without primary inflammation.

**phlebot'omist.** A bloodletter.

**phlebot'omize.** To perform phlebotomy.

**Phlebotomus** (flĕ-bot'o-mus) [ phlebo- + G. *tomos*, cutting ]. A genus of very small midges, or bloodsucking sand flies of the family Psychodidae.
  **P. argen'tipes,** the vector of kala azar in India.
  **P. chinen'sis,** the vector of kala azar in China.
  **P. flaviscutellatus,** the sand fly vector of chiclero's ulcer, a common form of cutaneous leishmaniasis in Mexico.
  **P. longipalpis,** a vector of kala azar in South America.
  **P. major,** a vector of kala azar in the Mediterranean region.
  **P. nogu'chi,** the transmitter of *Bartonella* organisms, the causal agent of Oroya fever.
  **P. orientalis,** a vector of kala azar in the Sudan.
  **P. papatasii,** transmits the virus of pappataci fever; also a vector of *Leishmania tropica* in the Mediterranean area.
  **P. perniciosus,** a vector of kala azar in the Mediterranean region.
  **P. sergen'ti,** a vector of *Leishmania tropica*, the cause of cutaneous leishmaniasis.
  **P. verruca'rum,** a form found in Peru which transmits *Bartonella* organisms, the causal agent of Oroya fever.

**phlebotomy** (flĕ-bot'o-mĭ) [ phlebo- + G. *tomē*, incision ]. Venesection; venotomy; incision into a vein for the purpose of drawing blood. See also bloodletting.
  **bloodless p.,** phlebostasis (2).

**phlegm** (flem) [ G. *phlegma*, inflammation. PHLEG- ]. 1. Mucus. 2. One of the four humors of the body, according to the ancients. 3. Self-restraint; calmness; apathy.

**phlegmasia** (fleg-ma'zĭ-ah) [ G. fr. *phlegma*, inflammation. PHLEG- ]. Inflammation, especially when acute and severe.
  **p. al'ba do'lens** [ L. *albus*, white; *dolens*, causing pain ], milk leg; puerperal phlebitis; an extreme edematous swelling of the leg following childbirth, due to thrombosis of the veins that drain the part.
  **cellulit'ic p.,** inflammatory swelling of the leg, following childbirth, due to septic inflammation of the connective tissue.
  **p. ceru'lea do'lens,** thrombosis of the veins of a limb, with sudden severe pain with swelling, cyanosis, and edema of the part, followed by circulatory collapse and shock.
  **p. do'lens,** cellulitic p.
  **p. malabar'ica,** elephantiasis.
  **thrombot'ic p.,** p. alba dolens.

**phlegmatic** (fleg-mat'ik) [ G. *phlegmatikos*, relating to phlegm ]. Relating to the heavy one of the four humors (see phlegm), and therefore calm, apathetic, unexcitable.

**phlegmon** (fleg'mon) [ G. *phlegmonē*, inflammation. PHLEG- ]. Acute suppurative inflammation of the subcutaneous connective tissue.
  **bronze p.,** a gaseous p., following a renal operation, marked by large, bronze-colored spots near the line of incision.
  **diffuse p.,** phlegmonous cellulitis; a diffuse inflammation of the subcutaneous tissues accompanied by constitutional symptoms of sepsis.
  **emphysematous p.,** gas p.

**gas p.,** emphysematous p.; gangrenous emphysema; a form attended with more or less extensive emphysema, due to the presence of *Clostridium perfringens* or other of the so-called gas bacilli; see also gas gangrene.

**phlegmonous** (fleg'mon-us). Relating to a phlegmon; denoting inflammation of the subcutaneous connective tissues.

**phlogiston** (flo-jis'ton) [ G. *phlogistos*, inflammable. PHLEG- ]. A hypothetical substance of negative mass that, according to the theory of Stahl (1660–1734), was given off by a substance when it underwent combustion thus accounting for the increase in mass of the ash over the starting substance. Abandoned when Lavoisier discovered oxygen.

**phlogocyte** (flo'go-sīt) [ G. *phlogōsis*, inflammation, + *kytos*, a hollow (cell) ]. One of a number of cells present in the tissues during the course of an inflammation; see also Türk's cell.

**phlogocytosis** (flo-go-si-to'sis). A blood state in which there are many phlogocytes in the peripheral circulation.

**phlogogenic, phlogogenous** (flo-go-jen'ik, flo-goj'ĕ-nus) [ G. *phlox* (*phlog-*), flame, + suffix *-gen*, producing ]. Exciting inflammation.

**phlo'gosin** [ G. *phlogōsis*, inflammation. PHLEG- ]. A substance, isolated from cultures of pus-producing cocci, injections of sterilized solutions of which will excite suppuration.

**phlogosis** (flo-go'sis) [ G. *phlogōsis*, a burning ]. 1. Inflammation. 2. Specifically, erysipelas.

**phlogotherapy** (flo'go-thĕr'ă-pī) [ G. *phlogōsis*, inflammation, + therapy ]. Nonspecific *therapy*.

**phlor'etin.** The aglucon of phlorizin; 2',4',6'-trihydroxy-3-(*p*-hydroxyphenyl)propiophenone.

**phlorhi'zin, phlorid'zin.** Phlorizin.

**phlorizin** (flōr'ī-zin, flo-ri'zin) [ G. *phloios*, bark, + *rhiza*, root ]. Phlorhizin, phloridzin; phlorrhizin; phloretin-2'-β-glucoside; obtained from the bark of the roots of apple, pear, plum, and cherry trees. When injected it produces glycosuria, and is used to induce glycosuria experimentally in animals. Formerly used as an antimalarial, but it is more dangerous than valuable.

**phloroglu'cin, phloroglu'cinol, phloroglu'col.** 1,3,5-Trihydroxybenzene; an isomer of pyrogallol, obtained from resorcinol by fusion with caustic soda; a whitish or yellowish crystalline powder. Used as a reagent with vanillin (Günzburg's reagent) as a test for hydrochloric acid, with which it gives a bright red color.

**phloropro'piophe'none.** LABRODAX; 2',4',6'-trihydroxypropiophenone; intestinal antispasmodic.

**phlor'rhizin.** Phlorizin.

**phloxine** (flok-sēn, -sin). Dichloro- or tetrachlorotetrabromofluorescein; a red acid dye used as a cytoplasmic stain in histology.

**phlyctena,** pl. **phlyctenae** (flik-te'nah, -ne) [ G. *phlyktaina,* a blister made by a burn ]. A small vesicle, especially one of a number of small blisters following a burn of the first degree.

**phlyctenar** (flik'te-nar). Phlyctenous; relating to or marked by the presence of phlyctenae.

**phlyctenoid** (flik'te-noyd) [ G. *phlyktaina,* blister, + *eidos,* resemblance ]. Resembling a phlyctena.

**phlyctenosis** (flik'te-no'sis). The occurrence of phlyctenae; a disease marked by a phlyctenar eruption.

**phlyctenous** (flik'te-nus). Phlyctenar.

**phlyctenula,** pl. **phlycten'ulae** (flik-ten'u-lah) [ Mod. L. dim. of G. *phlyktaina,* blister ]. A small red nodule of lymphoid cells, with ulcerated apex, occurring in the conjunctiva.

**phlyctenular** (flik-ten'u-lar). Relating to a phlyctenula.

**phlyc'tenule.** Phlyctenula.

**phlyctenulosis** (flik-ten'u-lo'sis). The presence of phlyctenulae.

**phlyzacium** (fli-za'sī-um) [ G. *phlyzakion,* a pimple, dim. of *phlyktaina,* a blister ]. 1. Phlyctena. 2. Ecthyma.

**PhNCS.** Abbreviation for phenylisothiocyanate.

**phobanthropy** (fo-ban'thro-pī) [ G. *phobos,* fear, + *anthrōpos,* man ]. Anthropophobia.

# PHOBIA

**phobia** (fo'bī-ah) [ G. *phobos,* fear ]. Any objectively unfounded morbid dread or fear. The word is used as a combining form in many terms expressing the object that inspires the fear.

**school p.,** a young child's sudden aversion to or fear of attending school, usually considered a manifestation of separation anxiety.

**Examples of other phobias:**
**air,** aerophobia.
**alcoholic beverages, alcoholism,** alcoholophobia.
**angina pectoris,** anginophobia.
**animals,** zoophobia.
**bacteria,** bacteriophobia, microbiophobia.
**bacilli,** bacillophobia.
**bees,** apiphobia, melissophobia.
**being afraid,** phobophobia, phobia.
**being alone,** autophobia, eremophobia, monophobia.
**being beaten,** rhabdophobia.
**being bound,** merinthophobia.
**being buried alive,** taphophobia.
**being dirty,** automysophobia.
**being egotistical,** autophobia.
**being locked in,** clithrophobia.
**being stared at,** scopophobia.
**blood,** hematophobia, hemophobia.
**blushing,** ereuthophobia.
**books,** bibliophobia.
**cancer,** cancerophobia; carcinomatophobia.
**cats,** ailurophobia, gatophobia.
**certain name,** onomatophobia.
**change,** kainophobia, kainotophobia, neophobia.
**childbirth,** tocophobia.
**children,** pediophobia.
**choking,** pnigophobia.
**climbing,** climacophobia.
**cold,** psychrophobia.
**colors,** chromatophobia.
**confinement,** claustrophobia.
**corpse,** necrophobia.
**crossing a bridge,** gephyrophobia.
**crowds,** ochlophobia.
**dampness** hygrophobia.
**darkness,** achluophobia, myctophobia, scotophobia.
**dawn,** eosophobia.
**daylight,** phengophobia.
**death,** necrophobia, thanatophobia.
**deep places,** bathophobia.
**deformity,** dysmorphophobia.
**devil,** demonophobia, satanophobia.
**dirt,** mysophobia, rhypophobia, rupophobia.
**disease,** nosophobia, pathophobia.
**disorder,** ataxiophobia.
**dogs,** cynophobia.
**dolls,** pediophobia.
**draft,** aerophobia, anemophobia.
**drinking,** dipsophobia.
**drugs,** pharmacophobia.
**eating,** phagophobia.
**electricity,** electrophobia.
**elevated places,** acrophobia.
**empty rooms,** cenophobia.
**enclosed space,** claustrophobia, clithrophobia.
**error,** harmatophobia.
**everything,** panophobia, panphobia, pantophobia.
**excrement,** coprophobia.
**eyes,** ommatophobia.
**fatigue,** ponophobia, kopophobia.
**fever,** pyrexiophobia.
**fire,** pyrophobia.
**fish,** ichthyophobia.
**flash,** selaphobia.
**floods,** antlophobia.
**flowers,** anthophobia.
**food,** sitophobia, cibophobia.

frogs, batrachophobia.
fur, doraphobia.
gaiety, cherophobia.
germs, microbiophobia, microphobia.
ghosts, phasmophobia.
glare, photaugiaphobia.
glass, crystallophobia, hyalophobia.
God, theophobia.
grave, taphophobia.
hair, trichophobia.
heart disease, cardiophobia.
heat, thermophobia.
heights, acrophobia, hypsophobia.
hell, stygiophobia, hadephobia.
home, returning to, nostophobia.
home surroundings, ecophobia, oikophobia.
house, domatophobia.
human beings, antropophobia.
ideas, ideophobia.
infection, molysmophobia, mysophobia.
injury, traumatophobia.
insanity, maniaphobia.
insects, entomophobia.
itch, acarophobia, scabiophobia.
jealousy, zelophobia.
left, levophobia.
leprosy, leprophobia.
lice, pediculophobia.
light, phengophobia, photophobia.
lightning, astrapophobia, keraunophobia.
love, in its physical expression, erotophobia.
machinery, mechanophobia.
making false statements, mythophobia.
many things, polyphobia.
marriage, gamophobia.
men (males), androphobia.
metal objects, metallophobia.
meteors, meteorophobia.
microbes, microbiophobia, microphobia.
microorganisms, bacteriophobia, microphobia, bacillo-
phobia.
mind, psychophobia.
mirrors, spectrophobia.
missiles, ballistophobia.
moisture, hygrophobia.
money, chrematophobia.
monstrosities, teratophobia.
nakedness, gymnophobia.
names, nomatophobia.
needles, belonophobia.
neglect or omission of some duty, paralipophobia.
night, nyctophobia.
noise or loud talking, phonophobia.
novelty, kainophobia, kainotophobia, neophobia.
odors, osmophobia.
odors, body, osphresiophobia, bromidrosiphobia.
oneself, autophobia.
open spaces, agoraphobia, cenophobia, kenophobia.
pain, algophobia, odynephobia.
parasites, parasitophobia; phthiriophobia, pediculophobia (lice); helminthophobia (worms).
pins, belonophobia.
phobias, phobophobia.
places, topophobia.
pleasure, hedonophobia.
pointed objects, aichmophobia.
poisoning, toxicophobia, iophobia.
poverty, peniaphobia.
precipices, cremnophobia.
pregnancy, maieusiophobia.
rabies, lyssophobia.
railways, siderodromophobia.
rain, ombrophobia.
rectal disease, proctophobia, rectophobia.
religious objects, hierophobia.
responsibility, hypengyophobia.
right (side), dextrophobia.
rivers, potamophobia.
robbers, harpaxophobia.
rod (punishment with), rhabdophobia.
rust, iophobia.

sacred things, hierophobia.
scabies, scabiphobia.
sea, thalassophobia.
self, autophobia.
semen, loss of, spermatophobia.
sermons, homilophobia.
sexual intercourse, coitophobia, cypridophobia.
sexual love, erotophobia.
sharp objects, belonophobia, aichmophobia.
sin, hamartophobia.
sinning, pecattiphobia.
skin diseases, dermatosiophobia.
skin of animals, doraphobia.
sleep, hypnophobia.
small objects, microphobia.
snakes, ophidiophobia.
society, anthropophobia.
solitude, eremophobia, autophobia, monophobia.
sounds, acousticophobia.
speaking, lalophobia.
spiders, arachnephobia.
spirits, demonophobia.
stairs, climacophobia.
standing upright, stasiphobia.
standing and walking, stasibasiphobia.
stealing, kleptophobia.
stillness, eremophobia
strangers, xenophobia.
streets, agyiophobia.
stuttering, laliophobia.
sun, heliophobia.
surgical operations, ergasiophobia.
tabes dorsalis, ataxiophobia, tabophobia.
tapeworms, taeniophobia; teniophobia.
teeth, odontophobia.
thinking, phronemophobia.
thirteen, triskaidekaphobia, triakaidekaphobia.
thunder, keraunophobia, ceraunophobia, tonitrophobia,
brontophobia.
time, chronophobia.
tomb, taphophobia.
touching or being touched, haphephobia.
trains, siderodromophobia.
trauma, traumatophobia.
traveling, hodophobia.
trembling, tremophobia.
trichinosis, trichinophobia.
tuberculosis, phthisiophobia, tuberculophobia.
uncleanliness, automysophobia.
uncovering the body, gymnophobia.
vaccination, vaccinophobia.
vehicles, amaxophobia.
venereal disease, cypridophobia, venereophobia.
vertigo, illyngophobia.
vomiting, emetophobia.
walking, basiphobia.
water, hydrophobia, aquaphobia.
weakness, asthenophobia.
wind, anemophobia.
wintry weather, cheimaphobia.
women, gynephobia.
work, ergasiophobia, ponophobia.
worms, helminthophobia.
writing, graphophobia.

---

**phobic** (fo'bik). Pertaining to or characterized by phobia.

**pho'bism.** The condition of being affected by a phobia.

**phobophobia** (fo-bo-fo'bĭ-ah) [ G. *phobos,* fear ]. A morbid dread of developing some phobia.

**Phocas** (fo-kah'), B. Gerasimo, French physician, 1861–1937. See P.'s *disease.*

**phocomelia** (fo-ko-me'lĭ-ah) [ G. *phōkē,* a seal, + *melos,* extremity ]. Phocomely; defective development of arms or legs, or both, so that the hands and feet are attached close to the body, resembling the flippers of a seal.

**phocomelus** (fo-kom'e-lus). A person with phocomelia.

**phocom'ely.** Phocomelia.

**pholcodine** (fol'ko-dēn) (BP). ETHNINE; 3-(2-morpholino-ethyl)morphine; a narcotic with little or no analgesic or europhorigenic activity, used mainly as an antitussive.

**pholedrine.** VERITOL; *p*-[ 2-(methylamino)propyl ]phenol; sympathomimetic for treatment of shock.

**Pho′ma.** A genus of rapidly growing saprophytic fungi that are common laboratory contaminants.

**phon-.** See phono-.

**phonacoscope** (fo-nak′o-skōp) [ phon- + G. *akouō*, to listen, + *skopeō*, to view ]. An instrument for increasing the intensity of the percussion note or of the voice sounds, the examiner's ear or the stethoscope being placed on the opposite side of the chest.

**phonacoscopy** (fo′nă-kos′ko-pĭ). Examination of the chest by means of the phonacoscope.

**phonal** (fo′nal). [ G. *phōnē*, voice ]. Relating to sound or to the voice.

**phonasthenia** (fo-nas-the′nĭ-ah) [ phon- + G. *astheneia*, weakness ]. Functional vocal fatigue; difficult or abnormal voice production, the enunciation being too high, too loud, or too hard.

**phonation** (fo-na′shun) [ G. *phōnē*, voice ]. The utterance of sounds by means of vocal cords.

  **subenerget′ic p.,** hypophonia.

  **superenerget′ic p.,** hyperphonia.

**phonatory** (fo′nă-tor-ĭ). Relating to phonation.

**phonautograph** (fōn-aw′to-graf) [ phon- + G. *autos*, self, + *graphō*, to record ]. An instrument for registering the vibrations of the voice or any other sound.

**phoneme** (fo′nēm) [ G. *phōnēma*, a voice ]. The smallest sound unit which, in terms of the phonetic sequences of sound, controls meaning.

**phone′mic.** Pertaining to or having the characteristics of a phoneme.

**phonendoscope** (fo-nend′o-skōp) [ phon- + G. *endon*, within, + *skopeō*, to view ]. A stethoscope which, by means of two parallel plates of guttapercha, one resting on the patient's chest or attached to a stethoscope tube, the other vibrating in unison with it, intensifies the auscultatory sounds.

**phonetic** (fo-net′ik) [ G. *phōnētikos* ]. Relating to speech or to the voice. See also phonic.

**phonetics** (fo-net′iks). Phonology; the science of speech and of pronunciation.

**phoniatrics** (fo-nĭ-at′riks) [ phon- + G. *iatrikos*, of the healing art ]. The study of speech habits; the science of speech.

**phonic** (fo′nik). Relating to sound or to the voice. See also phonetic.

**pho′nism.** Auditory synesthesia; a synesthetic auditory sensation.

**phono-, phon-** (fo′no-) [ G. *phone*, sound, voice ]. Combining forms relating to sound, speech, or voice sounds.

**phonocar′diogram.** A record of the heart sounds made by means of a phonocardiograph.

**phonocard′iograph.** An instrument for graphically recording the heart sounds. See phonocardiography.

  **linear p.,** one that records all chest wall vibrations resulting from cardiac activity with emphasis on low frequency vibrations.

  **logarithmic p.,** one that records only audible vibrations with emphasis on the higher frequencies.

  **spectral p.,** an instrument for recording the heart sounds in which the electrical changes created by the latter pass from a microphone through a series of filters, each of which is tuned to a particular frequency band. The output from each filter is led to and activates a separate light which shines with varying brightness according to the intensity of the sound transmitted through the corresponding filter. The lights are arranged vertically in descending order of frequencies. A record is obtained by photographing the vertical row of lights.

  **stethoscopic p.,** one that records all sound vibrations, audible and inaudible, conveyed by the stethoscope, but very slow vibrations are filtered out.

**phonocardiography** (fo′no-kar-dĭ-og′ră-fĭ) [ phono- + G. *kardia*, heart, + *graphō*, to record ]. Recording of the heart sounds, or the science of interpreting phonocardiograms. The sounds excite a microphone and are first amplified through an amplifier, then filtered, and finally displayed on an oscilloscope or recorded on a tracing ( *i.e.,* phonocardiogram).

**pho′nocath′eter.** A cardiac catheter with diminutive microphone housed in its tip, for recording sounds and murmurs from within the heart and great vessels.

**phonogram** (fo′no-gram) [ phono- + G. *gramma*, diagram ]. A graphic curve depicting the duration and intensity of a sound.

**phonology** (fo-nol′o-jĭ) [ phono- + G. *logos*, study ]. Phonetics.

**phonoma′nia** [ G. *phonos*, murder, + *mania*, frenzy ]. Homicidal mania.

**phonomassage** (fo-no-mă-sahzh′). The imparting of movements to the ossicles by means of loud noises directed into the external auditory meatus.

**phonometer** (fo-nom′e-ter) [ phono- + G. *metron*, measure ]. An instrument for measuring the pitch and intensity of sounds.

**phonomyoclonus** (fo-no-mi-ok′lo-nus) [ phono- + G. *mys*, muscle, + *klonos*, tumult ]. A condition in which fibrillary muscular contractions are present, as evidenced by the sound heard on auscultation, even though not visible.

**phonomyography** (fo-no-mi-og′ră-fĭ) [ phono- + G. *mys*, muscle, + *graphē*, drawing ]. The recording of the varying sounds made by contracting muscular tissue.

**phonopathy** (fo-nop′ă-thĭ) [ phono- + G. *pathos*, suffering ]. Any disease of the vocal organs affecting speech.

**phonophobia** (fo-no-fo′bĭ-ah) [ phono- + G. *phobos*, fear ]. Morbid fear of one's own voice, or of any sound.

**phonophore** (fo′no-fōr) [ phono- + G. *phoros*, carrying ]. A form of binaural stethoscope with a bell-shaped chest piece into which project the recurved extremities of the sound tubes.

**pho′nophotog′raphy** [ phono- + photography ]. The recording on a moving photographic plate of the movements imparted to a diaphragm by sound waves.

**phonopneumomassage** (fo′no-nu′mo-mă-sahzh′) [ phono- + G. *pneuma*, air, + massage ]. Phonomassage combined with the forcing of a jet of air into the external auditory meatus.

**phonopsia** (fo-nop′sĭ-ah) [ phono- + G. *opsis*, vision ]. A condition in which the hearing of certain sounds gives rise to a subjective sensation of color.

**pho′norecep′tor.** A receptor for sound stimuli.

**phonorenogram** (fo′no-re′no-gram). A sound tracing of the renal arterial pulse recorded by means of a phonocatheter placed in the renal pelvis.

**pho′noscope** (fo′no-skōp) [ phono- + G. *skopeō*, to view ]. An instrument for photographing the heart sounds; the vibrations are transmitted to a film of soap with a silvered glass thread attached, and the movements of the latter are recorded on a photographic plate.

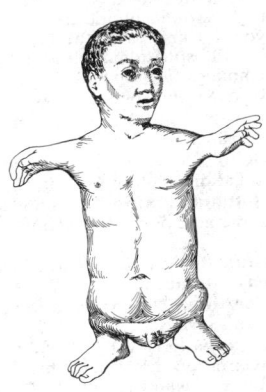

**Phocomelus**
(After Broman, from Patten, B. M.: *Human Embryology*, McGraw-Hill Book Co., New York, 1953.)

**phonoscopy** (fo-nos′ko-pī). The recording of the heart sounds by means of the phonoscope.

**phor-.** See phoro-.

**phoradendron** (fo-rä-den′dron) [ phor- + G. *dendron*, tree ]. American mistletoe, *Phoradendron flavescens* (family Loranthaceae); has been used as an oxytocic and emmenagogue.

**phorbin.** The parent hydrocarbon of the porphyrin derivative found in chlorophyll; differs from porphin in the presence of an isocyclic ring between the 6 position and the γ-methylidyne bridge, saturation of the 7–8 double bond, and shift of an H atom from N in ring IV to that in ring I (with realignment of conjugated double bonds).

**phoresis** (fōr′e-sis, fo-re′sis) [ G. *phorēsis*, a being borne ]. 1. The movement of ions under the influence of electric current; see also electrophoresis. 2. Epizoic commensalism; a biological association in which one animal is transported by another, as in the attachment of the eggs of *Dermatobia hominis*, a human and cattle botfly, to the legs of a mosquito, which transports them to the botfly (as well as the mosquito) host.

**phoria** (fōr′i-ah) [ G. *phora*, a carrying, motion. PHER- ]. The relative directions assumed by the eyes during binocular fixation of a given object in the absence of an adequate fusion stimulus; see anisophoria, cyclophoria, esophoria, exophoria, heterophoria, hyperphoria, hypophoria, orthophoria.

**phoriascope** (fōr′i-ă-skōp) [ G. *phora*, a carrying, motion, + *skopeō*, to view ]. An instrument containing prisms for use in visual training.

**Phor′mia regi′na.** The black blowfly, the larvae of which were formerly used in the treatment of septic wounds; they secrete a proteolytic enzyme that aids in the removal of dead tissue. This blowfly is also a frequent cause of maggot infestation of sheep, depositing eggs in the wool, and is a widely distributed cold weather species that lays its eggs on dead or decaying tissues.

**phoro-, phor-** (fōr′o-) [ G. *phoros*, carrying, bearing. PHER- ]. Combining forms meaning a carrying or bearing; denoting a carrier or bearer; or relating to phoria, *q.v.*

**phorocyte** (fōr′o-sīt) [ phoro- + G. *kytos*, cell ]. Obsolete designation for connective tissue cell.

**phorometer** (fo-rom′e-ter) [ phoro- + G. *metron*, measure ]. Originally, an apparatus to test oculomotor balance; now usually used as a synonym for phoro-optometer.

**phoro-optometer** (fo′ro-op-tom′e-ter). An instrument for determining phorias, ductions, and refractive states of the eyes.

**phoroscope** (fōr′o-skōp) [ phoro- + G. *skopeō*, to view ]. An instrument for reproducing an image, as a photograph, conveyed by electric or other procedures not necessarily optical, from a distance.

**phorotone** (fōr′o-tōn) [ phoro- + G. *tonos*, tension ]. A prism for exercising the eye muscles in cases of imbalance.

**phorozoon** (fōr′o-zo′on) [ phoro- + G. *zōon*, animal ]. The nonsexual generation in the life history of an animal organism which passes through several phases of existence.

**phos-** (fos-) [ G. *phōs*, light ]. Combined form denoting light.

**phose** (fōz) [ G. *phōs*, light ]. A subjective perception of a bright spot or patch.

**phosgene** (fos′jēn) [ G. *phōs*, light, + root GEN, to produce ]. Carbonyl chloride; $COCl_2$. At ordinary temperatures an extremely poisonous gas; below 8°C. (46.4°F.) a colorless liquid.

**phosgen′ic.** Light-producing.

**pho′sis.** Any condition causing the production of a phose.

**phosph-, phospho-, phosphor-.** Prefixes indicating presence of phosphorus in a compound. See also phospho- for specific usage of that prefix.

**phos′phagen.** Creatine phosphate.

**phos′phagen′ic.** Phosphate-producing.

**phospham′ic acid.** $R—NH—PO_3H$, one of the three types of "high energy" phosphate compounds. See also phosphoamide.

**phospham′idase.** Phosphoamidase.

**phosphastat** (fos′fă-stat) [ phosphate + L. *status*, a standing ]. Mechanism whereby the parathyroid hormone is increased when the levels of phosphorus increase above normal. A conceptual mechanism; there is as yet no satisfactory evidence for its existence.

**phos′phatase** (EC sub-subclass 3.1.3). Any of a group of enzymes that liberate inorganic phosphate from phosphoric esters.

**acid p.** (EC 3.1.3.2), a p. with an optimum pH of 5.4, notably present in prostate.

**alkaline p.** (EC 3.1.3.1), a p. with an optimum pH of 8.6, present ubiquitously.

**phosphorylase p.,** see under phosphorylase.

**phosphate** (fos′fāt). A salt or ester of phosphoric acid. For individual p.'s not listed here, see under the name of the base.

**alkaline p.,** the p. of sodium or of potassium; these are acid salts, but are called alkaline because they are salts of the alkali metals.

**bone p.,** calcium phosphate, tribasic.

**cyclic p.,** the salt form of a cyclic phosphoric acid; see also adenosine 3:5-cyclic phosphate.

**diba′sic p.,** a salt of phosphoric acid containing in its molecule two metal ions; *e.g.*, disodic p., $Na_2HPO_4$.

**dihydric p.,** dihydrogen p., *e.g.*, $NaH_2PO_4$.

**disodium p.,** alkaline sodium p., $Na_2HPO_4$.

**earthy p.,** a salt of phosphoric acid with one of the alkaline earths, *e.g.*, magnesium or calcium.

**energy-rich p.'s,** high-energy p.'s.

**high energy p.'s,** those p.'s which, on hydrolysis, yield an unusually high quantity of energy; *e.g.*, nucleotide polyphosphates such as ATP, enol p.'s such as phosphoenolpyruvate. See also high energy *compounds*.

**monobasic p.,** dihydric p.

**monohydric p.,** dibasic p.

**monosodic p., monosodium p.,** $NaH_2PO_4$; contains one atom of sodium; acid sodium p.; dihydric p.

**normal p.,** a salt of phosphoric acid in which all the hydrogen atoms are displaced; *e.g.*, $Na_3PO_4$, $Na_4P_2O_7$.

**organic p.,** an ester of phosphoric acid; *e.g.*, glycerophosphate, adenosine triphosphate, hexose p., etc.

**triple p.,** (1) magnesium ammonium p.; $MgNH_4PO_4$; (2) a crude phosphate fertilizer product from phosphate rock and phosphoric acid.

**phosphate acetyltransferase.** Phosphotransacetylase; phosphoacylase; enzyme (EC 2.3.1.8) catalyzing transfer of acetyl from acetyl-CoA to acetyl phosphate (phosphate from inorganic phosphate).

**phos′phated.** Containing phosphates.

**phosphatemia** (fos-fă-te′mi-ah) [ phosphate + G. *haima*, blood ]. An abnormally high concentration of inorganic phosphates in the blood.

**phosphat′ic.** Relating to or containing phosphates.

**phosphati′dal.** Condensation of acetal phosphatid(at)e; now termed alk-1-enylglycerol.

**phosphatidase.** Phospholipase $A_2$.

**phosphatidate.** A salt or ester of a phosphatidic acid.

**phosphatidic acid** (fos′fă-tid′ik). A phosphoglyceride; a derivative of glycerophosphoric acid in which the two remaining hydroxyl groups of the glycerol are esterified with fatty acids. Phosphatidic acids attached to choline are phosphatidylcholines (lecithins), etc.

**phosphatidolipase.** Phospholipase $A_2$.

**phosphatidyl.** The radical of a phosphatidic acid (*e.g.*, phosphatidylcholine).

**phosphati′dylcho′line.** Lecithin; the condensation product of a phosphatidic acid and choline.

**phosphati′dylethanol′amine.** The condensation product of a phosphatidic acid and ethanolamine; formerly called cephalin.

**phosphati′dylino′sitol.** Phosphoinositide; a phosphatidic acid combined with inositol.

**phosphati′dylser′ine.** The condensation product of phosphatidic acid and serine.

**phosphaturia** (fos′fă-tu′ri-ah) [ phosphate + G. *ouron*, urine ]. A condition in which there is an excessive excretion of phosphates in the urine.

**phosphene** (fos′fēn) [ G. *phōs*, light, + *phainō*, to show ]. Sensation of light produced by mechanical or electrical stimulation of the peripheral or central optic pathway of the nervous system.

**accommodation p.,** a p. occurring during accommodation, caused by sudden relaxation of the ciliary muscle.

**phosphide** (fos'fīd). A compound of phosphorus with valence −3 (*e.g.,* sodium phosphide, Na₃P).

**phosphine** (fos'fēn, -fin). Hydrogen phosphide; phosphureted hydrogen; PH₃; a colorless, poisonous gas with a characteristic odor.

**phosphin'ico.** The divalent radical HOP(O)< found in phosphodiesters and glycerophosphinicocholine (glycerophosphocholine); doubly substituted phosphinic acid, H₂P(O)OH.

**phos'phite.** A salt of phosphorous acid.

**phospho-.** 1. See phosph-. 2. Biochemical term for *O*-phosphono-, a prefix that may replace the suffix phosphate; *e.g.,* glucose phosphate is *O*-phosphonoglucose or phosphoglucose. (See also phosphoryl, incorrectly used in this situation.)

**phosphoac'ylase.** Phosphate acetyltransferase.

**phosphoamidase** (fos'fo-am'ĭ-dās) (EC 3.9.1.1). An enzyme catalyzing the hydrolysis of phosphorus-nitrogen bonds, notably the hydrolysis of phosphocreatine to creatine and phosphoric acid.

**phosphoam'ides.** Amides of phosphoric acid (phosphoramidates); salts or esters of phosphoramidic acid, (HO)₂PO—NH₂. The best known example is creatine phosphate.

**phosphoar'ginine.** A compound of arginine with phosphoric acid containing the phosphoamide bond; a source of energy in the contraction of muscle in invertebrates, corresponding to phosphocreatine in the muscles of vertebrates.

**phosphocho'line.** Phosphorylcholine; choline phosphate; (CH₃)₃N⁺—CH₂CH₂—OPO₃H⁻.

**phosphocre'atine.** Creatine phosphate.

**phosphocreosotic** (fos'fo-kre-o-sot'ik). Relating to the action of creosote-phosphate compounds.

**phosphodiester** (fos'fo-di-es'ter). A diesterified orthophosphoric acid, RO—(PO₂H)—OR', as in the nucleic acids.

**p. hydrolases,** phosphodiesterases.

**phosphodiesterases** (fos'fo-di-es'ter-a-sez). Phosphodiester hydrolases; enzymes (EC sub-subclass 3.1.4) cleaving phosphodiester bonds, such as those between nucleotides in nucleic acids, liberating smaller poly- or oligonucleotide units or mononucleotides but not inorganic phosphate. Ribonuclease and other nucleases are phosphodiesterases.

**spleen p.,** spleen *endonuclease.*

**phosphodihydrox'yac'etone.** CH₂OH—CO—CH₂—OPO₃H₂; one of the products of the splitting of fructose 1,6-bisphosphate under the catalytic influence of aldolase; an intermediate in glucose catabolism.

**phosphodis'mutase.** An enzyme that catalyzes the transfer of a phosphate residue from one compound to another; a phosphotransferase with regeneration of donor. See also phosphoglyceromutase, mutase.

**phosphoenolpyruvic acid** (fos'fo-e'nol-pi-ru'vik). CH₂=C(OPO₃H₂)—COOH. The phosphoric ester of pyruvic acid in the latter's *enol* form; an intermediate in the conversion of glucose to pyruvic acid and an example of a high energy phosphate ester.

**1-phosphofructal'dolase.** Fructose bisphosphate aldolase.

**1-phosphofruc'toki'nase.** Enzyme (EC 2.7.1.56) catalyzing phosphorylation of fructose 1-phosphate by ATP, etc., to fructose 1,6-bisphosphate.

**6-phosphofruc'toki'nase.** Phosphohexokinase; an enzyme (EC 2.7.1.11) that catalyzes the phosphorylation of fructose 6-phosphate by ATP or UTP, etc., to fructose 1,6-bisphosphate.

**phosphogalac'toisom'erase.** Hexose-1-phosphate uridylyltransferase.

**phosphoglu'coki'nase** (EC 2.7.1.10). Glucose-1-phosphate kinase; an enzyme that, in the presence of ATP, catalyzes the phosphorylation of glucose 1-phosphate to glucose 1,6-bisphosphate; found in yeast and muscle.

**phosphoglu'comu'tase** (EC 2.7.5.1). Glucose phosphomutase; an enzyme that catalyzes the reaction, glucose 1-phosphate → glucose 6-phosphate, with glucose 1,6-bisphosphate present.

**phosphoglu'conate dehydrogenase** (EC 1.1.1.43). 6-Phosphogluconic dehydrogenase; enzyme catalyzing dehydrogenation (to NADP) of 6-phosphogluconate to 6-phospho-2-ketogluconate (see Dickens *shunt*).

**phosphogluconate oxidation pathway.** Dickens *shunt.*

**phosphoglyceracetals** (fos'fo-glis'er-as'e-tals). Plasmalogens.

**phosphoglycerate kinase** (fos'fo-glis'er-āt) (EC 2.7.2.3). An enzyme catalyzing the formation of 1,3-diphosphoglyceric acid from 3-phosphoglyceric acid and ATP.

**phosphoglyceric acid** (fos'fo-glī-sĕr'ik, -glis'er-ik). Glyceroyl phosphoric acid; glyceroyl phosphate; acid anhydride between glyceric acid and phosphoric acid; CH₂OH—CHOH—CO—OPO₃H₂; contrast glycerophosphate (glycerol phosphate), phosphoglycerides.

**phosphoglyc'erides.** Phospholipids containing glycerol phosphate (glycerophosphoric acid); see phosphatidic acid.

**phosphoglyc'eromutase** (EC 2.7.5.3). An isomerizing enzyme catalyzing the interconversion of 2-phosphoglyceric acid and 3-phosphoglyceric acid with 2,3-diphosphoglyceric acid present.

**phosphohex'oki'nase.** 6-Phosphofructokinase.

**phosphohexomutase.** Glucosephosphate isomerase.

**phosphohex'ose isom'erase.** Glucosephosphate isomerase.

**phosphoino'sitide.** Phosphatidylinositol.

**phosphoke'topen'toep'imerase.** Ribulosephosphate 3-epimerase.

**phosphoki'nase.** Phosphotransferase or kinase.

**phospholip'ase.** Lecithinase; an enzyme that catalyzes the hydrolysis of a phospholipid.

**p. A₁** (EC 3.1.1.32), an enzyme converting a lecithin to a 2-acylphosphoglyceride by splitting off the 1-acyl residue.

**p. A₂** (EC 3.1.1.4), lecithinase A; phosphatidase; phosphatidolipase; enzyme catalyzing conversion of a lecithin to a lysolecithin; also acts on phosphatidylethanolamine, choline plasmalogen and phosphatides, removing fatty acid from 2-position.

**p. B,** lysophospholipase.

**p. C** (EC 3.1.4.3), lipophosphodiesterase I; lecithinase C; *Clostridium welchii* α-toxin; *Clostridium oedematiens* β- and γ-toxins; enzyme removing choline phosphate from a phosphatidylcholine; acts also on sphingomyelin.

**p. D** (EC 3.1.4.4), lipophosphodiesterase II; lecithinase D; choline phosphatase; enzyme removing choline from a phosphatidylcholine; also acts on other phosphatides.

**phospholip'id.** A lipid containing phosphorus, thus including the lecithins and other phosphatidic acids, sphingomyelin, and plasmalogens.

**phosphomu'tase.** See phosphodismutase.

**phosphonecrosis** (fos-fo-ne-kro'sis) [ phosphorus + G. *nekrōsis,* death (necrosis) ]. Phossy *jaw.*

**phospho'nium.** The radical PR₄⁺ (compare ammonium).

**O-phosphono-.** See phospho- (2).

**phosphopen'tose isom'erase.** Ribosephosphate isomerase.

**phosphoprotein** (fos-fo-pro'te-in). A protein containing phosphate groups attached directly to the side chains of its constituent amino acids, usually to the hydroxyl group of serine; casein and vitellin are p.'s.

**phosphopyr'uvate hy'dratase.** Enolase.

**phosphor** (fos'for) [ G. *phōs,* light, + *phoros,* bearing ]. A chemical substance that transforms incident electromagnetic or radioactive energy into light, as in scintillation radioactivity determinations.

**phosphor-, phosphoro-.** See phosph-.

**phos'phorated.** Phosphureted; forming a compound with phosphorus.

**phosphorescence** (fos-fo-res'ens) [ G. *phōs,* light, + *phoros,* bearing. PHER- ]. The quality or property of emitting light without active combustion or the production of heat, generally as the result of prior exposure to radiation.

**phosphores'cent.** Having the property of phosphorescence.

**phosphorhidrosis, phosphoridrosis** (fos'for-ĭ-dro'sis) [ G. *phōs*, light, + *phoros*, bearing, + *hidrōsis*, sweating ]. Phosphorescent *sweat*.

**phosphori'bosyl-gly'cineamide syn'thetase** (EC 6.3.1.3). An enzyme that adds glycine to ribosylamine 5-phosphate and cleaves ATP to ADP in the course of purine biosynthesis.

**5-phosphoribosyl 1-pyrophosphate.** Abbreviated PPRP, or PRPP; ribose carrying a phosphate group on ribose carbon-5 and a pyrophosphate group on ribose carbon-1; an intermediate in the formation of the pyrimidine nucleotides.

**phosphori'bosyltrans'ferase.** One of a group of enzymes (EC sub-subclass 2.4.2, pentosyltransferases) that transfers ribose 5-phosphate from 5-phospho-α-D-ribosyl 1-pyrophosphate to a purine, pyrimidine, or pyridine acceptor, forming a 5'-nucleotide and inorganic pyrophosphate; important in nucleotide biosynthesis. Specific p.'s are preceded by the name of the acceptor base, *e.g.*, uracil phosphoribosyltransferase (EC 2.4.2.9).

**phosphori'buloki'nase.** An enzyme (EC 2.7.1.19) that, in the presence of ATP, catalyzes the phosphorylation of ribulose 5-phosphate to ribulose 1,5-bisphosphate, a reaction of importance in the carbon dioxide fixation cycle of photosynthesis.

**phosphori'bulose ep'imerase.** Ribulosephosphate 3-epimerase.

**phosphoric acid** (fos-fōr'ik). A solvent; dilute solutions have been used as urinary acidifiers and as dressings to remove necrotic debris. $H_3PO_4$; the NF and BP specify 85.0 to 88.0 per cent and 90.0 per cent, w/w, respectively. In dentistry, it comprises about 60 per cent of the liquid used in zinc phosphate and silicate cements.

　**cyclic p. acid,** in general, a linear polymer of phosphoric acid residues in pyrophosphate linkage in which the α and ω residues are similarly linked to make one endless loop or cyclic compound. Specifically, a generic term applied to compounds in which one phosphoric acid residue is esterified to two hydroxyl groups of a single carbon chain, as in adenosine 3':5'-phosphoric acid, adenosine 2':3'-phosphoric acid, etc.

　**dilute p. acid** (NF), 10 per cent $H_3PO_4$; a solvent.

　**glacial p. acid,** $(HPO_3)_n$; metaphosphoric acid; used as a reagent, and in the manufacture of zinc oxyphosphate cement for dentistry.

**phos'phoridro'sis.** Phosphorhidrosis.

**phos'phorism.** Chronic poisoning with phosphorus.

**phos'phorized.** Containing phosphorus.

**phosphorolysis** (fos'fo-rol'ĭ-sis). A reaction analogous to hydrolysis except that the elements of phosphoric acid, rather than of water, are added in the course of splitting a bond; the conversion of glycogen to glucose 1-phosphate is an example.

**phosphorous** (fos'fo-rus, -fōr'us). Relating to, containing, or resembling phosphorus.

　**p. acid,** $H_3PO_3$; its salts are called phosphites.

**phosphoru'ria.** 1. The passage of phosphorescent urine. 2. Phosphaturia.

**phosphorus** (fos'fo-rus) [ G. *phosphoros*, fr. *phōs*, light, + *phoros*, bearing ]. A nonmetallic chemical element with symbol P, atomic no. 15, atomic weight 30.975, occurring extensively in nature, always in combination as phosphates, phosphites, etc., and in many animal tissues—bone, muscles, and nerves. Commercially, it comes usually in sticks, colorless, of soft solid consistence, with lustrous cut surface; it has a great affinity for oxygen, inflaming in air at a temperature only a little above 100°F. and burning with an intensely bright light and great heat; at ordinary temperatures it oxidizes slowly, being luminous in the dark. P. is extremely poisonous, causing intense inflammation and fatty degeneration; repeated inhalation of p. fumes may cause necrosis of the jaw (phossy jaw). It has been used in the treatment of rickets and other bone diseases, and in neurasthenia and sexual impotence. Its use is purely empirical and the use of p. as a therapeutic agent has ceased.

　**amorphous** or **red p.,** an allotropic form of p. formed by heating ordinary p., in the absence of oxygen, to 500°F.; it occurs as an amorphous dark red mass or powder,

nonpoisonous, and much less flammable than ordinary p.; it may be reconverted to the latter by heating to 850°F. in nitrogen gas.

**phos'phorus-32.** $^{32}P$; radioactive p. isotope with atomic weight of 32; beta emitter with half-life of 14.3 days; used as tracer in study of metabolism of nucleic acids, phospholipids, phosphorylated intermediates in carbohydrate catabolism, etc.; also used in the treatment of certain diseases of osseous and hematopoietic systems.

**phosphoryl** (fos'fo-ril). The radical, $PO\equiv$, as in phosphoryl chloride, $POCl_3$. Also used as prefix signifying a phosphate (*e.g.*, phosphorylserine) in place of the correct *O*-phosphono- or phospho- (*q.v.*), or esterification with phosphoric acid (*e.g.*, phosphorylation).

**phosphorylase** (fos-fōr'ĭ-lās). 1. General term for an enzyme transferring an inorganic phosphate group to some organic acceptor, hence belonging to the transferases (*e.g.*, the hexosyltransferases, EC sub-subclass 2.4.1). Phosphotransferases involving ATP, etc., are known as kinases. 2. An enzyme (EC 2.4.1.1) that cleaves a single glucose residue from a poly(1,4-α-glucose) as glucose 1-phosphate, the phosphate coming from inorganic orthophosphate. Also known as P enzyme; muscle phosphorylase *a;* amylphosphorylase; polyphosphorylase; glycogen phosphorylase.

　**p. a,** phosphorylase (2).

　**p. b,** cleavage product of p. *a;* see p. phosphatase.

　**p. phosphatase** (EC 3.1.3.17), phosphorylase-rupturing enzyme; PR enzyme (1); an enzyme catalyzing the conversion of muscle phosphorylase *a* into muscle phosphorylase *b* by splitting the former into halves, with release of four phosphates.

**phos'phoryla'tion.** The addition of phosphate to an organic compound, such as glucose to produce glucose monophosphate, through the action of a phosphotransferase (phosphorylase) or kinase.

　**oxidative p.,** the formation of "high energy" phosphoric bonds (*e.g.*, pyrophosphates) from the energy released by the dehydrogenation (*i.e.*, oxidation) of various substrates; most notably, isocitric acid, α-ketoglutaric acid, succinic acid, and malic acid in the tricarboxylic acid cycle.

**phos'phorylcho'line.** Phosphocholine.

**phosphoser'ine.** $H_2O_3P-OCH_2CH(NH_2)COOH$; the phosphoric ester of serine.

**phosphosphingosides** (fos'fo-sfing'go-sīdz). Sphingomyelins.

**phosphosug'ar.** Phosphorylated saccharide, *e.g.*, glucose phosphate. Any sugar containing an alcoholic group esterified with phosphoric acid.

**phosphotransacetylase** (fos'fo-trans'ā-set'ĭ-lās). Phosphate acetyltransferase.

**phosphotransferase** (fos'fo-trans'fer-ās) (EC subclass 2.7). A subclass of transferases (EC class 2) transferring phosphorus-containing groups. P.'s include the "kinases" (2.7.1) transferring phosphate to alcohols, to carboxyl groups (2.7.2), to nitrogenous groups (2.7.3), or to another phosphate group (2.7.4). Phosphomutases (2.7.5) catalyze apparent intramolecular transfers. Pyrophosphotransferases (2.7.6) catalyze transfer of the pyrophosphate group. Nucleotidyltransferases (2.7.7) catalyze transfer of the nucleotide (nucleotidyl) groups (this group includes polynucleotide phosphorylase) and other similar groups (2.7.8).

**phosphotri'ose isom'erase.** Triosephosphate isomerase.

**phosphotung'stic acid.** A mixture of phosphoric and tungstic acids. Approximately 24 $WO_3$, 2 $H_3PO_4$, 48 $H_2O$. Protein precipitant and reagent for arginine, lysine, histidine, and cystine.

**phosphuria** (fos-fu'rĭ-ah). Phosphaturia.

**phosvitin** (fos-vi'tin). A phosphoprotein isolated from the vitellin of egg yolk.

**phot-.** See photo-.

**phot** [ G. *phōs* (*phōt-*), light ]. A unit of illumination: 1 p. equals 1 lumen per sq. cm. of surface.

**photalgia** (fo-tal'jĭ-ah) [ photo- + G. *algos*, pain ]. Photodynia; pain caused by light; an extreme degree of photophobia.

**photaugiaphobia** (fo-taw'jĭ-ah-fo'bĭ-ah) [ G. *phōtaugeia,* glare of light, + *phobos,* fear ]. Shrinking from a glare of light.

**photechy** (fo'tek-ĭ) [ photo- + G. *ēchō,* echo ]. The law that an irradiated body produces the same effects as the source of the radiation itself.

**photerythrous** (fo'tĕ-rith'rŭs) [ photo- + G. *erythros,* red ]. Deuteranopic.

**photesthesia** (fo-tes-the'zĭ-ah) [ photo- + G. *aisthēsis,* sensation ]. 1. The perception of light. 2. Photophobia.

**photic** (fo'tik). Relating to light.

**pho'tism.** Pseudophotesthesia; the production of a sensation of light or color by a stimulus to another sense organ, such as of hearing, taste, or touch.

**photo-, phot-** [ G. *phōs* (*phōt-*), light. PHO- ]. Combining forms relating to light.

**photoactinic** (fo'to-ak-tin'ik) [ photo- + G. *aktis,* ray ]. Relating to radiation producing both luminous and chemical effects.

**photoallergy** (fo'to-al'er-jĭ). See photosensitization.

**photoautotroph** (fo'to-aw'to-trŏf) [ photo- + G. *autos,* self, + *trophē,* nourishment ]. An organism that depends on light for its energy and principally on carbon dioxide for its carbon.

**photoau'totroph'ic.** Pertaining to a photoautotroph.

**photobacteria** (fo'to-bak-tēr'ĭ-ah). A common term for members of the genus *Photobacterium* as well as for luminescent members of other genera, such as *Lucibacterium* and *Vibrio.*

**Photobacterium** (fo'to-bak-tēr'ĭ-um). A genus of motile and nonmotile, aerobic to facultatively anaerobic bacteria (family Pseudomonadaceae) containing Gram-negative coccobacilli and occasional rods; under adverse conditions pleomorphic forms frequently occur. Motile cells have polar flagella. The metabolism of these organisms is fermentative. They are usually luminescent and occur symbiotically in tissues of luminous organs of cephalopods and deep-sea fishes and on the skin and in the intestine of some marine fish. The type species is *P. phosphoreum.*

    P. **harveyi,** *Lucibacterium harveyi.*

    P. **phosphoreum,** a luminescent species found on dead fish and in sea water. It is the type species of the genus *P.*

**photobiology** (fo'to-bi-ol'o-jĭ). The study of the effects of light upon plants and animals.

**photobiotic** (fo'to-bi-ot'ik) [ photo- + G. *bios,* life ]. Living or flourishing only in the light.

**photocatalyst** (fo'to-kat'ă-list) [ photo- + G. *katalysis,* dissolution (catalysis) ]. A substance that helps bring about a light-catalyzed reaction; *e.g.,* chlorophyll.

**photocauterization** (fo'to-kaw'ter-ĭ-za'shun). Cauterization by using x-ray, radium, or other radioactive sources.

**photoceptor** (fo'to-sep'tor). Photoreceptor.

**photochem'istry.** The branch of chemistry that treats of the chemical changes caused by or involving light, as in photography.

**photochromogen** (fo'to-kro'mo-jen) [ photo- + G. *chrōma,* color, + suffix -*gen,* producing ]. See group I *mycobacteria.*

**photocinet'ic.** Photokinetic.

**photocoagulation** (fo'to-ko-ag'u-la'shun) [ photo- + L. *coagulo,* pp. -*atus,* to curdle ]. A method by which an intense light beam is directed to a desired area of the fundus under ophthalmoscopic control; localized coagulation results from absorption of light energy and its conversion to heat. Used for retinal detachment, peripheral degeneration, neovascularization, and angiomas.

**pho'tocoag'ulator.** The apparatus used in photocoagulation.

    **laser p.,** a prepared rod of synthetic ruby which, after priming by a xenon-arc flash bulb, delivers high energy monochromatic deep red light for 0.2 millisecond; requires 1 to 5 seconds for repetition.

    **xenon-arc p.,** a beam from a high pressure xenon-arc bulb delivers radiation from the entire visible and near-infrared spectrum; applied for ¼ to 1 second, and instantaneous repetition is possible.

**photodermatitis** (fo'to-der-mă-ti'tis) [ photo- + G. *derma,* skin, + suffix -*itis,* inflammation ]. Dermatitis

caused or elicited by exposure to ultraviolet light; may be phototoxic or photoallergic, and can result from topical application, ingestion, inhalation, or injection of mediating phototoxic or photoallergic material; see also photosensitization.

**photodromy** (fo-tod'ro-mĭ) [ photo- + G. *dromos,* a running ]. In the induced or spontaneous clarification of certain suspensions the particles settle on the side nearest the light (**positive p.**) or on the dark side (**negative p.**). Compare phototaxis, phototropism.

**photodynamic** (fo'to-di-nam'ik) [ photo- + G. *dynamis,* force ]. Relating to the energy or force exerted by light.

**photodynia** (fo-to-din'ĭ-ah) [ photo- + G. *odynē,* pain ]. Photalgia.

**photodysphoria** (fo-to-dis-fōr'ĭ-ah) [ photo- + G. *dysphoria,* extreme discomfort ]. Extreme photophobia.

**photoelectricity** (fo-to-e-lek-tris'ĭ-tĭ). Electricity produced by the action of light.

**photoelectrometer** (fo-to-e-lek-trom'e-ter). A device employing a photoelectric cell for measuring the concentration of substances in solution.

**photoelectron** (fo-to-e-lek'tron). An electron set free under the influence of a ray of light.

**photoerythema** (fo'to-ĕr'ĭ-the'mah) [ photo- + G. *erythēma,* flush ]. Erythema caused by sensitivity to light.

**photoesthetic** (fo'to-es-thet'ik) [ photo- + G. *aisthēsis,* sensation ]. Sensitive to light.

**photofluorography** (fo'to-flu'or-og'ră-fĭ) [ photo- + L. *fluor,* a flow, + G. *graphē,* a writing ]. Fluorography; fluororoentgenography; recording by photographs on film of fluoroscopic views; used in mass x-ray study of lungs.

**photogastroscope** (fo'to-gas'tro-skōp) [ photo- + G. *gastēr,* stomach, + *skopeō,* to view ]. An instrument for taking photographs of the interior of the stomach.

**photogen** (fo'to-jen) [ photo- + G. suffix *gen-,* producing ]. A microorganism that produces luminescence.

**photogene** (fo'to-jēn). Obsolete term for afterimage.

**photogenesis** (fo'to-jen'ĕ-sis) [ photo- + G. *genesis,* production ]. The production of light; phosphorescence.

**photogenic, photogenous** (fo'to-jen'ik, fo-toj'ĕ-nus). Light-producing; phosphorescent.

**photohemotachometer** (fo'to-he'mo-tă-kom'e-ter) [ photo- + G. *haima,* blood, + *tachos,* speed, + *metron,* measure ]. An appliance for recording photographically the rapidity of the blood current.

**photoheterotroph** (fo'to-het'er-o-trof, -trŏf) [ photo- + G. *heteros,* other, + *trophē,* nourishment ]. An organism that depends on light for its energy and principally on organic compounds for its carbon.

**pho'tohet'erotroph'ic.** Pertaining to a heterotroph.

**photokinetic** (fo'to-kĭ-net'ik) [ photo- + G. *kinētikos,* relating to movement ]. Photocinetic; relating to movement by light.

**photokymograph** (fo'to-ki'mo-graf) [ photo- + G. *kyma,* wave, + *graphō,* to record ]. A device for moving film at a constant speed so that a continuous record of a physiologic event may be obtained, as by a beam of light shining on the film.

**photology** (fo-tol'o-jĭ) [ photo- + G. *logos,* study ]. The science of light production and energy, especially in its therapeutic application.

**photoluminescent** (fo'to-lu-mĭ-nes'ent) [ photo- + L. *lumen,* light ]. Having the ability to become luminescent upon exposure to visible light.

**photoly'ase.** See deoxydipyrimidine photolyase.

**photolysis** (fo-tol'ĭ-sis) [ photo- + G. *lysis,* dissolution ]. Decomposition of a chemical compound by the action of light.

**photolyte** (fo'to-līt). Any product of decomposition by light.

**photolytic** (fo'to-lit'ik). Pertaining to photolysis.

**photomacrography** (fo'to-mă-krog'ră-fĭ) [ photo- + G. *makros,* large, + *graphō,* to write ]. A technique for investigating and recording conditions and procedures involving small objects which ordinarily would be inspected through a loupe rather than a microscope.

**photomania** (fo'to-ma'nĭ-ah) [ photo- + G. *mania,* frenzy ]. A morbid or exaggerated desire for light.

**photometer** (fo-tom'e-ter) [ photo- + G. *metron,* measure ]. An instrument designed to measure the intensity of light or to determine the light threshold.

   **Förster's p.,** photoptometer; an instrument for determining the light threshold (introduced by Förster in 1875); it regulated the intensity of light on the screen by an adjustable diaphragm.

   **Nagel's p.,** a modified p. (introduced in 1907) in which addition of perforated plates made it possible to reduce the original light intensity.

**photom'etry.** The measurement of the intensity of light.

**photomicrograph** (fo'to-mi'kro-graf) [ photo- + G. *mikros,* small, + *graphē,* a record ]. Micrograph; an enlarged photograph of an object viewed with a microscope; distinguished from microphotograph, *q. v.*

**photomicrography** (fo'to-mi-krog'ră-fĭ). The production of a photomicrograph.

**photomyoclonus** (fo'to-mi-ok'lo-nus) [ photo- + G. *mys,* muscle, + *klonos,* confused motion ]. Clonic spasms of muscles in response to visual stimuli.

   **hereditary p.,** p. associated with diabetes mellitus, deafness, nephropathy, and cerebral dyfunction.

**pho'ton.** 1. Troland. 2. In physics, a corpuscle or particle of light; a quantum of light.

**photoncia** (fo-ton'sĭ-ah) [ photo- + G. *onkos,* a mass (tumor) ]. Any swelling resulting from the intense action of light.

**photonosus** (fo-ton'o-sus) [ photo- + G. *nosos,* disease ]. Photopathy; any disease caused by prolonged exposure to intense light.

**photopathy** (fo-top'ă-thĭ) [ photo- + G. *pathos,* suffering ]. Photonosus.

**photoperceptive** (fo'to-per-sep'tiv). Capable of both receiving and perceiving light.

**photoperiodism** (fo'to-pēr'ĭ-o-dizm). The periodic (seasonal or diurnal) activities, behavior, or changes in plants or animals brought about by the action of light.

**photophobia** (fo'to-fo'bĭ-ah) [ photo- + G. *phobos,* fear ]. 1. Abnormal sensitiveness to light, especially of the eyes. 2. Morbid dread and avoidance of light places.

**photopho'bic.** Relating to or suffering from photophobia.

**photophore** (fo'to-fōr) [ photo- + G. *phoros,* bearing ]. A lamp with reflector used in laryngoscopy and in the examination of other internal parts of the body.

**photophos'phoryla'tion.** Formation of ATP as a result of absorption of light by chloroplast material.

**photophthalmia** (fo'tof-thal'mĭ-ah) [ photo- + G. *ophthalmos,* eye ]. The inflammatory reaction caused by short-waved light on the external parts of the eye, as in snow blindness, exposure to ultraviolet lamp, arc welding, or short circuit of a high tension electric current.

**photopia** (fo-to'pĭ-ah) [ photo- + G. *opsis,* vision ]. Photopic *vision.*

**photop'ic.** Pertaining to photopic vision, *q. v.* under vision.

**photopsia, photopsy** (fo-top'sĭ-ah, -top-sĭ) [ photo- + G. *opsis,* vision ]. A subjective sensation of lights, sparks, or colors due to retinal or cerebral disease; see also Moore's lightning *streaks.*

**photop'sin.** The protein moiety (opsin) of the pigment (iodopsin) in the cones of the retina.

**photoptarmosis** (fo'to-tar-mo'sis) [ photo- + G. *ptarmos,* a sneezing, + suffix -*osis,* condition ]. Reflex sneezing occurring when bright light reaches the retina.

**photoptometer** (fo'top-tom'e-ter) [ photo- + optometer ]. Förster's *photometer.*

**photoptometry** (fo'top-tom'e-trĭ) [ photo- + optometry ]. Determination of the light threshold; see also photometry.

**photoradiometer** (fo'to-ra-dĭ-om'e-ter) [ photo- + L. *radius,* a ray, + G. *metron,* measure ]. An instrument for determining the penetrating power of radiation.

**photoreaction** (fo'to-re-ak'shun). A reaction caused or affected by light, *e.g.,* a photochemical reaction, photolysis, photosynthesis, phototrophy, or thymine dimer formation.

**photoreactivation** (fo'to-re-ak-tĭ-va'shun). Activation by light of something or of some process previously inactive or inactivated; see photoreactivating *enzyme.*

**photoreceptive** (fo'to-re-sep'tiv). Functioning as a photoreceptor.

**photoreceptor** (fo'to-re-sep'tor) [ photo- + L. *re-cipio,* pp. -*ceptus,* to receive, fr. *capio,* to take ]. Photoceptor; a receptor that is sensitive to light, *e.g.,* a retinal rod or cone.

**photoretinitis** (fo'to-ret'ĭ-ni'tis). See photoretinopathy.

**photoretinopathy** (fo'to-ret'ĭ-nop'ă-thĭ) [ photo- + retina, + G. *pathos,* suffering ]. Electric or solar retinopathy; a macular burn from excessive exposure to sunlight or other intense light (as in the flash of a short circuit); characterized subjectively by a central positive scotoma. See also eclipse *amblyopia.*

**photoscan** (fo'to-skan). Scintiscan; gammagram; the photographic display of the distribution of an internally administered radiopharmaceutical.

**photoscope** (fo'to-skōp) [ photo- + G. *skopeō,* to view ]. Fluoroscope.

**photoscopy** (fo-tos'ko-pĭ). Fluoroscopy.

**pho'tosensitiza'tion.** 1. Sensitization of the skin to light, due, usually, to the action of certain drugs (or plants, or other substances); may occur shortly after administration of the drug (phototoxic sensitivity), or may occur only after a latent period of from days to months (photoallergic sensitivity, or photoallergy). 2. Photodynamic *sensitization.*

**photosen'sor.** Photocells, mounted on each side of a trial-frame cell, used as the eye-movement monitor in a method of oculography; see also photosensor *oculography.*

**photo-shootur.** Camelpox.

**photostable** (fo'to-sta'bl). Not subject to change upon exposure to light.

**photostethoscope** (fo'to-steth'o-skōp). A device that converts sound into flashes of light; used for continuous observation of the fetal heart.

**pho'tostress.** Exposure to intense light; see also p. *test.*

**photosynthesis** (fo-to-sin'thĕ-sis) [ photo- + G. *synthesis,* a putting together ]. The compounding or building up of chemical substances under the influence of light; in particular, the process by which green plants, using chlorophyll and the energy of sunlight, produce carbohydrate out of water and carbon dioxide, liberating molecular oxygen in the process.

**phototaxis** (fo'to-tak'sis) [ photo- + G. *taxis,* orderly arrangement ]. Reaction of living protoplasm to the stimulus of light, whereby the animal or plant is attracted (positive p.) or repelled (negative p.) by a luminous body; involving bodily motion of the organism (usually of microscopic size) toward or away from the stimulus.

**photother'apy.** Treatment of disease by means of light rays.

**photother'mal** [ photo- + G. *thermē,* heat ]. Relating to radiant heat.

**phototonus** (fo-tot'o-nus) [ photo- + G. *tonos,* tension ]. The sensitivity to light.

**phototox'ic.** Relating to, characterized by, or causing phototoxis.

**phototoxis** (fo'to-tok'sis) [ photo- + G. *toxikon,* poison ]. The condition resulting from an overexposure to ultraviolet light, or from the combination of exposure to certain wavelengths of light and a phototoxic substance. See also photosensitization.

**phototropism** (fo-tot'ro-pizm) [ photo- + G. *tropē,* a turning ]. The movement of an organism toward or away from light; differing from phototaxis in that the motion is of parts of the organism (leaves, stems) rather than of the organism as a whole.

**photronreflectometer** (fo'tron-re-flek-tom'e-ter). A device for measuring turbidity (turbidometric measurement).

**photuria** (fo-tu'rĭ-ah) [ photo- + G. *ouron,* urine ]. The passage of phosphorescent urine.

**phragmoplast** (frag'mo-plast) [ G. *phragma,* hedge, enclosure, + *plassō,* to form ]. Barrel-shaped enlargement of the spindle associated with formation of the new cell membrane during telophase in plant cells.

**phren** (fren) [ G. *phrēn,* the diaphragm, heart, seat of emotions, mind ]. 1. Diaphragma (2). 2. The mind.

**phren-** (fren-). See phreno-.

**phrenalgia** (frĕ-nal'jĭ-ah) [ phren- + G. *algos,* pain ]. 1. Psychalgia. 2. Pain in the diaphragm.

**phrenectomy** (frĕ-nek'to-mĭ). Phrenicectomy.

**phrenemphraxis** (fren'em-frak'sis) [ phren- + G. *emphraxis*, a stoppage ]. Phreniclasia.

**phrenetic** (frĕ-net'ik) [ G. *phrenitikos*, frenzied ]. 1. Frenzied; maniacal. 2. A maniac.

**phreni-, phrenico-** (fren'ĭ-, fren'ĭ-ko-). See phreno-.

**-phrenia** [ see phren ]. A suffix denoting relationship to (a) the diaphragm, (b) the mind.

**phrenic** (fren'ik). 1. Relating to the diaphragm. 2. Relating to the mind.

**phrenicectomy** (fren-ĭ-sek'to-mĭ) [ phreni- G. *ektomē*, excision ]. Phrenectomy; phreniconeurectomy; phrenicoexeresis; exsection of a portion of the phrenic nerve, to prevent reunion such as may follow phrenicotomy.

**phreniclasia** (fren-ĭ-kla'sĭ-ah) [ phreni- + G. *klasis*, a breaking away ]. Phrenicotripsy; crushing of a section of the phrenic nerve as a substitute for phrenicotomy.

**phrenicoexeresis** (fren-ĭ-ko-eks-er'ĕ-sis) [ phrenico- + G. *exairesis*, a taking out, fr. *haireo*, to take, grasp ]. Phrenicectomy.

**phreniconeurectomy** (fren'ĭ-ko-nu-rek'to-mĭ). Phrenicectomy.

**phrenicotomy** (fren-ĭ-kot'o-mĭ) [ phrenico- + G. *tomē*, incision ]. Section of the phrenic nerve in order to induce unilateral paralysis of the diaphragm, which is then pushed up by the abdominal viscera and exerts compression upon a diseased lung.

**phrenicotripsy** (fren'ĭ-ko-trip'sĭ) [ phrenico- + G. *tripsis*, a rubbing ]. Phreniclasia.

**phrenitis** (frĕ-ni'tis) [ phren- + suffix -*itis*, inflammation ]. 1. Encephalitis. 2. Delirium.

**phreno-, phren-, phreni-, phrenico-** (fren'o-) [ G. *phren*, (1) diaphragm; (2) mind, heart (as seat of emotions) ]. Combining forms meaning diaphragm, mind, phrenic (*e.g.*, phrenic nerve).

**phrenocardia** (fren'o-kar'dĭ-ah) [ phreno- + G. *kardia*, heart ]. Cardiophrenia; precordial pain and dyspnea of psychogenic origin, often a symptom of anxiety neurosis.

**phrenocolic** (fren'o-kol'ik) [ phreno- + G. *kolon*, colon ]. Relating to the diaphragm and the colon.

**phrenocolopexy** (fren'o-kol'o-pek'sĭ, -ko'lo-) [ phreno- + G. *kolon*, colon, + *pēxis*, fixation ]. Suture of a displaced or prolapsed transverse colon to the diaphragm.

**phrenogastric** (fren-o-gas'trik) [ phreno- + G. *gastēr*, stomach ]. Relating to the diaphragm and the stomach.

**phrenoglottic** (fren'o-glot'ik) [ phreno- + G. *glōttis*, glottis ]. Relating to the diaphragm and the glottis; denoting a spasm involving the diaphragm and the vocal cords.

**phrenograph** (fren'o-graf) [ phreno- + G. *graphō*, to record ]. An instrument for recording graphically the movements of the diaphragm.

**phrenohepatic** (fren'o-hĕ-pat'ik) [ phreno- + G. *hepar*, liver ]. Relating to the diaphragm and the liver.

**phrenol'ogist** [ see phrenology ]. One who claims to be able to diagnose mental and behavioral characteristics by a study of the external configuration of the skull.

**phrenology** (frĕ-nol'o-jĭ) [ phreno- + G. *logos*, study ]. Craniognomy; Gall's craniology; an obsolete doctrine, according to which each of the mental faculties is located in a definite part of the cerebral cortex, the size of which part varies in a direct ratio with the development of the corresponding faculty, this size being indicated by the external configuration of the skull.

**phrenopathy** (frĕ-nop'ă-thĭ) [ phren- + G. *pathos*, suffering ]. Any emotional or mental disorder.

**phrenoplegia** (fren'o-ple'jĭ-ah) [ phreno- + G. *plēgē*, stroke ]. 1. A psychosis of sudden onset. 2. Paralysis of the diaphragm.

**phrenoptosia** (fren-op-to'sĭ-ah) [ phreno- + G. *ptōsis*, a falling ]. An abnormal sinking down of the diaphragm.

**phrenosin** (fren'o-sin). Cerebron; cerebrin (2); a cerebroside abundant in white matter of the brain, composed of phrenosinic acid, galactose, and sphingosine.

**phrenosinic acid** (fren'o-sin'ik). Cerebronic acid.

**phrenospasm** (fren'o-spazm) [ phreno- + G. *spasmos*, spasm ]. Cardiospasm.

**phrenosplenic** (fren'o-splen'ik) [ phreno- + G. *splēn*, spleen ]. Relating to the diaphragm and the spleen.

**phrenotropic** (fren'o-trop'ik) [ phreno- + G. *tropē*, a turning ]. Affecting or working through the mind or brain; literally, turning brainward.

**phrictopathic** (frik'to-path'ik) [ G. *phriktos*, causing a shudder, fr. *phrissō*, to bristle, shudder, + *pathos*, suffering ]. Relating to a peculiar sensation, accompanied by shuddering, provoked by stimulation of a hysterical anesthetic area during the process of recovery.

**phry'nin** [ G. *phrynos*, toad ]. A substance contained in the skin secretion of the toad which is an intense irritant of the mucous membranes.

**phrynoderma** (frin'o-der'mah) [ G. *phrynos*, toad, + *derma*, skin ]. A follicular hyperkeratotic eruption thought to be due to deficiency of vitamin A.

**phrynolysin** (fri-nol'ĭ-sin) [ G. *phrynos*, toad, + *lysis*, solution ]. The poison of the fire-toad.

**PHS.** Abbreviation for Public Health Service (of the U. S. Department of Health, Education and Welfare); see under *health*.

**pH-stat.** A device for continuously sensing the pH of a solution and automatically adding acid or alkali as necessary to keep the pH constant; used to follow the time-course of reactions which liberate an acid or alkali.

**phthalein** (thal'e-in). One of a group of highly colored compounds of which phenolphthalein is the best known example.

**phthalic acid** (thal'ik). *o*-Benzenedicarboxylic acid; $C_6H_4(COOH)_2$.

**phthaline** (thal'ēn). One of a number of colorless compounds related to the phthaleins.

*N*-**phthaloyl-** (thal'o-il-). The radical of phthalic acid.

**phthal'ylhydrazines.** A group of tuberculostatic synthetic compounds, such as *N,N* ′-phthalylhydrazine.

**phthal'ylsulfacet'amide.** TALSUTIN; a sulfonamide that is not absorbed from the gastrointestinal tract but is diffused into the intestinal wall; used in the treatment of enteric infections.

**phthal'ylsulf'athi'azole** (BP). SULFATHALIDINE; 2-(*N*₄-phthalylsulfanilamido)thiazole. A sulfonamide for gastrointestinal antisepsis.

**phthinoid** (thin'oyd) [ G. *phthinōdēs*, consumptive. PHTH- ]. Wasting; consumptive; relating to or resembling phthisis.

**phthiocol** (thi'o-kol). 2-Methyl-3-hydroxy-1,4-naphthoquinone; a compound with slight antihemorrhagic activity isolated from *Mycobacterium tuberculosis*. This compound is also antituberculous.

**phthioic acid** (thi-o'ik). A mixture of methyl-branched long chain fatty acids obtained from tubercle bacilli.

**phthiremia** (thi-re'mĭ-ah) [ G. *phtheirō*, to destroy, corrupt, + *haima*, blood ]. A morbid state of the blood.

**phthiriasis** (thi-ri'ă-sis) [ G. *phtheiriasis*, fr. *phtheir*, a louse ]. Pediculosis.

 **p. cap'itis,** *pediculosis* capitis.

 **p. cor'poris,** *pediculosis* corporis.

 **p. pubis,** presence of crab lice.

**Phthirus** (thi'rus) [ L. *phthir*; G. *phtheir*, a louse ]. A genus of lice, family Pediculidae.

 **P. pu'bis,** *Pediculis pubis*; crab or pubic louse; a parasite infesting the pubis and neighboring hairy parts of the body. See fig. on p. 1084.

**phthisic** (tiz'ik) [ G. *phthisikos*, consumptive ]. Tisic. 1. Phthisis. 2. Formerly also asthma. 3. Relating to phthisis. 4. A sufferer from phthisis, or, formerly also, from asthma.

**phthisical** (tiz'ĭ-kal). Relating to or suffering from phthisis.

**phthisicky** (tiz'ĭ-kĭ). 1. Phthisical. 2. Asthmatic.

**phthisio-** (tiz'ĭ-o-) [ G. *phthisis*, a wasting. PHTH- ]. Combining form relating to phthisis, or to tuberculosis.

**phthisiologist** (tiz-ĭ-ol'o-jist). A phthisiotherapist; one versed in phthisiology; a specialist in the prevention and treatment of tuberculosis (phthisis).

**phthisiology** (tiz-ĭ-ol'-o-jĭ). The branch of medical science that treats of tuberculosis (phthisis) in all its relations.

**phthisiophobia** (tiz'-ĭ-o-fo'bĭ-ah). Morbid fear of tuberculosis.

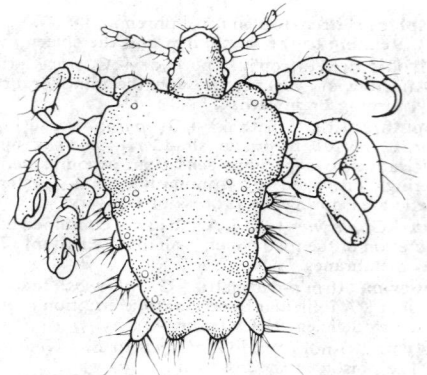

**Phthirus pubis, the Pubic Louse (×25)**
(From Najarian, H. H.: *Textbook of Medical Parasitology*,
The Williams & Wilkins Co., Baltimore, 1967.)

**phthisiotherapeutic** (tiz-ĭ-o-thĕr-ă-pu′tik). Relating to the treatment of tuberculosis (phthisis).

**phthisiotherapeutics** (tiz-ĭ-o-thĕr-ă-pu′tiks). Phthisiotherapy.

**phthisiotherapist** (tiz-ĭ-o-thĕr′ă-pist). Phthisiologist.

**phthisiotherapy** (tiz-ĭ-o-thĕr′ă-pī). Phthisiotherapeutics; the treatment of tuberculosis (phthisis).

**phthisis** (ti′sis, te′sis, thi′sis, the′sis) [ G. a wasting. PHTH- ]. 1. A wasting or atrophy, local or general. 2. An obsolete term for consumption, or specifically, tuberculosis of the lungs.

  **abdominal p.** intestinal tuberculosis; see *tabes* mesenterica.

  **aneurysmal p.,** the clinical picture of chest pain, cough with sputum, and hemoptysis sometimes produced by aortic aneurysm.

  **black p.,** anthracosis.

  **p. bulbi,** shrinking of the eyeball following uveitis or other inflammatory disease.

  **colliers′ p.,** anthracosis.

  **essential p. bulbi,** a softening of the eyeball (ophthalmomalacia) and reduction in size, not due to inflammation.

  **fibroid p.,** pulmonary tuberculosis with hyperplasia of connective tissue in the lung.

  **file cutters′ p.,** siderosis.

  **flax dressers′ p.,** pneumoconiosis; byssinosis.

  **p. flor′ida,** acute fulminant tuberculosis; so-called galloping consumption.

  **glandular p.,** cervical adenitis; tuberculous inflammation of the lymph glands, especially in the neck.

  **grinder′s p.,** siderosis; silicosis.

  **p. incip′iens,** the primary stage of pulmonary tuberculosis.

  **laryngeal p.,** tuberculosis of the larynx.

  **marble cutters′ p.,** calcicosis.

  **miners′ p.,** anthracosis.

  **p. nodo′sa,** miliary *tuberculosis.*

  **p. phlegmat′ica,** tuberculosis with little systemic reaction.

  **potters′ p.,** silicosis.

  **stonecutters′ p.,** pneumoconiosis.

  **p. ventric′uli,** tuberculosis of the stomach.

**phyco-** (fi′ko-) [ G. *phykos,* seaweed ]. Combining form relating to seaweed.

**phycobilins** (fi′ko-bil′inz, -bi′linz). Noncyclic tetrapyrroles, similar to bilirubin, found in chloroplasts of certain algae.

**phycochrome** (fi′ko-krōm) [ phyco- + G. *chrōma,* color ]. A bluish green coloring matter from certain algae.

**phy′cocy′anin** [ phyco- + G. *kyanos,* blue ]. A blue chromoprotein found in certain algae. The chromophore is a bile pigment.

**phy′coeryth′rin** [ phyco- + G. *erythros,* red ]. A red chromoprotein found in red algae. The chromophore is a bile pigment.

**Phycomycetes** (fi′ko-mi-se′tēz) [ phyco- + G. *mykēs,* fungus ]. Old name for Zygomycetes.

**phycomycetosis** (fi′ko-mi-se-to′sis). Infection by Phycomycetes (Zygomycetes); see also phycomycosis.

**phycomycosis** (fi′ko-mi-ko′sis). An infectious disease caused by fungi of the class Phycomycetes (Zygomycetes). Because these fungi are common saprophytes found in nature, infection is usually seen in patients with various predisposing conditions, such as diabetes mellitus, blood dyscrasias, malignancy, prolonged antibiotic or steroid therapy, etc. Species of the following genera may be involved: *Rhizopus, Mucor, Absidia,* and *Cunninghamella.* The genera *Entomophthora* and *Basidobolus* are causative agents.

**phygogalac′tic** [ G. *phygē,* flight, + *gala* (*galakt*-), milk ]. 1. Lactifuge; galactophygous; ischogalactic; checking the secretion of milk. 2. Lactifuge; an agent that lessens or arrests the secretion of milk.

**phylacagogic** (fi-lak-ă-goj′ik) [ G. *phylaxis,* a guarding, protection, + *agogos,* leading ]. Stimulating the production of protective antibodies.

**phylaxin** (fi-lak′sin) [ see phylaxis ]. Complement, or alexin.

**phylaxis** (fi-lak′sis) [ G. a guarding, protection ]. Protection against infection.

**phyletic** (fi-let′ik) [ G. *phyletikos,* tribal, fr. *phylōn,* a tribe ]. Denoting the mode of evolution characterized by sequential changes in a single line of descent without branching of lines; one species is transformed over a period of time to give rise to a single new species.

**phyllo-** (fil′o-) [ G. *phyllon,* leaf. PHYLL- ]. Combining form meaning leaf.

**phyllochromanol** (fil′o-kro′mă-nol). Naphthcopherol; the chroman form of reduced phylloquinone (*i.e.,* of phylloquinol).

**phyllode** (fil′ōd) [ G. *phyllōdēs,* like leaves, fr. *phyllon,* leaf, + *eidos,* resemblance ]. A flattened, leaflike petiole; a term applied to any structure resembling a leaf, especially to a cross section of a neoplasm with a foliated structure.

**phylloporphyrin** (fil′o-por′fī-rin). A porphyrin derived from chlorophyll; 1,3,5,8,γ-pentamethyl-2,4-diethylporphin-7-propionic acid (position 6 is unsubstituted and the γ-carbon is methylated).

**phyllopyrrole** (fil′o-pīr′ōl). A pyrrole derivative obtained by the reduction of chlorophyll; 3-ethyl-2,4,5-trimethylpyrrole.

**phylloquinone** (fil′o-kwin′ōn, -kwi-nōn). Phylloquinone K (abbreviation, K); vitamin $K_1$ or $K_1(20)$; phytonadione; phytomenadione; 2-methyl-3-phytyl-1,4-naphthoquinone; 3-phytylmenaquinone; isolated from alfalfa; also prepared synthetically; *cf.* menaquinone.

  **p. reductase,** NAD(P)H dehydrogenase (quinone).

**phylo-** (fi′lo-) [ G. *phylon,* tribe ]. Combining form relating to tribe, race, or phylum (*q. v.*).

**phy′loanal′ysis** [ phylo- + analysis ]. 1. The study of bioracial origins. 2. A method of investigating individual and collective behavioral disorders putatively arising from impaired tensional processes.

**phylogenesis** (fi-lo-jen′e-sis) [ phylo- + G. *genesis,* origin ]. The evolutionary development of any plant or animal species; ancestral history of the individual as opposed to ontogenesis, or the development of the individual.

**phy′logenet′ic, phy′logen′ic.** Relating to phylogenesis.

**phylogeny** (fi-loj′ĕ-nī). Phylogenesis.

**phylum,** pl. **phyla** (fi′lum, fi′lah) [ Mod. L. fr. G. *phylon,* tribe ]. One of the primary divisions of the animal or vegetable kingdom, such as the Chordata or the Bryophyta; it is the division next below the subkingdom and above the subphylum.

**phyma** (fi′mah) [ G. a tumor. PHYS-1 ]. A nodule or small rounded tumor of the skin.

**phy′matoid** [ G. *phyma,* a tumor, + *eidos,* resemblance ]. Resembling a neoplasm.

**phymatorrhysin** (fi′mă-tōr′ĭ-sin) [ G. *phyma* (*phymat*-), tumor, + *rhysis,* a flowing. RHE- ]. A variety of melanin obtained from certain melanotic neoplasms, and from hair and other heavily pigmented parts.

**phymatosis** (fi'mă-to'sis). The growth or the presence of phymas or small nodules in the skin.

**phy'one** [ G. *phyō*, to bring forth, produce ]. An obsolete term for the growth hormone of the anterior lobe of the pituitary.

**phys'alif'erous.** Physaliphorous.

**physaliform** (fi-sal'ĭ-form) [ G. *physallis*, bladder, bubble, + L. *forma*, form. PHYS-2 ]. Like a bubble or small bleb.

**physaliphore** (fi-sal'ĭ-fōr) [ G. *physallis*, bladder, bubble, + *phoros*, bearing ]. A brood cell, or giant cell containing a large vacuole, in a malignant growth.

**physaliphorous** (fis'ă-lif'er-us) [ G. *physallis*, bladder, bubble, + *phoros*, bearing ]. Physaliferous; having bubbles or vacuoles.

**Physalis** (fis'ă-lis) [ G. *physallis*, bladder, bubble. PHYS-2 ]. A genus of solanaceous herbs, several species of which are used medicinally in the regions where they grow.

**physalis** (fis'ă-lis) [ G. *physallis*, a bladder ]. A vacuole in a giant cell found in certain malignant neoplasms.

**Physaloptera** (fi'să-lop'ter-ah, fis-) [ G. *physallis*, bladder, + *pteron*, wing ]. A genus of spiruroid roundworms parasitic in the stomach and duodenum of vertebrates, especially birds and mammals. They are transmitted via insect and annelid intermediate hosts and are frequently pathogenic, causing erosions and catarrhal gastritis.

    **P. caucas'ica,** a species reported in man in southern Russia.

    **P. mor'dens,** a species from tropical Africa found only rarely in the esophagus, stomach, and intestine of man (probably cases of temporary infection from ingestion of infected insects).

**physi-.** See physio-.

**physiatrics** (fiz-ĭ-at'riks) [ G. *physis*, nature, + *iatrikos*, healing. PHYS-1 ]. 1. Physiotherapy. 2. Rehabilitation management.

**physiatrist** (fiz-i'ă-trist). A physician who specializes in physical medicine.

**physic** (fiz'ik) [ G. *physikos*, natural, physical. PHYS-1 ]. 1. The art of medicine. 2. A medicine, especially a cathartic; drugs in general.

    **Culver's p.,** leptandra.

    **p. nut,** the seed of *Jatropha curcas*, which furnishes a purgative oil.

**physical** (fiz'ĭ-kal) [ Mod. L. *physicalis*, fr. G. *physikos* ]. Relating to the body, as distinguished from the mind.

**physician** (fi-zish'un) [ Fr. *physicien*, a natural philosopher ]. A practitioner of medicine; a medical man; a doctor; a person fitted by knowledge, and licensed by the proper authorities, to examine and care for the sick.

    **house p.,** the senior resident in a hospital who runs the service during the absence of the attending p. and executes his orders.

    **osteopathic p.,** a practitioner of osteopathy.

**Physick,** Philip S., Philadelphia surgeon, 1768–1837. See P.'s *operation, pouches.*

**physicochemical** (fiz'ĭ-ko-kem'ĭ-kal). Relating to both physics and chemistry, *i.e.,* to the field of physical chemistry.

**physics** (fiz'iks) [ see physic ]. The branch of science that deals with the phenomena of matter, with the changes that matter undergoes without losing its chemical identity.

**physinosis** (fiz-ĭ-no'sis) [ irregularly from G. *physikos*, physical, + *nosos*, disease ]. A disease caused by physical agents.

**physio-, physi-** (fiz'ĭ-o-) [ G. *physis*, nature. PHYS-1 ]. Combining forms meaning physical (physiological) or natural (relating to physics).

**physiogenic** (fiz'ĭ-o-jen'ik) [ physio- + G. *genesis*, origin ]. Related to or caused by physiologic activity.

**physiognomy** (fiz'ĭ-og'no-mĭ) [ physio- + G. *gnōmōn*, a judge, GNO- ]. 1. The countenance, especially regarded as an indication of the character. 2. The estimation of one's character and mental qualities by a study of the face and general bodily carriage.

**physiognosis** (fiz-ĭ-og-no'sis) [ physio- + G. *gnōsis*, knowledge ]. Diagnosis of disease based upon a study of the facial expression.

**physiologic, physiological** (fiz-ĭ-o-loj'ik, -loj'ĭ-kal). 1. Relating to physiology. 2. Normal as opposed to pathologic; denoting the various vital processes. 3. Denoting the action of a drug when given to a healthy person, as distinguished from its therapeutic action.

**physiologicoanatomical** (fiz-ĭ-o-loj'ĭ-ko-an-ă-tom'ĭ-kal). Relating to both physiology and anatomy.

**physiologist** (fiz'ĭ-ol'o-jist). One having a special knowledge of, or whose vocation is the study of, physiology.

**physiology** (fiz'ĭ-ol'o-jĭ) [ L. or G. *physiologia*, fr. G. *physis*, nature, + *logos*, study ]. The science that deals with living things, with the normal vital processes of animal and vegetable organisms.

    **comparative p.,** the science dealing with the differences in the vital processes in different species of organisms, particularly with a view to the adaptation of the processes to the specific needs of the species, to illuminating the evolutionary relationships among different species, or to establishing other interspecific generalizations and relationships.

    **developmental p.,** the study of physiologic processes in relation to embryonic development.

    **general p.,** the science of the functions or vital processes common to almost all living things, whether animal or plant, as opposed to aspects of p. peculiar to particular types of animals or plants, or to the application of p. to applied sciences such as medicine and agriculture.

    **hom'inal p.,** p. as applied to the elucidation of the normal functions of the human being.

    **pathologic p.,** physiopathology; that part of the science of disease dealing with disordered function, as distinguished from anatomical lesions.

**physiomedical** (fiz-ĭ-o-med'ĭ-kal). Denoting the use of physical rather than medicinal measures in the treatment of disease.

**physiopathic** (fiz-ĭ-o-path'ik). In neurology, denoting a functional, nonorganic affection.

**physiopathologic** (fiz'ĭ-o-path-o-loj'ik). Relating to pathologic physiology.

**physiopathology** (fiz'ĭ-o-pă-thol'o-jĭ). Pathologic *physiology.*

**physiopsychic** (fiz'ĭ-o-si'kik). Pertaining to both mind and body.

**physiopyrexia** (fiz'ĭ-o-pi-rek'sĭah) [ physio- + G. *pyrexis*, feverishness ]. Fever produced by a physical agent.

**phys'iotherapeu'tic.** Pertaining to physiotherapy.

**physiotherapy** (fiz'ĭ-o-thĕr'ă-pĭ) [ physio- + G. *therapeia*, treatment ]. physiatrics (1); physical therapy; the use of natural forces in the treatment of disease: electro-, hydro-, aero-, and mechanotherapy, massage, and therapeutic exercises.

    **oral p.,** the use of a toothbrush, interdental stimulator, floss, irrigating device, or other adjunctive aid to maintain oral health.

**physique** (fi-zēk') [ Fr. ]. Biotype; constitutional type; the physical or bodily structure; the "build."

**physis** (fi'sis) [ G. growth. PHYS-1 ]. A term sometimes used in referring to the *cartilago* epiphysialis.

**physo-** (fi'so-) [ G. *physaō*, to inflate, distend. PHYS-2 ]. Combining form denoting (1) tendency to swell or inflate; (2) relation to air or gas.

**physocele** (fi'so-sēl) [ physo- + G. *kēlē*, tumor, hernia ]. 1. A gas tumor, a circumscribed swelling due to the presence of gas. 2. A hernial sac distended with gas.

**Physocephalus sexalatus** (fi'so-sef'ah-lus seks'a-la'tus). A small spiruroid nematode in the stomach of pigs, horses, camels, rabbits, and hares. It is worldwide in distribution, and is especially prevalent in hogs.

**physocephaly** (fi'so-sef'ă-lĭ) [ physo- + G. *kephalē*, head ]. Swelling of the head resulting from introduction of air into the subcutaneous tissues.

**physohematometra** (fi'so-he-mă-to-me'trah) [ physo- + G. *haima*, blood, + *mētra*, uterus ]. Distention of the cavity of the uterus with blood and gas.

**physohydrometra** (fi'so-hi-do-me-trah) [ physo- + G. *hydōr*, water, + *mētra*, uterus ]. Distention of the cavity of the uterus with gas and a serous fluid.

**physometra** (fi'so-me'trah) [ physo- + G. *mētra*, uterus ]. Distention of the uterine cavity with air or gas.

**physopyosalpinx** (fi'so-sal'pingks) [ physo- + G. *pyon*, pus, + *salpinx*, trumpet ]. Pyosalpinx accompanied by a formation of gas in the tube.

**physostig'ma** [ G. *physa*, bellows, + *stigma*, a mark, spot, (STIG-); so called because of the shape of the stigma ]. Calabar bean; ordeal bean; the dried seed of *Physostigma venenosum* (family Leguminosae), a vine of western Africa; it contains the alkaloids physostigmine (eserine), eseramine, eseridine (geneserine) and physovenine; in toxic doses it causes vomiting, colic, salivation, sweating, dyspnea, vertigo, slow pulse, and extreme prostration.

**physostigmine** (fi'so-stig'mēn, -min) (USP). Eserine; an alkaloid of physostigma; it is a reversible inhibitor of the cholinesterases, and prevents destruction of acetylcholine; used as a cholinergic agent, and experimentally to enhance the action of acetylcholine at any of its sites of liberation.

   **p. salic'ylate** (USP, BP), eserine salicylate; used by conjunctival instillation to reduce intraocular tension in glaucoma, in the treatment of postoperative intestinal atony and urinary retention, in the management of myasthenia gravis, and to counteract excessive doses of tubocurarine. P. sulfate, with the same uses as p. salicylate, is also available (USP).

Physostigmine salicylate

**phyt-.** See phyto-.

**phytal'bumose** [ G. *phyton*, plant ]. A vegetable albumose.

**phy'tanate.** The anion of phytanic acid.

**phy'tanate α-oxidase.** An enzyme that oxidizes phytanic acid, removing the carboxyl group.

**phytan'ic acid.** 3,7,11,15-Tetramethylhexadecanoic acid that accumulates in the serum and tissues of patients with Refsum's disease and is attributed to the hereditary absence of phytanate α-oxidase. It arises from phytol and acts as an inhibitor of the α-oxidation of palmitic (hexadecanoic) acid.

**6-phytase** (fi'tās). Phytase; enzyme (EC 3.1.3.26) hydrolyzing phytate (phytic acid), the hexaphosphoric acid ester of inositol, removing the 4-phosphoric group.

**phytic acid** (fi'tik). Inositol hexaphosphoric acid; the mixed salt with Mg and Ca is phytin.

**phy'tin.** The calcium magnesium salt of phytic acid; a dietary supplement used to provide calcium, organic phosphorus, and inositol.

**phyto-, phyt-** (fi'to-) [ G. *phyton*, a plant. PHYS-1 ]. Combining form denoting relation to plants.

**phytoagglutinin** (fi'to-ă-glu'tĭ-nin). 1. A lectin. 2. An agglutinin (1) formed in response to an effective contact or appropriate experience with antigenic material from a plant form.

**phytobezoar** (fi-to-be'zōr) [ phyto- + G. bezoar, *q.v.* ]. A gastric concretion formed of vegetable fibers, with the seeds and skins of fruits, and sometimes starch granules and fat globules.

**phytochemistry** (fi'to-kem'is-trī). The biochemical study of plants; concerned with the identification, biosynthesis, and metabolism of chemical constituents of plants.

**phytocholesterol** (fi-to-ko-les'ter-ol). Phytosterol.

**Phytoflagellata** (fi'to-flaj'e-la'tah) [ phyto- + L. *flagellum*, a whip ]. A subclass of Phytomastigophora, the members of which have yellow or green chromatophores.

**phytoflu'ene.** A hexahydrolycopene, and a possible colorless precursor of the plant carotenoids.

**phy'tohemagglu'tinin.** A lectin from plants that agglutinates red blood cells; abbreviated PHA.

**phy'tohor'mones.** Plant hormones; *e.g.*, auxins.

**phytoid** (fi'toyd) [ G. *phytōdēs*, fr. *phyton*, plant, + *eidos*, resemblance ]. Resembling a plant; denoting an animal having many of the biologic characteristics of a vegetable.

**phy'tol.** An unsaturated primary alcohol derived from the hydrolysis of chlorophyll (for structure, see phytyl); used for the synthesis of vitamins E and K1.

**Phytomastigina** (fi'to-mas'tĭ-ji'nah) [ phyto- + G. *mastix*, whip ]. Class of Mastigophora, the flagellates; termed Phytomastigophorea in a recent classification.

**Phytomastigophorea** (fi'to-mas'tĭ-gof'o-re'ah) [ phyto- + G. *mastix*, whip, + *phoros*, bearing ]. Phytomastigina.

**phytomenadione** (fi'to-men'ă-di'ōn) (BP). Phylloquinone.

**phytonadione** (fi'to-na'dĭ-ōn, -nad'-) (USP). Phylloquinone.

**phytonucle'ic acid.** Obsolete for ribonucleic acid.

**phytopathogen'ic.** Causing disease in a plant.

**phytopathology** (fi'to-pă-thol'o-jĭ) [ G. *phyton*, plant ]. Vegetable pathology; the science of plant diseases.

**phytophagous** (fi-tof'ă-gus) [ phyto- + G. *phagein*, to eat ]. Plant-eating; vegetarian.

**phytophar'macol'ogy.** A branch of pharmacology dealing with the effect of drugs on plant development.

**phytophlyctodermatitis** (fi'to-flik'to-der-mă-ti'tis) [ phyto- + G. *phlyktaina*, blister, + dermatitis ]. Meadow *dermatitis*.

**phytopneumoconiosis** (fi'to-nu'mo-ko-ne-o'sis) [ phyto- + pneumoconiosis ]. A chronic fibrous reaction in the lungs due to the inhalation of dust particles of vegetable origin.

**phy'toprecip'itin.** A precipitin formed in response to the injection of a vegetable antigen.

**phytosis** (fi-to'sis) [ phyto- + G. suffix -*osis*, condition ]. Any skin eruption caused by the presence of a fungus.

**phytosphingosine** (fi'to-sfing'go-sēn, -sin). 4-D-Hydroxysphinganine; 4-hydroxydihydrosphingosine; a sphingosine derivative isolated from various plants.

**phytostearin** (fi-to-ste'ă-rin). Phytosterol.

**phytosterin** (fi-tos'ter-in). Phytosterol.

**phytosterols** (fi-tos'ter-ols). A generic term for the sterols of plants (sitosterol, stigmasterol, etc.).

**phytotox'ic.** 1. Poisonous to plant life. 2. Pertaining to phytotoxin.

**phytotoxin** (fi'to-tok'sin) [ phyto- + G. *toxikon*, poison ]. Plant *toxin*.

**phytotrichobezoar** (fi'to-trik'o-be'zōr) [ phyto- + G. *thrix*, hair, + bezoar, *q.v.* ]. Trichophytobezoar.

**phytyl** (fi'til). The radical, $-CH_2-CH=C(CH_3)-CH_2\left[-CH_2-CH_2-CH(CH_3)-CH_2-\right]_3H$, found in phylloquinone (vitamin K1 (20)). A tetraprenyl radical, reduced in 3 of the 4 prenyl groups.

**pI.** The pH value for the isoelectric point of a given substance.

**pia** (pi'ah) [ L. fem. of *pius*, tender ]. Pia mater.

**pia-arachnitis** (pi'ah-ă-rak-ni'tis). Leptomeningitis.

**pia-arachnoid** (pi'ah-ă-rak'noyd). Leptomeninges.

**pi'al.** Relating to the pia mater.

**pi'alyn** [ G. *piar*, fat, + *lyo*, to dissolve ]. Lipase.

**pia mater** (pi'ah ma'ter) [ L. tender, affectionate mother ]. A delicate, vasculated fibrous membrane firmly adherent to the glial capsule of the brain and spinal cord (membrana limitans gliae); following exactly the outer markings of the cerebrum and also the ependymal lining of the choroid membranes and plexus, it invests the cerebellum but not so intimately as it does the cerebrum, not dipping down into all the smaller sulci. The pia mater and the arachnoid are collectively called leptomeninges, as distinguished from dura mater or pachymeninx.

**pian** (pe-an' or pi'an). Yaws.

   **p. bois,** bosch yaws; bush yaws; forest yaws; a mild chronic form of New World cutaneous leishmaniasis found in forested parts of French Guiana; the etiological agent, *Leishmania guyanensis* (or *L. tropica* var. *guyanensis*) is uncertainly characterized as yet and may not prove to be a distinct entity. The disease is typical of dermal leishmani-

asis with chronic sores from the bite of infected sandflies. A small proportion of cases are said to metastasize to the nasal mucosa to produce the espundia-like involvement.
 **hemorrhagic p.,** *verruga* peruana.
**piantic** (pi-an′tik) [ G. *piantikos,* fattening ]. An obsolete term denoting sensitized and readily agglutinative microorganisms, such as have been subjected to piantication.
**piantication** (pi-an-tĭ-ka′shun) [ see piantic ]. An obsolete term denoting exaggerated sensitization of bacteria by subculturing already sensitized organisms.
**piarachnoid** (pi′ă-rak′noyd). Leptomeninges.
**piarrhemia** (pi′ă-ra′mĭ-ah) [ G. *piar,* fat, + *haima,* blood ]. Obsolete term for lipemia.
**pica** (pi′kah, pe′kah) [ L. *pica,* magpie ]. A depraved or perverted appetite; a hunger for substances not fit for food. See also *cissa.*
**Picchini's syndrome.** See under syndrome.
**piceous** (pi′se-us, pis′e-us) [ L. *piceus,* fr. *pix* (*pic-*), pitch ]. Relating to or containing pitch.
**pichi** (pe′che). Fabiana.
**Pick,** A. G. See P.'s tubular *adenoma.*
**Pick,** Arnold, Prague psychiatrist, 1851–1924. See P.'s *atrophy, bundle, disease.*
**Pick,** Friedel, Prague physician, 1867–1926. See P.'s *bodies, disease, syndrome.*
**Pick,** Ludwig, German physician, 1868–1935. See P. *cell,* Niemann-P. *cell,* Niemann-P. *disease.*
**pick′ling.** In dentistry, the process of cleansing metallic surfaces of the products of oxidation and other impurities by immersion in acid.
**pico-** (pi′ko-) [ It. *piccolo,* small ]. 1. Combining form meaning small. 2. Bicro-; prefix denoting $10^{-12}$; symbol p (replacing $\mu\mu$).
**picogram** (pi-ko-gram). Formerly micromicrogram; $10^{-12}$ gram; abbreviated pg.
**pic′oline.** 2-Methylpyridine; a base found in tobacco smoke, coal tar and other substances.
**pic′olin′ic acid.** 2-Pyridinecarboxylic acid; an isomer of nicotinic acid.
**picolinuric acid** (pik-o-lĭ-nu′rik). *N*-Picolinoylglycine; the amide, with glycerol, of picolinic acid; hippuric acid analogue in which picolinic acid, rather than benzoic acid, is conjugated with glycine and excreted.
**picometer** (pi′ko-me-ter). Bicron; micromicron; $10^{-12}$ meter; abbreviated pm.
**picornavirus** (pi-kor-nah-vi′rus). See under virus.
**picram′ic acid.** 2-Amino-4,6-dinitrophenol; red crystals sometimes found in the blood of persons poisoned with picric acid; formed as a result of partial reduction of the latter.
**Picrasma** (pĭ-kraz′mah) [ L. fr. G. *pikrasmos,* bitterness ]. See quassia.
**pic′rate.** A salt of picric acid.
**pic′ric acid** [ G. *pikros,* bitter ]. 2,4,6-Trinitrophenol; nitroxanthic acid; carbazotic acid; $C_6H_2(NO_2)_3OH$; has been used as an application in burns, eczema, erysipelas, and pruritus.
**picrocarmine** (pik-ro-kar′min, -mēn). A stain made of carmine 1, ammonia 5, distilled water 50, aqueous solution of picric acid 50. Used in histology.
**pic′rofor′mol.** A fixative containing formalin and picric acid.
**pic′romy′cin.** Pikromycin; an antibiotic principle, $C_{25}H_{43}NO_7$, obtained from cultures of a species of *Actinomyces.*
**pic′roni′grosin.** An alcoholic solution of picric acid and nigrosin, used as a histologic stain.
**picropodophyllin** (pik′ro-po-dof′ĭ-lin, -po′do-fil′in). [ G. *pikros,* bitter ]. An intensely bitter substance, isomeric with podophyllotoxin; formed from podophyllotoxin-β-D-glucoside during extraction.
 **p. glucoside,** a constituent of Indian podophyllum.
**picrorhiza** (pik′ro-ri′zah). The rhizome of *Picrorhiza kurroa* (family Scrophulariaceae); antiperiodic, laxative, and tonic.
**pic′rotin.** $C_{15}H_{18}O_7$; a dilactone breakdown product of picrotoxin; it is pharmacologically inactive.

**pic′rotox′in** [ G. *pikros,* bitter, + *toxicon,* poison ] (NF, BP). Cocculin; a very bitter neutral principle derived from the fruit of *Anamirta cocculus* (family Menispermaceae) (see also cocculus). It is an equimolar mixture of picrotoxinin and picrotin. A central nervous system stimulant, used as an antidote for poisoning by barbiturates and certain other CNS-depressant drugs.
**pic′rotox′inin.** $C_{15}H_{16}O_6$; a dilactone breakdown product of picrotoxin; pharmacological properties resemble those of picrotoxin.
**picryl** (pik′ril). Trinitrophenyl; the organic radical derived from picric acid by removal of the hydroxyl group; thus, the replacement of the hydroxyl by a chlorine atom would result in the compound p. chloride.
**pictograph** (pik′to-graf). A vision test chart for illiterates.
**PID.** Abbreviation for pelvic inflammatory *disease.*
**piebaldness** (pi′bawld-ness). Albinismus conscriptus; a term usually used to describe patchy absence of pigment of scalp hair, giving a streaked appearance; patches of vitiligo may be present in other areas.
**piedra** (pe-a′drah) [ Sp. a stone ]. A fungus disease of the hair characterized by the presence on the hairs of numerous, waxy, small, hard, nodular masses. Also called trichosporosis, *q. v.*
 **black p.,** caused by *Piedraia hortai,* and found in South America, Southeast Asia, and Indonesia.
 **p. nostras,** a condition similar to p., but affecting the hair of the beard.
 **white p.,** caused by *Trichosporon beigelii,* and found in South America, Europe, and Japan.
**Piedraia** (pi′ĕ-dri′ah) [ see piedra ]. A genus of fungi, based on *P. hortai* which is probably the only species.
 **P. hortai,** a fungus which is parasitic on human hair and causes black piedra.
**pieds terminaux** (pe-a′ ter-me-no′) [ Fr., end feet ]. Axon *terminals.*
**Pierre Robin.** See Robin, Pierre.
**piesesthesia** (pi-es-es-the′zĭ-ah) [ G. *piesis,* pressure, + *aisthēsix,* sensation ]. Pressure *sense.*
**piesimeter, piesometer** (pi-ĕ-sim′e-ter, pi-ĕ-som′e-ter) [ G. *piesis,* pressure ]. Piezometer; an instrument for measuring the degree of pressure of a gas or a fluid.
 **Hales' p.,** a glass tube inserted into an artery at right angles to its axis, the pressure being shown by the height to which the blood ascends in the tube.
**piesis** (pi′ĕ-sis) [ G. pressure ]. Blood *pressure.*
**piezochemistry** (pi-ĕ-zo-kem′is-trĭ). The study of the effect of very high pressures on chemical reactions.
**piezoelectric** (pi-ĕ-zo-e-lek′trik). Pertaining to piezoelectricity.
**piezoelectricity** (pi′ĕ-zo-e-lek-tris′ĭ-tĭ) [ G. *piezō,* to press, squeeze, + *electricity* ]. Electric currents generated by pressure upon certain crystals, *e. g.,* quartz, mica, calcite.
**piezometer** (pi-ĕ-zom′e-ter). Piesimeter.
**piezotherapy** (pi′ĕ-zo-thĕr′ă-pī) [ G. *piezō,* to press, squeeze, + *therapeia,* therapy ]. Artificial pneumothorax.
**PIF.** Abbreviation for prolactin-inhibiting *factor.*
**pig′ment** [ L. *pigmentum,* paint ]. 1. Any organic coloring matter, as that of the red blood cells, of the hair, of the iris, etc. 2. A stain for histologic or bacteriologic work. 3. A medicinal preparation for external use, applied to the skin like paint.
 **hematog′enous p.,** a p. derived from the hemoglobin of the red blood cells.
 **hepatog′enous p.,** bile p. derived from the destruction of hemoglobin in the liver.
 **melanotic p.,** melanin.
 **malarial p.,** a dark brown to black hematin derivative produced from the hemoglobin of red cells by malarial parasites.
 **respiratory p.'s,** the oxygen-carrying (colored) substances in blood and tissues (hemoglobin, myoglobin, hemocyanin, etc.).
 **visual p.'s,** the photopigments in the retinal cones (photopsins) and rods (scotopsins) that absorb light and by photochemical processes initiate the phenomenon of vision.

**wear-and-tear p.,** lipofuscin that accumulates in aging or atrophic cells as residue of lysosomal digestion.

**pigmentary** (pig′men-tĕr′ĭ). Relating to a pigment.

**pigmentation** (pig′men-ta′shun). Coloration, either normal or pathologic, of the skin or tissues by a deposit of pigment.

**arsenic p.,** generalized but spotty increased melanin p. of the skin in chronic arsenic poisoning.

**exogenous p.,** discoloration of the skin or tissues by a pigment introduced from without, as in argyria.

**pig′mented.** Colored as the result of a deposit of pigment.

**pigmentolysin** (pig′men-tol′ĭ-sin) [ L. *pigmentum,* pigment, + G. *lysis,* a loosening ]. An antibody causing destruction of pigment.

**pigmentophage** (pig-men′to-fāj) [ L. *pigmentum,* pigment, + phagocyte ]. Chromophage.

**pigmentophore** (pig′men′to-fōr) [ L. *pigmentum,* pigment, + G. *phoros,* bearing ]. Chromatophore.

**pigmen′tum** [ L. ]. Pigment.

**p. ni′grum,** Melanin of the choroid coat of the eye.

**pigmy** (pig′mĭ). Pygmy.

**Pignet** (pin-ya′), Maurice-C. J., French surgeon, *1871. See P.'s *formula.*

**pik′romy′cin.** Picromycin.

**pil.** Abbreviation of L. *pilula,* pill.

**pi′lar, pil′ary** [ L. *pilus,* a hair ]. Relating to or covered with hair.

**pilas′ter** [ Mediev. L. *pilastrum,* dim. of L. *pila,* pillar ]. An abnormally prominent linea aspera on the femur, the bone being convex anteriorly.

**pila′tion** [ L. *pilus,* a hair ]. A capillary *fracture.*

**pile.** 1 [ L. *pila,* pillar ]. A series of plates of two different metals imposed alternately one on the other, separated by a sheet of cloth or paper moistened with a dilute acid solution, used to produce a current of electricity. 2 [ L. *pila,* ball ]. An individual hemorrhoidal tumor; see hemorrhoids.

**atomic p.,** term used to express the earliest self-sustaining nuclear reactors, which were constructed of uranium and graphite piled in alternate layers.

**sentinel p.,** a circumscribed thickening of the mucous membrane at the lower end of a fissure of the anus.

**thermoelectric p.,** thermopile.

**pileous** (pi′le-us) [ L. *pilus,* hair ]. Hairy.

**piles** [ L. *pila,* a ball ]. Hemorrhoids.

**pileus** (pi′le-us) [ L. *pileum* or *pileus,* a felt cap ]. A nipple *shield.*

**p. ventric′uli** [ L. cap of the stomach ], duodenal cap.

**pi′li** [ L. ] [ NA ]. Plural of pilus.

**pilig′anine** [ fr. the plant *piligan* ]. An alkaloid from *Lycopodium saururus* (family Lycopodiaceae), a plant of Argentina. Has spasmodic, miotic, and emetic action.

**pilimiction** (pi-lĭ-mik′shun) [ L. *pilus,* hair, + *mictio,* urination ]. 1. The passage of hairs in the urine, as has been observed in cases of dermoid tumors. 2. The passage of threads of mucus in the urine.

**pill** [ L. *pilula;* dim. of *pila,* ball ]. A small globular mass of some coherent but soluble substance, containing a medicinal substance to be swallowed.

**bread p.,** a placebo made of bread crumbs or other indifferent substances.

**enteric coated p.,** one with a coating that prevents its disintegration until it has entered the intestine.

**pep p.'s,** colloquialism for tablets containing a central nervous system stimulant, especially amphetamine.

**pil′lar** [ L. *pila* ]. A structure or part having a resemblance to a column or pillar.

**anterior p. of fauces,** *arcus* palatoglossus.

**Corti's p.'s,** pillar *cells.*

**p.'s of the fauces,** *arcus* palatini.

**p.'s of the fornix,** the anterior (columna fornicis) and posterior (crus fornicis) portions of the fornix in front of and behind the corpus fornicis.

**p. of the iris,** *ligamentum* pectinatum anguli iridocornealis.

**posterior p. of fauces,** *arcus* palatopharyngeus.

**pil′let.** Pellet; a small pill.

**pillion** (pil′yon) [ Gaelic *pill,* a cover ]. A temporary artificial leg.

**pillow, Frejka.** A p. used for malposition of hip in infants.

**pill-rolling.** A circular movement of the opposed tips of the thumb and the index finger appearing as a form of tremor in paralysis agitans.

**pilo-** (pi′lo-) [ L. *pilus,* hair ]. Combining form relating to hair.

**pilobezoar** (pi′lo-be′zōr) [ pilo- + bezoar ]. Trichobezoar.

**pilocar′pidine.** A liquid alkaloid, $C_{10}H_{14}N_2O_2$, obtained from the leaves of *Pilocarpus jaborandi.*

**pilocarpine** (pi-lo-kar′pēn). An alkaloid obtained from the leaves of pilocarpus; a parasympathomimetic agent used as a diaphoretic, sialogogue, and stimulant of intestinal motility; and externally as a miotic and in the treatment of glaucoma. The official salts of p. are the hydrochloride (USP) and the nitrate (USP, BP).

**pilocar′pus** [ G. *pilos,* a felt hat, + *karpos,* fruit ]. Jaborandi; the leaves of *Pilocarpus microphyllus* or *P. jaborandi* (family Rutaceae), shrubs of the West Indies and tropical America; the source of pilocarpine, pilocarpidine, isopilocarpine, jaborine, and jaboridine; diaphoretic.

**pilocereine** (pi-los′er-ēn) [ pilo- + L. *cereus,* waxen ]. An alkaloid from *Pilocereus sargentianus* (family Cactaceae), a species of cactus.

**pilocystic** (pi′lo-sis′tik) [ pilo- + G. *kystis,* bladder ]. Denoting a dermoid cyst containing hair.

**piloerection** (pi′lo-e-rek′shun). Erection of hair due to action of arrectores pilorum muscles.

**pi′loid** [ pilo- + G. *eidos,* resemblance ]. Hairlike; resembling hair.

**pilojection** (pi′lo-jek′shun) [ pilo- + injection ]. The process of shooting shafts of stiff mammalian hair into a saccular aneurysm in the brain in order to produce thrombosis.

**pilomatrixoma** (pi′lo-ma′trik-so′mah) [ pilo- + L. *matrix,* *q.v.,* + G. suffix *-oma,* tumor ]. Malherbe's calcifying *epithelioma.*

**pi′lomo′tor** [ pilo- + L. *motor,* mover ]. Moving the hair; denoting the arrectores pilorum muscles of the skin and the postganglionic sympathetic nerve fibers innervating these small smooth muscles.

**pilonidal** (pi′lo-ni′dal) [ pilo- + L. *nidus,* nest ]. Denoting a growth of hair in a dermoid cyst or in the deeper layers of the skin. In the latter instance the misplaced hair may result from an ingrowth of cutaneous hair.

**pi′lose** [ L. *pilosus* ]. Hairy; downy; furry; covered with hair.

**pilosebaceous** (pi′lo-se-ba′shus) [ pilo- + L. *sebum,* suet ]. Relating to the hair follicles and sebaceous glands.

**pilosis** (pi-lo′sis) [ pilo- + G. suffix *-osis,* condition ]. Hirsuties.

**Piltz,** Jan, Polish neurologist, 1870–1931. See Westphal-P. *phenomenon,* P. *reflex, sign.*

**pilula,** gen. and pl. **pilulae** (pil′u-lah, -le) [ L. dim. of *pila,* a ball ]. A pill or pilule.

**pil′ular.** Relating to a pill.

**pilule** (pil′ūl) [ L. *pilula* ]. A small pill.

**pi′lus,** pl. **pi′li** [ L. ]. 1 [ NA ]. Hair; one of the fine, threadlike appendages of the skin, covering more or less thickly the entire body, except the palms and soles and the flexor surfaces of the joints. A p. consists of *radix* or root, embedded in the hair follicle, and a free portion, *scapus,* stem or shaft. 2. Fimbria (2); a fine, filamentous appendage, somewhat analogous to the flagellum, that occurs on some bacteria. Pili are shorter, straighter, and much more numerous than flagella. They consist only of protein and may be chemically similar to flagella. F pili and I pili seem to mediate bacterial conjugation (see also F *agent*); the functions of other types of pili are not known for certain.

**pi′li annula′ti,** ringed *hair.*

**pili cuniculati,** ingrown *hairs.*

**F pili,** see pilus (2).

**I pili,** see pilus (2).

**pili incarnati,** ingrown *hairs.*

**pili multigem′ini,** the presence of several hairs in a single follicle.

**pi′li tor′ti,** twisted hairs; the shafts of the hairs are twisted on the long axis, probably as a result of self-inflicted trauma. Areas of alopecia may occur.

**pimar′icin.** $C_{34}H_{49}NO_{14}$; an antifungal antibiotic produced by *Streptomyces natalensis;* effective against *Aspergillus, Candida,* and *Mucor* species. It is poorly absorbed from the gastrointestinal tract, and may cause anorexia and nausea.

**pimelic acid** (pī-mel′ik). Heptanedioic acid; $HOOC-(CH_2)_5COOH$.

**pimeli′tis** (pim-ĕ-li′tis) [ pimelo- + G. suffix *-itis,* inflammation ]. Inflammation of adipose tissue.

**pimelo-, pimel-** [ G. *pimelē,* soft fat, lard, fr. *piar,* fat ]. Combining forms meaning fat or fatty.

**pimeloma** (pim′ē-lo-mah) [ pimelo- + G. suffix *-oma,* tumor ]. Lipoma.

**pimelopterygium** (pim′ē-lo-ter-ij′ī-um) [ pimelo- + pterygium, *q. v.* ]. A pterygium containing fat, composed in part of fatty tissue.

**pimelorrhea** (pim′ē-lo-re′ah) [ pimelo- + G. *rhoia,* a flux ]. Fatty *diarrhea.*

**pimelorthopnea** (pim′ē-lor-thop′ne-ah, -ne′ah) [ pimelo- + G. *orthos,* straight, + *pnoē,* breath ]. Piorthopnea; orthopnea, or difficulty in breathing in any but the erect posture, owing to excessive adiposity.

**pimelosis** (pim′ē-lo′sis) [ pimelo- + G. suffix *-osis,* condition ]. 1. Adiposity; obesity; lipomatosis. 2. Fatty *degeneration.*

**pimeluria** (pim′ē-lu′rī-ah) (pimelo- + G. *ouron,* urine ]. Lipuria.

**pimenta** (pī-men′tah) [ Sp. fr. L. *pigmentum,* paint (Mediev. L. meaning, spice) ]. Pimento; allspice; Jamaica pepper; the dried fruit of *Pimenta officinalis* (family Myrtaceae), a tree native in Jamaica and other parts of tropical America; used as a carminative and aromatic spice.

**p. oil,** comprises 3 to 4.5 per cent of the dried fruit.

**pimen′to.** Pimenta.

**pimin′odine esylate** (NF). ALVODINE ethanesulfonate; ethyl-4-phenyl-1-[ 3- (phenylamino) propyl ]-piperidine-4-carboxylate ethanesulfonate; an analgesic chemically related to meperidine, used to relieve severe pain; its duration of action is shorter than that of morphine; it has addiction liability.

**pim′ozide** (USAN). 1-[ 1-[ 4,4-bis(*p*-Fluorophenyl)-butyl ]-4-piperidyl ]-2-benzimidazolinone; a tranquilizing drug.

**pimple** (pim′pl). A papule or small pustule.

**pin.** A metal rod used in surgical treatment of fractures.

**Steinmann p.,** a p. that is used to transfix bone for traction of fixation.

**pinacolone** (pī-nak′o-lōn). 3,3-Dimethyl-2-butanone; a yellow liquid with peppermint odor.

**pinacyanol** (pin-ă-si′ă-nol). A basic dye, $C_{25}H_{25}N_2I$, used as a color sensitizer (violet red in water, blue in alcohol) in photography and for vital staining of leukocytes.

**Pinard** (pe-nar′), Adolphe, French obstetrician, 1844–1934. See P.'s *maneuver,* sign.

**pincement** (pans-mon′) [ Fr. pinching ]. A pinching manipulation in massage.

**pine** (pin). *Pinus.*

**p. oil,** the volatile oil from the wood of *Pinus palustris* and other species of *Pinus;* used as a deodorant and disinfectant.

**p.-needle oil** (NF), a volatile oil distilled with steam from the fresh leaf of *Pinus mugo;* used by inhalation and spray in catarrhal affections of the air passages, and locally in rheumatism; also used as a flavoring and in perfumery.

**p. tar** (NF), tar (BP); liquid pitch; obtained by the destructive distillation of the wood of *Pinus palustris* and other species of pine; used internally as an expectorant, and externally in the treatment of skin diseases.

**white p.,** (1) *Pinus alba;* (2) the dried inner bark of *Pinus strobus;* used as an ingredient in cough syrups.

**pinea** [ L. ] [ NA ]. Pineal.

**pineal** (pin′e-al) [ L. *pineus,* relating to the pine, *pinus* ]. 1. Piniform; shaped like a pine cone. 2. Pertaining to the corpus pineale.

**pinealectomy** (pin-ī-ă-lek′to-mī) [ pineal + G. *ektomē.* excision ]. Removal of the pineal body.

**pinealocyte** (pī-ne′al-o-sīt) [ pineal + G. *kytos,* cell ]. Chief cell or parenchymatous cell of the corpus pineale; a cell of the pineal body with long processes ending in bulbous expansions.

**pinealoma** (pin′e-ă-lo′mah) [ pineal + G. suffix *-oma,* tumor ]. A neoplasm derived from the pineal gland, and characterized by relatively large, round or polygonal cells with a large nucleus, as well as small cells that resemble lymphocytes. P.'s are relatively rare; they are usually discrete masses that may cause hydrocephalus, as a result of pressure on the aqueduct of Sylvius, or sometimes are apparently the cause of precocious puberty, as a result of pressure or other involvement of the hypothalamic region.

**ectopic p.,** extrapineal p.; an undifferentiated neoplasm resembling a p., usually found near the pituitary gland; believed by some to be an undifferentiated teratoma.

**extrapineal p.,** ectopic p.

**pinealopathy** (pin′e-ă-lop′ăthī) [ pineal + G. *pathos,* disease ]. Disease of the pineal gland.

**pineapple** (pīn′ap-pl). The fruit of *Ananas sativa* or *Bromelia ananas* (family Bromeliaceae); it contains a proteolytic and milk-clotting enzyme, bromelain.

**Pinel** (pe-nel′), Phillippe, French psychiatrist, 1745–1826. See P.'s *system.*

**pi′nene.** α-Pinene; a constituent of pine oil and turpentine: dextropinene from the American and levopinene from the European oil.

**pineoblastoma** (pin′e-o-blas-to′mah) [ pineal + G. *blastos,* germ, + suffix *-oma,* tumor ]. A poorly differentiated form of pinealoma.

**pinguecula, pinguicula** (ping-gwek′u-lah) [ L. *pinguiculus,* fattish, fr. *pinguis,* fat ]. A yellowish spot sometimes observed on either side of the cornea in the aged; it is a connective tissue (not fatty) thickening of the conjunctiva.

**piniform** (pin′ī-form, pi′nī-) [ L. *pinus,* pine, + *forma,* form ]. Pineal (1).

**pink′eye.** 1. Acute epidemic *conjunctivitis.* 2. Infectious bovine *keratitis.* 3. In horses, generally a form of equine viral enteritis.

**Pinkus** (pin′koos), Felix, German dermatologist, *1868. See P.'s *disease.*

**pin′ledge.** A dental restoration or technique that employs vertical parallel pins which are placed into the tooth or teeth to aid in retention.

**pinna,** pl. **pinnae** (pin′ah, pin′e) [ L. *pinna* or *penna,* a feather, in pl. a wing ]. 1 [ NA ]. Auricula. 2. A feather, wing, or fin.

**p. nasi,** *ala* nasi.

**pin′nal.** Relating to the pinna; auricular.

**pinocyte** (pin′o-sīt, pi′no-) [ G. *pineo,* to drink, + *kytos,* cell ]. A cell that exhibits pinocytosis.

**pinocytosis** (pin′o-si-to′sis, pi′no-) [ pinocyte + G. suffix *-osis,* condition ]. The cellular process of actively engulfing liquid, a phenomenon in which minute incuppings or invaginations are formed in the surface of the cell membrane and close to form fluid-filled vesicles. Resembles phagocytosis, which is the engulfing of solid particles.

**pi′nol.** A constituent present in turpentine oil obtained from *Pinus pinaster* or *P. maritima.*

**pinosome** (pin′o-sōm, pi′no-) [ G. *pineō,* to drink, + *sōma,* body ]. A fluid-filled vacuole formed by pinocytosis.

**pinother′apy** [ G. *peina,* hunger, + therapy ]. Hunger *therapy.*

**Pins,** Emil, Austrian physician, 1845–1913. See P.'s *sign,* syndrome.

**pint** (pīnt). A measure of quantity, containing 16 fluid-ounces, 28.875 cubic inches; 473.166 cc.

**imperial p.,** contains 20 fluidounces, 34.659 cubic inches; 567.94 cc.

**pinta** (pin′tah, pēn′tah) [ Sp. spot, blemish ]. Azul; spotted sickness; mal de los pintos; a disease caused by a spirochete, endemic in Mexico and Central America, marked by an eruption of patches of varying color that finally become white.

**pin'tids** [ pinta + suffix -id(1), *q. v.* ]. Eruptions of plaque-like lesions complicating pinta. The lesions, which vary in color, result in depigmentation.

**Pi'nus** [ L. a pine tree ]. A genus of evergreen coniferous trees (family *Pinaceae*) yielding tar, turpentine, resin, and volatile oils.

  **P. alba,** white *pine.*

  **P. canaden'sis,** red pine, *P. resinosa.*

  **P. maritima,** *P. pinaster;* one of the sources of turpentine oil.

  **P. mugo,** *P. montana; P. pumilio;* Swiss mountain pine; Scotch pine; dwarf pine; the source of dwarf pine-needle oil.

  **P. palus'tris,** long-leaved pine; a source of pine oil, pine tar rosin, and turpentine oil.

**pi'nus** [ L. a pine tree ]. *Corpus* pineale.

**pin'worm.** *Oxyuris,* or related nematodes of in the family Oxyuridae, abundant in a large variety of vertebrates.

  **horse p.,** *Oxyuris equi.*

  **human p.,** *Enterobius vermicularis.*

  **mouse p.,** see *Syphacia* and *Aspicularis.*

  **rabbit p.,** *Passalurus ambiguus.*

  **rat p.,** *Syphacia muris.*

**pioepithelium** (pi'o-ep-ĭ-the'lĭ-um) [ G. *pion,* fat, + epithelium ]. Fatty degenerated epithelium, or any epithelium containing fat globules.

**pionemia** (pi'o-ne'mĭ-ah) [ G. *pion,* fat, + *haima,* blood ]. Lipemia.

**Piophila casei** (pi-of'ĭ-lah ka'se-i) [ L. fr. G. *pion,* fat, + *philos,* fond; L. *caseus,* cheese ]. Cheese fly; the eggs of this muscoid fly are deposited on exposed cheese, cured meats, and other foods and are thus ingested, sometimes giving rise to temporary intestinal myiasis, with diarrhea, colicky pains, and vomiting.

**Piorkowski** (pyor-kov'ske), Max, German bacteriologist, *1859. See P.'s *stain* (for metachromatic granules).

**piorthopnea** (pi'or-thop'ne-ah, -ne'ah) [ G. *pion,* fat, + *orthos,* straight, + *pnoē,* breath ]. Pimelorthopnea.

**pipam'azine.** NOMETINE; 1-[ 3-(2-chlorophenothiazin-10-yl)propyl ]-isonipectoamide; antiemetic.

**pipam'perone** (USAN). PROPITAN; 1'-[ 3- (*p*-fluorobenzoyl)propyl ]-[ 1,4'-bipiperidine ]-4'-carboxamide; ataractic.

**pipazethate** (pĭ-paz'ĕ-thāt) (USAN). THERATUSS; 2-(2-piperidinoethoxy)ethyl 10*H*-pyridol[ 3,2-*b* ][ 1,4 ]benzothiazine-10-carboxylate; an antitussive agent chemically related to the phenothiazines; less effective than codeine for the suppression of coughing.

**pipecolic acid** (pip'e-ko'lik, -kol'ik). Pipecolinic acid; 2-piperidinecarboxylic acid; saturated picolinic acid; a carboxypiperidine; a heterocyclic intermediate in the catabolism of lysine.

**pipenzolate methylbromide** (pi-pen'zo-lāt). PIPTAL 1-ethyl-3-piperidyl benzilate methylbromide; an anticholinergic drug with predominantly peripheral atropine-like action; used as an adjunct in the treatment of peptic ulcers and to relieve spasms of the lower intestinal tract.

**Piper,** E. B. See P.'s *forceps.*

**pi'per** [ L. pepper ]. Black pepper; the dried unripe fruit of *Piper nigrum* (family Piperaceae), a climbing plant of the East Indies; used as a condiment, diaphoretic, stimulant, and carminative, and locally as a counterirritant.

**piperacet'azine** (NF). QUIDE; 10-{ 3-[ 4-(2-hydroxyethyl)-piperidino ]-propyl } phenothiazin-2-yl methyl ketone; antipsychotic agent.

**piperazine** (pĭ-pĕr'ă-zēn, -zin). Diethylenediamine; pyrazine hexahydride; its former use in gout was based upon its property of dissolving uric acid *in vitro,* but it is ineffective in increasing uric acid excretion. Its compounds are now used as anthelmintics in oxyuriasis and ascariasis.

  **p. adipate** (BP), a veterinary anthelmintic and filaricide.

  **p. calcium edetate** (USAN), PERIN; (ethylenedinitrilo)-tetraacetic acid piperazine calcium salt.

  **p. citrate** (USP, BP), a vermifuge for pinworms and roundworms.

  **p. estrone sulfate** (NF), SULTESTREX; a purified preparation of natural estrone sulfate. The p. acts as a buffer to increase the stability of estrone sulfate.

**piperidolate hydrochloride** (pĭ-pĕr'ĭ-do-lāt) (NF). DACTIL; 1-ethyl-3-piperidyl diphenylacetate hydrochloride; an anticholinergic, used as a gastrointestinal antispasmodic.

**piperilate** (pĭ-pĕr'ĭ-lāt). PIPETHANATE; SYCOTROL; *β*-piperidineethanol benzilate; a nonbarbiturate related chemically to benactyzine; a sedative and minor tranquilizer used to reduce anxiety and tension.

**piperine** (pip'er-ēn, -in). A feebly basic principle obtained from black pepper; in the presence of alkalies it is split into piperidine and piperic acid. Formerly used as a tonic and antiperiodic; now used as an insecticide.

**piperocaine hydrochloride** (pip'er-o-kān, pĭ-pĕr'o-kān). METYCAINE hydrochloride; 3-(2-methyl-1-piperidyl)propyl benzoate hydrochloride; a rapidly acting local anesthetic for infiltration and spinal anesthesia.

**piperonal** (pip'er-o-nal). $C_8H_6O_3$; heliotropin; methylene ether of protocatechuic aldehyde; colorless needles with a strong odor of heliotrope; used in perfumery and as a pediculicide.

**piperoxan hydrochloride** (pip'er-ok'san). BENODAINE hydrochloride; Fourneau 933; adrenergic (*α*-receptor) blocking agent of the Fourneau series of benzodioxanes; 2-(1-piperidylmethyl)-1,4-benzodioxane hydrochloride; used as a diagnostic test for pheochromocytoma.

**piper'ylon.** PALEROL; 4-ethyl-1-(1-methyl-4-piperidyl)-3-phenyl-3-pyrazolin-5-one; analgesic and antipyretic.

**pipet** (pĭ-pet'). Pipette.

**pipette** (pĭ-pet') [ Fr. dim. of *pipe,* pipe ]. Pipet; a tube used to transport small amounts of a gas or liquid in laboratory work; usually marked to deliver a particular volume of fluid with quantitative accuracy, so that one might speak of a 5-ml. p., a 100-ml. p., etc.

**pipobroman** (pip'o-bro'man) (NF). VERCYTE; 1,4-bis(3-bromopropionyl)piperazine; an alkylating agent used in polycythemia vera and chronic granulocytic leukemia.

**piposul'fan** (USAN). ANCYTE; 1,4-dihydracryloylpiperazine dimethanesulfonate; antineoplastic agent.

**pipradrol hydrochloride** (pip'rā-drol). MERATRAN hydrochloride; *α*-[ 2-piperidyl ]benzhydrol hydrochloride; a central nervous system stimulant.

**piprinhy'drinate.** MEPEDYL; *N*-methylpiperidyl 4-benzhydryl ether 8-chlorotheophyllinate; antihistaminic and antiemetic.

**piprozo'lin** (USAN). Ethyl 3-ethyl-4-oxo-5-piperidino-$Δ^{2,α}$-thiazolidineacetate; a choleretic agent.

**pipsyl-** (pip'sil-). *p*-Iodophenylsulfonyl-, the radical of p. chloride used to combine with $NH_2$ groups of amino acids and proteins.

**piquizil hydrochloride** (pik'wĭ-zil) (USAN). Isobutyl 4-(6,7-dimethoxy-4-quinazolinyl)-1-piperazinecarboxylate monohydrochloride; a bronchodilating drug.

**piqûre diabetique** (pe-kĕr') [ Fr. ]. Diabetic *puncture.*

**Piria** (pe're-ah), Raffaele, Italian chemist, 1815–1865. See P.'s *test.*

**pirid'ocaine hydrochloride.** LUCAINE hydrochloride; anthranilic acid 2-(2-piperidyl)ethyl ester hydrochloride; a local anesthetic of the piperidine type used by injection for regional anesthesia.

**Pirie** (peer'e), George A., Scottish radiologist, 20th century. See P.'s *bone.*

**piriform** (pĭr'ĭ-form, pi'rĭ-) [ L. *pirum,* pear, + *forma,* form ]. Pyriform; pear-shaped.

**pirifor'mis** [ L. ] [ NA ]. Piriform.

**pirini'tramide.** DIPIDOLOR; 1'-(3-cyano-3,3-diphenylpropyl)-[ 1,4'-bipiperidine ]-4'-carboxamide; analgesic.

**Pirogoff,** Nikolai I., Moscow surgeon, 1810–1881. See P.'s *amputation, angle, triangle.*

**piromen** (pĭr'o-men, pi'ro-). Pyromen; a sterile, nonprotein, nonanaphylactogenic extract of *Pseudomonas aeruginosa* and *Proteus vulgaris.* The active components are bacterial polysaccharides of low toxicity; used in the treatment of certain allergic, dermatologic, and ophthalmic disorders.

**Piroplasma** (pĭr'o-plaz'mah, pi'ro-) [ L. *pirum,* pear, + G. *plasma,* a thing formed ]. *Babesia.*

**Piroplasmi'da.** An order of sporozoan protozoa comprised of the families Babesiidae and Theileriidae.

**pir'oplasmo'sis.** Babesiosis.

**Pirquet von Cesenatico** (peer-ka'), Clemens P., Vienna physician, 1874–1929. See P.'s *reaction, test.*

**Pisces** (pis'ēz, pi'sēz) [ L. pl. of *piscis,* a fish ]. A superclass of vertebrates, generally known as fish; the term is sometimes confined to the bony fishes.

**piscicide** (pis'ĭ-sīd) [ L. *piscis,* fish + *caedo,* to kill ]. A substance that poisons or kills fish.

**piscidia** (pĭ-sid'ĭ-ah) [ L. *piscis,* fish, + *caedo,* to kill ]. Fishpoison tree; the bark of the root of Jamaica or white dogwood, *Piscidia erythrina* (family Leguminosae), a tree of Jamaica, Cuba, and southern Florida; used as an anodyne.

**pisiform** (pis'ĭ-form) [ L. *pisum,* pea, + *forma,* appearance ]. Pea-shaped or pea-sized.

**Piskacek,** Ludwig, Hungarian obstetrician, 1854–1933. See P.'s *uterus.*

**pit** [ L. *puteus* ]. 1. Any natural depression on the surface of the body, as the armpit or axilla; see also dimple. 2. One of the pinhead-sized, depressed scars following the pustule of acne, chickenpox, or smallpox; see also pockmark. 3. A sharp-pointed depression in the enamel surface of a tooth, due to faulty or incomplete calcification; the depression on the surface of a tooth formed by the confluent point of two or more lobes of enamel. 4. To indent, as by pressure of the finger on the edematous skin; to become indented, said of the edematous tissues when pressure is made with the fingertip.

    **anal p.,** proctodeum.

    **auditory p.'s,** paired depressions, one on either side of the head of the embryo, marking the location of the future auditory vesicles.

    **buccal p.,** a structural depression found on the buccal enamel of molars.

    **central p.,** *fovea* centralis retinae.

    **costal p. of transverse process,** *fovea* costalis transversalis.

    **gastric p.,** *foveola* gastrica.

    **granular p.,** *foveola* granularis.

    **inferior articular p. of atlas,** *fovea* articularis inferior atlantis.

    **inferior costal p.,** *fovea* costalis inferior.

    **lens p.'s,** the paired depressions formed in the superficial ectoderm of the embryonic head as the lens placodes sink in toward the optic cup. The external openings of the p.'s are closed as the lens vesicles are formed.

    **nasal p.'s;** olfactory p.'s; the paired depressions formed when the nasal placodes come to lie below the general external contour of the developing face as a result of the rapid growth of the adjacent nasal processes. The p.'s are the primordia of the rostral portions of the nasal chambers.

    **oblong p. of arytenoid cartilage,** *fovea* oblonga cartilaginis arytenoideae.

    **olfactory p.'s,** nasal p.'s.

    **primitive p.,** a small depression extending beneath Hensen's node from the most cephalic part of the primitive groove.

    **pterygoid p.,** *fovea* pterygoidea.

    **p. of the stomach,** *fossa* epigastrica.

    **sublingual p.,** *fovea* sublingualis.

    **superior articular p. of atlas,** *fovea* articularis superior atlantis.

    **superior costal p.,** *fovea* costalis superior.

    **trochlear p.,** *fovea* trochlearis.

**PITC.** Abbreviation for phenylisothiocyanate; PhNCS is preferred.

**pitch** [ L. *pix* ]. A resinous substance obtained from tar after the volatile substances have been expelled by boiling.

    **Burgundy p.,** white p.; a resinous exudation from the spruce fir or Norway spruce, *Picea excelsa.* Has been used as a counterirritant in the form of a plaster.

    **liquid p.,** pine tar.

**pitch'blende.** Uraninite; a substance of pitchlike appearance; chiefly uranium oxide, the main source of uranium and the elements (*i.e.,* radium) produced as a result of the radioactive breakdown of that element.

**Pitfield,** Robert L., American physician, 1870–1942. See P. *stain,* Smith-P. *stain.*

**pith** [ A.S. *pitha* ]. 1. The center of a hair. 2. The spinal cord and medulla oblongata. 3. To pierce the medulla of an animal with a sharp instrument introduced at the base of the skull.

**pithecoid** (pith'e-koyd) [ G. *pithēkos,* ape, + *eidos,* resemblance ]. Resembling an ape.

**pithiatic** (pith'ĭ-at'ik). Relating to pithiatism; curable by suggestion.

**pithiatism** (pĭ-thi'ă-tizm) [ G. *peithō,* to persuade, + *iatos,* curable ]. 1. A morbid condition curable by suggestion. 2. Pithiatry.

**pithiatric** (pith-ĭ-at'rik) [ G. *peithō,* persuade, + *iatrikos,* relating to medical treatment ]. Relating to pithiatry; curable by persuasion or suggestion.

**pithiatry** (pĭ-thi'ă-trĭ) [ G. *peithō,* persuade, + *iatros,* physician ]. Pithiatism (2); suggestive therapeutics.

**pithode** (pith'ōd) [ G. *pithōdēs,* like a jar, fr. *pithos,* earthenware wine-jar, + *eidos,* resemblance ]. The nuclear spindle in karyokinesis.

**Pitot,** Henri, French engineer, 1695–1771. See P. *tube.*

**Pitres** (pētr), Jean A., Bordeaux physician, 1848–1927. See P.'s *area, sign.*

**pit'ting.** In dentistry, the formation of well defined, relatively deep depressions in a surface, usually used in describing defects in surfaces (often golds, solder joints, or amalgam). It may arise from a variety of causes, although the clinical occurrence is often associated with corrosion.

**pituicyte** (pĭ-tu'ĭ-sit) [ pituitary + G. *kytos,* cell ]. The primary cell of the neurohypophysis or posterior pituitary body, a fusiform cell closely related to neuroglia.

**pituicytoma** (pĭ-tu'ĭ-si-to'mah) [ pituicyte + G. suffix *-oma,* tumor ]. A gliogenous neoplasm derived from pituicytes, occurring in the posterior lobe of the pituitary gland and characterized by cells with relatively small, round or oval nuclei and long branching processes that form a complex network of cytoplasmic material, in which numerous small droplets of fat may be demonstrated by means of osmic acid (and certain other special stains).

**pituita** (pĭ-tu'ĭ-tah) [ L. phlegm or thick mucous secretion. PITU- ] [ NA ]. Glairy mucus; a thick nasal secretion.

**pituitarism** (pĭ-tu'ĭ-tăr-izm). Pituitary dysfunction.

**pituita'rium** [ Mod. L. ]. Pituitary.

**pituitary** (pit-u'ĭ-tēr-ĭ) [ L. *pituita, q.v.* ]. Relating to the pituitary gland (hypophysis).

    **anterior p.,** the dried, partially defatted and powdered anterior lobe of the p. gland of cattle. sheep, or swine; now rarely used therapeutically.

    **pharyngeal p.,** the embryonic remnant of the oral end of Rathke's pouch that is cut off from the adenohypophysis by the developing sphenoid bone; it is composed chiefly of chromophobes, and under normal conditions it is considered physiologically inactive.

    **posterior p.,** hypophysis sicca; desiccated p.; the cleaned, dried, and powdered posterior lobe obtained from the p. body of domestic animals used for food by man; oxytocic, vasoconstrictor, antidiuretic, and a stimulant of intestinal motility.

**pitu'itec'tomy.** Obsolete synonym for hypophysectomy.

**pitu'itous.** Relating to pituita.

**pityriasic** (pit'ĭ-ri'ă-sik). Relating to or suffering from pityriasis.

**pityriasis** (pit'ĭ-ri'ă-sis) [ G. fr. *pityron,* bran, dandruff ]. A dermatosis marked by branny desquamation.

    **p. alba atroph'icans,** a scaling condition of the skin followed by atrophy.

    **p. cap'itis,** dandruff.

    **p. circina'ta,** p. rosea.

    **p. furfura'cea,** dandruff.

    **p. lichenoi'des,** maculopapular *erythroderma.*

    **p. lichenoi'des et variolifor'mis acu'ta,** a more or less acute dermal vasculitis that runs a relatively mild course and is self-limited; vesicles, papules, and crusted lesions eventually produce smallpox-like scars; also known as parapsoriasis lichenoides et varioliformis acuta; parapsoriasis varioliformis; Mucha-Habermann disease.

    **p. linguae,** geographical *tongue.*

    **p. macula'ta,** p. rosea.

    **p. ni'gra,** *tinea* nigra.

**p. ro'sea,** p. circinata; p. maculata; a self-limited eruption of macules or papules involving the trunk and extremities and rarely the face. The lesions are usually oval and follow the lines of cleavage of the skin. The onset is frequently preceded by a single larger lesion known as the herald patch.

**p. ru'bra,** exfoliative *dermatitis.*

**p. ru'bra pila'ris,** a chronic eruption of the hair follicles, which become firm, red, surmounted with a horny plug, and often confluent to form scaly plaques; it is most conspicuously noted on the dorsa of the fingers and on the elbows and knees, and is associated with erythema, thickening of the palms and soles, and opaque thickening of the nails.

**p. sic'ca,** dandruff.

**p. versic'olor,** *tinea* versicolor.

**pityroid** (pit'ĭ-royd) [ G. *pityrōdēs,* branlike, fr. *pityron,* bran, + *eidos,* resemblance ]. Branny; scaly; furfuraceous.

**Pityrosporum** (pit'ĭ-ros'po-rum, pit'ĭ-ro-spo'rum) [ G. *pityron,* bran, + *sporos,* seed ]. A genus of nonpathogenic fungi found in dandruff and seborrheic dermatitis.

**piv'alate.** USAN-approved contraction for trimethylacetate, $(CH_3)_3C—CO_2^-$.

**piv'alylbenzhy'drazine.** TERSAVID; pipalic acid 2-benzylhydrazide; monoamine oxidase inhibitor used for the treatment of angina pectoris.

**piv'ot.** A post upon which something hinges or turns.

**adjustable occlusal p.,** an occlusal p. which may be adjusted vertically by means of a screw or by other means.

**occlusal p.,** an elevation contrived on the occlusal surface, usually in the molar region, designed to act as a fulcrum and to induce sagittal mandibular rotation.

**pix,** gen. **pi'cis** [ L ]. Pitch; tar.

**pK.** The negative logarithm of the ionization constant ($K_a$) of an acid; the pH at which equal concentrations of the acid and basic forms of a substance (usually a buffer) are present.

**PKU.** Abbreviation for phenylketonuria.

**P.L.** Abbreviation for perception of light.

**placebo** (plă-se'bo) [ L. I will please, future of *placeo* ]. 1. An indifferent substance, in the form of a medicine, given for the suggestive effect. 2. An inert compound, identical in appearance with material being tested in experimental research, where the patient and the physician may or may not know which is which.

**placenta** (plă-sen'tah) [ L. a cake, PLAC- ] [ NA ]. The organ of metabolic interchange between fetus and mother. It has a portion of embryonic origin, derived from a highly developed area of the outermost embryonic membrane (chorion frondosum), and a maternal portion formed by a modification of the part of the uterine mucosa (decidua basalis) in which the chorionic vesicle is implanted. Within the placenta the chorionic villi with their contained capillaries carrying blood of the embryonic circulation are exposed to maternal blood in the sinusoidal spaces in the decidua basalis. There is no direct mixing of fetal and maternal blood, but the intervening tissue (the placental barrier) is sufficiently thin to permit the absorption of nutritive materials and oxygen into the fetal blood and the elimination of carbon dioxide and nitrogenous waste from it. The human placenta at term averages about $1/6$ to $1/7$ the weight of the fetus. It is disk-shaped, about an inch in thickness and 7 inches in diameter. Its fetal face is smooth, being formed by the adherent amnion. The umbilical cord is attached, normally, near the center of the fetal face. The maternal face of a detached placenta is rough because of the torn decidual tissue adhering to the chorion, and shows lobular elevations called cotyledons. After the delivery of the fetus the extruded placenta with the torn membranes adherent to its margins and the attached umbilical cord is called the "afterbirth."

**accessory p.,** supernumerary p.; succenturiate p.; a mass of placental tissue distinct from the main p.

**p. accre'ta,** the abnormal adherence of the chorionic villi to the myometrium, associated with partial or complete absence of the decidua basalis and, in particular, the stratum spongiosum.

**p. accreta vera,** the term applied when villi are in juxtaposition with the myometrium.

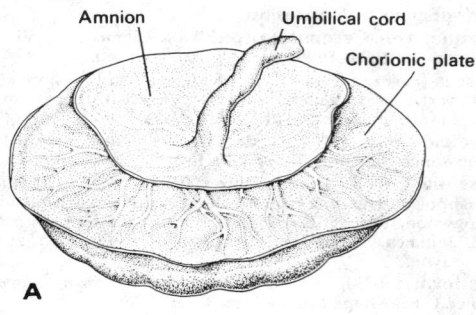

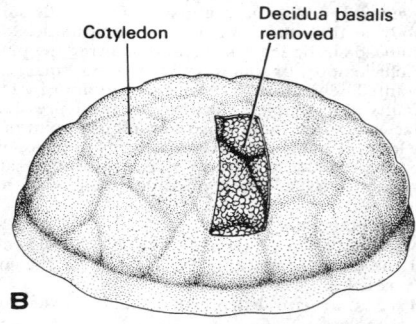

**A Full Term Placenta**

*A,* as seen from the fetal side: note that this side is covered by amnion. *B,* as seen from the maternal side: note the cotyledons; in one area the decidua has been removed. (From Langman, J.: *Medical Embryology,* Ed. 2, The Williams & Wilkins Co., Baltimore, 1969.)

**adherent p.,** one that fails to separate cleanly from the uterus after delivery.

**annular p.,** zonary p.; one in the form of a band encircling more or less completely the interior of the uterus.

**battledore p.,** one in which the umbilical cord is attached at the border.

**bidiscoidal p.,** chorioamnionic p.; a form of placentation in which the amnion is fused to the inside of the chorion, thus permitting interchange of water and electrolytes between mother and fetus.

**p. bilo'ba,** p. bipartita; a p. duplex in which the two parts are separated by a constriction.

**p. biparti'ta,** p. biloba.

**chorioallantoic p.,** a p. (such as that of primates) in which the chorion is formed by the fusion of the allantoic mesoderm and vessels to the inner face of the serosa.

**chorioamnionic p.,** bidiscoidal p.

**choriovitelline p.,** a p. (seen in some of the lower animals) in which the chorion is formed by the fusion of yolk-sac mesoderm and vessels to the inner face of the serosa.

**p. circumvalla'ta,** a cup-shaped p. with raised edges; a portion of the decidua separates the margin of the p. from its chorionic plate; there is a thick, round, white, opaque ring around the periphery of the p.; the remainder of the chorionic surface is normal in appearance but the fetal vessels are limited in their course across the p. by the ring. See also p. marginata and p. reflexa.

**cotyledonary p.,** a p. in which the substance is divided into lobes or cotyledons.

**dichorionic diamniotic p.,** see twin p.

**deciduate p.,** a p. in which the maternal decidua is cast off with the fetal p.

**p. diffusa,** p. membranaceae.

**p. dimidia'ta** [ L. *dimidiare,* to divide into halves ], p. duplex.

**disperse p.,** a p. in which the umbilical arteries divide dichotomously before entering the placental substance.

**p. duplex,** p. dimidiata; one consisting of two parts, almost entirely detached, being united only at the point of attachment of the cord.

**endothe'liochor'ial p.,** a p. in which the chorionic tissue penetrates to the endothelium of the maternal blood vessels.

**endothelio-endothelial p.,** a p. in which the endothelium of the maternal vessels comes in direct contact with the endothelium of the fetal vessels to form the placental barrier.

**epithe'liochor'ial p.,** a p. in which the chorion is merely in contact with, and does not erode, the endometrium.

**p. extrachora'les,** one in which the chorionic plate is limited by a thin, membranous fold at the edge.

**p. fenestra'ta,** one in which there are areas of thinning, sometimes extending to entire absence of placental tissue.

**fetal p., p. feta'lis,** *pars* fetalis placentae.

**hemochorial p.,** the type of p., as in man and some rodents, in which maternal blood is in direct contact with the chorion.

**he'moendothe'lial p.,** the type of p. (*e.g.,* rabbit), in which the trophoblast becomes so attenuated that, by light microscopy, maternal blood appears to be separated from fetal blood only by the endothelium of the chorionic capillaries.

**horseshoe p.,** an exaggerated p. reniformis curved in the form of a horseshoe.

**incarcerated p.,** trapped p.; a p. held in the uterus by a contracted cervix.

**p. incre'ta,** a form of p. accreta in which the chorionic villi invade the myometrium.

**labyrinthine p.,** one in which maternal blood circulates through channels within the fetal syncytiotrophoblast.

**Lobstein's p.,** p. velamentosa.

**p. margina'ta,** a p. with raised edges, less pronounced than the p. circumvallata; see also p. reflexa.

**maternal p.,** *Pars* uterina (2).

**p. membrana'cea,** p. diffusa; an abnormally thin p. covering an unusually large area of the uterine lining.

**monochorionic diamniotic p.,** see twin p.

**monochorionic monoamniotic p.,** see twin p.

**p. multilo'ba,** a p. having more than three lobes separated from each other by simple constrictions, the fetus being single.

**nondeciduous p.,** one in which the fetal p. is cast off,

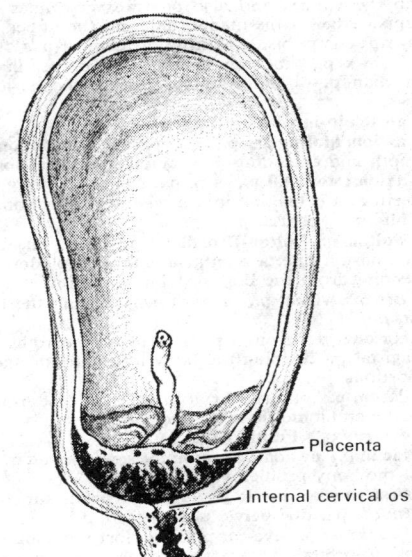

Placenta

Internal cervical os

**Total Placenta Previa**

(From Taylor, E. S.: *Beck's Obstetrical Practice*, Ed. 9, The Williams & Wilkins Co., Baltimore, 1971.)

leaving the uterine mucosa intact (*e.g.,* an epitheliochorial type).

**p. pandurafor'mis** [ L. *pandura,* a three-stringed musical instrument ], a form of p. dimidiata with the two halves placed side by side in a shape suggestive of a stringed musical instrument.

**p. percre'ta,** the term applied when the villi have invaded the full thickness of myometrium to or through the serosa of the uterus, causing incomplete or complete uterine rupture, respectively.

**p. pre'via** [ L. *praevius,* leading the way ], the condition in which the p. is implanted in the lower segment of the uterus, extending to the margin of the internal os of the cervix or partially or completely obstructing the os.

**p. pre'via centra'lis,** central or total p. previa; that form in which the p. entirely covers the internal os of the cervix.

**p. pre'via margina'lis,** a form in which the p. comes just to, but does not occlude, the os.

**p. pre'via partia'lis,** a form in which the internal os of the cervix is partially covered by placental tissue.

**p. reflex'a,** an anomaly of the p. in which the margin is thickened so as to appear turned back upon itself. See also p. circumvallata and p. marginata.

**p. renifor'mis,** a kidney-shaped p.

**retained p.,** incomplete separation of the p. and its failure to be expelled at the usual time after delivery of the child.

**Schultze's p.,** the p. appears at the vulva with the glistening fetal surface presenting.

**p. spu'ria,** a mass of placental tissue which has no vascular connection with the main p.

**succenturiate p.,** accessory p.

**supernumerary p.,** accessory p.

**syndesmochorial p.,** in ruminant animals, a type of p. in which the chorion is attached to maternal connective tissue.

**total p. previa,** p. previa centralis.

**trapped p.,** incarcerated p.

**p. tri'loba,** a p. tripartita in which the three parts form one mass separated by more or less deep constrictions.

**p. triparti'ta,** p. triplex; a p. consisting of three parts almost entirely separate, being joined together only by the blood vessels of the umbilical cord; the fetus is single.

**p. tri'plex,** p. tripartita.

**twin p.,** the placenta(s) of a twin pregnancy. If dizygotic, the p.'s may be separate or fused, the latter retaining two amniotic and two chorionic sacs (dichorionic diamniotic p.). If monozygotic, the p. may be monochorionic monoamniotic or monochorionic diamniotic, depending on the stage at which twinning took place, and only if this is very early may there be a fused p. with two chorionic and two amniotic membranes.

**p. uterina,** *pars* uterina (2).

**p. velamento'sa,** Lobstein's p.; a form in which the umbilical cord is attached on the adjoining membranes, with the umbilical vessels spread out and entering the p. independently.

**villous p.,** a p. in which the chorion forms villi.

**zo'nary p.,** annular p.

**placen'tal.** Relating to the placenta.

**Placentalia** (plas'en-ta'lĭ-ah) [ L. *placenta* ]. See Eutheria.

**placentascan** (plă-sen'tă-skan). A method of determining the location of the placenta by means of injected radioactive material and its localization and display by a scintillation detector.

**placentation** (plas'en-ta'shun). The structural organization and mode of attachment of fetal to maternal tissues in the formation of the placenta. Types of p. are defined under placenta.

**placentitis** (plas'en-ti'tis). Inflammation of the placenta.

**placentography** (plas'en-tog'ră-fĭ) [ placenta + G. *graphō,* to write ]. Roentgenography of the placenta following injection of a radiopaque substance.

**indirect p.,** roentgenographic determination of the presence of placenta praevia by estimating the distance between the presenting fetal part and the bladder filled with a radiopaque substance.

**placentolysin** (plas'en-tol'ĭ-sin). Syncytiolysin.

**placentoma** (plas'en-to'mah). Deciduoma.

**placentotherapy** (plă-sen'to-thĕr'ă-pĭ). The therapeutic use of an extract of placental tissue.

**Placido** (plah-se'do) da Costa, Antonio, Portuguese oculist, 1848–1916. See P.'s *disk.*

**placode** (plak'ōd) [ G. *plakōdēs*, fr. *plax*, anything flat or broad, + *eidos*, like ]. A local thickening in an embryonic epithelial layer. The cells of the p. ordinarily constitute a primordial group from which some organ or structure is later developed.

 **auditory p.'s**, otic p.'s; paired ectodermal p.'s that sink below the general level of the superficial ectoderm to form the auditory vesicles.

 **dorsolateral p.'s**, a series of p.'s forming the lateral line organs of certain aquatic vertebrates.

 **epibranchial p.'s**, ectodermal thickenings associated with the more dorsal parts of the embryonic branchial grooves. Their cells are believed to contribute to formation of the cranial ganglia, especially those of nerves IX and X.

 **lens p.'s**, optic p.'s; paired ectodermal p.'s that become invaginated to form the embryonic lens vesicles.

 **nasal p.'s**, olfactory p.'s.

 **olfactory p.'s**, nasal p.'s; paired ectodermal p.'s which come to lie in the bottom of the olfactory pits as the pits are deepened by the growth of the surrounding nasal processes.

 **optic p.'s**, lens p.'s.

 **otic p.'s**, auditory p.'s.

**pladaro'ma, pladaro'sis** [ G. *pladaros*, wet, damp, flaccid, + suffix *-oma*, tumor ]. A soft, wartlike growth on the eyelid.

**plagio-** (pla'ji-o-) [ G. *plagios*, oblique ]. Combining form meaning oblique, slanting.

**plagiocephalic** (pla'ji-o-sĕ-fal'ik). Relating to or marked by plagiocephaly.

**pla'gioceph'alism.** Plagiocephaly.

**pla'gioceph'alous.** Plagiocephalic.

**plagiocephaly** (pla'ji-o-sef'ă-li) [ G. *plagios*, oblique, + *kephalē*, head ]. Plagiocephalism; an asymmetric craniostenosis due to premature closure of the lambdoid and coronal sutures on one side; characterized by an oblique deformity of the skull.

**plague** (plāg) [ L. *plaga*, a stroke, injury, *cf.* G. *plēgē* ]. 1. Any disease of wide prevalence or of excessive mortality. 2. Pest; pestis; an acute infectious disease caused by Pasteurella pestis; it is marked clinically by high fever, toxemia, prostration, a petechial eruption, lymph node enlargement, and pneumonia, or hemorrhage from the mucous membranes; it is primarily a disease of rodents and is transmitted to man by fleas that have bitten infected animals.

 **ambulant p., ambulatory p.**, parapestis; pestis ambulans; pestis minor; larval plague; a mild form of bubonic p. characterized by symptoms such as mild fever and lymphadenitis.

 **black p.**, see black *death.*

 **bubonic p.**, pestis fulminans; pestis major; glandular p.; polyadenitis maligna; the usual form of p. marked by inflammatory enlargement of the lymphatic glands in the groins, axillae, or other parts.

 **cat p.**, panleukopenia.

 **cattle p.**, rinderpest.

 **fowl p.**, fowl pest; a highly fatal and highly transmissible virus disease of chickens.

 **glandular p.**, bubonic p.

 **hemorrhagic p.**, the hemorrhagic form of bubonic p.

 **larval p.**, ambulant *plague.*

 **Pahvant Valley p.**, tularemia.

 **pneumonic p.**, p. pneumonia; a frequently fatal form in which there are areas of pulmonary consolidation, with chill, pain in the side, bloody expectoration, and high fever.

 **septicemic p.**, pestis siderans; a generally fatal form in which there is an intense bacteremia with symptoms of profound toxemia.

 **swine p.**, a term seldom used today; formerly confused with hog cholera or swine fever, probably because the German word for hog cholera is *schweinepest* which means swine plague; when the word is used, modern writers are indicating an acute infection of the respiratory system, usually including pneumonia, associated with organisms of the *Pasteurella* group.

 **sylvatic p.**, bubonic p. in rats and other wild animals.

 **tar'bagan p.**, bubonic p. endemic in Eastern Siberia and Mongolia; so called because it attacks a species of rodent resembling a marmot, the local name of which is *tarbagan.*

 **white p.**, pulmonary *tuberculosis.*

**plak'albu'min.** The product of the action of the bacterial protease, subtilisin, upon egg albumin, removing a hexapeptide.

**pla'kins.** Bactericidal substances similar to leucins extracted from blood platelets.

**plan-.** See plano-.

**pla'na** [ L. ]. Plural of planum.

**plan'chet** [ Fr. *planchette*, dim. of *planche*, plank ]. A small, flat plate or dish used to support a sample for radioactivity determination. The sample is usually evaporated on (in) the p.

**Planck,** Max, German physicist, 1858–1947. See P.'s *constant, theory.*

# PLANE

**plane** (plān) [ L. *planus,* flat ]. 1. A flat surface; see planum. 2. An imaginary surface formed by extension through any axis or two definite points in reference especially to craniometry and to pelvimetry.

 **Addison's clinical p.'s.**, a series of p.'s used as landmarks in thoracoabdominal topography; the trunk is divided vertically by a *median line* from the upper border of the manubrium sterni to the symphysis pubis, by a *lateral line* drawn vertically on either side through a point half way between the anterior superior iliac spine and the median line, in a line drawn transversely across between the two anterior iliac spines, and by a *spinous line* passing vertically through the anterior superior iliac spine on either side; transversely the trunk is divided by a *transthoracic line* passing across the thorax 3.2 cm. above the lower border of the corpus sterni, by a *transpyloric line* midway between the jugular notch of the sternum and the pubic symphysis, corresponding to the disk between the first and second lumbar vertebrae, and by a *transtubercular line* passing on an average 5 cm. above the anterior superior iliac spine and 3.5 cm. below the highest part of the crista iliaca and cutting usually the fifth lumbar vertebra; the p.'s formed on these lines, and also on transverse lines cutting the upper edge of the manubrium and the upper edge of the symphysis pubis, constitute the clinical p.'s of Addison.

 **Aeby's p.**, in craniometry, a p. perpendicular to the median p. of the cranium, cutting the nasion and the basion.

 **auric'ulo-infraor'bital p.**, Frankfort p.

 **ax'iola'bioling'ual p.**, one parallel to the long axis of a tooth and extending in a labiolingual direction.

 **axiomesiodistal p.**, a p. parallel to the long axes of the teeth and extending in a mesiodistal direction.

 **bite p.**, occlusal p.

 **Bolton p., Bolton-Broadbent p., Bolton-nasion p.**, Bolton-nasion line; a roentgenographic cephalometric p. extending from the Bolton point to nasion.

 **Broca's visual p.**, a p. drawn through the two axes of vision.

 **cor'onal p.**, frontal p.; a vertical p. at right angles to a sagittal p., dividing the body into anterior and posterior portions.

 **datum p.**, an arbitrary p. used as a base from which to make craniometric measurements.

 **eye-ear p.**, Frankfort p.

 **facial p.**, nasion-pogonion measurement; a measurement of the bony profile of the face.

 **first parallel pelvic p.**, *apertura* pelvis superior.

 **fourth parallel pelvic p.**, *apertura* pelvis inferior.

 **Frankfort p.**, eye-ear p.; Frankfort horizontal p.; auriculo-infraorbital p.; a standard craniometric reference p. passing through the right and left porion and the left orbitale.

 **Frankfort horizontal p.**, Frankfort p.

 **frontal p.**, coronal p.

**guide p.,** (1) the p. developed in the occlusal surfaces of the occlusion rims (*viz.*, to position the mandible in centric relation); (2) a p. that guides movement.

**horizon'tal p.,** transverse p.; a p. across the body at right angles to the coronal and sagittal p.'s.

**p. of incidence,** the p. containing the incident light ray and the perpendicular to the surface at the point of incidence.

**p. of inlet,** *apertura* pelvis superior.

**labiolingual p.,** a p. parallel to the labial and lingual surfaces of the teeth.

**mean foundation p.,** the mean of the various irregularities in form and inclination of the basal seat. The ideal condition for denture stability exists when the mean foundation p. is most nearly at right angles to the direction of force.

**Meckel's p.,** a craniometric p. cutting the alveolar and the auricular points.

**me'dian p.** a vertical p. drawn through the midline of the body that divides the body into right and left halves.

**p. of midpelvis (least pelvic dimensions),** pelvic p. of least dimensions.

**midsag'ittal p.,** median p.

**Morton's p.,** a p. passing through the summits of the parietal and occipital protuberances.

**nasion-postcondylar p.,** a p. passing through the nasion anteriorly and to a point immediately behind each condylar process of the mandible, posteriorly.

**nuchal p.,** the external surface of the squamous part of the occipital bone below the superior nuchal line, giving attachment to the muscles of the back of the neck.

**occip'ital p.,** planum occipitale; the external surface of the occipital bone above the superior nuchal line.

**occlusal p.,** p. of occlusion; bite p.; an imaginary surface which is related anatomically to the cranium and which theoretically touches the incisal edges of the incisors and the tips of the occluding surfaces of the posterior teeth; it is not a p. in the true sense of the word but represents the mean of the curvature of the surface; see also *curve* of occlusion.

**or'bital p.,** planum orbitale; the orbital surface of the maxilla.

**p. of outlet,** *apertura* pelvis inferior.

**parasag'ittal p.,** any p. parallel to the sagittal p. or anteroposterior median p.

**p. of pelvic canal,** *axis* pelvis.

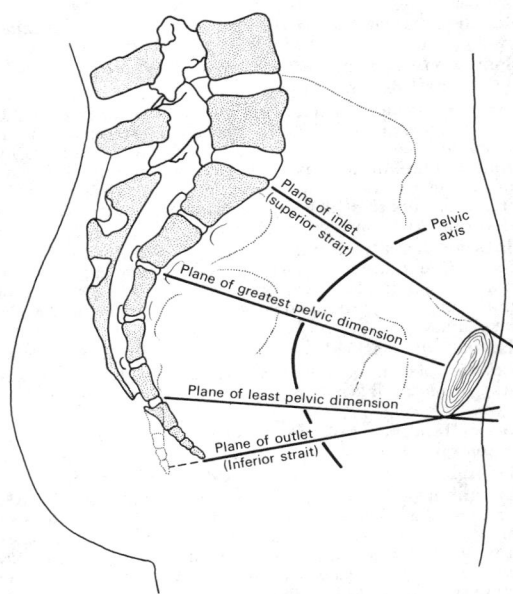

**The Pelvic Planes**

**pelvic p. of greatest dimensions,** second parallel pelvic p.; wide p.; the p. of greatest pelvic dimension, extends from the middle of the posterior surface of the pubic symphysis to the junction of the second and third sacral vertebrae, and laterally passes through the ischial bones over the middle of the acetabulum.

**pelvic p. of inlet,** *apertura* pelvis superior.

**pelvic p. of least dimensions,** third parallel pelvic p.; midplane; p. of midpelvis; p. of least pelvic dimension; it extends from the end of the sacrum to the inferior border of the pubic symphysis; it is bounded posteriorly by the end of the sacrum, laterally by the ischial spines, and anteriorly by the inferior border of the pubic symphysis.

**pelvic p. of outlet,** *apertura* pelvis inferior.

**popliteal p. of femur,** *facies* poplitea femoris.

**p.'s of reference,** p.'s which act as a guide to the location of other p.'s.

**p. of regard,** an imaginary p. through which the point of regard moves as the eyes are turned from side to side.

**sag'ittal p.,** the anteroposterior median p.; in a broad sense, it is used for any p. parallel to it.

**second parallel pelvic p.,** pelvic p. of greatest dimensions.

**sternal p.,** planum sternale; a p. indicated by the front surface of the sternum.

**subcos'tal p.,** a horizontal p. running through the lowest points of the 10th costal cartilages.

**su'praster'nal p.,** a horizontal p. passing through the body at the level of the clavicles.

**tangent p.,** perimeter (2).

**tem'poral p.,** planum temporale; a slightly depressed area on the side of the cranium, below the inferior temporal line, formed by the temporal and parietal bones, the greater wing of the sphenoid, and a part of the frontal bone.

**third parallel pelvic p.,** pelvic p. of least dimensions.

**tooth p.,** any one of the imaginary p.'s of section of a tooth, such as the axial, horizontal, or vertical.

**transpylor'ic p.,** see Addison's clinical p.'s.

**transverse p.,** horizontal p.

**wide p.,** pelvic p. of greatest dimensions.

---

**planigraphy** (plă-nig′ră-fĭ) [ L. *planum*, plane, + G. *graphē*, a writing ]. Tomography.

**planimeter** (plă-nim′e-ter) [ L. *planum*, plane, + G. *metron*, measure ]. An instrument formed of jointed levers with a recording index, used for measuring the area of any surface, by tracing its boundaries.

**planithorax** (plan′ĭ-tho′raks). A diagram of the chest showing the front and back in plane projection, after the manner of Mercator's projection of the earth's surface.

**plankter** (plangk′ter). Any type of plankton.

**plankton** (plangk′ton) [ G. *planktos*, wandering ]. A general term including many floating marine forms, mostly of microscopic or minute size, which are moved passively by winds, waves, tides, or currents. It includes diatoms, algae, copepods, and many protozoans, crustacea, mollusks, and worms.

**plankton'ic.** Relating to plankton; plankton-like.

**plano-, plan-, plani-.** 1 [ L. *planum*, plane; *planus*, flat ]. Combining form relating to a plane, or meaning flat or level. 2 [ G. *planos*, roaming, wandering ]. Combining form meaning wandering.

**planocellular** (pla′no-sel′u-lar) [ L. *planus*, flat, + cellular ]. Relating to or composed of flat cells.

**planoconcave** (pla′no-kon′kāv). Flat on one side and concave on the other; denoting a lens of that shape.

**planoconvex** (pla′no-kon′veks). Flat on one side and convex on the other; denoting a lens of that shape.

**planocyte** (plan′o-sīt) [ G. *planos*, wandering, + *kytos*, cell ]. Obsolete term for ameboid (wandering) cell.

**planocytosis** (plan′o-si-to′sis). The state of having an abnormally large number of planocytes.

**planog'raphy.** Planigraphy.

**planomania** (plan′o-ma′nĭ-ah) [ G. *planos*, wandering, + *mania*, frenzy ]. The morbid impulse to leave home and discard social restraints.

**planotopokinesia** (plan′o-top′o-kĭ-ni′zĭ-ah) [ G. *planos*, wandering, + *topos*, place, + *kinesis*, motion ]. Loss of orientation in space.

**pla'noval'gus** [ plano- + L. *valgus*, turned outward ]. A condition in which the longitudinal arch of the foot is flattened and everted.

**planta**, gen. and pl. **plantae** (plan'tah, plan'te) [ L. ] [ NA ]. P. pedis [ NA ]; the sole of the foot.

**planta'go** [ L. plantain ]. The root and leaves of the common or large-leaved plantain, *Plantago major* (family Plantaginaceae).

**p. ovata coating**, KONSYL; the separated outer mucilaginous layers of p. ovata seeds; used in simple constipation associated with lack of sufficient bulk.

**p. seed** (NF), plantain seed; psyllium seed, the dried ripe seed of *Plantago psyllium* or *P. arenaria* (*P. indica*) (Spanish or French psyllium seed), or of *P. ovata* (blond psyllium seed, or Indian plantago seed); light brown to chestnut brown ovate seeds. Used in the correction of intestinal sluggishness.

**plantalgia** (plan-tal'ji-ah) [ L. *planta*, sole of foot, + G. *algos*, pain ]. Pain in the sole of the foot.

**plan'tar** [ L. *plantaris* ]. Relating to the sole of the foot.

**planta'ris** [ L. ] [ NA ]. Plantar.

**planula**, pl. **planulae** (plan'u-lah, -le) [ L. dim. of *planum*, flat surface ]. The name given by Lankester to a coelenterate embryo when it consists of the two primary germ layers only, viz., ectoderm and endoderm.

**invag'inate p.**, gastrula.

**planum**, pl. **plana** (pla'num, pla'nah) [ L. plane ]. A plane or flat surface; see also plane.

**p. occipita'le**, occipital *plane*.

**p. orbita'le**, orbital *plane*.

**p. poplite'um**, *facies* poplitea femoris.

**p. semiluna'tum**, the area of epithelium bounding the sensory area of the crista ampullaris.

**p. sterna'le**, sternal *plane*.

**p. tempora'le**, temporal *plane*.

**planuria** (plē-nu'rī-ah) [ G. *planos*, wandering, + *ouron*, urine ]. 1. Extravasation of urine. 2. The voiding of urine from an abnormal opening.

**pla'nus** [ L. ] [ NA ]. Flat.

**plaque** (plak) [ Fr. a plate ]. 1. Platelet. 2. A patch or small differentiated area on a body surface (*e.g.*, skin, mucosa, or arterial endothelium) or on the cut surface of an organ such as the brain. 3. An area of clearing in a flat, confluent growth of bacteria or tissue cells, such as is caused by the lytic action of bacteriophage in an agar plate culture of bacteria, by the cytopathic effect (*q.v.*) of certain animal viruses in a sheet of cultured tissue cells, or by antibody (hemolysin) produced by lymphocytes cultured in the presence of erythrocytes and to which complement has been added. 4. A sharply defined zone of demyelination characteristic of multiple sclerosis.

**atheromatous p.**, a well demarcated yellow area or swelling on the intimal surface of an artery; produced by intimal lipid deposit.

**bacterial p.**, dental p.; mucous p.; mucinous p.; in dentistry, a mass of filamentous microorganisms and large variety of smaller forms attached to the surface of a tooth. Depending on bacterial activity and environmental factors, can give rise to caries, calculus, or inflammatory changes in adjacent tissue.

**dental p.**, bacterial p.

**Hollenhorst p.'s**, glittering, orange-yellow, atheromatous emboli in the retinal arterioles containing cholesterin crystals, an omen of disaster in the cardiovascular system.

**mucous p., mucinous p.**, bacterial p.

**-plasia** [ G. *plassō*, to form ]. Suffix meaning formation.

**plasm** (plazm). Plasma.

**plasma-, plasmat-, plasmato-, plasmo-** [ G. *plasma*, something formed. PLAS- ]. Combining forms relating to plasma.

**plasma** (plaz'mah) [ G. something formed. PLAS- ]. Plasm. 1. The fluid (noncellular) portion of the circulating blood, distinguished from the serum obtained after coagulation. 2. The fluid portion of the lymph. 3. Protoplasm. 4. A "fourth state of matter" in which, owing to elevated temperature (*ca.* 10⁶ degrees) atoms have broken down to form free electrons and more or less stripped nuclei; stars are composed of p. and p. is produced in the laboratory in connection with hydrogen fusion (thermonuclear) research.

**p. accelerator (ac)-globulin**, *factor* V.

**antihemophilic p. (human)** (USP), human p. in which the labile antihemophilic globulin component, present in fresh p., has been preserved. It is prepared from whole blood from 20 donors. Used to relieve temporarily dysfunction of the hemostatic mechanism in hemophilia.

**blood p.**, plasma (1).

**dried human p.** (BP), prepared like the USP product except that contributions from donors of A, O, and of B or AB groups respectively are represented in approximately the ratio 9:9:2.

**p. expander**, p. substitute.

**human p. protein fractions**, see under protein.

**p. hydrolysate**, an artificial digest of protein derived from bovine blood plasma prepared by a method of hydrolysis sufficient to provide more than half of the total nitrogen present in the form of α-amino nitrogen; used when high protein intake is indicated and cannot be accomplished through ordinary foods. See also *protein* hydrolysate.

**p. labile factor**, see under factor.

**p. mari'num**, sea water diluted to make it isotonic with p.

**muscle p.**, an alkaline fluid in muscle that is spontaneously coagulable, separating into myosin and muscle serum.

**normal human p.**, citrated normal human p.; sterile p. obtained by pooling approximately equal amounts of the liquid portion of citrated whole blood from eight or more adult humans who have been certified as free from any disease which is tranmissible by transfusion. It has been treated with ultraviolet irradiation for the purpose of destroying possible bacterial and viral contaminants.

**p. proteins**, see under protein.

**salted p.**, salted serum; the fluid portion of blood drawn from the vessels, which is prevented from coagulating by being drawn into a solution of sodium or magnesium sulfate.

**p. substitute**, p. expander; a solution of a substance such as dextran, used for transfusion in hemorrhage or shock as a substitute for p.

**thromboplastic p. component (TPC)**, *factor* VIII.

**p. thromboplastin antecedent**, *factor* XI.

**p. thromboplastin component**, *factor* IX.

**p. thromboplastin factor (PTF)**, *factor* VIII.

**p. thromboplastin factor B**, *factor* IX.

**plasmablast** (plaz'mah-blast) [ plasma + G. *blastos*, germ ]. Plasmacytoblast; precursor of the plasma cell.

**plasmacrit** (plaz'mah-krit) [ plasma + G. *krinō*, to separate ]. Blood volume × (100 − hematocrit/100).

**plasmacyte** (plaz'mah-sīt). A plasma *cell*.

**plas'macy'toblast**. Plasmablast.

**plasmacytoma** (plaz'mah-si-to'mah) [ plasmacyte + G. suffix -*oma*, tumor ]. Plasmocytoma; plasmoma; a term frequently used with reference to a discrete, presumably solitary mass of neoplastic plasma cells in bone or in one of various extramedullary sites. Such lesions are probably the initial phase of developing plasma cell myeloma, and they should be interpreted as malignant.

**plasmacytosis** (plaz'mah-si'to'sis) [ plasmacyte + G. suffix -*osis*, condition ]. Plasmocytosis. 1. The presence of plasma cells in the circulating blood. 2. The presence of unusually large proportions of plasma cells in the tissues or exudates.

**plasmagene** (plaz'mah-jēn) [ plasma + gene ]. Cytogene.

**plasmal** (plaz'mal). One of the long chain aldehydes occurring in plasmalogens; *e.g.*, stearaldehyde and palmitaldehyde.

**plas'malem'ma** [ plasma + G. *lemma*, husk ]. Plasma *membrane*.

**plasmalogen** (plaz-mal'o-jen). Alk-1-enylglycerol.

**plasmapheresis** (plaz'mah-fēr'ĕ-sis) [ plasma + G. *aphairesis*, a withdrawal ]. An experimental procedure in animals in which blood is removed and the corpuscles separated by centrifuging, suspended in Ringer's solution, and returned to the circulation, the plasma proteins of the animal being thus depleted.

**plas'mapheret'ic**. Relating to plasmapheresis.

**plasmatic** (plaz-mat′ik). Relating to plasma.

**plasmatogamy** (plaz′mă-tog′ă-mĭ). Plasmogamy.

**plasmatorrhexis** (plaz′mă-to-rek′sis) [ plasma + G. rhēxis, rupture ]. Plasmorrhexis; the splitting open of a cell from the pressure of the protoplasm.

**plasmic** (plaz′mik). Plasmatic.

**plasmid** (plaz′mid). Paragene.

**plasmin** (plaz′min). Fibrinolysin; fibrinase; enzyme (EC 3.4.21.7) hydrolyzing peptides and esters of arginine and histidine, and converting fibrin to soluble products. Occurs in plasma as plasminogen (profibrinolysin). Activated (to plasmin) by organic solvents, which remove an inhibitor, and by streptokinase, trypsin, and urokinase, all cleaving a single arginyl-valyl bond.

**plasminogen** (plaz-min′o-jen). See plasmin.

**plas′minoki′nase.** Streptokinase.

**plasminoplastin** (plaz′mĭ-no-plas′tin). Term proposed for activator agents that produce plasmin by direct action on plasminogen; cf. staphylokinase, urokinase.

**plasmo-.** See plasma-.

**plas′mocyte.** Plasma cell.

**plas′mocyto′ma.** Plasmacytoma.

**plasmocyto′sis.** Plasmacytosis.

**plasmodia** (plaz′mo′dĭ-ah) [ L. ]. Plural of plasmodium.

**plasmo′dial.** Relating to a plasmodium, or to any species of the genus Plasmodium.

**plasmodiotrophoblast** (plaz-mo′dĭ-o-tro′fo-blast) [ plasmodium + G. trophē, nourishment, + blastos, germ ]. Syncytiotrophoblast.

**plasmodium,** pl. **plasmodia** (plaz-mo′dĭ-um, -dĭ-ah) [ Mod. L. fr. G. plasma, something formed, + eidos, appearance ]. A protoplasmic mass containing several nuclei, resulting from multiplication of the nucleus without cell division.

  **placental p.,** syncytiotrophoblast.

**Plasmo′dium** (plaz-mo′dĭ-um) [ Mod. L. from G. plasma, something formed, + eidos, appearance ]. A genus of the class Sporozoa (phylum Protozoa), including the causal agents of malaria in man and other animals; the parasites have an asexual cycle in liver and red blood cells of vertebrates and a sexual cycle in mosquitoes; male and female gametocytes that have developed in the erythrocytes of the vertebrate host have a sexual cycle in the invertebrate host, which results in gamete release, fusion, zygote formation, motile ookinete, and sporocyst formation, after which numerous sporozoites are formed which concentrate in the salivary gland. The species that cause malaria in man are transmitted by various species of Anopheles mosquitoes.

  **P. ae′thio′picum,** probably a variant of P. falciparum.

  **P. brazilian′um,** a species found in monkeys in Brazil.

  **P. catheme′rium,** the cause of a highly fatal, anemic disease in canaries, but also infecting sparrows and other passerine birds.

  **P. cynomol′gi,** a species occurring naturally in the macaque, but man has been infected accidentally.

  **P. du′rae,** the cause of an acute and often fatal malaria of young turkeys in Africa.

  **P. falcip′arum,** the causal agent of falciparum or quotidian malaria; a young trophozoite is about one-fifth the size of an erythrocyte, but developing erythrocytic stages are rare in circulating blood, as they render infected cells sticky and they tend to concentrate in pulmonary capillaries; a schizont occupies about one-half to two-thirds of the red blood cell, and has fine, sparse granules (observed in peripheral blood only from moribund patients; the infected erythrocytes are normal or contracted in size and are likely to contain basophilic granules and red dots; multiple infection is extremely frequent, and causes bouts of fever somewhat irregularly every 36 to 48 hours.

  **P. falcip′arum quotidia′num,** a variant of P. falciparum.

  **P. gallina′ceum,** the cause of malaria in domestic chickens in southern Asia and Indonesia, sometimes with high mortality.

  **P. juxtanuclea′re,** a cause of chicken malaria in Mexico and South America.

  **P. kochi,** a malarial parasite that infects monkeys and has been reported from man. It is closely allied to P. vivax, the commonest agent of human malaria.

  **P. mala′riae,** the causal agent of quartan malaria; a ring-stage trophozoite is triangular, ovoid, or slightly bean-shaped, with fine or coarse black granules, and is approximately one-third the size of an erythrocyte; a schizont is oval or rounded, and nearly fills the red blood cell. Infected erythrocytes are normal or slightly contracted in size, usually with ɔ stippling (the two most important characteristics that distinguish it from P. vivax), although extremely fine Ziemann's dots may be observed. Multiple infection is extremely rare. Causes bouts of fever fairly regularly at 72-hour intervals.

  **P. ovale,** agent of the least common form of human malaria; though fairly common in West Africa, isolated cases are found in many other areas. The parasite resembles P. vivax in its earlier stages, but often modifies the cell membrane, causing it to form a fimbriated outline, and the cell often assumes an oval shape. Schüffner's dots are abundant and appear early; host cells are normal or only slightly enlarged; and only about 8 to 10 grapelike merozoites are produced. Fever is tertian (48-hour), relapses are infrequent, and the infection responds readily to treatment.

  **P. perni′cio′sum,** a variant of P. falciparum.

  **P. pith′eci,** a species found in the higher apes.

  **P. relic′tum,** a species of worldwide distribution found in pigeons, doves, ducks, swans and other birds. It is most pathogenic in pigeons, causing anemia, weakness and often death.

  **P. ten′ue,** a variant of P. falciparum, occurring in a malignant form of malaria in India.

  **P. vi′vax,** the more frequent of two species that cause tertian malaria; the early trophozoite is irregular and ameboid in shape, one-fourth to one-third the size of a red blood cell, and contains several fine granules; the schizont is irregular in shape, fills the enlarged erythrocyte, and contains numerous yellow-brown pigment granules. Affected red blood cells are pale, enlarged, and contain acidophilic granules (Schüffner's dots) in the later stages of infection. Multiple infection is common. Causes bouts of fever fairly regularly at 48-hour intervals.

  **P. vi′vax minu′ta,** probably a variant of P. ovale.

**Plasmodromata** (plaz-mo-dro′mă-tah) [ plasmo- + G. dromos, a running, a course ]. A division of Protozoa in which the nucleus is not separated into reproductive (micro-) and vegetative (macro-) portions.

**plasmogamy** (plaz-mog′ă-mĭ) [ plasmo- + G. gamos, marriage ]. Plasmatogamy; plastogamy; the union of two or more cells with preservation of the individual nuclei; the formation of a plasmodium.

**plasmogen** (plaz′mo-jen) [ plasmo- + G. suffix -gen, producing ]. Protoplasm.

**plas′minoki′nase.** Streptokinase, urokinase, or staphylokinase (see each).

**plasmokinin** (plaz′mo-ki′nin). See factor VIII.

**plasmolysis** (plaz-mol′ĭ-sis) [ plasmo- + G. lysis, dissolution ]. 1. The dissolution of cellular components. 2. The shrinking of plant cells by osmotic loss of cytoplasmic water.

**plasmolyt′ic.** Relating to plasmolysis.

**plasmolyzable** (plaz′mo-li′ză-bl). Denoting a cell in which, under certain conditions, the plasma may readily undergo dissolution.

**plas′molyze.** To cause the dissolution of the cell protoplasm.

**plasmoma** (plaz-mo′mah). Plasmacytoma.

**plasmon** (plaz′mon). Plasmotype; the total of the genetic properties of the cell cytoplasm.

**plasmoptysis** (plaz-mop′tĭ-sis) [ plasmo- + G. ptysis, a spitting, PTY- ]. The escape of protoplasm from a cell.

**plasmorrhexis** (plaz′mo-rek′sis). Plasmatorrhexis.

**plasmoschisis** (plaz-mos′kĭ-sis) [ plasmo- + G. schisis, a cleaving ]. Rapid disintegration of a red blood cell by breaking up into numerous particles resembling blood platelets.

**plas′mosin.** A highly viscous substance in cytoplasm containing discrete fibers of considerable length; regarded as the structural foundation of the cell; it is a nucleoprotein.

**plasmosome** (plaz′mo-sōm) [ plasmo- + G. *sōma,* body ]. Obsolete term for nucleolus.

**plasmotomy** (plaz-mot′o-mĭ) [ plasmo- + G. *tomē,* incision ]. A form of mitosis in multinuclear protozoan cells in which the cytoplasm divides into two or more masses, then reproducing later, in some cases by sporulation.

**plasmotrop′ic.** Pertaining to or manifesting plasmotropism.

**plasmotropism** (plaz-mot′ro-pizm) [ plasmo- + G. *tropē,* a turning ]. A condition in which the bone marrow, spleen, and liver contain strongly hemolytic bodies that cause the destruction of the erythrocytes, although the latter are not affected while in the circulating blood.

**plasmotype** (plaz′mo-tĭp). Plasmon.

**plasmozyme** (plaz′-zĭm) [ plasmo- + G. *zymē,* leaven ]. Prothrombin.

**plastein** (plas′te-in). Insoluble polypeptide formed through the random condensation of amino acid or peptides under the catalytic influence of a proteinase like chymotrypsin; molecular weights as high as 500,000 are reported.

**plas′ter** [ L. *emplastrum.* PLAS- ]. 1. A solid preparation which can be spread when heated, and which becomes adhesive at the temperature of the body; p.'s are used to keep the edges of a wound in apposition, to protect raw surfaces, and, when medicated, to redden or blister the skin or to apply drugs to the surface to obtain their systemic effects. 2. In dentistry, a colloquial term for p. of Paris.

    **p. of Paris,** exsiccated calcium sulfate; gypsum or calcium sulfate, from which the water of crystallization has been expelled by heat, but when mixed with water will form a paste which subsequently sets.

**plas′tic** [ G. *plastikos,* relating to molding ]. 1. Plasmic; plasmatic; formative. 2. Capable of being formed or molded. 3. A material, such as acrylic resin, that may be shaped by pressure to the form of a cavity or mold, sometimes with heat.

    **Bingham p.,** a material that, in the idealized case, does not flow until a critical stress (yield stress) is exceeded, and then flows at a rate proportional to the excess of stress over the yield stress; real materials probably only approach this ideal model.

    **modeling p.,** modeling composition; impression compound; modeling compound; a thermoplastic material usually composed of gum damar and prepared chalk, used especially for making dental impressions.

**plasticity** (plas-tis′ĭ-tĭ). The capability of being formed or molded; the quality of being plastic.

**plas′tics.** 1. Plastic *surgery.* 2. Plastic materials; see plastic (3).

**plastid** (plas′tid) [ G. *plastos,* formed, + suffix *-id* (2) ]. 1. One of the differentiated structures in cytoplasm of plant cells where photosynthesis or other cellular processes are carried on. 2. One of the granules of foreign or differentiated matter, food particles, fat, waste material, chromatophores, trichocysts, etc., in cells. 3. A self-duplicating virus-like particle that multiples within a host cell (such as kappa particles in certain paramecia).

    **blood p.,** any basic, morphologic unit in the biologic composition of blood, *e.g.,* an erythrocyte.

**plastochro′manol-3.** γ-Tocotrienol.

**plastochro′menol-8.** Solanochromene; the chromenol form of plastoquinone-9.

**plastogamy** (plas-tog′ă-mĭ). Plasmogamy.

**plastoquinone** (plas′to-kwin′ōn, -kwi′nōn). 2,3-Dimethyl-1,4-benzoquinone with a multiprenyl side chain; trivial name sometimes used for plastoquinone-9, one of a group of vitamins E and K and coenzymes Q.

**plastoquinone-9** (or **E₉**). 2,3-Dimethyl-6-nonaprenyl-1,4-benzoquinone; Kofler's quinone; abbreviated PQ-9; see also the isomeric form, plastochromenol-8.

**plas′tron** [ Fr. a breastplate. PLAS- ]. The sternum with costal cartilages attached.

**-plasty** [ G. *plastos,* formed, shaped ]. Suffix meaning molding or shaping or the result thereof, *e.g.,* of a surgical procedure.

**plas′ty** [ G. *plassō,* to fashion ]. A surgical procedure for repair of a defect and restoration of a part.

**plate** (plāt) [ O.Fr. *plat,* a flat object, fr. G. *platys,* flat, broad ]. 1. In anatomy, lamina; lamella; a thin, flat, differentiated structure. 2. A metal bar applied to a fractured bone in order to maintain the ends in apposition. 3. An undesirable term for denture. 4. The agar layer within a Petri dish or similar vessel. 5. To form a very thin layer of a bacterial culture by streaking it on the surface of an agar p. (usually within a Petri dish) in order to isolate individual organisms from which a colonial clone will develop.

    **alar p. of neural tube,** *lamina* alaris.

    **anal p.,** the anal portion of the cloacal p.

    **axial p.,** the primitive streak of an embryo.

    **basal p. of neural tube,** *lamina* basalis.

    **base p.,** see baseplate.

    **blood p.,** platelet.

    **bone p.,** a metal bar with perforations for the insertion of screws; used to immobilize fractured segments.

    **cardiogenic p.,** the thickened layer of mesoderm from which the cardiopericardial primordia of very young embryos are derived.

    **chorionic p.,** the chorion in the region of its uterine attachment at an early stage in the formation of the placenta; the developing chorion frondosum.

    **cloacal p.,** p. composed of a layer of cloacal entoderm in contact with a layer of proctodeal ectoderm. It subsequently ruptures, forming the anal and urogenital openings of the embryo.

    **crib′riform p.,** *lamina* cribrosa.

    **cutis p.,** dermatome (2).

    **end p.,** see endplate.

    **epiphysial p.,** *cartilago* epiphysialis.

    **equatorial p.,** the collected chromosomes at the equator of the spindle in the process of mitosis.

    **ethmovomerine p.,** the central portion of the ethmoid bone, forming a distinct element at birth.

    **floor p.,** ventral p.; the thin ventral portion of the embryonic neural tube which merges on either side with the basal portion of the lateral p.'s.

    **foot p.,** see footplate.

    **frontal p.,** in the fetus, a cartilage p. between the lateral parts of ethmoid cartilage and the developing sphenoid bone.

    **Kühne's p.,** the end-plate of a motor nerve fiber in a muscle spindle.

    **Lane's p.'s,** flattened, narrow, metal p.'s of various shapes and sizes, perforated for screws; used to hold the fragments of a fractured bone in apposition.

    **lateral p.,** a nonsegmented mass of mesoderm on the lateral periphery of the embryonic disk.

    **left p. of thyroid cartilage,** *lamina* sinistra cartilaginis thyroidea.

    **lingual p.,** a major partial denture connector formed as a lingual bar extended to cover the cingula of the lower anterior teeth.

    **medullary p.,** neural p.

    **p. of modiolus,** *lamina* modioli.

    **motor p.,** a motor end-plate.

    **muscle p.,** myotome (2).

    **nail p.,** unguis.

    **neural p.,** medullary p; the unpaired neuroectodermal region of the early embryo's dorsal surface which in later development is transformed into the neural tube and neural crest.

    **notochordal p.,** the sheet of notochordal cells that are intercalated in the entodermal roof of the primitive yolk sac.

    **oral p.,** a circumscribed area of fusion of foregut entoderm and stomodeal ectoderm in the embryo. It breaks through early in development to establish the oral opening.

    **or′bital p.,** *lamina* orbitalis ossis ethmoidalis.

    **paper** or **papyraceous p.,** *lamina* orbitalis ossis ethmoidalis.

    **parachordal p.,** the cartilage primordia of the base of the skull situated on either side of the cephalic part of the notochord.

**plate** 1099 **platyopic**

**pari′etal p.,** the outer of the two layers of the lateral mesoderm which becomes associated with the ectoderm. Together they constitute the somatopleure.

**perpendicular p. of ethmoid bone,** *lamina* perpendicularis.

**perpendicular p. of palate bone,** *lamina* perpendicularis ossis palatini.

**polar p.'s,** condensed platelike bodies at the ends of the spindle during mitosis of certain types of cells.

**prechordal p.,** prochordal p.

**prochordal p.,** prechordal p.; a small area immediately rostral to the cephalic tip of the notochord where ectoderm and entoderm are in contact. When turned under the growing head it forms the oral p. in the floor of the stomodeum.

**pterygoid p.'s,** *lamina* lateralis and *lamina* medialis processus pterygoidea.

**quadrigeminal p.,** *lamina* tecti mesencephali.

**right p. of thyroid cartilage,** *lamina* dextra cartilaginis thyroidea.

**roof p.,** roofplate; the thin layer of the embryonic neural tube connecting the lateral p.'s dorsally.

**secondary spiral p.,** *lamina* spiralis secundaria.

**segmental p.,** segmental *zone*.

**Sherman p.,** a chrome-cobalt alloy or stainless steel bone p. that can be affixed to a fracture site with screws; used in the open reduction of mandibular fractures.

**sieve p.,** *lamina* cribrosa ossis ethmoidalis.

**sole p.,** an obsolete term; the sole p. was considered to be the sarcoplasm in which the ending of a motor nerve is embedded. It has been shown by electron microscopy that the nerve fiber does not penetrate the sarcolemma.

**spiral p.,** *lamina* spiralis ossea of the cochlea.

**suction p.** in dentistry, one that is held in place by atmospheric pressure.

**tarsal p.'s,** *tarsus* superior and *tarsus* inferior.

**terminal p.,** *lamina* terminalis cerebri.

**trial p.,** trial *denture*.

**tympan′ic p.,** the bony p. between the anterior wall of the external acoustic meatus and the tympanic cavity and the posterior wall of the mandibular fossa.

**urethral p.,** an epithelial p. located ventromedially in the developing genital tubercle of a young embryo. It later becomes open to form the lining of the penile urethra.

**ventral p.,** floor p.

**vertical p. of ethmoid bone,** *lamina* perpendicularis.

**vis′ceral p.,** the inner of the two layers of the lateral mesoderm; the splanchnic mesoderm which becomes associated with the entoderm. Together they constitute the splanchnopleure.

**wing p.,** *lamina* alaris.

**plateau** (plă-tō′) [ Fr. ]. A flat elevated segment of a graphic record.

**ventricular p.,** a level portion of the intraventricular blood pressure curve, representing graphically the maintenance of contraction of the ventricle.

**platelet** (plāt′let). A little plate or plaque; specifically, a blood p.; an irregularly shaped disk, containing granules in the central part (the granulomere) and peripherally, clear protoplasm (the hyalomere), but no definite nucleus; about one-third to one-half the size of an erythrocyte, and containing no hemoglobin. The p.'s are more numerous than the leukocytes, numbering from 200,000 to 300,000 per cu. mm. Called also elementary particle; Zimmermann's corpuscle, granule, or elementary particle; Hayem's hematoblast; blood disk; blood plate; third corpuscle. See color plate 16.

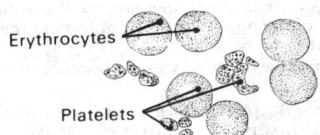

**Blood Platelets**
With erythrocytes for comparison of size (drawing taken from dry, stained smear of human blood).

**plating** (plāt′ing). 1. The sowing of bacteria on a solid medium in a Petri dish or similar container; the making of a plate culture. 2. The application of a metal strip to keep the ends of a fractured bone in apposition. 3. The electrolytic deposition of a metal.

**platin′ic.** Relating to platinum; denoting a compound containing platinum in its higher valency.

**plat′inous.** Relating to platinum; denoting a compound containing platinum in its lower valency.

**platinum** (plat′ĭ-num) [ Mod. ʟ., originally *platina*, fr. Sp. *plata*, silver ]. A metallic element, symbol Pt, atomic no. 78, atomic weight 195.09, of silver white color and of about the consistency of copper; it occurs usually as **spongy p.,** of gray color, soft and porous. It is used largely for making small parts for chemical apparatus because of its resistance to acids; in powdered form (**p. black**) it is an important catalyst in hydrogenation. Some of its salts have been used in the treatment of syphilis.

**p. foil,** see under foil.

**p. group,** a group of six amphoteric elements: palladium, platinum, osmium, iridium, ruthenium, and rhodium.

**platy-** (plat′ĭ-) [ G. *platys*, flat, broad ]. A combining form conveying the idea of width or flatness.

**platybasia** (plat′ĭ-ba′sĭ-ah) [ *platy-* + G. *basis*, ground ]. Basilar invagination; a developmental anomaly of the skull in which the floor of the posterior cranial fossa bulges upward in the region around the foramen magnum.

**platycephalic, platycephalous** (plat′ĭ-sĕ-fal′ik, -sef′ă-lus) [ *platy-* + G. *kephalē, head* ]. Having a flattened skull, one with a vertical index less than 70.

**platycephaly** (plat′ĭ-sef′ă-lĭ) [ *platy-* + G. *kephalē*, head ]. Flatness of the skull, a condition in which the vertical cranial index is below 70; platycrania.

**platycnemia** (plat′ik-ne′mĭ-ah) [ *platy-* + G. *knēmē*, leg ]. Platycnemism; a condition in which the tibia is abnormally broad and flat.

**platycnemic** (plat′ik-ne′mik). Relating to or marked by platycnemia.

**platycnemism** (plat′ik-ne′mizm). Platycnemia.

**platycoria** (plat′ĭ-ko′rĭ-ah) [ *platy-* + G. *korē*, pupil ]. Obsolete term for mydriasis.

**platycrania** (plat′ĭ-kra′nĭ-ah) [ *platy-* + G. *kranion*, skull ]. Platycephaly.

**platycyte** (plat′ĭ-sīt) [ *platy-* + G. *kytos*, cell ]. A relatively small giant cell sometimes formed in tubercles.

**platyglossal** (plat′ĭ-glos′al) [ *platy-* + G. *glōssa*, tongue ]. Having a broad, flattened tongue.

**platyhelminth** (plat′ĭ-hel′minth) [ *platy-* + G. *helmins, worm* ]. Common name for any flatworm of the phylum Platyhelminthes; any cestode (tapeworm) or trematode (fluke).

**Platyhelminthes** (plat′ĭ-hel-min′thēz) [ see platyhelminth ]. A phylum of flatworms that are bilaterally symmetric, flattened, and somewhat leaflike in contour, and without a true body cavity, as it is filled with a parenchymatous syncytium. This phylum is therefore considered in the acelom group, nematodes are in the pseudocelom group, and arthropods and vertebrates are combined in the celom group. There is no digestive tract in some platyhelminths (Cestoda) or the gut may be incomplete (without an anus) as in the Trematoda. Most of the forms are hermaphroditic. There are four classes, but the parasitic species of importance in man are included in the subclass Cestoda (the tapeworms) of the class Cestoidea, and in the subclass Digenea (the flukes) of the class Trematoda.

**platyhieric** (plat′ĭ-hi-ēr′ik) [ *platy-* + G. *heiron*, sacrum ]. Having a broad sacrum.

**platymeric** (plat′ĭ-me′rik, -mēr′ik) [ *platy-* + G. *meros*, thigh ]. Having a broad femur.

**platymorphia** (plat′ĭ-mor′fĭ-ah) [ *platy-* + G. *morphē*, shape ]. Having a flat shape; denoting an eye with a short anteroposterior axis.

**platyopia** (plat′ĭ-o′pĭ-ah) [ *platy-* + G. *ōps*, eye, face ]. Broadness of the face; denoting a condition in which the nasomalar index is less than 107.5.

**platyopic** (plat′ĭ-op′ik, -o′pik). Relating to or characterized by platyopia.

**platypellic** (plat'ĭ-pel'ik) [ platy- + G. *pellis*, bowl (pelvis) ]. Platypelloid; having a broad pelvis, with an index below 90°; see platypellic *pelvis*.

**platypel'loid.** Platypellic.

**platypodia** (plat'ĭ-po'dĭ-ah) [ platy- + G. *pous*, foot ]. *Talipes planus*.

**platyrrhine** (plat'ĭ-rin) [ platy- + G. *rhis*, nose ]. 1. Characterized by a nose of large width in proportion to its length. 2. Denoting a skull with a nasal index between 51.1 or 53, and 58.

**platyrrhiny** (plat'ĭ-ri-nĭ). A condition in which the nose is wide in proportion to its length.

**platysma,** pl. **platysmas, platysmata** (plă-tiz'mah) [ G. *platysma*, a flatplate ] [ NA ]. Musculus platysma; musculus platysma myoides; musculus subcutaneous colli; musculus tetragonus; panniculus carnosus muscle (2); *origin*, subcutaneous layer and fascia covering pectoralis major and deltoid at level of 1st or 2d rib; *insertion*, lower border of mandible, risorius and platysma of opposite side; *action*, depresses lower lip, wrinkles skin of neck and upper chest; *nerve supply*, cervical branch of facial.

**platyspondylia** (plat-ĭ-spon-dil'ĭ-ah) [ platy- + G. *spondylos*, vertebra ]. Flatness of the bodies of the vertebrae.

**plat'yspondyli'sis.** Platyspondylia.

**platystencephaly** (plă-tis'ten-sef'ă-lĭ) [ G. *platystos*, widest, superl. of *platys*, wide, + *enkephalē*, brain ]. Extreme width of the skull in the occipital region, with narrowing anteriorly and prognathism.

**Plaut** (plowt), Hugo K., Hamburg physician, 1858–1928. See P.'s *angina, bacillus, ulcer*.

**Pleasure,** Max A., U. S. dentist. See P. *curve*.

**plectridium** (plek-trid'ĭ-um) [ Mod. L. dim. of G. *plēktron*, an instrument to strike with. PLES- ]. A bacterial rod-shaped cell that contains a spore at one end, imparting a drumstick shape to the cell, such as the spore-containing cells in the organism causing tetanus, *Clostridium tetani*.

**pledget** (plej'et). A tuft of wool, cotton, or lint.

**plegaphonia** (pleg-ah-fo'ne-ah) [ G. *plēgē*, stroke (PLES-), + *aphōnia*, absence of voice ]. Tapping on the larynx or trachea, to take the place of the voice sounds in auscultation.

**-plegia** (-ple'jĭ-ah) [ G. *plēgē*, stroke. PLES- ]. Combining form (suffix) meaning paralysis.

**Plehn** (plān), Albert, German physician, 1861–1935. See P.'s karychromatophile *granules*.

**pleiades** (pli'ă-dēz) [ G. *Pleias*, pl. *Pleiades*, the group of small stars in the constellation *Taurus* ]. A collection of enlarged lymph nodes.

**pleio-** (pli'o-) [ G. *pleiōn*, more ]. Combining form meaning more; for words beginning thus, and not found here, see pleo-.

**pleiotropy, pleiotropia** (pli-ot'ro-pĭ, pli'o-tro'pĭ-ah) [ pleio- + G. *tropos*, turning ]. The production by a single mutant gene of apparently unrelated multiple effects at the clinical or phenotypic level; a pleiotropic gene produces a clinical syndrome.

**pleo-** (ple'o-) [ G. *pleiōn*, more ]. Combining form meaning more.

**pleochroic** (ple-o-kro'ik) [ pleo- + G. *chroa*, color ]. Pleochromatic.

**pleochroism** (ple-ok'ro-izm). Pleochromatism.

**pleochromatic** (ple-o-kro-mat'ik). Pleochroic; relating to pleochromatism.

**pleochromatism** (ple-o-kro'mă-tizm) [ pleo- + G. *chrōma*, color ]. Property of showing changes of color when illuminated along different axes, as certain crystals or liquids; chameleonism; pleochroism.

**pleochromocytoma** (ple-o-kro'mo-si-to'mah) [ pleo- + G. *chrōma*, color, + *kytos*, a hollow (cell), + suffix -*ōma*, tumor ]. A neoplasm consisting of cells that manifest varying pigmentation.

**pleocytosis** (ple'o-si-to'sis) [ pleo- + G. *kytos*, cell, + suffix -*ōsis*, condition ]. The presence anywhere of more cells than normal; often denotes leukocytosis and especially lymphocytosis or round cell infiltration. It orginally was applied to the lymphocytosis of the cerebrospinal fluid present in syphilis of the central nervous system.

**pleomas'tia** [ pleo- + G. *mastos*, breast ]. Polymastia.

**pleoma'zia** [ pleo- + G. *mazos*, breast ]. Polymastia.

**pleomorphic** (ple'o-mor'fik). 1. Pleomorphous; polymorphous; multiform; occurring in more than one morphological form. 2. Among fungi, having two or more spore forms; also used to describe a sterile mutant dermatophyte resulting from degenerative changes in culture.

**pleomorphism** (ple'o-mor'fizm) [ pleo- + G. *morphē*, form ]. Polymorphism; occurrence in more than one form; the existence of more than one morphological type in the same species or other natural group.

**pleomor'phous.** Pleomorphic (1).

**pleonasm** (ple'o-nazm) [ G. *pleonasmos*, exaggeration, excessive, fr. *pleiōn*, more ]. Redundancy of parts; excess in size.

**pleonectic** (ple-o-nek'tik). 1. Marked by pleonexia. 2. An obsolete term denoting specifically a blood that has a percentage saturation of oxygen above normal at any given pressure; see also mesectic and mionectic.

**pleonexia** (ple'o-nek'sĭ-ah) [ pleo- + G. *echō*, fut. *hexō*, to have ]. Excessive greediness.

**pleonosteosis** (ple'on-os'te-o'sis) [ pleo- + G. *osteon*, bone, + suffix -*osis*, condition ]. Superabundance of bone formation.

**Leri's p.,** a syndrome of precocious and excessive ossification resulting in short stature, upward slant of palpebral fissures, short spadelike hands with broad thumbs in valgus position, generalized limitation of joint mobility; autosomal dominant inheritance.

**pleoptics** (ple-op'tiks) [ pleo- + optics, *q. v.* ]. A term introduced by Bangerter to include all forms of treatment for amblyopia, particularly that associated with eccentric fixation.

**pleoptophor** (ple-op'to-fōr) [ pleo- + G. *optos*, visible, + *phoros*, bearing ]. An instrument for the treatment of amblyopia.

**plerocercoid** (ple-ro-ser'koyd) [ G. *plērēs*, full, complete, + *kerkos*, tail ]. A stage in the development of a tapeworm following the procercoid stage, which takes place in an animal serving as intermediate host. This form is a wormlike larva with an invaginated scolex at one end, such as the sparganum of infective p. in the flesh of various fishes, the ingestion of which transmits the broad fish tapeworm, *Diphyllobothrium latum*, to man.

**plesio-** (ple'sĭ-o-) [ G. *plēsios*, close, near ]. Combining form denoting nearness, or similarity.

**plesiomorphic** (ple'sĭ-o-mor'fik). Resembling in form.

**plesiomorphism** (ple'sĭ-o-mor'fizm) [ plesio- + G. *morphē*, form ]. Similarity in form.

**plesiomorphous** (ple'sĭ-o-mor'fus). Plesiomorphic.

**pless-, plessi-** [ G. *plessō*, to strike. PLES- ]. Combining forms denoting a striking, especially percussion.

**plessesthesia** (ples-es-the'zĭ-ah) [ G. *plēssō*, to strike, + *aisthēsis*, sensation ]. Palpatory *percussion*.

**plessimeter** (plĕ-sim'e-ter) [ G. *plēssō*, to strike, + *metron*, measure ]. Pleximeter; plexometer; an oblong plate of hard rubber, ivory, or other flexible substance, used in mediate percussion, being placed against the surface and struck with the plessor.

**ples'simet'ric.** Relating to a plessimeter.

**ples'sor** [ G. *plēssō*, to strike ]. Plexor; a small hammer, usually with soft rubber head, used to tap the part directly, or through the plesssimeter, in percussion of the chest or other part.

**plethora** (pleth'o-rah) [ G. *plēthōrē*, fullness, fr. *plēthō*, to become full ]. Repletion. 1. Hypervolemia. 2. An excess of any of the body fluids.

**p. apocop'tica,** a temporary increase in the volume of blood in the rest of the body, the result of forcing the blood from a limb that is to be amputated.

**hydremic p.,** increase in blood volume because of increase in its water content.

**plethoric** (plĕ-thor'ik, pleth'o-rik). Relating to plethora.

**plethysmograph** (plĕ-thiz'mo-graf) [ G. *plēthysmos*, increase, + *graphō*, to write ]. A device for measuring and recording changes in volume of a part, organ, or whole body.

**body p.,** aeroplethysmograph; a chamber apparatus surrounding the entire body, commonly used in studies of respiratory function.

**pressure p.,** (1) a p. applied to part of the body, *e.g.,* a limb segment, and arranged so that volume is measured during temporary application of sufficient pressure to the part to empty its blood vessels; (2) a body p. in which changes of body volume are measured in terms of the consequent changes in air pressure in the body p.

**volume-displacement p.,** a p., usually a body p., in which changes in volume displace a corresponding volume into or out of a very compliant measuring device, such as a pneometer or integrating flowmeter.

**plethysmography** (pleth'iz-mog'ră-fĭ) [ G. *plēthysmos,* increase, + *graphē,* a writing ]. Measuring and recording changes in volume of an organ or other part of the body by a plethysmograph.

    **impedance p.,** rheocardiography.

    **venous occlusion p.,** measurement of the rate of arterial inflow into an organ or limb segment by measuring its initial rate of increase in volume when its venous outflow is suddenly occluded.

**plethysmometry** (pleth'iz-mom'e-trĭ) [ G. *plēthysmos,* increase, + *metron,* measure ]. Measuring the fullness of a hollow organ or vessel, as of the pulse.

**pleur-, pleura-, pleuro-** (ploor-) [ G. *pleura,* a rib, the side. PLEUR- ] Combining forms denoting relationship to the rib, the side, or the pleura.

**pleura,** gen. and pl. **pleu'rae** (ploor'ah) [ G. *pleura,* a rib, pl. the side. PLEUR- ] [ NA ]. The serous membrane enveloping the lungs and lining the walls of the pleural cavity.

    **cervical p.,** *cupula pleurae.*

    **p. costa'lis** [ NA ], costal p.; the layer of parietal p. lining the chest walls.

    **p. diaphragmat'ica** [ NA ], diaphragmatic p.; the layer of parietal p. covering the upper surface of the diaphragm, except along its costal attachments and where it is covered with the pericardium.

    **p. mediastina'lis** [ NA ], mediastinal p.; the continuation of the costal p. passing from the sternum to the vertebral column which covers the side of the mediastinum.

    **p. parieta'lis** [ NA ], parietal p.; that which lines the different parts of the wall of the pleural cavity, called costal, diaphragmatic, mediastinal, and cervical according to the parts invested.

    **p. pericardi'aca,** pericardial p.; that portion of the mediastinal p. which is fused with the pericardium.

    **p. phren'ica,** p. diaphragmatica.

    **p. pulmona'lis** [ NA ], pulmonary p.; the layer investing the lungs and dipping into the fissures between the several lobes.

    **p. viscera'lis,** p. pulmonalis.

**pleuracentesis** (ploor'ă-sen-te'sis). Thoracentesis.

**pleuracotomy** (ploor'ă-kot'o-mĭ) [ pleura + G. *tomē,* a cutting ]. Thoracotomy.

**pleural** (ploor'al). Relating to the pleura.

**pleuralgia** (ploor-al'jĭ-ah) [ pleur- + G. *algos,* pain ]. Pleurodynia.

**pleural'gic.** Relating to pleuralgia.

**pleurapophysis** (ploor'ă-pof'ĭ-sis) [ pleur- + G. *apophysis,* process, offshoot. PHYS-1 ]. A rib, or the process on a cervical or lumbar vertebra corresponding thereto.

**pleurectomy** (ploor-ek'to-mĭ) [ pleur- + G. *ektomē,* excision ]. Excision of pleura.

**pleurisy** (ploor'ĭ-sĭ) [ L. *pleurisis,* fr. G. *pleuritis, q.v.* ]. Pleuritis; inflammation of the pleura.

    **adhesive p.,** dry p.

    **benign dry p.,** epidemic *pleurodynia.*

    **costal p.,** inflammation of the pleura lining the thoracic walls.

    **diaphragmat'ic p.,** epidemic *pleurodynia.*

    **dry p.,** p. with a fibrinous exudation, without an effusion of serum, resulting in more or less adhesion between the opposing surfaces of the pleura.

    **p. with effusion,** p. accompanied by serous exudation.

    **encys'ted p.,** a form of serofibrinous p., in which adhesions occur at various points, circumscribing the serous effusion.

    **epidemic benign dry p.,** Bornholm *disease.*

    **epidemic diaphragmat'ic p.,** Bornholm *disease.*

    **fi'brinous p.,** dry p.

    **hemorrhag'ic p.,** p. with an effusion of blood-stained serum.

    **interlob'ular p.,** inflammation more or less limited to the pleura in the sulci between the pulmonary lobes.

    **metapneumon'ic p.,** purulent p., or empyema, marked by the presence of the pneumococcus.

    **plastic p.,** dry p.

    **proliferating p.,** p. with a tendency for the proliferation of inflammatory exudate.

    **pulmonary p.,** visceral p.; inflammation of the pleura covering the lungs.

    **pu'rulent p.,** empyema.

    **sacculated p.,** p. with the inflammatory exudate divided into separate regions by adhesions or inflammatory changes.

    **serofi'brinous p.,** the more common form of p. characterized by a fibrinous exudate on the surface of the pleura and a more or less extensive effusion of serous fluid into the pleural cavity.

    **serous p.,** p. with effusion.

    **sup'purative p.,** empyema.

    **typhoid p.,** acute or subacute p. with typhoid symptoms.

    **vis'ceral p.,** pulmonary p.

    **wet p.,** p. with effusion.

**pleurisy root.** *Asclepias tuberosa.*

**pleuritic** (ploor-it'ik). Relating to pleura or suffering from pleurisy.

**pleuritis** (ploor-i'tis) [ G. fr. *pleura,* side, + suffix *-itis,* inflammation ]. Pleurisy.

**pleuritogenous** (ploor'ĭ-toj'ĕ-nus) [ G. *pleuritis,* pleurisy, + *genesis,* origin ]. Tending to produce pleurisy.

**pleuro-** (ploor'o-). See pleur-.

**pleurocele** (ploor'o-sēl) [ pleuro- + G. *kēlē,* hernia ]. Pneumonocele.

**pleurocentesis** (ploor'o-sen-te'sis) [ pleuro- + G. *kentēsis,* puncture ]. Thoracentesis.

**pleurocentrum** (ploor'o-sen'trum) [ pleuro- + G. *kentron,* center ]. One of the lateral halves of the body of a vertebra.

**pleuroclysis** (ploor-ok'lĭ-sis) [ pleuro- + G. *klysis,* a washing out ]. Washing out of the pleural cavity.

**pleurodynia** (ploor'o-din'ĭ-ah) [ pleuro- + G. *odynē,* pain ]. 1. Pleuritic pain in the chest. 2. Pleuralgia; a painful rheumatic affection of the tendinous attachments of the thoracic muscles, usually of one side only.

    **epidemic p.,** an acute infectious disease usually occurring in epidemic form and characterized by paroxysms of pain, usually in the chest; it is associated with strains of group B Coxsackie virus. Also called Bornholm, Balme, bamie, Daae's, or Sylvest's disease; devil's grip; myositis acuta epidemica; benign dry pleurisy; diaphragmatic pleurisy; epidemic transient diaphragmatic spasm; epidemic myalgia; epidemic myositis.

**pleurogenic, pleurogenous** (ploor'o-jen'ik, -oj'ĕ-nus) [ pleuro- + G. suffix *-gen,* producing ]. 1. Of pleural origin; beginning in the pleura. 2. Arising from a rib.

**pleurography** (ploor-og'ră-fĭ) [ pleuro- + G. *graphō,* to write ]. Roentgenography of the pleural cavity.

**pleurohepatitis** (ploor'o-hep-ă-ti'tis) [ pleuro- + G. *hēpar,* liver, + suffix *-itis,* inflammation ]. Hepatitis with extension of the inflammation to the neighboring portion of the pleura.

**pleurolith** (ploor'o-lith) [ pleuro- + G. *lithos,* stone ]. Pleural calculus; a concretion in the pleural cavity.

**pleurolysis** (ploor-ol'ĭ-sis) [ pleuro- + G. *lysis,* dissolution ]. Jacobaeus *operation.*

**pleuromelus** (ploor'o-me'lus) [ pleuro- + G. *melos,* limb ]. A congenitally abnormal individual with an accessory limb that arises from the thorax or flank.

**pleuroparietopexy** (ploor'o-pă-ri'e-to-pek'sĭ) [ pleuro- + parietal, *q.v.,* + G. *pēxis,* fixation ]. Suturing visceral pleura to thoracic wall.

**pleuropericardial** (ploor'o-pĕr-ĭ-kar'dĭ-al). Relating to both pleura and pericardium.

**pleuropericarditis** (ploor'o-pĕr'ĭ-kar-di'tis) [ pleuro- + pericardium + G. suffix *-itis,* inflammation ]. Combined inflammation of the pericardium and of the pleura.

**pleuroperitoneal** (ploor'o-pĕr-ĭ-to-ne'al). Relating to both pleura and peritoneum.

**pleuropneumonia** (ploor'o-nu-mo'nĭ-ah). A specific infectious disease in cattle, characterized by inflammation of the lungs and pleura; it occurs in Africa, Asia, and Australia and is caused by *Mycoplasma mycoides* subsp. *mycoides*.

**pleuropulmonary** (ploor'o-pul'mo-nĕr-ĭ). Relating to the pleura and the lungs.

**pleurorrhea** (ploor'o-re'ah) [ pleuro- + G. *rhoia*, a flow ]. Hydrothorax; a pleural effusion.

**pleurosoma** (ploor'o-so'mah) [ pleuro- + G. *sōma*, body ]. An individual with defects in the thoracic and upper abdominal walls accompanied by a variable amount of eventration; frequently involves imperfect development of the arm.

**pleurothotonos, pleurothotonus** (ploor'o-thot'o-nus) [ G. *pleurothen* (adv.), from the side, + *tonos*, tension ]. Tetanus lateralis; lateral bending of the body; formerly, but now rarely seen, a common symptom of conversion hysteria.

**pleurotomy** (ploor-ot'o-mĭ) [ pleuro- + G. *tomē*, incision ]. Thoracotomy.

**pleurotyphoid** (ploor'o-ti'foyd). Typhoid fever in which the early stage is masked by the physical signs of pleurisy.

**pleurovisceral** (ploor'o-vis'er-al). Visceropleural.

**plexal** (plek'sal). Relating to a plexus.

**plexalgia** (plek-sal'jĭ-ah) [ G. *plexis*, a stroke (PLES-), + *algos*, pain ]. A symptom complex observed in bodies of troops after prolonged exposure to cold and wet; it is characterized by multiple pains, paresthesia, general fatigue, excitability, and insomnia.

**plexectomy** (plek-sek'to-mĭ) [ plexus + G. *ektomē*, excision ]. Surgical section of a plexus.

**plexiform** (plek'sĭ-form) [ plexus + L. *forma*, form ]. Resembling or forming a plexus.

**pleximeter** (plek'sim'ĭ-ter) [ G. *plexis*, stroke (PLES-) ]. Plessimeter.

**plexitis** (plek'si'tis). Irritation of a plexus.

**plexometer** (plek-som'e-ter). Plessimeter.

**plexor** (plek'sor) [ G. *plexis*, a stroke ]. Plessor.

---

# PLEXUS

---

**plexus**, pl. (Eng.) **plexuses**, (Lat.) **plexus** (plek'sus) [ L. a braid. PLIC- ] [ NA ]. A network or interjoining of nerves and blood vessels or of lymphatic vessels.

    **abdominal aortic p.,** p. aorticus abdominalis.

    **an'nular p.,** p. annularis; a nerve p. near the corneoscleral junction from which myelinated and unmyelinated nerves pass to the cornea.

    **p. annula'ris,** annular p.

    **p. of anterior cerebral artery,** p. arteriae cerebri anterioris; an autonomic p. accompanying the anterior cerebral artery, derived from the internal carotid p.

    **anterior coronary p.,** the part of the cardiac p. that accompanies the coronary arteries on the anterior aspect of the heart.

    **aortic p.,** p. aorticus; a p. of lymph nodes and connecting vessels lying along the lower portion of the abdominal aorta.

    **p. aor'ticus,** aortic p.

    **p. aor'ticus abdomina'lis** [ NA ], abdominal aortic p.; an autonomic p. surrounding the abdominal aorta, directly continuous with the thoracic aortic p.

    **p. aor'ticus thora'cicus** [ NA ], thoracic aortic p.; an autonomic p. surrounding the thoracic aorta and passing with it through the aortic opening in the diaphragm, to become continous with the abdominal aortic p.

    **p. arte'riae cer'ebri ante'rioris,** p. of anterior cerebral artery.

    **p. arte'riae cer'ebri me'diae,** p. of middle cerebral artery.

    **p. arte'riae choroi'deae,** p. of choroid artery.

    **ascending pharyngeal p.,** p. pharyngeus ascendens; automatic p. on the artery of the same name, formed of fibers from the superior cervical ganglion.

    **Auerbach's p.,** p. myentericus.

    **p. auricula'ris poste'rior,** posterior auricular p.

    **autonomic p.'s,** p. autonomici.

    **p. autono'mici** [ NA ], autonomic p.'s; p.'s of nerves in relation to blood vessels and viscera, the component fibers of which are sympathetic, parasympathetic, and sensory.

    **p. axilla'ris,** axillary p.

    **axillary p.,** p. axillaris; a lymphatic p. formed of the lymph nodes, with their afferent and efferent vessels, in the axilla.

    **basilar p.,** p. basilaris.

    **p. basila'ris** [ NA ], basilar p.; sinus basilaris; a venous p. on the clivus, connected with the inferior petrosal and cavernous sinuses.

    **brachial p.,** p. brachialis.

    **p. brachia'lis** [ NA ], brachial p.; formed of the anterior rami of the fifth cervical to first thoracic nerves; the nerves converge in the posterior triangle of the neck between the scalenus anterior and medius and pass down on the lateral side of the subclavian artery behind the clavicle into the axilla.

    **cardiac p.,** p. cardiacus.

    **p. cardi'acus** [ NA ], cardiac p.; a wide-meshed network of anastomosing cords from the sympathetic and vagus nerves, surrounding the arch of the aorta and the pulmonary artery and continuing to the atria, ventricles, and coronary vessels.

    **p. cardi'acus profun'dus,** deep cardiac p.

    **p. cardi'acus superficia'lis,** superficial cardiac p.

    **p. carot'icus commu'nis** [ NA ], common carotid p.; an autonomic p. accompanying the artery of the same name formed by fibers from the middle cervical ganglion.

    **p. carot'icus exter'nus** [ NA ], external carotid p.; an autonomic p. formed by the external carotid nerves surrounding the artery of the same name, and giving origin to a number of secondary p.'s along the branches of this artery and to branches to the carotid body.

    **p. carot'icus inter'nus,** internal carotid p.; (1) [ NA ], an autonomic p. surrounding the internal carotid artery in the carotid canal and cavernous sinus, and sending branches to the tympanic p., sphenopalatine ganglion, abducens and oculomotor nerves, the cerebral vessels, and the ciliary ganglion; (2) p. venosus caroticus internus.

    **p. caverno'si concha'rum** [ NA ], cavernous p. of the conchae; corpus cavernosum conchae; erectile tissue in the mucous membrane covering the conchae of the nasal cavity.

    **p. caverno'sus,** cavernous p.

    **cavernous p.,** p. cavernosus; the portion of the internal carotid p. in the cavernous sinus.

    **cavernous p. of clitoris,** *nervi* cavernosi clitoridis.

    **cavernous p. of conchae,** p. cavernosi concharum.

    **cavernous p. of penis,** *nervi* cavernosi penis.

    **celiac p.,** p. celiacus.

    **p. celi'acus,** celiac p.; (1) [ NA ] solar p.; cerebrum abdominale; abdominal brain; Vieussens' ganglion; the largest of the autonomic p.'s lying in front of the aorta at the level of origin of the celiac artery, behind the stomach; it is formed by the splanchnic and the vagus nerves and cords from the celiac and superior mesenteric ganglia; through its connections with the other abdominal p.'s it sends branches to all the abdominal viscera; (2) a lymphatic p. formed of the superior mesenteric lymph nodes and the fifteen or twenty celiac nodes behind the stomach, duodenum, and pancreas, together with the connecting vessels.

    **cervical p.,** p. cervicalis.

    **p. cervica'lis** [ NA ], cervical p.; formed by loops joining the anterior rami of the first four cervical nerves and receiving gray communicating rami from the superior cervical ganglion; it lies beneath the sternocleidomastoid muscle, and sends out numerous cutaneous, muscular, and communicating rami.

    **choroid p.,** p. choroideus.

    **p. of choroid artery,** p. arteriae choroideae; an autonomic p. accompanying the artery of the same name, derived from the internal carotid p.

**choroid p. of fourth ventricle,** p. choroideus ventriculi quarti.

**choroid p. of lateral ventricle,** p. choroideus ventriculi lateralis.

**choroid p. of third ventricle,** p. choroideus ventriculi tertii.

**p. choroi'deus** [ NA ], choroid p.; a vascular proliferation or fringe of the tela choroidea in one of the cerebral ventricles; by secretion or absorption of cerebrospinal fluid the choroid p. serves to regulate the intraventricular pressure.

**p. choroi'deus ventric'uli latera'lis** [ NA ], choroid p. of the lateral ventricle; the vascular fringe that projects from the choroidal fissure into each lateral ventricle.

**p. choroi'deus ventric'uli quar'ti** [ NA ], choroid p. of the fourth ventricle; one of two vascular fringes of pia mater projecting on either side from the lower part of the roof of the fourth cerebral ventricle.

**p. choroi'deus ventric'uli ter'tii** [ NA ], choroid p. of the third ventricle; diaplexus; the double row of vascular projections from the undersurface of the tela choroidea where it roofs over the third ventricle.

**ciliary ganglionic p.,** p. gangliosus ciliaris; an autonomic p. lying on the ciliary muscle, derived from the oculomotor, trigeminal, and sympathetic.

**coccygeal p.,** p. coccygeus.

**p. coccyge'us** [ NA ], coccygeal p.; a small p. formed by the 5th sacral and the coccygeal nerves, usually regarded as forming part of the pudendal p.; it gives origin to the anococcygeal nerves.

**common carotid p.,** p. caroticus communis.

**p. corona'rius cor'dis,** coronary p. of the heart.

**coronary p. of the heart,** p. coronarius cordis; the continuation of the cardiac p. onto the coronary arteries.

**Cruveilhier's p.,** a nerve p. formed by communications between the posterior rami of the first three cervical nerves. It lies deep to the semispinalis capitis muscle.

**deep cardiac p.,** p. cardiacus profundus; the deeper part of the cardiac p.

**deferential p.,** p. deferentialis.

**p. deferentia'lis** [ NA ], deferential p.; an autonomic p. on the seminal vesicle and ampulla of the ductus deferens on each side, derived from the inferior hypogastric p.

**p. denta'lis infe'rior** [ NA ], inferior dental p.; formed by branches of the inferior alveolar nerve interlacing before they supply the teeth; it gives off dental branches (rami dentales inferiores) and branches to the gums (rami gingivales inferiores).

**p. denta'lis supe'rior** [ NA ], superior dental p.; formed by branches of the infraorbital nerve; it gives off dental branches (rami dentales superiores) and branches to the gums (rami gingivales superiores).

**enteric p.,** p. entericus.

**p. enter'icus** [ NA ], enteric p.; the autonomic p. in the wall of the intestine; it consists of three parts, p. submucosus, p. myentericus, and p. subserosus; ganglionic cells are scattered through the myenteric and submucous p.'s.

**esophageal p.,** p. esophageus.

**p. esophage'us** [ NA ], esophageal p.; p. gulae; one of two nervous p.'s, posterior and anterior on the walls of the esophagus; the first is formed by branches from the right vagus and left recurrent, the second by the anastomosing trunks of the vagus after leaving the pulmonary p.'s; branches supply the mucous and muscular coats of the esophagus.

**Exner's p.,** a p. formed by tangential nerve fibers in the superficial plexiform or molecular layer of the cerebral cortex.

**external carotid p.,** p. caroticus externus.

**external iliac p.,** p. iliacus externus; a lymphatic p. formed by the lymph nodes along the external iliac artery on either side, and their afferent and efferent vessels.

**external maxillary p.,** p. maxillaris externus; an autonomic p. on the facial artery, sending a branch to the submaxillary ganglion, derived from the external carotid p.

**femoral p.,** p. femoralis.

**p. femora'lis** [ NA ], femoral p.; an autonomic p. surrounding the femoral artery, derived from the iliac p.

**p. ganglio'sus cilia'ris,** ciliary ganglionic p.

**gastric p.'s of autonomic system,** p. gastrici systemati autonomici.

**p. gas'trici systema'ti autono'mici** [ NA ], gastric p.'s of the autonomic system; the p.'s along the greater and lesser curvatures of the stomach derived from the celiac p.; also known as inferior and superior p.

**p. gu'lae** [ L. *gula,* gullet ], p. esophageus.

**Haller's p.,** a nervous p. of sympathetic filaments and branches of the external laryngeal nerve on the surface of the inferior constrictor muscle of the pharynx.

**Heller's p.,** p. of small arteries in the wall of the intestine.

**hemorrhoidal p.,** p. venos ; rectalis; see also entries under p. rectales.

**hepatic p.,** p. hepaticus.

**p. hepat'icus** [ NA ], hepatic p.; an unpaired autonomic p. lying on the hepatc artery and its branches in the liver.

**p. hypogas'tricus infe'rior** [ NA ], p. pelvinus [ NA ]; inferior hypogastric p.; pelvic p.; the autonomic p. in the pelvis that is distributed to the pelvic viscera; it receives the hypogastric nerves and the pelvic splanchnic nerves.

**p. hypogas'tricus supe'rior** [ NA ], nervus presacralis [ NA ]; superior hypogastric p.; presacral nerve; the continuation of the aortic p. downward across the fifth lumbar vertebra into the pelvis where it divides into two hypogastric nerves at the sides of the rectum; these join the inferior hypogastric p.'s to supply pelvic viscera.

**iliac p.,** p. iliaci.

**p. ili'aci** [ NA ], iliac p.; the autonomic p. lying on the iliac arteries, derived from the aortic p.

**p. ili'acus exter'nus,** external iliac p.

**inferior dental p.,** p. dentalis inferior.

**inferior hemorrhoidal p.'s,** p. rectales inferiores.

**inferior hypogastric p.,** p. hypogastricus inferior.

**inferior mesenteric p.,** p. mesentericus inferior.

**inferior rectal p.'s,** p. rectales inferiores.

**inferior thyroid p.,** p. thyroideus inferior; an autonomic p. on the artery of this name, derived from the subclavian p.

**inferior vesical p.,** p. vesicalis inferior; a venous p. in the female corresponding to the prostatic venous p. in the male.

**inguinal p.,** p. inguinalis; a lymphatic p. formed of 10 to 15 lymph nodes with their connecting vessels lying superficially near the termination of the great saphenous vein and more deeply along the femoral artery and vein.

**p. inguina'lis,** inguinal p.

**intermesenteric p.** p. intermesentericus.

**p. intermesenter'icus** [ NA ], intermesenteric p.; the part of the aortic p. lying between the superior and inferior mesenteric p.'s.

**internal carotid p.,** p. caroticus internus.

**internal carotid venous p.,** p. venosus caroticus internus.

**internal mammary p.,** p. mammarius internus; an autonomic p. on the internal thoracic artery, derived from the subclavian p.

**internal maxillary p.,** p. maxillaris internus; the autonomic p. on the maxillary artery derived from the external carotid p.

**ischiadic p.,** p. sacralis.

**Jacobson's p.,** p. tympanicus.

**Jacques' p.,** a nerve p. within the muscular coat of the uterine (Fallopian) tube.

**jugular p.,** p. jugularis; a lymphatic p. formed of many lymph nodes, with their afferent and efferent vessels, extending along the internal jugular vein.

**p. jugula'ris,** jugular p.

**Leber's p.,** a small venous p. in the eye between the venous sinuses of the sclera (of Schlemm) and the spaces of the iridocorneal angle (of Fontana).

**p. liena'lis** [ NA ], splenic p.; the p. of autonomic nerves along the splenic artery.

**lingual p.,** p. lingualis; an autonomic p. on the artery of this name, derived from the external carotid p.

**p. lingua'lis,** lingual p.

**p. lumba'lis,** lumbar p.; (1) [ NA ], a nervous p., formed by the ventral rami of the first four lumbar nerves; it lies in the substance of the psoas muscle; (2) a lymphatic p. formed of about twenty lymph nodes and connecting vessels situated along the lower portion of the aorta and the common iliac vessels.

**lumbar p.,** p. lumbalis.

**lumbosacral p.,** p. lumbosacralis.

**p. lumbosacra'lis** [ NA ], lumbosacral p.; formed by the union of the anterior rami of the lumbar and sacral nerves; it is divided into lumbar and sacral p.'s.

**lymphatic p.,** p. lymphaticus.

**p. lymphat'icus** [ NA ], lymphatic plexus or network; a p. of lymphatic capillaries, usually without valves, that opens into one or more larger lymphatic vessels.

**p. mamma'rius,** mammary p.

**p. mamma'rius inter'nus,** internal mammary p.

**mammary p.,** p. mammarius; a lymphatic p., formed of small lymph nodes, with their vessels, situated along the course of the internal thoracic arteries.

**p. maxilla'ris exter'nus,** external maxillary p.

**p. maxilla'ris inter'nus,** internal maxillary p.

**Meissner's p.,** p. submucosus.

**meningeal p.,** p. meningeus.

**p. meninge'us,** meningeal p.; a nerve p. on the cerebral meninges, derived from the external carotid p.

**p. mesenter'icus infe'rior** [ NA ], inferior mesenteric p.; an autonomic p., derived from the aortic, surrounding the inferior mesenteric artery and sending branches to the descending colon, sigmoid, and rectum.

**p. mesenter'icus supe'rior** [ NA ], superior mesenteric p.; an autonomic p., a continuation or part of the celiac p., sending nerves to the intestines and forming with the vagus the subserous, myenteric, and submucous p.'s.

**p. of middle cerebral artery,** p. arteriae cerebri mediae; an autonomic p. accompanying the middle cerebral artery, derived from the internal carotid p.

**middle hemorrhoidal p.'s,** p. rectales medii.

**middle rectal p.'s,** p. rectales medii.

**middle sacral p.,** p. sacralis medius; a lymphatic p. formed of lymph nodes and connecting vessels situated chiefly in the mesorectum anterior and inferior to the promontory.

**myenteric p.,** p. myentericus.

**p. myenter'icus** [ NA ], myenteric p.; p. of Auerbach; a p. of unmyelinated fibers and postganglionic autonomic cell bodies lying in the muscular coat of the esophagus, stomach, and intestines; it communicates with the subserous and submucous p.'s, all subdivisions of the enteric p.

**nerve p.,** p. nervosus; a p. formed by the interlacing of nerves by means of numerous communicating branches.

**p. nervo'rum spina'lium** [ NA ], p. of spinal nerves; an intermingling of fiber fascicles from adjacent spinal nerves to form a network. The major p.'s are the cervical, brachial and lumbosacral.

**p. nervo'sus,** nerve p.

**occipital p.,** p. occipitalis; an autonomic p. on the artery of this name, derived from the external carotid p.

**ophthalmic p.,** p. ophthalmicus; an autonomic p., entering the orbit in company with the ophthalmic artery, derived from the internal carotid p.

**ovarian p.,** p. ovaricus.

**p. ova'ricus** [ NA ], ovarian p.; an autonomic p. derived from the aortic p. and accompanying the ovarian artery to the ovary, broad ligament, and uterine tube.

**pampiniform p.,** p. pampiniformis.

**p. pampinifor'mis** [ NA ], pampiniform p.; a p. formed, in the male, by veins from the testicle and epididymis, consisting of eight or ten veins lying in front of the ductus deferens and forming part of the spermatic cord; in the female the ovarian veins form this p. between the layers of the broad ligament.

**pancreatic p.,** p. pancreaticus.

**p. pancreat'icus** [ NA ], pancreatic p.; the autonomic p. that accompanies the pancretic arteries.

**parotid p.,** p. parotideus.

**p. parotide'us** [ NA ], parotid p.; pes anserinus (1); the diverging branches of the facial nerve passing through the substance of the parotid gland, connected by numerous looped anastomoses.

**pelvic p.,** p. hypogastricus inferior.

**p. pelvi'nus** [ NA ], official alternative name for p. hypogastricus inferior.

**periarterial p.,** p. periarterialis.

**p. periarteria'lis** [ NA ], periarterial p.; an autonomic p. that accompanies an artery.

**pharyngeal p.,** p. pharyngeus.

**p. pharyn'geus** [ NA ], pharyngeal p. (1) the p. of nerves including branches of the glossopharyngeal, vagus, and

accessory nerves, that lies along the posterior wall of the pharynx. (2) a venous p. on the posterolateral walls of the pharynx, emptying through the pharyngeal veins into the internal jugular.

**p. pharyn'geus ascen'dens,** ascending pharyngeal p.

**phrenic p.,** p. phrenicus; an autonomic p. surrounding the inferior phrenic artery.

**popliteal p.,** p. popliteus; a nerve p. surrounding the popliteal artery, derived from the femoral p.

**posterior auricular p.,** p. auricularis posterior; an autonomic p. on the artery of this name, derived from the external carotid p.

**posterior coronary p.,** the portion of the cardiac p. that accompanies branches of the coronary arteries on the posteroinferior surface of the heart.

**prostatic p.,** p. prostaticus.

**prostatic venous p.,** p. venosus prostaticus.

**prostaticovesical p.,** p. prostaticovesicalis; a venous p. around the prostate gland and neck of the bladder; it communicates with the vesical and pudendal p.'s, and empties by one or more efferent vessels into the internal iliac (hypogastric) vein; it corresponds to the inferior vesical p. in the female.

**p. prostat'icus** [ NA ], prostatic p.; an autonomic p. of nerves on the prostate, derived from the inferior hypogastric p.

**pterygoid p.,** p. pterygoideus.

**p. pterygoi'deus** [ NA ], pterygoid p.; a p. situated in the infratemporal fossa, receiving veins accompanying the branches of the maxillary artery, and terminating in the maxillary vein.

**p. pudenda'lis** p. venosus prostaticus.

**p. puden'dus nervo'sus,** *nervus* pudendus.

**p. pulmona'lis** [ NA ], pulmonary p.; one of two autonomic p.'s, anterior and posterior, at the hilus of each lung, formed by branches of the sympathetic and bronchial rami of the vagus nerve; from them various branches accompany the bronchi and arteries into the lung.

**pulmonary p.,** p. pulmonalis.

**Quénu's hemorrhoidal p.,** lymphatic p.'s in the skin about the anus.

**Ranvier's p.,** subbasal stroma p. of the cornea; see stroma p.

**rectal p.'s,** see entries under p. rectales.

**rectal venous p.,** p. venosus rectalis.

**p. recta'les inferio'res** [ NA ], inferior rectal p.'s; inferior hemorrhoidal p.'s; the autonomic p.'s along the anus derived from the inferior hypogastric p.

**p. recta'les me'dii** [ NA ], middle rectal p.'s; middle hemorrhoidal p.'s; the autonomic p.'s along the rectum derived from the inferior hypogastric p.

**p. recta'lis supe'rior** [ NA ], superior rectal p.; superior hemorrhoidal p.; the autonomic p. derived from the inferior mesenteric p. that accompanies the superior rectal artery.

**Remak's p.,** p. submucosus.

**renal p.,** p. renalis.

**p. rena'lis** [ NA ], renal p.; the autonomic p. surrounding the renal artery and extending with it into the substance of the kidney.

**sacral p.,** p. sacralis.

**sacral venous p.,** p. venosus sacralis.

**p. sacra'lis** [ NA ], sacral p.; sciatic p.; ischiadic p.; formed by the fourth and fifth lumbar and first, second, and third sacral nerves; it lies on the inner surface of the posterior wall of the pelvis; its nerves supply the lower limbs.

**p. sacra'lis me'dius,** middle sacral p.

**Sappey's p.,** a network of lymphatics in the areola of the nipple.

**sciatic p.,** p. sacralis.

**solar p.,** p. celiacus.

**spermatic p.,** p. testicularis.

**p. of spinal nerves,** p. nervorum spinalium.

**splenic p.,** p. lienalis.

**Stensen's p.,** the venous network surrounding the parotid (Stensen's) duct.

**stroma p.,** a p. of nerves in the parenchyma of the cornea consisting of the primary or deep p., in the substance of the cornea, and the subbasal or superficial p. just beneath the anterior limiting membrane.

**subclavian p.,** p. subclavius.

**p. subcla'vius** [ NA ], subclavian p.; the autonomic p. accompanying the artery of this name, formed by fibers from the cervico thoracic ganglion, and giving off secondary p.'s along the branches of the subclavian.

**submucosal p.,** p. submucosus.

**p. submuco'sus** [ NA ], submucosal p.; Meissner's or Remak's p.; a gangliated p. of unmyelinated nerve fibers, derived chiefly from the superior mesenteric p., ramifying in the intestinal submucosa.

**suboccipital venous p.,** p. venosus suboccipitalis.

**p. subsero'sus** [ NA ], subserous p.; the subserous part of the enteric plexus of autonomic nerves.

**subserous p.,** p. subserosus.

**superficial cardiac p.,** p. cardiacus superficialis; the superficial and smaller part of the cardiac p.

**superficial temporal p.,** p. temporalis superficialis; an autonomic p. of nerves on the artery of this name, derived from the external carotid p.

**superior dental p.,** p. dentalis superior.

**superior hemorrhoidal p.,** p. rectalis superior.

**superior hypogastric p.,** p. hypogastricus superior.

**superior mesenteric p.,** p. mesentericus superior.

**superior rectal p.,** p. rectalis superior.

**superior thyroid p.,** p. thyroideus superior; an autonomic p. on the artery of the same name, derived from the external carotid p.

**suprarenal p.,** p. suprarenalis.

**p. suprarenalis** [ NA ], suprarenal p.; an autonomic p. formed mainly by branches from the celiac ganglion, lying at the hilus of the suprarenal gland.

**sympathet'ic p.'s,** p. autonomici.

**p. temporalis superficialis,** superficial temporal p.

**testicular p.,** p. testicularis.

**p. testicula'ris** [ NA ], testicular p.; spermatic p.; the autonomic p. derived from the aortic p. and accompanying the testicular artery.

**thoracic aortic p.,** p. aorticus thoracicus.

**p. thyroid'eus im'par** [ NA ], a venous p. in front of the lower portion of the trachea formed by anastomoses between the inferior thyroid veins; it terminates in the unpaired vena thyroidea ima.

**p. thyroi'deus infe'rior,** inferior thyroid p.

**p. thyroi'deus supe'rior,** superior thyroid p.

**tympanic p.,** p. tympanicus.

**p. tympan'icus** [ NA ], tympanic p.; Jacobson's p.; a p. on the promontory of the labyrinthine wall of the tympanic cavity, formed by the tympanic nerve, an anastomotic branch of the facial, and sympathetic branches from the internal carotid p.; it supplies the mucosa of the middle ear, mastoid cells, and auditory (Eustachian) tube, and gives off the lesser petrosal nerve to the otic ganglion.

**ureteric p.,** p. uretericus.

**p. ureter'icus** [ NA ], ureteric p.; the autonomic p. derived from the celiac p. that accompanies the ureter.

**uterine venous p.,** p. venosus uterinus.

**uterovaginal p.,** p. uterovaginalis.

**p. uterovagina'lis** [ NA ], uterovaginal p.; Lee's or Frankenhäuser's ganglion; a gangliated autonomic p. on each side of the cervix uteri, derived from the inferior hypogastric p.

**vaginal venous p.,** p. venosus vaginalis.

**vascular p.,** p. vasculosus.

**p. vasculo'sus** [ NA ], vascular p.; a vascular network formed by frequent anastomoses between the blood vessels (arteries or veins) of a part.

**p. veno'sus** [ NA ], venous p.; a vascular network formed by numerous anastomoses between veins.

**p. veno'sus areola'ris** [ NA ], circulus venosus halleri; venous circle of the mammary gland; vascular circle (3); Haller's circle (2); a venous p. in the areola surrounding the nipple, formed by the mammary veins, and sending its blood to the lateral thoracic vein.

**p. veno'sus cana'lis hypoglos'si** [ NA ], venous p. of hypoglossal canal; circellus venosus hypoglossi; a small venous network around the hypoglossal nerve, connecting with the occipital sinus, inferior petrosal sinus and internal jugular vein.

**p. veno'sus carot'icus inter'nus** [ NA ], internal carotid venous p.; p. caroticus internus (2); a venous network around the internal carotid artery in the carotid canal of the temporal bone, connecting with the cavernous sinus and internal jugular vein.

**p. veno'sus foram'inis ova'lis** [ NA ], venous p. of the foramen ovale; a venous network around the mandibular nerve connecting the cavernous sinus and the pterygoid p.

**p. veno'sus prostat'icus** [ NA ], prostatic venous p.; p. pudendalis; a venous p., arising chiefly from the dorsal vein of the penis, situated at the base of the bladder and sides of the prostate.

**p. veno'sus recta'lis** [ NA ], rectal venous p.; hemorrhoidal p.; a venous p. resting upon the posterior and lateral walls of the rectum; it drains into the superior rectal vein to the portal, the middle rectal to the internal iliac and the inferior rectal to the internal pudendal.

**p. veno'sus sacra'lis** [ NA ], sacral venous p.; a venous p. on the anterior surface of the sacrum, formed by tributaries to the lateral sacral veins.

**p. veno'sus suboccipita'lis** [ NA ], suboccipital venous p.; the extensive p. of veins in the suboccipital region.

**p. veno'sus uteri'nus** [ NA ], uterine venous p.; the plexiform veins that lie along the sides of the uterus in the broad ligament.

**p. veno'sus vagina'lis** [ NA ], vaginal venous p.; the p. of veins that surrounds the vagina.

**p. veno'si vertebra'les** [ NA ], vertebral venous p.'s; venous networks on the outer and inner surfaces of the vertebral column; of the external p.'s the posterior are the larger, the anterior being well marked only in the neck; they empty into the intervertebral veins; the internal p.'s are found between the dura mater and periosteum the entire length of the vertebral canal.

**p. veno'sus vesica'lis** [ NA ], venous p. of the bladder; a p. of veins around the fundus and sides of the bladder.

**venous p.,** p. venosus.

**venous p. of bladder,** p. venosus vesicalis.

**venous p. of foramen ovale,** p. venosus foraminis ovalis.

**venous p. of hypoglossal canal,** p. venosus canalis hypoglossi.

**vertebral p.,** p. vertebralis.

**vertebral venous p.'s,** p. venosi vertebrales.

**p. vertebra'lis** [ NA ], vertebral p.; a p. of autonomic nerves on the artery of this name, derived from the subclavian p.

**vesical p.,** p. vesicalis.

**p. vesica'lis** [ NA ], vesical p.; an autonomic p. on the bladder, derived from the inferior hypogastric p.

**p. vesica'lis infe'rior,** inferior vesical p.

**Walther's p.,** cavernous p.

# PLICA

**plica,** gen. and pl. **plicae** (pli'kah, pli'se) [ Mod. L. a plait or fold. PLIC- ]. 1 [ NA ]. One of several anatomical structures in which there is a folding over of the parts. 2. False *membrane.*

**plicae adipo'sae,** adipose folds of the pleura; lobules of fat enveloped in the pleura, chiefly in the neighborhood of the costomediastinal sinus.

**plicae alares** [ NA ], alar folds; alar ligaments; winglike lateral fringes or expansions of the p. synovialis infrapatellaris.

**p. ampulla'ris,** one of the folds of mucous membrane at the fimbriated extremity of the uterine tube.

**p. aryepiglot'tica** [ NA ], aryepiglottic or arytenoepiglottidean fold; a prominent fold of mucous membrane stretching between the lateral margin of the epiglottis and the arytenoid cartilage on either side; it encloses the aryepiglottic muscle.

**p. axilla'ris** [ NA ], axillary fold; one of the folds of skin and muscular tissue bounding the axilla anteriorly (p. axillaris anterior) and posteriorly (p. axillaris posterior).

**plicae ceca'le** [ NA ], cecal folds; the two peritoneal folds that border the retrocecal fossa.

**p. cecalis vascula'ris** [ NA ], vascular fold of the cecum; a peritoneal fold that arches over a branch of the ileocolic artery and bounds in front a narrow recess, the superior ileocecal (or ileocolic) recess.

**p. chor'dae tym'pani** [ NA ], fold of the chorda tympani; the fold of mucosa that surrounds the chorda tympani nerve in its course through the tympanic cavity.

**p. choroid'ea,** an infolding of the choroid membrane in the embryo; from it the choroid plexus arises.

**plicae cilia'res** [ NA ], ciliary folds; a number of low ridges in the furrows between the ciliary processes; together with the processes they constitute the corona ciliaris.

**plicae circula'res** [ NA ], circular folds; valvulae conniventes; valves of Kerckring; the numerous folds of the mucous membrane of the small intestine, running transversely for about two-thirds of the circumference of the gut.

**p. duodena'lis infe'rior** [ NA ], p. duodenomesocolica [ NA ]; inferior duodenal fold; duodenomesocolic fold; a fold of peritoneum bounding the inferior duodenal fossa, or fossa of Treitz.

**p. duodena'lis supe'rior** [ NA ], p. duodenojejunalis [ NA ]; superior duodenal fold; duodenojejunal fold; a fold of peritoneum bounding the superior duodenal fossa.

**p. duodenojejuna'lis** [ NA ], p. duodenalis superior.

**p. duodenomesocol'ica** [ NA ], p. duodenalis inferior.

**p. epigas'trica,** p. umbilicalis lateralis.

**p. epiglot'tica,** one of the three folds of mucous membrane passing between the tongue and the epiglottis, p. glossoepiglottica lateralis on either side, and p. glossoepiglottica mediana.

**p. fimbria'ta** [ NA ], fimbriated fold; one of several folds running outward from the frenulum on the under surface of the tongue.

**plicae gas'tricae** [ NA ], gastric folds; characteristic folds of the gastric mucosa.

**plicae gas'tropancreat'icae** [ NA ], gastropancreatic folds; the folds of peritoneum in the omental bursa that encase the hepatic and left gastric arteries as these vessels pass toward their destinations.

**p. glossoepiglot'tica latera'lis** [ NA ], lateral glossoepiglottic fold; the fold of mucous membrane that extends from the margin of the epiglottis to the pharyngeal wall and base of the tongue on each side.

**p. glossoepiglot'tica media'na** [ NA ], middle glossoepiglottic fold; frenulum epiglottidis; a fold of mucous membrane in the midline that extends from the back of the tongue to the epiglottis.

**p. guberna'trix,** *ligamentum* genitoinguinale.

**p. hypogas'trica,** p. umbilicalis medialis.

**p. ileoceca'lis** [ NA ], ileocecal fold; a fold of peritoneum bounding the ileocecal or ileoappendicular fossa.

**p. in'cudis** [ NA ], incudal fold; a variable fold of mucosa that passes from the roof of the tympanic cavity to the body and short limb of the incus.

**p. inguina'lis,** inguinal fold; an embryonic mesodermal thickening that joins the caudal end of the urogenital ridge to the anterior abdominal wall; the gubernaculum of the testis develops in it.

**p. interdigita'lis,** one of the folds of skin, or rudimentary web, between the fingers and toes.

**p. interurete'rica** [ NA ], interureteric fold; p. ureterica; bar of bladder; Mercier's bar; a fold of mucous membrane extending from the orifice of the ureter of one side to that of the other side.

**plicae ir'idis** [ NA ], folds of the iris; numerous very fine, almost microscopic, radial folds on the posterior surface of the iris that extend around the pupillary margin.

**p. lacrima'lis** [ NA ], lacrimal fold; Bianchi's, Huschke's, or Rosenmüller's valve; Hasner's valve or fold; a fold of mucous membrane guarding the lower opening of the nasolacrimal duct.

**p. longitudina'lis duodeni** [ NA ], longitudinal fold of the duodenum; a fold of mucosa on the medial wall of the descending part of the duodenum above the papilla duodeni major, probably caused by the relation to the ductus choledochus.

**p. luna'ta,** p. semilunaris conjunctivae.

**p. mallea'ris** [ NA ], mallear fold; one of two ligamentous bands, anterior and posterior, making folds on the tympanic side of the tympanic membrane extending from each extremity of the tympanic notch to the malleolar promi-

nence; they mark the boundary between the tense and the flaccid portions of the tympanic membrane.

**p. membra'nae tym'pani,** p. mallearis.

**p. nervi laryngei** [ NA ], fold of the laryngeal nerve; the slight fold of mucosa in the piriform recess of the larynx that encloses the superior laryngeal nerve.

**p. neuropath'ica,** a twisting together of the hairs, forming a matted or feltlike condition; not due, as in p. polonica, to filth.

**p. palati'na transver'sa** [ NA ], transverse palatine ridge; a masticatory vestige on the hard palate; one of several irregular, sometimes branching, crests of soft tissue that radiate from the region of the incisive papillae at their most anterior parts and extend a slight distance backward, crossing the hard palate and reaching laterally for variable distances. In their entirety, sometimes called rugae.

**plicae palma'tae** [ NA ], palmate folds; arbor vitae uteri; lyra uterina; the two longitudinal ridges, anterior and posterior, in the mucous membrane lining the cervix uteri, from which numerous secondary folds, or rugae, branch off.

**p. palpebronasa'lis** [ NA ], epicanthus.

**p. paraduodena'lis** [ NA ], paraduodenal fold; a sickle-shaped fold of peritoneum sometimes found to the left of the duodenojejunal flexure; its right free edge contains the inferior mesenteric vein and a branch of the left colic artery.

**p. polon'ica,** a matted condition of the hair caused by filth and the presence of parasites.

**plicae recti,** plicae transversales recti.

**p. rectouteri'na** [ NA ], rectouterine fold; Douglas' fold; uterosacral ligament; Petit's ligament; a fold of peritoneum, containing the rectouterine muscle, passing from the rectum to the base of the broad ligament on either side, forming the lateral boundary of the rectouterine (Douglas') pouch.

**p. rectovagina'lis,** rectovaginal fold; the lower part of the p. rectouterina.

**p. salpin'gopalati'na** [ NA ], salpingopalatine fold; a ridge passing from the anterior border of the opening of the auditory (Eustachian) tube to the palate.

**p. salpin'gopharynge'a** [ NA ], salpingopharyngeal fold; a ridge of mucous membrane extending from the lower end of the tubal elevation along the wall of the pharynx overlying the salpingopharyngeal muscle.

**p. semiluna'ris** [ NA ], semilunar fold; the curved fold connecting the arcus palatoglossus and arcus palatopharyngeus above the fossa supratonsillaris; it always contains lymphoid tissue.

**p. semiluna'ris coli** [ NA ], semilunar fold of the colon; one of the folds of the wall of the colon between sacculations.

**p. semiluna'ris conjuncti'vae,** semilunar conjunctival fold; (1) [ NA ], the semilunar fold formed by the palpebral conjunctiva at the medial angle of the eye; (2) [ NAV ], palpebra III; palpebra tertia; third eyelid; nictitating membrane; membrana nictitans; a fold of the conjunctival mucous membrane found in many animals; normally partially hidden in the inner canthus of the eye when at rest, it may be extended to cover part or all of the cornea in a winking-like action to clean the cornea, as in birds.

**p. sigmoid'ea,** one of the transverse folds of mucous membrane in the cecum and colon.

**p. spira'lis duc'tus cys'tici** [ NA ], spiral fold of the cystic duct; valvula spiralis; valve of Heister or Amussat; a series of crescentic folds of mucous membrane in the upper part of the cystic duct, arranged in a somewhat spiral manner.

**p. stape'dia** [ NA ], stapedial fold; a reflection of the delicate mucous membrane from the posterior wall of the tympanic cavity that covers the stapes.

**p. sublingua'lis** [ NA ], sublingual fold; an elevation in the floor of the mouth beneath the tongue, on either side, marking the site of the sublingual gland.

**p. synovia'lis** [ NA ], synovial fold; a projection from the synovial membrane of a joint extending toward or between the two articular surfaces.

**p. synovia'lis infrapatella'ris** [ NA ], infrapatellar synovial fold; p. synovialis patellaris; ligamentum mucosum; a fold of synovial membrane extending from below the level of the articular surface of the patella to the anterior part of the intercondylar fossa.

**plicae transversa′les rec′ti** [ NA ], transverse folds of rectum; plicae recti; rectal valves; Houston's or Kohlrausch's valves; the three or four crescentic folds placed horizontally in the rectal mucous membrane. One fold is situated near the beginning of the rectum on the right side; a second one projects from the left side at a slightly lower level; a third is directed backwards from the anterior wall at the level of the fundus of the urinary bladder.

**p. triangula′ris** [ NA ], triangular fold; a fold of mucous membrane at the point of junction of the anterior pillar of the fauces with the tongue.

**plicae tuba′riae** [ NA ], many longitudinal folds in the mucous membrane of the uterine (Fallopian) tube.

**p. tubopalati′na,** p. salpingopalatina.

**plicae tu′nicae muco′sae ves′icae fel′leae** [ NA ], mucosal folds of the gallbladder; the interlacing folds of the mucosa that produce a honeycomb appearance in the interior of the gallbladder.

**p. umbilica′lis latera′lis** [ NA ], lateral umbilical fold; epigastric fold; the ridge on the peritoneal surface of the anterior abdominal wall formed by the inferior epigastric vessels.

**p. umbilica′lis me′dia,** p. umbilicalis mediana.

**p. umbilica′lis medialis** [ NA ], medial umbilical fold; a fold of peritoneum on the lower part of the anterior abdominal wall that covers the obliterated umbilical artery on either side of the urachus.

**p. umbilica′lis mediana** [ NA ], p. umbilicalis media; p. urachi; urachal fold or ligament; middle umbilical fold; a fold of peritoneum on the anterior wall of the abdomen covering the urachus, or remains of the allantoic stalk.

**p. u′rachi,** p. umbilicalis mediana.

**p. ureter′ica,** p. interureterica.

**p. uterovesica′lis,** vesicouterine *ligament.*

**p. ve′nae ca′vae sinis′trae** [ NA ], fold of the left vena cava; vestigial fold of Marshall; a pericardial fold lying between the left branch of the pulmonary artery and the left superior pulmonary vein containing the obliterated remains of the left common cardinal vein.

**p. ventricula′ris,** p. vestibularis.

**p. vesica′lis transver′sa** [ NA ], transverse vesical fold; a duplication of peritoneum passing over the empty bladder, but obliterated when the viscus is full.

**p. vesicouteri′na,** vesicouterine *ligament.*

**p. vestibula′ris** [ NA ], p. ventricularis; vestibular fold; ventricular fold or band; false vocal cord; one of the pair of folds of mucous membrane stretching across the laryngeal cavity from the angle of the thyroid cartilage to the arytenoid cartilage; they enclose a space called the rima vestibuli or false glottis.

**p. vestib′uli,** a fold of mucous membrane forming a ridge on the septum of the nose.

**p. villo′sa** [ NA ], one of the ridges of the mucous membrane of the stomach in the region of the pylorus.

**p. voca′lis** [ NA ], vocal fold; true vocal cord; chorda vocalis; labium vocale; one of Ferrein's cords; the sharp edge of a fold of mucous membrane stretching along either wall of the larynx from the angle between the laminae of the thyroid cartilage to the vocal process of the arytenoid cartilage; the vocal folds are the agents concerned in voice production.

---

**plicate** (pli′kāt). Folded; plaited; tucked.

**plication** (pli-ka′shun, plī-) [ L. *plico,* to fold. PLIC- ]. A folding or putting together in folds. Specifically, an operation for reducing the size of a hollow viscus by taking folds or tucks in its walls.

**plicotomy** (pli-kot′o-mĭ) [ plica + G. *tomē,* incision ]. Division of the plica mallearis.

**Plimmer,** Henry G., London protozoologist, 1857–1918. See P.'s *bodies.*

**Pliny the Elder** (plin′e). Roman writer on a number of scientific subjects, 23–79 A.D. His *Natural History* included thirteen books on medicine in which a great number of plants and drugs were described and many accounts given of and commentaries made on medical methods and customs of the times.

**-ploid** (-ployd) [ G. *-plo-,* -fold, + -ides, in form; L. *-ploideus* ]. An adjectival suffix meaning multiple in form. Its combinations are used both adjectively and substantively of a (specified) multiple of chromosomes.

**ploidy** (ploy′dĭ) [ see -ploid ]. The state of a cell nucleus with respect to the number of genomes it contains. Gametes normally contain a single set of chromosomes or one genome and are haploid; autosomal cells normally contain two genomes and are diploid; for higher multiples see polyploidy.

**plombage** (plom-bahzh′) [ Fr. lit. lead-work ]. The use of an inert body, *e.g.,* methylmethacrylate balls, in collapse of the lung in the surgical treatment of pulmonary tuberculosis.

**plo′sive.** Speech sound made by impounding the air stream for a moment and then suddenly releasing it.

**plototoxin.** A poison from the catfish (*Plotosus*).

**Plotz,** Harry, U. S. physician, 1890–1947. See P. *bacillus.*

**ploughshare** (plow-shār). Vomer.

**plug.** A peg or any mass filling a hole or closing an orifice.

**Dittrich's p.'s,** Traube's p.; minute, dirty-grayish, ill-smelling masses of bacteria and fatty acid crystals in the sputum in pulmonary gangrene and fetid bronchitis.

**epithelial p.,** a mass of epithelial cells temporarily occluding an embryonic opening; the term is most commonly used with reference to the external nares.

**mucous p.,** a mass of mucus and cells filling the cervical canal between periods or during pregnancy.

**Traube's p.'s,** Dittrich's p.'s.

**vaginal p.,** a p. formed by the coagulation of semen; found in the vagina after copulation in certain animals, such as the baboon, rat, and squirrel.

**yolk p.,** the mass of yolk crowded into the blastopore of amphibian embryos by the epiboly and involution of the outer cell layers during gastrulation.

**plug′ger.** Plugging instrument; used for condensing gold (foil), amalgam, or any plastic material in a cavity. May be operated by hand or mechanical means. **Gold foil p.'s** are serrated and usually used with a hand mallet, spring operated (automatic) mallet, pneumatic mallet, or engine driven mallets. **Amalgam p.'s** may be serrated mallets or smooth and may be energized by any of the above methods, but are usually used with hand pressure.

**automatic p.,** automatic condenser; a mechanically or electrically activated device used to provide condensing pressure in the placement of amalgam or gold foil in a cavity preparation.

**back-action p.,** an instrument for condensing gold foil or amalgam; the shank is bent through an angle of 180°. It is used with a pull stroke in the automatic mallet. When used with a hand mallet, the opposite end of the instrument is also bent through an angle of 180° for access to areas that cannot be reached directly.

**foot p.,** a p. for condensing gold foil, the shape of which resembles a foot. The working surface may be flat or curved in the heel-toe direction.

**gutta percha p.,** an instrument for forcing gutta percha into a root canal.

**Lentulo p.,** a spiral-shaped root canal instrument to be operated in a dental engine for conveying a cement or paste into a root canal or through the apical foramen.

**root canal p.,** fine-tapered root canal instrument, blunt at the tip, used for pressing or forcing a gutta percha cone into a root canal.

**plumbagin** (plum-ba′jin) [ L. *plumbago,* a plant, leadwort ]. 5-Hydroxy-2-methyl-1,4-naphthoquinone; an active principle extracted from the root of *Plumbago zeylanica* and *P. Rosea* (Indian evergreen shrubs), and *P. europea* and *P. officinalis* (family Plumbaginaceae); it has antihemorrhagic properties.

**plumbago** (plum-ba′go) [ L. *plumbago,* black lead ]. Graphite.

**plumbic** (plum′bik) [ L. *plumbum,* lead ]. 1. Relating to or containing lead. 2. Denoting the higher valence of lead ion, $Pb^{4+}$.

**plumbism** [ L. *plumbum,* lead ]. Lead *poisoning.*

**plum′bum** [ L. ]. Lead.

**plumieride** (plu-mi′ē-rīd, plu′mĭ-e-rīd). Agoniadin; $C_{21}H_{26}O_{12}$; a glucoside obtained from the bark of *Plumeria lancifolia* and other species of *Plumeria* (family Apocynaceae); used as a febrifuge in malaria.

**Plummer,** Henry S., American physician, 1874–1937. See P.'s *bag, dilator, disease,* P.-Vinson *syndrome.*

**plu′mose** [ L. *pluma,* feather ]. Feathery.

**plump′er.** An addition to the flange area of a denture to artificially fill out the lips or cheeks.

**pluri-** (ploor′ĭ-) [ L. *plus, pluris,* more ]. Combining form meaning several or more. For words beginning thus, but not found here, see also multi- and poly-.

**plu′ricau′sal.** Having two or more causes; used in reference to the etiology of a disease; often indicates that a given disease develops only when two or more causative factors are operative simultaneously.

**pluriceptor** (ploor′ĭ-sep′tor). A receptor having more than two complementophil groups.

**plu′ridyscrin′ia** [ pluri- + G. *dys-,* bad, + *krinō,* to separate, secrete ]. Obsolete term meaning disorder of several endocrine organs.

**plu′riglan′dular.** Polyglandular; denoting several glands or their secretions.

**plu′riloc′ular.** Multilocular.

**plu′rinu′clear.** Multinuclear.

**plurip′otent, plu′ripoten′tial.** 1. Having the capacity to affect more than one organ or tissue. 2. Not fixed as to potential development; see also pluripotent *cell.*

**plu′riresis′tant.** Having multiple aspects of resistance.

**plutomania** (plu′to-ma′nĭ-ah) [ G. *ploutos,* wealth, + *mania,* frenzy ]. An insane delusion that one has great wealth.

**plutonism** (plu′to-nizm). Effects produced, as demonstrated in experimental animals, by means of exposure to the radioactive element plutonium present in atomic piles; they consist of hepatic damage, bone changes, and graying of the hair.

**plutonium** (plu-to′nĭ-um) [ planet, *Pluto* ]. A transuranian radioactive element, symbol Pu, atomic no. 94. The half-life of the most stable known isotope (plutonium-244) is 70 million years; notable for use in atomic bomb and nuclear power plants. Pluronium-239 is formed by the $\beta$-decay of neptunium produced by the neutron bombardment of uranium-238. In a reactor, the neutrons come from fission of uranium-235.

**Pm.** Chemical symbol of the element promethium.

**P-mitrale.** An electrocardiographic syndrome consisting of broad, notched P waves in many leads and with a prominent late negative component to the P wave in lead $V_1$ and $V_2$, presumed to be characteristic of mitral valvular disease. (Although this term is extensively used in electrocardiographic literature, it is actually a misnomer and would be more appropriately called P-sinistrocardiale, as it results from overload of the left atrium regardless of the cause and may occur independently of disease of the mitral valve.)

**PMSG.** Abbreviation for pregnant mare's serum *gonadotropin.*

**PNA.** Abbreviation for *Paris Nomina Anatomica;* Paris anatomical nomenclature.

**pneo-** (ne′o-) [ G. *pneō,* to breathe. PN- ]. Combining form indicating relation to breath or respiration. See also pneum-.

**pneodynamics** (ne′o-di-nam′iks). Pneumodynamics.

**pneograph** (ne′o-graf). Pneumograph.

**pneom′eter** (ne-om′e-ter) [ pneo- + G. *metron,* measure ]. Pneumatometer; pulmometer; spirometer; an instrument for measuring the volume of respired air.

**pneometry** (ne-om′e-trī). Testing the air capacity of the lungs by means of a pneometer.

**pneoscope** (ne′o-skōp). Pneumatoscope.

**pneum-, pneuma-, pneumat-, pneumato-** [ G. *pneuma, pneumatos,* air, breath. PN- ]. Combining forms indicating presence of air or gas, or relation to the lungs or to breathing; see also pneo- and pneumo-.

**pneuma** (nu′mah) [ G. *pneuma,* air, breath. PN- ]. In ancient Greek philosophy and medicine: 1. Air or an all-pervading fiery essence in the air (which today would be identified with oxygen) which was the creative and animating spirit of the universe; drawn into the body through the lungs it generated and sustained the innate heat in the left ventricle of the heart and was distributed

by the arteries to the brain and all parts of the body. 2. Intelligence; breath; soul or psyche.

**pneumarthro′sis** (nu-mar-thro′sis) [ G. *pneuma,* air, + *arthron,* joint, + suffix *-osis,* condition ]. The presence of air in a joint.

**pneumat-, pneumato-** (nu-mat-, nu′mă-to-). See pneum- and pneumo-.

**pneumatic** (nu-mat′ik) [ G. *pneumatikos* ]. 1. Relating to air or gas, or to a structure filled with air. 2. Relating to respiration.

**pneumatics** (nu-mat′iks) [ G. *pneuma,* air or gas ]. The science that treats of the physical properties of air or gases.

**pneumaticus** (nu-mat′ĭ-kus) [ L. ] [ NA ]. Pneumatic (1).

**pneumatinuria** (nu-mă-tĭ-nu′rĭ-ah). Pneumaturia.

**pneumatism** (nu′mă-tizm). The doctrine of the pneuma.

**pneumatists** (nu′mă-tists). The followers of the school whose physiology centered around the pneuma and who conceived the causes of disease as distrubances of this vital principle.

**pneumatization** (nu′mă-tĭ-za′shun) [ G. *pneuma,* air ]. The development of air cells such as those of the mastoid and ethmoidal bones.

**pneumatized** (nu′mă-tīzd). Containing air.

**pneumatocardia** (nu′mă-to-kar′dĭ-ah). The presence of air bubbles or gas in the blood of the heart, produced by air embolism.

**pneumatocele** (nu′mă-to-sēl) [ G. *pneuma,* air, + *kēlē,* tumor, hernia ]. 1. Distention of the scrotum with gas. 2. An emphysematous or gaseous swelling. 3. Pneumonocele. 4. A thin-walled cavity forming within the lung, characteristic of staphylococcus pneumonia.

   **extracranial p.,** extracranial pneumocele; subgaleal emphysema; collection of gas beneath the galea aponeurotica, usually due to fracture into the paranasal sinuses.

   **intracranial p.,** a collection of gas within the skull, in the brain, or in the meninges.

**pneumatoenteric** (nu′mă-to-en-tĕr′ik). See pneumatoenteric *recess.*

**pneumatogram** (nu′mă-to-gram). Pneumogram (1).

**pneumatograph** (nu′mă-to-graf). Pneumograph.

**pneumatohemia** (nu-mă-to-he′mĭ-ah). Pneumohemia.

**pneumatology** (nu-mă-tol′o-jĭ) [ G. *pneuma,* air, + *logos,* study ]. The science dealing with air or gases, their physical and chemical properties, and their therapeutic application: for the control of pain (anesthesia), saving of life (resuscitation), and treatment of clinical disease (oxygen therapy).

**pneumatometer** (nu-mă-tom′e-ter). Pneometer.

**pneumatorrhachis** (nu-mă-tor′ă-kis) [ G. *pneuma,* air, + *rhachis,* spine ]. The presence of air or gas in the spinal canal.

**pneumatoscope** (nu′mă-to-skōp, nu-mat′o-skōp) [ G. *pneuma,* air, + *skopeō,* to examine ]. 1. Pneoscope; pneumoscope; an instrument for measuring the extent of the respiratory excursions of the chest. 2. An instrument for use in auscultatory percussion, the percussion sounds of the chest being heard at the mouth. 3. A device for determining the presence of air or of a liquid effusion in the mastoid cells, the principle being that a vibrating tuning fork is heard longer when in contact with the normal mastoid.

**pneumatosis** (nu-mă-to′sis) [ G. a blowing out ]. Abnormal accumulation of gas in any tissue or part of the body.

   **p. cystoi′des intestina′lis,** a condition characterized by the occurrence of gas cysts in the intestinal mucous membrane, especially of the small intestine, it is due to the presence of gas in the lymph spaces and probably from unknown causes.

**pneumatothorax** (nu′mă-to-tho′raks). Pneumothorax.

**pneumaturia** (nu-mă-tu′rĭ-ah) [ G. *pneuma,* air, + *ouron,* urine ]. Pneumatinuria; the passage of gas or air from the urethra during or after urination, resulting from decomposition of bladder urine, or more commonly from an intestinal fistula; pneumatinuria.

**pneumatype** (nu′mă-tīp) [ G. *pneuma,* breath, + *typos,* type ]. A device for determining the permeability of the nasal fossae by exhaling through the nose against a plate of cooled glass.

**pneumectomy** (nu-mek′to-mī). Pneumonectomy.

**pneumo-, pneumon-, pneumono-** (nu'mo-, nu'mōn-, nu'mo-no-) [ G. *pneumōn, pneumonos,* lung. PN- ]. Combining forms indicating relation to (1) the lung, the lungs; (2) air, gas, or breathing; (3) pneumonia. For some terms beginning with pneumo-, see also pneum-, pneumato-, pneo-.

**pneumoangiography** (nu'mo-an-jī-og'ră-fī) [ pneumo- + G. *angeion,* vessel, + *graphō,* to write ]. Contrast roentgenographic study of the pulmonary and bronchial blood vessels.

**pneumoarthrography** (nu'mo-ar-throg'ră-fī) [ G. *pneuma,* air, + *arthron,* joint, + *graphō,* to write ]. X-ray study of a joint after injection of air.

**pneumobacillin** (nu'mo-bā-sil'in). A toxin or toxic protein derived from cultures of the pneumobacillus (*Klebsiella pneumoniae*).

**pneumobacillus** (nu'mo-bā-sil'us). *Klebsiella pneumoniae.*

**pneumobacterine** (nu-mo-bak'ter-ēn). A stock vaccine made from killed cultures of the pneumococcus.

**pneumobulbar** (nu-mo-bul'bar) [ G. *penumōn,* lung, + L. *bulbus,* bulb ]. Relating to the lungs and their connection with the medulla oblongata by way of the vagus nerve.

**pneumocardial** (nu'mo-kar'dī-al). Cardiopulmonary.

**pneumocele** (nu'mo-sēl). 1. Pneumonocele. 2. Pneumatocele.

    **extracranial** and **intracranial p.'s,** see under pneumatocele.

**pneumocentesis** (nu'mo-sen-te'sis). Pneumonocentesis.

**pneumocephalus** (nu-mo-sef'ă-lus) [ G. *pneuma,* air, + *kephalē,* head ]. The presence of air or gas within the cranial cavity.

**pneumochirurgia** (nu-mo-ki-rur'jī-ah). Pneumonochirurgia.

**pneumocholecystitis** (nu'mo-ko'le-sis'ti'tis). Cholecystitis with gas-forming organisms giving rise to gas in the gallbladder.

**pneumococcal** (nu-mo-kok'al). Pertaining to or containing the pneumococcus.

**pneumococcemia** (nu-mo-kok-se'mī-ah) [ pneumococcus + G. *haima,* blood ]. The presence of pneumococci in the blood.

**pneumococcidal** (nu-mo-kok-sī'dal) [ pneumococcus + L. *caedo,* to kill ]. Destructive to pneumococci.

**pneumococcolysis** (nu-mo-kok-ol'ī-sis) [ pneumococcus + G. *lysis,* dissolution ]. Lysis or destruction of pneumococci.

**pneumococcosis** (nu'mo-kok-o'sis). Infection with the pneumococcus organisms.

**pneumococcosuria** (nu'mo-kok-o-su'rī-ah) [ pneumococcus + G. *ouron,* urine ]. The presence of pneumococci or their specific capsular substance in the urine.

**pneumococcus** (nu-mo-kok'us) [ G. *pneumōn,* lung, + *kokkos,* berry (coccus) ]. *Streptococcus pneumoniae.*

    **Fraenkel's p.,** *Streptococcus pneumoniae.*
    **Fraenkel-Weichselbaum p.,** *Streptococcus pneumoniae.*

**pneumocolon** (nu'mo-ko'lon) [ G. *pneuma,* air, + *kolon,* colon ]. Gas in the colon or interstitial gas in the wall of the colon.

**pneumoconiosis,** pl. **pneumoconioses** (nu'mo-ko-nī-o'sis, -sēz) [ G. *pneumōn,* lung, + *konis,* dust, + suffix -*osis,* condition ]. Pneumonoconiosis; inflammation commonly leading to fibrosis of the lungs due to the irritation caused by the inhalation of dust incident to various occupations, such as coal mining, knife grinding, stone cutting, etc.; the most prominent symptoms are: pain in the chest, cough, little or no expectoration, dyspnea, reduced thoracic excursion, sometimes cyanosis, and fatigue after slight exertion.

    **graphite p.,** p. occurring in graphite workers from inhalation of graphite dust.

    **p. siderot'ica,** siderosis.

    **talc p.,** p. due to the inhalation of talc-laden dust occurring in workers in the grinding and preparation of talc or in those whose occupation, *e.g.,* rubber manufacturing, entails the use of powdered talc.

**pneumocranium** (nu'mo-kra'nī-um) [ G. *pneuma,* air, + *kranion,* skull ]. The presence of air between the cranium and the dura mater.

**Pneumocystis carinii** (nu'mo-sis'tis kah-rī'ne-ī). A tiny parasite, probably a protozoan, characterized by basophilic, dotlike forms, 1 $\mu$ or less in diameter, frequently occurring as aggregates of 2 to 8 forms within a rounded cystlike structure with a visible wall; may be demonstrated by means of Giemsa and periodic acid-Schiff techniques with smears, and silver impregnation of sections of tissue (only faintly visible with hematoxylin and eosin). The organisms are the apparent cause of pneumocystosis.

**pneumocystography** (nu'mo-sis-tog'ră-fī) [ G. *pneuma,* air, + *kystis,* bladder, + *graphō,* to write ]. Roentgenography of the bladder following injection of air.

**pneumocystosis** (nu'mo-sis-to'sis). The disease resulting from infection with *Pneumocystis carinii;* interstitial plasmacellular pneumonia, particularly frequent in premature or debilitated babies during their first three months; reported from North America, and, more frequently, from Europe. The alveoli are filled with a peculiar, honeycomb-like or foamy network of acidophilic material (which is apparently not fibrin, and is not impregnable with silver), and the organisms are enmeshed, individually or in aggregates, within the network; throughout the alveolar walls and pulmonary sputums there is a diffuse infiltration of mononuclear inflammatory cells, chiefly plasma cells and macrophages, as well as a few lymphocytes. Patients may be only slightly febrile (or even afebrile), but are likely to be extremely weak, dyspneic, and cyanotic.

**pneumoderma** (nu-mo-der'mah) [ G. *pneuma,* air, + *derma,* skin ]. Subcutaneous emphysema.

**pneumodynamics** (nu'mo-di-nam'iks) [ G. *pneuma,* breath, + *dynamis,* force ]. Pneodynamics; the mechanics of respiration.

**pneumoempyema** (nu'mo-em'pi-e'mah). Pyopneumothorax.

**pneumoencephalitis** (nu'mo-en-sef'ă-li'tis). Newcastle disease.

**pneumoencephalogram** (nu'mo-en-sef'ă-lo-gram). The x-ray picture of the skull and its contents taken after introducing air or gas into the subarachnoid space.

**pneumoencephalography** (nu'mo-en-sef'ă-log'ră-fī) [ G. *pneuma,* air, + *enkephalos,* brain, + *graphō,* to write ]. Radiographic visualization of cerebral ventricles and subarachnoid spaces by use of gas such as air or oxygen.

**pneu'moenter'ic.** Pneumatoenteric; see under recess.

**pneumoenteritis** (nu'mo-en-ter-i'tis) [ G. *pneumōn,* lung, + *enteron,* intestine, + suffix -*itis,* inflammation ]. Pneumonia complicating or complicated by enteritis.

**pneumoerysipelas** (nu'mo-ĕr-ĭ-sip'e-las). Pneumonia complicating or complicated by erysipelas.

**pneumofasciogram** (nu-mo-fash'ĭ-o-gram) [ G. *pneuma,* air, + L. *fascia,* a band or fillet, + *gramma* a drawing ]. Roentgenogram of soft tissue following air injection of the fascial spaces.

**pneumogalactocele** (nu'mo-gă-lak'to-sēl) [ G. *pneuma,* air, + *gala,* milk, + *kēlē,* tumor ]. A swelling of the breast containing milk and gas.

**pneumogastric** (nu-mo-gas'trik) [ G. *pneumōn,* lung, + *gastēr,* stomach ]. Relating to the lungs and the stomach; denoting the p. nerve, nervus vagus.

**pneumogastrography** (nu'mo-gas-trog'ră-fī) [ G. *pneuma,* air, + *gastēr,* stomach, + *graphō,* to write ]. X-ray study of stomach after injection of air.

**pneumogram** (nu'mo-gram) [ G. *pneumōn,* lung, + *gramma,* a drawing ]. 1. Pneumatogram; record or tracing made by a pneumograph. 2. Roentgenogram following air injection as in encephalography.

**pneumograph** (nu'mo-graf) [ G. *pneumōn,* lung, + *graphō,* to write ]. Atmograph; pneograph; pneumatograph; an instrument for recording the force and rapidity of the respiratory movements.

**pneumography** (nu-mog'ră-fī) [ G. *pneumōn,* lung, + *graphō,* to write ]. Roentgenography of the lungs.

**pneumohemia** (nu'mo-he'mī-ah) [ G. *pneuma,* air, + *haima,* blood ]. Pneumatohemia; the presence of air in blood vessels; see also air *embolism.*

**pneumohemopericardium** (nu'mo-hēm'o-pĕr-ĭ-kar'dī-um). Hemopneumopericardium.

**pneumohemothorax** (nu'mo-hēmo-tho'raks). The presence of air or gas and blood in the thoracic cavity.

**pneumohydrometra** (nu'mo-hi'dro-me'trah) [ G. *pneuma*, air, + *hydōr* (*hydr-*), water, + *mētra*, uterus ]. The presence of gas and serum in the uterine cavity.

**pneumohydropericardium** (nu'mo-hi'dro-pĕr-ĭ-kar'dĭum). Hydropneumopericardium.

**pneumohydrothorax** (nu-mo-hi-dro-tho'raks). Hydropneumothorax.

**pneumohypoderma** (nu'mo-hi-po-der'mah) [ G. *pneuma*, air, + *hypo*, beneath, + *derma*, skin ]. Subcutaneous *emphysema*.

**pneumolith** (nu'mo-lith) [ G. *pneumōn*, lung, + *lithos*, stone ]. A calculus in the lung.

**pneumolithiasis.** Formation of calculi in the lungs.

**pneumology** (nu-mol'o-jī) [ G. *pneuma*, lung, + *logos*, study ]. Study of the lung.

**pneumolysis** (nu'mol'ī-sis) [ G. *pneumōn*, lung, + *lysis*, a loosening ]. Separation of the lung and costal pleura from the endothoracic fascia.

**pneumomalacia** (nu-mo-mal-a'shī-ah) [ G. *pneumōn*, lung, + *malakia*, softness ]. Softening of the lung tissue.

**pneumomassage** (nu'mo-mā-sahzh') [ G. *pneuma*, air, + massage ]. Compression and rarefaction of the air in the external auditory meatus, causing movement of the ossicles of the tympanum.

**pneumomediastinum** (nu'mo-me'dĭ-ā-sti'num) [ G. *pneuma*, air, + mediastinum, *q.v.* ]. The escape of air into mediastinal tissues, usually from interstitial emphysema or from a ruptured pulmonary bleb.

**pneumomelanosis** (nu'mo-mel-ā-no'sis) [ G. *pneumōn*, lung, + *melanosis*, a becoming black ]. Pneumonomelanosis; a blackening of the lung tissue from the inhalation of coal dust or other black particles.

**pneumometer** (nu-mom'e-ter). Pneometer.

**pneumometry** (nu-mom'e-trī). Pneometry.

**pneumomycosis** (nu'mo-mi-ko'sis) [ G. *pneumōn*, lung, + *mykēs*, fungus ]. Pneumonomycosis; any disease of the lungs caused by the presence of fungi.

**pneumomyelography** (nu'mo-mi'ē-log'rā-fī) [ G. *pneuma*, air, + *myelos*, marrow, + *graphō*, to write ]. X-ray examination of spinal canal after injection of air or gas into it.

**pneumon-, pneumono-.** See pneumo-.

**pneumonectomy** (nu'mo-nek'to-mī) [ G. *pneumōn*, lung, + *ektomē*, excision ]. Pneumectomy; operative removal of a portion of lung tissue.

**pneumonia** (nu-mo'nī-ah) [ G. fr. *pneumōn*, lung, + suffix *-ia*, condition ]. 1. Inflammation of the lungs; pneumonitis. 2. Lobar p.; specifically, an acute infectious disease.

**abortive p.,** p. that follows a mild and unusually short course.

**acute p.,** lobar p.

**acute intersti'tial p.,** a severe and usually fatal form of p. occurring in infants.

**p. alba,** white p.

**anthrax p.,** pulmonary *anthrax.*

**apex p.,** apical p.; p. of the apex or apices.

**apical p.,** apex p.

**aspiration p.,** deglutition p.; bronchopneumonia resulting from the entrance of a foreign body, usually food particles, into the bronchi.

**atypical p.,** virus p.

**bronchial p.,** bronchopneumonia.

**ca'seous p.,** cheesy p.; a form of pulmonary tuberculosis in which tubercles are absent, but there is a diffuse cellular infiltration which undergoes coagulation necrosis resulting in a more or less extensive area of caseation.

**catarrhal p.,** bronchopneumonia.

**central p.,** core p.; a form of p. in which exudation is confined for a time to the central portion of a lobe or the hilar region.

**cheesy p.,** caseous p.

**chemical p.,** caused by inhalation of war gas, *e.g.,* phosgene or chlorine. The lungs are edematous and hemorrhagic; large amounts of fluid are formed which fill the air passages and may literally drown the patient. If recovery occurs, permanent damage of the lungs remains, and recurrent pulmonary infections are the rule.

**chronic p.,** interstitial p.; see also Hamman-Rich syndrome.

**congenital p.,** p. in the newborn, infection being contracted prenatally.

**contusion p.,** inflammation of the lungs following a severe blow on or compression of the chest.

**core p.,** central p.

**croupous p.,** lobar p.

**degluti'tion p.,** aspiration p.

**desquam'ative p.,** parenchymatous p.

**desquamative interstitial p.,** diffuse proliferation of alveolar lining cells, which desquamate into the air sacs, producing a gradual onset of dyspnea and nonproductive cough, with x-ray changes.

**p. dis'secans,** p. interlobularis purulenta.

**double p.,** lobar p. involving both lungs.

**Eaton agent p.,** an acute pneumonitis produced by *Mycoplasma pneumoniae;* see also Eaton *agent.*

**embol'ic p.,** pneumonitis, congestion, and infarction following embolization of a pulmonary artery or arteries.

**ephem'eral p.,** pulmonary congestion; congestion of the lungs; the patient exhibits the symptoms and signs of p., but these disappear after 36 to 48 hours.

**fi'brinous p.,** lobar p.

**fibrous p.,** interstitial p.

**Friedländer's p.,** p. caused by infection with *Klebsiella pneumoniae* (Friedländer's bacillus); a severe form of lobar p. characterized by much swelling of the affected lobe which may be seen on roentgenograms.

**gangrenous p.,** pulmonary gangrene.

**giant cell p.,** a rare complication of measles, with the postmortem finding of multinucleated giant cells lining alveoli.

**hypostat'ic p.,** pulmonary congestion due to stagnation of blood in the dependent portions of the lungs in the aged or those debilitated by disease who lie in the same position for long periods.

**in'durative p.,** interstitial or parenchymatous p.

**influen'zal p.,** (1) p. complicating influenza; (2) p. due to *Haemophilus influenzae.*

**p. in'terlobula'ris purulen'ta,** p. dissecans; p. in which the lobules of the lung are separated by collections of purulent exudate.

**interstitial p.,** pneumonocirrhosis; fibrous p.; indurative p.; a chronic inflammation of the interstitial tissue of the lung resulting in compression of the air cells; see also Hamman-Rich *syndrome.*

**interstitial plasma cell p.,** a p. occurring in infants in which numerous plasma cells are found in the alveoli and pulmonary interstitial tissue.

**intrauterine p.,** fetal p. contracted *in utero* and manifesting itself in the early neonatal period.

**larval p.,** a pulmonary condition presenting the early symptoms of p. but terminating favorably in a day or two; abortive p.; congestion of the lungs.

**lipid p., lipoid p.,** oil p.; a pulmonary condition marked by inflammatory and fibrotic changes in the lungs due to the inhalation of various oily or fatty substances, particularly liquid petrolatum; or it may result from the accumulation in the lungs of endogenous lipid material. Phagocytes containing lipid are usually present.

**lobar p.,** p. (2); acute p.; croupous p.; pneumococcal p.; pleural p.; pleuritic p.; fibrinous p.; an acute, infectious disease, caused by one of the types of pneumococci; marked by fever, pleuritic pains, cough, and rusty or blood-stained sputum; it normally lasts about 9 days, and ends in crisis with profuse sweating; there is an abundant fibrinous exudation into the pulmonary alveoli, resulting in consolidation of the greater part or all of one or more lobes of the lungs, whence the term lobar p.

**lob'ular p.,** bronchopneumonia.

**Löffler's p.,** Löffler's *syndrome* (1).

**Marsh's ovine progressive p.,** pulmonary *adenomatosis* of sheep.

**metastat'ic p.,** a purulent inflammation of the lungs due to pyemic emboli.

**mi'gratory p.,** wandering p.; a form in which successive areas of the lung are invaded.

**monili'asis p.,** p. due to species of fungi of the genus *Candida*, usually *Candida albicans.*

**Montana chronic progressive p.,** a specific pulmonary disease of sheep similar to maedi and to pulmonary adenomatosis of sheep.

**mycoplasma p. of pigs,** virus p. of pigs; a worldwide, low grade p. usually involving only the anterior lobes; it seldom causes death but is responsible for much unthriftiness; it is believed to be caused by *Mycoplasma hypopneumoniae.*

**oil p.,** lipid p.

**organized p.,** unresolved p. in which fibrous tissue forms in the alveoli.

**parenchy'matous p.,** indurative p.; desquamative p.; chronic fibrinous or lobar p. with induration of the exudate and proliferation of the interstitial tissue.

**plague p.,** pneumonic *plague.*

**pleural p., pleurit'ic p.,** lobar p.

**pneumococ'cal p.,** lobar p.

**postoperative p.,** p. occurring after operation; may be an aspiration p. or p. due to ether anesthesia, or to atelectasis.

**rheumatic p.,** seen usually as a terminal event in acute rheumatic fever; pneumonic consolidation occurs, the lungs being of a rubbery consistency; nodules may be present in the fibrous septa of the lungs.

**secondary p.,** pulmonary inflammation, usually of bronchopneumonic type, occurring as a complication of some infectious disease and due to the microorganism of that affection or a microorganism from the flora of the nasopharynx.

**septic p.,** suppurative p.

**staphylococ'cal p.,** a form ushered in by chills, followed by high remittent fever; it commences as a bronchopneumonia and frequently leads to lung abscess. The sputum is yellowish and purulent, usually caused by *Staphylococcus aureus.*

**streptococ'cal p.,** a severe type occurring in epidemic form due to *Streptococcus pyogenes.*

**sup'purative p.,** septic p.; any p. associated with the formation of pus in the pulmonary tissue.

**terminal p.,** p. occurring in the course of some acute or chronic disease and materially hastening the fatal termination.

**traumatic p.,** inflammation of the lung following contusion of the chest or a wound of the lung itself.

**tulare'mic p.,** tularemia with pulmonary lesions.

**typhoid p.,** p. complicating typhoid fever, or accompanied with stupor and other evidences of profound depression.

**unresolved p.,** p. in which the alveolar exudate persists.

**uremic p.,** uremic lung; uremic pneumonitis; fibrinous pulmonary edema occurring in uremia; a characteristic butterfly type of shadow is seen in anterior and posterior x-rays; it is not a true p.

**virus p.,** atypical p.; an acute systemic disease due to a virus with involvement of the lungs, marked by high fever, cough, and relatively few physical signs.

**virus p. of pigs,** mycoplasma p. of pigs.

**wandering p.,** migratory p.

**white p.,** p. alba; syphilitic inflammation of the lungs in the newborn, characterized by a heavy infiltration of mononuclear cells and an increase in the connective tissue of the interalveolar septa.

**wool-sorter's p.,** pulmonary *anthrax.*

**pneumonic** (nu-mon'ik). 1. Pulmonary. 2. Relating to pneumonia.

**pneumonitis** (nu-mo-ni'tis) [ G. *pneumōn*, lung, + suffix *-itis*, inflammation ]. Inflammation of the lungs.

**feline p.,** an infectious pneumonia of domesticated cats caused by *Chlamydia psittaci.*

**uremic p.,** uremic *pneumonia.*

**pneumono-** (nu'mo-no-, nu'mon-o-) [ G. *pneumōn*, lung ]. Combining form denoting lung. For many words so beginning, see pneum- and pneumo-.

**pneumonocele** (nu'mo-no-sēl). Pneumocele; pleurocele; protrusion of a portion of the lung through a defect in the wall of the chest.

**pneumonocentesis** (nu'mo-no-sen-te'sis) [ G. *pneumōn*, lung, + *kentēsis*, puncture ]. Pneumocentesis; puncture of the lung in order to empty a pus-filled cavity.

**pneumonochirurgia** (nu'mo-no-ki-rur'ji-ah) [ G. *pneumōn*, lung, + *cheirourgia*, surgery ]. Pneumochirurgia; surgery of the lungs.

**pneumonococcus** (nu'mo-no-kok'us). Pneumococcus.

**pneumonoconiosis** (nu'mo-no-ko'nī-o'sis). Pneumoconiosis.

**pneumonocyte** (nu'mo-no-sīt) [ G. *pneumōn*, lung, + *kytos*, cell ]. A nonspecific term sometimes used in referring to cells characteristic of the respiratory part of the lung.

**pneumonomoniliasis** (nu'mo-no-mon'ī-li'ă-sis). Moniliasis (candidiasis) of the lung.

**pneumonopathy** (nu'mo-no-nop'ă-thī) [ G. *pneumōn*, lung, + *pathos*, suffering ]. Pneumopathy; any disease of the lungs.

**pneumonopexy** (nu'mo-no-pek'sī) [ G. *pneumōn*, lung, + *pēxis*, fixation ]. Pneumopexy; fixation of the lung by suturing the costal and pulmonary pleurae or otherwise causing adhesion of the two layers.

**pneumonopleuritis** (nu'mo-no-ploor-i'tis) [ G. *pneumōn*, lung, + *pleura*, side ]. Pneumopleuritis (2); inflammation of both lungs and pleura.

**pneumonorrhaphy** (nu'mo-nor'ă-fī) [ G. *pneumōn*, lung, + *rhaphē*, suture ]. Suture of a wound of the lung.

**pneumonotherapy** (nu'mo-no-thēr'ă-pī). Pneumotherapy.

**pneumonotomy** (nu'mo-not'o-mī) [ G. *pneumōn*, lung, + *tomē*, incision ]. Pneumotomy; incision of the lung for the evacuation of an abscess or for any other purpose.

**Pneumonyssoi'des cani'num.** A small mite (family Halarachnidae) inhabiting the sinuses and nasal passages of dogs. It causes relatively little trouble and the condition frequently is not diagnosed.

**Pneumonys'sus simic'ola.** A small mite (family Halarachnidae) that inhabits the lungs of monkeys.

**pneumo-orbitography** (nu'mo-or'bī-tog'ră-fī). Radiographic visualization of the orbital contents by injection of a gas, usually air.

**pneumo-oxygenator** (nu'mo-ok'sī-jě-na-tor). Apparatus for prolonged administration of oxygen.

**pneumopathy** (nu-mop'ă-thī). Pneumonopathy.

**pneumopericardium** (nu'mo-pěr-ī-kar'dī-um) [ G. *pneuma*, air, + *pericardium* ]. The presence of gas in the pericardial sac.

**pneumoperitoneum** (nu'mo-pěr-ī-to-ne'um) [ G. *pneuma*, air, + *peritoneum* ]. The presence of air or gas in the peritoneal cavity as a result of disease or produced artificially for the treatment of pulmonary or intestinal tuberculosis, bronchiectasis, tuberculous empyema, and certain other conditions.

**pneumoperitonitis** (nu'mo-pěr-ī-to-ni'tis) [ G. *pneuma*, air, + *peritonitis* ]. Inflammation of the peritoneum with an accumulation of gas in the peritoneal cavity.

**pneumopexy** (nu'mo-pek'sī). Pneumonopexy.

**pneumophagia** (nu'mo-fa'jī-ah). Aerophagia.

**pneumopleuritis** (nu'mo-ploor-i'tis). 1 [ G. *pneuma*, air ]. Pleurisy with air or gas in the pleural cavity. 2 [ G. *pneumōn*, lung ]. Pneumonopleuritis.

**pneumopyelography** (nu'mo-pi'ě-log'ră-fī) [ G. *pneuma*, air, + *pyelos*, pelvis, + *graphō*, to write ]. X-ray examination of the kidney after air or gas has been injected into the kidney pelvis.

**pneumopyothorax** (nu'mo-pi-o-tho'raks). Pyopneumothorax.

**pneumoradiography** (nu'mo-ra'dī-og'ră-fī). Pneumoroentgenography.

**pneumoresection** (nu'mo-re-sek'shun) [ G. *pneumōn*, lung, + *resection* ]. Excision of part of a lung.

**pneumoretroperitoneum** (nu'mo-ret'ro-pěr'ī-to-ne'um). The escape of air into the retroperitoneal tissues.

**pneumoroentgenography** (nu'mo-rent'gě-nog'ră-fī, -rěnt-jě-). Pneumoradiography; x-ray study of a region after air has been injected into it.

**pneumorrhachis** (nu-mor'ă-kis) [ G. *pneuma*, air, + *rachis*, spinal column ]. The presence of gas in the spinal canal.

**pneumorrhagia** (nu-mo-ra'jī-ah) [ G. *pneumōn*, lung, + *rhēgnymi*, to burst forth. RHAG- ]. 1. Hemorrhage from the lungs; see also hemoptysis. 2. Hemorrhage into the lung; see also pulmonary *apoplexy.*

**pneumoscope** (nu'mo-skōp). Pneumatoscope.

**pneumoserothorax** (nu'mo-se'ro-tho'raks). Hydropneumothorax.

**pneumosilicosis** (nu'mo-sil'ĭ-ko'sis). See silicosis.

**pneumotachogram** (nu'mo-tak'o-gram) [ G. *pneuma,* air, + *tachys,* swift, + *gramma,* something written ]. A recording of respired gas flow as a function of time, produced by a pneumotachograph.

**pneumotachograph** (nu-mo-tak'o-graf). Pneumotachometer; an instrument for measuring the instantaneous flow of respiratory gases.

**Fleisch p.,**   a p. that measures flow in terms of the proportional pressure drop across a resistance consisting of numerous capillary tubes in parallel.

**Silverman-Lilly p.,**   a p. that measures flow in terms of the proportional pressure drop across a resistance consisting of a very fine mesh screen.

**pneumotachometer** (nu'mo-tă-kom'e-ter) [ G. *pneuma,* air, + *tachys,* swift, + *metron,* measure ]. Pneumotachograph.

**pneumotherapy** (nu-mo-thĕr'ă-pī) [ G. *pneumōn,* lung, + *therapeia,* treatment ]. Pneumonotherapy; the treatment of pulmonary diseases.

**pneumothermomassage** (nu-mo-ther'mo-mă-sahzh') [ G. *pneuma,* air, + *thermē,* heat, + Fr. *massage* ]. The application to the body of hot air under varying degrees of pressure.

**pneumothorax** (nu-mo-tho'raks) [ G. *pneuma,* air, + *thorax* ]. The presence of air or gas in the pleural cavity.

**artificial p.,**   p. produced purposely by the injection of nitrogen gas into the pleural space; used in the treatment of tuberculosis to immobilize and collapse the involved lung.

**extrapleur'al p.,**   one in which air is present between the pleura and the thoracic wall, the parietal pleura being stripped off.

**open p.,**   one in which there is communication between the atmosphere and the pleural cavity, either through the lung or through the chest wall. Also called blowing, sucking, or traumatopneic wound.

**p. simplex,**   p. in apparently healthy persons without known cause.

**spontaneous p.,**   p. occurring from disease of the lung, *e.g.,* abscess, bullous emphysema, or from any natural (*i.e.,* nontherapeutic) cause.

**tension p.,**   valvular p.; p. in which a valve effect in the ruptured bleb or alveolar tissue permits air to enter the p. cavity during inspiration, but traps it during expiration, so that pressure builds up, displaces the mediastinum to the opposite side, and encroaches upon and distorts blood vessels.

**therapeutic p.,**   artificial p.

**val'vular p.,**   tension p.

**pneumotomy** (nu-mot'o-mī). Pneumonotomy.

**pneumoventricle** (nu'mo-ven'trĭ-kl). Air in the ventricular system of the brain; occurs as a complication of a fracture of the skull which passes through the accessory nasal sinuses.

**pneusis** (nu'sis) [ G. *pneuesthai,* to breathe ]. Breathing.

**pnigophobia** (ni-go-fo'bĭ-ah) [ G. *pnigos,* choking, + *phobos,* fear ]. A morbid fear of choking.

**PNPB.**   Abbreviation for positive-negative pressure *breathing.*

**Po.**   Chemical symbol of the element polonium.

**Po₂ or pO₂.**   Symbol for the partial pressure (tension) of oxygen; see partial *pressure.*

**pock** [ A.S. *poc,* a pustule ]. The specific pustular cutaneous lesion of smallpox.

**pock'et** [ Fr. *pochette* ]. 1. A cul-de-sac or pouchlike cavity. 2. A diseased gingival attachment; a space between the inflamed gum and the surface of a tooth, limited apically by an epithelial attachment. 3. To enclose the stump of the pedicle of an ovarian or other abdominal tumor between the lips of the external wound. 4. A collection of pus in a nearly closed sac.

**accessory p.,**   a p. formed by rupture of peptic ulcer.

**caval p.,**   used by Stewart and Rogoff in their method of determining the output of catecholamines by the adrenal glands. The inferior vena cava is temporarily clamped below the adrenal veins and again just below the diaphragm; all other veins entering the p. are ligated. Removal of the upper clamp at any moment desired permits the contained blood to enter the general circulation; any "adrenaline" which may be present is detected by means of the Meltzer-Auer test.

**gingival p.,**   a diseased gingival attachment in which the increased depth of the sulcus is due to an increase in the bulk of its gingival wall.

**infrabony p., intrabony p.,**   subcrestal p.

**periodontal p.,**   a pathologic deepening of the gingival sulcus resulting from detachment of the gingiva from the tooth.

**Rathke's p.,**   pituitary *diverticulum.*

**Seessel's p.,**   Seessel's pouch; the preoral gut; the part of the embryonic foregut that extends cephalic to the level of the oral plate.

**subcrestal p.,**   infrabony p.; intrabony p.; a p. extending apically below the level of the adjacent alveolar crest.

**Tröltsch's p.'s,**   *recessus* membranae tympani, anterior and posterior.

**pock'mark.**   The small depressed scar left after the healing of the smallpox pustule.

**pock'marked.**   Bearing on the skin of the face or elsewhere many scars of healed smallpox pustules.

**poculum** (pok'u-lum) [ L. ]. Cup.

**p. diogenis,**   Diogenes *cup.*

**pod-, podo-** [ G. *pous, podos,* foot. POD- ]. Combining forms meaning foot or foot-shaped.

**podagra** (po-dag'rah) [ G. fr. *pous,* foot, + *agra,* a seizure ]. Gout; especially typical gout in the great toe.

**pod'agral, podag'ric, pod'agrous.**   Gouty; relating to or suffering from gout.

**podalgia** (po-dal'jĭ-ah) [ pod- + G. *algos,* pain ]. Tarsalgia; pododynia; pain in the foot.

**podalic** (po-dal'ik) [ G. *pous* (*pod-*), foot ]. Relating to the foot.

**podarthritis** (pod-ar-thri'tis) [ pod- + arthritis ]. Inflammation of any of the tarsal or metatarsal joints.

**podedema** (pod'e-de'mah). Edema of the feet and ankles.

**podelcoma** (pod'el-ko'mah) [ pod- + G. *helkōma,* ulcer ]. Podhelcoma; rarely used term for mycetoma of the foot.

**podencephalus** (pod'en-sef'ă-lus) [ pod- + G. *enkephalos,* brain ]. A fetus with brain for the most part outside the cranium, attached only by a pedicle.

**podhelcoma** (pod'hel-ko'mah). Podelcoma.

**podiatrist** (po-di'ă-trist) [ pod- + G. *iatros,* physician ]. Chiropodist; a practitioner of podiatry.

**podiatry** (po-di'ă-trī) [ pod- + G. *iatreia,* medical treatment ]. Chiropody; the specialty that includes the diagnosis and/or medical, surgical, mechanical, physical, and adjunctive treatment of the diseases, injuries, and defects of the human foot.

**podismus** (po-diz'mus). Podospasm.

**poditis** (po-di'tis) [ pod- + G. suffix *-itis,* inflammation ]. An inflammatory disorder of the foot.

**tourniquet p.,**   postischemic acute inflammatory edema in the foot (or paw), as the result of complete obstruction of the circulation to that member by use of a tourniquet; produced experimentally in animals as a means of evaluating the anti-inflammatory efficacy of drugs.

**podo-.**   See pod-.

**podobromidrosis** (pod'o-bro-mĭ-dro'sis) [ podo- + G. *brōmos,* a foul smell, + *hidrōs,* sweat ]. Strong-smelling perspiration of the feet.

**pod'ocyte** [ podo- + G. *kytos,* a hollow (cell) ]. Epithelial cell of the renal glomerulus, attached to the outer surface of the glomerular capillary basement membrane by cytoplasmic foot processes, or pedicels.

**pod'oderm** [ podo- + G. *derma,* skin ]. Corium ungulae; the corium of the foot; that portion of the skin which lies under the hoof and secretes the horny structure. The regions of the p. are the periople (corium limbi), coronary band (corium coronae), wall (corium parietis), and sole (corium solae).

**pododermatitis** (pod'o-der'mă-ti'tis). Inflammation of the pododerm; see also laminitis (2).

**pododynamometer** (pod'o-di'nă-mom'e-ter) [ podo- + G. *dynamis*, force, + *metron*, measure ]. An instrument for measuring the strength of the muscles of the foot or leg.

**pododynia** (pod-o-din'ĭ-ah) [ podo- + G. *odynē*, pain ]. Podalgia.

**pod'ogram** *podo-* + G. *gramma*, something written ]. An imprint of the sole of the foot, showing the contour and the condition of the arch, or an outline tracing.

**pod'ograph** [ podo- + G. *graphō*, to write ]. A device for taking an outline at the foot and an imprint of the sole.

**pod'olite.** Dahllite.

**podologist** (po-dol'o-jist). Podiatrist.

**podology** (po-dol'o-jĭ) [ podo- + G. *logos*, study ]. Podiatry.

**podomechanotherapy** (pod'o-mek'ă-no-thĕr'ă-pĭ). Treatment of foot conditions with mechanical devices, *e.g.*, arch supports.

**podometer** (po-dom'e-ter) [ podo- + G. *metron*, measure ]. Pedometer (2).

**podophyllin** (pod'o-fil'in). Podophyllum resin; see under resin.

**podophyllotoxin** (pod'o-fil'o-tok'sin). A toxic, polycyclic substance, $C_{22}H_{22}O_8$, with cathartic properties present in podophyllum; has antineoplastic action.

**podophyllum** (pod'o-fil'um) (USP). May-apple; vegetable calomel; the rhizome of *Podophyllum peltatum* (family Berberidaceae), American mandrake, umbrella plant, duck's-foot; used as a laxative.
  **Indian p.,** the dried rhizome and roots of *P. emodi*, a Himalayan plant; cholagogue and cathartic.
  **p. resin,** see under resin.

**podospasm, podospasmus** (pod'o-spazm, -spaz-mus) [ podo- + G. *spasmos*, spasm ]. Podismus; spasm of the foot.

**podotrochilitis** (pod-o-trok-il-i'tis) [ G. *pous* (*pod*-), foot, + *trochilea*, pulley, fr. *trechō*, to run, + *-itis* ]. Navicular *disease*.

**Poehl** (pel), Alexander V. von, Russian physiological chemist, 1850–1908. See P.'s *test*.

**pogoniasis** (po-go-ni'ă-sis) [ G. *pōgōn*, beard, + suffix *-iasis*, condition ]. Growth of a beard on a woman, or excessive hairiness of the face in men.

**pogonion** (po-go'nĭ-on) [ G. dim. of *pōgōn*, beard ]. Mental point; in craniometry, the most anterior point on the mandible in the midline. See fig. under craniometric *point*.

**Pogonomyrmex** (po-go'no-mĭr'meks, -mer'meks) [ G. *pōgōn*, beard, + *myrmex*, ant ]. Harvester ants; a genus of ants that attack man and small animals. The venomous bites of large numbers of these ants have been known to kill young pigs.

**-poiesis** (-poy-e'sis) [ G. *poiēsis*, a making ]. Combining form meaning production.

**poikilo-, poikil-** (poy'kĭ-lo-, poy-kil'o-) [ G. *poikilos*, many colored, varied ]. Combining form meaning irregular or varied.

**poikiloblast** (poy'kĭ-lo-blast) [ poikilo- + G. *blastos*, germ ]. A nucleated red blood cell of irregular shape.

**poikilocyte** (poy'kĭ-lo-sīt) [ poikilo- + G. *kytos*, cell ]. A red blood cell of irregular shape.

**poikilocythemia** (poy'kĭ-lo-si-the'mĭ-ah) [ poikilocyte + G. *haima*, blood ]. Poikilocytosis.

**poikilocytosis** (poy'kĭ-lo-si-to'sis) [ poikilocyte + G. suffix *-osis*, condition ]. Poikilocythemia; the presence of poikilocytes in the peripheral blood.

**poikilodentosis** (poy'kĭ-lo-den-to'sis) [ poikilo- + L. *dens*, tooth, + suffix *-osis*, condition ]. Hypoplastic defects or mottling of enamel due to excessive fluoride in water supply.

**poikiloderma** (poy'kĭ-lo-der'mah) [ poikilo- + G. *derma*, skin ]. A variegated hyperpigmentation and telangiectasia of the skin, followed by atrophy.
  **p. atrophicans and cataract,** Rothmund's *syndrome*.
  **p. atroph'icans vascula're,** parapsoriasis lichenoides; a rare condition that simulates radiodermatitis in appearance; probably identical with mycosis fungoides.

**p. of Civatte,** Civatte's disease; reticulated pigmentation and telangiectasia of the sides of the cheeks and neck; common in middle-aged women.
  **p. congenita'le,** Rothmund's *syndrome*.

**poikilonymy** (poy'kĭ-lon'ĭ-mĭ) [ poikilo- + G. *onyma*, name ]. The use of two or more terms to indicate the same thing.

**poikilotherm** (poy'kĭ-lo-therm). Allotherm; a poikilothermal or cold-blooded animal.

**poikilothermal, poikilothermic, poikilothermous** (poy'kĭ-lo-ther'mal, -mik, -mus) [ poikilo- + G. *thermē*, heat ]. Cold-blooded; hematocryal. 1. Varying in temperature according to the temperature of the surrounding medium; denoting the so-called cold-blooded animals such as the reptiles and amphibians and the plants. 2. Capable of existence and growth in mediums of varying temperatures.

**poikilothermy, poikilothermism** (poy'kĭ-lo-ther'mĭ) [ poikilo- + G. *thermē*, heat ]. The condition of plants and cold-blooded animals, the temperature of which varies with the changes in the temperature of the surrounding medium.

**poikilothrombocyte** (poy'kĭ-lo-throm'bo-sīt) [ poikilo- + G. *thrombos*, clot, + *kytos*, cell ]. A blood platelet of abnormal shape.

**poikilothymia** (poy'kĭ-lo-thi'mĭ-ah) [ poikilo- + G. *thymos*, mind ]. A mental state marked by abnormal variations in mood.

**point** [ Fr.; L. *punctum*, fr. *pungo*, pp. *punctus*, to pierce ]. 1. Punctum (*q.v.*); a spot or small area. 2. A sharp end or apex. 3. A slight projection. 4. A stage or condition reached, as the boiling p. 5. To become ready to open, said of an abscess or boil the wall of which is becoming thin and is about to break.
  **p. A,** subspinale.
  **absorbent p.'s,** cones of paper or paper products used for drying or maintaining medicaments in conjunction with root canal therapy.
  **alveolar p.,** prosthion.
  **apoph'ysary p., apophys'ial p.,** (1) subnasal p.; (2) Trousseau's p.
  **auric'ular p.,** the midpoint of the opening of the external acoustic meatus.
  **p. B,** supramentale.
  **boiling p.,** the temperature at which the vapor pressure of a liquid equals the ambient atmospheric pressure; abbreviated b.p.
  **Bolton p.,** highest roentgenographic p. in the series of notches posterior to the occipital condyle.
  **Cap'uron's p.'s,** the iliopubic eminences and the sacroiliac joints, constituting four fixed p.'s in the pelvic inlet.
  **cardinal p.'s,** (1) the four p.'s in the pelvic inlet toward one of which the occiput of the baby is usually directed in case of head presentation, *viz.*, the two sacroiliac articulations and the two iliopectineal eminences corresponding to the acetabula; (2) six p.'s in the eye: the anterior focal p., where rays starting parallel from the retina are focused; the posterior focal p., the p. on the retina where parallel rays entering the eye are focused; the two principal p.'s; and the two nodal p.'s.
  **central-bearing p.,** the contact p. of a central-bearing device.
  **Clado's p.,** a p. at the junction of the interspinous and right semilunar lines, at the lateral border of the rectus abdominis muscle, where marked tenderness on pressure is felt in cases of appendicitis.
  **cold-rigor p.,** the degree of lowered temperature at which the activity of a cell ceases and it passes into the narcotic or hibernating state.
  **congruent p.'s,** a pair of p.'s in the two retinas referred to the same p. in the external stimulus.
  **contact p.,** the part of the proximal surface of a tooth that touches the adjacent tooth mesially or distally.
  **p.'s of convergence,** see under convergence.
  **craniomet'ric p.'s,** fixed p.'s on the skull used as landmarks in craniometry. See fig. on p. 1114.
  **critical p.,** a p. at which two phases become identical; thus, at a given critical temperature and critical pressure, the liquid and gaseous state of a particular substance can no longer be differentiated.

**Craniometric Points**

**dew p.,** the temperature at and below which moisture will condense for a specific humidity.

**end p.,** the completion of a reaction; usually evident by the first perceptible alteration of the color of an added indicator.

**Erb's p.,** a p. on the side of the neck where pressure can be made on the brachial plexus, giving rise to Erb's paralysis.

**far p.,** punctum remotum; the farthest p. of distinct vision.

**p. of fixation,** the p. on the retina at which the rays coming from an object regarded directly are focused.

**flash p.,** the lowest temperature at which vapors of a liquid may be ignited by a flame.

**freezing p.,** the temperature at which a liquid solidifies.

**fusing p. of metals,** see fusion *temperature.*

**fusion (dental) p.,** see fusion *temperature.*

**Guéneau de Mussy's p.,** a p., painful on pressure, at the junction of a line prolonging the left border of the sternum and a horizontal line at the level of end of the bony portion of the tenth rib; it is present in cases of diaphragmatic pleurisy.

**gutta percha p.'s,** cones of a gutta percha compound used for filling root canals in conjunction with a cement, paste, or plastic.

**Hallé's p.,** a p. at the intersection of a horizontal line touching the anterior superior spine of the ilium and a perpendicular line drawn from the spine of the pubis; here the ureter can be most readily palpated.

**heat-rigor p.,** the degree of elevated temperature at which coagulation of protoplasm occurs with death of the cell.

**hysterogenic p.'s,** hysterogenic *zones.*

**incisal p.,** the p. located between the incisal edges of the lower central incisors; the graphic projection of the excursions of the incisal p. in certain planes is generally used to illustrate the envelope of motion of mandibular movement.

**isoelec'tric p.,** the pH at which an amphoteric substance such as protein is electrically neutral. Below or above this pH, it acts as a base or acid, respectively. Protein is least soluble at or near the isoelectric p.

**isoionic p.,** the pH at which a zwitterion has an equal number of positive and negative charges; in water and in the absence of other solutes, this is the isoelectric p.

**J p.,** the S-T junction; the p. marking the end of the QRS complex and the beginning of the S-T segment in the electrocardiogram.

**ju'gal p.,** jugale.

**Lian's p.,** a p. at the junction of the outer and middle thirds of a line passing from the umbilicus to the anterior superior spine of the ilium, where the trocar may safely be introduced in paracentesis.

**ma'lar p.,** apex of the tuberosity of the zygomatic (malar) bone.

**p. of maximal impulse,** the p. on the chest wall at which the maximal cardiac impulse is seen and/or felt.

**maximum occip'ital p.,** the p. on the squama of the occipital bone farthest from the glabella.

**Mayo-Robson's p.,** a p. just above and to the right of the umbilicus, where tenderness on pressure exists in disease of the pancreas.

**McBurney's p.,** a p. between $1\frac{1}{2}$ and 2 inches above the anterior superior spine of the ilium, on a straight line joining that process and the umbilicus, where pressure of the finger elicits tenderness in acute appendicitis.

**median mandibular p.,** a p. on the anteroposterior center of the mandibular ridge in the median sagittal plane.

**melting p.,** the temperature at which a solid becomes a liquid.

**mental p.,** pogonion.

**metop'ic p.,** metopion.

**motor p.,** a p. on the skin where the application of an electrode will cause the contraction of a special muscle.

**Munro's p.,** a tender p. at the right edge of the rectus abdominis muscle, between the umbilicus and the anterior superior spine of the ilium, in appendicitis.

**nasal p.,** nasion.

**near p.,** punctum proximum; the nearest p. of distinct vision.

**neutral p.,** pH 7; the p. at which a solution is neither acid nor alkaline.

**nodal p.,** one of two p.'s in a compound optical system, so related that a ray directed toward the first before entering the system, will leave the system in a direction as if it had passed through the second p. parallel to its original direction.

**occip'ital p.,** the most prominent posterior p. on the occipital bone above the inion.

**painful p.,** see Valleix's p.'s.

**power p.,** in dentistry, the vertical dimension at which the greatest masticatory force may be registered.

**preauricular p.,** a p. of the posterior root of the zygomatic arch lying immediately in front of the upper end of the tragus.

**pressure p.,** the seat of the pressure sense; one of the p.'s in the skin where the nerve terminal organs are located.

**principal p.,** one of two p.'s in an optical system where the axis is cut by the two principal planes; lines drawn from these to corresponding p.'s on the object and the image will be parallel.

**p. of proximal contact,** the p. on the proximal (mesial or distal) surface of a tooth at which the next tooth in the same jaw makes contact.

**p. of regard,** the p. toward which the eye is directed.

**retention p.,** retention *area.*

**silver p.,** a solid core cone of silver used in filling root canals in conjunction with a cement or paste.

**p. source,** in photometry, a very small source of light which is regarded as a geometrical p. from which light emanates in straight lines in all direction.

**spinal p.,** subnasal p.

**subnasal p.,** the center of the root of the anterior nasal spine; apophysary p. (1); spinal p.

**Sudeck's critical p.,** region in the colon between the supply of the sigmoid arteries and that of the superior rectal artery.

**supra-auric'ular p.,** a craniometric p. on the posterior root of the zygomatic process of the temporal bone directly above the auricular p.

**supranasal p.,** ophryon.

**supraorbital p.,** ophryon.

**Sylvian p.,** the nearest p. on the skull to the lateral (Sylvian) fissure, about 30 mm. behind the zygomatic process of the frontal bone.

**tender p.'s,** Valleix's p.'s.

**trigger p.,** a specific p. on the body at which touch or pressure will give rise to pain.

**Trousseau's p.,** apophysary p. (2); a painful p., in neuralgia, at the spinous process of the vertebra below which arises the offending nerve.

**Valleix's p.'s,** various p.'s in the course of a nerve, pressure upon which is painful in cases of neuralgia; these p.'s are: where the nerve emerges from the bony canal; where it pierces a muscle or aponeurosis to reach the skin; where a superficial nerve rests upon a resisting surface where compression is easily made; where the nerve gives off one or more branches; where the nerve terminates in the skin.

**Vogt's p.,** Vogt-Hueter p.

**Vogt-Hueter p.,** Vogt's p.; a p. for the application of a trephine in case of hemorrhage from the middle meningeal artery; it is at the junction of a horizontal line two fingerbreadths above the zygomatic arch and a vertical line one fingerbreadth behind the nasal process of the malar bone.

**Voillemier's p.,** a p. in the linea alba, 2½ inches (6.25 cm.) below the level of a line joining the anterior superior spinal processes of the ilium, where a distended bladder can be safely punctured.

**Weber's p.,** a p. situated 1 cm. below the promontory of the sacrum representing the center of gravity of the body.

**zygomaxillary p.,** zygomaxillare.

**pointillage** (pwan-te-yazh') [ Fr. dotting, stippling ]. A massage manipulation with the tips of the fingers.

**point'ing.** Preparing to open spontaneously, said of an abscess or a boil.

**Poirier** (pwah-re-a'), Paul J., French surgeon, 1853–1907. See P.'s *gland, line.*

**poise** (poyz, pwahz) [ J. *Poiseuille* ]. The unit of viscosity in the CGS system equal to 1 dyne second per square centimeter.

**Poiseuille** (pwah-ze'e), Jean M., Paris physiologist and physicist, 1799–1869. See P.'s *coefficient, formula, law, space.*

**poison** (poy'zun) [ Fr. from L. *potio,* potion, draught ]. Any substance (either taken internally or applied externally) that is injurious to health or dangerous to life.

**acrid p.,** a p. which causes a destructive local irritation as well as systemic effects.

**bait p.'s,** poisonous substances used for the extermination of rats, mice, or other vermin.

**fugu p.** (foo'goo) [ Jap. *fugu,* a poisonous fish ], fish p.; a p. in the roe and other parts of various species of *Diodon, Triodon,* and *Tetradon,* fishes of eastern Asiatic water.

**Indian arrow p.,** curare.

**poisonberry.** Dulcamara.

**poisoning** (poy'zun-ing). 1. The administering of poison. 2. The state of being poisoned. For poisons not given as subentries here, see the specific substance.

**ack'ee p.,** vomiting sickness of Jamaica; an acute and frequently fatal vomiting disease associated with central nervous system symptoms and marked hypoglycemia caused by eating unripe ackee fruit of *Blighia spaida,* a tree common in Jamaica.

**alkali p.,** (1) milk sickness in cattle; (2) once applied to a paralytic disease of wild ducks, in some areas of the western part of the United States, thought to be due to the drinking of alkaline waters but now known to be botulism due to the type C organism.

**bacterial food p.,** commonly refers to conditions limited to enteritis or gastroenteritis (the enteric or typhoid fevers and the dysenteries being excluded) caused by bacterial multiplication *per se* or a soluble exotoxin.

**blood p.,** see septicemia; pyemia.

**bracken p.,** an acute fatal disease of cattle and horses caused by eating the common brake fern, *Pteridium latiusculum;* in horses, the disease is manifested by neurologic signs; in cattle, by pancytopenia.

**carbon disulfide p.,** acute or chronic intoxication by CS₂, an industrial condition encountered among rubber workers and makers of artificial silk (rayon) by the viscose process. Characterized by insomnia, listlessness, and irritability, followed by paralyses, impaired vision, peptic ulcer, and psychoses.

**carbon monoxide p.,** carboxyhemoglobinemia; a potentially fatal acute or chronic intoxication caused by inhalation of carbon monoxide gas which competes favorably with oxygen for binding with hemoglobin and thus interferes with the transportation of oxygen and carbon dioxide by the blood. Carbon monoxide is a colorless, odorless, and tasteless gas usually produced from incomplete combustion of carbon-containing fuels in a deficiency of air or oxygen.

**clay pigeon p.,** pitch p.

**crotalaria p.,** crotalism; p. of man and animals with alkaloids of the plants *Senecio* (ragwort), *Crotalaria* (rattle-

box), and *Heliotropum;* produces a veno-occlusive disease of the liver similar to Chiari's disease.

**cyanide p.,** a not uncommon disease of herbivorous animals, caused by eating cyanogenic plants containing glucosides which are hydrolyzed, yielding hydrocyanic acid; some farm chemicals, such as fungicides or insecticides, may be causes of cyanide p.

**Datura p.,** many plants of the order *Solanaceae* to which *Datura* belongs are used in the tropics to produce unconsciousness. The seeds contain hyoscine (scopoalamine), an alkaloid with an anticholinergic action similar to that of atropine.

**equisetum p.,** p. of horses from eating hay containing horsetail, *Equisetum arvense;* it is a paralytic disease from which recoveries occur if the poisonous feed is withdrawn before the paralytic symptoms are far advanced.

**food p.,** poisoning in which the active agent is contained in ingested food.

**forage p.,** a disease of horses, believed to be caused by ingestion of toxic agents in forage; in some cases the disease is botulism caused by *Clostridium botulinum* type C toxin, contained in damaged feed.

**jeng'hol p.,** djenkol; believed to result from eating an excessive amount of a bean, *Pitecolobium lobatum.* Symptoms are pain in the renal region, dysuria, and later anuria. The jenghol bean has a high vitamin B content and is used for food despite its toxic qualities.

**lead p.,** plumbism; saturnism; acute or chronic intoxication by lead or any of its salts. The symptoms of *acute* lead p. are usually those of acute gastroenteritis. *Chronic* lead p. (also called saturnine cachexia) is manifested chiefly by anemia, constipation, colicky abdominal pain, paralysis with wrist-drop involving the extensor muscles of the forearm, bluish lead line of the gums, convulsions, and coma.

**lechuguilla p.,** swellhead (1); a plant toxemia of sheep and goats in western Texas, southeastern New Mexico, and northern Mexico caused by eating *Agave lechuguilla;* there is liver damage resulting in icterus, sometimes hemoglobinuria and often death, and photosensitivity with edema, swelling, and crusting of the face and ears.

**mercury p.,** mercurialism; hydrargyria; hydrargyrism; a disease usually caused by the ingestion of mercury or mercury compounds. Such compounds are toxic in relation to their ability to produce mercuric ions. Acute poisoning is usually associated with ulcerations of the stomach and intestine and nephrotoxic changes in the renal tubules; it may be fatal. Chronic mercurialism may be related to metallic mercury and primarily involves the central nervous system, producing an intention tremor, increased tendon reflexes, and emotional instability.

**mushroom p.,** see subentries under mycetism.

**oxygen p.,** oxygen *toxicity.*

**pitch p.,** clay pigeon p.; a highly fatal disease of swine, usually caused by the ingestion of fragments of the clay pigeons used as targets by shooting clubs, some cases have been caused by consumption of other bituminous substances, such as road tar and tar paper.

**salmon p.,** a disease of dogs and other canids in the northwest coastal region of the United States; it results from their eating infected salmon and trout from streams flowing into the Pacific Ocean; these fish carry the encysted form of *Nanophytus salmincola,* which infects the intestine and carries with it *Neorickettsia helmintheca,* the actual agent of the disease.

**Salmonella food p.,** gastroenteritis caused by various strains of *Salmonella* that multiply freely in the gastrointestinal tract but do not produce septicemia; symptoms begin, usually, within 8 to 24 hours and include fever, headache, nausea, vomiting, diarrhea, and abdominal pain.

**salt p.,** an often fatal disease of animals, especially pigs fed on garbage, resulting from the ingestion of excessive quantities of ordinary table salt, sodium chloride; this usually does not occur if the animals have access to sufficient quantities of fresh drinking water.

**sausage p.,** allantiasis.

**selenium p.,** chronic p. of horses, cattle, and swine, caused by ingestion of grains and forage raised on soils high in selenium; it occurs only in arid regions, from eating certain plants which are selenium accumulators.

**silver p.,** argyria.

**Staphylococcus food p.,** outbreaks commonly caused by staphylococcal enterotoxin (*q. v.*) and characterized by an abrupt onset of gastroenteritis within several hours after ingestion of the food contaminated with the preformed exotoxin; vomiting is usually more severe and diarrhea less severe than in infectious forms of bacterial food p.

**sweet clover p.,** a hemorrhagic disease of herbivores, especially cattle, occurring as a result of consuming damaged hay or silage containing sweet clover, but never as a result of eating freshly cut plants or pasturing on sweet clover. The causative agent is the anticoagulant, dicumerol, which is formed in the spoilage process from the harmless coumarins.

**tetraethyl p.,** see tetraethyl lead.

**thallium p.,** a condition characterized by nephritis, formication in the hands and feet, pain in the extremities, insomnia, anorexia, loss of hair, keratoses on the hands and feet, white transverse streaks on the nails; similar to tabes and polyneuritis of arsenic, lead, mercury, or alcohol.

**wheat p.,** grass *tetany.*

**poison ivy, oak.** See *Rhus* and *Toxicodendron.*

**Poisson,** Siméon Denis, French mathematician, 1781–1840. See P. *distribution.*

**Poisson-Pearson formula.** See under formula.

**po′lar** [ Mod. L. *polaris,* fr. *polus,* pole ]. 1. Relating to a pole. 2. Having poles, said of certain nerve cells having one or more processes.

**polarimeter** (po′lar-im′e-ter) [ Mod. L. *polaris,* polar, + G. *metron,* measure ]. An instrument for measuring the angle of rotation in polarization or the amount of polarized light.

**po′larim′etry.** Measurement by polarimeter.

**polariscope** (po-lăr′ĭ-skōp) [ Mod. L. *polaris,* polar, + G. *skopeō,* to examine ]. An instrument for studying the phenomena of the polarization of light.

**polariscopic** (po-lăr-ĭ-skop′ik). Relating to the polariscope or to polariscopy.

**polariscopy** (po′lă-ris′ko-pī). Use of the polariscope in studying properties of polarized light.

**polarity** (po-lăr′ĭ-tī) [ Mod. L. *polaris,* polar ]. 1. The property of having two opposite poles, as that possessed by a magnet. 2. The possession of opposite properties or characteristics. 3. The direction or orientation of positivity relative to negativity.

**polarization** (po′lar-ĭ-za′shun). 1. In electricity, the coating of an electrode with a thick layer of hydrogen bubbles, with the result that the flow of current is weakened or arrested. 2. A change effected in a ray of light passing through certain media, whereby the transverse vibrations occur in one plane only, instead of in all planes as in the ordinary light ray. 3. The development of differences in potential between two points in living tissues, as between the inside and outside of the cell wall.

**po′larize.** To put into a state of polarization, referring either to light rays or to an electric battery.

**po′lari′zer.** The first element of a polariscope that polarizes the light, as distinguished from the analyzer, the second polarizing element.

**polarography** (po′lar-og′ră-fī) [ Mod. L. *polaris,* polar, + G. *graphō,* to write ]. That branch of electrochemistry dealing with the variation in current flowing through a solution as the voltage is varied. This will vary with the ionic concentration of reducible substances so that p. can be used in chemical analysis. P. is commonly employed in the form of a reduction at a dropping mercury electrode.

**poldine methylsulfate** (pōl′dēn) (NF, BP). NACTON; 2-benziloyloxymethyl-1,1-dimethylpyrrolidinium methylsulfate; an anticholinergic agent used as a smooth muscle antispasmodic.

**pole** [ L. *polus,* the end of an axis, pole, fr. G. *polos* ]. 1. One of the two points at the extremities of the axis of any body; see polus. 2. One of the two points on a sphere at the greatest distance from the equator. 3. One of the two points in a magnet or an electric battery or cell having the extremes of opposite properties, as of attraction or repulsion.

**abapical p.,** in an ovum, the p. opposite the animal p.

**animal p.,** germinal p.; the point in a telolecithal egg opposite the yolk, where most of the protoplasm is concentrated and where the nucleus is located. It is from this region that the polar bodies are extruded during maturation.

**anterior p. of eyeball,** *polus* anterior bulbi oculi.

**anterior p. of lens,** *polus* anterior lentis.

**cephalic p.,** the head end of the fetus.

**frontal p.,** *polus* frontalis cerebri.

**germinal p.,** animal p.

**inferior p.,** *extremitas* inferior.

**lateral p.,** *extremitas* tubaria.

**medial p.,** *extremitas* uterina.

**negative p.,** cathode.

**occipital p.,** *polus* occipitalis cerebri.

**pelvic p.,** the breech end of the fetus.

**positive p.,** anode.

**posterior p. of eyeball,** *polus* posterior bulbi oculi.

**posterior p. of lens,** *polus* posterior lentis.

**superior p.,** *extremitas* superior.

**temporal p.,** *polus* temporalis cerebri.

**vegetal p., vegetative p.,** the part of a telolecithal egg where the bulk of the yolk is situated.

**vitelline p.,** the vegetative p. of an ovum.

**Polenské number.** See under number.

**policeman** (po-lēs′man). An instrument for removing solid particles from a glass container—usually a rubber-tipped rod.

**policlinic** (pol′ĭ-klin′ik) [ G. *polis,* city, + *klinē,* bed ]. Polyclinic.

**polio-** (po′lī-o-) [ G. *polios,* gray ]. Combining form meaning gray; relating to the gray matter (substantia grisea).

**polioclastic** (po′lī-o-klas′tik) [ polio- + G. *klastos,* broken ]. Destructive to gray matter of the nervous system.

**po′liodystro′phia.** Poliodystrophy.

**p. cer′ebri progressi′va infanta′lis,** familial progressive spastic paresis of extremities with progressive mental deterioration, with development of seizures, blindness and deafness, beginning during the first year of life, and with destruction and disorganization of nerve cells of the cerebral cortex; also called Christensen-Krabbe disease, Alpers' disease, and progressive cerebral poliodystrophy.

**poliodystrophy** (po′lī-o-dis′tro-fī) [ polio- + G. prefix *dys-,* bad, + *trophē,* nourishment ]. Poliodystrophia; wasting of the gray matter of the nervous system.

**progressive cerebral p.,** *poliodystrophia* cerebri progressiva infantalis.

**polioencephalitis** (po′lī-o-en-sef′ă-li′tis) [ polio- + G. *enkephalos,* brain, + *-itis* ]. Inflammation of the gray matter of the brain, either of the cortex or of the central nuclei; an acute infectious disease marked at the onset by fever, headache, convulsions, or stupor, followed by ocular palsies, symptoms resembling those of bulbar paralysis, aphasia, or idiocy.

**p. infecti′va,** von Economo's *disease.*

**inferior p.,** p. with predominantly bulbar paralysis.

**superior p.,** p. with predominantly ophthalmoplegia.

**superior hemorrhagic p.,** Wernicke's *syndrome.*

**polioencephalomeningomyelitis** (po′lī-o-en-sef′ă-lo-mĕ-ning′go-mi-ĕ-li′tis) [ polio- + G. *enkephalos,* brain, + *mēninx,* membrane, + *myelon,* marrow, + *-itis* ]. Inflammation of the gray matter of the brain and spinal cord and of the meningeal covering of the parts.

**polioencephalomyelitis** (po′lī-o-en-sef′ă-lo-mi′e-li′tis). Poliomyeloencephalitis.

**polioencephalopathy** (po′lī-o-en-sef′ă-lop′ă-thī) [ polio- + G. *enkephalos,* brain, + *pathos,* suffering ]. Any disease of the gray matter of the brain.

**poliomyelencephalitis** (po′lī-o-mi′el-en-sef′ă-li′tis). Poliomyeloencephalitis.

**poliomyelitis** (po′lī-o-mi′ĕ-li′tis) [ polio- + G. *myelos,* marrow, + *-itis* ]. Inflammation of the gray matter of the spinal cord.

**acute anterior p.,** inflammation of the anterior cornua of the spinal cord; an acute infectious disease caused by the poliomyelitis virus and marked by fever, pains, and gastroenteric disturbances, followed by a flaccid paralysis of one or more muscular groups, and later by atrophy. Also called infantile paralysis; infantile spinal paralysis; acute atrophic or acute infectious paralysis; epidemic paralysis; Little's paralysis; Heine-Medin disease.

**acute bulbar p.,** poliomyelitis virus infection affecting nerve cells in the medulla oblongata.

**chronic anterior p.,** remitting spinal atrophy; muscular atrophy of the upper extremities and neck, in which there are long intermissions of quiescence or improvement; not to be confused with poliomyelitis virus infections.

**mouse p.,** mouse *encephalomyelitis*.

**poliomyeloencephalitis** (po'lĭ-o-mi'ĕ-lo-en-sef'ă-li'tis) [ polio- + G. *myelon*, marrow, + *enkephalos*, brain, + *-itis* ]. Polioencephalomyelitis; poliomyelencephalitis; acute anterior poliomyelitis with pronounced cerebral signs.

**poliomyelopathy** (po'lĭ-o-mi'ĕ-lop'ă-thĭ) [ polio- + G. *myelon*, marrow, + *pathos*, suffering ]. Any disease of the gray matter of the spinal cord.

**polioplasm** (po'lĭ-o-plazm) [ polio- + G. *plasma*, anything formed ]. An obsolete designation for granular protoplasm.

**poliosis** (po-lĭ-o'sis) [ G. fr. *polios*, gray ]. Canities.

**po'liovi'rus hom'inis.** See poliomyelitis *virus*.

**pol'ishing.** In dentistry, the act or process of making a restoration smooth and glossy.

**Pol'itzer,** Adam, Austrian otologist, 1835–1920. See *P. bag*, luminous *cone*, *method*.

**politzerization** (pol'it-zer-ĭ-za'shun). Inflation of the Eustachian tube and middle ear by the Politzer method.

**negative p.,** withdrawal of secretions from a cavity by suction, effected by attaching a compressed Politzer bag or rubber bulb to a tube inserted in the cavity.

**Pol'kissen of Zimmermann.** Juxtaglomerular *cells*.

**poll** (pōl). The occipital region of an animal, especially the horse; high point of the head between the ears.

**pollakidipsia** (pol'ă-kĭ-dip'sĭ-ah) [ G. *pollakis*, often, + *dipsa*, thirst ]. Unduly frequent thirst.

**pollakiuria** (pol'ă-kĭ-u'rĭ-ah) [ G. *pollakis*, often, + *ouron*, urine ]. Abnormally frequent micturition.

**pol'len** [ L. fine dust, fine flour ]. Microspores of seed plants carried by wind or insects prior to fertilization; important in the etiology of hay fever.

**polleno'sis.** Pollinosis.

**pollex,** gen. **pol'licis,** pl. **pollices** (pol'eks, pol'ĭ-sis, -sēz) [ L. ] [ NA ]. The thumb or first digit of the hand.

**p. exten'sus,** a deformity marked by backward deviation of the thumb.

**p. flexus,** a permanent flexion of the thumb.

**p. pe'dis,** hallux.

**p. superexten'sus,** p. extensus.

**p. valgus,** permanent deviation of the thumb to the ulnar side.

**p. varus,** permanent deviation of the thumb to the radial side.

**pollicization** (pol'ĭ-sĭ-za'shun) [ L. *pollex*, thumb, + suffix *-ize*, to make like, + suffix *-ation*, state ]. Construction of a substitute thumb from a portion of a finger and hand.

**pollinosis** (pol'ĭ-no'sis) [ L. *pollen*, pollen, + G. suffix, *-osis*, condition ]. Pollenosis; hay fever excited by the pollen of various plants.

**pollo'dic** [ G. *polloi*, many, + *hodos*, way ]. Panodic.

**pollution** (pŏ-lu'shun) [ L. *pollutio*, fr. *pol-luo*, pp. *-lutus*, to defile ]. 1. Defilement. 2. The discharge of semen, either voluntary or involuntary, other than during coitus.

**air p.,** contamination of air by smoke and harmful gases, mainly oxides of carbon, sulfur, and nitrogen, from automobile exhausts, industrial plants, and burning rubbish; see also *smog*.

**polocyte** (po'lo-sīt) [ G. *polos*, pole, + *kytos*, cell ]. A polar *body*.

**polonium** (po-lo'nĭ-um) [ L. fr. Polonia, Poland, the native country of Mme. Curie who with her husband discovered the substance ]. A radioactive element, isolated from pitchblende; it is one of the disintegration products of uranium; symbol Po, atomic no. 84; the longest-lived isotope is p.-210 with a half-life of 138.4 days.

**polox'alene.** POLYKOL; poloxalkol; an oxyalkylene polymer, nonionic surface-active agent similar in actions and uses to dioctyl sodium sulfasuccinate; used in constipation due to hard, dry stools.

**poltophagy** (pol-tof'ă-jĭ) [ G. *poltos*, porridge, + *phagein*, to eat ]. Fletcherism.

**po'lus,** pl. **po'li** [ L. pole ] [ NA ]. A pole; one of the two points at the extremities of the axis of any organ or body.

**p. anterior bulbi oculi** [ NA ], anterior pole of the eyeball; the center of the corneal curvature of the eye.

**p. anterior lentis** [ NA ], anterior pole of the lens; the central point on the anterior surface of the lens of the eye.

**p. fronta'lis cer'ebri** [ NA ], frontal pole; the most anterior promontory of each cerebral hemisphere.

**poli lienalis inferior et superior,** *extremitas* anterior; *extremitas* posterior.

**p. occipita'lis cer'ebri** [ NA ], occipital pole; the most posterior promontory of each cerebral hemisphere; the apex of the occipital lobe.

**p. posterior bulbi oculi** [ NA ], posterior pole of the eyeball; the center of the posterior curvature of the eye.

**p. posterior lentis** [ NA ], posterior pole of the lens; the central point on the posterior surface of the lens.

**poli renalis inferior et superior,** *extremitas* inferior; *extremitas* superior.

**p. tempora'lis cer'ebri** [ NA ], temporal pole; the most prominent part of the anterior extremity of the temporal lobe of each cerebral hemisphere, a short distance below the fissure of Sylvius.

**poly-** (pol'ĭ-) [ G. *polys*, much, many ]. 1. Prefix, in words formed from Greek roots, denoting multiplicity; corresponding to the Latin prefix *multi-*. For some words beginning thus; see also pluri- and multi-. 2. In chemistry, prefix meaning "polymer of," as in polypeptide, polysaccharide, polynucleotide; often used with symbols, as in poly(A) for poly(adenylic acid), poly(Lys) for poly(L-lysine).

**poly** (pol'ĭ). Abbreviation and colloquial name for polymorphonuclear leukocyte.

**Pólya,** Jenö (Eugene), Hungarian surgeon, 1876–1944. See P. *gastrectomy*, P.'s *operation*, Reichel-P. stomach *resection*.

**polyac'id.** An acid capable of liberating more than one hydrogen ion per molecule; *e.g.*, $H_2SO_4$ and citric acid. Not to be confused with polymer of an acid; see poly- (2).

**polyadenitis** (pol'ĭ-ă-de-ni'tis). Inflammation of many lymph nodes, especially with reference to the cervical group.

**p. malig'na,** bubonic *plague*.

**polyadenop'athy.** Adenopathy affecting many lymph nodes.

**polyadeno'sis.** Polyadenopathy.

**polyad'enous.** Pertaining to or involving many glands.

**polyalcohol.** An aliphatic or alicyclic molecule characterized by the presence of two or more hydroxyl groups; *e.g.*, glycerol, inositol. Not to be confused with poly(alchool), indicating a polymer of an alcohol; see poly- (2).

**polyam'ine.** Class name for substances of the general formula $H_2N(CH_2)_nNH_2$, $H_2N(CH_2)_nNH(CH_2)_nNH_2$, $H_2N(CH_2)_nNH(CH_2)_nNH(CH_2)_nNH_2$; n = 3, 4, or 5. Many p.'s arise by bacterial action on protein; many are normally occurring body constituents of wide distribution, or are essential growth factors for microorganisms. Putrescine, cadaverine, spermine, and spermidine are p.'s.

**poly(amine).** A polymer of an amine; see poly- (2).

**polyamine-methylene resin.** See under resin.

**poly(amino acids).** Polypeptides; polymers of aminoacyl groups.

**polyangiitis** (pol'ĭ-an'je-i'tis). Inflammation of multiple blood vessels involving more than one type of vessel, *e.g.*, arteries and veins, or arterioles and capillaries.

**polyan'tibiot'ic.** Composed of two or more antibiotics, referring to some pharmaceuticals.

**polyarteritis** (pol-ĭ-ar-ter-i'tis). Simultaneous inflammation of a number of arteries.

**p. nodo'sa,** Kussmaul's disease; periarteritis nodosa; segmental inflammation and necrosis of medium-sized or small arteries, most common in males, with varied symptoms related to involvement of arteries in the kidneys, muscles, gastrointestinal tract, and heart.

**polyar'thric.** Multiarticular.

**polyarthritis** (pol'ĭ-ar-thri'tis) [ poly- + G. *arthron*, joint, + suffix *-itis*, inflammation ]. Simultaneous inflammation of several joints.

**p. chron'ica,** rheumatoid *arthritis*.

**p. chron'ica villo'sa,** a chronic inflammation confined to the synovial membrane, involving a number of joints; it occurs in women at the menopause and in children.

**p. rheumat'ica acu'ta,** acute articular or inflammatory rheumatism; p. associated with rheumatic fever.

**tuber'culous p.,** pulmonary *osteoarthropathy.*

**ver'tebral p.,** inflammation of a number of the intervertebral disks without involvement of the vertebral bodies.

**polyartic'ular** [ poly- + L. *articulus,* joint ]. Multiarticular.

**polyavitaminosis** (pol'ĭ-a'vĭ'tă-mĭ-no'sis). Avitaminosis with multiple deficiencies.

**polyba'sic.** Having more than one replaceable hydrogen atom, denoting an acid with a basicity greater than 1.

**polybenzar'sol.** BENZODOL; a polymeric mixture containing formaldehyde, *p*-hydroxybenzenearsonic acid and sulfuric acid; amebicide.

**pol'yblast** [ poly- + G. *blastos,* germ ]. One of a group of ameboid, mononucleated wandering, phagocytic cells found in inflammatory exudates, derived from primitive wandering cells, histiocytes, monocytes, and lymphocytes.

**polyblen'nia** [ poly- + G. *blennos,* mucus ]. Excessive production of mucus.

**polycar'bophil** (NF). A polyacrylic acid cross-linked with divinyl glycol; used as a gastrointestinal absorbent.

**polycar'dia.** Tachycardia.

**polycen'tric.** Having several centers.

**polycheiria, polychiria** (pol-ĭ-ki'rĭ-ah) [ poly- + G. *cheir,* hand, + suffix -*ia,* condition ]. The condition of having supernumerary hands.

**pol'ychloru'ria.** Increased excretion of chloride in the urine.

**polycholia** (pol-ĭ-ko'lĭ-ah) [ poly- + G. *cholē,* bile, + suffix -*ia,* condition ]. The excretion of an excess of bile.

**polychondritis** (pol'ĭ-kon-dri'tis) [ poly- + G. *chondros,* cartilage, + suffix -*itis,* inflammation ]. A widespread disease of cartilage.

**chronic atrophic p.,** a degenerative disease of cartilage producing a bizarre form of arthritis: collapse of the ears, a cartilaginous portion of the nose, and the tracheaobronchial tree. The cause is unknown; perhaps a sensitivity mechanism is responsible. Death may occur from chronic infection or suffocation because of loss of stability in the tracheobronchial tree.

**polychromasia** (pol'ĭ-kro-ma'zĭ-ah). Polychromatophilia.

**polychromatia** (pol-ĭ-kro-ma'shyah). Polychromatophilia.

**polychromat'ic.** Multicolored.

**polychromatocyte** (pol-ĭ-kro'mă-to-sīt). Polychromatophil.

**polychromatophil, polychromatophile** (pol-ĭ-kro'mă-to-fil, -fīl) [ poly- + G. *chrōma,* color, + *phileō,* to love ]. Polychromophil. 1. Staining readily with acid, neutral, and basic dyes; denoting certain cells, especially certain red blood cells. 2. A young or degenerating erythrocyte that manifests acid and basic staining affinities.

**polychromatophilia** (pol-ĭ-kro'mă-to-fil'ĭ-ah) Polychromasia; polychromatia; polychromatosis; polychromophilia. 1. A tendency of certain cells, such as the red blood cells in pernicious anemia, to stain with basic and also acid dyes. 2. Condition characterized by the presence of many red blood cells that have an affinity for acid, basic, or neutral stains.

**polychro'matophil'ic.** Polychromatophil (1).

**polychro'mato'sis.** Polychromatophilia.

**polychromemia** (pol-ĭ-kro-me'mĭ-ah). An increase in the total amount of hemoglobin in the blood.

**polychromia** (pol-ĭ-kro'mĭ-ah). Increased pigmentation in any part.

**polychromophil** (pol-ĭ-kro'mo-fil). Polychromatophil.

**polychromophilia** (pol-ĭ-kro-mo-fil'ĭ-ah). Polychromatophilia.

**polychylia** (pol'ĭ-ki'lĭ-ah) [ poly- + G. *chylos,* chyle, + suffix -*ia,* condition ]. An increased production of chyle.

**polyclin'ic** [ poly- + G. *klinē,* bed ]. Policlinic; a dispensary for the treatment of diseases of all kinds and for their study.

**polyclonia** (pol'ĭ-klo'nĭ-ah) [ poly- + G. *klonos,* tumult ]. *Myoclonus* multiplex.

**polyco'ria.** 1 [ G. *korē,* pupil ]. The presence of two or more pupils in one iris. 2 [ G. *koros,* satiety, surfeit ]. The accumulation of reserve substances in an organ, thereby resulting in its enlargement; an obsolete usage.

**polycrot'ic.** Relating to or marked by polycrotism.

**polycrotism** (pol-ik'ro-tizm) [ poly- + G. *krotos,* a beat ]. A condition in which the sphygmographic tracing shows several upward breaks in the descending wave.

**polycyesis** (pol'ĭ-si-e'sis) [ poly- + G. *kyēsis,* pregnancy ]. Multiple pregnancy.

**polycys'tic.** Composed of many cysts.

**polycythemia** (pol'ĭ-si-the'mĭ-ah) [ poly- + G. *kytos,* cell, + *haima,* blood ]. An increase above the normal in the number of red cells in the blood; see also erythrocytosis and erythremia.

**compensatory p.,** a secondary p. resulting from anoxia, *e.g.,* in congenital heart disease, pulmonary emphysema, or prolonged residence at a high altitude.

**p. hyperton'ica,** Gaisböck's syndrome; p. associated with hypertension, but without splenomegaly.

**relative p.,** a relative increase in the number of red blood cells as a result of loss of the fluid portion of the blood.

**p. rubra,** erythremia.

**p. rubra vera,** erythremia.

**p. vera,** erythremia.

**polydactyl'ia.** Polydactyly.

**polydactylism** (pol'ĭ-dak'tĭ-lizm). Polydactyly.

**polydac'tylous.** Relating to polydactyly.

**polydactyly** (pol'ĭ-dak'tĭ-lī) [ poly- + G. *daktylos,* finger ]. Polydactylism; polydactylia; the presence of more than five digits on either hand or foot.

**polydentia** (pol'ĭ-den'shī-ah) [ poly- + L. *dens,* tooth ]. Polyodontia.

**polydip'sia** [ poly- + G. *dipsa,* thirst ]. Frequent drinking because of extreme thirst.

**p. ebrio'ria,** a craving for intoxicants.

**hysterical p.,** psychogenic p.; excessive fluid consumption resulting from a disorder of the personality, without demonstrable organic lesion.

**psychogenic p.,** hysterical p.

**polydispersoid** (pol'ĭ-dis-per'soyd). A colloid system in which the dispersed phase is composed of particles having different degrees of dispersion.

**polydysplasia** (pol'ĭ-dis-pla'zĭ-ah) [ poly- + G. prefix *dys-,* bad, + *plasis,* a molding ]. Tissue development abnormal in several respects.

**polydystro'phia.** Polydystrophy.

**polydystroph'ic.** Relating to polydystrophy.

**polydystrophy** (pol'ĭ-dis'tro-fī) [ poly- + dystrophy, *q.v.* ]. Polydystrophia; a condition characterized by the presence of many congenital anomalies of the connective tissues or mucopolysaccharides.

**polyembryony** (pol'ĭ-em'brī-o-nī) [ poly- + G. *embryon,* embryo ]. The condition of a zygote's giving rise to two or more embryos.

**polyene** (pol'ĭ-ēn). A chemical compound having a series of conjugated (alternating) double bonds; *e.g.,* the carotenoids.

**polyenic acids** (pol'ĭ-e'nik, -en'ik). Fatty acids with more than one double bond in the carbon chain; *e.g.,* linoleic acid, linolenic acid, arachidonic acid.

**polyergic** (pol-ĭ-er'jik) [ poly- + G. *ergon,* work ]. Capable of acting in several different ways.

**polyesthesia** (pol-ĭ-es-the'zĭ-ah) [ poly- + G. *aisthēsis,* sensation ]. A disorder of sensation in which a single touch or other stimulus is felt as several.

**polyestradi'ol phosphate** (NF). ESTRADURIN; estradiol phosphate polymer; used as long-acting estrogen for treatment of prostatic carcinoma.

**polyestrous** (pol'ĭ-es'trus). Having two or more estrous cycles in a mating season.

**polyethylene glycols.** CARBOWAX; poly(oxyethylene) glycols; condensation polymers of ethylene oxide and water, of the general formula HO—(CH$_2$CH$_2$O)$_n$—H; waxlike solids, soluble in water; used as ointment bases. Polyethylene glycols 300 and 1540 are listed in NF; polyethylene glycols 400 and 4000, in USP.

**polyfer′ose** (USAN). JEFRON; metallic iron sequestered within a polymerized carbohydrate; used in treatment of hypochromic anemia.

**polyfruc′tose.** Fructosan.

**polygalactia** (pol′ī-gă-lak′tī-ah, -shī-ah) [ poly- + G. *gala*, milk ]. An excessive secretion of milk, especially at the weaning period.

**polygalac′turonase** (EC 3.2.1.15). Pectinase; pectin depolymerase; hydrolase cleaving α-1,4-galacturonide links in pectate and other polygalacturonides.

**pol′yganglion′ic.** Containing or involving many ganglia.

**polygen** (pol′ī-jen). An element with two or more valences.

**polygene** (pol′ī-jēn). One of a group of genes acting together to produce quantitative variations of a particular character; for example, height.

**polygen′ic.** Polymeric (3); relating to a hereditary disease or normal characteristic controlled by interaction of genes at more than one locus.

**polyglan′dular.** Pluriglandular.

**poly-β-glucosaminidase.** Chitinase.

**poly(glutamic acid).** Polyglutamate; glutamic acid residues in the usual peptide linkage (α-carboxyl to α-amine); compare poly(γ-glutamic acid).

**poly(γ-glutamic acid).** A polypeptide formed of glutamic acid residues, the γ-carboxyl group of one glutamic acid being condensed to the amino group of its neighbor; occurs naturally in the anthrax bacillus capsule.

**poly(glycolic acid).** A polymer of glycolic acid, used as an absorbable surgical suture.

**polygnathus** (pol′i-nath′us, pō-lig′nă-thus) [ poly- + G. *gnathos*, jaw ]. Unequal conjoined twins in which the parasite is attached to the jaw of the autosite.

**polygraph** (pol′ī-graf) [ poly- + G. *graphō*, to write ]. 1. An instrument to obtain simultaneous tracings from several different pulsations; e.g., radial and jugular pulse, apex beat of the heart. 2. Lie detector; an instrument for recording changes in respiration, blood pressure, galvanic skin response, and other physiological changes while the person is questioned about some matter or asked to give associations to relevant and irrelevant words; the physiological changes are presumed to be indicators of emotional reactions, and thus whether the person is telling the truth.

  **Mackenzie's p.,** an instrument consisting of a system of tambours and a time-marker for recording simultaneously the jugular and arterial pulses and the apex beat. Used in the clinical investigation of cardiac arrhythmias.

**polygyria** (pol-ī-ji′rī-ah) [ poly- + G. *gyros*, circle, gyre ]. A condition in which the brain has an excessive number of convolutions.

**polyhe′dral** [ G. *polyedros*, many-sided, fr. poly- + G. *hedra*, seat, facet ]. Having many sides or facets.

**polyhidrosis** (pol′ī-hi-dro′sis). Hyperhidrosis.

**polyhybrid** (pol-ī-hi′brid) [ poly- + hybrid, q.v. ]. The offspring of parents differing from each other in more than three characters.

**polyhydramnios** (pol′ī-hi-dram′nī-os) [ poly- + G. *hydōr*, water, + amnion ]. An excess in the amount of amniotic fluid.

**polyhy′dric.** Containing more than one hydroxyl group, as polyhydric alcohols or polyhydric acids. Glycerol, $C_3H_5(OH)_3$ is an example of the former; *o*-phosphoric acid, $OP(OH)_3$, an example of the latter.

**polyhypermenorrhea** (pol′ī-hi′per-men-o-re′ah) [ poly- + G. *hyper*, above, + *mēn*, month, + *rhoia*, flow ]. Frequent and excessive menstruation.

**polyhypomenorrhea** (pol-ī-hi′po-men-o-re′ah) [ poly- + G. *hypo*, below, + *mēn*, month, + *rhoia*, a flow ]. Frequent but scanty menstruation.

**polyidrosis** (pol′ī-ī-dro′sis). Hyperhidrosis.

**polylep′tic** [ poly- + G. *lēpsis*, a seizing ]. Denoting a disease occurring in many paroxysms, e.g., malaria, epilepsy.

**polylogia** (pol′ī-lo′jī-ah) [ poly- + G. *logos*, word ]. Continuous and often incoherent speech.

**polymastia** (pol′ī-mas′tī-ah) [ poly- + G. *mastos*, breast ]. A condition in which, in the human, more than two breasts

are present. Also called polymazia; hypermastia; multimammae; pleomastia; pleomazia.

**polymastigote** (pol-ī-mas′tī-gōt). A mastigote having several flagella bunched together.

**polyma′zia** [ poly- + G. *mazos*, breast ]. Polymastia.

**polyme′lia** [ poly- + G. *melos*, limb ]. The presence of supernumerary limbs or parts of limbs.

**polyme′lus.** An individual exhibiting polymelia.

**polymenorrhea** (pol-ī-men-o-re′ah) [ poly- + G. *mēn*, month, + *rhoia*, flow ]. The occurrence of menstrual cycles of greater than usual frequency.

**polymer** (pol′ī-mer) [ poly- + suffix -mer, q.v. ]. A substance of high molecular weight, made up of a chain of identical, repeated "base units," sometimes called "mers," whence monomer, dimer, trimer, polymer, etc. Starch may be considered a p. of glucose.

  **cross-linked p.,** cross-linked resin; a p. in which long chain molecules are attached to each other, forming a three-dimensional network.

**polymerase** (pol′ī-mer-ās, po-lim′er-ās). Loosely, any enzyme catalyzing a polymerization, as of nucleotides to polynucleotides, thus belonging to EC class 2, the transferases.

**polymeria** (pol′ī-mēr′ī-ah) [ poly- + G. *meros*, part ]. A condition characterized by an excessive number of parts, limbs, or organs of the body.

**polymeric** (pol′ī-mēr′ik). 1. Having the properties of a polymer. 2. Relating to or characterized by polymeria. Rarely used synonym for polygenic.

**polym′erid.** Polymer.

**polymerization** (pol′ī-mer-ī-za′shun, po-lim′er-ī-). A reaction in which a high molecular weight product is produced by successive additions or condensations of a simpler compound; e.g., polystyrene may be produced from styrene, or rubber from isoprene, or a polynucleotide from a nucleotide.

**polymerize** (pol′ī-mer-īz, po-lim′er-īz). To bring about polymerization.

**polymetacarpa′lia, polymetacar′palism.** A congenital anomaly characterized by the presence of supernumerary metacarpal bones.

**polymetatarsa′lia, polymetatar′salism.** A congenital anomaly characterized by the presence of supernumerary metatarsal bones.

**polymicro′bial.** Polymicrobic.

**polymicrobic** (pol′ī-mi-kro′bik). Polymicrobial; indicating an infection by several kinds of microorganisms.

**pol′ymi′crolip′omato′sis** [ poly- + G. *mikros*, small, + lipoma, q.v., + suffix -osis, condition ]. The occurrence of multiple, small, nodular, fairly discrete masses of lipid in the subcutaneous connective tissue.

**polymitus** (pŏ-lim′ī-tus) [ poly- + G. *mitos*, thread ]. Exflagellation.

**pol′ymorph.** Colloquial term for polymorphonuclear *leukocyte.*

**polymorphic** (pol′ī-mor′fik) [ G. *polymorphos*, multiform ]. Pleomorphic; multiform; polymorphous; occurring in more than one morphologic form.

**polymorphism** (pol′ī-mor′fizm). Pleomorphism; occurrence in several forms; the existence in the same species or other natural group of several morphologic types.

  **lipoprotein p.,** heritable variations in low density β-lipoproteins; the variant lipoproteins exhibit different antigenic and chemical properties when compared with normal lipoproteins.

**polymor′phocel′lular** [ G. *polymorphos*, multiform, + L. *cellula*, cell ]. Relating to or formed of cells of several different kinds.

**polymorphonuclear** (pol′ī-mor-fo-nu′kle-ar) [ G. *polymorphos*, multiform, + L. *nucleus*, kernel ]. Having nuclei of varied forms; denoting a variety of leukocyte.

**polymor′phous.** Polymorphic.

**polymyalgia** (pol′ī-mi-al′jī-ah) [ poly- + G. *mys*, muscle, + *algos*, pain ]. Pain in several muscle groups.

  **p. arterit′ica,** p. rheumatica resulting from arteritis, especially disseminated giant cell arteritis.

  **p. rheumat′ica,** a syndrome within the group of collagen diseases different from spondylarthritis or from humeral scapular periarthritis by the presence of an elevated sedimentation rate; much commoner in women than in men.

**polymyocionus** (pol'ĭ-mi-ok'lo-nus). *Myoclonus* multiplex.

**polymyositis** (pol-ĭ-mi-o-si'tis) [ poly- + G. *mys*, muscle, + suffix *-itis*, inflammation ]. Inflammation of a number of voluntary muscles simultaneously.

**polymyx'in** (USP). A mixture of antibiotic substances obtained from cultures of *Bacillus polymyxa* (*B. aerosporus*), an organism found in water and soils; p. is obtainable as a crystalline hydrochloride. There are five different p.'s, designated A, B, C, D, and E, which are about equally effective against Gram-negative bacteria, but differ in toxicity, p. E (colistin) and p. B being the least toxic. The p.'s are polypeptides containing various amino acids and a branched chain fatty acid, (+)-6-methyloctanoic acid. See also colistin sulfate and colistimethate sodium.

   **p. B. sulfate** (USP, BP), AEROSPORIN; effective in tularemia, brucellosis, *Pseudomonas* infections, and urinary tract infections, but used systemically only for severe infections not responsive to less toxic agents; also used locally.

**polyne'sic** [ poly- + G. *nēsos*, island ]. Occurring in many separate foci; denoting certain forms of inflammation or infection.

**polyneu'ral** [ poly- + G. *neuron*, nerve ]. Relating to, supplied by, or affecting several nerves.

**polyneuralgia** (pol-ĭ-nu-ral'jĭ-ah). Neuralgia of several nerves simultaneously.

**polyneuritis** (pol-ĭ-nu-ri'tis). Multiple neuritis; simultaneous inflammation of a large number of the spinal nerves, marked by paralysis, pain, and wasting of muscles; see also nutritional *polyneuropathy*.

   **chronic familial p.,** irritation of nerves related to infiltration by amyloid.

   **erythredema p.,** a chronic disease of childhood; vasomotor changes are constant.

   **infectious p.,** Guillain-Barré *syndrome.*

**polyneuronitis** (pol'ĭ-nu'ro-ni'tis). Inflammation of several groups of nerve cells.

**polyneuropathy** (pol'ĭ-nu-rop'ă-thī) [ poly- + G. *neuron*, nerve, + *pathos*, disease ]. A disease process involving a number of peripheral nerves.

   **buckthorn p.,** ascending p. resulting from ingestion of the fruit of *Karwinskia humboldtiana, q.v.*

   **nutritional p.,** a disorder of multiple peripheral nerves; noted in beriberi, chronic alcoholism, and other clinical states characterized by thiamin deficiency.

   **uremic p.,** a distal sensory and motor p. without conspicuous inflammation and ascribed to the metabolic effects of chronic renal failure.

**polynox'ylin.** ANAFLEX; poly{methylenebis[ N,N'-di(hydroxymethyl)-urea ]}; topical antiseptic.

**polynuclear** (pol-ĭ-nu'kle-ar). Multinuclear.

**polynucleated** (pol-ĭ-nu'kle-a-ted). Multinuclear.

**polynucleo'sis.** Multinucleosis; the presence of numbers of polynuclear, or multinuclear, cells in the peripheral blood.

**polynu'cleoti'dase.** Enzyme catalyzing the hydrolysis of polynucleotides to oligonucleotides or to mononucleotides. See phosphodiesterase, nuclease.

**polynu'cleotide.** A linear polymer containing an indefinite (and usually large) number of nucleotides, linked from one ribose (or deoxyribose) to another *via* phosphoric residues.

   **p. phosphorylase,** polyribonucleotide nucleotidyltransferase.

**polyodontia** (pol'ĭ-o-don'shĭ-ah) [ poly- + G. *odous*, tooth ]. Polydentia; the presence of supernumerary teeth.

**polyol** (pol'ĭ-ol). Polyhydroxy alcohol; specifically, the sugar alcohols and inositols.

   **p. dehydrogenases,** oxidizing enzymes that catalyze the dehydrogenation of sugar alcohols to monosaccharides; dehydrogenases (EC class 1.1) named in terms of substrates.

**polyo'ma.** See polyoma *virus.*

**pol'yoncho'sis.** Polyoncosis.

**polyoncosis** (pol'ĭ-ong-ko'sis) [ poly- + G. *onkos*, tumor, + suffix *-osis*, condition ]. Polyonchosis; formation of multiple tumors.

   **hereditary cutaneomandibular p.,** basal cell nevus *syndrome.*

**polyonychia** (pol-ĭ-o-nik'ĭ-ah) [ poly- + G. *onyx*, nail ]. Polyunguia; the presence of supernumerary nails on fingers or toes.

**polyopia, polyopsia** (pol'ĭ-o'pī-ah, -op'sĭ-ah) [ poly- + G. *ōps*, eye ]. Double, or more correctly multiple, vision; the perception of several images of the same object.

**polyorchid** (pol'ĭ-or'kid). Polyorchis; an individual with polyorchism.

**polyorchidism** (pol-ĭ-or'kĭ-dizm). Polyorchism.

**polyorchis** (pol-ĭ-or'kis). Polyorchid.

**polyorchism** (pol-ĭ-or'kizm) [ poly- + G. *orchis*, testis ]. Polyorchidism; the presence of one or more supernumerary testes.

**polyorrhomeningitis** (pol-ĭ-or'ro-men-in-ji'tis) [ poly- + G. *orrhos*, serum, + meningitis, *q.v.* ]. Obsolete term for polyserositis.

**polyorrhomenitis** (pol-ĭ-or'ro-men-i'tis). Obsolete term for polyserositis.

**polyorrhomenosis** (pol-ĭ-or-ro-men-o'sis). Obsolete term for polyserositis.

**polyostotic** (pol'ĭ-os-tot'ik) [ poly- + G. *osteon*, bone ]. Involving more than one bone.

**polyotia** (pol-ĭ-o'shĭ-ah) [ poly- + G. *ous*, ear ]. The presence of a supernumerary auricle on one or both sides of the head.

**polyo'vulatory.** Discharging several ova in one ovulatory cycle.

**polyoxyl 40 stearate** (pol'ĭ-ok'sil) (USP). A mixture of the monostearate and distearate esters of a condensation polymer, $H(OCH_2CH_2)_n \cdot OCOC_{16}H_{32}CH_3$ ($n$ is approximately 40). It is a nonionic surface-active agent used as an emulsifying agent in hydrophilic ointment and other emulsions.

**polyp** (pol'ip) [ L. *polypus*; G. *polypous*, contr. fr. G. *polys*, many, + *pous*, foot ]. Polypus; a general, descriptive term used with reference to any mass of tissue that bulges or projects outward, or upward, from the normal surface level, thereby being macroscopically visible as a hemispheroidal, spheroidal, or irregularly moundlike structure growing from a relatively broad base or a slender stalk. P.'s may be neoplasms, foci of inflammation, degenerative lesions, or malformations.

   **adenomatous p.,** polypoid adenoma; cellular p.; a p. that consists of benign neoplastic tissue derived from glandular epithelium.

   **bleeding p.,** vascular p.

   **bronchial p.,** one growing from the bronchial mucosa.

   **cardiac p.,** usually a rounded thrombus attached to the endocardium.

   **cel'lular p.,** adenomatous p.

   **choanal p.,** a p. that extends into the nasopharynx.

   **cystic p.,** hydatid p.; a pedunculated cyst.

   **dental p.,** pulp p.; tooth p.; hyperplastic pulpal tissue growing out of a grossly decayed tooth with wide pulpal exposure.

   **fibrinous p.,** a misnomer for a mass of fibrin retained within the uterine cavity after childbirth.

   **fibrous p.,** one consisting chiefly of cellular fibrous tissue, frequently with foci of fairly dense collagen or hyaline material (or both).

   **fleshy p.,** myomatous p.

   **gelat'inous p.,** (1) one that consists of delicate, loose, edematous connective tissue; (2) a polypoid myxoma.

   **Hopmann's p.,** Hopmann's *papilloma.*

   **hydatid p.,** cystic p.

   **juvenile p.,** retention p.; a smoothly rounded mucosal hamartoma of the large bowel, which may be multiple and cause rectal bleeding, especially in the first decade of life; juvenile p.'s are not precancerous.

   **laryngeal p.,** a p. projecting from the surface of one of the vocal cords.

   **lipo'matous p.,** one consisting chiefly of adipose tissue; a lipoma that bulges from the surface or is attached by means of a stalk.

**lymphoid p.,** benign *lymphoma* of the rectum.

**mucous p.,** (1) an adenomatous p. in which conspicuous amounts of mucin are formed; (2) a polypoid cyst that contains mucus.

**myomatous p.,** fleshy p.; one that consists of benign neoplastic tissue derived from nonstriated (smooth) muscle; a submucous leiomyoma of the uterus that bulges or protrudes into the uterine cavity.

**nasal p.,** a p. that projects into the nasal cavity, arising from one of the paranasal sinuses.

**os'seous p.,** one consisting in part of bony tissue.

**pedunculated p.,** any form of p. that is attached to the base tissue by means of a slender stalk.

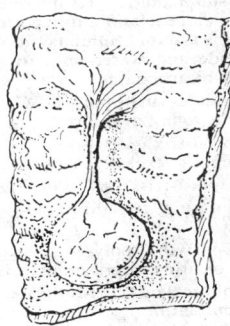

**Pedunculated Polyp of Rectal Mucosa**

**placental p.,** one developed from a piece of retained placenta.

**pulp p.,** dental p.

**rasp'berry p.,** a pedunculated, irregularly lobated mass of chronically inflamed granulation tissue in the external auditory meatus.

**retention p.,** juvenile p.

**sessile p.,** any form of p. that has a relatively broad base.

**spongy p.,** (1) mucous p.; (2) a pedunculated myxoma.

**tooth p.,** dental p.

**vas'cular p.,** bleeding p.; a bulging or protruding angioma of the nasal mucous membrane.

**polypapilloma** (pol'ĭ-pap'ĭ-lo'mah) [ poly- + papilloma ]. 1. Multiple papillomas. 2. Yaws.

**polyparesis** (pol'ĭ-pă-re'sis, -păr'e-sis) [ poly- + G. *paresis*, a slackening, weakness ]. General paralysis of the insane.

**pol'ypath'ia** [ poly- + G. *pathos*, disease ]. Multiplicity of diseases or disorders.

**polypec'tomy** [ polyp + G. *ektomē*, excision ]. Excision of a polyp.

**polypep'tide.** Poly(amino acid); a peptide formed by the union of an indefinite (usually large) number of amino acids.

**polypeptidemia** (pol-ĭ-pep-tĭd-e'mĭ-ah). The presence of polypeptides in the blood.

**polyphagia** (pol'ĭ-fa'jĭ-ah) [ poly- + G. *phagein*, to eat ]. Excessive eating; gluttony.

**polyphalangism** (pol'ĭ-fă-lan'jizm). Hyperphalangism.

**polyphallic** (pol'ĭ-fal'ik). Pertaining to the fantasy of possessing multiple phalli or penises.

**polyphar'macy.** The mixing of many drugs in one prescription; see also "shotgun" *prescription.*

**polyphe'nol oxidase.** Monophenol monooxygenase.

**polypho'bia** [ poly- + G. *phobos*, fear ]. Morbid fear of many things; a condition marked by the presence of many phobias.

**polyphos'phatase.** Endopolyphosphatase.

**polyphosphate depolymerase.** Endopolyphosphatase.

**polyphosphorylase.** Phosphorylase (2).

**polyphrasia** (pol'ĭ-fra'zĭ-ah) [ poly- + G. *phrasis*, speech ]. Extreme talkativeness.

**polyphyletic** (pol'ĭ-fi-let'ik). 1. Derived from more than one source, or having several lines of descent; opposed to monophyletic. 2. In hematology, relating to polyphyletism.

**polyphyletism** (pol-ĭ-fi'lĕ-tizm) [ poly- + G. *phylē*, tribe ]. Polyphyletic theory; in hematology, the theory based on the thesis that there are several stem cells.

**polyphyodont** (pol-ĭ-fi'o-dont) [ poly- + G. *phyō*, to produce, + *odous*(*odont-*), tooth ]. Having several sets of teeth formed in succession throughout life.

**pol'ypi.** Plural of polypus.

**polypiform** (po-lip'ĭ-form). Polypoid.

**polyplas'mia.** Hydremia.

**pol'yplast** [ poly- + G. *plastos*, formed ]. A polyplastic organism or individual; see polyplastic.

**polyplas'tic** [ poly- + G. *plastikos*, plastic ]. 1. Formed of several different structures. 2. Capable of assuming several forms.

**Polyplax** (pol'ĭ-plaks) [ poly- + G. *plax*, plate, plaque ]. A sucking louse (order Anoplura) of rats and mice.

**P. serra'tus,** the mouse louse, which has been shown experimentally to be capable of transmitting tularemia and may be also a vector for murine typhus and *Trypanosoma lewisi.*

**polyplegia** (pol'ĭ-ple'jĭ-ah) [ poly- + G. *plēgē*, a stroke ]. Paralysis of several muscles.

**polyploid** (pol'ĭ-ployd). Characterized by or pertaining to polyploidy.

**polyploidy** (pol'ĭ-ploy'dĭ) [ poly- + suffix -ploid, *q.v.* ]. The state of a cell nucleus containing three or a higher multiple of the haploid number of chromosomes. Cells containing three, four, five, or six multiples, are referred to, respectively, as triploid, tetraploid, pentaploid, or hexaploid; higher multiples may be expressed by using the appropriate Greek number.

**polypnea** (pol'ip-ne'ah) [ poly- + G. *pnoia*, breath ]. Tachypnea.

**polypo'dia.** The state of having supernumerary feet.

**polypoid** (pol'ĭ-poyd) [ polyp + G. *eidos*, resemblance ]. Polypiform; resembling a polyp in gross features.

**polyporous** (pol-ip'or-us) [ poly- + G. *poros*, pore ]. Cribriform.

**Polyporus** (pol-ip'or-us) [ poly- + G. *poros*, pore ]. A genus of mushrooms; see agaric.

**polyposia** (pol'ĭ-po'zĭ-ah) [ poly- + G. *posis*, drinking ]. Sustained, excessive drinking; see also hyperposia.

**polyposis** (pol'ĭ-po'sis) [ polyp + G. suffix *-osis*, condition ]. The presence of several polyps.

**p. coli,** multiple intestinal p. (1).

**familial intestinal p.,** multiple intestinal p.

**multiple intestinal p.,** familial intestinal p.; (1) p. coli; multiple p. of the colon; characterized by polyps of mucosa of colon only, with no associated lesions; the polyps begin to form usually in late childhood, increase in numbers, and may carpet the mucosal surface; there are symptoms of chronic colitis; carcinoma of the colon almost invariably develops in untreated cases; autosomal dominant inheritance; (2) multiple p. of small or large intestine is a feature of the following syndromes; Gardner's, Peutz-Jeghers, Turcot, Zollinger-Ellison.

**polypotome** (pol'ĭ-po-tōm) [ polyp + G. *tomos*, cutting ]. An instrument used for cutting away a polypus.

**polypotrite** (pol'ĭ-po-trit) [ polyp + L. *tero*, pp. *tritus*, to rub ]. A polyp crusher.

**pol'ypous.** Pertaining to, manifesting the gross features of, or characterized by the presence of a polyp or polyps.

**polypragmasy** (pol-ĭ-prag'mă-sĭ) [ poly- + G. *pragma*, a thing ]. The giving of many different remedies at the same time.

**polyptychial** (pol'ĭ-tik'ĭ-al) [ G. *polyptychos*, having many folds or layers, fr. poly- + *ptychē*, fold or layer ]. Folded or arranged so as to form more than one layer.

**polypus,** pl. **polypi** (pol'ĭ-pus, -pi) [ L. ]. Polyp.

**polyradic'uli'tis.** Inflammation of nerve roots.

**polyradic'ulomyopath'ia.** A combination of polyradiculitis (Guillain-Barré syndrome) with myositis.

**polyrhinia** (pol'ĭ-ri'nĭ-ah) [ poly- + G. *rhis*, nose ]. Duplication of the nose.

**polyribonucleotide nucleotidyltransferase.** Polynucleotide phosphorylase; enzyme (EC 2.7.7.8) catalyzing phosphorolysis of RNA, yielding nucleoside diphosphatase, or the reverse.

**polyribosomes** (pol'ĭ-ri'bo-sōmz). Polysomes; conceptually, two or more ribosomes connected by a molecule of messenger RNA; structures satisfying this concept can be seen in electron micrographs. They can be sedimented at rates consistent with aggregates of ribosomes, whence it is often, sometimes incorrectly, assumed that aggregates containing ribosomes are true polyribosomes. Polyribosomes are active in protein synthesis.

**polyrrhea** (pol'ĭ-re'ah) [ poly- + G. *rhoia,* a flow ]. A profuse discharge of serous or other fluid.

**polysaccharide** (pol-ĭ-sak'ă-rid, -rīd). A carbohydrate containing a large number of saccharide groups; $(C_6H_{10}O_5)_n$. Starch is the most familiar example.

    **pneumococcus p.,** see specific capsular *substance.*

    **specific soluble p.,** specific capsular *substance.*

**polyscelia** (pol-ĭ-se'lĭ-ah) [ poly- + G. *skelos,* leg, + suffix *-ia,* condition ]. A form of polymelia involving the presence of more than two legs.

**polyscelus** (pol-is'e-lus). A person with polyscelia.

**polyscope** (pol'ĭ-skōp). Diaphanoscope.

**polyserositis** (pol'ĭ-se'ro-si'tis) [ poly- + L. *serum,* serum, + G. suffix *-itis,* inflammation ]. Concato's disease; Bamberger's disease (2); chronic inflammation with effusions in several serous cavities resulting in fibrous thickening of the serosa and constrictive pericarditis.

    **familial paroxysmal p.,** transient recurring attacks of abdominal pain, fever, pleurisy, arthritis, and rash; the condition is asymptomatic between attacks; also known as benign paroxysmal peritonitis; familial recurring p.; familial Mediterranean fever; Mediterranean fever (2); periodic abdominalgia.

    **familial recurring p.,** familial paroxysmal p.

**polysialia** (pol'ĭ-si-a'lĭ-ah) [ poly- + G. *sialon,* saliva ]. Sialism.

**polysinuitis, polysinusitis** (pol'ĭ-sin-u-i'tis, -si'nus-i'tis). Simultaneous inflammation of two or more sinuses.

**polysomes** (pol'ĭ-sōmz). Polyribosomes.

**polysomia** (pol'ĭ-so'mĭ-ah) [ poly- + G. *sōma,* body ]. The condition exhibited by a fetal malformation involving two or more imperfect and partially fused bodies.

**polyso'mic.** Pertaining to or characterized by polysomy.

**polyso'mus.** An individual with polysomia.

**polysomy** (pol'ĭ-so'mĭ) [ poly- + G. *sōma,* body (chromosome) ]. State of a cell nucleus in which a specific chromosome is represented more than twice. Cells containing three, four, or five homologous chromosomes are referred to, respectively, as trisomic, tetrasomic, or pentasomic.

**polysor'bate 80** (USP). TWEEN 80; polyoxethylene (20) sorbitan monooleate; a "mixture of polyoxethylene ethers of mixed partial oleic esters of sorbitol anhydrides." Used as an emulsifier, as in the preparation of pharmacologic products.

**polyspermia, polyspermism** (pol-ĭ-sper'mĭ-ah, -sper'-mizm). 1. Polyspermy. 2. An abnormally profuse spermatic secretion.

**polyspermy** (pol'ĭ-sper'mĭ). Polyspermia (1); the entrance of more than one spermatozoon into the ovum.

**polysplenia** (pol'ĭ-sple'nĭ-ah) [ poly- + G. *splēn,* spleen ]. A condition in which splenic tissue is divided into two or more nearly equal masses.

**Polysporea** (pol'ĭ-spo're-ah) [ poly- + G. *sporos,* seed ]. A suborder of Myxosporidia in which the pansporoblast contains more than two spores; the latter are as a rule elongated.

**polysterax'ic.** Denoting behavior characterized by its socially provocative quality.

**polystichia** (pol-ĭ-stik'ĭ-ah) [ poly- + G. *stichos,* row ]. An arrangement of the eyelashes in two or more rows.

**polysul'fide rubber.** Synthetic rubber used as a dental impression material.

**polysuspensoid** (pol-ĭ-sus-pen'soyd). A colloid system compound of solid phases having different degrees of dispersion.

**polysymbrachydactyly** (pol'ĭ-sim-brak'ĭ-dak'tĭ-lĭ) [ poly- + symbrachydactyly ]. A congenital malformation

of the hand or foot in which the shortened digits are syndactylous and polydactylous.

**polysynaptic** (pol'ĭ-sĭ-nap'tik). Multisynaptic; referring to neural conduction pathways formed by a chain of many, synaptically connected, nerve cells, as distinguished from oligosynaptic conduction systems.

**polytendini'tis.** Inflammation of several tendons.

**polytene** (pol'ĭ-tēn). See polytene *chromosome.*

**polythe'lia** [ poly- + G. *thēlē,* nipple ]. The presence of supernumerary nipples, either on the breast or elsewhere on the body.

**polythi'azide** (NF). RENESE; 6-chloro-3,4-dihydro-2-methyl-3-[ (2,2,2-trifluoroethylthio)-methyl ]-2H-1,2,4-benzothiazine-7-sulfonamide 1,1-dioxide; a long-acting orally effective diuretic and antihypertensive agent of the benzothiadiazine group. It inhibits tubular reabsorption of sodium, chloride and water and, to a lesser extent, of potassium and bicarbonate.

**polytocous** (po-lit'o-kus) [ poly- + G. *tokos,* birth ]. Producing multiple young at a birth.

**polytrichia** (pol-ĭ-trik'ĭ-ah) [ poly- + G. *thrix* (*trich-*), hair ]. Polytrichosis; excessive hairiness.

**polytrichosis** (pol-ĭ-trī-ko'sis). Polytrichia.

**polyunguia** (pol'ĭ-ung'gwĭ-ah) [ poly- + L. *unguis,* nail ]. Polyonychia.

**polyuria** (pol-ĭ-u'rĭ-ah) [ poly- + G. *ouron,* urine ]. Excessive excretion of urine; profuse micturition; hydruria.

**polyvalent** (pol'ĭ-va'lent). 1. Multivalent. 2. Pertaining to a polyvalent *antiserum.*

**polyvidone** (pol'ĭ-vi'dōn). Povidone.

**polyvi'nyl.** Referring to a compound containing a number of vinyl groups in polymerized form.

    **p. alcohol,** $CH_2(CHOH)_n$; soluble in water; adhesive and emulsifier.

**polyvinylpyrrolidone** (pol'ĭ-vi'nil-pīr-rol'ĭ-dōn). Povidone.

    **p.-iodine complex,** povidone-iodine.

**polyzygot'ic** [ poly- + G. *zygōtos,* yoked ]. The discharge of more than two ova in one ovulatory cycle.

**pomade** (po-mād') [ Fr. *pomade,* fr. L. *pomum,* apple ]. Pomatum; an ointment or cream containing medicaments; usually used on the hair.

**poma'tum** [ Mod. L. ]. Pomade.

**pomegranate** (pum'gran-at) [ L. *pomum,* apple, + *granatus,* many seeded, fr. *granum,* grain or seed ]. Granatum; fruit of *Punica granatum* (family Punicaceae), a reddish yellow fruit the size of an orange, containing many seeds enclosed in a reddish acidic pulp. It is used in diarrhea for its astringent properties. The bark of the tree and of the root contains pelletierine and other alkaloids, and has been used as a teniacide.

**Pomeroy's operation.** See under operation.

**Pompe,** J. C. See P.'s *disease.*

**pompholyx** (pom'fo-liks) [ G. a bubble, fr. *pomphos,* a blister ]. Dyshidrosis.

**pomphus** (pom'fus) [ G. *pomphos,* blister ]. A wheal or blister.

**po'mum** [ L. ]. Apple.

    **p. ada'mi,** Adam's apple; *prominentia* laryngea.

**Poncet** (pawn-sa'), Antonin, French surgeon, 1849–1913. See P.'s *operation.*

**Ponfick,** Emil, German pathologist, 1844–1913. See P.'s *shadows.*

**pono-** (po'no-) [ G. *ponos,* toil, fatigue, pain ]. Combining form meaning bodily exertion, fatigue, overwork, pain.

**ponograph** (po'no-graf) [ pono- + G. *graphō,* to write ]. An instrument for recording graphically the progressive fatigue of a contracting muscle.

**ponopalmosis** (po'no-pal-mo'sis) [ pono- + G. *palmos,* palpitation. PALM-2 ]. A condition of irritable heart in which palpitation is excited by slight exertion.

**ponophobia** (po'no-fo'bĭ-ah) [ pono- + G. *phobos,* fear ]. Morbid fear of overwork or of becoming fatigued.

**ponos** (po'nos) [ G. toil, fatigue, pain ]. A disease occurring in young children in certain of the islands of Greece; it is characterized by enlargement of the spleen, hemorrhages, fever, and cachexia; possibly due to the presence of the Leishman-Donovan body.

**pons, pl. pontes** (ponz, pon'tēz) [ L. bridge ]. 1 [ NA ]. In neuroanatomy, the pons varolii or pons cerebelli; that part of the brainstem that is intermediate between the medulla oblongata caudally and the mesencephalon rostrally, and is composed of the pars basilaris pontis and the tegmentum pontis. On the ventral surface of the brain the pars basilaris appears as the large, white pontine protuberance, marked off from both the medulla oblongata and the mesencephalon by a distinct groove. 2. Any bridgelike formation connecting two more or less disjoined parts of the same structure or organ.

    **p. cerebel'li,** p. (1).

    **p. hep'atis,** a bridge of liver tissue that sometimes overlaps the fossa venae cavae, converting it into a canal.

    **p. varo'lii,** p. (1).

**pon'tes** [ L. ]. Plural of pons.

**pon'tic.** Dummy; an artificial tooth on a fixed partial denture; it replaces the lost natural tooth, restores its functions, and usually occupies the space previously occupied by the natural crown.

**ponticulus** (pon-tik'u-lus) [ L. dim. of *pons,* bridge ]. A vertical ridge on the eminentia conchae giving insertion to the auricularis posterior muscle.

    **p. hep'atis,** *pons* hepatis.

    **p. nasi,** bridge of the nose.

    **p. promonto'rii,** *subiculum* promontorii.

**pontile, pontine** (pon'tīl, -tēn, -tīn). Relating to a pons.

**Pool,** Eugene H., New York surgeon, 1874–1949. See P.'s *phenomenon,* P.-Schlesinger *sign.*

**pool** [ A.S. *pōl* ]. 1. A collection of blood in any region of the body, due to a dilation and retardation of the circulation in the capillaries and veins of the part. 2. A combination of resources.

    **abdom'inal p.,** the volume of blood within the abdomen, greatly increased in cases of shock, giving rise to the condition of exemia.

    **metabolic p.,** the quantity of a given chemical compound or group of related compounds participating in metabolic reactions; may constitute only a portion of the total bodily content of such compounds.

    **vaginal p.,** the mucoid secretions and cellular material that accumulate in the posterior fornix of the vagina; used as a cellular specimen, principally for hormonal evaluation and cancer detection.

**pop'lar.** *Populus.*

**poples** (pop'lēz) [ L. the ham of the knee ] [ NA ]. Ham (1); popliteus or popliteal region; the posterior region of the knee. See also *fossa poplitea.*

**popliteal** (pop-lit'e-al, pop-lī-te'al). Relating to the poples.

**poplite'us** [ L. ]. 1. Popliteal. 2. The poples. 3. *Musculus* popliteus.

**POPOP.** Abbreviation for 1,4-bis-2-(5-phenyloxazolyl)-benzene; see under phenyloxazolyl.

**poppy** (pop'ī). Papaver.

    **p. oil,** a fixed (drying) oil expressed from the seed of *Papaver somniferum;* sometimes used in the preparation of liniments and as a solvent of iodine in iodized oil.

**population** (pop-u-la'-shun) [ L. *populus,* a people, nation ]. A statistical term denoting all the objects, events, or subjects in a particular class.

**pop'ulin.** Benzoyl salicin; salicin benzoate; $C_{20}H_{22}O_8$; obtained from the bark and leaves of the aspen, *Populus tremula, P. nigra,* and *P. canadensis;* antipyretic.

**Pop'ulus** [ L. ]. A genus of trees of the family Salicinaceae, the poplars, aspens, and cottonwoods; the bark of several species possesses tonic properties, and the buds (poplar buds) have been used externally as a mild counterirritant and internally as a stimulating expectorant.

**por-.** See poro-.

**poradenitis** (pōr-ad'ē-ni'tis) [ G. *poros,* pore, + *aden,* gland, + suffix -*itis,* inflammation ]. Lymphogranulomatosis.

    **inguinal p.,** *lymphogranuloma* venereum.

**poradenolymphitis** (pōr-ad'ē-no-lim-fi'tis) [ G. *poros,* pore, + *adēn,* gland, + L. *lympha,* water, + suffix -*itis,* inflammation ]. *Lymphogranuloma* venereum.

**porcelain** (pōr'sĕ-lin). A powder composed of a clay, silica, and a flux which, when mixed with water, forms a paste that is molded to form artificial teeth, inlays, jacket crowns, and dentures. When heated, the materials fuse to form a ceramic.

    **high fusing p.,** dental p. having a fusing range of 2350°F. to 2500°F.

**porcine** (pōr'sīn, -sin) [ L. *porcinus,* fr. *porcus,* a hog ]. Relating to pigs.

**pore** (pōr) [ G. *poros,* passageway. POR-1 ]. A hole, perforation, or foramen; one of the minute openings of the sweat glands of the skin. Also see porus.

    **gustatory p.,** *porus* gustatorius.

    **interalveolar p.'s,** Kohn's p.'s; openings in the interalveolar septa of the lung.

    **Kohn's p.'s,** interalveolar p.'s.

    **nuclear p.'s,** the ultramicroscopic annular apertures in the nuclear envelope.

    **sweat p.,** *porus* sudoriferus.

    **taste p.,** *porus* gustatorius.

**porencephalia** (pōr'en-sĕ-fa'lī-ah). Porencephaly.

**porencephalic** (pōr'en-sĕ-fal'ik). Porencephalous; relating to or characterized by porencephaly.

**porencephalitis** (pōr'en-sef-ă-lī'tis) [ G. *poros,* pore, + *enkephalos,* brain, + suffix -*itis,* inflammation ]. Chronic inflammation of the brain with the formation of cavities in the substance of the organ.

**porencephalous** (pōr'en-sef'ă-lus). Porencephalic.

**porencephaly** (pōr'en-sef'ă-lī) [ G. *poros,* pore, + *enkephalos,* brain ]. Porencephalia; spelencephaly; the occurrence of cavities in the brain substance, communicating usually with the lateral ventricles.

**por'firomy'cin** (USAN). Antibiotic produced by *Streptomyces ardus;* antimicrobial agent.

**Porges** (por'ges), O., Vienna bacteriologist, *1879. See P. *method,* P.-Meier *test* P.-Salomon *test.*

**po'ri.** Plural of porus.

**poria** (pōr'ī-ah). Plural of porion.

**Porifera** (po-rif'er-ah) [ L. *porus,* pore, + *fero,* to bear ]. The sponges; a phylum of the Metazoa, comprising a group of sessile, aquatic animals possessing an endoskeleton and many branching canals, lined by flagellated collar cells. Communication of the canals with the surface is made through many pores or through larger openings and oscula.

**poriomania** (pōr'ī-o-ma'nī-ah) [ G. *poreia,* a journey (POR-1), + *mania,* frenzy ]. The morbid impulse to wander or journey away from home.

**porioma'niac.** One affected with poriomania.

**porion, pl. poria** (pōr'ī-on, pōr'ī-ah) [ G. *poros,* a passage ]. The central point on the upper margin of the porus acusticus externus. See fig. under craniometric *point.*

**pork** (pōrk). The meat from swine.

**pornography** (por-nog'ră-fī) [ G. *pornē,* a prostitute, + *graphō,* to write ]. Obscene or lust-arousing writing, drawing, or photography.

**pornolagnia** (por'no-lag'nī-ah) [ G. *pornē,* prostitute, + *lagneia,* lust ]. Sexual attraction toward prostitutes.

**poro-, por-** (po'ro-, pōr-) [ G. *poros* (L. *porus*), passageway (POR-1); G. *poreia,* a journey, passage (POR-1); G. *pōros,* a kind of marble, a stone (POR-2). Combining forms meaning, variously a pore, duct, or opening (see porus); a going or passing through; a callus or induration.

**porocele** (po'ro-sēl) [ G. *pōros,* callus, + *kēlē,* hernia ]. A hernia with indurated coverings.

**porocephaliasis, porocephalosis** (po'ro-sef'ă-li'ă-sis, -lo'sis) Infection with a species of *Porocephalus.* Larvae or nymphs are found in a great variety of vertebrates; adults usually in the lungs of reptiles.

**Porocephalidae** (po'ro-sĕ-fal'ī-de) [ G. *poros,* pore, + *kephalē,* head ]. A family of parasitic tongue worms (order Porocephalida in the class Pentastomida) characterized by four hooks arranged in a curved line on either side of the mouth. Adults are found in the lungs of reptiles, and larvae or nymphs are found in the tissues of a great variety of vertebrates, including man. See also Linguatulidae, and Arm*…!!!fer.*

**Porocephalus** (po'ro-sef'ă-lus) [ G. *poros*, pore, + *kephalē*, head ]. A genus of the family Porocephalidae, including certain wormlike arthropods, or their larvae, that cause porocephaliasis in a number of animals and in man.

**P. armilla'tus,** *Armillifer armillatus.*

**porokeratosis** (po'ro-kĕr'ă-to'sis) [ G. *poros*, pore, + keratosis ]. A rare dermatosis in which there is thickening of the stratum corneum and progressive centrifugal atrophy; also called Mibelli's disease; keratoderma eccentrica; hyperkeratosis eccentrica; hyperkeratosis figurata centrifuga atrophica, keratoatrophoderma.

**actinic p.,** a lesion which occurs on exposed areas of extremities primarily; bears a resemblance to actinic keratosis but the histologic features are those of p.

**poroma** (po-ro'mah) [ G. *pōrōma*, callus, fr. *pōros*, stone. POR-2 ]. 1. Callosity. 2. Exostosis. 3. Induration following a phlegmon.

**eccrine p.,** dermal duct tumor; a small, solitary, benign tumor, usually on the soles of the feet, belived to arise from the poral epithelium of sweat ducts running through the epidermis.

**porosis** pl. **poroses** (po-ro'sis, -sēz) 1 [ G. callus-formation. POR-2 ]. The formation of callus around the ends of a fractured bone. 2 [ L. *porosus*, porous ]. A porous condition.

**cer'ebral p.,** a porous condition of the brain caused by postmortem growth of *Clostridium perfringens* or other gas-forming organisms in the tissue.

**porosity** (po-ros'ĭ-tĭ) [ G. *poros*, pore ]. 1. A porous condition. 2. A perforation.

**p. in casting,** voids in metal castings caused by included gases or shrinkage during freezing.

**porotomy** (po-rot'o-mĭ) [ G. *poros*, passage, + *tomē*, incision ]. Meatotomy.

**porous** (po'rus). Having pores that pass directly or indirectly through the substance.

**porphin, porphine** (por'fin). The unsubstituted tetrapyrrole nucleus that is the basis of the porphyrins. (Compare phorbin, corrin.)

**Porphin**

**porphobilin** (por'fo-bi'lin). General term denoting intermediates between the monopyrrole, porphobilinogen, and the cyclic tetrapyrrole of heme (a porphin derivative). See bilin.

**porphobilinogen** (por'fo-bi-lin'o-jen). A porphyrin compound, 2-aminomethyl-4-(2'-carboxyethyl)-3-carboxymethylpyrrole; found in the urine in large quantities in cases of acute or congenital porphyria.

**p. synthase** (EC 4.2.1.24), δ-aminolevulinic dehydratase; a liver enzyme catalyzing the formation of porphobilinogen from 2 molecules of δ-levulinic acid; a reaction of importance in porphyrin biosynthesis.

**porphyria** (por-fir'ĭ-ah). A disorder of porphyrin metabolism; may be a heritable disease, of which four types have been described, or may be acquired, as from the effects of certain chemical agents (*e.g.,* hexachlorobenzene).

**acute p.,** intermittent acute p.

**congenital erythropoietic p.,** Günther's disease; formerly designated erythropoietic p.; porphyrin formation by erythroid cells in bone marrow is enhanced, leading to severe porphyrinuria, often in conjunction with hemolytic anemia and persistent cutaneous photosensitivity.

**p. cuta'nea tar'da,** symptomatic p.

**eryth'ropoietic p.,** (1) a relatively mild heritable form of p., characterized by enhanced formation of protoporphyrin III (9*a*), which leads to increased fecal excretion of this compound; acute solar urticaria or chronic solar eczema may be present, but the extent to which they are manifest varies considerably; (2) an older name for congenital erythropoietic p.

**p. hepatica,** intermittent acute p.

**intermittent acute p.,** acute p.; p. hepatica; caused by congenital hepatic overproduction of δ-aminolevulinic acid; urinary excretion of this compound and of porphobilinogen is greatly increased. The disease is characterized by hypertension, abdominal colic, psychosis, and peripheral and central neuropathy; no cutaneous photosensitivity develops. These characteristics are manifest intermittently, with frequency widely variable. Acute attacks follow use of a variety of drugs, during which attacks death may occur from respiratory paralysis.

**ovulocyclic p.,** acute episodic exacerbations of porphyria occurring in the premenstrual period.

**South African genetic p.,** variegate p.

**symptomatic p.,** p. cutanea tarda; p. occurring in middle-aged and elderly persons, usually with liver dysfunction; it is usually caused by alcoholism and is associated with porphyrinuria and bullous skin lesions.

**variegate p.,** protocoproporphyria hereditaria; South African genetic p.; a heritable disorder characterized by dermal sensitivity to light and mechanical trauma, and by increased fecal excretion of proto- and coproporphyrin. During acute attacks, usually caused by drugs or hepatotoxins, urinary excretion of δ-aminolevulinic acid, porphobilinogen, and porphyrins is increased.

**porphyrins** (por'fĭ-rinz). Pigments widely distributed throughout nature (*e.g.,* heme, bile pigments, cytochromes) consisting of four pyrrole nuclei joined in a ring (porphin) structure; they are substitution products of porphin and comprise several varieties, differing for the most part in the sidechains (methyl, ethyl, vinyl, formyl, carboxyethyl, carboxymethyl, etc.) present at the eight available positions on the pyrrole rings; depending on the nature of these, the prefixes etio-, meso-, proto-, copro-, uro-, deutero-, and hemato- are attached to p.; the distribution of these, within each of the seven classes, is given by type I, II, III, and IV. Protoporphyrin type III (or protoporphyrin IX), one of 15 possible isomers of protoporphyrin, is the only protoporphyrin found in nature, occurring in heme, etc. Of the others, only coproporphyrin and uroporphyrin occur in nature, usually as type III also. The p.'s combine with various metals (iron, copper, magnesium, etc.) to form metalloporphyrins, and with nitrogenous substances. See porphin.

**porphyrinuria** (por'fĭ-rin-u'rĭ-ah). Porphyruria; the excretions of porphyrins and related compounds in the urine.

**porphyrization** (por'fĭ-rĭ-za'shun). Grinding in a mortar (formerly on a slab of porphyry).

**porphyrop'sin** [ G. *porphyra*, purple, + *opsis*, sight ]. One of the two visual pigments (the other being rhodopsin) in the retinas of fresh-water fish and of marine fish that spawn in fresh water; it differs from rhodopsin in having its absorption maximum at about 522 mμ. True fresh-water fish have only p., not rhodopsin.

**porphyru'ria.** Porphyrinuria.

**porrigo** (po-ri'go) [ L. scurf, dandruff ]. Any disease of the scalp; *e.g.,* ringworm, favus, eczema.

**p. decal'vans** [ L. *decalvare* to make bald ], *alopecia areata.*

**p. favo'sa,** favus.

**p. fur'furans,** *tinea* tonsurans.

**p. larva'lis,** eczema of the scalp.

**p. lupino'sa** [ L. *lupinus*, relating to a wolf ], favus.

**p. scutula'ta,** favus.

**Porro,** Eduardo, Milan obstetrician, 1842–1902. See P. *hysterectomy, operation.*

**porrop'sia** [ G. *porrō*, at a distance, + *opsis*, vision ]. A condition in which objects look farther away than they are.

**porta,** pl. **portae** (pōr'tah, -te) [ L. gate ]. 1 [ NA ]. Hilus (1); the part of an organ where the vessels and nerves enter and the excretory ducts pass out. 2. *Foramen* interventriculare.

**p. hep'atis** [ NA ], portal fissure; a transverse fissure on the visceral surface of the liver between the caudate and quadrate lobes, lodging the portal vein, hepatic artery, hepatic nerve plexus, hepatic ducts, and lymphatic vessels.

**p. lie′nis,** *hilus* lienis.

**p. pulmo′nis,** *hilus* pulmonis.

**p. re′nis,** *hilus* renalis.

**portacaval** (pŏr′tă-ka′val). Concerning the portal vein and the inferior vena cava.

**portal** (pŏr′tal) [ L. *portalis,* pertaining to a porta (gate) ]. 1. Relating to any porta or hilus, specifically to the porta hepatis and the p. vein. 2. The point of entry into the body of a pathogenic microorganism.

    **intestinal p.'s,** in young embryos, the communications from the midgut to the foregut (**anterior intestinal p.**), or to the hindgut (**posterior intestinal p.**).

**portcaustic, portecaustique** (port-kaws′tik, port-kō-stēk′) [ Fr. *porter,* to carry, + caustic ]. Any form of handle, permanent or adjustable, for holding a stick of silver nitrate or other solid caustic.

**porteaiguille** (port-a-gü-e′e) [ Fr. *porter,* to carry, + *aiguille,* needle ]. A *needle-holder.*

**portemèche** (port-ĕ-mesh′) [ Fr. *porter,* to carry, + *mèche,* wick ]. A probe or sound with a notched extremity, used in introducing a drain or tent into a canal.

**portenoeud** (port-ĕ-në′) [ Fr. *porter,* to carry, + *noeud,* knot ]. An instrument used in carrying and tying a ligature around an artery or the stalk of a tumor.

**Porter,** Curt C., U. S. biochemist, \*1914. See P.-Silber *chromogens, reaction,* P.-Silber chromogens *test.*

**Porter,** Rodney R., British immunochemist, \*1917. Nobel laureate, 1972, with Gerald M. Edelman, for their studies in the basic structure of antibodies.

**Porter,** William H., Dublin surgeon, 1790–1861. See P.'s *fascia, sign.*

**Porter-Silber chromogens.** See under chromogen.

**portio,** pl. **portiones** (pŏr′shĭ-o, -o′nēz) [ L. portion ] [ NA ]. A part.

    **p. dura,** hard part; seventh nerve; nervus facialis; formerly regarded as forming one nerve with the eighth or acoustic, being distinguished from the latter as the harder of the two.

    **p. interme′dia,** *nervus* intermedius.

    **p. major nervi trigemini,** *radix* sensoria nervi trigemini.

    **p. minor nervi trigemini,** *radix* motoria nervi trigemini.

    **p. mol′lis,** soft part; eighth nerve; nervus acusticus; formerly regarded as forming one nerve with the seventh or facial, being distinguished from the latter as the softer of the two.

    **p. supravagina′lis** [ NA ], the part of the cervix uteri lying above the attachment of the vagina.

    **p. vagina′lis** [ NA ], the part of the cervix uteri contained within the vagina.

**por′tiplex′us.** The connection between the choroid plexuses of the lateral ventricles passing through the porta, or interventricular foramen (of Monro).

**portlig′ature, portelig′ature** [ Fr. *porter,* to carry ]. An appliance for passing a ligature in the depths of a wound or a cavity where the fingers cannot reach.

**porto-** (por′to-) [ L. *porta,* gate ]. Combining form meaning portal.

**por′tobil′ioarte′rial.** Relating to the portal vein, biliary ducts, and hepatic artery, which have similar distributions.

**por′togram** [ porto- G. *gramma,* a writing ]. X-ray film of the portal vein.

**portography** (pŏr-tog′ră-fī) [ porto- + G. *graphō,* to write ]. Delineation of the portal circulation by the use of x-ray films, using radiopaque material, usually introduced into the spleen or into the portal vein at operation.

**portosystemic** (pŏr′to-sis-tem′ik). Relating to connections between the portal and systemic venous systems.

**por′tovenog′raphy.** Portography.

**po′rus,** pl. **po′ri** [ L. fr. G. *poros,* passageway. POR-1 ] [ NA ]. A pore, meatus, or foramen.

    **p. acus′ticus externus** [ NA ], external acoustic or auditory pore or foramen; the orifice of the external acoustic meatus in the tympanic portion of the temporal bone.

    **p. acus′ticus internus** [ NA ], internal acoustic or auditory pore or foramen; a large round irregular opening on the posterior surface of the pyramid, or petrous portion

of the temporal bone, marking the inner termination of the internal acoustic meatus.

    **p. cro′taphy′tico-buc′cinator′ius,** a foramen formed in the sphenoid bone by ossification of a ligament below and lateral to the foramen ovale.

    **p. gustato′rius** [ NA ], gustatory or taste pore; the minute opening of a taste bud on the surface of the oral mucosa through which the gustatory hairs of the specialized neuroepithelial gustatory cells project.

    **p. op′ticus,** *discus* nervi optici.

    **p. sudorif′erus** [ NA ], sweat pore; the surface opening of the duct of a sweat gland.

**Posadas** (po-sah′dahs), Alejandro, Argentine parasitologist, 1870–1920. See P.'s *disease,* P.-Wernicke *disease.*

**posiomania** (po′sĭ-o-ma′nĭ-ah) [ G. *posis,* drinking, + *mania,* frenzy ]. Dipsomania or alcoholism.

---

# POSITION

---

**position** (po-zish′un) [ L. *positio,* a placing, position, fr. *pono,* pp. *positus,* to place ]. 1. Attitude; posture. 2. The place occupied. 3. Specifically, in obstetrics, the relation of some arbitrarily chosen position of the fetus to the right or left side of the mother; with each presentation there is one or other of two positions: right or left, the occiput, chin, and sacrum being the determining points in vertex, face, and breech presentations, respectively.

    **abdominoanterior p.,** a p. of the fetus *in utero,* with its abdomen turned toward the anterior abdominal wall of the mother.

    **abdominoposterior p.,** a p. of the fetus *in utero,* with its abdomen turned toward the back of the mother.

    **anatomical p.,** the erect p. of the body with the face directed forward, the arms at the side and the palms of the hands looking forward; the terms posterior, anterior, lateral, medial, etc., are applied to the parts as they stand related to each other and to the axis of the body when in this p.

    **Bonner's p.,** in irritation of hip joint, relaxation is obtained by flexion, abduction and external rotation of the thigh.

    **Bozeman's p.,** knee-elbow p., the patient being strapped to supports.

    **Brickner's p.,** by tying wrist to elevated head of bed, traction is obtained in abduction and external rotation.

    **Casselberry p.** a prone p. assumed when drinking, after intubation, in order to prevent the entrance of fluid into the tube.

    **centric p.,** the p. of the mandible in its most retruded relation to the maxillae; see also centric *relation.*

    **dorsal p.,** supine p.

    **dorsoanterior p.,** a p. of the fetus *in utero,* with its back directed toward the anterior abdominal wall of the mother.

    **dorsoposterior p.,** a p. of the fetus *in utero,* with its back toward the back of the mother.

    **dorsosacral p.,** lithotomy p.

    **eccentric p.,** eccentric *relation.*

    **Edebohls' p.,** for vaginal operations; the patient lies on her back, at the edge of the table, with hips and knees partly flexed, the feet being help up and apart by supports attached to the table.

    **Elliot's p.,** a p. to facilitate abdominal section, the patient resting upon a double inclined plane or on a single inclined plane with a cushion under the back at the level of the liver.

    **English p.,** Sims' p.

    **Fowler's p.,** an inclined p. obtained by raising the head of the bed from 2 to 2½ feet in order to ensure better dependent drainage after an abdominal operation.

    **frontoanterior p.'s,** p.'s of the fetus *in utero;* see left frontoanterior p. and right frontoanterior p.

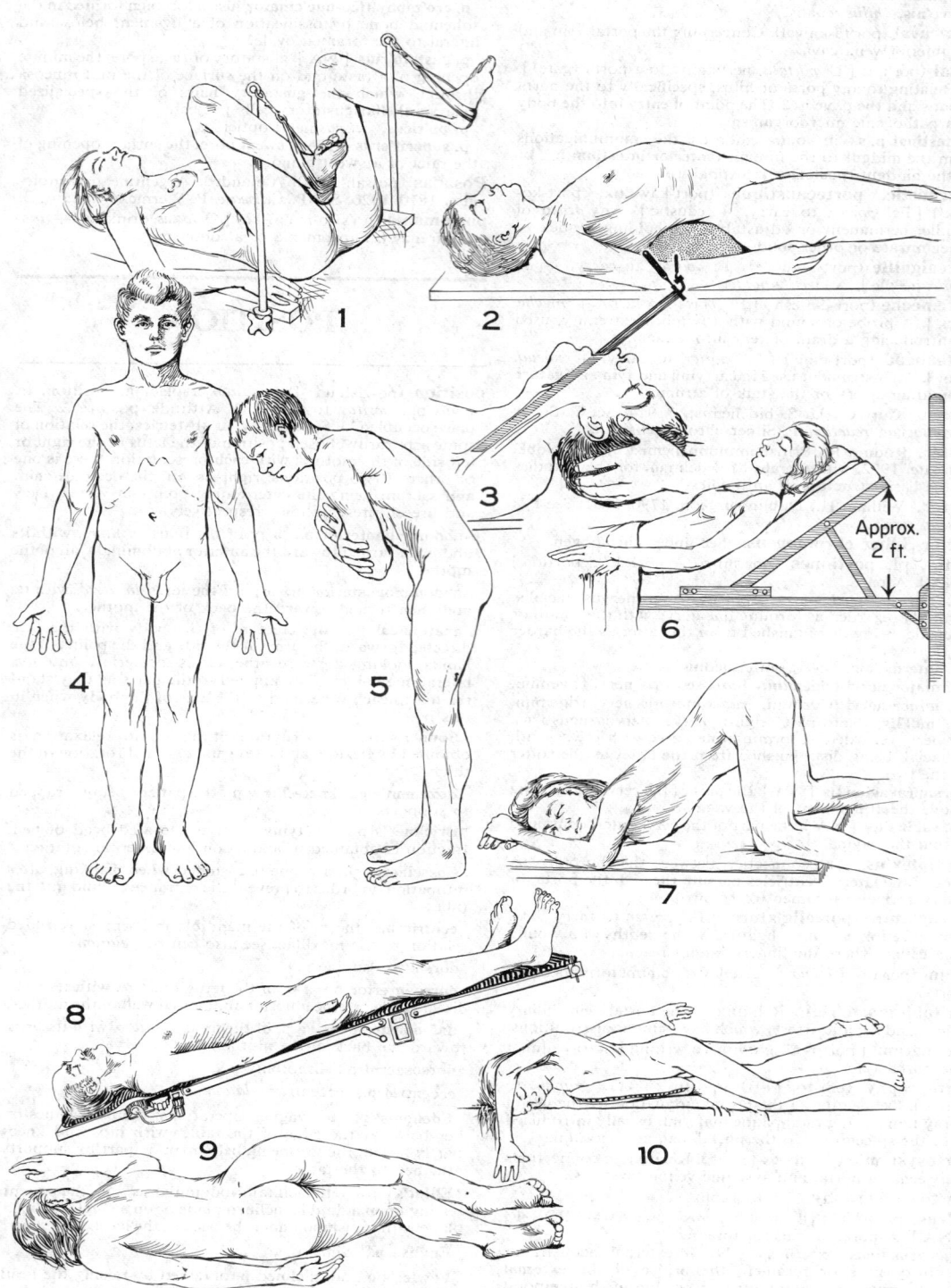

**Positions**

*1,* Lithotomy (dorsosacral) position; *2,* Robson's or Elliot's position; *3,* position for bronchoscopy; *4,* anatomical position; *5,* Noble's position; *6,* Fowler's position; *7,* knee-chest (genupectoral) position; *8,* Trendelenburg's position; *9,* Sim's (semiprone) position; *10,* tonsillectomy position (postoperative).

**frontoposterior p.'s,** p.'s of the fetus *in utero;* see left frontoposterior p. and right frontoposterior p.

**genucu'bital p.,** knee-elbow p.

**genupec'toral p.,** knee-chest p.

**heart p., electrical heart p.,** a description of the heart's electrical axis in the frontal plane, often based upon the form of the QRS complexes in leads aVL and aVF.

**hinge p.,** in dentistry, the orientation of parts in a manner permitting hinge movement between them.

**hinge p., condylar,** (1) the p. of the condyles in the temporomandibular joints at which a hinge movement of the mandible is possible; (2) the maxillomandibular relation from which a consciously stimulated true hinge movement can be executed.

**hinge p., mandibular,** any p. of the mandible which exists when the condyles are so situated in the temporomandibular joints that opening or closing movements can be made on the hinge axis.

**hinge p., terminal,** the mandibular hinge position from which further opening of the mandible would produce translatory rather than hinge movement.

**intercuspal p.,** the p. of the mandible when the cusps and sulci of the maxillary and mandibular teeth are in their greatest contact and the mandible is in its most closed position.

**knee-chest p.,** genupectoral p.; a prone posture resting on the knees and upper part of the chest, assumed for gynecologic or rectal examination.

**knee-elbow p.,** genucubital p.; a prone p. resting on the knees and elbows, assumed for rectal or vaginal examination or operation.

**lateral recumbent p.,** Sims' p.

**leapfrog p.,** a stooping p., such as that taken by boys in playing leapfrog, assumed for rectal examination.

**left dorsoanterior p.,** a p. of the fetus *in utero,* with its back toward the left side of the abdominal wall of the mother (a designation in shoulder or acromion presentation); abbreviated LDA.

**left dorsoposterior p.,** the p. of the fetus with its back toward the left side of the back of the mother (a designation in shoulder or acromion presentation); abbreviated LDP.

**left frontoanterior p.,** a presentation of the fetus with forehead directed toward the left acetabulum of the mother (more properly designated left mentoanterior); abbreviated LFA.

**left frontoposterior p.,** a presentation of the fetus with forehead directed toward the left sacroiliac articulation of the mother (more properly designated left mentoposterior); abbreviated LFP.

**left occipitoanterior p.,** occipitolevoanterior p.; a presentation with the occiput of the fetus being turned toward the left acetabulum of the mother; abbreviated LOA.

**left occipitoposterior p.,** occipitolevoposterior p.; a presentation with the occiput of the fetus being turned toward the left sacroiliac joint of the mother; abbreviated LOP.

**lithot'omy p.,** dorsosacral p.; the patient lying on the back with buttocks at the end of the operating table, the hips and knees being fully flexed with feet strapped in p.

**Mayo-Robson's p.,** the patient lies on the back with a thick pad under the loins, causing a marked lordosis in this region; used in operations on the gallbladder.

**mentoanterior p.,** a presentation of the fetus with its chin pointing to the right (right mentoanterior, abbreviated RMA) or to the left (left mentoanterior, abbreviated LMA) acetabulum of the mother.

**mentoposterior p.,** a presentation of the fetus with its chin pointing to the right (right mentoposterior, abbreviated RMP) or to the left (left mentoposterior, abbreviated LMP) sacroiliac articulation of the mother.

**Mercurio's p.,** an obstetrical p. similar to Walcher's.

**Noble's p.,** patient standing, with support by extended arms; useful for examination of kidney.

**obstetric p.,** the p. assumed by the parturient woman, either dorsal recumbent or lateral recumbent.

**occipitoanterior p.,** a variety of vertex presentation in which the occiput is directed to the anterior portion of the mother's pelvis.

**occipitoiliac p.,** occipitoposterior p.

**occipitolevoanterior p.,** left occipitoanterior p.

**occipitolevoposterior p.,** left occipitoposterior p.

**occipitoposterior p.,** occipitoiliac p.; the cephalic presentation in childbirth in which the occiput of the child points to one or the other iliac region of the mother.

**occlusal p.,** the relationship of the mandible and maxillae when the jaws are closed and the teeth are in contact. This position may or may not coincide with centric occlusion.

**physiologic rest p.,** postural p.; rest p.; the habitual postural p. of the mandible when the patient is resting comfortably in the upright p. and the condyles are in a neutral unstrained p. in the glenoid fossae; see also rest *relation.*

**postural p.,** physiologic rest p.

**prone p.,** lying face down.

**protrusive p.,** a forward p. of the mandible produced by muscular effort.

**rest p.,** physiologic rest p.

**right dorsoanterior p.,** a presentation of the fetus with its back toward the right acetabulum of the mother; abbreviated RDA.

**right dorsoposterior p.,** a presentation of the fetus with its back toward the rigth sacroiliac articulation of the mother; abbreviated RDP.

**right frontoanterior p.,** a fetal presentation with the forehead of the child directed toward the right acetabulum of the mother; abbreviated RFA.

**right frontoposterior p.,** a presentation of the fetus with the forehead directed toward the right sacroiliac articulation of the mother; abbreviated RFP.

**right occipitoanterior p.,** a presentation in which the occiput of the fetus is turned toward the right acetabulum of the mother; abbreviated ORA.

**right occipitoposterior p.,** a presentation with the occiput of the fetus turned toward the right sacroiliac joint of the mother; abbreviated ROP.

**Rose's p.,** the patient lies on his back with the head falling down over the end of the table; used in operations within the mouth, or the fauces, and on the fauciopharyngeal boundary.

**sacroanterior p.,** a breech presentation of the fetus with the sacrum directed toward the left (left sacroanterior, abbreviated LSA) or to the right (right sacroanterior, abbreviated RSA) acetabulum of the mother.

**sacroposterior p.,** a breech presentation of the fetus with the sacrum pointing to the left (left sacroposterior, abbreviated LSP) or to the right (right sacroposterior, abbreviated RSP) sacroiliac articulation of the mother.

**Scultetus' p.,** a p. of the patient on an inclined plane with head low, recommended by Scultetus for herniotomy and castration.

**semiprone p.,** Sims' p.; see also semiprone.

**Simon's p.,** a p. for vaginal examination, the woman lying on the back with hips elevated, thighs and legs flexed, and thighs widely separated.

**Sims' p.,** English p.; lateral recumbent p.; to facilitate a vaginal examination, the woman lying on the side with the under arm behind the back, the thighs flexed, the upper one more than the lower.

**supine p.,** dorsal p.; lying upon the back.

**tonsil p.,** semiprone p. with the under arm behind and a pillow in front; used to prevent aspiration during recovery from anesthesia.

**Trendelenburg's p.,** a supine p. on the operating table or the bed, inclined at an angle of 45°, so that the pelvis is higher than the head; used during and after operations in the pelvis or for shock.

**Valentine's p.,** a supine p. on a table with double inclined plane so as to cause flexion at the hips; used to facilitate urethral irrigation.

**Walcher p.,** a supine p. of the parturient woman with the lower extremities falling over the edge of the table.

---

**positive** (poz'ĭ-tiv) [ L. *positivus,* settled by arbitrary agreement, fr. *pono,* pp. *positus,* to set, place ]. Symbol, +. 1. Affirmative; definite; not negative. 2. In laboratory technique, denoting the occurrence of the reaction. 3. In diagnosis, denoting that examination reveals an abnormal condition. 4. In postmortem examinations, denoting that pathologic changes are present.

**positron** (poz'ĭ-tron). Positive electron; a subatomic particle of the same mass as the electron but of the opposite charge; this charge is the same, however, in magnitude as that of the electron.

**posologic** (po'so-loj'ik). Relating to posology.

**posology** (po-sol'o-jĭ) [ G. *posos*, how much, + *logos*, study ]. The branch of materia medica and therapeutics that has to do with a determination of the doses of remedies; the science of dosage.

**post-** (pōst-) [ L. *post*, after ]. Prefix to words derived from Latin roots, denoting after, behind, or posterior, corresponding to Greek, *meta-*.

**post** (pōst). In dentistry, a dowel or pin inserted into the root canal of a natural tooth as an attachment for an artificial crown.

**postacces'sual.** Occurring after an access or paroxysm of a disease.

**postacetab'ular.** Posterior to the acetabular cavity.

**postadoles'cence.** The period after adolescence or puberty.

**posta'nal.** Posterior to the anus.

**postanesthet'ic.** Occurring after anesthesia.

**postapoplec'tic.** Occurring after an attack of apoplexy.

**postax'ial.** 1. Posterior to the axis of the body or any limb, the latter being in the anatomical position. 2. Denoting the portion of a limb bud which lies caudal to the axis of the limb.

**postbra'chial.** On or in the posterior part of the upper arm.

**postcar'dinal.** Relating to the posterior cardinal veins.

**postcardiot'omy.** Following surgery that involved cutting through the muscle of the heart.

**postca'va.** *Vena* cava inferior.

**postca'val.** Relating to the inferior vena cava.

**postcen'tral.** Referring to the cerebral convolution forming the posterior bank of the central sulcus: the postcentral gyrus.

**postcibal** (pōst-si'bal) [ L. *cibum*, food ]. After a meal or the taking of food.

**postclavic'ular.** Posterior to the clavicle.

**postcoital** (pōst-ko'ĭ-tal). After coitus.

**postcoitus** (pōst-ko'ĭ-tus). The time immediately after coitus.

**postcor'dial** [ L. *cor* (*cord*-), heart ]. Posterior to the heart.

**postcos'tal.** Behind the ribs.

**postcrown.** A crown, replacing the natural crown, which is retained on the stump of the root of a tooth from which the pulp has been removed, by a post or pin integral with the crown. The post is sealed in the treated root canal with a cement.

**postcu'bital.** On or in the posterior or dorsal part of the forearm.

**post'dam.** Posterior palatal *seal.*

**postdiastol'ic.** Following the diastole of the heart.

**postdicrot'ic.** Following the dicrotic wave in a sphygmogram; denoting an additional interruption in the descending line of the pulse tracing.

**postdiph'therit'ic.** Following or occurring as a sequel of diphtheria.

**postdor'mital.** Relating to the postdormitum.

**postdor'mitum** [ L. *dormire*, to sleep ]. The period of increasing consciousness between sound sleep and waking.

**postduc'tal.** Relating to that part of tha aorta distal to the aortic opening of the ductus arteriosus.

**postenceph'ali'tic.** Following encephalitis.

**postepilep'tic.** Following an epileptic seizure.

**posterior** (pos-tēr'ĭ-or) [ L. comparative of *posterus*, following ]. 1 [ NA ]. Posticus; behind or after in place. 2. An undesirable and confusing substitute for caudal in quadrupeds; in veterinary anatomy, the term posterior is used only to denote some structures of the head.

**poste'rius** [ L. ]. Neuter of posterior.

**postero-** (pos'ter-o-) [ L. *posterior, q.v.* ]. Combining form meaning posterior.

**post'eroante'rior.** A term denoting the direction of view or progression, from posterior to anterior, through a part.

**post'eroclu'sion.** Posterior *occlusion.*

**post'eroexter'nal.** Posterolateral.

**post'erointer'nal.** Posteromedial.

**posterolat'eral.** Behind and to one side, specifically to the outer side.

**posterome'dial.** Behind and to the inner side.

**posterome'dian.** Occupying a central position posteriorly.

**posteropari'etal.** Relating to the posterior portion of the parietal lobe of the cerebrum.

**posterosupe'rior.** Situated behind and at the upper part.

**posterotem'poral.** Relating to or lying in the posterior portion of the temporal lobe of the cerebrum.

**postesophageal** (pōst'e-sof'ă-je'al, e-sō-faj'ĭ-al). Behind the esophagus.

**postes'trum.** Postestrus.

**postes'trus.** Postestrum; the period in the estrus cycle following estrus; sometimes called metestrus. It is characterized by the growth of the corpus luteum and physiologic changes related to the production of progesterone.

**postfe'brile.** Occurring after a fever.

**postganglion'ic.** Distal to or beyond a ganglion; referring to the unmyelinated nerve fibers originating from cells in an autonomic ganglion.

**postgrip'pal.** Postinfluenzal.

**posthemiplegic** (pōst'hem'ĭ-ple'jik). Following hemiplegia.

**posthemorrhagic** (pōst-hem-ŏ-raj'ik). Following a hemorrhage.

**posthepatic** (pōst-he-pat'ik). Behind the liver.

**posthetomy** (pos-thet'o-mĭ) [ G. *posthē*, prepuce, + *tomē*, incision ]. Circumcision.

**pos'thioplasty** [ G. *posthion*, dim. form of *posthē*, prepuce, + *plassō*, to form ]. Reparative or plastic surgery of the prepuce.

**posthitis** (pos-thi'tis) [ G. *posthē*, prepuce, + *-itis* ]. Acrobystitis; inflammation of the prepuce.

**pos'tholith** [ G. *posthē*, prepuce, + *lithos,* stone ]. A preputial *calculus.*

**posthyoid** (pōst-hi'oyd). Behind the hyoid bone.

**posthypnotic** (pōst-hip-not'ik). Following hypnotism.

**postic'tal.** Following a seizure, *e.g.*, epileptic.

**posticus** (pos-ti'kus) [ L. fr. *post,* after ]. Posterior; in the names of muscles the NA substitutes posterior for posticus, as musculus tibialis posterior instead of musculus tibialis posticus.

**postinfluen'zal.** Occurring as a sequel of influenza; postgrippal.

**postischial** (pōst-is'kĭ-al). Posterior to the ischium.

**postmala'rial.** Occurring as a sequel of malaria.

**postmas'toid.** Posterior to the mastoid process.

**postmature** (pōst'ma-tūr'). Remaining in the uterus longer than the normal gestational period.

**postme'dian.** Posterior to the median plane.

**postmediastinal** (pōst'me'dĭ-as'tĭ-nal, -me'dĭ-ă-sti'nal). 1. Posterior to the mediastinum. 2. Relating to the posterior mediastinum.

**postmediastinum** (pōst'me'dĭ-ă-sti'num). Posterior *mediastinum.*

**postmenopau'sal.** Relating to the period following the menopause.

**postmin'imus.** A small accessory appendage attached to the side of the fifth finger or toe; it may resemble a normal digit or be merely a fleshy mass.

**postmor'tal.** Postmortem.

**post mor'tem** [ L. *mors* (*mort*-), death ]. 1. After death. 2. Autopsy; necropsy; postmortem examination.

**postmor'tem.** Postmortal; pertaining to or occurring during the period after death.

**postna'rial.** Relating to the posterior nares or choanae; choanal.

**postna'ris.** Choana.

**postna'sal.** 1. Posterior to the nasal cavity. 2. Relating to the posterior portion of the nasal cavity.

**postna'tal** [ L. *natus*, birth ]. Occurring after birth.

**postnecrot'ic.** Subsequent to the death of a tissue or part of the body.

**postneurit'ic.** Following neuritis.

**postoc'ular** [ L. *oculus*, eye ]. Posterior to the eyeball.

**postop'erative.** Following a surgical operation.

**posto'ral** [ L. *os* (*or-*), mouth ]. In the posterior part of, or posterior to, the mouth.

**postor'bital.** Posterior to the orbit.

**postpal'atine.** Posterior to the palatine bones. Usually used to refer to the soft palate.

**postparalyt'ic.** Following or consequent upon paralysis.

**post par'tum** [ L. *partus*, birth (noun), fr. *pario*, pp. *partus*, to bring forth ]. After childbirth.

**postpar'tum.** Pertaining to, or occurring during, the period following childbirth or delivery.

**post'pericardiot'omy.** Following surgery that involved cutting through the pericardium.

**postpharyn'geal.** Posterior to the pharynx.

**postpneumonic** (pōst-nu-mon'ik). Following or occurring as a sequel of pneumonia.

**postpran'dial** [ L. *prandium*, breakfast ]. Following a meal.

**postpu'beral, postpu'bertal.** Postpubescent.

**postpu'berty.** The period after puberty.

**postpubescent** (pōst-pu-bes'ent). Subsequent to the period of puberty.

**postpyknotic** (pōst-pik-not'ik). Following the stage of pyknosis in a red cell, denoting the disappearance of the nucleus (chromatolysis).

**postrolan'dic.** Behind the fissure of Rolando, or central sulcus; see postcentral.

**postsa'cral.** Posterior or inferior to the sacrum; referring to the coccyx.

**postscapular** (pōst-skap'u-lar). Posterior to the scapula.

**postscarlatinal** (post-skar-lā-te'nal). Occurring as a sequel of scarlatina.

**postsphygmic** (post-sfig'mik). [ G. *sphygmos*, pulse ]. Occurring after the pulse wave.

**postsplen'ic.** Posterior to the spleen.

**postsynaptic** (post'si-nap-tik). Pertaining to the area on the distal side of a synaptic cleft.

**posttar'sal.** Relating to the posterior portion of the tarsus.

**posttecta.** Aboral to the pars tecta duodeni.

**posttib'ial.** Posterior to the tibia; situated in the posterior portion of the leg; sural.

**posttrans'verse.** Behind a transverse process.

**post'traumat'ic.** Temporally, and implied causally, related to a trauma.

**posttrematic** (post'tre-mat'ik) [ post- + G. *trēma*, perforation ]. Relating to the caudal surface of a branchial cleft.

**posttus'sis** [ L. *tussis*, cough ]. After coughing; referring usually to certain auscultatory sounds.

**postty'phoid.** Occurring as a sequel of typhoid fever.

**postulate** (pos'tu-lāt) [ L. *postulo*, pp. *-atus*, to demand ]. An unproved assertion or assumption; a statement or formula offered as the basis of a theory.

    **Ampère's p.,** Avogadro's *law.*

    **Avogadro's p.,** Avogadro's *law.*

    **Ehrlich's p.,** Ehrlich's side chain *theory.*

    **Koch's p.'s,** Koch's *law.*

**postural** (pos'tu-ral, pos'cher-al). Relating to or effected by posture, as the p. treatment of peritonitis (Fowler's position) or of a fracture.

**posture** (pos'tūr, pos'cher) [ L. *positura*, fr. *pono*, pp. *positus*, to place ]. Position of the body, as the erect p., the recumbent p., etc.; attitude.

    **Stern's p.,** in cases of tricuspid insufficiency the murmur is developed or made more distinct if the patient lies supine with the head extended and lowered over the end of the table.

**postuterine** (pōst-u'ter-in). Posterior to the uterus.

**postvaccinal** (post-vak'si-nal). After vaccination.

**postval'var, postval'vular.** Relating to a position distal to the pulmonary or aortic valves.

**potable** (po'tă-bl) [ L. *potabilis*, fr. *poto*, to drink ]. Drinkable; fit to drink.

**Potain** (pŏ-taṅ'), Pierre C. E., Paris physician, 1825–1901. See P.'s *sign.*

**potamophobia** (pot'ă-mo-fo'bǐ-ah) [ G. *potamos*, river, + *phobos*, fear ]. Morbid fears aroused by the sight, and sometimes thought, of a river or any stream.

**pot'ash** [ E. pot-ashes ]. Pearl-ash; impure potassium carbonate.

    **caustic p.,** potassium hydroxide.

    **sul'furated p.** (NF), liver of sulfur; a mixture composed chiefly of potassium polysulfides and potassium thiosulfate. Used externally in scabies, acne, and psoriasis.

**potas'sic.** Relating to or containing potassium.

**potas'siocu'pric.** Relating to or containing both potassium and copper.

**potas'siomercu'ric.** Relating to or containing both potassium and mercury.

**potassium** (po-tas'ĭ-um) [ Mod. L. fr. E. potash (fr. pot + ashes) + *-ium* ]. Kalium; an alkaline metallic element, symbol K (*kalium*), atomic no. 19, atomic weight 39.100, occurring abundantly in nature but always in combination. It is a soft, silvery white or gray, lustrous substance. Its salts are largely used in medicine. For some organic p. salts not listed below, see the name of the organic acid portion.

    **p. acetate,** sal diureticum; $KC_2H_3O_2$; a diuretic, diaphoretic, and systemic and urinary alkalizer.

    **p. alum,** aluminum potassium sulfate.

    **p. aminosalicylate,** see *p*-aminosalicylic acid.

    **p. antimonyltartrate,** antimony potassium tartrate.

    **p. bicarbonate** (BP), p. hydrogen carbonate; $KHCO_3$; used as a diuretic to decrease the acidity of the urine, and as an electrolyte replenisher.

    **p. bitartrate,** p. acid tartrate; cream of tartar; $KHC_4H_4O_6$; a diuretic and laxative.

    **p. bromide** (BP), KBr; a sedative and hypnotic (sodium bromide is usually preferred).

    **p. chlorate,** chlorate of potash; $KClO_3$; used as a mouthwash and gargle in stomatitis and follicular pharyngitis. It is incompatible in the dry state with all easily oxidizable substances.

    **p. chloride** (USP, BP), used to correct p. deficiency.

    **p. citrate** (NF, BP), Rivière's salt; $K_3C_6H_5O_7$; a deliquescent powder, soluble in water; used as a diuretic, diaphoretic, expectorant, and systemic and urinary alkalizer.

    **p. citrate, effervescent,** a mixture of p. citrate, citric acid, sodium bicarbonate, and tartaric acid; used as a gastric antacid and urinary alkalizer.

    **p. cyanide,** KCN; a commercial fumigant.

    **p. dichromate** or **bichromate,** $K_2Cr_2O_7$; used externally as an astringent, antiseptic, and caustic.

    **p. ferrocyanide,** yellow prussiate of potash; $K_4Fe(CN)_63\cdot H_2O$; used in the preparation of various cyanides and in medicine as an antidote to copper sulfate.

    **p. gluconate,** KAON; POTASORAL; KATORIN; gluconic acid potassium salt; used in hypokalemia as a replenisher.

    **p. guai'acolsulfonate,** THIOCOL; $C_6H_3OHOCH_3SO_3K$; used as a sedative expectorant in bronchitis and as an intestinal disinfectant.

    **p. hydroxide** (USP, BP), lye (*q.v.*); caustic potash; KOH; a strong, penetrating caustic.

    **p. hypophosphite,** $KH_2PO_2$; formerly believed to have a tonic effect upon the nervous system. An explosion may occur if it is triturated or heated with oxidizing agents.

    **p. i'odate,** $KIO_3$; an oxidizing agent and disinfectant.

    **p. iodide** (USP, BP), KI; used as an alterative and expectorant, and in certain mycoses.

    **p. metaphosphate** (NF), $KPO_3$; a pharmaceutical aid.

    **p. myronate,** sinigrin.

    **p. nitrate** (BP), niter; saltpeter; $KNO_3$; sometimes used as a diuretic and diaphoretic; formerly it was included in asthmatic powders containing stramonium leaves.

    **p. penicillin G** (USP), see under penicillin.

    **p. perchlorate,** PEROIDIN; $KClO_4$; occasionally used, as an alternative to a thiouracil derivative, in the control of hyperthyroidism; side effects may be minimized by keeping the daily dose low, but aplastic anemia has been reported.

    **p. permanganate** (USP, BP), $KMnO_4$; a strong oxidizing agent, used in solution as an antiseptic and deodorizing application for foul ulcers, cancer, and ozena, and as a gastric lavage in poisoning from morphine, strychnine, aconite, and picrotoxin.

**p. phosphate,** dipotassium phosphate; dibasic p. phosphate; $K_2HPO_4$; a mild saline cathartic and diuretic.

**p. phosphate, monobasic** (NF), $KH_2PO_4$; used as a urinary acidifier.

**p. sodium tartrate** (NF), sodium p. tartrate (BP); Rochelle salt; Seignette's salt; $KNaC_4H_4O_6$; a mild saline cathartic, used as an ingredient in compound effervescent powders.

**p. sorbate** (NF), BB powder; 2,4-hexadienoic acid potassium salt; a mold and yeast inhibitor, used as a preservative.

**p. suc'cinate,** a deliquescent powder used as a hemostatic.

**p. sulfate,** $K_2SO_4$; laxative.

**p. sulfocy'anate,** p. thiocyanate.

**p. tartrate,** soluble tartar; $K_2C_4H_4O_6 \cdot 1/2H_2O$; a mild purgative and diuretic.

**p. tartrate, acid,** p. bitartrate.

**p. thiocy'anate,** p. sulfocyanate; p. rhodanate; used in the treatment of essential hypertension and as a reagent in the detection of copper, iron, and silver.

**potassium-40.** $^{40}K$; naturally occurring (0.0119 per cent) radioactive p. isotope; beta emitter with half-life of 1.3 billion years; chief source of natural radioactivity of living tissue.

**potassium-42.** $^{42}K$; artificial isotope; beta emitter with half-life of 12.47 hours; used as tracer in studies of p. distribution in body fluid compartments.

**potency** (po'ten-sĭ) [ L. *potentia*, power ]. 1. Power, force, or strength; the condition or quality of being potent. 2. Specifically, sexual p., *q.v.* 3. In therapeutics, the pharmacological activity of a compound.

**sexual p.,** potentia coeundi; the ability to carry out and consummate the sexual act; applied mainly with reference to the male.

**po'tent.** 1. Possessing force, power, strength. 2. Indicating the ability of a primitive cell to differentiate; see also totipotent, pluripotent. 3. In psychiatry, possessing sexual potency.

**potentia** (po-ten'shĭ-ah) [ L. ]. Potency.

**p. coeundi** (ko-e-un'di) [ L. the power of cohabitating; *coeo*, to come together ], sexual *potency*.

**p. generan'di,** the ability to procreate.

**potential** (po-ten'shal) [ L. *potentia*, power, potency ]. 1. Capable of doing or being, although not yet doing or being; possible, but not actual. 2. A state of tension in an electric source enabling it to do work under suitable conditions; in relation to electricity the potential is analogous to the temperature in relation to heat; unit: volt.

**action p.,** the change in membrane p. occurring in nerve, muscle or other excitable tissue when excitation occurs.

**after-p.,** see afterpotential.

**bioelectric p.,** electrical p.'s occurring in living organisms.

**biotic p.,** a theoretical measurement of the capacity of a species to survive or to compete successfully.

**demarcation p.,** injury p.; the difference in p. recorded when one electrode is placed on intact nerve fibers or muscle fibers and the other electrode is placed on the injured ends of the same fibers. The intact portion is positive with reference to the injured portion.

**excitatory postsynaptic p.,** abbreviated EPSP; the change in p. which is produced in the membrane of the next neuron when an impulse which has an excitatory influence arrives at the synapse. It is a local change in the direction of depolarization. Summation of these p.'s can lead to discharge of an impulse by the neuron.

**inhibitory postsynaptic p.,** abbreviated IPSP; the change in p. produced in the membrane of the next neuron when an impulse which has an inhibitory influence arrives at the synapse. It is a local change in the direction of hyperpolarization. The frequency of discharge of a given neuron is determined by the extent to which impulses that lead to excitatory postsynaptic p.'s predominate over those that cause inhibitory postsynaptic p.'s.

**injury p.,** demarcation p.

**membrane p.,** transmembrane p.; the p. inside a cell membrane, measured relative to the fluid just outside; it is negative under resting conditions and becomes positive during an action p.

**oxidation-reduction p.,** redox p.; abbreviation, $E_h$; the p. in volts of an inert metallic electrode measured in a system of an arbitrarily chosen ratio of [ oxidant ] to [ reductant ] and referred to the normal hydrogen electrode at absolute temperature; it is calculated from the following equation:

$$E_h = E_0 + \frac{RT}{nF} \ln \frac{[\text{oxidant}]}{[\text{reductant}]},$$

where $R$ is the gas constant expressed in electrical units, $T$ the absolute temperature, $n$ the number of electrons transferred, $F$ the faraday and $E_0$ the normal p. of the system at pH 0.

**S p.,** prolonged, slow, depolarizing or hyperpolarizing responses to illumination; initiated between the photoreceptor and ganglion cell layers of the retina.

**spike p.,** the main wave in the action p. of a nerve; it is followed by negative and positive afterpotentials.

**thermodynamic p.,** see free *energy*.

**visual evoked p.,** the measurement that results from the recordings of an electroencephalogram from the occipital area of the scalp while the subject fixates a light flashing at 1/4-second intervals, as given by a computer that averages the electroencephalogram response of 100 consecutive flashes.

**transmembrane p.,** membrane p.

**potentiation** (po-ten'shĭ-a'shun). In chemotherapy, a degree of synergism that is greater than additive.

**potentiometer** (po-ten'shĭ-om'e-ter) [ L. *potentia*, power, + G. *metron*, measure ]. 1. An instrument used for measuring small differences in electrical potential. 2. An electrical resistor of fixed total resistance between two terminals, but with a third terminal attached to a slider which can make contact at any desired point along the resistance.

**potion** (po'shun) [ L. *potio, potus,* fr. *poto,* to drink ]. A draft or large dose of liquid medicine.

**potomania** (po'to-ma'nĭ-ah) [ L. *poto,* to drink, + G. *mania,* frenzy ]. *Delirium* tremens.

**Pott,** Percivall, English surgeon, 1713–1788. See P.'s *abscess, aneurysm, caries, curvature, disease, fracture, gangrene, paralysis, paraplegia,* puffy *tumor.*

**Potter,** E. L., U. S. pediatrician. See Potter's *disease, facies.*

**Potter,** Irving White, U. S. obstetrician, 1868–1956. See P. *version.*

**Potts,** Willis J., U. S. surgeon, *1895. See P.'s *anastomosis, operation.*

**pouch** (powch). Pocket; cul-de-sac.

**antral p.,** a p. made in the antrum of the stomach of experimental animals.

**branchial p.'s,** evaginations of embryonic pharyngeal entoderm between branchial arches; during development they give rise to epithelial tissues in the head and neck.

**Broca's p.,** pudendal *sac.*

**celomic p.'s,** lateral mesoderm-lined diverticula lying at either side of the notochord in the developing Amphioxus.

**Douglas' p.,** *excavatio* rectouterina.

**entodermal p.'s, endodermal p.'s,** pharyngeal p.'s.

**guttural p.,** a structure in the horse which is a diverticulum of the auditory (Eustachian) tube. Subject to chronic infections and inflammation and frequently necessitating surgery for relief.

**Hartmann's p.,** pelvis of the gallbladder; a spheroid or conical p. at the point of exit of the gallbladder into the cystic duct.

**Heidenhain p.,** a small sac or p. of the stomach closed off from the main cavity but with an opening through the abdominal wall, fashioned for the purpose of obtaining gastric juice and for studying gastric secretion in physiologic experiments.

**hepatorenal p.,** *recessus* hepatorenalis.

**laryn'geal p.,** *sacculus* laryngis.

**Morison's p.,** *recessus* hepatorenalis.

**paracys'tic p.,** the lateral portion of the uterovesical p.

**pararec'tal p.,** the lateral portion of the rectouterine p.

**paravesical p.,** the lateral portion of the uterovesical p.

**Pavlov p.,** Pavlov stomach; miniature stomach; a section

of the stomach of a dog, shut off from all communication with the main part of the organ and connected with the outside by a fistula; used in studies on the gastric secretions.

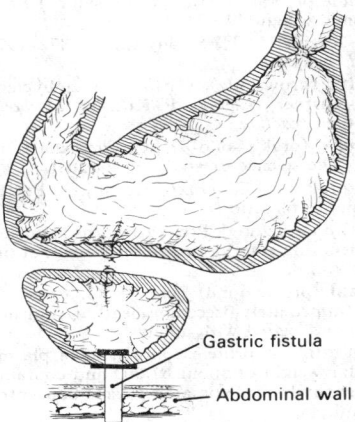

Cross Section of Heidenhain Pouch

— Gastric fistula

— Abdominal wall

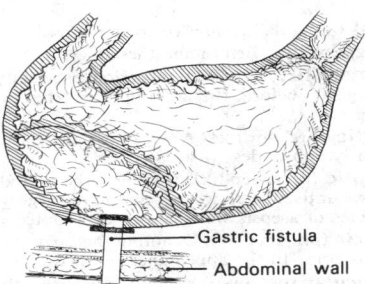

Cross Section of Pavlov Pouch

— Gastric fistula

— Abdominal wall

**pharyngeal p.'s,** entodermal p.'s; paired sacculations of the entodermal lining of the pharynx extending toward the corresponding ectodermally lined branchial grooves.

**Physick's p.'s,** proctitis with mucous discharge and burning pain, involving especially the sacculations between the rectal valves.

**Prussak's p.,** *recessus* membranae tympani superior.

**Rathke's p.,** pituitary *diverticulum.*

**rectou'terine p.,** *excavatio* rectouterina.

**rectovag'inal p.,** *excavatio* rectouterina.

**rectoves'ical p.,** *excavatio* rectovesicalis.

**Seessel's p.,** Seessel's *pocket.*

**ultimobranchial p.,** a transient fifth pharyngeal p.; it is now considered to be incorporated into the caudal pharyngeal complex, the cells of which become the parafollicular cells of the thyroid.

**uteroves'ical p.,** *excavatio* vesicouterina.

**vesicou'terine p.,** *excavatio* vesicouterina.

**Willis' p.,** *omentum* minus.

**poudrage** (poo-drahzh') [ F. ]. 1. Powdering. 2. Talc *operation.*

**pericardial p.,** talc *operation.*

**pleural p.,** covering the opposing pleural surfaces with a slightly irritating powder in order to secure adhesion.

**Poulet** (poo-la'), Alfred, French physician, 1848–1888. See P.'s *disease.*

**poultice** (pōl'tis) [ L. *puls* (*pult*-), a thick pap; G. *poltos* ]. Cataplasm; a soft magma or mush prepared by wetting various powders or other absorbent substances with oily or watery fluids, sometimes medicated, and usually applied hot to the surface. It exerts an emollient, relaxing, or stimulant, counterirritant effect upon the skin and underlying tissues.

**pound** (pownd) [ A.S. *pund;* L. *pondus,* weight ]. A unit of weight, containing 12 ounces, apothecaries' weight, or 16 ounces, avoirdupois.

**pound'al.** The force required to give a mass of 1 pound an acceleration of 1 foot per second per second.

**Poupart** (poo-par'), Franc·ois, French anatomist, 1616–1708. See P.'s *ligament, line.*

**povidone** (po'vĭ-dōn) (USP). PERISTON; polyvidone; polyvinylpyrrolidone; PVP; poly[ 1-(2-oxo-1-pyrrolidinyl)ethylene ]; a synthetic polymer consisting mainly of linear 1-vinyl-2-pyrrolidone groups, with mean molecular weights ranging from 10,000 to 70,000; used as a dispersing and suspending agents; p. with molecular weight between 20,000 and 40,000 has been used as a plasma extender. It is not metabolized, but is excreted unchanged by the kidney.

**po'vidone-i'odine** (USP). Polyvinylpyrrolidone-iodine complex; a topical antiinfective agent for the skin and mucous membranes; used for the prevention and control of infections susceptible to iodine.

**pow'der** [ Fr. *poudre;* L. *pulvis* ]. 1. A dry mass of minute separate particles of any substance. 2. In pharmaceutics, a homogenous dispersion of finely divided, relatively dry, particulate matter consisting of one or more substances; the degree of fineness of a p. is related to passage of the material through standard sieves. 3. A single dose of a powdered drug, enclosed in an envelope of folded paper. 4. To reduce a solid substance to a state of very fine division.

**bleaching p.,** chlorinated *lime.*

**pow'er.** 1. Potency. 2. In optics, the refractive vergence of a lens. 3. In physics and engineering, the rate at which work is done.

**back vertex p.,** effective p. of a lens as measured from surface toward eye; standard for measurement of ophthalmic lenses.

**equivalent p.,** that equal to an infinitely thin lens as measured on an optical bench.

**resolving p.,** definition of a lens; in a microscope objective lens it is calculated by dividing the wavelength of the light used by twice the numerical aperture of the objective; see also definition.

**pox** (poks) [ variant of the pl. of pock ]. 1. An eruptive disease; usually qualified by some term, as smallpox, cowpox, etc. 2. An eruption, first papular then pustular, occurring in chronic antimony poisoning. 3. Vulgarly, syphilis.

**camel p.,** see camelpox.

**chicken-p.,** see chickenpox.

**cow-p.,** cowpox; see vaccinia.

**fowl p.,** epithelioma contagiosum; a nodular eruption of viral origin, occurring in fowls and other birds.

**glass-p.,** alastrim.

**goat p.,** variola caprina; an acute infectious disease of goats caused by a virus and marked by generalized vesicular eruption on the skin and frequently the respiratory mucous membranes; occurs chiefly in southern and eastern Europe and North Africa.

**horse-p.,** see horsepox.

**Kaffir p.,** alastrim.

**milk p.,** alastrim.

**mouse p.,** ectromelia (2).

**rickett'sial p.,** Kew garden fever; an acute disease caused by *Rickettsia akari* transmitted by a mite (vector) which infests mice; a papule in the skin of a covered part of the body first appears which develops into a deep-seated vesicle and then shrinks to form a black eschar; symptoms develop about a week after the appearance of the papule and consist of fever, chills, headache, backache, sweating, and local adenitis; the first reported outbreak of the disease occurred in New York City.

**sheep-p.,** ovinia; a disease caused by a p. virus that is specific for sheep.

**small-p.,** see smallpox.

**swine-p.,** a disease of swine caused by a p. virus that is specific for swine. In America, the disease called swine-p. is not due to a true p. virus; it is really a pseudopox.

**water-p.,** varicella.

**white p.,** alastrim.

**poxvirus** (poks'vi'rus). See under virus.

**Pozzi** (pot'se), Samuel J., French gynecologist and anatomist, 1846–1918. See P.'s *muscle.*

**PP.** Abbreviation for pyrophosphate.

**PP**$_i$. Abbreviation for inorganic *pyrophosphate.*

**P.p.** Abbreviation for *punctum proximum* [ L. ]; see near *point.*

**PPCA.** Abbreviation for proserum prothrombin conversion *accelerator.*

**PPCF.** Abbreviation for plasmin prothrombin conversion *factor.*

**PPD.** Abbreviation for purified protein derivative of *tuberculin.*

**PPLO.** Abbreviation for pleuropneumonia-like *organisms.*

**p.p.m.** Abbreviation for parts per million.

**PPO.** Abbreviation for 2,5-diphenyloxazole.

**P-pulmonale.** An electrocardiographic syndrome of tall, narrow, peaked P waves in leads II, III, and aVF, and a prominent initial positive P wave component in $V_1$ and $V_2$, presumed to be characteristic of cor pulmonale. (Although this term is extensively used in the electrocardiographic literature, it is actually a misnomer and would be more appropriately called P-dextrocardiale, since it results from overload of the right atrium regardless of the cause, as in tricuspid stenosis, and may occur independently of cor pulmonale.)

**PQ-9.** Abbreviation for plastoquinone-9.

**Pr.** 1. Abbreviation for presbyopia. 2. Chemical symbol of the element praseodymium.

**P.r.** Abbreviation for *punctum remotum* [ L. ]; see far *point.*

**practice** (prak'tis) [ Mediev. L. *practica,* business, G. *praktikos,* pertaining to action, fr. *prassō,* to do. PRAG- ]. 1. The exercise of the profession of medicine. 2. To exercise the profession of medicine; to treat the sick.

  **extramural p.,** the delivery of health care services by university groups to persons beyond the confines of their respective medical centers.

  **intramural p.,** that type of p. by university faculties conducted within the confines of their respective medical centers.

**practitioner** (prak-tish'un-er). A person who practices medicine; a physician engaged in practice.

  **regular p.,** a physician who does not proclaim himself as the adherent of any school or sect in medicine or who does not follow exclusively any special system of therapeutics; a nonsectarian; sometimes called erroneously an allopathic p.

**prac'tolol** (USAN). 4'-[ 2-Hydroxy-3-(isopropylamino)-propoxy ]acetanilide; a β-receptor blocking drug for treatment of cardiac arrhythmias.

**Prader,** A. See P.-Willi *syndrome.*

**prae-.** For words beginning thus, see pre-.

**pragmatagnosia** (prag'mat-ag-no'si-ah) [ G. *pragma* (*pragmat-*), thing done, a deed, fr. *prassō,* to do, + *agnōsia,* ignorance. GN- ]. Loss of the power of recognizing objects.

**pragmatamnesia** (prag'mat-am-ne'zi-ah) [ G. *pragma,* a thing done, + *amnēsia,* forgetfulness ]. Loss of the memory of the appearance of objects.

**pragmatics** (prag-mat'iks) [ G. *pragmatikos,* fr. *pragma,* thing done ]. A branch of semiotics; the theory that deals with the relation between signs and their users, both senders and receivers.

**pragmatism** (prag'mă-tizm) [ G. *pragma* (*pragmat-*), thing done ]. A philosophy emphasizing practical applications and consequences of beliefs and theories, that the meaning of anything derives from its practicality.

**pralidoxime chloride** (pral'i-dok-sēm) (USP). PROTOPAM chloride; 2-formyl-1-methylpyridinium chloride oxime; used to restore the depressed cholinesterase activity resulting from organophosphate poisoning; has some limited value as an antagonist of the carbamate type of cholinesterase inhibitors that are used in the treatment of myasthenia gravis. Dizziness, blurred vision, drowsiness, nausea, tachycardia, and muscular weakness may occur.

**pramoxine hydrochloride** (prā-mok'sēn, -sin) (NF). TRONOTHANE hydrochloride; 4-[ 3-(*p*-butoxyphenoxy)propyl ]morpholine hydrochloride; a surface anesthetic agent for dermal and rectal use.

**prandial** (pran'di-al) [ L. *prandium,* breakfast ]. Relating to a meal.

**praseodymium** (pra-se-o-dim'i-um) [ G. *prasios,* leekgreen, fr. *prason,* a leek, + didymium ]. An element of the lanthanide or "rare earth" group; symbol Pr, atomic no. 59, atomic weight 140.92.

**Pratt,** Joseph H., U. S. physician, 1872–1956. See P.'s *method, symptom.*

**Prausnitz** (prows'nitz), Carl, German hygienist, *1876. See P.-Küstner *reaction,* P.-Kustner *antibody,* reversed P.-Küstner *reaction.*

**praxiology** (prak'si-ol'o-ji) [ G. *praxis,* action, + *logos,* study ]. The science or study of conduct.

**praxis** (prak'sis) [ G. *praxis,* action ]. 1. Practice. 2. The performance of action.

**pre-** [ L. *prae,* before ]. Prefix to words formed from Latin roots, denoting anterior or before, in space or time; see also ante-, pro-.

**preagonal** (pre-ag'o-nal) [ pre- + G. *agōn,* struggle (agony) ]. Immediately preceding death. (A misnomer: death is rarely associated with agony.)

**pre'albu'min.** A protein component of plasma having a molecular weight of about 61,000 and containing 1.3 per cent carbohydrate. Estimated plasma concentration is 0.3 g/100 ml.

  **thyroxine-binding p.,** a protein located in the "prealbumin" zone upon electrophoretic analysis of plasma proteins; its affinity for binding thyroxine is less than that of thyroxine-binding globulin but greater than that of albumin.

**preanal** (pre-a'nal). Anterior to the anus.

**pre'anesthet'ic.** Before anesthesia.

**pre'antisep'tic.** Denoting the period, especially in relation to surgery, before the adoption of the principles of antisepsis.

**preaortic** (pre'a-or'tik). Anterior to the aorta; denoting certain lymph nodes so situated.

**preaseptic** (pre-ă-sep'tik). Denoting the period, especially the early antiseptic period in relation to surgery, before the principles of asepsis were known or adopted.

**preataxic** (pre-ătak'sik). Denoting the early stages of tabes dorsalis prior to the appearance of ataxia.

**preauricular** (pre-aw-rik'u-lar). Anterior to the auricle of the ear; denoting lymphatic nodes so situated.

**preaxial** (pre-ak'si-al). Anterior to the axis of the body or a limb, the latter being in the anatomical position. 2. Denoting the portion of a limb bud which lies cranial to the axis of the limb.

**precancer** (pre-kan'ser). A lesion from which a malignant neoplasm is presumed to develop in a significant number of instances. A p. may or may not be recognizable clinically or by microscopic changes in the affected tissue.

**precan'cerous.** Premalignant; pertaining to any lesion that is interpreted as precancer.

**precap'illary.** Preceding a capillary; an arteriole or venule.

**precar'diac.** Precordial; anterior to the heart.

**precar'dinal.** Relating to the anterior cardinal veins.

**precar'tilage.** A closely packed aggregation of mesenchymal cells just prior to their differentiation into embryonic cartilage.

**preca'va.** *Vena* cava superior.

**precen'tral.** Referring to the cerebral convolution immediately anterior to the central sulcus: precentral gyrus.

**prechordal** (pre-kor'dal). Prochordal.

**precipitable** (pre-sip'i-tă-bl). Capable of being precipitated.

**precipitant** (pre-sip'i-tant). Anything causing a precipitation from a solution.

**precip'itate** [ L. *praecipito,* pp. -*atus,* to cast headlong, fr. *praeceps* (*praecipit-*), head foremost, fr. *prae* + *caput* head ]. 1. To cause a substance in solution to separate as a solid. 2. A solid separated out from a solution or suspension; a floc or clump (such as that resulting from the mixture of a specific antigen and its antibody). 3. A punctate opacity on the posterior surface of the cornea, apparently formed as a deposit from the aqueous.

**keratic p.'s,** lymphocytes deposited from the aqueous on the cornea, where they adhere; may be scattered over lower part of the cornea irregularly or in triangular arrangement of sharply defined spots; the condition is also called descemetitis, and is a finding in serous iridocyclitis.

**mutton-fat keratic p.'s,** coalescent p.'s forming small plaques that gradually become more translucent.

**pigmented keratic p.'s,** p.'s that occur in eyes with brown irides or after prolonged inflammation.

**red p.,** mercuric oxide, red.

**sweet p.,** mercurous chloride.

**white p.,** ammoniated mercury.

**yellow p.,** mercuric oxide, yellow.

**precipitation** (pre-sip′ĭ-ta′shun) [ see precipitate ]. 1. The act of precipitating. 2. The process of formation of solid matter previously held in solution or suspension in a liquid. 3. The phenomenon of clumping of proteins in serum produced by the addition of a specific precipitin.

**double antibody p.'s,** double antibody method or immunoassay; a method of separating antibody-bound antigen (*e.g.*, insulin) from free antigen by precipitating the former with antibody specific for immunoglobulin.

**hapten inhibition of p.,** inhibition of p. that occurs when the precipitin has combined with hapten of the same specificity as the subsequently added antigen.

**immune p.,** immunoprecipitation; the phenomenon of aggregation of sensitized antigen upon the addition of specific antibody (precipitin) to antigen in solution.

**precipitin** (pre-sip′ĭ-tin). Precipitating antibody; an antibody that under suitable conditions combines with and causes its specific and soluble antigen to precipitate from solution.

**precipitinogen** (pre-sip-ĭ-tin′o-jen) [ precipitin + G. suffix -gen, producing ]. 1. An antigen that stimulates the formation of specific precipitin when injected into an animal body. 2. A precipitable soluble antigen.

**precipitinogenoid** (pre-sip-ĭ-tin′o-jĕ-noyd). A precipitinogen that is altered by means of heating, thereby resulting in a substance that combines with the specific precipitin, but does not lead to the formation of a precipitate.

**precip′itogen.** Precipitinogen.

**precipitoid** (pre-sip′ĭ-toyd) [ precipitin + G. eidos, resemblance ]. A heat-treated precipitin that when mixed with specific precipitinogen does not cause a precipitate and also interferes with the precipitating effect of additional nonheated precipitin.

**precipitophore** (pre-sip′ĭ-to-fōr) [ precipitin + G. phoros, bearing ]. In Ehrlich's side chain theory, the portion of a precipitin molecule that is required in the formation of a precipitate, as distinguished from the haptophore group.

**preclin′ical.** 1. Before the onset of disease. 2. A period in medical education before the student deals with patients and clinical work.

**precocious** (pre-ko′shus) [ L. praecox, premature ]. Unusually early in development.

**precocity** (pre-kos′ĭ-tĭ) [ see precocious ]. Unusually early or rapid development of mental or physical traits.

**precognition** (pre′kog-nish′un) [ L. praecogito, to ponder before ]. Extrasensory perception of a future event.

**preconscious** (pre-kon′shus). In psychoanalysis, one of the three divisions of the psyche according to Freud's topographical psychology. The p. includes all ideas, thoughts, past experiences, and other memory impressions that with effort can be consciously recalled.

**preconvul′sive.** Denoting the stage in an epileptic paroxysm preceding convulsions.

**precor′dia** [ L. praecordia (ntr. pl. only), the diaphragm, the entrails, fr. prae, before, + cor (cord-), heart ]. Antecardium; fossa epigastrica; scrobiculus cordis; the epigastrium and anterior surface of the lower part of the thorax.

**precor′dial.** Relating to the precordia.

**precordialgia** (pre-kor′li-al′jĭ-ah) [ precordia + G. algos, pain ]. Pain in the precordial region.

**precor′dium.** Precordia.

**precos′tal** [ pre- + L. costa, rib ]. Anterior to the ribs.

**precrit′ical.** Relating to the phase before a crisis.

**precu′neal.** Anterior to the cuneus.

**precu′neate.** Relating to the precuneus.

**precu′neus** [ pre- + L. cuneus, a wedge ] ]NA ]. Quadrate lobe (3); quadrate lobule (2); lobulus quadratus (2); quader; a division of the medial surface of each cerebral hemisphere between the cuneus and the paracentral lobule; it lies above the subparietal sulcus and is bounded anteriorly by the pars marginalis of the sulcus cinguli and posteriorly by the parietooccipital sulcus.

**precursor** (pre-ker′ser) [ L. praecursor, fr. prae-, pre- + curro, to run ]. Anything that precedes another or from which another is derived, applied especially to a physiologically inactive substance that is converted to an active enzyme, vitamin, hormone, etc., or to a chemical substance that is built into a larger structure in the course of synthesizing the latter.

**predecidual** (pre′de-sid′u-al). Relating to the premenstrual or secretory phase of the menstrual cycle.

**preden′tin.** The organic fibrillar matrix of the dentin before its calcification.

**prediabetes** (pre-di-ah-be′tēz). A state in which one or a few of the abnormalities typical of diabetes mellitus can be observed episodically or persistently, and are often mild in nature.

**prediastole** (pre-di-as′to-le). Peridiastole; late systole; the interval in the cardiac rhythm immediately preceding the diastole.

**prediastol′ic.** Peridiastolic; late systolic; relating to the interval preceding the cardiac diastole.

**predicrot′ic.** Preceding the dicrotic notch.

**prediges′tion.** The artificial initiation of digestion of proteins (proteolysis) and starches (amylolysis) before they are eaten.

**predispose** (pre-dis-pōz′). To render susceptible.

**predisposition** (pre-dis-po-zish′un). A condition of special susceptibility to a disease.

**prednisolone** (pred-nis′o-lōn) (USP, BP). Δ-CORTEF; HY-DELTRA; METICORTELONE; METI-DERM; PARACORTOL; 11β,17,21-trihydroxy-1,4-pregnadiene-3,20-dione (for structure of pregnane, see steroids). A dehydrogenated analogue of cortisol with the same actions and uses as any compound exhibiting glucocorticoid activity; suitable for topical and oral administration; causes less electrolyte retention than cortisone.

**p. acetate** (USP), STERANE; prednisolone 21-acetate; same uses as p.; suitable for intramuscular administration.

**p. butylacetate,** HYDELTRA-T.B.A.; same actions and uses as p. but with longer duration of action and suitable for intrasynovial and soft tissue injection.

**p. sodium phosphate** (USP, BP), HYDELTRASOL; prednisolone 21-(disodium phosphate); more soluble than p. and the other p. esters and useful when a rapid onset or a short duration of action is desired. It is suitable for intrasynovial, parenteral, and topical administration.

**p. succinate** (USP), suitable for intramuscular, intravenous, or rectal administration.

**prednisone** (pred′nĭ-sōn) (USP, BP). DELTASONE; DELTRA; METICORTEN; PARACORT; 17,21-dihydroxy-1,4-pregnadiene-3,11,20-trione (for structure of pregnane, see steroids); a dehydrogenated analogue of cortisone with the same actions and uses, but produces less sodium retention.

**prednyl′idene.** DECORTILEN; 11β,17,21-trihydroxy-16-methylenepregna-1,4-diene-3,20-dione; glucocorticoid.

**predor′mital.** Pertaining to the predormitum.

**predor′mitum** [ pre- + L. dormire, to sleep ]. The stage of semi-unconsciousness preceding actual sleep.

**preduc′tal.** Relating to that part of the aorta proximal to the aortic opening of the ductus arteriosus.

**preeclampsia** (pre′e-klamp′sĭ-ah) [ pre- + G. eklampsis, a shining forth (eclampsia) ]. The development of hypertension with proteinuria or edema, or both, due to pregnancy or the influence of a recent pregnancy; it occurs after the 20th week of gestation but may develop before this time in the presence of trophoblastic disease; it is predominantly a disorder of primigravidas.

**superimposed p. or eclampsia** the development of p. or eclampsia in a patient with chronic hypertensive vascular or renal disease; when the hypertension antedates the pregnancy as established by previous blood pressure recordings, a rise in the systolic pressure of 30 mm Hg or a rise in the diastolic pressure of 15 mm Hg and the development of proteinuria or edema, or both, are required during pregnancy to establish the diagnosis.

**pre'epiglottic.** Anterior to the epiglottis.

**pre'eruptive.** Denoting the stage of an exanthematous disease preceding the eruption.

**pre'excita'tion.** Premature activation of part of the ventricular myocardium by an impulse that travels by an anomalous path and so avoids physiological delay in the atrioventricular junction; an intrinsic part of the Wolff-Parkinson-White syndrome.

**preforma'tion.** See preformation *theory.*

**prefron'tal.** Denoting the anterior portion of the frontal lobe of the cerebrum.

**preganglionic** (pre'gang-gli-on'ik). Situated proximal to or preceding a ganglion; referring specifically to the preganglionic motor neurons of the autonomic nervous system (located in the spinal cord and brainstem) and the preganglionic, myelinated nerve fibers by which they are connected to the autonomic ganglia.

**pregnancy** (preg'nan-sĭ) [ L. *praegnans* (*praegnant-*), pregnant, fr. *prae*, before, + *gnascor*, pp. *natus*, to be born. GEN- ]. Gestation; fetation; cyesis, cyophoria; graviditas; gravidity; the state of a female after conception until the birth of the baby. See also Table of Gestation Periods under gestation.

**abdominal p.,** abdominocyesis (1); the implantation and development of the ovum in the peritoneal cavity, usually secondary to an early rupture of a tubal p. Very rarely, primary implantation may occur in the peritoneal cavity.

**aborted ectopic p.,** tubal *abortion.*

**ampullar p.,** tubal p. situated near the midportion of the oviduct.

**bigeminal p.,** twin p.

**cervical p.,** the lodgment and development of the impregnated ovum in the cervical canal.

**combined p.,** coexisting uterine and ectopic p.

**compound p.,** development of a uterine p. in addition to a previously existing eccyesis, usually lithopedion.

**cornual p.,** the lodgment and development of the impregnated ovum in one of the cornua of the uterus.

**ectopic p.,** extrauterine p.; eccyesis; the development of an impregnated ovum outside the cavity of the uterus.

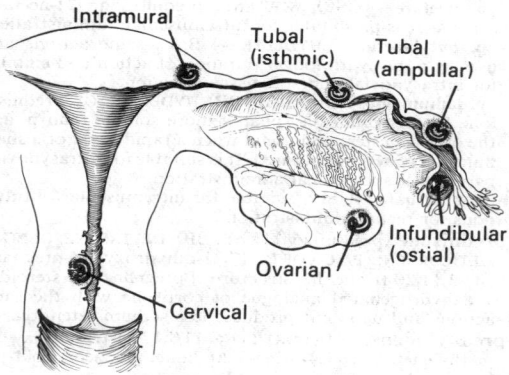

**Sites of Ectopic Pregnancy**

Sites of abnormal implantation and possible ectopic pregnancy.

**extraamniotic p.,** graviditas examnialis; a p. in which the chorion is intact, but the amnion has ruptured and shrunk.

**extrachorial p.,** graviditas exochorialis; p. in which the membranes rupture and shrink, causing the fetus to develop outside the chorionic sac but within the uterus.

**extramem'branous p.,** a p. in which during the course of gestation the fetus has broken through its envelopes, coming directly in contact with the uterine walls.

**extrau'terine p.,** ectopic p.

**Fallo'pian p.,** tubal p.

**false p.,** pseudocyesis.

**heterotopic p.,** a p. that is not in the uterine cavity.

**hydatid p.,** the presence of a hydatid mole in the pregnant uterus.

**interstitial p.,** intramural p.

**intraligamentary p.,** cyesis within the broad ligament.

**intramural p.,** interstitial p.; tubouterine p.; development of the fertilized ovum in the uterine portion of the Fallopian tube.

**intraperitone'al p.,** abdominal p.

**mesomet'ric p.,** ectopic p. beginning as a tubal p., the sac being eventually formed by the mesometrium.

**molar p.,** p. marked by a neoplasm within the uterus, whereby part or all of the chorionic villi are converted into a mass of clear vesicles.

**multiple p.,** the state of bearing two or more fetuses simultaneously.

**mural p.,** p. in uterine muscular wall.

**ovarian p.,** ovariocyesis; oothecocyesis; oocyesis; development of an impregnated ovum in an ovarian follicle; see also Spiegelberg's *criteria.*

**ovarioabdominal p.,** a beginning ovarian p. which, consequent upon growth of the embryo, later becomes abdominal.

**phantom p.,** pseudocyesis.

**plural p.,** multiple p.

**secondary abdominal p.,** abdominocyesis (2); a condition in which the embryo or fetus continues to grow in the abdominal cavity after its expulsion from the tube or other seat of its primary development.

**spurious p.,** pseudocyesis.

**tubal p.,** salpingocyesis; development of an impregnated ovum in the oviduct.

**tuboabdominal p.,** development of an ectopic p. partly in the tube and partly in the abdominal cavity.

**tubo-ovarian p.,** development of the ovum at the fimbriated extremity of the oviduct and involving the ovary.

**tubouterine p.,** intramural p.

**twin p.,** bigeminal p. that may result from the fertilization of two separate ova or of a single ovum; see also twin.

**uterine p.,** development of fetus within the uterus.

**uteroabdominal p.,** development of the ovum primarily in the uterus and later, in consequence of the rupture of the uterus, in the abdominal cavity.

**preg'nane.** Parent hydrocarbon of two series of steroids, stemming from 5α-pregnane (originally allopregnane) and 5β-pregnane (for structures, see steroids). 5β-Pregnane is the parent of the progesterones, pregnane alcohols, and ketones, and several adrenocortical hormones. 5α-Pregnane is found largely in urine as a metabolic product of 5β-pregnane compounds.

**pregnanediol** (preg'nan-di'ol). 5β-Pregnane-3α,20α-diol (for structure of pregnane, see steroids); a steroid metabolite, largely of progesterone; it is biologically inactive and occurs as pregnanediol glucuronidate in the urine.

**pregnanedione** (preg'nan-di'ōn). 5β-Pregnane-3,20-dione; 17α-[ 1-ketoethyl ]-etiocholane-3-one; a metabolite of progesterone, formed in relatively small quantities; occurs in 5α and 5β isomeric forms.

**pregnanetriol** (preg'nan-tri'ol). 5β-Pregnane-3α,17α,20α-triol (see steroids for pregnane structure); a urinary metabolite of 17-hydroxyprogesterone; a precursor in the biosynthesis of cortisol; its excretion is enhanced in certain diseases of the adrenal cortex and following administration of corticotropin.

**preg'nant** [ see pregnancy ]. Gravid; big with child; denoting a female bearing within her the product of conception.

**pregnene** (preg'nēn). An unsaturated steroid of primarily terminological importance; utilized in systematic nomenclature of appropriate 21-carbon steroids. See also steroids.

**preg'nenin'olone.** Ethisterone.

**pregnenolone** (preg-nēn'o-lōn). A steroid that serves as an intermediate in the biosynthesis of numerous hormones.

**p. succinate** (USAN), PRENOLON; corticosteroid used for the treatment of rheumatoid arthritis.

**prehal'lux** [ pre- + Mod. L. *hallux*, great toe ]. A supernumerary digit, usually only partial, attached to the medial border of the great toe.

**prehel'icine.** In front of the helix of the pinna.

**prehemiple'gic.** Preceding the occurrence of hemiplegia.

**prehen'sile** [ L. *prehendo,* pp. *-hensus,* to lay hold of, seize ]. Adapted for taking hold of or grasping.

**prehen'sion.** The act of grasping, or taking hold of.

**prehor'mone.** A glandular secretory product, having little or no inherent biological potency, that is converted peripherally to an active hormone in physiologically significant quantities.

**prehy'oid.** Anterior or superior to the hyoid bone; denoting certain accessory thyroid glands lying superior to the mylohyoid muscle.

**preictal** (pre-ik'tal) [ pre- + L. *ictus,* a stroke ]. Occurring before a convulsion or stroke.

**preinduction** (pre-in-duk'shun) [ L. *prae,* before, + *inductio,* a bringing in, fr. *in-duco,* to lead in ]. A modification in the third generation resulting from the action of environment on the germ cells of one or both individuals of the grandparental generation.

**Preisz** (prīz), Hugo von, Hungarian bacteriologist, 1860–1940. See P.-Nocard *bacillus.*

**prelac'rimal.** Anterior to the lacrimal sac.

**prelaryn'geal.** Anterior to the larynx; denoting especially one or two small lymphatic nodes.

**preleptotene** (pre-lep'to-tēn) [ pre- + leptotene, fr. G. *leptos,* slender, + *tainia,* band ]. The earliest stage of prophase in meiosis, characterized by physiochemical changes in cytoplasm and karyoplasm and beginning contraction of chromosomes.

**prelim'bic.** Anterior to the limbus of the fossa ovalis.

**pre'load.** The load to which a muscle is subjected before shortening.

**pre'lum** [ L. a press, fr. *premo,* pp. *pressus,* to press ]. Anything making strong compression.

   **p. abdomina'le,** the compression of the abdominal viscera caused by straining or bearing down.

**pre'luxa'tion.** Dislocation forward.

**premalig'nant.** Precancerous.

**premani'acal.** Preceding a manic attack.

**premature** (pre-mā-tūr', -chūr) [ L. *praematurus,* too early, fr. *prae-,* pre- + *maturus,* ripe (mature) ]. 1. Occurring before the usual or expected time. 2. Denoting an infant born after less than 37 weeks of gestation; birth weight is no longer considered a critical criterion for use of this designation.

**prematurity** (pre'mă-tūr'ĭ-tĭ). 1. The state of being premature. 2. In dentistry, deflective occlusal *contact,* interceptive occlusal *contact.*

**premaxilla** (pre'mak-sil'ah) [ pre- + L. *maxilla,* jawbone ]. *Os incisivum.*

**premaxillary** (pre-mak'sĭ-lĕr-ĭ). 1. Anterior to the maxilla. 2. Denoting the premaxilla.

**premedica'tion.** The administration of drugs prior to anesthesia to allay apprehension, produce sedation, and facilitate the administration of anesthesia to the patient.

**premelanosome** (pre-mel'ă-no-sōm). Precursor of a melanosome; contains no melanin granules. P.'s are prominent in melanocytes of albinos.

**premen'strual.** Relating to the period preceding menstruation.

**premenstruum** (pre-men'stroo-um) [ pre- + L. *menstruum,* ntr. of *menstruus,* monthly, pertaining to menstruation ]. The period preceding menstruation.

**premo'lar.** 1. Anterior to a molar tooth. 2. A bicuspid tooth.

**premon'ocyte.** Promonocyte; an immature monocyte not normally seen in the circulating blood.

**premor'bid** [ pre- + L. *morbidus,* ill, fr. *morbus,* disease ]. Preceding the occurrence of disease.

**premunition** (pre-mu-nish'un) [ Fr. fr. L. *praemunio,* pp. *-munitus,* to fortify beforehand ]. Infection immunity; a state in which an active, low grade infection establishes resistance to reinfection by a closely related microbe. The type of immunity established against tuberculosis by the BCG vaccine.

**premu'nitive.** Relating to premunition.

**premyeloblast** (pre-mi'ĕ-lo-blast). The earliest recognizable precursor of the myeloblast.

**premyelocyte** (pre-mi'ĕ-lo-sīt). Myeloblast.

**prena'ris,** pl. **prena'res.** One of the anterior nares; anterior opening of a nasal fossa; nostril.

**prena'tal** [ pre- + L. *natus,* born, pp. of *nascor,* to be born ]. Preceding birth; antenatal.

**preneoplastic** (pre-ne-o-plas'tik) [ pre- + G. *neos,* new, + *plastikos,* formative ]. Preceding the formation of any neoplasm, *i.e.,* benign or malignant. A p. condition is not always precancerous, although the term is frequently used erroneously in that sense.

**Prentice,** Charles F., American optician, 1854–1946. See P.'s *rule.*

**prenyl** (pren'il). 3-Methyl-2-buten-1-yl; —CH$_2$—CH=
$$\overset{\displaystyle \text{CH}_3}{\underset{\displaystyle}{|}}$$
C—CH$_3$; poly- or multiprenyl residues or derivatives thereof, apparently formed by end-to-end polymerization of isoprene molecules, are found in the so-called isoprenoids in nature (vitamins A, E, and K; coenzyme Q; tocopherols, carotenes, terpenes, rubber).

**prenyl'amine** (USAN). SEGONTIN; *N*-(3,3-diphenylpropyl)-α-methylphenethylamine; antianginal agent.

**preop'erative.** Preceding an operation.

**preop'tic.** Referring to the preoptic *region.*

**preoral** (pre-o'ral) [ pre- + L. *os* (*or*-), mouth ]. In front of the mouth.

**prepal'atal.** Relating to the anterior part of the palate, or anterior to the palate bone.

**preparalytic** (pre-păr-ă-lit'ik). Before the appearance of paralysis.

**preparation** (prep'ă-ra'shun) [ L. *praeparatio;* fr. *prae,* before, + *paro,* pp. *-atus,* to get ready ]. 1. A getting ready. 2. Something made ready, as a medicinal or other mixture, or a histologic specimen.

   **cavity p.,** the final form given an excavation in a tooth to enable it to retain a restoration, due consideration being given to the biological and mechanical requirements of the case.

   **corrosion p.,** one in which the hollow parts such as ducts, vessels or alveoli of the lung are filled with a substance that hardens and persists after dissolving the tissues by digestion.

   **cytologic filter p.,** a cytologic specimen made by depositing a watery sample (obtained by a variety of methods from many body sites) upon a filter having pores of uniform size smaller than the cellular material to be concentrated; this is followed by fixation and staining, usually with 95 per cent ethyl alcohol and Papanicolaou stain.

   **heart-lung p.,** an animal p. in which blood (rendered incoagulable) circulates through the heart and lungs and through an artificial system of vessels representing the systemic circulation. The latter is connected with the divided aorta on the one hand and with the superior vena cava on the other. Used in physiologic studies of the heart and circulation.

**prepatellar** (pre-pă-tel'ar). Anterior to the patella.

**pre'percep'tion.** Anticipation of, or a state of readiness for, a perception.

**pre'peritone'al.** Properitoneal; denoting a fatty layer between the peritoneum and the transversalis fascia in the lower anterior abdominal wall.

**prephenic acid** (pre-fe'nik, -fen'ik). An intermediate in the microbial conversion of shikimic acid to phenylalanine and tyrosine.

$$\text{HOOCCOCH}_2 \quad \text{COOH}$$

**Prephenic acid**

**pre'placen'tal.** Before formation of a placenta.

**prepotency** (pre-po'ten-sĭ) [ pre- + L. *potentia*, power ]. The ability or power possessed by one parent in greater degree than the other, of transmitting hereditable characteristics to the offspring.

**prepo'tent.** Possessing prepotency.

**prepoten'tial.** A gradual rise in potential between action potentials as a phasic swing in electric activity of the cell membrane, which establishes its rate of automatic activity, as in the ureter or cardiac pacemaker.

**prepsychotic** (pre'si-kot'ik). 1. Relating to the period antedating the onset of psychosis. 2. Denoting a potential for a psychotic episode, one that appears imminent under continued stress.

**prepu'beral, prepu'bertal.** Before puberty.

**prepubescent** (pre-pu-bes'ent). Immediately prior to the commencement of puberty.

**prepuce** (pre'pūs) [ L. *praeputium*, foreskin ]. Preputium.

**preputial** (pre-pu'shĭ-al). Relating to the prepuce.

**preputiotomy** (pre-pu'shĭ-ot'o-mĭ) [ preputium + G. *tomē*, incision ]. Incision of prepuce.

**preputium,** pl. **prepu'tia** (pre-pu'shĭ-um) [ L. *praeputium* ]. [ NA ]. Prepuce; foreskin; the free fold of skin that covers more or less completely the glans penis.

   **p. clitor'idis** [ NA ], the external fold of the labia minora, forming a cap over the clitoris.

**prepylor'ic.** Anterior to or preceding the pylorus; denoting a temporary constriction of the wall of the stomach separating the fundus from the antrum during digestion; prepyloric sphincter.

**prerec'tal.** Anterior to or preceding the rectum.

**pre'reduced.** Pertaining to bacteriological media that are boiled, tubed under oxygen-free gas with chemical reducing agents and colorimetric redox indicator in stopped tubes or bottles, and then sterilized.

**prere'nal** [ L. *ren*, kidney ]. Anterior to a kidney.

**pre'reproduc'tive.** Obsolete term denoting the period of life before puberty.

**preret'inal.** Anterior to the retina.

**presa'cral.** Anterior to or preceding the sacrum.

**presby-, presbyo-** (prez'bĭ-, prez'bĭ-o-) [ G. *presbys*, old man ]. Combining forms relating to old age.

**presbyacousia** (prez-bĭ-ă-koo'sĭ-ah). Presbyacusis.

**presbyacusis, presbyacusia** (prez'bĭ-ă-koo'sis) [ presby- + G. *akousis*, hearing ]. Presbyacousia; presbycusis; loss of ability to perceive or discriminate sounds as a part of the aging process; the pattern and age of onset may vary.

**presbyatrics** (prez-bĭ-at'riks) [ presby- + G. *iatreia*, medical treatment ]. Geriatrics.

**presbycusis** (prez-bĭ-koo'sis). Presbyacusis.

**presbyope** (prez'bĭ-ōp). A person with presbyopia.

**presbyophrenia** (prez-bĭ-o-fre'nĭ-ah) [ presbyo- + G. *phrēn*, mind ]. Presbyphrenia; one of the mental disorders of old age marked by loss of memory, disorientation, and confabulation, but with relative integrity of judgment.

**presbyopia** (prez-bĭ-o'pĭ-ah) [ presby- + G. *ōps*, eye ]. The physiologic change in accommodation power in the eyes in advancing age, said to begin when the near point has receded beyond 22 cm. (9 inches).

**presbyopic** (prez'bĭ-op'ik, -o'pik). Relating to or suffering from presbyopia.

**presbyphrenia** (prez'bĭ-fre'nĭ-ah). Presbyophrenia.

**presbytia** (prez-bish'ĭ-ah). Obsolete word for presbyopia.

**presbytiatrics** (prez-bĭ-tĭ-at'riks) [ G. *presbytēs*, an old man, + *iatreia*, medical treatment ]. Geriatrics.

**presbytism** (prez'bĭ-tizm). Obsolete word for presbyopia.

**prescribe** [ L. *prae-scribo*, pp. *-scriptus*, to write before ]. To give directions, either orally or in writing, for the preparation and administration of a remedy to be used in the treatment of any disease.

**prescrip'tion** [ L. *praescriptio;* see prescribe ]. 1. A written formula for the preparation and administration of any remedy. 2. A medicinal preparation compounded according to the directions formulated in a prescription. In the classical description of a p. it is said to consist of four parts: (a) the *superscription,* consisting of the word *recipe,* take, or its sign, ℞ ; (b) the *inscription,* or main part of the p., containing the names and amounts of the drugs ordered;

(c) the *subscription,* or directions for mixing the ingredients and designation of the form (pill, powder, solution, etc.) in which the drug is to be made; this usually begins with the word, *misce,* mix, or its abbreviation M.; and (d) the *signature,* or directions to the patient regarding the dose and times of taking the remedy; this is preceded by the word *signa,* designate, or its abbreviation S.

   **blun'derbuss p.,** shotgun p.

   **shotgun p.,** a p. containing many ingredients, some inert and all in a fixed dose relation one to another.

**pre'secre'tion.** Hormone.

**presenile** (pre-se'nil). Displaying presenility.

**presenility** (pre'sĕ-nil'ĭ-tĭ) [ pre- + L. *senilis,* old ]. Premature old age; the condition of an individual, not old in years, who displays the physical and mental characteristics of old age.

**prese'nium.** Period preceding old age.

**present** (pre-zent') [ L. *praesens* (-*sent*-), pres. p. of *praesum,* to be before, be at hand ]. To precede or appear first at the os uteri, said of the part of the fetus that is felt by the examining finger of the accoucheur.

**presentation** (pre'zen-ta'shun, prez'-) [ see present ]. The part of the body of the fetus which is in advance during birth. The occiput, chin, and sacrum are the determining points in vertex, face, and breech presentations, respectively. When the fetus lies with its long axis transversely the shoulder is the presenting part and the designation is shoulder p. See also position (3), and subentries under position.

   **acromion p.,** shoulder p.

   **breech p.,** p. of any part of the pelvic extremity of the fetus, the nates, knees, or feet; more properly only of the nates. When the fetus presents by the pelvic extremity, the thighs may be flexed and the legs extended over the anterior surfaces of the body (frank p.); or the thighs may be flexed on the abdomen and the legs upon the thighs (full breech p.); or the feet may be the lowest part (footling p.); or one leg may retain the position which is typical of one of the above-mentioned presentations, while the other foot or knee may present (incomplete foot or knee p.).

   **cephal'ic p.,** head p.; usually the head is sharply flexed so that the chin is in contact with the thorax (vertex p.); but more rarely, there may be degrees of deflexion so that the presenting part is the large fontanel (sincipital p.), the brow (brow p.), or the face (face p.).

   **footling p.,** foot p.; the descent of the fetus feet first.

   **pelvic p.,** a p. of the breech or any part of one or both lower extremities.

   **placen'tal p.,** *placenta* previa.

   **polar p.,** the p. of either pole of the fetal oval; cephalic or breech p.; longitudinal lie.

   **shoulder p.,** acromion p.; the fetus lies with its long axis transversely and the shoulder is the presenting part.

   **transverse p.,** transverse lie; shoulder p.

   **vertex p.,** the normal cephalic p.; p. of the upper and back part of the fetal head.

**preservative** (pre-zer'vă-tiv). A substance added to food products or to organic solution to preserve them from chemical change or bacterial action.

**presomite** (pre-so'mīt). Relating to the embryonic stage before the appearance of somites.

**presphenoid** (pre-sfe'noyd). In front of the sphenoid bone or cartilage.

**presphygmic** (pre-sfig'mik) [ pre- + G. *sphygmos,* pulse ]. Preceding the pulse beat; denoting a brief interval following the filling of the ventricles with blood before their contraction forces open the semilunar valves.

**prespi'nal.** Anterior to the spine.

**prespondylolisthesis** (pre-spon-dĭ-lo-lis'the-sis). A condition predisposing to spondylolisthesis, consisting in a defect in the laminae of a lumbar vertebra without as yet any displacement of the vertebral body.

**pres'sor** [ L. *premo,* pp. *pressus,* to press ]. Hypertensor; exciting to vasomotor activity; producing increased blood pressure; denoting afferent nerve fibers which, when stimulated, excite the vasoconstrictor center and lead to increased peripheral resistance.

**pres'sorecep'tive.** Pressosensitive; capable of receiving as

**Presentations**

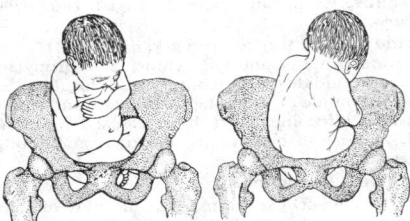

Breech presentation
Right sacroposterior     Right sacruanterior

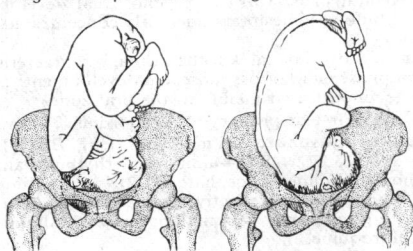

Vertex presentation
Right occipitoposterior     Right occipitoanterior

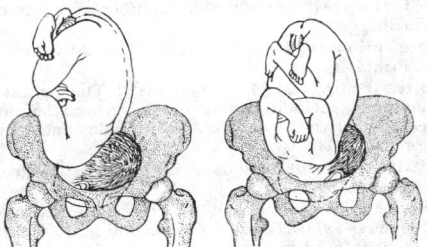

Face presentation
Right mentoposterior     Right mentoanterior

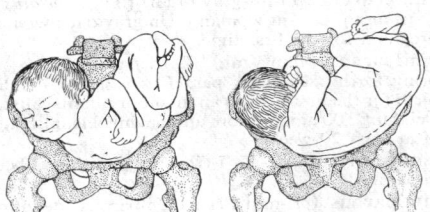

Transverse presentation
Right scapuloposterior     Right scapuloanterior

stimuli changes in pressure, especially changes of blood pressure.

**pres′sorecep′tor.** Baroreceptor.

**pres′sosen′sitive.** Pressoreceptive.

**pres′sosensitiv′ity.** The state of being able to perceive changes in pressure. See also pressoreceptive.

    **reflexogen′ic p.,** p. also capable of initiating the regulation of heart rate, vascular tone, and blood pressure.

**pressure** (presh′ur) [ L. *pressura*, fr. *premo*, pp. *pressus*, to press ]. 1. A stress or force acting in any direction against resistance. 2. Symbol P, frequently followed by a subscript indicating location; in physics and physiology, the force per unit area exerted by a gas or liquid against the walls of its container or that would be exerted on a wall immersed at that spot in the middle of a body of fluid. The p. can be considered either relative to some reference p., such as that of the ambient atmosphere (imagined to be on

the other side of the wall), or in absolute terms (relative to a perfect vacuum).

    **atmospheric p.,** barometric p.

    **back p.,** p. exerted upstream in the circulation as a result of obstruction to forward flow, as when congestion in the pulmonary circulation results from stenosis of the mitral valve or failure of the left ventricle.

    **barometric p.,** symbol $P_B$; atmospheric p.; the absolute p. of the ambient atmosphere, varying with weather, altitude, etc.; expressed in millibars (meteorology) or mm Hg or torr (respiratory physiology); at sea level it averages about 14.7 pounds per square inch, 1013.3 millibars, 1013 $\times 10^6$ dynes/cm², 760 mm Hg or torr; in SI units, 101,325 pascals (Pa).

    **biting p.,** occlusal p.

    **blood p.,** piesis; the p. or tension of the blood within the arteries, maintained by the contraction of the left ventricle, the resistance of the arterioles and capillaries, the elasticity of the arterial walls, as well as the viscosity and volume of the blood; blood p. is always expressed as relative to the ambient atmospheric p.

    **cerebrospinal p.,** tension of the cerebrospinal fluid, normally 100 to 150 mm. of water, relative to the ambient atmospheric p.

    **critical p.,** the minimal p. required to liquefy a gas at the critical temperature.

    **diastolic p.,** the p. during or resulting from diastolic relaxation of a cardiac chamber; more specifically, the lowest arterial blood p. reached during any given ventricular cycle.

    **differential blood p.,** the arterial blood p. at corresponding points on the two sides of the body.

    **Donders' p.,** an increase of about 6 mm. of mercury shown by a manometer connected with the trachea when the thorax of the dead body is opened; it is caused by the collapse of the lungs when air is admitted to the thorax.

    **effective osmotic p.,** that part of the total osmotic p. of a solution that governs the tendency of its solvent to pass across a boundary, usually a semipermeable membrane. It is commonly represented by the product of the total osmotic p. of the solution and the ratio (corrected for activities) of the number of dissolved particles that do not permeate the bounding membrane to the total number of particles in the solution. Equivalent in meaning to tonicity; commonly expressed in equivalent units of osmolality rather than p. per se.

    **hydrostatic p.,** the p. exerted by a liquid as a result of its potential energy, ignoring its kinetic energy; frequently used to distinguish a true p. from an osmotic p. or to emphasize the variation in p. in a column of fluid due to the effect of gravity.

    **hyperbaric p.,** p. of more than 1 atmosphere; used in therapy for shock, carbon monoxide poisoning, clostridial infections, and for some operations.

    **intracranial p.,** p. within the cranial cavity.

    **intraocular p.,** the p. (usually measured in millimeters of mercury) of the intraocular fluid within the eye, measured by means of a manometer.

    **negative p.,** p. less than that of the ambient atmosphere.

    **occlusal p.,** biting p.; any force exerted upon the occlusal surfaces of teeth.

    **oncotic p.,** osmotic p. exerted by colloids in solution.

    **osmotic p.,** the p. that must be applied to a solution to prevent the passage into it of solvent when solution and pure solvent are separated by a perfectly semipermeable membrane. (Sometimes less correctly viewed as the force with which the solution attracts solvent through the semipermeable membrane.)

    **partial p.,** the p. exerted by a single component of a mixture of gases, commonly expressed in mm Hg or torr; for a gas dissolved in a liquid, the partial p. is that of a gas that would be in equilibrium with the dissolved gas. Symbols: formerly, a lower case p followed by the chemical symbol in capital letters, *e.g.*, pCO₂, pO₂; now, in respiratory physiology, a capital P followed by subscripts denoting location and/or chemical species, *e.g.*, $PCO_2$, $PO_2$, $PA_{CO_2}$.

    **pleural p.,** the p. in the pleural space between the visceral and parietal pleurae.

**positive end-expiratory p.,** abbreviated PEEP; a technique used in respiratory therapy in which p. is maintained in the airway (*e.g.*, by having the patient expire through a tube that extends under water) so that the lungs empty less completely in expiration.

**pulmonary p.,** the blood p. in the pulmonary artery.

**pulse p.,** the variation in blood p. occurring in an artery during the cardiac cycle; it is the difference between the systolic or maximum and diastolic or minimum p.'s and varies normally between 25 and 50 mm. of mercury.

**selection p.,** see under selection.

**solution p.,** the force driving atoms or molecules to leave a solid particle and enter into solution (*i.e.*, to dissolve).

**standard p.,** the absolute p. to which gases are referred under standard conditions (STPD), *i.e.*, 760 mm Hg or 760 torr.

**systolic p.,** the p. during or resulting from systolic contraction of a cardiac chamber; more specifically, the highest arterial blood pressure reached during any given ventricular cycle.

**transmural p.,** the p. inside a vessel or hollow viscus, measured relative to the p. just outside its wall; thus, the p. difference across the wall.

**transpulmonary p.,** the difference between the p. of the respired gas at the mouth and the pleural p. around the lungs, measured when the airway is open; thus, it includes not only the transmural p. of the lung but also any drop in p. along the tracheobronchial tree during flow.

**transthoracic p.,** the p. in the pleural space measured relative to the p. of the ambient atmosphere outside the chest; the transmural p. across the chest wall.

**vapor p.,** the partial p. exerted by a vapor.

**wedge p.,** intravascular pressure obtained through a catheter placed in branches of the pulmonary or hepatic venous system.

**pre'ster'num.** *Manubrium* sterni.

**presuppurative** (pre-sup'-u-ra'tiv). Denoting an early stage in an inflammation prior to the formation of pus.

**presynaptic** (pre'sĭ-nap'tik). Pertaining to the area on the proximal side of a synaptic cleft.

**presystole** (pre-sis'to-le). Perisystole; late diastole; that part of diastole immediately preceding systole.

**presystol'ic.** Perisystolic; late diastolic; relating to the interval immediately preceding systole.

**pretar'sal.** Denoting the anterior, or inferior, portion of the tarsus.

**pretecta.** Orad to the pars tecta duodeni.

**pretec'tum.** Pretectal *area*.

**prethyroid, prethyroideal, prethyroidean** (pre-thi'-royd, -thi-roy'de-al, -thi-roy'de-an). Anterior to or preceding the thyroid gland or cartilage.

**pretib'ial.** Relating to the anterior portion of the leg; denoting especially certain muscles.

**pretrematic** (pre'tre-mat'ik) [ pre- + G. *trēma*, perforation ]. Relating to the cranial surface of a branchial cleft.

**pretympan'ic.** Anterior to the drum of the ear.

**preventive** (pre-ven'tiv) [ L. *prae-venio*, pp. *-ventus*, to come before, prevent ]. 1. Prophylactic; warding off disease. 2. A prophylactic, or anything that arrests the threatened onset of disease.

**preventorium** (pre-ven-to'rĭ-um) [ fr. prevent, formed on the model of sanatorium ]. An institution for the care of persons, especially children, of poor physique who are believed to be in danger of acquiring tuberculosis.

**prever'tebral.** Anterior to the body of a vertebra or of the vertebral column.

**preves'ical** [ pre- + L. *vesica*, bladder ]. Anterior to the bladder.

**previus** (pre'vĭ-us) [ L. *prae*, before, + *via*, way ]. In the way; referring usually to anything obstructing the passages in childbirth.

**pre'zone.** Prozone.

**priapism** (pri'ă-pizm) [ L. *priapus* (*q.v.*), penis ]. Persistent erection of the penis, especially when due to disease or excessive quantities of androgens, and not to sexual desire.

**priapitis** (pri-ă-pi'tis) [ L. *priapus*, penis, + G. suffix *-itis*, inflammation ]. Inflammation of the penis.

**priapus** (pri'ă-pus) [ L. fr. L. *Priapus* (G. *Priapos*), god of procreation ]. The penis.

**Price-Jones,** Cecil, English hematologist, 1863–1943. See P.-J. *curve*.

**prilocaine hydrochloride** (pril'o-kān) (NF). CITANEST hydrochloride; propitocaine hydrochloride; 2-(propylamino)-*o*-propionotoluidide hydrochloride; a local anesthetic agent of the amide type, related chemically and pharmacologically to lidocaine hydrochloride; used for peridural, caudal, and nerve blocks, and regional and infiltration anesthesia.

**pri'maclone.** Primidone.

**primacy** (pri'mă-sĭ) [ see primary ]. The state of being primary, or foremost in rank or importance.

**genital p.,** in psychoanalysis, the primary characteristic of the genital phase (*q.v.*) of psychosexual development; *i.e.*, the libido becomes preponderantly concentrated in the penis.

**oral p.,** in psychoanalysis, the primary characteristic of the oral phase (*q.v.*) of psychosexual development; *i.e.*, the libido is concentrated mainly in the oral zone.

**pri'mal.** 1. First or primary. 2. Primordial (2).

**primaquine phosphate** (pri'mă-kwin) (USP, BP). Plasmochin; SN 13,272; 8-[ (4-amino-1-methylbutyl)amino ]-6-methoxyquinoline phosphate (1:2); an antimalarial agent; found especially effective against *Plasmodium vivax*, terminating relapsing vivax malaria; usually administered with chloroquine.

**primary** (pri'mĕr-ĭ) [ L. *primarius*, fr. *primus*, first ]. 1. The first or foremost, as a disease or symptoms to which others may be secondary or occur as complications. 2. Relating to the first stage of growth or development; see primordial. 3. Principal.

**primate** (pri'māt) [ L. *primus*, first ]. An individual of the order Primates.

**Primates** (pri-ma'tēz) [ L. *primus*, first ]. The highest order of mammals, including man, monkeys, and lemurs embraced in the two suborders: Anthropoidea and Lemuroidea, or Prosimiae.

**pri'merite** [ L. *primus*, first, + G. *meris*, part ]. Protomerite.

**primidone** (USP, BP). MYSOLINE; primaclone; 5-ethyldihydro-5-phenyl-4,6-(1H,5H)-pyrimidenedione; an anticonvulsant drug used in the management of grand mal and psychomotor epilepsy; relatively free from serious toxic effects.

**primigravida** (pri-mĭ-grav'ĭ-dah) [ L. fr. *primus*, first, + *gravida*, a pregnant woman ]. Unigravida; a woman who is pregnant for the first time.

**primipara** (pri-mip'ă-rah) [ L. fr. *primus*, first, + *pario*, bring forth ]. Unipara; para I; a woman who has given birth for the first time to an infant or infants, alive or dead, weighing 500 gm. or more and having a length of gestation of at least 20 weeks.

**primiparity** (pri'mĭ-păr'ĭ-tĭ). The condition of being a primipara.

**primiparous** (pri-mip'ă-rus). Uniparous; denoting a primipara.

**pri'mite.** Protomerite.

**primitive** (prim'ĭ-tĭv) [ L. *primitivus*, fr. *primus*, first ]. Primordial (2).

**primocar'cin.** 5-Acetamide-4-oxo-5-hexamide; an antibiotic from *Nocardia fukaya;* possesses antineoplastic and antimicrobial activity.

**primor'dial.** 1. Relating to a primordium. 2. Primitive; primal (2); relating to a structure in its first or earliest stage of development.

**primor'dium** [ L. origin, fr. *primus*, first, + *ordior*, begin ]. Anlage (1), *q.v.;* an aggregation of cells in the embryo indicating the first trace of an organ or structure.

**primula** (prim'u-lah) [ Mediev. L. primrose, fem. of L. *primulus*, first ]. The rhizome and roots of a number of species of *Primula*, (family Primulaceae), primrose or cowslip. In some sensitive persons contact with the plant causes a rash; has been used as expectorant, diuretic, and anthelmintic.

**pri'mulin.** An acid yellow thiazole dye, $C_{21}H_{14}N_3O_3Na$, used as a fluorescent vital stain.

**pri'mus** [ L. ] [ NA ]. First; denoting the first of a series of similar structures.

**princeps,** pl. **principes** (prin'seps, -sĭ-pēz) [ L. chief, fr. *primus,* first, + *capio,* to take, choose ] [ NA ]. Principal; a term used to distinguish several arteries.

  **p. cervi'cis,** *ramus* descendens (2).

  **p. pol'licis,** *arteria* princeps pollicis.

**Princeteau** (praṅs-to'), L. R., French physician, *1884. See P.'s *tubercle.*

**principle** (prin'sĭ-pl) [ L. *principium,* a beginning, fr. *princeps,* chief ]. 1. A continuously acting power or force. 2. The essential ingredient in a drug or chemical compound.

  **active p.,** a constituent of a drug, usually an alkaloid or glycoside, upon the presence of which the characteristic therapeutic action of the substance largely depends.

  **antianemic p.,** the material in liver (and certain other tissues) that stimulates hemopoiesis in pernicious anemia; for practical purposes, the antianemic effect of extracts from such tissues is approximately equivalent to the content of vitamin $B_{12}$.

  **azygos vein p.,** low flow p.; based on the observation that animals can survive prolonged vena caval occlusion without sequelae: if blood from the azygos vein alone is permitted to enter the heart, patients are perfused during cardiac and pulmonary bypass at flows much less than the normal resting cardiac output.

  **Bernoulli's p.,** Bernoulli's *law.*

  **closure p.,** in psychology, the p. that when one views fragmentary stimuli forming a nearly complete figure (*e.g.,* an incomplete rectangle) one tends to ignore the missing parts and perceive the figure as whole.

  **consistency p.,** in psychology, the desire of the human being to be consistent, especially in his attitudes and beliefs; theories of attitude formation and change based on the consistency p. include balance theory, which suggests that the individual seeks to avoid incongruity in his various attitudes. See also cognitive dissonance *theory.*

  **Fick p.,** the basis of some indirect methods of measuring the output of the heart and of blood flow to some of the organs, *e.g.,* the kidneys. It can be used when arterial and venous concentrations of a substance can be measured and the amount of uptake or removal of the substance can be determined. Oxygen consumption is equal to the product of the blood flow and the difference in oxygen content of the arterial and mixed venous blood; usually rearranged so that $Q = \dot{V}O_2/(a - vO_2)$

  **follicle-stimulating p.,** follicle-stimulating *hormone.*

  **hematinic p.,** the p. previously thought to be produced by the action of the intrinsic factor of Castle upon an extrinsic factor in food, now recognized as vitamin $B_{12}$.

  **p. of inertia,** repetition-compulsion p.

  **low flow p.,** azygos vein p.

  **luteinizing p.,** luteinizing *hormone.*

  **melanophore-expanding p.,** melanocyte-stimulating *hormone.*

  **nirvana p.,** in psychoanalysis, the p. that expresses the tendency toward the death instinct.

  **organic p.,** proximate p.

  **pain p.,** an unconscious striving for pain and death.

  **pain-pleasure p.,** pleasure p.; a psychoanalytic concept that, in man's psychic functioning, he tends to seek pleasure and avoid pain.

  **Pauli's p.,** the theory limiting the number of electrons in the orbit or shell of an atom; it is not possible for any two electrons to have all four quantum numbers identical.

  **pleasure p.,** pain-pleasure p.

  **prox'imate p.,** in chemistry, an organic compound which may exist already formed as a part of some other more complex substance; various sugars, starches, and albumins belong to this class of substances.

  **reality p.,** the concept that the pleasure p. in personality development is modified by the demands of external reality; the p. or force that compels the growing child to adapt to the demands of external reality.

  **repetition-compulsion p.,** p. of inertia; in psychoanalysis, the impulse to redramatize or reenact earlier emotional experiences or situations.

  **ultimate p.,** one of the chemical elements.

**Pringle,** John J., English dermatologist, 1855–1922. See P.'s *disease,* Bourneville-P. *disease.*

**prism** (prizm) [ G. *prisma.* PRISM- ]. A solid whose sides are parallelograms and whose transverse section is a triangle; a triangular p. deflects the ray of light toward the base of the triangle and splits it up into its primary colors; it is used in spectacles to correct imbalance of the extrinsic ocular muscles.

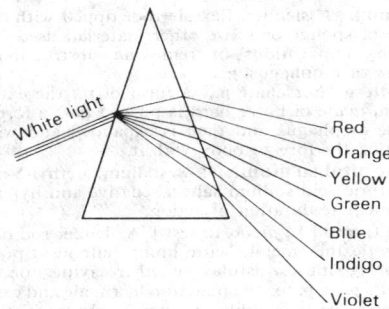

**Splitting of White Light by a Prism**

  **enamel p.'s,** *prismata adamantina.*

  **Maddox double p.,** two p.'s with their bases in close apposition, used in testing for cyclophoria.

  **Nicol p.,** a polarizing p. made by cutting through a p. of calcite or Iceland spar and reuniting the cut surfaces with Canada balsam; light passing through this p. is split, the ordinary rays being deflected by the layers of balsam, only the polarized light being transmitted.

  **Risley's rotary p.,** a p. with circular base that can be rotated in a metal frame marked with a scale, used in examination of imbalance of the ocular muscles.

**prisma,** pl. **prismata** (priz'mah, priz'mă-tah) [ G. something sawed, a prism ] [ NA ]. Prism.

  **prismata adamantina** [ NA ], enamel prisms, rods, or fibers; the calcified, microscopic rods radiating from the surface of the dentin, forming the substance of the enamel of a tooth.

**prismatic** (priz-mat'ik). Relating to or resembling a prism.

**prismoid** (priz'moyd). Resembling a prism; prismatic.

**prismosphere** (priz'mo-sfēr). A combined spherical lens and prism.

**privacy** (pri'vă-si). 1. Being apart from others; seclusion; secrecy. 2. Especially in psychiatry and clinical psychology, respect for the confidential nature of the therapist-patient relationship.

**p.r.n.** Abbreviation of L. *pro re nata,* according to the condition arising (born), according to needs; sometimes used in prescriptions or written orders.

**pro-** [ L. and G. *pro,* before ]. 1. Prefix denoting before or forward. 2. In chemistry, prefix indicating "precursor of"; see also suffix -gen.

**Pro.** Symbol for proline or its radicals.

**proaccelerin** (pro-ak-sel'er-in). *Factor* V.

**proacrosomal** (pro-ak'ro-so'mal). Relating to an early stage in the development of the acrosome.

**proactinium** (pro-ak-tin'ĭ-um). Protactinium.

**proactivator** (pro-ak'tĭ-va-tor). A substance that, when chemically split, yields a fragment (activator) capable of rendering another substance enzymically active.

  **C3 p.,** see cobra venom *cofactor,* and *properdin* factor B.

  **C3 p. convertase,** see under convertase.

**proagglutinoid** (pro-ă-glu'tĭ-noyd). A modified agglutinin that has a stronger affinity for agglutinogen than has agglutinin.

**pro'al.** Relating to a forward movement.

**proamnion** (pro-am'nĭ-on). An area of the extraembryonic membranes beneath, and in front of, the developing head of a young embryo which remains without mesoderm for some time.

**proatlas** (pro-at'las). A vertebral element intercalated between the atlas and occipital bone in *Crocodilia,* traces of which are sometimes seen as an anomaly on the undersurface of the occipital bone in man.

**probacteriophage** (pro-bak-tēr'ĭ-o-fāj). Prophage; the stage of a temperate bacteriophage in which the genome is incorporated in the genetic apparatus of the bacterial host.
  **defective p.,** see defective *bacteriophage.*

**pro'band** [ L. *probare,* to test, prove ]. Propositus (1); in human genetics, the patient or member of the family that brings a family under study.

**pro'bang.** A slender, flexible rod, tipped with a globular piece of sponge or some other material, used chiefly for making applications or removing obstructions in the larynx or esophagus.
  **bristle p., horsehair p.,** a form of p., the extremity of which, made of horse hair, is pushed past a foreign body in the esophagus and then is expanded and withdrawn, bringing the foreign body with it.

**probar'bital so'dium.** IPRAL sodium; 5-ethyl-5-isopropyl-barbituric acid sodium salt; a sedative and hypnotic with intermediate duration of action.

**probe** (prōb) [ L. *probo,* to test ]. A slender rod of silver or other flexible metal, with blunt bulbous tip, used for exploring sinuses, fistulas, or other cavities, or wounds.
  **Anel's p.,** a p. for the punctum lacrimale and canaliculae.
  **Bowman's p.,** a double-ended p. for the lacrimal duct, the body of the instrument being provided with a shield for convenience in manipulating.
  **electric p.,** Lilienthal's p.
  **Girdner's p.,** telephonic p.; one of the wires of a telephone receiver is attached to a metal p., the other to a metal plate; the latter is moistened and placed on the patient's body, with the receiver at the surgeon's ear; if the p. touches a bullet or piece of metal a click is heard.
  **Lilienthal's p.,** electric p.; two wires are attached to the tip of a p. composed of two or four pieces of metal insulated from the shank; these wires run to two plates, one of zinc and one of copper, placed above and below the examiner's tongue; if the p. touches a bullet or other piece of metal there will be a metallic taste produced in the mouth.
  **meer'schaum p.,** a bullet p. with meerschaum tip, which coming in contact with a leaden bullet will receive a mark.
  **periodontal p.,** a calibrated instrument used to measure the depth and topography of periodontal pockets.
  **telephon'ic p.,** Girdner's p.
  **ver'tebrated p.,** a p. made up of a series of short bits of metal hinged together, which readily accommodates itself to all the sinuosities of a fistula or other tract.

**probenecid** (pro-ben'e-sid) (USP, BP). Benemid; *p*-carboxy-*N,N*-diisopropylsulfonamide; a competitive inhibitor of the secretion of penicillin or *p*-aminohippurate by kidney tubules; a uricosuric agent used in chronic gouty arthritis.

**probilifuscins** (pro-bil'ĭ-fus'in). See bilirubinoids.

**probio'sis** [ pro- + G. *biōsis,* life ]. An association of two organisms that enhances the life processes of both, as contrasted with antibiosis.

**probiot'ic.** Relating to probiosis.

**prob'lem.** In the mental health professions, a term often used to denote life problems (the difficulties or challenges of life); sometimes used in preference to the terms mental illness or mental disorder.

**proboscis,** pl. **proboscides, proboscises** (pro-bos'is, pro-bos'ĭ-dēz, -sez) [ G. *proboskis,* a means of providing food, fr. pro- + *boskein,* to feed ]. 1. A long flexible snout such as that of a tapir or an elephant. 2. In teratology, a cylindrical protuberance of the face which, in cyclopia or ethmocephaly, represents the nose.

**Probstymay'ria vivip'ara.** Formerly *Oxyuris vivipara;* a nematode (family Atractidae) closely related to the true pinworms (family Oxyuridae) and still commonly considered the horse pinworm. It is distributed worldwide and found, often in tremendous numbers, in the colon of horses and other equids.

**procainamide hydrochloride** (pro-kān'ă-mīd, pro'kān-am'ĭd, -id) (USP, BP). *p*-Amino-*N*-[ 2-(diethylamino)-ethyl ]benzamide hydrochloride; differs chemically from procaine by containing the amide group (CONH) instead of the ester group (COO). It depresses the irritability of the cardiac muscle, having a quinidine-like action upon the heart, and is used in ventricular arrhythmias.

**procaine hydrochloride** (pro'kān) (USP, BP). Novocain hydrochloride; 2-diethylaminoethyl *p*-aminobenzoate

monohydrochloride; a local anesthetic used for infiltration and spinal anesthesia.

**pro'caine penicil'lin G.** See under penicillin.

**procar'bazine hydrochloride** (USP). MATULANE; *N*-iso-propyl-α-(2-methylhydrazino)-*p*-toluamide monohydrochloride; antineoplastic.

**procarbox'ypep'tidase.** Inactive precursor of a carboxy-peptidase.

**Procaryotae** (pro-kăr'ĭ-o'te) [ pro- + G. *karyon,* kernel, nut ]. A proposed kingdom of living microorganisms whose cells do not contain a limiting membrane around the nuclear material; this kingdom includes the divisions Cyanobacteria (the blue-green bacteria or cyanobacteria previously referred to as blue-green algae) and Bacteria. See also Protista; procaryote.

**procaryote** (pro-kăr'ĭ-ōt) [ pro- + G. *karyon,* kernel, nut ]. Prokaryote; a member of the Procaryotae, *q.v.;* a microorganismal cell that lacks mitochondria; its genome consists, seemingly, of a single large molecule of DNA not enclosed within a membrane, and does not undergo mitosis during replication. See also Protista.

**pro'caryot'ic.** Prokaryotic; pertaining to a procaryote.

**procatarctic** (pro-kă-tark'tik) [ G. *prokatarktikos,* beginning beforehand ]. Denoting the exciting cause of a disease.

**procatarxis** (pro-kă-tark'sis) [ G. a beginning beforehand, fr. *prokatararchō,* to begin first, fr. *pro,* before, + *kata,* upon, + *archō,* to begin ]. 1. Exciting cause. 2. The beginning of a disease under the influence of the exciting cause, a predisposition already existing.

**proce'dure.** Act or conduct of treatment or operation.
  **Ewart's p.,** elevation of the larynx between the thumb and forefinger to elicit tracheal tugging.
  **Noble-Collip p.,** induction of shock in rats by rotating them in a drum.
  **push-back p.,** a surgical maneuver designed to reposition the soft palate posteriorly and reestablish velopharyngeal competence.
  **Putti-Platt p.,** Putti-Platt *operation.*
  **shelf p.,** a graft from ilium is inserted into roof of acetabulum; for congenital dislocation of hip.
  **Stanley Way p.,** radical vulvectomy.
  **Vineberg p.,** implantation of the internal mammary artery into the myocardium to improve blood flow to the heart affected by coronary atherosclerosis.

**procelia** (pro-se'lĭ-ah) [ pro- + G. *koilia,* a hollow ]. A lateral ventricle of the brain; the hollow of the prosencephalon.

**procelous** (pro-se'lus) [ pro- + G. *koilos,* hollow ]. Concave anteriorly.

**procephalic** (pro-sĕ-fal'ik) [ pro- + G. *kephalē,* head ]. Relating to the anterior part of the head.

**procercoid** (pro-ser'koyd) [ pro- + G. *kerkos,* tail, + *eidos,* resemblance ]. An early stage in the aquatic life cycle of certain tapeworms. It develops into a tailed larva in the body cavity of a crustacean first intermediate host that ate the free-swimming embryo (coracidium). The next stage of development occurs after ingestion of the first intermediate host by a fish. The procercoid enters the new host's tissues and becomes a sparganum or plerocercoid—the infective stage to man and other fish-eating final hosts.

**proce'rus** [ L. long, stretched out ]. *Musculus procerus.*

# PROCESS

**process** (pros'es, pro'ses) [ L. *processus,* an advance, progress, process, fr. *pro-cedo,* pp. *-cessus,* to go forward ]. 1. A method or mode of action used in the attainment of a certain result. 2. An advance or progress, as of a disease; a pathologic p. 3. A projection or outgrowth; see processus. 4. In dentistry, a series of operations which convert a wax pattern, such as that of a denture base, into a solid denture base of another material; see also denture *curing.*
  **A.B.C. p.,** purification of water or deodorization of sewage by a mixture of *alum, blood,* and *charcoal.*

**accessory p.,** *processus* accessorius.

**acro′mial p.,** acromion.

**agene p.,** bleaching of flour with nitrogen trichloride (prohibited in the United States).

**a′lar p.,** *ala* cristae galli.

**alveolar p.,** *processus* alveolaris.

**anterior p. of malleus,** *processus* anterior mallei.

**apical p.,** apical dendrite; the dendritic p. extending from the apex of a pyramidal cell of the cerebral cortex toward the surface.

**articular p.,** *processus* articularis.

**ascending p.,** *processus* ascendens.

**au′ditory p.,** the roughened edge of the tympanic plate giving attachment to the cartilaginous portion of the external acoustic meatus.

**axonal p.,** axon.

**bas′ilar p.,** *pars* basilaris ossis occipitalis.

**Budde p.,** a method of sterilization of milk. To the fresh milk, hydrogen peroxide is added in proportion of 15 cc. of a 3 per cent solution to 1 liter of milk, and the mixture is heated to 51° or 52°C. (124°F.) for 3 hours; by this time the peroxide is decomposed and the nascent oxygen acts as an efficient germicide; the milk is now rapidly cooled and put into sealed bottles.

**Burns′ falciform p.,** *cornu* superius (2).

**caudate p.,** *processus* caudatus.

**ciliary p.,** *processus* ciliaris.

**Civinini′s p.,** *processus* pterygospinosus.

**clinoid p.,** *processus* clinoideus.

**cochleariform p.,** *processus* cochleariformis.

**complex learning p.'s,** those which require the use of symbolic manipulations, as in reasoning.

**condylar p.,** *processus* condylaris.

**con′dyloid p.,** *processus* condylaris.

**co′noid p.,** see *tuberculum* conoideum and *linea* trapezoidea.

**coracoid p.,** *processus* coracoideus.

**coronoid p.,** *processus* coronoideus.

**costal p.,** *processus* costarius.

**Deiters′ p.,** axon.

**dendrit′ic p.,** dendrite (1).

**dental p.,** *processus* alveolaris.

**en′siform p.,** *processus* xiphoideus.

**ethmoidal p.,** *processus* ethmoidalis.

**falciform p.,** *processus* falciformis.

**Folli′s p., Follian p.,** *processus* anterior mallei.

**foot p.,** pedicel.

**frontal p.,** *processus* frontalis.

**frontonasal p.,** in an embryo the medial elevation lying between the nasomedial p.'s and eventually merging with them to take part in the formation of the bridge of the nose and the underlying nasal septum.

**frontosphenoid′al p.,** *processus* frontalis (2).

**funic′ular p.,** the tunica vaginalis surrounding the spermatic cord.

**globular p.,** the primordial mass of tissue formed by the merging of the nasomedial p.'s of the embryo. It contributes to the primary palate and gives rise to the intermaxillary portion of the upper jaw and the prolabial portion of the upper lip.

**ham′ular p.,** hamulus.

**head p.,** the notochord.

**intrajugular p.,** *processus* intrajugularis.

**jugular p.,** *processus* jugularis.

**lacrimal p.,** *processus* lacrimalis.

**lateral p. of calcaneal tuberosity,** *processus* lateralis tuberis calcanei.

**lateral p. of malleus,** *processus* lateralis mallei.

**lateral nasal p.,** lateral nasal *fold.*

**lateral p. of talus,** *processus* lateralis tali.

**Lenhossék′s p.'s,** short p.'s ("aborted axons") possessed by some ganglion cells.

**lenticular p.,** *processus* lenticularis incudis.

**long p. of incus,** *crus* longum incudis.

**long p. of malleus,** *processus* anterior mallei.

**ma′lar p.,** *processus* zygomaticus (1).

**mamillary p.,** *processus* mamillaris.

**mandibular p.,** mandibular *arch.*

**mastoid p.,** *processus* mastoideus.

**maxillary p.,** *processus* maxillaris.

**maxillary p. (of embryo),** the part of the first pharyngeal arch that lies cranial to the stomodeum and then develops into the upper jaw.

**medial p. of calcaneal tuberosity,** *processus* medialis tuberis calcanei.

**medial nasal p.,** medial nasal *fold.*

**mental p.,** *protuberantia* mentalis.

**muscular p. of arytenoid cartilage,** *processus* muscularis cartilaginis arytenoidei.

**nasal p.,** *processus* frontalis (1).

**notochordal p.,** in the embryo, a midline column of cells migrating forward from Hensen's node to form the notochord.

**odontoid p.,** dens of second cervical vertebra.

**odon′toid p. of epistropheus,** dens.

**olec′ranon p.,** olecranon.

**orbic′ular p.,** *processus* lenticularis.

**orbital p.,** *processus* orbitalis.

**packing p.,** the method of placing denture base material in a flask for processing.

**palatal p.'s,** in the embryo, medially directed shelves from the oral surface of the maxillae; they develop into the palate after midline fusion.

**palatine p.,** *processus* palatinus.

**papillary p.,** *processus* papillaris.

**paramastoid p.,** *processus* paramastoideus.

**paroccipital p.,** *processus* paramastoideus.

**posterior p. of septal cartilage,** *processus* posterior cartilaginis septi nasi.

**primary p.,** in psychoanalysis, the mental p. directly related to the functions of the id and characteristic of unconscious mental activity; marked by unorganized, illogical thinking and by the tendency to seek immediate discharge and gratification of instinctual demands; *c.f.* secondary p.

**progressive p.'s,** those that continue after they no longer serve the needs of the organism, and after cessation of the stimulus that evoked the p.

**pterygoid p.,** *processus* pterygoideus.

**pterygospinous p.,** *processus* pterygospinosus.

**pyramidal p.,** *processus* pyramidalis.

**Rau′s p.,** *processus* anterior mallei.

**Ravius′ p.,** *processus* anterior mallei.

**secondary p.,** in psychoanalysis, the mental p. directly related to the functions of the ego and characteristic of conscious and preconscious mental activities; marked by logical thinking and by the tendency to delay gratification by regulation of the discharge of instinctual demands, *c.f.* primary p.

**sheath p. of sphenoid bone,** *processus* vaginalis ossis sphenoidalis.

**short p. of incus,** *crus* breve incudis.

**short p. of malleus,** *processus* lateralis mallei.

**slender p. of malleus,** *processus* anterior mallei.

**sphenoid p.,** see *processus* posterior cartilaginis septi nasi, and *processus* sphenoidalis (1).

**spi′nous p.,** (1) *spina* angularis; (2) *processus* spinosus.

**spinous p. of tibia,** *eminentia* intercondylaris.

**Stieda′s p.,** *processus* posterior tali.

**styloid p. of fibula,** *apex* capitis fibulae.

**styloid p. of radius,** *processus* styloideus radii.

**styloid p. of temporal bone,** *processus* styloideus ossis temporalis.

**styloid p. of third metacarpal bone,** *processus* styloideus ossis metacarpalis III.

**styloid p. of ulna,** *processus* styloideus ulnae.

**superior articular p. of sacrum,** *processus* articularis superior ossis sacri.

**supracondylar p.,** *processus* supracondylaris humeri.

**temporal p.,** *processus* temporalis.

**Tomes′ p.'s,** p.'s of the enamel cells.

**transverse p.,** *processus* transversus.

**troch′lear p.,** *trochlea* peronealis.

**unciform p.,** *processus* uncinatus.

**uncinate p.,** *processus* uncinatus.

**vag′inal p.,** *vagina* processus styloidei.

**vaginal p. of peritoneum,** *processus* vaginalis peritonei.

**vag′inal p. of the testis,** *processus* vaginalis peritonei.

**vermiform p.,** *appendix* vermiformis.

**xiphoid p.,** *processus* xiphoideus.

**zygomatic p.,** *processus* zygomaticus maxillae.

# PROCESSUS

**proces'sus,** pl. **proces'sus** [ L. see process ] [ NA ]. A process; in anatomy, a projection or outgrowth.

**p. accesso'rius** [ NA ], accessory process; accessory tubercle; a small apophysis at the posterior part of the base of the transverse process of each of the lumbar vertebrae.

**p. alveola'ris** [ NA ], alveolar process, ridge, or body; basal ridge (1); the projecting ridge on the undersurface of the body of the maxilla containing the tooth sockets; the term is sometimes applied to the upper border of the body of the mandible, containing the tooth sockets of the lower jaw. See also alveolar *bone* (2).

**p. anterior mallei** [ NA ], anterior or long process of the malleus; p. gracilis; Folli's, Rau's, or Ravius' process; p. ravii; a slender spur running anteriorward from the neck of the malleus toward the petrotympanic fissure.

**p. articula'ris** [ NA ], articular process; zygapophysis [ NA ]; one of the small flat projections on the superior and inferior surfaces of the arches of the vertebrae (**p. articularis superior** and **p. articularis inferior**), on either side, at the point where the pedicles and laminae join, forming the zygapophysial joint surfaces.

**p. articula'ris supe'rior os'sis sa'cri** [ NA ], superior articular process of the sacrum; the large process on each side of the sacrum posteriorly that articulates with the corresponding inferior articular process of the fifth lumbar vertebra.

**p. ascen'dens,** ascending process; an upward extension of the embryonic pterygoquadrate cartilage; it develops into the greater wing of the sphenoid bone.

**p. brev'is,** p. lateralis mallei.

**p. cauda'tus** [ NA ], caudate process; a narrow band of hepatic tissue connecting the caudate and right lobes of the liver, dividing the right sagittal fissure into two.

**p. cilia'ris** [ NA ], ciliary process; one of the radiating pigmented ridges, usually seventy in number, on the inner surface of the ciliary body, increasing in thickness as they advance from the orbiculus to the external border of the iris; these, together with the folds (plicae) in the furrows between them, constitute the corona ciliaris.

**p. clinoi'deus** [ NA ], clinoid process; clinoid; one of three pairs of bony projections from the sphenoid bone: the anterior (p. clinoideus anterior) is the recurved posterior angle of the lesser wing; the middle (p. clinoideus medius) is a little spur of bone on the body of the sphenoid, posterolateral to the tuberculum sellae; the posterior (p. clinoideus posterior) is a spur of bone at each superior angle of the dorsum sellae.

**p. cochlearifor'mis** [ NA ], cochleariform process; a bony angular process (the termination of the septum canalis musculotubarii) above the anterior end of the vestibular window, forming a pulley over which the tendon of the tensor tympani muscle plays.

**p. condyla'ris** [ NA ], condylar or condyloid process; mandibular condyle; the articular process of the ramus of the mandible; it contains the caput mandibulae, collum mandibulae, and fovea pterygoidea.

**p. coracoi'deus** [ NA ], coracoid process; a long curved projection from the neck of the scapula overhanging the glenoid cavity; it gives attachment to the short head of the biceps, the coracobrachialis, and the pectoralis minor muscles, and the conoid and coracoacromial ligaments.

**p. coronoi'deus** [ NA ], coronoid process; (1) the triangular anterior process of the mandibular ramus, giving attachment to the temporal muscle; (2) a bracket-like projection from the anterior portion of the proximal extremity of the ulna; its anterior surface gives attachment to the brachialis, its proximal surface enters into the formation of the trochlear notch.

**p. costa'rius** [ NA ], costal process; an apophysis extending laterally from the transverse process of a lumbar vertebra; it is the homologue of the rib.

**p. ethmoida'lis** [ NA ], ethmoidal process; a projection of the inferior concha, situated behind the lacrimal process and articulating with the uncinate process of the ethmoid.

**p. falcifor'mis** [ NA ], falciform process; falciform ligament; a continuation of the inner border of the sacrotuberous ligament upward and forward on the inner aspect of the ramus of the ischium.

**p. ferrei'ni,** *pars* radiata lobuli corticalis renis.

**p. fronta'lis** [ NA ], frontal process; (1) nasal process; the upward extension from the body of the maxilla, which articulates with the frontal bone; (2) frontosphenoidal process; the process of the zygomatic bone which extends upward to form the lateral margin of the orbit and articulates with the frontal bone and greater wing of the sphenoid bone.

**p. intrajugula'ris** [ NA ], intrajugular process; a small pointed process of bone extending from the middle of the jugular notch in both the occipital and the temporal bones, the two being joined by a ligament and dividing the jugular foramen into two portions.

**p. jugula'ris** [ NA ], jugular process; a short process jutting out from the posterior part of the condyle of the occipital bone, its anterior border forming the posterior boundary of the jugular foramen.

**p. lacrima'lis** [ NA ], lacrimal process; a projection from the anterior edge of the inferior concha which articulates with the lower border of the lacrimal bone.

**p. latera'lis mal'lei** [ NA ], lateral process of the malleus; p. brevis; tuberculum mallei; a short projection from the base of the manubrium of the malleus, attached firmly to the drum membrane.

**p. latera'lis ta'li** [ NA ], lateral process of the talus; a projection on the lateral side of the talus below the malleolar articular surface.

**p. latera'lis tu'beris calca'nei** [ NA ], lateral process of the calcaneal tuberosity; the lateral projection from the posterior part of the calcaneus.

**p. lenticula'ris in'cudis** [ NA ], lenticular process, apophysis, or bone; os orbiculare; os sylvii; (1) a knob at the tip of the long limb of the incus which articulates with the stapes; (2) an ossicle which, toward the end of fetal life, unites with the incus to form the lenticular process.

**p. mamilla'ris** [ NA ], mamillary process or tubercle; a small apophysis or tubercle on the dorsal margin of the superior articular process of each of the lumbar vertebrae and usually of the twelfth thoracic vertebra.

**p. mastoi'deus** [ NA ], mastoid process; mastoid bone; temporal apophysis; the nipple-like projection of the petrous part of the temporal bone.

**p. maxilla'ris** [ NA ], maxillary process; a thin plate of irregular form projecting from the middle of the upper border of the inferior concha, articulating with the maxilla bone and partly closing the orifice of the maxillary sinus.

**p. media'lis tu'beris calca'nei** [ NA ], medial process of the calcaneal tuberosity; the medial projection posteriorly from the calcaneus.

**p. muscula'ris cartila'ginis arytenoi'dei** [ NA ], muscular process of the arytenoid cartilage; the blunt lateral projection giving attachment to several intrinsic muscles of the larynx.

**p. orbita'lis** [ NA ], orbital process; the anterior and larger of the two processes at the upper extremity of the vertical plate of the palatine bone, articulating with the maxilla, ethmoid, and sphenoid bones.

**p. palati'nus** [ NA ], palatine process; the horizontal plate of the maxilla, forming with its fellow the anterior portion of the roof of the mouth.

**p. papilla'ris** [ NA ], papillary process; the left lower angle of the caudate lobe of the liver, opposite the caudate process.

**p. paramastoi'deus** [ NA ], paramastoid process; an occasional process of bone extending downward from the intrajugular process of the occipital bone in man.

**p. poste'rior cartila'ginis septi nasi** [ NA ], p. sphenoidalis cartilaginis septi nasi [ NA ]; posterior or sphenoid process of the septal cartilage; the tapering extension of the septal cartilage that lies between the perpendicular plate of the ethmoid and the vomer.

**p. poste'rior ta'li** [ NA ], Stieda's process; a process on the posterior aspect of the talus.

**p. pterygoi'deus** [ NA ], pterygoid process; a long process extending downward from the junction of the body and great wing of the sphenoid bone on either side; it is formed of two plates (*lamina lateralis* and *lamina medialis*), united anteriorly but separated below to form the pterygoid notch; the pterygoid fossa is formed by the divergence of these two plates posteriorly.

**p. pterygospino'sus** [ NA ], pterygospinous process; Civinini's process; a sharp projection from the posterior edge of the lateral pterygoid plate of the sphenoid bone.

**p. pyramida'lis** [ NA ], pyramidal process; the portion of the palatine bone passing lateral and posterior from the angle formed by the vertical and horizontal plates.

**p. ra'vii,** p. anterior mallei.

**p. retromandibula'ris,** that portion of the parotid salivary gland that is located behind the mandible and occupies the space between the ramus of the mandible and the mastoid process extending as far medially as the pharyngeal wall; also known as the p. retromandibularis glandulae parotidis.

**p. sphenoida'lis** [ NA ], sphenoid process; (1) the posterior and smaller of the two processes at the extremity of the vertical plate of the palatine bone; (2) p. posterior cartilaginis septi nasi.

**p. spinosus** [ NA ], spinous process; the dorsal projection from the center of a vertebral arch.

**p. styloi'deus os'sis metacarpa'lis III** [ NA ], styloid process of third metacarpal bone; a pointed projection from the dorsolateral angle of the base of the third metacarpal bone; it sometimes exists as a separate ossicle.

**p. styloi'deus os'sis tempora'lis** [ NA ], styloid process of temporal bone; a slender pointed projection running downward and slightly forward from the base of the inferior surface of the petrous portion of the temporal bone where it joins the tympanic portion; it gives attachment to the styloglossus, stylohyoid, and stylopharyngeus muscles and the stylohyoid and stylomandibular ligaments.

**p. styloi'deus ra'dii** [ NA ], styloid process of the radius; a thick; pointed projection on the lateral side of the distal extremity of the radius.

**p. styloi'deus ul'nae** [ NA ], styloid process of the ulna; a cylindrical, pointed projection from the medial and posterior aspect of the head of the ulna, to the tip of which is attached the radial collateral ligament of the wrist.

**p. supracondyla'ris hu'meri** [ NA ], supracondylar process; an occasional spine projecting from the anteromedial surface of the humerus about 5 cm. above the medial epicondyle to which it is joined by a fibrous band. The supracondylar foramen thus formed transmits the brachial artery and median nerve.

**p. tempora'lis** [ NA ], temporal process; the posterior projection of the zygomatic bone articulating with the zygomatic process of the temporal bone to form the zygomatic arch.

**p. transver'sus** [ NA ], transverse process; projecting on either side of the arch of a vertebra.

**p. trochlearis,** *trochlea* peronealis.

**p. uncina'tus os'sis ethmoida'lis** [ NA ], uncinate process of ethmoid bone; a sickle-shaped process of bone on the medial wall of the ethmoidal labyrinth below the middle concha; it articulates with the ethmoidal process of the inferior concha and partly closes the orifice of the maxillary sinus.

**p. uncina'tus pancre'atis** [ NA ], uncinate process of pancreas; lesser, small, uncinate, or unciform pancreas; pancreas of Willis or Winslow; a portion of the head of the pancreas that hooks around posterior to the superior mesenteric vessels.

**p. vagina'lis os'sis sphenoida'lis** [ NA ], sheath process of the sphenoid bone; a thin lamina of bone that extends medially under the body of the sphenoid bone from the medial lamina of the pterygoid process. It articulates with the vomer and the palatine bone.

**p. vagina'lis peritone'i** [ NA ], vaginal process of the peritoneum; a peritoneal diverticulum in the embryonic lower anterior abdominal wall that traverses the inguinal canal. It forms the tunica vaginalis testis and normally loses its connection with the peritoneal cavity. A persistent p. vaginalis in the female is known as the canal of Nuck.

**p. vermifor'mis,** *appendix* vermiformis.

**p. voca'lis cartila'ginis arytenoi'dei** [ NA ], the lower end of the anterior margin of the arytenoid cartilage to which the vocal cord is attached.

**p. xiphoid'eus** [ NA ], xiphoid or ensiform process or cartilage; ensisternum; metasternum; the cartilage at the lower end of the sternum.

**p. zygomat'icus** [ NA ], zygomatic process; (1) malar process; the rough projection from the maxilla that articulates with the zygomatic bone; (2) the massive projection of the frontal bone that joins the zygomatic bone to form the lateral margin of the orbit; (3) the anterior process of the temporal bone that articulates with the temporal process of the zygomatic bone to form the zygomatic arch.

**prochlorperazine** (pro'klōr-pěr'ă-zēn) (USP). COMPAZINE; 2-chloro-10-[ 3-(1-methyl-4-piperazinyl)propyl ]phenothiazine. A phenothiazine compound similar in structure, actions, and uses to chlorpromazine but more potent. A tranquilizer, used in the treatment of anxiety and tension and to combat nausea and vomiting.

**p. edisylate** (USP), same actions as p.; administered orally or intramuscularly.

**p. maleate** (USP, BP), COMPAZINE maleate; same actions and uses as p.; for oral administration.

**prochondral** (pro-kon'dral) [ pro- + G. *chondros,* cartilage ]. Denoting a developmental stage prior to the formation of cartilage.

**prochordal** (pro-kor'dal). Prechordal; located cephalic to the notochord.

**procidentia** (pros-ĭ-den'shĭ-ah, pro'sĭ-) [ L. a falling forward, fr. *procido,* to fall forward. CAD- ]. A sinking down or prolapse of any organ or part, as of the uterus.

**p. uteri,** see *prolapse* of the uterus.

**procollagen** (pro-kol'ă-jen). Soluble precursor of collagen, presumably formed by the fibroblast in the process of collagen synthesis.

**proconver'tin.** *Factor* VII.

**procreate** (pro'kre-āt) [ L. *pro-creo,* pp. -*creatus,* to beget ]. To beget; to produce by the sexual act; said usually of the male parent.

**procreation** (pro-kre-a'shun). The act of procreating or begetting.

**procreative** (pro'kre-a-tiv). Having the power to beget or procreate.

**proct-.** See procto-.

**proctagra** (prok'tag'rah) [ proct- + G. *agra,* a seizure ]. Proctalgia.

**proctalgia** (prok-tal'jĭ-ah) [ proct- + G. *algos,* pain ]. Proctagra; proctodynia; pain at the anus, or in the rectum.

**p. fugax,** anorectal spasm; painful spasm of the muscle about the anus without known cause; probably a neurosis.

**proctatresia** (prok'tă-tre'zĭ-ah) [ proct- + G. *a-* priv. + *trēsis,* a boring ]. Imperforate *anus.*

**proctectasia** (prok'tek-ta'zĭ-ah) [ proct- + G. *ektasis,* extension ]. Dilation of the anus or rectum.

**proctectomy** (prok-tek'to-mĭ) [ proct- + G. *ektomē,* excision ]. Exsection of the rectum.

**proctenclisis, proctencleisis** (prok'ten-kli'sis) [ proct- + G. *enkleisis,* enclosure ]. Stricture of the anus or rectum.

**procteurynter** (prok-tu-rin'tur) [ proct- + G. *eurynō,* to dilate, fr. *eurys,* wide ]. A dilatable bag for dilating the rectum.

**proctitis** (prok-ti'tis) [ proct- + G. suffix -*itis,* inflammation ]. Inflammation of the mucous membrane of the rectum.

**epidemic gangrenous p.,** caribi; Indian sickness; a generally fatal disease affecting chiefly children in the tropics, characterized by gangrenous ulceration of the rectum and anus, accompanied by frequent watery stools and tenesmus.

**idiopathic p.,** chronic ulcerative p.; probably a variant of ulcerative colitis, which in some cases progresses to involve the colon as well.

**procto-, proct-** (prok'to-) [ G. *prōktos,* anus ]. Combining forms signifying anus or, more frequently, rectum.

**proctocele** (prok'to-sēl) [ procto- + G. *kēlē,* tumor ]. Rectocele.

**proctoclysis,** pl. **proctoclyses** (prok-tok′lĭ-sis, -sēz) [ procto- + G. *klysis,* a washing out ]. Irrigation of the rectum and sigmoid colon by large amounts of saline solution usually by slow continuous drip. See also Murphy *method.*

**proctococcypexy** (prok-to-kok′sĭ-peks-ĭ) [ procto- + G. *kokkyx,* coccyx, + *pēxis,* fixation ]. Suture of a prolapsing rectum to the tissues anterior to the coccyx.

**proctocolitis** (prok′to-ko-li′tis). Coloproctitis.

**proctocolonoscopy** (prok′to-ko′lo-nos′ko-pĭ) [ procto- + G. *kolon,* colon, + *skopeō,* to view ]. Inspection of interior of rectum and colon.

**proctocolpoplasty** (prok′to-kol′po-plas-tĭ) [ procto- + G. *kolpos,* bosom (vagina), + *plassō,* to form ]. Proctoelytroplasty; plastic closure of a rectovaginal fistula.

**proctocystocele** (prok′to-sis′to-sēl) [ procto- + G. *kystis,* bladder, + *kēlē,* hernia ]. Herniation of the bladder into the rectum.

**proctocystoplasty** (prok′to-sis′to-plas-tĭ) [ procto- + G. *kystis,* bladder, + *plassō,* to form ]. Surgical closure of a rectovesical fistula.

**proctocystotomy** (prok′to-sis-tot′o-mĭ) [ procto- + G. *kystis,* bladder, + *tomē,* incision ]. Incision into the bladder from the rectum.

**proctodeum,** pl. **proctodea** (prok′to-de′um, -de′ah) [ L. fr. G. *prōktos,* anus + *hodaios,* on the way, fr. *hodos,* a way ]. 1. An ectodermally lined depression under the root of the tail, adjacent to the terminal part of the embryonic hindgut. At its bottom, proctodeal ectoderm and cloacal entoderm form the cloacal plate. When this epithelial plate ruptures, the anal and urogenital external orifices are established. 2. The terminal portion of the insect alimentary canal; it extends from the pylorus (area of Malpighian tubule attachment) to the anal opening. In certain diptera (flies) and other insects, it is divided into a tubular anterior intestine and an enlarged posterior intestine, or rectum, ending at the anus.

**proctodone** (prok′to-dōn). A substance postulated to be formed by the proctodeum, a portion of the anterior intestine in insects; it terminates the diapause, presumably by stimulating the insect brain to secrete brain hormone.

**proctodynia** (prok′to-din′ĭ-ah) [ procto- + G. *odynē,* pain ]. Proctalgia.

**proctoelytroplasty** (prok-to-el′ĭ-tro-plas-tĭ) [ procto- + G. *elytron,* sheath (vagina), + *plassō,* to form ]. Proctocolpoplasty.

**proctologic** (prok-to-loj′ik). Relating to proctology.

**proctologist** (prok-tol′o-jist). A specialist in proctology.

**proctology** (prok-tol′o-jĭ) [ procto- + G. *logos,* study ]. The branch of surgical science that deals with the anus and rectum and their diseases.

**proctomenia** (prok′to-me′nĭ-ah) [ procto- + G. *mēn,* month; L. pl. *menses, q. v.* ]. Vicarious menstruation involving the rectum.

**proctoparalysis** (prok′to-pă-ral′ĭ-sis). Paralysis of the anus, leading to incontinence of feces.

**proctoperineoplasty** (prok′to-pĕr-ĭ-ne′o-plas′tĭ) [ procto- + perineum, + G. *plassō,* to form ]. A plastic operation on anus and perineum.

**proctoperineorrhaphy** (prok′to-pĕr′ĭ-ne-or′ă-fĭ) [ procto- + perineum, + G. *rhaphē,* suture ]. Proctoperineoplasty.

**proctopexy** (prok′to-pek-sĭ) [ procto- + G. *pēxis,* fixation ]. Surgical fixation of a prolapsing rectum.

**proctophobia** (prok′to-fo′bĭ-ah) [ procto- + G. *phobos,* fear ]. Rectophobia; a morbid fear of rectal disease.

**proctoplasty** (prok′to-plas-tĭ) [ procto- + G. *plassō,* to form ]. Reparative or plastic surgery of the anus or of the rectum.

**proctoplegia** (prok′to-ple′jĭ-ah) [ procto- + G. *plēge,* stroke ]. Paralysis of the anus and rectum occurring with paraplegia.

**proctopolypus** (prok′to-pol′ĭ-pus). Polypus of the rectum.

**proctoptosia, proctoptosis** (prok-top-to′sĭ-ah, -to′sis) [ procto- + G. *ptōsis,* a falling ]. Prolapse of the rectum and anus.

**proctorrhagia** (proc-to-ra′jĭ-ah) [ procto- + G. *rhēgnymi,* to burst forth ]. State characterized by having a bloody discharge from the anus.

**proctorrhaphy** (prok-tor′ă-fĭ) [ procto- + G. *rhaphē,* suture ]. Repair by suture of a lacerated rectum or anus.

**proctorrhea** (prok-to-re′ah) [ procto- + G. *rhoia,* a flow ]. A mucoserous discharge from the rectum.

**proctoscope** (prok′to-skōp) [ procto- + G. *skopeō,* to view ]. A rectal speculum.
   **Tuttle's p.,** a tubular speculum with electric light at its distal extremity; after introduction the obturator is withdrawn and a glass window is inserted in the proximal end; then by means of a rubber bulb and tube connected with the p. the rectal ampulla may be inflated.

**proctoscopy** (prok-tos′ko-pĭ). Examination of the rectum and anus.

**proctosigmoidectomy** (prok′to-sig-moy-dek′to-mĭ) [ procto- + sigmoid, + G. *ektomē,* excision ]. Excision of the rectum and sigmoid colon.

**proctosigmoiditis** (prok′to-sig-moy-di′tis) [ procto- + sigmoid + G. suffix *-itis,* inflammation ]. Inflammation of the sigmoid colon and rectum.

**proctosigmoidoscopy** (prok′to-sig-moy-dos′ko-pĭ) [ procto- + sigmoid + G. *skopeō,* to view ]. Direct inspection through a sigmoidoscope of the rectum and sigmoid colon.

**proctospasm** (prok′to-spazm) [ procto- + G. *spasmos,* spasm ]. 1. Spasmodic stricture of the anus. 2. Spasmodic contraction of the rectum.

**proctostasis** (prok-tos′tă-sis) [ procto- + G. *stasis,* a standing ]. Constipation with stasis in the rectum and anus.

**proctostat** (prok′to-stat [ procto- + G. *statos,* standing ]. A tube containing radium for insertion through the anus in the treatment of rectal cancer.

**proctostenosis** (prok′to-stĕ-no′sis) [ procto- + G. *stenōsis,* a narrowing ]. Stricture of the rectum or anus.

**proctostomy** (prok-tos′to-mĭ) [ procto- + G. *stoma,* mouth ]. The formation of an articial opening into the rectum.

**proctotome** (prok′to-tōm). An instrument for use in proctotomy.

**proctotomy** (prok-tot′o-mĭ) [ procto- + G. *tomē,* incision ]. An incision, for the relief of a stricture or for any other purpose, into the rectum.

**proctotresia** (prok-to-tre′zĭ-ah) [ procto- + G. *trēsis,* a boring ]. Operation for the relief of an imperforate anus.

**proctovalvotomy** (prok′to-val-vot′o-mĭ). Incision of rectal valves.

**procumbent** (pro-kum′bent) [ L. *procumbens,* falling or leaning forward ]. In a prone position; lying face down.

**procurva′tion** [ L. *pro-curvo,* to bend forward ]. A bending forward.

**procyclidine hydrochloride** (pro-si′klĭ-dēn) (NF, BP). KEMADRIN; 1-cyclohexyl-1-phenyl-3-pyrrolidino-1-propanol hydrochloride; has predominantly atropine-like actions, exerting an antispasmodic effect on smooth and voluntary muscles; used in the treatment of paralysis agitans and drug-induced parkinsonism.

**procy′clidine methochloride.** ELORINE chloride; TRICOLOID chloride; tricyclamol chloride (BP); 1-(3-cyclohexyl-3-hydroxy-3-phenylpropyl) -1- methylpyrrolidinium chloride; an anticholinergic drug used in the treatment of functional gastrointestinal spasm.

**prodeco′nium bromide.** [ Decamethylenebis(oxyethylene) ]bis[ (carboxymethyl)dimethylammonium bromide ]-dipropyl ester; neuromuscular blocking agent.

**prodigiosin** (pro-dij′ĭ-o′sin). A blood-red antibiotic substance produced by *Chromobacterium prodigiosum* (*Serratia marcesens*), active against the anthrax bacillus, *Entamoeba histolytica,* and fungi.

**prodil′idine hydrochloride** (USAN). COGESIC; 1,2-dimethyl-3-phenyl-3-pyrrolidinol propionate (ester) hydrochloride; analgesic.

**α-prodine hydrochloride.** See alphaprodine hydrochloride.

**prodromal** (prod′ro-mal, pro-dro′mal). Prodromic; relating to a prodrome.

**prodrome** (pro′drōm) [ G. *prodromos,* a running before, fr. pro- + *dromos,* a running, a course ]. An early or premonitory symptom of a disease.

**prodrom'ic, prod'romous.** Prodromal.

**prod'romus,** pl. **prod'romi.** Prodrome.

**product** (prod'ukt) [ L. *productus,* fr. *pro-duco,* pp. *-ductus,* to lead forth. DUC- ]. Anything produced or made, either naturally or artificially.

    **cleavage p.,** a substance resulting from the splitting of a molecule into two or more simpler molecules.

    **fission p.,** an atomic species produced in the course of the fission of a massive atom such as U235.

    **spallation p.,** an atomic species produced in the course of the spallation of any atom.

    **substitution p.,** a p. obtained by replacing one atom or group in a molecule with another atom or group.

**productive** (pro-duk'tiv) [ see product ]. Producing or capable of producing; denoting especially an inflammation leading to the production of new tissue with or without an exudate.

**proemial** (pro-e'mĭ-al) [ L. *prooemium,* fr. G. *prooimion,* prelude ]. Prodromal.

**proencephalon** (pro-en-sef'ă-lon). Prosencephalon.

**proencephalus** (pro-en-sef'ă-lus) [ pro- + G. *enkephalos,* brain ]. A fetus with a large part of the brain protruding through a cranial defect in the frontal region.

**proenzyme** (pro-en'zim). Zymogen; proferment; the precursor of an enzyme, requiring some change (usually the hydrolysis of an inhibiting fragment that masks an active grouping) to render it active. Examples are pepsinogen, trypsinogen, and profibrolysin.

**proerythroblast** (pro'ĕ-rith'ro-blast). Pronormoblast; see discussion under erythroblast.

**proerythrocyte** (pro'ĕ-rith'ro-sīt). The precursor of an erythrocyte; an immature red blood cell with a nucleus.

**proestrogen** (pro-es'tro-jen). An estrogen that acts only after it has been metabolized in the body to an active compound.

**proestrum** (pro-es'trum). Proestrus.

**proestrus** (pro-es'trus) [ pro- + estrus, *q. v.* ]. Proestrum; the period in the estrus cycle preceding estrus. It is characterized by the growth of the Graafian follicles and physiologic changes related to estrogen production.

**profadol hydrochloride** (pro'fă-dōl) (USAN). *m*-(1-Methyl-3-propyl-3-pyrrolidinyl)phenol hydrochloride; an analgesic drug.

**profen'amine hydrochloride.** Ethopropazine hydrochloride.

**profer'ment.** Proenzyme.

**Profeta** (pro-fa'tah), Giuseppe, Italian dermatologist, 1840–1910. See P.'s *law.*

**profibrinolysin** (pro-fi'brĭ-nol'ĭ-sin). Plasminogen.

**Profichet** (pro-fe-sha'), Georges C., French physician, *1873. See P.'s *disease.*

**pro'file** [ It. *profilo,* fr. L. *pro,* forward, + *filum,* thread, line (contour) ]. 1. An outline or contour, especially one representing a side view of the human head. 2. A summary or brief account.

    **facial p.,** (1) the outline form of the face from a lateral view; (2) the sagittal outline form of the face.

    **personality p.,** (1) a method by which the results of psychological testing are presented in graphic form; (2) a vignette or brief personality description.

**profilometer** (pro'fĭ-lom'e-ter). An instrument for measuring the roughness of a surface, *e.g.,* of teeth.

**proflavine hem'isul'fate** (pro-fla'vin, -vēn) (BP). The neutral sulfate of 3,6-diaminoacridine; a compound closely allied to acriflavine, having similar antiseptic properties.

**pro'fondom'eter** [ Fr. *profondeur,* depth, + G. *metron,* measure ]. A device for fluoroscopically locating a foreign body by securing three lines of sight each of which passes through the foreign body.

**profunda** (pro-fun'dah) [ L. fem. of *profundus,* deep ]. A term applied to several arteries the course of which lies deep in the tissues; see under arteria.

**profundus** (pro-fun'dus) [ L. ] [ NA ]. Deep; profound.

**progas'ter** [ pro- + G. *gastēr,* belly ]. Old and rarely used term for archenteron.

**progas'trin.** Precursor of gastric secretion in the mucous membrane of the stomach.

**progenitalis** (pro-jen-ĭ-ta'lis) [ L. ]. On any of the exposed surfaces of the genitalia.

**progenitor** (pro-jen'ĭ-tor) [ L. ]. A precursor; ancestor; one who begets.

**progeny** (proj'ĕ-nĭ) [ L. *progenies,* fr. *progigno,* to beget ]. Offspring; descendents.

**progeria** (pro-je'rĭ-ah) [ pro- + G. *gēras,* old age ]. Hutchinson-Gilford disease or syndrome; progeria or premature senility syndrome; a condition in which a relatively young person has some physical characteristics of senility, particularly in regard to the face; in some dwarfs it is a manifestation of craniofacial anomalies.

    **p. with cataract, p. with microphthalmia,** see *dyscephalia* mandibulo-oculofacialis.

**progestational** (pro'jes-ta'shun-al). 1. Favoring pregnancy; conducive to gestation; having a stimulating effect upon the uterine changes essential for the implantation and growth of the fertilized ovum (secretory endometrium). 2. Referring to progesterone.

**progesterone** (pro-jes'ter-ōn) (USP, BP). Corpus luteum hormone; luteohormone; 4-pregnene-3,20-dione (for structure of pregnene, see steroids); a progestin; an antiestrogenic steroid believed to be the active principle of the corpus luteum, isolated from the corpus luteum and placenta or synthetically prepared. Used to correct abnormalities of the menstrual cycle.

**α-progesterone and β-progesterone.** Isomeric forms of progesterone with melting points 128°C. and 121°C., respectively. Occasionally referred to as luteosterone C and D or progestin B and C.

**progestin** (pro-jes'tin). 1. A hormone of the corpus luteum. 2. The generic term for any substance, natural or synthetic, that effects some or all of the biological changes produced by progesterone; a progestational substance.

**progestogen** (pro-jes'to-jen). 1. Any agent capable of producing biological effects similar to those of progesterone; most p.'s are steroids like the natural hormones. 2. A synthetic derivative from testosterone or progesterone that has some of the physiologic activity and pharmacologic effects of progesterone; progesterone is antiestrogenic, whereas some progestogens have estrogenic or androgenic properties in addition to progestational activity.

**proglos'sis** [ pro- + G. *glōssa,* tongue ]. The anterior portion, or tip, of the tongue.

**proglottid,** pl. **proglottids, proglottides** (pro-glot'id, -idz, -ĭ-dēz) [ pro- + G. *glōssa,* tongue ]. Proglottis; one of the segments of a tapeworm, containing the reproductive organs.

**proglot'tis.** Proglottid.

**prognathic** (prog-nath'ik) [ pro- + G. *gnathos,* jaw ]. Prognathous; having a projecting jaw; having a gnathic index above 103.

**prognathism** (prog'nă-thizm). The condition of being prognathic; abnormal projection foward of one or of both jaws.

    **basilar p.,** the concave facial profile, or forward position of the chin, resembling mandibular p., created by the prominence of the bone of the mandible at the chin or menton.

**prognathous** (prog'nă-thus). Prognathic.

**prognose** (prog-nōs', -nōz'). Prognosticate.

**prognosis** (prog-no'sis) [ G. *prognōsis,* fr. *pro,* before, + *gignōskō,* to know. GNO- ]. The foretelling of the probable course of a disease; a forecast of the outcome of a disease.

    **denture p.,** an opinion or judgment, given in advance of treatment, of the prospects for success in the construction and usefulness of a denture or restoration.

**prognostic** (prog-nos'tik) [ G. *prognōstikos* ]. 1. Relating to prognosis. 2. A symptom upon which a prognosis is based.

**prognosticate** (prog-nos'tĭ-kāt). Prognose; to give a prognosis.

**prognostician** (prog-nos-tish'un). One skilled in prognosis.

**progonoma** (pro'gon-o'mah) [ pro- + G. *gonos,* offspring (GEN-), + suffix *-oma,* tumor ]. A nodule or mass resulting from displacement of tissue when atavism (or reversion) occurs in embryonic development; a p. represents structures that do not occur in the normal individual of that species, but are observed in the ancestral forms of the species.

**p. of jaw,** melanotic neuroectodermal *tumor.*

**melanot'ic p.,** a pigmented hairy nevus.

**progranulocyte** (pro-gran′u-lo-sīt). Promyelocyte.

**progress** (prog′res) [ L. *pro-gredior,* pp. *-gressus,* to go forth, fr. *gradior,* to step, go, fr. *gradus,* a step ]. Advance; course of a disease.

**progress** (pro-gres′). To advance; to go forward; said of a disease, especially, when unqualified, of one taking an unfavorable course.

**progressive** (pro-gres′iv). Going forward; advancing; denoting the course of a disease, especially, when unqualified, an unfavorable course, as p. paralysis, p. atrophy.

**proguanil hydrochloride** (pro-gwah′nil) (BP). Chloroguanide hydrochloride.

**prohep'tazine.** DIMEPHEPRIMINE; hexahydro-1,3-dimethyl-4-phenylazepin-4-ol propionate; analgesic.

**pro′hor′mone.** 1. An intraglandular precursor of a hormone, such as proinsulin; not synonymous with prehormone, *q.v.* 2. An obsolete term formerly used to designate a substance developed in serum that antagonizes a specific antihormone, and thus enhances the action of the corresponding hormone.

**pro′insulin.** A single-chain precursor of insulin.

**proiosystole** (pro-ī-o-sis′to-lī) [ G. *prōios,* early, + *systolē,* a contracting ]. A heart beat occurring ahead of schedule; a premature systole; see hysterosystole.

**proiosystolia** (pro-ī-o-sis-to′lī-ah). Condition in which proiosystoles occur.

**projec′tio** [ L. ] [ NA ]. Projection (2).

**projec′tion** [ L. *projectio;* fr. *pro-jicio,* pp. *-jectus,* to throw before, fr. *jacio,* to throw ]. 1. A pushing out. 2. A prominence. 3. The referring of a sensation to the object producing it. 4. A defense mechanism involving the referring to another of a repressed complex in the individual, as when one reprobates in others faults to the commission of which he himself has a constant inclination. 5. The conception by the consciousness of a mental occurrence belonging to the self as of external origin. 6. Localization of visual impressions: straight ahead, right or left, above or below. 7. In neuroanatomy, the system or systems of nerve fibers by which a group of nerve cells discharges its nerve impulses ("projects") to one or more other cell groups.

**erroneous p.,** a miscalculation as to the exact position of an object, owing to a misjudgment of the effort required to focus it resulting from paresis of the eye muscles.

**projicient** (pro-jish′ent) [ L. *projicio,* to throw forth ]. Relating the organism to its environment.

**proka′ryote.** Procaryote.

**pro′karyot′ic.** Procaryotic.

**prola′bium** [ pro- + L. *labium,* lip ]. 1. The exposed carmine margin of the lip. 2. The small elevation at the termination of the philtrum.

**prolac′tin.** A hormone (a protein) of the anterior lobe of the hypophysis cerebri that stimulates the secretion of milk and possibly during pregnancy, breast growth; also lactogenic, mammogenic, or galactopoietic factor or hormone.

**prolamine** (pro-lam′ēn, pro′lă-mēn, -min). Protein insoluble in water or neutral salt solutions, soluble in dilute acids or alkalies, and in dilute (70 to 90 per cent) alcohol. Gliadin, hordein, and zein are p.'s.

**pro′lan.** An early, now obsolete, designation for urinary gonadotrophin.

**p. A,** a urinary gonadotrophin exhibiting follicle-stimulating hormone-like effects; obsolete usage.

**p. B,** a urinary gonadotrophin exhibiting luteinizing hormone-like effects; obsolete usage.

**prolapse** (pro-laps′) [ L. *prolapsus* (noun), a falling, fr. *pro-labor,* pp. *-lapsus,* to slide forward; *prolabi;* to fall forward ]. 1. To fall or sink down, said of an organ or other part. 2. A falling down of an organ or other part, especially its appearance at a natural or articicial orifice; procidentia; ptosis.

**p. of the corpus luteum,** ectropion of the corpus luteum, due to eversion of the granulosa membrane through the opening in the ruptured follicle; this occurs normally in certain animals.

**Morgagni's p.,** chronic inflammation of Morgagni's ventricle.

**p. of umbilical cord,** presentation of part of the umbilical cord ahead of the fetus; it may cause fetal death due to compression of the cord between the presenting part of the fetus and the maternal pelvis.

**p. of the uterus,** descensus uteri resulting from laxity and atony of the muscular and fascial structures of the pelvic floor, usually resulting from injuries of childbirth or advanced age. When the cervix of the prolapsed uterus is well within the vaginal orifice, it is spoken of as first degree; in second degree, the cervix is at or near the introitus; when the cervix protrudes well beyond the vaginal orifice, it is third degree (procidentia uteri).

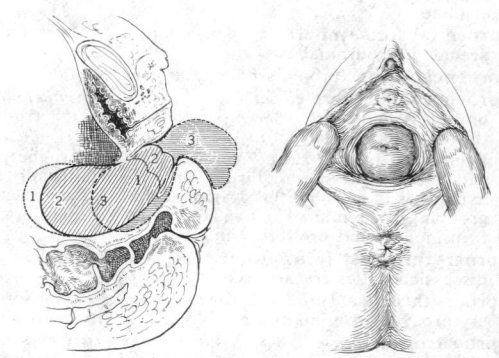

**Prolapse of the Uterus**

**prolap′sus** [ L. ]. Prolapse.

**prolepsis** (pro-lep′sis) [ G. *prolēpsis,* anticipation. LAB- ]. Recurrence of the paroxysm of a periodical disease at regularly shortening intervals.

**prolep′tic.** Relating to prolepsis.

**proleukemia** (pro-lu-ke′mī-ah). Leukanemia.

**proleukocyte** (pro-lu′ko-sīt). Leukoblast.

**pro′lidase.** Proline dipeptidase.

**prolif′erate** [ L. *proles,* offspring, + *fero,* to bear ]. To grow and increase in number by means of reproduction of similar forms.

**prolifera′tion.** Growth and reproduction of similar cells.

**gingival p.,** an overgrowth or hyperplastic change affecting the gingival tissues, usually resulting in a prominent gingival papilla.

**prolif′erative, prolif′erous.** Reproductive; increasing the numbers of similar forms.

**prolif′ic** [ L. *proles,* offspring, + *facio,* to make ]. Fruitful; bearing many children.

**proligerous** (pro-lij′er-us) [ L. *proles,* offspring, + *gero,* to bear ]. Germinating; producing offspring.

**pro′linase.** Prolyl dipeptidase.

**proline** (pro′lēn). An amino acid, 2-pyrrolidine carboxylic acid, found in proteins.

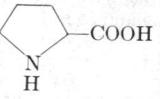

**Proline**

**p. aminopeptidase,** a hydrolase (EC 3.4.11.5) cleaving L-proline residues from N-terminal position in peptides.

**p. dehydrogenase,** pyrroline 5-carboxylate reductase; see also pyrroline 2-carboxylate reductase.

**p. dipeptidase,** prolidase; imidopeptidase; enzyme (EC 3.4.13.9) cleaving aminoacyl-proline bonds; distinct from prolyl dipeptidase.

**p. oxidase,** D-proline reductase.

**p. racemase,** an enzyme (EC 5.1.1.4) that converts D-proline to L-proline.

**D-proline reductase** (EC 1.4.1.6). Oxidoreductase cleaving D-proline (not the natural form) to 5-aminovalerate, with NADH as hydrogen donor.

**pro'lyl dipep'tidase.** Iminodipeptidase; prolinase; prolylglycine dipeptidase; enzyme (EC 3.4.13.8) cleaving L-prolyl-aminoacid bonds. Not the same as proline dipeptidase.

**prolylglycine dipeptidase.** Prolyl dipeptidase.

**promastigote** (pro-mas'tĭ-gōt) [ pro- + G. *mastix,* whip ]. Term now generally used instead of "leptomonad" or "leptomonad stage," to avoid confusion with the flagellate genus *Leptomonas.* It denotes the flagellate stage of a trypanosomatid protozoan in which the flagellum arises from a kinetoplast in front of the nucleus and emerges from the anterior end of the organism; usually an extracellular phase, as in the insect intermediate host (or in culture) of *Leishmania* parasites.

**pro'mazine hydrochloride** (NF, BP). SPARINE hydrochloride; 10-(3-dimethylaminopropyl)phenothiazine hydrochloride; it has the same actions and uses as chlorpromazine but appears to be of lower toxicity, except in the areas of seizures and hypotension; used as an antiemetic, as an adjuvant to obstetric anesthesia, and in various psychiatric disorders.

**promegaloblast** (pro-meg'ă-lo-blast). The earliest of four maturation stages of the megaloblast; see discussion under erythroblast.

**prometaphase** (pro-met'ă-fāz) [ pro- + metaphase, *q.v.* ]. The stage of mitosis or meiosis in which the nuclear membrane disintegrates, the centrioles reach the poles of the cell, and the chromosomes continue to contract.

**prometh'azine hydrochloride** (USP, BP). PHENERGAN; 10-(2-dimethylaminopropyl)phenothiazine hydrochloride; antihistaminic.

**prometh'azine theoclate** (BP). Promethiazine salt of 8-chlorotheophylline; an antihistaminic drug used for motion sickness.

**prometh'estrol dipro'pionate.** Dimethylhexestrol dipropionate; 4,4'-(1,2-diethylethylene)di-*o*-cresol dipropionate; a synthetic estrogen derived from stilbene.

**promethium** (pro-me'thĭ-um) [ *Prometheus,* Greek demigod ]. A radioactive element of the rare earth series; symbol Pm, atomic no. 61; half-life of its most stable isotope (p.-145) is 30 years; isolated in 1948 among the fission products of uranium-235.

**prominence** (prom'ĭ-nens) [ L. *prominentia* ]. Prominentia.

**canine p.,** canine *eminence.*

**hypothenar p.,** hypothenar *eminence.*

**thenar p.,** thenar (1).

**prom'inens** [ L. ] [ NA ]. Prominent; in anatomy, denoting a prominence or projection.

**prominentia,** pl. **prominentiae** (prom-ĭ-nen'shĭ-ah, -shĭ-e) [ L. fr. *promineo,* to jut out, be prominent ] [ NA ]. A prominence or projection.

**p. cana'lis facia'lis** [ NA ], prominence of the facial canal; the prominence on the medial wall of the tympanic cavity above the vestibular (oval) window produced by the presence of the facial canal.

**p. cana'lis semicircula'ris lateralis** [ NA ], prominence of the lateral semicircular canal; the slight bulge in the medial wall of the epitympanic recess caused by the proximity of the lateral semicircular canal.

**p. larynge'a** [ NA ], laryngeal prominence; Adam's apple; pomum Adami; thyroid eminence; the projection on the anterior portion of the neck formed by the thyroid cartilage of the larynx.

**p. mallea'ris** [ NA ], mallear prominence; a small prominence at the upper end of the stria mallearis produced by the lateral process of the malleus.

**p. spira'lis** [ NA ], a projecting portion of the ligamentum spirale cochleae, bounding the lower edge of the stria vascularis and containing within it a blood vessel, the vas prominens.

**p. styloid'ea** [ NA ], a rounded eminence on the posterior wall (paries mastoidea) of the tympanic cavity corresponding to the base of the styloid process.

**promon'ocyte.** Premonocyte.

**promontorium,** pl. **promontoria** (prom'on-to'rī-um, -rī-ah) [ L. a mountain ridge, a headland, fr. *promineo,* to jut out ] [ NA ]. 1. A projection of a part. 2. Pelvic promontory; promontory of the sacrum; the most prominent anterior projection of the base of the sacrum. 3. Tympanic promontory; tuber cochleae; a rounded eminence on the labyrinthine wall of the middle ear, caused by the first coil of the cochlea.

**promontory** (prom'on-to-rī) [ L. *promontorium* ]. An eminence or projection; see promontorium.

**double p.,** a deformity of the sacrum in which the second segment is bent backward, its body forming an external angle with that of the first segment; this second p. is called false p.

**false p.,** see double p.

**pelvic p.,** promontorium (2).

**p. of the sacrum,** promontorium (2).

**tympanic p.,** promontorium (3).

**promo'tor.** In chemistry, a substance that increases the activity of a catalyst. See fig. under protein.

**promox'olane.** DIMETHYLANE; 2,2-diisopropyl-1,3-dioxolane-4-methanol; skeletal muscle relaxant and antianxiety agent.

**promyelocyte** (pro-mi'ĕ-lo-sīt) [ pro- + G. *myelos,* marrow, + *kytos,* cell ]. 1. The developmental stage of a granular leukocyte between the myeloblast and myelocyte, when a few specific granules appear in addition to azurophilic ones. 2. A large uninuclear cell occurring in the circulating blood of persons with myelocytic leukemia. See color plate 14.

**pro'nate** [ L. *pronatus,* fr. *prono,* pp. *-atus,* to bend forward, fr. *pronus,* bent forward ]. To assume, or to be placed in, a prone position; see prone and pronation.

**prona'tion.** The condition of being prone; the act of assuming or of being placed in a prone position, *i.e.,* face down.

**p. of foot,** eversion and abduction of foot, causing a lowering of the medial edge.

**p. of forearm,** rotation of the forearm in such a way that the palm of the hand looks backward when the arm is in the anatomical position, or downward when the arm is extended at a right angle to the body.

**prona'tis** [ L. *pro,* before, + *nasce,* born ]. A baby born prematurely.

**prona'tor.** [ L. ] [ NA ]. A muscle which turns a part into the prone position. See under musculus.

**prone** (prōn) [ L. *pronus,* bending down or forward ]. Denoting the hand or foot when pronated; the body when lying face downward.

**pronephros,** pl. **pronephroi** (pro-nef'ros, -roy) [ pro- + G. *nephros,* kidney ]. 1. The head- or forekidney of primitive fishes. 2. In the embryos of higher vertebrates, a vestigial structure consisting of a series of tortuous tubules emptying into the cloaca by way of the primary nephric duct. It is a very rudimentary and temporary structure in the human embryo, being followed by the mesonephros and still later by the metanephros.

**pronethalol hydrochloride** (pro-neth'ă-lol). ALDERLIN; NETHALIDE; the hydrochloride of 2-isopropylamino-1-(2-naphthyl)ethanol; an adrenergic β-receptor blocking agent used as an antagonist of the cardiac action of epinephrine (not used in the United States). Large repeated doses can induce malignant tumors of the thymus in experimental animals.

**prong** [ Goth. *praggan,* to press ]. The conical root of a tooth.

**pronograde** (pro'no-grād) [ L. *pronus,* inclined forward, + *gradior,* to walk ]. Walking or resting with the body horizontal, denoting the posture of quadrupeds; opposed to orthograde.

**pronometer** (pro-nom'e-ter). An instrument for indicating the degree of pronation or supination of the forearm.

**pro'normoblast.** The earliest of four stages in development of the normoblast; see discussion under erythroblast, and color plate 15.

**pronucleus** (pro-nu'kle-us). 1. One of two nuclei undergoing fusion in karyogamy. 2. In embryology, the nuclear material of the head of the spermatozoon (**male p.**) or of the ovum (**female p.**), after the ovum has been penetrated by the spermatozoon. Each p. carries the haploid number of chromosomes. When the pronuclei merge in fertilization, the diploid number of chromosomes characteristic of the species is reestablished.

**prootic** (pro-o'tik) [ pro- + G. *ous*, ear ]. In front of the ear.

**propadi'ene.** Allene.

**prop'agate** [ L. *propago*, pp. *-atus*, to generate, reproduce ]. 1. To reproduce; to generate. 2. To move along a fiber, *e.g.*, propagation of the nerve impulse.

**propagation** (prop-ă-ga'shun). The act of propagating; see propagate.

**propagative** (prop'ă-ga'tiv). Relating to or concerned in propagation; denoting the sexual part of an animal or plant as distinguished from the soma.

**propalinal** (pro-pal'ĭ-nal) [ pro- + G. *palin*, backward ]. Back and forth; denoting a forward and backward movement.

**propam'idine.** 4,4'-Diamidino-1,3-diphenoxypropane; active against *Trypanosoma gambiensi* infections; also markedly bacteriostatic; used as a local anti-infective agent in 0.1 per cent aqueous solution, and against systemic fungal infections such as blastomycosis.

**pro'pane.** $CH_3CH_2CH_3$; one of the alkane series of hydrocarbons.

**propanetriol** (pro'păn-tri'ol). Glycerol.

**propan'idid** (USAN). EPONTOL; propyl{4-[ (diethylcarbamoyl)methoxy ]-3-methoxyphenyl}acetate; a short-acting eugenol used intravenously for induction of general anesthesia.

**propanoic acid** (pro'pă-no'ik). Propionic acid.

**propanol** (pro'pă-nol). Propyl alcohol.

**propantheline bromide** (pro-pan'thĕ-lēn) (USP, BP). PRO-BANTHINE bromide; β-diisopropylmethylaminoethyl-9-xanthine carboxylate bromide; the isopropyl analogue of methantheline bromide; an anticholinergic agent with the same uses as methantheline bromide, but more potent.

**proparacaine hydrochloride** (pro-păr'ă-kān) (USP). OPHTHAINE; proxymetacaine hydrochloride; 2-diethylaminoethyl-3-amino-4-propoxybenzoate hydrochloride; a surface anesthetic agent used in ophthalmology; it produces little or no irritation, stinging, burning, lacrimation, or hyperemia.

**pro'patyl nitrate** (USAN). VASONGOR; 2-ethyl-2-(hydroxymethyl)-1,3-propanediol trinitrate; coronary vasodilator.

**pro'pene.** Propylene.

**propentdyopents** (pro'pent-di'o-pentz). See bilirubinoids.

**propenyl** (pro'pĕ-nil). The radical, $—CH=CH—CH_3$.

**propep'sin.** Pepsinogen.

**propep'tone.** Secondary proteose; a mixture of intermediate products in the conversion of native protein into peptone.

**propeptonuria** (pro-pep'to-nu'rĭ-ah). The excretion of propeptone in the urine.

**proper'din.** A normal serum globulin, molecular weight 223,000, that participates, in conjunction with other factors, in an alternate pathway to the activation of the terminal components of complement; see also p. system, and component of *complement*.

    **p. factor A,** a component of the p. system, *q.v.*; seemingly a hydrazine-sensitive euglobulin, molecular weight about 180,000.

    **p. factor B,** C3 proactivator (C3PA); cobra venom cofactor; glycine-rich β-glycoprotein; $β_2$-glycoprotein II; a normal serum protein, molecular weight 100,000, and a component of the p. system. See also cobra venom *cofactor*.

    **p. factor D,** C3 proactivator convertase (C3PA convertase), a normal serum euglobulin, molecular weight about 35,000, required in the p. system.

    **p. factor E,** a serum protein, molecular weight 160,000, required for activation of C3 (third component of complement) by cobra venom factor; see also p. system.

    **p. system,** an immunological system composed of several distinct proteins that react in a serial manner and activate C3, the third component of complement (see under complement), seemingly without utilizing components C1, C4, and C2. In addition to properdin, the system includes

properdin factors A, B (C3 proactivator), D (C3 proactivator convertase), and perhaps at least one other, E (*q.v.*). The system can be activated by bacterial endotoxin and by a variety of polysaccharides and lipopolysaccharides; also, seemingly, by a component of cobra venom (see cobra venom *factor*) in which case factor A seems to be bypassed but another serum substance (designated factor E) may be required.

**proper'idine hydrochloride.** GEVELINA hydrochloride; 1-methyl-4-phenylisonipecotic acid isopropyl ester hydrochloride; analgesic.

**properitoneal** (pro'pĕr-ĭ-to-ne'al). In front of the peritoneum.

**prophage** (pro'fāj). Probacteriophage.

    **defective p.,** see defective *bacteriophage*.

**prophase** (pro'fāz) [ G. *prophasis*, from *prophainō*, to foreshadow ]. The first stage of mitosis or meiosis consisting of linear contraction and increase in thickness of the chromosomes (each composed of two chromatids) accompanied by division of the centriole and migration of the two daughter centrioles and their asters toward the poles of the cell. In meiosis p. is complex and can be subdivided into stages: preleptotene, leptotene, zygotene, pachytene, diplotene and diakinesis.

**prophenpyridamine maleate** (pro'fen-pĭ-rid'ă-mēn). Pheniramine maleate.

**prophlogistic** (pro-flo-jis'tik) [ pro- + G. *phlogōsis*, inflammation ]. Causing or producing tissue inflammation.

**prophylactic** (pro-fĭ-lak'tik) [ G. *prophylaktikos;* see prophylaxis ]. 1. Preventing disease; relating to prophylaxis. 2. An agent, *e.g.* diphtheria toxoid, typhoid vaccine, etc., that acts as a preventive against any disease.

**prophylaxis,** pl. **prophylaxes** (pro'fĭ-lak'sis, -sēz) [ Mod.L. fr. G. *pro-phylassō*, to guard before, take precaution ]. The prevention of disease.

    **active p.,** use of an antigenic (immunogenic) agent to actively stimulate the immunological mechanism.

    **chemical p.,** the administration of chemicals or drugs to members of a community to reduce the number of carriers of a disease and to prevent others contracting the disease, *e.g.*, the administration of sulfonamides to check the spread of meningococcal meningitis.

    **dental p.,** a series of procedures whereby calculus, stain, and other accretions are removed from the clinical crowns of the teeth, and the enamel surfaces are polished.

    **passive p.,** use of an antiserum from another person or animal to provide temporary (a week to 10 days) protection against a specific infectious or toxic agent.

**propicillin** (pro'pĭ-sil'in). ORICILLIN; CETACILLIN; α-phenoxypropylpenicillin potassium; a semisynthetic, acid-stable penicillin that may be more effective than penicillin G.

**pro'piolac'tone** (USAN). BETAPRONE; β-propiolactone; hydracrylic acid β-lactone; used to sterilize plasma, vaccines, and tissue grafts.

**propiomazine hydrochloride** (pro-pī-o'mah-zēn) (NF). LARGON; 1-[ 10-[ 2-(dimethylamino)propyl ]phenothiazin-2-yl ]- 1-propanone monohydrochloride; used intramuscularly or intravenously as a tranquilizer, sedative, and hypnotic.

**propion** (pro'pĭ-ōn). Diethyl ketone.

**propionate** (pro'pĭ-o-nāt). A salt or ester of propionic acid.

**Propionibacterium** (pro-pī-on-ĭ-bak-tēr'ĭ-um). A genus of nonmotile, nonsporeforming, anaerobic to aerotolerant bacteria (family Propionibacteriaceae) containing Gram-positive rods which are usually pleomorphic, diphtheroid, or club-shaped with one end rounded, the other tapered or pointed. Some cells may be coccoid, elongate, bifid, or even branched. The cells usually occur singly, in pairs, in V and Y configurations, short chains, or clumps in "Chinese character" arrangement. The metabolism of these organisms is fermentative, and the products of fermentation include combinations of propionic and acetic acids. These organisms occur in dairy products, on the skin of man, and in the intestinal tracts of man and other animals. They may be pathogenic. The type species is *P. freudenreichii*.

    **P. acnes,** a species of bacteria commonly found in acne pustules, although it occurs in other types of lesions in humans and even as a saprophyte in the intestine, skin, hair follicles, and in sewage.

**P. freudenreichii,** a species found in raw milk, Swiss cheese, and other dairy products; it is the type species of the genus *P.*

**P. jensenii,** a species found in dairy products, silage, and occasionally in infections.

**propion′ic acid.** Propanoic acid; methylacetic acid; ethylcarbonic acid; $CH_3CH_2COOH$; found in sweat.

**propionyl.** The acyl radical of propionic acid; $CH_3CH_2CO—.$

**propionylcholine.** A choline ester isolated from ox spleen; its actions are qualitatively similar to those of acetylcholine at most cholinergic sites.

**pro′pior** [ L. comparative of *propinquus,* near ] [ NA ]. Nearer.

**propitocaine hydrochloride.** Prilocaine hydrochloride.

**pro′pla′sia** [ pro- + G. *plassō,* to form ]. That state of cell or tissue in which activity is increased above that of euplasia (*i.e.,* characterized by stimulation, repair, or regeneration).

**proplex′us.** The choroid plexus in the lateral ventricle of the brain.

**pro′polis.** A resinous, waxlike substance that bees collect from plants to use as a glue or putty to line their hives and fill up cracks. Source of p. wax, p. resin, and p. balsam.

**propositus,** pl. **propos′iti,** fem. sing., **propos′ita** (pro′-poz′ĭ-tus) [ L. fr. *proponere,* to propound ]. 1. Proband. 2. A premise; an argument.

**propoxycaine hydrochloride** (pro-pok′sĭ-kān) (NF). RAVOCAINE; propoxyprocaine; 2′-diethylaminoethyl-2-propoxy-4-aminobenzoate hydrochloride; a local anesthetic once used by injection for conduction anesthesia.

**propoxyphene hydrochloride** (pro-pok′sĭ-fēn) (USP). DARVON; dextropropoxyphene hydrochloride; (+)-α-4-(dimethylamino)-3-methyl-1,2-diphenyl-2-butanol propionate hydrochloride; a nonantipyretic, orally effective analgesic structurally related to methadone and used for the relief of mild to moderate pain; it is less effective than codeine but with less liability for abuse; combination of p. with acetylsalicylic acid provides more effective analgesia than either agent given alone.

**propox′yphene napsylate** (USAN). DARVON-N; mono-2-naphthalenesulfonate monohydrate salt of propoxyphene; analgesic.

**propranolol hydrochloride** (pro-pran′o-lōl) (USP, BP). INDERAL; propanolol; A 464043; ICI 45,520; 1-(isopropylamino)-3-(1-naphthyloxy)-2-propanol; an adrenergic β-receptor blocking agent.

**proprietary name** (pro-pri′e-tĕr-ĭ) [ L. *proprietarius* ]. The protected brand name or trademark, registered with the U. S. Patent Office, under which a manufacturer markets his product. Proprietary names are written with a capital initial letter and are often further distinguished by a superscript R in a circle (®); in the *Stedman* definitions, they are printed in small capital letters. See also *generic name.*

**proprioceptive** (pro′pri-o-sep′tiv) [ L. *proprius,* one's own, + *capio,* to take ]. Capable of receiving stimuli originating in muscles, tendons, and other internal tissues.

**proprioceptor** (pro′pri-o-sep′tor). One of a variety of sensory end organs (such as the muscle spindle and Golgi's tendon organ) in muscles, tendons, and joint capsules.

**pro′priospi′nal.** Relating especially or wholly to the spinal cord; specifically, denoting those nerve cells and their fibers that connect the different segments of the spinal cord with each other.

**proptometer** (prop-tom′e-ter) [ pro- + G. + *ptōsis,* a falling, + *metron,* measure ]. Exophthalmometer.

**proptosis** (prop-to′sis) [ G. *proptōsis,* a falling forward ]. A forward displacement of any organ; specifically, exophthalmos or protrusion of the eyeball.

**proptot′ic.** Referring to proptosis.

**propulsion** (pro-pul′zhun) [ G. *pro-pello,* pp. *-pulsus,* to drive forth ]. The tendency to fall forward that causes the festination in paralysis agitans.

**propyl** (pro′pil). The radical of propyl alcohol or propane; $CH_3CH_2CH_2—.$

**pro′pyl alcohol.** Ethylcarbinol; propanol; $CH_3—CH_2—CH_2OH$; a solvent; more toxic than ethyl alcohol.

**pro′pylcar′binol.** Butyl alcohol.

**propylene** (pro′pĭ-lēn). Propene; a gaseous olefinic hydrocarbon; $CH_2=CHCH_3.$

**p. glycol** (USP, BP), 1,2-propanediol; 1,2-dihydroxypropane; $CH_3CHOHCH_2OH$; an ingredient of the official hydrophilic ointment; also used as a diluent, its toxicity being about the same as glycerin.

**propyl gallate** (BP). *n*-Propyl gallate; an antioxidant for emulsions.

**pro′pylhex′edrine** (NF). BENZEDREX; *N,*α-dimethylcyclohexaneethylamine; 1-cyclohexyl-2-methylaminopropane; a sympathomimetic and local vasoconstrictor. Available as an inhalant (NF).

**propyl hydroxybenzoate** (BP). Propylparaben.

**pro′pyli′odone** (USP, BP). DIONOSIL; propyl-3,5-diiodo-4-oxo-1(4*H*)pyridineacetate; a radiopaque material used for bronchography.

**pro′pylpar′aben** (USP). Propyl hydroxybenzoate (BP); *p*-hydroxybenzoic acid propyl ester; an antifungal agent and pharmaceutical preservative.

**propylthiouracil** (pro′pil-thi′o-u′rā-sil) (USP, BP). For action and uses, see thiouracil.

**pro′pylure.** 10-Propyl-*trans*-5,9-tridecadienyl acetate; the sex pheromone of the female pink bollworm moth. The sexually excitatory effects of p. can be reduced or wholly abolished by the presence of relatively small concentrations of the *cis* isomer of the pheromone.

**propyro′mazine.** DIASPASMYL; 1-methyl-1-[ 1-(phenothiazin-10-ylcarbonyl)ethyl ]pyrrolidinium bromide; intestinal antispasmodic with anticholinergic properties.

**pro re nata** (pro-ra-nah′tah) [ L. ]. "As the occasion arises"; used sometimes in the signature of a prescription, abbreviated usually to p.r.n.

**pror′sad** [ L. *prorsum,* forward, + *ad,* to ]. In a forward direction; cephalad.

**prorubricyte** (pro-ru′brĭ-sīt) [ pro- + rubricyte ]. Basophilic normoblast; see discussion under erythroblast.

**pernicious anemia type p.,** basophilic megaloblast; see discussion under erythroblast.

**proscillaridin** (pro′sĭ-lăr′ĭ-din) (USAN). TALUSIN; 14-hydroxy-3β-(rhamnosyloxy)bufa-4,20,22-trienolide; prepared from *Urginea maritima;* cardiotonic agent, used for the treatment of congestive heart failure.

**proscolex** (pro-sko′leks) [ pro- + G. *skōlex,* a worm ]. The embryonic form of a tapeworm or other species in the class *Cestoda.*

**prosecretin** (pro-se-kre′tin). Unactivated secretin.

**prosect** (pro-sekt′) [ L. *pro-seco,* pp. *-sectus,* to cut. SEC- ]. To dissect a cadaver or any part, that it may serve for a demonstration of anatomy before a class.

**prosector** (pro′sek′tor). One who prosects, or prepares the material for a demonstration of anatomy before a class.

**pro′secto′rium** [ L. ]. A dissecting room; a place in which anatomical preparations are made for demonstration or for preservation in a museum.

**prosencephalon** (pros′en-sef′ă-lon) [ G. *prosō,* forward, + *enkephalos,* brain ]. [ NA ]. The anterior primitive cerebral vesicle; the forebrain, dividing in further development into diencephalon and telencephalon, or cerebral hemisphere.

**proserine** (pro-sēr′in). Neostigmine.

**proserozyme** (pro-se′ro-zīm). 1. Unactivated serozyme (Factor VII) that is activated by the effects of calcium. 2. Prothrombin.

**Prosimiae** (pro-sim′ĭ-e) [ pro- + L. *simia,* ape ]. A suborder of Primates, the same as Lemuroidea.

**Proskauer** (pross′kow-er), Bernhard, German bacteriologist, 1851–1915. See Voges-P. *reaction.*

**prosodemic** (pros′o-dem′ik) [ G. *prosō,* forward, + *dēmos,* people ]. Denoting a disease that is transmitted directly from person to person.

**prosop-.** See prosopo-.

**prosopagnosia** (pros′o-pag-no′sĭ-ah) [ prosop- + G. *a-* priv. + *gnōsis,* recognition ]. Difficulty in recognizing familiar faces.

**prosop′agus.** Prosopopagus.

**prosopalgia** (pros'o-pal'jĭ-ah) [ prosop- + G. *algos*, pain ]. Trigeminal *neuralgia.*

**prosopal'gic.** Relating to or suffering from trigeminal neuralgia.

**prosopectasia** (pros'o-pek-ta'zĭ-ah) [ prosop- + G. *ektasis*, extension ]. Enlargement of the face, as in acromegaly.

**prosoplasia** (pros'o-pla'zĭ-ah) [ G. *prosō*, forward, + *plasis* a molding ]. Cytomorphosis. 1. Progressive transformation, such as the change of cells of the salivary ducts into secreting cells. 2. Differentiation exceeding the physiologic limits for the kind of cell in question.

**prosopo-, prosop-** (pros'o-po-) [ G. *prosōpon*, face, countenance ]. Combining forms relating to the face.

**prosopoanoschisis** (pros'o-po-ă-nos'kĭ-sis) [ prosopo- + G. *anō*, upward, + *schisis*, fissure ]. Facial *cleft.*

**prosopodiplegia** (pros'o-po-di-ple'jĭ-ah) [ prosopo- + diplegia, *q.v.* ]. Paralysis affecting both sides of the face.

**prosoponeuralgia** (pros'o-po-nu-ral'jĭ-ah). Trigeminal *neuralgia.*

**prosopopagus** (pros'o-pop'ă-gus) [ prosopo- + G. *pagos*, something fastened ]. Prosopagus; unequal conjoined twins in which the parasite, in the form of a tumor-like mass, is attached to the orbit or cheek of the autosite.

**prosopoplegia** (pros'o-po-ple'jĭ-ah) [ prosopo- + G. *plēgē*, stroke ]. Facial *palsy.*

**prosopoplegic** (pros'o-po-ple'jik). Relating to, or suffering from, facial paralysis.

**prosoposchisis** (pros-o-pos'kĭ-sis) [ prosopo- + G. *schisis*, fissure ]. Congenital facial cleft from mouth to orbit; oblique facial cleft.

**prosopospasm** (pros'o-po-spazm) [ prosopo- + G. *spasmos*, spasm ]. Facial *tic.*

**prosoposternodidymus** (pros'o-po-ster'no-did'ĭ-mus) [ prosopo- + G. *sternon*, chest, + *didymos*, twin ]. Conjoined twins, double in face and chest but single below.

**prosopothoracopagus** (pros'o-po-tho'rā-kop'ă-gus) [ prosopo- G. *thōrax*, chest, + *pagos*, something fastened ]. Conjoined twins attached by the face and chest; a variety of cephalothoracopagus.

**prosopotocia** (pros'o-po-to'sĭ-ah) [ prosopo- + G. *tokos*, birth ]. A face presentation in childbirth.

**prospermia** (pro-sper'mĭ-ah) [ pro- + G. *sperma*, seed ]. Premature *ejaculation.*

**prostaglandins** (pros'tă-glan'dinz). A class of physiologically active substances present in many tissues; among effects are those of vasodepressors, stimulation of intestinal smooth muscle, uterine stimulation, antagonism to hormones influencing lipid metabolism. The p.'s are prostanoic acids with ortho side chains of varying degrees of unsaturation and varying degrees of oxidation. Often abbreviated PGE, PGF, PGA, PGB, with numerical subscripts, according to structure.

   **p. E$_2$,** dinoprostone.

   **p. F$_{2\alpha}$,** dinoprost.

   **p. F$_{2\alpha}$ tromethamine,** dinoprost tromethamine.

**prostanoic acid** (pros'tă-no'ik). The 20-carbon acid that is the skeleton of the prostaglandins. It has the structure and arbitrary numbering shown in the figure; a systematic name is 7-[ 2-(1-octanyl)cyclopentyl ]heptanoic acid. The prostaglandins are prostanoic acids with various hydroxyl and keto substitutions at positions 9, 11, and 15, and dehydrogenations (double bonds) in the long aliphatic chains.

**Prostanoic acid**

*Inner numbering,* prostanoic acid; *outer numbering,* systematic.

**prostat-.** See prostato-.

**prostata** (pros'tah-tah) [ Mod. L. from G. *prostatēs*, one standing before. STA- ] [ NA ]. Prostate gland; glandula prostatica; the prostate; a chestnut-shaped body that surrounds the beginning of the urethra in the male; it consists of two lateral lobes that are connected anteriorly by an isthmus and posteriorly by a middle lobe lying above and between the ejaculatory ducts. In structure the prostate consists of 30 to 50 compound tubuloalveolar glands between which is abundant stroma consisting of collagen and elastic fibers and many smooth muscle bundles. The secretion of the glands is a milky fluid that is discharged by excretory ducts into the prostatic urethra at the time of the emission of semen.

**prostatalgia** (pros'tă-tal'jĭ-ah) [ prostat- + G. *algos*, pain ]. Prostadodynia; prostatic neuralgia; pain in the prostate gland.

**prostate** (pros'tăt). Prostata.

   **female p.,** term sometimes applied to the periurethral glands in the upper part of the urethra in the female.

**prostatectomy** (pros'tă-tek'to-mĭ) [ prostat- + G. *ektomē*, excision ]. Removal of a part or all of the prostate.

**prostatic** (pros-tat'ik). Relating to the prostate gland.

**prostat'icoves'ical.** Relating to the prostate gland and the bladder.

**pros'tatism.** The symptoms and general condition induced by hypertrophy or chronic disease of the prostate gland.

**prostatit'ic.** Relating to prostatitis.

**prostatitis** (pros'tă-ti'tis) [ prostat- + G. suffix *-itis*, inflammation ]. Inflammation of the prostate gland.

**prostato-, prostat-** (pros'tă-to-) [ L. *prostata, q.v.* ]. Combining forms relating to the prostate gland.

**prostatocystitis** (pros'tă-to-sis-ti'tis) [ prostato- + G. *kystis*, bladder, + suffix -*itis*, inflammation ]. Inflammation of the prostate and the bladder; cystitis by extension of inflammation from the prostatic urethra.

**prostatocystotomy** (pros'tă-to-sis-tot'o-mĭ) [ prostato- + G. *kystis*, bladder, + *tomē*, incision ]. Incision through the prostate and bladder wall with drainage through the perineum.

**prostatodynia** (pros'tă-to-din'ĭ-ah) [ prostato- + G. *odynē*, pain ]. Prostatalgia.

**prostatography** (pros'tă-tog'ră-fĭ) [ prostato- + G. *graphē*, a writing ]. X-ray of the prostate.

**prostatolith** (pros-tat'o-lith) [ prostato- + G. *lithos*, stone ]. Prostatic *calculus.*

**prostatolithotomy** (pros'tă-to-li-thot'o-mĭ, pros-tat'o-) [ prostato- + G. *lithos*, stone, + *tomē*, incision ]. Incision of prostate for removal of calculus.

**prostatomegaly** (pros'tă-to-meg'ă-lĭ) [ prostato- + G. *megas*, large ]. Prostatic enlargement or hypertrophy.

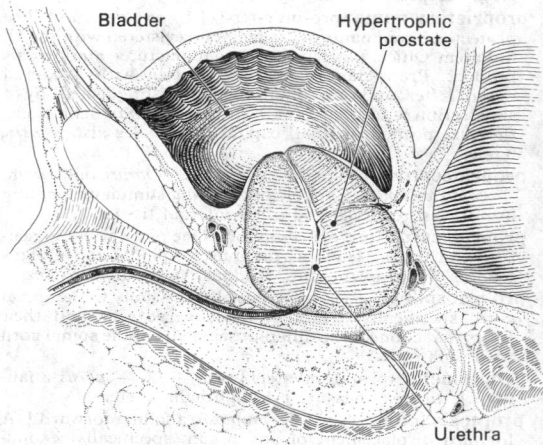

**Prostatomegaly**

**prostat'omy.** Prostatotomy.

**prostatomyomectomy** (pros'tă-to-mi-o-mek'to-mĭ) [ prostato- + myomectomy, *q.v.* ]. Surgical removal of a hypertrophied, or myomatous prostate.

**prostatorrhea** (pros'tă-to-re'ah) [ prostato- + G. *rhoia,* a flow ]. An abnormal discharge of prostatic fluid.

**pros'tatosem'inalvesiculec'tomy.** Prostatovesiculectomy.

**prostatotomy** (pros'tă-tot'o-mĭ) [ prostato- + G. *tomē,* incision ]. Prostatomy; an incision into the prostate.

**prostatotoxin** (pros'tă-to-tok'sin). A cytotoxin obtained by means of the injection of an emulsion of the prostate gland.

**prostatovesiculectomy** (pros'tă-to-vĕ-sik'u-lek'to-mĭ). Surgical removal of prostate and seminal vesicles.

**prostatovesiculitis** (pros'tă-to-vĕ-sik'u-li'tis). Inflammation of the prostate gland and seminal vesicles.

**pro'sterna'tion.** Camptocormia.

**pros'theon.** Prosthion.

**prosthesis,** pl. **prostheses** (pros'the-sis, pros-the'sis, -sēz) [ G. an addition. THE- ]. A fabricated substitute for a missing part of the body, as a limb, tooth, eye, or heart valve.

　**dental p.,** an artificial replacement of one or more teeth and/or associated structures; see also denture and subentries thereunder.

　**hybrid p.,** overlay *denture.*

　**Magovern-Cromie p.,** a ball-valve p. used to replace a diseased aortic valve.

　**ocular p.,** the use of an artificial eye or implant.

　**Sauerbruch's p.,** the use of an amputation stump to move an artificial limb.

　**Starr-Edwards ball valve p.,** artificial valve, consisting of a ball of solid silicone rubber in a cage of silicone-covered vitalium, used to replace diseased heart valves.

　**surgical p.,** an appliance prepared as an aid or as a part of a surgical proceeding such as a stent, heart valve, or cranial plate.

　**Vanghetti's p.,** an artificial limb in which movements are executed by means of plastic motors after cinematization.

**prosthetic** (pros-thet'ik). Relating to prosthesis or to an artificial limb or other part.

　**par'affin p.,** the restoration or change in the appearance of a facial part by the subcutaneous injection of a specially prepared melted paraffin.

**prosthet'ics.** The art and science of making and adjusting artificial parts of the human body.

　**dental p.,** prosthodontics.

**pros'thetist.** One skilled in constructing and fitting prostheses.

**prosthetophakia** (pros'thĕ-to-fak'ī-ah) [ G. *prosthesis,* an addition, + *phakos,* lens ]. Lenticulus.

**prosthion** (pros'thĭ-on) [ G. ntr. of *prosthios,* foremost ]. Prostheon; alveolar point; the most anterior point on the maxillary alveolar process in the midline. See fig. under craniometric *point.*

**prosthodontia** (pros'tho-don'shĭ-ah) [ L. ]. Prosthodontics.

**prosthodontics** (pros'tho-don'tiks) [ L. *prosthodontia,* fr. G. *prosthesis, q.v.,* + *odous* (*odont-*), tooth ]. Dental prosthetics; prosthetic dentistry; prosthodontia; the science of and art of providing suitable substitutes for the coronal portions of teeth, or for one or more lost or missing teeth and their associated parts, in order that impaired function, appearance, comfort, and health of the patient may be restored.

**pros'thodon'tist.** A dentist engaged in the practice of prosthodontics.

**Prosthogonimus macrorchis** (pros'tho-gon'ī-mus mak-ror'kis). A digenetic trematode (family Prosthogonimidae) located in the oviduct and bursa fabricii of poultry in North America, particularly common in states bordering the Great Lakes.

**prosthokeratoplasty** (pros'tho-kĕr'ă-to-plas-tĭ). The surgical technique involved in utilizing a keratoprosthesis.

**prostra'tion** [ L. *pro-sterno,* pp. -*stratus,* to strew before, overthrow ]. A marked loss of strength, as in exhaustion.

　**heat p.,** heat *exhaustion.*

　**nervous p.,** neurasthenia.

**prosympal.** 2-[ Diethylaminomethyl ]-1,4-benzodioxan; has been shown to competitively inhibit excitatory (α-receptor) responses of many smooth muscles to adrenergic stimuli; the blockade is relatively transient and affects responses to circulating mediators more readily than it affects sympathetic nerve activity responses.

**prot-.** See (1) proteo-; (2) proto-.

**protactinium** (pro-tak-tin'ī-um). A radioactive element, symbol Pa, atomic no. 91, atomic weight 231; its most long-lived isotope, p.-231, has a half-life of 34,000 years and is produced as an intermediate in the radioactive breakdown of uranium-235.

**pro'tagon.** A fatty substance, found chiefly in the white matter of the brain, consisting of a mixture of cerebrosides and sphingomyelin.

**protal'bumose.** Protoalbumose; intermediate products of protein digestion, derived from hemialbumose; soluble in water and not coagulable by heat, but precipitated by ammonium sulfate, cupric sulfate, and sodium chloride.

**protaminase.** Carboxypeptidase B.

**protamine** (pro'tă-mēn, -min). One of a group of proteins, highly basic because rich in arginine, much simpler in constitution than the albumins and globulins, etc., found in fish spermatozoa in combination with nucleic acid, *e.g.,* salmine (from salmon), sturine (from sturgeon). Neutralizes anticoagulant action of heparin.

　**p. sulfate** (USP), protamine sulphate injection (BP); a purified mixture of simple protein principles from the sperm or testes of suitable species of fish. It is a heparin antagonist used in certain hemorrhagic states associated with increased amounts of heparin-like substances in the circulation and for the treatment of heparin overdosage.

**protanomaly** (pro'tă-nom'ă-lĭ) [ G. *prōtos,* first, + *anōmalia,* anomaly ]. Partial color blindness in which appreciation of red (the first of the primary colors) is less than the normal.

**protanope** (pro'tă-nōp). A person with protanopia.

**protanopia** (pro'tă-no'pĭ-ah) [ G. *prōtos,* first, + *a-* priv. + *ōps* (*ōp-*) eye ]. Red blindness (red being the first of the primary colors); anerythropsia; a form of dichromatism characterized by decreased luminosity for long wavelengths and by the inability to differentiate red, orange, yellow, and green.

**protean** (pro'te-an) [ G. *Prōteus,* a god having the power to change his form ]. Ameboid; changeable in form; having the power to change form like the ameba.

**proteantigen** (pro-te-an'tĭ-jen). A protein, whether animal or vegetable, used as a therapeutic antigen.

**protease** (pro'te-ās). Descriptive term for proteolytic enzymes, both endopeptidases (proteinases, *e.g.,* pepsin, cathepsins, papain) and exopeptidases (carboxy- and aminopeptidases, dipeptidases).

　**gastric p.,** pepsin.

**protection** (pro-tek'shun) [ see protective ]. Protective *block.*

**protective** (pro-tek'tiv) [ L. *pro-tego,* pp. -*tectus,* to cover over, protect ]. 1. Prophylactic; preventing infection; conferring immunity. 2. A thin oil-silk tissue used in surgical dressings.

**proteid** (pro'te-id). Protein.

**protein** (pro'tēn, pro'te-in) [ G. *protein,* fr. *proteios,* primary ]. Macromolecules consisting of long sequences of α-amino acids in peptide linkage (elimination of $H_2O$ between the 2-$NH_2$ and 1-COOH of successive residues). Protein is three-fourths of the dry weight of most cell matter, and various p.'s are involved in structure (collagen, keratin), hormones, enzymes, muscle contraction, immunological responses, and other essential life functions (*e.g.,* all enzymes are p.'s). The amino acids involved are generally the 20 common "α-amino acids" (glycine, alanine, etc.). Cross-links yielding globular forms of p., are often effected through the —SH groups of the sulfur-containing amino acids, as well as by noncovalent forces (hydrogen bonds, lipophilic attractions, etc.). Simple or globular p.'s are classically grouped according to solubilities (see albumin, globulin, prolamine, protamine, histone); the insoluble ones are the fibrous p.'s (keratins, etc.). Complexes of p. with other materials are called conjugated p.'s.

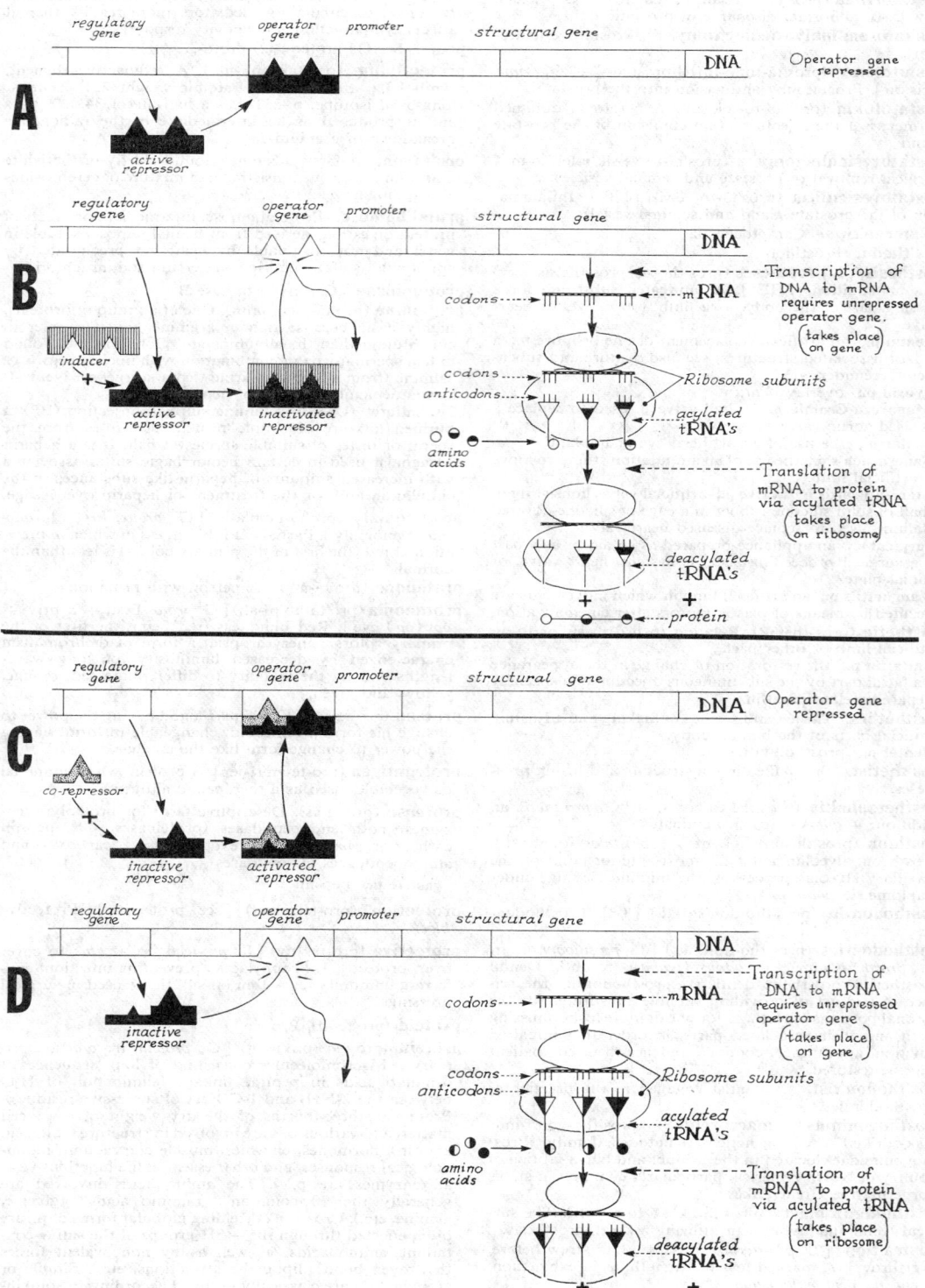

The operon concept for the regulation, in bacteria, of (*A, B*) inducible (negative control) and (*C, D*) repressible (positive control) protein synthesis.

1152

**acyl carrier p.,** see under acyl.

**alcohol-soluble p.,** prolamine.

**autol'ogous p.,** any p. found normally in the fluids or tissues of the body.

**Bence Jones p.,** p. with unusual thermosolubility (see Bence Jones *reaction*) found in the urine of patients with multiple myeloma and occasional persons with other diseases of the reticuloendothelial system; similar in size and physical properties to the light chains of the myeloma p. synthesized by a given patient. See also immunoglobulin.

**coag'ulated p.,** an insoluble product formed by the action of heat on p.; the white of an hard-boiled egg is an example.

**compound p.,** conjugated p.

**con'jugated p.,** p. attached to some other molecule or molecules (not amino acid in nature) otherwise than as a salt; the group contains the nucleoproteins, glycoproteins, phosphoproteins, lipoproteins, and chromoproteins or hemoglobins. See also prosthetic group, apoenzyme, holoenzyme. Opposed to simple p.

**corticosteroid-binding p.,** transcortin.

**C-reactive p.,** a β-globulin found in the serum of various persons with certain inflammatory, degenerative, and neoplastic diseases; although the p. is not a specific antibody, it precipitates *in vitro* the C carbohydrate that is present in all types of pneumococci.

**defensive p.,** an antibody; alexin; phylaxin.

**dena'tured p.,** a p. whose characteristics or properties have been altered in some way, as by heat, enzyme action, or chemicals. Coagulated p. is a denatured p.

**derived p.,** a derivative of the p. molecule effected by chemical change, *e.g.,* hydrolysis; (See albumin, peptone).

**p. factor,** the factor (6.25) by which the nitrogen content of a protein is multiplied to give the amount of protein.

**fibrous p.,** insoluble p.'s including the collagens, elastins, and keratins; all involved in structural or fibrous tissues.

**foreign p.,** one that differs from any contained in the blood, lymph, or tissues of the organism in question.

**globular p.,** p.'s soluble in water, usually with added acid, alkali, salt or ethanol, and roughly so classified (albumins, globulins, histones, protamines).

**heterol'ogous p.,** foreign p.

**human plasma p. fraction** (BP), a solution of the proteins of liquid human plasma that retain their solubility on heating; contains no bactericide or antibiotic, but is sterilized by filtration and heated at 59.5°C. to 60.5°C. for 10 hours to prevent the transmission of serum hepatitis.

**human plasma p. fraction, dried** (BP), freeze-dried human plasma protein fraction.

**p. hydrolysates (intravenous),** AMIGEN; PARENAMINE; a sterile solution of amino acids and short chain peptides prepared from a suitable protein by acid or enzymatic hydrolysis; used intravenously for the maintenance of positive nitrogen balance in severe illness and after surgery involving the alimentary tract.

**p. hydrolysates (oral),** CAMINOIDS; AMINONAT; used in the diets of infants allergic to milk, or as a supplement when high protein intake, from ordinary foods, cannot be accomplished.

**immune p.,** antitoxin.

**M p.,** the Streptococcus M antigen; see under antigen.

**native p.,** the concept of a p. in its natural state, in the cell, unaltered by heat, chemicals, enzyme action, or the exigencies of extraction.

**nonspecif'ic p.,** a p. substance that elicits a response not mediated by specific antigen-antibody reaction.

**phenylthiocarbamoyl p.,** PTC protein; formed by the reaction of phenylisothiocyanate with a terminal α-amino group of a peptide or protein.

**placenta p.,** human placental *lactogen.*

**plasma p.'s,** dissolved p.'s of blood plasma (normally 6 to 8 gm. per 100 ml.); they hold fluid in blood vessels by osmosis and include antibodies and blood-clotting p.'s.

**plasma p. fraction** (USP), a sterile solution of selected proteins derived from the blood plasma of adult human donors; contains 4.5 to 5.5 gm. of protein per 100 ml., of which 83 to 90 per cent is albumin and the remainder is α- and β-globulins. Used as a blood volume supporter.

**protective p.,** defensive p.

**PTC p.,** phenylthiocarbamoyl p.

**purified placental p.,** human placental *lactogen.*

**receptor p.,** an intracellular p. (or p. fraction) that has a high specific affinity for binding a known stimulus to cellular activity, such as a steroid hormone or adenosine 3':5'-cyclic phosphate (cyclic AMP).

**S p.,** the major fragment produced from pancreatic ribonuclease by the limited action of the bacterial proteinase subtilisin (from *B. subtilis*), which cleaves the ribonuclease between residues 20 and 21. The smaller fragment (residues 1-20) is termed the S peptide.

**silver p.,** see under silver.

**simple p.,** one that yields only α-amino acids or their derivatives by hydrolysis; the group contains albumins, globulins, glutelins, alcohol-soluble p.'s, albuminoids, histones, and protamines. Opposed to conjugated p.

**specific p.,** a p. that may act as an allergen.

**thyroxine-binding p.,** thyroxine-binding *globulin.*

**whey p.,** the soluble p. contained in the whey of milk clotted by rennin.

**proteinaceous** (pro'te-na'shus, pro'te-ĭ-na'shus) [ protein + L. adjectival suffix, *-aceus,* resembling or characterized by ]. Resembling a protein; possessing, to some degree, the physicochemical properties characteristic of proteins.

**proteinases** (pro'te-in-ās-ez) Enzymes (EC sub-subclasses 3.4.21 – 3.4.24) hydrolyzing native protein, or polypeptides, making internal cleavages (hence endopeptidases); they include pepsin, chymosin (rennin), trypsin, papain, etc.

**proteinosis** (pro'te-no'sis, pro'te-ĭ-no'sis) [ protein + G. suffix *-osis,* condition ]. A state characterized by disordered protein formation and distribution, particularly as manifested by the deposition of abnormal proteins in tissues.

**lipid p.,** Urbach-Wiethe disease; lipoidosis cutis et mucosae; a disturbance of lipid metabolism in which there are deposits of a protein-lipid complex on the labial mucosa and sublingual and faucial areas and characteristic papillomatous eyelid lesions; autosomal recessive inheritance.

**pulmonary alveolar p.,** a chronic progressive lung disease of adults, characterized by alveolar accumulation of granular proteinaceous material; there is little inflammatory cellular exudate and the cause is unknown.

**proteinuria** (pro'te-nu'rĭ-ah, pro'te-ĭ-nu'rĭ-ah) [ protein + G. *ouron,* urine ]. 1. The presence of urinary protein in concentrations greater than 0.3 gm. in a 24-hour urine collection or in concentrations greater than 1 gm. per liter (1+ to 2+ by standard turbidometric methods) in a random urine collection on two or more occasions at least 6 hours apart; the specimens must be clean, voided midstream, or obtained by catheterization. 2. Albuminuria.

**gestational p.,** the presence of p. during or under the influence of pregnancy in the absence of hypertension, edema, renal infection, or known intrinsic renovascular disease.

**or'thostat'ic p.,** orthostatic *albuminuria.*

**postural p.,** orthostatic *albuminuria.*

**proten'sity** [ L. *protendo* (*-tensum*), to extend ]. The time attribute of a mental process.

**proteo-, prot-, prote-** (pro'te-o-). Combining forms indicating protein.

**proteoclas'tic.** Proteolytic.

**proteohor'mone.** A hormone possessing protein structure; obsolete.

**proteolip'ids.** A class of lipid-soluble proteins found in brain, insoluble in water but soluble in chloroform-methanol-water mixtures.

**proteolysis** (pro'te-ol'ĭ-sis) [ proteo- + G. *lysis,* dissolution ]. Protein hydrolysis; the decomposition of protein.

**proteolyt'ic.** Relating to or effecting proteolysis.

**proteometabolic** (pro'te-o-met'ă-bol'ik). Relating to proteometabolism.

**proteometabolism** (pro'te-o-mĕ-tab'o-lizm). Protein metabolism.

**Proteomyxidia** (pro'te-o-mik-sid'ĭ-ah) [ *Proteus, q.v.,* + G. *myxa,* mucus ]. A subclass of Rhizopoda by some systemic arrangements (an order in others), characterized by the development of filopodia that frequently branch and adhere when they contact, the individual cells sometimes uniting to form plasmodia. Flagellated swarm cells are formed in the cycles of many; no test or shell is formed. A few species are parasitic in plants and in other protozoa.

**proteopec'tic, proteopex'ic.** Relating to proteopexis.

**proteopep'sis** [ proteo- + G. *pepsis*, digestion ]. The digestion of protein.

**proteopexis** (pro'te-o-pek'sis) [ proteo- + G. *pēxis*, fixation ]. The fixation of protein in the tissues.

**proteose** (pro'te-ōs). A descriptive term for protein derivatives resulting from further cleavage of metaprotein material; a mixture of intermediate products of proteolysis between protein and peptone.

　**primary p.,** the first result of hydrolysis of metaprotein; two stages, protoprotease and heteroprotease, have been distinguished; soluble in water.

　**secondary p.,** derived from primary p. by further hydrolysis.

**proteosemia** (pro'te-o-se'mī-ah) [ proteose + G. *haima*, blood ]. The presence of proteoses in the circulating blood.

**Proteosoma** (pro'te-o-so'mah). Nomenclature formerly used for a genus of protozoans, malarial parasites of birds; subsequently subdivided into a number of genera.

**proteosuria** (pro'te-o-su'rī-ah) [ proteose + G. *ouron*, urine ]. Albumosuria; the excretion of proteose in the urine.

**proteotoxin** (pro'te-o-tok'sin). A supposed toxic split-product resulting from the reaction of the serum of the host on a bacterial protein.

**pro'test.** An expression of objection, disapproval, or dissent.

　**masculine p.,** a term attributable to Adler used to describe the movement of individuals from passive to active roles in a desire to escape from the feminine role.

**Proteus** (pro'te-us) [ G. *Prōteus*, a sea-god, who had the power to change his form ]. 1. Formerly a genus of the Sarcodina, now termed *Amoeba*. 2. A genus of motile, peritrichous, nonsporeforming, aerobic to facultatively anaerobic bacteria (family Enterobacteriaceae) containing Gram-negative rods; coccoid forms, large irregular involution forms, filaments, and spheroplasts occur under certain conditions. The metabolism of these organisms is fermentative; they produce acid or acid and visible gas from glucose; lactose is not fermented. These organisms rapidly decompose urea and deaminate phenylalanine. They occur primarily in fecal matter and in putrefying materials. The type species is *P. vulgaris.*

　**P. inconstans,** a species found in urinary tract infections and in sporadic cases of diarrhea in man; some strains cause gastroenteritis.

　**P. mirab'ilis,** a species found in putrid meat, infusions, and abscesses; also reported to be a cause of gastroenteritis.

　**P. morgan'ii,** Morgan's bacillus; a species found in the intestinal canal and in normal and diarrhoeal stools.

　**P. rettgeri,** a species found in chicken cholera and human gastroenteritis.

　**P. vulgar'is,** a species found in putrefying materials and in abscesses. It is pathogenic for fish, dogs, guinea pigs, and mice. Certain strains, the X strains of Weil and Felix, are agglutinated by typhus serum and are therefore of great importance in the diagnosis of typhus. Strain X-19 is strongly agglutinated. See also Weil-Felix *reaction.* It is the type species of the genus *P.*

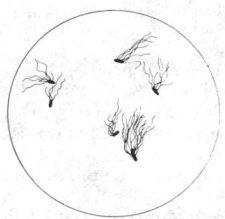

*Proteus vulgaris*

Cells stained to show flagella. Original magnification, ×1200.

**prothionamide.** TREVINTIX; 2-propylthioisonicotinamide; antituberculous agent.

**prothipendyl.** DOMINAL; 10-(3-dimethylaminopropyl)-10 *H*-pyrido-[ 3,2-*b* ][ 1,4 ]benzothiazine; sedative and antipsychotic agent.

**prothrombase** (pro-throm'bās). Prothrombinase.

**prothrombin** (pro-throm'bin). Factor II; plasmozyme; thrombinogen; thrombogen; a glycoprotein with a molecular weight of approximately 62,700, formed and stored in the parenchymal cells of the liver. This substance has been isolated from plasma and is present in blood in a concentration of approximately 20 mg. per 100 ml. In the presence of thromboplastin and calcium ion, p. is converted to thrombin, which in turn converts fibrinogen to fibrin, this process resulting in coagulation of the blood.

　**p. accelerator,** *factor* V.

　**component A of p.,** *factor* V.

　**p. conversion factor, p. converting factor,** *factor* VII.

　**serum p. conversion accelerator (SPCA),** *factor* VII.

**prothrombinase** (pro-throm'bī-nās). Prothrombase; *factor* V (*q. v.*); an enzyme (EC 3.4.16.5) hydrolyzing prothrombin to thrombin.

**prothrombinogen** (pro-throm'bī-no-jen). *Factor* VII.

**prothrom'binope'nia.** Hypoprothrombinemia.

**prothrombokinase.** *Factors* V and VIII.

**prothy'mia** [ G. eagerness, fr. *pro*, before, + *thymos*, mind. THYM-2 ]. Mental alertness.

**pro'tide.** Protein.

**protiodide** (pro-ti'o-dīd, -did). Protoiodide; the first of a series of compounds of iodine with a base, the one that contains the fewest iodine atoms.

**Protista** (pro-tis'tah) [ G. ntr. pl. of *protistos* (superl. of *protos*, first), the first of all ]. Haeckel's term for a proposed third kingdom of living things to include the lowest orders of the animal and vegetable kingdoms, the Protozoa and the Protophyta. On the basis of advances made possible by the electron microscope, it has been proposed that the Protista be divided into two groups according to complexity of structure: (1) The higher protists, including protozoa, fungi, and algae, resemble plants and animals in cell structure (*i.e.,* the cells are eucaryotic); nuclei include multiple chromosomes, are enclosed in a nuclear membrane, and undergo mitosis during replication; also, the cytoplasm contains mitochondria and vacuoles. The higher protists differ from plants and animals in being unicellular, or, if multicellular, in having cells that are all similar with little or none of the tissue differentiation that is characteristic of plants and animals. (2) The lower protists (procaryotes) include the bacteria and blue-green algae (Cyanophyta); the genome seems to consist of a single long molecule of DNA, is not surrounded by a "nuclear" membrane, and does not undergo mitosis during replication; there are no mitochondria. Viruses, although they have similar genomes, are, as a rule, not included among the procaryotes because they are considered not to be cells. See also procaryon; Procaryotae.

**protistologist** (pro-tis-tol'o-jist). One versed in protistology; a microbiologist.

**protistology** (pro-tis-tol'o-jī) [ G. *protistos*, first, + *logos*, study ]. Microbiology.

**protium** (pro'tī-um). The lighter and more common hydrogen isotope; hydrogen-1 in pure form.

**proto-** (pro'to-) [ G. *prōtos*, first ]. Prefix in words derived from Greek roots, denoting the first in a series or the highest in rank.

**protoactinium** (pro'to-ak-tin'ī-um). Protactinium.

**protoalbumose** (pro-to-al'bu-mōz). Protalbumose.

**protobe** (pro'tōb) [ proto- + G. *bios*, life ]. d'Herelle's term for the bacteriophage.

**protobiology** (pro-to-bi-ol'o-jī). Bacteriophagology.

**protocatechuic acid** (pro'to-kat'ē-chu'ik, -ku'ik). 3,4-Dihydroxybenzoic acid; 4-carboxycatechol; oxidation product of epinephrine.

**protochloride** (pro-to-klo'rīd, -rid). The first of a series of chlorine compounds, the one containing the fewest chlorine atoms.

**protocone** (pro'to-kōn) [ proto- + G. *kōnos*, cone ]. The mesiolingual cusp of an upper molar tooth in a mammal.

**protoconid** (pro'to-kon'id) [ proto- + -conid, *q. v.* ]. The mesiolingual cusp of a lower molar tooth in a mammal.

**protocoproporphyria** (pro'to-kop'ro-por-fir'i-ah). Enhanced fecal excretion of proto- and coproporphyrins.

**p. hereditaria,** variegate *porphyria*.

**pro'toderm** [ proto- + G. *derma*, skin ]. The undifferentiated cells of very young embryos from which the primary germ layers are destined to arise.

**protodiacrisis** (pro'to-di-ak'ri-sis) [ proto- + G. *diakrisis*, diacrisis (diagnosis) ]. Absence of a child's awareness of himself as distinct from his environment.

**protodiastolic** (pro'to-di-ă-stol'ik). Early diastolic; relating to the beginning of cardiac diastole.

**protoduodenum** (pro'to-du'o-de'num, -du-od'ē-num). The first part of the duodenum extending from the gastroduodenal pylorus as far as the papilla duodeni major; it has no plicae circulares and is the seat of the duodenal glands.

**protoerythrocyte** (pro'to-ē-rith'ro-sīt). A primitive erythroblast.

**pro'tofil'ament** [ proto- + L. *filum*, a thread ]. Basic element of a contractile flagellar microtubule, approximately 5 nm thick.

**protogala** (pro-tog'ă-lah) [ G. fr. proto- + *gala*, milk ]. Colostrum.

**protogen** (pro'to-jen). Lipoic acid.

**p. A,** lipoic acid; ovoprotogen.

**protoglobulose** (pro'to-glob'u-lōs). A product of the hydrolysis or digestion of a globulin.

**protogonoplasm** (pro'to-gon'o-plazm) [ proto- + G. *gonos*, seed, + *plasma*, a thing formed ]. A differentiated mass of cytoplasm in a protozoan, which forms the substance of later developing reproductive bodies.

**protoheme** (pro'to-hēm). Heme.

**protoiodide** (pro-to-i'o-dīd, -did). Protiodide.

**protokylol hydrochloride** (pro'to-ki'lōl). CAYTINE; α-[ (α-methyl-3,4-methylenedioxyphenethylamino)methyl ]-protocatechuyl alcohol hydrochloride; a derivative of isoproterenol with the selective β-receptor-stimulating activity of the parent compound. It is effective orally and is more stable in the body than isoproterenol. Used as a bronchodilator in the treatment of bronchial asthma and status asthmaticus.

**protoleukocyte** (pro-to-lu'ko-sīt). A primitive leukocyte; a leukocyte of the bone marrow.

**protolysate** (pro-tol'ĭ-sāt). A protein hydrolysate.

**protomerite** (pro-tom'er-it, pro'to-mēr'it) [ proto- + G. *meros*, part ]. Primerite; primite; the anterior portion of a gregarine cephalont, often with an anchoring structure, the epimerite, with which the cephalont adheres to the host tissue (usually the gut wall of an invertebrate host).

**protometrocyte** (pro-to-me'tro-sīt) [ proto- + G. *mētēr*, mother, + *kytos*, cell ]. The ancestor cell of the protoleukocyte and protoerythrocyte, or of the cells of the leukocytic and erythrocytic series.

**pro'ton** [ G. ntr. of *prōtos*, first ]. The positively charged unit of the nuclear mass; p.'s form part (or in hydrogen-1 the whole) of the nucleus of the atom around which the negative electrons revolve. See fig. under atom.

**protoneuron** (pro'to-nu'ron) [ proto- + G. *neuron*, nerve ]. A hypothetical primitive neuron lacking polarization.

**protopath'ic** [ proto- + G. *pathos*, suffering ]. Denoting a set or system of peripheral sensory nerve fibers furnishing a low order of sensibility, enabling one to appreciate pain and temperature to a not very delicate extent, and not definitely localized; distinguished from epicritic.

**protopec'tin.** See pectin.

**pro'topine.** Fumarine; $C_{20}H_{19}NO_5$; an alkaloid obtained in minute quantities from opium, other species of Papaveraceae, and species of Fumariaceae.

**protoplasm** (pro'to-plazm) [ proto- + G. *plasma*, thing formed. PLAS- ]. Living matter; the substance of which animal and vegetable cells are formed.

**totipoten'tial p.,** living matter with the least recognizable differentiation of structure but with the greatest potential, all cell organs being formable by it.

**protoplasmatic, protoplasmic** (pro'to-plaz-mat'ik, -plaz'mik). Relating to protoplasm.

**protoplasmolysis** (pro'to-plaz-mol'ĭ-sis). Achromatolysis.

**pro'toplast** [ proto- + G. *plastos*, formed ]. Archaic term meaning the first individual of a type or race.

**protoporphyria** (pro'to-por-fir'i-ah). Enhanced fecal excretion of protoporphyrin.

**erythropoietic p.,** a heritable disorder characterized by enhanced fecal excretion of protoporphyrin, and elevated quantities of protoporphyrin III in erythroid cells; acute solar urticaria or more chronic solar eczema develops quickly upon exposure to sunlight.

**protoporphyrin** (pro'to-por'fi-rin). 1,3,5,8-Tetramethyl-2,4-divinylporphin-6,7-dipropionic acid; the substituted porphin that, with iron, forms the heme of hemoglobin and the prosthetic groups of myoglobin, catalase, cytochromes, etc. The presence of 4 methyl groups, 2 vinyl groups, and 2 propionic acid side chains classifies it as a protoporphyrin; their locations (positions 1, 3, 5, and 8; 2 and 4; and 6 and 7) make it p. IX or p. type III.

**protoproteose** (pro-to-pro'tē-ōs). Primary proteose.

**pro'tosalt.** Acid *salt*.

**protospasm** (pro'to-spazm) [ proto- + G. *spasmos*, spasm ]. A spasm beginning in one limb or one muscle and gradually becoming more general.

**pro'tospore** [ proto- + G. *sporos*, seed ]. Initial product of progressive cleavage, in which a multinucleate spore is produced.

**Protostrongylus rufes'cens** (pro'to-stron'ji-lus) [ proto- + G. *strongylos*, round ]. The small lungworm of sheep, goats, deer, and occasionally other hosts that occurs in the smaller bronchioles, where it causes plugging of the air passages by its presence and the formation of multiple areas of bronchopneumonia. The symptoms produced generally are milder than those induced by the large lungworm, *Dictyocaulus filaria*.

**protosul'fate.** A compound of sulfuric acid with a protoxide of the metal.

**protosyphilis** (pro-to-sif'ĭ-lis). Primary *syphilis*.

**prototaxic** (pro-to-tak'sik) [ proto- + G. *taxis*, order, arrangement ]. In interpersonal psychiatry, a term referring to primitive illogical thought.

**prototoxin** (pro-to-tok'sin) [ proto- + G. *toxikon*, poison (toxin) ]. A hypothetical form of toxin in bacterial cultures possessing lethal properties and a very strong affinity for antitoxin.

**prototoxoid** (pro-to-tok'soyd) [ proto- + toxoid ]. A hypothetical substance in a bacterial culture, nonpoisonous, but with a stronger affinity than toxin for antitoxin.

**prototroph** (pro'to-trof, -trōf) [ proto- + G. *trophē*, nourishment ]. A bacterial strain that has the same nutritional requirements as the wild-type strain from which it was derived. See also wild-type *strain*.

**prototrophic** (pro'to-trof'ik). Pertaining to a prototroph.

**prototropy** (pro-tot'ro-pī) [ proto- + G. *tropē*, a turning ]. The formation of a tautomer through the shift of a hydrogen atom (prototropic shift).

**pro'totype** [ proto- + G. *typos*, type ]. The primitive form; the first form to which subsequent individuals of the class or species conform.

**protoveratrines A and B** (pro'to-věr'ă-trēn). VERALBA; a mixture of two alkaloids isolated from *Veratrum album*. They exert their main effect upon the cardiovascular system through the carotid sinus receptors and vagal sensory endings in the heart; they cause vasodilation and are thought to bring about a redistribution to all vascular beds and thus to induce a fall in blood pressure. Used in certain forms of hypertension. Protoveratrines A and B maleates (PROVELL) have the same actions.

**protovertebra** (pro'to-ver'te-brah). Provertebra. 1. In the older literature, a mesodermic somite. 2. More recently applied to the sclerotomal concentration which is the primordium of the centrum of a vertebra.

**protover'tebral.** Relating to a protovertebra.

**protox'ide.** Suboxide.

**protoxoid** (pro'tok'soyd). Prototoxoid.

**Protozoa** (pro-to-zo'ah) [ proto- + G. *zōon*, animal ]. A phylum (sometimes regarded as a subkingdom) of the animal kingdom, including all of the so-called unicellular forms. They consist of a single functional cell unit or of an aggregation of nondifferentiated cells, loosely held together and not forming tissues; distinguished from the Metazoa, which include all other animals. The Protozoa are divided into four classes: Sarcodina, Mastigophora, Sporozoa, and Ciliata, though new classifications employ higher taxa and a larger number of major subdivisions.

**protozo′al.** Protozoan (2).

**protozo′an.** 1. Protozoon; a member of the phylum Protozoa. 2. Relating to protozoa.

**protozoiasis** (pro′to-zo-i′ă-sis). Infestation with protozoans.

**protozoicide** (pro-to-zo′ĭ-sīd) [ protozoa + L. *caedo,* to kill ]. 1. Causing destruction of protozoan organisms. 2. An agent used to kill protozoa.

**protozoologist** (pro-to-zo-ol′o-jist). A biologist especially trained and experienced in protozoology.

**protozoology** (pro-to-zo-ol′o-jī) [ protozoa + G. *logos,* study ]. The science that treats of the *Protozoa.*

**protozoon,** pl. **protozoa** (pro-to-zo′on, -zo′ah). Protozoan (1).

**protozoophage** (pro-to-zo′o-fāj) [ protozoa + G. *phagein,* to eat ]. A phagocyte that ingests protozoa.

**protraction** (pro-trak′shun) [ see protractor ]. In dentistry, the extension of teeth or other maxillary or mandibular structures into a position anterior to normal.

   **mandibular p.,** a type of facial anomaly in which the gnathion lies anterior to the orbital plane.

   **maxillary p.,** a type of facial anomaly in which the subnasion lies anterior to the orbital plane.

**protrac′tor** [ L. *pro-traho,* pp. -*tractus,* to draw forth ]. 1. An instrument for extracting a bullet from a wound. 2. A muscle drawing a part forward, as antagonistic to a retractor.

**protrip′tyline hydrochloride** (NF). VIVACTIL; *N*-methyl-5*H*-dibenzo[ *a,d* ]cycloheptane-5-propylamine hydrochloride; antidepressant.

**protru′sio** [ L. ]. Protrusion.

   **p. acetab′uli,** Otto's *disease.*

**protrusion** (pro-tru′zhun) [ L. *protrusio* ]. 1. The state of being thrust forward. 2. In dentistry, a position of the mandible forward or lateral from centric position.

   **bimaxillary p.,** double p.; the projection of both the maxillae and the mandible forward of normal limits in relation to the cranial base; the positioning of the entire dentition forward with respect to the facial profile.

   **double p.,** bimaxillary p.

**protryp′sin.** Trypsinogen.

**protuberance** (pro-tu′ber-ans) [ Mod. L. *protuberantia, q. v.* ]. An outgrowth; a swelling; a knob. See also protuberantia.

   **Bichat's p.,** *corpus* adiposum buccae.

**protuberantia** (pro-tu-ber-an′shi-ah) [ Mod. L. fr. *protubero,* to swell out, fr. *tuber,* a swelling ] [ NA ]. Protuberance; prominence; eminence; projection.

   **p. larynge′a,** *prominentia* laryngea.

   **p. menta′lis** [ NA ], mental protuberance; mental prominence or process; the prominence of the chin at the anterior part of the mandible.

   **p. occipita′lis externa** [ NA ], external occipital protuberance; a prominence about the center of the outer surface of the squamous portion of the occipital bone, giving attachment to the ligamentum nuchae.

   **p. occipita′lis interna** [ NA ], internal occipital protuberance; a projection from about the center of the cruciform eminence on the inner surface of the occipital bone.

**Proust, P. T.,** French physician, 18th century. See P.'s *space.*

**Proust's law.** See under law.

**proventriculus** (pro-ven-trik′u-lus) [ L. *pro,* before, + *ventriculus,* dim. of *venter* ( *ventr*-) belly ]. 1 [ NAV ]. In birds, the thin-walled glandular stomach preceding the muscular gizzard. 2. In insects, the portion of the stomodeum that lies in front of the ventriculus or stomach; it is modified into a small proventricular valve in many diptera (flies).

**prover′tebra.** Protovertebra.

**Providencia** (prov′ĭ-den′sĭ-ah). A genus of motile, peritrichous, nonsporeforming, aerobic or facultatively anaerobic bacteria (family Enterobacteriaceae) containing Gram-negative rods. These organisms do not hydrolyze urea or produce hydrogen sulfide; they produce indole and grow on Simmons' citrate medium. They do not decarboxylate lysine, argine, or ornithine. These organisms occur in specimens from extraintestinal sources, particularly urinary tract infections; they have also been isolated from small outbreaks and sporadic cases of diarrheal disease. The type species is *P. alcalifaciens.*

   **P. alcalifa′ciens,** a species found in extraintestinal sources, particularly in urinary tract infections; it has also been isolated from small outbreaks and sporadic cases of diarrheal disease. It is the type species of *P.*

   **P. stuar′tii,** a species isolated from urinary tract infections, and from small outbreaks and sporadic cases of diarrheal disease.

**provirus** (pro-vi′rus). See under virus.

**provi′tamin.** A substance that may be converted into a vitamin (carotene, for example).

   **p. A,** a generic name for all carotenoids exhibiting qualitatively the biological activity of β-carotene; vitamin A precursors (α-, β-, and γ-carotene and cryptoxanthin). The provitamins A are contained in fish liver oils, spinach, carrots, egg yolk, milk products, and other green leaf or yellow vegetables and fruits.

   **p. $D_2$,** ergosterol.

   **p. $D_3$,** 7-dehydrocholesterol.

**Prowazek** (pro-vat′sek), Stanislas J. M. von, German protozoologist, 1876–1915. Gave his name to *Prowazekia.* See Halberstaedter–P. *bodies,* P.'s *bodies,* P.-Greeff *bodies.*

**Prowazekia** (pro-vă-ze′kĭ-ah) [ S. *Prowazek* ]. A genus of coprozoic flagellate protozoans, formerly included under the term Bodo; the organisms may be parasitic but are not, so far as known, pathogenic.

**prox-, proxi-.** See proximo-.

**proxemics** (prok-sem′iks) [ L. *proximus,* nearest, next ]. The scientific discipline that deals with the various aspects of urban overcrowding.

**proximad** (prok′sĭ-mad) [ L. *proximus,* nearest, next, + *ad,* to ]. In a direction toward a proximal part, or toward the center; not distad.

**prox′imal** [ Mod. L. *proximalis,* fr. L. *proximus,* nearest, next ]. 1. Nearest the trunk or the point of origin, said of part of a limb, of an artery or a nerve, etc., so situated. 2. In dentistry, mesial; opposed to distal. 3. In dental anatomy, denoting the surface of a tooth in relation with its neighbor, whether mesial or distal, *i.e.,* nearer to or farther from the anteroposterior median plane.

**proxima′lis** [ Mod. L. ] [ NA ], Proximal (1).

**prox′imate.** Immediate; next; proximal.

**proximo-, prox-, proxi-** (prok′sĭ-mo-) [ L. *proximus,* nearest, next (to) ]. Combining forms meaning proximal.

**proximoataxia** (prok′sĭ-mo-ă-tak′sĭ-ah) [ proximo- + ataxia, *q. v.* ]. Ataxia or lack of muscular coordination in the proximal portions of the extremities—arms and forearms, thighs and legs; opposed to acroataxia.

**proximobuccal** (prok′sĭ-mo-buk′al). Relating to the proximal and buccal surfaces of a tooth; denoting the angle formed by their junction.

**proximolabial** (prok′sĭ-mo-la′bĭ-al). Relating to the proximal and labial surfaces of a tooth; denoting the angle formed by their junction.

**proximolingual** (prok′sĭ-mo-ling′gwal). Relating to the proximal and lingual surfaces of a tooth; denoting the angle formed by their junction.

**proxymetacaine hydrochloride.** Proparacaine hydrochloride.

**prozone** (pro′zōn). Prezone; in the case of agglutination and of precipitation, the phenomenon in which visible reaction does not occur in mixtures of specific antigen and antibody because of either antibody excess or antigen excess.

**prozygosis** (pro-zi-go′sis) [ G. *pro,* before, + *zygōsis,* a yoking ]. Syncephaly.

**PRPP.** Abbreviation for 5′-phosphoribosyl 1-pyrophosphate.

**prune.** The dried ripe fruit of *Prunus domestica* (family Rosaceae), a tree cultivated in warm temperate regions; a food with laxative properties.

**prunetol.** Genistein.

**Pru'nus** [ L. a plum-tree ]. A genus of trees of the family Rosaceae.

   **P. amygdalus var. amara,** bitter almond.

   **P. amygdalus var. dulcis,** sweet almonds.

   **P. cerasus,** cherry.

   **P. domes'tica,** plum.

   **P. per'sica,** peach.

   **P. sero'tina,** wild black cherry; botanical source of wild cherry.

   **P. virginia'na,** (1) wild black cherry bark; the bark of *P. serotina.* Used as a tonic and in cough mixtures as a bronchial sedative; (2) choke cherry; chief substitute and adulterant of *P. serotina.*

**pruriginous** (pru-rij'ĭ-nus) [ L. *pruriginosus,* having the itch ]. Relating to or suffering from prurigo.

**prurigo** (pru-ri'go) [ L. itch, fr. *prurio,* to itch ]. A chronic disease of the skin marked by a persistent eruption of papules that itch intensely.

   **p. aestiva'lis,** summer p.; a form recurring each summer, and very severe as long as the hot weather continues.

   **p. a'gria** [ G. *agrios,* wild ]. Hebra's p.

   **Besnier's p.,** an atopic form which may be associated with asthma, hay fever, or other allergic conditions.

   **p. fe'rox** [ L. wild, cruel ], Hebra's p.

   **p. gestatio'nis,** a papular skin disease occurring in pregnant women.

   **Hebra's p.,** p. ferox; p. agria; a severe form of chronic dermatitis in which there are constantly recurring, intensely itchy papules and nodules.

   **p. infanti'lis,** *lichen* urticatus.

   **p. mi'tis,** a mild form of a chronic dermatitis characterized by recurring, intensely itching papules and nodules.

   **p. nodula'ris,** Hyde's disease; an eruption of hard nodules in the skin, accompanied by intense itching.

   **p. simplex,** a mild form having a pronounced tendency to relapse.

   **summer p.,** p. aestivalis.

**prurit'ic.** Itching; relating to pruritus.

**pruritus** (pru-ri'tus) [ L. an itching, fr. *prurio,* to itch ]. Itching.

   **p. aestiva'lis,** summer itch; p. occurring during hot weather; may be associated with prickly heat.

   **p. a'ni,** itching of varying degree at the anus; this symptom may be paroxysmal or constant; it may be associated with seborrheic dermatitis or moniliasis, or the may occur independently of any cutaneous lesions, in association with diabetes, intestinal carcinoma, or other systemic disease.

   **p. bal'nea,** bath p.

   **bath p.,** bath itch; p. balnea; itching produced by inadequate rinsing off of soap or by overdrying of skin from excessive bathing.

   **essential p.,** itching that occurs independently of skin lesions.

   **p. hiema'lis,** *dermatitis* hiemalis.

   **p. seni'lis,** senile p.; itching associated with degenerative changes in the skin of the aged.

   **symptomatic p.,** itching occurring as a symptom of some systemic illness such as gout, rheumatism, jaundice, gastrointestinal disturbances.

   **p. vul'vae,** itching of the external female genitalia.

**Prussak,** Alexander, Russian otologist, 1839–1897. See P.'s *fibers, pouch, space.*

**Prussian blue** (prush'an). *Berlin* blue.

**prussiate** (prush'e-āt, prus'e-āt). 1. A cyanide; a salt of hydrocyanic acid. 2. A ferricyanide or ferrocyanide.

**prus'sic acid.** Hydrocyanic acid.

**psalterial** (sahl-te'rĭ-al). Relating to the psalterium.

**psalterium,** pl. **psalteria** (sahl-te'rĭ-um, sahl-te'rĭ-ah) [ G. *psalterion,* harp ]. 1. *Commissura* fornicis. 2. Omasum.

**psammo-** (sam'o-) [ G. *psammos,* sand ]. Combining form meaning sand.

**psammocarcinoma** (sam'o-kar-sĭ-no'mah). A carcinoma that contains calcified foci resembling psammoma bodies.

**psammoma** (să-mo'mah) [ psammo- + G. suffix *-oma,* tumor ]. Angiolithic sarcoma; sand tumor; a firm, cellular neoplasm derived from fibrous tissue of the meninges, choroid plexus, and certain other structures associated with the brain; characterized by the formation of multiple, discrete, concentrically laminated, calcareous bodies (psammoma bodies). Most of these neoplasms are histologically benign, but may lead to severe symptoms as a result of compressing the brain.

   **Virchow's p.,** a group of small, nodular, fibrous neoplasms, originating from the pia mater or the vessels in the pia mater, and containing discrete foci of calcareous material; in some instances, the neoplasms were formerly termed angiolithic sarcoma.

**psammomatous** (să-mo'mă-tus). Possessing or characterized by the presence of psammoma bodies; refers usually to certain types of meningioma or to meningeal hyperplasia with psammoma bodies.

**psammotherapy** (sam'o-thĕr'ă-pĭ) [ psammo- + G. *therapeia,* treatment ]. Ammotherapy; sand treatment; arenation; the use of the sand bath in the treatment of certain rheumatic and other diseases.

**psammous** (sam'us) [ G. *psammos,* sand ]. Sandy.

**Psaume,** J., French physician. See Papillon-Léage and P. *syndrome.*

**pselaphesis, pselaphesia** (sĕ-laf'e-sis, sel'ă-fe'sis, -fe'zĭ-ah) [ G. *pselaphēsis,* a touching ]. The higher tactile sense, including the muscle sense.

**psellism** (sel'izm) [ G. *psellismos,* a stammering ]. Stammering, mispronunciation, or substitution of letter sounds.

**pseud-.** See pseudo-.

**pseudacromegaly** (su-dak-ro-meg'al-ĭ). Enlargement of the extremities and face, not caused by acromegaly.

**pseudactinomycosis** (su-dak'tĭ-no-mi-ko'sis). Para-actinomycosis; pulmonary tuberculosis in which the sputum contains forms that resemble *Actinomyces* organisms.

**pseudagraphia** (su-dă-graf'ĭ-ah) [ pseud- + G. *a-* priv. + *graphō,* to write ]. Pseudoagraphia; partial agraphia in which one can do no original writing, but can copy correctly.

**pseudalbuminuria** (su-dal-bu'mĭ-nu'rĭ-ah). Cyclic *albuminuria.*

**Pseudamphistomum** (su-dam-fis'to-mum) [ pseud- + G. *amphi,* two-sided, + *stoma,* mouth ]. A genus of digenetic flukes of the family Opisthorchiidae.

   **P. trunca'tum,** a species infecting the bile ducts of the dog and cat (rarely of man) in Europe and India.

**pseudangina** (su'dan-ji'nah, su-dan'jĭ-nah). *Angina* pectoris vasomotoria.

**pseudankylosis** (su-dang'kĭ-lo'sis). Fibrous *ankylosis.*

**pseudaphia** (su-daf'ĭ-ah) [ G. *haphē,* a touch ]. Paraphia.

**pseudarrhenia** (su'da-re'nĭ-ah) [ pseud- + G. *arrhēn,* male ]. Obsolete term for female pseudohermaphroditism.

**pseudarthritis** (su-dar-thri'tis). Conversion or neuromimetic disease of the joints.

**pseudarthrosis** (su-dar-thro'sis) [ pseud- + G. *arthrōsis,* a jointing ]. Pseudoarthrosis; neoarthrosis; nearthrosis; a false joint; motion in the shaft of a long bone between the two ends, following an ununited fracture. See fig. on p. 1158.

**pseudelminth** (su-del'minth) [ pseud- + G. *helmins,* worm ]. Anything having the appearance of an intestinal worm.

**pseudencephalus** (su-den-sef'ă-lus) [ pseud- + G. *enkephalos,* brain ]. A fetus with wide open cranial vault in which the brain is grossly defective, the cranium being filled with a vascular mass of ill-developed nervous tissue and meninges. The upper cervical vertebrae are usually cleft.

**pseudesthesia** (su-des-the'zĭ-ah) [ pseud- + G. *aisthēsis,* sensation ]. Pseudoesthesia. 1. Paraphia. 2. A subjective sensation not arising from an external simulus. 3. A sensation referred, after an amputation, to the absent member; see also stump *hallucination;* phantom *limb.*

**pseudinoma** (su-dĭ-no'mah) [ pseud- + G. *is* (*in*), fiber ]. 1. An indurated swelling that grossly resembles a fibroma. 2. A scirrhous tumefaction.

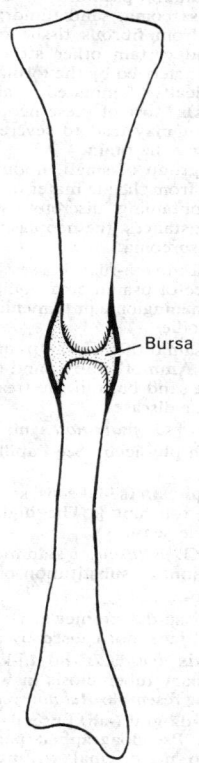

**Pseudarthrosis**

A false joint has formed between the fracture ligaments. (From Schultz, R. J.: *The Language of Fractures*, The Williams & Wilkins Co., Baltimore, 1972.)

**pseudo-, pseud-** (su'do-) [ G. *pseudēs*, false ]. Prefix denoting a resemblance, often deceptive, to the thing indicated by the second element of the compound. Before a vowel it is often contracted to pseud-.

**pseudoacanthosis nigricans** (su'do-ă-kan-tho'sis ni'-gri-kanz). Benign, hyperpigmented, velvety thickening of the skin in areas of maceration (*e.g.*, axilla and groin) in obese and dark-complexioned adults, or in association with endocrine disorders.

**pseudoacephalus** (su'do-ă-sef'ă-lus) [ pseudo- + G. *a*-priv. + *kephalē*, head ]. An apparently headless placental parasitic twin which, however, has rudimentary cephalic structures that can be demonstrated by dissection.

**pseudoachondropla'sia.** Dwarfism with short limbs and a relatively long trunk as in achondroplasia, but not evident at birth.

**pseudoaconitine** (su-do-ă-kon'ĭ-tēn). Acraconitine; an alkaloid from *Aconitum ferox*, said to be twice the strength of aconitine. Poisonous.

**pseudoagglutination** (su'do-ă-glu-tĭ-na'shun). False agglutination; agglomeration of particles in solution which does not involve antigen-antibody combination; in hematology, rouleaux *formation, q.v.*

**pseudoagrammatism** (su'do-ă-gram'ă-tizm) [ pseudo- + G. *a*- priv. + *gramma*, writing, + *-ismos*, condition ]. Paraphasia.

**pseudoagraphia** (su'do-ă-graf'ĭ-ah). Pseudagraphia.

**pseudo-ainhum** (su'do-in'yoom). Nonspontaneous amputation of a digit, caused by a variety of disorders, *e.g.*, neural leprosy, syringomyelia, palmoplantar keratoderma.

**pseudoalbuminuria** (su'do-al-bu'mĭ-nu'rĭ-ah). Cyclic *albuminuria*.

**pseudoallele** (su'do-ă-lēl') [ pseudo- + allele, *q. v.* ]. A gene exhibiting pseudoallelism.

**pseudoallelic** (su'do-ă-le'lik). Relating to pseudoallelism.

**pseudoallelism** (su'do-al'e-lizm). State of two or more genes that appear to occupy the same locus under certain conditions (*e.g.*, trans arrangement), but can be shown to occupy closely linked loci under other conditions (*e.g.*, cis arrangement).

**pseudo-alopecia areata** (su'do-al'o-pe'shĭ-ah ār'e-a'tah). Alopecia in which mild inflammatory changes develop at the orifices of the affected hair follicles.

**pseudoanaphylactic** (su'do-an-ă-fi-lak'tik). Relating to pseudoanaphylaxis; see also anaphylactoid.

**pseudoanaphylaxis** (su'do-an-ă-fi-lak'sis). A condition resembling anaphylaxis, but not due to specific antigen-antibody reaction.

**pseudoanemia** (su-do-ă-ne'mĭ-ah). False anemia; pallor of the skin and mucous membranes without the blood signs of anemia.

**pseudoaneurysm** (su'do-an'u-rizm). Aneurysmal dilation of an artery at the site of puncture as a complication of percutaneous arterial catheterization.

**pseudoangina** (su-do-an'jĭ-nah, -an-ji'nah). *Angina* pectoris vasomotoria.

**pseudoanodontia** (su'do-an'o-don'shĭ-ah) [ pseudo- + G. *an*- priv. + *odous*, tooth ]. Clinical absence of teeth due to a failure in eruption.

**pseudoapoplexy** (su-do-ap'o-plek-sĭ). Parapoplexy; pseudoplegia; a condition simulating apoplexy, not due to cerebral hemorrhage or thrombosis.

**pseudoappendicitis** (su-do-ă-pen-dĭ-si'tis). A symptom-complex simulating appendicitis without inflammation of the appendix.

**pseudoapraxia** (su-do-ă-prak'sĭ-ah). A condition of exaggerated awkwardness in which the person makes wrong use of objects.

**pseudoarthrosis.** Pseudarthrosis.

**pseudoasthma** (su-do-az'mah). Dyspnea.

**pseudoataxia** (su-do-ă-tax'ĭ-ah). Pseudotabes.

**pseudoauthenticity** (su'do-aw-then-tĭ'sĭ-tĭ) [ pseudo- + G. *authentikos*, original ]. False or copied expression of thoughts and feelings.

**pseudobacillus** (su-do-bă-sil'us). Any microscopic object, such as a poikilocyte, resembling a bacillus.

**pseudobacterium** (su'do-bak-tēr'ĭ-um). Any microscopic object resembling a small bacillary organism or other bacterial form.

**pseudoblepsia, pseudoblepsis** (su-do-blep'sĭ-ah, su-do-blep'sis) [ pseudo- + G. *blepsis*, vision ]. Pseudopsia.

**pseudobulbar** (su-do-bul'bar). Denoting a supranuclear paralysis of the bulbar nerves.

**pseudocartilaginous** (su-do-kar-tĭ-laj'ĭ-nus). Composed of a substance resembling cartilage in texture.

**pseudocast** (su'do-kast). False cast; mucous cast; spurious cast; mucous material in an elongated shred or epithelial cells in a cylindroid group, but not actually molded by the tubular structure.

**pseudocele** (su'do-sēl) [ pseudo- + G. *koilia*, cavity ]. *Cavum* septi pellucidi.

**pseudocelom** (su'do-se'lom). Partial or false celom; typical of Nemathelminthes (roundworms), in which the body cavity is lined by mesoderm only along one surface (hypodermis, under the cuticular body wall); *cf.* celom and acelom.

**pseudocephalocele** (su'do-sef'ă-lo-sēl) [ pseudo- + G. *kephalē*, head, + *kēlē*, tumor ]. Acquired herniation of intracranial tissues caused by injury or disease.

**pseudochalazion** (su-do-kal-a'zĭ-on). A tumor of the eyelid resembling a chalazion.

**pseudochancre** (su-do-shang'ker). A nonspecific indurated sore, usually located on the penis, resembling a chancre.

**pseudocholinesterase** (su'do-kol-ĭ-nes'ter-ās). Cholinesterase.

    **atypical p.,** a genetic variant of cholinesterase that fails to catalyze the hydrolysis of succinylcholine; the homozygous atypical form is present in 1 out of 2600 individuals, and the heterozygous atypical form in 4 per cent of the population; see also *dibucaine* number.

**"usual" p.,** a cholinesterase formed in the liver and present in plasma; it catalyzes the hydrolysis of succinylcholine, first into succinylmonocholine and choline, and then into choline and succinic acid.

**pseudochorea** (su-do-ko-re'ah). A spasmodic affection or extensive tic resembling chorea.

**pseudochromesthesia** (su'do-kro'-mes-the'zĭ-ah) [ pseudo- + G. *chrōma*, color, + *aisthēsis*, sensation ]. 1. An anomaly in which each vowel in the printed word is seen as colored; see also photism. 2. Color *hearing*.

**pseudochromhidrosis** (su'do-kro'mĭ-dro'sis) [ pseudo- + G. *chrōma*, color, + *hidrōs*, sweat ]. The presence of pigment on the skin in association with sweating, but due to the local action of pigment-forming bacteria and not to the excretion of colored sweat.

**pseudochylous** (su-do-ki'lus). Resembling chyle.

**pseudocirrhosis** (su-do-sĭ-ro'sis). Cardiac *cirrhosis*.

**pseudoclonus** (su'do-klo'nus). Clonic response of short duration despite continued force to elicit it.

**pseudocoarctation** (su'do-ko-ark-ta'shun). Buckled aorta; kinked aorta; distortion often with slight narrowing of the aortic arch at the level of insertion of the ligamentum arteriosum.

**pseudocodeine** (su'do-ko'dēn). The dextrorotatory stereoisomer of codeine, formed by the action of dilute sulfuric acid on codeine; it has narcotic action.

**pseudocolloid** (su-do-kol'oyd). A colloid-like or mucoid substance found in ovarian cysts, in the lips, and elsewhere.
  **p. of the lips,** Fordyce's *spots*.

**pseudocollusion** (su'do-col-lu'shun) [ pseudo- + Fr. *collusion*, fr. L. *colludere*, to play together ]. A merely apparent sense of closeness emanating from a transference.

**pseudocoloboma** (su-do-kol-o-bo'mah). An apparent coloboma, due to heterochromia of the iris.

**pseudocowpox** (su'do-kow'poks). Paravaccinia.

**pseudocoxalgia** (su'do-kok-sal'jĭ-ah) [ pseudo- + L. *coxa*, hip, + G. *algos*, pain ]. Epiphysial aseptic *necrosis* of the upper end of the femur.

**pseudocrisis** (su-do-kri'sis). A temporary fall of the temperature in pneumonia or other disease usually ending by crisis.

**pseudocroup** (su-do-kroop'). *Laryngismus* stridulus.

**pseudocryptorchism** (su'do-krip'tor-kizm) [ pseudo- + G. *kryptos*, hidden, + *orchis*, testis ]. A condition in which the testes descend to the scrotum but move up and down, rising high in the inguinal canal at one time and descending to the scrotum at another.

**pseudocumene** (su'do-ku'mēn). Pseudocumol; trimethyl benzene; a colorless liquid obtained from coal tar. Used in the sterilization of catgut.

**pseudocumol** (su'do-ku'mol). Pseudocumene.

**pseudocyesis** (su-do-si-e'sis) [ pseudo- + G. *kyēsis*, pregnancy ]. False, phantom, or spurious pregnancy; pseudopregnancy (1); a condition in which some of the signs and symptoms suggest pregnancy although the woman is not pregnant.

**pseudocylindroid** (su'do-sil'in-droyd). A shred of mucus or other substance in the urine resembling a renal cast.

**pseudocyst** (su'do-sist). 1. A false cyst; an accumulation of fluid in a cystlike locule, but without an epithelial or other membranous lining. 2. A mass of 50 or more *Toxoplasma* parasites, found within a host cell, frequently in the brain; the p. is now considered a true cyst enclosed in its own membrane within the host cell; it may rupture to release particles that form new cysts and apparently is infective to another vertebrate host; see also bradyzoite.

**pseu'dodeciduo'sis** [ pseudo- + L. *deciduus*, falling off ]. A decidual response of endometrium in the absence of pregnancy.

**pseudodementia** (su-do-de-men'shĭ-ah). A condition of exaggerated indifference to one's surroundings without actual mental impairment.

**pseudodiabetes** (su'do-di'ă-be'tēz). Subclinical *diabetes*.
  **stress p.,** subclinical *diabetes*.

**pseudodiastolic** (su-do-di-as-tol'ik). Seemingly associated with the cardiac diastole.

**pseudodiphtheria** (su'do-dif-thēr'ĭ-ah). Diphtheroid (1).

**pseudodipsia** (su'do-dip'sĭ-ah) [ pseudo- + G. *dipsa*, thirst ]. False *thirst*.

**pseudodiverticulum** (su'do-di-ver-tik'u-lum). An outpouching from the lumen into an area of central necrosis within a large smooth muscle tumor, along any part of the intestinal wall.

**pseudodysentery** (su-do-dis'en-tēr-ĭ). The occurrence of symptoms indistinguishable from those of bacillary dysentery, caused by dietetic errors, a chill, intestinal worms, or causes other than the presence of the specific microorganisms.

**pseudoedema** (su'do-e-de'ma) [ pseudo- + G. *oidēma*, a swelling (edema) ]. A puffiness of the skin not due to a fluid accumulation.

**pseudoemphysema** (su'do-em-fĭ-se'mah). A condition of the lung in which characteristic airflow changes of emphysema occur but without the typical parenchymal disruption of the lung tissue.

**pseudoephedrine hydrochloride** (su'do-e-fed'rin) (NF). SUDAFED; ISOEPHEDRINE; *d*-pseudoephedrine hydrochloride; the naturally occurring isomer of ephedrine; a sympathomimetic amine used as a bronchial dilator with supposedly lesser cardiovascular and central nervous system effects than ephedrine.

**pseudoerosion** (su'do-e-ro'zhun). Ectopia of the columnar epithelium of the cervix beyond the external os.

**pseudoerysipelas** (su'do-ēr'ĭ-sip'ē-las). Erysipeloid.

**pseudoesthesia** (su-do-es-the'zĭ-ah). Pseudesthesia.

**pseudoexfoliation** (su'do-eks-fo'lĭ-a'shun). A condition simulating exfoliation in some respects, but in which the surface layer is not actually detached.
  **p. of lens capsule,** a condition in which deposits on the lens resemble exfoliation of the lens capsule; it is frequently complicated by glaucoma.

**pseudofibrin** (su-do-fi'brin). A substance obtained by the precipitation of fibrinogen by sodium chloride; parafibrinogen.

**pseudofluctuation** (su-do-fluk-chu-a'shun). A wavelike sensation, resembling fluctuation, obtained by tapping muscular tissue.

**pseudofracture** (su'do-frak'chur). A condition in which an x-ray shows formation of new bone with thickening of periosteum at site of an injury to bone.

**pseudoganglion** (su-do-gang'glĭ-on). A localized thickening of a nerve trunk having the appearance of a ganglion.

**pseudogeusesthesia** (su'do-gu-ses-the'zĭ-ah) [ pseudo- + G. *geusis*, taste, + *aisthēsis*, sensation ]. Color *taste*.

**pseudogeusia** (su-do-gu'sĭ-ah) [ pseudo- + G. *geusis*, taste ]. A subjective taste sensation not produced by an external stimulus.

**pseudoglanders** (su'do-glan'derz). Melioidosis.

**pseudoglaucoma** (su'do-glaw-ko'mah). Glaucoma with physiologically normal intraocular pressure.

**pseudoglioma** (su-do-gli-o'mah). Any condition liable to be mistaken for retinoblastoma; *e.g.*, exudative retinitis, metastatic vitreous abscess, persistent tunica vasculosa lentis, retinopathy of prematurity, massive retinal fibrosis, or inflammatory retinal detachment.

**pseudoglobulin** (su-do-glob'u-lin). That fraction of the serum globulin not precipitated by saturation of its solution with sodium chloride but thrown out by saturation with magnesium sulfate or by half-saturation with ammonium sulfate. (Probably a mixture of $\alpha$ and $\beta$-globulins).

**pseudoglucosazone** (su-do-glu-ko'sā-zōn). A substance sometimes present in normal urine which gives a reaction in the phenylhydrazine test.

**pseudogout** (su'do-gowt). Articular *chondrocalcinosis*.

**pseudogynecomastia** (su'do-jin'e-ko-mas'tĭ-ah, -gi'ne-ko-) [ pseudo- + G. *gynē*, woman, + *mastos*, breast ]. Enlargement of the male breast by an excess of adipose tissue without any increase in breast tissue.

**pseudohematuria** (su'do-hem'ă-tu'rĭ-ah, -he'mă-tu'rĭ-ah). False hematuria; not actually hematuria, but a red pigmentation of urine caused by certain foods or drugs.

**pseudohemoglobin** (su'do-he'mo-glo'bin). A combination of oxygen and hemoglobin, intermediate between hemoglobin and oxyhemoglobin.

**pseudohemophilia** (su'do-he'mo-fil'ĭ-ah). False hemophilia; a noninherited hemophilia-like syndrome due to some specific disorder or disorders.

    **hereditary p.,** von Willebrand's *disease.*

**pseudohemoptysis** (su'do-he-mop'tĭ-sis) [ pseudo- + G. haima, blood, + *ptysis,* a spitting ]. Spitting of blood that does not come from the lungs or bronchial tubes.

**pseu'dohermaph'rodite** (su'do-her-maf'ro-dīt). An individual exhibiting pseudohermaphroditism.

**pseudohermaphroditism** (su'do-her-maf'ro-di-tizm). A state, somewhat resembling true hermaphroditism, in which the individual is distinctly of one sex (*i.e.,* possessing either testes or ovaries) although having somatic characteristics of both sexes.

    **female p.,** a condition in which an individual has ovaries, but possesses both male and female somatic characteristics.

    **male p.,** a condition in which an individual has testes, but possesses both male and female somatic characteristics.

**pseudohernia** (su-do-her'nĭ-ah). Inflammation of the scrotal tissues or of an inguinal gland, simulating a strangulated hernia.

**pseudoheterotopia** (su-do-het-er-o-to'pĭ-ah). A seeming displacement of certain tissues observed postmortem; actually an artifact, rather than a true heterotopia.

**pseudohydrocephaly** (su'do-hi-dro-sef'ă-lĭ). A condition characterized by an enlargement of the head without concomitant enlargement of the ventricular system.

**pseudohydronephrosis** (su-do-hi'dro-ne-fro'sis). The presence of a cyst near the kidney simulating hydronephrosis.

**pseudohyoscyamine** (su-do-hi-ō-si'ă-mēn, -min). Norhyoscyamine; an alkaloid occurring along with hyoscyamine and hyoscine in the leaf of *Duboisia myoporoides,* a tree of Australia and from the root of *Scopolia japonica.*

**pseudohypertrophic** (su-do-hi-per-trof'ik). Relating to or marked by pseudohypertrophy.

**pseudohypertrophy** (su'do-hi-per'tro-fĭ). False hypertrophy; increase in size of an organ or a part, due not to increase in size or number of the specific functional elements but to that of some other tissue, fatty or fibrous.

**pseudohypha** (su-do-hi'fah) [ pseudo- + G. *hyphē,* a web (hypha) ]. A chain of easily disrupted fungal cells that are intermediate between a chain of budding cells and a true hypha.

**pseudohypoparathyroidism** (su'do-hi'po-păr-ă-thi'-royd-izm). Seabright bantam syndrome; a heritable disorder resembling hypoparathyroidism, but the signs and symptoms of which are unresponsive to treatment with parathyroid hormone. Characterized by short stature, round face, achondroplasia, calcification of basal ganglia, true ectopic bone in fascial planes and skin, mental deficiency, hypocalcemia, hyperphosphatemia, and parathyroid tissue that is normal in appearance or hyperplastic; not infrequently associated with moniliasis and manifestations of diabetes mellitus; assumed to represent refractoriness of target tissues to parathyroid hormone.

**pseudohypothyroidism** (su'do-hi'po-thi'royd-izm). A rarely used synonym for pseudohypoparathyroidism or pseudo-pseudohypoparathyroidism. Because hypometabolism sometimes is present in these disorders, some believe that target tissue refractoriness to thyroid hormone also exists.

**pseudoicterus** (su-do-ik'ter-us). Pseudojaundice; discoloration of the skin not due to the bile pigments, as in Addison's disease.

**pseudoileus** (su-do-il'e-us). Absolute obstipation, stimulating ileus, due to paralysis of the intestinal wall.

**pseudoinfluenza** (su-do-in-flu-en'zah). An epidemic catarrh simulating influenza, but less severe.

**pseudointraligamentous** (su'do-in'trah-lig-ah-men'tus). Falsely giving the impression of lying within the broad ligament; for example, a p. tumor.

**pseudoisochromatic** (su'do-i'so-kro-mat'ik). Apparently of the same color; denoting certain charts containing colored spots mixed with figures printed in confusion colors; used in testing for color blindness.

**pseudojaundice** (su'do-jawn'dis). Pseudoicterus.

**pseudokeratin** (su'do-kĕr'ă-tin). A protein extracted from epidermis and nervous tissue (glial fibrils), probably involved in keratinization.

**pseudoleukemia** (su-do-lu-ke'mĭ-ah). An obsolete term for diseases marked by enlargement of the spleen and of the lymph nodes, the most prominent characteristic of which is a progressive anemia without leukemic changes in the blood.

    **p. cutis,** the occurrence of skin lesions of various forms in p.

    **infantile p.,** Jaksch's *disease.*

    **lymphat'ic p.,** p. without apparent participation of the spleen in the morbid process.

    **myelog'enous p.,** myelomatosis.

**pseudoleukocythemia** (su-do-lu'ko-si-the'mĭ-ah). Pseudoleukemia.

**pseudolipoma** (su-do-lĭ-po'mah). Any circumscribed, soft, smooth, usually movable swelling or tumefaction that grossly resembles a lipoma.

**pseudolithiasis** (su'do-lĭ-thi'ă-sis) [ pseudo- + G. *lithos,* stone ]. Disorder resembling one of the syndromes associated with stone in a hollow viscus or elsewhere.

**pseudologia** (su-do-lo'jĭ-ah) [ pseudo- + G. *logos,* word ]. Pathological lying in speech or writing.

    **p. phantastica,** an elaborate and often fantastic account of a patient's exploits, which are completely false but which the patient himself appears to believe.

**pseudoluxation** (su'do-luk-sa'shun). Incomplete dislocation.

**pseudolymphocyte** (su-do-lim'fo-sīt). A small neutropilic leukocyte.

**pseudolysogenic** (su'do-li'so-jen'ik). Pertaining to pseudolysogeny.

**pseudolysogeny** (su'do-li-soj'ē-nĭ). The condition in which a bacteriophage is maintained (carried) in a culture of a bacterial strain by infecting susceptible variants of the strain, in contradistinction to true lysogeny in which the bacteriophage genome multiplies as an integral part of the bacterial genome.

**pseudomamma** (su-do-mam'ah). A glandular structure resembling the mammary gland, occurring in dermoid cysts.

**pseudomania** (su-do-ma'nĭ-ah). 1. Feigned insanity. 2. A mental disorder in which the patient alleges to have committed a crime, but of which he is innocent. 3. Generally, the morbid impulse to falsify or lie, as in pseudologica.

**pseudomasturbation** (su'do-mas'ter-ba'shun). Peotillomania.

**pseudomelanosis** (su-do-mel-ă-no'sis) [ pseudo- + G. *melas,* black ]. A dark greenish or blackish postmortem discoloration of the surface of the abdominal viscera, resulting from the action of sulfureted hydrogen upon the iron of disintegrated hemoglobin.

**pseudomembrane** (su'do-mem'brān). False *membrane.*

**pseudomembranous** (su'do-mem'brā-nus). Relating to or marked by the presence of a false membrane.

**pseudomeningitis** (su-do-men-in-ji'tis). Meningism.

**pseudomenstruation** (su'do-men'stru-a'shun). Uterine bleeding without the typical premenstrual endometrial changes.

**pseudometaplasia** (su'do-met'ă-pla'zĭ-ah). Histologic *accomodation.*

**pseudomnesia** (su-dom-ne'zĭ-ah) [ pseudo- + G. *mnēsis,* memory. MNEM- ]. A subjective impression of memory of events that have not occurred.

**Pseudomonas** (su-do-mo'nas) [ pseudo- + G. *monas,* unit, monad ]. A genus of motile, polar flagellate, nonsporeforming, strictly aerobic bacteria (family Pseudomonadaceae) containing straight or curved, but not helical, Gram-negative rods which occur singly. The metabolism is respiratory, never fermentative. They occur commonly in soil and in fresh water and marine environments. Some species are plant pathogens. One species is a specialized mammalian parasite while others are occasionally pathogenic to animals. The type species is *P. aeruginosa.*

**P. acidovorans,** a species found in soil and occasionally in clinical specimens.

**P. aerugino'sa,** blue-pus organism; *P. pyocyanea;* a species found in soil, water, and commonly in clinical specimens (wound infections, infected burn lesions, urinary tract infections); the causative agent of blue pus; occasionally pathogenic for plants. It is the type species of the genus *P.*

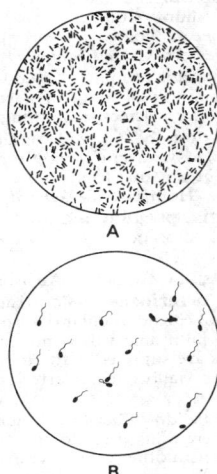

A

B

*Pseudomonas aeruginosa*

*A,* Gram-stained cells; *B,* cells stained to show flagella. Original magnification, ×1200

**P. cepacia,** a species found in rotted onions and in clinical specimens.

**P. diminuta,** a species found primarily in clinical specimens, rarely in water.

**P. fluorescens,** a species found in soil and water. It is frequently found in clinical specimens, and it is commonly associated with food spoilage (eggs, cured meats, fish, and milk).

**P. mallei,** *Actinobacillus mallei; Malleomyces mallei; Pfeifferella mallei;* Glander's bacillus; a species parasitic on horses and donkeys, causing the diseases glanders and farcy. It is the type species of the genera *Malleomyces* and *Pfeifferella.*

**P. maltophilia,** a species found primarily in clinical specimens but also in water, milk, and frozen food.

**P. pseudoalcaligenes,** a species found in a sinus discharge.

**P. pseudomallei,** *Malleomyces pseudomallei;* a species found in human and animal cases of melioidosis and in soil and water in tropical regions.

**P. pyocyan'ea,** *P. aeruginosa.*

**P. stutzeri,** a species found in soil and water, frequently in clinical specimens.

**P. vesiculare,** a species found in the medicinal leech (*Hirudo medicinalis*) and in water from a stream.

**pseudomorph** (su'do-morf) [ pseudo- + G. *morphē,* form ]. A mineral found crystallized in a form that is not proper to it but to some other mineral.

**pseudomorphine** (su-do-mor'fēn). 2,2′-Bimorphine; a non-narcotic derivative of morphine, having a chemical reaction practically the same as that of morphine.

**pseudomucin** (su'do-mu'sin). A gelatinous material resembling mucin, as found in certain ovarian cysts; see also paralbumin and metalbumin.

**pseudomucinous** (su'do-mu'sĭ-nus). Relating to pseudomucin.

**pseudomyopia** (su'do-mi-o'pī-ah). A condition simulating myopia and due to spasm of the ciliary muscle in spasm of accommodation.

**pseudomyxoma** (su'do-mik-so'mah). A gelatinous mass resembling a myxoma but composed of epithelial mucus.

**p. peritone'i,** hydrops spurius; the accumulation of large quantities of mucoid or mucinous material in the peritoneal cavity, as a result of (1) rupture of a mucocele of the appendix, or (2) rupture of benign or malignant cystic neoplasms of the ovary. P. peritonei will frequently persist because of the growth of mucus-secreting cells scattered on serosal surfaces, leading to intestinal adhesions and obstruction.

**pseudonarcotic** (su-do-nar-kot'ik). Inducing sleep by reason of a sedative effect, but not directly narcotic.

**pseudoneoplasm** (su-do-ne'o-plazm). Pseudotumor. 1. An enlargement of nonneoplastic character which clinically resembles a true neoplasm so closely as often to be mistaken for such. 2. A circumscribed fibrous exudate of inflammatory origin, temporary in character.

**pseudoneuritis** (su-do-nu-ri'tis). Congenital reddish appearance of the optic disk simulating optic neuritis.

**pseudoneuroma** (su-do-nu-ro'ma). traumatic n.

**pseudoneuronophagia** (su'do-nu'ro-no-fa'jĭ-ah) [ pseudo- + G. *neuron,* nerve, + *phagein,* to eat ]. An artifact falsely suggesting phagocytosis.

**pseudonystagmus** (su'do-nis-tag'mus). An accentuation of the normal oscillatory eye movements occurring on shifting fixation.

**pseudo-osteomalacia** (su-do-os'te-o-mă-la'shī-ah). Rachitic softening of bone.

**pseudo-osteomalacic** (su-do-os'te-o-mă-la'sik). Marked by pseudo-osteomalacia.

**pseudopapilledema** (su'do-pap'il-e-de'mah). Anomalous elevation of the optic disk; seen in high hyperopia and optic nerve drusen.

**pseudoparalysis** (su'do-pă-ral'ĭ-sis). Apparent paralysis due to voluntary inhibition of motion because of pain, to incoordination, or other cause, but without actual paralysis.

**arthritic general p.,** Klippel's disease; a disease, occurring in arthritic subjects, having symptoms resembling those of general paresis, the lesions of which consist of diffuse changes of a degenerative and noninflammatory character due to intracranial atheroma.

**congenital atonic p.,** *amytonia* congenita.

**pseudoparaplegia** (su'do-păr-ă-ple'jĭ-ah). Apparent paralysis in the lower extremities, in which the tendon and skin reflexes and the electrical reactions are normal; the condition is sometimes observed in rickets.

**Basedow's p.,** weakness in the thigh muscles in thyrotoxicosis which may occur suddenly and cause the patient to fall; a specific form of myopathy is fairly common in thyrotoxicosis.

**pseudoparasite** (su-do-păr'ă-sīt). A false parasite; may be either a commensal or a temporary parasite (the latter being an organism accidentally ingested that survives briefly in the intestine).

**pseudoparesis** (su'do-pă-re'sis, -păr'e-sis). 1. Pseudoparalysis. 2. A condition marked by the pupillary changes, tremors, and speech disturbances suggestive of early paresis, in which, however, the serologic tests are negative.

**pseudopelade** (su'do-pē-lahd) [ pseudo- + Fr. *pelade,* disease that causes sporadic falling of hair ]. A scarring type of alopecia; usually occurs in small areas preceded by folliculitis; assumed by many to be synonymous with folliculitis decalvans.

**pseudopericarditis** (su'do-pĕr'ĭ-kar-di'tis). An artifact of auscultation resembling a friction rub, but due to movement of the tissue in the intercostal space when the diapragm of the stethoscope is placed over the apex beat. It is not heard when a bell-type stethoscope is used.

**pseudoperitonitis** (su'do-pĕr'ĭ-to-ni'tis). Peritonism (2).

**pseudophakia** (su'do-fak'ĭ-ah) [ pseudo- + *phakos,* lentil (lens) ]. An eye in which a plastic lenticulus is substituted for the extracted cataract.

**pseudophlegmon** (su-do-fleg'mon) [ pseudo- + G. *phlegmonē,* inflammation ]. A noninflammatory circumscribed redness of the skin.

**Hamilton's p.,** a trophic affection of the subcutaneous connective tissue, marked by a circumscribed swelling which may become indurated and red, but never suppurates.

**pseudophotesthesia** (su-do-fo-tes-the'zī-ah) [ pseudo- + G. *phōs*, light, + *aisthēsis*, sensation ]. Photism.

**pseudophyllid** (su'do-fī'lid). Common name for members of the order Pseudophyllidea.

**Pseudophyllidea** (su'do-fī-lid'ī-ah) [ pseudo- + G. *phyllon*, leaf ]. An order of tapeworms with an aquatic life cycle, passing through coracidium, procercoid, and plerocercoid stages before developing into adults in fish, marine mammals, or fish-eating mammals; includes the broad fish tapeworm of man, *Diphyllobothrium latum*.

**pseudoplegia** (su-do-ple'jī-ah) [ pseudo- + G. *plēgē*, a stroke ]. Pseudoapoplexy.

**pseudopod** (su'do-pod). Pseudopodium.

**pseudopodium**, pl. **pseudopodia** (su-do-po'dī-um, -po'dī-ah) [ pseudo- + G. *pous*, foot ]. A temporary protoplasmic process, put forth by a protozoan for locomotion or for prehension of food.

**pseudopolydystrophy** (su'do-pol-ī-dis'tro-fī). Mucolipidosis III.

**pseudopolyp** (su'do-pol'ip). Inflammatory p.; a projecting mass of granulation tissue, large numbers of which may develop in ulcerative colitis; may become covered by regenerating epithelium.

**pseudopregnancy** (su'do-preg'nan-sī). 1. Pseudocyesis. 2. A condition in which symptoms resembling those of pregnancy are present, but which is not pregnancy. Occurs after sterile copulation in mammalian species in which copulation induces ovulation; also in dogs, in which the estrus cycle includes a marked luteal phase.

**pseudopremature** (su'do-pre'mă-tūr). Designating an infant delivered at term who has suffered growth retardation *in utero*.

**pseudo-pseudohypoparathyroidism** (su'do-su'do-hi'po-păr-ă-thi'royd-izm). Albright's syndrome (2); a heritable disorder that closely simulates pseudohypoparathyroidism; manifestations of hypoparathyroidism, however, are mild or absent. In particular, hypocalcemia is not present, or the consequences thereof, such as tetanic convulsions. The genetic defect responsible for this disorder is probably closely linked to that responsible for pseudohypoparathyroidism; patients exhibiting the latter disorder not infrequently are the offspring of mothers with pseudo-pseudohypoparathyroidism.

**pseudopsia** (su-dop'sī-ah) [ pseudo- + G. *opsis*, vision. OPO- ]. Pseudoblepsia; visual hallucinations, illusions, or false perceptions.

**pseudopterygium** (su'do-tĕ-rij'ī-um). Scar pterygium; a pterygium of irregular shape following diphtheria, a burn, or other injury of the conjunctiva; may occur at any part of the corneal margin.

**pseudoptosis** (su-do-to'sis, su-dop'to-sis) [ pseudo- + G. *ptōsis*, a falling ]. A condition resembling ptosis and due to blepharophimosis, blepharochalasis, or other affection.

**pseudopuberty** (su'do-pu'ber-tī). A condition characterized by the development of a varying number of the somatic and functional changes typical of puberty; commonly caused by the hormonal secretions of a tumor; arises typically before the chronological age of puberty.

   **precocious p.,** the development of p. in very young children; commonly characterized by secretion of gonadal hormones, without stimulation of gametogenesis.

**pseudorabies** (su'do-ra'bēz) [ pseudo- + rabies, *q. v.* ]. Aujeszky's disease.

**pseudoreaction** (su-do-re-ak'shun). A false reaction; one not due to specific causes in a given test.

**pseudoretinitis pigmentosa** (su'do-ret'ī-ni'tis pig'men-to'sah). A widespread pigmentary mottling of the retina that may follow serious eye trauma, especially from a penetrating injury.

**pseudorheumatism** (su-do-ru'mă-tizm). Rheumatoid arthritis, or other similar condition.

**pseudorickets** (su'do-rik'ets). Renal *rickets*.

**pseudorubella** (su'do-ru-bel'ah). *Exanthema* subitum.

**pseudoscarlatina** (su-do-skar-lă-te'nah). Erythema with fever, due to causes other than *Streptococcus pyogenes*.

**pseudosclerosis** (su'do-skle-ro'sis) [ pseudo- + G. *sklērosis*, hardening ]. 1. Inflammatory induration or fatty or other infiltration simulating fibrous thickening. 2. West-phal's p.; Westphal-Strümpell p.; the cerebral changes of hepatolenticular degeneration.

   **Westphal's p.,** pseudosclerosis (2).

   **Westphal-Strümpell p.,** pseudosclerosis (2).

**pseudosmallpox** (su'do-smawl'poks). Alastrim.

**pseudosmia** (su-doz'mī-ah) [ pseudo- + G. *osmē*, smell ]. A subjective sensation of an odor that is not present.

**Pseudostertagia bullosa** (su'do-ster-ta'jī-ah bul-o'sah). One of the medium stomach worms located in the abomasum of sheep, goats, and pronghorn; it is found chiefly in the western United States.

**pseudostoma** (su-dos'to-mah) [ pseudo- + G. *stoma*, mouth ]. An apparent opening in a cell, membrane, or other tissue, due to a defect in staining or other cause.

**pseudotabes** (su'do-ta'bēz). Pseudoataxia; Leyden's ataxia; peripheral tabes; a syndrome having the characteristics of tabes dorsalis but not due to syphilis.

   **papillotonic p.,** Holmes-Adie *syndrome*.

**pseudotrichinosis, pseudotrichiniasis** (su'do-trik'ī-no'sis, -trik'ī-ni'ă-sis) [ pseudo- + trichinosis, *q. v.* ]. Multiple myositis.

**pseudotropine** (su-do-tro'pēn). An isomer of tropine.

**pseudotruncus arteriosus** (su'do-trung'kus ar-tēr'ī-o'sus). A congenital cardiovascular deformity in which there is atresia of the pulmonic valve and no main pulmonary artery; the lungs are supplied with blood either through a patent ductus or via bronchial arteries arising from the aorta.

**pseudotubercle** (su'do-tu'ber-kl). A nodule histologically similar to a tuberculous granuloma; due to infection by some microorganism other than *Mycobacterium tuberculosis*.

**pseudotuberculosis** (su'do-tu-ber'ku-lo'sis). Occurs in rodents, mice, and sheep; characterized by nodules histologically similar to those of tuberculosis but due to a coccoid bacillus (guinea pigs) or to a diphtheroid bacillus (mice and sheep). P. occurs in man, rarely, as a result of infection by *Pasteurella pseudotuberculosis*.

**pseudotumor** (su'do-tu'mor). Pseudoneoplasm.

**pseudouridine** (su'do-u'rī-dēn, -din). 5-Ribosyluracil; symbols, $\psi$, $\psi$rd; a naturally occurring isomer of uridine found in transfer ribonucleic acids.

**pseudovacuole** (su-do-vak'u-ōl). An apparent vacuole in a cell, either an artifact or an intracellular parasite.

**pseudovariola** (su'do-vă-ri'o-lah) [ pseudo- + L. *variola*, smallpox ]. Alastrim.

**pseudoventricle** (su-do-ven'trī-kl). *Cavum* septi pellucidi.

**pseudovitamin** (su'do-vi'tă-min). A substance having a chemical structure closely similar to a given vitamin but lacking the usual physiologic action.

   **p. B$_{12}$,** vitamin B$_{12f}$; $\psi$ vitamin B$_{12}$; cobinamide cyanide phosphate, 3'-ester with 7-$\alpha$-D-ribofuranosyladenine, inner salt; vitamin B$_{12}$ with adenine replacing dimethylbenzimidazole; one of several substances produced during anaerobic fermentation by certain organisms in bovine rumen contents. Chemically closely similar to vitamin B$_{12}$ (cyancobalamin) but without the physiologic action of the vitamin, in man.

**pseudovomiting** (su'do-vom'ī-ting). Regurgitation of matter from the esophagus or stomach without expulsive effort.

**pseudoxanthoma elasticum** (su-do-zan-tho'mah e-las'tī-kum). Elastoma; slightly elevated yellowish plaques on the neck, axillae, abdomen, and thighs, associated with angioid streaks of the retina and similar elastic tissue degeneration in other organs.

**psicofuranine** (si'ko-fūr'ă-nēn). Antibiotic produced by *Streptomyces hygroscopicus;* possesses antineoplastic activity.

**D-psicose** (si'kōs). D-Ribo-2-hexulose; allulose; a ketohexose, isomeric with fructose. For structure, see sugars.

**psilocin** (si'lo-sin). Psilotsin; 3-[ 2-(dimethylamino)ethyl ]-indol-4-ol; a hallucinogenic agent related to psilocybin.

**Psilocybe mexicana.** A species of mushrooms (family Agaricaceae); the fruiting bodies are a source of the hallucinogen, psilocybin.

**psilocybin** (si'lo-si'bin, -sib'in). Teonanacath; psilotsibin; indocybin; 3-(2-dimethylamino)ethylindol-4-ol dihydrogen phosphate; the $N',N'$-dimethyl derivative of 4-hydroxytryptamine; obtained from the fruiting bodies of the Mexican hallucinogenic fungus *Psilocybe mexicana* and other species of *Psilocybe* and *Stropharia*. P. is a congener of 5-hydroxytryptamine with striking central effects. It is readily hydrolyzed to 4-hydroxybufotenine. Used as a hallucinogenic agent (and by Mexican aborigines to induce trances).

**psilosis** (si-lo'sis) [ G. *psilōsis*, a stripping, fr. *psilos*, bare ]. 1. Old term for sprue (1). 2. Falling of the hair.

**psilothin** (sil'o-thin). A depilatory plaster applied warm to a hairy surface, and torn off when cool, bringing with it the hairs.

**psilothron** (sil'o-thron) [ G. *psilōthron* ]. A depilatory.

**psilotic** (si-lot'ik). 1. Relating to psilosis. 2. Depilatory.

**P-sinis'trocardia'le.** An electrocardiographic syndrome characteristic of overloading of the left atrium; often erroneously called P-mitrale (*q.v.*), as the syndrome can result from any overloading of the left atrium and independently of disease of the mitral valve.

**psittacine** (sit'ă-sēn). Referring to birds of the parrot family (parrots, parakeets, and budgerigars).

**psittacosis** (sit-ă-ko'sis) [ G. *psittakos*, a parrot, + suffix *-osis*, condition ]. Parrot disease (1); parrot fever; an infectious disease of birds, especially parrots, characterized by diarrhea, loss of appetite, wasting, and ruffling of feathers; it is sometimes transmitted to man in whom the symptoms are headache, nausea, epistaxis, constipation, and fever preceded by a chill, and usually with added symptoms of bronchopneumonia. The causal agent is *Chlamydia psittaci*.

**psoas** (so'as) [ G. *psoa*, the muscles of the loins ]. See under musculus.

**psomophagia, psomophagy** (so-mo-fa'jī-ah, so-mof'a-jī) [ G. *psōmos*, morsel, bit, + *phagein*, to eat ]. The practice of swallowing the food without thorough mastication; bolting the food. The opposite of fletcherism.

**psora** (so'rah) [ G. *psōra*, itch ]. Psoriasis.

**psoralen** (so'ră-len). Furo[ 3,2-*g* ]coumarin; a phototoxic drug used by topical or oral administration for the treatment of vitiligo.

**psorelcosis** (so-rel-ko'sis) [ G. *psōra*, itch, + *helkōsis*, ulceration ]. Ulceration resulting from scabies.

**psorenteritis** (sor-en-ter-i'tis) [ G. *psōra*, itch (scabies), + *enteron*, intestine, + suffix *-itis*, inflammation ]. Inflammatory swelling of the solitary follicles of the intestine, in typhoid fever, cholera, and other affections.

**Psorergates** [ G. *psōra*, itch ]. A genus of itch mites (family Cheyletidae) parasitic on cattle, sheep and goats.

  **P. bos,** the itch mite of cattle; described in New Mexico.

  **P. o'vis,** the small itch mite of sheep in the United States, Australia, New Zealand, and South Africa.

**psoriasic** (so-rī-as'ik). Psoriatic.

**psoriasiform** (so-rī-as'ī-form). Resembling psoriasis.

**psoriasis** (so-ri'ă-sis) [ G. *psōriasis*, fr. *psōra*, the itch ]. Alphos; lepra alphos; psora; a condition characterized by the eruption of circumscribed, discrete and confluent, reddish, silvery-scaled maculopapules; the lesions occur preeminently on the elbows, knees, scalp, and trunk, and microscopically show characteristic parakeratosis and elongation of rete ridges.

  **p. annula'ris, p. annula'ta,** p. circinata.

  **p. arthrop'ica,** p. associated with severe arthritis resembling rheumatoid arthritis.

  **p. bucca'lis,** leukoplakia.

  **p. circina'ta,** Willan's lepra; p. annularis; p. annuata; p. orbicularis; p. in which healing is taking place at the center of the lesion while the process continues at the periphery, producing a ring-shaped or annular lesion.

  **p. diffu'sa,** diffused p.; a form with more or less coalescence of the lesions.

  **p. discoi'dea,** p. nummularis; p. in which the lesions are discrete and disklike.

  **p. geograph'ica,** p. gyrata in which the lesions suggest the coast outline on a map.

  **p. gutta'ta** [ L. *gutta*, drop ], p. occurring in round patches of small size, giving the appearance of a rain-bespattered surface.

  **p. gyra'ta,** p. circinata in which there is a coalescence of the rings giving rise to figures of various outlines.

  **p. invetera'ta,** a form in which the lesions are confluent, the affected skin being thickened, indurated, and scaly.

  **p. linguae,** leukoplakia.

  **p. nummula'ris,** p. discoidea.

  **p. orbicula'ris,** p. circinata.

  **p. ostrea'cea,** p. rupioides; p. with concentric tiers of scales which give the appearance of an oyster shell.

  **p. puncta'ta,** p. in which the individual lesions are papules, each red in color, and tipped with a single white scale.

  **pustular p.,** (1) an extensive exacerbation of p., with pustule formation in the normal and psoriatic skin, fever, and granulocytosis; sometime precipitated by oral steroids; (2) a local pustular eruption of the palms and soles, occurring most commonly in a patient with p.; it is difficult to distinguish it from acrodermatitis continua.

  **p. rupioi'des,** p. ostreacea.

  **p. spondylit'ica,** p. associated with an ankylosing spondylitis.

  **p. universa'lis,** generalized p.

**psoriatic** (so-rī-at'ik). Relating to psoriasis.

**psoric** (so'rik). Relating to scabies.

**psoroid** (so'royd) [ G. *psōra*, itch (scabies), + *eidos*, resemblance ]. Resembling scabies.

**psorophthalmia** (so-rof-thal'mī-ah) [ G. *psōra*, itch (scabies), + *ophthalmia*, *q.v.* ]. Blepharitis marginalis.

**Psoroptes** (so-rop'tēz) [ G. *psōra*, itch ]. A genus of itch or mange mites of the family Cheyletidae.

  **P. cunic'uli,** the scab mite of rabbits.

  **P. e'qui,** the mange or body mite of horses.

  **P. o'vis,** the common scab mite of sheep and cattle.

**psorous** (so'rus). Psoric.

**PSP.** Abbreviation for phenolsulfonphthalein.

**psych-, psyche-.** See psycho-.

**psychagogy** (si'kă-gō-jī) [ psych- + G. *agōgia*, a tutor's office ]. Psychotherapeutic reeducation stressing social adjustment of the individual.

**psychalgalia** (si-kal-ga'lī-ah). Psychalgia.

**psychalgia** (si-kal'jī-ah) [ psych- + G. *algos*, pain ]. Mind pain; soul pain; algopsychalia; phrenalgia; psychalgalia; distress attending a mental effort, noted especially in melancholia.

**psychalia** (si-ka-lī'-ah). An emotional condition characterized by auditory and visual hallucinations.

**psychanopsia** (si'kă-nop'sī-ah) [ psych- + G. *an-* priv, + *opsis*, vision ]. Mind *blindness*.

**psychataxia** (si-kă-tak'sī-ah) [ psych- + G. *ataxia*, confusion. TAX- ]. Mental confusion; inability to fix the attention or to make any continued mental effort.

**psyche** (si'ke) [ G. mind, soul. PSYCH- ]. An obsolete term for the subjective aspects of the mind and of the individual.

**psycheclampsia** (si-kĕ-klamp'sī-ah) [ psyche- + G. *eklampsis*, a flashing out ]. Psychlampsia; an emotional convulsion; acute mania.

**psychedelic** (si'kĕ-del'ik) [ psyche- + G. *dēloun*, to manifest ]. 1. Pertaining to a rather imprecise category of drugs with mainly central nervous system action, and with effects said to be the expansion or heightening of consciousness, *e.g.*, LSD, hashish, or mescaline. 2. A drug, visual display, music, or other sensory stimulus having such action.

**psychentonia** (si'ken-to'nī-ah) [ psych- + G. *en*, in, + *tonos*, tension ]. Mental tension.

**psychiatric** (si-kī-at'rik). Relating to psychiatry.

**psychiatrics** (si-kī-at'riks). Psychiatry.

**psychiatrist** (si-ki'ă-trist). A physician who specializes in psychiatry; the medical specialist in the diagnosis and treatment of mental diseases.

**psychiatry** (si-ki'ă-trī) [ psych- + G. *iatreia*, medical treatment ]. 1. The medical specialty dealing with mental disorders. 2. The diagnosis and treatment of mental diseases. For some types of p. not listed below, see also subentries under therapy, psychotherapy, and psychoanalysis.

  **analytic p.,** psychoanalytic p.

  **contractual p.,** psychiatric intervention voluntarily assumed by the patient who is prompted by his own personal difficulties or suffering, and who retains control over his participation with the psychiatrist.

**community p.,** p. focusing on the detection, prevention, and early treatment of emotional disorders and social deviance as they develop in the community rather than as they are encountered at large, centralized psychiatric facilities; particular emphasis is placed on the social-inter-personal-environmental factors that contribute to mental illness.

**dynamic p.,** psychoanalytic p.

**existential p.,** existential *therapy.*

**forensic p.,** legal p.; the application of p. in courts of law, as in determinations for commitment, fitness to stand trial, responsibility for crime, etc.

**legal p.,** forensic p.

**psychoanalytic p.,** analytic p.; dynamic p.; psychiatric theory and practice emphasizing psychoanalytic principles; see also psychoanalysis.

**social p.,** an approach to psychiatric theory and practice emphasizing the cultural and sociological aspects of mental disorder and treatment; the application of p. to social problems; see also community p.

**psychic** (si'kik) [ G. *psychikos* ]. 1. Relating to the phenomena of consciousness, mind, or soul; mental. 2. A person who is supposed to be endowed with the power of communicating with spirits; a spiritualistic medium.

**psychical** (si'ki-kal). Psychic (1).

**psychinosis** (si-ki-no'sis) [ psych- + G. *nosos,* disease ]. Psychopathy.

**psychism** (si'kizm) [ G. *psychē,* soul ]. The theory of a principle of life pervading all nature.

**psychlampsia** (si-klamp'sī-ah). Psycheclampsia.

**psycho-, psych-** (si'ko-) [ G. *psychē,* soul, mind. PSYCH- ]. Combining forms relating to the mind.

**psychoacoustics** (si'ko-ā-koos'tiks) [ psycho- + G. *akoustikos,* relating to hearing ]. The science pertaining to the psychologic factors that influence the individual's awareness of sound.

**psychoallergy** (si'ko-al'er-jī). A sensitization to emotionally charged symbols.

**psychoactive** (si'ko-ak'tiv). Possessing the ability to alter mood, anxiety, behavior, cognitive processes, or mental tension; usually applied to pharmacologic agents.

**psychoanalysis** (si'ko-ā-nal'ī-sis) [ psycho- + analysis, *q.v.* ]. 1. Psychoanalytic therapy; a method of psychotherapy, originated by Sigmund Freud, designed to bring preconscious and unconscious material to consciousness primarily through the analysis of transference and resistance. 2. A method of investigating the human mind and psychological functioning, especially through free association and dream analysis in the psychoanalytic situation. 3. An integrated body of observations and theories on personality development, motivation, and behavior. 4. An institutionalized school of psychotherapy, as in Freudian p.

**active p.,** that in which the analyst intervenes directly and actively in the patient's life, for example, by making prohibitions, assigning tasks, etc.

**Adlerian p.,** individual *psychology.*

**Jungian p.,** analytical psychology; the theory of psychopathology, and the practice of psychotherapy, according to the principles of Carl G. Jung; a system of psychology and psychotherapy emphasizing man's symbolic nature, and differing from Freudian p. especially in placing less significance upon instinctual (sexual) urges.

**psychoanalyst** (si-ko-an'ă-list). A psychotherapist, usually a psychiatrist, trained in psychoanalysis and employing its methods in the treatment of emotional disorders.

**psychoanalytic** (si'ko-an'ă-lit'ik). Pertaining to psychoanalysis.

**psychoasthenics** (si'ko-as-the'-niks) [ psycho- + G. *asthenia,* weakness ]. The study of intellectual deficiencies.

**psychoauditory** (si'ko-aw'dī-to-rī) [ psycho- + L. *auditorius,* relating to hearing ]. Relating to the mental perception and interpretation of sounds.

**psychobiology** (si'ko-bi-ol'o-jī). The study of the biology of the mind or psyche; Adolf Meyer's term for psychiatry.

**psychocatharsis** (si'ko-kă-thar'sis). Catharsis (2).

**psychochemistry** (si'ko-kem'is-trī). The alteration of affect or emotion by chemical means.

**psychochrome** (si'ko-krōm) [ psycho- + G. *chrōma,* color ]. A certain color mentally conceived in response to a sense impression; see also psychochromesthesia.

**psychochromesthesia** (si'ko-kro'mes-the'zī-ah) [ psycho- + G. *chrōma,* color, + *aisthēsis,* sensation ]. A form of synesthesia in which a certain stimulus to one of the special organs of sense produces the mental image of a color. See also pseudophotesthesia.

**psychodiagnosis** (si'ko-di'ag-no'sis). 1. Psychognosis; any method used to discover the factors which underlie behavior, especially malajusted or abnormal behavior. 2. A subspecialty within clinical psychology that emphasizes the use of psychological tests and techniques for assessing psychopathology.

**Psychodidae** (si-kod'ī-de). A family of small flies or gnats characterized by hairy, mothlike body and the presence of 7 to 11 long, parallel wing veins lacking cross-veins; includes the sand flies, *Phlebotomus,* vectors of leishmaniasis.

**psychodometry** (si-ko-dom'e-trī) [ psycho- + G. *hodos,* way, + *metron,* measure ]. The measurement of the rapidity of mental action.

**psychodrama** (si'ko-drah'mah). A method of psychotherapy in which patients act out their personal problems by taking roles in spontaneous dramatic performances.

**psychodynamics** (si-ko-di-nam'iks) [ psycho- + G. *dynamis,* force ]. The systematized study and theory of human behavior, emphasizing unconscious motivation and the functional significance of emotion.

**psychoendocrinology** (si'ko-en'do-kri-nol'o-jī). Study of the interrelationships between endocrine function and mental states.

**psychoexploration** (si'ko-eks'plor-a'shun). Study of the attitudes and emotional life of a person.

**psychogalvanic** (si'ko-gal-van'ik). Relating to changes in electric properties of the skin, as a change in skin resistance induced by psychologic stimulus.

**psychogalvanometer** (si'ko-gal'vă-nom'e-ter). A galvanometer which records changes in skin resistance related to emotional stress.

**psy'chogen'der.** The attitudes adopted by an individual related to his personal identification as either a male or a female. See also gender *role.*

**psychogenesis** (si-ko-jen'e-sis) [ psycho- + G. *genesis,* origin ]. Psychogeny; the origin and development of the psychic processes including mental, behavioral, personality, and related psychological processes.

**psychogenic, psychogenetic** (si'ko-jen'ik, -jē-net'ik). 1. Of mental origin or causation. 2. Relating to emotional development, or psychogenesis.

**psychogeny** (si-koj'ĕ-nī). Psychogenesis.

**psychogeusic** (si'ko-gu'sik) [ psycho- + G. *geusis,* taste ]. Pertaining to the mental perception and interpretation of taste.

**psychognosis** (si-kog-no'sis) [ psycho- + G. *gnōsis,* knowledge ]. Psychodiagnosis (1).

**psychognostic** (si-ko-nos'tik). Relating to psychognosis.

**psychogogic** (si-ko-goj'ik) [ psycho- + G. *agōgos,* a leading away ]. Acting as a stimulant to the emotions.

**psychogram** (si'ko-gram) [ psycho- + G. *gramma,* a writing ]. 1. Psychograph; a profile or graph indicating the personality traits of an individual. 2. A subjective visualization of a mental concept.

**psychograph** (si'ko-graf). Psychogram (1).

**psychographic** (si-ko-graf'ik). Relating to a psychogram or to psychography.

**psychography** (si-kog'rā-fī) [ psycho- + G. *graphē,* a writing ]. The literary characterization of an individual, real or fictional, that uses psychoanalytical and psychological categories and theories; a psychological biography or character description.

**psychohistory** (si'ko-his'to-rī). The combined use of psychology (especially psychoanalysis) and history in the writing especially of biography, *e.g.,* as in the work of Erik Erikson; see also psychography.

**psychokinesis, psychokinesia** (si'ko-kĭ-ne'sis, -ne'zĭ-ah) [ psycho- + G. *kinēsis*, movement ]. 1. Impulsive behavior. 2. The influence of mind upon matter.

**psychokym** (si'ko-kim) [ psycho- + G. *kyma*, wave ]. The physiologic substrate of psychic processes.

**psycholagny** (si-ko-lag'nĭ) [ psycho- + G. *lagneia*, lust ]. Sexual excitement and satisfaction from mental imagery.

**psycholepsy** (si'ko-lep'si) [ psycho- + G. *lepsis*, seizure ]. Sudden mood changes accompanied by feelings of hopelessness and inertia.

**psycholinguistics** (si'ko-lin-gwĭ'stiks) [ psycho- + L. *lingua*, tongue ]. The study of mental and intellectual factors that affect communication and understanding of language.

**psychologic, psychological** (si-ko-loj'ik, -loj'ĭ-kal). Relating to psychology; relating to the mind and its processes.

**psychologist** (si-kol'o-jist). A specialist in psychology licensed to practice professional psychology (*e.g.*, clinical p.), or certified to teach psychology as a scholarly discipline (academic p.), or whose scientific specialty is a subfield of psychology (research p.).

**psychology** (si'kol'o-jĭ) [ psycho- + G. *logos*, study ]. The profession (*e.g.*, clinical p.), scholarly discipline (academic p.), and science (research p.) concerned with the behavior of man and animals, and related mental and psysiological processes.

   **Adlerian p.,** individual p.

   **analytical p.,** Jungian *psychoanalysis.*

   **atomistic p.,** any psychologic system based on the doctrine that mental processes are built up through the combination of simple elements (*e.g.*, psychoanalysis, behaviorism); in contrast to holistic psychologies.

   **behavioral p.,** behaviorism.

   **clinical p.,** a branch of p. which specializes in both discovering new knowledge and in applying the art and science of p. to persons with emotional or behavioral disorders; subspecialties include clinical child p., pediatric p., and neuropsychology.

   **cognitive p.,** p. dealing with the process of thought as related to sensory stimuli.

   **community p.,** the application of p. to community programs, *e.g.*, in the schools, correctional and welfare systems, and community mental health centers.

   **compar'ative p.,** a branch of p. concerned with the study and comparison of the behavior of organisms at different levels of phylogenic development to discover developmental trends, as in the evolution of intelligence from ameba to man; often used synonymously with animal p.

   **constitutional p.,** the p. of the individual as related to body habitus.

   **criminal p.,** the study of the mind and its workings in relation to crime.

   **counseling p.,** p. with emphasis on facilitating the normal development and growth of the individual in coping with important problems of everyday living, as contrasted with clinical p.

   **depth p.,** the p. of the unconscious, especially in contrast with older (19th century) academic p. dealing only with conscious mentation; sometimes used synonymously with psychoanalysis.

   **developmental p.,** the study of the psychological changes in an organism which occur with aging.

   **dynamic p.,** an approach that concerns itself with the causes of behavior.

   **educational p.,** the application of p. to education, especially to problems of teaching and learning.

   **existential p.,** a theory of p., based on the philosophies of phenomenology and existentialism; it holds that the proper study of p. is man's experience of the sequence, spatiality, and organization of his existence in the world.

   **experimental p.,** a subdiscipline within the science of p. that is concerned with the study of conditioning, learning, perception, motivation, emotion, language, and thinking; (2) also used in relation to subject-matter areas in which experimental, in contrast to correlational or socio-experiential, methods are emphasized.

   **forensic p.,** the application of p. to legal matters in a court of law.

   **genetic p.,** a science dealing with the evolution of behavior and the relation to each other of the different types of mental activity.

   **gestalt p.,** see gestaltism.

   **holistic p.,** holism; any psychologic system which postulates that the human mind must be studied as a unit or gestalt, rather than as a sum of its individual parts or by attempts to break it down into hypothetical parts.

   **humanistic p.,** an existential approach to psychology which emphasizes man's uniqueness, his subjectivity, and his capacity for psychological growth.

   **individual p.,** Adlerian p.; Adlerian psychoanalysis; a theory of human behavior emphasizing man's social nature, his strivings for mastery, and his drive to overcome, by compensation, feelings of inferiority.

   **industrial p.,** the application of the principles of p. to problems in business and industry.

   **objective p.,** p. as studied by observation of the behavior and mental functions in others.

   **subjective p.,** the study of one's own mind and its various modes of action as a basis for psychologic deductions.

**psychometrics** (si-ko-mĕ'triks). Psychometry.

**psychometry** (si-kom'ĕ-trĭ) [ psycho- + G. *metron*, measure ]. Psychometrics; the disciplines pertaining to psychological and mental testing, and to any quantitative analysis of an individual's psychological traits or attitudes or mental processes.

**psychomotor** (si-ko-mo'tor). 1. Relating to the mental origin of muscular movement, to the production of voluntary movements. 2. Relating to the combination of psychic and motor events, including disturbances.

**psychoneurosis** (si-ko-nu-ro'sis) [ psycho- + G. *neuron*, nerve, + suffix -*osis*, condition ]. 1. A mental or behavioral disorder of mild or moderate severity. 2. Formerly a classification of neurosis including hysteria, psychasthenia, and neurasthenia.

   **p. maidica,** pellagra.

**psychoneurotic** (si-ko-nu-rot'ik). 1. Pertaining to psychoneurosis. 2. A patient suffering from a psychoneurosis.

**psychonomic.** Relating to psychonomy.

**psychonomy** (si-kon'o-mĭ) [ psycho- + G. *nomos*, law ]. The branch of psychology concerned with the laws of behavior.

**psychonosis** (si-ko-no'sis) [ psycho- + G. *nosos*, disease ]. Psychopathy.

**psychonosology** (si'ko-no-sol'o-jĭ) [ psycho- + G. *nosos*, disease, + *logos*, study ]. Psychiatric nosology; the classification of mental disorders.

**psychonoxious** (si-ko-nok'shus) [ psycho- + L. *noxius*, harmful ]. 1. Having an unfavorable effect on the emotional life and reactions mediated by higher levels of the central nervous system; may be endogenous or exogenous. 2. Denoting persons or situations that elicit fear, pain, or anxiety in an individual.

**psychoparesis** (si'ko-pă-re'sis, -păr'e-sis) [ psycho- + G. *paresis*, weakness ]. Mental or emotional weakness.

**psychopath** (si'ko-path). An obsolete term for personality disorders (*q. v.*), for any psychiatric patient, or for a sufferer of psychopathy; see also antisocial.

**psychopathia** (si-ko-path'ĭ-ah). Psychopathy.

   **p. martia'lis,** shell *shock.*

   **p. sexua'lis,** mental illness characterized by sex perversions.

**psychopathic** (si-ko-path'ik). Relating to psychopathy.

**psychopathist** (si-kop'ă-thist). Psychiatrist.

**psychopathologist** (si-ko-pă-thol'o-jist). One who specializes in psychopathology.

**psychopathology** (si-ko-pă-thol'o-jĭ) [ psycho- + G. *pathos*, disease, + *logos*, study ]. 1. The science that deals with the pathology of the psyche or mind. 2. The science of mental and behavioral disorders, including psychiatry and abnormal psychology.

**psychopathy** (si-kop'ă-thĭ) [ psycho- + G. *pathos*, disease ]. Psychopathia; psychinosis; psychonosis; psychosis; any mental or behavioral disorder, congenital or acquired.

**psychopharmaceuticals** (si-ko-far-mă-su'tĭ-kals). Drugs used in the treatment of emotional disorders.

**psychopharmacology** (si'ko-far'mă-kol'o-jĭ) [ psycho- + G. *pharmakon*, drug, + *logos*, study ]. Neuropsychopharmacology. 1. The use of drugs to influence affective and emotional states. 2. The science of drug-behavior relationships.

**psychophonasthenia** (si′ko-fo′nas-the′nĭ-ah). Phonasthenia of emotional origin.

**psychophysical** (si-ko-fiz′ĭ-kal). 1. Relating to the mental perception of physical stimuli. 2. Psychosomatic.

**psychophysics** (si-ko-fiz′iks). The science of the relation between the physical attributes of a stimulus and the measured, quantitative attributes of the mental perception of the same stimulus.

**psychophysiologic** (si′ko-fiz′ĭ-o-loj′ik). 1. Pertaining to psychophysiology. 2. Denoting a so-called psychosomatic illness, e.g., duodenal ulcer. 3. Denoting a somatic disorder with significant emotional or psychological etiology.

**psychophysiology** (si-ko-fiz-ĭ-ol′o-jĭ). The science of the relation between psychological and physiological processes, e.g., conscious elements of autonomic nervous system activity involved in emotion; see also biopsychology.

**psychoplegia** (si-ko-ple′jĭ-ah) [ psycho- + G. plēgē, stroke ]. Mental weakness or dementia of sudden onset.

**psychoplegic** (si-ko-ple′jik). 1. Relating to psychoplegia. 2. An agent that numbs mental action.

**psychopneumatology** (si′ko-nu′mă-tol′o-jĭ) [ psycho- + G. pneuma, breath, + logos, theory ]. Study of the interactions of mind and body.

**psychoprophylaxis** (si′ko-pro-fĭ-lak′sis) [ psycho- prophylaxis, q. v. ]. Psychotherapy directed toward the prevention of emotional disorder and the maintenance of mental health.

**psychoreaction** (si-ko-re-ak′shun). Much-Holzmann reaction.

**psychorelaxation** (si′ko-re-lak-sa′shun). A method of treating anxiety and tension by practicing general bodily relaxation, as in systematic desensitization.

**psychormic** (si-kor′mik) [ psycho- + G. horman, to set in motion ]. Pertaining to mind-rousing agents.

**psychorrhea** (si′ko-re′ah) [ psycho- + G. rhoia, flow ]. A psychiatric syndrome characterized by incoherent and strange philosophical theories; a manifestation of schizophrenia.

**psychorrhexis** (si′ko-rek′sis) [ psycho- + G. rhēxis, rupture ]. An especially intense or disabling type of anxiety reaction.

**psychorrhythmia, psychorhythmia** (si′ko-rith′mĭ-ah) [ psycho- + G. rhythmos, rhythm ]. Involuntary repetition of formerly voluntary acts.

**psychosensorial** (si-ko-sen-so′rĭ-al). Psychosensory.

**psychosensory** (si-ko-sen′so-rĭ). 1. Denoting the mental perception and interpretation of sensory stimuli. 2. Denoting a hallucination which the mind by an effort is able to distinguish from an actuality.

**psychosexual** (si′ko-sek′shu-al). Pertaining to the emotional or mental components of sex.

**psychosine** (si′ko-sēn). Galactosylsphingosine, a constituent of cerebrosides, formed from UDPgalactose and sphingosine by UDPgalactose-sphingosine β-galactosyltransferase (EC 2.4.1.23).

**psychosis,** pl. **psychoses** (si-ko′sis, -sez) [ G. an animating. PSYCH- ]. 1. A mental disorder causing gross distortion or disorganization of a person's mental capacity, affective response, and capacity to recognize reality, communicate, and relate to others to the degree of interfering with his capacity to cope with the ordinary demands of everyday life. The p. are divided into two major classifications according to their origins: p. associated with organic brain syndromes (e.g., Korsakoff's syndrome) and functional p. (e.g., the schizophrenias or manic-depressive p.). 2. A generic term for any of the insanities, the most common forms being the schizophrenias. 3. A severe emotional illness.

**affective p.,** manic-depressive p.

**alcoholic p.,** mental disorders that result from alcholism and that involve organic brain damage, such as in delirium tremens and Korsakoff's syndrome.

**arteriosclerotic p.,** psychotic disturbance in elderly persons suffering from cerebral arteriosclerosis.

**Cheyne-Stokes p.,** a mental state characterized by anxiety and restlessness, accompanying Cheyne-Stokes respiration.

**circular p.,** manic-depressive p.

**climacteric p.,** p. associated with the climacteric period; an involutional p.

**drug p.,** p. following or precipitated by ingestion of a drug, e.g., LSD.

**exhaustion p.,** a confusional emotional illness following a surgical operation, profuse hemorrhage, or other exhausting event.

**febrile p.,** infection-exhaustion p.

**gestational p.,** psychotic reaction associated with pregnancy.

**hysterical p.,** hysteropsychosis; hysterical insanity; (1) psychotic disturbance with predominantly hysterical symptoms; (2) a mental disorder resembling conversion hysteria but of psychotic severity.

**infection-exhaustion p.,** febrile p.; delirium; confusional insanity; a p. following an acute infection, shock, or chronic intoxication; it begins as delirium followed by pronounced mental confusion with hallucinations and unsystematized delusions and sometimes stupor.

**involutional p.,** mental disturbance occurring during the menopause or later life.

**Korsakoff's p.,** Korsakoff's syndrome.

**manic-depressive p.,** a major mental disorder or p. in which there are severe changes of mood and usually a tendency to remission and recurrance. In the manic state, the patient is over-elated and hyperactive; in the depressed state, he suffers from a depressed mood, anxiety, and possible physical slowing down that can lead to stupor. In the circular form of this disorder (circular p.), the patient has at least one of each type of episode. Also called affective, alternating, cyclic, circular, or periodic insanity or psychosis; cyclothymia; cyclophrenia.

**polyneurit′ic p.,** Korsakoff's syndrome.

**posthypnotic p.,** p. following or precipitated by hypnosis.

**postinfectious p.,** psychotic disturbance following acute febrile disease such as pneumonia or typhoid fever.

**postpartum p.,** puerperal mania; puerperal p.; acute mental disorder or p. in the mother following childbirth.

**posttraumatic p.,** p. following trauma, especially to the head; cf. traumatic p.

**prison p.,** a psychotic reaction to incarceration or the prospect thereof.

**puerperal p.,** postpartum p.

**schizo-affective p.,** psychotic disturbance in which there is a mixture of schizophrenic and manic-depressive symptoms.

**se′nile p.,** mental disturbance occurring in old age and related to degenerative cerebral processes.

**situational p.,** a transitory emotional disorder caused in a predisposed person by a seemingly unbearable situation.

**toxic p.,** a p. caused by some toxic substance, whether endogenous or exogenous.

**traumatic p.,** a p. resulting from physical injury or emotional shock; cf. posttraumatic p.

**Windigo (Wittigo) p.,** severe anxiety neurosis with special reference to food manifested in melancholia, violence, and obsessive cannibalism, occurring among Canadian Indians.

**psychosocial** (si′ko-so′shal). Involving both psychological and social aspects.

**psychosomatic** (si′ko-so-mat′ik) [ psycho- + G. soma, body ]. Pertaining to the influence of the mind or higher functions of the brain (emotions, fears, desires, etc.) upon the functions of the body, especially in relation to bodily disorders or disease. See also p. medicine.

**psychosomimetic** (si′ko-so-mĭ-met′ik). Psychotomimetic.

**psychosurgery** (si′ko-sur′jer-ĭ). The treatment of mental disorders by operation upon the brain, e.g., lobotomy.

**psychosynthesis** (si′ko-sin′the-sis) psycho- + synthesis, q. v. ]. A lay movement, the opposite of psychoanalysis, stressing therapy aimed at restoring useful inhibitions.

**psychotechnics** (si-ko-tek′niks) [ psycho- + G. technē, art, skill ]. The practical application of psychologic methods in the study of economics, sociology, and other problems.

**psychotherapeutics** (si′ko-thĕr-ă-pu′tiks). Psychotherapy.

**psychotherapist** (si′ko-ther′ă-pist). A person, usually a psychiatrist or clinical psychologist, professionally trained and engaged in psychotherapy.

**psychotherapy** (si′ko-thĕr′ă-pī) [ psycho- + G. *therapeia,* treatment ]. Treatment of emotional, behavioral, personality, and psychiatric disorders based primarily upon verbal or nonverbal communication with the patient, in contrast to treatments utilizing chemical and physical measures; for some types of p. not listed here, see also subentries under psychoanalysis, psychiatry, psychology, and therapy.

    **anaclitic p.,** a psychotherapeutic method characterized by encouragement and utilization of the patient's tendency to depend and lean upon the therapist as an authority figure; often contrasted with psychoanalytic therapy, which seeks to dissolve, rather than exploit, this phenomenon.

    **autonomous p.,** a type of psychoanalytic p. placing special emphasis on the value of the patient's self-determination in both the therapeutic situation and the patient's real life.

    **contractual p.,** p. based on a firm agreement, or "contract," between therapist and patient as to the role of each in the therapeutic situation.

    **directive p.,** utilizing the authority of the physician or psychologist to direct the course of the patient's therapy, as contrasted with nondirective p.

    **dyadic p.,** individual therapy; a psychotherapeutic session involving only two persons, the therapist and the patient.

    **dynamic p.,** psychoanalytic p.

    **existential p.,** a type of therapy based on existential analysis, emphasizing confrontation, primarily spontaneous interaction, and feeling experiences rather than rational thinking; less attention is given to patient resistances. The therapist is involved on the same level and to the same degree as the patient.

    **group p.,** a type of psychological treatment involving two or more patients participating together in the presence of one or more psychotherapists who facilitate both emotional and rational congnitive interaction to effect changes in the maladaptive behavior of the patient members in their everyday interpersonal exchanges. See also subentries under group.

    **heteronomous p.,** term embracing all forms of p. that foster the patient's dependence on others, especially dependence on the psychotherapist, in contrast to autonomous p.

    **hypnotic p.,** that based on hypnosis.

    **intensive p.,** p. involving an intensive exploration of the patient's life history and conflicts, often contrasted with superficial or supportive p.

    **marathon group p.,** a type of group p. characterized by prolonged sessions for periods of hours or days, with minimal interruptions for food and rest.

    **nondirective p.,** p. in which the therapist follows the lead of the patient during the interview rather than introducing his own theories and directing the course of the interview; this method is applied in both individual and group therapy. See also client-centered *therapy.*

    **psychoanalytic p.,** p. utilizing Freudian principles; see also psychoanalysis.

    **reconstructive p.,** a form of therapy, such as psychoanalysis, that seeks not only to alleviate symptoms but also to produce alterations in maladaptive character structure and to expedite new adaptive potentials; this aim is achieved by bringing into consciousness an awareness of and insight into conflicts, fears, inhibitions, and their manifestations.

    **regressive-inspirational group p.,** a form of group therapy in which group discussion and interaction is used to help seriously regressed group members to bolster their morale.

    **suggestive p.,** p. utilizing the influence and authority of the therapist; see also directive p.

    **supportive p.,** p. aiming at bolstering the patient's psychological defenses and providing him reassurance, rather than probing provacatively into his conflicts; crisis intervention is one form of supportive p.

    **transactional p.,** p. with central emphasis on the actual relations (transactions) between the patient and other people in his life.

**psychotic** (si-kot′ik). Relating to or affected by psychosis.

**psychotogen** (si-kot′o-jen) [ psychotic + G. suffix *-gen,* producing ]. A drug that produces psychotic manifestations.

**psychotogenic** (si-kot′o-jen′ik). Inducing psychosis; particulary used in reference to drugs of the LSD series and similar substances.

**psychotomimetic** (si′kot′o-mī-met′ik). 1. Psychosomimetic; a drug or substance that produces psychological and behavioral changes resembling those of psychosis *e.g.,* LSD. 2. Denoting such a drug or substance.

**psychotrine** (si′ko-trēn) [ *Psychotria,* a genus of gamopetalous plants ]. An alkaloid present in small amount in ipecac; it possesses low toxicity and poor amebicidal properties; a rapidly acting nauseant.

**psychotropic** (si′ko-trop′ik) [ psycho- + G. *tropē,* a turning ]. Affecting the psyche; denoting, specifically, drugs used in the treatment of mental illnesses.

**psychro-** (si′kro-) [ G. *psychros,* cold ]. Combining form relating to cold. See also cryo- and crymo-.

**psychroalgia** (si-kro-al′jī-ah) [ psychro- + G. *algos,* pain ]. A painful sensation of cold.

**psychroesthesia** (si-kro-es-the′zī-ah) [ psychro- + G. *aisthēsis,* sensation ]. 1. The form of sensation that perceives cold. 2. A sensation of cold although the body is warm; a chill.

**psychrometer** (si-krom′e-ter) [ psychro- + G. *metron,* measure ]. Hygrometer; wet-bulb thermometer; catathermometer; katathermometer; a device for measuring the humidity of the atmosphere by the difference in temperature between two thermometers, the bulk of one kept moist, the other dry. Evaporation from the moist bulb lowers the reading of that thermometer; the greater the difference in readings, the drier the air; no difference indicates 100 per cent relative humidity.

    **sling p.,** wet and dry bulb thermometers mounted on a hand sling, for use when a small portable psychrometer is required.

**psychrometry** (si-krom′e-trī) [ psychro- + G. *metron,* measure ]. Hygrometry; the calculation of relative humidity and water vapor pressures from wet and dry bulb temperatures and barometric pressure. Whereas relative humidity is the value ordinarily employed, the vapor pressure is the measurement of physiological significance. See fig. on p. 1168.

**psychrophilic** (si-kro-fil′ik) [ psychro- + G. *phileō,* to love ]. Preferring cold; thriving best at a low temperature, said of bacteria developing between the extremes of 0° and 30°C. (32° and 86°F.), with an optimum of 15° to 20°C. (59° to 68°F.).

**psychrophobia** (si-kro-fo′bī-ah) [ psychro- + G. *phobos,* fear ]. (1). Extreme sensitiveness to cold. 2. A morbid dread of cold.

**psychrophore** (si′kro-fōr) [ psychro- + G. *phoros,* bearing ]. An instrument in the form of a double catheter through which cold water is made to circulate in order to apply cold to the urethra or other canal or cavity.

**psyllium** (sil′ī-um) [ G. *psyllion,* flea-wort ]. 1. Plantain. 2. Plantago seed.

    **p. hydrophilic mucilloid,** METAMUCIL; the powdered mucilaginous outer epidermis of blond p. seeds; a demulcent laxative.

**Pt.** Chemical symbol of the element platinum.

**PTA.** Abbreviation for plasma thromboplastin antecedent; see *factor* XI.

**ptarmic** (tar′mik) [ G. *ptarmikos,* causing to sneeze, fr. *ptarmos,* a sneezing ]. 1. Causing sneezing. 2. A sternutatory; an agent that provokes sneezing.

**ptarmus** (tar′mus) [ G. *ptarmos,* a sneezing ]. Sneezing.

**PTC.** Abbreviation for (1) plasma thromboplastin component; see *factor* IX; (2) phenylthiocarbamide.

**PTC peptide, protein.** See the nouns.

**pter-, ptero-** [ G. *pteron,* wing, feather. PTER- ]. Combining forms meaning wing or feather.

**pteridine** (tĕr′ī-dēn, -din). A two-ring heterocyclic compound found as a component of pteroic acid and the

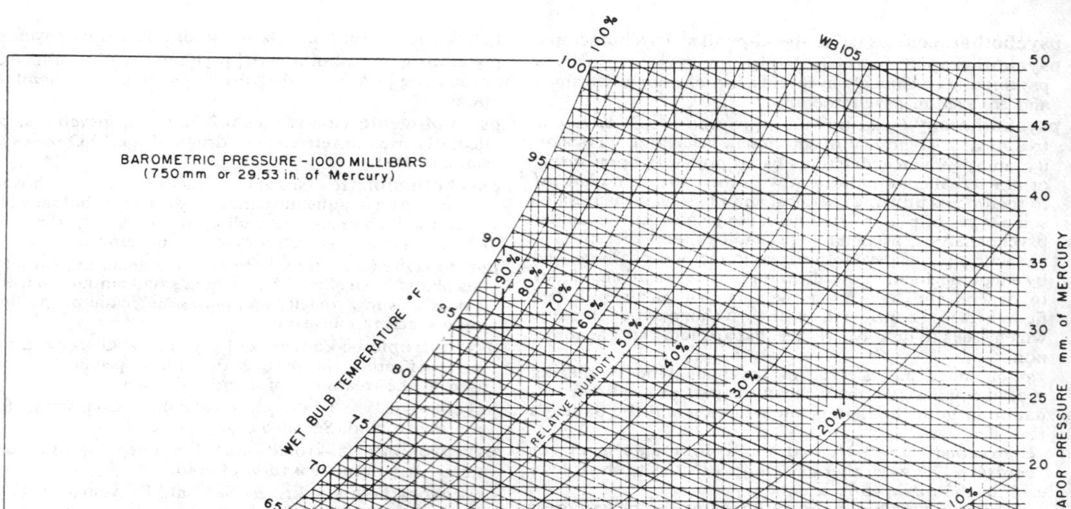

BAROMETRIC PRESSURE - 1000 MILLIBARS
(750mm or 29.53 in. of Mercury)

WET BULB TEMPERATURE °F

RELATIVE HUMIDITY

VAPOR PRESSURE mm of MERCURY

DRY BULB TEMPERATURE °F

**Psychrometric Chart**

Graph relating vapor pressure to dry and wet bulb temperature and percentage of relative humidity at a given barometric pressure.

pteroylglutamic acids (folic acids, pteropterin, etc.). Simple pteridine derivatives (xanthopterin, leucopterin) occur as pigments in butterfly wings, whence the name.

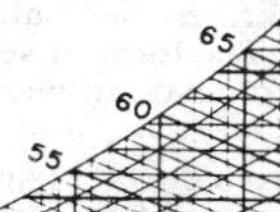

**Pteridine**

**pterin** (tĕr'in). Any of the compounds containing pteridine, but particularly those containing a 2-amino and 4-hydroxy group; specifically, 2-amino-4-hydroxypteridine. Most p.'s are named as pteridines; some (*e.g.*, xanthopterin, leucopterin) still retain the pterin root.

    **p. deaminase** (EC 3.5.4.11), aminohydrolase catalyzing hydrolytic deamination of a pterin to a lumazine.

**pterion** (te'rī-on) [ G. *pteron*, wing. PTER- ]. A craniometric point in the region of the sphenoid fontanelle, at the junction of the greater wing of the sphenoid, the squamous temporal, the frontal, and the parietal bones. See fig. under craniometric *point*.

**pternal'gia** (ter-nal'jĭ-ah) [ G. *pterna*, heel, + *algos*, pain ]. Talalgia.

**pteroic acid** (tĕ-ro'ik). A constituent of folic acid; it contains *p*-aminobenzoic acid and pteridine.

**pteropterin** (ter-op'ter-in). TEROPTERIN; pteroyltriglutamic acid; pteroyl-γ-glutamyl-γ-glutamyl-glutamic acid; folic acid conjugate; fermentation *Lactobacillus casei* factor; a principle chemically similar to folic acid except that it contains three molecules of glutamic acid instead of one.

**pteroylglutamic acid** (tĕr'o-il-glu-tam'ik). Folic acid.

**pteroyltriglutamic acid** (tĕr'o-il-tri'glu-tam'ik). Pteropterin.

**pterygium** (tĕ-rij'ĭ-um) [ G. *pterygion*, anything like a wing, a disease of the eye, dim. of *pteryx*, wing. PTER- ]. 1. Web

eye; a triangular patch of hypertrophied bulbar subconjunctival tissue, extending from the inner canthus to the border of the cornea or beyond, with apex pointing toward the pupil. 2. A forward growth of the eponychium with adherence to the proximal portion of the nail.

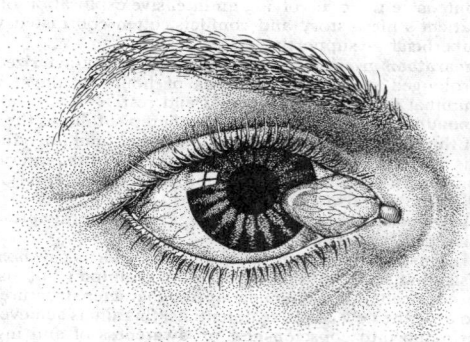

**Pterygium**

    **p. colli,** cervical patagium; a congenital web or tight band of skin of the neck extending from the acromion to the mastoid, usually bilateral.

    **scar p.,** pseudopterygium.

**pterygo-** (tĕr'ĭ-go-) [ G. *pteryx, pterygos,* wing. PTER- ]. Combining form meaning wing-shaped (pterygoid); relating, usually, to the pterygoid process.

**pterygoid** (tĕr'ĭ-goyd) [ G. *pteryx* (*pteryg*-), wing, + *eidos*, resemblance ]. Wing-shaped; alate; a term applied to various anatomical parts in the neighborhood of the sphenoid bone.

**pterygoma** (tĕr'ĭ-go'mah) [ G. *pteryx*, wing, + suffix *-oma*, tumor, swelling ]. 1 [ NA ]. The lobule of the auricle. 2. A persistent enlargement of the labia minora.

**pterygomandibular** (tĕr'ĭ-go-man-dib'u-lar). Relating to the pterygoid process and the mandible.

**pterygomaxillary** (tĕr'ĭ-go-mak'sĭ-lĕr-ĭ). Relating to the pterygoid process and the maxilla.

**pterygopalatine** (tĕr'ĭ-go-pal'ă-tin). Relating to the pterygoid process and the palatine bone.

**pterygoquadrate** (tĕr'ĭ-go-kwah'drāt). Relating to the pterygoid and quadrate bones in the upper jaw of lower vertebrates.

**pterygospinous** (tĕr-ĭ-go-spi'nus). *Processus* pterygospinosus.

**PTF.** Abbreviation for plasma thromboplastin factor; see *factor* VIII.

**PTH.** Abbreviation for (1) parathyroid *hormone;* (2) phenylthiohydantoin.

**ptilosis** (tĭ-lo'sis) [ G. *ptilōsis*, plumage, inflamed eyelids with falling lashes, fr. *ptilon*, soft feathers, down ]. Loss of the eyelashes.

**ptisan** (tiz'an) [ G. *ptisanē*, peeled barley, barley water, fr. *ptissō*, to peel ]. A decoction or "tea" of pleasant taste and little medicinal virtue.

**ptomaine** (to'mān) [ G. *ptōma*, a corpse. PTOM- ]. Ptomatine; a rather indefinite term applied to poisonous substances, *e.g.*, toxic amines, formed in the decomposition of protein by the decarboxylation of amino acids by bacterial action.

**ptomainemia** (to'ma-ne'mĭ-ah) [ ptomaine + G. *haima*, blood ]. A condition resulting from the presence of a ptomaine in the circulating blood.

**ptomatine** (to'mă-tēn). Ptomaine.

**ptomatropine** (to-mat'ro-pēn). A ptomaine characterized by poisonous properties similar to those of atropine, sometimes found in the tissues of persons who died of typhoid fever.

**ptosed** (tōzd) [ G. *ptosis*, a falling ]. Prolapsed; not held up in normal position or site.

**-ptosis** (-to'sis) [ G. *ptōsis*, a falling. PTOM- ]. Combining form, used in suffix position, to denote a falling or downward displacement of an organ.

**ptosis**, pl. **ptoses** (to'sis, to'sēz) [ G. *ptōsis*, a falling ]. 1. A falling or sinking down of any organ. 2. Specifically, a drooping of the upper eyelid, due to a fault of development or to paralysis of the levator palpebrae muscle, a weighting of the lid by a tumor, or recession of the eyeball.

   **p. adipo'sa,** blepharochalasis.

   **false p.,** pseudoptosis.

   **morning p., waking p.,** a functional paralysis of the upper lid, occurring temporarily after awakening in the anemic or neurotic.

   **p. sympathet'ica,** Horner's *syndrome*.

   **vis'ceral p.,** visceroptosis.

**ptotic** (tot'ik). Relating to or marked by ptosis.

**ptyal-, ptyalo-** [ G. *ptyalon*, saliva. PTY- ]. Combining form denoting relationship to saliva, or the salivary glands. For words beginning ptyal-, ptyalo- and not found here see also sial-, sialo-.

**ptyalagogue** (ti-al'ă-gog). Sialagogue.

**ptyalectasis** (ti'ă-lek'tă-sis) [ ptyal- + G. *ektasis*, a stretching out ]. Sialectasis.

**ptyalin** (ti'ă-lin). α-Amylase.

**ptyalism** (ti'ă-lizm) [ G. *ptyalismos*, spitting ]. Sialism.

**ptyalocele** (ti'ă-lo-sēl). Sialocele.

**ptyalography** (ti'ă-log'ră-fĭ). Sialography.

**ptyalolith** (ti'ă-lo-lith). Sialolith.

**ptyalolithiasis** (ti'ă-lo-lĭ-thi'ă-sis). Sialolithiasis.

**ptyalolithotomy** (ti'ă-lo-lĭ-thot-o-mĭ). Sialolithotomy.

**ptyaloreaction** (ti'ă-lo-re-ak'shun). A saliva test for pregnancy.

**ptyalorrhea** (ti'ă-lo-re'ah) [ ptyalo- + G. *rhoia*, a flow ]. Sialism.

**ptychotis oil** (ti-ko'tis). Ajowan oil.

**ptyocrinous** (ti-ok'rĭ-nus) [ G. *ptyo*, to spit out, + *krinō*, to separate ]. Secreting by discharge of the contents of the cell, as in mucous cells.

**Pu.** Chemical symbol of the element plutonium.

**pubarche** (pu-bar'ke) [ L. *pubertas*, puberty, + G. *archē*, beginning ]. The onset of puberty, particularly as manifested by the appearance of pubic hair.

**pu'beral, pu'bertal.** Relating to puberty.

**pubertas** (pu'ber-tas) [ L. ]. Puberty.

   **p. precox,** precocious *puberty.*

**puberty** (pu'ber-tĭ) [ L. *pubertas*, fr. *puber*, grown up ]. The sequence of events by which a child is transformed into a young adult. Gametogenesis begins, as well as secretion of gonadal hormones. Growth of secondary sexual characters occurs, reproductive functions begin, and sexual dimorphism is accentuated. The first signs of p. may be evident in girls at age 8 and the process is largely completed by age 16. In boys, p. commonly begins at ages 10 to 12 and is largely completed by age 18. Ethnic and geographical factors may influence the time at which various events typical of p. occur. In law, the ages of presumptive puberty are 12 years in girls and 14 years in boys.

   **Lipschutz law of p.,** see under law.

   **precocious p.,** pubertas precox; a state in which pubertal changes begin at an unexpectedly early age; often the result of a pathological process involving a gland capable of secreting estrogens or androgens (*e.g.*, the ovary or the adrenal cortex).

**puberu'lic acid.** $C_8H_6O_6$; antibiotic agent obtained from *Penicillium puberulum;* mildly active against Gram-positive bacteria.

**pubes** (pu'bēz) [ L. ]. Plural of pubis.

**pubescence** (pu-bes'ens). 1 [ L. *pubesco*, to attain puberty ]. The coming to the age of puberty or sexual maturity. 2 [ L. *pubes*, pubic hair ]. The presence of downy or fine, short hair.

**pubescent** (pu-bes'ent). Pertaining to pubescence; just coming to the age of puberty.

**pubic** (pu'bik). Relating to the os pubis.

**pubiotomy** (pu'bĭ-ot'o-mĭ) [ L. *pubis*, pubic bone, + G. *tomē*, incision ]. Hebotomy; severance of the pubic bone a few centimeters lateral to the symphysis, in order to increase the capacity of a contracted pelvis sufficiently to permit the passage of a living child.

**pubis,** pl. **pubes** (pu'bis, pu'bēz) [ L. *pubes*, the hair on the genitals; the genitals ]. 1. *Os* pubis. 2 [ NA ]. One of the pubic hairs; the hair of the pubic region just above the external genitals. 3 [ NA ]. The mons veneris; the pubic region.

**pubo-** (pu'bo-) [ L. *pubis, q. v.* ]. Combining form meaning pubis or pubic.

**pubocapsular** (pu'bo-kap'su-lar). Relating to the pubis and the capsule of the hip joint.

**pubococcygeal** (pu-bo-kok-sij'e-al). Relating to the pubis and the coccyx.

**pubofemoral** (pu'bo-fem'o-ral). Relating to the os pubis and the femur.

**pubomadesis** (pu'bo-mă-de'sis) [ L. *pubes*, pubic hair, + G. *madesis*, baldness ]. Pubic baldness; loss of pubic hair.

**puboprostatic** (pu'bo-pros-tat'ik). Relating to the pubic bone and the prostate gland.

**puborectal** (pu'bo-rek'tal). Relating to the pubis and the rectum.

**pubovesical** (pu'bo-ves'ĭ-kal). Relating to the pubic bone and the bladder.

**pudenda** (pu-den'dah) [ L. ]. Plural of pudendum.

**pudendagra** (pu'den-dag'rah) [ pudendum + G. *agra*, seizure ]. Pain in the female genitals.

**puden'dal.** Pudic; relating to the external genitals.

**pudendum,** pl. **pudenda** (pu-den'dum, -dah) [ L. ntr. of *pudendus*, particip. adj. of *pudeo*, to feel ashamed ]. The external genitals, especially the female genitals (vulva). Used also in the plural.

   **p. femini'num** [ NA ], vulva.

   **p. muliebre,** vulva.

**puden'dus** [ L. ] [ NA ]. Pudendal.

**pu'dic** [ L. *pudicus*, modest ]. Pudendal.

**puericulture** (pu'er-ĭ-kul-chur) [ L. *puer*, boy, child, + *cultura*, culture ]. 1. The care and training of children. 2. The antenatal care of the child by attention to the hygiene, mental and physical, of the pregnant woman.

**puerilism** (pu'er-ĭ-lizm) [ L. *puer*, child ]. 1. Childishness. 2. Second childhood; a mental disorder that sometimes accompanies old age.

**puerpera**, pl. **puerperae** (pu-er'per-ah, -per-e) [ L., fr. *puer*, child, + *pario*, to bring forth ]. Puerperant (2); a woman who has just given birth.

**puerperal** (pu-er'per-al). Puerperant (1); relating to the puerperium, or period after childbirth.

**puerperalism** (pu-er'per-ă-lizm). Any disorder consequent upon childbirth.

**puerperant** (pu-er'per-ant). 1. Puerperal. 2. A puerpera.

**puerperium**, pl. **puerperia** (pu'er-pēr'ĭ-um, -ĭ-ah) [ L. childbirth, fr. *puer*, child, + *pario*, to bring forth ]. The period from the termination of labor to complete involution of the uterus, usually defined as 42 days.

**puff.** A whiff; a short blowing sound heard on auscultation.

**veiled p.,** a faint pulmonary murmur, simulating the muffled flapping of a cloth in the wind.

**puff'ball.** *Lycoperdon.*

**pugillus** [ L. fr. *pugnus*, fist ]. A handful; a rough measure of quantity formerly used in directions for making an infusion or decoction of an innocuous drug.

**Pu'lex** [ L. flea ]. A genus of fleas (family Pulicidae, order Siphonaptera).

**P. che'opis,** former name for *Xenopsylla cheopis.*
**P. fascia'tus,** former name for *Nosopsyllus fasciatus.*
**P. ir'ritans,** a common flea that infests man and many domestic animals.

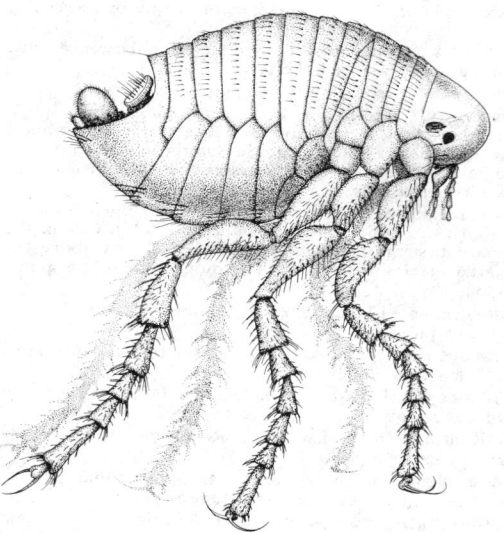

*Pulex irritans,* The Human Flea (× 25)

**P. pen'etrans,** incorrect name for *Tunga penetrans.*
**P. serra' ticeps,** former name for *Ctenophalides canis.*

**pulicicide, pulicide** (pu-lis'ĭ-sid, pu'lĭ-sid) [ L. *pulex (pulic-)*, flea, + *caedo*, to kill ]. Any agent destructive to fleas.

**pullet** (pŏo'let) [ O.Fr. *paulet* ]. A female chicken up to about one year of age.

**pulley.** See trochlea.

**pul'lulanase.** R enzyme; limit dextrinase; debranching enzyme (*q.v.*); a glucanohydrolase (EC 3.2.1.41) cleaving internal 1,6-α-glucosidic links in limit dextrins of amylopectin and glycogen; see also isoamylase; amylopectin 6-glucanohydrolase.

**pullulate** (pul'u-lāt) [ L. *pullulo*, pp. -*atus*, to sprout forth ]. To bud or sprout.

**pullulation** (pul-u-la'shun). The act of sprouting, or of budding as seen in yeast.

**pulmo**, gen. **pulmonis**, pl. **pulmones** (pul'mo, pul-mo'nis, -mo'nēz) [ L. ] [ NA ]. Lung.

**p. dex'ter** [ NA ], right lung.
**p. sinis'ter** [ NA ], left lung.

**pulmo-, pulmon-, pulmono-** [ L. *pulmo*, lung ]. Combining forms meaning lung, or pulmonary.

**pulmoaortic** (pul'mo-a-or'tik). Relating to the pulmonary artery and the aorta.

**pulmolith** (pul'mo-lith) [ L. *pulmo*, long, + G. *lithos*, stone ]. Stone in the parenchyma of the lung.

**pulmometer** (pul-mom'e-ter) [ L. *pulmo*, lung, + G. *metron*, measure ]. Pneometer.

**pulmometry** (pul-mom'e-trĭ). Pneometry.

**pulmonary** (pul'mo-něr-ĭ) [ L. *pulmonarius*, fr. *pulmo*, lung ]. Relating to the lungs, to the pulmonary artery, or to the aperture leading from the right ventricle into the pulmonary artery.

**pulmonectomy** (pul'mo-nek'to-mĭ) [ L. *pulmo (pulmon-)*, lung, + G. *ektomē*, excision ]. Pneumonectomy.

**pulmonic** (pul-mon'ik). 1. Pulmonary. 2. A sufferer from disease of the lungs. 3. A remedy for diseases of the lungs.

**pulmonitis** (pul'mo-ni'tis). Pneumonitis.

**pulmotor** (pul'mo-tor, pŏol-) [ L. *pulmo*, lung, + motor ]. An apparatus for supplying oxygen to the lungs and inducing artificial respiration in cases of asphyxiation by illuminating gas, drowning, etc.; oxygen under pressure is forced into the lungs and when the lungs are distended the action is automatically reversed and air is sucked out of the chest. The process is continued until natural respiration is established.

**pulp** [ L. *pulpa*, flesh ]. 1. A soft, moist, coherent solid. 2. *Pulpa* dentis. 3. Chyme.

**coronal p.,** *pulpa* coronale.
**dead p.,** nonvital p.; a p. that has died as a result of trauma, chemical action, or infection, and that gives no response to vitality tests such as the electric and thermal tests.
**dental p., den'tinal p.,** *pulpa* dentis.
**devital p., devitalized p.,** a p. that has been devitalized by trauma, by infection, or by chemical means such as arsenic or paraformaldehyde.
**digital p.,** p. of the finger.
**enamel p.,** a layer of stellate cells in the enamel organ.
**exposed p.,** one that has been exposed or laid bare by a pathologic process, trauma, or a dental instrument.
**p. of the finger,** the fleshy mass at the extremity of the finger.
**mum'mified p.,** a p. that has been destroyed by arsenic or other means, and has been preserved by an antiseptic paste.
**nonvital p.,** dead p.
**putrescent p.,** a decomposed p., often infected.
**radicular p.,** *pulpa* radicularis.
**red p.,** the splenic p. seen grossly as a reddish brown substance consisting of splenic sinuses and the tissue intervening between them called splenic cords.
**splenic p.,** *pulpa* lienis.
**tooth p.,** *pulpa* dentis.
**ver'tebral p.,** *nucleus* pulposus.
**vital p.,** a living p., either normal or diseased, that responds to the electric p. test and to heat and cold tests.
**white p.,** that part of the spleen that consists of nodules and other lymphatic concentrations.

**pulpa** (pul'pah) [ L. pulp ] [ NA ]. Pulp (1).

**p. corona'le** [ NA ]; coronal pulp; that portion of the p. dentis contained within the pulp chamber or crown cavity of the tooth.
**p. den'tis** [ NA ], dental pulp; tooth pulp; the soft tissue within the pulp cavity, consisting of connective tissue containing blood vessels, nerves and lymphatics, and at the periphery a layer of odontoblasts capable of internal repair of the dentin.
**p. lienis** [ NA ], splenic pulp; the soft substance of the spleen. See also red *pulp* and white *pulp.*
**p. radicula'ris** [ NA ], radicular pulp; that part of the p. dentis contained within the apical or root portion of the tooth.

**pul'pal.** Relating to the pulp.

**pulpalgia** (pul-pal'jĭ-ah) [ L. *pulpa*, pulp, + G. *algos*, pain ]. Pain of the pulp.

**pulpectomy** (pul-pek'to-mĭ) [ L. *pulpa*, pulp, + G. *ektomē*, excision ]. Removal of the entire pulp structure of a tooth, including the pulp tissue in the roots.

**pulpifaction** (pul'pĭ-fak'shun) [ L. *pulpa*, pulp, + *facio*, pp. *factus*, to make ]. Pulpation; the act of reducing to a pulpy condition.

**pul'piform.** Resembling pulp; pulpy.

**pul'pify.** To reduce to a pulpy state.

**pulpitis** (pul-pi'tis) [ L. *pulpa*, pulp, + G. suffix *-itis*, inflammation ]. Odontitis; inflammation of the pulp of a tooth.

   **hyperplastic p.,** a chronic inflammatory reaction of a young pulp in which there is an increase in the number of cells. The surface of the pulp is often covered with stratified squamous epithelium.

   **hypertrophic p.,** a misnomer for hyperplastic p.

   **serous p.,** an inflammation of the pulp, generally characterized by a sharp pain, which may be intermittent at first but becomes continuous.

   **suppurative p.,** an inflammation of the pulp giving rise to a severe pressure pain, often increased by heat and relieved by cold.

   **ulcerative p.,** a chronic inflammation of the pulp characterized by ulceration in the area of pulp exposure.

**pulp'less.** 1. Without a pulp. 2. Denoting a tooth in which the pulp has died or from which the pulp has been removed. 3. Denoting a tooth that gives no resonse to the electric pulp test and thermal test.

**pulpodontia** (pul'po-don'shĭ-ah) [ L. *pulpa*, pulp, + G. *odous*, tooth ]. The science of root canal therapy; see also endodontics.

**pulpo'sus** [ L. ] [ NA ]. Pulpy.

**pulpotomy** (pul-pot'o-mĭ) [ L. *pulpa*, pulp, + G. *tomē*, incision ]. Pulp amputation; removal of a portion of the pulp structure of a tooth. Usually refers to removal of the coronal portion of the pulp.

**pulpy** (pul'pĭ). In the condition of a soft, moist solid.

**pulque** (pool'ka) [ Sp. ]. A fermented drink from the juice of *Agave americana*; diuretic.

**pulsate** (pul'sāt) [ L. *pulso*, pp. *-atus*, to beat ]. To throb or beat rhythmically; said of the heart or an artery.

**pulsatile** (pul'să-til). Throbbing; beating.

**pulsatilla** (pul'să-til'ah) [ L. fr. *pulso*, to beat ]. Pasque flower; Easter flower; the herb *Anemone pulsatilla* and *A. pratensis* (family Ranunculaceae), collected soon after flowering; a powerful local irritant formerly used for a variety of diseases.

**pulsation** (pul-sa'shun) [ L. *pulsatio*, a beating ]. A throbbing or rhythmical beating, as of the pulse or the heart.

**pulsa'tor.** A machine or device that operates in a throbbing, vibrating, or rhythmic manner.

**pulse** (puls) [ L. *pulsus*, *q. v.* ]. The rhythmical dilation of an artery, produced by the increased volume of blood thrown into the vessel by the contraction of the heart. A p. may also at times occur in a vein or a vascular organ, as the liver. See also pulsus.

   **abdominal p.,** pulsus abdominalis; the soft, compressible, but usually regular pulse occurring in certain abdominal disorders.

   **alternating p.,** pulsus alternans; mechanical alternation; a pulse regular in time but with alternate beats stronger and weaker, often detectable only with the sphygmomanometer and usually indicating serious myocardial disease.

   **anacrot'ic p., anadicrot'ic p.,** a small slow rising p. with a perceptible notch or hesitation on the ascending limb, characteristic of aortic stenosis; plateau p.

   **bigeminal p.,** pulsus bigeminus; bigemina; coupled beats or p.; a p. in which the beats occur in pairs.

   **bulbar p.,** a jugular p. supposed to indicate tricuspid insufficiency.

   **cannonball p.,** water-hammer p.

   **capillary p.,** the alternate rhythmical reddening and blanching of a capillary area, well seen under the nails; a sign of arteriolar dilation, well seen in aortic insufficiency.

   **catacrotic p.,** pulsus catacrotus; a p. in which there is an upward notch interrupting the descending limb of the sphygmogram.

   **catadicrotic p.,** pulsus catadicrotus; a catacrotic p. in which there are two interrupting upward notches.

   **collapsing p.,** water-hammer p.

   **cordy p.,** tense p.

   **Corrigan's p.,** the water-hammer-type p. in aortic regurgitation or peripheral arterial dilation, characterized by an abrupt rise and rapid fall away.

   **coupled p.,** bigeminal p.

   **dicrot'ic p.,** a p. which is marked by a double beat, the second, due to a palpable dicrotic wave, being weaker than the first.

   **entop'tic p.,** an intermittent phose synchronous with the p.

   **filiform p.,** a thready p.

   **gaseous p.,** a soft, full, but feeble p.

   **gut'tural p.,** a pulsation felt in the throat.

   **hard p.,** pulsus durus; one that strikes forcibly against the tip of the finger and is with difficulty compressed, indicating arterial hypertension.

   **intermittent p.,** pulsus intercidens; irregularity of the heart due to extrasystoles which are too weak to open the semilunar valves. Owing to the long pause following the premature beat, extra long pauses equal to two regular cycles occur from time to time between p. beats.

   **jugular p.,** the p. in the right internal jugular vein at the root of the neck, due to waves transmitted in the blood stream from the right side of the heart.

   **Kussmaul's paradoxical p.,** see paradoxical p.

   **long p.,** one in which the impact is felt longer than usual.

   **monocrotic p.,** pulsus monocrotus; a p. without any perceptible dicrotism.

   **mousetail p.,** *pulsus* myurus.

   **movable p.,** the lateral movement of a strongly pulsating tortuous artery.

   **nail p.,** a capillary p. seen through the nail.

   **paradoxical p.,** an exaggeration of the normal variation in the p. volume with respiration, becoming weaker with inspiration and stronger with expiration; characteristic of constrictive pericarditis or pericardial effusion. So called because these changes are independent of changes in p. rate.

   **piston p.,** water-hammer p.

   **plateau p.,** the slow, sustained p. of aortic stenosis, producing a prolonged flat-topped curve in the sphygmogram.

   **pul'monary p.,** variation in intensity of the pulmonary second sound according to the tension in the pulmonary artery.

   **quadrigeminal p.,** pulsus quadrigeminus; one in which the beats are grouped in fours, a pause following every fourth beat.

   **Quincke's p.,** Quincke's sign; capillary pulsation, as shown by alternate reddening and blanching of the nailbed with each heart beat; a sign of arteriolar dilation and especially well seen in severe aortic insufficiency.

   **respiratory p.,** waxing and waning of venous pulsation produced by respiration.

   **reversed paradoxical p.,** amplitude of the p. increases with inspiration and decreases with expiration, as observed in some cases of tricuspid insufficiency.

   **Riegel's p.,** a p. that diminishes in volume during expiration.

   **soft p.,** one that is readily extinguished by pressure with the finger.

   **tense p.,** cordy p.; a hard full p. but without very wide excursions, resembling the vibration of a thick cord.

   **thready p.,** filiform p.; pulsus filiformis; a small fine p., feeling like a small cord or thread under the finger.

   **trigeminal p.,** pulsus trigeminus; one in which the beats occur in trios, a pause following every third beat.

   **trip'hammer p.,** water-hammer p.

   **undulating p.,** pulsus undulosus; pulsus fluens; a toneless p. in which there is a succession of waves without character or force.

   **vagus p.,** a slow p. due to the inhibitory action of the vagus nerve on the heart.

   **venous p.,** pulsus venosus; a pulsation occurring in the veins, especially the internal jugular.

**vermicular p.,** a small rapid p., giving a wormlike sensation to the finger.

**water-hammer p.,** Corrigan's p.; cannonball p.; collapsing p.; piston p.; triphammer p.; pulsus celerimus; one with forcible impulse but immediate collapse, characteristic of aortic incompetency.

**wiry p.,** a small, fine, incompressible p.

**pulsellum** (pul-sel'um) [ Mod. L. dim of L. *pulsus,* a stroking ]. A posterior flagellum constituting the organ of locomotion in certain protozoa.

**pulsim'eter, pulsom'eter** [ L. *pulsus,* pulse, + *metron,* measure ]. An instrument for measuring the force and rapidity of the pulse.

**pulsion** (pul'shun) [ L. *pulsio* ]. A pushing outward or swelling.

**pul'sus** [ L. a stroke, pulse, fr. *pello,* pp. *pulsus,* to beat ]. Pulse.

**p. abdomina'lis,** abdominal *pulse.*

**p. alter'nans,** alternating *pulse.*

**p. anadic'rotus,** anacrotic *pulse.*

**p. bigem'inus,** bigeminal *pulse.*

**p. bisfer'iens,** bisferious pulse; an arterial pulse with two palpable peaks, the second stronger than the first, as may be found in aortic insufficiency combined with aortic stenosis.

**p. cap'risans** [ L. capering ], a bounding leaping pulse, irregular in both force and rhythm.

**p. catac'rotus,** catacrotic *pulse.*

**p. catadic'rotus,** catadicrotic *pulse.*

**p. cel'er,** a pulse beat swift to rise and fall.

**p. celer'imus,** water-hammer *pulse.*

**p. cordis,** the apex beat of the heart.

**p. deb'ilis,** a weak pulse.

**p. differens,** a condition in which the pulses in the two radial arteries differ in strength.

**p. duplex,** dicrotic *pulse.*

**p. durus,** hard *pulse.*

**p. filifor'mis,** thready *pulse.*

**p. fluens,** undulating *pulse.*

**p. formi'cans** [ L. *formica,* ant ], a very small, nearly imperceptible pulse, the impression it gives to the finger being compared to formication.

**p. fortis,** a full strong pulse.

**p. frequens,** a rapid pulse.

**p. heterochron'icus,** an arrhythmic pulse.

**p. inaequa'lis,** a pulse irregular in rhythm and force.

**p. infre'quens,** a slow pulse.

**p. incongruens,** p. differens.

**p. inter'cidens,** intermittent *pulse.*

**p. intercur'rens,** an occasional strong dicrotic pulse wave giving the impression of an intercurrent ventricular contraction.

**p. irregula'ris perpet'uus,** permanently irregular pulse; a name formerly given to the condition now called atrial fibrillation, of which such pulse is characteristic.

**p. magnus,** a large full pulse.

**p. mollis,** a soft easily compressible pulse.

**p. monoc'rotus,** monocrotic *pulse.*

**p. myu'rus,** mousetail pulse; a pulse marked by a wave, the apex of which is reached suddenly and which then subsides very gradually.

**p. paradox'us,** paradoxical *pulse.*

**p. parvus,** a small pulse.

**p. quadrigem'inus,** quadrigeminal *pulse.*

**p. rarus,** p. tardus.

**p. respiratio'ne intermit'tens,** paradoxical *pulse.*

**p. tardus,** a pulse beat slow to rise and fall; see also plateau *pulse.*

**p. trem'ulus,** a feeble fluttering pulse.

**p. trigem'inus,** trigeminal *pulse.*

**p. undulosus,** undulating *pulse.*

**p. vac'uus,** a very weak pulse hardly distending the arterial wall.

**p. veno'sus,** venous *pulse.*

**pultaceous** (pul-ta'shus) [ G. *poltos,* porridge ]. Macerated; pulpy.

**pulv.** Abbreviation of L. *pulvis,* powder.

**pulveriza'tion.** Reduction to powder.

**pulverize** [ L. *pulverizo,* fr. *pulvis, pulveris,* dust ]. To reduce to a powder.

**pulverulent** (pul-věr'u-lent). In a state of powder; powdery.

**pulvinar** (pul-vi'nar) [ L. a couch made from cushions, fr. *pulvinus,* cushion ] [ NA ]. The posterior extremity of the thalamus which forms a cushion-like prominence slung over the posterior aspect of the internal capsule; see also *nucleus* lateralis thalami.

**pulvinate** (pul'vī-nāt) [ L. *pulvinus,* cushion ]. Raised or convex, denoting a form of surface elevation of a bacterial culture.

**pul'vis,** gen. **pul'veris,** pl. **pul'veres** [ L. dust ]. Powder.

**pumice** (pum'is) [ L. *pumex* (*pumic-*), a pumice stone ] (NF). Volcanic cinders ground to particles of varying sizes; used in dentistry for polishing restorations or teeth.

**pump.** 1. An apparatus for forcing a gas or liquid from or to any part. 2. Any mechanism for using metabolic energy to accomplish active transport of a substance.

**Alvegniat's p.,** a mercurial vacuum p. used to remove gases from the blood, for estimation of the contained amount.

**breast p.,** a suction instrument for withdrawing milk from the breast.

**Carrel-Lindbergh p.,** a perfusion device designed for use in culture of whole organs.

**dental p.,** a saliva ejector.

**jet ejector p.,** a suction p. in which fluid under high pressure is forced through a nozzle into an abruptly larger tube where a high velocity jet, at a low pressure in accordance with Bernoulli's law, entrains gas or liquid from a side tube opening just beyond the end of the nozzle to create suction; *e.g.,* the p. by which steam is used to evacuate an autoclave, a water aspirator.

**saliva p.,** dental p.

**sodium p.,** a p. that uses metabolic energy from ATP to achieve active transport of sodium across a membrane; sodium p.'s expel sodium from most cells of the body, sometimes coupled with the transport of other substances, and also serve to move sodium across multicellular membranes such as renal tubule walls.

**stomach p.,** an apparatus for removing the contents of the stomach by means of suction.

**pump-ox'ygena'tor.** A mechanical device that can substitute for both the heart (pump) and the lungs (oxygenator) during open heart surgery.

**puna** (poo'nah) [ Sp. a region in the Andes ]. Mountain *sickness.*

**punch** [ L. *pungo,* pp. *punctus,* to stick, to punch ]. An instrument for making a hole or indentation in some solid material or for driving out a foreign body inserted in a hole in such material.

**Murphy's kidney p.,** the determination of deep tenderness and rigidity in the region of the kidney by making jabbing movements with the thumb into the loin below the 12th rib.

**punch'drunk.** See punchdrunk *syndrome.*

**puncta** (pungk'tah) [ L. ]. Plural of punctum.

**punctate** (pungk'tāt) [ L. *punctum,* a point ]. 1. Marked with points or dots differentiated from the surrounding surface by color, elevation, or texture. 2. The matter withdrawn for examination by means of an exploratory puncture.

**punctiform** (pungk'tī-form) [ L. *punctum,* a point, + *forma,* shape ]. Very small but not microscopic, having a diameter of less than 1 mm.

**punctio** (pungk'shī-o) [ L. fr. *pungo,* to prick ]. The act of pricking or dotting.

**punctograph** (pungk'to-graf) [ L. *punctum,* point, + G. *graphō,* to write ]. A localizer, by x-ray, of a foreign body.

**punc'tum,** gen. **punc'ti,** pl. **punc'ta** (pungk'tum) [ L. a prick, point, pp. ntr. of *pungo,* to prick, used as noun ] [ NA ]. A point; the tip of a sharp process; a minute round spot differing in color or otherwise in appearance from the surrounding tissues.

**p. ce'cum,** the blind spot on the retina where the optic nerve enters the eyeball.

**p. coxa'le,** the highest point of the crest of the ilium.

**p. doloro'sum,** painful point; see Valleix's *points.*

**p. lacrima′le** [ NA ], lacrimal p. or opening; the minute circular opening of the lacrimal canaliculus, on the margin of each eyelid near the medial commissure.

**p. lu′teum,** *macula* retinae.

**p. prox′imum,** near *point.*

**p. remo′tum,** far *point.*

**p. vasculo′sum,** one of the minute dots seen on section of the brain, due to small drops of blood at the cut extremities of the arteries.

**punctu′ra** [ L. ]. Puncture.

**p. explorato′ria,** exploratory *puncture.*

**puncture** (pungk′chur) [ L. *punctura,* fr. *pungo,* pp. *punctus,* to prick ]. 1. To make a hole with a small pointed object, such as a needle. 2. A prick or small hole made with a pointed instrument.

**Bernard's p.,** diabetic p.

**cister′nal p.,** passage of a hollow needle through the posterior atlantooccipital membrane into the cisterna cerebellomedullaris.

**diabetic p.,** Bernard's p.; a p. at a point in the floor of the fourth ventricle of the brain which causes glycosuria.

**exploratory p.,** p. of a cavity or tumor with a hollow needle to determine the presence or absence of fluid or gas, and its nature, if present.

**lumbar p.,** a p. into the subarachnoid space of the lumbar region for diagnostic or therapeutic purposes; also referred to as Quincke's p.; spinal tap or p.; rachicentesis; rachiocentesis.

**Quincke's p.,** lumbar p.

**spinal p.,** lumbar p.

**sternal p.,** removal of bone marrow from the manubrium by needle.

**pungent** (pun′jent) [ L. *pungo,* pres. p. *-ens (-ent-),* to pierce ]. Sharp; acrid; said of the taste or odor of a substance.

**punicine** (pu′nĭ-sēn). Pelletierine.

**PUO.** Abbreviation for pyrexia of unknown (or uncertain) origin, a term applied to febrile illness before diagnosis has been established; also referred to as FUO (fever of unknown origin).

**pupa,** pl. **pupae** (pu′pah, pu′pe) [ L. *pupa,* doll ]. The stage of insect metamorphosis following the larva and preceding the imago.

**pu′pil** [ L. *pupilla, q. v.* ]. Pupilla.

**Argyll Robertson p.,** Argyll Robertson symptom; a form of reflex iridoplegia characterized by the loss of reflexes to light, direct and consensual, with normal pupillary contraction on accommodation and convergence; often present in tabes and general paresis.

**artificial p.,** an opening made by excision of a portion of the iris in order to improve the vision in cases of central opacity of the cornea or lens.

**bounding p.** a rapid dilation of the p. alternating with contraction, unassociated with illumination.

**Bumke's p.,** dilation of the p. in response to psychic stimuli.

**cat's-eye p.,** a distorted p. elongated in the vertical axis.

**cornpicker's p.,** mydriasis and cycloplegia, from picking corn in a field containing jimson weed.

**exclusion of the p.,** seclusion of the p.; the condition resulting from posterior annular synechia, in which the iris is bound down throughout the entire pupillary margin, but the p. is not occluded.

**fixed p.,** a stationary pupil unresponsive to all stimuli.

**Hutchinson's p.,** an immobile dilation of the p. on the side of the lesion, with contraction of the other p., occurring in meningeal hemorrhage compressing the third nerve at the base of the brain.

**keyhole p.,** a p. with an artificial coloboma on one side of the pupillary margin.

**occlusion of the p.,** the presence of an opaque membrane closing the pupillary area.

**paradoxical p.,** see paradoxical pupillary *reflex.*

**pinhole p.,** an extremely contracted p.

**Robertson p.,** Argyll Robertson p.

**seclusion of the p.,** exclusion of the p.

**skew p.'s,** deviation of the ocular axes, one passing upward, the other downward.

**stiff p.,** Argyll Robertson p.

**tonic p.,** Piltz sign; Westphal's pupillary reflex; Westphal-Piltz phenomenon; catatonic or mydriatic rigidity; a pupil, usually large, which responds very slowly, if at all, to light and accommodation. See also Holmes-Adie *syndrome.*

**pupilla,** pl. **pupillae** (pu-pil′ah, pu-pil′e) [ L. dim. of *pupa,* a girl or doll. PUP- ] [ NA ]. Pupil of the eye; the circular orifice in the center of the iris, through which the light rays enter the eye.

**pupilla′ris** [ L. ] [ NA ]. Pupillary.

**pupillary** (pu′pĭ-ler-ĭ). Relating to the pupil.

**pupillo-** [ L. *pupilla,* pupil. PUP- ]. Combining form relating to the pupils.

**pupillography** (pu′pĭ-log′rȧ-fĭ) [ pupillo- + G. *graphō,* to write ]. The recording of pupillary reactions.

**pupillometer** (pu′pĭ-lom′e-ter) [ pupillo- + G. *metron,* measure ]. An instrument for measuring the diameter of the pupil.

**pupillometry** (pu′pĭ-lom′e-trĭ). Measurement of the pupil.

**pupillomotor** (pu′pĭ-lo-mo′tor) [ pupillo- + L. *motor,* mover ]. Relating to the nerve fibers that supply the smooth muscle of the iris.

**pupilloplegia** (pu′pĭ-lo-ple′jĭ-ah) [ pupillo- + G. *plēgē,* stroke ]. A condition in which the pupil reacts slowly to light stimuli, as in Holmes-Adie syndrome.

**pupilloscopy** (pu′pĭ-los′ko-pĭ) [ pupillo- + G. *skopeō,* to view ]. Retinoscopy.

**pupillostatometer** (pu′pĭ-lo-stȧ-tom′e-ter) [ pupillo- + G. *statos,* placed, + *metron,* measure ]. An instrument for measuring the distance between the centers of the pupils.

**pupiparous** (pu-pip′ȧ-rus). Pupae-bearing; denoting those insects that give birth to pupae that have already passed their larval development within the body of the female.

**Purdy,** Charles W., American physician, 1846–1901. See P.'s *solution.*

**pure** (pūr) [ L. *purus* ]. 1. Unadulterated; free from admixture or contamination with any extraneous matter. 2. In genetics, referring to an inherited character which is transmitted without a break through an indefinite number of successive generations, or to an individual who is homozygous in respect to a particular pair of unit characters, not hybrid.

**pure′bred.** An animal whose ancestors on both sides have been members of a recognized breed, and usually registered.

**purgation** (pur-ga′shun) [ L. *purgatio* ]. Purging.

**purgative** (pur′gȧ-tiv) [ L. *purgativus,* purging ]. Cathartic.

**saline p.,** Epsom salt, Rochelle salt, or any salt having p. properties.

**purge** (purj) [ L. *purgo,* to cleanse, fr. *purus,* pure, + *ago,* to do ]. 1. To cause a copious evacuation of the bowels. 2. A cathartic remedy.

**purging** (pur′jing). Purgation; causing a free evacuation of the bowels by cathartics.

**pu′riform** [ L. *pus (pur-),* pus, + *forma,* form ]. Resembling pus.

**purine** (pu′rēn, -rin). The parent substance of adenine, guanine, and other naturally occurring purine bases; it is not known to exist as such in the body. There are three p. groups, *viz.,* oxypurines (hypoxanthine, xanthine, and uric acid); aminopurines (adenine and guanine); and methyl p.'s (caffeine, theophylline, and theobromine).

Purine

**p. am′idases,** see deaminases.

**p. base, p. body,** any purine.

**p. deam′idases,** see deaminases.

**p. nucleosidase,** nucleosidase.

**p. nucleoside phosphorylase** (EC 2.4.2.1), phosphorylase that catalyzes the phosphorolysis of a purine nucleoside to a purine and ribose 1-phosphate.

**purinemia** (pu'rī-ne'mī-ah) [ purine + G. *haima*, blood ]. The presence of purine or xanthine bases in the circulating blood.

**purinometer** (pu'rī-nom'e-ter) [ purine + G. *metron*, measure ]. A device for determining the amount of purine or xanthine bases in the urine.

**purity** (pu'rī-tī). The state of being pure.

**radiochemical p.**, the proportion of the total activity of a specific radionuclide in a specific chemical or biological form.

**radioisotopic p.**, a loose term commonly used to denote radionuclidic purity.

**radionuclidic p.**, the proportion of the total radioactivity that is present as a specific radionuclide.

**radiopharmaceutical p.**, the sterility and apyrogenicity of a radioactive tracer for human use.

**Purkinje** (poor-kin'zheh), Johannes E. von, Bohemian anatomist and physiologist, 1787–1869. See P.'s *cells, conduction, corpuscles, fibers, figures, images,* P.-Sanson *images,* P.'s *layer, network, phenomenon, shift, system.*

**Purmann,** Matthaeus G., German surgeon, 1648–1721. See P.'s *method.*

**purohepatitis** (pu'ro-hep-ă-ti'tis) [ L. *pus* (*pur*-), pus, + G. *hēpar*, liver, + suffix *-itis*, inflammation ]. Suppurative inflammation of the liver; hepatic abscess.

**puromucous** (pu'ro-mu'kus) [ L. *pus* (*pur*-), pus, + *mucus*, mucus ]. Mucopurulent; containing both pus and mucus.

**puromycin** (pu'ro-mi'sin) (USAN). STYLOMYCIN; 6-dimethylamino-9- (3'-*p*-methoxy-L-phenylalanylamino-β-D-ribofuranosyl) purine; an antibiotic produced by the growth of *Streptomyces alboniger;* effective in clinical trials in the treatment of amebiasis and trypanosomiasis.

**purple** (pur'pl) [ L. *purpura* ]. A color formed by a mixture of blue and red. For individual purple dyes see specific name.

**visual p.**, rhodopsin.

**purpura** (pur'pu-rah) [ L. fr. G. *porphyra,* purple. PORPH- ]. Peliosis; a condition characterized by hemorrhage into the skin. The appearance of the lesions varies with the type of p., the duration of the lesions, and the acuteness of the onset. The color is first red, becoming gradually darker, then purple, fading to a brownish yellow, and usually disappears in 2 or 3 weeks; the color of residual permanent pigmentation depends largely on the type of unabsorbed pigment of the extravasated blood; extravasations occur also into the mucous membranes and internal organs.

**acute vascular p.**, Henoch-Schönlein p.

**allergic p.**, anaphylactoid p. (1); nonthrombocytopenic p. due to foods, drugs, and insect bites.

**anaphylactoid p.**, (1) allergic p.; (2) Henoch-Schönlein p.

**p. angioneurot'ica**, an eruption marked by angioneurotic edema, petechiae, and hyperesthesia of the skin and gastric mucous membrane.

**p. annula'ris telangiecto'des**, Majocchi's disease; annular lesions, principally of the lower extremities, in which the peripheral portion is composed of purpura or petechiae with brawny staining of hemosiderin and minute telangiectasia.

**factitious p.**, self-induced, often painful, ecchymoses.

**fibrinoly'tic p.**, one in which the bleeding is associated with rapid fibrinolysis of the clot.

**p. ful'minans**, a severe and rapidly fatal form of p. hemorrhagica, occurring especially in children.

**p. hemorrhag'ica**, (1) idiopathic thrombocytopenic p.; (2) petechial fever (2); a noncontagious malady of horses, which occurs following suppurative infections, characterized by multiple hemorrhages and edema of the subcutaneous and submucous tissues.

**Henoch's p.**, Henoch-Schönlein p.

**Henoch-Schönlein p.**, an eruption of nonthrombocytopenic purpuric lesions associated with joint pains or swelling, colic, vomiting of blood, passage of bloody stools, and sometimes glomerulonephritis, most commonly occurring in male children. Also called Henoch's p.; Schönlein's p.; anaphylactoid p. (2); p. rheumatica; p.

nervosa; acute vascular p.; hemorrhagic exudative erythema.

**hyperglobulinemic p.**, Waldenström's *macroglobulinemia.*

**idiopathic thrombocytopenic p.**, a serious systemic illness characterized by extensive ecchymoses, hemorrhages from mucous membranes, deficiencies in platelet count, anemia, and prostration; it lasts from a few weeks to several months, and may be fatal; also known as land scurvy; purpura hemorrhagica (1); thrombopenic or thrombocytopenic purpura; Werlhoff's disease.

**p. iod'ica**, iodic p.; an eruption of discrete miliary petechiae, usually confined to the lower extremities, appearing in rare instances during the administration of any of the iodides.

**p. nau'tica**, scurvy.

**p. nervo'sa**, Henoch-Schönlein p.

**nonthrombocytopenic p.**, p. simplex.

**psychogenic p.**, autoerythrocyte *sensitization.*

**p. pu'licans, p. pulico'sa**, petechiae caused by the bites of insects and animal parasites.

**p. rheumat'ica**, Henoch-Schönlein p.

**Schönlein's p.**, Henoch-Schönlein p.

**p. scorbu'tica**, scurvy.

**p. seni'lis**, the occurrence of petechiae and ecchymoses on the legs in aged and debilitated subjects.

**p. simplex**, nonthrombocytopenic p.; the eruption of petechiae or larger ecchymoses, usually unaccompanied by constitutional symptoms and not associated with systemic illness.

**p. symptomat'ica**, a petechial eruption in scarlet fever and other exanthemas.

**thrombocytopenic p.**, idiopathic thrombocytopenic p.

**thrombopenic p.**, idiopathic thrombocytopenic p.

**thrombotic thrombocytopenic p.**, Moschowitz' disease; a rapidly fatal or occasionally protracted disease with varied symptoms in addition to p., including signs of central nervous system involvement, due to formation of fibrin or platelet thrombi in arterioles and capillaries in many organs.

**p. urti'cans**, p. simplex accompanied by an urticarial eruption.

**p. variolo'sa**, malignant smallpox.

**Waldenström's p.**, Waldenström's *macroglobulinemia.*

**purpurea glycosides A and B** (pur'pu-re'ah gli'ko-sīdz). The cardioactive precursor glycosides of *Digitalis* purpurea; they are structurally identical with desacetyl-lanatosides A and B, respectively. See also lanatoside.

**purpuric** (pur-pu'rik). Relating to or affected with purpura.

**purpuriferous** (pur'pu-rif'er-us) [ L. *purpura,* purple, + *fero,* to bear ]. Purpurigenous. 1. Forming a purple pigment. 2. Forming the visual purple.

**purpurigenous** (pur'pu-rij'ĕ-nus). [ L. *purpura,* purple, + G. suffix *-gen,* producing ]. Purpuriferous.

**purpurin** (pur'pu-rin). 1. Uroerythrin. 2. A violet stain related to alizarin.

**purpurinuria** (pur'pu-rī-nu'rī-ah). Porphyrinuria.

**purpuriparous** (pur'pu-rip'ă-rus) [ L. *purpura,* purple, + *pario,* to bring forth ]. Purpuriferous.

**purr.** A low vibratory murmur.

**purshianin.** Impure forms of one or more of the laxative constituents of cascara sagrada.

**Purtscher** (poor'cher), Otmar, German ophthalmologist, 1852–1927. See P.'s *disease.*

**purulence, purulency** (pu'ru-lens, pūr'u-lens, -len-sī) [ L. *purulentia,* a festering, fr. *pus* (*pur*-), pus ]. Suppuration; the condition of containing or forming pus.

**purulent** (pu'ru-lent). Suppurative; suppurating; containing or forming pus.

**puruloid** (pu'ru-loyd). Resembling pus.

**pus** [ L. ]. A fluid product of inflammation, consisting of a liquid (liquor puris) containing leukocytes (p. corpuscles) and the debris of dead cells and tissue elements liquefied by the proteolytic and histolytic enzymes (*e.g.,* leukoprotease) that are elaborated by polymorphonuclear leukocytes.

**blue p.**, p. tinged with pyocyanin, a product of *Pseudomonas aeruginosa.*

**p. bo'num et laudab'ile**, good and laudable p.; the old term for typical p. of thick creamy consistence and yellowish color, thought to indicate a healthy inflammatory process tending to recovery.

**cheesy p.,** a very thick almost solid p. resulting from the absorption of the liquor puris.

**curdy p.,** p. containing flakes of caseous matter.

**green p.,** blue p. when, as sometimes happens, it has more of a green hue.

**ich′orous p.,** thin p. containing shreds of sloughing tissue, and sometimes of a fetid odor; ichor.

**laudable p.,** typical creamy yellow p.

**sa′nious p.,** ichorous p. stained with blood.

**pustula** (pus′tu-lah) [ L. ]. Pustule.

**pustulant** (pus′tu-lant). 1. Causing a pustular eruption. 2. An agent producing pustules.

**pustular** (pus′tu-lar). Relating to or marked by pustules.

**pustulation** (pus′tu-la′shun). The formation or the presence of pustules.

**pustule** (pus′tūl) [ L. *pustula* ]. A small circumscribed elevation on the skin, containing pus.

**malignant p.,** cutaneous anthrax; a characteristic lesion that begins as a papule and soon becomes a vesicle and breaks, discharging a bloody serum; the seat of this vesicle, in about 36 hours, becomes a bluish black necrotic mass; the constitutional symptoms are severe—high fever, vomiting, profuse sweating, and extreme prostration; the affection is often fatal in its termination.

**postmor′tem p.,** an ulcer, on the knuckle usually, resulting from infection during a dissection or the performance of an autopsy.

**spongiform p. of Kogoj,** an epidermal p. formed by infiltration of neutrophils into necrotic epidermis in which the cell walls persist as a spongelike network; seen in pustular psoriasis.

**pustuliform** (pus′tu-lī-form). Having the appearance of a pustule.

**pustulocrustaceous** (pus′tu-lo-krus-ta′shus). Marked by pustules crusted with dry pus.

**pustulosis** (pus′tu-lo′sis) [ L. *pustula*, pustule, + G. suffix *-osis*, condition ]. 1. A more or less generalized eruption of pustules. 2. Occasionally used to designate acropustulosis.

**p. vaccin′iformis acu′ta,** *eczema* herpeticum.

**putamen** (pu-ta′men) [ L. that which falls off in pruning, fr. *puto*, to prune ] [ NA ]. The outer, larger, and darker gray of the three portions into which the nucleus lentiformis is divided by laminae of white fibers; it is connected with the caudate nucleus by intervening bands of gray substance that penetrate the internal capsule. Its histological structure is similar to that of the caudate nucleus with which together it composes the striatum. See also *corpus* striatum; *nucleus* lentiformis.

**Putnam,** James J., Boston neurologist, 1846–1918. See P.-Dana *syndrome*.

**putrefaction** (pu′tre-fak′shun) [ L. *putre-facio*, pp. *-factus*, to make rotten, fr. *puter* (*putr-*) rotten ]. Decomposition; rotting; the breakdown of organic matter usually by bacterial action, resulting in the formation of other substances of less complex constitution with the evolution of ammonia or its derivatives and hydrogen sulfide; characterized usually by the presence of toxic or malodorous products.

**putrefactive** (pu′trĭ-fak′tiv). Relating to or causing putrefaction.

**putrefy** (pu′trĭ-fi). 1. To cause to become putrid. 2. To become putrid; to rot.

**putrefying** (pu′trĭ-fi′ing). Undergoing putrefaction; rotting.

**putrescence** (pu-tres′ens). Decay; rottenness; putridity.

**putrescent** (pu-tres′ent) [ L. *putresco*, to grow rotten, fr. *puter*, rotten ]. Putrefying.

**putrescine** (pu-tres′ēn). A poisonous amine (polyamine), 1,4-diaminobutane, $NH_2(CH_2)_4NH_2$, formed from the amino acid, arginine, during putrefaction.

**pu′trid** [ L. *putridus* ]. Decayed; rotten.

**Putti-Platt procedure** or **operation.** See under operation.

**PVP.** Abbreviation for polyvinylpyrrolidone.

**pyarthrosis** (pi-ar-thro′sis) [ G. *pyon*, pus, + *arthrōsis*, a jointing ]. Suppurative *arthritis*.

**pycno-.** For words so beginning, see under pykno-.

**pyel-.** See pyelo-.

**pyelectasis, pyelectasia** (pi′e-lek′tă-sis, -ta′zī-ah) [ pyel- + G. *ektasis*, extension ]. Nephrectasia; dilation of the pelvis of the kidney.

**pyelit′ic.** Relating to pyelitis.

**pyelitis** (pi-ĕ-li′tis) [ pyel- + G. suffix *-itis*, inflammation ]. 1. Inflammation of the renal pelvis. 2. Obsolescent term for pyelonephritis.

**pyelo-, pyel-** (pi′ĕ-lo-) (G. *pyelos*, trough, tub, vat (pelvis). PYEL- ]. Combining forms meaning pelvis, relating usually to the renal pelvis.

**pyelocaliceal** (pi′ĕ-lo-kal′ĭ-se′al). Pyelocalyceal; relating to the renal pelvis and calices.

**pyelocaliectasis** (pi′e-lo-kal′ĭ-ek′tă-sis). Calicectasis.

**py′elocal′yce′al.** Pyelocaliceal.

**pyelocystitis** (pi-ĕ-lo-sis-ti′tis) [ pyelo- + G. *kystis*, bladder, + suffix *-itis*, inflammation ]. Inflammation of the renal pelvis and the bladder.

**pyelofluoroscopy** (pi′ĕ-lo-flu-or-os′ko-pī) [ pyelo- + L. *fluo*, to flow, + G. *skopeō*, to view ]. Fluoroscopic examination of the renal pelves, usually with a contrast medium.

**py′elogram.** A roentgenogram of the renal pelvis and ureter.

**pyelography** (pi′ĕ-log′ră-fī) [ pyelo- + G. *graphō*, to write ]. Radiography of the ureter and pelvis of the kidney; pelviureterography; ureteropyelography.

**pyelolithotomy** (pi′ĕ-lo-lĭ-thot′o-mī) [ pyelo- + G. *lithos*, stone, + *tomē*, incision ]. Pelvilithotomy.

**pyelolymphatic** (pi′ĕ-lo-lim-fat′ik). Pertaining to the lymphatics of the renal pelvis.

**pyelonephritis** (pi′ĕ-lo-ne-fri′tis) [ pyelo- + G. *nephros*, kidney, + suffix *-itis*, inflammation ]. Nephropyelitis; inflammation of the renal parenchyma and pelvis due to local bacterial infection.

**bacillary p. of cattle,** a specific, necrotizing inflammation of the kidney pelvis and ureters of cattle, caused by infection with *Corynebacterium renale*.

**xanthogranulomatous p.,** chronic p. with nodular infiltrations of the kidney and peripelvic and perirenal fat by lipid macrophages and multinucleated giant cells, usually associated with hydronephrosis and ureteral obstruction by calculi.

**pyelonephrosis** (pi′ĕ-lo-ne-fro′sis) [ pyelo- + G. *nephros*, kidney, + suffix *-osis*, condition ]. Any disease of the pelvis of the kidney.

**pyeloplasty** (pi′ĕ-lo-plas′tī) [ pyelo- + G. *plassō*, to fashion ]. A plastic operation on kidney pelvis.

**pyeloplication** (pi′ĕ-lo-pli-ka′shun) [ pyelo- + L. *plico*, to fold ]. Operation of taking tucks in the wall of the renal pelvis when unduly dilated by a hydronephrosis.

**pyeloscopy** (pi-ĕ-los′ko-pī) [ pyelo- + G. *skopeō*, to view ]. Fluoroscopic observation of the pelvis and calyces of the kidney after the injection through the ureter of an opaque solution.

**pyelostomy** (pi′ĕ-los′to-mī) [ pyelo- + G. *stoma*, mouth ]. Formation of an opening into the kidney pelvis.

**pyelotomy** (pi′ĕ-lot′o-mī) [ pyelo- + G. *tomē*, incision ]. Incision into the pelvis of the kidney.

**pyeloureterectasis** (pi′ĕ-lo-u-re′ter-ek′tă-sis) [ pyelo- + ureter + G. *ektasis*, a stretching ]. Dilation of kidney pelvis and ureter.

**pyeloureterography** (pi′ĕ-lo-u-re′ter-og′ră-fī). Pyelography.

**pyelovenous** (pi′ĕ-lo-ve′nus) [ pyelo- + venous ]. Usually with backflow, referring to the phenomenon of drainage from the renal pelvis into the renal veins and inferior vena cava resulting from increased pressure.

**pyemesis** (pi-em′e-sis) [ G. *pyon*, pus, + *emesis*, vomiting ]. The vomiting of pus.

**pyemia** (pi-e′mĭ-ah) [ G. *pyon*, pus, + *haima*, blood ]. Pyogenic fever; pyosapremia; pyohemia; septicemia due to pyogenic organisms causing multiple abscesses.

**cryptogen′ic p.,** a p. the source of which is not evident, the focus being concealed in the deeper tissues.

**portal p.,** suppurative pylephlebitis.

**pyemic** (pi-e′mik). Relating to or suffering from pyemia.

**pyencephalus** (pi-en-sef′ă-lus) [ G. *pyon*, pus, + *enkephalos*, brain ]. Pyocephalus.

**pyesis** (pi-e′sis) [ G. *pyon*, pus, + suffix *-esis*, condition or process ]. Suppuration.

**pyg-.** See pygo-.

**pygal** (pi′gal) [ G. *pygē*, buttocks ]. Relating to the buttocks.

**pygalgia** (pi-gal′jĭ-ah) [ pyg- + G. *algos*, pain ]. Rarely used term meaning pain in the buttocks.

**pygmalionism** (pig-māl′yon-izm) [ fr. Greek sculptor, Pygmalion, who fell in love with the form of a maid which he had carved and which was given life by Aphrodite ]. The state of being in love with an object of one's own creation.

**pygmy, pigmy** (pig′mĭ) [ G. *pygmaios*, dwarfish, fr. *pygmē*, fist, also a measure of length from elbow to knuckles ]. A physiologic dwarf; especially one of a race of similar beings, such as the p.'s of Central Africa.

**pygmyism** (pig′mĭ-izm). The state of being a pygmy.

**pygoamorphus** (pi′go-ă-mor′fus) [ pygo- + G. *a-* priv. + *morphē*, form ]. Conjoined twins in which the parasite, attached to the buttocks of the autosite, is reduced to a formless mass or embryoma.

**pygo-, pyg-** (pi′go-) [ G. *pygē*, buttocks ]. Combining forms relating to the buttocks.

**pygodidymus** (pi′go-did′ĭ-mus) [ pygo- + G. + *didymos*, twin ]. Conjoined twins fused in the cephalothoracic region but with the buttocks and parts below doubled; see also *duplicitas posterior*.

**pygomelus** (pi-gom′e-lus) [ pygo- + G. *melos*, part ]. Unequal conjoined twins in which the parasite is represented by a fleshy mass, or a more fully developed limb, attached to the sacral or coccygeal region of the autosite.

**pygopagus** (pi-gop′ă-gus) [ pygo- + G. *pagos*, something fixed ]. Conjoined twins in which the two individuals are joined at the buttocks, most often back to back.

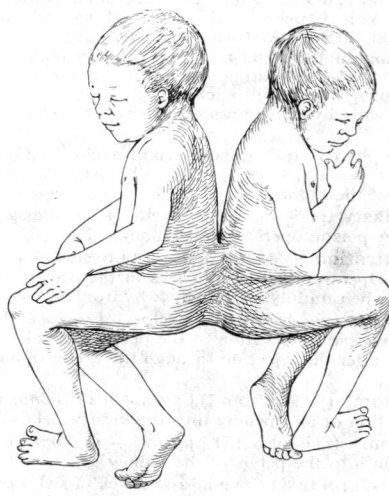

**Pygopagus**

**pyk-.** See pykno-.

**pyknemia** (pik-ne′mĭ-ah) [ pyk- + G. *haima*, blood ]. Obsolete term meaning for inspissation of the blood.

**pyknic** (pik′nik) [ G. *pyknos*, thick ]. Denoting a constitutional body type characterized by well rounded external contours and ample body cavities; virtually synonymous with endomorphic.

**pykno-, pyk-** [ G. *pyknos*, thick, dense ]. Combining forms meaning thick, dense, compact.

**pyknocytoma** (pik′no-si-to′mah). Oxyphil granular *adenoma*.

**pyknodysostosis** (pik′no-dis-os-to′sis) [ pykno- + G. prefix *dys-*, difficult, + *osteon*, bone, + suffix *-osis*, condition ]. Osteopetrosis acro-osteolytica; a condition characterized by short stature, delayed closure of the fontanelles, and hypoplasia of the terminal phalanges.

**pyknoepilepsy** (pik-no-ep′ĭ-lep-sĭ). Petit mal *epilepsy*.

**pyknohemia** (pik′no-he′mĭ-ah) [ pykno- + G. *haima*, blood ]. Obsolete term for inspissation of the blood.

**pyknolepsy** (pik′-no-lep-sĭ) [ pykno- + G. *lepsis*, seizure ]. Petit mal *epilepsy*.

**pyknometer** (pik-nom′e-ter) [ pykno- + G. *metron*, measure ]. An instrument for determining the specific gravity of any substance.

**pyknomorphous** (pik′no-mor′fus) [ pykno- + G. *morphē*, form, shape ]. Denoting a cell or tissue that stains deeply owing to the fact that the stainable material is closely packed.

**pyknophrasia** (pik′no-fra′zĭ-ah) [ pykno- + G. *phrasis*, speech ]. Thickness of utterance.

**pyknosis** (pik-no′sis) [ pykno- + G. suffix *-osis*, condition ]. Thickening; condensation; specifically, a condensation and reduction in size of the cell or its nucleus, usually associated with hyperchromatosis.

**pyknotic** (pik-not′ik). Relating to or characterized by pyknosis.

**pyla** (pi′lah) [ G. *pylē*, gate ]. The orifice of communication between the third ventricle and cerebral aqueduct (of Sylvius).

**py′lar.** Relating to the pyla.

**pylemphraxis** (pi′lem-frak′sis) [ G. *pylē*, gate, + *emphraxis*, a stoppage ]. Obstruction in some portion of the portal vein.

**py′lephlebecta′sia** [ G. *pylē*, gate, + *phleps* (*phleb-*), vein, + *ektasis*, extension ]. Dilation of the portal vein.

**pylephlebitis** (pi-le-flĕ-bi′tis) [ G. *pylē*, a gate, + *phleps*, vein, + suffix *-itis*, inflammation ]. Inflammation of the portal vein or any of its branches.

    **adhesive p.**, p. leading to thrombosis.

**pylethrombophlebitis** (pi′le-throm′bo-phlĕ-bi′tis) [ G. *pylē*, gate, + *thrombos*, a clot, + *phleps*, vein, + suffix *-itis*, inflammation ]. Inflammation of the portal vein with the formation of a thrombus.

**pylethrombo′sis** [ G. *pylē*, gate, + *thrombos*, a clot, + suffix *-osis*, condition ]. Thrombosis of the portal vein or any of its branches.

**pylic** (pi′lik). Portal; relating to the portal vein.

**pylon** (pi′lon) [ G. gateway ]. A temporary artificial leg; usually contains no joints.

**pylor-.** See pyloro-.

**pyloralgia** (pi-lo-ral′jĭ-ah) [ pylor- + G. *algos*, pain ]. Pain in the pyloric region of the stomach.

**pylorectomy** (pi′lo-rek′to-mĭ) [ pylor- + G. *ektomē*, excision ]. Excision of the pylorus; also called gastropylorectomy; pylorogastrectomy.

**pylori** (pi-lōr′i) [ L. ]. Plural of pylorus.

**pyloric** (pi-lōr′ik). Relating to the pylorus.

**pyloristenosis** (pi-lōr′ĭ-stĕ-no′sis) [ pylor- + G. *stenōsis*, narrowing ]. Pylorostenosis; stricture or narrowing of the orifice of the pylorus.

**pyloritis** (pi′lo-ri′tis) [ pylor- + G. suffix *-itis*, inflammation ]. Inflammation of the pyloric end of the stomach.

**pyloro-, pylor-** (pi-lōr′o-, pi-lor′o-) [ G. *pyloros*, gatekeeper (pylorus, *q. v.*) ]. Combining forms meaning pylorus.

**pylorodiosis** (pi-lōr′o-di-o′sis) [ pyloro- + G. *diōsis*, pushing apart ]. Operative dilation of the pylorus.

**pyloroduodenitis** (pi-lōr′o-du′o-dĕ-ni′tis) [ pyloro- + duodenitis ]. Inflammation involving the pyloric outlet of the stomach and the duodenum.

**pylorogastrectomy** (pi-lōr′o-gas-trek′to-mĭ). Pylorectomy.

**pyloromyotomy** (pi-lor′o-mi-ot′o-mĭ) [ pyloro- + G. *mys*, muscle, + *tomē*, incision ]. Fredet-Ramstedt operation; incision through the anterior wall of the pyloric canal to the level of the submucosa; used to treat hypertrophic pyloric stenosis.

**pyloroplasty** (pi-lōr′o-plas′tĭ) [ pyloro- + G. *plassō*, to form ]. An operation, commonly performed in conjunction with vagetectomy to treat peptic ulcer disease; an opening into pyloric canal is made in a longitudinal plane and closed transversely; the latter destroys the normal closing mechanism at the gastric outlet and facilitates prompt emptying of gastric contents into the duodenum.

**Finney p.,** longer incision extending into the duodenum and proximally into the gastric antrum; closure provides wider opening between stomach and duodenum.

**Heineke-Mikulicz p.,** p. in which a short longitudinal incision is made over the pylorus closed transversely, usually with one layer of nonabsorbable sutures.

**Jaboulay p.,** a side-to-side gastroduodenostomy which is especially valuable when the pylorus and proximal duodenum are extensively scarred or indurated by peptic ulcer disease.

**pyloroptosis, pyloroptosia** (pi-lōr'op-to'sis, -to'sĭ-ah) [ pyloro- + G. *ptōsis,* a falling ]. Downward displacement of the pyloric end of the stomach.

**pylorospasm** (pi-lōr'o-spazm). Spasmodic contraction of the pylorus.

**pylorostenosis** (pi-lōr'o-stĕ-no'sis). Pyloristenosis.

**pylorostomy** (pi'lo-ros'to-mĭ) [ pyloro- + G. *stoma,* mouth ]. Establishment of a fistula leading from the abdominal surface into the stomach near the pylorus.

**pylorotomy** (pi'lo-rot'o-mĭ) [ pyloro- + G. *tomē,* incision ]. Incision of the pylorus.

**pylorus,** pl. **pylori** (pi-lōr'us, pi-lōr'i) [ L. fr. G. *pylōros,* a gatekeeper, the pylorus, fr. *pylē,* gate, + *ouros,* a warder ] [ NA ]. 1. A muscular or myovascular device to open (musculus dilator) and to close (musculus sphincter) an orifice or the lumen of an organ. 2. The muscular tissue surrounding and controlling the aboral outlet of the stomach.

**Pym,** Sir William, English physician, 1772–1861. See P.'s *fever.*

**pyo-** (pi'o-) [ G. *pyon,* pus ]. Combining form denoting suppuration or an accumulation of pus.

**pyocele** (pi'o-sēl) [ pyo- + G. *kēlē,* tumor, hernia ]. An accumulation of pus in the scrotum.

**pyocelia** (pi'o-se'lĭ-ah) [ pyo- + G. *koilia,* a cavity ]. Pyoperitoneum.

**pyocephalus** (pi'o-sef'ă-lus) [ pyo- + G. *kephalē,* head ]. Pyencephalus; a purulent effusion within the cranium.

**circumscribed p.,** abscess of the brain.

**external p.,** meningeal suppuration.

**internal p.,** the presence of pus in the cerebrospinal fluid within the ventricles.

**pyochezia** (pi-o-ke'zĭ-ah) [ pyo- + G. *chezō,* to defecate ]. A discharge of pus from the bowel.

**pyocin** (pi'o-sin). Bacteriocin produced by strains of *Pseudomonas pyocyaneus.*

**pyococcus** (pi'o-kok'us) [ pyo- + G. *kokkos,* berry (coccus) ]. One of the cocci causing suppuration, especially *Streptococcus pyogenes.*

**pyocolpocele** (pi-o-kol'po-sēl) [ pyo- + G. *kolpos,* bosom (vagina), + *kēlē,* tumor, hernia ]. Pyocolpos.

**pyocolpos** (pi-o-kol'pos) [ pyo- + G. *kolpos,* bosom (vagina) ]. An accumulation of pus in the vagina.

**pyoculture** (pi'o-kul-chur) [ pyo- + L. *cultura,* tillage (culture) ]. Peptonized bouillon culture of pus compared with uncultured pus for the purpose of determining the effectiveness of the leukocytes toward the bacteria.

**pyocyanic** (pi'o-si-an'ik) [ pyo- + G. *kyanos,* blue ]. Relating to blue pus or the bacillus of blue pus, *Pseudomonas aeruginosa.*

**pyocyanin** (pi'o-si'ă-nin). $C_{13}H_{10}ON_2$; antibiotic crystalline substance isolated from peptone broth cultures of *Pseudomonas aeruginosa;* active against Gram-positive and Gram-negative bacteria, but highly toxic to animal tissues.

**pyocyanogenic** (pi'o-si'ă-no-jen'ik) [ pyo- + G. *kyanos,* blue, + suffix *-gen,* producing ]. Pyocyanic; causing blue pus; producing pyocyanin.

**pyocyanolysin** (pi'o-si-ă-nol'ĭ-sin). A hemolysin formed by *Pseudomonas aeruginosa.*

**pyocyst** (pi'o-sist) [ pyo- + G. *kystis,* bladder ]. A cyst with purulent contents.

**pyocyte** (pi'o-sīt) [ pyo- + G. *kytos,* cell ]. Pus *corpuscle.*

**pyoderma** (pi'o-der'mah) [ pyo- + G. *derma,* skin ]. Pyodermatitis; pyodermatosis; any pyogenic infection of the skin; may be primary, as impetigo contagiosa, or secondary to a previously existing condition.

**p. gangrenosum,** a chronic eruption of spreading, undermined ulcers showing central healing; often associated with ulcerative colitis.

**oral p.,** a mouth disease characterized by lesions involving the gingivae, mucobuccal folds or buccal mucosae; they are profuse in number, 2 to 7 mm. in size, grayish white to white to pale yellow in color, elevated, discrete, round or semicircular, soft, friable, easily detached, and somewhat necrotic appearing; resembles moniliasis.

**primary p.,** one such as impetigo, or sycosis vulgaris, in which pus formation is an essential part of the disease.

**secondary p.,** one in which the skin lesion (eczema, herpes, seborrheic dermatitis, etc.) becomes secondarily infected.

**p. vegetans,** *dermatitis* vegetans.

**pyodermatitis** (pi-o-der-mă-ti'tis) [ pyo- + G. *derma,* skin, + suffix *-itis,* inflammation ]. Pyoderma.

**pyodermatosis** (pi'o-der-mă-to'sis) [ pyo- + G. *derma,* skin, + suffix *-osis,* condition ]. Pyoderma.

**pyogen** (pi'o-jen) [ pyo- + G. suffix *-gen,* producing ]. An agent that causes pus formation.

**pyogenesis** (pi'o-jen'ĕ-sis) [ pyo- + G. *genesis,* production ]. Suppuration; the formation of pus.

**pyogenic, pyogenetic** (pi'o-jen'ik, -jĕ-net'ik). Pyogenous; pus-forming; relating to pus formation.

**pyogenous** (pi-oj'ĕ-nus). Pyogenic.

**pyohemia** (pi-o-he'mĭ-ah). Pyemia.

**pyohemothorax** (pi-o-he'mo-tho'raks) [ pyo- + G. *haima,* blood, + thorax ]. The presence of pus and blood in the pleural cavity.

**pyoid** (pi'oyd) [ G. *pyōdēs,* fr. *pyon,* pus, + *eidos,* resemblance ]. Resembling pus.

**pyolabyrinthitis** (pi-o-lab-ĭ-rin-thi'tis) [ pyo- + G. *labyrinthos,* labyrinth, + suffix *-itis,* inflammation ]. Suppurative inflammation of the labyrinth of the ear.

**pyometra** (pi'o-me'trah) [ pyo- + G. *mētra,* uterus ]. An accumulation of pus in the uterine cavity.

**pyometritis** (pi'o-me-tri'tis) [ pyo- + G. *mētra,* womb, + suffix *-itis,* inflammation ]. An inflammation of uterine musculature associated with pus in the uterine cavity.

**pyomyositis** (pi'o-mi-o-si'tis) [ pyo- + G. *mys,* muscle, + suffix *-itis,* inflammation ]. Abscesses, carbuncles, or infected sinuses lying deep in muscles.

**tropical p.,** *myositis* purulenta tropica.

**pyonephritis** (pi-o-ne-fri'tis) [ pyo- + G. *nephros,* kidney, + suffix *-itis,* inflammation ]. Suppurative inflammation of the kidney.

**pyonephrolithiasis** (pi'o-nef'ro-lĭ-thi'ă-sis) [ pyo- + G. *nephros,* kidney, + *lithos,* stone, + suffix *-iasis,* condition ]. Presence in the kidney of pus and calculi.

**pyonephrosis** (pi'o-ne-fro'sis) [ pyo- + G. *nephros,* kidney, + suffix *-osis,* condition ]. Distention of the pelvis and calices of the kidney with pus.

**pyonex** (pi'o-neks) [ pyo- + G. *ex,* out ]. Acupuncture; baunscheidtism; also the instrument, composed of a number of needles set in the extremity of a cylinder, used for performing acupuncture.

**pyoovarium** (pi'o-o-văr'ĭ-um). The presence of pus in the ovary; an ovarian abscess.

**pyopericarditis** (pi'o-pĕr-ĭ-kar-di'tis). Suppurative inflammation of the pericardium.

**pyopericardium** (pi'o-pĕr-ĭ-kar'di-um). Empyema of the pericardium; an accumulation of pus in the pericardial sac.

**pyoperitoneum** (pi'o-pĕr-ĭ-to-ne'um). [ G. *pyon,* pus ]. An accumulation of pus in the peritoneal cavity.

**pyoperitonitis** (pi'o-pĕr-ĭ-tŏ-ni'tis) [ pyo- + peritonitis ]. Suppurative inflammation of the peritoneum.

**pyophthalmia, pyophthalmitis** (pi'of-thal'mĭ-ah, pi'of-thal-mi'tis) [ pyo- + G. *ophthalmos,* eye, + suffix *-ia,* condition, or *-itis,* inflammation ]. Suppurative inflammation of the eye.

**pyophylactic** (pi'o-fi-lak'tik) [ pyo- + G. *phylaktikos,* guarding ]. Protecting against purulent infection or pus absorption; denoting a membrane lining the wall of an abscess.

**pyophysometra** (pi'o-fi'so-me'trah) [ pyo- + G. *physa*, air, + *mētra*, uterus ]. The presence of pus and gas in the uterine cavity.

**pyopneumocholecystitis** (pi'o-nu'mo-ko'le-sis-ti'tis) [ pyo- + G. *pneuma*, air, + cholecystitis ]. Combination of pus and gas in an inflamed gallbladder caused by gas-producing organisms or by the entry of air from the duodenum through the biliary tree.

**pyopneumohepatitis** (pi'o-nu'mo-hep-ă-ti'tis) [ pyo- + G. *pneuma*, air, + hepatitis ]. Combination of pus and air in the liver, usually in association with an abscess.

**pyopneumopericardium** (pi'o-nu'mo-pĕr-ĭ-kar'dĭ-um) [ pyo- + G. *pneuma*, air, + pericardium ]. The presence of pus and gas in the pericardial sac.

**pyopneumoperitoneum** (pi'o-nu'mo-pĕr-ĭ-tōne'um) [ pyo- + G. *pneuma*, air, + peritoneum ]. The presence of pus and gas in the peritoneal cavity.

**pyopneumoperitonitis** (pi'o-nu'mo-pĕr-ĭ-to-ni'tis) [ pyo- + G. *pneuma*, air, + peritonitis ]. Peritonitis with gas-forming organisms or with gas introduced from a ruptured bowel.

**pyopneumothorax** (pi'o-nu'mo-tho'raks) [ pyo- + G. *pneuma*, air, + thorax ]. Pneumopyothorax; pneumoempyema; the presence of gas together with a purulent effusion in the pleural cavity.

  **subdiaphragmat'ic p., subphren'ic p.,** subphrenic abscess associated with perforation of one of the hollow viscera, with gas in the chest, and abdomen.

**pyopoiesis** (pi'o-poy-e'sis) [ pyo- + G. *poiēsis*, a making ]. Suppuration.

**pyopoietic** (pi'o-poy-et'ik). Pus-producing.

**pyoptysis** (pi-op'tĭ-sis) [ pyo- + G. *ptysis*, a spitting ]. Purulent expectoration; spitting of pus.

**pyopyelectasis** (pi'o-pi-ĕ-lek'tă-sis) [ pyo- + G. *pyelos*, pelvis, + *ektasis*, a stretching ]. Dilation of the renal pelvis with pus-producing inflammation.

**pyorrhea** (pi-o-re'ah) [ pyo- + G. *rhoia*, a flow ]. A purulent discharge.

  **p. alveola'ris,** periodontitis.

**pyosalpingitis** (pi'o-sal-pin-ji'tis) [ pyo- + salpingitis ]. Suppurative inflammation of the Fallopian tube.

**pyosalpingo-oophoritis** (pi'o-sal'ping-go-o-of'o-ri'tis) [ pyo- + G. *salpinx*, trumpet (tube), + oophoritis ]. Pyosalpingo-oothecitis; suppurative inflammation of the Fallopian tube and the ovary.

**pyosalpingo-oothecitis** (pi'o-sal'ping-go-o-o-the-si'tis) [ pyo- + G. *salpinx* trumpet (tube), + Mod. L. *ootheca*, ovary, + suffix *-itis*, inflammation ]. Pyosalpingo-oophoritis.

**pyosalpinx** (pi-o-sal'pingks) [ pyo- + G. *salpinx*, trumpet (tube) ]. Pus tube; distention of a Fallopian tube with pus.

**pyosapremia** (pi'o-să-pre'mĭ-ah) [ pyo- + G. *sapros*, putrid, + *haima*, blood ]. Pyemia.

**pyosepticemia** (pi'o-sep-tĭ-se'mĭ-ah) [ pyo- + G. *sēptikos*, putrefying, + *haima*, blood ]. Infection of the blood with several forms of bacteria, so-called pyogenic and also nonpyogenic organisms.

**pyosis** (pi-o'sis) [ G ]. Suppuration.

  **Corlett's p.,** impetigo.

  **Manson's p.,** *pemphigus* contagiosus.

  **p. palma'ris,** an affection observed in children in the East Indies, characterized by the presence of numerous discrete pustules on the palms.

  **p. trop'ica,** Kurunegala ulcers; an affection observed by Castellani in Ceylon, marked by the presence of dirty yellowish or blackish lesions, covered with a crust, the removal of which leaves a shallow granulating ulcer.

**pyostatic** (pi'o-stat'ik) [ pyo- + G. *statikos*, causing to stand. STA- ]. 1. Arresting the formation of pus. 2. An agent that arrests the formation of pus.

**pyothorax** (pi'o-tho'raks). Empyema in a plural cavity.

**pyourachus** (pi-o-u'ră-kus). A purulent accumulation in the urachus.

**pyoureter** (pi-o-u-re'ter). Distention of a ureter with pus.

**pyoxanthin** (pi'o-zan'thin). A reddish yellow pigment obtained from blue pus by oxidation.

**pyoxanthose** (pi'o-zan'thōs). A yellowish pigment obtained from blue pus by oxidation; α-hydroxyphenazine; hemipyocyanine.

**pyr-** [ G. *pyr*, fire. PYR- ]. Combining form relating to fire or heat; see also pyreto- and pyro-.

**pyrabrom** (pīr'ă-brom) (USAN). GLYBROM; pyrilamine 8-bromotheophyllinate; antihistaminic-diuretic combination for treatment of Ménière's disease.

**pyracin** (pīr'ă-sin). Pyridoxolactone (the lactone of 4-pyridoxic acid, a metabolite of pyridoxal).

**pyramid** (pīr'ă-mid) [ G. *pyramis* (*pyramid*-), a pyramid ]. 1. A term applied to a number of anatomical structures having a more or less pyramidal shape. 2. An obsolete term denoting the petrous portion of the temporal bone.

  **anterior p.,** *pyramis* medullae oblongatae.

  **cerebellar p.,** *pyramis* vermis.

  **Ferrein's p.,** *pars* radiata lobuli corticalis renis.

  **Lalouette's p.,** *lobus* pyramidalis glandulae thyroideae.

  **p. of light,** a triangular area at the anterior inferior part of the drum membrane, running from the umbo to the periphery, where there is seen a bright reflection of light.

  **Malacarne's p.,** a lobule on the undersurface of the cerebellum, the posterior portion of the vermis.

  **Malpighian p.,** *pyramis* renalis.

  **olfactory p.,** a small area of gray matter situated between the roots of the olfactory tracts; it is continuous behind with the anterior perforated substance.

  **petrous p.,** *pars* petrosa ossis temporalis.

  **posterior p. of the medulla,** *fasciculus* gracilis.

  **renal p.,** *pyramis* renalis.

  **p. of the thyroid,** *lobus* pyramidalis glandulae thyroideae.

  **p. of the tym'panum,** *eminentia* pyramidalis.

  **p. of the ves'tibule,** *pyramis* vestibuli.

**pyramidal** (pī-ram'ĭ-dal). 1. Of the shape of a pyramid. 2. Relating to any anatomical structure called pyramid.

**pyramidale** (pi-ram-ĭ-da'le) [ Mod. L. ]. *Os* triquetrum.

**pyramida'lis.** See under musculus.

**pyramidotomy** (pī-ram'ĭ-dot'o-mī) [ G. *pyramis*, pyramid, + *tomē*, incision ]. Section of pyramidal tracts, in the spinal cord, for the relief of involuntary movements.

  **medullary p.,** a medullary pyramidal *tractotomy.*

  **spinal p.,** a spinal pyramidal *tractotomy.*

**pyramin** (pīr'ă-min). 4-Amino-5-hydroxymethyl-2-methylpyrimidine; one of the products resulting from the hydrolysis of thiamin by thiaminase and appearing in the urine.

**pyramis,** pl. **pyramides** (pīr'ă-mis, pī-ram'ĭ-dēz) [ G. pyramid ] [ NA ]. Pyramid.

  **p. medul'lae oblonga'tae** [ NA ], pyramid of the medulla oblongata; anterior column of medulla oblongata; anterior pyramid; an elongated, white prominence on the ventral surface of the medulla oblongata on either side along the anterior median fissure, corresponding to the pyramidal tract.

  **p. rena'lis,** pl. **pyramides rena'les** [ NA ], renal pyramid; Malpighian pyramid; medullary pyramid; one of a number of pyramidal masses seen on longitudinal section of the kidney; they contain part of the secreting tubules and the collecting tubules.

  **p. tym'pani,** *eminentia* pyramidalis.

  **p. ver'mis** [ NA ], cerebellar pyramid; a subdivision of the inferior vermis of the cerebellum anterior to the tuber, between it and the uvula.

  **p. vestib'uli** [ NA ], pyramid of the vestibule; the anterior triangular extremity of the crista vestibuli.

**pyran** (pi'ran). A cyclic compound that may be considered the parent substance of sugars with an oxygen bridge from carbon atoms 1 to 5 (the pyranoses). Compare furan.

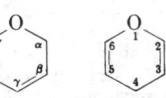

2*H*-pyran    4*H*-pyran
1,2-pyran    1,4-pyran
α-pyran    γ-pyran

**Pyran**

**pyranone** (pīr'ă-nōn, pī'-). Pyrone.

**pyranose** (pīr'ă-nōs, pī'-). A cyclic form of a sugar in which the oxygen bridge forms in such a way as to produce a ring made up of five carbon atoms and an oxygen atom; similar to pyran, whence the name. Compare furanose.

**pyran'tel pamoate** (USP). (*E*)-1,4,5,6-Tetrahydro-1-methyl-2-[ 2-(2-thienyl)vinyl ]pyrimidine 4,4'-methylene-bis[ 3-hydroxy-2-naphthoate ]; anthelmintic.

**pyrathiazine hydrochloride** (pīr'ă-thī'ă-zēn). PYR-ROLAZOTE; 10-[ 2-(1-pyrrolidyl)ethyl ]phenolthiazine hydrochloride; antihistaminic.

**pyrazinamide** (pīr'ă-zin'ă-mīd) (USP, BP). ALDINAMIDE; PZA; pyrazinoic acid amide; pyrazinecarboxamide; a moderately effective antituberculous agent; the rapid development of resistance is delayed when given in combination with isoniazid. P. may produce hepatic damage.

**pyrectic** (pi-rek'tik). Pyretic.

**pyrenemia** (pi'-re-ne'mī-ah) [ G. *pyrēn*, the pit of a fruit, + *haima*, blood ]. A condition characterized by the presence of nucleated red blood cells.

**pyrenoid** (pi're-noyd) [ G. *pyrēn*, pit of a fruit, + *eidos*, resemblance ]. One of the minute luminous bodies sometimes visualized in the chromatophores of some protozoa, such as *Euglena viridis*.

**pyrethrum** (pi-re'thrum) [ G. *pyrethron*, feverfew, fr. *pyr*, fire, from the hot-tasting root ]. Spanish chamomile; the root of *Anacyclus pyrethrum* (family Compositae), a shrub native of Morocco; has been used as a sialogogue; now used chiefly as an insecticide. Now used chiefly as an insecticide.

**pyretic** (pi-ret'ik) [ G. *pyretikos* ]. Feverish.

**pyreticosis** (pi-ret'ĭ-ko'sis) [ G. *pyretos*, fever, + suffix *-osis*, condition ]. Any fever.

**pyreto-, pyret-** (pi'rĕ-to-, pīr'ĕ-to-) [ G. *pyretos*, fever, fr. *pyr*, fire. PYR- ]. Combining forms meaning fever. For words beginning thus, and not found here, see also pyro-.

**pyretogen** (pi-ret'o-jen) [ pyreto- + G. suffix *-gen*, producing ]. Any agent that induces fever.

**pyretogenesis** (pi'rĕ-to-jen'ĕ-sis, pīr'ĕ-to-) [ pyreto- + G. *genesis*, origin ]. The origin and mode of production of fever.

**pyretogenet'ic, pyretogen'ic.** Pyrogenic.

**pyretogenin** (pi-rĕ-toj'ĕ-nin). A product of various pyretogenic bacteria, injection of which causes an elevation of body temperature.

**pyretogenous** (pi-rĕ-to'jĕ-nus). 1. Caused by fever. 2. Pyrogenic; causing fever.

**pyretotherapy** (pi're-to-thĕr'ă-pī) [ pyreto- + G. *therapeia*, treatment ]. 1. Malariotherapy; treatment of disease by raising the temperature of the body intermittently, either by diathermy or by inoculation of malarial organisms. 2. Treatment of fever.

**pyrexia** (pi-rek'sī-ah) [ G. *pyrexis*, feverishness. PYR- ]. Fever.

  **local p.,** acute inflammation.

**pyrexial** (pi-rek'sī-al). Febrile; pyretic; relating to fever.

**pyrexiophobia** (pi-rek'sī-o-fo'bī-ah) [ G. *pyrexis*, feverishness, + *phobos*, fear ]. A morbid fear of fever.

**pyri-** [ L. *pyrum*, pear ]. Combining form meaning pear, pear-shpaed; see also alternative spelling, piri-.

**pyriben'zyl methyl sulfate.** ACABEL; 2-(hydroxymethyl)-1,1-dimethylpiperidinium methyl sulfate benzylate; an intestinal antispasmodic with anticholinergic properties.

**pyridine** (pīr'ī-dēn, -din). $C_5H_5N$; a colorless volatile liquid of empyreumatic odor and burning taste, resulting from the dry distillation of organic matter containing nitrogen. Used as an industrial solvent, in analytical chemistry, and for denaturing alcohol.

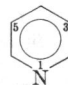

**Pyridine**

**2-pyridinecarboxylic acid** (pīr'ī-dēn-kar-bok-sil'ik). Picolinic acid.

**3-pyridinecarboxylic acid.** Nicotinic acid.

**4-pyridinecarboxylic acid.** Isonicotinic acid.

**pyridofylline.** ATHEROPHYLLINE; 7-(2-hydroxyethyl)-theophylline hydrogen sulfate compound with pyridoxol; coronary vasodilator.

**pyridostigmine bromide** (pīr'ī-do-stig'mēn) (USP, BP). MESTINON bromide; 3-hydroxy-1-methylpyridinium bromide dimethylcarbamate; a cholinesterase inhibitor useful in the treatment of myasthenia gravis. Gastrointestinal reactions may be less severe than those caused by neostigmine.

**pyridoxal** (pīr'ī-dok'sal). 4-Formyl-3-hydroxy-5-hydroxymethyl-2-methylpyridine; the aldehyde of pyridoxine, having a similar physiologic action.

  **p. kinase** (EC 2.7.1.35), an enzyme that catalyzes the phosphorylation by ATP of p. to p. 5'-phosphate codecarboxylase, thus converting the food factor to the active coenzyme.

**pyridoxal 5'-phosphate.** Codecarboxylase; a coenzyme essential to many reactions in tissue, notably transaminations and amino acid decarboxylations.

$$HO \quad \overset{CHO}{\underset{CH_3 \quad N}{\bigcirc}} \quad CH_2OPO_3H_2$$

**Pyridoxal phosphate**

**pyridoxamine** (pīr'ī-dok'să-mēn). The amine of pyridoxine (—$CH_2NH_2$ replacing —$CH_2OH$ at position 4), having a similar physiologic action.

**pyridoxamine 5'-phosphate.** Pyridoxamine phosphorylated on the 5-$CH_2OH$ group.

**pyridoxaminephosphate oxidase** (pīr'ī-dok'să-mēn-fos'fāt) (EC 1.4.3.5). Oxidoreductase catalyzing oxidative deamination of pyridoxamine 5'-phosphate (with $O_2$) to pyridoxal 5'-phosphate, $H_2O_2$, and $NH_3$.

**4-pyridoxic acid** (pīr'ī-dok'sik). The principal product of the metabolism of pyridoxal in man (—COOH replaces —CHO at position 4), appearing in the urine.

**pyridoxine** (pīr'ī-dok'sēn, -sin). 3-Hydroxy-4,5-bis(hydroxymethyl)-2-methylpyridine; the original vitamin $B_6$, which now includes pyridoxal and pyridoxamine. Also known as hexabione; pyridoxol; pyridoxonium (chloride); adermin(e); Y factor; yeast eluate factor. P. is associated with the utilization of unsaturated fatty acids. In rats, deficiency produces a nutritional dermatitis and acrodynia; in humans, deficiency may result in increased irritability, convulsions, and peripheral neuritis. It is used in the treatment of pyridoxine-responsive anemias and seborrheic dermatitis; when administered to human pellagrins it produces improvement in the neuromuscular symptoms; and there are indications that it is of importance in hemopoiesis. The hydrochloride is official in the USP and BP.

  **p. dehydrogenase** (EC 1.1.1.65), oxidoreductase catalyzing oxidation of pyridoxine to pyridoxal by NADP.

**pyriform** (pīr'ī-form) [ L. *pyrum* (prop. *pirum*), pear, + *forma*, form ]. Piriform.

**pyrifor'mis.** See under musculus.

**pyrilamine maleate** (pi-ril'ă-mēn, pīr-il-) (NF). NEO-ANTERGAN maleate; mepyramine maleate (BP); 2-[ (2-dimethylaminoethyl) (*p*-methoxybenzyl)amino ]-pyridine maleate; a histamine-antagonizing agent.

**pyrimethamine** (pīr'ī-meth'ă-mēn) (USP, BP). DARAPRIM; 2,4-diamino-5-*p*-chlorophenyl-6-ethylpyrimidine. A potent folic acid antagonist used as an antimalarial agent effective against *Plasmodium falciparum;* a valuable suppressant, active against the asexual erythrocytic and tissue forms; also used in the treatment of toxoplasmosis.

**pyrimidine** (pi-rim′ĭ-dēn). A heterocyclic substance, the parent substance of several "bases" present in nucleic acids (uracil, thymine, cytosine) as well as of the barbiturates.

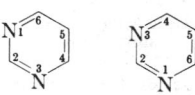

**Pyrimidine**

*Left*, original Fischer numbering system (*cf.* purine), now abandoned; *right*, current official numbering system.

**p. base,** pyrimidine.

**p. transferase,** thiamin pyridinylase.

**pyrithiamine** (pĭr′ĭ-thi′ă-mēn). A pyridine analogue of thiamin; when fed to mice induces symptoms of thiamin deficiency; also inhibits the growth of bacteria to which thiamin is essential.

**pyrithyldione** (pĭr′ĭ-thil-di′ōn). PRESIDON; PERSEDON; 3,3-diethyl-2,4-dioxotetrahydropyridine; a synthetic sedative and hypnotic drug; may cause agranulocytosis.

**pyro-** (pi′ro-) [ G. *pyr*, fire ]. 1. Combining form relating to fire, heat, or fever. 2. Used in chemistry to denote derivatives formed by removal of water (usually by heat) to form anhydrides (*cf.* anhydro-).

**pyrocalciferol** (pi′ro-kal-sif′er-ol). 10α-Ergosta-5,7,22-trien-3β-ol (for structure of ergostane, see steroids); thermal decomposition product of calciferol.

**pyrocatechase** (pi′ro-kat′ĕ-kās). Catechol 1,2-dioxygenase.

**pyrocatechin** (pi′ro-kat′ĕ-kin). Pyrocatechol.

**pyrocatechol** (pi′ro-kat′ĕ-kol). Catechol; pyrocatechin; *o*-diphenol; *o*-dihydroxybenzene; a constituent of epinephrine and norepinephrine (both "catecholamines") and dopa; used externally as an antiseptic to meet the same indications as resorcinol.

**pyrogallol** (pi′ro-gal′ol). Pyrogallic acid; $C_6H_3(OH)_3$; 1,2,3-trihydroxybenzene; used externally in the treatment of psoriasis, ringworm, and other skin affections.

**pyrogen** (pi′ro-jen) [ pyro- + suffix *-gen*, producing ]. An agent that causes a rise in temperature. Term used most commonly in referring to substances of unknown origin, but probably of a saccharide or protein in nature. P.'s are produced by bacteria, molds, viruses, and yeasts, and commonly occur in distilled water. Preparations for parenteral use can easily become contaminated with p.'s during their manufacture. See also pyrogen *test*.

**pyrogenic** (pi′ro-jen′ik). Pyretogenic; pyretogenetic; pyretogenous; causing fever.

**pyrolagnia** (pi′ro-lag′nĭ-ah) [ pyro- + G. *lagneia*, lust ]. Sexual gratification from setting fires.

**pyroligneous** (pi-ro-lig′ne-us) [ pyro- + L. *lignum*, wood ]. Relating to or produced by the dry distillation of wood.

**p. alcohol,** methyl alcohol.

**pyrolysis** (pi-rol′ĭ-sis) [ pyro- + G. *lysis*, dissolution ]. The decomposition of a substance by heat.

**pyromania** (pi-ro-ma′nĭ-ah) [ pyro- + G. *mania*, frenzy ]. Incendiarism; a morbid impulse to set fires.

**pyroma′niac.** One affected with pyromania.

**pyrometer** (pi-rom′e-ter) [ pyro- + G. *metron*, measure ]. An instrument for measuring very high degrees of heat, beyond the capacity of a mercurial thermometer.

**resistance p.,** resistance *thermometer*.

**pyrone** (pi′rōn). Pyranone; a keto derivative of pyran; *cf.* kojic acid and pyranose.

**pyronin** (pi′ro-nin). A basic red dye, the chloride of tetramethyldiaminoxanthene (pyronin G, Y) or tetraethyldiaminoxanthene (pyronin B).

**py′ronin B.** A red basic xanthine dye, $C_{21}H_{27}N_2OCl$, used in combination with methyl green for differential staining of ribonucleic acid (red) and deoxyribonucleic acid (green).

**pyroninophilia** (pi′ro-nin-o-fil′ĭ-ah) [ pyronin + G. *philos*, fond ]. An affinity for the basic pyronin dyes.

**pyrophobia** (pi′ro-fo′bĭ-ah) [ pyro- + G. *phobos*, fear ]. A morbid dread of fire.

**py′rophos′phatase.** Any enzyme cleaving a pyrophosphate between two phosphoric groups, leaving one on each of the two fragments. Examples are inorganic p., NAD+ p. (cleaves NAD, etc., to mononucleotides), ATP p. (cleaves inorganic pyrophosphate from ATP, leaving AMP).

**inorganic p.** (EC 3.6.1.1), phosphohydrolase catalyzing hydrolysis of inorganic pyrophosphate to orthophosphate.

**py′rophos′phate.** A salt of pyrophosphoric acid.

**pyrophos′phoki′nases.** Pyrophosphotransferases; enzymes transferring a pyrophosphoric group (*e.g.*, ribosephosphate pyrophosphokinase, EC 2.7.6.1).

**py′rophosphor′ic acid.** An acid, $H_4P_2O_7$, obtained by heating phosphoric acid to 213°C. (415°F.); it forms pyrophosphates with bases. Its esters are important in energy metabolism and in biosynthesis (*e.g.*, ATP).

**pyrophos′photrans′ferases.** Pyrophosphokinases.

**pyroptothymia** (pi-rop-to-thi′mĭ-ah) [ pyro- + G. *ptoein*, to frighten, + *thymos*, mind ]. A delusion in which one imagines being surrounded by flames.

**pyroscope** (pi′ro-skōp) [ pyro- + G. *skopeō*, to view ]. An instrument for measuring temperature by comparing the light of a heated object with a light standard.

**pyrosis** (pi-ro′sis) [ G. a burning ]. Heartburn; water pang; water brash; substernal pain or burning sensation, usually associated with regurgitation of acid-peptic gastric juice into the esophagus.

**py′rother′apy.** Treatment of disease by inducing an artificial fever in the patient.

**pyrot′ic.** 1. Relating to pyrosis. 2. Caustic.

**pyrotoxin** (pi′ro-tok′sin). A supposed toxic substance produced in the tissues during the progress of a fever.

**pyrovalerone hydrochloride** (pĭr′o-val′er-ōn) (USAN). CENTROTON; 4′-methyl-2-(1-pyrrolidinyl)valerophenone hydrochloride; analeptic.

**pyroxylin** (pi-rok′sĭ-lin) [ pyro- + G. *xylon* wood ] (USP, BP). Soluble gun cotton; nitrocellulose; dinitrocellulose; xyloidin; pyroxylon; consists chiefly of cellulose tetranitrate, obtained by the action of nitric and sulfuric acids on cotton; used in the preparation of collodion.

**pyrrobutamine phosphate** (pĭr′o-bu′tă-mēn) (NF). PYRONIL; 1-[ 4-(*p*-chlorophenyl)-3-phenyl-2-butenyl ]-pyrrolidine diphosphate; antihistamine with low incidence of side effects.

**pyrrocaine hydrochloride** (pĭr′o-kān) (USAN). ENDOCAINE; 1-pyrrolidineaceto-2′,6′-xylidide hydrochloride; a local anesthetic used in dentistry.

**pyrroetioporphyrin** (pĭr′o-e′tĭ-o-por′fĭ-rin). A porphyrin derivative, differing from etioporphyrin only in the absence of a side chain (replaced by H) in position 6; obtained after drastic degradation of the chlorophylls; 1,3,5,8-tetramethyl-2,4,7-triethylporphin.

**pyrrolase** (pĭr′o-lās). Tryptophan 2,3-dioxygenase.

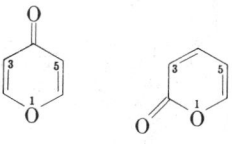

4-pyrone          2-pyrone
4*H*-pyran-4-one  2*H*-pyran-2-one
γ-pyrone          α-pyrone

**Pyrone**

**pyrrole** (pĭr′ōl). Azole; imidole; divinylenimine; a heterocyclic compound found in many biologically important substances (compare pyran, imidazole).

**p. nucleus,** of porphyrins (*i.e.*, porphin); a cyclic tetrapyrrole; four pyrrole groups joined into a ring structure by way of —CH= (methylidyne) bridges be-

H
N
1
α' 5 2 α
4 3
β' β

Pyrrole

tween α(2) position of one p. and α'(5) position of another p., the fourth p. being joined to the first.

**pyrrolidine** (pĭr-rol'ĭ-dēn). Tetrahydropyrrole; pyrrole to which four H atoms have been added. Basis of proline and hydroxyproline.

**pyrrolidone** (pĭr-rol'ĭ-dōn). 2-Ketopyrrolidine; 2-oxopyrrolidine.

**pyrroline** (pĭr'o-lēn). 2,5-Dihydropyrrole; pyrrole to which four H atoms have been added.

**pyrroline-2-carboxylate reductase.** Proline dehydrogenase; oxidoreductase (EC 1.5.1.1) reducing 1-pyrroline to L-proline with NAD(P)N₂.

**pyrroline-5-carboxylate reductase.** Proline dehydrogenase; oxidoreductase (EC 1.5.1.2) reducing 1-pyrroline to L-proline with NAD(P)H₂.

**pyr'rolni'trin** (USAN). 3-Chloro-4-(3-chloro-2-nitrophenyl)pyrrole; an antifungal agent.

**pyruval'dehyde.** Methylglyoxal.

**pyruvate** (pi-ru'vāt). A salt or ester of pyruvic acid.

**p. carboxylase** (EC 6.4.1.1), ligase catalyzing reaction of ATP, pyruvate, and CO₂, to form ADP, inorganic phosphate, and oxaloacetate. Biotin and acetyl-CoA are involved.

**p. decarboxylase** (EC 4.1.1.1), α-carboxylase (see carboxylase); a carboxy-lyase of yeast catalyzing decarboxylation of a 2-oxoacid (*e.g.,* pyruvate) to an aldehyde (*e.g.,* acetaldehyde) without oxidoreduction and without lipoate, in contrast to pyruvate dehydrogenase.

**p. dehydrogenase (cytochrome)** (EC 1.2.2.2), an oxidoreductase catalyzing reaction between ferricytochrome *b* and pyruvate to yield acetate and CO₂.

**p. dehydrogenase (lipoate)** (EC 1.2.4.1), an oxidoreductase catalyzing conversion of pyruvate and oxidized lipoate to CO₂ and S-acetyldihydrolipoate in two successive

reactions, the first between pyruvate and thiamin pyrophosphate to yield CO₂ and α-hydroxyethyl-thiamin pyrophosphate, the second between the last named and lipoamide to regain the thiamin pyrophosphate and yield acetylhydrolipoamide (6-S-acetylhydrolipoamide). The last named is the substrate for lipoate acetyltransferase, *q. v.*

**p. kinase** (EC 2.7.1.40), phosphoenolpyruvate kinase; phosphotransferase catalyzing transfer of phosphate from phosphoenolpyruvate to ADP, forming ATP and pyruvate. Other nucleoside phosphates can participate in the reaction.

**p. oxidase** (EC 1.2.3.3), oxidoreductase catalyzing the reaction of pyruvate, phosphate, and O₂ to yield acetylphosphate, CO₂, and H₂O₂. P. is a flavoprotein and requires thiamin phosphate.

**pyruvic acid** (pi-ru'vik). 2-Oxopropanoic acid; α-ketopropionic acid; CH₃—CO—COOH. An intermediate compound in the metabolism of carbohydrate; in thiamin deficiency, its oxidation is retarded and it accumulates in the tissues, especially in nervous structures. The enol form, enolpyruvic acid, CH₂=C(OH)—COOH, also plays a metabolic role (see phosphoenolpyruvic acid).

**pyruvic aldehyde.** Methylglyoxal.

**pyruvic-malic carboxylase.** Malate dehydrogenase.

**pyrvinium pamoate** (pĭr-vin'ĭ-um). (USP). POVAN; viprynium emboate (BP); 6-(dimethylamino)-2-[ 2-(2,5-dimethyl-1-phenylpyrrol-3-yl) -vinyl ]-1-methylquinolinium 4,4'- methylenebis [ 3-hydroxy-2-naphthoate ] (2:1); a highly effective drug used in the eradication (one to two doses) of human pinworms.

**Pythag'oras** of Samos, Greek philosopher, 580–489 B.C. Propounded the doctrine of the mystic power of numbers, a doctrine which probably influenced the Hippocratic teaching of crises and critical days in disease. He was the first to investigate the mathematical physics of sound and to state that the brain and not the heart was the seat of the emotions and the intellect.

**pythogenesis** (pi'tho-jen'ĕ-sis) [ G. *pythō,* to decay, + *genesis,* origin. PYTH- ]. 1. Origination from decaying matter. 2. The causation of decay.

**pythogen'ic.** Pythogenous; originating from filth or putrescence.

**pythogenous** (pi-thoj'ĕ-nus). Pythogenic.

**pyuria** (pi-u'rĭ-ah) [ G. *pyon,* pus, + *ouron,* urine ]. The presence of pus in the urine when voided.

# Q

**Q.** Symbol for (1) quantity; (2) coulomb.

**Q̇** [ quantity + an overdot denoting the time derivative ]. Symbol for blood *flow*.

**Q**$CO_2$. Symbol for the microliters of $CO_2$ given off per milligram of tissue per hour.

**Q**o or **Q**o$_2$. Symbols for oxygen *consumption* (1).

**Q**$_6$, **Q**$_{10}$. Q-6, Q-10; abbreviations for ubiquinone-6 and -10, or ubiquinone-Q$_6$ and -Q$_{10}$, respectively.

**Q**$_{10}$. Symbol for the increase in rate of a process produced by raising the temperature 10°C.

**q.d.** Abbreviation for L. *quaque die*, every day.

**q.h.** Abbreviation of L. *quaque hora*, every hour; q.2 h., *quaque secunda hora*, every second hour; q.3 h., *quaque tertia hora*, every third hour.

**q.i.d.** Abbreviation for L. *quater in die*, four times a day.

**q.l.** Abbreviation of L. *quantum libet*, as much as is desired.

**q.s.** Abbreviation of *quantum sufficit*, as much as is needed; or *quantum sufficiat*, as much as may be needed.

**quack** (kwak). Charlatan.

**quackery** (kwak'er-ĭ). Charlatanism.

**quader** (kwa'der) [ Ger. square ]. The precuneus.

**quadrangular** (kwah-drang'u-lar) [ L. *quadrangularis*, fr. *quadrangulum*, quadrangle ]. Having four angles.

**quadrang'ulum** [ L. ] [ NA ]. Quadrangle; a structure having four angles.

**quadrant** (kwah'drant) [ L. *quadrans*, a quarter ]. One quarter of a circle. In anatomy, roughly circular areas are divided for descriptive purposes into q.'s. The abdomen is divided into right upper and lower, and left upper and lower q.'s by a horizontal and a vertical line intersecting at the umbilicus. Q.'s of the fundus oculi (superior and inferior nasal, superior and inferior temporal) are demarcated by a horizontal and a vertical line intersecting at the optic disk. The tympanic membrane is divided into anterosuperior, anteroinferior, posterosuperior, and posteroinferior q.'s by a line drawn across the diameter of the drum in the axis of the handle of the malleus and another intersecting the first at right angles at the umbo.

    **Wilder's q.,** a small area on the ventral surface of the cerebral peduncle in the cat.

**quadrantanopsia** (kwah'drant-an-op'sĭ-ah) [ quadrant + anopsia ]. Quadrantic *hemianopsia*.

**quadrate** (kwah'drāt) [ L. *quadratus*, square. QUAD- ]. Having four equal sides; square.

**quadratus** (kwah-dra'tus) [ L. *square* ] [ NA ]. Denoting a structure that is more or less square in shape; see under musculus.

**quadri-** (kwah'drĭ-) [ L. *quattuor*, four. QUAD- ]. Combining form meaning four.

**quadribasic** (kwah'drĭ-ba'sik). Denoting an acid having four hydrogen atoms that are replaceable by atoms or radicals of a basic character.

**quadriceps** (kwah'drĭ-seps) [ L. fr. quadri- + *caput*, head ] [ NA ]. Having four heads, denoting a muscle of the thigh, musculus q. femoris, and one of the calf, musculus q. surae or the combined gastrocnemius (with two heads), soleus, and plantaris, more commonly called musculus triceps surae, the plantaris being counted as a separate muscle.

**quadricepsplasty** (kwah'drĭ-seps-plas'tĭ). A corrective surgical procedure on the quadriceps femoris.

**quadricuspid** (kwah'drĭ-kus'pid). Tetracuspid.

**quadridigitate** (kwah'drĭ-dij'ĭ-tāt) [ quadri- + L. *digitus*, digit ]. Tetradactyl.

**quadrifi'dins.** A group of unstable antibiotics obtained from cultures of *Coprinus quadrifidus.*

**quadrigeminal** (kwah'drĭ-jem'ĭ-nal) [ quadri- + L. *geminus*, twin ]. Four-fold.

**quadrigeminum** (kwah'drĭ-jem'ĭ-num). One of the corpora quadrigemina.

**quadrigem'inus** [ L. ]. Quadruplet.

**quadrigeminy** (kwah'drĭ-jem'ĭ-nĭ). Quadrigeminal *rhythm.*

**quadripara** (kwah-drip'ă-rah) [ quadri- + L. *pario*, to bear ]. Para IV; a woman who has given birth four times to an infant or infants, alive or dead, weighing 500 gm. or more or having a length of gestation of at least 20 weeks.

**quad'ripar'ity.** The state of being a quadripara.

**quadriparous** (kwah-drip'ă-rus). Denoting a quadripara.

**quadriplegia** (kwah'drĭ-ple'jĭ-ah) [ quadri- + G. *plēgē*, stroke ]. Tetraplegia; paralysis of all four limbs.

**quadriplegic** (kwah'drĭ-ple'jik). 1. A person with paralysis of all four limbs. 2. Pertaining to quadriplegia.

**quadripolar** (kwah'drĭ-po'lar). Having four poles.

**quadrisect** (kwah'drĭ-sekt) [ quadri- + L. *seco*, pp. *sectus*, to cut ]. To divide into four parts.

**quadrisection** (kwah'drĭ-sek'shun). Division into four parts.

**quadritubercular** (kwah'drĭ-tu-ber'ku-lar) [ quadri- + L. *tuberculum*, tubercle ]. Having four tubercles or cusps, as a molar tooth.

**quadriurate** (kwah'drĭ-u'rāt). (Obsolete); the urate forming the solid urine of birds and reptiles; the acid urate of human urine. A mixture of urate and uric acid, *i.e.*, partially neutralized uric acid, once thought to be a single compound.

**quadrivalent** (kwah'drĭ-va'lent, kwah-driv'ă-lent) [ quadri- + L. *valeo*, pres. p. *valens*, to have power ]. Having the combining power of four atoms of hydrogen.

**quadruped** (kwah'dru-ped) [ L. *quattuor*, four (QUAD-), + *pes* (*ped-*), foot ]. A four-footed animal.

**quadruplet** (kwah'drup-let, kwah-dru'plet) [ L. *quadruplus*, fourfold (see PLIC-) ]. Quadrigeminus; one of four children born at one birth.

**qualimeter** (kwah-lim'e-ter) [ L. *qualis*, of what kind, + G. *metron*, measure ]. A device for estimating the degree of hardness of x-rays.

**Quant's sign.** See under sign.

**quanta** (kwahn'tah) [ L. ]. Plural of quantum.

**quantimeter** (kwahn-tim'e-ter) [ L. *quantus*, how much, + G. *metron*, measure ]. A device for determining the quantity of x-rays generated by a Crookes or Coolidge tube.

**quantivalence** (kwahn-tiv'ă-lens) [ L. *quantus*, how much, + *valeo*, to have power ]. Valence.

**quantum,** pl. **quanta** (kwahn'tum, -tah) [ L. how much ]. 1. A unit of radiant energy ($\epsilon$) varying according to the frequency ($\nu$) of the radiation. 2. A certain definite amount.

    **q. li'bet,** as much as is desired; abbreviated q.l.

    **q. suf'ficit, q. suffic'iat,** as much as suffices, as much as may be needed; abbreviated in prescription writing to q.s. or quant. suff.

**quarantine** (kwahr'an-tēn) [ It. *quarantina* fr. L. *quadraginta*, forty. QUAD- ]. 1. A period (originally 40 days) of detention of vessels and their passengers coming from an area where an infectious disease prevails. 2. To detain such vessels and their passengers until the incubation period of the disease has passed. 3. A place where such vessels and their passengers are detained. 4. The isolation of a person with a contagious disease.

**quart** (kwort) [ L. *quartus*, fourth ]. 1. A measure of fluid capacity; the fourth part of a gallon; the equivalent of 0.9468 liter. 2. A dry measure holding a little more than the fluid measure.

    **imperial q.,** a liquid measure containing about 20 per cent more than the ordinary q., or 1.1359 liters.

**quartan** (kwor'tan) [ L. *quartanus*, relating to a fourth (thing) ]. Recurring every fourth day.

    **double q.,** infection with two independent groups of q. parasites, so that paroxysms occur on two successive days followed by one day without fever.

    **triple q.,** infection with three independent groups of q. parasites, so that a paroxysm occurs every day, resembling a double tertian or a quotidian fever.

**quarter** (kwor'ter) [ L. *quartus*, fourth ]. The lateral part of the wall of the hoof in the horse.

    **black q.,** blackleg.

**quar'ter-crack.** See sand-crack.

**quartipara** (kwor-tip'ă-rah) [ L. *quartus*, fourth, + *pario*, to bear ]. Quadripara.

**quartisect** (kwor'tĭ-sekt) [ L. *quartus*, fourth, + *seco*, pp. *sectus*, to cut ]. Quadrisect.

**quartz** (kworts). A form of silica used in dental casting investment.

**quassation** (kwah-sa'shun) [ L. *quassatio*, fr. *quasso*, pp. *-atus*, to shake violently, fr. *quatio*, to shake ]. The breaking up of crude drug materials, such as bark and woody stems, into small pieces to facilitate extraction and other treatment.

**quassia** (kwah'she-ah) [ named after *Quassi*, a resident of Surinam who used it as a tonic ]. *Quassiae lignum;* bitterwood; the heartwood of *Picrasma excelsa* (*Picraena excelsa*), or of *Quassia amara* (family Simarubaceae). It is marketed as Jamaica q. and Surinam q. It is a bitter tonic; the infusion has been administered by enema in the treatment of threadworms.

**quassin** (kwah'sin). The bitter principle of Surinam quassia, an amaroid. It is a molecular complex containing isoquassin and neoquassin.

**qua'ter in di'e** [ L. ]. Four times daily; abbreviated q.i.d.

**quaternary** (kwah'ter-nĕr'ĭ, kwah-ter'nē-rĭ) [ L. *quaternarius*, containing four, fr. *quattuor*, four ]. 1. Denoting a chemical compound containing four elements (*e.g.*, NaHSO₄). 2. Fourth in a series. 3. Relating to organic compounds in which some central atom is attached to four functional groups. Thus applied to the usually trivalent nitrogen in its "onium," q. state, $R_4N^+$, *e.g.*, "quaternary nitrogen."

**Quatrefages** (kă-tr-fazh'), J. L. A. de, French naturalist, 1810–1892. See Q.'s *angle*.

**quazodine** (kwa'zo-dēn) (USAN). 4-Ethyl-6,7-dimethoxyquinazoline; a cardiotonic drug with bronchodilating activity.

**quebrachamine** (ke-brah'chah-mēn). An alkaloid of quebracho, resembling quebrachine; obtained from the bark of *Aspidosperma quebracho blanco*.

**quebrachine** (ke-brah'chēn). An alkaloid, $C_{21}H_{26}N_2O_3$, from quebracho; identical with yohimbine. Formerly used in cardiac dyspnea.

**quebracho** (ke-brah'cho) [ Port. *quebrahacho*, fr. *quebrar*, to break, + *hacha*, axe, referring to the hardness of the wood ]. See *Aspidosperma*.

**red q.,** q. colorado; schinopsis; dried heartwood of *Schinopsis lorentzii* and *S. balansae (family Anacardiaceae).*

**white q.,** q. blanco; the dried bark has been used as respiratory stimulant in emphysema, dyspnea, and chronic bronchitis. The two chief alkaloids are aspidospermine and quebrachine.

**Queckenstedt** (kvek'en-stet), Hans, German physician, 1887–1918. See Q.-Stookey *test*.

**queen** (kwēn). A female cat of breeding age.

**quenching** (kwench'ing). 1. The process of extinguishing, removing, or diminishing a physical property such as heat or light; *e.g.*, the cooling of a hot metal rapidly by plunging it into water or oil. 2. In beta liquid scintillation counting, the shifting of the energy spectrum from a true to a lower energy; it is caused by a variety of interfering materials in the counting solution, including foreign chemicals and coloring agent.

**fluorescence q.,** a technique used in investigations dealing with binding of antigens (haptens) by purified antibodies, applicable in cases in which the bound antigen (hapten) absorbs (quenches) light emitted during fluorescence of protein (antibody) excited by ultraviolet light.

**Quénu** (ka-nü'), Eduard A. V. A., French surgeon and anatomist, 1852–1933. See Q.'s hemorrhoidal *plexus*, Q.-Muret *sign*, Q.'s *thoracoplasty*.

**quercetin** (kwer'se-tin). 3,3',4',5,7-Pentahydroxyflavone; an aglucon of quercitrin, rutin, and other glycosides; occurs usually as the 3-rhamnoside, quercitrin, as in rutin. Used in the treatment of abnormal capillary fragility.

**quercin** (kwer'sin). A crystalline *muco*-inositol contained in acorns and oak bark.

**quercit** (kwer'sit). *d*-Quercitol.

**d-quercitol** (kwer'si-tol). Quercit; 1,2,3,4,5-cyclohexanepentol; D-1-deoxy-*muco*-inositol; a crystalline substance obtained from acorns.

**quercitrin** (kwer-sit'rin). The 3-rhamnoside derivative of quercetin; present in oak bark, tea leaves, hops, and other plants.

**quercus** (kwer'kus) [ L. oak ]. 1. An important genus of hardwood trees and shrubs of the family Fagaceae. 2. The bark of *Quercus alba*, white oak, stone oak; was used as an astringent.

**querulent** (kwĕr'u-lent) [ L. *querulus*, complaining, fr. *queror*, to complain ]. Denoting one who is ever suspicious, always opposing any suggestion, complaining of ill treatment and of being slighted or misunderstood, easily enraged, and dissatisfied; the condition is characteristic of paranoid personalities.

**Quervain,** Fritz de. See de Quervain.

**Queyrat** (ki-rah'), Auguste, French dermatologist, *1872. See *erythroplasia* of Q.

**Quick,** Armand J., American physician, *1894. See Q.'s *method*, *test*.

**quick** (kwik) [ A.S. *cwic*, living ]. 1. Pregnant with a child the movement of which is felt. 2. A sensitive part, painful to touch. 3. Eponychium.

**quick'ening** [ A.S. *cwic*, living ]. The signs of life felt by the mother as a result of the fetal movements, usually noted first in the fourth or fifth month of pregnancy.

**quick'lime.** Unslaked lime; see lime (2).

**quick'silver.** Mercury.

**quiescent** (kwĭ-es'ent). At rest or inactive.

**quillaja** (kwil-lah'yah) [ Chilian ] (BP). Soap bark; Panama bark; the inner bark of *Quillaja saponaria* (family Rosaceae), a large tree of Chile; an irritant and detergent, has no pharmaceutical uses.

**quin-, quino-.** Root of quinoline and quinone, hence used in many names of substances containing these structures (*e.g.*, quinine, quinol).

**quina** (ke'nah, kwe'nah) [ Sp. fr. Peruv. *quina* or *kina*, cinchona ]. Cinchona bark.

**quinacrine hydrochloride** (kwin'ă-krēn, -krin) (USP). ATABRINE; ATEBRIN; ACRIQUINE; mepacrine hydrochloride; an acridine derivative, $C_{23}H_{30}ClN_3O \cdot 2HCl \cdot 2H_2O$; an antimalarial that destroys the trophozoites of *Plasmodium vivax* and *P. falciparum*, but does not affect the gametocytes, sporozoites, or exoerythrocytic stage of parasites; also used as an anthelmintic (cestode infections).

**quinalbarbitone sodium** (kwin'al-bar'bĭ-tōn) (BP). Secobarbital sodium.

**quinaldic acid** (kwin-al'dik). Quinaldinic acid; quinoline-2-carboxylic acid; a product of tryptophan catabolism, via kynurenic acid, found in human urine.

**quinal'dine.** 2-Methylquinoline.

**quinamine** (kwin'ă-mēn, kwĭ-nam'ēn). An alkaloid, $C_{19}H_{24}N_2O_2$, obtained from cinchona bark.

**quinapyramine** (kwin'ă-pīr'ă-mēn). ANTRYCIDE; 4-amino-6-[ (2-amino-6-methyl-4-pyrimidinyl)amino ]-1-methylquinaldinium methosalts; a trypanocidal agent that gives effective prophylaxis for two to three months.

**quinaquina** (ke'nah-ke'nah, kwin'ah-kwin'ah) [ a reduplication of Sp. *quina*, cinchona ]. Cinchona bark.

**quinate** (kwi'nāt, kwin'āt). A salt or ester of quinic acid.

**q. dehydrogenase** (EC 1.1.1.24), oxidoreductase catalyzing reaction of quinate and NAD to form 5-dehydroquinate.

**quin'bolone** (USAN). ANABOLICUM VISTER; 17β-(1-cyclopenten-1-yloxy)androsta-1,4-dien-3-one; anabolic agent.

**quince** (kwints). The edible fruit of *Cydonia oblongata* (family Rosaceae); the seeds have demulcent properties.

**Quincke** (kvin'keh), Heinrich I., German physician, 1842–1922. See Q.'s *disease*, *edema*, Q.'s *pulse*, Q.'s *puncture*, *sign*.

**quin'estradi'ol.** PENTOVIS; 3-(cyclopentyloxy)estra-1,3,5(10)-triene-16α,17β-diol; an estrogen.

**quineth'azone.** HYDROMAX; 7-chloro-2-ethyl-1,2,3,4-tetrahydro-4-oxo-6-quinazolinesulfonamide; an orally effective diuretic and antihypertensive agent.

**quinetolate** (kwĭ-net'o-lāt) (USAN). VENTAIRE; 6-(diethyl-carbamoyl)-3-cyclohexene-1-carbolic acid compound with 4-[ (2-dimethylaminoethyl)amino ]-6-methoxyquinoline; antiasthmatic agent.

**quinges'tanol acetate** (USAN). 3-(Cyclopentyloxy)-19-nor-17α-pregna-3,5-dien-20-yn-17-ol acetate; a progestational agent.

**quingestrone** (kwin-jes'trōn) (USAN). ENOL LUTEOVIS; progesterone cyclopentyl-3-enol ether; progestogen.

**quinhydrone** (kwin-hi'drōn). A mixture of equimolecular quantities of quinone and hydroquinone; used in pH determinations.

**quinic acid** (kwin'ik). Chinic acid; kinic acid; 1,3,4,5-tetrahydroxycyclohexanecarboxylic acid; hexahydro-1,3,4,5-tetrahydroxybenzoic acid; found in cinchona bark and elsewhere in plants. 5-Dehydroquinic acid is an intermediate in the biosynthesis of phenylalanine, tyrosine, and tryptophan from carbohydrate precursors (see quinate).

**quinicine** (kwin'ĭ-sēn). Quinotoxine; an amorphous alkaloid isomeric with quinine and quinidine.

**quinidine** (kwin'ĭ-dēn, -din). Conquinine; β-quinine; one of the alkaloids of cinchona, a stereoisomer of quinine; used as an antimalarial; also used in the treatment of atrial fibrillation and flutter, and paroxysmal ventricular tachycardia.

**quinine** (kwi'nīn, -nēn, kwin'-īn, -ēn). Quinina; Jesuit's bark; Cardinal's bark; the most important of the alkaloids derived from cinchona (family Rubiaceae); $C_{20}H_{24}N_2O_3 3H_2O$. An antimalarial effective against the asexual and erythrocytic forms; it has no effect on the exoerythrocytic (tissue) forms of the parasite; it does not produce a radical cure of malaria produced by *Plasmodium vivax*, *P. malariae*, or *P. ovale*. It is used in the treatment of cerebral malaria and other severe attacks of malignant tertian malaria, and in malaria produced by chloroquine-resistant strains of *P. falciparum*. Q. is also used as an antipyretic, analgesic, sclerosing agent, stomachic, and oxytocic (occasionally), and in the treatment of atrial fibrillation, myotonia congenita, and other myopathies.

  **q. and urea hydrochloride,** contains not less than 58 per cent and not more than 65 per cent of anhydrous q.; sclerosing agent for treatment of internal hemorrhoids, hydrocele, and varicose veins.

  **q. bisulfate** q. bisulphate (BP); the acid sulfate of q.; acicular crystals or white crystalline powder of bitter taste; very soluble in water.

  **q. carbacryclic resin,** see under resin.

  **q. dihydrochloride** (NF, BP), white, bitter powder, soluble in water or alcohol.

  **q. ethylcarbonate,** EUQUININE; euchinine; an almost tasteless form of q.; it is poorly absorbed from the intestinal tract.

  **q. phosphate,** white crystals or white crystalline powder of bitter taste.

  **q. sulfate** (USP), q. sulphate (BP); white, lustrous, silky, needle-shaped crystals of bitter taste; the most frequently prescribed salt of q.

  **q. urethan,** a mixture of urethan and q. hydrochloride; sclerosing agent for treatment of varicose veins.

**quininism** (kwi'nī-nizm, kwin'ī-). Cinchonism.

**Quinlan's test.** See under test.

**quinocide hydrochloride** (kwin'o-sīd). CHINOCIDE; 8-(4-aminopentylamino)-6-methoxyquinoline hydrochloride; an antimalarial comparable to primaquine in effectiveness and scope.

**quinol.** Hydroquinone.

Quinoline

**quinoline** (kwin'o-lēn, -lin). Chinoleine; leucoline; a volatile nitrogenous base obtained by the distillation of coal tar, bones, alkaloids, etc. Has been used in malaria.

**quinolinic acid** (kwin'o-lin'ik). Pyridine-2,3-dicarboxylic acid; a catabolite of tryptophan and a precursor of nicotinic acid.

**quinology** (kwin-ol'o-jī) [ Sp. *quina*, cinchona, + G. *logos*, study ]. The botany, chemistry, pharmacology, and therapeutics of cinchona and its alkaloids.

**quinone** (kwin'ōn, kwi'nōn). 1. An aromatic nucleus bearing two oxygens in place of two hydrogens, usually in the *para* position; the oxidation product of a hydroquinone. See also 1,4-benzoquinone and 1,4-naphthoquinone, which occur in vitamins E and K and in coenzyme Q. 2. Also used as a synonym for 1,4-benzoquinone.

**quinone reductase.** NAD(P)H dehydrogenase (quinone).

**quinotoxine** (kwin-o-tok'sin). Quinicine.

**quinovin** (kwin'o-vin). A glycoside obtained from cinchona bark, devoid of antipyretic and antimalarial properties.

**quinovose** (kwin'o-vōs). 6-Deoxy-D-glucose.

**Quinquaud** (kaṅ-ko'), Charles E., French physician, 1841–1894. See Q.'s *disease*.

**quinquedigitate** (kwin'kwe-dij'ī-tāt) [ L. *quinque*, five, + *digitus*, digit ]. Pentadactyl.

**quinquetubercular** (kwin-kwe-tu-ber'ku-lar) [ L. *quinque*, five, + *tuberculum*, tubercle, dim. of *tuber*, a swelling ]. Having five tubercles or cusps, as certain molar teeth.

**quinquevalent** (kwin'kwe-va'lent, kwin-kwev'ă-lent) [ L. *quinque*, five, + *valeo*, to have power ]. Pentavalent.

**quinquina** (kwin-kwi'nah). Cinchona bark.

**quinquivalent** (kwin-kwiv'ă-lent). Pentavalent.

**quinsy** (kwin'zī) [ M.E. *quinsie* (*quinesie*), a corruption of L. *cynanche*, sore throat. CYN- ]. Peritonsillar *abscess*.

  **lingual q.,** phlegmonous inflammation of the lingual tonsil and neighboring structures.

**quintan** (kwin'tan) [ L. *quintus*, fifth ]. Recurring every fifth day; *i.e.*, after a free interval of three days.

**quinter'enol sulfate** (USAN). 8-Hydroxy-α-[ (isopropylamino)methyl ]-5-quinolinemethanol sulfate; a bronchodilator drug.

**quintipara** (kwin-tip'ă-rah) [ L. *quintus*, fifth, + *pario*, to bear ]. Para V; a woman who has given birth five times to an infant or infants, alive or dead, weighing 500 gm. or more or having a length of gestation of at least 20 weeks.

**quintiparity** (kwin'tī-păr'ī-tī). The state of being a quintipara.

**quintiparous** (kwin-tip'ă-rus). Relating to quintiparity or to a quintipara.

**quintuplet** (kwin'tu-plet, kwin-tu'plet) [ L. *quintuplex*, fivefold (see PLIC-) ]. One of five children born at one birth.

**quinuronium sulfate** (kwin'u-ro'nĭ-um). ACAPRIN; 1,3-di-6-quinolylurea; an effective drug for treating *Babesia* infections in animals.

**quittor** (kwit'or) [ ME. *quetaur*, a boiling ]. A fistulous tract leading from the coronet to the lateral cartilage of the horse. It is due to an injury, followed by bacterial infection, followed by massive necrosis of cartilage and other tissues. The necrotic process may involve the joint capsule.

**quotidian** (kwo-tid'ī-an) [ L. *quotidianus*, daily, fr. *quot*, as many as, + *dies*, day ]. Amphemerous; daily; occurring every day.

**quotient** (kwo'shent) [ L. *quoties*, how often ]. The number of times one amount is contained in another. See also ratio, and index.

  **achievement q.,** a percentile rating of the amount a child has learned in relation to his age, level of education, or peers.

  **Ayala's quotient,** Ayala's *index*.

  **blood q.,** see color *index*.

  **caloric q.,** the heat evolved (in calories) divided by the oxygen consumed (in milligrams).

  **D:N q.,** the ratio of glucose to nitrogen in the urine.

  **growth q.,** the fractional part or percentage of the entire food energy which is utilized for growth in the young animal.

  **intelligence q.,** abbreviated IQ; the psychologist's index of measured intelligence as one part of a two-part determination of intelligence; the other part, an index of adaptive behavior, includes such criteria as school grades or work performance. Intelligence q. is a score or similar quantitative index, used by psychologists and educators to denote a person's standing relative to his age peers on a test of general ability, ordinarily expressed as a ratio between the person's score on a given test and the score which the average individual his age attained on the same test; the ratio being computed by the psychologist or determined from a table of age norms, such as the various Wechsler intelligence scales.

**protein q.,** a figure obtained by dividing the amount of the globulin by that of the albumin in a specimen of blood plasma.

**respiratory q.,** abbreviated R.Q.; the steady state ratio of carbon dioxide produced by tissue metabolism to oxygen consumed in the same metabolism; for the whole body, normally about 0.82 under basal conditions; in the steady state, the respiratory q. is equal to the respiratory exchange *ratio, q.v.*

**spinal q.,** Ayala's *index.*

**q.v.** 1. Abbreviation of L. *quantum vis,* as much as you wish. 2. Abbreviation of L. *quod vide,* which see.

# R

**R.** Abbreviation or symbol for gas *constant*, ohm, radical (usually an alkyl or aryl group, *e.g.*, ROH is an alcohol, RNH₂ an amine), Re'amur, L. *recipe*, respiration, respiratory exchange *ratio*, the remainder of a chemical formula, and the unit of resistance in the cardiovascular system.

**Rf.** Symbol denoting movement of a substance in paper chromatography relative to the solvent *front*.

**r.** 1. Abbreviation for "racemic," occasionally used in naming compounds in place of the more common "*dl*," as "r-alanine" (also rac.). 2. Abbreviation for roentgen.

**Ra.** Chemical symbol of the element radium.

**rab'beting** [ Fr. *raboter*, to plane ]. Making congruous stepwise cuts on apposing bone surfaces for stability after impaction.

**rab'ic.** Rabid.

**rab'id** [ L. *rabidus*, raving, mad ]. Relating to or suffering from rabies.

**rabies** (ra'bēz) [ L. rage, fury, fr. *rabio*, to rave, to be mad. RAB- ]. Hydrophobia; lyssa (Fr.); tollwut (Ger.); a highly fatal infectious disease that may affect all species of warm-blooded animals, including man. It is transmitted almost exclusively by the bite of carnivorous animals (dogs, cats, wolves, foxes, bats, skunks, etc.). It is caused by a neurotropic virus that occurs in the central nervous system and the salivary glands. The symptoms are those of a profound disturbance of the nervous system—excitement, aggressiveness, and madness, followed by paralysis and death. Characteristic cytoplasmic inclusion bodies (Negri bodies) found in many of the neurons are an aid to rapid laboratory diagnosis.

**dumb r.,** paralytic r.

**fixed virus r.,** r. caused by fixed r. virus (*q. v.*).

**furious r.,** spasmodic r.; the form or stage of r. in which the animal is wildly excited, running aimlessly about and snapping at objects, whether living or not, in its way.

**paralytic r.,** a form or stage marked by an ascending paralysis; also called dumb r.; sullen r.; drop jaw (named from characteristic symptom); dumb madness.

**spasmodic r.,** furious r.

**street virus r.,** r. in a domestic animal that has contracted the disease in the usual way, from the bite or scratch of another animal.

**sullen r.,** paralytic r.

**ra'biform.** Resembling rabies.

**race.** A class of animals or individuals having common somatic inherited characteristics.

**racefemine fumarate.** DYSMALGINE; *dl*-threo-α-methyl-*N*-(1-methyl-2-phenoxyethyl)phenethylamine fumarate; used as uterine relaxant for relief of postpartum pain.

**racemase** (ra'se-mās). An enzyme capable of catalyzing racemization, *i.e.*, inversions of asymmetric groups. When more than one center of asymmetry is present, "epimerase" is used (*e.g.*, hydroxyproline, ribulosephosphate). EC Class 5.1 includes racemases interconverting the D and L forms of alanine, lysine, and other amino acids (EC 5.1.1), of lactate and mandelate (EC 5.1.2.1 and 2).

**ra'cemate** (ra'se-māt). A racemic compound; also, the salt or ester of such a compound. See also racemic.

**raceme** (ra-sēm'). An optically inactive chemical compound. See also racemic.

**racemic** (ra-se'mik, -sem'ik). Denoting a mixture that is optically inactive, being composed of an equal number of dextro- and levorotatory substances, which are separable. Those compounds internally compensated, and therefore not separable into D and L forms, are termed "meso," not racemic.

**racemic acid.** DL (or *dl* or (+) )-tartaric acid.

**racemization** (ra'se-mī-za'shun, ras-). The partial conversion of one enantiomorph into another (as an L-amino acid to the corresponding D-amino acid) so that the specific optical rotation is decreased, or even reduced to zero, in the resulting racemate.

**racemose** (ras'e-mōs) [ L. *racemosus*, full of clusters ]. Branching, with nodular terminations, resembling a bunch of grapes.

**racephedrine hydrochloride** (rās'e-fed'rin, ras-). *dl*-Ephedrine hydrochloride; a sympathomimetic drug with peripheral effects similar to those of epinephrine, and with the same actions and uses as ephedrine.

**rachi-, rachio-** (ra'ki-, ra'kī-o-) [ G. *rhachis*, spine, backbone. RHACH- ]. Combining form meaning spine.

**rachial** (ra'kī-al). Spinal.

**rachialbuminimeter** (ra'kī-al-bu'min-im'e-ter) [ rachi- + albumin + G. *metron*, measure ]. A graduated test tube used to determine the amount of albumin or globulin (precipitated by means of heat and acid) in a specimen of cerebrospinal fluid.

**rachialbuminimetry** (ra'kī-al-bu'min-im'e-trĭ). Determination of the albumin (globulin) content of the spinal fluid.

**rachialgia** (ra-kī-al'jī-ah) [ rachi- + G. *algos*, pain ]. Rachiodynia; spondylalgia; spondylodynia; spinalgia; pain in the spine.

**rachicentesis** (ra-kī-sen-te'sis) [ rachi- + G. *kentēsis*, puncture ]. Lumbar *puncture*.

**rachidial** (rā-kid'ī-al). Spinal.

**rachidian** (rā-kid'ī-an). Spinal.

**rachigraph** (ra'kī-graf) [ rachi- + G. *graphō*, to write ]. A graph for recording the curves of the vertebrae.

**rachilysis** (rā-kil'ī-sis) [ rachi- + G. *lysis*, a loosening ]. Forcible correction of lateral curvature by lateral pressure against the convexity of the curve.

**rachio-.** See rachi-.

**rachiocampsis** (ra-kī-o-kamp'sis) [ rachio- + G. *kampsis*, a bending ]. Spinal *curvature*.

**rachiocentesis** (ra-kī-o-sen-te'sis) [ rachio- + G. *kentēsis*, puncture ]. Lumbar *puncture*.

**rachiochysis** (ra-kī-ok'ī-sis) [ rachio- + G. *chysis*, a pouring out. CHY- ]. A subarachnoid effusion of fluid in the spinal canal.

**rachiodynia** (ra'kī-o-din'ī-ah) [ rachio- + G. *odynē*, pain ]. Rachialgia.

**rachiometer** (ra-kī-om'e-ter) [ rachio- + G. *metron*, measure ]. An instrument for measuring the curvature, natural or pathologic, of the spinal column.

**rachiomyelitis** (ra-kī-o-mi-ĕ-li'tis). Myelitis.

**rachiopagus** (ra'kī-op'ā-gus) [ rachio- + G. *pagos*, something fixed ]. Rachipagus; conjoined twins united back to back in such a manner that the fusion involves the spinal column.

**rachiopathy** (ra-kī-op'ā-thĭ) [ rachio- + G. *pathos*, suffering ]. Spondylopathy; any disease of the spinal column.

**rachioplegia** (ra-kī-o-ple'jī-ah) [ rachio- + G. *plēgē*, stroke ]. Spinal *paralysis*.

**rachioscoliosis** (ra-kī-o-sko-lī-o'sis). Scoliosis.

**rachiotome** (ra'kī-o-tōm) [ rachio- + G. *tomē*, incision ]. Rachitome; a specially devised instrument for dividing the laminae of the vertebrae.

**rachiotomy** (ra-kī-ot'o-mĭ) [ rachio- + G. *tomē*, incision ]. Laminectomy. 2. Spondylotomy (1).

**rachipagus** (rā-kip'ā-gus). Rachiopagus.

**rachiresistance** (ra'kī-re-zis'tans). Failure of spinal anesthesia, ascribed to resistance of spinal nerves to the effects of the local anesthetics.

**rachis,** pl. **rachides, rachises** (ra'kis, ra'kī-dēz, rak-) [ G. spine, backbone. RHACH- ]. *Columna* vertebralis.

**rachischisis** (rā-kis'kī-sis) [ G. *rhachis*, spine, + *schisis*, division ]. Spondyloschisis.

**r. partia'lis,** merorachischisis.

**posterior r., r. posterior,** spondyloschisis of the entire vertebral column.

**r. tota'lis,** holorachischisis.

**rachitic** (rākit'ic). Relating to, or suffering from, rachitis.

**rachitis** (rā-ki'tis) [ G. *rhachitis*. RHACH- ]. Rickets.

**r. feta'lis annula'ris,** a congenital enlargement of the epiphyses of the long bones.

**r. feta'lis micromel'ica,** a congenital condition in which the long bones are deficiently developed.

**r. intrauteri'na, r. uteri'na,** r. fetalis.

**r. tarda,** adult *rickets.*

**rachitism** (rak'ĭ-tizm). A rachitic state or tendency.

**rachitogenic** (ră-kit-o-jen'ik) [ rachitis + G. *genesis,* production ]. Producing or causing rickets.

**rachitome** (rak'ĭ-tōm). Rachiotome.

**rachitomy** (ră-kit'o-mĭ). Rachiotomy.

**Racine,** W. See R.'s *syndrome.*

**raclage** (ră-klahzh') [ Fr. ]. Curettage.

**racoma** (ra-ko'mah) [ G. *rhakōma; rhakoō,* to tear in strips, fr. *rhakos,* a rag ]. An excoriation.

**rad.** 1. A measure of the dose absorbed from ionizing radiation equivalent to 100 ergs of energy per gm. 2. Abbreviation for L. *radix,* root. 3. Symbol for radian (unit of plane angle) in the SI system.

**radarkymography** (ra'dar-ki-mog'ră-fĭ). Video tracking of heart motion by means of image intensification and closed circuit television during fluoroscopy; enables cardiac motion to be measured by reproducible linear graphic tracing.

**radectomy** (ra-dek'to-mĭ) [ L. *radix,* root, + G. *ektomē,* excision ]. Removal of a part or the whole of the root of a tooth.

**Radford nomogram.** See under nomogram.

**radiability** (ra-dĭ-ă-bil'ĭ-tĭ). The property of being radiable.

**radiable** (ra'dĭ-ă-bl). Capable of being penetrated or examined by rays, especially x-rays.

**radiad** (ra'dĭ-ad). In a direction toward the radial side.

**radial** (ra'dĭ-al) [ L. *radialis,* fr. *radius,* ray, exterior bone of the forearm. RADI- ]. 1. Relating to the radius (bone of the forearm), to any structures named from it, or to the radial or lateral aspect of the upper limb as compared to the ulnar or medial aspect. 2. Relating to any radius. 3. Radiating; diverging in all directions from any given center.

**radialis** (ra-dĭ-a'lis) [ Mod. L. ] [ NA ]. Radial.

**radiant** (ra'dĭ-ant). 1. Giving out rays. 2. A point from which light radiates to the eye.

**radiate** (ra'dĭ-āt) [ L. *radio,* pp. *-atus,* to shine ]. 1. To spread out in all directions from a center. 2. To emit radiation.

**radiatio,** pl. **radiationes** (ra-dĭ-a'shĭ-o, -shi-o'nēz) [ L. ] [ NA ]. Radiation (3); in neuroanatomy, a term applied to any one of the thalamocortical fiber systems that together compose the corona radiata of the cerebral hemisphere's white matter (*e.g.,* radiatio optica, acustica, etc.).

**r. acus'tica** [ NA ], acoustic radiation; the fibers that pass from the medial geniculate body to the transverse temporal gyri of the cerebral cortex. They form part of the sublentiform part of the internal capsule.

**r. cor'poris callo'si** [ NA ], radiation of the corpus callosum; the spreading out of the fibers of the corpus callosum in the centrum semiovale of each cerebral hemisphere.

**r. op'tica** [ NA ], optic radiation; occipitothalamic radiation; geniculocalcarine radiation or tract; Gratiolet's radiation or fibers; Wernicke's radiation; the massive, fanlike fiber system passing from the lateral geniculate body of the thalamus to the visual cortex (striate or calcarine cortex, area 17 of Brodmann); the fibers follow the retrolenticular and sublenticular limbs of the internal capsule into the corona radiata in which they curve back sharply along the lateral wall of the temporal and occipital horns of the lateral ventricle to the striate cortex on the medial surface and pole of the occipital lobe.

**r. pyramida'lis,** pyramidal radiation; white fibers passing from the cortex to the pyramidal tract.

**radiation** (ra'dĭ-a'shun) [ L. *radiatio,* fr. *radius,* ray, beam ]. 1. The act or condition of diverging in all directions from a center. 2. The sending forth of light, short radio waves, ultraviolet or x-rays, or any other rays for treatment or diagnosis or for other purpose; irradiation. 3. Radiatio. 4. A ray. 5. Radiant energy or a radiant beam.

**acoustic r.,** *radiatio* acustica.

**beta r.,** radiant energy from a source of beta rays.

**Cerenkov r.,** light given off by a high energy particle speeding through a transparent medium at a velocity greater than that of light in that medium.

**r. of corpus callosum,** *radiatio* corporis callosi.

**electromagnetic r.,** r. originating in a varying electromagnetic field; *e.g.,* visible light, radio waves, x-radiation, etc.

**geniculocalcarine r.,** *radiatio* optica.

**Gratiolet's r.,** *radiatio* optica.

**K-r.,** a very penetrating form of r. excited by cathode rays (high speed electrons) impinging upon a metal anticathode; it is about 300 times harder than the L-r.

**L-r.,** a r. of slight penetrating power (300 times softer than the K-r.) excited by cathode rays (high speed electrons) impinging on a metal anticathode.

**mitogenet'ic r.,** the production of force by rays emanating from a cell during its mitosis.

**occipitothalamic r.,** *radiatio* optica.

**optic r.,** *radiatio* optica.

**pyramidal r.,** *radiatio* pyramidalis.

**Wernicke's r.,** *radiatio* optica.

**x-r.,** radiant energy from an x-ray tube; see also x-ray (under ray).

**radical** (rad'ĭ-kal) [ L. *radix* (*radic-*), root ]. 1. In chemistry, a group of elements or atoms usually passing intact from one compound to another, but usually incapable of prolonged existence in a free state; in chemical formulas a r. is often distinguished by being enclosed in parentheses or brackets. Methyl, ethyl, sulfate, cyanide, etc., are radicals. 2. The haptophore group of an antibody. 3. Relating to the root or cause; thorough; *e.g.,* a r. operation, one that removes every trace of possibly diseased tissue, or makes recurrence impossible.

**acid r.,** a r. formed from an acid by loss of one or more hydrogen ions; *e.g.,* $SO_4^-$, $NO_3^-$.

**color r.,** chromophore (2).

**free r.,** a radical in its (usually transient) uncombined state; an atom or atom group carrying an unpaired electron and no charge; *e.g.,* hydroxyl (·Ö:H) and methyl

$$\left( \begin{array}{c} H \\ H : \ddot{C} \cdot \\ \ddot{H} \end{array} \right)$$

Free r.'s may be involved as short-lived, highly active intermediates in various reactions in living tissue, notably in photosynthesis.

**radi'ces.** Plural of radix.

**radicle** (rad'ĭ-kl) [ L. *radicula,* dim. of *radix,* root ]. A rootlet or structure resembling one, as the r. of a *vein,* a minute veinlet joining with others to form a vein, or the r. of a *nerve,* a nerve fiber which joins others to form a nerve.

**radicotomy** (rad'ĭ-kot'o-mĭ) [ L. *radix* (*radic-*), root, + G. *tomē,* incision ]. Rhizotomy.

**radicul-.** See radiculo-.

**radicula** (ră-dik'u-lah) [ L. dim. of *radix,* root ]. A spinal nerve root; radix.

**radiculalgia** (ră-dik'u-lal'jĭ-ah) [ radicul- + G. *algos,* pain ]. Neuralgia due to irritation of the sensory root of a spinal nerve.

**radicular** (ră-dik'u-lar). 1. Relating to a radicle. 2. Pertaining to the root of a tooth.

**radiculectomy** (ră-dik'u-lek'to-mĭ) [ radicul- + G. *ektomē,* excision ]. Rhizotomy.

**radiculitis** (ră-dik-u-li'tis) [ radicul- + G. suffix *-itis,* inflammation ]. Inflammation of the intradural portion of a spinal nerve root prior to its entrance into the intervertebral foramen or of the portion between that foramen and the nerve plexus.

**radiculo-, radicul-** (ră-dik'u-lo-) [ L. *radicula,* radicle, dim. of *radix,* root ]. Combining forms meaning radicle, radicular.

**radiculoganglionitis** (ră-dik'u-lo-gang'glĭ-o-ni'tis). Guillain-Barré *syndrome.*

**radiculomeningomyelitis** (ră-dik'u-lo-mĕ-ning'go-mi'ĕ-li'tis). Rhizomeningomyelitis.

**radiculomyelopathy** (ră-dik'u-lo-mi'ĕ-lop'ă-thĭ). Myeloradiculopathy.

**radiculoneuropathy** (ră-dik'u-lo-nu-rop'ă-thĭ). Disease of the spinal nerve roots and nerves.

**radiculopathy** (ră-dik'u-lop'ă-thǐ) [ radiculo- + G. *pathos,* suffering ]. Disease of the spinal nerve roots.

**radif'erous.** Containing radium.

**radii** (ra'dǐ-i) [ L. ]. Plural of radius.

**radio-** (ra'dǐ-o-) [ L. *radius,* ray. RADI- ]. Combining form (1) relating to radiation; denoting chiefly (in medicine) x-ray; (2) denoting the radioactive isotope of the element to which it is prefixed; (3) relating to the radius.

**radioactinium** (ra'dǐ-o-ak-tin'ǐ-um). Thorium-227; a disintegration product of actinium, giving off alpha rays with a half-life of 18.4 days; its disintegration product is actinium X (radium-223).

**ra'dioac'tive.** Possessing radioactivity.
  **r. "cow,"** see radionuclide *generator.*

**radioactivity** (ra'dǐ-o-ak-tiv'ǐ-tǐ). The property of some atomic nuclei of spontaneously emitting rays or subatomic particles of matter with the release of large amounts of energy.
  **artificial r.,** induced r.; the r. of isotopes that exist only because man-made through the bombardment of naturally occurring isotopes by subatomic particles, or high levels of x- or gamma radiation.
  **induced r.,** artificial r.

**radioanaphylaxis** (ra'dǐ-o-an'ă-fi-lak'sis). Sensitivity to radiant energy.

**radioautogram** (ra'dǐ-o-aw'to-gram). Autoradiogram; the graphic record obtained by placing a radioactive material (*e.g.,* thyroid tissue after the administration of radioiodine) in contact with or in close proximity to a photographic emulsion and developing the exposed film or plate.

**radioautography** (ra'dǐ-o-aw-tog'rä-fǐ). The making of a radioautogram.

**radiobicipital** (ra'dǐ-o-bi-sip'ǐ-tal). Relating to the radius and the biceps muscle.

**ra'diobiol'ogy.** The biologic study of the effects of ionizing radiation upon living things.

**ra'diocal'cium.** A radioisotope of calcium, particularly calcium-45, *q. v.*

**ra'diocar'bon.** Radioactive isotope of carbon, *e.g.,* ¹⁴C; see entries under carbon.

**ra'diocar'diogram.** A graphic record of the concentration of injected radioisotope within the cardiac chambers.

**ra'diocardiog'raphy.** The technique of recording or interpreting radiocardiograms.

**ra'diocar'pal.** 1. Relating to the radius and the bones of the carpus. 2. On the radial or lateral side of the carpus.

**radiochemistry** (ra'dǐ-o-kem'is-trǐ). The science that uses radionuclides and their properties to study chemical applications and problems.

**ra'diochlo'rine.** Radioactive isotope of chlorine, *e.g.,* ³⁶Cl.

**radiochrometer** (ra'dǐ-o-krom'e-ter) [ radio- + G. *chroma,* color, + *metron,* measure ]. An instrument for measuring the penetrating power of x-rays.

**radiocinematography** (ra'dǐ-o-sǐ-ne-mă-tog'rä-fǐ) [ radio- + G. *kinēma,* motion, + *graphō,* to write ]. Actinocinematography; taking a moving picture of the movements of organs as revealed by an x-ray examination.

**ra'dioco'balt.** Any radioactive isotope of cobalt; see cobalt-58, cobalt-60.

**radiocurable** (ra'dǐ-o-kūr'ă-bl). Curable by irradiation.

**radiode** (ra'dǐ-ōd) [ radium + G. *hodos,* way ]. A metal container for radium.

**ra'diodermati'tis.** Dermatitis due to excessive exposure to x- or gamma rays.

**ra'diodiagno'sis.** Diagnosis by means of x-rays.

**radiodigital** (ra'dǐ-o-dij'ǐ-tal). Relating to the fingers on the radial or lateral side of the hand.

**radiodontia** (ra-dǐ-o-don'shǐ-ah) [ radio- + G. *odous* (*odont-*), tooth ]. Radioscopic examination of the alveoli and roots of the teeth.

**radioelec'trophysiol'ogram.** A record obtained by means of the radioelectrophysiolograph.

**radioelectrophysiolograph** (ra'dǐ-o-e-lek'tro-fiz-ǐ-ol'o-graf). An apparatus carried by a mobile subject by means of which changes in electrical potential from brain or heart can be picked up and radio-transmitted to an electroencephalograph or an electrocardiograph. An electroenceph-

alogram or an electrocardiogram can thus be obtained from a subject who is unrestricted in his movements by the usual wires.

**radioelectrophysiology** (ra'dǐ-o-e-lek'tro-fiz'ǐ-o-log'rä-fǐ). Recording the changes in the electrical potential of brain or heart by means of the radioelectrophysiolograph.

**ra'dioel'ement.** Any element possessing radioactivity.

**ra'dioep'idermi'tis.** Destructive changes in the epidermis produced by ionizing radiation.

**ra'dioep'itheli'tis.** Destructive changes in epithelium produced by ionizing radiation.

**radiofrequency** (ra'dǐ-o-fre'kwen-sǐ). Radiant energy of a certain frequency; *e.g.,* radio and television employ radiant energy having a frequency between 10⁵ and 10¹¹ cycles per second while diagnostic x-rays have a frequency of 3 × 10¹⁸ cycles per second.

**ra'diogal'lium.** Radioactive gallium; see gallium-68.

**radiogenesis** (ra'dǐ-o-jen'ĕ-sis) [ radio- + G. *genesis,* production ]. The formation or production of radioactivity resulting from radioactive transformation or disintegration of radioactive substances.

**ra'diogen'ic.** Actinogenic. 1. Producing rays of any sort, especially dynamic rays. 2. Caused by x- or gamma rays.

**ra'diogen'ics.** Actinogenics; the science of radiation.

**radiogold colloid.** ¹⁹⁸Au colloid; colloidal radioactive gold; AURCOLOID; AUREOTOPE; a radioactive isotope of gold emitting negative beta particles and gamma radiation; half-life is 2.7 days. Used for irradiation of closed serous cavities in the palliative treatment of ascites and pleural effusion due to metastatic malignancies, and for liver scans.

**radiogram** (ra'dǐ-o-gram) [ radio- + G. *gramma,* something written ]. A record made by means of x-rays or by a radioactive body or substance; also called actinogram; skiagram; roentgenogram.

**radiograph** (ra'dǐ-o-graf) [ radio- + G. *graphō,* to write ]. Any apparatus used for making a radiogram.
  **bite-wing r.,** intraoral dental film adapted to show the coronal portion and cervical third of the root of the teeth in near occlusion; especially useful in detecting interproximal caries and determining alveolar septal height.
  **occlusal r.,** intraoral section film positioned on the occlusal plane and used in visualizing entire sections of the jaw bones; especially useful in exploring calcifications of the sublingual salivary glands.

**radiography** (ra'dǐ-og'rä-fǐ). The making of a radiogram. See roentgenography.
  **electron r.,** a radiographic imaging process in which the incident x-radiation is converted to a latent charge image subsequently developed by a special printing process; it improves detail enhancement by the virtual absence of background fog and image noise.

**ra'diohu'meral.** Relating to the radius and the humerus; denoting the articulation between them.

**radioimmunity** (ra'dǐ-o-ǐ-mu'nǐ-tǐ). Lessened sensitivity to radiation.

**radioimmunoassay** (ra'dǐ-o-im'u-no-as-sa). An immunological (immunochemical) procedure in which radioisotope-labeled antigen (hormone or other substance) is reacted with (1) specific antiserum and (2) an aliquant part of the same antiserum previously treated with test fluid; any specific hormone or other substance in the test fluid sample (2) would have reacted with antibody and, accordingly, a greater quantity of free, labeled antigen (hormone) in the test fluid, with reference to the specific antiserum (1), would be a measure of hormone in the test fluid sample.

**radioimmunodiffusion** (ra'dǐ-o-im'u-no-dǐ-fu'zhun). A method for the study of antigen-antibody reactions by gel diffusion using radioisotope-labeled antigen or antibody.

**radioimmunoelectrophoresis** (ra'dǐ-o-im'u-no-e-lek'-tro-fo-re'sis). Immunoelectrophoresis (*q. v.*) in which the antigen or antibody is labeled with a radioisotope, as, for example, in testing for insulin-binding antibodies by treating the test serum with radioactive iodine-labeled insulin, subjecting the mixture (antigen) to electrophoresis, precipitating the separated immunoglobulins with immunoglobulin-specific antiserum, and, then, with radiosensitive film, testing for bound insulin in the precipitates.

**radioiodinated** (ra'dī-o-i'o-din-a'ted). Treated or combined with radioiodine.

   **r. serum albumin,** see iodinated serum *albumin.*

**radioiodine** (ra'dī-o-i'o-dīn). See radioactive *iodine.*

**radioiron** (ra'dī-o-i'ern). Radioactive iron; see iron-55, iron-59.

**radioisotope** (ra'dī-o-i'so-tōp). An unstable isotope that decays to a stable state by emitting characteristic radiation.

**radiolead** (ra'dī-o-led'). Radioactive lead; see lead-206, -207, and -208.

**radiolesion** (ra'dī-o-le'zhun). A lesion produced by ionizing radiation.

**radiologic, radiological** (ra'dī'o-loj'ĭk, -loj'ĭ-kal). Pertaining to radiology.

**radiologist** (ra'dī-ol'o-jist). One skilled in the diagnostic and therapeutic use of x-rays and other forms of radiant energy.

**radiology** (ra'dī-ol'o-jī) [ radio- + G. *logos,* study ]. Actinology; the science that treats of radiant energy; of the chemical and other actions of rays proceeding from luminous bodies, from radium and other radioactive substances, and from x-rays; and of the sources of these rays.

**radiolucency** (ra-dī-o-lu'sen-sī). The state of being radiolucent.

**radiolucent** (ra-dī-o-lu'sent) [ radio- + L. *lucens,* shining ]. Neither wholly penetrable nor wholly impenetrable by x-rays or other forms of radiation.

**radiolus** (ra-di'o-lus) [ L. dim. of *radius,* spoke. RADI- ]. A probe or sound.

**radiometer** (ra'dī-om'e-ter) [ radio- + G. *metron,* measure ]. A device for determining the penetrative power of x-rays.

   **pastil r.,** see Sabouraud's *pastil.*

**ra'diomicrom'eter.** A sensitive thermopile designed for the measurement of minute changes in radiant energy.

**radiomimetic** (ra'dī-o-mī-met'ik) [ radio- + G. *mimētikos,* imitative ]. Imitating the action of radiation, as in the case of chemicals such as nitrogen mustards which affect cells as high energy radiation does.

**ra'diomus'cular.** Relating to the radius and the neighboring muscles; denoting certain nerves and muscular branches of the radial artery.

**ra'dionecro'sis.** Necrosis due to radiation; for instance, after excessive exposure to x- or gamma rays.

**radioneuritis** (ra'dī-o-nu-ri'tis). Actinoneuritis.

**ra'dioni'trogen.** A radioisotope of nitrogen; see entries under nitrogen.

**radiopacity** (ra-dī-o-pas'ĭ-tī). State of being radiopaque.

**ra'diopal'mar.** Relating to the radial or lateral side of the palm.

**radiopaque** (ra-dī-o-pāk') [ radio- + Fr. opaque fr. L. *opacus,* shady ]. Exhibiting opacity to or impenetrability by x-rays or any other form of radiation.

**radioparency** (ra-dī-o-pār'en-sī). State of being radioparent.

**radioparent** (ra-dī-o-pār'ent). Transparent to or penetrable by x-rays or other forms of radiation.

**ra'diopathol'ogy.** A branch of radiology or pathology that deals with the effects of radioactive substances on cells and tissues.

**ra'diopelvim'etry.** Measurement of the pelvis by means of roentgen rays.

**radiopharmaceuticals** (ra'dī-o-far-mă-su'tĭ-kalz). Radioactive chemical or pharmaceutical preparations, used as diagnostic or therapeutic agents.

**radiophobia** (ra'dī-o-fo'bī-ah) [ radio- + G. *phobos,* fear ]. Morbid fear of x-ray or nuclear energy.

**ra'diophos'phorus.** Radioactive phosphorus, *e.g.,* phosphorus-32, *q. v.*

**radiophylaxis** (ra'dī-o-fi-lak'sis) [ radio- + G. *phylaxis,* protection ]. The lessened effect of radiation after a previous small dose of radiation.

**radiopill.** Radiotelemetering *capsule.*

**ra'diopotas'sium.** A radioactive isotope of potassium, *e.g.,* potassium-40 and potassium-42, *q. v.*

**ra'dioprax'is** [ radio- + G. *praxis,* a doing ]. Actinopraxis; the use of light rays, x-rays, or radium in diagnosis or treatment.

**radiopulmonography** (ra'dī-o-pul'mo-nog'rā-fī). A method for simultaneous estimation of individual lung function.

**radioreaction** (ra'dī-o-re-ak'shun). A reaction of the body to radiation.

**ra'diorecep'tor.** A receptor that normally responds to radiant energy such as light or heat.

**ra'dioresis'tant.** Indicating cells, *e.g.,* of a new growth, that are not destroyed by exposure to radiations.

**radiosclerometer** (ra'dī-o-skle-rom'e-ter) [ radio- + G. *skleros,* hard, + *metron,* measure ]. Penetrometer.

**ra'dioscope.** An instrument for detecting radiant energy.

**radioscopy** (ra'dī-os'ko-pī) [ radio- + G. *skopeō, to view* ]. Examination of the tissues and deep structures of the body by x-ray; actinoscopy; fluoroscopy; roentgenoscopy.

**radiosens'itive.** Affected by radiation.

**ra'diosensitiv'ity.** The condition of being readily acted upon by radioactive forces.

**ra'dioso'dium.** A radioactive isotope of sodium; see sodium-24.

**radiostereoscopy** (ra'dī-o-stēr'e-os'ko-pī) [ radio- + G. *stereos,* solid, + *skopeō,* to view ]. The observation of two roentgenograms, taken at slightly different angles, in a specially designed box so that one picture is seen by the left eye, the other by the right eye. By the application in this way of the principles of stereoscopic vision, one sees an x-ray picture in three dimensions instead of two. Thus it can be determined whether one opaque object lies in front of or behind the other.

**ra'diostron'tium.** A radioisotope of strontium; see strontium-89, strontium-90.

**ra'diosul'fur.** A radioisotope of sulfur; see sulfur-35.

**ra'diosur'gery.** Use of radium in surgical treatment.

**ra'diotelem'etry.** See telemetry and biotelemetry.

**ra'diotherapeu'tic.** Relating to radiotherapy or to radiotherapeutics.

**ra'diotherapeu'tics.** The study and use of radiotherapeutic agents.

**ra'diother'apist.** One who practices radiotherapy or is versed in radiotherapeutics.

**ra'diother'apy.** Actinotherapy; that specialty of the practice of medicine which relates to the use of electromagnetic or particulate radiations in the treatment of disease.

**ra'diother'my** [ radio- + G. *thermē,* heat ]. Diathermy effected by heat from radiant sources.

**radiothorium** (ra-dī-o-tho'rī-um). Thorium-228; a disintegration product of the thorium series, arising from the disintegration of actinium-228 (mesothorium-II) and itself producing alpha particles, disintegrating to radium-224 (thorium X) with a half-life of 1.91 years; see also thorium, thorium-230, and thorium X.

**radiothyroidectomy** (ra'dī-o-thi'roy-dek'to-mī). Jargon for the destruction of thyroid tissue by administration of radioactive iodine.

**ra'diothyrox'in.** Radioactive *thyroxin.*

**radiotoxemia** (ra'dī-o-tok-se'mī-ah) [ radio- + G. *toxikon,* poison, + *haima,* blood ]. Radiation sickness caused by the products of disintegration produced by the action of x-rays or other forms of activity and by the depletion of certain cells and enzyme systems from the organism.

**ra'diotranspar'ent.** Allowing transmission of radiant energy.

**ra'diotrop'ic** [ radio- + G. *tropē,* a turning ]. Affected by radiation.

**radioulnar** (ra'dī-o-ul'nar). Relating to both radius and ulna.

**ra'dium** [ L. *radius,* ray ]. A metallic element, symbol Ra, atomic no. 88, atomic weight 226.05, extracted in very minute quantities from pitchblende; its longest lived isotope, radium-226, is produced as an intermediate in the uranium series, being formed by the emission of an alpha particle by thorium-230 (ionium); it emits alpha particles itself, breaking down to radon-222 (radium emanation) with a half-life of 1,620 years; chemically, it is an alkaline earth metal with properties similar to barium. Its therapeutic action is similar to that of x-rays. It is applied in the form of one of its salts, the bromide, carbonate, chloride, and sulfate being those in common use. It causes extensive "burns" of the skin and other tissues when applied too long and without a proper shield.

**radiumization** (ra-dī-um-i-za'shun). Exposure of a part to radium rays; external radium therapy.

**radius,** gen. and pl. **radii** (ra'dī-us, ra'dī-i) [ L. spoke of a wheel, rod, ray. RADI- ]. 1. A straight line passing from the center to the periphery of a circle. 2 [ NA ]. The lateral and shorter of the two bones of the forearm.

**r. curvus,** Madelung's *deformity.*

**r. fixus,** a line passing from the hormion to the inion.

**ra'dii len'tis** [ NA ], lens sutures; lens stars; 9 to 12 faint lines on the anterior and posterior surfaces of the lens that radiate from the poles toward the equator; they mark the lines along which the ends of lens fibers abut.

**radix,** gen. **radicis,** pl. **radices** (ra'diks, ra-di'sis, ra'dī-sēz or ra-di'sēz) [ L. ] [ NA ]. Root; the primary or beginning portion of any part, as of a nerve at its origin from the brain or spinal cord.

**r. ante'rior,** r. ventralis.

**r. ar'cus ver'tebrae,** *pediculus* arcus vertebrae.

**r. bre'vis gan'glii cilia'ris,** r. oculomotoria ganglii ciliaris.

**r. clin'ica** [ NA ], clinical root; that portion of a tooth embedded in the investing structures; the portion of a tooth not visible in the oral cavity.

**r. cochlea'ris** [ NA ], cochlear root of the vestibulocochlear nerve; see *nervus* vestibulocochlearis.

**radices crania'les** [ NA ], cranial roots; the roots of the accessory nerve which arise from the medulla.

**r. den'tis** [ NA ], root of a tooth; that part below the neck, covered by cementum, which is fixed in the alveolus.

**r. dorsa'lis** [ NA ], dorsal root; r. posterior; posterior root; the sensory root of a spinal nerve.

**r. facia'lis** [ NA ], *nervus* canalis pterygoidei.

**r. infe'rior an'sae cervica'lis** [ NA ], inferior root of cervical loop; descendens cervicalis; fibers from the second and third cervical nerves that pass forward and downward along the internal jugular vein; they contribute to the ansa cervicalis and innervate the infrahyoid muscles.

**r. infe'rior ner'vi vestibulocochlea'ris** [ NA ], inferior root of vestibulocochlear nerve; see *nervus* vestibulocochlearis.

**r. latera'lis ner'vi media'ni** [ NA ], lateral root of the median nerve; the part of the median nerve arising from the lateral cord of the brachial plexus.

**r. latera'lis trac'tus op'tici** [ NA ], lateral root of the optic tract; the larger division of the posterior end of the optic tract that terminates in the lateral geniculate body.

**r. lin'guae** [ NA ], root or base of the tongue; the posterior attached portion of the tongue.

**r. lon'ga gan'glii cilia'ris,** *ramus* communicans cum nervo nasociliari.

**r. media'lis ner'vi mediani** [ NA ], medial root of the median nerve; the part coming from the medial cord of the brachial plexus.

**r. media'lis trac'tus op'tici** [ NA ], medial root of the optic tract; also called *brachium* colliculi superioris, *q.v.*

**r. mesenter'ii** [ NA ], root of the mesentery; the origin of the mesentery of the small intestine (jejunum and ileum) from the posterior parietal peritoneum.

**r. moto'ria ner'vi trigem'ini** [ NA ], motor root of the trigeminal nerve; portio minor nervi trigemini; masticator nerve; the smaller root of the trigeminal nerve, composed of fibers originating from the trigeminal motor nucleus and emerging from the pons medial to the much larger sensory root, to join the mandibular nerve; it carries motor and proprioceptive fibers to the muscles of mastication.

**r. na'si** [ NA ], root of the nose; the upper portion of the external nose situated between the two orbits.

**r. ner'vi facia'lis,** root of the facial nerve; fibers running from the facial motor nucleus upward to the colliculus facialis where they curve around the abducens nucleus and then pass outward, between the superior olive and sensory nucleus of the trigeminal, to emerge as the facial nerve from the pontomedullary groove.

**radices ner'vi trigem'ini,** roots of the trigeminal nerve; collective term for the r. sensoria nervi trigemini and r. motoria nervi trigemini.

**r. oculomoto'ria gan'glii cilia'ris** [ NA ], r. brevis ganglii ciliaris; motor root of the ciliary ganglion; short root of the ciliary ganglion; a branch of the oculomotor nerve supplying preganglionic nerve fibers to the ciliary ganglion.

**r. pe'nis** [ NA ], root of the penis; the proximal attached part of the penis, including the two crura and the bulb.

**r. pi'li** [ NA ], hair root; the part of a hair which is embedded in the hair follicle; its lower succulent extremity, capping the papilla of the follicle, is called the bulb.

**r. poste'rior,** r. dorsalis.

**r. pulmo'nis** [ NA ], root of the lung; all the structures entering or leaving the lung at the hilus, forming a pedicle invested with the pleura.

**r. senso'ria ner'vi trigem'ini** [ NA ], sensory root of the trigeminal nerve; portio major nervi trigemini; the large sensory root of the trigeminal (or fifth cranial) nerve, extending from the semilunar ganglion of Gasser into the pons through the middle cerebellar peduncle or brachium pontis, immediately lateral to the small r. motoria or portio minor.

**radices spina'les** [ NA ], spinal roots; the roots of the accessory nerve which arise from the ventrolateral part of the first five segments of the spinal cord.

**r. supe'rior an'sae cervica'lis** [ NA ], superior root of cervical loop; descendens hypoglossi; the fibers that arise from the first and second cervical nerves, accompany the hypoglossal nerve, then branch off to meet the inferior root in the ansa cervicalis. They innervate the infrahyoid muscles.

**r. supe'rior ner'vi vestibulocochlea'ris** [ NA ], superior root of the vestibulocochlear nerve; see *nervus* vestibulocochlearis.

**r. un'guis** [ NA ], root of the nail; the proximal end of the nail, concealed under a fold of skin.

**r. ventra'lis** [ NA ], ventral root; r. anterior; anterior root; the motor root of a spinal nerve.

**r. vestibula'ris** [ NA ], vestibular root of the vestibulocochlear nerve; see *nervus* vestibulocochlearis.

**ra'don.** Niton; radium emanation; symbol Rn, atomic no. 86, atomic weight 222.

**radon-219** (²¹⁹Rn). Actinon; the inert gas intermediate of the uranium-235 radioactive series; an alpha-emitter with a half-life of 3.9 seconds.

**radon-220** (²²⁰Rn). Thoron; the inert gas intermediate of the thorium-232 series; an alpha-emitter with a half-life of 52 seconds.

**radon-222** (²²²Rn). The inert gas intermediate of the uranium-238 series; an alpha-emitter with a half-life of 3.825 days.

**Raeder,** Georg Johan. Norwegian ophthalmologist, 1889–1956. See R.'s paratrigeminal *syndrome.*

**raf'finose.** Melitose; melitriose; gossypose; a dextrorotatory trisaccharide occurring in cotton seed and in the molasses of beet root; composed of D-galactose, D-glucose, and D-fructose and formed by transfer of galactose from UDP-galactose to sucrose.

**rage** (rāj). Violent anger; a total discharge of the sympathetic portion of the autonomic system.

**sham r.,** a quasi-emotional state, characterized by manifestations of fear and anger upon trifling provocation; produced in animals by the removal of the cerebral cortex (decortication).

**Raillietina** (ri-lī-ĕ-te'nah). A genus of tapeworms (family Davaineidae, order Gyelophyllidea), three species of which, *R. madagascariensis* or *R. demerariensis* (*Davainea madagascariensis*), *R. asiatica,* and *R. formsana,* have been found in man. However, the identification of many of these worms found in man has been questioned.

**Rainey,** George, English anatomist, 1801–1884. See R.'s *corpuscles.*

**rale** (rahl) [ Fr. rattle ]. A small rhonchus; an adventitious sound, of varied character, heard on auscultation of the chest in many cases of disease of the lungs or bronchi.

**amphoric r.,** sound heard through the stethoscope associated with the movement of fluid in a lung cavity communicating with a bronchus.

**atelectatic r.,** transitory light crackling sound that disappears after deep breathing or coughing.

**border r.,** atelectatic r.

**bubbling r.,** moist sound heard through the stethoscope, sometimes associated with resolving pneumonia or small lung cavities.

**cavernous r.,** a hollow bubbling sound caused by air entering a cavity partly filled with fluid.

**clicking r.,** short sticking sound usually associated with opening of small bronchi on deep breathing, sometimes heard in early pulmonary tuberculosis.

**consonating r.,** a resonant r. produced in a bronchial tube and heard through consolidated lung tissue.

**crepitant r.,** a fine bubbling or crackling sound produced by the presence of a very thin secretion in the smaller bronchial tubes.

**dry r.,** a sound produced by a constriction in a bronchial tube or the presence of a viscid secretion narrowing the lumen.

**gurgling r.,** coarse sound heard over large cavities or over trachea nearly filled with secretions.

**guttural r.,** sound heard over the lung but resulting from upper airway obstruction.

**marginal r.,** atelectatic r.

**metallic r.,** one of metallic quality caused by resonance in a large cavity.

**moist r.,** one of a bubbling character caused by the pressure of a fluid secretion in the bronchial tubes or a cavity.

**mucous r.,** a bubbling sound heard on auscultation over bronchial tubes containing mucus.

**palpable r.,** a vibration sometimes accompanying a low-pitched sonorous r.

**sibilant r.,** a whistling sound caused by the presence of a viscid secretion narrowing the lumen of a bronchus.

**Skoda's r.,** a r. in a bronchus heard through an area of consolidated tissue in pneumonia.

**sonorous r.,** a cooing or snoring sound often produced by the vibration of a projecting mass of viscid secretion in a large bronchus.

**subcrepitant r.,** a very fine crepitant r.

**vesicular r.,** crepitant r.

**whistling r.,** sibilant r.

**ram** [ A.S. ]. A male sheep of breeding age.

**ra′mal.** Relating to a ramus.

**Raman effect.** See under effect.

**ra′mex** [ L. hernia; pl. blood vessels of the lungs, fr. *ramus,* a branch ]. Hernia, varicocele, or any scrotal tumor.

**rami** (ra′mi) [ L. ]. Plural of ramus.

**Ramibacterium** (ra′mi-bak-tēr′ĭ-um) [ L. *ramus,* branch, + *bacterium* ]. An obsolete genus of bacteria, the type species of which, *R. ramosum,* is presently placed in the genus *Clostridium.*

**R. ramosum,** *Clostridium ramosum.*

**ramicotomy** (ram′ĭ-kot′o-mĭ) [ L. *ramus,* branch, + G. *tomē,* incision ]. Ramisection.

**ramification** (ram′ĭ-fĭ-ka′shun). A branching.

**ramify** (ram′ĭ-fi) [ L. *ramus,* branch, + *facio,* to make ]. To branch.

**ramisection** (ram-ĭ-sek′shun) [ L. *ramus,* branch, + L. *sectio,* section ]. Ramicotomy; section of the rami communicantes of the sympathetic nervous system.

**rami′tis** [ L. *ramus,* branch, + G. suffix *-itis,* inflammation ]. Inflammation of a ramus.

**Ramon y Cajal** (rah-mōn′ e kah-hahl′) See Cajal.

**ramose, ramous** (ra′mōs, ra′mus) [ L. *ramosus,* fr. *ramus,* a branch ]. Branching.

**Ramsay Hunt.** See Hunt, James Ramsay.

**Ramsden,** Jesse, English optician, 1735–1800. See R.'s *ocular.*

**Ramstedt** (rahm′stet), Conrad, German surgeon, *1867. See R. *operation,* Fredet-R. *operation.*

**ramulus,** pl. **ramuli** (ram′u-lus, -li) [ L. dim. of *ramus,* a branch ]. A small branch or twig; one of the terminal divisions of a ramus.

# RAMUS

**ra′mus,** pl. **ra′mi** [ L. ] [ NA ]. 1. A branch. 2. One of the primary divisions of a nerve or blood vessel. Arterial and nerve branches are also given under the major nerve or artery; see arteria and nervus. 3. A part of an irregularly shaped bone (less slender than a "process") which forms an angle with the main body. 4. One of the primary divisions of a cerebral sulcus.

**r. acetabula′ris arte′riae circumflex′ae fem′oris media′lis** [ NA ], acetabular branch of the medial femoral circumflex artery.

**r. acetabula′ris arte′riae obturato′riae** [ NA ], arteria acetabuli; acetabular artery; *origin,* obturator artery; *distribution,* ligamentum capitis femoris and head of femur.

**r. acromia′lis arte′riae thoracoacromia′lis** [ NA ], acromial artery; a branch of the thoracoacromial artery that runs over the coracoid process and under the deltoid muscle.

**rami ad pon′tem** [ NA ], pontine branches; arterial branches of the basilar artery to the pons.

**rami alveola′res superio′res anterio′res** [ NA ], anterior superior alveolar branches of superior alveolar nerves.

**r. alveola′ris supe′rior me′dius** [ NA ], middle superior alveolar branch (of superior alveolar nerves, of infraorbital nerve, of maxillary nerve, of trigeminal nerve).

**rami alveola′res superio′res posterio′res** [ NA ], posterior superior alveolar branches of superior alveolar nerves.

**r. anastomot′icus,** anastomotic branch; a blood vessel that interconnects two neighboring vessels. It should not be used for the nervous system, because there is no analogy between a vascular anastomosing branch and a connection between nerves or their subdivisions.

**r. anastomot′icus cum lacrima′li** [ NA ], anastomosing branch of the middle meningeal artery with the lacrimal artery.

**r. anterior** [ NA ], anterior branch; each of the following structures has a branch so named; (1) great auricular nerve; (2) lateral cerebral sulcus; (3) left and right superior pulmonary veins; (4) medial cutaneous nerve of the forearm; (5) obturator artery; (6) obturator nerve; (7) renal artery; (8) right branch of portal vein; (9) right hepatic duct; (10) superior thyroid artery; (11) ulnar recurrent artery.

**r. ante′rior ascen′dens** [ NA ], ascending anterior branch (of left pulmonary artery; of right pulmonary artery).

**r. ante′rior descen′dens** [ NA ], descending anterior branch (of right pulmonary artery; of left pulmonary artery).

**r. ante′rior latera′lis,** lateral anterior branch; the former name for the ascending anterior branch of the left pulmonary artery.

**r. apica′lis** [ NA ], apical branch; each of the following has a branch so named; (1) left and right inferior pulmonary veins; (2) left and right pulmonary arteries; (3) left superior pulmonary vein.

**r. apica′lis lobi inferio′ris** [ NA ], apical branch of the inferior lobe (of right and left pulmonary arteries); r. superior lobi inferioris is the alternative term.

**r. apicoposte′rior** [ NA ], apicoposterior branch of left superior pulmonary vein.

**rami articula′res** [ NA ], articular branches of descending genicular artery.

**r. ascen′dens** [ NA ], ascending branch (of deep circumflex iliac artery; of lateral cerebral sulcus; of lateral circumflex femoral artery).

**r. atrioventricula′ris,** atrioventricular branch; nodal branch; the small artery supplying the atrioventricular node; it usually arises from the right coronary artery where it turns to run in the posterior interventricular sulcus.

**rami auricula′res anteriores** [ NA ], anterior auricular branches (of superficial temporal artery).

**r. auricula′ris arte′riae occipita′lis** [ NA ], auricular branch of occipital artery.

**r. auricula′ris va′gi** [ NA ], auricular r. of the vagus; Arnold's nerve; a branch of the superior ganglion of the vagus, supplying the back of the pinna and the external acoustic meatus.

**r. basa'lis ante'rior** [ NA ], anterior basal branch; each of the following has a branch so named; (1) left and right pulmonary arteries; (2) left and right inferior pulmonary veins.

**r. basa'lis latera'lis** [ NA ], lateral basal branch (of basal part of right pulmonary artery; of basal part of left pulmonary artery).

**r. basa'lis media'lis** [ NA ], medial basal branch (of basal part of left pulmonary artery; of basal part of right pulmonary artery).

**r. basa'lis poste'rior** [ NA ], posterior basal branch (of basal part of left pulmonary artery; of basal part of right pulmonary artery).

**rami bronchia'les aor'tae thorac'icae** [ NA ], bronchial branches of thoracic aorta; bronchial arteries; the nutrient arteries of the lungs, usually two on the left and one on the right, that arise from the aorta.

**rami bronchia'les segmento'rum** [ NA ], branches of segmental bronchi.

**rami bucca'les** [ NA ], buccal branches (of facial nerves).

**rami calca'nei** [ NA ], calcaneal branches; branches to the structures in the calcaneal region from (1) the posterior tibial artery and (2) the peroneal artery.

**rami calca'nei latera'les** [ NA ], lateral calcaneal branches (of sural nerve).

**rami calca'nei media'les** [ NA ], medial calcaneal branches (of tibial nerve).

**rami capsula'res** [ NA ], capsular branches (of renal artery).

**r. cardi'acus** [ NA ], official alternative for r. basalis medialis.

**rami cardi'aci cervica'les inferio'res** [ NA ], inferior cervical cardiac branches (of vagus nerve).

**rami cardi'aci cervica'les superio'res** [ NA ], superior cervical cardiac branches (of vagus nerve).

**rami cardi'aci thora'cici** [ NA ], thoracic cardiac branches (of vagus nerve).

**rami caroticotympan'ici** [ NA ], caroticotympanic branches; small branches of the internal carotid that enter the tympanic cavity from the carotid canal.

**r. car'peus dorsa'lis arte'riae radia'lis** [ NA ], dorsal carpal branch of radial artery; it passes to the back of the carpus to join the dorsal carpal rete.

**r. car'peus dorsa'lis arte'riae ulna'ris** [ NA ], dorsal carpal branch of the ulnar artery; a branch that passes to the dorsal side of the carpus to enter the dorsal carpal rete.

**r. car'peus palma'ris arte'riae radia'lis** [ NA ], palmar carpal branch of radial artery; a small artery that passes medially across the wrist to supply the carpal joints; it anastomoses with the anterior carpal branch of the ulnar artery.

**r. car'peus palma'ris arte'riae ulna'ris** [ NA ], palmar carpal branch of ulnar artery; it supplies the carpal joints and communicates with the anterior carpal branch of the radial artery.

**rami cauda'ti** [ NA ], caudate branches of transverse part of left branch of portal vein.

**rami celi'aci** [ NA ], celiac branches of vagus nerve.

**rami centra'les** [ NA ], central branches (of anterior cerebral artery; of middle cerebral artery; of posterior cerebral artery).

**r. choroi'deus** [ NA ], choroid branch of the posterior cerebral artery; also officialy referred to as rami choroidei posteriores, because there are usually several of these branches, which must be differentiated from the anterior choroidal artery.

**rami choroi'dei posterio'res** [ NA ], posterior choroid branches; official alternative term for r. choroideus.

**r. circumflex'us** [ NA ], circumflex branch (of left coronary artery).

**r. circumflex'us fib'ulae** [ NA ], circumflex fibular branch; a branch of the posterior tibial artery; which winds around the neck of the fibula and joins the anastomoses around the knee joint.

**r. clavicula'ris** [ NA ], clavicular branch of thoracoacromial artery.

**r. cochlea'ris** [ NA ], cochlear branch of labyrinthine artery.

**r. collatera'lis** [ NA ], collateral branch of posterior intercostal arteries.

**r. col'li**, [ NA ], cervical branch of facial nerve.

**rami communican'tes**, sing. **ramus communicans** [ NA ], communicating branches; bundles of nerve fibers passing from one nerve to join another, *e.g.*, from the autonomic to the central nervous system. The term "ramus communicans" is used to replace the inadequate "ramus anastomoticus" in the nervous system.

**r. commu'nicans arte'riae perone'ae** [ NA ], r. communicans arteriae fibularis; communicating branch of the peroneal (fibular) artery.

**r. commu'nicans cum chorda tym'pani** [ NA ], communicating branch with tympanic chord; (1) a small branch of the lingual nerve which joins the chorda tympani; (2) a small branch from the otic ganglion to the chorda tympani.

**r. commu'nicans cum gan'glio cilia'ri** [ NA ], communicating branch of nasociliary nerve with ciliary ganglion.

**r. commu'nicans cum ner'vo auriculotempora'li** [ NA ], communicating branch of otic ganglion with auriculotemporal nerve.

**rami communican'tes cum nervo facia'li** [ NA ], communicating branches of mandibular nerve with facial nerve.

**r. communicans cum nervo glossopharyn'geo** [ NA ], communicating branch with glossopharyngeal nerve; (1) a small branch from the digastric branch of the facial nerve to the glossopharyngeal nerve; (2) a small branch from the auricular branch of the vagus to the glossopharyngeal nerve.

**rami communican'tes cum nervo hypoglos'so** [ NA ], communicating branches between mandibular nerve (from the trigeminal nerve) and hypoglossal nerve.

**r. commu'nicans cum nervo laryn'geo inferio're** [ NA ], communicating branch (of internal branch of superior laryngeal nerve) with inferior laryngeal nerve.

**rami communican'tes cum nervo lingua'li** [ NA ], communicating branches between submandibular ganglion and lingual nerve (of trigeminal nerve).

**r. commu'nicans cum nervo nasocilia'ri** [ NA ], communicating branch of ciliary ganglion with nasociliary nerve; radix longa ganglii ciliaris; sensory or long root of the ciliary ganglion; sensory fibers passing from the eyeball through the ciliary ganglion to the trigeminal ganglion.

**r. commu'nicans cum nervo ulna'ri** [ NA ], communicating branch of median nerve with ulnar nerve.

**r. commu'nicans cum nervo zygomat'ico** [ NA ], communicating branch of lacrimal nerve with zygomatic nerve.

**r. commu'nicans cum plexu tympan'ico** [ NA ], communicating branch of facial nerve with tympanic plexus.

**r. commu'nicans cum ra'mo auricula'ri nervi va'gi** [ NA ], communicating branch of glossopharyngeal nerve with auricular branch of the vagus nerve.

**r. commu'nicans cum ra'mo laryn'geo interno** [ NA ], communicating branch of inferior laryngeal nerve with internal laryngeal branch of superior laryngeal nerve.

**r. commu'nicans cum ra'mo menin'geo** [ NA ], communicating branch of otic ganglion with meningeal branch of mandibular nerve.

**rami communican'tes nervorum spina'lium** [ NA ], communicating branches of spinal nerves; small bundles of nerve fibers connecting spinal nerves with sympathetic ganglia; the fibers passing from the ganglion to the spinal nerve are nonmyelinated and are called gray rami communicantes, those passing in the reverse direction are myelinated and are called white rami communicantes; see also sympathetic nervous *system*.

**r. commu'nicans perone'us** [ NA ], r. communicans fibularis; peroneal anastomotic r.; nervus communicans fibularis or peroneus; peroneal (fibular) communicating branch of common peroneal, or fibular, nerve; arises from the common peroneal nerve in the popliteal space and passes over the lateral head of the gastrocnemius to the middle third of the leg, where it unites with the nervus cutaneus surae medialis to form the sural nerve.

**r. commu'nicans ulna'ris** [ NA ], ulnar communicating branch of superficial branch of radial nerve.

**rami cortica'les** [ NA ], cortical branches (of anterior cerebral artery; of middle cerebral artery; of posterior cerebral artery).

**r. costa'lis latera'lis** [ NA ], lateral costal branch of internal thoracic artery.

**r. cricothyroi'deus** [ NA ], cricothyroid branch; a small branch of the superior thyroid artery that supplies the cricothyroid muscle.

**rami cuta'nei anterio'res ner'vi femora'lis** [ NA ], anterior cutaneous branches of femoral nerve.

**r. cuta'neus ante'rior ner'vi iliohypogas'trica** [ NA ], anterior cutaneous branch of iliohypogastric nerve.

**r. cuta'neus anterior (pectora'lis et abdomina'lis) nervo'rum thoracico'rum** [ NA ], anterior cutaneous branch (pectoral and abdominal) of thoracic nerves.

**rami cuta'nei cru'ris media'les ner'vi saphe'ni** [ NA ], medial crural cutaneous branches of saphenous nerve.

**r. cuta'neus latera'lis** [ NA ], lateral cutaneous branch (of iliohypogastric nerve; of dorsal branch of thoracic nerves; of dorsal branch of posterior intercostal arteries).

**r. cuta'neus media'lis** [ NA ], medial cutaneous branch (of dorsal branch of thoracic nerves; of dorsal branch of posterior intercostal arteries).

**r. cuta'neus rami anterio'ris ner'vi obturato'rii** [ NA ], cutaneous branch of anterior branch of obturator nerve.

**r. deltoi'deus** [ NA ], deltoid branch of thoracoacromial artery.

**rami denta'les** [ NA ], dental branches (of anterior superior alveolar arteries; of inferior alveolar artery; of posterior superior alveolar artery).

**rami denta'les inferio'res** [ NA ], inferior dental branches of inferior dental plexus.

**rami denta'les superio'res** [ NA ], superior dental branches of superior dental plexus.

**r. descen'dens** [ NA ], (1) descending branch of the lateral femoral circumflex artery; (2) princeps cervicis; descending branch of the occipital artery.

**r. dexter** [ NA ], right branch (of portal vein; of proper hepatic artery).

**r. digas'tricus** [ NA ], digastric branch of the facial nerve.

**rami dorsa'les** [ NA ], dorsal branches (of cervical nerves; of coccygeal nerve; of lumbar nerves; of posterior intercostal arteries I and II; of sacral nerves; of thoracic nerves).

**r. dorsa'lis** [ NA ], dorsal branch (of lumbar artery; of posterior intercostal arteries; of posterior intercostal veins; of spinal nerves, *q.v.*, under r. dorsalis nervorum spinalium; of subcostal artery; of ulnar nerve).

**rami dorsa'les lin'guae** [ NA ], dorsal lingual branches of the lingual artery.

**r. dorsa'lis nervo'rum spina'lium** [ NA ], dorsal ramus of spinal nerves; posterior primary division; the smaller division of each spinal nerve that innervates posterior axial musculature and part of the skin of the back.

**rami duodena'les** [ NA ], duodenal branches of superior pancreaticoduodenal arteries.

**rami epiplo'ici** [ NA ], epiploic branches (of right gastroepiploic artery; of left gastroepiploic artery).

**rami esophage'i** [ NA ], esophageal branches (of inferior thyroid artery; of left gastric artery; of recurrent laryngeal nerve; of thoracic aorta).

**r. externus** [ NA ], external branch (of accessory nerve; of superior laryngeal nerve).

**r. femora'lis** [ NA ], femoral branch of genitofemoral nerve.

**rami fronta'les** [ NA ], frontal branches (of cortical branches of anterior cerebral artery; of middle cerebral artery).

**r. fronta'lis** [ NA ], frontal branch of superficial temporal artery.

**rami gas'trici ner'vi va'gi** [ NA ], gastric branches of the vagus; these consist of two sets of branches (**r. gastrici anteriores** and **r. gastrici posteriores**) that pass directly to the wall of the stomach from the anterior and posterior vagal trunks.

**r. genita'lis** [ NA ], nervus spermaticus externus; genital branch of genitofemoral nerve.

**rami gingiva'les inferio'res** [ NA ], inferior gingival branches of inferior dental plexus.

**rami gingiva'les superio'res** [ NA ], superior gingival branches of superior dental plexus.

**rami glandula'res** [ NA ], glandular branches (of vessels and nerves; of facial artery; of inferior thyroid artery; of submandibular ganglion).

**rami hepat'ici** [ NA ], hepatic branches of vagus nerve.

**r. ili'acus** [ NA ], iliac branch of iliolumbar artery.

**r. infe'rior** [ NA ], inferior branch (of oculomotor nerve; of pubic bone; of superior gluteal artery).

**rami inferio'res ner'vi transver'si col'li** [ NA ], inferior branches of the transverse nerve of the neck (of cervical plexus).

**r. infrahyoi'deus** [ NA ], infrahyoid branch of superior thyroid artery.

**r. infrapatella'ris** [ NA ], infrapatellar branch of saphenous nerve.

**rami inguina'les** [ NA ], inguinal branches of external pudendal arteries.

**rami intercosta'les anterio'res** [ NA ], anterior intercostal branches or arteries; two branches of the internal thoracic artery in each of the upper six intercostal spaces.

**rami interngangliona'res** [ NA ], interganglionic branches; the nerve strands interconnecting the ganglia of the sympathetic trunk; they consist of pre- or postganglionic fibers passing to higher or lower levels of the trunk.

**r. internus** [ NA ], internal branch (of accessory nerve; of superior laryngeal nerve).

**r. interventricula'ris anterior** [ NA ], anterior interventricular branch of left coronary artery.

**r. interventricula'ris posterior** [ NA ], posterior interventricular branch of right coronary artery.

**ischiopubic r.,** the inferior r. of the os pubis and the r. of the ischium continuous with it.

**rami isth'mi fau'cium** [ NA ], branches of the isthmus of the fauces of lingual nerve.

**rami labia'les anterio'res** [ NA ], anterior labial branches; anterior labial arteries; *origin*, external pudendal artery; *distribution*, labius majus.

**rami labia'les inferio'res** [ NA ], inferior labial branches of mental nerve.

**rami labia'les posterio'res** [ NA ], posterior labial branches; posterior labial arteries; *origin*, internal pudendal artery; *distribution*, labium majus.

**rami labia'les superio'res** [ NA ], superior labial branches of infraorbital nerve.

**rami laryngopharyn'gei** [ NA ], laryngopharyngeal branches of superior cervical ganglion.

**rami latera'les** [ NA ], lateral branches (of the umbilical part of left branch of portal vein).

**r. latera'lis** [ NA ], lateral branch (of the branch of the middle lobe of right pulmonary artery; of dorsal branches of cervical nerves; of dorsal branches of lumbar nerves; of left hepatic duct; of supraorbital nerve).

**rami liena'les** [ NA ], lienal or splenic branches of lienal, or splenic, artery.

**rami lingua'les** [ NA ], lingual branches (of hypoglossal nerve; of lingual nerve).

**r. lingua'lis** [ NA ], lingual branch (inconstant) of the facial nerve.

**r. lingula'ris** [ NA ], lingular branch (of left pulmonary artery; of left pulmonary ven).

**r. lingula'ris infe'rior** [ NA ], inferior lingular branch (of lingular branch of left pulmonary artery).

**r. lingula'ris supe'rior** [ NA ], superior lingular branch (of lingular branch of left pulmonary artery).

**r. lo'bi me'dii** [ NA ], branch of the middle lobe (of the right pulmonary artery; of the right superior pulmonary vein).

**r. lumba'lis** [ NA ], lumbar branch of iliolumbar artery.

**rami malleola'res latera'les** [ NA ], lateral malleolar branches of peroneal artery.

**rami malleola'res media'les** [ NA ], medial malleolar branches of posterior tibial artery.

**rami mamma'rii** [ NA ], mammary branches (of lateral cutaneous branch of posterior intercostal arteries III to XI; of perforating branches of internal thoracic artery).

**rami mamma'rii latera'les** [ NA ], lateral mammary branches (of lateral thoracic artery; of intercostal nerve).

**rami mamma'rii media'les** [ NA ], medial mammary branches of thoracic nerve.

**r. mandib'ulae** [ NA ], r. of the mandible; the upturned perpendicular extremity of the mandible on either side; it gives attachment on its lateral surface to the masseter muscle.

**r. margina'lis mandib'ulae** [ NA ], marginal branch of the mandible (of facial nerve).

**rami mastoi'dei** [ NA ], mastoid branches of posterior auricular artery.

**r. mastoi'deus** [ NA ], mastoid branch of occipital artery.

**rami media'les** [ NA ], medial branches of umbilical part of left branch of portal vein.

**r. media'lis** [ NA ], medial branch (of branch of the middle lobe of right pulmonary artery; of dorsal branches of cervical nerves; of dorsal branches of lumbar nerves; of left hepatic duct; of supraorbital nerve).

**rami mediastina'les** [ NA ], mediastinal branches (of internal thoracic artery; of thoracic aorta).

**r. membra'nae tym'pani** [ NA ], nerve of the tympanic membrane; a branch of the auriculotemporal nerve supplying the tympanic membrane.

**r. meninge'us** [ NA ]meningeal branch (of occipital artery; of vertebral artery).

**r. meninge'us accesso'rius** [ NA ], accessory meningeal branch of middle meningeal artery.

**r. meninge'us (me'dius) ner'vi maxilla'ris** [ NA ], meningeal branch of maxillary nerve; a small branch that supplies the meninges of the middle cranial fossa.

**r. meninge'us ner'vi mandibula'ris** [ NA ], meningeal branch of the mandibular nerve; nervus spinosus; recurrent nerve; a small branch of the mandibular that reenters the skull through the foramen spinosum to supply the meninges.

**r. meninge'us nervo'rum spina'lium** [ NA ], meningeal branch of spinal nerves; sinuvertebral nerve; a small filament or plexus that passes from the proximal part of each spinal nerve back through the intervertebral foramen to supply the spinal meninges, ligaments and periosteum within the vertebral canal.

**r. meninge'us nervi va'gi** [ NA ], meningeal r. of the vagus nerve; recurrent branch of the vagus; a branch from the superior ganglion of the vagus to supply the dura mater of the posterior cranial fossa.

**rami menta'les** [ NA ], mental branches of mental nerve.

**rami muscula'res** [ NA ], branches of nerves or vessels that supply the muscles.

**r. mus'culi stylopharyn'gei** [ NA ], branch to the stylopharyngeal muscle (of the glossopharyngeal nerve).

**r. mylohyoi'deus** [ NA ], branch to the mylohyoid muscle (of maxillary artery).

**rami nasa'les** [ NA ], nasal branches of anterior ethmoidal nerve.

**rami nasa'les exter'ni** [ NA ], external nasal branches (of infraorbital nerve; of nasociliary nerve).

**rami nasa'les inter'ni** [ NA ], internal nasal branches (of infraorbital nerve; of nasociliary nerve).

**rami nasa'les latera'les** [ NA ], lateral nasal branches of nasociliary nerve.

**rami nasa'les media'les** [ NA ], medial nasal branches of nasociliary nerve.

**rami nasa'les posterio'res inferio'res latera'les** [ NA ], lateral inferior posterior nasal branches of pterygopalatine ganglion.

**rami nasa'les posterio'res superio'res latera'les** [ NA ], lateral superior posterior nasal branches of pterygopalatine ganglion.

**rami nasa'les posterio'res superio'res media'les** [ NA ], medial superior posterior nasal branches of major palatine nerve of pterygopalatine ganglion.

**r. obturato'rius** [ NA ], obturator branch of pubic branch of inferior epigastric artery.

**rami occipita'les** [ NA ], occipital branches (of cortical branches of posterior cerebral artery; of occipital artery).

**r. occipita'lis** [ NA ], occipital branch (of posterior auricular artery; of posterior auricular nerve).

**rami orbita'les** [ NA ], orbital branches (of anterior cerebral artery; of middle cerebral artery; of pterygopalatine ganglion).

**r. os'sis is'chii** [ NA ], branch of the ischial bone; formerly called inferior branch of the ischium; the portion of the bone that passes forward from the ischial tuberosity to join the inferior r. of the pubic bone.

**r. ova'ricus** [ NA ], ovarian branch of uterine artery.

**r. palma'ris ner'vi media'ni** [ NA ], palmar branch of median nerve.

**r. palma'ris ner'vi ulna'ris** [ NA ], palmar branch of ulnar nerve.

**r. palma'ris profun'dus arte'riae ulna'ris** [ NA ], deep palmar branch of the ulnar artery; it supplies the hypothenar muscles then passes deep into the palm to the flexor

tendons and anastomoses with the deep palmar arch from the radial artery.

**r. palma'ris superficia'lis arte'riae radia'lis** [ NA ], superficial palmar branch of radial artery; it supplies the thenar muscles then enters the palm to communicate with the superficial palmar arch from the ulnar artery.

**rami palpebra'les** [ NA ], palpebral branches of infratrochlear nerve.

**rami pancreat'ici** [ NA ], pancreatic branches (of lienal artery; of superior pancreaticoduodenal arteries).

**rami parieta'les** [ NA ], parietal branches (of anterior cerebral artery; of middle cerebral artery; of middle meningeal artery).

**r. parieta'lis** [ NA ], parietal branch of superficial temporal artery.

**r. parietooccipita'lis** [ NA ], parietooccipital branch of cortical branches of posterior cerebral artery.

**rami parotide'i** [ NA ], parotid branches (of auriculotemporal nerve; of facial vein; of superficial temporal artery).

**rami pectora'les** [ NA ], pectoral branches of thoracoacromial artery.

**rami perforan'tes arte'riae metacarpa'lium palma'res** [ NA ], perforating branches of palmar metacarpal arteries; three small arteries that pass dorsally through the second, third, and fourth interosseous spaces from the deep palmar arch.

**rami perforan'tes arte'riae metatarsea'rum planta'res** [ NA ], perforating branches of plantar metatarsal arteries of lateral plantar artery; three branches of the plantar arch that passes dorsally through the second, third, and fourth interosseous spaces.

**r. per'forans** [ NA ], perforating branch of peroneal artery.

**rami perforan'tes** [ NA ], perforating branches (of internal thoracic artery; of palmar metacarpal arteries; of plantar metatarsal arteries).

**rami pericardi'aci aor'tae thora'cicae** [ NA ], pericardiac branches of thoracic aorta.

**r. pericardi'acus ner'vi phren'ici** [ NA ], pericardiac branch of phrenic nerve.

**rami perinea'les** [ NA ], perineal branches of posterior femoral cutaneous nerve.

**r. petro'sus** [ NA ], petrous branch of middle meningeal artery.

**rami pharyn'gei** [ NA ], pharyngeal branches (of ascending pharyngeal artery; of glossopharyngeal nerve; of inferior thyroid artery; of vagus nerve).

**r. pharyn'geus** [ NA ], Bock's nerve; nervus pharyngeus; pharyngeal branch of pterygopalatine ganglion.

**rami phrenicoabdomina'les** [ NA ], phrenicoabdominal branches of phrenic nerve.

**r. planta'ris profun'dus** [ NA ], deep plantar branch of arcuate artery.

**r. poste'rior** [ NA ], posterior branch (of great auricular nerve; of lateral sulcus; of left pulmonary artery; of obturator artery; of obturator nerve; of recurrent ulnar artery; of right branch of portal vein; of right hepatic duct; of right superior pulmonary vein; of superior thyroid artery; of left hepatic duct; of right branch of portal vein; of renal artery).

**r. poste'rior ascen'dens** [ NA ], ascending posterior branch of right pulmonary artery.

**r. poste'rior descen'dens** [ NA ], descending posterior branch of right pulmonary artery.

**r. profun'dus** [ NA ], deep branch (of lateral plantar nerve; of medial femoral circumflex artery; of medial plantar artery; of radial nerve; of superior gluteal artery; of ulnar nerve).

**r. profun'dus arte'ria scapula'ris descen'dens** [ NA ], r. profundus arteriae transversae colli (official alternative term); deep branch of the transverse artery of the neck.

**rami pterygoi'dei** [ NA ], pterygoid branches of middle meningeal artery.

**pubic rami,** see *os pubis.*

**pu'bicus arte'riae epigas'tricae inferio'ris** [ NA ], pubic branch of inferior epigastric artery; it communicates with pubic branch of obturator artery and frequently replaces obturator artery.

**r. pu'bicus arte'riae obturato'riae** [ NA ], pubic branch of obturator artery; *distribution,* inner part of pubic bone; *anastomoses,* pubic branch of inferior epigastric.

**rami pulmona'les** [ NA ], pulmonary branches of thoracic portion of autonomic system.

**rami rena'les ner'vi va'gi** [ NA ], renal branches of vagus nerve.

**r. rena'lis par'tis thora'cicae system'atis autono'mici** [ NA ], renal branch of thoracic portion of autonomic system.

**r. saphe'nus** [ NA ], saphenous branch of descending genicular artery.

**rami scrota'les anterio'res** [ NA ], anterior scrotal branches; *origin,* external pudendal arteries; *distribution,* skin of the scrotum.

**rami scrota'les posterio'res** [ NA ], posterior scrotal branches; *origin,* perineal branch of internal pudendal; *distribution,* skin of scrotum.

**r. sinis'ter** [ NA ], left branch (of portal vein; of proper hepatic artery).

**r. si'nus carot'ici ner'vi glossopharyn'gei** [ NA ], carotid sinus branch of the glossopharyngeal nerve; sinus nerve of Hering; an afferent branch of the glossopharyngeal nerve the peripheral endings of which are in the wall of the carotid sinus. The fibers of the nerve are activated by a rise in the intracarotid arterial pressure, and by their central connections with the medulla oblongata elicit a reflex vasodilation and decrease of the heart rate, both of which tend to lower the blood pressure. In its functional characteristics the sinus nerve is entirely comparable to the aortic nerve of Ludwig (depressor nerve).

**rami spina'les** [ NA ], spinal branches; (1) branches of the following arteries which supply the meninges and spinal cord: (a) vertebral, (b) ascending cervical, (c) dorsal branch of posterior intercostal I to XI (also called arteries of Adamkiewicz), (d) dorsal branch of subcostal, (e) dorsal branch of lumbar arteries, (f) lumbar branch of iliolumbar, (g) lateral sacral; (2) veins draining the meninges and spinal cord, tributaries of the intervertebral veins.

**r. stape'dius** [ NA ], stapedial branch of posterior tympanic artery.

**rami sterna'les** [ NA ], sternal branches of internal thoracic artery.

**rami ster'noclei'domastoi'dei** [ NA ], sternocleidomastoid branches of occipital artery.

**r. sternocleidomastoi'deus** [ NA ], sternocleidomastoid branch of superior thyroid artery.

**rami stria'ti arte'riae cer'ebri me'diae** [ NA ], striate branches of central branches of middle cerebral artery; lateral or medial striate arteries; *distribution,* internal capsule and basal ganglia.

**r. stylohyoi'deus** [ NA ], stylohyoid branch of facial nerve.

**r. subapica'lis** [ NA ]r. subsuperior [ NA ]; subapical or subsuperior branch (of basal part of left pulmonary artery; of basal part of right pulmonary artery).

**rami subscapula'res** [ NA ], subscapular branches of axillary artery.

**r. subsupe'rior** [ NA ], r. subapicalis.

**r. superficia'lis** [ NA ], superficial branch (of lateral plantar nerve; of medial plantar artery; of radial nerve; of superior gluteal artery; of ulnar nerve).

**r. superficia'lis arteriae transver'sae col'li** [ NA ], superficial branch of transverse artery of the neck; the official alternative term is arteria cervicalis superficialis.

**r. supe'rior** [ NA ], (1) superior branch (of deep branch of superior gluteal artery; of ischial bone; of oculomotor nerve; of pubic bone); (2) r. apicalis (1).

**r. superior lobi inferioris** [ NA ], official alternative term for r. apicalis lobi inferioris.

**rami superio'res ner'vi transver'si col'li** [ NA ], superior branches of transverse nerve of neck.

**r. suprahyoi'deus** [ NA ], suprahyoid branch of lingual artery.

**r. sympath'icus ad ganglion cilia're** [ NA ], sympathetic branch to ciliary ganglion.

**r. sympath'icus ad ganglion submandibula're** [ NA ], sympathetic branch to the submandibular ganglion.

**rami tempora'les** [ NA ], temporal branches (of facial nerve; of middle cerebral artery; of posterior cerebral artery).

**rami tempora'les superficia'les ner'vi auriculotempora'lis** [ NA ], superficial temporal branches of auriculotemporal nerve.

**r. tentor'ii** [ NA ], tentorial branch; nervus tentorii; tentorial nerve; a branch of the ophthalmic nerve supplying the tentorium.

**rami thy'mici** [ NA ], thymic branches of internal thoracic artery.

**r. thyrohyoi'deus** [ NA ], thyrohyoid branch; a branch of the cervical ansa containing fibers of the first and second cervical nerves that accompany the hypoglossal nerve, then branch from it to reach the thyrohyoid muscle.

**r. tonsilla'ris** [ NA ], tonsillar branch of facial artery.

**rami tonsilla'res** [ NA ], tonsillar branches of glossopharyngeal nerve.

**rami trachea'les** [ NA ], tracheal branches (of inferior thyroid artery; of recurrent laryngeal nerve).

**r. transver'sus** [ NA ], transverse branch (of lateral femoral circumflex artery; of medial femoral circumflex artery).

**r. tuba'rius** [ NA ], tubal branch (of tympanic nerve; of uterine artery).

**r. ulna'ris** [ NA ], ulnar branch of medial cutaneous nerve of forearm.

**rami ureter'ici** [ NA ], ureteral or ureteric branches (of artery of ductus deferens; of ovarian artery; of renal artery; of testicular artery).

**rami ventra'les (nervi intercosta'les) nervo'rum thora'cicum** [ NA ], ventral branches (intercostal nerves) of thoracic nerves.

**r. ventra'lis ner'vi spina'lis** [ NA ], ventral r. of a spinal nerve; anterior primary division; the major division of each spinal nerve that contributes to the innervation of the limbs and the anterolateral parts of the body wall; the major plexuses (cervical, brachial and lumbosacral) are formed by the ventral rami.

**rami ventra'les nervo'rum cervica'lium** [ NA ], ventral branches of cervical nerves.

**rami ventra'les nervo'rum lumba'lium** [ NA ], ventral branches of lumbar nerves.

**rami ventra'les nervorum sacra'lium** [ NA ], ventral branches of sacral nerves.

**rami vestibula'res** [ NA ], vestibular branches of labyrinthine artery.

**rami zygomat'ici** [ NA ], zygomatic branches of facial nerve.

**r. zygomaticofacia'lis** [ NA ], zygomaticofacial branch of zygomatic nerve.

**r. zygomaticotempora'lis** [ NA ], zygomaticotemporal branch of zygomatic nerve.

---

**ramy'cin.** Fusidic acid.

**Rana** (ra'nah) [ L. frog ]. The frogs; a genus of the family Ranidae, order Salienta.

**rancid** (ran'sid) [ L. *rancidus,* stinking, rank ]. Having a disagreeable odor and taste, usually characterizing fat that is undergoing oxidation or bacterial decomposition to more volatile, odiferous substances.

**rancidify** (ran-sid'ĭ-fi). To make or become rancid.

**rancidity** (ran-sid'ĭ-tĭ). State of being rancid.

**Rand,** M. J. See Burn and R. *theory.*

**Raney Nickel.** Raney catalyst; proprietary name for a finely powdered nickel catalyst made from Raney alloy (*q.v.,* under alloy) by dissolving out the aluminum by means of alkali; used in the hydrogenation of organic substances.

**range.** A statistical measure of the dispersion or variation of values determined by the endpoint values; *e.g.,* in a group of children aged 6, 8, 9, 10, 13, and 16, the r. would be 10 (16 minus 6).

**Ranidae** (ran'ĭ-de) [ Mod. L. fr. L. *rana,* a frog ]. Family of frogs.

**ran'imy'cin** (USAN). An antibiotic produced by *Streptomyces lincolnensis.*

**ranine** (ra'nĭn) [ L. *rana,* a frog ]. 1. Relating to the frog. 2. Relating to the undersurface of the tongue.

**Ran'ke,** H. Rudolph, Dutch anatomist, 1849–1887. See R.'s *angle.*

**Ran'ke,** Karl E. von, German chemist, 1870–1926. See R.'s *formula.*

**Rankin,** Fred Wharton, U. S. surgeon, 1886–1954. See R.'s *clamp.*

**Rankine scale.** See under scale.

**Ransohoff,** Joseph, American surgeon, 1853–1921. See R.'s *sign.*

**ranula** (ran'u-lah) [ L. tadpole, dim. of *rana,* frog ]. 1. Hypoglottis. 2. Sublingual cyst or ptyalocele; a cystic tumor of the floor of the mouth, due to obstruction of the duct of the sublingual glands; any cystic tumor of the undersurface of the tongue or floor of the mouth.

  **r. pancreat'ica,** a cystic tumor caused by obstruction of the pancreatic duct.

**ran'ular.** Relating to a ranula.

**Ranvier** (roṅ-ve-a'), Louis A., French pathologist, 1835–1922. See R.'s *crosses, disks, node, plexus, segment.*

**Raoult** (rah-ol'), François, M., French physicist, 1830–1899. See R.'s *law.*

**rape** (rāp) [ L. *rapio,* to seize, to drag away ]. 1. To ravish, to perform the act of raping. 2. Sexual intercourse with a woman by force or without her legal consent.

**rape'seed** [ L. *rapio,* turnip ]. The seed of *Brassica campestris* (family *Cruciferae*).

  **r. oil,** the compressed oil of rapeseeds; used in the manufacture of soaps, margarine, and lubricants.

**raphania** (rā-fa'nĭ-ah). Rhaphania; a spasmodic disease supposed to be due to poisoning by the seeds of *Rhaphanus rhaphanistrum,* or wild radish.

**raphe** (raf'e) [ G. *rhaphē,* suture, seam. RHAPH- ] [ NA ]. The line of union of two contiguous, bilaterally symmetrical structures.

  **amniotic r.,** the line of fusion of the amniotic folds over the embryo in reptiles, birds and certain mammals.

  **r. anococcyge'a,** *ligamentum* anococcygeum.

  **anogenital r.,** in the male embryo the line of closure of the genital folds and swellings extending from the anus to the tip of the penis; it is differentiated in the adult into three regions: perineal r., scrotal r., and penile r.

  **r. cor'poris callo'si,** a slight anteroposterior furrow on the median line of the upper surface of the corpus callosum.

  **r. lin'guae,** *sulcus* medianus linguae.

  **median longitudinal r. of tongue.** *sulcus* medianus linguae.

  **r. medul'lae oblonga'tae** [ NA ], the seamlike median zone of the medulla oblongata, marked by intercrossing fiber bundles among which lie scattered neuronal cell bodies.

  **r. nuclei,** see *nuclei* raphes.

  **r. pala'ti** [ NA ], palatine r.; palatine ridge; a rather narrow, low elevation in the center of the hard palate that extends from the incisive papilla posteriorly over the entire length of the hard palate.

  **r. palpebra'lis latera'lis** [ NA ], lateral palpebral r.; lateral tarsal ligament; a narrow fibrous band attached to the zygomatic bone and to the margins of the upper and lower tarsi.

  **r. pe'nis** [ NA ], the continuation of the r. of the scrotum onto the under side of the penis.

  **r. perine'i** [ NA ], the central anteroposterior line of the perineum, most marked in the male, being continuous with the r. of the scrotum.

  **r. pharyn'gis** [ NA ], the central line of the pharynx posteriorly where the muscular fibers meet and partly interlace.

  **r. pon'tis** [ NA ], the continuation of the r. medullae oblongatae into the pars dorsalis (or tegmentum) pontis.

  **r. pterygomandibula'ris** [ NA ], pterygomandibular ligament; a tendinous thickening of the buccopharyngeal fascia, separating the buccinator muscle from the superior constrictor of the pharynx.

  **r. scro'ti** [ NA ], a central line, like a cord, running over the scrotum from the anus to the root of the penis; it marks the position of the septum scroti.

  **Stilling's r.,** the transverse interdigitations of fiber bundles across the anterior median fissure of the medulla oblongata at the decussation of the pyramidal tracts.

**rapport** (rap-or') [ Fr. ]. A feeling of relationship, especially when characterized by emotional affinity.

**rapture of the deep.** A psychosis seen in deep-sea divers and others subjected to sensory deprivation and disorientation, and excessive blood levels of nitrogen.

**rap'tus** [ L. ]. Any sudden, violent seizure or attack.

  **r. mani'acus,** a violent attack of overactivity.

  **r. melanchol'icus,** an attack of extreme agitation or frenzy occurring in the course of depression.

  **r. nervo'rum,** a sudden violent attack of nervousness or anxiety.

**rarefaction** (rār'e-fak'shun) [ L. *rarus,* thin, + *facio,* to make ]. Expansion; the process of becoming light or less dense; the condition of being light; opposed to condensation.

**rarefy** (rār'e-fi). To become light or less dense.

**RAS.** Abbreviation for reticular activating *system.*

**rasceta** (rā-se'tah) [ Mod. L. *raseta,* fr. Ar. *rāhah,* palm of hand ]. The transverse wrinkling on the anterior surface of the wrist.

**Rasch,** Hermann, German obstetrician, *1873. See R.'s *sign.*

**rash** [ O. Fr. *rasche,* skin eruption, fr. L. *rado,* pp. *rasus,* to scratch, scrape ]. Lay term for a cutaneous eruption.

  **ammonia r.,** diaper *dermatitis.*

  **an'iline r.,** a dermatitis due to aniline.

  **antitox'in r.,** a serum r. following an injection of antitoxin.

  **ast'acoid r.,** a r., massive exfoliation, sometimes occurring in malignant smallpox, the color of which resembles that of a boiled lobster.

  **black currant r.,** that seen in xeroderma pigmentosa.

  **butterfly r.,** butterfly (2).

  **cable r.,** a popular r. due to irritation by halowax (β-chlornaphthalene) used to waterproof cables.

  **canker r.,** scarlatina.

  **caterpillar r.,** caterpillar *dermatitis.*

  **crystal r.,** *miliaria* crystallina.

  **diaper r.,** diaper *dermatitis.*

  **drug r.,** drug *eruption.*

  **enema r.,** a generalized erythema, with pruritus, sometimes occurring after the administration of a soapsuds enema.

  **flannel r.,** pityriasis or dermatitis seborrheica of the chest and back.

  **gum r.,** *miliaria* rubra.

  **heat r.,** *miliaria* rubra.

  **hydatid r.,** toxic eruption following occasionally on rupture of hydatid cyst.

  **lily r.,** a form of dermatitis affecting flower pickers, especially those handling daffodils and narcissuses; it is a papular, vesicular, or pustular eruption on an erythematous base.

  **medicinal r.,** drug *eruption.*

  **mulberry r.,** a morbilliform r. occasionally seen in typhus fever.

  **napkin r.,** diaper *dermatitis.*

  **nettle r.,** urticaria.

  **rose r.,** roseola.

  **rose r. of children,** *exanthema* subitum.

  **scarlet r.,** (1) roseola; (2) scarlatina.

  **serum r.,** cutaneous manifestation of serum disease.

  **summer r.,** *miliaria* rubra.

  **tooth r.,** *miliaria* rubra.

  **wandering r.,** geographical *tongue.*

  **wildfire r.,** *miliaria* rubra.

**rasion** (ra'zhun) [ L. *rasio,* a scraping, fr. *rado,* pp. *rasus,* to scrape, shave ]. The subdivision of a crude drug by a rasp to prepare it for extraction.

**Rasmussen,** Fritz W., Danish physician, 1834–1881. See R.'s *aneurysm.*

**raspatory** (ras'pă-tōr'ĭ) [ L. *raspatorium* ]. An instrument used for scraping a bone.

**raspberry** (raz'bĕr-ĭ). The fruit of *Rubis idaeus* or *R. strigosus* (family Rosaceae).

  **r. juice,** the juice expressed from the fresh ripe fruit; a flavoring agent.

**rat.** A rodent of the genus *Rattus* (family Muridae), involved in the spread of diseases, including bubonic plague. There are more species of r.'s than of any other genus of mammals; several species are frequently found in or near human habitations.

  **albino r.,** one with white fur and pink eyes; used extensively in laboratory experiments.

  **black r.,** *Rattus rattus.*

**Wistar r.'s,** a well known line of white r.'s developed at the Wistar Institute for use in experimental biology and medicine.

**rate** (rāt) [ L. *ratum,* a reckoning (see ratio) ]. Record of the measurement of an event or process in terms of its relation to some fixed standard; measurement expressed as the ratio of one quantity to another (*e.g.,* velocity, which is distance per unit time).

**abortion r.,** the number of abortions per 1000 terminated pregnancies during a given period of time.

**basal metabolic r.,** basal *metabolism.*

**birth r.,** the precise number of births for a year related to an exact population and place.

**critical r.,** a heart r. at which aberration or incomplete block will occur; a result of shortening of cycle length so that it barely includes the refractory period.

**death r.,** mortality r.

**erythrocyte sedimentation r.,** ESR; the rate of settling of red blood cells in anticoagulated blood. Since many factors influence the erythrocyte sedimentation r., it is important to utilize a standardized test method such as that of Wintrobe and Landsberg or of Westergren. Increased rates are often associated with anemia or inflammatory states in the individual tested.

**fatality r.,** mortality r.

**glomerular filtration r.,** abbreviated GFR; the volume of water filtered out of the plasma through glomerular capillary walls into Bowman's capsules per unit time; it is considered to be equivalent to inulin clearance.

**growth r.,** absolute or relative growth increase, expressed in units of time.

**heart r.,** r. of the heart's beat, invariably recorded as the number of beats per minute.

**lethality r.,** mortality r.

**maternal death r.,** the number of maternal deaths that occur as the direct result of the reproductive process per 100,000 live births; see also maternal *death.*

**morbidity r.,** the proportion of patients with a particular disease during a given year per given unit of population.

**mortality r.,** death r., fatality r.; lethality r.; the ratio of the total number of deaths to the total population of a given community, usually expressed as deaths per 1000, 10,000, or 100,000 population.

**pulse r.,** r. of the pulse as observed in an artery; invariably recorded as beats per minute.

**repetition r.,** the number of pulses per minute.

**respiration r.,** frequency of breathing, recorded as the number of breaths per minute.

**sedimentation r.,** see under sedimentation.

**shear r.,** the change in velocity of parallel planes in a flowing fluid separated by unit distance; units: seconds$^{-1}$.

**steroid metabolic clearance r.,** a measure of the r. of metabolism of a given steroid within the body, usually expressed as liters per day; abbreviated MCR.

**steroid production r.,** the total quantity of a given steroid formed in the body, usually expressed as milligrams per day; represents the sum of the glandular secretion of the steroid and extraglandular formation of it from various steroid precursors.

**steroid secretory r.,** the r. of glandular secretion of a given steroid, usually expressed as milligrams per day; does not include any amount of the steroid that might be formed extraglandularly.

**rat-fish.** Chimera (5).

**Rathke** (raht′keh), Martin H., German anatomist, 1793–1860. See R.'s cleft *cyst,* R.'s *diverticulum, pocket, pouch,* R.'s pouch *tumor.*

**ratio** (ra′shĭ-o) [ L. *ratio* (*ration-*) a reckoning, reason, fr. *reor,* pp. *ratus,* to reckon, compute ]. Proportion; rate; an expression of the relation of one quantity to another. See also index and quotient.

**absolute terminal innervation r.,** the number of motor endplates divided by the number of terminal axons related to them.

**AC/A r.,** the r. of accommodative convergence to accommodation, expressed as the quotient of accommodative convergence in prism diopters divided by the accommodate response in diopters.

**A/G r.,** abbreviation for albumin-globulin r.

**albumin-globulin r.,** abbreviated A/G r.; the r. of albumin to globulin in the serum or in the urine in kidney disease; the normal r. in the serum is approximately 1.55.

**body-weight r.,** body weight (in grams) divided by stature (in centimeters).

**cardiothoracic r.,** the transverse diameter of the heart by x-ray compared with that of the thoracic cage.

**cell-color r.,** a figure obtained by dividing the number of red blood cells in a cubic millimeter (5,000,000 being the normal) by the percentage of hemoglobin.

**D:N r.,** dextrose to nitrogen r.; see G:N r.

**extraction r.,** abbreviated E; the fraction of a substance removed from the blood flowing through the kidney; it is calculated from the formula $(A - V)/A$, where $A$ and $V$, respectively, are the concentrations of the substance in arterial and renal venous plasma.

**flux r.,** the r. of the two unidirectional fluxes through a particular boundary layer or membrane.

**functional terminal innervation r.,** the number of muscle fibers divided by the number of axons that innervate them.

**G:N r.,** glucose to nitrogen r.; D:N r. (dextrose to nitrogen r.); the r. of glucose to nitrogen in the urine in diabetes; it has a value of approximately 3.65.

**hand r.,** the r. of the length of the hand (measured on the dorsum from the styloid process of the ulna to the tip of the third finger) to the width across the knuckles.

**K:A r.,** abbreviation for ketogenic-antiketogenic r.

**ketogen′ic-an′tiketogen′ic r.,** the proportion between substances that form ketones in the body and those that form glucose.

**Mendelian r.,** the r. of contrasting phenotypes or genotypes expected in accordance with genetic principles among the offspring of matings specified as to genotype.

**nuclear-cytoplasmic r.,** r. of volume of nucleus to volume of cytoplasm; the nuclear-cytoplasmic r. is fairly constant for a particular cell type, and is usually increased in malignant neoplasms.

**nutritive r.,** the ratio or proportion of digestible protein to digestible non-nitrogenous nutrients in a ration for livestock.

**P/O r.,** the r. of phosphate radicals esterified (to form adenosine triphosphate from adenosine diphosphate) to atoms of oxygen consumed by mitochondria; normally, the r. is 3.

**respiratory exchange r.,** symbol R; the r. of the net output of carbon dioxide to the simultaneous net uptake of oxygen at a given site, both expressed as moles or STPD volumes per unit time; in the steady state, respiratory exchange r. is equal to the respiratory quotient (*q.v.*) of metabolic processes.

**therapeutic r.,** the r. of the maximally tolerated dose of a drug to the minimal curative or effective dose; LD$_{50}$ divided by ED$_{50}$.

**rational** (rash′un-al) [ L. *rationalis,* fr. *ratio,* reason ]. 1. Pertaining to reasoning or to the higher thought processes. 2. Influenced by reasoning rather than by emotion. 3. Having the reasoning faculties; not delirious or comatose.

**rationalization** (ra̤-shun-al-i-za′shun) [ L. *ratio,* reason ]. In psychoanalysis, a postulated defense mechanism through which irrational behavior, motives, or feelings are made to appear reasonable.

**rats′bane.** Arsenic.

**rat′tlesnake.** See *Crotalus.*

**Rat′tus.** The rats, a genus of rodents, family Muridae; see rat.

**R. hawaiien′sis,** a species inhabiting Hawaii, responsible for the spread of rodent plague there.

**R. rat′tus,** black r.; the rat most commonly responsible for transmitting plague to man by means of its flea, *Xenopsylla cheopis;* it is smaller and darker in color than the brown rat (*Rattus norvegicus*) and has longer ears and tail.

**Rau** (row), Johann J., Dutch anatomist, 1668–1719. See R.'s *process.*

**Rauber** (row′ber), August A., German anatomist, 1845–1917. See R.'s *layer.*

**rauschbrand** (rowsh′brahnt) [ Ger. ]. Blackleg or symptomatic anthrax.

**Rauwolf,** Leonhard, German botanist, 16th century. Gave his name to *Rauwolfia.*

**Rauwolfia** (row-wŏŏl'fĭ-ah, raw-, rah-) [ L. *Rauwolf*]. A genus of the family Apocyanaceae, dogbane.

    **R. root,** the powdered whole root of *Rauwolfia serpentina;* the component alkaloids produce the sedative-antihypertensive-bradycrotic action. Approximately 50 per cent of the total activity is due to reserpine.

    **R. serpentina** (NF), yields the hypotensive principle reserpine; it has been used for centuries in India for various medicinal purposes, and is now extensively used as a hypotensive and sedative.

**Ravius.** Latinized form of Rau. See Rau's *process; processus* ravii.

**Ray,** Isaac, 1807–1881, pioneer U. S. forensic psychiatrist.

**ray** [ L. *radius*]. 1. A line of light, heat, or other form of radiation. The r.'s from radium and other radioactive substances are produced by a spontaneous disintegration of the atom; they are material particles, electrically charged, or electromagnetic waves of extremely short wavelength. 2. A part or line that extends radially from a structure.

    **actin'ic r.,** a light r. toward and beyond the violet end of the spectrum that acts upon a photograph plate and produces other chemical effects.

    **alpha r.'s,** fast-moving streams of minute particles of matter consisting of helium nuclei, containing two protons and two neutrons, and consequently carrying a double positive charge, emitted from radioactive bodies with enormous velocity; they have less penetrative power than beta r.'s, and like them are deflected by a magnet.

    **anode r.'s,** positive r.'s; those originating in a gas discharge tube and moving in a direction opposite to that of cathode r.'s; made up of positively charged ions.

    **Becquerel r.'s,** radiations given off by uranium and other radioactive substances; discovered first by Henri Becquerel; these include alpha, beta, and gamma r.'s.

    **beta r.'s,** electrons emitted with great velocity in radioactive decomposition; they have properties identical with the cathode r.'s emitted from a Crookes tube; they have greater penetrative power than the alpha r.'s, and like them are deflected by a magnet.

    **borderline r.'s,** grenz r.'s; very soft x-r.'s, closely allied to the ultraviolet r.'s in their wavelength and in their biologic action upon tissues; they are produced by an especially built vacuum tube with a hot cathode operating from a transformer delivering not more than 8 kw.

    **Bucky's r.'s,** borderline r.'s.

    **canal r.'s,** r.'s observed back of the cathode in a Crookes tube; they are analogous to the alpha r.'s but of much lower velocity.

    **cathode r.'s,** a stream of electrons emitted from the negative electrode (cathode) in a Crookes tube; their bombardment of the glass wall of the tube or of the anode gives rise to the x-r.'s or roentgen r.'s.

    **chemical r.,** actinic r.

    **cosmic r.'s,** high velocity particles of enormous energies, bombarding earth from outer space; the "primary radiation" consists of protons and more complex atomic nuclei, which on striking the atmosphere give rise to neutrons, mesons, and other less energetic "secondary radiation."

    **direct r.'s,** primary r.'s (2).

    **Dorno r.'s,** the ultraviolet r.'s with wavelengths below 289 m$\mu$; those biologically active.

    **dynamic r.'s,** physically or therapeutically active r.'s.

    **gamma r.'s,** electromagnetic radiation emitted from radioactive substances; analogous to the x-r.'s but originate from the nucleus rather than the orbital shell and are not deflected by a magnet.

    **glass r.'s,** those formed by cathode r.'s striking the wall of an x-ray tube.

    **grenz r.** (grents) [ Ger. borderline, boundary ], long wavelength x-ray; borderline r.

    **H r.'s,** a stream of hydrogen nuclei; *i.e.,* protons.

    **hard r.'s,** r.'s of short wavelength and great penetrability.

    **Hertzian r.'s,** radio waves.

    **incident r.,** the r. that strikes the surface before reflection.

    **indirect r.'s,** x-r.'s generated at the surface of the glass of the tube.

    **infrared r.,** see infrared.

    **intermediate r.'s,** those between ultraviolet and x-rays.

    **ion'ic r.'s,** alpha r.'s.

    **medullary r.,** *pars* radiata lobuli corticalis renis.

    **monochromatic r.'s,** light r.'s of a very narrow band of wavelengths (ideally, of a single wavelength).

    **Niewenglowski r.'s,** radiation emitted from a phosphorescent body after exposure to sunlight.

    **parallel r.'s,** r.'s parallel to the axis of an optical system.

    **positive r.'s,** anode r.'s.

    **primary r.'s,** (1) cosmic r.'s in the form in which they first strike the atmosphere; (2) x-r.'s generated at the focal point of the tube.

    **reflected r.,** a r. of light or other form of radiant energy which is thrown back from a nonpermeable or nonabsorbing surface; the r. which strikes the surface before reflection is the incident r.

    **roentgen r.'s,** x-r.'s.

    **Sagnac r.'s,** secondary r.'s produced when x-r.'s or gamma r.'s impinge upon the surface of any body; they resemble or are identical with the beta r.'s.

    **Schumann r.'s,** r.'s of various wavelengths between 1850 and 1230 Å.

    **secondary r.'s,** r.'s generated when primary r.'s impinge upon matter.

    **soft r.'s,** r.'s of relatively long wavelength and slight penetrability.

    **supersonic r.'s,** r.'s with a wavelength higher than that perceptible to the human ear, above 20,000 cycles per second.

    **transition r.'s,** borderline r.'s.

    **ultrasonic r.'s,** see ultrasonic.

    **ultravi'olet r.'s,** see ultraviolet.

    **W r.'s,** intermediate r.'s.

    **x-r.'s,** the electromagnetic radiation emitted from a highly evacuated tube, excited by the bombardment of the target anode with a stream of electrons from a heated cathode.

**rayage** (ra'ej). The dosage in radiotherapeutics.

**Rayer** (ra-yär'), Pierre F., French physician, 1793–1867. See R.'s *disease.*

**Raygat's test.** See under test.

**Rayleigh,** Lord John W. S., English physicist, 1842–1919. See R. *test.*

**Raymond** (ra-mon'), Fulgence, French neurologist, 1844–1910. See R. type of *apoplexy.*

**Raynaud** (ra-no'), Maurice, Paris physician, 1834–1881. See R.'s *disease, phenomenon.*

**Raynier's white mycetoma.** See under mycetoma.

**Rb.** Chemical symbol of the element rubidium.

**rbc, RBC.** Abbreviation for red blood *cells.*

**RBF.** Abbreviation for renal blood flow; see effective renal blood *flow.*

**R.C.P.** Abbreviation for Royal College of Physicians (England).

**R.C.P.E.** Abbreviation for Royal College of Physicians (Edinburgh).

**R.C.S.** Abbreviation for Royal College of Surgeons (England).

**R.C.S.I.** Abbreviation for Royal College of Surgeons (Ireland).

**RD.** Abbreviation for reaction of *degeneration.*

**Re.** Chemical symbol of the element rhenium.

**R.E.** Abbreviation for right eye.

**re-.** Prefix fr. L. meaning again or backward.

**react** (re-akt) [ Mod. L. *reactus.* ACT- ]. To take part in or to undergo a chemical reaction.

**reactance** (re-ak'tans). Inductive resistance; the weakening of an alternating electric current by passage through a coil of wire or a condenser; symbol X.

**reactant** (re-ak'tant). A substance taking part in a chemical reaction.

# REACTION

**reaction** (re-ak'shun) [ L. prefix *re-,* again, backward, + *actio,* action. ACT- ]. 1. The response of a muscle or other living tissue to a stimulus. 2. The color change effected in litmus and certain other organic pigments by contact with various substances (acids or alkalies); also the property that such substances possess of producing this change. 3. In chemistry, the intermolecular action of two or more substances upon each other, whereby these substances are caused to disappear, new ones being formed in their place (chemical reaction).

**Abderhalden's r.,** Abderhalden's *test.*

**accelerated r.,** vaccinoid r.

**acid r.,** (1) the change of blue litmus paper to red, indicating that the liquid or gas with which it is brought into contact is acid; (2) an excess of hydrogen ions over hydroxide ions in aqueous solution indicated by a pH value less than 7.

**Adamkiewicz' protein r.,** various protein solutions are stained violet by a mixture of concentrated sulfuric acid 1 and glacial acetic acid 2 and, when diluted, show an absorption band between green and blue in the spectrum.

**alarm r.,** the various phenomena, *e.g.,* stimulated endocrine activity, which the body exhibits as an adaptive response to injury or stress; first phase of the general adaptation syndrome.

**aldehyde r.,** Ehrlich r.; the r. of the indole derivatives with aromatic aldehydes (*e.g.,* tryptophan and *p*-dimethylaminobenaldehyde in $H_2SO_4$ give a red-violet color useful in assaying proteins for tryptophan content).

**al'kaline r.,** (1) the change of red litmus paper to blue, indicating that the liquid or gas with which the paper is brought in contact is alkaline; (2) an excess of hydroxyl ions in aqueous solution as indicated by a pH value greater than 7.

**allergic r.,** a local or general r. of the organism to contact, internal or external, with a specific allergen to which the subject has been previously sensitized; synonymous with immune r. in smallpox vaccination; more specifically, allergic r. refers to the idiosyncratic type of immune (sensitivity) r., (*e.g.* hay fever, urticaria, food sensitivity) associated with the Prausnitz-Küstner (IgE class) antibody.

Gell and Coombs classify allergic r.'s as follows: *type I,* those resulting from antigen (allergen) combining with cell-fixed, cytophilic antibody—anaphylaxis and r.'s associated with Prausnitz-Küstner (IgE) antibodies; see idiosyncrasy (2); *type II,* those resulting from specific, noncytophilic antibody combining with cellular antigen or cell-fixed antigen (or hapten) and frequently, but not always, requiring complement—cytotoxic r.'s; *type III,* those resulting from deposition of antigen-antibody complexes in or around the small blood vessels, in blood vessel walls basement membranes (*e.g.,* such as occurs in the Arthus phenomenon); *type IV,* those associated with infiltration of mononuclear cells after injection of antigen (allergen)—skin r.'s (see skin *test*) of the delayed kind.

**amphoteric r.,** a double r. possessed by certain fluids, such as freshly drawn milk, which turns blue litmus paper red and red litmus paper blue.

**anamnestic r.,** augmented production of an antibody due to previous response of the subject to stimulus by the same antigen.

**anergastic r.,** a psychosis related to organic brain injury.

**anterior pituitary r.'s,** abbreviated APR; obsolete r.'s: (1) APR I, the finding of mature but unruptured follicles in ovaries of mice in the Ascheim-Zondek test; (2) APR II, the finding of hemorrhagic follicles (*Blutpunkte*) in the Ascheim-Zondek test; (3) APR III, the development of corpora lutea in the Ascheim-Zondek test.

**antigen-antibody r.,** the phenomenon of antibody combining with antigen of the type that stimulated the formation of the antibody, thereby resulting in agglutination, precipitation, complement-fixation, greater susceptibility to ingestion and destruction by phagocytes, or neutralization of exotoxin; may occur *in vitro* or *in vivo.* See also skin *test.*

**anxiety r.,** a psychological r. or experience involving the apprehension of danger accompanied by a feeling of dread and such physical symptoms as restlessness and tachycardia, in the absence of a clearly identifiable fear stimulus; when chronic, it is called anxiety neurosis.

**arousal r.,** change in pattern of the brain waves when the subject is suddenly awakened and becomes alert.

**Arthus r.,** Arthus *phenomenon.*

**Ascoli r.,** a method for confirming the diagnosis of anthrax by means of a precipitin r.; material from a dead animal (*e.g.,* spleen or hide) is boiled for 5 to 10 min. in physiologic saline solution, cooled, filtered, and carefully layered over antiserum from a rabbit previously immunized with encapsulated *Bacillus anthracis,* a zone of precipitate at the interface of the fluid indicates the presence of heat-stable *B. anthracis* antigen (probably specific capsular polypeptide) in the extracted tissue. See also miostagmin r.

**associative r.,** a secondary or side r.

**Beierinck's r.,** cholera-red r.

**Bence Jones r.,** the classic means of identifying Bence Jones protein, which *precipitates* when urine (from patients with this type of proteinuria) is gradually warmed to 45 to 70°C. and *redissolves* as the urine is heated to near boiling; as the specimen cools, the Bence Jones protein *precipitates* in the indicated range of temperature, and *redissolves* as the temperature of the specimen becomes less than 30 to 35°C. See also Bence Jones *protein.*

**bi-bi r.,** a r. catalyzed by a single enzyme in which two substrates and two products are involved. The ping-pong mechanism (*q.v.,* under mechanism) may be involved in such a r.

**Bittorf's r.,** in cases of renal colic the pain on squeezing the testicle or pressing the ovary radiates to the kidney.

**biuret r.,** a r. for polypeptides (from tripeptides to proteins) based upon the formation of biuret ($NH_2CONH$-$CONH_2$), which gives a violet color with $CuSO_4$ in strongly alkaline solution. Dipeptides and amino acids (except histidine, serine, and threonine) do not so react. The b.r. is used to detect and to quantitate protein.

**Bloch's r.,** dopa r.

**Brahn r.,** the increased absorption of water through the skin of the frog when the animal is injected with pituitrin and immersed in water.

**Brieger's r.,** the r. by which is calculated the antitryptic index.

**Burchard-Liebermann r.,** acetic anhydride produces a blue-green color with cholesterol dissolved in chloroform, when a few drops of concentrated sulfuric acid are added.

**Cannizzaro's r.,** the formation of an acid and an alcohol by the simultaneous oxidation of one aldehyde molecule and reduction of another. A dismutation: 2 RCHO → RCOOH + RCH$_2$OH.

**catalatic r.,** decomposition of $H_2O_2$ to $O_2$ and $H_2O$, as in the action of catalase; analogous to peroxidatic r.

**catastrophic r.,** the disorganized behavior that is the response to a severe shock or threatening situation with which the person cannot cope.

**cell-mediated r.,** immunological r. of the delayed kind; see also skin *test.*

**chain r.,** a self-perpetuating r., because a product of one step in the r. itself serves to bring about the next step in the r., and so on until a stable product eventuates; *c.f.* autocatalysis.

**Chantemesse r.,** ophthalmoreaction, especially as applied to typhoid.

**cholera-red r.,** Beierinck's r.; Poehl's test; upon adding 3 or 4 drops of sulfuric acid (concentrated, chemically pure) to an 18-hour-old bouillon or peptone culture of the cholera vibrio, a color from rose-pink to claret is produced.

**circular r.,** in sensorimotor theory, the tendency of an organism to repeat novel experiences.

**cocarde r.,** see Romer's *test.*

**cockade r.,** see Römer's *test.*

**complement-fixation r.,** see complement fixation, under complement.

**conjunctival r.,** ophthalmoreaction; ophthalmic test; conjunctival test; r. analogous to a skin r. when specific antigen (allergen) is placed on the conjunctiva of a subject sensitive to the allergen, convalescent from the specific disease, or chronically infected.

**consensual r.,** indirect pupillary r.; consensual light reflex; contraction of the pupil of the shaded eye when light is directed into the other.

**constitutional r.,** a generalized r. in contrast to a focal or local r.; in allergy the immediate or delayed response, following the introduction of an allergen, occurring at sites remote from that of injection.

conversion r., conversion *hysteria.*

cross r., a specific r. between an antiserum and an antigen complex other than the antigen complex that evoked the various specific antibodies of the antiserum, due to the two complexes including among their respective antigenic determinants at least one that is included also among the determinants of the other complex.

cuta'neous r., cutireaction.

cu'tituber'culin r., a form of tuberculin test proposed by Lignières in which undiluted tuberculin is rubbed on the skin with a pledget of cotton.

Dale r., see Schultz-Dale r.

dark r., in photosynthesis, the fixation of $CO_2$ into carbohydrate, which is independent in place and time of the absorption of light.

decidual r., the cellular and vascular changes occurring in the endometrium at the time of implantation.

r. of degeneration, see under degeneration.

delayed r., a local or generalized response that begins 24 to 48 hours after exposure to an antigen (allergen, immunogen) to which the person or animal has been sensitized (immunized); see also skin *test.*

depot r., reddening of the skin at the point where the needle entered, in the subcutaneous tuberculin test.

der'motuber'culin r., Pirquet's *test.*

diazo r., Ehrlich's diazo r.; an obsolete r. that is the basis of the van den Bergh *test q.v.*

digitonin r., the r. of naturally occurring steroids with $3\beta$-hydroxyl groups with digitonin, a steroid glyoside, resulting in the formation of an insoluble precipitate, useful in determining the presence of cholesterol and ergosterol.

Dische r., the assay of DNA by means of the blue color formed with diphenylamine in acid.

dissociative r., r. characterized by such dissociative behavior as amnesia, fugues, sleepwalking, and dream states.

dopa r., Bloch's r.; a 1:1000 solution of dopa applied to fresh tissue sections causes a dark staining presumably due to the presence of dopa oxidase in the protoplasm of certain cells.

Ebbecke's r., dermatographism.

echo r., echolalia.

Ehrlich's benzaldehyde r., a test for urobilinogen in the urine; 2 g. of dimethyl-*p*-aminobenzaldehyde are dissolved in 100 cc. of 5 per cent hydrochloric acid; 10 to 15 drops of this reagent are added to 10 cc. of urine. A red color in the cold indicates the presence of an excessive amount of urobilinogen.

Ehrlich's diazo r., diazo r.

endergonic r.'s, those requiring the addition of energy in order to proceed. Most syntheses are of this type. See endothermal r.; contrast exergonic r.

endothermal r., endother'mic r., a chemical r. in which heat is absorbed.

eosinope'nic r., reduction in the numbers of circulating eosinophils by the adrenocorticotrophic hormone or by adrenal corticoids.

erythrophore r., fish test; a reddish coloration (nuptial coloration) caused in certain male fishes (bitterling) by the injection of the gonad hormone.

exergonic r.'s, those liberating energy as they proceed. Most catabolic r.'s are of this type. See exothermal r.; contrast endergonic r.

exother'mal r., exother'mic r., a chemical r. in which heat is evolved, as in ordinary combustion.

false-negative r., an erroneous or mistakenly negative response.

false-positive r., an erroneous or mistakenly positive response.

fatigue r., the rise in temperature of a tuberculous subject caused by exercise.

ferric chloride r. of epinephrine, Vulpian r.; an intense emerald green color in a neutral or slightly acid solution of epinephrine when ferric chloride is added to it. A reaction typical of catechols.

Feulgen r., see Feulgen *test.*

first-order r., a r. the rate of which is proportional to the concentration of the single substance undergoing change. Radioactive decay is a first-order process, defined by the equation $-(dN/dt) = kN$, where $N$ is the number of atoms subject to decay (reaction), $t$ is time, and $k$ is the first-order decay (reaction) constant, *i.e.,* the fraction of all atoms decaying per unit of time. See also radioactive *constant.*

fixation r., see complement *fixation.*

floccula'tion r., a form of precipitin r. in which precipitation occurs over a narrow range of antigen-antibody ratio, due chiefly to peculiarities of the antibody (precipitin).

Florence's r., Florence's *test.*

focal r., a r. which occurs at the point of entrance of an infecting organism or of an injection, as in the Arthus phenomenon.

Folin's r., the r. of amino acids in alkaline solution with 1,2-naphthoquinone-4-sulfonate to yield a red color, useful for quantitative assay.

r. formation, see under formation.

Forssman r., Forssman antigen-antibody r.

Forssman antigen-antibody r., Forssman r.; the combination of Forssman antibody with heterogenetic antigen of the Forssman type, as in the agglutination of sheep erythrocytes (which contain Forssman antigen) by serum from a person with infectious mononucleosis which contains Forssman antibody.

Frei-Hoffman r., Frei *test.*

fright r., after section and degeneration of the facial nerve of an animal, the denervated facial muscles contract if the animal is frightened or becomes angry; due to the release of acetylcholine into the circulation.

fuchsinophil r., the property possessed by certain elements, when stained with acid fuchsin, of retaining the stain when treated with picric acid alcohol.

fur'furol r., production of a red color on addition of furfurol to a solution of aniline.

galvanic skin r., galvanic skin *response.*

gel diffusion r.'s, see gel diffusion precipitin *tests.*

Gell and Coombs r.'s, see allergic r.'s.

gemistocytic r., a r. to injury resulting in the proliferation of reactive, protoplastic, or gemistocytic astrocytes.

general adaptation r., see general adaptation *syndrome.*

Gerhardt's r., Gerhardt's *test* for acetoacetic acid.

glyoxylic acid r., glyoxylic acid *test.*

graft versus host r., graft versus host *disease.*

group r., a r. with an agglutinin or other antibody that is common (though usually in varying concentrations) to an entire group of related bacteria, *e.g.,* the coli group.

Gruber's r., Widal r.

Gruber-Widal r., Widal r.

Günning's r., the formation of iodoform from acetone by iodine and ammonia in alcohol.

harlequin r., sudden blanching of the lower half of the body of an infant lying on its side, leaving the remaining half of the body the normal pink color.

heel-tap r., see heel *tap.*

hemiop'ic r., Wernicke's r.

hemiop'ic pupillary r., Wernicke's r.

hemoclas'tic r., hemolysis as observed in the laking of the blood.

Henle's r., dark brown staining of the medullary cells of the adrenal bodies when treated with the salts of chromium, the cortical cells remaining unstained; see chromaffin.

Herxheimer's r., Jarisch-Herxheimer r.; an inflammatory r. in syphilitic tissues (skin, mucous membrane, nervous system, or viscera) induced in certain cases by specific treatment with Salvarsan, mercury, or antibiotics; believed to be due to a rapid release of treponemal antigen with an associated allergic reaction in the patient.

Hill r., that portion of the photosynthesis r. that involves the photolysis of water and the liberation of oxygen and does not include carbon dioxide fixation. It involves the addition of oxidants (quinones or ferricyanide) to chloroplasts; upon illumination, $O_2$ is evolved and the added oxidant is reduced.

hunting r., hunting phenomenon; an unusual r. of digital blood vessels exposed to cold; vasoconstriction is alternated with vasodilation in irregular repeated sequences, in an apparent "hunting" of equilibrium of skin temperature.

hypomanic r., hyperkinetic *syndrome.*

r. of identity, see gel diffusion precipitin tests in two dimensions (under test).

immediate r., a local or generalized response that begins within a few minutes to about an hour after exposure to an antigen (allergen, immunogen) to which the person or animal has been sensitized (immunized); see also skin *test.*

**immune r.,** antigen-antibody r. indicating a certain degree of resistance usually in reference to the 36- to 48-hour reaction in vaccination against smallpox; because the degree of resistance indicated by the r. is not true immunity and may disappear relatively rapidly there is a tendency to refer to the immune r. as an allergic r. (*q.v.*).

**IMViC r.,** a mnemonic referring to indole production, the methyl red test, the Voges-Proskauer r., and the ability to utilize citrate as a sole source of carbon (the lower case *i* is inserted for euphony). Used primarily with reference to *Escherichia coli, Enterobacter aerogenes,* and related organisms.

**incompatible blood transfusion r.,** a syndrome due to intravascular hemolysis of transfused blood by serum antibodies of the recipient, which react with an antigen of the donor red cells. The syndrome consists of chills, fever, backache or muscle cramps, hemoglobinemia, hemoglobinuria, and oliguria which may result in acute renal failure.

**indirect pupillary r.,** consensual r.

**intracutaneous r.,** a r. following the injection of antigen into the skin of a sensitive subject, such as in the case of the tuberculin test.

**i'odate r. of epinephrine,** depends upon the oxidation of epinephrine by iodine liberated from iodate, which is decomposed by the hormone; a faint pink color results; Krauss test.

**iodine r. of epinephrine,** resulting from the oxidation of the hormone, a faint pink color appearing upon the addition of iodine.

**irreversible r.,** a r. or response by the tissues to a pathogenic agent characterized by a permanent pathologic change.

**Jarisch-Herxheimer r.,** Herxheimer's r.

**Jolly's r.,** myasthenic r.; rapid loss of response to faradic stimulation of a muscle, the galvanic response and the power of voluntary contraction being retained.

**Knaus' r.,** the excised uterus of an animal (rabbit) does not respond to Pituitrin (posterior pituitary extract) if the animal previously has been treated with corpus luteum hormone (*i.e.,* progesterone).

**Kraus' r.,** the formation of a precipitate by antiserum obtained by inoculating animals with cultures of whole bacteria when the antiserum is added to a filtrate of a culture of the bacterium.

**late r.,** delayed r.

**lengthening r.,** in the decerebrate animal, the rather sudden relaxation with lengthening of the extensor muscles when a limb is passively flexed; associated with clasp-knife spasticity.

**lepromin r.,** Mitsuda r.; a persisting nodule at the site of intradermal injection of a boiled extract of leprous tissue; positive in tuberculoid leprosy.

**leuke'moid r.,** see the major entry, *leukemoid reaction,* following leukemoid.

**local r.,** focal r.

**local anesthetic r.,** a toxic r. due to absorption of local anesthetic drug in conduction anesthesia, ranging from drowsiness to convulsions and cardiovascular collapse.

**Loewenthal's r.,** the agglutinative r. in relapsing fever.

**lymphat'ic r.,** see glandular *fever.*

**magnet r.,** seen in an animal deprived of its cerebellum. When the animal is placed upon its back and the head strongly flexed, the four limbs become flexed in all their joints. Light pressure made upon a toe-pad with the finger causes (due to stimulation of receptors in the deep layers of the skin) reflex contraction of the limb extensors. The limb is thus pressed gently against the finger and when the finger is withdrawn slightly, the experimenter has the sensation that his finger is raising the limb or drawing it out as by a magnet.

**Marchi's r.,** failure of the myelin sheath of a nerve to blacken when submitted to the action of osmic acid.

**Meltzer's r.,** paradoxical pupillary r.

**microbiallergic r.,** see microbiallergic.

**Millon r.,** the r. of phenolic compounds (*e.g.,* tyrosine in protein) with $Hg(NO_3)_2$ in $HNO_3$ (and a trace of $HNO_2$) to give a red color.

**miostag'min r.,** a physiochemical immunity test, designed by Ascoli, consisting in determination of the surface tension of an immune serum to which its specific antigen has been added, before and after incubation at 37°C. for 2 hours. In case of a positive r. the surface tension, as measured by the stalagmometer, is lowered.

**Mitsuda r.,** lepromin r.

**mixed agglutination r.,** mixed agglutination; immune agglutination in which the aggregates contain cells of two different kinds but with common antigenic determinants; when used to identify isoantigens, the test cells are exposed to appropriate isoantibody, washed, and then mixed with indicator erythrocytes that combine with free sites on the test cell-attached isoantibody.

**mixed lymphocyte culture r.,** see mixed lymphocyte culture *test.*

**monomolecular r.,** unimolecular r.; a r. involving a single molecule, *e.g.,* decomposition, intramolecular rearrangement, intramolecular oxidation or reduction. A r. is considered monomolecular even if a catalytic agent, such as acid or alkali, is present in large excess, on a molecular basis, or is not rate determining. Monomolecular r.'s are usually of the first order, *i.e.,* the rate is proportional to the concentration of one reactant. Radioactive decay is a good example.

**Much's r.,** Much-Holzmann r.

**Much-Holzmann r.,** Much's r.; psychoreaction; the alleged property of the serum from a person suffering from dementia precox or from manic-depressive insanity of inhibiting hemolysis by cobra venom.

**myasthen'ic r.,** Jolly's r.

**Nadi r.,** peroxidase r.

**Neufeld r.,** Neufeld capsular *swelling.*

**neurotonic r.,** muscular contraction continuing well after cessation of stimulation.

**neutral r.,** pH of 7.00; H and OH ion concentrations equal at $10^{-7}$ M.

**ninhy'drin r.,** a test for proteins, peptones, peptides, and amino acids possessing free carboxyl and α-amino groups. To 5 ml. of a neutral solution of protein 0.5 ml. of a 0.3 per cent solution of triketohydrindene hydrate is added. A blue color, caused by the linking of 2 molecules of the reagent through the N of the amino group, develops if the mixture is heated to boiling for 2 minutes and then allowed to cool. From α-amino acids, $CO_2$ (from the —COOH group) is evolved, also quantitatively. The color reaction is widely used to quantitate free amino acids (*e.g.,* after hydrolysis and separation of the amino acids of a protein).

**nitritoid r.,** a severe r. resembling that following the administration of nitrites; it sometimes follows the intravenous administration of arsphenamine and consists of flushing of the face, edema of the tongue and lips, vomiting, profuse sweating, a fall in blood pressure, and sometimes death; such r.'s occurring after the injection of organic arsenicals have been thought to be due to the formation of minute pulmonary emboli.

**r. of nonidentity,** see gel diffusion precipitin tests in two dimensions (under test).

**nuclear r.,** the interaction of two atomic nuclei or of one such with a subatomic particle, or of the subatomic particles within an atomic nucleus, resulting in a change in the nature of the nuclei concerned or in the energy content of the nuclei or both, usually manifested by transmutation (accompanied by emission of α-, β-, or γ-rays) or by fission or fusion of the nuclei.

**ophthal'mic r.,** conjunctival r.

**orcinol r.,** see orcinol *test.*

**oxidase r.,** (1) the formation of indol blue when a blood smear containing myeloid leukocytes is treated with a mixture of α-naphthol and *p*-dimethylaniline sulfate; the myeloid leukocytes contain an oxidase that catalyzes this r., the lymphoid leukocytes do not (*cf.* peroxidase r.); (2) a r. in bacteriology that depends on the presence of certain oxidases in some bacteria that catalyze the transport of electrons between electron donors in the bacteria and an oxidation-reduction dye, such as tetramethyl-*p*-phenylenediamine; the dye is reduced to a blue or black color.

**oxidation-reduction r.,** see oxidation-reduction.

**pain r.,** dilation of the pupil or any other involuntary act occurring in response to a stimulus causing sharp pain anywhere.

**Pandy's r.,** Pandy's test; to determine the presence of proteins (chiefly globulins) in the spinal fluid; one drop of spinal fluid is added to 1 ml. of (1) a solution of 1 part carbolic acid crystals in 15 parts distilled water, (2) a 4 per cent solution of cresol, or (3) a 10 per cent solution of pyrogallic acid; the r. varies from a faint turbidity to a dense "milky" precipitate according to the degree of protein content.

**paradoxical pupillary r.,** Meltzer's r.; the greatly increased response of the pupil to the dilator action of epinephrine (1:1000) after excision of the superior cervical ganglion of the superior sympathetic cervical ganglion. See also Meltzer-Auer *test.*

**r. of partial identity,** see gel diffusion precipitin tests in two dimensions (under test).

**Paul's r.,** Paul's test; pus is rubbed into a scarification on a rabbit's eye; if the pus is from a variolous or vaccinal pustule a condition of epitheliosis develops in from 36 to 48 hours; the sputum of a smallpox patient is said to cause the same r.

**Pauly r.,** the coupling r. of compounds containing or capable of producing an imidazole ring with diazobenzenesulfonic acid to give red substitution product; useful in the colorimetric estimation of histidine and tyrosine.

**perox'idase r.,** Nadi r.; formation of indophenol blue by the action of an oxidizing enzyme present in certain cells and tissues when these are treated with a solution of $\alpha$-naphthol and dimethylparaphenylenediamine. By this method cells of the myelocyte series, which give a positive r., may be distinguished from those of the lymphocyte series, which give a negative r. Endothelial leukocytes give a variable r., probably positive when they have phagocytized the debris of myeloid cells. This has caused some authors to feel that endothelial leukocytes may originate in the bone marrow.

**phosphoroclastic r.,** cleavage of C—C bonds that involves phosphate transfer but not, as in phosphorolysis, directly to one of the products. An example is the decomposition of pyruvate to acetate + $CO_2$, in which $P_i$ is added to ADP to form ATP.

**Pirquet's r.,** Pirquet's *test.*

**Porter-Silber r.,** the basis of the 17-hydroxycorticosteroid test; C-21 adrenocorticosteroids, which contain a dihydroxyacetone group at carbons 19, 20, and 21, react with phenylhydrazine.

**Prausnitz-Küstner r.,** a test based on passive transfer of allergic sensitivity; blood serum from an allergic individual is injected into the skin of a normal person; 48 hours later the injected site shows an urticarial r. when injected with antigens to which the donor is allergic, other parts of the recipient's skin show no response.

**precip'itin r.,** see precipitin and precipitin *test.*

**primary r.,** vaccinia (2).

**prozone r.,** see prozone.

**psychogalvanic r.,** galvanic skin *response.*

**psychogalvanic skin r.** galvanic skin *response.*

**quellung r.** [ Ger. swelling ], Neufeld capsular *swelling.*

**reversed Prausnitz-Küstner r.,** the appearance of an urticarial r. at the site of injection when serum containing reaginic antibody is injected into the skin of a person in whom the allergen is already present.

**reversible r.,** a chemical r. that takes place either from left to right or from right to left. Ionization is such a reaction; so are, by definition, reactions in which an enzyme (a catalyst) is involved.

**Sachs-Georgi r.,** see Sachs-Georgi *test.*

**Sakaguchi r.,** guanidines in alkaline solution develop an intense red color when treated with $\alpha$-naphthol and sodium hypochlorite; a qualitative test for arginine, free or in a protein.

**Schardinger r.,** the reduction of methylene blue to methylene white by formaldehyde is rapidly catalyzed by fresh milk but not by boiled milk; the catalyzing agent is xanthine oxidase; an example of oxidation in the absence of $O_2$ with an organic hydrogen acceptor (the dye).

**Schultz-Charlton r.,** Schultz-Charlton phenomenon; the specific blanching of a scarlatinal rash at the site of intracutaneous injection of scarlatina antiserum.

**Schultz-Dale r.,** the contraction of an excised intestinal loop (Schultz) or of an excised strip of virginal uterus

(Dale) from a sensitized animal (guinea pig) which occurs when the tissue is exposed to the specific antigen.

**sedimentation r.,** sedimentation *rate.*

**serum r.,** seroreaction.

**shortening r.,** the adaptive shortening of the extensor muscles of the limb of a decerebrate animal when the limb is extended after it has been flexed; *cf.* lengthening r.

**Shwartzman r.,** Shwartzman *phenomenon.*

**skin r.,** skin *test.*

**specific r.,** the phenomena produced by an agent that is identical with or immunologically related to the one that has already caused an alteration in capacity of the tissue to react.

**startle r.,** a reflex response to a sudden intense stimulus, consisting of a diffuse motor response involving flexion movements of trunk and extremities together with a sudden increase in the level of consciousness; see also startle *reflex.*

**Straus r.,** a diagnostic test for glanders. Male guinea pigs are inoculated intraperitoneally with suspected material. If the glanders organism is present it will usually set up a necrotizing inflammation in the scrotal sac within a few days. The animals are sacrificed and the presence of the specific organism confirmed bacteriologically.

**stress r.,** acute situational r.; an acute emotional r. related to extreme environmental stress.

**supporting r.'s,** supporting reflexes; described by Magnus, who distinguishes two types: *positive* and *negative.* Positive supporting r.'s consist of those reflex muscular contractions whereby the body is supported against gravity. The negative supporting r. consists of inhibition of the extensor muscles and unfixing of the joints which thus enable the limb to be flexed and moved into a new position. The positive supporting r.'s are seen in an exaggerated form in the decerebrate animal.

**symptomatic r.,** an allergic response similar to the original one, but occurring after the use of a test or therapeutic dose of an allergen or atopen.

**thermoprecip'itin r.,** the throwing down of a precipitate on the application of heat, as in the case of albuminous urine.

**thymergastic r.,** abnormal affective behavior; see thymergasia.

**Tollens' r.,** (1) phoroglucinol and HCl react with galactose, glycuronic acids and pentoses to give a red color; (2) naphthoresorcinol and HCl react with glucuronate to give a colored compound.

**Treponema pallidum immobilization r.,** *Treponema pallidum* immobilization *test.*

**triketohydrindene r.,** ninhydrin r.

**unimolec'ular r.,** monomolecular r.

**vaccinoid r.,** accelerated r.; the local r. to vaccination in a person with partial immunity from a previous vaccination or attack of smallpox intermediate to the primary and immune r.'s.

**Voges-Proskauer r.,** a chemical r. used in testing for the production of acetyl methyl carbinol by various bacteria; 5 ml. of a 10 per cent solution of potassium hydroxide are added to 5 ml. of a 24-hr. culture in a suitable medium (*e.g.*, peptone 7 gm., dextrose 5 gm., and dipotassium phosphate 5 gm. in 1000 ml. of water), and thoroughly mixed; the treated culture is permitted to stand (exposed to air), and is observed at intervals of 2, 12, and 24 hr.; a positive r. consists of the development of an eosin-like pink color. The color is due to the production of acetyl-methyl-carbonol, which in the presence of alkali and oxygen is oxidized to diacetyl.

**Wassermann r.,** Wassermann *test.*

**Weidel's r.,** showing the presence of xanthine bodies; a solution of the suspected substance in chlorine water with a little nitric acid is evaporated in a water bath, and then exposed to the vapor of ammonia; the presence of the xanthine bodies is indicated when a red or purple color develops.

**Weil-Felix r.,** the agglutination of the X-strains of *Proteus vulgaris;* especially X-19, with serum of patients with certain rickettsial diseases *e.g.,* typhus fever.

**Weinberg's r.,** a complement fixation test of the presence of hydatid disease.

**Wernicke's r.,** Wernicke's sign; hemiopic r.; in hemianopsia due to injury of the optic tract; it consists in loss of the light reflex when the light is thrown on the blind side of the retina, with preservation of the same when the light strikes the sensitive side.

**Widal's r.,** agglutination r. as applied to the diagnosis of typhoid.

**xan'thoprote'ic r.,** xanthoproteic *test.*

**Yorke's autolytic r.,** a test for paroxysmal hemoglobinuria; serum is placed in the ice chest and kept at O°C. for 5 to 7 minutes, then in an incubator at 37°C. with erythrocytes for 1 hour, at which time, if the r. is positive, hemolysis occurs; if the serum is kept at 1°C. for an hour and then placed in the incubator with erythrocytes there is little hemolysis.

**zero-order r.,** a r. that proceeds at a particular rate independently of the concentration of the reactant or reactants.

**Zimmermann r.,** Zimmermann test; a chemical r. between metadinitrobenzene and an active methylene group (carbon-16) of 17-ketosteroids; it is the basis of the 17-ketosteroid assay t.

**reactivate** (re-ak'tĭ-vāt). To render active again; said of an inactivated immune serum to which normal serum (complement) is added.

**reactivation** (re-ak-tĭ-va'shun). The restoration of the lytic activity of an inactivated serum by means of the addition of complement.

**reactivity** (re-ak-tiv'ĭ-tĭ). 1. The property of reacting, chemically or in any other sense. 2. The process of reacting.

**reagent** (re-a'jent) [ Mod. L. *reagens.* ACT- ]. Any substance added to a solution of another substance to participate in a chemical reaction.

**Benedict-Hopkins-Cole r.,** magnesium glyoxalate, made from a mixture of oxalic acid and magnesium, used for testing proteins for the presence of tryptophan; see also Hopkins-Cole *test.*

**biuret r.,** an alkaline solution of copper sulfate.

**Cleland's r.,** dithioerythritol or dithiothreitol; HS—$CH_2(CHOH)_2CH_2SH$.

**diazo r.,** Ehrlich's diazo r.; two solutions, one of sodium nitrite, the other of acidified sulfanilic acid, used in bringing about diazotization.

**Edlefsen's r.,** an alkaline permanganate solution used in the determination of sugar in the urine.

**Edman's r.,** phenylisothiocyanate, $C_6H_5NCS$.

**Erdmann's r.,** a mixture of sulfuric and nitric acids, used in testing alkaloids.

**Esbach's r.,** picric acid 1, citric acid 2, water 97; used as a test for albumin in urine.

**Exton's r.,** a r. used as a test for albumin; consists of 50 gm. of sulfosalicylic acid and 200 gm. of $Na_2SO_4 \cdot 10H_2O$ in a liter of water.

**Fehling's r.,** Fehling's *solution.*

**Fouchet's r.,** a 25 per cent solution of trichloroacetic acid, containing 0.9 per cent ferric chloride; a drop of the r. added at the surface line of barium chloride-impregnated filter paper which has been dipped in urine for 10 seconds will give a green color if bilirubin is present.

**Froehde's r.,** sodium molybdate 1, in strong sulfuric acid 1000; gives various color reactions with alkaloids.

**Frohn's r.,** bismuth subnitrate 1.5, water 20.0; heat to boiling and add hydrochloric acid 10.0, and potassium iodide 7.0; a test for alkaloids and for sugar.

**Girard's r.,** the hydrazine of betaine chloride, used to extract ketonic steroids by forming water-soluble hydrazones with them.

**Hahn's oxine r.,** an alcoholic solution of 8-hydroxyquinoline used in the determination of zinc, aluminum, magnesium, etc.

**Haines' r.,** copper sulfate 2, potassium hydroxide 7.5, glycerin 15, distilled water 150; used in Trommer's test.

**Hammarsten's r.,** a mixture of 1 part of a 25 per cent solution of nitric acid and 19 parts of a 25 per cent solution of hydrochloric acid; the addition of a few drops to a mixture of 1 part of this r. and 4 parts of alcohol will give a green color if bile is present.

**il'osvay r.,** sulfanilic acid 0.5, dissolved in dilute acetic acid 150, is mixed with naphthylamine 1, dissolved in boiling water 20; the blue sediment which forms is dissolved in dilute acetic acid 150; a few drops of this r.

added to water, saliva, or other fluid to be tested will produce a red color if nitrites are present.

**Lloyd's r.,** precipitated aluminum silicate, used in the determination of alkaloids.

**Mandelin's r.,** a solution of ammonium vanadate in sulfuric acid, used in color tests for alkaloids.

**Marme's r.,** a solution of potassium iodide and cadmium iodide used in testing for alkaloids.

**Marquis' r.,** a solution of formaldehyde in sulfuric acid used in color tests for formaldehyde.

**Mecke's r.,** a solution of selenous acid in sulfuric acid, used for color tests of alkaloids.

**Meyer's r.,** a solution of phenolphthalein 0.032, in decinormal sodium hydroxide 21, with water (distilled from glass) sufficient to make 100; in the presence of minute traces of blood, the solution becomes purple or blue-red.

**Millon's r.,** mercuric nitrate and nitric acid (see Millon *reaction).*

**Nessler's r.,** a solution of potassium hydroxide, mercuric iodide, and potassium iodide; it yields a yellow color with ammonia (a brown precipitate with larger amounts) that can be used for quantitive assay.

**Pavy's r.,** potassium hydroxide and potassium sodium tartrate, of each 20.4, copper sulfate 4.158, ammonia (sp. gr. 0.880) 300, water 1000; used in place of Fehling's solution for the quantitative estimation of sugar in the urine, 10 cc. of the solution being decolorized by 5 mg. of sugar.

**Rosenthaler-Turk r.,** a solution of potassium arsenate in sulfuric acid used in obtaining color tests for various opium alkaloids.

**Sanger's r.,** 2,4-dinitrofluorobenzene.

**Schaer's r.,** an alcoholic or aqueous solution of chloral hydrate used as an extraction medium in investigations of alkaloids.

**Scheibler's r.,** a solution of sodium tungstate in phosphoric acid used in tests for alkaloids.

**Schiff's r.,** see Schiff's *test* (4).

**Scott-Wilson r.,** an alkaline solution of mercuric cyanide and silver nitrate used in the detection of acetone.

**Soldaini's r.,** copper carbonate 15, potassium bicarbonate 416, water 1400; one part of this r. boiled with two parts or urine will result in the formation of a yellow precipitate if the urine contains glucose.

**Spiegler's r.,** mercuric chloride 8, tartaric acid and sodium chloride each 4, glycerin 20, distilled water 200; one or two drops of urine, acidified with acetic acid and filtered, are run down the side of a test tube containing this r., and, where the two fluids touch, there will be a sharply defined gray-white ring if the urine contains even a slight trace (1:250,000) of albumin.

**Stokes' r.,** a solution of ammonium ferrotartrate (or citrate) used as a test for hemoglobin.

**Sulkowitch's r.,** for the detection of calcium in the urine; it consists of oxalic acid 2.5 gm., ammonium oxalate 2.5 gm., glacial acetic acid 5 cc., and distilled water to make 150 cc. A milky precipitate of calcium oxalate is formed when the r. is added to urine that contains calcium.

**Tanret's r.,** a r. for albumin in the urine; potassium iodide 3.32, mercuric chloride 1.35, acetic acid 20, water 64; it forms a white precipitate when added to albuminous urine.

**Uffelmann's r.,** a solution of 3 drops each of concentrated phenol and liquid ferric chloride in 300 drops of water. The solution is of an amethyst blue color, which turns lemon yellow in the presence of lactic acid, assumes an opaline tint in butyric acid, and is decolorized by hydrochloric acid.

**Wurster's r.,** filter paper impregnated with tetramethyl-*p*-phenylenediamine, which turns blue in the presence of ozone or hydrogen peroxide.

**reagin** (re-a'jin). 1. Wolff-Eisner's term for antibody. 2. An old term for the "Wassermann" antibody; not to be confused with the Prausnitz-Küstner antibody of the IgE class.

**atopic r.,** Prausnitz-Küstner *antibody.*

**reaginic** (re'a-jin'ik). Pertaining to a reagin.

**realgar** (re-al'gar) [ Ar. *rahj al- ghār,* powder of the mine ]. Arsenic disulfide, $As_2S_2$.

**reality** (re-al'ĭ-tĭ) [ L. *res,* thing, fact ]. That which exists objectively and in fact, and can be consensually validated.

**reality testing.** In psychiatry, the ego function by which the objective or real world and one's relationship to it are evaluated and appreciated.

**reamer** (re′mer) [ A.S. *ryman,* to widen ]. 1. A rotating instrument with spirally turned blades, used for enlarging root canals of teeth. 2. A twist drill for enlarging root canals.

    **engine r.,** an engine-mounted spirally-bladed instrument, used for enlarging the root canals of teeth.

**Réaumur** (ra-o-mür′), René A. F. de, French physicist, 1683–1757. See R.'s *scale.*

**re′attach′ment.** The reimbedding of periodontal fibers into newly formed cementum at tooth surfaces denuded by periodontal disease.

**re′base.** In dentistry, to refit a denture by replacing the denture-base material without changing the occlusal relationship of the teeth; see also reline.

**recalcification** (re-kal-sĭ-fĭ-ka′shun). The restoration to the tissues of lost calcium salts.

**re′call.** The process of remembering thoughts, words, and actions of a past event in an attempt to recapture actual happenings.

**Récamier** (ra-kam-e-a′), Joseph C. A., French gynecologist, 1774–1852. See R.'s *operation.*

**recan′aliza′tion.** Restoration of a lumen in a blood vessel following thrombotic occlusion, by organization of the thrombus with formation of new capillaries.

**recapitulation** (re′kă-pit′u-la′shun). See recapitulation *theory.*

**receiver** (re-se′ver) [ L. *receptor, q.v.* ]. In chemistry, a vessel attached to a condenser to receive the product of distillation.

**receptaculum,** pl. **receptacula** (re′sep-tak′u-lum, -lah) [ L. fr. *re-cipio,* pp. *-ceptus,* to receive, fr. *capio,* to take ]. A receptacle.

    **r. chy′li,** *cisterna* chyli.

    **r. gan′glii petro′si,** *fossula* petrosa.

    **r. Pecquet′i,** *cisterna* chyli.

**recepto′ma.** Chemodectoma; see also paraganglioma.

**receptor** (re-sep′tor) [ L. receiver, fr. *recipio,* to receive ]. 1. In Ehrlich's theory of immunity, one of the side chains of the cell which combine with foreign substances, conceived as being of three orders, first, second, and third (see subentries). 2. Sherrington's term for any one of the various sensory nerve endings in the skin, deep tissues, viscera, and special sense organs.

    **adrenergic r.'s,** adrenoreceptors; postulated reactive components of effector tissues, most of which are innervated by adrenergic postganglionic fibers of the sympathetic nervous system. Such r.'s can be activated by norepinephrine and/or epinephrine and by various adrenergic drugs; r. activation results in a change in effector tissue function, such as contraction of arteriolar muscles or relaxation of bronchial muscles; adrenergic r.'s are divided into α-r.'s and β-r.'s, on the basis of their response to various adrenergic activating and blocking agents.

    **α-adrenergic r.'s,** postulated adrenergic r.'s in effector tissues capable of selective activation and blockade by drugs; conceptually derived from the ability of certain agents, such as phenoxybenzamine, to block only some adrenergic r.'s and of other agents, such as methoxamine, to activate only the same adrenergic r.'s. Such r.'s are designated as α-receptors. Their activation results in physiological responses such as increased peripheral vascular resistance, mydriasis, and contraction of pilomotor muscles.

    **β-adrenergic r.'s,** postulated adrenergic r.'s in effector tissues capable of selective activation and blockade by drugs; conceptually derived from the ability of certain agents, such as propranolol, to block only some adrenergic r.'s and of other agents, such as isoproterenol, to activate only the same adrenergic r.'s. Such r.'s are designated as β-receptors. Their activation results in physiological responses such as relaxation of bronchial muscles and increases in cardiac rate and force of contraction.

    **cholinergic r.'s,** chemical sites in effector cells or at synapses through which acetylcholine exerts its action.

    **r. of the first order,** a r. that possesses only a haptophore group and can therefore merely bind the toxin or a food molecule, but provides no ferment for the digestion of the latter; antitoxin is a r. of the first order.

    **r. of the second order,** a r. that has two groups, a haptophore group for the anchoring of the foreign molecule and a zymophore group for its digestion; precipitins and agglutinins are r.'s of the second order.

    **sensory r.'s,** peripheral endings of afferent neurons.

    **sessile r.,** in Ehrlich's side chain theory, a r. of peculiar construction that cannot be cast off to form an antibody.

    **stretch r.'s,** r.'s that are sensitive to elongation, especially those in Golgi tendon organs and muscle spindles, but also those found in visceral organs such as stomach, small intestine, and urinary bladder. These r.'s have the function of detecting elongation, and this distinguishes them from baroreceptors, which are activated by stretching of the wall of the blood vessel but whose function is to elicit central reflex mechanism reducing the arterial blood pressure.

    **r. of the third order,** a r. that has two combining groups, a haptophore group for the anchoring of the foreign molecule and a complementophile group that binds the complement that carries the zymotoxic principle; these r.'s are different from those of the second order in that the digesting principle is not a component part of the r., but is available to it in the complement; the cytolysins (hemolysins, bacteriolysins) are castoff r.'s of the third order.

**recess** (re′ses) [ L. *recessus, q.v.* ]. Recessus.

    **anterior r. of tympanic membrane,** *recessus* membranae tympani anterior.

    **cecal r.,** *recessus* retrocecalis.

    **cerebellopontine r.,** pontocerebellar r.; the angle formed where the cerebellum and the pons meet.

    **cochlear r.,** *recessus* cochlearis.

    **costodiaphragmatic r. of pleura,** *recessus* costodiaphragmaticus pleurae.

    **costomediastinal r.,** *recessus* costomediastinalis.

    **duodenojejunal r.,** *recessus* duodenalis superior.

    **elliptical r.,** *recessus* ellipticus.

    **epitympanic r.,** *recessus* epitympanicus.

    **hepatoenteric r.,** a peritoneal r. at the caudal end of the embryonic pneumatoenteric r.; it separates the developing liver and stomach.

    **hepatorenal r.,** *recessus* hepatorenalis.

    **Hyrtl's epitympanic r.,** *recessus* epitympanicus.

    **inferior duodenal r.,** *recessus* duodenalis inferior.

    **inferior ileocecal r.,** *recessus* ileocecalis inferior.

    **inferior omental r.,** *recessus* inferior omentalis.

    **infundibular r.,** *recessus* infundibuli.

    **intersigmoid r.,** *recessus* intersigmoideus.

    **Jacquemet's r.,** a pouch of peritoneum between the gallbladder and the liver.

    **lateral r. of fourth ventricle,** *recessus* lateralis ventriculi quarti.

    **mesentericoparietal r.,** parajejunal *fossa.*

    **optic r.,** *recessus* opticus.

    **pancreaticoenteric r.,** a r. of the embryonic peritoneal cavity that develops into the adult omental bursa.

    **paracolic r.'s,** *sulci* paracolici.

    **paraduodenal r.,** *recessus* paraduodenalis.

    **parotid r.,** recessus parotideus; a deep hollow on the side of the head below and in front of the mastoid; it lodges the parotid gland.

    **pineal r.,** *recessus* pinealis.

    **piriform r.,** *recessus* piriformis.

    **pleural r.'s,** *recessus* pleurales.

    **pneumatoenteric r.,** pneumoenteric r.; a r. of the embryonic celum between the right lung bud and the gut; it is normally largely obliterated before birth, leaving only the superior r. of the vestibule of the lesser peritoneal sac as a vestige.

    **pneumoenteric r.,** pneumatoenteric r.

    **pontocerebellar r.,** cerebellopontine r.

    **posterior r. of tympanic membrane,** *recessus* membranae tympani posterior.

    **Reichert's cochlear r.,** *recessus* cochlearis.

    **retrocecal r.,** *recessus* retrocecalis.

    **retroduodenal r.,** *recessus* retroduodenalis.

    **Rosenmüller's r.,** *recessus* pharyngeus.

    **sacciform r.,** *recessus* sacciformis.

    **sphenoethmoidal r.,** *recessus* sphenoethmoidalis.

**spherical r.,** *recessus* sphericus.

**splenic r.,** *recessus* lienalis.

**subhepatic r.,** *recessus* subhepatici.

**subphrenic r.'s,** *recessus* subphrenici.

**subpopliteal r.,** *recessus* subpopliteus.

**superior duodenal r.,** *recessus* duodenalis superior.

**superior ileocecal r.,** *recessus* ileocecalis superior.

**superior r. of lesser peritoneal sac,** see pneumatoenteric r.

**superior omental r.,** *recessus* superior omentalis.

**superior r. of tympanic membrane,** *recessus* membranae tympani superior.

**suprapineal r.,** *recessus* suprapinealis.

**supratonsillar r.,** *fossa* supratonsillaris.

**triangular r.,** recessus triangularis; an occasional evagination of the anterior wall of the third ventricle of the brain between the anterior commissure and the diverging pillars of the fornix.

**Tröltsch's r.'s,** *recessus* membranae tympani, anterior and posterior.

**tubotympanic r.,** the dorsal portion of the embryonic first entodermal pharyngeal pouch; it develops into the middle ear cavity.

**recession** (re-sesh'un) [ L. *recessio* (see recessus) ]. Retraction; the act of drawing away or retiring.

**gingival r.,** apical migration of gingiva along tooth surface, with exposure of tooth surface.

**tendon r.,** surgical displacement of the tendon of an eye muscle posteriorly.

**reces'sive.** Drawing away; not dominant.

**recessus,** pl. **recessus** (re-ses'sus) [ L. a withdrawing, a receding ] [ NA ]. Recess; a small hollow or indentation.

**r. ante'rior,** a circumscript deepening of the interpeduncular fossa in the direction of the mamillary bodies.

**r. cochlea'ris** [ NA ], cochlear recess; Reichert's cochlear recess; a small depression on the inner wall of the vestibule of the labyrinth at the portion of the pyramis vestibuli, between the two limbs into which the vestibular crest divides posteriorly; it is perforated by foramina giving passage to fibers which the cochlear branch of the vestibulocochlear nerve sends to the posterior extremity of the cochlear duct.

**r. costodiaphragmat'icus pleu'rae** [ NA ], costodiaphragmatic recess of pleura; the cleftlike extension of the pleural cavity between the diaphragm and the rib cage.

**r. costomediastina'lis** [ NA ], costomediastinal recess or sinus; the recess of the pleural cavity between the costal cartilages and the mediastinum.

**r. duodena'lis infe'rior** [ NA ], inferior duodenal recess; Gruber-Landzert fossa; the variable peritoneal recess which lies behind the inferior duodenal fold and along the ascending part of the duodenum.

**r. duodena'lis supe'rior** [ NA ], superior duodenal recess; Jonnesco's fossa; duodenojejunal fossa; a peritoneal recess extending upward behind the superior duodenal fold.

**r. ellip'ticus** [ NA ], elliptical recess; fovea hemielliptica; an oval depression in the roof and inner wall of the vestibule of the labyrinth, lodging the utriculus.

**r. epitympan'icus** [ NA ], epitympanic recess; epitympanum; tympanic attic; the upper portion of the tympanic cavity above the tympanic membrane; it contains the head of the malleus and the body of the incus.

**r. hep'atorena'lis** [ NA ], hepatorenal recess; the deep recess of the peritoneal cavity on the right side extending upward between the liver in front and the kidney and suprarenal behind.

**r. ileoceca'lis infe'rior** [ NA ], inferior ileocecal recess; a deep fossa sometimes found between the ileocecal fold, the mesoappendix, and the cecum.

**r. ileoceca'lis supe'rior** [ NA ], superior ileocecal recess; a shallow pouch occasionally existing between the terminal ileum, the cecum, and the ileocolic artery when the latter is present.

**r. infe'rior omenta'lis** [ NA ], inferior omental recess; a recess of the omental bursa extending into the great omentum.

**r. infundib'uli** [ NA ], infundibular recess; a funnel-shaped diverticulum leading down from the anterior portion of the third ventricle into the infundibulum of the hypophysis.

**r. infundibulifor'mis,** r. pharyngeus.

**r. intersigmoi'deus** [ NA ], intersigmoid recess; a peritoneal recess behind and below the sigmoid colon created by the attachment of the sigmoid mesocolon ascending across the left psoas then turning sharply to descend into the pelvis. The left ureter (pars tecta ureterica) passes posterior to this recess.

**r. latera'lis ventric'uli quar'ti** [ NA ], lateral recess of the fourth ventricle; the narrow recess of the ventricle that extends laterally over, and down along the side of, the inferior cerebellar peduncle and the overlying cochlear nuclei; at its tip it opens by way of Luschka's foramen into the cisterna basalis of the subarachnoid space.

**r. liena'lis** [ NA ], splenic recess; the extension of the omental bursa toward the hilus of the spleen.

**r. membra'nae tym'pani ante'rior** [ NA ], anterior recess of tympanic membrane; a slitlike space on the tympanic wall between the anterior malleolar fold and the tympanic membrane.

**r. membra'nae tym'pani poste'rior** [ NA ], posterior recess of tympanic membrane; a narrow pocket in the tympanic wall between the posterior malleolar fold and the tympanic membrane.

**r. membra'nae tym'pani supe'rior** [ NA ], superior recess of tympanic membrane; a space in the mucous membrane on the inner surface of the tympanic membrane between the flaccid part of the membrane and the neck of the malleus.

**r. op'ticus** [ NA ], optic recess; a diverticulum extending forward from the anterior part of the third ventricle above the optic chiasm.

**r. paraduodena'lis** [ NA ], paraduodenal recess; paraduodenal fossa; fossa venosa; an occasional recess in the peritoneum to the left of the terminal portion of the duodenum located behind a fold containing the inferior mesenteric vein.

**r. pharyn'geus** [ NA ], pharyngeal recess; r. infundibuliformis; Rosenmüller's recess or fossa; a slitlike depression in the pharyngeal wall behind the opening of the auditory (Eustachian) tube.

**r. pinea'lis** [ NA ], pineal recess; a diverticulum from the posterior part of the third ventricle extending back between the posterior commissure and the habenular commissure.

**r. pirifor'mis** [ NA ], piriform recess; piriform fossa; a recess in the pharynx on each side of the opening of the larynx.

**r. pleura'les** [ NA ], pleural recesses; two recesses of the pleural cavity, one behind the sternum and costal cartilages (r. costomediastinalis) and the other between the diaphragm and chest wall (r. costodiaphragmaticus).

**r. poste'rior,** a deepening of the interpeduncular fossa toward the pons.

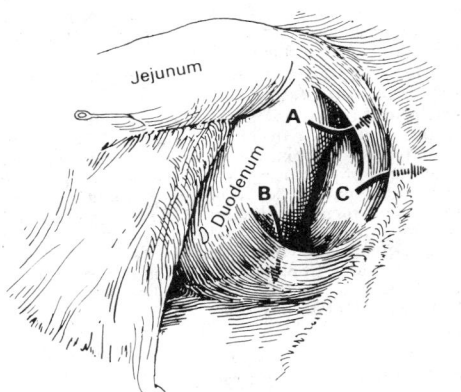

**Duodenal Recess**

*A,* superior duodenal recess; *B,* inferior duodenal recess; *C,* paraduodenal recess.

**r. retroceca'lis** [ NA ], retrocecal recess; one of several small pockets sometimes found extending alongside the right margin of the ascending colon near the cecum.

**r. retroduodena'lis** [ NA ], retroduodenal recess; a peritoneal recess occasionally found behind the third part of the duodenum, between it and the aorta.

**r. sacciform'is**, sacciform recess; (1) [ NA ], an extension of the cavity of the distal radioulnar articulation between the two bones; (2) an extension of the capsule of the elbow joint at the neck of the radius.

**r. sphenoethmoida'lis** [ NA ], sphenoethmoidal recess; a small cleftlike pocket in the superior meatus of the nasal cavity above the superior concha.

**r. spher'icus** [ NA ], spherical recess; fovea hemispherica; a rounded depression on the inner wall of the vestibule of the labyrinth, lodging the sacculus.

**r. subhepatici** [ NA ], subhepatic recess; the part of the peritoneal cavity between the visceral surface of the liver and the transverse colon.

**r. subphren'ici** [ NA ], subphrenic recesses; suprahepatic spaces; the recesses in the peritoneal cavity between the anterior part of the liver and the diaphragm, separated into right and left by the falciform ligament.

**r. subpoplite'us** [ NA ], subpopliteal recess; bursa of popliteus; the extension of the cavity of the knee joint between the tendon of the popliteus and lateral condyle of the femur.

**r. supe'rior omenta'lis** [ NA ], superior omental recess; a portion of the vestibule of the bursa omentalis that extends upward between the inferior vena cava and the esophagus.

**r. suprapinea'lis** [ NA ], suprapineal recess; a variable diverticulum from the posterior portion of the third ventricle of the brain, running backward some distance above and beyond the pineal r.

**r. triangula'ris**, triangular *recess.*

**recidivation** (re-sid-ī-va'shun) [ L. *recidivus,* falling back, recurring, fr. *re-cido,* to fall back, fr. *cado,* to fall ]. Relapse of a disease, a symptom or a behavioral pattern, such as an illegal activity for which one was previously hospitalized or imprisoned.

**recidivism** (re-sid'ī-vizm) [ L. *recidivus,* recurring ]. The tendency of an individual toward recidivation.

**recidivist** (re-sid'ī-vist). A person who tends toward recidivation.

**recipe** (res'ī-pī) [ L. imperative *recipio,* to receive ]. 1. Take; the superscription of a prescription, usually indicated by the sign ℞. 2. A prescription or formula.

**recipiomotor** (re-sip'ī-o-mo'tor) [ L. *recipio,* to receive, + *motor,* mover ]. Relating to the reception of motor stimuli.

**reciprocation** (re-sip'ro-ka'shun) [ L. *reciprocare,* pp. *reciprocatus,* to move back and forth ]. In prosthodontics, the means by which one part of an appliance is made to counter the effect created by another part.

**Recklinghausen** (rek'ling-how-sen), Friedrich D. von, German histologist and pathologist, 1833–1910. See R.'s *disease,* R.'s *disease* of bone, R.'s *tumor.*

**reclination** (rek'lī-na'shun) [ L. *reclino,* pp. *-atus,* to bend back. CLIM- ]. Turning the cataractous lens over into the vitreous to remove it from the line of vision; distinguished from couching, in which the lens is simply depressed into the vitreous.

**recollection** (re'kŏ-lek'shun) [ re- + L. *collectus,* pp. of *colligo,* to collect ]. In renal physiology, a technique in which a known fluid is infused into a renal tubule lumen at one point and collected for analysis by a second micropipette further downstream.

**recombinant** (re-kom'bi-nant). 1. A microbe, or strain, that has received chromosomal parts from different parental strains. 2. Pertaining to or denoting such organisms.

**recombination** (re-kom'bī-na'shun). The process of reuniting of parts that had become separated.

**genetic r.,** in microbial genetics, the inclusion of a chromosomal part or extrachromosomal element of one microbial strain in the chromosome of another; the interchange of chromosomal parts between different microbial strains.

**recon** (re'kon). In genetics, the smallest unit (corresponding to a single DNA nucleotide) of recombination or crossing-over between two homologous chromosomes.

**re'constitu'tion.** 1. The restitution or return to an original state of a substance, or combination of parts to make a whole. 2. In the case of a lower organism, the restoration of a part of the body by regeneration.

**rec'ord.** In dentistry, a registration of desired jaw relations in a plastic material or on a device in order that such relations may be transferred to an articulator.

**face-bow r.,** a registration by means of a face-bow of the position of the hinge axis and/or the condyles; the face-bow r. is used to orient the maxillary cast to the opening and closing axis of the articulator.

**functional chew-in r.,** a r. of the natural chewing movements of the mandible made on an occlusion rim by teeth or scribing studs.

**interocclusal r.,** a r. of the positional relationship of the teeth or jaws to each other. It is recorded by placing a plastic material which hardens, such as plaster of Paris, wax, etc., between the occlusal surfaces of the rims or teeth. The hardened material serves as the r. It may be registered in centric or eccentric positions.

**maxillomandibular r.,** biscuit bite; maxillomandibular registration; (1) a r. of the relation of the mandible to the maxillae; (2) the act of recording the relation of the mandible to the maxillae.

**occluding centric relation r.,** a registration of centric relation made at the established occlusal vertical dimension.

**pre-extraction r.,** preoperative r.

**preoperative r.,** pre-extraction r.; any r. made for the purpose of study or treatment planning; see also cast.

**profile r.,** a registration or r. of the profile of a patient.

**protrusive r.,** a registration of a forward position of the mandible with reference to the maxillae.

**terminal jaw relation r.,** a r. of the relationship of the mandible to the maxillae made at the vertical relation of occlusion and at the centric position.

**three-dimensional r.,** a maxillomandibular r. made at the occluding relation.

**record'ing.** Preserving the results of a study.

**depth r.,** study of subcortical cerebral electrical activity after placing microelectrodes in these areas.

**recov'ery.** 1. Regaining of health or function after disease or disability. 2. Emergence from general anesthesia.

**spontaneous r.,** the return of the conditioned response, after apparent extinction, in the presence of the conditioned stimulus without the unconditioned stimulus also being present.

**recrement** (rek're-ment) [ L. *recrementum,* refuse, filth, fr. re- + *cerno,* to separate ]. A secretion, like the saliva and in part the bile, that is reabsorbed after having performed its function.

**recrementitious** (rek're-men-tish'us). Of the nature of a recrement.

**recrudescence** (re-kru-des'ens) [ L. *re-crudesco,* to become raw again, break out afresh, fr. *crudus,* raw, harsh ]. A lighting up again of a morbid process or its symptoms after a period of improvement.

**recrudescent** (re-kru-des'ent). Becoming active again, relating to a recrudescence.

**recruitment** (re-kroot'ment) [ Fr. *recrutement,* fr. L. *re-cresco,* pp. *-cretus,* to grow again. CRES- ]. 1. A term used in the testing of hearing: the unequal reaction of the ear to equal steps of increasing intensity, measured in decibels, when such inequality of response results in a greater than normal increment of loudness. 2. Recruiting response; the bringing into activity of additional motor neurons and thus causing greater activity in response to increased duration of the stimulus applied to a given receptor or afferent nerve. See also irradiation (4). 3. The adding of parallel channels of flow in any system.

**rect-.** See recto-.

**rectal** (rek'tal). Relating to the rectum.

**rectalgia** (rek-tal'jī-ah). Proctalgia.

**rectectomy** (rek-tek'to-mī). Proctectomy.

**rectify** (rek'tī-fi) [ L. *rectus,* right, straight ]. 1. To correct. 2. To purify or refine by distillation; usually implies repeated distillations.

**rectitis** (rek-ti'tis). Proctitis.

**recto-, rect-** (rek'to-) [ L. *rectum,* fr. *rectus,* straight. REG- ]. Combining forms relating to the rectum; for words so beginning and not found here, see also procto-.

**rec'toabdom'inal.** Relating to the rectum and the abdomen; denoting a bimanual method of examination with one hand on the abdominal wall and a finger of the other hand, or on occasion the whole hand, in the rectum.

**rectocele** (rek'to-sēl) [ recto- + G. *kēlē,* tumor, hernia ]. Proctocele; prolapse or herniation of the rectum.

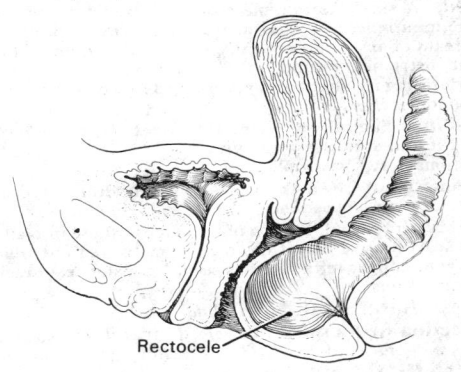

Rectocele

**Rectocele**

**rectoclysis** (rek-tok'lĭ-sis). Proctoclysis.

**rectococcygeal** (rek-to-kok-sij'e-al). Relating to the rectum and the coccyx.

**rectococcypexy** (rek'to-kok'sĭ-pek-sĭ). Proctococcypexy.

**rectocolitis** (rek'to-ko-li'tis). Proctocolitis.

**rectocystotomy** (rek'to-sis-tot'o-mĭ). Proctocystotomy.

**rectoperineal** (rek'to-pĕr-ĭ-ne'al). Relating to the rectum and perineum.

**rectoperineorrhaphy** (rek'to-pĕr'ĭ-ne-or'ă-fĭ). Proctoperineoplasty.

**rectopexy** (rek'to-pek'sĭ). Proctopexy.

**rectophobia** (rek'to-fo'bĭ-ah) [ recto- + G. *phobos,* fear ]. Proctophobia.

**rectoplasty** (rek'to-plas'tĭ). Proctoplasty.

**rectoromanoscope** (rek'to-ro-man'o-skōp) [ recto- + S romanum (sigmoid colon), + G. *skopeō,* to view ]. A form of speculum or endoscope for aid in examining the rectum and sigmoid colon.

**rectorrhaphy** (rek-tor'ră-fĭ). Proctorrhaphy.

**rectoscope** (rek'to-skōp). Proctoscope.

**rectoscopy** (rek-tos'ko-pĭ). Proctoscopy.

**rectosigmoid** (rek'to-sig'moyd). The rectum and sigmoid colon considered as a unit; the term is also applied to the junction of the sigmoid colon and rectum.

**rectostenosis** (rek'to-stĕ-no'sis). Proctostenosis.

**rectostomy** (rek-tos'to-mĭ). Proctostomy.

**rectotome** (rek'to-tōm). Proctotome.

**rectotomy** (rek-tot'o-mĭ). Proctotomy.

**rectourethral** (rek-to-u-re'thral). Relating to the rectum and the urethra.

**rectouterine** (rek-to-u'ter-in). Relating to the rectum and the uterus.

**rectovaginal** (rek-to-vaj'ĭ-nal). Relating to the rectum and the vagina.

**rectovesical** (rek-to-ves'ĭ-kal). Relating to the rectum and the bladder.

**rectovestibular** (rek'to-ves-tib'u-lar). Relating to the rectum and the vestibule of the vagina.

**rectum,** pl. **rectums** or **recta** (rek'tum) [ L. *rectus,* straight, pp. of *rego,* to make straight. REG- ] [ NA ]. The terminal portion of the digestive tube, extending from the sigmoid colon to the anal canal.

**rec'tus** [ L. ] [ NA ]. Straight; see under musculus.

**recumbent** (re-kum'bent) [ L. *recumbo,* to lie back, recline, fr. *re-,* back, + *cubo,* to lie ]. 1. Lying down. 2. Leaning against another part.

**recuperate** (re-ku'per-āt) [ L. *recupero* (or *recip-*), pp. *-atus,* to take again, recover ]. To recover; to regain health and strength.

**recuperation** (re-ku'per-a'shun) [ L. *recuperatio* (see recuperate) ]. Recovery; restoration to the normal state.

**recurrence** (re-kŭr'ens) [ L. *re-curro,* to run back, recur ]. 1. A return of the symptoms, occurring as a phenomenon in the natural history of the disease, as seen in recurrent fever. 2. Relapse; a return of the symptoms after convalescence had begun.

**recur'rens** [ L. ] [ NA ]. Recurrent (1).

**recurrent** (re-kŭr'ent). 1. In anatomy, turning back on itself. 2. Returned; denoting symptoms or lesions reappearing after an intermission or remission.

**recurvation** (re-ker-va'shun) [ L. *re-curvus,* bent back ]. A backward bending or flexure.

**red** [ A.S. *réad* ]. One of the primary colors, occupying the lower extremity of the spectrum at the other end from violet. For individual red dyes not listed below, see specific name.

**oil r. O,** a weakly acid disazo dye, $C_{26}H_{24}N_4O$, used as a fat stain.

**vital r.,** C.I. Direct Red 34; trisodium salt of a sulfonated diazo dye, $C_{34}H_{25}N_6Na_7O_9S_3$; it is used as a vital stain and also may be injected into the blood stream to determine the blood volume.

**Red Cross.** A red Geneva cross on a white background, a sign of neutrality for the protection of the sick and wounded and the physicians and nurses caring for them in time of war.

**R. C. Society,** an international society established for the purpose of caring for the sick and wounded in war and for giving aid in times of famine, earthquake, fire, and other public calamities.

**Redi** (ra'de), Francesco, Italian naturalist, 1626–1697. Demonstrated to the scientific world the fallacy of the theory of spontaneous generation; in decaying meat protected from flies by means of wire gauze no maggots appeared, whereas unprotected meat was soon swarming with larvae.

**redia,** pl. **rediae** (re'dĭ-ah, re'dĭ-e) [ F. *Redi* ]. Larva of a trematode following the stage of the sporocyst. Rediae are produced from cells within the sporocyst and are liberated from the latter. They are elongated, saclike, muscular

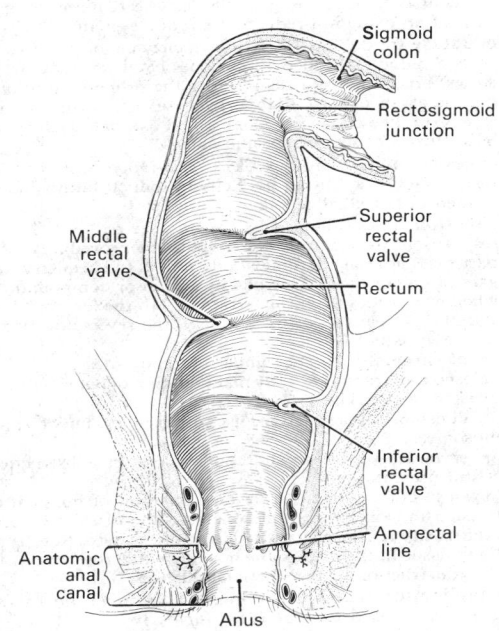

The Rectum

organisms with a mouth and gut. The rediae may produce another one or two generations of rediae or the next developmental state, the cercaria. See also sporocyst (1).

**redifferentiation** (re′dif′er-en′shī-a′shun). The return to a fully specialized condition for the performance of a particular function after a period of nonspecific activity.

**redigitalization** (re′dij′ĭ-tal-ĭ-za′shun). A now disapproved idea that excessive diuresis mobilizes digitalis from edema fluid, leading to increased effects of digitonin, sometimes with intoxication.

**redintegration** (re-din′te-gra′shun) [ L. *red-integro*, pp. *-atus*, to make whole again, renew, fr. *integer*, untouched, entire ]. 1. The restoration of lost or injured parts. 2. Restoration to health. 3. The recalling of a whole experience on the basis of a stimulus representing some item or portion of the original circumstances of the experience.

**Redlich**, E., Austrian neurologist, 1866–1930. See Obersteiner-R. *line, zone.*

**red-out.** Term sometimes applied to the effect upon the circulation of a pilot of an airplane when he makes a turn at high velocity with his head directed outward, that is, toward the circumference of the circling movement. A symptom characteristic of obstruction of the superior vena cava. The blood is forced toward the head. There is severe throbbing pain in the head; the eyes feel as if they were being forced from their sockets; cerebral confusion or unconsciousness may result. See also blackout.

**redox.** Coinage meaning oxidation-reduction, *q.v.*

**redressement** (rë-dres-man′) [ Fr. ]. Redressment.

   **r. forcé** (for-sa′), the straightening by force of a deformed part, as of a knock-knee.

**redress′ment.** 1. Correction of a deformity; putting a part straight. 2. A renewed dressing of a wound.

**reduce** (re-dūs′) [ L. *re-duco*, pp. *-ductus*, to lead back, restore, reduce ]. 1. To replace, as the bowel in a hernia, the ends of a fractured bone, or a dislocation. 2. In chemistry, to initiate a reaction involving a gain of electrons by the substance in question, as when a metal oxide is converted to the metal itself, or when hydrogen is added to the double bond of an organic compound, or when an aldehyde is converted to an alcohol. The substance supplying the electrons or the hydrogen, or removing the oxygen, is itself oxidized in so doing.

**reducible** (re′du′sĭ-bl). Capable of being reduced.

**reductant** (re-duk′tant). The substance that is oxidized in the course of performing reduction; the reduced component of an oxidation-reduction enzyme system.

**reductase** (re-duk′tās). A reducing enzyme; one that catalyzes a reduction. Since all enzymes catalyze reactions in either direction, any r. can, under the proper conditions, behave as an oxidase (dehydrogenases are oxidases) and *vice versa.* The class (EC 1) is termed oxidoreductase. For individual r.'s, see the specific names.

**reductic acid** (re-duk′tik). 2,3-Dihydroxy-2-cyclo-penten-1-one; a strong reducing product (antioxidant) formed in hot alkaline sugar solutions.

**reduction** (re-duk′shun) [ L. *reductio*, see reduce ]. 1. The restoration, by surgical or manipulative procedures, of a part to its normal anatomical relation. 2. In chemistry, the gain of one or more electrons by an ion or compound, as when iron passes from the ferric $(3+)$ to the ferrous $(2+)$ state $(+ =$ electropositive charge); the reverse of oxidation. See reduce (2).

   **r. of chromosomes,** see under chromosome.

   **closed r. of fractures,** r. by manipulation of bone, without incision in the skin.

   **r. division,** see reduction of chromosomes, under chromosome.

   **r. en masse,** r. of sac and contents, so that obstruction is still present.

   **open r. of fractures,** r. by manipulation of bone, after incision in skin and muscle over the site of the fracture.

   **tuberosity r.,** the surgical excision of excessive fibrous or bony tissue in the area of the maxillary tuberosity prior to the construction of prosthetic appliances.

**reduplication** (re-du′plĭ-ka′shun) [ L. *reduplicatio*, fr. *re-,* again, + *duplico*, to double, fr. *duplex*, two-fold. PLIC- ]. 1. A redoubling. 2. A doubling, as of the sounds of the heart in certain morbid states. 3. A fold or duplicature.

**Reed,** Charles A. L., U. S. gynecologist, 1856–1928. See R.'s *operation.*

**Reed,** Dorothy R., American pathologist, *1874. See R.-Sternberg *cells.*

**Reed,** Walter, American army surgeon, 1851–1902. Noted for his researches into yellow fever in Cuba; he and his associates proved that the disease was caused by a filterable virus transmitted to man by the mosquito *Aëdes* (*Stegomyia*) *aegypti.*

**reed.** A small flexible piece of cane or metal attached to the mouthpiece of wind instruments; when vibrated by a stream of air, it subsequently vibrates the column of air in the instrument's tube.

   **vibrating r.,** an aerosol generator designed for producing monodisperse aerosols.

**reef′ing.** Sugically reducing the extent of a tissue by folding it and securing with sutures.

   **stomach r.,** gastroplication.

**reenactment** (re-en-akt′ment). In psychodrama, the acting out of a past experience.

**reentry** (re′en′trī). Return of the same impulse into an area of heart muscle that it has recently activated but which is now no longer refractory, as seen, for instance, in reciprocal rhythms.

**Rees,** H. M. See R.-Ecker *fluid.*

**refection** (re-fek′shun) [ L. *refectio*, fr. *reficere*, to restore, fr. *re-* + *facio*, to do. FAC- ]. A restoring to normal state.

**Refetoff,** S. See R. *syndrome.*

**refine** (re-fin′). To free from impurities.

**reflect** (re-flekt′) [ L. *re-flecto*, pp. *-flexus*, to bend back. FLECT- ]. 1. To bend back. 2. To throw back, as the rays of light from a mirror. 3. To meditate; to think over a matter. 4. To send back a motor impulse in response to a sensory stimulus.

**reflection** (re-flek′shun) [ L. *reflexio*, a bending back ]. 1. A bending back. 2. The throwing back of a ray of light or other form of radiant energy from a surface. 3. Meditation.

**reflector** (re-flek′tor). Any surface that reflects the waves of light, heat, or sound.

# REFLEX

**reflex** (re′fleks) [ L. *reflexus*, pp. of *re-flecto*, to bend back. FLECT- ]. 1. A reaction; an involuntary movement or exercise of function in a part, excited in response to a stimulus applied to the periphery and transmitted to the nervous centers in the brain or spinal cord; see also phenomenon. 2. A reflection. Most of the deep r.'s listed in this table are stretch or myotatic r.'s, striking a tendon or bone causing stretching, often very slight, of the muscle which then contracts as a result of the stimulus applied to its proprioceptors.

   **abdominal r.'s,** contraction of the muscles of the abdominal wall upon stimulation of the skin or tapping neighboring bony structures. The former are called **superficial abdominal r.'s.;** the latter are known as **deep abdominal r.'s.**

   **abdom′inocar′diac r.,** mechanical stimulation of the abdominal viscera causes changes in heart rate, usually slowing, or the occurrence of extrasystoles.

   **Abrams' heart r.,** a contraction of the myocardium when the skin of the precordial region is irritated.

   **Abrams' lung r.,** increase in the pulmonary area following irritation of the skin of the thorax or upper abdominal region.

   **accommodation r.,** near r.; constriction of the pupil, convergence of the eyes, and increased convexity of the lens (due to contraction of the ciliary muscle and relaxation of the suspensory ligament) when the eyes view a near object.

   **Achilles r., Achilles tendon r.,** ankle jerk or r.; triceps surae r.; a contraction of the calf muscles when the tendo calcaneus is sharply struck.

   **acous′ticopal′pebral r.,** cochleopalpebral r.

**acquired r.,** conditioned r.

**acro′mial r.,** contraction of the biceps muscle caused by a tap on the acromion or the coracoid process.

**adductor r.,** contraction of the adductors of the thigh caused by tapping the tendon of the adductor magnus muscle while the thigh is abducted.

**allied r.'s,** r.'s which, acting toward a common purpose, can traverse the final common path together.

**anal r.,** contraction of the internal sphincter gripping the finger passed into the rectum.

**ankle r.,** Achilles r.

**antagonistic r.'s,** r.'s which do not act toward a common purpose, and cannot together traverse the final common path.

**aor′tic r.,** cardiac depressor r.

**aponeurot′ic r.,** plantar flexion of the foot and toes elicited by tapping the sole near its outer edge; has the same significance as the Rossolimo toe flexion r.; also called Guillain-Barrér.; Reimer's r.; Weingrow's r.; sole-tap r.

**Aschner's r.,** oculocardiac r.

**Aschner-Dagnini r.,** oculocardiac r.

**attention r. of the pupil,** Piltz r.

**attitu′dinal r.'s,** statotonic r.'s.

**auditory r.,** any r. occurring in response to a sound, *e.g.,* cochleopalpebral r.

**auditory oc′ulogy′ric r.,** the turning of the two eyes toward the source of a sudden sound.

**auric′ular r.,** a movement of the ears in animals in response to a sound; part of the investigatory r.

**auric′ulopal′pebral r.,** Kisch's r.

**auriculopres′sor r.,** Pavlov's r.; peripheral vasoconstriction and a rise in blood pressure in response to a fall in pressure in the great veins.

**aur′opal′pebral r.,** cochleopalpebral r.

**axon r.,** an effect brought about by the passage of the nerve impulses from a sensory ending to the effector organ along divisions of a nerve fiber without traversing a nerve cell, *e.g.,* as in the vasodilation resulting from stimulation of the skin or the irritation of the conjunctiva; the reaction occurs though the nerve fiber has been sectioned and thus isolated from the nervous centers.

**Babinski's r.,** Babinski's *sign* (1).

**back (dorsum) of foot r.,** Mendel's instep r.

**Bainbridge r.,** an increase in heart rate caused by a rise in pressure of the blood in the great veins at the entrance to the right atrium.

**Balduzzi's r.,** almost identical with Bing's r.

**Barkman's r.,** contraction of the ipsilateral rectus muscle in response to a stimulus applied to the skin below a nipple.

**basal joint r.,** opposition and adduction of the thumb with flexion at its metacarpophalangeal joint and extension at its interphalangeal joint, when firm passive flexion of the 3rd, 4th, or 5th finger is made. The r. is present normally but is absent in pyramidal lesions. Also known as finger-thumb r. or Mayer's r.

**Bechterew-Mendel r.,** Mendel-Bechterew r.; dorsum pedis r.; percussion of the dorsum of the foot causes flexion of the toes; present in a pyramidal lesion.

**behavior r.,** conditioned r.

**Benedek's r.,** plantar flexion of the foot by tapping the anterior margin of the lower part of the fibula, while the foot is slightly dorsiflexed.

**Bezold-Jarisch r.,** a r. with afferent and efferent pathways in the vagus, originating in unidentified chemoreceptors in the heart and resulting in sinus bradycardia, hypotension, and probable peripheral vasodilation.

**biceps r.,** contraction of the biceps muscle when its tendon is struck.

**biceps fem′oris r.,** contraction of the biceps femoris upon tapping its lower part, just above its attachment to the head of the fibula, while the limb is partly flexed at hip and knee.

**Bing's r.,** when the foot is passively dorsiflexed, plantar flexion occurs if any point on the ankle between the two malleoli is tapped.

**bladder r.,** micturition r.

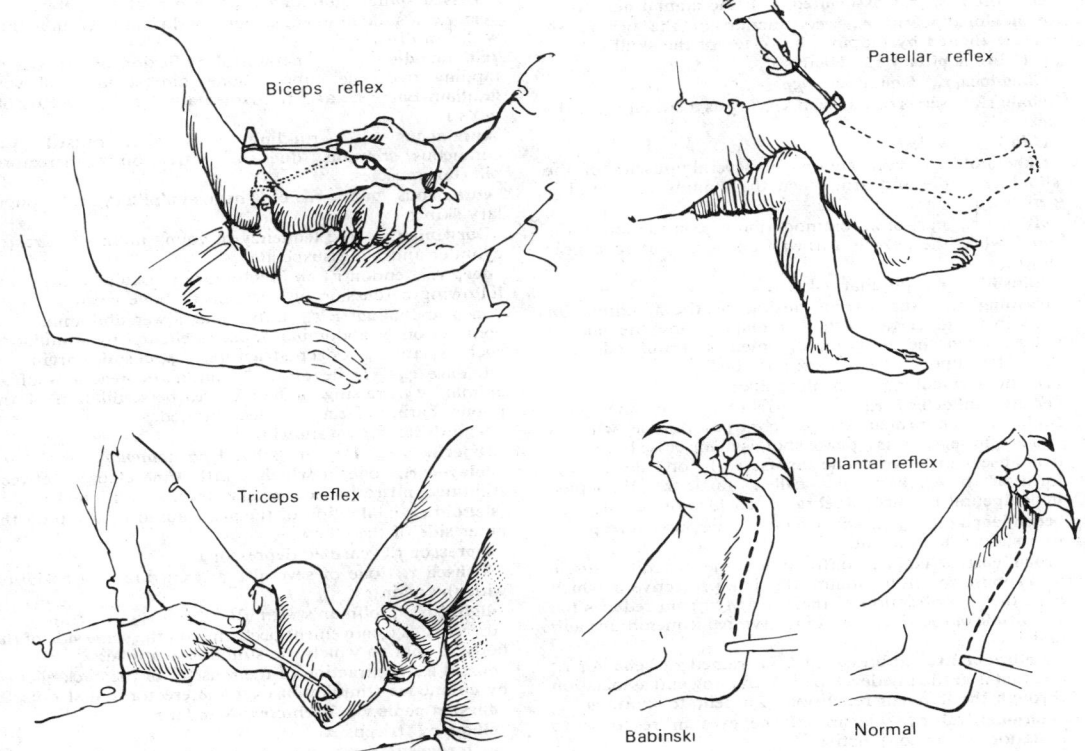

Biceps reflex

Patellar reflex

Triceps reflex

Plantar reflex

Babinski

Normal

**Reflexes**

**body righting r.'s,** stimulation of pressoreceptors in the body wall by contact with the ground causes r. effects upon the neck muscles which bring the head into the correct position in space.

**bone r.,** a r. excited by a stimulus applied to a bone.

**bra'chiora'dial r.,** with the arm supinated to 45° a tap near the lower end of the radius causes contraction of the brachioradial (supinator longus) muscle; also called supinator jerk or r., styloradial r., supinator longus r., radioperiosteal r.

**Brain's r.,** quadripedal extensor r.

**breg'mocar'diac r.,** in infants, pressure upon the anterior fontanelle causes cardiac slowing.

**Brissaud's r.,** tickling the sole causes a contraction of the tensor fasciae femoris, even when there is no responsive movement of the toes.

**Brudzinski's r.,** Brudzinski's *sign.*

**bulbocav'ernous r.,** virile r.

**bulbomimic r.,** facial r.; Mondonesi's r.; in a case of coma from severe apoplexy, pressure on the eyeballs causes contraction of the facial muscles of expression on the side opposite to the lesion; in coma due to diabetes, uremia, or other toxic cause the r. is present on both sides.

**Capps' r.,** vasomotor collapse at the time of crisis in pneumonia.

**cardiac r.,** decrease in the area of cardiac dullness in response to stimulation of the skin of the chest wall overlying the heart.

**cardiac depressor r.,** aortic r.; depressor r.; a fall in blood pressure due to peripheral vasodilation and cardiac inhibition by stimulations of terminations of cardiac depressor nerve in aortic arch and base of heart.

**carot'id si'nus r.,** carotid sinus *syndrome.*

**celiac plexus r.,** (1) a progressive fall in blood pressure in some pregnant women upon assuming the dorsal recumbent position; due to pressure upon the structures related to the celiac plexus by the enlarged uterus; (2) arterial hypotension coincident with surgical manipulations in the upper abdomen during general anesthesia.

**cephalic r.'s,** r.'s associated with the cranial nerves.

**ceph'alopal'pebral r.,** contraction of the orbicularis muscle elicited by tapping the vertex of the skull.

**cer'ebropu'pillary r.,** Haab's r.

**Chaddock r.,** Chaddock *sign.*

**chain r.,** a series of r.s, each serving as a stimulus for the next.

**chin r.,** jaw *jerk.*

**Chodzko's r.,** contractions of several muscles of the shoulder girdle and arm when the manubrium sterni is percussed.

**cil'iary r.,** part of accommodation r.; contraction of the pupil when the gaze is turned from a distant to a near object.

**ciliospi'nal r.,** pupillary-skin r.

**clasping r.,** the strong flexion of the forelimbs of amphibia and certain other animals during the mating season when the chest or abdomen is stimulated. It is dependent upon the male sex hormone.

**cochleo-orbicular r.,** cochleopalpebral r.

**cochleopal'pebral r.,** a contraction, sometimes very slight, of the orbicularis palpebrarum muscle when a sudden noise, such as a pistol shot, is made close to the ear; it is absent in labyrinthine disease with total deafness; a form of the wink r.; also called startle r. (2); acousticopalpebral r.; auropalpebral r.; cochleo-orbicular r.

**coch'leopu'pillary r.,** constriction of the pupil in response to a sudden loud sound.

**coch'leostape'dial r.,** contraction of the stapedius muscle in response to a loud sound; this is a protective r. which with the r. contraction of the tensor tympani reduces the amplitude of the vibrations of the tympanic membrane and ossicles.

**conditioned r.,** abbreviated CR; trained r.; behavior r.; one that is gradually developed by training and association through the frequent repetition of a definite stimulus.

**conjuncti'val r.,** closure of the eyes in response to irritation of the conjunctiva.

**consen'sual light r.,** consensual *reaction.*

**contralat'eral r.,** Brudzinski's *sign.*

**convulsive r.,** an incoordinated r. in which muscles, even those opposing one another as in strychnine poisoning, contract.

**coordinated r.,** one in which several muscles take part to perform a purposeful act.

**corneal r.,** (1) lid r.; a contraction of the eyelids when the cornea is lightly touched with a camel's hair pencil; (2) reflection of light from the surface of the cornea.

**coronary r.,** the increase in the rate of the heart in the heart-lung preparation in response to an increase in the venous inflow; due to decreased vagal tone.

**corticopu'pillary r.,** Haab's r.

**costal arch r.,** contraction of the rectus abdominus muscle by tapping the costal margin inside the mammary line.

**cos'topec'toral r.,** pectoral r.

**cough r.,** irritation of the mucous membrane of the larynx or tracheobronchial tree causes coughing.

**craniocardiac r.,** stimulation of nerve endings of certain cranial nerves (*e.g.,* olfactory, ophthalmic branch of trigeminal), with resultant cardiac depressor r., manifested by bradycardia and hypotension, through the cardiac branch of the vagus.

**cremaster'ic r.,** a drawing up of the scrotum and testicle of the same side when the skin over Scarpa's triangle or on the inner side of the thigh is scratched.

**crossed r.,** a stimulus applied to one side of the body causes a r. movement on the opposite side.

**crossed adductor r.,** contraction of the adductors of the thigh and inward rotation of the limb elicited by tapping the sole.

**crossed extension r.,** extension of the contralateral hind limb when the paw of an animal is painfully stimulated or the central cut end of an afferent nerve, *e.g.,* the peroneal, is stimulated. Sometimes occurs in man upon tapping the skin.

**crossed r. of the pelvis,** crossed spino-adductor r.; contraction of the contralateral adductors of the thigh upon tapping the anterior superior iliac spine.

**crossed spino-adductor r.,** crossed r. of the pelvis.

**cry r.,** a sudden unconscious cry during sleep in a child with hip disease.

**cuboid'odig'ital r.,** metatarsal r.; flexion of the toes on tapping over the cuboid bone; almost identical with Guillain-Barré r., and fundamentally similar to Rossolimo's r.

**cuta'neous r.,** wrinkling of the skin, caused by a cutaneous stimulus, due to contraction of arrectores pilorum muscles.

**cuta'neous pupil r., cuta'neous-pu'pillary r.,** pupillary-skin r.

**Darwinian r.,** the tendency of young infants to grasp a cylinder and hang suspended.

**deep r.,** tendon r.; an involuntary muscular contraction following percussion of a tendon or bone.

**deep abdominal r.'s,** upper and lower abdominal r.'s; contraction of abdominal muscles elicited by stimulation such as tapping a deep structure, *e.g.,* costal margin.

**defense r.,** (1) flexor r. (2) automatic reactions of an animal, *e.g.,* raising of hair or feathers, dilation of the pupils, baring of claws, when alarmed.

**deglutit'ion r.,** swallowing r.

**Déjérine's r.,** Déjérine's hand *phenomenon.*

**delayed r.,** one in which a little time elapses between stimulus and response. See also trace conditioned r.

**deltoid r.,** abduction of the arm caused by a tap on the outer side of the elbow.

**depressor r.,** cardiac depressor r.

**diffused r.,** one of several r.'s occurring in association with the main r.

**digital r.,** Hoffman's *sign* (2).

**direct r.,** a r. movement occurring on the same side of the body as that to which the stimulus is applied.

**dorsal r.,** contraction of the muscles of the back elicited by cutaneous stimulation over the erector spinal muscle.

**dorsum pedis r.,** Bechterew-Mendel r.

**elbow r.,** triceps r.

**en'terogas'tric r.,** peristaltic contraction of the small intestine induced by the entrance of food into the stomach; see also gastrocolic r.

**epigas′tric r.,** a contraction of the upper portion of the rectus abdominis muscle when the skin of the epigastrium above is scratched.

**erector-spinal r.,** a contraction of part of the erector spinae muscle following scratching of the skin on its outer border.

**esoph′agosal′ivary r.,** Roger's r.; salivation caused by irritation of the lower end of the esophagus, as by carcinoma in this situation.

**external oblique r.,** contraction of the external oblique and rectus abdominus muscles upon tapping the anterior and outer part of the lower thoracic wall.

**eye r.,** fundus r.

**eye-closure r.,** wink r.

**facial r.,** bulbomimic r.

**faucial r.,** gag r.

**fem′oral r.,** scratching the skin of the upper part of the front of the thigh causes extension of the knee and flexion of the foot.

**fem′oroabdominal r.,** hypogastric r.; contraction of the abdominal muscles upon stroking the inner aspect of the thigh; it accompanies the cremasteric r.

**finger-thumb r.,** basal joint r.

**flexor r.,** withdrawal r.; nociceptive r.; defense r. (1); flexion of ankle, knee, and hip when the foot is painfully stimulated: the crossed extension r. occurs in association with it.

**forced grasping r.,** grasping r.

**front-tap r.,** periosteal r. (1); contraction of the gastrocnemius muscle when the shin is struck.

**fundus r.,** the red glow seen in the pupil of the human eye during ophthalmoscopic examination.

**gag r.,** faucial r.; contact of a foreign body with the mucous membrane of the fauces causes retching or gagging.

**Galant's r.,** lower abdominal periosteal r.; contraction of the abdominal muscles on tapping the anterior superior iliac spine; lower abdominal r.; a deep abdominal r.

**galvanic skin r.,** galvanic skin *response.*

**gastrocolic r.,** a mass movement of the contents of the colon, frequently preceded by a similar movement in the small intestine, that sometimes occurs immediately following the entrance of food into the stomach.

**gastroileac r.,** entrance of food into the stomach causes opening of the ileocolic valve.

**Geigel's r.,** on gently stroking the inner side of the thigh there is a contraction of the muscular fibers at the upper edge of Poupart's ligament; analogue in woman of the cremasteric r.

**Gifford's r.,** contraction of the pupils when an attempt is made to close the eyes while the lids are held open.

**glu′teal r.,** contraction of the gluteal muscles following irritation of the skin of the buttocks.

**Gordon r.,** paradoxical flexor r.; dorsal flexion of the great toe produced by firm lateral pressure on the calf muscles.

**grasp r.,** grasping r.

**grasping r.,** grasp r.; forced grasping r.; usually associated with frontal lobe lesions, an involuntary flexion of the fingers to tactile or tendon stimulation on the palm of the hand, producing an uncontrollable grasp.

**great-toe r.,** Babinski's *sign* (1).

**Guillain-Barré r.,** aponeurotic r.

**gus′tatory-sudorif′ic r.,** sweating, especially over the face, when chewing food; see also auriculotemporal *syndrome.*

**H r.,** a monosynaptic r. obtained by stimulating the tibial nerve. It short-circuits the neuromuscular spindle.

**Haab's r.,** corticopupillary r.; cerebropupillary r.; constriction of the pupils when the subject who has been in a dark room for some time turns the eyes and without accommodation looks at a bright object.

**heart r.,** reduction of the cardiac area when the skin of the precordial region is irritated.

**hepatojugular r.,** see hepatojugular *reflux.*

**Hering-Breuer r.,** the effects of afferent impulses from the pulmonary vagi in the control of respiration, *e.g.,* inflation of the lungs arrests inspiration, expiration then ensuing, while deflation brings on inspiration.

**Hirschberg's r.,** tickling the sole of the foot at the base of the great toe is followed by adduction of the foot.

**Hoffmann's r.,** Hoffmann's *sign* (2).

**hypochon′drial r.,** sharp pressure beneath the costal margin causes a quick inspiration.

**hy′pogas′tric r.,** femoroabdominal r.

**innate r.,** unconditioned r.

**intrinsic r.,** a r. muscular contraction elicited by the application of a stimulus, usually stretching, to the muscle itself as opposed to a muscular contraction caused by an extrinsic stimulus, *e.g.,* skin, as in the abdominal skin r.'s.

**inverted r.,** paradoxical r.

**inverted radial r.,** flexion of the fingers without flexion of the forearm, on tapping the lower end of the radius; regarded as indicating a lesion of the fifth cervical segment of the spinal cord.

**investiga′tory r.,** orienting r.

**ipsilat′eral r.,** one in which the response occurs on the side of the body that is stimulated.

**Jacobson's r.,** flexion of the fingers elicited by tapping the flexor tendons over the wrist joint or the lower end of the radius.

**jaw r.,** jaw *jerk.*

**jaw-working r.,** see jaw-winking *syndrome.*

**Joffroy's r.,** hip phenomenon; twitching of the glutei muscles when firm pressure is made on the nates, in cases of spastic paralysis.

**Kisch's r.,** closure of the eye in response to stimulation of the skin at the depth of the external auditory meatus.

**knee r.,** patellar r.

**knee-jerk r.,** patellar r.

**labyrin′thine r.,** r.'s initiated through stimulation of receptors in the utricle or semicircular canals. See also statotonic, statokinetic, and righting r.'s.

**labyrin′thine righting r.'s,** stimulation of the proprioceptors of the labyrinth causes changes in tone of the neck muscles which bring the head into its natural position in space.

**lac′rimal r.,** discharge of tears when the conjunctiva is irritated.

**lac′rimo-gus′tatory r.,** chewing of food causes secretion of tears; see also crocodile tears *syndrome.*

**larynge′al r.,** cough r.

**laryngospastic r.,** laryngospasm.

**la′tent r.,** a r. which must be considered a normal one but which, as a rule, appears only under some pathologic circumstance that lowers its threshold.

**laughter r.,** uncontrollable laughter excited by tickling.

**lid r.,** corneal r. (1).

**Liddel-Sherrington r.,** myotatic r.

**light r.,** (1) pupillary r.; (2) a red glow reflected from the fundus of the eye when a light is cast upon the retina, as in retinoscopy; (3) *cone* of light.

**lip r.,** a pouting movement of the lips provoked in young infants by tapping near the angle of the mouth.

**lordosis r.,** adoption of a copulatory posture when touched on the back; exhibited by female animals of certain species but only during the time of estrus.

**Loven r.,** a reaction in which a local dilation of vessels accompanies a general vasoconstriction. For example, when the central end of an afferent nerve to an organ is suitably stimulated, its efferent vasomotor fibers remaining intact, a general rise in blood pressure occurs together with a dilation of the vessels of the organ.

**lower abdominal perios′teal r.,** Galant's r.

**lung r.,** increase in the pulmonary area following irritation of the skin of the thorax or upper abdomen.

**magnet r.,** see magnet *reaction.*

**mandib′ular r.,** jaw *jerk.*

**mass r.,** in cases of gross injury to the spinal cord, as the stage of r. activity follows the primary flaccidity of the shock, a condition arises in which a strong stimulus to any part of one of the paralyzed limbs will be followed by contraction of the hip, knee, and ankle of the same side and often, when the stimulus is applied to the middle line of the body, of both sides, as well as of the abdominal wall, and even evacuation of the bladder and sweating over an area corresponding to the level of the lesion.

**mas′seter r.,** jaw *jerk.*

**Mayer's r.,** basal joint r.

**McCarthy's r.'s,** (1) spino-adductor r.; (2) supraorbital r.

**me′diopu′bic r.,** contraction of the adductors of the thigh upon tapping the pubic bone near the symphysis.

**Mendel's instep r.,** back (dorsum) of foot r.; the foot being firmly supported on its inner side, a sharp tap on the dorsal tendons causes extension of the toes from the second to the fifth.

**Mendel-Bechterew r.,** Bechterew-Mendel r.

**metacar′pohypothe′nar r.,** flexion of the little finger on tapping the dorsum of the hand; seen in pyramidal tract lesions and is similar to Sterling's r.

**metacar′pothe′nar r.,** thumb r.

**metatarsal r.,** cuboidodigital r.

**micturition r.,** bladder r.; urinary r.; contraction of the walls of the bladder and relaxation of the trigone and urethral sphincter in response to a rise in pressure within the bladder; the r. can be voluntarily inhibited; the inhibition is readily abolished in turn by an effort of the will when micturition automatically follows.

**milk-ejection r.,** release of milk from the breast following tactile stimulation of the nipple. Afferent path is postulated to exist from the nipple to the hypothalamus; efferent limb is represented by the neurohypophysial release of oxytocin into the systemic circulation; contraction of myoepithelial elements within the breast, caused by oxytocin, moves milk into the collecting ducts and toward the nipple.

**Mondonesi's r.,** bulbomimic r.

**Moro's r.,** startle r. (1).

**myenter′ic r.,** law of intestine; contraction above and relaxation below a stimulated point in the intestine.

**myotat′ic r.,** stretch r.; Liddell-Sherrington r.; tonic contraction of the muscles in response to a stretching force, due to stimulation of muscle proprioceptors.

**nasal r.,** sneezing caused by irritation of the nasal mucous membrane.

**nasomental r.,** contraction of the mentalis muscle following a tap on the side of the nose.

**near r.,** accommodation r.

**neck r.'s,** changes in position of the head cause alterations in tone of the neck muscles through stimulation of proprioceptors in the labyrinth which bring the head into its correct position in space. Stimulation of proprioceptors in the neck muscles causes in turn r. movements of the limbs which bring the animal into the normal position in relation to the head.

**nocicep′tive r.,** flexor r.

**nocifen′sor r.,** vascular dilation in a part surrounding or in the neighborhood of an injury.

**nose-bridge-lid r.,** orbicularis oculi r.

**nose-eye r.,** orbicularis oculi r.

**oc′ulocar′diac r.,** Aschner's r.; Aschner's phenomenon; Aschner-Dagnini r.; Ashley's phenomenon; a change in the pulse rate, usually a slowing, following compression of the eyeball.

**oculocephalic r.,** oculocephalogyric r.

**oc′uloceph′alogy′ric r.,** turning of the eyes and head toward the source of an auditory, visual, or other form of stimulation.

**oculopharyn′geal r.,** relating to the eye and the pharynx; denoting a r. marked by rapid deglutition following the instillation of a solution of one of several chemical substances into the eye, especially if of a low temperature.

**olec′ranon r.,** paradoxical triceps r.; flexion of the forearm caused by tapping the olecranon.

**Onanoff's r.,** Onanoff's *sign.*

**Oppenheim's r.,** extension of the toes following scratching of the inner side of the leg, or following sudden flexion of the thigh on the abdomen and the leg on the thigh; it is a sign of cerebral irritation.

**optical righting r.'s,** visual stimuli that enable an animal to maintain the correct position of the head in space, by bringing about movements of the muscles of the neck and limbs.

**op′ticofa′cial r.,** wink r.

**orbicularis oculi r.,** contraction of the orbicularis oculi muscles upon tapping the margin of the orbit, the bridge or tip of the nose; also called nose-bridge-lid r. or nose-eye r.

**orbicularis pupillary r.,** Galassi's pupillary phenomenon; contraction followed by dilation of the pupil upon forcible closure of the eyelids, or upon the attempt to close them while they are held apart.

**orienting r.,** investigatory r.; orienting response; an aspect of attending in which an organism's initial response

to a change or to a novel stimulus is such that the organism becomes more sensitive to the stimulation; *e.g.,* dilation of the pupil of the eye in response to dim light.

**pal′atal r., palatine r.,** swallowing r. induced by stimulation of the palate.

**palmar r.,** flexion of the fingers following tickling of the palm.

**palm-chin r.,** palmomental r.

**pal′momen′tal r.,** palm-chin r.; unilateral (sometimes bilateral) contraction of the mentalis and orbicularis oris muscles caused by a brisk scratch made on the palm of the ipsilateral hand.

**paradox′ical r.,** any r. in which the usual response is reversed or does not conform to the pattern characteristic of the particular r.; inverted r.

**paradox′ical extensor r.,** Babinski's *sign* (1).

**paradox′ical flexor r.,** Gordon r.

**paradox′ical patellar r.,** (1) a tap on the patellar tendon causes contraction of the adductor; (2) sudden passive extension of the leg causes a contraction of the extensor muscles of the leg.

**paradox′ical pu′pillary r.,** paradoxical pupillary phenomenon; a pupillary response to light, which is the reverse of that expected, *e.g.,* to photic stimulation the pupil dilates.

**paradox′ical triceps r.,** olecranon r.

**patellar r.,** a sudden contraction of the anterior muscles of the thigh, caused by a smart tap on the patellar tendon while the leg hangs loosely at a right angle with the thigh; also called patellar-tendon r., knee jerk or r., quadriceps r.

**patellar-tendon r.,** patellar r.

**patello-adductor r.,** crossed adduction of the leg on tapping the quadriceps tendon.

**Pavlov's r.,** auriculopressor r.

**pec′toral r.,** costopectoral r.; contraction of the pectoralis major muscle elicited by tapping the seventh rib between the anterior and the medial axillary lines while the arm is abducted; contraction of the deltoid and biceps may also occur.

**penile r.,** virile r.

**Perez r.,** an infant is held supported in a prone position; when a finger is run down the spine the whole body normally becomes extended.

**pericardial r.,** a vagal r. seen during operations involving pericardial manipulation; characterized by signs of vagal stimulation (bradycardia and arterial hypotension).

**perios′teal r.,** (1) front-tap r.; (2) a muscular contraction in the arm following a tap on the radius or ulna.

**pharyn′geal r.,** (1) swallowing r.; (2) vomiting r.

**phasic r.,** a coordinated complex response such as the scratch r. in the spinal animal.

**Phillipson's r.,** a contraction of the extensors of the knee when the extensors of the opposite knee are inhibited.

**pilomo′tor r.,** contraction of the smooth muscle of the skin resulting in "gooseflesh" caused by mild application of a tactile stimulus or by local cooling.

**Piltz r.,** change in the size of the pupils when one's attention is suddenly attracted to some object.

**plantar r.,** sole r.; the response to tactile plantar stimulation, normally plantar flexion of the toes. Extension and abduction of the toes, Babinski's sign, is evidence of extrapyramidal tract involvement.

**plantar muscle r.,** Rossolimo's r. (1).

**pneocardiac r.** (ne-o-kar′dĭ-ak) [ G. *pneō,* to breathe, + *kardia,* heart ], a modification in the blood pressure or heart rhythm caused by the inhalation of an irritating vapor.

**pneopneic r.** (ne-op-ne′ik) [ G. *pneō,* to breathe ], a modification of the respiratory rhythm caused by the inhalation of an irritating vapor.

**postural r.,** static r.; responses that control the position of the trunk and extremities; see also righting r.

**pressoreceptor r.,** carotid sinus *syndrome.*

**prona′tor r.,** ulnar r.

**proprioceptive r.'s,** any r. brought about by stimulation of proprioceptors, *e.g.,* in labyrinth, muscles, or carotid sinus.

**protective laryngeal r.,** closure of the glottis to prevent entry of foreign substances into the respiratory tract, usually abolished in the second state of anesthesia.

**psychocardiac r.,** a change in the circulatory rate and the consciousness of heart thumping resulting from a memory of, or a subconscious dream state recollection of, an emotional impression or experience.

**psychogalvanic r.,** galvanic skin *response.*

**psychogalvanic skin r.,** galvanic skin *response.*

**pulmonocor'onary r.,** r. constriction of the coronary arteries as a result of vagal stimuli arising in the lungs, as in pulmonary embolism.

**pu'pillary r.,** change in diameter of the pupil as a reflex response to any type of stimulus, *e.g.,* constriction caused by light.

**pu'pillary-skin r.,** ciliospinal r.; dilation of the pupil following scratching of the skin of the neck.

**quad'riceps r.,** patellar r.

**quadripedal extensor r.,** Brain's r.; extension of the arm of a hemiplegic patient when turned prone as if on all fours.

**radial r.,** on tapping the lower end of the radius, flexion of the forearm occurs, and sometimes, on strong percussion, flexion of the fingers; see also inverted radial r.

**ra'diobicip'ital r.,** contraction of the biceps muscle which sometimes occurs in the elicitation of the brachioradial r.

**ra'dioperios'teal r.,** brachioradial r.

**rectal r.,** the entrance of fecal matter into the rectum from the sigmoid colon causes an impulse to defecate.

**rectocardiac r.,** a parasympathetic r. producing bradycardia and hypotension upon stimulation of the pelvic nerve, the afferent limb being the sacral outflow of the parasympathetic division of the autonomic nervous system, and the efferent limb, the cardiac vagus.

**rectolaryngeal r.,** laryngeal spasm precipitated during general anesthesia by stretching the anal sphincter.

**Reimer's r.,** aponeurotic r.

**Remak's r.,** stroking of the upper anterior surface of the thigh causes plantar flexion of the first three toes and sometimes of the foot, with extension of the knee; it occurs when the conducting paths in the cord are interrupted.

**renal r.,** anuria caused by injury to a remote part of the body, or by disease or injury to one kidney or ureter.

**righting r.'s,** static r.'s; r.'s which through various receptors, in labyrinth, eyes, muscles, or skin, tend to bring an animal's body into its normal position in space and which resist any force acting to put it into a false position, *e.g.,* on its back. See also neck r.'s; labyrinthine righting r.'s, optical righting r.'s, body righting r.'s.

**Roger's r.,** esophagosalivary r.

**Rossolimo's r.,** Rossolimo's sign; (1) flicking the tops of the toes from the plantar surface causes flexion of the toes; it is a stretch r. of the flexors of the toes and is seen in lesions of the pyramidal tracts; (2) flexion of the fingers by tapping the tips of the fingers on their volar surfaces.

**scap'ular r.,** contraction of the upper muscles of the back by stimulation between the scapulae; interscapular r.

**scap'ulohu'meral r.,** scapuloperiosteal r.; contraction of muscles of the shoulder girdle and arm caused by tapping the lower part of the unilateral border of the scapula; the muscles which respond vary according to their degree of stretching at the time.

**scap'uloperio'steal r.,** scapulohumeral r.

**Schäffer's r.,** in cases of injury to the corticospinal tract, the great toe is dorsiflexed when the skin over the Achilles tendon is pinched.

**scratch r. in dogs,** stimulus applied to the skin of a saddle-shaped area of the back, sides, and flanks produces a scratching movement of the hind leg of the side stimulated.

**sem'imembrano'sus and sem'itendino'sus r.,** contraction of these muscles by tapping in the region of the tuberosity of the tibia.

**senile r.,** a grayish r. from the pupil of the aged due to the normal senile hardening of the lens.

**shot-silk r.,** shot-silk phenomenon; shimmering reflections like those of watered silk, sometimes seen in the retina in childhood.

**sinus r.,** see carotid sinus *syndrome.*

**skin r.'s,** skin-muscle r.'s.

**skin-muscle r.'s,** superficial or cutaneous r.'s, such as the superficial abdominal r.'s.

**skin-pu'pillary r.,** pupillary-skin r.

**snapping r.,** Hoffmann's *sign* (2).

**snout r.,** light tapping of closed lips near the midline causes pouting or pursing of the lips; it is seen in defective pyramidal innervation of facial musculature.

**sole r.,** plantar r.

**sole tap r.,** aponeurotic r.

**spinal r.,** a r. arc involving the spinal cord; see reflex *arc.*

**spino-adductor r.,** McCarthy's r. (1); contraction of the adductors of the thigh upon tapping the spinal column.

**Starling's r.,** tapping the volar surfaces of the fingers causes flexion of the fingers; analogous to Rossolimo's r., for the toes.

**startle r.,** (1) Moro's r.; startle reaction; the r. response of an infant (contraction of the limb and neck muscles) when allowed to drop a short distance through the air or startled by a sudden noise or jolt; (2) cochleopalpebral r.

**static r.,** postural or righting r.

**statokinetic r.,** that which, through stimulation of the receptors in the neck muscles and semicircular canals, brings about movements of the limbs and eyes appropriate to a given movement of the head in space.

**statotonic r.'s,** attitudinal r.'s; r.'s which through labyrinthine (utricular) and muscle receptors influence the tone of the limb muscles; the former are brought about by alterations in the position of the head in space, the latter by changes in the position of the head in relation to the body.

**stepping r.,** if the plantar surface of a hind foot of a dog is pressed gently, a movement of extension of the limb will follow accompanied sometimes by flexion of the opposite hind limb.

**ster'nobra'chial r.,** contraction of the adductors of the arm when the sternum is tapped.

**stretch r.,** myotatic r.

**Strümpell's r.,** stroking the abdomen or thigh causes flexion of the leg and adduction of the foot.

**sty'lora'dial r.,** brachioradial r.

**suckling r.,** the r. liberation of prolactin from the anterior lobe of the hypophysis evoked by stimulation of nerves in the nipple during the act of suckling by the newborn animal.

**superficial r.,** any r., *e.g.,* the abdominal r. or the cremasteric r., which is elicited by stimulation of the skin.

**supinator r., supination r.,** brachioradial r.

**su'pinator longus r.,** brachioradial r.

**supporting r.'s,** supporting *reactions.*

**supraor'bital r.,** McCarthy's r. (2); trigeminofacial r.; tapping the supraorbital nerve causes a contraction of the orbicularis oculi muscle.

**suprapatellar r.,** a tap on the quadriceps tendon above the patella causes the patella to rise.

**supraumbilical r.,** (1) epigastric r.; (2) abdominal r.

**swallowing r.,** deglutition r.; pharyngeal r. (1); the act of swallowing (second stage) induced by stimulation of the palate, fauces or posterior pharyngeal wall.

**syn'chronous r.,** subsidiary r. actions occurring in association with the main or leading r.

**tape'tal light r.,** the red glow from the eyes of certain carnivorous animals in the dark when a light illumines the retina. Due to the relection of the light from the tapetum, an iridescent layer (containing guanidine crystals) in the choroid coat.

**tarsophalangeal r.,** extension of all the toes except the first, when the outer part of the tarsus is tapped; in certain cerebral diseases the reverse takes place, the toes being flexed.

**tendo Achil'lis r.,** Achilles r.

**tendon r.,** deep r.

**thumb r.,** metacarpothenar r.; flexion of the thumb upon tapping the dorsum of the hand.

**toe r.,** (1) strong passive flexion of the great toe excites contraction of the flexor muscles in the leg; (2) toe *clonus;* (3) Babinski's *sign* (1).

**tonic r.,** Gordon's symptom; the occurrence of an appreciable interval after the production of a r. before relaxation, *e.g.,* the leg hangs up after the knee jerk.

**trace conditioned r.,** a conditioned r. established by applying the stimulus a short time before reinforcement; in the conditioned r. of the animal prepared in this way the response occurs at the same interval of time after the application of the stimulus as during the period of training.

**trained r.,** conditioned r.

**triceps r.,** elbow jerk; elbow r.; a sudden contraction of the triceps muscle caused by a smart tap on its tendon when the forearm hangs loosely at a right angle with the arm.

**triceps surae r.,** Achilles r.

**trigem'inofa'cial r.,** supraorbital r.

**trochan'ter r.,** contraction of the adductor muscles of the thigh elicited by a tap on the trochanter.

**Trömmer's r.,** a modified Rossolimo r.; with the fingers of the patient partially flexed, tapping the volar aspect of the tip of the middle or index finger causes flexion of all four fingers and thumb; seen in pyramidal tract lesions with moderate spasticity.

**ulnar r.,** pronator r.; pronation and adduction of the hand caused by tapping the styloid process of the ulna.

**unconditioned r.,** innate r.; an instinctive r. not dependent on previous learning or experience.

**upper abdominal perios'teal r.,** deep abdominal r.

**urinary r.,** micturition r.

**utricular r.'s,** see statotonic r.'s.

**vagovagal r.,** a cardiac r. originating from stimulation of the respiratory tract, both the afferent and efferent limbs of the r. arc being the vagus nerve; may be precipitated by laryngeal or tracheal irritation during the introduction of an endotracheal tube during the administration of a vagus-stimulating anesthetic agent such as cyclopropane or intravenous barbiturate.

**va'sopres'sor r.,** vasoconstriction caused by stimulation of certain afferent fibers, *e.g.,* in vagus nerve.

**venorespiratory r.,** stimulation of respiration and increased pulmonary ventilation in response to an increase in venous pressure at the right auricle.

**ver'tebra prom'inens r.,** pressure upon the last cervical vertebra of an animal, especially of one whose labyrinths have been destroyed and the vestibular nuclei isolated, causes relaxation or reduced tone of all four limbs.

**vesical r.,** the desire to urinate caused by moderate distention of the bladder.

**vestibulospinal r.,** the influence of vestibular stimulation on body posture.

**virile r.,** bulbocavernous r.; penile r.; a movement of contraction of the bulbous portion of the urethra caused by tapping the under surface or side of the penis close to the scrotum.

**visceral traction r.,** laryngeal spasm precipitated during general anesthesia by traction on the stomach, gallbladder, or appendiceal mesentery.

**viscerogen'ic r.,** any of a number of r.'s, such as headache, cough, disturbed pulse, etc., caused by disordered conditions of any of the viscera.

**visceromo'tor r.,** contraction of the muscles of the thorax or abdomen in response to a stimulus from one of the contained viscera.

**vis'ceropannic'ular r.,** contraction of the panniculus carnosus muscle in the cat and certain other animals, in response to a stimulus applied to an abdominal viscus. The center for the r. is in the spinal cord; the afferent pathway in the splanchnic nerves.

**viscerosen'sory r.,** an area of pain or sensitiveness to pressure in the external body wall due to disease of one of the viscera; see also Head's *lines.*

**viscerotroph'ic r.,** a degenerative change in the skeletal soft tissues consequent upon a chronic inflammatory condition of any of the thoracic or abdominal viscera.

**visual orbicula'ris r.,** contraction of the orbicularis oculi muscle caused by a sudden visual stimulus; see also wink r.

**vomiting r.,** pharyngeal r. (2); vomiting (contraction of the abdominal muscles with relaxation of the cardiac sphincter of the stomach and of the muscles of the throat) elicited by a variety of stimuli, especially one applied to the region of the fauces.

**Weingrow's r.,** aponeurotic r.

**Weiss' r.,** a crescentic light r. seen in the retina to the inner, nasal, side of the papilla; regarded as a sign of myopia.

**Westphal's pu'pillary r.,** tonic *pupil.*

**wink r.,** general term for r. closure of eyelids caused by any stimulus; also called eye-closure r., opticofacial r.

**withdrawal r.,** flexor r.

**wrist clonus r.,** sudden extension of the wrist induces a sustained clonic movement.

---

**reflexogenic** (re-flek'so-jen'ik). Causing a reflex.

**reflexogenous** (re'flek-soj'ĕ-nus). Reflexogenic.

**reflexograph** (re-flek'so-graf) [ reflex + G. *graphō,* to write ]. An instrument for graphically recording a reflex.

**reflexology** (re'flek-sol'o-jĭ) [ reflex + G. *logos,* study ]. The study of reflexes.

**reflexometer** (re'flek-som'e-ter) [ reflex + G. *metron,* measure ]. An instrument for measuring the force necessary to excite a reflex.

**reflexophil, reflexophile** (re-fleks'o-fil, -fīl) [ reflex + G. *phileō,* to love ]. Having exaggerated reflexes.

**reflexotherapy** (re-flek'so-thĕr'ă-pī). Reflex *therapy.*

**reflux** (re'fluks) [ L. re-, back, + *fluxus,* a flow, fr. *fluo,* pp. *fluxus,* to flow ]. 1. A backward flow; regurgitation. 2. In chemistry, to boil without loss of vapor because of the presence of a condenser that returns vapor as liquid.

**abdominojugular r.,** hepatojugular r.

**hepatojugular r.,** abdominojugular r.; an elevation of venous pressure visible in the jugular veins and measurable in the veins of the arm, produced in active or impending congestive heart failure by firm pressure with the flat hand over the abdomen; sometimes mistakenly called hepatojugular reflex.

**ure'terore'nal r.,** the backward flow of urine from ureter into renal pelvis.

**ves'icoure'teral r.,** the backward flow of urine from bladder into ureter.

**refract** (re-frakt') [ L. *refringo,* pp. *-fractus,* to break up. FRA- ]. 1. To bend a ray of light. 2. To detect an error of refraction in the media of the eye and to correct it by means of lenses.

**refrac'ta do'si** [ Mod. L. in broken dose ]. In divided doses; denoting a definite quantity of a drug taken within a certain time in a number of equal fractional parts.

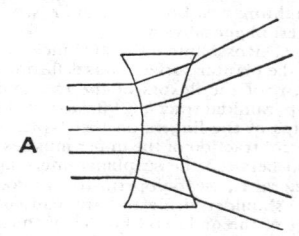

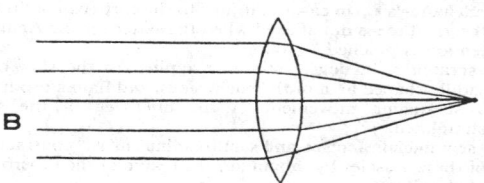

**Refraction of Parallel Rays**
*A,* by a concave lens; *B,* by a convex lens

**refraction** (re-frak'shun) [ L. *refractio* (see refract) ]. 1. The deflection of a ray of light when it passes from one medium into another of different optical density; in passing from a denser into a rarer medium it is deflected away from a line perpendicular to the surface of the refracting medium, in passing from a rarer to a denser medium it is bent toward this perpendicular line. 2. The act of determining the nature and degree of the refractive errors in the eye and correction of the same by lenses.

**angle of r.,** see under angle.

double r., the property of having more than one refractive index according to the direction of the transmitted light; birefringence.

dynamic r., r. of the eye during accommodation.

index of r., see refractive *index.*

law of r., see under law.

static r., r. under suspension of accommodation.

**refractionist** (re-frak'shun-ist). One skilled in the art of measuring the degree of refraction in the eye and who scientifically determines the proper corrective lenses.

**refractionometer** (re'frak-shun-om'e-ter). Refractometer.

**refractive** (re-frak'tiv). Pertaining to refraction.

**refractivity** (re'frak-tiv'i-tī). Ability of a substance to refract rays of light.

**refractometer** (re'frak-tom'e-ter) [ refraction + G. *metron,* measure ]. Objective optometer; refractionometer; an instrument for measuring the degree of refraction in translucent substances, especially the eye media; see refractive *index.*

**refractometry** (re'frak-tom'e-trī). 1. Measurement of index of refraction. 2. Use of a refractometer in determining the refractive error of the eye.

**refractory** (re-frak'to-rī) [ L. *refractarius,* fr. *refringo,* pp. *-fractus,* to break in pieces. FRA- ]. Obstinate; not yielding readily to treatment.

**refracture** (re-frak'chur) [ re- + fracture ]. The breaking again of a bone that has united, after a previous fracture, in a bad position.

**refrangible** (re-fran'jī-bl) [ L. *refringo,* to break in pieces ]. Capable of being refracted.

**refresh** (re-fresh') [ O. Fr. *re-frescher* ]. 1. To renew; to cause to recuperate. 2. To freshen; to pare or scrape two opposing surfaces of an old wound so that they may unite.

**refrigerant** (re-frij'er-ant) [ L. *re-frigero,* pp. *-atus,* pr. p. *-ans,* to make cold, fr. *frigus (frigor-),* cold ]. 1. Cooling; reducing slight fever. 2. An agent that gives a sensation of coolness or relieves feverishness.

**refrigeration** (re-frij'er-a'shun) [ L. *refrigeratio* (see refrigerant) ]. The act of cooling or reducing fever.

**refringence** (re-frin'jens). Refraction.

**refringent** (re-frin'jent). Refractive.

**Refsum,** Sigvald, Norwegian physician, 20th century. See R.'s *disease, syndrome.*

**refusion** (re-fu'zhun) [ L. *re-fundo,* pp. *-fusus,* to pour back ]. The return to the circulation of blood which has been temporarily cut off by ligature of a limb.

**regenerate** (re-jen'er-āt) [ L. *re-genero,* pp. *-atus,* to reproduce, fr. *genus (gener-),* birth, race. GEN- ]. To renew; to reproduce.

**regeneration** (re'jen-er-a'shun) [ L. *regeneratio* (see regenerate) ]. 1. Reproduction or reconstitution of a lost or injured part. 2. A form of asexual reproduction; *e.g.,* when a worm is divided into two or more parts, each segment is regenerated into a new individual.

**regimen** (rej'ī-men) [ L. direction, rule. REG- ]. 1. A regulation of the mode of living, diet, sleep, exercise, etc., for a hygienic or therapeutic purpose; sometimes mistakenly called regime. 2. Diet. 3. Hygiene.

**regio,** gen. **regionis,** pl. **regiones** (re'jī-o, -o'nis, -o'nēz) [ L. ]. Region. 1 [ NA ]. A more or less arbitrarily limited portion (*e.g.,* area, space, zone) of the surface of the body. 2. See region (2).

**regiones abdo'minis** [ NA ], regions of the abdomen; abdominal zones; the topographical subdivisions of the abdomen, including the right and left hypochondriac, right and left lateral, right and left inguinal, and the unpaired epigastric, umbilical and pubic regions.

r. ana'lis [ NA ], anal region or triangle; the posterior portion of the perineal region through which the anal canal opens.

r. antebra'chii ante'rior [ NA ], anterior region of the forearm; the area between the radial and ulnar borders of the forearm anteriorly.

r. antebra'chii poste'rior [ NA ], posterior region of the forearm; the area between the radial and ulnar borders of the forearm posteriorly.

r. axilla'ris [ NA ], axillary region; the region of the axilla, including the axillary fossa.

r. bra'chii ante'rior [ NA ], the anterior region of the arm.

r. bra'chii poste'rior [ NA ], the posterior region of the arm.

r. bucca'lis [ NA ], buccal region; the region of the cheek, corresponding approximately to the outlines of the underlying buccinator muscle.

r. calca'nea [ NA ], calcaneal region; the region of the heel.

**regiones cap'itis** [ NA ], regions of the head; the topographical division of the cranium in relation to the bones of the cranial vault. The regions include frontal, parietal, occipital, temporal and infratemporal.

**regiones col'li** [ NA ], regions of the neck; the topographical subdivisions of the neck, including the r. colli anterior, r. sternocleidomastoidea, r. colli lateralis and r. colli posterior.

r. col'li ante'rior [ NA ], anterior region of the neck; the area of the neck anterior to the sternocleidomastoid muscles; it includes on each side a submandibular and carotid triangle.

r. col'li latera'lis [ NA ], lateral region of the neck; posterior triangle of the neck; the region of the neck bounded by the sternocleidomastoid muscle, the trapezius muscle and the upper border of the clavicle, including the omoclavicular triangle.

r. col'li poste'rior [ NA ], posterior region of the neck; the back of the neck.

**regiones cor'poris** [ NA ], regions of the body; the topographical divisions of the body.

r. cru'ris ante'rior [ NA ], the anterior region of the leg.

r. cru'ris poste'rior [ NA ], the posterior region of the leg.

r. cu'biti ante'rior [ NA ], anterior cubital region; the area in front of the elbow, including the cubital fossa.

r. cu'biti poste'rior [ NA ], posterior cubital region; the posterior part of the elbow.

r. deltoi'dea [ NA ], deltoid region; the lateral aspect of the shoulder demarcated by the outlines of the deltoid muscle.

**regiones dor'si** [ NA ], regions of the back; the topographical regions of the back of the trunk, including the r. vertebralis, r. sacralis, r. scapularis, r. infrascapularis and r. lumbalis.

r. epigas'trica [ NA ], epigastrium [ NA ]; epigastric region; the upper central region of the abdomen.

**regiones fa'ciei** [ NA ], regions of the face; the topographical subdivisions of the face, including nasal, oral, mental, orbital, infraorbital, buccal, zygomatic and parotideomassesteric regions.

r. fem'oris ante'rior [ NA ], the anterior region of the thigh, including the femoral triangle.

r. fem'oris poste'rior [ NA ], the posterior region of the thigh.

r. fronta'lis [ NA ], frontal region; the surface region of the head corresponding to the outlines of the frontal bone.

r. ge'nus ante'rior [ NA ], the anterior region of the knee.

r. ge'nus posterior [ NA ], the posterior region of the knee, including the popliteal fossa.

r. glutea [ NA ], gluteal region; the region of the buttocks.

r. hypochondri'aca [ NA ], hypochondriac region; the region on each side of the abdomen overlying the costal cartilages. It is lateral to the epigastric region.

r. infraclavicula'ris [ NA ], infraclavicular region or fossa; Mohrenheim's fossa; the area inferior to the clavicle on each side.

r. infraorbita'lis [ NA ], infraorbital region; the region of the face below the orbit and alongside the nose on each side.

r. infrascapula'ris [ NA ], infrascapular region; the region of the back lateral to the vertebral region and below the scapula.

r. infratempora'lis [ NA ], infratemporal region; the region of the head corresponding to the fossa infratemporalis.

r. inguina'lis [ NA ], inguinal region; inguen; the topographical area of the abdomen related to the inguinal canal, lateral to the pubic region; the groin, which may indicate, sometimes, just the crease in the junction of the thigh with the trunk.

**r. latera'lis abdom'inis** [ NA ], lateral region of the abdomen; the area of the abdomen on each side of the umbilical region.

**r. lumba'lis** [ NA ], lumbar region; flank; the region of the back lateral to the vertebral region and between the rib cage and the pelvis.

**r. mamma'ria** [ NA ], mammary region; the region of the breast.

**regiones mem'bri inferio'ris** [ NA ], regions of the inferior limb; the topographical divisions of the lower limb, including the r. glutea, r. femoris anterior, r. femoris posterior, r. genus anterior, r. genus posterior, r. cruris anterior, r. cruris posterior, r. calcanea, dorsum pedis and planta pedis.

**regiones mem'bri superio'ris** [ NA ], regions of the superior limb; the topographical divisions of the upper limb, including the r. deltoidea, r. brachii anterior, r. brachii posterior, r. cubiti anterior, r. cubiti posterior, t. antebrachii anterior, r. antebrachii posterior, dorsum manus, and palma manus.

**r. menta'lis** [ NA ], mental region; the region of the chin.

**r. nasa'lis** [ NA ], nasal region; the region of the nose.

**r. occipita'lis** [ NA ], occipital region; the surface region of the head corresponding to the outlines of the occipital bone.

**r. olfacto'ria tu'nicae muco'sae na'si** [ NA ], olfactory region of the tunica mucosa of the nose; Schultze's membrane; the specialized olfactory receptive area that includes the upper one-third of the nasal septum and the lateral wall above the superior concha. It is lined with olfactory epithelium containing nerve cells whose axons form the filaments of the olfactory nerve. The lamina propria contains numerous olfactory glands (Bowman) that open to the surface.

**r. ora'lis** [ NA ], oral region; the region of the face including the lips and mouth.

**r. orbita'lis** [ NA ], orbital region; the region about the orbit.

**r. parieta'lis** [ NA ], parietal region; the surface region of the head corresponding to the outlines of the underlying parietal bone.

**r. parotideomasseter'ica** [ NA ], parotideomasseteric region; the area overlying the parotid gland and the masseter muscle on each side of the face.

**regiones pecto'ris** [ NA ], regions of the chest; the topographical divisions of the pectoral region, including the infraclavicular, mammary and axillary regions.

**r. perinea'lis** [ NA ], perineal region; the r. at the lower end of the trunk, anterior to the sacral region between the thighs; it is divided into the anal region posteriorly and the urogenital region or perineum anteriorly.

**r. pu'bica** [ NA ], hypogastrium [ NA ]; pubic region; the lower central region of the abdomen below the umbilical region.

**r. respirato'ria tu'nicae muco'sae** [ NA ], respiratory region of the tunica mucosa of the nose; it consists of pseudostratified ciliated columnar epithelium with goblet cells and a lamina propria containing, in addition to connective tissue, numerous seromucous glands and in some regions many thin-walled veins.

**r. sacra'lis** [ NA ], sacral region; the area of the back overlying the sacrum.

**r. scapula'ris** [ NA ], scapular region; the area of the back corresponding to the outlines of the scapula.

**r. sternocleidomastoi'dea** [ NA ], sternocleidomastoid region; the region overlying the sternocleidomastoid muscle, including the lesser supraclavicular fossa.

**r. tempora'lis** [ NA ], temporal region; the surface region of the head corresponding approximately to the outlines of the temporal bone.

**r. umbilica'lis** [ NA ], umbilical region; the central region of the abdomen about the umbilicus.

**r. urogenita'lis** [ NA ], urogenital region or triangle; the anterior portion of the perineal region containing the openings of the urethra and vagina in the female and the urethra and root structures of the penis in the male.

**r. vertebra'lis** [ NA ], vertebral region; the central region of the back, corresponding to the underlying vertebral column.

**r. zygomat'ica** [ NA ], zygomatic region; the region of the face outlined by the zygomatic bone; the prominence above the cheek.

**region** (re'jun) [ L. *regio*. REG- ]. 1. Regio. 2. A portion of the body having a special nervous or vascular supply, or a part of an organ having a special function.

**abdominal r.'s,** *regiones* abdominis.

**anal r.,** *regio* analis.

**anterior r. of arm,** *regio* brachii anterior.

**anterior cubital r.,** *regio* cubiti anterior.

**anterior r. of forearm,** *regio* antebrachii anterior.

**anterior r. of knee,** *regio* genus anterior.

**anterior r. of leg,** *regio* cruris anterior.

**anterior r. of neck,** *regio* colli anterior.

**anterior r. of thigh,** *regio* femoris anterior.

**axillary r.,** *regio* axillaris.

**r.'s of back,** *regiones* dorsi.

**r.'s of body,** *regiones* corporis.

**buccal r.,** *regio* buccalis.

**calcaneal r.,** *regio* calcanea.

**r. of cheek,** *regio* buccalis.

**r.'s of chest,** *regiones* pectoris.

**deltoid r.,** *regio* deltoidea.

**ecphylactic r.,** a focus of infection envisioned as being impregnable to the action of the defensive fluids, by reason of the virulence of the infection and the quantity of radiating toxins.

**epigastric r.,** *regio* epigastrica.

**r.'s of face,** *regiones* faciei.

**frontal r.,** *regio* frontalis.

**gluteal r.,** *regio* glutea.

**r.'s of head,** *regiones* capitis.

**hypochondriac r.,** *regio* hypochondriaca.

**iliac r.,** *regio* inguinalis.

**r.'s of inferior limb,** *regiones* membri inferioris.

**infraclavicular r.,** *regio* infraclavicularis.

**infraorbital r.,** *regio* infraorbitalis.

**infrascapular r.,** *regio* infrascapularis.

**infratemporal r.,** *regio* infratemporalis.

**inguinal r.,** *regio* inguinalis.

**K r.,** carbons 9 and 10 of the phenanthrene ring system; thought by some to be the reactive spot in the various hydrocarbon carcinogens.

**lateral r. of abdomen,** *regio* lateralis abdominis.

**lateral r. of neck,** *regio* colli lateralis.

**lumbar r.,** *regio* lumbalis.

**mammary r.,** *regio* mammaria.

**mental r.,** *regio* mentalis.

**nasal r.,** *regio* nasalis.

**r.'s of neck,** *regiones* colli.

**occipital r.,** *regio* occipitalis.

**olfactory r. of tunica mucosa of nose,** *regio* olfactoria tunicae mucosae nasi.

**oral r.,** *regio* oralis.

**orbital r.,** *regio* orbitalis.

**parietal r.,** *regio* parietalis.

**parotideomasseteric r.,** *regio* parotideomasseterica.

**perineal r.,** *regio* perinealis.

**posterior r. of arm,** *regio* brachii posterior.

**posterior cubital r.,** *regio* cubiti posterior.

**posterior r. of forearm,** *regio* antebrachii posterior.

**posterior r. of knee,** *regio* genus posterior.

**posterior r. of leg,** *regio* cruris posterior.

**posterior r. of neck,** *regio* colli posterior.

**posterior r. of thigh,** *regio* femoris posterior.

**preoptic r.,** preoptic area; the most anterior part of the hypothalamus surrounding the anterior or preoptic part of the third ventricle and including the lamina terminalis; containing the lateral and medial preoptic nucleus continuous caudally with, respectively, the lateral and anterior hypothalamic nucleus; rostrally the preoptic r. is continuous with the precommissural septum, laterally with the substantia innominata.

**presumptive r.,** in experimental embryology, the r. from which a specific structure or organ may be expected to develop.

**pretectal r.,** prectectal *area*.

**pubic r.,** *regio* pubica.

**respiratory r. of tunica mucosa of nose,** *regio* respiratoria tunicae mucosae.

**sacral r.,** *regio* sacralis.

**scapular r.,** *regio* scapularis.
**sternocleidomastoid r.,** *regio* sternocleidomastoidea.
**r.'s of superior limb,** *regiones* membri superioris.
**temporal r.,** *regio* temporalis.
**umbilical r.,** *regio* umbilicalis.
**urogenital r.,** *regio* urogenitalis.
**vertebral r.,** *regio* vertebralis.
**Wernicke's r.,** Wernicke's *center.*
**zygomatic r.,** *regio* zygomatica.

**regional** (re'jun-al). Relating to a region.

**regiones** (re'ji-o'nēz) [ L. ]. Plural of regio.

**registrant** (rej'is-trant). A nurse who is entered on the books of the registry as ready to take charge of a case.

**registration** (rej'is-tra'shun). In dentistry, a record.
**maxillomandibular r.,** maxillomandibular *record.*
**tissue r.,** in dentistry, (1) the accurate r. of the shape of tissues under any condition by means of a suitable material; (2) an impression.

**regnancy** (reg'nan-sī) [ L. *regnant-, regnans,* pres. p. of *regnare,* to rule ]. The briefest unit of experience.

**regression** (re-gresh'un) [ L. *re-gredior,* pp. *-gressus,* to go back ]. 1. Recession; a subsidence of symptoms. 2. A relapse; return of symptoms. 3. Any retrograde movement or action. 4. Return to a more primitive mode of behavior due to an inability to function adequately at a more adult level. 5. An unconscious defense mechanism by which there occurs a return to earlier patterns of adaptation.
**phonemic r.,** a decrease in intelligibility of speech associated with an increase in loudness.

**regres'sive.** Relating to or characterized by regression.

**regulation** (reg'u-la'shun) [ L. *regula,* a rule ]. 1. The control of the rate or manner in which a process progresses or a product is formed. 2. In experimental embryology, the power of what remains of a very young embryo, after part of it has been destroyed, to restore its normal structure.

**regurgitant** (re-ger'ji-tant). Regurgitating; flowing backward.

**regurgitate** (re-ger'ji-tāt) [ L. *re-,* back, + *gurgito,* pp. *-atus,* to flood, fr. *gurges (gurgit-),* a whirlpool ]. 1. To flow backward. 2. To expel the contents of the stomach in small amounts, short of vomiting.

**regurgitation** (re-ger'ji-ta'shun) [ L. *regurgitatio* (see regurgitate) ]. 1. A backward flow, as of blood through an incompetent valve of the heart. 2. The return of gas or small amounts of food from the stomach.
**aortic r.,** Corrigan's disease; reflux of blood through an incompetent aortic valve into the left ventricle during ventricular diastole.
**mitral r.,** reflux of blood through an imcompetent mitral valve.

**rehabilitation** (re-hă-bil'ĭ-ta'shun) [ L. *rehabilitare,* pp. *-tatus,* to make fit, fr. *re-* + *habilitas,* ability ]. Restoration, following disease, illness, or injury, of ability to function in a normal or near normal manner.
**mouth r.,** restoration of the form and function of the masticatory apparatus to as nearly a normal condition as possible.

**Rehfuss** (ra'foos), Martin E., American physician, 1887–1964. See R. *method,* stomach *tube.*

**rehydration** (re-hi-dra'shun). The return of water to a system after its loss.

**Reichel-Pólya stomach resection.** See under resection.

**Reichert** (ri'khert), Karl B., Berlin anatomist, 1811–1884. See R.'s *cartilage,* cochlear *recess,* R.-Meissl *number,* R.'s *scar.*

**Reichstein** (rīkh'stīn), Tadeus, Polish biochemist in Switzerland, *1897. Nobel laureate, 1950, with Philip S. Hench and Edward C. Kendall, for their discoveries relating to the hormones of the adrenal cortex, their structure and biological effects. See R.'s *substances.*

**Reid,** Robert W., Scottish anatomist, 1851–1938. See R.'s base *line.*

**Reid Hunt.** See Hunt.

**Reil** (ril), Johann C., German physician, neurologist, and histologist, 1759–1813. See R.'s *ansa, band, island, ribbon, sulcus, triangle.*

**Reimer's reflex.** See under reflex.

**reimplantation** (re'im-plan-ta'shun). Replacement of an organ to its natural position, as a tooth to its socket, or as in present-day experimental surgery, lung to the chest cavity.

**re'infec'tion.** A second infection by the same microorganism, after recovery from or during the course of a primary infection.

**re'inforce'ment.** 1. An increase of force or strength; denoting specifically the increased sharpness of the patellar reflex when the patient at the same time closes the fist tightly or pulls against the flexed fingers or contracts some other set of muscles; see also Jendrassik's *maneuver.* 2. In dentistry, a structural addition or inclusion used to give additional strength in function; *e.g.,* bars in plastic denture base, or wire in silicate or amalgam. 3. In conditioning, the totality of the process in which the conditioned stimulus is followed by presentation of the unconditioned stimulus which, itself, elicits the response to be conditioned. See also reinforcer.
**primary r.,** satisfaction of physiological needs or drives, such as that supplied by food or sleep.
**secondary r.,** r. through something which, while it does not satisfy the need directly, has been associated with direct satisfaction of the need.

**re'inforcer.** Reward; in conditioning, a satisfaction-yielding or unsatisfying stimulus, object, or stimulus event that is obtained upon the performance of a desired or predetermined operant. See also reinforcement (3).
**negative r.,** one which is unpleasant, unsatisfying, or painful to the recipient.
**positive r.,** one which is pleasant or satisying to the recipient.

**Reinke's crystalloids.** See under crystalloid.

**reinnervation** (re-in-ner-va'shun). The restoration of nerve control of a paralyzed muscle or organ by means of regrowth of nerve fibers either spontaneously or after anastomosis.

**reinoculation** (re'ī-nok'u-la'shun). A reinfection by means of inoculation.

**Reinsch's test.** See under test.

**reintegration** (re'in-te-gra'shun). In psychiatry, the return to well adjusted functioning following disturbances due to mental illness.

**re'inver'sion.** The correction, spontaneous or operative, of an inversion, as of the uterus.

**Reisseissen** (ris'is-en), Franz D., Berlin anatomist, 1773–1828. See R.'s *muscles.*

**Reissner** (ris'ner), Ernst, German anatomist, 1824–1878. See R.'s *fiber, membrane.*

**Reiter** (ri'ter), Hans, German bacteriologist, 1881–1969. See R.'s *disease, syndrome.*

**Reiter test.** See under test.

**rejection** (re-jek'shun) [ L. *rejectio,* a throwing back. JAC- ]. 1. The immunological response to an incompatible transplanted organ (generally a homograft); failure of the graft to "take" results in necrosis. 2. A refusal to accept, recognize, or grant; a denial.
**parental r.,** parental withholding or unacceptance of affection or attention from a child.

**rejuvenescence** (re-ju've-nes'ens) [ L. *re-,* again, + *juvenesco,* to grow young, fr. *juvenis,* a youth ]. A renewal of youth; the return of a cell or tissue to a state in which it was in an earlier stage of existence.

**Rekoss disk.** See under disk.

**relapse** (re'laps) [ L. *re-labor,* pp. *-lapsus,* to slide back ]. The return of a disease after it has once spent its course.

**relap'sing.** Recurring; said of a disease that returns in a new attack after convalescence has begun.

**relation** (re-la'shun) [ L. *relatio,* a bringing back ]. 1. An association or connection between or among people or objects; see also relationship and subentries there. 2. In dentistry, term used to denote mode of contact of teeth or positional relationship of oral structures.
**acentric r.,** eccentric r.
**buccolingual r.,** the position of a space or tooth in r. to the tongue and the cheek.
**centric r.,** centric jaw r.
**centric r., acquired,** see eccentric r., centric jaw r.

**centric jaw r.,** centric r.; median r.; median retruded r.; (1) the most retruded physiologic r. of the mandible to the maxillae to and from which the individual can make lateral movements; it is a condition which can exist at various degrees of jaw separation; it occurs around the terminal hinge axis; (2) the most posterior r. of the mandible to the maxillae at the established vertical r.; see also eccentric r.

**dynamic r.'s,** relative movements between two objects, *e.g.,* the relationship of the mandible to the maxillae.

**eccentric r.,** acentric r.; eccentric position; any r. of the mandible to the maxillae other than centric r.

**eccentric r., acquired,** an eccentric r. that is assumed by habit in order to bring the teeth into occlusion.

**intermaxillary r.,** maxillomandibular r.

**maxillomandibular r.,** any one of the many r.'s of the mandible to the maxillae, *e.g.,* centric jaw r., eccentric r., intermaxillary r.

**median r.,** centric jaw r.

**median retruded r.,** centric jaw r.

**occluding r.,** the jaw r. at which the opposing teeth occlude.

**protrusive r.,** the r. of the mandible to the maxillae when the lower jaw is thrust forward.

**protrusive jaw r.,** a jaw r. resulting from a protrusion of the mandible.

**rest r.,** rest jaw r.; the postural r. of the mandible to the maxillae when the patient is resting comfortably in the upright position and the condyles are in a neutral unstrained position in the glenoid fossa.

**rest jaw r.,** rest r.

**ridge r.,** the positional r. of the mandibular ridge to the maxillary ridge.

**static r.'s,** relationship between two parts that are not in motion.

**unstrained jaw r.,** (1) the r. of the mandible to the skull when a state of balanced tonus exists between all of the muscles involved; (2) any jaw r. which is attained without undue or unnatural force and which causes no undue distortion of the temporomandibular joints.

**relationship** (re-la′shun-ship). The state of being related, associated, or connected; see also relation.

**coefficient of r.,** see under coefficient.

**hypnotic r.,** r. between hypnotizer or hypnotist (the person inducing the hypnosis) and the hypnotized or hypnotee (the person undergoing hypnosis).

**object r.,** in psychiatry, the emotional bond between an individual and another person, as opposed to the individual's interest in himself (narcissism).

**sadomasochistic r.,** one characterized by the complementary enjoyment of inflicting and suffering pain.

**relax** (re-laks′) [ L. *re-laxo,* to loosen ]. 1. To loosen; to slacken. 2. To cause a movement of the bowels.

**relax′ant.** 1. Relaxing; causing relaxing; reducing tension (especially muscular tension). 2. An agent that reduces muscular tension; usually referred to as muscle r., *q. v.*

**muscle r.,** an agent or drug, such as curare or succinylcholine, that produces relaxation of striated muscle by interruption of the transmission of nervous impulses at the myoneural junction.

**smooth muscle r.,** an agent (such as an antispasmodic, bronchodilator, or vasodilator) that reduces the tension or tone of a smooth (involuntary) muscle.

**relaxation** (re′lak-sa′shun) [ L. *relaxatio* (see relax) ]. Dilation; loosening; lengthening or lessening of tension in a muscle.

**cardioesophageal r.,** achalasia of the cardia.

**isometric r.,** decrease in tension of a muscle while the length remains constant due to fixation of the ends.

**isovolumetric r.,** isovolumic r.

**isovulumic r.,** isovolumetric r.; that part of the cardiac cycle between the time of aortic valve closure and mitral opening, during which the ventricular muscle decreases its tension without lengthening so that ventricular volume remains unaltered.

**relax′in.** A polypeptide hormone isolated from the corpus luteum with the specific capacity to relax the symphysis pubis of guinea pig, gopher, or mouse; active only when injected into an animal in estrus.

**re′learning.** The process of regaining a skill or ability that has been partially or entirely lost. The savings involved in

r., as compared with original learning, gives an index of the degree of retention.

**reli′abil′ity.** In psychology, the consistency of measurement or degree of dependability of a measuring instrument.

**equivalent form r.,** in psychology, the consistency of measurement based on the correlation between scores on two similar forms of the same test taken by the same individual; see also reliability *coefficient.*

**interjudge r.,** in psychology, the consistency of measurement obtained when different judges or examiners independently administer the same test to the same individual.

**test-retest r.,** in psychology, the consistency of measurement based on the correlation between test and retest scores for the same individual; see also reliability *coefficient.*

**relief** (re-lēf′) [ see relieve ]. 1. The removal of pain or distress, physical or mental. 2. In dentistry, the reduction or elimination of pressure from a specific area under a denture base; see also r. *area,* r. *chamber.*

**relieve** (re-lēv′) [ thru O. Fr. fr. L. *re-levo,* to lift up, lighten ]. To free wholly or partly from pain or discomfort, either physical or mental.

**reline** (re′lin′). In dentistry, to resurface the tissue side of a denture with new base material to make it fit more accurately; see also rebase.

**REM.** Abbreviation for rapid eye *movement.*

**rem.** Abbreviation for roentgen-equivalent-man; see under roentgen.

**Remak** (ra′mahk), Ernst J., German neurologist, 1848–1911. See R.'s *paralysis, reflex, sign.*

**Remak** (ra′mahk), Robert, German anatomist and histologist, 1815–1865. See R.'s nuclear *division, fibers, ganglia, plexus.*

**remediable** (rĕ-me′dĭ-a-bl) [ L. *remediabilis,* fr. *remedio,* to cure ]. Curable.

**remedial** (rĕ-me′dĭ-al). Curative.

**remedy** (rem′e-dĭ) [ L. *remedium,* fr. *re-,* again, + *medior,* or cure ]. An agent that cures disease or alleviates its symptoms.

**remineralization** (re′min′er-al-ĭ-za′shun). The return to the body of necessary mineral constituents lost through disease or dietary deficiencies; a term commonly used in referring to the content of calcium salts in bone; also used in reference to tooth structure as a defensive mechanism against dental caries.

**reminiscence** (rem-ĭ-nis′sens). In the psychology of learning, an improvement in recall of incompletely leaned material after an interval without practice.

**remission** (re-mish′un) [ L. *remissio,* fr. *re-mitto,* pp. -*missus,* to send back, slacken, relax ]. 1. Abatement or lessening in severity of the symptoms of a disease. 2. The period during which such abatement occurs.

**spontaneous r.,** in psychiatry and clinical psychology, disappearance of symptoms without formal treatment; causes of their disappearance are assumed to exist but are not known.

**remit** (re-mit′) [ see remission ]. To become less severe for a time without absolutely ceasing.

**remit′tence.** A temporary amelioration, without actual cessation, of symptoms.

**remit′tent.** Characterized by temporary remissions or periods of abatement of the symptoms.

**ren,** gen. **renis,** pl. **renes** (ren, re′nis, re′nēz) [ L. ] [ NA ]. Kidney.

**re′nal.** Relating to a kidney or the kidneys.

**rena′lis** [ L. ] [ NA ]. Renal.

**renculus** (ren′ku-lus). Reniculus.

**Rendu** (roṅ-dü′), Henri J. L. M., French physician, 1844–1902. See R.-Osler-Weber *disease, syndrome.*

**reni-, ren-.** See reno-.

**renicapsule** (ren′ĭ-kap′sūl) [ reni- + L. *capsula,* capsule ]. The capsule of the kidney.

**ren′icar′diac** [ reni- + G. *kardia,* heart ]. Cardiorenal.

**reniculus,** pl. **reniculi** (rĕ-nik′u-lus, -li [ L. dim. of *ren,* kidney ]. Renculus; renunculus. 1. *Lobulus* corticalis renalis. 2. A lobe of the human fetal kidney and that of some lower animals in which fibrous septa subdivide the organ.

**ren'ifleur'** [ Fr. ]. A sniffer; a person who is sexually excited by odors.

**ren'iform.** Kidney-shaped.

**re'nin.** Term originally used for a pressor substance obtained from rabbits' kidneys. Once thought to be a unique enzyme that, acting upon the hypertensinogen (or angiotensinogen) of plasma, forms hypertensin I, precursor of hypertensin II (angiotonin or angiotensin). Not to be confused with rennin.

    **r. activator,** the name previously given to angiotonin precursor or hypertensinogen.

**ren'ipor'tal** [ reni- + L. *porta,* gate ]. 1. Relating to the hilus of the kidney. 2. Relating to the portal, or venous capillary circulation in the kidney.

**ren'ipunc'ture.** Incision of the capsule of the kidney followed by the multiple puncture of the substance of the organ, performed for the relief of tension and the cure of albuminuria.

**ren'net.** Rennin.

**ren'nin.** 1 (EC 3.4.18.4). Rennet; chymosin; chymase; pexin (not to be confused with renin); proteinase present as such (or as a zymogen) in the chief cells of the gastric tubules. 2. The partially purified milk-curdling enzyme obtained from the glandular layer of the stomach of the calf. Ingredient of pepsin and r. elixir.

**renninogen** (rĕ-nin'o-jen) [ rennin + G. suffix *-gen,* producing ]. Rennogen; prorennin; prochymosin; pexinogen; the precursor of rennin.

**rennogen** (ren'o-jen). Renninogen.

**reno-, reni-, ren-** (re'no-, ren'ĭ-) [ L. *ren,* kidney ]. Combining form relating to the kidney; see also nephr-.

**renocutaneous** (re'no-ku-ta'ne-us) [ reno- + L. *cutis,* skin ]. Relating to the kidneys and the skin.

**re'nogas'tric** [ reno- + G. *gastēr,* stomach ]. Relating to the kidneys and the stomach.

**renogenic** (re'no-jen'ik). Originating in or from the kidney.

**re'nogram.** The assessment of renal function by external radiation detectors after the administration of a radiopharmaceutical with renotropic characteristics.

**renography** (re'nog'rä-fĭ). Radiography of the kidney.

**re'nointes'tinal.** Relating to the kidneys and the intestine.

**renomegaly** (re'no-meg'ä-lĭ). Enlargement of the kidney.

**Rénon,** L., French physician, 1863–1922. See R.-Delille *syndrome.*

**renopathy** (re-nop'ä-thĭ). Nephropathy.

**renoprival** (re'no-pri'val) [ reno- + L. *privus,* deprived of ]. Relating to removal or absence of kidneys.

**re'nopul'monary.** Relating to the kidneys and the lungs.

**renotrophic** (re'no-trof'ik) [ reno- + G. *trophē,* nourishment ]. Renotropic; nephrotropic; nephrotropic; relating to any agent influencing the growth or nutrition of the kidney or to the action of such an agent.

**renotrophin** (re'no-tro'fin). Renotropin; an agent affecting the growth or nutrition of the kidney.

**renotropic** (re'no-trop'ik) [ reno- + G. *tropē,* a turning ]. Renotrophic.

**renotropin** (re'no-tro'pin). Renotrophin.

**re'novas'cular.** Pertaining to the blood vessels of the kidney, particular in the sense of disease of these vessels.

**Renshaw cells.** See under cell.

**renunculus** (re-nun'ku-lus). [ L. dim. of *ren* ]. Reniculus.

**reovirus** (re'o-vi'rus). See under virus.

**rep.** Abbreviation for roentgen-equivalent-physical (*q.v.* under roentgen); see also rad.

**repand'** [ L. *repandus,* bent or turned back, fr. *re-,* back, + *pandus,* curved ]. Denoting a bacterial colony with edges marked by a series of slightly concave segments with angular projections at their points of union.

**repel'lent** [ L. *re-pello,* pp. *-pulsus,* to drive back ]. 1. Capable of driving off or repelling; repulsive. 2. An agent that drives away or prevents annoyance or irritation by insect pests. 3. An astringent or other agent that reduces swelling.

**repetition-compulsion** (rep'e-tish'un-kom-pul'zhun). In psychoanalysis, the tendency to repeat earlier experiences or actions, in an unconscious effort to achieve belated mastery over them.

**replantation** (re'plan-ta'shun) [ G. *re-,* again, + *planto,* pp. *-atus,* to plant, fr. *planta,* a sprout, slip ]. 1. Removing an organ or other part of the body, replacing it, and reestablishing its circulation by vascular anastomosis; reimplantation. 2. In dentistry, reimplantation.

    **intentional r.,** removal of a tooth from its socket, resecting the roots, obturating the root canals, and replanting the tooth in its socket. An effort is made to keep the periodontal membrane viable while the tooth is out of the socket.

**repletion** (re-ple'shun) [ L. *repletio,* fr. *re-pleo,* pp. *-pletus,* to fill up ]. Plethora.

**replicate** (rep'lĭ-kāt). 1. One of several identical processes or observations. 2. To repeat; to produce an exact copy.

**replication** (rep'lĭ-ka'shun) [ L. *replicatio,* a reply, fr. *re-plico,* pp. *-atus,* to fold back. PLIC- ]. 1. Repeating a process or observation; a word commonly used in describing experimental work. 2. Autoreproduction.

**rep'licon.** A segment of a chromosome (or of the DNA of a chromosome or similar entity) that can replicate, with its own initiation and termination points, independently of the chromosome in which it may be located, and that has a unique function.

**repolarization** (re'po-lar-ĭ-za'shun). The process whereby the membrane, cell, or fiber, after depolarization, is polarized again, with positive charges on the outer and negative charges on the inner surface.

**reposal.** REPOSAMAL; 5-bicyclo[ 3.2.1 ]octen-2-yl-5-ethylbarbituric acid; a short-acting hypnotic.

**repositioning** (re'po-zish'un-ing). Reduction; the return of a part to its normal place.

    **jaw r.,** the changing of any relative position of the mandible to the maxillae, by altering the occlusion of the natural or artificial teeth or by surgical means.

    **muscle r.,** the surgical replacement of a muscle attachment into a more acceptable functional position.

**repositor** (re-poz'ĭ-tor). An instrument used to replace a dislocated part, especially a prolapsed uterus.

**repressed** (re-prest'). Subjected to repression.

    **return of the r.,** in psychoanalysis, the return to consciousness of an idea, feeling, or impulse that had been repressed into the sphere of the unconscious.

**repression** (re-presh'un) [ L. *re-primo,* pp. *-pressus,* to press back, repress ]. In psychoanalysis, the defense mechanism by which ideas, impulses, and affects once available to conscious thought are removed from consciousness.

    **primal r.,** r. of material never in conscious thought.

**repres'sor.** The product of a regulator or repressor gene. See fig. under protein.

    **active r.,** a r. that combines directly with an operator gene to repress activity of the operator and its structural genes, thus repressing enzyme synthesis; active r. may be inactivated by an inducer, with resulting activation of enzyme synthesis; a homeostatic mechanism for regulation of inducible enzyme systems.

    **inactive r.,** aporepressor; a r. that is unable to combine with an operator gene until it has been activated by combination with a corepressor molecule (usually a product of an enzyme pathway); after activation the r. stops production of the enzymes controlled by the operator gene; a homeostatic mechanism for regulation of repressible enzyme systems.

**reproduction** (re'pro-duk'shun) [ L. *re-,* again, + *pro-duco,* pp. *-ductus,* to lead forth, produce ]. 1. The recall and presentation in the mind of the steps of a former impression. 2. Procreation; the production of a new generation of living beings.

    **asexual r.,** r. other than by union of male and female sex cells.

    **cytogenic r.,** r. by means of unicellular germ cells; includes both sexual r. and asexual r. by means of spores.

    **sexual r.,** r. by union of male and female gametes to form a zygote.

    **somatic r.,** asexual r. by fission or budding of somatic cells.

**reproductive** (re'pro-duk'tiv). Relating to reproduction.

**Reptilia** (rep-til'ĭ-ah) [ L. *reptilis,* ntr. *-e,* creeping; ntr. as n., reptile ]. A class of vertebrates comprising the alligators, crocodiles, lizards, turtles, tortoises, and snakes.

**repullulation** (re-pul-u-la'shun) [ L. *re-*, again, + *pullulo*, pp. *-atus*, to sprout ]. Renewed germination; the return of a morbid process or growth.

**repulsion** (re-pul'shun) [ L. *re-pello*, pp. *-pulsus*, to drive back ]. 1. The act of repelling or driving apart; opposed to attraction. 2. Aversion.

**resaz'urin.** A blue α-hydroxyphenoxazone dye, $C_{12}H_7NO_4$, used as a redox indicator in the reductase test of milk; it is also used as a pH indicator, orange at 3.8, violet at 6.5.

**re-Schick.** A second Schick test made after an immunizing injection of diphtheria toxin (or toxoid)-antitoxin.

**rescinnamine** (re-sin'ā-mēn, -min). MODERIL; 3,4,5-trimethoxycinnamic acid ester of methyl reserpate; a purified ester alkaloid of the alseroxylon fraction of species of *Rauwolfia.* It is chemically and pharmacologically related to reserpine, and used in mild hypertension and as a tranquilizing agent.

**resect** (re-sekt') [ L. *re-seco*, pp. *sectus*, to cut off ]. 1. To cut off, especially to cut off the articular ends of one or both bones forming a joint. 2. To excise a segment of a part, as of the intestine.

**resectable** (re-sek'tā-bl). Amenable to surgical removal.

**resection** (re-sek'shun). 1. Removal of the articular ends of one or both bones forming a joint. 2. Excision of a segment of any part, such as the intestine.

    **gum r.,** gingivectomy.

    **Miles' r.,** Miles' *operation.*

    **Reichel-Pólya stomach r.,** retrocolic implantation of the open stomach into the jejunum.

    **root r.,** apicoectomy.

    **transurethral r.,** r. of prostatic obstruction by an instrument inserted into the urethra.

    **wedge r.,** removal of a wedge-shaped portion of the ovary; used in the treatment of virilizing disorders of ovarian origin, such as the Stein-Leventhal syndrome.

**resectoscope** (re-sek'to-skōp). An endoscope for transurethral resection of prostatic obstruction.

**reserpine** (re-ser'pēn, -pin) (USP, BP). RAULOYDIN; RAU-RINE; RAU-SED; RESERPOID; SANDRIL; SERPASIL; SERPATE; VIO-SERPINE; an ester alkaloid isolated from the root of certain species of *Rauwolfia.* It decreases the 5-hydroxytryptamine and catecholamine concentrations in the central nervous system and in peripheral tissues. Used in the management of mild hypertension associated with anxiety and, in conjunction with other hypotensive agents, in essential hypertension. It is useful as a tranquilizer in psychotic states.

**reserve** (re-zerv') [ L. *re-servo*, to keep back, reserve ]. Something available, but held back for later use, *e.g.*, r. strength or carbohydrate r.

    **alkali r.,** the sum total of the basic ions (mainly bicarbonates) of the blood and other body fluids which, acting as buffers, maintain the normal pH of the blood.

    **breathing r.,** the difference between the pulmonary ventilation (*i.e.,* the volume of air breathed under ordinary resting conditions) and the maximum breathing capacity.

    **cardiac r.,** the work which the heart is able to perform beyond that required under the ordinary circumstances of daily life. It depends upon the state of the myocardium and the degree to which, within physiologic limits, the cardiac muscle fibers can be stretched by the volume of blood reaching the heart during diastole.

**reservoir** (rez'er-vwor) [ Fr. ]. Receptaculum.

    **Pecquet's r.,** *cisterna* chyli.

    **r. of spermatozoa,** the site where spermatozoa are stored, that is, the distal portion of the tail of the epididymis and the beginning of the ductus deferens.

    **vitelline r.,** vitellarium.

**resibu'fogenin.** RESPIGON; 14,15β-epoxy-3β-hydroxy-5β-bufa-20,22-dienolide; cardiotonic agent.

**resident** (rez'ĭ-dent) [ L. *resideo*, to reside ]. House officer attached to a hospital for clinical training after the intern year. Formerly, actually a resident in the hospital.

**residual** (re-zid'u-al). Relating to or of the nature of a residue; left behind.

**residue** (rez'ĭ-du) [ L. *residuum, q.v.* ]. Remainder; rest.

    **day r.,** psychoanalytic term for a dream related to an experience of the previous day.

**residuum,** pl. **residua** (re-zid'u-um, -u-ah) [ L. ntr. of *residuus,* left behind, remaining, fr. *re-sideo,* to sit back, remain behind, fr. *sedeo,* to sit ]. Residue.

**resilience** (re-zil'yens) [ L. *resilio,* to spring back, rebound ]. 1. Energy per unit of volume released upon unloading. 2. Springiness; elasticity.

**resin** (rez'in). 1. An amorphous, brittle substance consisting of the hardened secretion of a number of plants, probably derived from a volatile oil and similar to a stearoptene. 2. Rosin; a r. official in the NF and BP (colophony). 3. A precipitate formed by the addition of water to certain tinctures. 4. A broad term used to indicate organic substances soluble in ether, etc., but not in water; these monomers are named according to their chemical composition, physical structure, and means for activation or curing, *e.g.,* acrylic r., autopolymer r.

    **r. acids,** rosin acids; a class of organic compounds derived from various natural plant r.'s; diterpenes containing a phenanthrene ring system; *e.g.,* abietic acid, pimaric acid, ester gums.

    **acrylic r.,** a general term applied to a resinous material of the various esters of acrylic acid; used as a denture-base material, for other dental restorations, and for trays.

    **activated r.,** autopolymer r.

    **anion-exchange r.,** see anion exchange and anion exchanger.

    **autopolymer r.,** activated r.; cold cure r.; cold-curing r.; quick cure r.; autopolymerizing r.; self-curing r.; any r. which can be polymerized by chemical catalysis rather than by the application of heat. Used in dentistry for dental restoration, denture repair, and impression trays.

    **autopolymerizing r.,** autopolymer r.

    **carbacryl'amine r.'s,** a mixture of the cation-exchange r.'s, carbacrylic r. and potassium carbacrylic r. (87.5 per cent) and of the anion-exchange r., polyamine-methylene r. (12.5 per cent). Used to increase the fecal excretion of sodium in edema associated with excessive sodium retention by the kidneys, *e.g.,* in congestive heart failure, cirrhosis of the liver, and nephrosis.

    **cation-exchange r.,** see cation exchange and cation exchanger.

    **cholestyramine r.** (USP), DOWEX 1-X2-Cl; CUEMID; QUESTRAN; a strongly basic anion-exchange r. in the chloride form, consisting of styrene-divinylbenzene copolymer with quaternary ammonium functional groups; lowers the blood cholesterol by binding the bile acids in the intestine, thus promoting their excretion in the feces instead of reabsorption from the bowel. Used in the treatment of hypercholesterolemia, xanthomatous biliary cirrhosis, and other forms of xanthomatosis.

    **cold cure r.,** autopolymer r.

    **cold-curing r.,** autopolymer r.

    **copolymer r.,** a synthetic r. which is the product of the concurrent and joint polymerization of two or more different monomers or polymers.

    **cross-linked r.,** cross-linked polymer.

    **direct filling r.,** an autopolymerizing r. especially designed as a dental restorative material.

    **epoxy r.,** any thermosetting r. based on the reactivity of the epoxy group (*q.v.*); used as adhesives, protective coatings, and embedding media for electron microscopy.

    **gum r.,** the dry exudate from a number of plants, consisting of a mixture of a gum and a r., the former soluble in water but not alcohol, the latter soluble in alcohol but not water.

    **heat-curing r.,** a r. that requires heat to initiate polymerization.

    **Indian podophyllum r.,** r. from *Podophyllum emodi;* cathartic and cholagogue.

    **ion-exchange r.,** see ion exchange and ion exchanger.

    **ipomea r.,** Mexican scammony r.; obtained from the dried root of *Ipomoea orizabensis;* a cathartic.

    **jalap r.,** r. extracted from the dried tuberous root of *Exogonium purga;* purgative.

    **mel'amine r.,** melamine formaldehyde; a plastic material used mixed with plaster of Paris for casts. Such a cast is lighter and stronger than one made with plaster of Paris alone.

    **methac'rylate r.,** polymerized methacrylic acid; a translucent plastic material, used for the manufacture of various medical appliances and surgical instruments. It possesses the optical properties of fused quartz; it is readily molded when heated.

**podophyllum r.** (USP, BP), podophyllin; a mixture of r.'s obtained from the dried rhizomes and roots of *Podophyllum peltatum*. The BP also recognizes *P. hexandrum* as a source of the r.; used as a laxative.

**polyamine-methylene r.**, RESINAT; a synthetic acid-binding r. that withdraws acids from solution by molecular attraction; a gastric antacid.

**quick cure r.**, autopolymer r.

**quinine carbacry′lic r.**, the quinine salt of a polyacryalic carboxylic acid r. containing about 1.85 per cent of quininium ion. Used as a test for gastric anacidity without withdrawal of the gastric contents. The compound is displaced by hydrogen ions in the gastric contents, and 1 per cent of the quinine is excreted in the urine within 2 hours after ingestion of the resin. A stimulant to gastric secretion (*e.g.*, histamine) is given 1 hour before the resin is administered. The urine is analyzed for quinine 2 hours later; the presence or absence of quinine in the urine indicates the presence or absence of free hydrochloric acid in the stomach.

**self-curing r.**, autopolymer r.

**resi′na** [ L. ]. 1. Resin. 2. Rosin.

**resinoid** (rez′ĭ-noyd). 1. Resembling rosin. 2. An extract obtained by evaporating a tincture. 3. A substance containing a resin or resembling one.

**resinous** (rez′ĭ-nus). Relating to or derived from a resin.

**resistance** (re-zis′tans) [ L. *re-sisto*, to stand back, withstand ]. 1. A passive force exerted in opposition to another and active force. 2. The opposition in a conductor to the passage of a current of electricity, whereby there is a loss of energy and a production of heat. 3. In psychoanalysis, opposition to the uncovering of the unconscious. 4. The power residing in the red blood cells to resist hemolysis and to preserve their shape under varying degrees of osmotic pressure in the liquor sanguinis.

**bacteriophage r.**, r. of a bacterial mutant to infection by a bacteriophage to which the parent (wild type) strain is susceptible; the r. is due to bacterial surface changes that prevent adsorption by the phage, in contrast to bacteriophage *immunity* (*q.v.*), which depends on lysogeny.

**expiratory r.**, r. to flow of gas out of the lungs or the total r. to flow of gas during the expiratory phase of the respiratory cycle.

**impact r.**, the ability of a lens for eyewear to withstand shattering or breakage upon impact, *i.e.*, of a $^3/_8$-inch steel ball dropped 50 feet; criteria for determination of impact r. are specified by United States law.

**inductive r.**, reactance.

**peripheral r.**, total peripheral r.

**synaptic r.**, the ease or difficulty with which a nerve impulse can cross a synapse.

**total peripheral r.**, peripheral r.; the total r. to flow of blood in the systemic circuit; it is the driving pressure (mean arterial pressure minus mean right atrial pressure) divided by the mean cardiac output.

**resistor** (re-zis′tor). An element included in an electrical circuit to provide resistance to the flow of current.

**res′odec.** An ion-exchange resin used in congestive heart failure with edema, to restrict sodium absorption.

**resolution** (rez′o-lu′shun) [ L. *resolutio*, a slackening, fr. *re-solvo*, pp. *-solutus*, to loosen, relax ]. 1. The arrest of an inflammatory process without suppuration; the absorption or breaking down and removal of the products of inflammation, as in pneumonia, or of a new growth. 2. The ability optically to distinguish detail such as the separation of closely approximated objects.

**resolve** (re-zolv′) [ L. *resolvo*, to loosen ]. To return or cause to return to the normal without suppuration, said of a phlegmon or other form of inflammation.

**resolvent** (re-zol′vent). 1. Discutient; causing resolution. 2. An agent that arrests an inflammatory process or causes the absorption of a neoplasm.

**resonance** (rez′o-nans) [ L. *resonantia*, echo, fr. *re-sono*, to resound, to echo ]. 1. The sound obtained on percussing a part that can vibrate freely. 2. The intensification and hollow character of the voice sound obtained on auscultating over a cavity. 3. In chemistry, the manner in which electrons or electric charge are distributed among the

atoms in compounds which are planar and symmetrical, particularly those with conjugated (alternating) double bonds; the existence of r. in the latter case lowers the energy content and increases the stability of a compound. 4. The natural or inherent frequency of any oscillating system (see electron spin r., nuclear magnetic r.).

**amphor′ic r.**, cavernous r.; a percussion sound like that produced by blowing across the neck of an empty bottle, obtained by percussing over a pulmonary cavity, the patient's mouth being open.

**bandbox r.**, vesiculotympanitic r.

**bellmetal r.**, a clear metallic sound obtained by striking a coin, held against the chest, by another coin, in cases of a large pulmonary cavity or of pneumothorax; coin test.

**cavernous r.**, amphoric r.

**cracked-pot r.**, a peculiar sound, resembling that heard on striking a cracked pot, elicited on percussing over a pulmonary cavity that commmunicates with a bronchial tube, the patient having the mouth open.

**electron spin r.**, abbreviated ESR; a spectrometric method, based on measurement of electron spins and magnetic moments, for detecting and estimating free radicals in organic reactions.

**hydat′id r.**, a peculiar vibratile r. heard on auscultatory percussion over a hydatid cyst.

**nuclear magnetic r.**, abbreviated NMR; a method for defining the character of covalent bonds by measuring the magnetic moment of the atomic nuclei involved.

**Skodaic r.**, a peculiar, high-pitched sound, less musical than that obtained over a cavity, elicited by percussion just above the level of a pleuritic effusion.

**tympanit′ic r.**, a drumlike r. obtained by percussion over a large space filled with air, as the stomach or intestine or a large pulmonary cavity.

**vesic′ular r.**, the sound obtained on percussing over the normal lungs.

**vesic′ulotympanit′ic r.**, bandbox r.; wooden r.; a peculiar, partly tympanitic, partly vesicular sound, obtained on percussion in cases of pulmonary emphysema.

**vocal r.**, the voice sounds as heard on auscultation of the chest.

**wooden r.**, vesiculotympanitic r.

**resonator** (rez′o-na′tor). A device for employing inductance to create an electrical current of very high potential and small volume.

**resorb** (re-sorb′) [ L. *re-sorbeo*, to suck back ]. To reabsorb; to absorb what has been excreted, as an exudate or pus.

**resorcin** (re-zor′sin). Resorcinol.

**resorcinol** (re-zor′sĭ-nol) (USP, BP). Resorcin; *m*-dihydroxybenzene; used internally for the relief of nausea, asthma, whooping cough, and diarrhea, but chiefly as an external antiseptic in psoriasis, eczema, seborrhea, and ringworm. Pyrocatechol and hydroquinone are isomers of r.

**r. monoac′etate** (NF), used externally in the treatment of acne, sycosis, seborrhea, and alopecia.

**r. phthal′ic anhy′dride**, fluorescein.

**resorcinolphthalein** (re-zor′sĭ-nol-thal′e-in). 1. Fluorescein. 2. Fluorescin.

**resorption** (re-sorp′shun). 1. The act of resorbing; the removal of an exudate, a blood clot, pus, etc., by absorption. 2. A loss of substance by lysis. 3. A loss of substance by physiologic or pathologic means.

**bone r.**, the removal of osseous tissue.

**gingival r.**, gingival *recession.*

**internal r.**, a loss of tooth structure originating within the pulp cavity.

**ridge r.**, a loss in the volume and size of the alveolar portion of the mandible or maxillae.

**root r.**, dissolution of the root of a tooth, generally the apical portion.

**respirable** (rĕ-spir′ă-bl, res′pĭ-rā-bl). Capable of being breathed.

**respira′tio** [ L. ] [ NA ]. Respiration.

**respiration** (res′pĭ-ra′shun) [ L. *respiratio*, fr. *re-spiro*, pp. *-atus*, to exhale, breathe ]. 1. A function common to all living plants or animals, consisting in the taking in of oxygen and the throwing off of the products of oxidation in the tissues, mainly carbon dioxide and water. 2. Breathing.

**abdominal r.,** breathing effected mainly by the action of the diaphragm.

**aerobic r.,** a form of r. in which molecular oxygen is consumed and carbon dioxide and water are produced.

**amphor'ic r.,** a sound like that made by blowing across the mouth of a bottle, heard on auscultation in some cases in which a large pulmonary cavity exists, or occasionally in pneumothorax.

**anaerobic r.,** a form of r. in which molecular oxygen is not consumed; e.g., glycolysis, in which glucose is broken down to lactic acid.

**artificial r.,** the maintenance of pulmonary ventilation by artificial means in cases of apnea of hypoventilation.

**assisted r.,** artificial augmentation of inhalation during spontaneous breathing when ventilation is inadequate for maintenance of normal exchange of carbon dioxide and oxygen; usually accomplished by application of positive pressure to the airway during inhalation, with exhalation by passive recoil.

**Biot's r.,** Biot's *breathing*.

**Bouchut's r.,** a form of r. in children with bronchopneumonia, in which expiration is longer than inspiration.

**bronchial r.,** tubular r.; a tubular blowing sound caused by the passage of air through a bronchus in an area of consolidated lung tissue.

**bronchovesic'ular r.,** combined bronchial and vesicular r.

**cavernous r.,** a hollow reverberating sound heard on auscultation over a cavity in the lung.

**Cheyne-Stokes r.,** the pattern of breathing with gradual increase in depth and sometimes in rate to a maximum, followed by a decrease resulting in apnea. The cycles ordinarily are 30 seconds to a minute in length; characteristically seen in coma from affection of the nervous centers of respiration.

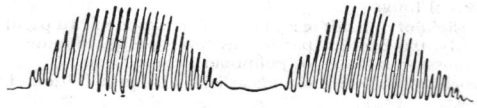

**Cheyne-Stokes Respiration**

**cogwheel r.,** jerky or interrupted r., the inspiratory sound being broken into two or three by silent intervals.

**controlled r.,** artificial ventilation with elimination of spontaneous efforts to breathe; usually achieved by application of positive pressure to the airway to produce artificial inhalation, with exhalation by passive recoil.

**costal r.,** thoracic r.

**diffusion r.,** apneic oxygenation; maintenance of oxygenation by intratracheal insufflation of oxygen at high flow rates.

**elec'trophre'nic r.,** the term given to the rhythmical electrical stimulation of the phrenic nerve by an electrode applied to the skin at the motor points of the phrenic nerve; it is used in paralysis of the respiratory center resulting from acute bulbar poliomyelitis.

**external r.,** the exchange of respiratory gases in the lungs as distinguished from the exchange in the tissues, or internal r.

**forced r.,** voluntary hyperventilation.

**internal r.,** tissue r.

**interrupted r.,** cogwheel r.

**jerky r.,** cogwheel r.

**Kussmaul r.,** deep, rapid r. characteristic of the air hunger of diabetic acidosis or coma.

**Kussmaul-Kien r.,** Kussmaul r.

**meningitic r.,** Biot's *breathing*.

**mouth-to-mouth r.,** the most effective and simplest method of artificial r.; it involves an overlap of the patient's mouth (and nose in small children) with the operator's mouth, to inflate the patient's lungs by blowing, followed by an unassisted expiratory phase brought about by elastic recoil of the patient's chest and lungs; repeated 12 to 16 times a minute.

**paradoxical r.,** deflation of the lung during inspiration, and inflation of the lung during the phase of expiration; seen in the lung on the side of an open pneumothorax.

**physiologic r.,** metabolism; the giving off of waste material and the formation of new protoplasm.

**positive pressure r.,** positive pressure *breathing*.

**puerile r.,** an exaggeration of the normal respiratory sounds, heard in children and in adults after exertion.

**thorac'ic r.,** r. effected chiefly by the action of the intercostal and other muscles that raise the ribs, causing expansion of the chest.

**tidal r.,** Cheyne-Stokes r.

**tissue r.,** internal r.; the interchange of gases between the blood and the tissues.

**tubular r.,** high-pitched bronchial r.

**vesic'ular r.,** vesicular murmur; the respiratory murmur heard on auscultating over the normal lung.

**vesiculocav'ernous r.,** cavernous r., due to the presence of a cavity, mingled with the vesicular murmur of the surrounding normal lung tissue.

**vicarious r.,** increased respiratory action in one lung when that in the other lung is diminished or abolished.

**res'pira'tor.** 1. An appliance fitting over the mouth and nose, used for the purpose of excluding dust, smoke, etc., or of otherwise altering the air before it enters the respiratory passages. 2. An apparatus for administering artificial respiration, especially for a prolonged period, in cases of paralysis of the respiratory muscles, e.g., in poliomyelitis or during anesthesia.

**cuirass r.,** one of several types of r.'s producing alternating negative pressure about the thoracic cage.

**Drinker r.,** a mechanical r. in which the whole body except the head is encased within a metal tank, which is sealed with an airtight gasket; artificial respiration is induced by making the air pressure inside alternatively negative and positive; also called iron lung.

**pressure-controlled r.,** a r. that provides a predetermined pressure to gases during inhalation, the volume of gas moved being variable, depending upon resistance.

**volume-controlled r.,** a r. that provides a predetermined volume of gases during inhalation, with the pressure required to move that volume remaining variable, depending upon resistance.

**respiratory** (rĕ-spīr'ă-to-rĭ, res'pĭ-ră-to-rĭ). Relating to respiration.

**respire** (rĕ-spīr') [ L. *respiro,* to breathe ]. 1. To breathe. 2. To consume oxygen and produce carbon dioxide by metabolism.

**respirometer** (res'pĭ-rom'e-ter) [ L. *respiro,* to breathe, + G. *metron,* measure ]. 1. An instrument for measuring the extent of the respiratory movements. 2. An instrument for measuring oxygen consumption or carbon dioxide production, usually of an isolated tissue.

**Drager r.,** an inferential meter to measure tidal and minute volume from the number of revolutions of a vane rotated by the gas stream as the latter passes through two light-weight lozenge-shaped meshing rotors.

**Wright r.,** an inferential meter to measure tidal and minute volume from the number of revolutions of a vane rotated by the gas stream as the latter passes through 10 tangential slots in a cylindrical stator ring to turn a flat two-bladed rotor.

**response** (re-spons') [ L. *responsus* (noun), an answer ]. 1. The reaction of a muscle or other part to any stimulus. 2. Operant behavior; any act or behavior, or its constituents, that an animal or human is capable of emitting. Reflexes are usually excluded because they are typically elicited by a specifiable (unconditioned or natural) stimulus rather than emitted under circumstances in which the stimulus was not specifiable.

**conditioned r.,** a r. already in an individual's repertoire but which, through repeated pairings with its natural stimulus, has been acquired or conditioned anew to a previously neutral or conditioned stimulus; cf. unconditioned r.

**depletion r.,** subnormal metabolic r. to trauma in a person whose physiologic processes are already depressed by disease.

**evoked r.,** an alteration in the electrical activity of a particular part of the nervous system produced by an incoming sensory stimulus.

**galvanic skin r.,** abbreviated GSR; the change in electrical resistance in the skin, due to vasomotor or secretory activity, associated with certain mental and emotional reactions to a stimulus; it is used (e.g., in a polygraph) as a measurement of a person's response to certain stimuli, by the amount of resistance (perspiration) in his skin to electrical current; also called psychogalvanic or psychogalvanic skin r. and galvanic skin, psychogalvanic, or psychogalvanic skin reaction or reflex.

**immune r.,** (1) the r. of previously sensitized tissue to an antigen; in the case of antigens produced by microbes and other parasitic organisms, the immune r. tends to resist infection; (2) the r. of the immunological mechanism to an antigen (immunogen) that leads to the condition of induced sensitivity (*q.v.*), especially from the viewpoint of antibody (immunoglobulin) production; the immune r. to the initial antigenic exposure (primary immune r.) is serologically detectable, as a rule, only after a lag period of from several days to two weeks or more and is initiated by transient production of 19 S (IgM) immunoglobulins, followed by production of 7 S (mostly IgG) antibodies; the immune r. to a subsequent stimulus (secondary immune r.) by the same antigen (even in relatively small amounts) is more rapid than in the case of the primary immune r., and the antibodies produced reach higher titers, persist for a much longer period of time, and have a greater affinity for the antigen.

**isomorphic r.,** Köbner's *phenomenon.*
**oculomotor r.,** widespread myogenic potential evoked by visual stimuli.
**orienting r.,** orienting *reflex.*
**psychogalvanic r.** (PGR), galvanic skin r.
**psychogalvanic skin r.,** galvanic skin r.
**recruiting r.,** recruitment (2).
**sonomotor r.,** widespread myogenic potential evoked by click stimulation.
**target r.,** operant.
**triple r.,** the triphasic r. to the firm stroking of the skin: Phase 1 is the sharply demarcated erythema that follows a momentary blanching of the skin, and is the result of release of histamine from the mast cells. Phase 2 is the intense red flare extending beyond the margins of the line of pressure but in the same configuration, and is the result of arteriolar dilation; also called axon flare because it is mediated by axon reflex. Phase 3 is the appearance of a line wheal in the configuration of the original stroking.
**unconditioned r.,** a r. such as salvation which is a part of the animal or human repertoire; *cf.* conditioned r.

**rest.** 1 [ A.S. *raest* ]. Quiet; repose. 2 [ A.S. *raestan* ]. To repose; to cease from work. 3 [ L. *restare,* to remain ]. A group of cells or a portion of fetal tissue that has become displaced and lies embedded in tissue of another character; it was formerly believed that under certain conditions this embryonic structure may begin renewed growth and develop into a neoplasm called also embryonal r. 4. In dentistry, an extension from a prosthesis that affords vertical support for a restoration.
**adrenal r.,** accessory *adrenal.*
**incisal r.,** the portion of a removable partial denture supported by an incisal edge.
**lingual r.,** a metallic extension onto the lingual surface of a tooth to provide support or indirect retention for a removable partial denture.
**lug r.,** the portion of a removable partial denture that seats in a box-shaped preparation in an abutment tooth or crown to provide support.
**Malassez' epithelial r.'s,** epithelial remains of Hertwig's sheath in the alveolodental periosteum near the cementum; occasionally they develop into dental cysts or cancer of the jaw.
**mesonephric r.,** Wolffian r.
**precision r.,** a r. consisting of closely interlocking parts.
**Walthard's cell r.,** a nest of epithelial cells occurring in the uterine tubes or ovary; probably derived from the pelvic peritoneum and, when neoplastic, possibly comprising one of the components of the Brenner tumor.
**Wolffian r.,** mesonephric r.; remnants of the Wolffian duct in the female genital tract that give rise to cysts; *e.g.,* Gartner's duct cyst.

**re'stenosis** [ L. prefix *re-,* again, + G. *stenōsis,* a narrowing ]. Recurrence of stenosis after corrective surgery on the heart valve.
**res'tiform** [ L. *restis,* rope, + *forma,* form ]. Ropelike; rope-shaped; referring to the restiform body (pedunculus cerebellaris inferior).

**restitution** (res'tĭ-tu'shun) [ L. *restitutio,* act of restoring ]. In obstetrics, the return of the rotated head of the fetus to its natural relation with the shoulders after its emergence from the vulva.
**restoration** (res'to-ra'shun) [ L. *restauro,* pp. *-atus,* to restore, to repair ]. 1. In dentistry, a prosthetic r. or appliance; broad terms applied to any inlay, crown, bridge, partial denture, or complete denture which restores or replaces lost tooth structure, teeth, or oral tissues. 2. That portion of a tooth replaced by amalgam, gold foil, or synthetic porcelain.
**restor'ative.** 1. Renewing health and strength. 2. An agent that promotes a renewal of health or strength.
**restraint** (re-strānt') [ O. Fr. *restrainte* ]. In psychiatry, an intervention (by means of a straitjacket or camisole, or other methods) to prevent an excited or violent patient from doing harm to himself or others.
**resu'pinate.** 1. To supinate; to turn on the back. 2. Supinated; supine; lying on the back.
**resupina'tion.** Supination; lying, or turning over, on the back.
**resuscitate** (re-sus'ĭ-tāt) [ L. *re-suscito,* pp. *-atus,* to raise up again, revive, fr. *re-,* again, + *sub,* under, + *cito,* to rouse ]. To revive; to restore to life after apparent death.
**resuscitation** (re-sus'ĭ-ta'shun) [ L. *resuscitatio* ]. Restoration to life after apparent death. See also artificial *respiration.*
**resus'citator.** An apparatus that forces gas (usually O₂) into lungs to produce artificial respiration.
**retain'er.** Any type of clasp, attachment, or device used for the fixation or stabilization of a prosthesis; an appliance used to prevent the shifting of teeth following orthodontic treatment.
**continuous bar r.,** continuous clasp; a metal bar, usually resting on lingual surfaces of teeth, to aid in their stabilization and to act as indirect r.'s.
**direct r.,** a clasp or attachment applied to an abutment tooth for the purpose of maintaining a removable appliance in position.
**extracoronal r.,** a r. that depends upon contact with the outer circumference of the crown of a tooth for its retentive qualities.
**indirect r.,** a part of a removable partial denture which assists the direct r.'s in preventing displacement of free end denture bases by functioning through lever action on the opposite side of the fulcrum line.
**intracoronal r.,** a r. that depends upon components placed within the crown portion of a tooth for its retentive qualities.
**space r.,** space *maintainer.*
**ret'amine.** An alkaloid from *Spartium junceum,* or *Genista hispanica,* Spanish broom, or from *Genista sphaerocarpa,* resembling in its action sparteine.
**retar'date** [ L. *retardo,* to delay, hinder ]. A person who has mental retardation.
**retardation** (re-tar-da'shun). A slowness or limitation of development.
**mental r.,** subaverage general intellectual functioning which originates during the develomental period and is associated with impairment in adaptive behavior. The American Association on Mental Deficiency lists 8 medical classifications and 5 psychological classifications (see table); the latter five replace the former classifications of moron, imbecile, and idiot. The definition of mental r. requires assignment of an index for performance relative to one's peers on two interrelated criteria: measured intelli-

*Psychological classifications of mental retardation*

| Classification | Stanford-Binet IQ | Wechsler IQ |
|---|---|---|
| Borderline | 68-83 | 70-84 |
| Mild | 52-67 | 55-69 |
| Moderate | 36-51 | 40-54 |
| Severe | 20-35 | 25-39 |
| Profound | below 20 | below 25 |

gence (IQ) and overall socio-adaptive behavior (a judgmental rating of the individual's relative level of performance in school, at work, at home, and in the community).

**psychomotor r.,** slowed psychic activity or motor activity, or both.

**retch** [ A.S. *hraecan*, to hawk ]. To make an involuntary effort to vomit.

**retch'ing.** Vomiturition; making movements of vomiting without effect.

**rete,** pl. **re'tia** (re'te, re'shĭ-ah, -tĭ-ah) [ L. a net. RET- ] [ NA ]. 1. A network of nerve fibers or small vessels. 2. A structure composed of a fibrous network or mesh.

**r. acromia'le** [ NA ], acromial network; a vascular network between the acromion and the skin of the shoulder, formed by anastomoses of the acromial branch of the suprascapular artery with the acromial branch of the thoracoacromialis.

**r. arterio'sum** [ NA ], arterial network; a vascular network formed by anastomoses between minute arteries just before they become capillaries.

**r. articula're,** a r. vasculosum in the neighborhood of a joint, where such arrangements are common.

**r. articula're cu'biti** [ NA ], articular network of the elbow; vascular networks in the region of the elbow, composed of anastomoses between branches of the radial and middle collateral, superior and inferior ulnar collateral, radial recurrent, interosseous recurrent, and recurrent ulnar arteries.

**r. articula're ge'nus** [ NA ], articular network of the knee; an arterial network over the front and sides of the knee, formed by branches of the genu suprema, of the five genual (articular) arteries from the popliteal, of the recurrens tibialis anterior and posterior, and of the tibialis posterior.

**r. calca'neum** [ NA ], network of the heel; a superficial network over the calcaneus, formed by branches of the peroneal and posterior tibial arteries and twigs from the malleolar retia.

**r. cana'lis hypoglos'si,** *plexus* venosus canalis hypoglossi.

**r. carpi dorsa'le** [ NA ], dorsal carpal network; r. carpi posterius; a vascular network over the dorsal surface of the carpal joints, formed by anastomoses of branches of the dorsal and palmar interosseous, and dorsal carpal branches of the radial and ulnar arteries.

**r. carpi poste'rius,** r. carpi dorsale.

**r. cutaneum corii,** the network of vessels parallel to the surface between the corium and the tela subcutanea.

**r. foram'inis ova'lis,** *plexus* venosus foraminis ovalis.

**Haller's r., r. hal'leri,** r. testis.

**r. malleola're latera'le** [ NA ] a network over the lateral malleolus formed by branches of the posterior lateral malleolar, anterior lateral malleolar, peroneal, lateral tarsal, and dorsalis pedis arteries.

**r. malleola're media'le** [ NA ], a network over the medial malleolus formed by branches from the anterior and posterior medial malleolar and medial tarsal arteries.

**Malpighian r.,** *stratum* germinativum.

**r. mirab'ile** [ NA ], a vascular network interrupting the continuity of an artery or vein, such as occurs in the glomeruli of the kidney (arterial) or in the liver (venous).

**r. muco'sum,** *stratum* germinativum.

**r. ova'rii,** a transient network of cells in the developing ovary; homologous to the r. testis.

**r. patel'lae** [ NA ], patellar network; the superficial portion of the r. articulare genus.

**r. subpapillare,** the network of vessels between the papillary and reticular strata of the corium.

**r. tes'tis** [ NA ], Haller's r.; r. vasculosum halleri; the network of canals at the termination of the straight tubules in the mediastinum testis.

**r. vasculo'sum halleri,** r. testis.

**r. veno'sum** [ NA ], venous network.

**r. veno'sum dorsa'le ma'nus** [ NA ], dorsal venous network of the hand; a superficial network of veins on the dorsum of the hand emptying into the cephalic and the basilic veins.

**r. veno'sum dorsa'le pe'dis** [ NA ], dorsal venous network of the foot; a superficial network of fine veins on the dorsum of the foot.

**r. veno'sum planta're** [ NA ], plantar venous network; a fine superficial venous network in the sole of the foot.

**retention** (re-ten'shun) [ L. *retentio*, a holding back, see retain ]. 1. The keeping in the body of what normally belongs there, especially the retaining of food and drink in the stomach. 2. The keeping in the body of what normally should be discharged, as urine or feces. 3. Memory; retaining that which has been learned so that it can be utilized later as in recall, recognition, or, if r. is partial, relearning. 4. Resistance to dislodgement.

**area, groove, or point,** see under *area*.

**denture r.,** the means by which dentures are held in position in the mouth.

**direct r.,** r. obtained in a removable partial denture by the use of attachments or clasps which resist their removal from the abutment teeth.

**indirect r.,** r. obtained in a removable partial denture through the use of indirect retainers.

**partial denture r.,** the fixation of a removable partial denture by the use of clasps, indirect retainers, or precision attachments.

**re'tia** [ L. ]. Plural of rete.

**retial** (re'shĭ-al). Relating to a rete.

**reticul-.** See reticulo-.

**retic'ula** [ L. ]. Plural of recticulum.

**reticular** (re-tik'u-lar). Relating to a reticulum; netlike; cancellar.

**reticularis, fetal.** Term sometimes used as a synonym for fetal *cortex*.

**reticulated** (re-tik'u-la'ted) [ L. *reticulatus*, netlike, fr. *reticulum*, q.v. ]. Reticular.

**reticulation** (re-tik-u-la'shun). The presence or formation of a reticulum or network, such as that observed in the red blood cells during active regeneration of blood.

**retic'ulin.** 1. An albuminoid or scleroprotein present in the connective tissue framework of the lymphatic tissues. 2. Hydroxystreptomycin.

**reticulitis** (re-tik'u-li'tis) [ reticul- + G. suffix -*itis*, inflammation ]. Inflammation of the reticulum of ruminant animals.

**reticulo-, reticul-** (re-tik'u-lo-) [ L. *reticulum*, a small net, dim. of *rete*, a net. RET- ]. Combining forms meaning reticulum, reticular.

**reticulocyte** (re-tik'u-lo-sit) [ reticulo- + G. *kytos*, cell ]. Reticulated corpuscle; a young red blood cell with a network of precipitated basophilic substance, and occurring during the process of active blood regeneration. See also the discussion under erythroblast, and color plate 15.

**reticulocytopenia** (re-tik'u-lo-si-to-pe'nĭ-ah) [ reticulocyte + G. *penia*, poverty ]. Paucity of reticulocytes in the blood.

**reticulocytosis** (re-tik'u-lo-si-to'sis) [ reticulocyte + G. suffix -*osis*, condition ]. An increase in the number of circulating reticulocytes above the normal, which is less than 1 per cent of total number of red blood cells; it occurs during active blood regeneration (stimulation of red bone marrow) and in certain anemias, especially congenital hemolytic anemia.

**reticuloendothelial** (re-tik'u-lo-en-do-the'lĭ-al). Denoting or referring to reticuloendothelium.

**reticuloendothelioma** (re-tik'u-lo-en'do-the-lĭ-o'mah) [ reticuloendothelium + G. suffix -*oma*, tumor ]. A localized reticuloendotheliosis, or neoplasm derived from reticuloendothelial tissue.

**reticuloendotheliosis** (re-tik'u-lo-en'do-the-lĭ-o'sis) [ reticuloendothelium + G. suffix -*osis*, condition ]. Hyperplasia of the reticuloendothelium in any of the organs or tissues.

**avian r.,** a virus infection of fowl which causes a leukosis-like disease.

**leukemic r.,** a not clearly defined condition in which neoplastic disease of reticuloendothelial tissue (*e.g.*, certain types of lymphoma) is intimately associated with frank leukemia or abnormal findings that are virtually indistinguishable from those of leukemia.

**reticuloendothelium** (re-tik'u-lo-en-do-the'lĭ-um) [ reticulo- + endothelium, q.v. ]. Reticuloendothelial system; system of macrophages; phagocytic macrophages which actively take up particles and dyes; they are present in linings of sinuses and in reticulum of various organs and tissues (spleen, liver, lymph nodes, bone marrow, connective tissue, etc.).

**reticulogen** (re-tik'u-lo-jen) [ reticulo- + G. suffix -gen, producing ]. Hematinic *principle.*

**reticulohistiocytosis** (re-tik'u-lo-his'to-si'to'sis). See reticuloendotheliosis.

**reticulopenia** (re-tik'u-lo-pe'nĭ-ah). Reticulocytopenia.

**reticulosis** (re-tik'u-lo'sis) [ reticulo- + G. suffix -osis, condition ]. An increase in histiocytes, monocytes, or other reticuloendothelial elements.

**benign inoculation r.,** cat-scratch *disease.*

**histiocytic medullary r.,** a rapidly fatal form of lymphoma, characterized by fever, jaundice, pancytopenia, and enlargement of the liver, spleen and lymph nodes. The affected organs show focal necrosis and hemorrhage, with proliferation of histiocytes and phagocytosis of red blood cells.

**leuke'mic r.,** monocytic *leukemia.*

**lipomelan'ic r.,** dermatopathic *lymphadenopathy.*

**my'eloid r.,** r. involving the bone marrow in which giant cells with a reticulated nucleus are found; they are thought to be derived from reticular cells of the reticuloendothelial system.

**retic'ulospi'nal.** Pertaining to the *tractus* reticulospinales.

**reticulotomy** (re-tik'u-lot'o-mĭ) [ reticulo- + G. tomē, incision ]. Production of lesions in the reticular formation.

**reticulum,** pl. **reticula** (re-tik'u-lum, -lah) [ L. dim of *rete,* a net. RET- ]. 1 [ NA ]. A fine network formed by cells, or formed of certain structures within cells or of connective tissue fibers between cells. 2. Neuroglia. 3 [ NAV ]. The second compartment of the stomach of a ruminant, sometimes called the honeycomb, because of the characteristic structure of its wall. It is a comparatively small chamber communicating with the rumen.

**agranular cytoplasmic r.,** smooth-surfaced cytoplasmic r.; cytoplasmic r. that is lacking in ribosomal granules and is characteristic of cells that secrete steroid hormones.

**cytoplasmic r.,** the network of tubules or flattened sacs (cisternae) with or without ribosomes on the surface of their membranes; originally, the cytoplasmic r. was thought to occur only in the endoplasm of cells, hence it was called endoplasmic r.

**Ebner's r.,** a network of nucleated cells in the seminiferous tubules.

**endoplasmic r.,** cytoplasmic r.

**Golgi internal r.,** Golgi *apparatus.*

**granular cytoplasmic r.,** rough-surfaced cytoplasmic r.; ergastoplasm; chromidial substance; cytoplasmic r. in which ribosomal granules are applied to the cytoplasmic surface of the cisternae; this type of cytoplasmic r. is concerned in secretion of protein and peptides.

**Kölliker's r.,** neuroglia.

**rough-surfaced cytoplasmic r.,** granular cytoplasmic r.

**sarcoplasmic r.,** the cytoplasmic r. of skeletal and cardiac muscle; the vesicles and tubules forming a continuous structure around striated myofibrils, with a repetition of structure within each sarcomere.

**smooth-surfaced cytoplasmic r.,** agranular cytoplasmic r.

**stellate r.,** a network of cells in the center of the enamel organ between the outer and inner enamel epithelium.

**ret'iform** [ L. *rete,* network ]. Resembling a net or network.

**retin-.** See retino-.

**retina** (ret'ĭ-nah) [ Mediev. L. prob. fr. L. *rete,* a net. RET- ] [ NA ]. Tunica interna bulbi; optomeninx; nervous tunic of eyeball; grossly, the r. consists of a stratum pigmenti attached to the inner surface of the choroid, ciliary body, and iris, and an inner layer, the stratum cerebrale. The r. comprises three parts: (1) pars optica retinae, the physiologic portion that receives the visual rays; (2) pars ciliaris retinae; (3) pars iridica retinae. The optic part has the following layers: (1) pigment layer; (2) layer of rods and cones; (3) external limiting membrane, actually a row of junctional complexes; (4) outer nuclear layer; (5) outer plexiform layer; (6) inner nuclear layer; (7) inner plexiform layer; (8) layer of ganglion cells; (9) layer of nerve fibers; (10) internal limiting membrane. At the posterior pole of the visual axis is the macula, in the center of which is the fovea, the area of acute vision. Here layers

6, 7, 8, and 9 and blood vessels are absent, and only elongated cones are present. About 3 mm. medial to the macula is the optic disk, where axons of the ganglionic cells converge to form the optic nerve.

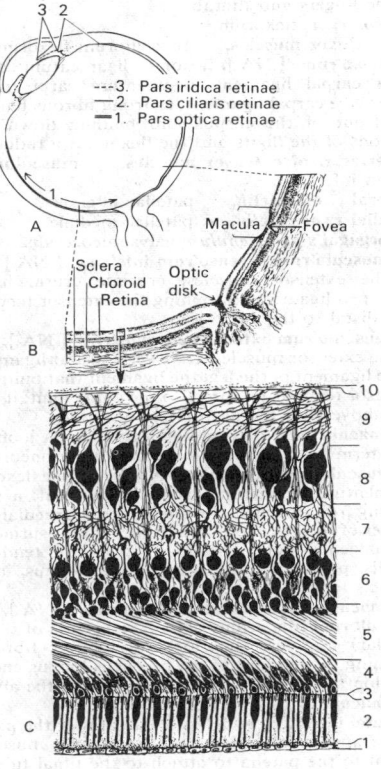

- - -3. Pars iridica retinae
— 2. Pars ciliaris retinae
— 1. Pars optica retinae

**The Retina**

*A,* horizontal, meridional section of the eye, showing subdivisions of the retina; *B,* a posterior sector of the eye which includes the macula and optic disk; *C,* the layers of the pars optica retinae (after Polyak). For identification of layers, see definition of retina.

**ablatio retinae, amotio retinae,** detachment of the r; see under detachment.

**coarc'tate r.,** a ringlike effusion of fluid between the choroid and r., giving the latter a funnel shape.

**commotio retinae,** *concussion* of retina.

**detachment of the r.,** see under detachment.

**dialysis retinae,** disinsertion (2).

**leopard r.,** tesselated *fundus.*

**shot-silk r.,** the appearance of numerous wavelike, glistening reflexes, like the shimmer of silk, observed sometimes in the r. of a young person.

**tigroid r.,** tesselated *fundus.*

**retinaculum,** gen. **retinaculi,** pl. **retinacula** (ret'ĭ-nak'u-lum, -li, -lah) [ L. a band, a halter, fr. *retineo,* to hold back ] [ NA ]. A frenum, or a retaining band or ligament.

**r. cap'sulae articula'ris cox'ae,** one of several longitudinal folds of the articular capsule of the hip joint reflected onto the femoral neck.

**caudal r.,** r. caudale.

**r. cauda'le** [ NA ], caudal r.; ligamentum caudale; fibrous bands that extend from the skin to the coccyx, forming the coccygeal fovea.

**r. cu'tis** [ NA ], r. of the skin; one of the numerous small fibrous strands that attaches the dermis to the underlying tela subcutanea. These are particularly well developed over the breast where they are known as ligamenta suspensoria mammae or suspensory ligaments of Cooper.

**extensor r.,** r. extensorum.

**retinacula of extensor muscles,** r. musculorum extensorum inferius and superius.

**r. extenso'rum** [ NA ], extensor r.; dorsal carpal ligament; a strong fibrous band stretching obliquely across the back of the wrist and binding down the extensor tendons of the fingers and thumb.

**flexor r.** r. flexorum.

**r. of flexor muscles,** r. musculorum flexorum.

**r. flexo'rum** [ NA ], flexor r.; ligamentum carpi volare; volar carpal ligament; ligamentum carpi transversum; transverse carpal ligament; a strong fibrous band crossing the front of the carpus and binding down the flexor tendons of the digits and the flexor carpi radialis tendon. **inferior. of extensor muscles,** r. musculorum extensorum inferius.

**lateral r. of patella,** r. patellae laterale.

**medial r. of patella,** r. patellae mediale.

**Morgagni's r.,** *frenulum* valvae ileocecalis.

**r. musculo'rum extenso'rum infe'rius** [ NA ], inferior r. of the extensor muscles; cruciate crural ligament; a V-shaped ligament restraining the extensor tendons of the foot distal to the ankle joint.

**r. musculo'rum extenso'rum supe'rius** [ NA ], superior r. of the extensor muscles; transverse crural ligament; transverse ligament of the leg; the ligament that binds down the extensor tendons proximal to the ankle joint; it is continuous above with the deep fascia of the leg.

**retinacula musculo'rum fibula'rium** [ NA ], official alternate term for retinacula musculorum peroneorum.

**r. musculo'rum flexo'rum** [ NA ], r. of the flexor muscles; ligamentum laciniatum; laciniate ligament; a wide band passing from the medial malleolus to the medial and upper border of the calcaneus and to the plantar surface as far as the navicular bone; it holds in place the tendons of the tibialis posterior, flexor digitorum longus, and flexor hallucis longus.

**retinacula musculo'rum peroneo'rum** [ NA ], retinacula musculorum fibularium [ NA ]; retinacula of the peroneal (fibular) muscles; superior and inferior fibrous bands retaining the tendons of the peroneus longus and brevis in position as they cross the lateral side of the ankle.

**retinacula of nail,** retinacula unguis.

**r. patel'lae latera'le** [ NA ], lateral r. of the patella; part of the aponeurosis of the vastus lateralis muscle passing lateral to the patella to attach to the tibial tuberosity.

**r. patel'lae media'le,** medial r. of the patella; part of the aponeurosis of the vastus medialis muscle passing medial to the patella to attach to the medial condyle of the tibia.

**retinacula of peroneal muscles,** retinacula musculorum peroneorum.

**r. of skin,** r. cutis.

**superior r. of extensor muscles,** r. musculorum extensorum superius.

**r. ten'dinum,** the annular ligament of the ankle or wrist.

**retinacula un'guis** [ NA ], retinacula of the nail; fibrous attachments of the nail-bed to the underlying phalanx.

**retinal** (ret'ĭ-nal). Relating to the retina.

**ret'inal.** Retinaldehyde.

**11-*cis*-retinal.** The isomer of retinaldehyde that can combine with opsin to form rhodopsin; 11-*cis*-retinal is formed from all-*trans*-retinal trans-retinal by retinal isomerase.

***trans*-retinal, all-*trans*-retinal.** Visual yellow; xanthopsin (obsolete); metarhodopsin II or *trans*-retinal plus opsin; the orange pigment resulting from action of light on the visual purple (rhodopsin) of the retina, which converts the 11-*cis*-retinal component of the rhodopsin to all -*trans*-retinal plus the protein, opsin.

**retinal'dehyde.** Retinal; retinene (retinene-1); vitamin A (A$_1$) aldehyde; 11-*cis*-retinal; axophtheral (obsolete); retinol oxidized to a terminal aldehyde. A carotene released (as all-*trans*-retinal(dehyde)) in the bleaching of rhodopsin (visual purple) by light and the dissociation of the protein, opsin.

**r. dehydrogenase,** an oxidoreductase (EC 1.2.1.36) catalyzing the interconversion of retinaldehyde and retinoic acid.

**r. isomerase** (EC 5.2.1.3), retinene isomerase; an isomerase that catalyzes the *cis*–*trans* conversion of all-*trans*-retinal(dehyde) to 11-*cis*-retinal(dehyde); a reaction of importance in the visual cycle.

**r. reductase,** retinol dehydrogenase.

**retinene** (ret'ĭ-nēn). Retinaldehyde.

**r. isomerase,** retinaldehyde isomerase.

**r. reductase,** retinol dehydrogenase.

**retinene-1.** Retinaldehyde.

**retinene-2.** Dehydroretinaldehyde.

**retinitis** (ret'ĭ-ni'tis) [ retina + G. suffix -*itis, inflammation* ]. Inflammation of the retina.

**apoplectic r.,** thrombosis of the central retinal vein.

**central angiospastic r.,** central serous *retinopathy.*

**cir'cinate r.,** see circinate *retinopathy.*

**diabetic r.,** see diabetic *retinopathy.*

**ex'udative r.,** r. exudativa; Coats' disease; a chronic inflammatory condition characterized by the appearance of white or yellowish raised areas encircling the optic disk due to the accumulation of edematous fluid beneath the retina; retinal detachment may occur.

**gravid'ic r.,** see toxemic *retinopathy* of pregnancy.

**leuke'mic r.,** see leukemic *retinopathy.*

**metastat'ic r.,** purulent r. resulting from the arrest of septic emboli in the retinal vessels.

**r. pigmento'sa,** pigmentary retinopathy; a progressive abiotrophy of the neuroepithelium, with atrophy and pigmentary infiltration of the inner layers.

**r. proliferans,** neovascularization of the retina extending into the vitreous.

**punctate r.,** see punctata albescens *retinopathy.*

**r. sclopedaria,** a severe traumatic lesion of the retina.

**serous r.,** simple r.; edema of the retina; a mild inflammation of the superficial layers of the retina.

**r. stellata,** exudate in the retina in stellate form.

**r. syphilit'ica,** syphilitic r.; vasculitis retinae syphilitica; often associated with syphilitic choroiditis, especially in congenital syphilis.

**retino-, retin-** (ret'ĭ-no-) [ Mediev. L. *retina.* RET- ]. Combining forms relating to the retina.

**retinoblastoma** (ret'ĭ-no-blas-to'mah) [ retino- + G. *blastos,* germ, + suffix -*oma,* tumor ]. A malignant neoplasm composed of primitive retinal cells, occurring often bilaterally, usually before the third year of life, and exhibiting a familial tendency. R.'s are characterized by small, round cells with deeply staining nuclei, and elongate cells forming rosettes. They usually cause death by local invasion, especially along the optic nerves.

**retinochoroid** (ret'ĭ-no-ko'royd). Chorioretinal; relating to the retina and the choroid.

**retinochoroiditis** (ret'ĭ-no-ko-roy-di'tis) [ retinochoroid + G. suffix -*itis,* inflammation ]. Chorioretinitis; inflammation of the retina and the choroid.

**r. juxtapapilla'ris,** Jensen's disease; inflammation on the fundus, close to the papilla.

**retinodialysis** (ret'ĭ-no-di-al'ĭ-sis) [ retino- + G. *dialysis,* separation ]. Disinsertion (2).

**retinography** (ret'ĭ-nog'ră-fi) [ retino- + G. *graphō,* to write ]. Photography of the fundus of the eye.

**retinoic acid** (ret'ĭ-no'ik). Vitamin A$_1$ acid; retinaldehyde in which the terminal —CHO has been oxidized to a —COOH; *cf.* dehydroretinoic acid.

**retinoid** (ret'ĭ-noyd). 1 [ G. *retinē,* resin, + *eidos,* resemblance ]. Resembling a resin; resinous. 2 [ Mediev. L. *retina* ]. Resembling the retina.

**retinol** (ret'ĭ-nol). Vitamin A (original); vitamin A$_1$; vitamin A or A$_1$ alcohol; axerophtherol (obsolete); axerol (obsolete); 2,6,6-trimethyl-1-(9'-hydroxy-3',7'-dimethyl-nona-1',3',5',7'-tetraenyl)cyclohex-1-ene; a half-carotene bearing the β (or β-ionone) form of the cyclic end group (see carotenoids for β structure) and a CH$_2$OH at the C-15 position (numbering as in carotenoids) or 9' position (numbering as a nonyl side chain on a cyclohexene ring). See also dehydroretinol.

**r. dehydrogenase** retinaldehyde reductase; retinene reductase; an oxidoreductase (EC 1.1.1.105) catalyzing interconversion of retinaldehyde and retinol, a reaction of importance in the chemistry of rod vision.

**11-*cis*-retinol.** Neoretinene B; retinol with *cis*-configuration at 11-position (carotenoid numbering) or 5'-position (retinol numbering) of side chain.

**retinomalacia** (ret′ĭ-no-mă-la′shĭ-ah) [ retino- + G. *malakia*, a softness ]. Retinosis; noninflammatory degeneration of the retina.

**retinopapillitis** (ret′ĭ-no-pap′ĭ-li′tis). Papilloretinitis.

**r. of premature infants,** *retinopathy* of prematurity.

**retinopathy** (ret′ĭ-nop′ă-thĭ) [ retino- + G. *pathos*, suffering ]. Noninflammatory degenerative disease of the retina, as distinguished from retinitis.

**arteriosclerotic r.,** r. distinguished by attenuated retinal arterioles with increased tortuosity, copper- or silver-wire appearance, perivascular sheathing, irregularity of lumen and scattered small hemorrhages, and small, sharp-edged exudates without surrounding edema.

**central angiospastic r.,** central serous r.

**central serous r.,** central angiospastic r. or retinitis; a restricted edema of macula showing grayish spots occasionally and often encircled by a light reflex; usually unilateral with subjective symptoms of misty vision and frequently a positive central scotoma.

**chloroquine r.,** pigmentary degeneration and visual impairment associated with prolonged administration of chloroquine.

**circinate r.,** a retinal degeneration marked by a girdle of sharply defined white exudates around a grayish macula; the disease is usually bilateral and typically affects the aged.

**diabetic r.,** retinal changes occurring in diabetes of long standing, marked by punctate hemorrhages, microaneurysms, and sharply defined waxy exudates; preretinal hemorrhages may cause retinitis proliferans.

**eclamptic r.,** toxemic r. of pregnancy.

**electric r.,** photoretinopathy.

**gravidic r.,** toxemic r. of pregnancy.

**hypertensive r.,** a retinal picture occurring in malignant hypertension, marked by arteriolar constriction, flame-shaped hemorrhages, cotton-wool exudates, increased severity of star-figure edema at macula, and papilledema.

**Leber's idiopathic stellate r.,** a condition of unknown origin, showing unilaterally macular star with papilledema and spontaneous regression in 1 to 3 months.

**leukemic r.,** retinal picture in all types of leukemia, characterized by a yellow-orange fundus, engorgement and tortuosity of veins, scattered hemorrhages, and edema of the retina and disk.

**macular r.,** maculopathy.

**photo r.,** see photoretinopathy.

**pigmentary r.,** *retinitis* pigmentosa.

**r. of prematurity,** retrolental fibroplasia (*q. v.*); Terry's syndrome; a bilateral retinal disorder of premature infants placed in a high oxygen environment; marked by vascular proliferation, intraocular hemorrhage, retinal edema and detachment, and formation of a fibrous retrolental membrane.

**punctata albescens r.,** a familial disease in which both fundi show numerous white dots through the retina; causes night blindness.

**renal r.,** hypertensive r. associated with chronic glomerulonephritis or nephrosclerosis.

**rubella r.,** pigmentary retinal changes in congenital rubella, not affecting visual function.

**sickle cell r.,** a condition marked by dilation and tortuosity of retinal veins, and by microaneurysms and retinal hemorrhages; advanced stages may show sea fan neovascularization, vitreous hemorrhage, or retinal detachment.

**solar r.,** photoretinopathy.

**stellate r.,** a retinal picture resembling hypertensive r., occurring as the result of trauma or obstruction of a retinal vessel.

**thioridazine r.,** pigmentary degeneration and visual impairment associated with large doses of this phenothiazine derivative.

**toxemic r. of pregnancy,** gravidic or eclamptic r.; sudden angiospasm of retinal arterioles, later followed by the picture of advanced hypertensive retinopathy; restitution rapidly follows the termination of pregnancy.

**venous-stasis r.,** a uniocular diabetes-like retinopathy associated with spontaneous occlusion of the carotid artery or of the ophthalmic artery.

**vitreo-r.,** see vitreoretinopathy.

**retinopiesis** (ret′ĭ-no-pi-e′sis) [ retino- + G. *piesis*, pressure ]. Replacement of detached retina by pressing it into position by air, saline, spinal fluid, or preserved vitreous.

**retinoschisis** (ret′ĭ-nos′kĭ-sis) [ retino- + G. *schisis*, division ]. Splitting of the retina due to degeneration, with cyst formation between the two layers.

**juvenile r.,** r. occurring before 10 years of age and within the nerve-fiber layer, with frequent macular involvement; at first, the inner wall is a translucent veil-like membrane, but becomes more dense and may render the retina white; x-linked recessive inheritance.

**senile r.,** r. occurring most often after 40 years of age and affecting the outer plexiform layer; it starts in the extreme inferotemporal periphery and is not significantly progressive; vision usually is good.

**retinoscopy** (ret′ĭ-nos′ko-pĭ) [ retino- + G. *skopeō*, to view ]. Shadow test; skiascopy (1); Cuignet's method; a method of detecting errors of refraction by illuminating the retina and noting the direction of movement of the light when the mirror is rotated.

**retinosis** (ret′ĭ-no′sis). Retinomalacia.

**retoperithelium** (re′to-pĕr-ĭ-the′lĭ-um) [ L. *rete*, net, + G. *peri*, around, + Mod. L. *thelium*, fr. G. *thēlē*, nipple ]. The reticular cells related to the reticular fiber network, as in the stroma of lymphatic tissue.

**retort** (re-tort′) [ Mediev. L. *retorta*, fem. pp. of *re-torqueo*, pp. *-tortus*, to twist or bend back. TORS- ]. A flasklike vessel with a long neck passing outward, once used in distilling.

**Retortamo′nas.** A genus of protozoan flagellates, one species of which, *R. intestinalis,* is found occasionally in the human intestine, although it is nonpathogenic and infrequently reported.

**retothelioma** (re′to-the′lĭ-o′mah). A neoplasm derived from reticular cells of the reticuloendothelial system.

**retract** (re-trakt′) [ L. *re-traho*, pp. *-tractus*, a drawing back ]. 1. To shrink. 2. To draw back.

**retractile** (re-trak′tĭl). Retractable; capable of being drawn back.

**retraction** (re-trak′shun) [ L. *retractio*, a drawing back ]. 1. A shrinking. 2. A drawing back. 3. The state of being drawn back.

**gingival r.,** a pulling away of the gingival margin from the tooth surface and indicative of underlying pocket formation or inflammation; a displacement of the marginal gingivae away from the tooth by mechanical, chemical, or surgical means.

**mandibular r.,** a type of facial anomaly in which the gnathion lies posterior to the orbital plane.

**retractor** (re-trak′tor). 1. An instrument for drawing aside the lips of a wound. 2. A muscle that draws a part backward.

**re′trad** [ L. *retro*, backward, + *ad*, to ]. Backward; toward the back part; caudad.

**retrahens aurem, retrahens auriculam** (re′tra-henz aw′-rem, aw-rik′u-lam) [ L. drawing back the ear, or auricle ]. See *musculus* auricularis posterior.

**retreat from reality.** Substitution of imaginary satisfactions for relations with the real world.

**retrench′ment** [ F. *re-*, back, + *trancher*, to cut ]. The cutting away of superfluous tissue.

**retro-** (ret′ro-, re′tro-) [ L. back, backward ]. Prefix in words formed from Latin roots, denoting backward or behind.

**retroauricular** (ret′ro-aw-rik′u-lar). Behind the auricle.

**retrobuccal** (ret′ro-buk′al). Relating to the back part of, or behind, the cheek.

**ret′robul′bar.** Behind the eyeball.

**retrocalcaneobursitis** (ret′ro-kal-ka′ne-o-bur-si′tis) [ retro- + L. *calcaneum* heel, + bursitis ]. Achillobursitis.

**retrocecal** (ret′ro-se′kal). Posterior to the cecum.

**retrocervical** (ret′ro-ser′vĭ-kal). Posterior to the cervix uteri.

**retrocession** (ret′ro-sesh′un). [ L. *retro-cedo*, pp. *-cessus*, to go back, retire ]. 1. A going back; a relapse. 2. The cessation of the external symptoms of a disease followed by signs of involvement of some internal organ or part. 3.

Denoting a position of the uterus or other organ further back than is normal.

**retroclusion** (ret'ro-klu'zhun) [ retro- + L. *claudo* (*cludo*) to close. CLAUS- ]. A form of acupressure for the arrest of bleeding; the needle is passed through the tissues over the cut end of the artery, is turned around and then passed backward beneath the vessel.

**retrocolic** (ret'ro-kol'ik) [ retro- + G. *kolon*, colon ]. Posterior to the colon.

**retrocollic** (ret'ro-kol'ik) [ retro- + L. *collum*, neck ]. Relating to the back of the neck; drawing back the head.

**retrocollis** (ret'ro-kol'is). Retrocollic *spasm.*

**retroconduction** (ret'ro-kon-duk'shun). Retrograde *conduction.*

**retrocursive** (ret'ro-ker'siv) [ retro- + L. *cursus*, a running ]. Running backward.

**retrodeviation** (ret'ro-de'vi-a'shun). A backward bending or inclining.

**ret'rodisplace'ment.** Any backward displacement, such as retroversion or retroflexion of the uterus.

**retroesophageal** (ret'ro-e-sof'ā-je'al). Posterior to the esophagus.

**retroflected** (ret'ro-flek'ted). Retroflexed.

**retroflection** (ret'ro-flek'shun). Retroflexion.

**retroflexed** (re-tro-flekst') [ retro- + L. *flecto*, pp. *flexus*, to bend ]. Bent backward or posteriorly.

**retroflexion** (ret'ro-flek'shun). Retroflection; backward bending, as of the uterus when the corpus is bent back, forming an angle with the cervix.

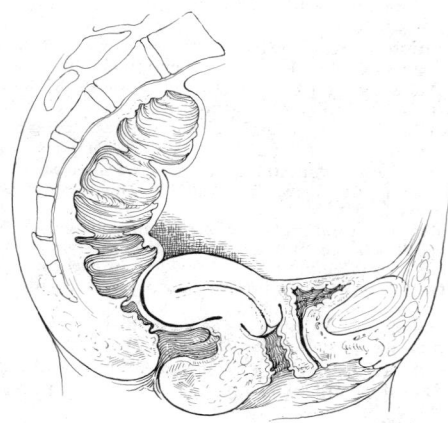

**Retroflexion of the Uterus**

**retroflex'us** [ L. ] [ NA ]. Retroflexed.

**retrognathia** (ret'ro-nath'i-ah, re'trog-na'thi-ah) [ retro- + G. *gnathos*, jaw ]. Underdevelopment of the maxillae or mandible, or both.

**retrograde** (ret'ro-grād) [ L. *retrogradus*, fr. retro- + *gradior*, to go ]. 1. Moving backward. 2. Degenerating; reversing the normal order of growth and development.

**retrography** (re-trog'rā-fi) [ retro- + G. *graphō*, to write ]. Mirror-writing.

**retrogression** (ret'ro-gresh'un) [ L. *retrogressus* (noun), fr. *retro-gradior*, to go backwards ]. Catabolism (2).

**retroiridian** (ret'ro-i-rid'i-an). Posterior to the iris.

**retrojection** (ret'ro-jek'shun) [ L. *retro*, backward, + *jacio*, to throw. JAC- ]. The washing out of a cavity by the backward flow of an injected fluid.

**ret'rojec'tor.** A form of syringe with long tubular attachment to the nozzle, used in retrojection.

**ret'rolen'tal.** Retrolenticular (1) posterior to the lens of the eye.

**retrolenticular** (ret'ro-len-tik'u-lar). 1. Retrolental. 2. Behind the lentiform nucleus of the brain.

**retrolingual** (ret'ro-ling'gwal) [ retro- + L. *lingua*, tongue ]. Relating to the back part of the tongue; posterior to the tongue.

**retromammary** (ret'ro-mam'ā-ri). Posterior to the mamma.

**retromandibular** (ret'ro-man-dib'u-lar) [ retro- + L. *mandibula*, lower jaw ]. Posterior to the lower jaw.

**retromastoid** (ret'ro-mas'toyd). Posterior to the mastoid process; relating to the posterior mastoid cells.

**retromolar** (ret'ro-mo'lar). Distal (or posterior) to the last erupted (or present) molar tooth.

**retromorphosis** (ret'ro-mor'fo-sis, -mor-fo'sis) [ retro- + G. *morphōsis*, process of forming ]. Catabolism (2).

**retronasal** (ret'ro-na'zal). Posterior nasal; relating to the posterior nares.

**retro-ocular** (ret'ro-ok'u-lar). Retrobulbar (1).

**retroperitoneal** (ret'ro-pĕr'i-to-ne'al). External or posterior to the peritoneum.

**retroperitoneum** (ret'ro-pĕr'i-to-ne'um) [ retro- + peritoneum ]. *Spatium* retroperitonealis.

**retroperitonitis** (ret'ro-pĕr'i-to-ni'tis). Inflammation of the cellular tissue behind the peritoneum.

**retropharyngeal** (ret'ro-fā-rin'je-al). Posterior to the pharynx.

**retropharynx** (ret'ro-fār'ingks). The posterior part of the pharynx.

**retroplacental** (ret'ro-pla-sen'tal). Behind the placenta.

**retroplasia** (ret'ro-pla'zi-ah) [ retro- + G. *plasis*, a molding ]. That state of cell or tissue in which activity is decreased below that of euplasia; associated with retrogressive changes (*e.g.,* injury, degeneration, death, necrosis).

**retroposed** (ret'ro-pōzd) [ retro- + L. *pono*, pp. *positus*, to place ]. Displaced backward, but not inclined or bent, neither retroverted nor retroflexed.

**retroposition** (ret'ro-po-zish'un) [ retro- + L. *positio*, a placing ]. Simple backward displacement of a structure or organ, as the uterus, without retroversion or retroflexion.

**retropulsion** (ret'ro-pul'shun) [ retro- + L. *pulsio*, a pushing, fr. *pello*, pp. *pulsus*, beat, drive ]. An involuntary backward walking or running, occurring in patients with the parkinsonian syndrome. 2. A pushing back of any part.

**retrospection** (ret'ro-spek'shun) [ retro- + L. *specto*, pp. *-spectatus*, to look at ]. The act or process of surveying the past.

**retrospective** (ret'ro-spek'tiv). Relating to retrospection.

**retrospondylolisthesis** (ret'ro-spon'di-lo-lis-the'sis) [ retro- + G. *spondylos*, vertebra, + *olisthēsis*, a slipping ]. Slipping backward of the body of a vertebra, bringing it out of line with the vertebra above and below.

**ret'roster'nal.** Posterior to the sternum.

**retrosteroid** (ret'ro-stēr'oyd, -stěr-). A term sometimes used to designate a steroid in which the orientations of the substituents at carbons 9 and 10 are the opposite of those of the reference or "parent" compound; see also steroids.

**ret'rotar'sal.** Posterior to the tarsus, or edge of the eyelid.

**retrouterine** (ret'ro-u'ter-in). Posterior to the uterus.

**retroversioflexion** (ret'ro-ver'si-o-flek'shun, -ver'zho-). Combined retroversion and retroflexion of the uterus.

**retroversion** (ret'ro-ver'zhun) [ retro- + L. *verto*, pp. *versus*, to turn ]. 1. A turning backward, as of the uterus, without flexing or bending the organ. 2. A condition in which the teeth are located in a more posterior position than is normal.

**ret'rovert'ed.** Turned or inclined backward, without being bent.

**retrusion** (re-tru'zhun) [ L. *re-trudo*, pp. *-trusus*, to push back ]. 1. Retraction of the mandible from any given point. 2. The backward movement of the mandible.

**Retzius,** Anders A., Swedish anatomist, 1796–1860. See R.'s *cavity, fibers, gyrus, ligament, ligamentum* Retzii, *space, veins.*

**Retzius,** Magnus G., Swedish histologist, 1842–1919. See Key-R. *corpuscles,* R.'s *foramen,* Key-R. *foramen, lines of* R., R.'s *striae, sheath of* Key-R.

**reunient** (re-u'ni-ent) [ L. *re-*, again, + *unio*, pp. *unitus*, to unite ] . Connecting; denoting the ductus reuniens.

**Reuss** (roys), August R. von, Vienna ophthalmologist, 1841–1924. See R.'s *formula*, color *tables*, *test*.

**revaccination** (re'vak-sǐ-na'shun). Vaccination of a person previously successfully vaccinated.

**revascularization** (re-vas'ku-lăr-ǐ-za'shun). Reestablishment of blood supply to a part by blood vessel graft.

**revellent** (re-vel'ent) [ L. *re-vello*, pp. -*vulsus*, to pluck or pull away ]. Revulsive.

**Reverdin** (rĕ-ver-daṅ'), Jacques L., Swiss surgeon, 1842–1908. See R.'s *method*.

**reversal** (re-ver'sal) [ L. *re-verto*, pp. -*versus*, to turn back or about ]. 1. A turning in the opposite direction, as of a disease, symptom, or a state; *e.g.*, sex reversal or a chemical reaction. 2. The changing of a dark line or a bright one of the spectrum into its opposite. 3. Denoting the difficulty of some persons in distinguishing the lower case printed or written letter *p* from *q* or *g, b* from *d*, or *s* from *z* 4. In psychoanalysis, the change of an instinct or affect into its opposite, as from love into hate.

    **epinephrine r.,** see under epinephrine.

    **sex r.,** a process whereby the sexual identity of an individual is changed from one sex to that of the other. Sex r. may be accomplished by transsexual procedures. It may figure also in the life history of pseudohermaphroditic individuals whose sex at birth was uncertain; initially reared as members of one sex, such individuals may, upon subsequent medical examination and advice, be reared thereafter as members of the opposite sex.

**reversible** (re-ver'sǐ-bl). Capable of reversal; said of diseases or chemical reactions.

**reversion** (re-ver'zhun) [ L. *reversio* (see reversal) ]. 1. The cropping out in an individual of certain characteristics peculiar to a remote ancestor, which characteristics have been in abeyance during one or more of the intermediate generations. 2. The return to the original phenotype, either by reinstatement of the original genotype (true r.) or by a mutation at a site different from that of the first mutation and which cancels the effect of the first mutation (suppressor mutation).

    **true r.,** see r. (2).

**Revilliod** (rĕ-ve-yo'), Léon, Swiss physician, 1835–1919. See R.'s *sign*.

**revivescence** (re-vi-ves'ens) [ L. *re-vivesco*, to come to life again, fr. *vivo*, to live ]. Revivification (1).

**revivification** (re-viv'ǐ-fi-ka'shun) [ L. *re*, again, + *vivo*, to live, + *facio*, to make ]. 1. Revivescence; renewal of life and strength. 2. Vivification (2); freshening the edges of a wound by paring or scraping to promote union.

**revul'sant** [ see revellent ]. 1. Revulsive; derivative; revellent. 2. A counterirritant.

**revulsion** (re-vul'shun) [ L. *revulsio*, art of pulling away, fr. *re-vello*, pp. -*vulsus*, to pluck or pull away ]. Counterirritation; derivation.

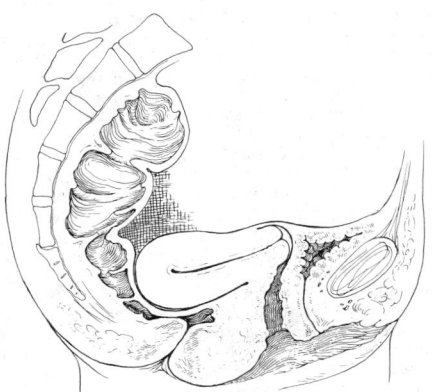

**Retroversion of the Uterus**

**revul'sive.** 1. Causing revulsion. 2. A revulsant or counterirritant.

**reward'.** Reinforcer.

**rewarm'ing.** The application of heat to raise the body temperature in the technique of intentional hypothermia.

**Reye,** R. D. K. See R.'s *syndrome*.

**Reymond,** Emil Du Bois. See under Du Bois.

**Reynals' factor.** See under factor.

**Reynier** (ra-ne-a'), J. B., French orthopedist, 19th century. See R.'s *mycetoma*.

**RF.** Abbreviation for (1) releasing *factor;* (2) rheumatoid *factor;* (3) replicative *form*.

**RH.** Abbreviation for releasing hormone (synonym for releasing *factor, q.v.*).

**Rh.** 1. Chemical symbol of the element rhodium. 2. See Rh blood group, in appendix 2. 3. See Rh *hapten*.

**rhabar'berone.** Aloe-emodin.

**rhabd-.** See rhabdo-.

**Rhabditis** (rab-di'tis) [ G. *rhabdos*, a rod ]. A genus of small, oxyurid-like, nematodes (family Rhabditidae, order Rhabditida); some are free-living, others are parasitic on plants and animals.

    **R. genita'lis,** *R. pellio.*

    **R. niel'lyi,** a species observed by Nielly of Brest in a case of vesicopapular eruption on the skin.

    **R. pel'lio,** *R. genitalis;* a species found in the vagina in one instance.

    **R. strongyloi'des,** a saprophytic organism in the soil which may under certain conditions cause dermatitis in cattle, dogs, and probably other animals.

**rhabdo-, rhabd-** (rab'do-) [ G. *rhabdos*, rod ]. Combining forms meaning rod, rod-shaped (rhabdoid).

**rhabdocyte** (rab'do-sīt) [ rhabdo- + G. *kytos*, cell ]. A rarely used term for band cell or metamyelocyte.

**rhabdoid** (rab'doyd) [ rhabdo- + G. *eidos*, resemblance ]. Rod-shaped.

**rhabdomyolysis** (rab'do-mi-ol'ǐ-sis) [ rhabdo- + G. *mys*, muscle, + *lysis*, loosening ]. An acute, fulminating, potentially fatal disease of skeletal muscle; entails destruction of skeletal muscle as evidenced by myoglobinemia and myoglobinuria.

    **exertional r.,** r. produced in susceptible individuals by muscular exercise.

    **familial paroxysmal r.,** postulated to be a heritable disease in which excessive phosphorylase activity in skeletal muscle results in r.

**rhabdomyoma** (rab-do-mi-o'mah) [ rhabdo- + G. *mys*, muscle, + suffix -*oma*, tumor ]. A benign neoplasm derived from striated muscle.

    **r. sarcomato'sum,** rhabdomyosarcoma.

**rhabdomyosarcoma** (rab'do-mi'o-sar-ko'mah) [ rhabdo- + G. *mys,* muscle, + *sarkōma,* sarcoma ]. Rhabdomyoma sarcomatosum; rhabdosarcoma; a malignant neoplasm derived from skeletal (striated) muscle; characterized by poorly differentiated, bizarre, polygonal and oblong, as well as rounded and bizarre cells with large hyperchromatic nuclei; the cytoplasm is usually granular and structures that resemble cross striations may be observed.

    **embryonal r.'s,** malignant neoplasms occurring in children, consisting of loose, spindle-celled tissue with rare cross-striations, and arising in many parts of the body in addition to skeletal muscles.

**rhabdophobia** (rab'do-fo'bǐ-ah) [ rhabdo- + G. *phobos,* fear ]. Morbid fear of the rod (or switch) as an instrument of punishment.

**rhabdosarcoma** (rab'do-sar-ko'mah). Rhabdomyosarcoma.

**rhabdosphincter** (rab'do-sfingk'ter) [ rhabdo- + G. *sphinktēr,* sphincter ]. A sphincter made up of striated musculature.

**rhachi-.** For words so beginning, see rachi-.

**rhagades** (rag'ă-dēz) [ G. *rhagas,* pl. *rhagades,* a crack. RHAG- ]. Chaps, cracks, or fissures occurring at mucocutaneous junctions; seen in vitamin deficiencies and in congenital syphilis.

**rhagadiformis** (rā-gad-ǐ-for'mis) [ G. *rhagas* (*rhagad-*), crack, + L. *forma,* shape ]. Fissured.

**-rhagia.** See -rrhagia.

β-L-**rham′nose.** 6-Deoxy-L-mannose; isodulcit; a methyl-pentose present in a number of plant glycosides free in poison sumac, in lipopolysaccharides of *Enterobacteriaceae*, in rutinose (a disaccharide). For structure, see sugars.

**rham′noside.** A glycoside of rhamnose upon hydrolysis.

**rhamnoxanthin** (ram′no-zan′thin). Frangulin.

**Rhamnus** (ram′nus) [ G. *rhamnos*, buckthorn ]. A genus of shrubs and trees of the family Rhamnaceae.

    **R. cathar′tica,** purging buckthorn; a shrub of southern Europe the bark and berries of which are cathartic.

    **R. fran′gula,** alder buckthorn; its bark, frangula, is cathartic.

    **R. purshia′na,** the source of the bark cascara sagrada.

**rhaniket.** See Newcastle *disease.*

**rhapha′nia.** Raphania.

**rha′phe.** Raphe.

**-rhaphy.** See -rrhaphy.

**rhatany** (rat′ă-nǐ) [ Peruv. *ratana* ]. Krameria.

**rhathymia** (ră-thi′mǐ-ah) [ G. *rhathymein*, to take a holiday, be relaxed ]. Outgoing, carefree behavior.

**Rhazes,** Persian physician, *c.* 860–932 A.D. Noted for his accurate clinical accounts of disease. His encyclopedic work on medicine, the *Continens,* written in Arabic, was an authoritative source of medical knowledge throughout the Middle Ages.

**rhe** (re) [ G. *rheos*, a stream ]. The absolute unit of fluidity, the reciprocal of the unit of viscosity.

**-rhea.** See -rrhea.

**rheboscelia** (re′bo-se′lǐ-ah) [ G. *rhaibos*, crooked, + *skelos*, leg ]. Rhebosis; a condition characterized by bowlegs or crooked legs.

**rhebosis** (re-bo′sis). Rheboscelia.

**rhegma** (reg-mah) [ G. breakage. RHAG- ]. A rent or fissure.

**rhegmatogenous** (reg-mă-toj′ē-nus) [ G. *rhegma*, breakage, + suffix -*gen*, producing ]. Arising from a bursting or fractionating of an organ. See r. retinal *detachment.*

**rheic** (re′ik). Relating to rheum, or rhubarb.

**rhe′in.** A crystalline substance of little or no activity, obtained from rhubarb.

**Rheinberg microscope.** See under microscope.

**rhembasmus** (rem-baz′mus) [ G. *rhembasmos*, mental indecision, fr. *rhembō*, to roam ]. Indecision; mental uncertainty.

**rhenium** (re′nǐ-um) [ Mod. L., fr. L. *Rhenus*, Rhine river ]. A metal of the platinum group; symbol Re, atomic weight 186.22; atomic no. 75.

**rheo-** (re′o-) [ G. *rheos*, stream, current, flow. RHE- ]. A combining form usually indicating blood flow or electrical current.

**rheobase** (re′o-bās) [ rheo- + G. *basis*, a base ]. Galvanic threshold; the minimal strength of an electrical stimulus of indefinite duration that is able to cause excitation of a tissue, *e.g.,* muscle or nerve. See also chronaxie.

**rheobasic** (re-o-ba′sik). Pertaining to or having the characteristics of a rheobase.

**rheocardiography** (re′o-kar-dǐ-og′ră-phǐ) [ rheo- + cardiography ]. Dielectrography; impedance plethysmography; the technique of measuring and recording rhythmic changes in body impedance.

**rheoencephalogram** (re′o-en-sef′ă-lo-gram). Graphic registration of the changes in conductivity of tissue of the head caused by vascular factors.

**rheoencephalography** (re′o-en-sef-ă-log′ră-fǐ) [ rheo- + encephalography ]. The technique of measuring blood flow of the brain. Commonly used to denote impedance r. which uses (inaptly) the changes in electrical impedance and resistance as a measure of flow.

**rheogram** (re′o-gram) [ rheo- + G. *gramma*, something written ]. A plot of the shear stress *versus* the shear rate for a fluid.

**rheologist** (re-ol′o-jist). One versed in some branch of rheology.

**rheology** (re-ol′o-jǐ) [ rheo- + G. *logos*, study ]. The study of the deformation and flow of materials.

**rheometer** (re-om′e-ter) [ rheo- + G. *metron*, measure ]. 1. An instrument for measurement of the rheologic properties of materials, *e.g.,* of blood. 2. A galvanometer.

**rheom′etry.** The measurement of electrical current or blood flow.

**rheostat** (re′o-stat) [ rheo- + G. *statos*, stationary ]. A variable resistor used to adjust the current in an electrical circuit.

**rheostosis** (re-os-to′sis) [ rheo- + G. *osteon*, bone, + suffix -*osis*, condition ]. Streak or flowing hyperostosis; a hypertrophying and condensing osteitis which tends to run in longitudinal streaks or columns and involves a number of the long bones.

**rheotachygraphy** (re-o-tă-kig′ră-fǐ) [ rheo- + G. *tachys*, swift, + *graphō*, to write ]. Recording graphically the variations of electromotive force in a muscle.

**rheotannic acid** (re′o-tan′ik). A glucoside, $C_{26}H_{26}O_{14}$; the form of tannin occurring in rhubarb.

**rheotaxis** (re′o-tak′sis) [ rheo- + G. *taxis*, orderly arrangement ]. A form of positive barotaxis, in which a microorganism is impelled to move contrary to the direction of the current in a fluid in which it is.

**rheotropism** (re-ot′ro-pizm) [ rheo- + G. *tropos*, a turning ]. A movement contrary to the motion of a current, involving part of an organism, rather than, as in rheotaxis, the organism as a whole.

**rhestocythemia** (res′to-si-the′mǐ-ah) [ G. *rhaiō*, to destroy, + *kytos*, a hollow (a cell), + *haima*, blood ]. The presence of broken down red blood cells in the peripheral circulation.

**rhesus** (re′sus) [ Mod. L. arbit. use of L. *Rhesus*, G. *Rhesos*, a mythical king of Thrace ]. A species of Catarrhine monkey of India and China of the genus *Macaca.* Also called macaques. See *Macaca.*

**rheum** (re′um) [ G. *rhēon* ]. Rhubarb.

    **r. emodin,** emodin.

**rheum** (room) [ G. *rheuma*, a flux. RHE- ]. A mucous or watery discharge.

    **epidemic r.,** influenza.

**rheumapyra** (roo-map′ǐ-rah) [ G. *rheuma*, flux, + *pyr*, fire ]. Rheumatic *fever.*

**rheumarthritis** (roo-mar-thri′tis) [ G. *rheuma*, flux, + *arthron*, joint, + -*itis* ]. Articular *rheumatism.*

**rheumarthrosis** (roo-mar-thro′sis). Rheumarthritis.

**rheumatalgia** (roo-mă-tal′jǐ-ah) [ G. *rheuma*, flux, + *algos*, pain ]. Rheumatic pain.

**rheumatic** (roo-mat′ik) [ G. *rheumatikos*, subject to flux, fr. *rheuma*, flux ]. Rheumatismal; relating to or suffering from rheumatism.

**rheumatid** [ G. *rheum*, flux, + -*id* (1), *q.v.* ]. Rheumatic nodules or other eruptions which may accompany rheumatism.

**rheumatism** (roo′mă-tizm) [ G. *rheumatismos*, rheuma, a flux ]. 1. Obsolete term for rheumatic *fever.* 2. An indefinite term applied to various conditions with pain or other symptoms which are of articular origin or related to other elements of the musculoskeletal system.

    **acute artic′ular r., acute inflammatory r.,** *polyarthritis* rheumatica acuta.

    **chronic r.,** a nonspecific affection of the joints, slow in progress, producing a painful thickening and contraction of the fibrous structures, interfering with motion, and causing more or less deformity.

    **desert r.,** coccidioidomycosis.

    **gonorrhe′al r.,** an arthritis, often a polyarthritis, caused by systemic infection with the gonococcus.

    **inflammatory r.,** *polyarthritis* rheumatica acuta.

    **lumbar r.,** lumbago.

    **Macleod's r.,** rheumatoid arthritis with abundant serous effusion in the affected joints.

    **muscular r.,** fibrositis.

    **nodose r.,** (1) rheumatoid *arthritis;* (2) an acute or subacute articular r., accompanied by the formation of nodules on the tendons, ligaments, and periosteum in the neighborhood of the affected joints.

    **osseous r.,** rheumatoid *arthritis.*

    **subacute r.,** a mild, but usually protracted form of acute rheumatic fever, often rebellious to treatment.

**tuberculous r.,** an inflammatory condition of the joints or fibrous tissues during the course of tuberculosis.

**rheumatismal** (roo-mă-tiz′mal). Rheumatic.

**rheumatocelis** (roo′mă-to-se′lis) [ G. *rheuma,* flux, + *kē-lis,* spot ]. Henoch-Schönlein *purpura.*

**rheumatoid** (roo′mă-toyd) [ G. *rheuma,* flux, + *eidos,* resemblance ]. Resembling rheumatism in one or more features.

**rheumatologist** (roo′mă-tol′o-jist). One skilled in the diagnosis and treatment of rheumatic conditions.

**rheumatopyra** (roo-mă-top′ĭ-rah). Rheumatic *fever.*

**rhexis** (rek′sis) [ G. *rhēxis,* rupture. RHAG- ]. Bursting or rupture of an organ or vessel.

**rhigosis** (rĭ-go′sis) [ G. *rhigoun,* to be cold, + suffix *-osis,* condition ]. The perception of cold.

**rhigotic** (rĭ-got′ik). Pertaining to rhigosis.

**rhin-, rhino-** [ G. *rhis,* nose. RHIN- ]. Combiningform denoting the nose.

**rhinal** (ri′nal). Nasal.

**rhinalgia** (ri-nal′jĭ-ah) [ rhin- + G. *algos,* pain ]. Rhinodynia; pain in the nose.

**rhina′rium,** pl. **rhina′ria.** The area of hairless skin surrounding the nostrils in some mammals.

**rhinedema** (ri′ne-de′mah) [ rhin- + G. *oidema,* swelling ]. Swelling of the nasal mucous membrane.

**rhinencephalic** (ri′nen-sē-fal′ik). Relating to the rhinencephalon.

**rhinencephalon** (ri′nen-sef′ă-lon) [ rhin- + G. *enkephalos,* brain ]. Olfactory brain; smell brain; collective term denoting the parts of the cerebral hemisphere directly related to the sense of smell: the olfactory bulb, olfactory peduncle (together still listed as the first cranial nerve or olfactory nerve despite the fact that they form part of the central nervous system), olfactory tubercle, and olfactory or piriform cortex including the cortical nucleus of the amygdala. The term originally also encompassed the hippocampus, the entire amygdala, and the gyrus fornicatus, which are no longer believed to be specifically related to the sense of smell. See also limbic *system.*

**rhinencephalus** (ri′nen-sef′ă-lus). Rhinocephalus.

**rhinenchysis** (ri-nen′kĭ-sis) [ rhin- + G. *enchysis,* a pouring in. CHY- ]. A nasal douche; washing out the nasal cavities.

**rhineurynter** (ri-nu-rin′ter) [ rhin- + G. *eurynō,* to dilate, fr. *eurys,* wide ]. A dilatable bag used to make pressure within the nostril to arrest a profuse epistaxis.

**rhinion** (rin′ĭ-on) [ G. *rhinion,* nostril, dim. of *rhis* (*rhin-*), nose ]. A craniometric point: the lower end of the internasal suture; see fig. under craniometric *point.*

**rhinism** (ri′nizm). Rhinolalia.

**rhinitis** (ri-ni′tis) [ rhin- + G. suffix *-itis,* inflammation ]. Nasal catarrh; inflammation of the nasal mucous membrane.

   **acute r.,** coryza; cold in the head; an acute catarrhal inflammation of the mucous membrane of the nose, marked by sneezing, lacrimation, and a profuse secretion of watery mucus.

   **allergic r.,** pale, boggy swelling of nasal mucosa associated with sneezing and watery discharge, attributable to hypersensitivity to foreign substances.

   **atrophic r.,** chronic r. with thinning of the mucous membrane; often associated with crusts and foul-smelling discharge.

   **atrophic r. of swine,** a disease of uncertain etiology, manifested by atrophy, shrinkage, and often almost complete disappearance of the turbinate bones; it is accompanied by distortion of the facial bones, sneezing, and stunting of the growth of young animals.

   **r. caseo′sa,** caseous r.; a form of chronic r. in which the nasal cavities are more or less completely filled with an ill smelling cheesy material.

   **chronic r.,** a protracted sluggish inflammation of the nasal mucous membrane; in the later stages the mucous membrane with its glands may be thickened (hypertrophic r.) or thinned (atrophic r.).

   **croupous r.,** membranous r.

   **fi′brinous r.,** membranous r.

   **gan′grenous r.,** cancrum nasi.

   **hypertroph′ic r.,** chronic r. with permanent thickening of the mucous membrane.

   **r. medicamento′sa,** inflammation of the nasal mucosa secondary to excessive or improper topical medication.

   **mem′branous r.,** a chronic inflammation of the nasal mucous membrane attended with a fibrinous or pseudomembranous exudate; croupous r.; fibrinous r.; pseudomembranous r.

   **necrotic r. of pigs,** bullnose; an infection of the subcutaneous structures of the snout of swine which causes malformation of the face; it is frequently due to infection of wounds made for the insertion of metal rings to discourage or prevent the animal from rooting in the soil; the necrosis bacillus (*Actinomyces necrophorous*) plays an important role in this disease.

   **r. nervo′sa,** hay *fever.*

   **pseudomem′branous r.,** membranous r.

   **r. purulen′ta,** purulent r.; a chronic r. in which pus formation is excessive.

   **scrof′ulous r.,** tuberculous infection of the nasal mucous membrane.

   **r. sicca,** a form of chronic r. with little or no secretion.

   **vasomotor r.,** congestion of nasal mucosa without infection or allergy.

**rhino-** (ri′no-) [ G. *rhis,* nose. RHIN- ]. Combining form relating to the nose.

**rhinoanemometer** (ri′no-an′e-mom′e-ter) [ rhino- + G. *anemos,* wind, + *metron,* measure ]. A variation of the pneumotachometer, used for measuring nasal air flow and nasal resistance to air flow.

**rhinoantritis** (ri′no-an-tri′tis) [ rhino- G. *antron,* cave (antrum) + suffix *-itis,* inflammation ]. Inflammation of the nasal cavities and one or both maxillary antrums.

**rhinobyon** (ri-no′bi-on) [ rhino- + G. *byō,* to stuff, plug ]. A nasal plug or tampon.

**rhinocanthectomy** (ri′no-kan-thek′to-mī) [ rhino- + G. *kanthos,* canthus, + *ektomē,* excision ]. Excision of the inner canthus of the eye.

**rhinocele, rhinocoele** (ri′no-sēl) [ rhino- + G. *koilia,* a hollow ]. The cavity or ventricle of the rhinencephalon or primitive olfactory part of the telencephalon.

**rhinocephalia** (ri′no-sē-fa′lĭ-ah). Rhinocephaly.

**rhinocephalus** (ri′no-sef′ă-lus). An individual with rhinocephaly.

**rhinocephaly** (ri′no-sef′ă-lī) [ rhino- + G. *kephalē,* head ]. Rhinencephaly; a form of cyclopia in which the nose is represented by a fleshy, proboscis-like protuberance arising above the slitlike orbits, and the rhinencephalic lobes of the telencephalon are poorly developed and show more or less tendency to become fused together.

**rhinochiloplasty** (ri-no-ki′lo-plas-tī) [ rhino- + G. *cheilos,* lip, + *plassō,* to form ]. Plastic or reparative surgery of the nose and upper lip.

**rhinocleisis** (ri-no-kli′sis) [ rhino- + G. *kleisis,* a closure ]. Rhinostenosis.

**rhinodacryolith** (ri-no-dak′rĭ-o-lith) [ rhino- + G. *dakryon,* tear (duct), + *lithos,* stone ]. A calculus in the nasolacrimal duct.

**rhinodymia** (ri′no-dim′ĭ-ah) [ rhino- + G. suffix *-dymos,* fold ]. Duplication of the nose on an otherwise normal face.

**rhinodynia** (ri-no-din′ĭ-ah) [ rhino- + G. *odynē,* pain ]. Rhinalgia.

**rhinogenous** (ri-noj′ē-nus) [ rhino- + G. suffix *-gen,* producing ]. Originating in the nose.

**rhinokyphectomy** (ri′no-ki-fek′to-mī) [ rhino- + G. *kyphōsis,* humped condition, + *ektomē,* excision ]. A plastic operation for rhinokyphosis.

**rhinokyphosis** (ri′no-ki-fo′sis) [ rhino- + G. *kyphōsis,* humped condition ]. A humpback deformity of the nose.

**rhinolalia** (ri′no-la′lĭ-ah) [ rhino- + G. *lalia,* talking ]. Nasalized speech.

   **r. aperta,** abnormal phonation attributable to inadequate velopharyngeal closure.

   **r. clau′sa,** abnormal phonation attributable to nasal obstruction.

**rhinolaryngitis** (ri′no-lăr′in-ji′tis) [ rhino- + G. *larynx,* larynx, + suffix *-itis,* inflammation ]. Inflammation of the nasal and laryngeal mucous membranes.

**rhinolaryngology** (ri′no-lăr-ing-gol′o-jī). Rhinology and laryngology combined.

**rhinolite** (ri′no-lit). Rhinolith.

**rhinolith** (ri′no-lith) [ rhino- + G. *lithos*, stone ]. Nasal calculus; a calcareous concretion in the nasal cavity.

**rhinolithiasis** (ri′no-lĭ-thi′ă-sis) [ rhinolith + G. suffix *-iasis*, condition ]. The presence of a nasal calculus.

**rhinologic** (ri-no-loj′ik). Relating to rhinology.

**rhinologist** (ri-nol′o-jist). One versed in rhinology; a specialist in diseases of the nose.

**rhinology** (ri-nol′o-jī) [ rhino- + G. *logos*, study ]. The branch of medical science that has to do with the nose and its diseases.

**rhinomanometer** (ri′no-mă-nom′ĕ-ter) [ rhino- + manometer ]. A manometer used to determine the presence and amount of nasal obstruction, and the nasal air pressure and flow relationships.

**rhinomanometry** (ri′no-mă-nom′ĕ-trī). 1. The use of a rhinomanometer. 2. The study and measurement of nasal air flow and pressures.

**rhinomucormycosis** (ri′no-mu′kor-mi-ko′sis) [ rhino- + mucormycosis, *q.v.* ]. Mucormycosis involving the nose, paranasal sinuses, the eye, and, sometimes, the cranial cavity.

**rhinomycosis** (ri′no-mi-ko′sis) [ rhino- + mycosis ]. Fungus infection of the nasal mucous membranes.

**rhinonecrosis** (ri′no-ne-kro′sis) [ rhino- + necrosis ]. Necrosis of the bones of the nose.

**rhinopathy** (ri-nop′ă-thī) [ rhino- + G. *pathos*, suffering ]. Disease of the nose.

**rhinopharyngeal** (ri′no-fă-rin′je-al). 1. Relating to the nose and the pharynx. 2. Relating to the rhinopharynx.

**rhinopharyngitis** (ri′no-făr′in-ji′tis) [ rhino- + pharynx, + G. suffix *-itis*, inflammation ]. Nasopharyngitis; inflammation of the mucous membrane of the upper part of the pharynx and posterior nares.

   **r. mu′tilans,** gangosa.

**rhinopharyngolith** (ri′no-fă-ring′go-lith) [ rhinopharynx + G. *lithos*, stone ]. A concretion in the rhinopharynx.

**rhinopharynx, ri′no-făr′ingks)** [ rhino- + pharynx ]. Pars nasalis pharyngis.

**rhinophonia** (ri′no-fo′nĭ-ah) [ rhino- + G. *phōnē*, voice ]. Rhinolalia.

**rhinophyma** (ri′no-fi′mah) [ rhino- G. *phyma*, tumor, growth ]. Permanent thickening of connective tissues and hypertrophy of the sebaceous glands of the nose, with resulting enlargement and dilation; also called hypertrophic rosacea, copper nose, rum nose, brandy nose, hammer nose, toper's nose, rum-blossom.

**rhinoplasty** (ri′no-plas-tī) [ rhino- + G. *plassō*, to form ]. Reparative or plastic surgery of the nose; the supplying of a partial or complete defect of the nose by tissue taken from elsewhere.

   **English r.,** r. by means of a flap from the cheek.

   **Indian r.,** Carpue's method; r. by means of a flap from the forehead.

**rhinopneumonitis** (ri′no-nu′mo-ni′tis) [ rhino- + G. *pneumōn*, lung, + suffix *-itis*, inflammation ]. Obsolete term for inflammatory condition involving the mucous membranes of the nose and lung.

   **equine r.,** equine virus *abortion.*

**rhinopsia** (ri-nop′sĭ-ah) [ rhino- + G. *opis*, vision ]. Esotropia.

**rhinoreaction** (ri′no-re-ak′shun). Moeller's test; a form of tuberculin test, utilizing nasal mucous membrane.

**rhinorrhagia** (ri-no-ra′jī-ah) [ rhino- + G. *rhēgnymi*, to burst forth ]. Epistaxis; nosebleed; especially if profuse.

**rhinorrhea** (ri-no-re′ah) [ rhino- + G. *rhoia*, flow ]. Nasal hydrorrhea; a discharge from the nasal mucous membrane.

   **cerebrospi′nal fluid r.,** a discharge of cerebrospinal fluid from the nose.

   **gustatory r.,** watery nasal discharge associated with stimulation of the sense of taste.

**rhinosalpingitis** (ri′no-sal′pin-ji′tis) [ rhino- + G. *salpinx*, tube, + suffix *-itis*, inflammation ]. Inflammation of the mucous membrane of the nose and Eustachian tube.

**rhinoscleroma** (ri′no-skle-ro′mah) [ rhino- + G. *sklērōma*, an induration (scleroma) ]. A chronic granulo-

matous process involving the nose, upper lip, mouth, and upper air passages; starts usually as a growth of hard, smooth nodules in the anterior nares which spreads backward into the pharynx, larynx, trachea, and even into the bronchi; it may involve the external auditory meatus. It is believed to be due to a specific bacillus, possibly a strain of *Klebsiella.* Streptomycin has been used successfully in its treatment.

**rhinoscope** (ri′no-skōp). Nasoscope; a small mirror attached at a suitable angle to a rodlike handle, used in posterior rhinoscopy.

**rhinoscopic** (ri′no-skop′ik). Relating to the rhinoscope or to rhinoscopy.

**rhinoscopy** (ri-nos′ko-pī) [ rhino- + G. *skopeō*, to view ]. Inspection of the nasal cavity.

   **anterior r.,** inspection of the anterior portion of the nasal cavity with or without the aid of a nasal speculum.

   **median r.,** inspection of the roof of the nasal cavity and openings of the posterior ethmoid cells and sphenoidal sinus by means of a long-bladed nasal speculum or nasopharyngoscope.

   **posterior r.,** inspection of the nasopharynx and posterior portion of the nasal cavity by means of the rhinoscope, or with a nasopharyngoscope.

**rhinosporidiosis** (′no-spo-rid-ī-o′sis). Invasion of the nasal cavity by a species of *Rhinosporidium*, found in natives of North and South America as well as India and Ceylon.

**Rhinosporidium seebe′ri** (ri′no-spo-rid′ī-um) [ rhino- + G. *sporidion*, dim. of *sporos*, seed ]. A yeastlike organism of the order Haplosporidia, found in certain vascular raspberry-like tumors of the septum nasi in natives of India.

**rhinostenosis** (ri′no-stĕ-no′sis) [ rhino- + G. *stenōsis*, a narrowing ]. Rhinocleisis; nasal obstruction.

**rhinotomy** (ri-not′o-mī) [ rhino- + G. *tomē*, incision, cutting ]. 1. Any cutting operation on the nose. 2. Operative procedure in which the nose is incised along one side so that it may be turned away to provide full vision of the nasal passages for radical sinus operations.

**rhinotracheitis** (ri′no-tra-ke-i′tis) [ rhino- + trachea + suffix *-itis*, inflammation ]. Inflammation of the nasal cavities and trachea.

   **infectious bovine r.,** a specific infectious disease of cattle, caused by a virus; manifested by severe inflammation and ulceration of the nasal cavities and trachea, frequently followed by pneumonia.

**rhinovirus** (ri′no-vi′rus). See under virus.

**Rhipicephalus** (ri′pĭ-sef′ă-lus) [ G. *rhipis*, fan, + *kephalē*, head ]. A genus of inornate hard ticks (family Ixodidae) consisting of about 50 species, all of which are Old World except *R. sanguineus.* Eyes and festoons are present in both sexes; short palpi and ventral plates are present only in the male. The genus includes important vectors of diseases in man and domestic animals.

   **R. appendicula′tus,** a brown tick transmitting *Theileria parva,* agent of East Coast fever, and *Theileria mutans,* agent of benign bovine theileriosis.

   **R. bur′sa,** a species that transmits *Theileria ovis,* agent of benign and malignant ovine theileriosis, and probably *Theileria hirci,* agent of benign and malignant caprine theileriosis.

   **R. capen′sis,** an African species found on cattle and horses, and one of the ticks that transmits East Coast fever and theileriosis.

   **R. evert′si,** African red t.; a species supposed to transmit *Borrelia theileri,* the cause of a relapsing fever in cattle, *Theileria ovis,* agent of benign ovine and caprine theileriosis, and *Theileria mutans,* agent of benign bovine theileriosis.

   **R. sanguin′eus,** brown dog tick; probably the most common and cosmopolitan species found on dogs in the United States; it may attack other animals but rarely attacks man; it is the chief vector of Rocky Mountain spotted fever in Mexico, the vector of canine babesiosis, and probably important in the spread of the rickettsia of boutonneuse fever.

   **R. si′mus,** black-pitted tick; a species which, like *R. appendiculatus,* transmits *Theileria parva.*

**rhizo-** (ri′zo-) [ G. *rhiza*, root ]. Combining form meaning root.

**rhizoid** (ri′zoyd) [ rhizo- + G. *eidos*, resemblance ]. 1. Rootlike. 2. Irregularly branching, like a root; denoting a form of bacterial growth.

**rhizome** (ri′zōm) [ G. *rhizōma*, mass of roots, fr. *rhiza*, root, + suffix -*oma*, mass ]. The creeping underground stem of plants such as iris, calamus, and sanguinaria.

**rhizomelic** (ri-zo-mel′ik) [ rhizo- + G. *melos*, limb ]. Relating to the "roots" of the limbs; *i.e.*, to the hips and shoulders, as in r. spondylosis.

**rhizomeningomyelitis** (ri′zo-mĕ-ning′go-mi-ĕ-li′tis) [ rhizo- + G. *mēninx*, membrane, + *myelon*, marrow, + suffix -*itis*, inflammation ]. Radiculomeningomyelitis; inflammation of the nerve roots, the meninges, and the spinal cord.

**rhizoplast** (ri′zo-plast) [ rhizo- + G. *plastos*, formed ]. A fine connection between the flagellum or blepharoplast of a protozoan and the nucleus of the cell.

**Rhizopodea** (ri′zo-po′de-ah) [ rhizo- + G. *pous* (*pod*-), foot ]. A class of the superclass Sarcodina, having pseudopodia of various forms, but without axial filaments; the amebae of man belong to this class.

**rhizopterin** (ri-zop′ter-in). Formylpteroic acid, a folic acid factor.

**Rhizopus** (ri-zo′pus). A genus of fungi belonging to the class Phycomycetes (Zygomycetes) and the family Mucoraceae; they may cause phycomycosis in man.

**rhizotomy** (ri-zot′o-mī) [ G. *rhiza*, root, + *tomē*, section ]. Radiculectomy; radicotomy; section of the spinal nerve roots for the relief of pain or spastic paralysis.

    **anterior r.,** section of anterior spinal root.

    **posterior r.,** Dana's operation; section of posterior spinal root.

    **trigeminal r.,** retrogasserian neurectomy and neurotomy; division or section of a sensory root of the fifth cranial nerve, accomplished through a subtemporal (Frazier-Spiller operation), suboccipital (Dandy operation), or transtentorial approach.

**rhod-.** See rhodo-.

**rhodamine B** (ro′dă-mēn, -min). A fluorescent red dye, tetraethylrhodamine chloride, used as a stain in histology.

**rhodanate** (ro′dă-nāt). Thiocyanate.

**rhodanese** (ro′dă-nēz). Thiosulfate sulfurtransferase.

**rhodanic acid** (ro-dan′ik). Thiocyanic acid.

**rhodeose** (ro′de-ōs). D-Fucose.

**rhodin** (ro′din). A dihydroporphyrin derivative (the two additional hydrogens being at positions 7 and 8) of the type found in the chlorophyll b molecule; *i.e.*, with a formyl group on position 3, rather than a methyl group as in a chlorin.

**rhodium** (ro′dī-um) [ Mod. L. fr. G. *rhodon*, a rose ]. A metallic element, symbol Rh, atomic no. 45, atomic weight 102.91.

**rhodo-, rhod-** (ro′do-) [ G. *rhodon*, rose ]. Combining forms indicating a rose or red color.

**rhodogenesis** (ro′do-jen′ĕ-sis) [ rhodopsin + G. *genesis*, production ]. The reproduction of a visual purple (rhodopsin) by combination of 11-*cis*-retinal and opsin in the dark.

**rhodomycin** (ro′do-mi′sin). An antibiotic obtained from *Streptomyces purpurascens.* The hydrochloride and phosphate give red solutions in water; active against *Staphylococcus aureus in vitro.* Consists of r. A and r. B.

**rho′dophylac′tic.** Relating to rhodophylaxis.

**rhodophylaxis** (ro-do-fi-lak′sis) [ rhodopsin + G. *phylaxis*, a guarding ]. The action of the pigment cells of the choroid in preserving or facilitating the reproduction of rhodopsin.

**rhodopsin** (ro-dop′sin). Visual purple; erythropsin; a red thermolabile protein, MW ca. 40,000, found in the external segments of the rods of the retina; it is bleached by the action of light, which converts it to opsin and *trans*-retinal (formerly retinene or vitamin $A_1$ aldehyde), and restored in the dark (see rhodogenesis).

    **lumi-r.,** see lumirhodopsin.

    *meta*-**rhodopsin I and II.** Formed from lumirhodopsin in the visual cycle; the immediate precursors of opsin and *trans*-retinal.

**rhoeadine** (re′ă-dēn). An alkaloid obtained from *Papaver rhoeas* (corn poppy); nonpoisonous.

**rhombencephalon** (rom′ben-sef′ă-lon) [ rhombo- + G. *enkephalos*, brain ]. [ NA ]. The hindbrain or afterbrain, divided secondarily into metencephalon and myelencephalon; it includes the pons, cerebellum, and medulla oblongata.

**rhombic** (rom′bik). 1. Rhomboid. 2. Relating to the rhombencephalon.

**rhomb′inin.** Anagyrine.

**rhombo-, rhomb-** (rom′bo-) [ G. *rhombos*, a rhomb or rhombus ]. Combining forms meaning rhombic, rhomboid.

**rhomboatloideus** (rom′bo-at-lo-id′e-us). See under musculus.

**rhombocele** (rom′bo-sēl) [ rhombo- + G. *koilia*, a hollow ]. Rhomboidal *sinus.*

**rhomboid, rhomboidal** (rom′boyd, rom-boy′dal) [ rhombo- + G. *eidos*, appearance ]. Rhombic (1); resembling a rhomb; *i.e.*, an oblique parallelogram, but having unequal sides; in anatomy, denoting especially a ligament and two muscles.

**rhomboi′des** [ L. ] [ NA ]. Rhomboid.

**rhomboideus** (rom-bo-id′e-us). See under musculus.

**rhombomere** (rom′bo-mēr) [ rhombo- + G. *meros*, part ]. Neuromere.

**rhonchal, rhonchial** (rong′kal, rong′kī-al). Relating to a rhonchus.

**rhonchus**, pl. **rhonchi** (rong′kus, -ki) [ L. fr. G. *rhenchos*, a snoring ]. A loud rale; especially a whistling or sonorous (snoring) rale produced in the larger bronchi or the trachea.

    **cavernous r.,** cavernous *rale.*

**rhopheocytosis** (ro′fi-o-si-to′sis) [ G. *rhophein*, to gulp down, or aspirate, + *kytos*, cell, + suffix -*osis*, condition ]. The formation of vacuoles at a cell surface without prior formation of cytoplasmic projections, by which the cell appears to aspirate surrounding material. See also pinocytosis.

**rhoptries**, sing. **rhoptry** (rōp′trēs) [ G. *rhopalon*, club ]. Paired organelles; club-shaped, electron-dense structures in the anterior portion of sporozoites and merozoites of protozoa in the subphylum Apicomplexa (Sporozoa); they are paired in sporozoites of *Plasmodium* and in merozoites of *Isospora*, and *Eimeria;* in other related genera, more than two rhoptries are found. They appear to have a glandular, perhaps proteolytic, function as part of the activity of the conoid.

**rhotacism** (ro′tă-sizm) [ G. *rhō*, the letter r ]. The too frequent use or incorrect pronunciation of the letter r.

**rhubarb** (ru′barb). Any plant of the genus *Rheum* (family Polygonaceae), especially *R. rhaponticum*, garden rhubarb, pieplant, and *R. officinale* or *R. palmatum.* The last two species or their hybrids, deprived of periderm tissues, dried and powdered, are used for their astringent, tonic, and laxative effects. R. is listed in the BP.

**Rhus** (rōōs, rŭs) [ L. fr. G. *rhous*, sumac ]. A genus of trees and shrubs of the family Anacardiaceae, containing various species that are used for their ornamental foliage; formerly used in tanning.

    **R. caus′tica,** a South American irritant species.

    **R. glabra,** sumac berries; brown, hard, globular or somewhat reinform, dry berries, inodorous, with acidulous and astringent taste. Used as an astringent in diarrhea, and in infusion as a gargle in chronic pharyngitis.

    **R. meto′pium,** poisonwood; coral sumac; a poisonous species of the West Indies and southern Florida.

    **R. pu′mila,** dwarf sumac; poisonous.

    **R. toxicoden′dron,** (1) poison ivy; climbing sumac; (2) *Toxicodendron quercifolium.*

    **R. venena′ta,** *Toxicodendron vernix.*

**rhyparia** (ri-pa′rī-ah) [ G. filth, fr. *rhypos*, filth ]. Sordes.

**rhypophagy** (ri-pof′ă-jī) [ G. *rhypos*, filth, + *phagein*, to eat ]. Scatophagy.

**rhypophobia** (ri-po-fo′bī-ah) [ G. *rhypos*, filth, + *phobos*, fear ]. An exaggerated and morbid fear of dirt or filth.

**rhythm** (rithm) [ G. *rhythmos* ]. 1. Measured time or motion; the regular alternation of two different or opposite states; especially applied to the pattern of the heart's beat, regular and irregular. 2. Denoting the cyclical intermenstrual periods of fertility and sterility, advantage of which is taken in natural birth control. 3. A regular occurrence of an electrical event in the electroencephalogram. See also subentries under wave.

**agonal r.,** an idioventricular r., characterized by unusually wide and bizarre ventricular complexes, often seen in moribund patients.

**alpha r.,** Berger r.; alpha wave; a recurring wave pattern in the encephalogram in the frequency band of 8 to 13 cycles per second.

**at′rioventric′ular r.,** A-V nodal r.

**A-V nodal r.,** nodal bradycardia; nodal r.; the cardiac r. when the heart is controlled by the A-V node; arising in the A-V node, the impulse ascends to the atria and descends to the ventricles more or less simultaneously. In **upper nodal r.,** the P′ wave precedes the QRS complex; in **lower nodal r.** it follows the QRS complex; and in **midnodal r.** it is lost within the QRS complex.

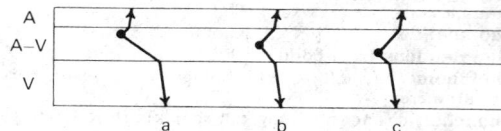

**A-V Nodal Rhythms**
*a,* Upper nodal rhythm; *b,* midnodal rhythm; *c,* lower nodal rhythm.

**Berger r.,** alpha r.

**beta r.,** beta wave; the frequency band of the electroencephalogram from 18 to 30 cycles per second.

**bigeminal r.,** bigeminy; coupling; coupled r.; that cardiac r. when each sinus beat is followed by a premature beat, with the result that the heart beats occur in pairs.

**cantering r.,** gallop (2).

**circadian r.,** see circadian.

**circus r.,** circus *movement.*

**coronary nodal r.,** applied by some authorities to the electrocardiographic pattern of normal upright P waves in leads I and II with a short P-R interval.

**coronary sinus r.,** an ectopic atrial r. supposedly originating from a pacemaker at the mouth of the coronary sinus; recognized in the electrocardiogram by a P-wave pattern similar to that of A-V nodal r. but with a normal or prolonged P-R interval.

**coupled r.,** bigeminal r.

**delta r.,** delta wave (2); a wave pattern in the electroencephalogram that lies in the frequency band of $1\frac{1}{2}$ to 4 cycles per second.

**diurnal r.,** see diurnal.

**ectopic r.,** any cardiac r. arising from a center other than the normal pacemaker, the sinus node.

**fast r.,** a wave pattern in the electroencephalogram in the frequency bands above 13 cycles per second.

**gallop r.,** gallop (2).

**idiono′dal r.,** an independent ventricular r., the ventricles being under control of the A-V node.

**idioventric′ular r.,** ventricular r.; a slow independent ventricular r. under control of an ectopic ventricular center.

**nodal r.,** A-V nodal r.

**pendulum r.,** embryocardia.

**quadrigem′inal r.,** quadrigeminy; a cardiac dysrhythmia in which the heart beats are grouped in fours, each usually composed of one sinus beat followed by three extrasystoles.

**quadruple r.,** trainwheel r.; a quadruple cadence to the heart sounds due to the easy audibility of both third and fourth heart sounds, indicative of serious myocardial disease.

**reciprocal r.,** echo beat; reciprocal beat; a cardiac dysrhythmia in which the impulse arising in the A-V junction descends to and activates the ventricles and simultaneously ascends toward the atria; before reaching the atria, however, the impulse is reflected downward and again activates the ventricles, the reciprocal beat. Recognized in the electrocardiogram by the presence of an inverted P wave sandwiched between two normal ventricular complexes.

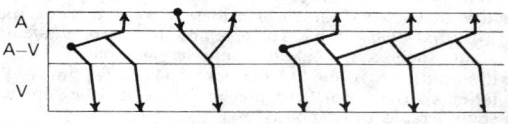

**Reciprocal and Reciprocating Rhythms**
*Left,* reciprocal; *center,* reversed reciprocal; *right,* reciprocating.

**reciprocating r.,** a cardiac dysrhythmia initiated by an A-V nodal beat followed in turn by a reciprocal beat; the descending impulse of the reciprocal beat, before reaching the ventricles, is also reflected backward to the atria, but before reaching the atria is reflected downward again to the ventricles, and so on.

**reversed reciprocal r.,** a normal sinus impulse, before reaching the ventricles is reflected backward to the atria; thus in the electrocardiogram a ventricular complex is sandwiched between a normal sinus P wave and a retrograde P wave; if the dysrhythmia continues, subsequent cycles are similar to those of reciprocating r.

**sinus r.,** normal cardiac r. proceeding from the sinoatrial node.

**theta r.,** theta wave; the frequency band in the electroencephalogram from 4 to 7 cycles per second.

**tic-tac r.,** embryocardia.

**trainwheel r.,** quadruple r.

**trigeminal r.,** trigeminy; a cardiac dysrhythmia in which the heart beats are grouped in trios, usually composed of a sinus beat followed by two extrasystoles.

**triple r.,** a triple cadence to the heart sounds at any rate, due to the easy audibility of a third or fourth heart sound.

**ventricular r.,** idioventricular r.

**rhythmeur** (rēt-mër′ or rith′mur) [ Fr. ]. An apparatus for securing rhythmic interruptions of the electric current in an x-ray machine.

**rhytidectomy** (rit-ĭ-dek′to-mĭ) [ G. *rhytis* (*rhytid-*), a wrinkle ]. The operative removal of wrinkles.

**rhytidoplasty** (rit′ĭ-do-plas′tĭ) [ G. *rhytis,* a wrinkle, + *plassō,* to fashion ]. Surgery for elimination of wrinkles.

**rhytidosis** (rit′ĭ-do′sis) [ G. a wrinkling, fr. *rhytis,* a wrinkle, + suffix *-osis,* condition ]. Rutidosis. 1. Wrinkling of the face to a degree disproportionate to age. 2. Laxity and wrinkling of the cornea, an indication of approaching death.

**Rib.** Symbol for ribose.

**rib-.** See ribo-.

**rib** [ A.S. *ribb* ]. Costa.

**beading of the r.'s,** rachitic *rosary.*

**bicip′ital r.,** fusion of first thoracic r. with cervical vertebra.

**bifid r.,** one in which the body bifurcates.

**cervical r.,** an occasional short r., unattached anteriorly, in the neck above the first r.; see also cervical rib *syndrome.*

**false r.'s,** *costae* spuriae.

**floating r.,** costa fluctuans; vertebral r.; one of the two lower r.'s on either side that are not attached anteriorly.

**lumbar r.,** an occasional r. articulating with the transverse process of the first lumbar vertebra.

**slipping r.,** subluxation of a r. cartilage.

**true r.'s,** *costae* verae.

**vertebral r.,** floating r.

**vertebrochondral r.'s,** *costae* spuriae.

**vertebrosternal r.'s,** *costae* verae.

**α-ribazole(phosphate)** (ri′bă-zōl). The benzimidazole nucleoside (nucleotide) in vitamin B₁₂; α-(5,6-dimethylbenzimidazolyl) ribonucleoside(phosphate).

**Ribbert,** Moritz W. H., German pathologist, 1855–1920. See R.'s *theory.*

**rib′bon** [ M. E. *riban* ]. A ribbon-shaped structure.

**Reil's r.,** *lemniscus* medialis.

**Ribera y Sans,** Jose, Spanish surgeon, 1853–1912. See R.'s *method.*

**Ribes** (rēb), Franc·ois, French physician, 1800–1864. See R.'s *ganglion.*

**ribitol** (ri'bĭ-tol). $CH_2OH(CHOH)_3CH_2OH$; reduction product of ribose (—CHO at position 1 reduced to $CH_2OH$).

**ribityl** (ri'bĭ-til). The radical of ribitol; found in riboflavin.

**ribo-** (ri'bo-). 1. Root of ribose, and thus part of its derivatives, e.g., ribofuranose, ribopyranose. 2. As an italicized prefix to the systematic name of a monosaccharide, *ribo*- indicates that the configuration of a set of three consecutive, but not necessarily contiguous, CHOH (or asymmetric) groups is that of ribose; e.g., D-ribose, a trivial name, is D-*ribo*-pentose in systematic nomenclature.

**riboflavin, riboflavine** (ri'bo-fla'vin). (USP, BP). Lactoflavin; or 7,8-dimethyl-10-(1'-D-ribityl)isoalloxazine; one of the heat-stable factors of the vitamin B complex, vitamin $B_2$ or G. It is part of the structure of the isoalloxazine nucleotides which are coenzymes of the flavodehydrogenases. The daily human requirement is 1 to 2 mg, with higher daily requirement during pregnancy and lactation. Dietary sources include green vegetables, liver, kidneys, wheat germ, milk, eggs, and cheese. Deficiency causes cheilosis, glossitis, keratitis, seborrheic dermatitis, and other symptoms of a still controversial nature. R. is used as replacement therapy in araboflavinosis and general vitamin B complex deficiencies.

Riboflavin

**r. kinase** (EC 2.7.1.26), flavokinase; an enzyme catalyzing the formation of flavin mononucleotide (riboflavin phosphate) from riboflavin, utilizing ATP or ADP as phosphorylating agent.

**meth'ylol r.**, a mixture of methylol derivatives of r. formed by the action of formaldehyde on r. in weakly alkaline solution. It has the same action as r., but is preferred for parenteral administration.

**riboflavin 5'-phosphate.** Flavin mononucleotide.

**ribofuranose** (ri'bo-fūr'ă-nōs). The 1,4 cyclic form of ribose; for structure, see sugars.

**ri'bofuran'osylad'enine.** Adenosine.

**ri'bofuran'osylcy'tosine.** Cytidine.

**ri'bofuran'osylgua'nine.** Guanosine.

**ri'bofuran'osylthy'mine.** Ribothymidine.

**ri'bofuran'osylu'racil.** Uridine.

**ribonuclease** (ri'bo-nu'kle-ās). Transferases or phosphodiesterases that catalyze the hydrolysis of ribonucleic acid.

**r. I** (EC 3.1.4.22), pancreatic r.; alkaline r.; transfers 3'-phosphate of a pyrimidine ribonucleotide residue in a polynucleotide from the 5'-position of the adjoining nucleotide to the 2'-position of the pyrimidine nucleotide itself (a transferase, endonuclease action), forming a pyrimidine 2':3'-cyclic phosphate, then (or independently), hydrolyzes this phosphodiester to leave a pyrimidine nucleoside 3'-phosphate residue (phosphodiesterase action; transfers the phosphate from the 2'-position to water.

**r. II** (EC 3.1.4.23), TAKADIASTASE; plant r.; acid r.; *Escherichia coli* r.; acts similarly to r. I, but adjacent to purine nucleosides as well, thus producing nucleoside cyclic phosphates and then nucleoside 3'-phosphates.

**acid r.,** r. II.

**alkaline r.,** r. I.

**r. B,** r. I in more purified state.

**Escherichia coli r.,** r. II.

**pancreatic r.,** r. I.

**plant r.,** r. II.

**r. T₁,** guanyloribonuclease.

**r. T₂,** r. II.

**ribonucleic acid** (ri'bo-nu-kle'ik). RNA; at various times, but no longer, called phytonucleic (plant) acid, zymonucleic acid, yeast nucleic acid. A macromolecule consisting of ribonucleoside residues connected by phosphate from the 3' hydroxyl of one to the 5' hydroxyl of the next nucleoside. Found in all cells, in both nuclei and cytoplasm, and in particulate and nonparticulate form, also in many viruses. Various RNA fractions are identified by location, form or function as listed below. Polynucleotides made *in vitro* are generally called such, not ribonucleic acids, which are more properly called macromolecules.

**aminoacyl-tRNA,** generic term for those compounds in which amino acids are esterified through their COOH groups to the 3' (or 2') OH's of the terminal adenosine residues of transfer RNA's. The individual compounds are named alanyl-tRNA, glycyl-tRNA, etc., and each involves one or a small number of tRNA's of specific chemical structure (see transfer RNA).

**informational RNA,** messenger RNA.

**messenger RNA,** mRNA; informational RNA; template RNA; conceived to be the RNA reflecting the exact nucleoside sequence of the genetically active DNA and carrying the "message" of the latter coded in its sequence to the cytoplasmic areas where protein is made in amino acid sequences specified by the mRNA, and hence primarily by the DNA. Viral RNA's are considered to be natural messengers.

**nuclear RNA,** nRNA; RNA found in nuclei, or associated with DNA, or with nuclear structures (nucleoli).

**RNA polymerase,** see nucleotidyltransferase.

**ribosomal RNA,** rRNA; the RNA of ribosomes and polyribosomes.

**soluble RNA,** sRNA; now known as transfer RNA (tRNA).

**template RNA,** messenger RNA.

**transfer RNA,** tRNA; formerly soluble RNA (soluble in molar salt); short chain RNA molecules present in cells in at least 20 varieties, each variety capable of combining with a specific amino acid. By joining (through their anticodons) with particular spots (codons) along the messenger RNA molecule and carrying their amino acids along, they serve to form protein molecules with a specific amino acid arrangement—the one ultimately dictated by a segment of DNA in the chromosomes. tRNA's have about 80 nucleotides each, molecular weight about 25,000. The exact primary chemical structures of many are known. Most of the 20 varieties occur in multiple "isoacceptor" forms, separable by chromatography. Further subvarieties exist in different strains of an organism, in subcellular organelles, in different metabolic states, etc.

**ribonucleinase** (ri'bo-nu'kle-ĭ-nās). Ribonuclease.

**ribonucleoprotein** (ri'bo-nu'kle-o-pro'te-in, -pro'tēn). A combination of protein and ribonucleic acid.

**ri'bonu'cleoside.** A nucleoside in which the sugar component is ribose; some common r.'s are adenosine, guanosine, cytidine, uridine.

**ri'bonu'cleotide.** A nucleotide (nucleoside phosphate) in which the sugar component is ribose; the most common r.'s are adenylic acid, guanylic acid; cytidylic acid, and uridylic acid of ribonucleic acids, nicotinamide ribonucleotide of NAD and NADP.

**ri'boprine** (USAN). N-(3-Methyl-2-butenyl)adenosine; an antineoplastic drug.

**ri'bopyr'anose.** The 1,5 cyclic form of ribose (β form shown under riboside).

**D-ribose** (ri'bōs). The pentose present in ribonucleic acid. For structure, see sugars.

**riboside** (ri'bo-sĭd). The product formed by replacement of the H of the C-1 OH of ribose by an alcohol residue (which may be another sugar); differs from ribosyl compounds and does *not* occur in ribonucleic acids (common error), where the radical is a ribosyl (1-OH missing entirely). See structure for methyl β-D-ribofuranoside on p. 1236.

**ri'boso'mal RNA.** See under ribonucleic acid.

**ribosome** (ri'bo-sōm). Palade granule; a granule of ribonucleoprotein, 120 to 150 Å in diameter.

**ribosuria** (ri'bo-su'ri-ah) [ ribose + G. *ouron,* urine ]. The enhanced urinary excretion of D-ribose; commonly one manifestation of muscular dystrophy.

**ribosyl** (ri'bo-sil). The radical formed by loss of the hemiacetal OH group from either of the two cyclic forms of ribose (yielding ribofuranosyl and ribopyranosyl compounds), by combination with an H of —NH— or —CH— groups. The natural nucleosides are ribosyl compounds, not ribosides (see adenosine and *cf.* riboside), as the bond between ribose and aglycon is C—N, not —C—O—X—.

**1-ribosylorotic acid** (ri'bo-sil-o-rot'ik). See orotidine.

**ri'bothy'midine.** 5-Methyluridine; ribosylthymine; the ribosyl analogue of thymidine (deoxyribosylthymine); found in small amounts in ribonucleic acids. Symbols, Thd, T.

**ribotide** (ri'bo-tīd). Double corruption of riboside, by analogy with nucleoside-nucleotide, to mean ribonucleotide.

**ribovirus** (ri'bo-vi'rus). See RNA viruses, under virus.

**ribulose** (ri'bu-lōs). D-*erythro*-2-Pentulose; the 2-keto isomer of ribose (see structures under sugars). As the 5-phosphate, participates in the Dickens shunt. As the 1,5-bisphosphate, it combines with $CO_2$ at the start of the photosynthetic process in green plants (the "carbon dioxide trap").

**ribulosebisphosphate carboxylase** (EC 4.1.1.39). Carboxydismutase; a dimerizing carboxy-lyase; an enzyme that catalyzes the addition of carbon dioxide to ribulose 1,5-bisphosphate and the hydrolysis of the addition product to two molecules of 3-phosphoglyceric acid. This is a key reaction in the fixation of $CO_2$ in photosynthesis.

**ribulosephosphate 3-epimerase** (EC 5.1.3.1). Phosphoribulose epimerase; phosphoketopentoepimerase; an enzyme catalyzing the interconversion of xylulose 5-phosphate and its isomer, ribulose 5-phosphate.

**Ricard,** Alfred Louis, French surgeon, *1858. See R.'s *amputation.*

**Ricco's law.** See under law.

**rice** [ G. *oryza* ]. The grain of *Oryza sativa* (family Gramineae), the rice plant; a food; also used, finely pulverized, as a dusting powder.

**Rich,** Arnold R., U. S. pathologist, *1893. See Hamman-R. *syndrome.*

**Richard** (re-shar'), F. Adolphe, Paris surgeon, 1822–1872. See R.'s *fringe.*

**Richards,** Dickinson W., U. S. physician, *1895. Nobel laureate, 1956, with André F. Cournand and Werner T. O. Forsmann, for their discoveries concerning heart catheterization and pathological changes in the circulatory system.

**Richardson,** J. C., Canadian neurologist. See Steele-R.-Olszewski *syndrome.*

**Richet** (re-sha'), Charles Robert, French physiologist, 1850–1935. Nobel laureate, 1913, for his work on anaphylaxis.

**Richmond,** C. M., American dentist, 1835–1902. See R. *crown.*

**Richter** (rikh'ter), August G., German surgeon, 1742–1812. See R.'s *hernia,* R.-Monro *line,* Monro-R. *line,* R.'s *suture.*

**ricin** (ri'sin, ris'in). A phytotoxic protein occurring in the seeds of the castor oil plant, *Ricinus sanguineus;* it acts as a violent irritant and may be fatal.

**ricinine** (ris'in-ēn). 3-Cyano-4-methoxy-1-methyl-2-oxopyyridine; a toxic principle obtained from the castor oil bean.

**ricinism** (ris'i-nizm). Poisoning with castor oil or its potent ingredient, ricin.

**ricinoleate** (ris'i-no'le-āt). A salt of ricinoleic acid.

Methyl β-ᴅ-ribofuranoside

**sodium r.,** see under sodium.

**ricinoleated** (ris'i-no'le-a'ted). Treated with sodium ricinoleate; referring to a bacterial vaccine detoxicated with this substance.

**ricinoleic acid** (ris'i-no-le'ik, ri'sī-). $C_{18}H_{34}O_3$; an unsaturated hydroxy acid present in castor oil.

**Ricinus** (ris'i-nus) [ L. ]. A genus of plants with one species, *R. communis,* (family Euphorbiaceae), the castor oil plant, the source of castor oil; the leaves are said to be galactagogue.

**rickets** (rik'ets) [ E. *wrick,* to twist ]. Rachitis; a calcium-deficiency disease occurring in infants and young children; it is characterized by softening of the bones, with associated skeletal deformities, enlargement of the liver and spleen, profuse sweating, and general tenderness of the body when touched.

**acute r.,** hemorrhagic r.

**adult r.,** late r.; rachitis tarda; a disease resembling r. in many of its features, occurring in adult life.

**ce'liac r.,** arrested growth, and osseous deformities associated with defective absorption of fat and calcium in celiac disease.

**familial vitamin D-resistant r. with hypophosphatemia,** see vitamin D-resistant r.

**hemorrhagic r.,** acute r.; bone changes seen in infantile scurvy, consisting of subperiosteal hemorrhage and deficient osteoid tissue formation.

**late r.,** adult r.

**renal r.,** renal fibrocystic osteosis; renal osteitis fibrosa; renal infantilism; pseudorickets; a form of r. occurring in children in association with and apparently caused by renal disease with hyperphosphatemia.

**scurvy r.,** infantile scurvy.

**vitamin D-resistant r.,** a heritable form of r., characterized by hypophosphatemia due to defective renal tubular reabsorption of phosphate and subnormal absorption of dietary calcium; not responsive to standard therapeutic doses of vitamin D, but does respond to very large doses of phosphate and of vitamin D.

**Ricketts,** Howard T., american pathologist, 1871–1910. Gave his name to *Rickettsia.*

**Rickettsia** (ri-ket'si-ah) [ H. T. *Ricketts* ]. A genus of bacteria (order Rickettsiales) containing small (nonfilterable), often pleomorphic coccoid to rod-shaped, Gram-negative organisms which usually occur intracytoplasmically in lice, fleas, ticks, and mites. They do not grow in cell-free media. Pathogenic species are parasitic on man and other animals. They cause epidemic typhus, murine or endemic typhus, Rocky Mountain spotted fever, tsutsugamushi disease, rickettsial pox, and other diseases. The type species is *R. prowazekii.*

**R. ak'ari,** a species that causes human rickettsial pox (vesicular rickettsiosis); transmitted by a mite that infests mice.

**R. austral'is,** a species causing a spotted fever, in which the patient's serum contains a different antibody from that reacting with *R. rickettsii, R. prowazekii,* and others; the disease is presumed (but not known) to be transmitted by a tick.

**R. burnet'ii,** *Coxiella burnetti.*

**R. conor'ii,** a species causing boutonneuse fever in man (also known as eruptive Mediterranean or Marseilles fever and probably Indian tick typhus, Kenya typhus, and perhaps as South African tick bite fever); transmitted by ticks.

**R. prowazek'ii,** a species causing epidemic typhus fever; transmitted by the body louse.

**R. psitta'ci,** *Chlamydia psittaci.*

**R. quinta'na,** *R. wolhynica;* a species causing trench fever (Wolhynian fever, shin bone fever, 5-day fever); transmitted by the human body louse.

**R. ricketts'ii,** a species causing Rocky Mountain spotted fever, São Paulo exanthematic typhus of Brazil, Tobia fever of Colombia, and spotted fevers of Minas Gerais and Mexico; transmitted by infected ticks.

**R. tsutsugamushi,** a species causing tsutsugamuchi disease and scrub typhus; transmitted by trombiculid mites.

**R. typhi,** a species causing murine or endemic typhus fever; it is transmitted by the rat flea.

R. **wolhynica,** *R. quintana.*

**rickettsial** (rĭ-ket′sĭ-al). Pertaining to or caused by rickettsiae.

**rickettsiosis** (rĭ-ket′sĭ-o′sis). Infection with rickettsiae.

**rickettsiostatic** (rĭ-ket′sĭ-o-stat′ik) [ *Rickettsia* + G. *statikos,* bringing to a standstill ]. An agent inhibitory to the growth of *Rickettsia.*

**rick′ety.** Rachitic; suffering from rickets.

**Rideal** (rid′el), Samuel, English chemist and bacteriologist, 1863–1929. See R.-Walker *coefficient, method.*

**Ridell's operation.** See under operation.

**ridge** (rij) [ A. S. *hyrcg,* back, spine ]. 1. A (usually rough) linear elevation; see also crest, and crista. 2. In dentistry, any linear elevation on the surface of a tooth. 3. The remainder of the alveolar process and its soft tissue covering after the teeth are removed.

**alveolar r.,** *processus alveolaris.*

**apical ectodermal r.,** the layer of surface ectodermal cells at the apex of the embryonic limb bud; they are considered to exert an inductive influence on the condensation of underlying mesenchyme.

**basal r.,** (1) *processus* alveolaris; (2) cingulum (3).

**bicip′ital r.'s,** *crista* tuberculi majoris and minoris.

**buccocervical r.,** a convexity within the cervical third of the buccal surface of molars.

**buccogin′gival r.,** a distinct r. on the buccal surface of a deciduous molar tooth, close to the gingival margin.

**bulbar r.,** a spiral subendocardial thickening in the embryonic bulbus cordis; when fused with its partner it divides the bulbus into the aorta and pulmonary artery.

**bulboventricular r.,** an elevation on the inner surface of the 4- to 5-week-old embryonic heart; it indicates the division between the developing ventricles and the bulbus cordis.

**center of r.,** the buccolingual midline of the residual r.

**crest of r.,** the highest continuous surface of the r., but not necessarily the center of the r.; the top of a residual or alveolar r.

**dental r.,** the prominent border of a cusp or margin of a tooth.

**dermal r.'s,** *cristae* cutis.

**epicon′dylar r.,** supracondylar r.; the distal portion of the medial and lateral margins of the humerus.

**epipericardial r.,** an elevation separating the developing pharyngeal region from the embryonic pericardium.

**external oblique r.,** a horizontal bony crest on the external surface of the mandibular corpus, inferior to the alveolar bone, marking the site of attachment of the buccinator muscle.

**ganglion r.,** neural *crest.*

**genital r.,** gonadial r.

**gluteal r.,** *tuberositas* glutea.

**gonadial r.,** genital r.; an elevation of thickened mesothelium and underlying mesenchyme on the ventromedial border of the embryonic mesonephros. The primordial germ cells become embedded in it, establishing it as the primordium of the testis or ovary.

**interpapillary r.'s,** rete r.'s.

**linguocer′vical r.,** linguogingival r.

**linguogin′gival r.,** linguocervical r.; a r. occurring on the lingual surface, near the gum, of the incisor and cuspid teeth.

**lower r. slope,** the slope of the mandibular residual r. in the second and third molar as seen from the buccal side.

**Mall's r.'s,** pulmonary r.'s.

**mammary r.,** mammary fold; milk r.; milk line; a bandlike thickening of ectoderm in the embryo extending on either side from just below the axilla to the inguinal region. In human embryos the mammary glands arise from primordia in the thoracic part of the r., the balance of the r. disappearing. In the lower mammals which give birth to a litter of young, several milk glands develop along these lines.

**marginal r.,** *crista* marginalis.

**mesoneph′ric r.,** urogenital r.

**milk r.,** mammary r.

**mylohy′oid r.,** *linea* mylohyoidea.

**r. of nose,** *agger* nasi.

**oblique r.,** a r. on the masticatory surface of an upper molar tooth from the mesiolingual to the distobuccal cusp.

**oblique r. of trapezium,** *tuberculum* ossis trapezii.

**palatine r.,** *raphe* palati.

**Passavant's r.,** Passavant's *cushion.*

**pec′toral r.,** *crista* tuberculi majoris.

**primitive r.,** one of the paired r.'s on either side of the primitive groove.

**prona′tor r.,** an oblique r. on the anterior surface of the ulna, giving attachment to the pronator quadratus muscle.

**pter′ygoid r.,** *crista* infratemporalis.

**pulmonary r.'s,** Mall's r.'s; a pair of r.'s overlying the common cardinal veins and bulging from the lateral body wall into the embryonic celom; so called because they give early indication of where the pleuroperitoneal folds will develop.

**residual r.,** that portion of the processus alveolaris remaining in the edentulous mouth following resorption of the section containing the alveoli.

**rete r.'s,** rete pegs; interpapillary r.'s; downward thickenings of the epidermis between the dermal papillae; peg is a misnomer because the dermal papillae are cylindrical but the epidermal thickening between papillae is not.

**skin r.'s,** *cristae* cutis.

**supercil′iary r.,** *arcus* superciliaris.

**supplemental r.,** a r. on the surface of a tooth that is not normally present.

**supracon′dylar r.,** epicondylar r.

**supraor′bital r.,** *margo* supraorbitalis.

**taste r.,** one of the r.'s surrounding the vallate papillae of the tongue.

**temporal r.,** *linea* temporalis.

**transverse r.,** *crista* transversalis.

**transverse palatine r.,** *plica* palatina transversa.

**trap′ezoid r.,** *linea* trapezoidea.

**triangular r.,** *crista* triangularis.

**urogenital r.,** genital fold; mesonephric r. or fold; Wolffian r.; one of the paired longitudinal r.'s developing in the dorsal body-wall of the embryo on either side of the dorsal mesentery. The r. is formed at first by the growing mesonephros and later by the mesonephros and the gonad.

**Wolffian r.,** urogenital r.

**ridgling** (rij′ling) [ Dial. ]. A male horse in which one or both testes have failed to descend into the scrotum; a cryptorchid.

**Ridley,** Humphrey, English anatomist, 1653–1708. See *circulus* venosus ridleyi, R.'s *circle, sinus.*

**Riedel** (re′del), Bernhard M. C. L., German surgeon, 1846–1916. See R.'s *disease, lobe, struma.*

**Rieder** (re′der), Hermann, German pathologist, 1858–1932. See R.'s *cells, lymphocyte.*

**Riegel** (re′gel), Franz, German physician, 1843–1904. See R.'s *pulse, test.*

**Rieger,** H., German ophthalmologist. See R.'s *anomaly, syndrome.*

**Riehl** (reel), Gustav, Austrian dermatologist, 1855–1943. See R.'s *melanosis.*

**rif′ampin** (USP). RIMACTANE; 3-(4-methylpiperazinyliminomethyl) rifamycin SV; an antibacterial agent.

**rifamycin** (rif′ă-mi′sin). Rifomycin; a complex antibiotic, isolated from the fermentation broth of *Streptomyces mediterranei,* that is active against *Mycobacterium tuberculosis* and *Staphylococcus aureus.* It is poorly absorbed from the gastrointestinal tract, and often causes irritation and severe pain at the sites of injection.

**Riga** (re′gah), Antonio, Italian physician, 1832–1919. See R.'s *disease.*

**Riggs,** John M., American dentist, 1810–1885. See R.'s *disease.*

**right-eyed.** Seeing more distinctly with the right eye, or using that eye instinctively, as when sighting a gun.

**right-handed.** Using the right hand for writing and most manual operations habitually or with greater ease than the left.

**rigidity** (rĭ-jid′ĭ-tĭ) [ L. *rigidus,* rigid, inflexible ]. 1. Rigor (1). 2. In psychiatry and clinical psychology, an aspect of personality characterized by an individual's resistance to change.

**anatomic r.,** r. of the cervix uteri in labor, not due to any pathologic infiltration.

**cadav'eric r.,** *rigor* mortis.

**catatonic r.,** tonic *pupil.*

**cerebellar r.,** increased tone of the extensor muscles, related to injury of the vermis of the cerebellum.

**clasp-knife r.,** clasp-knife *spasticity.*

**cogwheel r.,** a type of r. seen as part of Parkinson's disease in which, upon applying force to bend the limb, the muscles yield jerkily giving a feeling to the examiner as of cogwheels moving upon one another.

**decer'ebrate r.,** rigid contraction of the extensor and other muscles which maintain an animal in the standing position (antigravity muscles) following transection of the brain anywhere below the anterior corpora quadrigemina but above the vestibular nuclei.

**lead-pipe r.,** the plastic type of r. resembling that offered by a bar or pipe of lead seen in certain forms of parkinsonism.

**mydriat'ic r.,** tonic *pupil.*

**pathologic r.,** r. of the cervix uteri in labor, due to fibrosis, scarring, cancer, or other condition.

**postmortem r.,** *rigor* mortis.

**rigor** (rig'or) [ L. stiffness ]. 1. Rigidity (1). 2. A chill.

**acid r.,** coagulation of muscle protein induced by acids.

**calcium r.,** arrest of the heart in the fully contracted state as a result of poisoning with calcium.

**heat r.,** coagulation of muscle protein induced by heat.

**r. mortis** [ L. *mors* (gen. *mortis*), death ], stiffening of the body, from 1 to 7 hours after death, from hardening of the muscular tissues in consequence of the coagulation of the myosinogen and paramyosinogen; it disappears after from 1 to 5 or 6 days, or when decomposition begins.

**r. nervo'rum,** tetanus.

**r. tre'mens,** *paralysis* agitans.

**Riley,** Henry A., American physician, \*1887. See R.-Day *syndrome.*

**rim.** A margin, border, or edge, usually circular in form.

**bite r.,** occlusion r.

**occlusal r.,** occlusion r.

**occlusion r.,** bite block; bite r. occlusal r.; record r.; occluding surfaces built on temporary or permanent denture bases for the purpose of making maxillomandibular relation records and for arranging teeth.

**record r.,** occlusion r.

**rima,** gen. and pl. **rimae** (ri'mah, ri'me) [ L. a slit ] [ NA ]. A slit or fissure, or narrow elongated opening between two symmetrical parts.

**r. cornea'lis,** corneal cleft; a groove in the sclera into which the edge of the cornea fits.

**r. glot'tidis** [ NA ], glottis vera; true glottis; the interval between the true vocal cords.

**r. o'ris** [ NA ]. the mouth slit; the aperture of the mouth.

**r. palpebra'rum** [ NA ], the lid slit, or fissure between the eye lids.

**r. puden'di** [ NA ], r. vulvae; pudendal or vulvar slit; urogenital cleft; pudendal cleavage; the cleft between the labia majora.

**r. respirato'ria,** r. vestibuli.

**r. vestib'uli** [ NA ], glottis spuria; false glottis; the interval between the false vocal cords or ventricular folds.

**r. voca'lis,** r. glottidis.

**r. vulvae,** r. pudendi.

**Rimini's test.** See under test.

**rimose** (ri'mōs) [ L. *rimosus,* fr. *rima,* a fissure ]. Fissured; marked by cracks in all directions, like the crackle of porcelain.

**rimula** (rim'u-lah) [ L. dim. of *rima* ]. A minute slit or fissure.

**rinderpest** (rin'der-pest) [ Ger. *rinder,* cattle ]. Cattle plague; an acute, contagious, highly destructive disease of cattle caused by a virus and characterized by severe necrotizing inflammation of the alimentary canal and severe diarrhea. The death rate among western cattle ordinarily is greater than 90 per cent.

**Rindfleisch** (rint'flish), Georg E., German physician, 1836–1908. See R.'s *cells, folds.*

**ring** [ A.S. *hring* ]. 1. A circular band surrounding a wide central opening. 2. In anatomy, anulus; any approximately circular structure surrounding an opening or a level area. 3. The closed (*i.e.,* endless) chain of atoms in a cyclic compound; commonly used for "cyclic" or "cycle." 4.

Marginal growth on the upper surface of a broth culture of bacteria, adhering to the sides of the test tube in the form of a r.

**abdominal r.,** *anulus* inguinalis profundus.

**Albl's r.,** dark r. seen in radiogram of skull due to calcification of aneurysmal sac of cerebral artery.

**amnion r.,** the r. formed by the attachment of the amnion to the umbilical cord at its point of emergence from the umbilicus.

**annular r.'s,** pleural r.'s; an opaque area on x-ray of lung, indicating cavity of tuberculosis.

**anterior limiting r.,** Schwalbe's r. (1); the periphery of the cornea thickened by a bundle of circular connective and elastic fibers, in front of or in the termination of the lamina limitans posterior corneae, to which the ligamentum pectinatum anguli iridocornealis is attached; a white translucent, refractile r., an important landmark in gonioscopy.

**Bandl's r.,** pathologic retraction r.

**benzene r.,** see under benzene.

**Bickel's r.,** lymphoid r.

**Cannon's r.,** a tonically contracted muscular band in the transverse colon close to the hepatic flexure.

**carbocy'clic r.,** see carbocyclic *compound.*

**casting r.,** refractory *flask.*

**cil'iary r.,** *orbiculus* ciliaris.

**conjuncti'val r.,** *anulus* conjunctivae.

**constriction r.,** true spastic stricture of the uterine cavity resulting when a zone of muscle goes into local tetanic contraction and forms a tight constriction about some part of the fetus.

**crural r.,** *anulus* femoralis.

**deep inguinal r.,** *anulus* inguinalis profundus.

**Döllinger's tendinous r.,** a thickening of Descemet's membrane, forming an elastic r. around the circumference of the cornea.

**Donders' r.'s,** the colored r.'s seen in glaucoma.

**external inguinal r.,** *anulus* inguinalis superficialis.

**femoral r.,** *anulus* femoralis.

**Fleischer's r.,** an incomplete ring often present at the base of the keratoconus cone; it may be yellow or greenish from deposition of hemosiderin.

**Flieringa's r.,** a stainless steel r. sutured around the cornea; used to prevent collapse of globe in hazardous intraocular operations.

**glauco'matous r.,** glaucomatous *halo.*

**Graefenberg r.,** a silver or silkworm gut r. designed for insertion into the uterine cavity as a means of contraception.

**heterocy'clic r.,** see heterocyclic *compound.*

**homocyclic r.,** see isocyclic *compound.*

**Imlach's r.,** that part of the inguinal canal which lodges the round ligament of the uterus.

**r. of iris,** *anulus* iridis.

**isocy'clic r.,** see isocyclic *compound.*

**Kayser-Fleischer r.,** a greenish yellow pigmented r. encircling the cornea just within the corneoscleral margin, seen in Wilson's syndrome.

**Liesegang r.'s,** colored r.'s of precipitated silver chromate formed when a drop of concentrated silver nitrate is added to the surface of a gel (such as gelatin, agar, or silica gel) containing potassium dichromate.

**Löwe's r.,** Maxwell's *spot.*

**Lower's r.,** *anulus* fibrosus (1).

**lym'phoid r.,** tonsillar r.; Waldeyer's throat r.; Bickel's r.; the broken r. of lymphoid tissue, formed of the lingual, faucial, and pharyngeal tonsils.

**Maxwell's r.,** Maxwell's *spot.*

**pathologic retraction r.,** Bandl's r.; a constriction located at the junction of the thinned lower uterine segment with the thick retracted upper uterine segment, resulting from obstructed labor; this is one of the classic signs of threatened rupture of the uterus.

**physiologic retraction r.,** a ridge on the inner uterine surface at the boundary line between the upper and lower uterine segment that occurs in the course of normal labor.

**pleural r.'s,** annular r.'s.

**polar r.,** an osmiophilic thickening formed by the inner membranous layer of the pellicle of sporozoan protozoa in their sporozoite and merozoite stages; one polar r. is present in most genera; there are two in *Isospora* and a few similar genera, and three in *Plasmodium* merozoites.

**posterior limiting r.,** Schwalbe's r. (2); a circular bundle of the sclera at the level of the termination of the deep trabeculae (trabecular zone).

**Schwalbe's r.'s,** (1) anterior limiting r.; (2) posterior limiting r.

**signet r.,** the early stage of trophozoite development of the malaria parasite in the red blood cell; the parasite cytoplasm stains blue around its circular margin, and the nucleus stains red in Romanovsky stains, while the central vacuole is clear, giving the ringlike appearance.

**subcutaneous r.,** *anulus* inguinalis superficialis.

**superficial inguinal r.,** *anulus* inguinalis superficialis.

**tonsillar r.,** lymphoid r.

**tra'cheal r.,** *cartilago* trachealis.

**tympanic r.,** *anulus* tympanicus.

**umbilical r.,** *anulus* umbilicalis.

**vascular r.,** anomalous arteries congenitally encircling the trachea and esophagus, at times producing pressure symptoms.

**Vieussens' r.,** *limbus* fossae ovalis.

**Vossius' lenticular r.,** a ring-shaped opacity found on the anterior lens capsule after contusion of the eye; due to pigment and blood.

**Waldeyer's throat r.,** lymphoid r.

**Zinn's r.,** *anulus* tendineus communis.

**ring'bone.** A term applied to exostoses involving either the first or second phalanx of the horse. Sometimes they are differentiated into high and low r. The condition is usually found in the fore leg. Lameness may or may not result.

**false r.,** an exostosis on the middle or upper part of the long pastern bone in the horse.

**Ringer,** Sidney, English physiologist, 1835–1910. See R.'s *injection,* lactated R.'s *injection,* R.'s *solution,* lactated R.'s *solution,* Krebs-R. *solution,* Locke-R. *solution.*

**ring-knife.** Spoke-shave; a circular or oval ring of steel with internal cutting edge, on the model of the carpenter's spoke-shave, used for shaving off tumors in the nasal and other cavities.

**ring'worm.** Tinea.

**r. of the beard,** *tinea* sycosis.

**black-dot r.,** tinea capitis due to *Trichophyton.*

**r. of the body,** *tinea* circinata.

**Bowditch Island r.,** *tinea* imbricata.

**Burmese r.,** *tinea* imbricata.

**Chinese r.,** *tinea* imbricata.

**crusted r.,** favus.

**r. of the foot,** *tinea* pedis.

**r. of the genitocru'ral region,** *tinea* cruris.

**honeycomb r.,** favus.

**hypertroph'ic r.,** *granuloma* trichophyticum.

**India r.,** *tinea* imbricata.

**r. of the nails,** onychomycosis.

**Oriental r.,** *tinea* imbricata.

**r. of the scalp,** *tinea* tonsurans.

**scaly r.,** *tinea* imbricata.

**Tokelau r.,** *tinea* imbricata.

**Rinne** (rin'neh), Heinrich A., German otologist, 1819–1868. See R.'s *test.*

**Riolan** (re-o-lahn'), Jean, French anatomist and botanist, 1577–1657. See R.'s *anastomosis, arcade, bones, bouquet, muscle.*

**ripa'rian.** Relating to a ripa; marginal.

**Ripault** (re-po'), Louis H. A., French physician, 1807–1856. See R.'s *sign.*

**Risley,** Samuel D., Philadelphia ophthalmologist, 1845–1920. See R.'s rotary *prism.*

**risorius** (rĭ-so'rĭ-us) [ L. *risor,* a laughter, fr. *rideo,* pp. *risus,* to laugh ]. See under musculus.

**ristocetin** (ris'to-se'tin). SPONTIN; an antibiotic produced by the fermentation of *Nocardia lurida.* The antibiotic is made up of two substances: r. A and r. B. Useful against staphylococcic and enterococcic infections refractory to other antibiotics. A number of serious side effects have been reported.

**ri'sus** [ L. ]. A laugh.

**r. cani'nus, r. sardon'icus,** the semblance of a grin caused by facial spasm, especially in tetanus. Also called canine or cynic spasm; sardonic grin; trismus sardonicus.

**Ritgen,** Ferdinand August Marie Franz von, German obstetrician, 1787–1867. See R.'s *maneuver.*

**ritodrine** (USAN). PREMAR; *erythro-p-*hydroxy-α-{ 1-[ (p-hydroxyphenethyl)amino ]ethyl ]benzyl alcohol; a smooth muscle relaxant.

**Ritter,** Gottfried R. von Rittershain, German physician, 1820–1883. See R.'s *disease.*

**Ritter,** Johann W., German physicist, 1776–1810. See R.'s *law,* R.-Rollett *phenomenon,* R.'s opening *tetanus.*

**ritual** (rich'u-al) [ L. *ritualis,* fr. *ritus,* rite ]. In psychiatry and psychology, any psychomotor activity sustained by an individual to relieve anxiety or forestall its development; typically seen in obsessive-compulsive neurosis.

**rivalry** (ri'val-ri) [ L. *rivalis,* competitor, rival ]. Competition between two or more individuals for the same object or goal.

**binocular r.,** alteration of perception of portions of the visual field when the two eyes are simultaneously and rapidly exposed to targets containing dissimilar colors or borders.

**sibling r.,** jealous competition among children, especially for the attention, affection, and esteem of their parents; by extension, sibling r. is a factor in both normal and abnormal competitiveness throughout life.

**Rivea corymbosa.** Mexican morning glory; heavenly blue; flower of the virgin; Mexican bindweed; ololiuqui; a plant of the family Convulvulaceae. The seeds were used in ceremonies by Aztec Indians in Mexico; they contain lysergic acid amide, isolysergic acid, lysergic acid monoethylamide, chanoclavine and other indole alkaloids. Several hundred seeds must be ingested to produce hallucinatory and euphoric effects.

**Riverius.** See Rivière.

**Rivers,** William H., English physician, 1864–1922. See R.'s *cocktail.*

**Rivière** (re-ve-air'), Lazare (Riverius, Lazarus), French physician, 1589–1655. See R.'s *salt.*

**Rivinus** (re-ve'noos), August Q. (R. is the Latin form of Bachmann), German anatomist, 1652–1723. See R.'s *canals, ducts, foramen, glands, incisure, membrane, notch.*

**ri'vus lacrima'lis** [ L. *rivus,* stream, + Mediev. L. *lacrimalis,* fr. L. *lacrima,* a tear ] [ NA ]. Ferrein's canal; a space between the closed lids and the eyeball through which the tears flow to the punctum lacrimale.

**riz'iform** [ Fr. *riz,* rice ]. Resembling rice grains.

**Rn.** Chemical symbol of the element radon.

**R.N.** Abbreviation for registered nurse.

**RNA.** Abbreviation for ribonucleic acid; for terms bearing this abbreviation, see subentries under ribonucleic acid.

**RNase.** Abbreviation for ribonuclease.

**RNP.** Abbreviation for ribonucleoprotein.

**Roach,** F. Ewing, Chicago dentist. See R. *clasp.*

**roach** (rōch) [ Dial. ]. To clip the mane of a horse short, so the hairs stand erect in an arc from withers to poll.

**roarer** (rōr'er). A horse suffering from roaring.

**roaring** (rōr'ing). A loud, rough, whistling or roaring sound emitted upon inspiration during active exercise by a horse that is suffering from laryngeal hemiplegia. It is caused by unilateral or bilateral paralysis of certain laryngeal muscles due to injury of the recurrent laryngeal nerve.

**Robbins,** Frederick C., U. S. pediatrician, *1916. Nobel laureate, 1954, with John F. Enders and Thomas H. Weller, for their discovery of the ability of poliomyelitis viruses to grow in cultures of various types of tissue.

**Robert,** Heinrich, L. F., German gynecologist, 1814–1878. See R.'s *pelvis.*

**Robertson,** Douglas Argyll, Scottish ophthalmologist, 1837–1909. See R. (or Argyll Robertson) *pupil, symptom.*

**Robin** (rō-baň'), Charles P., Paris physician, 1821–1885. See R.'s *myeloplaxes,* Virchow-R. *space.*

**Robin,** Pierre, French pediatrician. See Pierre Robin *syndrome.*

**Robinson,** Andrew R., New York dermatologist, 1845–1924. See R.'s *disease.*

**Robinson,** Robert A., American orthopaedic surgeon, *1914. See Smith-R. *operation.*

**Robinson-Kepler-Power test.** See under test.
**Robison,** Robert, British chemist, 1884–1941. See R. *ester,* R.-Embden *ester,* R. ester *dehydrogenase.*
**Robles,** Rudolfo. See R.'s *disease.*
**rob′orant** [ L. *roboro,* to strengthen, fr. *robur* (*robor-*), oak tree, strength ]. 1. Tonic; strength-giving. 2. A strengthening agent; a tonic.
**Robson.** See Mayo-Robson.
**roccellin** (rok′sel-in). Archil.
**Rocher** (rush-a′), Henri G. L., Bordeaux surgeon, *1876. See R.'s *sign.*
**rock oil.** Petroleum.
**rod** [ A.S. *rōd* ]. 1. A straight slender cylindrical formation. 2. The photosensitive, outward-directed process of a rhodopsin-containing rod cell in the external granular layer of the retina; many millions of such rods, together with the cones, form the photoreceptive layer of rods and cones; see fig. under retina.
  **analyzing r.,** a device used with a surveyor to determine the relative positions of parallel surfaces and undercuts when designing removable partial dentures.
  **basal r.,** costa (2).
  **Corti's r.'s,** pillar *cells.*
  **enamel r.'s,** *prismata* adamantina.
  **germinal r.,** sporozoite.
  **Maddox's r.,** a glass r., or series of parallel glass r.'s, set in the center of an opaque disk; when held in front of one eye it converts the image of a light source into a streak of light perpendicular to the axis of the rod; the position of this streak in relation to the image of the light source seen by the other eye indicates the presence and degree of heterophoria.
**Rodentia** (ro-den′shĭ-ah) [ Mod. L. fr. L. *rodo,* pres. p. *rodens,* to gnaw ]. The rodents; the largest order of placental mammals; included in this order are the mouse, rat, squirrel, beaver, and many more. They all possess chisel-like incisors for gnawing and flat-crowned premolars and molars for grinding. The rodents are ground-dwellers, for the most part, and are found in all parts of the world.
**rodenticide** (ro-den′tĭ-sīd) [ rodent + L. *caedo,* to kill ]. An agent lethal to rodents.
**rodonalgia** (ro-don-al′jĭ-ah) [ G. *rhodon,* rose, + *algos,* pain ]. Erythromelalgia.
**Roederer** (rĕ′der-er), Johann G., German obstetrician, 1727–1763. See R.'s *ecchymoses.*
**Roenne** (rĕn′eh), Henning K. T., Danish ophthalmologist, 1878–1947. See R.'s nasal *step.*
**Roentgen** (rĕnt′gen), Wilhelm K., German physicist, 1845–1923. Gave his name to roentgen. See R. *rays.*
**roentgen** (rent′gen, -jen, rĕnt′gen) [ W. K. *Roentgen* ]. Abbreviated r or R; the international unit of x- or gamma-radiation. From the Second International Congress of Radiology: "The roentgen shall be the quantity of x- or gamma-radiation such that the associated corpuscular emission per 0.001293 gm. of air produces, in air, ions carrying 1 electrostatic unit (e.s.u.) of quantity of electricity of either sign."
  **r.-equivalent-man,** unit of dose equal to that quantity of ionizing radiation of any type that produces in man the same biologic effect as one r. of x-rays or gamma rays. It is equal to the absorbed dose, measured in rads, multiplied by the relative biologic effectiveness of the radiation in question. Abbreviated rem.
  **r.-equivalent-physical,** rep; that quantity of ionizing radiation of any kind which, upon absorption by living tissue, produces an energy gain per gram of tissue equivalent to that produced by 1 r. of x-rays or gamma-rays.
**roent′gencinematog′raphy.** Roentgenocinematography.
**roentgenism** (rent′gĕ-nizm). 1. The use of roentgen rays in the diagnosis and treatment of disease. 2. Any untoward effects of roentgen rays on the tissues.
**roentgenization** (rent′gen-ī-za′shun). Roentgenism (1).
**roentgenkymogram** (rent′gen-ki′mo-gram). A record of the heart's movements taken with the roentgenkymograph.
**roentgenkymograph** (rent′gen-ki′mo-graf). An x-ray apparatus for recording the movements of the heart and great

vessels on a single film. It consists essentially of a large lead sheet, called the grid, in which narrow horizontal slits, 0.4 mm. wide, are cut at 12-mm. intervals.
**roentgenkymography** (rent′gen-ki-mog′rä-fĭ). Recording the movements of the heart by means of the roentgenkymograph.
**roentgenocinematography** (rent′gen-o-sin′e-mă-tog′rä-fĭ). Roentgenography of movements of the internal organs.
**roentgenogram** (rent′gen-o-gram). The shadow picture made on a sensitized film or plate by roentgen rays; radiogram.
  **cephalometric r.,** cephalogram; a roentgenographic view of the jaws and skull, for taking measurements.
  **lateral oblique r.,** oblique lateral jaw r.; a roentgenographic view of the mandible, unilaterally revealing the mandible from symphysis to condyle.
  **lateral ramus r.,** a roentgenographic view of the mandibular ramus and condyle.
  **lateral skull r.,** a roentgenographic view of the sinuses and lateral aspects of the skeletal structures of the cranium.
  **maxillary sinus r.,** Waters' view r.; a roentgenographic view of the maxillary sinuses and the zygomas; enables direct comparison of the sides.
  **oblique lateral jaw r.,** lateral oblique r.
  **panoramic r.,** a roentgenographic view of the maxilla and mandible extending from the left to the right glenoid fossae.
  **periapical r.,** a roentgenographic view of one or several teeth and adjacent bony structures.
  **submental vertex r.,** a roentgenographic view used to visualize lateral movements of the condyle, lateral displacement of the condyle or coronoid process, or both, and the contour of the zygomatic arches.
  **Towne projection r.,** a roentgenographic view of the mandibular condyles and the midfacial skeleton.
  **transcranial r.,** a roentgenographic view of the temporomandibular articulation.
  **Waters' view r.,** maxillary sinus r.
**roentgenograph** (rent′gen-o-graf). To make a roentgenogram.
**roentgenography** (rent′gen-og′rä-fĭ). Examination of any part of the body for diagnostic purposes by means of roentgen rays, the record of the findings being impressed upon a photographic plate; radiography.
  **mucosal relief r.,** after a barium enema has been evacuated and a small quantity of air has been injected into rectum, x-ray shows fine detail of mucosa.
  **sectional r.,** tomography.
  **serial r.,** several x-ray exposures, over a period of time, of a region under study.
  **spot-film r.,** an x-ray of a localized region under study by fluoroscopy.
**roentgenologist** (rent′gen-ol′o-jist). One skilled in the diagnostic or therapeutic application of roentgen rays.
**roentgenology** (rent′gen-ol′o-jĭ). The study of the roentgen rays in all their applications.
**roentgenometer** (rent′gen-om′e-ter). Radiometer.
**roentgenometry** (rent-gen-om′e-trĭ). Measurement of the roentgenotherapeutic dosage and of the penetrating power of x-rays; x-ray dosimetry.
**roentgenoscope** (rent′gen-o-scōp). An apparatus for examination by means of the shadow picture produced by roentgen rays on a fluorescent screen; fluoroscope.
**roentgenoscopy** (rent-gen-os′ko-pĭ). Examination of any part of the body for diagnostic purposes by means of roentgen rays projected upon a fluorescent screen; fluoroscopy.
**roentgenotherapy** (rent′gen-o-thĕr-ă-pĭ). The treatment of disease by means of roentgen rays.
**roetheln, röteln** (rĕ-teln) [ see röteln ]. Rubella.
**Roger** (rō-zha′), Georges Henri, French physiologist, 1860–1946. See R.'s *reflex.*
**Roger** (rō-zha′), Henri L., Paris physician, 1809–1891. See *bruit* de R., R.'s *disease, maladie* de R., R.'s *murmur.*
**Roger-Anderson appliance.** See under appliance.
**Rogers,** Oscar H., New York physician, *1857. See R.'s *sphygmomanometer.*
**Rohr,** Karl, German anatomist, *1863. See R.'s *stria.*
**Röhrer's index.** See under index.

**Rokitan'sky,** Carl F. von, Austrian pathologist, 1804–1878. See R.'s *disease, diverticulum, hernia, kidney, pelvis,* R.-Aschoff *sinus,* R.'s *tumor.*

**Rolan'dic.** Relating to or described by Luigi Rolando.

**Rolan'do,** Luigi, Italian anatomist, 1773–1831. See R.'s *angle, area, cells, column, fissure,* gelatinous *substance, tubercle.*

**role** (rōl) [ Fr. ]. The pattern of behavior that a person exhibits in relationship to significant persons in his life; it has its roots in childhood and is influenced by significant people with whom the person had primary relationships.

    **complementary r.,** one in which the behavior pattern conforms with the expectations and demands of other people.

    **gender r.,** the sex of a child assigned by a parent; when it is opposite to the child's anatomical sex, *e.g.,* due to genital ambiguity at birth or to the parents' strong wish for a child of the opposite sex, the basis is set for postpubertal dysfunctions such as transsexualism.

    **noncomplementary r.,** one that does not conform with the expectations and demands of other people.

    **sick r.,** in sociology, a term designating that the individual is regarded, by himself or others, as a patient; the sick role may be assumed voluntarily or it may be imposed on a person against his will.

**role-playing.** A psychotherapeutic method used in psychodrama to understand and treat emotional conflicts through the enactment of stressful interpersonal events; see also role *conflict.*

**rolicyprine** (ro'lĭ-si'prēn) (USAN). CYPROMIN; 5-oxo-*N*-(D-*trans*- 2-phenylcyclopropyl) -L-2-pyrrolidinecarboxamide; antidepressant.

**rolitetracycline** (ro'lĭ-tet'ră-si'klēn) (NF). SYNTETRIN; VELACYCLINE; *N*-(pyrrolidinomethyl)-tetracycline; a more soluble and less irritating derivative of tetracycline. Uses and effectiveness are similar to those of tetracycline. It may be administered intravenously or intramuscularly, which makes it useful when oral administration of a tetracycline is impossible or impracticable.

**roll** (rōl). A mass or structure in the shape of a roll.

    **iliac r.,** sigmoid sausage; a sausage-shaped, often painful, nonfluctuating mass, with convexity to the right, palpable in the left iliac fossa, due to induration of the walls of the sigmoid flexure.

    **sausage-shaped r.,** iliac r.

    **scleral r.,** scleral *spur.*

**Roller,** Christian F. W., German alienist, 1802–1878. See R.'s *nucleus.*

**roller** (ro'ler). Roller *bandage.*

**Rolleston's rule.** See under rule.

**Rollet,** Alexander, Austrian physiologist, 1834–1903. See Ritter-R. *phenomenon,* R.'s *stroma.*

**Romanov'sky,** Dimitri L., Russian physician, 1861–1921. See R.'s chromatin *stain.*

**Romberg,** Moritz H., Berlin physician, 1795–1873. See R.'s *disease, sign, syndrome, symptom,* R.-Howship *symptom,* R.'s *trophoneurosis.*

**rom'bergism.** Romberg's *sign.*

**Römer** (rĕ'mer), Paul H., German bacteriologist, 1876–1916. See R.'s *experiment, test.*

**Rommelaere,** Guillaume, Belgian physician, 1836–1916. See R.'s *sign.*

**rongeur** (rawn-zhër') [ Fr. *ronger,* to gnaw ]. A strong biting forceps for gouging away bone.

**roni'dazole** (USAN). DUGRO; 1-methyl-5-nitroimidazole-2-methanol carbamate ester; an antiprotozoal drug for veterinary use.

**roof** [ A.S. *hrōf*]. Tegmen; tectum.

    **r. of fourth ventricle,** *tegmen* ventriculi quarti.

    **r. of mouth,** palatum.

    **r. of orbit,** *paries* superior orbitae.

    **r. of skull,** calvaria.

    **r. of tympanum,** *tegmen* tympani.

**roof'plate.** See roof *plate.*

**room.** In hospitals, an enclosed area set apart for special equipment and procedures.

    **recovery r.,** a hospital facility with special equipment and personnel for the immediate postoperative care of patients as they recover from anesthesia and surgery; abbreviated RR.

**root** [ A.S. rot ]. 1. In anatomy, the base, foundation, or beginning of any part; see also radix. 2. *Radix* dentis. 3. The descending underground portion of a plant; it absorbs water and nutrients, provides support, and stores nutrients; for r.'s of pharmacological significance not listed below, see specific names.

    **anatomical r.,** that portion of a tooth extending from the cervical line to its apical extremity.

    **anterior r.,** *radix* ventralis.

    **clinical r.,** *radix* clinica.

    **cochlear r. of vestibulocochlear nerve,** see *nervus* vestibulocochlearis. (2).

    **cranial r.'s,** *radices* craniales.

    **Culver's r.,** leptandra.

    **dorsal r.,** *radix* dorsalis.

    **facial r.,** *nervus* canalis pterygoidei.

    **r. of facial nerve,** *radix* nervi facialis.

    **r. of the foot,** tarsus.

    **hair r.,** *radix* pili.

    **inferior r. of cervical loop,** *radix* inferior ansae cervicalis.

    **inferior r. of vestibulocochlear nerve,** see *nervus* vestibulocochlearis.

    **lateral r. of the median nerve,** *radix* lateralis nervi mediani.

    **lateral r. of the optic tract,** *radix* lateralis tractus optici.

    **long r. of ciliary ganglion,** *ramus* communicans cum nervo nasociliari.

    **r. of the lung,** *radix* pulmonis.

    **medial r. of the median nerve,** *radix* medialis nervi mediani.

    **medial r. of the optic tract,** *radix* medialis tractus optici; also called *brachium* colliculus superioris, *q.v.*

    **r. of the mesentry,** *radix* mesenterii.

    **motor r. of the ciliary ganglion,** *radix* oculomotoria ganglii ciliaris.

    **motor r. of the trigeminal nerve,** *radix* motoria nervi trigemini.

    **r. of the nail,** *radix* unguis.

    **nerve r.,** one of the two bundles of nerve fibers (dorsal and ventral r.'s) emerging from the spinal cord which join to form a single segmented spinal nerve. Some of the cranial nerves are similarly formed by the union of two r.'s, in particular the fifth or nervus trigeminus. In the case of the eighth cranial (vestibulocochlear) nerve, each of its two components (nervus vestibularis or radix dorsalis and nervus cochlearis or radix ventralis) is referred to as a root even though they do not join each other.

    **r. of the nose,** *radix* nasi.

    **olfactory r.,** *stria* olfactoria.

    **r.'s of olfactory tract, lateral and medial,** the two fiber bands that form the caudal continuation of the olfactory tract and, diverging, enclose the olfactory tubercle.

    **r. of the penis,** *radix* penis.

    **posterior r.,** *radix* dorsalis.

    **sensory r. of ciliary ganglion,** *ramus* communicans cum nervo nasociliari.

    **sensory r. of the trigeminal nerve,** *radix* sensoria nervi trigemini.

    **short r. of the ciliary ganglion,** *radix* oculomotoria ganglii ciliaris.

    **spinal r.'s,** *radices* spinales.

    **superior r. of cervical loop,** *radix* superior ansae cervicalis.

    **superior r. of the vestibulocochlear nerve,** see *nervus* vestibulocochlearis.

    **r. of the tongue,** *radix* linguae.

    **r. of a tooth,** *radix* dentis.

    **r.'s of trigeminal nerve,** *radices* nervi trigemini.

    **tuberous r.,** a r. that is swollen for food storage; tuberous primary r.'s occur in aconite, beet, and carrot; tuberous secondary r.'s occur in plants of the Umbelliferae; and tuberous adventitious roots occur in jalap and sweet potato.

    **ventral r.,** *radix* ventralis.

    **vestibular r. of vestibulocochlear nerve,** see *nervus* vestibulocochlearis.

**root'lets.** In neuroanatomy, refers to the nerve rootlets, or fila radicularis, *q.v.* under filum.

**ropalocytosis** (ro-pal'o-si-to'sĭs) [ G. *ropalon*, club, + *kytos*, cell, + suffix *-osis*, condition ]. Formation of numerous processes of erythroid cells, which in ultrathin sections appear club-shaped; it is associated with cytoplasmic vesicles and found in some diseases of the blood.

**Ror'schach**, Hermann, Swiss psychiatrist, 1884–1922. See R. *test*.

**Rosa** (ro'zah) [ L. rose ]. A genus of plants including the roses (family Rosaceae); several varieties are the sources of rose oil: *R. alba*, cottage rose; *R. centifolia*, the pale rose or cabbage rose (source of official rose oil); *R. damascena*, damask rose; and *R. gallica*, red rose or French rose.

**rosacea** (ro-za'she-ah) [ L. *rosaceus*, rosy ]. Acne rosacea; acne erythematosa; vascular and follicular dilation involving the nose and contiguous portions of cheeks; may vary from very mild but persistent erythema to extensive hyperplasia of the sebaceous glands with deep-seated papules and pustules of the affected erythematous sites.

    **hypertrophic r.**, rhinophyma.

**rosanilin** (ro-zan'ĭ-lin). Aminotolyldi(aminophenyl)-methyl chloride; together with pararosanilin it is a component of the red stain, basic fuchsin.

    **r. dyes**, triphenylmethane dyes.

**rosary** (ro'zĕr-ĭ). A beadlike arrangement or structure.

    **rachitic r.**, rachitic beads; beading of the ribs; a row of beading at the junction of the ribs with their cartilages, often seen in rachitic children.

**Roscoe**, Sir Henry E., English chemist, 1833–1915. See Bunsen-R. *law*.

**Rose**, Anton R., U. S. biochemist, 1877–1948. See Exton-R. *test*.

**Rose** (ro'zeh), Edmund, Berlin physician, 1836–1914. See R.'s cephalic *tetanus*.

**Rose**, Frank A., London surgeon. See R.'s *position*.

**Rose** (ro'zeh), Heinrich, German chemist, 1796–1864. See R.'s *metal*.

**rose** (rōz) [ L. *rosa* ]. 1. Erysipelas. 2. Red r.; the petals of *Rosa gallica*, collected before expanding; used for its agreeable odor.

    **r. bengal**, the sodium salt of tetraiodotetrachlorfluorescein, $C_{20}H_2O_5I_4Cl_4Na_2$; a coarse dark red powder. Used as a stain for bacteria and as a stain (1 per cent aqueous solution) in the diagnosis of keratitis sicca.

    **r. oil** (NF), oleum rosae; attar of rose; a volatile oil from *Rosa centifolia;* used in perfumery and in ointments.

**rosemary oil** (rōz'mĕr-ĭ). The volatile oil distilled with steam from the fresh flowering tops of *Rosmarinus officinalis* (family Labiatae); used as a flavoring and in perfumery.

**Rosenbach** (ro'zen-bahkh), Ottomar, Berlin physician, 1851–1907. See R.'s *disease, law, sign, test*, R.-Gmelin *test*.

**Rosenblueth**, Arturo S., Mexican neurophysiologist, *1900. See R.-Cannon *test*.

**Rosenheim**, O., British physician, *1871. See Acree-R. *test* (for protein).

**Rosenmüller** (ro'zen-mü-ler), Johann C., German anatomist, 1771–1820. See R.'s fossa, gland, node, organ, recess, valve.

**Rosenow** (ro'zen-ow), Edward C., American bacteriologist, *1875. See R.'s *stain* (for capsules).

**Rosenthal** (ro'zen-tahl), Friedrich C., German anatomist, 1780–1829. See R.'s *vein*, basal *vein* of R.

**Rosenthal** (ro'zen-tahl), Isidor, German physiologist, 1836–1915. See R.'s *canal*.

**Rosenthaler-Turk reagent.** See under reagent.

**roseola** (ro-ze'o-lah) [ Mod. L. dim. of L. *roseus*, rosy ]. Rose rash; scarlet rash; macular erythema; a symmetrical eruption of small closely aggregated patches of rose-red color.

    **epidemic r.**, rubella.

    **idiopathic r.**, r. not occurring as a symptom of a recognized general disease.

    **r. infan'tilis**, *exanthema* subitum.

    **r. infan'tum**, *exanthema* subitum.

    **symptomatic r.**, a rash symptomatic of typhoid fever, measles, or other eruptive fever.

    **syphilitic r.**, macular or erythematous syphilid; usually the first eruption of syphilis, occurring 6 to 12 weeks after the initial lesion.

**roseolous** (ro-ze'o-lus). Relating to or resembling roseola.

**Roser**, Wilhelm, German surgeon, 1817–1888. See R.-Nélaton *line*.

**rosette** (ro-zet') [ Fr. a little rose ]. 1. The quartan malarial parasite of *Plasmodium malariae* in its segmented or mature phase. 2. A grouping of cells characteristic of neoplasms of neuroblastic or neuroectodermal origin; a number of nuclei form a ring from which neurofibrils, which can be demonstrated by silver impregnation, extend to interlace in the center.

    **Wintersteiner r.'s**, found only in retinal embryonic tumors; the r. is formed by a group of columnar cells with a peripheral basement membrane arranged in a radial manner around a central cavity, the spokes corresponding to the rods and cones.

**Rose-Waaler test.** See under test.

**Rosicrucians** (ro-zĭ-krö'shĭ-anz) [ Latinized form of the supposed name of the mythical founder of the sect, *Rosenkreuz*, from L. *rosa*, a rose, + *crux* (*cruc-*), a cross ]. Brethren or Knights of the Rosy Cross; a sect of physicians of the 15th and 16th centuries steeped in astrology, alchemy, and Eastern sorcery who applied their mystic rites to the treatment of the sick.

**rosin** (roz'in) (USP). Resin (*q.v.*); colophony; the solid resin obtained from *Pinus palustris* and from other species of *Pinus* (family Pinaceae); used in plasters to render them adhesive, and also in ointments to render them locally stimulating.

***p*-rosolic acid** (ro'sol'ik). Aurin.

**Ross**, Sir Ronald, English physician and Officer in the Indian Medical Service, 1957–1932. Nobel laureate, 1902, for his work on malaria.

**Ross-Jones test.** See under test.

**Rosso.** See Russo.

**Rossolimo** (ros-o-le'mo), Grigoriy I., Russian neurologist, 1860–1928. See R.'s *reflex, sign*.

**rostellum** (ros-tel'um) [ L. dim. of *rostrum*, a beak ]. The anterior portion of the scolex of a tapeworm, frequently provided with a row (or several rows) of hooks.

**ros'tral** [ L. *rostralis*, fr. *rostrum*, beak ]. 1. Relating to any rostrum or anatomical structure resembling a beak. 2. Cephalad; oral; situated at or directed toward the anterior (snout) end of an organism; depending on context, the term can be synonymous with anterior or superior; its antonym is caudal.

**rostrate** [ L. *rostratus* ]. Having a beak or hook.

**ros'triform** [ L. *rostrum*, beak ]. Beak-shaped.

**rostrum**, pl. **rostra, rostrums** (ros'trum, -trah) [ L. a beak ] [ NA ]. Any beak-shaped structure.

    **r. cor'poris callo'si** [ NA ], beak of the corpus callosum; the recurved portion of the corpus callosum passing backward from the genu to the anterior commissure.

    **r. sphenoida'le** [ NA ], the anterior projecting part of the body of the sphenoid bone which articulates with the vomer.

**rot** [ A.S. *rotian* ]. 1. To decay. 2. Decay; a process of decomposition. Used specifically of wood and leather.

    **Bar'coo r.** [ *Barcoo*, a river in S. Australia ], desert *sore*.

    **foot r.**, (1) in sheep, a contagious disease characterized by chronic inflammation of the foot, softening of the hoof, discharge of a fetid odor, lameness, and lip and leg ulceration; (2) fouls.

    **grinder's r.**, siderosis.

    **liver r.**, a disease of the liver in sheep and cattle caused by the liver fluke *Fasciola hepatica* or *Fasciola gigantica*.

**rotameter** (ro'tam'e-ter) [ L. *rota*, wheel, + G. *metron*, measure ]. Device for measuring flow of gas or fluid.

**rotation** (ro-ta'shun) [ L. *rotatio*, fr. *roto*, pp. *rotatus*, to revolve, rotate ]. 1. Turning or movement of a body round its axis. 2. A recurrence in regular order of certain events, such as the symptoms of a periodical disease.

    **intestinal r.**, see malrotation.

    **molecular r.**, $1/100$ of the product of the specific r. of an optically active compound and its molecular weight.

    **optical r.**, the change in the plane of polarization of polarized light upon passing through optically active substances; measured in terms of specific rotation (*q.v.*) by polarimetry; an important tool in organic chemical structural work, especially on carbohydrates.

**specific r.,** the arc through which the plane of polarized light is rotated by 1 gram of a substance per milliliter of water when the length of the layer of the solution is 1 decimeter. Symbol [ α ].

**rotator** [ L. See rotation ]. A muscle by which a part can be turned circularly; see *musculi rotatores.*

**Rotch,** Thomas M., Boston physician, 1848–1914. See R.'s *sign.*

**röteln, roetheln** (rë'teln) [ Ger. dim. of *röte*, redness ]. Rubella.

**ro'tenone.** The principal insecticidal component of derris root, *Derris elliptica, D. malaccensis,* and other species of *Derris,* and from *Lonchocarpus nicou* (family Leguminosae); used externally for the treatment of scabies and infestation with chiggers, and in veterinary medicine for follicular mange and infestation with lice, fleas, and ticks.

**Roth,** Moritz, Swiss physician and pathologist, 1839–1914. See R.'s *spots,* R.'s *vas* aberrans.

**Roth** (rōt), Vladimir K., Russian neurologist, 1848–1916. See R.'s *disease,* R.-Bernhardt *disease,* B.-Roth *syndrome.*

**Rothera,** Arthur C. H., English biochemist, 1880–1915. See R.'s nitroprusside *test.*

**Rothia** (roth'i-ah) [ G. D. *Roth* ]. A genus of nonmotile, nonsporeforming, non-acid fast, aerobic to facultatively anaerobic bacteria (family Actinomycetaceae) containing Gram-positive, coccoid, diphtheroid, or filamentous cells. Microcolonies are smooth and growth is best anaerobically. The metabolism of these organisms is fermentative. Glucose fermentation yields primarily lactic acid and no propionic acid. The cell walls do not contain diaminopimelic acid or arabinose. These organisms are commonly found in the oral cavity of man. The type species is *R. dentocariosa.*

**R. dentocariosa,** a species commonly found in the oral cavity of man. Pathogenicity has not been demonstrated for this organism. It is the type species of the genus *R.*

**Rothmund,** August von, German physician, 1830–1906. See R.'s *syndrome.*

**rotoscoliosis** (ro'to-sko-lī-o'sis) [ L. *roto,* to rotate, + G. *skoliōsis,* crookedness ]. Curvature of the vertebral column by turning on its axis.

**rotox'amine tartrate** (NF). TWISTON tartrate; (—)-2-[ *p*-chloro-α-(2-dimethylaminoethoxy)benzyl ]pyridine lactate; antihistaminic.

**rotun'dus** [ L. ] [ NA ]. Round.

**Rouget** (roo-zha'), Antoine D., French physiologist, 19th century. See R.'s *bulb, muscle.*

**Rouget** (roo-zha'), Charles M. B., French physiologist, 1824–1904. See R.'s *cells,* R.-Neumann *sheath.*

**rough** (ruf). Not smooth; denoting the irregular, coarsely granular surface of a certain bacterial colony type.

**roughage** (ruf'ij). 1. Anything in the diet, *e.g.,* bran, serving as an intestinal irritant to excite peristalsis. 2. Hay or other coarse feed fed to cattle and other herbivores.

**Rougnon** (roon-yon'), Nicholas F., French physician, 1727–1799. See R.-Heberden *disease.*

**Roughton,** Francis J. W., British scientist, 1899–1972. See R.-Scholander *apparatus, syringe.*

**round'worm.** A nematode member of the phylum Nemathelminthes, commonly confined to the parasitic forms.

**roup** (roop). An old name for any suppurative inflammation of the nares and infraorbital sinuses of birds. See avian diphtheria; fowlpox.

**Rous** (rows), F. Peyton, American physician, 1879–1970. Nobel laureate, 1966, with Charles Huggins, for their investigations of cancer. See R. *sarcoma, tumor.*

**Roussy** (roo-se'), Gustave, French pathologist, 1874–1948. See R.-Lévy *disease, syndrome,* Déjèrine-R. *syndrome.*

**Roux** (roo), César, Swiss surgeon, 1857–1926. See R.-en-Y *operation.*

**Roux** (roo), Philibert J., Paris surgeon, 1780–1854. See R.'s *method.*

**Roux** (roo), Pierre P. E., Paris bacteriologist, 1853–1933. See R. *spatula, stain.*

**Rovsing,** Niels T., Copenhagen surgeon, 1862–1927. See R.'s *sign.*

**Rowntree,** Leonard G., American physician, *1883. See R. and Geraghty's *test.*

**RPF.** Abbreviation for renal plasma flow; see effective renal plasma *flow.*

**r.p.m.** Abbreviation for revolutions per minute.

**R.Q.** Abbreviation for respiratory *quotient.*

**-rrhagia** [ G. *rhēgnymi,* to burst forth. RHAG- ]. A combining form (suffix) indicating excessive or unusual discharge.

**-rrhaphy** [ G. *rhaphē,* suture. RHAPH- ]. A comgining form (suffix) indicating surgical suturing.

**-rrhea** (re'ah) [ G. *rhoia,* a flow. RHE- ]. Combining form, used as a suffix, meaning a flowing or flux.

**rRNA.** Abbreviation for ribosomal RNA; see under ribonucleic acid.

**Ru.** Chemical symbol of the element ruthenium.

**rub.** Friction encountered in moving one body over another.

**friction r.,** friction *sound.*

**pericar'dial r.,** a friction sound produced by the rubbing together of inflamed or roughened pericardial surfaces.

**pleurit'ic r.,** a friction sound produced by the rubbing together of the roughened surfaces of the costal and visceral pleurae.

**Rubarth,** Sven, Swedish veterinarian, 20th century. See R.'s *disease.*

**rub'ber.** Caoutchouc.

**rubber policeman.** See policeman.

**rubedo** (ru-be'do) [ L. redness, fr. *ruber,* red ]. A temporary redness of the skin.

**rubefacient** (ru-be-fa'shent) [ L. *rubi-facio,* fr. *ruber,* red, + *facio,* to make ]. 1. Causing a reddening of the skin. 2. A counterirritant that produces erythema when applied to the skin surface.

**rubefaction** (ru'be-fak'shun) [ see rubifacient ]. Erythema of the skin caused by local application of a counterirritant.

**rubella** (ru-bel'ah) [ L. *rubellus,* fem. -*a,* reddish, dim. of *ruber,* red ]. German or three-day measles; röteln; epidemic roseola; rubeola notha; third disease; an acute exanthematous disease caused by an RNA virus, and marked by enlargement of lymph nodes, but usually with little fever or constitutional reaction; of importance because of the high incidence of abnormalities of children from infection during first several months of fetal life.

**rubel'lin.** A cardiac glycoside with a digitalis-like action, obtained from *Urginia rubella* (family Liliaceae).

**rubeola** (ru-be'o-lah) [ Mod. L. dim. of *ruber,* red, reddish ]. R. has been used as a synonym for two different virus diseases of man, namely measles (morbilli) and rubella. Presently, r. is often used as a synonym for measles (morbilli); however, the term should be avoided because of the confusion which exists.

**r. no'tha** [ L. *nothus,* spurious ], rubella.

**rubeosis** (ru'be-o'sis) [ L. *ruber,* red, + G. suffix -*osis,* condition ]. Reddish discoloration, as of skin.

**r. i'ridis diabet'ica,** neovascularization of anterior surface of iris, seen in chronic severe diabetes.

**ru'ber** [ L. *ruber* (*rubr-*). RUB- ] [ NA ]. Red.

**rubescent** (ru-bes'ent) [ L. *rubesco,* pr. p. *rubescens* (-*scent-*), to become red ]. Reddening.

**rubidium** (ru-bid'i-um) [ L. *rubidus,* reddish, dark red, fr. *rubeo,* to be red ]. An alkali element, symbol Rb, atomic no. 37, atomic weight 85.48, a silvery white metal. The salts of r. have been used in medicine for the same purposes as the corresponding sodium or potassium salts.

**Rubin,** Isidor C., U. S. gynecologist, 1883–1958. See R.'s *test.*

**ru'bin, ru'bine.** Fuchsin.

**Rubinstein,** J. H. See R.-Taybi *syndrome.*

**Rubner** (roob'ner), Max, Berlin hygienist and biochemist, 1854–1932. See R.'s *laws* (of growth), R.'s *test.*

**ru'bor** [ L. ]. Redness; one of the classical signs of inflammation.

**ru'briblast** [ L. *ruber,* red, + G. *blastos,* germ ]. Pronormoblast; see discussion under erythroblast.

**pernicious anemia type r.,** promegaloblast; see discussion under erythroblast.

**ru'bricyte** [ L. *ruber,* red, + *kytos,* cell ]. Polychromatic normoblast; see discussion under erythroblast.

**ru′brogliocla′din.** An antibiotic obtained from cultures of *Gliocladium roseum.* It is the quinhydrone of aurantiogliocladin.

**ru′brospi′nal.** Relating to the nerve fibers passing from the red nucleus to the spinal cord: the *tractus* rubrospinalis.

**Ru′bus** [ L. blackberry bush or bramble bush ]. A genus of plants of the family Rosaceae; *R. idaeus* and *R. strigosus* are botanical sources of raspberry juice.

**ructus** (ruk′tus) [ L. fr. *ructo,* pp. *-atus,* to belch ]. Eructation.

**rudiment** (ru′dĭ-ment) [ L. *rudimentum, q. v.* ]. An organ or structure which is incompletely developed.

**ru′dimen′tary.** Imperfectly developed; vestigial.

**rudimentum,** pl. **rudimenta** (ru′dĭ-men′tum, -tah) [ L. a beginning, fr. *rudis,* unformed ] [ NA ]. Rudiment; a term included in the *Nomina Anatomica* only for the first indication of a structure in the course of ontogeny.
  **r. hippocam′pi,** tenia tecta; see *indusium* griseum.

**Ruffini** (roo-fe′ne), Angelo, Italian anatomist, 1864–1929. See R.'s *corpuscles,* flower-spray *organ.*

**Ruffmann's test.** See under test.

**rufous** (ru′fus) [ L. *rufus,* reddish ]. Erythristic.

**Rufus** of Ephesus, Roman surgeon, first century A.D. Described the capsule of the crystalline lens, erysipelas, the optic chiasm, epithelioma, and bubonic plague; wrote an extensive work on anatomical nomenclature.

**ruga,** pl. **rugae** (ru′gah, ru′ge) [ L. a wrinkle ] [ NA ]. A fold, ridge, or crease; a wrinkle.
  **r. gas′trica,** one of the folds of the mucous membrane of the stomach when the organ is contracted.
  **r. palati′na,** *plica* palatina transversa.
  **rugae vagina′les** [ NA ], a number of transverse ridges in the mucous membrane of the vagina.

**rugine** (ru-zhĕn′) [ Fr. ]. 1. Periosteum *elevator.* 2. Raspatory.

**rugitus** (ru′jĭ-tus) [ L. a roaring, fr. *rugio,* to roar ]. Borborygmus; intestinal rumbling.

**rugose** (ru′gōs) [ L. *rugosus* ]. Marked by rugae; wrinkled.

**rugosity** (ru-gos′ĭ-tĭ). 1. The state of being thrown into folds or wrinkles. 2. A ruga.

**rugous** (ru′gus). Rugose.

**rule** (rūl) [ O. Fr. *reule,* fr. L. *regula,* a guide, pattern ]. Criterion; standard; guide.
  **Abegg's r.,** the tendency of the sum of the maximum positive and maximum negative valence of a particular element to equal 8; e.g., carbon may have a valence of $+4$ and $-4$, oxygen of $+6$ and $-2$, and so on. Sometimes loosely stated as all atoms have the same number of valences. A consequence of the tendency of valence electron shells to be filled to 8.
  **American Law Institute r.,** a 1962 test of criminal responsibility; it states that "a person is not responsible for criminal conduct if at the time of such conduct as a result of mental disease or defect he lacks substantial capacity either to appreciate the wrongfulness of his conduct or to conform his conduct to the requirements of law."
  **Bartholomew's r. of fourths,** the duration of pregnancy can be obtained by measuring the height of the fundus of the uterus above the pubic symphysis.
  **Clark's weight r.,** an approximate child's dose (for patients 2 years of age or over) is obtained by dividing the child's weight in pounds by 150 and multiplying the result by the adult dose.
  **Cowling's r.,** the dose of any drug for a child is that fraction of the adult dose obtained by dividing the age of the child at the nearest birthday by 24. See also Young's r.
  **Durham r.,** an American test (1954) of criminal responsibility; it states that "an accused is not criminally responsible if his unlawful act was the product of mental disease or mental defect."
  **Goriaew's r.,** a r. of a blood counting field by which it is marked off in a series of squares, some of which are again subdivided into sixteen smaller ones.
  **Haase's r.,** the length of the fetus in centimeters, divided by 5, is the duration of pregnancy in months, *i.e.,* the age of the fetus.
  **His' r.,** the duration of pregnancy is to be reckoned from the first day of the first omitted menstrual period.

**isoprene r.,** the classical, outmoded statment that naturally occurring terpenes are build up by condensation of isoprene units by either a 1-4 linkage ("head to tail") or a 4-4 linkage ("tail to tail").
  **Jackson's r.,** after an epileptic attack, simple and quasiautomatic functions are less affected and more rapidly recovered than the more complex ones.
  **Le Bel-van't Hoff r.,** the number of stereoisomers of an organic compound is $2^n$ where $n$ represents the number of asymmetric carbon atoms. A corollary of their simultaneously announced conclusions, in 1874, that the most probable orientation of the bonds of a carbon atom linked to four groups or atoms is toward the apexes of a tetrahedron, and that this accounted for all then-known phenomena of molecular asymmetry (which involved a carbon atom bearing four different atoms or groups). See also stereoisomerism.
  **Liebermeister's r.,** in febrile tachycardia in the adult, about eight pulse beats correspond to an increase of 1°C.
  **M'Naghten r.,** the classic English test of criminal responsibility (1843); it states that "to establish a defense on the ground of insanity, it must be clearly proved that, at the time of committing the act, the party accused was laboring under such a defect of reasoning, from disease of the mind, as not to know the nature and quality of the act he was doing, or if he did know it, that he did not know he was doing what was wrong."
  **Nägele's r.,** means of estimating date of delivery by counting back three months from the first day of the last menstrual period and adding seven days.
  **New Hampshire r.,** pioneering American test of criminal responsibility (1871); it states that "if the [ criminal ] act was the offspring of insanity–a criminal intent did not produce it."
  **Ogino-Knaus r.,** pertains to the time in the menstrual period when conception is most likely to occur, namely, at about midway between two menstrual periods; fertilization of the ovum is least likely just before or just after menstruation; the basis for "rhythm" method of contraception.
  **r. of outlet,** an obstetric r. for determining whether the pelvic outlet will permit the passage of a fetus; the sum of the posterior sagittal diameter (internal) and the transverse diameter (external) of the outlet must equal at least 15 cm. if a normal-sized baby is to pass.
  **phase r.,** an expression of the relationships existing between systems in equilibrium: $P + V = C + 2$, where $P$ is the number of phases, $V$ the variance or degrees of freedom, and $C$ the number of components; it also follows that the variance is, $V = C + 2 - P$. For $H_2O$ at its triple point, $V = 1 + 2 - 3 = 0$, *i.e.,* both temperature and pressure are fixed.
  **Prentice's r.,** for every centimeter of decentration of a lens, the effect is 1 prism diopter for every diopter of lens power.
  **Rolleston's r.,** the ideal adult systolic blood pressure is 100 plus half the age, whereas the maximal physiologic pressure is 100 plus the age.
  **Schutz' r.,** (or law); the rate of an enzyme reaction is proportional to the square root of the enzyme concentration; applied specifically to pepsin within a limited range.
  **Young's r.,** a r. to determine the dose of a medicine suitable for a child; 12 is added to the child's age and the sum is divided by the age; the adult dose divided by the figure so obtained gives the proper dose for the child. Thus, for a child of 6 years: $6 + 12 = 18 \div 6 = 3$; the adult dose divided by 3 is the proper dose for the child.

**ru′ler.** A calibrated strip for measuring plane surfaces.
  **isometric r.,** isometric *scale.*

**rum.** A spirit distilled from the fermented juice of the sugar cane.

**rum-blossom.** Rhinophyma.

**rumen,** pl. **rumina** (ru′men, ru′mĭ-nah) [ L. gullet, throat ]. [ NAV ]. The largest compartment of the stomach, or paunch, of a ruminant.

**rumenitis** (ru′mĕ-ni′tis) [ rumen + G. suffix *-itis,* inflammation ]. Inflammation of the rumen of ruminant animals.

**rumenotomy** (ru′mĕ-not′o-mĭ) [ rumen + G. *tomē,* incision ]. Incision into the rumen.

**ru'mex** [ L. sorrel ]. Dock; the root of *Rumex crispus* or *R. obtusifolius* (family Polygonaceae), curly or yellow dock; has been used as a laxative, astringent, and in the treatment of various chronic skin diseases.

**ru'minant.** An animal that chews the cud, *e.g.*, the sheep, cow, deer, or antelope.

**rumina'tion** [ L. *ruminatio*, fr. *rumino*, to chew the cud, think over, fr. *rumen*, throat ]. 1. The physiologic process in ruminant animals in which coarse, hastily eaten food is regurgitated from the rumen and thoroughly rechewed. The food is reduced to finer particles, mixed with saliva, and reswallowed. 2. Periodic reconsideration of the same subject.

**ru'mina'tive.** Characterized by a preoccupation with certain thoughts and ideas.

**ruminoreticulum** (ru'mĭ-no-rĕ-tik'u-lum) [ NAV ]. The rumen and reticulum of the ruminant stomach taken together since they freely communicate via the ruminoreticular orifice.

**rump.** The buttocks or gluteal region.

**Rumpel** (room'pel), Theodor, German physician, 1862–1923. See R.-Leede *sign, test.*

**Rumpf,** Theodor, German physician, *1851. See R.'s *symptom.*

**runaround, runround.** Colloquialism for paronychia.

**Runeberg** (roo'na-berg), Johan W., Finnish physician, 1843–1918. See R.'s *anemia, formula.*

**runt** [ A.S. ]. A stunted animal, occurring most frequently in species which give birth to large litters.

**Ruotte** (roo-ott'), Paul, French surgeon, *1862. See R.'s *operation.*

**rupia** (ru'pĭ-ah) [ G. *rhypos*, filth ]. 1. Ulcers of late secondary syphilis, covered with yellowish or brown crusts which have been compared in their appearance to oyster shells. 2. Yaws. 3. Occasionally also used to designate a very scaly and secondarily infected psoriatic lesion.

   **r. escharot'ica,** *dermatitis* gangrenosa infantum.

**ru'pial.** Relating to rupia.

**rupioid** (ru'pĭ-oyd) [ G. *rhypos*, filth (rupia), + *eidos*, resemblance ]. Resembling rupia.

**rupophobia** (ru-po-fo'bĭ-ah). Rhypophobia.

**rupture** (rup'chur) [ L. *ruptura*, a fracture (of limb or vein), fr. *rumpo*, pp. *ruptus*, to break ]. 1. Hernia. 2. A tear or solution of continuity; a break of any organ or other of the soft parts.

**Russell,** J. S. Risien, *1894. See hook *bundle* of R., uncinate *bundle* of R.

**Russell,** William, Edinburgh physician, 1852–1940. See R. *bodies.*

**Russell effect.** See under effect.

**Russell traction.** See under traction.

**Russell's viper** and **viper venom.** See the nouns.

**Rust,** Johann N., Berlin surgeon, 1775–1840. See R.'s *disease, phenomenon.*

**rut** [ O. F. *ruit*, roaring of deer in the breeding season ]. A period of sexual desire in the males of certain mammals, such as deer, camels, and elephants, which occurs seasonally. It is only during this season that spermatogenesis occurs and the males will mate; in most mammalian males spermatogenesis is continuous and breeding occurs whenever the females will accept the males; *c.f.* estrus.

**ruthenium** (ru-the'nĭ-um) [ Mediev. L. *Ruthenia*, Russia, where the metal was first obtained ]. A metallic element, symbol Ru, atomic no. 44, atomic weight 101.1; a metal of the platinum group.

   **r. red,** ammoniated r. oxychloride; $Ru_2(OH)_2Cl_4 \cdot 7NH_3 \cdot 3H_2O$; used in histology as a stain for certain complex polysaccharides.

**Rutherford,** Ernest, British physicist, 1871–1937. Gave his name to rutherford.

**rutherford.** A unit of radioactivity, representing that quantity of radioactive material in which a million disintegrations are taking place per second; 37 r. equal 1 mc.

**ru'tido'sis.** Rhytidosis.

**ru'tin.** Rutoside; quercetin-3-rutinoside; quercetin-3-rhamnoglucoside; melin; phytomelin; sophorin; eldrin; and others. A flavonoid obtained from buckwheat, having an action similar to the so-called vitamin P, causing increased capillary resistance. See also bioflavonoids; hesperidin.

**rutinose** (ru'tĭ-nōs). 6-(β-1-L-Rhamnosido)-D-glucose, a disaccharide of glucose and rhamnose; it is a component of rutin.

**Ruysch** (rīsh), Frederik, Dutch anatomist, 1638–1731. See R.'s *membrane, muscle, tube, veins.*

**RV.** Abbreviation for residual *volume.*

**rye smut.** Ergot.

**Ryle,** John A., British physician, *1889. See R.'s *tube.*

# S

σ. The 18th letter of the Greek alphabet, sigma, *q. v.*

**S.** 1. Abbreviation of L. *signa.* 2. Abbreviation of spherical, or spherical *lens.* 3. Chemical symbol of the element sulfur. 4. Designation of a rare human antigen (hemagglutinogen) related genetically to the MNSs blood group; see appendix 2, MNSs blood group. 5. Abbreviation for Svedberg *unit.* 6. Symbol for entropy in thermodynamics. 7. Symbol for substrate in Michaelis-Menton hypothesis. 8. Symbol for percentage saturation of hemoglobin, when followed by subscript $O_2$ or $CO_2$; see also saturation.

**$S_f$.** Symbol for flotation *constant.*

**s.** 1. Abbreviation of L. *sinister,* left, and L. *semis,* half. 2. As a subscript, denotes steady *state.*

**sabadilla** (sab'ă-dil'ah) [ Sp. *cevadilla,* ult. fr. L. *cibus,* food ]. Cevadilla; the seed of *Schoenocaulon officinale* (family Liliaceae), a plant of the shores of the Gulf of Mexico and Caribbean Sea; it yields cevadine, veratridine, and several other alkaloids; has been used externally as a parasiticide.

**Sabin,** Albert B., U. S. virologist, *1906. See S.'s *vaccine.*

**Sabin,** Florence Rena, American hematologist and anatomist, 1871–1954. Described the three different stages in the development of the erythroblast and myelocyte, *q. v.*

**Sabin-Feldman dye test.** See under test.

**sabi'na** [ L. (sc. *herba*), a kind of juniper, the savin, fem. of *Sabinus,* Sabine ]. Savin; the tops of *Juniperus sabina* (family Pinaceae); formerly used for rheumatism, gout, and amenorrhea, and locally for certain skin disorders.

**Sabouraud** (să-boo-ro'), Raymond J. A., French dermatologist, 1864–1938. See S.'s *agar,* S.-Noiré *instrument,* S.'s *pastilles.*

**sab'ulous** [ L. *sabulosus,* fr. *sabulum,* coarse sand ]. Sandy; gritty.

**sabulum** (sab'u-lum) [ L. coarse sand ]. Psammoma *bodies* (1).

**sabur'ra** [ L. sand ]. 1. Decomposition of the food in the stomach. 2. Sordes.

**sabur'ral.** Relating to saburra.

**sac** (sak) [ L. *saccus,* a bag ]. 1. A pouch; a bursa; see saccus and sacculus. 2. An encysted abscess at the root of a tooth. 3. The capsule of a tumor, or envelope of a cyst.

  **abdominal s.,**  the part of the embryonic coelom that becomes the abdominal cavity.

  **air s.,** *sacculus* alveolaris.

  **allantoic s.,** the dilated distal portion of the allantois.

  **alveolar s.,** *sacculus* alveolaris.

  **amniotic s.,** amnion.

  **anal s.,** a vesicular cutaneous invagination opening by a duct on each side of the anal canal in carnivores (best developed in skunks, but absent in some bears, the raccoon dog, kinkajou, coati, and sea otter). Each anal s. lies between the external and internal anal sphincter muscles, which aid in emptying the contents. The s. stores odoriferous scent markers produced by glands that line its wall or duct. Frequently the s. becomes impacted in the dog or cat, requiring manual emptying. The anal s. may be mistakenly referred to as the anal gland.

  **aneurysmal s.,** the dilated wall of an artery in a saccular aneurysm.

  **aortic s.,** in mammalian embryos, the endothelially lined dilation just distal to the truncus arteriosus. It is the primordial vascular channel from which the aortic arches arise and which becomes reshaped to form the ventral aortic roots.

  **chorionic s.,** chorion.

  **conjuncti'val s.,** *saccus* conjunctivae.

  **cupular blind s.,** *cecum* cupulare.

  **dental s.,** the outer, connective-tissue envelope surrounding a developing tooth; also applied to the mesenchymal concentration that is the primordium of the s.

  **endolymphatic s.,** *saccus* endolymphaticus.

  **greater peritoneal s.,** *cavum* peritonei.

  **heart s.,** pericardium.

  **hernial s.,** the peritoneal envelope of a hernia.

  **Hilton's s.,** *sacculus* laryngis.

  **lac'rimal s.,** *saccus* lacrimalis.

  **lesser peritoneal s.,** *bursa* omentalis.

  **lymph s.'s,** the earliest lymphatic vessels formed in the embryo.

  **nasal s.'s,** deepened nasal pits that develop into definitive nasal cavities.

  **omental s.,** *bursa* omentalis.

  **preputial s.,** the space between the prepuce and the glans penis.

  **puden'dal s.,** Broca's pouch; a pear-shaped encapsulated collection of connective tissue and fat in each labium majus.

  **tear s.,** *saccus* lacrimalis.

  **tooth s.,** a capsule that encloses the developing tooth.

  **vestibular blind s.,** *cecum* vestibulare.

  **vitelline s.,** yolk s.

  **yolk s.,** vitelline s.; umbilical vesicle; the highly vascular layer of splanchnopleure surrounding the yolk of an embryo.

**sac'brood.** A viral disease affecting the larvae of bees.

**saccadic** (să-kad'ik) [ Fr. *saccade,* sudden check of a horse ]. Jerky; see saccadic *movement.*

**saccate** (sak'āt) [ L. *saccus,* sac ]. Relating to a sac; pouched; saccular.

**sacchar-, sacchari-.** See saccharo-.

**saccharase** (sak'ă-rās). β-Fructofuranosidase.

**saccharate** (sak'ă-rāt). A salt or ester of saccharic acid.

**saccharated** (sak'ă-ra-ted). Sweetened.

**saccharephidrosis** (sak-ar-ef-ĭ-dro'sis) [ sacchar- + G. *ephidrōsis,* a slight perspiration ]. The presence of sugar in the sweat.

**saccharic** (să-kăr'ik). Relating to sugar.

  **s. acid,** D-glucaric acid; D-glucosaccharic acid; D-tetrahydroxyadipic acid; obtained from glucose by oxidation of C-1 and C-6 to —COOH's. Also used to denote the class of dicarboxy sugar acids.

**saccharide** (sak'ă-rīd). Sugar; carbohydrate.

**sacchariferous** (sak'ă-rif'er-us). Producing sugar.

**saccharification** (să-kăr'ĭ-fĭ-ka'shun). The process of saccharifying.

**saccharify** (să-kăr'ĭ-fī) [ sacchari- + L. *facio,* to make ]. To convert starch into sugar.

**saccharimeter** (sak-ă-rim'e-ter) (sacchari- + G. *metron,* measure ]. An instrument for determining the amount of sugar in a solution; it may be a polarimeter, a hygrometer, or container in which the solution is fermented and the amount estimated by the volume of $CO_2$ produced.

  **Einhorn's s.,** an instrument once used for carrying out the fermentation test for sugar in the urine.

  **Lohnstein's s.,** an apparatus for making a quantitative fermentation test of sugar in the urine.

**saccharin** (sak'ă-rin) (USP, BP). GLUSIDE; benzosulfimide; *o*-sulfobenzimide; in dilute aqueous solution it is 300 to 500 times sweeter than sucrose; used as a sweetening agent (sugar substitute). Also available are s. sodium (NF, BP) and s. calcium (NF), with the same use.

Saccharin

**saccharine** (sak'ă-rēn, -rin, -rīn). Relating to sugar; sweet.

**saccharo-, sacchar-, sacchari-** (sak'ă-ro) [ G. *sakcharon,* sugar. SACCH- ]. Combining forms relating to sugar (saccharide).

**saccharogalactorrhea** (sak'ă-ro-gă-lak'to-re'ah) [ saccharo- + G. *gala,* milk, + *rhoia,* a flow ]. Excessive secretion of lactose in milk.

**sac'charogen amylase.** β-Amylase.

**saccharolytic** (sak'ă-ro-lit'ik) [ saccharo- + G. *lysis*, loosening ]. Capable of hydrolyzing or otherwise breaking down a sugar molecule.

**saccharometabolic** (sak'ă-ro-met'ă-bol'ik). Relating to saccharometabolism.

**saccharometabolism** (sak-ă-ro-mĕ-tab'o-lizm). The process of utilization of sugar in cells.

**saccharometer** (sak-ă-rom'e-ter). Saccharimeter.

**Saccharomyces** (sak-ă-ro-mi'sēz) [ saccharo- + G. *mykēs*, fungus ]. Fungus yeast; yeast fungi; a genus of budding yeasts belonging to the family Saccharomycetaceae; a type of ascomycete.

  **S. al'bicans,** Old name for *Candida albicans.*

  **S. busse,** a species isolated by O. Busse in a patient with visceral and osseous lesions; probably synonymous with *Cryptococcus neoformans.*

  **S. capilit'ii,** a form found on the scalp, probably not pathogenic.

  **S. cerevi'siae** beer yeast; ordinary yeast; bread yeast.

  **S. hom'inis,** old synonym for *Cryptococcus neoformans.*

  **S. neofor'mans,** a blastomycete regarded by Sanfelice as pathogenic for man; old name for *Cryptococcus neoformans.*

  **S. subcuta'neus tumefa'ciens,** a species isolated in a case of multiple tumors; pathogenic for certain animals but not a recognized pathogen for man.

  **S. tumefa'ciens al'bus,** a form isolated in a few cases of pharyngitis; pathogenic for certain animals but not a recognized pathogen for man.

**Saccharomycetaceae** (sak'ă-ro-mi'se-ta'se-e). The family of yeasts; that group of fungi comprising the ascomycetes which possess a predominantly unicellular thallus, which reproduce asexually by budding, transverse division, or both, and which produce ascospores in an ascus, originating from a zygote or pathogenetically from a single somatic cell. Yeasts are widely distributed in substrates which contain sugars (such as fruits) and also in soil, animal excreta, the vegetative part of plants, etc. Because of the ability to ferment carbohydrates, some are important to the brewing and baking industries. One member, *Lipomyces neoformans,* believed to be the perfect stage of *Cryptococcus neoformans,* is the cause of cryptococcosis in man. A number of asporogenous yeasts (usually classified with the deuteromycetes) are also pathogenic for man.

**Saccharomycetales** (sak'ă-ro-mi'se-ta'lēz). An order of the *Ascomycetes* which includes the yeasts.

**saccharomycetic** (sak'ă-ro-mi-se'tik, -set'ik). Relating to or caused by the yeast fungus.

**saccharomycosis** (sak'ă-ro-mi-ko'sis) [ *Saccharomyces* + G. suffix *-osis,* condition ]. An old term for cryptococcosis or European blastomycosis.

**saccharorrhea** (sak'ă-ro-re'ah) [ saccharo- + G. *rhoia,* a flow ]. Obsolete term for glycosuria.

**saccharose** (sak'ă-rōs). Sucrose.

**saccharosuria** (sak'ă-ro-su'rĭ-ah) [ saccharose + G. *ouron,* urine ]. The excretion of saccharose in the urine; obsolete.

**saccharum** (sak'ă-rum) [ Mod. L. fr. G. *sakcharon* ]. Sucrose.

  **s. canaden'se,** maple sugar.

  **s. lactis,** lactose.

**saccharuria** (sak'ă-ru'rĭ-ah) [ saccharo- + G. *ouron,* urine ]. Excretion of sugar in the urine; glycosuria.

**sacciform** (sak'sĭ-form) [ L. *saccus,* sack, + *forma,* form ]. Saccate; pouched; sac-shaped; saccular.

**saccular** (sak'u-lar). Sacciform.

**sacculated** (sak'u-la'ted). Sacciform.

**sacculation** (sak'u-la'shun). 1. A structure formed by a group of sacs. 2. The formation of a sac or pouch.

**saccule** (sak'ūl) [ L. *sacculus, q.v.* ]. Sacculus; a small sac.

**sacculocochlear** (sak'u-lo-kok'le-ar). Relating to the sacculus (2) and the membranous cochlea.

**sacculus,** pl. **sacculi** (sak'u-lus, -li) [ L. dim. of *saccus,* sac ]. Saccule. 1 [ NA ]. A small sac or pouch. 2 [ NA ]. The smaller of the two membranous sacs in the vestibule of the labyrinth, lying in the spherical recess; it is connected with the cochlear duct by a very short tube, the ductus reuniens, and with the utriculus by the beginning of the ductus endolymphaticus and the ductus utriculosaccularis which joins it.

  **s. alveola'ris,** pl. **sacculi alveola'res** [ NA ], alveolar sac; air sac; dilation of the ductuli alveolares which give rise to the alveoli of the lung; a small air chamber in the pulmonary tissue from which the pulmonary alveoli project like bays and into which an alveolar duct opens.

  **s. commu'nis,** utriculus.

  **s. endolymphat'icus,** *saccus* endolymphaticus.

  **s. lacrima'lis,** *saccus* lacrimalis.

  **s. laryn'gis** [ NA ], saccule of the larynx; appendix ventriculi laryngis; a small diverticulum extending upward from the ventricle of the larynx between the ventricular fold and the lamina of the thyroid cartilage.

  **s. pro'prius,** s. (2).

  **s. vestibu'uli,** s. (2).

**saccus,** pl. **sacci** (sak'us, sak'si) [ L. a bag, sack. SACC- ] [ NA ]. A sac.

  **s. conjuncti'vae** [ NA ], conjunctival sac; the space bound by the conjunctival membrane between the palpebral and bulbar conjunctiva; it opens anteriorly between the eyelids.

  **s. endolymphat'icus** [ NA ], endolymphatic sac; Böttcher's or Cotunnius' space; the dilated blind extremity of the ductus endolymphaticus.

  **s. lacrima'lis** [ NA ], lacrimal sac; dacryocyst; the upper portion of the nasolacrimal duct into which empty the two lacrimal canaliculi. See fig. under *apparatus* lacrimalis.

  **s. reu'niens,** *sinus* venosus.

  **s. vagina'lis,** an embryonic peritoneal fossa indicating the site where the processus vaginalis extends through the anterior abdominal wall during descent of the testis.

**Sachs,** Bernard, U. S. neurologist, 1858–1944. See Tay-S. *disease.*

**Sachs,** Hans, German bacteriologist, 1877–1945. See S.-Georgi *reaction, test.*

**Sacks,** Benjamin, U. S. physician, *1896. See Libman-S. *endocarditis, syndrome.*

**sacr-.** See sacro-.

**sacrad** (sa'krad) [ sacr- + L. *ad,* to ]. In the direction of the sacrum.

**sacral** (sa'kral). Relating to or in the neighborhood of the sacrum.

**sacralgia** (sa-kral'jĭ-ah) [ sacr- + G. *algos,* pain ]. Sacrodynia; pain in the sacral region.

**sacralization** (sa'kral-ĭ-za'shun). An anomaly of the fifth lumbar vertebra that tends to conform it to the type of the upper sacral vertebra, the spinous processes of the upper sacral and lower lumbar vertebrae being fused to it.

**sacrectomy** (sa-krek'to-mī) [ sacr- + G. *ektomē,* excision ]. Sacrotomy; resection of a portion of the sacrum to facilitate excision of the rectum.

**sacro-, sacr-** (sa'kro-) [ L. *sacrum, q.v.* ]. Combining forms relating to the sacrum.

**sacrococcygeal** (sa-kro-kok-sij'e-al). Relating to both sacrum and coccyx.

**sacrococcygeus** (sa'ko-kok-sĭ-je'us). See under musculus.

**sacrodynia** (sa'kro-din'ĭ-ah) [ sacro- + G. *odyne,* pain ]. Sacralgia.

**sacroiliac** (sa-kro-il'ĭ-ak). Relating to the sacrum and the ilium.

**sacrolisthesis** (sa'kro-lis'the-sis) [ sacro- + G. *olisthēsis,* a slipping and falling ]. A forward displacement of the fifth lumbar vertebra on the sacrum.

**sacrolumbalis** (sa'kro-lum-ba'lis). The musculus iliocostalis lumborum.

**sa'crolum'bar.** Lumbosacral; relating to both the sacrum and the lumbar region.

**sacrosciatic** (sa'kro-si-at'ik). Relating to both sacrum and ischium.

**sacrospinal** (sa'kro-spi'nal). Relating to the sacrum and the vertebral column above.

**sacrospinalis** (sa'kro-spi-na'lis). See under musculus.

**sacrotomy** (sa-krot'o-mī) [ sacro- + G. *tome,* incision ]. Sacrectomy.

**sacrovertebral** (sa'kro-ver'te-bral). Relating to the sacrum and the vertebrae above.

**sacrum,** pl. **sacra** (sa'krum, sa'krah) [ L. (lit. sacred bone), neuter of *sacer* (*sacr-*), sacred ]. *Os* sacrum.

**assimila'tion s.,** one which is composed of six segments, the last lumbar vertebra assuming the appearance of a sacral segment; or one which is composed of but four segments, the first sacral being free and having the characteristics of a lumbar vertebra.

**sactosalpinx** (sak'to-sal'pingks) [ G. *saktos*, stuffed, fr. *sattō*, to load, + *salpinx*, trumpet. SALP- ]. Obsolete term for hydrosalpinx or pyosalpinx.

**saddle** (sad'l). 1. Sella; a structure shaped like, or suggestive of, a seat or saddle used in riding horseback. 2. Denture *base*.

**Turkish s.,** *sella* turcica.

**sadism** (sa'dizm) [ after the Marquis de *Sade*, 1740–1814, who was confessedly addicted to the practice ]. A form of sexual perversion in which the subject finds pleasure in inflicting pain; algolagnia; the opposite of masochism.

**sa'dist.** One who practices sadism.

**sadis'tic.** Pertaining to or characterized by sadism.

**Sadler,** Michael T., English obstetrician, 1834–1923. See Hofacker-S. *laws.*

**sadomasochism** (sa'do-mas'o-kizm, sad'o-) [ sadism + masochism ]. A form of sexual perversion marked by love of cruelty in its active and/or passive form.

**Saemisch** (za'mish), Edwin T., German ophthalmologist, 1833-1909. See S.'s *operation, section, ulcer.*

**Saenger** (zeng'er), Alfred, German neurologist, 1860–1921. See S.'s *sign.*

**Saenger** (zeng'er), M., Prague obstetrician, 1853–1903. See S.'s *macula, operation.*

**saf'flower** [ Ar. *safrā,* yellow ]. *Carthamus tinctorius* (family Compositae); source of s. oil.

**s. oil,** an oil extracted from the seeds of *Carthamus tinctorius;* contains 74.5 per cent linoleic acid and 6.6 per cent saturated fatty acids; used in hypercholesteremia, myocardial infarction, and coronary insufficiency.

**saffron** [ Ar. *zafarān,* fr. *safrā,* yellow ]. Crocus.

**meadow s.,** colchicum.

**saf'ranin O.** A mixture of dimethyl- and trimethyl-phenosafranin chloride, a basic red dye used in histology and microbiology.

**safranophil, safranophile** (saf'rā-no-fil, -fil). Staining readily with safranin; denoting certain cells and tissues.

**saf'role.** The methylene ether of allyl pyrocatechol; $C_{10}H_{10}O_2$; contained in oil of sassafras, oil of camphor, and various other volatile oils; it is obtained chiefly from oil of camphor by fractional distillation. Tonic and carminative. Prolonged administration causes fatty degeneration.

**sage** (sāj) [ L. *salvia,* the sage plant, fr. *salvus,* safe ]. Salvia.

**sagitta** (saj'ĭ-tah). See statoconia.

**sagittal** (saj'ĭ-tal) [ L. *sagitta,* an arrow ]. Resembling an arrow; in the line of an arrow shot from a bow, *i.e.,* in an anteroposterior direction.

**sagitta'lis** [ L. ] [ NA ]. Sagittal; referring to a sagittal plane or direction.

**Sagnac rays.** See under ray.

**sa'go** [ Malay, *sāgu* ]. A pearly starch made from the pith of several species of palms, the sago palms, *Metroxylon laevis, M. rumphii,* or *Arenga saccharifera* (family Palmae); the s. of commerce is often tapioca.

**Sahli** (sah'le), Hermann, Swiss physician, 1856–1933. See S.'s *test.*

**Saint's triad.** See under triad.

**Saint Martin,** Alexis. A French-Canadian hunter who, having sustained a gunshot wound which left a fistulous opening through the abdominal wall into the stomach, was the subject in 1825 and following years of William Beaumont's experiments upon gastric digestion.

**Sakaguchi reaction.** See under reaction.

**sal,** pl. **sal'es** [ L. salt ]. Salt.

**s. alem'broth** [ an alchemist's term of unknown origin ], salt of wisdom; the product obtained by crystallization from a solution of equal parts of ammonium chloride and mercuric chloride.

**s. ammo'niac,** ammonium chloride.

**s. diuret'icum,** potassium acetate.

**s. soda,** sodium carbonate.

**s. volatile,** smelling salts; see under salt.

**Salah's needle.** See under needle.

**salazosulfadimidine.** AZUDIMIDINE; 5-{ p-[ (4,6-dimeth-yl-2-pyrimidinyl)-sulfamoyl ]phenylazo}salicyclic acid; antimicrobial agent used for the treatment of chronic ulcerative colitis.

**salazosulf'amide.** LUTAZOL; 5-(p-sulfamoylphenylazo)-salicyclic acid; antimicrobial agent used in treatment of trachoma.

**salbu'tamol** (BP). Albuterol.

**salicin** (sal'ĭ-sin). Salicoside; saligenin-β-D-glucopyrano-side; a glucoside of o-hydroxybenzylalcohol, obtained from the bark of several species of *Salix* (willow) and *Populus* (poplar); s. is hydrolyzed to glucose and saligenin (salicyl alcohol. Formerly used in rheumatoid arthritis.

**salicyl** (sal'ĭ-sil). The acyl radical of salicylic acid (o-hy-droxybenzoic acid).

**s. alcohol,** saligenin; o-hydroxybenzyl alcohol; obtained by the hydrolysis of salicin.

**s. aldehyde,** salicylic aldehyde; o-hydroxybenzaldehyde; $HOC_6H_4CHO$; obtained from *Spirea ulmaria* (meadow sweet), and made synthetically; diuretic and antiseptic.

**salicyl'amide.** The amide of salicylic acid, o-hydroxyben-zamide; an analgesic, antipyretic and antiarthritic, similar in action to acetylsalicylic acid.

**sal'icylan'ilide.** N-Phenylsalicylamide; an antifungal agent especially useful in the treatment of tinea capitis caused by *Microsporon audouini.*

**salicylate** (sā-lis'ĭ-lāt, sal-ĭ-sil'āt). 1. A salt of salicylic acid. 2. To salicylize; to treat foodstuffs with salicylic acid as a preservative.

**sal'icylated.** Treated by the addition of salicylic acid as a preservative.

**sal'icylaz'osulfapyr'idine** (NF). AZULFIDINE; SALAZOPY-RIN; 5-[ p-(2-pyridylsulfamyl)phenylazo ]salicyclic acid; a sulfonamide used in chronic ulcerative colitis; it is broken down in the body to amino salicylic acid and sulfapyridine. An acid-azosulfa compound with a marked affinity for connective tissues, especially for those rich in elastin.

**salicylic** (sal'ĭ-sil'ik). Derived from salicin; containing the radical salicyl.

**s. acid** (USP, BP), o-hydroxybenzoic acid; $HOC_6H_4-COOH$; used externally as a keratolytic agent, antiseptic, and fungicide.

**s. aldehyde,** salicyl aldehyde.

**salicylism** (sal'ĭ-sĭ-lizm). Poisoning by salicylic acid or any of its compounds.

**sal'icylize.** To salicylate.

**salicylsalicylic acid** (sal'ĭ-sil-sal'ĭ-sil'ik). SALYSAL; the salicylic ester of salicylic acid; antipyretic, analgesic, and antirheumatic.

**sal'icylsulfon'ic acid.** Sulfosalicylic acid.

**salicyluric acid** (sal'ĭ-sil-u'rik). The conjugation product of glycine with salicylic acid; excreted in urine after the administration of salicylic acid or some of its compounds.

**salient** (sāl'yent) [ L. *salio,* to leap or spring up ]. Promi-nence; projection.

**pulmonary s.,** the middle of the three convexities forming the left cardiovascular border in the teleroentgenogram or on fluoroscopy; it is composed of the main pulmonary artery and its left main branch.

**salifiable** (sal-ĭ-fi'a-bl). Capable of being made into salts; said of a base that combines with acids to make salts.

**sal'ify.** To convert into a salt.

**saligen'in.** Salicyl alcohol.

**salimeter** (sā-lim'e-ter). A hydrometer used to determine the specific gravity, or the concentration, of a saline solution.

**saline** (sa'lēn, -līn). Relating to, of the nature of, or contain-ing salt; salty.

**physiological s.,** an isotonic aqueous solution of salts in which cells will remain alive for a time; contains 0.9 per cent sodium chloride.

**sal'ini'grin.** A glycoside of p-hydroxyacetophenone; $CH_3COC_6H_4OC_6H_{11}O_5$; needle-shaped crystals, obtained from the bark of *Salix discolor* (family Salicaceae) and from needles and sprouts of plants of the family Coniferae; has been used as a substitute for salicin.

**salinometer** (sal'ĭ-nom'e-ter). [ G. *metron,* measure ]. A hydrometer so calibrated as to give a direct reading of the percentage of a particular salt present in solution.

**sal'it.** The salicylic-acid ester of borneol, bornyl, or borneol salicylate; an oily liquid, insoluble in water. Has been used externally in gout and rheumatism, neuralgia, and other painful conditions.

**saliva** (sā-li'vah) [ L. akin to G. *sialon* ] [ NA ]. Spittle; a clear, tasteless, odorless, slightly acid (pH 6.8) viscid fluid, consisting of the secretion from the parotid, sublingual, and submaxillary salivary glands and the mucous glands of the oral cavity; its function is to keep the mucous membrane of the mouth moist, to lubricate the food during mastication, and, in a measure, to convert starch into maltose, the latter action being effected by a diastatic enzyme, ptyalin.

    **chorda s.,** the secretion of the submaxillary gland obtained by stimulation of the chorda tympani nerve.

    **ganglion'ic s.,** submaxillary s. obtained by direct irritation of the gland.

    **resting s.,** the s. found in the mouth in the intervals of food taking and mastication.

    **sympathetic s.,** submaxillary s. obtained by stimulation of the sympathetic fibers innervating the gland.

**sal'ivant.** 1. Causing a flow of saliva. 2. Salivator; an agent that increases the flow of saliva.

**salivary** (sal'ĭ-věr-ĭ) [ L. *salivarius* ]. Relating to saliva.

**sal'ivate.** To cause an excessive flow of saliva.

**salivation** (sal'ĭ-va'shun). Sialism.

**sal'ivator.** Salivant (2).

**sali'volithi'asis.** Sialolithiasis.

**Salk,** Jonas, American immunologist, *1914. See S. *vaccine.*

**sal-lamziekte** (sal-lahm'zĕk-teh). Botulism.

**sal'man.** A hydrolysis product of salmine formed under the catalytic influence of carboxypeptidase B; differs from salmine in the loss of two arginine residues at the C-terminal.

**sal'mine.** A protamine present in the salmon sperm; made up of some 70 amino acid residues, of which most are arginine.

**Salmon,** Daniel E., American pathologist, 1850–1914. Gave his name to *Salmonella.*

**Salmonella** (sal'mo-nel'ah) [ D. *Salmon* ]. A genus of aerobic to facultatively anaerobic bacteria (family Enterobacteriaceae) containing Gram-negative rods that are either motile or nonmotile. Motile cells are peritrichous. These organisms do not liquefy gelatin or produce indole; they vary in their production of hydrogen sulfide. The metabolism of these organisms is fermentative. They produce acid and usually gas from glucose, but they do not attack lactose. Most of these organisms are aerogenic, but *S. typhi* never produces gas. They utilize citrate as a sole source of carbon. They are pathogenic for man and other animals. The type species is *S. choleraesuis.*

    **S. aborti'voequina,** a species causing abortion in mares; also infects guinea pigs, rabbits, goats, and cows, producing abortion.

    **S. abor'tusovis,** a species causing abortion in sheep.

    **S. chol'eraesu'is,** hog cholera bacillus; a species which occurs in pigs, where it is an important secondary invader in the virus disease hog cholera; does not occur as a natural pathogen in other animals; occasionally causes acute gastroenteritis and enteric fever in humans. It is the type species of the genus *S.*

    **S. enterit'idis,** Gärtner's bacillus; a species which is widely distributed. It occurs in humans and in domestic and wild animals, especially rodents.

    **S. gallina'rum,** a species causing fowl typhoid; it causes white diarrhea in young chicks and occasionally causes food poisoning or gastroenteritis in man.

    **S. hirschfeld'ii** (L. *Hirschfeld*), a species causing enteric fever in man.

    **S. paraty'phi,** a species causing enteric fever in man; not known to be pathogenic for other animals.

    **S. schottmuelleri** (H. *Schottmüller*), a species causing enteric fever in man; found rarely in cattle, sheep, swine, chickens, and lower primates.

    **S. typhi,** *S. typhosa;* Eberth's bacillus; a species found in human cases of typhoid fever and in contaminated water and food; it was found once in a chicken. The name *S. typhi* has been conserved over *S. typhosa* in an opinion issued by the Judicial Commission of the International Committee on Systematic Bacteriology.

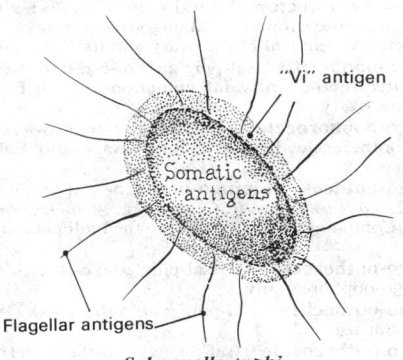

*Salmonella typhi*

Antigenic structure

    **S. ty'phimu'rium,** a species causing food poisoning in humans; it is a natural pathogen of all warm-blooded animals and is also found in snakes.

    **S. typho'sa,** *S. typhi.*

**salmonellosis** (sal'mo-nel-o'sis) [ *Salmonella* + G. suffix *-osis,* condition ]. Infection with organisms of the genus *Salmonella.*

**sal'ol.** Phenyl salicylate.

**salping-.** See salpingo-.

**salpingectomy** (sal'pin-jek'to-mĭ) [ salping- + G. *ektomē,* excision ]. Removal of the Fallopian tube.

    **abdominal s.,** celiosalpingectomy; laparosalpingectomy; removal of one or both Fallopian tubes through an abdominal incision.

**salpingemphraxis** (sal'pin-jem-frak'sis) [ salping- + G. *emphraxis,* a stopping ]. Obstruction of the Eustachian or of the Fallopian tube.

**salpingian** (sal-pin'jĭ-an). Relating to the uterine (Fallopian) tube or to the auditory (Eustachian) tube.

**salpingioma** (sal-pin'jĭ-o'mah) [ salping- + G. suffix *-oma,* tumor ]. Any tumor arising in the tissues of a uterine tube.

**salpingitic** (sal'pin-jit'ik). Relating to salpingitis.

**salpingitis** (sal'pin-ji'tis) [ salping- + G. suffix *-itis,* inflammation ]. Inflammation of the Fallopian tube, or of the Eustachian tube.

    **chronic interstitial s.,** s. in which fibrosis or mononuclear cell infiltration involves all layers of the Fallopian or Eustachian tube.

    **foreign body s.,** s. in which giant cells form in the tissue, as a result of introduction of foreign material into the Fallopian tube.

    **gonorrheal s.,** inflammation of the Fallopian tube following acute gonorrheal infection.

    **s. isth'mica nodo'sa,** adenosalpingitis; a condition of the Fallopian tube characterized by nodular thickening of the tunica muscularis of the isthmic portion of the tube.

    **pyogenic s.,** a form of acute s. usually occurring with puerperal infection.

**salpingo-, salping-** [ G. *salpinx,* trumpet (tube). SALP- ]. Combining form meaning tube, denoting usually the Fallopian or Eustachian tubes; see also tubo-.

**salpingocele** (sal-ping'go-sēl) [ salpingo- + G. *kēle,* hernia ]. Hernia of a Fallopian tube.

**salpingocyesis** (sal-ping'go-si-e'sis) [ salpingo- + G. *kyēsis,* pregnancy ]. Tubal *pregnancy.*

**salpingography** (sal'ping-gog'rä-fĭ) [ salpingo- + G. *graphō,* to write ]. Radiographic demonstration of the uterine tubes after the injection of a solution of a radiopaque compound.

**salpingolysis** (sal'ping-gol'ĭ-sis) [ salpingo- + G. *lysis*, loosening ]. Freeing the Fallopian tube from adhesions.

**salpingo-oophor-, salpingo-oophoro-** [ salpingo- + Mod. L. *oophoron*, ovary, fr. G. *ōophoros*, egg-bearing. OO- ]. Combining forms relating to the Fallopian tube and ovary.

**salpingo-oophorectomy** (sal-ping'go-o'of'o-rek'to-mĭ). Salpingo-oothecectomy; salpingo-ovariectomy; tubo-ovariectomy; removal of the ovary and its Fallopian tube.

**salpingo-oophoritis** (sal-ping'go-o'of-o-ri'tis). Salpingo-oothecitis; tubo-ovaritis; inflammation of both Fallopian tube and ovary.

**salpingo-oophorocele** (sal-ping'go-o-of'o-ro-sēl). Salpingo-oothecocele; hernia of both ovary and Fallopian tube.

**salpingo-oothec-, salpingo-ootheco-** [ salpingo- + Mod. L. *ootheca*, ovary, fr. G. *ōon*, egg, + *thēkē*, box, case. OO- ]. Combining forms relating to the Fallopian tube and ovary.

**salpingo-oothecectomy** (sal-ping'go-o'o-the-sek'to-mĭ). Salpingo-oophorectomy.

**salpingo-oothecitis** (sal-ping'go-o'o-the-si'tis). Salpingo-oophoritis.

**salpingo-oothecocele** (sal-ping'go-o'o-the'ko-sēl). Salpingo-oophorocele.

**salpingo-ovariectomy** (sal-ping'go-o-vār'ĭ-ek'to-mĭ). Salpingo-oophorectomy.

**salpingoperitonitis** (sal-ping'go-pĕr'-ĭ-to-ni'tis) [ salpingo- + peritonitis ]. Inflammation of the Fallopian tube, perisalpinx, and peritoneum.

**salpingopexy** (sal'ping-go-pek-sĭ) [ salpingo- + G. *pēxis*, fixation ]. The operative fixation of an oviduct.

**salpingopharyngeal** (sal-ping'go-fă-rin'je-al). Relating to the auditory (Eustachian) tube and pharynx.

**salpingopharyngeus** (sal-ping'go-făr-in-je'us) [ L. ]. See under musculus.

**salpingoplasty** (sal-ping'go-plas'tĭ) [ salpingo- + G. *plassō*, to fashion ]. Tuboplasty; plastic operation upon the uterine tubes.

**salpingorrhagia** (sal-ping'go-ra'jĭ-ah) [ salpingo- + G. *rhēgnymi*, to burst forth ]. Hemorrhage from a Fallopian tube.

**salpingorrhaphy** (sal'ping-gor'ă-fĭ) [ salpingo- + G. *rhaphē*, stitching ]. Suture of the Fallopian tube.

**salpingoscopy** (sal'ping-gos'ko-pĭ) [ salpingo- + G. *skopeō*, to view ]. Visualization of tubes, usually by x-ray or by means of a culdoscope.

**salpingostomatomy** (sal-ping'go-sto-mat'o-mĭ) [ salpingo- + G. *stoma*, mouth, + *tomē*, incision ]. Salpingostomy.

**salpingostomy** (sal'ping-gos'to-mĭ) [ salpingo- + G. *stoma*, mouth ]. Salpingostomatomy; establishment of an artificial opening in a Fallopian tube in cases in which the fimbriated extremity has been closed by inflammation.

**salpingotomy** (sal'ping-got'o-mĭ) [ salpingo- + G. *tomē*, incision ]. Incision into a Fallopian tube.

  **abdominal s.,** celiosalpingotomy; laparosalpingotomy; incision into the Fallopian tube (for tubal pregnancy, salpingitis, etc.) through an opening in the abdominal wall.

**salpingysterocyesis** (sal'pin-jis'ter-o-si-e'sis) [ salpingo- + G. *hystera*, uterus, + *kyēsis*, pregnancy ]. Ectopic pregnancy in the intramural or interstitial portion of the Fallopian tube.

**salpinx**, pl. **salpinges** (sal'pingks, sal-pin'jēz) [ G. a trumpet (tube) ]. SALP- ]. 1. *Tuba uterina*. 2. *Tuba auditiva*.

**salt.** 1. A compound formed by the interaction of an acid and a base, the hydrogen atoms of the acid being replaced by the positive ion of the base. 2. Sodium chloride, the prototypical salt.

  **acid s.,** bisalt; a s. in which all of the hydrogen of the acid is not replaced by the electropositive element; *e.g.*, NaHSO$_4$, KH$_2$PO$_4$.

  **artificial Carlsbad s.,** potassium sulfate 2, sodium chloride 18, sodium bicarbonate 36, dried sodium sulfate 44. Laxative.

  **artificial Kissingen s.,** potassium chloride 17, sodium chloride 357, anhydrous magnesium sulfate 59, sodium bicarbonate 107. Antacid and laxative.

  **artificial Vichy s.,** sodium bicarbonate 846, anhydrous magnesium sulfate 38.5, potassium carbonate 38.5, sodium chloride 77. Antacid.

  **basic s.,** one in which there are one or more hydroxy ions not replaced by the electronegative element of an acid; *e.g.*, Fe(OH)$_2$Cl.

  **binary s.,** a s., such as sodium chloride, that contains only two elements.

  **bone s.,** see bone-salt.

  **double s.,** one in which two different positive ions are bonded to the same negative ion, or vice versa, *e.g.*, NaKSO$_4$.

  **effervescent s.'s,** preparations made by adding sodium bicarbonate and tartaric and citric acids to the active s.; when thrown into water the acids break up the sodium bicarbonate, setting free the carbonic acid gas.

  **effervescent artificial Carlsbad s.,** made by the addition to the artificial Carlsbad salt 250, of sodium bicarbonate 400, tartaric acid 157, and citric acid 250.

  **effervescent artificial Kissingen s.,** made by the addition to the artificial Kissingen salt 400, sodium bicarbonate 406, tartaric acid 94, citric acid 250.

  **effervescent artificial Vichy s.,** artificial Vichy s. 250, sodium bicarbonate 485.5, tartaric acid 164.5, citric acid 250.

  **Epsom s.,** magnesium sulfate.

  **Glauber's s.,** sodium sulfate.

  **Rivière's s.,** potassium citrate.

  **Rochelle s.,** potassium sodium tartrate.

  **Seignette's s.,** potassium sodium tartrate.

  **smelling s.'s,** sal volatile; ammonium carbonate, scented with aromatic oils (lavender, nutmeg, etc.); sniffed as a general stimulant.

  **s. of wisdom,** sal alembroth.

**saltation** (sal-ta'shun) [ L. *saltatio*, fr. *salto*, pp. -*atus*, to dance, fr. *salio*, to leap ]. Dancing; leaping.

**Salter,** Sir Samuel J. A., English dentist, 1825–1897. See S.'s incremental *lines*.

**salt'ing out.** The precipitation of a protein from its solution by saturation or partial saturation with such neutral salts as sodium chloride, magnesium sulfate, or ammonium sulfate.

**saltpe'ter.** Potassium nitrate.

  **Chil'ean s.,** sodium nitrate.

**salubrious** (să-lu'brĭ-us) [ L. *salubris*, healthy, fr. *salus*, health ]. Healthful, usually in reference to climate.

**salubrity** (să-lu'brĭ-tĭ). State of being salubrious.

**saluresis** (sal'u-re'sis) [ L. *sal*, salt, + G. *ourēsis*, uresis (urination) ]. Excretion of sodium in the urine.

**saluretic** (sal'u-ret'ik) Facilitating the renal excretion of sodium.

**salutarium** (sal'u-ta'rĭ-um) [ L. *salutaris*, healthful, fr. *salus* (*salut-*), health ]. Sanitarium.

**salutary** (sal'u-tēr-ĭ) [ L. *salutaris* ]. Healthful; wholesome.

**Sal'varsan** [ L. *salvare*, to preserve, + *sanitas*, health ]. Historic proprietary name for arsphenamine.

**salve** (sav) [ A.S. *sealf* ]. An ointment or cerate.

**sal'verine.** MONTAMED; 2-[ 2-(diethylamino)ethoxy ]benzanilide; intestinal antispasmodic.

**salvia** (sal'vĭ-ah) [ L. ]. Sage; the dried leaves of *Salvia officinalis* (family Labiatae), garden sage or meadow sage; it inhibits secretory activity, especially of the sweat glands, and is also used in bronchitis and inflammation of the throat.

**Salzer** (zahlt'ser), Fritz A., Utrecht surgeon, *1858. See S.'s *operation*.

**Salzmann** (zahlts'mahn), Maximilian, Austrian ophthalmologist, 1862–1954. See S.'s *dystrophy*.

**samarium** (să-mēr'ĭ-um) [ bands indicating its presence first found in the spectrum of *samarskite*, a mineral named after Col. Samarski ]. A grayish white metallic element of the lanthanide, or rare earth, group, symbol Sm, atomic no. 62, atomic weight 150.35.

**sambu'cus** [ L. an elder-tree ]. Elder flowers; the dried flowers of *Sambucus canadensis* or *S. nigra* (family Caprifoliaceae), the common elder or black elder; slightly laxative.

**sam'ple.** In statistics, a portion of a population (*q. v.*) selected, often randomly, for research.

**random s.,** a selection on the basis of chance of individuals or items in a population for research; selection is made in such a way that all members presumably have the same chance of being selected.

**Sampson,** John A., U. S. gynecologist, 1873–1946. See S.'s *cyst.*

**Sanarel′li,** Giuseppe, Italian bacteriologist, 1864–1940. See S. *phenomenon,* S.-Shwartzman *phenomenon.*

**san′ative** [ L. *sano,* to cure, heal ]. Curative; healing.

**sanatorium** (san′ă-tōr′ĭ-um) [ Mod. L. neuter of *sanatorius,* curative, fr. *sano,* to cure, heal ]. An institution for the treatment of chronic diseases, such as tuberculosis, nervous disorders, chronic rheumatism, etc., and as a place for recuperation under medical supervision; often improperly called sanitarium.

**san′atory** [ Mod. L. *sanatorius* ]. Health-giving; curative.

**sancy′cline** (USAN). BONOMYCIN; 6-demethyl-6-deoxytetracycline; antimicrobial agent.

**sand** [ A.S. ]. The fine detritus of quartz and other crystalline rocks.

    **brain s.,** psammoma *bodies* (1).

    **hydatid s.,** the scoleces of *Echinococcus* tapeworms in the fluid within a primary or daughter hydatid cyst.

    **intestinal s.,** minute calculi or gritty material occurring in feces, composed of soaps, bile pigment, cholesterol, magnesium salts, succinic acid, etc.

**san′dalwood oil.** Santal oil.

**sand-crack.** A crack or fissure in the hoof of the horse, occurring usually on the inside of the forefoot (quarter-crack) or in the forepart of the hindfoot (toe-crack); when the crack is deep enough to expose the sensitive laminae, or when it extends to the coronary band, lameness results.

**Sandison-Clark chamber.** See under chamber.

**sand′paper.** Used for finishing and smoothing dental restorations. Available in various grits, and in disks on strips. The strips usually have a cloth backing.

**Sandström** (sahn′strĕm), I., Swedish physician, 1852–1889. See S.'s *bodies.*

**sand′worm.** Any of the various dog and cat hookworms whose larvae cause cutaneous larva migrans.

**sane** [ L. *sanus* ]. Denoting sanity.

**Sanfilippo,** Sylvester J. See S.'s *syndrome.*

**Sanger's reagent.** See under reagent.

**Sanger-Brown ataxia.** See under ataxia.

**sangui-, sanguin-, sanguino-** [ G. *sanguis,* blood. SANG- ]. Combining forms meaning blood, bloody.

**sanguifacient** (sang′gwĭ-fa′shĭ-ent) [ sangui- + L. *facio,* to make ]. Hemopoietic.

**sanguiferous** (sang-gwif′er-us) [ sangui- + L. *fero,* to carry ]. Circulatory; conveying blood.

**sanguification** (sang′gwĭ-fĭ-ka′shun) [ sangui- + L. *facio,* to make ]. Hemopoiesis.

**sanguinaria** (sang′gwĭ-nĕr′ĭ-ah) [ L. a herb that stanches blood, fr. *sanguis,* blood ]. The rhizome of *Sanguinaria canadensis* (family Papaveraceae); bloodroot; tetterwort; a common wild flower of eastern North America; formerly used as an expectorant.

**sanguinarine** (sang-gwin′ă-rēn, -rin). An alkaloid from sanguinaria; $C_{20}H_{15}NO_5.$

**sanguine** (sang′gwin) [ L. *sanguineus* ]. 1. Plethoric. 2. hopeful; full of vitality.

**sanguineous** (sang-gwin′e-us) [ L. *sanguineus* ]. 1. Relating to blood; bloody. 2. Plethoric.

**sanguinolent** (sang-gwin′o-lent) [ L. *sanguinolentus* ]. Bloody; tinged with blood.

**sanguinopurulent** (sang′gwĭ-no-pu′ru-lent) [ sanguino- + L. *purulentus,* festering (suppurative), fr. *pus,* pus ]. Denoting exudate or matter containing blood and pus.

**sanguinous** (sang′gwĭ-nus). Sanguineous.

**sanguis** (sang′gwis) [ L. ] [ NA ]. Blood.

**Sanguisuga** (sang-gwi-su′gah) [ L. a leech, fr. *sanguis,* blood, + *sugo,* pp. *suctus,* to suck ]. Former name for a genus of leeches, now called *Hirudo.*

**sanguivorous** (sang′gwiv′er-us) [ sangui- + L. *voro,* to devour ]. Bloodsucking, as applied to certain bats, leeches, insects, etc.

**sanies** (sa′nĭ-ēz) [ L. See SANG- ]. A thin, blood-stained, purulent discharge.

**saniopurulent** (sa′nĭ-o-pu′ru-lent) [ L. *sanies,* thin, bloody matter, + *purulentus,* festering (suppurative), fr. *pus,* pus ]. Characterized by bloody pus.

**sa′niose′rous.** Characterized by blood-tinged serum.

**sanious** (sa′nĭ-us). Relating to sanies; ichorous and blood-stained.

**sanitarian** (san′ĭ-tĕr′ĭ-an) [ L. *sanitas,* health, fr. *sanus,* sound ]. A hygienist; one versed in the science of public health.

**sanitarium** (san′ĭ-tĕr′ĭ-um) [ L. *sanitas,* health ]. A health resort; not to be confused with sanatorium.

**sanitary** (san′ĭ-tĕr-ĭ) [ L. *sanitus,* health ]. Healthful; conducive to health.

**sanitation** (san′ĭ-ta′shun) [ L. *sanitas,* health ]. The use of measures designed to promote health and prevent disease; the development and establishment of conditions in the environment favorable to health.

**sanitization** (san′ĭ-tĭ-za′shun). The process of making something sanitary, as in the sterilization of eating utensils.

**sanity** (san′ĭ-tĭ) [ L. *sanitas,* health ]. Soundness of mind, emotions, and behavior; mental health.

**Sansom,** Arthur E., English physician, 1838–1907. See S.'s *sign.*

**Sanson** (sahn-son′), Louis J., French physician, 1790–1841. See Purkinje-S. *images,* S. *images.*

**san′tal oil.** Sandalwood oil; East Indian sandalwood oil; a volatile oil distilled from the wood of *Santalum album* (family Santalaceae), a tree of India; used in subacute bronchitis and in gonorrhea.

**san′talol.** Two isomeric sesquiterpene alcohols, $C_{15}H_{24}O;$ the α-santalol is tricyclic and the β-santalol is bicyclic, forming almost the entire part of sandalwood (santal) oil; used as a urinary antiseptic.

**Santini's booming sound.** See under sound.

**santon′ica** [ G. *santonikon,* wormwood ]. Levant wormseed; semen-contra; the unexpanded flower heads of *Artemisia cina* (family Compositae), a shrub growing in Turkestan; the source of santonin.

**san′tonin.** The inner anhydride or lactone of santoninic acid; obtained from the unexpanded flower heads of *Artemisia cina* and other species of *Artemisia* (family Compositae); has been used to effect expulsion of roundworms (*Ascaris lumbricoides*), and in the treatment of urinary incontinence.

**Santorini** (sahn-to-re′ne), Giovanni D., Italian anatomist, 1681–1737. See S.'s *canal, cartilage,* major and minor *caruncle, concha, duct, fissures, incisure, labyrinth, muscle, tubercle, veins.*

**san′tyl.** Santalyl salicylate; salicylic acid ester of santalol; has been used as a urinary antiseptic.

**sap.** The juice or tissue fluid of a living organism.

    **nuclear s.,** karyolymph.

**saphena** (să-fe′nah) [ Med. L. attributed by some as derived fr. Ar. *safin,* standing; by others, fr. G. *saphēnēs,* manifest, clearly visible ]. See *vena* saphena.

**saphenectomy** (saf′e-nek′to-mĭ) [ saphena + G. *ektomē,* excision ]. Excision of a saphenous vein.

**saphenous** (să-fe′nus) [ see saphena ]. Relating to or associated with a saphenous vein; denoting a number of structures in the leg.

**sa′po** [ L. fr. ancient Ger. ]. Soap.

**sapo-, sapon-** [ L. *sapo,* soap ]. Combining forms relating to soap.

**sapogenin** (să-poj′ĕ-nin). The aglycone of a saponin; one of a family of steroids of the spirostan type (*i.e.,* a 16,22:22,26-diepoxycholestane; see structure XI under steroids).

**saponaceous** (sap′o-na′shus). Soapy; relating to or resembling soap.

**sapona′tus** [ L. ]. Mixed with soap.

**saponification** (să-pon′ĭ-fĭ-ka′shun) [ L. *sapo* (*sapon-*), soap, + *facio,* to make ]. Conversion into soap; denoting the hydrolytic action of an alkali upon fat.

    **s. number,** the number of milligrams of KOH required to saponify 1 gm. of fat; it is a roughly approximate measure of the average molecular weight of a fat, with which it varies inversely.

**sapon'ify.** To make into soap.

**sap'onins.** A class of non-nitrogenous glycosides found in many plants which possess the common property of foaming, or making suds, when strongly agitated in aqueous solution; they can hold resinous and fatty substances in suspension in water; they are amorphous bodies as a rule, though a few are crystallizable, and possess the properties of glycosides; they are irritants when applied to the skin or mucous membranes, and given internally cause nausea and vomiting.

**sapota** (sah-po'tah) [ Sp. *zapote* ]. The fruit of *Achras sapota* (family Sapotaceae), a tree of tropical America, having diuretic properties. The dried latex is known as Mexican chicle. Used in making chewing gum.

**sapotoxin** (sap'o-tok'sin). A glycosidal principle from quillaia, or soap-bark; a saponin.

**sappan** (să-pan') [ Malay ]. Indian redwood; false sandalwood. The heart-wood of *Caesalpinia sappan* (family Leguminosae); used to make a dye, and in medicine as an astringent, similarly to hematoxylon.

**Sappey** (sap-a'), Marie P. C., French anatomist, 1810–1896. See S.'s *fibers, ligament, plexus, veins.*

**sapphism** (saf'izm) [ *Sappho*, homosexual Greek poetess, queen of the island of Lesbos ]. Lesbianism.

**sapr-.** See sapro-.

**sapremia** (să-pre'mĭ-ah) [ sapr- + G. *haima*, blood ]. Septicemia.

**sapre'mic.** Relating to or suffering from sapremia.

**sap'rine.** A ptomaine from the putrefying abdominal viscera.

**sapro-, sapr-** (sap'ro-) [ G. *sapros*, rotten ]. Combining forms meaning rotten or putrid; decaying; decayed.

**saprocyclozoonosis** (sap-ro-si'klo-zo-o-no'sis). See saprozoonosis and cyclozoonosis.

**saprodontia** (sap'ro-don'shĭ-ah) [ sapro- + G. *odous*, tooth ]. Dental *caries.*

**saprogen** (sap'ro-jen) [ sapro- + G. suffix -*gen*, producing ]. An organism living on dead organic matter and causing the decay thereof.

**saprogenic, saprogenous** (sa-pro-jen'ik, să-proj'en-us). Causing or resulting from decay.

**saprometazoonosis** (sap-ro-met'ah-zo-o-no'sis). See saprozoonosis and metazoonosis.

**saprophilous** (să-prof'ĭ-lus) [ sapro- + G. *philos*, fond ]. Thriving on decaying organic matter.

**saprophyte** (sap'ro-fit) [ sapro- + G. *phyton*, plant ]. Necroparasite; an organism that grows on dead organic matter, plant or animal.

    **facultative s.,** an organism which is usually parasitic but which may, on occasion, live and grow as a s.

**saprophytic** (sap-ro-fit'ik). Relating to a saprophyte; obtaining nourishment from dead organic matter.

**sapropyra** (sap'ro-pi'rah) [ sapro- + G. *pyr*, fire ]. Typhus.

**sap'roty'phus.** Typhus.

**saprozoic** (sap'ro-zo'ik) [ sapro- + G. *zōikos*, relating to animals ]. Living in decaying organic matter; denoting especially certain protozoa.

**saprozoonosis** (sap'ro-zo-o-no'sis) [ sapro- + G. *zōon*, animal, + *nosos*, disease ]. A zoonosis the agent of which requires both a vertebrate host and a nonanimal (food, soil, plant) reservoir or developmental site for completion of its cycle. Combination terms may be used, such as saprometazoonoses for flukes whose metacercariae encyst on plants, or saprocyclozoonoses for ticks with more than one host, part of whose life cycles are passed on the soil.

**sarapus** (săr'ă-pus) [ G. *sarapous*, splay-footed ]. A flat-footed person.

**Sarcina** (sar'sĭ-nah) [ L. *sarcina*, a pack, bundle, fr. *sarcio*, to mend, patch ]. A genus of nonmotile, strictly anaerobic bacteria (family Micrococcaceae) containing Gram-positive cocci, 1.8 to 3.0 μm in diameter, which divide in three perpendicular planes, producing regular packets of eight or more cells. The metabolism of these chemoorganotrophic organisms is fermentative. Saprophytic and facultatively parasitic species occur. The type species is *S. ventriculi.*

**S. maxima,** a species from the hull or outer coat of cereal grains such as wheat, oat, rice, and rye, and from horse manure and soil.

**S. ventric'uli,** a species found in soil, mud, the contents of a diseased human stomach, rabbit and guinea pig stomach contents, and on the surfaces of cereal seeds. It is the type species of the genus *S.*

**sar'cine.** 1. Hypoxanthine. 2. A packet of cocci of the genus *Sarcina.*

**sarcin'ic.** Relating to the genus *Sarcina.*

**sarcitis** (sar-si'tis) [ G. *sarx*, flesh, + suffix -*itis*, inflammation ]. Myositis.

**sarco-** (sar'ko-) [ G. *sarx* (*sark*-), flesh. SARC- ]. Combining form denoting muscular substance or a resemblance to flesh.

**sar'coadeno'ma.** Adenosarcoma.

**sar'coblast** [ sarco- + G. *blastos*, germ ]. Myoblast.

**sar'cocarcino'ma.** Carcinosarcoma.

**sarcocele** (sar'ko-sēl) [ sarco- + G. *kēlē*, tumor ]. A fleshy tumor or sarcoma of the testis.

**Sarcocystis** (sar'ko-sis'tis) [ sarco- + G. *kystis*, bladder ]. A genus of protozoan parasites, related to the sporozoan genera *Toxoplasma* and *Besnoitea*, placed in a separate order (Toxoplasmida) or combined with the true coccidia (*e.g., Eimeria, Isospora, Tyzerria*) in a single suborder (Eimeriorina); recent discoveries show closer similarities and probable relationship among *Eimeria, Toxoplasma,* and *S.* Tissue stages of *S.* are usually seen as thick-walled cylindrical or fusiform cycts (Miescher's tubes) in reptile, bird or mammal striated muscles. Cysts are smooth in the house mouse form or with radial spines (cytophaneres) in sheep or rabbit cysts; contents may be compartmentalized by septa. Variably-shaped spores (Rainey's corpuscles) probably are peripheral, rounded cells (sporoblasts, cytomeres) that divide to form mature "spores" (bradyzoites), 5 to 12 μ by 1 to 4 μ, that are motile bodies when released from the cyst; sexual stages have been described in tissue cultures. These parasites are not of pathogenic significance.

**S. fusifor'mis,** found in the striated and heart muscle of cattle and water buffalo.

**S. lindeman'ni,** species described from man by Lindemann in 1868 and named by Rivolta in 1878; it has been described on rare occasions from the striated and heart muscles of man, but it is probably an infection from domestic animals and not a distinct species from man.

**S. miescheria'na,** a common species of worldwide distribution that is found in the striated and heart muscle of pigs; it is the type species of the genus *S.*

**S. tenel'la,** an extremely common species of worldwide distribution that is found in the striated and heart muscle of sheep and goats.

**sarcocystosis** (sar'ko-sis-to'sis). Infection with *Sarcocystis.*

**sarcode** (sar'kōd) [ sarco- + G. *eidos*, resemblance ]. A term of historical interest (1835), applied to the protoplasm of Protista before the term protoplasm was coined.

**Sarcodina** (sar'ko-di'nah, -de'nah) [ Mod. L. fr. G. *sarx*, flesh ]. A superclass of protozoa in the subphylum Sarcomastigophora, possessing pseudopodia for locomotion, *e.g.,* ameba.

**sarcoenchondroma** (sar'ko-en-kon-dro'mah). Chondrosarcoma.

**sarcoglia** (sar-kog'lĭ-ah) [ sarco- + G. *glia*, glue ]. The accumulation of neurolemma cells at the motor end-plate.

**sarcoid** (sar'koyd) [ sarco- + G. *eidos*, resemblance ]. 1. Sarcoidosis. 2. A tumor resembling a sarcoma.

    **Boeck's s.** 1, sarcoidosis.

**sarcoidosis** (sar'koy-do'sis) [ sarcoid + G. suffix -*osis*, condition ]. Sarcoid; Boeck's sarcoid; Besnier-Boeck-Schaumann syndrome or disease; a systemic granulomatous disease of unknown cause, especially involving the lungs with resulting fibrosis, also involving lymph nodes, skin, liver, spleen, eyes, phalangeal bones, and parotid glands. The granulomas are composed of epithelioid and multinucleated giant cells with little or no necrosis. The Kveim test is often positive, the tuberculin test negative, and hypercalcemia and hyperglobulinemia are common.

    **hypercalcemic s.,** s. with hypercalcemia of unknown cause, not necessarily associated with detectable bone involvement by s.; found in about one fifth of patients with s. and responsive to corticosteroids.

**sar'colac'tic acid.** L-Lactic acid.

**sarcolemma** (sar'ko-lem'ah) [ sarco- + G. *lemma*, husk ]. The plasma membrane of a muscle fiber; formerly, the delicate connective tissue of the endomysium was included under this term by some.

**sarcolem'mal, sarcolem'mic, sarcolem'mous.** Relating to the sarcolemma.

**sarcology** (sar'kol'o-jĭ) [ sarco- + G. *logos*, study ]. 1. Myology. 2. The anatomy of the soft parts, as distinguished from osteology.

**sar'coly'sine.** Merphalan.

**sarcoma** (sar-ko'mah) [ G. *sarkōma*, a fleshy excrescence, fr. *sarx*, flesh, + suffix *-oma*, tumor ]. A tumor, usually highly malignant, formed by proliferation of mesodermal cells; a malignant connective tissue neoplasm.

    **Abernethy's s.,** a variety of neoplasm, consisting of malignant fat cells (liposarcoma), found chiefly on the trunk.

    **alveolar soft part s.,** a tumor formed of a reticular stroma of connective tissue enclosing numerous, large, round or polygonal cells; occurs in subcutaneous and fibromuscular tissues.

    **angiolith'ic s.,** psammoma.

    **s. botryoides, botryoid s.,** a polypoid form of rhabdomyosarcoma that occurs in children, most frequently in the urogenital tract; characterized by the formation of grossly apparent grapelike clusters of neoplastic tissue that consists of rhabdomyoblasts, spindle, and stellate cells in a myxomatous stroma; the neoplasms of this type grow relatively rapidly and are highly malignant, chiefly as a result of their position and invasiveness (but metastases may occur).

    **decid'uocel'lular s.,** choriocarcinoma.

    **enceph'aloid s.,** round cell s.

    **endometrial stromal s.,** stromal endometriosis; stromatosis; a term sometimes used for a relatively rare sarcoma believed to be a form of endometriosis in which the lesions form multiple foci in the myometrium and in vascular spaces in other sites, and consisting of histologic and cytologic elements that resemble those of the endometrial stroma.

    **Ewing's s.,** Ewing's *tumor.*

    **fascic'ular s.,** spindle cell s.

    **giant cell s.,** a malignant giant cell *tumor* of bone.

    **Jensen's s.,** a mouse tumor transmissible by inoculation.

    **juxtacortical osteogenic s.,** a form of osteogenic s. of relatively low malignancy; probably arising from the periosteum and initially involving cortical bone and adjacent connective tissue; occurs in middle-aged as well as young adults, and most commonly affects the lower part of the femoral shaft.

    **Kaposi's s.,** multiple idiopathic hemorrhagic s.; a multifocal malignant or benign neoplasm of primitive vasoformative tissue, occurring in the skin and sometimes in lymph nodes or viscera; consists of spindle cells and small vascular spaces, frequently infiltrated by hemosiderin-pigmented macrophages.

    **leukocyt'ic s.,** leukemia.

    **lymphatic s.,** lymphosarcoma.

    **med'ullary s.,** a soft, extremely vascular, malignant growth.

    **melanot'ic s.,** a malignant melonoma; see melanoma.

    **multiple idiopath'ic hemorrhag'ic s.,** Kaposi's s.

    **myelogen'ic s.,** one originating in the bone marrow.

    **my'eloid s.,** a mixed s. containing both round and spindle cells.

    **osteogen'ic s.,** osteosarcoma; osteoma sarcomatosum; the most common and malignant of bone s.'s; it arises from bone-forming cells and affects chiefly the ends of long bones. Its greatest incidence is in the age group between 10 and 25 years.

    **os'teoid s.,** a s. containing bony tissue.

    **reticulum cell s.,** a malignant lymphoma composed of reticulum cells, sometimes limited to a single organ, or disseminated in lymphoid tissues.

    **round cell s.,** encephaloid s.; an undifferentiated malignant neoplasm, believed to be of mesenchymal origin, composed chiefly of closely packed round cells.

**Rous s.,** a fibrosarcoma originally from a Plymouth Rock hen and shown in 1910 by Peyton Rous to be caused by a virus; it is now thought to be an expression of infection by the avian leukosis-sarcoma virus.

    **spindle cell s.,** fascicular s.; a malignant neoplasm, believed to be of mesenchymal origin, composed of elongated, spindle-shaped cells.

    **synovial s.,** malignant synovioma; a rare malignant tumor of synovial origin, composed of spindle cells usually enclosing slits or pseudoglandular spaces that may be lined by radially disposed epithelial-like cells; radioresistant and usually involving the knee joint.

**sarcomatoid** (sar-ko'mă-toyd) [ sarcoma + G. *eidos*, resemblance ]. Resembling a sarcoma.

**sarcomatosis** (sar-ko'mă-to'sis) [ sarcoma + G. suffix *-osis*, condition ]. The occurrence of several sarcomatous growths on different parts of the body.

    **s. genera'lis,** *mycosis* fungoides.

**sarcomatous** (sar-ko'mă-tus). Relating to or of the nature of sarcoma.

**sarcomere** (sar'ko-mēr) [ sarco- + G. *meros*, part ]. The part of a cross-striated muscle fiber between two adjacent Z lines.

**sarcomphalocele** (sar-kom'fă-lo-sēl) [ sarco- + G. *omphalos*, umbilicus, + *kēlē*, tumor ]. A hard fleshy tumor at or near the umbilicus.

**sarcomyces** (sar-ko-mi'sēz) [ sarco- + G. *mykēs*, fungus ]. A fungous fleshy growth.

**sar'coneme** [ sarco- + G. *nema*, thread ]. Microneme.

**sarcoplasm** (sar'ko-plazm) [ sarco- + G. *plasma*, a thing formed ]. The nonfibrillar cytoplasm of a muscle fiber.

**sarcoplas'mic.** Relating to sarcoplasm.

**sar'coplast** [ sarco- + G. *plastos*, formed ]. One of the rounded interfibrillary cells in a muscle fiber.

**sarcopoietic** (sar'ko-poy-et'ik) [ sarco- + G. *poiēsis*, a making ]. Forming muscle.

**Sarcopsyl'la pen'etrans.** Incorrect name for *Tunga penetrans.*

**Sarcopsyllidae** (sar-kop-sil'lĭ-de) [ sarco- + G. *psylla*, flea ]. A family of fleas, containing the species *Tunga penetrans* or jigger.

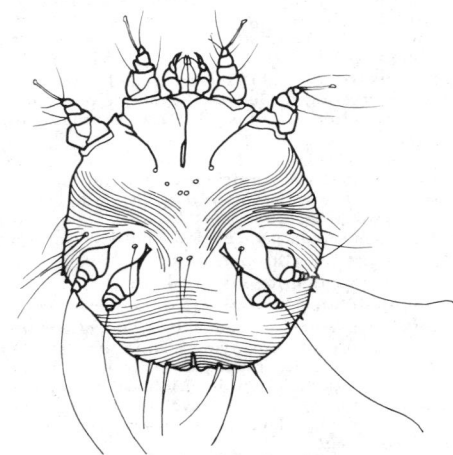

***Sarcoptes scabiei*, Scabies or Itch Mite** (×100)
(From Najarian, H. H.: *Textbook of Medical Parasitology,*
The Williams & Wilkins Co., Baltimore, 1967.)

**Sarcoptes scabiei** (sar-kop'tez ska'bĭ-i) [ sarco- + G. *koptō*, to cut; L. *scabies*, scurf ]. Itch mite; varieties are distributed worldwide and affect man, horses, cattle, swine, sheep, dogs, cats, and many wild animals. Serious and fatal infections are not uncommon in untreated animals. Although considered to belong to a single species, they do not readily pass from one host to another of a different animal species; transitory infections of this type do occur, however, especially from various animals to man, and are spread by direct contact. The mite burrows into the skin and lays eggs within the burrow; intense itching and rash (probably a sensitization response) develop near the burrow in about a month. See scabies, mange.

**sar'cosine.** CH₃NHCH₂COOH; *N*-methylglycine.

**sarcosis** (sar-ko'sis) [ G. *sarkōsis*, the growth of flesh, fr. *sarx*, flesh ]. 1. An abnormal increase of flesh. 2. A multiple growth of fleshy tumors. 3. A diffuse sarcoma involving the whole of an organ.

**sarcosome** (sar'ko-sōm) [ sarco- + G. *soma*, body ]. 1. Formerly, any granule in a muscle fiber. 2. Sometimes now used synonymously with myomitochondrion.

**sarcostosis** (sar'kos-to'sis) [ sarco- + G. *osteon*, bone, + suffix -*osis*, condition ]. Ossification of muscular tissue.

**sarcostyle** (sar'ko-stīl) [ sarco- + G. *stylos*, pillar ]. An obsolete term formerly applied to a bundle of myofibrils by some, and to a single fibril by others.

**sarcot'ic.** 1. Relating to sarcosis. 2. Causing an increase of flesh.

**sar'cotrip'sy** [ sarco- + G. *tripsis*, a rubbing ]. Use of a crushing forceps to stop hemorrhage.

**sarcotubules** (sar'ko-tu'būlz). The continuous system of membranous tubules in striated muscle which corresponds to the smooth endoplasmic reticulum of other cells.

**sar'cous** [ G. *sarx*, flesh ]. Relating to muscular tissue; muscular; fleshy.

**sardon'ic grin** [ G. *sardanios*, (later) *sardonios*, an adj. used only as an epithet of bitter, scornful laughter ]. *Risus sardonicus* or *caninus*.

**sarin** (zah-rēn') [ Ger. ]. Isopropyl methylphosphonofluoridate; a nerve poison similar to diisopropylfluorophosphate and tetraethylpyrophosphate; a very potent irreversible cholinesterase inhibitor. It is a more toxic nerve gas than tabun or soman.

**sarmassa'tion** [ G. *sarx*, flesh, + *massein*, to knead ]. Erotic squeezing, kneading, or caressing of female tissues and organs.

**sarsaparilla** (sar'sah-per-il'ah, sas'per-il'ah) [ Sp. *zarza*, a bramble ]. The dried root of *Smilax aristolochioefolia* (Mexican s.), *S. regelii* (Honduras s.), *S. febrifuga* (Ecuadorian s.), or of undetermined species of *Smilax* (family Liliaceae), a thorny vine widely distributed throughout the tropical and semitropical world. It has been used in psoriasis, gout, rheumatism, and syphilis, and popularly as a "blood purifier."

**sartorius** (sar-to'rī-us) [ L. *sartor*, a tailor, the muscle being used in crossing the legs in the tailor's position, fr. *sarcio*, pp. *sartus*, to patch, mend ]. See under *musculus*.

**sassafras** (sas'ă-fras). The dried bark of the root of *Sassafras albidum* (family Lauraceae), a tree of the eastern United States; a flavoring agent, diuretic, and diaphoretic.

**s. oil,** a volatile oil obtained by distillation from the bark of *Sassafras albidum* and *S. variifolium;* carminative, topical antiseptic, pediculicide, and flavoring agent.

**sas'sy bark.** Erythrophleum.

**sat.** Abbreviation for saturated.

**sa'tanopho'bia.** Morbid fear of the devil (Satan).

**satellite** (sat'ĕ-lit) [ L. *satelles* (*sattelit-*), attendant ]. A minor structure accompanying a more important or larger one, as a vein accompanying an artery, or a small or secondary skin lesion in the neighborhood of a larger one; a small structure or body revolving around a larger one, *e.g.,* a secondary planet or space system revolving around a primary one.

**chromosome s.,** see under *chromosome*.

**nucleolar s.,** term originally given by Murray Barr to a small dot of chromatin found adjacent to the nucleolus in nerve cells of females but not in those of males; see sex chromatin.

**perineuronal s.,** an oligodendroglia cell surrounding the neuron.

**satellitosis** (sat'ĕ-lī-to'sis) [ L. *satelles* (*satellit-*), attendant, + G. -*ōsis* ]. A condition marked by an accumulation of neuroglia cells around the neurons of the central nervous system; often as a prelude to neuronophagia.

**satiation** (sa'shī-a'shun) [ L. *satio*, pp. -*atus*, to fill, satisfy ]. The state produced by having had a specific need fulfilled, such as hunger or thirst.

**sat. sol.** Abbreviation for saturated solution.

**Sattler,** Hubert, Austrian ophthalmologist, 1844–1928. See S.'s elastic *layer*, S.'s *veil.*

**saturate** (satch'u-rāt) [ L. *saturo*, pp. -*atus*, to fill, fr. *satur*, sated ]. 1. To impregnate to the greatest possible extent. 2. To neutralize; to satisfy all the chemical affinities of a substance (as by converting all double bonds to single bonds). 3. To dissolve a substance up to that concentration beyond which the addition of more results in two phases.

**saturation** (satch'u-ra'shun). 1. Impregnation of one substance by another to the greatest possible degree, as a liquid by a soluble salt or the atmosphere by vapor. 2. Neutralization, as of an acid by an alkali. 3. In optics, see saturated *color*. 4. That concentration of a dissolved substance that cannot be exceeded. 5. Filling of all the available sites on an enzyme molecule by its substrate, or on a hemoglobin molecule by oxygen (symbol $SO_2$) or carbon monoxide (symbol $SCO$).

**secondary s.,** a technique of nitrous oxide anesthesia that consists of an abrupt curtailment of the oxygen in the inhaled mixture in order to produce a deep or even profound plane of anesthesia, following which oxygen is administered to correct overdosage and produce muscular relaxation.

**saturnine** (sat'ur-nīn) [ Mediev. L. *saturninus*, fr. *saturnus*, lead, fr. L. *saturnis*, the god and planet Saturn ]. 1. Relating to lead. 2. Due to or symptomatic of lead poisoning.

**saturnism** (sat'ur-nizm) [ Mediev. L. *saturnus*, the alchemical term for lead ]. Lead *poisoning*.

**satyriasis** (sat-ī-ri'ă-sis) [ G. *satyros*, a satyr ]. Satyrism; satyromania; excessive sexual excitement and behavior in the male; formerly, the alleged condition in the male of being oversexed.

**satyrism** (sat'ī-rizm). Satyriasis.

**satyromania** (sat'ī-ro-ma'nī-ah) [ G. *satyros*, satyr, + *mania*, frenzy ]. Satyriasis.

**saucerization** (saw'ser-ī-za'shun). 1. Excision of tissue to form a shallow depression, in wound treatment. 2. The appearance presented by a crushed vertebra which often shows a saucer-like collapse on its horizontal surface.

**Sauerbruch** (zow'er-brookh), Ferdinand, Munich surgeon, 1875–1951. See S.'s *cabinet, prosthesis.*

**sauna** (sow'nah) [ Finn. ]. Finnish bath; steam bath of Finland followed by plunge in snow.

**Saundby,** Robert, English physician, 1849–1918. See S.'s *test.*

**sauriasis** (saw-ri'as-is) [ G. *sauros*, lizard, + suffix -*iasis*, condition ]. Ichthyosis.

**sauriderma** (saw'rī-der'mah) [ G. *sauros*, lizard, + *derma*, skin ]. Ichthyosis.

**sauriosis** (saw'rī-o'sis) [ G. *sauros*, lizard, + suffix -*osis*, condition ]. Ichthyosis.

**sauroderma** (saw'ro-der'mah) [ G. *sauros*, lizard, + *derma*, skin ]. Ichthyosis.

**sauropsida** (saw-rop'sī-dah) [ G. *sauros*, lizard, + *opsis*, appearance. OPO- ]. A vertebrate group which includes the birds and reptiles.

**Savage,** Henry, English anatomist and gynecologist, 1810–1900. See S.'s perineal *body.*

**Sav'ill,** Thomas D., London physician, 1856–1910. See S.'s *disease.*

**saw** [ A.S. *saga* ]. An instrument having an edge of sharp, toothlike projections; used in surgery for cutting bone.

**Gigli's s.,** a chain s. for use in craniotomy or pubiotomy.

**Shrady's subcutaneous s.,** an instrument consisting of a trocar and fenestrated cannula; when it has been introduced alongside the bone the trocar is withdrawn and a s. set in a shaft of the same diameter as the trocar, is introduced in its place.

**subcuta'neous s.,** Shrady's s.

**saw-palmet'to.** Serenoa.

**saxifragant** (sak-sīf'rā-gant) [ L. fr. *saxum*, stone, + *frango*, p.p. *fractus*, to break ]. Lithotriptic; possessing the power of dissolving or of crushing calculi.

**sax'itox'in.** A potent neurotoxin found in shellfish such as the mussel or the clam. It is produced by the dinoflagellate *Gonyaulax catenella,* which is ingested by the shellfish.

**Saxtorph,** Matthias, †1771. See S.'s *maneuver.*

**Sayre,** Lewis A., New York surgeon, 1820–1900. See S.'s suspension *apparatus*, S.'s *jacket*.

**Sb.** Chemical symbol of the element antimony (stibium).

**Sc.** Chemical symbol of the element scandium.

**s.c.** Abbreviation for subcutaneous, or subcutaneously.

**scab** (skab) [ A.S. *scaeb*]. A crust formed by coagulation of blood, pus, serum, or a combination of these, on the surface of an ulcer, erosion, or other type of wound.

**scabicidal** (ska′bĭ-si-dal). Destructive to itch mites.

**scabicide** (ska′bĭ-sīd). An agent lethal to itch mites.

**scabies** (ska′beez) [ L. fr. *scabo*, to scratch ]. 1. Seven-year itch; an eruption due to *Sarcoptes scabiei* var. *hominis*. The female of the species burrows into the skin, producing a vesicular eruption, with intense pruritus, between the fingers, on the male genitalia, buttocks, and elsewhere on the trunk and extremities. 2. In animals, the term scabies or scab is usually applied to cutaneous ascariasis in sheep, which may be caused by *Sarcoptes*, *Psoroptes* and *Chorioptes*. Mite infections causing dermatitis in wild and domestic animals, including sheep, are more commonly called mange, and may be caused by species and varieties of the genera listed above and of others such as *Demodex*, *Notoedres* and *Otodectes*. See mange.

    **Norwegian s.,** Norway itch; a severe form of s. caused by *Sarcoptes scabiei* var. *crustosae*.

**scabieticide** (ska-bĭ-et′ĭ-sīd). Scabicide.

**scabious** (ska′bĭ-us). Relating to or suffering from scabies.

**scabrities** (ska-brish′ĭ-ēz) [ L. fr. *scaber*, scurfy ]. Roughness of the skin.

    **s. un′guium,** thickening and distortion of the nails.

**scab′wort.** Elecampane.

**scala,** pl. **scalae** (ska′lah, -le) [ L. a stairway ] [ NA ]. One of the cavities of the cochlea winding spirally around the modiolus.

    **Löwenberg′s s.,** *ductus* cochlearis.

    **s. me′dia,** *ductus* cochlearis.

    **s. tym′pani** [ NA ], tympanic stairway; the division of the spiral canal of the cochlea lying below the lamina spiralis. See fig. under cochlea.

    **s. vestib′uli** [ NA ], vestibular canal; the division of the spiral canal of the cochlea lying above the lamina spiralis and vestibular membrane. See fig. under cochlea.

**scald** (skawld) [ L. *excaldo*, to wash in hot water ]. 1. To burn by contact with a hot liquid or steam. 2. The lesion resulting from such contact. 3 [ see scall ]. Any crusted or scaly lesion of the scalp, such as favus.

**scalding** (skawl′ding). A burning pain in urinating.

**scale** (skāl) [ 1. L. *scala*, a stairway. 2. O. E. *scealu*, fr. O. Fr. *escale*, shell, husk ]. 1. A strip of metal, glass, or other substance, marked off in lines, for measuring. 2. Squama. 3. A small thin plate of horny epithelium, resembling a fish s., cast off from the skin. 4. To desquamate. 5. To remove tartar from the teeth. 5. A standardized test for measuring psychological, personality, or behavioral characteristics; see also subentries under test.

    **absolute s.,** Kelvin s.

    **Ångström′s s.,** a table of wavelengths of a large number of light rays corresponding to as many Fraunhofer′s lines in the spectrum.

    **Baumé s.,** one of two hydrometer s.′s for determining the specific gravity of liquids heavier and lighter than water, respectively. To read the Baumé s. in terms of specific gravity: for liquids lighter than water divide 140 by 130 plus the Baumé degree; for liquids heavier than water divide 145 by 145 minus the Baumé degree.

    **Benois′ s.,** a s. for measuring penetrability of x-rays.

    **Binet s.,** a measure of intelligence designed for both children and adults.

    **Binet-Simon s.,** forerunner of individual intelligence tests, particularly the Stanford-Binet intelligence s.

    **Bloch′s s.,** a series of tubes with varying amounts of tincture of benzoin diluted in glycerolated water; the resulting turbid mixtures are used as a means of quantitatively estimating the amount of albumin precipitated from urine (or other body fluid) by means of heating or treatment with nitric acid.

    **Celsius s.,** centigrade s.

    **centigrade s.,** Celsius s.; the temperature s. in which there are 100 degrees (100°C.) between ice (0°C.) and boiling water at sea level (100°C.).

    **Charrière s.,** the French s. for grading the sizes of urethral catheters or sounds; the size of any instrument is determined by Charrière′s *filière*, a metal plate perforated with 30 holes varying in diameter from 1/3 to 1 cm., each differing from the next above or below in the scale by 1/3 mm.

    **Dunfermline s.** (dun-furm′lin) [ *Dunfermline*, a city in Scotland where the system was developed ], a s. of classification of children according to their condition of nutrition, as (1) superior, (2) passable, (3) requiring supervision, and (4) requiring medical care.

    **Fahrenheit s.,** a temperature thermometer s., in which the freezing point of water is 32° and the boiling point of water 212°; the zero indicates the lowest temperature Fahrenheit could obtain by a mixture of ice and salt. A degree Fahrenheit (abbreviated °F.) is 5/9 of a degree Celsius, 4/9 of a degree Rèaumur. See also appendix 8.

    **French s.,** usually abbreviated Fr.; a s. used in measuring catheters. See also Charrière s.

    **Gaffky s.,** Gaffky *table*.

    **hardness s.,** Mohs s.; a qualitative s. in which minerals are classified in order of their increasing hardness. It is based on the fact that the harder of two materials will scratch the softer, and will not be scratched by it. The new Mohs scale lists 15 substances: 1, talc; 2, gypsum; 3, calcite; 4, fluorite; 5, apatite; 6, orthoclase, periclase; 7, vitreous pure silica; 8, quartz, stellite; 9, topaz; 10, garnet; 11, tantalum carbide, fused zirconia; 13, silicon carbide; 14, boron carbide; 15, diamond.

    **homigrade s.,** a special thermometer s. in which 100° indicates the normal temperature of man (98.5°F., 37°C.), zero the freezing point, 270° the boiling point (212°F., 100°C.)

    **interval s.,** like a temperature s. in centigrade or Fahrenheit units, a s. on which the intervals are equal but which has an arbitrary zero point; *e.g.,* intelligence quotient values are values along an interval s.

    **isometric s.,** isometric ruler; a radiopaque strip of metal calibrated in centimeters and placed in the midsagittal plane of the patient; since it is subject to the same distortions as the pelvic diameters, it can be used to measure these diameters directly.

    **Kelvin s.,** absolute s.; temperature measured in degrees Centigrade from absolute zero (−273.16°C.).

    **masculinity-femininity s.,** any s. on a psychological test that assesses the relative masculinity or femininity of an individual; s.′s vary and may focus, for example, on basic identification with either sex or preference for a particular sex role.

    **Mohs s.,** hardness s.

    **pH s.,** Sorensen s.

    **Rankine s.,** a temperature thermometer s. in which each degree Rankine (abbreviated °Rank.) is equal to the Fahrenheit but applied to the absolute temperature s. with its zero point at absolute zero. See also appendix 8.

    **ratio s.,** one that involves physical units and demonstrates their relations; *e.g.,* that person A is twice as strong as person B.

    **Réaumur s.,** a temperature thermometer s. in which each degree Réaumur (abbreviated °R.) is 1/80 of the temperature difference between the freezing point and boiling point of pure water at 1 atmosphere pressure, with 0°R. set at the freezing point of water and 80°R. set at the boiling point of water. A degree Réaumur is equal to 1.25 degrees Celsius and 2.25 degrees Fahrenheit. See also appendix 8.

    **Shipley-Hartford s.,** a test of conceptual facility and flexibility.

    **Sorensen s.,** the pH scale; the negative logarithms of the hydrogen ion concentration used as a s. for expressing acidity and alkalinity. See also pH.

    **Stanford-Binet intelligence s.,** Binet test; Binet-Simon test; a standardized test for the measurement of intelligence consisting of a series of questions, graded according to the intelligence of normal children at different ages, the answers to which indicate the mental age of the person tested; it is used primarily with children, but also contains norms for adults.

**Tallqvist's hemoglobin s.,** a chromolithograph of graduated blood tints showing the varying color of samples of blood containing from 10 to 100 per cent of the normal content of hemoglobin; a piece of filter paper is moistened with a drop of the blood to be examined and its color is then compared with those of the s., the corresponding tint on the s. indicating the percentage of hemoglobin.

**thermometer s.,** a s. used to indicate the degree of heat registered by a thermometer; there are three of these in more or less common use, the *centigrade,* the *Fahrenheit,* and the *Réaumur,* the s. for measuring the absolute temperature is a centigrade s., the freezing point on which is marked 273° and the boiling point (100°C.) 373°. See the comparative thermometer s.'s in appendix 8.

**Wechsler-Bellevue s.,** a measure of general intelligence superceded by the Wechsler adult intelligence s.; see also Wechsler intelligence s.'s.

**Wechsler intelligence s.'s,** standardized s.'s for the measurement of general intelligence in preschool children (Wechsler preschool and primary s. of intelligence), in children (Wechsler intelligence s. for children), and in adults (Wechsler adult intelligence s., the successor to the Wechsler Bellevue s.).

**scalene** (ska'lēn) [ G. *skalēnos,* uneven ]. 1. Having sides of unequal length, said of a triangle so formed. 2. One of several muscles; see scalenus under musculus.

**scalenectomy** (ska'le-nek'to-mĭ) [ scalene + G. *ektomē,* excision ]. Resection of the scalene muscles.

**scalenotomy** (ska'le-not'o-mĭ) [ scalene + G. *tomē,* incision ]. Division or section of the anterior scalene muscle.

**scale'nus** [ L. ] [ NA ]. Scalene (1).

**scaler** (ska'ler). 1. An instrument for removing tartar from the teeth. 2. Device for counting electrical impulses, as in the assay of radioactive materials.

**hoe s.,** a hoe-shaped s. with a very short blade.

**scaling** (ska'ling). In dentistry, removal of accretions from the crowns and roots of teeth by use of special instruments.

**scall** (skawl) [ Ice. *skalli,* bald-head ]. A pustular, scaly eruption of the skin or scalp.

**honeycomb s.,** archaic term for an eruption of minute contiguous ulcers separated by raised edges.

**milk s.,** *crusta* lactea.

**scalp** (skălp) [ M. E. fr. Scand. *skalpr,* sheath ]. The skin covering the cranium.

**bulldog s.,** rarely used term for *cutis* verticis gyrata.

**scalpel** (skal-pel) [ L. *scalpellum;* dim. of *scalprum,* a knife ]. A pointed knife with convex edge. See fig. under knife.

**scalping** (skal'ping). A defect of a horse's gait in which the front surface of the fetlock joint of a hind leg is struck by the toe (or shoe) of the front foot.

**scalpriform** (skal'prĭ-form) [ L. *scalprum,* chisel, + *forma,* shape ]. Like a chisel.

**scalprum** (skal'prum) [ L. chisel, penknife, fr. *scalpo,* pp. *scalptus,* to carve ]. 1. A large strong scalpel. 2. A raspatory.

**scaly** (ska'lĭ). 1. Scurfy. 2. Squamous.

**scammony** (skam'o-nĭ) [ G. *skammōnia* ]. The plant, *Convolvulus scammonia* (family Convolvulaceae), the dried root of which contains a cathartic resin.

**Mexican s.,** ipomea.

**scandium** (skan'dĭ-um) [ L. *Scandia,* Scandinavia; discovered in Scand. mineral euxenite ]. A metallic element, symbol Sc, atomic no. 21, atomic weight 44.96.

**scanning** (skan'ing) [ L. *scando,* to climb ]. 1. Determination of the distribution of a specific radioactive element or compound in the body by recording the emitted ray on a photographic film; scintiscanning. 2. See under speech.

**scintillation s.,** see scintiscan.

**scansorius** (skan-so'rĭ-us) [ L. relating to climbing, fr. *scando,* to climb ]. See under musculus.

**Scanzoni** (skahnt-so'ne), Friedrich W., German obstetrician, 1821–1891. See S.'s *maneuver,* second *os.*

**scapha** (skaf'ah, ska'fah) [ L. fr. G. *skaphē,* skiff ] [ NA ]. 1. A boat-shaped structure. 2. Fossa of the helix; scaphoid fossa; the longitudinal furrow between the helix and the antihelix of the auricle.

**scapho-** (skaf'o-) [ G. *skaphē,* skiff, boat ]. Combining form meaning scapha or scaphoid.

**scaphocephalic** (skaf'o-sē-fal'ik). Denoting a long narrow skull with a more or less prominent ridge along the prematurely ossified sagittal suture.

**scaphocephalism** (skaf'o-sef'ă-lizm). The state of having a scaphocephalic skull.

**scaphocephalous** (skaf'o-sef'ă-lus). Scaphocephalic.

**scaphocephaly** (skaf'o-sef'ă-lĭ) [ scapho- + G. *kephalē,* head ]. Scaphocephalism.

**scaphohydrocephalus, scaphohydrocephaly** (skaf'o-hi'dro-sef'ă-lus, -lĭ). The occurrence of hydrocephalus in a scaphocephalic individual.

**scaphoid** (skaf'oyd) [ scapho- + G. *eidos,* resemblance ]. Boat-shaped; navicular; hollowed.

**scapula,** gen. and pl. **scapulae** (skap'u-lah, -le) [ L. *scapulae,* the shoulder blades ] [ NA ]. The shoulder blade; blade bone; a large triangular flattened bone lying over the ribs, posteriorly on either side, articulating laterally with the clavicle and the humerus.

**s. ala'ta,** winged s.

**s. eleva'ta,** Sprengel's *deformity.*

**scaphoid s.,** one in which the vertebral border below the level of the spine presents a more or less marked concavity in place of the normal convexity; the **scaphoid type of s.** (Graves) is one in which the vertebral border between the spine and the teres major process is straight or somewhat concave.

**winged s.,** s. alata; condition wherein the medial border of the scapula protrudes away from the thorax; the protrusion is posterior and lateral, as the scapula rotates out.

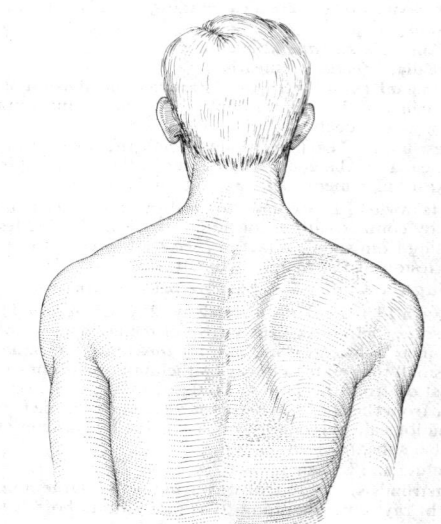

**Winged Scapula**

**scapulalgia** (skap'u-lal'jĭ-ah) [ scapula + G. *algos,* pain ]. Scapulodynia; rarely used term meaning pain in the shoulder blades.

**scapular** (skap'u-lar). Relating to the scapula.

**scapulary** (skap'u-lĕr-ĭ). A form of brace or suspender for keeping a belt or body bandage in place.

**scapulectomy** (skap'u-lek'to-mĭ) [ scapula + G. *ektomē,* excision ]. Excision of the scapula.

**scapulo-, scapul-** (skap'u-lo-) [ L. *scapulae,* shoulder blades ]. Combining forms meaning scapula or scapular.

**scapuloclavicular** (skap'u-lo-klă-vik'u-lar). Acromioclavicular or coracoclavicular.

**scapulodynia** (skap'u-lo-din'ĭ-ah) [ scapulo- + G. *odynē,* pain ]. Scapulalgia.

**scapulohumeral** (skap'u-lo-hu'mer-al). Relating to both scapula and humerus.

**scapulopexy** (skap'u-lo-pek'sĭ) [ scapulo- + G. *pēxis*, fixation ]. Operative fixation of the scapula to the chest wall.

**scapus,** pl. **scapi** (ska'pus, -pi) [ L. shaft, stalk ] [ NA ]. A shaft or stem.

    **s. penis,** *corpus* penis.

    **s. pili** [ NA ], hair shaft; see pilus (1).

**scar** (skar) [ G. *eschara*, scab ]. Cicatrix.

    **cigarette-paper s.'s,** papyraceous s.'s; atrophic s.'s in the skin over the knees, shins, and elbows of persons with Ehlers-Danlos syndrome.

    **papyraceous s.'s,** cigarette-paper s.'s.

    **Reichert's s.,** a small area on the impregnated ovum, where decidual tissue is absent, its place being taken by a fibrinous membrane formed from a blood clot at its point of entrance into the mucous membrane.

    **shilling s.'s,** round, well healed s.'s that follow involution of rupial syphilids.

**Scarff,** John E., U. S. neurosurgeon, *1898. See Stookey-S. *operation.*

**scarification** (skăr'ĭ-fĭ-ka'shun) [ L. *scarifico,* to scratch, fr. G. *skariphos,* a style for sketching ]. The act of scarifying; the condition of being scarified.

**scarificator** (skăr'ĭ-fĭ-ka'tor). An instrument for scarifying; it consists of a number of concealed cutting blades, set near together, which are projected at will by a spring.

**scarify** (skăr'ĭ-fi). To make a number of superficial incisions in the skin.

**scarlatina** (skar'lă-te'nah) [ through It. fr. Mediev. L. *scarlatum,* scarlet, a scarlet cloth ]. Scarlet fever; an acute exanthematous disease, caused by the streptococcal erythrogenic toxin, and marked by fever and other constitutional disturbances, and a generalized eruption of closely aggregated points or small macules of a bright red color, followed by desquamation in large scales, shreds, or sheets. The mucous membrane of the mouth and fauces is usually also involved.

    **anginose s., s. anginosa,** a form of s. in which the throat affection is unusually severe.

    **s. hemorrhag'ica,** a form in which blood extravasates into the skin and mucous membranes, giving to the eruption a dusky hue; there is frequently also bleeding from the nose and into the intestine.

    **s. la'tens,** latent s.; a form in which the rash is absent, the action of the specific poison being manifested in acute nephritis.

    **s. malig'na,** a severe scarlet fever in which the patient is early overcome with the intensity of the systemic intoxication.

    **s. rheumat'ica,** dengue.

    **s. simplex,** a mild form of the disease.

**scarlatinal** (skar-lă-te'nal). Relating to scarlatina.

**scarlatinella** (skar-lătĭ-nel'ah) [ dim. of scarlatina ]. Fourth *disease.*

**scarlatiniform** (skar'lă-te'nĭ-form, -tin'ĭ-form). Resembling scarlatina; denoting a rash.

**scarlatinoid** (skar'lă-te'noyd, skar-lat'ĭ-noyd) [ scarlatina + G. *eidos,* resemblance ]. 1. Scarlatiniform. 2. Fourth *disease.*

**scarlet** (skar'let) [ Mediev. L. *scarlatum,* scarlet cloth ]. Of a bright red color tending toward orange.

    **Biebrich s. red,** s. red.

    **s. red,** s. red, medicinal; scharlach red; Sudan IV; Biebrich red; *o*-tolylazo-*o*-tolylazo-*β*-naphthol. An azo dye; a dark, brownish red powder, soluble in oils, fats, and chloroform; insoluble in water. Used in medicine as a vulnerary and in histology as a stain to color fat in tissue sections.

    **s. red, medicinal,** s. red.

    **s. red sulfonate,** an azo dye that has been used to stimulate healing of chronic superficial wounds and ulcers.

**Scarpa,** Antonio, Venice anatomist, orthopedist, and ophthalmologist, 1747–1832. See S.'s *fascia, fluid, foramina, fossa* (scarpae major), S.'s *ganglion, habenula, hiatus, liquor, membrane, method, sheath, shoe, staphyloma, triangle.*

**scatacratia** (skat-ă-kra'shĭ-ah) [ scato- + G. *akratia,* lack of control ]. Incontinence of feces.

**scatemia** (skă-te'mĭ-ah) [ scato- + G. *haima,* blood ]. Intestinal autointoxication.

**scato-, scat-** (skat'o-) [ G. *skōr* (*skat*-), feces, excrement ]. Combining forms relating to feces.

**scatologic** (skat-o-loj'ik). Pertaining to scatology.

**scatology** (skă-tol'o-jĭ) [ scato- + G. *logos,* study ]. 1. Coprology; the scientific study and analysis of the feces, for physiologic and diagnostic purposes; skatology; 2. The study relating to the psychiatric aspects of excrement or the excremental (anal) function.

**scatoma** (skă-to'mah) [ scato- + G. suffix *-oma,* tumor ]. Coproma.

**scatophagy** (skă-tof'ă-jĭ) [ scato- + G. *phagein,* to eat ]. Eating of excrement; rhypophagy.

**scatoscopy** (skă-tos'ko-pĭ) [ scato- + G. *skopeō,* to view ]. Skatoscopy; examination of the feces for purposes of diagnosis.

**scat'ter.** A change in direction of a photon or subatomic particle, as the result of a collision or interaction.

**scatula** (skat'u-lah) [ Mediev. L. a rectangular figure whose width is one-tenth of its length ]. A square pillbox.

**scelalgia** (sĕ-lal'jĭ-ah) [ G. *skelos,* leg, + *algos,* pain ]. Pain in the leg.

**scele'tus** [ L. fr. G. *skeletos* (see skeleton) ] [ NA ]. Skeletal.

**scelotyrbe** (sel-o-tur'be) [ G. *skelos,* leg, + *tyrbē,* disorder ]. Spastic paralysis of the legs.

**scene** (sēn). A display of strong emotion and improper behavior, usually in a public place.

    **primal s.,** in psychoanalysis, the actual or fantasied observation by a child of sexual intercourse, particularly between the parents.

**Schacher** (shah'kher), Polycarp G., German physician, 1674–1737. See S.'s *ganglion.*

**Schachowa** (shah'kho-vah), Seraphina, Russian histologist in Berne, 19th century. See S.'s *tube.*

**Schaer's reagent.** See under reagent.

**Schäfer,** Sir Edward A. Sharpey-, British physiologist and histologist, 1850–1935. See S.'s *method.*

**Schäffer,** Max, German neurologist, 1852–1923. See S.'s *reflex.*

**Schaffer's test.** See under test.

**Schamberg,** Jay F., Philadelphia dermatologist, 1870–1934. See S.'s *disease, dermatitis.*

**Schanz** (shahnts), Alfred, German orthopedic surgeon, 1868–1931. See S.'s *syndrome.*

**Schapiro,** Heinrich, Russian physician, 1852–1901. See S.'s *sign.*

**Schardinger enzyme, reaction.** See the nouns.

**scharlach red** (shar'lak). *Scarlet* red.

**Schaudinn,** Fritz R., German bacteriologist, 1871–1906. See S.'s *fixative.*

**Schaumann,** Jörgen, Swedish physician, 1879–1953. See Besnier-Boeck-S.'s *disease, syndrome,* S.'s *bodies, lymphogranuloma, syndrome.*

**Schauta-Amreich vaginal operation.** See under operation.

**Schede** (sha'deh), Max, German surgeon, 1844–1902. See S.'s *clot, method.*

**schedule** (sked'jūl) [ L. *scheda,* fr. *scida,* a strip of papyrus, leaf of paper ]. A procedural plan for a proposed objective, especially the sequence and time allotted for each item or operation required for its completion.

    **s.'s of reinforcement,** in the psychology of conditioning, established procedures or sequences for reinforcing operant behavior. Thus, in a lever pressing situation, every displacement of the lever will bring a reinforcer (continuous reinforcement s.); or the reinforcer will come at every 5 seconds, regardless of how many displacements occur earlier (fixed-interval reinforcement s.), at every 10th displacement (fixed-ratio reinforcement s.), or on an average of every 5 seconds (variable-interval reinforcement s.; or the reinforcer will come in a noncontinuous fashion in which less than 100 per cent of the displacements bring a reinforcer (intermittent reinforcement s.).

**Scheele** (sha'leh, usually sheel), Karl W., Swedish chemist, 1742–1786. See S.'s *green.*

**Scheibler's reagent.** See under reagent.

**Scheie,** Harold G., U. S. ophthalmologist, *1909. See S.'s *syndrome.*

**Scheiner** (shi'ner), Christoph, German physicist, 1575–1650. See S.'s *experiment.*

**Schellong,** Fritz, German physician, *1891. See S.-Strisower *phenomenon,* S. *test.*

**schema,** pl. **schemata** (ske'mah, skĕ-mă'tah) [ G. *schēma,* shape, form ]. 1. Scheme; a plan, outline, or arrangement. 2. In sensorimotor theory, the organized unit of cognitive experience.

   **body s.,** body *image.*

**schematic** (ske-mat'ik) [ G. *schēmatikos,* in outward show, fr. *schēma,* shape, form ]. Made after a definite type of formula; representing in general, but not with absolute exactness; denoting an anatomical drawing or model.

**schematograph** (ske-mat'o-graf) [ G. *schēma,* form, + *graphō,* to write ]. An instrument for making a tracing in reduced size of the outline of the body.

**scheme** (skēm). Schema (1).

   **occlusal s.,** occlusal *system.*

**Schenck** (shenk), Benjamin R., American surgeon, 1873–1920. See S.'s *disease.*

**Scheu'ermann,** Holger W., Danish surgeon, 1877–1960. See S.'s *disease.*

**Schick** (shik), Bela, Vienna and New York pediatrician, *1877. See S. *control, method, test.*

**Schiff,** Hugo, German chemist in Florence, 1834–1915. See S.'s *base, tests,* periodic acid-S. *stain.*

**Schiff,** Moritz, German physiologist, 1923–1896. See S.-Sherrington *phenomenon.*

**Schilder** (shil'der), Paul, German-American psychiatrist, 1886–1940. See Flatau-S. *disease,* S.'s *disease.*

**Schiller,** Walter, Austrian pathologist in U. S., 1887–1960. See S.'s *test.*

**Schilling,** Victor, German hematologist, 1883–1960. See S.'s *blood count,* band *cell, index, tests,* S. type of monocytic *leukemia.*

**Schimmelbusch** (shim'el-boosh), Curt, German surgeon, 1860–1895. See S.'s *bacillus, disease.*

**schindylesis** (skin-di-le'sis) [ G. *schindylēsis,* splintering. SCHI- ]. Schindyletic joint; a form of fibrous joint in which the sharp edge of one bone is received in a cleft in the edge of the other, as in the articulation of the vomer with the rostrum of the sphenoid.

**Schiötz** (shūts), Hjalmar, Norwegian physician, 1850–1927. See S.'s *tonometer.*

**Schirmer,** R. See S.'s *syndrome, test.*

**schisto-** (skis'to-) [ G. *schistos,* split. SCHI- ]. Combining form meaning split or cleft.

**schistocelia** (skis-to-se'lī-ah) [ schisto- + G. *koilia,* a hollow ]. A congenital fissure of the abdominal wall.

**schistocephalus** (skis-to-sef'ă-lus) [ schisto- + G. *kephalē,* head ]. A fetus with unclosed cranium.

**schistocormia** (skis-to-kor'mī-ah) [ schisto- + G. *kormos,* trunk of a tree ]. Schistosomia; a congenital cleft of the trunk, the lower extremities of the fetus usually being imperfectly developed.

**schistocormus** (skis-to-kor'mus). Schistosomus; an individual with schistocormia.

**schistocystis** (skis'to-sis'tis) [ schisto- + G. *kystis,* bladder ]. Fissure of the bladder.

**schistocyte** (skis'to-sīt) [ schisto- + G. *kytos,* cell ]. 1. Microcyte; it was so called because it has the appearance of having been produced by budding from an ordinary red blood cell. 2. A dividing or fragmented red blood cell.

**schistocytosis** (skis-to-si-to'sis). The occurrence of many schistocytes in the blood.

**schistoglossia** (skis-to-glos'ī-ah) [ schisto- + G. *glōssa,* tongue ]. A congenital fissure or cleft of the tongue.

**schistomelus** (skis-tom'e-lus) [ schisto- + G. *melos,* limb ]. An individual with one or more cleft limbs.

**schistoprosopus** (skis-to-pros'o-pus, -pros-o'pus) [ schisto- + G. *prosōpon,* face ]. An individual with a more or less extensive cleft of the face.

**schistorrhachis** (skis-tor'ă-kis) [ schisto- + G. *rhachis,* spine ]. *Spina bifida.*

**Schistosoma** (skis-to-so'mah) [ schisto- + G. *sōma,* body ]. Formerly called *Bilharzia;* a genus of digenetic trematodes, including the important blood flukes of man and domestic animals, that cause schistosomiasis. They are characterized by elongate shape, separate sexes with marked sexual dimorphism, and their unusual location in the smaller mesenteric and portal blood vessels of their host.

**S. bo'vis,** infects sheep and cattle in S. Africa; characterized by long, narrow eggs with a terminal spine; the intermediate host is the aquatic snail, *Physopsis nusata.*

**S. haemato'bium,** formerly called *Distoma haematobium* and *Bilharzia haematobia,* a species with terminally spined eggs that occurs as a parasite in the portal system and mesenteric the veins of the bladder and rectum; it is common in the Nile delta but is found along waterways, irrigation ditches, or streams throughout Africa and in parts of the Middle East; the intermediate host is *Bulinus truncatus* in Egypt; elsewhere, other snails of the subfamily Bulininae ( *Bulinus, Physopsis, Pyrgophysa* ) are involved; this species is the cause of human schistosomiasis haematobium.

**S. in'dicum,** occurs in the portal mesenteric and other veins of cattle, sheep, goats, horses and camels; first described in India, later in Rhodesia.

**S. intercala'tum,** a blood fluke related to *S. haematobium* and found in natives of the Congo; symptoms are usually mild dysentery and abdominal pains, with enlargement of spleen and liver; a physid snail ( *Physopis africana* ) serves as the intermediate host.

**S. japon'icum,** a species of human blood fluke, having eggs without spines (or at most a small knob), that causes schistosomiasis japonicum and also extensive pathology resulting from encapsulation of the eggs; this species is the most pathogenic of the three schistosomes of man, owing to the greater egg production per female worm, and is also the most intractable to treatment and the most difficult to control; the intermediate hosts are amphibious snails (species of *Oncomelania,* family Amnicolidae) that can leave the water to avoid molluscicides; many other animals, such as pigs, oxen, cattle, dogs, serve as reservoir hosts; where night soil is still extensively used, control is an extremely difficult public health problem.

**S. manso'ni,** a common species infecting man in Africa, parts of the Middle East, the West Indies, and South America; characterized by large eggs with a strong lateral spine, transmitted by planorbid snails of the genus *Biomphalaria,* and the cause of human schistosomiasis mansoni.

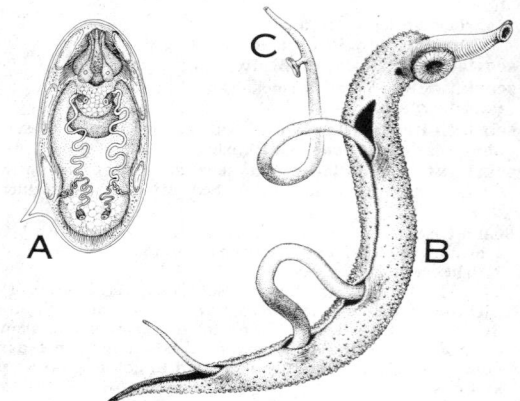

*Schistosoma mansoni*

A, egg containing miracidium (×200); B, adult male (×8); C, adult female (×8).

**S. mat'theei,** a species found in the portal mesenteric vein of sheep in South Africa; may also infect man.

**S. spinda'le,** a species parasitic in the mesenteric vein of cattle, zebu, sheep, goats and dogs in India and Southeast Asia.

**schistosome** (skis'to-sōm). Common name for a member of the genus *Schistosoma*.

**schistosomia** (skis-to-so'mĭ-ah) [ schisto- + G. *sōma*, body ]. Schistocormia.

**schistosomiasis** (skis-to-so-mi'ă-sis). Bilharziasis; snail fever; infection with a species of *Schistosoma*. Possibly the most rapidly spreading helminthic infection of man, involving some 200,000,000 persons in tropical and subtropical regions of Africa, the Middle East, the Orient, South America, and the Caribbean. It is often chronic and debilitating; manifestations vary with the infecting species but depend in large measure upon tissue reaction (granulation and scars) to the eggs deposited in venules. See also schistosome *dermatitis*.

**Asiatic s.,** s. japonicum.
**bladder s.,** s. haematobium.
**s. haematobium,** urinary or bladder s.; endemic or Egyptian hamaturia; infestation with *Schistosoma haematobium*, the eggs of which invade the urinary tract, causing cystitis and hematuria.
**intestinal s.,** s. mansoni.
**Japanese s.,** s. japonicum.
**s. japonicum,** infection with *Schistosoma japonicum*, characterized by dysenteric symptoms, painful enlargement of liver and spleen, dropsy, urticaria, and progressive anemia. Also called Asiatic, Oriental, or Japanese s.; Katayama disease; urticarial fever; kabure; kabure itch.
**s. mansoni,** Manson's s. or Manson's disease; intestinal s.; infection with *Schistosoma mansoni*, the eggs of which invade the wall of the large intestine and the liver, causing irritation, inflammation, and ultimately fibrosis of those parts.
**Oriental s.,** s. japonicum.
**urinary s.,** s. haematobium.

**schistosomus** (skis-to-so'mus). Schistocormus.

**schistosternia** (skis-to-ster'nĭ-ah) [ schisto- + G. *sternon*, sternum ]. A congenital cleft of the sternum.

**schistothorax** (skis-to-tho'raks) [ schisto- + G. *thorāx*, thorax ]. Congenital cleft of the chest wall.

**schistotrachelus** (skis-to-trā-ke'lus) [ schisto- + G. *trachēlos*, neck ]. An individual with a cleft of the neck.

**schiz-.** See schizo-.

**schizamnion** (skiz-am'nĭ-on) [ schiz- + amnion, *q.v.* ]. An amnion developing, as in the human embryo, by the formation of a cavity within the inner cell mass.

**schizaxon** (skiz-ak'son) [ schiz- + G. *axōn*, axis ]. A neuraxon divided into two branches.

**schizencephaly** (skiz'en-sef'ă-lĭ) [ schiz- + G. *enkephalos*, brain ]. Abnormal divisions or clefts of the brain substance.

**schizo-, schiz-** (skiz'o-) [ G. *schizō*, to split or cleave. SCHI- ]. Combining forms indicating split, cleft, or division.

**schizocyte** (skiz'o-sīt) [ schizo- + G. *kytos*, cell ]. Schistocyte.

**schizocytosis** (skiz-o-si-to'sis). Schistocytosis.

**schizogenesis** (skiz'o-jen'e-sis) [ schizo- + G. *genesis*, origin ]. Fissiparity; scissiparity; origin by fission.

**schizogony** (skī-zog'o-nĭ) [ schizo- + G. *gonē*, generation ]. 1. Multiple fission in which the nucleus first divides into several and then the cell divides into as many parts as there are nuclei. 2. Agamocytogeny; a stage in the asexual cycle of the malarial parasite occurring in the blood of man. The organism at the beginning of this stage is about a quarter of the diameter of the red blood cell, round, and actively ameboid, but increases to a diameter equal to or (in vivax malaria) greater than that of a red blood cell.

**schizogyria** (skiz-o-ji'rĭ-ah, -jir'ĭ-ah) [ schizo- + G. *gyros*, circle (convolution) ]. A deformity of the cerebral convolutions marked by occasional interruptions of continuity.

**schizoid** (skit'zoyd) [ schizo(phrenia), + G. *eidos*, resemblance ]. 1. Schizophrenia-like; resembling the personality characteristic of schizophrenia, but in milder form. 2. Also used to describe the withdrawal or "shut-in-ness" of the introverted personality.

**schizoidism** (skit'zoy-dizm). A schizoid state; the manifestation of schizoid tendencies.

**schizokinesis** (skiz'o-kī-ne'sis) [ schizo- + G. *kinēsis*, movement ]. Differential susceptibility of different systems in the body for learning, retention, and recall, so that in a given situation one may overreact and another underreact.

**schizomycete** (skiz'o-mi-sēt). A member of the class Schizomycetes; a bacterium.

**Schizomycetes** (skiz-o-mi-se'tēz) [ schizo- + G. *mykēs*, fungus ]. A name, used in some classification systems, for a class to include all of the bacteria.

**schizomycetic** (skiz-o-mi-se'tik). Relating to or caused by fission fungi (bacteria).

**schizomycosis** (skiz-o-mi-ko'sis). Any schizomycetic or bacterial disease.

**schizont** (skiz'ont) [ schizo- + G. *ōn* (*ont-*), a being ]. Agamont; a sporozoan trophozoite (vegetative form) that reproduces by schizogony, producing a varied number of daughter trophozoites or merozoites; see also segmenter.

**schizonticide, schizontocide** (skī-zon'tĭ-sid, -o'sid) [ schizont + L. *caedo*, to kill ]. An agent that kills schizonts.

**schizonychia** (skiz-o-nik'ĭ-ah) [ schizo- + G. *onyx*, nail ]. Splitting of the nails.

**schizophasia** (skiz'o-fa'zĭ-ah) [ schizo- + G. *phasis*, speech ]. The disordered speech of the schizophrenic person; "word-salad."

**schizophrene** (skit'so-frēn, skiz'o-). A person with schizophrenia or with a schizophrenic tendency.

**schizophrenia** (skit'so-fre'nĭ-ah, skiz'o-) [ schizo- + G. *phrēn*, mind ]. A term, coined by Bleuler, synonymous with and replacing dementia precox; the most common type of psychosis, characterized by a disorder in the thinking processes, such as delusions and halucinations, and extensive withdrawal of the individual's interest from other people and the outside world, and the investment of it in his own. S. is now considered a group of mental disorders rather than as a single entity, and distinction is made between process and reactive s.'s (*q. v.*).

**ambulatory s.,** a milder form of s. in which the patient is capable of maintaining himself in society and need not be hospitalized.

**catatonic s.,** s. characterized by marked disturbances in activity, with either generalized inhibition or excessive activity.

**latent s.,** a preexisting susceptibility for developing overt s. under strong emotional stress.

**hebephrenic s.,** hebephrenia.

**paranoid s.,** s. characterized predominantly by delusions of persecution and megalomania.

**process s.,** those forms of severe schizophrenic disorders in which chronic and progressive organic brain changes are considered to be the primary cause and in which prognosis is poor, as contrasted with reactive s.

**pseudoneurotic s.,** a form in which the underlying psychotic process is masked by complaints ordinarily regarded as neurotic.

**reactive s.,** those forms of severe schizophrenic disorders which are distinguished from process s. by their more acute onset, greater relation to environmental stress, and better prognosis.

**simple s.,** s. characterized by withdrawal, apathy, indifference, and impoverishment of human relationships.

**schizophrenic** (skit'so-fren'ik, -fre'nik, skiz'o-). Relating to or suffering from one of the schizophrenias.

**schizothemia** (skiz-o-the'mĭ-ah) [ schizo- + G. *thema*, theme ]. Repeated interruptions in a conversation by the speaker himself introducing other suggested topics.

**schizotonia** (skiz'o-to'nĭ-ah) [ schizo- + G. *tonos*, tension, tone ]. Division of the distribution of tone in the muscles.

**schizotrichia** (skiz-o-trik'ĭ-ah) [ schizo- + G. *thrix*, hair ]. Scissura pilorum; a splitting of the hairs at their ends.

**Schizotry'panum cru'zi** [ schizo- + G. *trypanon*, a borer, an auger ]. A distinct generic designation used for *Trypanosoma cruzi*, especially by workers in the endemic area of South American trypanosomiasis.

**schizozoite** (skiz'o-zo-īt) [ schizo- + G. *zōn*, animal ]. Merozoite.

**Schlatter,** Carl, Zurich surgeon, 1864–1934. See Osgood-S. *disease.*

**Schleiden** (shli′den), Matthias J., German botanist and microscopist, 1804–1881; among the first to see that plant tissues consist of cells and, along with Schwann, helped to establish the cell theory.

**Schlemm,** Friedrich S., German anatomist, 1795–1858. See S.'s *canal.*

**Schlesinger** (shla′zing-er), Hermann, Austrian physician, 1868–1934. See Pool-S. *sign,* S.'s *sign.*

**Schlösser** (shlës′er), Karl, German oculist, 1857–1925. See S.'s *method.*

**Schmid,** Rudi, Swiss-American internist and biochemist, *1922. See McArdle-S.-Pearson *disease.*

**Schmid,** W. See S.-Fraccaro *syndrome.*

**Schmidel** (shme′del), Casimir C., German anatomist, 1718–1792. See S.'s *anastomoses.*

**Schmidt,** Eduard Oskar, German anatomist, 1823–1886. See S.'s *fibrinoplastin.*

**Schmidt,** Gerhard, U. S. biochemist, *1900. See S.-Thannhauser *method.*

**Schmidt,** Henry D., American anatomist and pathologist, 1823–1888. See S.-Lantermann *clefts, incisures.*

**Schmidt,** Johann F. M., German laryngologist, 1838–1907. See S.'s *syndrome.*

**Schmidt,** Martin Benno, German physician, 1863–1949. See S.'s *syndrome.*

**Schmincke** (shmin′ka), Alexander, German pathologist, 1877–1953. See S.'s *tumors.*

**Schmorl,** Christian G., German pathologist, 1861–1932. See S.'s *bacillus, furrow, nodule.*

**Schneider,** Conrad V., German anatomist, 1610–1680. See Schneiderian *membrane.*

**Schneider,** Franz C., German chemist, 1813–1897. See S.'s *carmine.*

**Schneidersitz** (shni′der-zitz) [ Ger. ]. A typical sitting position exhibited by severely defective patients with phenylketonuria; resembles the position commonly attributed to tailors.

**Scholander,** Per F., Norwegian physiologist. See Roughton-S. *apparatus, syringe;* S. *apparatus.*

**Scholz,** Willibald, German neurologist, *1889. See S.'s *disease, theory.*

**Schönbein** (shën′bīn), Christian F., German chemist, 1799–1868. See S. *tests.*

**Schönlein** (shën′līn), Johann L., German physician, 1793–1864. See S.'s *disease,* Henoch-S. *purpura,* S.'s *purpura.*

**school** (skool) [ O. E. *scōl* ]. A set of beliefs, teachings, methods, etc.

   **dogmatic s.,** ancient Greek s. or tradition in medicine whose members were the successors to or followers of Hippocrates. They based their conceptions of disease upon the humoral theory and their practice upon experience and sound reasoning; they were comparatively free from fads, speculative theories, and dogma, which the term dogmatic falsely implies.

   **dynamic s.,** a group of theorists founded by Stahl, who professed the belief that all vital action is the result of an internal force independent of anything external to the body.

   **Hippocrat′ic s.,** the followers of the teachings of Hippocrates. See also Hippocrates.

   **iatromathematical s.,** mechanistic s.; a group of academicians, of whom Descartes was one of the foremost proponents, who maintained that all physiologic processes were the result of physical laws.

   **mechanistic s.,** iatromathematical s.

**Schott,** August, 1839?–1886, and Theodor, 1852–1920, German physicians in Bad Nauheim. See S. *treatment.*

**Schottmüller** (shot′mül-er), Hugo A. G., Hamburg physician, 1867–1936. See S.'s *bacillus, disease.*

**Schramm's phenomenon.** See under phenomenon.

**Schreger** (shra′ger), Christian H. T., Danish anatomist, 1768–1833. See S.'s *lines.*

**Schreiner's base.** See under base.

**Schridde** (shrid′eh), Hermann, German pathologist, *1875. See S.'s cancer *hairs.*

**Schröder** (shrë′der), Robert, German physician, 1884–1959. See S.'s *disease.*

**Schroeder** (shrë′der), Karl L. E., German gynecologist, 1838–1887. See S.'s *operation.*

**Schuchardt,** Karl A., German surgeon, 1856–1901. See S.'s *operation.*

**Schuegner's granules.** See under granule.

**Schüffner** (shüf′ner), Wilhelm, German pathologist in Sumatra, 1867–1949. See S.'s *granules.*

**Schüle** (shü′leh), Heinrich, German psychiatrist, 1839–1916. See S.'s *sign.*

**Schüller,** Artur, Austrian neurologist, *1874. See S.'s *disease,* Hand-S.-Christian *disease,* S.'s *phenomenon, syndrome.*

**Schüller** (shü′ler), Karl H. M., German surgeon, 1843–1907. See S.'s *ducts.*

**Schulte-Tigges,** Hugo, German bacteriologist, *1885. See S.-T. *stain.*

**Schultz,** Werner, Berlin internist, 1878–1947. See S.-Charlton *reaction,* S.-Charlton *phenomenon,* S.-Dale *reaction.*

**Schultze,** Bernhard S., German obstetrician, 1827–1919. See S.'s *fold, mechanism, phantom, placenta.*

**Schultze,** Max J., German histologist and zoologist, 1825–1874. See S.'s *cells, membrane, sign,* comma *bundle* of S., comma *tract* of S.

**Schultze's monochord.** See under monochord.

**Schumann rays.** See under ray.

**Schütz,** Erich, German biochemist, *1902. See S.'s *rule.*

**Schütz,** H., German anatomist. See S.'s *bundle.*

**Schütz** (shüts), Johann W., German veterinarian, 1839–1920. See S.'s *micrococcus.*

**Schwabach** (shvah′bahkh), Dagobert, Berlin otologist, 1846–1920. See S. *test.*

**Schwalbe** (shvahl′beh), Gustav A., German anatomist, 1844–1916. See S.'s *corpuscles, nucleus, rings, space.*

**Schwann** (shvahn), Theodor, German histologist and physiologist, 1810–1882. Founder with Schleiden of the cell theory. See S. *cells* S.'s *sheath,* white *substance, tumor.*

**schwannoma** (shwah-no′mah, shvah-). 1. Neurofibroma. 2. Neurilemoma.

   **acoustic s.,** acoustic *neurinoma.*

**schwannosis** (shwah-no′sis). A non-neoplastic proliferation of Schwann cells in the perivascular spaces of the spinal cord; seen particularly in older patients, especially those with diabetes mellitus.

**Schwartz** (shvarts), Charles E., French surgeon, *1852. See S.'s *method.*

**Schwartz,** Henry, U. S. neurosurgeon, *1909. See S. *tractotomy.*

**Schwartze** (shvart′seh), Hermann, German otologist, 1837–1910. See S. *operation,* S.-Stacke *operation.*

**Schwarz,** Karl L. H., German chemist, 1824–1890. See S.'s *test.*

**Schweigger-Seidel** (shvī′ger-sī′del), Franz, German physiologist, 1834–1871. See *sheath* of S.-S.

**Schweninger,** E. See S.-Buzzi *anetoderma.*

**sciage** (se-ahzh′) [ Fr. *scie,* saw ]. A to-and-fro sawlike movement of the hand in massage.

**sciatic** (si-at′ik) [ Mediev. L. *sciaticus,* a corruption of G. *ischiadikos,* fr. *ischion,* the hip joint. ISCHI- ]. 1. Relating to or situated in the neighborhood of the ischium or hip; ischiatic. 2. Relating to sciatica.

**sciatica** (si-at′ĭ-kah) [ see sciatic ]. Cotunnius' disease; neuralgia of the sciatic nerve, felt at the back of the thigh, usually due to herniated lumbar disc, but occasionally to sciatic neuritis.

**scilla** (sil′ah) [ G. ]. Squill.

**scillaren** (sil′lar-en). A mixture of glycosides, possessing digitalis-like actions, present in squill.

   **s. A.,** a crystalline steroidal glycoside present in squill. Can be hydrolyzed to glucose and proscillaridin A; the latter can be hydrolyzed to rhamnose and the steroid aglycone scillaridin A. Same actions and uses as digitalis glycosides.

   **s. B,** an amorphous glycosidal fraction obtained from squill, consisting of at least seven cardioactive glycosides:

glucoscillaren A, scillipheoside, glucoscillipheoside, scillicryptoside, scilliglaucoside, scillicyanoside and scillazuroside.

**scintigram** (sin'tĭ-gram) [ fr. L. *scintilla*, spark, + G. *gramma*, something written ]. Automatically obtained record on paper or film indicating the intensity, location, and distribution of radioactivity in tissue following the use of radioactive tracer substances; gammagram.

**scintillascope** (sin-til'ă-skōp) [ L. *scintilla*, spark, + G. *skopeō*, to observe ]. Scintillation *counter*.

**scintillation** (sin'tĭ-la'shun) [ L. *scintilla*, a spark ]. 1. A flashing or sparkling; a subjective sensation as of sparks or flashes of light. 2. In nuclear medicine the light emitted when an x- or gamma ray is absorbed by a crystal or liquid radiation detector.

**scintillator** (sin'tĭ-la'tor). Scintillation *counter*.

**scintillometer** (sin'tĭ-lom'e-ter) [ L. *scintilla*, spark, + G. *metron*, measure ]. Scintillation *counter*.

**scintiphotography** (sin'tĭ-fo-tog'ră-fi). The process of obtaining a photographic recording (scintiphotograph) of the distribution of an internally administered radiopharmaceutical with the use of a stationary scintillation detector device, a gamma camera.

**scintiscan** (sin'tĭ-skan). Photoscan.

**scintiscanner** (sin'tĭ-skan'er). Apparatus used to scintiscan.

**scion** (si'on) [ O. Fr. *sion*, shoot, sprig, fr. L. *seco*, to cut ]. In experimental embryology an embryonic tissue or part, grafted to another embryo of the same or of another species. See also chimera.

**scios'ophy** [ G. *skia*, shadow, + *sophia*, wisdom ]. A system of beliefs that are claimed to be facts but are not supported by scientific data.

**scirrhencanthis** (skĭr'en-kan'this, sĭr'en-) [ G. *skirrhos*, hard, a hard tumor, + *en*, in, + *kanthos*, canthus ]. An indurated tumor of the lacrimal gland.

**scirrhoblepharoncus** (skĭr'o-blef-ă-rong'kus, sĭr'o-) [ G. *skirrhos*, hard, + *blepharon*, eyelid, + *onkus*, mass ]. A scirrhous cancer of the eyelid.

**scirrhophthalmia** (skĭr'of-thal'mĭ-ah, sĭr'of-) [ G. *skirrhos*, hard, + *ophthalmos*, eye ]. A scirrhous tumor of the eye.

**scirrhosity** (skĭr-os'ĭ-tĭ, sĭr-). A scirrhous state or hardness of a tumor.

**scirrhous** (skĭr'us, sĭr-). Hard; relating to a scirrhus.

**scirrhus** (skĭr'us, sĭr-) [ G. *skirrhos*, hard, a hard tumor ]. An obsolete term meaning any fibrous indurated area, especially an indurated carcinoma.

**scission** (sish'un) [ L. *scissio*, fr. *scindo*, pp. *scissus*, to cleave ]. Fission; cleavage.

**scissiparity** (sis-ĭ-păr'ĭ-tĭ) [ L. *scissio*, cleavage, + *pario*, to bring forth ]. Schizogenesis.

**scissors** (siz'erz) [ L. *scindo*, pp. *scissus*, to cut ]. An instrument with two blades moving on a pivot cutting against each other.

**de Wecker's s.,** small s. with sharp points for intraocular cutting of iris and lens capsule.

**Smellie's s.,** lance-pointed shears, with external cutting edges, used in craniotomy.

**scissura,** pl. **scissurae** (sĭ-su'rah, -re) [ L. ]. Scissure. 1. A cleft or fissure. 2. A splitting.

**s. pilo'rum,** schizotrichia.

**scissure** (sish'ūr). Scissura.

**scler-.** See sclero-.

**sclera,** pl. **scleras, sclerae** (sklēr'ah, sklēr'e) [ Mod. L. fr. G. *sklēros*, hard. SCLER- ] [ NA ]. Sclerotica; sclerotic coat; white of the eye; a fibrous tunic forming the outer envelope of the eye, except for its anterior sixth which is occupied by the cornea.

**scleradenitis** (sklēr-ad-en-i'tis) [ scler- + G. *adēn*, gland, + suffix *-itis*, inflammation ]. Inflammatory induration of a gland.

**scleral** (sklēr'al). Relating to the sclera.

**scleratogenous** (sklēr'ă-toj'ĕ-nus). Sclerogenous.

**sclerectasia** (sklēr-ek-ta'zĭ-ah) [ scler- + G. *ektasis*, an extension ]. A protrusion or bulging of the sclera.

**sclerectoiridectomy** (skle-rek'to-ĭr-ĭ-dek'to-mĭ). A combined sclerectomy and iridectomy used in glaucoma to form a filtering cicatrix.

**sclerectoiridodialysis** (skle-rek'to-ĭr'ĭ-do-di-al'ĭ-sis). A combined operation of sclerectomy and iridodialysis for the relief of glaucoma.

**sclerectomy** (skle-rek'to-mĭ) [ scler- + G. *ektomē*, excision ]. 1. Excision of a portion of the sclera. 2. Removal of the fibrous adhesions formed in chronic otitis media.

**scleredema** (sklēr'e-de'mah) [ scler- + G. *oidēma* a swelling (edema) ]. Hard, nonpitting edema of the skin, giving a waxy appearance and no sharp demarcation.

**s. adulto'rum,** Buschke's disease (1); benign spreading induration of the skin and subcutaneous tissue that usually follows a febrile illness, usually streptococcal; it begins usually on the head and neck and spreads over the trunk.

**sclerema** (skle-re'mah) [ scler- + edema ]. Induration of the subcutaneous fat.

**s. adiposum,** s. neonatorum.

**s. neonato'rum,** s. of newborn, adiponecrosis neonatorum; s. adiposum; subcutaneous fat necrosis of the newborn; Underwood's disease; appears at birth or in early infancy as indurated plaques, sharply demarcated and yellowish white; usually occurs in premature and debilitated infants. If lesions are widespread prognosis is poor. Localized lesions may resolve slowly over a period of many months; usually involves cheeks, buttocks, shoulders, and calves. The subcutaneous fat may have a low oleic acid content. Microscopically, there is necrosis of subcutaneous fat with thickening of interlobular connective tissue and formation of fatty acid crystals and foreign body giant cells.

**sclerencephaly, sclerencephalia** (sklēr-en-sef'ă-lĭ, -en-sĕ-fa'lĭ-ah) [ scler- + G. *enkephalos*, brain ]. Sclerosis and shrinkage of the brain substance.

**scleriasis** (skle-ri'ă-sis) [ scler- + G. suffix *-iasis*, condition ]. Diffuse, symmetrical scleroderma.

**scleriritomy** (sklēr'ĭ-rit'o-mĭ). The operation of incising the iris and sclera.

**scleritis** (skle-ri'tis). Inflammation of the sclera.

**annular s.,** a protracted inflammation involving the sclera in a ring around the limbus of the cornea.

**anterior s.,** an inflammation of the sclera adjoining the limbus of the cornea, appearing as a dark red or bluish swelling.

**brawny s.,** a gelatinous-appearing swelling surrounding the limbus with a tendency to involve the periphery of the cornea.

**posterior s.,** s. with a tendency to extend posteriorly Tenon's capsule and causing chemosis.

**sclero-, scler-** (skle'ro-) [ G. *skleros*, hard. SCLER- ]. Combining forms meaning hard, or denoting relationship to the sclera.

**scleroblastema** (skle-ro-blas-te'mah) [ sclero- + G. *blastēma*, sprout ]. The embryonic tissue entering into the formation of bone.

**scle'rocat'aract.** Obsolete term for hard cataract.

**sclerochoroidal** (skle'ro-ko-roy'dal). Relating to both the sclera and the choroid.

**sclerochoroiditis** (skle-ro-ko-roy-di'tis). Inflammation of the sclerotic and choroid coats of the eye.

**s. anterior,** a secondary involvement of the sclera by an extension of a process from the uvea.

**s. posterior,** posterior *staphyloma*.

**scleroconjunctival** (skle'ro-kon'jungk-ti'val). Relating to the sclera and the conjunctiva.

**sclerocornea** (skle'ro-kor'ne-ah). 1. The cornea and sclera regarded as forming together the hard outer coat of the eye, the tunica fibrosa bulbi. 2. A congenital anomaly in which the whole or part of the cornea is opaque and resembles the sclera; other ocular abnormalities are frequently present.

**sclerodactyly, sclerodactylia** (skle'ro-dak'tĭ-lĭ, -dak-til'ĭ-ah) [ sclero- + G. *daktylos*, finger or toe ]. Scleroderma of the digits of the hands or feet.

**scleroderma** (skle'ro-der'mah) [ sclero- + G. *derma*, skin ]. Dermatosclerosis; sclerosis cutanea; sclerosis corii; hidebound or skinbound disease; thickening of the skin caused by swelling and thickening of fibrous tissue, with eventual atrophy of the epidermis; a manifestation of progressive systemic *sclerosis* (*q. v.*) and used synonymously for that disease.

**circumscribed s.,** morphea.

**scle'rodermati'tis.** Inflammation and thickening of the skin.

**sclerogenic** (skle'ro-jen'ik). Sclerogenous.

**sclerogenous** (skle-roj'ĕ-nus) [ sclero- + G. suffix -*gen*, producing ]. Scleratogenous; sclerogenic; producing hard or sclerotic tissue; causing sclerosis.

**scleroid** (skle'royd) [ sclero- + G. *eidos*, resemblance ]. Sclerous; of unusually firm texture.

**scleroiritis** (skle-ro-i-ri'tis). Inflammation of both sclera and iris.

**sclerokeratitis** (skle'ro-kĕr-ă-ti'tis) [ sclero- + G. *keras*, horn ]. Inflammatory cellular infiltration of the sclera and cornea.

**sclerokeratoiritis** (skle-ro-kĕr'ă-to-i-ri'tis). Inflammation of sclera, cornea, and iris.

**sclerokeratosis** (skle'ro-kĕr'ă-to'sis). 1. *Scleroperikeratitis* progressiva. 2. Sclerokeratitis.

**scleroma** (skle-ro'mah) [ G. *sklērōma*, an induration ]. A circumscribed indurated focus of granulation tissue in the skin or mucous membrane.

**respiratory s.,** rhinoscleroma in which the lesion involves the mucous membrane of the greater part or all of the upper respiratory tract.

**scleromalacia** (skle'ro-mă-la'shī-ah) [ sclero- + G. *malakia*, a softening ]. Degenerative thinning of the sclera, occurring in persons with rheumatoid arthritis.

**scleromeninx** (skle'ro-me'ningks, -men'ingks) [ sclero- + G. *mēninx*, membrane ]. Dura mater.

**scleromere** (skle'ro-mēr) [ sclero- + G. *meros*, part ]. Any metamere of the skeleton, such as a vertebral segment.

**sclerometer** (skle-rom'e-ter) [ sclero- + G. *metron*, measure ]. A form of penetrometer for determining the density or hardness of any substance.

**scleromyxedema** (skle'ro-mik'se-de'mah). *Lichen myxedematosus.*

**scleronychia** (skle'ro-nik'ī-ah) [ sclero- + G. *onyx*, nail, + suffix -*ia*, condition ]. Induration and thickening of the nails.

**scleronyxis** (skle'ro-nik'sis) [ sclero- + G. *nyxis*, a pricking ]. Scleroticopuncture; scleroticotomy; an operative procedure, no longer used, involving puncture of the sclera with a view to couching or needling the lens.

**sclero-oophoritis** (skle'ro-o-of'o-ri'tis) [ sclero- + Mod. L. *oophoron*, ovary + G. suffix -*itis*, inflammation ]. Sclero-oothecitis; inflammatory induration of the ovary.

**sclero-oothecitis** (skle'ro-o'o-the-si'tis) [ sclero- + Mod. L. *ootheca*, ovary, + G. suffix -*itis*, inflammation ]. Sclero-oophoritis.

**scleroper'ikerati'tis progres'siva.** Obsolete term for tuberculosis of the sclera and cornea.

**sclerophthalmia** (sklēr'of-thal'mī-ah) [ sclero- + G. *opthalmos*, eye ]. A congenital condition in which the opacity of the sclera has advanced over the edge of the cornea so that only a small central area of the latter remains transparent; it may be unilateral, one-half of the cornea being normal.

**scleroplasty** (skle'ro-plas'tī) [ sclero- + G. *plassō*, to fashion ]. Plastic surgery on the sclera.

**scle'ropro'tein.** Albuminoid (3); see also fibrous *protein*.

**sclerosal** (skle-ro'sal). Sclerous.

**sclerose** (skle-rōz'). To harden; to undergo sclerosis.

**sclerosis** (skle-ro'sis) [ G. *sklērōsis*, hardness ]. Induration or hardening of chronic inflammatory origin; especially induration of nervous and other structures by a hyperplasia of the interstitial fibrous or glial connective tissue.

**Alzheimer's s.,** hyaline degeneration of the medium and smaller blood vessels of the brain.

**amyotrophic lateral s.,** Charcot's disease (1); a disease of the motor tracts of the lateral columns and anterior horns of the spinal cord, causing progressive muscular atrophy, increased reflexes, fibrillary twitching, and spastic irritability of muscles.

**arterial s.,** arteriosclerosis.

**arteriocapillary s.,** arteriosclerosis, especially of the finer vessels.

**arteriolar s.,** arteriolosclerosis.

**bone s.,** eburnation.

**Canavan's s.,** spongy *degeneration*.

**central areolar choroidal s.,** areolar *choroidopathy*.

**combined s.,** a form of s. of the spinal cord involving both posterior and lateral columns, often associated with severe anemia, particularly pernicious anemia.

**s. co'rii,** scleroderma.

**s. cuta'nea,** scleroderma.

**diffuse s.,** *encephalitis* periaxialis diffusa.

**diffuse infantile familial s.,** Krabbe's disease; globoid cell leukodystrophy; a form marked by generalized demyelination of the cerebrum in infants, and often affecting members of the same family.

**disseminated s.,** multiple s.

**endocardial s.,** endomyocardial *fibroelastosis*.

**focal s.,** multiple s.

**hippocampal s.,** a loss of cortical neurons and a reactive astrocytosis in the hippocampal regions of some persons with epilepsy.

**idiopathic hypercalcemic s. of infants,** see idiopathic *hypercalcemia* of infants.

**insular s.,** multiple s.

**laminar cortical s.,** a degeneration of nerve fibers in the corona radiata in a laminar pattern.

**lateral spinal s.,** a degenerative state of the lateral tracts of the spinal cord causing spastic paraplegia; a clinical variant of amyotrophic lateral s.

**lobar s.,** s. of the brain involving the greater part or all of a lobe; typically caused by perinatal hypoxia.

**mantle s.,** a common cerebral lesion in the palsied states of early life characterized by nodular cortical atrophy.

**menstrual s.,** physiologic s.

**Mönckeberg's s.,** Mönckeberg's *arteriosclerosis*.

**multiple s.,** disseminated, focal, or insular s.; the occurrence of patches of s. (plaques) in the brain and spinal cord, causing more or less paralysis, tremor, nystagmus, and disturbances of speech, the various symptoms depending upon the seat of the lesions; it occurs chiefly in early adult life, with characteristic exacerbations and remissions.

**nodular s.,** atherosclerosis.

**ovulational s.,** physiologic s.

**physiologic s.,** menstrual or ovulational s.; a slowly progressive s. in the walls of the ovarian arteries which commences after puberty, that is, at the commencement of the menstrual cycles.

**posterior s.,** *tabes* dorsalis.

**posterior spinal s.,** *tabes* dorsalis.

**progressive systemic s.,** scleroderma (*q. v.*); a systemic disease characterized by formation of hyalinized and thickened collagenous fibrous tissue, with thickening of the skin and adhesion to underlying tissues, especially of the hands and face; dysphagia due to loss of peristalsis and submucosal fibrosis of the esophagus; dyspnea due to pulmonary fibrosis; myocardial fibrosis; and renal vascular changes resembling those of malignant hypertension. Raynaud's phenomenon, atrophy of the soft tissues, and osteoporosis of the distal phalanges (acrosclerosis) are common findings.

**tuberous s.,** epiloia; Bourneville's disease; multisystem hamartomas producing the typical triad of seizures, mental retardation, and skin nodules of the face, originally considered to be sebaceous adenomas but since shown to be angiofibromas; the cerebral and retinal lesions are glial nodules; other skin lesions are white macules, shagreen patches, and periungual fibromas.

**unicellular s.,** a growth of fibrous tissue between and isolating the individual cells of a part.

**vascular s.,** arteriosclerosis.

**s. ventric'uli,** sclerotic *gastritis*.

**s. of white matter,** leukodystrophy.

**sclerostenosis** (skle'ro-stĕ-no'sis) [ sclero- + G. *stenōsis*, a narrowing ]. Induration and contraction of the tissues.

**Sclerostoma** (skle-ros'to-mah) [ sclero- + G. *stoma*, mouth ]. A genus of strongyle (hookworm) nematode worms, formerly used for the trichostrongyle worms of horses, now replaced by other genera but still used as a collective term for this group.

**S. duodena'le,** now replaced by *Ancylostoma duodenale*.

**S. syn'gamus,** now replaced by *Syngamus trachea*.

**sclerostomy** (skle-ros'to-mĭ) [ sclero- + G. *stoma,* mouth ]. Surgical perforation of the sclera, as for the relief of glaucoma.

**scle'rother'apy.** The treatment of varicose veins by the injection of an agent such as sodium ricinoleate which obliterates the lumen of the vessel.

**sclerothrix** (sklēr'o-thriks) [ sclero- + G. *thrix,* hair ]. Sclerotrichia; induration and brittleness of the hair.

**sclerotic** (skle-rot'ik). 1. Relating to or characterized by sclerosis. 2. Relating to the sclera.

**sclerot'ica** [ Mod. L. *scleroticus,* hard ]. Sclera.

**scleroticochoroiditis** (skle-rot'ĭ-ko-ko-roy-di'tis). Inflammation of the sclerotic and choroid coats of the eye.

**sclerotitis** (sklēr'o-ti'tis). 1. Scleritis. 2. Otosclerosis.

**sclerotome** (sklēr'o-tōm) [ sclero- + G. *tomos,* a cutting ]. 1. A knife used in sclerotomy. 2. The group of mesenchymal cells emerging from the ventromesial part of a mesodermic somite and migrating toward the notochord. Sclerotomal cells from adjacent somites become merged in intersomitically located masses that are the primordia of the centra of the vertebrae.

**sclerotomy** (skle-rot'o-mĭ) [ sclero- + G. *tome,* incision ]. An incision through the sclerotic coat of the eye.

    **anterior s.,** incision into the anterior chamber of the eye.

    **posterior s.,** incision through the sclera into the vitreous humor.

**sclerotrichia** (skle-ro-trik'ĭ-ah). Sclerothrix.

**sclerous** (sklēr'us) [ G. *skleros,* hard ]. Indurated; leatherlike in consistency; scarred.

**scoleciasis** (sko-le-si'a-sis) [ G. *skōlēx,* worm, + suffix *-iasis,* condition ]. Infestation of the intestine by larvae.

**scoleciform** (sko-le'sĭ-form). Scolecoid; vermiform.

**scolecitis** (sko-le-si'tis) [ G. *skōlēx,* worm, + suffix *-itis,* inflammation ]. Inflammation of the vermiform appendix.

**scolecoid** (sko'le-koyd) [ G. *skōlēkoeidēs,* fr. *skōlēx,* worm, + *eidos,* appearance ]. 1. Wormlike; vermiform. 2. Resembling a scolex.

**scolecoidectomy** (sko'le-koy-dek'to-mĭ) [ scolecoid + G. *ektome,* excision ]. Appendectomy.

**scolecoiditis** (sko'le-koy-di'tis) [ scolecoid + G. suffix *-itis,* inflammation ]. Inflammation of the vermiform appendix; appendicitis.

**scolecology** (sko'le-kol'o-jĭ) [ G. *skōlēx,* worm, + *logos,* study ]. Helminthology.

**scolec'tomy.** Appendectomy.

**scolex,** pl. **scoleces** or **scolices** (sko'leks, sko-le'sēz, sko'lĭ-sēz) [ G. *skōlēx,* a worm ]. The head of a tapeworm by which it is attached to the wall of the intestine; it is formed in the interior of the daughter cyst in an echinococcus hydatid cyst, or within the cysticercus or cysticercoid in the case of a *Taenia* or *Hymenolepis* tapeworm, respectively.

**scoliokyphosis** (sko'lĭ-o-ki-fo'sis) [ G. *scolios,* curved, + G. *kyphōsis,* kyphosis ]. Lateral and posterior curvature of the spine.

**scoliometer** (sko'lĭ-om'e-ter) [ G. *skolios,* curved, + *metron,* measure ]. An instrument for measuring curves, especially those in lateral curvature of the spine.

**scoliosis** (sko'lĭ-o'sis) [ G. *skoliōsis,* a crookedness ]. Lateral curvature of the spine. Depending on the etiology, there may be just one curve, or primary and secondary compensatory curves. S. may be "fixed" as a result of muscle and/or bone deformity, or "mobile" as a result of unequal muscle contraction.

    **coxit'ic s.,** s. in the lumbar spine resulting from tilting of the pelvis in a case of hip disease.

    **empye'mic s.,** s. due to retraction of one side of the chest following an empyema.

    **habit s.,** one supposed to be due to habitual standing or sitting in an improper position.

    **myopath'ic s.,** lateral curvature due to weakness of the spinal muscles.

    **ocular s., ophthalmic s.,** s. supposed to be due to head tilting, caused by ophthalmological dysfunction.

    **osteopathic s.,** lateral curvature due to vertebral disease.

    **paralytic s.,** lateral curvature of spine due to paralysis of spinal muscles.

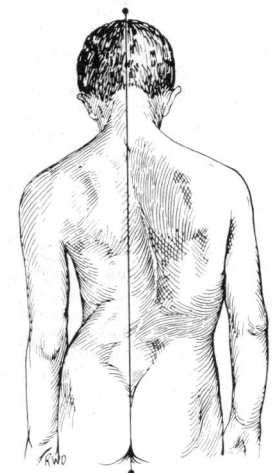

Scoliosis

    **rachitic s.,** s. occurring as a result of rickets.

    **sciatic s.,** s. caused by asymmetric spasm of spinal muscles usually associated with sciatica.

    **static s.,** lateral spinal curvature due to inequality in length of the two legs.

**scoliotic** (sko'lĭ-ot'ik). Relating to or suffering from scoliosis.

**scoliotone** (sko'lĭ-o-tōn) [ G. *skolios,* crooked, + *tonos,* tension ]. An apparatus for stretching the spine and reducing the curve in scoliosis.

**Scolopendra** (sko'lo-pen'drah) [ Mod. L. fr. G. *skōlopendra,* multipede ]. A genus of centipedes characterized by 21 to 23 pairs of legs. Common United States species are *S. heros* (the western house centipede) and *S. morsitans.*

**scom'brine** [ G. *skombros,* mackerel ]. A protamine found in spermatozoa of mackerel.

**scoop** (skōōp) [ A.S. *skopa* ]. A narrow, spoonlike instrument for extracting the contents of cavities or cysts.

**scoparin** (sko'pă-rin). A glycoside from scoparius; believed to be a diuretic by some investigators; others state that it is physiologically inert.

**scoparius** (sko-pa'rĭ-us) [ L. *scopa,* a broom ]. Broom; besom; the dried tops of *Cytisus scoparius* (family Leguminosae), a shrub of Europe and northwestern Asia, containing sparteine; cathartic and diuretic.

**-scope** [ G. *skopeō,* to view. SCOP- ]. Suffix generally indicating an instrument for viewing but including other methods of examination.

**sco'pine.** Scopolamine less the tropic acid side chain, *i.e.,* 6,7-epoxytropine, or 6,7-epoxy-3-hydroxytropane.

**scopolamine** (sko-pol'ă-mēn, -min). Hyoscine; atroscine; scopine tropate; an alkaloid found in the leaves and seeds of *Hyoscyamus niger, Duboisia myoproides, Scopola japonica, Scopolia carniolica, Atropa belladonna,* and other solanaceous plants. S. is the 6,7-epoxide of atropine, *i.e.,* 6,7-epoxytropine tropate. For structure, see tropine.

    **s. hydrobro'mide** (USP), hyoscine hydrobromide (BP); anticholinergic action is similar to that of atropine; sedative and mild analgesic, used in obstetrics to produce twilight sleep.

    **s. methylbromide,** a quaternary ammonium derivative of s.; used when spasmolytic or antisecretory effects are desired.

**Scopoli,** Giovanni A., Italian naturalist, 1723–1788. Gave his name to *Scopolia.*

**scopolia** (sko-po'lĭ-ah) [ G. A. *Scopoli* ]. The dried rhizome and roots of *Scopolia carniolica* (family Solanaceae), a herb of Austria and neighboring countries of Europe; it resembles belladonna in pharmacologic action.

    **s. japon'ica,** Japanese belladonna; the leaves, root, and seeds contain scopolamine.

**scopoline** (sko'po-lēn, -lin). Oscine; 3,6-epoxy-7-hydroxy-tropane; a decompostion product of scopolamine, and an isomer of scopine, in that the epoxy and hydroxyl groups are in different locations.

**scopometer** (sko-pom'e-ter) [ G. *skopeō*, to view, + *metron*, measure ]. A device for determining the density of a precipitate by the degree of translucency of a fluid containing it; see nephelometer.

**scopomorphinism** (sko'po-mor'fi-nizm). Associated chronic addiction to scopolamine and morphine.

**scopophilia** (sko'po-fil'ī-ah) [ G. *skopeō*, to view, + *philos*, fond ]. Voyeurism.

**scopophobia** (sko'po-fo'bī-ah) [ G. *skopeō*, to view, + *phobos*, fear ]. A dread of being looked at.

**Scopulariopsis** (sko-pu-lār-ī-op'sis) [ Mod. L. *scopula*, a small broom, + G. *opsis*, appearance ]. A genus of filamentous fungi related to *Penicillium*, and like the latter found in certain cases of otomycosis.

**scoracratia** (skōr-ă-kra'shī-ah) [ G. *skōr*, dung, + G. *akratia*, lack of control ]. Scatacratia.

**scorbutic** (skor-bu'tik). Relating to or suffering from scorbutus or scurvy.

**scorbu'tigen'ic.** Scurvy-producing.

**scorbutus** (skor-bu'tus) [ Mediev. L. form of the Teutonic word for scurvy, *schorbuyck* ]. Scurvy.

**scordinema** (skor'dī-ne'mah) [ G. *skordinēma*, yawning ]. Heaviness of the head with yawning and stretching, occurring as a prodrome of an infectious disease.

**score** (skōr) [ M. E. *scor*, notch, tally ]. An evaluation, usually expressed numerically, of status, achievement, or condition in a given set of circumstances.

   **Apgar s.**, evaluation of a newborn infant's physical status by assigning numerical values (0 to 2) to each of five criteria: heart rate, respiratory effort, muscle tone, response to stimulation, and skin color. A score of 10 indicates the best possible condition.

   **recovery s.**, a number expressing the condition of an infant at various stipulated intervals greater than 1 minute after birth and based on the same features assessed by the Apgar s. at 60 seconds after birth.

   **standard s.**, a derived s. representing the deviation of a raw score from its mean in standard deviation units.

**scoretemia** (skōr-ĕ-te'mī-ah) [ G. *skōr*, dung, + *haima*, blood ]. Intestinal autointoxication.

**scor'ings.** On x-ray, small dark lines in the metaphysis, due to delay in growth.

**scorpion** (skor'pī-on) [ G. *skorpios* ]. A member of the order Scorpionida, *q. v.*

   **devil s.**, *Vejovis*.

   **hairy s.**, *Hadrurus*.

**Scorpionida** (skor'pī-on'ī-dah). An order of venomous, predaceous, arachnid arthropods, the scorpions, characterized by a bony, distinctly segmented abdomen terminating in a sharply recurved stinging spine equipped with a poison gland; causes a severely painful but rarely fatal sting. North American genera include *Centruroides*, *Hadrurus*, and *Vejovis*, which see.

**scoto-** (sko'to-) [ G. *skotos*, darkness ]. Combining form meaning darkness.

**scotochromogen** (sko'to-kro'mo-jen) [ scoto- + G. + *chrōma*, color, + suffix -*gen*, producing ]. See group II mycobacteria.

**scotodinia** (sko-to-din'ī-ah) [ scoto- + G. *dinē*, a whirling ]. Vertigo; faintness.

**scotograph** (sko'to-graf) [ scoto- + G. *graphō*, to write ]. 1. An appliance for aiding one to write in straight lines in the dark or for aiding the blind to write. 2. An impression made on a photographic plate by a radioactive substance without the intervention of any opaque object other than the screen of the plate.

**scotoma** (sko-to'mah) [ G. *skotōma*, vertigo, fr. *skotos*, darkness ]. 1. An isolated area of varying size and shape, within the visual field, in which vision is absent or depressed. 2. A blind spot in psychological awareness.

   **an'nular s.**, ring s.; a circular s. surrounding the center of the field of vision.

   **Bjerrum's s.**, Bjerrum's sign; a comet-shaped s., occurring in glaucoma, attached at the temporal end to the blind

spot or separated from it by a narrow gap. As the defect pushes up and nasally it broadens in width, curving around the fixation spot, and then abruptly swerves downward to end sharply at the nasal horizontal meridian.

   **cecocentral s.**, a s. involving the optic disk area (blind spot) and the papillomacular fibers. There are three special forms: (1) the cecocentral defect which extends from the blind spot toward or into the fixation area; (2) angioscotoma; (3) glaucomatous nerve-fiber bundle s., due to compression of nerve-fiber bundles at the edge of the optic disk; see also Bjerrum's s., and Roenne's nasal *step*.

   **central s.**, a s. involving the macula of the retina.

   **color s.**, an area of color blindness in the visual field.

   **flittering s.**, scintillating s.

   **insular s.**, a small spot of blindness surrounded by an area of good vision.

   **mental s.**, blind spot (2); absence of insight into, or inability to grasp, a mental problem.

   **negative s.**, one that is not ordinarily perceived, but is detected only on examination of the visual field.

   **paracen'tral s.**, one that is only partly central, the fixation point not being entirely obscured.

   **periph'eral s.**, a s. within the field of vision outside of the point of fixation.

   **physiological s.**, blind spot (1); a negative scotoma in the visual field, corresponding to the optic disk.

   **positive s.**, one that is perceived subjectively as a black spot within the field of vision.

   **relative s.**, one in which vision is impaired but not entirely destroyed.

   **ring s.**, annular s.

   **scintillating s.**, fortification spectrum; teichopsia; flittering s.; the appearance of a dark patch with bright zigzag outline in the visual field of one or both eyes; usually a prodromal symptom of migraine.

   **Seidel's s.**, a type of Bjerrum s.; see also Seidel's *sign*.

**scotomagraph** (sko-to'mă-graf) [ scotoma + G. *graphō*, to write ]. An instrument for automatically recording the size and shape of a scotoma.

**scotomatous** (sko-to'mă-tus). Relating to scotoma.

**scotometer** (sko-tom'e-ter). An instrument for measuring the size of a scotoma.

**scotometry** (sko-tom'e-trī) [ scoto- + G. *metron*, measure ]. The plotting and measuring of a scotoma.

**scotophilia** (sko-to-fil'ī-ah) [ scoto- + G. *philos*, fond ]. Nyctophilia; preference for night time, or for the dark.

**scotophobia** (sko-to-fo'bī-ah) [ scoto- + G. *phobos*, fear ]. Fear of the dark.

**scotopia** (sko-to'pī-ah) [ scoto- + G. *opsis*, vision ]. Scotopic *vision*.

**scotopic** (sko-to'pik, -top'ik). Referring to low illumination to which the eye is dark-adapted; see scotopic *vision*.

**scotopsin** (sko-top'sin). The protein moiety of the pigment in the rods of the retina.

**scotoscopy** (sko-tos'ko-pī) [ scoto- + G. *skopeō*, to view ]. Retinoscopy.

**Scott-Wilson,** H., English scientist. See S.-W. *reagent*.

**scours** (skowrz). A term used for severe diarrhea in an animal.

**scrape** (skrāp). A specimen scraped from a lesion or specific site, for cytological examination. See also smear and subentries.

**scrapie** (skrap'e, skra'pe). A disease of sheep and goats, manifested by various nervous symptoms and usually leading to death. It is contagious, but the nature of the causative agent remains in doubt (it is believed to be a virus) and the method of transmission is unknown.

**scratch'es.** Grease *heel* (2).

**screen** [ Fr. *écran* ]. 1. A thin sheet of any substance used to shield an object from any influence, such as heat, light, x-rays, etc. 2. A sheet upon which a picture is projected. 3. To make a fluoroscopic examination. 4. In psychoanalysis, a term meaning concealment, one image or memory concealing another; see also screen *memory*. 5. See screening.

   **fluores'cent s.**, a s. coated with crystals of calcium tungstate used in the fluoroscope.

**screen'ing.** 1. See screen. 2. The process of examining a population (usually a high risk population) for a given disease or state such as cancer, diabetes, tuberculosis. 3. In psychiatry, initial patient evaluation that includes medical and psychiatric history, mental status evaluation, and diagnostic formulation to determine the patient's suitability or a particular treatment modality.

**cytologic s.,** for the detection of early disease, usually cancer, thorough microscopic examination of a cellular specimen by inspecting each cell and structure present, usually at ×100 magnification with a mechanical stage, so that all areas are screened. The findings are evaluated and significant abnormalities are flagged (*e.g.*, by dotting the cover slip) for further evaluation by a cytopathologist. This screening usually is performed by an experienced cytotechnologist, but at times there is automated machine prescreening.

**screw** (skru). A helically grooved cylinder for fastening two objects together or for adjusting the position of an object resting on one end of the s.

**afterloading s.,** a device for setting the length at which a contracting muscle encounters an afterload.

**screw'worm.** The larva of the fly, *Callitroga hominivorax*, that causes human myiasis.

**primary s.,** one that can initiate a wound and invade the skin directly.

**secondary s.,** one that enters a prior wound or supporated condition and feeds on infected rather than intact tissues.

**scrobiculate** (skro-bik'u-lāt) [ L. *scrobiculus*; dim. of *scrobis*, a trench ]. Pitted; marked with minute depressions.

**scrobic'ulus cordis** [ L. pit or fossa of the heart ]. *Fossa* epigastrica.

**scrofula** (skrof'u-lah) [ L. *scrofulae* (pl. only), a glandular swelling, scrofula, fr. *scrofa*, a breeding sow ]. Obsolete term for tuberculous cervical *lymphadenitis*.

**scrofuloderma** (skrof'u-lo-der'mah) [ scrofula + G. *derma*, skin ]. Cutaneous *tuberculosis*.

**s. gummo'sa,** a deep cutaneous tuberculous lesion.

**pap'ular s.,** papular *tuberculid*.

**tuber'culous s.,** scrofulotuberculosis; ulcerative s.; a granulating ulcer surrounding the orifice of a sinus leading down to a tuberculous gland or focus of bone tuberculosis.

**ul'cerative s.,** tuberculous s.

**verr'ucous s.,** *tuberculosis* cutis verrucosa.

**scrofulophyma** (skrof'u-lo-fi'mah) [ scrofula + G. *phyma*, a growth ]. *Tuberculosis* cutis verrucosa.

**scrofulosis** (skrof'u-lo'sis). Scrofula.

**scrof'ulotuberculo'sis.** Tuberculous *scrofuloderma*.

**scrof'ulous.** Relating to or suffering from scrofula.

**scrotal** (skro'tal). Relating to the scrotum; oscheal.

**scrotectomy** (skro-tek'to-mī) [ scrotum, + G. *ektomē*, excision ]. Removal of part of scrotum.

**scro'tiform.** Having the shape or form of a scrotum.

**scrotitis** (skro-ti'tis). Inflammation of the scrotum.

**scrotocele** (skro'to-sēl) [ scrotum + G. *kēlē*, hernia ]. Scrotal *hernia*.

**scro'toplas'ty** [ scrotum + G. *plassō*, to form ]. Oscheoplasty; reparative or plastic surgery of the scrotum.

**scrotum,** pl. **scrota, scrotums** (skro'tum, -tah) [ L. ] [ NA ]. A musculocutaneous sac containing the testes; it is formed of skin, containing a network of nonstriated muscular fibers (the dartos), cremasteric fascia, cremaster muscle, and the serous coverings of the testes and epididymides.

**lymph s.,** stasis of the scrotal lymphatics; elephantiasis of the scrotum; also called chyloderma.

**watering-can s.,** urinary sinuses in scrotum and perineum, resulting from rupture of perineal urethra.

**scruff of the neck.** Nucha.

**scruple** (skru'pl) [ L. *scrupulus*, a small sharp stone, a weight, the 24th part of an ounce, a scruple, dim. of *scrupus*, a sharp stone ]. An apothecaries' weight of 20 grains or one-third of a dram.

**SCUBA.** Acronym for self-contained underwater breathing apparatus.

**Scultetus (Scultet),** originally Schultes, Johann, German surgeon, 1595–1645. See S.'s *bandage, position.*

**scum** (skum) [ M. E. ]. Epistasis; a film of insoluble mate-

rial that rises to the surface of a liquid; that which sinks to the bottom of a liquid is the sediment or hypostasis.

**scurf** [ A.S. ]. Dandruff.

**scurf'skin.** Epidermis.

**scurvy** (skur'vī) [ fr. A. S. scurf ]. A disease marked by inanition, debility, anemia, edema of the dependent parts, a spongy condition, sometimes with ulceration, of the gums, and hemorrhages into the skin and from the mucous membranes; the disease is due to a monotonous diet of salt meats, and the lack of fresh vegetables, fruits, and other sources of vitamin C in the diet.

**Alpine s.,** pellagra.

**infantile s.,** Barlow's disease; Brinton's disease (2); Cheadle's disease; acute rickets; a cachectic condition, resulting from the use of improper food, in infants; marked by pallor, fetid breath, coated tongue, diarrhea, and subperiosteal hemorrhages.

**land s.,** idiopathic thrombocytopenic *purpura*.

**sea s.,** s.

**scur'vy-grass.** *Cochlearia officinalis* (family Cruciferae), a cress used as a salad and as a remedy for scurvy.

**scutate** (sku'tāt). Scutiform.

**scute** (skūt) [ L. *scutum*, shield ]. Scutum (1); squama; a thin lamina or plate.

**tympan'ic s.,** the thin bony plate separating the epitympanic recess from the mastoid cells.

**scu'tiform** [ L. *scutum*, shield, + *forma*, form ]. Scutate; shield-shaped.

**Scutigera** (sku-tij'er-ah). A genus of centipedes commonly found in the eastern United States; the eastern house centipede is a member of the species *S. cleopatra*.

**scutular** (sku'tu-lar). Relating to a scutulum.

**scutulum,** pl. **scutula** (sku'tu-lum, sku'chu-lum, -lah) [ L. dim. of *scutum*, shield ]. A yellow saucer-shaped crust, the characteristic lesion of favus, consisting of a mass of hyphae and spores.

**scutum,** pl. **scuta** (sku'tum, -tah) [ L. shield ]. 1. Scute. 2. In ixodid (hard) ticks, a plate that largely or entirely covers the dorsum of the male and forms an anterior shield behind the capitulum of the female or immature ticks.

**scybala** (sib'ă-lah). Plural of scybalum.

**scybalous** (sib'ă-lus). Relating to scybala.

**scybalum,** pl. **scybala** (sib'ă-lum, -lah) [ G. *skybalon*, excrement ]. A hard round mass of inspissated feces.

**scyllitol** (sil'ĭ-tol). *scyllo*-Inositol; isomeric to the *myo*-inositol commonly found in nature; found in dogfish liver and cartilage.

**scyphiform** (si'fĭ-form) [ G. *skyphos*, goblet, cup, + L. *forma*, form ]. Scyphoid.

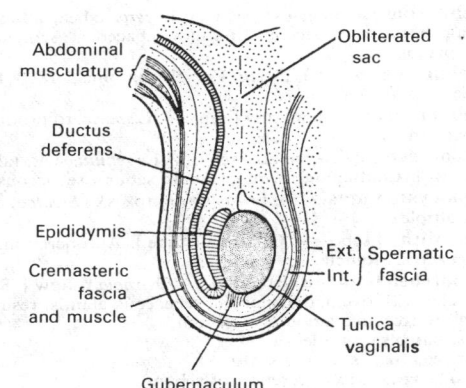

**Scrotum**

Diagrammatic drawing of the testis, epididymis, ductus deferens, and the various layers of the abdominal wall that surround the testis in the scrotum. (From Langman, J.: *Medical Embryology*, Ed. 2, The Williams & Wilkins Co., Baltimore, 1969.)

**scyphoid** (si'foyd) [ G. *skyphos*, cup, + *eidos*, resemblance ]. Cup-shaped.

**scytitis** (si-ti'tis) [ G. *skytos*, skin, + *-itis* ]. Dermatitis.

**SD.** Abbreviation for (1) streptodornase, (2) standard *deviation*.

**SDA.** Abbreviation for specific dynamic *action.*

**Se.** Chemical symbol of the element selenium.

**seal** (sēl). 1. An airtight closure. 2. To effect an airtight closure.

**border s.,** peripheral s.; the contact of the denture border with the underlying or adjacent tissues to prevent the passage of air or other substances.

**palatal s.,** posterior palatal s.

**peripheral s.** border s.

**posterior palatal s.,** postdam; palatal s.; postpalatal s.; the s. at the posterior border of a denture; see also posterior palatal s. *area.*

**postpalatal s.,** posterior palatal s.

**sealant** (se'lant). A material used to effect an airtight closure.

**fissure s.,** a dental material, comprised of bisphenol A glycidyl methacrylate, used to seal nonfused, noncarious fissures on the occlusal surfaces of teeth.

**searcher** (ser'cher). A form of sound used to determine the presence of a calculus in the bladder.

**Searl's ulcer.** See under *ulcer.*

**Seashore,** Carl E., American psychologist, 1866–1949. See S. *test.*

**seasickness** (se'sik-nes). Naupathia; mal de mer; a form of motion sickness caused by the motion of a floating platform (ship, raft, etc.) and commonly characterized by pallor, sweating, nausea, and vomiting which may lead to incapacitation.

**season** (se'zon). A particular phase of some slow cyclic phenomenon, especially the annual weather cycle.

**mating s.,** the period of "heat" during which an animal will mate, *i.e.*, the period during which estrus occurs.

**seat** (sēt). A surface against which an object may rest to gain support.

**basal s.,** denture *foundation.*

**rest s.,** rest *area.*

**sea urchin.** A member of the class Echinoidea (*q. v.*); see also sea urchin *granuloma;* sea urchin *sting.*

**seb-, sebi-.** See sebo-.

**sebaceous** (se-ba'shus) [ L. *sebaceus* ]. Relating to sebum; oily; fatty.

**seba'ceus** [ L. ] [ NA ]. Sebaceous.

**sebastomania** (sē-bas'to-ma'nī-ah) [ Gr. *sebastos*, worthy of reverence, + *mania*, frenzy ]. Theomania.

**sebiagogic** (seb-ī-ă-goj'ik) [ sebi- + G. *agōgos*, leading ]. Sebiferous.

**sebiferous** (se-bif'er-us) [ sebi- + L. *fero*, to bear ]. Producing fatty or sebaceous matter; sebaceous; sebiparous; sebiagogic.

**Sebileau** (seb-e-lo'), Pierre, French anatomist, 1860–1953. See S.'s *hollow, muscle.*

**sebiparous** (se-bip'ar-rus) [ sebi- + L. *pario*, to produce ]. Sebiferous.

**sebo-, seb-, sebi-** (se'bo-, seb'o-) [ L. *sebum*, suet, tallow. SEB- ]. Combining forms meaning sebum, sebaceous.

**sebocystomatosis** (se'bo-sis'to-mă-to'sis). *Steatocystoma* multiplex.

**seb'olith** [ sebo- + G. *lithos*, stone ]. A concretion in a sebaceous follicle.

**seborrhea** (seb-o-re'ah) [ sebo- + G. *rhoia*, a flow ]. Steatorrhea (2); overactivity of the sebaceous glands, resulting in an excessive amount of sebum.

**s. adipo'sa,** s. oleosa.

**s. cap'itis,** s. of the scalp.

**s. ce'rea,** waxy secretion of sebum.

**concrete s.,** thick, oily crusts on scalp and eyebrows.

**s. cor'poris,** seborrheic *dermatitis.*

**eczematoid s.,** seborrheic eczema in which lesions have lost definition and have become confluent, usually as a result of trauma and overzealous use of soap and medication.

**s. faciei,** s. of the face; s. oleosa affecting especially the nose and forehead.

**s. furfura'cea,** s. sicca (1).

**s. ni'gra,** a form of s. characterized by a pigmented secretion.

**s. oleo'sa,** a greasy condition of the skin due to excessive secretion of the sebaceous glands; also called s. adiposa; cutis unctuosa; acne sebacea; hyperhidrosis oleosa.

**s. sic'ca** [ L. *siccus*, dry ], (1) s. furfuracea; an accumulation on the skin, especially the scalp, of dry scales; (2) dandruff.

**s. squamo'sa neonato'rum,** seborrheic dermatitis in infants.

**seborrheic** (seb-o-re'ik). Relating to seborrhea.

**se'bum** [ L. tallow. SEB- ] [ NA ]. Smegma; the secretions of the sebaceous glands.

**s. cuta'neum,** cutaneous fatty secretion.

**s. palpebra'le,** lema; secretion of the Meibomian glands.

**s. preputia'le,** *smegma* preputii.

**seca'dera.** In South America, the name for a nagana-like trypanosomiasis, the pathogenic agent of which is *Trypanosoma vivax.*

**secobarbital** (se'ko-bar'bī-tal, sek'o-) (USP). SECONAL; 5-allyl-5-(1-methylbutyl)barbituric acid; sedative and short-acting hypnotic.

**secodont** (sek'o-dont, se'ko-) [ L. *seco*, to cut, + G. *odous* (*odont-*), tooth ]. Denoting an animal in which the tubercles of the molar teeth have cutting edges.

**secondaries** (sek'on-dēr-iz). The lesions of secondary syphilis.

**secreta** (se-kre'tah) [ L. neuter pl. of *secretus*, pp. of *se-cerno*, to separate. CRET- ]. Secretions.

**secretagogue** (se-kre'tă-gog) [ secreta + G. *agōgos*, drawing forth ]. Secretogogue; an agent that promotes secretion.

**secrete** (se-krēt') [ L. *se-cerno*, pp. *-cretus*, to separate. CRET- ]. To elaborate or produce some physiologically useful substance (*e.g.*, enzyme, hormone, metabolite) by a cell, and to deliver it into sap, blood, or body cavity, either by direct diffusion or by means of a duct.

**secre'tin.** A hormone, formed by the epithelial cells of the duodenum under the stimulus of acid contents from the stomach, that incites secretion of pancreatic juice.

**gastric s.,** gastrin.

**secre'tinase.** Descriptive name for the agent in serum that destroys the activity of secretin.

**secretion** (se-kre'shun) [ L. *se-cerno*, pp. *-cretus*, to separate ]. 1. The production by a cell or aggregation of cells (a gland) of some substance differing in chemical and physical properties from the body from which or by which it is produced. 2. The product, solid, liquid, or gaseous, of cellular or glandular activity. A secretion is stored up in or utilized by the animal or plant in which it is produced, thereby differing from an excretion, which is intended to be expelled from the body.

**biliary s.,** (1) the bile; (2) the s. of bile.

**internal s.'s,** hormones.

**neurohumoral s.,** transmission of a nerve impulse across a synapse or to an end-organ by s. of a minute amount of a chemical transmitter such as acetylcholine.

**secretogogue** (se'kre'to-gog). Secretagogue.

**secre'tomo'tor, secre'tomo'tory.** Stimulating secretion.

**secre'tor.** An individual whose saliva and other body fluids contain a water-soluble form of the antigens of the ABO blood group found in his erythrocytes.

**secre'tory.** Relating to secretion or the secretions.

**secre'tum** [ L. ] [ NA ]. Secretion; separation.

**sectile** (sek'til) [ L. *sectilis*, fr. *seco*, to cut ]. 1. Capable of being cut or divided. 2. Having the appearance of being divided.

**sectio,** pl. **sectio'nes** (sek'shī-o) [ L. ] [ NA ]. Section; in anatomy, a subdivision or segment.

**s. alta,** the high operation for stone, suprapubic lithotomy, or cystotomy.

**s. cadav'eris,** autopsy.

**s. latera'lis,** lateral *lithotomy.*

**s. media'na,** median *lithotomy.*

**section** (sek'shun) [ L. *sectio*, a cutting, fr. *seco*, to cut ]. The act of cutting. 2. A cut or division. 3. A segment or part of any organ or structure delimited from the remainder. 4. A cut surface. 5. A thin slice of tissue, cells, microorganisms, or any material for examination under the microscope.

**abdominal s.,** celiotomy.

**attached cranial s.,** attached *craniotomy.*

**cesarean s.** [ so called not because performed at the birth of Julius Caesar (100 B.C.), but because included under *lex cesarea,* Roman law (715 B.C.) ], cesarean operation; incision through the abdominal wall and the uterus (abdominohysterotomy) for extraction of the fetus.

**cor'onal s.,** a vertical s. of the skull at right angles to the sagittal s.

**detached cranial s.,** detached *craniotomy.*

**frozen s.,** a thin slice of tissue cut from a frozen specimen.

**Latzko's cesarean s.,** a cesarean s. in which the uterus is entered by paravesical blunt dissection without entering the peritoneal cavity.

**microscop'ic s.,** s. (5).

**perine'al s.,** any s. through the perineum, either lateral or median lithotomy or external urethrotomy.

**pituitary stalk s.,** transection of the neurovascular connection between the hypothalamus and the pituitary gland.

**Saemisch's s.,** procedure of transfixing the cornea beneath an ulcer and then cutting from within outward through the base.

**sag'ittal s.,** a vertical s. of the skull or part of the body in an anteroposterior direction, dividing it into two lateral halves.

**serial s.,** one of a number of consecutive microscopic s.'s.

**sectorial** (sek-to'rĭ-al) [ L. *sector,* cutter ]. 1. Relating to a sector. 2. Cutting or adapted for cutting; denoting the carnassial or shearing molar and premolar teeth of carnivores.

**secundigravida** (sē-kun'dĭ-grav'ĭ-dah) [ L. *secundus,* second, + *gravida,* pregnant ]. A woman in her second pregnancy.

**secundina, pl. secundinae** (sek'un-di'nah, -ne) [ L. *secundinae,* the afterbirth, fr. *secundus,* second ]. The afterbirth.

**secundines** (sek'un-dēnz) [ L. *secundinae,* the afterbirth ]. The afterbirth.

**secundipara** (sek'un-dip'ă-rah) [ L. *secundus,* second, + *pario,* to give birth ]. Para II; a woman who has given birth for the second time to an infant or infants, alive or dead, weighing 500 gm. or more or having a length of gestation of at least 20 weeks.

**secundiparity** (sē-kun'dĭ-păr'ĭ-tĭ). The state of being a secundipara.

**sedate** (sē-dāt) [ L. *sedatus;* see sedation ]. To bring under the influence of a sedative.

**sedation** (sē-da'shun) [ L. *sedatio,* fr. *sedo,* pp. *-atus,* to calm, allay, fr. *sedeo,* to sit ]. The act of calming, especially by the administration of a sedative drug; the state of being calm.

**sedative** (sed'ă-tiv) [ L. *sedatious;* see sedation ]. 1. Calming; quieting. 2. An agent that quiets nervous excitement; the s.'s are designated, according to the part or the organ upon which their specific action is exerted, cardiac, cerebral, nervous, respiratory, spinal, etc.

**sedigitate** (sē-dij'ĭ-tāt) [ L. *sex,* six, + *digitus,* digit ]. Sexdigitate.

**sediment** (sed'ĭ-ment) [ L. *sedimentum* a settling, fr. *sideo,* to sit, settle down ]. Hypostasis; sedimentum; insoluble material that sinks to the bottom of a liquid; that which rises to the surface is called epistasis or scum.

**sedimentation** (sed'ĭ-men-ta'shun). The formation of a sediment.

**s. constant,** the constant *s* in Svedberg's equation for estimating the molecular weight of a protein from the rate of movement in a centrifugal field:

$$M = s\,\frac{RT}{D(1 - Vp)}$$

where *M* is the molecular weight, *R* the gas constant, *T* the absolute temperature, *D* the diffusion constant (in square centimeters per second), *V* the partial specific volume of the protein, *p* the density of the solvent. The

constant *s,* with dimensions of time per unit of field force, is usually between $1 \times 10^{-13}$ and $200 \times 10^{-13}$ second. The Svedberg unit (S) is fixed at $1 \times 10^{-13}$ second and is often used to describe the sedimentation rate of macromolecules.

**s. rate,** sinking velocity of the blood cells, *i.e.,* the degree of rapidity with which the red cells sink in a mass of drawn blood.

**sed'imentator.** A centrifuge.

**sedimentometer** (sed-ĭ-men-tom'e-ter) [ sediment + G. *metron,* measure ]. A photographic apparatus for the automatic recording of blood sedimentation rate.

**sedimen'tum** [ L. ]. Sediment.

**s. laterit'ium,** brickdust *deposit.*

**sedoheptulose** (se'do-hep'tu-lōs). D-*altro*-2-Heptulose; a 2-ketoheptulose formed metabolically (as the 7-phosphate) by condensation of xylulose (5-phosphate) and ribose (5-phosphate), splitting out glyceraldehyde (3-phosphate). See structures under sugars.

**seed** [ A.S. *soed* ]. 1. The reproductive body of a flowering plant; the mature ovule. 2. In bacteriology, to inoculate a culture medium with microorganisms.

**millet s.,** the s. of a grass, *Panicum miliaceum,* used as a rough designation of size of cutaneous and other lesions; it is the equivalent of about 2 mm., or $^1/_{12}$ inch, in diameter.

**Seeligmüller** (za'likh-mü-ler), Otto L. G. A., German neurologist, 1837–1912. See S.'s *sign.*

**Seessel** (za'sel), Albert, American embryologist, 1850–1910. See S.'s *pocket, pouch.*

**seg'ment** [ L. *segmentum,* fr. *seco,* to cut. SEC- ]. 1. Segmentum. 2. Metamere. 3. To divide and redivide into minute equal parts.

**anterior s.,** *segmentum* anterius.

**anterior basal s.,** *segmentum* basale anterius.

**anterior inferior s.,** *segmentum* anterius inferius.

**anterior superior s.,** *segmentum* anterius superius.

**apical s.,** *segmentum* apicale.

**apicoposterior s.,** *segmentum* apicoposterius.

**bronchopulmonary s.,** *segmentum* bronchopulmonalis.

**cardiac s.,** *segmentum* cardiacum.

**hepatic s.'s,** segmenta hepatis; segments of the liver; territories of the liver with independent portobilioarterial distribution or independent venous drainage. See *segmentum* anterius (1), laterale (1), mediale (1), posterius (1).

**inferior s.,** *segmentum* inferius.

**inferior lingular s.,** *segmentum* lingulare inferius.

**interan'ular s.,** internodal s.

**internodal s.,** segmentum internodale; interanular s.; Ranvier's s.; internode; the portion of a myelinated nerve fiber between two successive nodes.

**Lantermann's s.'s,** the divisions of the nerve fiber between the Schmidt-Lantermann incisures.

**lateral s.,** *segmentum* laterale.

**lateral basal s.,** *segmentum* basale laterale.

**lower uterine s.,** the inferior portion or isthmus of the uterus, the lower extremity of which joins with the cervical canal and, during pregnancy, expands to become the lower part of the uterine cavity.

**medial s.,** *segmentum* mediale.

**medial basal s.,** *segmentum* basale mediale.

**mesoblastic s.,** somite.

**neural s.,** neuromere.

**P-R s.,** that part of the electrocardiographic curve between the end of the P wave and the beginning of the QRS complex.

**posterior s.,** *segmentum* posterius.

**posterior basal s.,** *segmentum* basale posterius.

**Ranvier's s.,** internodal s.

**renal s.'s,** *segmenta* renalia.

**RS-T s.,** the part of the electrocardiogram between the QRS complex and T wave.

**s. of the spinal cord,** a portion of the spinal cord corresponding to the line of attachment of one pair of spinal nerves. See fig. under medulla spinalis.

**s.'s of the spleen,** segmenta lienis; splenic territories receiving independent arterial supply or drained by independent roots of the splenic vein.

**S-T s.,** that part of the electrocardiographic tracing immediately following the QRS complex and merging into the T wave.

**subapical s.,** *segmentum* subapicale.

**subsuperior s.,** *segmentum* subsuperius.

**superior s.,** *segmentum* superius (1).

**superior lingular s.,** *segmentum* lingulare superius.

**sympathetic s.,** a divison of the sympathetic trunks based on the origins of the gray rami communicantes.

**upper uterine s.,** the main portion of the body of the gravid uterus, the contraction of which furnishes the chief force of expulsion in labor.

**venous s.'s of the kidney,** segmenta renalia drained by main roots of the renal veins.

**venous s.'s of the liver,** hepatic venous segments; each of the four territories of the liver separately drained by the hepatic veins.

**segmen'ta.** Plural of segmentum.

**segmen'tal.** Relating to a segment.

**segmentation** (seg'men-ta'shun). 1. The act of dividing into segments; the state of being divided into segments. 2. Cleavage (1).

**seg'menter.** Schizont (*q.v.*); usually applied to the malaria parasite developing in a red blood cell having undergone nuclear and cytoplasmic division, just before cell rupture and release of the merozoites.

**segmentum,** pl. **segmenta** (seg-men'tum, -tah) [ L. segment, *q.v.* ] [ NA ]. Segment. 1. A section; a part of an organ or other structure delinited naturally, artificially, or in the imagination from the remainder. 2. A territory of an organ having independent function, supply, or drainage.

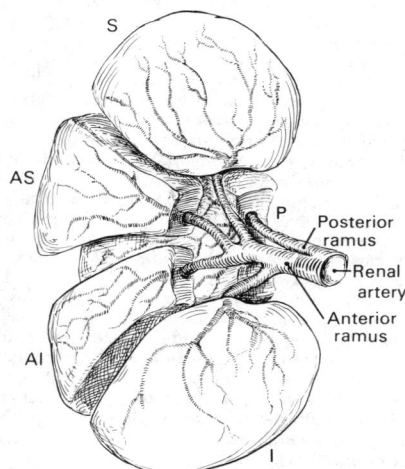

**Renal Segments (Segmenta Renalia)**

Shown with segmental arteries that supply them. *S*, superior; *AS*, anterosuperior; *AI*, anteroinferior; *I*, inferior; *P*, posterior.

**s. ante'rius** [ NA ], anterior segment; (1) of the right lobe of the liver; (2) of the superior lobe of right and left lungs.

**s. ante'rius infe'rius** [ NA ], anterior inferior segment (of kidney).

**s. ante'rius supe'rius** [ NA ], anterior superior segment (of kidney).

**s. apica'le** [ NA ], apical segment; (1) apical segment of the superior lobe of the right lung; (2) s. superius (2); apical segment of the inferior lobe of the right and left lungs.

**s. apicoposte'rius** [ NA ], apicoposterior segment (of superior lobe of left lung).

**s. basa'le ante'rius** [ NA ], anterior basal segment (of inferior lobe of right and left lung).

**s. basa'le latera'le** [ NA ], lateral basal segment (of inferior lobe of right and left lung).

**s. basa'le media'le** [ NA ], medial basal segment (of inferior lobe of right and left lung).

**s. basa'le poste'rius** [ NA ], posterior basal segment (of inferior lobe of right and left lungs).

**s. bronchopulmona'lis** [ NA ], bronchopulmonary segment; the largest subdivision of a lobe of the lung; it is supplied by a direct branch of a lobar bronchus and is separated from adjacent segments by connective tissue septa. See fig. under bronchus.

**s. cardi'acum** [ NA ], cardiac segment; official alternative term for s. basale mediale.

**segmenta hep'atis,** hepatic *segments.*

**s. infe'rius** [ NA ], inferior segment (of kidney).

**s. internoda'le,** internodal *segment.*

**s. latera'le** [ NA ], lateral segment; (1) of the left lobe of the liver; (2) of the middle lobe of the right lung.

**segmenta lien'is,** *segments* of the spleen.

**s. lingula're infe'rius** [ NA ], inferior lingular segment (of superior lobe of left lung).

**s. lingula're supe'rius** [ NA ], superior lingular segment (of the superior lobe of the left lung).

**s. media'le** [ NA ], medial segment; (1) of the left lobe of the liver; (2) of the middle lobe of the right lung.

**s. poste'rius** [ NA ], posterior segment; (1) of the right lobe of the liver; (2) of the superior lobe of the right lung; (3) of the kidney.

**segmenta rena'lia** [ NA ], renal segments; arterial segments of the kidney; s.r. having independent blood supply and isolated arterial distribution.

**s. subapica'le** [ NA ], subapical segment; s. subsuperius; an inconstant segment of the inferior lobe of the right and left lungs.

**s. subsupe'rius** [ NA ], subsuperior segment; official alternative term for s. subapicale.

**s. supe'rius** [ NA ], (1) superior segment (of kidney); (2) official alternative term for s. apicale (2).

**segregation** (seg-re-ga'shun) [ L. *segrego*, pp. *-atus*, to set apart from the flock, separate, fr. *se-*, apart, + *grex (greg-)*, flock ]. 1. Separation; removal of certain parts from a mass. 2. The separation of contrasting characters in the offspring of heterozygotes.

**seg'regator.** A separator; a device by means of which the portions of urine entering the bladder from the two ureters are collected separately without being allowed to mingle.

**Harris s.,** Harris *separator.*

**Seidel,** Erich, German ophthalmologist, 1882–1946. See S.'s *scotoma, sign.*

**Seignette** (sayn-yet'), Pierre, Rochelle apothecary, 1660–1719. See S.'s *salt.*

**Seiler** (si'ler), Carl, Swiss Laryngologist and anatomist in America, 1849–1905. See S.'s *cartilage.*

**seismotherapy** (sīz-mo-thĕr'ă-pī) [ G. *seismos*, a shaking, vibration ]. Vibratory *massage.*

**seizure** (se'zhur) [ O. Fr. *seisir*, Med. L. *sacire*, to grasp, take possession of ]. An attack; the sudden onset of a disease or of certain symptoms, such as convulsions.

**anosognosic s.,** an attack of which the patient is unaware.

**psychic s.,** an attack of morbid sensations, such as fullness in the head, vertigo, palpitation, etc., with temporary disturbance of consciousness, not amounting to unconsciousness.

**sejunction** (se-jungk'shun) [ L. *se-jungo*, pp. *-junctus*, to disjoin ]. A separation; a breaking of continuity in the mental processes.

**selachyl alcohol** (sel'ă-kil). A glyceryl ether, found in shark oil, of the structure $CH_2OH$—$CHOH$—$CH_2$—$O$—$(CH_2)_8CH$ = $CH(CH_2)_7CH_3$.

**selaphobia** (se'lă-fo'bĭ-ah) [ G. *selas*, light, + *phobos*, fear ]. Morbid fear of a flash of light.

**selection** (se-lek'shun) [ L. *se-ligo*, to separate, select, fr. *se*, apart + *lego*, to pick out ]. Differential and nonrandom reproduction of individuals of different genotypes, resulting in a change in gene frequency in the population; *e.g.*, death during childhood of individuals homozygous for the recessive gene causing Tay-Sachs disease tends to slowly reduce the frequency of this gene in the population.

**artificial s.,** interference by man with natural s. by purposeful breeding of animals or plants of specific genotype or phenotype to produce a strain with desired characteristics; *e.g.*, breeding of dairy herds for high milk production.

**s. coefficient,** a quantitative measure of the intensity of s. expressed as *s*, the proportional reduction in production of progeny by one genotype as compared with a standard genotype, usually the most favored; the reproductive contribution of the standard genotype is taken as 1, and that of the genotype selected against is (1 − *s*); this expresses the fitness of one genotype relative to another.

**medical s.,** the preservation, by medical care and treatment, of individuals of pathologic genotypes who would not otherwise reproduce, thus tending to increase the frequency of pathologic genes in the population. Medical s. can also reduce the frequency of pathologic genes by preventing reproduction of individuals of specified genotype by surgical sterilization or other means.

**natural s.,** "survival of the fittest"; the process in nature whereby those individuals best able to adapt to their environment survive and reproduce, while those less able die without progeny; the genes carried by the survivors will increase in frequency; this is a major mechanism of evolution.

**s. pressure,** the intensity of s., usually measured as the change in frequency per generation due to s.

**sexual s.,** a form of natural s. in which, according to Darwin's theory, the male or female is attracted by certain characteristics, form, color, behavior, etc., in the opposite sex; thus modifications of a special nature are brought about in the species.

**selene unguium** (se-le'ne ung'gwī-um) [ G. *selēnē*, moon; gen. pl. of L. *unguis*, nail ]. Lunula.

**selenium** (sĕ-le'nĭ-um) [ G. *selēnē*, moon ]. A metallic element, symbol Se, atomic no. 34, atomic weight 78.96; chemically similar to sulfur.

**s. sulfide** (USP, NF), a mixture of crystalline s. monosulfide and solid solutions of s. and sulfur in an amorphous form, containing 52 to 55.5 per cent Se; used in the treatment of seborrhea of the scalp or dandruff; it is applied to the scalp as a suspension containing 4.5 per cent of the agent.

**selenocystine** (sĕ-le'no-sis'tēn). Cystine containing Se in place of one S atom, found in traces in naturally occurring amino acids and, at least in part, responsible for the curative effects of cystine which respect to liver necrosis in rats fed experimental diets deficient in tocopherol and cystine.

**selenodont** (sĕ-le'no-dont) [ G. *selēnē*, moon, + *odous* (*odont*-), tooth ]. Denoting an animal, or man, having teeth, as the human molars, with longitudinal crescent-shaped ridges.

**sele'nomethi'onine.** Methionine containing Se in place of S.

**self.** 1. A sum of the attitudes and behavioral predispositions that make up the personality (*q.v.*). 2. The individual as represented in his own awareness and in his environment.

**subliminal s.,** subconscious mind; the sum of the mental processes which take place without the conscious knowledge of the individual.

**self-accusation.** A common psychiatric symptom, encountered most characteristically in agitated depression.

**self-analysis.** Autoanalysis.

**self-awareness.** Realization of one's ongoing emotional experience; a major goal of all psychotherapy.

**self-commitment.** Voluntary mental hospitalization.

**self-differentiation.** Differentiation resulting from the action of intrinsic causes.

**self-discovery.** In psychoanalysis, the freeing of the repressed ego in a person raised to be submissive to those around him.

**self-fertilization.** The fecundation of the ovules by the pollen of the same flower; or of the ova by the spermatozoa of the same animal, in hermaphrodite forms; denoting an extreme type of inbreeding seen in certain plants and animal forms (hermaphroditic earthworm and the parasitic flatworms) which produce both male and female gametes.

**self-hypnosis.** Autohypnosis.

**self-infection.** Autoinfection.

**self-limited.** Denoting a disease that tends to cease after a definite period, as a result of its own processes; *e.g.,* pneumonia.

**self-poisoning.** Exogenic or endogenic autointoxication.

**Selivanoff** (sel-iv-ah'nof), Feodor, Russian chemist, *1859. See S.'s *test.*

**sella** (sel'ah) [ L. saddle ]. The sella turcica.

**empty s.,** jargon for a condition, demonstrable at operation or by pneumoencephalography, in which the sella turcica contains no discernible pituitary gland; commonly occurs in association with enlargement of the sella turcica and varying degrees of pituitary dysfunction.

**s. tur'cica** [ L. Turkish saddle ] [ NA ], pars sellaris; a saddle-like prominence on the upper surface of the sphenoid bone, situated in the middle cranial fossa and dividing it into two halves.

**sel'lar.** Relating to the sella turcica.

**Sellick's maneuver.** See under maneuver.

**Selter** (zel'ter), Paul, German pediatrician, *1866. See S.'s *disease.*

**Selye,** Hans, Canadian endocrinologist, *1907. See S.-Schenker *test.*

**seman'tics** [ G. *sēmainein,* to show ]. A branch of semiotics: 1. The study of the significance and development of the meaning of words. 2. The study dealing with the relations between signs and what they refer to (referents); the relations between the signs of a system; and human behavioral reaction to signs, including unconscious attitudes, influences of social institutions, and epistomological and linguistic assumptions.

**semeio-.** For words beginning thus, see semio-.

**semelincident** (sem'el-in'sī-dent) [ L. *semel,* once, + *incido,* to happen, fr. *cado,* to fall. CAD- ]. Happening once only; said of an infectious disease, one attack of which confers permanent immunity.

**se'men,** pl. **semi'na, semens** [ L. *semen* (*semin*-), seed (of plants, men, animals) ]. 1 [ NA ]. Seminal fluid; sperm; the penile ejaculate; a thick, yellowish white, viscid fluid containing spermatozoa; it is a mixture of the secretions of the testes, seminal vesicles, prostate, and bulbourethral glands. 2. A seed.

**semenuria** (se'mĕ-nu'rĭ-ah). The excretion of urine containing semen.

**semi-** (sem'ĭ-) [ L. *semis,* half ]. Prefix denoting one-half or partly; used with words derived from Latin roots; the corresponding Greek prefix is *hemi-.*

**semial'dehyde.** The monoaldehyde of a dicarboxylic acid; so called because half the COOH groups of the original acid are reduced to the aldehyde while the other half are unchanged; glutamic acid s. (CHO—$CH_2CH_2$—$CHNH_2$—COOH) is an example. Many semialdehydes are intermediates in the biosynthesis and metabolic degradation of amino acids (*e.g.,* lysine, aspartate, glutamate, valine).

**sem'icanal.** Semicanalis.

**semicanalis,** pl. **semicanales** (sem'ĭ-kă-nal'is, -ēz) [ L. ]. Semicanal; a half canal; a deep groove on the edge of a bone which, uniting with a similar groove or part of an adjoining bone, forms a complete canal.

**s. mus'culi tensor'is tym'pani** [ NA ], semicanal of the tensor muscle of the tympanum; the superior division of the canalis musculotubarius containing the tensor tympani muscle.

**s. tu'bae auditi'vae** [ NA ], semicanal of the auditory tube; the inferior division of the canalis musculotubarius which forms the bony part of the auditory (Eustachian) tube.

**semicartilaginous** (sem'ĭ-kar-tĭ-laj'ĭ-nus). Composed partly of cartilage.

**semicir'cular.** Forming a half circle or an incomplete circle.

**semico'ma.** A mild degree of coma from which it is possible to arouse the patient; see also consciousness.

**semico'matose.** In a condition of unconsciousness from which one can be aroused.

**semiconscious** (sem'ĭ-kon'shus). Partly conscious.

**semicrista** (sem'ĭ-kris'tah) [ semi- + L. *crista,* crest, tuft ]. A small or imperfect ridge or crest.

**s. incisi'va,** *crista* nasalis.

**semidecussation** (sem'ĭ-de-kus-sa'shun). Incomplete decussation such as occurs in the human optic chiasm.

**semiflexion** (sem'ĭ-flek'shun). The position of a joint or segment of a limb midway between extension and flexion.

**semilu'nar** [ semi- + L. *luna*, moon ]. Half-moon-shaped; crescentic.

**semilunare** (sem-ĭ-lu-nah're). *Os* lunatum.

**semiluxa'tion.** Subluxation.

**sem'imembrano'sus.** See under musculus.

**semimem'branous.** Consisting partly of membrane; denoting the musculus semimembranosus.

**sem'inal.** Relating to the semen.

**semina'tion.** Insemination.

**seminiferous** (sem'ĭ-nif'er-us) [ L. *semen*, seed (semen) + *fero*, to carry ]. Carrying or conducting the semen; denoting the tubules of the testis.

**seminoma** (sem'ĭ-no'mah) [ L. *semen*, seed (semen) + G. suffix *-oma*, tumor ]. A malignant testicular neoplasm arising from the sex cells in young male adults; they metastasize to paraortic lymph nodes, but may be cured by orchiectomy and abdominal irradiation. See also dysgerminoma.

**semino'matous.** Relating to a seminoma.

**seminor'mal.** One-half of the normal; denoting a solution one-half the strength of a normal solution; abbreviated N/2 or 0.5 N.

**seminuria** (se'mĭ-nu'rĭ-ah). Semenuria.

**semiography, semeiography** (se-mĭ-og'rä-fĭ) [ G. *sēmeion*, sign, + *graphē*, a description ]. A treatise on symptomatology; a description of the symptoms of a disease.

**semiologic, semeiologic** (se-mĭ-o-loj'ik). Symptomatic.

**semiology, semeiology** (se'mĭ-ol'o-jĭ) [ G. *sēmeion*, sign, + *logos*, study ]. Symptomatology.

**semiopathic, semeiopathic** (se'mĭ-o-path'ik) [ G. *sēmeion*, sign, + *pathos*, disease ]. Denoting the disordered use of symbols.

**semiorbic'ular.** Semicircular; hemispherical.

**semiosis, semeiosis** (se'mĭ-o'sis) [ G. *sēmeiōsis*, fr. *sēmeion*, sign ]. The mental or symbolic process in which something functions as a sign for the organism.

**semiotic, semeiotic** (sem'ĭ-ot'ik) [ G. *sēmeiōtikos*, fr. *sēmeion*, sign ]. 1. Relating to semiotics. 2. Relating to signs, linguistic or bodily.

**semiotics, semeiotics** (sem'ĭ-ot'iks) [ see semiotic ]. 1. Symptomatology or semiology. 2. The general philosophical theory of signs and symbols; comprises three branches (syntactics, semantics, and pragmatics).

**semipen'niform.** Penniform on one side; denoting a muscle the fibers of which are obliquely attached to one side of a tendon.

**semiper'meable.** Permeable to certain molecules, but not to others. See under membrane.

**semiplacenta** (sem'ĭ-pla-sen'tah). The type of placenta in ruminants, horse and pig, in which the maternal and fetal placentas do not grow together but can be easily separated without tearing; an apposed or contact placenta.

**semiprona'tion.** 1. A semiprone position; see semiprone. 2. The act of assuming or being placed in a semiprone position.

**semiprone** (sem-ĭ-prōn'). Halfway between the midposition and pronation; three-quarters prone. See also Sims' *position*.

**semiqui'none.** A free radical resulting from the removal of one hydrogen atom with its electron during the process of dehydrogenation of a hydroquinone to quinone (whence the name) or similar compound (flavin mononucleotide, for example).

**se'mis** [ L. ]. One-half; denoted in prescriptions by *ss.*

**semisideratio** (sem'ĭ-sid-ĕ-ra'shĭ-oh) [ semi- + L. *sideratio*, stroke ]. Hemiplegia.

**semisom'nus.** Semicoma.

**semispi'nal.** Half spinal; denoting muscles attached in part to the spinous processes of the vertebrae.

**semisulcus** (sem'ĭ-sul'kus). A slight groove on the edge of a bone or other structure, which, uniting with a similar groove on the corresponding adjoining structure, forms a complete sulcus.

**semisupine** (sem-ĭ-su-pīn'). Halfway between the midposition and supination; three-quarters supine.

**semisynthet'ic.** Describing the process of synthesizing a particular chemical utilizing a naturally occurring complex chemical as a starting material, thus obviating part of a total synthesis. The conversion of cholesterol, obtained from a natural source, into a corticosteroid is a semisynthetic process.

**semisystematic name** (sem'ĭ-sis'tĕ-mat'ik). Semitrivial name; a name of a chemical of which at least one part is systematic and at least one part is not (*i.e.*, is trivial). For example, calciferol includes the -ol suffix denoting an -OH radical, while calcif-, which has no systematic meaning whatsoever, is used only in this word. Cortisone contains the -one suffix, indicating an aldehyde group, but the rest of the term derives from cortex (adrenal). Hippuric acid (trivial) may be defined as *N*-benzoylglycine (semitrivial name); benzoyl is systematic for the $C_6H_5$—CO— radical, whereas glycine is the trivial name for α-aminoacetic (or 2-aminoethanoic, to be completely systematic) acid, and the *N* signifies that the benzoyl is attached to the N in the glycine. From this, the structure $C_6H_5$—CO—NH—$CH_2$—COOH is uniquely defined. Many generic or nonproprietary names of drugs, including USAN names, hormones, etc., are semitrivial in this chemical sense, although often termed trivial names. The distinction between trivial and semitrivial is not often made.

**semitendino'sus** [ L. ]. Semitendinous.

**semitendinous** (sem'ĭ-ten'dĭ-nus) [ L. *semitendinosus* ]. Composed in part of tendon; denoting the musculus semitendinosus.

**semitertian** (sem-ĭ-ter'shĭ-an, -shun). Partly tertian, partly quotidian; denoting a malarial fever in which two paroxysms occur on one day and one on the succeeding day.

**semitrivial name** (sem'ĭ-triv'ĭ-al). Semisystematic name.

**semiva'lent.** The ability to form a one-electron bond.

**Semon,** Richard W., German biologist, 1859–1908. See S.-Hering *theory*.

**Semon,** Sir Felix, London laryngologist, 1849–1921. See Gerhardt-S. *law*, S.'s *law*.

**Semple,** Sir David, English physician, 1856–1937. See S. *vaccine*.

**Senear,** Francis E., U. S. dermatologist, 1889–1958. See S.-Usher *disease, syndrome.*

**Senecio** (sĕ-ne'sĭ-o, -shĭ-o) [ L. a plant, groundsel, fr. *senecio*, an old man ]. 1. A large genus of the Compositae; many of its species contain alkaloids that produce hepatic necrosis. 2. *Senecio aureus*, life-root; squaw-weed; ragwort; a common weed of the eastern United States; formerly used in the treatment of amenorrhea and other menstrual irregularities.

**senecio'ic acid.** 3,3-Dimethylacrylic acid; methylcrotonic acid; $(CH_3)_2C$=CH—COOH; a precursor of isoprenoid and terpene compounds; intermediate in leucine degradation; polymer precursor.

**seneciosis** (sĕ-ne'sĭ-o'sis). Liver degeneration and necrosis caused by ingestion of plants of the genus *Senecio*, such as ragwort and groundsel. Similar hepatotoxic properties have been observed after ingestion of some kinds of *Crotalaria* and *Heliotropium*.

**senega** (sen'e-gah) [ *Seneca*, an Indian tribe ]. Seneca snakeroot; the dried root of *Polygala senega* (family Polygalaceae), a herb of eastern and central North America; expectorant.

**senegin** (sen'e-jin). The active principle, a saponin, of senega, occurring in the drug in a mixture with polygalic acid.

**senescence** (se-nes'ens) [ L. *senesco*, to grow old, fr. *senex*, old ]. The state of growing old; beginning old age.

**dental s.,** that condition of the teeth and associated structures in which there is deterioration due to aging or premature aging processes.

**senescent** (se-nes'ent). Growing old.

**Sengstaken-Blakemore tube.** See under tube.

**senicul'ture** [ L. *senex*, old, + *cultura*, culture ]. The hygiene of old age.

**senile** (se'nīl, sen'īl) [ L. *senilis* ]. Relating to or characteristic of old age.

**se'nilism.** Premature senility.

**senil'ity.** Old age; the sum of the physical and mental changes occurring in advanced life.

**se'nium** [ L. the feebleness of age, fr. *seneo,* to be old, feeble ]. Old age; especially the debility of the aged.

   **s. precox,** premature senility.

**senna** (sen'ah) [ Ar. *senā* ] (NF, BP). The dried leaflets of *Cassia acutifolia* (Alexandrine s.) and *C. angustifolia* (Tinnevelly or Indian s.), family Leguminosae; laxative.

   **Alexan'drine s.,** *Cassia acutifolia.*

   **s. fruit** (BP), s. pod; the dried legumes of *Cassia acutifolia* and *C. angustifolia;* laxative, but milder than the leaf.

   **Indian s.,** *Cassia angustifolia.*

   **s. pod,** s. fruit.

   **Tin'nevelly s.,** *Cassia angustifolia.*

**sen'nosides A and B** (NF). Two anthraquinone glucosides which are the laxative principles of senna.

**senopia** (se-no'pi-ah) [ L. *senilis,* senile, + G. *ōps,* eye ]. Second *sight.*

**sensation** (sen-sa'shun) [ L. *sensatio,* perception, feeling, fr. *sentio,* to perceive, feel ]. A feeling; the translation into consciousness of the effects of a stimulus exciting any of the organs of sense.

   **after-s.,** see aftersensation.

   **cincture s.,** zonesthesia.

   **delayed s.,** a s. that is not perceived until the lapse of an appreciable interval following the application of the stimulus.

   **general s.,** one referred to the body as a whole and not to any particular external object.

   **girdle s.,** zonesthesia.

   **objective s.,** a s. caused by some material object.

   **primary s.,** s. that is the direct result of a stimulus.

   **referred s.,** reflex or transferred s.; a s. felt in one place in response to a stimulus applied in another.

   **reflex s.,** referred s.

   **special s.,** one referred to a stimulus produced by an external body and acting on any of the sense organs.

   **subjective s.,** a s. not readily referrable to verifiable external stimulus, as contrasted with objective s.

   **transferred s.,** referred s.

**sense** (sens) [ L. *sentio,* pp. *sensus,* to feel, to perceive ]. Feeling; sensation; consciousness; the faculty of perceiving any stimulus.

   **color s.,** the ability to perceive variations in color.

   **s. of equilibrium,** static s.; the s. that makes possible a normal physiologic posture.

   **joint s.,** articular *sensibility.*

   **kinesthet'ic s.,** myesthesia.

   **light s.,** the ability to perceive variations in the degree of light or brightness.

   **muscular s.,** myesthesia.

   **obstacle s.,** the ability, often found in the blind, to avoid objects without visual warning.

   **posture s.,** the ability to recognize the position in which a limb is passively placed, the subject's eyes being closed.

   **pressure s.,** baresthesia; piesesthesia; the faculty of discriminating various degrees of pressure on the surface.

   **seventh s.,** visceral s.

   **sixth s.,** cenesthesia.

   **space s.,** the faculty of perceiving the relative positions of objects in the external world.

   **special s.,** one of the five senses related to the organs of sight, hearing, smell, taste, and touch.

   **static s.,** s. of equilibrium.

   **tactile s.,** touch (1).

   **temperature s.,** thermoesthesia.

   **thermal s., thermic s.,** thermoesthesia.

   **time s.,** the faculty by which the passage of time is appreciated.

   **visceral s.,** seventh s.; splanchnesthesia; splanchnesthetic sensibility; the perception of the existence of the internal organs.

**sensibility** (sen'si-bil'i-ti) [ L. *sensibilitas* ]. The consciousness of sensation; the capability of perceiving sensible stimuli.

   **articular s.,** arthresthesia; joint sense; appreciation of sensation in joint surfaces.

   **bone s.,** pallesthesia.

   **cortical s.,** the integration of sensory stimuli by the cerebral cortex.

   **deep s.,** myesthesia.

   **dissociation s.,** the loss of the pain and the thermal senses with preservation of tactile sensibility.

   **electromuscular s.,** s. of muscular tissue to stimulation by electricity.

   **epicritic s.,** see epicritic.

   **mesoblas'tic s.,** myesthesia.

   **pallesthetic s.,** pallesthesia.

   **proprioceptive s.,** see proprioceptive.

   **protopathic s.,** see protopathic.

   **splanchnesthetic s.,** visceral *sense.*

   **vibratory s.,** pallesthesia.

**sensible** (sen'si-bl) [ L. *sensibilis,* fr. *sentio,* to feel, perceive ]. 1. Perceptible to the senses. 2. Capable of sensation. 3. Sensitive. 4. Having reason or judgment; intelligent.

**sensif'erous** [ L. *sensus,* sense, + *fero,* to carry ]. Conducting a sensation.

**sensigenous** (sen-sij'en-us) [ L. *sensus,* sense, + G. suffix *-gen,* to produce ]. Giving rise to sensation.

**sensim'eter** [ L. *sensus,* sense, + G. *metron,* measure ]. An instrument that measures degrees of cutaneous sensation.

**sensitive** (sen'si-tiv). 1. Capable of perceiving sensations. 2. Responding to a stimulus. 3. Acutely perceptive of interpersonal situations. 4. One who is readily hypnotizable. 5. One supposed to receive communications from spirits; a psychic. 6. Readily undergoing a chemical change, with but slight change in environmental conditions, as a s. reagent. 7. In immunology, denoting (1) a sensitized *antigen* (*q.v.*), and (2) a person (or animal) who has been rendered susceptible to immunological reactions (especially those reactions not associated directly with resistance to infection) by previous exposure of the immunological system to the antigen concerned.

**sensitivity** (sen-si-tiv'i-ti) [ L. *sentio,* pp. *sensus,* to feel ]. The state of being sensitive.

   **acquired (induced) s.,** hypersensitiveness (2); allergy; the immunological state induced in a susceptible subject by an antigen; acquired (induced) s. is characterized by a marked change in the subject's reactivity; on the subject's initial contact with it, the antigen is seemingly immunologically inert, but after a latent period of several days to two weeks or so, the subject becomes sensitive (even to antigen that persists from the initial inoculation, as in serum *disease, q.v.*), and thereafter antigen evokes a reaction, within minutes or hours, the severity of which depends upon quantitative relationships and route of antigen inoculation. See also anaphylactic *shock;* allergy; and skin *test.*

   **idiosyncratic s.,** idiosyncrasy (2).

   **pacemaker s.,** the minimum cardiac activity required to consistently trigger a pulse generator.

   **photoallergic s.,** see photosensitization.

   **phototoxic s.,** see photosensitization.

   **primaquine s.,** nonimmunological inborn s. to primaquine, causing hemolysis on exposure to the drug, due to deficiency of glucose 6-phosphate dehydrogenase in red cells.

   **salt s.,** the tendency of certain bacterial suspensions to agglutinate spontaneously in physiological saline solution.

**sensitiza'tion.** Immunization, especially with reference to antigens (immunogens) not associated with infection; the induction of acquired *sensitivity* (*q.v.*), or allergy.

   **aut'oeryth'rocyte s.,** psychogenic purpura; a peculiar and unusual condition in which various persons, usually women, are easily bruised (purpura simplex), and the ecchymoses are likely to enlarge and involve adjacent tissues, and result in pain in the affected parts. So-called because similar lesions are produced by the inoculation of the subject's own blood and is assumed to be a form of autosensitization although no specific antibodies have been demonstrable; in at least some of the subjects there seems to be a psychogenic mechanism.

   **photodynamic s.,** the action by which certain substances, notably fluorescing dyes (acridine, eosin, methylene blue, rose bengal) absorb visible light and emit the energy at wavelengths that are deleterious to microbes or other organisms in the dye-containing suspension.

**sen'sitize.** To render sensitive (7); to induce acquired sensitivity, to immunize; see also sensitized *antigen.*

**sen'sitizer.** 1. Antibody. 2. A substance that causes dermatitis only after sensitization of the skin by previous exposure.

**sensomo'bile.** Capable of movement in response to a stimulus.

**sensomobil'ity.** The state of being sensomobile.

**sensomo'tor.** Sensorimotor.

**sensori-** (sen'so-rĭ-) [ L. *sensorius*, sensory ]. Combining form meaning sensory.

**senso'rial.** Relating to the sensorium.

**sen'soriglan'dular.** Relating to glandular secretion excited by stimulation of the sensory nerves.

**sen'sorimetab'olism.** Metabolism activated by stimulation of the sensory nerves; obsolete usage.

**sen'sorimo'tor.** Both sensory and motor; denoting a mixed nerve with afferent and efferent fibers.

**sen'sorimus'cular.** Denoting muscular contraction in response to a sensory stimulus.

**sensorium, pl. sensoria, sensoriums** (sen-so'rĭ-um, -ah) [ Late L. ]. 1. [ NA ]. An organ of sensation. 2. Perceptorium; the hypothetical "seat of sensation." 3. In psychiatry, synonymous with consciousness; also sometimes used as a generic term for the intellectual functions.

**sen'sorivas'cular.** Sensorivasomotor.

**sen'sorivasomo'tor.** Sensorivascular; denoting contraction or dilation of the blood vessels occurring as a sensory reflex.

**sensory** (sen'so-rĭ) [ L. *sensorius*, fr. *sensus*, sense ]. Relating to sensation.

**sensualism** (sen'shu-al-izm) [ L. *sensualis*, endowed with feeling, fr. *sentio*, to feel ]. Sensuality; domination by the emotions.

**sen'sus** [ L. ] [ NA ]. Sense.

**sentient** (sen'chent, sen'chĭ-ent) [ L. *sentiens*, pres. p. of *sentio*, to feel, perceive ]. Sensitive; capable of sensation.

**sentiment** (sen'tĭ-ment) [ L. *sentio*, to feel ]. 1. Feeling or emotion in relation to one idea. 2. A complex disposition or organization of a person with reference to a given object, whether a person, thing, or abstract idea, that makes the object what it is for him.

**sentisec'tion.** Vivisection of an animal that is not anesthetized.

**separation, jaw.** The amount of space between the jaws at any degree of opening.

**sep'arator** [ L. *se-paro*, pp. -*atus*, to separate, fr. *se*, apart, + *paro*, to prepare ]. Anything that separates two or more substances or prevents them from mingling. 1. Specifically, a device by means of which the portions of urine entering the bladder from the two ureters are prevented from mingling; a segregator. 2. In dentistry, an instrument for forcing two teeth apart, so as to gain access to adjacent proximal walls.

   **Harris s.,** Harris segregator; a double catheter the beaks of which are separated when in the bladder, a ridge being formed between the two by a sound in the rectum making upward pressure; the urine from each kidney thus collects in its own pouch and is aspirated out through the catheter on that side.

   **Luys' s.,** a diaphragm attached to a curved and doubly tunneled sound, by means of which the cavity of the bladder is divided into two compartments, so that the urine entering from each ureter may be collected separately.

**separato'rium.** Archaic term for periosteal *elevator*.

**se'pedogen'esis** [ G. *sēpedōn*, rottenness, + *genesis*, origin, production ]. Sepedonogenesis; the origin or causation of sepsis.

**se'pedon** [ G. *sēpedōn*, rottenness. SEP- ]. Putrescence; putridity.

**se'pedonogen'esis.** Sepedogenesis.

**Sephadex.** Proprietary name for polymers (gels) composed of cross-linked dextrans and sold in the form of beads suitable for packing into columns for use as molecular sieves.

**sep'sine.** A ptomaine formed in putrefying animal matter.

**sepsis, pl. sepses** (sep'sis, -ēz) [ G. *sēpsis*, putrefaction. SEP- ]. The presence of various pus-forming and other pathogenic organisms, or their toxins, in the blood or tissues; septicemia is a common type of s.

   **intestinal s.,** s. associated with autointoxication of the intestinal origin.

   **s. lenta,** a slowly developing and more or less localized infection.

   **puer'peral s.,** puerperal *fever*.

**sept-.** See (1) septi-; (2) septico-; (3) septo-.

**septa** (sep'tah) [ L. ]. Plural of septum.

**sep'tal.** Relating to a septum.

**sep'tan** [ L. *septem*, seven ]. Denoting a malarial fever the paroxysms of which recur every seventh day.

**sep'tate** [ L. *saeptum*, septum ]. Having a septum; divided into compartments.

**septectomy** (sep-tek'to-mĭ) [ L. *saeptum*, septum, + G. *ektomē*, excision ]. Operative removal of the whole or a part of a septum, specifically of the nasal septum.

**septe'mia.** Septicemia.

**septi-, sept-** [ L. *septem*, seven. SEPT-2 ]. Combining forms meaning seven.

**septic** (sep'tik). Relating to or caused by sepsis.

**septicemia** (sep'tĭ-se'mĭ-ah) [ G. *sēpsis*, putrefaction, + *haima*, blood ]. Septemia; sapremia; septic fever; hematosepsis; septic intoxication; systemic disease caused by the multiplication of microorganisms in the circulating blood. See also pyemia.

   **acute fulminating meningococcal s.,** Waterhouse-Friderichsen *syndrome*.

   **ap'oplec'tiform s.,** a specific infectious disease of chickens and other birds, caused by *Streptococcus gallinarum*.

   **cryptogen'ic s.,** a form of s. in which no primary focus of infection can be found.

   **hemorrhagic s.,** disease in animals caused by members of the *Pasteurella* group of bacteria. The disease occurs in cattle, sheep, swine, rabbits, and fowls.

   **s. meliten'sis,** undulant *fever*.

   **mouse s.,** a disease of mice caused by *Pasteurella muriseptica*.

   **s. pluriform'is,** hemorrhagic s.

   **puer'peral s.,** a severe blood stream infection resulting from an obstetric delivery or procedure.

   **rabbit s.,** a disease in rabbits caused by *Pasteurella cuniculicida*.

   **typhoid s.,** typhoid during the phase when the organism can be cultured from the blood.

**septice'mic.** Relating to, suffering from, or resulting from septicemia.

**sep'ticine.** A ptomaine from decaying animal matter.

**septico-, septic-** [ G. *sēptikos*, putrifying, fr. *sēpsis*, putrefaction. SEP- ]. Combining form meaning sepsis, septic.

**septicophlebitis** (sep-tĭ-ko-fle-bi'tis) [ septico- + phlebitis ]. Septic inflammation of a vein.

**septicopyemia** (sep-tĭ-ko-pi-e'mĭ-ah). Pyemia and septicemia occurring together.

**septicopye'mic.** Relating to septicopyemia.

**septigravida** (sep'tĭ-grav'ĭ-dah) [ L. *septem*, seven, + *gravida*, pregnant woman ]. A woman who is pregnant for the seventh time.

**sep'timetri'tis** [ G. *sēptikos*, septic, + *mētra*, uterus, + -*itis* ]. Septic inflammation of the uterus.

**septip'ara** [ L. *septem*, seven, + *pario*, to bear ]. A woman who has borne seven children in as many pregnancies.

**septivalent** (sep'tĭ-va'lent, sep-tiv'ă-lent) [ L. *septem*, seven, + *valentia*, strength ]. Having a valency of seven, e.g., Mn in $KMnO_4$.

**septo-, sept-** [ L. *saeptum*, septum (*q. v.*). SEPT-1 ]. Combining forms meaning septum.

**septomarginal** (sep'to-mar'jĭ-nal). Relating to the margin of a septum, or to both a septum and a margin.

**sep'tona'sal.** Relating to the nasal septum.

**sep'toplas'ty** [ septo- + G. *plassō*, to fashion ]. An operation to correct defects or deformities of the nasal septum, often by alteration or partial removal of supporting structures.

**septorhinoplasty** (sep'to-ri'no-plas'tĭ) [ septo- + G. *rhis*, nose, + *plassō*, to fashion ]. A combined operation to repair defects or deformities of the nasal septum and of the external nasal pyramid.

**septostomy** (sep-tos'to-mĭ) [ septo- + G. *stoma*, mouth ]. The surgical creation of a septal defect.

**septotomy** [ septo- + G. *tomē*, incision ]. Incision of a septum, specifically of the nasal septum.

**septulum,** pl. **septula** (sep'tu-lum, -lah) [ Mod. L. dim. of *septum* ]. [ NA ]. A minute septum.

**s. tes'tis** [ NA ], trabecula testis; one of the trabeculae of the testis; imperfect septa and fibrous cords radiating toward the surface of the gland from the mediastinum testis.

---

# SEPTUM

---

**septum,** gen. **septi,** pl. **septa** (sep'tum, -ti, -tah) [ L. *saeptum,* a partition. SEPT-1 ]. 1 [ NA ]. A thin wall dividing two cavities or masses of softer tissue. 2. In neuroanatomy, the septal *area; septum* pellucidum.

**s. accesso'rium,** an additional ridge forming the lower border of the limbus fossae ovalis.

**alveolar s.,** s. interalveolare.

**aortopulmonary s.,** the spiral s. which, during development, separates the truncus arteriosus into a ventral pulmonary trunk and dorsal aorta.

**atrioventricular s.,** s. atrioventriculare.

**s. atrioventricula're** [ NA ], atrioventricular s.; the small part of the membranous s. of the heart just above the septal cusp of the tricuspid valve that separates the right atrium from the left ventricle.

**s. of auditory tube,** s. canalis musculotubarii.

**Bigelow's s.,** *calcar* femorale.

**bony nasal s.,** s. nasi osseum.

**bulbar s.,** a s. dividing the embryonic bulbus cordis into pulmonary and aortic outflow tracts from the developing heart. The distal bulbar s. is derived from the right and left endocardial cushions and so separates the pulmonary and aortic orifices. The proximal bulbar s. is the portion of the bulbar s. that is incorporated into the membranous part of the interventricular s.

**s. bul'bi ure'thrae,** a fibrous s. in the interior of the bulb of the penis which divides it into two hemispheres.

**s. cana'lis musculotuba'rii** [ NA ], s. of the musculotubal canal; s. tubae; s. of the auditory tube; a very thin horizontal plate of bone forming two semicanals, the upper, smaller, for the tensor tympani muscle, the lower, larger for the auditory (Eustachian) tube. Its termination in the middle ear is the processus cochleariformis.

**cartilaginous s.,** *pars* cartilaginea septi nasi.

**s. cervica'le interme'dium** [ NA ], a thin s. composed of glia fiber and leptomeningeal connective tissue, in the cervical spinal cord marking the border between the fasciculi gracilis and cuneatus of the dorsal funiculus.

**s. clit'oridis,** an incomplete fibrous pectiniform s. separating the two corpora cavernosa of the clitoris.

**Cloquet's s.,** s. femorale.

**comblike s.,** pectiniform s.

**s. corpo'rum cavernoso'rum** [ NA ], an incomplete fibrous s. between the corpora cavernosa of the clitoris.

**crural s.,** s. femorale.

**distal bulbar s.,** see bulbar s.

**endovenous s.,** s. endovenosum.

**s. endoveno'sum,** endovenous s.; a remnant of the primitive separation between veins which fused to form the definitive trunk, such as the left common iliac and the left renal veins.

**femoral s.,** s. femorale.

**s. femora'le** [ NA ], femoral s.; crural s.; Cloquet's s.; the delicate fibrous membrane that closes the femoral ring at the base of the femoral canal.

**s. of frontal sinuses,** s. sinuum frontalium.

**gingival s., gum s.,** interdental *papilla.*

**s. glan'dis** [ NA ], s. of the glans; a fibrous partition extending through the glans penis from the lower surface of the tunica albuginea to the urethra.

**s. of glans,** s. glandis.

**hanging s.,** the deformity caused by an abnormal width of the septal portion of the alar cartilages.

**interalveolar s.,** (1) the tissue intervening between two adjacent pulmonary alveoli; it consists of a close-meshed capillary network covered on both surfaces by very thin alveolar epithelial cells; (2) s. interalveolare.

**s. interalveola're,** pl. **septa interalveola'ria** [ NA ], interalveolar s. (2); alveolar s.; one of the interalveolar septa; the bony partitions between the tooth sockets.

**interatrial s.,** s. interatriale.

**s. interatria'le** [ NA ], interatrial s.; the wall between the atria of the heart. See also s. primum and s. secundum.

**interdental s.,** the bony portion separating two adjacent teeth in a dental arch.

**s. interme'dium,** old term for the s. of the atrioventricular canal of the embryonic heart formed by the fusion of the dorsal and ventral atrioventricular endocardial cushions.

**intermuscular s.,** s. intermusculare.

**s. intermuscula're** [ NA ], intermuscular s.; a term applied to aponeurotic sheets separating various muscles of the extremities; these are anterior and posterior crural, lateral and medial femoral, lateral and medial humeral.

**interradicular septa,** septa interradicularia.

**sep'ta interradicula'ria** [ NA ], interradicular septa; the bony partitions that project into the alveoli between the roots of the molar teeth.

**interventricular s.,** s. interventriculare.

**s. interventricula're** [ NA ], interventricular s.; the wall between the ventricles of the heart.

**s. lin'guae** [ NA ], lingual s.; nucleus fibrosus linguae; the median vertical fibrous partition of the tongue merging posteriorly into the transverse hypoglossal membrane.

**s. lu'cidum,** s. pellucidum.

**s. mediastina'le,** mediastinum.

**s. membrana'ceum ventriculo'rum,** *pars* membranacea septi interventricularis.

**membranous s.,** (1) *pars* membranacea septi nasi; (2) *pars* membranacea septi interventricularis.

**s. mobile nasi,** *pars* mobilis septi nasi.

**s. muscula're ventriculo'rum,** *pars* muscularis septi interventricularis.

**s. of musculotubal canal,** s. canalis musculotubarii.

**nasal s.,** s. nasi.

**s. na'si** [ NA ], nasal s.; the wall dividing the nasal cavity into halves; it is composed of a central supporting skeleton covered on each side by a mucous membrane.

**s. na'si oss'eum** [ NA ], bony nasal s.; the bones supporting the pars ossea septi nasi; these are the perpendicular plate of the ethmoid, the vomer, the sphenoidal rostrum, the crest of the nasal bones, the frontal spine, and the median crest formed by the apposition of the maxillary and palatine bones.

**s. orbita'le** [ NA ], a fibrous membrane attached to the margin of the orbit and extending into the lids, constituting in great part the posterior fascia of the musculus orbicularis oculi.

**pectin'iform s.,** s. pectiniforme; comblike s.; the anterior portion of the s. penis which is broken by a number of slitlike perforations.

**s. pellu'cidum** [ NA ], transparent s.; s. lucidum; a thin plate of brain tissue, containing nerve cells and numerous nerve fibers, that is stretched like a flat, vertical sheet between the columna and corpus fornicis below, the corpus callosum above and anteriorly. It is usually fused in the median plane with its partner on the opposite side so as to form a thin, median partition between the left and right frontal horn of the lateral ventricles; in less than 10 per cent of humans there is a blind, slitlike, fluid-filled space between the two septa pellucidi, the cavum septi pellucidi. The s. pellucidum is continuous ventralward through the interval between the corpus callosum and the anterior commissure with the precommissural septum, gyrus subcallosus or corpus paraterminale. See also *cavum* septi pellucidi; septal *area.*

**s. pe'nis** [ NA ], the portion of the tunica albuginea separating the two corpora cavernosa of the penis.

**placental septa,** incomplete avascular partitions between placental cotyledons; they are covered with trophoblast and contain a core of maternal tissue.

**precommissural s.,** see septal *area.*

**s. primum,** a crescentic s. in the embryonic heart that arises on the dorsocephalic wall of the originally single atrium and initiates its partitioning into right and left chambers. The tips of the s. primum grow toward and soon become fused with the atrioventricular canal cushions.

**proximal bulbar s.,** see bulbar s.

**rectovaginal s.,** s. rectovaginale.

**s. rectovagina'le** [ NA ], rectovaginal s.; the fascial layer between the vagina and the lower part of the rectum.
**rectovesical s.,** s. rectovesicale.
**s. rectovesica'le** [ NA ], rectovesical s.; rectovesical fascia; Denonvilliers' aponeurosis; Tyrrell's fascia; a fascial layer that extends from the central tendon of the perineum to the peritoneum between the prostate and rectum.
**scrotal s.,** s. scroti.
**s. scro'ti** [ NA ], scrotal s.; an incomplete wall of connective tissue and nonstriated muscle dividing the scrotum into two sacs, each containing a testis.
**s. secun'dum,** the second of two major septal structures involved in the partitioning of the atrium, it arises later than s. primum, is more heavily muscular, and lies to the right of it. Like s. primum s. secundum is crescentic but its tips are directed toward the sinus venosus. It remains an incomplete partition until after birth, with its unclosed area constituting the foramen ovale.
**sinus s.,** a small fold forming the medial end of the valve of the inferior vena cava; it is developed from the dorsal wall of the embryonic sinus venosus.
**s. sin'uum fronta'lium** [ NA ], s. of the frontal sinuses; the bony partition between the two frontal sinuses; it is often deflected to one side of the middle line.
**s. sin'uum sphenoida'lium** [ NA ], s. of the sphenoidal sinuses; the bony partition between the two sphenoidal sinuses, often deflected to one side of the middle line.
**s. of sphenoidal sinuses,** s. sinuum sphenoidalium.
**s. spu'rium** [ L. *spurius,* false ], a s. in the right atrium of the embryonic heart formed by the right venous valve and its continuation onto the dorsocephalic wall of the atrium. In human embryos, it reaches the height of its development during the third month and then undergoes regression, taking no part in atrial partitioning (hence its designation as false). Reduced portions of it persist as the valve of the inferior vena cava and the valve of the coronary sinus.
**s. of tongue,** s. linguae.
**transparent s.,** s. pellucidum.
**transverse s.,** (1) *crista* ampullaris; (2) the fibromuscular layer that forms on the cephalic surface of the embryonic liver; its upper face is clothed with mesothelium and forms the floor of the pericardial cavity; it constitutes the primordium for the more ventral portions of the diaphragm.
**s. tu'bae,** *septum* canalis musculotubarii.
**urogenital s.,** the coronally placed ridge formed by the caudal portion of the urogenital ridges fusing in the midline of the embryo; it lies between the hindgut dorsally and the bladder ventrally.
**urorec'tal s.,** urorectal fold; in embryos, a partition dividing the cloaca into a dorsal, rectal portion and a ventral portion called the urogenital sinus. Reaching the cloacal membrane at about the time of its disintegration the urorectal s. divides the cloacal exit into an anal and a urogenital orifice.
**ventricular s.,** s. interventriculare.

---

**sequela,** pl. **sequelae** (se-kwel'ah, se-kwel'e) [ L. *sequela,* a sequel, fr. *sequor,* to follow ]. A morbid condition following as a consequence of a disease.
**sequence** (se'kwens) [ L. *sequor,* to follow ]. 1. The succession, or following, of one thing or event after another. 2. A sequel or sequela.
**sequential** (se-kwen'shal). Occurring in sequence.
**sequester** (se-kwes'ter). Sequestrum.
**sequestral** (se-kwes'tral). Relating to a sequestrum.
**sequestration** (se-kwes-tra'shun) [ L. *sequestratio,* fr. *sequestro,* pp. *-atus,* to lay aside ]. 1. Isolation; separation from others, as in the case of one with a contagious disease. 2. The formation of a sequestrum.
**bron'chopul'monary s.,** a congenital anomaly in which a mass of lung tissue or a cyst with an independent bronchial branch exists separated from the rest of the lung; it is supplied by a large systemic artery derived from the thoracic aorta.
**sequestrectomy** (se-kwes-trek'to-mi) [ sequestrum + G. *ektome,* excision ]. Sequestrotomy; the operative removal of a sequestrum.
**sequestrotomy** (se'kwes-trot'o-mi) [ sequestrum + G. *tome, incision* ]. Sequestrectomy.

**sequestrum,** pl. **sequestra** (se-kwes'trum, -trah) [ Mod. L. use of Mediev. L. *sequestrum,* something laid aside, fr. L. *sequestro,* to lay aside, separate ]. A piece of necrosed tissue, usually bone, that has become separated from the surrounding healthy tissue.
**primary s.,** a completely detached s.
**Ser.** Symbol for serine and its aminoacyl (seryl) form.
**sera** (ser'ah). One of the plural forms of serum.
**seralbumin** (ser'al-bu'min). Serum *albumin.*
**serangitis** (se'ran-ji'tis) [ G. *seranx, serangos,* cavern, + *-itis,* inflammation ]. Cavernitis.
**serendipity** (se-ren-dip'i-ti) [ coined by Horace Walpole and relates to *The Three Princes of Serendip,* fr. alternate spelling of *Serendib,* ancient name for Ceylon ]. Accidental discovery; finding one thing while looking for something else, as in Fleming's dicovery of penicillin.
**serenoa** (ser'e-no'ah). Sabal; the partially dried fruit of *Serenoa serrulata,* saw-palmetto; has been used in cystitis.
**Sergent** (sair-zhahn'), Emile, French physician, 1867–1943. See S.'s white *line,* Bernard-S. *syndrome.*
**sericeps** (ser'i-seps) [ L. *sericum,* silk, + *caput,* head ]. A bandage or sort of reversed cap, made of ribbon, used to make traction on the fetal head during parturition.
**sericin** (ser'i-sin). The protective covering of fibroin strands of silk; the second secretion which joins the two strands of fibroin just prior to ejection through the spinneret.
**series,** pl. **series** (ser'ez) [ L. fr. *sero,* to join together ]. 1. A succession of similar objects following one another in space or time. 2. In chemistry, a group of substances, either elements or compounds, having similar properties or differing from each other in composition by a constant ratio.
**aromat'ic s.,** all the compounds derived from benzene, or similar cyclic compounds, distinguished from those compounds that are acyclic or that contain rings that lack the unsaturated conjugated double bond structure characteristic of benzene.
**eryth'rocyt'ic s.,** the cells in the various stages of development in the red bone marrow leading to the formation of the erythrocyte, *e.g.,* erythroblasts, normoblasts, erythrocytes.
**fatty s.,** the alkanes; all the acyclic compounds in the methane, ethane, propane, etc., group, distinguished from the aromatic s.
**gran'ulocyt'ic s.,** the cells in the several stages of development in the bone marrow leading to the mature granulocyte of the circulation, *e.g.,* myeloblasts, different stages of the myelocyte, granulocytes.
**Hofmeister s.,** lyotropic s.; specifically, the series of cations $Mg^{2+}$, $Ca^{2+}$, $Sr^{2+}$, $Ba^{2+}$, $Li^+$, $Na^+$, $K^+$, $Rb^+$, $Cs^+$, and of anions $citrate^{3-}$, $tartrate^{2-}$, $SO_4{}^{2-}$, $acetate^-$, $NO_3^-$, $ClO_3^-$, $I^-$, $CNS^-$ (among others), each series arranged in order of decreasing ability (a) to precipatate the dispersed substance of lyophilic sols, (b) to "salt out" organic substances (*e.g.,* aniline, ethyl acetate) from aqueous solutions, or (c) to inhibit the swelling of gels. These effects, among other related ones, are most probably ascribable to the abstraction and binding of water by these ions(*i.e.,* hydration), which also decreases in the orders given, so that (in the monovalent cation series) $Li^+$ with the smallest crystal radius, has the largest hydrated radius, and *vice versa* for $Cs^+$.
**homol'ogous s.,** a s. of organic compounds, the succeeding members of which differ from each other by the radical $CH_2$ (as in the fatty series).
**lymphocyt'ic s.,** the cells at various states in the development in lymphoid tissue of the mature lymphocytes, *e.g.,* lymphoblasts, young lymphocytes, mature lymphocytes.
**lymphoid s.,** lymphocytic s.
**lyotropic s.,** Hofmeister s.
**my'eloid s.,** granulocytic and erythrocytic s.
**thrombocyt'ic s.,** the cells of successive stages in thrombocytic development in the bone marrow, *e.g.,* thromboblasts, thrombocytes.
**seriflux** (ser'i-fluks) [ serum + L. *fluxus,* a flow ]. Orrhorrhea; a profuse serous discharge.

**se'rine.** α-Amino-β-hydroxypropionic acid; 2-amino-3-hydroxypropanoic acid; $CH_2OH$—$CH_2$—$NH_2COOH$; one of the amino acids occurring in proteins.

**s. deaminase,** L-serine dehydratase or threonine dehydratase.

**s. dehydrase,** L-serine dehydratase or threonine dehydratase.

**s. sulfhydrase,** cystathionine β-synthase.

**L-serine dehydratase** (EC 4.2.1.13). Serine dehydrase; serine deaminase; a deaminating hydro-lyase converting L-serine to pyruvate and $NH_3$. See also threonine dehydratase.

**seriograph** (sēr'ĭ-o-graf) [ series + G. *graphō*, to write ]. An instrument for taking a series of radiographs of 6 or 8 exposures in from 4.5 to 6 seconds. Used in cerebral angiography.

**seriography** (sēr'ĭ-og'ră-fĭ). The taking of a series of radiographs by means of the seriograph.

**serioscopy** (sēr'ĭ-os'ko-pĭ) [ series + G. *skopeō*, to view ]. A series of x-rays of a region taken in various directions, and later matched to coincide on a desired spot.

**seriscission** (sēr-ĭ-sish'un) [ L. *sericum*, silk, + *scissio*, a cleaving ]. Division of the pedicle of a tumor or other tissue by a silk ligature.

**sero-** (sēr'o-) [ L. *serum*, whey. SER- ]. Combining form meaning serum or serous.

**seroalbuminuria** (sēr'o-al-bu'mĭ-nu'rĭ-ah). Serous *albuminuria.*

**serocolitis** (sēr'o-ko-li'tis) [ Mod. L. *serosa*, serous membrane, + colitis ]. Pericolitis.

**serocystic** (sēr'o-sis'tik). Relating to one or more serous cysts.

**se'rodiagno'sis.** Diagnosis by means of a reaction in the blood serum or other serous fluids in the body.

**seroenteritis** (sēr'o-en-ter-i'tis) [ Mod. L. *serosa*, serous membrane, + enteritis ]. Perienteritis.

**se'rofast.** Serum-fast.

**serofibrinous** (sēr-o-fi'brĭ-nus). Denoting an exudate composed of serum and fibrin.

**serofibrous** (sēr-o-fi'brus). Relating to a serous membrane and a fibrous tissue.

**serologic** (sēr'o-loj'ik). Relating to serology.

**serology** (se-rol'o-jĭ) [ sero- + G. *logos*, study ]. The branch of science dealing with serum, especially with specific immune or lytic serums.

**serolysin** (se-rol'ĭ-sin). A bactericidal substance in the blood serum.

**seroma** (se-ro'mah) [ sero- + G. suffix -*oma*, tumor ]. A mass or tumefaction caused by the localized accumulation of serum within a tissue or organ.

**seromembranous** (sēr'o-mem'bră-nus). Relating to a serous membrane.

**seromucous** (sēr'o-mu'kus). Pertaining to a mixture of watery and mucinous material such as that of certain glands.

**seropurulent** (sēr'o-pu'ru-lent). Composed of or containing both serum and pus; denoting a discharge of thin, watery pus, or seropus.

**seropus** (sēr'o-pus). Purulent serum; pus largely diluted with serum.

**seroreaction** (sēr'o-re-ak'shun). Serum reaction. 1. Serum *disease.* 2. Any reaction occurring in serum, such as deflection of the complement.

**serosa,** pl. **serosae** (se-ro'sah, -se) [ fem. of Mod. L. *serosus*, serous. SER- ]. 1. *Tunica* serosa. 2. Membrana serosa; the outermost of the extraembryonic membranes that encloses the embryo and all its other membranes; it consists of somatopleure, *i.e.*, ectoderm reinforced by somatic mesoderm; the serosa of mammalian embryos is frequently called the trophoderm.

**serosamucin** (se-ro'sah-mu'sin). Mucoid material found in serous fluids: ascitic, synovial, etc.

**serosanguineous** (sēr'o-sang-gwin'e-us). Denoting an exudate or a discharge composed of or containing serum and also blood.

**seroserous** (sēr'o-sēr'us). Relating to two serous surfaces; denoting a suture, as of the intestine, in which the edges of

the wound are infolded so as to bring the two serous surfaces in apposition.

**serositis** (sēr'o-si'tis). Orrhomeningitis; oromeningitis; inflammation of a serous membrane.

**multiple s.,** polyserositis.

**serosity** (se-ros'ĭ-tĭ). 1. A serous fluid; serum. 2. The condition of being serous. 3. The serous quality of a liquid.

**serosynovial** (sēr'o-sĭ-no'vĭ-al). Relating to serum and also synovia.

**serosynovitis** (sēr'o-sin-o-vi'tis). Synovitis attended with a copious serous effusion.

**serotaxis** (sēr'o-tak'sis) [ sero- + G. *taxis*, an arranging ]. Edema of the skin induced by the application of a strong cutaneous irritant.

**serotherapy** (sēr'o-thĕr'ă-pĭ). Treatment of an infectious disease by the injection of an antitoxin or specific serum.

**serotho'rax.** Hydrothorax.

**serotina** (sēr'o-ti'nah) [ L. fem. of *serotinus*, late ]. See under decidua.

**seroti'nus** [ L. ] [ NA ]. Late; appearing later than similar related structures.

**serotonin** (sēr-o-to'nin, sēr-). 5-Hydroxytryptamine; enteramine; thrombocytin; thrombotonin; 5-(2-aminoethyl)-5-indolol; a vasoconstrictor liberated by the blood platelets. It is present in relatively high concentrations in some areas of the central nervous system (hypothalamus, basal ganglia), and occurs in many peripheral tissues and cells and in carcinoid tumors. It is also present in many nonmammalian organisms (in the clam, *Mercenaria mercenaria*, it is a neurotransmitter). Its precursor is 5-hydroxytryptophan. When liberated from the bound state, it is rapidly deaminated by monoamine oxidase (the major catabolite is 5-hydroxyindoleacetic acid). S. inhibits gastric secretion and stimulates smooth muscle.

**serotype** (sēr'o-tĭp). A subdivision of a species or subspecies distinguishable from other strains therein on the basis of antigenic character.

**serous** (sēr'us). Relating to, containing, or producing serum or a substance having a watery consistency.

**serovaccination** (sēr'o-vak'sĭ-na'shun). A process for producing mixed immunity by the injection of a serum, to secure passive immunity, and by vaccination with a modified or killed culture to acquire active immunity later.

**serozyme** (sēr'o-zim). See *factor* VII.

**serpenta'ria** (ser-pen-ta'rĭ-ah, -tăr'ĭ-ah) [ L. snakeweed ]. The dried rhizome and roots of *Aristolochia serpentaria*, Virginia snakeroot, or of *A. reticulata*, Texas snakeroot (family Aristolochiaceae); a stomachic.

**serpiginous** (ser-pij'ĭ-nus) [ Mediev. L. *serpigo- (-gin)*, ringworm, fr. L. *serpo*, to creep ]. Creeping; denoting an ulcer or other cutaneous lesion that extends with an arciform border; the margin has a wavy or serpent-like border.

**serpigo** (ser-pi'go) [ Mediev. L. *serpigo (-gin)*, ringworm, fr. L. *serpo*, to creep ]. 1. Tinea. 2. Herpes. 3. Any creeping or serpiginous eruption.

**serrate, serrated** (sēr'at, -a'ted) [ L. *serratus*, fr. *serra*, a saw ]. Notched; dentate; toothed.

**Serrati** (sĕ-rah'te). Serafino, Italian physicist, 18th century. Gave his name to *Serratia.*

**Serratia** (sĕ-ra'shĭ-ah) [ S. *Serrati* ]. A genus of motile, peritrichous, aerobic to facultatively anaerobic bacteria (family Enterobacteriaceae) which contains small, Gram-negative rods. Some strains are encapsulated. Many strains produce a pink, red, or magenta pigment. The metabolism of these organisms is fermentative. They are saprophytic on decaying plant and animal materials. The type species is *S. marcescens.*

**S. marces'cens,** a species found in water, soil, milk, foods, silkworms, and other insects. It is the type species of the genus *S.*

**serration** (sĕ-ra'shun) [ L. *serra*, saw ]. 1. The state of being serrated or notched. 2. Any one of the processes in a serrate or dentate formation.

**serratus** (sĕ-ra'tus) [ L. ] [ NA ]. Serrate.

**serrefine** (sair-fēn') [ Fr. ]. A small spring forceps, usually made of wire, used for approximating the edges of a wound or for closing the cut end of an artery during an operation.

**serrenoeud** (sair-në') [ Fr. *serrer*, to press, + *noeud*, knot ]. An instrument for tightening a ligature.

**Serres** (sair), Antoine E. R. A., Paris physician, 1786–1868. See S.'s *angle, glands.*

**serrulate, serrulated** (sĕr'u-lāt, -la'ted) [ L. *serrula*, a small saw, dim. of *serra* ]. Finely serrated.

**Serto'li**, Enrico, Italian histologist, 1842–1910. See S.'s *cells, columns,* S. cell *tumor.*

**serum,** pl. **serums** or **sera** (sēr'um, sēr'ah) [ L. whey. SER- ]. 1 [ NA ]. A clear watery fluid, especially that moistening surface of serous membranes, or exuded in inflammation of any of those serous membranes. 2. The fluid portion of the blood obtained after removal of the fibrin clot and blood cells, distinguished from the plasma in circulating blood; sometimes used as a synonym for antiserum (*q. v.*) or antitoxin (*q. v.*).

    **an'ticomplemen'tary s.,** one that destroys or inactivates complement.

    **an'tiepithe'lial s.,** an antiserum (cytotoxin) for epithelial cells.

    **antilymphocyte,** antiserum against lymphoid tissue, used to suppress rejection of grafts or organ transplants; when used in man, the globulin fraction of the heterologous s. (prepared in horse or other animals) is usually used in conjunction with other immunosuppressive agents (drugs or chemicals) and for a limited period of time.

    **antirabies s.** (USP); a sterile solution containing antiviral substances obtained from the blood s. or plasma of a healthy animal, usually the horse, that has been immunized against rabies by means of vaccine. Administered immediately after severe or multiple bites by domestic animals suspected to be rabid and in all wild animal bites, to be followed by a regimen of rabies vaccine.

    **an'tiretic'ular cytotox'ic s.,** an antiserum specific for cells of the reticuloendothelial system.

    **antitox'ic s.,** an antitoxin.

    **bacteriolyt'ic s.,** an antiserum (bacteriolysin) that sensitizes a bacterium to the lytic action of complement.

    **blood s.,** see s. (2).

    **convalescent s.,** s. from patients recently recovered from a disease; useful in preventing or modifying by passive immunization the same disease in exposed susceptible individuals.

    **dried human s.** (BP), prepared by drying liquid human s. by freeze-drying or by any other method that will avoid denaturation of the proteins and will yield a product readily soluble in a quantity of water equal to the volume of liquid human s. from which it was prepared.

    **foreign s.,** a s. derived from an animal and injected into an animal of another species or into man.

    **gastrotoxic s.,** a s. prepared by injecting and emulsion of the gastric cells of one animal into another animal.

    **human measles immune s.,** measles convalescent s.; obtained from the blood of a healthy person who has survived an attack of measles.

    **human pertussis immune s.,** the sterile s. prepared from the pooled blood of healthy adult human beings who have received repeated courses of phase I pertussis vaccine. Administered intravenously or intramuscularly for the prophylaxis or treatment of whooping cough.

    **human scarlet fever immune s.,** scarlet fever convalescent s.; obtained from healthy persons who have survived an attack of scarlet fever.

    **immune s.,** an antibody-containing s.; *i.e.,* an antiserum.

    **s. lactis,** whey.

    **liquid human s.,** the pool of fluids separated from blood withdrawn from human subjects and allowed to clot in the absence of any anticoagulant. Not more than 10 separate donations are pooled; the contributions from donors of A, O and either B or AB groups are represented in approximately the ratio 9:9:2.

    **muscle s.,** the fluid remaining after the coagulation of muscle plasma and the separation of myosin.

    **normal s.,** a nonimmune s., usually with reference to a s. obtained previously to immunization.

    **normal horse s.,** the sterile and filtered s. of a healthy horse.

    **normal human s.,** human s.; sterile s. obtained by pooling approximately equal amounts of the liquid portion of

coagulated whole blood from eight or more persons who are free from any disease transmissible by transfusion.

    **polyva'lent s.,** an antiserum obtained by inoculating an animal with several species or strains of the bacterium in question.

    **pooled s.,** pooled blood s.; the mixed s. from a number of individuals.

    **s. prothrombin conversion accelerator (SPCA),** see factor VII.

    **specific s.,** a monovalent *antiserum.*

    **thyrotoxic s.,** an antiserum obtained by injecting into animals the nucleoproteins of the thyroid gland.

    **truth s.,** a drug such as amobarbital sodium or thiopental sodium, intravenously injected for the purpose of eliciting information from the subject under its influence (narcotherapy); the term "truth serum" is false and misleading, because the subject's revelations may or may not be factually true, and their legal status and use is open to serious moral and judicial questions.

**serumal** (sēr'um-al). Relating to or derived from serum.

**serum-fast.** Serofast; pertaining to a serum in which there is little or no change in the titer of antibody, even under conditions of treatment or immunologic stimulation.

**serumuria** (sēr'um-u'rĭ-ah). Obsolete term for albuminuria.

**serva'tion.** The use or function of an organ; see also *propriation.*

**Serve'tus (Servet; Servide),** Miguel, Spanish anatomist and theologian, 1509–1553. See S.'s *circulation.*

**servomechanism** (ser'vo-mek'ā-nizm) [ L. *servus*, servant, + G. *mēchanē*, contrivance ]. 1. A control system using negative feedback to operate another system. 2. A process that behaves as a self-regulatory device; *e.g.,* the reaction of the pupil to light.

**seryl** (sēr'il, sĕr'il). A radical of serine.

**sesame** (ses'ā-me) [ G. *sēsamē*, sesame, an eastern leguminous plant ]. Benne plant; a herb, *Sesamum indicum* (family pedaliaceae), the seeds of which are used as a food, and which are the source of sesame oil.

    **s. oil** (USP, BP), benne oil; teel oil; gingili oil; the refined fixed oil obtained from the seed of one or more cultivated varieties of *Sesamum indicum;* a solvent for intramuscular injections.

**sesamoid** (ses'ā-moyd) [ G. *sēsamoeidēs*, like sesame ]. 1. Resembling in size or shape a grain of sesame. 2. Denoting the sesamoid bone (*os sesamoideum*).

**sesamoi'des** [ L. ] [ NA ]. Sesamoid.

**sesamoiditis** (ses-ā-moy-di'tis). Inflammation of the proximal sesamoid bones in the horse.

**sesqui-** (ses'kwĭ-) [ L. ]. Prefix denoting $1^1/2$; at one time used in chemistry to indicate a ratio of 3 to 2 between the two parts of a compound (*e.g.,* sesquisulfide, sesquibasic), but presently used only for sesquihydrates, *i.e.,* compounds crystallizing with 1.5 molecules of water.

**sesquiterpenes** (ses'kwĭ-ter'pēnz). Hydrocarbons or their derivatives consisting of condensation of three isoprene units and containing, therefore, 15 carbon atoms; *e.g.,* farnesol.

**sessile** (ses'il) [ L. *sessilis*, low-growing, fr. *sedeo*, pp. *sessus*, to sit ]. Having a broad base of attachment; not pedunculated.

**set.** A readiness to perceive or to respond in some way; an attitude which facilitates or predetermines an outcome. Prejudice or bigotry are examples of a s. to respond independently of the merits of the stimulus.

    **learning s.,** a readiness or predisposition to learn developed from previous learning experiences, as when an organism learns to solve each successive problem (of equal or increasing difficulty) in fewer trials.

    **postural s.,** an overall motor readiness to respond, as in a runner instructed to get set and on the mark.

**seta,** pl. **setae** (se'tah, -te) [ L. *saeta* or *seta,* a stiff hair or bristle ]. Chaeta. 1. A bristle. 2. A slender, stiff, bristle-like structure.

**setaceous** (se-ta'shus) [ L. *seta,* a bristle ]. 1. Having bristles. 2. Resembling a bristle.

**Setaria** (se-ta'rĭ-ah, -tăr'ĭ-ah) [ L. *seta,* a bristle ]. A nematode genus of the family Stephanofilariidae (superfamily Filarioidea). Adults are long and thin, typically occur in the peritoneal cavity, and produce sheathed microfilariae in the blood that are transmitted to other hosts after cyclical development in appropriate mosquito hosts. They are parasitic in cattle or equines (wild or domestic) and generally are nonpathogenic, although occasionally young worms may wander into the anterior chamber of the eye.

**S. cer'vi,** occurs in the abdominal cavity of cattle, buffalo, bison, yak, and various deer but rarely sheep.

**S. equi'na,** a common parasite of horses and other equids in all parts of the world; these worms are slender whitish filaments, several inches in length, usually found free in the peritoneal cavity, but occasionally reported in the pleural cavity, lungs, scrotum, eye, and intestine.

**setariasis** (se'tă-rĭ-ă-sis) [ *Setaria* + G. suffix *-iasis,* condition ]. Infestation with *Setaria.*

**set'back.** A surgical operation involving a bilateral cleft of the palate in which the premaxilla is moved posteriorly; the procedure is often accompanied by bone grafting.

**Setchenoff.** See Siechenoff.

**setiferous** (se-tif'er-us) [ L. *seta,* bristle, + *fero,* to carry ]. Bristly; having bristles.

**setigerous** (sĕ-tij'er-us) [ L. *seta,* bristle, + *gero,* to bear ]. Setiferous.

**se'ton** [ L. *seta,* bristle ]. A wisp of threads or a strip of gauze passed through the subcutaneous tissues, forming an issue.

**set'ting.** Hardening, as of amalgam ( *q. v.* ).

**set-up.** The arrangement of teeth on a trial denture base.

**Severinghaus,** John W., U. S. physiologist and anesthesiologist, *1922. See S. *electrode.*

**se'voflu'rane** (USAN). Fluoromethyl 2,2,2-trifluoro-1-(trifluoromethyl)ethyl ether; a halogenated ether for inhalation anesthesia.

**se'vum** [ L. SEB- ]. Suet or tallow.

**sex** [ L. *sexus* ]. 1. The character or quality that distinguishes between male and female as expressed in the nature of the sex chromosomes, the gonads, and the accessory genital organs, as contrasted with gender role. 2. The physiological and psychological processes within an individual which prompt behavior related to procreation and/or erotic pleasure.

**sexdigitate** (seks-dij'ĭ-tāt) [ L. *sex,* six, + *digitus,* finger or toe ]. Sedigitate; having six digits on one or both hands or feet.

**sex'duction.** F *duction.*

**sexivalent** (sek'sī-va'lent, sek-siv'ă-lent) [ L. *sex,* six, + *valeo,* to have strength ]. Having a combining power equal to six atoms of hydrogen.

**sex-limited.** Occurring in one sex only.

**sex-linked.** See sex *linkage;* also sex-linked *gene.*

**sexology** (sek-sol'o-jī) [ L. *sexus,* sex, + G. *logos,* study ]. The study of all aspects of sex and, in particular, sexual behavior.

**sex'tan** [ L. *sextus,* sixth ]. Denoting a malarial fever the paroxysms of which recur every sixth day.

**sextigravida** (seks-tĭ-grav'ĭ-dah) [ L. *sextus,* sixth, + *gravida,* pregnant woman ]. A woman in her sixth pregnancy.

**sextipara** (seks-tip'ă-rah) [ L. *sextus,* sixth, + *pario,* to bear ]. Para VI; a woman who has given birth six times to an infant or infants, alive or dead, weighing 500 gm. or more or having a length of gestation of at least 20 weeks.

**sextiparity** (seks'tĭ-păr'ĭ-tĭ). The state of being a sextipara.

**sextiparous** (seks-tip'ă-rus). Relating to sextiparity or to a sextipara.

**sexual** (sek'shu-al) [ L. *sexualis,* fr. *sexus,* sex ]. 1. Relating to sex; erotic; genital. 2. A person considered in his or her s. relation or tendencies.

**contrary s.,** (1) an invert; (2) a homosexual.

**sexuality** (sek'shu-al'ĭ-tĭ). Sex; the sum of a person's sexual behaviors and tendencies, and the strength of sexual tendencies; the quality of having sexual functions or implications.

**infantile s.,** in psychoanalytic personality theory, the concept concerning the psychosexual development in infants and children; infantile s. encompasses the overlapping oral, anal, and phallic phases of psychosexual development during the first 5 years of life.

**sexualization** (sek'shu-al-ĭ-za'shun). 1. The state characterized by the presence of sexual energy or drive. 2. The act of being sexualized (acquiring sexual energy or drive).

**sex'valent.** Sexivalent.

**Sézary,** A. See S. *cell, syndrome.*

**S.G.O.** Abbreviation for Surgeon General's Office.

**SGOT.** Abbreviation for serum glutamic-oxaloacetic transaminase, now known as aspartate aminotransferase.

**SGPT.** Abbreviation for serum glutamic-pyruvic transaminase, now known as alanine aminotransferase.

**SH.** Abbreviation for serum *hepatitis.*

**shadow** (shad'o). 1. Achromocyte. 2. In Jungian psychology, the archtype consisting of collective animal instincts.

**Gumprecht's s.'s,** smudge *cells.*

**Ponfick's s.,** achromocyte.

**shadow-casting.** Deposition of a film of carbon or certain metals such as palladium, platinum or chromium on a contoured microscopic object in order to allow the object to be seen in relief with the electron microscope or sometimes with the light microscope.

**Shaffer,** Philip A., American biochemist, *1881. See Coleman-S. *diet.*

**Shaffer-Hartman method.** See under method.

**shaft** [ A.S. *sceaft* ]. An elongated rodlike structure, as the part of a long bone between the epiphysial extremities.

**s. of femur,** *corpus* femoris.

**hair s.,** *scapus* pili.

**s. of humerus,** *corpus* humeri.

**s. of radius,** *corpus* radii.

**s. of tibia,** *corpus* tibiae.

**shakes.** Ague; malarial chill.

**shank** [ A.S. *sceanca* ]. 1. The tibia; the shin; the leg. 2. The portion of an instrument that connects the cutting or functional portion to a handle; with rotary tools, such as burs or stones, it is the end that fits into the chuck.

**shaping.** In operant conditioning, when the operant is not in the organism's repertoire, a procedure in which the experimenter breaks down the operant into those parts which appear most frequently, beings reinforcing them, and then slowly and successively withholds the reinforcer until more and more of the operant is emitted.

**shark live▸ oil.** Oil extracted from the livers of sharks, mainly of the species *Hypoprion brevirostris;* a rich source of vitamins A and D.

**Sharpey,** William, Scottish physiologist and histologist, 1802–1880. See S.'s *fibers.*

**Shea-Anthony antral balloon.** See under balloon.

**shear** (shēr) [ A.S. ]. The distortion of a body by two oppositely directed parallel forces. The distortion consists of a sliding over one another of imaginary planes (within the body) parallel to the planes of the forces.

**shears** (shērz). Scissors.

**Dubois' s.,** strong s. used for decapitation of the fetus.

**Liston's s.,** strong s. for cutting plaster of Paris bandages.

**sheath** (shēth) [ A.S. *scaeth* ]. 1. Any enveloping structure, such as the membranous covering of a muscle, nerve, or blood vessel. 2. Vagina (1). 3. The prepuce of male animals, especially of the horse.

**caudal s.,** a group of microtubules arranged cylindrically around the caudal pole of the nucleus in a developing spermatozoon.

**crural s.,** femoral s.

**dentinal s.,** Neumann's s.; a layer of tissue relatively resistant to the action of acids, which forms the walls of the dentinal tubules. It is possibly composed of a form of keratin. Its discrete existence is in dispute; some investigators impute its apparent presence to surface refraction from tubular walls.

**dural s.,** an extension of the dura mater which ensheathes the roots of spinal nerves or, more particularly, the vagina externa nervi optici.

**enamel rod s.,** organic covering of the individual enamel rod.

**femoral s.,** crural or infundibuliform s.; the fascia enclosing the femoral vessels, formed by the fascia transversalis anteriorly and the fascia iliaca posteriorly; two septa divide the s. into three compartments, the lateral of which contains the femoral artery and the femoral branch of the genitofemoral nerve, the middle the femoral vein, and the medial is the femoral canal.

**fibrous s.'s,** see entries under *vagina* fibrosa.

**Henle's s.,** endoneurium.

**Hertwig's s.,** the merged outer and inner epithelial layers of the enamel organ, extending beyond the region of the crown to invest the upper part of the root of a developing tooth. It atrophies as the root is formed, but when any of the cells persist they receive the name of Malassez' epithelial rests.

**infundibuliform s.,** femoral s.

**s. of Key and Retzius,** endoneurium.

**Mauthner's s.,** axolemma.

**medullary s.,** myelin s.

**microfilarial s.,** the membrane surrounding the embryos of certain blood-borne microfilariae, such as *Wuchereria, Brugia,* and *Loa* of man; thought to be derived from the vitelline membrane.

**mitochondrial s.,** the spirally arranged mitochondria in the middle piece of a spermatozoon.

**mucous s. of a tendon,** *vagina* synovialis tendinis.

**myelin s.,** medullary s.; the lipoproteinaceous envelope in vertebrates surrounding most axons of more than 0.5-micron diameter. It consists of a double plasma membrane wound tightly around the axon in a variable number of turns, and supplied by oligodendroglia cells (in the brain and spinal cord) or Schwann cells (in peripheral nerves); unwound, the double membrane would appear as a sheetlike cell expansion that is empty of cytoplasm but for a few narrow cytoplasmic strands corresponding to apparent interruptions of the regular myelin structure, the incisures of Schmidt-Lantermann. The myelin s. of each axon is composed of a fairly regular longitudinal sequence of segments, each corresponding to the length of s. supplied by a single oligodendroglia or Schwann cell; in the short interval between each two neighboring segments, the nodes of Ranvier, the axon is unmyelinated even though enclosed by complex finger-like plasmatic expansions of the neighboring oligodendroglia or Schwann cells.

**Neumann's s.,** dentinal s.

**notochordal s.,** the fibrous outer covering of the notochord.

**root s.,** one of the epidermic layers of the hair follicle; the external root s. is continuous with the stratum basale and stratum spinosum of the epidermis; the internal root s. comprises the cuticle of the internal roots, Huxley's layer and Henle's layer.

**Rouget-Neumann s.,** the amorphous ground substance between an osteocyte and the lacunar or canalicular wall.

**Scarpa's s.,** *fascia* cremasterica.

**s. of Schwann,** neurolemma.

**s. of Schweigger-Seidel,** a sheath of reticular cells surrounding the endothelium of the sheathed artery of the splenic pulp.

**synovial s.,** *vagina* synovialis.

**tail s.,** the protoplasmic envelope in the tail of a spermatozoon.

**Sheehan,** H. L., English pathologist, 20th century. See S.'s *syndrome.*

**sheet.** A large, rectangular piece of material, usually thin, used as a bedcovering. See also draw-sheet and drip-sheet.

**Macintosh s.,** a s. made of rubberized waterproof cloth.

**Sheldon,** J. H. See Freeman-S. *syndrome.*

**shelf.** In anatomy, a structure resembling a shelf.

**Blumer's s.,** rectal s.

**dental s.,** dental *ledge.*

**palatal s.,** a medially directed outgrowth of the embryonic maxilla; when fused with its opposite number it forms the secondary palate.

**rectal s.,** Blumer's s.; a s. in the rectum felt above and behind the prostate from metastatic tumors, often of the stomach.

**vocal s.,** *plica* vocalis.

**shell.** An outer covering.

**cytotrophoblastic s.,** the external layer of fetally derived trophoblastic cells on the maternal surface of the placenta.

**diffusion s.,** a small vessel made of a semipermeable membrane through which peptone, but not serum albumin, can pass; used in performing the Abderhalden test.

**shellac** (shĕ-lak') (NF). Lacca; a resinous excretion of an insect, *Laccifer (Tachardia) lacca* (family Coccidae); the insects suck the juice of various resiniferous Asiatic (chiefly Indian) trees and excrete and deposit "stick-lac." S. softens at a low temperature. It has many nonmedicinal uses; it is also used to coat confections and tablets and in dental materials, *e.g.,* impression compound and denture base plates.

**shel'ter.** A tent with open front in which a sanatorium patient may obtain sun baths with considerable privacy.

**Shenton,** Thomas, English radiologist. See S.'s *arch, line.*

**Shepherd,** Francis J., Canadian surgeon, 1851–1929. See S.'s *fracture.*

**Sherman,** Henry C., American biochemist, 1875–1955. See S. *unit,* S.-Bourquin *unit,* S.-Munsell *unit.*

**Sherman plate.** See under plate.

**Sherrington,** Charles S., English physiologist, 1857–1952. Nobel laureate, 1932, with Edgar D. Adrian, for their discoveries regarding the functions of neurons. See S.'s *law, phenomenon,* Schiff-S. *phenomenon,* Liddel-S. *reflex.*

**shield** (shēld) [ A.S. *scild* ]. A protecting screen. 1. A lead sheet for protecting the operator from the x-rays. 2. A watchglass sealed over the sound eye to protect it in a case of gonorrheal ophthalmia.

**Buller's s.,** a watchglass in a frame of adhesive plaster, used to protect the unaffected eye in cases of purulent ophthalmia.

**embryon'ic s.,** a thickened area of the embryonic blastoderm within which the primitive streak appears.

**nipple s.,** A cap or dome placed over the nipple to protect it during nursing.

**shift.** Transfer; change. See also deviation.

**axis s.,** axis *deviation.*

**chloride s.,** see under chloride.

**Doppler s.,** the magnitude of the frequency change in cycles per second when sound and observer are in relative motion away from or toward each other. See also Doppler *effect.*

**Purkinje s.,** Purkinje's *phenomenon.*

**s. to the left,** in hematology, the bone marrow with its immature myeloid cells is visualized on the left, while on the right is the circulating blood with its mature neutrophils; when the percentage of immature cells in the circulating blood increases, the blood picture is shifting to the left.

**s. to the right,** in a differential count of white blood cells in the peripheral blood, the absence of young and immature forms.

**threshold s.,** hearing loss in terms of a decibel s. from a previous audiogram; see also hearing loss, under hearing.

**Shiga** (she'gah), Kiyoshi, Japanese bacteriologist, 1870–1957. Gave his name to *Shigella.* See S. *bacillus,* S.-Kruse *bacillus.*

**Shigella** (she-gel'lah) [ K. *Shiga* ]. A genus of nonmotile, aerobic to facultatively anaerobic bacteria (family Enterobacteriaceae) containing Gram-negative nonencapsulated rods. These organisms cannot use citrate as a sole source of carbon. The growth of these organisms is inhibited by potassium cyanide. Their metabolism is fermentative. They ferment glucose and other carbohydrates with the production of acid but not gas; lactose is ordinarily not fermented, although it is sometimes slowly attacked. The normal habitat is the intestinal tract of man and of higher monkeys. All of the species produce dysentery. The type species is *S. dysenteriae.*

**S. boydii,** a species found only in feces of the sick; occurs in a low proportion of cases of bacillary dysentery.

**S. dysenter'iae,** a species causing dysentery in humans and in monkeys; found only in feces of the sick. It is the type species of the genus *S.*

**S. flexneri,** Flexner's bacillus; paradysentery bacillus; *S. paradysenteriae;* a species found in the feces of the sick and of convalescents or carriers; the most common cause of dysentery epidemics and sometimes of infantile gastroenteritis.

**S. paradysenter'iae,** *S. flexneri.*

**S. son'nei,** a species causing mild dysentery in man and summer diarrhea in children.

**shigellosis** (shig'ĕ-lo'sis). Bacillary dysentery caused by bacteria of the genus *Shigella*, often occurring in epidemic patterns.

**shikimate dehydrogenase** (shī-kim'āt) (EC 1.1.1.25). Oxidoreductase reducing 5-dehydroshikimate to shikimate, by transfer of hydrogens from NADPH, in phenylalanine and tyrosine biosynthesis.

**shikimic acid** (shī-kim'ik). 3,4,5-Trihydroxy-1-cyclohexene-1-carboxylic acid, a cyclic trihydroxy acid; an intermediate in the bacterial synthesis of phenylalanine and tyrosine.

Shikimic acid

**shin** [ A.S. *scina* ]. The anterior portion of the leg.
  **bucked s.'s,** sore s.'s.
  **saber s.,** the sharp-edged anteriorly convex tibia in hereditary syphilis.
  **sore s.'s,** bucked s.'s; a condition seen most frequently in young thoroughbreds during early training, and characterized by periostitis of the dorsal surface of the third metacarpal or metatarsal bone.
  **toasted s.'s,** *erythema* caloricum.
  **trench s.,** trench leg; a disease marked by fever, headache, and dull, aching pain in the tibiae and tibiales antici muscles; there is present also a polymorphonuclear leukocytosis; an affection observed chiefly in soldiers serving in the trenches; it is believed to be an infectious fibrositis affecting chiefly the tibiae.

**shingles** (shing'glz) [ L. *cingulum*, girdle ]. *Herpes* zoster.

**shin-splints.** Tenderness and pain with induration and swelling of pretibial muscles, following athletic overexertion by the untrained; it may be a mild form of anterior tibial compartment syndrome.

**ship.** A ship-shaped structure.
  **Fabricius' s.,** the outline of the sphenoid, occipital, and frontal bones from the supposed resemblance to the lines of a s.

**Shipley-Hartford scale.** See under scale.

**Shirodkar operation.** See under operation.

**shiv'er.** 1. To shake or tremble, especially from cold. 2. A tremor; a slight chill.

**shiv'ering.** 1. Trembling from cold or fear. 2. A spasmodic affection, resembling chorea, affecting the thigh muscles of the horse.

**shoat** (shōt). Shote; a young hog.

**shock.** 1. A sudden physical or mental disturbance. 2. A state of profound mental and physical depression consequent upon severe physical injury or an emotional disturbance. 3. The abnormally palpable impact, appreciated by a hand on the chest wall, of an accentuated heart sound; see diastolic s. and systolic s.
  **anaphylac'tic s.,** the antithesis of prophylaxis, an exaggerated or extreme form of anaphylactic reaction that may be induced in various animal species (notably guinea pigs, rabbits, and dogs) as the result of the injection of even a small dose of foreign material (antigen); incubation period of 10 to 14 days, and then the injection of a second, larger dose of the same material (usually termed the *shocking dose*) promptly results in anaphylactic s., which is associated with pathologic changes that are variable, but characteristic for individual species of animals. The route of injection of the sensitizing dose is not critical, but the shocking dose is more effective when administered intravenously. Development of anaphylaxis varies with species, *i.e.*, guinea pigs may be sensitized by a single dose, whereas a series of fairly widely spaced sensitizing doses is required in rabbits; similarly, the degree of anaphylaxis and intensity of anaphylactic s. (including death) vary with the species of animal, the type of antigen, and the shocking dose. Anaphylaxis is an "artificial" phenomenon that

occurs only under conditions provided by man, *i.e.*, in experimental animals, and rarely as an accident in serum therapy in man; true anaphylaxis is not observed in naturally occurring infections. Anaphylactic s. is presently thought to result from a reaction between antigen and specific antibody that is "fixed" to tissue cells.
  **anaphylac'toid s.,** anaphylactoid *crisis;* see also anaphylactoid.
  **anesthetic s.,** s. produced by the administration of an anesthetic drug or drugs, usually in relative overdosage.
  **break s.,** the s. produced by breaking a constant current passing through the body.
  **cardiogenic s.,** s. resulting from decline in cardiac output secondary to serious heart disease, usually myocardial infarction.
  **chronic s.,** the state of peripheral circulatory insufficiency that develops in elderly patients with some debilitating disease, *e.g.*, carcinoma. There is a subnormal blood volume and the patient is susceptible to hemorrhagic s. as a result of a moderate blood loss as may occur during an operation.
  **colloidoclas'tic s.,** anaphylactoid *crisis.*
  **counter-s.,** see countershock.
  **cultural s.,** a form of stress associated with an individual's assimilation into a new culture vastly different from that in which he was raised.
  **declamping s.,** declamping *phenomenon.*
  **deferred s., delayed s.,** a state of s. coming on at a considerable interval after the receipt of the injury.
  **delirious s.,** erethistic s.
  **diastolic s.,** the abnormally palpable impact, appreciated by a hand on the chest wall, of an accentuated second heart sound.
  **drum s.,** s. produced by rotating the animal in a Noble-Collip drum.
  **electric s.,** a sudden violent impression caused by the passage of a current of electricity through any portion of the body.
  **endotoxin s.,** s. produced by bacterial endotoxins, especially of *Escherichia coli.*
  **erethistic s.,** traumatic or toxic delirium following s.
  **hemorrhagic s.,** hypovolemic s. resulting from acute hemorrhage, characterized by hypotension, tachycardia, pale, cold, and clammy skin, and oliguria.
  **histamine s.,** the s. state produced in animals by the injection of histamine; bronchiolar spasm in the guinea pig, constriction of hepatic veins in the dog.
  **hypovolemic s.,** s. caused by a reduction in volume of blood, *e.g.*, that resulting from hemorrhage.
  **insulin s.,** wet s.; hypoglycemic s. produced by administration of insulin; the chief symptoms are sweating, tremor, anxiety, vertigo, and diplopia, followed by delirium, convulsions, and collapse.
  **irreversible s.,** that which has progressed beyond the stage when it will respond to transfusion or other form of treatment, and recovery is impossible.
  **nitroid s.,** a syndrome resembling that produced by the administration of a large dose of a nitrite, sometimes caused by a too rapid intravenous injection of arsphenamine or some other drug; see nitritoid.
  **oligemic s.,** s. associated with pronounced fall in blood volume, sometimes resulting from increased permeability of blood vessels.
  **osmotic s.,** a sudden change in the osmotic pressure to which a cell (or virus particle) is subjected, usually in order to cause it to lyse and lose its contents.
  **pleural s.,** a condition marked by pallor, loss of consciousness, cyanosis, irregular pulse and respiration, and dilated pupils, sometimes following thoracentesis.
  **primary s.,** s. mainly nervous in nature, from pain, anxiety, etc., which ensues almost immediately upon the receipt of a severe injury.
  **protein s.,** the systemic reaction following the parenteral administration of a protein.
  **reversible s.,** s. that will respond to treatment and from which recovery is possible.
  **secondary s.,** surgical s.
  **septic s.,** s. resulting from acute infection; particularly with septicemia or infection by Gram-negative bacilli. See also endotoxin s.

**serum s.,** anaphylactic or anaphylactoid s. caused by the injection of antitoxic or other foreign serum.

**shell s.,** sinistrosis; psychopathia martialis; a euphemistic term used especially during and after World War I to denote psychiatric illness consequent to battle; a type of traumatic neurosis. See also war *neurosis.*

**surgical s.,** secondary s.; s. that comes on 3 to 5 hours after a severe injury; its chief features are marked fall in blood pressure, low venous pressure, reduced cardiac output, pallor, coldness of the extremities, and other signs of collapse.

**systolic s.,** the abnormally palpable impact, appreciated by a hand on the chest wall, of an accentuated first heart sound.

**vasogenic s.,** s. resulting from depressed activity of the higher vasomotor centers in the brain stem and the medulla, producing vasodilation without loss of fluid so that the container is disproportionately large. In oligemic s. blood volume is reduced; in both, return of venous blood is inadequate.

**wet s.,** insulin s.

**shoe.** A covering or appliance for the foot.

**Scarpa's s.,** a metal support preventing plantar extension of the foot beyond a right angle, used in the treatment of talipes equinus.

**Shone,** John D. See S.'s *anomaly.*

**shook jong.** Koro.

**Shope,** Richard E., American pathologist, *1902. See S. *fibroma, papilloma,* fibroma *virus.*

**shortsightedness.** Myopia.

**shote.** Shoat.

**shot-feel.** A peculiar sensation as of a nervous discharge or electric shock passing rapidly from the top of the head to the feet, sometimes described as a sensation of rolling of shot down the body, occurring in acromegaly.

**shoulder** (shōl'der) [ A.S. *sculder*]. 1. The lateral portion of the scapular region, where the scapula joins with the clavicle and humerus and is covered by the rounded mass of the deltoid muscle. 2. In dentistry, the ledge formed by the junction of the gingival and axial walls in extracoronal restorative preparations.

**s. blade,** scapula.

**frozen s.,** a condition in which there is restriction of glenohumeral and scapulothoracic motion and in which there is pain both on motion and at rest; not caused by infection or neoplasm.

**sugar loaf s.,** a conical deformity of the s. caused by dislocation at the acromioclavicular joint with overriding of the acromion by the clavicle.

**show** (sho) [ A.S. *sceáwe*]. An appearance; specifically, the first appearance of blood in beginning menstruation or a sign of impending labor; characterized by the discharge from the vagina of a small amount of blood-tinged mucus that represents the extrusion of the mucous plug which has filled the cervical canal during pregnancy.

**Shrady,** George F., New York surgeon, 1837–1907. See S.'s *subcutaneous saw.*

**Shrapnell,** Henry J., English anatomist, 1761–1841. See S.'s *membrane.*

**shud'der.** A convulsive or involuntary tremor.

**carotid s.,** vibrations at the height of the carotid pulse tracing, seen in aortic stenosis.

**shunt.** 1. To change direction; to divert. 2. Diversion of accumulations of fluid to an absorbing or excreting system by fistulation or a mechanical device to establish a communication between the origin and the terminus. For the relief of hydrocephalus, the sites of origin are the intracranial cavities and the termini are various absorbing or excreting systems usually in the thorax and abdomen. The nomenclature commonly includes origin and terminus, *e.g.,* ventriculocisternal (Torkildsen), ventriculoatrial, ventriculoperitoneal, subarachnoid ureterostomy (Heile operation, Matson operation), third ventriculostomy (Dandy operation, Stookey-Scarff operation), and ventriculomastoid.

**arteriovenous s.,** derivative circulation; the passage of blood directly from arteries to veins, without going through the capillary network.

**dialysis s.,** arteriovenous s. connecting the arterial and venous cannulas in arm or leg.

**Dickens s.,** phosphogluconate oxidation pathway; hexose monophosphate s.; Warburg-Dickens-Lipmann pathway; the oxidative conversion of glucose 6-phosphate to glyceraldehyde 3-phosphate with the formation of three molecules of $CO_2$; a major route of carbohydrate catabolism in tissues other than liver and brain.

**jejunoileal s.,** jejunoileal *bypass.*

**left-to-right s.,** a diversion of blood from the left side of the heart to right (as through a septal defect), or from the systemic circulation to the pulmonary (as through a patent ductus arteriosus).

**mesocaval s.,** anastomosis of the side of the superior mesenteric vein to the proximal end of the divided inferior vena cava, for portable hypertension.

**portaca'val s.,** any communication or anastomosis between portal vein and general circulation, as paraumbilical, azygos or esophageal veins; surgical anastomosis between portal vein and vena cava; see also Eck *fistula.*

**portasystemic vascular s.,** a s. between portal and systemic blood supplies.

**renal-splenic venous s.,** splenorenal s.

**reversed s.,** right-to-left s.

**right-to-left s.,** reversed s.; the passage of blood from the right side of the heart into the left (as through a septal defect), or from the pulmonary artery into the aorta (as through a patent ductus arteriosus); such a shunt can occur only when the pressure in the right heart exceeds that in the left, as in advanced pulmonic stenosis, or when the pulmonary artery pressure exceeds aortic pressure, as in one form of Eisenmenger's syndrome.

**splenorenal s.,** renal-splenic venous s.; anastomosis of the splenic vein to the left renal vein, usually end-to-side, for portable hypertension.

**Torkildsen s.,** a ventriculocisternal s.; see s. (2).

**Warburg-Lipmann-Dickens S.,** Dickens s.

**Shwartzman** (shvarts'mahn), Gregory, New York physician, *1896. See S. *phenomenon, reaction,* Sanarelli-S. *phenomenon,* generalized S. *phenomenon.*

**Shy,** G. Milton, U. S. neurologist, 1919–1967. See S.-Drager *syndrome.*

**Si.** Chemical symbol of the element silicon.

**SI.** Abbreviation for International System of Units; see under International.

**siagonantritis** (si-ă-gon-an-tri'tis) [ G. *siagōn,* jaw, + *antron,* cave, + *-itis* ]. Inflammation of the maxillary sinus.

**sial-.** See sialo-.

**sialaden** (si-al'ă-den) [ sial- + G. *adēn,* gland ]. A salivary gland.

**sialadenitis** (si-al-ad-ē-ni'tis) [ sial- + G. *adēn,* gland, + suffix *-itis,* inflammation ]. Sialoadenitis; inflammation of a salivary gland.

**sialadenoncus** (si'al-ad-ē-nong'kus) [ sial- + G. *adēn,* gland, + *onkos,* bulk (tumor) ]. A neoplasm of salivary tissue.

**sialadenotropic** (si'al-ad'ē-no-trop'ik) [ sial- + G. *adēn,* gland, + *tropē,* a turning ]. Having an influence on the salivary glands.

**sialagogue** (si-al'ă-gog) [ sial- + G. *agōgos,* drawing forth ]. Sialogogue; ptyalagogue. 1. Promoting the flow of saliva. 2. An agent having this action.

**sialaporia** (si'al-ă-po'rī-ah) [ sial- + G. *aporia,* difficulty of passage. POR-1 ]. A deficient secretion of saliva.

**sialectasis** (si'ă-lek'tă-sis) [ sial- + G. *ektasis,* a stretching ]. Ptyalectasis; dilation of a salivary duct.

**sialemesis, sialemesia** (si'al-em'e-sis, -ē-me'zī-ah) [ sial- + G. *emesis,* vomiting ]. Vomiting of saliva, or vomiting caused by or accompanying an excessive secretion of saliva.

**sialic** (si-al'ik). Salivary.

**s. acid,** term for esters and other derivatives of *N*-acetylneuraminic acid; a component of various mucoproteins. The radical of a sialic acid is sialoyl, if the OH of the COOH is removed, and sialosyl, if the OH comes from the anomeric carbon (C-2) of the cyclic structure.

**sialidase** (si-al'ī-dās). Neuraminidase.

**si'aline.** Sialic.

**sialism, sialismus** (si'ă-lizm, si'ă-liz'mus) [ G. *sialismos* ]. Ptyalism; ptyalorrhea; salivation; sialorrhea; an excess secretion of saliva.

**sialo-, sial-** (si'ă-lo-) [ G. *sialon*, saliva ]. Combining forms indicating saliva or salivary gland. See also ptyalo-.

**sialoadenectomy** (si'ă-lo-ad-ĕ-nek'to-mĭ) [ sialo- + G. *adēn*, gland, + *ektomē*, excision ]. Excision of a salivary gland.

**sialoadenitis** (si'ă-lo-ad-ĕ-ni'tis). Sialadenitis.

**sialoadenotomy** (si'ă-lo-ad-ĕ-not'o-mĭ) [ sialo- + G. *adēn*, gland, + *tomē*, incision ]. Incision of a salivary gland.

**sialoaerophagy** (si'ă-lo-a-er-of'ă-jĭ) [ sialo- + G. *aēr*, air, + *phagein*, to eat ]. Aerosialophagy; a habit of frequent swallowing whereby quantities of saliva and air are taken into the stomach.

**sialoangiectasis** (si'ă-lo-an-jĭ-ek'tă-sis) [ sialo- + G. *angeion*, vessel, + *ektasis*, a stretching ]. Dilation of salivary ducts.

**sialoangiitis** (si'ă-lo-an-je-i'tis) [ sialo- + G. *angeion*, vessel, + suffix *-itis*, inflammation ]. Inflammation of a salivary duct.

**sialocele** (si'ă-lo-sēl) [ sialo- + G. *kēlē*, tumor ]. Ptyalocele; sublingual cyst; see also ranula (2).

**sialodochitis** (si'ă-lo-do-ki'tis) [ sialo- + G. *dochē*, receptacle (DOCH-), + suffix *-itis*, inflammation ]. Inflammation of the duct of a salivary gland.

**sialodochoplasty** (si'ă-lo-do'ko-plas'tĭ) [ sialo- + G. *dochē*, receptacle (DOCH-), + *plassō*, to fashion ]. Repair of a salivary duct.

**sialogenous** (si'ă-loj'ĕ-nus) [ sialo- + G. suffix *-gen*, producing ]. Producing saliva. See also sialagogue.

**sialogogue** (si-al'ă-gog). Sialagogue.

**sialogram** (si-al'o-gram) [ sialo- + G. *gramma*, a writing ]. A roentgenogram of one or more of the salivary ducts.

**sialography** (si'ă-log'ră-fĭ) [ sialo- + G. *graphō*, to write ]. Ptyalography; x-ray examination of the salivary glands and ducts after the introduction of a radiopaque material into the ducts; ptyalography.

**sialolith** (si'ă-lo-lith) [ sialo- + G. *lithos*, stone ]. Ptyalolith; a salivary calculus.

**sialolithiasis** (si'ă-lo-lĭ-thi'ă-sis) [ sialolith + G. suffix *-iasis*, condition ]. Ptyalolithiasis; salivolithiasis; the formation or presence of a salivary calculus.

**sialolithotomy** (si'ă-lo-lĭ-thot'o-mĭ) [ sialolith + G. *tomē*, incision ]. Ptyalolithotomy; incision of a salivary duct or gland to remove a calculus.

**sialometry** (si'ă-lom-ĕ-trĭ) [ sialo- + G. *metron*, measure ]. A measurement of salivary secretion function, generally for a comparison of a denervated or diseased gland with its healthy counterpart.

**sialorrhea,** (si'ă-lo-re'ah) [ sialo- + G. *rhoia*, a flow ]. Sialism.

**sialoschesis** (si'ă-los'ke-sis) [ sialo- + G. *schesis*, retention ]. Suppression of the secretion of saliva.

**sialosemiology, sialosemeiology** (sī-ă-lo-se-mī-ol'o-jĭ) [ sialo- + G. *sēmeion*, sign, + *logos*, study ]. The study and analysis of the saliva as an aid to diagnosis.

**sialosis** (si'ă-lo'sis). Salivation.

**sialostenosis** (si'ă-lo-stĕ-no'sis) [ sialo- + G. *stenōsis*, a narrowing ]. Stricture of a salivary duct.

**sialosyrinx** (si'ă-lo-sĭr'ingks) [ sialo- + G. *syrinx*, a pipe, fistula ]. A salivary fistula; a pathologic communication between the outside via the skin or the oral tissues and the salivary gland or duct.

**sib.** Sibling.

**sib'ilant** (sib'ĭ-lant) [ L. *sibilans* (*-ant-*), pres. p. of *sibilo*, to hiss ]. Hissing or whistling in character; denoting a form of rale.

**sib'ilus** [ L. a hissing ]. A sibilant rale.

**sib'ling** [ A. S. *sib*, relation, + *-ling*, diminutive ]. Sib; one of two or more children of the same parents.

**sib'ship** [ A.S. *sib*, relationship ]. Relationship, as between children of the same parents.

**Sibson,** Francis, English anatomist, 1814–1876. See S.'s *aponeurosis, fascia, groove, muscle,* and aortic *vestibule.*

**siccant** (sik'ant) [ L. *siccans* (*-ant-*), pres. p. of *sicco,* pp. *-atus,* to dry ]. Siccative; drying.

**siccative** (sik'ă-tiv). Siccant.

**sicchasia** (sĭ-ka'zĭ-ah) [ G. *sikchasia,* loathing, fr. *sicchos,* squeamish ]. 1. Nausea. 2. The nausea of pregnancy. 3. Loathing for food.

**siccolabile** (sik'o-la'bil, -bĭl) [ L. *siccus,* dry, + *labilis,* perishable ]. Subject to alteration or destruction on drying.

**siccostabile, siccostable** (sik'o-sta'bil, -bĭl, -bl) [ L. *siccus,* dry, + *stabilis,* stable ]. Not subject to alteration or destruction on drying.

**siccus** (sik'us) [ L. ]. Dry.

**sick** [ A.S. *seóc* ]. 1. Ill; unwell; suffering from disease. 2. Nauseated.

**sickle-form** (sik'el). Malarial *crescent.*

**sickle-hocked.** In a normal horse, the plantar part of the hind leg should be relatively straight from the point of the hock to the fetlock. When it is bowed so the foot is carried too far forward, the animal is said to be sickle-hocked.

**sicklemia** (sik-le'mĭ-ah). Presence of sickle- or crescent-shaped erythrocytes in peripheral blood; seen in sickle cell anemia and sickle cell trait.

**sick'ling.** Production of sickle-shaped erythrocytes in the circulation, as in sickle cell anemia.

**sick'ness.** 1. Disease. 2. Nausea.

   **African horse s.,** a disease of horses and other equids in South Africa, caused by a virus which is transmitted by biting gnats of several species.

   **African sleeping s.,** African trypanosomiasis; an endemic disease in tropical Africa caused by the presence in the blood and cerebrospinal fluid of *Trypanosoma gambiense,* a protozoan introduced by the bite of a species of tsetse fly, *Glossina palpalis.* The symptoms consist of mental deterioration, an increasing tendency to drowse or sleep, tremors, enlargement of the lymphatic glands, emaciation, an evening elevation of temperature, and a rapid pulse. The disease is uniformly fatal, if untreated, but recovery has been observed after the use of organic arsenic compounds.

   **air s.,** a condition resembling seasickness or other forms of motion s. occurring in airplane flight as a result of vibration, deflections from linear flight, and gravitational forces.

   **altitude s.,** hypobaropathy; mountain fever; mountain s.; altitude anoxia; the syndrome of giddiness, nausea, dyspnea, headache, thirst, malaise, and sometimes a slight elevation of temperature, resulting from reduced oxygen intake in the presence of reduced atmospheric pressure in those ascending in planes, climbing mountains, or ascending to great heights. See also caisson *disease.*

   **black s.,** visceral *leishmaniasis.*

   **bush s.,** an anemia of sheep and cattle in Australia due to deficiency of iron and cobalt.

   **car s.,** a form of motion s. similar to seasickness and caused by riding on a railway or in an automobile with resultant nausea, dizziness, and, sometimes, vomiting.

   **decompression s.,** caisson *disease.*

   **duck s.,** botulism.

   **falling s.,** epilepsy.

   **gall s.,** anaplasmosis.

   **green s.,** chlorosis.

   **Indian s.,** epidemic gangrenous *proctitis.*

   **lambing s.,** pregnancy *disease* of sheep.

   **laughing s.,** see pseudobulbar *paralysis.*

   **milk s.,** a disease of man caused by ingesting milk from cows suffering from the trembles; see milk fever.

   **Monday morning s.,** *azoturia* of horses.

   **morning s.,** the nausea and vomiting of early pregnancy.

   **motion s.,** kinesia; the syndrome of pallow, nausea, weakness, and malaise which may progress to vomiting and incapacitation, caused by the stimulation of the semicircular canals during travel or motion as on a boat, plane, swing, or rotating amusement ride.

   **mountain s.,** see altitude s.

   **radiation s.,** the condition that follows x-irradiation, whether therapeutic, industrial, or military. In mild forms there are anorexia, nausea, vomiting, malaise, and leukopenia. In more severe forms there are reduction or disappearance of platelets with bleeding, reduction or disappearance of leukocytes with risk of infection, and reduction of new red cells leading to anemia.

   **sea s.,** see seasickness.

**serum s.,** serum disease; serum eruption; local and general symptoms (urticaria, fever, general glandular enlargement, edema, pains in the joints, and occasionally albuminuria) appearing 8 to 12 days after an injection of a foreign serum; the immediate occurrence of the symptoms is regarded as anaphylactic in character, denoting sensitization by a previous injection of the same kind of serum (see anaphylactic *shock*); recovery takes place after a variable period or, in exceptional cases, symptoms of collapse appear and sudden death may occur.

**spotted s.,** pinta.

**stiff sickness,** ephemeral fever of cattle; see under fever.

**sweating s.,** an acute febrile disease of young cattle in South Africa. It is transmitted by the tick, *Hyalomma transiens,* but the precise causative agent has not been identified.

**three-day s.,** ephemeral fever of cattle; see under fever.

**side** [ A.S. *sīde* ]. One of the two lateral margins or surfaces of a body, midway between the front and back.

**balancing s.,** in dentistry, the side opposite the working s. of the dentition or denture. See also working s.

**working s.,** in dentistry, the lateral segment of a denture or dentition toward which the mandible is moved. See also balancing s.

**side′bones.** Ossification of the lateral cartilages of the horse's foot, seen most often in the forefeet of the heavier working breeds; exostoses often appear, and may be seen and palpated above the hoof line.

**side-effect.** A result of drug or other therapy in addition to or in extension of the desired therapeutic effect. While technically the therapeutic effect carried beyond the desired limit (*e.g.,* a hemorrhage from an anticoagulant) is a s., the term more often refers to pharmacologic results of therapy unrelated to the usual objective (*e.g.,* a development of signs of Cushing's syndrome with steroid therapy). The term usually, but not necessarily, connotes an undesirable effect.

**sid′erans** [ L. (see sideration) ]. Fulminating.

**sideration** (sid′er-a′shun) [ L. *sideror,* pp. *sideratus,* to be blasted or palsied by a constellation, fr. *sidus* (*sider-*), a constellation, the heavens ]. Any sudden attack, as of apoplexy.

**siderism** (sid′er-izm) [ G. *sidēros,* iron ]. Metallotherapy.

**sidero-** (sid′er-o-) [ G. *sidērōs,* iron ]. Combining form relating to iron.

**sideroblast** (sid′er-o-blast). An erythroblast containing granules of ferritin stained by the Prussian blue reaction.

**siderocyte** (sid′er-o-sit) [ sidero- + G. *kytos,* cell ]. An erythrocyte containing granules of free iron, as detected by the Prussian blue reaction, in the blood of normal fetuses; they constitute from 0.10 to 4.5 per cent of the erythrocytes.

**sideroderma** (sid′er-o-der′mah) [ sidero- + G. *derma,* skin ]. Brownish discoloration of skin of legs due to hemosiderin deposits.

**siderodromophobia** (sid′er-o-drom-o-fo′bi-ah) [ sidero- + G. *dromos,* a running, a course, + *phobos,* fear ]. Morbid fear aroused by the sight, or sometimes thought, of a railway, a locomotive, or a train of cars.

**siderofibrosis** (sid′er-o-fi′bro′sis). Fibrosis associated with small foci in which iron is deposited.

**siderogenous** (sid′er-oj′e-nus) [ sidero- + G. suffix *-gen,* producing ]. Iron-forming.

**sideropenia** (sid′er-o-pe′ni-ah) [ sidero- + G. *penia,* poverty ]. Hyposiderosis; iron deficiency; an abnormally low level of serum iron.

**sid′erope′nic.** Characterized by iron deficiency.

**siderophil, siderophile** (sid′er-o-fil, -fīl) [ sidero- + G. *philos,* fond ]. 1. Absorbing iron. 2. A cell or tissue that contains iron.

**siderophilin** (sid′er-o-fil′in, sid′er-of′ī-lin). Transferrin.

**siderophilous** (sid′er-of′ī-lus). Siderophil (1).

**siderophone** (sid′er-o-fōn, sī-dēr′o-fōn) [ sidero- + G. *phōnē,* sound ]. An electrical device for detecting a bit of iron in the eyeball, its presence causing the instrument to sound.

**siderophore** (sid′er-o-fōr) [ sidero- + G. *phoros,* bearing ]. A macrophage in the lung containing hemosiderin; also known as "heart failure" cell.

**sideroscope** (sid′er-o-skōp) [ sidero- + G. *skopeō,* to view ]. A very delicately poised magnetic needle for the detection of the presence and location of a particle of iron or steel imbedded in the eyeball.

**siderosilicosis** (sid′er-o-sil′ī-ko′sis) [ sidero- + silicosis, *q. v.* ]. Silicosis produced by exposure to iron-containing dust.

**siderosis** (sid-er-o′sis) [ sidero- + G. suffix *-osis,* condition ]. 1. Steel grinder's disease, arc-welder's disease, scissors grinder's disease, grinder's asthma; a form of pneumoconiosis due to the presence of iron dust. 2. Discoloration of any part by an iron pigment; when the iron is derived from the blood it is called hemosiderosis; when derived from an iron foreign body it is called transfusional or exogenous s. 3. An excess of iron in the circulating blood. 4. A reddish brown or greenish discoloration of the iris and lens caused by the presence of a particle of iron in the vitreous.

**Siebold** (ze′bolt), Carl C. von, German surgeon, 1736–1807. See S.'s *operation.*

**Siegert,** Ferdinand, German pediatrician, 1865–1946. See S.'s *sign.*

**Siegle** (ze′gleh), Emil, German otologist, 1833–1900. See S.'s *otoscope.*

**Siemens,** Hermann Werner, German dermatologist, *1891. See Christ-S. *syndrome.*

**sieve** (siv) [ O.E. *sive* ]. A meshed or perforated device for separating fine particles from coarser ones.

**molecular s.,** a gel-like material with pore sizes of such ranges as to exclude molecules above certain sizes; used in fractionating or purifying macromolecules; see also Sephadex.

**sig.** Abbreviation of L. *signa, q. v.*

**Sigault** (se-go′), Jean-René, French obstetrician, *1740. See S.'s *operation.*

**Siggaard-Andersen nomogram.** See under nomogram.

**sigh** [ A.S. *sican* ]. 1. To make an audible inspiration and expiration under the influence of some emotion. 2. A deep inspiration, made involuntarily under the influence of some emotion, followed by an audible expiration.

**sight** [ A.S. *gesiht* ]. Vision; the ability or faculty of seeing.

**day s.,** nyctalopia.

**far s.,** hyperopia.

**long s.,** hyperopia.

**near s.,** myopia.

**night s.,** hemeralopia.

**old s.,** presbyopia.

**second s.,** prodromal myopia; senile lenticular myopia; gerontopia; senopia; an improvement in near vision in the aged caused by the myopia of increasing lenticular nuclear sclerosis, a precursor of eventual nuclear cataract.

**short s.,** myopia.

**sigma.** The 18th letter of the Greek alphabet (σ); used as a symbol for reflection coefficient.

**sigmatism** (sig′mă-tizm) [ G. *sigma,* the letter S ]. A form of stammering in which pronunciation of the letter s is imperfect.

**sigmoid** (sig′moyd) [ G. *sigma,* the letter S, + *eidos,* resemblance ]. Resembling in outline the letter S or one of the forms of the Greek sigma.

**sigmoid-.** See sigmoido-.

**sigmoidectomy** (sig′moy-dek′to-mī) [ sigmoid- + G. *ektomē,* excision ]. Excision of the sigmoid flexure.

**sigmoi′deus** [ L. ] [ NA ]. Sigmoid.

**sigmoiditis** (sig-moy-di′tis) [ sigmoid- + G. suffix *-itis,* inflammation ]. Inflammation of the sigmoid flexure.

**sigmoido-, sigmoid-** (sig-moy′do-) [ G. *sigma,* the letter S, + *eidos,* resemblance ]. Combining forms meaning S-shaped (sigmoid) and relating, usually, to the sigmoid colon.

**sigmoidopexy** (sig-moy′do-pek-sī) [ sigmoido- + G. *pēxis,* fixation ]. Operative attachment of the sigmoid colon to the belly wall for the relief of prolapse of the rectum.

**sigmoidoproctostomy** (sig-moy′do-prok-tos′to-mī) [ sigmoido- + G. *prōktos,* anus, + *stoma,* mouth ]. Establishment of an artificial anus by opening into the junction of the sigmoid colon and the rectum.

**sigmoidorectostomy** (sig-moy-do-rek-tos'to-mĭ). Sigmoidoproctostomy.

**sigmoidoscope** (sig-moy'do-skōp) [ sigmoido- + G. *skopeō*, to view ]. A speculum for viewing the cavity of the sigmoid colon.

**sigmoidoscopy** (sig'moy-dos'ko-pĭ). Inspection, through a speculum, of the interior of the sigmoid colon.

**sigmoidostomy** (sig'moy-dos'to-mĭ) [ sigmoido- + G. *stoma*, mouth ]. Establishment of an artificial anus by opening into the sigmoid colon.

**sigmoidotomy** (sig'moy-dot'o-mĭ) [ sigmoido- + G. *tomē*, incision ]. Surgical opening of the sigmoid.

**sigmoscope** (sig'mo-skōp). Sigmoidoscope.

---

# SIGN

---

**sign** (sīn) [ L. *signum*, mark ]. 1. Any abnormality indicative of disease, discoverable by the physician at his examination of the patient; a sign is an objective symptom of disease; a symptom is a subjective sign of disease. 2. An abbreviation or symbol. 3. In psychology, any object or artifact (stimulus) that represents a specific thing or conveys a specific idea to the person who perceives it; see also conventional s., iconic s., and indexical s.

**Aaron's s.,** a referred pain or feeling of distress in the epigastrium or precordial region, on continuous firm pressure over McBurney's point, in acute appendicitis.

**Abadie's s. of exophthalmic goiter,** spasm of the levator palpebrae superioris in Graves' disease.

**Abadie's s. of tabes dorsalis,** insensibility to pressure over the tendo Achillis.

**Abrahams' s.,** (1) rales and other adventitious sounds, changes in the respiratory murmurs, and increase in the whispered sounds can be heard on auscultation over the acromial end of the clavicle some time before they become audible at the apex; (2) a dull-flat note, *i.e.*, one between the normal dullness at the right apex and absolute flatness, heard on percussion in that region, indicating the progress from incipient to advanced tuberculosis.

**accessory s.,** a symptom usually though not always present in a disease.

**Ahlfeld's s.,** Braxton Hicks' s.

**Allis' s.,** in fracture of the neck of the femur, the trochanter rides up relaxing the fascia lata so that the finger can be sunk deeply between the great trochanter and the iliac crest.

**Amoss' s.,** when a patient is told to sit up in bed, he does so by extending his arms and supporting himself with the hands far behind him in cases in which flexion of the spine is painful.

**Anghelescu's s.,** in cases of vertebral tuberculosis, when the patient lies on his back, bending the spine so that he rests on the heels and occiput only is painful or impossible.

**antecedent s.,** prodromic s.

**Arroyo's s.,** asthenocoria.

**assi'dent s.,** accessory s.

**Auenbrugger's s.,** an epigastric prominence seen in cases of marked pericardial effusion.

**Aufrecht's s.,** diminished breath sounds in the trachea just above the jugular notch, in cases of stenosis.

**Babinski's s.,** (1) extension of the great toe instead of the normal flexion reflex to plantar stimulation, considered indicative of pyramidal tract involvement; also called Babinski's reflex or phenomenon; "positive" Babinski; paradoxical extensor reflex; great toe reflex; toe phenomenon; (2) in hemiplegia, weakness of the platysma muscle on the affected side, as is evident in such actions as blowing or opening the mouth; (3) when the patient is lying upon his back with arms crossed on the front of his chest, and attempts to assume the sitting posture, the thigh on the side of an *organic* paralysis is flexed and the heel raised, whereas the limb on the sound side remains flat; (4) in

hemiplegia the forearm on the affected side when placed in a position of supination turns into the pronated position.

**Baccelli's s.,** good conduction of the whisper in nonpurulent pleural effusions.

**Ballance's s.,** the presence of a dull percussion note in both flanks, constant on the left side but shifting with change of position on the right, said to indicate ruptured spleen; the dullness is due to the presence of blood, fluid on the right side but coagulated on the left.

**Ballet's s.,** partial or complete external ophthalmoplegia without internal ophthalmoplegia, in Graves' disease.

**Bamberger's s.,** (1) jugular pulse in tricuspid insufficiency; (2) allesthesia; (3) dullness on percussion at the angle of the scapula, clearing up as the patient leans forward, indicating pericarditis with effusion.

**bandage s.,** Rumpel-Leede *test*.

**Bárány's s.,** in cases of ear disease, in which the vestibule is healthy, injection into the external auditory canal of water below the body temperature (65°F. or lower) will cause rotary nystagmus toward the opposite side; when the injected fluid is above the body temperature (106°F. or higher) the nystagmus will be toward the injected side; if the labyrinth is diseased there is no nystagmus.

**Bard's s.,** increased rapidity of the oscillations, in organic nystagmus, in fixating a moving target.

**Barré's s.,** if the hemiplegic is placed in the prone position with the limbs flexed at the knees, he is unable to maintain the flexed position on the side of the lesion but extends the leg.

**Bassler's s.,** in chronic appendicitis pinching the appendix between the thumb of the operator and the iliacus muscle causes sharp pain; the tip of the thumb is pressed into the abdominal wall halfway between the umbilicus and the anterior superior spine of the ilium and is then pushed to the right.

**Bastedo's s.,** pain and tenderness in the right iliac fossa on inflation of the colon with air, in cases of chronic appendicitis.

**Battle's s.,** postauricular ecchymosis in cases of fracture of the base of the skull.

**Beccaria's s.,** a painful sense of pulsation in the occiput in pregnancy.

**Bechterew's s.,** paralysis of automatic facial movements, the power of voluntary movement being retained.

**Beevor's s.,** with paralysis of the lower portions of the recti abdominis muscles the umbilicus moves upward.

**Bezold's s.,** Bezold's *symptom*.

**Biederman's s.,** a dusky redness of the lower portion of the anterior pillars of the fauces in certain cases of syphilis.

**Bielschowsky's s.,** in paralysis of a superior oblique muscle, tilting the head to the side of the involved eye causes that eye to make an upward movement.

**Biermer's s.,** Gerhardt's s.

**Biernacki's s.,** analgesia of the ulnar nerve (the "funny-bone" sensation being absent) in tabes dorsalis and dementia paralytica.

**Bird's s.,** the presence of a zone of dullness on percussion with absence of respiratory s.'s in hydatid cyst of the lung.

**Bjerrum's s.,** Bjerrum's *scotoma*.

**Bonhoeffer's s.,** loss of normal muscle tone in chorea.

**Boston's s.,** jerky lowering of upper eyelid on downward rotation of the eye, characteristic of Graves' disease when present.

**Bouveret's s.,** (1) an absence of concordance between the limits of a bilocular stomach as indicated by clapotage and by insufflation; (2) a tumor in the right iliac fossa in cases of obstruction in the colon.

**Bozzolo's s.,** pulsating vessels in the nasal mucous membrane, noted occasionally in thoracic aneurysm.

**Branham's s.,** slowing of the heart rate following compression or excision of an arteriovenous fistula.

**Braun von Fernwald's s.,** asymmetrical enlargement of the uterus in early pregnancy, one side being greater than the other, a perceptible furrow separating the two; a congenital defect.

**Braxton Hicks' s.,** Hicks' s.; Ahlfeld's s.; irregular uterine contractions occurring after the third month of pregnancy.

**Broadbent's s.,** a retraction of the thoracic wall, synchronous with cardiac systole, visible in the left posterior axillary line; a s. of adherent pericardium.

**Brudzinski's s.,** (1) contralateral reflex or s.; in meningitis on passive flexion of the leg on one side, a similar movement occurs in the opposite leg; (2) neck s.; in meningitis if the neck is passively flexed, flexion of the legs occurs.

**Bryant's s.,** abnormal position of axillary folds in dislocation of the shoulder.

**burning drops s.,** a sensation as of drops of hot liquid falling into the abdominal cavity or as of a stream of intensely hot liquid being poured into the cavity; noted in certain cases of perforated gastric ulcer.

**Calkins' s.,** the change of shape of the uterus from discoid to ovoid indicates placental separation from the uterine wall.

**Cantelli's s.,** see doll's eye s.

**Cardarelli's s.,** tracheal *tugging.*

**Carnett's s.,** includes two maneuvers: (1) the disappearance of abdominal tenderness to palpation when the anterior abdominal muscles are contracted indicates pain of intraabdominal origin; its persistence suggests a source in the abdominal wall; (2) the latter is also indicated when tenderness is caused by gently pinching a fold of skin and fat between thumb and forefinger.

**Carvallo's s.,** increase in the intensity of the pansystolic murmur of tricuspid regurgitation during or at the end of inspiration.

**Castellani-Low s.,** a fine tremor of the tongue observed in sleeping sickness.

**Chaddock s.,** Chaddock reflex; external malleolar s.; when the external malleolar skin area is irritated extension of the great toe occurs in cases of organic disease of the corticospinal reflex paths.

**Chadwick's s.,** Jacquemier's s.

**Chaussier's s.,** severe pain in the epigastrium, a prodrome of eclampsia. May be of central origin or caused by distention of the capsule of liver by hemorrhage.

**Chvostek's s.,** Weiss' s.; facial irritability in tetany, unilateral spasm being excited by a slight tap over the facial nerve.

**Claybrook's s.,** transmission of breath and heart sounds through abdominal wall in rupture of abdominal viscus.

**Cleemann's s.,** wrinkling of the skin just above the patella, in fracture of the femur with overriding of the fragments.

**clenched fist s.,** the eloquent gesture of the patient with angina pectoris when he presses his clenched fist against his chest to indicate the constricting, pressing quality of his pain.

**Cloquet's s.,** an obsolete s. in which a bright needle is not quickly rusted when passed into the muscular tissue, if life is extinct.

**Codman's s.,** hunching of shoulder when deltoid contracts in absence of rotator cuff function.

**coin s.,** bellmetal *resonance.*

**Coles's s.,** deformity of duodenum on x-ray indicates ulcer.

**Comby's s.,** an early s. of measles, consisting in thin whitish patches on the gums and buccal mucous membrane, formed of degenerated squamous epithelium.

**commemorative s.,** a phenomenon pointing to the previous existence of some disease other than the one present at the time.

**Comolli's s.,** a typical triangular cushion-like swelling, corresponding to the outline of the scapula, in cases of fracture of that bone.

**contralat′eral s.,** Brudzinski's s. (1).

**conventional s.'s,** s.'s that acquire their function through social (linguistic) custom; also called symbols; *e.g.,* words or mathematical symbols.

**Coopernail's s.,** ecchymosis of the perineum and scrotum, or labia, in fracture of the pelvis.

**Courvoisier's s.,** see Courvoisier's *law.*

**Crichton-Browne's s.,** a slight tremor at the angles of the mouth and at the outer canthus of each eye in general paresis.

**Cruveilhier's s.,** *caput* medusae.

**Cullen's s.,** periumbilical darkening of the skin from blood, a s. of intraperitoneal hemorrhage especially in ruptured ectopic pregnancy.

**cushingoid s.'s,** s.'s characterizing Cushing's disease or Cushing's syndrome; buffalo hump obesity, striations, adiposity, hypertension, diabetes, and osteoporosis.

**Dalrymple's s.,** in Graves' disease, abnormal wideness of the palpebral fissures, the upper lid being retracted.

**Dance's s.,** a slight retraction in the neighborhood of the right iliac fossa in some cases of intussusception.

**Danforth's s.,** shoulder pain on inspiration, due to hemoperitoneum in ruptured eccyesis.

**Davidsohn's s.,** absence of illumination of the pupil when an electric light is placed in the mouth, indicating the presence of fluid or a solid tumor in the antrum of Highmore on the darkened side.

**Dawbarn's s.,** pain of subacromial bursitis disappears when arm is abducted.

**Déjérine's s.,** aggravation of symptoms of radiculitis by raising intraspinal pressure through the acts of coughing, sneezing, or straining at stool.

**Delbet's s.,** in a case of aneurysm of a main artery, if the nutrition of the part below is well maintained despite the fact that the pulse has disappeared, the collateral circulation is efficient.

**D'Espine's s.,** (1) bronchophony over the spinous processes heard, at a lower level than in health, in pulmonary tuberculosis; (2) an echoed whisper following a spoken word, heard in the stethoscope placed over the seventh cervical or first or second dorsal spine, in cases of tuberculosis of the mediastinal glands.

**doll's eye s.,** dissociation between the movements of the eyes and those of the head, the eyes being lowered as the head is raised, and the reverse (Cantelli); protrusion of the eyeballs and sluggish movements of the eyes and lids (Widowitz). Both s.'s may occur in diphtheria.

**Dorendorf's s.,** fullness of one supraclavicular groove in aneurysm of the aortic arch.

**drawer s.,** see drawer *test.*

**Drummond's s.,** a puffing sound, synchronous with the cardiac systole, heard from the nostrils, the mouth being closed, in certain cases of aortic aneurysm.

**Duchenne's s.,** falling in of the epigastrium during inspiration in paralysis of the diaphragm.

**Dupuytren's s.,** (1) free up and down movement of the head of the femur, upon intermittent traction, in cases of congenital dislocation; (2) a crackling sensation on pressure over the bone in certain cases of sarcoma.

**ear s.,** the ears are not involved in cases of subcutaneous inflammation, because of the close adhesion of the skin and cartilage, but in erysipelas and other skin inflammations the ears do not escape.

**Ebstein's s.,** obtuseness of the cardiohepatic angle on percussion in pericardial effusion.

**s. of edema of the lower lid,** swelling of the lower lid found in congestive failure, myxedema, or nephrosis.

**Enroth's s.,** edema of the eyelids, especially of the upper lid near the supraorbital margin, in Graves' disease.

**Erb's s.,** (1) increased electric excitability of the muscles to the galvanic current, and frequently to the faradic, in tetany; (2) Erb-Westphal s.

**Erb-Westphal s.,** abolition of the patellar tendon reflex, in tabes and certain other diseases of the spinal cord, and occasionally also in brain disease.

**Erichsen's s.,** when sudden pressure is made approximating the iliac bones, pain is caused in the case of sacroiliac disease, but not in that of hip disease.

**Escherich's s.,** in hypoparathyroidism (latent tetany) tapping the skin at the angle of the mouth causes protrusion of the lips.

**Ewart's s.,** Pins' s.; in large pericardial effusions, an area of dullness with bronchial breathing and bronchophony below the angle of the left scapula.

**Ewing's s.,** (1) dullness on percussion to the inner side of the angle of the left scapula, denoting an accumulation of fluid in the pericardium behind the heart; (2) tenderness at the upper inner angle of the orbit at the point of attachment of the pulley of the superior oblique muscle, denoting closure of the outlet of the frontal sinus.

**eyelash s.,** in a case of apparent unconsciousness due to functional disease, such as conversion hysteria, stroking the eyelashes will occasion movement of the lids, but no such reflex will occur in case of severe organic brain lesion such as apoplexy, fracture of the skull, or other traumatism.

**fabere s.**, (acronym formed from the words flexion, abduction, external rotation and extension); see Patrick's *test.*

**Faget's s.**, a slow pulse with an elevated temperature, often seen in yellow fever.

**fan s.**, the spreading apart of the toes in the complete Babinski's sign.

**Fischer's s.**, in a case of tuberculosis of the bronchial glands, if one bends the child's head as far back as possible, auscultation over the manubrium sterni will sometimes reveal a continuous loud murmur caused by the pressure of the enlarged glands on the vena anonyma.

**Forchheimer's s.**, the presence, in German measles, of a reddish maculopapular eruption on the soft palate.

**Fothergill's s.**, finding with rectus sheath hematoma; the hematoma produces a mass which does not cross the midline and remains palpable when the rectus muscle is tense.

**Friedreich's s.**, sudden collapse of the previously distended veins of the neck at each diastole of the heart; it occurs in cases of adherent pericardium.

**Froment's s.**, flexion of the distal phalanx of the thumb when a sheet of paper is held between the thumb and index finger in ulnar nerve palsy.

**Gaenslen's s.**, pain on hyperextension of hip with pelvis fixed by flexion of opposite hip; causes a torsion stress at the sacroiliac and lumbosacral joints.

**Garel's s.**, when an electric bulb is placed in the mouth the light is not perceived by the eye on the side of an empyema or tumor of the antrum of Highmore.

**Gauss' s.**, marked mobility of the uterus in the early weeks of pregnancy.

**Gerhardt's s.**, complete bilateral paralysis of the adductor muscles of the larynx with severe inspiratory dyspnea.

**Gifford's s.**, difficulty in everting the upper eyelid in Graves' disease.

**Glasgow's s.**, a systolic murmur heard over the brachial artery in aneurysm of the aorta.

**Goggia's s.**, the fibrillation of the biceps muscle, when pinched and tapped, is confined to a limited area in cases of debilitating disease, whereas in health it is general.

**Goldstein's toe s.**, increased space between the great toe and its neighbor, seen in mongolism and occasionally in cretinism.

**Goldthwait's s.**, in sprain of sacroiliac ligaments, flexion of hip with extended knee elicits pain in sacroiliac region; not now considered specific.

**Goodell's s.**, softening of the cervix and vagina as being usually indicative of pregnancy.

**Gordon s.**, finger *phenomenon.*

**Gorlin's s.**, unusual ease in touching the tip of the nose with the tongue; seen in Ehlers-Danlos syndrome.

**Gould's s.**, bowing of the head in order to obtain better vision in cases of retinitis pigmentosa.

**Graefe's s., von Graefe's s.**, in Graves' disease with exophthalmos, the upper eyelid does not follow evenly the movement of the eyeball downward, but lags or moves jerkily.

**Grasset's s.**, normal contraction of the sternocleidomastoid muscle on the paralyzed side in cases of hemiplegia.

**Grey Turner's s.**, local areas of discoloration about the umbilicus and in the region of the loins, in acute hemorrhagic pancreatitis.

**Grisolle's s.**, the papules of smallpox do not disappear when the skin is stretched; they remain palpable.

**Grocco's s.**, (1) acute dilation of the heart following a muscular effort, noted in Graves' disease. (2) extension of the liver dullness several centimeters to the left of the midspinal line in cases of enlargement of that organ; (3) Grocco's *triangle.*

**Gunn's s.**, Marcus Gunn's s.; the compression of the underlying vein at arteriovenous crossings seen ophthalmoscopically in arteriolar sclerosis.

**Guyon's s.**, (1) ballottement of the kidney in cases of nephroptosia, especially when there is also a renal tumor; (2) the hypoglossal nerve lies directly upon the external carotid artery, whereby this vessel may be distinguished from the internal carotid when ligation is necessary.

**halo s.**, elevation of the subcutaneous fat layer over the fetal skull in a dead or dying fetus; said to be the commonest radiologic sign of fetal death.

**halo s. of death,** in a fetus, roentgenographic evidence of thickening of soft tissues between the fat layer of the scalp and the cranial bones; due to an accumulation of fluid.

**halo s. of hydrops,** a discredited roentgenographic s. of fetal hydrops caused by scalp edema so that a definite corona surrounds the skull.

**Hamman's s.**, crunching, rasping sound, synchronous with heart beat, heard over the precordium and sometimes at a distance from the chest in interstitial emphysema of the lungs.

**Hegar's s.**, softening and compressibility of the lower segment of the uterus in early pregnancy (about the seventh week); on bimanual examination it feels to the finger in the vagina as though the neck and body of the uterus were separated, or connected by only a thin band of tissue.

**Heim-Kreysig s.**, Kreysig's.; an indrawing of the intercostal spaces, synchronous with the cardiac systole, in cases of adherent pericardium.

**Heryng's s.**, absence of illumination of the orbit when an electric light is placed in the mouth, in case of empyema or tumor of the antrum of Highmore.

**Hicks' s.**, Braxton Hicks s.

**Hill's s.**, in aortic insufficiency, the exaggerated excess of femoral over brachial artery systolic pressure; in normal persons the arterial systolic pressure in the leg is 10 to 20 mm. of Hg above that in the arm, whereas in aortic insufficiency the difference may be 60 to 100 mm. of Hg.

**Hoffmann's s.'s,** (1) in latent tetany mild mechanical stimulation of the trigeminal nerve causes severe pain; (2) Hoffmann's reflex; digital reflex; snapping reflex; flexion of the terminal phalanx of the thumb and of the second and third phalanges of one or more of the fingers when the volar surface of the terminal phalanx of the fingers is flicked.

**Homans' s.**, slight pain at the back of the knee or calf when the ankle is forcibly dorsiflexed, indicative of incipient or established thrombosis in the veins of the leg.

**Hoover's s.'s,** (1) a person lying supine on a couch, when asked to raise one leg, involuntarily makes counterpressure with the heel of the other leg; if this leg is paralyzed, whatever muscular power is preserved in it will be exerted in this way; or if the patient attempts to lift contour paralyzed limb, counterpressure will be made with the other heel, whether any movement occurs in the paralyzed leg or not; not present in hysteria or malingering; (2) a modification in the movement of the costal margins during respiration, caused by a flattening of the diaphragm; it is suggestive of empyema or other intrathoracic condition causing a change in the countour of the diaphragm.

**Hueter's s.**, when the soft parts intervene, in a case of fracture, the vibration, on tapping the bone, is not transmitted.

**iconic s.'s,** s.'s that acquires their function through similarity to what they signify; *e.g.*, a photograph as a s. of the person in the picture.

**indexical s.'s,** s.'s that acquire their function through a causal connection with what they signify; *e.g.*, smoke as a s. of fire.

**Itard-Cholewa s.**, anesthesia of the membrana tympani in otosclerosis.

**Jackson's s.** (Chevalier Q.), asthmoid wheeze; a puffing sound heard on listening before the patient's open mouth in a case of foreign body in the trachea or a bronchus.

**Jackson's s.** (John Hughlings), during quiet respiration the movement of the paralyzed side of the chest may be greater than that of the opposite side, while in forced respiration the paralyzed side moves less than the other.

**Jacquemier's s.**, Kluge's s.; Chadwick's s.; dark bluish or purplish discoloration of the vaginal mucous membrane; a presumptive s. of pregnancy.

**Jellinek's s.**, a brownish pigmentation of the eyelids, especially the upper, in Graves' disease.

**Joffroy's s.**, (1) immobility of the facial muscles when the eyeballs are rolled upward, in exophthalmic goiter; (2) disorder of the arithmetical faculty (the person being unable to do simple sums in addition or multiplication) in the early stages of organic brain disease.

**Jorissenne's s.,** the pulse rate is not quickened on rising from the recumbent position, in the early months of pregnancy.

**Kahn-Falta s.,** in latent tetany, while Trousseau's s. is being elicited, there occurs vasoconstriction with ischemia of the fingers.

**Keen's s.,** increased width at the malleoli in Pott's fracture.

**Kehr's s.,** violent pain in the left shoulder in a case of rupture of the spleen.

**Kernig's s.,** when the subject lies upon the back and the thigh is flexed to a right angle with the axis of the trunk, complete extension of the leg on the thigh is impossible; present in various forms of meningitis.

**Kluge's s.,** Jacquemier's s.

**Kocher's s.,** in Graves' disease, if the examiner's hand is placed on a level with the patient's eyes and then suddenly raised higher, the upper lids move upward more rapidly than the eyeballs, giving the appearance of globe lag.

**Kreysig's s.,** Heim-Kreysig s.

**Kussmaul's s.,** the paradoxical increase in venous distention and pressure during inspiration seen in patients with cardiac tampanade.

**Küstner's s.,** dermoid cysts of the ovary are often found anterior to the uterus, contrary to the usual position of ovarian cysts in lateral and posterior locations.

**Ladin's s.,** an area of elasticity, felt on palpation through the vagina as early as the fifth or sixth week of uterine pregnancy; it is on the anterior face of the uterus just above the cervix; the area grows larger as pregnancy progresses.

**Lancisi's s.,** a large systolic jugular venous wave caused by tricuspid regurgitation replacing the normal negative systolic trough ("x" descent).

**Landolfi's s.,** systolic contraction and diastolic dilation of the pupil, seen in aortic insufficiency.

**Lasègue's s.,** when patient is supine with hip flexed, dorsiflexion of the ankle causing pain or muscle spasm in the posterior thigh indicates lumbar root or sciatic nerve irritation.

**Laugier's s.,** in fracture of the lower portion of the radius, the styloid processes of the radius and of the ulna are on the same level.

**Legendre's s.,** in facial hemiplegia of central origin, when the examiner raises the lids of the actively closed eyes the resistance is less on the affected side.

**Leichtenstern's s.,** Leichtenstern's phenomenon; tapping gently one of the bones of the extremities causes the patient to draw back violently, sometimes with a loud cry; noted in cases of cerebrospinal meningitis.

**Leri's s.,** voluntary flexion of the elbow is impossible in a case of hemiplegia when the wrist on that side is passively flexed.

**Leser-Trélat s.,** sudden appearance of large numbers of keratoses; associated with internal malignancy.

**Lhermitte's s.,** sudden electric-like shocks extending down the spine when the patient flexes his head; a s. of meningeal irritation.

**Lichtheim's s.,** Déjérine-L. phenomenon; in subcortical aphasia, the patient can indicate by his fingers the number of syllables of the word he has in mind but cannot speak.

**lig′ature s.,** in cases of hemophilia, the application of a ligature, not very tightly drawn, around a limb will cause the production of ecchymoses in the peripheral portion of the member.

**local s.,** the characteristic of a sensation that permits it to be distinguished from another sensation in respect to position in space.

**Loenen's s.,** Ladin's s.

**Lorenz′ s.,** stiffness of the thoracic spine in early pulmonary tuberculosis.

**Ludloff's s.,** (1) swelling and ecchymosis at the base of Scarpa's triangle in traumatic separation of the epiphysis of the small trochanter; (2) inability to raise the thigh when in the sitting posture in case of the same accident.

**Lust's s.,** in latent tetany, tapping over the peroneal nerve causes contraction of muscles of the leg.

**Macewen's s.,** Macewen's symptom; percussion of the skull gives a cracked-pot sound in cases of hydrocephalus.

**Magendie-Hertwig s.,** Magendi-Hertwig syndrome; skew deviation of the eyes in acute cerebellar lesions.

**Magnan's s.,** paresthesia in the psychosis of cocaine addicts, who imagine they have a foreign body, in the shape of a powder or fine sand, under the skin, and that it is constantly changing its position.

**Magnus′ s. of death,** constriction of a limb or one of its segments is not followed by venous congestion of the distal part.

**Mahler's s.,** a gradual increase in the rapidity of the pulse, without change in temperature, in venous thrombosis in the puerperium.

**Mannkopf's s.,** acceleration of the pulse when a painful point is pressed upon.

**Marcus Gunn's s.,** Gunn's s.

**Masini's s.,** a marked degree of dorsal extension of the fingers on the metacarpals and of the toes on the metatarsals, noted in children of mental instability.

**McClintock's s.,** a pulse rate of over 100, an hour or more after childbirth, indicative of postpartum hemorrhage.

**menis′cus s.,** in the case of a gastric ulcer on or near the lesser curvature in the vertical portion of the stomach, radioscopy shows the crater of the ulcer as a crescentic shadow with convexity directed outward; when the ulcer is distal to the angular incisure, the crescentic shadow has its convexity directed downward.

**Mirchamp's s.,** a premonitory symptom of mumps; if a strongly flavored substance is placed on the tongue a painful reflex secretion of saliva occurs in the gland which is the seat of the incipient affection.

**Möbius′ s.,** impairment of ocular convergence in Graves' disease.

**Müller's s.,** rhythmical pulsatory movements of the uvula, with swelling and redness of the velum palati and tonsils, synchronous with the heart's action, in aortic insufficiency.

**Musset's s.,** rhythmical nodding of the head, synchronous with the heart beat, occurring in incompetence of the aortic valve.

**neck s.,** Brudzinski's s. (2).

**Néri's s.,** in hemiplegia, the knee bends spontaneously when the leg is passively extended.

**Nikolsky's s.,** a peculiar vulnerability of the skin in pemphigus vulgaris: the apparently normal epidermis may be rubbed off with slight trauma.

**objective s.,** one that is evident to the examiner.

**Oliver's s.,** tracheal *tugging.*

**Oliver-Cardarelli s.,** tracheal *tugging.*

**Onanoff's s.,** Onanoff's reflex; a sharp contraction of the ischiocavernosus and bulbocavernosus muscles when the glans penis is suddenly compressed.

**s. of the orbicula′ris,** Revilliod's s.; inability of a hemiplegic voluntarily to close the eye upon the paralyzed side except in conjunction with closure of the other eye.

**Osler's s.,** circumscribed painful erythematous swellings, from the size of a pinhead to that of a pea, in the skin and subcutaneous tissues of the hands and feet, in cases of malignant endocarditis.

**Pastia's s.,** the presence of pink or red transverse lines at the bend of the elbow in the preeruptive stage of scarlatina; they persist through the eruptive stage and remain as pigmented lines after desquamation.

**Payr's s.,** pain on pressure over the sole of the foot; a s. of thrombophlebitis.

**Perez′ s.,** rales audible over the upper part of the chest when the arms are alternately raised and lowered, a common occurrence in cases of fibrous mediastinitis and also of aneurysm of the aortic arch.

**Pfuhl's s.,** the pressure of pus within a subphrenic abscess rises during inspiration and falls during expiration; the reverse of what happens in the case of a purulent collection above the diaphragm; when the diaphragm is paralyzed this distinction is lost.

**physical s.,** one that is elicited by auscultation, percussion, or palpation.

**Piltz s.,** tonic *pupil.*

**Pinard's s.,** pain on pressure over the fundus uteri toward the end of pregnancy, said to denote a breech presentation.

**Pins′ s.,** Ewart's s.

**Pitres′ s.,** (1) the axis of the sternum is marked on the chest wall, then a string is stretched between the center of the sternal notch and the symphysis pubis; normally this line coincides with the line of the sternal axis; if it does not, in cases of pleurisy, the angle that it forms with the sternal line indicates the degree of pleural effusion in the chest; (2) haphalgesia; (3) diminished sensation in the testes and scrotum in tabes dorsalis.

**placental s.,** slight endometrial oozing of blood which occurs in certain animals and sometimes in women at the time of implantation of the fertilized ovum. If when, in women, blood appears externally it may be mistaken for a scanty menstrual period.

**Pool-Schlesinger s.,** Pool's *phenomenon* (1).

**Porter's s.,** tracheal *tugging.*

**Potain's s.,** in dilation of the aorta, dullness on percussion is found extending from the manubrium sterni toward the second intercostal space and the third costal cartilage on the right, the upper limit extending from the base of the sternum in the segment of a circle to the right.

**prodromic s.,** antecedent s.; a s. that appears during the prodrome of a disease.

**pseudo-Graefe s.,** a phenomenon similar to Graefe's s., due to aberrant regeneration of fibers of the oculomotor nerve following its paresis or paralysis.

**puddle s.,** a s. of free abdominal fluid detected by having the patient assume a position on all fours. One flank is percussed by repeated light flicking of constant intensity. The Bowles type stethoscope is placed over the most dependent portion of the abdomen and gradually moved towards the flank opposite the percussion. A sharp increase in the intensity of the sound picked up by the stethoscope indicates the level of fluid.

**pyramid s.,** any of the symptoms indicating a morbid condition of the pyramidal tracts, such as the Babinski or Gordon s., spastic paralysis, foot clonus, etc.

**Quant's s.,** a T-shaped depression on the occipital bone occurring in many cases of rickets.

**Quénu-Muret s.,** in a case of aneurysm, the main artery of the limb is compressed and then a puncture is made at the periphery; if blood issues it is assumed that the collateral circulation is well maintained.

**Quincke's s.,** Quincke's *pulse.*

**Ransohoff's s.,** yellow pigmentation in the umbilical region in rupture of the common bile duct.

**Rasch's s.,** fluctuation in the lower segment of the uterus when the organ is pressed down against the examining fingers in the vagina; a s. of pregnancy in the early months.

**Remak's s.,** the dissociation of the sensations of touch and of pain in tabes dorsalis and polyneuritis.

**Revilliod's s.,** s. of the orbicularis.

**Ripault's s.,** a s. of death, consisting in a permanent change in the shape of the pupil produced by unilateral pressure on the eyeball.

**Rocher's s.,** signe du tiroir; drawer s.; if one lies supine with knees flexed, the soles of the feet resting flat on the table, and then grasps the tibia pushing it forward, as in closing a drawer, it will slide freely over the femoral surface if the crucial ligaments have been injured.

**Romberg's s.,** rombergism; Romberg's symptom (1); station test; if a patient standing is more unsteady with the eyes closed it indicates a loss of proprioceptive control.

**Rommelaere's s.,** diminution of the phosphates, sodium chloride, and nitrogen in the urine in cancer.

**Rosenbach's s.,** (1) fine tremor of the upper lids, when the eyes are gently closed, in Graves' disease; (2) loss of the abdominal reflex in cases of acute inflammation of the viscera.

**Rossolimo's s.,** Rossolimo's *reflex.*

**Rotch's s.,** percussion dullness in the fifth intercostal space on the right, in cases of pericardial effusion.

**Rovsing's s.,** pain at McBurney's point induced in cases of appendicitis, by pressure exerted over the descending colon.

**Rumpel-Leede s.,** Rumpel-Leede *test.*

**Saenger's s.,** a lost light reflex of the pupil returns after a short time in the dark, noted in cerebral syphilis but absent in tabes dorsalis.

**Sansom's s.,** reduplication of the second heart sound in mitral stenosis.

**Schapiro's s.,** no slowing of the pulse occurs when the patient lies down, in cases of myocardial weakness.

**Schlesinger's s.,** in tetany, if the lower limb, kept extended at the knee, is strongly flexed at the hip, a spasm quickly occurs in the extensors of the knee.

**Schüle's s.,** *omega* melancholicum.

**Schultze's s.,** tongue phenomenon; in latent tetany, tapping the tongue causes its depression with a concave dorsum.

**Seeligmüller's s.,** contraction of the pupil on the affected side in facial neuralgia.

**Seidel's s.,** a sickle-shaped scotoma appearing as an upward or downward extension of the blind spot.

**Siegert's s.,** shortness and inward curvature of the terminal phalanges of the fifth fingers in mongolism.

**Signorelli's s.,** tenderness on pressure in the glenoid fossa in front of the mastoid process in meningitis.

**Simon's s.,** in incipient meningitis in children, the movements of the diaphragm are dissociated from those of the thorax.

**Sisto's s.,** continuous crying of infants suffering from heredosyphilis.

**Skoda's s.,** Skodaic *resonance.*

**spinal s.,** the spinal muscles are in a state of tonic contraction on the affected side in pleurisy.

**spine s.,** resistance to flexion of the spine in cases of poliomyelitis.

**Steinberg thumb s.,** in Marfan's syndrome, when the thumb is held across the palm of the same hand, it projects well beyond the ulnar surface of the hand.

**Stellwag's s.,** infrequent and incomplete blinking in Graves' disease.

**Stewart-Holmes s.,** rebound phenomenon; the inability to check a movement when passive resistance is suddenly released, present in cerebellar deficit.

**Stierlin's s.,** constant emptying of the cecum, with barium remaining in the terminal part of the ileum and in the transverse colon; due to irritation of the cecum, frequently by tuberculosis.

**Straus' s.,** in case of facial paralysis, if an injection of pilocarpine is followed by sweating on the affected side later than on the other, the lesion is peripheral.

**subjective s.,** one that is perceived only by the patient; not objective.

**Sumner's s.,** a slight increase in tonus of the abdominal muscles, an early indication of inflammation of the appendix, stone in the kidney or ureter, or a twisted pedicle of an ovarian cyst; it is detected by exceedingly gentle palpation of the right or left iliac fossa.

**Ten Horn's s.,** pain caused by gentle traction on the right spermatic cord, pointing to appendicitis.

**Testivin's s.,** an obsolete s.; the formation of a thin pellicle, like gold-beaters' skin, on albumin-free urine after treatment with an acid and ether, alleged by the author to be a prodromal sign of an infectious disease.

**Thomson's s.,** Pastia's s.

**Tinel's s.,** a sensation of tingling, or "pins and needles," felt in the distal extremity of a limb when percussion is made over the site of an injured nerve; it indicates a partial lesion or early regeneration in the nerve. It is sometimes called "distal tingling on percussion" (abbreviated DTP).

**Toma's s.,** to distinguish between inflammatory and noninflammatory ascites; in inflammatory conditions of the peritoneum the mesentery contracts, drawing the intestines over to the right side; consequently, when the patient lies on his back, tympany is elicited on the right side, dullness on the left.

**Topalanski's s.,** congestion of the pericorneal region of the eye in Graves' disease.

**Tournay s.,** dilation of the pupil in the abducting eye on extreme lateral fixation.

**Trélat's s.,** an obsolete s.; the presence of disseminated yellowish spots in the neighborhood of tuberculous ulcers of the mouth; they are minute tubercles or miliary abscesses.

**Trendelenburg's s.,** in congenital dislocation of the hip, or in hip abductor weakness, if the patient stands on the dislocated leg and flexes the hip and knee on the other side the pelvis on this side will sag, whereas if normal, it will be raised on the side of the flexed hip and knee.

**Tresilian's s.,** a reddish prominence at the orifice of Stenson's duct, noted in mumps.

**Trousseau's s.,** in latent tetany, typical attitude of the hand that is assumed when the upper arm is compressed, as by a tourniquet, or blood pressure armlet.

**Vanzetti's s.,** sciatic scoliosis; scoliosis as a symptom of sciatica.

**Vipond's s.,** a generalized adenopathy occurring during the period of incubation of various of the exanthemas of childhood, affording an early diagnostic s. in a case of known exposure.

**vital s.'s,** manifestation of breathing, heart beat, and sustained blood pressure.

**Voltolini-Heryng s.,** Heryng's s.

**Weber's s.,** Weber's *syndrome.*

**Wegner's s.,** broadening, roughening, and discoloration of the epiphysial line, observed post mortem in infants dead of hereditary syphilis.

**Weiss' s.,** Chvostek's s.

**Wernicke's s.,** Wernicke's *reaction.*

**Westphal's s.,** Westphal's phenomenon; Westphal-Erb s.; abolition of the patellar reflex.

**Westphal-Erb s.,** Westphal's s.

**Widowitz' s.,** see doll's eye s.

**Wilder's s.,** a slight twitch of the eyeball when changing its movement from abduction to adduction or the reverse, noted in Graves' disease.

**Winterbottom's s.,** swelling of the posterior cervical lymph nodes, characteristic of early stages of African sleeping sickness; useful for surveys or control of migrations of persons with preclinical infections.

**Wreden's s.,** in the case of a stillborn child a gelatinous material more or less completely fills the external auditory meatus.

**wrist s.,** in Marfan's syndrome, when the wrist is gripped with the opposite hand, the thumb and fifth finger overlap appreciably.

**signa** (sig'nah) [ imperative of L. *signo,* pp. *-atus,* to set a mark upon ]. Term used to introduce the signature in a prescription; abbreviated S or sig.

**signature** (sig'nă-chūr, -tūr) [ Mediev. L. *signatura,* fr. L. *signum,* a sign, mark ]. 1. The part of a prescription containing the directions to the patient. 2. Some marking on, or the color or shape of, a plant or mineral, supposed to be symbolic or indicative of its therapeutic virtues.

**doctrine of s.'s,** a belief that there were specific therapeutic essences, a cure for every disease, to be found in plants, minerals, or chemicals with a clue to their specificity.

**significant** (sig-nif'ĭ-kant) [ L. *significo,* to make known, signify, fr. *signum,* sign, + *facio,* to make ]. In statistics, denoting the reliability of a finding or, conversely, the probability of the finding being the result of chance; the probability that the finding may be due to chance is generally less than 5 per cent.

**Signorelli** (se-nyor-el'le), Angelo, Italian physician, 1876–1952. See S.'s *sign.*

**silan'drone** (USAN). 17β-(Trimethylsiloxy)androst-4-en-3-one; an androgen.

**Silas'tic.** Trade name for siliconized rubber, or elastic, biologically inert polymer used in surgery.

**Silber,** Robert H., U. S. biochemist, *1915. See Porter-S. *chromogens, reaction,* Porter-S. chromogens *test.*

**silica** (sil'ĭ-kah) [ Mod. L. fr. L. *silex* (*silic-*), flint ]. Silicon dioxide; silicic anhydride; $SiO_2$.

**s. gel** (USP), precipitated form of silicic acid, used for adsorption of various vapors.

**s. gel pearl,** used in cataract extraction; the lens adheres to the pearl, which is grasped in an extractor, and thus removed.

**sil'icate.** 1. A salt of silicic acid. 2. The term sometimes applied to dental restorations of synthetic porcelain.

**siliceous** (sĭ-lish'us). Silicious; containing silica.

**silicic** (sĭ-lis'ik). Relating to silica or silicon.

**s. acid,** $Si(OH)_4$; obtained in water as a colloid by treating silicates. Precipitated s. acid is silica gel.

**s. anhydride,** silica.

**silicious** (sĭ-lish'us). Siliceous.

**silicofluoride** (sil'ĭ-ko-flu'o-rid). A compound of silicon and fluorine with another element.

**silicon** (sil'ĭ-kon). A very abundant nonmetallic element, symbol Si, atomic no. 14, atomic weight 28.09. In pure form it is used as a semiconductor, and in solar batteries. $SiO_2$ is the chief constituent of sand, hence of glass.

**s. dioxide, colloidal** (NF), a submicroscopic fumed silica prepared by the vapor-phase hydrolysis of a s. compound; used as a tablet diluent and as a suspending and thickening agent.

**silicone** (sil'ĭ-kōn). A plastic, based on silicon, with a variety of uses: (1) used as a grease or sealing substance; (2) used in the form of tubes to anastomose vessels, since it has less effect than other materials in causing coagulation of blood; (3) used to coat the interior of glass vessels for the collection of blood; (4) in dentistry, serves as a viscous impression material that sets to an elastic but firm state; setting is accomplished by catalytic action with a chemical accelerator such as tin octoate; (5) in ophthalmology, used in the scleral buckling operation and in plastic procedures such as lengthening the medial rectus muscle.

**silicosiderosis** (sil'ĭ-ko-sid'er-o'sis). Fibrosis of lungs produced by dust containing silica and iron.

**silicosis** [ L. *silex,* flint, + suffix *-osis,* condition ]. Stone-mason's disease; a form of pneumoconiosis, due to the inhalation of stone dust or quartz.

**silicotuberculosis** (sil'ĭ-ko-tu-ber-ku-lo'sis). Silicosis associated with tuberculous pulmonary lesions.

**sil'iqua oli'vae** [ L. the husk of the olive ]. The arcuate fibers, which appear to encircle the inferior olive in the medulla oblongata.

**siliquose** (sil'ĭ-kwōs). Resembling a silique, or long slender pod; denoting a form of cataract resulting in shriveling of the lens with calcareous deposit in the capsule.

**silk.** The fibers or filaments obtained from the cocoon of the silkworm.

**floss s.,** dental *floss.*

**surgical s.,** chorda serica chirurgicalis; thread prepared from the cocoon filaments of glutinous gum which are spun by the mulberry silkworm *Bombyx mori;* used as suture material in surgical operations in 14 sizes from 0.025 mm. to 1.016 mm. in diameter and numbered accordingly from 7-0 to 7.

**virgin s.,** an extremely fine ophthalmic suture material consisting of 2 to 7 natural s. filaments bonded together by the natural adhesive, sericin.

**silk'weed.** *Asclepias tuberosa.*

**sil'ver** [ A.S. *seolfor* ]. Argentum; symbol Ag; a metallic element of lustrous white color, specific gravity of 10.4 to 10.7, atomic no. 47, atomic weight 107.873.

**s. chloride,** used in the preparation of antiseptic silver preparations.

**s. fluoride,** $AgF_2 \cdot H_2O$; antiseptic.

**s. iodate,** a reagent for the determination of chloride.

**s. iodide, colloidal,** an antiseptic; used for treatment of inflammation of the mucous membranes.

**s. lactate,** ACTOL; has been used as an astringent and antiseptic.

**s. nitrate** (USP, BP), an antiseptic and astringent; used externally in solution in the prevention of ophthalmia neonatorum.

**s. nitrate, fused,** s. nitrate, toughened.

**s. nitrate, toughened** (USP, BP), fused s. nitrate; lunar caustic; s. nitrate pencil; lapis imperialis; escharotic and germicide for local application.

**s. oxide,** has been used in epilepsy and chorea; it is explosive when mixed with readily combustible substances.

**s. picrate,** PICROTOL; an ionizable salt of s., used in the treatment of trichomoniasis and moniliasis of the vagina.

**s. protein, mild,** ARGYROL; mild PROTARGIN; rendered colloidal by the presence of or combination with protein; it contains not less than 19 and not more than 23 per cent of s.; used externally as an antiseptic devoid of irritating properties.

**s. protein, strong,** PROTARGOL; a compound of s. and protein containing not less than 7.5 and not more than 8.5 per cent of s.; used externally as an antiseptic, devoid of astringent and nearly so of irritant properties.

**Silverman,** Leslie, U. S. engineer, 1914–1966. See S.-Lilly *pneumotachograph.*

**Silverman,** William A., U. S. pediatrician. See Caffey-S. *syndrome.*

**Silverskiöld's syndrome.** See under syndrome.

**Simchowicz,** T., Polish physician. See S. *granules.*

**simeth'icone** (NF). MYLICON; a mixture of dimethyl polysiloxanes and silica gel; antiflatulent.

**simil'ia simil'ibus curan'tur** [ L. likes are cured by likes ]. The homeopathic formula expressing the law of similars, or the doctrine that any drug which is capable of producing morbid symptoms in the healthy will remove similar symptoms occurring as an expression of disease. Another reading of the formula, the one employed by Hahnemann, the founder of homeopathy, is *similia similibus curentur,* let likes be cured by likes.

**simil'imum, simil'limum** [ L. *simillimus,* most like, superl. of *similis,* like ]. In homeopathy, the remedy indicated in a certain case because the same drug, when given to a healthy person, will produce the symptom complex most nearly approaching that of the disease in question.

**Simmonds,** Morris, Hamburg physician, 1855–1925. See S.'s *disease.*

**Simmons,** J. S. See S.'s citrate *medium.*

**Simon** (si'mon), Charles E., American physician, 1866–1927. See S.'s *sign.*

**Simon** (ze'mon), Gustav, German surgeon, 1824–1876. See S.'s *operation, position.*

**Simon** (se-mawn'), Théodore, French physician, *1873. See Binet-S. *scale, test.*

**Simonart** (se-mon-ar'), Pierre J. C., Belgian obstetrician, 1817–1847. See S.'s *bands, ligaments, threads.*

**Simo'nea folliculo'rum.** *Demodex folliculorum.*

**Simons,** Arthur, German physician, *1877. See S.'s *disease.*

**simple** (sim'pl) [ L. *simplex.* PLIC- ]. 1. Not complex or compound. 2. In anatomy, composed of a minimum number of parts. 3. A medicinal herb.

**sim'pler, sim'plist.** An herb doctor; one who treats disease with simples.

**sim'plex** [ L. ] [ NA ]. Simple (1).

**Simpson,** Sir James Y., Scottish obstetrician, 1811–1870. See S.'s *forceps.*

**Simpson,** William S., British civil engineer, †1917. See S. *light.*

**Sims,** J. Marion, U. S. gynecologist, 1813–1883. See S.'s *position, speculum.*

**si'mul** [ L. ]. At once; at the same time; a term used in the signature of a prescription.

**simulation** (sim'u-la'shun) [ L. *simulatio,* fr. *simulo,* pp. -*atus,* to imitate, fr. *similis,* like ]. 1. Imitation; said of a disease or symptom that resembles another. 2. Malingering; feigning illness.

    **computer s.,** computer *model.*

**sim'ulator.** An apparatus designed to produce effects simulating those of specific environmental conditions; used in experimentation and training.

    **space s.'s,** closed cabins or chambers, hermetically sealed and holding human or animal subjects at ground level, used to study some of the effects of spacecraft.

**Simulium** (si-mu'li-um) [ L. *simulo,* to simulate ]. A genus of biting gnats or midges, the black flies, humpbacked flies, or buffalo gnats in the dipteran family Simuliidae. The aquatic larvae require swift-flowing streams or highly oxygenated waters for their development; a critical epidemiological factor in the role of these flies as disease vectors. In Central America, Mexico, and Central Africa, various species transmit *Onchocerca volvulus,* agent of human onchocerciasis; in North America, *Onchocerca gutterosa* and other onchocercid infections of cattle, horses, and various wild ruminants.

    **S. av'idum,** a vector of onchocerciasis in Guatemala.

    **S. damno'sum,** an important vector of onchocerciasis in Central Africa.

    **S. nae'vei,** an important vector of onchocerciasis in east and central Africa where its larvae and pupae are confined to the shells of crabs of the genus *Potamonautes.*

    **S. occidenta'le,** transmits *Leucocytozoon smithi,* agent of leucocytozoonosis in turkeys in the United States.

    **S. ochra'ceum,** vector of onchocerciasis in South America.

    **S. orna'tum,** vector of bovine onchocerciasis in Australia.

    **S. ruggle'si,** vector of *Leucocytozoon simondi* in Canada and the northern United States.

**sinal'bin.** Sinapine glucosinalb(in)ate; a glycoside present in white mustard, which on enzymatic hydrolysis yields glucose, *p*-hydroxybenzylisothiocyanate, choline, and sinap(in)ic acid.

**sinapic acid** (si-na'pik). 4-Hydroxy-3,5-dimethoxycinnamic acid; see sinapine.

**sin'apine.** Choline sinapate; the choline ester of sinapic acid; the base itself is unstable, existing as a sulfocyanate in mustard.

**Sinapis** (si-na'pis) [ L. fr. G. *sinapi,* mustard ]. A subgenus of *Brassica* (family Cruciferae), including mustard.

    **S. alba,** white *mustard.*

    **S. nigra,** black *mustard.*

**sinapiscopy** (sin'ă-pis'ko-pī) [ G. *sinapi,* mustard, + *skopeō,* to examine ]. The testing of disorders of sensation by the application of mustard to the skin.

**sin'apism.** Application of a mustard poultice or plaster.

**sin'caline.** See choline.

**sincipital** (sin-sip'ĭ-tal). Relating to the sinciput.

**sinciput,** pl. **sincipita, sinciputs** (sin'sĭ-put, sin-sip'ĭ-tah) [ L. half of the head. CAP-1 ] [ NA ]. 1. The upper half of the cranium; in a restricted sense, the anterior part of the head just above and including the forehead. 2. Bregma.

**sin'ew** [ A.S. *sinu* ]. A tendon.

**sing.** Abbreviation of singular, and of L. *singulorum,* of each.

**singula'ris** [ L. ] [ NA ]. Singular; solitary.

**singultation** (sing'gul-ta'shun) [ L. *singulto,* pp. -*atus,* to hiccup ]. Hiccupping.

**singultous** (sing-gul'tus). Relating to hiccups.

**singultus** (sing-gul'tus) [ L. ]. A hiccup.

**sinigrase.** Thioglucosidase.

**sin'igrin.** Sinigroside; potassium myronate; myronate potassium; the β-glucopyranoside of black mustard seeds and of horseradish root (*Alliaria officinalis,* family Cruciferae).

**sinigrinase** (sin'ĭ-grĭ-nās). Thioglucosidase.

**sinis'ter** [ L. ] [ NA ]. Left.

**sinistrad** (sin'is-trad, sĭ-nis'trad) [ L. *sinister,* left, + *ad,* to ]. Toward the left side.

**sinistral** (sin'is-tral, sĭ-nis'tral). 1. Relating to the left side. 2. A left-handed person.

**sin'istral'ity.** Left-handedness.

**sinistro-, sinistr-** (sin'is-tro-, sĭ-nis'tro-) [ L. *sinister,* left ]. Combining form indicating left, or toward the left.

**sinistrocardia** (sin'is-tro-kar'dĭ-ah) [ sinistro- + G. *kardia,* heart ]. Displacement of the heart beyond the normal position on the left side.

**sinistrocer'ebral** (sin'is-tro-sĕr'ĕ-bral) [ sinistro- + L. *cerebrum,* brain ]. Relating to the left cerebral hemisphere.

**sinistrocular** (sin'is-trok'u-lar) [ sinistro- + L. *oculus,* eye ]. Left-eyed; denoting one who uses the left eye by preference in monocular work, such as the use of the microscope.

**sinistrogyration** (sin'is-tro-ji-ra'shun) [ sinistro- + L. *gyratio,* a turning around (gyration) ]. Sinistrotorsion.

**sinistromanual** (sin'is-tro-man'u-al) [ sinistro- + L. *manus,* hand ]. Left-handed.

**sinistropedal** (sin'is-trop'ĕdal) [ sinistro- + L. *pes* (*ped*-), foot ]. Left-footed; denoting one who uses the left leg by preference, in hopping for instance.

**sinistrophobia** (sin'is-tro-fo'bĭ-ah) [ sinistro- + G. *phobos,* fear ]. Morbid fear of things on the left side.

**sinistrorotation** (sin'is-tro-ro-ta'shun). Sinistrotorsion.

**sinistrorse** (sin'is-trors) [ L. *sinistrorsus,* on the left side, fr. *sinister,* left, + *verto,* pp. *versus,* to turn ]. Turned or twisted to the left.

**sinistro'sis** [ L. *sinister,* unlucky (malign) + G. suffix -*osis,* condition ]. Shell *shock.*

**sinistrotorsion** (sin'is-tro-tor'shun) [ sinistro- + L. *torsio,* a twisting (torsion) ]. Sinistrogyration; sinistrorotation; a turning or twisting to the left.

**sinistrous** (sin'is-trus, sĭ-nis'trus). Sinistral.

**sinoatrial** (si'no-a'trĭ-al). Sinuatrial; relating to the sinus venosus and the right atrium of the heart.

**sinography** (si-nog'rā-fĭ) [ sinus + G. *graphō*, to write ]. Radiographic study in which a contrasting medium is to visualize a sinus tract, as in infections or abdominal wounds.

**si'nopul'monary.** Relating to the paranasal sinuses and the pulmonary airway.

**sinovaginal** (si'no-vaj'ĭ-nal). Relating to that part of the vagina derived from the urogenital sinus.

**sin'ter** [ Ger. dross, slag ]. To heat a powdered substance without thoroughly melting it, causing it to fuse into a solid but porous mass.

**sinuatrial** (sin'u-a'trĭ-al, si'nu-). Sinoatrial.

**sinuitis** (sin'u-i'tis, si'nu-). Sinusitis.

**sinuotomy** (sin'u-ot'o-mĭ-si'nu-). Sinusotomy.

# SINUS

**si'nus**, pl. (Lat.) **si'nus**, (Eng.) **si'nuses** [ L. *sinus*, cavity, channel, hollow. SINU- ]. 1 [ NA ]. A channel for the passage of blood or lymph, which has not the coats of an ordinary vessel; such are the blood passages in the gravid uterus or those in the cerebral meninges. 2 [ NA ]. A hollow in bone or other tissue; antrum. 3. A fistula or tract leading to a suppurating cavity.

**accessory nasal s.'s,** s. paranasales.
**s. a'lae par'vae,** s. sphenoparietalis.
**anal s.'s,** s. anales.
**s. ana'les,** (1) [ NA ], anal or rectal s.'s; Morgagni's crypts; the grooves between the anal columns; (2) [ NAV ], anal s.'s; pockets or crypts in the columnar zone of the anal canal between the anocutaneous line and the anorectal line; the s.'s give the mucosa a scalloped appearance.
**s. aor'tae** [ NA ], aortic s.; s. of Valsalva; the space between each semilunar valve and the wall of the aorta.
**aortic s.,** s. aortae.
**Arlt's s.,** an inconstant depression on the internal surface of the lacrimal sac.
**barber's pilonidal s.,** pilonidal s. occurring in barbers, usually in the web between fingers, due to the burying of hairs by the alternate loosening and tightening of tissues of the hand by the manipulation of scissors.
**basilar s.,** *plexus* basilaris.
**Breschet's s.,** s. sphenoparietalis.
**s. carot'icus** [ NA ], carotid s.; carotid bulb; a slight dilation of the common carotid artery at its bifurcation into external and internal carotids. It contains baroreceptors which, when stimulated, cause slowing of the heart, vasodilation, and a fall in blood pressure.
**carotid s.,** s. caroticus.
**s. caverno'sus** [ NA ], cavernous s.; a paired dural s. on either side of the sella turcica, the two being connected by anastomoses, the anterior and posterior intercavernous s., in front of and behind the hypophysis, respectively, making thus the circular s.
**cavernous s.,** s. cavernosus.
**cerebral s.'s,** s. durae matris.
**cervical s.,** precervical s.; in young mammalian embryos a depression in the nuchal region caudal to the hyoid arch, with the third and fourth branchial arches and grooves in its floor. Normally it is obliterated after the second month, but occasionally cervical fistulae persist as vestiges of it.
**circular s.,** s. circularis.
**s. circula'ris,** circular s.; (1) circulus venosus ridleyi; Ridley's circle or s.; a venous ring around the hypophysis, formed by the cavernous and the two intercavernous s.'s; (2) a venous s. at the periphery of the placenta; (3) s. venosus sclerae.
**coccygeal s.,** a fistula opening in the region of the coccyx, being the result of incomplete closure of the caudal end of the neural tube; see also pilonidal s.
**s. corona'rius** [ NA ], coronary s.; a short trunk receiving most of the veins of the heart, running in the posterior part of the coronary sulcus and emptying into the right atrium

between the inferior vena cava and the atrioventricular orifice.
**coronary s.,** s. coronarius.
**costomedias'tinal s.,** *recessus* costomediastinalis.
**cranial s.'s,** s. durae matris.
**dermal s.,** one lined with epidermis and skin appendages extending from the skin to some deeper-lying structure, most frequently the spinal cord.
**s.'s of dura mater,** s. durae matris.
**s. du'rae ma'tris** [ NA ], s.'s of the dura mater; dural s.'s; cerebral s.'s; endothelium-lined venous channels in the dura mater.
**dural s.'s,** s. durae matris.
**Englisch's s.,** s. petrosus inferior.
**s. epididym'idis** [ NA ], a narrow space between the body of the epididymis and the testis.
**ethmoidal s.,** s. ethmoidalis.
**s. ethmoida'lis** [ NA ], ethmoidal s.; antrum ethmoidale; evaginations of the mucous membrane of the middle and superior meatuses of the nasal cavity considered as one s. on each side; it is subdivided into *cellulae* anteriores, *cellulae* mediae, and *cellulae* posteriores, *q. v.*
**Forssell's s.,** a smooth area in the stomach wall, hemmed in by folds of the mucosa, shown by x-ray examination.
**frontal s.,** s. frontalis.
**s. fronta'lis** [ NA ], frontal s.; a hollow formed on either side in the lower part of the squama of the frontal bone; it communicates by the infundibulum with the middle meatus of the nasal cavity of the same side.
**Guérin's s.,** a cul-de-sac or diverticulum behind the valvula fossae navicularis.
**Huguier's s.,** a small fossa in the tympanic cavity between the fenestra vestibuli and the fenestra cochleae.
**inferior longitudinal s.,** s. sagittalis inferior.
**inferior petrosal s.,** s. petrosus inferior.
**inferior sagittal s.,** s. sagittalis inferior.
**s. intercaverno'si** [ NA ], intercavernous s.'s; the anterior and posterior anastomoses between the cavernous s.'s.
**intercav'ernous s.,** s. intercavernosus.
**jug'ular s.,** s. jugularis; one of three enlargements of the jugular veins; that of the external jugular (*s. j. externae*) is between the two sets of valves; those of the internal jugular (*s. j. internae*) are at the origin (superior bulb) and near the termination (inferior bulb).
**s. lactif'eri** [ NA ], lactiferous s.; ampulla of milk duct; ampulla lactiferi; a circumscribed spindle-shaped dilation of the lactiferous duct just before it enters the nipple.
**lactiferous s.,** s. lactiferi.
**laryn'geal s.,** *ventriculus* laryngis.
**s. laryngeus,** *ventriculus* laryngis.
**lateral s.,** s. transversus.
**s. lie'nis** [ NA ], splenic sinuses; dilated venous channels, lined by rod-shaped reticuloendothelial cells, that connect splenic capillaries with collecting venules and serve to convey blood through the splenic pulp.
**longitu'dinal s.,** s. sagittalis.
**Luschka's s.,** venous s. in the petrosquamous suture.
**lymph s.,** lymphatic s.
**lymphatic s.,** lymph s.; the channels in a lymph node crossed by a reticulum of cells and fibers and bounded by littoral cells; there are subcapsular, trabecular, and medullary s.'s.
**Maier's s.,** an infundibuliform depression on the internal surface of the lacrimal sac which receives the lacrimal canaliculi.
**marginal s. of placenta,** discontinuous venous lakes at the margin of the placenta.
**mastoid s.,** *cellula* mastoidea.
**s. maxilla'ris** [ NA ], maxillary s.; antrum of Highmore; maxillary antrum; an air cavity in the body of the maxilla, communicating with the middle meatus of the nose.
**maxillary s.,** s. maxillaris.
**Meyer's s.,** a small concavity in the floor of the external auditory canal near the membrana tympani.
**Morgagni's s.,** (1) s. analis; (2) *utriculus* prostaticus; (3) *ventriculus* laryngis.
**s. of nail,** s. unguis.
**oblique s. of pericardium,** s. obliquus pericardii.
**s. obli'quus pericardii** [ NA ], oblique s. of the pericardium; the recess in the pericardial cavity behind the heart

bounded by the pericardial reflections on the pulmonary veins and inferior vena cava.

**occipital s.,** s. occipitalis.

**s. occipita′lis** [ NA ], occipital s.; an unpaired cerebral s. commencing at the confluens sinuum and passing downward in the base of the falx cerebelli to the foramen magnum.

**Palfyn′s s.,** a space within the crista galli of the ethmoid described as communicating with the ethmoidal and frontal s.'s.

**paranasal s.'s,** s. paranasales.

**s. paranasa′les** [ NA ], paranasal s.'s; accessory nasal s.'s; the cavities in the bones of the face lined by mucous membrane continuous with that of the nasal cavity; these s.'s are the frontal, sphenoidal, maxillary, and ethmoidal.

**parasinoidal s.'s,** *lacunae* laterales.

**Petit′s s.,** s. aortae.

**petrosal s.,** s. petrosus.

**s. petro′sus infe′rior** [ NA ], inferior petrosal s.; a paired s. of the dura mater running in the groove on the petrooccipital fissure connecting the cavernous s. with the superior bulb of the internal jugular vein.

**s. petro′sus supe′rior** [ NA ], superior petrosal s.; a paired s. of the dura mater in the groove on the superior margin of the petrous part of the temporal bone, connecting the cavernous s. with the transverse s.

**phrenicocos′tal s.,** *recessus* costodiaphragmaticus pleurae.

**pilonidal s.,** congenital fistula or pit in the sacral region, communicating with the exterior, containing hair which may act as a foreign body producing chronic inflammation.

**pir′iform s.,** *recessus* piriformis.

**pleural s.'s** *recessus* pleurae.

**s. pocula′ris** [ cup-cavity ], *utriculus* prostaticus.

**s. poste′rior** [ NA ], a deep groove above the pyramidal eminence in the posterior wall of the tympanic cavity.

**precervical s.,** cervical s.

**prostatic s.,** s. prostaticus.

**s. prostat′icus** [ NA ], prostatic s.; the groove on either side of the urethral crest in the prostatic part of the urethra.

**rectal s.'s,** s. anales.

**s. rec′tus** [ NA ], straight s.; tentorial s.; an unpaired s. of the dura mater in the posterior part of the falx cerebri where it is attached to the tentorium cerebelli; it passes horizontally to the confluens sinuum.

**renal s.,** s. renalis.

**s. rena′lis** [ NA ], renal s.; the cavity of the kidney, containing the calyces and pelvis.

**s. reu′niens,** archaic term for s. venosus.

**rhom′boidal s.,** s. rhomboidalis; rhombocele; a dilation of the central canal of the spinal cord in the lumbar region.

**Ridley′s s.,** s. circularis (1).

**Rokitansky-Aschoff s.'s,** small outpocketings of the mucosa of the gallbladder which extend through the muscular layer. They may be congenital but are often involved in chronic cholecystitis.

**s. sagitta′lis infe′rior** [ NA ], inferior sagittal s.; inferior longitudinal s.; an unpaired dural s. in the lower margin of the falx cerebri, running parallel to the superior saggital s. and emptying into the straight s.

**s. sagitta′lis supe′rior** [ NA ], superior sagittal s.; superior longitudinal s.; an unpaired dural s. in the sagittal groove, beginning at the foramen caecum and terminating at the confluens sinuum.

**sigmoid s.,** s. sigmoideus.

**s. sigmoi′deus** [ NA ], sigmoid s.; the S-shaped dural s. lying on the mastoid process of the temporal bone and the jugular process of the occipital bone; it is continuous with the transverse s. and empties into the internal jugular vein.

**sphenoidal s.,** [ NA ], sphenoidalis.

**s. sphenoida′lis** [ NA ], sphenoidal s.; one of a pair of cavities in the body of the sphenoid bone communicating with the nasal cavity.

**sphenoparietal s.,** s. sphenoparietalis.

**s. sphenoparieta′lis** [ NA ], sphenoparietal s.; s. alae parvae; a paired s. of the dura mater beginning on the parietal bone, running along the posterior margin of the lesser wing of the sphenoid, and emptying into the cavernous s.

**splenic s.'s,** s. lienis.

**straight s.,** s. rectus.

**superior petrosal s.,** s. petrosus superior.

**superior sagittal s.,** s. sagittalis superior.

**tarsal s.,** s. tarsi.

**s. tar′si** [ NA ], tarsal s.; a hollow or canal formed by the groove of the talus, and the groove of the calcaneus.

**tentorial s.,** s. rectus.

**terminal s.,** s. terminalis; the vein bounding the area vasculosa in the blastoderm.

**s. tonsilla′ris,** *fossa* tonsillaris.

**Tourtual′s s.,** *fossa* supratonsillaris.

**transverse s.,** s. transversus.

**transverse s. of pericardium,** s. transversus pericardii.

**s. transver′sus** [ NA ], transverse s.; lateral s.; a paired dural s. that begins at the confluens sinuum and terminates in the sigmoid s.

**s. transver′sus pericar′dii** [ NA ], transverse s. of the pericardium; a passage in the pericardium between the origins of the great vessels and the atria.

**s. trun′ci pulmona′lis** [ NA ], the space at the origin of the pulmonary trunk between the wall of the vessel and each cusp of the semilunar valve.

**s. tym′pani** [ NA ], tympanic s.; a depression in the tympanic cavity posterior to the tympanic promontory.

**tympanic s.,** s. tympani.

**s. un′guis** [ NA ], s. of the nail; the deep cleft housing the root of the nail.

**urogenital s.,** s. urogenitalis.

**s. urogenita′lis,** (1) [ NA ], urogenital s.; the ventral part of the cloaca after its separation from the rectum by the growth of the urorectal septum. It gives rise to the lower part of the bladder in both sexes, to the prostatic portion of the male urethra, and to the urethra and vestibule in the female; (2) persistent *cloaca.*

**uterine s.,** uterine sinusoid; a small irregular vascular channel in the endometrium.

**uteroplacental s.,** irregular vascular spaces in the zone of the chorionic attachment to the decidua basalis.

**Valsalva′s s.,** s. aortae.

**s. vena′rum cava′rum** [ NA ], the portion of the cavity of the right atrium of the heart that receives the blood from the venae cavae; it is separated from the rest of the atrium by the crista terminalis.

**s. veno′sus** [ NA ], cavity at the caudal end of the embryonic cardiac tube in which the veins from the intra- and extraembryonic circulatory arcs unite. In the course of development it forms the portion of the right atrium known in adult anatomy as the sinus venarum cavarum.

**s. veno′sus scle′rae** [ NA ], venous s. of the sclera; canal of Schlemm or of Lauth; Fontana's canal; a ringlike vein in the sclera, near its anterior edge, encircling the cornea.

**venous s.,** s. durae matris.

**venous s. of sclera,** s. venosus sclerae.

**s. vertebra′les longitudina′les,** portions of the internal vertebral venous plexus lying on the posterior surfaces of the vertebral bodies on either side of the posterior longitudinal ligament.

---

**sinusitis** (si′nus-i′tis) [ sinus + G. suffix *-itis,* inflammation ]. Sinuitis; inflammation of the lining membrane of any sinus, especially of one of the paranasal sinuses.

**s. abscen′dens,** s. complicated with caries or necrosis of the bony wall directly beneath the affected portion of the mucous lining of the sinus.

**frontal s.,** infection in one or both frontal sinuses.

**infectious s. of turkeys,** see chronic respiratory *disease.*

**sinusoid** (si′nus-oyd) [ sinus + G. *eidos,* resemblance ]. 1. Resembling a sinus. 2. A blood channel in certain organs (as the spleen, liver, red bone marrow) which is lined by reticuloendothelium.

**uterine s.,** uterine *sinus.*

**sinusoidal** (si-nus-oy′dal). Relating to a sinusoid.

**sinusotomy** (sin-us-ot′o-mǐ) [ sinus + G. *tomē,* incision ]. Sinuotomy; incision into a sinus.

**siphon** (si′fon) [ G. *siphōn,* tube ]. 1. A bent tube or pipe having legs of unequal length; when the shorter leg is immersed in a liquid and suction is applied to the longer leg so as to bring the liquid over the bend into the longer leg, the liquid will continue to flow through the s. until the shorter leg no longer reaches the surface of the liquid. 2. A bottle containing a liquid charged with carbonic acid, with a glass tube running to the bottom of the bottle; when a stopcock at the upper end of the tube is opened, the presence of the carbonic acid gas forces the liquid out.

**Downes' separate-urine s.,** an instrument for obtaining the urine from each ureter separately; it consits of a lever in the rectum which is pressed against the bladder, making a central ridge; on each side of this ridge is a perforated curved beak attached to a catheter through which the urine on that side is siphoned away as soon as it enters the bladder.

**siphonage** (si'fon-ej). Washing out the stomach or other cavity by means of a siphon.

**Siphona irritans** (si-fo'nah) [ G. *siphōn*, tube ]. The horn fly, a bloodsucking muscoid fly that causes great irritation and annoyance to cattle.

**Siphonaptera** (si'fo-nap'tĕ-rah) [ G. *siphōn*, tube, + G. *a-* priv. + *pteron*, wing ]. The fleas, an order of wingless insect ectoparasites highly adapted for survival in mammalian fur; they are flattened laterally, spined, and equipped with well developed metathoracic legs for jumping.

**siphonoma** (si'fo-no'mah) [ G. *siphōn*, tube, + suffix *-oma*, tumor ]. A neoplasm of tubular structure.

**Sipple,** J. H. See S.'s *syndrome*.

**Sippy,** Bertram W., Chicago physician, 1866–1924. See S.'s *method*.

**siren'iform.** Denoting a malformation with the appearance of sirenomelia.

**sirenin** (si-ren'in). A female plant hormone that exerts a chemotactic attraction for male gametes; it is an oxygenated sesquiterpene, having a molecular weight of 236, and is inactivated by the male gametes.

**sirenomelia** (si'rĕ-no-me'lī-ah) [ L. *siren*, G. *seirēn*, a siren, in G. and L. myth, a sea-nymph, half woman and half fish ]. Mermaid deformity; symmelia; in teratology, union of the legs with partial or complete fusion of the feet; see also sympus.

**sirenomelus** (si-rĕ-nom'ĕ-lus). Symelus; symmelus; uromelus; an individual with sirenomelia.

**siriasis** (si-ri'ă-sis) [ G. *seiriasis*, from *seiriaō*, to be hot ]. Sunstroke.

**sirup.** Syrup.

**sismother'apy** [ G. *seismos*, a shaking, fr. *seiō*, fut. *seisō*, to shake ]. Vibratory *massage*.

**sis'ter.** In Great Britain (a) the title of a head nurse in a public hospital or in a ward or the operating room of a hospital; (b) any registered nurse in private practice.

**Sisto,** Genaro, Argentine pediatrician, †1923. See S.'s *sign*.

**site** [ L. *situs* ]. Place; seat; situation; location. See also subentries under situs.

**active s.,** that portion of an enzyme molecule at which the actual reaction proceeds. The active s. is considered to consist of one or more residues or atoms in a spatial arrangement that permits interaction with the substrate to effect the reaction of the latter.

**allosteric s.,** postulated as the place on an enzyme where a nonsubstrate, which may be the product of the biosynthetic pathway involving the enzyme, may bind and influence the activity of the enzyme. The influence of CTP on aspartate carbamoyl transferase activity exemplifies the concept of an allosteric site on an allosteric protein.

**receptor s.,** point of attachment of viruses to cell membranes.

**sit'fast.** A small, hard, cutaneous callus on the back of a horse, often resulting from the rubbing of a badly fitted collar or saddle.

**sitieirgia** (sit-ī-īr'jī-ah) [ G. *sitos*, food, + *eirgō*, to shut out, abstain from ]. Refusal to take food.

**sitiology** (sit'ī-ol'o-jī). Sitology.

**sito-** [ G. *sitos, sition*, food, grain. SIT- ]. Combining form relating to food or grain.

**sitology** (si-tol'o-jī) [ sito- + G. *logos*, study ]. Dietetics.

**sitomania** (si'to-ma'nī-ah) [ sito- + G. *mania*, frenzy ]. Bulimia; morbid increase in appetite.

**sitophobia** (si'to-fo'bī-ah) [ sito- + G. *phobos*, fear ]. Morbid fear of taking food.

**sitostane** (si-tos'tān, si'to-stān). Stigmastane.

**β-sitosterol.** Cinchol; 5-stigmasten-3β-ol; (24 *R*)-24-ethyl-5-cholesten-3β-ol (for structure of stigmastane and cholestane, see steroids).

**sitosterols** (si-tos'ter-olz, si'to-stēr'olz, -stēr'olz). The principal sterols of plant oils; they differ from cholesterol chiefly in the presence of an additional ethyl group in the C-17 side chain. S.'s increase fecal excretion of cholesterol by interfering with the absorption of exogenous and reabsorption of endogenous cholesterol. Used in the treatment of hypercholesteremia. The NF preparation contains not less than 95 per cent of unsaturated sterols.

**sitotaxis** (si'to-tak'sis) [ sito- + G. *taxis*, orderly arrangement ]. Sitotropism.

**sitotherapy** (si'to-thĕr'ă-pī). Dietotherapy.

**si'totox'in** [ sito- + G. *toxikon*, poison ]. Any food poison, especially one developing in grain.

**sitotoxism** (si'to-tok'sizm) [ sito- + G. *toxikon*, poison ]. 1. Poisoning by spoiled or fungous grain. 2. Food poisoning in general.

**sitotropism** (si-tot'ro-pizm) [ sito- + G. *tropē*, a turning ]. Sitotaxis; turning of living cells to or away from food.

**situation** (sich-u-a'shun). The aggregate of biological, psychological, and sociological factors that affect an individual's behavioral pattern.

**psychoanalytic s.,** the relationship, characteristically restricted to the therapist's office, between patient and therapist.

**si'tus** [ L. ]. Site (*q. v.*).

**s. inver'sus,** s. transversus; a transposition of the viscera, the liver being on the left side, the heart on the right, etc.

**s. perver'sus,** malposition of any viscus.

**s. transver'sus,** s. inversus.

**Siwe** (se'veh), Sture A., German pediatrician, 19th century. See Letterer-S. *disease*.

**size, aerodynamic.** In aerosols, the particle size with unit density which best represents the aerodynamic behavior of a particle.

**Sjögren** (syeh'gren), Henrik S. C., Stockholm ophthalmologist, *1899. See S.'s *disease*, Gougerot-S. *disease*, S.-Mikulicz *syndrome*, S. *syndrome*.

**Sjögren** (syeh'gren), Torsten, Swedish physician, 1859–1939. See S.-Larsson *syndrome*, Torsten S.'s *syndrome*, Marinesco-S. *syndrome*.

**Sjöqvist** (sho'kwist), O., Swedish neurosurgeon, 1901–1954. See S.'s *tractotomy*.

**SK.** Abbreviation for streptokinase.

**skato-** [ G. *skōr, skatos*, dung ]. Obsolescent spelling of combining form relating to feces; for such terms not listed here, see scato-; see also copro-.

**ska'tole.** 3-Methylindole; formed in the intestine by the bacterial decomposition of tryptophan; found in fecal matter, to which it imparts its characteristic odor.

**skatox'yl.** 3-Hydroxymethylindole; formed in the intestine by the oxidation of skatole. Some undergoes conjugation in the body with sulfuric or gluronic acids and is excreted in the urine in conjugated form.

**skein** (skān) [ Gael. *sgeinnidh*, hempen thread ]. The coiled threads of chromatin seen in the prophase of mitosis.

**choroid s.,** *glomus* choroideum.

**test s.'s,** s.'s of wool of various colors used in testing for color blindness by Holmgren's method.

**skelalgia** (ske-lal'jī-ah) [ G. *skelos*, leg, + *algos*, pain ]. Pain in the leg.

**skelasthenia** (ske-las-the'nī-ah) [ G. *skelos*, leg, + *astheneia*, weakness ]. Rarely used term meaning weakness of the legs.

**skeletal** (skel'ĕ-tal). Relating to the skeleton.

**skeletization** (skel'ĕ-tī-za'shun). Extreme emaciation; "reduced to a skeleton."

**skeletogenous** (ske-lĕ-toj'ĕ-nus). Producing a skeleton or bony framework; osteogenic.

**skeletology** (skel'ĕ-tol'o-jī). The branch of anatomy and of mechanics dealing with the skeleton.

**skeleton** (skel'ĕ-ton) [ G. *skeletos*, dried, ntr. *skeleton*, a mummy, a skeleton. SKEL- ]. 1. The bony framework of the body in vertebrates (endoskeleton) or the hard outer envelope of insects (exoskeleton or dermoskeleton). 2. All the dry parts remaining after the destruction and removal of the soft parts; this includes ligaments and cartilages as well as bones. 3. All the bones of the body taken collectively. See color plates 17 and 18.

**appendic'ular s.,** the s. of the limbs.

**articulated s.,** mounted s., one with the various parts connected in such a way as to allow of motion as in the living body.

**ax'ial s.,** the s. of the head and trunk.

**cardiac s.,** the dense supporting connective tissue of the heart; it consists of the four anuli fibrosi from which some of the myocardial fibers take origin, the right and left trigona fibrosa, and the membranous part of the interventricular septum.

**s. of free inferior limb,** s. membri inferioris liberi.

**s. of free superior limb,** s. membri superioris liberi.

**gill arch s.,** cartilages associated with the visceral portion of the embryonic mammalian chondrocranium, representing the gill arch (branchial) skeletons as seen in shark-type fishes; they are the primordia of Meckel's cartilage, styloid, hyoid, cricoid, thyroid, and arytenoid cartilages and the auditory ossicles. See also branchial *arch*.

**jaw s.,** viscerocranium.

**s. membri inferioris liberi** [ NA ], s. of the free inferior limb; the bones of the lower limb except the hip bones.

**s. membri superioris liberi** [ NA ], s. of the free superior limb; the bones of the upper limb except the scapula and clavicle.

**vis'ceral s.,** Visceroskeleton (2).

**Skene,** Alexander J. C., American gynecologist, 1838 –1900. See S.'s *glands, tubules.*

**skeneitis, skenitis** (ske-ni'tis). Inflammation of Skene's glands.

**skeneoscope** (skēn'o-skōp). A form of endoscope for inspecting Skene's glands.

**skeocytosis** (ske-o-si-to'sis) [ G. *skaios*, left, + *kytos*, cell, + suffix *-osos*, condition ]. Neocytosis.

**skeptophylaxis** (skep'to-fi-lak'sis) [ G. *skēptos*, stroke of lightning, + *phylaxis*, a guarding ]. 1. The rapid development of resistance against a nocuous agent. 2. Hyposensitization or temporary deallergization by repeated microshocks resulting from administrations, parenterally or orally, of small quantities of specific antigen (allergen).

**skew.** Departure from symmetry of a frequency distribution.

**skia-** (ski'ah-) [ G. *skia*, shadow ]. Combining form denoting shadow, sometimes used as synonyms of radiological terms. For words beginning thus and not listed here, see radio-, roentgeno-.

**ski'agram.** Obsolete term for radiogram.

**ski'agraph.** Obsolete term for radiograph.

**skiagraphy** (ski-ag'rǎ-fī). Obsolete term for radiography.

**skiameter** (ski-am'e-ter). Obsolete term for radiometer.

**ski'ascope.** Obsolete term for radioscope.

**skiascopy** (ski-as'ko-pī). Obsolete term for (1) retinoscopy; (2) fluoroscopy.

**skiascotometry** (ski'ah-sko-tom'e-trī) [ G. *skia*, shadow, + scotometry, *q.v.* ]. A method of plotting scotomas in the visual field by using an adaptation of the Goldmann perimeter.

**Skillern's fracture.** See under fracture.

**skimmetin.** Umbelliferone.

**skim'min.** 7-Hydroxycoumarin-7-glucoside; umbelliferone glucoside; see umbelliferone.

**skin** [ A.S. *scinn* ]. Cutis.

**alligator s.,** ichthyosis.

**bronzed s.,** the dark s. in Addison's disease.

**decid'uous s.,** keratolysis (2).

**elastic s.,** *cutis* hyperelastica.

**farmer's s.,** sailor's s.; sailor-farmer s.; dry wrinkled s. with presence of dry premalignant keratoses; observed most commonly in fair-skinned, blue-eyed persons who are exposed to sunshine for prolonged periods.

**fish s.,** ichthyosis.

**glabrous s.,** s. that is devoid of hair.

**glossy s.,** atrophoderma neuriticum; shiny atrophy of the s., usually of the hands, following nerve injury.

**loose s.,** *cutis* laxa.

**nail s.,** eponychium (2).

**parchment s.,** parchment-like appearance of the s. caused by loss of underlying connective and elastic tissue, or by the relatively rapid and persistent loss of water from the horny layer.

**piebald s.,** vitiligo.

**pig s.,** soft s. in which follicles are widely dilated; seen in pretibial myxedema.

**porcupine s.,** epidermolytic *hyperkeratosis.*

**sailor's s.,** see farmer's s.

**scarf s., scurf s.,** epidermis; cuticle.

**sex s.,** the s. of the genital regions of the *Macaca mulatta* and other primates which becomes hyperemic during estrus; at the same time the dermis becomes gelatinous and the epidermis thickened.

**shagreen s.,** paving-stone nevus; oval-shaped, slightly yellowish or buff-colored plaques that are irregularly nodular or crinkled; associated with tuberous sclerosis.

**veal s.,** a s. eruption resembling veal in color and texture.

**yellow s.,** xanthoderma.

**Skinner,** Burrhus, American psychologist, *1904. See S. *box, conditioning.*

**Sklowsky** (sklov'ske), E. L., German physician. See S. *symptom.*

**Skoda,** Joseph, Bohemian clinician in Vienna, 1805–1881. See S.'s *rale,* Skodaic *resonance,* S.'s *sign, tympany.*

**Skoda'ic.** Relating to Skoda.

**skull** [ Early Eng. *skulle*, a bowl ]. Cranium.

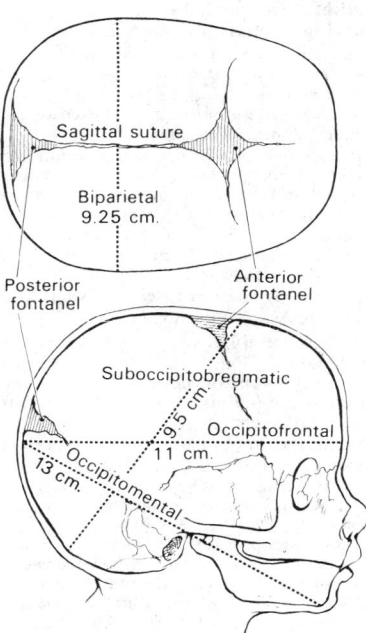

Diameters of the Fetal Skull

**maplike s.,** various defects in the s., especially in the temporal bone, the anterior fossa, and orbits, forming irregular outlines resembling the national boundaries on an atlas.

**natiform s.,** the appearance presented by the occurrence of two periostitic syphilitic nodes on the outer table of the s.

**steeple s.,** oxycephaly.

**tower s.,** oxycephaly.

**skull'cap.** Calvaria.

**sl.** Abbreviation for slyke.

**slab-off.** A process by which prism base-up is produced in the reading field of a spectacle lens through bicentric grinding.

**Slater factor.** See under factor.

**sleep** [ A.S. *slaep* ]. A physiologic state of relative unconsciousness and inaction of the voluntary muscles, the need for which recurs periodically. The number of hours in the 24 given to s. varies from 6 or 7 in the aged to 12 or 14 in the infant; the average for the male adult is 8 and for the female adult 9.

**crescendo s.,** normal s., marked by a gradual increase in movements of the sleeper during the course of the night.

**electric s.,** a condition of unconsciousness induced by the passage of an electric current through the brain.

**electrotherapeutic s.,** see electrotherapeutic s. *therapy.*

**hypnotic s.,** hypnosis.

**paradoxical s.,** a deep s., with a brain wave pattern more like that of waking states than of other states of sleep, which occurs during the rapid eye movement state of s.

**paroxys'mal s.,** narcolepsy.

**rapid eye movement s.,** rapid eye movement state; that state of deep s. in which rapid eye movements are exhibited; several central and autonomic functions are distinctive during this state; abbreviated REM s.

**twilight s.,** a previously popular method of producing analgesia and amnesia with a combination of morphine and scopolamine.

**winter s.,** hibernation.

**sleep'iness.** Somnolence; an inclination to sleep.

**sleep'lessness.** Insomnia.

**sleep-producing.** Soporific.

**sleep'talking.** 1. Somniloquence. 2. Somniloquy.

**sleep'walker.** Somnambulist.

**sleep'walking.** Somnambulism (1).

**slide.** An oblong glass plate on which is placed an object to be examined under the microscope.

**sling.** A supporting bandage, such as a loop suspended from the neck and supporting the flexed forearm.

**lentic'ular s.,** *ansa* lenticularis.

**slit'lamp.** An instrument presenting a diaphragm with a narrow slit through which a thin, intense beam of light is projected obliquely; used in examination of the eye through a microscope; see also biomicroscope.

**slough** (sluf). 1. Necrosed tissue separated from the living structure. 2. To separate from the living tissue, said of a dead or necrosed part.

**sludge.** A muddy sediment; see also sludged *blood.*

**sluiceway** (slūs'way). Spillway.

**slur'ry.** A thin, semifluid suspension of a solid in a liquid.

**slyke** [ Donald D. Van Slyke ]. Abbreviated sl; a unit of buffer value, the slope of the acid-base titration curve of a solution; it is the millimoles of strong acid that must be added per unit of change in pH.

**Sm.** Chemical symbol of the element samarium.

**small'pox** [ E. *small pocks,* or pustules ]. Variola; pestis variolosa; an acute eruptive contagious disease caused by a DNA poxvirus and marked at the onset by chills, high fever, backache, and headache; in from 2 to 5 days the constitutional symptoms subside and the eruption appears; this is at first papular, the papules become vesicles, and the latter pustules; the vesicles are umbilicated; the pustules dry and form scabs which on falling off leave a permanent marking of the skin (pock marks). The average incubation period is 8 to 14 days.

**con'fluent s.,** a severe form in which the lesions run into each other, forming large suppurating areas.

**discrete s.,** the usual form in which the lesions are separate and distinct from each other.

**hemorrhag'ic s.,** a severe form of s. accompanied by extravasation of blood into the skin in the early stage, or into the pustules at a later stage, accompanied often by nosebleed and hemorrhage from other orifices of the body.

**modified s.,** varioloid (2).

**varicel'loid s.,** varioloid (2).

**West Indian s.,** alastrim.

**smear** (smēr). Spread; cellular or cytologic spread; a thin specimen for examination; it is usually prepared by spreading material uniformly onto a glass slide, fixing it, and staining it before examination.

**alimentary tract s.,** a group of cytologic specimens containing material from the mouth (oral s.) esophagus, stomach (gastric s.), duodenum (paraduodenal s.), and colon, obtained by specialized lavage techniques; used principally for the diagnosis of cancer of those areas.

**bronchoscopic s.,** lower respiratory tract s.

**buccal s.,** a cytologic s. containing material obtained by scraping the lateral buccal mucosa above the dentate line, smearing, and fixing immediately; used principally for determining somatic sex as indicated by the presence of the sex chromocenter (Barr body).

**cervical s.,** a generic name for different types of FGT (female genital tract) smears of the cervix uteri, *e.g.,* ectocervical, endocervical, pancervical; used principally for cervical screening.

**colonic s.,** see alimentary tract s.

**cul-de-sac s.,** an FGT (female genital tract) cytologic specimen of material obtained by aspirating the pouch of Douglas from the posterior vaginal fornix and prepared by smearing, centrifuging, or filtering; used principally for ovarian cancer.

**cytologic s.,** cytosmear; a type of cytologic specimen made by smearing a sample (obtained by a variety of methods from a number of sites), then fixing it and straining it, usually with 95 per cent ethyl alcohol and Papanicolaou stain.

**duodenal s.,** see alimentary tract s.

**ectocervical s.,** a cytologic s. of material obtained from the ectocervix, usually by scraping; used principally for the diagnosis of late cervical cancers involving the ectocervix.

**endocervical s.,** a cytologic s. of material obtained from the endocervical canal by swab, aspiration, or scraping; used principally for the detection of early cervical cancer.

**endometrial s.,** a group of FGT (female genital tract) cytologic s.'s containing material obtained directly from the endometrium by aspiration, lavage, or brushing of the uterine cavity.

**esophageal s.,** see alimentary tract s.

**fast s.,** an FGT (female genital tract) cytologic smear containing material from the vaginal pool and pancervical scrapings, mixed and prepared on one microscopic slide, smeared, and fixed immediately; used principally for routine FGT screening of ovaries, endometrium, cervix, vagina, and hormonal states.

**FGT cytologic s.,** any cytologic s. obtained from the female genital tract.

**gastric s.,** see alimentary tract s.

**lateral vaginal wall s.,** a cytologic s. containing material obtained by scraping the lateral wall of the vagina near the junction of its upper and middle third; used for cytohormonal evaluation.

**lower respiratory tract s.,** bronchoscopic s.; sputum s.; a group of cytologic specimens containing material from the lower respiratory tract and consisting mainly of sputum (spontaneous, induced) and material obtained at bronchoscopy (aspirated, lavaged, brushed); used for cytologic study of cancer and other diseases of the lungs.

**oral s.,** see alimentary tract s.

**pancervical s.,** a cytologic s. of material obtained from the endocervical canal, external os, and ectocervix by scraping these areas with a properly designed cervical spatula; used principally for early cervical cancer detection.

**Papanicolaou s.,** see cytologic *examination.*

**sputum s.,** lower respiratory tract s.

**urinary s.,** a group of cytologic specimens containing processed urine obtained from bladder, ureters, or renal pelvis; used for cytologic study of cancer and other diseases of the urinary tract.

**vaginal s.,** a s. of debris from the vaginal lumen of mammals, used to determine the stage of their reproductive cycle. It is most useful in subprimate mammals having short estrous cycles; nucleated epithelial cells and leukocytes prevail in the s. during diestrus and proestrus, and cornified cells during estrus.

**VCE s.,** a cytologic s. of material obtained from the vagina, ectocervix, and endocervix, smeared separately (in that order) on one slide, and fixed immediately; used principally for the detection of cervical cancer and identification of the sites of diseases of those areas, and for hormonal evaluation.

**smegma** (smeg'mah) [ G. unguent ]. Sebum.

**s. clitor'idis,** the secretion of the apocrine glands of the clitoris, in combination with desquamating epithelial cells.

**s. prepu'tii,** sebum preputiale; whitish secretion that collects under the prepuce of the foreskin of the penis or of the clitoris; it is comprised chiefly of desquamating epithelial cells.

**smegmalith** (smeg'mă-lith) [ smegma + G. *lithos*, stone ]. A calcareous concretion in the smegma.

**smell.** 1. To scent; to perceive by means of the olfactory apparatus. 2. Olfaction (1). 3. An odor; a scent.

**smell-brain.** Rhinencephalon.

**Smellie,** William, London obstetrician, 1697–1763. See S.'s *scissors.*

**Smi'lax** [ G. ]. A genus of plants of the family Liliaceae; the root of several tropical American species yields sarsaparilla.

**Smith,** Erwin F., American plant pathologist, 1854–1927. Gave his name to *Erwinia.*

**Smith,** G. W., American neurosurgeon. See S.-Robinson *operation.*

**Smith,** Henry, British military surgeon (born in Ireland), 1862–1948. See S.'s *operation,* S.'Indian *operation.*

**Smith,** John B., Irish pathologist, 1865–1928. See S.-Pitfield *stain.*

**Smith,** Robert W., Irish surgeon, 1807–1873. See S.'s *fracture.*

**Smith,** Theobald, American pathologist, 1859–1934. See Theobald S.'s *phenomenon.*

**Smith,** Walter G., irish physician, 1844–1932. See S.'s *test.*

**Smith,** William H., American bacteriologist. See S.'s *stain* (for pneumococci in sputum).

**Smith-Petersen,** Marius N., U. S. surgeon, 1886–1953. See S.-P. *nail.*

**Smith-Smith test.** See under test.

**smog.** Hazy and often highly irritating atmosphere resulting from a mixture of smoke and other air pollutants, and fog. See also air *pollution.*

**smudging** (smuj'ing). Scamping speech in which the more difficult consonants are dropped.

**Sn.** Chemical symbol of the element tin (L. *stannum*).

**sn-.** Prefix meaning stereospecifically numbered; a system of numbering the glycerol carbon atoms in lipids.

**snake'root.** Serpentaria.

    **black s.,** cimicifuga.

    **Canada s.,** *Asarum canadense.*

    **European s.,** *Asarum europaeum.*

    **Seneca s.,** senega.

    **smaller white s.,** *Eupatorium aromaticum.*

    **Texas s.,** *Aristolochia reticulata;* botanical source of serpentaria.

    **Virginia s.,** *Aristolochia serpentaria;* botanical source of serpentaria.

    **white s.,** *Eupatorium ageratoides* or *E. urticaefolium;* suspected to cause trembles or milk sickness in cattle.

**snap.** A short sharp sound; a click; said especially of cardiac sounds.

    **closing s.,** the accentuated first heart sound of mitral stenosis, related to closure of the abnormal valve.

    **opening s.,** a sharp, highpitched click in early diastole, usually best heard between the cardiac apex and the lower left sternal border, related to opening of the abnormal valve in cases of mitral stenosis.

**snare** [ A.S. *snear,* a cord ]. An instrument for use in removing polyps and other projections from any surface, especially one within a cavity; it consists of a wire loop that is passed around the base of the tumor and gradually tightened.

    **cold s.,** the ordinary unheated s.

    **galvanocaus'tic s., hot s.,** a s. the wire of which is raised to a red or white heat by the galvanic current.

    **Jarvis' s.,** a wire s., tightened by a screw in the handle, used for the cutting off of polyps and other sessile growths in the nose and other accessible cavities.

**Sneddon,** I. B. See S.-Wilkinson *disease.*

**sneeze** [ A.S. *fneōsan* ]. 1. To expel air from the nose and mouth by an involuntary spasmodic contraction of the muscles of expiration. 2. An act of sneezing; a reflex excited by an irritation of the mucous membrane of the nose or, sometimes, by a bright light striking the eye.

**Snell,** Simeon, English ophthalmologist, 1851–1909. See S.'s *law.*

**Snellen,** Hermann, Dutch ophthalmologist, 1834–1908. See S.'s reform *eye,* S.'s *test–types.*

**snore** [ A.S. *snora* ]. 1. A rough, rattling, inspiratory noise produced by vibration of the pendulous palate, or sometimes of the vocal cords, during sleep or coma; see also stertor and rhonchus. 2. To breathe noisily, or with a s.

**snout** [ M.E. ]. In veterinary anatomy, the rostral extremity of the face and rhinarium, frequently elongate and related to specialized feeding habits as in the gar, soft-shelled turtle, echidna, pig, etc.

**snow.** See carbon dioxide snow (under carbon).

**snow'berry.** Cahinca.

**snuff.** 1. To inhale forcibly through the nose. 2. Finely powdered tobacco used by inhalation through the nose or applied to the gums. 3. Any medicated powder applied by insufflation to the nasal mucous membrane; see also errhine.

**snuff bean.** Dipteryx.

**snuff-box.** See *anatomical* snuff-box.

**snuffles** (snuf'lz). Obstructed nasal respiration, especially in the newborn infant, sometimes due to congenital syphilis.

    **rabbit s.,** acute inflammation of the upper nasal passages, usually associated with *Pasteurella* organisms. In outbreaks of s. in rabitries there usually are some deaths from pneumonia.

**Snyder,** M. L. See S.'s *test.*

**soap** [ A.S. *sape,* L. *sapo,* G. *sapōn* ]. The sodium or potassium salts of long chain fatty acids (*e.g.,* sodium stearate); used for cleansing purposes and as an excipient in the making of pills and suppositories.

    **animal s.,** tallow s.; curd s.; domestic s.; s. made with sodium hydroxide and a purified animal fat consisting chiefly of stearin; used in pharmacy in the preparation of certain liniments.

    **Castile s.,** hard s.

    **curd s.,** animal s.

    **domestic s.,** animal s.

    **green s.** (NF), medicinal soft s.

    **hard s.,** Castile s.; a s. made with olive oil, or some other suitable oil or fat, and sodium hydroxide. Used as a detergent, as an antidote in poisoning by mineral acids, and in the form of a suppository or soapsuds enema for constipation; used also as an excipient in pills.

    **insoluble s.,** s. made with a fatty acid and an earthy or metallic base.

    **marine s.,** a s. made of palm or cocoanut oil for use with sea water in which it is soluble.

    **medicinal soft s.,** soft s.; green s.; made with vegetable oils, potassium hydroxide, oleic acid, glycerin, and purified water. Used as a stimulant in chronic skin diseases.

    **salt water s.,** marine s.

    **soft s.** (BP). medicinal soft s.

    **soluble s.,** any s. made with potassium, sodium or ammonium hydroxide: ordinary animal s., Castile s., green s., etc.

    **superfatted s.,** a s. containing an excess (3 to 5 per cent) of fat above that necessary to neutralize completely all the alkali. Used in the manufacture of medicated s., and in the treatment of skin diseases.

    **tallow s.,** animal s.

**soap bark.** Quillaja.

**soap'stone.** Talc.

**socaloin** (sok-al'o-in). An aloin obtained from socotrine aloes.

**socialization** (so'shă-lĭ-za'shun) [ L. *socia,* partner, companion ]. 1. The process of learning interpersonal and interactional skills which are in conformity with the values of one's society. 2. In a group therapy setting, s. includes a member's way of learning to effectively participate in the group.

**so'cia parot'idis** [ L. companion of the parotid; fem. of *socius* ]. *Glandula* parotis accessoria.

**socio-** (so'si-o-, so'shi-o-) [ L. *socius,* companion ]. Combining form meaning social, relating to society.

**sociocentric** (so'sī-o-sen'trik) [ socio- + L. *centrum,* center ]. Outgoing; reactive to the culture.

**so'ciocen'trism.** Taking one's own social group as the standard of excellence.

**sociocosm** (so'sī-o-kozm) [ socio- + G. *kosmos*, universe ]. The totality that includes human society, human thought, and the relationship of man to nature.

**sociogenesis** (so'sī-o-jen'ē-sis) [ socio- + G. *genesis*, origin ]. The origin of social behavior from past interpersonal experiences.

**sociogram** (so'sī-o-gram) [ socio- + G. *gramma*, something written ]. A diagrammatic representation of the interpersonal interactions of members of a group.

**sociomedical** (so'sī-o-med'ī-kal). Pertaining to the relation of the practice of medicine to society.

**sociometry** (so'sī-om'e-trī) [ socio- + G. *metron*, measure ]. The study of interpersonal relationships in a group.

**sociopath** (so'sī-o-path) [ socio- + G. *pathos*, suffering ]. Psychopath.

**sock'et** [ thr. O. Fr. fr. L. *soccus*, a shoe, a sock ]. 1. The hollow part of a joint; the excavation in one bone of a joint which receives the articular end of the other bone. 2. Any hollow or concavity into which another part fits, as the eye s.

   **dry s.,** alveoalgia.

   **tooth s.,** *alveolus* dentalis.

**soda** (so'dah) [ It., possibly fr. Mediev. L. barilla plant ]. Sodium carbonate.

   **baking s.,** sodium bicarbonate.

   **caustic s.,** sodium hydroxide.

   **s. lime** (BP), a mixture of calcium hydroxide with sodium or potassium hydroxide or both. Used to absorb carbon dioxide and moisture in metabolism determinations, in anesthesia, and in oxygen administrations. It may contain an indicator which is inert and which changes color when the absorption capacity for carbon dioxide is exhausted.

   **washing s.,** commercial sodium carbonate.

**so'dic.** Relating to or containing soda or sodium.

**sodio-.** A prefix denoting a compound containing sodium; as sodiocitrate, sodiotartrate, a citrate or tartrate of some element containing sodium in addition.

# SODIUM

**sodium** (so'dī-um) [ Mod. L. fr. *soda* ]. A metallic element, symbol Na (Mod. L. *natrium*), atomic no. 11, atomic weight 22.991; a silvery-white, lustrous alkali metal of the consistency of wax, oxidizing readily in air or water; it is very caustic. The salts of s. are extensively used in medicine. For organic sodium salts not listed below, see under the name of the organic acid portion.

   **s. acetate** (USP, BP), $CH_3COONa \cdot 3H_2O$; systemic and urinary alkalizer, expectorant, and diuretic.

   **s. acid citrate** (BP), s. citrate.

   **s. acid phosphate** (BP), s. biphosphate.

   **s. alginate** (NF), algin.

   **s. _p_-aminohippurate,** used intravenously in renal function tests, to determine the renal plasma flow and the tubular excretion.

   **s. _p_-aminophenylarsonate,** ATOXYL; s. arsanilate; $H_2N—C_6H_4—AsO(OH)(ONa) \cdot 3H_2O$; this compound is of historical interest as being one of the first modern pentavalent arsenicals.

   **s. aminosalicylate** (USP, BP), s. _p_-aminosalicylate; $C_6H_3$-($p$-$NH_2$)($o$-OH)—$COONa \cdot 2H_2O$; used for the same purposes as aminosalicylic acid.

   **s. antimonylgluconate** (BP), stibogluconate sodium, trivalent.

   **s. ascorbate** (USP), same actions and uses as ascorbic acid. It is preferred for intramuscular administration.

   **s. aurothiomalate** (BP), gold sodium thiomalate.

   **s. aurothiosulfate,** gold sodium thiosulfate.

   **s. benzoate** (USP, BP), $C_6H_5COONa$; used in chronic and acute rheumatism and as a liver function test.

   **s. benzosulfimide,** saccharin sodium.

   **s. bicarbonate** (USP, BP), baking soda; s. acid carbonate; s. hydrogen carbonate; $NaHCO_3$; used as a gastric and

systemic antacid, to alkalize urine and for washes of body cavities.

   **s. biphosphate** (USP), sodium acid phosphate (BP); s. dihydrogenphosphate; primary s. phosphate; $NaH_2PO_4 \cdot H_2O$; used to increase urinary acidity.

   **s. bisulfite** (USP), s. metabisulphite (BP); s. pyrosulfite; s. hydrogen sulfite; acid s. sulfite; $NaHSO_3$; used in gastric and intestinal fermentation, externally in the treatment of parasitic diseases and as an antioxidant in certain injections.

   **s. borate** (USP), borax; s. pyroborate; s. tetraborate; $Na_2B_4O_7 \cdot 10H_2O$; used in lotions, gargles, mouthwashes, and as a detergent.

   **s. bromide** (BP), NaBr; hypnotic and sedative; used in epilepsy and other functional disorders of the nervous system.

   **s. cacodylate,** s. dimethylarsenate; $(CH_3)_2AsOONa \cdot 3H_2O$; used in anemia, leukemia, and malaria.

   **s. calcium edetate** (BP), edetate calcium disodium.

   **s. carbonate** (USP), sal soda; washing soda; $Na_2CO_3 \cdot 10H_2O$; used in the treatment of scaly skin diseases; otherwise rarely used in medicine because of its irritant action.

   **s. carboxymethyl cellulose** (USP), CM-cellulose sodium; sodium carboxymethyl cellulose and microcrystalline cellulose (NF); the sodium salt of a polycarboxymethyl ether of cellulose; used as a gastric antacid and laxative.

   **s. chloride** (USP, BP), common salt; table salt; NaCl; one of its most important medical uses is in making isotonic and physiological salt solutions; also used as an emetic and in the treatment of salt depletion, and topically for inflammatory lesions.

   **s. chromate Cr 51** (USP, BP), RACHROMATE; s. chromate $^{51}$Cr; anionic hexavalent radioactive chromium in the form of s. chromate ($NA_2^{51}CrO$) with a half-life of 27.8 days; used for the determination of circulating red cell volume and red cell survival time.

   **s. citrate** (USP), sodium acid citrate (BP); $Na_3C_6H_5O_7 \cdot 2H_2O$; trisodium citrate; used as diuretic, antilithic, systemic and urinary alkalizer, expectorant, and anticoagulant (*in vitro*).

   **s. citrate, acid** (BP), disodium hydrogen citrate; $C_6H_6O_7Na \cdot 1^1/_2H_2O$; same actions and uses as s. citrate; in addition, it may be used in solutions of glucose without producing caramelization of the latter during autoclaving.

   **s. cloxacillin,** cloxacillin sodium.

   **s. cromoglycate** (BP), cromolyn sodium.

   **s. cyclamate,** (BP), s. cyclohexylsulfamate dihydrate; s. salt of cyclamic acid; a synthetic food sweetener for use by diabetics and others who must restrict carbohydrate intake. It was banned as a food additive in the United States in 1969 because of a reported association with bladder carcinoma in rats.

   **s. dehydrocholate,** DECHOLIN s.; cholagogue; also used to determine circulation time.

   **s. diatrizoate** (USP, BP), HYPAQUE s.; s. 3,5-diacetamido-2,4,6-triiodobenzoate; a water-soluble organic iodine compound used for intravenous excretory urography.

   **s. dodecyl sulfate,** widely used detergent, identical with s. lauryl sulfate.

   **s. ethacrynate,** see ethacrynate sodium.

   **s. ethylsulfate,** s. sulfovinate; $Na(C_2H_5SO_4) \cdot H_2O$; a laxative.

   **s. fluoride** (USP, BP), used as a dental prophylactic in drinking water, and topically as a 2 per cent solution applied on the teeth.

   **s. fluosilicate,** s. hexafluorosilicate.

   **s. folate,** the s. salt of folic acid; s. pteroylglutamate; its action and uses are the same as those of folic acid, but it is preferred for parenteral administration.

   **s. fusidate** (BP), fusidate sodium.

   **s. glutamate,** GLUTAVENE; monosodium L-glutamate; used intravenously as an adjunct in the treatment of encephalopathies associated with liver diseases and ammoniacal azotemia.

   **s. glycerophosphate,** $C_3H_5(OH)_2PO_4Na$; has been used as a tonic.

   **s. group,** the alkali metals, lithium, sodium, potassium, rubidium, and cesium.

**s. hexafluorosilicate,** SALUFER; s. fluosilicate; s. silico-fluoride; $Na_2SiF_6$; used (in dilute solutions) as an antiseptic and deodorant, and for fluoridation of drinking water.

**s. hydroxide** (USP, BP), caustic soda; NaOH; used externally as a caustic.

**s. hypophosphite,** $NaPH_2O_2 \cdot H_2O$; formerly used as a nerve tonic.

**s. hyposulfite,** s. thiosulfate.

**s. ichthyolsulfonate,** alterative and antiseptic.

**s. indigotindisulfonate** (USP), indigo carmine (BP); disodium indigotin-5,5'-disulfonate; FD & C Blue No. 2; occurs in the form of a blue powder or a soft, purple mass. Used as a stain in microscopy and as a kidney function test.

**s. iodide** (USP, BP), NaI; used as a source of iodine.

**s. iodide I 131** (USP, BP), prepared from radioactive iodine ($^{131}$I); practically carrier-free, with a half-life of 8.0 days; used as a diagnostic agent in suspected thyroid disease and in the treatment of selected thyroid diseases.

**s. iodipamide** (USP), see iodipamide sodium.

**s. iodoacetate,** the sodium salt of iodoacetic acid, *q.v.*

**s. o-iodohippurate,** see iodohippurate sodium.

**s. iodomethamate,** see under iodomethamate.

**s. iothalamate** (USP), see iothalamate sodium.

**s. lactate** (USP), $C_3H_5NaO_3$; a systemic and urinary alkalizer.

**s. lauryl sulfate** (USP), s. lauryl sulphate (BP); $CH_3(CH_2)_{10}CH_2OSO_3Na$; a surface-active agent of the anionic type.

**s. levothyroxine** (USP), 3,3',5,5'-tetraiodothyronine pentahydrate. It is twice as effective as the racemic form. Used in the treatment of cretinism, myxedema and milder forms of hypothyroidism.

**s. liothyronine** (USP, BP), CYTOMEL; s. L-triiodothyronine, the physiologically active isomer of triiodothyronine, is twice as active as the racemic form; used in the treatment of hypothyroidism, metabolic insufficiency, and certain reproductive disorders.

**s. metabisulfite** (NF), s. metabisulphite (BP); $Na_2S_2O_5$; used as an antioxidant in injectable solutions.

**s. methicillin** (USP), see under methicillin.

**s. methiodal,** contains not less than 98 per cent of iodine equivalent, and not more than 102 per cent of $CH_2INaO_3S$; a radiopaque medium.

**s. methylarsonate,** disodium monomethyl arsonate; $CH_3H_5O(ONa)_2 \cdot 5H_2O$; used in tuberculosis, chorea, and other affections in which the cacodylates are used.

**s. morrhuate,** the s. salts of the fatty acids of cod liver oil; a sclerosing agent, used in the treatment of varicose veins, mixed with a local anesthetic; official in the USP as the injection.

**s. nitrate,** cubic niter; Chilean saltpeter; $NaNO_3$; formerly used for dysentery and as a diuretic.

**s. nitrite** (USP), $NaNO_2$; used to lower systemic blood pressure, to relieve local vasomotor spasms, especially in angina pectoris and Raynaud's disease, to relax bronchial and intestinal spasms, and as an antidote for cyanide poisoning.

**s. nitroprusside** (USP), s. nitroferricyanide; $(Na_2\text{-}FeCCN)_5NO \cdot 5H_2O$; used as a reagent for detection of organic compounds in the urine.

**s. nucleate, s. nucleinate,** s. salts of yeast acids, used in the treatment of anemias, rheumatism, and gout.

**s. oxacillin** (USP), see oxacillin sodium.

**s. perborate,** $NaBO_2H_2O_2 \cdot 3H_2O$; used in the extemporaneous preparation of hydrogen peroxide. A 2 per cent solution is equivalent in germicidal action to 0.4 per cent of hydrogen peroxide.

**s. peroxide,** $Na_2O_2$; used externally as a paste or soap in the treatment of comedones and acne.

**s. phenolsulfonate,** s. sulfocarbolate; has been used in tonsillitis and as an intestinal antiseptic; has no antiseptic properties.

**s. phosphate** (USP, BP), s. orthophosphate; dibasic s. phosphate; secondary s. phosphate; $Na_2HPO_4 \cdot H_2O$; laxative.

**s. phosphate, effervescent** (NF), exsiccated s. phosphate 200, s. bicarbonate 477, tartaric acid 252, citric acid 162, mixed and passed through a sieve to make a granular salt.

**s. phosphate P 32** (USP, BP), anionic radioactive phosphorus in the form of a solution of s. acid phosphate and s. basic phosphate; a beta emitter with a half-life of

14.3; pH between 5.0 and 6.0. After administration, highest concentrations are found in rapidly proliferating tissues with high phosphorus content. Used in the treatment of polycythemia vera and chronic myelogenous leukemia, and in colloid form to control malignant pleural or peritoneal effusions.

**s. polyanhydromannuronic acid sulfate,** an anticoagulant drug prepared from alginic acid and having an action similar to that of heparin.

**s. polystyrene sulfonate** (USP), RESONIUM A; KAYEXALATE; a cationic exchange resin used in hyperpotassemia.

**s. potassium tartrate** (BP), see potassium sodium tartrate.

**s. propionate** (NF), the s. salt of propionic acid; used for fungus infections of the skin, usually in combination with calcium propionate.

**s. psylliate,** the s. salt of the liquid fatty acids of psyllium oil, prepared by dissolving the fatty acid in dilute s. hydroxide solution. Used like s. morrhuate as a sclerosing agent in the treatment of varicose veins.

**s. pyroborate,** s. borate.

**s. rhodanate,** s. thiocyanate.

**s. ricinoleate,** s. ricinate; the s. salt of ricinoleic acid; a sclerosing agent similar in its action to that of s. morrhuate.

**s. salicylate** (BP), used as an analgesic, antipyretic, and antirheumatic.

**s. silicate,** soluble glass; water glass; made by fusing together s. carbonate and powdered quartz; a solution is used to impregnate bandages for applying fixed dressings; it has also been given internally in gout and tuberculosis.

**s. silicofluoride,** s. hexafluorosilicate.

**s. stearate** (USP, NF), a mixture of stearate with varying proportions of s. palmitate; used externally in sycosis and parasitic skin diseases, and as an ingredient in greaseless ointments or vanishing creams and in glycerin suppositories.

**s. stibogluconate** (BP), see stibogluconate sodium.

**s. succinate,** disodium succinate; used as an analeptic in barbiturate poisoning, and as a hepatic stimulant, urinary alkalizer, and diuretic; also used to measure circulation time.

**s. sulfabromomethazine,** an antibacterial used in veterinary medicine for infections such as shipping fever, pneumonia, foot rot, metritis and acute mastitis in cattle, and coccidiosis in cattle and sheep.

**s. sulfate** (USP, BP), Glauber's salt; $Na_2SO_4 \cdot 10H_2O$; it is an ingredient of many of the natural laxative waters, and is used as a hydragogue cathartic.

**s. sulfite,** $Na_2SO_3 \cdot 7H_2O$; has been used for the relief of intestinal fermentation, and externally for aphthous stomatitis.

**s. sulfite, exsiccated,** anhydrous s. sulfite; used as a preservative of pharmaceutical preparations.

**s. sulfocyanate,** s. thiocyanate.

**s. sulforicinate, s. sulforicinoleate,** made by combining castor oil, sulfuric acid, and s. hydroxide and chloride; used as a solvent for iodine, iodoform, resorcinol, pyrogallol, and a number of other substances for external use.

**s. sulfovinate,** s. ethylsulfate.

**s. tartrate,** $Na_2C_4H_4O_6 \cdot 2H_2O$; laxative.

**s. taurocholate,** the sodium salt of taurocholic acid, extracted from the bile of carnivora; cholagogue.

**s. tetraborate,** s. borate.

**s. tetradecyl sulfate,** an anionic surface-active agent used for its wetting properties to enhance the surface action of certain antiseptic solutions; also used as a sclerosing agent similar to s. morrhuate in the treatment of varicose veins.

**s. tetraiodophthalein,** iodophthalein sodium.

**s. thiocyanate,** NaSCN; s. sulfocyanate; s. rhodanate; used in the management of essential hypertension.

**s. thiosulfate** (USP), s. hyposulfite; $Na_2S_2O_3 \cdot 5H_2O$. An antidote in cyanide poisoning in conjunction with s. nitrite. Used as a prophylactic agent against ringworm infections in swimming pools and baths, and to measure the extracellular fluid volume of the body.

---

**sodium-24** ($^{24}$Na). The isotope of sodium with an atomic weight of 24, and a half-life of 14.8 hours; it emits beta and gamma rays. It is more easily prepared than the longer-lived positron-emitting $^{22}$Na (half-life, 2.6 years). Incorporated into sodium compounds, $^{24}$Na is used in the treatment of malignant growths, especially of the bladder, a balloon being inserted into the bladder and filled with a solution of the radioactive salt. It is also used to measure the extracellular fluid, and, injected intravenously, to follow the course of the blood through the heart in abnormal cardiac conditions, a shielded counter being used.

**sodo'ku** [ Jap. rat poison ]. Rat-bite *fever.*

**sod'omist, sod'omite** [ G. *sodomitēs,* an inhabitant of the biblical city of Sodom, which was destroyed by fire because of the wickedness of its people ]. One who practices sodomy.

**sod'omy** [ see sodomist ]. A term denoting a variety of sexual practices considered abnormal, especially copulation of man and animal (bestiality), fellatio, and anal intercourse.

**Soemmering** (zë'mer-ing), Samuel T. von, German anatomist, 1755–1830. See S.'s *foramen, ganglion, ligament, muscle, spot.*

**Soffer,** Louis J., U. S. internist, *1904. See Sohval-S. *syndrome.*

**softening** (sof'ĕ-ning). Malacia; mollities; the act of becoming or state of being soft; a diminution of the normal consistence of a tissue.

**Sohval,** Arthur R., U. S. internist, *1904. See S.-Soffer *syndrome.*

**soja** (so'yah). Soybean.

**soko'sho** [ Jap. *so,* rat, + *ko,* bite, + *sho,* malady ]. Rat-bite *fever.*

**sol.** 1. A colloidal dispersion of a solid in a liquid; *cf.* gel. 2. Abbreviation for solution.

**Solanaceae** (so'lă-na'se-e). A family of plants that includes the genus *Solanum.* There are some 84 other genera comprising 1800 species.

**solanaceous** (so'lă-na'shus, sol'-). Pertaining to plants of the family Solanaceae, or to drugs derived from them.

**solanidine** (so-lan'ĭ-dēn, -din). Solatubine; a crystallizable alkaloid, $C_{27}H_{43}NO$; see solanine.

**solanine** (so'lă-nēn, -nin, sol'-). Solatunine; $C_{45}H_{73}NO_{15}$; a glycosidal alkaloid obtained from potato sprouts, woody nightshade, and tomato. The trisaccharide moiety, rhamnose, galactose, and glucose, is linked to one molecule of the aglycone solanidine.

**solanochromene** (sol'ă-no-kro'mēn). Plastochromenol-8.

**solanoid** (sol'ă-noyd) [ L. *solanum,* nightshade, + G. *eidos,* resemblance ]. Resembling a potato in texture, said of certain malignant growths.

**solanoma** (sol'ă-no'mah) [ L. *solanum, q.v.,* + G. suffix *-oma,* tumor ]. A solanoid neoplasm.

**Sola'num** (so-la'num) [ L. nightshade ]. A genus of plants of the family Solanaceae, including various species of nightshade as well as the potato.

    **S. carolinen'se,** horse-nettle; apple of Sodom; a North American plant. The dried ripe fruit has been used in epilepsy.

    **S. dulcama'ra,** see dulcamara.

    **S. lycoper'sicum,** the tomato plant.

    **S. melonge'na,** eggplant; a solution of the dried fruit and leaves has been used to reduce the cholesterol of the blood in hypercholesterolemia.

    **S. nigrum,** black nightshade.

    **S. tubero'sum,** the potato plant.

**solap'sone** (BP). Solasulfone.

**solasulf'one.** Solapsone (BP); SULPHETRONE; CIMEDONE; 1,1'- [ sulfonylbis(*p*-phenyleneimino) ] bis [ 3-phenyl-1,3-propanedisulfonic acid ]tetrasodium salt; leprostatic agent.

**solation** (sol-a'shun). In colloidal chemistry, the transformation of a gel into a sol as by melting gelatin.

**Soldaini** (sol-dah-e'ne), Arturo, Italian chemist, 19th century. See S.'s *reagent.*

**solder** (sod'er) [ L. *solidare,* to make solid, through Fr., various forms ]. A fusible metal alloy used to join pieces of metal. Alloys classified as hard s.'s are usually used in dentistry to connect noble metal alloys.

    **hard s.,** in dentistry, hard s.'s are of higher melting range and stronger than the soft lead tin s.'s; they are usually alloys with either gold or silver as their main constituent.

**soldering** (sod'er-ing). The joining of metal parts by an alloy whose fusing temperature is lower than that of the components to be connected. (In dentistry no distinction is made between s. and brazing.)

**sole** [ A.S. ]. The under part of the foot; the plantar surface; planta.

**Solenoglypha** (so'lĕ-nog'lĭ-fah) [ L. fr. G. *sōlēn,* pipe channel, + *glyphein,* to carve ]. A major category of snakes including the viper and rattlesnake families.

**so'lenoid.** A spiral coil of wire energized electrically to produce a magnetic field, which induces current in any conductor placed within or near the coil.

**Solenopo'tes capilla'tus** [ G. *solen,* pipe, + *potos,* a drinking ]. A sucking louse of cattle, called the little blue cattle louse in the United States and the tubercle-bearing louse in Australia.

**solenop'sin A.** *trans*-2-Methyl-6-*n*-undecylpiperidine; one of several, probably five, alkaloidal constituents present in the venom of the imported fire ant, *Solenopis saevissima;* the venom has necrotoxic, hemolytic, insecticidal, and antibiotic properties.

**sole'us** [ Mod. L. fr. L. *solea,* a sandal, sole of the foot (of animals), fr. *solum,* bottom, floor, ground ]. See under musculus.

**sol'id** [ L. *solidus* ]. 1. Firm; compact; not fluid; without interstices or cavities; not cancellous. 2. A body that retains its form when not confined; one that is not fluid, neither liquid nor gaseous.

**Solida'go** [ Mediev. L. fr. L. *solidus,* solid ]. A genus of plants of the family Compositae, the goldenrods. *S. odora* (sweet or fragrant goldenrod) and *S. virgaurea* (Aaron's rod, woundwort) have carminative and astringent properties.

**sol'idism.** Methodism; the theory propounded by Asclepiades and his followers that disease was due to an imbalance between solid particles (atoms) of the body and the spaces (pores) between them, a doctrine which opposed the humoral conception of Hippocrates.

**sol'idist.** An adherent of the doctrine of solidism.

**solidis'tic.** Relating to solidism.

**sol'idus.** The line on a constitution diagram below which temperature all metal is solid.

**soliped** (sol'ĭ-ped) [ L. *solus,* alone, + *pes,* foot ]. A solid-hoofed animal such as the horse.

**solipsism** (so'lip-sizm, sol'ip-sizm) [ L. *solus,* alone, + *ipse,* self ]. A philosophical concept that only one's own experience is real.

**solubility** (sol'u-bil'ĭ-tĭ). The property of being soluble.

**soluble** (sol'u-bl) [ L. *solubilis,* fr. *solvo,* to dissolve. SOL- ]. Capable of being dissolved.

**soluble-RNA.** See under ribonucleic acid.

**so'lum** [ L. ] [ NA ]. Bottom; floor; the lowest part.

**solute** (so-lūt') [ L. *solutus,* dissolved, pp. of *solvo,* to dissolve ]. The dissolved substance in a solution.

**solutio** (so-lu'shĭ-o) [ L. ]. Solution.

**solution** (so-lu'shun) [ L. *solutio* ]. 1. The incorporation of a solid, a liquid, or a gas in a liquid or noncrystalline solid resulting in a homogeneous single phase; see dispersion and suspension. 2. Generally, an aqueous s. of a nonvolatile substance. 3. In the language of the Pharmacopeia, an aqueous s. of a nonvolatile substance is called a solution or liquor; an aqueous s. of a volatile substance is a water (aqua); an alcoholic s. of a nonvolatile substance is a tincture (tinctura), an alcoholic s. of a volatile substance is a spirit (spiritus); a s. in vinegar is a vinegar (acetum); a s. in glycerin is a glycerite (glyceritum); a s. in wine is a wine (vinum); a s. of sugar in water is a syrup (syrupus); a s. of a mucilaginous substance is a mucilage (mucilago); a s. of an alkaloid or metallic oxide in olieic acid is an oleate (oleatum). 4. The termination of a disease by crisis. 5. A break, cut, or laceration of the solid tissues; see s. of contiguity, and s. of continuity.

    **acetic s.,** a vinegar.

    **alcoholic s.,** a tincture.

    **aniline-water s.,** Koch-Ehrlich *stain.*

**Benedict's s.,** see Benedict's test for glucose in the urine.

**Bouin's s.,** Bouin's *fluid.*

**buffer salts s.,** a s. of buffer salts given by injection for the relief of either acidosis or alkalosis.

**centinor'mal s.,** see centinormal.

**chemical s.,** solution (1).

**colloid s.,** a dispersoid, emulsoid or suspensoid.

**s. of contiguity,** the breaking of contiguity; a dislocation or displacement of two normally contiguous parts.

**s. of continuity,** dieresis; division of bones or soft parts that are normally continuous, as by a fracture, a laceration, or an incision.

**decanormal s.,** see decanormal.

**decinormal s.,** see decinormal.

**disclosing s.,** a s. that selectively stains the mucinous plaque that adheres to the tooth surface.

**Earle's s.,** a tissue culture medium; contains $CaCl_2$, $MgSO_4$, KCl, $NaHCO_3$, NaCl, $NaH_2PO_4 \cdot H_2O$, and glucose.

**ethereal s.,** a s. of any substance in ether.

**Fehling's s.,** used for detection of reducing sugars; (*a*) crystallized copper sulfate 40, distilled water 160; (*b*) sodium hydroxide 130, neutral potassium tartrate 160, distilled water 600; mix the two s.'s at the time of using. Glucose 50 mg will reduce 10 ml. of the solution, giving a precipitate of cuprous oxide.

**Flemming's s.,** Flemming's *fluid.*

**Fonio's s.,** a diluent used for stained smears of blood platelets: magnesium sulfate 14 gm., water to make 100 cc.

**Gabbet's s.,** Gabbet's *stain.*

**Gey's s.,** a salt s. usually used in combination with naturally occurring body substances (*e.g.,* blood serum, tissue extracts) and/or more complex chemically defined nutritive s.'s for culturing animal cells.

**Golgi's osmiobichromate s.,** 1 per cent osmic acid s. 2 parts, 8 per cent potassium bichromate s. 1 part.

**Hanks' s.,** a salt s. usually used in combination with naturally occurring body substances (*e.g.,* blood serum, tissue extracts) and/or more complex chemically defined nutritive s.'s for culturing animal cells; two variations contain $CaCl_2$, $MgSO_4 \cdot 7H_2O$, KCl, $KH_2PO_4$, $NaHCO_3$, NaCl, $NaH_2PO_4 \cdot 2H_2O$, and glucose.

**Hartman's s.,** a s. used to desensitize dentin in dental operations; contains thymol, ethyl alcohol, and sulfuric ether.

**Hayem's s.,** composed of mercuric chloride 0.5, sodium chloride 1, sodium sulfate 5, distilled water 200; it is used for diluting blood prior to counting the red blood cells.

**hemoglobin Ringer s.,** a s. of hemoglobin in Ringer's s.; used in animal experiments during World War II, with a view to its possible use as a blood substitute for transfusion purposes.

**Hucker-Conn s.,** 20 ml. of 10 per cent alcoholic crystal violet mixed with 80 ml. of 1 per cent aqueous ammonium oxalate; used in the Gram stain.

**hyperbaric s.,** a s. with specific gravity greater than that of spinal fluid.

**hypertonic salt s.,** a s. of sodium chloride having a greater osmotic pressure than that of the blood.

**hypobaric s.,** see hypobaric.

**hypotonic salt s.,** one having an osmotic pressure less than that of blood (less than that of 0.154 M NaCl).

**isobaric s.,** a s. having the same specific gravity as spinal fluid.

**isotonic sodium chloride s.,** physiologic salt s.; one having a concentration of 0.154 M NaCl or equivalent, equal in osmotic pressure to that of plasma.

**Krebs-Ringer s.,** a modification of Ringer's s., prepared by mixing 100 parts by volume of 0.154 M NaCl, 4 parts of 0.154 M KCl, 3 parts of 0.11 M $CaCl_3$, 1 part of 0.154 M $MgSO_4$, and 21 parts of 0.16 M phosphate buffer, pH 7.4.

**Kronecker's s.,** a 5 per cent sodium chloride s. rendered faintly alkaline with sodium carbonate, for use in the examination of fresh tissues under the microscope.

**lactated Ringer's s.,** 600 mg. of sodium chloride, 310 mg. of sodium lactate, 20 mg. of calcium chloride (dihydrate), and 30 mg. of potassium chloride in each 100 ml. of distilled water; used for the same purposes as Ringer's s.

**Lange's s.,** colloidal gold s.: to 500 ml. of hot distilled water add 5 ml. of a 1 per cent solution of gold chloride and 5 ml. of a 2 per cent solution of potassium carbonate,

and then heat rapidly to the boiling point; then add 5 ml. of a 1 per cent dilution of formalin and shake until the s. is of a clear red color.

**Locke's s.'s,** s.'s containing, in varying amounts, sodium chloride, calcium chloride, potassium chloride, sodium bicarbonate, glucose, and distilled water; used for irrigating mammalian heart and other tissues, in laboratory experiments; also used in combination with naturally occurring body substances (*e.g.,* blood serum, tissue extracts) and/or more complex chemically defined nutritive s.'s for culturing animal cells.

**Locke-Ringer s.,** sodium chloride 9 gm., calcium chloride 0.24 gm., potassium chloride 0.42 gm., magnesium chloride 0.2 gm., sodium bicarbonate 0.5 gm., glucose 0.5 gm., and water to make 1000 ml.; used in the laboratory for physiological and pharmacological experiments.

**Loeffler's caustic s.,** an aqueous s. of tannin and ferrous sulfate with the addition of an alcoholic fuchsin s.; used to stain flagella.

**millinormal s.,** see millinormal.

**molal s.,** see molal.

**molar s.,** see molar (4).

**molecular dispersed s.,** dispersoid.

**normal s.,** see normal (3).

**ophthalmic s.'s,** sterile s.'s, free from foreign particles and suitably compounded and dispensed for instillation into the eye; the inherent toxicity of the drug itself, the osmotic pressure, the need for buffering agents, a preservative, and sterilization must be taken into consideration.

**physiologic salt s.,** isotonic sodium chloride s.

**Purdy's s.,** a modified Fehling's s., consisting of copper sulfate 4.752, potassium hydroxide 23.5, stronger ammonia water 350, glycerol 38, distilled water to make 1000.

**Ringer's s.'s,** (1) (NF) a s. resembling the blood serum in its salt constituents; it contains sodium chloride 8.6 gm., potassium chloride 0.3 gm., and calcium chloride 0.33 gm. in each 1000 ml. of distilled water; used topically for burns and wounds; (2), a salt s. usually used in combination with naturally occurring body substances (*e.g.,* blood serum, tissue extracts) and/or more complex chemically defined nutritive s.'s for culturing animal cells; (3) see Ringer's *injections.*

**saline s.,** (1) salt s.; a s. of any salt; (2) specifically, isotonic sodium chloride s. (usually called "saline").

**salt s.,** saline s. (1).

**saturated s.,** one that contains all of a substance capable of dissolving; a solution of a substance in equilibrium with excess, undissolved substance.

**seminormal s.,** see seminormal.

**standard s., standardized s.,** a s. of known concentration, used as a standard of comparison or analysis.

**supersaturated s.,** a s. containing more of the solid than the menstruum would ordinarily dissolve; it is made by heating the solvent when the substance is added, and on cooling the latter is retained without precipitation.

**Takayama's s.,** a s. used for the identification of blood stains; it consists of pyridine 10 per cent, s. of sodium hydrate and saturated s. of dextrose each 3, distilled water 7; a small drop of this s. added to a minute fragment of a scraping of a suspected blood stain on a clean slide will, if positive, result in the formation of hemochromogen crystals.

**test s.,** a s. of some reagent, in definite strength, used in chemical analysis or testing.

**Toison's s.,** a blood diluent and leukocyte stain; methyl violet 0.025, sodium chloride 1, sodium sulfate 8, glycerin 30, water to 200. Used for erythrocyte counts.

**Tyrode's s.,** a modified Lock's s.; it contains the chlorides of sodium 8 gm., potassium 0.2 gm., calcium 0.2 gm., magnesium 0.1 gm., sodium biphosphate 0.05 gm., sodium bicarbonate 1 gm., glucose 1 gm., and water to make 1000 ml.; used to irrigate the peritoneal cavity, and in laboratory work.

**Weigert's iodine s.,** iodine 1 part, potassium iodide 2 parts, water 100 parts.

**Ziehl's s.,** carbolic fuchsin; carbol-fuchsin; fuchsin 1, absolute alcohol 10, 5 per cent phenol solution 100; used as a stain for the tubercle bacillus.

**solv.** Abbreviation for L. *solve,* dissolve.

**solvate** (sol'vāt). A nonaqueous solution or dispersoid in which there is a noncovalent or easily reversible combination between solvent and solute, or dispersion means and disperse phase; when water is the solvent or dispersion medium, it is called a hydrate.

**solvation** (sol-va′shun). Noncovalent or easily reversible combination of a solvent with solute, or of a dispersion means with the disperse phase. If the solvent is $H_2O$, s. is called hydration. S. affects the size of ions in solution. Thus $Na^+$ is much larger in $H_2O$ than in solid NaCl.

**sol′vent** [ L. *solvens*, pres. p. of *solvo*, to dissolve ]. 1. Capable of dissolving a substance. 2. A menstruum; a liquid that holds another substance in solution, *i.e.*, dissolves it.

**amphiprotic s.,** a s. ($H_2O$ is the commonest and best example) capable of acting as an acid or a base; see solvolysis and hydrolysis.

**fat s.'s,** nonpolar s.'s; organic liquids, notable for their ability to dissolve lipids; *e.g.*, diethyl ether, carbon tetrachloride, carbon disulfide, gasoline. Usually, but not always, immiscible in water.

**nonpolar s.'s,** fat s.'s.

**polar s.'s,** s.'s (like $H_2O$, $NH_3$, HF, alcohols, and acids) that exhibit polar forces on solutes, due to high dipole moment, wide separation of charges, or tight association.

**universal s.,** a substance sought by the alchemists, and claimed by some to have been found, supposedly capable of dissolving all substances. Sometimes, in a physiological sense, applied to water.

**solvolysis** (sol-vol′ĭ-sis). The reaction of a dissolved salt with the solvent to form an acid and a base; lyolysis; the (partial) reverse of neutralization. If the solvent is $H_2O$, an amphiprotic solvent, s. is called hydrolysis.

**soma** (so′mah) [ G. *sōma*, body. SOM- ]. 1. The axial part of the body, *i.e.*, head, neck, trunk, and tail. 2. All of an organism with the exception of the germ cells.

**so′man.** Methylphosphonofluoridic acid 1,2,2-trimethylpropyl ester; an extremely potent cholinesterase inhibitor; see also sarin and tabun.

**somasthenia** (so-mas-the′nĭ-ah). Somatasthenia.

**somat-.** See somato-.

**somatagnosia** (so′mă-tag-no′sĭ-ah) [ somat- + G. *a-* priv. + *gnōsis*, recognition ]. Inability of the patient to identify parts of his own body and parts of the observer's body.

**somatalgia** (so′mă-tal′jĭ-ah) [ somat- + G. *algos*, pain ]. 1. Pain in the body. 2. Pain due to organic causes, as opposed to psychalgia, or psychogenic pain.

**somatasthenia** (so′mă-tas-the′nĭ-ah) [ somat- + G. *asthenia*, weakness ]. A condition of chronic physical weakness and fatigability.

**somatesthesia** (so′mă-tes-the′zĭ-ah) [ somat- + G. *aisthēsis*, sensation ]. Bodily sensation, the consciousness of the body.

**somatesthet′ic.** Relating to somatesthesia.

**somatic** (so-mat′ik) [ G. *sōmatikos*, bodily ]. 1. Relating to the soma or trunk. 2. Relating to the wall of the body cavity; parietal. 3. Relating to the body; corporeal; physical. 4. Relating to the vegetative as distinguished from the generative, functions.

**somaticosplanchnic** (so-mat-ĭ-ko-splangk′nik) [ G. *sōmatikos*, relating to the body, + *splanchnikos*, relating to the viscera ]. Relating to the body and the viscera.

**somaticovisceral** (so-mat-ĭ-ko-vis′er-al). Somaticosplanchnic.

**so′matist.** One who considers that neuroses and psychoses are manifestations of organic disease.

**so′matiza′tion.** The conversion of anxiety into physical symptoms.

**somato-, somat-, somatico-** (so′mă-to-, so-mat′o-) [ G. *sōma*, body. SOM- ]. Combining forms meaning body.

**somatochrome** (so′mă-to-krōm) [ somato- + G. *chrōma*, color ]. Denoting the group of neurons or nerve cells in which there is an abundance of cytoplasm completely surrounding the nucleus.

**somatogenic** (so′mă-to-jen′ik) [ somato- + G. *genesis*, origin ]. Originating in the soma or body under the influence of external forces.

**so′matolib′erin.** Somatotropin-releasing factor; growth hormone-releasing factor or hormone; a decapeptide released by the hypothalamus; it induces the release of

human growth hormone (somatotropin); isolated human growth hormone deficiency is probably caused by lack of this releasing factor.

**somatology** (so′mă-tol′o-jĭ) [ somato- + G. *logos*, study ]. The science that deals with the body, including both anatomy and physiology.

**somatome** (so′mă-tōm) [ somato- + G. *tomos*, cutting. TOM- ]. 1. An instrument for cutting the trunk in embryotomy. 2. A segment of the body (metamere).

**so′matome′din.** Sulfation factor; a peptide with a molecular weight of about 4,000, synthesized in the liver and probably in the kidney; it is capable of stimulating certain anabolic processes in bone and cartilage, such as synthesis of DNA, RNA, and protein (including chondromucoprotein), and the sulfation of mucopolysaccharides; it has been detected in both serum and hard tissues; secretion and/or biological activity of s. is known to be dependent on growth hormone (somatotropin).

**somatomegaly** (so′mă-to-meg′ă-lĭ) [ somato- + G. *megas* (*megal-*), great ]. Gigantism.

**somatometry** (so′mă-tom′e-trĭ) [ somato- + G. *metron*, measure ]. The classification of persons according to body form, and relation of the types to physiologic and psychologic characteristics.

**somatopagus** (so′mă-top′ă-gus) [ somato- + G. *pagos*, something fixed ]. Conjoined twins united in their body regions.

**somatopathic** (so-mă-to-path′ik) [ somato- + G. *pathos*, suffering ]. Relating to bodily or organic illness, as distinguished from nervous (neurologic) or mental (psychologic) disorder.

**somatopathy** (so′mă-top′ă-thĭ) [ somato- + G. *pathos*, suffering ]. Disease of the body.

**somatophrenia** (so′mă-to-fre′nĭ-ah) [ somato- + G. *phrēn*, mind ]. A tendency to imagine or exaggerate body ills.

**somatoplasm** (so′mă-to-plazm, so-mat′o-) [ somato- + G. *plasma*, something formed ]. The aggregate of all the forms of specialized protoplasm entering into the composition of the body, other than germ plasm.

**somatopleural** (so′mă-to-ploor′al). Relating to the somatopleure.

**somatopleure** (so′mă-to-ploor) [ somato- + G. *pleura*, side ]. The embryonic layer formed by the association of the parietal layer of the lateral mesoderm with the ectoderm.

**somatopsychic** (so′mă-to-si′kik) [ somato- + G. *psychē*, soul ]. Relating to the body-mind relationship; the study of the effects of the body upon the mind.

**somatopsychosis** (so′mă-to-si-ko′sis) [ somato- + G. *psychōsis*, an animating ]. An emotional disorder associated with an organic disease.

**somatoscopy** (so′mă-tos′ko-pĭ) [ somato- + G. *skopeō*, to view ]. Examination of the body.

**so′matosex′ual.** Denoting the somatic aspects of sexuality and distinguishing them from its psychosexual aspects.

**so′matostatin.** Somatotropin release-inhibiting factor; a tetradecapeptide capable of inhibiting the release of growth hormone (somatotropin) by the anterior lobe of the pituitary gland.

**so′matother′apy.** 1. Therapy directed at bodily or physical disorders. 2. In psychiatry, a variety of therapeutic interventions employing chemical or physical (as opposed to psychological) methods.

**somatotonia** (so′mă-to′nĭ-ah) [ somato- + G. *tonos*, tension ]. Term for a personality type characterized by vigorous activity and assertiveness.

**somatotroph** (so′mă-to-trof). A cell of the adenohypophysis that produces somatotropin (growth hormone).

**somatotrophic** (so′mă-to-trof′ik) [ somato- + G. *trophē*, nourishment ]. Somatotropic.

**somatotropic** (so′mă-to-trop′ik) [ somato- + G. *tropē*, a turning ]. Somatotrophic; having a stimulating effect on body growth.

**somatotropin** (so′mă-to-tro′pin). Growth hormone; somatotropic hormone; pituitary growth hormone; a protein hormone of the anterior lobe of the pituitary, produced by the acidophil cells; it promotes body growth, fat mobilization, and inhibition of glucose utilization; diabetogenic when present in excess.

**so'matotype.** 1. The constitutional or body type of an individual. 2. The particular constitutional or body type associated with a particular personality type.

**somatotypology** (so'mă-to-ti-pol'o-jĭ) [ somato- + G. *typos*, form, + *logos*, study ]. The study of somatotypes.

**somesthesia** (so'mes-the'zĭ-ah). Somatesthesia.

**somite** (so'mĭt) [ G. *sōma*, body, + suffix *-ite, q. v.* ]. Mesoblastic segment; one of the paired, metamerically arranged cell masses formed in the early embryonic paraxial mesoderm. Commencing in the third or early fourth week in the region of the hindbrain, they develop in a caudal direction until 42 pairs are formed. Their presence is considered to provide evidence that metameric segmentation is a vertebrate characteristic.

  **occipital s.,** one of the four most rostral s.'s which become incorporated into the occipital region of the embryonic skull.

**somnam'bulance.** Somnambulism.

**somnambulism** (som-nam'bu-lizm) [ L. *somnus,* sleep, + *ambulo,* to walk ]. 1. Sleepwalking; somnambulance; hypnobatia; oneirodynia activa; a disorder of sleep, involving complex motor acts, that occurs primarily during the first third of the night but not during rapid eye movement sleep. 2. A form of hysteria in which purposeful behavior is forgotten.

**somnam'bulist.** Sleepwalker; hypnobat; one who is subject to somnambulism.

**somnifacient** (som'nĭ-fa'shent) [ L. *somnus,* sleep, + *facio,* to make ]. Soporific.

**somniferous** (som-nif'er-us) [ L. *somnus,* sleep, + *fero,* to bring ]. Soporific (1).

**somnif'ic.** Soporific (1).

**somnifugous** (som-nif'u-gus) [ L. *somnus,* sleep, + *fugo,* to put to flight ]. Dispelling sleep.

**somniloquence, somniloquism** (som-nil'o-kwens, som-nil'o-kwizm) [ L. *somnus,* sleep, + *loquor,* to talk ]. 1. Talking in one's sleep. 2. Somniloquy.

**somniloquist** (som-nil'o-kwist). A habitual sleep-talker.

**somniloquy** (som-nil'o-kwĭ) [ L. *somnus,* sleep, + *loquor,* to speak ]. Talking under the influence of hypnotic suggestion.

**somnip'athist.** One affected by or under the influence of somnipathy.

**somnipathy** (som-nip'ă-thĭ) [ L. *somnus,* sleep, + G. *pathos,* suffering ]. 1. Any disorder of sleep. 2. Hypnotism.

**somnocinematograph** (som'no-sin'e-mat'o-graf) [ L. *somnos,* sleep, + G. *kinēma,* motion, + G. *graphō,* to write ]. Somnokinematograph; hypnokinematograph; a device for recording the movements made by sleepers.

**somnokinematograph** (som'no-kin'e-mat'o-graf). Somnocinematograph.

**som'nolence, som'nolency** [ L. *somnolentia* ]. 1. Drowsiness; sleepiness. 2. A condition of semiconsciousness approaching coma.

**som'nolent** [ L. *somnus,* sleep ]. 1. Sleepy; drowsy; having an inclination to sleep. 2. In a condition of incomplete sleep; semicomatose.

**somnolentia** (som-no-len'shĭi-ah) [ L. ]. 1. Somnolence. 2. Sleep *drunkenness.*

**somnolescent** (som-no-les'ent). Inclined to sleep; drowsy.

**som'nolism.** Hypnotism.

**som'nus** [ L. ]. Sleep.

**Somogyi,** Michael, American biochemist, *1883. See S. *effect,* S.-Shaffer-Hartman *method,* S. *unit.*

**sone** (sōn) [ L. *sonus,* sound ]. A unit of loudness; a pure tone of 1000 c.p.s. at 40 db. above normal threshold of audibility has a loudness of 1 sone.

**sonic** (son'ik) [ L. *sonus,* sound ]. Of, pertaining to, or determined by sound; *e.g.,* s. *vibration* or s. *boom.*

**Sonne** (sun'eh), Carl, Danish bacteriologist, 1882–1948. See S. *bacillus.*

**son'ochemistry.** The branch of chemistry that treats of chemical changes caused by, or involving, sound, particularly ultrasound.

**sonomo'tor.** See sonomotor *response.*

**sontoquine** (son'to-kwēn, -kwĭn). SONTOCHIN; 7-chloro-4-(4-diethylamino-1-methylbutylamino)-3-methylquinoline; a congener of chloroquine used in the treatment of malaria; it is not as well tolerated as chloroquine.

**sophisticate** (so-fis'tĭ-kāt) [ Mod. L. *sophisticare,* pp. *sophisticatus,* to alter deceptively, fr. G. *sophistikos,* deceitful ]. To adulterate.

**sophomania** (sof'o-ma'nĭ-ah) [ G. *sophos,* wise, + *mania,* insanity ]. An exaggerated opinion of one's own intelligence.

**Sophora** (so-fōr'ah) [ Mod. L. fr. Ar. ]. A genus of plants of the family Leguminosae.

  **S. japonica,** Chinese scholar or pagoda tree; the flower buds yield several times as much rutin as buckwheat.

  **S. secundiflo'ra,** coral bean, a Texas species containing sophorine.

**sophor'icoside.** Genistein 4'-glucoside.

**soph'orine.** An amorphous alkaloid from *Sophora secundiflora* and other species of *Sophora;* see also ulexine.

**so'pient** [ L. pres. act. part. of *sopire,* to lull to sleep ]. Soporific.

**so'por** [ L. ]. Stupor; an unnaturally deep sleep.

**soporif'erous** (so'pōr-if'er-us, sop'ōr-) [ L. *soporifer,* fr. *sopor,* deep sleep, + *fero,* to bring ]. Soporific (1).

**soporific** (so'pōr-if'ik, sop'ōr-) [ L. *sopor,* deep sleep, + *facio,* to make ]. 1. Somnifacient, somniferous; somnific; soporiferous; hypnotic; causing sleep. 2. An agent that produces sleep.

**so'porose, so'porous** [ L. *sopor,* deep sleep ]. Relating to or causing sopor; comatose; stuporous.

**Sora'nus** of Ephesus, Roman physician, 2nd century A.D. Wrote works on gynecology, obstetrics, and pediatrics which were the authorities on these subjects for more than fifteen centuries.

**sorbefacient** (sor'be-fa'shent) [ L. *sorbeo,* to suck up, + *facio,* to make ]. 1. Causing absorption. 2. An agent that causes or facilitates absorption.

**sor'bic acid** (NF). 2,4-Hexadienoic acid; obtained from berries of the mountain ash, *Pyrus Sorbus aucuparia* (family Rosaceae), or prepared synthetically; it inhibits growth of yeast and mold and is nearly nontoxic to humans; used as a preservative.

**sor'binose.** D-Sorbose.

**sor'bitan.** Sorbitol or sorbose and related compounds in ester combination with fatty acids (to form Span detergents) and polyoxyethylenes (to form Tween detergents, *e.g.,* polysorbate 80).

**sor'bite.** Sorbitol.

**sor'bitol** (USP, BP). D-Sorbitol; D-glucitol; L-gulitol; sorbite; reduction product of glucose found in the berries of the mountain ash, *Sorbus aucuparia* (family Rosaceae), and in many fruits and seaweeds. It has many industrial and pharmaceutical uses; medicinally, it is used as a diuretic and as a sweetening agent. It is almost completely metabolized to $CO_2$).

**sorbitol dehydrogenase.** Ketose reductase.

**D-sorbitol-6-phosphate dehydrogenase.** Ketose reductase.

**sor'bitose.** D-Sorbose.

**D-sor'bose.** Sorbitose; sorbin; sorbinose; a very sweet reducing but not fermentable 2-ketohexose obtained from the berries of the mountain ash, *Sorbus aucuparia* (family Rosaceae), and from sorbitol by fermentation with *Acetobacter suboxydans.* It is isomeric with fructose (see structures under sugars). Used in manufacture of vitamin C.

**sordes** (sor'dēz) [ L. fifth, fr. *sordeo,* to be foul ]. Rhyparia; a dark brown or blackish crustlike collection on the lips, teeth, and gums of a person with dehydration in chronic debilitating disease.

**sore** (sōr) [ A.S. *sār* ]. 1. A wound, ulcer, or any open skin lesion. 2. Painful.

  **bed s.,** decubitus *ulcer.*

  **canker s.'s,** ulcerative *stomatitis.*

  **cold s.,** colloquialism for *herpes* simplex.

  **desert s.,** Barcoo rot; veldt s.; any of a variety of chronic, nonspecific cutaneous ulcers, probably pyogenic, that occur in tropical desert areas.

  **fungating s.,** a granulating chancroid.

**hard s.,** chancre.

**Oriental s.,** the dermal lesion of cutaneous leishmaniasis, *q.v.*

**pressure s.,** decubitus *ulcer.*

**recurrent canker s.'s,** recurrent ulcerative *stomatitis.*

**soft s.,** chancroid.

**summer s.'s.,** cutaneous *habronemiasis.*

**tropical s.,** Oriental s.; see cutaneous *leishmaniasis.*

**veldt s.,** desert s.

**venereal s.,** chancroid.

**water s.,** cutaneous *ancylostomiasis.*

**sore′head.** Filarial *dermatosis.*

**sore′mouth.** Contagious *ecthyma.*

**soremuzzle** (sōr′muz-ul). Bluetongue.

**Sorenson scale.** See under scale.

**Soret** (so-ra′), C., French radiologist, †1931. See S.'s *band, phenomenon.*

**sororiation** (so-ror′ĭ-a′shun) [ L. *sororio,* to increase in size together (said of the female breasts), fr. *soror,* sister ]. Obsolete term meaning growth of the breasts at puberty.

**sorption** (sorp′shun). Adsorption or absorption.

**Sorsby,** A. See S.'s macular *degeneration.*

**S.O.S.** Abbreviation of *si opus sit,* if necessary, if occasion requires. Appears on written orders, *e.g.,* from physician to nurse.

**so′talol hydrochloride** (USAN). 4′-[ 1-Hydroxy-2-(iso-propylamino)ethyl ]methanesulfonanilide monohydrochloride; a β-receptor blocking agent for the treatment of cardiac arrhythmias.

**Sottas,** J., French neurologist, 1866–1943. See Déjérine-S. *disease.*

**souffle** (soo′fl) [ Fr. *souffler,* to blow ]. A soft blowing sound heard on ausculation.

**cardiac s.,** a soft puffing heart murmur.

**fetal s., funic s., funicular s.,** a blowing murmur, synchronous with the fetal heart beat, sometimes only systolic and sometimes continuous, heard on ausculation over the pregnant uterus.

**mammary s.,** a blowing murmur heard late in pregnancy and during lacatation at the medial border of the breast, sometimes only systolic and sometimes continuous.

**placental s.,** uterine s.

**umbil′ical s.,** fetal s.

**u′terine s.,** a blowing sound, synchronous with the cardiac systole of the mother, heard on auscultation of the pregnant uterus.

**souma** (soo′mah). A nagana-like trypanosomiasis of horses in West Africa and the Sudan; the pathogenic agent is *Trypanosoma vivax.*

**sound.** 1. Noise; the vibrations produced by a sounding body, transmitted by the air or other medium, and perceived by the internal ear. 2. An elongated, cylindrical, usually curved instrument of metal, used for exploring the bladder or other cavities of the body or for dilating strictures in the urethra or other canal. 3. To explore a cavity by means of a s. 4. Whole; healthy; not diseased or injured.

**after-s.,** see aftersound.

**amphoric voice s.,** see amphoric *voice.*

**anvil s.,** bellmetal *resonance.*

**atrial s.,** fourth heart s.; see cardiac s.

**auscul′tatory s.,** a rale, murmur, bruit, fremitus, or other s. heard on auscultation of the chest or abdomen.

**bell s.,** bellmetal *resonance.*

**Belloc's s.,** Belloc's *cannula.*

**Béniqué's s.,** a s. of lead or block tin of wide curve used to dilate strictures in the male urethra.

**cannon s.,** *bruit de canon.*

**cardiac s., heart s.,** one of the s.'s heard on auscultation over the region of the heart; the **first heart s.,** occurs with ventricular systole and is mainly produced by closure of the atrioventricular valves; the **second heart s.** signifies the beginning of diastole and is due to closure of the semilunar valves; the **third heart s.** occurs in early diastole and corresponds with the first phase of rapid ventricular filling; the **fourth heart s.** occurs in late diastole and corresponds with atrial contraction and is rarely audible in normal hearts.

**cavernous voice s.,** the hollow or metallic voice s. heard over a pulmonary cavity.

**coconut s.,** a s. like that produced when a cracked coconut is tapped; it is elicited by percussing the skull of a patient with osteitis deformans (Paget's disease).

**cracked-pot s.,** see under resonance.

**double-shock s.,** *bruit de rappel.*

**eddy s.'s,** s.'s that punctuate the continuous murmur of patent ductus arteriosus, imparting to it a characteristically "uneven" quality.

**ejection s.,** a sharp s. heard in early systole over the aortic or pulmonic area when the aorta or pulmonary artery is dilated.

**friction s.,** the s., heard on auscultation, made by the rubbing of two opposed serous surfaces roughened by an inflammatory exudate.

**gallop s.,** the abnormal third or fourth heart s. which, when added to the first and second s.'s, produces the triple cadence of gallop rhythm; see also gallop (2).

**Hippocratic succussion s.,** a splashing s. elicited by shaking a patient with hydro- or pyopneumothorax, the physician's ear being applied to the chest.

**infrasonic s.'s,** s.'s whose frequencies lie below the human range of hearing.

**intensity of s.,** the objective measurement of the amplitude of vibration of a sound wave.

**Korotkoff s.'s,** the s.'s heard over an artery when blood pressure is determined by the auscultatory method.

**Mercier's s.,** a catheter the beak of which is short and bent almost at a right angle.

**muscle s.,** a fine murmur heard on auscultation over the belly of a contracting muscle.

**percussion s.,** any s. elicited on percussing over one of the cavities of the body.

**pericardial friction s.,** a to-and-fro creaking s. heard over the heart in some cases of pericarditis, due to rubbing of the inflamed pericardial surfaces as the heart contracts and relaxes; pericardial friction rub.

**pistol-shot femoral s.,** a shotlike systolic s. heard over the femoral artery in high output states, especially aortic insufficiency, and presumably due to sudden stretching of the elastic wall of the artery.

**posttussis suction s.,** a s. produced by the falling back of a drop of mucus or pus into a pulmonary cavity after the latter has been emptied by coughing.

**respiratory s.,** a murmur, bruit, fremitus, or rale heard on auscultation over the lungs or any part of the respiratory tract.

**Santini's booming s.,** a sonorous booming s. heard on auscultatory percussion of a hydatid cyst.

**sail s.,** a s., likened to the snapping of a sail, heard in early systole in some patients with Ebstein's anomaly.

**tambour s.,** a heart s., usually the aortic or pulmonic valve closure s. when it has a booming and ringing quality like that of a tambour or drum; the aortic s. commonly has a tambour quality in systemic hypertension, the pulmonary s. in pulmonary hypertension.

**tic-tac s.'s,** see embryocardia.

**water-whistle s.,** a bubbling whistle heard on auscultation over a bronchial or pulmonary fistula.

**Winternitz' s.,** a double-current catheter in which water at any desired temperature circulates.

**xiphisternal crunching s.,** see Hamman's *sign.*

**Southey,** Reginald S., English physician, 1835–1899. See S.'s *tubes.*

**sow** [ M.E. ]. A female hog of breeding age.

**soya** (soy′ah) [ Hind. *soyā,* fennel ]. Soybean.

**soybean** (soy′bēn) [ Hind. *soyā,* fennel ]. Chinese pea; soya; soja; the bean of the climbing herb *Glycine soja* or *G. hispida* (family Leguminosae); a bean rich in protein and containing little starch; it is the source of soybean oil. Soybean flour is used in preparing a bread for diabetics, in feeding formulas for infants who are unable to tolerate cow's milk, and for adults allergic to cow's milk.

**s. oil,** obtained from soybeans by expression or solvent extraction; contains triglycerides of linoleic acid, oleic acid, linolenic acid, and saturated fatty acids; used as a food and in the manufacture of margarine and other food products; also has many industrial uses.

**so′zin** [ G. *sōzō*, to preserve ]. Complement or alexin; an old term for protective substances normally present in blood serum.

**sp.** Abbreviation of L. *spiritus*, spirit.

**spa** (spah) [ *Spa*, a mineral spring health resort in Belgium ]. A health resort where there are one or more mineral springs the waters of which possess therapeutic properties. These waters are classified as: (1) alkaline (sulfated, borated, or muriated); (2) alkaline-saline (sulfated, borrated, or muriated); (3) saline (sulfated or muriated); (4) acid (sulfated, muriated, or silicious); (5) neutral or indifferent.

# SPACE

**space** (spās) [ L. *spatium*, room, space ]. Spatium (*q. v.*); any demarcated portion of the body, either an area of the surface, a segment of the tissues, or a cavity; see also area, region, zone.

**anatomical dead s.,** the part of the respiratory tract possessing relatively thick walls, *i.e.*, from the nostrils to the terminal bronchioles, between which and the blood no interchange of oxygen and carbon dioxide can take place; *cf.* physiologic dead s.

**antecubital s.,** *fossa* cubitalis.

**apical s.,** the s. between the alveolar wall and the apex of the root of a tooth where an alveolar abscess usually has its origin.

**axillary s.,** axilla.

**Bogros' s.,** *spatium* retroinguinale.

**Böttcher's.,** *saccus* endolymphaticus.

**Burns' s.,** suprasternal s.

**capsular s.,** filtration s.; the slitlike s. between the visceral and parietal layers of the capsule of the renal corpuscle; it opens into the proximal tubule of the nephron at the neck of the tubule.

**car′tilage s.,** cartilage *lacuna*.

**Chassaignac's s.,** s. between the pectoralis major and the mammary gland.

**Cloquet's s.,** a s. between the zonula ciliaris and the vitreous body.

**Colles' s.,** *spatium* perinei superficiale.

**corneal s.,** lacuna (4); one of the stellate s.'s in interstitial cement substance connecting the lamellae of the cornea, each of which contains a cell or corneal corpuscle.

**Cotunnius' s.,** *saccus* endolymphaticus.

**dead s.,** (1) a cavity remaining after the closure of a wound which is not obliterated by the pressure of the dressings; (2) see anatomical dead s. and physiologic dead s.

**deep perineal s.,** *spatium* perinei profundum.

**denture s.,** (1) that portion of the oral cavity which is, or may be, occupied by maxillary and/or mandibular denture(s); (2) the s. between the residual ridges which is available for dentures; see also interarch *distance*.

**Disse's s.,** perisinusoidal s.

**s. of Donders,** the space between the dorsum of the tongue and the hard palate when the mandible is in rest position following the expiratory cycle of respiration.

**epidu′ral s.,** *cavum* epidurale.

**episcleral s.,** *spatium* episclerale.

**epitympan′ic s.,** *recessus* epitympanicus.

**Faraday s.,** a dark s. between the positive column and the negative glow when a current is passed through a partially exhausted tube.

**filtration s.,** capsular s.

**Fontana's s.'s,** *spatia* anguli iridocornealis.

**free-way s.,** interocclusal *distance*.

**gingival s.,** gingival *sulcus*.

**H s.,** retrocardiac s.; prevertebral s.; the central of three clear lung fields in an x-ray picture of the chest, when the rays are projected from the left posteriorly to the right anteriorly.

**Haversian s.'s,** s.'s in bone formed by the enlargement of Haversian canals.

**Henke's s.,** a s., filled with connective tissue, between the vertebral column and the pharynx and esophagus.

**His' s.'s,** the perivascular s.'s in the pia mater.

**interalveolar s.,** interarch *distance*.

**intercos′tal s.,** *spatium* intercostale.

**interfascial s.,** *spatium* episclerale.

**interglob′ular s.,** *spatium* interglobulare.

**interglobular s. of Owen,** *spatium* interglobulare.

**interocclusal rest s.,** interocclusal *distance*.

**interpleu′ral s.,** mediastinum.

**interprox′imal s.,** the s. between adjacent teeth in a dental arch; it is divided into the embrasure occlusal to the contact point and the septal s. gingival to the contact point.

**interradicular s.,** the s. between the roots of multirooted teeth.

**interseptovalvular s.,** the interval in the developing embryonic heart between the septum primum and the left valve of the sinus venosus.

**intersheath s.'s of optic nerve,** *spatia* intervaginalia nervi optici.

**intervillous s.'s,** the s.'s between placental villi containing maternal blood.

**intraretinal s.,** the potential cleft between the pigmented and nervous layers of the retina; it represents the cavity of the embryonic optic vesicle.

**s.'s of iridocorneal angle,** *spatia* anguli iridocornealis.

**Kiernan's s.,** interlobular s. in the liver.

**Kretschmann's s.,** a slight depression in the epitympanic recess below the recessus membranae tympani superior.

**Kuhnt's s.'s,** shallow diverticula or recesses between the ciliary bodies of the posterior chamber of the eye.

**lymph s.,** a s., in tissue or a vessel, filled with lymph.

**Magendie's s.'s,** s.'s between the pia and arachnoid at the level of the fissures of the brain.

**Malacarne's s.,** *substantia* perforata posterior.

**Meckel's s.,** *cavum* trigeminale.

**medias′tinal s.,** mediastinum.

**medullary s.,** the central cavity and the cellular intervals between the trabeculae of bone, filled with marrow.

**Mohrenheim's s.,** Mohrenheim's *fossa*.

**Nuel's s.,** an interval in the spiral organ (of Corti) between the outer pillar cells on one side and the phalangeal cells and hair cells on the other.

**palmar s.,** one of fascial s.'s in the palm; one, toward the ulnar side is called the middle palmar s., the other toward the radial side is called the thenar s.

**parapharyngeal s.,** pharyngomaxillary s.

**Parona's s.,** a s. between the deep muscles of the forearm.

**perforated s.,** *substantia* perforata.

**perichoroid s.,** *spatium* perichoroideale.

**perilymphatic s.,** *spatium* perilymphaticum.

**perineal s.'s,** see *spatium* perinei profundum and *spatium* perinei superficiale.

**perinuclear s.,** the s. between the two membranes of the nuclear envelope as seen with the electron microscope.

**periportal s. of Mall,** a tissue s. between the limiting lamina and the portal canal in the liver.

**perisinusoidal s.,** Disse's s.; the potential extravascular s. between the liver sinusoids and liver cells.

**perivitelline s.,** the s. between the vitelline membrane and the zona pellucida, appearing in an ovum immediately following fertilization.

**pharyngeal s.,** the area occupied by the pharynx (naso-, oro-, and laryngopharynx). Not to be confused with the retropharyngeal s.

**pharyngomaxillary s.,** parapharyngeal s.; the s. limited by the lateral wall of the pharynx, the cervical vertebrae, and the musculus pterygoideus medialis.

**physiologic dead s.,** symbol $V_D$; the dead s. calculated when the carbon dioxide pressure in systemic arterial blood is used instead of that of alveolar gas in Bohr's equation; it is a virtual or apparent volume that takes into account the impairment of gas exchange because of uneven distributions of lung ventilation and perfusion.

**plantar s.,** one of four areas between fascial layers in the foot, where pus may be confined when the foot is infected.

**pleural s.,** *cavum* plurae.

**pneumatic s.,** any one of the paranasal sinuses.

**Poiseuille's s.,** still *layer*.

**poplit′eal s.,** *fossa* poplitea.

**postpharyngeal s.,** retropharyngeal s.

**Proust's s.,** *excavatio* rectovesicalis.

**Prussak's s.,** *recessus* membranae tympani superior.

**pterygomandibular s.,** the area between the ramus mandibulae and the processus pterygoideus ossi sphenoidalis.

**retroin'guinal s.,** *spatium* retroinguinale.

**retromylohyoid s.,** the sulcus at the posterior end of the mylohyoid ridge.

**retroperitone'al s.,** *spatium* retroperitoneale.

**retropharyn'geal s.,** the s. posterior to the pharynx, filled with loose areolar tissue.

**retropubic s.,** *spatium* retropubicum.

**Retzius' s.,** *spatium* retropubicum.

**Schwalbe's s.'s,** *spatia* intervaginalia nervi optici.

**subarach'noid s.,** *cavum* subarachnoidale.

**subchorial s.,** subchorial lake; the part of the placenta adjacently beneath the chorion.

**subdu'ral s.,** subdural cavity; cavum subdurale; the very narrow interval between the dura mater and the arachnoid. It contains only sufficient fluid to moisten the opposing surfaces of the two membranes.

**subgin'gival s.,** the s. between a tooth and the free margin of the gums; sulcus.

**suprahepatic s.'s,** *recessus* subphrenici.

**supraster'nal s.,** Burn's s.; narrow interval between the deep and superficial layers of the cervical fascia above the manubrium sterni through which pass the anterior jugular veins.

**Tarin's s.,** that part of the basal subarachnoid cistern that lies between the left and right cerebral peduncles.

**Tenon's s.,** *spatium* episclerale.

**the'nar s.,** see palmar s.

**Traube's s.,** a semilunar s. about 12 cm. wide, bounded medially by the left border of the sternum, above by an oblique line from the sixth costal cartilage to the lower border of the eighth or ninth rib, and below by the costal margin; the percussion note here is normally tympanitic, because of the underlying stomach, but is modified by pulmonary emphysema or a pleural effusion.

**Trautmann's triangular s.,** area bounded by the sinus sigmoideus, the sinus petrosus inferior, and the seventh cranial nerve.

**Virchow-Robin s.,** a tunnel-like extension of the subarachnoid s. surrounding blood vessels that pass into the brain or spinal cord from the subarachnoid s.; the lining of the channel is composed of pia and glial feet of astrocytes; a continuation of the s. around capillaries and nerve cells probably does not occur.

**Westberg's s.,** the s. surrounding the origin of the aorta which is invested with the pericardium.

**zon'ular s.'s,** *spatia* zonularia.

---

**spade.** Spay.

**spagiric** (spä-jīr'ik) [ G. *spao̅*, to tear open, + *ageiro*, to collect ]. Relating to the Paracelsian or alchemical system of medicine.

**spagirist** (spaj'ī-rist). A physician of the 16th century, a follower of the teachings of Paracelsus who believed in the essential importance of chemical or alchemical knowledge in the understanding and treatment of disease.

**Spallanzani,** Lazaro, Italian priest and scientist, 1729–1799. See S.'s *law.*

**spallation** (spaw-la'shun) [ M.E. *spalle*, fragment ]. A nuclear reaction in which nuclei, on being bombarded by high energy particles, liberate a number of protons and alpha particles with the final nucleus possessing a mass number 10 to 20 less than the original.

**span.** The amount, distance, or length between two points; the full extent or reach of anything.

**memory s.,** the maximum number of items recalled after a single presentation, whether presented in an auditory or visual manner.

**Span'nungs-P.** Prominent prolonged and high voltage P waves recorded in electrocardiograms of patients with hypertrophy of both atria, particularly in those with congenital heart disease; see also P-congenitale.

**spanomenorrhea** (span'o-men-o-re'ah) [ G. *spanos*, rare, + *me̅n*, month, + *rhoia*, flow ]. Scanty menstruation.

**sparer** (spär'er). A substance capable of exerting a sparing action (see under action).

**sparganoma** (spar-gă-no'mah). A localized mass resulting from sparganosis.

**sparganosis** (spar-gă-no'sis). Infection with the plerocercoid or sparganum of a pseudophyllidean tapeworm.

**ocular s.,** infestation of the orbits with the sparganum of *Spirometra mansoni;* characterized by redness and edema of the eyelids, lacrimation, and ptosis; caused by application of infected raw frog flesh against the eye as a poultice.

**Sparganum** (spar'gă-num) [ G. *sparganon*, a swathing band, fr. *spargo*, to swathe ]. The plerocercoid larva of pseudophyllid tapeworms of the genus *Spirometra* that develop in the flesh of aquatic animals (fish, amphibians, reptiles, and amphibious mammals) as a result of ingesting infected water fleas (minute aquatic Crustacea) such as *Cyclops* or *Diaptomus*, or other vertebrates harboring the sparganum; originally described as a genus, now restricted to the plerocercoid form of the worm. See *Spirometra mansoni.*

**spargo'sis** [ G. fr. *spargao̅*, to be full to bursting ]. 1. Distention of the breasts with milk. 2. Swelling or thickening of the skin.

**sparteine** (spar'te-ēn, -te-in). *l*-Sparteine; lupinidine; an alkaloid obtained from scoparius, *Cytisus scoparius* and *Lupinus luteus.*

**s. sulfate** (USAN), used as an oxytocic drug.

**spasm** (spazm) [ G. *spasmos.* SPA- ]. 1. An involuntary muscular contraction; if painful, usually referred to as a cramp; if violent, a convulsion. 2. Increased muscular tension and shortness which cannot be released voluntarily and which prevent lengthening of the muscles involved; s. is due to pain stimuli to the lower motor neuron.

**s. of accommodation,** excessive contraction of the ciliary muscle.

**affect s.'s,** spasmodic attacks of laughing, weeping, and screaming, accompanied by marked tachypnea.

**Bell's s.,** facial *tic.*

**cadav'eric s.,** rigor mortis occurring irregularly in the different muscles, causing movements of the limbs.

**canine s.,** *risus* caninus.

**carpopedal s.,** s. of the feet and hands observed in hyperventilation, calcium deprivation, and tetany: flexion of the hands at the wrists and of the fingers at the metacarpophalangeal joints and extension of the fingers at the phalangeal joints; the feet are dorsiflexed at the ankles and the toes plantar flexed.

**clonic s.,** alternate involuntary contraction and relaxation of a muscle.

**cynic s.,** *risus* caninus.

**dancing s.,** saltatory s.

**epidemic transient diaphragmatic s.,** epidemic *pleurodynia.*

**facial s.,** facial *tic.*

**functional s.,** an occupation neurosis, such as writer's cramp.

**habit s.,** tic.

**histrion'ic s.,** facial *tic.*

**intention s.,** a spasmodic contraction of the muscles occurring when a voluntary movement is attempted.

**masticatory s.,** involuntary convulsive muscular contraction affecting the muscles of mastication.

**milker's s.,** an occupation neurosis, occurring occasionally in milkmaids.

**mimic s.,** facial *tic.*

**mobile s.,** a tonic s. occurring in spastic infantile hemiplegia on attempted movement.

**muscle s.,** spasm (2).

**nic'titating s.,** winking s.; spasmus nictitans; involuntary spasmodic winking.

**nodding s.,** salaam s.; convulsion spasmus nutans; in adults, a psychogenic nodding of the head from clonic s.'s of the sternomastoid muscles; in babies, a similar nodding of the head from side to side.

**occupation s., professional s.,** occupation or professional *neurosis.*

**phonic s.,** *dysphonia* spastica.

**progressive torsion s. of childhood,** *dystonia* musculorum deformans.

**retrocollic s.,** retrocollis; torticollis in which the s. affects the posterior neck muscles.

**rotatory s.,** spasmodic *torticollis.*

**salaam s.,** nodding s.

**saltatory s.,** Gower's disease (1); Bamberger's disease (1); static convulsion; a spasmodic affection of the muscles of the lower extremities.

**sewing s.,** seamstress's *cramp.*

**synclon'ic s.,** clonic s. of two or more muscles.

**tailor's s.,** tailor's *cramp.*

**tonic s.,** entasis; a continuous involuntary muscular contraction.

**tonoclonic s.,** convulsive contraction of muscles.

**tooth s.'s,** infantile convulsions associated with teething.

**torsion s.,** a spasmodic twisting of the body and pelvis.

**vasomotor s.,** spasmodic contraction of the smaller arteries.

**winking s.,** nictitating s.

**spasmo-** (spaz'mo-) [ G. *spasmos,* spasm. SPA- ]. Combining form denoting spasm.

**spasmodic** (spaz-mod'ik) [ G. *spasmōdes,* convulsive, fr. *spasmos, Ā eidos,* form ]. Relating to or marked by spasm.

**spasmogen** (spaz'mo-jen). A substance causing contraction of smooth muscle; *e.g.,* histamine, bradykinin, serotonin, slow-reacting substance.

**spasmogenic** (spaz'mo-jen'ik) [ spasmo- + G. suffix *-gen,* producing ]. Causing spasms.

**spasmology** (spaz-mol'o-jī) [ spasmo- + G. *logos,* study ]. Study of the nature, causation, and means of relief of spasms.

**spasmolygmus** (spaz'mo-lig'mus) [ spasmo- + G. *lygmos,* a sobbing, hiccup, fr. *lyzō,* to hiccup, sob ]. 1. Spasmodic sobbing. 2. Spasmodic hiccup.

**spasmolysis** (spaz-mol'ī-sis) [ spasmo- + G. *lysis,* dissolution ]. The arrest of a spasm or convulsion.

**spasmolytic** (spaz'mo-lit'ik). 1. Relating to spasmolysis. 2. Antispasmodic; denoting a chemical agent that relieves smooth muscle spasms.

**spasmophemia** (spaz-mo-fe'mī-ah) [ spasmo- + G. *phēmē,* speech ]. Stuttering.

**spasmophilia** (spaz'mo-fil'ī-ah) [ spasmo- + G. *phileō,* to love ]. Spasmophilic *diathesis.*

**spasmophilic** (spaz'mo-fil'ik). Relating to spasmophilic *diathesis.*

**spasmotoxin** (spaz'mo-tok'sin). *Bacillus tetani* exotoxin.

**spasmus** (spaz'mus) [ L. fr. G. *spasmos,* spasm ]. Spasm.

**s. agi'tans,** parkinsonism (1).

**s. cani'nus,** *risus* sardonicus.

**s. coordina'tus,** compulsive movements, such as imitative or mimic tics, festination, etc.

**s. glot'tidis,** *laryngismus* stridulus.

**s. nic'titans,** nictitating *spasm.*

**s. nu'tans,** nodding *spasm.*

**spastic** (spas'tik) [ L. *spasticus,* fr. G. *spastikos,* drawing in. SPA- ]. 1. Hypertonic (1). 2. Relating to spasm or to spasticity.

**spasticity** (spas-tis'ī-tī). A state of increased muscular tone with exaggeration of the tendon reflexes.

**clasp-knife s.,** clasp-knife effect or rigidity; rigidity of the extensor muscles of a joint which thus offer resistance to passive flexion up to a point, when they give way rather suddenly allowing the joint then to be easily flexed; the rigidity is due to an exaggeration of the stretch reflex; see also lengthening reaction.

**s. of conjugate gaze,** an oblique or horizontal deviation of the eyes evoked (1) during forceable lid closure or (2) while fixating on an object 30 or 40 cm. in front, the eyelids are opened and closed at 4- to 5-second intervals; it is usually associated with a temporal lesion opposite to the direction of deviation.

**spatia** (spa'shī-ah) [ L. ]. Plural of spatium.

**spatial** (spa'shal). Relating to space or a space.

**spatium,** pl. **spatia** (spa'shī-um, -shī-ah) [ L. ] [ NA ]. A space.

**spatia an'guli iridocornea'lis** [ NA ], spaces of the iridocorneal angle; spaces of Fontana; ciliary canals; irregularly shaped endothelium-lined spaces within the trabecular meshwork.

**s. episclera'le** [ NA ], episcleral space; s. intervaginale bulbi oculi; Tenon's space; interfascial space; s. interfasciale; the space between the vagina bulbi and the sclera.

**s. intercosta'le** [ NA ], intercostal space; an interval between the ribs.

**s. interfascia'le,** s. episclerale.

**s. interglobula're, pl. spatia interglobula'ria** [ NA ], interglobular s.; interglobular s. of Owen; one of a number of irregularly branched spaces near the periphery of the dentin of the crown of a tooth, through which pass the ramifications of the tubules. They are caused by failure of calcification of the dentin.

**spatia interos'sea metacar'pi** [ NA ], the spaces between the metacarpal bones in the hand.

**spatia interos'sea metatar'si** [ NA ], the spaces between the metatarsal bones in the foot.

**s. intervagina'le bulb'i oc'uli,** s. episclerale.

**spatia intervagina'lia ner'vi op'tici** [ NA ], intersheath spaces of the optic nerve; Schwalbe's spaces; the spaces between the internal and external vaginae of the optic nerve, filled with cerebrospinal fluid and continuous with the subarachnoid space.

**s. perichoroidea'le** [ NA ], perichoroid space; the interval between the choroid and the sclera filled by the loose meshes of the lamina fusca and the lamina suprachoroidea.

**s. perilymphat'icum** [ NA ], perilymphatic space; cisterna perilymphatica; space between the bony and membranous portions of the labyrinth.

**s. perine'i profun'dum** [ NA ], deep perineal space or pouch; the cleft between the superior and inferior fascial layers of the urogenital diaphragm occupied by the membranous part of the urethra, the bulbourethral gland (in the male), the deep transverse perineal and sphincter urethrae muscles and the dorsal nerve and artery of the penis or clitoris.

**s. perine'i superficia'le** [ NA ], superficial compartment of the perineum; the space bounded above by the perineal membrane (inferior fascia of the urogenital diaphragm) and below by the superficial perineal fascia (Colles' fascia). It contains the root structure of the penis or clitoris.

**s. retroinguina'le,** Bogros' space; a triangular space between the peritoneum and the transversalis fascia, at the lower angle of which is the inguinal ligament; it contains the lower portion of the external iliac artery.

**s. retroperitonea'le** [ NA ], the space between the parietal peritoneum and the muscles and bones of the posterior abdominal wall.

**s. retropu'bicum** [ NA ], retropubic space; cavum retzii; space of Retzius; the area of loose connective tissue between the bladder with its related fascia and the pubis and anterior abdominal wall.

**spatia zonula'ria** [ NA ], zonular spaces; Petit's canals; the spaces between the fibers of the zonula ciliaris at the equator of the lens of the eye.

**spatula** (spach'u-lah) [ L. dim. of *spatha,* a broad, flat wooden instrument, fr. G. *spathē* ]. A flat blade like a knife blade, with no sharp edge, used in pharmacy for spreading plasters and ointments.

**Roux s.,** a very small nickeled steel s. used to transfer bits of infected material, such as diphtheritic membrane, to culture tubes.

**spatulate, spatulated** (spach'u-lāt, -la'ted). 1. Spatulated; shaped like a spatula. 2. To manipulate or mix with a spatula.

**spatulation** (spach'u-la'shun). The manipulation of material with a spatula.

**spav'in** [ M.E. *spavayne,* swelling fr. O. Fr. *esparvain* ]. A disease of the tarsal joints of the horse.

**blood s.,** a distention of the veins in the vicinity of the tarsus in a horse, due to pressure from the swelling of bog s. impeding the return flow of blood.

**bog s.,** a chronic synovitis of the tibiotarsal joint in the horse resulting in distention of the joint capsule with fluid; it usually causes little or no lameness.

**bone s.,** a rarefying osteitis involving the bones of the tarsus of the horse, usually those on the medial surface, resulting in exostoses and ankylosis.

**spavined** (spav'ind). Affected with spavin.

**spay** [ Gael. *spoth,* castrate, or G. *spadōn,* eunuch(00 ]. Spade; to remove the ovaries of an animal.

**SPCA.** Abbreviation for serum prothrombin conversion accelerator (factor VII).

**spear'mint** (NF). The leaves and flowering tops of *Mentha viridis* (green garden or lamb mint) or *Mentha cardiaca* (family Labiatae); carminative and flavoring agent.

**s. oil** (NF), the volatile oil, distilled with steam from the fresh, overground parts of the flowering plant of *Mentha viridis* or *Mentha cardiaca;* a flavoring agent.

**specialism** (spesh'ă-lizm) [ see specialty ]. In medicine, the study and treatment of a particular group of diseases, as of the eye, the nervous system, or of children.

**specialist** (spesh'ă-list). One who devotes himself to the study and treatment of a particular group of diseases.

**specialization** (spesh'ă-lĭ-za'shun). Confining attention to a single disease, region of the body, age, or sex of a patient for study, research, and treatment. 2. Differentiation (1).

**specialize** (spesh'ă-līz). To devote one's special study and attention to one subject or group of subjects.

**specialty** (spesh'al-tĭ) [ L. *specialitas* fr. *specialis,* special ]. The particular group of diseases or branch of medical science to which one devotes his time and attention.

**speciation** (spe'she-a'shun). The evolutionary process by which new species of animals or plants are formed from preexisting species.

**species,** pl. **species** (spe'shēz) [ L. appearance, form, kind, fr. *specio,* to look at ]. 1. A biological division between the genus and a variety or the individual; a group of organisms which generally bear a close resemblance to one another in the more essential features of their organization, and with sexual forms which produce fertile progeny. 2. A class of pharmaceutical preparations consisting of a mixture of dried plants, not pulverized, but in sufficiently fine division to be conveniently used in the making of extemporaneous decoctions or infusions; a tea.

**aromatic s.,** aromatic tea, composed of peppermint leaves, wild thyme, and lavender flowers, each 2 parts; cloves and cubeb, each 1 part.

**diuretic s.,** diuretic tea, composed of levisticum root, ononis root, licorice root, and juniper berries each 1 part.

**emol'lient s.,** composed of althaea leaves, malva leaves, melilot (wild laburnum), German chamomile flowers, and flaxseed, each 1 part.

**laxati've s.,** laxative tea; St. Germain tea; composed of senna 160, elder flowers 100, fennel and anise each 50, potassium tartrate 25, tartaric acid 15.

**pectoral s.,** pectoral tea; composed of marshmallow root 8, licorice root 3, orris root 1, colt's foot leaves 4, mullein flowers 2, anise 2.

**type s.,** the name of the single s. or of one of the s. of a genus or subgenus when the name of the genus or subgenus was originally validly published.

**species-specific.** Indicating a serum that is produced by the injection of cells, protein, or other material into an animal, and that acts only upon the cells, protein, etc., of a member of the same species as that from which the original antigen was obtained.

**specific** (spe-sif'ik) [ L. *specificus* fr. *species, q.v.,* + *facio,* to make ]. 1. Relating to a species; see also s. *epithet.* 2. Relating to an individual infectious disease, one caused by a special microorganism; in a special restricted sense, syphilitic. 3. A remedy having a definite curative action in relation to a particular disease or symptom, as quinine in relation to malaria, or mercury to syphilis.

**specificity** (spes'ĭ-fis'ĭ-tĭ). The condition or state of being specific, of having a fixed relation to a single cause, or to a definite result, as the case may be; specificity is manifested in the relation of a disease to its pathogenic microorganism, of a reaction to a certain chemical union, or of an antibody to its antigen, or the reverse.

**specillum,** pl. **specilla** (spē-sil'um, -lah) [ L. a probe, fr. *specio,* to look at ]. A probe or small sound.

**specimen** (spes'ĭ-men) [ L. fr. *specio,* to look at ]. A small part, or sample, of any substance or material (specifically, tissue) obtained for testing.

**cytologic s.,** a s. obtainable by a variety of methods from many areas of the body, including the female genital tract, respiratory tract, urinary tract, alimentary tract, and body cavities; used for cytologic examination and diagnosis (*e.g.,* cytologic smears, filter preparations, centrifuged buttons).

**spectacles** (spek'tĭ-klz) [ L. *specto,* pp. *-atus,* to watch, observe, fr. *specio,* to look at ]. Lenses set in a frame which holds them in front of the eyes, used to correct errors of vision or to protect the eyes from the glare of the sun or electric light. The parts of the s. are the *lenses;* the *bridge* between the lenses, resting on the nose; the *rims* or *frames,* encircling the lenses, sometimes omitted, the bridge and the shoulders being riveted directly to the lenses; the *sides* or *temples,* wires passing on either side of the head to the ears; the *bows,* the curved extremities of the sides over the roots of the auricles; the *shoulders,* short bars attached to the rims or riveted to the lenses and jointed with the sides.

**bifo'cal s.,** s. with bifocal lenses; see under lens.

**clerical s.,** half-glass s.

**Franklin s.,** divided s.; an early form of bifocal s. in which the lower half of the lens is for near, the upper half for distant vision.

**half-glass s.,** s., used for reading, in which the top halves of the lenses are cut off. Also called clerical, pantoscopic, or pulpit s.

**Masselon's s.,** s. with little offsets of metal with smooth edges, which engage below the upper eyelid and keep it raised above the pupil in cases of paralytic ptosis.

**pantoscop'ic s.,** half-glass s.

**prismatic s.'s,** spectacle frame holding prisms for correction of phorias; also for reading in bed.

**pulpit s.,** half-glass s.

**stenopeic s., stenopaic s.,** (1) s. with disks of wood or metal, with narrow slits in the center allowing only a minimum amount of light to enter; used as a protection against snow blindness; (2) s. having opaque disks with multiple perforations used to aid vision in incipient cataract and in discrete opacities of the cornea; occasionally used as a substitute for corrective lenses or sunglasses.

**spectinomycin hydrochloride** (spek'tĭ-no-mi'sin) (USP). TROBICIN; decahydro-4a,7,9-trihydroxy-2-methyl-6,8-bis-(methylamino)-4*H*-pyrano [ 2,3-*b* ] [ 1,4 ] -benzodioxin-4-one dihydrochloride; an antibacterial agent.

**spectra** (spek'trah) [ L. ]. Plural of spectrum.

**spectral** (spek'tral). Relating to a spectrum.

**spectro-** (spek'tro-) [ L. *spectrum,* an image ]. Combining form relating to a spectrum.

**spectrochemistry** (spek'tro-kem'is-trĭ). The study of chemical substances and their identification by means of spectroscopy, *i.e.,* by light emitted or absorbed; see spectrum.

**spec'trocolorim'eter.** A colorimeter using a source of light from a selected portion of the spectrum, *i.e.,* of a selected wavelength.

**spectrogram** (spek'tro-gram) [ spectro- + G. *gramma,* something written ]. A photograph or representation of a spectrum.

**spectrograph** (spek'tro-graf). An instrument used in spectography.

**mass s.,** an instrument that subjects charged and accelerated ions (atomic or molecular) to a magnetic field that imparts a curved path that differs for each mass to charge ratio, thus separating individual species. Used in detecting and assaying isotopic ratios and in molecular structure determinations.

**spectrography** (spek-trog'ră-fĭ) [ spectro- + G. *graphō,* to write ]. The procedure of photographing or tracing a spectrum.

**spectrometer** (spek-trom'e-ter) [ spectro- + G. *metron,* measure ]. An instrument for determining the wavelength or energy of light or other electromagnetic emission.

**spectrometry** (spek-trom'e-trĭ). The procedure of observing and measuring the wavelengths of light and other electromagnetic rays.

**clinical s.,** biospectrometry.

**spectrophobia** (spek'tro-fo'bĭ-ah) [ spectro- + G. *phobos,* fear ]. Morbid fear of mirrors or of one's mirrored image.

**spectrophotofluorimetry** (spek'tro-fo'to-flu-or-im'e-trĭ). Measurement of the intensity and quality of fluorescence by spectrophotometric means.

**spectrophotometer** (spek'tro-fo-tom'e-ter) [ spectro- + photometer ]. An instrument for measuring the intensity of various wavelengths of light transmitted by a substance or a solution, giving rise to a spectrum of light absorbed.

**spectrophotometry** (spek'tro-fo-tom'e-trĭ). Spectrophotometric *analysis.*

**spectropolarimeter** (spek'tro-po'lar-im'e-ter) [ spectro-
+ polarimeter ]. An instrument for measuring the rotation
of light of specific wavelength upon passage through a
solution or translucent solid.

**spectroscope** (spek'tro-skōp) [ spectro- + G. *skopeō*, to
view ]. An instrument for resolving light from any luminous body into its spectrum, and for the observation of the
spectrum so formed. It consists of a prism that refracts the
light or a grating for diffraction of the light, an arrangement for rendering the rays parallel, and a telescope that
magnifies the spectrum.

    **direct vision s.,** one consisting of a single tube containing
a series of prisms; one end of the tube is placed in as close
contact as possible with the substance to be examined
while the observer places his eye at the opposite end. Can
be employed to make a spectroscopic examination of the
blood *in vivo*, as in the ear lobe or web of the thumb.

**spec'troscop'ic.** Relating to or performed by means of a
spectroscope.

**spectroscopy** (spek-tros'ko-pĭ). The observation and study
of spectrums of absorbed or emitted light by means of a
spectroscope or spectrophotometer. See also spectrometry.

    **clinical s.,** see biospectroscopy.

    **infrared s.,** the study of the specific absorption in the
infrared region of the electromagnetic spectrum; used in
the study of the chemical nature of various atomic
groupings within molecules.

**spectrum,** pl. **spectra, spectrums** (spek'trum, -ah) [ L.
an image, fr. *specio*, to look at ]. 1. The color picture
presented when white light is resolved into its constituent
colors by being passed through a prism or through a
diffraction grating. The colors of the s., arranged according
to the increasing frequency of vibration or decreasing
wavelength, are red, orange, yellow, green, blue, indigo,
and violet. 2. Applied in a figurative sense to the
pathogenic microorganisms against which an antibiotic, or
other antibacterial agent, is active. 3. The plot of intensity
*vs.* wavelength of light emitted or absorbed by a substance,
usually characteristic of the substance and used in qualitative and quantitative analysis.

    **absorption s.,** the s. observed after light has passed
through, and been partially absorbed by a solution or
translucent substance. Many molecular groupings have
characterisitic light absorption patterns, which can be used
for detection and quantitative assay.

    **an'timicro'bial s.,** see s. (2).

    **broad s.,** a term indicating a broad range of activity of
an antibiotic against a wide variety of microorganisms.

    **chromatic s.,** color s.; the continuum of colors that white
light forms on passing through a prism or diffraction
grating.

    **color s.,** chromatic s.

    **continuous s.,** one in which there are no absorption bands
or lines.

    **fortification s.,** scintillating *scotoma.*

    **invisible s.,** the radiation lying to either side of the
chromatic s.; for example, the infrared and ultraviolet
radiation.

    **thermal s.,** infrared s.; the invisible part of the s. outside
of the red rays.

    **toxin s.,** a figure in the form of a s. used by Ehrlich to
represent the neutralizing power of antitoxin in the
presence of toxin, prototoxoid, toxone, etc.

    **visible s.,** that part of the spectrum that is visible to the
human eye; it extends from extreme red, 7606 Å, to
extreme violet, 3934 Å.

    **wide s.,** see s. (3).

**speculum,** pl. **specula** (spek'u-lum, -lah) [ L. a mirror, fr.
*specio*, to look at ]. An instrument for enlarging the
opening of any canal or cavity in order to facilitate
inspection of its interior.

    **Barnes' s.,** a form of vaginal s.

    **Boucheron s.,** an ear s.

    **Bozeman's s.,** a bivalve vaginal s., the long blades of
which remain parallel when separated so that the vagina is
evenly dilated.

    **Brinkerhoff's s.,** a conical tubular s. for rectal examina-
tion, with closed extremity but with a sliding bar on one
side the opening of which gives a window of any desired
size.

    **Cooke's s.,** a three-pronged s. for rectal examinations and
operations.

    **Cusco's s.,** a bivalve duckbill vaginal s.

    **duckbill s.,** a bivalve s., the blades of which are broad and
flattened, resembling a duck's bill, used in inspection of the
vagina and cervix.

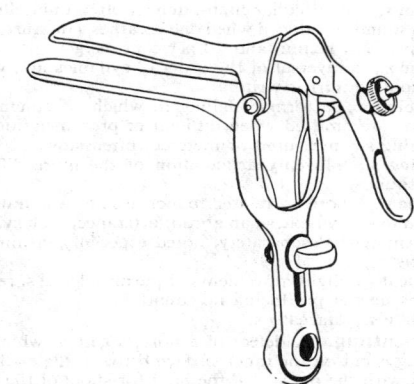

**Duckbill Speculum**

    **eye s.,** blepharostat; an instrument for keeping the eyelids
apart during inspection of or operation on the eye.

    **Fergusson's s.,** a cylindrical vaginal s. of silvered glass
with a coating of caoutchouc.

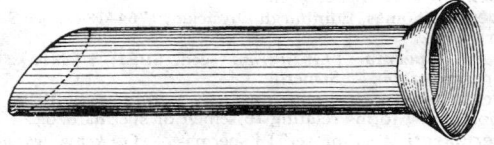

**Fergusson's Speculum**

    **Huffman s.,** a bivalve vaginal s. used in the examination
of adolescents.

    **Fraenkel's s.,** a nasal s., sometimes fenestrated.

    **Kelly's rectal s.,** a tubular s. with obturator, for rectal
examination.

    **Martin's s.,** a conicocylindrical s. with obturator for
rectal examination.

    **Mathew's s.,** a four-pronged s. for rectal examination.

    **mouth s.,** an instrument which, when fitted between the
upper and lower incisor teeth of horses, will force and hold
open the animal's mouth.

    **Pedersen's.,** a narrow flat s. used in vaginas with a small
introitus.

    **Sims' s.,** a double duckbill vaginal s.

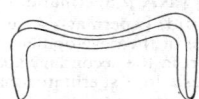

**Sims' Speculum**

    **stop-s.,** a dilating s., as for example a s. of the eyelids,
which is provided with a catch to prevent its being opened
too wide.

    **Trélat's s.,** a bivalve rectal s.

**Spee,** Ferdinand Graf von, German embryologist,
1855–1937. See S.'s *curve.*

**speech** [ A.S. *spaec* ]. Speaking; talk; the use of the voice
in conveying ideas.

    **cerebel'lar s.,** an explosive type of utterance, with
slurring of words.

**clipped s.,** scamping s.

**echo s.,** echolalia.

**esophageal s.,** a technique for speaking following total laryngectomy; consists of swallowing air and regurgitating it, producing a vibration in the hypopharynx.

**explosive s.,** logospasm; loud, sudden s. related to injury of the nervous system.

**helium s.,** the peculiar high-pitched, often unintelligible speech sounds produced when one breathes a mixture of up to 80 per cent helium and 20 per cent oxygen.

**mirror s.,** a reversal of the order of syllables in a word, analogous to mirror writing.

**scamping s.,** a form of lalling in which consonants or syllables are omitted when difficult of pronunciation.

**scanning s.,** measured or metered, often slow s.

**slurring s.,** slovenly articulation of the more difficult letter sounds.

**spastic s.,** labored s. related to increased tone of muscles.

**stacca'to s.,** syllabic s.; an abrupt utterance, each syllable being enunciated separately; noted especially in multiple sclerosis.

**subvocal s.,** slight movements of the muscles of s. related to thinking but producing no sound.

**syllab'ic s.,** staccato s.

**speedy-cutting.** A defect of a horse's gait in which the hind leg is cut on the inner surface between the hock and fetlock with the outside of the hoof (or shoe) of the front foot of the same side.

**spelencephaly** (spe'len-sef'ă-lĭ) [ *spēlaion*, cave, + *enkephalos*, brain ]. Porencephaly.

**speleostomy** (spe'le-os'to-mĭ) [ G. *spēlaion*, cave, + *stoma*, mouth ]. Cavernostomy.

**Spemann,** Hans, German embryologist, 1869–1941. Nobel laureate, 1935, for his discovery of the organizer effect in embryonic development. See S.'s concept of *induction.*

**Spencer Wells.** See Wells.

**Spens,** Thomas, Edinburgh physician, 1764–1842. See S.'s *syndrome.*

**sperm, sperma** [ G. *sperma*, seed. SPER- ] [ NA ]. 1. Spermatozoon. 2. Semen.

**sperm-, spermato-, spermo-** [ G. *sperma*, seed. SPER- ]. Combining forms relating to semen or spermatozoon.

**spermaceti** (sper'mă-set'ĭ) [ sperma- + G. *ketos, whale* ] (USP). Cetaceum; a peculiar fatty, waxy substance, chiefly cetin (cetyl palmitate), obtained from the head of the sperm whale, *Physeter macrocephalus.* Used to impart firmness to ointment bases.

**sperm'agglu'tina'tion.** The agglutination of spermatozoa.

**sperm-aster** [ sperm + G. *astēr,* a star (aster) ]. A cytocentrum with astral rays in the cytoplasm of an inseminated ovum; it is brought in by the penetrating spermatozoon and gives rise to the mitotic spindle of the first cleavage division.

**spermatacrasia** (sper-mat'ă-kra'zĭ-ah) [ spermat- + G. *akrasia,* incontinence ]. Obsolete term for spermatorrhea.

**spermatemphraxis** (sper'mat-em-frak'sis) [ spermat- + G. *emphraxis,* stoppage ]. An impediment to the discharge of semen.

**spermat'ic.** Relating to the sperm or semen.

**spermat'icus** [ L. ] [ NA ]. Spermatic.

**spermatid** (sper'mă-tid) [ spermat- + suffix -*id* (2), *q. v.* ]. A cell in a late stage of the development of the spermatozoon; it is derived from the secondary spermatocyte gives rise by spermiogenesis to a spermatozoon.

**sper'matin.** An albuminoid in the seminal fluid.

**spermatitis** (sper'mă-ti'tis). Deferentitis.

**spermato-** (sper'mă-to-). See sperm-.

**sper'matoblast** [ spermato- + G. *blastos,* germ ]. Spermatogonium.

**spermatocele** (sper'mă-to-sēl) [ spermato- + G. *kēlē,* tumor ]. A cyst of the epididymis containing spermatozoa.

**spermatocidal** (sper'mă-to-si'dal). Spermicidal; destructive to spermatozoa.

**spermatocide** (sper'mă-to-sīd) [ spermato- + L. *caedo,* to kill ]. Spermicide; an agent destructive to spermatozoa.

**spermatocyst** (sper'mă-to-sist) [ spermato- + G. *kystis,* bladder ]. 1. *Vesicula seminalis.* 2. Spermatocele.

**spermatocystectomy** (sper'mă-to-sis-tek'to-mĭ) [ spermatocyst + G. *ektomē,* excision ]. Surgical removal of the seminal vesicles.

**spermatocystitis** (sper'mă-to-sis-ti'tis) [ spermatocyst + G. suffix -*itis,* inflammation ]. Inflammation of a seminal vesicle.

**spermatocystotomy** (sper'mă-to-sis-tot'o-mĭ) [ spermatocyst + G. *tomē,* incision ]. Incision into a seminal vesicle.

**sper'matocy'tal.** Relating to spermatocytes.

**spermatocyte** (sper'mă-to-sīt) [ spermato- + G. *kytos,* cell ]. A cell arising from a spermatogonium and destined to give rise to spermatozoa.

**primary s.,** the s. arising by a growth phase from a spermatogonium.

**secondary s.,** the s. derived from a primary s. by the first meiotic division; each secondary s. gives rise by the second meiotic division to two spermatids.

**spermatocytogenesis** (sper'mă-to-si'to-jen'ĕ-sis). Spermatogenesis.

**spermatogenesis** (sper'mă-to-jen'ĕ-sis) [ spermato- + G. *genesis,* production ]. Spermatocytogenesis; spermatogeny; the process of formation and development of the spermatozoon. See also spermiogenesis, spermatogonium, spermatocyte, and spermatid.

**sper'matogenet'ic.** Spermatogenic.

**spermatogenic** (sper'mă-to-jen'ik). Spermatogenetic; spermatogenous; relating to spermatogenesis; sperm-producing.

**spermatogenous** (sper-mă-toj'ĕ-nus). Spermatogenic.

**spermatogeny** (sper-mă-toj'ĕ-nĭ). Spermatogenesis.

**spermatogone** (sper'mă-to-gōn). Spermatogonium.

**spermatogonium** (sper'mă-to-go'nĭ-um) [ spermato- + G. *gonē,* generation ]. Spermatoblast; spermatogone; the primitive sperm cell derived by mitotic division from the germ cell; increasing several times in size, s.'s become primary spermatocytes.

**spermatoid** (sper'mă-toyd) [ spermato- + G. *eidos,* resemblance ]. Resembling semen.

**spermatology** (sper'mă-tol'o-jĭ) [ spermato- + G. *logos,* study ]. The branch of histology, physiology, and embryology dealing with the seminal secretion.

**spermatolysin** (sper'mă-tol'ĭ-sin). A specific lysin (antibody) formed in response to the repeated injection of spermatozoa.

**spermatolysis** (sper'mă-tol'ĭ-sis) [ spermato- + G. *lysis,* dissolution ]. Spermolysis; destruction, with dissolution, of the spermatozoa.

**sper'matolyt'ic.** Relating to spermatolysis.

**sper'matop'athy, sper'matopath'ia** [ spermato- + G. *pathos,* suffering ]. Any morbid change in the seminal secretion.

**spermatopho'bia** (sper'mă-to-fo'bĭ-ah) [ spermato- + G. *phobos,* fear ]. Abnormal fear of spermatorrhea or loss of semen.

**spermatophore** (sper'mă-to-fōr) [ spermato- + G. *phoros,* bearing ]. A capsule containing spermatozoa; found in a number of invertebrates.

**Spermatophyta** (sper'mă-tof'ĭ-tah) [ spermato- + G. *phyton,* plant ]. A division of the plant kingdom containing the plants which reproduce by means of seeds. Two subdivisions, the gymnosperms and the angiosperms, comprise the S.

**spermatopoietic** (sper'mă-to-poy-et'ik) [ spermato- + G. *poieō,* to make ]. 1. Spermatogenic. 2. Relating to the production of semen; secreting semen.

**spermatorrhea** (sper'mă-to-re'ah) [ spermato- + G. *rhoia,* a flow ]. An involuntary discharge of semen, without orgasm.

**spermatoschesis** (sper'mă-tos'kĕ-sis) [ spermato- + G. *schesis,* retention ]. Nonsecretion of semen.

**sper'matox'in.** Spermotoxin; a cytotoxic antibody specific for spermatozoa.

**spermatozoa** (sper'mă-to-zo'ah). Plural of spermatozoon.

**sper'matozo'al, sper'matozo'an.** Relating to spermatozoa.

**spermatozoon,** pl. **spermatozoa** (spur'mah-to-zo'on) [ G. *sperma,* seed, + *zoön,* animal ]. Sperm; sperma; the male gamete or sex cell; the human s. is composed of a head and a tail. The tail is divisible into a neck, a middle piece, a principal piece, and end piece. The head, which is 4 to 6 $\mu$ in length, is a broadly oval, flattened body containing the nucleus. The tail measures about 55 $\mu$ in length. The spermatozoon contains the genetic information to be transmitted by the male, exhibits autokinesia, and is able to effect zygosis with an ovum.

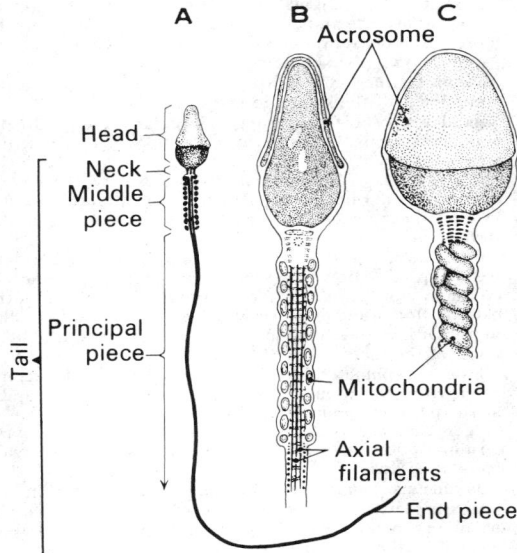

**Human Spermatozoon**

*A,* at magnification of $\times 720$; *B,* diagram of longitudinal section of head, as seen with the electron microscope; *C,* head viewed from its flattened surface, as seen with electron microscope. (Slightly modified from Patten, B. M.: *Human Embryology,* Ed. 3, McGraw-Hill Book Co., New York, 1968. Used with permission.)

**spermaturia** (sper'mă-tu'rĭ-ah). Semenuria.

**spermectomy** (sper-mek'to-mĭ). Surgical removal of a part of a spermatic cord.

**spermia** (sper'mĭ-ah). Plural of spermium.

**spermicidal** (sper'mĭ-si'dal). Spermatocidal.

**spermicide** (sper'mĭ-sīd). Spermatocide.

**sper'midine.** $NH_2(CH_2)_4NH(CH_2)_3NH_2$; a polyamine found along with spermine in a wide variety of organisms and tissues.
   **s. oxidase,** amine oxidase (flavin-containing).

**sper'miduct.** 1. *Ductus* deferens. 2. *Ductus* ejaculatorius.

**spermine.** $NH_2(CH_2)_3NH(CH_2)_4NH(CH_2)_3NH_2$; see spermidine.
   **s. oxidase,** amine oxidase (flavin-containing).

**spermiogenesis** (sper'mĭ-o-jen'ĕ-sis) [ sperm- + G. *genesis,* production ]. That segment of spermatogenesis during which nonmotile spermatids are changed into motile spermatozoa.

**spermism** (sper'mizm). The belief by preformationists that the male sex cell (sperm) contains a miniature preformed body called the homunculus.

**sper'mist.** A preformationist who believed in the concept of spermism.

**spermium, pl. spermia** (sper'mĭ-um, -ah). Waldeyer's term for the mature male germ cell or spermatozoon.

**spermo-** (sper'mo-). See sperm-.

**sper'molith** [ spermo- + G. *lithos,* stone ]. A concretion in the ductus deferens.

**spermol'ysis.** Spermatolysis.

**spermoneuralgia** (sper'mo-nu-ral'jĭ-ah). Neuralgia of the spermatic cord.

**spermophlebectasia** (sper'mo-flĕ-bek-ta'zĭ-ah) [ spermo- + G. *phleps,* vein, + *ektasis,* extension ]. Dilation of the spermatic veins.

**spermotox'in.** Spermatoxin.

**spes phthisica** (spēz (or spās)-tiz'ĭ-kah) [ L. *spes,* hope; G. *phthisikos,* consumptive ]. The feeling of hopefulness and confidence of recovery experienced by many sufferers from tuberculosis even in the later stages of the disease.

**spew** [ A.S. *spiwan* ]. Vomit.

**sp. gr.** Abbreviation for specific *gravity.*

**sph.** Abbreviation for spherical, or spherical *lens.*

**sphacelate** (sfas'ĕ-lāt) [ G. *sphakelos,* gangrene ]. To slough; to become gangrenous.

**sphacelation** (sfas-ĕ-la'shun) [ G. *sphakelos,* gangrene ]. 1. The process of becoming gangrenous. 2. Necrosis; gangrene.

**sphacelism** (sfas'ĕ-lizm). Sphacelation.

**sphaceloderma** (sfas'ĕ-lo-der'mah) [ G. *sphakelos,* gangrene, + *derma,* skin ]. Gangrene of the skin.

**sphacelous** (sfas'ĕ-lus). Necrotic; gangrenous; sloughing.

**sphacelus** (sfas'ĕ-lus) [ G. *sphakelos,* gangrene ]. 1. Moist *gangrene.* 2. A slough; soft mass of necrotic matter.

**Sphaerophorus** (sfe-rof'er-us) [ L. fr. G. *sphaira,* sphere, + *phoros,* bearing ]. *Spherophorus; Fusobacterium;* an illegitimate bacterial generic name; organisms previously placed in this genus have been transferred to *Fusobacterium* or *Bacteroides.* The type species, *S. necrophorus,* has been transferred to *Fusobacterium.*
   **S. mortiferus,** *Fusobacterium mortiferum.*
   **S. necrophorus,** *Fusobacterium necrophorum;* it is the type species of the genus *S.*

**sphenethmoid** (sfe-neth'moyd). Sphenoethmoid.

**sphenion** (sfe'nĭ-on) [ Mod. L. fr. G. *sphēn,* wedge, + dim. suffix *-iōn* ]. The tip of the sphenoidal angle of the parietal bone; a craniometric point.

**spheno-** (sfe'no-) [ G. *sphēn,* wedge ]. Combining form meaning wedge or wedge-shaped, or relating to the sphenoid bone.

**sphenobasilar** (sfe-no-bas'ĭ-lar). Relating to the sphenoid bone and the basilar process of the occipital bone.

**sphenoccipital** (sfe'nok-sip'ĭ-tal). Sphenobasilar.

**sphenocephalus** (sfe'no-sef'ă-lus). An individual with sphenocephaly.

**sphenocephaly** (sfe'no-sef'ă-lĭ) [ spheno- + G. *kephalē,* head ]. The state of having a wedge-shaped head.

**sphenoethmoid** (sfe-no-eth'moyd). Relating to the sphenoid and ethmoid bones.

**sphenofrontal** (sfe'no-fron'tal). Relating to the sphenoid and frontal bones.

**sphenoid** (sfe'noyd) [ G. *sphēnoeidēs,* fr. *sphēn,* wedge, + *eidos,* resemblance ]. Wedge-shaped; sphenoidal.

**sphenoidal** (sfe-noy'dal). Sphenoid. 1. Relating to the sphenoid bone. 2. Wedge-shaped.

**sphenoida'lis** [ L. ] [ NA ]. Sphenoidal (1).

**sphenoiditis** (sfe-noy-di'tis) [ sphenoid + G. suffix *-itis,* inflammation ]. 1. Inflammation of the sphenoid sinus. 2. Necrosis of the sphenoid bone.

**sphenoidostomy** (sfe'noy-dos'to-mĭ) [ sphenoid + G. *stoma,* mouth ]. An operative opening made in the anterior wall of the sphenoid sinus.

**sphenoidotomy** (sfe'noy-dot'o-mĭ) [ sphenoid + G. *tomē,* a cutting ]. Surgical creation of an opening in the anterior wall of the sphenoid sinus.

**sphenomalar** (sfe'no-ma'lar). Sphenozygomatic.

**sphenomaxillary** (sfe'no-mak'sĭ-lĕr-ĭ). Relating to the sphenoid bone and the maxilla.

**spheno-occipital** (sfe'no-ok-sip'ĭ-tal). Sphenobasilar.

**sphenopalatine** (sfe'no-pal'ă-tin). Relating to the sphenoid and the palate bones.

**sphenoparietal** (sfe'no-pă-ri'ă-tal). Relating to the sphenoid and the parietal bones.

**sphenopetrosal** (sfe'no-pe-tro'sal). Relating to the sphenoid bone and the petrous portion of the temporal bone.

**sphenorbital** (sfe-nor'bĭ-tal). Denoting the portions of the sphenoid bone in relation with the orbits.

**sphenosalpingostaphylinus** (sfe'no-sal-ping'go-staf-ĭ-li'-nus) [ L. ]. See under musculus.

**sphenosis** (sfe-no'sis) [ G. sphēnōsis, a wedging together ]. Impaction of the fetus in the pelvic canal during labor.

**sphenosquamosal** (sfe'no-skwa-mo'sal). Relating to the sphenoid bone and the squama of the temporal bone.

**sphenotemporal** (sfe'no-tem'po-ral). Relating to the sphenoid and the temporal bones.

**sphenotic** (sfe-no'tik) [ spheno- + G. ous, ear ]. Relating to the sphenoid bone and the bony case of the ear.

**sphenotresia** (sfe-no-tre'zĭ-ah) [ spheno- + G. trēsis, perforation. TREM- ]. Boring through the base of the skull, in order to facilitate its crushing, in craniotomy.

**sphenotribe** (sfe'no-trīb) [ spheno- + G. tribō, to rub, bruise ]. An instrument for crushing the base of the skull after sphenotresia.

**sphenotripsy** (sfe'no-trip'sĭ) [ spheno- + G. tripsis, a rubbing ]. Crushing the base of the skull after sphenotresia.

**sphenoturbinal** (sfe'no-tur'bĭ-nal). Denoting the concha sphenoidalis.

**sphenovomerine** (sfe'ι,o-vo'mer-ēn, -in). Relating to the sphenoid bone and the vomer.

**sphenozygomatic** (sfe'no-zi-go-mat'ik). Relating to the sphenoid and the zygomatic bones.

**sphere** (sfēr) [ G. sphaira ]. A ball or globular body.
  **attraction s.,** astrosphere.
  **Morgagni's s.'s,** Morgagni's globules.
  **segmenta'tion s.,** archaic term for morula.

**spheresthesia** (sfēr'es-the'zĭ-ah) [ G. sphaira, sphere, + aisthēsis, sensation ]. Globus hystericus.

**spherical** (sfēr'ĭ-kal, sfer-). Pertaining to, or shaped like, a sphere.

**sphe'ricus** [ L. ] [ NA ]. Spherical.

**sphero-, spher-** (sfēr'o-) [ G. sphaira, globe, sphere ]. Combining forms relating to sphere.

**spherocylinder** (sfēr'o-sil'in-der). A spherocylindrical lens.

**spherocyte** (sfēr'o-sit) [ sphero- + G. kytos, cell ]. Microcyte; a small, spherical red blood cell.

**spherocytosis** (sfēr'o-si-to'sis) [ spherocyte + G. suffix -osis, condition ]. The presence of sphere-shaped red blood cells in the blood, a feature of familial hemolytic anemia.
  **hereditary s.,** a congenital defect of the erythrocyte cell membrane, which is abnormally permeable to sodium, resulting in erythrocytes that are thickened and almost spherical in shape. The erythrocytes are fragile, susceptible to spontaneous hemolysis, and their survival in the circulation is decreased. This results in chronic anemia with reticulocytosis, episodes of mild jaundice due to hemolysis, and acute crises with fever and abdominal pain; symptomatology is highly variable; autosomal dominant inheritance. Synonymous terms are: congenital hemolytic jaundice, icterus, or anemia; chronic familial jaundice or icterus; spherocytic, icterohemolytic, or globe-cell anemia; acholuric jaundice.

**spheroid** (sfēr'oyd, sfer'oyd) [ L. spheroideus ]. Shaped like a sphere.

**spheroi'deus** [ L. ] [ NA ]. Spheroid.

**spheroma** (sfēr-o'mah). A tumor of spherical shape.

**spherometer** (sfēr-om'e-ter) [ sphero- + G. metron, measure ]. An instrument for determining the degree of convexity of the surface of a sphere or a spherical lens.

**spherophakia** (sfēr'o-fa'kĭ-ah) [ sphero- + G. phakos, lens ]. Microphakia; microlentia; a congenital bilateral aberration in which the lenses are small, spherical, and subject to subluxation; may occur as an independent anomaly or may be associated with the Marchesani syndrome.

**Spheroph'orus.** Sphaerophorus.

**spheroprism** (sfēr'o-prizm). A spherical lens decentered to produce a prismatic effect, or a combined spherical lens and prism.

**spherospermia** (sfēr'o-sper'mĭ-ah) [ sphero- + G. sperma, seed ]. Spermatozoa having no elongated tail, such as those of the nematodes; in contrast to nematospermia.

**spher'ule.** A sproangium-like structure in Coccidiodes that contains endospores.

**sphincter** (sfingk'ter) [ G. sphinktēr, a band or lace. SPHIN- ]. Musculus sphincter.
  **anatomical s.,** an accumulation of muscular circular fibers or specially arranged oblique fibers the function of which is to reduce partially or totally the lumen of a tube, the orifice of an organ, or the cavity of a viscus; the closing component of a pylorus.
  **s. angula'ris,** angular s.; thickening of the circular muscular layer forming the so-called s. intermedius at the level of the incisura angularis of the stomach.
  **s. ani,** musculus sphincter ani.
  **s. ani tertius,** the third s. of the anus, the closing component of the sigmoidorectal pylorus.
  **annular s.,** short thickening of circular muscular fibers, similar to a ring; ring-shaped s. as opposed to segmental s.
  **s. an'tri,** s. of the antrum; antral s.; s. of the gastric antrum; s. intermedius; a portion of the circular muscular layer of the stomach acting as a s. between the corpus and the antrum.
  **artificial s.,** a s. produced by surgical procedures to reduce speed of flow in the digestive system or to maintain continence of the intestine; by removal of 1 to 2 cm. of the external longitudinal muscular layer the internal circular muscular layer predominates, causing reduction or obliteration of the lumen.
  **basal s.,** sphincteroid tract of the ileum; the thickening of the circular muscular coat at the base of the ileal papilla at the terminal ileum.
  **bicanalic'ular s.,** a s. encircling two canals, such as the terminal portions of the common bile duct and the main pancreatic duct.
  **Boyden's s.,** musculus sphincter ductus choledochi.
  **canalic'ular s.,** a s. located somewhere along the course of an organ, a tube, or a duct as opposed to ostial s., located at the level of an orifice.
  **Cannon, Boehm, and Roith's s.,** Cannon's ring.
  **choledochal s.,** musculus sphincter ductus choledochi.
  **colic s.,** one of the s.'s of the colon.
  **s. of common bile duct,** musculus sphincter ductus choledochi.
  **s. constrictor cardiae,** the s. of the esophagogastric junction.
  **s. detrusor foecium superior,** an old name for the closing mechanism at the sigmoidorectal junction.
  **duodenal s.,** one of the s.'s described in the duodenum.
  **duodenojejunal s.,** the s. supposedly present at the duodenojejunal flexure.
  **extrinsic s.,** a s. provided by circular muscular fibers extraneous to the organ.
  **first duodenal s.,** the s. supposedly located at the level of the aboral extremity of the duodenal bulb.
  **Glisson's s.,** musculus sphincter ampullae hepatopancreaticae.
  **s. of hepatic flexure of colon,** s. at the level of the flexura coli dextra.
  **Hyrtl's s.,** a band, generally incomplete, of circular muscular fibers in the rectum about 4 inches above the anus.
  **ileal s.,** ileocecocolic s.; marginal s.; a thickening of circular musculature at the free margin of the ileal papilla.
  **ileocecocolic s.,** ileal s.
  **s. intermedius,** s. antri.
  **intrinsic s.,** a thickening of the circular fibers of the tunica muscularis of an organ.
  **macroscopic s.,** a s. visible to the naked eye.
  **marginal s.,** ileal s.
  **mediocolic s.,** a s. located midway in the ascending colon.
  **microscopic s.,** a s. visible only under the microscope.
  **midgastric transverse s.,** a s. described at the level of the junction between the body of the stomach and the antrum.
  **midsigmoid s.,** iliopelvic s.; the s. midway in the sigmoid colon.
  **myovascular s.,** a s. having a muscular and a vascular (usually venous) component.
  **myovenous s.,** a s. having a muscular and a venous component, e.g., at the pharyngoesophageal junction and anal canal.

**Nélaton's s.,** Nélaton's fibers; an inconstant band of circular muscular fibers in the wall of the rectum between three and four inches above the anus.

**O'Beirne's s.,** a circular band of muscular fibers in the upper part of the rectum.

**s. oc'uli,** *musculus* orbicularis oculi.

**Oddi's s.,** *musculus* sphincter ampullae hepatopancreaticae.

**s. o'ris,** *musculus* orbicularis oris.

**ostial s.,** a thickening of circular muscular fibers at the level of an orifice.

**pancreatic s.,** a s. at the level of the termination of the main and of the accessory pancreatic duct.

**pathologic s.,** a thickening of circular musculature caused by disease.

**pelvirectal s.,** sigmoidorectal s.

**physiological s.,** functional s.; radiological s.; a s. seen in radiograms taken from living individuals and not recognizable in surgical specimens or during necroscopy either by dissection or by histological techniques, probably because the s. assumes a resting arrangement which cannot be differentiated from adjacent tissues during anesthesia, after removal, or after death.

**postpyloric s.,** the duodenal portion of the s. or closing mechanism of the gastroduodenal pylorus.

**prepapillary s.,** a s. of duodenum described in the location oral to the major duodenal papilla.

**prepylor'ic s.,** a band of circular muscular fibers in the wall of the stomach near the gastroduodenal pylorus.

**s. pupil'lae,** *musculus* sphincter pupillae.

**pylor'ic s.,** *musculus* sphincter pylori.

**radiological s.,** physiological s.

**rectosigmoid s.,** sigmoidorectal s.

**segmental s.,** a s. of a segment of an organ, a tube, or a canal, and longer than an annular s.

**smooth muscular s.,** lissosphincter.

**striated muscular s.,** rhabdosphincter.

**s. of third portion of duodenum,** a s. supposedly located at the horizontal (inferior) portion of the duodenum.

**unicanalicular s.,** a s. limited to one visceral canal or tube.

**s. ure'thrae,** *musculus* sphincter urethrae.

**s. vagi'nae,** *musculus* bulbocavernosus.

**Varolius' s.,** operculum ilei; the sphincter muscle at the terminal ileum.

**s. vesi'cae,** *musculus* sphincter vesicae.

**s. vesicae felleae,** the s. of the gallbladder, at the transition between the neck of the gallbladder and the cystic duct.

**sphincteral** (sfingk'ter-al). Sphincterial; sphincteric; relating to a sphincter.

**sphincteralgia** (sfingk'ter-al'ji-ah) [ sphincter + G. *algos*, pain ]. Pain in the sphincter ani muscles.

**sphincterectomy** (sfingk'ter-ek'to-mī) [ sphincter + G. *ektomē*, excision ]. 1. Excision of a portion of the pupillary border of the iris. 2. Dissecting away any sphincter muscle.

**sphincte'rial, sphincter'ic.** Sphincteral.

**sphincterismus** (sfingk'ter-iz'mus). Spasmodic contraction of the sphincter ani muscles.

**sphincteritis** (sfingk'ter-i'tis). Inflammation of any sphincter.

**sphincteroid** (sfingk'ter-oyd) [ sphincter + G. *eidos*, resemblance ]. Denoting similarity to a musculus sphincter.

**sphinctero'lysis** (sfingk'ter-ol'ĭ-sis) [ sphincter, + G. *lysis*, loosening ]. Operation for freeing the iris from the cornea in anterior synechia involving only the pupillary border.

**sphincteroplasty** (sfingk'ter-o-plas'tī) [ sphincter + G. *plassō*, to form ]. Reparative or plastic surgery of any sphincter muscle.

**sphincteroscope** (sfingk'ter-o-skōp) [ sphincter + G. *skopeō*, to view ]. A speculum to facilitate inspection of the internal sphincter ani muscle.

**sphincteroscopy** (sfingk'ter-os'ko-pī). Visual examination of a sphincter.

**sphincterotome** (sfingk'ter-o-tōm). An instrument for incising a sphincter.

**sphincterotomy** (sfingk'ter-ot'o-mī) [ sphincter + G. *tomē*, incision ]. Division of a sphincter muscle.

**transduodenal s.,** division of the sphincter of Oddi, performed through a duodenotomy in the lateral wall of the duodenum adjacent to the papilla of Vater; an operation used to open the lower end of the common duct to remove impacted stones or to relieve spasm or stricture of the terminal bile and pancreatic ducts.

**sphinganine** (sfing'gă-nēn). Dihydrosphingosine; 2-aminoöctadecane-1,3-diol.

**4-sphin'genine.** Sphingosine.

**sphingoine** (sfing'go-ēn). A leukomaine found in brain substance.

**sphingol.** Sphingosine.

**sphingolipid** (sfing'go-lip'id). Any lipid containing a long chain base (like sphingosine), such as ceramides, cerebrosides, gangliosides, and sphingomyelins.

**sphingolipidosis** (sfing'go-lip'ĭ-do'sis). Collective designation for a variety of diseases characterized by abnormal sphingolipid metabolism, such as gangliosidosis, Gaucher's disease, and Niemann-Pick disease.

**cerebral s.,** formerly termed amaurotic familial idiocy; any one of a group of inherited diseases characterized by failure to thrive, hypertonicity, progressive spastic paralysis, loss of vision and occurrence of blindness usually with macular degeneration and optic atrophy, convulsions, and mental deterioration; associated with abnormal storage of sphingomyelin and related lipids in the brain. Four types are recognized as clinically and genetically distinct: infantile type (Tay-Sachs disease, $G_{M2}$ gangliosidosis); early juvenile type (Jansky-Bielschowsky disease); late juvenile type (Spielmeyer-Vogt disease; Batten-Mayou disease; ceroid lipofuscinosis); and adult type (Kufs' disease).

**sphingomyelinase** (sfing'go-mi'ē-lī-nās). Sphingomyelin phosphodiesterase.

**sphingomyelin phosphodiesterase.** Sphingomyelinase; an enzyme (EC 3.1.4.12) catalyzing hydrolysis of sphingomyelin to ceramide and phosphocholine.

**sphingomyelins** (sfing'go-mi'ē-linz). Phosphosphingosides; a group of phospholipids found in brain, spinal cord, kidney, and egg yolk, containing 1-phosphocholine (choline phosphate) combined with a ceramide (an *N*-acyl long chain base, such as sphingosine).

**sphingosine** (sfing'go-sēn). $CH—(CH_2)_{12}CH=CHCH(OH)CH(NH_2)CH_2OH$; 4-sphingenine; 2-aminoöctadec-4-ene-1,3-diol; principal long chain base found in sphingolipids.

**sphygm-.** See sphygmo-.

**sphygmic** (sfig'mik). Relating to the pulse.

**sphygmo-, sphygm-** (sfig'mo-) [ G. *sphygmos*, pulse. SPHYG- ]. Combining forms relating to pulse.

**sphygmobolometer** (sfig'mo-bo-lom'e-ter) [ sphygmo- + G. *bolos*, a throw, a cast, + *metron*, measure ]. Sphygmodynamometer; used in sphygmobolometry.

**sphygmobolometry** (sfig-mo-bo-lom'e-trī). The technique of measuring the force of the pulse wave and so indirectly of cardiac systole.

**sphygmocardiograph** (sfig'mo-kar'dī-o-graf) [ sphygmo- + G. *kardia*, heart, + *graphō*, to write ]. Sphygmocardioscope; a polygraph recording both the heart beat and the radial pulse.

**sphygmocardioscope** (sfig'mo-kar'dī-o-skōp) [ sphygmo- + G. *skopeō*, to view ]. Sphygmocardiograph.

**sphygmochronograph** (sfig'mo-kron'o-graf) [ sphygmo- + G. *chronos*, time, + *graphō*, to write ]. A modified sphygmograph that represents graphically the time relations between the beat of the heart and the pulse; one recording the character of the pulse as well as its rapidity.

**sphygmodynamometer** (sfig'mo-di'nă-mom'e-ter) [ sphygmo- + G. *dynamis*, force, + *metron*, measure ]. Sphygmobolometer.

**sphygmogram** (sfig'mo-gram) [ sphygmo- + G. *gramma*, something written ]. Pulse curve; the graphic curve made by a sphygmograph.

**sphygmograph** (sfig'mo-graf) [ sphygmo- + G. *graphō*, to write ]. An instrument consisting of a lever, the short end of which rests on the radial artery at the wrist, its long end being provided with a stylet which records on a moving ribbon of smoked paper the excursions of the pulse.

**sphyg′mograph′ic.**  Relating to or made by a sphygmograph; denoting the s. tracing, or sphygmogram.

**sphygmography** (sfig-mog′ră-fĭ). 1. The use of the sphygmograph in recording the character of the pulse. 2. A treatise on or description of the pulse.

**sphygmoid** (sfig′moyd) [ sphygmo- + G. *eidos*, resemblance ]. Pulselike; resembling the pulse.

**sphygmology** (sfig-mol′o-jĭ) [ sphygmo- + G. *logos*, study ]. The scientific study of the pulse and the knowledge derived therefrom.

**sphygmomanometer** (sfig′mo-mă-nom′e-ter) [ sphygmo- + G. *manos*, thin, scanty, + *metron*, measure ]. Sphygmometer; an instrument for measuring the blood pressure.
    **Mosso′s s.,** an apparatus for measuring the blood pressure in the digital arteries.
    **Rogers′ s.,** one constructed with the usual arm sleeve and inflating bulb, but with an aneroid barometer gauge instead of the mercury manometer, as in the Janeway apparatus.

**sphygmomanometry** (sfig′mo-mă-nom′e-trĭ). The determination of the blood pressure by means of a sphygmomanometer.

**sphygmometer** (sfig-mom′e-ter). Sphygmomanometer.

**sphygmometroscope** (sfig-mo-met′ro-skōp) [ sphygmo- + G. *metron*, measure, + *skopeō*, to view ]. An instrument for auscultating the pulse, used especially in the auscultatory method of reading the blood pressure, more particularly the diastolic pressure.

**sphygmo-oscillometer** (sfig′mo-os′ĭ-lom′e-ter) [ sphygmo- + L. *oscillo*, to swing, + G. *metron*, measure ]. An instrument resembling an aneroid sphygmomanometer used in the measurement of the systolic and diastolic blood pressure.

**sphymopalpation** (sfig′mo-pal-pa′shun) [ sphygmo- + L. *palpatio*, palpation ]. Feeling the pulse.

**sphygmophone** (sfig′mo-fōn) [ sphygmo- + G. *phōnē*, sound ]. An instrument by which a sound is produced with each beat of the pulse.

**sphygmoscope** (sfig′mo-skōp) [ sphygmo- + G. *skopeō*, to view ]. An instrument by which the pulse beats are made visible by causing fluid to rise in a glass tube, by means of a mirror projecting a beam of light, or simply by a moving lever as in the sphygmograph.
    **Bishop′s s.,** an instrument for measuring the blood pressure, with special reference to diastolic pressure. The tube is filled with a solution of cadmium borotungstate, and the scale is the reverse of that of a mercurial manometer, the pressure being made directly by the weight of the liquid and not by compressed air.

**sphygmoscopy** (sfig-mos′ko-pĭ) [ sphygmo- + G. *skopeō*, to view ]. Examination of the pulse.

**sphygmosystole** (sfig-mo-sis′to-le) [ sphygmo- + G. *systolē*, a contracting ]. The segment of the pulse wave corresponding to the cardiac systole.

**sphygmotonograph** (sfig-mo-to′no-graf) [ sphygmo- + G. *tonos*, tension, + *graphō*, to write ]. An instrument for recording graphically both the pulse and the blood pressure.

**sphygmotonometer** (sfig-mo-to-nom′e-ter) [ sphygmo- + G. *tonos*, tension, + *metron*, measure ]. An instrument, like the sphygmotonograph, for determining the degree of blood pressure.

**sphygmoviscosimetry** (sfig-mo-vis-ko-sim′e-trĭ). Measurement of the pressure and the viscosity of the blood.

**sphyrectomy** (sfi′rek′to-mĭ) [ G. *sphyra*, malleus, + *ektomē*, excision ]. Exsection of the malleus.

**sphyrotomy** (sfi-rot′o-mĭ) [ G. *sphyra*, malleus, + *tomē*, incision ]. Section of the handle or other part of the malleus.

**spica**, pl. **spicae** (spi′kah, spi′ke) [ L. a point, an ear of grain ]. See under bandage.

**spicula** (spik′u-lah) [ L. ]. Plural of spiculum.

**spicular** (spik′u-lar). Relating to or having spicules.

**spicule** (spik′ūl) [ L. *spiculum*, dim. of *spica*, or *spicum*, a point ]. A small, needle-shaped body.

**spiculum**, pl. **spicula** (spik′u-lum, -lah) [ L. ]. A spicule or small spike.

**spi′der** [ O. E. *spinnan*, to spin ]. 1. An arthropod of the order Araneida (subclass Arachnida) characterized by four pairs of legs, a cephalothorax, globose, smooth abdomen, and a complex of web-spinning spinnerets. Among the venomous s.′s found in the New World are the black widow s., *Latrodectus mactans;* red-legged widow s., *Latrodectus bishopi;* pruning s., or Peruvian tarantula, *Glyptocranium gasteracanthoides;* Chilean brown s., *Loxosceles laeta;* Peruvian brown s., *Loxosceles rufiper;* brown recluse s. of North America, *Loxosceles reclusus.* 2. Arterial s. 3. An obstructive growth in the teat of a cow.
    **arterial s.,** a telangiectatic arteriole in the skin with radiating capillary branches simulating the legs of a s.; characteristic of parenchymatous liver disease, but also seen in pregnancy and at times in normal persons. Also called vascular spider; spider angioma; nevus arachnoideus; nevus araneus; spider nevus; spider mole; spider telangiectasia.
    **vascular s.,** arterial s.

**spider-burst.** Radiating dull red capillary lines on the skin of the leg, usually without any visible or palpable varicose veins, but nevertheless due to deep-seated venous dilation; called also skyrocket capillary ectasis.

**Spiegel.** See Spigelius.

**Spiegelberg,** O. See S.′s *criteria.*

**Spiegler** (spe′gler), Edward, Vienna dermatologist, 1860–1908. See S.′s *reagent.*

**Spielmeyer,** Walter, Munich neurologist, 1879–1935. See S.-Stock *disease,* S.-Vogt *disease,* S.′s acute *swelling.*

**spigelia** (spi-je′lĭ-ah) [ *Spigelius* ]. Pinkroot; the rhizome and roots of *Spigelia marilandica* (family Loganiaceae); a herb of the southern United States; anthelmintic.

**Spige′lian.** Relating to or described by Spigelius.

**spi′geline.** A toxic volatile alkaloid of spigelia.

**Spigelius** (spe-ga′le-oos), Adrian (properly van der Spieghel), Belgian anatomist in Padua, 1578–1625. See Spigelian *hernia,* S.′s *line,* S.′s *lobe.*

**spike.** A brief electrical event of 3 to 25 milliseconds′ duration that gives the appearance in the electroencephalogram of a rising and falling vertical line.

**spill.** An overflow; a scattering of fluid or finely divided matter.
    **cellular s.,** a dissemination of cells through the lymph or blood, thereby resulting in metastases or implantation of foreign tissue in any part or organ.

**Spiller,** W. G., U. S. neurologist, 1864–1940. See Frazier-S. *operation.*

**spill′way.** Sluiceway; a groove or channel through which food may pass from the occlusal surfaces of teeth during the masticatory process.

**spiloma** (spi-lo′mah) [ G. *spilos*, spot, + suffix *-oma*, tumor ]. Nevus.

**spiloplaxia** (spi′lo-plak′sĭ-ah) [ G. *spilos*, spot, + *plax*, plaque, plate ]. A red spot observed in leprosy or pellagra.

**spi′lus** [ Mod. L. fr. G. *spilos*, a spot ]. Nevus.

**spin-.** See spino-.

**spina**, gen. and pl. **spinae** (spi′nah, -ne) [ L. a thorn, the backbone, spine ] 1 [ NA ]. Any spine or sharp thornlike process. 2. *Columna* vertebralis.
    **s. angula′ris,** s. ossis sphenoidalis.
    **s. bif′ida** (or **bi′fida**), schistorrhachis; limited defect in the spinal column, consisting in absence of the vertebral arches, through which the spinal membranes, with or without spinal cord tissue, may protrude. See fig. on p. 1313.
    **s. bifida aper′ta,** s. bifida occulta.
    **s. bifida cys′tica,** a form associated with a meningocele.
    **s. bifida manifes′ta,** a form in which the vertebral defect is apparent and may be associated with a meningeal or myelic anomaly.
    **s. bifida occul′ta,** cryptomerorachischis; s. bifida aperta; a form in which there is a spinal defect, but no protrusion of the cord or its membrane, although often some abnormality in their development.
    **s. dorsa′lis,** *columna* vertebralis.
    **s. fronta′lis,** s, nasalis ossis frontalis.
    **s. hel′icis** [ NA ], spine of the helix; apophysis helicis; an

anteriorly directed spine at the extremity of the crus of the helix of the auricle.

**s. ili′aca ante′rior infe′rior** [ NA ], anterior inferior iliac spine; spine on the anterior border of the ilium between the s. iliaca anterior superior and the acetabulum.

**s. ili′aca ante′rior supe′rior** [ NA ], anterior superior iliac spine; the anterior extremity of the iliac crest.

**s. ili′aca poste′rior infe′rior** [ NA ], posterior inferior iliac spine; spine on the posterior border of the ilium between the s. iliaca posterior superior and the greater sciatic notch.

**s. ili′aca poste′rior supe′rior** [ NA ], posterior superior iliac spine; the posterior extremity of the iliac crest.

**s. ischiad′ica** [ NA ], sciatic spine; spine of the ischium; a pointed process from the posterior border of the ischium on a level with the lower border of the acetabulum.

**s. mea′tus,** s. supra meatum.

**s. menta′lis** [ NA ], mental spine; genial tubercle; a slight projection, sometimes two, in the middle line of the posterior surface of the body of the mandible, giving attachment to the geniohyoid muscle (below) and the genioglossus (above).

**s. nasa′lis ante′rior** [ NA ], anterior nasal spine; a pointed projection at the anterior extremity of the intermaxillary suture.

**s. nasa′lis os′sis fronta′lis** [ NA ], nasal spine of the frontal bone; a projection from the center of the nasal part of the frontal bone, which lies between and articulates with the nasal bones and the perpendicular plate of the ethmoid.

**s. nasa′lis poste′rior** [ NA ], posterior nasal spine; posterior palatine spine; the sharp posterior extremity of the nasal crest.

**s. os′sis sphenoida′lis** [ NA ], sphenoidal spine; angular spine; a posterior and downward projection from the greater wing of the sphenoid bone on either side.

**spinae palati′nae** [ NA ], palatine spines; the longitudinal ridges on the inferior surface of the palatine process of the maxilla.

**s. pedis,** a corn.

**s. peronea′lis,** *trochlea* peronealis.

**s. pu′bis,** *tuberculum* pubicum.

**s. scap′ulae** [ NA ], spine of the scapula; the prominent triangular ridge on the dorsal aspect of the scapula.

**s. su′pramea′tum** [ NA ], suprameatal spine; Henle's spine; a small bony prominence anterior to the supramastoid fossa at the posterosuperior margin of the bony external acoustic meatus.

**s. trochlea′ris** [ NA ], trochlear spine; a spicule of bone arising from the edge of the fovea trochlearis, giving attachment to the pulley of the superior oblique muscle of the eyeball.

**s. tympan′ica major** [ NA ], greater tympanic spine; the anterior edge of the notch of Rivinus, or incisura tympanica.

**s. tympan′ica minor** [ NA ], lesser tympanic spine; the posterior edge of the tympanic notch (of Rivinus).

**s. vento′sa,** a condition occasionally seen in tuberculosis or cancer of bone, in which there is absorption of bone bordering the medulla, with a new deposit under the periosteum, resulting in a change that is suggestive of bone being inflated with gas.

**spinacene** (spin′ă-sēn). Squalene.

**spi′nal** [ L. *spinalis* ]. 1. Relating to any spine or spinous process. 2. Relating to the vertebral column.

**spinal′gia.** Rachialgia.

**spina′lis** [ L. ]. Spinal.

**spi′nant.** An agent increasing the reflex irritability of the spinal cord.

**spinast′erol.** A sterol obtained from spinach, then from animal tissues. β-Spinasterol is 5α-stigmasga-7,22-dien-3β-ol, an isomer of stigmasterol (for structure of stigmastane, see steroids), and is identical with hitodesterol.

**spi′nate.** Spined; having spines.

**spindle** (spin′dl) [ A.S. ]. 1. In anatomy and pathology, any fusiform cell or structure. 2. The fusiform figure characteristic of a dividing cell formed by the microtubules extending between the two asters and attached to the chromosomes; part of the amphiaster.

**aortic s.,** His' s.; a fusiform dilation of the aorta immediately beyond the isthmus.

**central s.,** see s. (2).

**cleavage s.,** see s. (2).

**His' s.,** aortic s.

**Krukenberg's s.,** a vertical fusiform area of melanin pigmentation on the posterior surface of the cornea in the pupillary area.

**Kühne's s.,** neuromuscular s.

**muscle s.,** neuromuscular s.

**neuromuscular s.,** muscle s.; Kühne's s.; a fusiform end organ in skeletal muscle in which afferent and a few efferent nerve fibers terminate; it contains from 3 to 10 striated muscle fibers (intrafusal fibers) which are much

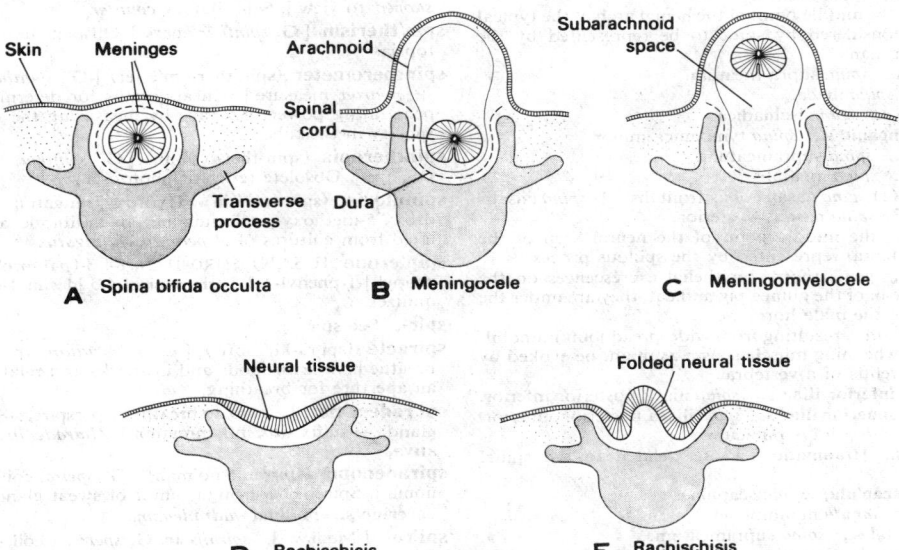

**Spina Bifida**
Schematic drawings showing the various types. (From Langman, J.: *Medical Embryology*, Ed. 2, The Williams & Wilkins Co., Baltimore, 1969.)

smaller than the ordinary muscle fibers, are separated from them by a capsule that encloses the organ, and are innervated by the thin axon of a gamma motoneuron (gamma motor fiber). The sensory endings that occur on the intrafusal fibers are either annulospiral or flower spray endings (see under ending). This sensory end organ is particularly sensitive to passive stitch of the muscle in which it is enclosed.

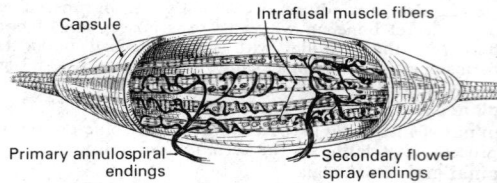

Capsule      Intrafusal muscle fibers

Primary annulospiral endings     Secondary flower spray endings

**Neuromuscular Spindle, with Capsule Cut Open**

**neurotendinous s.,** Golgi tendon *organ.*
**nuclear s.,** s. (2).
**sleep s.,** waves of a frequency of 14 per second rising and falling in amplitude, appearing in the electroencephalogram during sleep.
**spine** [ L. *spina* ]. 1. A short sharp process of bone; a spinous process. 2. *Columna* vertebralis. 3. The bar or stay in a horse's hoof.
   **a'lar s., angular s.,** *spina* ossis sphenoidalis.
   **anterior inferior iliac s.,** *spina* iliaca anterior inferior.
   **anterior superior iliac s.,** *spina* iliaca anterior superior.
   **cleft s.,** rachischisis.
   **dendritic s.'s,** gemmules (2); dendritic thorns; variably long excrescences of nerve cell dendrites, varying in shape from small knobs to thornlike or filamentous processes, usually more numerous on distal dendrite arborizations than on the proximal part of dendritic trunks. They are a preferential site of synaptic axodendritic contact. Sparse or absent in some types of nerve cells (motor neurons; the large cells of the globus pallidus; stellate cells of the cerebral cortex), they are exceedingly numerous in others such as the pyramidal cells of the cerebral cortex and the Purkinje cells of the cerebellar cortex.
   **dorsal s.,** *columna* vertebralis.
   **greater tympanic s.,** *spina* tympanica major.
   **s. of helix,** *spina* helicis.
   **hemal s.,** the middle point of the hemal arch of the typical vertebra; considered by some to be represented by the sternum in man.
   **Henle's s.,** *spina* supra meatum.
   **il'iac s.,** *spina* iliaca.
   **ischiad'ic s.,** *spina* ischiadica.
   **lesser tympanic s.,** *spina* tympanica minor.
   **me'atal s.,** *spina* suprameatum.
   **mental s.,** *spina* mentalis.
   **nasal s.,** (1) *spina* nasalis ossis frontalis; (2) *spina* nasalis anterior; (3) *spina* nasalis posterior.
   **neural s.,** the middle point of the neural arch of the typical vertebra, represented by the spinous process.
   **penis s.'s,** penis thorns; epithelial excrescences on the glans of the p. of the guinea pig and cat; they are under the influence of the male hormone.
   **poker s.,** stiff s. resulting from widespread joint immobility or overwhelming muscle spasm as might be evoked by an osteomyelitis of a vertebra.
   **posterior inferior iliac s.,** *spina* iliaca posterior inferior.
   **posterior superior iliac s.,** *spina* iliaca posterior superior.
   **pubic s.,** *tuberculum* pubicum.
   **railway s.,** traumatic neurosis related to the spinal column.
   **s. of the scap'ula,** *spina* scapulae.
   **Spix's s.,** *lingula* mandibulae.
   **suprame'atal s.,** *spina* suprameatum.
   **thoracic s.,** the thoracic region of the columna vertebralis; the vertebrae thoracicae as a whole; that part of the vertebral column which enters into the formation of the thorax.
   **troch'lear s.,** *spina* trochlearis.

   **typhoid s.,** spondylitis typhosa; weakness and hyperesthesia of the spinal column occasionally noted as a sequel of typhoid fever.
**Spinel'li,** Pier G., Italian gynecologist, 1862–1929. See S. *operation.*
**spinifugal** (spi-nif'u-gal) [ spine + L. *fugio,* to flee ]. Conducting in a direction away from the spinal cord; denoting the efferent fibers of the spinal nerves.
**spinipetal** (spi-nip'ĕ-tal) [ spine + L. *peto,* to seek ]. Conducting in a direction toward the spinal cord; denoting the afferent fibers of the spinal nerves.
**spinnbarkheit** (spin'bahr-kīt) [ Ger. "spinnability" ]. Designating the stringy, elastic character of cervical mucus during the ovulatory period. In contrast to other times in the menstrual cycle, cervical secretions at midcycle are clear, abundant, and of low viscosity.
**spino-, spin-, spina-** (spi'no-) [ L. *spina, q. v.* ]. Combining forms (1) relating to the spine; (2) meaning spinous.
**spi'nobul'bar.** Relating to the spinal cord and the medulla oblongata.
**spi'nocollic'ular.** Spinotectal.
**spi'nocosta'lis** [ L. ]. The superior and inferior serratus posterior muscles regarded as one.
**spi'nogalvaniza'tion.** The application of the constant electrical current to the spinal cord.
**spi'nogle'noid.** Relating to the spine and the glenoid cavity of the scapula.
**spi'nomus'cular.** Relating to the spinal cord and the muscles supplied by the spinal nerves.
**spinoneural** (spi-no-nu'ral). Relating to the spinal cord and the nerves given off from it.
**spi'nose.** Spinous.
**spinotectal** (spi-no-tek'tal). Spinocollicular; passing upward from the spinal cord to the tectum.
**spi'notransversa'rius.** The splenius and obliquus capitis major muscles regarded as one.
**spinous** (spi'nus). Relating to, shaped like, or having a spine or spines.
**spintharicon** (spin-thăr'ĭ-kon) [ G. *spinthēr,* spark ]. A spark chamber device used to record the distribution of low energy emissions from radiopharmaceuticals administered internally, especially for thyroid scans using iodine-125.
**spinthariscope** (spin-thăr'ĭ-skōp) [ G. *spinthēr,* spark, + *skopeō,* to view ]. Scintillation *counter.*
**spin'therism** [ G. *spinthēr,* spark ]. Obsolete term for photopsia.
**spintherometer** (spin'ther-om'e-ter) [ G. *spinthēr,* spark, + *metron,* measure ]. An apparatus for determining the penetrating power of x-rays by measuring the degree of vacuity in the tube.
**spintheropia** (spin-ther-o'pī-ah) [ G. *spinthēr,* spark, + *ōps,* eye ]. Obsolete term for photopsia.
**spinulosin** (spi-nu-lo'sin). Hydroxyfumigatin; 3,6-dihydroxy-5-methoxy-*p*-toluquinone; an antibiotic agent isolated from cultures of *Aspergillus fumigatus.*
**spip'erone** (USAN). SPIROPITAN; 8-[ 3-(*p*-fluorobenzoyl)-propyl ]-1-phenyl-1,3,8-triazaspiro[ 4.5 ]decan-4-one; tranquilizer.
**spir-.** See spiro-.
**spiracle** (spi'rā-kl, spīr-) [ L. *spiraculum,* fr. *spiro,* to breathe ]. In arthropods and in sharks and related fishes, an aperture for breathing.
**spi'radeni'tis** [ L. *spiro,* to breathe or perspire, + G. *adēn,* gland, + suffix -*itis,* inflammation ]. *Hidradenitis* suppurativa.
**spiradenoma** (spi-rad'ĕ-no'mah) [ G. *speira,* coil, + adenoma ]. Spiroma; a benign tumor of sweat glands.
   **eccrine s.,** nodular *hidradenoma.*
**spi'ral** [ Mediev. L. *spiralis,* fr. G. *speira,* a coil. SPIR-1). 1. Coiled; winding around a center like a watch spring; winding and ascending like a wire spring. 2. A structure in the shape of a coil.
   **Curschmann's s.'s,** spirally twisted masses of mucus occurring in the sputum in bronchial asthma.

**spiramycin** (spīr'ă-mi'sin) (USAN). ROVAMYCIN; antibiotic substance produced by *Streptomyces ambofaciens;* antimicrobial agent.

**spirem, spireme** (spi'rem, spi'rēm) [ G. *speirēma,* a coil. SPIR-1 ]. Term formerly applied to first stage of mitosis when extended chromosome filaments have appearance of loose ball of yarn, under incorrect hypothesis that the filaments were continuous and later broke apart to form individual chromosomes.

**spiril'la.** Plural of *Spirillum.*

**Spirillaceae** (spi-rī-la'se-e) [ see *Spirillum* ]. A family of usually motile, aerobic to facultatively anaerobic bacteria (order Pseudomonadales) containing Gram-negative, rod-shaped cells which are curved or spirally twisted. Motile cells contain a single polar flagellum or a tuft of polar flagella. These organisms are primarily water forms, although some are parasitic or pathogenic on man and other higher animals. The type genus is *Spirillum.*

**spirillicidal** (spi-ril-ĭ-si'dal) [ spirilla + L. *caedo,* to kill ]. Destructive to spirilla or spirochetes.

**spirillosis** (spi'rĭ-lo'sis). Any disease caused by the presence of spirilla in the blood or tissues.

**Spirillum** (spi-ril'um) [ Mod. L. dim. of L. *spira,* coil, fr. G. *speira* ]. A genus of large (1.4 to 1.7 μm in diameter), rigid, helical, Gram-negative bacteria (family Spirillaceae) which are motile by means of bipolar fascicles of flagella. These organisms are obligately microaerophilic and chemoorganotrophic, possessing a strictly respiratory metabolism; they neither oxidize nor ferment carbohydrates. The habitat of these organisms is fresh water. This genus contains only a single species, *S. volutans,* the type species.

   **S. un'dula,** a species formerly regarded as the type species of *S.;* this and other species formerly placed in this genus have been transferred to the genus *Aquaspirillum* or to *Oceanospirillum.*

   **S. vol'utans,** a species found in fresh water; it is the type species of *S.*

**spiril'lum,** pl. **spiril'la.** A member of the genus *Spirillum.*

   **Obermeier's s.** *Borrelia recurrentis.*

   **Vincent's s.,** the s. or spirochete found in association with Vincent's bacillus.

**spirit** (spīr'it) [ L. *spiritus,* a breathing, life soul, fr. *spiro,* to breathe. SPIR-2 ]. 1. An alcoholic liquor stronger than wine, obtained by distillation. 2. Any distilled liquid. 3. An alcoholic or hydroalcoholic solution of volatile substances; some s.'s are used as flavoring agents, others have medicinal value.

   **ardent s.'s,** brandy, whiskey, and other forms of distilled alcoholic liquors.

   **industrial methylated s.** (BP), denatured *alcohol.*

   **meth'ylated s.,** denatured *alcohol.*

   **proof s.,** spiritus tenuior; dilute alcohol of a specific gravity of 0.920, containing 49.5 per cent by weight (57.27 per cent by volume) of $C_2H_5OH$ at 15.56°C. Originally in England it was the weakest alcohol which would permit ignition of gunpowder moistened with it. British proof s. has a specific gravity of 0.9198 and contains 49.2 per cent $C_2H_5OH$ by weight, or 57.1 per cent by volume at the temperature of 51°F.

   **pyrolig'neous s.,** methyl alcohol (see under methyl).

   **pyroxyl'ic s.,** methyl alcohol.

   **rectified s.,** alcohol (2).

   **vital s.'s,** in the Galenical teachings, a vital essence or principle supposed to be generated from the air or pneuma in the left ventricle of the heart; carried in the blood to the brain, it was converted to animal s.'s which then flowed along the nerves to all parts of the body. See also Galen.

   **wine s.,** ethyl alcohol (see under ethyl).

   **wood s.,** methyl alcohol (see under methyl).

**spirituous** (spīr'ĭ-tu-us). Alcoholic; containing alcohol in large amount, denoting liquors.

**spiritus,** gen. and pl. **spiritus** (spīr'ĭ-tus) [ L. ]. Spirit.

   **s. frumen'ti,** whisky.

   **s. tenuior** [ L. weaker spirit ], proof *spirit.*

   **s. vini rectifica'tus,** alcohol.

   **s. vini vitis,** brandy.

**spiro-, spir-** (spi'ro-). 1 [ G. *speira,* a coil. SPIR-1 ]. Combining forms meaning coil or coil-shaped. 2 [ L. *spiro,* to breathe. SPIR-2 ]. Combining forms relating to breathing.

**spirobarbit'urate.** A barbiturate with an alkyl substitution at position 5 that forms a ring structure.

**Spirocerca lupi** (spi'ro-ser'kah lu'pi) [ L. fr. G. *speira,* coil, + G. *kerkos,* tail; L. *lupus,* wolf ]. The esophageal worm of dogs and other carnivores, a bright red spiruroid nematode that occurs in nodules in the wall of the esophagus, stomach, and aorta of dogs, foxes, and wolves; clinical symptoms occur only in very heavy infestations. Intermediate hosts are various coprophagous beetles.

**Spirochaeta** (spi'ro-ke'tah) [ Mod. L. fr. G. *speira,* a coil, + *chaitē,* hair ]. A genus of motile bacteria (order Spirochaetales) containing presumably Gram-negative, flexible, undulating, spiral-shaped rods which may or may not possess flagelliform, tapering ends. The protoplast is spirally wound around an axial filament. No obvious periplast membrane or cross-striations occur. These organisms are motile by means of a creeping motion over the surfaces of supporting objects. They are not parasitic, but are found free-living in fresh or sea water slime; they are commonly found in sewage and foul waters. At present there are five species in this genus. The type species is *S. plicatilis.*

   **S. obermei'eri,** *Borrelia recurrentis.*

   **S. plicat'ilis,** a very large species (sometimes as long as 200 μm) of bacteria. It is nonparasitic, so far as known. It is the type species of the genus *S.*

**Spirochaetaceae** (spi-ro-ke-ta'se-e) [ see *Spirochaeta* ]. A family of bacteria (order Spirochaetales) consisting of coarse, spiral cells, 30 to 50 μm in length and possessing definite protoplasmic structures. These organisms occur in stagnant, fresh or salt water and in the intestinal tracts of bivalve molluscs. The type genus is *Spirochaeta.*

**Spirochaetales** (spi-ro-ke-ta'lēz). An order of motile bacteria containing slender, flexuous cells, 6 to 500 μm in length, in the form of spirals with at least one complete turn. Some species may have an axial filament, a lateral crista, or ridge, or transverse striations. All of these organisms are motile, whirling or spinning about the long axis, thus driving the organism forward or backward. Free-living, saprophytic, and parasitic forms occur. The type family is *Spirochaetaceae.*

**spirochetal** (spi-ro-kē'tal). Relating to spirochetes, especially to infection with such organisms.

**spirochete** (spi'ro-kēt). Any individual of the genus *Spirochaeta.*

**spirocheticide** (spi-ro-ke'tĭ-sīd) [ spirochete + L. *caedo,* to kill ]. An agent destructive to spirochetes.

**spirochetolysis** (spi-ro-ke-tol'ĭ-sis) [ spirochete + G. *lysis,* a loosening ]. Destruction of spirochetes, by chemotherapy or by specific antibodies.

**spirochetosis** (spi-ro-ke-to'sis). Any disease caused by a spirochete.

   **avian s.,** a very highly fatal disease of chickens, turkeys and pheasants caused by *Borrelia anserina* and transmitted chiefly by the fowl tick, *Argas persicus.*

   **bronchopulmonary s.,** hemorrhagic *bronchitis.*

**spirochetotic** (spi-ro-ke-tot'ik). Relating to or marked by spirochetosis.

**spi'rogram.** The tracing made by the spirograph.

**spi'rograph** [ L. *spiro,* to breathe, + G. *graphō,* to write ]. Anapnograph; a device for representing graphically the depth and rapidity of respiratory movements.

**spiro-index.** The vital capacity divided by the height.

**spiro'ma.** Spiradenoma.

**spirometer** (spi-rom'e-ter) [ L. *spiro,* to breathe, + G. *metron,* measure ]. Pneometer.

**Spirome'tra** [ G. *speira,* coil, + *metra,* womb (uterus) ]. A genus of pseudophyllid tapeworms.

   **S. manso'ni,** a species of pseudophyllid tapeworm of wild and feral cats, but the larval form (sparganum) may survive in human tissues; *S. mansoni* has been commonly found in man in the Orient, but is also reported from widely scattered areas elsewhere; infection of man with the sparganum occurs from active migration of the larva from the fresh split infected frogs used as a poultice for wounds, sore eyes (see ocular *sparganosis*), bruises, or ulcerations; it is also likely that man may be infected with sparganum larvae from eating any vertebrate harboring these plerocercoids.

**S. mansonoi'des,** a species of pseudophyllid tapeworm from North America, whose larva (sparganum) may be a cause of sparganosis of man in Florida and the Gulf States.

**spirometry** (spi-rom'e-tri). Pneometry.

**spironolactone** (spi'ro-no-lak'tōn). (USP, BP). ALDAC-TONE-A; 3-(3-oxo-7α-acetylthio-17β-hydroxy-4-andros-ten-17α-yl)propionic acid-α-lactone; a diuretic agent that blocks the renal tubular actions of aldosterone. It increases the urinary excretion of sodium and chloride, decreases the excretion of potassium and ammonium, and reduces the titratable acidity of the urine. It is most effectively used to potentiate the natriuretic action and reduce the potassium excretion produced by other diuretics. Its toxicity appears to be minimal. Used in the treatment of edema associated with hepatic cirrhosis, congestive heart failure, idiopathic edema, and the nephrotic syndrome.

**spirophore** (spi'ro-fōr) [ L. *spiro,* to breathe, + G. *phoros,* bearing ]. A pneumatic cabinet used for artificial respira-tion; the patient is placed in the cabinet, with his head outside, and as the air within is alternately exhausted and under pressure the patient is made to inhale and exhale.

**spiroscope** (spi'ro-skōp) [ L. *spiro,* to breathe, + G. *skopeō,* to view ]. A device for measuring the air capacity of the lungs.

**spi'rostan.** A 16,22;22,26-diepoxycholestane (for struc-ture, see steroids).

**spirothiobar'bital** SPIROTHAL; 1-ethyl-2,4-dimethyl-8-thio-7,9-diazaspiro[ 4,5 ]decane-6,8,10-trione; hypnotic.

**spiruroid** (spi'ru-royd). Common name for a member of the superfamily Spiruroidea.

**Spiruroidea** (Spi-ru-roy'dī-ah). A superfamily of nema-todes including the genera *Gnathostoma, Gongylonema, Habronema, Physaloptera, Physocephalus, Spirocerca,* and *Thelazia.*

**spis'sated** [ L. *spisso,* pp. *spissatus,* to thicken ]. Inspis-sated; thickened.

**spis'situde** [ L. *spissitudo,* fr. *spissus,* thick ]. The state of being inspissated; denoting the condition of a fluid thickened almost to a solid by evaporation or inspissation.

**spit'ting.** Expectoration.

**spittle** (spit'l) [ A.S. *spātl* ]. Saliva.

**Spitzer's theory.** See under theory.

**Spitz'ka,** Edward C., New York neurologist, 1852–1914. See S.'s *nucleus,* marginal *tract,* marginal *zone.*

**Spix,** Johann B., German anatomist, 1781–1826. See S.'s *spine.*

**splanchn-.** See splanchno-.

**splanchnapophysial, -physeal** (splangk'nă-po-fiz'ī-al). Relating to a splanchnapophysis.

**splanchnapophysis** (splangk'nă-pof'ī-sis) [ splanchn- + G. *apophysis,* offshoot ]. An apophysis of the typical vertebra, on the side opposite to the neural apophysis, and enclosing any viscera.

**splanchnectopia** (splangk'nek-to'pī-ah) [ splanchn- + G. *ektopos,* out of place ]. Splanchnodiastasis; displacement of any of the viscera.

**splanchnemphraxis** (splangk'nem-frak'sis) [ splanchn- + G. *emphraxis,* a stoppage ]. Intestinal obstruction.

**splanchnesthesia** (splangk'nes-the'zī-ah) [ splanch- + G. *aisthēsis,* sensation ]. Visceral *sense.*

**splanchnic** (splangk'nik). Visceral.

**splanchnicectomy** (splangk-nī-sek'to-mī) [ splanchni- + G. *ektomē,* excision ]. Resection of the splanchnic nerves and usually of the celiac ganglion as well.

**splanchnicotomy** (splangk-nī-kot'o-mī) [ splanchni- + G. *tomē,* incision ]. Section of a splanchnic nerve or nerves, a surgical procedure used in the treatment of arterial hypertension.

**splanchno-, splanchn-, splanchni-** (splangk'no-) [ G. *splanchnon,* viscus. SPLAN- ]. Combining forms relating to the viscera. See also viscero-.

**splanchnocele** (splangk'no-sēl). 1 [ G. *koilos,* hollow ]. The primitive body cavity or celom in the embryo. 2 [ G. *kēlē,* hernia ]. Hernia of any of the abdominal viscera.

**splanchnocramium** (splangk'no-kra'nī-um). Viscerocra-nium.

**splanchnodiastasis** (splangk'no-di-as'tă-sis) [ splanchno- + G. *diastasis,* separation ]. Splanchnectopia.

**splanchnography** (splangk-nog'ră-fī) [ splanchno- + G. *graphō,* to write ]. A treatise on or description of the viscera.

**splanchnolith** (splangk'no-lith) [ splanchno- + G. *lithos,* stone ]. An intestinal calculus.

**splanchnologia** (splangk'no-lo'jī-ah) [ NA ]. Splanchnol-ogy.

**splanchnology** (splangk-nol'ŏ-jī) [ splanchno- + G. *logos,* study ]. The branch of medical science dealing with the viscera.

**splanchnomegaly** (splangk-no-meg'ă-lī) [ splanchno- + G. *megas,* large ]. Visceromegaly.

**splanchnomicria** (splangk'no-mi'krī-ah) [ splanchno- + G. *mikros,* small ]. A condition in which the splanchnic organs are of smaller than normal size.

**splanchnopathy** (splangk-nop'ă-thī) [ splanchno- + G. *pathos,* disease ]. Disease of the abdominal viscera.

**splanchnopleural** (splangk'no-ploor'al). Splanchnopleu-ric.

**splanchnopleure** (splangk'no-ploor) [ splanchno- + G. *pleura,* side ]. The embryonic layer formed by the associa-tion of the visceral layer of the lateral mesoderm with the entoderm.

**splanchnopleuric** (splangk'no-ploor'ik). Splanchno-pleural; relating to the splanchnopleure.

**splanchnoptosis, splanchnoptosia** (splangk'nop-to'sis, -to'sī-ah) [ splanchno- + G. *ptosis,* a falling ]. Visceropto-sis.

**splanchnosclerosis** (splangk'no-skle-ro'sis) [ splanchno- + G. *sklērōsis,* hardening ]. Hardening, through connec-tive tissue overgrowth, of any of the viscera.

**splanchnoscopy** (splangk-nos'ko-pī) [ splanchno- + G. *skopeō,* to view ]. Examination of the viscera by roentgen rays.

**splanchnoskeletal** (splangk'no-skel'ē-tal). Visceroskele-tal.

**splanchnoskeleton** (splangk'no-skel'ē-ton). Visceroskele-ton.

**splanchnosomatic** (splangk'no-so-mat'ik) [ splanchno- + G. *sōma,* body ]. Viscerosomatic.

**splanchnotomy** (splangk-not'o-mī) [ splanchno- + G. *tomē,* a cutting ]. Visceral *anatomy.*

**splanchnotribe** (splangk'no-trīb) [ splanchno- + G. *tribō,* to rub, bruise ]. An instrument resembling a large angio-tribe used for occluding the intestine temporarily, prior to resection.

**splay.** The rounding of the corner on the graph relating rate of renal tubular secretion or reabsorption of a substance to its arterial plasma concentration, due primar-ily to the fact that some nephrons reach their tubular maximum before others do.

**splay'foot.** *Talipes* planus.

**spleen** [ G. *splēn.* SPLEN- ]. Lien; a large vascular lym-phatic organ lying in the upper part of the abdominal cavity on the left side, between the stomach and dia-phragm. It is composed of white pulp consisting of lymphatic nodules and diffuse lymphatic tissue and of red pulp consisting of venous sinusoids between which are splenic cords. The stroma of both red and white pulp is reticular fibers and cells. A framework of fibroelastic trabeculae extending from the capsule subdivides the structure into poorly defined lobules. The spleen is a blood-forming organ in early life. It is a storage organ for red corpuscles, and, because of the large number of macrophages, acts as a blood filter.

**accessory s.,** splenule; spleneolus; an additional isolated body, composed of splenic tissue, found usually in one of the peritoneal folds or elsewhere.

**bacon s.,** lardaceous s.; amyloid degeneration of the s.

**diffuse waxy s.,** a condition of amyloid degeneration of the s., affecting chiefly the extrasinusoidal tissue spaces of the pulp.

**floating s.,** movable s.; a s. that is palpable because of excessive mobility from a relaxed or lengthened pedicle rather than because of enlargement.

**larda'ceous s.,** waxy s.

**movable s.,** floating s.

**sago s.,** amyloidosis in the s. affecting chiefly the Malpighian bodies.

**sugar-coated s.,** hyaloserositis (*q. v.*) involving the s.

**waxy s.,** amyloidosis of the s.

**splen-.** See spleno-.

**splenadenoma** (splen'ad-ē-no'mah) [ splen- + G. *adēn*, gland, + suffix *-oma*, tumor ]. Enlargement of the spleen as a result of hyperplasia of the pulp.

**splenalgia** (sple-nal'jī-ah) [ splen- + G. *algos*, pain ]. Splenodynia; a painful condition of the spleen.

**splenauxe** (sple-nawk'se) [ splen- + G. *auxē*, increase ]. Splenomegaly.

**Splendore,** A. See Lutz-S.-Almeida *disease.*

**splenectasia** (splen'ek-ta'zī-ah) [ splen- + G. *ektasis*, extension ]. Enlargement of the spleen.

**splenectomize** (sple-nek'to-mīz). To perform splenectomy on.

**splenectomy** (sple-nek'to-mī) [ splen- + G. *ektomē*, excision ]. Removal of the spleen.

**splenectopia, splenectopy** (splen'ek-to'pī-ah, sple-nek'-to-pī) [ splen- + G. *ektopos*, out of place ]. 1. Displacement of the spleen, as in a floating spleen. 2. The presence of rests of splenic tissue, usually in the region of the spleen.

**splenelcosis** (splen'el-ko'sis) [ splen- + G. *helkōsis*, ulceration ]. Abscess of the spleen.

**splenemia** (sple-ne'mī-ah). Splenic *leukemia.*

**splenemphraxis** (splen'em-frak'sis, sple'nem-) [ splen- + G. *emphraxis*, stoppage ]. Congestion of the spleen.

**spleneolus** (sple-ne'o-lus) [ Mod. L. dim. of G. *splēn* ]. Accessory *spleen.*

**splenepatitis** (splen'ep'ā-ti'tis) [ splen- + G. *hēpar* (*hēpat-*), liver, + suffix *-itis*, inflammation ]. Inflammation of both spleen and liver.

**splenetic** (sple-net'ik). 1. Splenic; relating to the spleen. 2. Suffering from chronic disease of the spleen. 3. Fretful; surly.

**sple'nial** [ G. *splēnion*, bandage ]. 1. Relating to the splenium. 2. Relating to a splenius muscle.

**splen'ic.** Relating to the spleen.

**splenicterus** (sple-nik'ter-us) [ splen- + G. *ikteros*, jaundice (icterus) ]. Jaundice associated with splenitis.

**spleniculus** (sple-nik'u-lus) [ Mod. L. ]. Accessory *spleen.*

**splen'ifica'tion.** Obsolete term for red *hepatization.*

**spleniform** (splen'ī-form, sple'nī-). Splenoid.

**spleniserrate** (splen'ī-sĕr'āt). Relating to the splenius and serratus muscles.

**splenitis** (sple-ni'tis) [ splen- + G. suffix *-itis*, inflammation ]. Lienitis; inflammation of the spleen.

**splenium, pl. splenia** (sple'nī-um, -ah) [ Mod. L. fr. G. *splēnion*, bandage ]. 1. A compress or bandage. 2 [ NA ]. A structure resembling a bandaged part.

**s. cor'poris callo'si** [ NA ], tuber corporis callosi; the thickened posterior extremity of the corpus callosum.

**splenius** (sple'nī-us) [ Mod. L. fr. G. *splēnion*, a bandage ]. See under musculus.

**splenization** (splen'ī-za'shun). Obsolete term for red *hepatization.*

**spleno-, splen-** (sple'no-) [ G. *splēn*, spleen. SPLEN- ]. Combining forms relating to the spleen.

**splenocele** (sple'no-sēl) [ spleno- + G. *kēlē*, tumor, hernia ]. Lienocele. 1. A splenic tumor. 2. A splenic hernia.

**splenocleisis** (sple'no-kli'sis) [ spleno- + G. *kleisis*, closure ]. Inducing the formation of new fibrous tissue on the surface of the spleen by friction or wrapping with gauze.

**splenocolic** (sple'no-kol'ik). Relating to the spleen and the colon; denoting a ligament or fold of peritoneum passing between the two viscera.

**splenocyte** (sple'no-sit) [ spleno- + G. *kytos*, cell ]. A phagocytic mononuclear leukocyte of the spleen.

**splenodynia** (sple'no-din'ī-ah) [ spleno- + G. *odynē*, pain ]. Splenalgia.

**splenography** (sple-nog'rā-fī) [ spleno- + G. *graphō*, to write ]. 1. Splenic venography; X-ray of the spleen after injection of contrast material into it. 2. A treatise on or description of the spleen.

**sple'nohe'mia.** Splenic *leukemia.*

**splenohepatomegaly, splenohepatomegalia** (sple'no-hep'ă-to-meg'ā-lī, -mē-ga'lī-ah) [ spleno- + G. *hēpar*, liver, + *megas*, large ]. Enlargement of both spleen and liver.

**splenoid** (sple'noyd) [ spleno- + G. *eidos*, resemblance ]. Spleniform; resembling the spleen.

**splenokeratosis** (sple'no-kĕr'ā-to'sis) [ spleno- + keratosis, *q. v.* ]. Induration of the spleen.

**sple'nolaparot'omy.** Laparosplenotomy.

**splenology** (sple-nol'o-jī) [ spleno- + G. *logos*, study ]. The branch of medical science that has to do with the spleen.

**sple'nolymphat'ic.** Relating to the spleen and the lymph nodes.

**splenol'ysin.** A specific antibody destructive to the splenic cells, obtained by means of injection of splenic pulp into an animal.

**splenolysis** (sple-nol'ī-sis) [ spleno- + G. *lysis*, dissolution ]. Destruction of the splenic tissue.

**splenoma** (sple-no'mah) [ spleno- + G. suffix *-oma*, tumor ]. Splenocele (1); splenoncus; a general, nonspecific term for an enlarged spleen.

**splenomalacia** (sple'no-mă-la'shī-ah) [ spleno- + G. *malakia*, softness ]. Lienomalacia; softening of the spleen.

**sple'nomed'ullary** [ spleno- + L. *medulla*, marrow ]. Splenomyelogenous.

**splenomegalia** (sple'no-mē-ga'lī-ah). Splenomegaly.

**splenomegaly** (sple'no-meg'ă-lī) [ spleno- + G. *megas* ( *megal-*), large ]. DéBove's disease; splenomegalia; megalosplenia; splenauxe; enlargement of the spleen.

**congestive s.,** enlargement of the spleen due to passive congestion; sometimes used as a synonym for Banti's syndrome.

**Egyptian s.,** term sometimes used as a synonym for schistosomiasis mansoni, although hepatomegaly and fibrosis are more consistently found than is an enlarged spleen.

**hemolyt'ic s.,** s. associated with congenital hemolytic jaundice.

**spodogenous s.,** enlargement of the spleen supposed to be due to an accumulation of degenerated erythrocytes in the organ.

**tropical s.,** visceral *leishmaniasis.*

**splenomyelogenous** (sple'no-mi'ē-loj'ē-nus) [ spleno- + G. *myelos*, marrow, + suffix *-gen*, producing ]. Splenomedullary; lienomedullary; lienomyelogenous; originating in the spleen and bone marrow; denoting a form of leukemia.

**splenomyelomalacia** (sple'no-mi'ē-lo-mă-la'shī-ah) [ spleno- + G. *myelos*, marrow, + *malakia*, softness ]. Lienomyelomalacia; pathologic softening of the spleen and bone marrow.

**splenoncus** (sple-nong'kus) [ spleno- + G. *onkos*, mass ]. Splenoma.

**splenonephric** (sple'no-nef'rik) [ spleno- + G. *nephros*, kidney ]. Lienorenal; relating to the spleen and the kidney.

**splenopancreatic** (sple'no-pan-kre-at'ik). Lienopancreatic; relating to the spleen and the pancreas.

**splenoparectasia** (sple'no-păr-ek-ta'zī-ah) [ spleno- + G. *parektasis*, a stretching out ]. Extreme enlargement of the spleen.

**splenopathy** (sple-nop'ă-thī) [ spleno- + G. *pathos*, suffering ]. Any disease of the spleen; lienopathy.

**splenopexy, splenopexia** (sple'no-pek'sī, -pek'sī-ah) [ spleno- + G. *pēxis*, fixation ]. Suturing in place an ectopic or wandering spleen.

**splenophrenic** (sple'no-fren'ik) [ spleno- + G. *phrēn*, diaphragm ]. Relating to the spleen and the diaphragm; denoting a ligament or fold of peritoneum extending between the two structures.

**splenopneumonia** (sple-no-nu-mo'nī-ah). Pneumonia with extensive splenization of the lung, the exudate filling the smaller bronchi as well as the alveoli.

**sple'nopor'togram.** An outline of the portal vascular bed obtained at x-ray by the injection of radiopaque material into the spleen.

**splenoportography** (sple'no-pōr-tog'rā-fī) [ spleno- + portography, *q. v.* ]. The introduction of radiopaque material into the spleen to obtain an x-ray delineation of the portal vessel of the portal circulation.

**splenoptosis, splenoptosia** (sple'nop-to'sis, -to'sĭ-ah) [ spleno- + G. *ptōsis*, falling ]. Downward displacement of the spleen, as in a floating spleen.

**splenorrhagia** (sple'no-ra'jĭ-ah) [ spleno- + G. *rhēgnymi*, to burst forth ]. Hemorrhage from a ruptured spleen.

**splenorrhaphy** (sple-nor'ră-fĭ) [ spleno- + G. *rhaphē*, suture ]. 1. Suturing a ruptured spleen. 2. Splenopexia.

**spleno'sis.** Hypersplenism; overactivity of splenic function, especially with regard to its supposedly destructive action on the platelets or erythrocytes.

**splenotomy** (sple-not'o-mĭ) [ spleno- + G. *tomē*, incision ]. 1. Anatomy or dissection of the spleen. 2. A surgical operation on the spleen.

**sple'notox'in** [ spleno- + G. *toxikon*, poison ]. A cytotoxin specific for cells of the spleen; lienotoxin.

**splenulus,** pl. **splenuli** (splen'u-lus, -li) [ Mod. L. dim. of L. *splen*, spleen. SPLEN- ]. Accessory *spleen*.

**splenunculus,** pl. **splenunculi** (sple-nung'ku-lus, -li) [ Mod. L. dim. of L. *splen*, spleen ]. Accessory *spleen*.

**splint** [ Middle Dutch *splinte* ]. 1. An appliance for preventing movement of a joint or for the fixation of displaced or movable parts. 2. The s. bone, or fibula.

  **airplane s.,** one that keeps the arm at shoulder level.

  **anchor s.,** one used for fracture of jaw, with wires around teeth and held in place by a rod.

  **Anderson s.,** a skeletal traction s., with pins inserted into proximal and distal ends of a fracture and reduction obtained by an external plate attached to the pins.

  **Balkan s.,** see Balkan *frame*.

  **banjo s.,** see fig.

  **Bava'rian s.,** a s. made of plaster of Paris between two layers of flannel; when it is in place, adapted to the limb, the plaster is moistened and sets into a firm, perfectly fitting s.

  **Cabot's s.,** a metal frame placed posterior to thigh and leg.

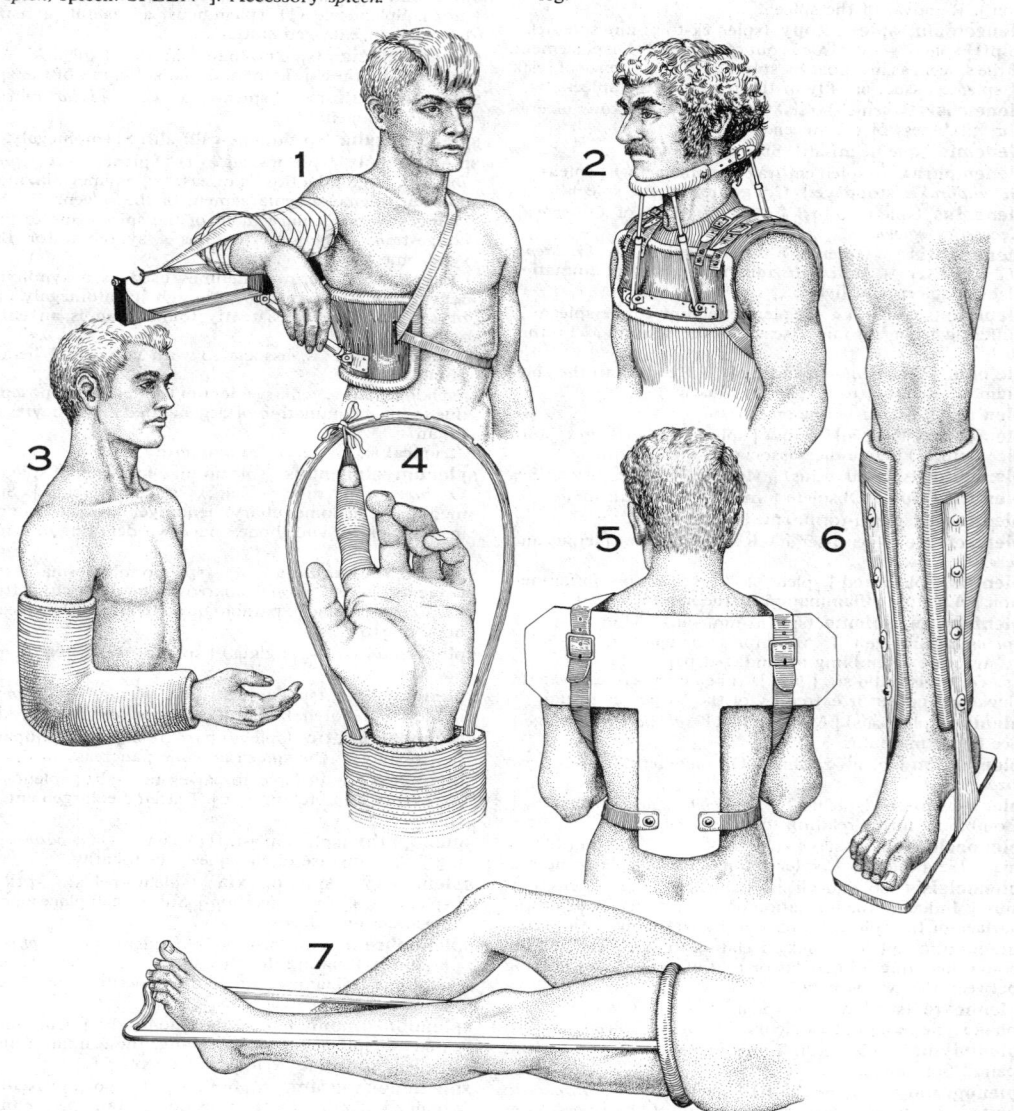

**Types of Splint**

*1,* Airplane splint; *2,* cervical splint; *3,* plaster splint; *4,* banjo splint; *5,* "T" splint; *6,* short convalescent splint; *7,* Hodgen's splint.

**cap s.,** a plastic or metallic fracture appliance designed to cover the crowns of the teeth and usually cemented to them.

**coapta'tion s.,** a short s. designed to prevent overriding of the ends of a fractured bone, usually supplemented by a longer s. to fix the entire limb.

**contact s.,** a slotted plate, held by screws, used in the treatment of fracture of long bones.

**Cramer's s.,** a flexible s., consisting of two stout wires, parallel, with fine cross wires, resembling a ladder.

**Denis-Browne s.,** a light aluminum s. applied to the lateral aspect of the leg and foot; used for clubfoot.

**DePuy's s.,** a brace for fracture of the clavicle.

**dynamic s.,** functional s. (1); one that aids in the movements initiated by the patient; controls the plane and range of motion.

**Essig-type s.,** a stainless steel wire passed labially and lingually around a segment of the dental arch and held in position by individual ligature wires around the contact areas of the teeth; used to stabilize fractured or repositioned teeth and the involved alveolar bone.

**functional s.,** (1) dynamic s.; (2) the joining of two or more teeth into a rigid unit by means of fixed restorations that cover all or part of the abutment teeth.

**Gordon's s.,** a s. for fracture of the distal end of the radius.

**Gunning's s.,** a prosthesis fabricated from models of endentulous maxillary and mandibular arches in order to aid in reduction and fixation of a fracture.

**Hodgen's s.,** a s. for fractures of the middle or lower end of the femur; it offers a supportive role for traction.

**interden'tal s.,** a s. for a fractured jaw, consisting of two metal or acrylic resin bands wired to the teeth of the upper and lower jaws, respectively, and then fastened together to keep the jaws immovable.

**Kingsley s.,** a winged maxillary s. used to apply traction to reduce maxillary fractures as well as immobilize them by having the wings attached to a head appliance by elastics; also called reverse Kingsley s.

**labial s.,** an appliance of plastic, metal, or in combination, made to conform to the outer aspect of the dental arch and used in the management of jaw and facial injuries.

**lingual s.,** one similar to the labial s., but conforming to the inner aspect of the dental arch.

**Liston's s.,** a long s. extending from the axilla to the sole of the foot.

**plaster s.,** a s. constructed of bandages impregnated with plaster of Paris.

**reverse Kingsley s.,** see Kingsley s.

**shin s.'s,** see shin-splints.

**Stader s.,** with metal pins through proximal and distal segments of a long bone fracture, the fixation of the pins is maintained by the apparatus which is external to the limb.

**Stromeyer's s.,** a hinged s. for the knee, admitting of being set at any angle.

**surgical s.,** one of many devices used to maintain tissues in a new position following surgery.

**T s.,** see fig.

**Taylor's s.,** Taylor's *apparatus.*

**Thomas' s.,** (1) rigid s., made of steel bars curved to the shape of the limb and retained by plaster of Paris bandages, used in the treatment of chronic joint diseases; with modification, called a Tobruk s. (2) a rigid bar metal s. extending from a ring at the hip to beyond the foot, allowing traction to a fractured leg, for emergencies and transportation.

**Tobruk s.,** a modification of the Thomas s., in which the limb is partially encased in plaster which goes circumferentially around the s. and the limb to prevent lateral displacement; probably named after the port of Tobruk, where, during World War II, it was used to immobilize the limb during hazardous conditions such as transport from small boats to large boats.

**Volkmann's s.,** a s. for fractures of the lower extremity, consisting of a guttered splint with a footpiece with two lateral supports to prevent turning.

**wire s.,** a device to stabilize teeth loosened by accident or by a periodontal condition in the maxilla or mandible; a device to reduce and stabilize maxillary or mandibular fractures by applying it to both jaws and connecting it by intermaxillary wires or rubber bands.

**splint'ing.** In dentistry, the joining of two or more teeth into a rigid unit by means of fixed or removable restorations or appliances.

**splints** [ see splint ]. Exostoses occurring along the course of the small metacarpal and metatarsal bones of the horse.

**"splitters."** Those who classify diseases into many small groups according to differences, rather than into a few large groups because of similarities ("lumpers").

**split'ting.** In chemistry, the cleavage of a covalent bond, fragmenting the molecule involved.

**spodiomyelitis** (spod'ĭ-o-mi-ĕ-li'tis) [ G. *spodios,* gray (ash-colored), + myelitis, *q.v.* ]. Poliomyelitis.

**spodogenous** (spō-doj'ĕ-nus) [ G. *spodos,* ashes, + suffix -*gen,* producing ]. Caused by waste material.

**spo'dogram** [ G. *spodos,* ashes, + *gramma,* a drawing ]. The pattern of ash residue formed by microincineration of a minute tissue specimen, usually a thin section.

**spodography** (spo-dog'-rä-fī) [ G. *spodos,* ashes, + *graphō,* to write ]. Microincineration.

**spodophagous** (spo-dof'ä-gus) [ G. *spodos,* ashes, + *phagein,* to eat ]. Eating the waste materials of the body.

**spodophorous** (spō-dof'o-rus) [ G. *spodos,* ashes, + *phoros,* bearing ]. Removing or carrying off waste materials from the body.

**spoke-shave.** Ring-knife.

**sponda'ic.** Relating to spondee.

**spon'dees** [ Fr. ]. Bisyllabic words with generally equivalent stress on the two syllables; used in the testing of speech hearing.

**spondyl-.** See spondylo-.

**spondylalgia** (spon'dī-lal'jī-ah) [ spondyl- + G. *algos,* pain ]. Rachialgia.

**spondylarthritis** (spon-dil-ar-thri'tis) [ spondyl- + G. *arthron,* joint, + suffix -*itis,* inflammation ]. Inflammation of the intervertebral articulations.

**spondylarthrocace** (spon-dil-ar-throk'ă-se) [ spondyl- + G. *arthron,* joint, + kakē, badness ]. Spondylocace. 1. Tuberculous *spondylitis.* 2. Rust's *disease.*

**spondylexarthrosis** (spon'dil-eks'ar-thro'sis) [ spondyl- + G. *ex,* out of, + *arthron,* joint, + suffix -*osis,* inflammation ]. Obsolete term for dislocation of a vertebra.

**spondylitic** (spon'dī-lit'ik). Relating to spondylitis.

**spondylitis** (spon-dī-li'tis) [ spondyl- + G. suffix -*itis,* inflammation ]. Inflammation of one or more of the vertebrae.

**ankylosing s.,** arthritis of the spine, resembling rheumatoid arthritis, that may progress to bony ankylosis with lipping of vertebral margins; the disease is more common in the male and rheumatoid factor is often absent; also known as Marie's disease; Strümpell-Marie or Marie-Strümpell disease; rheumatoid s.; rhizomelic spondylosis; s. rhizomelica.

**s. defor'mans,** poker back; Bechterew's disease; Strümpell's disease (1); arthritis and osteitis deformans involving the spinal column; it is marked by nodular deposits at the edges of the intervertebral disks, with ossification of the ligaments and bony ankylosis of the intervertebral articulations, and results in a rounded kyphosis with rigidity.

**Kümmell's s.,** Kümmell's *disease.*

**rheumatoid s.,** ankylosing s.

**s. rhizomel'ica,** ankylosing s.

**tuberculous s.,** tuberculous infection of the spine; also called Pott's disease; Pott's caries; spinal caries; trachelocyrtosis; trachelokyphosis; spondylarthrocace.

**s. typho'sa,** typhoid *spine.*

**spondylo-, spondyl-** (spon'dī-lo-) [ G. *spondylos,* vertebra ]. Combining forms relating to the vertebrae.

**spondylocace** (spon-dī-lok'ă-se) [ spondylo- + G. *kakē,* badness ]. Spondylarthrocace.

**spondylodynia** (spon'dī-lo-din'ī-ah) [ spondylo- + G. *odynē,* pain ]. Rachialgia.

**spondylolisthesis** (spon'dī-lo-lis-the'sis) [ spondylo- + G. *olisthēsis,* a slipping and falling ]. Spondyloptosis; forward movement of the body of one of the lower lumbar vertebrae on the vertebra below it, or upon the sacrum.

**spondylolisthetic** (spon'dī-lo-lis-thet'ĭk). Relating to or marked by spondylolisthesis.

**spondylolysis** (spon-dī-lol'ī-sis) [ spondylo- + G. *lysis*, loosening ]. 1. Breaking down or dissolution of the body of a vertebra. 2. A cleft formation in the vertebral body. 3. A loosening of the firm attachment of the contiguous vertebrae.

**spondylomalacia** (spon'dī-lo-mă-la'shī-ah) [ spondylo- + G. *malakia*, softness ]. Softening of vertebrae.

**spondylopathy** (spon'dī-lop'ă-thī) [ spondylo- + G. *pathos*, suffering ]. Rachiopathy; any disease of the vertebrae.

   **traumatic s.,** Kümmell's *disease.*

**spondyloptosis** (spon'dī-lop-to'sis, -lo-to'sis) [ spondylo- + G. *ptosis*, a falling ]. Spondylolisthesis.

**spondylopyosis** (spon'dī-lo-pi-o'sis) [ spondylo- + G. *pyosis*, suppuration ]. Suppurative inflammation of one or more of the vertebral bodies.

**spondyloschisis** (spon'dī-los'kī-sis) [ spondylo- + G. *schisis*, fissure ]. Rachischisis; congenital fissure of one or more of the vertebral arches.

**spondylo'sis** [ G. *spondylos*, vertebra ]. Vertebral ankylosis; this term is also often applied nonspecifically to any lesion of the spine of a degenerative nature.

   **cervical s.,** a general term indicating reactive changes in the vertebral bodies about the interspace, usually associated with chronic discopathy.

   **hyperostotic s.,** hypertrophic deformity of vertebrae, usually in old age.

   **rhizomel'ic s.,** ankylosing *spondylitis.*

**spondylosyndesis** (spon'dī-lo-sin-de'sis) [ spondylo- + G. *syndesis*, binding together ]. Spinal *fusion.*

**spondylothoracic** (spon'dī-lo-tho-ras'ik). Relating to the vertebra and the thorax.

**spondylotomy** (spon'dī-lot'o-mī) [ spondylo- + G. *tomē*, incision ]. 1. Rachiotomy; section of the spine of the fetus to facilitate delivery in case of impaction. 2. Laminectomy.

**spon'dylous.** Vertebral; relating to a vertebra.

**sponge** (spunj) [ G. *spongia* ]. 1. The fibrous skeleton of an aquatic organism from which all cellular matter has been removed, used in surgery for mopping away blood and other fluids during an operation; now usually replaced by 2. 2. Any absorbent material, such as gauze or prepared cotton, used in lieu of a s. in surgical operations.

   **absorbable gelatin s.** (USP, BP), a sterile, absorbable, water insoluble gelatin base s., employed to control capillary bleeding in surgical operations. It is left *in situ* and is absorbed in from 4 to 6 weeks.

   **Bernays' s.,** a compressed disk of aseptic cotton that swells when moistened; used in packing cavities.

   **bronchoscop'ic s.,** a small fold of gauze used on a long applicator to apply medication or remove secretions through a bronchoscope.

   **compressed s.,** a s. is impregnated with thin mucilage of acacia, wrapped with twine to the desired shape, and then dried; used to dilate sinuses, the os uteri, etc., the dried s. absorbing moisture after insertion.

   **decol'orized or bleached s.,** a s. treated successively with potassium permanganate, sodium thiosulfate, diluted hydrochloric acid, and sodium carbonate.

   **waxed s.,** purified s. cut to the desired shape and dipped in melted wax.

**spongia** (spun'jī-ah) [ G. ]. Sponge.

**spongiform** (spun'jī-form). Having the appearance of a sponge.

**spongin** (spun'jin). The fibrous or horny constituent of sponges; a scleroprotein.

**spongio-, spongi-** (spun'jī-o-) [ G. *spongia*, sponge ]. Combining forms meaning sponge, sponge-like, spongy.

**spongioblast** (spun'jī-o-blast) [ spongio- + G. *blastos*, germ ]. A filiform ependyma cell extending across the entire thickness of the wall of the brain or spinal cord, *i.e.*, from the internal to the external limiting membrane.

**spongioblastoma** (spun'jī-o-blas-to'mah) [ spongioblast + G. suffix -*oma* tumor ]. A glioma derived from spongioblasts, *i.e.*, immature forms of the astrocytic series. Sometimes termed gliosarcoma. See also glioblastoma, astrocytoma grade IV.

   **s. multiform'e,** glioblastoma multiforme; a glioma consisting chiefly of undifferentiated, anaplastic cells that

are precursors of astrocytes; the cells vary greatly in size, shape, and staining reactions; frequently, they are arranged radially about an irregular focus of necrosis, and pseudorosettes are sometimes formed. These neoplasms grow rapidly and invade extensively, and occur most frequently in the cerebrum of adult persons. Sometimes termed astrocytoma, grade IV.

   **s. polare, s. unipolare,** a glioma consisting of cells that resemble the embryonic spongioblasts occurring normally around the neural canal of the human embryo; the neoplastic cells are elongated, spindle-shaped, and sometimes pleomorphic, with one or two fibrillary processes. These neoplasms grow relatively slowly, usually originating in the brainstem, optic chiasm, or infundibulum, and infiltrate adjacent structures or cause compression of the third or fourth ventricle.

**spongiocyte** (spun'jī-o-sīt) [ spongio- + G. *kytos*, cell ]. 1. A neuroglial cell. 2. A cell in the zona fasciculata of the adrenal containing many droplets of lipid material which, after staining with hematoxylin and eosin, show pronounced vacuolization.

**spongioid** (spun'jī-oyd) [ spongio- + G. *eidos*, resemblance ]. Spongiform.

**spongiose** (spun'jī-ōs) [ L. *spongiosus* ]. Spongy; porous; resembling a sponge.

**spongiosis** (spun'jī-o'sis). Intercellular edema of the epidermis.

**spongiositis** (spun-jī-o-si'tis). Inflammation of the corpus spongiosum, or corpus cavernosum urethrae.

**spongio'sus** [ L. ] [ NA ]. Spongiose.

**spongy** (spun'jī). Of sponge-like texture; spongiform; spongioid.

**spontaneous** (spon-ta'ne-us) [ L. *spontaneus*, voluntary, capricious ]. Without apparent cause; said of disease processes or remissions.

**spoon** [ A.S. *spōn*, chip ]. An instrument consisting of a rod with a small bowl or cup-shaped extremity.

   **cataract s.,** a small spoon-shaped instrument for removing a cataractous lens.

   **Daviel's s.,** a small spoonlike instrument for removing the remains of a cataract after discission.

   **sharp s.,** an instrument with a small cup-shaped extremity having sharpened edges, used for scraping skin lesions.

   **Volkmann's s.,** a sharp s. for scraping away carious bone or other diseased tissue.

**spor-, spori-.** See sporo-.

**sporadic** (spo-rad'ik) [ G. *sporadikos*, scattered. SPER- ]. Occurring singly, not grouped; neither epidemic nor endemic.

**sporangiophore** (spo-ran'jī-o-fōr) [ sporangium + G. *phoros*, bearing ]. In fungi, a threadlike structure that bears a sporangium at its tip.

**sporangium,** pl. **sporangia** (spo-ran'ji-um, -ah) [ L. fr. G. *sporos*, seed, + *angeion*, vessel ]. An organ, within a plant or fungus, containing asexual spores.

**spore** (spōr) [ G. *sporos*, seed. SPER- ]. The reproductive cell of a protozoan Sporozoa or of a cryptogamous plant; a cell of a plant lower in organization than the seed-bearing spermatophytic plants; a resistant form of certain species of bacteria.

   **black s.,** a degenerating malarial or other blood parasite in the body of the mosquito.

**sporicidal** (spōr'ī-si'dal) [ spori- + L. *caedo*, to kill ]. Destructive to spores.

**sporicide** (spōr'ī-sīd). 1. Sporicidal. 2. An agent that kills spores.

**sporidium,** pl. **sporidia** (spo-rid'ī-um, -ah) [ Mod. L. dim. fr. G. *sporos*, seed ]. A protozoan spore; an embryonic protozoan organism.

**sporo-, spori-, spor-** [ G. *sporos*, seed. SPER- ]. Combining forms denoting seed or spore.

**sporoagglutination** (spōr'o-ă-glu-tī-na'shun). A diagnostic method in relation to the mycoses, based upon the fact that the blood of sufferers from diseases caused by fungi contains specific agglutinins that cause clumping of the spores of these organisms.

**sporoblast** (spōr'o-blast) [ sporo- + G. *blastos*, germ ]. An early stage in the development of a sporocyst prior to differentiation of the sporozoites. See also sporocyst (2).

**sporocyst** (spōr'o-sist) [ sporo- + G. *kystis*, bladder ]. 1. A larval form of digenetic trematode (fluke) that develops in the body of its intermediate host, usually a snail. The s. forms a simple, saclike structure with germinal cells that bud off internally and develop into other larval types that continue this process of larval multiplication within the snail (considered to be a form of polyembryony). See also miracidium, redia, and cercaria. 2. A secondary cyst that develops within the oocyst of Coccidia, a group of Sporozoa that includes many of the most important disease agents of domestic animals and fowl. The s., developing from a sporoblast, in turn produces within itself one or several sporozoites, the actual infective agents for subsequent infection and multiplication.

**Sporocystinea** (spōr'o-sis-tin'e-ah). A suborder of Coccidia in which the sporoblasts have sporocysts.

**sporodin** (spōr'o-din). Parasitic trophozoite stage of a gregarine in the host intestine, with the epimerite usually attached. In the intestinal wall where the cephalont was attached.

**sporogenesis** (spōr'o-jen'ĕ-sis) [ sporo- + G. *genesis*, production ]. Sporogony; sporogeny. 1. Reproduction by means of spores. 2. The process of spore production.

**sporogenous** (spo-roj'ĕ-nus). Relating to or involved in sporogenesis.

**sporogeny** (spo-roj'ĕ-nĭ). Sporogenesis.

**sporogony** (spo-rog'o-nĭ). Sporogenesis.

**sporont** (spōr'ont) [ sporo- + G. *ōn* (*ont-*), being ]. A sexually mature protozoan sporozoan parasite that has become detached from its host, leavng its attaching organ behind; it produces anisospores that conjugate to form the zygote, this developing into the schizont that begins the nonsexual cycle.

**spor'ophore** [ sporo- + G. *phoros*, bearing ]. A spore-bearing structure in fungi.

**sporoplasm** (spōr'o-plazm) [ sporo- + G. *plasma*, thing formed ]. The protoplasm of a spore.

**sporotheca** (spōr'o-the'kah) [ sporo- + G. *thēkē*, case ]. The envelope enclosing the minute needle-like spores of certain Sporozoa.

**Sporothrix** (spo'ro-thriks) [ Mod. L. fr. G. *sporos*, seed, + *thrix*, hair ]. A genus of imperfect fungi, of which *S. schenkii* (formerly *Sporotrichum schenkii*) is the causative agent of sporotrichosis in man and animals.

**Sporotrichinaceae** (spōr'o-trĭ-kĭ-na'se-e). An obsolete family name for fungi of the genus *Sporotrichum*. The proper family name is now Moniliaceae.

**sporotrichosis** (spōr'o-trĭ-ko'sis). A cutaneous and subcutaneous mycosis (affecting also the mucous membrane of the mouth and pharynx) caused by *Sporothrix (Sporotrichum) schenkii*. Three forms are described: a disseminated gummatous form (Beurmann's disease), a gummatous lymphangitis (Schenck's disease), and a hematogenous form characterized by the presence of multiple abscesses.

**Sporotrichum** (spo-rot'rĭ-kum) [ Mod. L. fr. G. *sporos*, seed, + *thrix*, hair ]. A genus of imperfect fungi that formerly included *S. schenkii;* see Sporothrix.

**Sporozoa** (spōr'o-zo'ah) [ Mod. L. fr. G. *sporos*, seed, + *zoōn*, animal ]. A subphylum (or class) of the phylum Protozoa, including parasitic forms that have no organs of locomotion, and reproduce chiefly by means of sexual or nonsexual formation of spores.

**sporozoan** (spōr'o-zo'an). 1. Relating to the Sporozoa. 2. An individual cell of the Sporozoa; a sporozoon.

**sporozoite** (spōr'o-zo'ĭt) [ sporo- + G. *zoōn*, animal ]. One of the minute elongated bodies resulting from the repeated division of the oocyst; in the case of the malarial parasite, it is the form which is concentrated in the salivary glands and introduced into the blood by the bite of a mosquito and enters the liver cells and eventually the red blood cells, there to develop into the mature schizont, which reproduces cyclically, producing vast numbers of merozoites and gametocytes which ultimately, if successful, reproduce sexually in the mosquito.

**sporozooid** (spōr'o-zo'oyd) [ sporo- + G. *zoōn*, animal, + *eidos*, resemblance ]. A falciform figure seen in certain cancerous tumors, regarded by some as a sporozoan spore or sporozoite.

**sporozoon** (spōr'o-zo'on) An individual sporozoan organism.

**sport** (spōrt). An organism varying in whole or in part, without apparent reason, from others of its type; this variation may be transmitted to the descendants or the latter may revert to the original type.

**sporular** (spōr'u-lar). Relating to a spore or sporule.

**sporulation** (spōr'u-la'shun). Multiple *fission*.

**sporule** (spōr'ūl) [ Mod. L. *sporula;* dim. of G. *sporos*, seed ]. A spore; a small spore.

**spot.** 1. Macula. 2. To lose a slight amount of blood *per vaginam*, sufficient to "spot" the napkin.

  **acous'tic s.'s**, see *macula* utriculi and *macula* sacculi.

  **Bitot's s.'s**, small, circumscribed, lusterless, grayish white, foamy, greasy, triangular deposits on the bulbar conjunctiva adjacent to the cornea in the area of the palpebral fissure of both eyes. Children and adults always give a history of malnutrition due to vitamin A deficiency.

  **blind s.**, (1) physiologic *scotoma;* (2) mental *scotoma;* (3) *discus* nervi optici.

  **blood s.'s**, hemorrhagic Graafian follicles seen in ovaries of mice, caused by injection of urine of pregnant women; positive result of Aschheim-Zondek test for pregnancy.

  **blue s.**, (1) *macula* cerulea; (2) mongolian s.

  **Brushfield's s.'s**, mottled or marbled or speckled s.'s on iris in mongolism.

  **café au lait s.'s** (kaf-a'o-la'), uniformly light brown, sharply defined, and usually oval-shaped patches of the skin that are characteristic of neurofibromatosis, but also found in normal individuals.

  **cherry-red s.**, Tay's cherry-red s.

  **corneal s.**, *macula* corneae.

  **cotton-wool s.'s**, scattered areas of white exudate in the retina, usually in posterior segment; seen in diseases causing ischemia of the precapillary retinal vessels.

  **De Morgan's s.'s**, senile *hemangioma.*

  **diffusion s.**, diffusion *circle.*

  **Elschnig's s.'s**, isolated bright yellow or red s.'s with black pigment flecks at their borders, seen ophthalmoscopically in advanced hypertensive retinopathy.

  **Filatov's s.'s**, Koplik's s.'s.

  **flame s.'s**, hemorrhagic areas in the eyegrounds, occurring in the nerve fiber layer.

  **Fordyce's s.'s**, Fordyce's disease or granules; pseudocolloid of the lips; a condition marked by the presence of numerous small, yellowish white bodies or granules on the inner surface and vermilion border of the lips; histologically the lesions are ectopic sebaceous glands.

  **germinal s.**, macula germinativa; archaic terms for the nucleolus in the nucleus of an ovum.

  **Graefe's s.'s**, small areas over the vertebrae or near the supraorbital foramen, pressure upon which causes relaxation of blepharofacial spasm.

  **hypnogenic s.**, a pressure-sensitive point on the body of certain susceptible persons, which, when pressed, causes the induction of sleep.

  **hysterogen'ic s.'s**, hysterogenic *zones.*

  **Koplik's s.'s**, Filatov's s.'s; small red s.'s on the buccal mucous membrane, in the center,of each of which may be seen, in a strong light, a minute bluish white speck; they occur early in measles (morbilli), before the skin eruption, and are regarded as a pathognomonic sign of the disease.

  **liver s.**, senile *lentigo.*

  **Mariotte's blind s.**, *discus* nervi optici.

  **Maxwell's s.**, Maxwell's ring; Löwe's ring; entoptic projection of macula and fovea, elicited by a dichromic purple filter and an alternating neutral filter while the patient is gazing at transilluminated opal glass; aids in maintaining precise fixation in visual field studies.

  **milk s.'s**, (1) soldier's patches; white plaques of hyalinized fibrous tissue situated in the epicardium overlying the right ventricle of the heart where it is not covered by lung; (2) white macroscopic areas in the omentum, due to accumulation of macrophages and lymphocytes.

  **mongolian s.'s**, mongolian maculae; dark bluish or mulberry-colored s.'s on the sacral region, observed as a congenital condition in children under 4 or 5 years old; the s.'s are rounded or oval, and do not disappear on pressure. The lesions usually disappear spontaneously.

**mulberry s.'s,** the abdominal eruption in typhus fever.

**pelvic s.,** phlebolith.

**rose s.'s,** characteristic exanthema of typhoid fever.

**Roth's s.'s,** round white s.'s surrounded by hemorrhage, observed in the retina in some cases of bacterial endocarditis, probably of embolic origin.

**ruby s.'s,** senile *hemangioma.*

**saccular s.,** *macula* sacculi.

**Soemmering's s.,** *macula* retinae.

**spongy s.,** *zona* vasculosa.

**Tay's cherry-red s.,** cherry-red s.; the choroid appearing as a red s. through the fovea centralis surrounded by a contrasting white edema; noted in cases of infantile cerebral sphingolipidosis.

**temperature s.,** one of a number of definitely arranged s.'s on the skin sensitive to heat and cold, but not to ordinary pressure or pain stimuli.

**ten'dinous s.,** *macula* albida.

**Trousseau's s.,** meningitic *streak.*

**utricular s.,** *macula* utriculi.

**white s.,** *macula* albida.

**yellow s.,** *macula* retinae.

**sprain** (sprān). 1. An injury to a joint, with possible rupture of some of the ligaments or tendons, but without dislocation or fracture. 2. To cause a s. of a joint.

**vertebral cervical s.,** a temporary subluxation that has resulted in stretching or rupture of ligaments.

**spray.** A jet of liquid in fine drops, coarser than a vapor; it is produced by forcing the liquid from the minute opening of an atomizer, mixed with air.

**spreader** (spred′er). An instrument used to distribute parts over a broader surface or area.

**rib s.,** an instrument for widening the space between ribs in intrathoracic operations.

**root canal s.,** a tapered instrument utilized for condensing root filling materials laterally.

**Sprengel,** Otto G. K., German surgeon, 1852–1915. See S.'s *deformity.*

**Sprinz-Nelson syndrome.** See under syndrome.

**sprout.** A structure resembling the s. of a plant.

**syncytial s.,** syncytial *knot.*

**sprue** (spru) [ D. *spruw* ]. 1. Psilosis; primary intestinal malabsorption with steatorrhea. 2. In dentistry, wax or metal used to form the aperture or apertures for molten metal to flow into a mold to make a casting; also, the metal that later fills the s. hole or holes.

**nontropical s.,** s. occurring in persons away from the tropics; usually associated with sensitivity to gluten and atrophy of intestinal mucous villi; in children, nontropical s. is called celiac *disease, q. v.*

**tropical s.,** aphthae orientalis or tropicae; Cochin China diarrhea; stomatitis tropica; tropical diarrhea; s. occurring in the tropics and associated with macrocytic anemia.

**sprue-former.** The base to which the sprue (2) is attached while the wax pattern is being invested in a refractory investment in a casting flask; it is sometimes referred to as a crucible-former.

**spur** [ A.S. *spora* ]. Calcar.

**Morand's s.,** *calcar* avis.

**scleral s.,** scleral roll; a ridge of the sclera at the internal scleral sulcus from which ciliary muscle fibers take origin.

**vascular s.,** partial septum between vessels (arteries and veins) at the level of fusion or branching at acute angle.

**spu'rious** [ L. *spurius* ]. False; not genuine.

**spu'rius** [ L. ] [ NA ]. Spurious.

**sputa** (spu′tah). Plural of sputum.

**sputum,** pl. **sputa** (spu′tum, -tah) [ L. *sputum,* fr. *spuo,* pp. *sputus,* to spit ]. 1. Expectorated matter, especially mucus or mucopurulent matter expectorated in diseases of the air passages. 2. An individual mass of such matter.

**s. aerogeno'sum,** green s.; a green expectoration seen occasionally in jaundice.

**albuminoid s.,** the frothy expectoration of pulmonary edema.

**s. coctum,** the opaque purulent s. of the later stage of bronchitis.

**s. crudum,** the clear, viscid mucous expectoration of the early stages of bronchitis.

**s. cruen'tum,** bloody expectoration.

**globular s.,** nummular s.

**green s.,** s. aeruginosum.

**num′mular s.,** globular s.; a thick, coherent mass expectorated in globular shape which does not run at the bottom of the cup but forms a discoid mass resembling a coin.

**prune-juice s.,** prune-juice expectoration; a thin reddish expectoration, characteristic of gangrene or cancer of the lung and certain cases of peneumonia.

**rusty s.,** a reddish brown, blood-stained expectoration characterisitc of croupous pneumonia.

**squalene** (skwa′lēn). A hexaisoprenoid triterpenoid hydrocarbon found in shark oil and in some plants; intermediate in the biosynthesis of cholesterol.

Squalene

**squama,** pl. **squamae** (skwa′mah, skwa′me) [ L. a scale ]. Squame, scale. 1 [ NA ]. A thin plate of bone. 2. An epidermic scale.

**s. fronta′lis** [ NA ], frontal s.; the broad curved portion of the frontal bone forming the forehead.

**s. occipita′lis** [ NA ], the tabular or squamous portion of occipital bone.

**s. tempora′lis,** *pars* squamosa ossis temporalis.

**squamate** (skwa′māt). Squamous.

**squamatization** (skwa′mā-tĭ-za′shun). The transformation of other types of cells into squamous cells. See also squamous *metaplasia.*

**squame** (skwām). Squama.

**squamo-** (skwa′mo-) [ L. *squama,* a scale ]. Combining form meaning squama or squamous.

**squamocellular** (skwa′mo-sel′u-lar). Relating to or having squamous epithelium.

**squamocolumnar** (skwa′mo-kol′um-nar). Pertaining to the junction between a stratified squamous epithelial surface and one lined by columnar epithelium, *e.g.,* the cardia or anus.

**squamofrontal** (skwa′mo-fron′tal). Relating to the squama frontalis.

**squamomastoid** (skwa′mo-mas′toyd). Relating to the squamous and petrous portions of the temporal bone.

**squamo-occipital** (skwa′mo-ok-sip′ĭ-tal). Relating to the squamous portion of the occipital bone, developing partly in membrane and partly in cartilage.

**squamoparietal** (skwa′mo-pă-ri′e-tal). Relating to the parietal bone and the squamous portion of the temporal bone.

**squamopetrosal** (skwa′mo-pe-tro′sal). Relating to the squamous and petrous portions of the temporal bone.

**squamosa,** pl. **squamosae** (skwa-mo′sah, -se) [ L. *squamosus,* scaly, fr. *squama,* scale ]. The squama of the frontal, occipital, or temporal bone, especially the latter.

**squamosal** (skwa-mo′sal). Squamous; relating to the squama of the temporal bone.

**squamosphenoid** (skwa′mo-sfe′noyd). Sphenosquamosal; relating to the sphenoid bone and the squama of the temporal bone.

**squamotemporal** (skwa′mo-tem′po-ral). Relating to the pars squamosa ossis temporalis.

**squamous** (skwa′mus) [ L. *squamosus* ]. Squamate; squamosal; scale-like; scaly; relating to or covered with scales; relating to a squama.

**squamozygomatic** (skwa′mo-zi-go-mat′ik). Relating to the squama and the zygomatic process of the temporal bone.

**squarrose, squarrous** (skwar′ōs, skwar′us) [ L. *squarrosus* ]. Scaly; scurfy.

**squill** (skwil) [ L. *squilla* or *scilla* ]. Scilla; the cut and dried fleshy inner scales of the bulb of the white variety of *Urginea maritima* or of *Urginea indica* (family Liliaceae). The central portion of the bulb is excluded during its processing. It contains cardiac glycosides (scillaren-A and scillaren-B). Red s. is sometimes used as a rat poison; rats poisoned with it go into clonic convulsions and die of respiratory failure. White s. is a diuretic and nauseant.

**Indian s.,** *Urginea indica.*

**Mediterranean s.,** *Urginea maritima.*

**white s.,** *Urginea maritima.*

**squint** (skwint). 1. Strabismus. 2. To suffer from strabismus.

**Sr.** Chemical symbol of the element strontium.

**SRF.** Abbreviation for somatotropin-releasing factor (somatoliberin, *q. v.*).

**SRIF.** Abbreviation for somatotropin release-inhibiting factor (somatostatin, *q. v.*).

**sRNA.** Abbreviation for soluble RNA; now known as transfer RNA (tRNA); see under ribonucleic acid.

**S roma′num.** *Colon* sigmoideum.

**SRS, SRS-A.** Abbreviation for slow-reacting substance (or slow-reacting substance of anaphylaxis); see under substance.

**ss.** Abbreviation of L. *semis,* half; in prescription writing, *cum semisse,* with (or and) a half, *e.g.,* iiss, *duo cum semisse,* two and a half.

**SSS.** Abbreviation for soluble specific *substance.*

**stab** [ Gael. *stob*]. 1. To pierce with a narrow pointed instrument, as a knife or dagger. 2. Stab wound; a wound made by stabbing. 3. A stab *culture.*

**stabile** (sta′bil, -bil) [ L. *stabilis.* STA- ]. Stable; steady; fixed; the opposite of labile; denoting (1) certain constituents of serum unaffected by ordinary degrees of heat, etc., and (2) an electrode held steadily on a part during the passage of an electric current.

**stabilimeter** (sta′bĭ-lim′e-ter) [ L. *stabilitas,* firmness, + G. *metron,* measure ]. An instrument to measure the sway of the body when standing with feet together and usually with eyes closed.

**stability** (stă-bil′ĭ-tĭ). The condition of being stabile or resistant to change.

    **denture s.,** stabilization (2); the quality of a denture to be firm, steady, constant, and resist change of position when functional forces are applied.

    **dimensional s.,** the property of a material to retain its size and form.

    **suspension s.,** a very slow sedimentation rate.

**stabilization** (sta′bĭ-lĭ-za′shun). 1. The accomplishment of a stabile state. 2. Denture *stability.*

**sta′bilizer.** 1. Something that renders something else more stable. 2. An agent that retards the effect of an accelerator, thus preserving a chemical equilibrium. 3. A part possessing the quality of rigidity or creating rigidity when added to another part.

    **endodontic s.,** a pin implant passing through the apex of a tooth from its root canal and extending well into the underlying bone to provide immobilization of periodontally involved teeth.

**stable** (sta′bl). Stabile; steady; not varying.

**stachydrine** (stak′ĭ-drēn). Hydric acid methyl betaine; the betaine of proline; found in hay and in leaves of the orange tree.

**stachyose** (stak′ĭ-ōs). A raffinosegalactopyranoside; a tetrasaccharide that yields glucose, fructose, and 2 moles of galactose upon hydrolysis; present in certain tubers and other plant tissues.

**Stacke** (stah′keh), Ludwig, German otologist, 1859–1918. See S. *operation,* Schwartze-S. *operation.*

**stactometer** (stak-tom′e-ter) [ G. *staktos,* dropping, fr. *stazō,* to let fall by drops, + *metron,* measure ]. Stalagmometer.

**Stader splint.** See under splint.

**Staderini** (stah-der-e′ne), Rutilio, Italian neuroanatomist, 19th century. See S.'s *nucleus.*

**stadiometer** (sta′dĭ-om′e-ter) [ L. *stadium, q. v.,* + G. *metron,* measure ]. An instrument for measuring standing or sitting height.

**sta′dium,** pl. **sta′dia** [ L. fr. G. *stadion,* a fixed standard length. STA- ]. A stage in the course of a disease, especially of an acute pyretic disease; see also stage, and period.

    **s. acmes,** the acme or height of a disease.

    **s. augmen′ti,** the stage of rising temperature.

    **s. calo′ris,** the feverish stage in a malarial paroxysm.

    **s. decremen′ti,** the stage of falling temperature or defervescence.

    **s. defervescen′tiae,** s. decrementi.

    **s. deflorescen′tiae,** the stage of disappearing eruption in an exanthematous disease.

    **s. florescen′tiae,** the eruptive stage in an exanthematous disease.

    **s. fri′goris,** (1) the cold stage or stage of chill in a malarial paroxysm; (2) the algid stage in cholera.

    **s. incrementi,** s. augmenti.

    **s. invasio′nis,** the prodromal or incubative stage of an infectious disease.

    **s. sudo′ris,** the sweating stage in a malarial paroxysm.

**staff** [ A.S. *staef* ]. 1. An instrument, usually in the form of a grooved probe or sound, designed for guiding the knife of the operator in slitting open a sinus, or in the operation of external urethrotomy; also called a director or guide. 2. A specific group of workers.

    **s. of Aescula′pius,** see under Aesculapius.

    **consulting s.,** the body of specialists attached to a hospital who do not make stated visits, but serve in an advisory capacity when called upon for counsel by members of the attending s.

    **house s.,** the junior physicians and surgeons attached to a hospital who care for the patients under the direction of the attending s.

**stag** [ M.E. ]. 1. The male of certain species of deer. 2. A male horse, ox, or hog which was castrated so late that marked masculine characteristics are retained.

**stage** (stāj) [ M.E. thr. O. Fr. *estage,* standing-place, fr. L. *sto,* pp. *status,* to stand ]. 1. Stadium; a period in the course of a disease; see also period. 2. The part of a microscope on which the microslide bears the object to be examined. 3. A particular step, phase, or position in a developmental process. For psychosexual s.'s, see subentries under phase.

    **algid s.,** the cold s. or s. of collapse in cholera.

    **amphibol′ic s.,** amphibolic period; the s. following the acme of a disease in which the outcome, whether recovery or death, is in doubt.

    **Arneth s.'s,** a differential grouping of polymorphonuclear neutrophils in accordance with the number of lobes in their nuclei, *i.e.,* cells with 1, 2, 3, 4, or 5 (or more) lobes are designated, respectively, as class I, II, and so on. See also Arneth formula.

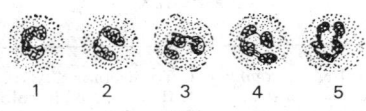

**Arneth Stages**

    **cap s.,** the second s. in the proliferative phase of tooth development.

    **cold s.,** *stadium* frigoris.

    **deferves′cent s.,** the s. of falling temperature.

    **end s.,** the late, fully developed phase of a disease; *e.g.,* the end-stage shrunken kidney that may result from a variety of chronic diseases which become indistinguishable in their effect on the kidney.

    **eruptive s.,** *stadium* fluorescentiae.

    **ex′oeryth′rocytic s.,** developmental s. of the malaria parasite(*Plasmodium*) outside of the red blood cells of the vertebrate host, usually in liver parenchyma cells; referred to as the tissue or pre-erythrocytic s. (before erythrocytes are invaded) or the secondary or para-erythrocytic s. (after invasion of the erythrocytes).

    **imperfect s.,** a mycological term used to describe the asexual life cycle phase of a fungus.

    **incubative s.,** the primary s. of certain infectious diseases during which the prodromal symptoms are appearing, and usually synchronous with the induction of sensitivity.

**intuitive s.,** in psychology, a s. of development, usually occurring between 4 and 7 years of age, in which a child's thought processes are determined by the most prominent aspects of the stimuli to which he is exposed, rather than by some form of logical thought.

**s. of invasion,** incubative s.

**s.'s of labor,** see under labor.

**latent s.,** incubative s.

**perfect s.,** a mycological term used to describe the sexual life cycle phase of a fungus in which spores are formed after nuclear fusion.

**preconceptual s.,** in psychology, the s. of development in an infant's life, prior to actual conceptual thinking, in which sensorimotor activity predominates.

**prodromal s.,** incubative s.

**resting s.,** the quiescent s. of a cell or its nucleus in which no karyokinetic changes are taking place; vegetative s.

**sweating s.,** *stadium* sudoris.

**trypanosome s.,** see trypomastigote.

**vegetative s.,** resting s.

**stag′ger.** To walk unsteadily; to reel.

**stag′gers.** 1. A form of caisson disease in which vertigo, mental confusion, and muscular weakness are the chief symptoms. 2. Sturdy; gid; a disease in sheep, marked by swaying and uncertain gait, caused by the presence of the larva of *Multiceps multiceps* in the brain, or by other cerebral lesions.

**blind s.,** mad s.; acute selenium poisoning in animals.

**bracken s.,** a condition occurring in horses as a result of eating bracken; characterized by locomotor incoordination; it is due to thiamine deficiency (bracken contains thiaminase) and is cured by the administration of vitamin B₁.

**grass s.,** grass *tetany.*

**mad s.,** blind s.

**stagnation** (stag-na′shun) [ L. *stagnum,* a pool ]. The retardation or cessation of flow of blood in the vessels; passive congestion; accumulation in any part of a normally circulating fluid.

**Stahl,** Friedrich K., German physician, 1811–1873. See S.'s *ear.*

**Stahl,** George E., German physician and chemist, 1660–1734. He promulgated the phlogiston theory and the concept of a vital force or sensitive soul which he supposed motivated all activities of the human body.

**Stähli,** Jean, Swiss ophthalmologist, *1890. See Hudson-S. *line,* Stahl's *line.*

---

# STAIN

**stain** (stān) [ M.E. *steinen* ]. 1. To discolor. 2. To color; to dye. 3. A discoloration. 4. A dye used in histologic and bacteriologic technique. 5. A procedure in which a dye or combination of dyes and reagents is used to color the constituents of cells and tissues. Types of staining procedures are listed in the subentries below; for individual dyes or staining substances, see the specific names.

**Abbott's s. for spores,** the specimen is covered with alkaline methylene blue and brought to a boil several times, decolorized in 2 per cent nitric acid in 80 per cent alcohol, and finally dipped in a saturated alcoholic solution of eosin 10, in water 90; spores are stained blue; bodies of the bacilli pink.

**acid s.,** a dye in which the anion is the colored component of the dye molecule, *e.g.,* sodium eosinate (eosin).

**Albert's s.,** used as a s. for diphtheria bacilli; contains toluidine blue, methyl green, glacial acetic acid, alcohol, and distilled water.

**Babès′ s.,** a solution of safranin O in 2 per cent aniline water.

**basic s.,** nuclear s.; a dye in which the cation is the colored component of the dye molecule, *e.g.,* methylene blue chloride.

**Baumgarten's s.,** for distinguishing *Mycobacterium leprae* from *M. tuberculosis* on the basis of relative acid-fastness;

smears are fixed by heat, stained in dilute alcoholic solution of basic fuchsin for 5 minutes, decolorized for 30 to 60 seconds in 10 per cent concentrated nitric acid in alcohol, counterstained in methylene blue, washed in water, and dried; most strains of the leprosy bacillus are stained red, whereas most strains of tubercle bacilli are stained blue, the latter being relatively less acid-fast.

**Beale's s.,** a fluid of carmine 1, ammonia 3, glycerin 96, distilled water 96, 95 per cent alcohol 24.

**Benian's s.,** a procedure for demonstrating spirochetal, treponemal, and other flexuous spiral bacteria, unstained, against a background of Congo red.

**Best's carmine s.,** a method for the demonstration of glycogen in tissues; consists of carmine 2 gm., potassium carbonate 1 gm., potassium chloride 5 gm., distilled water 60 ml.; the mixture is gently boiled until the color darkens, is then permitted to cool, and 20 ml. of concentrated solution of ammonium hydroxide are added (used after "ripening" for 24 hours).

**Biondi-Heidenhain s.,** a s. for spirochetes using acid fuchsin and orange G.

**Birch-Hirschfeld s.,** for demonstrating amyloid; sections are treated for 5 minutes in 2 per cent alcoholic Bismarck brown, washed in alcohol and then in distilled water, placed in 2 per cent aqueous crystal violet for 5 to 10 minutes, and, finally, decolorized in dilute acetic acid. Amyloid is usually stained a bright ruby red, whereas the cytoplasm of cells is not stained and nuclei are brown.

**Borrel's blue s.,** a s. for demonstrating spirochetes, treponemes, and Borrelia organisms; a black precipitate of silver oxide (prepared by means of mixing solutions of silver nitrate and sodium bicarbonate) is added to a saturated aqueous solution of methylene blue; after thoroughly mixing the preparation (by means of vigorous shaking), it is permitted to stand for 10 to 14 days, and the blue supernatant fluid is used as a s.

**Bostroem's s.,** a method for staining actinomyces, using crystal violet and picrocarmine.

**Buchner's s.,** a s. for spores of bacteria; after treating the film for thirty seconds in concentrated sulfuric acid, s. with carbol-fuchsin.

**Buerger's s.,** for demonstrating the capsules of bacteria; the smear is fixed in Müller's fluid, washed in water, then alcohol, and covered with tincture of iodine for 1 to 3 minutes; it is then again washed in alcohol, dried, stained for 2 to 5 seconds in aniline water-crystal violet, and finally washed and examined in 2 per cent salt solution.

**Bunge-Trantenroth s.,** for differentiating tubercle and smegma bacilli; wash with alcohol, treat with chromic acid, stain with hot carbolfuchsin, decolorize with 16 per cent sulfuric acid, counterstain with alcoholic methylene blue, and wash in water; tubercle bacilli stain red, smegma bacilli are decolorized.

**Cajal's astrocyte s.,** a method for demonstrating astrocytes by impregnation in a solution containing gold chloride and mercuric chloride.

**contrast s.,** differential s.; a dye used to color one portion of a tissue or cell which remained unaffected when the other part was stained by a dye of different color.

**Cross s.,** for phagocytes and bacteria; to a 2 per cent solution of phenol in alcohol (95 per cent) and glycerin, each 20 ml., and distilled water 100 ml. are added crystal violet 0.06, and pyronin 0.20; the cytoplasm is stained lavender, the nuclei violet, and the bacteria a dark purple.

**Czaplewski's s.,** coloring the tubercle bacillus with carbolic fuchsin, and counterstaining by dipping the specimen in a solution of fluorescein 1, and methylene blue 5, in alcohol 100, and then several times in a 5 per cent methylene blue alcoholic solution without fluorescein.

**differential s.,** contrast s.

**Dorset's s.,** for the tubercle bacillus; Sudan red III; a fat s.

**double s.,** a mixture of two dyes, each of which stains different portions of a tissue or cell.

**Ehrlich's aniline-oil s.,** Koch-Ehrlich s.

**Ehrlich's triacid s.,** a mixture of saturated solutions of orange G, acid fuchsin, and methyl green; a differential leukocytic s.

**Ehrlich's triple s.,** a mixture of indulin, eosin Y, and aurantia.

**Fiocca's s.,** a method for staining bacterial spores.

**Flemming's triple s.,** fix section in acetic alcohol, s. 1 hour in saturated aqueous safranin solution, wash and s. $^1/_2$ hour in saturated aqueous methyl violet solution; wash and flood with orange G acetone.

**fluorescent s.,** a s. (or staining procedure) involving the use of a fluorescent dye or substance that will combine selectively with certain tissue components and that will then fluoresce upon irradiation with ultraviolet light.

**Fontana's s.,** a method for silver-impregnation of treponemes and other spirochetal forms; after fixing in glacial acetic acid 1, formalin 20, and water 100, the films are stained in 1 per cent aqueous phenol solution containing tannic acid 5 per cent, and then covered with a 0.25 per cent aqueous solution of silver nitrate to which a dilute ammonium hydrate solution has been added drop by drop until a slight turbidity occurs.

**Fraenken-Gabbet s.,** staining tubercle bacilli with carbolic fuchsin, the contrast color being obtained by immersing in an acidulated solution of methylene blue.

**Friedländer's s. for capsules.** (1) treat the film fixed on coverglass with 1 per cent acetic acid solution, s. with aniline water-gentian violet solution; (2) for sections, immerse for 24 hours in acetic acid 10 parts, concentrated alcoholic gentian violet solution 50 parts, distilled water 100 parts, differentiate in 1 per cent acetic acid solution.

**Gabbet's s.,** a method for staining acid-fast bacilli, including *Mycobacterium tuberculosis;* the cover glass preparation, fixed by heat, is dipped in Ziehl's solution and warmed until vapor arises, then washed and immersed for 2 to 4 minutes in a solution containing methylene blue 1, sulfuric acid 25, water 75.

**Gasis' s.,** a s. for acid-fast bacteria using eosin and methylene blue.

**Giemsa s.,** a s. for demonstrating Negri bodies, the malarial organisms, spirochetes and protozoans, and for differential staining of blood smears; compound of azur II-eosin 30, azur II 0.8, chemically pure glycerin and chemically pure methyl alcohol each 250.0.

**Goldhorn's s.,** a modified Romanovsky s. in which the methylene blue is polychromed by heating in solution with lithium carbonate.

**Golgi's s.,** any of several methods for staining nerve cells and their processes, nerve fibers, and neuroglia; using fixation and hardening in formalin-osmic-dichromate combinations for various times, followed by impregnation in 0.75 per cent silver nitrate for 1 to 2 days.

**Goodpasture's s. for Gram-negative bacteria,** basic fuchsin 0.6, aniline and phenol crystals of each 1.0, and 50 per cent alcohol 100.

**Goodpasture's polychrome s.,** methylene blue and potassium carbonate of each 1 gm., in distilled water 400 ml.; boil for 5 minutes and when cool add glacial acetic acid 3 ml.; simmer down to 200 ml.

**Gram's s.,** a method for differential staining of bacteria; smears are fixed by flaming, stained for 1 minute in Hucker-Conn solution of crystal violet, rinsed with water, covered with Gram's solution of iodine for 1 minute; rinsed, decolorized with 95 per cent alcohol for 30 to 60 seconds, rinsed, counterstained with 0.25 per cent safranin O for 1 minute, rinsed, blotted, and dried. Gram-positive organisms are purple black; Gram-negative organisms are pink. The Gram s. is not only useful in bacterial taxonomy and identification, but also in indicating fundamental differences in cell wall structure.

**green s.,** a deposit, produced by chromogenic bacteria, found on the cervicolabial portions of the teeth, usually in children; see also brown *pellicle.*

**Guenther's s.,** a s. for spirochetes; the film is dried with gentle heat (not flamed), covered with a 5 per cent acetic acid solution for 30 seconds, then exposed to ammonia fumes for a few seconds, and, after washing, stained with Ehrlich's aniline gentian violet for 8 to 10 minutes.

**Hasting's s.,** a modified Romanovsky s.

**Hauser's s. for spores,** staining with 10 ml. of aqueous solution of fuchsin, passing the cover glass repeatedly through the flame and renewing the s. from time to time.

**Heidenhain's s.,** Heidenhain's iron-hematoxylin; I, iron alum 2, distilled water 100; II, hematoxylin crystals 1, 95 per cent alcohol 10, distilled water 90. Sections are mordanted in I, stained in II, and differentiated in I.

**hematoxylin and eosin s.,** probably the most generally useful of all staining methods for tissues. If tissues are fixed in a fluid that contains mercuric chloride (*e.g.,* Zenker's or Helly's fluid), remove paraffin from sections and treat for 1 to 2 minutes with dilute solution of iodine in 70 per cent alcohol, wash in distilled water, bleach in a 5 or 10 per cent aqueous solution of sodium thiosulfate, and then wash again in distilled water. If tissues are fixed in 10 per cent formalin, the s.'s may be applied without the above treatment. S. with full strength Harris' hematoxylin for 12 to 15 minutes; "blue" in tap water or in distilled water plus a few drops of saturated aqueous solution of lithium carbonate for 5 to 10 minutes; s. in 0.2 per cent aqueous solution of eosin for 1 minute; rinse in distilled water and 95 per cent alcohol; dehydrate in absolute alcohol, clear in xylene, and mount. Nuclei are stained deeply blue, and cytoplasm is pink. Delafield's alum hematoxylin or Ehrlich's acid hematoxylin may be used instead of Harris' hematoxylin.

**Hewlett's s.,** a capsule s. using carbol-fuchsin and gentian violet.

**Hiss' s.,** for demonstrating the capsules of microorganisms; (1) a saturated alcoholic solution of fuchsin or crystal violet 5, in water 95, is poured on the dried cover glass preparation and heated, and is then washed off with a 20 per cent solution of copper sulfate; (2) the fixed specimen is covered for a few seconds with crystal violet solution and then washed off with a 0.25 per cent solution of potassium carbonate.

**immunofluorescent s.,** s. resulting from combination of fluorescent antibody with antigen specific for the antibody portion of the fluorochrome conjugate.

**intravital s.,** a s. which is taken up by living cells after parenteral administration, *e.g.,* intravenously or subcutaneously.

**Israel's s.,** for actinomyces; immerse in a strong solution of orcein in dilute acetic acid for several hours, then wash and treat with absolute alcohol for a few seconds.

**Jenner's s.,** a 1.2 per cent aqueous solution of eosin is mixed with equal parts of a 1 per cent aqueous solution of methylene blue; at the end of 24 hours the precipitate is filtered out and washed with water; to make the s., 0.5 gm. of the dry precipitate is dissolved in 100 ml. of methyl alcohol.

**Johne's s.,** a capsule s. using crystal violet followed by decolorization in dilute acetic acid.

**Kaufmann's s.,** a capsule s. using methylene blue followed by silver nitrate, then fuchsin.

**Kieffer's s.,** a s. for acid fast bacteria using a mixture of carbol-fuchsin and carbol-methyl violet.

**Klein's s.,** a s. for spores; add a solution of carbol-fuchsin to an equal quantity of an emulsion of the spore containing solution; spread the mixture on a cover glass and fix in the flame; decolorize with 1 per cent sulfuric acid, and then s. in dilute methylene blue solution.

**Koch-Ehrlich s.,** add 2 ml. of aniline oil to 98 ml. of distilled water, shake, and filter; then add 75 ml. of this filtrate to 25 ml. of a concentrated alcoholic solution of fuchsin, gentian violet, or methylene blue.

**Laveran's s.,** (1) for Gram-negative bacteria; after immersion in 0.5 per cent aqueous solution of eosin for 1 minute, the film is exposed for 30 seconds to a saturated aqueous solution of methylene blue; (2) for hematozoa: Borrel's blue 1, 1 per cent solution of eosin 5, distilled water 4.

**Leishman's s.,** an eosin-methylene blue s. used in the examination of blood films.

**Lillie's allochrome s.,** a procedure using PAS, picric acid, and methylene blue during which the color of certain connective tissue elements changes from red to blue.

**Lillie's azure-eosin s.,** a s. in which an azure eosinate solution is used.

**Loeffler's, s.** a s. for flagella; the specimen is treated with a mixture of ferrous sulfate, tannic acid, and alcoholic fuchsin, then stained with aniline-water fuchsin or gentian violet made alkaline with 0.1 per cent sodium hydroxide solution.

**MacNeal's tetrachrome s.,** a s. for blood smears; methylene blue 1, azure A 0.6, methylene violet 0.2, eosin Y 1.

**Malassez' s.,** a method for staining neuroglia with ammoniacal picrocarmine.

**Mallory's s. for actinomyces,** s. in alum hematoxylin; immerse for 10 minutes in a 5 per cent solution of eosin, wash, and immerse in Ehrlich's aniline crystal violet for 2 to 5 minutes, wash in saline, then treat for 1 minute with Weigert's iodine solution, wash again, blot, differentiate in aniline oil, and clear in xylol.

**Mallory's aniline blue s.,** a method especially suitable for studying connective tissue. Fix in Zenker's fluid, embed in paraffin or celloidin. Remove mercury (see hematoxylin and eosin s.) and then stain in 0.5 per cent aqueous solution of acid fuchsin for 1 to 5 minutes; drain excess s. and place in aniline blue-orange G solution (*i.e.,* water soluble aniline blue 0.5 gm., orange G 2 gm., 1 per cent aqueous solution of phosphotungstic acid 100 ml.) for 20 minutes or more; rinse in 2 or 3 changes of 95 per cent alcohol, dehydrate in absolute alcohol, clear in xylene, and mount in neutral balsam; for celloidin sections, reduce staining time and pass from 95 per cent alcohol to terpineol and mount in balsam. Fibrils of collagen are blue; fibroglia, neuroglia, and muscle fibers are red; fibrils of elastin are pink or yellow.

**Mallory's triple s.,** a connective tissue s.; see Mallory's aniline blue s.

**Marx's s.,** a s. composed of eosin, potassium hydrate, and quinine.

**metachromat'ic s.,** a s., such as methylene blue, which manifests different colors under specific conditions.

**Moeller's s.,** a s. for spores; fix on cover glass and treat with 5 per cent chromic acid solution, wash, and s. with an aqueous solution of methylene blue.

**Much-Weiss s.,** Weiss s.

**multiple s.,** a mixture of several dyes each having an independent selective action on one or more portions of the tissue.

**negative s.,** s. forming an opaque or colored background against which the object to be demonstrated appears as a translucent or colorless area.

**Neisser's s.,** a s. for the polar nuclei of the diphtheria bacillus; a mixture of 2 parts of solution *a* (methylene blue 1, absolute alcohol 20, distilled water 1000 glacial acetic acid 50) and 1 part solution *b* (crystal violet 1, absolute alcohol 10, distilled water 300); after-s. with chrysoidin.

**neutral s.,** a compound of an acid s. and a basic s., such as the eosinate of methylene blue, in which the anion and cation each contains a chromophore group.

**Nicolle's s. for capsules,** s. in a mixture of a saturated solution of gentian violet, in 95 per cent alcohol 10 parts, and a 1 per cent solution of phenol 100 parts, then wash off in a mixture of 1 part acetone in 2 parts absolute alcohol.

**Nissl's s.,** (1) a method for staining nerve cells with basic fuchsin; (2) a method for staining chromophil substance in nerve cells, with methylene blue, now largely replaced by thionine and toluidine blue.

**Nocht's s.,** a modified Romanovsky s.; a solution is made of 1 per cent methylene blue and 1/2 per cent sodium carbonate and kept for a few days at 60°C. Then to 2 ml. of water in a watch glass 2 or 3 drops of a 1 per cent eosin solution are added, and to this, drop by drop, the first solution is added until the eosin tint just disappears.

**nuclear s.,** basic s.

**Nuttall's s. for capsules,** same as Welch's s.

**Orth's s.,** a s. for nerve cells and their processes; carmine 2.5, saturated solution of lithium carbonate 97.

**Paltauf's s.,** a modified Gram s. containing crystal violet and aniline oil.

**panop'tic s.,** a method of blood staining; the film is flooded with Jenner's s. for 3 minutes; then with a mixture of Jenner's 1, and distilled water 20, for 1 minute; then with Giemsa's s. 1, and distilled water 20, for 30 minutes; finally with distilled water for 5 to 30 minutes.

**Papanicolaou s.,** a multichromatic s. used principally on cytologic specimens; it is based on aqueous solutions with multiple counterstaining dyes in 95 per cent ethyl alcohol, giving great transparency and delicacy of detail.

**Pappenheim's s.,** a method for differentiating tubercle and smegma bacilli; the preparation is stained with hot carbol-fuchsin solution, then treated with an alcoholic solution of rosolic acid and methylene blue to which

glycerin is added; tubercle bacilli are stained bright red, but smegma bacilli are decolorized.

**periodic acid-Schiff s.,** PAS s.; a tissue-staining procedure in which 1,2-glycol groupings are first oxidized with periodic acid to aldehydes, which then react with the sulfite leukofuchsin reagent of Schiff, and become colored red; strong staining occurs with polysaccharides such as glycogen, and mucopolysaccharides of epithelial mucins, basement membranes, and connective tissue.

**Piorkowski's s. for metachromat'ic granules,** s. with alkaline methylene blue, slightly heating; decolorize in alcohol containing 3 per cent hydrochloric acid, and then s. in 1 per cent solution of aqueous eosin.

**Pitfield s.,** Smith-Pitfield s.

**plasma s., plasmat'ic s., plasmic s.,** a s. whose principal affinity is for the cytoplasm of cells.

**port-wine s.,** *nevus* flammeus.

**Romanovsky's s.,** prototype of the eosin-methylene blue s.'s for blood smears; aqueous solutions are made of methylene blue (saturated) and of eosin (1 per cent), and a mixture is made of 1 part of the first to 2 parts of the second at the time of staining.

**Rosenow's s.,** a s. for capsules; immerse the film, when nearly dry, in a 10 per cent tannic acid solution for 15 seconds, wash and s. by steaming with aniline crystal violet for 45 seconds, again wash and apply Lugol's solution for 45 seconds, decolorize with 95 per cent alcohol, and finally s. with an alcoholic solution of eosin.

**Roux's s.,** a double s. for diphtheria bacilli; compound of crystal violet or dahlia 0.5, methyl green 1.5, distilled water 200.

**Schulte-Tigges s.,** a s. for acid-fast bacteria using carbol-fuchsin, decolorization with sodium sulfite, and counterstaining with picronitric acid.

**selective s.,** a s. that colors one portion of a tissue or cell exclusively or more deeply than the remaining portions.

**Smith's s.,** a modified Gram s. for pneumococci in sputum.

**Smith-Pitfield s.,** a method for demonstrating flagella; a mordant is made by saturating a hot, saturated solution of corrosive sublimate with ammonia alum, then mixing with an equal part of 10 per cent tannic acid solution and adding one-half part 5 per cent carbol-fuchsin solution; the preparation is treated with this mixture and then stained with a saturated alcoholic solution of crystal violet 1, in a saturated ammonium alum solution 10.

**Stirling's modification of Gram's s.,** crystal violet, 5 gm., is ground in a mortar with 10 ml. of 95 per cent alcohol; when dissolved, aniline oil, 2 ml., is added and then distilled water, 88 ml.

**supravi'tal s.,** a procedure in which living cells are placed in a nontoxic dye solution so that their vital processes may be studied.

**Taenzer's s.,** an orcein solution used for staining elastic tissue.

**trichrome s.,** see Mallory's triple s.

**Türk's s.,** a weak iodine-potassium iodide solution for staining polymorphonuclear basophile leukocytes.

**Unna's s.,** alkaline methylene blue s., 1 part each of methylene blue and potassium carbonate in 100 parts of water.

**Unna-Pappenheim s.,** a contrast s. for gonococci consisting of a methyl green-pyronin solution.

**Unna-Taenzer s.,** Taenzer's s.

**Van Gieson's s.,** acid fuchsin 0.05, saturated picric acid solution 100.

**vital s.,** a s. applied to cells or parts of cells while they are still living.

**von Kossa s.,** a s. for calcium, utilizing a 5 per cent aqueous silver nitrate solution followed by 5 per cent sodium thiosulfate.

**Wadsworth's s.,** a method for demonstrating the capsules of bacteria; smears are fixed by immersion in 40 per cent formalin for 2 to 5 minutes, then stained in 5 per cent solution of crystal violet in aniline water, or by Gram's s.

**Warthin-Starry silver s.,** a s. for spirochetes in which preparations are incubated in 1 per cent silver nitrate solution followed by a developer.

**Weigert's s.'s,** (1) *elastin:* a solution of fuchsin, resorcin, and ferric chloride s.'s elastic fibers blue-black; (2) *fibrin:* stain in aniline-crystal violet solution, treat with iodine-potassium iodide solution, decolorize in aniline oil and xylol; the fibrin is stained a dark blue; (3) *myelin:* stained with ferric chloride and hematoxylin a deep blue, degenerated portions taking a light yellowish color; (4) *neuroglia:* a complicated process in which the final treatment is like that for staining fibrin; neuroglia and nuclei stain blue; (5) *copper hematoxylin:* a s. especially for the nervous tissues; (6) *actinomyces:* immerse for 1 hour in a dark red orsellin solution in alcohol 20. acetic acid 5, distilled water 40 then wash and stain in 1 per cent aqueous crystal-violet solution, decolorizing in 60 per cent alcohol; (7) *iron hematoxylin:* a solution containing hematoxylin, ferric chloride, and hydrochloric acid; useful as a s. for nuclei.

**Weigert-Gram s. for bacteria in tissues,** s. sections in alum-hematoxylin, wash, and treat for 1 to 5 minutes with a 1 per cent aqueous solution of eosin, wash again and treat with aniline methyl violet for 30 to 60 minutes, wash and apply Lugol's solution for 1 or 2 minutes, then clear in equal parts of xylol and aniline.

**Weiss' s.,** a combined s. for both acid-fast and non-acid-fast microorganisms; keep for 24 hours in methyl violet solution 25, carbol-fuchsin 75, then in Lugol's solution 10 minutes, in 5 per cent nitric acid 1 minute, in 3 per cent hydrochloric acid 10 seconds, and in acetone alcohol until no more color comes off; then dry with filter paper and s. for 1 minute in 10 per cent Bismarck brown.

**Welch's s.,** a method of demonstrating the capsules of microorganisms; apply glacial acetic acid for a few seconds; draw off and add aminine water-crystal violet solution; then wash in 1 or 2 per cent sodium chloride solution.

**Williams' s.,** a s. for Negri bodies; the fixed films (1 per cent picric acid in neutral methyl alcohol) are stained with a saturated alcoholic solution of fuchsin (0.5), a saturated alcoholic solution of methylene blue (10.0), and distilled water (50.0); the smear is flooded with the stain, heated over the flame until vapor rises, then washed and blotted; the Negri bodies are magenta and the granules blue, the nerve cells blue, and the erythrocytes yellowish.

**Wright's s.,** the dry s. is a mixture of eosinates of polychromed methylene blue. Originally a 0.5 per cent solution of the dry s. in pure methanol was called for.

**Ziehl-Neelsen s.,** a method for staining acid-fast bacteria in Ziehl's solution, decolorizing in acid alcohol, counterstaining with methylene blue; acid-fast organisms stain red, other tissue elements light blue.

---

**stain′ing.** 1. The act of applying a stain. Types of staining procedures are listed under stain. 2. In dentistry, modification of the color of the tooth or denture base.

**staircase** (stăr′kās). A series of reactions that follow one another in progressively increasing or decreasing intensity, so that a chart shows a continuous rise or fall.

**stal′agom′eter** [ G. *stalagma*, a drop, + *metron*, measure ]. Stactometer; an instrument for determining exactly the number of drops in a given quantity of liquid; used as a measure of the surface tension of a fluid, for the lower the tension the smaller the drops, and consequently the more numerous in the given quantity of the fluid.

**stalk** (stawk). A narrowed connection with a structure or organ.

**allantoic s.,** the narrow connection between the intraembryonic portion of the allantois and the extraembryonic allantoic vesicle.

**body s.,** the extraembryonic precursor of the connecting s. or umbilical cord by which the embryo is attached to its trophoblastic chorion.

**optic s.,** the constricted proximal portion of the optic vesicle in the embryo; it develops into the optic nerve.

**pineal s.,** the attachment of the pineal body to the roof of the third ventricle; it contains the pineal recess of the third ventricle.

**yolk s.,** omphalomesenteric duct; ductus omphalomesentericus; the narrowed connection between the intraembryonic gut and the yolk sac; its walls are splanchnopleure.

**stallion** (stal′yon) [ O. fr. *estalion* ]. An uncastrated male horse, usually kept for breeding purposes.

**stal′tic** [ G. *staltikos*, contractile. STAL- ]. Styptic.

**stam′mer** [ A.S. *stamur* ]. 1. To hesitate in speech, halt, repeat, and mispronounce, by reason of embarrassment, agitation, or unfamiliarity with the subject; distinguish from stutter. 2. To mispronounce or transpose certain consonants in speech.

**stam′mering.** Dysarthria literalis; a speech disorder characterized by (1) hesitation and repetition of words, or (2) mispronunciation or transposition of certain consonants, especially *l, r,* and *s.* Lisping, lalling, rhotacism, and idioglossia are varieties of the second form of s.

**Stamnoso′ma** [ G. *stamnos,* a jar, + *sōma,* body ]. A genus of flukes of the family Heterophyidae, possibly identical with *Centrocestus.* Two species are described as sometimes infecting man, *S. armatum* and *S. formosanum.*

**stanch, staunch** [ L. *stagno,* to stagnate ]. To arrest bleeding.

**stan′dardiza′tion.** 1. The making of a solution of definite strength so that it may be used for comparison and in tests. 2. Making any drug or other preparation conform to the type or standard.

**s. of a test,** in psychology, following definite procedures for administering, scoring, and evaluating the results of a new test which is under development.

**stand′still.** Arrest; cessation of activity.

**atrial s.,** auricular s.; cessation of atrial contractions, marked by absence of atrial waves in the electrocardiogram.

**auricular s.,** atrial s.

**sinus s.,** cessation of sinus node activity, marked by absence of normal P waves in the electrocardiogram.

**ventricular s.,** cessation of ventricular contractions, marked by absence of ventricular complexes in the electrocardiogram.

**Stanley,** Edward, London surgeon, 1793–1862. See S.'s cervical *ligaments.*

**Stanley Way.** See Way, Stanley.

**stan′nic** [ L. *stannum,* tin ]. Relating to tin, especially when in combination in its higher valency.

**s. chloride,** SnCl₄; a fuming liquid (fuming spirit of Libavius), specific gravity 2.23, boiling point 115°C.; it forms several hydrates. The pentahydrate (butter of tin) is used for mordanting and "loading" or "weighting" silk.

**s. oxide,** tin oxide; SnO₂; used in industry; it is a cause of pneumoconiosis.

**Stannius,** Herman F., German biologist, 1808–1883. See S.'s *ligature.*

**stan′nous** [ L. *stannum,* tin ]. Relating to tin; especially denoting compounds ocntaining tin in its lower valency.

**s. fluoride** (USP, NF), contains not less than 71.2 per cent of stannous tin and not less than 22.3 per cent and not more than 25.5 per cent of fluoride; used as a prophylactic in dentistry.

**stan′num** [ L. ]. Tin; a metallic element, symbol Sn, atomic no. 50, atomic weight 119.

**stanolone** (stan′o-lōn). NEODROL; 17β-hydroxy-5α-androstane-3-one (for androstane structure, see steroids); an androgen with the same actions and uses as testosterone; used for its anabolic and tumor-suppressing effects, specifically, in carcinoma of the breast.

**stanozolol** (stă-no′zo-lol, -lōl) (USAN). WINSTROL; STROMBA; 17α-methyl-5α-androstan-17β-ol carrying a pyrazole ring (=CH—NH—N=) attached to C-2 and C-3 (see steroids for androstane structure). A semisynthetic, orally effective, anabolic steroid that may promote nitrogen retention when combined with an adequate diet. However, effective doses may produce virilization and other untoward effects associated with androgenic hormones.

**stapedectomy** (sta-pe-dek′to-mĭ) [ stapes, *q.v.,* + G. *ek-tomē,* excision ]. Removal of the stapes.

**stapedial** (sta-pe′dī-al). Relating to the stapes.

**stapediotenotomy** (sta-pe′dī-o-tĕ-not′o-mĭ) [ stapedius, *q.v.,* + G. *tenōn,* tendon, + *tomē,* incision ]. Division of the tendon of the stapedius muscle.

**stapediovestibular** (sta-pe′dī-o-ves-tib′u-lar). Relating to the stapes and the vestibule of the ear.

**stapedius,** pl. **stapedii** (sta-pe′dī-us, sta-pe′dī-i) [ Mod. L. ]. See *musculus* stapedius.

**stapes,** pl. **stapes, stapedes** (sta′pēz, sta′pe-dēz) [ Mod.

L. stirrup ] [ NA ]. Stirrup (so named from its shape); the smallest of the three auditory ossicles; its base, or foot-piece, fits into the vestibular (oval) window, while its head is articulated with the lenticular process of the long limb of the incus.

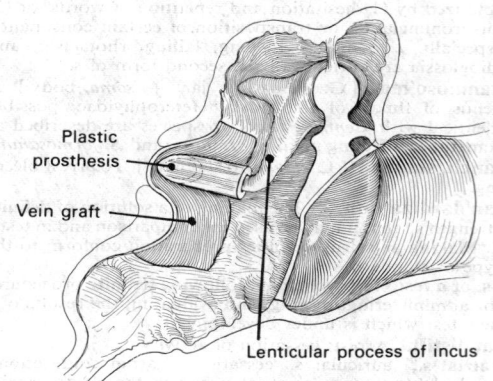

Plastic prosthesis

Vein graft

Lenticular process of incus

**Stapedectomy**

Stapes and oval window membrane have been replaced with a vein graft; plastic prosthesis connects graft with incus. This is only one of many techniques for correction of lesion produced by otosclerosis or other injury.

**staphyl-.**  See staphylo-.

**staphylagra** (staf'ĭ-lag'rah) [ staphyl- + G. *agra,* seizure ]. A forceps for holding the uvula.

**staphylectomy** (staf'ĭ-lek'to-mī) [ staphyl- + G. *ektomē,* excision ]. Uvulectomy.

**staphyledema** (staf'il-e-de'mah) [ staphyl- + G. *oidēma,* swelling (edema) ]. Edema of the uvula.

**staphyline** (staf'ĭ-lĭn, -lēn). 1. Botryoid; resembling a bunch of grapes. 2. Obsolete synonym for uvular.

**staphyli'nus.**  See under musculus.

**staphylion** (stă-fil'ĭ-on) [ G. dim. of *staphylē,* a bunch of grapes ]. A craniometric point; the midpoint of the posterior edge of the hard palate.

**staphylitis** (staf'ĭ-li'tis) [ staphyl- + G. suffix *-itis,* inflammation ]. Uvulitis.

**staphylo-, staphyl-** (staf'ĭ-lo-) [ G. *staphylē,* a bunch of grapes. STAPH- ]. Combining forms denoting resemblance to a grape or a bunch of grapes, hence relating usually to staphylococci, or (in obsolete or obsolescent terms) to the uvula palatina; for the latter, see also uvulo-.

**staphylococcal** (staf'ĭ-lo-kok'al). Relating to or caused by any organism of the genus *Staphylococcus.*

**staphylococcemia** (staf'ĭ-lo-kok-se'mĭ-ah) [ staphylo- + G. *haima,* blood ]. Staphylohemia; staphylococcic sepsis; the presence of staphylococci in the circulating blood.

**staphylococci** (staf'ĭ-lo-kok'si). Plural of staphylococcus.

**staphylococcia** (staf'ĭ-lo-kok'sĭ-ah). Any staphylococcic infection.

**staphylococcic** (staf'ĭ-lo-kok'sik). Relating to or caused by any species of *Staphylococcus.*

**staph'ylococcol'ysin.**  Staphylolysin.

**staphylococcolysis** (staf'ĭ-lo-kok-ol'ĭ-sis) [ staphylo- + G. *lysis,* dissolution ]. Lysis or destruction of staphylococci.

**Staphylococcus** (staf'ĭ-lo-kok'us) [ staphylo- + G. *kokkos,* a berry ]. A genus of nonmotile, nonsporeforming, aerobic to facultatively anaerobic bacteria (family Micrococcaceae) containing Gram-positive, spherical cells, 0.5 to 1.5 $\mu$m in diameter, which divide in more than one plane to form irregular clusters. These organisms are chemoorganotrophic, and their metabolism is respiratory and fermentative. Under anaerobic conditions, lactic acid is produced from glucose; under aerobic conditions, acetic acid and small amounts of $CO_2$ are produced. Coagu-

lase-positive strains produce a variety of toxins and are therefore potentially pathogenic and may cause food poisoning. These organisms are usually sensitive to antibiotics such as the $\beta$-lactam and macrolide antibiotics, tetracyclines, novobiocin, and chloramphenicol, but are resistant to polymyxin and polyenes. They are sensitive to antibacterials such as phenols and their derivatives, surface-active compounds, salicylanilides, carbanilides, and halogens (chlorine and iodine) and their derivatives such as chloramines and iodophors. They are found on the skin, in skin glands, on the nasal and other mucous membranes of warm-blooded animals, and in a variety of food products. The type species is *S. aureus.*

**S. au'reus,** a common species found especially on nasal mucous membrane and skin (hair follicles); it causes furunculosis, pyemia, osteomyelitis, suppuration of wounds, and food poisoning. It is the type species of the genus *S.*

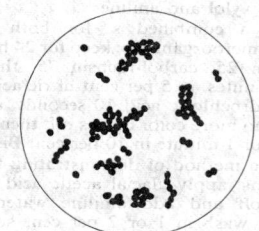

*Staphylococcus aureus*

(Original magnification, $\times 2000$)

**S. epider'midis,** a species, originally found in small stitch abscesses and other skin wounds, which occurs on parasitic skin and mucous membranes of man and other animals; it is parasitic rather than pathogenic.

**S. pyog'enes albus,** *S. aureus;* a name formerly applied to the organisms which are now regarded as the mutants of *S. aureus* which form white colonies.

**S. pyog'enes au'reus,** *S. aureus.*

**staphyloderma** (staf'ĭ-lo-der'mah) [ staphylo- + G. *derma,* skin ]. Pyoderma due to staphylococci.

**staphylodermatitis** (staf'ĭ-lo-der'mă-ti'tis). Inflammation of the skin due to the action of staphylococci.

**staphylodialysis** (staf'ĭ-lo-di-al'ĭ-sis) [ staphylo- + G. *dialysis,* a separation ]. Uvuloptosis.

**staph'ylohe'mia.**  Staphylococcemia.

**staph'ylohemol'ysin.**  Staphylolysin.

**staph'yloki'nase.**  A proteinase (EC 3.4.99.22) with action similar to that of urokinase and streptokinase.

**staphylolysin** (staf'ĭ-lol'ĭ-sin). 1. A hemolysin elaborated by a staphylococcus. 2. An antibody causing lysis of staphylococci.

**staphyloma** (staf'ĭ-lo'mah) [ G. See STAPH- ]. A bulging of the cornea or sclera due to inflammatory softening, usually containing adherent uveal tissue.

**annular s.,** a s. extending around the periphery of the cornea.

**anterior s.,** corneal s.; a bulging near the anterior pole of the eyeball.

**corneal s.,** anterior s.

**cil'iary s.,** scleral s. occurring in the region of the ciliary body.

**equato'rial s.,** a scleral s. occurring in the area of exit of the vortex veins.

**intercal'ary s.,** a scleral s. occurring between the insertion of the ciliary body and the root of the iris.

**posterior s.,** Scarpa's s.; posterior sclerochoroiditis; a bulging of a weakened sclera, from loss of the choroid lining, at the posterior of the eyeball due to degenerative changes in high myopia.

**Scarpa's s.,** posterior s.

**scleral s.,** equatorial s.

**u'veal s.,** protrusion of the iris through a rupture of the sclera.

**staphylo'matous.** Relating to or marked by staphyloma.

**staphyloncus** (staf'ĭ-long'kus) [ staphylo- + G. *onkos*, mass ]. Tumor or enlargement of the uvula.

**staphylopharyngorrhaphy** (staf'ĭ-lo-făr'ing-or'ă-fĭ) [ staphylo- + pharynx + G. *rhaphē*, suture ]. Palato-pharyngorrhaphy; surgical repair of defects in the uvula or soft palate and the pharynx.

**staph'yloplas'min.** Staphylotoxin.

**staphyloplasty** (staf'ĭ-lo-plas'tĭ) [ staphylo- + G. *plassō*, to form ]. Palatoplasty.

**staphyloplegia** (staf'ĭ-lo-ple'jĭ-ah). Palatoplegia.

**staphyloptosis** (staf'ĭ-lop-to'sis) [ staphylo- + G. *ptōsis*, a falling ]. Uvuloptosis.

**staphylorrhaphy** (staf'ĭ-lor'ă-fĭ) [ staphylo- + G. *rhaphē*, suture ]. Palatorrhaphy.

**staphyloschisis** (staf'ĭ-los'kĭ-sis) [ staphylo- + G. *schisis*, fissure ]. Bifid uvula with or without cleft of soft palate.

**staphylotome** (staf'ĭ-lo-tōm). Uvulotome.

**staphylotomy** (staf'ĭ-lot'o-mĭ) [ staphylo- + G. *tomē*, incision ]. 1. Uvulotomy. 2. Cutting away a staphyloma.

**staphylotoxin** (staf'ĭ-lo-tok'sin) [ staphylo- + G. *toxikon*, poison ]. Staphyloplasmin; the toxin elaborated by any species of *Staphylococcus.*

**star** [ A.S. *steorra* ]. Any star-shaped structure; aster. See also astrosphere.

    **daughter s.,** polar s.; one of the figures forming the diaster.

    **dental s.,** a spot of deeper yellow in the center of the dentine of a horse's incisor tooth, between the central enamel and the anterior border of the table; it varies considerably with the age of the animal.

    **lens s.'s.** (1) *radii* lentis; (2) congenital cataracts with opacities along the suture lines of the lens; may be anterior or posterior, or both.

    **mother s.,** monaster.

    **polar s.,** daughter s.

    **venous s.,** a small, red nodule formed by a dilated vein in the skin; caused by increased venous pressure.

    **Verheyen's s.'s,** *venulae* stellatae.

    **Winslow's s.'s,** *stellulae* winslowii.

**starch** [ A.S. *stearc*, strong ]. A polysaccharide built up of glucose residues in α-1,4 linkage; differs from cellulose in the presence of α- rather than β-glucoside linkages. It exists more or less throughout the vegetable kingdom, its chief commercial sources being the cereals and potatoes. commercial s. is a white, tasteless, odorless powder or mass consisting of minute rounded or ovoid granules that split into layers when heated. The granules swell and form a pasty mass in water. When subjected to the action of dry heat, s. is converted into dextrin; it is converted into dextrin and glucose by amylases and glucoamylases in saliva and pancreatic juice. S. is used as a dusting powder, an ingredient of ointments, an excipient, diluent, and disintegrant for tablets. It is an important raw material for the manufacture of alcohol, acetone, *n*-butanol, lactic acid, citric acid, glycerine, and gluconic acid by fermentation. An aqueous dispersion is useful as an antidote in iodine poisoning. The USP recognizes the following forms: starch, flowable starch; potato starch, and pregelatinized starch; the BP recognizes s. from maize (corn), rice, wheat, and potato.

    **animal s.,** glycogen.

    **s. equivalent,** the amount of oxygen consumed in the combustion of a given weight of fat as compared with that consumed in the combustion of an equal weight of starch; the figure is about 2.38, that for starch being taken as 1.

    **liver s.,** glycogen.

    **soluble s.,** a high molecular weight dextrin produced by the partial acid hydrolysis of s., water-soluble and useful in iodimetry, producing as it does an easily visible purple-black end point in the presence of free iodine.

    **s. sugar,** glucose.

**stare** [ A.S. *starian* ]. 1. To look intently or fixedly with wide-open eyes at any point. 2. An intent gaze.

    **postbasic s.,** a peculiar appearance in children with posterior basic meningitis, due to a retraction of the upper eyelid and a rolling down of the eyeball.

**star-fishes.** Members of the class Asteroidea with star-shaped bodies comprising five tapering arms. They

posses an endoskeleton. At the tip of each arm is a soft, tactile tentacle and a light-sensitive organ or eye spot. The mouth lies in the center of the under surface of the body.

**Stargardt,** Karl, German ophthalmologist, 1875–1927. See S.'s *disease.*

**Starling,** Ernest H., English physiologist, 1866–1927. See S.'s *curve, hypothesis, law, reflex.*

**Starr-Edwards ball valve prosthesis.** See under prosthesis.

**starva'tion.** Suffering from long-continued deprivation of food.

**starve** [ A.S. *steorfan*, to die ]. 1. To suffer from lack of food. 2. To deprive of food so as to cause suffering or death. 3. Formerly, to die of cold.

**Stas** (stahs), Jean-Servais, Belgian chemist, 1813–1891. See S.-Otto *method.*

**stasibasiphobia** (stas'ĭ-ba-sĭ-fo'bĭ-ah) [ G. *stasis*, a standing still, + *basis*, step, + *phobos*, fear ]. Morbid fear of standing and walking; see astasia-abasia.

**stasimorphia** (stas'ĭ-mor'fĭ-ah) [ G. *stasis*, a standing still, + *morphē*, shape ]. Deformity due to arrested development.

**stasiphobia** (stas'ĭ-fo'bĭ-ah) [ G. *stasis*, a standing still, + *phobos*, fear ]. Morbid fear of standing up.

**stasis,** pl. **stases** (sta'sis, stas'is, -ēz) [ G. a standing still. STA- ]. Stagnation of the blood or other fluids.

    **papillary s.,** papilledema.

    **pressure s.,** traumatic *asphyxia*; ecchymotic *mask.*

**stat.** Abbreviation for statim.

**-stat** [ G. *statēs*, stationary ]. Suffix indicating an agent intended to keep something from changing or moving.

**statam'pere** [ G. *statos*, standing (stationary), + ampere ]. The electrostatic unit of current; the flow of 1 electrostatic unit of charge (1 statcoulomb) per second; equal to $3.3 \times 10^{-10}$ ampere.

**statcou'lomb** [ G. *statos*, standing (stationary), + coulomb ]. The electrostatic unit of charge, such that two objects, each carrying such a charge and separated (center to center) by 1 cm. in a vacuum, will repel each other with a force of 1 dyne (or $10^{-5}$ newton); equal to $3.3 \times 10^{10}$ coulomb.

**state** [ L. *status*, condition, state. STA- ]. Condition; situation; status.

    **anxiety s.,** anxiety *neurosis.*

    **carrier s.,** the s. of being a carrier of pathogenic organisms; *i.e.,* one who is infected but free of disease.

    **central excitatory s.,** the building up of excitatory influences produced by individual impuses finally causes firing of the next neuron.

    **convulsive s.,** a clinical condition characterized by one or more transient episodes of altered consciousness or other neurologic dysfunction, often associated with jerking of the extremities and trunk, due to paroxysmal neuronal discharge; see also epilepsy.

    **dreamy s.,** the semiconscious s. associated with an epileptic attack.

    **eunuchoid s.,** an imprecisely delineated condition; a term applied to any individual showing signs of inadequate androgen secretion, regardless of the cause.

    **ground s.,** the normal, inactivated s. of an atom from which, on activation, the triplet and other excited s.'s are derived.

    **hypnotic s.,** hypnosis.

    **hypometabolic s.,** a rare s. of reduced metabolism with symptoms resembling hypothyroidism but with some tests for thyroid gland function normal; an imprecisely delineated disorder of uncertain occurrence.

    **local excitatory s.,** increased irritability of a nerve fiber or muscle fiber which is produced by an ineffective electrical stimulus. Summation of it may occur to result in a propagated impulse if two or more subliminal stimuli are applied in rapid succession.

    **multiple ego s.'s,** various psychological organizational s.'s reflecting different life experiences.

    **rapid eye movement s.,** rapid eye movement *sleep.*

    **refractory s.,** subnormal excitability immediately following a response to previous excitation. It is divided into absolute and relative phases.

**singlet s.,** a transient, excited s. of a molecule, *e.g.,* of chlorophyll, upon absorbing light. The excited (singlet) s. can release its energy as heat or light (fluorescence) and thus return to its initial (ground) s. It may alternatively assume a slightly more stable, but still excited s. (triplet s.), with an electron still dislocated as before but with reversed spin.

**steady s.,** symbol s as a subscript; a s. obtained in moderate muscular exercise, when the removal of lactic acid by oxidation keeps pace with its production, the oxygen supply being adequate, and the muscles do not go into debt for oxygen; more generally, any condition in which the formation of substances just keeps pace with their destruction so that all volumes, concentrations, pressures, and flows remain constant.

**triplet s.,** a second excited s. of a molecule (*e.g.,* chlorophyll) produced by absorption of light to produce the singlet s., then loss of some energy (fluorescence) to arrive at the longer-lived triplet s. The molecule may remain sufficiently long in the triplet s. for a second activating light quantum to be effective in producing a "second triplet" s., obviously at still a higher level of excitation, hence reactivity. Alternatively, it may lose the triplet s. energy directly and return to the ground s.

**twilight s.,** a condition of disordered consciousness during which actions may be performed without the conscious volition of the individual and without any remembrance of them being retained.

**statfar'ad.** The electrostatic unit of capacitance, equal to $1.1 \times 10^{-12}$ farad.

**stathen'ry.** Electrostatic unit of inductance, equal to $9 \times 10^{11}$ henries.

**sta'tim** [ L. ]. Abbreviated stat.; at once; immediately.

**statistics** (stă-tis'tiks). A collection of facts numerically grouped into definite classes.

**descriptive s.,** numerical values which describe the chief features of a group of scores, without regard to a larger population; *e.g.,* mean, median, mode.

**inferential s.,** s. from which an inference is made about the nature of a population; the purpose is to generalize about the population, based upon data from the sample selected from the population.

**vital s.,** biostatistics; the branch of s. that deals with data concerning human birth, health, disease, and death.

**statoacoustic** (stat'o-ā-koo'stik) [ G. *statos,* standing, + *akoustikos,* acoustic ]. Vestibulochochlear (1); relating to equilibrium and hearing.

**statoconia,** singular **statoconium** (stat'o-ko'nĭ-ah, -nĭ-um) [ L. fr. G. *statos,* standing, *konis,* dust ] [ NA ]. Statoliths; otoconia; otoliths; sagitta; crystalline particles of calcium carbonate and a protein adhering to the gelatinous membrane of the maculae of the utricle and saccule.

**stat'okinet'ic.** Pertaining to statokinetics.

**statokinetics** (stat'o-kĭ-net'iks) [ G. *statos,* standing, + *kinēsis,* movement ]. The adjustment made by the body in motion to maintain stable equilibrium.

**stat'oliths** [ G. *statos,* standing, + *lithos,* stone ]. Statoconia.

**statometer** (stă-tom'e-ter) [ G. *statos,* standing, + *metron,* measure ]. Exophthalmometer.

**statosphere** (stat'o-sfēr). Centrosphere.

**stature** (statch'ur) [ L. *statura,* fr. *statuo,* pp. *statutus,* to cause to stand. STA- ]. The height of a person.

**status** (sta'tus, stat'us) [ L. a way of standing. STA- ] [ NA ]. State; condition.

**s. anginosus,** prolonged angina pectoris refractory to treatment.

**s. arthrit'icus,** gouty diathesis or predisposition.

**s. asthmat'icus,** a condition of severe, prolonged asthma.

**s. cholera'icus,** the cold stage of shock and depression in cholera characterized by weak pulse, cold clammy skin, hebetude, and depression.

**s. chore'icus,** a very severe form of chorea in which the persistence of the movements prevents sleep and the patient may die of exhaustion.

**s. convul'sivus,** see convulsive *state.*

**s. cribro'sus,** a condition marked by dilations of the perivascular spaces in the brain.

**s. crit'icus,** a very severe and persistent form of crisis in tabes dorsalis.

**s. dysmyelinisa'tus,** a condition marked by disease of myelinated fibers in the globus pallidus and substantia nigra with accumulation of iron pigment in the cells. The children affected show motor disturbances (dyskinesias) and often mental deficiency.

**s. dysra'phicus,** a condition in which there is failure of fusion of midline structures; related to syringomyelia and perhaps to Marfan's syndrome or arachnodactyly.

**s. epilep'ticus,** a condition in which one major attack of epilepsy succeeds another with little or no intermission.

**s. hemicra'nicus,** a condition in which attacks of migraine succeed each other with such short intervals as to be almost continuous.

**s. hypnot'icus,** hypnosis.

**s. lacuna'ris,** a condition, occurring in cerebral arteriosclerosis, in which there are numerous small areas of degeneration in the brain.

**s. lymphat'icus,** s. thymicolymphaticus.

**s. mac'robiot'icus multip'arus,** heredofamilial *tremor.*

**s. marmora'tus,** a congenital condition due to maldevelopment of the corpus striatum associated with choreoathetosis, in which the striate nuclei have a marble-like appearance caused by altered myelination.

**s. nervo'sus,** s. typhosus.

**s. prae'sens,** the present state; the part of the anamnesis or history of a case, describing the condition of the patient at the time when he comes under observation.

**s. rap'tus,** ecstasy.

**s. spongio'sus,** multiple fluid-filled spaces of microscopic size in the cerebral white matter; seen in certain hypoxic, toxic, and metabolic diseases.

**s. thymicolymphat'icus,** s. lymphaticus; s. thymicus; supposed enlargement of the thymus and lymph nodes in infants and children, formerly believed to be associated with unexplained sudden death. It was erroneously believed that pressure of the thymus on the trachea might cause death during anesthesia. Prominence of these structures is now considered normal in young children, including those who have died suddenly without preceding illnesses that might lead to atrophy of lymphoid tissue. See also crib *death,* and sudden death *syndrome.*

**s. thy'micus,** s. thymicolymphaticus.

**s. typho'sus,** s. nervosus; an erethistic or typhoidal state.

**s. vertigino'sus,** chronic vertigo; a condition in which attacks of vertigo occur in rapid succession.

**statuvolence** (stat'u-vo'lens, stă-tu'vo-lens) [ status (hypnoticus) + L. *volens,* pres. p. of *volo,* to wish ]. Autohypnosis.

**statuvo'lent.** Relating to statuvolence; denoting a person capable of self-hypnotism.

**stat'volt** [ G. *statos,* standing (stationary), + volt ]. The electrostatic unit of potential or electromotive force, equal to 300 volts.

**Staub,** Hans, Swiss internist, *1890. See S.-Traugott *effect.*

**staurion** (staw'rĭ-on) [ G. dim. of *stauros,* cross ]. A craniometric point at the intersection of the median and transverse palatine sutures.

**stauroplegia** (staw-ro-ple'jĭ-ah) [ G. *stauros,* cross, + *plēgē,* stroke ]. Alternate *hemiplegia.*

**staxis** (stak'sis) [ G. a dripping, fr. *stazō,* to let fall by drops ]. Stillicidium.

**steal** (stēl). Diversion of blood via collaterals or reversed flow, from a vascularized tissue to one deprived by local arterial obstruction.

**external carotid s.,** see external carotid steal *syndrome.*

**iliac s.,** the decrease in flow in one common iliac artery when an occlusion of the other common iliac artery is released.

**renal-splanchnic s.,** diversion of blood from the right renal artery via the inferior adrenal branch into splanchnic collaterals distal to a stenosis of the celiac axis.

**subclavian s.,** obstruction of the subclavian artery proximal to the origin of the vertebral artery, with the result that the blood flow through the vertebral artery is reversed and the subclavian artery thus "steals" cerebral blood, causing symptoms of cerebrovascular insufficiency (subclavian steal syndrome).

**steapsin** (ste-ap'sin). Triacylglycerol lipase.

**stear-.** See stearo-.

**stearal** (ste'ă-ral). The aldehyde of stearic acid; stearaldehyde.

**stearate** (ste'ă-rāt). A salt of stearic acid.

**stearic acid** (ste'ă-rik) (USP). Octadecanoic acid; one of the most abundant fatty acids found in animal lipids. Used in pharmaceutical preparations, ointments, soaps, and suppositories.

**stearin** (ste'ă-rin). Tristearin; tristearoylglycerol; the "triglyceride" of stearic acid present in solid animal fats and in some vegetable fats; source of stearic acid.

**Stearns,** A. Warren, American physician, 1885–1959. See S.'s alcoholic *amentia.*

**stearo-, stear-** (ste'ă-ro-) [ G. *stear,* tallow ]. Combining forms relating to fat; see also steato-.

**stearoderma** (ste'ă-ro-der'mah) [ stearo- + G. *derma,* skin ]. Steatosis (3).

**stearoptene** (ste'ă-rop'tēn). A tough, crystalline solid that separates out from a volatile oil which has been standing for some time or has been subjected to cold; sometimes called a camphor.

**stearrhea** (ste'ă-re'ah). Steatorrhea.

**stearyl alcohol** (ste'ă-ril) (USP). Octadecyl alcohol; octadecanol; $CH_3(CH_2)_{16}CH_2OH$; ingredient of hydrophilic ointment and hydrophilic petrolatum; also used in the preparation of creams.

**steatite** (ste'ă-tit). Talc in the form of a mass.

**steatitis** (ste-ă-ti'tis) [ G. *stear(steat-),* tallow, + suffix *-itis,* inflammation ]. 1. Inflammation of adipose tissue. 2. A disease of young mink, characterized by a brownish yellow discoloration of the adipose tissues. It is believed to be caused by feeding diets containing too much of unsaturated fatty acids and too little vitamin E.

**steato-** (ste'ă-to-) [ G. *stear (steat-),* tallow ]. Combining form relating to fat.

**steatocryptosis** (ste'ă-to-krip-to'sis) [ steato- + G. *kryptē,* crypt ]. Dysfunction of the sebaceous glands.

**steatocystoma** (ste'ă-to-sis-to'mah). 1. A cyst with sebaceous gland cells in its wall. 2. Sebaceous *cyst.*

  **s. mul'tiplex,** steatomatosis; sebocystomatosis; widespread, multiple, thin-walled cysts of the skin that are lined by squamous epithelium, including lobules of sebaceous cells.

**steatogenesis** (ste'ă-to-jen'e-sis) [ steato- + G. *genesis,* production ]. Biosynthesis of lipids; term is used specifically to designate lipid accumulation in the testes of

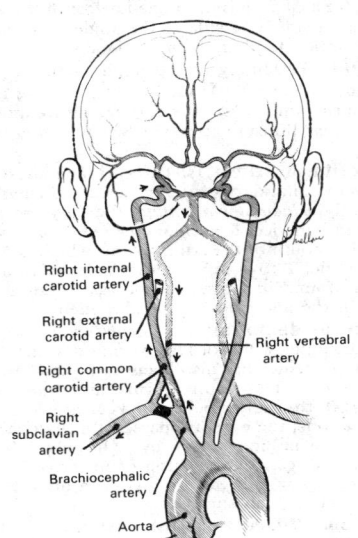

**Subclavian "Steal"**

Abnormal flow of blood due to occlusion in the subclavian artery proximal to the origin of the vertebral artery.

Right internal carotid artery

Right external carotid artery

Right vertebral artery

Right common carotid artery

Right subclavian artery

Brachiocephalic artery

Aorta

nonmammalian vertebrates on completion of spermatogenesis in the breeding period.

**steatogenous** (ste-ă-toj'ĕ-nus) [ steato- + G. suffix *-gen,* producing ]. 1. Causing fatty defeneration. 2. Causing any disease of the sebaceous glands.

**steatolysis** (ste-ă-tol'ĭ-sis) [ steato- + G. *lysis,* dissolution ]. The hydrolysis or emulsion of fat in the process of digestion.

**steatolytic** (ste-ă-to-lit'ik). Relating to steatolysis.

**steatoma** (ste-ă-to'mah) [ G. a sebaceous tumor, fr. steato- + suffix *-oma,* tumor ]. 1. A benign neoplasm derived from adipose tissue, *i.e.,* a lipoma. 2. Any mass or tumefaction consisting chiefly of lipid.

  **Müller's s.,** *lipoma* fibrosum.

**steatomatosis** (ste'ă-to-mă-to'sis). *Steatocystoma* multiplex.

**steatonecrosis** (ste'ă-to-ne-kro'sis) [ steato- + G. *nekrōsis,* death ]. Fat *necrosis.*

**steatopathy** (ste-ă-top'ă-thī) [ steato- + G. *pathos,* disease ]. Disease of sebaceous apparatus.

**steatopyga, steatopygia** (ste-ă-to-pi'ga, -pij'ĭ-ah) [ steato- + G. *pygē,* buttocks ]. An excessive accumulation of fat on the buttocks.

**ste'atop'ygous.** Having excessively fat buttocks.

**steatorrhea** (ste-ă-to-re'ah) [ steato- + G. *rhoia,* a flow ]. 1. Fatty stools; the passage of fat in large amounts in the feces, as noted in pancreatic disease and the malabsorption syndrome. 2. Seborrhea.

  **biliary s.,** s. due to the absence of bile from the intestine; usually accompanied by jaundice.

  **intestinal s.,** s. due to malabsorption resulting from intestinal disease; see also sprue, and celiac *disease.*

  **pancreatic s.,** s. due to the absence of pancreatic juice from the intestine.

**steatosis** (ste-ă-to'sis) [ steato- + G. suffix *-osis,* condition ]. 1. Adiposis. 2. Fatty *degeneration.* 3. Stearoderma; any disease of the sebaceous glands.

  **s. cordis,** fatty degeneration of the heart.

**steatozoon** (ste-ă-to-zo'on) [ steato- + G. *zōon,* animal ]. *Demodex folliculorum.*

**steel** [ A.S. *style* ]. An alloy of iron, usually with carbon ($1/4$ to 3 per cent).

  **stainless s.,** rustless metal alloys of iron containing sufficient chromium to passivate the surface under usual service.

**Steele,** J., Canadian neurologist. See S.-Richardson-Olszewski *syndrome.*

**Steell.** See Graham Steell.

**Steenbock,** Harry, American physiologist and chemist, *1886. See S. *unit.*

**steer** [ M.E. ]. A castrated male bovine.

**stef'fimy'cin** (USAN). Antibiotic substance produced by *Streptomyces steffisburgensis;* possesses antibacterial and antiviral activity.

**stege** (ste'ge) [ G. *stegos,* roof, a house ]. The internal pillar of Corti's organ.

**stegnosis** (steg-no'sis) [ G. stoppage ]. 1. A stoppage of any of the secretions or excretions. 2. Constriction; stenosis.

**stegnot'ic.** 1. Astringent; constipating. 2. An astringent agent; one checking secretion or causing constipation.

**Steidele,** Ralph. Viennese obstetrician. See S.'s *complex.*

**Stein,** Irving F., U. S. gynecologist, *1887. See S.-Leventhal *syndrome.*

**Stein,** Stanislav A. F. von, Russian otologist, *1855. See S.'s *test.*

**Steinberg,** I. See S. thumb *sign.*

**Steinbrinck,** W. See Chediak-S.-Higashi *anomaly, syndrome.*

**Steiner,** Gabriel, German neurologist, *1883. See S.'s *tumors.*

**Steinert,** Bruno, German physician, 19th century. See S.'s *disease.*

**Steinmann,** Fritz, Swiss surgeon, 1872–1932. See S. *pin.*

**stella,** pl. **stellae** (stel'ah, stel'e) [ Mod. L. ]. 1. A star. 2 [ NA ]. A star-shaped figure.

  **s. lentis hyaloi'dea,** the posterior pole of the lens; see *radii* lentis.

**s. lentis irid'ica,** the anterior pole of the lens; see *radii* lentis.

**stellate** (stel'āt) [ L. *stella,* a star ]. Star-shaped.

**stellectomy** (stel-ek'to-mī). Stellate ganglionectomy.

**stellula,** pl. **stellulae** (stel'u-lah, -le) [ L. dim. of *stella,* star ]. A small star or star-shaped figure.

**stel'lulae vasculo'sae,** stellulae winslowii.

**stellulae verheyen'ii,** *venulae* stellatae.

**stellulae winslowii,** Winslow's stars; stellulae vasculosae; capillary whorls in the lamina choroidocapillaris from which arise the venae vorticosae.

**Stellwag** (stel'vahgh), Carl von C., Vienna ophthalmologist, 1823–1904. See S.'s *sign.*

**Stender,** Wilhelm P., Leipzig manufacturer of scientific apparatus. See S. *dish.*

**Stenger test.** See under test.

**stenion** (sten'ī-on) [ G. *stenos,* narrow, + dim. suffix *-iōn* ]. The termination in either temporal fossa of the shortest transverse diameter of the skull; a craniometric point.

**Steno.** See Stensen.

**steno-** (sten'o-) [ G. *stenos,* narrow ]. Combining form denoting narrowness or constriction.

**stenobregmatic** (sten'o-breg-mat'ik) [ steno- + G. *bregma, q.v.* ]. Denoting a skull narrow anteriorly, at the part where the bregma is.

**stenocardia** (sten'o-kar'dī-ah) [ steno- + G. *kardia,* heart ]. *Angina* pectoris.

**sten'ocepha'lia.** Stenocephaly.

**stenocephalic** (sten'o-sē-fal'ik). Stenocephalous.

**stenocephalous** (sten'o-sef'ă-lus). Denoting one with a narrow head, marked by stenocephaly.

**stenocephaly** (sten'o-sef'ă-lī) [ steno- + G. *kephalē,* head ]. Stenocephalia; marked narrowness of the head.

**stenochoria** (sten-o-ko'rī-ah) [ G. *stenochōria,* narrowness, fr. steno- + *chōra,* place, room ]. Abnormal contraction of any canal or orifice, especially of the lacrimal ducts.

**ste'nocompres'sor.** An instrument for compressing the ducts of the parotid glands (Stensen's duct) in order to keep back the saliva during dental operations.

**stenocoriasis** (sten'o-ko-ri'ă-sis) [ steno- + G. *korē,* pupil ]. Obsolete term for miosis (2).

**stenocrotaphy, stenocrotaphia** (sten'o-krot'ă-fī, -krota'fī-ah) [ steno- + G. *krotaphos,* temple ]. Narrowness of the skull in the temporal region; the condition of a stenobregmate skull.

**Stenon** [ *Stenonius,* Latin form of Stensen ]. See Stensen.

**stenope'ic, stenopa'ic** [ steno- + G. *opē,* opening ]. Provided with a narrow opening or slit.

**stenosal** (stē-no'sal). Relating to stenosis.

**stenosed** (sten'ōzd'). Narrowed; contracted: strictured.

**stenosis,** pl. **stenoses** (stē-no'sis, -sēz) [ G. *stenōsis,* a narrowing ]. A narrowing of any canal; a stricture; especially a narrowing of one of the cardiac valves.

**aortic s.,** pathologic narrowing of the aortic valve orifice.

**buttonhole s.,** extreme narrowing, usually of the mitral valve.

**calcific nodular aortic s.,** the commonest type of aortic s., occurring usually in elderly men; the cusps contain calcified fibrous nodules on both surfaces. The causes are not certainly known, but include rheumatic fever (especially when the mitral valve is also deformed), atherosclerosis, and hypertension.

**congenital pyloric s.,** hypertrophic pyloric s.

**coronary ostial s.,** narrowing of the mouths of the coronary arteries, usually as a result of syphilitic aortitis.

**Dittrich's s.,** infundibular s.

**double aortic s.,** subaortic s. associated with s. of the valve itself, both lesions being congenital.

**fishmouth mitral s.,** extreme mitral s.

**hypertrophic pyloric s.,** congenital pyloric s.; muscular hypertrophy of the pyloric sphincter, associated with projectile vomiting appearing in the second or third week of life, usually in males.

**idiopathic hypertrophic subaortic s.,** muscular subaortic a.; left ventricular outflow obstruction due to hypertrophy of the ventricular septum; of unknown cause.

**infundibular s.,** Dittrich's s.; narrowing of the outflow tract of the right ventricle below the pulmonic valve; this may be due to a localized fibrous diaphragm just below the valve, or more commonly to a long narrow fibromuscular channel.

**mitral s.,** pathologic narrowing of the orifice of the mitral valve.

**muscular subaortic s.,** idiopathic hypertrophic subaortic s.

**pulmonary s.,** narrowing of the opening into the pulmonary artery from the right ventricle.

**pyloric s.,** narrowing of the gastric pylorus, especially by congenital muscular hypertrophy or scarring resulting from a peptic ulcer; see also hypertrophic pyloric s.

**subaortic s.** congenital narrowing of the outflow tract of the left ventricle by a ring of fibrous tissue or by hypertrophy of the muscular septum shortly below the aortic valve.

**subvalvular s.,** narrowing of the aorta above the aortic valve by a constricting ring or shelf, or by coarctation or hypoplasia of the ascending aorta.

**tricuspid s.,** pathologic narrowing of the orifice of the tricuspid valve.

**stenostenosis** (ste'no-stē-no'sis). Stricture of the parotid duct (Steno's or Stensen's duct).

**stenostomia** (sten'o-sto'mī-ah) [ steno- + G. *stoma,* mouth ]. Narrowness of the oral cavity.

**sten'other'mal** [ steno- + G. *thermē,* heat ]. Thermostable through a small range; able to withstand only slight changes in temperature.

**sten'otho'rax** [ steno- + thorax ]. A narrow contracted chest.

**stenot'ic.** Narrowed; affected with stenosis.

**Stensen** (Steno; Stenon; Stenonius), Nicholaus or Niels, Danish anatomist, 1638–1686. See S.'s *duct, experiment, foramen, plexus, veins.*

**Stent,** C., English dentist, 19th century. Gave his name to stent.

**stent** [ C. *Stent* ]. A device used to maintain a bodily orifice or cavity during skin grafting.

**step.** 1. In dentistry, a dove-tailed or similarly shaped projection of a cavity prepared in a tooth into a surface perpendicular to the main part of the cavity for the purpose of preventing displacement of the restoration (filling) by the force of mastication. 2. A change in direction resembling a stair-step in a line, a surface, or the construction of a solid body.

**Krönig's s.'s,** extension of the lower part of the right border of absolute cardiac dullness in hypertrophy of the right heart.

**Roenne's nasal s.,** a right-angled defect of the visual field on the nasal side, one side of the angle corresponding to the horizontal meridian, seen in glaucoma.

**stepha'nial,** Pertaining to the stephanion.

**stephanion** (stē-fa'nī-on) [ G. dim. of *stephanos,* crown ]. A craniometric point where the coronal suture intersects the temporal crest (linea temporalis). See fig. under craniometric *point.*

**Stephanofilaria stilesi** (stef'ă-no-fī-lär'ī-ah sti-le'sī). A skin-infecting filaria, parasitic in cattle and transmitted by the horn fly, *Haematobia irritans;* the only species known to occur in America. It is characterized by a row of spines behind the mouth of the adult worm, which is 6 to 8 mm. in the female, 2 to 3 mm. in the male. Both adults and larvae are found in granulomatous skin lesions in cattle, usually on the underside of the abdomen.

**Stephanu'rus denta'tus** [ G. *stephanos,* crown, + *oura,* tail ]. The kidney worm or lard worm of swine; a strongyle nematode parasite that also occurs, though rarely, in the liver of cattle. The adult worms in swine live in the perirenal fat, the kidney pelvis, or as erratic forms in many other locations; the eggs are passed through the urine; as many as one million a day by a heavily infected hog. Infection is direct, by ingestion of infective larvae or by skin infection, or indirect, by ingestion of earthworms in which the larvae can survive.

**Stephenson,** William, Scottish obstetrician, 1837–1908. See S.'s *wave.*

**step'page** [ Fr. ]. The peculiar gait of sufferers from neuritis of the peroneal nerve and from tabes dorsalis; in consequence of this, dorsal flexion of the foot is impossible, and the patient in walking is obliged to raise the foot very high in order to clear the ground with the drooping toes.

**steradion** (stĕ-ra'dĭ-on) [ G. *stereos*, solid, + *radion*, radius ]. The unit of a solid angle; the solid angle that encloses an area on the surface of a sphere equivalent to the square of the radius of the sphere.

**sterane** (stĕr'ān, stĕr'ăn). The hypothetical parent molecule for any steroid hormone. S.'s are saturated hydrocarbon compounds, such as pregnane, that contain no oxygen. Originally conceived to achieve forms of systematic nomenclature. Supplanted by the fundamental variants: gonane, estrane, androstane, norandrostane (etiane), cholane, cholestane, ergostane, and stigmastane, described under steroids.

**sterco-** (ster'ko-) [ L. *stercus*, feces, excrement ]. Combining form relating to feces.

**stercobilin** (ster'ko-bi'lin, -bil'in). A brown degradation product of hemoglobin, present in the feces. See also bilirubinoids.

*l*-**stercobilinogen** (ster'ko-bi-lin'o-jen). Reduction product of *l*-urobilinogen, precursor of *l*-stercobilin in the final stages of bilirubin metabolism. It is excreted in feces, wherein it is oxidized to stercobilin. See also bilirubinoids.

**stercolith** (ster'ko-lith) [ sterco- + G. *lithos*, stone ]. Fecalith.

**stercoporphyrin** (ster'ko-por'fĭ-rin). Coproporphyrin.

**stercoraceous** (ster'ko-ra'shus). Fecal; stercoral; stercorous; relating to or containing feces.

**stercoral** (ster'ko-ral). Stercoraceous.

**stercorin** (ster'ko-rin). Coprosterol.

**stercoroma** (ster'ko-ro'mah) [ stereo- + G. suffix *-oma*, tumor ]. Coproma.

**stercorous** (ster'ko-rus). Stercoraceous.

**sterculia gum** (ster-ku'lĭ-ah). See under gum.

**sterculic acid** (ster-ku'lik). 2-Octylcycloprop-1-ene-1-octanoic acid; a fatty acid of plant origin, notable for the presence of a cyclopropene ring.

**stercus** (ster'kus) [ L. feces, excrement ]. Feces.

**stere** (stēr, stair) [ Fr. fr. G. *stereos*, solid ]. A measure of capacity; a cubic meter; a kiloliter.

**stereo-** (stĕr'e-o-, stĕr'e-o-) [ G. *stereos*, solid ]. 1. Combining form denoting a solid, or a solid condition or state. 2. Prefix denoting spatial qualities, three-dimensionality.

**stereoagnosis** (stĕr'e-o-ag-no'sis). Astereognosis.

**stereoanesthesia** (stĕr'e-o-an-es-the'zĭ-ah) [ stereo- + G. *an-* priv. + *aisthēsis*, sensation ]. Astereognosis.

**stereoarthrolysis** (stĕr'e-o-ar-throl'ĭ-sis) [ stereo- + G. *arthron*, joint, + *lysis*, loosening ]. The production of a new joint with mobility in cases of bony ankylosis.

**stereoauscultation** (stĕr'e-o-aws-kul-ta'shun). Auscultation with the symballophone.

**stereoblastula** (stĕr'e-o-blas'tu-lah). Archaic term for a solid blastula, now more properly called a morula.

**stereocampimeter** (stĕr'e-o-kam-pim'e-ter) [ stereo- + L. *campus*, field, + G. *metron*, measure ]. An apparatus for studying the central visual fields.

**stereochemical** (stĕr'e-o-kem'ĭ-kal). Relating to stereochemistry.

**stereochemistry** (stĕr-e-o-kem'is-trĭ). The branch of chemistry dealing with atoms in their spatial, three-dimensional relations; defining the positions the atoms in a compound bear in relation to one another in space; see stereoisomer.

**stereocilium,** pl. **stereocilia** (stĕr'e-o-sil'ĭ-um, -ah) [ stereo- + cilium, *q.v.* ]. Nonmotile cilium; long microvillus.

**stereocinefluorography** (ster'e-o-sīn'e-flu'or-og'rä-fĭ). Motion picture recording of x-ray pictures obtained by stereoscopic fluoroscopy; three-dimensional views are obtained.

**stereocolpogram** (stĕr'e-o-kol'po-gram). Picture taken with the stereocolposcope.

**stereocolposcope** (stĕr'e-o-kol'po-skōp) [ stereo- + G. *kolpos*, a hollow (vagina), *skopeō*, to view ]. An instrument that provides the observer with a magnified three-dimensional gross inspection of the vagina and cervix.

**stereoencephalometry** (stĕr'e-o-en-sef'ă-log'rä-fĭ). The localization of brain structures by use of three-dimensional coordinates.

**stereoencephalotomy** (stĕr'e-o-en-sef'ă-lot'o-mĭ) [ stereo- + G. *encephalos*, brain, + *tomē*, a cutting ]. Stereotaxy.

**stereognosis** (stĕr'e-og'no'sis) [ stereo- + G. *gnōsis*, knowledge ]. The appreciation of the form of an object by means of touch.

**stereognos'tic.** Relating to stereognosis.

**ster'eogram.** A stereoscopic x-ray picture.

**ster'eograph.** A stereoscopic x-ray apparatus.

**stereoisomer** (stĕr'e-o-i'so-mer) [ stereo- + G. *isos*, equal, + *meros*, part ]. A molecule containing the same number and kind of atom groupings as another but in a different arrangement in space, by virtue of which it exhibits different properties. Many enzymes distinguish between stereoisomers, as *e.g.*, between D and L amino acids, D and L sugars, 5α and 5β steroids, etc.; see stereoisomerism.

**stereoisomeric** (stĕr'e-o-i-so-mĕr'ik). Relating to stereoisomerism.

**stereoisomerism** (stĕr'e-o-i-som'er-izm). Stereochemical isomerism; molecular asymmetry; isomerism involving different spatial arrangement of the same groups (*e.g.*, androsterone and isoandrosterone, differing only in that one has a 3α OH, the other a 3β OH). See also stereoisomer, and LeBel-van't Hoff *rule*.

**stereology** (stĕr'e-ol'o-jĭ) [ stereo- + G. *logos*, study ]. A study of the three-dimensional aspects of a cell or microscopic structure.

**stereometer** (stĕr-e-om'e-ter) [ stereo- + G. *metron*, measure ]. 1. An instrument for measuring the capacity of a vessel or the size of a solid body. 2. An instrument for determining the specific gravity of a liquid.

**ster'eom'etry.** 1. The measurement of a solid object or the cubic capacity of a vessel. 2. Determination of the specific gravity of a liquid.

**stereo-ophthalmoscope** (stĕr'e-o-of-thal'mo-skōp). A binocular *ophthalmoscope.*

**stereo-orthopter** (stĕr'e-o-or'thop-ter) [ stereo- + G. *orthos*, straight, + *optikos*, optical ]. A type of stereoscope used in visual training.

**stereopathy** (stĕr'e-o-op'ă-thĭ). Persistent stereotyped thinking.

**stereophantoscope** (stĕr'e-o-fan'to-skōp) [ stereo- + G. *phantos*, visible, + *skopeō*, to view ]. A stereophoroscope with rotating disks of different colors instead of pictures, used to import motion to the views.

**stereophorometer** (stĕr'e-o-fo-rom'e-ter). A phorometer with stereoscopic attachment.

**stereophoroscope** (stĕr'e-o-fōr'o-skōp) [ stereo- + G. *phoros*, bearing, *skopeō*, to view ]. A stereoscope producing images in apparent motion.

**stereophotomicrograph** (stĕr'e-o-fo'to-mi'kro-graf). A stereoscopic photomicrograph which, when viewed with a stereoscope, appears three-dimensional.

**stereopsis** (stĕr'e-op'sis) [ stereo- + G. *opsis*, vision ]. Stereoscopic *vision.*

**stereoradiography** (stĕr'e-o-ra-dĭ-og'rä-fĭ). Stereoroentgenography.

**stereoroentgenography** (stĕr'e-o-rent'gen-og'rä-fĭ, -rĕnt-jen). Stereoskiagraphy; stereoradiography; the taking of an x-ray picture from two slightly different positions so as to obtain a stereoscopic effect.

**stereoscope** (stĕr'e-o-skōp) [ stereo- + G. *skopeō*, to view ]. An instrument by means of which two images of the same object, as seen from slightly different viewpoints, are blended into one, giving an appearance of relief to the picture. See fig. on p. 1334.

**reflecting s.,** Wheatstone s.

**Wheatstone s.,** reflecting s.; an instrument fitted with mirrors so placed that reflections of identical images (targets) seen individually by each eye are merged and projected as a single spatial image.

**ster'eoscop'ic.** Relating to a stereoscope or to the appearance of relief presented by a solid body.

**stereospecific** (stĕr'e-o-spe-sif'ik). Denoting generally the characteristic of a reaction that meets with one or both of

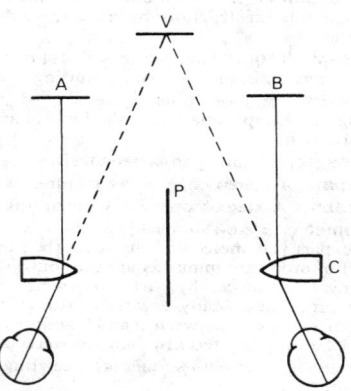

**Diagram Illustrating the Principle of the Stereoscope**
*A* and *B* represent photographs of two views taken from slightly different angles; *C*, prisms; *P*, partition to prevent one eye seeing the picture opposite the other eye; *V*, the image formed when the two views are fused by the instrument appears to be at *V*.

the following conditions: (1) a given product is obtained preferentially or exclusively from only one of two or more conceivable stereoisomeric precursors; (2) a given compound yields preferentially or exclusively one of two or more possible stereoisomeric products. Two recent proposals to restrict the meaning of stereospecific and to differentiate it from stereoselective are mutually incompatible; neither has met with general acceptance.

**stereotactic** (stĕr'e-o-tak'tik). Stereotaxic.

**stereotaxic** (stĕr'e-o-tak'sik). Stereotactic; relating to stereotaxis or stereotaxy.

**stereotaxis** (stĕr'e-o-tak'sis) [ stereo- + G. *taxis*, orderly arrangement ]. 1. Three-dimensional arrangement. 2. Stereotropism, but applied more exactly where the organism as a whole, rather than a part only, reacts. 3. Stereotaxy.

**stereotaxy** (stĕr'e-o-tak'sĭ). Stereotaxis (3); stereoencephalotomy; stereotactic surgery; a precise method of destroying deep-seated brain structures located by use of three-dimensional coordinates.

**ster'eotrop'ic.** Relating to or exhibiting stereotropism.

**stereotropism** (stĕr'e-ot'ro-pizm) [ stereo- + G. *tropos*, a turning ]. Growth or movement of a plant or animal toward (**positive s.**) or away from (**negative s.**) a solid body, usually applied where a part of the organism rather than the whole reacts.

**stereotypy** (stĕr'e-o-ti-pī) [ stereo- + G. *typos*, impression, type ]. 1. The maintenance of one attitude for a long period. 2. The constant repetition of certain meaningless gestures or movements.

    **oral s.,** verbigeration.

**steric** (stĕr'ik, stēr-). Pertaining to stereochemistry.

    **s. hindrance,** interference or inhibition of an otherwise feasible reaction (usually synthetic) because the size of one or another reactant prevents approach to the required distance.

**sterids** (stĕr'idz, stēr-). Steroids.

**sterig'ma** [ G. *stērigma*, a support ]. A stalk or narrow, pointed structure from a cell that supports a spore or conidium; among the Basidiomycetes, a slender stalk at the top of the basidium, from the tips of which the basidiospores are formed.

**sterile** (stĕr'il) [ L. *sterilis*, barren ]. Relating to or characterized by sterility.

**sterility** (stĕ-ril'ĭ-tĭ) [ L. *sterilitas* ]. 1. In general, the inability to produce progeny; see female s.; male s. 2. The state of being aseptic, or free from all living microorganisms and their spores.

    **adolescent s.,** a period following the menarche, and lasting up to approximately 18 months, during which

menstrual cycles may be markedly irregular and are often anovulatory.

    **aspermatogen'ic s.,** s. due to a failure to produce living spermatozoa.

    **dys'spermatogen'ic s.,** male s. due to some abnormality in production of spermatozoa.

    **female s.,** absolute s.; the inability of the female to conceive, due to inadequacy in structure or function of the genital organs.

    **male s.,** the inability of the male to fertilize the ovum; it may or may not be associated with impotence.

    **normospermatogen'ic s.,** male s. due to some cause other than failure to produce live, normal spermatozoa, *e.g.,* blockage of the seminiferous passages.

    **one-child s.,** s. occurring in a woman who has borne one child and has no more.

    **relative s.,** infertility.

**sterilization** (stĕr'ĭ-lĭ-za'shun). 1. The act or process of making any person or thing sterile. 2. Castration. 3. The destruction of all microorganisms in or about an object.

    **discontin'uous s.,** fractional s.

    **electron'ic s.,** s. of surgical instruments, dressings, sutures, etc., by means of high velocity electrons generated by a specially designed electron accelerating apparatus with an anode voltage of from 2 to 3 million volts.

    **s. by ethylene oxide,** a form of gaseous s. which is nondestructive of materials and highly bactericidal, with excellent ability to penetrate but with the major disadvantage of being very slow.

    **s. by flowing steam,** s. by exposure in an unsealed vessel to the action of steam at a temperature of 100°C. (212°F.).

    **fractional s.,** tyndallization; discontinuous s.; exposure to a temperature 100°C. **(flowing steam)** for a definite period, usually an hour, on each of several days; at each heating the developed bacteria are destroyed; the spores which are unaffected germinate during the intervening period.

    **intermit'tent s.,** fractional s. or discontinuous s.

    **s. by steam under pressure,** s. effected by exposure to the action of superheated steam in an autoclave.

**sterilize** (stĕr'ĭ-liz). To render sterile.

**sterilizer** (stĕr'ĭ-li-zer). An apparatus for making anything aseptic or germ-free.

    **glass bead s.,** a s. for root canal equipment; the heat is transmitted to the instruments, absorbent points, or cotton pellets by means of glass beads.

    **hot salt s.,** a s. for endodontic equipment in which table salt is heated in a container at 425 to 475°F.; the dry heat is transmitted to root canal instruments, absorbent points, or cotton pellets for their rapid (5 to 10 seconds) sterilization.

**Stern,** Heinrich, New York physician, 1868–1918. See S.'s *posture.*

**stern-.** See sterno-.

**ster'na.** Plural of sternum.

**ster'nad.** In a direction toward the sternum.

**ster'nal.** Relating to the sternum.

**sternalgia** ster-nal'jĭ-ah) [ stern- + G. *algos*, pain ]. Sternodynia; pain in the sternum or the sternal region.

**sterna'lis.** See under musculus.

**Sternberg,** George M., American bacteriologist, 1838–1915. See S. *cells,* Reed-S. *cells.*

**Sternberg,** Karl, German pathologist, 1872–1935. See S. *disease,* Paltauf-S. *disease.*

**sternebra,** pl. **sternebrae** (ster'ne-brah, -bre) [ Mod. L. fr. stern(um) + (vert)ebra ]. One of the four segments of the primordial sternum of the embryo by the fusion of which the body of the adult sternum is formed.

**ster'nen** (stern- + G. *en*, in ]. Relating to the sternum independent of any other structures.

**sterno-, stern-** (ster'no-) [ G. *sternon*, chest (sternum). STERN- ]. Combining form relating to the sternum.

**sternochondroscapularis** (ster'no-kon'dro-skap-u-la'ris) [ Mod. L. ]. See under musculus.

**sternoclavicular** (ster'no-klā-vik'u-lar). Relating to the sternum and the clavicle.

**ster'noclavicula'ris.** See under musculus.

**sternocleidal** (ster'no-kli'dal) [ sterno- + G. *kleis*, key (clavicle) ]. Relating to the sternum and the clavicle.

**sternocleidomastoid** (ster'no-kli'do-mas'toyd). Relating to sternum, clavicle, and mastoid process.

**sternocleidomastoideus** (ster'no-kli'do-mas-to-id'-e-us) [ Mod. L. ]. See under musculus.

**sternocostal** (ster'no-kos'tal). [ L. *costa*, rib ]. Relating to the sternum and the ribs.

**sternodynia** (ster'no-din'ĭ-ah) [ sterno- + G. *odynē*, pain ]. Sternalgia.

**sternofascialis** (stur'no-fă-shĭ-al'is). See under musculus.

**sternoglossal** (ster'no-glos'al). Denoting muscular fibers which occasionally pass from the sternohyoid muscle to join the hyoglossal muscle.

**sternohyoideus** (ster'no-hi'o-id'e-us) [ Mod. L. ]. See under musculus.

**sternoid** (ster'noyd) [ sterno- + G. *eidos*, resemblance ]. Resembling the sternum.

**sternomastoid** (ster'no-mas'toyd). Relating to the sternum and the mastoid process of the temporal bone; applied to the musculus sternocleidomastoideus.

**sternopagia** (ster'no-pa'jĭ-ah) [ sterno- + G. *pagos*, something fixed, + suffix -ia, condition ]. The condition shown by conjoined twins united at the sterna or more extensively at the ventral walls of the chest.

**sternopagus** (ster-nop'ă-gus) [ sterno- + G. *pagos*, something fixed ]. An individual with sternopagia.

**sternopericardial** (ster'no-pĕr'ĭ-kar'dĭ-al). Relating to the sternum and the pericardium.

**sternoschisis** (ster-nos'kĭ-sis) [ sterno- + G. *schisis*, a cleaving ]. Congenital cleft of the sternum.

**sternothyroideus** (ster'no-thi-ro-id'e-us) [ Mod. L. ]. See under musculus.

**sternotomy** (ster-not'o-mĭ) [ sterno- + G. *tomē*, incision ]. Incision into or through the sternum.

**sternotracheal** (ster'no-tra'ke-al). Relating to the sternum and the trachea.

**sternotrypesis** (ster'no-tri-pe'sis) [ sterno- + G. *trypēsis*, a boring ]. Trephining of the sternum.

**sternovertebral** (ster'no-ver'te-bral). Vetebrosternal; relating to the sternum and the vertebrae; denoting the true ribs, or the seven upper ribs on either side, which articulate with the vertebrae and with the sternum.

**sternum**, gen. **sterni**, pl. **sterna** (ster'num, -ni, -nah) [ Mod. L. fr. G. *sternon*, the chest ] [ NA ]. The breast bone; a long flat bone, articulating with the cartilages of the first seven ribs and with the clavicle, forming the middle part of the anterior wall of the thorax; it consists of three portions: the corpus or body, the manubrium, and the xiphoid process.

**sternutatio** (ster'nu-ta'shĭ-o) [ L. ]. Sternutation.

**s. convulsi'va**, paroxysmal sneezing; the sneezing of hay fever.

**sternutation** (ster'nu-ta'shun) [ L. *sternutatio*, fr. *sternuo* (*sternuto*), pp. *sternutatus*, to sneeze ]. The act of sneezing; see sneeze.

**ster'nuta'tor.** Sneezing gas; diphenylchlorarsine.

**sternu'tatory.** Errhine.

**steroid** (stēr'oyd, stĕr'oyd). 1. Steroidal; pertaining to the steroids. 2. One of the steroids; see steroids. 3. A generic designation for compounds closely related in structure to steroids, such as sterols, bile acids, cardiac glycosides, and precursors of the vitamins D. 4. Jargon for a compound having biological actions similar to a steroid hormone, of semisynthetic or synthetic origin, and whose structure may or may not resemble that of a steroid.

**s. hydroxylases**, s. monooxygenases.

**s. monooxygenases**, s. hydroxylases; enzymes catalyzing addition of hydroxyl groups to the steroid rings utilizing $O_2$. They are differentiated into steroid $11\beta$-monooxygenase (EC 1.14.15.4), steroid $17\alpha$-monooxygenase (EC 1.14.99.9), and steroid 21-monooxygenase (EC 1.14.99.10), in accordance with the position of the catalytically introduced hydroxyl group. Included in the group of steroid monooxygenases are estradiol $6\beta$-monooxygenase; progesterone $11\alpha$-monooxygenase; androstene 3,17-monooxygenase; methylsterol monooxygenase; and corticosterone 18-monooxygenase.

**s. nucleus,** tetracyclic s. nucleus.

**tetracyclic s. nucleus,** perhydrocyclopenta[ *a* ]phenanthrene; perhydrocyclopentenophenanthrene; cyclopentanoperhydrophenanthrene; the group of four fused rings forming the framework or parent substance of the steroids. The correct systematic name is cyclopenta[ *a* ]phenanthrene (see steroids).

**steroidogenesis** (ste'roy'do-jen'ē-sis). [ steroid + G. *genesis*, production ]. The formation of steroids; term is commonly used to refer to the biological synthesis of steroid hormones, but not to the production of such compounds in a chemical laboratory.

**steroids** (stēr'oydz, stĕr'oydz). A large family of chemical substances, comprising many hormones, vitamins, body constituents, and drugs, each containing the tetracyclic cyclopenta[ *a* ]phenanthrene skeleton. Formula I of the accompanying page of structures shows the numbering and lettering of the rings, which are retained even if, in a given compound, any of the atoms shown are absent or involved in ring closures, or if rings are expanded ("homo," see below) or contracted ("nor," see below). Stereoisomerism among steroids is not only common but of critical biological significance, and the isomeric groups are usually represented as shown in II. The conventions are that the nucleus is presented as if projected onto the plane of the paper, with groups then lying upward being denoted by thickened bonds and called $\beta$, those then lying downward by broken bonds and called $\alpha$. The letter $\xi$ indicates unknown or unspecified orientation. Depending on the situation at C-5, the molecule is sometimes represented in perspective as in III and IV; $5\alpha$, $5\beta$, or $5\xi$ is usually included in the name. Unless otherwise stated, it is assumed that atoms or groups attached to the other ring-junctions 8, 9, 10, 13, 14) are as in II, *i.e.*, $8\beta$, $9\alpha$, $10\beta$, $13\beta$, $14\alpha$.

The principal classes of steroids, with names for the unsubstituted, saturated hydrocarbon forms that are clearly related to physiological functions or sources, are shown in V, VI, VII, and VIII. The digitaloid lactone derivatives known as cardanolides have the basic structure IX. The squill-toad poison group of lactones are called bufanolides (X). Spirostans and furostans (the basic structures of many "genins," including the sapogenins) are derived from XI and XII, respectively.

The natural and synthetic derivatives are named by adding conventional chemical prefixes and suffixes for substituents (for example, -ol for a hydroxyl group, -one) for a keto group, -al for an aldehyde group, etc.). "Nor" indicates loss of a —CH₂— group; "homo," the addition of a —CH₂— group; each is preceded by the letter indicating which ring is contracted or expanded, respectively, or, in the case where the —CH₂— is lost from a methyl group, the number of the carbon atom lost (see 18-norandrostane, formula XV). "Seco" indicates fission of a ring with addition of hydrogen atoms at the positions indicated by numerals preceding the term (see cholecalciferol and ergocalciferol in the table on p. 1337). Unsaturation is denoted, as usual, by substituting appropriate terms (for example, -en(e), -yn(e), -adien(e)) for the -ane or -an parts of the hydrocarbon or parent class names, with numerals indicating locations of the unsaturated bonds. The locations of double bonds are specified by the lower of the two (consecutive) numbers of the carbon atoms involved. When a double bond is formed between two nonconsecutive carbon atoms, the second is indicated in parentheses after the first; *e.g.*, estriol and the estradiols (see table) possess three double bonds, between C1 and C2, between C3 and C4, and between C5 and C10, respectively.

Steroid alkaloids may be named from the steroid parent, as above, or from trivial family names usually ending in -anine if the steroid is saturated or in -enine, -adienine, etc., if it is not saturated (*e.g.*, conanine, tomatanine).

Some individual steroids of significant biological activity are defined systematically in the accompanying table (see p. 1337).

**sterol** (stēr'ol). A steroid of 27 or more carbon atoms with one OH (alcohol) group; the systematic names contain

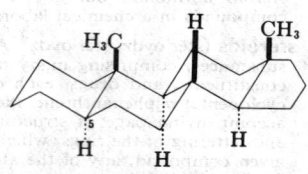

I. Numbering of atoms and rings of steroids and conventional orientation.

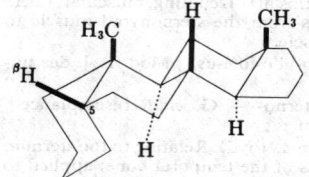

II. Depiction of α and β exocyclic atoms of steroids. These orientations are assumed to prevail in a steroid unless specifically otherwise indicated in the name.

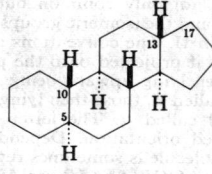

III. Perspective view of a 5α-steroid

IV. Perspective view of a 5β-steroid

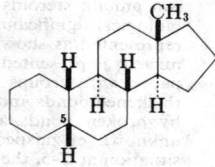

V. 5α-gonane    VI. 5β-estrane    VII. 5α-18-norandrostane (= 10-methyl-5α-gonane)

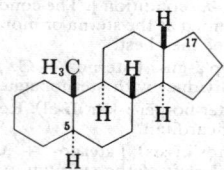

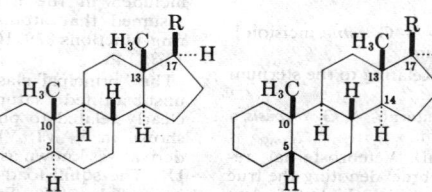

VIII. Steroids with methyl groups at both C-10 and C-13. *Left*, 5α series; *right*, 5β series. The names listed below are used for these steroids.

| R (at position 17) | 5α Series | 5β Series |
|---|---|---|
| H | 5α-Androstane (*not* etioallocholane) | 5β-Androstane (*not* testane or etiocholane or etiane) |
| $C_2H_5$ | 5α-Pregnane (*not* allopregnane) | 5β-Pregnane |
| $CH(CH_3)CH_2CH_2CH_3$ | 5α-Cholane (*not* allocholane) | 5β-Cholane |
| $CH(CH_3)CH_2CH_2CH_2CH(CH_3)_2$ | 5α-Cholestane | 5β-Cholestane (*not* coprostane) |
| $CH(CH_3)CH_2CH_2CH(CH_3)CH(CH_3)_2$ | 5α-Ergostane | 5β-Ergostane |
| $CH(CH_3)CH_2CH_2CH(C_2H_5)CH(CH_3)_2$ | 5α-Stigmastane | 5β-Stigmastane |
| COOH | 5α-Etianic Acid | 5β-Etianic Acid |

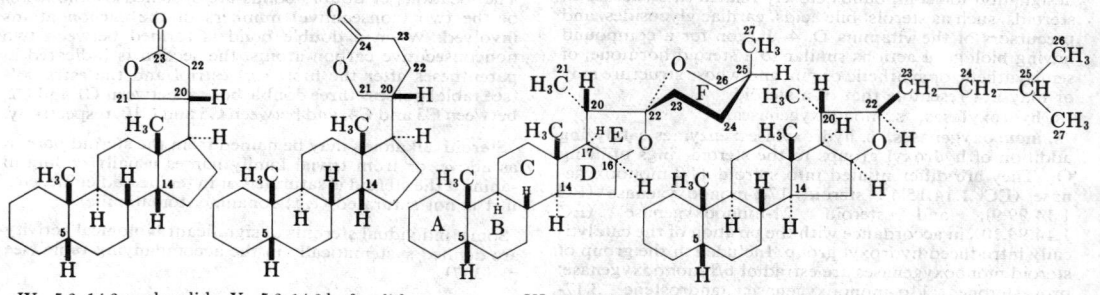

IX. 5β, 14β-cardanolide    X. 5β, 14β-bufanolide    XI. 5β-spirostan    XII. 5β-furostan

**Steroids**

either the prefix hydroxy- or the suffix -ol, *e.g.,* cholesterol, ergosterol.

**plant s.'s,** phytosterols; see also sitosterols.

**s. X,** lumisterol.

*Some trivial names for biologically important steroids*

| Trivial name | Systematic name |
| --- | --- |
| Aldosterone | 18,11-Hemiacetal of 11$\beta$,21-dihydroxy-3,20-dioxo-4-pregnen-18-al |
| Androsterone | 3$\alpha$-Hydroxy-5$\alpha$-androstan-17-one |
| Cholecalciferol | *9,10-Seco-5,7,10(19)-cholestatrien-3$\beta$-ol |
| Cholesterol | 5-Cholesten-3$\beta$-ol |
| Cholic acid | 3$\alpha$,7$\alpha$,12$\alpha$-Trihydroxy-5$\beta$-cholan-24-oic acid |
| Corticosterone | 11$\beta$,21-Dihydroxy-4-pregnene-3,20-dione |
| Cortisol | 11$\beta$,17,21-Trihydroxy-4-pregnene-3,20-dione |
| Cortisol acetate | Cortisol 21-acetate |
| Cortisone | 17,21-Dihydroxy-4-pregnene-3,11,20-trione |
| Cortisone acetate | Cortisone 21-acetate |
| Deoxycorticosterone | 21-Hydroxy-4-pregnene-3,20-dione (*i.e.,* the 11-deoxy derivative of corticosterone) |
| Ergocalciferol | *9,10-Seco-5,7,10(19),22-ergostatetraen-3$\beta$-ol |
| Ergosterol | 5,7,22-Ergostatrien-3$\beta$-ol |
| Estradiol-17$\alpha$ | 1,3,5(10)-Estratriene-3,17$\alpha$-diol |
| Estradiol-17$\beta$ | 1,3,5(10)-Estratriene-3,17$\beta$-diol |
| Estriol | 1,3,5(10)-Estratriene-3,16$\alpha$,17$\beta$-triol |
| Estrone | 3-Hydroxy-1,3,5(10)-estratrien-17-one |
| Lanosterol | 8,24-Lanostadien-3$\beta$-ol |
| Lithocholic acid | 3$\alpha$-Hydroxy-5$\beta$-cholan-24-oic acid |
| Progesterone | 4-Pregnene-3,20-dione |
| Testosterone | 17$\beta$-Hydroxy-4-androsten-3-one |

* "Seco" indicates fission of a ring with addition of a hydrogen at the places indicated by the numerals preceding the term.

**ster'tor** [ L. *sterto,* to snore ]. A snore; a noisy inspiration occurring in coma or deep sleep.

**hen-cluck s.,** a breath sound like the clucking of a hen, sometimes heard in cases of postpharyngeal abscess.

**ster'torous.** Relating to or characterized by stertor or snoring.

**steth-.** See stetho-.

**stethalgia** (stĕ-thal'jī-ah) [ steth- + G. *algos,* pain ]. Pain in the chest.

**stetharteritis** (steth-ar-ter-i'tis) [ steth- + arteritis ]. Inflammation of the aorta or other arteries in the chest.

**stethemia** (stĕ-the'mī-ah) [ steth- + G. *haima,* blood ]. Pulmonary congestion.

**stethendoscope** (steth'en'do-skōp) [ steth- + endoscope ]. A fluoroscope for examination of the chest.

**stetho-, steth-** (steth'o-) [ G. *stēthos,* chest ]. Combining forms relating to the chest.

**stethocatharsis** (steth'o-kă-thar'sis) [ stetho- + G. *katharsis,* a purging ]. Expectoration.

**stethocyrtograph** (steth'o-sur'to-graf) [ stetho- + G. *kyrtos,* bent, + *graphō,* to write ]. Stethokyrtograph; an apparatus for measuring and recording the curvatures of the thorax.

**stethocyrtometer** (steth'o-sur-tom'e-ter) [ stetho- + G. *kyrtos,* bent, + *metron,* measure ]. An instrument for measuring curvature or deformity of the vertebral column in kyphosis.

**stethogoniometer** (steth'o-go'nĭ-om'e-ter) [ stetho- + G. *gōnia,* angle, + *metron,* measure ]. An apparatus for measuring the curvatures of the thorax.

**stethograph** (steth'o-graf) [ stetho- + G. *graphō,* to write ]. An apparatus for recording the respiratory movements of the chest.

**stethokyrtograph** (steth'o-kur'to-graf). Stethocyrtograph.

**stethomenia** (steth'o-me'nī-ah) [ stetho- + G. *mēn,* month ]. Hemoptysis occurring as a form of vicarious menstruation.

**stethometer** (stĕ-thom'e-ter) [ stetho- + G. *metron,* measure ]. Thoracometer; an instrument for measuring the circumference of the chest and its variations in respiration.

**stethomyitis, stethomyositis** (steth-o-mi-i'tis, steth-o-mi-o-si'tis) [ stetho- + G. *mys,* muscle, + suffix *-itis,* inflammation ]. Inflammation of the muscles of the chest wall.

**stethoparalysis** (steth'o-pă-ral'ī-sis). Paralysis of the respiratory muscles.

**steth'ophone** [ stetho- + G. *phōnē,* sound ]. Stethoscope.

**stethophonometer** (steth'o-fo-nom'e-ter) [ stetho- + G. *phōnē,* sound, + *metron,* measure ]. A device for measuring the intensity of the sounds heard on auscultation or of the percussion note.

**stethopolyscope** (steth'o-pol'ĭ-skōp) [ stetho- + G. *polys,* many, + *skopeō,* to view ]. A stethoscope with a number of flexible ear tubes, so that several persons can listen at the same time to the same auscultatory sound.

**stethoscope** (steth'o-skōp) [ stetho- + G. *skopeō,* to view ]. Stethophone; an instrument originally devised by Laennec for aid in hearing the respiratory and cardiac sounds in the chest; now modified in various ways and used in auscultation of any of the vascular or other sounds in the body anywhere.

**binau'ral s.,** a s. in which the two ear pieces connect with a single bell.

**Bowles type s.,** a s. in which the chest piece is a shallow metal cup about 4.5 cm. in diameter, the mouth of which is covered by a hard rubber or celluloid diaphragm.

**differential s.,** one having two chest pieces so that two sounds in different parts of the chest may be heard simultaneously and compared.

**head s.,** one which by means of a metal T-plate is brought into contact with the examiner's forehead; hearing by air conduction through ear pieces is thus aided by bone conduction.

**steth'oscop'ic.** 1. Relating to or effected by means of a stethoscope. 2. Relating to an examination of the chest.

**stethoscopy** (stĕ-thos'ko-pī). 1. Examination of the chest by means of auscultation, either mediate or immediate, and percussion. 2. Mediate auscultation with the stethoscope.

**stethospasm** (steth'o-spazm). Spasm of the chest.

**Stevens,** Albert M., American pediatrician, 1884–1945. See S.-Johnson *syndrome.*

**Stewart,** Fred D. See S.-Treves *syndrome.*

**Stewart,** R. M., English physician, 20th century. See S.-Morel *syndrome.*

**Stewart-Holmes sign.** See under sign.

**Stewart's test.** See under test.

**STH.** Abbreviation for somatotropic (growth) hormone, or somatotropin, *q. v.*

**sthenia** (sthe′nĭ-ah) [ G. *sthenos*, strength, + suffix -*ia*, condition ]. A condition of activity and apparent force, as in an acute sthenic fever.

**sthen′ic.** Strong; active; marked by sthenia; said of a fever with strong bounding pulse, high temperature, and active delirium.

**stheno-, sthen-** (sthen′o-) [ G. *sthenos*, strength. STHEN- ]. Combining forms denoting strength, force, or power.

**sthenometer** (sthĕ-nom′e-ter) [ stheno- + G. *metron*, measure ]. An instrument for measuring muscular strength.

**sthenom′etry.** The measurement of muscular strength.

**stib′amine glu′coside** A pentavalent antimony compound; a nitrogen glycoside of sodium *p*-aminobenzenestibonate; has been used in kala azar and certain other tropical diseases (no longer marketed).

**stibenyl** (stib′ĕ-nil). Sodium 4-acetamidobenzenestibonate; the first pentavalent antimonial used in the treatment of kala azar.

**stibialism** (stib′ĭ-ă-lizm) [ L. *stibium*, antimony ]. Chronic antimonial poisoning.

**stib′iated.** Impregnated with or containing antimony.

**stibiation** (stib′ĭ-a′shun). Impregnation with antimony.

**stib′ium** [ L. fr. G. *stibi* ]. Antimony.

**stib′ocap′tate.** Antimony dimercaptosuccinate.

**stib′oglu′conate sodium.** 1 (USP, BP). PENTOSTAN; MYOSTIBIN; pentavalent antimony sodium gluconate; pentavalent sodium stibogluconate; used in the treatment of all types of leishmaniasis. 2. TRIOSTAM; trivalent antimony sodium gluconate; trivalent sodium stibogluconate; sodium antimonylgluconate; used in the treatment of schistosomiasis. For both forms, toxic effects are frequent.

**stibonium** (stĭ-bo′nĭ-um). The hypothetical radical, $SbH_4^+$, analogous to ammonium.

**stib′ophen** (USP, BP). FUADIN; pentasodium bis[ 4,5-dihydroxybenz-1,3-disulfonate ]antimonate · $7H_2O$; an organic trivalent antimony compound; used in the treatment of schistosomiasis, filariasis, leishmaniasis, and lymphogranuloma inguinale.

**stichochrome** (stik′o-krōm) [ G. *stichos*, a row, + *chrōma*, color ]. Denoting a nerve cell in which the chromophil substance, or stainable material, is arranged in roughly parallel rows or lines.

**Sticker,** Georg, German physician, *1860. See S.'s *disease.*

**Stickler,** G. B. See S. *syndrome.*

**stictacne** (stikt-ak′ne) [ G. *stiktos*, pricked, + acne ]. Acne with punctate scar formation.

**Stieda** (ste′dah), Alfred, German surgeon, *1869. See S.'s *fracture.*

**Stieda** (ste′dah), Ludwig, German anatomist, 1837–1918. See S.'s *process.*

**Stierlin,** Eduard, German surgeon, 1878–1919. See S.'s *sign.*

**Stifel's figure.** See under figure.

**stifle** (sti′fl). Stifle *joint.*

**stigma,** pl. **stigmas** or **stigmata** (stig′mah, stig′mă-tah) [ G. a mark, fr. *stizō*, to prick. STIG- ]. 1. Visible evidence of a disease. 2. Stoma (3); the interval between the endothelial cells in the wall of a capillary or lymph channel. 3. The point of rupture of a Graafian follicle on the surface of the ovary. 4. Any spot or blemish on the skin. 5. A bleeding spot on the skin which is considered a manifestation of conversion hysteria. 6. The orange pigmented eyespot of certain chlorophyll-bearing protozoa, such as *Euglena viridis*; it serves as a light filter, absorbing certain wavelengths. 7. A mark of shame or discredit.

**s. of degeneration,** one of a number of physical, nervous, or psychic abnormalities occurring solely, or with preponderating frequency, in degenerate constitution.

**Giuffrida-Ruggieri s.,** an archaic eponym denoting extreme shallowness of the glenoid fossa.

**Koplik's s. of degeneration,** a prominence over the pisiform bone observed in certain cases of sporadic cretinism.

**Malpighian s.'s,** the points of entrance of the smaller veins into the larger veins of the spleen.

**s. ventric′uli,** one of a number of miliary ecchymoses of the gastric mucosa.

**stig′mal.** Stigmatic.

**stigmas′tane.** Sitostane; parent substance of sitosterols and stigmasterols (for structure, see steroids).

**stigmast′erol.** Anti-stiffness factor (*q. v.*); stigmasta-5,22-dien-3β-ol (for structure of stigmastane, see steroids); a sterol obtained from the oil of *Physostigma* (calabar bean) and from soybean oil.

**stig′mata.** Alternate plural of stigma.

**stig′mata maydis.** Corn silk; see zea.

**stigmat′ic.** Relating to or marked by a stigma.

**stig′matism.** The condition of having stigmas.

**stigmatization** (stig′mă-tĭ-za′shun). 1. Stigmatism. 2. The production of stigmas, especially of hysterical stigmas. 3. The debasement of a person by attributing a stigma to him.

**stig′matom′eter.** Astigmatometer.

**stilbam′idine.** Stilbene-4,4′-dicarbonamidine; a compound used in the treatment of kala azar, in infections due to *Blastomyces dermatitidis*, and in actinomycosis; also used in multiple myeloma for the relief of bone pain.

**stilbaz′ium iodide** (USAN). MONOPAR; 1-ethyl-2,6-bis[ *p*-(1-pyrrolidinyl)styryl ]-pyridinium iodide; anthelmintic.

**stil′bene.** *trans*-α,β-Diphenylethylene; $C_6H_5CHCHC_6H_5$; an unsaturated hydrocarbon, the nucleus of stilbestrol and other synthetic estrogenic compounds.

**stilbes′trol.** Diethylstilbestrol.

**Stiles,** W. S., British physiologist. See S.-Crawford *effect.*

**stilet, stilette** (sti′let, sti-let′). Stylet.

**Still,** Sir George F., English physician, 1868–1941. See S.'s *disease*, S.-Chauffard *syndrome.*

**Still's murmur.** See under murmur.

**still′birth.** The birth of an infant who shows no evidence of life after birth; see also stillborn *infant.*

**still′born.** Born dead; see stillborn *infant.*

**stillicidium** (stil′ĭ-sid′ĭ-um) [ L. the trickling of rain; *stilla*, drop, + *cado*, to fall ]. Staxis; a dripping, dribbling, or falling of a liquid drop by drop.

**s. lacrima′rum,** obsolete term for epiphora.

**s. uri′nae,** incontinence of urine in cases of distended bladder.

**Stilling,** Benedict, German anatomist, 1810–1879. See S.'s *canal, column, fibers, fleece, nucleus, raphe*, gelatinous *substance.*

**Stilling,** Jakob, German ophthalmologist, 1842–1915. See S.'s color *tables.*

**sti′lus,** pl. **sti′li** [ L. a stake, a style used for writing ]. Stylus.

**stimulant** (stim′u-lant) [ L. *stimulans*, pres. p. of *stimulo*, pp. -*atus*, to goad, incite, fr. *stimulus*, a goad ]. 1. Stimulating; exciting to action. 2. Stimulator; an agent that arouses organic activity, strengthens the action of the heart, increases vitality, and promotes a sense of well-being. S.'s are classified, according to the parts upon which they chiefly act, as cardiac, respiratory, stomachic, hepatic, cerebral, spinal, vascular, genital, etc. See also stimulus.

**diffu′sible s.,** one that produces a rapid but temporary effect.

**general s.,** one that affects the entire body.

**local s.,** one whose action is confined to the part to which it is applied.

**stimulation** (stim′u-la′shun) [ see stimulant ]. 1. The arousing of the body or any of its parts or organs to increased functional activity. 2. The condition of being stimulated.

**photic s.,** the use of a flickering light to influence the pattern of the electroencephalogram and also to bring out latent abnormalities.

**stimulator** (stim′u-la-tor). Stimulant (2).

**long-acting thyroid s.,** abbreviated LATS; a substance found in the blood of hyperthyroid patients that exerts a prolonged stimulatory effect on the thyroid gland. It is associated in plasma with the immunoglobulin G (7S γ-globulin) fraction; may be an antibody; believed not to be formed in the pituitary gland, and is clearly not identical with thyrotropin.

**stimuli** (stim′u-li). Plural of stimulus.

**stimulin** (stim'u-lin). 1. A substance said to be present in fresh gastric juice which stimulates the gastric glands to renewed secretion. 2. The term given by Metchnikoff to phagocytosis-enhancing substances in serum, now known to be antibodies.

**stimulus,** pl. **stimuli** (stim'u-lus, -li) [ L. a goad ]. 1. A stimulant. 2. Anything internal or from the external environment that can elicit or evoke action (response) in a muscle, nerve, gland or other excitable tissue, or cause an augmenting action upon any function or metabolic process.

**adequate s.,** one to which a particular receptor responds effectively and which gives rise to the characteristic sensation, *e.g.,* light and sound waves that stimulate, respectively, visual and auditory receptors.

**conditioned s.,** (1) a s. applied to one of the sense organs, *e.g.,* receptors of vision, hearing, touch, etc., which are an essential and integral part of the neural mechanism underlying a conditioned reflex; (2) a neutral s., when paired with the unconditioned s. in simultaneous presentation to an organism, capable of eliciting a given response.

**discriminant s.,** a s. which can be differentiated from all other s. in the environment because it has been, and continues to serve as, an indicator of a potential reinforcer.

**heterol'ogous s.,** a s. that acts upon any part of the sensory apparatus or nerve tract.

**homol'ogous s.,** one that acts only upon the nerve terminations in a special sense organ.

**inadequate s.,** subthreshold s.; subliminal s.; one that is too weak to evoke a response.

**lim'inal s.,** threshold s.

**max'imal s.,** one strong enough to evoke a maximal response.

**square wave stimuli,** electrical stimulation in which the intensity of the current is brought suddenly to a given level and maintained at that level until it suddenly is cut off; this type of s. is particularly useful in obtaining a strength-duration curve.

**subliminal s.,** inadequate s.

**subthreshold s.,** inadequate s.

**summation of stimuli,** see under summation.

**supramaximal s.,** a s. having a strength significantly above that which is barely sufficient to activate all of the nerve fibers or muscle fibers under the electrode. It is used when it is desired that all will respond despite some degree of decrease in irritability of the fibers.

**threshold s.,** liminal s.; one of threshold strength, *i.e.,* that is just strong enough to excite. See also adequate s.

**unconditioned s.,** a s. that elicits an unconditioned response; *e.g.,* food is an unconditioned s. for salivation, an unconditioned response in a hungry animal.

**stimulus word.** The word used in association tests to evoke a response.

**sting.** 1. Sharp momentary pain, most commonly produced by the puncture of the skin by many species of arthropods, including hexapods, myriapods, and arachnids. Stinging sensation can also be produced by jellyfish, sea urchins, sponges, mollusks, and several species of venomous fish, such as the stingray, toadfish, rabbitfish, and catfish. See also bites. 2. The venom apparatus of a stinging animal; it consists of a chitinous spicule or bony spine and a venom gland or sac. 3. To introduce (or the process of introducing) a venom by stinging.

**sea urchin s.,** severe pain and variable swelling from injection of venom (neurotoxin) of a great variety of sea urchins, most notably the genera *Anosoma* and *Asthmosoma.*

**stip'pling.** Punctate basophilia; a speckling of a blood cell or other structure with fine dots when exposed to the action of a basic stain, due to the presence of free basophil granules in the cell protoplasm.

**geographic s. of nails,** regularly arranged longitudinal s. found commonly in psoriasis and occasionally in alopecia areata.

**Ziemann's s.,** fine dots sometimes seen in erythrocytes in quartan malaria.

**Stirling,** William, British histologist and physiologist, 1851–1932. See S.'s modification of Gram's stain (under stain).

**stirp** (sturp) [ L. *stirps,* stem, stock, race ]. 1. A race or family. 2. Galton's term for the aggregation or sum total of gemmules or organic units in the fertilized ovum.

**stirrup** (stur'up, stĭr'up) [ A.S. *stīrāp* ]. Stapes.

**stitch** [ A.S. *stice,* a pricking ]. 1. A sharp sticking pain of momentary duration. 2. A suture.

**Stock,** Wolfgang, Jena ophthalmologist, *1874. See Spielmeyer-S. *disease.*

**stock** [ A.S. *stoc* ]. The source from which a line or race is descended, a race or family of animals or plants.

**Stocker,** Frederick William, American ophthalmologist, *1893. See S.'s *line.*

**stock'ing.** Edema of the leg in the horse.

**Stoerk,** Karl, Vienna laryngologist, 1832–1899. See S.'s *blenorrhea.*

**Stoffel,** Adolf, German orthopedic surgeon, 1880–1937. See S.'s *operation.*

**stoichiology** (stoy-kĭ-ol'-o-jĭ) [ G. *stoicheion,* element (lit. one of a row), fr. *stoichos,* a row, + *logos,* study ]. The science that deals with the elements or principles in any branch of knowledge, as in chemistry, in anatomy, or in physiology; cellular physiology; histology of the cells. See stoichiometry.

**stoichiometer** (stoy-kĭ-om'e-ter). Instrument used in stoichiometry.

**stoichiometry** (stoy-kĭ-om'e-trĭ) [ G. *stoicheion,* element, + *metron,* measure ]. The determination of the relative quantities of the substances concerned in any chemical reaction; dealing with the laws of definite proportions in chemistry, as in the molar proportions in a reaction.

**stoke** [ Sir George Gabriel Stokes ]. A unit of kinematic viscosity, that of a fluid with a viscosity of 1 poise and a density of 1 gm. per ml.

**Stokes,** Sir George Gabriel, British mathematician and physicist, 1819–1903. Gave his name to stoke.

**Stokes,** Sir William, Irish surgeon, 1839–1900. See S.'s *amputation.*

**Stokes,** William, Irish physician, 1804–1878. See Cheyne-S. *asthma,* S.'s *law,* Cheyne-S. *psychosis, respiration,* Adams-S. or Morgagni-Adams-S. or S.-Adams *disease* or *syndrome.*

**Stokes,** William R., American pathologist, 1870–1930. See S.'s *reagent.*

**Stoltz,** Joseph, French gynecologist, 1803–1896. See S.'s *operation.*

**stom-, stoma-.** See stomato-.

**stoma,** pl. **stomas** or **stomata** (sto'mah, sto'mă-tah) [ G. a mouth. STOM- ]. 1 [ NA ]. A minute opening or pore. 2 [ NA ]. The mouth. 3. Stigma (2). 4. An artificial opening between two cavities or canals, or between such and the surface of the body.

**Fuchs' s.'s,** small depression on the surface of the iris near the margin of the pupil.

**stomacace** (sto-mak'a-se). Ulcerative *stomatitis.*

**stomach** (stum'uk) [ G. *stomachos,* L. *stomachus.* STOM- ]. 1. Ventriculus (1); gaster; a large irregularly piriform sac between the esophagus and the small intestine, lying just beneath the diaphragm; when distended it is 10 or 11 inches in length and 4 to 4¹/₂ inches in its greatest diameter, and has a capacity of about 1 quart. Its wall has four coats or tunics: mucous, submucous, muscular, and peritoneal; the muscular coat is composed of three layers, the fibers running longitudinally in the outer, circularly in the middle, and obliquely in the inner layer.

**biloc'ular s.,** hourglass s.

**cascade s.,** a radiographic diagnosis in which the upper stomach serves as a barium reservoir until sufficient volume is present to spill ("cascade") into the antrum; said to cause symptoms of postprandial distention and inability to belch.

**drain-trap s.,** water-trap s.

**hourglass s.,** a condition in which there is a central constriction of the wall of the s. dividing it more or less completely into two cavities, a cardiac and a pyloric.

**leather-bottle s.,** marked thickening and rigidity of the s. wall, with reduced capacity of the lumen although often

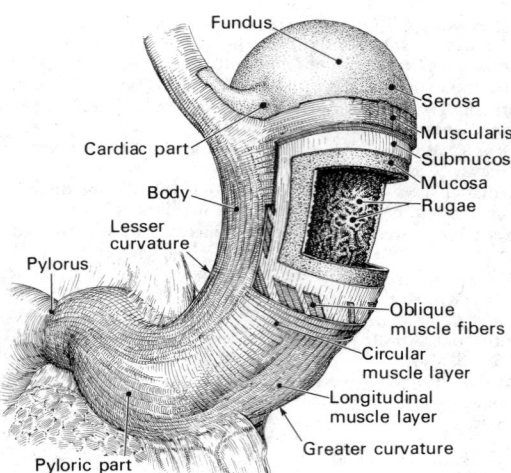

**Parts of Human Stomach**

without obstruction; nearly always due to scirrhous carcinoma. See also *linitis* plastica.

**miniature s.,** Pavlov *pouch.*

**Pavlov s.,** Pavlov *pouch.*

**powdered s.,** the dried and powdered defatted wall of the s. of the hog, *Sus scrofa*; it contains thermolabile factors including native vitamin $B_{12}$ and intrinsic factor; has been used in the treatment of pernicious anemia.

**sclerotic s.,** leather-bottle s.

**thoracic s.,** s. partly or wholly contained within the thorax; may be a variant of hiatal hernia.

**trifid s.,** a condition in which the s. is divided by two constrictions into three pouches.

**wallet s.,** a form of dilated s. in which there is a general baglike distention, the antrum and fundus being indistinguishable.

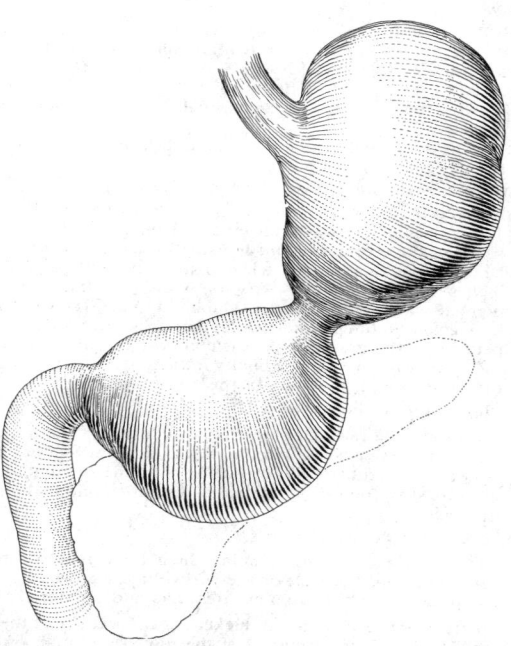

**Hourglass Stomach**

**water-trap s.,** a ptotic and dilated s., having a relatively high (though normally placed) pyloric outlet which is held up by the gastrohepatic ligament.

**stomachache** (stum′uk-āk). Gastralgia; gastrodynia; stomachalgia; stomachodynia; pain in the stomach.

**stomachal** (stum′ă-kal). Relating to the stomach.

**stomachalgia** (stum′ă-kal′jī-ah) [ stomach + G. *algos*, pain ]. Stomachache.

**stomachic** (sto′mak′ik). 1. Stomachal. 2. An agent that improves appetite and digestion.

**stomachodynia** (stum′ă-ko-din′ĭ-ah) [ stomach + G. *odynē*, pain ]. Stomachache.

**sto′mal.** Relating to a stoma.

**stomat-.** See stomato-.

**sto′mata.** Alternate plural of stoma.

**sto′matal.** Relating to a stoma.

**stomatalgia** (sto′mă-tal′jī-ah) [ stomat- + G. *algos*, pain ]. Pain in the mouth.

**stomatic** (sto-mat′ik). Relating to the mouth; oral.

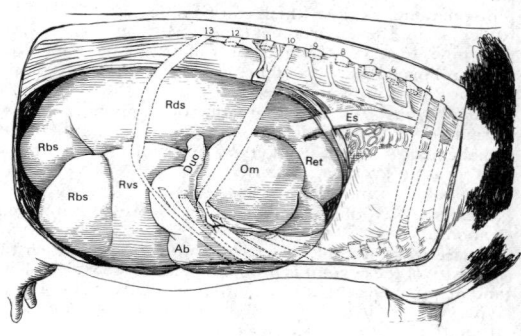

**Stomach of Cow**

*Es*, esophagus; *Ret*, reticulum; *Rds*, dorsal sac of rumen; *Rvs*, ventral sac of rumen; *Rbs*, posterior blind sacs; *Om*, omasum; *Ab*, abomasum; *Duo*, duodenum.

**stomatitis** (sto′mă-ti′tis) [ stomat- + G. suffix -*itis*, inflammation ]. Inflammation of the mucous membrane of the mouth.

**angular s.,** an inflammation at the corners of the mouth usually superimposed over a wrinkled or fissured epithelium, stopping at the mucocutaneous junction and not involving the mucosa; many etiologic factors may be involved.

**aphthobullous s.,** the type of s. occurring in foot and mouth disease, characterized by vesication and ulceration.

**contagious pustular s.,** contagious *ecthyma*.

**epidemic s.,** foot and mouth *disease.*

**equine contagious pustular s.,** horsepox.

**gan′grenous s.,** noma.

**lead s.,** deposition of lead sulfide in inflamed marginal gingiva with production of bluish black line due to increased lead absorption.

**maculofibrinous s.,** recurrent ulcerative s.

**s. medicamento′sa,** inflammatory oral changes due to the use of a medication.

**membranous s.,** inflammatory oral changes characterized by membrane formation.

**mercurial s.,** s. associated with mercury poisoning; see mercurial *line.*

**mycotic s.,** a form of ulcerative s., usually accompanied by dermatitis and lameness, which occurs in cattle during the pasture season; it does not appear to be contagious and the cause is not known; the name originated from the early belief that fungi growing on pasture vegetation were the cause.

**s. neurot′ica chron′ica,** pemphigus neuroticus occurring in the mouth.

**primary herpetic s.,** first infection of oral tissues with herpes simplex virus; characterized by gingival inflammation, vesicles, and ulcers.

**recurrent aphthous s.,** recurrent ulcerative s.

**recurrent herpetic s.,** reactivation of herpes simplex virus; characterized by vesicles and ulceration; see ulcerative s., recurrent.

**recurrent ulcerative s.,** an oral disease with clinical characteristics of chronically recurring, painful, mucosal ulcerations, single or multiple in number, 1 mm. to 2 cm. in size, round or oval in shape, flat or slightly depressed, with a gray to grayish yellow coating, and surrounded by a narrow zone of inflammation; also known as dyspeptic ulcer; habitual aphthosis; maculofibrinous s.; recurrent aphthous s.; recurrent canker sores.

**s. simplex,** nonulcerating inflammation of the oral mucous membranes.

**s. trop'ica,** tropical *sprue*.

**ulcerative s.,** canker sores; stomacace; stomatocace; stomatitis ulcerosa; a destructive ulceration of the mucous membrane of the mouth; see also recurrent ulcerative s.

**s. ulcero'sa,** ulcerative s.

**s. ulcero'sa chron'ica,** periodontitis.

**s. venena'ta,** inflammation of the oral mucous membrane caused by irritants such as poison ivy and various chemicals.

**vesicular s.,** an acute vesicular disease of horses, cattle, and swine, caused by a virus; in horses and cattle the disease usually causes mouth vesicles, in cattle these cannot be certainly differentiated from those of foot-and-mouth disease by inspection alone; this disease is not as highly contagious as foot-and-mouth disease, and apparently arthropods play a role in its transmission; this disease is transmissible to man; see also ulcerative s., recurrent.

**Vincent's s.,** Vincent's *disease*.

**stomato-, stom-, stomat-** [ G. *stoma*, mouth. STOM- ]. Combining forms denoting mouth.

**stomatocace** (sto-mă-tok'a-se) [ stomato- + G. *kakē*, badness ]. Ulcerative *stomatitis*.

**stomatocatharsis** (sto'mă-to-kă-thar'sis) stomato- + G. *katharsis*, purgation, cleansing ]. Disinfection of the oral cavity.

**stomatodeum** (sto'mă-to-de'um). Stomodeum.

**stomatodynia** (sto'mă-to-din'ĭ-ah) [ stomato- + G. *odynē*, pain ]. Stomatalgia.

**stomatodysodia** (sto'mă-to-dĭ-so'dĭ-ah) [ stomato- + G. *dysōdia*, bad odor ]. A bad odor or stench from the mouth.

**stomatognathic** (sto'mă-tog-nath'ik) [ stomato- + G. *gnathos*, jaw ]. Pertaining to the physiology of the mouth; see s. system.

**stomatologic** (sto-mă-to-loj'ik). Relating to stomatology.

**stomatol'ogist.** A dentist with medical background.

**stomatology** (sto'mă-tol'o-jĭ) [ stomato- + G. *logos*, study ]. The study of the structures, functions, and diseases of the mouth.

**stomatomalacia** (sto-mă-to-mal-a'shĭ-ah) [ stomato- + G. *malakia*, softness ]. Pathologic softening of any of the structures of the mouth.

**stomatomenia** (sto'mă-to-me'nĭ-ah) [ stomato- + G. *mēn*, month ]. Stomenorrhagia; bleeding from the gums as a form of vicarious menstruation.

**stomat'omy.** Stomatotomy.

**stomatomycosis** (sto'mă-to-mi-ko'sis) [ stomato- + G. *mykēs*, fungus, + suffix -*osis*, condition ]. Disease of the mouth due to the presence of a microscopic fungus.

**stomatonecrosis** (sto'mă-to-ne-kro'sis) [ stomato- + G. *nekrōsis*, death ]. Noma.

**stomatonoma** (sto'mă-to-no'mah) [ stomato- + G. *nomē*, a spreading (sore) ]. Noma.

**stomatopathy** (sto'mă-to-top'ă-thĭ) [ stomato- + G. *pathos*, suffering ]. Any disease of the mouth.

**sto'matoplas'tic.** Relating to stomatoplasty.

**stomatoplasty** (sto'mă-to-plas'tĭ) [ stomato- + G. *plassō*, to form ]. Reconstructive or plastic surgery of the mouth.

**stomatorrhagia** (sto'mă-to-ra'jĭ-ah) [ stomato- + G. *rhēgnymi*, to burst forth ]. Bleeding from the gums or other part of the oral cavity.

**stomatoscope** (sto'mă-to-skōp) [ stomato- + G. *skopeō*, to view ]. An apparatus for illuminating the interior of the mouth to facilitate examination.

**sto'mato'sis** [ stomato- + G. suffix -*osis*, condition ]. Any disease of the oral cavity.

**stomatotomy** (sto'mă-tot'o-mĭ) [ stomato- + G. *tomē*, incision ]. Stomatomy; surgical incision of the cervix uteri to facilitate labor.

**stomenorrhagia** (sto'men-o-ra'jĭ-ah). Stomatomenia.

**stomocephalus** (sto'mo-sef'ă-lus) [ G. *stoma*, mouth, + *kephalē*, head ]. A malformed individual with undeveloped jaw and a snoutlike mouth; likely to be combined with an ethmocephalic type of cyclopia.

**stomodeal** (sto'mo-de'al). Relating to a stomodeum.

**sto'mode'um** [ Mod. L. fr. G. *stoma*, mouth, + *hodaios*, on the way, fr. *hodos*, a way. HOD- ]. 1. A midline ectodermal depression ventral to the embryonic brain; it is surrounded by the mandibular arch; when the buccopharyngeal membrane disappears it becomes continuous with the foregot and forms the mouth. 2. The anterior portion of the insect alimentary canal, consisting of mouth, buccal cavity, pharynx, esophagus, crop (frequently a diverticulum), and the proventriculus.

**Stomox'ys cal'citrans** [ Mod. L. fr. G. *stoma*, mouth, + *oxys*, sharp; L. pres. p. of *calcitro*, to kick, fr. *calx*, the heel ]. Stable fly; a species of biting fly, resembling in size and general appearance the common housefly. It is an annoying pest of man and domestic animals worldwide and is implicated in the mechanical transmission of diseases, such as trypanosomiasis, anthrax, and vesicular stomatitis; a role similar to that of horseflies of the genus *Tabanus*. These flies are especially important in the spread of surra by transmitting *Trypanosoma evansi*. They also serve as intermediate hosts for *Habronema*, when infected flies are ingested by horses, for the deer filaria, *Setaria cervi*, and for the chicken tapeworm, *Hymenolepis carioca*.

**-stomy** [ G. *stoma*, mouth ]. Combining form denoting artificial or surgical opening.

**stone** [ A.S. *stān* ]. 1. Calculus. 2. An English unit of weight of the human body, equal to 14 pounds. 3. Denoting a complete loss of any of the senses or of life; as s. blind, s. deaf, s. dead.

**Arkansas s.,** a natural s. that is utilized as a whetstone.

**artificial s.,** a specially calcined gypsum derivative similar to plaster of Paris, but stronger, because the grains are nonporous.

**blue s.,** cupric sulfate.

**dendritic s.,** dendritic *calculus*.

**philosopher's s.,** grand magistery; a s. sought by the alchemists of the Middle Ages which was able, so it was supposed, to transmute base metals into gold, to make precious s.'s, and to cure all ills, and thus confer longevity. It was also believed to be a universal solvent.

**pulp s.,** pulp nodule; a calcified mass of dentin within the pulp or projected into it from the cavity wall; it generally lies within the pulp chamber.

**rotten s.,** pumice.

**skin s.'s,** *calcinosis* cutis.

**tear s.,** dacryolith.

**vein s.,** phlebolith.

**womb s.,** (1) a calcified myoma of the uterus; (2) a uterine calculus.

**Stookey,** Byron, American neurosurgeon, *1887. See S.-Scarff *operation*, Queckenstedt-S. *test*.

**stool** [ A.S. *stōl*, seat ]. 1. An evacuation of the bowels. 2. Feces; the matter discharged at one movement of the bowels.

**butter s.'s,** fatty s.'s, occurring especially in steatorrhea.

**rice-water s.,** a watery fluid containing whitish flocculi, discharged from the bowel in Asiatic cholera, and occasionally in other cases of serous diarrhea.

**spinach s.'s,** dark greenish porridge-like s.'s, resembling chopped spinach.

**Trélat's s.'s,** glairy s.'s streaked with blood in proctitis.

**sto'rax** [ G. *styrax*, a sweet-smelling gum ] (USP). Styrax; liquid s.; a liquid balsam obtained from the wood and inner bark of *Liquidamber orientalis*, a tree of Asia Minor, or *L. styraciflua* (family Hamamelidaceae); has been used in the treatment of chronic inflammation of the mucous membranes, and externally for scabies.

**storesinol** (sto-rez'ĭ-nol). Storesin; an amorphous alcohol resin, $C_{35}H_{55}(OH)_3$, present in two forms, alpha and beta, both free or in the form of a cinnamic ester. The predominant constituent of storax.

**storm.** An exacerbation of symptoms or a crisis in the course of a disease.

   **thyroid s.,** thyrotoxic *crisis.*

**Stormont test.** See under test.

**stoss'therapy** [ Ger. *Stoss,* shove, + therapy ]. Treatment by use of a single massive dose.

**Stout's wiring.** See under wiring.

**STP.** See 2,5-dimethoxy-4-methylamphetamine.

**STPD.** Symbol indicating that a gas volume has been expressed as if it were at standard temperature (0°C.), standard pressure (760 mm Hg absolute), dry; under these conditions a mole of gas occupies 22.4 liters.

**strabismal, strabismic** (strā-biz'mal, -mik). Relating to or affected with strabismus.

**strabismometer** (strā-biz-mom'e-ter) [ G. *strabismos,* a squinting, + *metron,* measure ]. Strabometer; a plate with upper margin curved, to conform with the lower lid, and marked in millimeters or fractions of an inch, used to measure the lateral deviation in squint.

**strabismus** (strā-biz'mus) [ Mod. L. fr. G. *strabismos,* a squinting, fr. *strabos,* distorted, fr. *strephō,* to twist. STREP- ]. Heterotropia; squint; a constant lack of parallelism of the visual axes of the eyes.

   **accommodative s.,** overconvergence caused by strong or excessive accommodation.

   **alternating s.,** a form of s. in which either eye fixes.

   **concomitant s.,** s. in which the deviating eye follows the other in its movements, the angle between the visual axes remaining the same.

   **convergent s.,** esotropia.

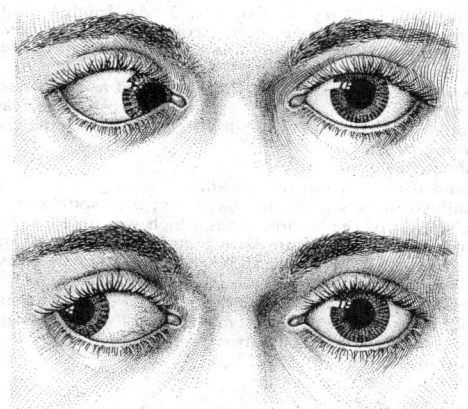

**Strabismus**
*Upper,* convergent; *lower,* divergent

   **s. deor'sum vergens,** hypotropia; vertical s. in which the visual axis of one eye deviates downward.

   **divergent s.,** exotropia.

   **external s.,** exotropia.

   **internal s.,** esotropia.

   **kinetic s.,** s. due to spasm of an extraocular muscle.

   **mechanical s.,** s. due to a pressure on the eye from within the orbit.

   **monocular s.,** uniocular s.; s. in which one eye only fixes; that is, when one eye is covered both eyes move; when the other eye is covered both remain steady.

   **s. sursum vergens,** hypertropia; vertical s. in which the visual axis of one eye deviates upward.

   **unioc'ular s.,** monocular s.

   **vertical s.,** a form in which the visual axis of one eye deviates upward (s. sursum vergens) or downward (s. deorsum vergens).

**strabometer** (strā-bom'e-ter ]. Strabismometer.

**straboscopic** (strab'o-skop'ik) [ G. *strabos,* distorted, + *skopeō,* to view ]. Causing distorted visual perception; see straboscopic *disk.*

**strabotome** (strab'o-tōm). A knife for use in performing strabotomy.

**strabotomy** (strā-bot'o-mĭ) [ G. *strabismos,* strabismus, + *tomē,* a cutting ]. Division of one or more of the ocular muscles or their tendons for the correction of squint.

**strain** (strān) [ A.S. *stryand; streōnan,* to beget ]. 1. A race or stock; in bacteriology, the set of descendants that originates from a common ancestor and retains the characteristics of the ancestor; members of a s. that subsequently differ from the original isolate are regarded as belonging either to a substrain of the original s., or to a new s. 2. A hereditary tendency. 3 [ L. *stringere,* to bind ]. To make an effort to the limit of one's strength. 4. To injure by overuse or improper use. 5. An act of straining. 6. Injury resulting from s. or overuse. 7. The change in shape that a body undergoes when acted upon by an external force. 8. To filter; to percolate.

   **auxotrophic s.'s,** s.'s which are derived from the prototrophic s. but which require extra growth factors.

   **carrier s.,** pseudolysogenic s.; a bacterial s. that is contaminated with a bacteriophage of low infectivity.

   **cell s.,** in tissue culture, cells derived from a single cell (clone) and possessing a specific feature such as a marker chromosome, antigen, or resistance to a virus.

   **HFR s.,** Hfr s.; high frequency of recombination s.; an $F^+$ (male) bacterial s. that exhibits a high rate of recombination with $F^-$ s.'s but does not transfer the F agent.

   **isogenic s.,** a s. of animals inbred for many generations, homozygous for certain specified genes; pure line.

   **neotype s.,** a s. accepted by international agreement to replace a type s. which is no longer in existance or to serve as the type s. if a type s. was not designated and if no s.'s exist which can be designated as the type.

   **prototrophic s.'s,** s.'s that have the same nutritional requirements as the wild-type s.

   **pseudolysogenic s.,** carrier s.

   **recombinant s.,** see recombinant.

   **stock s.,** a bacterial (or other microbial) s. that has been maintained under laboratory conditions as representative of its type.

   **type s.,** the nomenclatural type of a species or subspecies.

   **vertebral cervical s.,** minor stretching of ligaments or tendons with minimal damage.

   **wild-type s.,** a s. found in nature or a standard s.; see also auxotrophic s.'s and protrophic s.'s.

**strain'er.** A filter or percolator.

**strait** (strāt) [ M.E. *streit* thr. O. Fr. fr. L. *strictus,* drawn together, tight ]. In obstetrics, (1) the upper opening (superior s. or inlet), or (2) the lower opening (inferior s. or outlet), of the pelvic canal.

   **inferior s.,** *apertura* pelvis inferior.

   **superior s.,** *apertura* pelvis superior.

**straitjacket** (strāt'jak-et). Straight jacket; camisole; a garment-like device with long sleeves used to restrain a violently disturbed person.

**stramonium** (strā-mo'nĭ-um) [ Mod. L. ] (BP). Thorn-apple; Jamestown or Jimson weed; stink-weed; the dried leaves and flowering or fruiting tops with branches of *Datura stramonium* (family Solanaceae); a herb abounding in temperate and subtropical countries. It contains an alkaloid, daturine, identical with hyoscyamine. Antispasmodic; has been used in the treatment of asthma and parkinsonism. When abused or taken inadvertently may cause an atropine-like toxic psychosis.

**strand.** In microbiology, a filamentous or threadlike structure.

   **complementary s.,** see replicative *form.*

   **minus s.,** see replicative *form.*

   **plus s.,** see replicative *form.*

   **viral s.,** see replicative *form.*

**Strandberg,** J. V. See Grönblad-S. *syndrome.*

**strangalesthesia** (strang'gal-es-the'zĭ-ah) [ G. *strangalē,* halter, + *aisthēsis,* sensation ]. Zonesthesia.

**strangle** (strang'gl) [ G. *strangaloō,* to choke, fr. *strangalē,* a halter ]. To suffocate; to choke; to compress the trachea so as to prevent respiration.

**strangles** (strang'glz). Distemper (3); an acute infectious disease in the horse, marked by mucopurulent nasal catarrh and edematous and hemorrhagic nasal and pharyngeal respiratory passages with enlargement and suppuration of associated lymph nodes; it is caused by *Streptococcus equi*, and affects chiefly horses under the age of five years.

**strangulated** (strang'gu-la-ted) [ L. *strangulo*, pp. *-atus*, to choke, fr. G. *strangaloō*, to choke (strangle) ]. Constricted so as to prevent the passage of air, denoting the trachea; or so as to cut off the blood supply, denoting a hernia or any part encircled by a tight band.

**strangulation** (strang'gu-la'shun). The act of strangulating or the condition of being strangulated, in any sense.

**strangury** (strang'gu-rī) [ G. *stranx* (*strang-*), something squeezed out, a drop, + *ouron*, urine ]. Difficulty in micturition, the urine being passed drop by drop with pain and tenesmus.

**strap** [ A.S. *stropp* ]. 1. A strip of adhesive plaster. 2. To apply overlapping strips of adhesive plaster.

**cribbing s.,** a s. placed on the neck of a horse to prevent cribbing; it limits the arching of the neck necessary for the animal to swallow air.

**Strassburg** (strahs'boorg), Gustav A., German physiologist, *1848. See S.'s *test*.

**Strassman,** Paul F., German gynecologist, 1866–1938. See S.'s *phenomenon*.

**strata** (stra'tah, strat'ah). Plural of stratum.

**stratification** (strat'ĭ-fĭ-ka'shun) [ L. *stratum*, layer, + *facio*, to make ]. An arrangement in the form of layers or strata.

**strat'ified.** Arranged in the form of layers or strata.

**stratigraphy** (stră-tig'ră-fĭ) [ L. *stratum*, layer, + G. *graphē*, a writing ]. Sectional roentgenography; tomography.

# STRATUM

**stratum,** gen. **strati,** pl. **strata** (stra'tum, strat'um, -ah) [ L. *sterno*, pp. *stratus*, to spread out, strew, ntr. of pp. as noun, *stratum*, a bed cover, layer ] [ NA ]. One of the layers of differentiated tissue, the aggregate of which forms any given structure, such as the retina or the skin.

**s. aculea'tum,** obsolete term for s. spinosum.

**s. al'bum profun'dum,** a layer of myelinated fibers, the deepest layer of the colliculus superior, delimiting the latter from the central gray substance surrounding the cerebral aqueduct.

**s. basa'le,** (1) the outermost layer of the endometrium which undergoes only minimal changes during the menstrual cycle; (2) s. basale epidermidis.

**s. basa'le epider'midis** [ NA ], s. cylindricum [ NA ]; palisade, columnar, or basal cell layer; the deepest layer of the epidermis; see fig. under epidermis.

**s. cerebra'le ret'inae** [ NA ], pars optica retinae [ NA ]; cerebral or neural layer of the retina; optic part of the retina; the internal layer of the retina containing the neural elements, as distinguished from the outer leaf of the retina, or stratum pigmenti.

**s. cine'reum collic'uli superio'ris,** s. griseum colliculi superioris.

**s. circula're membra'nae tym'pani** [ NA ], circular layer of the tympanic membrane; circular fibers deep to the radiate layer of the membrane which are more abundant near the periphery. They are not present in the pars flaccida.

**s. circula're tu'nicae muscula'ris co'li** [ NA ], circular layer of the muscular tunic of the colon.

**s. circula're tu'nicae muscula'ris intesti'ni ten'uis** [ NA ], circular layer of the muscular tunic of the small intestine.

**s. circula're tu'nicae muscula'ris rec'ti** [ NA ], circular layer of the muscular tunic of the rectum.

**s. circula're tu'nicae muscula'ris ventric'uli** [ NA ], circular layer of the muscular tunic of the stomach.

**s. compac'tum,** compacta; the superficial layer of decidual tissue in the pregnant uterus, in which the interglandular tissue preponderates.

**s. cor'neum epider'midis** [ NA ], corneal layer of epidermis; horny layer; the outer layer of the epidermis, consisting of several layers of flat keratinized nonnucleated cells. See fig. under epidermis.

**s. cor'neum un'guis** [ NA ], cornified layer of the nail; the outer, horny layer of the nail.

**s. cuta'neum membra'nae tym'pani** [ NA ], cutaneous layer of the tympanic membrane; the thin cuticular layer on the external surface of the tympanic membrane.

**s. cylin'dricum** [ NA ], s. basale epidermidis.

**s. disjunc'tum,** the layer of partly detached cells on the free surface of the s. corneum.

**s. fibro'sum,** *membrana* fibrosa.

**s. functiona'le,** the endometrium except for the s. basale; it formerly was believed to be lost during menstruation but is now considered to be only partially disrupted.

**s. gangliona're ner'vi op'tici** [ NA ], ganglionic layer of the optic nerve; the inner layer of multipolar neurons in the retina consisting of the relatively large neurons that give rise to the fibers of the optic nerve.

**s. gangliona're ret'inae** [ NA ], ganglionic layer of the retina; stratum nucleare retinae; inner granular layer of the retina; the intermediate layer of neurons in the retina composed largely of bipolar cells; see also granular *layers* of retina.

**s. ganglio'sum cerebel'li,** ganglionic layer of the cerebellar cortex; Purkinje's layer; the layer of Purkinje cells formerly described as an individual s. of the cerebellar cortex but currently included in the NA term, s. moleculare cerebelli.

**s. germinati'vum,** the combined s. basale epidermidis and s. spinosum epidermidis. Also called Malpighian layer, stratum, or rete; germinative layer; stratum mucosum.

**s. germinati'vum un'guis** [ NA ], germinative layer of the nail; the deeper layer of the nail that is continuous with the s. germinativum of the surrounding skin; from it the nail plate or stratum corneum is continuously formed.

**s. granulo'sum cerebel'li** [ NA ], granular layer of the cerebellar cortex; the deeper of the two layers of the cortex. It contains large numbers of granule cells, the dendrites of which synapse with incoming mossy fibers whereas their thin, unmyelinated axons ascend perpendicularly into the s. moleculare in which they bifurcate into the parallel fibers coursing parallel to the long axis of the cerebellar folia and forming numerous synapses with the dendrites of Purkinje cells, basket cells, and stellate cells.

**s. granulo'sum epider'midis** [ NA ], granular layer of epidermis; a layer of somewhat flattened cells containing granules of keratohyalin and eleidin, lying just above the s. spinosum of the epidermis. See fig. under epidermis.

**s. granulo'sum follic'uli ova'rici vesiculo'si** [ NA ], s. granulosum ovarii; granulosa; membrana granulosa; the layer of small cells that forms the wall of an ovarian follicle.

**s. granulo'sum ova'rii,** s. granulosum folliculi ovarici vesiculosi.

**s. gris'eum collic'uli superio'ris** [ NA ], gray layer(s) of the superior colliculus; stratum cinereum colliculi superioris; term applied to any one of the three gray layers of gray matter of the superior colliculus that alternate with layers composed chiefly of nerve fibers: (1) the *s. griseum superficiale* or superficial gray layer, above the largely white layer of the incoming fibers of the optic tract (s. opticum); (2) the *s. griseum medium,* placed between the s. opticum and a more deeply located layer of fibers, the s. lemnisci; (3) the *s. griseum profundum,* between the s. lemnisci and the central gray substance surrounding the cerebral aqueduct, and containing the large nerve cells from which most of the colliculus descending connections (tractus tectobulbaris, tectopontinus, and tectospinalis) originate.

**s. gris'eum me'dium,** see s. griseum colliculi superioris.

**s. gris'eum profun'dum,** see s. griseum colliculi superioris.

**s. gris'eum superficia'le,** see s. griseum colliculi superioris.

**s. interoliva're lemnis'ci,** the medial region of the medulla oblongata between the left and right olivary nucleus, traversed lengthwise by the left and right medial lemniscus, and transversally by the decussating olivocerebellar fibers.

**s. lemnis'ci,** fillet layer; a largely fibrous (hence whitish) layer of the superior colliculus separating the s. griseum medium from the s. griseum profundum and containing, among others, fibers from the spinal and trigeminal lemnisci.

**s. longitudina'le tu'nicae muscula'ris co'li** [ NA ], longitudinal layer of the muscular tunic of the colon.

**s. longitudina'le tu'nicae muscula'ris intesti'ni ten'uis** [ NA ], longitudinal layer of the muscular tunic of the small intestine.

**s. longitudina'le tu'nicae muscula'ris rec'ti** [ NA ], longitudinal layer of the muscular tunic of the rectum.

**s. longitudina'le tu'nicae muscula'ris ventric'uli** [ NA ], longitudinal layer of the muscular tunic of the stomach.

**s. lu'cidum** [ NA ], clear layer; the layer of the epidermis just beneath the s. corneum; it consists of two or three layers of flat clear cells with atrophied nuclei. See fig. under epidermis.

**Malpighian s.,** s. germinativum.

**s. molecula're,** plexiform layer; term applied to any layer of brain tissue that contains few nerve-cell bodies and is composed largely of terminal arborizations of dendrites and axons. Notable examples: the superficial layer of the cerebral cortex (see *cortex* cerebri, layer 1), the s. moleculare cerebelli, and the s. moleculare retinae.

**s. molecula're cerebel'li** [ NA ], molecular layer of the cerebellar cortex; the outer lamina of the cortex, containing the cell bodies and dendrites of Purkinje cells, the axons of the granule cells, and the cell bodies, dendrites, and axons of basket cells.

**s. molecula're ret'inae,** molecular or plexiform layer of the retina; name applied to each of two layers of the retina that are composed largely of interlacing dendrites and axons of the cells of the adjoining granular layers: an outer molecular layer (plexiform layer) between the outer and inner granular layers, and an inner molecular layer (plexiform layer) between the inner granular layer and the ganglionic layer (s. ganglionare nervi optici).

**s. muco'sum,** s. germinativum.

**s. muco'sum membra'nae tym'pani** [ NA ], mucosal layer of the tympanic membrane; the mucosal lining of the internal surface of the tympanic membrane.

**s. neuroepithelia'le ret'inae** [ NA ], neuroepithelial layer of the retina; the outermost layer of the pars optica retinae, composed of the primary receptor cells of the retina; the s. consists of two sublayers: (1) an external layer made up of the rods and cones, the photosensitive processes of the receptor cells, and (2) the external granular layer containing the cell bodies of these cells; the external limiting membrane forms a perforated supporting plate between the two sublayers. The name refers to the fact that the retinal receptor cells are a specialized form of (epithelial) ependyma cell and thus, in a sense, are comparable to the neuroepithelial cells (*e.g.,* hair cells) of other sense organs.

**s. nuclea're retinae,** s. ganglionare retinae.

**s. op'ticum,** optic layer; (1) a layer of white matter interspersed with nerve-cell bodies, immediately below the s. griseum superficialis of the superior colliculus, composed largely of myelinated fibers originating in the retina; (2) the inner layer of the retina, consisting of the fibers originating from the cells of the s. ganglionare nervi optici; in their further course these fibers combine to form the optic nerve or optic tract.

**s. papilla're corii** [ NA ], papillary layer; corpus papillare; the more superficial layer of the corium whose papillae interdigitate with the epidermis. See figs. under corium and epidermis.

**s. pigmen'ti bul'bi,** s. pigmenti retinae.

**s. pigmen'ti cor'poris cilia'ris** [ NA ], pigmented layer of the ciliary body; the continuation of the pigment layer of the retina onto the posterior aspect of the ciliary body.

**s. pigmen'ti i'ridis** [ NA ], pigmented layer of the iris; the double layer of pigmented epithelium on the posterior surface of the iris.

**s. pigmen'ti ret'inae** [ NA ], s. pigmenti bulbi; tapetum nigrum; tapetum oculi; the outer layer of the retina, consisting of pigmented epithelium.

**s. radia'tum membra'nae tym'pani** [ NA ], radiate layer of the tympanic membrane; the connective tissue layer of the tympanic membrane beneath the stratum cutaneum, the fibers of which radiate from the manubrium of the

malleus to the peripheral fibrocartilaginous ring of the membrane. This layer is absent from the pars flaccida.

**s. reticula're co'rii** [ NA ], s. reticulare cutis; reticular layer of the corium; tunica propria corii; the thicker, deep layer of the corium consisting of dense, irregularly arranged connective tissue. See figs. under corium and epidermis.

**s. reticula're cutis,** s. reticulare corii.

**s. spino'sum epider'midis** [ NA ], spinous layer; prickle-cell layer; the layer of polyhedral cells in the epidermis; the intercellular bridges give the cells a spiny or prickly appearance; see fig. under epidermis.

**s. spongio'sum,** the middle layer of the decidua, formed chiefly of dilated glandular structures.

**s. subcuta'neum,** *tela* subcutanea.

**s. synovia'le,** *membrana* synovialis.

**s. zona'le** [ NA ], zonular layer; (1) a thin layer of white substance covering the upper surface of the thalamus and forming part of the floor of the central portion of the lateral ventricle; (2) a layer of white substance seen on the surface of a section of the lamina tecti mesencephali.

---

**Straus,** Isidore, Paris physician, 1845–1896. See S. *reaction,* S.'s *sign.*

**Strauss,** Hermann, Berlin physician, 1868–1944. See S.'s *test.*

**streak** (strēk) [ A.S. *strica* ]. A line, stria, or stripe, especially one that is more or less indistinct or evanescent.

**Knapp's s.'s,** Knapp's *striae.*

**meningit'ic s.,** Trousseau's spot; tache méningéale; tache cérébrale; a line of redness following the drawing of the nail or a pencil point across the skin, marked especially in cases of meningitis.

**Moore's lightning s.'s,** a special form of photopsia manifested by vertical flashes of light, seen usually on the temporal side of the affected eye, accompanied by a crop of vitreous opacities; may occur recurrently for a few days or for a period of up to 20 years, and is caused by the senile shrunken vitreous striking the retina on ocular motion; the condition is not of serious portent.

**primitive s.,** an ectodermal ridge in the midline at the caudal end of the embryonic disk from which arises the intraembryonic mesoderm; this is achieved by inward and then lateral migration of cells; in human embryos it first appears on day 15 and thus gives a cephalocaudal axis to the developing embryo.

**stream.** Flumen.

**blood s.,** see *blood stream.*

**hair s.'s,** *flumina* pilorum.

**streblodactyly** (streb'lo-dak'tĭ-lĭ) [ G. *streblos,* twisted, + *daktylos,* finger ]. Campylodactyly.

**Streeter,** George L., U. S. embryologist, 1873–1948. See S.'s *bands,* S. *horizons.*

**Streiff,** E. B., French ophthalmologist. See Hallermann-S. *syndrome.*

**stremma** (strem'ah) [ G. a twist, fr. *strephō,* to twist. STREP- ]. Sprain.

**strength.** 1. The quality of being strong or powerful. 2. The degree of intensity. 3. The property of materials by which they endure the application of force without yielding or breaking.

**associative s.,** in psychology, the s. of a stimulus response linkage as measured by the frequency with which a stimulus elicits a particular response.

**biting s.,** *force* of mastication.

**compressive s.,** same as tensile s., except that the stress is in compression.

**ionic s.,** see under ionic.

**tensile s.,** the maximum tensile stress or load that a material is capable of sustaining; usually expressed in pounds per square inch.

**strephosymbolia** (stref-o-sim-bo'lĭ-ah) [ G. *strephō,* to turn, + *symbolon,* a mark or sign ]. 1. The perception of objects reversed as if in a mirror. 2. Specifically, difficulty in distinguishing written or printed letters that extend in opposite directions but are otherwise similar, such as *p* and *d,* or related kinds of mirror reversal.

**strephotome** (stref'o-tōm) [ G. *strephō,* to turn, twist, + *tomē,* incision ]. A corkscrew-shaped instrument, with flat ribbon-like spirals, formerly used in the radical cure of inguinal hernia; the instrument was introduced, encircling the canal, the walls of which were thus brought together, and was left in situ until obliterating adhesions had formed.

**strepitus** (strep′ĭ-tus) [ L. ]. A noise; usually, an auscultatory sound; see also sound.

**strepogenin** (strep′o-jen′in). A peptide that exhibits growth-promoting properties in connection with microorganisms.

**Strepsic′eros spek′ei.** Formerly called *Limnotragus spekei;* the African antelope (bush buck, kudu, nyala); a reservoir host of trypanosomes (*e.g., Trypanosoma brucei*) that are pathogenic to domestic animals.

**strepticemia** (strep-tĭ-se′mĭ-ah). Streptococcemia.

**strep′tidine.** 1,3-Diguanidinocyclohexane-2,4,5,6-tetrol; a constituent of streptomycin, consisting of an inositol and two guanidine residues.

**strepto-** (strep′to-) [ G. *streptos,* twisted, fr. *strephō,* to twist. STREP- ]. Combining form meaning curved or twisted; relating, usually, to organisms thus described, *e.g.,* streptococci.

**Streptobacillus** (strep-to-bă-sil′us) [ strepto- + bacillus ]. A genus of nonmotile, nonsporeforming, aerobic to facultatively anaerobic bacteria (family Bacteroidaceae) containing Gram-negative, pleomorphic cells which vary from short rods to long, interwoven filaments which have a tendency to fragment into chains of bacillary and coccobacillary elements. These organisms are parasitic to pathogenic for rats, mice, and other mammals. The type species is *S. moniliformis.*

    **S. monilifor′mis,** *Haverhillia multiformis;* a species commonly found as an inhabitant of the nasopharynx of rats. It occurs as the etiological agent of an epizootic septic polyarthritis in mice and of one type of ratbite fever. It is the type species of the genus *S.*

**strep′tobio′samine.** A methylamino disaccharide (streptose + *N*-methyl-L-glucosamine); with streptidine, forms streptomycin. The oxygen link is between C-2 of streptose and C-1 of the glucosamine.

**strep′tobi′ose.** Older term for streptose.

**streptococcal** (strep-to-kok′al). Relating to or caused by any organism of the genus *Streptococcus.*

**streptococcal fibrinolysin.** Streptokinase.

**streptococcal proteinase** (EC 3.4.22.10). Formerly *Streptococcus* peptidase A; a proteinase, formed from an inactive zymogen by proteolysis (see streptokinase).

**streptococcemia** (strep′to-kok-se′-mĭ-ah) [ streptococcus + G. *haima,* blood ]. Strepticemia; streptosepticemia; streptococcus infection or sepsis; the presence of streptococci in the blood.

**streptococci** (strep′to-kok′sī). Plural of streptococcus.

**streptococcosis** (strep′to-kok-ko′sis). Any streptococcal infection.

**Streptococcus** (strep-to-kok′us) [ strepto- + G. *kokkus,* berry (coccus) ]. A genus of nonmotile (with few exceptions), nonsporeforming, aerobic to facultatively anaerobic bacteria (family Lactobacillaceae) containing Gram-positive, spherical or ovoid cells which occur in pairs or short or long chains. Dextrorotatory lactic acid is the main product of carbohydrate fermentation. These organisms occur regularly in the mouth and intestines of man and other animals, in dairy and other food products, and in fermenting plant juices. Some species are pathogenic. The type species is *S. pyogenes.*

    **S. acidominimus,** a species found in the bovine vagina and on the skin of calves.

    **S. agalactiae,** a species found in the milk and tissues from udders of cows with mastitis; also reported to be associated with a variety of human infections, especially those of the urogenital tract.

    **S. angino′sus,** a species found in the human throat, sinuses, abscesses, vagina, skin, and feces; this organism has been associated with glomerular nephritis and various types of mild respiratory diseases.

    **S. bo′vis,** a species found in the bovine alimentary tract; this organism may also be found in blood and heart lesions in cases of subacute endocarditis.

**S. dur′ans,** a species found in dried milk powder, and in human and animal intestines.

**S. dysgalactiae,** a species found in the milk and udder of cows with acute mastitis; also found in various tissues and organs of lambs with suppurative polyarthritis.

**S. e′qui,** a species causing strangles in horses.

**S. equi′nus,** a species which is the predominant organism in the intestines of horses.

**S. equisimilis,** a species found in the normal human nose and throat, vagina, and skin; sometimes found in the respiratory tract of domestic animals; ocassionally associated with erysipelas and puerperal fever.

**S. faeca′lis,** a species found in human feces and in the intestines of many warm-blooded animals; occasionally found in urinary infections and in blood and heart lesions in cases of subacute endocarditis; associated with European foul brood of bees and with mild outbreaks of food poisoning.

**S. lactis,** a species found commonly as a contaminant in milk and dairy products; a common cause of the souring and coagulation of milk; some strains produce nisin, a powerful antibiotic that inhibits the growth of many other Gram-positive organisms.

**S. mitis,** a species found in the human mouth, throat, and nasopharynx; ordinarily, it is not considered to be pathogenic, but this organism may be recovered from ulcerated teeth and sinuses and from blood and heart lesions in cases of subacute endocarditis.

**S. pneumo′niae,** *Diplococcus pneumoniae;* pneumococcus; this species is the most common pathogenic microorganism of lobar pneumonia. Thirty-two types are recognized on the basis of agglutination with immune sera. The principal types are types I, II, and III; type III is distinguished sharply from the others by morphological and cultural differences; group IV presents a heterogenous group of organisms that are not agglutinated by either type I, II, or III serum. It contains the remaining 28 types which are responsible for 40 to 60 per cent of cases of pneumonia, varying with age, locality, season, and year; these are generally considered less virulent; type III is generally the most virulent; type I probably causes the greatest number of cases in adults, but responds best to serum treatment. It is the type species of the genus *Diplococcus, q.v.*

**S. pyog′enes,** a species found in the human mouth, throat, and respiratory tract and in inflammatory exudates, blood stream, and lesions in human diseases. It is sometimes found in the udders of cows, and in dust from sickrooms, hospital wards, schools, theaters, and other public places. It causes the formation of pus or even fatal septicemias. It is the type species of the genus *S.*

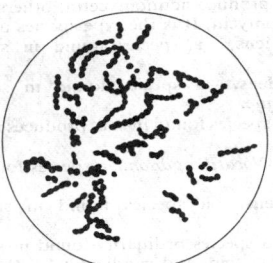

*Streptococcus pyogenes*
(Original magnification, ×2650)

**S. saliva′rius,** a species found in the human mouth, throat, and nasopharynx.

**S. sanguis,** a species originally found in the so-called vegetation on heart valves from cases of subacute bacterial endocarditis; occasionally found in infected sinuses and teeth and in house dust.

**S. uberis,** a species found in bovine udder infections.

**S. zooepidemicus,** a species found in diseased animals, but not in man.

**streptococcus** (strep′to-kok′us). A term used to refer to any member of the genus *Streptococcus.*

α **streptococci,** streptococci that form a green variety of reduced hemoglobin in the area of the colony on a blood agar medium.

**s. erythrogenic toxin,** see under toxin.

β-**hemolytic streptococci,** hemolytic streptococci; those that produce active hemolysins (O and S) which cause a zone of clear hemolysis on the blood agar medium in the area of the colony; Lancefield group A β-hemolytic streptococci include most strains pathogenic for man.

**hemolytic streptococci,** β-hemolytic streptococci.

**Lancefield classification of streptococci,** see under classification.

**s. peptidase A,** former name for streptococcal proteinase.

**streptoder'ma.** Pyoderma due to streptococci.

**streptodermatitis** (strep-to-der-mă-ti'tis). Inflammation of the skin caused by the action of streptococci.

**streptodor'nase.** A "dornase" (deoxyribonuclease) obtained from streptococci; used with streptokinase to facilitate drainage in septic surgical conditions.

**streptofu'ranose.** Streptose.

**streptoki'nase.** Streptococcal fibrinolysin; plasminokinase; an extracellular enzyme activator present in the cultures of certain strains of streptococci; cleaves plasminogen, producing plasmin, which causes the liquefaction of fibrin (same activity as staphylokinase and urokinase). Used clinically to dissolve fibrinous adhesions, to break down blood clots, or in meningitis to remove fibrinous blocks that prevent the free circulation of cerebrospinal fluid; used usually in conjunction with streptodornase.

**streptokinase-streptodornase.** VARIDASE; contains streptokinase, streptodornase, and other proteolytic enzymes; used by topical application or by injection into body cavities to remove clotted blood and fibrinous and purulent accumulations of exudate.

**streptolydigin.** PORTAMYCIN; antibiotic substance produced by *Streptomyces lydicus;* possesses antimicrobial activity.

**streptolysin** (strep-tol'ĭ-sin). A hemolysin produced by streptococci.

**s. O,** s. that is reversibly inactivated by oxygen.

**Streptomyces** (strep'to-mi'sēz) [ strepto- + G. *mykēs,* fungus ]. A genus of nonmotile, aerobic, Gram-positive bacteria (family Streptomycetaceae) that grow in the form of a much-branched mycelium; conidia are produced in chains on aerial hyphae. These organisms are predominantly saprophytic soil forms; some are parasitic on plants or animals. Many streptomycetes produce antibiotics. There are over 150 species in this genus. The type species is *S. albus.*

**S. albus,** a species found in dust, soil, grains, and straw. Some strains produce actinomycetin; others produce thiolutin or endomycin. It is the type species of the genus *S.*

**S. an'tibiot'icus,** a species found in soil; produces actinomycin.

**S. aureofaciens,** a species found in soil; produces chlortetracycline.

**S. fradiae,** a species found in soil; produces neomycin and fradicin.

**S. gibsonii,** *Nocardia gibsonii;* a species found in human infections.

**S. griseoluteus,** a species found in soil; produces griseolutein.

**S. gris'eus,** a species ordinarily found in soil; produces streptomycin, grisein, and candicidin.

**S. noursei,** a species found in soil; produces nystatin and phalamycin.

**S. rimo'sus,** a species found in soil; produces oxytetracycline, an amphoteric substance active against various bacteria, rickettsiae, and the larger viruses; also produces rimocidin, an antifungal agent.

**Streptomycetaceae** (strep'to-mi'sē-ta'se-e). A family of aerobic, Gram-positive bacteria (order Actinomycetales) that produce a vegetative mycelium which does not fragment into bacillary or coccoid forms; they produce conidia which are borne on sporophores. These organisms occur primarily in the soil; some are thermophiles which are found in rotting manure. A few species are parasitic, and many produce antibiotics. The type genus is *Streptomyces.*

**streptomycete** (strep'to-mi'sēt). A term used to refer to a member of the genus *Streptomyces;* it is sometimes improperly used to refer to any member of the family Streptomycetaceae.

**streptomy'cin.** An antibiotic agent obtained from the soil organism, *Streptomyces griseus;* active against the tubercle bacillus and a large number of Gram-positive and Gram-negative bacteria. It is a glucoside and contains streptidine and streptobiosamine linked by an oxygen bridge between C-4 of the inositol residue and C-1 of the streptose residue. Can be administered intramusculularly, intravenously, or subcutaneously; also used in the form of dihydrostreptomycin. S.

**streptomycosis** (strep'to-mi-ko'sis) [ strepto- + G. *mykēs,* fungus, + suffix -*osis,* condition ]. An old term for streptococcemia.

**strep'tonivi'cin.** Novobiocin.

**strep'tose.** Streptofuranose; formerly called streptobiose; an unusual pentose (3-aldehydo-5-deoxyfuranose), a component of streptobiosamine, hence of streptomycin. For structure, see sugars.

**streptosepticemia** (strep'to-sep-tĭ-se'mĭ-ah). Streptococcemia.

**streptothrichosis** (strep'to-thrĭ-ko'sis). Streptotrichosis.

**streptothricin** (strep'to-thri'sin). An antibiotic agent obtained from cultures of *Actinomyces lavendulae.*

**Strep'tothrix.** An obsolete generic name of bacteria. The type species, *S. fosteri,* isolated from a concretion in a tear duct, is not recognizable by modern standards. A number of the pathogenic species that were placed in this genus have subsequently been transferred to other genera (*e.g.,* *Actinomyces israelii, Nocardia madurae,* and *Streptobacillus moniliformis*).

**streptotrichiasis** (strep'to-trĭ-ki'ă-sis). Streptotrichosis.

**streptotrichosis** (strep'to-trĭ-ko'sis). Streptothrichosis; streptotrichiasis. 1. An infectious disease caused by one or more species of *Streptothrix,* most of which are now classed in other genera, *e.g., Streptobacillus, Actinomyces, Actinobacillus,* and so on; the condition is frequently characterized by a chronic suppurative inflammation, the pus containing granules composed chiefly of colonies of the causal microorganism. 2. An old term for actinomycosis.

**streptovaricin** (strep'to-văr'ĭ-sin). DALACIN; a mixture of several antibiotic substances (streptovaricin A, B, C, D, and E) produced by *Streptomyces spectabilis.*

**stress** [ L. *strictus,* tight, fr. *stringo,* to draw together ]. 1. The reactions of the animal body to forces of a deleterious nature, infections and various abnormal states that tend to disturb its normal physiologic equilibrium (homeostasis). 2. The resisting force set up in a body as a result of an externally applied force. 3. In dentistry, the forces set up in teeth, their supporting structures, and structures restoring or replacing teeth as a result of the force of mastication. 4. The force or pressure applied or exerted between portions of a body or bodies, generally expressed in pounds per square inch. 5. In rheology, the force in a material transmitted per unit area to adjacent layers. 6. In psychology, a physical or psychological stimulus which, when impinging upon an individual, produces strain or disequilibrium.

**shear s.,** the force acting in shear flow expressed in force per unit area; units in the CGS system: dynes/cm².

**tensile s.,** a s. acting on a body per unit cross-sectional area so as to elongate the body.

**yield s.,** the critical s. that must be applied to a material before it begins to flow, as in a Bingham plastic.

**stress breaker.** A device that relieves the abutment teeth, to which a fixed or removable partial denture is attached, of all or part of the forces generated by occlusal function.

**stretch'er** [ A.S. *streccan,* to stretch ]. A sheet of canvas stretched to a frame with four handles, used for transporting the sick or wounded; a litter.

**stria,** gen. and pl. **striae** (stri'ah, stri'e) [ L. channel, furrow ]. 1. [ NA ]. A stripe, band, streak, or line, distinguished by color, texture, depression, or elevation from the tissue in which it is found. 2. *Striae* cutis distensae.

**acoustic striae,** striae medullares ventriculi quarti.

**striae atroph'icae,** striae cutis distensae.

**auditory striae,** striae medullares ventriculi quarti.

brown striae, Retzius' striae.

striae cu'tis disten'sae, bands of thin, wrinkled skin, initially red but becoming purple and white; they occur commonly on the abdomen, buttocks, and thighs during and following pregnancy, and result from atrophy of the dermis and overextension of the skin; they are associated with ascites and Cushing's syndrome; also known as linea albicans or atrophica; linear or traction atrophy; striae (2); striae gravidarum.

s. for'nicis, s. medullaris thalami.

Gennari's s., Gennari's *line*.

striae gravida'rum, striae cutis distensae resulting from pregnancy.

Knapp's striae, angioid streaks of the retina; associated with pseudoxanthoma elasticum (of the skin) and Paget's disease (of the bone).

striae lancisi, the s. longitudinalis lateralis and the s. longitudinalis medialis.

Langhan's s., fibrinoid that accumulates on the chorionic plate between the bases of placental villi during the first half of pregnancy.

lateral longitudinal s., s. longitudinalis lateralis.

s. longitudina'lis latera'lis [ NA ], lateral longitudinal s.; s. tecta; a thin longitudinal band of nerve fibers accompanied by gray matter, near each outer edge of the upper surface of the corpus callosum under cover of the gyrus cinguli.

s. longitudina'lis media'lis [ NA ], medial longitudinal s.; a thin longitudinal band of nerve fibers accompanied by gray matter, running along the surface of the corpus callosum on either side of the median line. Together with the s. longitudinalis lateralis it forms part of a thin layer of gray matter on the dorsal surface of the corpus callosum, the indusium griseum, a rudimentary component of the hippocampus.

s. mallea'ris [ NA ], mallear stripe; a bright line seen through the membrana tympani, produced by the attachment of the manubrium of the malleus.

medial longitudinal s., s. longitudinalis medialis.

s. medulla'ris thal'ami [ NA ], medullary s. of the thalamus; s. fornicis; s. ventriculi tertii; a narrow, compact fiber bundle that extends along the line of attachment of the roof of the third ventricle to the thalamus on each side and terminates posteriorly in the habenular nucleus. It is composed of fibers originating in the septal area, the substantia perforata anterior, the lateral preoptic nucleus, and the medial segment of the globus pallidus.

striae medulla'res ventric'uli quar'ti [ NA ], medullary striae of the fourth ventricle; acoustic or auditory striae; teniae acusticae; medullary teniae; Bergmann's cords; slender fascicles of fibers extending transversally below the ependymal floor of the ventricle from the median sulcus to enter the inferior cerebellar peduncle. They arise from the arcuate nuclei of the medulla oblongata.

Nitabuch's s., Nitabuch's *membrane*.

striae olfacto'riae [ NA ], olfactory striae; three more or less distinct fiber bands (s. medialis, s. intermedia, s. lateralis) that extend the olfactory peduncle (olfactory nerve) caudalward beyond its attachment to the olfactory trigone. The medial s. curves dorsally into the tenia tecta; the intermediate, often barely visible, extends straight back and terminates in the olfactory tubercle; the lateral olfactory s., the largest of the three, passes along the lateral side of the olfactory tubercle, curving laterally as far as the limen insulae, then sharply medialward to reach the uncus of the parahippocampal gyrus where it terminates in the plexiform layer of the olfactory cortex. See also s. longitudinalis medialis.

olfactory striae, striae olfactoriae.

striae parallelae, Retzius' striae.

Retzius' striae, striae parallelae; brown striae; dark concentric lines crossing the enamel prisms of the teeth, seen in axial cross sections of the enamel.

Rohr's s., layer of fibrinoid in the intervillous spaces of the placenta.

s. spino'sa, Lucas' groove; a faint groove occasionally caused by the chorda tympani nerve on the spine of the sphenoid.

s. tec'ta, s. longitudinalis lateralis.

terminal s., s. terminalis.

s. termina'lis [ NA ], terminal s.; tenia semicircularis; Foville's fasciculus; Tarin's tenia; a slender, compact fiber bundle that connects the amygdala (corpus amygdaloideum) with the hypothalamus and other basal forebrain regions. Originating from the amygdala, the bundle passes first caudalward in the roof of the temporal horn of the lateral ventricle; it follows the medial side of the caudate nucleus forward in the floor of the ventricle's pars centralis (or body) until it reaches the interventricular foramen, in the posterior wall of which it steeply curves down to enter the hypothalamus, in part passing behind the anterior commissure, in part curving over and around the commissure. Coursing caudalward in the medial part of the hypothalamus, the bundle terminates in the anterior and ventromedial hypothalamic nuclei.

s. vascula'ris duc'tus cochlea'ris [ NA ], vascular stripe; psalterial cord; the stratified epithelium lining the upper part of the ligamentum spirale cochleae; it is penetrated by capillaries and is believed to be the site of production of endolymph.

s. ventric'uli ter'tii, s. medullaris thalami.

Wickham's striae, whitish lines on the surface of lichen planus papules.

striae of Zahn, *lines* of Zahn.

**striatal** (stri-ā-tal). Relating to the corpus striatum.

**stri·ate, stri'ated** [ L. *striatus*, furrowed ]. Striped; marked by striae.

**striation** (stri-a'shun). 1. Stria; striae. 2. A striate appearance. 3. The act of streaking or making striae.

basal s.'s, the vertical infranuclear s.'s due to the infolded plasma membrane and mitochondria; they are seen in kidney tubules and certain intralobular salivary ducts.

tabby-cat s. tigroid s.

tigroid s., linear whitish or yellowish markings on the fatty degenerated heart muscle.

**striatonigral** (stri-a-to-ni'gral). Referring to the efferent connection of the striatum with the substantia nigra (*q. v.*).

**striatum** (stri-a'tum) [ L. neut. of *striatus*, furrowed ]. Collective name for the caudate nucleus and putamen which together with the globus pallidus or pallidum form the corpus striatum.

**stricture** (strik'chur) [ L. *strictura*, fr. *stringo*, pp. *strictus*, to draw tight, bind ]. A circumscribed narrowing or stenosis of a tubular structure.

annular s., a ringlike constriction encircling the wall of a canal.

bridle s., narrowing of a canal by a band of tissue stretching across part of its lumen.

contractile s., recurrent s.

functional s., spasmodic s.

Hunner's s., bladder s. produced by Hunner's ulcer.

organic s., permanent s.; one due to the presence of cicatricial or other new tissue, not spasmodic.

permanent s., organic s.

recurrent s., contractile s.; a s. due to the presence of contractile tissue which may be dilated but soon returns.

spasmodic s., functional s.; temporary s.; a s. due to localized spasm of muscular fibers in the wall of the canal.

temporary s., spasmodic s.

**stricturotome** (strik'chur-o-tōm). A stricture knife; an instrument for use in dividing a stricture.

**stricturotomy** (strik'chur-ot'o-mī) [ stricture + G. *tomē*, incision ]. Surgical division of a stricture.

**stri'dent** [ L. *stridens*, pres. p. of *strideo*, to creak ]. Creaking; grating; harsh-sounding; denoting an auscultatory sound or rale.

**stri'dor** [ L. a harsh, creaking sound ]. A high-pitched, noisy respiration, like the blowing of the wind; a sign of respiratory obstruction, especially in the trachea or larynx.

congenital s., laryngeal s.; crowing inspiration occurring at birth or within the first few months of life; sometimes without apparent cause and sometimes due to abnormal flaccidity of epiglottis or arytenoids.

s. den'tium, grinding of the teeth.

expiratory s., a singing sound during general anesthesia due to the semi-approximated vocal cords offering resistance to the escape of air; usually arises in response to somatic sensory stimulation and is in effect a vocal protest against insufficient anesthesia.

**inspiratory s.,** a crowing sound during the inspiratory phase of respiration due to relaxation during general anesthesia of those laryngeal muscles that maintain vocal cord abduction; some air passes between the cords unimpeded at the commencement of inspiration, but as the cords approximate, a phonating vibratory sound is emitted.

**laryn'geal s.,** congenital s.

**s. serrat'icus,** a rough grating like the sound of a saw.

**stridulous** (strid'u-lus) [ L. *stridulus*, fr. *strideo*, to creak, to hiss ]. Having a shrill or creaking sound.

**strike.** Myiasis.

**stringhalt** (string'hawlt) [ A.S. *streng*, cord, + *healt*, lame ]. A myoclonic affection, characterized by spasmodic overflexion of the hind legs of a horse while walking or running. It occurs in all breeds of horses. Its cause is unknown.

**strip** [ A.S. *strypan*, to rob ]. 1. To express the contents from a flexible tube or canal, such as the urethra, by running the finger along it. 2. Subcutaneous excision of a vein in its longitudinal axis, performed with a special instrument, a stripper.

**stripe.** In anatomy, a streak, line, band, or stria.

**s. of Gennari,** *line* of Gennari.

**Hensen's s.,** a band on the undersurface of the membrana tectoria of the cochlear duct.

**Mees' s.'s,** Mees' *lines*.

**stro'bila,** pl. **stro'bilae** [ G. *stobilē*, a twist of lint. STREP-. ]. A chain of segments, less the scolex and unsegmented neck portion, of a tapeworm. In some cestode groups, it may consist of a single proglottid.

**Strobilocercus** (stro'bi-lo-ser-kus) [ G. *stobilē*, a twist of lint, + *kerkos*, tail ]. A taenioid tapeworm larva of the cysticercus type, but with a conspicuous segmented neck, small terminal bladder, and everted scolex. It is the larval form of *Taenia taeniaeformis* called *Cysticercus fasciolaris*.

**strob'iloid** [ G. *strobilē*, strobile, + *eidos*, resemblance ]. Resembling a chain of segments of a tapeworm.

**stro'boscope.** 1. An electronic instrument that produces intermittent light flashes of controlled frequency; used to influence electrical activity of the cerebral cortex. 2. Zoescope; an instrument for producing motionless pictures of periodic or varying motion by means of light periodically interrupted.

**stro'boscop'ic** [ G. *strobos*, a twisting around, fr. *strephō*, to twist, + *skopeō*, to view ]. Pertaining to the illusion of motion, retarded or accelerated, produced by a series of visual exposures viewed in rapid succession.

**Stroganoff,** Vasili V., Russian obstetrician, 1857–1938. See S.'s *method.*

**stroke** [ A.S. *strāc* ]. 1. A blow; coup; hence a sudden attack, as a sunstroke or paralytic s. See also apoplexy. 2. A pulsation. 3. To pass the hand or any instrument gently over a surface; see also stroking. 4. A gliding movement over a surface.

**heart s.,** (1) impact of the apex of the heart against the wall of the chest; (2) *angina* pectoris.

**heat s.,** a severe illness produced by exposure to excessively high temperatures, beginning with headache, vertigo, confusion, and slight temperature rise; in severe cases there are collapse and coma, fever as high as 110°F., tachycardia, and hot dry skin. In civil life it usually occurs among older people who are forced to remain in quarters where the night temperature does not permit them to cool off adequately.

**sun s.,** see sunstroke.

**water-s.,** serous *apoplexy.*

**stroking.** The nonverbal fondling and nurturance accorded infants or the nonverbal and verbal forms of acceptance, reassurance, and positive reinforcement accorded to children and adults either by an individual to himself or to another person in order to satisfy a basic biopsychological need of all developing humans; various psychopathological conditions are believed to result when such s. is absent or faulty.

**stroma,** pl. **stromata** (stro'mah, stro'mă-tah) [ G. *strōma*, bed ]. [ NA ]. The framework, usually of connective tissue,

of an organ, gland, or other structure; distinguished from the parenchyma or specific substance of the part.

**s. glan'dulae thyroid'eae** [ NA ], framework of the thyroid gland; the connective tissue that supports the lobules and follicles of the gland.

**s. i'ridis** [ NA ], s. of the iris; the delicate vascular connective tissue that lies between the anterior surface of the iris and the pars iridica retinae.

**lymphatic s.,** the network of reticular fibers and associated reticular cells of lymphatic tissue.

**s. ova'rii** [ NA ], framework of the ovary; the fibrous tissue of the medulla of the ovary.

**Rollet's s.,** the colorless s. of the red blood cells.

**s. vit'reum** [ NA ], s. of the vitreous; the delicate framework of the vitreous body.

**stro'mal.** Relating to the stroma of an organ or other structure; stromatic.

**stromat'ic.** Stromal.

**stro'matin.** An insoluble protein in the stroma of erythrocytes.

**stromatolysis** (stro-mă-tol'ĭ-sis) [ stroma + G. *lysis*, solution ]. Solution of the enveloping membrane of a bacterial or other cell, the cell body not being affected.

**stromato'sis.** See endometrial stromal *sarcoma.*

**Stromeyer,** Georg F. L., German surgeon, 1804–1876. See S.-Little *operation*, S.'s *splint.*

**stromuhr** (stro'moor) [ Ger. *Strom*, stream, + *Uhr*, clock ]. An instrument for measuring the quantity of blood that flows per unit of time through a blood vessel.

**Ludwig's s.,** one of the first devices for measuring flow in blood vessels.

**thermo-s.,** consists of a heating element between two thermocouples, which are applied to the outside of a vessel. The blood flow is calculated from the difference in the temperatures recorded by the proximal and distal thermocouples.

**Strong,** Edward K., Jr., American psychologist, °1884. See S. vocational interest *test.*

**strongyle** (stron'jīl). Common name for members of the family Strongylidae.

**Strongylidae** (stron-jīl'ĭ-de) [ see *Strongyloides* ]. A family of parasitic nematode worms (order Strongyloidea) including the genera *Strongylus* and *Oesophagostomum.*

**Strongyloidea** (stron'jĭ-loy'de-ah) [ see strongyloides ]. An order of parasitic nematode worms including the genera *Ancyclostoma, Necator, Ostertagia, Haemonchus,* and *Strongylus,* as well as the gapeworms of fowl, the lungworms of carnivores, and some of the most important helminth pathogens of man and domestic animals.

**Strongyloides** (stron'jĭ-loy'dēz) [ G. *strongylus*, round, + *eidos*, resemblance ]. Threadworm; a genus of small nematode parasites (superfamily Rhabditoidea) commonly found in the small intestine of mammals, particularly ruminants. They are characterized by an unusual life cycle that involves a generation of free-living adult worms.

**S. bo'vis,** *Cooperia punctata.*

**S. fullebor'ni,** occurs in primates.

**S. papillo'sus,** occurs in cattle, sheep, and goats.

**S. ranso'mi,** occurs in swine.

**S. stercora'lis,** occurs in dogs and causes strongyloidiasis in man.

**S. weste'ri,** occurs in horses.

**strongyloidiasis, strongyloidosis** (stron-jĭ-loy-di'ă-sis, -do'sis). Infection with the nematode *Strongyloides stercoralis;* considered to be a parthenogenetic female. Larvae passed to the soil form free-living adults or develop directly into infective third stage strongyliform or filariform larvae, which penetrate the skin or buccal mucosa via drinking water. Infection can occur by larvae of a new generation developed in the soil (indirect cycle), by infective larvae developed without an intervening adult stage (direct cycle), or by larvae that develop directly in the feces in the intestine of the host, penetrate the mucosa, and pass by blood-lung migration back to the intestine (autoreinfection). Most serious human infections and nearly all fatalities result from autoreinfection.

**strongyloplasm** (stron'jĭ-lo-plazm) [ G. *strongylos*, round, + *plasma*, something formed ]. A filtrable virus; an old term for the minute bodies found in inclusion bodies; see virus (2).

**strongylosis** (stron-jĭ-lo'sis). Disease caused by infection with a species of *Strongylus*; effects may be extreme from worm-caused lesions, nodules and aneurisms.

**Strongylus** (stron'jĭ-lus) [ G. *strongylos*, round ]. Palisade worm; a genus of large strongyle nematodes (subfamily Strongylinae, family Strongylidae) parasitic in horses and other equids, and the cause of strongylosis.

**S. asi'ni**, occurs in the large intestine of the ass and other wild equids.

**S. edenta'tus**, a bloodsucking worm occurring in the cecum and colon of the horse, ass, mule, and zebra.

**S. equi'nus**, a cosmopolitan bloodsucking worm found in the cecum and (rarely) colon of horses and other equids.

**S. vulga'ris**, a bloodsucking worm found chiefly in the cecum of horses and other equids; in the course of their migration, larvae commonly lodge in the wall of the posterior aorta, causing wall damage and the development of verminous aneurysms in this vessel and especially in the anterior mesenteric arteries.

**strontium** (stron'she-um) [ *Strontian*, a town in Scotland ]. A metallic element, symbol Sr, atomic no. 38; atomic weight 87.63; of dark yellow color; one of the alkaline earth series and similar to calcium in chemical properties.

**s. bromide**, $SrBr_2 \cdot 6H_2O$; used to meet the same indications as the other bromides.

**s. iodide**, $SrI_2 \cdot 6H_2O$; used for the same purposes as the other iodides.

**s. lactate**, has been used in albuminuria and in osteoporosis.

**s. peroxide**, insoluble in water but decomposed in it to hydrogen peroxide; has been used externally as a dusting powder and in the form of an ointment.

**strontium-89** ($^{89}Sr$). Radioactive strontium isotope; beta emitter with half-life of 54 days; used as tracer in studies of strontium absorption by body, strontium incorporation in bone, etc.

**strontium-90** ($^{90}Sr$). Radioactive s. isotope; beta emitter with half-life of 28 years; a major component (about 5 per cent) of the uranium fission products; it is incorporated into bone tissue where turnover is slow and where its relatively long half-life makes it a continuing factor in possibly deleterious radiation effects.

**strophanthin** (stro-fan'thin). K-strophanthin; a glycoside or mixture of glycosides from *Strophanthus kombé*; a cardiac tonic, like ouabain; extremely toxic.

**G-s.**, ouabain.

**K-s.**, see s.

**Strophanthus** (stro-fan'thus) [ G. *strophos*, a twisted cord, + *anthos*, flower ]. A genus of vines of east Africa (family Apocynaceae); the dried ripe seeds of *S. kombé* or *S. hispidus* contain the cardiac glycoside strophanthin, and were used as an arrow poison; the seeds of *S. gratus* are the botanical source of ouabain.

**strophocephalus** (strof'o-sef'ă-lus). An individual with strophocephaly.

**strophocephaly** (strof'o-sef'ă-lĭ) [ G. *strophē*, a twist, fr. *strephō*, to twist, + *kephalē*, head ]. A condition characterized by a congenitally distorted head and face, in which there is a tendency toward cyclopia and malformation of the oral region.

**strophosomia** (strof'o-so-mī-ah) [ G. *strophē*, a twist, + *sōma*, body ]. A severe form of a congenital ventral fissure, extremely rare in man.

**strophulus** (strof'u-lus) [ Mod. L. dim. of G. *strophus*, colic. STREP- ]. *Miliaria* rubra.

**s. can'didus** [ L. dazzling white ], a form in which the papules are colorless and shining.

**s. intertinc'tus, s. prurigino'sus**, a form marked by an eruption of itching papules.

**Stroud**, Bert B., American physiologist, anatomist, and zoologist, 19th century. See S.'s pectinated *area*.

**struck.** A disease of adult sheep in England caused by *Clostridium perfringens* type C.

**struc'tural.** Relating to the structure of a part; having a structure.

**structuralism** (struk'chur-al-ism) A branch of psychology interested in the basic structure of the mind, including intellect and feeling, and behavior of man, as contrasted with functionalism, *q.v.*

**structure** (struk'chur) [ L. *structura*, fr. *struo*, pp. *structus*, to build ]. 1. The arrangement of the details of a part; the manner of formation of a part. 2. A tissue or formation made up of different but related parts. 3. In chemistry, the specific connections of the atoms in a given molecule.

**brush heap s.**, haphazard interlocking of fibrils in a gel or hydrocolloid impression material.

**crystal s.**, the arrangement in space and the interatomic distances and angles of the atoms in crystals, usually determined by x-ray diffraction measurements.

**denture-supporting s.'s**, the tissues, teeth, and/or residual ridges, which serve as the foundation for removable partial or complete dentures.

**fine s.**, see ultrastructure.

**gel s.**, brush heap s. of fibrils giving firmness to hydrocolloids.

**struma**, pl. **strumae** (stru'mah, -me) [ L. a scrofulous tumor, fr. *struo*, to pile up, build ]. 1. Scrofula (obs.). 2. Goiter. 3. Formerly, any enlargement.

**s. aberra'ta**, a goitrous tumor of an accessory thyroid gland.

**adre'nal s.**, hyperplasia of adrenal glands.

**s. aneurysmat'ica**, s. pulsans; vascular goiter with dilated vessels.

**s. ba'seous lin'guae**, a mass of thyroid tissue at the base of the tongue derived from a remnant of the oral end of the thyroglossal duct.

**s. calculo'sa**, a calcified goiter with atrophy of the parenchyma.

**cast iron s.**, Riedel's s.

**s. colloid'es**, colloid goiter; s. gelatinosa; enlargement of the thyroid gland with an increase in colloid due to degeneration of the glandular epithelium.

**s. colloid'es cys'tica**, colloid goiter in which the increased colloid occurs in the form of cystic collections.

**s. cys'tica os'sea**, cystic goiter with calcification in the hyaline connective tissue.

**s. endothorac'ica**, enlargement of a deeply lying thyroid or of an accessory thyroid in the anterior mediastinum.

**s. fibro'sa**, s. hyperplastica; enlargment of the thyroid due to hyperplasia of the interstitial connective tissue, often with atrophy of the parenchyma.

**s. follicula'ris**, colloid parenchymatous goiter.

**s. gelatino'sa**, s. colloides.

**Hashimoto's s.**, Hashimoto's *disease.*

**s. hyperplas'tica**, s. fibrosa.

**lig'neous s.**, Riedel's s.

**s. lipomato'des aberra'ta re'nis**, renal *adenocarcinoma*.

**s. lymphomato'sa**, Hashimoto's *disease.*

**s. malig'na**, cancer of the thyroid gland.

**s. medic'amento'sa**, goiter due to the use of some remedy, *e.g.*, sulfocyanate for hypertension.

**s. mollis**, soft or colloid goiter.

**s. nodo'sa**, adenoma of the thyroid.

**s. ova'rii**, thyroid tumor of the ovary; a rare ovarian tumor, regarded as teratomatous, in which thyroid tissue has surpassed the other elements; occasionally associated with hyperthyroidism.

**parathy'roid s.**, an adenoma of the parathyroid gland, with microscopic structures that resemble those of thyroid glandular tissue.

**s. parenchymato'sa**, enlargement of the thyroid due to hyperplasia of the parenchyma.

**s. petro'sa**, hard or fibrous goiter.

**pituitary s.**, s. pituitaria; obsolete terms meaning enlargment of the hypophysis.

**s. postbranchia'lis**, Getsowa's *adenoma.*

**s. pulsans**, s. aneurysmatica.

**retroster'nal s.**, substernal s.

**Riedel's s.**, Riedel's disease or thyroiditis; ligneous s. or thyroiditis; cast iron s.; a rare fibrous induration of the thyroid, with adhesion to adjacent structures, that may cause tracheal compression; possibly an end state of Hashimoto's disease.

**subster'nal s.**, retrosternal s.; a goiter with a prolongation downward behind the sternum.

**s. supraren'alis**, fatty tumor of the suprarenal body.

**s. thy'mica,** enlargement of the thymus, or persistence of this gland after the period at which it usually undergoes atrophy.

**s. thy'micolymphat'ica,** thymic s. associated with status thymicolymphaticus (*q. v.*); probably a misnomer based on failure to realize the size of the normal thymus gland.

**strumectomy** (stru-mek'to-mĭ) [ struma + G. *ektomē*, excision ]. 1. Excision of a scrofulous gland. 2. Surgical removal of all or a portion of a goitrous tumor.

**median s.,** isthmectomy; removal of a median goiter or an enlarged isthmus of the thyroid gland.

**stru'miform** [ struma + L. *forma*, form ]. 1. Resembling scrofula. 2. Resembling a goiter.

**strumipriv'ic, strumip'rivous.** Strumiprivus.

**strumiprivus,** fem. **strumipriva** (stru-mĭ-pre'-vus) [ Mod. L. fr. struma + L. *privo*, to deprive ]. Strumiprivic; strumiprivous; relating to the removal of a goiter.

**strumitis** (stru-mi'tus) [ struma + G. suffix -*itis*, inflammation ]. Inflammation of a goitrous tumor; inflammation, with swelling, of the thyroid gland. See also thyroiditis.

**stru'mous.** Goitrous; relating to a struma.

**Strümpell,** Adolf von, German physician, 1853–1925. See S.'s *disease, phenomenon, reflex,* S.-Marie, Marie-S., S.-Westphal *disease,* Westphal-S. *pseudosclerosis.*

**strychnine** (strik'nin, -nēn, -nīn). An alkaloid from *Strychnos nux- vomica;* C$_{21}$H$_{22}$N$_2$O$_2$; colorless crystals of intensely bitter taste, nearly insoluble in water. It stimulates all parts of the central nervous system, and is used as a stomachic, an antidote for depressant poisons, and in the treatment of myocardities; its therapeutic popularity is unwarranted, however. The commonly used salts of s. are s. hydrochloride, s. phosphate, and s. sulfate. It is a potent chemical capable of producing acute or chronic poisoning of man or animals.

**strychninism** (strik'nĭ-nizm). Chronic strychnine poisoning.

**strychninomania** (strik'nĭ-no-ma'nĭ-ah). Addiction to the use of strychnine.

**Strychnos** (strik'nos) [ G. nighshade ]. A genus of tropical shrubs or trees of the family Loganiaceae. Most South American species contain chiefly quaternary neuromuscular blocking alkaloids; the African, Asiatic, and Australian species contain tertiary strychnine-like alkaloids.

**S. castelnaei,** source of curare.

**s. crevauxii,** source of curare.

**S. igna'tii,** the source of ignatia.

**S. nux-vom'ica,** the source of nux vomica and of the alkaloids brucine and strychnine.

**S. toxifera,** source of curare.

**Stryker,** Garold V., U. S. pathologist, *1896. See S.-Halbeisen *syndrome.*

**Stryker frame.** See under frame.

**Stuart-Prower factor.** See under factor.

**stud** [ M.E. ]. 1. A male horse used for breeding; stallion. 2. An establishment that maintains a number of stallions especially for breeding purposes.

**stud'y** [ L. *studium*, study, inquiry ]. Research, detailed examination, and/or analysis of an organism, object, or phenomena.

**longitudinal s.,** an examination of the important events of a long time period or segment of a whole life, in contrast to concentration on one cross-sectional time period.

**multivariate s.'s,** simultaneous investigations of the influence of several variables.

**stump.** The extremity of a limb left after amputation; the pedicle remaining after removal of the tumor which was attached to it.

**stun** [ A.S. *stunian*, to make a loud noise ]. To stupefy; to render unconscious by cerebral trauma.

**stupe** (stūp) [ L. stupa, oakum, tow ]. A compress or cloth wrung out of hot water, usually impregnated with turpentine or other irritant, applied to the surface to produce counterirritation.

**stupefa'cient, stupefac'tive** [ L. *stupefacio* ]. Causing stupor; narcotic.

**stu'por** [ L. fr. *stupeo*, to be stunned ]. Lethargy; torpor; unconsciousness. See also consciousness.

**benign s.,** a stuporous syndrome from which recovery is the rule, as opposed to malignant s.; also called depressive s.

**catatonic s.,** s. associated with catatonic schizophrenia.

**depressive s.,** benign s.

**malignant s.,** a stuporous condition from which recovery is infrequent, as opposed to benign s.

**stu'porous.** Relating to or marked by stupor.

**stur'dy.** Staggers (2).

**Sturge,** William A., English physician, 1850–1919. See S.'s *disease,* S.-Kalischer-Weber *syndrome.*

**stu'rine.** A protamine in the sperm of the sturgeon.

**Sturm** (stoorm), Johann C., 1635–1703. See S.'s *conoid, interval.*

**Sturmdorf,** A., U. S. gynecologist, 1861–1934. See S.'s *operation.*

**stut'ter** [ frequentative of *stut*, from Goth. *stautan*, to strike ]. To enunciate certain words with difficulty and with frequent halting and repetition of the initial consonant of a word or syllable.

**stut'tering.** Dysarthria syllabaris spasmodica; a spasmodic dysphemia; phonatory or articulatory disorder, characteristically beginning in childhood, with intense anxiety about the efficiency of oral communications.

**urinary s.,** stammering of the bladder; frequent involuntary interruption occurring during the act of urination.

**sty, stye,** pl. **sties, styes** (sti, stiz). *Hordeolum* externum.

**Meibo'mian s.,** *hordeolum* internum.

**Zeisian s.,** inflammation of one of Zeis' glands.

**style** (stil). Stylet.

**stylet, stylette** (sti'let, sti-let') [ It. *stilletto*, a dagger; dim. of L. *stilus* or *stylus*, a stake, a pen ]. Stylus (3); style. 1. A wire contained in the lumen of a flexible catheter used to stiffen it and give it form during its passage; see also mandrel; mandrin. 2. A slender probe.

**endotracheal s.,** a rod of malleable metal used to maintain the desired curve of an endotracheal tube for its insertion into the trachea.

**styliform** (sti'lĭ-form) [ L. *stilus* (*stylus*), a stake, + *forma*, form ]. Styloid.

**stylo-** (sti'lo-) [ G. *stylos*, pillar, post ]. Relating to a styloid process; specifically, to the styloid process of the temporal bone.

**styloauricularis** (sti'lo-aw-rik-u-la'ris). See under musculus.

**styloglossus** (sti'lo-glos'us). Relating to the styloid process and the tongue; see under musculus.

**stylohyal** (sti-lo-hi'al). Relating to the styloid process of the temporal bone and to the hyoid bone.

**stylohyoid** (sti-lo-hi'oyd). 1. Stylohyal. 2. Relating to the musculus stylohyoideus.

**styloid** (sti'loyd) [ stylo- + G. *eidos*, resemblance ]. Peg-shaped; styliform; denoting one of several slender bony processes; see *processus* styloideus.

**styloiditis** (sti'loy-di'tis). Inflammation of a styloid process.

**stylolaryngeus** (sti'lo-lăr-in-je'us). See under musculus.

**stylomandib'ular.** Relating to the styloid process of the temporal bone and the mandible; denoting the ligamentum stylomandibulare.

**stylomas'toid.** Relating to the styloid and the mastoid processes of the temporal bone; denoting especially a small artery and a foramen.

**stylomax'illary.** Stylomandibular.

**stylopharynge'us.** See under musculus.

**stylopodium** (sti'lo-po'dĭ-um) [ stylo- + G. *podion*, small foot ]. The proximal intermediate segment of the limb skeleton, *viz.*, humerus and femur.

**stylostaphyline** (sti-lo-staf'ĭ-lĭn). Relating to the styloid process of the temporal bone and the uvula.

**stylosteophyte** (sti-los'te-o-fīt) [ G. *stylos*, post, + *osteon*, bone, + *phyton*, growth ]. A peg-shaped bony outgrowth.

**sty'lus** [ L. *stilus* or *stylus*, a stake or pen ]. 1 [ NA ]. Any pencil-shaped structure. 2. A pencil-shaped medicinal preparation for external application; *e.g.*, a medicated bougie, or a pencil or stick of silver nitrate or other caustic. 3. A stylet.

**stymato'sis** [ G. *styma*, priapism ]. Obsolete term meaning painful priapism.

**stype** (stip) [ G. *stypē*, tow ]. A tampon.

**stypsis** (stip'sis) [ G. See STYP- ]. 1. Astringency. 2. The application of a styptic.

**styp'tic** [ G. *styptikos*. STYP- ]. 1. Having an astringent or hemostatic effect. 2. An astringent hemostatic agent used externally to stop the flow of blood.

**sty'racin.** Cinnamyl cinnamate; $C_{18}H_{16}O_2$; a crystalline constituent of storax.

**sty'ramate.** SINAXAR; carbamic acid $\beta$-hydroxyphenethyl ester; an orally effective skeletal muscle relaxant with a relatively long duration of action.

**sty'rax.** Storax.

**sty'rene.** Styrol; cinnamene; vinylbenzene; phenylethylene; $C_6H_5CH=CH_2$; contained in storax; the monomer from which polystyrenes are made. Together with divinylbenzene (for cross-linking) it is the basis of many synthetic ion exchangers.

**sty'rol.** Styrene.

**sty'rone.** Cinnamic alcohol; cinnamyl alcohol; $C_9H_{10}O$; obtained from storax by distillation with potassium hydroxide. Used as a deodorant in 12 per cent glycerin solution, and as a decolorizing agent in histology.

**sub-** [ L. *sub*, under ]. Prefix to words formed from Latin roots, denoting beneath; less than the normal or typical; inferior; it corresponds to the Greek prefix *hypo-*.

**subabdom'inal.** Below the abdomen.

**subabdominoperitoneal** (sub-ab-dom'ĭ-no-pĕr-ĭ-to-ne'-al). Beneath the abdominal, as distinguished from the pelvic, peritoneum.

**subacetate** (sub-as'e-tāt). An acetate containing one or more atoms of the base still capable of combining with the acid to form higher salts; a basic acetate; a mixture or complex of a base and its acetate.

**subacid'ity.** Slight acidity.

**subacro'mial.** Beneath the acromion process.

**subacute** (sub-ă-kūt'). A zone between acute and chronic; denoting the course of a disease.

**subalimenta'tion.** A condition of insufficient nourishment.

**suba'nal.** Below the anus.

**subaortic** (sub'a-or'tik). Below the aorta.

**subap'ical.** Below the apex of any part.

**subaponeurot'ic.** Beneath an aponeurosis.

**subarachnoid** (sub-ă-rak'noyd). Underneath the arachnoid membrane.

**subar'cuate.** Slightly arcuate or bowed.

**subareolar** (sub-a-re'o-lar). Beneath an areola; especially the areola of the mamma.

**subastrag'alar.** Beneath the calcaneus (astragalus).

**subatom'ic.** Pertaining to particles making up the intraatomic structure (*e.g.*, protons, electrons, neutrons).

**subaural** (sub-aw'ral). Below the ear; subauricular.

**subauricular** (sub-aw-rik'u-lar). Below an auricle; especially the concha or pinna of the ear.

**subax'ial.** Below the axis of the body or any part.

**subax'illary.** Beneath the axilla.

**subbasal** (sub-ba'sal). Beneath any base or basal membrane.

**subbrachycephalic** (sub-brak-ĭ-sĕ-fal'ik). Slightly brachycephalic; having a cephalic index of 80.01 to 83.33.

**subcal'carine.** Below the calcarine fissure; denoting the gyrus lingualis.

**subcallo'sal.** Below the corpus callosum; denoting either the gyrus or the fasciculus subcallosus.

**subcap'sular.** Beneath any capsule.

**subcar'bonate.** A basic carbonate; a complex of a base and its carbonate. Azurite (blue malachite), 2 $CuCO_3 \cdot$ $Cu(OH)_2$ is an example.

**subcar'dinal.** Lying ventral to the anterior or posterior cardinal veins in the embryo.

**subcartilaginous** (sub-kar-tĭ-laj'ĭ-nus). 1. Partly cartilaginous. 2. Beneath a cartilage.

**subcecal** (sub-se'kal). Below the cecum; denoting a fossa.

**subception** (sub-sep'shun) [ sub- + L. *-ceptum*, perceived ]. The reaction to a stimulus not fully perceived.

**subchlo'ride.** The chloride of a series that contains proportionally the greatest amount of the other element in the compound; s. of mercury is $Hg_2Cl_2$; chloride or perchloride of mercury is $HgCl_2$. Silver s. is a solid solution of Ag in AgCl, with composition approximately $Ag_2Cl$. Alkaline earth s.'s are known (*e.g.*, $CaCl$ or $Ca_2Cl_2$).

**subchondral** (sub-kon'dral). Subcartilaginous; beneath or below the cartilages of the ribs.

**subchorionic** (sub-ko-rĭ-on'ik). Beneath the chorion.

**subchoroid'al** (sub-ko-roy'dal). Beneath the choroid coat of the eye.

**sub'class.** In biological classification, an occasional division between the class and the order.

**subclavian** (sub-kla'vĭ-an). 1. Beneath the clavicle. 2. Pertaining to the s. artery.

**subclavic'ular.** Subclavian.

**subcla'vius.** See under musculus.

**subclinical** (sub-klin'ĭ-kal). Denoting a period prior to the appearance of manifest symptoms in the evolution of a disease.

**subcollat'eral.** Below the collateral fissure; denoting a cerebral convolution, or gyrus.

**subconjuncti'val.** Beneath the conjunctiva.

**subconscious** (sub-kon'shus). 1. Not wholly conscious. 2. Denoting an idea or impression which is present in the mind, but of which there is at the time no conscious knowledge or realization.

**subconsciousness** (sub-kon'shus-nes). 1. Partial unconsciousness. 2. The state in which mental processes take place without the conscious perception of the individual.

**subcor'acoid.** Beneath the coracoid process.

**subcor'tex.** Any part of the brain lying below the cerebral cortex, and not itself organized as cortex.

**subcor'tical.** Relating to the subcortex; beneath the cerebral cortex.

**subcos'tal.** Beneath the ribs; denoting a number of arteries and grooves.

**subcostalgia** (sub'kos-tal'jĭ-ah) [ subcostal + G. *algos*, pain ]. Subcostal pain.

**subcos'toster'nal.** Below or beneath the ribs and sternum.

**subcra'nial.** Beneath or below the cranium.

**subcrep'itant.** Nearly, but not frankly, crepitant; denoting a rale.

**subcrepita'tion.** 1. The presence of subcrepitant rales. 2. A sound approaching crepitation in character.

**subcrure'us, subcrura'lis** [ sub- + L. *crus*, leg ]. *Musculus* articularis genu.

**subcul'ture.** 1. A culture made by transferring to a fresh medium microorganisms from a previous culture; a method used to prolong the life of a particular strain where there is a tendency to degeneration in older cultures. 2. To make a fresh culture with material obtained from a previous one.

**subcur'ative** (sub-kūr'ă-tiv). Denoting a dose less than that necessary for a curative effect.

**subcutaneous** (sub'ku-ta'ne-us) [ sub- + L. *cutis*, skin ]. Beneath the skin; hypodermic.

**subcutic'ular.** Subepidermal; subepidermic; beneath the cuticle or epidermis.

**subcu'tis.** *Tela* subcutanea.

**subdelir'ium.** Slight or not continuous delirium.

**subdel'toid.** Beneath the deltoid muscle; denoting a bursa.

**subden'tal.** Beneath the roots of the teeth.

**subder'mic.** Subcutaneous.

**subdiaphragmatic** (sub'di-ă-frag-mat'ik). Beneath the diaphragm.

**subdor'sal.** Below the dorsal region.

**subduce, subduct** (sub-dūs', sub-dukt') [ L. *sub-duco*, pp. *-ductus*, to lead away ]. To pull or draw downward.

**subdu'ral.** Beneath the dura mater, between it and the arachnoid.

**subendocar'dial.** Beneath the endocardium.

**subendothe'lial.** Beneath endothelium.

**subendothe'lium.** The connective tissue between the endothelium and inner elastic membrane in the intima of arteries.

**suben'dymal, subepen'dymal.** Beneath the endyma, or ependyma.

**subepider'mal, subepider'mic.** Subcuticular.

**subepithe'lial.** Beneath the epithelium.

**subepithe'lium.** Any structure beneath the epithelium.

**suberic acid.** $HOOC(CH_2)_6COOH$.

**su'berin** [ L. *suber*, cork ]. The modified cellulose in cork.

**suberosis** (su-ber-o'sis) [ L. *suber*, cork, + G. suffix *-osis*, condition ]. Extrinsic allergic alveolitis caused by inhalation of mold spores from contaminated cork.

*N*α-**su'berylar'ginine.** Compound between suberic acid and arginine; $HOOC(CH_2)_6CO—NHCH(COOH)(CH_2)_3-NHC(NH)NH_2$; found in bufotoxin.

**subfam'ily.** In biologic classification, an occasional division between the family and the tribe.

**subfascial** (sub-fash'i-al). Beneath a fascia.

**sub'fertil'ity.** A less than normal capacity for reproduction.

**subfis'sure.** A cerebral fissure beneath the surface, concealed by overlapping convolutions.

**subfo'lium.** A secondary division of a cerebellar folium.

**subgal'late.** A salt of gallic acid having one or more atoms of the base unneutralized; a basic gallate, *e.g.*, bismuth s.

**subgem'mal.** Below a gemma or bud (*e.g.*, a taste bud).

**subge'nus.** In biologic classification the division between the genus and the species.

**subgingival** (sub-jin'ji-val). Below the gingival margin.

**subgle'noid.** Infraglenoid; below the glenoid fossa or glenoid cavity.

**subglos'sal.** Sublingual; hypoglossal; below or beneath the tongue.

**subglossitis** (sub-glos-si'tis). Inflammation of the tissues beneath the tongue, or of the undersurface of the tongue.

**subglot'tic.** Below the glottic opening between the vocal cords.

**subgran'ular.** Slightly granular.

**subgrunda'tion** [ sub- + A.S. *grund*, bottom, foundation ]. The depression of one fragment of a broken cranial bone below the other.

**subhepat'ic.** Beneath the liver.

**subhyaloid** (sub-hi'ā-loyd). Beneath, on the vitreous side of, the hyaloid membrane.

**subhy'oid, subhyoid'ean.** Below the hyoid bone.

**subicteric** (sub-ik'ter-ik). [ sub- + G. *ikterikos*, jaundiced ]. Slightly jaundiced.

**subicular** (su-bik'u-lar). Relating to the subiculum.

**subiculum,** pl. **subicula** (su-bik'u-lum, -lah) [ L. dim. of *subex*, support ]. 1. A support or prop. 2. The zone of transition between the parahippocampal gyrus and Ammon's horn of the hippocampus.

  **s. promonto'rii** [ NA ], support of the promontory; a bony ridge bounding the fossula fenestrae cochleae posteriorly.

**subiliac** (sub-il'ī-ak). 1. Below the ilium. 2. Relating to the subilium.

**subilium** (sub-il'ī-um). The portion of the ilium contributing to the acetabulum.

**subinfec'tion.** A secondary infection occurring in one exposed to and successfully resisting an epidemic of another infectious disease.

**subinflam'matory.** Very slightly inflammatory; showing irritation of the tissues.

**subinteg'umen'tal.** Subcutaneous.

**subin'timal.** Beneath the intima.

**subin'trant** [ L. *sub-intro*, pres. p. *-ans*, to enter by stealth ]. Proleptic.

**subinvolu'tion.** An arrest in the normal involution of the uterus following childbirth, the organ remaining abnormally large.

**subiodide** (sub-i'o-dīd). That one of a series of iodine compounds with a given cation containing the least iodine. See subchloride.

**subja'cent** [ L. *sub-jaceo*, to lie under ]. Below or beneath another part.

**subject** (sub'jekt) [ L. *subjectus*, lying beneath ]. An organism which is the object of medical or surgical treatment, experimentation, or dissection.

**subjec'tive** [ L. *subjectivus*, fr. *subjicio*, to throw under ]. Perceived by the individual only and not evident to the examiner; said of certain symptoms, such as pain.

**subjec'toscope** [ L. *subjectus*, subject, + *skopeō*, to examine ]. An instrument for examination of subjective vision.

**subju'gal.** Below the zygomatic (jugal) bone.

**subking'dom.** A large or primary division of a kingdom, either animal or vegetable; it is not a definite division, some naturalists recognizing more, some fewer, s.'s.

**sublatio** (sub-la'shī-o) [ L. ]. Sublation.

**sublation** (sub-la'shun) [ L. *sublatio*, a lifting up ]. Detachment, elevation, or removal of a part.

**suble'thal.** Not quite lethal.

**subleukemia** (sub-lu-ke'mī-ah). Hypoleukemia.

**sublimate** (sub'lim-āt) [ L. *sublimo*, pp. *-atus*, to raise on high, fr. *sublimis*, high ]. 1. To convert a solid into a gas or vapor and back to a solid without passing through the liquid state (*e.g.*, solid $CO_2 \rightarrow$ gaseous $CO_2$), usually to free it from nonvaporizable impurities. 2. Any substance that has been submitted to sublimation. 3. In psychoanalysis, to accomplish sublimation.

  **corrosive s.,** mercuric chloride.

**sublima'tion.** 1. The process of vaporizing a solid substance without passing through a liquid state; analogous to distillation. 2. In psychoanalysis, an unconscious defense mechanism in which unacceptable instinctual drives and wishes are modified into more personally and socially acceptable channels.

**sublime** (sub-līm'). 1. To sublimate. 2. To undergo a process of sublimation.

**subliminal** (sub-lim'ī-nal) [ sub- + L. *limen* (*limin-*), threshold ]. Below the limit of sensory perception; below the limit or threshold of consciousness; subconscious.

**subli'mis** [ L. ]. At the top; on the surface; superficial.

**sublingual** (sub-ling'gwal). Subglossal.

**sublinguitis** (sub-ling-gwi'tis). Inflammation of the sublingual salivary gland.

**sublob'ular.** Beneath a lobule, as of the liver.

**sublum'bar.** Below the lumbar region.

**sublu'minal.** Below or beneath the structure facing the lumen of an organ.

**subluxation** (sub-luk-sa'shun) [ sub- + L. *locatio*, luxation

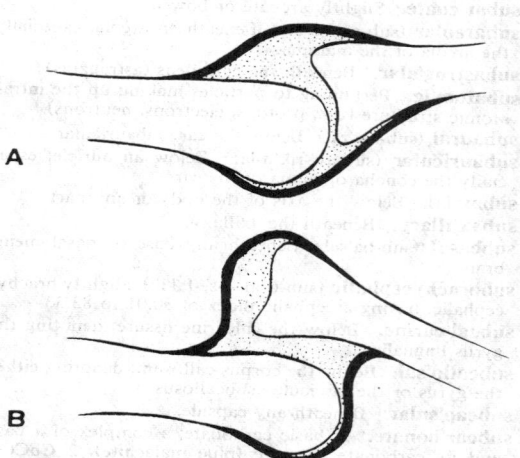

**Subluxation**
Diagram of subluxation (*A*) shows partial contact of apposing articular surfaces; in dislocation (*B*) there is complete loss of contact. (From Schultz, R. J.: *The Language of Fractures*, The Williams & Wilkins Co., Baltimore, 1972.)

(dislocation) ]. Semiluxation; an imcomplete luxation or dislocation; though a relationship is altered, contact between joint surfaces remains.

**vertebral cervical s.,** an incomplete dislocation in which normal relationship is disturbed but articular surfaces are partially in contact.

**Volkmann's s.,** s. of the knee, due probably to tuberculous arthritis.

**sublymphemia** (sub-lim-fe'mĭ-ah) [ sub- + L. *lympha,* lymph, + G. *haima,* blood ]. A blood state in which there is a great increase in the proportion of lymphocytes although the total number of white cells is normal.

**submam'mary.** Below or beneath the mammary gland.

**submandib'ular.** Submaxillary (2); beneath the lower jaw.

**submar'ginal.** Near the margin of any part.

**submaxil'la.** Mandibula.

**submaxillaritis** (sub-mak'sĭ-lă-ri'tis) [ sub- + maxilla, *q.v.,* + G. suffix *-itis,* inflammation ]. Submaxillitis; inflammation, usually due to mumps virus, affecting the submaxillary salivary gland.

**submax'illary.** 1. Mandibular. 2. Submandibular; an old term for various structures now named submandibular.

**submaxillitis** (sub-mak'sĭ-li'tis). Submaxillaritis.

**subme'dial, subme'dian.** Almost, but not exactly in the middle.

**submem'branous.** Partly or nearly membranous.

**submen'tal.** Beneath the chin.

**submerged** (sub-merjd'). In dentistry, describing a field of operation covered by saliva.

**submetacen'tric.** See s. chromosome.

**submicron'ic.** Smaller than 1 micron in size.

**submicroscop'ic.** Too minute to be visible under the most powerful light microscope.

**submor'phous.** Neither definitely amorphous nor definitely crystalline; denoting the structure of certain calculi.

**submuco'sa.** A layer of tissue beneath a mucous membrane.

**submu'cous.** Beneath a mucous membrane.

**subnarcot'ic.** Slightly narcotic.

**subna'sal.** Under the nose.

**subneu'ral.** Below the neural axis.

**subni'trate.** A basic nitrate; a salt of nitric acid having one or more atoms of the base still capable of combining with the acid.

**subnor'mal.** Below the normal.

**subnormal'ity.** The state of being below normal.

**subnu'cleus.** A secondary nucleus.

**subnutrition** (sub-nu-trish'un). A mild degree of innutrition.

**suboccipital** (sub-ok-sip'ĭ-tal). Below the occiput or the occipital bone.

**subop'timal.** Below optimum.

**subor'bital.** Beneath the orbit.

**subor'der.** In zoologic classification, an occasional division between the order and the family.

**suboxida'tion.** Deficient oxidation.

**subox'ide.** That of a series of oxides which contains the least oxygen.

**subpap'ular.** Denoting the eruption of few and scattered paules, in which the lesions are very slightly elevated, being scarcely more than macules.

**subparietal** (sub-pă-ri'ĕ-tal). Below or beneath any structure called parietal: bone, lobe, layer of a serous membrane, etc.

**subpatel'lar.** Beneath the patella.

**subpec'toral.** Beneath the pectoralis muscle.

**subpel'viperitone'al.** Beneath the pelvic, as distinguished from the abdominal peritoneum.

**subpericar'dial.** Beneath the pericardium.

**subperiosteal** (sub-pĕr-ĭ-os'te-al). Beneath the periosteum.

**subperitoneal** (sub-pĕr-ĭ-to-ne'al). Beneath the peritoneum.

**subperitone'oabdom'inal.** Subabdominoperitoneal.

**subperitone'opel'vic.** Subpelviperitoneal.

**subpetro'sal.** Inferior petrosal; denoting a cerebral sinus.

**subpharyngeal** (sub-fă-rin'je-al). Below the pharynx.

**subphren'ic** (sub-frenik). Subdiaphragmatic.

**subphylum** (sub-fi'lum). In biological classification, the division between the phylum and the class.

**subpi'al.** Beneath the pia mater.

**subplacen'tal.** Beneath the placenta; denoting the decidua basalis.

**subpleural** (sub-plu'ral). Beneath the pleura.

**subplex'al.** Below or beneath any plexus.

**subpreputial** (sub-pre-pu'shĭ-al). Beneath the prepuce.

**subpu'bic.** Beneath the pubic arch; denoting a ligament, ligamentum arcuatum pubis, connecting the two pubic bones below the arch.

**subpul'monary.** Below the lungs.

**subpyramidal** (sub-pī-ram'ĭ-dal). 1. Below any pyramid; denoting especially the sinus tympani. 2. Nearly pyramidal in shape.

**subret'inal.** Beneath, on the outer side of, the retina.

**sub'salt.** A basic salt, one in which the base has not been completely neutralized by the acid.

**subsarto'rial.** Beneath the sartorius muscle; denoting a nerve plexus.

**subscap'ular.** Beneath or below the scapula.

**subscapula'ris.** See under musculus.

**subscle'ral.** Beneath the sclera of the eye, *i.e.,* on the choroidal side of this layer.

**subsclerot'ic.** 1. Subscleral. 2. Partly or slightly sclerotic or sclerosed.

**subscription** (sub-skrip'shun) [ L. *subscriptio,* fr. *subscribo,* pp. *-scriptus,* to write under, subscribe ]. The part of a prescription preceding the signature, in which are the directions for compounding.

**subse'rous, subsero'sal.** Beneath a serous membrane.

**subsibilant** (sub-sib'ĭ-lant) Denoting a rale with a quality between blowing and whistling.

**subspina'le.** point A; in cephalometrics, the most posterior midline p. of the premaxilla between the angle ANS (SNA) and the prosthion.

**subspi'nous.** Infraspinous. 1. Beneath any spine, as of the scapula, of a vertebra, etc. 2. Beneath, or anterior to, the spinal column.

**substage** (sub'stāj). An attachment to a microscope, below the stage, supporting the condenser or other accessory.

**substance** (sub'stans) [ L. *substantia,* essence, material, fr. *sub-sto,* to stand under, be present. STA- ]. Matter; stuff; material. See also substantia.

**s. 248,** toxisterol.

**alpha s.,** reticular s. (1).

**anterior perforated s.,** *substantia* perforata anterior.

**anterior-pituitary-like s.,** chorionic *gonadotropin.*

**bacteriotropic s.,** opsonin or other s. that alters bacterial cells in such a manner that they are more susceptible to phagocytic action.

**basophil s.,** chromophil s.

**beta s.,** Heinz *bodies.*

**blood group specific s.'s A and B,** see under blood.

**cement s.,** a hypothetical material that was thought to bind tissue elements together, as in intercellular cements of epithelium.

**central gray s.,** *substantia* grisea centralis.

**chromidial s.,** granular cytoplasmic *reticulum.*

**chromophil s.,** the material consisting of granular cytoplasmic reticulum and ribosomes which occurs in nerve cell bodies and dendrites; also called Nissl s., granules, or bodies; tigroid s. or bodies; basophil s.; substantia basophilia.

**cortical s.,** *substantia* corticalis.

**exophthalmos-producing s.,** a pituitary hormone, possibly separate from thyrotrophic hormone, responsible for exophthalmos in hyperthyroidism; has been demonstrated by assays on the Atlantic minnow.

**s. Fa, Reichstein's,** cortisone.

**filar s.,** reticular s. (1).

**s. G, Reichstein's,** adrenosterone.

**gelatinous s. of Rolando,** *substantia* gelatinosa.

**gelatinous s. of Stilling,** *substantia* intermedia centralis et lateralis.

**glandular s. of prostate,** *substantia* glandularis prostatae.

**gray s.,** *substantia* grisea.

**ground s.,** substantia fundamentalis; the amorphous material in which structural elements occur; in connective tissue it is composed of protein polysaccharides, tissue fluids, and metabolites present between cells and fibers.

**H s.,** designation given by Sir Thomas Lewis to a diffusible s. in skin which is indistinguishable in action from histamine. Liberated by injury and causes the triple response; released s.

**s. H, Reichstein's,** corticosterone.

**innominate s.,** *substantia* innominata.

**interspon'gioplas'tic s.,** obsolete term for cytochylema.

**s. M, Reichstein's,** hydrocortisone.

**medullary s.,** (1) Schwann's white s.; the fatty material present in the myelin sheath of nerve fibers; (2) medulla of bones and other organs.

**muscular s. of prostate,** *substantia* muscularis prostatae.

**neurosecretory s.,** the secretion of nerve cell bodies located in the hypothalamus; it is transported by way of the fibers of the hypothalamo-hypophysial tract into the neurohypophysis; there the terminals of the nerve fibers containing the secretion are in relation to capillaries. The secretion in the fibers and terminals is seen with the light microscope as Herring bodies.

**Nissl s.,** chromophil s.

**s. P,** a polypeptide present in minute quantities in the brain and intestines of man and various animals; it is one of the most potent compounds affecting smooth muscle (dilation of blood vessels and contraction of intestine); believed by some to be the transmitter of pain impulses.

**posterior perforated s.,** *substantia* perforata posterior.

**pressor s.,** pressor *base*.

**pump s.,** postulated s. which, by combining with sodium ion, brings about its diffusion out of the cell, setting up an electric potential which maintains a high potassium ion concentration within the cell; it has been suggested that histamine is the pump s.

**s. Q, Reichstein's,** deoxycorticosterone.

**Reichstein's s.'s,** see s. Fa, G, H, M, Q, and S.

**released s.,** H s.

**retic'ular s.,** (1) substantia reticulofilamentosa; filar mass; filar structure; alpha s.; filar s.; a filamentous plasmatic material, beaded with granules, demonstrable by means of vital staining in the immature red blood cells; (2) *formatio* reticularis.

**Rolando's s., Rolando's gelatinous s.,** *substantia* gelatinosa.

**s. S, Reichstein's,** 11-deoxycortisol.

**Schwann's white s.,** medullary s. (1).

**sensitizing s.,** complement-fixing *antibody*.

**slow-reacting s.,** slow-reacting s. of anaphylaxis (abbreviated SRS and SRS-A); an unidentified s. released in anaphylactic shock which produces slower and more prolonged contraction of muscle than does histamine.

**soluble specific s.,** specific capsular s.

**specific capsular s.,** soluble specific s. (SSS); specific-soluble polysaccharide; pneumococcus polysaccharide; specific soluble sugar; a soluble type specific polysaccharide produced during active growth of virulent pneumococci composing a large part of the capsule.

**Stilling's gelatinous s.,** *substantia* intermedia centralis et lateralis.

**threshold s.,** threshold *body*.

**tigroid s.,** chromophil s.

**transmitter s.,** transmittor s.; a chemical s. synthesized by nerve cells and subserving the transmission of nerve impulses across the synaptic junction; see also synapse.

**white s.,** *substantia* alba.

**zymoplastic s.,** thromboplastin.

**substantia,** pl. **substan'tiae** (sub-stan'shĭ-ah) [ NA. ] [ NA ]. Substance.

**s. adamanti'na,** enamelum.

**s. al'ba** [ NA ], alba; white substance; white matter; those regions of the brain and spinal cord which are largely or entirely composed of nerve fibers and contain few or no neuronal cell bodies or dendrites.

**s. basophilia,** basophil *substance*.

**s. cine'rea,** s. grisea.

**s. compac'ta** [ NA ], substantia compacta ossium; compact bone; the compact, noncancellous portion of bone

that consists largely of concentric lamellar osteons and interstitial lamellae.

**s. cortica'lis** [ NA ], cortical bone or substance; cortex; specifically, the superficial thin layer of compact bone.

**s. ebur'nea,** dentinum.

**s. ferrugin'ea** [ NA ], *locus* ceruleus.

**s. fundamenta'lis,** ground *substance*.

**s. gelatino'sa** [ NA ], gelatinous substance of Rolando; Rolando's substance; the apical part of the posterior horn (dorsal horn; posterior gray column) of the spinal cord's gray matter, composed largely of very small nerve cells; its gelatinous appearance is due to its very low content of myelinated nerve fibers. See fig. under *medulla* spinalis.

**s. gelatino'sa centra'lis,** s. intermedia centralis et lateralis.

**s. glandula'ris prosta'tae** [ NA ], the glandular substance of the prostate, consisting of numerous compound tubuloalveolar glands interspersed through the fibromuscular tissue of the gland and draining into the urethra through 20 or more ductules.

**s. gris'ea** [ NA ], s. cinerea; gray substance; gray matter; those regions of the brain and spinal cord which are made up primarily of the cell bodies and dendrites of nerve cells rather than myelinated axons.

**s. gris'ea centra'lis** [ NA ], central gray substance; (1) in general: the predominantly small-celled gray matter adjoining or surrounding the central canal of the spinal cord and the third and fourth ventricles of the brainstem; (2) in particular: the thick sleeve of gray matter surrounding the cerebral aqueduct of Sylvius in the midbrain, rostrally continuous with the posterior nucleus of the hypothalamus; in sections stained for myelin it stands out from the adjoining tectum and tegmentum by its poverty in myelinated fibers.

**s. innomina'ta,** innominate substance; the region of the forebrain that lies ventral to the anterior half or so of the lentiform nucleus, extending in the frontal plane from the lateral preopticohypothalamic zone laterally over the optic tract to the amygdala (corpus amygdaloideum); rostrally it tapers off over the dorsal border of the olfactory tubercle, caudally it ends where the internal capsule reaches the surface to form the cerebral peduncle or pes pedunculi. Notable among its polymorphic cell population is the large-celled nucleus basalis of Ganser; it is traversed by the ansa peduncularis.

**s. interme'dia centra'lis et latera'lis** [ NA ], Stilling's gelatinous substance; s. gelatinosa centralis; commissura anterior and posterior grisea; the central gray matter of the spinal cord surrounding the central canal.

**s. len'tis** [ NA ], substance of the lens of the eye.

**s. medulla'ris,** (1) medulla; (2) medullary *substance*.

**s. metachromat'icogranula'ris,** Heinz *bodies*.

**s. muscula'ris prosta'tae** [ NA ], muscular substance of the prostate; musculus prostatae; the smooth muscle in the stroma of the prostate.

**s. ni'gra** [ NA ], nucleus niger, locus niger; nigra; ganglion of Soemmering; a large cell mass, crescentic on transverse section, extending forward over the dorsal surface of the pes pedunculi from the rostral border of the pons into the subthalamus; it is composed of a dorsal stratum of closely spaced pigmented (*i.e.,* melanin-containing) cells, the pars compacta, and a larger ventral region of widely scattered cells, the pars reticulata. The pars compacta in particular includes numerous cells that project forward to the striatum (caudate nucleus and putamen) and contain dopamine, which presumably acts as the transmitter substance at their synaptic endings; other, apparently non-dopaminergic cells of the s. nigra project to a rostral part of the nucleus ventralis thalami. The nigrostriatal projection is reciprocated by a massive striatonigral fiber system; no other afferent connection of the s. nigra is known. Destruction or dysfunction of the s. nigra is associated with Parkinson's disease.

**s. os'sea den'tis,** cementum.

**s. perfora'ta ante'rior** [ NA ], anterior perforated substance; olfactory area; area olfactoria; locus perforatus anticus; a region at the base of the brain through which numerous small branches of the anterior and middle cerebral arteries (lenticulostriate arteries) enter the depth of the cerebral hemisphere; it is bordered medially by the optic chasm and anterior half of the optic tract, rostrally and laterally by the lateral olfactory stria; its anteromedial part corresponds to the olfactory tubercle.

**s. perfora'ta poste'rior** [ NA ], posterior perforated substance; locus perforatus posticus; the bottom of the interpeduncular fossa at the base of the midbrain, extending from the anterior border of the pons forward to the mamillary bodies, and containing numerous openings for the passage of branches of the posterior cerebral arteries.

**s. pro'pria cor'neae** [ NA ], the proper substance of the cornea, consisting of modified transparent connective tissue, between the layers of which are open spaces or lacunae nearly filled with the corneal cells or corpuscles.

**s. pro'pria membra'nae tym'pani,** the layer of radial and circular collagenous fibers of the tympanic membrane.

**s. pro'pria scle'rae** [ NA ], proper substance of the sclera; the dense white fibrous tissue arranged in interlacing bundles that forms the main mass of the sclera, continuous anteriorly with the substantia propria corneae.

**s. reticula'ris,** *formatio* reticularis.

**s. reticulofilamento'sa,** reticular *substance* (1).

**s. spongio'sa** [ NA ], spongy, cancellous, or trabecular bone; bone in which the spicules or trabeculae form a three-dimensional latticework (cancellus) with the interstices filled with embryonal connective tissue or bone marrow.

**s. vitrea,** enamelum.

**subster'nal.** Beneath the sternum.

**subster'nomas'toid.** Beneath the sternomastoid muscle; denoting a group of deep cervical lymph nodes.

**sub'stitute.** In psychology, a surrogate (*q. v.*).

**substitution** (sub'stĭ-tu'shun) [ L. *substitutio,* to put in place of another ]. 1. In chemistry, the replacement of an atom or group in a compound by another atom or group (*e.g.,* s. of H by Cl in CH₄ to give CH₃Cl). 2. In psychiatry, an unconscious defense mechanism by which an unacceptable or unattainable goal, object, or emotion is replaced by one that is more acceptable or attainable; the process is more acute and direct, and less subtle, than sublimation.

**stimulus s.,** classical *conditioning.*

**symptom s.,** symptom formation; unconscious psychological process by which a repressed impulse is indirectly manifested through a particular symptom, *e.g.,* anxiety, compulsion, depression, hallucination, obsession.

**sub'strate** [ L. *sub-sterno,* pp. *-stratus,* to spread under ]. The substance acted upon and changed by an enzyme; the reactant considered to be attacked in a chemical reaction.

**substra'tum** [ L. see substrate ]. Any layer or stratum lying beneath another.

**substruc'ture.** A tissue or structure wholly or partly beneath the surface.

**implant denture s.,** the metal framework which is placed beneath the soft tissues in contact with, or embedded into, bone for the purpose of supporting an implant denture superstructure.

**subsul'fate.** A basic sulfate; one that contains some base unneutralized and still capable of combining with the acid. The mineral alunite (alum stone), K₂Al₆(OH)₁₂(SO₄)₄, is an example.

**subsul'tus** [ L. *subsilio,* pp. *-sultus,* to leap up, fr. *salio,* to leap ]. A twitching or jerking.

**s. clonus,** s. tendinum.

**s. ten'dinum,** s. clonus; tremor tendinum; a twitching of the tendons, especially noticeable at the wrist, occurring in low fevers.

**subtar'sal.** Below the tarsus.

**subtegumen'tal.** Subcutaneous; hypodermic.

**subtento'rial.** Beneath the tentorium cerebelli.

**subter'minal.** Situated near the end or extremity of an oval or rod-shaped body.

**subtetan'ic.** Not quite tetanic; denoting tonic muscular spasms or convulsions that are not entirely sustained but have brief remissions.

**subthalam'ic.** Related to the subthalamus or to the subthalamic nucleus.

**subthal'amus.** That part of the diencephalon that lies wedged between the thalamus on the dorsal side and the cerebral peduncle ventrally, lateral to the dorsal half of the hypothalamus from which it cannot be sharply delineated. It is composed of the nucleus subthalamicus (corpus luysi),

the zona incerta, and the fields of Forel; laterally it expands in a winglike fashion into the nucleus reticularis thalami; caudally it is continuous with the midbrain tegmentum.

**subthyroideus** (sub-thi-ro-id'e-us). A muscular bundle formed of fibers derived from the thyroarytenoideus and the vocalis muscles.

**sub'tilin.** An antibiotic peptide obtained from cultures of *Bacillus subtilis;* it is bacteriostatic and bacteriolytic to the tubercle bacillus and other organisms. It is active against heat-resistant spore formers that are important in the canning industry.

**subtilisin** (sub-tĭ-li'sin) (EC 3.4.16.12). Subtilopeptidase; a peptidase formed by *Bacillus subtilis, Aspergillus flavus-oryzae* (aspergillopeptidase B) and *Bacillus amyloliquefaciens* (a serine proteinase catalyzing the hydrolysis of a few specific peptide bonds in certain proteins, converting chymotrypsinogen to chymotrypsin and egg albumin to plakalbumin in this manner. Cleaves pancreatic ribonuclease into S-peptide and S-protein.

**subtrapezial** (sub-trä-pe'zĭ-al). Beneath the trapezius muscle; denoting a nerve plexus.

**sub'tribe.** In zoologic classification, an indefinite division of a tribe.

**subtrochanteric** (sub-tro-kan-tĕr'ik). Below any trochanter.

**subtrochlear** (sub-trok'le-ar). Below any trochlea.

**subtu'beral.** Lying below any tuber.

**subtympan'ic.** Below the tympanic cavity.

**subumbil'ical.** Below the umbilicus.

**subungual, subunguial** (sub-ung'gwal, sub-ung'gwĭ-al) [ L. *unguis,* nail ]. Hyponychial; beneath the (toe or finger) nail.

**subvaginal** (sub-vaj'ĭ-nal). 1. Below the vagina. 2. On the inner side of any tubular membrane serving as a sheath.

**subval'var, subval'vular.** Below the valve.

**subver'tebral.** Beneath, or on the ventral side, of a vertebra or the vertebral column; subspinal.

**subvirile** (sub-vĭr'il). More or less lacking in virility.

**subvit'rinal.** Beneath the vitreous body.

**subvolu'tion** [ L. *sub,* under, + *volvo,* pp. *volutus,* to turn ]. Turning over a flap of mucous membrane, as in the operation for pterygium, to prevent adhesion.

**subwa'king.** Hypnoidal.

**subzo'nal.** Below or beneath any zona or zone, such as the zona radiata or zona pellucida.

**subzygomat'ic.** Below or beneath the zygomatic bone or arch.

**succagogue** (suk'ă-gog) [ L. *succus,* juice, + G. *agōgos,* leading ]. 1. Stimulating the flow of juice. 2. An agent that stimulates the flow of juice.

**succedaneous** (suk-se-da'ne-us) [ see succedaneum ]. Relating to a succedaneum; used as a substitute.

**succedaneum** (suk-se-da'ne-um) [ L. *succedaneus,* following after, substituting, fr. *suc-cedo,* to follow, to take the place of, fr. *sub,* under, + *cedo,* to go ]. A substitute; a drug or any therapeutic agent that has the properties of and can be used in place of another.

**succenturiate** (suk-sen-tu'rĭ-āt) [ L. *suc-centurio,* pp. *-atus,* to substitute ]. Substituting; accessory.

**succinate** (suk'sĭ-nāt). A salt of succinic acid.

**s. dehydrogenase,** a flavoenzyme (EC 1.3.99.1) that catalyzes the removal of hydrogen from succinic acid and converts it into fumaric acid; see also fumarate reductase.

**succinchlorimide** (suk'sin-klōr'ĭ-mīd). *N*-Chlorosuccinimide; a chlorinating agent.

**succinic acid** (suk-sin'ik). 1,4-Butanedioic acid; ethylenedicarboxylic acid; COOH(CH₂)₂COOH; an intermediate in the tricarboxylic acid cycle. Several of its salts have been variously used in medicine.

**s. acid cycle,** see under cycle.

**succinic dehydrogenase.** Succinate dehydrogenase.

**succinic thiokinase.** Succinyl-CoA synthetase.

**suc'cinite.** Amber.

**suc'cinous.** Relating to amber.

**suc'cinox'idase.** See succinate dehydrogenase; fumarate reductase.

**suc'cinylcho'line bromide.** Suxamethonium bromide; an alternate preparation for the chloride, *q.v.*

**suc'cinylcho'line chloride** (USP). ANECTINE; suxamethonium chloride; choline chloride succinate; a muscle-relaxing drug that produces persistent depolarization of the motor end-plate (phase I block), which is followed by a curare-like, nondepolarizing block (phase II block); used to produce muscle relaxation during surgical anesthesia and electroconvulsive therapy.

**succinyl-CoA.** Abbreviation for succinylcoenzyme A.

**succinyl-CoA synthetase.** Succinic thiokinase. 1. A ligase (EC 6.2.1.5) combining succinate and CoA with the splitting of ATP to ADP and inorganic phosphate. 2. A ligase (EC 6.2.1.4) similar to (1), but able to use itaconate as well as succinate and GTP (or ITP) in place of ATP.

**succinylocoenzyme A** (suk'sī-nil-ko-en'zīm). Succinyl-CoA; "active succinate"; the condensation product of succinic acid and CoA; one of the intermediates of the tricarboxylic acid cycle.

**suc'cinylmon'ocho'line.** The initial metabolite of succinyl(bis)choline; it has only a fraction of the neuromuscular blocking action of the parent compound, and has a predominantly competitive action.

**suc'cinylsul'fathi'azole** (USP, BP). SULFASUXIDINE; 4'-(2-thiazolylsulfamoyl)succinanilic acid; the most effective of the poorly absorbed bacteriostatic sulfonamides used for sterilization of the intestinal tract.

**succisul'fone iminodiethanol.** EXOSULFONYL; 4'-sulfanilylsuccinanilic acid 2,2'-iminodiethanol salt; antimicrobial agent.

**succorrhea** (suk'o-re'ah) [ L. *succus*, juice, + G. *rhoia*, a flow ]. An abnormal increase in the secretion of a digestive fluid, such as the saliva or gastric juice.

**succuba** (suk'u-bah). Succubus.

**succubus** (suk'u-bus) [ L. *succubo*, to lie under. CUB- ]. Succuba; a demon, in female form, believed to have sexual intercourse with a man during sleep, as contrasted with incubus.

**succus,** gen. and pl. **succi** (suk'us, suk'si) [ L. ]. Juice. 1 [ NA ]. The fluid constituents of the body tissues. 2 [ NA ]. A fluid secretion, especially the digestive fluid. 3. Formerly, a pharmacopeial preparation obtained by expressing the juice of a plant and adding to it sufficient alcohol (1 part to 3 of juice) to preserve it; see also juice.
  **s. cerasi,** cherry juice or other preservative.
  **s. enter'icus,** intestinal *juice.*
  **s. gas'tricus,** gastric *juice.*
  **s. pancreat'icus,** pancreatic *juice.*
  **s. prostat'icus,** prostatic *fluid.*
  **s. thebaicus,** opium.

**succuss** (sū-kus'). To make succussion.

**succussion** (sŭ-kush'un) [ L. *suceussio,* fr. *suc-cutio* (*subc-*), pp. *-cussus,* to shake up, fr. *quatio,* to shake ]. A diagnostic procedure that consists in shaking the body so as to elicit a splashing sound in a cavity containing both gas and fluid.
  **Hippocratic s.,** a splashing noise produced by shaking the body when there is gas or air and fluid in the stomach or intestine, or free in the peritoneum, thorax, and rarely the pericardium.

**suck** [ A.S. *sūcan* ]. 1. To draw a fluid through a tube by exhausting the air in front. 2. To draw a fluid into the mouth; specifically, to draw milk from the breast.

**suckle** (suk'l). 1. To nurse; to feed by milk from the breast. 2. To suck; to draw sustenance from the breast.

**Sucquet** (sü-ka'), J. P., French anatomist, 1840–1870. See S.'s *canals.*

**su'crase.** β-Fructofuranosidase.

**su'crate.** A compound of sucrose.

**su'crol.** Dulcin; *p*-phenetol carbamide; 4-ethoxyphenylurea; has been used as a substitute for sugar, being 200 times as sweet as cane sugar. Because of hydrolysis to aminophenol, it may produce an injurious effect when used over long periods of time.

**su'crose** (USP, BP). Sucrosum; saccharum; cane sugar; a saccharose; a nonreducing disaccharide, $C_{12}H_{22}O_{11}$, made up of glucose and fructose, obtained from sugar cane, *Saccharum officinarum* (family Gramineae), from several species of sorghum, and from the sugar beet, *Beta vulgaris*

(family Chenopodiaceae). Used in pharmacy in the manufacture of syrup, confections, etc.
  **s. octaacetate** (NF), used as an alcohol denaturant.

**sucrosemia** (su-kro-se'mī-ah) [ sucrose + G. *haima,* blood ]. The presence of sucrose in the blood.

**sucrosuria** (su-kro-su'rī-ah) [ sucrose + G. *ouron,* urine ]. The excretion of sucrose in the urine.

**suction** (suk'shun) [ L. *sugo,* pp. *suctus,* to suck ]. Aspiration; the act or process of sucking.
  **posttussive s.,** a s. sound heard on auscultation over a pulmonary cavity at the end of a cough.
  **Wangensteen s.,** Wangensteen tube; a modified siphon that maintains constant negative pressure used with duodenal tube for the relief of gastric and intestinal distention.

**suctorial** (suk-to'rī-al). Relating to suction, or the act of sucking; adapted for sucking.

**sudamen,** pl. *sudamina* (su-da'men, -dam'ī-nah) [ Mod. L. fr. *sudo,* to sweat ]. A minute vesicle due to retention of fluid in a sweat follicle, or in the epidermis.

**sudam'ina.** 1. Plural of sudamen. 2. *Miliaria* crystallina.

**sudam'inal.** Relating to sudamina.

**Sudan** (su-dan'). A name given to several fat dyes.
  **S. black B,** a disazo dye, $C_{29}H_{24}N_6$, used as a stain for fats.
  **S. brown,** $(C_{10}H_7)N = N(C_{10}H_6)OH$, derived from α-naphthylamine; a brown stain for fats.
  **S. III, S. red III,** $(C_6H_5)N = N(C_6H_4)N = N(C_{10}H_6)OH$; a red stain for neutral fat in histologic technique; it also stains the fatty envelope of the tubercle bacillus.
  **S. IV,** scarlet red.
  **S. yellow G,** metadioxyazobenzene; a yellow stain for fats.

**sudanophilia** (su-dan'o-fil'ī-ah) [ sudan (dye) + G. *phileo,* to love ]. 1. Affinity for a Sudan stain. 2. A condition in which the leukocytes contain minute fat droplets which take a brilliant red stain when treated with 0.2 per cent Sudan III and 0.1 per cent cresyl blue in absolute alcohol.

**sudation** (su-da'shun) [ L. *sudatio,* fr. *sudo,* pp. *-atus,* to sweat ]. Sweating.

**sudato'ria** [ L. *sudatorius,* relating to sweating ]. 1. Ephidrosis. 2. Hyperidrosis.

**sudatorium** (su'dā-to'rī-um) [ L. a sweating room, fr. *sudo,* pp. *-atus,* to sweat ]. A hot air or Turkish bath to induce profuse perspiration.

**Sudeck** (soo'dek), Paul H. M., German surgeon, 1866–1938. See S.'s critical *point,* S.'s *syndrome.*

**sudomo'tor** [ L. *sudor,* sweat, + *motor,* mover ]. Sudoriferous; denoting especially the nerves that stimulate the sweat glands to activity.

**su'dor** [ L. ] [ NA ]. Sweat; perspiration.
  **s. an'glicus,** miliary *fever.*
  **s. sanguin'eus,** hematidrosis.
  **s. urino'sus,** uridrosis.

**sudor-** (su'dor-) [ L. *sudor,* sweat. SUD- ]. Combining form relating to sweat, perspiration.

**su'doral.** Relating to perspiration.

**sudoresis** (su'do-re'sis) [ sudor- G. suffix -*ēsis,* condition ]. Profuse sweating.

**sudoriferous** (su'do-rif'er-us) [ sudor- L. *fero,* to bear ]. Carrying or producing sweat.

**sudorific** (su'do-rif'ik) [ sudor- + L. *facio,* to make ]. Diaphoretic; sudoriferous; sudoriparous; causing perspiration.

**sudorikeratosis** (su'dor-ī-kĕr-a-to'sis). Keratosis of the sudoriferous ducts.

**sudoriparous** (su'do-rip'ă-rus) [ sudo- + L. *pario,* to produce ]. Producing sweat.

**sudorometer** (su'do-rom'e-ter) [ sudor- + G. *metron,* measure ]. An instrument for measuring the amount of perspiration.

**sudorrhea** (su'do-re'ah) [ sudor- + G. *rhoia,* a flow ]. Hyperhidrosis.

**su'et.** The hard fat around the kidneys of cattle and sheep. When rendered it yields tallow.
  **prepared s.,** prepared mutton tallow; the internal fat of the abdomen of the sheep, *Ovis aries,* purified by melting and straining; used in pharmacy in making ointments.

Actual        Fischer projection

**suffocate** (suf'o-kāt) [ L. *suffoco*(*subf-*), pp. -*atus*, to choke, strangle, fr. *faux* (*fauc-*), the pharynx ]. 1. To impede respiration; to asphyxiate. 2. To suffer from want of oxygen; to be unable to breathe.

**suffocation** (suf'o-ka'shun). The act or condition of suffocating; asphyxiation.

**suffusion** (suf-fu'zhun) [ L. *suffusio*, fr. *suffundo*(*subf-*), to pour out ]. 1. The act of pouring a fluid over the body. 2. Reddening of the surface. 3. The condition of being wet with a fluid. 4. An extravasation.

**sugar** (shŏŏg'ar) [ G. *sakcharon*; L. *saccharum* ]. 1. A carbohydrate; a saccharide; see also sugars. 2. Sucrose. 3. Pharmaceutical forms are: compressible sugar (USP) and confectioner's sugar (USP).

  **s. acids,** acids such as gluconic, glycuronic, and saccharic, produced by the oxidation of glucose.

  **s. alcohol,** a polyalcohol resulting from the reduction of the carbonyl group in a monosaccharide to a hydroxyl group.

  **amino s.'s,** s.'s that contain an amino group, such as glucosamine.

  **beech-wood s.,** xylose.

  **beet s.,** sucrose extracted from beet root.

  **blood s.,** glucose.

  **brain s.,** D-galactose.

  **cane s.,** sucrose extracted from the sugarcane; saccharum.

  **deoxy s.'s,** see under deoxy.

  **fruit s.,** D-Fructose.

  **gelatin s.,** glycine.

  **grape s.,** glucose.

  **invert s.,** a mixture of equal parts of glucose and fructose. See also inversion (2).

  **s. of lead,** lead acetate.

  **malt s.,** maltose.

  **maple s.,** saccharum canadense; sucrose extracted from the sap of the sugar maple, *Acer saccharinum.*

  **milk s.,** lactose.

  **nucleoside diphosphate s.'s,** see under nucleoside.

  **reducing s.,** one that has the property of reducing various inorganic ions, notably the cupric ion of Benedict's solution to cuprous ion, this being a test of long standing for reducing s. such as glucose in urine.

  **specific soluble s.,** specific capsular *substance.*

  **starch s.,** glucose.

  **wood s.,** xylose.

**su'gars.** Saccharides; carbohydrates; those substances having the general composition $(CH_2O)_n$ (whence the class name, carbo(n)hydrate) and simple derivatives thereof. While the structures are often written as polyhydroxy aldehydes or ketones, *e.g.*, $CH_2OH$—$(CHOH)_4$—$CHO$ for aldohexoses (*e.g.*, glucose) or $CH_2OH$—$(CHOH)_3$—$CO$—$CH_2OH$ for 2-ketoses (*e.g.*, fructose), cyclization can give rise to varied structures as described below. S.'s are generally identifiable by the ending -ose or, if in combination with a nonsugar (aglycon), -oside or -osyl. S.'s, especially glucose, are the chief source of energy, by oxidation, in nature, and they and their derivatives (*e.g.*, glucosamine, glucuronic acid), in polymeric form, are major constituents of mucoproteins, bacterial cell walls, and plant structural material (*e.g.*, cellulose). S.'s are often found in combination with steroids (steroid glycosides) and other aglycons.

  **Fischer projection formulas of s.'s,** representations, by projection, of acyclic or cyclic s.'s, or derivatives thereof, in which the carbon chain is depicted vertically. The lowest numbered asymmetric carbon atom is drawn at the top, and the rest of the carbon atoms of the chain are drawn in sequence below the top carbon atom. For each carbon atom, depicted in projection as lying in the plane of the paper, the carbon-to-carbon (bond or) bonds, which actually point away from the viewer, are drawn as vertical lines. The left-hand and right-hand bonds of each carbon atom, which actually point toward the viewer, are, in projection, depicted as horizontal lines.

  The conventions of the Fischer formulas of cyclic s.'s are: (1) carbon atoms (excluding the highest-numbered one)

having O to the right are D carbon atoms (*i.e.*, related in configuration to D-glyceraldehyde, the prototype); (2) on C-1, an OH, or substituted OH that lies to the right, with the OH of the highest numbered asymmetric carbon atom to the right, is α; if to the left, with the OH of the highest numbered asymmetric carbon atom to the right, it is β; the reverse applies if the OH of the highest numbered asymmetric carbon atom is to the left; (3) if the highest-numbered asymmetric C-atom has the OH (or its replacement) lying to the right, as is the 2-OH of D-glyceraldehyde, the sugar has the D configuration; if to the left, it is L; (4) the orientation of a terminal $CH_2OH$ group carries no configurational significance. Fischer projection formulas for various s.'s are shown in the accompanying composite (p. 1358), compared with Haworth formulas.

  **Haworth perspective formulas of cyclic s.'s,** perspective representations of furanose or pyranose structures as pentagons or hexagons, respectively, with the connecting bonds so shaded as to make them appear as though the plane of the ring is at an angle of 30° to the plane of the paper, and the bonds of H and OH are at right angles to the plane of the ring. These formulas depict the planar conformation, a situation not usually met. Other conformational formulas (see Haworth conformational formulas of cyclic s.'s) attempt to depict the many deviations from planarity. (See also Fischer projection formulas.)

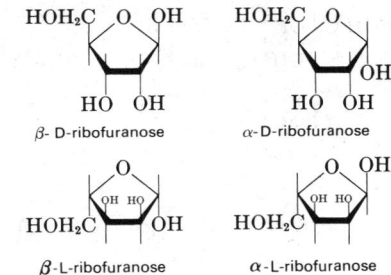

β- D-ribofuranose    α-D-ribofuranose

β-L-ribofuranose    α -L-ribofuranose

  The basic conventions in Haworth formulas of cyclic aldoses are: (1) carbon atoms (other than C-1 or that bearing the final $CH_2OH$) having O atoms below the plane of the ring are D carbons (*i.e.*, are configurationally identical to D-glyceraldehyde, the prototype), whereas those having O atoms above the plane are L; (2) if the highest numbered asymmetric carbon atom is D α and β hydroxyl groups at C-1 are situated below and above the plane of the ring, respectively; the reverse applies if the highest numbered asymmetric carbon atom is L. The L-ribofuranose formulas are formally derivable from the D formulas shown by reversing the up or down direction of all of the groups. Haworth perspective formulas for various sugars are shown in the accompanying composite (p. 1359).

  **Haworth conformational formulas of cyclic s.'s,** for the pyranoses, these depict those shapes (conformations) in which none, one, or two ring-atoms lie outside the plane of the ring. If there are two such atoms *para* to each other, they can lie (1) on opposite sides of the plane (*trans*), giving

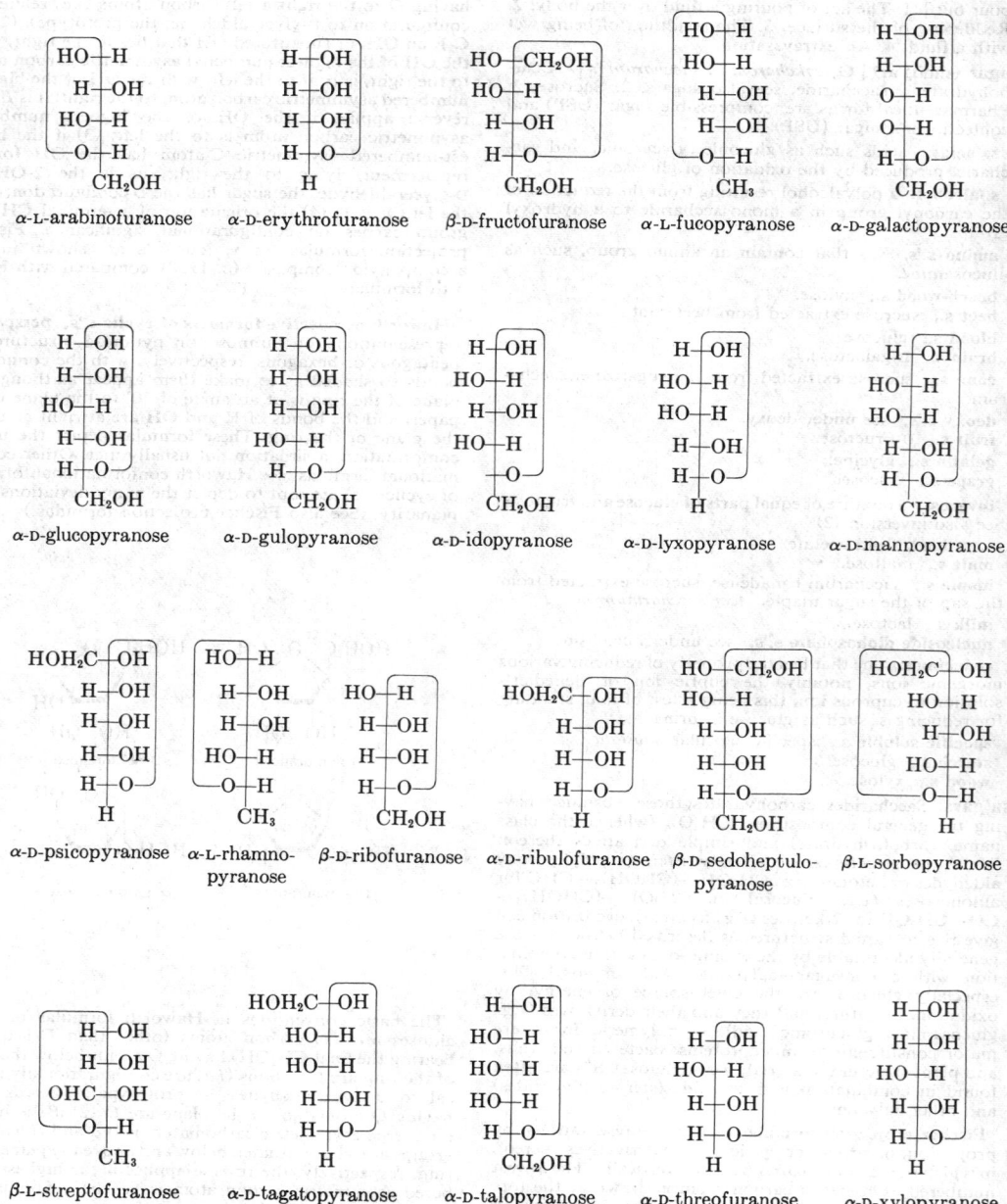

Fischer projection formulas for sugars

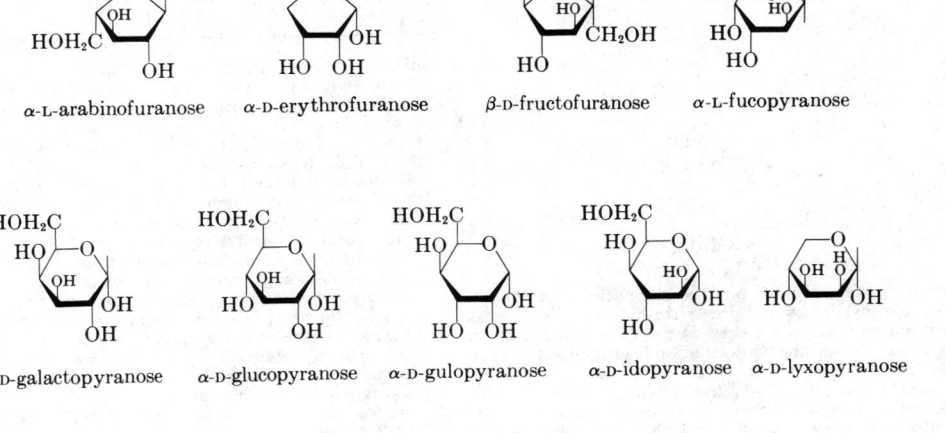

α-L-arabinofuranose     α-D-erythrofuranose     β-D-fructofuranose     α-L-fucopyranose

α-D-galactopyranose     α-D-glucopyranose     α-D-gulopyranose     α-D-idopyranose     α-D-lyxopyranose

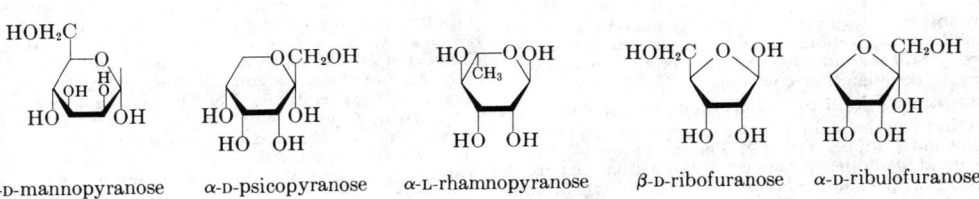

α-D-mannopyranose     α-D-psicopyranose     α-L-rhamnopyranose     β-D-ribofuranose     α-D-ribulofuranose

β-D-sedoheptulopyranose     β-L-sorbopyranose     β-L-streptofuranose     α-D-tagatopyranose

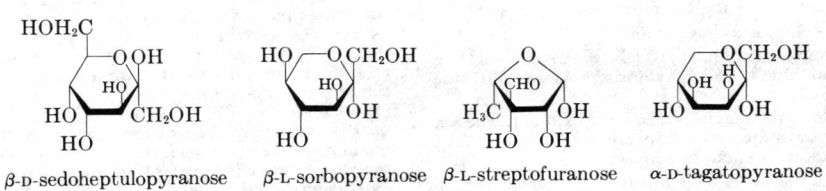

α-D-talopyranose     α-D-threofuranose     α-D-xylopyranose

**Haworth perspective formulas for cyclic sugars**

chair forms, or (2) on the same side of the plane (*cis*), giving boat forms. For β-D-ribopyranose, the two chair forms (*C1* and *1C*) are depicted.

C1(D)

1C(D)

Similarly, there are six boat conformations. If the two (*trans*) exoplanar atoms are *meta* to each other, the conformation is termed a skew form; if the two atoms are *ortho* to each other, the conformation is termed a half-chair form.

For the furanoses, the envelope conformations have one ring-atom exoplanar. If there are three adjacent, coplanar ring-atoms (the two exoplanar ring atoms on opposite sides of the plane), the conformations are termed twist forms.

**suggestibility** (sug-jes′tĭ-bil′ĭ-tĭ). Responsiveness or susceptibility to a psychological process whereby an idea is induced into, or adopted by, an individual without argument, command, or coercion.

**suggestible** (sug-jes′tĭ-bl). Susceptible to suggestion.

**suggestion** (sug-jes′chun) [ L. *sug-gero* (*subg-*), pp. *-gestus*, to bring under, supply. GEST- ]. The implanting of an idea in the mind of another by some word or act on the part of the operator, the subject being more or less influenced in his conduct or physical condition by such implanted idea. See also autosuggestion.

posthypnotic s., s. given to a subject who is under hypnosis for certain actions to be performed by him after he is "awakened" from the hypnotic trance.

**sugges′tive.** Relating to suggestion.

**suggillation** (sug′jĭ-la′shun, suj′i-) [ L. *sugillo*, pp. *-atus*, to beat black and blue ]. 1. Ecchymosis; a black and blue mark. 2. A livedo.

**suicide** (su′ĭ-sīd) [ L. *sui*, self, + *caedō*, to kill ]. 1. The act of taking one's own life voluntarily and intentionally. 2. A person who commits such an act.

**suicidology** (su′ĭ-si-dol′o-jĭ) [ suicide + G. *logos*, study ]. A branch of the behavioral sciences devoted to the study of the nature, causes, socioeconomic correlates, and prevention of suicide.

**suigen′derism** [ L. *sui*, self-, + Fr. *gendre*, fr. L. *generis*, sort, kind ]. A rarely used term for nonerotic relationships between persons of the same sex.

**suint** (swint) [ Fr. wool-grease ]. The natural grease in sheep's wool, from which the official wool fat is extracted.

**suit** (sūt). An outer garment designed for protection against specific environmental conditions.

anti-G s., a garment with bladders that expand to apply external pressure to the abdomen and lower extremities during positive G maneuvers in flight or on a human centrifuge; the anti-G s. is worn to prevent the pooling of blood and serves to increase the wearer's ability to withstand exposure to higher G forces.

space s., flexible or partially flexible garment designed to protect the wearer from some of the untoward effects of space travel; see anti-G s.

**sulcal** (sul′kal). Relating to a sulcus.

**sulcate, sulcated** (sul′kāt, -ka-ted). Grooved; furrowed; marked by a sulcus or sulci.

**sulciform** (sul-sī-form). Having the form of a groove or sulcus.

**sulculus**, pl. **sulculi** (sul′ku-lus, -li) [ Mod. L. dim. of L. *sulcus*, furrow ]. A small sulcus.

# SULCUS

**sulcus**, gen. and pl. **sulci** (sul′kus, sul′si) [ L. a furrow or ditch. SULC- ]. 1 [ NA ]. One of the grooves or furrows on the surface of the brain, bounding the several convolutions or gyri; a fissure. 2 [ NA ]. Any long narrow groove, furrow, or slight depression. 3. A groove or depression in the oral cavity or on the surface of a tooth.

s. aboma′si [ NAV ], abomasal groove; that portion of the gastric groove which courses along the inner surface of the lesser curvature of the abomasum; it extends from the omasoabomasal orifice to the pylorus.

alveolobuccal s., alveolobuccal *groove*.

alveololabial s., alveololabial *groove*.

alveololingual s., alveololingual *groove*.

s. ampulla′ris [ NA ], ampullary s.; the groove on the external surface of the ampulla of each semicircular duct where the nerve enters the crista ampullaris.

ampullary s., s. ampullaris.

s. angula′ris, incisura angularis.

anterior parolfactory s., s. parolfactorius anterior.

anterolateral s., s. lateralis anterior.

s. anthel′icis transver′sus [ NA ], a deep groove on the cranial surface of the auricle separating the eminences of the triangular fossa and of the concha.

aor′tic s., s. aorticus; a broad deep groove on the medial aspect of the left lung above and behind the hilus receiving the arch of the aorta and the thoracic aorta.

s. arte′riae occipita′lis [ NA ], s. of the occipital artery; a narrow groove medial to the mastoid notch of the temporal bone that lodges the occipital artery.

s. arte′riae subcla′viae [ NA ], groove for the subclavian artery; a groove immediately posterior to the scalene tubercle on the upper surface of the first rib across which the subclavian artery passes.

s. arte′riae tempora′lis me′diae [ NA ], s. for the middle temporal artery; a vertical groove located above the external acoustic meatus on the external surface of the squamous part of the temporal bone.

s. arte′riae vertebra′lis [ NA ], s. for the vertebral artery; the s. on the superior aspect of the posterior arch of the atlas that transmits the vertebral artery medially toward the foramen magnum.

sulci arterio′si [ NA ], arterial grooves; branching sulci on the interior surface of the cranial vault in which the meningeal arteries course, the most prominent of which are related to branches of the middle meningeal artery.

atrioventricular s., s. coronarius.

s. auric′ulae anterior, incisura anterior auris.

s. auric′ulae posterior [ NA ], posterior auricular groove; the s. between the antitragus and cauda helicis overlying the antitragicohelicine fissure.

basilar s., s. basilaris pontis.

s. basila′ris pon′tis [ NA ], basilar s.; a median groove on the ventral surface of the pons varolii in which lies the basilar artery.

s. bicipita′lis latera′lis [ NA ], lateral bicipital groove; the groove separating the biceps brachii and brachialis muscles on the lateral side.

s. bicipita′lis media′lis [ NA ], medial bicipital groove; the groove separating the biceps brachii and brachialis muscles on the medial side.

calcaneal s., s. calcanei.

s. calca′nei [ NA ], calcaneal s.; interosseous groove; the groove on the upper part of the calcaneus, which with a corresponding groove on the talus forms the sinus tarsi.

calcarine s., s. calcarinus.

s. calcari′nus [ NA ], calcarine s.; calcarine or posthippocampal fissure; fissura calcarina; a deep fissure on the medial aspect of the cerebral cortex, extending on an arched line from the isthmus of the fornicate gyrus back to the occipital pole, marking the border between the lingual gyrus below and the cuneus above it. The cortex at its bottom corresponds to the horizontal meridian of the contralateral half of the total field of vision.

**callosal s.,** s. corporis callosi.

**s. callosomargina'lis,** s. cinguli.

**s. carot'icus** [ NA ], carotid s.; the groove on the body of the sphenoid bone in which the internal carotid artery lies in its course through the cavernous sinus.

**carotid s.,** s. caroticus.

**s. car'pi** [ NA ], carpal groove; carpal canal; the concavity on the anterior surface of the arch formed by the carpal bones.

**central s.,** s. centralis.

**s. centra'lis** [ NA ], central s.; fissure of Rolando; a double-S-shaped fissure extending obliquely upward and backward on the lateral surface of each cerebral hemisphere at the border between the frontal and parietal lobes.

**cerebellar sulci,** grooves between the folia cerebelli.

**cerebral sulci,** sulci cerebri.

**sulci cer'ebri** [ NA ], cerebral sulci; the grooves between the cerebral gyri or convolutions.

**chiasmatic s.,** s. chiasmatis.

**s. chias'matis** [ NA ], chiasmatic s.; optic groove; a groove on the upper surface of the sphenoid bone between the optic canals in which the optic chiasm lies.

**s. cin'guli** [ NA ], s. of the cingulum; s. callosomarginalis; callosomarginal fissure; a fissure on the mesial surface of the cerebral hemisphere, bounding the upper surface of the gyrus cinguli (callosal convolution); the anterior portion is called the pars subfrontalis; the posterior portion which curves up to the superomedial margin of the hemisphere and borders the paracentral lobule posteriorly, the pars marginalis.

**s. of cingulum,** s. cinguli.

**circular s. of Reil,** s. circularis insulae.

**s. circula'ris in'sulae** [ NA ], circular or limiting s. of Reil; a semicircular fissure demarcating the insula from the opercula above, below, and behind.

**collateral s.,** s. collateralis.

**s. collatera'lis** [ NA ], s. occipitotemporalis [ NA ], collateral or occipitotemporal s.; collateral fissure; fissura collateralis; a long and deep sagittal fissure on the undersurface of the temporal lobe, marking the border between the fusiform gyrus on its lateral side and the hippocampal and lingual gyri on its medial side. The great depth of the s. collateralis results in a bulging of the floor of the occipital and temporal horn of the lateral ventricle, the eminentia collateralis.

**s. corona'rius** [ NA ], coronary s.; atrioventricular s. or groove; a groove on the outer surface of the heart marking the division between the atria and the ventricles.

**coronary s.,** s. coronarius.

**s. cor'poris callo'si** [ NA ], s. of the corpus callosum; callosal s.; the fissure between the corpus callosum and the gyrus cinguli.

**s. of corpus collasum,** s. corporis callosi.

**s. cos'tae** [ NA ], costal groove; a groove in the lower inner border of the rib, lodging the intercostal vessels and nerve.

**s. cru'ris heli'cis** [ NA ], groove of the crus of the helix; a transverse fissure on the cranial surface of the auricle corresponding to the crus of the helix.

**sulci cu'tis** [ NA ], grooves of the skin; the numerous grooves of variable depth on the surface of the epidermis.

**s. ethmoida'lis** [ NA ], ethmoidal groove; a groove on the inner surface of each nasal bone, lodging the external nasal branch of the anterior ethmoid nerve.

**external spiral s.,** s. spiralis externus.

**fimbrioden'tate s.,** s. fimbriodentatus; a shallow groove between the fimbria and the dentate fascia of the hippocampus.

**s. fronta'lis infe'rior** [ NA ], inferior frontal s.; a sagittal fissure on the outer surface of each frontal lobe of the cerebrum demarcating the middle from the inferior frontal gyrus.

**s. fronta'lis me'dius,** middle or median frontal s.; a relatively shallow sagittal fissure dividing the middle frontal convolution into an upper and lower part; this s. is

found only in man and the anthropoid apes; at its anterior extremity it bifurcates, the two branches spreading out laterally and constituting the frontomarginal s.

**s. fronta'lis supe'rior** [ NA ], superior frontal s.; a sagittal fissure on the superior surface of each frontal lobe of the cerebrum starting from the precentral or anterior border of the anterior central s.; it forms the lateral boundary of the superior frontal convolution.

**s. frontomargina'lis,** see s. frontalis medius.

**gingival s.,** gingival crevice; the space between the surface of the tooth and the free gingiva.

**gingivobuc'cal s.,** alveolobuccal *groove.*

**gingivolabial s.,** alveololabial *groove.*

**gingivolingual s.,** alveololingual *groove.*

**s. glute'us** [ NA ], gluteal furrow; the furrow between the buttock and thigh.

**s. for greater palatine nerve,** (1) s. palatinus major maxillae; (2) s. palatinus major ossis palatini.

**s. ham'uli pterygoi'dei** [ NA ], s. of pterygoid hamulus; a groove at the base of the hamular process which forms a pulley for the tendon of the tensor veli palatini.

**s. hippocam'pi** [ NA ], hippocampal fissure; fissura hippocampi; dentate fissure; fissura dentata; a shallow groove between the gyrus dentatus (dentate gyrus or fascia dentata) and the parahippocampal gyrus; the remains of a fissure that extended deep into the hippocampus between Ammon's horn and the dentate gyrus, but became obliterated during fetal development.

**hypothalamic s.,** s. hypothalamicus.

**s. hypothalam'icus** [ NA ], hypothalamic s.; s. of Monro; a groove in the lateral wall of the third ventricle on either side leading from the interventricular foramen to the aditus ad aqueductum cerebri.

**inferior frontal s.,** s. frontalis inferior.

**inferior petrosal s.,** s. sinus petrosi inferioris.

**inferior temporal s.,** s. temporalis inferior.

**s. infraorbita'lis** [ NA ], infraorbital groove; a gradually deepening groove on the orbital surface of the maxilla, which leads to the infraorbital canal.

**s. infrapalpebra'lis** [ NA ], the hollow or furrow below the lower eyelid.

**s. interme'dius ante'rior,** anterior paramedian groove; a furrow occasionally seen in the adult between the anterior median fissure and the anterior lateral s. of the spinal cord but usually present only in the fetus. It indicates the lateral border of the anterior corticospinal fasciculus.

**s. interme'dius poste'rior,** posterior intermediate groove; a longitudinal furrow between the posterior median and the posterior lateral sulci of the spinal cord in the cervical region, marking the funiculus gracilis from the funiculus cuneatus.

**internal spiral s.,** s. spiralis internus.

**interparietal s.,** s. intraparietalis.

**intertubercular s.,** s. intertubercularis.

**s. intertubercula'ris** [ NA ], intertubercular s.; intertubercular groove; bicipital groove; a furrow running down the shaft of the humerus between the two tubercles, lodging the tendon of the long head of the biceps, and giving attachment in its floor to the latissimus dorsi muscle.

**s. interventricula'ris ante'rior** [ NA ], anterior interventricular groove; crena cordis; a groove on the anterosuperior surface of the heart, marking the location of the septum between the two ventricles.

**s. interventricula'ris cor'dis,** see s. interventricularis anterior and s. interventricularis posterior.

**s. interventricula'ris poste'rior** [ NA ], posterior interventricular groove; crena cordis; a groove on the diaphragmatic surface of the heart, marking the location of the septum between the two ventricles.

**s. intragra'cilis,** a fissure between the gracilis minor and gracilis posterior lobuli of the cerebellum.

**intraparietal s.,** s. intraparietalis.

**intraparietal s. of Turner,** s. intraparietalis.

**s. intraparieta'lis** [ NA ], intraparietal or interparietal s.; Turner's s.; intraparietal s. of Turner; a horizontal s. extending back from the postcentral s. over some distance, then dividing perpendicularly into two branches so as to form, with the postcentral s., a figure H. It divides the parietal lobe into a superior and inferior parietal lobule.

**labial s.,** lip s.; a furrow between the developing lip and gum.

**s. lacrima'lis** [ NA ], lacrimal groove; (1) the hollow in the lacrimal bone; (2) the groove in the nasal surface of the maxilla which, together with (1) forms the fossa for the lacrimal sac.

**lateral cerebral s.,** s. lateralis cerebri.

**lateral occipital s.,** s. occipitalis lateralis; one of several variable sulci on the lateral aspect of the occipital lobe of each cerebral hemisphere, bounding the lateral occipital convolutions.

**s. latera'lis ante'rior** [ NA ], anterolateral groove or s.; an indistinct furrow on the ventral surface of the spinal cord and medulla oblongata, on either side marking the line of exit of the anterior nerve roots.

**s. latera'lis cer'ebri** [ NA ], lateral cerebral s. or fissure; fissura cerebri lateralis; fissure of Sylvius; the deepest and most prominent of the cortical fissures, extending from the anterior perforated substance first laterally at the deep incisure between the frontal and temporal lobes, then back and slightly upward over the lateral aspect of the cerebral hemisphere, with the superior temporal gyrus as its lower bank, the insula forming its greatly expanded floor. Two short side branches, the ramus anterior and ramus ascendens, divide the inferior frontal gyrus into a pars orbitalis, pars triangularis, and pars opercularis.

**s. latera'lis poste'rior** [ NA ], posterolateral groove or s.; a longitudinal furrow on either side of the posterior median s. of the spinal cord and medulla oblongata, marking the line of entrance of the posterior nerve roots.

**s. lim'itans** [ NA ], the medial longitudinal groove on the inner surface of the neural tube.

**s. lim'itans fos'sae rhomboi'deae** [ NA ], limiting s. of rhomboid fossa; a lateral groove running the whole length of the floor of the rhomboid fossa on either side of the midline, the remains of the s. demarcating the alar from the basal plate of the embryonic rhombencephalon.

**limiting s. of Reil,** s. circularis insulae.

**limiting s. of rhomboid fossa,** s. limitans fossae rhomboideae.

**lip s.,** labial s.

**longitudinal s. of heart,** *crena* cordis.

**lunate s.,** s. lunatus cerebri.

**s. luna'tus cer'ebri** [ NA ], ape, lunate, or simian fissure; lunate sulcus; Affenspalte; a small, inconstant semilunar groove on the cortical convexity near the occipital pole, marking the anterior border of the striate cortex (area 17) and considered homologous with the major sulcus of the same name that is a more constant feature of the cerebral cortex in monkeys and apes.

**malleolar s.,** s. malleolaris.

**s. malleola'ris** [ NA ], malleolar s.; a broad groove on the posterior surface of the medial malleolus, through which the tendon of the tibialis posterior muscle runs.

**s. ma'tricis un'guis** [ NA ], groove of the nail matrix; the cutaneous furrow in which the lateral border of the nail is situated.

**s. media'lis cru'ris cer'ebri** [ NA ], s. nervi oculomotorii; a groove in the lateral wall of the interpeduncular fossa of the midbrain from which emerge the rootlets of the oculomotor nerve.

**median s. of fourth ventricle,** s. medianus ventriculi quarti.

**median frontal s.,** s. frontalis medius.

**s. media'nus lin'guae** [ NA ], median groove of the tongue; raphe linguae; a slight longitudinal depression running forward on the dorsal surface of the tongue from the foramen cecum.

**s. media'nus poste'rior medul'lae oblonga'tae** [ NA ], posterior median s. or fissure of the medulla oblongata; the longitudinal groove marking the posterior midline of the medulla oblongata; continuous below with the posterior median s. of the spinal cord.

**s. media'nus poste'rior medul'lae spina'lis** [ NA ], posterior median s. or fissure of the spinal cord; fissure; a shallow furrow in the median line of the posterior surface of the spinal cord.

**s. media'nus ventric'uli quar'ti** [ NA ], median s. of the fourth ventricle; the shallow midline groove in the floor of the ventricle.

**s. mentolabia'lis** [ NA ], the mentolabial furrow; the indistinct line separating the lower lip from the chin.

**middle frontal s.,** s. frontalis medius.

**middle temporal s.,** s. temporalis medius.

**s. for middle temporal artery,** s. arteriae temporalis mediae.

**Monro's s.,** s. hypothalamicus.

**s. mylohyoi'deus** [ NA ], mylohyoid groove; a groove on the medial surface of the ramus of the mandible beginning at the lingula; it lodges the mylohyoid artery and nerve.

**s. nasolabia'lis** [ NA ], nasolabial groove; a furrow between the ala nasi and the lip.

**s. ner'vi oculomoto'rii,** s. medialis cruris cerebri.

**s. ner'vi petro'si majo'ris** [ NA ], groove of the greater petrosal nerve; the groove on the anterior surface of the petrous part of the temporal bone that lodges the greater petrosal nerve.

**s. ner'vi petro'si mino'ris** [ NA ], groove of the lesser petrosal nerve; the groove on the anterior surface of the petrous part of the temporal bone that accommodates the lesser petrosal nerve in its course to the otic ganglion.

**s. ner'vi radia'lis** [ NA ], groove for radial nerve; musculospiral groove; the shallow groove that passes around the shaft of the humerus. It lodges the radial nerve and deep brachial artery.

**s. ner'vi spina'lis** [ NA ], groove for spinal nerve; the laterally directed groove on the superior surface of the transverse processes of typical cervical vertebrae between the anterior and posterior tubercles along which the emerging spinal nerve passes.

**s. ner'vi ulna'ris** [ NA ], groove for ulnar nerve; a furrow on the posterior surface of the medial epicondyle of the humerus, lodging the ulnar nerve.

**nymphocaruncular s.,** nymphohymenal s.; s. nymphocaruncularis; a groove between the labium minus and the border of the remains of the hymen, in which is the opening of the duct of the glandula vestibularis major (Bartholin's gland) on either side.

**nymphohymenal s.,** nymphocaruncular s.

**s. obturato'rius** [ NA ], obturator groove; a deep groove on the inner surface of the superior ramus of the pubis.

**s. of occipital artery,** s. arteriae occipitalis.

**s. occipita'lis latera'lis,** lateral occipital s.

**s. occipita'lis supe'rior,** superior occipital s.

**s. occipita'lis transver'sus** [ NA ], transverse occipital s.; the posterior, vertical limb of the intraparietal s.

**occipitotemporal s.,** s. collateralis.

**s. occipitotempora'lis** [ NA ], s. collateralis [ NA ].

**s. olfacto'rius** [ NA ], olfactory s.; the sagittal s. on the inferior or orbital surface of each frontal lobe of the cerebrum, demarcating the gyrus rectus from the orbital gyri, and covered on the orbital surface by the bulbus and tractus olfactorii.

**s. olfacto'rius na'si** [ NA ], olfactory s. of nose; the narrow groove in the nasal cavity above the agger nasi that leads from the atrium to the olfactory area.

**olfactory s.,** s. olfactorius.

**olfactory s. of nose,** s. olfactorius nasi.

**s. oma'si** [ NAV ], omasal groove; a portion of the gastric groove that extends from the reticulo-omasal orifice to the omasoabomasal orifice; it lies on the inner surface of the base of the omasum and represents the shortest path for ingesta to pass from the rumen and reticulum to the abomasum.

**orbital sulci,** sulci orbitales.

**sulci orbita'les** [ NA ], orbital sulci; a number of irregularly disposed, variable sulci dividing the inferior or orbital surface of each frontal lobe of the cerebrum into the orbital gyri.

**s. palati'nus,** pl. **sulci palati'ni** [ NA ], palatine groove; one of a number of grooves on the lower surface of the palatine process of the maxilla in which the palatine vessels and nerves lie.

**s. palati'nus ma'jor maxil'lae** [ NA ], s. for the greater palatine nerve; together with a corresponding groove on the palatine bone it forms the canal for the greater palatine nerve and artery (formerly called pterygopalatine canal).

**s. palati'nus ma'jor os'sis palati'ni** [ NA ], s. for the greater palatine nerve; converted into a canal by a corresponding s. on the maxilla.

**s. palatovagina'lis** [ NA ], palatovaginal groove; a furrow on the inferior aspect of the vaginal process of the sphenoid bone that is bridged below by the sphenoidal process of the palatine bone to form the palatovaginal canal.

**sulci paraco'lici** [ NA ], paracolic recesses; the grooves between the lateral aspect of the ascending or descending colon and the abdominal wall.

**paraglenoid s.,** preauricular *groove*.

**s. paraglenoida'lis,** preauricular *groove*.

**parietooccipital s.,** s. parietooccipitalis.

**s. parietooccipita'lis** [ NA ], parietooccipital fissure or s.; fissura parietooccipitalis; a very deep, almost vertically oriented fissure on the medial surface of the cerebral cortex, marking the border between the parietal lobe and the cuneus of the occipital lobe; its lower part curves forward and fuses with the anterior extent of the calcarine fissure (sulcus calcarinus); the great depth of this combined fissure causes a bulge in the medial wall of the occipital horn of the lateral ventricle, the calcar avis.

**s. parolfacto'rius ante'rior,** anterior parolfactory s.; a fissure marking the anterior border of the parolfactory area.

**s. parolfacto'rius poste'rior,** posterior parolfactory s.; a shallow groove on the medial surface of the hemisphere demarcating the subcallosal gyrus or precommissural septum from the parolfactory area.

**periconchal s.,** *fossa* anthelicis.

**s. poplite'us,** popliteal *groove*.

**postcentral s.,** s. postcentralis.

**s. postcentra'lis** [ NA ], postcentral sulcus; the s. that demarcates the postcentral gyrus from the superior and inferior parietal lobules.

**posterior median s. of medulla oblongata,** s. medianus posterior medullae oblongatae.

**posterior median s. of spinal cord,** s. medianus posterior medullae spinalis.

**posterior parolfactory s.,** s. parolfactorius posterior.

**posterolateral s.,** s. lateralis posterior.

**preauricular s.,** preauricular *groove*.

**precentral s.,** s. precentralis.

**s. precentra'lis** [ NA ], precentral s.; s. verticalis; an interrupted fissure anterior to and in general parallel with the s. centralis, marking the anterior border of the precentral gyrus.

**s. promonto'rii** [ NA ], a narrow branched groove running vertically over the surface of the promontory in the middle ear, lodging the tympanic plexus.

**s. of pterygoid hamulus,** s. hamuli pterygoidei.

**s. pterygopalati'nus,** s. palatinus major.

**s. pulmona'lis** [ NA ], pulmonary s.; the deep recess on either side of the vertebral column formed by the posterior sweep of the curvature of the ribs.

**pulmonary s.,** s. pulmonalis.

**Reil's circular** or **limiting s.,** s. circularis insulae.

**s. retic'uli** [ NAV ], reticular or esophageal groove; a spiraling segment of the gastric groove, with thickened lips; it extends from the cardia to the reticulo-omasal orifice.

**rhinal s.,** s. rhinalis.

**s. rhina'lis** [ NA ], rhinal s. or fissure; the shallow s. that delimits the anterior part of the hippocampal gyrus from the fusiform or lateral occipitotemporal gyrus. One of the oldest sulci of the pallium, it marks the border between the neocortex and the allocortical (olfactory) and juxtallocortical areas medial to it.

**sag'ittal s.,** s. sinus sagittalis superioris.

**s. of sclera,** s. sclerae.

**s. scle'rae** [ NA ], s. of the sclera; a slight groove on the external surface of the eyeball indicating the line of union of the sclera and cornea.

**sigmoid s.,** s. sinus sigmoidei.

**s. si'nus petro'si inferio'ris** [ NA ], inferior petrosal s.; a groove lodging the inferior petrosal sinus, formed by union of similarly named grooves in the petrous part of the temporal bone and the basilar part of the occipital bone.

**s. si'nus petro'si superio'ris** [ NA ], superior petrosal s.; a groove on the superior border of the petrous portion of the temporal bone in which rests the superior petrosal sinus.

**s. si'nus sagitta'lis superio'ris** [ NA ], sagittal s.; groove for the superior sagittal sinus; superior longitudinal s.; the

groove in the midline of the inner table of the calvaria lodging the superior sagittal sinus; it is composed of a groove with the same name in the frontal, parietal, and occipital bones.

**s. si'nus sigmoi'dei** [ NA ], sigmoid s.; sigmoid fossa or groove; a broad groove in the posterior cranial fossa, first situated on the lateral portion of the occipital bone, then curving around the jugular process on to the mastoid portion of the temporal bone, and finally turning sharply on the posterior inferior angle of the parietal bone and becoming continuous with the transverse groove; it lodges the transverse sinus.

**s. si'nus transver'si** [ NA ], s. for the transverse sinus; the groove on the inner surface of the occipital bone marking the course of the transverse sinus. The tentorium is attached to its margins.

**s. spino'sus,** *stria* spinosa.

**s. spira'lis exter'nus** [ NA ], external spiral s.; a concavity in the outer wall of the cochlear duct between the prominentia spiralis and the spiral organ.

**s. spira'lis inter'nus** [ NA ], internal spiral s.; a concavity in the floor of the cochlear duct formed by the overhanging labium vestibulare.

**s. subcla'vius,** a groove on the surface of the lung just below the apex, corresponding to the course of the subclavian artery.

**subparietal s.,** s. subparietalis.

**s. subparieta'lis** [ NA ], subparietal s.; a s. continuing the direction of the s. cinguli from where the pars marginalis of that fissure bends upward; it forms the upper boundary of the posterior portion of the gyrus cinguli.

**superior frontal s.,** s. frontalis superior.

**superior longitudinal s.,** s. sinus sagittalis superioris.

**superior occipital s.,** s. occipitalis superior; one of several small and variable sulci bordering the superior occipital gyri on the upper aspect of the occipital lobe of the cerebrum.

**superior petrosal s.,** s. sinus petrosi superioris.

**superior temporal s.,** s. temporalis superior.

**talar s.,** s. tali.

**s. ta'li** [ NA ], talar s.; interosseous groove; the groove on the inferior surface of the talus which with a corresponding groove on the calcaneus forms the sinus tarsi.

**s. tempora'lis infe'rior** [ NA ], inferior temporal s.; Clevenger's fissure; the s. on the basal aspect of the temporal lobe that separates the fusiform gyrus from the inferior temporal gyrus on its lateral side.

**s. tempora'lis me'dius,** middle temporal s.; the s. between the gyrus temporalis medius and gyrus temporalis inferior.

**s. tempora'lis supe'rior** [ NA ], superior temporal s.; the longitudinal s. that separates the superior and middle temporal gyri.

**sulci tempora'les transver'si** [ NA ], transverse temporal sulci; the shallow sulci that demarcate the transverse temporal gyri on the opercular surface of the superior temporal gyrus.

**s. ten'dinis mus'culi fibula'ris lon'gi** [ NA ], official alternate term for s. tendinis peronei longi.

**s. ten'dinis mus'culi flexo'ris hal'lucis lon'gi** [ NA ], groove for the tendon of the flexor hallucis longus; a vertical s. on the posterior process of the talus continuous with a similar groove on the under side of the sustentaculum tali of the calcaneus.

**s. ten'dinis mus'culi perone'i lon'gi** [ NA ], s. tendinis musculi fibularis longi [ NA ], groove for the tendon of the long peroneal (fibular) muscle; (1) the groove below the peroneal trochlea of the calcaneus; (2) the groove distal to the tuberosity of the cuboid bone.

**terminal s.,** s. terminalis.

**s. termina'lis** [ NA ], terminal s.; (1) a V-shaped groove, with apex pointing backward, on the surface of the tongue, marking the separation between the oral, or horizontal, and the pharyngeal, or vertical, parts; (2) a groove on the surface of the right atrium of the heart, marking the junction of the primitive sinus venosus with the atrium.

**tonsillolingual s.,** the space between the palatine tonsil and the tongue.

**transverse occipital s.,** s. occipitalis transversus.

**s. for transverse sinus,** s. sinus transversi.

**transverse temporal sulci,** sulci temporales transversi.

**s. tu'bae auditi'vae** [ NA ], groove for the auditory tube; a furrow on the inner surface of the posterior border of the greater wing of the sphenoid bone, for the cartilaginous auditory (Eustachian) tube.

**Turner's s.,** s. intraparietalis.

**s. tympan'icus** [ NA ], tympanic groove; the s. on the inner aspect of the tympanic part of the temporal bone in which the tympanic membrane is fixed.

**s. for vena cava,** s. venae cavae.

**s. ve'nae ca'vae** [ NA ], s. for the vena cava; fossa for the vena cava; a groove on the posterior surface of the liver between the caudate lobe and the right lobe which gives passage to the inferior vena cava.

**s. ve'nae ca'vae crania'lis,** a groove on the surface of the right lung, above the hilus, in which runs the superior vena cava.

**s. ve'nae subcla'viae** [ NA ], groove for the subclavian vein; a groove just anterior to the scalene tubercle of the first rib marking the course of the subclavian vein across the rib.

**s. ve'nae umbilica'lis** [ NA ], the s. on the fetal liver occupied by the umbilical vein.

**sulci veno'si** [ NA ], venous grooves; grooves occasionally found on the internal surface of the parietal bone, in which veins lie.

**s. ventra'lis,** *fissura* mediana anterior medullae spinalis.

**s. ventric'ulus** [ NAV ], gastric groove; the internal groove along the lesser curvature of the stomach; in ruminants the gastric groove is divided into three segments that correspond with divisions of the compound stomach: the s. reticuli (reticular groove), s. omasi (omasal groove), and s. abomasi (abomasal groove).

**s. for vertebral artery,** s. arteriae vertebralis.

**s. vertica'lis,** s. precentralis.

**s. vomerovagina'lis** [ NA ], vomerovaginal groove; a s. on the inferior aspect of the vaginal process of the sphenoid bone that, together with ala of the vomer forms the vomerovaginal canal.

---

**sulf-, sulfo-.** A prefix denoting that the compound to the name of which it is attached contains a sulfur atom. This spelling (rather than sulph-, sulpho-) is preferred by the American Chemical Society and has been adopted by the USP and NF, but not by the BP. The British (BP) spellings are usually listed as alternative spellings within the definitions.

**sulfa** (sul'fah). Denoting the sulfa drugs, or sulfonamides, *q. v.*

**sulfacet'amide** (NF). *N*-Sulfanilylacetamide; *N*1-acetyl-sulfanilamide; a sulfonamide drug; used in the treatment of urinary tract infections and widely used as a component of the three-sulfonamide mixture with sulfadiazine and sulfa-merazine.

**s. sodium** (USP), sulphacetamide sodium (BP); same uses as s.; also used locally for eye infections and for prevention of gonorrheal ophthalmia in newborn infants.

**sulfachloropyrid'azine.** SONILYN; *N*1-(6-chloro-3-pyridazinyl)sulfanilamide; antimicrobial agent used for treatment of genitourinary system.

**sulfacid** (sulf-as'id). Thioacid.

**sulfadi'azine** (USP). ESKADIAZINE; sulphadiazine (BP); *N*1-2-pyrimidinylsulfanilamide; one of a group of diazine derivatives of sulfanilamide, the pyrimidine analogue of sulfapyridine and sulfathiazole. Highly effective against pneumococcal, staphylococcal, and streptococcal infections, also against infections with *Escherichia coli, Klebsiella pneumoniae,* and in acute gonococcal arthritis.

**s. sodium** (USP), sulphadiazine sodium (BP); same uses as those of s.

**sulfadi'cramide.** SULFIRGAMIDE; IRGAMIDE; 3-methyl-*N*-sulfanilylcrotonamide; an antibacterial sulfonamide.

**sulfadimethoxine** (sul'fā-di'mē-thok'sēn) (NF). MADRI-BON; sulphadimethoxine (BP); 2,4-dimethoxy-6-sulfanila-mide-1,3-diazine; a long-acting sulfonamide that is rapidly absorbed after oral administration and is slowly excreted by the kidney. It accumulates in the tissue, and requires lower doses to attain effective tissue concentrations than do the other sulfonamides.

**sulfadimidine.** Sulfamethazine.

**sulfadox'ine** (USAN). FANASIL; sulformethoxine; *N*1-(5,6-dimethoxy-4-pyrimidyl)sulfanilamide; a long-acting sulfonamide, used with quinine and pyrimethamine to reduce the relapse rate of malaria.

**sulfaethidole** (sul'fā-eth'ī-dōl) (NF). GLOBUCID; *N*1-(5-ethyl-1,3,4-thiadiazole-2-yl)sulfanilamide; a sulfonamide used in the treatment of systemic and urinary tract infections.

**sulfafu'razole.** Sulfisoxazole.

**sulfagua'nidine.** Sulfanilylguanidine; the guanidine derivative of sulfanilamide. It is poorly absorbed from the gastroenteric tract; useful for bacterial infections of the lower intestinal tract and for preoperative sterilization of the intestinal tract.

**sulfalene** (sul'fā-lēn) (USAN). KELFIZINA; *N*1-(3-methoxy-2-pyrimidyl)sulfanilamide; a very long-acting sulfonamide that enhances, as do other sulfonamides and sulfones, the effectiveness of antimalarial agents such as pyrimethamine, chloroguanide, or cycloguanil. Believed to act by interference with the utilization of folic acid.

**sulfamer'azine** (USP). *N*1-(4-Methyl-2-pyrimidinyl)sul-fanilamide; a bacteriostatic agent of the sulfanilamide group; one of the components of mixtures of two or three sulfonamides. Used in the treatment of meningococcal infections. The sodium salt is suitable for intravenous administration.

**sulf'ame'ter** (USAN). SULLA; sulfamethoxydiazine; sul-phamethoxydiazine (BP); 2-(4-aminobenzenesulfon-amido)-5-methoxypyrimidine; a slowly excreted sulfon-amide used in the treatment of acute and chronic urinary tract infections.

**sulfameth'azine** (USP). DIAZIL; sulfadimidine; sul-phadimidine (BP); *N*1-(4,6-dimethyl-2-pyrimidinyl)sul-fanilamide; an antibacterial agent of the sulfonamide group. It is active against hemolytic streptococci, staphylo-cocci, pneumococci, meningococci, *Escherichia coli, Pseu-domonas aeruginosa, Aerobacter aerogenes,* and *Proteus vulgaris.* One of the components of the three-sulfonamide mixture; sulfadiazine and sulfamerazine are the other components.

**sulfameth'izole** (NF). THIOSULFIL; sulphamethizole (BP); *N*1-(5-methyl-1,3,4-thiadiazol-2-yl)sulfanilamide; because of its high solubility, a sulfonamide useful for the treatment of urinary tract infection.

**sulfamethox'azole** (NF, USAN). GANTANOL; sulphame-thoxazole (BP); *N*1-(5-methyl-3-isoxazoyl)sulfanilamide; a sulfonamide related chemically to sulfisoxazole with a similar antibacterial spectrum. Its rate of absorption from the gastrointestinal tract and urinary excretion is slower. Its effectiveness in meningitis, streptococcal infection, pneumonia and gonorrhea has not been proved.

**sulfamethox'ydia'zine.** Sulfameter.

**sulfamethox'ypyrid'azine.** KYNEX; MIDICEL; sulphame-thoxypyridazine (BP); a long-acting sulfonamide that requires a single daily dose for maintaining effective tissue concentrations.

**acetyl s.,** KYNEX acetyl; well suited for pediatric use because it is tasteless; also used to enhance the actions of quinine and other supressants in the chemoprophylaxis of malaria.

**sulfameth'ylthi'azole.** SULFAZOLE; ULTRASEPTYL; 4-methyl-2-sulfanilamidothiazole; a sulfonamide suggested for the treatment of staphylococcal infections.

**sulfamipyr'ine.** MELUBRIN; sodium 1-phenyl-2,3-dime-thylpyrazolone-4-aminomethanesulfonate; an antipyretic and analgesic, used for the treatment of neuralgia and acute articular rheumatism.

**sulfamox'ole** (USAN). DEPOMIDE; *N*1-(4,5-dimethyl-2-oxazolyl)sulfanilamide; antimicrobial agent.

*p*-**sulfamylacetanilide.** *N*4-Acetylsulfanilamide; an inter-mediate in the synthesis of sulfanilamide; formed in animal body by acetylation of sulfanilamide.

**sulfanilamide** (sul'fā-nil'ā-mīd). *p*-Aminobenzenesulfona-mide; white crystals or a crystalline powder, soluble in 125 parts of water or 37 parts of alcohol. It was the first sulfonamide used for its chemotherapeutic effect in infec-tions caused by some β-hemolytic streptococci, meningo-cocci, gonococci, *Clostridium welchii,* and in certain infections of the urinary tract, especially those due to

*Escherichia coli* and *Proteus vulgaris*. It is less effective than sulfapyridine in the treatment of penumococcic, staphylococcic, and Friedlander's bacillus infections. Some toxic manifestations are acidosis, cyanosis, hemolytic anemia, and agranulocytosis.

$$H_2N - \bigcirc - SO_2NH_2$$

Sulfanilamide

**sulfan'ilate.** A salt of sulfanilic acid.

**sulfanil'ic acid.** *p*-Aminobenzenesulfonic acid; used in the synthesis of sulfonamides and indicators.

**N-sulfan'ilylben'zamide.** SULFABENZIDE; antimicrobial agent.

**sulfan'ilylsulfanil'amide.** DISULON; used in treatment of streptococcal and gonococcal infections. May cause neuritis.

**sulfan'ilylure'a.** URACTYL; N-sulfanilylcarbamide; antimicrobial agent.

**sulfani'tran** (USAN). POLYSTAT; 4'-[ (*p*-nitrophenyl)sulfamoyl ]acetanilide; antimicrobial agent.

**sulfaphen'azole.** ORISUL; a long-acting sulfonamide that is rapidly absorbed after oral administration; one dose is sufficient to maintain effective tissue concentration for 24 hours.

**sulfapyrazine** (sulf-ă-pīr'ă-zēn). 2-Sulfanilamidopyrazine; a diazine derivative of sulfanilamide, the pyrazine analogue of sulfapyridine and sulfathiazole. Highly effective against pneumococcal, streptococcal, and gonococcal infections.

**sulfapyridine** (sulf-ăpīr'ĭ-dēn) (USP). DAGENAN; M & B 693; sulphapyridine (BP); N 1-2-pyridylsulfanilamide; used in the treatment of pneumonia caused by certain types of pneumococci, but has been largely replaced by less toxic agents. It is useful in the treatment of dermatitis herpetiformis.

**sul'faquinox'aline.** Used in the treatment and prevention of coccidiosis in chickens.

**sulfar'side.** BEMARSIDE; 4-sulfamoyl-*o*-arsanilic acid; amebicide.

**sulfatase** (sul'fă-tās). Trivial name for enzymes in EC group 3.1.6, sulfohydrolases catalyzing the hydrolysis of sulfate esters to the corresponding alcohol plus inorganic sulfate. The group includes aryl-, sterol, glycol-, chondroitin, choline-, cellulose, cerebroside, and chondro- sulfatases (EC 3.1.6.1 to .10).

**sul'fate.** A salt or ester of sulfuric acid $(H_2SO_4)$.

active s., adenosine 3'-phosphate 5'-phosphosulfate (3'-phosphoadenosine 5'-phosphosulfate); general esterification agent in the biosynthesis of sulfuric esters.

**sulfathi'azole.** 2-Sulfanilylaminothiazole; 2-(*p*-aminobenzenesulfonamido)thiazole; a sulfanilamide compound efficacious against the same organisms as sulfanilamide, probably more effective and less toxic. It is more useful against staphylococcal infections than sulfapyridine and sulfanilamide, and is effective in combination with a vasoconstrictor drug as nose drops in acute and chronic nasopharyngitis and sinusitis. Also available as the sodium salt.

**sulfathi'oure'a.** FONTAMIDE; 1-sulfanilyl-2-thiourea; antimicrobial agent.

**sulfatidates.** Sulfatides; cerebroside sulfuric esters; cerebrosides containing sulfate groups in the sugar portion of the molecule.

**sul'fatides.** Sulfatidates.

**sulfatidosis** (sul'fă-ti-do'sis). Metachromatic *leukodystrophy*.

**sulfaz'amat** (USAN). VESULONG; methyl-1-phenylpyrazol-5-yl)sulfanilamide; an antibacterial drug.

**sulfhemoglobin** (sulf-he'mo-glo-bin). Sulfmethemoglobin.

**sulfhe'moglobine'mia.** A morbid condition due to the presence of sulfhemoglobin in the blood; it is marked by a persistent cyanosis, but the blood count does not reveal any special abnormality in that fluid; it is thought to be

caused by the action of hydrogen sulfide absorbed from the intestine.

**sulfhy'drate.** A hydrosulfide; a compound containing the ion $HS^-$.

**sulfhy'dryl.** The radical —SH; mercapto- or thiol-; it is contained in glutathione, cysteine, coenzyme A, lipoamide (all in the reduced state), and in mercaptans (R—SH).

**sul'fide.** A compound of sulfur in which the sulfur has a valence of −2; *e.g.,* $Na_2S$, HgS.

**sul'findigot'ic acid.** $C_8H_5NOSO_3$; formed by the action of sulfuric acid on indigo, a reaction that also yields indigo-carmine or sodium indigotindisulfonate.

**sulfinpyrazone** (sul'fin-pīr'ă-zōn) (USP). ANTURANE; sulphinpyrazone (BP); 1,2-diphenyl-4-(2-phenylsulfinylethyl)pyrazolidine-3,5-dione; an analgesic and uricosuric agent; promotes the excretion of uric acid probably by interfering with the tubular reabsorption of uric acid.

**β-sulfinylpyruvic acid** (sul'fī-nil-pi-ru'vik). $HO_2S$—$CH_2$—$CO$—$COOH$, an intermediate product of cysteine catabolism in mammalian tissue.

**sulfisomidine** (sul'fī-so'mī-dēn). ELKOSIN; N1-(2,6-dimethyl-4-pyrimidinyl)sulfanilamide. The structural isomer of sulfamethazine. Used in the treatment of systemic and urinary tract infections.

**sulfisox'azole** (USP). GANTRISIN; sulfafurazole; sulphafurazole (BP); N1-(3,4-dimethyl-5-isoxazolyl)sulfanilamide; a sulfonamide used chiefly in bacterial infections of the urinary tract.

acetyl s. (USP), GANTRISIN acetyl; same use as s.

s. diolamine (NF), the 2,2'-iminodiethanol salt of s.; used for intravenous, subcutaneous, or intramuscular administration.

**sul'fite.** A salt of sulfurous acid $(H_2SO_3)$.

s. dehydrogenase (EC 1.8.2.1), an oxidoreductase catalyzing oxidation of sulfite to sulfate with the reduction of ferricytochrome *c*.

s. oxidase (EC 1.8.3.1), a liver oxidoreductase (a hemoprotein) catalyzing the oxidation of inorganic sulfite ion to sulfate ion with $O_2$ and producing $H_2O_2$.

s. reductase (EC 1.8.99.1), oxidoreductase catalyzing reduction of sulfite to $H_2S$.

**sulfmethemoglobin** (sulf-met-he'mo-glo-bin). Sulfhemoglobin; the complex formed by $H_2S$ (or sulfides) and ferric ion in methemoglobin.

**sulfo-.** See sulf-.

**sulfoacid** (sul'fo-as-id). 1. Thioacid. 2. Sulfonic *acid.*

**sulfobromophthalein sodium** (sul'fo-bro'mo-thal'e-in) (USP). BROMSULPHALEIN; sulphobromophthalein sodium (BP); bromosulfophthalein; bromsulfophthalein; BSP; a triphenylmethane derivative. It is excreted by the liver and is used in testing hepatic function, particularly of the reticuloendothelial cells.

**sulfocy'anate.** Thiocyanate.

**sulfocyan'ic acid.** Thiocyanic acid.

**sulfogel** (sul'fo-jel). Same as hydrogel, with sulfuric acid instead of water as the dispersion means.

**sulfohy'drate.** Sulfhydrate.

**sulfol'ysis.** A lysis brought on or accelerated by sulfuric acid.

**sulfomu'cin.** A mucin containing sulfate esters in its mucopolysaccharides or glycoproteins.

**sulfomyx'in sodium.** Solphomyxin sodium (BP); a mixture of sulfomethylated polymyxin B and sodium bisulfite.

**sulfon'amides.** The so-called sulfa drugs; a group of bacteriostatic drugs containing the sulfanilamide group (sulfanilamide, sulfapyridine, sulfathiazole, sulfadiazine, and other sulfanilamide derivatives).

**sul'fonate.** The salt or ester of sulfonic acid.

**sul'fone.** A compound of the general structure R'—$SO_2$—R''.

**sulfonethylmethane** (sul'fōn-eth'il-meth'ān). TRIONAL; methylsulfonal; 2,2-bis(ethylsulfonyl)butane; a hypnotic.

**sulfon'ic acids.** Compounds in which a hydrogen atom of a CH group is replaced by the sulfonic acid group —$SO_3H$; general formula, R—$SO_3H$.

**sulfonium ion** (sul-fo'nī-um). A compound in which a sulfur atom has three single covalent bonds and therefore has a positive charge analogous to the nitrogen of an ammonium ion; a notable example is S-adenosylmethionine, an important intermediate in transmethylation processes.

**sulfonmethane** (sul'fōn-meth'ān). SULFONAL; 2,2-bis-(ethylsulfanyl)propane; a hypnotic.

**sulfonylurea compounds** (sul'fo-nil-u-re'ah). Sulfonylureas; derivatives of isopropylthiodiazylsulfanilamide, chemically related to the sulfonamides, which possess hypoglycemic action. Belonging to this series are acetohexamide, azepinamide, chlorpropamide, fluphenmepramide, glymidine, hydroxyhexamide, heptolamide, indylamide, thiohexamide, tolazamide, and tolbutamide.

**sulfopro'tein.** A protein molecule containing sulfate groups.

**6-sulfoquinovosyl monoglyceride** (sul'fo-kwi'no-vo-sil, -kwin'o). The sulfolipid occurring in all photosynthetic tissues; quinovose containing an $SO_3H$ on C-6 and a doubly substituted glycerol on C-1.

**sulformethox'ine.** Sulfadoxine.

**sulfosalicylic acid** (sul'fo-sal'ĭ-sil'ik) (USP). Salicylsulfonic acid; 3-carboxy-4-hydroxybenzenesulfonic acid; $C_6H_3SO_3H(OH)(COOH)$; used as a test for albumin and ferric ion.

**sul'fosol.** Same as hydrosol, with sulfuric acid instead of water as the dispersion means.

**sulfotrans'ferase.** Generic term for enzymes (EC sub-subclass 2.8.2) catalyzing the transfer of a sulfate group from 3'-phosphoadenylyl sulfate to the hydroxyl group of an acceptor.

**sulfox'ide.** The sulfur analogue of a ketone, R'—SO—R''.

**sulfox'one sodium.** DIASONE sodium; disodium sulfonylbis(p-phenyleneimino) dimethanesulfinate; antileprotic.

**sul'fur** [ L. *sulfur* or *sulphur*, brimstone, sulfur ]. Brimstone; an element, symbol S, atomic no. 16, atomic weight 32.066, occurring in native state in volcanic countries. It is of bright yellow color and occurs as a crystalline solid or as an amorphous powder; it combines with oxygen to form s. dioxide and s. trioxide, and with many of the metals and nonmetallic elements to form sulfides. It is mildly laxative; has been used in rheumatism, gout, and bronchitis; externally it is used in the treatment of skin diseases.

**s. dioxide** (USP), sulfurous oxide; a colorless, nonflammable gas with a strong, suffocating odor; a powerful reducing agent used to prevent oxidative deterioration of food and medicinal products. A saturated solution in water, about 6 per cent $SO_2$, is known as sulfurous acid and has been used externally for its parasiticidal effect in various skin diseases.

**flowers of s.,** sublimed s.

**s. group,** the elements sulfur, selenium, and tellurium; they form dibasic acids with hydrogen, and their oxyacids are also dibasic.

**s. iodide,** has been used in the treatment of certain skin diseases.

**liver of s.,** sulfurated potash.

**milk of s.,** precipitated s.

**precipitated s.** (USP, BP), milk of s.; sublimed s. boiled with lime water, the lime being removed from the precipitate by washing with diluted hydrochloric acid; used in preparing s. ointment and in the treatment of various skin disorders.

**roll s.,** brimstone; sublimed s. melted and cast in cylindrical molds.

**soft s.,** an allotropic form obtained by dropping very hot melted s. into water; it is then temporarily of a viscid or waxy consistency.

**sublimed s.** (NF), flowers of s.; used in preparing s. ointment and in the treatment of various skin disorders.

**s. trioxide,** $SO_3$; sulfuric oxide; forms sulfuric acid, $H_2SO_4$, by its reaction with water.

**vegetable s.,** lycopodium.

**washed s.,** sublimed s. macerated in diluted ammonia water to remove the free acid; same therapeutic uses as sublimed s.

**wettable s.,** prepared from calcium polysulfide solution containing a protective colloid such as casein. This s. is easily dispersed and suspended in water.

**sulfur-35** ($^{35}S$). Radioactive s. isotope; beta emitter with half-life of 87.1 days; used as a tracer in study of metabolism of cysteine, cystine, methionine, etc.

**sul'furet.** Sulfide.

**sulfu'ric acid.** Oil of vitriol; $H_2SO_4$; a colorless, nearly odorless, heavy, oily, corrosive liquid containing 96 per cent of absolute acid. Used occasionally as a caustic. Caution.

**fuming s. acid,** Nordhausen s. acid.

**Nordhausen s. acid** [ named for *Nordhausen*, a town in Saxony where it was first prepared ], fuming s. acid; s. acid containing sulfurous acid gas in solution.

**sulfuric ether.** Diethyl ether.

**sul'furize.** To sulfurate; to combine with sulfur.

**sulfurous** (sul'fu-rus). Designating a sulfur compound in which sulfur has a valence of +4 as contrasted to sulfuric compounds in which sulfur has a valence of +6.

**s. acid,** $H_2SO_3$; a solution of about 6 per cent sulfur dioxide in water; used chiefly as a disinfectant and bleaching agent, and occasionally as a spray in tonsillitis.

**sulfuryl** (sul'fu-ril). The bivalent radical $SO_2$.

**sulfy'drate.** Sulfohydrate; a compound of SH-.

**sul'isoben'zone** (USAN). UVAL; 5-benzoyl-4-hydroxy-2-methoxybenzene sulfonic acid; sunscreen agent.

**Sulkowitch,** Hirsh W., American physician, *1906. See S.'s reagent.

**sulph-.** See sulf-; for BP terms and other words beginning thus, and not found here, see those beginning with sulf-.

**sul'piride** (USAN). DOGMATYL; N-[ (1-ethyl-2-pyrrolidinyl)methyl ]-5-sulfamoyl-*o*-anisamide; an antidepressant.

**sulthiame** (sul'thi-ām) (BP, USAN). CONTRAVUL; CONADIL; p-tetrahydro-2H-1,2-thiazin-2-yl)benzenesulfonamide, *S,S*-dioxide; an anticonvulsant used in the treatment of temporal lobe epilepsy and grand mal with psychomotor seizures. May cause ataxia, paresthesias, and psychotic episodes.

**Sulzberger,** Marion B., American dermatologist, *1895. See Bloch-S *disease*, S.-Garbe *disease, syndrome*.

**sum.** Abbreviation of L. *sume*, take, or *sumendus*, sumendum, to be taken (a direction in the signature of a prescription), fr. *sumo*, pp. *sumptus*, to take.

**sumac, sumach** (su'mak) [ Ar. *summaq* ]. Rhus glabra.

**fragrant s.,** Rhus aromatica.

**sum'bul** [ Hindu word ]. Sumbul root; musk root; the dried rhizome and roots of *Ferula sumbul* and of other closely related species of *Ferula* (family Umbelliferae); formerly used as a sedative.

**summation** (sum-a'shun) [ Mediev. L. *summatio*, fr. *summo*, pp. *-atus*, to sum up, fr. L. *summa*, sum ]. The aggregation of a number of similars; totality.

**s. of stimuli,** muscular or neural effects produced by the frequent repetition of slight stimuli, one of which alone might be without evident response.

**Sumner,** F. W., British surgeon, 20th century. See S.'s *sign*.

**sun'burn.** Erythema solare; erythema caused by exposure to critical amounts of ultraviolet light, usually within the range of 2600 to 3200 Å.

**sun'flower seed oil.** Oil from the seeds of *Helianthus annuus* (family Compositae); the glycerides consist mainly of the mixed triglycerides, each containing one or two linoleic acid radicals; used as a food, and in dietary supplements.

**sun'stroke.** Insolation; siriasis; thermoplegia; a form of heatstroke resulting from undue exposure to the sun's rays, probably caused by the action of the actinic rays combined with the high temperature. The symptoms are those of heatstroke, but there is often an absence of fever, with extreme prostration and collapse.

**super-** [ L. *super*, above, beyond ]. Prefix to words of Latin derivation, signifying in excess, above, superior, or in the upper part of; often the same as *supra*; it corresponds to the Greek prefix *hyper-*; for some words beginning with super- and not found here, see hyper-.

**superabduc'tion.** Abduction of a limb beyond the normal limit.

**superacid'ity.** Hyperacidity; hyperchlorhydria; an excess of acid; specifically excessive acidity of the gastric juice.

**superacro'mial.** Above the acromion process.

**superactiv'ity.** Hyperactivity; abnormally great activity.

**superacute** (su'per-ă-kūt'). Extremely acute; marked by great severity of symptoms and rapid progress; denoting the course of a disease.

**superalbu'mino'sis.** Hyperalbuminosis.

**superalimenta'tion.** Hyperalimentation.

**superalkalin'ity.** Excessive alkalinity.

**supercil'iary.** Relating to or in the region of the eyebrow.

**supercilium,** pl. **supercilia** (su'per-sil'ī-um, -ah) [ L. fr. *super*, above, + *cilium*, eyelid ] [ NA ]. 1. Eyebrow; the crescentic line of hairs at the superior edge of the orbit. 2. An individual hair of the eyebrow.

**superdicrot'ic.** Hyperdicrotic.

**su'perdisten'tion.** Hyperdistention.

**superduct'** [ L. *super-duco*, pp. *-ductus*, to lead over ]. To elevate or draw upward.

**supere'go.** In psychoanalytic theory, an outgrowth of the ego that has identified itself unconsciously with important persons, such as the parents, from early life, and which results from incorporating the values and wishes of these persons as part of one's own standards to form the "conscience."

**superexcita'tion.** Surexcitation. 1. The act of exciting or stimulating unduly. 2. Overstimulation; a condition of extreme excitement.

**superexten'sion.** Hyperextension.

**superfat'ted.** With additional fat added, as in the case of soap.

**superfecundation** (su'per-fe-kun-da'shun) [ super- + L. *fecundus*, fertile ]. The impregnation of two or more ova, liberated at the same ovulation, by successive acts of coitus.

**superfeta'tion.** Hypercyesis; the presence of two fetuses of different ages, not twins, in the uterus; due to the impregnation of two ova liberated at successive periods of ovulation.

**superfi'brina'tion.** The presence of an excessive amount of fibrin or fibrinogen in the blood or other body fluids.

**superficial** (su'per-fish'al) [ L. *superficialis*, fr. *superficies*, surface ]. 1. On, near, or relating to the surface; sublimis. 2. Cursory; not thorough.

**superficia'lis** [ L. ] [ NA ]. Superficial; denoting a number of nerves, arteries, veins, and other structures near the surface of the body.

    **s. vo'lae,** *ramus* palmaris superficialis arteriae radialis.

**superficies** (su-per-fish'ī-ēz) [ L. the top surface, fr. *super*, above, + *facies*, figure, form ]. Outer surface; facies.

**superflex'ion.** Hyperflexion.

**supergen'ual.** Above the knee or any genu.

**superimpregna'tion.** 1. Superfecundation. 2. Superfeta-tion.

**superinduce** (su'per-in-dūs). To induce or bring on in addition to something already existing.

**superinfection** (su-per-in-fek'shun). A fresh infection added to one of the same nature already present.

**superinvolu'tion.** Hyperinvolution; an extreme reduction in size of the uterus, after childbirth, below the normal size of the nongravid organ.

**superior** (su-pēr'ī-or) [ L. comparative of *superus*, above ] [ NA ]. Above in relation to another structure; higher; cephalic.

**superlacta'tion.** Hyperlaction; the continuance of lactation beyond the normal period.

**superliga'men** [ L. *ligamen*, bandage ]. A retentive dressing; a bandage retaining a surgical dressing in place.

**superme'dial.** Above the middle of any part.

**su'permotil'ity.** Hyperkinesis; the capability of motion in excess of the normal.

**su'pernate.** Jargon for supernatant fluid.

**supernumerary** (su'per-nu'mer-ēr-ī) [ super- + L. *numerus*, number ]. Accessory; epactal; exceeding the normal number.

**supernutrition** (su-per-nu-trish'un). Hypernutrition; overeating leading to obesity.

**superolat'eral.** At the side and above.

**su'perovula'tion.** Ovulation of a greater than normal number of ova; usually the result of the administration of exogenous gonadotropins.

**superox'ide.** The molecule $HO_2$, a strong acid, hence often written as $H^+ + \cdot O_2^-$, the latter being the superoxide radical.

    **s. dismutase,** the enzyme (EC 1.15.1.1) decomposing the superoxide radical to $O_2 + H_2O_2$ (with consumption of hydrogen ion); a metalloprotein (also known as erythrocuprein, hemocuprein, or cytocuprein).

**superpar'asite.** A member of a large population of parasites living on a host, usually a parasitic hymenopteran larva in its insect host.

**superpar'asitism.** 1. Association between parasitic Hymenoptera and their insect hosts. 2. An excess of parasites in a host, overtaxing the defense mechanism to the degree that disease results.

**superpetro'sal.** Above or at the upper part of the petrous portion of the temporal bone.

**superphos'phate.** A mixture of calcium phosphate and calcium sulfate, in much use as a fertilizer.

**superpigmenta'tion.** Hyperpigmentation.

**supersat'urate.** To make a solution hold more of a salt or other substance in solution than it will dissolve when in equilibrium with that salt in the solid phase. Supersaturated solutions are usually unstable with respect to becoming saturated.

**superscription** (su'per-skrip'shun) [ L. *super-scribo*, pp. *-scriptus*, to write upon or over ]. The beginning of a prescription, consisting of the injunction, *recipe*, take, usually denoted by the sign ℞.

**supersonic** (su'per-son'ik) [ super- + L. *sonus*, sound ]. 1. Pertaining to or characterized by a speed greater than the speed of sound; see also hypersonic. 2. Pertaining to sound vibrations of high frequency above the level of human audibility; see also ultrasonic.

**superstruc'ture.** A structure above the surface.

    **implant denture s.,** the denture which is retained and stabilized by the implant denture substructure.

**superten'sion.** Extreme tension; incorrectly used as a synonym of high blood pressure, or hyperpiesis.

**supervenos'ity.** A state of incomplete oxidation of the blood.

**supervoltage.** High kilovoltage above 1000 kv.

**supinate** (su'pī-nāt) [ L. *supino*, pp. *-atus*, to bend backwards, place on back, fr. *supinus*, supine ]. To turn the forearm and hand palmar side uppermost.

**supination** (su'pī-na'shun). The act of supinating; the state of being supinated, or turned palmar side upward, referring to the hand, or with the face and abdomen upward, referring to the body; opposite of pronation.

**su'pinator.** A muscle that produces supination of the forearm; see under musculus.

**supine** (su-pīn') [ L. *supinus* ]. Lying on the back; supinated or in a position of supination.

**supi'nus** [ L. ] [ NA ]. Supine.

**suppedanium,** pl. **suppedania** (sup'e-da'nī-um, -ah) [ Late L. a footstool, fr. L. *sub*, beneath, + *pes*, foot ]. An application to the sole of the foot.

**support** (su-port') [ L. *supporto*, to carry ]. In dentistry, a term used to denote resistance to vertical components of masticatory force.

**suppository** (su-poz'ī-tōr-ī) [ L. *suppositorium*, fr. *suppositorius*, placed underneath ]. A small solid body shaped for ready introduction into one of the orifices of the body other than the oral cavity, made of a substance, usually medicated, which is solid at ordinary temperatures but melts at body temperature. S. bases usually used are theobroma oil, glycerinated gelatin, hydrogenated vegetable oils, mixtures of polyethylene glycols of various molecular weights and fatty acid esters of polyethylene glycol.

    **evacuant s.,** a s. made for insertion into the rectum for stimulation thereof, to result in evacuation of its contents.

    **rectal s.,** a cone- or spindle-shaped s., weighing about 2.0 gm.

    **urethral s.,** urethral bougie; a pencil-shaped s., pointed at one extremity, either 2.8 in. (7 cm.) or 5.6 in. (14 cm.)

in length, and weighing 2.0 or 4.0 gm. when made of glycerinated gelatin.

**vaginal s.,** a globular or egg-shaped s., weighing about 5.0 gm.

**suppression** (sŭ-presh'un) [ L. *sub-primo* (*subp*-), pp. -*pressus*, to press down, fr. *premo*, to press ]. 1. Deliberately excluding from conscious thought, as distinguished from repression (*q.v.*). 2. Arrest of the secretion of a fluid, as urine or bile, to be distinguished from retention, in which secretion occurs but the discharge from the body is prevented. 3. Checking of an abnormal flow or discharge, as in s. of a hemorrhage. 4. The effect of a second mutation, that cancels a phenotypic change caused by a previous mutation at a different point on the chromosome.

**sup'purant** [ L. *suppurans*, causing suppuration ]. 1. Causing or inducing suppuration. 2. An agent with this action.

**sup'purate** [ L. *sup-puro* (*subp*-), pp. -*atus*, to form *pus* (*pur*), pus ]. To form pus.

**suppuration** (sup'u-ra'shun) [ L. *suppuratio* (see suppurate) ]. Pyesis; pyosis; pyopoiesis; pyogenesis; the formation of pus.

**sup'purative.** Forming pus.

**supra-** (su'prah-) [ L. above ]. Prefix denoting a position above the part indicated by the word to which it is joined; often signifying the same as super-.

**supra-acro'mial.** Superacromial.

**supra-a'nal.** Superanal; above the anus.

**supra-auric'ular.** Above the auricle or pinna of the ear.

**supra-ax'illary.** Above the axilla.

**suprabuc'cal.** Above the cheek.

**suprabulge** (su'prah-bulj'). The portion of the crown of a tooth that converges toward the occlusal surface of the tooth.

**supracar'dinal.** Lying dorsal to the anterior or posterior cardinal veins in the embryo.

**supracerebel'lar.** On or above the surface of the cerebellum.

**supracer'ebral.** On or above the surface of the cerebrum.

**suprachoroid** (su-prah-ko'royd). On the outer side of the choroid of the eye.

**suprachoroidea** (su'prah-ko-roy'dĭ-ah). *Lamina* suprachoroidea.

**supracil'iary.** Superciliary.

**supraclavic'ular.** Above the clavicle.

**supraclavicula'ris.** See under musculus.

**supracon'dylar, supracon'dyloid.** Above a condyle.

**supracos'tal.** Above the ribs.

**supracot'yloid.** Above the cotyloid cavity, or acetabulum.

**supracris'tal.** Above a crest.

**supradiaphragmat'ic.** Above the diaphragm.

**supraduc'tion.** Sursumduction; the moving upward of one eye independently of its fellow by base-down prisms.

**supraep'icon'dylar.** Above an epicondyle.

**supragle'noid.** Above the glenoid cavity or fossa.

**supraglot'tic.** Above the glottis.

**suprahepat'ic.** Above the liver.

**suprahy'oid.** Above the hyoid bone.

**suprain'guinal.** Above the inguinal region, or groin.

**supraintes'tinal.** Above the intestine.

**supraliminal** (su'prah-lim'ĭ-nal) [ supra- + L. *limen*, threshold ]. More than just perceptible; above the threshold for conscious awareness.

**supralum'bar.** Above the lumbar region.

**supramalle'olar.** Above a malleolus.

**supramam'mary.** Above the mammary gland.

**supramandib'ular.** Above the mandible.

**supramar'ginal.** Above any margin; denoting especially the s. gyrus.

**supramas'toid.** Above the mastoid process of the temporal bone.

**supramaxil'la.** The maxilla.

**supramax'illary.** Relating to the maxilla.

**supramen'tal.** Above the chin.

**supramenta'le** [ supra- + L. *mentum*, chin ]. Point B; in cephalometrics, the most posterior midline point, above the chin, on the mandibula between the infradentate and the pogonion.

**suprana'sal.** Above the nose.

**supraneu'ral.** Above the neural axis.

**supranuclear** (su'prah-nu'kle-ar). Above (cranial to) the level of the motor neurons of the spinal or cranial nerves. The term is used in clinical neurology to indicate disorders of movement caused by destruction or functional impairment of brain structures other than the motor neurons, such as the motor cortex, pyramidal tract, or corpus striatum; *e.g.*, supranuclear palsy, as distinguished from the nuclear (or flaccid, or "lower motor neuron") paralysis that results from destruction or functional impairment of the motor neurons or their axons in a peripheral nerve.

**supraocclusion** (su'pro-o-klu'zhun). An occlusal relationship in which a tooth extends beyond the occlusal plane.

**supraor'bital.** Above the orbit, either on the face or within the cranium; denoting numerous structures, see canalis, foramen, incisura, nerve, etc.

**suprapatel'lar.** Above the patella.

**suprapel'vic.** Above the pelvis.

**suprapu'bic.** Above the pubic arch.

**suprarenal** (su'prah-re'nal) [ supra- + L. *ren*, kidney ]. 1. Above the kidney. 2. Pertaining to the glandula suprarenalis.

**suprare'nalec'tomy.** Adrenalectomy.

**suprarenogenic** (su-prah-re-no-jen'ik). Obsolete term for adrenogenic.

**suprarenopathy** (su-prah-re-nop'a-thĭ). Obsolete term for adrenalopathy.

**suprarenotrophic** (su'prah-re-no-trof'ic). Obsolete term for adrenocorticotrophic.

**suprascap'ular.** Above the scapula.

**suprascle'ral.** On the outer side of the sclera, denoting the s. or perisclerotic space between the sclera and the fascia bulbi.

**suprasel'lar.** Above or over the sella turcica.

**supraspi'nal.** Above the vertebral column or any spine.

**supraspina'lis.** See under musculus.

**supraspina'tus.** See under musculus.

**supraspi'nous.** Above any spine; especially above one or more of the vertebral spines or the spine of the scapula.

**suprastape'dial.** Above the stapes.

**supraster'nal.** Above the sternum; episternal.

**suprasterol I and II** (su'pra-stēr'ol). Two products (isomers) among many produced in the irradiation of ergosterol, calciferol, or toxisterol.

**suprasyl'vian.** Above the fissure of Sylvius.

**suprasymphysary** (su-prah-sim-phiz'ā-rĭ). Above the symphysis pubis.

**supratem'poral.** Supertemporal.

**suprathoracic** (su-prah-tho-ras'ik). Above or in the upper part of the thorax.

**supraton'sillar.** Above the tonsil; denoting a recess above and slightly back of the tonsil.

**supratrochlear** (su-prah-trok'le-ar). Above a trochlea.

**supratur'binal.** *Concha* nasalis suprema.

**supratympan'ic.** Above the tympanic cavity.

**supravaginal** (su-prah-vaj'ĭ-nal). Above the vagina, or above any sheath.

**supraval'var, supraval'vular.** Above the valves, either pulmonary or aortic.

**supraventric'ular.** Above the ventricles; especially applied to rhythms originating from centers proximal to the ventricles, namely in the atrium or A-V node, in contrast to rhythms arising in the ventricles themselves.

**supravergence** (su'prah-ver'jens) [ supra- + L. *vergo*, to incline or turn ]. Sursumvergence; upward rotation of an eye, the other eye remaining stationary.

**supraversion** (su'prah-ver'zhun) [ supra- + L. *verto*, pp. *versus*, to turn ]. 1. A turning (version) upward. 2. In dentistry, the position of a tooth when it is out of the line of occlusion in an occlusal direction; a deep overbite. 3. In ophthalmology, binocular conjugate movement upward.

**sura** (su'rah) [ L. ] [ NA ]. Calf of the leg; the muscular swelling of the back of the leg below the knee, formed chiefly by the bellies of the gastrocnemius and soleus muscles.

**su'ral.** Relating to the calf of the leg.

**suralimentation** (sur-al'ī-man-ta'shun) [ Fr. *sur*, fr. L. *super*, above ]. Superalimentation.

**su'ramin sodium** (USP). Suramin (BP); sodium suramin (NF); ANTRYPOL; GERMANIN; NAPHURIDE; BAYER 205; NAGANOL; a complex derivative of urea; $C_{51}H_{34}N_6O_{23}S_6\cdot Na_6$; used in the treatment of trypanosomiasis, onchocerciasis, and pemphigus.

**sur'dity** [ L. *surditas*, fr. *surdu*, deaf ]. Deafness.

**sur'domute.** 1. Deaf and dumb. 2. A deafmute.

**sur'excita'tion** [ Fr. *sur*; L. *super*, above ]. Superexcitation.

**sur'face** [ F. fr. L. *superficius*, see superficial ]. The outer part of any solid; see also facies.

acromial articular s. of clavicle, *facies* articularis acromialis claviculae.

s. of acromion, *facies* articularis acromii.

anterior s., *facies* anterior.

anterior articular s. of dens, *facies* articularis anterior dentis.

anterior s. of eyelid, *facies anterior palpebrarum.*

anterior s. of maxilla, *facies* anterior maxillae.

anterior s. of patella, *facies* anterior patellae.

anterior s. of petrous part of temporal bone, *facies* anterior partis petrosae.

articular s., *facies* articularis.

articular s. of head of fibula, *facies* articularis capitis fibulae.

articular s. of head of rib, *facies* articularis capitis costae.

articular s. of patella, *facies* articularis patellae.

articular s. of tubercle of rib, *facies* articularis tuberculi costae.

arytenoidal articular s., *facies* articularis arytenoidea.

auricular s. of ilium, *facies* auricularis ossis ilii.

auricular s. of sacrum, *facies* auricularis ossis sacri.

axial s., the s. of a tooth parallel with its long axis; the axial s.'s are the vestibular (labial or buccal), lingual, and contact (mesial or distal).

balancing occlusal s., balancing *contact.*

basal s., the s. of the denture of which the detail is determined by the impression and which rests upon the basal seat.

buccal s., (1) *facies* vestibularis; (2) the mucosa of the cheek; (3) in prosthodontics, the side of a denture adjacent to the cheek.

calcaneal articular s. of talus, *facies* articularis calcanea tali.

carpal articular s. of radius, *facies* articularis carpea radii.

cerebral s., *facies* cerebralis.

cerebral s. of greater wing of sphenoid, *facies* cerebralis alae majoris.

cerebral s. of squamous part of temporal bone, *facies* cerebralis partis squamosae.

colic s., *facies* colica.

contact s., *facies* contactus.

costal s. of lung, *facies* costalis pulmonis.

costal s. of scapula, *facies* costalis scapulae.

cuboidal articular s. of calcaneus, *facies* articularis cuboidea calcanei.

denture basal s., denture foundation s.

denture foundation s., denture basal s.; that portion of the s. of a denture which has its contour determined by the impression and bears the greater part of the occlusal load.

denture impression s., that portion of the s. of a denture which has its contour determined by the impression. It includes the borders of the denture and extends to the polished s.

denture occlusal s., occlusal s. (2); that portion of the s. of a denture that makes contact or near contact with the corresponding s. of an opposing denture or facies masticatoria.

denture polished s., that portion of the denture which extends in an occlusal direction from the border of the denture and includes the palatal s.; it is the part of the denture base which is usually polished and includes the buccal and lingual s.'s of the teeth.

diaphragmatic s. of heart, *facies* diaphragmatica cordis.

diaphragmatic s. of liver, *facies* diaphragmatica hepatis.

diaphragmatic s. of lung, *facies* diaphragmatica pulmonis.

distal s., *facies* distalis.

dorsal s. of sacrum, *facies* dorsalis ossis sacri.

dorsal s. of scapula *facies* dorsalis scapulae.

external s. of frontal bone, *facies* externa ossis frontalis.

external s. of parietal bone, *facies* externa ossis parietalis.

facial s., *facies* vestibularis.

fibular s., *facies* fibularis.

fibular articular s. of tibia, *facies* articularis fibularis tibiae.

gastric s., *facies* gastrica.

glenoid s., *cavitas* glenoidalis.

gluteal s. of ilium, *facies* glutea ossis ilii.

grinding s., *facies* occlusalis.

incisal s., incisal *edge.*

inferior articular s. of tibia, *facies* articularis inferior tibiae.

inferior s. of cerebellar hemisphere, *facies* inferior hemispherii cerebelli.

inferior s. of petrous part of temporal bone, *facies* inferior partis petrosae.

inferior s. of tongue, *facies* inferior linguae.

infratemporal s. of maxilla, *facies* infratemporalis maxillae.

interlobar s.'s of lung, *facies* interlobares pulmonis.

internal s. of frontal bone, *facies* interna ossis frontalis.

internal s. of parietal bone, *facies* interna ossis parietalis.

intestinal s. of uterus, *facies* intestinalis uteri.

labial s., (1) of a tooth, *facies* vestibularis; (2) the inner s. of the lip itself.

lateral s., *facies* lateralis.

lateral malleolar s., *facies* malleolaris lateralis.

lingual s., *facies* lingualis.

lunate s. of acetabulum, *facies* lunata acetabuli.

malleolar s., *facies* malleolaris.

malleolar articular s. of fibula, *facies* articularis malleoli fibulae.

malleolar articular s. of tibia, *facies* articularis malleoli tibiae.

masticating s., *facies* occlusalis.

masticatory s., *facies* occlusalis.

maxillary s., *facies* maxillaris.

maxillary s. of palatine bone, *facies* maxillaris ossis palatini.

maxillary s. of sphenoid bone, *facies* maxillaris ossis sphenoidalis.

medial s., *facies* medialis.

medial s. of cerebral hemisphere, *facies* medialis cerebri.

medial s. of lung, *facies* medialis pulmonis.

medial malleolar s., *facies* malleolaris medialis.

mesial s., *facies* mesialis.

nasal s. of maxilla, *facies* nasalis maxillae.

navicular articular s. of talus, *facies* articularis navicularis tali.

occlusal s., (1) *facies* occlusalis; (2) denture occlusal s.

orbital s. of maxilla, *facies* orbitalis maxillae.

palatine s., *facies* palatina.

palmar s., *facies* palmaris.

patellar s. of femur, *facies* patellaris femoris.

pelvic s. of sacrum, *facies* pelvina ossis sacri.

plantar s., *facies* plantaris.

popliteal s. of femur, *facies* poplitea femoris.

posterior s., *facies* posterior.

posterior articular s. of dens, *facies* articularis posterior dentis.

posterior s. of eyelid, *facies* posterior palpebrarum.

posterior s. of petrous part of temporal bone, *facies* posterior partis petrosae.

pulmonary s. of heart, *facies* pulmonalis cordis.

radial s., *facies* radialis.

renal s., *facies* renalis.

sacropelvic s. of ilium, *facies* sacropelvina ossis ilii.

sternal articular s. of clavicle, *facies* articularis sternalis claviculae.

sternocostal s. of heart, *facies* sternocostalis cordis.

subocclusal s., a portion of the occlusal s. of a tooth which is below the level of the occluding portion of the tooth.

**superior s.,** *facies* superior.

**superior articular s. of tibia,** *facies* articularis superior tibiae.

**superior s. of cerebellar hemisphere,** *facies* superior hemispherii cerebelli.

**superolateral s. of cerebrum,** *facies* superolateralis cerebri.

**symphysial s. of pubis,** *facies* symphysialis.

**talar articular s. of calcaneus,** *facies* articularis talaris calcanei.

**temporal s.,** *facies* temporalis.

**thyroidal articular s.,** *facies* articularis thyroidea.

**tibial s.,** *facies* tibialis.

**ulnar s.,** *facies* ulnaris.

**urethral s. of penis,** *facies* urethralis penis.

**vesical s. of uterus,** *facies* vesicalis uteri.

**vestibular s.,** *facies* vestibularis.

**visceral s. of liver,** *facies* visceralis hepatis.

**visceral s. of the spleen,** *facies* visceralis lienis.

**working occlusal s.'s,** the s.'s of teeth upon which mastication can occur.

**surface-active.** Indicating the property of certain agents of altering the physicochemical nature of surfaces and interfaces, bringing about lowering of interfacial tension. surface-active compounds (*e.g.*, detergents) usually possess both lipophilic and hydrophilic groups. See also surfactant.

**surfactant** (sur-fak′tant). A surface-active agent. 1. Includes substances commonly referred to as wetting agents, surface tension depressants, detergents, dispersing agents, emulsifiers, quaternary ammonium antiseptics, etc. 2. Term in current use to describe those surface-active agents forming a monomolecular layer over pulmonary alveolar surfaces. It stabilizes alveolar volume by reducing surface tension and altering the relationship between surface tension and surface area.

**surgeon** (sur′jun) [ G. *cheirourgos;* L. *chirurgus.* CHIR- ]. 1. A physician who treats disease or injury by operation or manipulation. 2. In England, formerly a general practitioner, one without a degree of M.D. but with the license of the Royal College of Surgeons.

**acting assistant s.,** a noncommissioned s. in one of the public services who has the duties of an assistant s., but is not in line of promotion.

**assistant s.,** a member of the junior grade of s.'s in one of the public services, a newly appointed member of the medical corps.

**dental s.,** dentist.

**house s.,** the senior member of the house staff on the surgical side, who is responsible for the execution of the orders of the attending s. and who acts in his place when the latter is absent.

**oral s.,** a kind of dentist; a specialist in the surgery of the soft tissue and bony areas of the mouth. The term should not be identified with dentist unmodified.

**passed assistant s.,** an assistant s. in one of the public services who has passed the examination entitling him to the rank of s. when a vacancy occurs.

**surgeon-apothecary.** In England, a general practitioner who has not the M.D. degree, but has the license of the Royal College of Surgeons and the Apothecaries' Hall.

**surgeon-general.** The chief medical officer in the United States Army, Navy, Air Force, or Public Health Service. In some foreign military services any member of the medical corps who has the rank of general, not necessarily the chief medical officer.

**surgery** (sur′je̅-rī) [ L. *chirurgia;* G. *cheir,* hand, + *ergon,* work. CHIR- ]. The branch of medicine that is concerned with therapy of diseases or injuries by operation or manipulation.

**aseptic s.,** the performance of an operation, in a field free from pyogenic or septic germs, with sterilized hands, instruments, etc., preventing the introduction of germs from without.

**closed s.,** s. without incision into skin, *e.g.,* reduction of a fracture or dislocation.

**conservative s.,** surgical treatment that aims to preserve and restore injured or diseased parts, avoiding operative mutilation or removal.

**dental s.,** oral s.

**featural s.,** plastic s. of the face, having for its object th‹ correction of congenital defects in the nose and othe‹ features.

**major s.,** operative s. in which the operation itself i‹ hazardous, as in amputation above the ankle or wrist‹ abdominal and cerebral s., the removal of large tumors‹ etc.

**minor s.,** s. that has to do with slight and not hazardou‹ operations, the application of splints, bandages, etc.

**open heart s.,** direct vision correction of intracardia‹ disease.

**oral s.,** dental s.; the branch of dentistry devoted to th‹ treatment of oral disorders by surgical means.

**orificial s.,** Pratt's method; an obsolete therapeuti‹ system based on the notion that many morbid condition‹ are caused by reflexes originating at the anus or othe‹ orifices, and that they can be relieved by dilation or othe‹ forms of treatment of these body openings.

**orthopaedic s.,** the branch of s. that embraces th‹ treatment of deformities and of chronic joint diseases. Se‹ also orthopaedics.

**plastic s.,** the branch of operative s. that has to do wit‹ the repair of defects, the results of loss of tissue, o‹ extensive cicatrices, etc., by direct union of parts, b‹ grafting, the transfer of tissue from one part to another, etc.

**stereotactic s., stereotaxic s.,** Stereotaxy.

**transsexual s.,** transsexualism (2); procedures designed‹ to alter a patient's external sexual characteristics so that‹ they resemble those of the other sex.

**veterinary s.,** s. dealing with the diseases and injuries of‹ animals other than man.

**surgical** (sur′ji̅-kal). Relating to surgery.

**surra** (soor′ah) [ East Indian name ]. A disease of horses, mules, and cattle in Mauritius, Africa, Southern Asia, and the Philippines, caused by the presence in the blood of *Trypanosoma evansi,* infection probably occurring through mechanical transmission by a bloodsucking species of *Stomoxys* or *Tabanus,* or both. The symptoms are anemia, ecchymoses, edema, and emaciation; the disease is pathogenic to all domestic animals. The effect on the host depends upon the virulence of the strain of pathogen and the susceptibility of the host. Camels are severely affected, as are horses in North Africa but not in the Sudan; in dogs, the course of infection is acute; laboratory animals rapidly succumb. See also murrina.

**surrenal** (su̅r-re′nal). Suprarenal (1).

**surrogate** (sur′o-ga̅t) [ L. *surrogare,* to put in another's place ]. 1. A person who functions in another's life as a substitute for some third person. 2. A person who reminds one of another person so that one uses the first as an emotional substitute for the second.

**mother s.,** one who substitutes for or takes the place of the mother.

**sursa′nure** [ Fr. fr. L. *super,* over, + *sanus,* healthy ]. A superficially healed ulcer, with pus beneath the surface.

**sursumduction** (sur′sum-duk′shun) [ L. *sursum,* upward, + *duco,* pp. -*ductus,* to draw ]. Supraduction.

**sursumvergence** (sur-sum-ver′jens) [ L. *sursum,* upward, + *vergo,* to bend ]. Supravergence.

**sursumversion** (sur-sum-ver′zhun) [ L. *sursum,* upward, + *verto,* pp. *versus,* to turn ]. The act of moving the eyes upward.

**surveying** (sur-va′ing). In dentistry, the procedure of locating and delineating the contour and position of the abutment teeth and associated structures before designing a removable partial denture.

**survey′or** (sur-va′or). In dentistry, the instrument used in surveying.

**survival** (sur-vi′val). Continued existence.

**five-year s.,** s. for five years after diagnosis or commencing treatment, with no evidence of the continued presence of disease; this does not necessarily mean that the patient is cured.

**suscitate** (sus′i̅-ta̅t) [ L. *suscito,* pp. *suscitatus,* to excite ]. To stimulate; to arouse to increased activity.

**suscitation** (sus′i̅-ta′shun). Excitation.

**susotoxin** (sus′o-tok′sin) [ L. *sus,* hog, + G. *toxikon,* poison ]. A toxin extracted from a pure culture of the hog cholera bacillus.

**suspen′sion** [ L. *suspensio*, fr. *sus-pendo*, pp. *-pensus*, to hang up, suspend, fr. *sub*, under, + *pendo*, to hang ]. 1. A temporary interruption of any function. 2. A hanging from a support, as used in the treatment of spinal curvatures or during the application of a plaster jacket. 3. Fixation of an organ, *e.g.*, uterus, to other tissue for support. 4. The dispersion through a liquid of a solid in finely divided particles of a size large enough to be detected by purely optical means. If the particles are too small to be seen by microscope but still large enough to scatter light (Tyndall phenomenon) they will remain dispersed indefinitely and are then called a colloidal s. 5. A class of pharmacopeial preparations of finely divided, undissolved drugs (*e.g.*, powders for s.) dispersed in liquid vehicles for oral or parenteral use; s.'s for parenteral use are sterile.

   **Coffey s.**, an operative technique following partial excision of the cornu as in salpingectomy whereby the broad and the round ligament are sutured over the cornual wound in order to reperitonize the area and to suspend the uterus on the operated side.

**suspensoid** (sus-pen′soyd) [ suspension + G. *eidos*, resemblance ]. Suspension colloid; a colloid solution in which the disperse particles are solid and lyophobe or hydrophobe, and are therefore sharply demarcated from the fluid in which they are suspended; distinguished from emulsoid.

**suspen′sory**. 1. Suspending; supporting; denoting a ligament, a muscle, or other structure the office of which is to keep an organ or other part in place. 2. Denoting a bandage applied as a support to a dependent part, such as the scrotum or a pendulous breast.

**sustentac′ular**. Relating to a sustentaculum; supporting.

**sustentaculum,** pl. **sustentacula** (sus′ten-tak′u-lum, -lah) [ L. a prop, fr. *sustento*, to hold upright ] [ NA ]. A structure that serves as a stay or support to another.

   **s. li′enis**, *ligamentum* phrenicocolicum.

   **s. ta′li** [ NA ], support of the talus; a bracket-like lateral projection from the medial surface of the calcaneus, the upper surface of which presents a facet for articulation with the talus.

**susur′rus** [ L. ]. Murmur.

   **s. aurium**, murmur in the ear.

**Sutherland,** Earl W., U. S. pharmacologist, 1915–1974. Nobel laureate, 1971, for his study in mechanisms of hormone actions.

**Sutter blood group.** See appendix 2, Blood Groups.

**Sutton,** Henry G., English physician, 1837–1891. See Gull-S. *disease.*

**Sutton,** Richard L., U. S. dermatologist, 1878–1952. See S.'s *disease, nevus.*

**Sutton,** Richard L., Jr., U. S. dermatologist, *1908. See S.'s *disease, ulcer.*

# SUTURA

**sutura,** pl. **suturae** (su′tu′rah, -re) [ L. a sewing, a suture, fr. *suo*, pp. *sutus*, to sew ]. 1. A suture in any sense. 2 [ NA ]. Suture joint; a form of fibrous joint in which two bones formed in membrane are united by a fibrous membrane continuous with the periosteum. See fig. under joint.

   **s. corona′lis** [ NA ], coronal suture; the line of junction of the frontal with the two parietal bones of the skull.

   **suturae cra′nii** [ NA ], cranial sutures; the sutures between the bones of the skull. See color plates 19 and 20.

   **s. ethmoidomaxilla′ris** [ NA ], ethmoidomaxillary suture; line of apposition of the orbital surface of the body of the maxilla with the orbital plate of the ethmoid bone.

   **s. fronta′lis** [ NA ], frontal suture; the suture between the two halves of the frontal bone, usually obliterated by about the sixth year; if persistent it is called s. metopica.

   **s. frontoethmoida′lis** [ NA ], frontoethmoidal suture; line of union between the cribriform plate of the ethmoid and the orbital plate and posterior margin of the nasal process of the frontal bone.

   **s. frontolacrima′lis** [ NA ], frontolacrimal suture; line of union between the upper margin of the lacrimal and the orbital plate of the frontal bone.

   **s. frontomaxilla′ris** [ NA ], frontomaxillary suture; articulation of the frontal process of the maxilla with the frontal bone.

   **s. frontonasa′lis** [ NA ], frontonasal suture; line of union of the frontal and of the two nasal bones.

   **s. frontozygomat′ica** [ NA ], frontozygomatic suture; line of union between the zygomatic process of the frontal and the frontal process of the zygomatic bone.

   **s. inci′siva** [ NA ], incisive suture; premaxillary suture; line of union of the two portions of the maxilla (pre- and postmaxilla); it is present at birth but may persist into old age.

   **s. infraorbita′lis** [ NA ], an inconstant suture running from the infraorbital foramen to the infraorbital groove.

   **s. intermaxilla′ris** [ NA ], intermaxillary suture; the line of union of the two maxillae.

   **s. internasa′lis** [ NA ], internasal suture; line of union between the two nasal bones.

   **s. interparieta′lis**, s. sagittalis.

   **s. lacrimoconcha′lis** [ NA ], lacrimoconchal suture; line of union of the lacrimal bone with the inferior nasal concha.

   **s. lacrimomaxilla′ris** [ NA ], lacrimomaxillary suture; line of union, on the medial wall of the orbit, between the anterior and inferior margin of the lacrimal bone and the maxilla.

   **s. lambdoi′dea** [ NA ], lambdoid suture; line of union between the occipital and the parietal bones.

   **s. meto′pica** [ NA ], metopic suture; a persistent frontal suture, sometimes discernible a short distance above s. frontonasalis.

   **s. nasofronta′lis**, s. frontonasalis.

   **s. nasomaxilla′ris** [ NA ], nasomaxillary suture; line of union of the lateral margin of the nasal bone with the frontal process of the maxilla.

   **s. notha** (no′tah) [ G. fem. of *nothos*, spurious ], false *suture.*

   **s. occipitomastoi′dea** [ NA ], occipitomastoid suture; continuation of the lambdoid suture between the posterior border of the mastoid portion of the temporal bone and the occipital.

   **s. palati′na media′na** [ NA ], median palatine suture; line of union between the horizontal plates of the palate bones, continuing the intermaxillary suture posteriorly.

   **s. palati′na transversa** [ NA ], transverse palatine suture; line of union of the palatine processes of the maxillae with the horizontal plates of the palatine bones.

   **s. palatoethmoida′lis** [ NA ], palatoethmoidal suture; line of junction of the orbital process of the palatine bone and the orbital plate of the ethmoid.

   **s. palatomaxilla′ris** [ NA ], palatomaxillary suture; line of union, in the floor of the orbit, between the orbital process of the palatine bone and the orbital surface of the maxilla.

   **s. parietomastoi′dea** [ NA ], parietomastoid suture; articulation of the posterior inferior angle of the parietal with the mastoid process of the temporal bone.

   **s. pla′na** [ NA ], plane suture; harmonic suture; a simple firm apposition of two smooth surfaces of bones, without overlap, as seen in the lacrimomaxillary suture.

   **s. sagitta′lis** [ NA ], sagittal suture; line of union between the two parietal bones.

   **s. serra′ta** [ NA ], serrate suture; one whose opposing margins present deep sawlike indentations, as most of the sagittal suture.

   **s. sphenoethmoida′lis** [ NA ], sphenoethmoidal suture; line of union between the crest of the sphenoid bone and the perpendicular and cribriform plates of the ethmoid.

   **s. sphenofronta′lis** [ NA ], sphenofrontal suture; line of union between the orbital plate of the frontal and the lesser wings of the sphenoid on either side.

   **s. sphenomaxilla′ris** [ NA ], sphenomaxillary suture; an inconstant suture between the pterygoid process of the sphenoid bone and the body of the maxilla.

   **s. sphenoparieta′lis** [ NA ], sphenoparietal suture; line of union of the lower border of the parietal with the upper edge of the greater wing of the sphenoid.

**s. sphenosquamo'sa** [ NA ], sphenosquamous suture; articulation of the greater wing of the sphenoid with the squamous portion of the temporal bone.

**s. sphenozygoma'tica** [ NA ], sphenozygomatic suture; junction of the zygomatic bone and greater wing of the sphenoid.

**s. squamo'sa** [ NA ], squamous suture; (1) a scalelike suture, one whose opposing margins are scalelike and overlapping; (2) specifically, the articulation of the parietal with the squamous portion of the temporal bone.

**s. squamosomastoi'dea** [ NA ], squamomastoid suture; petrosquamous suture; line of union of the squamous and petrous portions of the temporal bone during development; it sometimes persists in the region of the mastoid process.

**s. temporozygomat'ica** [ NA ], temporozygomatic suture; line of junction of the zygomatic process of the temporal and the temporal process of the zygomatic bone.

**s. zygomaticofronta'lis,** s. frontozygomatica.

**s. zygomaticomaxilla'ris** [ NA ], zygomaticomaxillary suture; articulation of the zygomatic bone with the zygomatic process of the maxilla.

**s. zygomaticotempora'lis,** s. temporozygomatica.

**sutural** (su'chur-al). Relating to a suture in any sense.
**sutura'tion.** The act of suturing.

# SUTURE

**suture** (su'chŭr) [ L. *sutura,* a seam ]. 1. Sutura. 2. The surgical uniting of two surfaces by means of stitches. 3. Chorda chirurgicalis; the material, silk thread, wire, catgut, etc., by means of which the two surfaces are kept in apposition. 4. The seam so formed, a surgical s.

**absorbable surgical s.** (1) a surgical s. material prepared from a substance that can be digested by the tissues of the wound and is therefore not permanent; see catgut; (2) (USP), a sterile strand prepared from collagen derived from healthy animals; various diameters and tensile strengths are available. May be absorbed by living mammalian tissue, may be treated to modify its resistance to absorption, and may be impregnated with antimicrobial agents. There are two types: type A (a plain s.) and type C (a chromic s. treated to resist absorption); both types are supplied in boilable and nonboilable forms.

**Albert's s.,** a modified Czerny s., the first row of stitches passing through the entire thickness of the wall of the gut.

**apposition s.,** coaptation s.; a s. of the skin only.

**approxima'tion s.,** one involving the deep tissues.

**atraumatic s.,** a s. onto the end of which an eyeless needle is swaged.

**blanket s.,** a continuous lock-stitch used to approximate the skin of a long wound.

**Bunnell's s.,** a method of tenorrhaphy using a pull-out wire affixed to buttons.

**buried s.,** any s. placed entirely below the surface of the skin.

**button s.,** one in which the threads are passed through the eyes of a button and then tied; used when there is danger of the threads cutting through the flesh.

**catgut s.,** a surgical s. material made from the collage fibers of the submucosa of the small intestine of sheep; it is completely digested by the activity of the wound tissues and therefore impermanent; see also catgut.

**coapta'tion s.,** apposition s.

**cobbler's s.,** one made with a thread having a needle at each end.

**continuous s.,** a long, back-and-forth series of stitches using one long piece of s. material fastened at each end by a knot.

**Connell's s.,** a continuous s. used for inverting the gastric or intestinal walls in performing an anastomosis.

**cor'onal s.,** *sutura coronalis.*

**cranial s.'s,** *suturae cranii.*

**Cushing's s.,** a continuous intestinal s.

**Sutures**

*Skin sutures: 1,* blanket; *2,* continuous, *3,* vertical mattress; *4,* interrupted; *5,* Halsted subcuticular. *Fascial sutures; 6,* near-and-far; *7,* figure-of-8. *Tendon suture: 8,* Bunnell wire pull-out. *Intestinal sutures: 9,* Connell; *10,* Lembert, continuous; *11,* Lembert, interrupted; *12,* Parker-Kerr; *13,* purse-string.

**Czerny's s.,** the first row of the Czerny-Lembert intestinal s.; the needle enters the serosa and passes out through the submucosa or muscularis, and then enters the submucosa or muscularis of the opposite side and emerges from the serosa. The second row is the Lembert s.

**Czerny-Lembert s.,** an intestinal s. in two rows combining the Czerny and the Lembert s.'s.

**delayed s.,** a suturing of a wound after an interval of days.

**dentate s.,** *sutura serrata.*

**doubly armed s.,** a s. armed with a needle at both ends.

**Dupuytren's s.,** a continuous Lembert s. (2).

**end-on mattress s.,** a vertical mattress stitch used for exact skin approximation.

**ethmoidomaxillary s.,** *sutura ethmoidomaxillaris.*

**false s.,** sutura notha; one whose opposing margins are smooth or present only a few ill-defined projections.

**far-and-near s.,** a stitch used to approximate fascial edges.

**figure-of-8 s.,** a stitch used to approximate fascial edges.

**frontal s.,** *sutura* frontalis.

**frontoethmoidal s.,** *sutura* frontoethmoidalis.

**frontolacrimal s.,** *sutura* frontolacrimalis.

**frontomaxillary s.,** *sutura* frontomaxillaris.

**frontonasal s.,** *sutura* frontonasalis.

**frontozygomatic s.,** *sutura* frontozygomatica.

**Gély's s.,** a cobbler's s. used in closing intestinal wounds.

**glover's s.,** a continuous s. in which each stitch is passed through the loop of the preceding one.

**Gould's s.,** an intestinal mattress s. in which each loop is invaginated in such a way that the tissue at the loop is bulged out, becoming convex instead of concave.

**Gussenbauer's s.,** a figure-of-8 s. for the intestine, resembling the Czerny-Lembert but not including the mucous membrane.

**Halsted's s.,** a stitch placed through the subcuticular fascia; used for exact skin approximation.

**harelip s.,** obsolete term for a s. formerly used for repairing cleft palate.

**harmon'ic s.,** *sutura* plana.

**implanted s.,** a pin is passed through each lip of the wound parallel to the line of incision and the pins are then tied together.

**incisive s.,** *sutura* incisiva.

**infraorbital s.,** *sutura* infraorbitalis.

**intermaxillary s.,** *sutura* intermaxillaris.

**internasal s.,** *sutura* internasalis.

**interpari'etal s.,** *sutura* sagittalis.

**interrupted s.,** a single stitch fixed by tying ends together.

**Jobert de Lamballe's s.,** an interrupted intestinal s., used for invaginating the margins of the intestines in circular enterorrhaphy.

**lacrimoconchal s.,** *sutura* lacrimoconchalis.

**lacrimomaxillary s.,** *sutura* lacrimomaxillaris.

**lambdoid s.,** *sutura* lambdoidea.

**Lembert s.,** an inverting s. for intestinal surgery, used either as a continuous s. or interrupted, producing serosal apposition and including the collagenous submucosal layer but not entering the lumen of the intestine.

**lens s.'s,** *radii* lentis.

**mattress s.,** quilted s.; a double stitch that forms a loop about the tissue on both sides of a wound, producing eversion of the edges when tied.

**median palatine s.,** *sutura* palatina mediana.

**meto'pic s.,** *sutura* metopica.

**nasomaxillary s.,** *sutura* nasomaxillaris.

**nerve s.,** neurorrhaphy.

**neurocentral s.,** neurocentral *synchondrosis*.

**nonabsorbable surgical s.'s,** suturing materials that are relatively unaffected by the cells and biological activities of the tissues of the body, and are therefore permanent unless removed; included are stainless steel, silk, cotton, nylon, and other synthetic materials.

**occipitomastoid s.,** *sutura* occipitomastoidea.

**palatoethmoidal s.,** *sutura* palatoethmoidalis.

**palatomaxillary s.,** *sutura* palatomaxillaris.

**Pancoast's s.,** union of two edges, in plastic surgery, by a tongue-and-groove arrangement.

**Paré's s.,** the approximation of the edges of a wound by pasting strips of cloth to the surface and stitching them instead of the skin.

**parietomastoid s.,** *sutura* parietomastoidea.

**Parker-Kerr s.,** a continuous inverting s. used to close an open end of intestine.

**petrosquam'ous s.,** see *fissura* petrosquamosa and *sutura* squamosomastoidea.

**plane s.,** *sutura* plana.

**premax'illary s.,** *sutura* incisiva.

**primo-secondary s.,** a s. passed through the edges of a wound, but not tied until the third day, when no evidences of infection have shown themselves.

**purse-string s.,** a continuous s. placed in a circular manner either for inversion (as for an appendiceal stump) or closure (as for a hernia).

**quilled s.,** one in which the threads are tied over a quill on either side of the line of incision, to prevent tearing out when there is much tension.

**quilted s.,** mattress s.

**relaxa'tion s.,** one so arranged that it may be loosened if the tension of the wound becomes excessive.

**Richter's s.,** an interrupted silver s. for wounds of the intestine.

**sagittal s.,** *sutura* sagittalis.

**secondary s.,** delayed closure of a wound.

**serrate s.,** *sutura* serrata.

**shotted s.,** one in which the ends are fastened by passing through a split shot which is then compressed.

**sphenoethmoidal s.,** *sutura* sphenoethmoidalis.

**sphenofrontal s.,** *sutura* sphenofrontalis.

**sphenomaxillary s.,** *sutura* sphenomaxillaris.

**sphenooccipital s.,** *synchondrosis* sphenooccipitalis.

**sphenoor'bital s.,** sutura sphenoorbitalis; articulation between the orbital process of the palatine bone and the outer surface of the body of the sphenoid.

**sphenoparietal s.,** *sutura* sphenoparietalis.

**sphenosquamous s.,** *sutura* sphenosquamosa.

**sphenozygomatic s.,** *sutura* sphenozygomatica.

**spiral s.,** a continuous s.

**squamomastoid s.,** *sutura* squamosomastoidea.

**squamopari'etal s.,** *sutura* squamosa (2).

**squamous s.,** *sutura* squamosa.

**subcutic'ular s.,** see Halsted s.

**temporozygomatic s.,** *sutura* temporozygomatica.

**tendon s.,** tenorrhaphy.

**tension s.,** a large stitch of heavy material placed through and through both sides of a wound in order to prevent disruption caused by undue stress.

**transfixion s.,** a criss-cross stitch so placed as to control bleeding from a tissue surface or small vessel when tied tightly.

**transverse palatine s.,** *sutura* palatina transversa.

**tympanomastoid s.,** the s. line at the junction of the tympanic and mastoid portions of the temporal bones.

**uninterrupted s.,** a continuous s.

**Wölfler's s.,** an interrupted s. by which broad layers of the serosa are united, the knots being tied on the inner surface of the bowel.

**zygomaticomaxillary s.,** *sutura* zygomaticomaxillaris.

**suxametho'nium bromide** (BP). Succinylcholine bromide.

**suxametho'nium chloride** (BP). Succinylcholine chloride.

**Suzanne** (su-zahn'), Jean G., French physician, *1859. See S.'s *gland*.

**SV.** Abbreviation for simian *virus*.

**Svedberg,** Theodor, Swedish chemist, *1884. See *Svedberg* of flotation, S. *unit*.

**Svedberg of flotation.** Flotation *constant*.

**swab** (swob). A tuft of cotton, ball of gauze, or the like, attached to the end of a stock or wire; used for cleansing cavities, applying remedies to the walls of cavities, or getting a bit of secretion for bacteriologic examination.

**swage** [ Old F. *souage* ]. 1. To fuse suture thread to suture needles. 2. To shape metal by hammering or adapting it onto a die, often by using a counterdie.

**swallow** (swol'o) [ A.S. *swelgan* ]. To pass anything through the fauces, pharynx, and esophagus into the stomach; to perform deglutition.

**swarm'ing** [ A.S. *swearm* ]. A progressive spreading by motile bacteria over the surface of a solid medium.

**swarm-spore.** In certain fungi, one of a large number of active motile individuals resulting from the sporulation or multiple fission of the parent cell.

**sway-back.** Lordosis, or sinking down of the back, in quadrupeds.

**sweat** (swet) [ *A.S. swāt* ]. 1. Sudor; perspiration (3); especially sensible perspiration. 2. To perspire.

**bloody s.,** hematidrosis.

**colliq'uative s.,** profuse clammy s.

**colored s.,** chromidrosis.

**excessive s.,** hyperhidrosis.

**fetid s.,** bromidrosis.

**night s.'s,** profuse sweating at night, occurring in pulmonary tuberculosis and other chronic debilitating affections.

**phosphores'cent s.,** phosphorhidrosis; the secretion of luminous s.

**profuse s.,** hidrosis; sudoresis; hyperhidrosis.

**red s.,** reddening of s., especially in the axilla, due to pigment produced by *Rhodococcus roseofulvis.* See also chromidrosis.

**scanty s.,** hypohidrosis.

**sweat'ing.** Perspiration (1).

**Swediauer** (shva'de-ow-er), Francois X., Austrian physician, 1748–1824. See S.'s *disease.*

**sween'y** [ Dial. ]. Swinny; atrophy of the supraspinatus and infraspinatus muscles of the horse, resulting in shrinkage of the shoulder region; the condition is believed to be due to mechanical injury to the suprascapular nerve by a blow, or pressure from an ill-fitting collar.

**sweet'bread.** The thymus gland (**neck s., throat s.**) or the pancreas (**stomach s., abdominal s.**) of an animal used for food.

**sweet'wood bark.** Cascarilla.

**swell'head.** 1. Of sheep and goats, lechuguilla *poisoning.* 2. Of turkeys, distention of the sinuses due to accumulation of exudate in infectious sinusitis.

**swell'ing.** 1. An enlargement, *e.g.*, a protuberance or tumor. 2. In embryology, a primordial elevation that develops into a fold, ridge, or process.

**albu'minous s.,** cloudy s.

**arytenoid s.,** paired primordial elevations, on either side of the embryonic larynx, within which the arytenoid cartilages are formed.

**brain s.,** a pathologic entity characterized by an increase in bulk of brain tissue, due to expansion of the intravascular (congestion) or extravascular (edema) compartments. These may coexist or may occur separately and be clinically indistinguishable. The process may be localized or generalized. Clinical manifestations depend on disturbed neuronal function due to local swelling, shifting of intracranial structures, and the effects of intracranial hypertension or circulatory disturbance.

**Calabar s.,** loiasis.

**cloudy s.,** albuminous, granular, floccular, or parenchymatous degeneration; s. of cells due to injury to the membranes affecting ionic transfer; it causes an accumulation of intracellular water.

**fugitive s.,** loiasis.

**genital s.'s,** labioscrotal s.'s; paired primordial elevations flanking the genital tubercle and the urogenital orifice of the embryo. They develop into the labioscrotal folds which become the labia majora in the female, and unite to form the scrotal pouch of the male.

**glassy s.,** amyloid *degeneration.*

**hunger s.,** starvation edema caused by many factors, of which reduced serum albumin is prominent.

**labial s.,** the female embryonic genital s. which elongates to become the definitive labium majus; see also genital s.'s.

**labioscrotal s.'s,** genital s.'s.

**lateral lingual s.'s,** in the embryo, paired oval elevations that appear in the floor of the mouth at mandibular arch level. The primordial elevations, composed of mesenchyme covered by ectoderm of stomodeal origin, merge to form the greater part of the body of the tongue.

**levator s.,** *torus* levatorius.

**Neufeld capsular s.,** Neufeld reaction; quellung phenomenon; increase in opacity and visibility of the capsule of capsulated organisms exposed to specific agglutinating anticapsular antibodies.

**scrotal s.,** the embryonic genital s. after it has become spherical and has migrated caudally to the base of the penis; just before birth the testis comes to lie within it.

**Spielmeyer's acute s.,** a form of degeneration of nerve cells in which the cell body and its processes swell and stain palely and diffusely.

**white s.,** gonyocele; gonyoncus; tumor albus; tuberculous arthritis, with thickening of synovium by granulomas and formation of pannus.

**Swift,** W., Australian physician, 20th century. See S.'s *disease.*

**swine** [ A.S. *swin* ]. Hog; pig; a quadruped mammal of the family Suidae.

**swine'pox.** 1. A disease occurring in swine, caused by a DNA poxvirus, usually mild, characterized by papulopustular lesions and usually transmitted by lice. 2. A poxlike disease in swine caused by vaccinia.

**swin'ny.** Rarely used alternative spelling for sweeny.

**swoon.** A faint; syncope.

**sycoma** (si'ko'mah) [ G. *sykōma,* fr. *sykon,* fig, + suffix *-oma,* tumor ]. A pendulous figlike growth; a large soft wart.

**syco'siform.** Resembling sycosis.

**sycosis** (si-ko'sis) [ G. *sykōsis,* fr. *sykōn,* fig, + suffix *-osis,* condition ]. Mentagra; ficosis; a pustular folliculitis, particularly of the bearded area.

**chronic coccogen'ic s.,** *tinea* sycosis.

**s. contagio'sa,** *tinea* sycosis.

**s. framboesifor'mis,** acne *keloid.*

**lupoid s.,** ulerythema sycosiforme; a papular or pustular inflammation of the hair follicles of the beard, followed by punctuate scarring and loss of the hair.

**nonparasit'ic s.,** *tinea* sycosis.

**s. nuchae necroti'sans,** acne keloid on the back of the neck at the hairline.

**parasitic s.,** *tinea* sycosis.

**s. staphylog'enes,** *tinea* sycosis.

**s. vulga'ris,** *tinea* sycosis.

**Sydenham,** Thomas, English physician, 1624–1689. See S.'s *chorea, disease.*

**syl'lable-stumb'ling** [ L. *syllabē,* several letters or sounds taken together. LAB- ]. Dyssyllabia; a form of stuttering in which the patient halts before certain syllables that he finds difficult to enunciate.

**syllepsiology** (sī-lep'sī-ol'o-jī) [ G. *syllēpsis,* pregnancy, + *logos,* study ]. The science that treats of conception and of the period of pregnancy.

**syllepsis** (sī-lep'sis) [ G. ]. Pregnancy.

**Sylvest,** Ejnar, Danish physician. See S.'s *disease.*

**Syl'vian.** Relating to Franciscus or Jacobus Sylvius or to any of the structures described by either of them.

**syl'vic acid.** Abietic acid.

**Syl'vius,** Franciscus, Latinized form of François Dubois (or de le Boe), physician, anatomist, and physiologist, 1614–1672. Professor of medicine at Leyden; follower of the iatrochemical school; pointed out the importance of the saliva and the pancreatic juice in digestion which he recognized to be a chemical (fermentative) process. He introduced bedside instruction into medical teaching. See Sylvian *angle, fissure, fossa, line, point, ventricle.*

**Syl'vius,** Jacobus, Latinized form of Jacques Dubois, French anatomist, 1478–1555. Teacher of Vesalius at Paris but later bitterly opposed his pupil's teachings. See Sylvian *aqueduct, os* sylvii.

**sym-.** See syn-.

**symballophone** (sim-bal'o-fōn) [ G. *symballō,* to throw together, + *phōnē,* sound ]. A stethoscope having two bells or chest pieces, each of which leads to one ear, with a length of tubing adjusted to accentuate the difference in the time of arrival of sounds in the two ears. Designed by William Kerr to lateralize sound producing an auditory effect comparable to stereoscopic vision.

**symbion, symbiont** (sim'bī-on, -ont) [ G. *symbiōn,* of *symbiōs,* living together ]. Mutualist; an organism associated with another in symbiosis.

**symbiosis** (sim'bī-o'sis) [ G. *symbiōsis,* state of living together, fr. sym- *bios,* life, + suffix *-osis,* condition ]. 1. The mutually advantageous association of two or more organisms; for example: (a) the growth of certain rumen bacteria within the cow's rumen, a relationship whereby the cellulose consumed by the cow is partially digested and made available nutritionally to the cow by the bacteria, which in turn find a satisfactory environment; (b) the intimate association of alga and fungus to form the morphologically distinct combination plants, the lichens. 2. In psychiatry, the mutual cooperation or interdependence of two persons, as mother and infant, or husband and wife; the term is sometimes used to denote excessive or pathological interdependence of two persons.

**dyadic s.,** s. between a child and one parent.

**triadic s.,** s. between a child and both parents.

**symbiote** (sim'bī-ōt). Symbion.

**symbiotic** (sim'bī-ot'ik). Relating to symbiosis.

**symblepharon** (sim-blef'ā-ron) [ sym- + G. *blepharon*, eyelid ]. Atretoblepharia; adhesion of one or both lids to the eyeball.

**anterior s.,** union between the lid and eyeball by a fibrous band not involving the fornix.

**complete s.,** adhesion involving the entire surface between the lid and eyeball.

**partial s.,** anterior or posterior s.; incomplete s.

**posterior s.,** adhesion between the eyeball and lid involving the fornix.

**total s.,** complete s.

**symblepharopterygium** (sim-blef'ā-ro-tē-rij'ī-um) [ symblepharon + pterygium ]. Union of the lid to the eyeball through a pterygium-like cicatricial band.

**symbol** (sim'bol) [ G. *symbolon*, a mark or sign, fr. *symballō*, to throw together ]. 1. A conventional sign (*q.v.*) serving as an abbreviation, such as the ℞ at the beginning of a prescription. 2. In chemistry, an abbreviation (the initial and usually one other letter) of the name of an element, radical, or compound, expressing in chemical formulas, one atom or molecule of that element. 3. In psychiatry, an object or action that is interpreted to represent some repressed or unconscious desire, often sexual. 4. A philosophical-linguistic sign; see iconic *sign* and indexical *sign*.

**symbo'lia** [ G. *symbolon*, a mark or sign ]. The power of recognizing the form and nature of an object by touch.

**symbolism** (sim'bo-lizm). 1. In psychoanalysis, the process involved in the disguised representation in consciousness of unconscious or repressed contents or events. 2. A mental state in which everything that happens is regarded by the individual as symbolic of his own thoughts. 3. The description of the emotional life and experiences in abstract terms.

**symbolization** (sim'bo-lī-za'shun). An unconscious mental mechanism whereby one object or idea is represented by another.

**symbrachydactyly** (sim-brak'ī-dak'tī-lī) [ sym- + G. *brachys*, short, + *daktylos*, finger ]. A condition in which abnormally short fingers are more or less joined or webbed in their proximal portions.

**Syme,** James, Scottish surgeon, 1799–1870. See S.'s *amputation, operation.*

**sym'elus.** Sirenomelus.

**Symington,** Johnson, Scottish anatomist, 1851–1924. See S.'s anococcygeal *body.*

**symmelia** (sī-me'lī-ah) [ sym- + G. *melos*, limb ]. Sirenomelia.

**symmelus** (sim'e-lus). Sirenomelus.

**Symmers,** Douglas, American pathologist, *1879. See Brill-S. *disease.*

**symmetry** (sim'ē-trī) [ G. *symmetria*, fr. sym- + *metron*, measure ]. Equality or correspondence in form of parts distributed around a center or an axis, at the two extremities or poles, or on the two opposite sides of any body.

**inverse s.,** correspondence of the right or left side of an asymmetrical individual to the left or right side of another.

**sympath-, sympathetic-, sympathico-, sympatho-** [ see sympathetic ]. Combining forms relating to the sympathetic part of the autonomic nervous system. The various spellings are used more or less interchangeably.

**sympathec'tomy, sympathetec'tomy** [ sympath- + G. *ektomē*, excision ]. Excision of a segment of a sympathetic nerve or of one or more sympathetic ganglia.

**chemical s.,** destruction of the periarterial sympathetic nerves, as in Doppler's operation, by a corrosive such as phenol.

**periarte'rial s.,** histonectomy; Leriche's operation; sympathetic denervation by arterial decortication.

**presacral s.,** presacral *neurectomy.*

**sympathet'ic** [ G. *sympathētikos*, fr. *sympatheō*, to feel with, sympathise, fr. *syn*, with, + *pathos*, suffering ]. Sympathic. 1. Relating to or exhibiting sympathy. 2.

Denoting the sympathetic part of the autonomic nervous system.

**sympathet'oblast.** Sympathoblast.

**sympathet'oblasto'ma.** Sympathoblastoma.

**sympath'ic.** Sympathetic.

**sympathicectomy** (sim-path'ī-sek'to-mī). Sympathectomy.

**sympathico-** See sympath-.

**sympath'icoblast.** Sympathoblast.

**sympath'icoblasto'ma.** Sympathoblastoma.

**sympath'icogonio'ma.** Sympathogonioma.

**sympath'icolyt'ic.** Sympatholytic.

**sympath'icomimet'ic.** Sympathomimetic.

**sympathiconeuritis** (sim-path'ī-ko-nu-ri'tis). Inflammation of the autonomic nerves.

**sympathicopathy** (sim-path-ī-kop'ā-thī) [ sympathico- + G. *pathos*, suffering ]. A disease resulting from disordered action of the autonomic nervous system.

**sympathicotonia** (sim-path'ī-ko-to'nī-ah) [ sympathico- + G. *tonos*, tone, tension ]. A condition in which there is increased tonus of the sympathetic system and a marked tendency to vascular spasm and high blood pressure; opposed to vagotonia.

**sympath'icoton'ic.** Relating to or characterized by sympathicotonia.

**sympathicotripsy** (sim-path'ī-ko-trip'sī) [ sympathico- + G. *tripsis*, a rubbing ]. Operation of crushing the sympathetic ganglion.

**sympathicotropic** (sim-path'ī-ko-trop'ik) [ sympathico- + G. *tropikos*, inclined, fr. *tropē*, a turning ]. Having a special affinity for the sympathetic nervous system.

**sympath'icus** [ L. ] [ NA ]. Sympathetic (2).

**sympathin** (sim'pā-thin). The substance diffusing into circulation from sympathetic nerve terminals when they are active. The term was introduced by W. B. Cannon, who thought that this substance differed from the mediator produced by the nerve ending. This is now known to be incorrect. The mediator itself (norepinephrine) diffuses into circulation.

**s. E,** excitatory s.; vasoconstrictor (possibly identical with norepinephrine).

**s. I,** inhibitory s.; vasodilator.

**two-s. theory,** see under theory.

**sympathism** (sim'pā-thizm) [ G. *sympatheia*, sympathy ]. Suggestibility.

**sym'pathist.** One susceptible to sympathism.

**sympathizer** (sim'pā-thī'zer). 1. An eye affected with sympathetic ophthalmia. 2. A person who exhibits sympathy.

**sympatho-** See sympath-.

**sym'pathoadre'nal.** Relating to the sympathetic part of the autonomic nervous system and the medulla of the adrenal gland, as the postganglionic neurons.

**sympathoblast** (sim'pā-tho-blast) [ sympatho- + G. *blastos*, sprout ]. A primitive cell derived from the neural crest glia; with the pheochromoblasts, s.'s enter into the formation of the adrenal medulla.

**sym'pathoblasto'ma** [ sympathoblast + G. suffix -*oma*, tumor ]. Sympathicoblastoma; sympatheticoblastoma; sympathogonioma; neuroblastoma sympatheticum embryonale; a tumor composed of sympathoblasts; a completely undifferentiated malignant tumor which originates from embryonal cells of the sympathetic nervous system.

**sympathogonia** (sim'pā-tho-go'nī-ah) [ sympatho- + G. *gonē*, seed ]. The completely undifferentiated cells of the sympathetic nervous system.

**sympathogonioma** (sim'pā-tho-go-nī-o'mah) [ sympathogonia + G. suffix -*oma*, tumor ]. Sympathoblastoma.

**sympatholytic** (sim'pā-tho-lit'ik) [ sympatho- + G. *lysis*, a loosening ]. Sympathoparalytic; sympathicolytic; denoting antagonism to or inhibition of adrenergic nerve activity; see also adrenergic blocking *agent.*

**sympathomimetic** (sim-pāth-o-mī-met'ik) [ sympatho- + G. *mimikos*, imitating ]. Sympathicomimetic; denoting mimicking of action of the sympathetic system; see also adrenomimetic.

**sym'pathoparalyt'ic.** Sympatholytic.

**sympathy** (sim′pă-thĭ) [ G. *sympatheia*, fr. sym- + *pathos*, suffering ]. 1. The mutual relation, physiologic or pathologic, between two organs, systems, or parts of the body. 2. Mental contagion, as seen in the spread of chorea or other nervous disease through a school, or in the yawning induced by seeing another person yawn. 3. An expressed sensitive appreciation or emotional concern for and sharing of the mental and emotional state of another person, as distinguished from empathy (1).

**symperitoneal** (sim′pĕr-ĭ-to-ne′al). Relating to the surgical induction of adhesion between two portions of the peritoneum, as in Talma's operation.

**sympexis** (sim-pek′sis) [ G. concretion. PAG- ]. A term proposed by Heidenhain to denote the deposition of red blood cells according to the laws of surface tension.

**symphalangism, symphalangy** (sim-fal′an-jizm, simfal′-an-jĭ) [ sym- + phalanx, *q.v.* ]. 1. Syndactyly. 2. Ankylosis of the finger or toe joints.

**symphyogenetic** (sim′fĭ-o-jĕ-net′ik) [ G. *symphyēs*, grown together, + *genesis*, origin ]. Relating to the combined effects of hereditary and environmental factors in determining the structure and function of the organism.

**symphysial, symphyseal** (sim-fiz′e-al). Relating to a symphysis; grown together; fused.

**symphysic** (sim-fiz′ik). Symphysial.

**symphysion** (sim-fiz′ĭ-on). A craniometric point, the most anterior point of the alveolar process of the mandible.

**symphysiorrhaphy, symphyseorrhaphy** (sim-fiz′ĭ-or′ă-fĭ) [ symphysis + G. *rhaphē*, suture ]. The fastening together of the parts of a divided symphysis.

**symphysiotome, symphyseotome** (sim-fiz′ĭ-o-tōm). An instrument for use in symphysiotomy.

**symphysiotomy, symphyseotomy** (sim-fiz′ĭ-ot′o-mĭ) [ symphysis + G. *tomē*, incision ]. Division of the pubic joint, by means of a wire saw, to increase the capacity of a contracted pelvis sufficiently to permit the passage of a living child.

**symphysis,** gen. **symphyses** (sim′fĭ-sis, -sēz) [ G. a growing together. PHYS-1 ]. 1. [ NA ]. A form of cartilaginous joint in which union between two bones is effected by means of fibrocartilage. See fig. under joint. 2. A union, meeting point, or commissure of any two structures. 3. A pathologic adhesion or growing together.

    **cardiac s.,** adhesion between the parietal and visceral layers of the pericardium.

    **s. mandib′ulae,** s. menti; a vertical ridge in the midline of the lower jaw, indicating the line of union of its embryonic primordia.

    **s. men′ti,** s. mandibulae.

    **s. pelvi′na** [ NAV ], the combined rami of the s. pubica and s. ischiadica in domestic mammals.

    **s. pu′bica** [ NA ], pubic s.; the firm cartilaginous joint between the two pubic bones.

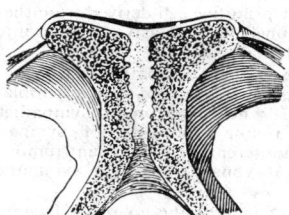

**Symphysis Pubica**

    **s. sacrococcygea,** *junctura* sacrococcygea.

**symphysodactyly, symphysodactylia** (sim′fĭ-so-dak′tĭ-lĭ, -dak-til′ĭ-ah) [ G. *symphysis*, fusion, + *daktylos*, finger ]. Syndactyly.

**symplasmatic** (sim′plaz-mat′ik) [ G. *sym-plassō*, to mold together. PLAS- ]. Relating to the union of protoplasm as in giant cell formation.

**symplast** (sim′plast) [ sym- + G. *plastos*, formed ]. A multinucleated cell which has formed by fusion of separate cells.

**sympodia** (sim-po′dĭ-ah) [ sym- + G. *pous,* foot ]. A condition characterized by union of the feet; see also sirenomelia and sympus.

**symptom** (simp′tom) [ G. *symptōma;* see PTOM- ]. Any morbid phenomenon or departure from the normal in function, appearance, or sensation, experienced by the patient and indicative of disease. For the various s.'s and varieties of S.'s, see below and also under phenomenon, reflex, sign, and syndrome.

    **ab′stinence s.,** withdrawal s.

    **accessory s.,** assident s.; one that usually but not always accompanies a certain disease; distinguished from a pathognomonic s.

    **accidental s.,** any morbid phenomenon occurring in the course of a disease, but having no relation with it.

    **Argyll Robertson s.,** Argyll Robertson *pupil.*

    **as′sident s.,** accessory s.

    **Baumès′ s.,** pain behind the sternum in angina pectoris.

    **Bezold's s.,** inflammatory edema at the tip of the mastoid process in mastoiditis.

    **Bolognini's s.,** a feeling of crepitation on gradually increasing pressure on the abdomen in cases of measles.

    **cardinal s.,** primary or major s.

    **concom′itant s.,** accessory s.

    **constitutional s.,** a s. indicating that the disease has become general.

    **deficiency s.,** the manifestation of a lack, in varying degrees, of some substance (*e.g.,* a hormone, a vitamin, or a mineral) necessary for normal structure and function of an organism.

    **Demarquay's s.,** absence of elevation of the larynx during deglutition, said to indicate syphilitic induration of the trachea.

    **Duroziez′ s.,** Duroziez′ murmur; a double murmur (systolic and diastolic) heard over the femoral artery, when compressed by the stethoscope, in cases of aortic insufficiency.

    **Epstein's s.,** a lid s., resembling Graefe's, occurring in neurotic nurslings; it gives a frightened expression to the infant, characterized by Epstein as a "wild glance."

    **equiv′ocal s.,** one that points definitely to no special disease, being associated with any one of a number of morbid states.

    **esophagosal′ivary s.,** an excessive secretion of saliva occurring sometimes in cancer of the esophagus.

    **Fischer's s.,** a presystolic nonvalvular murmur audible in cases of pericardial adhesions.

    **Frenkel's s.,** lowered muscular tonus in tabes dorsalis.

    **Gordon's s.,** tonic *reflex.*

    **Griesinger's s.,** edema of the superficial tissues at the tip of the mastoid process in cases of thrombosis of the sigmoid sinus.

    **Haenel's s.,** absence of sensation on pressure of the eyeball in tabes.

    **Howship's s.,** pain or paresthesia on the inner side of the thigh in cases of obturator hernia.

    **incarceration s.,** Dietl's *crisis.*

    **induced s.,** one excited by a drug, exercise, or other means, often intentionally for diagnostic purposes.

    **Kerandel's s.,** deep-seated hyperesthesia observed in cases of sleeping sickness.

    **Kussmaul's s.,** filling of the veins of the neck during inspiration in cases of pericardial effusion or constrictive pericarditis.

    **local s.,** one of limited extent caused by disease of a particular organ or part.

    **localizing s.,** one indicating clearly the seat of the morbid process.

    **Macewen's s.,** Macewen's *sign.*

    **objective s.,** one that is evident to the observer.

    **Oehler's s.,** a sudden pallor and coldness in the arm with slight disability, occurring on lifting of a heavy weight.

    **pathognomon′ic s.,** one that, when present, points unmistakably to a certain definite disease.

    **Pel-Ebstein s.,** intermittent fever seen in Hodgkin's disease.

    **Pratt's s.,** rigidity in the muscles of an injured limb, which precedes the occurrence of gangrene.

    **rainbow s.,** glaucomatous *halo.*

    **reflex s.,** a disturbance of sensation or function in an organ or part more or less remote from the morbid condition giving rise to it, as vertigo or headache due to eyestrain.

**Robertson s.,** Argyll Robertson s.

**Romberg's s.,** (1) Romberg's *sign;* (2) Romberg-Howship s.

**Romberg-Howship s.,** Romberg's s. (2); lancinating pains along the inner side of the thigh to the knee, or even down the leg to the foot, in cases of incarcerated obturator hernia; caused by compression of the obturator nerve.

**Rumpf's s.,** (1) pressure over a painful point, in cases of emotional disturbance, will accelerate the pulse from 10 to 20 beats in the minute; (2) fibrillary twitching in traumatic neuroses.

**Sklowsky s.,** very slight pressure with the finger on a varicella vesicle will cause its rupture, greater pressure being necessary to break the vesicles of smallpox, herpes, or other affections.

**subjective s.,** one apparent only to the patient himself.

**sympathet'ic s.,** reflex s.

**Trendelenburg's s.,** a waddling gait in paresis of the gluteal muscles, as in progressive muscular dystrophy.

**Trunecek's s.,** palpable impulse of the subclavian artery near the point of origin of the sternomastoid muscle in cases of aortic sclerosis.

**Wartenberg's s.,** (1) intense pruritus of the tip of the nose and nostrils in cases of cerebral tumor; (2) flexion of the thumb when the patient attempts to flex the four fingers against resistance, a "pyramid sign."

**withdrawal s.'s,** abstinence s.'s; a group of morbid s.'s, predominantly erethistic, occurring in an addict who is deprived of his accustomed dose of the addicting agent.

**symptomatic** (simp'to-mat'ik). Indicative; semiologic; relating to or constituting the semiology of symptoms of a disease.

**symptomatology** (simp'to-mă-tol'o-jĭ) [ symptom + G. *logos,* study ]. 1. Semiology; the science of the symptoms of disease, their production, and the indications they furnish. 2. The aggregate of symptoms of a disease.

**symptomatolytic** (simp'to-mat'o-lit'ik) [ symptom + G. *lytikos,* dissolving ]. Symptomolytic; removing symptoms.

**symptomes complices** (samp-tōm' kom-plēs') [ Fr. accessory symptoms ]. In roentgenography of the gastroenteric tract, a group of symptoms, recognized in part by the use of the roentgen ray, usually by fluoroscopic examination, that help to establish the diagnosis.

**symp'tomless.** Asymptomatic; without symptoms.

**symptomolytic** (simp-to-mo-lit'ik). Symptomatolytic.

**symptosis** (simp-to'sis) [ G. a falling together, collapse, fr. *syn,* together, + *ptōsis,* a falling ]. Marasmus; atrophy, either local or general.

**sympus** (sim'pus) [ G. *sympous,* fr. sym- + *pous,* foot ]. A sirenomelus in which the fusion of the legs has extended to involve the feet.

**s. a'pus,** a sirenomelus without feet.

**s. di'pus,** a sirenomelus with both feet more or less distinct.

**s. mo'nopus,** a sirenomelus with but one foot externally visible.

**Syms,** Parker, New York surgeon, 1860–1933. See S.'s *tractor.*

**syn-** [ G. *syn,* with, together ]. A prefix to words of Greek derivation, indicating together, with, joined; it corresponds to the Latin *con-.* Appears as sym- before b, p, ph, or m.

**synadelphus** (sin-ă-del'fus) [ syn- + G. *adelphos,* brother ]. Cephalothoracoiliopagus; conjoined twins with single head, partially united trunk, and four upper and four lower limbs.

**synalbu'min.** A postulated insulin antagonist, present in the blood of some diabetics, that is associated with the albumin fraction; believed to be a polypeptide and possibly closely related in structure to the B chain of insulin.

**synalgia** (sĭ-nal'jĭ-ah) [ syn- + G. *algos,* pain ]. Reflex or referred pain; pain felt at a part more or less remote from the seat of the causative lesion.

**synal'gic.** Relating to or marked by reflex or referred pain.

**syn'anastomo'sis.** An anastomosis between several blood vessels.

**synanche** (sĭ-nang'ke). Cynanche.

**synandrogenic** (sin-an-dro-jen'ik). Relating to any agent or condition that enhances the effects of androgens.

**synanthem, synanthema** (sĭ-nan'them, sin'an-the'mah) [ G. *syn-antheō,* to blossom together. ANTH- ]. An exanthem consisting of several different forms of eruption.

**synaphocep'tors** [ G. *synaphe,* contact, + L. *recipio,* to receive ]. Receptors stimulated by direct contact.

**synapse,** pl. **synapses** (sin'aps, sĭ-naps', sĭ-nap'sēz) [ syn- + G. *haptein,* to clasp; *cf.* synapsis ]. Term coined by Sherrington to denote the functional, membrane-to-membrane contact of the nerve cell with another nerve cell, an effector (muscle, gland) cell, or a sensory receptor cell. The s. subserves the transmission of nerve impulses, commonly from a variably large (1 to 12 μ), generally knob-shaped or club-shaped axon terminal (the presynaptic element) to the circumscript patch of the receiving cell's plasma membrane (the postsynaptic element) on which the s. occurs. In most cases the impulse is transmitted by means of a chemical transmitter substance (such as acetylcholine, γ-aminobutyric acid, dopamine, norepinephrine, etc.) released into a synaptic cleft (150 to 500 Å wide) which separates the presynaptic from the postsynaptic membrane; the transmitter is stored in quantal form in synaptic vesicles: round or ellipsoid, membrane-bound vacuoles (100 to 500 Å in diameter) in the presynaptic element. In other s.'s transmission takes place by direct propagation of the bioelectrical potential from the presynaptic to the postsynaptic membrane; in such electrotonic s.'s ("gap junctions"), the synaptic cleft is no more than about 20 Å wide. In most cases, transmission can take place in only one direction ("dynamic polarity" of the s.), but in some s.'s synaptic vesicles occur on both sides of the synaptic cleft, suggesting the possibility of reciprocal chemical transmission.

**axoaxonic s.,** the synaptic junction between an axon terminal of one neuron and either the initial axon segment or an axon terminal of another nerve cell.

**axodendritic s.,** the synaptic contact between an axon terminal of one nerve cell and a dendrite of another nerve cell.

**axosomatic s.,** pericorpuscular s.; the synaptic junction of an axon terminal of one nerve cell to the cell body of another nerve cell.

**electrotonic s.,** gap *junction;* see also synapse.

**pericorpuscular s.,** axosomatic s.

**synapsis** (sĭ-nap'sis) [ G. a connection, junction ]. The point for point pairing of homologous chromosomes during the prophase of meiosis.

**synaptase** (sĭ-nap'tās). Emulsin.

**synap'tic.** Relating to (1) the synapse, and (2) synapsis.

**synaptology** (sin'ap-tol'o-jĭ). Study of the synapse.

**synarthrodia** (sin'ar-thro'dĭ-ah). *Junctura* fibrosa.

**synarthro'dial.** Relating to synarthrosis; denoting an (almost) immovable articulation between two bones.

**synarthrophysis** (sin-ar'thro-fi'sis) [ syn- + G. *arthron,* joint, + *physis,* growth ]. The process of ankylosis.

**synarthrosis,** pl. **synarthroses** (sin'ar-thro'sis, -sēz) [ G. fr. *syn,* together, + *arthrōsis,* articulation ]. In the BNA this class of joints included those that in the NA are classified as *junctura* fibrosa and *junctura* cartilaginea, *q. v.*

**synathresis** (sin'ă-thre'sis) [ G. *synathroisis,* a gathering together, fr. *syn- athroizō,* to gather together ]. 1. Congestion. 2. Bier's method of induced hyperemia.

**syncanthus** (sin-kan'thus) [ syn- + L. *canthus,* wheel ]. Adhesion of the eyeball to orbital structures.

**syncar'yon.** Synkaryon.

**syncephalus** (sin-sef'ă-lus) [ syn- + G. *kephalē,* head ]. Monocephalus; monocranius; conjoined twins having a single head with two bodies; *cf.* craniopagus, janiceps.

**s. asymmetros,** *janiceps* asymmetrus.

**syncephaly** (sin-sef'ă-lĭ). The condition exhibited by a syncephalus.

**syncheilia, synchilia** (sin-ki'lĭ-ah) [ syn- + G. *cheilos,* lip ]. A more or less complete adhesion of the lips; atresia of the mouth.

**syncheiria, synchiria** (sin-ki'rĭ-ah) [ syn- + G. *cheir,* hand ]. A form of dyscheiria in which the subject refers a stimulus applied to one side of the body to both sides.

**synchondroseotomy** (sin-kon'dro-se-ot'o-mī) [ synchondrosis + G. tomē, cutting ]. Operation of cutting through a synchondrosis; specifically, Trendelenburg's operation, cutting through the sacroiliac ligaments and forcibly closing the arch of the pubes in the treatment of exstrophy of the bladder

**synchondrosis,** pl. **synchondro'ses** (sin'kon-dro'sis, -sēz) [ Mod. L. fr. G. syn, together, + chondros, cartilage, + suffix -osis, condition ] [ NA ]. Synchondrodial joint; a union between two bones formed either by hyaline cartilage or fibrocartilage. See fig. under joint.
  **s. arycornicula'ta,** the junction of the corniculate cartilage (of Santorini) with the arytenoid.
  **cranial synchondroses,** synchondroses cranii.
  **synchondroses cranii** [ NA ], cranial synchondroses; the cartilaginous joints of the skull; these include s. sphenooccipitalis, s. sphenopetrosa, s. petrooccipitalis, s. intraoccipitalis anterior, and s. intraoccipitalis posterior.
  **s. epiphy'seos,** linea epiphysialis.
  **synchrondoses interssternebra'les** [ NAV ], interssternebral joints; in some domestic animals such as the dog the osseous sternebral elements are separated from one another throughout life by cartilage; see also synchondroses sternales (2).
  **s. intraoccipita'lis ante'rior** [ NA ], anterior intraoccipital joint; cartilaginous union in the newborn between the lateral and the basilar portions of the occipital bone.
  **s. intraoccipita'lis poste'rior** [ NA ], posterior intraoccipital joint; Budin's obstetrical joint; cartilaginous union between the squamous and lateral parts of the occipital bone in the newborn.
  **s. manubriostern'a'lis** [ NA ], manubriosternal joint; the cartilaginous union between the manubrium and the body of the sternum.
  **neurocentral s.,** neurocentral joint; neurocentral suture; the cartilaginous union on either side between the body and arch of a vertebra in the young child.
  **s. petrooccipita'lis** [ NA ], petrooccipital joint; fibrocartilage filling the petrooccipital fissure.
  **s. sphenooccipita'lis** [ NA ], sphenooccipital joint; cartilaginous union between the body of the sphenoid and the basilar portion of the occipital; it fuses by the 20th year.
  **s. sphenopetro'sa** [ NA ], sphenopetrous or sphenopetrosal s.; fibrocartilage filling the sphenopetrosal fissure.
  **sternal synchondroses,** synchondroses sternales.
  **synchondroses sterna'les,** (1) [ NA ], sternal synchondroses; sternal joints; the cartilaginous junctions between the manubrium and body of the sternum; (2) [ NAV ], in domestic animals, the sternebral joints; there may be several, e.g., s. manubriosternalis, s. interssternebralis, and s. xiphosternalis.
  **s. xiphosterna'lis** [ NA ], xiphisternal joint; the cartilaginous union between the xiphoid process and the body of the sternum.

**synchondrotomy** (sin'kon-drot'o-mī). Symphysiotomy.

**synchorial** (sin-ko'rī-al) [ syn- + chorion, q.v. ]. Relating to fused chorions.

**synchronia** (sin-kro'nī-ah) [ syn- + G. chronos, time ]. 1. Synchronism. 2. The origin, development, involution, or functioning of tissues or organs at the usual time for such an event; opposed to heterochronia.

**synchronism** (sin'kro-nizm) [ syn- + G. chronos, time ]. Sychronia (1); occurrence of two or more events at the same time; the condition of being simultaneous.

**synchronous** (sin'kro-nus) [ G. synchronos ]. Occurring simultaneously.

**synchrony** (sin'kro-nī) [ syn- + G. chronos, time ]. The simultaneous appearance of two separate events.
  **bilateral s.,** the simultaneous appearance on two sides of the head in homologous points of some normal or abnormal activity as seen in the electroencephalogram.

**synchrotron** (sin'kro-tron). A machine for generating high speed electrons or protons.

**synchysis** (sin'kī-sis) [ G. a mixing together, fr. syn- + chysis, a pouring ]. A fluid condition of the vitreous humor of the eye.
  **s. scintil'lans,** an appearance of glistening spots in the eye, due to cholesterol crystals floating in a fluid vitreous.

**syncine'sis.** Synkinesis.

**synclinal** (sin'klī-nal) [ G. syn- klinō, to incline together. CLIM- ]. Denoting two structures inclined one toward the other.

**synclit'ic.** Relating to or marked by synclitism.

**synclitism** (sin'klī-tizm) [ G. syn-klinō, to incline together ]. A condition of parallelism between the planes of the fetal head and of the pelvis, respectively.

**synclonus** (sin'klo-nus) [ syn- + G. klonos, tumult ]. Clonic spasm or tremor of several muscles.

**syncopal** (sin'ko-pal). Relating to syncope.

**syncope** (sin'ko-pe) [ G. synkopē, a cutting short, a swoon ]. Fainting; deliquium; deliquium animi; a swoon; a sudden fall of blood pressure or failure of the cardiac systole, resulting in cerebral anemia and more or less complete loss of consciousness.
  **carotid sinus s.,** s. resulting from overactivity of the carotid sinus; attacks may be spontaneous or result from pressure on a sensitive carotid sinus or from emotion.
  **hysterical s.,** fainting due to, or to avoid, emotional stress.
  **laryn'geal s.,** a paroxysmal neurosis characterized by attacks of coughing, with unusual sensations, as of tickling, in the throat, followed by a brief period of unconsciousness; sometimes called laryngeal vertigo or Charcot's vertigo.
  **local s.,** limited numbness in a part, especially of the fingers; one of the symptoms, usually associated with local asphyxia, of Raynaud's disease.
  **micturition s.,** fainting or s. occurring in association with the act of emptying the bladder; also called psychomotor epilepsy associated with micturition.
  **postural s.,** s. upon assuming an upright position caused by inadequate blood flow to the brain resulting from failure of normal vasconstrictive mechanisms.
  **vasovagal s.,** vagal attack.

**syncop'ic.** Syncopal.

**syncretio** (sin-kre'shī-o) [ L. a growing together ]. Development of adhesion between inflamed opposing surfaces.

**syncyanin** (sin-si'ā-nin). A blue pigment produced by Pseudomonas syncyanea.

**syncytial** (sin-sish'al, -sish'ī-al, -sit'ī-al). Relating to a syncytium.

**syncytiolysin** (sin-sish'ī-ol'ī-sin, -sit'ī-). Placentolysin; a cytolysin formed in response to injections of emulsions of placental tissue.

**syncytioma** (sin-sish'ī-o'mah, -sit'ī-). Obsolete term for chorioma.
  **s. benig'num,** obsolete term for hydatidiform mole.
  **s. malig'num,** obsolete term for choriocarcinoma.

**syncytiotoxin** (sin-sish'ī-o-tok'sin, -sit'ī-). A cytotoxin specific for the cells of the syncytium.

**syncytiotrophoblast** (sin-sish'ī-o-tro'fo-blast) [ syncytium + trophoblast ]. Syntrophoblast; plasmodiotrophoblast; plasmodial or syncytial trophoblast; placental plasmodium; the syncytial outer layer of the trophoblast; see also trophoblast.

**syncytium,** pl. **syncytia** (sin-sish'ī-um, -sit'ī-um, -ah) [ Mod. L. fr. syn- + G. kytos, cell ]. 1. A multinucleated protoplasmic mass formed by the secondary union of originally separate cells.

**syndac'tyl, syndac'tyle.** Syndactylous.

**syndactyl'ia, syndac'tylism.** Syndactyly.

**syndac'tylous.** Having fused or webbed fingers or toes.

**syndactylus** (sin-dak'tī-lus). A person with fused or webbed fingers or toes.

**syndactyly** (sin-dak'tī-lī) [ syn- + G. daktylos, finger or toe ]. Syndactylia; syndactylism; symphalangism(1); symphysodactyly; any degree of webbing or fusion of fingers or toes, involving soft parts only or including bone structure; usually autosomal dominant inheritance, with marked tendency for repetition of similar anatomical defects within family.

**syndectomy** (sin-dek'to-mī) [ G. syn-desmos, a binding together (conjunctiva), + ektomē, excision ]. Obsolescent term for peritomy.

**syndesis** (sin-de'sis) [ G. fr. syn- + G. desis, a binding ]. 1. Synapsis. 2. Arthrodesis.

**syndesm-.** See syndesmo-.

**syndesmectomy** (sin-dez-mek′to-mī) [ syndesm- + G. *ektomē,* excision ]. Cutting away a section of a ligament.

**syndesmectopia** (sin-dez-mek-to′pī-ah) [ syndesm- + G. *ektopos,* out of place ]. Displacement of a ligament.

**syndesmitis** (sin-dez-mi′tis) [ syndesm- + suffix *-itis,* inflammation ]. Inflammation of a ligament.

    **s. metatar′sea,** inflammation of the metatarsal ligaments.

**syndesmo-, syndesm-** (sin-dez′mo-, sin-des′mo-) [ G. *syndesmos,* a fastening, fr. *syndeo-,* to bind ]. Combining forms meaning ligament (*q.v.*), or ligamentous.

**syndesmochorial** (sin-dez′mo-ko′rī-al) [ syndesmo- + G. *chorion,* membrane ]. Relating to the placenta in ruminant animals; see s. *placenta.*

**syndesmography** (sin-dez-mog′ră-fī) [ syndesmo- + G. *graphō,* to write ]. A treatise on or description of the ligaments.

**syndesmologia** (sin-dez′mo-lo′jī-ah) [ NA ]. Syndesmology.

**syndesmology** (sin-dez-mol′o-jī) [ syndesmo- + G. *logos,* study ]. The branch of anatomy that has to do with the ligaments and the related joints.

**syndesmoma** (sin′dez-mo′mah) [ syndesmo- + G. suffix *-oma,* tumor ]. Obsolete term meaning a connective tissue tumor.

**syndesmopexy** (sin-dez′mo-pek′sī) [ syndesmo- + G. *pēxis,* fixation ]. The joining of two ligaments, or attachment of a ligament in a new place.

**syndesmoplasty** (sin-dez′mo-plas′tī) [ syndesmo- + G. *plassō,* to form ]. Plastic surgery on a ligament.

**syndesmorrhaphy** (sin′dez-mor′ă-fī) [ syndesmo- + G. *rhaphē,* suture ]. Suture of ligaments.

**syndesmosis,** pl. **syndesmoses** (sin′dez-mo′sis, -sēz) [ syndesmo- + G. suffix *-osis,* condition ] [ NA ]. Syndesmodial or syndesmotic joint; a form of fibrous joint in which opposing surfaces that are relatively far apart are united by ligaments; *e.g.,* the union of the styloid process of the temporal bone and the hyoid bone via the stylohyoid ligament, and the union between the distal ends of the tibia and fibula. See fig. under joint.

    **s. tibiofibula′ris** [ NA ], tibiofibular s.; inferior tibiofibular articulation; the union between the distal ends of the fibula and tibia.

    **s. tym′panostape′dia** [ NA ], tympanostapedial junction; the connection of the base or foot-plate of the stapes with the vestibular (oval) window.

**syndesmotomy** (sin′dez-mot′o-mī) [ syndesmo- + G. *tomē,* incision ]. Surgical division of a ligament.

# SYNDROME

**syndrome** (sin′drōm) [ G. *syndromē,* a running together, tumultous concourse; (in med.) a concurrence of symptoms, fr. *syn,* together, + *dromos,* a running ]. The aggregate of signs and symptoms associated with any morbid process, and constituting together the picture of the disease. See also sign and symptom.

    **Abderhalden-Fanconi s.,** cystinosis.

    **abdominal muscle deficiency s.,** a congenital condition with partial or complete absence of abdominal muscles.

    **Achard s.,** arachnodactyly with small receding mandible, broad skull, and joint laxity limited to the hands and feet.

    **Achard-Thiers s.,** diabetes of bearded women; one form of a virilizing disorder of adrenocortical origin in women, characterized by masculinization and menstrual disorders in association with manifestations of diabetes mellitus, such as glucosuria.

    **acrofacial s.,** acrofacial *dysostosis.*

    **ac′roparesthe′sia s.,** abnormal sensation such as numbness and tingling in the extremities.

    **acute radiation s.,** caused by exposure of the body to large amounts of radiation as in certain forms of therapy, accidents, and nuclear explosions. The s. consists of vomiting commencing with 12 hours after exposure and followed 24 hours later by prostration, fever, and diarrhea.

Petechial and purpuric spots appear. In about 5 days extreme weakness develops, accompanied by hypotension, tachycardia, profuse diarrhea becoming bloody, and severe dehydration. Death occurs in 7 to 10 days.

    **Adams-Stokes s.,** Adams-Stokes disease; Stokes-Adams s.; Morgagni's disease; Morgagni-Adams-Stokes s.; Spens' s.; a s. characterized by slow or absent pulse, vertigo, syncope, convulsions, and sometimes Cheyne-Stokes respiration, usually as a result of heart block.

    **adherence s.,** the adherence of fascial sheaths of lateral rectus and inferior oblique muscles, or of medial rectus and superior oblique muscles.

    **Adie s.,** Holmes-Adie s.

    **adipo′sogen′ital s.,** *dystrophia* adiposogenitalis.

    **adrenal cortical s.,** an inexact (and obsolete) term that has been applied to Cushing's s., Addison's disease, or the adrenogenital s.

    **adrenal virilizing s.,** adrenal *virilism.*

    **adrenogen′ic s.,** suprarenogenic s.; adrenalism marked by pigmentation, adiposity, hirsuties, and, in women, amenorrhea; obsolete usage.

    **adre′nogen′ital s.,** generic designation for a group of disorders caused by adrenocortical hyperplasia or malignant tumors; characterized by masculinization of women, feminization of men, or precocious sexual development of children; representative of excessive or abnormal secretory patterns of adrenocortical steroids.

    **afferent loop s.,** acute or chronic obstruction of the duodenum and jejunum proximal to the gastrojejunostomy performed in a Billroth II type gastrectomy; a distended afferent loop causes symptoms of pain and fullness.

    **aglossia-adactylia s.,** congenital absence or hypoplasia of the tongue, associated with absence of the digits.

    **Ahumada-Del Castillo s.,** Argonz-Del Castillo s.; lactation-amenorrhea s. unrelated to a previous pregnancy.

    **Albright's s.,** (1) Albright's *disease;* (2) pseudo-pseudohypoparathyroidism.

    **Aldrich s.,** a heritable disorder occurring in male infants and caused by antibody deficiency associated with dysgammaglobulinemia; thrombocytopenia, eczema, and melena are present in association with susceptibility to bacterial infection; death commonly occurs within a few months.

    **Alice in Wonderland s.,** the illusion of dreams, feelings of levitation, and alteration in the sense of the passage of time, sometimes associated with migraine, epilepsy, and various diseases of the parietal lobe of the brain.

    **Alport's s.,** progressive nephropathy and nerve deafness, sometimes with ocular defects; autosomal dominant inheritance.

    **Alström's s.,** retinal degeneration with nystagmus and loss of central vision, associated with obesity in childhood; nerve deafness and diabetes mellitus usually occur after age 10; autosomal recessive inheritance.

    **amnestic s.,** Korsakoff's *syndrome.*

    **amniotic fluid s.,** pulmonary embolic phenomena due to infusion of a considerable volume of amniotic fluid containing epithelial squames into maternal blood vessels; shock ensues and sudden death may occur.

    **Angelucci's s.,** extreme excitability, vasomotor disturbances, and palpitation, associated with vernal conjunctivitis.

    **angio-osteohypertrophy s.,** Klippel-Trenaunay-Weber s.

    **ankyloglossia superior s.,** a congenital condition in which the tongue adheres to the hard palate.

    **anorectal s.,** soreness, burning, itching, or other irritation of the rectum together with redness about the anus, and sometimes accompanied by diarrhea, occurring as a toxic effect of the oral administration of certain broad spectrum antibiotics.

    **anterior chamber cleavage s.,** Peters' anomaly; a congenital disorder originating from faulty cleavage of embryonic structures; it results in bilateral central corneal opacities, with an anterior ring attachment of the iridic pupillary border and anterior polar cataracts.

    **anterior tibial compartment s.,** ischemic necrosis of the muscles of the anterior tibial compartment of the leg, presumed due to compression of arteries by swollen muscles following unaccustomed exertion.

**antibody deficiency s.,** the group of symptoms associated with a defective mechanism of humoral immunity, chief of which is an increased susceptibility to infection by various cocci, especially Gram-positive cocci; see also agammaglobulinemia.

**Anton's s.,** in cortical blindness, lack of awareness of being completely blind.

**anxiety s.,** tachycardia, difficulty in breathing, and sweating accompanying panic in the absence of a clearly discernable fear-producing stimulus.

**aortic arch s.,** Martorell's s.; thrombotic obliteration of the branches of the arch of the aorta leading to dimished or absent pulses in the neck and arms; see also pulseless *disease,* reversed *coarctation.*

**Apert's s.,** typical (type I) *acrocephalosyndactyly.*

**s. of approximate answers,** Ganser s.

**argent'affin s.,** carcinoid s.

**Argonz-Del Castillo s.,** Ahumada-Del Castillo s.

**Arndt-Gottron s.,** a variant of lichen myxedematosus.

**Arnold-Chiari s.,** Arnold-Chiari *deformity.*

**Ascher's s.,** a condition in which a congenital double lip is associated with blepharochalasis and nontoxic thyroid gland enlargement.

**auric'ulotemporal nerve s.,** gustatory sweating s.; Frey's s.; localized flushing and sweating of the ear and cheek in response to eating.

**Avellis' s.,** jugular foramen s.; unilateral paralysis of the larynx and velum palati, with contralateral loss of pain and temperature sensibility in the parts below.

**Axenfeld's s.,** a congenital ocular dysgenesis expressed as widened trabecular meshwork, large iridial bands, and glaucoma.

**Balint's s.,** ocular motor apraxia with no ability for voluntary visual fixation, especially for objects in the peripheral field.

**Banti's s.,** Banti's disease; chronic congestive splenomegaly that occurs as a sequel to hypertension in the portal or splenic veins (as a result of cirrhosis of the liver, or thrombosis of the veins); anemia, splenomegaly, and irregular episodes of gastrointestinal bleeding are usually observed, and ascites, jaundice, leukopenia, and thrombocytopenia may develop in various instances.

**Bardet-Biedl s.,** Laurence-Biedl s.

**Barrett s.,** chronic peptic ulcer of a lower esophagus which is lined by columnar epithelium resembling the mucosa of the gastric cardia.

**Bartter's s.,** primary juxtaglomerular cell hyperplasia with secondary hyperaldosteronism. The s. has been reported in children with hypokalemic alkalosis and elevated renin or angiotensin levels; however, the blood pressure is low or normal, and growth is retarded.

**basal cell nevus s.,** hereditary cutaneomandibular polyoncosis; a s. of myriad basal cell carcinoma of the skin, cysts of the jaw bones, erythematous pitting of the palms and soles, calcification of the cerebral falx, and frequently skeletal anomalies, particularly ribs that are bifid or broadened anteriorly.

**Bassen-Kornzweig s.,** abetalipoproteinemia.

**battered child s.,** various injuries to the skeleton, soft tissues, or organs of a child sustained as a result of repeated mistreatment or beating, usually by a parent or step-parent.

**Beckwith-Wiedemann s.,** EMG s.

**Behçet's s.,** Behçet's disease; uveo-encephalitic s.; triple symptom complex; cutaneomucouveal s.; characterized by simultaneously or successively occurring recurrent attacks of genital and oral ulcerations (aphthae) and uveitis or iridocyclitis with hypopyon; a phase of a generalized disorder showing in some cases fewer and in others additional manifestations such as cutaneous ulcerations, erythema nodosum, thrombophlebitis, and cerebral involvement.

**Benedikt's s.,** hemiplegia with clonic spasm or tremor and oculomotor paralysis on the opposite side.

**Bernard-Horner s.,** Horner's s.

**Bernard-Sergent s.,** acute adrenocortical *insufficiency.*

**Bernhardt-Roth s.,** *meralgia* paraesthetica.

**Bernheim's s.,** right heart failure (enlarged liver, distended neck veins, and edema) without pulmonary congestion, in subjects with left ventricular enlargement from any cause, *e.g.,* hypertension. Post mortem, reduction in the size of the right ventricular cavity is found due to encroachment by the hypertrophied septum.

**Besnier-Boeck-Schaumann s.,** sarcoidosis.

**Blatin's s.,** hydatid *thrill.*

**blind loop s.,** usually occurs in the small intestine following operations which produce a blind loop; stagnation of intestinal contents results in the formation of a toxic substance which interferes with absorption of fat, vitamin K, and other nutrients.

**Bloom's s.,** congenital telangiectatic erythema primarily in butterfly distribution of face and occasionally of hands and forearms; sensitivity of skin lesions; dwarfism with normal body proportions except for narrow face and dolichocephalic skull; autosomal recessive inheritance.

**Bogorad's s.,** crocodile tears s.

**Bonnevie-Ullrich s.,** see Turner's s.

**Bonnier's s.,** s. due to a lesion of Deiters' nucleus and its connection. The symptoms include ocular disturbances, *e.g.,* paralysis of accommodation, nystagmus, diplopia, as well as deafness, nausea, thirst, anorexia, and symptoms referable to the involvement of the vagus centers.

**Böök s.,** PHC s.; congenitally associated premolar aplasia, hyperhidrosis, and canities prematura.

**Börjeson-Forssman-Lehmann s.,** a hereditary condition characterized by microcephaly, hypogonadism, short stature, and mental deficiency; transmitted as an x-linked recessive trait.

**brain s., acute,** abnormalities of cerebral function developing suddenly and of relatively short duration; see also neuropsychologic disorder, under disorder.

**brain s., chronic,** disturbances of cerebral function of long duration; see also neuropsychologic disorder.

**Briquet's s.,** aphonia and shortness of breath, due to hysterical paralysis of the diaphragm.

**Brissaud-Marie s.,** unilateral spasm of the tongue and lips, of hysterical nature.

**Brock's s.,** middle lobe s.

**Brown-Séquard's s.,** hemiparaplegia and hyperesthesia, but with loss of joint and muscle sense on the side of the lesion, and hemianesthesia of the opposite side, in case of a unilateral involvement of the spinal cord.

**Brugsch's s.,** acropachyderma.

**Budd's s.,** Chiari's s.

**Bürger-Grütz s.,** type I familial *hyperlipoproteinemia.*

**Burnett's s.,** milk-alkali s.

**Caffey's s.,** infantile cortical *hyperostosis.*

**Caffey-Silverman s.,** infantile cortical *hyperostosis.*

**Capgras' s.,** illusion of doubles; failure to recognize a familiar person and instead believing him to be a "double."

**Caplan's s.,** intrapulmonary nodules, histologically similar to subcutaneous rheumatoid nodules, associated with rheumatoid arthritis and pneumoconiosis in coal workers.

**carcinoid s.,** malignant carcinoid s.; metastatic carcinoid s.; vasculocardiac s. of hyperserotoninemia; argentaffin s.; a combination of symptoms and lesions presumably produced by the release of serotonin from carcinoid tumors in the small intestine which have metastasized to the liver. It consists of irregular mottled blushing, angiomas of the skin, acquired tricuspid and pulmonary stenosis with some minor involvement of valves on the left side of the heart, diarrhea, bronchial spasm, mental aberration, and the excretion of large quantities of 5-hydroxyindoleacetic acid.

**carotid sinus s.,** Charcot-Weiss-Baker s.; pressoreceptor reflex; carotid sinus reflex; stimulation of a hyperactive carotid sinus, causing a marked fall in blood pressure due to vasodilation and cardiac slowing; syncope with or without convulsions or heart block may occur.

**carpal tunnel s.,** pain and paresthesia (tingling, burning, and numbness) in the hand in the area of distribution of the median nerve. Caused by compression of the median nerve by fibers of the flexor retinaculum.

**Carpenter's s.** [ C. C. J. Carpenter ], the association of primary hypothyroidism, primary adrenocortical insufficiency, and diabetes mellitus.

**Carpenter's s.** [ G. Carpenter ], acrocephalopolysyndactyly.

**cataract-oligophrenia s.,** Marinesco-Sjögren s.

**cat-cry s.,** cri-du-chat s.

**cat's-eye s.,** Schmid-Fraccaro s.; a s. characterized by iris colobomas (resembling the vertical pupils of a cat) and anal atresia, associated with an additional acrocentric chromosome; other malformations and mental retardation may be present.

**cauda equina s.,** dull pain in upper sacral region with anesthesia or analgesia in buttocks, genitalia or thigh; disturbed bowel and bladder function.

**cavernous s.,** a s. caused by thrombosis of the cavernous intracranial sinus characterized by edema of eyelids and conjunctivae, and paralysis of the 3rd, 4th and 6th nerves.

**celiac s.,** celiac *disease.*

**cellular immunity deficiency s.,** a s. marked by increased susceptibility to infection, especially to viral infection, associated with defective functioning of the mechanism responsible for acquired immunity of the cell-mediated kind.

**cerebel'lar s.,** the signs and symptoms of cerebellar deficiency: dysmetria, dysarthria, asynergia, nystagmus, ataxia, staggering gait, and adiadochokinesia.

**cerebellomedullary malformation s.,** Arnold-Chiari *deformity.*

**cerebellopontine angle s.,** a s. due most commonly to an acoustic tumor in the region between the cerebellum and pons, and marked by ataxia and hypotension of muscles on the side of the lesion together with nystagmus, tinnitus, deafness, disturbances of labyrinth function, and also involvement of the 5th, 6th, 7th, 9th, or 10th cranial nerves.

**cerebrohepatorenal s.,** Zellweger s.; a rare s. characterized by muscular hypotonia, incomplete myelinization of nervous tissue, craniofacial malformations, hepatomegaly, and small glomerular cysts of the kidney; possibly autosomal recessive inheritance.

**cervical compression s.,** cervical disc s.

**cervical disc s.,** cervical compression s.; pain, paresthesias, and muscular spasms in the area of the distribution of the cervical spinal nerve roots, due to pressure of a protruded cervical intervertebral disc.

**cervical fusion s.,** Klippel-Feil s.

**cervical rib s.,** symptoms due to pressure upon nerves of brachial plexus by a supernumerary rib which arises from the seventh cervical vertebra. The chief symptoms are pain and tingling along the forearm and hand over the distribution of the first thoracic nerve root and, later, anesthesia with cyanosis and coldness over the ulnar area of the hand. Wasting of the intrinsic muscles of the hand may occur.

**cervical tension s.,** posttraumatic neck s.

**cervico-oculo-acoustic s.,** a congenital short neck associated with paralysis of the external ocular muscles and with perceptive deafness.

**Cestan-Chenais s.,** contralateral hemiplegia, hemianesthesia, and loss of pain and temperature sensibility, with ipsilateral hemiasynergia and lateropulsion, paralysis of the larynx and soft palate, enophthalmia, miosis, and ptosis, due to lesions of the brain stem.

**chancriform s.,** an ulcerative lesion at the site of primary infection by microorganisms, with regional lymph node enlargement; it occurs not only in chancroid infections but also in various bacterial and fungal infections.

**Charcot's s.,** intermittent *claudication.*

**Charcot-Weiss-Baker s.,** carotid sinus s.

**Chauffard's s.,** Still-Chauffard s.; the symptoms of Still's disease in one suffering from bovine or other nonhuman form of tuberculosis.

**Chédiak-Steinbrinck-Higashi s.,** Chédiak-Steinbrinck-Higashi anomaly; Chédiak-Higashi disease; Béguez César disease; abnormalities of granulation and nuclear structure of all types of leukocytes with gigantic and monstrous malformation of peroxidase-positive granules, cytoplasmic inclusions and Döhle bodies, often with hepatosplenomegaly, lymphadenopathy, anemia, thrombocytopenia, roentgenologic changes of bones, lungs and heart, skin and psychomotor abnormalities, and susceptibility to infection, usually resulting in death in childhood. Autosomal recessive inheritance.

**Chiari's s.,** thrombosis of the hepatic vein with great enlargement of the liver and extensive development of collateral vessels, intractable ascites, and great portal hypertension. Also called Rokitansky's disease (2); Chiari-Budd s.; Budd-Chiari s.; Budd's s.

**Chiari II s.,** elongation of medulla and cerebellar tonsils and vermis with displacement through the foramen magnum into the upper spinal canal; often associated with other cerebral anomalies.

**Chiari-Frommel s.,** the lactation-amenorrhea s. that is an abnormal prolongation of postpregnancy lactation.

**chias'ma s.,** s. characterized by central scotoma, with unilateral or bilateral visual defect due to a lesion in or about the chiasm.

**Chilaiditi's s.,** interposition of the colon between the liver and the diaphragm.

**"Chinese restaurant" s.,** development of chest pain, feelings of facial pressure, and sensation of burning over variable portions of the body surface after dining in Chinese restaurants; these effects can be produced by administration of monosodium L-glutamate, although size of effective oral doses vary substantially from one individual to another. Sufferers from this syndrome are assumed to be unusually sensitive to the effects of this food additive.

**choleriform s.,** infection resembling cholera.

**Christ-Siemens s.,** anhidrotic ectodermal *dysplasia.*

**Christian's s.,** Hand-Schüller-Christian *disease.*

**chronic hyperventila'tion s.,** reduced $CO_2$ content of the blood (acapnia) as a result of hyperpnea of prolonged duration. May occur in psychotic or nervous subjects or be caused by some chronic organic, usually cardiovascular, disease. It is marked by disorders of respiration, *e.g.,* sighing, and often quite obvious hyperpnea which is increased upon slight provocation. Paresthesia, muscular termors, or even mild tetany may occur.

**Clarke-Hadfield s.,** viscidosis.

**Claude's s.,** midbrain s. with oculomotor palsy on one side and incoordination on the other.

**climacteric s.,** menopausal s.

**Cockayne's s.,** Cockayne's disease; dwarfism, precociously senile appearance, pigmentary degeneration of the retina, optic atrophy, deafness, sensitivity to sunlight, mental retardation; autosomal recessive inheritance.

**Cogan's s.,** oculovestibulo-auditory s.

**compression s.,** crush s. (1).

**Conn's s.,** primary *aldosteronism.*

**Cooke-Apert-Gallais s.,** an imprecise and obsolete designation of various types of female virilization, arising from excessive or abnormal adrenocortical secretions.

**Cornelia de Lange s.,** de Lange s.

**corpus luteum deficiency s.,** functional disturbances due to insufficient ovarian luteinization; they include palpitation, tachycardia, dermographia, dyspnea, hypertension, and blotchy flushing in the facial, cervical, and thoracic regions.

**Costen's s.,** temporomandibular s.

**costochond'ral s.,** pain in the chest with tenderness over one or more costochondral junctions; there is anxiety or apprehension, the patient attributing the pain to some abnormality of the heart; the pain disappears when he is reassured by his physician. The s. is usually the result of some minor injury to the chest.

**costoclavicular s.,** a s. resulting from compression of the neurovascular bundle between the medial portions of the clavicle and the first rib.

**Cotard's s.,** a form of depressive insanity with delusions of negation and suicidal impulse.

**cri-du-chat s.,** cat-cry s.; a disorder due to partial deletion of chromosome 5, characterized by microcephaly, antimongoloid palpebral fissures, epicanthal folds, micrognathia, strabismus, mental and physical retardation, and a characteristic high-pitched catlike whine.

**Crigler-Najjar s.,** Crigler-Najjar disease; defect in ability to form bilirubin glucuronide; a rare entity characterized by familial nonhemolytic jaundice and, in its severe form, by irreversible brain damage that resembles kernicterus and may be fatal. Autosomal recessive inheritance.

**crocodile tears s.,** Bogorad's s.; residual facial paralysis with profuse lacrimation during eating; caused by a lesion of the 7th nerve central to the geniculate ganglion. There is misdirection of regenerating autonomic fibers which formerly innervated the salivary gland to the lacrimal glands.

**Cronkhite-Canada s.,** gastrointestinal polyps with diffuse alopecia and nail dystrophy.

**CRST s.,** a s. characterized by calcinosis cutis, Raynaud's phenomenon, sclerodactyly, and telangiectasia; usually due to scleroderma.

**crush s.,** (1) compression s.; the shocklike state that follows release of a limb or limbs or the trunk and pelvis after a prolonged period of compression, as by a beam, earth, masonry, or other heavy objects; the condition is characterized by suppression of urine, probably the result of damage to the renal tubules by myoglobin from the damaged muscles; (2) delayed complications of electric shock therapy.

**Cruveilhier-Baumgarten s.,** Cruveilhier-Baumgarten disease; cirrhosis of the liver with patent umbilical or paraumbilical veins and varicose periumbilical veins (caput medusae).

**cryptophthalmus s.,** Fraser's s.

**Cushing's s.,** a disorder resulting from increased adrenocortical secretion of cortisol; it is caused by ACTH-dependent adrenocortical hyperplasia or tumor, ectopic ACTH-secreting tumor, or ACTH-independent adrenocortical tumor or nodular hyperplasia; it is characterized by centripetal obesity, moon face, acne, abdominal striae, hypertension, decreased carbohydrate tolerance, protein catabolism, psychiatric disturbances, and amenorrhea and hirsutism in females; Cushing's s. associated with a pituitary adenoma is sometimes called Cushing's disease.

**Cushing's s. medicamentosus,** a variable number of the signs and symptoms of Cushing's s.; produced by the chronic administration of large doses of any steroid that is a potent glucocorticoid.

**cutaneomucouveal s.,** Behçet's s.

**Da Costa's s., neurocirculatory** *asthenia.*

**Dandy-Walker s.,** hydrocephalus in infants associated with atresia of the foramen of Magendie.

**dead fetus s.,** s. characterized by lengthy intrauterine retention of a dead fetus and loss of incoagulable blood; persistent tachycardia is usually present before hemorrhage occurs; fibrinogen levels are usually chronically depressed.

**Degos' s.,** malignant atrophic *papulosis.*

**Déjérine-Roussy s.,** thalamic s.

**de Lange s.,** Cornelia de Lange s.; typus degenerativus amstelodamensis; growth failure, mental retardation, characteristic facies with eyebrows growing across base of nose and hairline well down on forehead, depressed bridge of nose with uptilted tip of nose, small head with low-set ears, hands flat and spadelike, with short tapering fingers.

**De Sanctis-Cacchione s.,** xeroderma pigmentosum with neurological complications.

**De Toni-Fanconi s.,** cystinosis.

**s. of deviously relevant answers,** Ganser s.

**dialysis disequilibrium s.,** nausea, vomiting, and hypertension, occasionally with convulsions, developing within several hours after starting hemodialysis for renal failure; apparently caused by too rapid removal of urea from the extracellular fluid compartment, with movement of water into cells, and cerebral edema.

**diencephalic s. of infancy,** profound emaciation after initial normal growth, locomotor hyperactivity and euphoria, usually with skin pallow, hypotension and hypoglycemia; usually due to neoplasm involving the anterior hypothalamus.

**Di George s.,** third and fourth pharyngeal pouch s.; congenital absence of the thymus and parathyroid glands, without agammaglobulinemia but with frequent infections and delayed development.

**Di Guglielmo's s.,** acute erythremic *myelosis.*

**disc s.,** low back pain, pain in the thigh, sometimes wasting and loss of knee and ankle jerks; the result of a compressive radiculopathy from intervertebral disc pressure.

**dorsalgic-gynecologic s.,** in patients with functional gynecologic problems, thoracic and lumbosacral pain associated with menstrual dysfunction and mastalgia, flattening of the thoracic vertebrae, and probably hemisacralization or sacralization.

**Down's s.,** a syndrome of mental retardation associated with a variable constellation of abnormalities caused by representation of at least a critical portion of chromosome 21 three times instead of twice in some or all cells; no single physical sign is diagnostic and most stigmata are found in some normal persons; the abnormalities include retarded growth, flat hypoplastic face with short nose, prominent epicanthic skin folds, protruding lower lip, small rounded ears with prominent antihelix, fissured and thickened tongue, laxness of joint ligaments, pelvic dysplasia, broad hands and feet, stubby fingers usually with dysplasia of the middle phalanx of the fifth finger, transverse palmar crease, dermatoglyphic changes including distal displacement of the palmar axial triradius, dry rough skin in older patients and abundant slack neck skin in newborns, and muscle hypotonia and absence of Moro reflex in newborns; most patients are trisomic for chromosome 21 as a result of nondisjunction; some patients are mosaic, with both normal and trisomic cell lines; a few patients have 46 chromosomes but are effectively trisomic because of translocation of a major portion of chromosome 21 to another chromosome; in rare patients no chromosome abnormality can be detected; also called mongolism; mongolian or mongoloid idiocy; trisomy 21 syndrome.

**Duane's s.,** retraction s.

**Dubin-Johnson s.,** recurrence of mild jaundice, impaired dye excretion, iron free pigment from hepatic cells, Bromsulphalein retention, nonvisualization of gallbladder; originally discovered by Sprinz and Nelson; also called maverohepatic *icterus.*

**Dubreuil-Chambardel s.,** simultaneous caries of the upper incisor teeth occurring in either sex between the ages of 14 and 17; after an interval of varying length the other teeth are also attacked.

**Duchenne's s.,** subacute or chronic anterior spinal paralysis combined with multiple neuritis.

**dumping s.,** postgastrectomy s.; the s. that occurs after eating in patients with shunts of the upper alimentary canal; characterized by flushing, sweating, dizziness, weakness, and vasomotor collapse; occasionally with pain and headache.

**dysmnesic s.,** Korsakoff's s.

**dystocia-dystrophia s.,** a condition characterized by failure of the fetal head to engage; maternal pelvic measurements are less than normal, cyesis is apt to be prolonged, and cephalopelvic disproportion exists.

**ectopic ACTH s.,** the association of Cushing's s. with a neoplasm, usually a lung carcinoma that produces ACTH.

**Edwards' s.,** trisomy E s.

**effort s.,** neurocirculatory *asthenia.*

**egg-white injury s.,** dermatitis, loss of hair and loss of muscle coordination, produced in rats by diets containing large amounts of raw egg white, the avidin of which combines with biotin producing a deficiency of the latter.

**Ehlers-Danlos s.,** a developmental mesenchymal dysplasia characterized by overelasticity and friability of the skin, excessive extensibility of the joints, fragility of the cutaneous blood vessels and sometimes large arteries, due to deficient quality or quantity of collagen; there are several types, the most common of which is inherited as an autosomal dominant.

**Eisenlohr's s.,** numbness and weakness in the extremities, paralysis of the lips, tongue, and palate, and dysarthria.

**Eisenmenger s.,** the pathophysiologic s. resulting when pulmonary hypertension is associated with a congenital communication between the two circulations (*e.g.*, atrial or ventricular septal defect, patent ductus arteriosus) so that a right-to-left shunt results.

**Ekbom s.,** restless legs s.

**Ellis-van Creveld s.,** chondroectodermal *dysplasia.*

**EMG s.,** Beckwith-Wiedemann s.; exomphalos, macroglossia, and gigantism, often with neonatal hypoglycemia, flame nevus of the face, or ear lobe anomalies; autosomal recessive inheritance.

**enceph'alotrigem'inal vascular s.,** angiomatosis of the brain accompanied by nevi in the trigeminal area.

**endocrine polyglandular s.,** multiple endocrinopathy; multiple endocrine tumors involving the pancreatic islets, the parathyroid, and the pituitary.

**extrapyramidal s.,** abnormalities of movement related to injury of motor pathways other than the pyramidal tract.

**external carotid steal s.,** characterized by brief ischemic attacks during which dizziness and loss of balance are experienced; caused by vertebrobasilar insufficiency resulting from siphoning of blood from the vertebral artery to the external carotid artery.

**Faber's s., achlorhydric** *anemia.*

**Fanconi's s.,** (1) Fanconi's *anemia;* (2) a group of conditions with characteristic disorders of renal tubular function, which may be classified as: (*a*) cystinosis (*q.v.*), also termed Lignac-Fanconi, De Toni-Fanconi, or Abderholden-Fanconi s.; a recessive hereditary disease of early childhood; (*b*) *adult Fanconi s.,* a rare hereditary form, probably due to a different recessive gene than cystinosis, characterized by the tubular malfunction seen in cystinosis and by osteomalacia, but cystine deposit in tissues is absent; and (*c*) *acquired Fanconi s.,* which may be associated with multiple myeloma, or result from chemical poisoning, injury, or persisting damage of proximal tubular epithelium due to various causes, leading to multiple defects of tubular function.

**Felty's s.,** rheumatoid arthritis with splenomegaly and leukopenia.

**female prostatic obstructing s.,** obstruction of the bladder neck in a female, usually caused by muscular hypertrophy with fibrous contraction due to nonspecific inflammation of the mucosa and glands which may represent homologues of the prostate.

**fetal aspiration s.,** a s. resulting from uterine aspiration by the fetus and characterized by meconium-stained fetal skin and nails, coarse and irregular streaks of interstitial markings, and areas of aeration focal irregularities.

**fibrinogen-fibrin conversion s.,** a s. characterized by hypofibrinogenemia with incoagulable blood; it may be seen in abruptio placentae, prolonged retention of a dead fetus in an Rh-isosensitized mother, Sheehan's syndrome, hemolytic blood reactions, bilateral renal cortical necrosis, and cases of trauma.

**Figueira's s.,** weakness of the neck muscles with slight spasticity of the muscles of the lower extremities and increased tendon reflexes; supposed to be an attenuated sporadic form of acute poliomyelitis.

**first arch s.,** generic term including s.'s of malformations involving derivatives of the first branchial arch, with or without associated malformations; includes mandibulofacial dysostosis, micrognathia with peromelia, otomandibular dystosis, acrofacial dysostosis and others.

**Fisher's s.,** ophthalmoplegia, ataxia, areflexia; a form of polyneuroradiculitis.

**Fitz-Hugh and Curtis s.,** gonococcal perihepatitis in women with a history of gonorrheal salpingitis.

**floppy valve s.,** incompetence of the mitral valve (in women) or aortic valve (in men) due to fibromyxomatous degeneration of the valve leaflets.

**Flynn-Aird s.,** a familial s. characterized by muscle wasting, ataxia, dementia, skin atrophy, and ocular anomalies.

**Forbes-Albright s.,** pituitary tumor in a patient without acromegaly which secretes excessive amounts of prolactin (LTH) and produces persistent lactation.

**Foster Kennedy's s.,** Kennedy's s.; ipsilateral optic atrophy with central scotoma and contralateral choked disk or papilledema, cause by a meningioma of the ipsilateral optic nerve.

**Foville's s.,** alternating hemiplegia; abducens paralysis on one side, paralysis of the extremities on the other.

**Franceschetti's s.,** see mandibulofacial *dysostosis.*

**Fraser's s.,** cryptophthalmus s.; an association of cryptophthalmus with multiple anomalies, including middle and outer ear malformations, cleft palate, laryngeal deformity, displacement of umbilicus and nipples, digital malformations, separation of symphysis pubis, maldevelopment of kidneys, and masculinization of genitalia in females; probably autosomal recessive inheritance.

**Freeman-Sheldon s.,** craniocarpotarsal *dystrophy.*

**Frenkel's anterior ocular traumatic s.,** mydriasis, hyphema, small iris tears near the pupil, discrete punctate opacities of lens, and occasionally iridodialysis.

**Frey's s.,** auriculotemporal nerve s.

**Friderichsen-Waterhouse s.,** see Waterhouse-Friderichsen s.

**Fröhlich's s.,** Launois-Cléret s.; dystrophia adiposogenitalis (*q.v.*) caused by an adenohypophysial tumor.

**Froin's s.,** loculation s.; an alteration in the cerebrospinal fluid, which is yellowish in hue and coagulates spontaneously in a few seconds after withdrawal, owing to its greatly increased protein (albumin and globulin) content; noted in loculated portions of the subarachnoid space isolated from spinal fluid circulation by an inflammatory or neoplastic obstruction.

**Fuchs' s.,** unilateral heterochromia of the iris, iridocyclitis, keratitic precipitates and cataract; a congenital progressive disease of unknown origin.

**functional prepubertal castration s.,** characterized by the absence of testes from the scrotum but in their place Wolffian duct derivatives, pronounced gynecomastia, and increased urinary excretion of gonadotrophins. The clinical manifestations are those of a boy surgically castrated before puberty, namely, failure in the development of the sex organs and of the secondary sex characters.

**Gaisböck's s.,** *polycythemia* hypertonica.

**Ganser's s.,** s. of approximate relevant answers; s. of deviously relevant answers; nonsense s.; a psychotic-like condition, without the symptoms and signs of a traditional psychosis, occurring typically in prisoners who feign insanity; *e.g.,* such a person, when asked to multiply 6 by 4, will give 23 as the answer, or he will call a key a lock.

**Gardner's s.,** the development of multiple tumors, inherited as a dominant trait, including osteomas of the skull, epidermoid cysts, fibromas and scattered polyps of the colon.

**gastrocardiac s.,** disturbances of the heart's action due to faulty action of the digestive system, especially of the stomach.

**gastrojejunal loop obstruction s.,** afferent loop s.

**Gee-Herter s.,** celiac *disease.*

**Gélineau's s.,** narcolepsy.

**general-adaptation s.,** term given by Selye to the nonspecific reactions of organisms to organic and mental injury or stress. It comprises three stages: (1) alarm reaction; (2) stage of resistance, which includes all those nonspecific systemic adaptive reactions called forth by prolonged exposure to injurious stimuli; (3) state of exhaustion, in which the adaptation can no longer be maintained.

**Gerstmann s.,** finger agnosia, agraphia, confusion of laterality of body, and acalculia; caused by lesions between the occipital area and the angular gyrus.

**Gianotti-Crosti s.,** an exanthem comprised of dusky papules on the legs, buttocks, and extensors of the arms; it lasts 2 to 8 weeks and is associated with adenopathy and malaise.

**Gilles de la Tourette s.,** Gilles de la Tourette *disease.*

**glomangiomatous osseous malformation s.,** a congenital association of glomus tumors with osteoporosis of limb bones.

**Goldberg-Maxwell s.,** testicular feminization s.

**Goldenhar's s.,** oculoauriculovertebral *dysplasia.*

**Goodpasture's s.,** glomerulonephritis associated with or preceded by hemoptysis. The nephritis usually progresses to produce death from renal failure, and the lungs at autopsy show extensive hemosiderosis or recent hemorrhage.

**Gorlin-Chaudhry-Moss s.,** a very rare congenital condition in which are associated craniofacial dysostosis, patent ductus arteriosus, hypertrichosis, hypoplasia of labia majora, and dental and ocular abnormalities.

**Gowers' s.,** vagal *attack.*

**gracilis s.,** osteonecrosis of the pubic bone following trauma.

**Gradenigo's s.,** petrositis with abducens paralysis and pain in the temporal region, due to localized meningitis involving the fifth and sixth nerves.

**Greig's s.,** ocular *hypertelorism.*

**Grönblad-Strandberg s.,** angioid streaks of the retina together with pseudoxanthoma elasticum of the skin.

**Gruber's s.,** *dysencephalia* splanchnocystica.

**Gubler's s.,** alternate *hemiplegia.*

**Guillain-Barré s.,** myeloradiculopolyneuronitis; radiculoganglionitis; so-called infectious polyneuritis; a neurologic s. of unknown cause, but probably due to a virus, or sensitivity to a virus; marked by paresthesias of the limbs and muscular weakness or a flaccid paralysis. The characteristic laboratory finding is increased protein in the cerebrospinal fluid without increase in cell count.

**Gunn's s.,** jaw-winking s.

**gustatory sweating s.,** auriculotemporal nerve s.

**Hallermann-Streiff s.,** *dyscephalia* mandibulo-oculofacialis.

**Hallervorden s.,** a pathologic process in which the nerve fibers connecting the striatum and pallidum are completely demyelinated.

**Hamman s.,** Hamman's disease; spontaneous mediastinal emphysema, resulting from rupture of alveoli.

**Hamman-Rich s.,** acute or chronic interstitial fibrosis of the lung, giving rise to serious right-sided heart failure and cor pulmonale. The cuase is unknown; there may be multiple etiologies.

**hand-and-foot s.,** sickle cell dactylitis; recurrent painful swelling of the hands and feet occurring in infants and young children with sickle cell anemia.

**Hanhart's s.,** *micrognathia* with peromelia.

**Harada's s.,** Harada's disease; uveoencephalitis; uveomeningitis s.; bilateral fundal edema, uveitis, choroiditis, and retinal detachment, with temporary or permanent loss of hearing and visual acuity, graying of the hair, and alopecia; related to the Vogt-Koyanagi s. and sympathetic ophthalmia.

**harlequin color change s.,** a unilateral flushing reaction seen sometimes in newbown or young infants.

**Hartnup s.,** Hartnup *disease.*

**Hayem-Widal s.,** Widal's s.; icteroanemia; acquired hemolytic icterus; a s. in which icterus and anemia occur in association with a moderate degree of splenomegaly, increased fragility of red blood cells, and increased amounts of urobilin in the urine.

**hemangioma-thrombocytopenia s.,** a rare congenital association of vascular tumors with thrombocytopenic purpura.

**hemolytic-uremic s.,** acute renal failure, hemolytic anemia, and thrombocytopenia.

**hemopleuropneumonia s.,** hemoptysis, sudden dyspnea, moderate tachycardia, and a fever, with tubular breathing over the middle zone of the chest and dullness at the base, indicating a pneumonia combined with hemothorax in cases of puncture wounds of the chest.

**Henoch-Schönlein s.,** Henoch-Schönlein *purpura.*

**hepatonephric s.,** hepatorenal s.

**hepatorenal s.,** the occurrence of acute renal failure in patients with disease of the liver or biliary tract. Apart from special conditions which damage both organs, such as carbon tetrachloride poisoning and leptosprosis, there is disagreement whether the kidneys of patients with obstructive jaundice or cirrhosis are more susceptible than usual to the common causes of acute renal failure such as hypotension. Animal experiments suggest that conjugated bilirubin may increase renal damage resulting from ischemia.

**holiday s.,** regression, development of diffuse anxiety, feelings of helplessness, irritability, and depression; said to occur in certain psychoanalytic patients before Thanksgiving and continuing into the Christmas holiday season, ending a few days after January first.

**Holmes-Adie s.,** a condition of unknown etiology and pathology characterized by tonic pupillary reactions (see tonic *pupil*); the tendon reflexes may be absent or diminished. Also called Adie s.; papillotonic pseudotabes.

**Holt-Oram s.,** atriodigital dysplasia; a hereditary and congenital s. consisting of a secundum atrial septal defect in association with fingerized or absent thumb and other deformities of the forearm.

**Horner's s.,** ptosis sympathetica; Bernard-Horner s.; ptosis, miosis, anidrosis, and enophthalmos due to paralysis of the cervical sympathetic.

**Houssay s.,** the amelioration of diabetes mellitus by a destructive lesion in, or surgical removal of, the pituitary gland.

**Hunt's s.'s,** Ramsay Hunt's s.'s; (1) progressive cerebellar tremor; dyssynergia cerebellaris progressiva; an intention tremor beginning in one extremity, gradually increasing in intensity, and subsequently involving other parts of the body; (2) facial paralysis, otalgia, and herpes zoster resulting from viral infection of the seventh cranial nerve and geniculate ganglion; (3) paleostriatal or pallidal s.; a form of juvenile paralysis agitans associated with primary atrophy of the pallidal system.

**Hunter's s.,** mucopolysaccharidosis type II; gargoylism (X-linked recessive type); an error of mucopolysaccharide metabolism with excretion of chondroitin sulfate B and heparitin sulfate in the urine; clinically similar to Hurler's

s. (*q. v.*), but distinguished by less severe skeletal changes, no corneal clouding, and X-linked recessive inheritance.

**Hurler's s.,** an error of mucopolysaccharide metabolism characterized by a deficiency of α-L-iduronidase, an accumulation of an abnormal intracellular material, and excretion of chondroitin sulfate B and heparitin sulfate in the urine; severe abnormality in development of skeletal cartilage and bone, with dwarfism, kyphosis, deformed limbs, limitation of joint motion, spadelike hand, corneal clouding, hepatosplenomegaly, mental retardation, and gargoyl-like facies; autosomal recessive inheritance; also known as dysostosis multiplex; gargoylism (autosomal recessive type); Hurler's disease; lipochondrodystrophy; mucopolysaccharidosis type I; Pflaundler-Hurler s.; see also mucolipidosis.

**Hutchinson-Gilford s.,** progeria.

**Hutchison s.,** adrenal neuroblastoma of infants with metastasis to the orbit; at one time erroneously believed to arise predominantly from the left adrenal gland; see also Pepper s.

**hydralazine s.,** a s. simulating disseminated lupus erythematosus and rheumatoid arthritis, occurring during protracted therapy of hypertension with hydralazine; LE phenomenon may be positive.

**17-hydroxylase deficiency s.,** congenital deficiency of adrenocortical, and possibly ovarian, steroid C-17α hydroxylase; the resulting excessive secretion of corticosterone and deoxycorticosterone produces hypertension and hypokalemic alkalosis; absence of aldosterone secretion in such patients may indicate a multiple enzymic deficiency.

**hyperabduction s.,** pain running down the arm, numbness, paresthesias, and erythema, with weakness of the hands; due to abduction of the arm for a prolonged period (*e.g.,* during sleep or necessitated by occupation) which stretches the axillary vessels and the nerves of the brachial plexus.

**hyperkinetic s.,** hypomanic reaction; a condition marked by pathologically excessive energy; seen sometimes in young children with brain injury or mental defect and in epileptics; hypermotility and emotional instability are the chief characteristics. Distractibility, inattention, lack of shyness and of fear are common accompaniments.

**hypersensitive xiphoid s.,** abnormal tenderness of the xiphoid, often associated with spontaneous pains in the chest, upper abdomen, and shoulders.

**hypertrophied frenula s.,** a condition marked by abnormal frenula, pseudoclefts in lip, tongue and palate, mental retardation, and syndactyly.

**hyperventilation s.,** hyperpnea and dyspnea in anxious or depressed individuals, leading to alkalosis and the symptoms incident thereto.

**hyperviscosity s.,** a s. resulting from increased viscosity of the blood; an increase in serum proteins may be associated with bleeding from mucous membranes, retinopathy, and neurological symptoms, and is sometimes seen in Waldenström's macroglobulinemia and in multiple myeloma; an increased viscosity secondary to polycythemia may be associated with organ congestion and decreased capillary perfusion.

**hypometabolic s.,** a clinical situation suggesting hypothyroidism or myxedema, in which some tests of thyroid function may be normal and the gland is not obviously atrophic or diseased; suggests a failure of the body to react to thyroid hormone. An imprecisely delineated s. of uncertain occurrence.

**hypoparathyroidism s.,** a s. characterized by fatigue, muscular weakness, paresthesia and cramps of the extremities, tetany, and laryngeal stridor; it may be idiopathic, postoperative, or caused by organic lesions of the parathyroids.

**hypophysis s.,** *dystrophia* adiposogenitalis.

**hypoplastic left heart s.,** the association of underdevelopment of the left heart chambers with atresia or stenosis of the aortic and/or mitral valve and hypoplasia of the ascending aorta.

**immunological deficiency s.,** immunodeficiency s.; a s. associated with an immunological deficiency or disorder, chief among the symptoms of which is an increased susceptibility to infection, the pattern of susceptibility being dependent upon the kind of deficiency; see also immunodeficiency.

**indifference to pain s.,** congenital insensitivity to pain, possibly due to an absence of organized nerve endings in the skin.

**internal capsule s.,** hemianopsia with contralateral hemianesthesia of the face.

**inversed jaw-winking s.,** when there are supranuclear lesions of the trigeminal nerve, touching the cornea may produce a brisk movement of the mandible to the opposite side.

**Irvine's s.,** edema of macula that occasionally follows cataract extraction.

**Ivemark's s.,** splenic agenesis s.

**Jackson's s.,** unilateral paralysis of the larynx, velum palati, and tongue.

**Jadassohn-Lewandowsky s.,** *pachyonychia* congenita.

**Jahnke's s.,** Sturge-Weber s. without glaucoma.

**jaw-winking s.,** an increase in the width of the eye lids during chewing, sometimes with a rhythmic elevation of the upper lid when the mouth is open and ptosis when the mouth is closed. Also called jaw-winking phenomenon; Gunn's (or Marcus Gunn) phenomenon or syndrome; jaw-working reflex.

**Jeghers-Peutz s.,** Peutz-Jeghers s.

**Jervell and Lange-Nielsen s.,** a heritable disorder characterized by deafmutism and electrocardiographically by a prolonged Q-T interval. Syncopal episodes develop and death from cardiac standstill occurs, usually within the first decade of life. Commonly, no organic heart disease is found at autopsy. May represent a congenital disorder of myocardial metabolism.

**Job s.** [ after *Job*, biblical character ], multiple abscesses of the skin and viscera due to increased susceptibility, of unknown cause, to staphylococcal infection.

**jugular foramen s.,** Avellis' s.

**Kallmann's s.,** hypogonadism with anosmia; see under hypogonadism.

**Kanner's s.,** infantile *autism*.

**Kartagener's s.,** complete situs inversus associated with bronchiectasis and chronic sinusitis. Bronchiectasis is a common finding in persons with situs inversus, compared with the general population.

**Kasabach-Merritt s.,** capillary hemangioma associated with thrombocytopenic purpura.

**Katayama s.,** *schistosomiasis* japonicum.

**Kennedy's s.,** Foster Kennedy's s.

**Kimmelstiel-Wilson s.,** Kimmelstiel-Wilson *disease.*

**Klinefelter's s.,** XXY; a chromosomal anomaly with chromosome count 47, XXY sex chromosome constitution; buccal and other cells are usually sex chromatin-positive; patients are male in development, but with seminiferous tubule dysgenesis, elevated urinary gonadotropins, variable gynecomastia, eunuchoid habitus; some patients are chromosomal mosaics, with two or more cell lines of different chromosome constitution.

**Klippel-Feil s.,** cervical fusion s.; a congenital defect manifest as a short neck, extensive fusion of the cervical vertebrae, and abnormalities of the brain stem and cerebellum.

**Klippel-Trenaunay-Weber s.,** an anomaly of the extremity in which there is a combination of angiomatosis and anomalous development of the underlying bone and muscle, sometimes associated with localized gigantism; to be differentiated from Maffucci's syndrome; also known as angio-osteohypertrophy syndrome; congenital dysplastic angiectasis; elephantiasis congenita angiomatosa; hemangiectatic hypertrophy.

**Klumpke-Déjérine s.,** Klumpke's *paralysis.*

**Klüver-Bucy s.,** a s. characterized by psychic blindness or hyperreactivity to visual stimuli, increased oral and sexual activity, and depressed drive and emotional reactions; reported in monkeys after bilateral temporal lobe ablation, but rarely reported in man.

**Koenig's s.,** alternating attacks of constipation and diarrhea, with colic, meteorism, and gurgling in the right iliac fossa, said to be symptomatic of cecal tuberculosis.

**Korsakoff's s.,** Korsakoff's psychosis; polyneuritic, amnestic, or dysmnesic psychosis; cerebropathia psychica toxemica; a s. characterized by confusion and severe impairment of memory, especially for recent events, for which the patient compensates by confabulation; typically encountered in chronic alcoholics. Delirium tremens may

precede the s., and Wernicke's s. often coexists. Treatment with thiamin and glucose is helpful, but less so than in Wernicke's s. The precise pathogenesis is uncertain, but direct toxic effects of alcohol are probably less important than severe nutritional deficiencies often associated with chronic alcoholism.

**Krabbe's s.,** an incomplete form of Sturge-Weber s. consisting of angiomas of face and meninges only; not to be confused with Krabbe's disease.

**Kuskokwim s.,** congenital joint contractures resembling arthrogryposis, found in Eskimos of the Kuskokwim river delta in Alaska.

**Laband's s.,** hereditary fibromatosis of the gingivae, associated with lysis of the distal phalanges, nail dysplasia, and sometimes hepatosplenomegaly; autosomal dominant inheritance.

**Labbé's neurocirculatory s.,** an anxiety neurosis that may occur in Basedow's disease but may be associated with tachycardia and exophthalmos without increase of basal metabolic rate or other evidence of hyperthyroidism.

**lactation-amenorrhea s.,** abnormal postpartum milk production, plus amenorrhea, in a woman who is not nursing.

**Lambert-Eaton s.,** carcinomatous myopathy; progressive proximal muscle weakness in patients with carcinoma, in the absence of cutaneous lesions of dermatomyositis.

**Larsen's s.,** a s. characterized by multiple congenital dislocations with osseous anomalies, including characteristic flattened facies and cleft soft palate.

**Lasègue's s.,** inability to move the anesthetic limb, except under control of the sight, in conversion hysteria.

**Launois-Cléret s.,** Fröhlich's s.

**Laurence-Biedl s.,** an inherited (autosomal recessive) disorder characterized by some or all of the following: mental defects, dystrophia adiposogenitalis, polydactylism, visual disturbances such as retinitis pigmentosa and optic nerve atrophy, and various anomalies of infrequent occurrence; also called Bardet-Biedl s.; Laurence-Moon-Biedl s.; Laurence-Moon-Bardet-Biedl s.

**Laurence-Moon-Bardet-Biedl s.,** Laurence-Biedl s.

**Laurence-Moon-Biedl s.,** Laurence-Biedl s.

**Lawford's s.,** an incomplete form of Sturge-Weber s. consisting of angiomas of face and choroid only, with late glaucoma.

**Leri-Weill s.,** dyschondrosteosis.

**Leriche's s.,** aortoiliac occlusive *disease.*

**Lermoyez' s.,** increasing deafness, interrupted by a sudden attack of dizziness, after which the hearing improves.

**Lesch-Nyhan s.,** a heritable disorder that occurs only in males and is characterized by hyperuricemia, choreoathetosis, mental retardation and compulsive self-mutilation. Associated with failure to form hypoxanthine-guanine phosphoribosyl transferase.

**Libman-Sacks s.,** Libman-Sacks *endocarditis.*

**Lignac-Fanconi s.,** cystinosis.

**Lobstein's s.,** the coexistence in one patient of brittle bones, blue sclera, and otosclerosis, all three of which are common findings in osteogenesis imperfecta, *q. v.*

**loculation s.,** Froin's s.

**Löffler's s.,** (1) eosinophilia with migratory opacities in the lungs, sometimes associated with fever, cough, breathlessness, anorexia, and weight loss; postmortem examination or lung biopsy reveals scattered areas of increased density in the lungs that show granulomatous tissue and many eosinophils; (2) Löffler's *endocarditis.*

**Lorain-Lévi s.,** pituitary *dwarfism.*

**Louis-Bar s.,** *ataxia* telangiectasia.

**low salt s.,** a s. resulting from salt restriction in treatment of congestive heart failure and hypertension; occurs also in cirrhosis of the liver with ascites and in adrenal insufficiency. It is characterized by weakness, drowsiness, muscle cramps, and a reduction in glomerular filtration with consequent nitrogen retention, renal failure, and death.

**low sodium s.,** low salt s.

**Lowe's s.,** oculocerebrorenal s.

**Lowe-Terrey-MacLachlan s.,** oculocerebrorenal s.

**Lown-Ganong-Levine s.,** electrocardiographic s. of a short P-R interval with normal duration of the QRS complex; it lacks the slurred Δ wave of the Wolff-Parkinson-White s., but resembles it in its frequent association with paroxysmal tachycardia.

**Lutembacher's s.,** a congenital cardiac abnormality consisting of a defect of the interatrial septum, mitral stenosis, and enlarged right atrium.

**MacEod s.,** a unilateral pulmonary condition characterized clinically by decreased breath sounds and radiographically with increased radiolucency and decreased lung markings on the affected side. The lung is normal or decreased in size and the bronchi are not obstructed.

**Macleod's s.,** abnormal transradiancy of one lung associated with diminished breath sounds and diminished movement of the diaphragm on that side, apparently secondary to airway obstruction.

**Maffucci's s.,** dyschondroplasia with hemangiomas; enchondromatosis with multiple cavernous hemangiomas.

**Magendie-Hertwig s.,** Magendie-Hertwig *sign.*

**malabsorption s.,** a state characterized by diverse features such as diarrhea, weakness, edema, lassitude, weight loss, poor appetite, protuberant abdomen, pallor, bleeding tendencies, paresthesias, muscle cramps, etc., caused by any of several conditions in which there is ineffective absorption of nutrients, *e.g.,* sprue, gastroileostomy, tuberculosis, and certain fistulas.

**malignant carcinoid s.,** carcinoid s.

**Mallory-Weiss s.,** laceration of the lower end of the esophagus associated with bleeding, or penetration into the mediastinum, with subsequent mediastinitis; caused usually by the incoordinate and severe retching and vomiting of a person when drunk.

**mandibulofacial dysotosis s.,** mandibulofacial *dysostosis.*

**mandibulo-oculofacial s.,** *dyscephalia* mandibulo-oculofacialis.

**Marchesani s.,** spherophakia-brachymorphia s.

**Marchiafava-Micheli s.,** paroxysmal nocturnal *hemoglobinuria.*

**Marcus Gunn s.,** jaw-winking s.

**Marfan's s.,** a hereditary condition due to congenital changes in the mesodermal and ectodermal tissues, skeletal changes (arachnodactyly, excessive length of extremities, laxness of joints), bilateral ectopia lentis, and vascular defects (particularly aneurysm of the aorta, dissecting or diffuse); iris transillumination is marked due to a deficiency of posterior epithelium pigment; autosomal dominant inheritance.

**Marie-Robinson s.,** insomnia and mild melancholia associated with alimentary levulosuria.

**Marinesco-Garland s.,** Marinesco-Sjögren s.

**Marinesco-Sjögren s.,** a rare, inherited (autosomal recessive) neurologic disorder characterized by cerebellolental degeneration with mental retardation; also called Marinesco-Garland s.; Torsten Sjögren's s.; cataract-oligophrenia s.

**Maroteaux-Lamy s.,** type VI mucopolysaccharidosis; polydystrophic dwarfism; an error of mucopolysaccharide metabolism with excretion of chondroitin sulfate B in the urine; growth retardation, lumbar kyphosis, sternal protrusion, genu valgum, usually hepatosplenomegaly, no mental retardation; onset occurs after the age of 2 years; autosomal recessive inheritance.

**Martorell's s.,** aortic arch s.

**massive bowel resection s.,** the state of malabsorption which follows extensive resection of the bowel, particularly the small intestine, characterized by diarrhea, steatorrhea, hypoproteinemia, and malnutrition.

**meconium blockage s.,** low intestinal obstruction in newborn infants resulting from blockage of meconium.

**megacystic s.,** large, smooth, thin-walled bladder, vesicoureteral regurgitation, dilated ureters.

**Meigs' s.,** fibromyoma of the ovary associated with hydroperitoneum and hydrothorax.

**Melkersson's s.,** a rare triad of recurrent facial paralysis, facial edema, and lingua plicata.

**Mendelson's s.,** aspiration of gastric contents into the lungs which often follows vomiting or regurgitation in obstetrical patients still under the effects of anesthetic, or in a stupor.

**Menétrièr's s.,** Menétrièr's *disease.*

**Ménière's s.,** Ménière's *disease.*

**Menkes' s.,** kinky-hair *disease.*

**menopausal s.,** climacteric s.; recurring symptoms experienced by some women during the climacteric period; they include hot flashes, chills, headache, irritability, and depression.

**metastatic carcinoid s.,** carcinoid s.

**Meyenburg-Altherr-Uehlinger s.,** relapsing *perichondritis.*

**Meyer-Schwickerath and Weyers s.,** oculodentodigital *dysplasia.*

**micrognathia with peromelia (s. of),** see under micrognathia.

**middle lobe s.,** Brock's s.; atelectasis with chronic pneumonitis of the middle lobe of the (right) lung. The chief symptoms are chronic cough, wheezing, recurrent respiratory infections, hemoptysis, chest pain, malaise, easy fatigability, and loss of weight. Sometimes confused with interlobar accumulation of fluid.

**Mikulicz' s.,** the symptoms characteristic of Mikulicz' disease occurring as a complication of some other disease, such as lymphosarcoma, leukemia, or uveoparotid fever.

**milk-alkali s.,** a chronic nephrosis-like disorder of the kidneys, reversible in its early stages, induced by protracted therapy of peptic ulcer with alkalis and a high milk regimen.

**Milkman's s.,** osteoporosis with multiple fractures; occurs most frequently in middle-aged women.

**Millard-Gubler s.,** alternate *hemiplegia.*

**Milles' s.,** an incomplete form of Sturge-Weber s. consisting of angiomas of face and choroid, without glaucoma.

**Möbius s.,** congenital facial diplegia; a developmental bilateral facial paralysis usually associated with oculomotor or other neurological disorders.

**Monakow's s.,** contralateral hemiplegia, hemianesthesia, and homonomous hemianopsia due to occlusion of the anterior choroidal artery.

**Morgagni's s.,** Stewart-Morel s.; metabolic craniopathy; hyperostosis frontalis interna in elderly women, with virilism and obesity of uncertain cause.

**Morgagni-Adams-Stokes s.,** Adams-Stokes s.

**Morquio's s.,** mucopolysaccharidosis type IV; Morquio disease; Morquio-Ullrich disease; Brailsford-Morquio disease; an error of mucopolysaccharide metabolism with excretion of keratosulfate in urine; characterized by severe skeletal defects with short neck, severe deformity of spine and thorax, long bones with irregular epiphyses but with shafts of normal length, enlarged joints, flaccid ligaments, and waddling gait; autosomal recessive inheritance.

**Morris s.,** testicular feminization s.

**Morton's s.,** congenital shortening of the first metatarsal; supposed to cause metatarsalgia.

**Muckle-Wells s.,** urticaria, deafness and amyloidosis; familial amyloidosis with febrile urticaria and deafness; a syndrome characterized by amyloidosis, notably involving the kidneys, progressive hearing loss of neural origin and unknown cause, and periods of febrile urticaria associated with pain in joints and muscles of the extremities; autosomal dominant inheritance.

**multiple mucosal neuroma s.,** multiple submucosal neuromas or neurofibromas of the tongue, lips, and eyelids in young persons; sometimes associated with tumors of the thyroid or adrenal medulla, or with subcutaneous neurofibromatosis.

**Munchausen s.,** the fabrication by an itinerant malingerer of a clinically convincing simulation of disease. It may include self-induced hemorrhage, addiction to unnecessary operation, simulated fits, faints, spells, anesthesias, hallucinations, or delusions.

**my'eloprolif'erative s.'s,** a group of conditions that result from a disorder in the rate of formation of cells of the bone marrow, including chronic granulocytic (myelocytic) leukemia, polycythemia vera (erythremia), myelosclerosis, panmyelosis, and Di Guglielmo's s. (erythremic myelosis and erythroleukemia).

**myofacial pain-dysfunction s.,** temporomandibular joint pain-dysfunction s.

**Naffziger s.,** scalenus-anticus s.

**nail-patella s.,** arthro-onychodysplasia; hereditary arthrodysplasia; bilateral hypoplasia or aplasia of the patella, deformity and luxation of the head of the radius, posterior iliac spurs and dystrophy of the finger nails; autosomal dominant inheritance.

**Nelson s.,** postadrenalectomy s.; a s. of hyperpigmentation, third nerve damage, and enlarging sella turcica caused by development of a pituitary tumor after adrenalectomy for Cushing's s.

**nephritic s.,** the clinical symptoms of nephritis, particularly hematuria, hypertension, and renal failure.

**nephrot'ic s.,** a clinical state characterized by edema, albuminuria, decreased plasma albumin, doubly refractile bodies in the urine, and usually increased blood cholesterol. Lipid droplets may be present in the cells of the renal tubules, but the basic lesion is increased permeability of the glomerular capillary basement membranes, of unknown cause or resulting from glomerulonephritis, diabetic glomerulosclerosis, systemic lupus erythematosus, amyloidosis, renal vein thrombosis, or hypersensitivity to various toxic agents.

**Netherton's s.,** ichthyosiform erythroderma in females, characterized by sparse brittle hair, bamboo hair, and some symptoms of atrophy.

**s. neuroane'mique,** subacute combined *degeneration* of the spinal cord.

**neurocuta'neous s.,** the occurrence of nevi and sometimes various skeletal deformities with symptoms pointing to gliosis or abiotrophy of the central nervous system.

**Nezelof s.,** Nezelof type of thymic alymphoplasia; failure of development of the thymus, with defective cellular and humoral immunity; immunoglobin levels are normal and germinal centers and plasma cells are present.

**nonsense s.,** Ganser s.

**Noonan's.,** a triad consisting of low set ears, antimongoloid slant to eyes, and valvar pulmonic stenosis.

**Nothnagel's s.,** dizziness, staggering, and rolling gait, with irregular forms of oculomotor paralysis and often nystagmus, seen in cases of tumor of the midbrain.

**ocular-mucous membrane s.,** a s. consisting of erythema multiforme with ocular lesions (conjunctivitis, panophthalmitis, iritis), oral lesions (bullae, erosions, superficial ulcers), and genital lesions (urethritis, balanitis circinata, blebs).

**oculobuccogenital s.,** Behçet's s.

**oculocerebrorenal s.,** Lowe's s; Lowe-Terrey-MacLachlan s.; a congenital, sex-linked s. consisting of metabolic defects, involvement of the central nervous system (mental retardation), cataracts, glaucoma, corneal streaks, and renal defects (proteinuria, acidosis, hyperaminoaciduria).

**oculocutaneous s.,** Vogt-Koyanagi s.

**oculodentodigital s.,** oculodentodigital *dysplasia*.

**oculopharyngeal s.,** a myopathic disorder producing a slowly progressive ptosis and dysphagia beginning late in life; transmitted dominantly.

**oculovertebral s.,** oculovertebral *dysplasia*.

**oculovestibulo-auditory s.,** Cogan's s.; a nonsyphilitic interstitial keratitis characterized by an abrupt onset with vertigo and tinnitus followed by deafness; about 50 per cent of patients have an associated systemic disease, most commonly polyarteritis nodosa.

**OFD s.,** abbreviation for oral-facial-digital s. (orodigitofacial *dysostosis*, q.v.).

**Oppenheim's s.,** *amyotonia* congenita.

**oral-facial-digital s.,** orodigitofacial *dysostosis*.

**orodigitofacial s.,** orodigitofacial *dysostosis*.

**os'teomy'elofibrot'ic s.,** myelofibrosis.

**Othello s.,** a delusional belief in the infidelity of the spouse.

**otomandibular s.,** otomandibular *dysostosis*.

**otopalatodigital s.,** familial deafness and cleft palate occurring in males, with facies characterized by frontal bossing and a small open mouth, and with various skeletal abnormalities, including toes resembling those of a frog.

**pachydermoperiostosis s.,** see pachydermoperiostosis.

**painful-bruising s.,** an intense inflammatory reaction to slight extravasation of blood, due to an allergic sensitivity to red blood cells; more commonly seen in adult women.

**paleostriatal s.,** Hunt's s. (3).

**pallidal s.,** Hunt's s. (3).

**Pancoast s.,** pain and tingling of the arm over the area of distribution of the ulnar nerve, constriction of the pupil, and paralysis of the levator palpebrae superioris muscle, due to pressure on the brachial plexus by a malignant tumor (as shown by x-rays) in the region of the superior pulmonary sulcus.

**papillary muscle s.,** papillary muscle *dysfunction*.

**Papillon-Léage and Psaume s.,** orodigitofacial *dysostosis*.

**Papillon-Lefèvre s.,** a congenital hyperkeratosis of the palms and soles, with gradual destruction of the teeth beginning at about 3 years of age.

**Parinaud's s.,** paralysis of conjugate upward gaze with a lesion at the level of the superior colliculi; Bell's phenomenon is present.

**Patau's s.,** trisomy D s.

**Paterson-Kelly s.,** iron-deficiency anemia with dysphagia, due to a constricting esophageal web in the postcricoid region.

**Pellizzi's s.,** *macrogenitosomia* precox.

**Pendred's s.,** congenital nerve deafness with goiter (usually small) due to defective organic binding of iodine in the thyroid; afflicted individuals are usually euthyroid; inherited as a recessive trait.

**Pepper s.,** neuroblastoma of the adrenal gland with metastases in the liver; formerly believed to occur more frequently when the primary tumor was in the right adrenal, whereas tumors of the left adrenal tended to metastasize to the skull (Hutchison's syndrome).

**pericol'ic membrane s.,** a symptom complex simulating chronic appendictis, caused by congenital constricting pericolic membranes.

**Peutz' s.,** Peutz-Jeghers s.

**Peutz-Jeghers s.,** Peutz' s.; generalized multiple polyposis of the intestinal tract, consistently involving the jejunum, associated with melanin spots of the lips, buccal mucosa, and fingers; autosomal dominant inheritance.

**Pfaundler-Hurler s.,** Hurler's s.

**PHC s.,** Böök s.

**Picchini's s.,** a form of polyserositis involving the three great serosae in contact with the diaphragm, sometimes also the meninges, tunica vaginalis testis, synovial sheaths, and bursae, caused by the presence of a trypanosome.

**Pick's s.,** Pick's *disease*.

**Pickwickian s.** [ after the "fat boy" in Dickens' *Pickwick Papers* ], a combination of grotesque and deforming obesity, hypoventilation, and general debility, theoretically resulting from the respiratory disability induced by extreme fatness. The cause is in doubt since pulmonary lesions impairing pulmonary function have been found in many persons said to have the Pickwickian syndrome.

**Pierre Robin s.,** Robin's s.; micrognathia and abnormal smallness of tongue, with cleft palate in about two-thirds of cases, often with bilateral eye defects including high myopia, congenital glaucoma and retinal detachment.

**pincer nail s.,** unique idiopathic distortion in the shape of the nail which produces excessive transverse curvature of the nail plate, causing pinching and loss of soft tissue.

**Pins' s.,** dullness, diminution of vocal fremitus and of the vesicular murmur, and a slight distant blowing sound, heard in the posteroinferior region of the chest on the left side, in cases of pericardial effusion; there is sometimes also a fine rale in this region, but all the adventitious auscultatory signs disappear when the patient assumes the genupectoral position.

**placental dysfunction s.,** fetal malnutrition and hypoxia resulting from impaired transfer of oxygen and various nutritive materials from mother to fetus.

**Plummer-Vinson s.,** sideropenic dysphagia; dysphagia due to degeneration of the muscle of the esophagus, atrophy of the papillae of the tongue, and hypochromic anemia.

**PNP s.** (psychogenic nocturnal polydipsia), emotionally induced excessive water drinking at night.

**polycystic ovary s.,** Stein-Leventhal s.; sclerocystic disease of the ovary; commonly characterized by hirsutism, obesity, menstrual abnormalities, infertility, and enlarged ovaries; thought to reflect excessive androgen secretion of ovarian, and possibly adrenocortical, origin; often ameliorated by ovarian wedge resection.

**postadrenalectomy s.,** Nelson s.

**postcardiotomy s.,** postpericardiotomy s.

**postcholecystectomy s.,** the unhappy persistence of signs and symptoms which lead to removal of the gallbladder remaining as a sequel to cholecystectomy. Sometimes associated with a regeneration or enlargement of the stump of the gallbladder.

**postcommissurotomy s.,** a s. of uncertain cause appearing abruptly within a few weeks after cardiac valvular surgery; it is characterized by fever, chest pain, pericardial rub or effusion, and pleural rub or effusion, and clears spontaneously in one or two weeks without sequelae.

**postconcussion s.,** see posttraumatic s.

**posterior inferior cerebellar artery s.,** Wallenberg's s.; due usually to thrombosis and marked by hypotonia, asthenia, and incoordination of voluntary movement on the ipsilateral side, together with staggering gait and often nystagmus, vertigo, and loss of pain and temperature senses on the side of the body opposite to the lesion.

**postgastrec'tomy s.,** dumping s.

**postmyocardial infarction s.,** a complication developing several days to several weeks after myocardial infarction; its clinical features are fever, chest pain, evidence of pericarditis, pleurisy and pneumonitis, and a tendency to recurrence.

**postpartum pituitary necrosis s.,** Sheehan's s.

**postpericardiotomy s.,** postcardiotomy s.; the occurrence of the symptoms of pericarditis with or without fever, often in repeated episodes, two weeks to several months after cardiac surgery.

**postphlebitic s.,** a state characterized by edema, pain, stasis dermatitis, cellulitis, and varicose veins, and ending in protracted ulceration of the lower leg, developing as a sequel to deep venous thrombosis of the lower extremity.

**postrubella s.,** a group of congenital defects resulting from maternal rubella during the first trimester of pregnancy and including microphthalmos, cataracts, deafness, mental retardation, patent ductus arteriosus, and pulmonary arterial stenosis.

**posttraumatic s.,** traumatic neurasthenia; a clinical complex, caused by injury to the head, characterized by headache, dizziness, neurasthenia, hypersensitivity to stimuli, and diminished concentration.

**posttraumatic neck s.,** a clinical complex of pain, tenderness, tight neck musculature, vasomotor instability, and ill-defined symptoms such as dizziness and blurred vision. Also variously termed occipital or suboccipital neuralgia or neutritis, tension headache, cervical tension s., cervical myospasm, cervical myositis, and cervical fibrositis.

**Prader-Willi s.,** mental deficiency, short stature, marked obesity, and sexual infantilism; the muscular hypotonia and swallowing difficulty in infancy.

**precordial catch s.,** a benign s. of uncertain origin, characterized by intense pain in the region of the cardiac apex on inspiration, yet usually relieved by forcing a deeper breath.

**preexcitation s.,** Wolff-Parkinson-White s.

**preinfarction s.,** the situation when angina pectoris abruptly develops, or when existing angina abruptly worsens by increasing its frequency or becoming more severe; often the herald of myocardial infarction.

**premature senility s.,** progeria.

**premenstrual salivary s.,** Racine's s.; glandular abnormalities occurring prior to the onset of menses, including swelling of the breast tissues and enlargement of the salivary glands.

**premen'strual tension s.,** in women of reproductive age, the regular monthly experience of physiological and emotional distress, usually during the several days preceding menses, typically involving fatigue, edema, irritability, tension, anxiety, and depression.

**premo'tor s.,** hemiplegia with spasticity, Rossolimo's reflex, but not the Babinski response, together with forced grasping and vasomotor disturbances.

**progeria s.,** progeria.

**"prune belly" s.,** congenital absence of abdominal musculature.

**pseudo-Turner's s.,** characterized by short stature and a webbed neck; unlike Turner's s., patients with this disorder may be of either sex, have normal chromosomes, have no renal abnormalities, are often mentally retarded, and have various forms of congenital heart disease.

**pulmonary dysmaturity s.,** Wilson-Mikity s.; a respiratory disorder occurring in small, premature infants who are incapable of normal pulmonary ventilation and who often die of hypoxia after an illness of 6 to 8 weeks. The lungs

contain widespread focal emphysematous blebs and the parenchyma thickened alveolar walls. Diagnosed principally on the basis of the clinical history, chest radiographic findings, and the findings at autopsy, which must include the absence of pathological changes characteristic of other pulmonary disorders commonly encountered in this age group.

**punchdrunk s.,** a condition seen in boxers and alcoholics, presumably caused by repeated cerebral concussions; it is characterized by weakness in lower limbs, unsteadiness of gait, slowness of muscular movements, tremors of hands, hesitancy of speech, and slow cerebration.

**Putnam-Dana s.,** subacute combined *degeneration* of the spinal cord.

**Racine's s.,** premenstrual salivary s.

**radicular s.,** a group of symptoms resulting from any interference with the intradural portion of one or more spinal nerve roots; the chief symptoms are pain, paresthesia, hypesthesia, or hyperesthesia, motor, trophic, and reflex disturbances.

**Raeder's paratrigeminal s.,** an incomplete Horner's s. with cranial nerve disturbance caused by involvement of carotid sympathetic plexus.

**Ramsay Hunt's s.'s,** Hunt's s.'s.

**Refetoff s.,** a condition characterized by goiter, elevated serum level of thyroid hormones without true tissue thyrotoxicosis, and target organ unresponsiveness to thyroid hormones.

**Refsum's s.,** Refsum's *disease;* degradation of phytanic acid; autosomal recessive inheritance.

**Rieger's s.,** iridocorneal mesodermal *dysgenesis.*

**Reiter's s.,** Reiter's disease; a triad of urethritis, iridocyclitis, and arthritis which appear in that order; one or more of these conditions may recur at intervals of months or years.

**Rendu-Osler-Weber s.,** hereditary hemorrhagic *telangiectasia.*

**Rénon-Delille s.,** a thyroid-ovarian deficiency associated with hypophysial hyperactivity and resulting in hypotension, tachycardia, hyperhidrosis, heat intolerance, and oliguria.

**residual ovary s.,** the development of a pelvic mass, pelvic pain, and occasionally dyspareunia following hysterectomy without removal of both ovaries.

**restless legs s.,** Ekbom s.; jimmy legs; jitter legs; restless legs; anxietas tibiarum; a sense of indescribable uneasiness, twitching, or restlessness that occurs in the legs after going to bed, frequently leading to insomnia. It may be relieved temporarily by walking about. It is thought to be caused by inadequate circulation, and is most common in neurotic patients.

**retraction s.,** Duane's s.; inability to abduct the affected eye with retraction of globe and pseudoptosis on attempted adduction; due to a paradoxical innervation of the horizontal recti causing simultaneous contraction of both muscles on adduction and relaxation on abduction. More rarely, the vertical muscles are similarly affected, producing a vertical retraction syndrome.

**Reye's s.,** sudden loss of consciousness in children following a prodromal infection, usually resulting in death with cerebral edema and marked fatty change in the liver and renal tubules.

**right ovarian vein s.,** right ureteral obstruction from an aberrant right ovarian vein.

**Riley-Day s.,** familial *dysautonomia.*

**Robin's s.,** see Pierre Robin s.

**Romberg's s.,** facial *hemiatrophy.*

**Rothmund's s.,** Rothmund-Thomson s.; poikiloderma congenitale; poikiloderma atrophicans and cataract; atrophy, pigmentation, and telangiectasia of the skin, usually with juvenile cataract, saddle nose, congenital bone defects, disturbance of hair growth, hypogonadism; autosomal recessive inheritance.

**Rothmund-Thomson s.,** Rothmund's s.

**Roussy-Lévy s.,** Roussy-Lévy *disease.*

**Rubinstein-Taybi s.,** a constellation of congenital defects including broad thumb and great toe, antimongoloid slant to the eyes, thin and beaked nose, prominent forehead, low set ears, high arched palate, and cardiac anomaly.

**salt depletion s.,** low salt s.

**Sanfilippo's s.,** mucopolysaccharidosis type III; an error of mucopolysaccharide metabolism, with excretion of large amounts of heparitin sulfate in the urine; severe mental retardation with hepatomegaly; skeleton may be normal or may present mild changes similar to those in Hurler's s.; autosomal recessive inheritance.

**Sassoon hospital s.,** epidemic polyuria caused by a phycomycetous fungus, a strain of the common bread mold *Rhizopus nigricans,* found in millet grains in Maharashtra, India.

**scalded skin s.,** toxic epidermal *necrolysis.*

**scale'nus-anti'cus s.,** Naffziger s.; an affection having symptoms identical with those of cervical rib but due to compression of the brachial plexus and subclavian artery against the first thoracic rib by a hypertonic scalenus anticus muscle; pressure upon sympathetic nerves may cause vascular spasm resembling Raynaud's disease.

**scapulocos'tal s.,** pain of insidious development in the upper or posterior part of the shoulder radiating into the neck and occiput with severe headache, down the arm or around the chest; there may be numbness or tingling in the fingers. It is attributed to an alteration from the normal relationship between the scapula and posterior wall of the thorax.

**Schanz' s.,** spinal muscle weakness, marked by early fatigue, pain on pressure over the spinous processes, pain produced by the prone position, and a tendency to curvature of the spine.

**Schaumann's s.,** sarcoidosis.

**Scheie's s.,** type IS mucopolysaccharidosis; a variant of Hurler's syndrome characterized by α-L-iduronidase deficiency, corneal clouding, deformity of the hands, aortic valve involvement, and normal intelligence; formerly also called type V mucopolysaccharidosis.

**Schirmer's s.,** an incomplete form of Sturge-Weber syndrome consisting of angiomas of face and choroid only, with early glaucoma (buphthalmia).

**Schmid-Fraccaro s.,** cat's-eye s.

**Schmidt's s.** [ J. F. M. Schmidt ], unilateral paralysis of a vocal cord, the velum palati, trapezius, and sternocleidomastoid.

**Schmidt's s.** [ M. B. Schmidt ], the association of primary hypothyroidism and primary adrenocortical insufficiency.

**Schönlein-Henoch s.,** Henoch-Schönlein *purpura.*

**Schüller's s.,** Hand-Schüller-Christian *disease.*

**scimitar s.,** malformation of pulmonary venous system associated with hypoplasia of the right lung with bronchial anomalies, dextroposition and/or dextrorotation of the heart, hypoplasia of the right pulmonary artery, and anomylous subdiaphragmatic systemic arterial supply to the right lower lobe. Its name is taken from the shape of the frontal thoracic roetngenogram of anomylous pulmonary vein entering the vena cava.

**Seabright bantam s.** [ from the appearance of female plumage in the tail feathers of the Seabright bantam rooster ], pseudohypoparathyroidism.

**Senear-Usher s.,** *pemphigus* erythematosus.

**"Sertoli cell only" s.,** the absence from the seminiferous tubules of the testes of germinal epithelium, Sertoli cells alone being present. There is sterility due to azoospermia but no other sexual abnormality. Leydig cells are normal; the output of gonadotrophins in the urine is increased. Probably represents one form of seminiferous tubule dysgenesis.

**Sézary s.,** exfoliative dermatitis with intense pruritus, associated with cutaneous infiltration by atypical mononuclear cells also found in the peripheral blood.

**Sheehan's s.,** postpartum pituitary necrosis s.; thyrohypophysial s.; hypopituitarism arising from a severe circulatory collapse post partum, with resultant pituitary necrosis.

**shoulder-hand s.,** pain and limited motion in both shoulder and hand; usually late trophic changes in hand; may be seen after neck, upper extremity injury or myocardial infarction. Autonomic system hyperfunction is present as a secondarily evoked phenomenon.

**Shy-Drager s.,** a progressive encephalomyelopathy involving the autonomic system, characterized by hypotension, external ophthalmoparesis, atrophy of iris, incontinence, anhidrosis, impotence, tremor, and muscle wasting.

**sicca s.,** Sjögren's s.

**sick sinus s.,** chaotic atrial activity characterized by continual changes in P wave configuration, with bradycardia alternating with recurring ectopic beats and runs of supraventricular tachycardia.

**sickle cell s.,** sickle cell *anemia.*

**Silverskiöld's s.,** a type of osteochondrodystrophy with only slight vertebral changes but with shortened and curved long bones of the extremities.

**Sipple's s.,** a heritable disorder characterized by the development of pheochromocytoma and medullary thyroid carcinoma with amyloid stroma. In some such families, parathyroid adenomas may also occur.

**Sjögren's s.** [ H. S. C. Sjögren ], Sjögren's disease; Sjögren-Mikulicz s.; Gougerot-Sjögren disease; sicca s.; keratoconjunctivitis sicca, dryness of mucous membranes, telangiectases or purpuric spots on the face, and bilateral parotid enlargement, seen in menopausal woman, often associated with rheumatoid arthritis, Raynaud's phenomenon, and dental caries. There are changes in the lacrimal and salivary glands resembling those of Mikulicz' disease.

**Sjögren's s.** [ Torsten Sjögren ], see Torsten Sjögren's s.

**Sjögren-Larsson s.,** congenital icthyosiform erythroderma in association with oligophrenia and spastic disorders typical of Little's disease; autosomal recessive inheritance.

**Sjögren-Mikulicz s.,** Sjögren's s.

**smoker's respiratory s.,** a triad of symptoms seen in smokers, consisting of chronic pharyngitis, wheezing and dyspnea, and a susceptibility to respiratory infections. Small lymphoid nodules may appear in the pharynx. There is also often cough, pain in the chest, and hoarseness of the voice; edema of the vocal cords and later an edematous fibroma may be found.

**Sohval-Soffer s.,** a condition characterized by hypogonadism, gynecomastia, skeletal anomalies, and mental retardation without chromosomal abnormality.

**spastic s. in cattle,** Krämpfigkeit [ Ger. ]; a disease of the nervous system manifested by spastic contractions of the muscles of one or both hind legs, most common in old bulls; the cramps usually become more frequent and severe, eventually resulting in decreasing the usefulness of the animal.

**Spens' s.,** Adams-Stokes s.; it was described by Spens in 1792.

**spherophakia-brachymorphia s.,** Marchesani s.; Weill-Marchesani s.; ectopia lentis (lens abnormally round and small), short stature, brachydactyly; autosomal inheritance, incompletely recessive.

**splenic flexure s.,** symptoms of pain, gas, bloating, a sense of fullness experienced in the left upper abdominal quadrant, sometimes beneath the ribs, in some instances radiating upward, and in some instances producing anterior chest pain central or predominantly on the left. It may be induced experimentally by the introduction and trapping of air in the splenic flexure.

**Sprinz-Nelson s.,** see Dubin-Johnson *syndrome.*

**Steele-Richardson-Olszewski s.,** a progressive neurologic disorder in the sixth decade characterized by paralysis of downward gaze rendering ambulation impossible, retraction of lids, exophoria under cover, dysarthria and dementia.

**Stein-Leventhal s.,** polycystic ovary s.

**steroid withdrawal s.,** a condition exhibited by persons who have been receiving large doses of glucocorticoid hormones for long periods of time to suppress the manifestations of a responsive disease; when hormonal therapy is stopped, pituitary-adrenocortical insufficiency is manifested, particularly during stress, for as long as a year thereafter; in addition, patients may exhibit varying degrees of emotional disturbance.

**Stevens-Johnson s.,** *erythema* multiforme exudativum.

**Stewart-Morel s.,** Morgagni's s.

**Stewart-Treves s.,** lymphangiosarcoma arising in arms affected by postmastectomy lymphedema.

**Stickler s.,** hereditary progressive *arthro-ophthalmopathy.*

**stiff-man s.,** a chronic, progressing but variable disorder associated with fluctuating muscle spasm and stiffness. Biopsy of muscle may show nothing but some atrophy; the cause is unknown.

**Still-Chauffard s.,** Chauffard s.

**Stokes-Adams s.,** Adams-Stokes s.

**straight back s.,** loss of the normal anterior concavity of the thoracic spine with resulting compression of the heart between spine and sternum and consequent prominent precordial pulsations, an ejection murmur, and radiologic evidence of a widened cardiac silhouette.

**Stryker-Halbeisen s.,** reddish, scaling, macular eruption on head and upper trunk due to vitamin B complex deficiency; associated with macrocytic anemia.

**Sturge-Kalischer-Weber s.,** Sturge-Weber s.

**Sturge-Weber s.,** the full s. is a triad: congenital cutaneous angioma (flame nevus) in distribution of trigeminal nerve, usually unilateral; homolateral meningeal angioma with intracranial calcification and neurologic signs; angioma of choroid, often with secondary glaucoma. Incomplete forms of the s. may exhibit any two of the major features in variable degree, occasionally with angiomas elsewhere. Also called cephalotrigeminal, encephalotrigeminal, or encephalofacial angiomatosis; Sturge-Kalischer-Weber s.; Sturge's disease; Sturge-Weber disease.

**subclavian steal s.,** symptoms of cerebrovascular insufficiency resulting from subclavian *steal, q.v.*

**sudden death s.,** (1) crib *death;* (2) abrupt and inexplicable death of an apparently healthy individual; various theories have been advanced to explain such deaths (for example, laryngospasm or overwhelming infectious disease) but none has been generally accepted.

**Sudeck's s.,** acute reflex bone atrophy; an acute atrophy of a bone, more commonly one of the tarsal or carpal bones, following a slight injury such as a strain or a sprain.

**Sulzberger-Garbe s.,** Sulzberger-Garbe *disease.*

**superior cerebellar artery s.,** s. due to thrombosis of the superior cerebellar artery which supplies the spinothalamic tract and the peduncle; there is incoordination in performing skilled movements, with loss of pain and temperature senses on the side of the face and body opposite to that of the lesion.

**superior mesenteric artery s.,** Wilkie's disease; partial or complete block of third segment of duodenum, with pain and vomiting.

**superior vena caval s.,** obstruction of the superior vena cava or its main tributaries by bronchogenic carcinoma, mediastinal neoplasm or lymphoma, or, rarely, substernal goiter, causing edema and engorgement of the vessels of the face, neck, and arms, nonproductive cough, and dyspnea. Bluish looking venous stars may be found in the early phases, overlying the large veins to which they are tributary. Venous stars tend to diminish in size and disappear after collateral circulation has been reestablished.

**supersonic s.,** multiple injuries occurring in fliers who bail out at speeds of 650 miles per hour or more.

**supine hypotensive s.,** in the pregnant woman, a condition due to obstruction of the inferior vena cava by the gravid uterus, particularly immediately after the administration of spinal or epidural anesthesia.

**suprarenogenic s.,** adrenogenic s.

**supraspinatus s.,** pain on abduction of the shoulder and tenderness upon deep pressure over the supraspinatus tendon; due to pressure of an injured tendon or inflamed subacromial bursa coming into contact or pressing upon the overlying acromial process when the arm is abducted within an arc of 60° to 120°.

**supravalvular aortic stenosis s.,** a constellation of congenital abnormalities associated with supravalvular stenosis and including strabismus, hyperteleorism, hypoplastic mandible, pouting lips, and mental retardation.

**Takayashu's s.,** pulseless *disease.*

**Tapia's s.,** unilateral paralysis of the larynx, the velum palati, and the tongue, with atrophy of the later.

**tarsal tunnel s.,** s. produced by entrapment neuropathy of posterior tibial nerve.

**Taussig-Bing s.,** Taussig-Bing disease; complete transposition of the aorta which arises from the right ventricle with a left sided pulmonary artery overriding the left ventricle with high ventricular septal defect, right ventricular hypertrophy, anteriorly situated aorta, and posteriorly situated pulmonary artery; compatible with fairly long life.

**tegmen'tal s.,** caused by a lesion in the tegmentum of the midbrain marked by hemiplegia together with paresis or paralysis of the extrinsic ocular muscles.

**temporomandibular s.,** Costen's s.; those various symptoms of discomfort, pain, or pathosis stated to be caused by loss of vertical dimension, lack of posterior occlusion, or other malocclusion, trismus, muscle tremor, arthritis, or direct trauma to the temporomandibular joint.

**temporomandibular joint pain-dysfunction s.,** myofacial pain-dysfunction s.; a myofacial s. consisting of the symptoms of facial pain and mandibular dysfunction in the form of either clicking, limitation, subluxation, or dislocation.

**tendon sheath s.,** shortening of the effective tendon of the superior oblique muscle, producing a condition that simulates paresis of inferior oblique muscle.

**Terry's s.,** *retinopathy* of prematurity.

**testicular feminization s.,** Goldberg-Maxwell s.; Morris s.; a type of male pseudohermaphroditism characterized when complete by female external genitalia, incompletely developed vagina often with rudimentary uterus and Fallopian tubes, female habitus at puberty but with scanty or absent axillary and pubic hair and amenorrhea; testes are present within the abdomen or in the inguinal canals or labia majora; epididymis and vas deferens are usually present. The genitalia may be ambiguous when the s. is incomplete. Both androgens and estrogens are formed; however, target tissues are largely unresponsive to androgens. Patients are sex chromatin-negative and have a normal male karyotype; the s. is familial and is transmitted through the female line.

**thalam'ic s.,** Déjérine-Roussy s.; disturbances of cortical sensation, or hemiparesis together with hyperesthesia and severe spontaneous pain. Pleasant as well as unpleasant sensations or feelings are exaggerated.

**third and fourth pharyngeal pouch s.,** Di George s.

**thoracic outlet s.,** compression of brachial plexus and subclavian artery by the region of the first rib and clavical.

**Thorn's s.,** salt-losing *nephritis.*

**Thornwaldt's s.,** nasopharyngeal discharge, occipital headache, and stiffness of posterior cervical muscles, with halitosis due to chronic infection of the pharyngeal bursa.

**thrombopathic s.,** a nondescript term to describe any of a number of bleeding diseases in which clot formation is deficient rather than those in which there is an organic fault of blood vessels.

**thyrohypophysial s.,** Sheehan's s.

**Tietze's s.,** a painful, benign, nonsuppurative swelling of the costochondral junction.

**time-zone s.,** a result of subsonic or hypersonic migration through a varied number of time zones, leading to extreme tiredness, tenseness, and irritability; an imbalance of normal circadian rhythm.

**tooth-and-nail s.,** hypodontia associated with absent or very small nails at birth.

**Torre's s.,** multiple sebaceous gland tumors associated with visceral malignancy and long survival.

**Torsten Sjögren's s.,** Marinesco-Sjögren s.

**transplant lung s.,** a s. associated with fever and diffuse bilateral pulmonary infiltration mainly at the base or at the hilum of the lung. It may accompany rejection of an organ (kidney) transplant, or following a reduction in dosage of the immunosuppressive drug.

**Treacher Collins' s.,** an incomplete form of mandibulofacial dysostosis with notching of outer third of lower eyelids and deficient malar bones.

**trichorhinophalangeal s.,** a condition characterized by sparse fine hair, broad nose with a long philtrum, swollen middle phalanges with cone-shaped epiphyses, and growth retardation.

**trisomy D s.,** a variable s. of malformations in infants with 47 chromosomes, the extra chromosome being of group D, no. 13, 14 or 15, usually fatal within two years; more than 30 signs have been described, including apparent mental retardation and malformed ears in all patients, and in most cleft palate or lip, microphthalmia or coloboma, small mandible, polydactyly, cardiac defects, convulsions, renal anomalies, umbilical hernia, malrotation of intestines, and dermatoglyphic anomalies; also called trisomy $D_1$ s.; trisomy 13 s.; trisomy 13-15 s.; Patau's s.

**trisomy D₁ s.,** trisomy D s.

**trisomy E s.,** a variable s. of malformations in infants with 47 chromosomes, the extra chromosome being of group E, probably no. 17 or 18, usually fatal within 2 to 3 years; more than 30 signs have been described, including mental retardation, abnormal skull shape, lowset and malformed ears, small mandible, cardiac defects, short sternum, diaphragmatic or inguinal hernia, Meckel's diverticulum, abnormal flexion of fingers, and dermatoglyphic anomalies; also called trisomy E₁ s.; trisomy 17–18 s.; trisomy 17 s.; trisomy 18 s.; Edwards' s.

**trisomy E₁ s.,** trisomy D s.

**trisomy 13 s.,** trisomy D s.

**trisomy 13–15 s.,** trisomy D s.

**trisomy 17 s.,** trisomy E s.

**trisomy 17–18 s.,** trisomy E s.

**trisomy 18 s.,** trisomy E s.

**trisomy 21 s.,** Down's s.

**trochanteric s.,** tendonitis and bursitis about the trochanter major.

**Trousseau's s.,** (1) Hodgkin's *disease;* (2) gastric *vertigo;* (3) thrombophlebitis migrans associated with visceral cancer.

**Turcot s.,** the development of polyps of the colon and brain tumors; inherited as a recessive trait.

**Turner's s.,** XO s.; a chromosomal anomaly with chromosome count 45, including only a single X chromosome (XO sex chromosome constitution); buccal and other cells are usually sex chromatin-negative; anomalies include dwarfism, webbed neck, valgus of elbows, shield-shaped chest, infantile sexual development, amenorrhea; the ovary has no primordial follicles and may be represented only by a fibrous streak; some patients are chromosomal mosaic, with two or more cell lines of different chromosome constitution.

**Uehlinger's s.,** acropachyderma.

**Ulysses s.** [ Ulysses, G. mythological hero ], the ill effects of extensive diagnostic investigations conducted because of a false-positive result in the course of routine laboratory screening.

**Usher's s.,** congenital nerve deafness and retinitis pigmentosa; autosomal recessive inheritance.

**uveocutaneous s.,** Vogt-Koyanagi s.

**uveo-encephalitic s.,** Behçet's s.

**uveomeningitis s.,** Harada's s.

**Van Buchem's s.,** generalized cortical hyperostosis; an inherited skeletal dysplasia, with mandibular enlargement and thickening of the diaphyses and calvaria; the serum alkaline phosphatase is increased.

**vasculocardiac s. of hyperserotoninemia,** carcinoid s.

**va'sova'gal s.,** vagal *attack.*

**Vernet's s.,** a s. characterized by paralysis of the motor components of the glossopharyngeal, vagus, and accessory cranial nerves as they lie in the posterior fossa; it is most commonly the result of head injury.

**vertical retraction s.,** see retraction s.

**vitreoretinal traction s.,** a complication of posterior vitreous separation marked by blurred vision, photopsia, micropsia, positive scotoma, and metamorphopsia caused by traction on the internal limiting membrane of retina by adherent vitreous fibrils.

**Vogt s.,** spastic diplegia with athetosis and pseudobulbar paralysis associated with a lesion of the caudate nucleus and putamen.

**Vogt-Koyanagi s.,** oculocutaneous s.; uveocutaneous s.; bilateral uveitis with iritis and glaucoma, premature graying of the hair, and alopecia, vitiligo, and dysacusia; related to Harada's s. and sympathetic ophthalmia.

**vulnerable child s.,** a reaction characterized by disturbance in psychosocial development, often occurring in children whose parents expect them to die prematurely.

**Waardenburg s.,** a dominant autosomal familial disease characterized by lateral dystopia of medial canthi and lacrimal punctae, increased width of root of nose, heterochromia or hypochromia iridis, unilateral deafness, white forelock, and synophrys.

**Waldenström's s.,** Waldenström's *macroglobulinemia.*

**Wallenberg's s.,** posterior inferior cerebellar artery s.

**Waterhouse-Friderichsen s.,** a fulminating meningococcal septicemia occurring mainly in children under 10 years of age, characterized by vomiting, diarrhea, extensive purpura, cyanosis, toniclonic convulsions and circulatory collapse, and usually hemorrhage into the adrenal glands.

**Weber's s.,** Weber's sign; paralysis of the oculomotor nerve on the side of the lesion and of the extremities and of the face and tongue on the opposite side due to a lesion in the ventral and internal part of a cerebral peduncle.

**Weil's s.,** neuromuscular hemihyperesthesia associated with other disorders of central and peripheral sensibility, said to occur frequently in the tuberculous.

**Weill-Marchesani s.,** spherophakia-brachymorphia s.

**Wermer's s.,** familial polyendocrine *adenomatosis.*

**Werner's s.,** a rare familial disorder in which sclerodermatous alterations of the extremities, bilateral juvenile cataracts, progeria, hypogonadism, and a tendency to diabetes mellitus occur together.

**Wernicke's s.,** Wernicke's disease; Wernicke's encephalopathy; superior hemorrhagic polioencephalitis; a condition, frequently encountered in chronic alcoholics, characterized by disturbances in ocular motility, pupillary alterations, nystagmus, and ataxia with tremors; an organic-toxic psychosis is often an associated finding; thiamin deficiency is largely responsible for the condition; treatment with thiamin and glucose is helpful, but does not reverse symptoms that are due to irreversible changes in the brain; Korsakoff's s. often coexists.

**Weyers-Thier s.,** oculovertebral *dysplasia.*

**whistling face s.,** craniocarpotarsal *dystrophy.*

**white-out s.,** a psychosis which occurs in Arctic explorers or others similarly exposed to the stimulus deprivation of a snow-clad environment; see also sensory *deprivation.*

**Widal's s.,** Hayem-Widal s.

**Wilson's s.,** hepatolenticular *degeneration.*

**Wilson-Mikity s.,** pulmonary dysmaturity s.

**Wiskott-Aldrich s.,** Aldrich s.

**Wolff-Parkinson-White s.,** preexcitation s.; an electrocardiographic pattern sometimes associated with paroxysmal tachycardia; it consists of short P-R interval (0.1 second or less) together with a prolonged QRS complex with a slurred initial component (delta wave).

**XO s.,** Turner's s.

**XXY s.,** Klinefelter's s.

**yellow nail s.,** the complete or almost complete cessation of all nail growth, with thickening of the nails, increase in the convexity, loss of cuticles, and yellowing in color; the resulting onycholysis can cause loss of some of the nails, usually permanent, although the nails can occasionally become normal. The s. is caused by peripheral or universal lymphedema.

**Zellweger s.,** cerebrohepatorenal s.

**Zieve's s.,** transient jaundice, hemolytic anemia, and hyperlipemia associated with acute alcoholism in patients with cirrhosis or a fatty liver.

**Zollinger-Ellison s.,** peptic ulceration with gastric hypersecretion and non-beta cell tumor of the pancreatic islets.

---

**syndromic** (sin-drom'ik, -dro'mik). Relating to a syndrome.

**synechia,** pl. **synechiae** (sĭ-nek'ĭ-ah, sĭ-ne'kĭ-ah, -kĭ-e) [ G. *synecheia,* continuity, fr. *syn,* together, + *echō,* to have, hold. ECT- ]. Any adhesion; specifically adhesion of the iris to the cornea (**anterior s.**) or to the capsule of the lens (**posterior s.**).

**annular s.,** adhesion of the entire pupillary margin of the iris to the capsule of the lens.

**s. pericar'dii,** *concretio* cordis.

**total s.,** adhesion of the entire surface of the iris to the lens capsule.

**synechiotomy** (sĭ-nek'ĭ-ot'o-mĭ) [ synechia + G. *tomē,* incision ]. Division of the adhesions in synechia.

**synechotome** (sĭ-nek'o-tōm). A small knife for use in synechiotomy.

**synectenterotomy** (sĭ-nek'ten-ter-ot'o-mĭ) [ G. *synektos,* held together (see synechia), + *enteron,* intestine, + *tomē,* incision ]. The separation of intestinal adhesions.

**synencephalocele** (sin-en-sef'ā-lo-sēl) [ syn- + G. *enkephalos,* brain, + *kēlē,* hernia ]. Protrusion of brain substance through a defect in the skull, with adhesions preventing reduction.

**syneph′rine tartrate.** SYMPATOL; *p*-hydroxy-α-{ (methylamino)methyl ]benzyl alcohol tartrate; sympathomimetic agent used for treatment of shock.

**syneresis** (si-nĕr′ĕ-sis) [ G. *synairesis*, a taking or drawing together ]. The contraction of a gel, *e.g.*, a blood clot, by which part of the dispersion medium is squeezed out.

**synergetic** (sin-er-jet′ik). Synergistic.

**synergia** (si-ner′ji-ah). Synergy.

**synergic** (si-ner′jik). Synergistic.

**synergism** (sin′er-jizm). Synergy.

**synergist** (sin′er-jist). 1. An adjuvant; a structure or drug that aids the action of another. 2. A muscle or organ that assists another in its action; *e.g.*, the flexor muscles of a part are s.'s one of another; the reverse of antagonist.

**synergistic** (sin′er-jis′tik). Synergic; synergetic. 1. Pertaining to synergy. 2. Denoting a synergist.

**synergy** (sin′er-ji) [ G. *synergia*, fr. *syn*, together, + *ergon*, work ]. Synergia; synergism. 1. Coordinated or correlated action by two or more structures or drugs. 2. Coordination of muscules or organs by the nervous system so that specific actions can be performed.

    **s. of ventricular contraction,** the temporal sequence of ventricular contraction with integrated inward movement during ejection.

**synesthesia** (sin-es-the′zi-ah) [ syn- + G. *aisthēsis*, sensation ]. A condition in which a stimulus, in addition to exciting the usual and normally located sensation, gives rise to a subjective sensation of different character or localization; color-hearing and color-taste are forms of synesthesia.

    **s. al′gica,** synesthesialgia.

    **auditory s.,** phonism.

**synesthesialgia** (sin-es-the-zi-al′ji-ah). Synesthesia algica; painful synesthesia.

**Syngam′idae** [ see *Syngamus* ]. A family of parasitic nematodes (order Stongyloidea) including the genera *Cyathostoma, Mammomonogamus*, and *Syngamus*.

**Syngamus** (sin′gă-mus) [ syn- + G. *gamos*, marriage ]. A genus of moderate-sized, bloodsucking, strongyle nematodes (family Syngamidae) that live in the bronchi and tracheae of birds, and are called gapeworms because the host often gapes with open mouth due to the presence of the worms in the throat; also called forked worms, as the male is permanently attached to the midregion of the female, where the bursa of the male is clasped over the female vulva. They are especially important parasites of gallinaceous birds.

    **S. tra′chea,** gapeworm; throatworm; formerly called *S. trachealis* or *Sclerostoma syngamus*, a worldwide parasite of the trachea of fowls and many wild birds, causing the disease called gapes, which is particularly severe in young birds. Infection is either direct, by ingestion of infective eggs, or indirect, by ingestion of land snails, slugs, or earthworms that fed on the eggs; these transport hosts can harbor infective larvae for long periods of time, up to 3.5 years in earthworms.

**syngamy** (sin′gă-mi) [ syn- + G. *gamos*, marriage ]. Conjugation of the gametes in fertilization.

**syngeneic** (sin′jĕ-ne′ik). Isologous.

**syngenesioplasty** (sin-jĕ-ne′zi-o-plas′ti) [ syn- + G. *genesis*, origin, + *plassō*, to form ]. Plastic surgery in which donor and recipient of a graft are closely related, *e.g.*, mother and child, or siblings.

**syngenesiotransplantation** (sin-jĕ-ne′zi-o-trans-plan-ta′-shun). See syngenesioplasty.

**syngenesis** (sin-jen′ĕ-sis) [ syn- + G. *genesis*, production ]. Sexual *reproduction*.

**syngenetic** (sin-jĕ-net′ik). Relating to syngenesis.

**syngenic** (sin-jen′ik) [ G. *syngenēs*, congenital ]. 1. Alternative spelling of syngeneic (*i.e.*, isologous). 2. Obsolete synonym for congenital.

**syngnathia** (sing-nath′i-ah) [ syn- + G. *gnathos*, jaw ]. Congenital ankylosis of the jaw.

**synidrosis** (sin′i-dro′sis) [ syn- + G. *hidrosis*, sweating ]. A diseased state in which excessive sweating is part of the picture.

**synizesis** (sin′i-ze′sis) [ G. collapse ]. 1. Closure or obliteration of the pupil. 2. The massing of chromatin at one side

of the nucleus that occurs usually at the beginning of synapsis.

**synkaryon** (sin-kār′i-on) [ syn- + G. *karyon*, kernel (nucleus) ]. The nucleus formed by the fusion of the two pronuclei in karyogamy.

**synkinesis** (sin′ki-ne′sis) [ syn- + G. *kinēsis*, movement ]. Syncinesis; involuntary movement accompanying a voluntary one; as the movement of a closed eye following that of the uncovered one, or the movement occurring in a paralyzed muscle accompanying motion in another part.

**synkinet′ic.** Relating to or marked by synkinesis.

**synnematin B.** Cephalosporin N.

**syn′onym.** In biological nomenclature, a term used to denote one of two or more names for the same species or taxonomic group. For species names, with rare exceptions, the earliest published of the two or more available s.'s (senior s.) is used as the correct name.

**synophrys** (sin-of′ris) [ syn- + G. *ophrys*, eyebrow ]. The growing together of the eyebrows.

**synophthalmia, synophthalmus** (sin′of-thal′mi-ah, -mus) [ syn- + G. *ophthalmos*, eye ]. Cyclopia.

**synoptophore** (sin-op′to-fōr) [ syn- + G. *ōps*, eye, + *phoros*, bearing ]. A modified form of Wheatstone stereoscope used in orthoptic training.

**synorchidism, synorchism** (sin-or′ki-dizm, sin-or′kizm) [ syn- + G. *orchis*, testis ]. Congenital fusion of the testes in the abdominal cavity.

**synoscheos** (sin-os′ke-os) [ syn- + G. *oschē*, scrotum ]. Partial or complete adhesion of the penis and scrotum, a malformation in hermaphroditism.

**synosteology** (sin-os′te-ol′o-ji) [ syn- + G. *osteon*, bone, + *logos*, study ]. Arthrology.

**synosteosis** (sin-os′te-o′sis). Synostosis.

**synosteotomy** (sin-os′te-ot′o-mi) [ syn- + G. *osteon*, bone, + *tomē*, incision ]. Arthrotomy.

**synostosis** (sin′os-to′sis) [ syn- + G. *osteon*, bone, + suffix *-osis*, condition ]. Bony ankylosis; true ankylosis; osseous union between the bones forming a joint.

    **tribasilar s.,** fusion in early life of the three bones at the base of the skull, resulting in interference with the development of the brain.

**synostotic** (sin′os-tot′ik). Relating to synostosis.

**synotia** (si-no′shi-ah) [ syn- + G. *ous*, ear, + suffix *-ia*, condition ]. Fusion or abnormal approximation of the lobes of the ears in otocephaly.

**synotus** (si-no′tus). Cyclotus; an individual with synotia.

**synovectomy** (sin′o-vek′to-mi) [ synovial membrane + G. *ektomē*, excision ]. Exsection of a portion or all of the synovial membrane of a joint.

**synovia** (si-no′vi-ah) [ Mod. L., a word invented by Paracelsus, fr. G. *syn*, together, + *ōon* (L. *ovum*), egg ] [ NA ]. Joint oil; a clear, thixotropic fluid the function of which is to serve as a lubricant in a joint, tendon sheath, or bursa. It consists mainly of mucin with some albumin, fat, epithelium, and leukocytes.

**synovial** (si-no′vi-al). 1. Relating to, containing, or consisting of synovia. 2. Relating to the membrana synovialis.

**synovioma** (si-no′vi-o′mah) [ sinovia + G. suffix *-oma*, tumor ]. A tumor of synovial origin involving joint or tendon sheath.

    **malignant s.,** synovial *sarcoma*.

**synoviparous** (sin′o-vip′ă-rus) [ synovia + L. *pario*, to produce ]. Synovial (1); producing synovia.

**synovitis** (sin′o-vi′tis) [ synovial membrane + G. suffix *-itis*, inflammation ]. Arthromeningitis; inflammation of a synovial membrane, especially that of a joint; in general, when unqualified, the same as arthritis.

    **bursal s.,** bursitis.

    **chronic hemorrhagic villous s.,** pigmented villonodular s.

    **dry s.,** s. with little serous or purulent effusion.

    **fila′rial s.,** s. due to microfilariae in the joint, which cause inflammation followed often by fibrotic ankylosis.

    **fungous s.,** *arthritis* fungosa.

    **pigmented villonodular s.,** chronic hemorrhagic villous s.; diffuse outgrowths of synovial membrane of a joint, usually the knee, composed of synovial villi and fibrous nodules infiltrated by hemosiderin- and lipid-containing macrophages and multinucleated giant cells; the condition may be inflammatory, although recurrence is likely to follow incomplete removal.

**pu'rulent s.,** suppurative *arthritis.*

**serous s.,** hydrarthrosis; hydrops articuli; s. with a large effusion of nonpurulent fluid.

**s. sicca,** dry s.

**sup'purative s.,** suppurative *arthritis.*

**tendinous s.,** tenosynovitis.

**vaginal s.,** tenosynovitis.

**syntactics** (sin-tak'tiks) [ syn- + G. *taxis,* order ]. A branch of semiotics that deals with the formal relations between signs, in abstraction from their signification (meaning) and their interpreters.

**syntality** (sin-tal'ĭ-tĭ) [ prob. telescoped from syn- + mentality ]. The consistent and predictable behavior of a social group.

**syntec'tic.** Pertaining to or marked by syntexis.

**synteresis** (sin'ter-e'sis) [ G. preservation, fr. *syn-tēreō,* to watch over, preserve ]. Prophylaxis.

**syntex'is** [ G. *syn-tēxis,* a melting together, fr. *syn-tēkō,* fut. *-tēxō,* to melt together ]. Emaciation; wasting; phthisis.

**synthase** (sin'thās). Trivial name used (in Enzyme Commission Report) for a lyase reaction going in the reverse direction; *cf. synthetase.* For individual s.'s, see the specific names.

**synthermal** (sin-ther'mal) [ syn- + G. *thermē,* heat ]. Having the same temperature.

**synthesis,** pl. **syntheses** (sin'the-sis, -sēz) [ G. fr. *syn,* together, + *thesis,* a placing, arranging. THE- ]. 1. A building up; a putting together; composition. 2. In chemistry, the formation of compounds by the union of simpler compounds or elements.

**s. of continuity,** healing of the edges of a wound or fracture.

**enzymatic s.,** s. by enzymes; *cf.* biosynthesis.

**protein s.,** see fig. under protein.

**syn'thesize.** To make something by synthesis (*i.e.,* synthetically).

**synthetase** (sin'the-tās). An enzyme catalyzing the synthesis of a specific substance. S. is limited, in the Enzyme Commission Report (rule 29), to use as a trivial name for the ligases (class 6), which in turn are those synthesizing enzymes that require the cleavage of a pyrophosphate linkage in ATP or in similar compound. Reversal of lyase (class 4) reactions, producing a synthesis, is indicated (in trivial names) by synthase (rule 24); such reactions do not involve pyrophosphate cleavage. For individual s.'s, see the specific names.

**synthet'ic.** Relating to or made by synthesis.

**synthorax** (sin-tho'raks). Thoracopagus.

**syntonic** (sin-ton'ik) [ G. *syntonos,* in harmony, fr. *syn,* together, + *tonos,* tone ]. Having even tone.

**syn'tonin.** Acid *albumin.*

**syntoxoid** (sin-tok'soyd). A toxoid having the same degree of affinity for an antitoxin that the toxin has.

**syntrip'sis** [ syn- + G. *tripsis,* a rubbing ]. Obsolete term for comminuted fracture, or its production.

**syntrophism** (sin'tro-fizm) [ syn- + G. *trophē,* nourishment ]. State of mutual dependence, with reference to food supply, of organs or cells of a plant or an animal.

**syntrophoblast** (sin-tro'fo-blast, -trof'o-). Syncytiotrophoblast.

**syntrophus** (sin'tro-fus) [ G. *syntrophos,* brought up or nursed together, fr. syn- + *trophē,* nourishment ]. A congenital disease.

**syntrop'ic.** Relating to syntropy.

**syntropy** (sin'tro-pĭ) [ syn- + G. *tropē,* a turning ]. 1. The tendency sometimes seen in two diseases to coalesce into one. 2. The state of wholesome association with others. 3. In anatomy, a number of similar structures inclined in one general direction, as the spinous processes of a series of vertebrae, or the ribs.

**inverse s.,** a situation in which the presence of one disease tends to decrease the possibility of another.

**synulosis** (sin'u-lo'sis) [ G. *synoulōsis.* UL-1 ]. Cicatrization.

**synulot'ic.** 1. Promoting cicatrization. 2. An agent with this action.

**Syphacia** (si-fa'shĭ-ah) [ fr. L. *siphon,* tube ]. Genus of oxyurid nematode pinworms of rodents; *S. obvelata* is the common cecal pinworm of mice, and *S. muris,* of rats. See also *Aspiculuris tetraptera.*

**syphilelcosis** (sif'ĭ-lel-ko'sis) [ syphilis + G. *helkōsis,* ulceration ]. Syphilitic ulceration.

**syphilelcus** (sif'ĭ-lel'kus) [ syphilis + G. *helkos,* ulcer ]. An old term for syphilitic ulcer.

**syphilemia** (sif'ĭ-le'mĭ-ah) [ syphilis + G. *haima,* blood ]. A state in which the specific organism, *Treponema pallidum,* is present in the blood stream.

**syphilid** (sif'ĭ-lid) [ syphilis + suffix *-id (1), q.v.* ]. Syphiloderm; an eruption comprised of one or many cutaneous lesions caused by syphilis.

**ac'neform s.,** pustular s.

**acu'minate pap'ular s.,** follicular s.

**an'nular s.,** cutaneous lesions of secondary syphilis in which the papules form annular lesions with raised papular borders and clear central portions.

**bullous s.,** pemphigoid s.; a rare manifestation of congenital syphilis.

**corym'bose s.,** a secondary syphilitic eruption consisting of a large central papule surrounded by a more or less complete ring of smaller papules.

**ecthy'matous s.,** pustular s.

**erythem'atous s.,** syphilitic *roseola.*

**flat papular s.,** lenticular s.

**follic'ular s.,** lichen syphiliticus; acuminate papular s.; miliary papular s.; secondary eruption of small follicular papules, usually appearing as groups of lesions.

**frambe'siform s.,** rupial s.

**gum'matous s.,** gumma.

**impetiginous s.,** pustular s.

**lentic'ular s.,** an eruption of flattened, dull reddish papules, 5 mm. to 1 cm. in diameter, occurring in secondary syphilis.

**mac'ular s.,** syphilitic *roseola.*

**miliary papular s.,** follicular s.

**nod'ular s.,** gumma.

**nummular s.,** flat, disk-shaped papules of secondary syphilis.

**palmar s.,** occurring in secondary syphilis, with dull red paules in the palms.

**papular s.,** see follicular s. and lenticular s.

**papulosquamous s.,** scaling papules of secondary syphilis.

**pem'phigoid s.,** bullous s.

**pig'mentary s.,** lesions of secondary syphilis consisting of rounded white macules on the trunk.

**plantar s.,** dull red papules on the soles in secondary syphilis.

**pus'tular s.,** acne syphilitica; acneform, impetiginous, varioliform, or ecthymatous s.; a type of pustular eruption occurring in secondary syphilis.

**ru'pial s.,** frambesiform s.; lesions appear granulomatous and crusted, resembling the lesions of yaws.

**secondary s.,** one of the skin lesions of secondary syphilis.

**serpig'inous s.,** a spreading eruption consisting of nodules or ulcers associated with late syphilis. Lesions are gummas.

**ter'tiary s.,** a syphilitic skin lesion peculiar to the third stage of the disease.

**tuber'cular s.,** gumma.

**vario'liform s.,** pustular s.

**syphilidography** (sif'ĭ-lĭ-dog'ră-fĭ). Syphilography.

**syphilimetry** (sif'ĭ-lim'e-trĭ) [ syphilis + G. *metron,* measure ]. Test designed to determine intensity of syphilitic infection, *e.g.,* titered serologic test.

**syphilionthus** (sif'ĭ-lĭ-on'thus) [ syphilid + G. *ionthos,* acne of adolescence ]. A copper-colored syphilid with branny scales.

**syphilipher** (sĭ-fil'ĭ-fur) [ G. *pherō,* to carry ]. A syphilis carrier; one who has syphilis in the infectious stage.

**syphilis** (sif'ĭ-lis) [ Mod. L. *syphilis* (*syphilid-*), orig. the title of a poem, *Syphilis sive Morbus Gallicus,* published by Fracastorius, *Syphilus* being the name of a shepherd, the principal character in the poem; ultimate etymology unknown ]. Lues venera; malum venereum; an acute and chronic infectious disease caused by *Treponema pallidum* (*Spirochaeta pallida*) and transmitted by direct contact, usually through sexual intercourse. After an incubation period of 12 to 30 days, the first symptom is the chancre, followed by slight fever and other constitutional symptoms, and a skin eruption of various appearances with mucous patches; this constitutes the second stage. The third stage is marked by the formation of gummas and cardiovascular and central nervous system lesions.

**congenital s.,** s. acquired by the fetus *in utero*, thus present at birth.

**s. d'emblée** (dom-bla') [ Fr. right away ], s. occurring without an initial sore.

**s. econom'ica,** s. innocentium in which infection occurs through the medium of table utensils, towels, and other articles of domestic use.

**equine s.,** dourine.

**s. heredita'ria, hereditary s.,** congenital s.

**s. heredita'ria tarda,** s., supposed to be congenital, that does not manifest itself until several years after birth.

**s. innocen'tium,** s. acquired in other ways than by coitus or other sexual practices.

**meningovascular s.,** a rare manifestation of secondary or tertiary s. characterized by mild, nonsuppurative, chronic inflammation of the leptomeninges and an intracranial angiitis.

**noduloulcerative s.,** a form of tertiary (late) cutaneous s., gummatous pattern.

**primary s.,** protosyphilis; the first stage of the disease from the development of the chancre to the appearance of the eruption.

**quaternary s.,** parasyphilis.

**secondary s.,** mesosyphilis; the second stage of the disease, beginning with the appearance of the eruption and lasting an indefinite period.

**tertiary s.,** the final stage of the disease, of indefinite beginning and ending, marked by the formation of gummas and cellular infiltration.

**syphilitic** (sif'ĭ-lit'ik). Relating to, caused by, or suffering from syphilis.

**syphilization** (sif'ĭ-lĭ-za'shun). Inoculation with chancre material, with prophylactic or curative intent.

**syphilo-, syphil-, syphili-** [ see syphilis ]. Combining forms relating to syphilis.

**syphiloderm, syphiloderma** (sif'il-o-derm, -der'mah) [ syphilo- + G. *derma*, skin ]. Syphilid.

**syphilogenesis, syphilogeny** (sif'ĭ-lo-jen'ĕ-sis, sif'ĭ-loj'ĕ-nĭ) [ syphilo- + G. *genesis*, production ]. The origin and progressive course of syphilis.

**syphilographer** (sif'ĭ-log'rā-fer). A writer on syphilis.

**syphilography** (sif'ĭ-log'rā-fĭ) [ syphilo- + G. *graphō*, to write ]. Syphilidography; a treatise on or description of syphilis.

**syphiloid** (sif'ĭ-loyd) [ syphilo- + G. *eidos*, resemblance ]. Resembling syphilis.

**syphilologist** (sif'ĭ-lol'o-jist). 1. One versed in the knowledge of syphilis.

**syphilology** (sif'ĭ-lol'o-jĭ) [ syphilo- + G. *logos*, study ]. The branch of medical science that has to do with syphilis in all its relations.

**syphiloma** (sif'ĭ-lo'mah) [ syphilo- + G. suffix -*oma*, tumor ]. Gumma; syphilophyma; a syphilitic tumor.

**syphilomatous** (sif'ĭ-lo'mă-tus). Relating to a syphiloma.

**syphilophobia** (sif'ĭ-lo-fo'bĭ-ah) [ syphilo- + G. *phobos*, fear ]. A morbid fear of acquiring syphilis.

**syphilophyma** (sif'ĭ-lo-fi'mah) [ syphilo- + G. *phyma*, a tumor ]. Syphiloma; gumma.

**syr.** Abbreviation of Mod. L. *syrupus*, syrup.

**syrigmophonia** (sĭ-rig'mo-fo'nĭ-ah) [ G. *syrigmos*, a hissing, + *phōnē*, sound, voice ]. A sibilant rale.

**syrigmus** (sĭ-rig'mus) [ L. fr. G. *syrigmos*, a hissing ]. *Tinnitus aurium*.

**syring-.** See syringo-.

**syringadenoma** (sĭr'ing-ad-ĕ-no'mah) [ syring- + G. *adēn*, gland, + suffix -*oma*, tumor ]. A benign sweat gland tumor showing glandular differentiation.

**syringadenosus** (sĭr'ing-ad-ĕ-no'sus) [ L. fr. syring- + G. *adēn*, gland ]. Relating to the sweat glands.

**syringe** (sĭ-rinj', sĭr'inj) [ G. *syrinx*, pipe or tube. SYRI- ]. An instrument used for injecting fluids.

**chip s.,** a tapered metal tube through which air is forced from a rubber bulb or pressure tank to blow debris from, or to dry, a cavity in preparing teeth for restoration.

**Davidson s.,** a rubber tube, armed with an appropriate nozzle, intersected with a compressible bulb, with valves so arranged that compression forces the fluid, into which one end of the tube is inserted, forward to the nozzle end.

**dental s.,** a breech-loading metal cartridge s. into which fits a hermetically sealed glass cartridge containing the anesthetic solution.

**fountain s.,** an apparatus consisting of a reservoir for holding fluid, to the bottom of which is attached a tube armed with a suitable nozzle; used for vaginal or rectal injections, irrigating wounds, etc., the force of the flow being regulated by the height of the reservoir above the point of discharge.

**hypodermic s.,** a small s., armed with a hollow needle in place of a nozzle, for use in giving remedies by the subcutaneous method.

**Luer s.,** a glass s. with airtight glass piston, for hypodermic and intravenous use.

**Roughton-Scholander s.,** Roughton-Scholander *apparatus*.

**rubber-bulb s.,** a s. with a hollow rubber bulb in place of a cylinder and piston. The cannula is usually of metal and provided with a check valve. Used to obtain a jet of air or water.

**syringeal** (si-rin'je-al). Relating to a syrinx.

**syringectomy** (sĭr'in-jek'to-mĭ) [ syring- + G. *ektomē*, excision ]. Fistulectomy.

**syringin** (sĭ-rin'jin). Syringoside; ligustrin; methoxyconiferin; 4-(3-hydroxypropenyl)-2,6-dimethoxyphenyl D-glucoside; present in the bark and leaves of *Syringa vulgaris* or lilac (family Oleaceae) and various other plants; formerly used as a tonic and antiperiodic.

**syringitis** (sĭr'in-ji'tis) [ syring- + G. suffix -*itis*, inflammation ]. Inflammation of the Eustachian tube.

**syringo-, syring-** [ G. *syrinx*, pipe or tube. SYRI- ]. Combining forms relating to a syrinx.

**syringobulbia** (sĭ-ring'go-bul'bĭ-ah) [ syringo- + L. *bulbus*, bulb (medulla oblongata) ]. A fluid-filled cavity of the brainstem, analogous to syringomyelia.

**syringocarcinoma** (sĭ-ring'go-kar'sĭ-no'mah) [ syringo- + carcinoma ]. A malignant epithelial neoplasm which has undergone cystic change (cystic carcinoma); a carcinoma with a tubular structure or fistula usually caused by degeneration and necrosis.

**syringocele** (sĭ-ring'go-sēl) [ syringo- + G. *koilia*, a hollow ]. 1. *Canalis* centralis. 2. A meningomyelocele in which there is a cavity in the ectopic spinal cord.

**syringocystadenoma** (sĭ-ring'go-sis-tad-ĕ-no'mah) [ syringo- + cystadenoma ]. A multiple nodular growth due to dilation and epithelial proliferation of the sweat glands; a form of multiple benign cystic neoplasm.

**s. papilliferum,** one that is characterized by numerous finger-like projections of the proliferated, neoplastic epithelial cells in two layers on a stromal core of fibrous connective tissue.

**syringocystoma** (sĭ-ring'go-sis-to'mah) [ syringo- + cystoma ]. A cystic tumor composed of cylindrical celled epithelium, originating from the hair follicles.

**syringoencephalomyelia** (sĭ-ring'go-en-sef'ă-lo-mi-e'lĭ-ah) [ syringo- + G. *enkephalos*, brain, + *myelos*, marrow ]. A tubular cavity, involving both brain and spinal cord, and etiologically unrelated to vascular insufficiency.

**syringoid** (sĭ-ring'goyd) [ syringo- + G. *eidos*, resemblance ]. Resembling a tube; fistulous.

**syringoma** (sĭr'ing-go'mah) [ syringo- + G. suffix -*oma*, tumor ]. A benign neoplasm of the sweat glands.

**syringomeningocele** (sĭ-ring'go-mĕ-ning'go-sēl) [ syringo- + meningocele ]. A form of spina bifida in which the dorsal sac consists chiefly of membranes, with very little cord substance, enclosing a cavity that communicates with a syringomyelic cavity.

**syringomyelia** (sĭ-ring'go-mi-e'lĭ-ah) [ syringo- + G. *myelos*, marrow ]. Hydrosyringomyelia; Morvan's disease; myelosyringosis; syringomyelus; the presence in the spinal cord of longitudinal cavities lined by dense, gliogenous tissue, and not caused by vascular insufficiency; it is marked clinically by pain and paresthesia followed by muscular atrophy of the hands; there is analgesia with thermoanesthesia of the hands and arms, but the tactile sense is preserved. Later, painless whitlows are seen, spastic paralysis appears in the lower extremities, and scoliosis of the lumbar spine occurs. Some cases are associated with low grade astrocytomas or vascular malformations of the spinal cord.

**syringomyelocele** (sĭ-ring′mi′ē-lo-sēl) [ syringo- + myelocele ]. A form of spina bifida, consisting in a protrusion of the membranes and spinal cord through a dorsal defect in the vertebral column, the fluid of the syrinx of the cord being increased and expanding the cord tissue into a thin-walled sac which then expands through the vertebral defect.

**syringomyelus** (sĭ-ring′go-mi′ē-lus) [ syringo- + G. myelos, marrow ]. Syringomyelia.

**syringopontia** (sĭ-ring′go-pon′shĭ-ah) [ syringo- + L. pons, bridge ]. A condition of cavity formation in the pons, of the same nature as syringomyelia.

**syringosystrophy** (sĭ-ring′go-sis′tro-fĭ) [ syringo- + G. systrophē, a twisting together. STREP- ]. Tubotorsion.

**syringotome** (sĭ-ring′o-tōm). Fistulatome.

**syringotomy** (sĭr′ing-got′o-mĭ). Fistulotomy.

**syrinx,** pl. **syringes** (sĭr′ingks, sĭ-rin′jēz) [ G. a tube, pipe. SYRI- ]. 1. A fistula. 2. A pathologic tube-shaped cavity in the brain or spinal cord. 3. The vocal organ of birds.

**syrosingopine** (sĭr′o-sin′go-pēn). SINGOSERP; carbethoxy-syringoyl methyl reserpate; prepared from reserpine by hydrolysis and reesterification; used in the treatment of hypertension.

**syrup** (sur′up, sĭr′up) [ Mod. L. syrupus, fr. Ar. sharāb ]. 1. Refined molasses; the uncrystallizable saccharine solution left after the refining of sugar. 2. Any sweet fluid; a solution of sugar in water in any proportion. 3. A liquid preparation of medicinal or flavoring substances in a concentrated aqueous solution of a sugar, usually sucrose; other polyols such as glycerin or sorbitol, may be present to retard crystallization of sucrose or to increase the solubility of added ingredients. When the s. contains a medicinal substance, it is termed a medicated s.; a s. may contain antimicrobial agents to prevent bacterial and mold growth.

**syr′upus** [ Mod. L. ]. Syrup.

**syrupy** (sur′uh-pĭ, sĭr′-). Relating to syrup; of the consistency of syrup.

**syssarcosic** (sis′ar-ko′sik). Syssarcotic.

**syssarcosis** (sis′ar-ko′sis) [ G. syssarkōsis, a being overgrown with flesh, fr. syn, with, + sarx, flesh ]. Union of bones by muscle; a muscular articulation; in man examples of s. are the muscular connections of the hyoid bone, of the patella, and of other sesamoid bones.

**syssarcotic** (sis′ar-kot′ik). Relating to or characterized by syssarcosis.

**syssomus** (sĭ-so′mus) [ G. fr. syn, together, + sōma, body ]. Obsolete term for dicephalus.

**systaltic** (sis-tahl′tik, -tal′tik) [ G. systaltikos, contractile. STAL- ]. Pulsating; alternately contracting and dilating; denoting the action of the heart.

# SYSTEM

**system** (sis′tem) [ G. systēma, an organized whole. STA- ]. A consistent and complex whole made up of correlated and semi-independent parts. Specifically: 1. The entire organism. 2. Any complex of structures anatomically related, e.g., the vascular s. 3. Any complex of structures functionally related, e.g., the digestive s. 4. A scheme of medical theory, e.g., the Brunonian s. 5. An encyclopedic treatise on medicine or any of its branches, the work of several authors, arranged systematically according to subjects. 6. A progressive course of instruction, arranged according to a definite plan. 7. See also apparatus and systema.

  **absolute s. of units,** see under unit.

  **absorbent s.,** systema lymphaticum.

  **alimentary s.**

  **association s.,** tractus digestorius. necting different or tracts of nerve fibers interconsubdivision of tns of one and the same major various areas of the nervous system, such as the of the spinal cordral cortex or the various segments

  **autonomic nervou**

    **blood group s.'s,** systema nervosum autonomicum.

    **blood-vascular s.,** endix 2, Blood Groups.

  **Brunonian s.,** basvascular s. theory that disease rebrunonianism, the obsolete stimulus. from a lack or an excess of

  **bulbosacral s.,** the autonomic nervous systempathetic division of the the central, preganglionmname refers to the fact that localized to the brainstesympathetic neurons are fourth sacral segments of tbus) and the second to nervosum autonomicum. al cord. See also systema

  **cardiovascular s.,** blood-va vessels considered as a whole.; the heart and blood

  **caudal neurosecretory s.,** ui

  **centimeter-gram-second s.,** aphysis. internationally accepted scientted CGS or cgs; the fundamental physical units of lei of expressing the those units derived from them, inmass, and time, and seconds (see, for example, dyneneters, grams, and replaced by the Système Internatio. Currently being or International System of Units (q. Unités (hence SI), based on the meter, the kilogram, ar International), 

  **central nervous s.,** systema nervost second. 

  **cerebrospinal s.,** the combined centrale. peripheral nervous s. ervous s. and

  **chromaffin s.,** the cells of the body chromium salts and occur in the medulla stain with adrenal body, paraganglia, and in relrtion of the sympathetic nerves. to certain

  **circulatory s.,** vascular s.

  **colloid s.,** a combination of the two phase external, of a colloid solution; the various srnal and liquid (foam); gas + solid (meerschaum); l, gas + (fog); solid + gas (smoke); solid + liquid (so+ gas solid (gel); liquid + liquid (emulsion); solid + (colored glass). solid

  **conducting s. of the heart,** the s. of atypica muscle fibers comprising the sinoatrial node, iniiac tracts, atrioventricular node and bundle, the dal branches, and their terminal ramifications into tlle kinje network; sometimes also called cardionector.r-

  **dermal s., dermoid s.,** the skin and its appendage. nails and hair.

  **digestive s.,** apparatus digestorius.

  **ecological s.,** ecosystem.

  **endocrine s.,** collective designation for those tissu capable of secreting hormones.

  **esthesiodic s.,** see esthesiodic.

  **exterofective s.,** name applied by Cannon to the somatic nervous s. as opposed to the interofective or autonomic s.

  **extrapyramidal motor s.,** literally: all of the brain structures affecting bodily (somatic) movement, excluding the motor neurons, the motor cortex, and the pyramidal (corticobulbar and corticospinal) tract. Despite its very wide literal connotation, the term is commonly used to denote in particular the corpus striatum (basal ganglia), its associated structures (substantia nigra; subthalamic nucleus), and its descending connections with the midbrain and, indirectly, with the rhombencephalic and spinal motor neurons.

  **feedback s.,** see feedback.

  **Galton's s. of classification of fingerprints,** see under fingerprint.

  **gamma motor s.,** the small motor neurons that innervate the muscle spindles or neuromuscular spindles of skeletal (striated) muscles.

  **genital s.,** reproductive s.; the complex s. consisting of the male or female gonads, associated ducts, and external genitalia dedicated to the function of reproducing the species.

  **genitourinary s.,** apparatus urogenitalis.

  **glandular s.,** all the glands of the body collectively.

  **Haversian s.,** osteon.

organs, principally
**hematopoietic s.,** the blood-*f*
the bone marrow and lymph / various distinct and
**heterogeneous s.,** one that *c*ses, *e.g.,* a suspension
mechanically separable parts
or an emulsion.                           resulting if the lines of
**hexaxial reference s.,** th*e*ds of the electrocardio-
derivation of the unipolar *f*erence s., *q.v.*
gram are added to the tri. of interlacing Purkinje
**His-Tawara s.,** the co*r*yocardium; see also con-
fibers within the ventri*c*
ducting s. of the heart. arts cannot be mechanically
**homogeneous s.,** one *v*e uniform throughout and
separated, which is *f*tically physical properties; a
possesses in every p*a*oride, is such a s.
solution, *e.g.,* of sod*i***portal s.,** a s. of veins that
**hypothalamohypop***y* tufts of the median eminence,
originate from the *e* stalk and pars tuberalis of the
pass downward al*e* anterior lobe of the hypophysis
hypophysis, and *e*nto a secondary capillary bed, the
in which they ar*t*ese portal vessels convey to the
capillary sinuso*i*sing factors," chemical transmitters
anterior lobe th*a* neurons of the hypothalamus. See
synthesized by*t*ian *eminence.*
also hypophys.,   a device designed to produce an
**hypoxia wa***r*al at a predetermined level of oxygen
audio or visu*i*deally, the system would warn of
partial pre*s*a in time for corrective action to be
impending
taken.       .he use in microscopy of a layer of liquid,
**immersi***c*er, between the object lens and the object
either oil *i*d, thereby correcting the dispersion and
to be e*y*working distance.
increasi*r* a combination of antigen cellular or other
**immu***r*ptor and complement.
with a*r*ary s., the skin and its associated derivatives;
**inte***fl* from ectoderm and subjacent mesoderm.
it is *i*ary s.'s., interstitial *lamellae.*
**int***f*onal s. of units, see under International.
**In***r*ctive s., term applied by Cannon to the auto-
i*r*ervous s. as opposed to the somatic nervous s. or
n*e*ctive s.
*e*untary nervous s., *systema* nervosum autonomicum.
**siodic s.,** see kinesiodic.
etic s., (1) a term proposed by Crile to denote the
*i*n of organs through which latent energy is transformed
*i*o motion and heat: it includes the brain, the thyroid, the
*i*renals, the liver, the pancreas, and the muscles; (2) that
*a*rt of the neuromuscular s. whereby active movements
*i*re effected; distinguished from the static s.
**lateral line s.,** a series of sense organs that detect pressure
or vibrations along the head and side of cyclostomes,
fishes, and some amphibians.
**limbic s.,** visceral brain; collective term denoting a
heterogeneous array of brain structures at or near the edge
(limbus) of the medial wall of the cerebral hemisphere, in
particular the hippocampus, amygdala, and gyrus fornicatus; the term is often used so as to include also the
interconnections of these structures, as well as their
connections with the septal area, the hypothalamus, and a
medial zone of mesencephalic tegmentum. By way of the
latter connections, the limbic s. exerts an important
influence upon the endocrine and autonomic motor s.'s; its
functions also appear to affect motivational and mood
states.
**lymphatic s.,** *systema* lymphaticum.
**masticatory s.,** masticatory apparatus (1); dental apparatus; the muscles of mastication (see also musculus temporalis,
masseter, and pterygoideus); the organs and structures
primarily functioning in mastication. They are: jaws, teeth
with their supporting structures, temporomandibular articulation, mandibular musculature, tongue, lips, cheeks,
and oral mucosa.
**metameric nervous s.,** paleencephalon (or paleoencephalon); that part of the nervous s. which innervates body
structures that developed in ontogeny from the segmentally arranged somites or, in the head region, branchial
arches. The term somewhat vaguely refers to the neural
mechanisms intrinsic to the spinal cord and brainstem
(represented by the sensory nuclei, motoneuronal cell
groups, and their associated interneurons in the reticular

formation); by strict definition it should exclude the
autonomic nervous system.
**metric s.,** a s. of weights and measures, based upon the
meter as a unit. It is the universal s. for scientific use and
is employed commercially in most countries except those
of English speaking people; it is legalized in the United
States and allowable in England. The unit, the meter, was
originally intended to be one ten-millionth of a quadrant
of the earth's meridian, the equivalent of 39.37 inches.
Fractions of a meter are expressed in Latin numerals:
decimeter, $1/10$; centimeter, $1/100$; millimeter, $1/1000$; multiples
in Greek numerals: decameter, 10; hectometer, 100; kilometer, 1000. The unit of weight is the gram which is the
weight of one cubic centimeter of distilled water, equivalent to 15.432 + grains. The unit of volume is the liter or
one cubic decimeter, equal to 1.056 quarts; a cubic
centimeter is about 15 minims. See also International
System of Units.
**muscular s.,** all the muscles of the body collectively.
**neokinetic s.,** see neokinetic.
**nervous s.,** *systema* nervosum.
**neuromuscular s.,** the muscles of the body collectively
and the nerves supplying them.
**nonspecific s.,** see reticular activating s. and *formatio*
reticularis.
**occlusal s.,** occlusal scheme; the form or design and
arrangement of the occlusal and incisal units of a dentition
or the teeth on a denture.
**oculomotor s.,** that part of the central nervous s. that has
to do with eye movements; it is composed of pathways
connecting various regions of the cerebrum, brainstem,
and ocular nuclei, utilizing multisynaptic articulations.
**O-R s.,** abbreviation for oxidation-reduction s.
**oxidation-reduction s.,** O-R s.; redox s.; an enzyme s. in
the tissues by which oxidation and reduction proceed
simultaneously through the transference of hydrogen or of
one or more electrons from one metabolite to another; see
also oxidation-reduction.
**paleokinetic s.,** see paleokinetic.
**parasympathetic nervous s.,** pars parasympathica systematis nervosi autonomici [ NA ]; the parasympathetic part
of the autonomic nervous system; see also *systema* nervosum autonomicum; bulbosacral s.
**pedal s.,** efferent fibers connecting the forebrain with
more caudal structures.
**periodic s.,** the arrangement of the chemical elements in
a definite order as indicated by their respective atomic
numbers in such a way that groups of elements with similar
chemical properties (similar valence shell electron number)
are grouped together. See Mendeléeff's *law.*
**peripheral nervous s.,** *systema* nervosum periphericum.
**Pinel's s.,** the abolition of forcible restraint in the
treatment of the mental hospital patient.
**portal s.,** a s. of vessels in which blood, after passing
through one capillary bed, is conveyed through a second
capillary network, as in the hepatic portal system in which
blood from the intestines passes through the liver sinusoids.
**preconscious s.,** see preconscious.
**pressoreceptor s.,** the pressoreceptive areas which with
their afferent fibers and connections with the autonomic
system react to a rise in arterial blood pressure and serve
to buffer it by inhibiting the heart rate and vascular tone.
See also baroreceptor.
**projection s.,** the s. of axons carrying stimuli from one
portion of the nervous system to other portions.
**properdin s.,** see under properdin.
**Purkinje s.,** terminal ramifications in the ventricles of the
specialized conducting s. of the heart.
**redox s.,** oxidation-reduction s.
**reproductive s.,** genital s.
**renin-angiotensin s.,** a selective regulator of the aldosterone biosynthetic pathway that acts by increasing aldosterone production and sodium retention during volume
depletion; see also angiotensin; renin.
**respiratory s.,** *apparatus* respiratorius.
**reticular activating s.** abbreviated RAS; nonspecific s.; a
physiological term denoting that part of the brainstem
reticular formation that plays a central role in the
organism's bodily and behavorial alertness. It extends as a
diffusely organized neural apparatus through the central

region of the brainstem into the subthalamus and the intralaminar nuclei of the thalamus; by its ascending connections it affects the function of the cerebral cortex in the sense of behavioral responsiveness; its descending (reticulospinal) connections transmit its activating influence upon bodily posture and reflex mechanisms (*e.g.*, muscle tonus), in part by way of the gamma motor neurons. See also *formatio* reticularis.

**reticuloendothelial s.,** the s. of macrophages; collectively, the cells in different organs chiefly concerned with phagocytosis. They may occur as a reticulum in lymphatic structures or form the lining of sinusoids in such organs as the liver, spleen and bone marrow. In connective tissue they are termed histiocytes and in nervous tissue, microglia.

**second signaling s.,** Pavlovian term for speech in which words are considered to be the "second signals" capable of producing conditioned responses.

**somesthetic s.,** the sensory data from skin, muscles, and body organs in distinction to the special senses.

**static s.,** that part of the neuromuscular s. whereby the animal organism is maintained in posture and equilibrium, and counteracts the forces of gravity and atmospheric pressure; distinguished from the kinetic s. (2).

**stomatognathic s.,** masticatory apparatus (2); all of the structures involved in speech and in the receiving, mastication, and deglutition of food; see also masticatory s.

**sympathetic nervous s.,** (1) originally, the entire autonomic nervous s.; (2) now applied only to the thoracolumbar portion of the autonomic nervous system; also known as pars sympathica systematis nervosi autonomici [ NA ]. See *systema* nervosum autonomicum.

**T s.,** the transverse component of the sarcoplasmic reticulum of skeletal muscle; see also T *tubule.*

**thoracolumbar s.,** the sympathetic division of the autonomic nervous system; see *systema* nervosum autonomicum.

**triaxial reference s.,** the figure resulting from rearranging the lines of derivation of the three standard limb leads of the electrocardiogram (as represented in Einthoven's triangle) so that, instead of forming the sides of an equilateral triangle, they bisect one another.

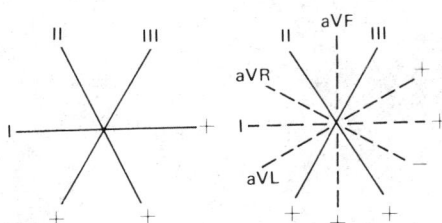

**Triaxial (*left*) and Hexaxial (*right*) Reference Systems**

**urinary s.,** urinary apparatus; the kidneys, ureters, bladder, and urethra.

**urogenital s.,** *apparatus* urogenitalis.

**uropoietic s.,** the organs concerned in the secretion and excretion of urine, viz., the kidneys, the ureters, the bladder, and the urethra.

**vascular s.,** circulatory s.; the cardiovascular and lymphatic s.'s collectively.

**vegetative nervous s.,** *systema* nervosum autonomicum.

**vertebral-basilar s.,** the arterial complex comprising the two vertebral arteries joining to form the basilar artery, and their immediate branches.

**vertebral venous s.,** *plexus* venosi vertebrales.

**visceral nervous s.,** *systema* nervosum autonomicum.

---

**systema** (sis′te′mah) [ L. fr. G. systēma. STA- ] [ NA. System; apparatus; a complex of anatomical structures functionally related.

**s. digesto′rium** [ NA ], official alternate term for *apparatus* digestorius.

**s. lymphat′icu**
of lymphatic ve⟨ ], the lymphatic system, consisting into the veins atdes, and lymphoid tissue; it empties thorax. See colorel of the superior aperture of the

**s. nervo′sum** [ ⟩.
apparatus, composervous system; the entire nerve ganglia.      e brain, spinal cord, nerves, and

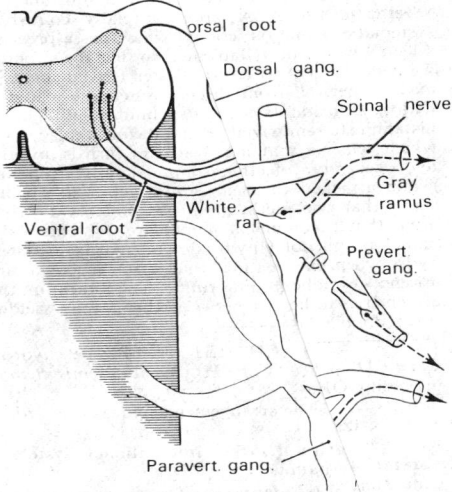

**Systema Nervosum Autonomicum (Auto⟨    Nervous System)**

Diagram of the efferent fibers of the sympa⟨     (thoraco-lumbar) division.

**s. nervo′sum autonom′icum** [ NA ], autonon system; sympathetic nervous system (1); involu⟨vous vous system; vegetative nervous system; viscera⟨ner-system; that part of the nervous system which r⟨ious the motor innervation of the internal organs, spe⟨ts the latter's smooth muscle, cardiac muscle (in the⟨lly the heart), and gland cells. It consists of two phys⟨f cally and anatomically distinct, by-and-large mur antagonistic components: the sympathetic or thoraco. bar system, and the parasympathetic or bulbosa system. In both of these subsystems the pathway innervation consists of a synaptic sequence of two mot neurons, one of which lies in the spinal cord or brainste⟨ as the preganglionic motor neuron, the thin but myelinate⟨ axon of which (preganglionic fiber, B fiber) emerges with an outgoing spinal or cranial nerve and synapses with one or more of the postganglionic (or, more strictly, ganglionic) motor neurons composing the autonomic ganglia; the unmyelinated postganglionic fibers originating in these ganglia in turn innervate the muscle or gland cells of the internal organs. The preganglionic neurons of the sympathetic lie in the columna lateralis of the thoracic and upper two lumbar segments of the spinal gray matter; those of the parasympathetic compose the visceral motor (visceral efferent) nuclei of the brainstem (dorsal motor nucleus of the vagus, salivatory nuclei, and nucleus of Edinger-Westphal) as well as the lateral column of the second to fourth sacral segments of the spinal cord. The autonomic ganglia of the sympathetic are the paravertebral ganglia of the sympathetic trunk, and the prevertebral or collateral ganglia (celiac ganglion); those of the parasympathetic lie either near the organ to be innervated (juxtamural ganglia, *e.g.* submandibular ganglion for the salivary and lachrymal glands, ciliary ganglion for the eye, cardiac (Wrisberg's) ganglion for the heart, pelvic ganglion for the pelvic organs) or even as intramural ganglia within the organ itself (*e.g.* Auerbach's and Meissner's plexus in the wall of the intestinal tract).

**s. nervo′sum centra′le** [ NA ], the central nervous system: the brain and spinal cord.

the peripheral ner-
**s. nervo'sum peripher'icum** d ganglia.
vous system, composed of ne| alternate term for
**s. respirato'rium** [ NA ],
*apparatus* respiratorius. ernate term for *appara-*
**s. urogenita'le** [ NA ], off'
*tus* urogenitalis. ing to a system in any
**systematic** (sis'tĕ-mat'ik),ystem.

sense; arranged accordin'to chemical substances, a
**systematic name.** As id of specially coined or
systematic name is cich of which has a precisely
selected words or syllaeaning, so that the structure
defined chemical strucame. Water (trivial name) is
may be derived from c). The systematic name of
hydrogen oxide (syne, q.v.) is imidazolethylamine,
histamine (a semitriiical of imidazole replaces one
which tells us thatnine, which in turn is an ethyl
hydrogen atom ofmine group. Dimethyl sulfoxide
group attached t(radicals are attached to a sulfur
states that holdsitritival atom. Carbolic acid (trivial
atom that holdsnitrivial name) are, systematically,
name) or phenienylhydroxide or hydroxycyclohex-
hydroxybenzenndicating that six carbon atoms,
atriene (cyclqe, are in a ring; triene indicating that
attached as ith occur between them, thus yielding
three double

CH—CH = CH, or benzene; hydroxy
CH = CH place of one H). See also *semisystematic*
indicating
*name.* on. The arrangement of ideas into orderly
**system'ai**
sequenc**ernational.** See International System of
**Systèm**International).
Units **s**-tem'ik). Relating to a system; specifically so-
**systen**ng to the entire organism as distinguished from
mati(ndividual parts.
any **d.** Resembling a system; denoting a tumor of
**sys't**structure resembling an organ.
co**r**sis'to-le) [ G. *systolē,* a contracting, STAL- ]. The
**sys**ical contraction of the heart, especially of the
r'les, by which the blood is driven through the aorta

and pulmonary artery to traverse the systemic and pulmonary circulations, respectively; its occurrence is indicated
physically by the first sound of the heart heard on
auscultation, by the palpable apex beat and by the arterial
pulse.
  **aborted s.,** a loss of the systolic beat in the radial pulse
through weakness of the ventricular contraction.
  **s. alter'nans,** hemisystole.
  **arterial s.,** the contraction of an artery following its
dilation by the pulse wave.
  **atrial s.,** auricular s.; contraction of the atria.
  **auricular s.,** atrial s.
  **electromechanical s.,** Q-S$_2$ interval; the period from the
beginning of the QRS complex to the first vibration of the
second heart sound.
  **extra-s.,** see extrasystole.
  **late s.;** prediastole.
  **premature s.,** extrasystole.
  **ventricular s.,** contraction of the ventricles.
**systol'ic.** Relating to, or occurring during cardiac systole.
**systolometer** (sis'to-lom'e-ter) [ systole + G. *metron,*
measure ]. 1. An apparatus for determining the force of the
cardiac contraction. 2. An instrument for analyzing the
sounds of the heart.
**systrem'ma** [ G. anything twisted. STREP- ]. A muscular
cramp in the calf of the leg, the contracted muscles forming
a hard ball.
**syzygial** (sĭ-zij'ĭ-al). Relating to syzygy.
**syzygiology** (sĭ-zij'ĭ-ol'o-jĭ) [ G. *syzygios,* yoked (see syzygy), + *logos,* study ]. The study of interrelationships, or
interdependencies, especially of the whole, as opposed to
the study of separate parts or isolated functions.
**syzygium** (sĭ-zij'ĭ-um). Syzygy.
**syzygy** (siz'ĭ-jĭ) [ G. *syzygios,* yoked, bound together, fr.
*syn,* together, + *zygon,* a yoke ]. Syzygium. 1. The
association of varying members of gregarine protozoans
end-to-end or in lateral pairing (without sexual fusion). 2.
Pairing of chromosomes in meiosis.
**Szent-Gyorgyi** (sent-jur'je), Albert, Hungarian biochemist in the U. S., *1893. Nobel laureate, 1937, for discoveries
in connection with biological combustion processes.

# T

**T.** Symbol for: 1. Tension; T+, increased tension; T−, diminished tension. 2. Absolute *temperature*. 3. Ribothymidine. 4. As a subscript, refers to tidal *volume*.

**T$_m$.** Symbol for *temperature* midpoint or melting *temperature*.

**t.** Abbreviation for: 1. Lat. *ter*, three times. 2. Metric ton. 3. Temperature, on the Centigrade scale.

**T$_3$.** Symbol for 3,5,3-triiodothyronine.

**T-1824.** *Evans* blue.

**Ta.** Chemical symbol of the element tantalum.

**tabanid** (tab′ă-nid) [ L. *tabanus*, gadfly ]. Common name for flies of the family Tabanidae.

**Tabanidae** (tă-ban′ĭ-de) [ see *tabanus* ]. a family of blood-sucking flies that includes the genera *Tabanus* (horsefly) and *Chrysops* (deerfly and mango fly), which are involved in transmission of several blood-borne parasites.

**Tabanus** (tă-ba′nus) [ L. a gadfly ]. the gadflies and horse-flies, a genus of biting flies, some species of which transmit surra, infectious equine anemia, anthrax, and other diseases.

**tabardillo** (tah-bar-de′yo). The Mexican term for typhus fever.

**tabasheer** (tab′ă-shēr′) [ Hindu word ]. An excretion found at the joints of the bamboo in India and Brazil. Used as a tonic and cough remedy.

**tabatière anatomique** (tab-ah-te-ār′ an-ah-to-mēk) [ Fr. snuffbox ]. Anatomical snuffbox; see under anatomical.

**tabefaction** (ta-be-fak′shun) [ L. *tabe-facio*, pp. *-factus*, to melt, fr. *tabes*, a wasting away, + *facio*, to make ]. Tabescence; emaciation; atrophy; tabes.

**tabella**, pl. **tabellae** (tă-bel′lah) [ L. dim. of *tabula*, tablet ]. A medicated tablet or lozenge.

**tab′ernamonta′nain.** A proteolytic enzyme from *Tabernaemontana grandiflora*; anthelminthic, digesting *Trichina* and *Ancylostoma*.

**tabes** (ta′bēz) [ L. a wasting away ]. Progressive wasting or emaciation.

   **t. diabet′ica**, diabetic neuropathy, especially of the motor nerves of the lower extremities, marked by muscular atrophy and a steppage gait.

   **t. dorsa′lis**, locomotor ataxia (2); posterior spinal sclerosis; t. spinalis; spinal atrophy; Duchenne's disease (1); a chronic inflammation and progressive sclerosis of the posterior proximal spinal roots, the posterior columns of the spinal cord, and the peripheral nerves; the symptoms include ataxia, or muscular incoordination, anesthesia, neuralgia, lacinating pains, visceral crises, and muscular atrophy; atrophy of the optic nerve is not uncommon, trophic disorders of the joints (arthropathies) are frequent, and paralysis is a late symptom; the disease begins usually in middle life and is a tertiary form of syphilis.

   **t. ergot′ica**, ataxia, amyotrophy, and neuralgic pain seen in ergot intoxication.

   **t. heredita′ria**, hereditary spinal *ataxia*.

   **t. mesenter′ica**, tuberculosis of the mesenteric and retroperitoneal lymph nodes.

   **peripheral t.**, pseudotabes.

   **t. spasmod′ica**, spastic *diplegia*.

   **t. spina′lis**, t. dorsalis.

**tabescence** (ta-bes′ens). The state of progressive wasting away.

**tabescent** (ta-bes′ent) [ L. *tabesco*, to waste away, fr. *tabes*, a wasting away ]. Progressively emaciating; tabetic; phthisical.

**tabet′ic.** Relating to or suffering from tabes, especially tabes dorsalis.

**tabet′iform** [ irreg. formed fr. L. *tabes*, a wasting, + *forma*, form ]. Resembling tabes dorsalis.

**tab′ic.** Tabetic.

**tab′id** [ L. *tabidus*, wasting away ]. Tabetic; tabic; emaciating; wasting away.

**tablature** (tab-lă-tūr) [ L. *tabula*, tablet ]. The state of division of the cranial bones into two plates separated by the diploë.

**ta′ble** [ L. *tabula* ]. 1. One of the two plates or laminae, separated by the diploë, into which the cranial bones are divided. 2. An arrangement of the data of a clinical history, the steps of an experiment, etc., in parallel columns, showing the essential facts in a readily appreciable form.

   **Aub-DuBois t.**, t. of basal metabolic rates in calories per square meter of body surface per hour or day for different ages.

   **examining t.**, a t. on which the patient lies during a medical examination.

   **Gaffky t.**, Gaffky scale; a numerical rating for the classification of tuberculosis according to the number of tubercle bacilli in the sputum, ranging from 1 (one to four organisms in the whole preparation) to 9 (an average of 100 per field).

   **inner t. of skull**, *lamina* interna cranii.

   **occlusal t.**, the occlusal or grinding surfaces of the bicuspid and molar teeth.

   **operating t.**, a t. on which the patient lies during a surgical operation.

   **outer t. of skull**, *lamina* externa cranii.

   **Reuss' color t.'s**, Stilling color t.'s; charts in which colored letters are printed on colored backgrounds in such combination that some of them are invisible to a color-blind person.

   **Stilling color t.'s**, Reuss' color t.'s.

   **tilt-t.**, a t. with a top capable of being rotated on its transverse axis so that a subject lying upon it can be brought into the erect position as desired. Used in experimental investigation and in certain conditions (*e.g.*, prevention of bedsores).

   **vit′reous t.**, the inner t. of one of the cranial bones; it is more compact and harder than the outer t.

**ta′blespoon.** A large spoon, used as a measure of the dose of a medicine, equivalent to about 4 fluidrams or $^1/_2$ fluidounce or 15 ml.

**tab′let** [ Fr. *tablette*, L. *tabula* ]. A solid dosage form containing medicinal substances with or without suitable diluents. May vary in shape, size, and weight. May be classed according to the method of manufacture, as molded t. and compressed t.

   **buccal t.**, usually a small, flat t. intended to be inserted in the buccal pouch, where the active ingredient is absorbed directly through the oral mucosa; such a t. dissolves or erodes slowly.

   **compressed t.**, a t. prepared, usually as a large-scale production, by means of great pressure; most compressed t.'s consist of the active ingredient and a diluent, binder, disintegrator, and lubricant.

   **dispensing t.**, prepared by molding or by compression; used by the dispensing pharmacist for obtaining certain potent substances in a convenient form for accurate compounding.

   **hypodermic t.**, a compressed or molded t. that dissolves completely in water (for injection) to form an injectable solution.

   **sublingual t.**, usually a small, flat t. intended to be inserted beneath the tongue, where the active ingredient is absorbed directly through the oral mucosa; such a t. dissolves very promptly.

   **t. triturate**, a small, usually cylindrical, molded or compressed disk of varying size, containing a diluent usually consisting of dextrose (glucose) or of a mixture of lactose and powdered sucrose and a moistening agent or excipient, such as dilute alcohol.

**taboo, tabu** (tă-boo′) [ Tongan, set apart ]. Restricted, prohibited, or forbidden; set apart for religious or ceremonial purposes (as, for example, a sacred interdiction).

**taboparesis** (ta′bo-pă-re′sis, -păr′e-sis). A condition in which the symptoms of tabes dorsalis and general paresis are associated.

**tabular** (tab′u-lar) [ L. *tabularis*, fr. *tabula*, table ]. 1. Laminar; table-like. 2. Arranged in the form of a table (2).

**tabule** (tab′ūl) [ L. *tabula* ]. Tablet.

**ta′bun.** Dimethylphosphoramidocyanidic acid, ethyl ester; an extremely potent cholinesterase inhibitor; the lethal dose for man is believed to be as low as 0.01 mg. per kg.

**tache** (tash) [ Fr. spot ]. A macule; a freckle; a circumscribed discoloration of the skin or mucous membrane.

    **t. blanche** (blahṅsh), *macula albida.*

    **t. bleuatre** (blĕ-atr′), *macula* cerulea.

    **t. cérébrale** (sa-ra-bral′), meningitic *streak.*

    **t. laiteuse** (la-tĕz′), (1) milk *spot;* (2) *macula* albida.

    **t. méningéale** (ma-naṅ-zha-al′), meningitic *streak.*

    **t. noir** (nwahr) [ Fr. black ], necrotic area covered with black crust characteristic of the tick bite lesion in certain tick-borne diseases.

    **t. spina′le,** a trophic bulla forming on the skin in certain cases of disease of the spinal cord.

    **t. vièrge** (vī-airzh′), one of a number of small circular areas on the surface of a bacterial culture, assumed by d'Herelle to be evidence of the action of a bacteriophage.

**tachetic** (tă-ket′ik) [ F. *tache,* spot ]. Marked by bluish or brownish spots.

**tachistesthesia** (tă-kis′tes-the′zī-ah) [ G. *tachistos,* very rapid, from *tachys,* rapid, + *aesthēsis,* perception. TACH- ]. Recognition of light flicker.

**tachistoscope** (tă-kis′to-skōp) [ G. *tachistos,* very rapid, fr. *tachys,* rapid, + *skopeō,* to view. TACH- ]. An instrument used in experimental optics to determine the shortest exposure capable of making a conscious impression on the retina; it is on the plan of the movable shutter used in photography.

**tachogram** (tak′o-gram) [ G. *tachos,* speed, + *gramma,* mark ]. Record made by a tachometer.

**tachography** (tă-kog′ră-fī) [ G. *tachos,* speed, + *graphō,* to write ]. The recording of the speed or rate of something.

**tachometer** (tă-kom′e-ter) [ G. *tachos,* speed, + *metron,* measure ]. An instrument for measuring the speed or rate of something; *e.g.,* revolutions of a shaft, heart rate (cardiotachometer), arterial blood flow (hemotachometer), respiratory gas flow (pneumotachometer).

**tachy-** (tak′ī-) [ G. *tachys,* quick, rapid. TACH- ]. Combining form meaning rapid.

**tachyarrhythmia** (tak′ī-ă-rith′mī-ah) [ tachy- + G. *a-* priv. + *rhythmos,* rhythm ]. Any disturbance of the heart's rhythm, regular or irregular, resulting in a rate over 100 beats per minute.

**tachyauxesis** (tak′ī-awk-se′sis) [ tachy- + G. *auxō,* to increase ]. Type of growth in which a part grows more rapidly than the whole.

**tachycardia** (tak′ī-kar′dī-ah) [ tachy- + G. *kardia,* heart ]. Heart hurry; polycardia; tachysystole; rapid beating of the heart, usually applied to rates over 100 per minute.

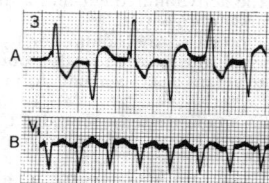

**Tachycardia**
*A,* bidirectional ventricular tachycardia; *B,* double tachycardia.

    **atrial t.,** auricular t.; paroxysmal t. originating in an ectopic focus in the atrium.

    **auric′ular t.,** atrial t.

    **A-V nodal t.,** nodal t.; originating in the A-V junction.

    **bidirectional ventricular t.,** ventricular t. in which the QRS complexes in the electrocardiogram are alternately mainly positive and mainly negative; many such cases may in fact represent A-V t. with alternating forms of aberrant ventricular conduction.

    **double t.,** the simultaneous presence of two ectopic t.'s, *e.g.,* atrial and A-V nodal.

    **ectopic t.,** a t. originating in a focus other than the sinus node, *e.g.,* atrial, A-V nodal, or ventricular.

    **essential t.,** persistent rapid action of the heart due to no discoverable organic lesion.

    **t. exophthal′mica,** the rapid heart action occurring as one of the symptoms of exophthalmic goiter.

    **fetal t.,** a fetal heart rate of 160 or more beats per minute.

    **nodal t.,** A-V nodal t.

    **paroxys′mal t.,** recurrent attacks of t., with abrupt onset and termination, originating from an ectopic focus which may be atrial, A-V nodal, or ventricular.

    **sinus t.,** t. originating in the sinus node.

    **ventricular t.,** paroxysmal t. originating in an ectopic focus in the ventricle.

**tachycar′diac.** Relating to or suffering from excessively rapid action of the heart.

**tachycrotic** (tak′ī-krot′ik) [ tachy- + G. *krotos,* a striking ]. Relating to, causing, or characterized by a rapid pulse.

**tachyla′lia** [ tachy- + G. *lalia,* talking ]. Tachylogia.

**tachylogia** (tak-ī-lo′jī-ah) [ tachy- + G. *logos,* word ]. Rapid or voluble speech; also called tachylalia, tachyphasia, tachyphemia, tachyphrasia.

**tachyphagia** (tak-ī-fa′jī-ah) [ tachy- + G. *phagein,* to eat ]. Rapid eating; bolting of food.

**tachyphasia** (tak-ī-fa′zī-ah) [ tachy- + G. *phasis,* speaking ]. Tachylogia.

**tachyphemia** (tak-ī-fe′mī-ah) [ tachy- + G. *phēme* ], speech ]. Tachylogia.

**tachyphrasia** (tak-ī-fra′zī-ah) [ tachy- + G. *phrasis,* speaking ]. Tachylogia.

**tachyphrenia** (tak-ī-fre′nī-ah) [ tachy- + G. *phrēn,* mind ]. Rapidity of the mental processes.

**tachyphylaxis** (tak-ī-fi-lak′sis) [ tachy- + G. *phylaxis,* protection ]. Rapid appearance of progressive decrease in response following repetitive administration of a pharmacologically or physiologically active substance.

**tachypnea** (tak-ip-ne′ah) [ tachy- + G. *pnoē (pnoiē),* breathing ]. Very rapid breathing; polypnea.

**tachypsychia** (tak-ī-si′kī-ah) [ tachy- + G. *psychē,* mind ]. Abnormally rapid action of psychological processes.

**tachyrhythmia** (tak-ī-rith′mī-ah) [ tachy- + G. *rhythmos,* rhythm ]. Tachycardia.

**tachysterol** (tă-kis′ter-ōl). A sterol formed upon ultraviolet irradiation of ergosterol or lumisterol.

**tachysystole** (tak-ī-sis′to-le) [ tachy- + G. *systolē,* contracting ]. Tachycardia.

**tachyzoite** (tak-ī-zo′īt) [ tachy- + G. *zōon,* animal ]. A rapidly multiplying stage of *Toxoplasma gondii* found in acute infections of toxoplasmosis.

**tac′rine.** ROMOTAL; 9-amino-1,2,3,4-tetrahydroacridine; anticholinesterase agent.

**tactile** (tak′til) [ L. *tactilis,* fr. *tango,* pp. *tactus,* to touch ]. Relating to touch or to the sense of touch.

**taction** (tak′shun) [ L. *tactio,* fr. *tango,* see prec. ]. 1. The sense of touch. 2. The act of touching.

**tactom′eter** [ L. *tactus,* touch, + G. *metron,* measure ]. Esthesiometer.

**tactor** [ L. one who or that which touches ]. A tactile end organ.

**tac′tual.** Relating to or caused by touch.

**tac′tus** [ L. ] [ NA ]. Touch; the sense of touch.

    **t. erudi′tus,** t. expertus; the trained sense of touch in a diagnostician or obstetrician.

    **t. exper′tus,** t. eruditus.

**taenia** (te′nī-ah) [ L. fr. G. *tainia,* band, tape, a tapeworm. TEN- ]. 1. A coiled, bandlike anatomical structure; see tenia (1). 2. Tapeworm; see *Taenia.*

**Taenia** (te′nī-ah) [ see taenia ]. A genus of cestodes that formerly included most of the tapeworms, but is now restricted to those species infecting carnivores with cysticercus found in tissues of various herbivores, rodents, and other animals of prey; see also tapeworm.

    **T. africa′na,** a tapeworm found in native Africans, the cysticercus of which is unknown.

    **T. arma′ta,** *T. solium.*

    **T. confu′sa,** a rare tapeworm, the cysticercus of which is unknown.

    **T. crassic′ollis,** *T. taeniformis.*

    **T. cucurbiti′na,** *T. solium.*

**T. demerarien'sis,** *Davainea madagascariensis.*

**T. denta'ta,** *T. solium.*

**T. diminu'ta,** *Hymenolepis nana.*

**T. equi'na,** *Anoplocephala perfoliata.*

**T. hom'inis,** unusual form of *T. saginata.*

**T. hydatig'ena,** a tapeworm of dogs, cats, wolves, foxes, and other carnivores; the larva is known as *Cysticercus tenuicollis* (*q.v.*), and the adult is the largest tapeworm of dogs.

**T. iner'mis,** *T. saginata.*

**T. lata,** *Diphyllobothrium latum.*

**T. lophoso'ma,** an abnormal form of *T. saginata.*

**T. madagascarien'sis,** *Davainea madagascariensis.*

**T. mediocanella'ta,** *T. saginata.*

**T. min'ima,** *Hymenolepis nana.*

**T. pellu'cida,** *T. solium.*

**T. philippi'na,** atypical form of *T. saginata.*

**T. pisifor'mis,** a common tapeworm of dogs, foxes, and other carnivores; the larval form is *Cysticercus pisiformis;* adult worms were formerly called *T. serrata.*

**T. sagina'ta,** beef tapeworm of man, acquired by eating insufficiently cooked flesh of cattle infected with *Cysticercus bovis.*

**T. so'lium,** pork tapeworm of man, acquired by eating insufficiently cooked pork infected with *Cysticercus cellulosae.* Hatching of ova within the human intestine may result in establishment of cysticerci in human tissues, resulting in cysticercosis.

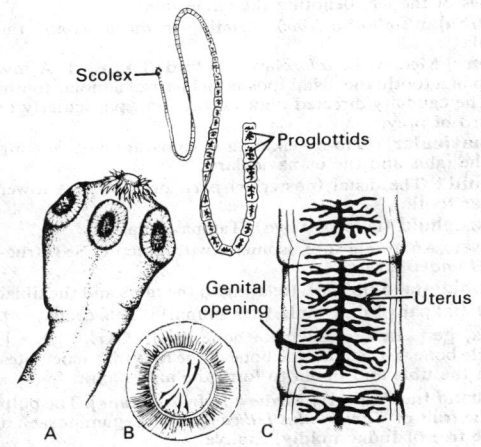

**Taenia solium,** the pork tapeworm

A, enlarged scolex (×18); B, egg (×375); C, enlarged proglottid (×1.5).

**T. taeniaefor'mis,** *Hydatigera taeniaeformis; T. crassicollis;* one of the common tapeworms of household cats; the larval form is called *Cysticercus fasciolaris.*

**Taeniarhynchus** (te'nĭ-ă-ring'kus) [ G. *tainia*, band, + *rhynchos*, snout ]. A genus established for the *Taenia* species having a rudimentary rostellum but lacking the rostellar hooklets typical of *Taenia.* The best known example is *Taeniarhynchus saginatus*, but the older name, *Taenia saginata*, is more commonly used.

**taeniid** (te-ni'id). Common name for a member of the family Taeniidae.

**Taeniidae** (te-ni'ĭ-de). A family of parasitic cestodes (order Cyclophyllidea) that includes the genera *Taenia, Taeniarhynchus, Multiceps,* and *Echinococcus.*

**Taeniorhynchus** (te-nĭ-o-ring'kus) [ G. *tainia*, band, + *rhynchos*, snout ]. A genus and subgenus of mosquitoes now considered synonymous with *Mansonia.*

**Taenzer** (ten'zer), Paul R., German dermatologist, 1858–1919. See T.'s *stain,* Unna-T. *stain.*

**tag.** 1. Label; tracer; to incorporate into a compound an element or other substance that is more readily detected,

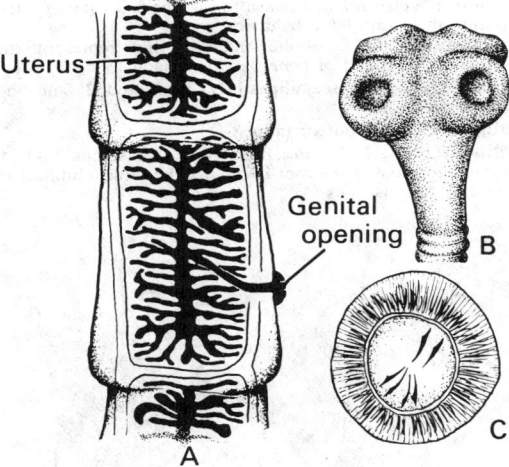

**Taenia saginata,** the beef tapeworm

A, proglottid or body segment showing reproductive organs (×1.7); B, scolex (×12); C, egg (×550).

such as a heavy or radioactive isotope, whereby the compound can be detected and its metabolic or chemical history followed; see also tagged. 2. A small outgrowth or polyp.

    **anal skin t.,** a fibrous polyp of the anus, probably resulting from thrombosis and organization of a hemorrhoid.

    **sentinel t.,** projecting edematous skin at the lower end of an anal fissure.

    **skin t.,** acrochordon; fibroma molluscum (2); soft wart; senile fibroma; fibroepithelial papilloma; an outgrowth of both epidermal and dermal fibrovascular tissue.

**tag'atose.** A ketohexose isomeric with fructose. For structure, see sugars.

**tagged** (tagd). Labeled; indicating a compound in which a radioactive isotope or other substance readily detected has been incorporated; the metabolism of the tagged material can thus be followed.

**Tagliacozzi** (tal-yah-cot'se), Gaspara, Italian surgeon, 1546–1599. See Tagliacotian *operation.*

**tail** (tāl) [ A.S. *taegl* ]. Cauda.

    **t. of caudate nucleus,** *cauda* nuclei caudati.

    **t. of dentate gyrus,** uncus *band* of Giacomini.

    **t. of epididymis,** *cauda* epididymidis.

**tail'gut.** Postanal gut.

**Tait,** Robert L., English gynecologist, 1845–1899. See T.'s *knot, law, operation.*

**Takahara,** Shigeo, Japanese physician. See T.'s *disease.*

**Takayama** (tah-kah-yah'mah), Masao, Japanese physician, \*1871. See T.'s *solution.*

**Takayashu** (alternative spellings: Takayasu, Takayoshu), Michishige, Japanese physician, \*1872. See T.'s *disease, syndrome.*

**take.** A successful grafting operation or vaccination.

**talalgia** (tă-lal'jĭ-ah) [ L. *talus*, heel, + G. *algos*, pain ]. Plernalgia; pain in the heel.

**ta'lar.** Relating to the talus.

**tal'butal** (NF). LOTUSATE; 5-allyl-5-*sec*-butylbarbituric acid; short-acting hypnotic and sedative.

**talc** (tălk) [ Ar. *talq* ]. (USP, BP). Talcum; soapstone, steatite, French chalk; purified t.; native hydrous magnesium silicate, sometimes containing small proportions of aluminum silicate. Purified by boiling powdered t. with hydrochloric acid in water. Used in pharmacy as a filter aid, as a dusting powder, and in cosmetic preparations.

**talcosis** (tal-ko'sis). Pulmonary disorder related to silicosis, occurring in workers in the talc industry exposed to talc mixed with silicates; characterized by restrictive or obstructive disorders of breathing or the two in combination.

**talcum** (tal'kum) [ L. ]. Talc.

**tal'ion** [ Welsh *tal,* compensation ]. The principle of retribution in intrapsychic behavior.

**t. dread,** the symbolic anxieties that represent the unconscious dread of penalties for an act.

**taliped** (tal'ĭ-ped) [ see talipes ]. 1. Clubfooted. 2. One who has a clubfoot.

**taliped'ic.** Clubfooted; taliped (1).

**talipes** (tal'ĭ-pēz) [ L. *talus,* heel, ankle, + *pes,* foot. TAL- ]. Any deformity of the foot involving the talus; clubfoot in general; see also pes (4).

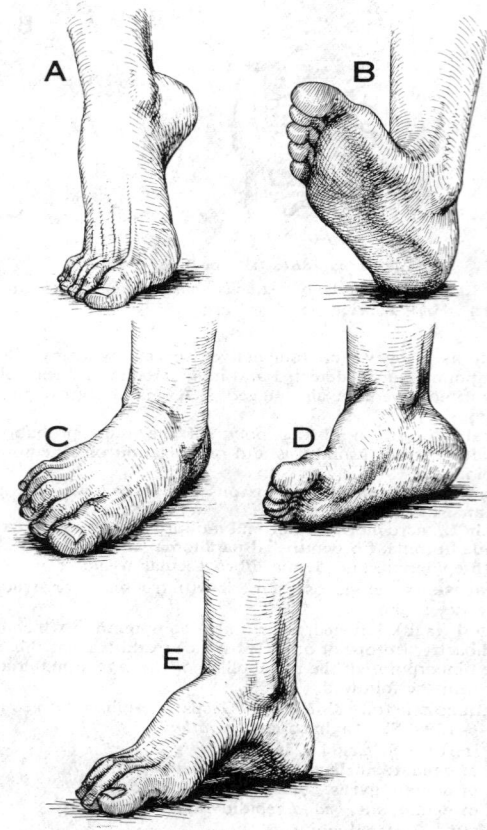

**Talipes**
*A,* equinus; *B,* calcaneus; *C,* valgus; *D,* varus; *E,* cavus.

**t. arcua'tus,** t. cavus.

**t. calca'neoval'gus,** t. calcaneus and t. valgus combined; the clubfoot is dorsiflexed, everted, and abducted.

**t. calca'neova'rus,** t. calcaneus and t. varus combined; the clubfoot is dorsiflexed, inverted, and adducted.

**t. calca'neus,** permanent dorsal flexion of the foot, so that the weight of the body rests on the heel only.

**t. cavus,** hollow foot; cross foot; t. arcuatus; t. plantaris; pes cavus; an exaggeration of the normal arch of the foot.

**t. equi'noval'gus,** pes equinovalgus; t. equinus and t. valgus combined; the clubfoot is plantarflexed, everted, and abducted.

**t. equi'nova'rus,** pes equinovarus; t. equinus and t. varus combined; the clubfoot is plantarflexed, inverted, and adducted.

**t. equi'nus,** tip foot; permanent extension of the foot so that only the ball rests on the ground; it is commonly combined with t. varus.

**t. planta'ris,** t. cavus.

**t. pla'nus,** flatfoot; splayfoot; platypodia; pes planus; a condition in which the arch of the foot is broken down, the entire sole touching the ground.

**t. spasmod'icus,** a temporary distortion of the foot, usually t. equinus, due to muscular spasm.

**t. transver'sopla'nus,** *metatarsus* latus.

**t. valgus,** pes pronatus, valgus, or abductus; permanent eversion of the foot, the inner side alone of the sole resting on the ground; it is usually combined with a breaking down of the plantar arch.

**t. va'rus,** pes adductus; pes varus; inversion of the foot, the outer side of the sole only touching the ground; there is usually more or less t. equinus associated with it, and often t. cavus.

**talipomanus** (tal'ĭ-pom'ă-nus, -po-ma'nus) [ Mod. L. *talipes* + L. *manus,* hand ]. Clubhand; a fixed deformity of the hand, either congenital or acquired. The spatial relationship of the hand to the forearm determines the names of the conditions. See subentries under manus.

**Tallerman,** Lewis A., English inventor, 19th century. See T. *apparatus.*

**tallow** (tal'o). Adeps ovillus; the rendered fat from mutton suet.

**Tallqvist** (tahl'kvist), Theodor W., Finnish physician, 1871–1927. See T.'s hemoglobin *scale.*

**Talma,** Sape, Dutch physician, 1847–1918. See T.'s *disease, operation.*

**talo-** (ta'lo-) [ L. *talus,* ankle, ankle bone. TAL- ]. Combining form for talus (ankle or ankle bone).

**talocalcaneal, talocalcanean** (ta-lo-kal-ka'ne-al, ta-lo-kal-ka'ne-an). Relating to the talus and the calcaneus.

**talocrural** (ta-lo-kru'ral). Relating to the talus and the bones of the leg; denoting the ankle joint.

**talofibular** (ta-lo-fib'u-lar). Relating to the talus and the fibula.

**tal'on** [ Mediev. L. *talo,* claw of a bird. TAL- ]. 1. A low cusp of a tooth; the distal (posterior) part of a molar tooth. 2. The caudally directed digit on the foot, particularly of a bird of prey.

**talonavicular** (ta-lo-nă-vik'u-lar). Taloscaphoid; relating to the talus and the os naviculare.

**tal'onid.** The distal (posterior) part, or heel, of a lower molar tooth.

**taloscaphoid** (ta-lo-skaf'oyd). Talonavicular.

**tal'ose.** An aldohexose, isomeric with glucose. See structures under sugars.

**talotibial** (ta'lo-tib'ĭ-al). Relating to the talus and the tibia.

**talpa** (tal'pah) [ L. a mole (the animal) ]. Sebaceous *cyst.*

**ta'lus,** gen. **ta'li** [ L. ankle bone, heel. TAL- ] [ NA ]. Ankle bone; astragalus; the bone of the foot that articulates with the tibia and fibula to form the ankle joint.

**tamarind** (tam'ă-rind) [ Mediev. L. fr. Ar. *tamr* ]. The pulp of the fruit of *Tamarindus indica* (family Leguminosae), a large tree of India; mildly laxative.

**tambour** (tahm-boor') [ Fr. drum ]. The recording part of a graphic apparatus, such as a sphygmograph, consisting of a membrane stretched across the open end of a cylinder and the recording stile attached to it.

**tam'picin.** A resin from *Ipomoea simulans* (family Convolvulaceae), Tampico jalap. Laxative in small doses, purgative in large ones.

**tam'pon** [ O. Fr. ]. 1. A cylinder or ball of cotton-wool, gauze, or other loose substance; used as a plug in a canal or cavity to restrain hemorrhage, absorb secretions, or maintain a displaced organ, such as the uterus, in position. 2. To insert a tampon; to plug a canal with gauze, cotton-wool, or other substance.

**Corner's t.,** a plug of omentum stuffed into a wound of the stomach or intestine as a temporary t.

**tamponade, tamponage** (tam-pŏ-nād', tam'pŏ-nij). The insertion of a tampon.

**cardiac t.,** compression of the heart resulting from accumulation of fluid within the pericardial sac.

**tam'poning, tampon'ment.** The act of inserting a tampon.

**tanace'tol.** Thujone.

**tanace'tone.** Thujone.

**tangentiality** (tan-jen'shī-al'ĭ-tī) [ L. *tangeno,* to touch, take away ]. A disturbance in the associative thought processes in which the patient is unable to express his idea;

in contrast to circumstantiality (*q.v.*), the digression in t. is such that the central idea is not communicated. T. is observed in schizophrenia and certain types of organic brain disorders.

**tang'hinin.** $C_{32}H_{46}O_{10}$; a glycoside found in the seed of *Tanghinia venenifera* (family Apocynaceae), an ordeal tree of Madagascar, and related species.

**tan'nase** (EC 3.1.1.20). Tannin acyl-hydrolase; an enzyme produced in cultures of *Penicillium glaucum* and found in certain tannin-forming plants; it hydrolyzes digallate to gallate, also acts on ester links in other tannins.

**tan'nate.** A salt of tannic acid.

**tan'nic.** Relating to tan (tan-bark) or to tannin.

   **t. acid** (BP), tannin (*q.v.*) ; $C_{76}H_{52}O_{46}$; occurs in many plants, particularly in the bark of oaks and other members of the *Fagaceae;* used as a styptic and astringent, and in the treatment of diarrhea. Available also as tannic acid glycerite (NF).

**tan'nin.** Tannic acid; one of a group of complex, nonuniform plant constituents that can be classified into hydrolyzable t.'s (esters of a sugar, usually glucose, and one or several trihydroxybenzenecarboxylic acids) and condensed t.'s (derivatives of flavonols). T.'s are used in tanning, dyeing, photography, and as clarifying agents for beer and wine; for medicinal uses see tannic acid.

**tan'noform.** HELGOTAN; methyleneditannin; astringent.

**Tanret** (tahn-ra'), Charles, French physician, 1847–1917. See T.'s *reagent.*

**Tansini** (tahn-se'ne), Iginio, Italian surgeon, 1855–1943. See T.'s *operation.*

**tan'talum** [ mythical king *Tantalus* ]. A heavy metal of the vanadium group, atomic no. 73, atomic weight 180.95. It is used surgically; since it does not corrode, it can be introduced into the tissues for the repair of various defects, *e.g.*, as a plate in the skull bone, or as a wire mesh to fill in layer defects in the abdominal wall.

**tan'trum.** Temper tantrum; a fit of bad temper, especially in children.

**tanypho'nia** [ G. *tanyō,* to stretch, + *phonē,* sound ]. A thin, weak voice resulting from tension of vocal muscles.

**tap.** 1. To withdraw fluid from a cavity by means of a trocar and cannula or a hollow needle. 2. To strike lightly with the finger or a hammer-like instrument in percussion or to elicit a tendon reflex. 3. A light blow. 4. An East Indian fever of undetermined nature.

   **heel t.,** pertaining to a reflex movement of the toes when the heel is tapped, present in multiple sclerosis and other diseases of the pyramidal tract.

   **mitral t.,** the palpable equivalent of the opening snap of the mitral valve.

   **spinal t.,** lumbar *puncture.*

**tape** (tāp). A long, thin and flat strip of fascia or tendon, or of synthetic material, used as a tie or suture.

   **adhesive t.,** fabric or film evenly coated on one side with a pressure-sensitive adhesive mixture.

**tapeino-.** For words beginning thus, see tapino-.

**tapetochoroidal** (tă-pe'to-ko-roy'dal). Relating to the tapetum and the choroid.

**tape'toret'inal.** 26 Relating to the tapetum and retina.

**tape'toretinop'athy** [ tapetum + retinopathy ]. Hereditary degeneration of the retina and pigmentary epithelium and of the retinal neurepithelium; seen in pigmentary retinopathy, choroideremia gyrate atrophy, congenital nyctalopia, congenital amaurosis, and heredomacular degeneration.

**tapetum,** pl. **tapeta** (tă-pe'tum, -tah) [ L. *tapēte,* a carpet ]. 1. In general, any membranous layer or covering. 2. In neuroanatomy, a thin sheet of fibers in the lateral wall of the temporal horn of the lateral ventricle, continuous with the fasciculus subcallosus, and largely composed of fibers passing from the temporal cortex to the caudate nucleus; also known as membrana versicolor; Fielding's membrane. 3. A dense layer in the choroidea of the eye of many mammalian species, including cat and dog, but not man; it forms a discrete or diffuse area of reflective cells, rodlets, and fibers; its strong light-reflecting properties cause the familiar light-glow of such eyes in the dark.

   **t. alve'oli,** periodontium.

   **t. cellulo'sum,** a layer of polygonal cells in the choroid coat of the eye in carnivores, believed responsible for the light reflection as seen in the cat's eyes in the dark; ultramicroscopic rodlets may be present.

   **t. fibro'sum,** a layer of wavy connective tissue fibers in the choroid of ungulates, giving a metallic hue to the eye and reflecting light in the dark.

   **t. lu'cidum** [ NAV ], collective term for the cellular and fibrous tapeta of the choroid, with any accompanying rodlets or crystals; see also t. (3).

   **t. ni'grum,** *stratum* pigmenti retinae.

   **t. oc'uli,** *stratum* pigmenti retinae.

**tape'worm.** An intestinal parasitic worm, adults of which are found in the intestine of vertebrates; the term is commonly restricted to members of the class Cestoda, subclass Eucestoda. T.'s consist of a scolex, variously equipped with spined or sucking structures by which the worm is attached to the intestinal wall of the host, and strobila having several to many proglottids, but they lack a digestive tract at any stage of development. The ovum, entering the intestine of an appropriate intermediate host, hatches and the hexacanth penetrates the gut wall and develops into a specific larval form (*e.g.*, cysticercoid, cysticercus, hydatid, strobilocercus), which develops into an adult when the intermediate host is ingested by the proper final host. A three-host cycle with a swimming coracidium, procercoid and plerocercoid (sparganium) larva, and adult intestinal worm is found in aquatic life cycles, as in *Diphyllobothrium latum* and other pseudophyllid cestodes.

   **armed t.,** *Taenia solium.*

   **beef t.,** *Taenia saginata.*

   **broad t.,** *Diphyllobothrium latum.*

   **broad fish t.,** *Diphyllobothrium latum.*

   **dwarf t., dwarf mouse t.,** *Hymenolepis nana.*

   **fringed t. of sheep,** *Thysanosoma actinoides.*

   **hookless t.,** *Taenia saginata.*

   **hy'datid t.,** *Echinococcus granulosus.*

   **pork t.,** *Taenia solium.*

   **solitary t.,** *Taenia solium.*

   **unarmed t.,** *Taenia saginata.*

**taphophilia** (taf'o-fil'ĭ-ah) [ G. *taphos,* grave, + *phileō,* to love ]. Morbid attraction for graves.

**taphophobia** (taf'o-fo'bĭ-ah) [ G. *taphos,* the grave, + *phobos,* fear ]. A morbid fear of being buried alive.

**Tapia,** Antonio, Spanish otolaryngologist, 1875–1950. See T.'s *syndrome.*

**tapinocephalic** (tă-pi'no-sē-fal'ik). Having a low flat head; relating to tapinocephaly.

**tapinocephaly** (tă-pi-no-sef'ă-lĭ) [ G. *tapeinos,* low, + *kephalē,* head ]. A condition of flat head in which the skull has a vertical index below 72; similar to chamecephaly.

**tapioca** (tap'ĭ-o'kah) [ Braz. *tipioca* ]. Cassava starch; amylum manihot; a starch from the root of *Janipha manihot* and other species of *J.* (family Euphorbiaceae), plants of tropical America; an easily digested starch, free of irritant properties.

**ta'piroid** [ tapir + G. *eidos,* resemblance ]. Resembling a tapir's snout; a term sometimes applied to an elongated cervix uteri.

**tapotage** (tă-pū-tazh'). A loose cough excited in certain pulmonary diseases by strong percussion in the supraclavicular space.

**tapotement** (tă-put-mon') [ Fr. fr. *tapoter,* to tap ]. Tapping (1); a massage movement consisting in striking with the side of the hand, usually with partly flexed fingers.

**tap'ping.** 1. Tapotement. 2. Paracentesis.

**tar.** A thick, semisolid, blackish brown mass, of complex composition, obtained by the destructive distillation of the wood of various species of pine, juniper, and other trees, and of bituminous coal. For individual t.'s, see specific names.

   **rectified t. oil,** a volatile oil distilled from pine t.; used externally in the treatment of various scaly skin diseases.

**Taractogenos** (tăr'ak-toj'ē-nos) [ G. *taraktēs,* a disturber (of the stomach), + suffix -*gen,* producing ]. A genus of trees (family Bixaceae) from a species of which, *T. kurzii,* chaulmoogra oil is obtained.

**tar′antism.** [ fr. It. city, Taranto, where people were afflicted with a dancing mania attributed to the bite of a tarantula ]. A nervous affliction marked by stupor, melancholia, and uncontrolled dancing mania.

**tarantula** (tă-ran′tu-lah) [ tarantism (*q. v.*) ]. A very large, hairy spider, considered highly venomous and often greatly feared, but usually the bite is no more harmful than a bee sting, and the creature is relatively inoffensive.

**American t.,** *Eurypelma hentzii*, the Arkansas t.; although greatly feared, its bite is relatively uncommon and harmless to man.

**black t.,** *Sericopelma communis*, a large black t. of Panama and the Canal Zone, whose bite is poisonous although the effect is localized.

**European t.,** *Lycosa tarentula*, the large European wolf spider or true t. Its bite was once believed to cause madness, which inspired frenzied contortions and dancing to rid the body of the venom, though the bite is, in fact, harmless, as is that of most of the large, hairy "tarantula spiders" of the tropics.

**taraxacum** (tă-rak′să-kum). Dandelion; lion's tooth; the dried rhizome and root of *Taraxacum officinale* (family Compositae), a wild plant of wide distribution throughout the temperate regions of the northern hemisphere; tonic and hepatic stimulant.

**taraxein** (tă-rak′se-in). A copper-containing protein obtained from the serum of some schizophrenics; it allegedly produces psychotic symptoms when injected into normal people.

**Tardieu** (tar-de-ë′), Auguste A., French physician, 1818–1879. See T.'s *ecchymoses*.

**tardive** (tar′div). Late; tardy.

**tare.** In commerce, an allowance made for the weight of a box or other vessel containing the goods; hence, in chemistry, a weight used to counterbalance the vessel holding the substance being weighed.

**tar′entism.** Tarantism.

**tar′get** [ It. *targhetta*, a small shield ]. 1. An object of fixation. 2. In the ophthalmometer, the mire. 3. Target *organ*.

**tarichatoxin** (tăr′ĭ-kă-tok′sin). A potent neurotoxin found in the newt *Taricha torosa* and other closely related newts. It is identical with tetrodotoxin.

**Tarin** (tăran′), Pierre, French anatomist, 1725–1761. See T.'s *fascia, foramen, fossa, space, tenia, valve, valvula semilunaris tarini, velum* tarini.

**tariric acid** (tă-ri′rik). An 18-carbon acid, notable for the presence of a triple bond; $CH_3(CH_2)_{10}C{\equiv}C(CH_2)_4COOH$.

**Tarlov,** Isadore Max, U. S. surgeon, *1905. See T.'s *cyst*.

**Tarnier** (tar-ne-a′), Etienne S., French obstetrician, 1828–1897. See T.'s *forceps*.

**tar′ragon oil.** Estragon oil; a volatile oil distilled from the leaves of *Artemisia dranculus* (family Compositae); a flavoring.

**tars-.** See tarso-.

**tarsadenitis** (tar′sad-ĕ-ni′tis) [ tarsus + G. *adēn*, gland, + suffix -*itis*, inflammation ]. Inflammation of the tarsal borders of the eyelids and of the Meibomian glands.

**tar′sal.** Relating to a tarsus in any sense.

**tarsale,** pl. **tarsa′lia** (tar-sa′le) [ Mod. L. fr. G. *tarsos*, sole of the foot ]. Any tarsal bone.

**tarsal′gia** [ tarsus + G. *algos*, pain ]. Podalgia.

**tarsa′lis.** See under musculus.

**tarsec′tomy** [ tarsus + G. *ektomē*, excision ]. Excision of the tarsus of the foot or of a segment of the tarsus of an eyelid.

**tarsecto′pia, tarsec′topy** [ tarsus + G. *ektopos*, out of place ]. Subluxation of one or more tarsal bones.

**tarsen** [ tarsus + G. *en*, in ]. Within the tarsus; relating to the tarsus independent of other structures.

**tarsi′tis.** 1. Inflammation of the tarsus of the foot. 2. Inflammation of the tarsal border of an eyelid.

**tarso-, tars-** [ Mod. L. *tarsus, q.v.* TAR- ]. Combining forms relating to a tarsus.

**tarsochiloplasty** (tar-so-ki′lo-plas-tĭ) [ tarso- + G. *cheilos*, lip, + *plassō*, to form ]. Marginal blepharoplasty.

**tarsoclasia, tarsoclasis** (tar′so-kla′zĭ-ah, tar-sok′lă-sis) [ tarso- + G. *klasis*, a breaking ]. Instrumental fracture of the tarsus, for the correction of clubfoot.

**tarsomalacia** (tar′so-mă-la′shĭ-ah) [ tarso- + G. *malakia*, softness ]. Softening of the tarsal cartilages of the eyelids.

**tarsomegaly** (tar′so-meg′ă-lĭ) [ tarso- + G. *megas*, large ]. Dysplasia epiphysialis hemimelia; a congenital maldevelopment and overgrowth of a tarsal or carpal bone.

**tarsomet′atar′sal.** Relating to the tarsal and metatarsal bones; denoting the articulations between the two sets of bones, and the ligaments in relation thereto.

**tarsomet′atar′sus.** The lowermost long bone or shank in the leg of a bird; the distal tarsal elements fuse with the metatarsals, resulting in a compound bone unlike that in mammals.

**tar′so-or′bital.** Relating to the eyelids and the orbit.

**tarsophalangeal** (tar-so-fă-lan′je-al). Relating to the tarsus and the phalanges.

**tarsophyma** (tar-so-fi′mah) [ tarso- + G. *phyma*, a tumor, boil ]. Any tarsal growth or tumor.

**tarsopla′sia, tar′soplasty.** Blepharoplasty.

**tarsopto′sia** [ tarso- + G. *ptōsis*, a falling ]. Obsolete term for talipes planus.

**tarsorrhaphy** (tar-sor′ă-fĭ) [ tarso- + G. *rhaphē*, suture ]. Blepharorrhaphy; the suturing together of the eyelid margins, partially or completely, to shorten the palpebral fissure or to protect the cornea in case of chronic ulcer or paralysis of the orbicularis muscle.

**tarsotar′sal.** Mediotarsal.

**tarsotib′ial.** Relating to the tarsal bones and the tibia; tibiotarsal; talotibial.

**tarsotomy** (tar-sot′o-mĭ) [ tarso- + G. *tomē*, incision ]. 1. Incision of the tarsal cartilage of an eyelid. 2. Any operation on the tarsus of the foot.

**tar′sus,** gen. and pl. **tar′si** [ G. *tarsos*, a flat surface, sole of the foot, edge of eyelid. TAR- ] [ NA ]. 1. The root of the foot, or instep; as a division of the skeleton, the seven bones of the instep, *viz.*, talus, calcaneus, navicular, three cuneiform (wedge) bones, and the cuboid. 2. The fibrous plates giving solidity and form to the edges of the eyelids; they are often erroneously called tarsal or ciliary cartilages.

**t. infe′rior** [ NA ], the fibrous plate in the lower eyelid.

**t. supe′rior** [ NA ], the fibrous plate in the upper eyelid.

**tar′tar** [ Mediev. L. *tartarum*, ult. etym. unknown ]. 1. A crust on the interior of wine casks, consisting essentially of potassium bitartrate. 2. A white, brown, or yellow-brown deposit at or below the gingival margin of teeth, chiefly hydroxyapatite in an organic matrix.

**cream of t.,** postassium bitartrate.

**t. emet′ic,** antimony potassium tartrate.

**soluble t.,** potassium tartrate.

**tartar′ic acid** (NF, BP). Dihydroxysuccinic acid; HOOC—CHOH—CHOH—COOH; made from crude tartar; laxative and refrigerant; used in the manufacture of various effervescing powders, tablets, and granules.

***p*-tartaric acid.** Racemic acid; an isomer of tartaric acid and occurring with the latter in some grapes.

**tar′trate.** A salt of tartaric acid.

**acid t.,** bitartrate; a salt of tartaric acid which contains an acid group still capable of combining with a base.

**normal t.,** one that contains no uncombined acid groups.

**tar′trated.** Combined with or containing tartar or tartaric acid.

**tar′trazine.** A yellow acid dye, $C_{16}H_9N_4O_9S_2Na_3$, used as a stain in histology and pathology.

**taste** [ It. *tastare*; L. *tango*, to touch ]. 1. To perceive through the medium of the gustatory nerves. 2. The sensation produced by a suitable stimulus applied to the gustatory nerve endings in the tongue.

**after-t.,** see aftertaste.

**color t.,** pseudogeusesthesia; a form of synesthesia in which the color sense and t. are associated, stimulation of either inducing a subjective sensation on the part of the other as well.

**franklin′ic t.,** voltaic t.; a metallic or sour t. produced by the application of static electricity to the tongue.

**volta′ic t.,** franklinic t.

**tattoo** (tă-too') [ Tahiti, *tatu* ]. 1. A tinctorial and pictorial effect of deliberate (and occasionally accidental) implanting or injecting of indelible pigments into the skin. 2. To produce such an effect.

**Tatum** (ta'tem), Edward L., U. S. biochemist, *1909. Nobel laureate, 1958, with George W. Beadle and Joshua Lederberg for his discovery that genes act by regulating definite chemical events.

**taurine** (taw'rin, -rēn). A crystallizable substance, $NH_2CH_2CH_2SO_3H$, formed by the decomposition of taurocholic acid.

**taurocholate** (taw-ro-ko'lāt). A salt of taurocholic acid.

**taurocholic acid** (taw-ro-ko'lik). Cholaic acid; cholytaurine; a compound of cholic acid and taurine, involving the —COOH group of the former and the $NH_2$— of the latter.

**tau'rocy'amine.** *N*-Amidinotaurine; $NH_2C(=NH)$-$NHCH_2SO_3H$; a glycocyamine analogue, with taurine replacing glycine, having the function of glycocyamine in some annelids.

**taurodontism** (taw'ro-don'tizm) [ L. *taurus*, bull, + G. *odous*, tooth ]. A condition in which the bodies of molar teeth are elongated.

**Taussig,** Helen B., American pediatrician, *1898. See Blalock-T. *operation*, T.-Bing *disease, syndrome.*

**tautomenial** (taw-to-me'nī-al) [ G. *tautos*, the same, + *mēn*, month ]. Relating to the same menstrual period.

**tautomeric** (taw-to-mer'ik) [ G. *tautos*, the same, + *meros*, part ]. 1. Relating to the same part; denoting certain nerve fibers of the spinal cord that do not extend beyond the limits of the spinal cord segment in which they originate. 2. Relating to or marked by tautomerism.

**tautomerism** (taw-tom'er-izm) [ G. *tautos*, the same, + *meros*, part ]. A phenomenon in which a chemical compound exists in two forms of different structure (isomers), in equilibrium, the two forms differing, usually, in the position of a hydrogen atom, as in keto-enol tautomerism,

$$R—CH_2—C(O)—R' \rightleftarrows R—CH=C(OH)—R',$$

or lactam-lactim or amino-imino tautomerism.

**Tawara** (tah-wah'rah), K. Sunao, Japanese physician, *1873. See T.'s *node*, His-T. *system.*

**taxa** (tak'sah). Plural of taxon.

**taxis** (tak'sis) [ G. orderly arrangement. TAX- ]. 1. Reduction of a hernia or of a dislocation of any part by means of manipulation. 2. Systematic classification or orderly arrangement. 3. The reaction of protoplasm to a stimulus, by virtue of which animals and plants are led to move or act in certain definite ways in relation to their environment; the various kinds of t. are designated by prefixing a word denoting the stimulus governing them; see chemotaxis, electrotaxis, thermotaxis.
　**bipolar t.,** the reposition of a retroverted uterus by making traction on the cervix in the vagina, and pushing up the fundus by the finger in the rectum.
　**negative t.,** the repulsion of protoplasm away from a stimulus.
　**positive t.,** the attraction of protoplasm toward a stimulus.

**taxology** (tak-sol'o-jī) [ G. *taxis*, arrangement, + *logos*, study ]. Taxonomy.

**tax'on,** pl. **tax'a.** A level of grouping in a systematic classification of natural objects (*i.e.*, genus, species). See also taxonomy.

**taxonom'ic.** Relating to taxonomy.

**taxonomy** (tak-son'o-mī) [ G. *taxis*, orderly arrangement, + *nomos*, law ]. Taxology, the classification of various plants and animals. The plant and animal kingdoms are divided into the following subdivisions in descending order: Phyla, Classes, Orders, Families, Genera (sing. Genus), Species, and Varieties.

**Tax'us** [ L. fr. G. *taxos*, the yew tree ]. A genus of coniferous trees, the yews (family Taxaceae); the leaves, seeds, and bark of several species contain alkaloids, taxines, a glycoside, taxicatin, and ephedrine.

**Tay,** Warren, English physician, 1843–1927. See T.'s *choroiditis, disease*, T.-Sachs *disease*, T.'s *cherry red spot.*

**Taybi,** H. See Rubinstein-T. *syndrome.*

**Taylor,** Charles F., New York orthopaedic surgeon, 1827–1899. See T.'s *apparatus, splint.*

**Taylor,** Robert W., U. S. dermatologist, 1842–1908. See T.'s *disease.*

**Tb.** Chemical symbol of the element terbium.

**tb.** Abbreviation for tuberculosis and tubercle bacillus.

**TBG.** Abbreviation for thyroxine-binding *globulin.*

**TBP.** Abbreviation for thyroxine-binding *protein.*

**Tc.** Chemical symbol of the element technetium.

**TDP.** Abbreviation for ribothymidine 5'-diphosphate. The thymidine analogue is dTDP.

**t.d.s.** Abbreviation of L. *ter die sumendum*, to be taken three times a day; see also t.i.d.

**Te.** 1. Abbreviation in electrodiagnosis denoting tetanic contraction. 2. Chemical symbol of the element tellurium.

**tea** (tē) [ of Chinese derivation ]. 1. The dried leaves of various genera of the family Theaceae, including *Thea* (*T. senensis*), *Camellia*, and *Gordonia*. There are 16 genera with approximately 175 species. The shrub is indigenous to China, southern and southeastern Asia, and Japan. Its chief constituent, upon which its stimulating action largely depends, is the alkaloid theine (caffeine), which is present in amount of 1 to 4 per cent. 2. The infusion made by pouring boiling water upon tea leaves. 3. Any infusion or decoction made extemporaneously; see also species (2).
　**black t.,** thea nigra; prepared by allowing the leaves to wilt and ferment before drying.
　**green t.,** thea viridis; prepared by drying the leaves rapidly immediately after picking, without allowing them to wilt and ferment.
　**Hottentot t.,** buchu.
　**Jesuit t.,** chenopodium.
　**Mexican t.,** chenopodium.
　**Paraguay t.,** maté.

**TEAE-cellulose.** See under cellulose.

**teak** (tēk). The tree *Tectona grandis* (family Verbenaceae), of eastern and southern Asia, furnishing a timber wood. The leaves are astringent and the flowers are diuretic.

**Teale,** Thomas P., English surgeon, 1801–1868. See T.'s *amputation.*

**tear** (tēr) [ A.S. *teár* ]. A drop of the fluid secreted by the lacrimal glands by means of which the conjunctiva is kept moist.
　**crocodile t.'s,** see crocodile t.'s *syndrome.*

**tear** (tār). Laceration; a discontinuity in substance of a structure.
　**bucket-handle t.,** a t. in the central part of a semilunar cartilage; also called (rarely) bucket-handle fracture.

**tease** (tēz) [ A. S. *taesan* ]. To separate the structural parts of a tissue by means of a needle, in order to prepare it for microscopic examination.

**tea'spoon.** A small spoon, holding about 1 dram (or about 4 ml.) of liquid; used as a measure in the dosage of fluid medicines.

**teat** (tēt) [ A.S. *tit* ]. 1. *Papilla* mammae. 2. Breast; mamma. 3. Papilla.

**teb'utate.** USAN-approved contraction for tertiary butylacetate, $(CH_3)_3C—CH_2—CO_2^-$.

**technetium** (tek-ne'shī-um) [ G. *technetos*, artificial ]. A radioactive element, symbol Tc, atomic no. 43; half-life of its most stable known isotope (technetium-99) is 215,000 years; artificially produced in 1937 by bombardment of molybdenum by deutrons. Does not exist in nature.

**technetium-99.** $^{99}Tc$; a radioisotope of technetium which is the decay product of technetium-99m and has a weak beta emission and a physical half-life of $2.1 \times 10^5$ years.

**technetium-99m.** $^{99m}Tc$; a radioisotope of technetium which decays by isomeric transition emitting an essentially monoenergetic gamma ray of 140 Kev with a physical half-life of 6 hours. It is usually obtained from a radionuclide generator of molybdenum-99 and is used to prepare radiopharmaceuticals for scanning the brain, parotid, thyroid, lungs, blood pool, liver, spleen, kidney, lacrimal drainage apparatus, and bone marrow.

**technic** (tek-nēk'). Technique.

**tech'nical.** 1. Relating to technique. 2. Pertaining to some particular art, science, or trade. 3. Used in connection with a chemical substance, it indicates that the substance contains appreciable quantities of impurities.

**technician** (tek-nish'un) [ G. *technē,* an art ]. Technologist.

**technique** (tek-nēk') [ Fr. from G. *technikos,* relating to *technē,* art, skill ]. Technic; the manner of performance, or the details, of any surgical operation, experiment, or mechanical act.

    **airbrasive t.,** a method of grinding or cutting tooth structure, now little used, by means of a device utilizing a gas-impelled jet of fine $Al_2O_3$ particles which, after striking the tooth, are removed by a powerful aspirator.

    **atrial-well t.,** a closed surgical t. for repairing atrial septal defects.

    **Barcroft-Warburg t.,** see Warburg *apparatus.*

    **Begg light wire differential force t.,** see light wire *appliance.*

    **Coutard's t.,** the giving of a heavy dose (6 to 8 erythema doses), utilizing 190 kilovolts, 2 mm. of zinc filter, 5 milliamperes of current, and a target skin distance of 50 cm., the application being divided into ten equal sittings.

    **direct t.,** see direct *method.*

    **flicker fusion frequency t.,** flicker *perimetry.*

    **fluorescent antibody t.,** antiserums are conjugated with a fluor to obtain a solution of fluor-labeled proteins and antibodies. When allowed to react with antigen in tissue, antibody is precipitated where antigen is located and these sites may then be located with the fluorescence microscope.

    **flush t.,** a t. for determining the systolic blood pressure in infants; the elevated limb is "milked" of blood from the hand or foot proximally; the blood pressure cuff is then inflated above the likely systolic pressure and the limb lowered; the cuff pressure is then gradually released until the blanched limb flushes.

    **Hampton t.,** atraumatic, nonpalpation, fluoroscopic examination of the upper gastrointestinal tract in peptic ulcer disease with acute hemorrhage.

    **Hartel t.,** a method of reaching the Gasserian ganglion by passing the needle from the mouth, inserting it about the level of the upper midmolar tooth, and passing it inward until the point reaches the bone in front and to the outer side of the foramen ovale, enabling an alcohol injection to be made for the relief of trigeminal neuralgia.

    **implant t.,** implant *denture.*

    **indirect t.,** indirect *method* for making inlays.

    **Kristeller t.,** expression of the child by force applied to the fundus uteri through the abdominal wall, the fingers of the two hands being behind and the thumbs in front, and the force being exerted during a uterine contraction.

    **long cone t.,** the use of a cone distance of 14 inches or more in making oral roentgenographs.

    **McGoon's t.,** plastic reconstruction of the incompetent mitral valve, when the cause of the incompetence is rupture of chordae to the posterior leaflet, by plication of the leaflet.

    **Merendino's t.,** plastic reconstruction of the incompetent mitral valve using heavy silk sutures to narrow the anulus in the region of the medial commissure.

    **Mohs' chemosurgery t.,** excision of superficial cancers after fixation *in vivo* with an escharotic such as zinc chloride.

    **opsonic t.,** the sum of the manipulations used in relation to opsonic therapy: preparation of bacterial vaccines, determination of the opsonic index, injection of vaccines, etc.

    **Papanicolaou vaginal smear t.,** see cytologic *examination.*

    **rebreathing t.,** a method of producing hypoxia by rebreathing air with carbon dioxide replacing oxygen in the breathing mixture.

    **sealed jar t.,** a t. for producing suspended animation in small experimental animals, consisting of sealing the animal in a jar which is then refrigerated.

    **supersonic vibration t.,** an oscillatory method used for the fragmentation of bacteria and spermatozoa preparatory to study of their antigenic composition.

    **washed field t.,** the cutting of cavity preparations in teeth utilizing a constant irrigant which is immediately removed from the mouth by means of a vacuum device.

    **Weir's t.,** sterilization of the hands by scrubbing for 5 minutes with green soap, friction with calx chlorinata for

5 minutes, and washing off with carbonate of soda and running water.

**technocausis** (tek-no-kaw'sis) [ G. *technē,* art, + *kausis,* a burning ]. Actual *cautery.*

**technol'ogist.** Technician; one trained in and using the techniques of a profession, art, or science.

**technology** (tek-nol'o-jī) [ G. *technē,* an art, + *logos,* study ]. The knowledge and use of the techniques of a profession, art, or science.

**teclothi'azide.** Tetrachlormethiazide.

**tec'tal.** Relating to a tectum.

**tec'tiform.** Roof-shaped.

**tectocephalic** (tek'to-sē-fal'ik). [ L. *tectum,* roof, + G. *kephalē,* head ]. Scaphocephalic.

**tectocephaly** (tek'to-sef'ă-lī). Scaphocephalism.

**tectology** (tek-tol'o-jī) [ G. *tektōn,* builder, + -*logia* ]. Structural morphology.

**tecton'ic** [ G. *tektonikos,* relating to building ]. Relating to plastic surgery or to the restoration of lost parts by grafting.

**tectorial** (tek-to'rī-al). 1. Relating to a tectorium. 2. Forming a roof or cover.

**tectorium** (tek-to'rī-um) [ L. a covering, fr. *tego,* pp. *tectus,* to cover ]. 1. Any rooflike structure. 2. *Membrana* tectoria ductus cochlearis.

**tectospi'nal.** Indicating nerve fibers that pass from the tectum down to the spinal cord.

**tectum,** pl. **tecta** (tek'tum, tek'tah) [ L. roof, fr. *tego,* pp. *tectus,* to cover ] [ NA ]. Tectorium; tegmen; any covering or roofing structure.

    **t. mesenceph'ali** [ NA ], *lamina* tecti mesencephali.

**teel oil.** Sesame oil.

**teeth.** Dentes; plural of tooth. For table of teeth, see under tooth.

**teeth'ing.** Odontiasis; the eruption or "cutting" of the teeth, especially of the dens decidua.

**Teflon.** A proprietary synthetic fabric used for surgical implantation.

**tef'lurane** (USAN). TERFLURANE; 2-bromo-1,1,1,2-tetrafluoroethane; nonexplosive and nonflammable inhalation anesthetic of moderate potency.

**teg'men,** gen. **teg'minis,** pl. **teg'mina** [ L. a cover, roof, fr. *tego,* to cover ] [ NA ]. A structure that covers or roofs over a part.

    **t. cru'ris,** old term for *tegmentum* mesencephali.

    **t. mastoid'eum,** the lamina of bone roofing over the mastoid cells.

    **t. tym'pani** [ NA ], roof of the middle ear, formed by the thinned anterior surface of the petrous portion of the temporal bone.

    **t. ventric'uli quar'ti** [ NA ], roof of the fourth ventricle, formed in its upper part by the superior, or anterior, medullary velum stretching between the two brachia conjunctiva, in its lower part by the inferior medullary velum composed of the choroid membrane choroid plexus of the fourth ventricle.

**tegmen'tal.** 1. Relating to any tegmentum or covering. 2. Superior; placed or oriented toward the tegmen or cover.

**tegmentotomy** (teg-men-tot'o-mī) [ tegmentum + G. *tome,* incision ]. Production of lesions in the reticular formation of the midbrain tegmentum.

**tegmen'tum,** pl. **tegmen'ta** [ L. cover, fr. *tego,* to cover ] [ NA ]. 1. A covering structure. 2. The t. mesencephali.

    **t. mesenceph'ali,** tegmentum (2); mesencephalic or midbrain t.; that major part of the substance of the mesencephalon or midbrain that lies between the lamina tecti mesencephali (lamina quadrigemina) dorsally and the pedunculus cerebri (basis pedunculi) ventrally.

    **mesencephalic t.,** t. mesencephali.

    **midbrain t.,** t. mesencephali.

    **t. of pons,** *pars* dorsalis pontis; see also t. rhombencephali.

    **t. rhombenceph'ali** [ NA ], t. of the rhombencephalon; the portion of the pons and medulla oblongata continuous with the tegmentum of the mesencephalon; it consists of reticular formation, tracts, and cranial nerve nuclei, and forms the dorsal part of the pons (pars dorsalis pontis) as well as that part of the medulla oblongata that lies dorsal to the pyramids.

**t. of rhombencephalon,** t. rhombencephali.

**tegument** (teg'u-ment) [ L. *tegumentum,* a collat. form of *tegmentum* ]. Integument.

**tegumen'tal.** Relating to the integument.

**tegumen'tary.** Tegumental.

**Teichmann** (tikh'mahn), Ludwig, German histologist, 1823–1895. See T.'s *crystals.*

**teichoic acids** (ti-ko'ik). One of two classes (the other being the muramic acids or mucopeptides) of polymers constituting the cell walls of Gram-positive bacteria (the teichoic acids are also found intracellularly), linear polymers of a polyol (ribitol or glycerol phosphate) carrying D-alanine residues esterified to OH groups and glycosidically linked sugars. Many variants are known.

**teichopsia** (ti-kop'sī-ah) [ G. *teichos,* wall, + *opsis,* vision ]. A transient visual sensation of bright shimmering colors; such as the fortification spectrum associated with a scintillating scotoma.

**tel-, tele-, telo-** [ G. *tēle,* distant, *telos,* end ]. Combining forms denoting distance, end, or other end.

**te'la,** gen. and pl. **te'lae** [ L. a web ] [ NA ]. 1. Any thin weblike structure. 2. A tissue; especially one of delicate formation.

**choroid t. of fourth ventricle,** t. choroidea ventriculi quarti.

**choroid t. of third ventricle,** t. choroidea ventriculi tertii.

**t. choroid'ea,** that portion of the pia mater which covers the ependymal roof or, in the case of the lateral ventricle, medial wall of a cerebral ventricle.

**t. choroid'ea inferior,** t. choroidea ventriculi quarti.

**t. choroid'ea superior,** t. choroidea ventriculi tertii.

**t. choroid'ea ventric'uli quar'ti** [ NA ], choroid t. of the fourth ventricle; t. choroidea inferior; the sheet of pia mater covering the lower part of the ependymal roof of the fourth ventricle.

**t. choroid'ea ventric'uli ter'tii** [ NA ], choroid t. of the third ventricle; t. choroidea superior; velum interpositum or triangulare; diatela; a double fold of pia mater, enclosing subarachnoid traveculae, between the fornix above and the epithelial roof of the third ventricle and the thalami below; at each lateral margin is a vascular fringe projecting into the fissura choroidea of the lateral ventricle; on its undersurface are several small vascular projections filling the folds of the ependymal roof of the third ventricle.

**t. conjuncti'va,** connective *tissue.*

**t. elas'tica,** elastic *tissue.*

**t. subcuta'nea** [ NA ], superficial fascia; subcutis; stratum subcutaneum; hypoderm; hypodermis; a loose fibrous envelope beneath the skin, containing more or less fat in its meshes (panniculus adiposus) or fasciculi of muscular tissue (panniculus carnosus); it contains the cutaneous vessels and nerves and is in relation by its undersurface with the deep fascia.

**t. submuco'sa** [ NA ], tunica submucosa; the layer of connective tissue beneath the tunica mucosa.

**t. submuco'sa pharyn'gis** *fascia* pharyngobasilaris.

**t. subsero'sa** [ NA ], the layer of connective tissue beneath a serous membrane.

**t. vasculo'sa,** *plexus* choroideus.

**Te'ladorsa'gia davtian'i.** One of the medium stomach worms (family Trichostrongylidae) of sheep, goats, and deer occurring in the abomasum; it is similar to *Ostertagia trifurcata.*

**telalgia** (tel-al'jī-ah) [ G. *tēle,* distant, + *algos,* pain ]. Referred *pain.*

**telangiectasia** (tel-an'jī-ek-ta'zī-ah) [ G. *telos,* end, + *angeion,* vessel, + *ektasis,* a stretching out. TEN- ]. Dilation of the previously existing small or terminal vessels of a part.

**cephalo-oculocutaneous t.,** an angioma involving the skin of the face, orbit, meninges, and brain; see also Sturge-Weber *syndrome.*

**essential t.,** (1) localized capillary dilation of undetermined origin; may be due to trauma; (2) *angioma* serpiginosum.

**hered'itary hemorrhag'ic t.,** Osler's disease; Rendu-Osler-Weber disease or syndrome; a familial disease appearing after puberty, marked by telangiectases and

aneurysmal venules developing slowly on the face and body and in the gastrointestinal tract. Severe anemia may be caused by repeated hemorrhages.

**t. lymphat'ica,** lymphangiectasia.

**t. macula'ris erupti'va per'stans,** a diseminated eruption of telangiectases associated with erythematous and edematous macules.

**spider t.,** arterial *spider.*

**t. verruco'sa,** angiokeratoma.

**telangiectasis,** pl. **telangiectases** (tel-an'jī-ek'tă-sis, -sēz). Telangiectasia.

**telangiectat'ic.** Relating to or marked by telangiectasia.

**telangiectodes** (tel-an-jī-ek-to'dēz) [ telangiectasis + suffix *-odes,* fr. G. *eidos,* resemblance ]. A term used to qualify highly vascular tumors.

**telangioma** (tel-an'jī-o-mah). Angioma due to dilation of the capillaries or terminal arterioles.

**telangion** (tel-an'jī-on) [ G. *telos,* end, + *angeion,* vessel ]. Trichangion; one of the terminal arterioles or a capillary vessel.

**telangiosis** (tel-an'jī-o'sis). Any disease of the capillaries and terminal arterioles.

**tele-.** See tel-.

**telecanthus** (tel'e-kan'thus) [ G. *tēle,* distant, + *kanthos,* canthus ]. Canthal hypertelorism; increased breadth between the medial canthi of the eyelids.

**telecar'diogram.** Telelectrocardiogram.

**telecar'diophone** [ G. *tēle,* distant, + *kardia,* heart, + *phōnē,* sound ]. A specially constructed stethoscope by means of which heart sounds can be heard by listeners at a distance from the patient.

**telecobalt** (tel'e-ko'bawlt). Radioactive cobalt for use at a long distance from the region being treated.

**tel'ediagno'sis.** The detection of a disease by evaluation of data transmitted to a receiving station. The process normally involves patient-monitoring instruments and a transfer link to a diagnostic center at some distance from the patient, such as an airplane or spacecraft to ground link or an intensive care unit to a central monitoring station.

**telediastol'ic** [ G. *telos,* end, + *diastolē,* dilation ]. Pertaining to or occurring toward the cardiac diastole.

**telelectrocardiogram** (tel'e-lek'tro-kar'dī-o-gram) [ G. *tēle,* distant, + electrocardiogram ]. Telecardiogram; an electrocardiogram recorded at a distance from the subject being tested. Examples include the electrocardiogram obtained through telemetry or as with a galvanometer in the laboratory being connected by a wire with the patient in another room.

**telem'eter** [ G. *tēle,* distant, + *metron,* measure ]. An electronic instrument that senses and measures a quantity, then transmits radio signals to a distant station for recording and interpretation.

**telem'etry.** The science of measuring a quantity, transmitting the results to a distant station, and there interpreting, indicating, and/or recording the results; see also biotelemetry.

**cardiac t.,** the transmission of electrocardiographic signals to a receiving location where the electrocardiogram is displayed for monitoring.

**telemnemonike** (tel-e-ne-mon'ī-ke) [ G. *tēle,* distant, + *mnēmonikos,* relating to memory ]. Acquiring consciousness of matters held in the memory of another person.

**telencephalic** (tel'en-sē-fal'ik). Relating to the telencephalon or endbrain.

**telenceph'aliza'tion.** Corticalization.

**telencephalon** (tel'en-sef'ă-lon) [ G. *telos,* end, + *enkephalos,* brain ] [ NA ]. Endbrain; the anterior division of the prosencephalon corresponding to the cerebral hemispheres. Together with the diencephalon it composes the prosencephalon or forebrain.

**teleology** (tel'e-ol'o-jī) [ G. *telos,* end, + *logos,* study ]. The philosophical doctrine according to which events, especially in biology, are explained in part by reference to final causes or end goals, as, for example, in vitalism.

**teleomitosis** (tel'e-o-mi-to'sis) [ G. *teleos,* complete, + mitosis, *q. v.* ]. A completed mitosis.

**tel'eonomic.** 1. Pertaining to teleonomy. 2. In psychology, pertaining to those patterns of behavior which are a function of an inferred purpose or motive; *e.g.*, a child's behavior pattern may be classified by an observer teleonomically as attention-getting.

**teleonomy** (tel'e-on-o-mī) [ G. *telos*, end, + *nomos*, law ]. The doctrine that life is characterized by endowment with a project or purpose; *i.e.*, the existence in an organism of a structure or function implies that it has had evolutionary survival value.

**teleopsia** (tel'e-op'sī-ah) [ G. *tēle*, distant, + *opsis*, vision ]. A perceptual disturbance in which close objects appear far away.

**teleorgan'ic** [ G. *teleos*, complete, + *organikos*, organic ]. Vital; manifesting life.

**tel'eost** [ G. *teleos*, complete, perfect, + *osteon*, bone ]. One of the bony or true fishes.

**telepathine.** Harmine.

**telep'athy** [ G. *tēle*, distant, + *pathos*, feeling ]. Extrasensory thought transference; mind-reading; see also extrasensory *perception*.

**teleradiog'raphy** [ G. *tēle*, distant, + radiography ]. Roentgenography with the tube held about 2 meters (6½ ft.) from the body, thereby securing practical parallelism of the rays.

**teleradium** (tel'e-ra'dī-um). See teleradium *therapy*.

**telerecep'tor.** An organ, such as the eye, that can receive sense stimuli from a distance.

**telergy** (tel'ur-jī) [ G. *tēle*, far off, + *ergon*, work ]. Automatism.

**teleroentgenogram** (tel-e-rĕnt'gen-o-gram). The picture obtained by teleroentgenography.

**teleroentgenography** (tel'e-rĕnt-gen-og'rā-fī). Teleradiography.

**teleroentgentherapy** (tel'e-rĕnt'gen-thĕr'ā-pī). X-ray therapy administered at a distance from the body; teletherapy (3).

**tele'sis** [ G. *telos*, end, + suffix *-sis*, condition ]. A goal to be attained by planned conduct.

**telesystolic** (tel'e-sis-tol'ik) [ G. *telos*, end, + *systolē*, a contracting ]. Relating to the end of cardiac systole.

**teletac'tor** [ G. *telos*, end, + L. *tactus*, touch ]. An instrument to transmit sound waves to the skin.

**telether'apy** [ G. *tēle*, distant, + *therapeia*, treatment ]. Treatment with radiations from a distance.

**TeLinde,** Richard W., U. S. gynecologist, *1894. See T. *operation*.

**tel'lurate.** A salt of telluric acid.

**tellu'ric** [ L. *tellus* (*tellur*-), the earth ]. 1. Relating to or originating in the earth. 2. Relating to the element tellurium.

**tellurism** (tel'u-rizm) [ L. *tellus* (*tellur*-), the earth ]. The alleged influence of soil emanations in producing disease.

**tellurium** (tel-u'rī-um) [ L. *tellus* (*tellur*-), the earth ]. A rare semimetallic element, symbol Te, atomic no. 52, atomic weight 127.61, belonging to the sulfur group; in its pure state it is a lustrous white, brittle substance.

**teloden'dron** [ G. *telos*, end, + *dendron*, tree ]. End-brush; the terminal arborization of an axon.

**tel'ogen** [ G. *telos*, end, + suffix *-gen*, producing ]. Resting phase of hair cycle.

**teloglia** (tĕ-log'lī-ah) [ G. *telos*, end, + *glia*, glue ]. The accumulation of neurolemmal cells at the myoneural junction.

**telognosis** (tel'og-no'sis) [ G. *tēle*, distant, + *gnosis*, a knowing ]. Diagnosis by means of roentgenograms or other diagnostic tests transmitted by telephone or radio; see also telediagnosis.

**telokinesia** (tel'o-kī-ne'zī-ah) [ G. *telos*, end, + *kinēsis*, movement ]. Telophase.

**telolecithal** (tel-o-les'ī-thal) [ G. *telos*, end, + G. *lekithos*, yolk ]. Denoting an ovum in which a considerable amount of deutoplasm accumulates at one pole, as in the eggs of birds and reptiles.

**tel'omere** [ G. *telos*, end, + *meros*, part ]. The distal extremity of a chromosome arm.

**telopep'tide.** A peptide covalently bound in or on a protein, protruding therefrom and therefore subject to enzyme

attack and maturation modifiction or cross-linking, and conferring immunogenic specificity.

**telophase** (tel'o-fāz) [ G. *telos*, end, + *phasis*, appearance ]. The final stage of mitosis or meiosis beginning when migration of chromosomes to the poles of the cell is complete. The chromosomes progressively lose their state of condensation and lengthen while the nuclear membranes of the two daughter nuclei are reconstructed and the cytoplasm becomes divided at the equator by formation of cell membrane to complete the separation of the two daughter cells.

**telophragma** (tel-o-frag'mah) [ G. *telos*, end, + *phragma*, fence, screen ]. Z *line*.

**Telosporidia** (tel'o-spo-rid'ī-ah) [ G. *telos*, end, + *sporos*, seed ]. A class of Sporozoa in which the reproductive spore-producing phase follows the trophic phase and is distinct from it. Sexual and asexual reproduction are found; flagellated microgametes are found in some groups. Includes the gregarines and coccidia; the latter includes the Haemosporidia, which in turn includes the malarias of man.

**telosynapsis** (tel'o-sī-nap'sis) [ G. *telos*, end, + *synapsis*, a connection, junction ]. An obsolete term referring to the supposed union of chromosomes end to end during synapsis.

**tel'otism** [ G. *telos*, end ]. The perfect performance of a function, as that of sight or hearing.

**tel'son** [ G. limit ]. The terminal point of a crustacean, such as the sting of a scorpion.

**TEM.** Abbreviation for triethylene melamine.

**tem'per.** 1. Mood; disposition; temperament; in general, any characteristic or particular state of mind. 2. A display of irritation or anger; see tantrum. 3. To treat metal by application of heat, as in annealing or quenching (see both).

    **epileptic t.,** sudden and unreasonable outburst of temper in an epileptic subject, classed by some as an epileptic equivalent (*q. v.*, under equivalent).

**temperament** (tem'per-ā-ment) [ L. *temperamentum*, proper measure, moderation, disposition. TEMP- ]. The psychophysical organization peculiar to the individual, including his character or personality predispositions, which influence his manner of thought and action, and general views of life.

    **atrabil'ious t.,** melancholic t.

    **bilious t.,** one marked by more or less general pigmentation, high blood pressure, slow pulse, well developed muscle, strong appetites, tenacity of purpose, and a choleric temper.

    **choleric t.,** bilious t.

    **melancholic t.,** one marked by emaciation, irritability, and a pessimistic outlook on the world.

    **nervous t.,** one in which the subject overly mentally and physically alert, with rapid pulse, excitability, often volubility, but not always fixity of purpose.

    **san'guine t., sanguin'eous t.,** one the subject of which has a fresh complexion, light hair and eyes, a full pulse, good digestion, and a quick but not lasting temper.

**tem'perance** [ L. *temperantia*, moderation ]. 1. Moderation in eating, drinking, exercise, and all things else. 2. In a special and restricted sense, abstinence from the use of alcoholic beverages.

**tem'perate.** Moderate; restrained in the indulgence of any of the appetites, in thought, or in action.

**temperature** (tem'per-ā-chur) [ L. *temperatura*, due measure, temperature, fr. *tempero*, to proportion duly. TEMP- ]. The sensible intensity of heat of any substance; the measure of the average kinetic energy of the molecules making up a substance. See also entries under scale.

    **absolute t.,** t. reckoned in Celsius degrees from the absolute zero.

    **t. coefficient,** see under coefficient.

    **critical t.,** the t. of a gas above which it is no longer possible by use of any pressure, however great, to reduce it to liquid form.

    **effective t.,** a comfort index or scale which takes into account the t. of air, its moisture content, and movement.

    **equivalent t.,** of a thermally nonuniform enclosure is defined as the t. of a thermally uniform enclosure in which, under still air conditions, a "sizable" black body loses heat at the same rate as in the nonuniform environment.

**eutectic t.,** the t. at which a eutectic mixture becomes fluid (melts).

**fusion t. (wire method),** the recorded t. at which a 20-gauge metal wire will collapse under a 3-ounce load; the recorded t. at which porcelain becomes glazed.

**maximum t.,** in bacteriology, denoting a t. above which growth will not take place.

**mean t.,** the average atmospheric t. in any locality for a designated period of time, as a month or a year.

**mean radiant t.,** represents the sum of all positive and negative radiations.

**melting t.,** t. midpoint.

**t. midpoint,** symbol $T_m$; melting t.; the midpoint in the change in optical properties (absorbance, rotation) of a structured polymer (e.g., DNA) with increasing t.

**minimum t.,** in bacteriology, denoting a t. below which growth will not take place.

**optimum t.,** the t. at which any operation, such as the culture of any special microorganism, is best carried on.

**room t.,** the ordinary t. (65° to 80°F.) of the atmosphere in the laboratory; a culture kept at room t. is one kept in the laboratory, not in an incubator.

**sensible t.,** the atmospheric t. as felt by the individual, supposed to be that recorded by the wet bulb thermometer.

**standard t.,** a t. of 0°C. or 273° absolute.

**tem'plate.** 1. A pattern or guide that determines the shape of a substance. Used metaphorically to indicate the specifying nature of a nucleic acid or polynucleotide with respect to the primary structure of the nucleic acid or polynucleotide or protein made from it *in vivo* or *in vitro*. 2. In dentistry, a curved or flat plate utilized as an aid in setting teeth. 3. A pattern or guide that determines the specificity of antibody globulins.

**t. RNA,** see under *ribonucleic* acid.

**surgical t.,** (1) a thin, transparent, resin base shaped to duplicate the form of the impression surface of an immediate denture, used as a guide for surgically shaping the alveolar process to fit an immediate denture; (2) a guide for various osteotomy procedures.

**temple** (tem'pl) [ L. *tempus* (*tempor-*), time, the temple. TEMP- ]. 1. The area of the temporal fossa on the side of the head above the zygomatic arch. 2. The part of a spectacle frame passing from the rim backward over the ear.

**tempolabile** (tem'po-la'bil) [ L. *tempus*, time, + *labilis*, perishable ]. Undergoing spontaneous change or destruction during the passage of time.

**tempora** (tem'po-rah) [ L. pl. of *tempus* ] [ NA ]. The temples.

**tem'poral** [ L. *temporalis*, fr. *tempus* (*tempor-*), time, temple ]. 1. Relating to time; limited in time; temporary. 2. Relating to the temple.

**tempora'lis** [ L. ]. See under musculus.

**tem'poro-** [ L. *temporalis*, temporal. TEMP- ]. Combining form meaning temporal.

**temporoauricular** (tem'po-ro-aw-rik'u-lar). Relating to the temporal region and the auricle.

**temporohyoid** (tem'po-ro-hi'oyd). Relating to the temporal and the hyoid bones or regions.

**temporoma'lar.** Temporozygomatic.

**tem'poromandib'ular.** Relating to the temporal bone and the mandible; denoting the articulation of the lower jaw.

**tem'poromax'illary.** 1. Relating to the regions of the temporal and maxillary bones. 2. Temporomandibular.

**temporo-occipital** (tem'po-ro-ok-sip'ĭ-tal). Relating to the temporal and the occipital bones or regions.

**temporoparietal** (tem'po-ro-pă-ri'e-tal). Relating to the temporal and the parietal bones or regions.

**temporopon'tine.** Referring to the relationship of the temporal lobe of the cerebral cortex with the pars ventralis pontis.

**temporosphenoid** (tem'po-ro-sfe'noyd). Relating to the temporal and sphenoid bones.

**temporozygomatic** (tem'po-ro-zi'go-mat'ik). Relating to the temporal and zygomatic bones or regions.

**tempostabile, tempostable** (tem'po-sta'bil, tem-po-sta'bl) [ L. *tempus*, time + *stabilis*, stable ]. Not subject to spontaneous alteration or destruction.

**temps utile** [ Fr. service or utilization time ]. Utilization time.

**tem'pus,** gen. **tem'poris,** pl. **tem'pora** [ L. See TEMP- ]. 1 [ NA ]. The temple. 2. Time.

**tem'ulence** [ L. *temulentia* ]. Drunkenness.

**TEN.** Abbreviation for toxic epidermal *necrolysis*.

**tenacious** (tĕ-na'shus) [ L. *tenax* (*tenac-*), fr. *teneo*, to hold ]. Sticky; glutinous; viscid; not easily diverted.

**tenacity** (tĕ-nas'ĭ-tĭ) [ L. *tenacitas*, fr. *teneo*, to hold ]. Adhesiveness; the character of holding fast.

**cellular t.,** the inherent property of all cells to persist in a given form or direction of activity.

**tenaculum,** pl. **tenacula** (tĕ-nak'u-lum, -lah) [ L. a holder, fr. *teneo*, to hold ]. 1. A sharp-pointed wire hook set in a handle: used for picking up the divided end of an artery, or bits of tissue during an operation. 2. A fibrous band that holds a part in position.

**tenacula ten'dinum,** *vincula* tendinum.

**tenalgia** (tĕ-nal'jĭ-ah) [ G. *tenōn*, tendon, + *algos*, pain ]. Tenontodynia; tenodynia; pain referred to a tendon.

**t. crep'itans,** *tenosynovitis* crepitans.

**ten'der** [ L. *tener*, soft, delicate ]. Sensitive; painful on pressure or contact.

**ten'derness.** The condition of being tender; painfulness to pressure or contact.

**pencil t.,** strictly localized t., elicited by pressure with the rubber tip of a pencil, *e.g.*, in cases of incomplete or subperiosteal fracture.

**rebound t.,** t. felt when pressure, particularly abdominal pressure, is suddenly released.

**tendini'tis.** Tenontitis.

**ten'dinoplas'ty** [ Mediev. L. *tendo* (*tendin-*), tendon, + G. *plassō*, to form ]. Tenontoplasty.

**ten'dinosu'ture.** Tenorrhaphy.

**ten'dinous.** Relating to, composed of, or resembling a tendon.

**tendo-** [ L. *tendo*, tendon. TEN- ]. Combining form meaning tendon; see also teno-.

**tendo,** gen. **tendinis,** pl. **tendines** (ten'do, -dĭ-nis, -dĭ-nēz) [ Mediev. L. fr. L. *tendo*, to stretch out, extend. TEN- ] [ NA ]. Tendon; a fibrous cord or band of variable length that connects a muscle with its bony attachment; it may unite with the muscle at its extremity or may run along the side or in the center of the muscle for a longer or shorter distance, receiving the muscular fibers along its lateral border. For histological description, see tendon.

**t. achil'lis** [ NA ], official alternative term for calcaneus.

**t. calca'neus** [ NA ], calcanean tendon; t. achillis; chorda magna; the tendon of insertion of the triceps surae (gastrocnemius and soleus) into the tuberosity of the calcaneus.

**t. calca'neus commu'nis** [ NAV ], see hamstring (2).

**t. conjuncti'vus** [ NA ], official alternate term for *falx* inguinalis.

**t. cricoesophage'us** [ NA ], cricoesophageal tendon; suspensory ligament of the esophagus; Gillette's suspensory ligament; longitudinal fiber of the esophagus that attaches to the posterior aspect of the cricoid cartilage of the larynx.

**t. oc'uli,** *ligamentum* palpebrale mediale.

**t. palpebra'rum,** *ligamentum* palpebrale mediale.

**tendolysis** (ten-dol'ĭ-sis) [ tendo- + G. *lysis*, dissolution ]. Tenolysis; release of a tendon from adhesions.

**tendomucin, tendomucoid** (ten'do-mu'sin, -mu'koyd). A form of mucin in tendon.

**ten'don** [ L. *tendo, q.v.* ]. A fibrous cord or band that connects a muscle to a bone or other structure; it consists of fascicles of very densely arranged, almost parallel collagenous fibers, rows of elongated tendon cells, and a minimal of ground substance. For gross anatomical definition, see tendo.

**Achilles t.,** *tendo* calcaneus.

**bowed t.,** a condition caused by severe strain of the digital flexor tendons, the outer osseus (suspensory ligament), or the accessory ligament (distal cheek ligament) of the horse's limb and characterized by swelling, pain, and lameness; it occurs most frequently in race horses under stress of running.

**calcanean t.,** *tendo* calcaneus.

**central t. of the diaphragm,** *centrum* tendineum.

**central t. of perineum,** *centrum* tendineum perinei.

**conjoined** or **conjoint t.,** *falx* inguinalis.

**contracted t.,** a condition of young horses, probably hereditary in some instances, in which the flexor t.'s of the leg are shortened.

**coronary t.,** *anulus* fibrosus (1).

**Gerlach's annular t.,** *anulus* fibrocartilagineus membranae tympani.

**hamstring t.,** see hamstring.

**heel t.,** *tendo* calcaneus.

**kangaroo t.,** a t. from the tail of the kangaroo-rat or wallaby, fibers of which are used as a ligature material.

**rider's t.,** traumatic state ranging from sprain to a tear of adductor t. of thigh.

**slipped t.,** see perosis.

**subpelvic t.,** a heavy plate of fibrous tissue, found in the ox and dog, which attaches the pelvic symphysis proximally and ends in a convex border distally. Several of the medial muscles of the thigh arise from its lateral surface.

**Todaro's t.,** an inconstant tendinous structure that extends from the right fibrous trigone of the heart toward the valve of the inferior vena cava.

**trefoil t.,** *centrum* tendineum.

**Zinn's t.,** *anulus* tendineus communis.

**tendoni′tis.** Tenontitis.

**tendoph′ony.** Tenophony.

**ten′doplasty.** Tenontoplasty.

**tendosynovitis** (ten′do-sĭ-no-vi′tis). Tenosynovitis.

**ten′dotome.** Tenotome.

**tendot′omy.** Tenotomy.

**tendovaginal** (ten-do-vaj′ĭ-nal) [ tendo- + L. *vagina*, sheath ]. Relating to a tendon and its sheath.

**tendovaginitis** (ten-do-vaj-ĭ-ni′tis) [ tendo- + L. *vagina*, sheath, + G. suffix *-itis*, inflammation ]. Tenosynovitis.

**radial styloid t.,** de Quervain's *disease*.

**tenectomy** (tĕ-nek′to-mĭ) [ G. *tenōn*, tendon, + *ektomē*, excision ]. Tenonectomy; resection of part of a tendon.

**tenesmic** (tĕ-nez′mik). Relating to or marked by tenesmus.

**tenesmus** (tĕ-nez′mus) [ G. *teinesmos*, ineffectual effort to defecate, fr. *teinō*, to stretch ]. A painful spasm of the anal sphincter with an urgent desire to evacuate the bowel or bladder, involuntary straining, and the passage of but little fecal matter or urine.

**Ten Horn's sign.** See under sign.

**tenia,** pl. **teniae** (te′nĭ-ah, te′nĭ-e) [ L. fr. G. *tainia*, band, tape, a tapeworm. TEN- ]. 1 [ NA ]. Any anatomical bandlike structure. 2. A genus of tapeworm; see *Taenia*.

**teniae acus′ticae,** *striae* medullares ventriculi quarti.

**t. choroid′ea** [ NA ], tenia telae [ NA ]; the somewhat thickened line along which a choroid membrane or plexus is attached to the rim of a brain ventricle.

**teniae co′li** [ NA ], bands of the colon; colic teniae; teniae of Valsalva; the three bands in which the longitudinal muscular fibers of the large intestine, except the rectum, are collected; these are called, respectively, t. mesocolica, situated at the place corresponding to the mesenteric attachment; t. libera, free band, opposite the mesocolic band; and t. omentalis, at the place corresponding to the site of adhesion of the greater omentum to the transverse colon.

**colic teniae,** teniae coli.

**t. fim′briae,** t. fornicis.

**t. for′nicis** [ NA ], t. of the fornix; t. fimbriae; the line of attachment of the choroid plexus of the lateral ventricle to the fornix.

**t. of the fornix,** t. fornicis.

**t. of fourth ventricle,** t. ventriculi quarti.

**t. hippocam′pi,** *fimbria* hippocampi.

**t. lib′era** [ NA ], see teniae coli.

**medullary teniae,** *striae* medullares ventriculi quarti.

**t. mesocol′ica,** [ NA ], see teniae coli.

**t. omenta′lis,** [ NA ], see teniae coli.

**t. semicircula′ris,** *stria* terminalis.

**Tarin's t.,** *stria* terminalis.

**t. tec′ta,** rudimentum hippocampi; see *indusium* griseum.

**t. te′lae** [ NA ], t. choroidea [ NA ].

**t. termina′lis,** *crista* terminalis.

**t. thal′ami** [ NA ], t. of the thalamus; thalamic t.; t. ventriculi tertii; the sharp edge or angle between the superior and medial surface of the thalamus on either side; to it is attached the epithelial lamina forming the lining of the roof of the third ventricle.

**thalamic t.,** t. thalami.

**teniae of Valsalva,** teniae coli.

**t. ventric′uli quar′ti** [ NA ], t. of the fourth ventricle; the line of attachment of the choroid roof to the rim of the fourth ventricle.

**t. ventric′uli ter′tii,** t. thalami.

**teniacide** (te′nĭ-ă-sid) [ L. *taenia*, tapeworm, + *caedo*, to kill ]. A remedy destructive to tapeworms.

**teniafuge** (te′nĭ-ă-fūj) [ L. *taenia*, tapeworm, + *fugo*, to put to flight ]. 1. Having the power to expel tapeworms. 2. An agent that causes the expulsion of tapeworms.

**te′nial.** 1. Relating to a tapeworm. 2. Relating to one of the structures called tenia.

**teniasis** (te-ni′ă-sis). The presence of a tapeworm in the intestine.

**somat′ic t.,** invasion of the body by the cysticercus of a tenioid worm.

**ten′icide.** Teniacide.

**ten′iform.** Tenioid.

**tenif′ugal.** Teniafuge (1).

**ten′ifuge.** Teniafuge.

**tenioid** (te′nĭ-oyd) [ G. *tainia*, a tape, + *eidos*, resemblance ]. Teniform. 1. Band-shaped; ribbon-shaped. 2. Resembling a tapeworm.

**teniola** (te-ni′o-lah) [ L. dim. of *taenia*, ribbon ]. A slender tenia or bandlike structure.

**t. cor′poris callo′si,** *lamina* rostralis.

**teno-, tenon-, tenonto-** [ G. *tenōn*, tendon. TEN- ]. Combining forms meaning tendon. See also tendo-.

**tenodesis** (tĕ-nod′e-sis, ten′o-de′sis) [ teno- + G. *desis*, a binding ]. Implantation of a tendon; transferring a tendon to a new point of attachment.

**tenodynia** (ten′o-din′ĭ-ah) [ teno- + G. *odynē*, pain ]. Tenalgia.

**tenofibril** (ten′o-fi′bril) [ teno- + Mod. L. *fibrilla*, a small fiber ]. Tonofibril.

**tenol′ysis.** Tendolysis.

**tenomyoplasty** (ten′o-mi′o-plas-tĭ). Tenontomyoplasty.

**tenomyotomy** (ten′o-mi-ot′o-mĭ). Myotenotomy.

**Tenon,** Jacques R., French anatomist and oculist, 1724–1816. See T.'s *capsule, space.*

**tenon-, tenont-.** See teno-.

**tenonectomy** (ten′o-nek′to-mĭ) [ tenon- + G. *ektomē*, excision ]. Tenectomy.

**tenoni′tis.** 1. Inflammation of Tenon's capsule or the connective tissue within Tenon's space. 2. Tenontitis.

**tenonom′eter.** Tonometer.

**tenontagra** (ten′on-tag′rah) [ tenont- + G. *agra*, a seizure ]. Gouty inflammation of a tendon.

**tenontitis** (ten′on-ti′tis) [ tenont- + G. suffix *-itis*, inflammation ]. Inflammation of a tendon; also called tenonitis; tendinitis; tenositis.

**tenonto-.** See teno-.

**tenontodynia** (tĕ-non′to-din′ĭ-ah). Tenalgia.

**tenontography** (ten′on-tog′ră-fĭ) [ tenonto- + G. *graphē*, description ]. A treatise on or description of the tendons.

**tenontolemmitis** (tĕ-non′to-lem-mi′tis) [ tenonto- + G. *lemma*, husk, + *-itis* ]. Tenosynovitis.

**tenontology** (ten′on-tol′o-jĭ) [ tenonto- + G. *logos*, study ]. The branch of science that has to do with the tendons.

**tenontomyoplasty** (tĕ-non′to-mi′o-plas-tĭ) [ tenonto- + G. *mys*, muscle, + *plassō*, to form ]. Tenomyoplasty; a combined tenontoplasty and myoplasty, used in the radical cure of hernia.

**tenontomyotomy** (tĕ-non′to-mi-ot′o-mĭ). Myotenotomy.

**tenontophyma** (tĕ-non′to-fi′mah) [ tenonto- + G. *phyma*, growth ]. A neoplasm connected with a tendon.

**tenon′toplas′tic.** Relating to tenontoplasty.

**tenontoplasty** (tĕ-non'to-plas'tĭ) [ tenonto- + G. *plassō*, to form ]. Tenoplasty; tendinoplasty; tendoplasty; reparative or plastic surgery of the tendons.

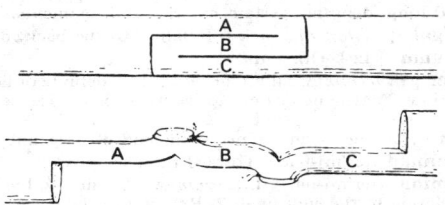

**One Type of Tenontoplasty**

**tenontothecitis** (tĕ-non'to-the-si'tis) [ tenonto- + G. *thēkē*, case, box, + *-itis* ]. Tenosynovitis.

**tenophony** (tĕ-nof'o-nĭ) [ teno- + G. *phōnē*, sound ]. Tendophony; a heart murmur assumed to be due to an abnormal condition of the chordae tendineae; tendophony.

**tenophyte** (ten'o-fīt) [ teno- + G. *phyton*, plant ]. Bony or cartilaginous growth in or on a tendon.

**tenoplas'tic.** Relating to tenoplasty.

**ten'oplasty.** Tenontoplasty.

**ten'orecep'tor.** Receptor in a tendon; it is activated by increased tension.

**tenorrhaphy** (tĕ-nor'ă-fī) [ teno- + G. *raphē*, suture ]. Tendinosuture; tenosuture; suture of the divided ends of a tendon.

**tenosi'tis.** Tenonitis.

**tenostosis** (ten'os-to'sis) [ teno- + G. *osteon*, bone, + suffix *-osis*, condition ]. Ossification of a tendon.

**ten'osuspen'sion.** Using a tendon as a suspensory ligament, sometimes as a free graft or in continuity.

**ten'osu'ture.** Tenorrhaphy.

**tenosynovectomy** (ten'o-sin-o-vek'to-mī) [ teno- + synovia + G. *ektomē*, excision ]. Excision of a tendon sheath.

**tenosynovitis** (ten'o-sin-o-vi'tis) [ teno- + synovia + G. suffix *-itis*, inflammation ]. Inflammation of a tendon and its enveloping sheath; also called tendosynovitis; tendovaginitis; tenontothecitis; tenontolemmitis; vaginal or tendinous synovitis.

**t. crep'itans,** inflammation of a tendon sheath in which movement of the tendon is accompanied by a cracking sound.

**localized nodular t.,** giant cell *tumor* of tendon sheath.

**villonodular pigmented t.,** villous t.

**villous t.,** villonodular pigmented t.; a condition resembling pigmented villonodular synovitis but arising in periarticular soft tissue rather than in joint synovia; occurs most commonly in the hands.

**ten'otomc.** Tendotome; a knife used in tenotomy.

**tenot'omize.** To perform tenotomy upon.

**tenotomy** (tĕ-not'o-mī) [ teno- + G. *tomē*, incision ]. Tendotomy; the surgical division of a tendon for the relief of a deformity caused by congenital or acquired shortening of a muscle, as in clubfoot or squint.

**curb t.,** excision of the tendon of the shortened muscle in squint, and fixation of the same farther back on the aponeurosis of the globe.

**graduated t.,** partial incisions of the tendon of an eye muscle for the relief of a slight degree of strabismus.

**tenovaginitis** (ten'o-vaj-ĭ-ni'tis) [ teno- + L. *vagina*, sheath, + G. suffix *-itis*, inflammation ]. Tenosynovitis.

**tense** [ L. *tensus*, pp. of *tendo*, to stretch. TEN- ]. Tight; rigid; strained; anxious.

**tensiom'eter** [ L. *tensio*, tension, + G. *metron*, measure ]. A device for measuring tension.

**tension** [ L. *tensio*, fr. *tendo*, pp. *tensus*, to stretch. TEN- ]. 1. The act of stretching. 2. The condition of being stretched or tense. 3. The partial pressure of a gas, especially that of a gas dissolved in a liquid such as blood. 4. Mental, emotional, or nervous strain; strained relations or barely controlled hostility between persons or groups.

**arte'rial t.,** the blood pressure within an artery.

**interfacial surface t.,** the t. or resistance to separation possessed by the film of liquid between two well adapted surfaces, *viz.,* the thin film of saliva between the denture base and the tissues.

**intraocular t.,** the resistance of the tunics of the eye to indentation; it can be estimated digitally or by means of a tonometer.

**surface t.,** a condition of intermolecular attraction at the surface of a liquid, in contact with air or another gas, a solid, or another immiscible liquid, tending to pull the molecules inward from the surface. Dimensional formula: $mt^2$.

**tissue t.,** a theoretical condition of equilibrium or balance between the tissues and cells whereby overaction of any part is restrained by the pull of the mass.

**ten'sor,** pl. **tenso'res** [ Mod. L. fr. L. *tendo*, pp. *tensus*, to stretch ] [ NA ]. A muscle the function of which is to render a part firm and tense.

**tent** [ L. *tenta*, a probe, fr. *tento*, to feel, to test. TEN- ]. 1. A protective canopy used in various types of inhalation therapy. 2. A cylinder of some material, usually an absorbent material (such as laminaria, tupelo, compressed sponge, or absorbent cotton), introduced into a canal or sinus to maintain its patency or to dilate it.

**oxygen t.,** a transparent enclosure, suspended over the bed and enclosing the patient, used to supply a high concentration of oxygen.

**sponge t.,** compressed *sponge.*

**tentacle** (ten'tă-kl) [ Mod. L. *tentaculum*, a feeler, fr. *tento*, to feel ]. A slender process for feeling, prehension, or locomotion in invertebrates.

**tentiginous** (ten-tij'ĭ-nus) [ L. *tentigo*, lust ]. Lustful; lascivious.

**tenti'go** [ L. ]. Lust.

**tento'rial.** Relating to a tentorium.

**tentorium,** pl. **tentoria** (ten-to'rĭ-um, -rĭ-ah) [ L. tent, fr. *tendo*, to stretch. TEN- ] [ NA ]. A membranous cover or horizontal partition.

**t. cerebel'li** [ NA ], a strong fold of dura mater roofing over the posterior cranial fossa but for an anterior median opening, the incisura tentorii, through which the midbrain passes; the t. cerebelli is attached along the midline to the falx cerebri and separates the cerebellum from the basal surface of the occipital and temporal lobes of the cerebral cortex.

**t. of hypophysis,** *diaphragma* sellae.

**te'nuis** [ L. tenuous ] [ NA ]. Slender; delicate.

**t. mater,** *pia* mater.

**tephromalacia** (tef'ro-mă-la'shĭ-ah) [ G. *tephros*, ashen-gray, + *malakia*, softness ]. Softening of the gray matter of the brain or spinal cord.

**tephrylometer** (tef'rĭ-lom'e-ter) [ G. *tephros*, ashen, + *hylē*, stuff, + *metron*, measure ]. An instrument for measuring the thickness of the cerebral cortex; it consists of a graduated tube of thin glass which is plunged into the brain substance, the depth of the gray matter being read off on the scale.

**TEPP.** Abbreviation for tetraethylpyrophosphate.

**ter** [ L. ]. Three times; thrice.

**t. in di'e** [ L. *dies*, day ], three times a day; abbreviation, t.i.d.

**tera-** (tĕr'ah-) [ G. *teras*, monster ]. 1. A prefix used in the metric system to signify one trillion ($10^{12}$). 2. A combining form relating to a teras.

**teras,** pl. **terata** (tĕr'as, tĕr'ă-tah) [ G. ]. A monster (*q. v.*); a fetus with deficient, redundant, misplaced or grossly misshapen parts.

**terat'ic.** Relating to a teras.

**teratism** (tĕr'ă-tizm) [ G. *teratisma*, fr. *teras* ]. Teratosis.

**terato-** (tĕr'ă-to-). See tera- (2).

**ter'atoblasto'ma** [ terato- + G. *blastos*, germ, + suffix *-oma*, tumor ]. Teratoma.

**ter'atocarcino'ma.** 1. A malignant teratoma, occurring most commonly in the testis. 2. A malignant epithelial tumor arising in a teratoma.

**teratogen** (tĕr'ă-to-jen) [ terato- + G. suffix -gen, producing ]. A drug or other agent that causes abnormal development.

**teratogenesis** (tĕr'ă-to-jen'ĕ-sis) [ terato- + G. genesis, origin ]. Teratogeny; the origin or mode of production of a malformed fetus; the disturbed growth processes involved in the production of a malformed fetus.

**teratogenetic** (tĕr'ă-to-jĕ-net'ik). Teratogenic.

**teratogenic** (tĕr'ă-to-jen'ik). Teratogenetic. 1. Relating to teratogenesis. 2. Causing abnormal development.

**teratogeny** (tĕr'ă-toj'ĕ-nĭ). Teratogenesis.

**teratoid** (tĕr'ă-toyd) [ G. teratōdēs, fr. teras (terat-), monster, + eidos, resemblance ]. Resembling a teras.

**teratologic** (tĕr'ă-to-loj'ik). Relating to teratology.

**teratology** (tĕr'ă-tol'o-jĭ) [ terato- + G. logos, study ]. The branch of science that deals with the production, the development, the anatomy, and the classification of malformed fetuses.

**teratoma** (tĕr'ă-to'mah) [ terato- + G. suffix -oma, tumor ]. A neoplasm composed of multiple tissues, including tissues not normally found in the organ in which it arises. Derivatives of all three germ layers may be found on careful search. T.'s occur most frequently in the ovary, where they are usually benign and form dermoid cysts; they also occur in the testis, where they are usually malignant, and, uncommonly, in other sites, especially the midline of the body.

   **t. orbitae,** orbitopagus.

   **t. strumo'sum thryoidea'le ova'rii,** a t. of the ovary composed largely of thyroid gland tissue.

   **triphyllomatous t.,** a tumor composed of tissues derived from all three gern layers.

**teratomatous** (tĕr'ă-to'mă-tus). Relating to or of the nature of a teratoma.

**teratophobia** (tĕr'ă-to-fo'bĭ-ah) [ terato- + G. phobos, fear ]. Morbid fear on the part of a pregnant woman lest she give birth to a malformed fetus.

**teratosis** (tĕr'ă-to'sis) [ terato- + G. suffix -osis, condition ]. Teratism; an anomaly producing a teras.

   **atre'sic t.,** one in which any of the normal openings, as the nares, mouth, anus, or vagina, is imperforate.

   **ceas'mic t.,** a malformation in which there is a failure of the lateral halves of a part to unite, as in cleft palate.

   **ectogen'ic t.,** one in which there is a deficiency of parts.

   **ectop'ic t.,** one in which the organs or other parts are misplaced.

   **hypergen'ic t.,** one in which there is a redundancy of parts.

   **symphys'ic t.,** one in which there is a fusion of normally separated parts.

**teratospermia** (tĕr'ă-to-sper'mĭ-ah) [ terato- + G. sperma, seed ]. A condition characterized by the presence of malformed spermatozoa in the semen.

**ter'bium** [ fr. Ytterby, a place in Sweden ]. A metallic element of the lanthanide or "rare earth" series, symbol Tb, atomic no. 65, atomic weight 158.93.

**terbu'taline sulfate** (USAN). α-[ (tert-butylamino)-methyl ]-3,5-dihydroxybenzyl alcohol sulfate; a bronchodilating drug.

**terebene** (tĕr'ĕ-bēn). A thin, colorless liquid of an aromatic odor and taste, a mixture of terpene hydrocarbons, chiefly dipentene and terpinene, obtained from oil of turpentine. Used as an expectorant and in cystitis and urethritis.

**terebinth** (tĕr'ĕ-binth) [ G. terebinthos, the terebinth or turpentine-tree ]. The tree, Pistacia terebinthus (family Pinaceae), from which Chian turpentine is obtained; it is native to the shores of the eastern Mediterranean.

**terebinthinate** (tĕr-ĕ-bin'thĭ-nāt). Terebinthine. 1. Containing or impregnated with turpentine. 2. A preparation containing turpentine.

**terebinthine** (tĕr-ĕ-bin'thin). Terebinthinate.

**terebin'thinism.** Turpentine poisoning.

**terebrachesis** (te're-bră-ke'sis) [ L. teres, round, + G. brachys, short ]. A surgical procedure for shortening the round ligaments of the uterus.

**terebrant, terebrating** (tĕr'ĕ-brant, -bra-ting) [ L. terebro, pp. -atus, to bore, fr. terebra, an auger ]. Boring; piercing; used figuratively, as in the term t. pain.

**terebration** (tĕr-ĕ-bra'shun) [ L. terebro, to bore, fr. terebra, an auger ]. 1. The act of boring, or of trephining. 2. A boring pain.

**teres,** gen. **teretis,** pl. **teretes** (tĕr'ēz, tĕr'e-tis, tĕr'e-tēz, -tĕr-) [ L. round, smooth, fr. tero, to rub ] [ NA ]. Round and long; denoting certain muscles and ligaments.

**ter'gal** [ L. tergum, back ]. Relating to the back; dorsal.

**ter'gum** [ L. ]. Dorsum.

**term** [ L. terminus, a limit, an end ]. 1. A definite or limited period. 2. A name or descriptive word or phrase; see also terminus.

   **at t.,** at the normal time, at the end of pregnancy.

**terminad** (ter'mĭ-nad). Toward the terminus.

**terminal** (ter'mĭ-nal) [ L. terminus, a boundary, limit ]. 1. Relating to the end; final. 2. Relating to the extremity or end of any body. 3. A termination, extremity, end, or ending.

   **axon t.'s,** end-feet; terminal boutons; boutons terminaux; pieds terminaux; axonal terminal boutons; synaptic endings or t.'s; neuropodia; the somewhat enlarged, often club-shaped endings by which axons make synaptic contacts with other nerve cells or with effector cells (muscle or gland cells); see also synapse.

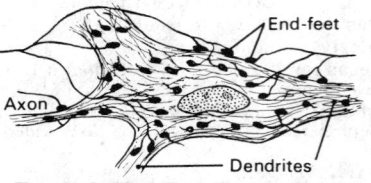

**Axon Terminals (End-Feet; Boutons Terminaux)**

   Arborizations of axons terminate as end-feet (synaptic endings or terminal boutons) on the cell body, dendrites, and proximal part of the axon of another neuron to form axo-somatic, axodendritic, and axoaxonic synapses, respectively.

   **synaptic t.'s,** axon t.'s.

**termina'lis** [ L. ] [ NA ]. Terminal (2).

**terminatio,** pl. **terminationes** (ter'mĭ-na-shĭ-o, -o'nēz) [ L. ] [ NA ]. A termination or ending, particularly a nerve ending; see also ending.

   **terminatio'nes nervo'rum li'berae** [ NA ], free nerve endings; a form of peripheral ending of sensory nerve fibers in which the terminal filaments end freely in the tissue.

**termination** (ter'mĭ-na'shun) [ L. terminatio ]. An end or ending; see terminatio, and ending.

**terminatio'nes** [ L. ]. Plural of terminatio.

**terminus,** pl. **ter'mini** (ter'mĭ-nus) [ L. ]. 1 [ NA ]. Term; a descriptive expression or word. 2. A boundary or limit.

   **termini ad mem'bra spectan'tes** [ NA ], terms specific to the limbs.

   **termini genera'les** [ NA ], general terms; words that are of general use in descriptive anatomy.

   **termini ontogenet'ici** [ NA ], developmental (ontogenetic) terms.

   **termini si'tum et directio'nem par'tium corpo'ris indican'tes** [ NA ], terms indicating location and direction of the parts of the body.

**ter'mone.** A type of ectohormone, secreted by some invertebrate organisms, that stimulates gametogenesis.

**terms.** Menses.

**ter'nary** [ L. ternarius, of three ]. Denoting a chemical compound containing three elements, or a complex formed by three molecules.

**terox'ide.** Trioxide.

**ter'pene.** One of a class of unsaturated hydrocarbons with an empirical formula of $C_{10}H_{16}$, occurring in essential oils and resins. The acyclic terpenes may be regarded as isomers and polymers of diisoprene, [ $(CH_3)_2C=CH-CH$ ]$_2$ (cf. carotenoids, tocopherols). Cyclic forms include menthane (cf. terpin), bornane, camphene. Terpenes containing 15, 20, 30, 40, etc., atoms are called sesquiterpenes, diterpenes, triterpenes, tetraterpenes, etc.

***p*-terphenyl** (ter'fĕ-nil). $C_6H_5$—$C6H_4$—$C_6H_5$; useful as a scintillator in scintillation counting (of radioactive decompositions).

**ter'pin.** *p*-Menthane-1,8-diol; a cyclic terpene alcohol, $C_{10}H_{18}(OH)_2$, obtained by the action of nitric acid and dilute sulfuric acid on pine oil.

    **t. hydrate** (NF), terpinol; monohydrate of terpin; an expectorant.

**terpineol** (ter-pin'e-ol). *p*-Menth-1-ene-8-ol; an unsaturated, alcoholic terpene obtained by heating terpin hydrate with diluted phosphoric acid; an active antiseptic and a perfume.

**ter'pinol.** Terpin hydrate.

**terra** (ter'rah) [ L. ]. Earth; soil.

    **t. alba,** (1) barium sulfate; (2) kaolin.

    **t. japon'ica,** gambir.

    **t. ponderosa,** barium sulfate.

    **t. sigilla'ta,** a form of clay from Asia Minor.

**ter'race** [ thr. O. Fr. fr. L. *terra,* earth ]. To suture in several rows, in closing a wound through a considerable thickness of tissue.

**terrac'inoic acid.** A crystalline tribasic acid obtained from axytetracycline by hydrolysis with aqueous alkali in the presence of zinc.

**Terrey,** Mary. See Lowe-T.-MacLachlan *syndrome.*

**Terrier** (ter-e-a'), Louis F., Paris surgeon, 1837–1908. See T.'s *valve.*

**Terrillon** (ter-e-yawn'), Octave R. S., French surgeon, 1844–1895. See T.'s *operation.*

**territoriality** (tĕr'ĭ-to-rĭ-al'ĭ-tĭ). 1. The tendency of individuals or groups to defend a particular domain or sphere of interest or influence. 2. The tendency of an individual animal to define a finite space as his own habitat from which he will fight off trespassing animals of his own species.

**Terry,** Theodore L., U. S. opthalmologist, 1899–1946. See T.'s *syndrome.*

**Terson,** Albert, Paris ophthalmologist, 1867–1935. See T.'s *glands.*

**tertian** (ter'shăn) [ L. *tertianus,* fr. *tertius,* third ]. 1. Occurring every third day (by inclusive reckoning); actually, occurring every 48 hours or every other day. 2. A variety of malaria with chills and fever occurring every other day; see malaria.

    **double t.,** infections with two different sets of malarial organisms producing daily chills. See also quotidian *malaria.*

**tertiarism, tertiarismus** (ter'shĭ-ā-rizm, -riz'mus). All the symptoms of the tertiary stage of syphilis taken collectively.

    **t. d'emblèe** (don-bla'), the occurrance of tertiary syphilitic symptoms, without distinct secondaries, in the mother of a child with taint from a syphilitic father.

**tertigravida** (ter'shĭ-grav'ĭ-dah) [ L. *tertius,* third, + *gravida,* a pregnant woman ]. A woman who has been pregnant three times.

**tertipara** (ter-tip'ă-rah) [ L. *tertius,* third, + *pario,* to bear ]. Para III; a woman who has given birth for the third time to an infant or infants, alive or dead, weighing 500 gm. or more or having a length of gestation of at least 20 weeks.

**ter'tipar'ity.** The state of being a tertipara.

**tertip'arous.** Relating to tertiparity or to a tertipara.

**tes'sellated** [ L. *tessella,* a small square stone ]. Made up of small squares; checkered.

# TEST

**test** [ L. *testum,* an earthen vessel. TEST-1 ]. 1. To try a substance; to prove; to determine the chemical nature of a substance by means of reagents. 2. A method of examination to determine the presence or absence of a definite disease, as the tuberculin t.; or the presence or absence of some substance in any of the fluids or excretions of the body, as a t. for albumin or sugar in the urine. 3. A substance used in making a t., a reagent. 4. Testa. (For t.'s not included in this table, see also reaction.)

    **Abderhalden's t.,** protective ferment; Abderhalden's reaction; dialysis t.; optical t.; an obsolete t. of historical interest, formerly used to determine the presence of protective enzymes ("ferments") in the blood; the "ferments" were thought to be specific for the various proteins that stimulate their production; suggested for the detection of pregnancy, malignant disease, and various other conditions.

    **abortus-Bang-ring t.,** ABR t., in the United States commonly known as the milk-ring t. (MR t.), essentially a special form of agglutination t. done on the mixed milk of many cows, usually entire herds, for the detection of herds containing individuals infected with bovine brucellosis.

    **ABR t.,** abbreviation for abortus-Bang-ring t.

    **acetone t.,** a t. for ketonuria; the suspected urine is shaken up with a few drops of sodium nitroprusside, and strong ammonia water is then gently poured over the mixture; if acetone is present, a magenta ring forms at the line of contact; tablets containing sodium nitroprusside and alkali are now more commonly used.

    **achievement t.,** a standardized t. used by psychologists and educators to measure acquired learning, *e.g.,* competence in a specific subject area, in contrast to an intelligence t. which is a useful index of potential learning; the Stanford achievement t. and Iowa achievement t. are examples.

    **acidified serum t.,** Ham's t.; lysis of the patient's red cells in acidified fresh serum, specific for paroxysmal nocturnal hemoglobinuria.

    **acid phosphatase t. for semen,** a screening t. for semen by determining acid phosphatase content; because seminal fluid contains high concentrations of acid phosphatase, while other body fluids and extraneous foreign materials have very low concentrations, high values of acid phosphatase on vaginal aspirate or lavage, or on wash fluid from stains, render positive identification of semen, even if the male is aspermic.

    **Acree-Rosenheim t.,** a qualitative t. for protein; mix 5 to 10 drops of a 1:5000 solution of formaldehyde with the suspected fluid in a test tube, then trickle a little sulfuric acid down the side of the tube; if protein is present the line of contact will show a violet coloration.

    **active rosette t.,** a t. for rosette-forming cells (T-lymphocytes) in which these cells and sheep erythrocytes, suspended in serum, are incubated and centrifuged lightly, then examined under a microscope for rosette formation.

    **adhesion t.,** immune adhesion t.; red cell adherence t.; erythrocyte adherence t.; the diagnostic application of the immune adhesion phenomenon, as, for example, the identification of serologic types of leptospira, the identification of antibodies to *Treponema pallidum,* or the differentiation of leukocytes.

    **Adler's t.,** benzidine t.

    **adrenal ascorbic acid depletion t.,** used to measure the quantity of corticotrophin in tissue, blood, or urine.

    **Adson's t.,** for thoracic outlet syndrome; patient is seated, with head extended and turned to the side of the lesion; with deep inspiration there is a diminution or total loss of radial pulse on the affected side.

    **Albarran's t.,** the drinking of large quantities of water will cause a proportionate increase in the urinary excretion if the kidneys are sound, but not if the epithelium of the secreting tubules is damaged.

    **Allen's t. for glucose in urine,** an obsolete t.; if urine is added to boiling Fehling's solution, turbidity develops as the mixture is cooled.

    **Allen's t. for phenol,** upon the addition of 5 or 6 drops of hydrochloric acid and then 1 of nitric acid to the suspected fluid, a red color develops.

    **Allen's t. for strychnine,** fluid is extracted with ether, which is then evaporated by means of "drop-by-drop" pipetting into a warmed porcelain dish or crucible; the residue is treated with a small bit of manganese dioxide and dilute sulfuric acid; a red-blue or violet color develops if strychnine is present.

    **Allen-Doisy t. for estrogenic activity,** the material to be investigated is injected repeatedly into immature or spayed rats or mice; the disappearance of leukocytes from the vaginal smear and the appearance of cornified cells constitutes a positive reaction.

**Almén's t. for blood,** Schönbein's t.; van Deen's t.; glacial acetic acid, gum guaiac solution, and hydrogen peroxide are added to an aqueous suspension of the suspected stain; if occult blood or blood pigment is present, a blue color develops.

**Anderson-Collip t.,** a procedure for evaluating the thyrotropic activity of an extract of the anterior lobe of the pituitary gland, as indicated by an increased basal metabolic rate or histologic evidence of stimulation of the thyroid gland in a hypophysectomized rat injected with the test extract.

**anoxemia t.,** hypoxemia t.; a t. for coronary insufficiency; the patient breathes a mixture of 10 per cent oxygen and 90 per cent nitrogen; if anginal pain or electrocardiographic abnormalities are induced, the t. is positive.

**antiglob'ulin t.,** Coombs' t.

**anti-human glob'ulin t.,** Coombs' t.

**anti-insulin t.,** a t. of glucocorticoid activity; male mice are divided into two groups of 20 animals each. At the beginning of a 6-hour fast the animals of one group are given the t. material in oil; at the end of the fast the animals of both groups are given 2 units of insulin per kilogram of body weight, and maintained at a temperature of 34°C. The percentage of animals protected from insulin convulsion by the material under t. is taken as a measure of its activity.

**aptitude t.,** an occupation-oriented intelligence t. used to evaluate a person's abilities, interests, talents, and skills; it is particularly valuable in vocational counseling.

**Arnold's t.,** an obsolete t. for diacetic acid in urine.

**Aschheim-Zondek t.,** an obsolete t. for pregnancy; repeated injections of small quantities of urine voided during the first months of pregnancy produce in infantile mice, within 100 hours, (1) minute intrafollicular ovarian hemorrhages, and (2) the development of lutein cells.

**association t.,** a word (the stimulus word) is spoken to the subject, who replies immediately with another word (the reaction word) suggested to him by the first; it is used as an aid in diagnosis, clues being given by the length of time (association time) between the stimulus and reaction words, and also by the nature of the reaction words.

**Astwood's t.,** metrotrophic t.

**at'ropine t.,** Dehio's t.

**augmented histamine t.,** histamine t.

**aussage t.** (aus'zah-guh) [ Ger. a declaration ], a t. of ability to reproduce correctly something that has been seen for a brief interval.

**A.-Z. t.,** Aschheim-Zondek t.

**Babcock's t.,** a t. to determine the amount of milk fat, by centrifuging equal parts of milk and sulfuric acid.

**Bachman-Pettit t.,** a modification of Kober's t. for the detection of estradiol and similar estrogenic hormones in urine.

**BALB t.** (binaural alternate loudness balance t.), a t. for recruitment in one ear; the comparison of relative loudness of a series of intensities presented alternately to either ear.

**Bárány's caloric t.,** nystagmus t.; a t. for vestibular function, made by irrigating the external auditory meatus with either hot or cold water. This normally causes stimulation of the vestibular apparatus resulting in nystagmus and past-pointing. In vestibular disease, the response fails relatively or entirely.

**Becker's t.,** a t. for astigmatism, using a diagram of lines radiating in different meridians, in sets of three. See fig. under astigmatism.

**BEI t.,** butanol-extractable iodine t.

**belt t.,** firm upward pressure on the lower part of the abdomen will remove the feeling of discomfort in cases of enteroptosia.

**Bender Gestalt t.,** a psychological t. used by neurologists and clinical psychologists to measure a person's ability to visually copy a set of geometric designs; it is useful for measuring visuomotor coordination to detect brain damage.

**Benedict's t. for glucose,** a copper-reduction t. for glucose in urine, which involves thiocyanate in addition to copper sulfate for qualitative or quantitative use.

**ben'zidine t.,** Adler's t.; a t. for blood; the suspected fluid is treated with glacial acetic acid and ether, and the latter is then decanted and treated with hydrogen peroxide and

a solution of benzidine in acetic acid; the presence of blood is indicated by a bluish color turning to purple.

**Berson t.,** a t. of thyroid clearance of $^{131}$I from the plasma by the thyroid gland.

**Bettendorff's t.,** a t. for arsenic; after mixing the suspected fluid with hydrochloric acid a solution of stannous chloride is added; when a piece of tin foil is then added, a brown precipitate forms.

**Bial's t.,** a t. for pentoses with orcinol.

**Binet t.,** Stanford-Binet intelligence *scale.*

**Binet-Simon t.,** Stanford-Binet intelligence *scale.*

**Binz' t.,** a t. for quinine in the urine; a precipitate is thrown down on the addition of iodine 2, potassium iodide 1, in water 40, if quinine is present.

**biuret t.,** a t. for the determination of serum proteins; based on the reaction of an alkaline copper reagent with substances containing two or more peptide bonds to produce a violet-blue color.

**blind t.,** a method of testing in which an independent observer records the results of any t., drug, placebo, or procedure without knowing the identity of the samples or what result might be expected.

**block design t.,** a performance t. using colored blocks to match standard designs; one of the subtests of the Wechsler intelligence scales.

**Bodal's t.,** a t. for color vision, involving the sorting of variously colored blocks.

**Boedeker's t.,** an obsolete t. for albumin in urine.

**Bordet's t.,** precipitin t.

**Bordet's serologic t.,** a t. for identifying the species of animal from which unknown protein material is derived by means of precipitation when mixed with known specific antiserums.

**Bragard's t.,** pain along the sciatic nerve when the foot is dorsiflexed during straight leg raising.

**breath-holding t.,** a rough index of cardiopulmonary reserve measured by the length of time that a subject can hold his breath; the normal duration is in excess of 30 seconds, whereas a patient with diminished cardiac or pulmonary reserve cannot hold his breath for more than 20 seconds.

**bromphenol t.,** a colorimetric t. for measurement of protein, albumin, and globulin in urine by use of reagent strips.

**Bromsulphalein t.,** BSP t., a t. for liver function (hepatic excretory capacity) in which a known amount of dye, usually 5 mg. per kg. of body weight, is injected intravenously. Subsequently (usually after 45 minutes elapsed time), the amount of dye remaining in the serum is measured. A concentration of 0.4 mg. or less of Bromsulphalein per 100 ml. of serum or less than 4 per cent of the injected dye is considered normal. Bromsulphalein retention may follow decreased hepatic blood flow or biliary obstruction as well as hepatic cell damage.

**butanol-extractable iodine t.,** BEI t.; a t. for thyroid function, applicable in patients who have received large amounts of iodine or iodized products.

**California psychological inventory t.,** a personality inventory, used with normal persons, in which emphasis is upon social interaction variables.

**Calmette t.,** conjuctival reaction to tuberculin.

**caloric t.,** Bárány's caloric t.

**Cannon's t.,** a t. for endogenous epinephrine; the denervated heart (cardiac vagus and sympathetic fibers severed) responds by acceleration to the liberation of epinephrine from the adrenal glands.

**Cannon and La Paz t.,** a t. for epinephrine; Langley's t.

**capillary fragility t.,** capillary resistance t.; a modified tourniquet t.; a circle 2.5 cm. in diameter, the upper edge of which is 4 cm. below the crease of the elbow, is drawn on the inner aspect of the forearm. Pressure midway between the systolic and diastolic blood pressure is applied above the elbow for 15 minutes. A count of petechiae within the circle is made; normal 10, marginal zone 10 to 20, abnormal over 20. Positive in vitamin C deficiency.

**capillary resistance t.,** capillary fragility t.

**capon-comb-growth t.,** comb-growth t.

**Carr-Price t.,** antimony trichloride t.; a quantitative color t. for assay of vitamin A content of oils.

**Castellani's absorption t.,** misnomer for what is actually an adsorption t.; an early application of immune adsorption to separate antibodies for specific antigens from those for group antigens.

**catator'ulin t.,** an assay method for thiamine based upon its effect in increasing the uptake of oxygen by incubated slices of brain tissue to which it has been added.

**catecholamine t.,** total catecholamine t.

**Chick-Martin t.,** a method of testing the *in vitro* efficiency of a bactericidal agent; a standard culture of *Salmonella typhi* which has been added to a fixed amount of sterilized feces or yeast is tested for a fixed period (30 minutes), against various concentrations of phenol solution and various concentrations of the disinfectant. The result is expressed as a ratio: the phenol coefficient. This is the highest dilution of the disinfectant under t. at which the bacteria are killed divided by the highest dilution of phenol which sterilizes the solution in the same length of time.

**Clauberg t.,** a t. for progestational activity; immature rabbits are treated with 8 daily injections of estrogen and then given 5 daily injections of the t. substance. The amount required to produce definite progestational changes in the endometrium is taken as the unit; it is equivalent to 0.75 mg. of progesterone.

**coccidioi'din t.,** an intracutaneous t. for determining presence of infection with the fungus *Coccidioides immitis.* A positive t. indicates a reaction of delayed hypersensitivity and is interpreted as meaning past or present infection with the fungus.

**Cohn's t.,** a t. for color vision, by means of a comparison of embroidery patterns of different colors.

**coin t.,** see bellmetal *resonance.*

**cold t.,** a t. for adrenal cortical hormones; based upon the fact that adrenalectomized animals are usually susceptible to cold. Adrenalectomized rats are kept at a temperature between $-5°C.$ and $+2°C.$ They are given injections of the substance to be tested at 2-hour intervals over a period of 6 hours. The number surviving are compared with the number surviving in a control group of adrenalectomized animals. A unit of cortical hormone is defined as the minimum amount which maintains alive 6 out of 9 rats when 6 out of 9 untreated control rats are dead.

**cold bend t.,** a t. of the ability of a wire to be shaped; performed by counting the number of times a wire can be bent to a right angle and reversed at the same point before breaking; important in establishing specifications for orthodontic wires.

**colorimetric caries susceptibility t.,** Snyder's t.; a procedure for determining the density of acid producing organisms in saliva by the usage of bromcresol green in a culture medium.

**comb-growth t.,** a t. for androgenic activity, based upon the stimulation of comb growth in capons (castrated cockerels) or immature roosters.

**Comessatti t.,** see sublimate reaction of epinephrine, under reaction.

**complement-fixation t.,** an immunological t. for determining the presence of a particular antigen or antibody when one of the two is known to be present, based on the fact that complement is "fixed" in the presence of antigen and its specific antibody. See also Bordet-Gengou *phenomenon.*

**conjunctival t.,** conjunctival *reaction.*

**Coombs' t.,** antiglobulin t.; a t. for antibodies; the so-called anti-human globulin t. using either the direct or indirect Coombs' t.'s, *q.v.*

**Corner-Allen t.,** a t. for progestational activity; adult female rabbits are mated during estrus and spayed 18 hours later; the t. substance is injected subcutaneously on 5 successive days; the minimal amount required to produce complete progestational proliferation of the endometrium is taken as a unit. The latter is equivalent to 1.25 mg. of progesterone.

**CO₂-withdrawal seizure t.,** hyperventilation t.; utilization of hyperventilation to demonstrate abnormalities in the brain waves or even to precipitate a convulsion.

**Crampton t.,** a record is made of the pulse and the blood pressure in the recumbent and in the standing position. The difference is graded from the theoretical perfection of 100 (seldom attained) downward; a reading of 75 is considered to be excellent, but 65 is poor. High values indicate a good physical resistance but low ones are said to indicate weakness and a liability to shock after an operation.

**t.'s of criminal responsibility,** in forensic psychiatry, legal precedents upon which are based decisions concerning insanity in criminals; see also American Law Institute *rule,* Durham *rule,* M'Naghten *rule,* and New Hampshire *rule.*

**Cuboni t.,** Kober t.

**Cunisset's t.,** a t. for bile in the urine; a yellow color develops when chloroform is added and the mixture is shaken.

**cutaneous t.,** skin t.

**cutaneous tuberculin t.,** see tuberculin t.

**cutireaction t.,** skin t.

**Cutler-Power-Wilder t.,** a rarely used t. for adrenal insufficiency, in which the intake of sodium is restricted and that of potassium is increased. The t. is positive if signs of adrenal insufficiency appear. The t. is dangerous in Addison's disease, since a crisis may be precipitated; it should be performed with caution.

**cytophilic antibody t.,** a rosette t. for macrophage cytophilic antibody; monolayers of macrophages are exposed first to antibody cytophilic for macrophages, then to the antigen (for which the antibody is specific), and indicator sheep erythrocytes. If the antibody is specific for sheep erythrocytes the latter will form a rosette around the macrophages directly, but if not, and the antigen is soluble, the antigen must be coupled to the sheep erythrocytes by an agent such as bis-diazotized benzidine.

**DA pregnancy t.,** direct agglutination latex t. for pregnancy; see immunologic pregnancy t.

**Davy's t.,** a t. for carbolic acid; to a few drops of the suspected fluid, add double the quantity of a mixture of molybdic acid 1, and sulfuric acid 15; the presence of carbolic acid is indicated by a brown color that changes to purple.

**Day's t.,** a t. for blood; add to the suspected fluid, or the washing of a suspected stain, tincture of guaiac and then hydrogen peroxide; the presence of blood results in a blue color.

**deciduo'ma t.,** a t. for progestational activity; the endometrium of animals (rats, guinea pigs) which have been pretreated with an estrogen, responds to local irritation by the development of a deciduoma, if the t. material injected has progestational activity.

**Dehio's t.,** atropine t.; if an injection of atropine relieves bradycardia, the condition is due to action of the vagus; if it does not, the condition is due to an affection of the heart itself.

**dehydrocho'late t.,** a method of determining the speed of the blood circulation; a solution of sodium dehydrocholate is injected intravenously, and the time that elapses before a bitter taste is noted in the mouth is recorded; the average of this time if 13 seconds, more or less.

**denervated eye (iris) t.,** a t. for epinephrine; see Meltzer-Auer t.

**dial'ysis t.,** Abderhalden t.

**Dick t.,** Dick method; an intracutaneous t. of susceptibility to the erythrogenic toxin of *Streptococcus pyogenes* responsible for the rash and other manifestations of scarlet fever.

**direct Coombs' t.,** a t. for detecting sensitized erythrocytes in erythroblastosis fetalis and in cases of acquired hemolytic anemia; the patient's erythrocytes (2 per cent suspension) are washed with saline to remove serum and unattached antibody protein, then incubated with Coombs' anti-human globulin (usually serum from a rabbit or goat previously immunized with human globulin). After incubation the system is centrifuged and examined for agglutination. Agglutination indicates the presence of so-called incomplete or univalent antibodies on the surface of the erythrocytes.

**Doerfler-Stewart t.,** D-S t.; examination of the patient's ability to respond to spondee words in the presence of a masking noise of the saw-tooth type. Used especially in differentiating between functional and organic hearing loss.

**Donders' t.,** a t. for color vision, by means of lanterns with colored glass sides.

**double (gel) diffusion precipitin t. in one dimension,** see gel diffusion precipitin t.'s in one dimension.

**double (gel) diffusion precipitin t. in two dimensions,** see gel diffusion precipitin t.'s in two dimensions.

**Dragendorff's t.,** a qualitative t. for bile; a play of colors is produced by adding a drop of nitric acid to white filter paper or unglazed porcelain, moistened with a fluid containing bile pigments. The t. is essentially the same as Gmelin's t. for bile in urine.

**drawer t.,** patient sits with knee flexed to 90°. Upper end of leg is grasped with one hand and foot is stabilized with examiner's other hand. Force is applied to axis of femur forward and backward. If tibia moves distally on femur to an abnormal degree, anterior cruciate ligament is relaxed or torn. If movement is proximal, posterior cruciate ligament is involved. Compare with opposite knee for individual variations.

**Duane's t.,** a black screen is held for a moment between the light and the eye to be examined and then is suddenly shifted in front of the other eye; if there is imbalance of the muscles of the first eye the image of the light will be displaced.

**Dugas' t.,** in the case of an injured shoulder, if the elbow cannot be made to touch the chest while the hand rests on the opposite shoulder the injury is a dislocation and not a fracture of the humerus.

**Ebbinghaus t.,** a psychological t. in which the patient is asked to complete certain sentences from which several words have been left out.

**Ellsworth-Howard t.,** measurement of serum and urinary phosphorus after intravenous administration of parathyroid extract; used in the diagnosis of pseudohypoparathyroidism.

**Emmens' S/L t.,** a t. for distinguishing estrogenic precursors from active estrogens; a number of mice are divided into two groups, one of which is treated subcutaneously with the estrogen; the other group receives the estrogen intravaginally. The systemic and local effective doses are expressed as a ratio (S/L). The ratio is unity for the precursors but much greater than unity for active estrogens.

**erythrocyte adherence t.,** adhesion t.

**ether t.,** a t. to determine arm-to-lung circulation time; diluted ether is injected intravenously and the end point taken when the subject coughs or tastes ether or the observer smells ether on the subject's breath.

**exercise t.,** two-step exercise t.

**Exton-Rose t.,** a glucose tolerance t. in which glucose, instead of being given in a single dose, is administered in two 50-gm. doses 30 minutes apart; blood sugar determinations are made 30 minutes after each dose. In normal persons the blood sugar level in the second sample is less than, the same as, or not more than 5 mg. higher than the first; in diabetes the sugar of the blood rises steeply after the second dose.

**fatigue t.,** fatigue *reaction.*

**fern t.,** an obsolete, nonspecific t. for estrogenic activity; cervical mucus smears form a fern pattern at times when estrogen secretion is elevated, as at the time of ovulation.

**ferric chloride t.,** Several modifications of this screening t. are available. The t.'s depend upon the production of a green or blue-green color when ferric chloride is added to urine containing phenylpyruvic acid. These t.'s for phenylketonuria have largely been replaced by other t. procedures such as the Guthrie t. or fluorometric determinations performed on blood for increased levels of phenylalanine.

**Feulgen's t.,** a t. for the presence of deoxyribonucleic acid in tissue sections, based upon the purple color that appears when, after hydrolysis with dilute hydrochloric acid, Schiff's reagent is added.

**Fevold t.,** a t. for relaxin; based on the degree of relaxation of the pelvic ligaments of the guinea pig upon injection of extracts of the corpus luteum.

**Finckh t.,** a psychological t. in which the patient is asked to explain certain proverbial expressions, such as "burn the candle at both ends," "the early bird catches the worm," etc.

**fish t.,** erythrophore *reaction.*

**fistula t.,** compression or rarefaction of the air in the external auditory canal excites nystagmus when there is an erosion of the inner bony wall of the tympanum, so long as the labyrinth is still capable of functioning; when the tympanic wall is intact, no nystagmus occurs.

**FIT t.,** fusion-inferred threshold t.

**Fleitmann's t.,** a t. for arsenic; hydrogen is generated in a t. tube containing the suspected fluid; the fluid is heated and a piece of filter paper moistened with silver nitrate solution is held over the top; if arsenic is present the moistened paper is blackened.

**flocculation t.,** see flocculation *reaction.*

**Florence's t.,** Florence's reaction; a screening t. for semen (now largely replaced by the acid phosphate t.) in which the presence of choline in seminal secretions or stains is determined by adding an iodine-potassium iodide reagent; in a positive t., crystals of periodide of choline are found.

**fluorescein string t.,** a string t. in which fluorescein is given intravenously. When the string fluoresces after removal it is known that it has been contaminated by blood that has appeared since injection of the fluorescein.

**fluorescent t.,** a t. for epinephrine; see Gaddum and Schild t.

**fluorescent treponemal antibody-absorption t.,** FTA-ABS t.; a sensitive and specific serologic t. for syphilis using a suspension of the Nichols strain of *Treponema pallidum* as antigen; the presence or absence of antibody in the patient's serum is indicated by an indirect fluorescent antibody technique.

**Folin's t.,** (1) a quantitative t. for uric acid by means of the color produced with phosphotungstic acid and a base. (2) a quantitative t. for urea; the urea is decomposed by boiling with magnesium chloride, and the freed ammonia is measured.

**Folin-Looney t.,** a t. for tyrosine which gives a blue color in alkaline solution with a reagent consisting of sodium tungstate, phosphomolybdic acid, and phosphoric acid.

**Foshay t.,** an intradermal t. for cat-scratch disease, using material prepared from suppurative lymph nodes of persons known to have had the disease.

**fragility t.,** the erythrocyte fragility t. measures the resistance of erythrocytes to hemolysis in hypotonic saline solutions. Erythrocytes to be tested are added to varying concentrations of saline, usually ranging from 0.85 to 0.10 per cent sodium chloride with 0.05 per cent increments. Beginning and complete hemolysis are measured. Normal erythrocytes show initial hemolysis at concentrations of 0.45 to 0.39 per cent and complete hemolysis at 0.33 to 0.30 per cent. In hereditary spherocytosis the fragility of the erythrocytes is markedly increased, whereas in thalassemia, sickle cell anemia, and obstructive jaundice the fragility of the erythrocytes is usually reduced.

**Frei t.,** Frei-Hoffman reaction; an intracutaneous diagnostic t. for lymphogranuloma venereum, based on reaction to an antigen prepared by means of (1) aspirating exudate from a softened, partially liquefied bubo (in a person known to have the disease), (2) mixing the material with physiologic saline solution, and then (3) heating the suspension in order to kill the chlamydiae. If the patient in question has lymphogranuloma venereum, intracutaneous injection of 0.1 ml. of the antigen results in a red, indurated area at least 7 mm. in diameter within 24 to 48 hours. This reaction of delayed hypersensitivity is interpreted as indicative of past or present infection; however, the t. is only group-specific and will be positive in infections with related organisms such as psittacosis. Modern Frei antigen is usually a yolk sac preparation of the chlamydiae.

**Fridenberg's stigmomet'ric card t.,** a t. using a card containing a series of dots and squares, of definite and graduated size, arranged in groups; these dots are to be counted at various distances as a t. of vision and accommodation in illiterates.

**Friedman t.,** Friedman-Lapham t.; an obsolete modification (using rabbits) of the Aschheim-Zondek t. for pregnancy.

**Friedman-Lapham t.,** Friedman t.

**FTA-ABS t.,** fluorescent treponemal antibody-absorption t.

**Funkenstein t.,** a t. of autonomic reactivity.

**fusion-inferred threshold (FIT) t.,** employment of the phenomenon of cerebral fusion of binaural sounds to substitute for conventional masking in hearing testing.

**Gaddum and Schild t.,** a sensitive method for identification of epinephrine in tissue or other material, based on the fluorescence of epinephrine when it is exposed to ultraviolet light in the presence of alkali and oxygen. The sensitivity ranges from 1:50 to 1:100 million.

**galactose tolerance t.,** a liver function t., based on the ability of the liver to convert galactose to glycogen, measured by the rate of excretion of galactose following ingestion or intravenous injection of a known amount; normally, less than 3 gm. appear in the urine within 5 hours after the ingestion of 40 gm.

**Galli-Mainini t.,** an obsolete t. for pregnancy.

**Geissler t.,** a t. for albumin in the urine; two bits of filter paper, impregnated, respectively, with citric acid and with a mixture of corrosive sublimate and potassium iodide, are dropped into the urine; albumin, if present, will be precipitated.

**gel diffusion precipitin t.'s,** gel diffusion reactions; precipitin t.'s in which the immune precipitate forms in a gel medium (usually agar) into which one or both reactants have diffused. These t.'s are generally classified in two types, gel diffusion in one dimension, and gel diffusion in two dimensions, defined in the following subentries.

**gel diffusion precipitin t.'s in one dimension,** precipitin t.'s in which antigen solution and antibody incorporated in agar are layered in tubes (permitting effective diffusion in the vertical dimension); the antibody-containing agar may be overlaid directly with antigen solution (*single (gel) diffusion in one dimension*), or the antigen (fluid or in agar) layer and the antibody-containing agar layer may be separated by a layer of plain agar into which both antigen and antibody diffuse (*double (gel) diffusion in one dimension*).

**gel diffusion precipitin t.'s in two dimensions,** precipitin t.'s made in a uniform, flat layer of agar that permits radial diffusion (*i.e.,* in both of the horizontal dimensions) of one or both reactants. *Single (gel) diffusion in two dimensions* is a precipitin t. in which antibody is incorporated in the agar and antigen solutions are placed in wells from which the agar has been removed. *Double (gel) diffusion in two dimensions* (the Ouchterlony test, technique, or method) is a precipitin t. in which antigen and antibody solutions are placed in separate wells in a sheet of plain agar, permitting radial diffusion of both reactants. This method is widely used to determine antigenic relationships; the bands of precipitate that form where the reactants meet in optimal concentration are of three patterns, referred to as *reaction of identity, reaction of partial identity* (*cross reaction*), and *reaction of nonidentity.*

**Gellé t.,** a vibrating tuning fork is applied over the mastoid process; if it is heard, the air in the external auditory canal is compressed, by means of a rubber tube inserted into the canal and a hand bulb, thereby fixing the stapes in the oval window, and the sound ceases to be heard, but is again perceived if the air pressure is removed; a t. of the mobility of the ossicles.

**Geraghty's t.,** phenolsulfonphthalein t.

**Gerhardt's t. for acetoacetic acid,** Gerhardt's reaction; in fresh urine a red color develops upon addition of FeCl₃; no color develops if the urine has first been boiled; this t. has low specificity and sensitivity.

**Gerhardt's t. for urobilin in the urine,** the urobilin is extracted with chloroform and then treated with iodine and potassium hydrate, a fluorescent green color being produced.

**glucose oxidase paper strip t.,** a qualitative t. for glucose in urine, in which glucose is oxidized to gluconic acid by glucose oxidase; a specific t., unless ascorbic acid is present.

**glucose tolerance t.,** a t. for diabetes, based upon the ability of the normal liver to absorb and store excessive amounts of glucose as glycogen. Following ingestion of 100 gm. of glucose the fasting blood sugar promptly rises, then falls to normal within 2 hours. In a diabetic patient the increase is greater and the return to normal unusually prolonged.

**glyoxyl'ic acid t.,** Hopkins-Cole t.; a t. for protein; the protein solution containing a salt of glyoxylic acid is stratified above concentrated sulfuric acid; a violet ring appears at the junction of the two liquids; it depends upon the tryptophan group containing the indole ring.

**Gmelin's t.,** Rosenbach-Gmelin t.; a t. for bile in the urine or other body fluid; nitric acid, with a little nitrous acid,

is cautiously added to a few milliliters of the material to be tested; if bile (bilirubin) is present, it is oxidized to varying degrees, thereby resulting in disklike zones that are (from the interface outward) yellow, red, violet, blue, and green; development of green and violet layers is issential to the validity of the t.

**Gofman t.,** a t. for various serum lipoproteins that contain cholesterol, as an index of the tendency to the development of atheromatous lesions and arteriosclerosis; the t. is based on the differential flotation of molecules of various sizes when the serum is treated in an ultracentrifuge.

**Goldscheider's t.,** determination of the temperature sense by touching the skin with a sharp-pointed metallic rod, heated to varying degrees.

**gold sol t.,** Lange's t.

**Göthlin's t.,** a capillary fragility t. to determine the presence or absence of scurvy.

**Graefe's t.,** a t. for heterophoria; a prism of 10 Δ is held base up or down before one eye; this produces two images of the object looked at; in orthophoria one image is directly above the other, in lateral heterophoria there is a lateral displacement of one image.

**group t.,** in psychology, a t. designed to be administered to more than one individual at a time; *e.g.,* scholastic achievement t., medical college admissions t.

**guai'ac t.,** Almén's t. for blood.

**Guthrie t.,** detection of a raised level of phenylalanine in a drop of blood dried on filter paper; positive in phenylketonuria.

**Gutzeit's t.,** a t. for arsenic; a piece of zinc and a little sulfuric acid are added to the suspected liquid which is then boiled; a bit of filter paper with a silver nitrate solution is held in the vapor and will turn yellow if arsenic is present.

**Habel t.,** a method of determining the antigenic efficacy of inactivated rabies vaccines.

**Hallion's t.,** Tuffier's t.; when the main artery and vein of a limb are compressed, in a case of aneurysm, swelling of the veins of the hand or foot will take place only when the collateral circulation is free.

**Ham's t.,** acidified serum t.

**Hamilton's t.,** in axillary dislocation of the shoulder a rod will touch both the acromion process and the outer condyle of the humerus.

**Hamilton-Swartz t.,** a qualitative t. for parathyroid hormone in a biological fluid, based upon the fact that calcium enhances the effect of the parathyroid hormone upon the serum calcium. Rabbits are given calcium by stomach tube at 0, 1, 3, and 5 hour intervals and a curve drawn of the serum calcium levels. The last dose has little effect. On the other hand, if a fluid containing parathyroid hormone is given before the administration of calcium there is a definite rise in the serum calcium after the last dose of calcium.

**Harrington-Flocks t.,** for rapid measurement of central visual fields, a screening device in which single patters are presented tachistoscopically to the fixating eye; the patterns are visible only when illuminated by a flash of ultraviolet light.

**Harris t.,** Harris and Ray t.

**Harris and Ray t.,** a t. for vitamin C in urine; a microtitration t. of urine against a known amount of 0.05 per cent aqueous solution of the dye 2, 6-dichlorophenol indophenol in 10 per cent acetic acid (usually 0.05 cc. of dye is used, roughly equivalent to 0.025 mg. of ascorbic acid).

**head-dropping t.,** a t. used in the diagnosis of disease of the extrapyramidal or striatal system (*e.g.,* parkinsonism, Wilson's disease). With the patient supine, relaxed, and his attention diverted, the examiner briskly lifts the patient's head with the right hand and then allows it to drop upon the palm of his left hand. The head of a normal person drops suddenly like a dead weight, whereas, in the subject of striatal disease the head falls slowly, gently and almost hesitantly.

**heat coagulation t.,** a t. for measurement of protein in urine; albumin and globulin are coagulated by heat at an acid pH, and the amount of turbidity present provides a qualitative estimation of the degree of proteinuria.

**heel-tap t.,** see heel *tap.*

**hemadsorption virus t.,** a procedure for titratig viral antibodies in a serum (using a known virus), or for identifying a virus (using a known antiserum); the t. is based on the fact that some viruses are adsorbed on the surface of red blood cells during an appropriate incubation period, and cells treated in this manner may be used in an agglutination t. with serum that contains antibody for the virus that is on the surface of the erythrocytes.

**Hering's t.,** one looks through an apparatus having at the farther end a thread about which a little ball is dropped; if binocular vision is present the observer is able to tell whether the ball is in front of or behind the thread; with monocular vision this is not possible.

**Hess' t.,** Rumpel-Leede t.

**Heynsius' t.,** a t. for albumin in the urine; the urine is acidulated with acetic acid and then boiled with the addition of common salt; if albumin is present a white cloud will form.

**Hindenlang's t.,** a t. for albumin in the urine; a precipitate is formed on the addition of metaphosphoric acid if albumin is present.

**Hinton t.,** a formerly widely used precipitin (flocculation) t. for syphilis in which the "antigen" consisted of glycerol, cholesterol, and beef heart extract.

**HISTALOG t.,** maximal HISTALOG t.; a t. for measurement of maximal production of gastric acidity or anacidity; it is similar to the histamine t. (*q.v.*), but uses HISTALOG (betazole hydrochloride), an analogue of histamine.

**histamine t.,** augmented histamine t.; a t. for maximal production of gastric acidity or anacidity; after preliminary administration of an antihistamine, histamine acid phosphate is injected subcutaneously in a dose of 0.04 mg. per kg. of body weight, followed by analysis of gastric contents; see also Histalog t.

**histo-latex t.,** an antigen-antibody t. for histoplasmosis; latex particles are sensitized with antigen and this reagent is used in a flocculation reaction with the patient's serum.

**Hogben t.,** Xenopus t.

**Hollander t.,** insulin t. for intact nerve fibers after vagal operation for peptic ulcer.

**Holmgrèn's t.,** a t. for color blindness by having the subject pick out and match variously colored skeins of worsted.

**homovanillic acid t.,** HVA t.; a t. for HVA based upon the fact that dopamine is present in sympathetic nervous tissue as precursor of norepinephrine; since norepinephrine has a metabolic pathway which yields HVA, tumors such as neuroblastomas and ganglioneuromas may cause elevations of urinary dopamine and HVA.

**Hooker-Forbes t.,** a t. for compounds with progestational activity; such compounds cause hypertrophy of the stromal nuclei of the endometrium in uteri obtained from spayed mice; a sensitive t. capable of detecting 0.0002 $\mu$g. of progesterone.

**Hopkins-Cole t.,** glyoxylic acid t.

**Hoppe-Seyler t.,** a rarely used screening t. for carbon monoxide; a t. for carbon monoxide in the blood; on adding to the blood twice the volume of sodium hydrate solution (1.3 sp. gr.) the red color of blood is preserved if carbon monoxide is present; normal blood is colored a greenish brown.

**hormone t.'s for pregnancy,** see pregnancy t.

**Horsley's t.,** a t. for sugar in the urine, the presence of which is indicated when a green color is produced by boiling with potassic hydrate and potassium chromate.

**Houghton's t.,** the former official biological assay for ergot; the preparation of ergot to be assayed and a standard preparation of ergotoxine ethanesulfonate were injected into white Leghorn cocks, producing a characteristic darkening of the comb.

**Huggins' t.,** see Huggins-Miller-Jensen t.

**Huggins-Miller-Jensen t.,** an invalid t. of historical interest only, for cancer using iodoacetic acid; the serums of patients with malignant growths, but only a small proportion of others, show deficient heat coagulation when treated with iodoacetic acid.

**Huhner t.,** determination of sperm quantity and motility in specimens obtained from the vaginal seminal pool and the cervical canal following coitus.

**HVA t.,** homovanillic acid t.

**hydrostatic t.,** Raygat's t.

**17-hydroxycorticosteroid t.,** 17-OH-corticoids t.; Porter-Silber chromogens t.; a t., dependent on the Porter-Silber reaction, that is used as a measure of adrenocortical function; it may be performed on blood or urine. Low values are seen in Addison's disease and hypopituitarism; high values are seen in Cushing's syndrome and extreme stress.

**hypere'mia t.,** Moszkowicz' t.

**hyperventilation t.,** $CO_2$-withdrawal seizure t.

**hypoxemia t.,** see anoxemia t.

**$^{131}$I uptake t.,** radioactive iodide uptake t.; RAI t.; a t. of thyroid function in which $^{131}$I-iodide is given orally; after 24 hours, the amount present in the thyroid gland is measured and compared with normal values.

**immune adhesion t.,** adhesion t.

**immunologic pregnancy t.,** urine to be tested for the presence of human chorionic gonadotropin (HCG) is mixed with antiserum specific for HCG, and the mixture is then tested with latex particles coated with HCG; if the urine contained HCG, the antibodies would have combined with it and would not be available to agglutinate the coated latex particles; accordingly, inhibition of agglutination of the latex particles is an indication that HCG was in the urine.

**indirect t.,** see Prausnitz-Küstner *reaction.*

**indirect Coombs' t.,** a t. routinely performed in cross-matching blood or in the investigation of transfusion reactions; test or patient's serum is incubated with a suspension of donor erythrocytes; if specific antibodies are present, they become attached to the antigen in donor's cells. After a washing with saline, Coombs' anti-human globulin is added; agglutination at this point indicates that antibodies present in the original test serum had indeed become attached to donor erythrocytes.

**intelligence t.,** a t., using well researched items and involving a systematic method of administration and scoring, used by psychologists and educators to assess an individual's global aptitude or level of competence, in contrast to an achievement t.; types of intelligence t.'s include verbal versus performance, child versus adult forms, and those requiring individual administration (Wechsler adult intelligence scale) versus group administration (medical college admissions t.).

**iodate t.,** a t. for epinephrine; see iodate *reaction* of epinephrine.

**iodine t.,** a t. for epinephrine; see iodine *reaction* of epinephrine.

**Ishihara's t.,** a t. for color blindness which utilizes a series of pseudoisochromatic cards; all of the figures or letters are easily read by the normal person but not by one with defective color vision.

**Jacquemin's t.,** a t. for phenol; to the suspected fluid an equal amount of aniline is added, and, after thorough admixture, a little solution of sodium hypochlorite; if phenol is present the fluid becomes blue in color.

**Jaffe's t.,** a t. for indican; to 10 cc. of urine add an equal amount of hydrochloric acid after shaking, add 1 to 2 cc. of a weak solution of calcium chloride and 3 or 4 cc. of chloroform; if the urine contains indican the droplets of chloroform which sink to the bottom of the tube have a blue or purplish color.

**Janet's t.,** the patient is told to say "yes" or "no" according as he feels or does not feel the touch of the examiner's finger; in the case of functional anesthesia he may say "no" when an anesthetic area is touched (the eyes being closed), but will say nothing, being unaware that he is touched, in cases of organic anesthesia.

**Jolles' t.,** a t. for bile; a precipitate is obtained by agitation with chloroform, a solution of barium chloride, and hydrochloric acid; the precipitate is removed and the addition of a drop or two of sulfuric acid will produce a play of color if bile pigments are present.

**Kahn t.,** a modification of the Meinicke precipitin (flocculation) t. for syphilis, the chief innovation being use of a greatly increased quantity of lipoidal antigen (alcoholic extract of powdered dry beef heart previously extracted with ether); introduced in 1922, the Kahn t., with various modifications, was a standard t. for several decades but has been supplanted by the VDRL t.

**Kathrein's t.,** Maréchal's t.; Smith's t.; Trousseau's t.; a 1 per cent alcoholic solution of iodine is poured gently over urine in a t. tube; if bile pigment is present an emerald green color appears at the line of contact.

**Kelling's t.,** a t. for lactic acid in gastric contents; the addition of a drop or two of a 5 per cent solution of ferric chloride to the diluted gastric contents will produce a greenish yellow color if lactic acid is present.

**ketogenic corticoids t.,** 17-ketogenic steroid assay t.

**17-ketogenic steroid assay t.,** ketogenic corticoids t.; a t. (performed on urine) that is valuable in diagnosis of adrenogenital syndrome and in some cases of Cushing's syndrome; it provides a better assessment of adrenocorticoid secretion than the 17-hydroxycorticosteroid t.

**17-ketosteroid assay t.,** a colorimetric t., based on the Zimmermann reaction, that indicates metabolites or adrenal and testicular steroids excreted as 17-ketones in the urine; increased values are most striking in adrenocortical tumors, decreased values in Addison's disease or in panhypopituitarism.

**Kober t.,** a t. for naturally occurring estrogens, based upon the production of a pink color (absorption maximum: 520 m$\mu$) when an estrogen is heated in a mixture of phenol and sulfuric acid.

**Kolmer t.,** a quantitative method for the Wassermann t. that, with numerous modifications (especially as to antigen), served as a standard for almost half a century.

**Korotkoff's t.,** while the artery above an aneurysm is compressed, the blood pressure in the distal circulation is estimated; if it is fairly high the collateral circulation is good.

**Krauss t.,** iodate *reaction* of epinephrine.

**Kurzrok-Ratner t.,** a t. for estrogens in urine; the urine is extracted with ethyl acetate; after purification the extract is subjected to bio-assay as in the Allen-Doisy t.

**Kveim t.,** an intradermal t. for the detection of sarcoidosis, done by injecting 0.1 cc. of Kveim antigen (obtained from lymph nodes of persons with sarcoidosis), and requiring skin biopsies after three and six weeks. Positive t. is indicated by typical tubercles and giant cell formation; Nickerson-Kveim t.

**Ladendorff's t.,** an obsolete t. for blood; upon adding ticture of guaiac and oil of eucalyptus to the suspected fluid and allowing the mixture to stand, the presence of blood will be indicated by a blue coloration below and a purplish one above.

**Landsteiner-Donath t.,** see Donath-Landsteiner *phenomenon.*

**Lange's t.,** gold sol t.; Zsigmondy's t.; an obsolete, nonspecific t. for altered proteins in spinal fluid. As originally used by Lange in 1912, the t. was thought to be specific for neurosyphilis; however, this proved to be incorrect. Dilutions of spinal fluid are made in saline and to these a colloidal gold solution is added; if altered proteins are present, there is a color change or precipitate formed. At present, its chief use is to demonstrate cerebrospinal fluid protein abnormalities in multiple sclerosis.

**Langley's t.,** a t. for epinephrine; the movements of a loop of rabbit's intestine suspended in oxygenated Locke's solution are inhibited by adrenaline.

**latex t.,** a procedure that is useful in the diagnosis of rheumatoid arthritis; monodisperse polystyrene latex particles are suspended in a dilute solution of $\gamma$-globulin and incubated (at 56°C. for 30 minutes) with equal aliquots of serial dilutions of the patient's serum; if the latter contains "rheumatoid factor" (a macroglobulin that includes a hexose, hexosamine, and sialic acid), the latex particles are agglutinated; the t. yields positive results in most examples of rheumatoid arthritis, and relatively few nonspecific reactions are observed in other diseases.

**Legal's t.,** a t. for acetone; the urine is rendered alkaline by a few drops of a solution of potassium hydroxide, and to this are added 2 or 3 drops of a freshly prepared 10 per cent solution of sodium nitroprusside; it is colored red, then yellow; then a few drops of acetic acid are trickled down the side of the t. tube and at the line of junction of the two fluids is formed a carmine or purple ring.

**Liebermann-Burchard t.,** a colorimetric t. for unsaturated sterols, notably cholesterol; a blue-green color develops when such substances are added to acetic anhydride and sulfuric acid in chloroform.

**line t.,** a t. for rickets, based on observation of the lines of calcification in the growing ends of rachitic long bones in rats given vitamin D preparations under standard test, condition; used in biological assay of vitamin D by the U.S.P.

**Lombard voice-reflex t.,** the observation of fluctuations in the intensity of a patient's voice when a masking noise is increased or decreased; a t. useful in assessing functional hearing loss.

**Lücke's t.,** a t. for hippuric acid; add hot nitric acid to the urine and evaporate to dryness; the presence of hippuric acid is indicating by an odor of nitrobenzol upon further heating.

**Machado-Guerreiro t.,** a complement-fixation t. for infection with *Trypanosoma cruzi.*

**macrophage migration inhibition t.,** migration inhibition t.

**MacWilliam's t.,** on the additon of a few cyrstals of salicylsulfonic acid to 30 drops of urine in a small test tube, a precipitate not dissipated on heating indicates albumin; if boiling clears the urine the precipitate is albumose.

**male frog t.,** the urine or serum of a woman injected into male *Rana pipiens* (frogs) causes excretion of spermatozoa if the woman is pregnant.

**Malerba's t.,** a t. for acetone, the presence of which is indicated by the appearance of a red color on the addition of dimethylparaphenylenediamine.

**Maly's t.,** van der Velden's t. for free hydrochloric acid; the presence of hydrochloric acid will change the color of a solution of methylene blue from violet to blue or bluish green.

**Mantoux t.,** the intracutaneous tuberculin t.

**Maréchal's t.,** Kathrein's t.

**Markee t.,** an obsolete t. for pregnancy, based upon the vascular reaction of a scrap of endometrium transplanted into the anterior chamber of the eye of a rabbit when injected with the serum of a pregnant woman.

**Master's t., Master's two-step exercise t.,** see two-step exercise t.

**Mauthner's t.,** a t. for color perception similar to Holmgrèn's, but made with vials filled with pigments instead of with skeins of worsted.

**maximal HISTALOG t.,** HISTALOG t.

**McMurray t.,** test for rotation of tibia on femur for injury to meniscal structures.

**McPhail t.,** a t. for progesterone and like substances; immature female rabbits are treated with 150 international units of estrone over a period of 6 days; the t. material is then given in five daily subcutaneous doses; progestational proliferation of the endometrium is noted and the results estimated according to a scale from 0 to + + + +. The unit is taken as the amount required to produce an average (+ +) response; it is equivalent to 0.25 mg. of progesterone.

**Meinicke t.,** the first successful application (1917-1918) of immune precipitation to diagnosis of syphilis, but now obsolete, based on the phenomenon that flocculation occurs when lipoidal antigen (alcoholic tissue extract) diluted $1/8$ with distilled water is added to serum and that when salt solution is then added the precipitate of normal serum redissolves whereas that of syphilitic serum remains insoluble; there were several modifications, the last of which (1919) introduced precipitin test antigen prepared from dried heart muscle previously extracted with ether.

**melanoflocculation t.,** an obsolete, nonspecific serologic t. for malaria; flocculation occurs when a suspension of melanin is added to malarial serum; believed to depend upon an increase of euglobulin in the serum. At present, the t. has only historical value.

**Meltzer-Auer t.,** a t. for epinephrine; after excision of the superior cervical sympathetic ganglion the dilator response of the iris of the rabbit to epinephrine is greatly enhanced; see also paradoxical pupillary *reaction.*

**Meltzer-Lyon t.,** used in diagnosis of gallbladder conditions; 25 cc. of a 25 per cent solution of magnesium sulfate are delivered into the region of the sphincter of Oddi through a duodenal tube. This causes contraction of the gallbladder, relaxation of the sphincter, and the expulsion of bile from the common duct and gallbladder. The bile from the common duct is pale and is expelled first, that from the gallbladder follows. The samples are examined for pus cells, pigment granules, epithelial cells, cholesterol, etc.

**3-methoxy-4-hydroxymandelic acid t.,** vanillylmandelic acid t.

**methylene blue t.,** Achard-Castaigne method; an obsolete t. for renal permeability impairment.

**metrotroph'ic t.,** Astwood's t.; a t. for the assay of estrogenic substances; immature female rats (25 to 49 gm.) are injected subcutaneously with the hormone and killed after 6 hours, when the increase in uterine weight (due largely to imbibation of water) is taken as the criterion of estrogenic activity.

**microprecipitation t.,** a precipitation t. in which reduced quantities of t. reagents are used.

**migration inhibition t.,** macrophage migration inhibition t.; an *in vitro* method of testing for cellular (delayed type) sensitivity; when specific antigen is present, peritoneal exudate cells (macrophages) from a sensitized animal do not migrate from the capillary tube in which they have been packed, or from a well in agar, in the manner characteristic of similar cells from a normal animal.

**milk-ring t.,** MR t., see abortus-Bang-ring t.

**Millon-Nasse t.,** a t. for protein, the tyrosine of which reacts with nitrite after a brief treatment with mercuric ion in acid to give a color.

**Minnesota multiphasic personality inventory t.,** a questionnaire type of psychological test for ages 16 and over, with 550 true-false statements coded in 14 personality scales in both individual and group forms; abbreviated MMPI.

**mixed agglutination t.,** see mixed agglutination *reaction.*

**mixed lymphocyte culture t.,** a t. for histocompatibility in which donor and recipient lymphocytes are mixed in culture; the degree of incompatibility is indicated by the number of cells that have undergone transformation and mitosis, or by the uptake of radioactive thymidine.

**Molisch's t.,** a color t. for sugar, which condenses with α-naphthol or thymol in the presence of strong sulfuric acid, which converts the sugar to furfural derivatives.

**Moloney's t.,** a t. to detect a high degree of sensitivity to diphtheria toxoid; more than a minimal local reaction to diluted ($1/_{20}$) toxoid given intradermally indicates that prophylactic toxoid should be inoculated in fractional doses at suitable intervals.

**Morelli's t.,** an obsolete t. of historical value, used to distinguish between an exudate and a transudate; a few drops of the suspected fluid are added to a saturated solution of mercuric chloride in a t. tube; if the result is a flaky precipitate the fluid is a transudate; if a cohesive clot forms it is an exudate.

**Morner's t.,** (1) for cysteine, which gives a brilliant purple color with sodium nitroprusside; (2) for tyrosine, gives a green color on boiling with sulfuric acid containing formaldehyde.

**Moszkowicz' t.,** hyperemia t.; a lower limb is made anemic by means of an Esmarch bandage, which is removed at the end of 5 minutes; one then notes the return of color, which normally reaches the tips of the toes in a few seconds, but in arteriosclerosis the color returns slowly, requiring sometimes several minutes to involve the entire limb.

**MR t.,** milk-ring t.

**multiple puncture tuberculin t.,** a kind of tine t.; see tuberculin t.

**mumps sensitivity t.,** a skin t. for sensitivity to mumps, in which inactivated mumps virus is used as antigen.

**Nagel's t.,** a t. for color vision in which one-half the field in an anomaloscope is illuminated with standard yellow, and the other half is matched with the yellow by the person tested by mixing red and green.

**Napier's aldehyde t.,** an obsolete, nonspecific diagnostic t. of historical interest, used as an initial indicator for kala azar; 5 ml. of blood are drawn from a vein and allowed to stand until the serum separates, 1 ml. of which is then placed in a t. tube and 1 drop of formalin added. In a certain proportion of kala azar cases jellification of the serum occurs within a few minutes (3 to 20), whereas normal serum remains fluid.

**neutraliza'tion t.,** protection t.

**Nickerson-Kveim t.,** Kveim t.

**Nicklè's t.,** a t. for cane sugar; heating with carbon tetrachloride to the boiling point produces a black color if the sugar is cane sugar (sucrose), but not if it is glucose.

**nic'titating membrane t.,** a t. for ephinephrine; see Cannon t.

**nitroprusside t.,** free sulfhydryl groups give a red color with sodium nitroprusside, $Na_2(NO)Fe(CN)_5\cdot2H_2O$, in ammoniacal solution.

**Nothnagel's t.,** a t. to determine the direction of the intestine in abdominal operation; one places a small crystal of sodium chloride on the peritoneal surface of the gut; this causes ascending peristalsis, or antiperistalsis.

**nystagmus t.,** Bárány's caloric t.

**Obermayer's t.,** a t. for indican; precipitate the solids in the urine by means of a 20 per cent solution of acetate of lead, filter, and add to the filtrate fuming hydrochloric acid containing a small amount of ferric chloride solution; the addition now of chloroform causes the formation of indigo, indicated by the blue color, if indican is present.

**17-OH-corticoids t.,** 17-hydroxycorticosteroid t.

**ophthalmic t.,** conjunctival *reaction.*

**optical t.,** Abderhalden t.

**orcin t., orcinol t.,** Bial's t.

**Ott's t.,** a t. for "conjugated protein" (presumably nucleoprotein) in the urine; involving precipitation with tannic acid in strong salt solution.

**Ouchterlony t.,** double gel diffusion t. in two dimensions (see gel diffusion precipitin t. in two dimensions).

**ovarian ascorbic acid depletion t.,** used to measure the quantity of luteinizing hormone in tissue, blood, or urine.

**ovarian hypere'mia t.,** an obsolete t. for activity of the lutein stimulating hormone (LSH) of the hypophysis, and as a pregnancy t., in which infantile female rats are used.

**P and P t.,** prothrombin and proconvertin t.

**Pachon's t.,** determination of the collateral circulation, in a case of aneurysm, by estimation of the blood pressure.

**Palmer acid t. for peptic ulcer,** in duodenal ulcer, the administration of acid by duodenal tube causes severe pain.

**palmin t., palmitin t.,** a t. of pancreatic efficiency, based upon the fact that the presence of fat in the stomach causes the pylorus to open and admit the pancreatic juice; this splits the palmin so that an examination of the stomach contents, after a t. meal containing palmin, will reveal the presence of fatty acids.

**pancreozymin-secretin t.,** see secretin t.

**Pandy's t.,** Pandy's *reaction.*

**Papanicolaou smear t.,** see cytologic *examination.*

**parallax t.,** see phi *phenomenon.*

**patch t.,** a t. of skin sensitiveness; a small piece of blotting paper or cloth, wet with the t. fluid, is applied to the skin and on removal of the patch the area previously covered is compared with the uncovered surface.

**Patrick's t.,** fabere sign; a t. to distinguish arthritis of the hip from sciatica; with the patient supine the thigh and knee are flexed and the external malleolus is placed above the patella of the opposite leg; except in advanced cases this can ordinarily be done without pain, but on depressing the knee, pain is promptly elicited if the case is one of arthritis of the hip.

**Paul's t.,** Paul's *reaction.*

**PBI t.,** protein-bound iodine t.

**performance t.,** a t., such as five of the eleven Wechsler adult intelligence scale subtests, requiring little or no verbal instruction from the examiner and virtually no verbal response by the examinee.

**Perls' t.,** a t. for hemosiderin, the presence of which is indicated by a blue color on the addition of potassium ferrocyanide and hydrochloric acid.

**personality t.,** any of the category of psychological t.'s designed to test the characteristics of the personality, emotional status, mental disorder, etc., in contrast to intelligence t.

**Perthes' t.,** a t. for patency of deep femoral vein; with the patient standing, a tourniquet is applied above the knee. After walking, if deep circulation is competent, the superficial varicosities remain unchanged and legs become painful.

**phe'nolsul'fonphtha'lein t.,** Geraghty t.; phthalein t.; red t.; Rowntree and Geraghty t.; a t. for renal function; the patient having drunk a glass or two of water, 1 cc. of a 0.6 per cent solution of dye is injected hypodermically; the time between this injection and the appearance of a pink tinge in the urine as it falls into an alkaline solution is noted; the amount excreted in each of the next 2 hours is then estimated colorimetrically.

**phe'noltet'rachlorphtha'lein t.,** a t. of the functional activity of the liver; the dye in a specially prepared solution is injected intravenously, and the stools are then collected for 48 hours and the urine for 24, and examined to determine the amount of the dye excreted; a diminution of the amount normally recovered from the feces offers a presumption of disease of the liver.

**phentol'amine t.,** a t. for pheochromocytoma; phentolamine (5 mg. intravenously) administration reduces hypertension due to a pheochromocytoma but not that due to other causes, *e.g.,* essential hypertension; the blood pressure is raised by the drug in the latter form of hypertension.

**phloroglu'cin-HCl t.,** Tollens' *reaction.*

**photostress t.,** prolongation of visual blurring after a timed exposure to intense light reveals macular dysfunction.

**phrenic pressure t.,** pressure is made on the phrenic nerve on each side, above the clavicles where the nerve passes over the scalenus anticus muscle; if pain is felt, the patient inclining the head to the painful side, the trouble is in the pleural space; if the head does not incline to one side, the trouble is in the abdominal cavity.

**phthalein t.,** phenolsulfonphthalein t.

**pineapple t.,** a t. for butyric acid in the stomach; if a few drops of a strong sulfuric acid and alcohol are added to a dried ethereal extract of the gastric juice, a pineapple odor (ethyl butyrate) will be given off if butyric acid was present.

**Piria's t.,** a t. for tyrosine; concentrated sulfuric acid forms tyrosine-sulfuric acid; this is neutralized with barium carbonate, filtered, and treated with $FeCl_3$, when a violet color appears.

**Pirquet's t.,** Pirquet's reaction; a cutaneous tuberculin t.; see tuberculin t.

**plasmacrit t.,** a serologic screening method as an aid in the diagnosis of syphilis, based on the use of only a few drops of heparinized blood (the latter being collected in a special capillary tube after pricking a finger) the capillary tube is centrifuged in order to collect plasma, which is then mixed with a 0.01-ml. drop of antigen (cardiolipin previously treated with choline chloride as an antiinhibitor, in order to avoid falsely negative results that may occur with nonheated plasma or serum). After mechanically agitating the antigen-plasma mixture for 4 min., the presence or absence of flocculation is observed. A positive result should not be regarded as conclusively diagnostic, but a negative result excludes the likelihood of syphilis.

**Poehl's t.,** cholera-red *reaction.*

**polyuria t.,** Albarran's t.

**Porges-Meier t.,** an early flocculation t. for syphilis; of significance in having introduced as antigens acetone-insoluble, alcohol-soluble fractions of tissue, and lecithin.

**Porges-Salomon t.,** an early, obsolete, flocculation t. for syphilis in which sodium glycocholate served as "antigen".

**Porter-Silber chromogens t.,** 17-hydroxycorticosteroid t.

**precip'itin t.,** Bordet's t.; an *in vitro* t. in which antigen is in soluble form and precipitates when it combines with added specific antibody in the presence of an electrolyte. See also gel diffusion precipitin t.'s and ring precipitin t.

**pregnancy t.'s,** see immunologic pregnancy t.; also Aschheim-Zondek, ovarian hyperemia, Xenopus, Friedman, and Markee t.'s.

**prism vergence t.,** measurement of amplitude of fusion by placing prisms of gradually increasing power in the direction tested until diplopia results.

**projective t.,** a loosely structured psychological t. containing many ambiguous stimuli that require the subject to reveal his own feelings, personality, or psychopathology in response to them; *e.g.,* the Rorschach and thematic apperception t.'s.

**protection t.,** neutralization t.; a t. to determine the antimicrobial activity of a serum by inoculating a susceptible animal with a mixture of the serum and the virus or other microbe being tested.

**protein-bound iodine t.,** PBI t.; a widely used t. of thyroid function; serum protein-bound iodine is measured to provide an estimate of hormone bound to protein in peripheral blood.

**prothrom'bin t.,** Quick's t.; a quantitative t. for prothrombin in blood based on the clotting time of oxalated blood plasma in the presence of thromboplastin and calcium chloride. See also prothrombin *time.*

**prothrombin and proconvertin t.,** P and P t.; a t. used by some to control anticoagulant therapy with bishydroxycoumarin and indandione drugs.

**provocative t.,** a t. for pheochromocytoma, *e.g.,* histamine t., which when positive provokes a paroxysm of hypertension.

**provocative Wassermann t.,** an obsolete t. of historical interest only; the employment of the Wassermann test one or two days up to one or two weeks after the administration of arsphenamine or neoarsphenamine; the result may then be positive when before the giving of arsphenamine it was negative.

**psychological t.'s,** t.'s designed to measure a person's achievements, intelligence, skills, personality, or individual and occupational characteristics, or potentialities; see also subentries under scale.

**psychomotor t.'s,** psychological t.'s which, although based on other psychological processes (*e.g.,* sensory, perceptual), require a motor reaction such as copying designs, building blocks, or manipulating controls.

**pulp t.,** vitality t.

**pyrogen t.,** a t. for the presence of pyrogens in a fluid prepared for parenteral use. Healthy rabbits, weighting 1500 gm. or more, which have been kept for a week on a uniform, unrestricted diet, are used. After removing each animal from its cage 15 min. is allowed to elapse when its rectal temperature is taken. This control temperature should not be lower then 38.9°C. nor higher than 39.8°C. Food is withheld for 1 hr. before the t. and until the t. is completed. The material to be tested should be warmed to 37°C. and 10 cc. per kg. of body weight injected within 15 min. of taking the control temperature. The rectal temperature is recorded hourly for 3 hr. after the injection. Three rabbits are used for each t.; if two, or all three rabbits show a rise of 0.6°C. or more, the t. is positive (*i.e.,* the material contains pyrogen). If one animal shows a rise of 0.6°C. or more, or if the sum of the temperatures of the three rabbits exceeds 1.4°C., the t. is repeated with five rabbits; if two or more show a rise of 0.6°C. or over, the t. is positive. All syringes, needles, etc., used for the injections must be rendered pyrogen-free by a suitable method.

**Queckenstedt-Stookey t.,** compression of the jugular vein in a healthy person causes a rapid increase in the pressure of the spinal fluid within 10 to 12 seconds, and an equally rapid fall to normal on release of the pressure of the vein; when there is a block of subarachnoid channels, compression of the vein causes little or no increase of pressure in the cerebrospinal fluid.

**Quick's t.'s,** prothrombin t.

**quinine carbacryl'ic resin t.,** a t. for gastric anacidity. See quinine carbacrylic *resin.*

**Quinlan's t.,** a t. for bile; when a thin layer of bile is examined through a spectroscope, absorption lines appear in the violet.

**radial compression t. of Allen,** a t. for patency of the ulnar artery and the palmar arterial arch; the examiner occludes the radial artery at the wrist while the patient squeezes the blood out of his hand by clenching his fist; while radial compression is maintained, the patient relaxes his hand; if color fails to return to the hand within 3 seconds, occlusion of the ulnar artery or ulnar side of the palmar arch is probable.

**radioactive colloidal gold (198Au) t.,** a t. of liver function in which the t. agent is removed from the blood by reticuloendothelial cells of the liver and other organs; scintillation scanning of the liver allows determination of size and contour of the liver, as well as the presence of space-occupying masses; this t. is used in preference to the rose bengal radioactive (131I) t. in patients with cirrhosis of the liver.

**radioactive iodide uptake t.,** 131I uptake t.

**RAI t.,** 131I uptake t.

**rapid plasma reagin t. for treponematoses,** RPR t.; a group of serologic t.'s for syphilis in which unheated serum or plasma is reacted with a standard test antigen containing charcoal particles. Positive t.'s yield a flocculation. One modification called the RPR (circle) card t. is widely used as a screening t.

**Raygat's t.,** if the lungs of a dead infant float in water it is a sign that the child was born alive; called also the hydrostatic t.

**Rayleigh t.,** a t. for color vision similar to that used in the anomaloscope. If the subject's appreciation of red is defective he adds more red than does a normal person to the yellow light; if his color vision is defective in respect to green, he adds more of this color.

**red t.,** phenolsulfonphthalein t.

**red cell adherence t.,** adhesion t.

**Reinsch's t.,** a strip of copper is placed in the suspected fluid, which is then acidulated with hydrochloric acid and boiled; if arsenic is present a gray deposit occurs on the copper, and this deposit on heating is sublimated and deposited as a crystalline layer on a piece of glass held above the copper strip.

**Reiter t.,** a complement-fixation test for syphilis using as antigen material prepared from the Reiter strain of *Treponema pallidum;* the t. has been largely replaced in laboratory medicine by the fluorescent treponemal antibody-absorption (FTA-ABS) t.

**resor'cinol-HCl t.,** Selivanoff's t.

**Reuss' t.,** a t. for atropine; the addition of oxidizing agents and sulfuric acid to a liquid containing atropine produces an odor of orange-flowers and roses.

**Rh blocking t.,** a t. for nonagglutinating Rh antibodies. An Rh agglutination t. is first carried out. If the t. for Rh agglutinins is negative, then 1 drop of anti-$Rh_0$ agglutinating serum of moderate titer is mixed with the patient's serum containing Rh-positive t. cells. If after incubating for from 1 to 2 hr. at 37°C. no agglutination occurs, $Rh_0$-blocking antibodies are assumed to be present in the patient's serum.

**Riegel's t.,** a t. for rennin; 5 cc. of neutralized gastric juice are added to 10 cc. of milk, and if coagulation occurs after incubation for 15 minutes rennin is present.

**Rimini's t.,** a t. for formaldehyde in urine, milk, and other fluids, by the use of dilute solution of phenylhydrazine hydrochloride, sodium nitroprusside, and sodium hydroxide.

**ring t.,** ring precipitin t.

**ring precipitin t.,** ring t.; a precipitin t. in which antigen solution is carefully layered over antibody solution in a tube; as diffusion proceeds a disk of precipitate forms where the antibody ratio is optimal.

**Rinne's t.,** (1) *positive t.:* a vibrating tuning fork is held in contact with the skull (usually the mastoid process) until the sound is lost, its prongs are then brought close to the auditory orifice when, if the hearing is normal, a faint sound will again be heard; (2) *negative t.:* a vibrating tuning fork is heard longer and louder when in contact with the skull than when held near the auditory orifice, indicating some disorder of the sound conducting apparatus.

**Robinson-Kepler-Power t.,** a rarely used t. for adrenal insufficiency based upon the delayed diuresis after drinking water which occurs in this condition; a dangerous t. because of the risk of water intoxication.

**Römer's t.,** a t. of historical interest only; tuberculin, either pure or diluted, is injected intracutaneously into a guinea pig; if the animal is tuberculous a large papule with a necrotic hemorrhagic center appears in about 24 hours; this is called the cocarde or cockade reaction.

**Rorschach t.,** a projective psychological t. in which the subject reveals his attitudes, emotions, and personality by responding to a series of 10 inkblot pictures.

**rose bengal radioactive (131I) t.,** a t. of liver function used as a means of measuring hepatic blood flow and for scintillation scanning of the liver to determine size and contour of the liver, or the presence of space-occupying masses in the liver; see also radioactive colloidal gold (198Au) t.

**Rose-Waaler t.,** a t. of historical interest only; when sheep red cells are suspended in a concentration of antiserum to sheep red cells which is too low to cause agglutination, the addition of serum from a patient with rheumatoid arthritis will cause agglutination.

**Rosenbach's t.,** a t. for bile in the urine; the suspected urine is passed several times through the same filter paper,

this is then dried and touched with a drop of slightly fuming nitric acid when the play of colors characteristic of the bile pigments is produced, *viz.,* a yellow spot surrounded by rings of red, violet, blue, and green.

**Rosenbach-Gmelin t.,** Gmelin's t.

**Rosenblueth and Cannon t.,** a t. for epinephrine; the nictitating membrane of the cat contracts in response to a minute dose of epinephrine.

**Ross-Jones t.,** a t. for an excess of globulin in the cerebrospinal fluid; 1 ml. of cerebrospinal fluid is carefully floated over 2 ml. of a concentrated ammonium sulfate solution and if globulin is present in excess a fine white ring appears at the line of junction in about 3 minutes.

**Rothera's nitroprusside t.,** 5 ml. of fresh urine are saturated with solid ammonium sulfate and mixed with 10 drops of freshly prepared 2 per cent sodium nitroprusside solution, which is the mixed with 10 drops of concentrated ammonia water and allowed to stand for 15 min. The presence of acetoacetic acid, or of larger concentrations of acetone, is indicated by the development of a blue-purple color. Hence, a test for ketone bodies.

**Rowntree and Geraghty t.,** phenolsulfonphthalein t.

**RPR t.,** rapid plasma reagin t.

**rubella HI t.,** hemagglutination-inhibiting (HI) t. for rubella; see hemagglutination *inhibition.*

**Rubin t.,** a t. of patency of the Fallopian tubes. A cannula is introduced into the cervix uteri, slight pressure being made so that the cervix is tightly closed. Carbon dioxide gas is passed through the cannula by means of a syringe with manometer attachment. Carbon dioxide in pressures up to 200 mm. Hg is forced out into the Fallopian tubes; if they are patent, the escape of gas into the abdominal cavity is evidenced by a high-pitched bubbling sound heard on auscultation over the lower abdomen. A tracing may be made on a kymograph. The patient may have shoulder pain from diaphragmatic irritation, or free gas under the diaphragm can be demonstrated by x-ray.

**Rubner's t.,** acetate of lead is added to the suspected urine and the latter is filtered; ammonia is added until a permanent precipitate is formed; if lactose is present, the precipitate will take on a pink to red color when the fluid is heated; if there is glucose, the color will be yellow to brown.

**Ruffmann t.,** a t. for epinephrine based upon the oxidation of the hormone by iodine liberated from iodate; the addition of sulfanilic acid and corrosive sublimate makes the iodate reaction more sensitive; see Krauss and Comessatti t.'s. This t. will detect 1 part of epinephrine in 400,000,000.

**Rumpel-Leede t.,** Rumple-Leede sign; bandage sign; Hess' t.; a tourniquet t. for capillary fragility.

**Sabin-Feldman dye t.,** a method for the detection of anti-toxoplasma antibody in serum, based on the fact that *Toxoplasma gondii* cells (from peritoneal exudate in mice) are fairly well stained with alkaline methylene blue, whereas organisms in a serum that contains specific antibody have no affinity for the dye; furthermore, normal toxoplasma cells become rounded, and the nucleus and cytoplasm deeply stained, when treated with the methylene blue; on the other hand, when dye is mixed with organisms and antibody, the cells retain their crescent shape and only the shrunken nuclear endosome is stained.

**Sachs-Georgi t.,** the first precipitin t. for syphilis of diagnostic practicality, the significant innovation having been the addition of cholesterol to the lipoidal antigen (alcoholic tissue extract) used in the earlier Meinicke t.

**Sahli's t.,** the salol t. of pancreatic efficiency; salol is decomposed into phenol and salicylic acid by the action of the pancreatic juice; therefore if these substances cannot be found in the urine 2 hours after the administration of 30 grains of salol, the pancreatic function is presumably in abeyance.

**salol t.,** Ewald's t. of the motility of the stomach; the patient swallows a tablet of salol, which is not decomposed until it reaches the intestine; hence the time of the appearance of phenol in the urine is a measure of the rapidity with which the salol was passed through the stomach.

**Saundby's t.,** a t. for blood in the stools; on the addition of 30 drops of a 20-volume hydrogen peroxide solution to a mixture of 10 drops of a saturated benzidine solution and a small quantity of feces in a test tube, a persistent dark blue color denotes the presence of blood.

**scarification t.,** a t., *e.g.,* Pirquet's t., in which a material is pricked or scratched into the skin.

**Schaffer's t.,** decolorize the fluid with animal charcoal and then add 4 cc. of a 10 per cent solution of acetic acid and 3 drops of a 5 per cent solution of potassium ferrocyanide; if nitrites are present an intense yellow color will be produced.

**Schellong t.,** the subject is required to stand for 10 to 20 minutes, during which time the blood pressure is measured continuously; a fall of systolic pressure of 20 mm. Hg or more indicates poor circulatory function.

**Schick t.,** Schick method; a t. for susceptibility to *Corynebacterium diphtheriae* toxin; 0.1 ml. of Schick test toxin is injected into the skin of one forearm (test site) and the same quantity of the same, but heat-inactivated, material into the skin of the other forearm (control site); subjects with toxin-neutralizing antibodies either will have no reaction at either injection site (negative test) or may have a pseudoreaction due to antibodies for substances (antigens) in the test materials other than diphtheria toxin *per se*—pale red areas of the delayed kind of induced sensitivity (immune) reaction reaching a maximum within 48 hours and then receding; subjects lacking toxin-neutralizing antibodies either may have a simple positive reaction (a red area that appears at the test site only and increases in intensity, in contrast to the pseudoreaction) for 5 or more days, or this positive reaction may occur along with a pseudoreaction (combined reaction).

**Schiff's t.,** (1) for sugar in the urine; a piece of filter paper impregnated with xylidine and glacial acetic acid is exposed to the vapor of urine heated with sulfuric acid; if sugar is present the paper is reddened; (2) for urea; when furfurol and hydrochloric acid are added to a liquid containing urea a purple color is produced; (3) for uric acid; filter paper impregnated with silver nitrate and dipped in an alkaline liquid containing uric acid turns brown; (4) for aldehyde; a blue or purple color appears when an aqueous solution of fuchsin (0.25 gm. in 1000 cc.), decolorized by sulfur dioxide, is added to a material containing aldehyde.

**Schiller's t.,** a test for non-glycogen-containing areas of the portio vaginalis of the cervix, which may be the site of early carcinoma; such areas fail to stain dark brown with iodine solution; loss of glycogen due to erosion and other benign conditions may also give a positive result.

**Schilling t.,** a procedure for determining the amount of vitamin $B_{12}$ excreted in the urine using cyanocobalamine tagged with a radioisotope of cobalt.

**Schirmer t.,** a paper strip test for tear production.

**Schönbein's t.,** Almén's t. for blood.

**Schwabach t.,** a series of five tuning forks of different tones is used and the number of seconds is noted in which the patient can hear each by air and bone conduction.

**Schwarz's t.,** a t. for sulfonmethane, heating of which with charcoal gives rise to the odor of mercaptan.

**scratch t.,** a form of skin t. in which antigen is applied through a scratch in the skin.

**screening t.,** any testing procedure designed to separate people or objects according to a fixed characteristic or property.

**Seashore t.,** a t. of innate musical ability in which sense of pitch, intensity, rhythm, and other components of musical "talent" are measured.

**secretin t.,** a test of pancreatic exocrine function, variably performed and standardized, in which the bicarbonate, amylase and volume of the duodenal aspirate are measured after intravenous administration of secretion.

**sedimentation t.,** the use in gastric roentgenology of a nonsuspended mixture of a contrast salt, such as barium or bismuth, in water; the salt sediments rapidly and can be spread over all parts of the stomach wall, thus giving information as to shape and movement of the organ, and also bringing into view lesions on the anterior or posterior wall invisible when the stomach is full.

**Seidlitz powder t.,** distention of the stomach in a case of suspected diaphragmatic hernia by means of a Seidlitz powder, thus rendering the herniated loop of stomach visible roentgenologically.

**Selivanoff's t.,** a t. for fructose in urine, which gives a color when heated with resorcinol in acid.

**Selye and Schenker t.,** see cold t.

**serum t.,** precipitation t. for serum.

**sexual receptivity t.,** a t. for progestational substances; ovariectomized virgin guinea pigs, previously treated with estrogen, give the copulatory or lordosis reflex (raising of the pudenda, arching and straightening of the back) in response to stimulation of the vulva, if a progestogen has been administered.

**shadow t.,** retinoscopy.

**sickle cell t,** in an anaerobic wet preparation containing equal amounts of blood and 2 per cent sodium bisulfite, erythrocytes containing hemoglobin S undergo a change in shape to a sickle cell form; the number of sickled red cells per 1000 red blood cells is determined, and expressed as a percentage.

**single (gel) diffusion precipitin t. in one dimension,** see gel diffusion precipitin t.'s in one dimension.

**single (gel) diffusion precipitin t. in two dimensions,** see gel diffusion precipitin t.'s in two dimensions.

**SISI t.** (small increment sensitivity index), the sounding of a tone 20 db. above threshold, followed by a series of 200 millisecond tones 1 db. louder; perception of these is indicative of cochlear damage.

**situational t.,** in psychology and psychiatry, a t. situation in which a subject is observed as he performs a daily task or an actual sample of the job or role he will fill.

**skin t.,** skin reaction; cutireaction t.; cutaneous t.; a commonly used method for determining induced sensitivity (allergy) by applying an antigen (allergen) to, or inoculating it into, the skin; induced sensitivity (allergy) to the specific antigen is indicated by an inflammatory reaction of one or other of two general kinds: immediate or delayed (microbial). The former appears in minutes to an hour or so and in general is dependent upon circulating immunoglobulins (antibodies), whereas the latter is not dependent upon these soluble substances but upon leukocytic infiltration.

**skin-puncture t.** (for Behçet's syndrome), after pricking the skin with a sterile needle, pustulation follows within 24 hours owing to the dermal sensitivity in this disease.

**smear t.,** see smear.

**Smith's t.,** Kathrein's t.

**Smith-Smith t.,** a t. for urinary estrogen; the conjugated folliculoids are first hydrolyzed and the resulting free, more active estrogens concentrated and purified, then dissolved in oil and assayed by the vaginal smear t. upon spayed rats.

**Snyder's t.,** colorimetric caries susceptibility t.

**spironolactone t.,** the administration of spironolactone, 400 mg. orally, for 4 consecutive days; an increase in serum potassium during the t., and a decrease afterward, strongly suggest primary aldosteronism.

**standing t.,** a t. for the effect of a hypotensive drug, carried out by the patient himself. He is advised after taking the drug to stand perfectly still for 1 minute commencing from the time that the maximal action of the drug should be manifested; if the dose is adequate the patient should experience a slight hypotensive reaction.

**station t.,** Romberg's *sign.*

**Stein's t.,** in cases of labyrinthine disease the patient is unable to stand or to hop on one foot with his eyes shut.

**Stenger t.,** a test for detecting simulation of unilateral deafness.

**Stewart's t.,** estimation of the amount of collateral circulation, in case of an aneurysm of the main artery of a limb, by means of a calorimeter.

**Stormont t.,** a modification of the intradermal tuberculin t. in its application to cattle; two injections are made into the same skin site, the second 7 days after the first, and the reactions are judged 24 hours after the second injection; the t. receives its name from the Irish experiment station at Stormont, where it was first used.

**Strasburg's t.,** a t. for bile in the urine; albumin, if present, is precipitated, then cane sugar is added and filter paper is dipped in the fluid and dried; if bile pigments are present in the urine sulfuric acid will turn the filter paper a reddish violet color.

**Strauss' t.,** an obsolete t. of historical interest only, for lactic acid in the contents of the stomach, by means of a solution of ferric chloride and ether.

**string t.,** in gastrointestinal hemorrhage a string is swallowed and removed, each time allowing the string to go further down the gut. If blood is encountered a rough estimate of the location of the blood is possible. See also fluorescein string t.

**Strong vocational interest t.,** a t. that matches an individual's interests to those characteristic of persons working in a number of vocations.

**sulfosalicylic acid turbidity t.,** a t. for measurement of protein in urine; sulfosalicylic acid precipitates protein in urine with a turbidity that is approximately proportional to the concentration of protein in a solution.

**sweat t.,** a test for cystic fibrosis of the pancreas, revealing abnormal elevation of sodium chloride content.

**sweating t.,** a t. for locating the level of a lesion in the spinal cord; when the body is heated or the patient is given a diaphoretic, sweat secretion is absent below the level of the lesion.

**swimming t.,** a t. for activity of adrenal cortical preparations. Rats, two days after adrenalectomy, are placed in water and the time during which they can swim recorded. They are then injected with the material to be tested. The response is termed "positive" if the swimming time is doubled.

**swordfish t.,** *Xiphophorus* t.; a rarely used t. for androgenic activity, based upon the fact that androgens cause the development of the sword, a male structure, in female swordfish (*Xiphophorus helleri*).

**T3 uptake t.,** triiodothyronine uptake t.; a radioiodine t. of thyroid function in which radioiodine is added to the patient's serum *in vitro;* the t. measures the relative affinities of serum proteins and of an added competitive substance for radioactive T3; higher T3 uptakes are associated with hyperthyroidism; administration of iodides does not seem to affect the t.

**t t.,** a statistical method that is analogous to the calculation of the normal deviate, both of which are t.'s of significance; the formula for the *t* t. is $t = (x - \bar{x})/s$, where the numerator is the deviation from the mean, and the denominator is the standard deviation for sample sizes of less than 30 cases.

**thematic apperception t.,** a projective psychological t. in which the subject is asked to tell a story about standard ambiguous pictures depicting life-situations to reveal his own attitudes and feelings; abbreviated TAT.

**thermostable opsonin t.,** a t. for opsonic activity of antibody in the absence of effect of heat-labile complement.

**Thompson's t.,** two-glass t.; the urine, in a case of gonorrhea, is passed into two glasses; if the gonococci and gonorrheal threads are found only in the first glass the probability is that the process is limited to the anterior urethra.

**Thormählen's t.,** a t. for melanin; the suspected liquid is treated with sodium nitroprusside, caustic potash, and acetic acid; if melanin is present the solution takes on a deep blue color.

**Thorn t.,** a putative t. of adrenal cortical function; stimulation of a normally functioning adrenal cortex by the adrenocorticotrophic hormone is followed by a reduction in the number of circulating eosinophils and lymphocytes and an increase in the excretion of uric acid. The t. lacks sufficient specificity and is rarely used.

**three-glass t.,** Valentine's t.; the bladder is emptied by passing urine into a series of 3-ounce test tubes, and the contents of the first and the last examined; the first tube contains the washings from the anterior urethra, the second, material from the bladder, and the last, material from the posterior urethra, prostate, and seminal vesicles.

**Thudichum's t.,** a t. for creatinine; a mixture of the suspected fluid with dilute ferric chloride solution will turn dark red on heating, if creatinine is present.

**thymol turbidity t.,** an obsolete procedure that may be used as a laboratory aid in the diagnosis of hepatic dysfunction, based on the fact that a certain amount of turbidity occurs when normal serum is mixed with a saturated solution of thymol, but greater degrees of turbidity are observed with serum from patients who have hepatitis; the amount of turbidity may be measured with a photoelectric colorimeter or by means of comparison with artificial standards. The t. does not indicate a specific dysfunction, and may be positive in other diseases.

**thyroid-stimulating hormone t.,** TSH t.; a t. that measures the uptake of $^{131}$I in the thyroid gland before and after administration of a thyroid-stimulating hormone; this t. is useful in the study of patients with pituitary myxedema, primary myxedema, or postthyroidectomy states.

**tine t.,** see tuberculin t.

**Tizzoni's t.,** a t. for iron in the tissue; it consists in treating the tissue with a 2 per cent solution of potassium ferrocyanide and then with a 0.5 per cent solution of hydrochloric acid; a blue coloration indicates the presence of iron.

**tone decay t.,** the sounding of a continuous tone at threshold for 1 min. if the intensity must be increased by more than 5 db. for continued perception it is thought to be a sign of retrocochlear damage.

**Töpfer's t.,** an obsolete t. for free hydrochloric acid in the gastric contents; by means of the indicator, dimethylaminoazobenzene.

**total catecholamine t.,** catecholamine t.; a fluorometric determination of catecholamines in 24-hour urine specimens; elevated values are seen in patients with pheochromocytoma and neuroblastoma; spurious elevations may be seen due to excretion products of medication containing adrenaline, tetracyclines, quinidine, and some antihypertensive agents; false positive elevations may be seen in persons with extensive burns, in vigorous exercise, or in progressive muscular dystrophy.

**tourniquet t.,** capillary fragility t.

**TPI t.,** abbreviation for *Treponema pallidum* immobilization t.

**transverse t.,** a t. for measuring resistance of plastics to bending.

**Trendelenburg's t.,** the leg is raised above the level of the heart until the veins are empty; it is then rapidly lowered and in case of varicosity and incompetence of the valves the veins will at once become distended.

**Treponema pallidum immobilization t.,** *Treponema pallidum* immobilization reaction; abbreviated TPI t.; a t. based upon the fact that an antibody other than Wassermann antibody is present in the serum of a syphilitic patient and which in the presence of complement causes the immobilization of actively motile *Treponema pallidum* obtained from testes of a rabbit infected with syphilis.

**triiodothyronine uptake t.,** T3 uptake t.

**Trommer's t.,** a t. for reducing sugar with alkaline copper sulfate solution.

**Trousseau's t.,** Kathrein's t.

**TSH t.,** thyroid-stimulating hormone t.

**tuberculin t.,** application of the skin t. to the diagnosis of infection by *Mycobacterium tuberculosis* in which tuberculin or its "purified" protein derivative serves as an antigen (allergen); injection of graduated doses of tuberculin or of purified protein derivative into the skin, most often by means of a needle and syringe (Mantoux t.) or by means of tines (tine t.); t. material may also be applied by means of a "patch" in which it is absorbed but this method (patch t.) is viewed as being less reliable; the t. is read on the basis of induration and erythema, the former being considered the more diagnostic of infection with the tubercle bacillus (*M. tuberculosis*); the t. does not distinguish between infection in a resistant person without disease and an individual with clinical manifestations of disease.

**Tuffier's t.,** Hallion's t.

**two-glass t.,** Thompson's t.

**two-step exercise t.,** Master's t.; exercise t.; a t. for coronary insufficiency; the subject makes two steps 9 inches high repeatedly for $1^1/_2$ minutes. The total number of steps to be made in the time is determined by the age, weight, and sex of the subject. Significant depression of RS-T in the electrocardiogram is considered abnormal and suggests coronary disease.

**Tzank t.,** the characteristic finding, in the fluid in bullae of pemphigus vulgaris, of Tzank cells, altered epithelial cells, rounded and devoid of intercellular attachments. The periphery is basophilic and the nucleus is spherical and enlarged with prominent nucleoli.

**Unterberger's t.,** with eyes closed, patient marks time for 1 minute; turning more than 60 degrees to one side suggests peripheral vestibular damage on that side.

**urea clearance t.,** a t. of renal function based on urea clearance.

**vaginal cornifica'tion t.,** a t. for estrogenic activity, in which the appearance of cornified epithelial cells in a vaginal smear of a test animal is an indication of the action of an estrogen.

**vaginal mucifica'tion t.,** a t. for progestational activity; stimulation of mucus production by the vaginal epithelium in rats, guinea pigs, or mice by progestogens.

**Valentine's t.,** three-glass t.

**Valsalva t.,** the heart is observed fluoroscopically while the patient performs the Valsalva maneuver; in normal persons the heart becomes smaller, but in the patient with impaired myocardial reserve it may dilate.

**van Deen's t.,** Almén's t. for blood.

**van den Bergh's t.,** a t. for bile pigments (bilirubin) by reaction with diazotized sulfanilic acid (Ehrlich's diazoreagent).

**van der Velden's t.,** a t. for free hydrochloric acid, the presence of which turns an added solution of methylene blue from violet to green; called also Maly's t.

**vanillylmandelic acid t.,** VMA t.; 3-methoxy-4-hydroxymandelic acid t.; a t. for catecholamine-secreting tumors (pheochromocytoma and neuroblastoma) performed on a 24-hour urine specimen; it is based on the fact that vanillylmandelic acid is the major urinary metabolite of norepinephrine and epinephrine.

**VDRL t.,** a flocculation t. for syphilis, using cardiolipin-lecithin-cholesterol antigen as developed by the venereal Disease Research Laboratory of the United States Public Health Service.

**vitality t.,** pulp t.; a test to help in determining whether a dental pulp is alive, diseased, or dead; usually some form of electrical stimulation is used.

**vitamin C t.,** capillary fragility t.

**VMA t.,** vanillylmandelic acid t.

**Volhard's t.,** the patient drinks 1500 cc. (about 3 pints) of water on an empty stomach; if the kidneys are normal all this fluid will be excreted by the end of 4 hours, the specific gravity of the urine being from 1001 to 1004.

**Vollmer's t.,** tuberculin "patch" t.

**Vulpian's t.,** see (1) ferric chloride *reaction* of epinephrine; (2) iodine *reaction* of epinephrine.

**Waldenström's t.,** a t. for porphyrin in the urine; 2 cc. of urine are mixed with an equal amount of a 2 per cent dimethyl-*p*-aminobenzaldehyde in 50/100 HCl. A red color appears if urobilinogen or porphobilinogen is present. The t. for urobilinogen is also known as Ehrlich's benzaldehyde reaction.

**Wang's t.,** a quantitative t. for indican, which is transformed into indigo-sulfuric acid and then titrated by a solution of potassium permanganate.

**Warren's t.,** Trommer's t.

**Wassén t.,** a t. for the diagnosis of lymphogranuloma venereum; it consists of causing a fatal encephalitis in mice by the injection of the chlamydia of the human disease. This is not a specific diagnostic t.

**Wassermann t.,** Wassermann reaction; a complement-fixation t. used in the diagnosis of syphilis. Originally the "antigen" was an extract of liver from a syphilitic fetus, but later the active substance was found to be present in normal tissues, including heart, is referred to as cardiolipin, and has been identified as a diphosphatidylglycerol.

**water-gurgle t.,** a gurgling sound heard on auscultation of the throat when the patient swallows, in cases of esophageal stricture.

**Weber's t. for hearing,** the application of a vibrating tuning fork to one of several points in the midline of the head or face, to ascertain in which ear the sound is heard best by bone conduction, that ear being the affected one if the sound-conducting apparatus (middle ear) is at fault (positive t.), but probably the normal one if the neurosensory apparatus is diseased (negative t.).

**Webster's t.,** a t. for trinitrotoluene in the urine.

**Weil's t.,** an obsolete t. based on the observation that washed red blood cells of syphilitic subjects are resistant to the hemolytic action of cobra venom.

**Wheeler-Johnson t.,** cystosine or uracil when treated with bromine yields dialuric acid which gives a green color with excess of barium hydroxide.

**Wormley's t.,** a t. for alkaloids, by treating the solution with picric acid or a dilute iodine-potassium-iodide solu-

tion, the presence of alkaloids being shown by a color reaction.

**worsted t.,** Holmgrèn's t.

**Wurster's t.,** a t. for tyrosine; the substance is dissolved in boiling water and quinone is added; if tyrosine is present a ruby colored reaction takes place, the solution changing to brown after a few hours.

**Wyle's t.,** a t. for creatinine; production of a ruby-red color in urine or a solution of creatinine treated with sodium nitroprusside and NaOH, the color soon changes to yellow.

**xan'thoprote'ic t.,** a t. for protein with which concentrated nitric acid gives a yellow solution as a result of nitration of tyrosine and tryptophan. The color changes in alkaline solution.

**Xenopus t.,** Hogben t.; an obsolete t. for pregnancy, in which *Xenopus laevis* is the test animal.

**Xiphoph'orus t.,** swordfish t.

**xylose t.,** a procedure used as a laboratory aid in diagnosing the alimentary type of pentosuria, and that occurring as a result of an inborn error of metabolism (*i.e.,* primary pentosuria). Xylose is the pentose that is excreted, and it may be identified as follows: (1) reduces Benedict's solution rapidly; (2) is not fermented by yeasts; (3) yields a positive Bial's t. for pentose.

**Yvon's t.,** (1) a t. for alkaloids; to the suspected solution is added a mixture of bismuth subnitrate, potassium iodide, and hydrochloric acid in water; a positive reaction is indicated by the appearance of a red color; (2) a t. for acetanilid in the urine; extract the suspected fluid with chloroform and heat with yellow nitrate of nercury; if acetanilid is present the fluid will be colored green.

**Ziehen t.,** the patient is asked to explain the difference between certain contrasted objects, such as water and ice, child and dwarf, or horse and ox.

**Zimmermann t.,** Zimmermann *reaction.*

**Zondek-Aschheim t.,** Aschheim-Zondek t.

**Zsigmondy's t.,** Lange's t.

**Zwenger's t.,** if a crystal of cholesterol is dropped into a mixture of 5 parts sulfuric acid and 1 part water, a red ring, changing to violet, will form.

---

**testa** (tes'tah) [ L. shell; TEST-1 ]. 1. A shell; egg shell. 2. In protozoology, usually termed test; an envelope of certain forms of protozoa, consisting of various earthy materials cemented to a chitinous base. 3. In botany, the outer, sometimes the only, coat of the seed.

**Testacea** (tes'ta'she-ah) [ L. *testa,* shell ]. A group of Sarcodina (amebae), in which the cells are provided with a firm chitinous envelope, often containing earthy material, with an opening through which the pseudopodia are protruded. Now generally divided among several taxa of amebae.

**testal'gia** [ testis + G. *algos,* pain ]. Orchialgia.

**tes'tane.** 5β-Androstane.

**testec'tomy** [ testis + G. G. *ektomē,* excision ]. Orchiectomy.

**testes** (tes'tēz) [ L. ]. Plural of testis.

**testicle** (tes'tĭ-kl) [ L. *testiculus,* dim. of *testis* ]. Testis.

**tes'ticond** [ testis + L. *condo,* to hide ]. A person having undescended testes.

**testicular** (tes-tik'u-lar). Relating to the testes.

**testic'ulus** [ L. ]. Testicle.

**testis,** pl. **testes** (tes'tis, -tēz) [ L. See TEST-2 ] [ NA ]. Testicle; one of the two male reproductive glands, located in the cavity of the scrotum.

**ectopic t.,** ectopia testis; parorchidium; (1) a condition in which the t. has descended but occupies an abnormal position, *e.g.,* in a superficial abdominal, inguinal, or femoral position; (2) a state in which one or both testes are abnormally situated.

**inverted t.,** one that is rotated in the scrotum, the epididymis being anterior.

**irritable t.,** neuralgia of the t.

**pulpy t.,** medullary sarcoma of the t.

**t. redux,** a condition in which there is a tendency in the testis to ascend to the upper part of the scrotum or into the inguinal canal.

**retained t.,** undescended t.

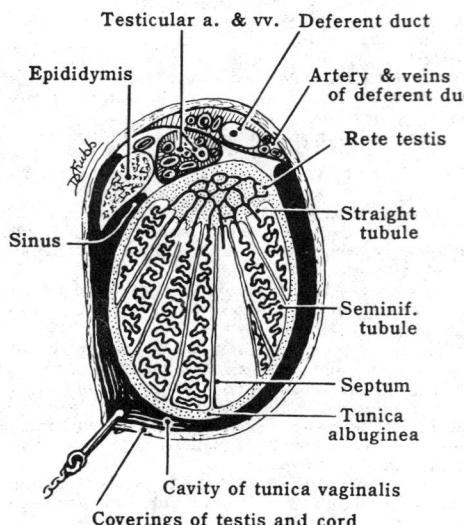

**Right Testis (Transverse Section)**
(From Grant, J. C. B.: *Grant's Atlas of Anatomy*, Ed. 5,
The Williams & Wilkins Co., Baltimore, 1962.)

**undescended t.,** retained t.; failure of the t. to descend
into the scrotum, it being retained in the abdomen or
inguinal canal.

**testi′tis.** Orchitis.

**Testivin's sign.** See under sign.

**tes′tocor′ticoid.** A postulated steroid principle in the
adrenal cortex that influences the growth and functional
activity of the testes. No such compound has as yet been
identified.

**tes′tocor′ticotroph′ic.** Indicating a postulated action of
the anterior lobe of the hypophysis which influences,
through the adrenal cortex, the growth and functional
activity of the testes. No such action has as yet been
demonstrated.

**testoid** (tes′toyd) [ testis + G. *eidos*, resemblance ]. 1. Androgenic. 2. An androgen.

**testolac′tone** (NF). TESLAC; 17α-oxo-D-homo-1,4-andros-
tadiene-3,17-dione; used as antineoplastic agent for treatment of mammary carcinoma.

**testop′athy** [ testis + G. *pathos*, disease ]. Orchiopathy.

**testos′terone.** 17β-Hydroxy-4-androstene-3-one (for
structure of androstane, see steroids); the male hormone;
the most potent naturally occurring androgen. It is formed
in greatest quantities by the interstitial cells of the testes;
possibly secreted also by the ovary and adrenal cortex; may
be produced in nonglandular tissues from precursors such
as androstenedione. The official preparation (NF and BP)
is obtained in pure crystalline form from the tissue of the
testes, and is used in the treatment of hypogonadism,
cryptorchism, certain carcinomas, and menorrhagia.

   **t. cypionate** (USP), t. cyclopentylpropionate; same
actions and uses as t. propionate, but with a prolonged
duration of action.

   **t. enanthate** (USP), DELATESTRYL; same actions and uses
as t., but with a prolonged duration of action, being
administered in oil.

   **t. phenylpropionate** (BP), an alternate preparation for the
propionate.

   **t. propionate** (USP, BP), has an action similar to but
more pronounced and prolonged than that of t. Used in the
treatment of undescended testes and in menorrhagia.

**test types.** Letters of various sizes printed on a card used
to test the acuity of vision.

   **Jaeger's t. t.'s,** lines of type of different sizes, printed on
a card, used for testing the acuteness of near vision.

   **point system t. t.'s,** a near-vision test chart in which the
various type bodies are multiples of a point ($1/_{72}$ inch), with

the lower-case letters being half the designated point size;
reading 4-point at 16 inches is normal, and is designated
N-4.

   **Snellen's t. t.'s,** square black letters printed on a card,
employed in testing the acuteness of distant vision; the
letters vary in size in such a way that each one subtends
a visual angle of 5′ at the distance at which the normal eye
should be able to distinguish it.

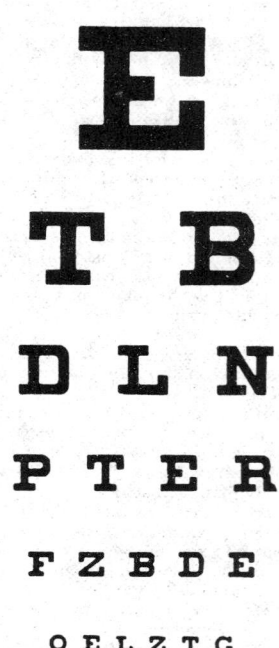

Snellen's Test Types

**tetan-.** See tetano-.

**teta′nia** (tē-ta′nĭ-ah). Tetany.

   **t. epidem′ica,** rheumatic *tetany*.

   **t. gas′trica,** gastric *tetany*.

   **t. gravida′rum,** tetany in pregnant women.

   **t. neonatorium,** neonatal *tetany*.

   **t. parathyreopri′va,** parathyroid *tetany*.

   **t. rheumat′ica,** rheumatic *tetany*.

**tetanic** (tē-tan′ĭk) [ G. *tetanikos* ]. 1. Relating to or marked
by tetanus. 2. An agent, such as strychnine, that in
poisonous doses produces tonic muscular spasm.

**tetan′iform.** Resembling tetanus.

**tetanigenous** (tet′ă-nij′ĕ-nus) [ tetanus + G. suffix *-gen*,
producing ]. Causing tetanus or tetaniform spasms.

**tetanilla** (tet′ă-nil′ah) [ Mod. L. dim. of L. *tetanus* ]. 1.
Fibrillary *myoclonia*. 2. Tetany.

**tet′anin.** Tetanotoxin.

**tetanism** (tet′ă-nizm). Neonatal *tetany*.

**tetanization** (tet′ă-nĭ-za′shun). 1. The act of tetanizing the
muscles. 2. A condition of tetaniform spasm.

**tet′anize.** To stimulate a muscle by a rapid series of stimuli
so that the individual muscular responses (contractions)
are fused into a sustained contraction; to cause tetanus (2)
in a muscle.

**tetano-, tetan-** (tet′ă-no-) [ G. *tetanos*, convulsive tension.
TEN- ]. Combining forms relating to tetanus or tetany.

**tet′anode** [ G. *tetanōdēs* ]. 1. Tetanoid. 2. Denoting the
quiet interval between the recurrent tonic spasms in
tetanus.

**tetanoid** (tet'ă-noyd) [ tetano- + G. *eidos*, resemblance ]. 1. Resembling or of the nature of tetanus; tetaniform. 2. Resembling tetany.

**tetanolysin** (tet'ă-nol'ĭ-sin). A hemolytic principle elaborated by *Clostridium tetani*. See also tetanospasmin.

**tetanometer** (tet'ă-nom'e-ter) [ tetano- + G. *metron*, measure ]. An instrument for measuring the force of tonic muscular spasms.

**tetanomotor** (tet'ă-no-mo'tor) [ tetano- + L. *motor*, a mover ]. An instrument by means of which tonic spasms are produced by the mechanical irritation of a hammer striking the motor nerve of the muscle affected.

**tetanospasmin** (tet'ă-no-spaz'min). The neurotoxin of *Clostridium tetani;* causes the characteristic signs and symptoms of tetanus. The chief action is on the anterior horn cells, and the spasms seem to be due to action at inhibitory synapses.

**tetanotoxin** (tet'ă-no-tok'sin) [ tetano- + G. *toxikon*, poison ]. Tetanin; the heat-labile, true exotoxin formed by *Clostridium tetani;* although there are several agglutinable types of the organism, the toxins are identical. See also tetanolysin and tetanospasmin.

**tetanus** (tet'ă-nus) [ L. fr. G. *tetanos*, convulsive tension. TEN- ]. 1. A disease marked by painful tonic muscular contractions; it is caused by the toxin (tetanospasmin) of *Clostridium tetani* acting upon the central nervous sytem; see emprosthotonos, opisthotonos, and pleurothotonos. 2. A sustained muscular contraction caused by a series of stimuli repeated so rapidly that the individual muscular responses are fused. Motor impulses reach intact muscles in the body at such a rate, usually, as to produce a tetanic contraction.

    **acous'tic t.**, experimental t. induced by a faradic current, the speed of which is estimated by the pitch of the vibrations.

    **anodal closure t.**, abbreviated ACTe; a tetanic muscular contraction occurring during the time the circuit is closed, the current then running, while the positive pole is applied.

    **anodal duration t.**, AnDTe; the period of muscular contraction occurring at the anode when the electric circuit is closed.

    **anodal opening t.**, a tonic contraction in a muscle, to which the anode is applied, when the circuit is opened.

    **t. anti'cus**, emprosthotonos.

    **apyret'ic t.**, benign t.; tetany.

    **cathodal closure t.**, abbreviated CCTe; a tetanic muscular contraction occurring during the time the circuit is closed, the current then running, while the negative pole is applied.

    **cathodal duration t.**, abbreviated CaDTe; a tetanic contraction occurring on application of the cathode or negative pole, while the circuit is closed.

    **cathodal opening t.**, abbreviated COTe; a tonic contraction in a muscle, to which the cathode is applied, when the circuit is opened.

    **cephal'ic t.**, cerebral t. (1); head t.; hydrophobic t.; Rose's cephalic t.; tonic spasms in the face and throat due to a wound of the head, usually injuring the facial nerve.

    **cer'ebral t.**, (1) cephalic t.; (2) experimental t. produced in animals by an injection of tetanospasmin into the brain substance.

    **t. comple'tus**, generalized t.; t. involving most of the muscles of the body.

    **t. dorsa'lis**, opisthotonos.

    **drug t.**, toxic t.; tonic spasms caused by strychnine or other tetanic.

    **extensor t.**, t. affecting chiefly the extensor muscles.

    **flexor t.**, t. affecting chiefly the flexor muscles.

    **head t.**, cephalic t.

    **hydropho'bic t.**, cephalic t.

    **idiopath'ic t.**, t. occurring without any visible wound to serve as a portal of entry for the specific bacillus.

    **imitative t.**, conversion hysteria that resembles t.

    **intermit'tent t.**, tetany.

    **t. latera'lis**, pleurothotonos.

    **local t.**, a form of the disease without generalized convulsions, a group of muscles in close proximity to an infected wound and resulting from action of the neurotoxin on the anterior horn cells at that level.

    **medical t.**, idiopathic t.

    **modified t.**, local t.

    **t. neonato'rum**, a form of t. affecting newborn infants, usually due to infection through the open end of the severed umbilical cord.

    **t. posti'cus**, opisthotonos.

    **postpartum t.**, puerperal t.

    **puer'peral t.**, t. occurring during the puerperium from infection of the obstetric wound.

    **rheumatic t.**, idiopathic t.

    **Ritter's opening t.**, the tetanic contraction which occasionally occurs when a strong current, passing through a long stretch of nerve, starts to flow.

    **Rose's cephal'ic t.**, cephalic t.

    **toxic t.**, drug t.

    **traumatic t.**, t. following infection of a wound.

    **uterine t.**, puerperal t.

**tetany** (tet'ă-nĭ) [ G. *tetanos*, tetanus. TEN- ]. A disorder marked by intermittent tonic muscular contractions, accompanied by fibrillary tremors, paresthesias, and muscular pains; the hands are usually first affected, the spasm occurring later in the face, trunk, and sometimes the laryngeal muscles; there is increased irritability of the motor and sensory nerves to electrical and mechanical stimuli; the disorder occurs with gastric and intestinal troubles, alkalosis, or a deficiency of calcium salts.

    **t. of alkalosis**, t. due to a loss of acid from the body or an increase in alkali, resulting in a reduction of ionized calcium in serum and body fluids, *e.g.*, hyperventilation t. (loss of $CO_2$), gastric t. (loss of HCl by vomiting), or injection or ingestion of excessive amounts of sodium bicarbonate.

    **duration t.**, a tonic spasm occurring in degenerated muscles upon application of a strong galvanic current.

    **epidemic t.**, rheumatic t.

    **gastric t.**, tetania gastrica; a form associated with gastric disorder affecting the muscles of the extremities and of respiration.

    **grass t.**, grass staggers; wheat poisoning; a highly fatal disease of cows and sheep occurring generally during the first two weeks in the spring after the animals have been out on lush pastures; it is characterized by convulsions, loss of consciousness, hypomagnesemia, and usually hypocalcemia.

    **guan'idine t.**, t. due to guanidine poisoning; it is usually an experimental condition induced by the injection of guanidine.

    **hy'perventila'tion t.**, t. caused by forced breathing, due to a reduction in the carbon dioxide of blood; see t. of alkalosis.

    **hy'poparathy'roid t.**, parathyroid t.

    **infantile t.**, t. of infants occurring usually in rickets in the healing stage when the blood calcium is reduced; also sometimes called idiopathic t.

    **latent t.**, t. that is made manifest only when certain procedures are used; see Trousseau's *sign*, Chvostek's *sign*, and Erb's *sign*.

    **t. of magnesium deficiency**, t. seen in grazing animals due to a lack of magnesium in the pasturage.

    **manifest t.**, t. from any cause in which the symptoms (as under main title) referable to neuromuscular hyperexcitability are clearly evident, as opposed to latent t.

    **neonatal t.**, tetania neonatorum; tetanism; myotonia neonatorum; a more or less continuous general muscular hypertonicity in neonates or young infants.

    **parathyroid t.**, (1) t. following excision of the parathyroid glands; (2) postoperative t.

    **parathyroprival t.**, parathyroid t.

    **phosphate t.**, t. due to the ingestion of an excess of alkaline phosphates ($Na_2HPO_4$ or $K_2HPO_4$). Most commonly produced experimentally in animals by the injection of alkaline phosphate which reduces the ionized calcium of the blood.

    **postoperative t.**, parathyroid t. caused by injury to or excision of the parathyroids in the operation for thyroid removal.

    **rheumatic t.**, tetania rheumatica; tetania epidemica; an acute epidemic form of t., of several weeks' duration, occurring chiefly in winter.

    **transport t.**, an acute disease seen in cattle and sheep during and shortly after shipping; it appears most often in females in advanced pregnancy and is believed to be precipitated by stress, lack of food and water, and perhaps heat; it is often associated with hypocalcemia.

**tet'artano'pia.** Tetartanopsia.

**tetartanopsia** (tĕ-tar'tă-nop'sĭ-ah) [ G. *tetartos*, fourth, + *an-* priv. + *ōps*, eye, fr. *opsis*, vision ]. Tetarnopia; loss of vision in a homonymous quadrant in each field; quadrantic hemianopsia.

**teth'elin** [ G. *tethēlōs*, pp. of *thallō*, to flourish ]. Obsolete term for growth *hormone*.

**tet'mil.** Ten millimeters.

**tetra-** (tet'rah-) [ G. prefix *tetra-*, four ]. Prefix to words formed from Greek roots, meaning four.

**tetra-amelia** (tet'rah-ă-me'lĭ-ah) [ tetra- + G. *a-* priv. + *melos*, limb ]. Complete amelia; absence of upper and lower limbs.

**tetrabar'bital** BUTYSAL; 5-ethyl-5-(1-ethylbutyl)barbituric acid; hypnotic and sedative.

**tetraba'sic.** Denoting an acid having four acid groups and thereby being able to neutralize four equivalents of base.

**tetraben'azine.** NITOMAN; 2-oxo-3-isobutyl-9,10-dimethoxy-1,2,3,4,6,7-hexahydro-11b*H*-benzo[ α ]quinolizine; a tranquilizer resembling reserpine in effect. It releases serotonin and norepinephrine in the brain. It is a serotonin antagonist, an antianxiety agent, and an antipsychotic agent. May cause excessive sedation, potentiation of barbiturates and anesthetics, parkinsonism, and loss of appetite.

**tetrabo'ric acid.** Pyroboric acid.

**tetrabrachius** (tet'rah-bra'kĭ-us) [ tetra- + G. *brachion*, arm ]. A malformed individual with four arms.

**tetrabromophenolphthalein sodium** (tet'rah-bro'mo-fe'-nol-thal'e-in). The sodium salt of a dibasic dye; has been used for x-ray examination of the gallbladder.

**tetracaine hydrochloride** (tet'rah-kān) (USP). PENTOCAINE hydrochloride; amethocaine hydrochloride; 2-(dimethylamino)ethyl *p*-(butylamino)benzoate monohydrochloride; used as a topical or spinal anesthetic agent. The base is listed in NF.

**tetrachirus** (tet-rah-ki'rus) [ tetra- + G. *cheir*, hand ]. A malformed individual having four hands.

**tetrachlorethylene** (tet-rah-klōr-eth'ĭ-lēn) (USP, BP). Tetrachloroethylene; carbon dichloride; ethylene tetrachloride; anthelmintic against hookworm and other nematodes.

**tetrachlo'ride.** A compound containing four atoms of chlorine to one atom of the other element or one radical equivalent; *e.g.*, carbon t., CCl₄.

**tetrachlormeth'ane.** Carbon tetrachloride.

**tetrachlormethi'azide.** DEPLEIL; teclothiazide; 6-chloro-3,4-dihydro-3-trichloromethyl-2*H*-1,2,4-benzothiadiazine-7-sulfonamide 1,1-dioxide; diuretic.

**tetrachloroethane** (tet'ra-klo'ro-eth'ān). Acetylene tetrachloride; cellon; Cl₂HC—CHCl₂. Nonflammable solvent for fats, oils, waxes, resins, etc. Used in the manufacture of paint and varnish removers, photographic films, lacquers, and insecticides. Its toxicity exceeds that of chloroform and carbon tetrachloride; it produces narcosis, liver damage, kidney damage, and gastroenteritis.

**tetrachlo'roeth'ylene.** Tetrachlorethylene.

**tetrachromic** (tet'rah-kro'mik) [ tetra- + G. *chromos*, color ]. Pertaining to vision that is normal for four colors.

**tetracoccus,** pl. **tetracocci** (tet'rah-kok'us, -kok'si) [ tetra- + G. *kokkos*, berry ]. A spherical bacterium that divides in two planes and characteristically forms groups of four cells.

**tetracosactide.** SYNACTHEN; β1-24-corticotropin; synthetic corticotrophic agent.

**tetracosanoic acid** (tet'ra-ko-să-no'ik). Lignoceric acid.

**tetracrotic** (tet'rah-krot'ik) [ tetra- + G. *krotos*, a striking ]. Denoting a pulse curve with four upstrokes in the cycle.

**tetracus'pid.** Quadricuspid; having four cusps.

**tetracyclic steroid nucleus** (tet'rah-si'klik, -sik'lik). See under steroid.

**tetracycline** (tet'rah-si'klēn, -klin) (USP). A broad spectrum antibiotic (a naphthacene derivative), the parent of oxytetracycline, *q.v.;* prepared from chlortetracycline, also

obtained from the culture filtrate of several species of *Streptomyces* originally found in soil from Texas. Also available as t. hydrochloride (USP, BP), and t. phosphate complex (NF); the latter is more rapidly absorbed than the base or the hydrochloride.

**Tetracycline**

**tet'rad** [ G. *tetras* (*tetrad-*), the number four ]. 1. A collection of four things having something in common. 2. In chemistry, a quadrivalent element. 3. In heredity, a bivalent chromosome that divides into four during meiosis.

**Fallot's t.,** Fallot's *tetralogy.*

**narcoleptic t.,** uncontrollable sleep, cataplexy, and hypnagogic hallucinations.

**tetradactyl** (tet'rah-dak'til) [ tetra- + G. *daktylos*, finger or toe ]. Having only four fingers or toes on a hand or foot.

**tetradehydro-doisynolic acid** Bisdehydrodoisynolic acid; a synthetic compound, closely resembling a steroid, with potent estrogenic activity.

**Tetradehydro-doisynolic acid**

**tetrad'ic.** Relating to a tetrad.

**tetraethylammonium chloride** (tet'rah-eth'ĭl-ă-mo'nĭ-um). ETAMON chloride; (C₂H₅)₄N⁺Cl⁻; a quaternary ammonium compound that partially blocks transmission of impulses through parasympathetic and sympathetic ganglia. Neostigmine counteracts this effect. Its clinical usefulness is limited. It is used occasionally in the management of peripheral vascular diseases.

**tetraethyl lead** (tet'rah-eth'ĭl). Pb(C₂H₅)₄; an anti-knock compound added to motor fuel; has a toxic action causing anorexia, nausea, vomiting, diarrhea, tremors, muscular weakness, insomnia, irritability, nervousness, and anxiety; death may occur, but otherwise recovery is complete.

**tetraethylmonothionopyrophosphate.** An anticholinesterase agent used in the treatment of glaucoma.

**tetraethylpyrophosphate** (tet'rah-eth-il-pi'ro-fos'făt). TEPP; Et₄P₂O₇; (EtO)₂PO—O—PO(OEt)₂; (C₂H₅)₄P₂O₇; an organic phosphorus compound used as an insecticide. It is toxic to man, being, like isopropylfluorophosphate, a powerful, irreversible cholinesterase inhibitor; its effects are therefore those of acetylcholine; the antidotes are atropine, pralidoxime, or similar reactivators of cholinesterases. T. has been used in the treatment of myasthenia gravis and topically in glaucoma.

**tetraethylthiuram disul'fide** (tet'rah-eth'ĭl-thi'u-ram). Disulfiram.

**tetraglycine hydroperiodide** (tet'rah-gli'sēn hi'droper-i'o-did). GLOBALINE; (NH₂CH₂COOH)₄HI·11/₄I₂; dissolves in water to the extent of 380 gm. per liter; used for the emergency disinfection of drinking water in amounts to yield 8 p.p.m. of active iodine.

**tet'ragon, tetrago'num** [ tetra- + G. *gōnia*, angle ]. Quadrangle.

**t. lumba'le,** lumbar quadrangle; a space bounded laterally by the obliquus externus abdominis muscle, medially by the erector spinae, above by the serratus posterior inferior, and below by the obliquus internus abdominis.

**tetrago′nus.** Quadrangular; a name given to the platysma.

**tetrahy′dric.** Denoting a compound containing four ionizable hydrogen atoms (four acid groups).

**tetrahydro-** (tet′rah-hi′dro-). Prefix denoting attachment of four hydrogen atoms (e.g., tetrahydrofolate, $H_4$folate).

**tetrahydrocannabinol** (tet′rah-hi′dro-kă-nab′ĭ-nol). $C_{21}H_{30}O_2$; several isomers have been synthesized. The $\Delta^{1-3,4}$-trans isomer and the $\Delta^{6-3,4}$-trans isomer are believed to be the active isomers present in Cannabis; the $\Delta^{1-3,4}$-trans isomer has been isolated from marihuana. See also Cannabis.

Tetrahydrocannabinol
(Dotted lines indicate $\Delta^1$ and $\Delta^6$ isomers)

**tetrahydrozoline hydrochloride** (tet′rah-hi′dro-zo′lēn) (USP). TYZINE; a sympathomimetic agent related to ephedrine; used as a topical nasal decongestant; must be used sparingly as excessive amounts may convert an acute congestion into a chronic reactive hyperemia.

**Tetrahymena pyriformis.** A ciliate belonging to a large group characterized by three membranes on one side of the buccal cavity and one on the other; it somewhat resembles the paramecium and, like it, is readily cultured and used extensively for experimental studies.

**tetraiodophthalein sodium** (tet-rah-i′o-do-thal′e-in). Iodophthalein.

**tetralogy** (tet′ral′o-jī) [ G. tetralogia ]. Tetrad (1).
  Eisenmenger′s t., Eisenmenger′s complex.
  Fallot′s t., Fallot′s tetrad; the most common form of cyanotic congenital heart disease, the t. consisting of pulmonic stenosis, ventricular septal defect, dextroposition of the aorta, and right ventricular hypertrophy.

**tetramastia** (tet′rah-mas′tĭ-ah) [ tetra- + G. mastos, breast ]. The presence of four breasts on an individual.

**tetramastigote** (tet′rah-mas′tĭ-gōt) [ tetra- + G. mastix, whip ]. A protozoan or other microorganism provided with four flagella.

**tetramas′tous.** Having four breasts.

**tetramelus** (tĕ-tram′e-lus) [ tetra- + G. melos, limb ]. A conjoined twin possessing four arms (tetrabrachius), or four legs (tetrascelus).

**Tetrameres** (tet-ram′er-ēz) [ see tetrameric ]. A genus of stomach-infecting parasitic nematodes (family Spiruridae) of birds. When filled with eggs, the female worm is enormously enlarged and has a globular, blood-red appearance.
  T. america′na, found in the proventriculus of chickens, turkeys, grouse, and quail and transmitted by infected cockroaches and grasshoppers; it is sometimes severely pathogenic in young chicks.
  T. fissis′pina, found in the proventriculus of ducks, geese, wild waterfowl, pigeons, and doves but rarely in gallinaceous birds.

**tetrameric, tetramerous** (tet′rah-měr′ik, tĕ-tram′er-us) [ tetra- + G. meros, part ]. Having four parts, or parts arranged in groups of four, or capable of existing in four forms.

**tetrameth′ylammo′nium iodide.** $(CH_3)_4NI_3$; dissolves in water to the extent of 0.25 gm. per liter. Used for the emergency disinfection of drinking water.

**tetrameth′ylputres′cine.** A derivative of putrescine, $C_8H_{20}N_2$, similar in its action to muscarine.

**tetrani′trol.** Erythrityl tetranitrate.

**tetranope** (tet′ră-nōp). A person who exhibits tetartanopsia.

**tetranop′sia, tetrano′pia.** Obsolete terms for tetartanopsia.

**tetranu′cleotide.** A compound of four nucleotides; once thought to represent the actual structure of nucleic acid (tetranucleotide theory).

**tetrapep′tide.** A compound of four amino acids in peptide linkage.

**tetraperomelia** (tet′rah-pe′ro-me′lĭ-ah) [ tetra- + G. peros, maimed, + melos, limb ]. Peromelia involving all four extremities.

**tetraphocomelia** (tet′rah-fo′ko-me′lĭ-ah). Phocomelia involving all four limbs.

**tetraplegia** (tet′rah-ple′jĭ-ah) [ tetra- + G. plēgē, stroke ]. Quadriplegia.

**tetraple′gic.** Quadriplegic.

**tetraploid** (tet′rah-ployd) [ G. tetraploos, fourfold, + eidos, form ]. See polyploidy.

**tet′rapod** [ tetra- + G. pous, foot ]. A vertebrate with four limbs; quadruped.

**tetrapus** (tet′rah-pus) [ G. tetrapous, fr. tetra- + pous, foot ]. A malformed individual with four feet.

**tet′rapyr′rol.** A molecule of four pyrrol nuclei, as in porphyrin.

**tet′rasac′charide.** A sugar containing four molecules of a monosaccharide, e.g., stachyose.

**tetrascelus** (tĕ-tras′ĕ-lus) [ tetra- + G. skelos, leg ]. A malformed individual with four legs.

**tetraso′mic** (tet′rah-so′mik) [ tetra- + chromosome ]. Relating to a cell nucleus in which one chromosome is represented four times while all others are present in the normal number.

**tetras′ter** [ tetra- G. astēr, star ]. A figure exceptionally and abnormally occurring in mitosis, in which there are four asters.

**tetrastichiasis** (tet-rah-stī-ki′ă-sis) [ tetra- + G. stichos, row ]. A duplication of the growth of the eyelashes (in four rows).

**tetrater′penes.** Hydrocarbons or their derivatives formed by the condensation of eight isoprene units (i.e., four terpenes) and containing, therefore, 40 carbon atoms; e.g., various carotenoids.

**tetratom′ic** [ tetra- + G. atomos, atom ]. Denoting a quadrivalent element or radical; tetradic.

**Tet′ratrichom′onas** [ tetra- + Trichomonas ]. A genus of parasitic protozoan flagellates, formerly part of the genus Trichomonas but now separated into a distinct genus by the presence of four anterior and one trailing flagella, a pelta, and a disc-shaped parabasal body; see Trichomonas.
  T. gallina′rum, formerly Trichomonas gallinarum; occurs in the ceca and sometimes in the liver of the turkey, chicken, guinea fowl, and other gallinaceous birds and is the probable cause of trichomoniasis of the lower intestine, with symptoms of diarrhea and loss of appetite, condition, and weight.
  T. o′vis, formerly Trichomonas ovis; occurs in the cecum or rumen of domestic sheep.

**tetravaccine** (tet-rah-vak′sēn). A vaccine recommended by Castellani, consisting of a mixture of dead cultures of typhoid, paratyphoid A, paratyphoid B, and cholera.

**tetravalent** (tet′rah-va′lent, tĕ-trav′ă-lent) [ tetra- + L. valens, pres. p. of valeo, to have power ]. Quadrivalent.

**tet′razole.** The compound $CN_4H_2$ with the structure of tetrazolium.

**tetrazo′lium.** Any of a group of organic salts having the general structure

$$R-C\overset{5}{\underset{}{}}\begin{array}{c} N\overset{3}{=}N-R \\ \\ N\underset{2}{=}N-R \end{array}\overset{+}{}$$
$$Cl^-$$

which on reduction (cleaving the 2,3 bond) yields a colored insoluble formazan (q.v.); used as a reagent in oxidative enzyme histochemistry. The structure shown, if R = C₆H₅, is triphenyltetrazolium chloride.

**tetrelle** (tĕ-trel′) [ Fr. dim. of *tetin*, nipple ]. An appliance by means of which the feeble sucking of a weakly infant is made effectual by supplementary suction of the mother.

**tetrodotoxin** (tet′ro-do-tok′sin). A potent neurotoxin found in the liver and ovaries of the Japanese pufferfish, *Sphoeroides rubripes*, and other species of pufferfish and also certain newts. It produces axonal blocks of the preganglionic cholinergic fibers and the somatic motor nerves. It is a nonprotein compound having a hemilactal structure, and is identical with tarichatoxin, found in three genera of newts.

**tetrophthalmos, tetrophthalmus** (tet′rof-thal′mus) [ tetra- + G. *ophthalmos*, eye ]. A malformed individual with four eyes.

**tet′rose.** A monosaccharide containing only four carbon atoms in the main chain; *e.g.*, erythrose, threose.

**tetro′tus** (tĕ-tro′tus) [ tetra- + G. *ous* (ōt-), ear ]. A malformed individual with four ears.

**tetrox′ide.** An oxide containing four oxygen atoms; *e.g.*, OsO₄.

**tetry′damine** (USAN). 4,5,6,7-Tetrahydro-2-methyl-3-(methylamino)-2*H*-indazole; an analgesic with anti-inflammatory action.

**tet′ter** [ A.S. *teter* ]. A colloquial term, popularly applied to ringworm and eczema, and occasionally applied to other eruptions.

**branny t.,** dandruff; *seborrhea* capitis.
**crusted t.,** impetigo.
**dry t.,** eczema.
**honeycomb t.,** favus.
**humid t.,** *eczema* madidans.
**milk t.,** *crusta* lactea.
**moist t.,** *eczema* madidans.
**scaly t.,** eczema.
**wet t.,** *eczema* madidans.

**Teutleben's ligament.** See under ligament.

**texis** (tek′sis) [ G. fr. *tiktō*, fut *texō*, to bring forth ]. Childbearing.

**textiform** (teks′tĭ-form) [ L. *textum*, something woven ]. Reticular; weblike.

**textural** (teks′chur-al). Relating to the texture of the tissues.

**texture** (teks′chur) [ L. *textura*, fr. *texo*, pp. *textus*, to weave ]. The composition or structure of a tissue or organ.

**tex′tus** [ L. ]. A tissue.

**TF.** Abbreviation for transfer *factor*.

**Th.** Chemical symbol of the element thorium.

**thalam-.** See thalamo-.

**thalamectomy** (tha′ă-mek′to-mĭ) [ thalamus + G. *ektomē*, excision ]. See chemothalamectomy.

**thal′amencephal′ic.** Relating to the thalamencephalon.

**thalamencephalon** (thal′ă-men-sef′ă-lon) [ thalamus + G. *enkephalos*, brain ]. [ NA ]. Diencephalon.

**thalamic** (thă-lam′ik). Relating to the thalamus.

**thalamo-, thalam-** [ G. *thalamos*, bedroom (thalamus) ]. Combining forms relating to the thalamus.

**thalamocortical** (thal′ă-mo-kor′tĭ-kal). Relating to the efferent connections of the thalamus with the cerebral cortex.

**thalamotomy** (thal′ă-mot′o-mĭ) [ thalamus + G. *tomē*, incision ]. Destruction of a selected portion of the thalamus by stereotaxy for the relief of pain, involuntary movements, epilepsy, and, rarely, emotional disturbances; it produces few, if any neurologic deficits or unpleasant personality changes.

**thalamus,** pl. **thalami** (thal′ă-mus, -mi) [ G. *thalamos*, a bed, a bedroom ] [ NA ]. The large, ovoid mass of gray matter that forms the larger dorsal subdivision of the diencephalon; it is placed medial to the internal capsule and the body and tail of the caudate nucleus. Its medial aspect forms the dorsal half of the lateral wall of the third ventricle; its dorsal surface can be subdivided into a lateral triangle forming the floor of the body (pars centralis) of the lateral ventricle, and a medial triangle covered by the velum interpositum; its tail-like caudal part curves ventralward around the posterolateral aspect of the cerebral peduncle and ends in the lateral geniculate body. The t. is composed of a large number of anatomically and functionally distinct cell groups or nuclei, usually classified as (1) sensory relay nuclei (nucleus ventralis posterior, corpus geniculatum laterale and mediale) each receiving a modally specific sensory conduction system and in turn projecting each to the corresponding primary sensory area of the cortex; (2) "secondary" relay nuclei (nucleus ventralis lateralis and ventralis anterior) receiving fibers from the medial segment of the globus pallidus as well as cerebello-thalamic fibers and projecting to the precentral motor cortex; (3) a nucleus associated with the limbic system: the composite nucleus anterior receiving the mamillothalamic tract and projecting to the gyrus fornicatus; (4) association nuclei (nucleus medialis dorsalis, nucleus lateralis including the large pulvinar) each projecting to a large expanse to association cortex; (5) the midline and intralaminar nuclei or "nonspecific" nuclei (nucleus centromedianus, centralis lateralis, paracentralis, reuniens); and (6) the habenula or nucleus habenularis. See also relevant subentries under *nucleus; corpus; cortex* cerebri.

**thal′assane′mia.** Thalassemia.

**thalassemia** (thal′ă-se′mĭ-ah) [ G. *thalassa*, the sea, + *haima*, blood ]. Any of a group of inherited disorders of hemoglobin metabolism in which there is a decrease in net synthesis of a particular globin chain without change in the structure of that chain; several genetic types exist, and the corresponding clinical picture may vary from barely detectable hematologic abnormality to severe and fatal anemia. The hemoglobin Lepore syndromes are clinically indistinguishable, but the non-α-globin chains are structurally altered (see under hemoglobin). Various examples of thalassemic disorders have been known as Mediterranean anemia, hereditary leptocytosis, Cooley's anemia, erythroblastic anemia, target cell anemia, familial microcytic anemia, and other terms.

**A₂ t., β t.,** heterozygous state.

**α t.,** t. due to one of two or more genes that depress, severely and moderately, synthesis of α-globin chains by the chromosome with the abnormal gene. Heterozygous state, severe type: t. minor with 5 to 15 per cent of Hb Barts at birth, only traces of Hb Barts in adult; mild type, 1 to 2 per cent of Hb Barts at birth, not detectable in adult. Homozygous state: severe type, erythroblastosis fetalis and fetal death, only Hb Barts and Hb H present; mild type not clinically defined. See also *hemoglobin* H.

**α t. intermedia,** hemoglobin H disease; see *hemoglobin* H.

**β t.,** t. due to one of two or more genes that depress (partially or completely) synthesis of β-globin chains by the chromosome bearing the abnormal gene. Heterozygous state: t. minor with Hb A₂ increased, Hb F normal or variably increased, Hb A normal or slightly reduced. Homozygous state: t. major with Hb A reduced to very low but variable levels, Hb F very high level.

**β-δ t.,** F t.; t. due to a gene that depresses synthesis of both β- and δ- globin chains by the chromosome bearing the abnormal gene. Heterozygous state: t. minor with Hb F comprising 5 to 30 per cent of total hemoglobin but distributed unevenly among cells, Hb A₂ reduced or normal. Homozygous state: moderate anemia with only Hb F present, no Hb A or Hb A₂.

**F t., β-δ t.**

**Lepore t.,** t. syndrome due to production of abnormally structured Lepore hemoglobin (*q. v.*). Heterozygous state: t. minor with about 10 per cent Hb Lepore, Hb F moderately increased, Hb A₂ normal. Homozygous state: t. major with only Hb F and Hb Lepore produced, no Hb A or Hb A₂.

**t. major,** Cooley's anemia; primary erythroblastic anemia; the syndrome of severe anemia resulting from the homozygous state of one of the t. genes or one of the hemoglobin Lepore genes; onset, in infancy or childhood, of pallor, icterus, weakness, splenomegaly, cardiac enlargement, thinning of inner and outer tables of skull, microcytic hopochromic anemia with poikilocytosis, anisocytosis, stippled cells, target cells, nucleated erythrocytes; types of hemoglobin are variable and depend on gene involved.

**t. minor,** the heterozygous state of a t. gene or a hemoglobin Lepore gene; usually asymptomatic, quite variable hematologically, with leptocytosis, mold hypochromic microcytosis, often slightly reduced hemoglobin level with slightly increased erythrocyte count; types of hemoglobin are variable and depend on gene involved.

**thalassophobia** (thal'ă-so-fo'bĭ-ah, thă-las'o-) [ G. *thalassa*, the sea, + *phobos*, fear ]. Morbid fear of the sea.

**thalassoposia** (thal'ă-so-po'zĭ-ah, thă-las'o-) [ G. *thalassa*, the sea, + *posis*, drinking ]. Mariposia.

**thal'assother'apy** [ G. *thalassa*, the sea ]. Treatment of disease by residence at the seashore, by sea bathing, or by a sea voyage.

**thalidomide** (thă-lid'o-mid). α-Phthalimidoglutarimide; 2,6-dioxo-3-phthalimidopiperidine; a hypnotic drug which, if taken in early pregnancy, may cause the birth of infants with phocomelia and other defects.

Thalidomide

**thallium** (thal'ĭ-um) [ G. *thallos*, a green shoot (it gives a green line in the spectrum) ]. A soft, lustrous white metallic element, symbol Tl, atomic no. 81, atomic weight 204.39.

**Thallophyta** (thă-lof'ĭ-tah) [ G. *thallos*, a green shoot, + *phyton*, plant ]. In older classification systems, a primary division of the plant kingdom whose members, with a few exceptions, are devoid of true roots, stems, and leaves. It included bacteria, fungi, and algae.

**thallophyte** (thal'o-fīt). A member of the division Thallophyta.

**Thallosporales** (thal'o-spo-ra'lēz) [ G. *thallos*, green shoot, + *sporos*, seed ]. An order of the Fungi Imperfecti, characterized by the formation of thallospores, as in the genera *Trichophyton*, *Epidermophyton*, and the like.

**thallospore** (thal'o-spōr) [ G. *thallos*, a green twig, + *sporos*, seed ]. A reproductive asexual type of spore formed as an integral part of the thallus or mycelium, in contrast to a conidium formed on a specialized hypha. T.'s are of three types: (1) blastospores, formed by means of a budding process from the cells of the mycelium; (2) chlamydospores, formed as the result of a cell becoming enlarged and developing a thick wall at the end of a hypha or along its course; and (3) arthrospores, formed by means of segmentation of a hypha, resulting in a rectangular, "cut-off," thick-walled body.

**thallotoxicosis** (thal'o-tok-sĭ-ko'sis) [ thallium + G. *toxikon*, poison, + suffix *-osis*, condition ]. Poisoning by thallium, marked by stomatitis, gastroenteritis, peripheral and retrobulbar neuritis, endocrine disorders, and alopecia.

**thal'lus** [ G. *thallos*, a young shoot ]. A simple plant or fungus body which is devoid of roots, stems, and leaves.

**Thalmann's agar.** See under agar.

**thamu'ria** [ G. *thama*, often, + *ouron*, urine ]. Pollakiuria; frequent micturition.

**thanato-** (than'ă-to-) [ G. *thanatos*, death ]. Combining form relating to death.

**thanatobiologic** (than'ă-to-bi-o-loj'ik) [ thanato- + G. *bios*, life, + *logos*, study ]. Relating to the processes concerned in life and death.

**thanatognomonic** (than'ă-to-no-mon'ik) [ thanato- + G. *gnōmē*, a sign. GNO- ]. Of fatal prognosis, indicating the approach of death.

**thanatography** (than'ă-tog'ră-fī) [ thanato- + G. *graphē*, a writing ]. 1. A description of one's symptoms and thoughts while dying. 2. A treatise on death.

**thanatoid** (than'ă-toyd) [ thanato- + G. *eidos*, resemblance ]. 1. Resembling death. 2. Mortal; deadly.

**thanatology** (than'ă-tol'o-jī) [ thanato- + G. *logos*, study ]. The branch of science that treats of death in all its aspects.

**thanatomania** (than'ă-to-ma'nĭ-ah) [ thanato- + G. *mania*, frenzy ]. Illness or death resulting from belief in the efficacy of magic; a phenomenon observed among those primitive societies or illiterate and superstitious people who believe in the power of evil spirits, spells, curses, and individuals over one's bodily processes, with such belief and resulting fear manifesting themselves as psychosomatic illness and even death.

**thanatometer** (than'ă-tom'e-ter) [ thanato- + G. *metron*, measure ]. An instrument to determine the presence of death; one form is a thermometer for taking the internal temperature.

**thanatophidia** (than'ă-to-fid'ĭ-ah) [ thanato- + G. *ophidion*, dim. of *ophis*, a serpent ]. Venomous snakes.

**thanatophobia** (than'ă-to-fo'bĭ-ah) [ thanato- + G. *phobos*, fear ]. Morbid fear of death.

**thanatophoric** (than'ă-to-fōr'ik) [ thanato- + G. *phoros*, bearing ]. Lethal; leading to death.

**thanatopsy, thanatopsia** (than'ă-top'si, -top'sĭ-ah) [ thanato- + G. *opsis*, view ]. Autopsy.

**thanatos** (than'ă-tos) [ G. death ]. In psychoanalysis, the death principle, representing all instinctual tendencies toward senescence and death, as opposed to eros. See also subentries under instinct.

**Thane,** Sir George D., English anatomist, 1850–1930. See T.'s *method.*

**thaumatropy** (thaw-mat'ro-pī) [ G. *thauma* (*thaumat-*), a wonder, + *tropē*, a turning ]. The transforming of one form of tissue into another.

**Thd.** Symbol for ribothymidine (5-methyluridine).

**thea** (the'ah) [ Mod. L. ]. Tea.
  **t. ni'gra,** black *tea.*
  **t. vir'idis,** green *tea.*

**theaism** (the'ah-izm). Theinism.

**theater** (the'a-ter) [ G. *theatron*, a place for seeing, theater, fr. *theomai*, to look at ]. The operating room of a public hospital or one in which invited guests or the general surgical public are permitted to see the operations.

**thebaic** (the-ba'ik) [ L. *Thebaicus*, relating to Thebes, whence opium was formerly obtained ]. Relating to or derived from opium.

**thebaine** (the-ba'ēn, -in). Paramorphine; $C_{19}H_{21}NO_3$; an alkaloid obtained from opium (0.3 to 1.5 per cent). It causes tetanic convulsions, resembling strychnine in its action.

**thebaism** (the'bah-izm). Opium *addiction.*

**Thebesius,** Adam C., German physician, 1686–1732. See Thebesian *foramina, valve, veins.*

**theca,** pl. **the'cae** (the'kah) [ G. *thēkē*, a box ]. [ NA ]. A sheath or capsule.
  **t. cordis,** pericardium.
  **t. externa,** *tunica* externa thecae folliculi.
  **t. follic'uli** [ NA ], the wall of a vesicular ovarian follicle; see *tunica* externa and *tunica* interna thecae folliculi.
  **t. interna,** *tunica* interna thecae folliculi.
  **t. ten'dinis,** *vagina* synovialis tendinis.
  **t. vertebra'lis,** *dura mater* spinalis.

**thecal** (the'kal) [ see theca ]. Relating to a sheath, especially a tendon sheath.

**thecitis** (the-si'tis) [ G. *thēkē*, box (sheath), + suffix *-itis*, inflammation ]. Inflammation of the sheath of a tendon; tendovaginitis.

**thecodont** (the'ko-dont) [ G. *thēkē*, box, + *odous* (*odont-*), tooth ]. Having the teeth inserted in alveoli.

**thecoma** (the-ko'mah) [ G. *thēkē*, box (theca), + suffix *-oma*, tumor ]. Theca cell tumor; a neoplasm derived from ovarian mesenchyme, and consisting chiefly of spindle-shaped cells that frequently contain small droplets of fat (*i.e.,* small clear vacuoles when observed in routine preparations). These neoplasms generally manifest gross features that resemble those of granulosa cell tumore, *i.e.,* firm, yellow, encapsulated masses, ordinarily about 10 cm. or less in diameter. T.'s may form considerable quantities of estrogens, thereby resulting in (1) precocious development of secondary sexual features in prepubertal girls, or (2) hyperplasia of the endometrium in older patients. Thus, the clinical findings are similar to those of granulosa call tumor, except that t.'s tend to be less malignant.

**theco'mato'sis.** A stromal hyperplasia or increase in the number of connective tissue elements of an ovary.

**thecostegnosia, thecostegnosis** (the'ko-stegno'sĭ-ah, the'ko-steg-no'sis) [ G. *thēkē*, box (sheath), + *stegnōsis*, a narrowing ]. Constriction of a tendon sheath.

**Theden** (ta'den), Johann C. A., German surgeon, 1714–1797. See T.'s *method.*

**the'ic** [ Mod. L. *thea*, tea ]. An intemperate tea-drinker.

**Theile** (ti'leh), Friedrich W., German anatomist, 1801–1879. See T.'s *canal, glands, muscle.*

**Theiler** (ti'ler), Max, South African microbiologist in the U. S., 1899–1972. Nobel laureate, 1951, for his discoveries concerning yellow fever and how to combat it. See T.'s *disease, virus.*

**Theileria** (thi-lēr'ĭ-ah) [ A. *Theiler* ]. A genus of sporozoan protozoa (family Theileriidae) that are tick-borne parasites and among the most important pathogens of domestic animals. They multiply asexually in lymphocytes or other cells and then invade the erythrocytes, where they remain without multiplying until ingested by a transmitting tick.

**T. annula'ta,** causes Transcaucasian fever, a disease similar to East Coast fever, in Africa, Mediterranean countries, Transcaucasia and Turkistan.

**T. hir'ci,** agent of malignant ovine and caprine theileriosis in the Mediterranean region, southern USSR, and India.

**T. lawren'ci,** *T. parva.*

**T. mu'tans,** the cause of benign bovine theileriosis in Africa and other parts of the world, including the United States; in Africa, the infection is also called Tzaneen disease.

**T. o'vis,** causes benign ovine and caprine theileriosis chiefly in countries near the Mediterranean, but also in India, Ceylon, and the USSR.

**T. par'va,** *T. lawrenci;* the causative agent of the most severe theileriosis of cattle, East Coast fever.

**theileriasis** (thi'le-rī'ă-sis). Theileriosis.

**Theile'riidae.** A family of sporozoan protozoa (order Piroplasmida) comprised of two genera, *Theileria* and *Haematoxenus.*

**theileriosis** (thi-lēr'ĭ-o'sis). Theileriasis; disease of cattle, sheep and goats caused by infection with *Theileria,* and transmitted chiefly by ticks of the genera *Rhipicephalus* and *Hyalomma.*

**benign bovine t.,** mild gallsickness; caused by *Theileria mutans* and transmitted by *Rhipicephalus appendiculatus* and *Rhipicephalus evertsi;* occurs in cattle in Africa and other parts of the world, including the United States.

**bovine t.,** East Coast *fever.*

**benign ovine and caprine t.,** occurs in sheep and goats chiefly in countries near the Mediterranean, but also in the USSR, India, and Ceylon; it is caused by *Theileria ovis* and transmitted chiefly by *Rhipicephalus bursa* and *Rhipicephalus evertsi.*

**malignant ovine and caprine t.,** a highly pathogenic disease of sheep and goats in the Mediterranean region, southern USSR, and India that kills 50 to 100 percent of the affected animals but is seldom fatal to young lambs and kids; it is caused by *Theileria hirci* and probably transmitted by *Rhipicephalus bursa.*

**thein** (the'in, te'in). Caffeine.

**theinism, theism** (the'ĭ-nizm, the'izm, te'-) [ Mod. L. *thea,* tea ]. Theaism; chronic poisoning resulting from immoderate tea-drinking, marked by palpitation, insomnia, nervousness, headache, and dyspepsia.

**thel-.** See thelo-.

**thelalgia** (the-lal'jĭ-ah) [ thel- + G. *algos,* pain ]. Pain in the nipple.

**thelarche** (the-lar'ke) [ thel- + G. *archē,* beginning ]. A form of precocious sexual maturation occurring in girls before the age of 8 years; characterized by breast development and, in some cases, by changes in the vaginal epithelium of a type produced by estrogenic stimulation.

**Thelazia** (the-la'zĭ-ah) [ G. *thēlazō,* to suck ]. The eye worms, a genus of spirurid nematodes that inhabit the lacrimal ducts and surface of the eyes of various domestic and wild animals, but rarely man; a number of species have been reported from wild birds. Cyclic development occurs in muscoid flies; infective larvae emerge from the fly mouthparts while the fly is feeding on or near the eyes of the host. Infection by species of *T.* is called thelaziasis.

**T. californien'sis,** occurs in the tear ducts, conjunctival sac, or under the nictitating membrane of dogs, coyotes, black bears, sheep, deer, jack rabbits, and (rarely) man and cats in the western and southwestern United States; heavy infections cause photophobia, lacrimation, eyelid edema, conjunctivitis, and possibly blindness.

**T. callip'aeda,** reported from man in Southeast Asia and California; the worm, embedded in a subconjunctival tumor or swimming in the aqueous humor after penetrating the limbus, causes pain, photophobia, and tearing.

**thelaziasis** (the'lă-zī-ă-sis, thel'-ă-zī-ă-sis). Infection or infestation with *Thelazia.*

**the'le** [ G. ]. *Papilla* mammae.

**theleplasty** (the'le-plas'tĭ) [ thel- + G. *plassō,* to form ]. Mammillaplasty; reparative or plastic surgery of the nipple.

**thelerethism** (the-ler'ĕ-thizm) [ thel- + G. *erethismos,* irritation ]. Thelothism; erection of the nipple.

**thelitis** (the-li'tis) [ thel- + G. suffix -*itis,* inflammation ]. Mammillitis; inflammation of the nipple.

**thelium,** pl. **thelia** (the'lĭ-um, -lĭ-ah) [ Mod. L. fr. G. *thēlē,* nipple ]. 1. A papilla. 2. A cellular layer. 3. *Papilla* mammae.

**thelo-, thel-** (the'lo-) [ G. *thēlē,* nipple. THEL- ]. Combining form relating to the nipples.

**theloncus** (the-long'kus) [ thelo- + G. *onkos,* a mass ]. A neoplasm involving the nipple.

**thelophlebostemma** (the'lo-fleb'o-stem'ah) [ thelo- + G. *phleps,* vein, + *stemma,* a wreath ]. A venous circle surrounding the nipple.

**thelorrhagia** (the'lo-ra'jĭ-ah) [ thelo- + G. *rhēgnymi,* burst forth ]. Bleeding from the nipple.

**the'lothism.** Thelerethism.

**thelygenic** (thel'ĭ-jen'ik) [ G. *thelys,* female, + suffix -*gen,* producing ]. Producing only female offspring.

**thelygonia** (thel'ĭ-go'nĭ-ah) [ G. *thelygonia,* generation of females, fr. *thelys,* female, + *gonos,* offspring. GEN- ]. Procreation of female offspring.

**thelyplasty** (thel'ĭ-plas'tĭ) [ G. *thēlys,* female, + *plassō,* to form ]. Theleplasty.

**thelytocia** (thel'ĭ-to'sĭ-ah) [ G. *thēlys,* female, + *tokos,* birth ]. State of giving birth only to females.

**the'nad** [ G. *thenar,* the palm of the hand, + L. *ad,* to ]. Toward the thenar or lateral side of the palm of the hand.

**the'nal.** Thenar (2).

**thenal'dine tartrate.** SANDOSTENE tartrate; 1-methyl-4-*N*-2-thenylanilinopiperidine tartrate; antihistaminic and antipruritic agent.

**the'nar** [ G. the palm of the hand ]. 1 [ NA ]. The fleshy mass on the lateral side of the palm; the radial palm; the ball of the thumb. 2. Applied to any structure in relation with this part.

**the'nen** [ G. *thenar,* palm, + *en,* in ]. Relating only to the palm; specifically to the radial side of the palm.

**then'yl.** The radical of 2-methylthiophene, $(SC_4H_3)CH_2—$; contrast thienyl.

**thenyldi'amine hydrochloride.** Thenfadil; Tenfidil; $C_{14}H_{19}N_3S$ HCl; 2-[ (2-dimethylaminoethyl)-3-thenylamino ]pyridine hydrochloride; an antihistaminic.

**theobro'ma** [ G. *theos,* a god, + *brōma,* food ]. Cacao.

**t. oil** (USP, BP), cacao oil; cacao butter; cocoa butter; the fat obtained from the wasted seed of *Theobroma cacao* (family Sterculiaceae); it contains the glycerides of stearic, palmitic, oleic, arichidic, and linoleic acids; used as a base for suppositories and ointments and, in operative dentistry, as a lubricant and protective.

**theobro'mic acid.** A waxy substance reported to be a constituent of theobroma oil.

**theobro'mine.** 3,7-Dimethyl-2,6-dihydroxypurine; 3,7-dimethylxanthine; an alkaloid resembling caffeine in its action, prepared from the dried ripe seed of *Theobroma cacao* or made synthetically; used as a diuretic, myocardial stimulant, dilator of coronary arteries, and smooth muscle relaxant. Compounds with calcium gluconate, calcium salicylate, sodium acetate, sodium lactate, and sodium salicylate have been listed.

**theomania** (the′o-ma′nĭ-ah) [ G. *theos*, god, + *mania*, frenzy ]. Sebastomania; religious insanity; insanity in which the subject believes that he is God.

**theophobia** (the′o-fo′bĭ-ah) [ G. *theos*, god, + *phobos*, fear ]. A morbid fear of God.

**theophylline** (the-of′ĭ-lēn, -lin). (USP, BP). 1,3-Dimethylxanthine; an alkaloid found with thein (caffeine) in tea leaves (commercial t. is prepared synthetically); a smooth muscle relaxant, diuretic, cardiac stimulant, and vasodilator; used in angina pectoris, peripheral vascular disease, and bronchial asthma.

    **t. calcium salicylate,** PHYLLICIN; a mixture of calcium t. and sodium salicylate in molecular proportion; has the same actions and uses as t.

    **t. cholinate,** choline theophyllinate.

    **t. ethanolamine,** MONOTHEAMIN; t. monoethanolamine; same actions and uses as t.

    **t. eth′ylenedi′amine,** aminophylline.

    **t. isopropanolamine,** THEOPROPANOL; same actions and uses as aminophylline but has a more rapid onset and a longer duration of action.

    **t. sodium acetate,** THEOCIN soluble; t. sodium and sodium acetate; contains 60 per cent of t. and has the same uses as t.

    **t. sodium gly′cinate** (NF), equilibrium mixture containing t. sodium and glycine in approximately molecular proportions, buffered with an additional mole of glycine. Similar in action and uses to aminophylline but more stable in air, and less irritating to the gastric mucosa.

**Theorell** (ta′o-rel), A. Hugo, Swedish biochemist, *1903. Nobel laureate, 1955, for his discoveries concerning the nature and mode of action of oxidative enzymes.

**theorem** (the′o-rem). A proposition that can be proved, and so is established as a law or principle.

    **Bernoulli's t.,** Bernoulli's *law.*

    **Ehrlich's t.,** every specific microorganism has a specific chemical affinity which, when found and injected intravenously or intramuscularly into the infected host, will cure the disease caused by the microorganism.

    **Gibbs' t.,** substances that lower the surface tension of the pure dispersion medium tend to collect in its surface, whereas substances that raise the surface tension tend to remain out of the surface film.

# THEORY

**theory** (the′o-rī) [ G. *theōria*, a beholding, speculation, theory, fr. *theōros*, a beholder ]. A reasoned explanation of the manner in which something occurs or has been produced or will be produced; lacking absolute proof, but more nearly established than hypothesis, which is closer to speculation.

    **adsorption t. of narcosis,** drug becomes concentrated at the surface of the cell as a result of adsorption, and thus alters permeability and metabolism.

    **Altmann's t.,** that protoplasm is composed of a number of granular elements (bioblasts) surrounded by an indifferent substance.

    **Arrhenius-Madsen t.,** that the reaction of an antigen with its antibody is a reversible reaction—the equilibrium being determined according to the law of mass action, by the concentrations of the reacting substances.

    **atomic t.,** that chemical compounds are formed by the union of atoms in certain definite proportions; in its modern form, first advanced in 1803 by the British chemist, John Dalton.

    **Baeyer's t.,** that carbon bonds are set at fixed angles (109°) and that those carbon rings are most stable which least distort those angles. It is for this reason that planar rings composed of 5 or 6 carbon atoms (*e.g.,* cyclopentane, benzene) are so much more common than rings containing less than 5 or more than 6 carbon atoms.

    **balance t.,** in social psychology, a t. which assumes that steady and unsteady states can be specified for cognitive units, such as an individual and his attitudes or acts, and that such units tend to seek steady states (balance); *e.g.,* balance exists when both parts of a unit are evaluated the same, but disequilibrium arises when both parts are not evaluated the same, which causes either cognitive reevaluation of the parts or their segregation; see also cognitive dissonance t. and consistency *principle.*

    **balance t. of sex,** a t. of sex determination that attributes female differentiation of the embryo to a 1:1 balance of X chromosomes to haploid autosome sets (*i.e.,* 2 X chromosomes + 2 sets of autosomes = female), male differentiation to a 1:2 balance (*i.e.,* 1 X chromosome + 2 autosome sets = male), and intersexual development to ratios other than 1:1 and 1:2. This t. is apparently correct for certain animals but is probably incorrect for man. The Y chromosome seems essential for male differentiation in man.

    **beta-oxidation-condensation t.,** that the two carbon fragments split from the fatty acid molecule by beta-oxidation are converted to acetic acid and then condensed to acetoacetic acid.

    **Bohr's t.,** that spectrum lines are produced, (1) by the emission of radiant energy when electrons drop from an orbit of higher to one of lower energy (energy level); or (2) by absorption of radiation when an electron rises from a lower to a higher energy level.

    **Bordeau t., Bordeu t.,** see de Bordeau t.

    **Bowman's t.,** that the urine is formed by passive filtration through the glomeruli and secretion by the epithelium of the tubules, the water and salts being separated from the plasma in the former situation, the urea and other urinary constituents in the latter. Parts of this t. are now known to be wrong.

    **Brønsted t.,** defines an acid as a substance, charged or uncharged, liberating hydrogen ions in solution, a base as a substance that removes them from solution; thus, $NH_3$, $CH_3COO^-$, and $SO_4^=$ are bases; $NH_4{}^+$, $CH_3COOH$, and $H_2SO_4{}^-$ are acids. Useful in the concept of weak electrolytes and buffers.

    **Burn and Rand t.,** stimulation of sympathetic fibers results first in the production of acetylcholine in the postganglionic nerve endings, which then release norepinephrine to act on the active site of the effector cell.

    **Cannon's t.,** emergency t.

    **Cannon-Bard t.,** the view that the feeling aspect of emotion and the pattern of emotional behavior are controlled by the hypothalamus.

    **celomic metaplasia t. of endometrio′sis,** that endometrial tissue arises directly from the peritoneal mesothelium.

    **cloacal t.,** the belief sometimes held by neurotics or children that a child is born, as a stool is passed, from a common opening.

    **clonal selection t.,** that mutation of stem cells produces all possible templates for antibody production. Exposure to a specific antigen will then selectively stimulate proliferation of the cell with the appropriate template to form a clone or colony of specific antibody-forming cells.

    **cognitive dissonance t.,** a t. of attitude formation and behavior which indicates that persons try to achieve consistency (consonance) and avoid dissonance which, when it arises, may be coped with by changing one's attitudes, rationalizing, selective perception, and other means; see also balance t. and consistency *principle.*

    **Cohnheim's t.,** emigration t.; that neoplasms originate from various cell rests, *i.e.,* embryonal cells thought to persist in various sites after the development of the fetal organs and tissues.

    **colloid t. of narcosis,** coagulation or flocculation of protein causes dehydration and reduction of metabolism.

    **Darwinian t.,** see Darwin.

    **de Bordeau t.,** Bordeau or Bordeu t.; that each organ of the body manufactured a specific humor which it secreted into the blood stream.

    **decay t.,** a t. of forgetting based on the premise that an engram deteriorates progressively with time during the interval when it is not activated.

    **De Vries' t.,** see mutation (2).

    **Dieulafoy's t.,** that appendicitis is always the result of the transformation of the appendicular canal into a closed cavity.

**dipole t.,** a t. in which the activation current of the heart is conceived as a moving dipole, the positive pole leading.

**duplicity t. of vision,** that the cones of the retina function in bright light and are sensitive to color while the rods function in dim light and give sensations of black and white.

**Edridge-Green t. of color blindness,** that light and color are transmitted to two independent centers in the brain. The light center is primitive, the color center evolving later. Color blindness is considered atavistic, resulting from central failure of development.

**Ehrlich's t.,** see side chain t.

**Ehrlich's side chain t.,** see side chain t.

**t. of electrolytic dissociation,** see Arrhenius' *doctrine*.

**emergency t.,** the theory advanced by Cannon that the rate of secretion from the adrenal medulla is negligible except during conditions which may threaten the life or well-being of the individual.

**emigration t.,** Cohnheim's t.

**enzyme inhibition t. of narcosis,** narcotics inhibit respiratory enzymes by suppression of the formation of high energy phosphate bonds within the cell.

**Flourens' t.,** that thought is a process depending upon the action of the entire cerebrum.

**Frerich's t.,** that uremia represents a toxic condition caused by ammonium carbonate, which is formed as the result of the action of a plasma enzyme on the increased amounts of urea.

**Freud's t.,** a comprehensive t. of how personality is formed and develops in normal and emotionally disturbed individuals, *e.g.,* that an attack of conversion hysteria is due to a psychic trauma which was not adequately reacted to at the time it was received, and persists as an affect memory; see also psychoanalysis.

**Galen's t.'s,** see under Galen.

**gam'etoid t.,** that the malignancy of a tumor results from the neoplastic cells having developed sexual characteristics, by means of which they multiply and grow autonomously as parasites on the host's tissues.

**gastrea t.,** Haeckel's gastrea t.

**gate t.,** the hypothesis that a control mechanism exists within the spinal cord that modulates afferent stimuli before they evoke the sensation of pain.

**germ layer t.,** the concept that young embryos differentiate three primary germ layers (ectoderm, mesoderm and entoderm), each of which has the potentiality of forming different characteristic structures and organs in the developing body.

**germ t.,** the t., now a doctrine, that infectious diseases are due to the presence and functional activity within the body of microorganisms.

**Gestalt t.,** see gestaltism.

**Haeckel's gastrea t.,** that the two-layered gastrula is the ancestral form of all multicellular animals.

**Helmholtz t. of accommodation,** that for near vision the ciliary muscle relaxes and allows the anterior aspect of the crystalline lens to become more convex.

**Helmholtz t. of color vision,** Young-Helmholtz t. of color vision.

**Helmholtz t. of hearing,** resonance t. of hearing.

**Helmholtz-Gibbs t.,** see Gibbs-Helmholtz *equation*.

**hematogenous t. of endometriosis,** that endometrial tissue is carried, like metastases of a malignant tumor, through the blood stream.

**Hering's t. of color blindness,** that there are three opponent visual substances in the retina: blue-yellow, red-green, and white-black; the absence of one of these substances results in inability to perceive the corresponding colors.

**Huguier's t.,** that in the great majority of cases prolapse of the uterus is due to a primary elongation of the supravaginal portion of the cervix.

**humoral t.,** humoral *doctrine*.

**hydrate microcrystal t. of anesthesia,** Pauling's t.; a t. of narcosis pertaining to non-hydrogen-bonding agents; postulates the interaction of the molecules of the anesthetic drug with water molecules in the brain.

**implantation t. of the production of endometriosis,** that at the time of menstruation cells of the uterine mucosa pass through the uterine tubes and escape into the pelvic cavity where they implant themselves on the periotoneum.

**information t.,** in the behavioral sciences, a system for studying the communication process; it involves the detailed analysis, often mathematical, of all aspects of the process including the encoding, transmission, and decoding of signals but is not concerned in any direct sense with the meaning of a message.

**incasement t.,** preformation t.

**James-Lange t.,** the t. that bodily changes, such as tachycardia or sweating, precede rather than follow the conscious perception of an emotion and by themselves evoke the emotional feeling.

**kern-plasma relation t.,** a t. enunciated by Hertwig (1903) that a definite relation as to size normally exists in every cell between the mass of nuclear material and that of the protoplasm.

**Knoop's t.,** that the catabolism of fatty acids occurs in stages in each of which there is a loss of two carbon atoms as a result of oxidation at the $\beta$-carbon atom, *e.g.,*

$$C_6H_5\overset{\beta}{-}CH_2\overset{\alpha}{-}CH_2-COOH \rightarrow C_6H_5-COOH.$$

**Ladd-Franklin t.,** molecular dissociation t.

**Lamarckian t.,** that acquired characteristics may be transmitted to the descendants.

**learning t.,** any of several prominent theories designed to explain learning, especially those promulgated by Pavlov, Thorndike, Guthrie, Hull, Kohler, Spence, Miller, Skinner, and their modern followers; see also conditioning.

**libido t.,** that man's psychic life results mainly from instinctual or libidinal needs and the attempts to satisfy them.

**Liebig's t.,** that the hydrocarbons that oxidize readily and burn are aliments that produce the greatest quantity of animal heat.

**lipoid t. of narcosis,** Meyer-Overton t. of narcosis; narcotic efficiency parallels the coefficient of partition between oil and water, and lipoids in the cell and on the cell membrane absorb the drug because of this great affinity.

**lymphatic dissemination t. of endometriosis,** that endometrial tissue is transmitted by the lymphatic channels.

**mass action t.,** that large areas of brain tissue function as a whole in learned or intelligent action.

**t. of medicine,** the science, as distinguished from the art, or practice, of medicine.

**Metchnikoff's t.,** the phagocytic t., that the body is protected against infection by the leukocytes and other cells that engulf and destroy the invading microorganisms.

**Meyer-Overton t. of narcosis,** lipoid t. of narcosis.

**migration t.,** the t. of Leber that sympathetic ophthalmia is caused by a transportation of the pathogenic agent through the lymph channels of the optic nerve.

**mnemic t.,** mnemic *hypothesis*.

**molecular dissociation t.,** Ladd-Franklin t.; a t., pertaining to color vision, that gray is the earliest of color sensations, from which are derived, by molecular change, two paired substances that, respectively, detect yellow and blue, and that the yellow gives rise to paired substances for detection of red and green.

**monophyletic t.,** monophyletism.

**myoelastic t.,** a t. stating that sound of the human voice is produced by vibrations of the vocal cords resulting from folding upward due to air pressure below, and subsequent movement downward due to elastic tension of cords.

**myogen'ic t.,** that the cardiac movements are due mainly to stimuli originating in the heart muscle itself, and that the heart does not act solely in response to nerve stimulation.

**Nernst's t.,** that the passage of an electric current through the tissues causes a dissociation of the ions, with consequent concentration of salts in the solution bathing the cell membranes, the electric stimulus being thereby effected.

**neurochronaxic t.,** t. stating that variations in pitch of the human voice are produced by active muscular contractions synchronized with cycles per second of pitch, no longer believed to be true.

**neurogenic t.,** that the cardiac movements are due solely to stimuli conveyed by the nerves; opposed to the myogenic t.

**Ollier's t.,** a t. of compensatory growth; after resection of the articular extremity of a bone, the articular cartilage of the other bone entering into the structure of the joint takes on an increased growth.

**omega-oxidation t.,** that the oxidation of fatty acids commences at the $CH_3$ group, that is, the terminal or omega-group; beta-oxidation then proceeds at both ends of the fatty acid chain; see also Knoop's t.

**overproduction t.,** Weigert's *law.*

**oxygen deprivation t. of narcosis,** narcotics inhibit oxidation, which causes the cell to be narcotized.

**Pasteur's t.,** that immunity produced by an attack of a disease or vaccination is due to exhaustion of the soil necessary for the growth of the specific microorganism.

**Pauling's t.,** hydrate microcrystal t. of anesthesia.

**permeability t. of narcosis,** permeability of the cell membrane is decreased by narcotic concentrations of aliphatic and other central nervous system depressants.

**phlogiston t.,** see phlogiston; see also Stahl, George E.

**pithecoid t.,** the t. of man's descent with the ape from a common ancestor.

**place t.,** a t. of pitch perception which states that the perception of the pitch of a sound depends upon the level or region of the basilar membrane of the cochlea which is set into vibration by the sound waves. See also resonance t.

**Planck's t.,** quantum t.

**polyphyletic t.,** polyphyletism.

**preformation t.,** incasement t.; old t. that the embryo was fully formed in miniature within a gamete at the time of conception. See also homunculus.

**proteomorphic t.,** the t. that the mechanism of immunity against bacterial disease resides in the hemopoietic system, and secondarily in all the cells of the body, the liver being the excretory organ for the waste products resulting from the immunizing process.

**quantum t.,** Planck's t.; that energy can be emitted, transmitted and absorbed only in discrete quantities (quanta), so that atoms and subatomic particles can exist only in certain energy states.

**recapitulation t.,** the t. formulated by Haeckel that individuals in their embryonic development pass through stages similar in general structural plan to the stages their species passed through in its evolution; more technically phrased, the t. that ontogeny is an abbreviated recapitulation of phylogeny; also called law of recapitulation, Haeckel's law; biogenetic law.

**reed instrument t.,** a no longer tenable t. stating that in human voice production the larynx functions in a manner similar to a reed musical instrument.

**reentry t.,** the t. that extrasystoles are due to reentry of the sinus impulse, to which the extrasystole is coupled, into the ectopic focus.

**resonance t. of hearing,** that the basilar membrane of the cochlea acts as a resonating structure, recording low tones from its apical turns and high tones from its basal turns.

**Ribbert's t.,** the t. that a neoplasm may result when a reduction in tension (exerted by adjacent tissues) leads to conditions favorable to uncontrolled growth of cell rests.

**Scholz' t.,** see pathoclisis.

**Semon-Hering t.,** mnemic *hypothesis.*

**sensorimotor t.,** in the developmental t. of Piaget, the postulation that during the first 18 months of life there occurs a transformation of action into thought; at first there is a gradual shift from inborn to acquired behavior, then from body-centered to object-centered activity, ultimately permitting intentional behavior and inventive thinking.

**side chain t.,** the t. advanced by Ehrlich to explain the phenomena of infection, immunity, nutrition, etc.; it assumes that the protoplasmic molecule is analogous in constitution to the benzene molecule, or benzene nucleus, with its linked hydrogen atoms capable of being displaced by various groups to form side chains. So, linked to the protoplasmic molecule are numerous "side chains," or receptors, capable of seizing upon certain bodies, such as food stuffs or poisons, and incorporating them in the molecule; see receptor.

**somatic mutation t. of cancer,** the t. that cancer is caused by a mutation or mutations in the body cells (as opposed to germ cells), especially nonlethal mutations associated with increased multiplication of the mutant cells.

**Spitzer's t.,** an interpretation of the partitioning of the heart of mammalian embryos primarily on the basis of recapitulations of the adult structural pattern of lower forms. Most frequently cited in relation to the partitioning of the truncus arteriosus to form ascending aorta and pulmonary trunk.

**Stahl's t.,** see Stahl, George E.

**stringed instrument t.,** a no longer tenable t. stating that in human voice production the vocal cords function in a manner similar to the strings in a stringed muscial instrument.

**surface tension t. of narcosis,** substances that lower surface tension of water pass more readily into the cell and cause narcosis by decreasing metabolism.

**telephone t.,** a t. of pitch perception which states that the cochlea possesses no faculty of sound analysis, but that the frequency of the impulses transmitted over the auditory nerve fibers corresponds to the frequency of the sound vibrations, and is the sole basis for pitch discrimination.

**thermodynamic t. of narcosis,** interposition of narcotic molecules in nonaqueous cellular phase causes changes that interfere with facilitation of ionic exchange.

**two-sympathin t.,** the t. advanced by Cannon and Rosenblueth that two different types of substances diffuse into circulation when adrenergic nerves are stimulated, although the mediator itself is the same. See also sympathin E and sympathin I.

**van't Hoff's t.,** that substances in dilute solution obey the gas laws.

**Warburg's t.,** that the development of cancer is due to irreversible damage to the respiratory mechanism of cells, leading to the selective multiplication of cells with increased glycolytic metabolism, both aerobic and anaerobic.

**Weismann's t.,** that the vehicle of inheritance is the germ plasm transmitted from one generation to another, and that modifications in the offspring can be effected only by the mingling of the germ plasm of the parents; acquired characters, which affect only the somatic cells, are never transmitted since the somatic cells are mortal and perish with the individual, only the germ cells passing down the succeeding generations and transmitting the inheritance.

**Wollaston's t.,** semidecussation of optic nerves, proved by the hemianopsia in brain lesions.

**Young-Helmholtz t. of color vision,** that there are three sets of color-perceiving elements in the retina, for red, green, and violet, respectively, the perception of the other colors arising from the combined stimulation of these elements. The loss of any one of these elements results in inability to perceive that primary color and a misperception of any other color of which it forms a part.

**zymotic t.,** zymotic *doctrine.*

---

**theother'apy** [ G. *theos*, god, + *therapeia*, therapy ]. Treatment of disease by prayer or religious exercises.

**thèque** (tek) [ Fr. a small box ]. A nest or aggregation of nevi or other cells in the epidermis.

**therapei'a** [ G. See THER- ]. Therapy.

**therapeusis** (thĕr-ă-pu'sis). Therapeutics; therapy.

**therapeutic** (thĕr-ă-pu'tik) [ G. *therapeutikos* ]. Relating to therapeutics, or the treatment of disease.

**therapeutics** (thĕr-ă-pu'tiks) [ G. *therapeutikē*, medical practice. THER- ]. The practical branch of medicine dealing with the treatment of disease.

　**empir'ical t.,** see empirical *treatment.*

　**massive sterilizing t.,** therapia magna sterilisans; "one-shot" cure; the treatment of an infectious disease, especially one of protozoal origin, by one large dose of a suitable remedy, large enough to sterilize all the tissues and to destroy the microorganisms contained therein.

　**mediate t.,** treatment of a nursing infant by administering remedies to the mother.

　**rational t.,** rational *medicine.*

　**ray t.,** radiotherapy.

　**specific t.,** specific *treatment.*

　**suggestive t.,** pithiatry; treatment of disease by means of suggestion.

**therapeu'tist.** One skilled in therapeutics.

**therapia** (ther-ah-pe'ah) [ L. fr. G. *therapeia*, therapy ]. 1. Therapy. 2. Therapeutics.

**t. magna sterili'sans,** massive sterilizing *therapeutics.*

**t. sterili'sans cover'gens,** in chemotherapy, a rapid decrease in the number of the parasites, following the administration of the remedy.

**t. sterili'sans diver'gens,** Browning's phenomenon; in chemotherapy a primary increase in the number of the parasites preceding their final disappearance; see also anamnestic *reaction.*

**t. sterili'sans fractiona'ta,** in chemotherapy, the use of small repeated doses of a microparasiticide when the organism does not become refractory to the drug so given.

**therapist** (thĕr'ă-pist). One skilled in the practice of some type of therapy.

**behavior t.,** a psychotherapist who practices behavior therapy.

**physical t.,** one skilled in the practice of physical therapy; one who has graduated from a course in physical therapy.

**therapy** (thĕr'ă-pī) [ G. *therapeia,* medical treatment. THER- ]. 1. The treatment of disease by various methods; see also therapeutics. 2. In psychiatry, and clinical psychology, used as a short form for psychotherapy; see also subentries under psychotherapy, psychiatry, psychology, and psychoanalysis.

**alimentary t.,** dietotherapy.

**alkali t.,** alkalotherapy.

**analytic t.,** short term for psychoanalytic t.; see psychoanalysis (1).

**anticoagulant t.,** the use of anticoagulant drugs in order to reduce or prevent any tendency toward intravascular or intracardiac clotting.

**autoserum t.,** t. with serum obtained from the patient's own blood.

**beam t.,** chromotherapy; exposure of the patient to one of the colors of the spectrum, especially red or blue.

**behavior t.,** an offshoot of psychotherapy involving the use of procedures and techniques associated with research in the fields of conditioning and learning for the treatment of a variety of psychological conditions; systematic desensitization, flooding, counter-conditioning, and biofeedback are some of the therapeutic techniques employed. Behavior t. is distinguished from psychotherapy because specific symptoms (*e.g.,* phobia, enuresis, high blood pressure) are selected as the target for change, planned interventions or remedial steps to extinguish or modify these symptoms are then employed, and the progress of changes are continuously and quantitatively monitored.

**client-centered t.,** a system of nondirective psychotherapy based on the assumption that the client (patient) both has the internal resources to improve and is in the best position to resolve his own personality dysfunction, provided that the therapist can establish a permissive, accepting, and genuine atmosphere in which the client feels free to discuss his problems and to obtain insight into them in order to achieve self-actualization.

**collapse t.,** the surgical treatment of pulmonary tuberculosis whereby the diseased lung is placed, totally or partially, temporarily or permanently, in a state of retraction and immobilization.

**conjoint t.,** a type of marriage t. in which a therapist sees the partners together in joint sessions.

**depot t.,** injection of a drug together with a substance that slows the release and prolongs the action of the drug.

**diathermic t.,** treatment of lupus, cancer, and other lesions by means of diathermy.

**diet t.,** dietotherapy; see also diet.

**electric shock t.,** electroshock t.

**electroconvulsive t.,** electroshock t.

**electroshock t.,** electric shock t.; electroconvulsive t.; a form of treatment of mental disorders in which convulsions are produced by the passage of an electric current through the brain.

**electrotherapeutic sleep t.,** treatment by inducing sleep by means of nonconvulsive electric stimulation of the brain.

**extended family t.,** a type of family t. that involves family members outside the nuclear family and who are closely associated with it and affect it.

**family t.,** a type of group psychotherapy in which a family in conflict meets as a group with the therapist and explores its relationships and processes; focus is on the resolution of current interactions between members rather than on individual members.

**fango t.,** treatment of rheumatic, gouty, and other diseases by applications of fango or other muds.

**fever t.,** treatment by inducing artificial fever.

**foreign protein t.,** protein shock t.

**geriatric t.,** gerontotherapy.

**Gestalt t.,** a type of psychotherapy, used with individuals or groups, that emphasizes treatment of the person as a whole: his biological component parts and their organic functioning, his perceptual configuration, and his interrelationships with the external world; it focuses on the sensory awareness of the person's immediate experiences rather than on past recollections or future expectations, and employs role playing and other techniques to promote the patient's growth process and to develop his full potential.

**heterovaccine t.,** t. with a vaccine obtained from organisms not directly concerned with the disorder being treated.

**hunger t.,** limotherapy; pinotherapy; nestiatria; nestitherapy; hunger cure; treatment of disease by a restricted diet or absolute fasting.

**hyperbaric oxygen t.,** treatment in which oxygen is provided in a compression chamber at an ambient pressure greater than 1 atmosphere; see also hyperbaric *oxygenation.*

**implosive t.,** a type of behavior t. using implosion (*q. v.*).

**individual t.,** dyadic *psychotherapy.*

**inhalation t.,** the therapeutic use of gases or aerosols by inhalation.

**insulin shock t.,** see insulin shock *treatment.*

**larval t.,** maggot t.

**maggot t.,** larval t.; the application of maggots to open suppurative wounds of bones or soft tissues to remove necrotic tissue.

**maintenance drug t.,** in chemotherapy, systematic dosage reduction to a level at which protection against exacerbation is minimally maintained.

**malarial t.,** malariotherapy.

**marriage t.,** a type of family t. that involves both husband and wife and focuses on the marital relationship as it affects the individual psychopathologies of the partners; the rationale for this method is the assumption that psychopathological processes within the family structure and in the social matrix of the marriage perpetuate individual pathological personality structures, which find expression in the disturbed marriage and are aggravated by the feedback between partners.

**microwave t.,** microkymatotherapy.

**milieu t.,** psychiatric treatment employing manipulation of the social environment for the benefit of the patient.

**nonspecific t.,** the injection of a foreign protein, typhoid vaccine, etc., to induce fever in the treatment of certain diseases, especially those of a parasyphilitic nature.

**occupational t.,** a form of psychiatric t. in which the patient is encouraged to perform vocational or avocational tasks, usually in a social setting; sometimes considered an expressive t., as in art t. or dance t.

**opsonic t.,** vaccine t.; treatment of disease by stimulating the tissues to the production of specific opsonins.

**orthodontic t.,** see orthodontics.

**orthodontic t., functional,** the treatment of malocclusion by utilizing the forces of occlusion or muscular exercise as orthodontic forces.

**orthomolecular t.,** treatment designed to remedy deficiencies in any of the normal chemical constituents of the body.

**oxygen t.,** treatment in which an increased supply of oxygen is made available for breathing, through a nasal catheter, an oxygen tent, oxygen chamber, or oxygen mask.

**paren'teral t.,** t. introduced usually by a needle through some other route than the alimentary canal.

**physical t.,** physiotherapy.

**plasma t.,** treatment with plasma.

**play t.,** a type of t. used with children in which the young patient reveals his problems and fantasies by playing with dolls, clay, or other toys.

**protein shock t.,** the injection of a foreign protein to induce fever as a means of treating certain diseases.

**psychedelic t.,** psychiatric t. utilizing psychedelic drugs; see psychedelic.

**psychoanalytic t.,** analytic t.; psychoanalysis (1).

**quadrangular t.,** marriage t. involving the husband and wife and their respective therapists.

**radium beam t.,** see teleradium t.

**rational t.,** therapeutic procedures based on the premise that lack of information or illogical thought patterns are basic causes of the patient's difficulties; it is assumed that the patient can be assisted in overcoming his problems by a direct, prescriptive, advice-giving approach by the therapist.

**reflex t.,** reflexotherapy; treatment of some morbid condition by exciting a reflex action, as in the household treatment of nosebleed by a piece of ice applied to the cervical spine.

**replacement t.,** t. designed to compensate for a lack or deficiency arising from inadequate nutrition, from certain dysfunctions (such as glandular hyposecretion), or from losses (such as hemorrhage); replacement may be physiological or may entail administration of a substitute (for example, a synthetic estrogen in place of estradiol).

**root canal t.,** dental t. involving sterilization and filling of the root canal.

**sclerosing t.,** sclerotherapy.

**serum t.,** serotherapy.

**shock t.,** see shock *treatment.*

**social t.,** a psychiatric rehabilitative t. to improve a patient's social functioning.

**social network t.,** a type of t. involving the assembling of all persons emotionally or functionally important to the patient; *cf.* extended family t.

**solar t.,** heliotherapy.

**specific t.,** specific *treatment.*

**substitution t.,** replacement t., particularly when replacement is not physiological but a substitute is used (*e.g.,* the use of dextran to correct temporarily hemorrhagic blood loss).

**substitutive t.,** allopathy.

**teleradium t.,** therapeutic use of radium rays the source of which is a large quantity of radium situated at a distant from the patient; also called radium beam t.

**thyroid t.,** (1) the treatment of hypothyroidism; (2) the use of thyroid hormones to promote weight loss.

**total push t.,** the application of all available t.'s to the treatment of a psychiatric patient in a hospital setting.

**ultrasonic t.,** see ultrasonic.

**vaccine t.,** opsonic t.

**therencephalous** (thĕr'en-sef'ă-lus, -thĕr-) [ G. *thēr*, wild beast, + *enkephalos*, brain ]. Denoting a skull in which the angle at the hormion, formed by lines converging from the inion and nasion, measures from 116° to 129°.

**theriaca** (the-ri'ă-kah) [ L. antidote to snake bite, fr. G. *thēriakos*, pertaining to wild beasts ]. A mixture containing a great number of ingredients, used in the Middle Ages and believed to possess antidotal and curative powers to an almost miraculous degree.

**theriatrics** (thĕr'ī-at'ri-ks) [ G. *thērion*, beast, + *iatrikē*, medical treatment ]. 1. The medical treatment of animals in a zoo or menagerie. 2. Veterinary medicine in general.

**therio-** (thĕr'ī-o-) [ G. *thēr, thērion*, beast ]. Combining form relating to animals.

**theriogenology** (thĕr'ī-o-jen-ol'o-jī) [ therio- + G. *genos* birth, + *logos*, study ]. The study of reproduction in animals, especially domestic animals. This veterinary specialty includes the study of veterinary obstetrics and genital diseases in male and female animals, as well as the physiology of animal reproduction.

**therioma** (thĕr'ī-o'mah) [ G. *thērion*, beast, + suffix *-oma*, tumor ]. Old term for a malignant neoplasm.

**theriomorphism** (thĕr'ī-o-mor'fizm) [ G. *thērion*, beast, + *morphē*, form ]. The ascription of animal characteristics to human beings, as contrasted with anthropomorphism.

**theriotherapy** (thĕr'ī-o-thĕr'ă-pī) [ G. *thērion*, beast, + *therapeia*, treatment ]. Veterinary therapeutics.

**therm** [ G. *thermē*, heat ]. An uncertain term for a heat unit used indiscriminately for (1) a small calorie, (2) a large calorie, (3) 1000 large calories, (4) 100,000 British thermal units.

**therm-.** See thermo-.

**thermacogenesis** (ther'mă-ko-jen'ĕ-sis) [ G. *thermē,* heat, + *pharmakon,* drug, + *genesis,* production ]. The elevation of body temperature by drug action.

**thermae** (ther'me) [ G. *thermai,* pl. of *thermē,* heat ]. Hot springs.

**thermaerotherapy** (ther-ma'er-o-thĕr'ă-pī) [ therm- + G. *aēr,* air, + *therapeia,* treatment ]. The treatment of disease by means of heated air.

**ther'mal.** Pertaining to heat.

**thermalgesia** (ther-mal-je'zī-ah) [ therm- + G. *algēsis,* sense of pain ]. Thermoalgesia; excessive sensibility to heat; pain caused by slight degree of heat.

**thermalgia** (ther-mal'jī-ah) [ therm- + G. *algos,* pain ]. Burning pain; see also causalgia.

**thermanalgesia** (therm'an-al-je'zī-ah) [ therm- + analgesia ]. Thermoanesthesia.

**thermanesthesia** (therm'an-es-the'zī-ah). Thermoanesthesia.

**thermatology** (ther'mă-tol'o-jī) [ therm- + G. *logos,* study ]. The branch of therapeutics dealing with the application of heat; see also thermotherapy.

**thermelometer** (ther'mĕ-lom'e-ter) [ therm- + electric + G. *metron,* measure ]. An electric thermometer, especially used for recording slight variations of temperature.

**thermesthesia** (therm'es-the'zī-ah). Thermoesthesia.

**therm'esthesiom'eter.** Thermoesthesiometer.

**ther'min.** Tetrahydro-β-naphthylamine hydrochloride; a psychotomimetic agent resembling amphetamine; it elevates the body temperature.

**ther'mistor** [ G. *thermē,* heat ]. A device for determining temperature; may be extremely small and also may be used to establish and maintain temperature.

**thermo-, therm-** (ther'mo-) [ G. *therme,* heat; *thermos,* warm or hot ]. Combining forms relating to heat.

**thermoalgesia** (ther'mo-al-je'zī-ah). Thermalgesia.

**thermoanalgesia** (ther'mo-an'al-je'zī-ah). Thermoanesthesia.

**thermoanesthesia** (ther'mo-an-es-the'zī-ah) [ thermo- + G. *an-* priv. + *aisthēsis,* sensation ]. Ardanesthesia; thermanesthesia; thermoanalgesia; thermalgesia; loss of the temperature sense or of the ability to distinguish between heat and cold; insensibility to heat or to temperature changes.

**thermocauterectomy** (ther'mo-kaw-ter-ek'to-mī) [ thermocautery + G. *ektomē,* excision ]. Removal of a part by means of the thermocautery.

**thermocautery** (ther'mo-kaw'ter-ī) [ thermo- + G. *kautērion,* branding iron (cautery) ]. The actual cautery; thermoelectric cautery; specifically the Paquelin cautery.

**thermochem'istry.** The interrelation of chemical action and heat.

**thermochroic** (ther-mo-kro'ik). 1. Relating to thermochrose. 2. Exerting a selective action on heat rays.

**thermochroism** (ther-mok'ro-izm). Thermochrosis.

**thermochrose** (ther'mo-krōz) [ thermo- + G. *chrōsis,* coloring ]. The property possessed by heat rays of reflection, refraction, and absorption, similar to that of light rays.

**thermochrosis** (ther-mo-kro'sis) [ thermo- + G. *chrōsis,* coloring ]. The selective action of certain substances on radiant heat, absorbing some of the rays, reflecting and transmitting others.

**thermochrosy** (ther-mok'ro-sī). Thermochrose.

**thermocoagulation** (ther'mo-ko-ag-u-la'shun). The process of gelling tissue by heat.

**thermocouple** (ther-mo-kup'l). Thermopile; a device for measuring slight changes in temperature, consisting of two wires of different metals, *e.g.,* iron and constantan, one wire being kept at a certain low temperature, the other in the tissue or other material whose temperature is to be measured. A thermoelectric current is set up which is measured by a potentiometer.

**thermocur'rent.** A current of thermoelectricity.

**thermodiffusion** (ther'mo-dī-fu'zhun). The diffusion of fluids, either gaseous or liquid, as influenced by the temperature of the fluid.

**thermodilution** (ther'mo-dī-lu'shun). Reduction in temperature in a liquid which occurs when it is introduced into a colder liquid. The volume of the latter liquid can be calculated from the amount of rise in its temperature.

**thermoduric** (ther'mo-du'rik) [ thermo- + L. *durus*, hard, enduring ]. Resistant to the effects of exposure to high temperature; a term used especially with reference to microorganisms.

**thermodynamics** (ther'mo-di-nam'iks) [ thermo- + G. *dynamis*, force ]. 1. The branch of physicochemical science that deals with heat and energy and their conversions one into the other involving mechanical work. 2. The study of the flow of heat.

    **second law of t.,** see under law.

**ther'moelec'tric.** Relating to thermoelectricity.

**thermoelectricity** (ther'mo-e-lek-tris'ĭ-tĭ). An electrical current generated in a circuit of two or more metallic substances, such as antimony and bismuth, when the junction of the two is heated.

**thermoesthesia** (ther'mo-es-the'zĭ-ah) [ thermo- + G. *aisthēsis*, sensation ]. Thermesthesia; thermal or thermic sense; temperature sense; the ability to distinguish differences of temperature.

**thermoesthesiometer** (ther'mo-es-the'zĭ-om'e-ter) [ thermo- + G. *aisthēsis*, sensation, + *metron*, measure ]. Thermesthesiometer; an instrument for testing the temperature sense, consisting of a metal disk with thermometer attached, by which the exact temperature of the disk at the time of application may be known.

**thermoexcitory** (ther'mo-ek-si'to-rĭ). Stimulating the production of heat.

**thermogenesis** (ther'mo-jen'ĕ-sis) [ thermo- + G. *genesis*, production ]. The production of heat; specifically the physiologic process of heat production in the body.

**thermogenet'ic, thermogen'ic.** Thermogenous; relating to thermogenesis.

**thermogen'ics.** The science of heat production.

**thermogenous** (ther-moj'ĕ-nus). Thermogenetic.

**ther'mogram** [ thermo- + G. *gramma*, a writing ]. 1. A regional temperature map of a body or organ obtained, without direct contact, by infrared sensing devices. It measures radiant heat, and thus the blood flow, if the environment is constant. 2. The record made by a thermograph.

**ther'mograph** [ thermo- + G. *graphō*, to write ]. A registering thermometer, one form of which records every variation of temperature by means of a style, moving with the mercury in the tube, and registering its rise and fall upon a circular temperature chart turned by clockwork.

**thermography** (ther-mog'rǎ-fĭ). A process for measuring temperature by means of a thermograph.

    **infrared t.,** measurement of the heat of the regional skin temperature by an infrared technique.

**thermohyperalgesia** (ther'mo-hi'per-al-je'zĭ-ah) [ thermo- + G. *hyper*, over, *algēsis*, sense of pain ]. Excessive thermalgesia.

**thermohyperesthesia** (ther-mo-hi'per-es-the'zĭ-ah) [ thermo- + G. *hyper*, over, + *aisthēsis*, sensation ]. Very acute thermoesthesia or temperature sense.

**thermohypesthesia** (ther'mo-hip'es-the'zĭ-ah) [ thermo- + G. *hypo*, under, + *aisthēsis*, sensation ]. Thermohypoesthesia; diminished heat perception.

**thermohypoesthesia** (ther-mo-hi'po-es-the'zĭ-ah). Thermohypesthesia.

**thermoinhibitory** (ther-mo-in-hib'ĭ-to-rĭ). Inhibiting or arresting thermogenesis.

**thermointegrator** (ther'mo-in'te-gra'tor). A radiation-convection device proposed as an indicator of environmental warmth consisting of a hollow cylinder 8 inches in diameter and 24 inches high, with hemispherical ends, evacuated and heated from within by a wire filament furnishing heat at the rate of 17.5 B.T.U. per sq. ft. per hour. Surface temperature is recorded by means of thermocouples distributed over the surface of the instrument.

**thermojunc'tion.** Thermocouple.

**thermoker'atoplasty** [ thermo- + G. *keras*, horn, + *plassō*, to form ]. A treatment of keratoconus, based on the hydrothermal shrinkage of collagen fibers; corneal flattening (up to 19 diopters) occurs after a heating instrument at 130°C. is applied to the cornea for a few seconds.

**thermolabile** (ther'mo-la-bil) [ thermo- + L. *labilis*, perishable ]. Subject to alteration or destruction by heat.

**ther'molamp.** A lamp used to give heat treatment.

**thermology** (ther-mol'o-jĭ) [ thermo- + G. *logos*, study ]. Thermotics; the science of heat.

**thermolysis** (ther-mol'ĭ-sis) [ thermo- + G. *lysis*, dissolution ]. 1. The loss of body heat by evaporation, radiation, etc. 2. Chemical decomposition by heat.

**thermolyt'ic.** 1. Relating to thermolysis. 2. An agent promoting heat dissipation.

**thermomassage** (ther'mo-mǎ-sahzh'). Combination of heat and massage in physical therapy.

**thermometer** (ther-mom'e-ter) [ thermo- + G. *metron*, measure ]. An instrument for indicating the temperature of any substance. The ordinary t. is a sealed vacuum tube, expanded into a bulb at its lower extremity, and containing mercury; the latter expands with heat and contracts with cold, its level accordingly rising or falling in the tube, the exact degree of variation of level being indicated by a scale etched on the glass of the tube or marked on the frame which holds the tube. For measuring extreme degrees of cold, a t. filled with alcohol instead of mercury is used (**spirit t.**). High temperatures are measured by means of a vessel containing dry air or gas (**air** or **gas t.**), the expansion or increased pressure of which indicates the degree of heat. For measuring excessive heat, such as that of a furnace or pottery kiln, a special form of t., in the shape of a metallic bar or other contrivance is used; this is termed a pyrometer.

    **absolute, Celsius, centigrade, Fahrenheit, homigrade, Kelvin, Rankine, Réaumur t. scales,** see under scale.

    **clinical t.,** a small, self-registering t., consisting of a simple glass tube without frame, used for taking the temperature of the body.

    **heated globe t.,** a radiation-convection instrument proposed as an indicator of environmental warmth, consisting of an outer 6-inch sphere with a t. bulb adjacent to its inner surface and an inner 4-inch sphere electrically heated to produce a heat loss per sq. ft. of the outer sphere equivalent to that of an ordinary human under sedentary conditions (15.3 B.T.U. per sq. ft. per hour).

    **maximum t.,** see self-registering t.

    **resistance t.,** resistance pyrometer; a device measuring temperature by the change of the electrical resistance of a metal wire.

    **self-registering t.,** one in which the maximum or minimum temperature, during the period of observation, is registered by means of a special appliance; in the clinical t. only the highest temperature is registered; this is effected usually by a steel bar above the column of mercury, or by a segment of the mercury separated from the main column by a bubble of air; after the maximum temperature is registered, the bar or segment of mercury remains in place as the column of mercury continues.

    **surface t.,** a clinical t. the bulb of which is flattened in the form of a disk which indicates roughly the temperature of the portion of the skin to which it is applied.

    **wet-bulb t.,** psychrometer.

**thermomet'ric.** Relating to thermometry or to a thermometer reading.

**thermom'etry** [ thermo- + G. *metron*, measure ]. The measurement of temperature.

**thermoneurosis** (ther-mo-nu-ro'sis). An elevation of the temperature of the body due to emotional influence.

**thermonuclear** (ther'mo-nu'kle-ar). Pertaining to nuclear reactions brought about by high temperatures; *e.g.*, the fusion of hydrogen to helium at temperatures of over 100,000,000°C. (the reaction in the "hydrogen bomb").

**thermopenetra'tion.** Medical diathermy.

**thermophagy** (ther-mof'ǎ-jĭ) [ thermo- + G. *phagein*, to eat ]. The eating of hot food.

**thermophile, thermophil** (ther'mo-fil, -fil) [ thermo- + G. *phileō*, to love ]. An organism which grows best at a temperature of 50°C. or higher.

**thermophil'ic.** Pertaining to a thermophile.

**thermopho'bia** [ thermo- + G. *phobos*, fear ]. Morbid fear of heat.

**thermophore** (ther'mo-fōr) [ thermo- + G. *phoros*, bearing ]. 1. An arrangement for applying heat to a part; it consists of a water heater, a tube conveying hot water to a coil, and another tube conducting the water back to the heater. 2. A flat bag containing certain salts that produce heat when moistened; used as a substitute for the hot-water bag. 3. An appliance for preventing cooling of the mask in ether inhalations.

**thermophylic** (ther-mo-fi'lik) [ thermo- + G. *phylaxis,* protection ]. Resistant to heat; denoting certain microorganisms; see also thermostable and thermoduric.

**thermopile** (ther'mo-pīl) [ thermo- + pile ]. A thermoelectric battery, consisting usually of a series of bars of antimony and bismuth joined together; used as a thermoscope, heating of the bars at their junctions giving rise to an electric current.

**thermoplacentography** (ther'mo-plă-sen-tog'ră-fī) [ thermo- + L. *placenta,* placenta, + G. *graphō,* to write ]. Determination of placental position by detection of infrared rays from the large amounts of blood flowing through the placenta.

**Thermoplasma** (ther'mo-plaz'mah) [ thermo- + G. *plasma,* something formed ]. A genus of bacteria (order Mycoplasmatales) which possess the same characteristics as the organisms in the genus *Mycoplasma* except that the thermoplasmas do not require sterol for growth, have an optimal temperature of 55 to 59°C., have an optimal pH of 1.0 to 2.0, and reproduce by budding. The type species is *T. acidophilum.*

  **T. acidophilum,** a species found in a coal refuse pile which had undergone self-heating; it is also found in acid hot springs. It is the type species of the genus *T.*

**thermoplas'tic.** A classification for materials that can be made soft by the application of heat and harden upon cooling.

**thermoplegia** (ther'mo-ple'jī-ah) [ thermo- + G. *plēgē,* stroke ]. Heat stroke; sunstroke.

**thermopolypnea** (ther'mo-pol'ip-ne'ah) [ thermo- + G. *polys,* much, + *pnoia,* breath ]. Rapid respiration caused by fever.

**ther'morecep'tor.** A receptor that is sensitive to heat.

**ther'moregula'tion.** Temperature control.

**thermoreg'ulator.** Thermostat.

**ther'moscope** [ thermo- + G. *skopeō,* to view ]. Differential thermometer; an instrument for indicating slight differences of temperature, without registering or recording them.

**ther'moset.** A classification for materials that become hardened or cured by the application of heat.

**thermostabile, thermostable** (ther'mo-sta'bil, -sta'bl) [ thermo- + L. *stabilis,* stable ]. Not subject to alteration or destruction by heat.

**ther'mostat** [ thermo- + G. *statos,* standing ]. An apparatus for the automatic regulation of heat, as in an incubator.

**thermosteresis** (ther-mo-stě-re'sis) [ thermo- + G. *steresis,* deprivation, loss ]. The abstraction or deprivation of heat.

**thermostrom'uhr.** See under stromuhr.

**thermosystaltic** (ther'mo-sis-tal'tik) [ thermo- + G. *systaltikos,* contractile. STAL- ]. Relating to thermosystaltism.

**thermosystaltism** (ther'mo-sis'tal-tizm) [ see thermosystaltic ]. Contraction, as of the muscles, under the influence of heat.

**thermotac'tic, thermotax'ic.** Relating to thermotaxis.

**thermotaxis** (ther'mo-tak'sis) [ thermo- + G. *taxis,* orderly arrangement ]. 1. Reaction of living protoplasm to the stimulus of heat; distinguished from thermotropism in that the latter refers to the movement of parts of an organism, as leaves, whereas t. refers to the movement of the organism as a whole. 2. Regulation of the temperature of the body.

  **negative t.,** repulsion of a plant or animal from heat.
  **positive t.,** attraction of a plant or animal to heat.

**thermotherapy** (ther'mo-thěr'a-pī) [ thermo- + G. *therapeia,* treatment ]. Treatment of disease by the application of heat in any way.

**thermot'ic.** Relating to thermotics.

**thermot'ics** [ G. *thermotēs,* heat ]. Thermology.

**thermotonometer** (ther'mo-to-nom'e-ter) [ thermo- + G. *tonos,* tone, tension, + *metron,* measure ]. An instrument for measuring the degree of thermosystaltism, or muscular contraction under the influence of heat.

**thermotox'in.** A toxin or poison supposedly formed in the tissues under the influence of excessive heat.

**thermotracheotomy** (ther'mo-tra-ke-ot'o-mī). Tracheotomy performed by means of the thermocautery.

**thermotropism** (ther-mot'ro-pizm) [ thermo- + G. *trope,* a turning ]. The motion toward or away from a source of heat on the part of a portion of an organism, such as leaves or stems; see also thermotaxis.

**the'roid** [ G. *thēr,* a wild beast, + *eidos,* resemblance ]. Resembling an animal in instincts or propensities.

**therology** (the-rol'o-jī) [ G. *thēr,* a wild beast, + *logos,* study ]. The study of mammals.

**thesaurismosis** (the'saw-riz-mo'sis) [ G. *thesauros,* store, storehouse, + G. suffix *-osis,* condition ]. A metabolic disorder in which a substance accumulates or is stored in certain cells, usually in large amounts.

**thesaurismotic** (the'saw-riz-mot'ik). Pertaining to thesaurismosis.

**thesaurosis** (the'saw-ro'sis) [ G. *thesauros,* store, storehouse ]. Abnormal or excessive storage in the body of normal or foreign substances.

**thesis,** pl. **theses** (the'sis, -sēz) [ G. a placing, a position, thesis. THE- ]. 1. An essay on a medical topic prepared by the graduating student. 2. A proposition submitted by the candidate for a doctorate degree in some universities, that must be sustained by argument against any objections offered. 3. Any theory or hypothesis advanced as a basis for discussion.

**the'tins.** Methyl sulfonium compounds in which the *S*-methyl group is "active," and that therefore act as methyl donors in some plants. Dimethylpropiothetin, $(CH_3)_2S^+$—$CH_2$—$CH_2$—$COO^-$, is an example. T.'s are abundant in marine algae.

**Theve'tia.** A genus of plants of the family Apocynaceae, or dogbanes.

  **T. ahou'ai** and **T. neriifo'lia,** species containing the glycosides thevetin A and thevetin B, and thevetoxin; they are fish poisons of Brazil.

  **T. yccot'li,** a Mexican species, containing the glycosides cerberin and thevetoxin. Cerberin (the aglycone is digitoxigenin) combines a digitalis-like action with a paralyzing effect on sympathetic nerves and stimulation of smooth muscles.

**thev'etin A.** A glycoside present in *Thevetia.* The aglycone thevetigenin is digitoxigenin.

**thev'etin B.** THEVANIL; cerberoside; a glycoside of *Thevetia;* has digitalis-like action.

**thia-.** Prefix indicating the replacement of carbon of sulfur in a ring or chain.

**thiaben'dazole** (USP). MINTEZOL; 2-(4-thiazolyl)benzimidazole; a broad spectrum anthelmintic especially effective against roundworms in animals and man.

**thiacetazone** (thi'ă-set'ă-zōn, -ă-se'tă-zōn). Amithiozone.

**thialbarbital.** KEMITHAL; thialbarbitone; 5-allyl-5-(2-cyclohexen-1-yl)-2-thiobarbituric acid; used as the sodium salt; an ultra-short acting thiobarbiturate for induction of general anesthesia by intravenous injection.

**thiambu'tosine** (BP). 4-Butoxy-4'-(dimethylamino)thiocarbanilide; an antileprotic agent.

**thi'amin.** Thiamine (USP, BP); vitamin $B_1$; aneurine; antineuritic vitamin or factor; antiberiberi vitamin or factor; B-P (beriberi-preventive) vitamin; a heat-labile vitamin, contained in milk, yeast, and in the germ and husk of grains, also artifically synthesized. It is essential for growth.

Thiamin

**t. hydrochloride,** thiamine hydrochloride (USP, (BP); aneurine hydrochloride; a coenzyme, used in the prevention of beriberi and other conditions associated with a deficiency of t. in the diet.

**t. mononitrate** thiamine mononitrate (USP); same action as t. hydrochloride.

**t. pyridinylase,** thiaminase I; pyrimidine transferase; enzyme (EC 2.5.1.2) catalyzing transfer of a pyridine or other bases into the position of the pyrimidine in thiamin.

**t. pyrophosphate,** TPP; diphosphothiamin; cocarboxylase; the diphosphoric acid ester of t.; coenzyme of several (de)carboxylases.

**thiam'inase.** 1. An enzyme present in raw fish that destroys thiamin and may produce thiamin deficiency in animals on a diet largely composed of raw fish. 2. Thiaminase II; a hydrolase (EC 3.5.99.2) cleaving thiamin into a pyrimidine moiety and a thiazole moiety; the pyrimidine moiety may appear in the urine as pyramin.

**t. I,** thiamin pyridinylase.

**t. II,** thiaminase (2).

**thi'amine** (USP, BP). Thiamin.

**thi'amphen'icol** (USAN). THIOCYMETIN; D-(+)-threo-2,2-dichloro-$N$-[ $\beta$-hydroxy-$\alpha$-(hydroxymethyl)-$p$-(methylsulfonyl)phenethyl ]acetamide; an antibacterial drug.

**thiam'ylal sodium.** SURITAL sodium; sodium 5-allyl-5-(1-methylbutyl)-2-thiobarbiturate. Prepared as a mixture with sodium bicarbonate. A short-acting barbiturate, used intravenously to produce anesthesia of short duration.

**thi'azin.** Iminothiodiphenylimine; $C_{12}H_{10}SN_2$; parent substance of a family of biological dyes; e.g., methylene blue, thionin, toluidine blue.

**thiazolsul'fone.** PROMIZOLE; 2-amino-5-sulfanylthiazole; same uses as glucosulfone sodium. It is less toxic but also less effective in the treatment of leprosy.

**thiemia** (thi-e'mĭ-ă) [ G. theion, sulfur, + haima, blood ]. The presence of sulfur in the circulating blood.

**thi'enyl.** The radical of thiophene, $SC_4H_3$—; contrast thenyl.

**thienylalanine** (thi'ĕ-nil-al'ă-nēn). 3-(3-Thienyl)alanine; a compound structurally similar to phenylalanine and inhibiting the growth of Escherichia coli, presumably by competitive inhibition of enzymes for which phenylalanine is substrate.

**Thier,** Carl Jorg. See Weyers-T. syndrome.

**Thiers,** Joseph, French physician, *1885. See Achard-T. syndrome.

**Thiersch** (teersh), Karl, German surgeon, 1822–1895. See T.'s canaliculi, graft, knife, method.

**thiethazone** TEBACYL; 1-ethyl-3-($p$-formylphenyl)urea thiosemicarbazone; tuberculostatic agent.

**thiethylperazine maleate** (thi-eth'il-pĕr'ă-zēn) (NF). TORECAN maleate; 2-ethyl-mercapto-10-3-(1-methyl-4-piperazinyl)propyl phenothiazine dimaleate; an antiemetic agent with mild tranquilizing activity. It is used to control nausea and vomiting associated with vertigo, the administration of general anesthetics, and with several other clinical conditions. It also has weak hypotensive, spasmolytic, antihistaminic, and hypothermic actions.

**thigh** (thi). The part of the inferior limb, between the hip and the knee.

**driver's t.,** neuralgia or neuritis of the sciatic nerve, due to pressure on the nerve produced by the long-continued use of the accelerator pedal in driving a motor car.

**Heilbronner's t.,** flattened and broadening of the t., when the patient lies supine on a hard mattress, in cases of organic paralysis; absent in hysterical paralysis.

**thigmesthesia** (thig'mes-the'zĭ-ah) [ G. thigma, touch, + aisthēsis, sensation ]. Sensibility to touch.

**thigmotaxis** (thig'mo-tak'sis) [ G. thigma, touch, + taxis, orderly arrangement ]. A form of barotaxis; denoting the reaction of plant or animal protoplasm to contact with a solid body.

**thigmotropism** (thig-mot'ro-pizm) [ G. thigma, touch, + tropē, a turning ]. A movement toward or away from a touch stimulus on the part of a portion of an organism, such as leaves or tendrils; see thigmotaxis.

**thihex'inol methylbromide.** ENTOQUEL methylbromide; [ 4-(hydroxydi-2-thienylmethyl)cyclohexyl ] trimethylam-

monium bromide; an anticholinergic and gastrointestinal antispasmodic.

**thimer'fonate sodium** (USAN). SULFO-MERTHIOLATE; sodium $p$-ethylmercurithiophenylsulfonate; antiseptic.

**thimer'osal** (NF). MERTHIOLATE sodium; thiomersalate; thimersal; [ (o-carboxyphenyl)thio ]ethylmercury sodium salt; antiseptic.

**think'ing.** The act of reasoning.

**abstract t.,** t. in terms of concepts and general principles (e.g., a table and a chair are both furniture), as contrasted with concrete t.

**archaic-paralogical t.,** prelogical t.

**concrete t.,** t. of objects as specific or disparate items (e.g., one eats at a table and sits on a chair), as contrasted with abstract t.

**creative t.,** productive t., with novel rather than routine results.

**magical t.,** the irrational equating of t. with doing.

**prelogical t.,** archaic-paralogical t.; prelogical mind; a concrete type of t., characteristic of children and primitives, to which schizophrenic persons are sometimes said to regress.

**thinking through.** The psychological process of understanding, with insight, one's own behavior.

**thinning.** Causing a decrease in viscosity by chemical means, as by the addition of a solvent, or mechanical means, as in shear t.

**shear t.,** decreasing the viscosity of a polymer or macromolecule or gel by increasing the rate of shear; not ordinarily a function of time. See also thixotropy.

**thio-** (thi'o-). A prefix denoting that sulfur has replaced oxygen in the compound to the name of which it is attached.

**thioacid** (thi-o-as'id). Sulfacid; sulfoacid; an organic acid in which one or more of the oxygen atoms have been replaced by sulfur atoms.

**thioal'cohol.** Mercaptan.

**thioam'ide.** An amide in which S replaces O.

**thioate** (thi'o-āt). A salt or ester of a thioic acid.

**thioaurin** (thi-o-aw'rin). $C_{14}H_{12}O_4N_4S_4$; an orange-yellow antibiotic active against both Gram-positive and Gram-negative bacteria, produced by an unidentified Streptomyces species.

**thiobar'bital.** An antithyroid agent with double the potency of thiouracil, but more toxic.

**thiobarbit'urates.** Hypnotics of the barbiturate group, e.g., thiopental, in which the oxygen atom at carbon-2 is replaced by sulfur.

**thiocar'bamide.** Thiourea.

**thi'ocar'lide.** ISOXYL; AMIXYL; 4,4'-di(isoamyloxy)thiocarbanilide; a synthetic compound whose molecule contains the three antituberculous groups $p$-aminosalicylic acid, $p$-aminobenzaldehyde thiosemicarbazone, and the thiocarbamide group; antitubercular agent.

**thiochrome** (thi'o-krōm). A fluorescent compound, $C_{12}H_{14}N_4OS$, produced by the oxidation of thiamin; used in methods for detection and determination of thiamin.

**thioctic acid** (thi-ok'tik). Lipoic acid.

**thiocy'anate.** Rhodanate; a salt of thiocyanic, or sulfocyanic, acid.

**thiocyan'ic acid.** H—S—C≡N; hydrogen thiocyanate.

**thiocyanogen number** (thi'o-si-an'o-jen). Thiocyanogen value; the number of grams of thiocyanogen taken up by 100 gm. of fat; analogous to the iodine number, except that thiocyanogen will not add to all the double bonds in polyunsaturated fatty acids as will iodine.

**thiodi'phenyl'amine.** Phenothiazine.

**thioethanolamine acetyltransferase.** Thiotransacetylase B; enzyme (EC 2.3.1.11) transferring acetyl from acetyl-CoA to the sulfur atom of thioethanolamine.

**thioether** (thi-o-e'ther). Sulfide; an ether in which the oxygen is replaced by sulfur; a sulfur ether.

**thiofla'vin S.** A methylated and sulfonated derivative of primulin; a yellowish dye used in fluorescence microscopy.

**thioglu'cosi'dase** (EC 3.2.3.1). Myrosinase; sinigrinase; sinigrase; an enzyme in mustard seed that converts thioglycosides into thiols plus sugars (e.g., hydrolyzes sinalbin and sinigrin of mustard seeds).

**thi'oglyc'erol.** See monothioglycerol.

**thioglycolate, thioglycollate** (thi-o-gli'ko-lāt). A salt or ester of thioglycolic acid. Frequently used in bacterial media to reduce the oxygen content of the medium so as to create favorable conditions for the growth of anaerobes; the t. will also inactivate any mercurial that might be carried over with the inoculum.

**thioglycol'ic acid.** Mercaptoacetic acid; $HSCH_2COOH$; used as a reagent for the detection of metals such as iron, molybdenum, silver, and tin. The ammonium and sodium salts are used in home permanents, the calcium salt as a depilatory.

**thioguanine** (thi-o-gwah'nēn) (USP, NF). 6-TG; 2-amino-purine-6-thiol; an antineoplastic agent used for leukemias and nephrosis.

**-thioic acid** (-thi-o'ik). Suffix denoting the radical, —C(S)OH or —C(O)SH, the sulfur analogue of a carboxylic acid; a thiocarboxylic acid.

**thioki'nases.** Acyl-CoA synthetase; see under acyl-coenzyme A.

**thi'ol.** 1. The monovalent radical —SH when attached to carbon; a hydrosulfide; a compound containing this group. 2. A mixture of sulfurated and sulfonated petroleum oils purified with ammonia; used in the treatment of skin diseases.

**thi'olase.** Acetyl-CoA acetyltransferase.

**thiolhistidylbetaine** (thi-ol-his'tĭ-dil-ba'tā-ēn). Ergothioneine.

**thioltransacetylase A** (thi'ol-trans-ă-set'ĭ-lās). Lipoate acetyltransferase.

**thiolysis** (thi-ol'ĭ-sis). The cleavage of a chemical bond with the addition to one part of coenzyme A; a term analogous to hydrolysis and phosphorolysis.

**thiomersal** (BP). Thimerosal.

**thiomer'salate.** Thimerosal.

**thiometh'yladen'osine.** Methylthioadenosine.

**β-thionase.** Cystathionine β-synthase.

**-thione.** Suffix denoting the radical >C=S, the sulfur analogue of a ketone; a thiocarbonyl group.

**thioneine** (thi'o-ne'in). Ergothioneine.

**thion'ic** Relating to sulfur.
  **t. acid,** see -thioic acid.

**thi'onine.** Amidophenthiazine; Lauth's violet; a dark green powder, giving a purple solution in water. Used as a stain in bacteriology and histology.

**thiono-.** Prefix sometimes used for thioxo-.

**thiopan'ic acid.** Pantoyltaurine; pantothenic acid in which the carboxyl group is replaced by a sulfonic acid group.

**thiopen'tal sodium** (USP). PENTOTHAL sodium; thiopentone sodium; sodium 5-ethyl-5-(1-methylbutyl)-2-thiobarbiturate; an ultra-short-acting barbiturate administered intravenously or rectally for induction of anesthesia or for general anesthesia of short duration.

**thiopen'tone sodium** (BP). Thiopental sodium.

**thioper'azine.** VONTIL; thioproperazine; N,N-dimethyl-10-[ 3- (4-methyl-1-piperazinyl) propyl ]phenothiazine-2-sulfonamide; antiemetic and antianxiety agent.

**thi'ophene.** The fundamental ring compound

S—CH=CH—CH=CH
1    2    3    4    5

**thiophorases.** CoA transferases.

**thiopro'pazate hydrochloride.** DARTAL dihydrochloride; 2-chloro-10-{3-[ 4-(2-acetoxyethyl)piperazinyl ]propyl}phenothiazine dihydrochloride; a phenothiazine derivative related chemically and pharmacologically to prochlorperazine and perphenazine; antipsychotic agent.

**thioproper'azine.** Thioperazine.

**thioridazine hydrochloride** (thi'o-rid'ă-zēn) (USP, BP). MELLARIL; 10-[ 2-(1-methyl-2-piperidyl)ethyl ]-2-(methylthio)phenothiazine monohydrochloride; an antipsychotic agent with action similar to that of chlorpromazine; side

effects are reported to be generally less than those of other phenothiazine derivatives.

**thiosemicar'bazide.** One of the group of thiosemicarbazones with a tuberculostatic action. Used as a reagent in the detection of metals.

**thiosemicar'bazone.** 1. A compound containing the thiosemicarbazide radical, =N—NH—C(S)—NH$_2$. 2. One of a group of tuberculostatic drugs which includes thiosemicarbazide, benzaldehyde thiosemicarbazone, and 4-aminoacetylbenzaldehyde thiosemicarbazone. 3. Thioacetazone.

**thiosinamine** (thi'o-sin-am'ēn). (NH$_2$)CSNHCH$_2$CHCH$_2$; allyl sulfocarbamide; allylthiourea; has been used as a resolvent of scar tissue, uterine fibroids, and fibrous adhesions in joints.

**thiosul'fate.** $S_2O_3=$; a salt of thiosulfuric acid.
  **t. cyanide transsulfurase,** t. sulfurtransferase.
  **t. sulfurtransferase,** rhodanese; thiosulfate thiotransferase; thiosulfate cyanide transsulfurase; a transferase (EC 2.8.1.1) that catalyzes the formation of thiocyanate and sulfite from cyanide and thiosulfate.
  **t. thiotransferase,** t. sulfurtransferase.

**thiosulfu'ric acid.** Sulfuric acid in which an atom of oxygen has been replaced by one of sulfur; $H_2S_2O_3$.

**thio-TEPA** (thi'o-tep'ah) (BP). Triethylenethiophosphoramide.

**thiothix'ene** (NF). NAVANE; N,N-dimethyl-9-[ 3-(4-methyl-1-piperazinyl)-propylidene ]thioxanthene-2-sulfonamide; antipsychotic agent.

**thiotransacetylase B.** Thioethanolamine acetyltransferase.

**2-thiouracil** (thi'o-u'ră-sil). 2-Mercapto-4-pyrimidinone; a thioamide derivative that inhibits the synthesis of thyroid hormones; produces hypothyroidism which results in hyperplasia and increased vascularity. It is used in the treatment of hyperthyroidism, either to induce permanent remission or prior to thyroidectomy. Side effects are common; agranulocytosis may occur. Propylthiouracil, methimazole, and carbimazole are less toxic.

2-Thiouracil

**4-thiouracil.** Uracil with S replacing O in position 4; isomeric with 2-thiouracil.

**thiourea** (thi-o-u-re'ah). Thiocarbamide; SC(NH$_2$)$_2$; an antithyroid compound of the thioamide group; for actions and uses, see thiouracil. Several derivatives of t. are useful in the treatment of leprosy.

**thi'oxan'thene.** A class of tricyclic compounds resembling phenothiazine, but with the central ring nitrogen replaced by a carbon atom; current use emphasizes the antipsychotic and antiemetic properties of this class.

**thioxo-.** Prefix indicating =S in a thioketone (see also -thione, the suffix form).

**thiox'olone.** STEPIN; 4-hydroxy-1,3(2H)-benzoxathiol-2-one; antiseborrheic agent.

**thiphen'amil hydrochloride** (USAN). TROCINATE; diphenylthioacetic acid S-(2-diethylaminoethyl)ester hydrochloride; used as genitourinary and intestinal antispasmodic.

**thirst** [ A.S. *thurst*]. A desire to drink associated with uncomfortable sensations in the mouth and pharynx.
  **absence of t.,** adipsia; aposia.
  **excessive t.,** polydipsia.
  **false t.,** pseudodipsia; t. that is not satisfied by drinking or taking water; t. associated with a dry mouth but not with a bodily need for water.
  **morbid t.,** dipsosis.
  **true t.,** t. that can be satisfied by drinking water.

twilight t., hypodipsia.

**Thiry** (tē're), Ludwig, Austrian physiologist, 1817–1897. See T.'s *fistula,* T.-Vella *fistula.*

**thixola'bile.** Exhibiting thixotropy.

**thixotrop'ic.** Exhibiting thixotropy.

**thixotropy** (thik-sot'ro-pī) [ G. *thixis,* a touching, + *trope,* turning ]. The property of certain gels of becoming less viscous when shaken or subjected to shearing forces and returning to the original viscosity upon standing; *e.g.,* synovial fluid, ferrous hydroxide gel. It is a characteristic of a system exhibiting a decrease in viscosity with an increase in the rate of shear, usually a function of time.

**thlipsencephalus** (thlip'sen-sef'ă-lus) [ G. *thlipsis,* pressure, fr. *thlibō,* fut. *thlipsō,* to press, + *enkephalos,* brain ]. An anencephalic fetus in which the brain is represented by a spongy mass which extrudes through a defect in the upper cervical spine and back of the skull.

**thob'bling** [ fr. init. letters of *think, opine, believe* + *-ing* ]. Thinking that is affected by bias, prejudice, or related predispositions; emotional thinking.

**Thoma** (to'mah), Richard, German histologist, 1847–1923. See T.'s *ampulla,* counting *chamber, fluid,* T.-Zeiss *hemocytometer,* T.'s *laws.*

**Thomas,** Hugh O., British surgeon, 1834–1891. See T.'s *splints.*

**Thompson,** Sir Henry, London surgeon, 1820–1904. See T.'s *test.*

**Thomsen,** Asmus J., Danish physician, 1815–1896. See T.'s *disease.*

**Thomson,** F. H., English physician, 1867–1938. See T.'s *sign.*

**Thomson,** M. S. See Rothmund-T. *syndrome.*

**thonzo'nium bromide** (USAN). THONZIDE; hexadecyl [ 2-[ (*p*-methoxybenzyl) -2-pyrimidinylamino ]ethyl ]dimethylammonium bromide; a detergent used for pharmaceuticals.

**thonzyl'amine hydrochloride.** NEOHETRAMINE hydrochloride; 2-[ (2-dimethylaminoethyl)(*p*-methoxybenzyl)-amino ]pyrimidine hydrochloride; a histamine-antagonizing agent.

**thorac-, thoracico-.** See thoraco-.

**tho'racal.** Thoracic.

**thoracalgia** (tho'ră-kal'jī-ah) [ thoraco- + G. *algos,* pain ]. Pleurodynia; thoracodynia; pain in the chest.

**thoracectomy** (tho'ră-sek'to-mī) [ thoraco- + G. *ektome,* excision ]. Resection of a portion of a rib.

**thoracentesis** (thor'ră-sen-te'sis) [ thoraco- + G. *kentesis,* puncture ]. Pleuracentesis; pleurocentesis; thoracocentesis; insertion of a hollow needle or a trocar and cannula into the pleural cavity.

**thoracic** (tho-ras'ik). Relating to the thorax.

**thoracico-** (tho-ras'ī-ko-). See thoraco-.

**thoracicoabdom'inal.** Relating to the thorax and the abdomen.

**thoracicoacro'mial.** Acromiothoracic.

**thoracicohu'meral.** Relating to the thorax and the humerus.

**thoraco-, thorac-, thoracico-** (tho-ră-ko-) [ G. *thorax,* chest ]. Combining forms relating to the chest (thorax).

**thoracoabdom'inal.** Thoracicoabdominal.

**thoracoacro'mial.** Acromiothoracic.

**thoracoceloschisis** (tho'ră-ko-se-los'kī-sis) [ thoraco- + G. *koilia,* belly, + *schisis,* fissure ]. Thoracogastroschisis; a congenital fissure of the trunk embracing both the thoracic and abdominal cavities.

**thoracocente'sis.** Thoracentesis.

**thoracocyllosis** (tho'ră-ko-sī-lo'sis) [ thoraco- + G. *kyllosis,* a crippling ]. Any deformity of the chest walls.

**thoracocyrtosis** (tho'ră-ko-ser'to'sis) [ thoraco- + G. *kyrtōsis,* a being crooked ]. Abnormally wide curvature of the chest wall.

**tho'racodel'phus.** Thoradelphus.

**thoracodyn'ia** [ thoraco- + G. *odyne,* pain ]. Thoracalgia.

**thoracogastroschisis** (tho'ră-ko-gas-tros'kī-sis) [ thoraco- + G. *gastēr,* belly, + *schisis,* fissure ]. Thoracoceloschisis.

**tho'racograph** [ thoraco- + G. *graphō,* to record ]. An instrument for obtaining the horizontal contour of the chest.

**tho'racolap'arot'omy** [ thoraco- + laparotomy ]. Exposure of diaphragmatic region by an incision that opens both thorax and abdomen.

**thoracolum'bar.** 1. Relating to the thoracic and lumbar portions of the vertebral column. 2. Relating to the sympathetic division of the autonomic nervous system; see *systema* nervosum autonomicum.

**thoracolysis** (tho-ră-kol'ī-sis) [ thoraco- + G. *lysis,* dissolution ]. Breaking up of pleural adhesions.

**thoracomelus** (tho'ră-kom'e-lus) [ thoraco- + G. *melos,* limb ]. Unequal conjoined twins in which the parasite, often only a single arm or leg, is attached to the thorax of the autosite.

**thoracom'eter** [ thoraco- + G. *metron,* measure ]. Stethometer.

**thoracomyodynia** (tho'ră-ko-mi-o-din'ī-ah) [ thoraco- + G. *mys,* muscle, + *odyne,* pain ]. Pain in the muscles of the chest wall.

**thoracopagus** (tho'ră-kop'ă-gus) [ thoraco- + G. *pagos,* something fastened ]. Synthorax; conjoined twins with fusion in the thoracic region.

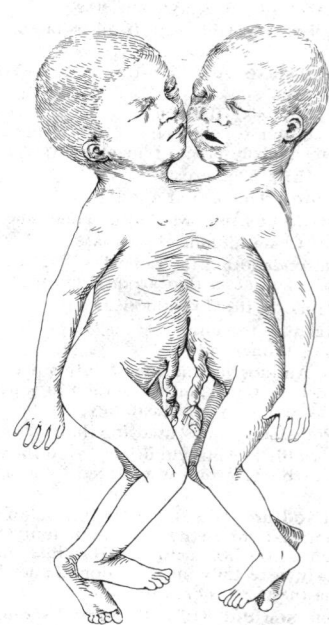

**Thoracopagus**

**thoracoparacephalus** (tho'ră-ko-păr'ă-sef'ă-lus) [ thoraco- + G. *para,* beside, + *kephale,* head ]. Unequal conjoined twins in which a rudimentary parasitic head is attached to the thorax of the autosite.

**thoracopathy** (tho'ră-kop'ă-thī) [ thoraco- + G. *pathos,* suffering ]. Any disease of the thoracic organs or tissues.

**thoracoplasty** (tho'ră-ko-plas'tī) [ thoraco- + G. *plassō,* to form ]. Reparative or plastic surgery of the thorax. **Quénu's t.,** resection of the ribs to allow retraction of the thorax in the treatment of empyema.

**thoracopneumoplasty** (tho'ră-ko-nu'mo-plas-tī) [ thoraco- + G. *pneumōn,* lung, + *plassō,* to form ]. Reparative or plastic surgery of the chest in which the lung is also involved.

**thoracoschisis** (tho-ră-kos'kī-sis) [ thoraco- + G. *schisis,* fissure ]. Congenital fissure of the chest wall.

**thorac'oscope** [ thoraco- + G. *skopeō,* to view ]. Stethoscope.

**thoracoscopy** (tho'ră-kos'ko-pĭ) [ thoraco- + G. *skopeō*, to view ]. Examination of the pleural cavity by means of an endoscope introduced through a cannula.

**thoracosteno'sis** [ thoraco- + G. *stenōsis*, narrowing ]. Narrowness of the chest.

**thoracostomy** (tho'ră-kos'to-mĭ) [ thoraco- + G. *stoma*, mouth ]. The establishment of an opening into the cavity of the chest, as for the drainage of an empyema; or resection of a portion of a rib over a greatly hypertrophied heart.

**thoracotomy** (tho'ră-kot'o-mĭ) [ thoraco- + G. *tome*, incision ]. Pleuracotomy; pleurotomy; any cutting operation upon the chest wall.

**thoradelphus** (tho'ră-del'fus) [ thoraco- + G. *adelphos*, brother ]. Thoracodelphus; conjoined twins belonging to the class of duplicitas posterior in which, from the navel upward, the two individuals are fused into one.

**thorax,** gen. **thora'cis,** pl. **thoraces** (tho'raks, tho'ră-sēz, -ra'sēz) [ L. fr. G. *thōrax,* breastplate, the chest, fr. *thōrēssō,* to arm ] [ NA ]. The chest; the upper part of the trunk between the neck and the abdomen; it is formed by the 12 thoracic vertebrae, the 12 pairs of ribs, the sternum, and the muscles and fasciae attached to these; below it is separated from the abdomen by the diaphragm; it contains the chief organs of the circulatory and respiratory systems, as distinguished from the abdomen which encloses those of the digestive apparatus.

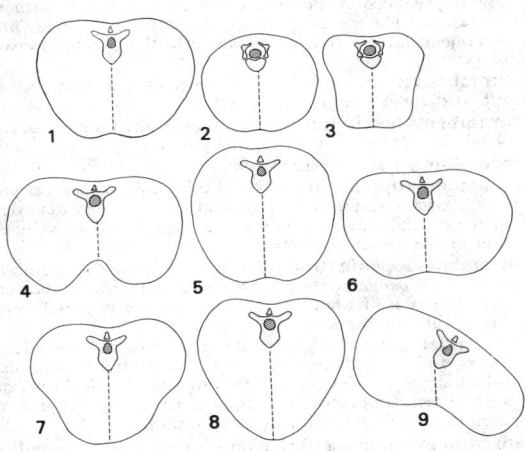

**Thorax**

Types of abnormal thorax compared with normals in cross section: *1,* normal adult; *2,* normal infant; *3,* rachitic; *4,* funnel breast; *5,* emphysematous; *6,* phthisical; *7,* unilaterally retracted; *8,* pigeon breast; *9,* in scoliosis.

**Peyrot's t.,** an obliquely oval deformity of the chest in cases of a very large pleural effusion.

**thorium** (tho'rĭ-um) [ Thor, the Norse god of thunder ]. A metallic element, symbol Th, atomic no. 90, atomic weight 232.05; it is radioactive; the one naturally occurring nuclide being t.-232, with a half-life of 14,000,000,000 years; see also radiothorium.

**thorium-230.** Part of the uranium-238 radioactive series, formed through the breakdown of uranium-234 (uranium II); decays by way of alpha particle emisssion to form radium-226, its half-life being $7.5 \times 10^4$ years. Formerly termed ionium.

**thorium X.** An early radioactive breakdown product of thorium; identified as the radium isotope, $^{224}$Ra.

**Thormählen** (tor'ma-len), Johann, German physician, 19th century. See T.'s *test.*

**Thorn** George W., American physician, *1906. See T.'s *syndrome, test.*

**thorn.** In anatomy, a thornlike or spinous structure.
  **dendritic t.'s,** dendritic *spines.*
  **penis t.'s,** penis *spines.*

**Thornwaldt,** G. L., German physician, 1843–1910. See T.'s *abscess, cyst, syndrome.*

**tho'ron.** Radon-220.

**thoroughbred** (thur'o-bred). A breed of light horses used for racing purposes. This term is often used erroneously for purebred.

**thorough-pin** (thur'o-pin). Synovial distention of the sheath of the flexor perforans tendon of the horse, causing a swelling on each side of the hollow of the hock.

**thought reading.** Telepathy.

**thought transference.** Telepathy.

**Thr.** Symbol for threonine or its radical forms.

**thread** (thred). 1. Suture material. 2. A thread-shaped structure.
  **Pagenstecher's t.,** celluloid yarn; linen t. impregnated with celluloid; used as a suture material, especially in intestinal work.
  **Simonart's t.'s,** amniotic *bands.*
  **terminal t.,** *filum* terminale.

**thread'worm.** Common name for species of the genus *Strongyloides;* sometimes applied to any of the smaller parasitic nematodes.

**thready** (thred'ĭ). Filamentous; filiform.

**threon'ic acid.** The acid derived by oxidation of the —CHO group of threose to COOH; a product of the oxidation of ascorbic acid by hypoiodite.

**thre'onine.** $CH_3$—CHOH—$CHNH_2$—COOH; 2-amino-3-hydroxybutyric acid; one of the naturally occurring amino acids, included in the structure of most proteins, and essential to the diet of man and other mammals.
  **t. deaminase,** t. dehydratase.
  **t. dehydratase** (EC 4.2.1.16), t. deaminase; an enzyme catalyzing the anaerobic deamination of t. to 2-ketobutyric acid, possibly identical with serine dehydratase.

**thre'ose.** One of the two aldoses (the other is erythrose) containing four carbon atoms; an aldotetrose. See structures under sugars.

**threpsol'ogy** [ G. *threpsis,* nourishment (TREPH-), + *logos,* study ]. The science of nutrition.

**threshold** (thresh'old) [ A.S. *therxold* ]. 1. The point where a stimulus begins to produce a sensation, the lower limit of perception of a stimulus. 2. The minimal stimulus eliciting a motor response. 3. Limen.
  **absolute t.,** stimulus t.; the lowest limit of any perception whatever; distinguished from differential t.
  **achromatic t.,** visual t.
  **auditory t.,** the intensity of any barely perceptible sound.
  **brightness difference t.,** light difference (2); the smallest difference that can be perceived as a difference in brightness.
  **t. of consciousness,** the lowest point at which a stimulus sensation can be perceived.
  **convulsant t.,** the smallest amount of stimulation, electric current, or drug required to induce a convulsion.
  **differen'tial t.,** the lowest limit at which two stimuli can be differentiated.
  **displacement t.,** the least distinguishable break in the contour of a line.
  **double-point t.,** the least degree of separation of two points applied to the body surface that permits of their being felt as two.
  **erythe'ma t.,** the point where erythema of the skin is produced by irradiation with ultraviolet or other kinds of rays.
  **galvanic t.,** rheobase.
  **ketogenic t.,** the ketogenic-antiketogenic ratio at which ketosis appears.
  **ketosis t.,** the critical level in the blood of ketones at which they appear in the urine.
  **light t.,** visual t.
  **relational t.,** the smallest degree of difference between two stimuli that permits them to be perceived as different.
  **renal t.,** concentration of plasma substance above which the substance appears in the urine.
  **stimulus t.,** absolute t.
  **swallowing t.,** (1) the moment that the act of swallowing begins after the mastication of food; (2) the critical moment

of reflex action initiated by minimum stimulation, prior to the act of deglutition.

**visual t.,** t. of visual sensation; light t.; achromatic t.; the minimal light intensity evoking a visual sensation; it varies with adaptation, size and color of stimulus, and diameter of pupil.

**t. of visual sensation,** visual t.

**thrill.** The vibration accompanying a cardiac or vascular murmur, which can be felt on palpation; see also fremitus.

**diastol′ic t.,** a t. felt over the precordium or over a blood vessel during ventricular diastole.

**hydatid t.,** the peculiar trembling or vibratory sensation felt on palpation of a hydatid cyst.

**presystol′ic t.,** a t. sometimes felt, on palpation over the apex of the heart, immediately preceding the ventricular contraction.

**systol′ic t.,** a t. felt over the precordium or over a blood vessel during ventricular systole.

**thrix** [ G. ]. Hair.

**t. annula′ta,** ringed *hair.*

**throat** (thrōt) [ A.S. *throtu* ]. 1. The gullet; the fauces and pharynx. 2. The anterior aspect of the neck; jugulum. 3. Any narrowed entrance into a hollow part.

**putrid sore t.,** gangrenous *pharyngitis.*

**septic sore t.,** a severe pseudomembranous inflammation of the fauces and tonsils, usually occurring in epidemic form, caused by the hemolytic Streptococcus transmitted in an infected milk supply.

**sore t.,** odynphagia; angina; a condition characterized by pain or discomfort on swallowing; it may be any of a variety of inflammations of the tonsils, pharynx, or larynx.

**ulcerated sore t.,** gangrenous *pharyngitis.*

**throat′worm.** *Syngamus trachea.*

**throb.** 1. To pulsate. 2. A beating or pulsation.

**throe** (thro) [ A.S. *thrāw* ]. 1. A severe pain or pang. 2. The pain of childbirth.

**thromb-.** See thrombo-.

**throm′base.** Thrombin.

**thrombasthenia** (throm′bas-the′nĭ-ah) [ thromb- + G. *asthenia,* weakness ]. Glanzmann's t.

**Glanzmann's t.,** Glanzmann's disease; constitutional thrombopathy (2); hereditary hemorrhagic t.; a hemorrhagic diathesis characterized by normal or prolonged bleeding time, normal coagulation time, defective clot retraction, normal platelet count but morphologic or functional abnormality of platelets; several different kinds of platelet abnormalities have been described.

**hereditary hemorrhagic t.,** Glanzmann's t.

**thrombectomy** (throm-bek′to-mĭ) [ thromb- + G. *ektomē,* excision ]. The excision of a thrombus.

**thrombelas′togram.** Registration of coagulation process by a thrombelastograph.

**thrombelastograph** (thromb′e-las′to-graf) [ thromb- + G. *elastreō,* to push, + *graphō,* to write ]. Apparatus for registering elastic variations of a thrombus during the process of coagulation.

**throm′bi.** Plural of thrombus.

**throm′bin.** Thrombosin; thrombase; fibrinogenase. 1. An enzyme (a proteinase, EC 3.4.21.5) formed in the blood, after this is shed, that converts fibrinogen into fibrin by hydrolyzing peptides (and amides and esters) of L-arginine; it is formed from prothrombin by the action of prothrombinase (factor XA), another proteinase. 2 (USP). Sterile protein substance prepared from prothrombin of bovine origin through interaction with thromboplastin in the presence of calcium. It causes clotting of whole blood, plasma, or a fibrinogen solution. Used as a topical hemostatic for capillary bleeding with or without fibrin foam in general and plastic surgical procedures.

**human t.** (BP), obtained from human plasma by precipitation with suitable salts and organic solvents; same uses as t.

**thrombinogen** (throm-bin′o-jen). Prothrombin.

**thrombinogenesis** (throm′bĭ-no-jen′ĕ-sis). Thrombin production.

**throm′bintimec′tomy** [ thromb- + L. *intima* (*tunica*), innermost tunic, + G. *ektomē,* excision ]. Old term for thromboendarterectomy.

**thrombo-, thromb-** (throm′bo-) [ G. *thrombos,* clot (thrombus). TREPH- ]. Combining forms denoting blood clot or relation thereto.

**thromboangiitis** (throm-bo-an-jī-i′tis) [ thrombo- + G. *angeion,* vessel, + suffix, *-itis,* inflammation ]. Inflammation of the intima of a vessel, with thrombosis.

**t. oblit′erans,** Buerger's disease; Winiwarter-Buerger disease; inflammation of the entire wall and connective tissue surrounding medium-sized arteries and veins, especially of the legs of young and middle-aged men; associated with thrombotic occlusion and commonly resulting in gangrene.

**thromboarteritis** (throm-bo-ar-ter-i′tis). Thromboangiitis affecting an artery.

**throm′boasthe′nia.** Thrombasthenia.

**throm′boblast** [ thrombo- + G. *blastos,* germ ]. The precursor of the blood platelet (or thrombocyte), *i.e.,* a megakaryocyte.

**thromboclasis** (throm-bok′lă-sis) [ thrombo- + G. *klasis,* a breaking ]. Thrombolysis.

**thromboclas′tic.** Thrombolytic.

**thrombocyst, thrombocystis** (throm′bo-sist, -sis′tis) [ thrombo- + G. *kystis,* a bladder ]. A membranous sac enclosing a thrombus.

**thrombocytasthenia** (throm′bo-si′tas-the′nĭ-ah) [ thrombocyte + G. *astheneia,* weakness ]. A term for a group of hemorrhagic disorders in which the platelets may be only slightly reduced in number (or even within the normal range), but (1) are morphologically abnormal, or (2) are lacking in factors that are effective in the coagulation of blood.

**thrombocyte** (throm′bo-sit) [ thrombo- + G. *kytos,* cell ]. Blood platelet (see platelet).

**thrombocythemia** (throm′bo-si-the′mĭ-ah) [ thrombocyte + G. *haima,* blood ]. Thrombocytosis.

**throm′bocy′tin.** Serotonin.

**thrombocytopathy** (throm′bo-si-top′ă-thĭ) [ thrombocyte + G. *pathos,* suffering ]. A general germ for any disorder of the coagulating mechanism that results from dysfunction of the blood platelets.

**thrombocytopenia** (throm-bo-si-to-pe′nĭ-ah) [ thrombocyte + G. *penia,* poverty ]. Thrombopenia; a condition in which there is an abnormally small number of platelets in the circulating blood.

**essential t.,** a primary form of t., in contrast to secondary forms that are associated with metastatic neoplasms, tuberculosis, and leukemia involving the bone marrow, or with direct suppression of bone marrow by the use of chemical agents, or with other conditions.

**thrombocytopoiesis** (throm′bo-si-to-poy-e′sis) [ thrombocyte + G. *poiēsis,* a making ]. The process of formation of thrombocytes or platelets.

**thrombocytosis** (throm′bo-si′to′sis) [ thrombocyte + G. suffix *-osis,* condition ]. Thrombocythemia; an increase in the number of platelets in the circulating blood.

**thromboembolectomy** (throm′bo-em-bo-lek′to-mĭ) [ thrombo- + G. *embolos,* embolus (*q.v.*), + *ektomē,* excision ]. Extraction of an embolic thrombus.

**thromboembolism** (throm′bo-em′bo-lizm) [ thrombo- + G. *embolismos,* embolism (*q.v.*) ]. Embolism from a thrombus dislodged from a vein.

**throm′boendar′terec′tomy** [ thrombo- + endarterectomy ]. The operation that involves opening an artery and removing an occluding thrombus.

**thromboendocarditis** (throm′bo-en′do-kar-di′tis). Nonbacterial thrombotic *endocarditis.*

**thrombogen** (throm′bo-jen) [ thrombo- + G. suffix *-gen,* producing ]. Prothrombin.

**thrombogene** (throm′bo-jēn). See factor V.

**thrombogenic** (throm′bo-jen′ik) [ thrombo- + G. suffix *-gen,* producing ]. 1. Relating to thrombogen. 2. Causing thrombosis or coagulation of the blood.

**thromboid** (throm′boyd) [ thrombo- + G. *eidos,* resemblance ]. Resembling a thrombus.

**throm′bokatil′ysin.** See factor VIII.

**thrombokinase** (throm′bo-ki′nās). Thromboplastin.

**thrombol′ic.** Relating to a thrombolus.

**throm'bolus** [ thrombo- + G. *embolos*, embolus ]. An embolus composed of agglutinated platelets.

**thrombolymphangitis** (throm-bo-lim-fan-ji'tis). Inflammation of a lymphatic vessel with the formation of a lymph clot.

**thrombolysis** (throm-bol'ĭ-sis) [ thrombo- + G. *lysis*, a dissolving ]. Thromboclasis; fluidifying or dissolving of a thrombus.

**thrombolytic** (throm-bo-lit'ik). Thromboclastic; breaking up or dissolving a thrombus.

**throm'bon.** An all-inclusive term for circulating thrombocytes (blood platelets) and the cellular forms from which they arise (thromboblasts or megakaryocytes). It is analogous to erythron and leukon of the red and white blood cells, respectively.

**thrombonecrosis** (throm'bo-ne-kro'sis). Necrosis of the walls of a blood vessel with thrombosis in the lumen.

**thrombopathy** (throm-bop'ă-thĭ) [ thrombo- + G. *pathos*, disease ]. A nonspecific term applied to disorders of blood platelets resulting in defective thromboplastin, without obvious change in the appearance or number of platelets.
   **constitutional t.,** (1) von Willebrand's *disease;* (2) Glanzmann's *thrombasthenia.*

**thrombope'nia.** Thrombocytopenia.

**thrombophilia** (throm-bo-fil'ĭ-ah) [ thrombo- + G. *philos*, fond ]. A disorder of the hemopoietic system in which there is a tendency to the occurrence of thrombosis.

**thrombophlebitis** (throm'bo-flĕ-bi'tis) [ thrombo- + G. *phleps*, vein, + suffix *-itis*, inflammation ]. Inflammation of a vein with secondary thrombus formation.
   **t. mi'grans,** creeping or slowly advancing t.; t. appearing in first one vein and then another.
   **t. saltans,** t. occurring in the same vein, but at a distance from the original lesion, or appearing suddenly in a distant vein.

**thromboplas'tid** [ thrombo- + plastid, *q.v.* ]. 1. Blood platelet (see platelet). 2. A nucleated spindle cell in submammalian blood.

**throm'boplast'in.** Thrombozyme; platelet tissue factor; zymoplastic substance; thrombokinase; a substance present in tissues, platelets, and leukocytes necessary for the coagulation of blood; in the presence of calcium ions it is necessary for the conversion of prothrombin to thrombin, which conversion is an important step in coagulation of blood. It is now generally believed that t. activity may be developed through blood (intrinsic) or tissue (extrinsic) systems. Tissue t. (factor III) interacts with factor VII and calcium to activate factor X; active factor X combines with factor V in the presence of calcium and phospholipid to produce t. activity (also commonly called t.).
   **cofactor of t.,** *factor* V.
   **tissue t.,** factor III; see thromboplastin.

**thromboplastinogen** (throm'bo-plas-tin'o-jen). *Factor* VIII.

**thromboplastinogenase** (throm'bo-plas-tin'o-jĕ-nās, -tĭ-noj'ĕ-nās). An enzyme in blood that catalyzes the conversion of inactive thromboplastinogen to thromboplastin.

**thromboplastinogenemia** (throm'bo-plas-tin'o-jĕ-ne'mia) [ thromboplastinogen + G. *haima*, blood ]. The presence of thromboplastinogen in the circulating blood.

**thrombopoiesis** (throm-bo-poy-e'sis) [ thrombo- + G. *poiēsis*, a making ]. Precisely, the process of a clot forming in blood, but generally used with reference to the formation of blood platelets (thrombocytes).

**thrombosed** (throm'bōzd). 1. Clotted, 2. Denoting a blood vessel that is the seat of thrombosis.

**throm'bosin.** Thrombin.

**thrombosis,** pl. **thromboses** (throm-bo'sis, -sēz) [ G. *thrombōsis*, a clotting, fr. *thrombos*, clot ]. 1. The formation of a thrombus. 2. The presence of a thrombus.
   **atroph'ic t.,** marantic t.; t. due to feebleness of the circulation, in marasmus for example.
   **cerebral t.,** clotting of blood in a cerebral vessel.
   **compression t.,** t. due to arrest of the circulation in a vessel by compression, as from a tumor.
   **coronary t.,** coronary occlusion by thrombus formation, usually the result of atheromatous changes in the arterial wall and usually leading to myocardial infarction.

   **creeping t.,** a gradually increasing t. involving one section of a vein after another in continuity.
   **dilation t.,** t. due to slowed circulation consequent upon dilation of a vein.
   **jumping t.,** t. occurring in one vein and another in different regions.
   **maran'tic t., maras'mic t.,** atrophic t.
   **mural t.,** the formation of a thrombus in contact with the endocardial lining of a cardiac chamber.
   **placen'tal t.,** t. of the veins of the uterus at the placental site.
   **plate t., platelet t.,** t. due to an abnormal accumulation of platelets.
   **posttraumatic arterial** or **venous t.,** intravascular clotting due to injury to a vessel wall.

**thrombostasis** (throm'bos'tă-sis) [ thrombo- + G. *stasis*, a standing ]. Local arrest of the circulation caused by thrombosis.

**thrombot'ic.** Relating to, caused by, or characterized by thrombosis.

**thromboto'nin.** Serotonin.

**thrombozyme** (throm'bo-zīm). Thromboplastin.

**throm'bus,** pl. **throm'bi** [ L. fr. G. *thrombos*, a clot. TREPH- ]. A clot in a blood vessel or in one of the cavities of the heart, formed during life from constituents of blood; it may be occlusive or attached to the vessel or heart wall without obstructing the lumen (mural t.).
   **agglu'tinative t.,** hyaline t.
   **agony t.,** a heart clot formed during the act of dying after prolonged heart failure.
   **antemor'tem t.,** a clot formed in the circulation during life.
   **ball t.,** a white antemortem t. found in the left atrium in certain cases of mitral stenosis.
   **ball-valve t.,** ball t. intermittently occluding the mitral orifice.
   **bile t.,** an intracanalicular deposit of bile, usually a result of obstruction to bile drainage.
   **ferment t.,** a t. supposed to be formed because of the liberation of fibrin ferment into the circulating blood.
   **fibrin t.,** one formed by repeated deposits of fibrin from the circulating blood; it usually does not completely occlude the vessel.
   **globular t.,** one of a number of thrombi of varying size, from a pea to a walnut, within the heart cavity, connected by a delicate fibrinous network; they are usually cystic in character, the interior having broken down into a thick fluid mass.
   **hy'aline t.,** agglutination t.; a translucent colorless plug, partly or completely filling a capillary or small artery or vein; it is formed by an agglutination of red blood corpuscles which lose their hemoglobin.
   **infective t.,** one formed in septic phlebitis.
   **Laënnec's t.,** an antemortem heart clot.
   **lam'inated t.,** one formed gradually by clotting of the blood in successive layers.
   **maran'tic t., maras'mic t.,** a t. formed in cases of marasmus or general debility.
   **mixed t.,** laminated t., the layers of different ages being of different color or consistency.
   **mural t.,** a t. formed on and attached to a diseased patch of endocardium, not on a valve or on one side of a vessel.
   **obstructive t.,** one due to obstruction in the vessel from compression or other cause.
   **pale t.,** white t.
   **pari'etal t.,** an arterial t. which has been in large part absorbed, the remains adhering to one side of the wall of the vessel.
   **postmortem t.,** a clot formed within the heart or in a blood vessel after death.
   **prop'agated t.,** see creeping *thrombosis.*
   **red t.,** one formed rapidly by the coagulation of stagnating blood.
   **secondary t.,** one formed about an embolus as a nucleus.
   **stratified t.,** mixed t.
   **val'vular t.,** a parietal t. that projects into the lumen of the vessel.
   **white t.,** pale t.; a clot of opaque, dull white color, in the heart or any vessel, composed essentially of blood platelets.

**throw'back.** Atavus.

**thrush** [ fr. the thrush fungus, *Candida albicans* ]. 1. Infection of the oral tissues with *Candida albicans*. Oral thrush may show lesions similar to aphthous ulcers and many believe *Candida albicans* is one cause of aphthae. 2. A foul-smelling infective process of the horse's foot, involving the frog and sole. The affected parts degenerate and soften, and a black exudate is present. Generally occurs when horses are made to stand in wet, unhygienic stalls.

**thrypsis** (thrip'sis) [ G. a breaking in pieces, fr. *thyrptō*, fut. *thrypsō*, to break in pieces ]. A comminuted *fracture*.

**Thudichum** (too'de-khoom), Johann L. W., German physician in London, 1829–1901. See T.'s *test*.

**thuja** (thoo'jah, -yah) [ G. *thyia*, an African tree with sweet-smelling wood ]. Thuya; the fresh tops of *Thuja occidentalis* (family Pinaceae) an ornamental evergreen tree (one of the arborvitae) of eastern North America, source of cedar leaf oil. Has been used internally as an expectorant, emmenagogue, and anthelmintic, and externally as a mild counterirritant.

    **t. oil,** cedar leaf oil.

**thu'jol.** Thujone.

**thu'jone.** Thujol; thuyol; thuyone; absinthol; tanacetol; tanacetone; $C_{10}H_{16}O$; chief constituent of cedar leaf oil; a stimulant similar to camphor.

**thulium** (thu'li-um) [ L. *Thule*, an island in extreme north of Europe ]. A metallic element of the lanthanide series, symbol Tm, atomic no. 69, atomic weight 168.94.

**thumb** [ A.S. *thuma* ]. Pollex; the first digit on the radial side of the hand.

    **gamekeeper's t.,** a subluxation of the metacarpophalangeal joint of the t.

    **stave of the t.,** Bennett's *fracture*.

    **tennis t.,** tendinitis with calcification in the tendon of the long flexor of the t. (flexor pollicis longus) caused by friction and strain as in tennis playing, but it also occurs in other exercises in which the t. is subject to much pressure or strain.

**thumps.** 1. Spasmodic contractions of the diaphragm, or hiccups. Occasionally seen in animals. 2. In swine, a type of irregular, jerky breathing seen in swine influenza, in severely anemic pigs, and in young pigs when ascarid larvae are migrating through the tissues.

**thus,** gen. **thu'ris** (thus, thūs) [ L. incense ]. Olibanum.

**thuya** (thu'yah). Thuja.

**thu'yol, thu'yone.** Thujone.

**thylacitis** (thi'lă-si'tis) [ G. *thylax*, bag, + suffix -*itis*, inflammation ]. Inflammation of the sebaceous glands of the skin.

**thym-.** See thymo-.

**thyme** (tim) [ G. *thymon*, thyme. THYM-1 ] (NF). The dried leaves and flowering tops of *Thymus vulgaris* (family Labiatae), sweet t.; garden t.; used as a condiment; it contains a volatile oil, t. oil, and is a source of thymol.

    **t. oil,** a volatile oil distilled from the flowering plants of *Thymus vulgaris* or *T. zygis*; a flavor.

**thymectomize** (thi-mek'to-mīz). To perform a thymectomy.

**thymectomy** (thi-mek'to-mī) [ thymus + G. *ektomē*, excision ]. Removal of the thymus gland.

**thymelcosis** (thi'mel-ko'sis) [ thymus + G. *helkōsis*, ulceration ]. Suppuration of the thymus gland.

**thymeme** (ti'mēn). A colorless volatile oil, $C_{10}H_{16}$, derived from oil of thyme, possessing antiseptic properties. It is identical with levo-α-pinene.

**thymergasia** (thi'mer-ga'zī-ah) [ G. *thymos*, mind, + *ergazesthai*, to work ]. An emotional disorder characterized by excitement or depression.

**-thymia** [ G. *thymos*, the mind or heart as the seat of strong feelings or passion. THYM-2 ]. A suffix denoting relation to the mind, soul, or emotions. See also thymo-.

**thymic** (thi'mik). Relating to the thymus gland.

**thymicolymphatic** (thi'mī-ko-lim-fat'ik). Relating to the thymus and the lymphatic system; see *status* thymicolymphaticus.

**thy'midine.** Thymine deoxyribonucleoside; 1-(2-deoxyribosyl)thymine; one of the four major nucleosides in DNA.

    **t. phosphorylase** (EC 2.4.2.4), phosphorylase that catalyzes the phosphorolysis of t.

    **tritiated t.,** t. containing the hydrogen radioisotope, tritium; used as a radioactive marker in cell and tissue studies for new formation of DNA, in which it is incorporated.

**thymidylate synthetase** (thi'mī-dil'āt). Enzyme catalyzing conversion of deoxyuridine 5'-phosphate to thymidine 5'-phosphate, the methyl group coming from methylene tetrahydrofolate.

**thymidylic acid** (thi'mī-dil'ik). Thymidine phosphoric acid; a hydrolysis product of DNA.

**thymine** (thi'mēn, -min). 5-Methyluracil; a constituent of thymidylic acid and DNA.

**Thymine**

*Inner numbering,* official international (IUPAC); *outer numbering,* original Fischer (abandoned).

    **t. dimer,** a product of ultraviolet irradiation of thymine (free in ice or bound in nucleic acids) in which two thymine residues become linked by formation of a cyclobutane ring involving both C-5's and both C-6's at the expense of the two 5-6 double bonds. Several stereoisomeric forms are possible.

    **t. nucleotide,** thymidylic acid.

**thymion** (thi'mī-on) [ G. dim. of *thymos*, a warty excrescence. THYM-1 ]. A wart.

**thymiosis** (thi'mī-o'sis) [ G. *thymion*, a wart ]. 1. A warty condition. 2. Yaws.

**thymitis** (thi-mi'tis). Inflammation of the thymus gland.

**thymo-, thym-, thymi-** (thi'mo-). 1 [ G. *thymos*, thymus. THYM- ]. Combining forms relating to the thymus. 2 [ G. *thymos*, the mind as the seat of strong feelings or passions. THYM-2 ]. Combining forms denoting relation to the mind, soul, or emotions.

**thymocyte** (thi'mo-sīt) [ thymus + G. *kytos*, cell ]. A cell that develops in the thymus, seemingly from a stem cell of bone marrow and of fetal liver, and is the precursor of the thymus-derived lymphocyte (T lymphocyte) that effects cell-mediated (delayed type) sensitivity.

**thymogenic** (thi'mo-jen'ik) [ G. *thymos*, mind, + *genesis*, origin ]. Of affective origin.

**thymokinetic** (thi'mo-kī-net'ik) [ thymus + G. *kinēsis*, movement ]. Activating the thymus gland.

**thy'mol** (USP, BP). 1-Methyl-3-hydroxy-4-isopropylbenzene; thymic acid; thyme camphor; $C_{10}H_{14}O$; a phenol present in the volatile oil of *Thymus vulgaris* (thyme), *Monarda punctata* (horsemint), and other volatile oils; used externally and internally as an antiseptic, as a deodorizer of offensive discharges, and as a specific for ancylostomiasis.

    **t. blue,** an acid-base indicator with a pK value at 1.7 and another at 8.9; red at pH values below 1.2, yellow between 2.8 and 8.0, and blue above 9.6

    **t. i'odide,** ARISTOL; $C_{20}H_{24}I_2O_2$; has been used as a substitute for iodoform in skin diseases, wounds, ulcers, purulent rhinitis, otitis, etc.

**thymoma** (thi-mo'mah) [ thymus + G. suffix -*oma*, tumor ]. A neoplasm in the anterior mediastinum, apparently originating from thymic tissue, usually benign, and frequently encapsulated; occasionally invasive, but metastases are extremely rare. Histologically, t.'s consist of cellular elements that are normally present, *e.g.,* lymphocytes (sometimes termed thymocytes), spindle cells or others that resemble the stromal elements, and epithelial cells, but they vary considerably in arrangement and proportions. Approximately 15 per cent of patients with myasthenia gravis have an associated thymic neoplasm, but the relation of the latter to the neuromuscular dysfunction is not known; at any rate, such neoplasms are characterized by (1) large, pale epithelial cells that are loosely mixed with lymphocytes, and (2) frequently tend to be arranged in cords or clusters about the blood vessels, thereby being somewhat suggestive of an endocrine function. Malignant lymphoma that involves the thymus, *e.g.*, lymphosarcoma, Hodgkin's disease (previously termed granulomatous t.) and the like, should not be regarded as t., and most neoplasms formerly classified as thymic carcinoma seem to be examples of mediastinal seminoma.

**thymopathy** (thi-mop′ă-thī). 1. Any disease of the thymus gland. 2. An emotional illness.

**thymoprival, thymoprivic, thymoprivous** (thi′mo-pri′-val, -priv′ik, -pri′vus) [ thymus + L. *privus*, deprived of ]. Relating to or marked by premature atrophy or removal of the thymus.

**thymopsyche** (thi′mo-si′ke) [ G. *thymos*, the mind (emotions), + *psychē*, soul ]. The affective processes.

**thy′mosin.** Thymic lymphopoietic *factor*.

**thymox′amine hydrochloride.** OPILON; 5-(2-dimethylaminoethoxy)carvacrol acetate hydrochloride; used as alpha-adrenergic blocking agent for treatment of peripheral vascular disease.

**thymus,** pl. **thymuses, thymi** (thi′mus, thi′mi) [ G. *thymos*, excrescence, sweetbread. THYM-1 ]. 1 [ NA ]. A lymphoid organ located in the superior mediastinum and lower part of the neck; it is a structure of early life, necessary for the normal development of immunological function. It reaches its greatest relative weight shortly after birth, and its greatest absolute weight at puberty. It then begins to involute; much of the lymphoid tissue is replaced by fat, and the organ is small in the adult. The t. consists of two irregularly shaped parts united by a connective tissue capsule. Each part is partially subdivided by connective tissue septa into lobules 0.5 to 2 mm. in diameter. A lobule consists of an inner medullary portion, continuous with the medullae of adjacent lobules, and an outer cortical portion. It is supplied by the inferior thyroid and internal thoracic arteries, and its nerves are derived from the vagus and sympathetic. 2. The t. of the calf or lamb is the sweetbread, called also the throat sweetbread, the pancreas being the stomach sweetbread.

**thyr-.** See thyro-.

**thyrasthenia** (thi-ras-the′nī-ah) [ thyr- + G. *astheneia*, weakness ]. A neurosis related to deficient thyroid secretion.

**thyremphraxis** (thi′rem-frak′sis) [ thyr- + G. *emphraxis*, a stoppage ]. Obsolete designation for diminished or arrested function of the thyroid gland.

**thyreo-.** For words beginning thus, see thyro-.

**thyrine** (thi′rēn). Obsolete designation for the active principle of the thyroid gland secretion.

**thyro-, thyr-** (thi′ro-) [ see thyroid ]. combining form relating to the thyroid gland.

**thy′roace′tic acid.** A degradation product of thyronine (alanine side chain reduced to acetic acid), itself a degradation product (or precursor) of thyroxine.

**thyroadenitis** (thi-ro-ad-e-ni′tis) [ thyro- + G. *adēn*, gland, + suffix -*itis*, inflammation ]. Inflammation of the thyroid gland.

**thyroaplasia** (thi′ro-ă-pla′zī-ah) [ thyro- + G. *a*- priv. + *plasis*, a molding ]. The anomalies observed in cases of congenital defects of the thyroid gland and deficiency of its secretion.

**thyroarytenoid** (thi′ro-ăr′ĭ-te′noyd). Relating to the thyroid and arytenoid cartilages.

**thyrocalcitonin** (thi′ro-kal′sĭ-to′nin). A hypocalcemic hormone secreted by the thyroid gland and also by the ultimobranchial bodies of some submammalian vertebrates. Believed to inhibit the resorption of bone. Sometimes called calcitonin, *q.v.*

**thyrocardiac** (thi′ro-kar′dī-ak). Affecting the heart as a result of hyperthyroidism.

**thyrocele** (thi′ro-sēl) [ thyro- + G. *kēlē*, tumor ]. Enlargement of the thyroid gland.

**thy′rocer′vical.** Relating to the thyroid gland and the neck.

**thyrochondrotomy** (thi′ro-kon-drot′o-mĭ) [ thyro- + G. *chondros*, cartilage, + *tomē*, incision ]. Laryngofissure.

**thyrocol′loid.** A colloid substance in the thyroid gland.

**thyrocricotomy** (thi′ro-kri-kot′o-mĭ). Division of the cricothyroid membrane.

**thyroepiglottic** (thi′ro-ep-ĭ-glot′ik). Relating to the thyroid cartilage and the epiglottis.

**thy′roesophage′us.** A small inconstant band of muscular fibers passing between the esophagus and the thyroid cartilage.

**thyrofissure** (thi′ro-fish′ur). Laryngofissure.

**thyrogenic** (thi-ro-jen′ik) [ thyro- + G. suffix -*gen*, producing ]. Thyrogenous; of thyroid gland origin.

**thyrogenous** (thi-roj′ē-nus). Thyrogenic.

**thyroglob′ulin.** 1. Iodoglobulin; a thyroid hormone-containing protein, usually stored in the colloid within the thyroid follicles. The biosynthesis of thyroid hormone entails iodination of the tyrosine moieties of this protein and the combination of two iodotyrosines to form thyroxine, the fully iodinated thyronine. Secretion of thyroid hormone requires proteolytic degradation of t., with the attendant release of free hormone. 2 (NF). PROLOID; a substance obtained by the fractionation of thyroid glands from the hog, *Sus scrofa*, containing not less than 0.7 per cent of total iodine; used as a thyroid hormone in the treatment of hypothyroidism.

**thyroglos′sal.** Thyrolingual; relating to the thyroid gland and the tongue.

**thyrohy′al.** The greater cornu of the hyoid bone.

**thyrohy′oid.** Relating to the thyroid cartilage and the hyoid bone, hyothyroid; see musculus thyrohyoideus.

**thyroid** (thi′royd) [ G. *thyreoeidēs*, fr. *thyreos*, an oblong shield, + *eidos*, form. THYR- ]. 1. Resembling a shield, scutiform; denoting a gland (glandula thyroidea) and a cartilage of the larynx (cartilago thyroidea). 2 (USP, BP). Dried t. gland; the cleaned, dried, and powdered t. gland obtained from one of the domesticated animals used for food; a yellowish amorphous powder of a slight characteristic odor. It contains 0.17 to 0.23 per cent of iodine. Used in the treatment of cretinism and myxedema, in certain cases of obesity, and in skin disorders.

  **acces′sory t.,** *glandula* thyroidea accessoria.

  **t. peroxidase** (EC 1.11.1.7), see peroxidases.

**thyroi′dea.** *Glandula* thyroidea.

  **t. accesso′ria, t. ima,** *glandula* thyroidea accessoria.

**thyroidectomize** (thi′roy-dek′to-mīz). To remove the thyroid gland.

**thyroidectomy** (thi′roy-dek′to-mĭ) [ thyroid + G. *ektomē*, excision ]. Removal of the thyroid gland.

  **"chemical" t.,** jargon for the reduction of thyroid function produced by the administration of antithyroid drugs. See also radiothyroidectomy.

**thyroidism** (thi′roy-dizm). Obsolete designation for (1) hyperthyroidism, and (2) poisoning by overdoses of a thyroid extract.

**thyroiditis** (thi-roy-di′tis) [ thyroid + G. suffix -*itis*, inflammation ]. Inflammation of the thyroid gland.

  **chronic atrophic t.,** replacement of the thyroid gland by fibrous tissue; the commonest cause of myxedema in older persons; the thyroid weighs only 4 to 8 gm.

  **de Quervain's t.,** subacute granulomatous t.

  **focal lymphocytic t.,** focal infiltration of the thyroid by lymphocytes and plasma cells; see also Hashimoto's *disease*.

  **Hashimoto's t.,** Hashimoto's *disease*.

  **lig′neous t.,** Riedel's *struma*.

  **parasit′ic t.,** chronic South American trypanosomiasis with involvement of the thyroid gland causing myxedema.

  **subacute granulomatous t.,** de Quervain's t.; t. with round cell (usually lymphocytes) infiltration, obstruction of thyroid cells, giant cell proliferation, and evidence of regeneration. Thought by some to be a reflection of a systemic infection and not an example of true chronic t.

**thyroidization** (thi′roy-dī-za′shun). Obsolete term meaning the therapeutic use of a thyroid gland preparation.

**thyroidology** (thi′roy-dol′o-jĭ) [ thyroid + G. *logos*, study ]. The study of the thyroid gland, both normal and pathological.

**thyroidomania** (thi'roy-do-ma'nĭ-ah) [ thyroid + G. *mania*, frenzy ]. Emotional disturbance related to hyperthyroidism.

**thyroidotomy** (thi'roy-dot'o-mĭ) [ thyroid + G. *tomē*, incision ]. Laryngofissure.

**thyrolaryngeal** (thi'ro-lă-rin'je-al). Relating to the thyroid gland or cartilage and the larynx.

**thyrolingual** (thi'ro-ling'gwal) [ thyro- + L. *lingua*, tongue ]. Thyroglossal.

**thyrolytic** (thi'ro-lit'ik) [ thyro- + G. *lytikos*, dissolving ]. Causing destruction of thyroid gland cells.

**thyromegaly** (thi'ro-meg'ă-lĭ) [ thyro- + G. *megas*, large ]. Enlargement of the thyroid gland.

**thyroncus** (thi-rong'kus) [ thyro- + G. *onkos*, a mass (tumor) ]. Obsolete term for goiter.

**thyronine** (thi'ro-nēn, -nin). HOC$_6$H$_4$—O—C$_6$H$_4$—CH$_2$—CHNH$_2$—COOH; an amino acid with a diphenyl ether group in the side chain; occurs in proteins only in the form of iodinated derivatives (iodothyronines) such as, notably, thyroxine.

**thyropal'atine.** Denoting the musculus palatopharyngeus.

**thyroparathyroidectomy** (thi'ro-păr'ă-thi'roy-dek'to-mĭ). Surgical excision of thyroid and parathyroid glands.

**thyropathy** (thi-rop'ă-thĭ) [ thyro- + G. *pathos*, suffering ]. Disorder of the thyroid gland.

**thyrope'nia** [ thyro- + G. *penia*, poverty ]. Obsolete term meaning reduced activity of the thyroid gland.

**thyropharyngeal** (thi-ro-fă-rin'je-al). Denoting the thyropharyngeal portion of the musculus constrictor pharyngis inferior.

**thyrophyma** (thi'ro-fi'mah) [ thyro- + G. *phyma*, a tumor ]. A thyroid tumor.

**thyroprival** (thi'ro-pri'val) [ thyro- + L. *privus*, deprived of ]. Thyroprivic; thyroprivous; thyroprivus; strumiprivus; relating to thyroprivia; denoting hypothyroidism produced by disease or thyroidectomy.

**thyroprivia** (thi'ro-priv'ĭ-ah). State characterized by reduced activity of the thyroid.

**thyroprivic** (thi-ro-priv'ik). Thyroprival.

**thyroprivous** (thi'ro-pri'vus). Thyroprival.

**thyropro'tein.** 1. Thyroglobulin. 2. Iodinated protein, usually casein, which has thyroxine activity; once used in hypothyroidism.

**thyroptosis** (thi-rop-to'sis) [ thyro- + G. *ptōsis*, a falling ]. Downward dislocation of the thyroid gland.

**thyrosis** (thi-ro'sis) [ thyro- + G. suffix *-osis*, condition ]. Obsolete designation for any disorder caused by abnormal thyroid activity.

**thyrother'apy.** Obsolete term meaning the use of desiccated thyroid in therapy.

**thyrotomy** (thi'rot'o-mĭ) [ thyro- + G. *tomē*, a cutting ]. Any cutting operation on the thyroid gland.

**thyrotox'ic.** Designating the state produced by excessive quantities of endogenous or exogenous thyroid hormone.

**thyrotoxicosis** (thi-ro-tok-sĭ-ko'sis) [ thyro- + G. *toxikon*, poison, + suffix *-osis*, condition ]. The state produced by excessive quantities of endogenous or exogenous thyroid hormone.

apathetic t., chronic, low grade t., presenting as cardiac disease or as a wasting syndrome, with weakness of proximal muscles but few of the more typical clinical manifestations of t.

**thyrotox'in.** 1. A substance formerly postulated to be an abnormal product of diffusely hyperplastic thyroid glands in persons with Graves' disease, and presumed to be the cause of the distinctive signs and symptoms of that condition (in contrast to simple hyperthyroidism). 2. A complement-fixing antigenic factor associated with certain diseases of the thyroid gland; see also thyrotoxic complement-fixation *factor*. 3. Used infrequently with reference to any material that is toxic to thyroidal tissue.

**thy'rotroph.** A cell in the anterior lobe of the pituitary that produces thyrotropic hormone (TSH).

**thyrotrophic** (thi'ro-trof'ik) [ thyro- + G. *trophē*, nourishment ]. Thyrotropic.

**thyrotrophin** (thi-rot'ro-fin, thi'ro-tro'fin). Thyrotropin.

**thyrotropic** (thi'ro-trop'ik) [ thyro- + G. *tropē*, a turning ]. Thyrotrophic; stimulating or nurturing the thyroid gland.

**thyrotropin** (thi-rot'ro-pin, thi'ro-tro'pin). Thyrotrophin; thyrotropic hormone; a glycoprotein hormone produced by the anterior pituitary gland; it stimulates the growth and function of the thyroid gland, and is used as a diagnostic test to differentiate primary and secondary hypothyroidism.

**thyrotropism** (thi-rot'ro-pizm) [ thyro- + G. *tropē*, a turning ]. A type of endocrine constitution in which the thyroid exercises a dominating influence; a conceptually obscure, and obsolete, designation.

**thyroxine, thyroxin** (thi-rok'sēn, -sin). 3,3',5,5'-Tetraiodothyronine; β-[ (3,5-diiodo-4-hydroxyphenoxy)-3,5-diiodophenyl ]alanine; the active iodine compound existing normally in the thyroid gland and extracted therefrom in crystalline form for therapeutic use. It is also prepared synthetically. It is used for the relief of hypothyroidism, cretinism, and myxedema.

radioactive t., t. in which a radioisotope of iodine ($^{125}$I or $^{131}$I) is incorporated into its molecule. Used in experiments tracing the metabolism of t.

t. sodium (BP), a preparation obtained by the action of a limited amount of sodium carbonate upon t.; it contains between 61 and 65 per cent of iodine. See sodium levothyroxine and sodium liothyronine.

**Thysanoso'ma actinoi'des** (this-ă-no-so'mah). Fringed tapeworm of sheep; a relatively short, thick tapeworm (family Anocephalidae) in which the posterior borders of the proglottids are fringed. It inhabits the small intestine, but often invades the bile ducts and causes many livers to be condemned for human food. It is essentially nonpathogenic and is common in stock-raising countries, where it infects a wide variety of ruminants; oribatid mites are probably the vectors.

**Ti.** Chemical symbol of the element titanium.

**tibia,** gen. and pl. **tibiae** (tib'ĭ-ah, tib'ĭ-e) [ L. the large shinbone ] [ NA ]. Shin bone; shank bone (2); the medial and larger of the two bones of the leg, articulating with the femur, fibula, and talus.

sabre t., deformity of the t. occurring in tertiary syphilis or yaws, the bone having a marked forward convexity as a result of the formation of gummas and periostitis.

t. valga, *genu* valgum.

t. vara, *genu* varum.

**tibiad** (tib'ĭ-ad) [ tibia + L. *ad*, to ]. In a direction toward the tibia.

**tibial** (tib'ĭ-al) [ L. *tibialis* ]. Relating to the tibia.

**tibia'le posti'cum.** *Os* tibiale posterius.

**tibialgia** (tib'ĭ-al'jĭ-ah) [ tibia + G. *algos*, pain ]. Pain in the shin.

**tibia'lis** [ L. ] [ NA ]. Tibial; relating to the tibia or to any structure named from it; also denoting the medial or tibial aspect of the lower limb.

**tibio-** (tib'ĭ-o-) [ L. *tibia*, the large shinbone ]. Combining form relating to the tibia.

**tibiocalcanean** (tib'ĭ-o-kal-ka'ne-an). Relating to the tibia and the calcaneus.

**tibiofascia'lis.** See under musculus.

**tibiofem'oral.** Relating to the tibia and the femur.

**tibiofib'ular.** Relating to both tibia and fibula.

**tibionavic'ular.** Relating to the tibia and the navicular bone of the tarsus.

**tibioperoneal** (tib'ĭ-o-pĕr'o-ne'al). Tibiofibular.

**tibioscaphoid** (tib'ĭ-o-skaf'oyd). Tibionavicular.

**tibiotar'sal.** Tarsotibial.

**tib'olone** (USAN). 17-Hydroxy-7α-methyl-19-nor-17α-pregn-5(10)-en-20-6n-3-one; an anabolic drug.

**ti'brofan** (USAN). 4,4'5-Tribromo-2-thiophenecarboxanilide; a disinfectant.

**tic** [ Fr. ]. Habit chorea; a more or less involuntary repeated contraction of a certain group of associated muscles; a habitual spasmodic movement of any part; a habit contraction. See also spasm.

convulsive t., facial t.

t. douloureux (doo-loo-rĕ') [ Fr. painful ], trigeminal *neuralgia*.

**facial t.,** involuntary twitching of the facial muscles, sometimes unilateral. Also variously referred to as convulsive or mimic t.; palmus; facial, histrionic, or Bell's spasm; prosospasm; mimic convulsion.

**habit t.,** a habitual repetition of some grimace, shrug of the shoulder, twisting or jerking of the head, or the like.

**local t.,** a t. of very limited extent, as the winking of an eye or a twitch of a finger.

**mimic t.,** facial t.

**t. nondouloureux,** myoclonus.

**t. de pensée** (dë pahn-sa') [ Fr. of thought ], the habit of involuntarily giving expression to any thought that happens to be present in the mind.

**psychic t.,** a gesture or ejaculation made under the influence of an irresistible morbid impulse.

**ro'tatory t.,** spasmodic *torticollis.*

**spasmod'ic t.,** Henoch's chorea; a disorder in which sudden spasmodic coordinated movements of certain muscles or groups of physiologically related muscles occur at irregular intervals.

**tick.** An acarine of the families Ixodidae (hard t.'s) or Argasidae (soft t.'s), which contain many bloodsucking species that are important pests of man and domestic birds and mammals, and that probably exceed all other arthropods in the number and variety of disease agents that they transmit. T.'s are differentiated from the much smaller true mites by possession of an armed hypostome and a pair of tracheal spiracular openings located behind the basal segment of the third or fourth pair of walking legs; the larva (seed t.) has six legs, and after molting appears as an eight-limbed nymph.

**adobe t.,** *Argas persicus.*
**African red t.,** *Rhipicephalus everti.*
**African relapsing fever t.,** *Ornithodoros moubata.*
**American dog t.,** *Dermacentor variabilis;* also known, along with *D. andersoni* and *D. occidentalis,* as wood t.
**bird t.,** *Haemaphysalis chordeilis* or other haemaphysalid t.'s.
**black-legged t.,** *Ixodes scapularis.*
**black-pitted t.,** *Rhipicephalus simus.*
**bont t.,** *Amblyomma hebraeum.*
**brown dog t.,** *Rhipicephalus sanguineus.*
**California black-legged t.,** *Ixodes pacificus.*
**castor bean t.,** *Ixodes ricinus.*
**cattle t.,** see *Boophilus.*
**dog t.,** see brown dog t. and American dog t.
**fowl t.,** *Argas persicus.*
**horse t.,** *Dermacentor albopictus.*
**Lone Star t.,** *Amblyomma americanum.*
**Pacific t.,** *Dermacentor occidentalis.*
**pajaroel'lo t.,** *Ornithodoros coriaceus.*
**paralysis t.,** *Ixodes pilosus.*
**Persian t.,** *Argas persicus.*
**pigeon t.,** *Argas reflexus.*
**rabbit t.,** *Haemaphysalis leporispalustris.*
**Rocky Mountain t.,** *Dermacentor andersoni.*
**shoulder t.,** *Ixodes scapularis.*
**spotted-fever t.,** *Dermacentor andersoni.*
**tampan t.,** *Ornithodoros moubata.*
**tropical horse t.,** *Dermacentor nitens.*
**winter t.,** *Dermacentor albopictus.*
**wood t.,** *Dermacentor andersoni, D. variabilis,* and *D. occidentalis.*

**tickle** (tik'l). To cause a peculiar and intolerable sensation by repeated light stimulation of the cutaneous nerve endings; to titillate.

**tick'ling.** Titillation; a peculiar disagreeable sensation, caused by repeated light stimulation of the skin; it is accompanied by laughing.

**tictology** (tik-tol'o-jī) [ G. *tiktō,* to bear young, + *logos,* study ]. Obstetrics.

**t.i.d.** Abbreviation of L. *ter in die,* three times a day; see also t.d.s.

**ti'dal.** Relating to or resembling the tides, alternately rising and falling.

**tide** [ A.S. *tīd,* time ]. An alternate rise and fall, ebb and flow, or an increase or a decrease.

**acid t.,** acid wave; a temporary increase in the acidity of the urine occurring during fasting.

**alkaline t.,** alkaline wave; a period of urinary neutrality or even alkalinity after meals due to withdrawal of hydrogen ion for the purpose of secretion of the highly acid gastric juice.

**fat t.,** an increase in the fat content of blood and lymph following a meal.

**tie** [ A.S. ]. An area of skin of the back of a fat animal that adheres to the vertebrae, forming a dimple-like drpression. A show cattle term.

**Tiedemann** (te'deh-mahn), Friedrich, German anatomist, 1781–1861. See T.'s *gland, nerve.*

**Tietze** (teets), Alexander, German surgeon, 1864–1927. See T.'s *syndrome.*

**tiges'tol** (USAN). 19-Nor-17α-pregn-5(10)-en-20-yn-17-ol; a progestational agent.

**tig'late.** A salt of tiglic acid.

**tig'lic acid.** *trans*-2-Methyl-2-butenoic acid; $CH_3CH = C(CH_3)COOH$; an unsaturated fatty acid present in glycerides in croton oil.

**tig'lium.** *Croton tiglium,* the source of croton oil.

**tigretier** (te-grē-tya') [ Fr. ]. A form of saltatory chorea or dancing mania occurring in certain parts of Abyssinia.

**ti'groid** [ G. *tigroeidēs,* fr. *tigris,* tiger, + *eidos,* appearance ]. See chromophil *substance.*

**tigrolysis** (ti-grol'ĭ-sis) [ tigroid + G. *lysis,* dissolution ]. Chromatolysis; chromolysis; chromophilysis; disintegration and dissolution of the tigroid masses (Nissl substance, or ribosomal matter) in a neuron.

**tilet'amine hydrochloride** (USAN). 2-(Ethylamino)-2-(2-thienyl)cyclohexanone hydrochloride; a general anesthetic with anticonvulsant activity.

**til'idine hydrochloride** (USAN). (+)-Ethyl *trans*-2-(dimethylamino)-1-phenyl-3-cyclohexene-1-carboxylate hydrochloride; an analgesic drug.

**Tillaux** (te-lo'), Paul J., Paris surgeon, 1834–1904. See T.'s *disease.*

**til'mus** [ G. *tilmos,* plucking, tearing ]. Floccillation.

**timbre** (tam'br, tim'br) [ Fr. ]. Tone color; the distinguishing quality of a sound, by which one may determine its source.

**time** [ A.S. *tima* ]. 1. That relation of events which is expressed by the terms past, present, and future, and measured by units such as minutes, hours, days, months, or years. 2. A certain period during which something definite or determined is done.

**association t.,** t. elasping between a stimulus and the verbalized mental association.

**biologic t.,** the concept that our appreciation of t. varies with age and is governed by the neural organization of the individual; it obeys a logarithmic rather than an arithmetic law.

**bleeding t.,** as originally described by Duke and shown in the illustration, the t. interval between the appearance of the first drop and the removal of the last drop following puncture of the lobe of the ear or the finger, usually 1 to 3 minutes. It is prolonged in cases with thrombocytopenia, diminished prothrombin, phosphorus poisoning or chloroform poisoning, and in some liver diseases. It is normal in hemophilia. Since the earlier techniques were not well controlled, better controlled modifications such as that of Ivy are now employed to determine the bleeding.

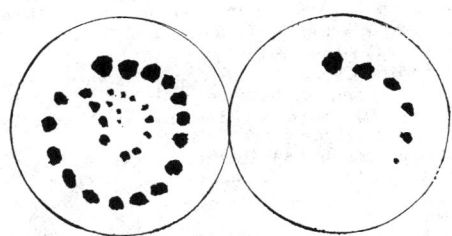

**Bleeding Time**
*Right,* normal; *left,* in thrombocytopenic purpura; blood samples at 20-second intervals. (After Quick.)

**calcium t.,** the t. required for the coagulation of blood to which calcium chloride has been dded. If this t. is less than the coagulation t. for the same blood without the added calcium, then the delay is probably the result of a deficiency of calcium in the patient.

**circulation t.,** the t. taken for the blood to pass through a given circuit of the vascular system, *e.g.,* the pulmonary or systemic circulation, from one arm to another, from arm to tongue, from arm to lung, etc. It is measured by the injection into an arm vein of a substance, such as Decholin, ether, fluorescein, histamine, or a radium salt, which can be detected when it arrives at another point in the vascular system.

**clot retraction t.,** the t. required for a blood clot to separate from the tube wall and express serum, usually completed in 18 to 24 hours, but retarded or absent in persons with thrombocytopenic purpura.

**clotting t.,** coagulation t.

**coagulation t.,** clotting t.; the t. required for blood to coagulate. It is prolonged in hemophilia and in the presence of obstructive jaundice, some anemias and leukemias, and some of the infectious diseases.

**fading t.,** the t. required for a constant stimulus applied to a fixed area of the peripheral visual field to fade and cease.

**half-t.,** see half-time.

**iner'tia t.,** the interval elapsing between the reception of the stimulus from a nerve and the contraction of the muscle.

**left ventricular ejection t.,** abbreviated LVET; the t. measured from onset to incisural notch of the carotid pulse.

**prothrombin t.** when thromboplastin and calcium are added in optimal amounts to blood of normal fibrinogen content, the only factor that can vary the clotting t. is an inadequate concentration of prothrombin; if prothrombin is diminished, the clotting t. increases. See also prothrombin *test.*

**reaction t.,** the interval between the presentation of a stimulus and the responsive reaction to it.

**recognition t.,** the interval between the application of a stimulus and the recognition of its nature.

**rise t.,** the t. required for a pulse to rise from 10 per cent to 90 per cent of its peak amplitude.

**sensation t.,** the minimal t. a visual image must be exposed to be perceived.

**survival t.,** (1) the period elapsing between the completion or institution of any procedure, *e.g.,* removal of the adrenal glands, or the withdrawal from the diet of an essential constituent, and death; (2) the life span of biologically or physically marked erythrocytes or other cells.

**utilization t.,** temps utile; the minimum duration of a stimulus of rheobasic strength that is just sufficient to produce excitation.

**tin.** Sn; a metallic element, stannum; atomic no. 50, atomic weight 118.70.

**tin-113.** $^{113}$Sn; a radioisotope of tin with a physical half-life of 115 days; used in the manufacture of radionuclide generators for the production of indium-113m.

**Tinbergen,** Nikolaas, Dutch zoologist, *1907. Nobel laureate, 1973, with Karl Ritter von Frisch and Konrad Lorenz, for their discoveries concerning organization and elicitation of individual and social behavior patterns.

**tinct.** Abbreviation of L. *tinctura,* tincture.

**tinc'table.** Stainable.

**tinction** (tink'shun) [ L. *tingo,* pp. *tinctus,* to dye ]. 1. A stain; a preparation for staining. 2. The act of staining.

**tinctorial** (tingk-tōr'ĭ-al) [ L. *tinctorius,* fr. *tingo,* to dye ]. Relating to coloring or staining.

**tinctura,** gen. and pl. **tincturae** (tingk-tu'rah, -re) [ L. a dyeing, fr. *tingo,* pp. *tinctus,* to dye ]. Tincture.

**tinc'tura'tion.** The making of a tincture from a crude drug.

**tincture** (tingk'chur) [ see *tinctura* ]. An alcoholic or hydroalcoholic solution prepared from vegetable materials or from chemical substances; most t.'s are prepared by percolation or by maceration. The proportions of drug represented in the different t.'s are not uniform, but vary according to the established standards for each. T.'s of potent drugs essentially represent the activity of 10 gm. of the drug in each 100 ml. of t., the potency being adjusted after assay; most other t.'s represent 20 gm. of drug in each 100 ml. of t. Compound t.'s are made according to long-established formulas.

**alcoholic t.,** a t. made with undiluted alcohol.

**ammoniated t.,** a t. made with ammoniated.

**ethereal t.,** a class of preparations consisting of 10 per cent percolations of drugs in a menstruum of ether 1 and alcohol 2.

**t. of fresh drugs,** the general formula for these is to macerate 500 gm. of the cut, bruised or crushed fresh drug in alcohol, 1000 cc., for 14 days, then strongly express the liquid and filter it through paper. Lemon t. and sweet orange peel t. are prepared from fresh drugs.

**glycerinated t.,** a t. made with diluted alcohol to which glycerin is added to facilitate the extraction or to preserve the preparation.

**hydroalcoholic t.,** a t. made with diluted alcohol in various proportions with water.

**tine** (tin) [ A.S. *tind,* a prong ]. 1. In dentistry, the slender, pointed end of an explorer. 2. An instrument used to introduce antigen such as tuberculin into the skin, and usually containing several individual t.'s.

**tinea** (tin'e-ah) [ L. worm, moth ]. Ringworm; Saint Aignan's disease; serpigo (1); a fungus infection of the skin and its appendages; among the common genera of fungi causing cutaneous infection are *Microsporum, Trichophyton, Epidermophyton,* and *Keratinomyces.*

**t. amianta'cea,** an inflammatory condition of the scalp in which heavy scales extend onto the hairs and bind the proximal portions together; it is not caused by a fungus.

**t. axilla'ris,** t. imbricata of the axilla.

**t. bar'bae,** t. sycosis.

**t. cap'itis,** t. tonsurans.

**t. cilio'rum,** fungus infection of the eyelashes.

**t. circina'ta,** t. corporis; trichophytosis corporis; herpes tonsurans; ringworm of the body; a well defined, scaling, macular eruption that frequently forms annular lesions and may appear on any part of the body.

**t. circina'ta trop'ica,** t. imbricata.

**t. corporis,** t. circinata.

**t. cru'ris,** t. inguinalis; trichyphytosis cruris; dhobie itch; jock itch; eczema marginatum; ringworm (t. imbricata, *q.v.*) of the genitocrural region, including the inner side of the thighs, the perineal region, and the groin.

**t. favo'sa,** favus.

**t. flava,** a form which is very common in tropical Asia, due to *Malassezia tropica.*

**t. furfura'cea,** t. versicolor.

**t. gal'li,** a fungal infection involving chiefly the combs of chickens and turkeys, forming dull white patches; also called whitecomb.

**t. glabro'sa,** ringworm or fungus infection of the hairless skin.

**t. imbrica'ta** [ L. overlapping like tiles ], an eruption consisting of a number of concentric rings of overlapping scales forming papulosquamous patches scattered over the body; it occurs in tropical climates and is caused by the fungus *Endodermophyton,* or, more commonly, *Trichophyton concentricum;* the disease is known by many names, among which are: herpes desquamans; Burmese, Chinese, India, Tokelau, Oriental, or Bowditch Island ringworm; scaly ringworm; lota tokelau; t. circinata tropica; t. tropicalis; Malabar itch.

**t. inguina'lis,** t. cruris.

**t. ke'rion** [ G. *kērion,* honeycomb ], Celsus' kerion; inflammatory fungus infection of the scalp and beard, marked by pustules and a boggy infiltration of the surrounding parts; most commonly caused by *Microsporum audouini* and *Microsporum canis.*

**t. nigra,** pityriasis nigra; a fungus infection due to *Cladosporium werneckii;* lesions occur most commonly on the hands.

**t. ni'grocircina'ta,** t. caused by *Trichophyton ceylonense;* the lesions are annular, with elevated margins and central blackish areas; they occur on the neck and scrotum.

**t. pe'dis,** dermatomycosis pedis; dermatophytosis of the feet; athlete's foot; Hong Kong foot; Hong Kong toe; ringworm of the foot; epidermophytosis interdigitalis pedum; an infection of the feet, especially of the skin between the toes, caused by one of the dermatophytes. The disease consists of small vesicles, fissures, scaling, maceration, and eroded areas between the toes and on the plantar surfaces of the feet. Other skin areas may be involved.

**t. profun'da,** pustules with deep follicular lesions occurring in some patients with a superficial mycotic infection.

**t. syco'sis** [ G. *sykon,* a fig ], ringworm of the beard, occurring as a follicular infection or as a granulomatous lesion. The primary lesions are papules and pustules. Also called t. sycosis; barber's itch; folliculitis barbae; chronic coccogenic sycosis; parasitic or nonparasitic sycosis; sycosis contagiosa; sycosis staphylogenes; sycosis vulgaris; sycosis tinea; trichophytosis barbae.

**t. tar'si,** fungus infection of eyelids.

**t. tondens,** t. tonsurans.

**t. tonsu'rans,** ringworm of the scalp; herpes tonsurans; t. tondens; t. capitis; porrigo furfurans; trichonosus furfuracea; trichophytosis capitis; a fungus infection caused by species of *Microsporum* or *Trichophyton.*

**t. trichophyti'na,** ringworm; trichophytosis; a disease of the skin, hair, and nails, due to invasion of a fungus of the genus *Trichophyton.*

**t. tropica'lis,** t. imbricata.

**t. un'guium,** onychomycosis.

**t. vera,** favus.

**t. versic'olor,** Eichstedt's disease; t. furfuracea; pityriasis versicolor; chromophytosis; an eruption of tan or brown, branny patches on the skin of the trunk, and appearing white in contrast with hyperpigmented skin after exposure to the summer sun; caused by *Malassezia furfur.*

**Tinel** (te-nel'), Jules, French neurologist, 1879–1952. See T.'s *sign.*

**tingibility** (tin'ji-bil'i-ti). The property of being tingible.

**tingible** (tin'ji-bl) [ L. *tingo,* to dye ]. Capable of being stained.

**tingle** (ting'gl). To feel a peculiar pricking sensation.

**ting'ling.** A peculiar pricking thrill, caused by cold, by an emotional shock, or striking a nerve, such as the ulnar at the elbow (the "funny bone").

**tinid'azole** (USAN). 1-[ 2-(Ethylsulfonyl)ethyl ]-2-methyl-5-nitroimidazole; an antiprotozoal agent.

**tinkle** (tingk'l) [ an imitative word ]. 1. To make a metallic clinking sound like that of a coin or a small bell. 2. A tinkling; a clinking metallic sound sometimes heard on auscultation over a pneumothorax or a large pulmonary cavity.

**tinnitus** (ti-ni'tus) [ L. a jingling, fr. *tinnio,* pp. *tinnitus,* to jingle, clink ]. Noises (ringing, whistling, booming, etc.) in the ears; also called t. aurium.

**t. aurium,** sensation of sound in one or both ears associated with disease in the middle ear, the inner ear, or the central auditory apparatus.

**t. cerebri,** subjective sensation of noise in head rather than ears.

**clicking t.,** an objective clicking sound in the ear in cases of chronic catarrhal otitis media; it may be audible to the bystander as well as to the patient and is supposed to be due to an opening and closing of the mouth of the Eustachian tube, or to a rhythmical spasm of the velum palati.

**Leudet's t.,** a dry spasmodic click, audible also through the otoscope, heard in catarrhal inflammation of the Eustachian tube; caused by reflex spasm of the tensor palati muscle.

**tint** [ L. *tingo,* pp. *tinctus,* to dye ]. A shade of color varying according to the amount of white admixed with the pigment.

**t. B,** in x-ray measurement by the Sabouraud-Noire instrument, a color of the pastille indicating the quantity of radiation that will cause the hair to fall; about four-fifths of the erythema dose.

**tintometer** (tin-tom'e-ter) [ tint + G. *metron,* measure ]. A scale of colors of different shades, used to determine by comparison the intensity of color of the blood (hemoglobinometer) or of other fluids.

**tint'omet'ric.** Pertaining to tintometry.

**tintometry** (tin-tom'e-tri) [ tint + G. *metron,* measure ]. Estimation of the intensity of color in a fluid by means of comparison with a standard color scale.

**tip.** 1. A point; a more or less sharp extremity. 2. A separate, but attached, piece of the same or another structure, forming the extremity of a part.

**t. of auricle,** *apex* auriculae.

**t. of horn,** *apex* cornus posterioris.

**t. of nose,** *apex* nasi.

**root t.,** a portion of the root of a tooth nearest the apex.

**t. of tongue,** *apex* linguae.

**Woolner's t.,** the extremity of the helix of the auricle.

**tipren'olol hydrochloride** (USAN). (+)-1-(Isopropylamino)-3-[ *o*-(methylthio)phenoxy ]-2-propanol hydrochloride; a β-receptor blocking agent.

**tiqueur** (te-kër') [ Fr. ]. One who suffers from a tic.

**tire** (tīr) [ A.S. *teorian* ]. 1. To fatigue. 2. To become fatigued.

**tireballe** (tēr-bal') [ Fr. *tirer,* to pull, + *balle,* ball ]. An instrument in the form of a screw or spiral, designed for extracting a bullet or other foreign body from the tissues.

**tirefond** (tēr-fawn') [ Fr. *tirer,* to pull, + *fond,* bottom ]. An instrument in the form of a conical screw, designed for raising depressed bone as in fracture of the skull.

**tiring** (tīr'ing). Fixing the fragments of a broken bone by fastening a wire around them.

**Tiselius** (te-sa'lī-us). Arne, Swedish biochemist, *1902. See T. *apparatus,* electrophoresis *cell.*

**tisic.** Phthisic.

**tissue** (tish'u) [ Fr. *tissu,* woven, fr. L. *texo,* to weave ]. A collection of similar cells and the intercellular substances surrounding them. There are four basic tissues in the body: (1) epithelium; (2) the connective tissues, including blood, bone, and cartilage; (3) muscle tissue; and (4) nerve tissue.

**adenoid t.,** lymphatic t.

**ad'ipose t.,** fat (1); white fat (1); a connective t. consisting chiefly of fat cells surrounded by reticular fibers and arranged in lobular groups or along the course of one of the smaller blood vessels.

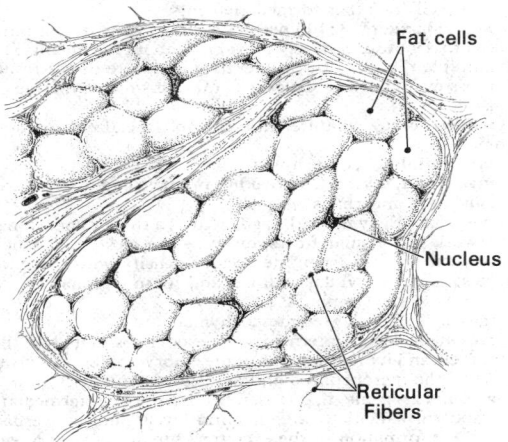

Fat cells

Nucleus

Reticular Fibers

**Adipose Tissue**

**are'olar t.,** loose, irregularly arranged connective t.; it consists of collagenous and elastic fibers; a protein polysaccharide ground substance, and connective t. cells (fibroblasts, macrophages, mast cells, and sometimes fat cells, plasma cells, leukocytes, and pigment cells).

**bone t.,** osseous t.

**can'cellous t.,** lattice-like or spongy osseous t.

**cardiac muscle t.,** see cardiac *muscle.*

**cartilaginous t.,** see cartilage.

**cav'ernous t.,** erectile t.

**chondroid t.,** (1) fibrohyaline t.; in an adult, t. resembling cartilage; (2) in an embryo, an early stage in cartilage formation.

**chromaffin t.,** a cellular t., vascular and well supplied with nerves, made up chiefly of chromaffin cells; it is found in the medulla of the suprarenal glands and, in smaller collections, in the paraganglia.

**compression of t.,** t. displaceability.

**connective t.,** interstitial t.; the supporting or framework t. of the animal body, formed of fibrous and ground substance with more or less numerous cells of various kinds. It is derived from the mesenchyme, and this in turn from the mesoderm. The varieties of connective t. are: areolar or loose; adipose; dense, regular or irregular, white fibrous; elastic; mucous; and lymphoid t.; cartilage; and bone. The blood and lymph may be regarded as connective t.'s the ground substance of which is a liquid.

**dartoic t.,** t. resembling tunica dartos.

**elastic t.,** a form of connective t. in which the elastic fibers predominate; it constitutes the ligamenta flava of the vertebrae and the ligamentum nuchae, especially of quadrupeds; it occurs also in the walls of the arteries and of the bronchial tree, and connects the cartilages of the larynx.

**epithe′lial t.,** see epithelium.

**erectile t.,** cavernous t.; a t. with numerous vascular spaces which may become engorged with blood.

**fatty t.,** (1) adipose t.; (2) in some animals, brown *fat.*

**fibrohyaline t.,** chondroid t. (1).

**fibrous t.,** a t. composed of bundles of collagenous white fibers between which are rows of connective t. cells; the tendons, ligaments, aponeuroses, and some of the membranes, such as the dura mater.

**flabby t.,** hyperplastic t. (2).

**Gamgee t.,** a material consisting of a thick layer of absorbent cotton between two layers of absorbent gauze, used in surgical dressings.

**gelat′inous t.,** mucous connective t.

**gingival t.'s,** see gingiva.

**granulation t.,** vascular connective t. forming granular projections on the surface of a healing wound, ulcer, or inflamed t. surface. See also granulation.

**Haller's vascular t.,** *lamina* vasculosa choroideae.

**hard t.,** (1) t. that has become mineralized; (2) t. having a firm intercellular substance, *e.g.,* cartilage and bone.

**hemopoietic t.,** t. in which there is a development of blood cells or other formed elements.

**hyperplastic t.,** (1) hyperplasia; (2) in dentistry, a term used to denote excessively movable t. about the maxillae or mandible that may be proliferative in nature or the result of loss of supporting structures; (3) t. in which hyperplasia has occurred.

**indifferent t.,** undifferentiated, nonspecialized, embryonic t.

**interstitial t.,** connective t.

**investing t.'s,** the t.'s covering or enclosing a structure.

**islet t.,** Langerhans' *islands.*

**lymphatic t.,** lymphoid t.; adenoid t.; a three-dimensional network of reticular fibers and cells the meshes of which are occupied in varying degrees of density with lymphocytes; there is nodular, diffuse, and loose lymphatic t.

**lymphoid t.,** lymphatic t.

**mesen′chymal t.,** see mesenchyme.

**mesonephric t.,** intermediate mesoderm situated in the thoracic and lumbar regions of the embryo or fetus; it gives rise to the mesonephros and associated structures.

**metanephrogenic t.,** t. derived from the intermediate mesoderm caudal to mesonephric levels, and concerned with the formation of the excretory tubules of permanent kidney, or metanephros.

**mucous connective t.,** gelatinous t.; a type of connective t. but little differentiated beyond the mesenchymal stage. Its ground substance of protein polysaccharide is abundant and contains fine collagenous fibers and fibroblasts. In its most characteristic form it appears in the umbilical cord supporting the vessels and is called Wharton's jelly.

**multilocular adipose t.,** brown *fat.*

**muscular t.,** a t. characterized by the ability to contract upon stimulation; its three varities are skeletal, cardiac, and smooth. Skeletal and cardiac muscle fibers are marked by transverse lines in their fibrils, whence the term striated or striped muscle; smooth muscle fibers are spindle-shaped, uninuclear cells with very fine fibrils with no cross striations. All varieties are held together by a close-meshed network of connective t. See also muscle.

**myeloid t.,** bone marrow consisting of the developmental and adult stages of erythrocytes, granulocytes and mega-

karyocytes in a stroma of reticular cells and fibers, with vascular channels lined with reticuloendothelium.

**nephrogen′ic t.,** the t. from which the pronephros, mesonephros and metanephros develop.

**nervous t.,** a highly differentiated t. composed of nerve cells, nerve fibers, dendrites, and a supporting t., the neuroglia.

**nodal t.,** see *nodus* atrioventricularis and *nodus* sinuatrialis.

**os′seous t.,** bone t.; a connective t., the matrix of which consists of collagen fibers and ground substance and in which are deposited calcium salts (phosphate, carbonate, and some fluoride) in the form of an apatite.

**osteogen′ic t.,** a connective t. with the property of forming osseous t.

**osteoid t.,** osseous t. prior to calcification.

**periap′ical t.,** the structures adjacent to a root apex, particularly the periodontal ligament and bone.

**reticular t., retiform t.,** a t. in which the argyrophilic fibers form a network and which usually has a network of reticular cells associated with the fibers.

**rubber t.,** a thin sheet of caoutchouc used as a protective in surgical dressings.

**skeletal muscle t.,** see skeletal *muscle.*

**smooth muscle t.,** see smooth *muscle.*

**subcutaneous t.,** a layer of loose, irregular, connective t. immediately beneath the skin and closely attached to the corium by coarse fibrous bands, the retinacula cutis; it contains fat cells except in the auricles, eyelids, penis, and scrotum.

**tissue-trimming.** Border *molding.*

**tissular** (tish′u-lar). Relating or pertaining to a tissue.

**titanium** (ti-ta′nĭ-um) [ *Titan,* one of the primitive gods of antiquity ]. A metallic element, symbol Ti, atomic no. 22, atomic weight 47.90.

**t. dioxide** (USP), $TiO_2$; contains not less than 99.0 per cent and not more than 100.5 per cent of $TiO_2$, calculated on the dry basis; used in creams and powders as a protectant against external irritations and solar rays.

**ti′ter** [ Fr. *titre,* standard ]. The standard of strength of a volumetric test solution; assay value of an unknown measure by volumetric means.

**TITh.** Abbreviation for triiodothyronine.

**titillation** (tit′ĭ-la′shun) [ L. *titillatio,* fr. *titillo,* pp. -*atus,* tickle ]. Tickling.

**ti′trant.** In chemistry, the solution that is added (titrated with) in a titration.

**ti′trate.** To analyze volumetrically by a solution (the titrant) of known strength to an end point.

**titration** (ti-tra′shun) [ Fr. *titre,* standard ]. Volumetric analysis by means of the addition of definite amounts of a test solution to a solution of the substance being assayed.

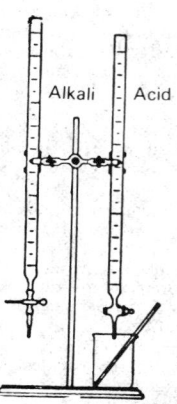

Alkali    Acid

**Burettes for Titrating**

**colorimetric t.,** a t. in which the end point is marked by a sudden color change.

**formol t.,** a method of titrating the amino group of amino acids, by adding formaldehyde to the neutral solution. The formaldehyde reacts with the $NH_3^+$ group, liberating an equivalent quantity of $H^+$, which may then be estimated by t. with NaOH.

**potentiometric t.,** a t. during which the pH is continually measured with some value of the pH serving as end point.

**titubation** (tit′u-ba′shun) [ L. *titubo*, pp. -*atus*, to stagger ]. 1. A staggering or stumbling in trying to walk. 2. Restlessness.

**lingual t.,** stammering; stuttering.

**Tizzoni** (tid-zo′ne), Guido, Italian physician 1853–1932. See T.'s *test*.

**Tl.** Chemical symbol of the element thallium.

**TLC.** Abbreviation for (1) thin-layer *chromatography*; (2) total lung *capacity*.

**TLE.** Abbreviation for thin-layer *electrophoresis*.

**Tm.** 1. Chemical symbol of the element thulium. 2. Symbol for transport or tubular *maximum*.

**TMP.** Abbreviation for ribothymidine 5′-phosphate (thymidine 5′-phosphate is dTMP).

**T-mycoplasma.** *Ureaplasma.*

**Tn.** Abbreviation for intraocular *tension.*

**TNT.** Abbreviation for trinitrotoluene.

**TO.** Abbreviation for Theiler's Original, which refers to Theiler's original strain of virus.

**tocamphyl** (to-kam′fil) (USAN). LICARBIN; camphoric acid *p*-α-dimethylbenzyl ester diethanolamine salt; choleretic.

**toco-** (to′ko-, tok′o-) [ G. *tokos*, birth ]. Combining form relating to childbirth.

**tocochromanol-3** (to′ko-kro′mă-nol). α-Tocotrienol.

**tocodynagraph** (to′ko-di′nă-graf, tok′o-) [ toco- + G. *dynamis*, force, + *graphē*, a writing ]. Tokodynagraph; tocograph; tokograph; a recording of the force of uterine contractions.

**tocodynamometer** (to′ko-di′nă-mom′e-ter, tok′o-) [ toco- + G. *dynamis*, force, + *metron*, measure ]. Tokodynamometer; tocometer; an instrument for measuring the force of uterine contractions.

**tocography** (to-kog′ră-fĭ) [ toko- + G. *graphō*, to write ]. Tokography; the process of recording uterine contractions.

**to′col.** Fundamental unit of the tocopherols (methyltocols); 6-phytylhydroquinone (see structure *A*, below) in the chromanol form; 2-methyl-2-(4,8,12-trimethyltridecyl)-chroman-6-ol (structure *B*). Compare tocotrienol; phyllochromanol.

(A)          (B)

$$R = +(CH_2)_2 - \overset{\overset{\displaystyle CH_3}{|}}{CH} - CH_2 \}_3 H$$

Tocol

**tocology** (to-kol′o-jĭ) [ toco- + G. *logos*, study ]. Obstetrics.

**tocomania** (to′ko-ma′nĭ-ah, tok′o-) [ toco- + G. *mania*, frenzy ]. Puerperal *mania*.

**tocometer** (to-kom′e-ter). Tocodynamometer.

**tocopepantic** (to′ko-pe-pan′tik) [ toco- + G. *pepanos*, ripe ]. Ready for childbearing.

**tocopherol** (tok-of′er-ōl). Abbreviation, T. 1. Name given to vitamin E (*q. v.*) by its discoverer; now a generic term for vitamin E and compounds chemically related to it, with or without biological activity. Similar in chemical structure and properties to vitamins K and coenzyme Q; also known as methyltocols. Vitamin E is essential for normal reproduction in rats. Used in "stiff lamb" disease and "white muscle" disease in calves. 2. A methylated tocol or methylated tocotrienol; see α-tocopherol, etc., below, also tocol.

**mixed t.'s concentrate,** a source of vitamin E, obtained by vacuum distillation of edible vegetable oils or their by-products.

**α-tocopherol.** 2,5,7,8-Tetramethyl-2-(4′,8′,12′-trimethyltridecyl)-6-chromanol; 5,7,8-trimethyltocol (see tocol, structure *B*); vitamin E; abbreviated α-T. A light yellow, viscous, odorless, oily liquid which deteriorates on exposure to light. It is obtained from wheat germ oil or by synthesis and biologically exhibits the most vitamin E activity of the tocopherols. It is an antioxidant retarding rancidity by interfering with the autoxidation of fats. *dl*-α-Tocopherol is prepared synthetically. Also available are *d*-α-tocopherol acetate, *dl*-α-tocopherol acetate, *d*-α-tocopheryl acid succinate (NF), and *d*-α-tocopherol acetate concentrate. See also vitamin E.

**β-tocopherol.** 5,8-Dimethyltocol; abbreviated β-T. A lower homologue of α-tocopherol, containing one less methyl group in the aromatic nucleus and less active biologically. Accompanies α-T and γ-T.

**γ-tocopherol.** 7,8-Dimethyltocol; abbreviated γ-T; biologically less active than α-T. Corn oil is rich in γ-T.

**δ-tocopherol.** 8-Methyltocol; abbreviated δ-T. Soybean oil is rich in δ-T.

**ε-tocopherol.** β-Tocotrienol; abbreviated β-T-3.

**ζ₁- or ζ₂-tocopherol.** α-Tocotrienol; abbreviated α-T-3.

**η-tocopherol.** γ-Tocotrienol; abbreviated γ-T-3.

**tocoph′erolqui′none.** Tocoquinone; tocopherylquinone; an oxidized tocopherol, from the isomeric 2-methyl-2-phytyl-6-chromenol with methyl groups in one or more of positions 5,7, and 8 by migration of H atom from 6-OH to C-4 position, which yields a 1,4-benzoquinone. Abbreviation, TQ preceded by α, β, etc., as in tocopherols; see also tocol.

**tocoph′erylqui′none.** Tocopherolquinone.

**tocophobia** (to′ko-fo′bĭ-ah, tok′o-) [ toco- + G. *phobos*, fear ]. Morbid dread of childbirth.

**to′coqui′none.** Tocopherolquinone.

**tocoquinone-10** (E₁₀). 2,3,5-Trimethyl-6-decaprenyl-1,4-benzoquinone; vitamin E₂(50); *cf.* tocopherolquinone, tocotrienolquinone, ubiquinone-10.

**to′cotri′enol.** Similar to tocol, but with three additional double bonds in the phytyl chain, thus a 6-(3′,7′,11′,15′-tetramethyl-2′,6′,10′,14′-hexadecatetraenyl) -1,4- hydroquinone or a 2-methyl-2-(4,8,12-trimethyltrideca-3,7,11-trienyl)chroman-6-ol; a tocol with three double bonds in the side chain. The natural products carry methyls at one or more of positions 5, 7, and 8 of the chromanol and are thus identical, except for the unsaturation in the phytyl-like side chain, to the tocopherols. Also analogous is the cyclization to form a chromanol derivative and oxidation to form the tocotrienolquinones (or chromenols). Abbreviated, T-*n* (hydroquinone form) or TQ-*n* (quinone form), preceded by α-, β-, etc., as in the tocopherols, to indicate degree of methylation (the *n* indicates the number of intact isoprene or prenyl units remaining in the chromanol or chromenol form). The tocotrienol terminology is used to indicate relationships to tocols and tocoenols (vitamin E-like), the chromanol terminology to indicate relationship to the isoprenoidal compounds of the vitamin K and coenzyme Q series.

**α-tocotrienol.** 5,7,8-Trimethyltocotrienol (chromanol numbering); 2,3,5-trimethyl-6-triprenyl-1,4-hydroquinone; ζ₁- or ζ₂-tocopherol; tocochromanol-3 (or E₃); abbreviated α-T-3.

**β-tocotrienol.** 5,8-Dimethyltocotrienol; ε-tocopherol; abbreviated β-T-3.

**γ-tocotrienol.** 7,8-Dimethyltocotrienol (chromanol numbering); 2,3-dimethyl-6-triprenyl-1,4-hydroquinone; η-tocopherol; plastochromanol-3 (or E₃); abbreviated PQ-3 (or PQ₃).

**δ-tocotrienol.** 8-Methyltocotrienol.

**to'cotri'enolqui'none.** A tocotrienol in which the hydroquinone has been oxidized to a quinone (the chromanol has become a chromenol); the t.'s carry α, β, γ and δ prefixes in accordance with the degree of methylation (see tocotrienol).

**Tod's muscle.** See under muscle.

**Todaro** (to-dah'ro), Francesco, Italian anatomist, 1839–1918. See T.'s *tendon.*

**Todd,** Robert B., English physician, 1809–1860. See T.'s *paralysis.*

**toe** [ A.S. *ta* ]. Digitus pedis; one of the digits of the feet.

**t. drop,** a drooping of the anterior portion of the foot, owing to paralysis of the muscles that dorsally flex the foot.

**great t.,** hallux.

**hammer t.,** permanent flexion at the midphalangeal joint of one or more of the t.'s. See fig. under hallux.

**Hong Kong t.,** *tinea* pedis.

**pheasant hunter's t.,** gout caused by trauma, fatigue, excess calories, and pheasant meat containing purine bodies.

**pigeon t.'s,** nonspecific term for a condition in which the t.'s are directoward the midsagittal plane of the body. When fixed, the condition may arise from an angular deformity in the foot or a rotational deformity higher in the extremity. When functional, it is present only when the patient walks, in which case it is the result of muscle imbalance.

**seedy t.,** in the horse, a separation of the horn of the wall from that of the sole at the t. It frequently follows laminitis.

**stiff t.,** *hallux* rigidus.

**webbed t.'s,** syndactyly involving the toes.

**toe-crack.** See sand-crack.

**toe'nail.** Unguis.

**ingrowing t.,** see ingrown *nail.*

**tofen'acin hydrochloride** (USAN). *N*-Methyl-2-[ (*o*-methyl-α -phenylbenzyl)oxy ]ethylamine hydrochloride; an anticholinergic drug.

**toilet** (toy'let) [ Fr. *toilette* ]. The cleansing of the parts after childbirth or of a wound after an operation preparatory to the application of the dressing.

**Toison** (twah-zawn'), J., French histologist, 1858–1950. See T.'s *solution.*

**toko-** [ G. *tokos,* birth ]. For words so beginning, see toco-.

**tola'zamide** (USP). TOLINASE; 1-(hexahydro-1 *H*-azeprin-1-yl)-3-(*p*-tolylsulfonyl)urea; an oral hypoglycemic agent that stimulates pancreatic secretion of insulin; most useful therapeutically in mild cases of maturity-onset diabetes mellitus.

**tolaz'oline hydrochloride** (NF, BP). PRISCOLINE hydrochloride; 2-benzyl-2-imidazoline hydrochloride; an adrenergic α-receptor blocking agent used to augment blood flow in peripheral vascular disorders.

**tolbox'ane.** CLARMIL; *p*-tolueneboronic acid cyclic 2-methyl-2-propyltrimethylene ester; antianxiety agent.

**tolbu'tamide** (USP, BP). ORINASE; 1-butyl-3-*p*-tolylsulfonylurea; an orally active hypoglycemic agent used in the management of certain cases of diabetes mellitus. It appears to stimulate the synthesis and release of endogenous insulin from functional islets. islets. Available as t. sodium (USP) for injection.

**tolcy'clamide.** DIABORAL; tolhexamide; 1-cyclohexyl-3-*p*-tolylsulfonylurea; oral hypoglycemic agent.

**Toldt** (tōlt), Karl, Austrian anatomist, 1840–1920. See T.'s *fascia, membrane.*

**tol'erance** [ L. *tolero,* pp. - *atus,* to endure ]. Toleration; the power of resisting the action of a poison, or of taking a drug continuously or in large doses without injurious effects.

**acoustic t.,** the maximum sound pressure level (SPL) that can be experienced without producing pain of permanent defect of hearing in a normal individual.

**cross t.,** the resistance to one or several effects of a compound as a result of t. developed to a pharmacologically similar compound.

**frustration t.,** the level of an individual's ability to withstand frustration without developing inadequate modes of response, such as "going to pieces" emotionally or becoming neurotic.

**g-tolerance,** the t. of a person or a piece of equipment to forces that develop as a result of acceleration or deceleration.

**immunological t.,** immunotolerance; acquired, specific failure of the immunological mechanism to respond, induced by exposure to the given antigen.

**individual t.,** t. to a drug that the subject has never received before.

**species t.,** the insensitivity to a particular drug exhibited by a particular species.

**split t.,** immune *deviation.*

**vibration t.,** the maximum vibratory or oscillatory movements that an individual can experience and bear without pain; the limit of t. is a function of amplitude and frequency of the vibration and varies with the direction of application.

**tol'erant.** Having the property of tolerance.

**tolerogenic** (tol'er-o-jen'ik). Producing immunologic tolerance.

**tolhex'amide.** Tolcyclamide.

**Tollens,** Bernard C. G., German chemist, 1841–1918. See T.'s *reaction.*

**tol'metin** (USAN). TOLECTIN; 1-methyl-5-*p*-toluoylpyrrole-2-acetic acid; an anti-inflammatory drug.

**tolnaf'tate** (USP, BP). FOCUSAN; SPORILINE; TINACTIN; *O*-2-naphthyl *m*,*N*-dimethylthiocarbanilate; a topical antifungal agent.

**tolonium chloride** (to-lo'nī-um). BLUTENE chloride; 3-amino-7-dimethylamino-2-methylphenazothionium chloride; toluidine blue O. See also toluidine blue.

**tolpro'pamine.** TYLAGEL; *N*,*N*-dimethyl-3-phenyl-3-*p*-tolylpropylamine; topical antipruritic agent.

**toluene** (tol'u-ēn). Toluol; methylbenzene; by the dry distillation of tolu and other resinous bodies, and also derived from coal tar; its physical and chemical properties resemble those of benzene. Used in explosives and dyes, and in the extraction of various principles from plants.

**toluidine** (tol-u'ī-dēn, -din). Aminotoluene, one of three isomeric substances, $CH_3C_6H_4NH_2$, derived from toluene. May cause hematuria.

**t. blue O,** a blue basic dye, $C_{15}H_{16}N_3SCl$, used as an antibacterial agent; it also antagonizes the anticoagulant action of heparin; used as a nuclear stain and to stain (metachromatically) certain structures, such as the granules in mast cells which are believed to give rise to heparin. The medicinal grade is known as tolonium chloride (*q. v.*).

**toluol** (tol'u-ol). Toluene.

**toluoyl** (tol-u'o-il). The radical of toluic acid, $CH_3C_6H_4CO-$.

**toluylene** (tol-u'ī-lēn). Stilbene.

**to'lycaine hydrochloride.** BAYCAIN; 2-(2-diethylaminoacetamido)-*m*-toluic acid methyl ester hydrochloride; local anesthetic.

**tolyl** (tol'il). A univalent radical, $CH_3C_6H_4-$.

**tom.** 1. A male cat of breeding age. 2. A male turkey of breeding age; a turkey gobbler.

**Toma's sign.** See under sign.

**tomatine** (to'mă-tēn). LYCORSICIN; $C_{50}H_{83}NO_{21}$; a mixture of glycosides present in the leaves and stems of wild tomato plants; partial hydrolysis yields α-tomatine (the major constituent), β-tomatine, $β_2$-tomatine, γ-tomatine, and δ-tomatine. α-Tomatine is made up of 1 mol of tomatidine linked to a tetrasaccharide (2 mols of D-glucose, 1 mol of D-xylose, and 1 mol of D-galactose). It has antifungal and anti-inflammatory properties; is capable of antagonizing bradykinin and other substances believed to be involved in the development of allergic reactions; and is used as a precipitating agent for steroids, as an alternate to digitonin.

**-tome** [ G. *tomos,* cutting, sharp; a cutting (section or segment). TOM- ]. A termination denoting (1) a cutting instrument, the first element in the compound usually indicating the part that the instrument is designed to cut, and (2), a segment, part, or section.

**tomen'tum, tomen'tum cer'ebri** [ L. a stuffing for cushions ]. The numerous small blood vessels passing between the cerebral surface of the pia mater and the cortex of the brain.

**Tomes,** Sir John, English dentist and anatomist, 1815–1895. See T.'s *fibers,* granular *layer, processes.*

**Tommaselli,** Salvatore, Italian physician, 1834–1906. See T.'s *disease.*

**tomogram** (to′mo-gram) [ G. *tomos,* a cutting (section) + *gramma,* a writing ]. The roentgenogram obtained with a tomograph.

**tomograph** (to′mo-graf) [ G. *tomos,* a cutting (section), + *graphō,* to write ]. A device for taking sectional roentgenograms. By giving the x-ray tube a curvilinear motion during exposure synchronous with the recording plate but in the opposite direction, the shadow of the selected plane remains stationary on the moving film while the shadows of all other planes have a relative displacement on the film and are therefore obliterated or blurred.

**tomography** (to-mog′ră-fĭ). Sectional roentgenography; planigraphy; stratigraphy; laminagraphy; see tomograph.

**tomolevel** (to′mo-lev-el). The level at which tomography is performed.

**tomomania** (to′mo-ma′nĭ-ah) [ G. *tomos,* cutting, + *mania,* frenzy ]. An irrational desire to use surgery, by a doctor or a patient.

**tomoto′cia** [ G. *tomos,* cutting, + *tokos,* birth ]. Cesarean section; extraction of a child by hysterotomy.

**-tomy** [ G. *tomē,* incision. TOM- ]. A termination denoting a cutting operation.

**tonaphasia** (to′nă-fa′zĭ-ah) [ G. *tonos,* tone, + *a-* priv. + *phasis,* speech ]. Loss, through cerebral lesion, of the ability to remember tunes.

**tone** (tōn) [ G. *tonos,* tone, or a tone. TEN- ]. 1. A musical sound. 2. The character of the voice expressing an emotion. 3. The tension present in resting muscles. 4. Firmness of the tissues; normal functioning of all the organs; strength. 5. See toning.
   **affective t.,** feeling t.
   **emotional t.,** feeling t.
   **feeling t.,** the mental state (pleasure, repugnance, etc.) that accompanies every act or thought; emotional t; affective t.; affectivity.
   **fundamental t.,** the component of lowest frequency in a complex t.
   **Traube's double t.,** a double sound heard on auscultation over the femoral vessels in cases of aortic and tricuspid insufficiency.

**to′ner.** A solution used in toning.

**tongue** (tung) [ A.S. *tunge* ]. Lingua.
   **baked t.,** the dry, blackish t. noted when patients with typhoid fever and other disorders are allowed to become dehydrated.
   **bald t.,** atrophic *glossitis.*
   **beet-t.,** sometimes used of the t. in pellagra, where intense erythema appears, first at the tip, then along the edges, and finally over the dorsum. There may be pain and increased elevation. The shiny appearance results from edema, not atrophy, except in chronic pellagra.
   **bifid t.,** cleft t.; one whose extremity is divided longitudinally for a greater or lesser distance.
   **black t.,** nigrities linguae; glossophytia; glossitis parasitica; melanoglossia; lingua nigra; the presence of a blackish to yellowish brown patch or patches on the t., accompanied by elongation of the papillae; due to a fungal infection and sometimes seen after the use of antibiotic lozenges.
   **blue t.,** see bluetongue.
   **t. of cerebellum,** *lingula* cerebelli.
   **cleft t.,** bifid t.
   **coated t.,** furred t.; one with a whitish layer on its upper surface, composed of epithelial debris, food particles, and bacteria; it is often an indication of indigestion or of fever.
   **dotted t.,** stippled t.; one in which each separate papilla is capped with a whitish deposit.
   **fissured t.,** *lingua* fissurata.
   **fluted t.,** furrowed t.
   **frog t.,** ranula.
   **furred t.,** coated t.
   **furrowed t.,** fluted, grooved, ribbed, or wrinkled t.; lingua plicata; a t. marked by numerous longitudinal grooves on the dorsal surface, caused by splitting apart or separation of the papillae.

   **geographical t.,** the occurrence on the dorsum of the t. of peripherally spreading patches of temporary papillary atrophy; transitory benign migrating plaques. Coalescence of the lesions produces an irregular maplike appearance. Also called benign migratory glossitis; lingua geographica or dissecta; mappy t.; pityriasis linguae; exfoliatio areata linguae; glossitis areata exfoliativa; erythema migrans; erythema migrans linguae.
   **grooved t.,** furrowed t.
   **hairy t.,** glossotrichia; trichoglossia; a t. with black hairlike elongations of the papillae; sometimes found in patients who have sucked lozenges containing penicillin or other antibiotics.
   **hobnail t.,** interstitial glossitis with hypertrophy and verrucous changes in papillae; seen in some cases of late acquired syphilis.
   **magenta t.,** purplish red coloration of the t. with edema and flattening of the filiform papillae, occurring in riboflavin deficiency; not to be confused with cyanosis.
   **mappy t.,** geographical t.
   **raspberry t.,** strawberry t. that is a dark red color.
   **ribbed t.,** furrowed t.
   **scrotal t.,** a chronic glossitis marked by multiple deep fissures on its surface.
   **smoker's t.,** leukoplakia.
   **stippled t.,** dotted t.
   **strawberry t.,** a t. with a whitish coat through which the enlarged papillae project as red points, characteristic of scarlet fever.
   **wooden t. of cattle,** actinobacillosis.
   **wrinkled t.,** furrowed t.

**tongue-swallowing.** A slipping back of the tongue against the pharynx, causing choking.

**tongue-tie.** Ankyloglossia; abnormal shortness of the frenulum linguae.

**tonic** (ton′ik) [ G. *tonikos,* fr. *tonos,* tone. TEN- ]. 1. In a state of continuous unremitting action; denoting especially a muscular contraction. 2. Invigorating; increasing physical or mental tone or strength. 3. A remedy that restores enfeebled function and promotes vigor and a sense of well being; t.'s are qualified, according to the organ or system on which they act, as cardiac, digestive, hematic, vascular, nervine, uterine, general, etc.
   **bitter t.,** a t. of bitter taste, such as quinine, gentian, quassia, etc., which acts chiefly by stimulating the appetite and improving digestion.

**tonicity** (to-nis′ĭ-tĭ) [ G. *tonos,* tone. TEN- ]. 1. Tonus; a state of normal tension of the tissues by virtue of which the parts are kept in shape, alert, and ready to function in response to a suitable stimulus. In the case of muscle, it refers to a state of continuous activity or tension beyond that related to the physical properties; *i.e.,* it is active resistance to stretch. In skeletal muscle it is dependent upon the efferent innervation. 2. The osmotic pressure or tension of a solution, usually relative to that of blood; see also isotonicity.

**tonicoclonic** (ton′ĭ-ko-klon′ik). Tonoclonic; both tonic and clonic, referring to muscular spasms.

**to′ning.** The replacing of a silver deposit with one of gold in an impregnated histologic section, by treatment with a solution of gold chloride.

**tonitrophobia** (to-nĭ-tro-fo-bĭ′ah) [ L. *tonitrus,* thunder, fr. *tono,* to thunder, + G. *phobos,* fear ]. Morbid fear of thunder.

**tonka bean.** Dipteryx.

**tono-** [ G. *tonos,* tone, tension. TEN- ]. Combining form relating to tone, tension, pressure.

**tonoclonic** (ton′o-klon′ik). Tonicoclonic.

**tonofibril** (ton′o-fi′bril). One of a system of fibers, found in the cytoplasm of epithelial cells; see cytoskeleton.

**tonofilament** (ton′o-fil′ă-ment). A structural cytoplasmic protein, bundles of which together form a tonofibril. The protein of epidermal t.'s is keratin.

**ton′ofilm.** A natural latex membrane molded as a sheath to slide over the Schiötz tonometer footplate and plunger, to assure sterility.

**ton′ografilm.** A natural latex membrane, approximately 0.0012 inch thick, molded as a sheath to slide over the footplate and plunger of a Mueller electric tonometer.

**tonograph** (ton'o-graf, to'no-) [ tono- + G. *graphō*, to write ]. An instrument for recording the blood pressure.

**tonography** (to-nog'ră-fĭ). Continuous measurement of intraocular pressure by means of a recording tonometer, for determining the facility of aqueous outflow; a coefficient of 0.14 is indicative of open-angle glaucoma.

**tonometer** (to-nom'e-ter) [ tono- + G. *metron*, measure ]. 1. Tenonometer; an instrument for determining pressure or tension. 2. Ophthalmotonometer; an instrument for determining intraocular tension. 3. A vessel for equilibrating a liquid (*e.g.*, blood) with a gas, usually at a controlled temperature. Originally so named because it was used with a very small gas/blood ratio so that the gas would approach the blood oxygen tension and thus serve as a measure of it, it is now commonly used with a very large gas/blood ratio to adjust the blood to the oxygen pressure of the gas. 4. To equilibrate a liquid with a gas in such a t.

**applanation t.,** an instrument for determining intraocular tension by application of a small flat disk to the cornea.

**Gärtner's t.,** an apparatus for estimating the blood pressure by noting the force, expressed by the height of a column of mercury, needed to arrest pulsation in a finger encircled by a compressing ring.

**Goldmann's applanation t.,** an applanation t. that flattens but 3 sq. mm. of cornea, used with a slitlamp; values are not affected by variations of ocular rigidity or corneal curvature.

**Mackay-Marg t.,** a recording electronic applanation t.; gives accurate readings in scarred, irregular corneas.

**Maklakoff applanation t.,** a type of applanation t. developed and still standard in Russia.

**Mueller electronic t.,** a Schiötz type t. to which is attached an electronic device in the form of a helix for indicating the extent of corneal indentation; it may also have an attached recorder for continuous pressure readings (tonography).

**pneumatic t.,** a recording applanation t., operated by a gas supply from liquefied Freon.

**Schiötz t.,** an instrument that measures the indentation of the cornea produced by a metallic plunger of known weight 3 mm. in diameter. The plunger protrudes through a concave foot-plate which is flatter than the normal cornea.

**tonometry** (to-nom'e-trĭ). 1. The measurement of the tension of a part, *e.g.*, intravascular tension or blood pressure. 2. Ophthalmotonometry; the measurement of intraocular tension.

**tonophant** (to'no-fant, ton'o-) [ tono- + G. *phainō*, to appear. PHAN- ]. An instrument for visualizing sound waves.

**tonoplast** (to'no-plast, ton'o-) [ tono- + G. *plastos*, formed ]. An intracellular structure or vacuole.

**tonoscillograph** (to-nos'ĭ-lo-graf) [ tono- + L. *oscillo*, to swing, + G. *graphō*, to write ]. An instrument that produces graphic records of arterial and capillary pressures as well as of individual pulse characters.

**tonquinol** (ton'kwĭ-nol). Artificial musk; trinitroisobutyltoluene.

**ton'sil** [ L. *tonsilla*, a stake, in pl. the tonsils. TONS- ]. 1. Tonsilla. 2. *Tonsilla palatina*.

**cerebellar t.,** *tonsilla cerebelli*.
**Eustachian t.,** *tonsilla tubaria*.
**fau'cial t.,** *tonsilla palatina*.
**Gerlach's t.,** *tonsilla palatina*.
**laryn'geal t.'s,** *folliculi* lymphatici laryngei.
**lingual t.,** *tonsilla lingualis*.
**Luschka's t.,** *tonsilla pharyngea*.
**pal'atine t.,** *tonsilla palatina*.
**pharyn'geal t.,** *tonsilla pharyngea*.
**submerged t.,** a faucial t. that is flat and lying below the level of the pillars of the fauces.
**third t.,** *tonsilla pharyngea*.
**tubal t.,** *tonsilla tubaria*.

**tonsilla,** pl. **tonsillae** (ton-sil'ah, ton-sil'e) [ L. (see tonsil) ] [ NA ]. Tonsil; amygdala (2); any collection of lymphoid tissue.

**t. cerebel'li** [ NA ], cerebellar tonsil; amygdala cerebelli; a rounded lobule on the undersurface of each cerebellar

hemisphere, continuous medially with the uvula of the vermis.

**t. intestina'lis,** see *folliculi* lymphatici aggregati.

**t. lingua'lis** [ NA ], lingual tonsil; a collection of lymphoid follicles on the posterior or pharyngeal portion of the dorsum of the tongue.

**t. palati'na** [ NA ], faucial or palatine tonsil; a large oval mass of lymphoid tissue embedded in the lateral wall of the oral pharynx on either side between the pillars of the fauces.

**t. pharynge'a** [ NA ], pharyngeal tonsil; third tonsil; Luschka's tonsil; Luschka's gland (1); a collection of more or less closely aggregated lymphoid nodules on the posterior wall of the nasopharynx, the hypertrophy of which constitutes the morbid condition called adenoids.

**t. tuba'ria** [ NA ], tubal tonsil; Eustachian tonsil; a collection of lymphoid nodules near the pharyngeal opening of the auditory tube.

**ton'sillar, ton'sillary.** Amygdaline; relating to a tonsil, especially the palatine tonsil.

**tonsillectomy** (ton'sĭ-lek'to-mĭ) [ tonsil + G. *ektomē*, excision ]. Removal of the entire tonsil.

**ton'sillith.** Tonsillolith.

**tonsillitis** (ton'sĭ-li'tis) [ tonsil + G. suffix -*itis*, inflammation ]. Inflammation of a tonsil, especially of the palatine tonsil.

**lacu'nar t.,** inflammation of the mucous membrane lining the tonsillar crypts.

**parenchy'matous t.,** inflammation of the entire substance of the faucial tonsil, often passing into quinsy.

**superficial t.,** inflammation simply of the mucous membrane covering the tonsil.

**Vincent's t.,** angina limited chiefly to the tonsils, caused by Vincent's organisms (bacillus and spirillum).

**tonsillo-, tonsill-** [ L. *tonsilla*, tonsil. TONS- ]. Combining form denoting tonsil.

**tonsillolith** (ton-sil'o-lith) [ tonsillo- + G. *lithos*, stone ]. Tonsillar calculus; a calcareous concretion in a distended tonsillar crypt.

**tonsillopathy** (ton'sĭ-lop'ă-thĭ) [ tonsillo- + G. *pathos*, suffering ]. Disease of the tonsil.

**tonsillotome** (ton-sil'o-tōm) [ tonsillo- + G. *tomos*, cutting ]. An instrument, sometimes modelled after a guillotine, for use in cutting away a portion of a hypertrophied tonsil.

**tonsillotomy** (ton'sĭ-lot'o-mĭ) [ tonsillo- + G. *tomē*, incision ]. The cutting away of a portion of a hypertrophied faucial tonsil.

**to'nus** [ L. fr. G. *tonos*. TEN- ]. Tonicity (1).

**Tooth,** Howard H., English physician, 1856–1925. See Charcot-Marie-T. *disease*.

---

# TOOTH

---

**tooth,** pl. **teeth** [ A.S. *tōth* ]. Dens; one of the hard, conical structures set in the alveoli of the upper and lower jaws, used in mastication and assisting also in articulation. A t. is a dermal structure, not bone; it is composed of dentin (dentinum) encased in cement (cementum) on the covered portion, and enamel (enamelum) on its exposed portion. It consists of a root (radix) buried in the alveolus, a neck (collum) covered by the gum, and a crown (corona), the exposed portion. In the center is a hollow, the pulp cavity (cavum dentis), filled with a connective tissue reticulum containing a jelly-like substance (pulpa dentis) and blood vessels and nerves which enter through a canal at the apex of the root. The 20 milk teeth or deciduous teeth appear between the 6th or 9th and the 24th months of life. These exfoliate and are replaced by the 32 permanent teeth appearing from the 5th or 7th to the 17th or 23rd years. There are four kinds of teeth; incisor (dens incisivus), canine (dens caninus), premolar (dens premolaris), and molar (dens molaris). See also subentries under dens.

**acrylic resin t.,** a t. made of acrylic resin.

**anatomic teeth,** artificial teeth which more or less

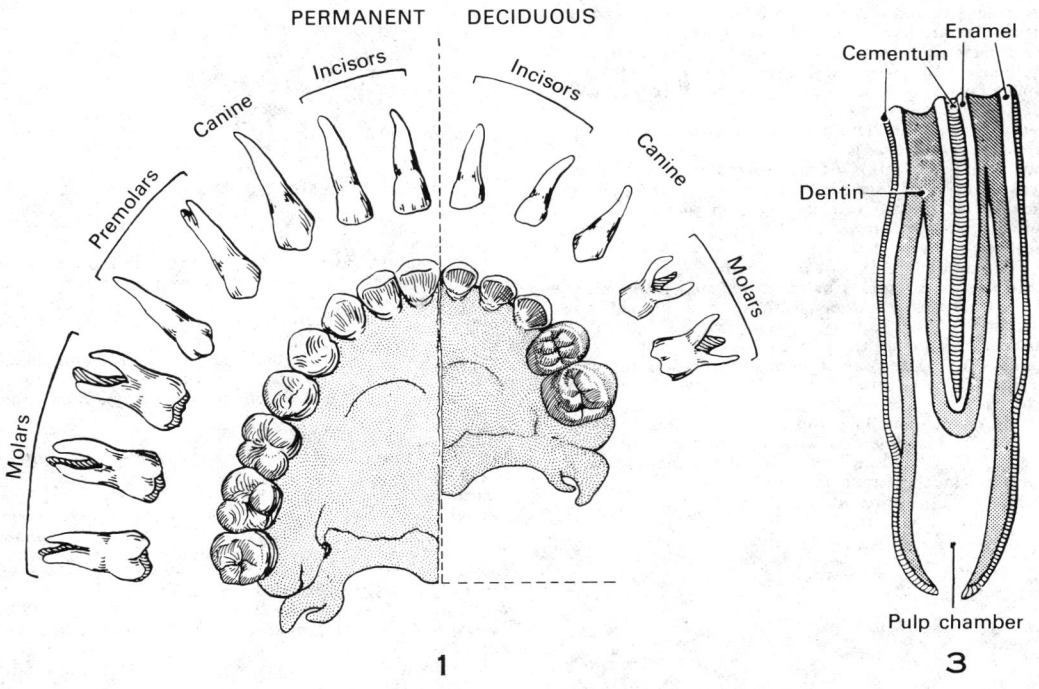

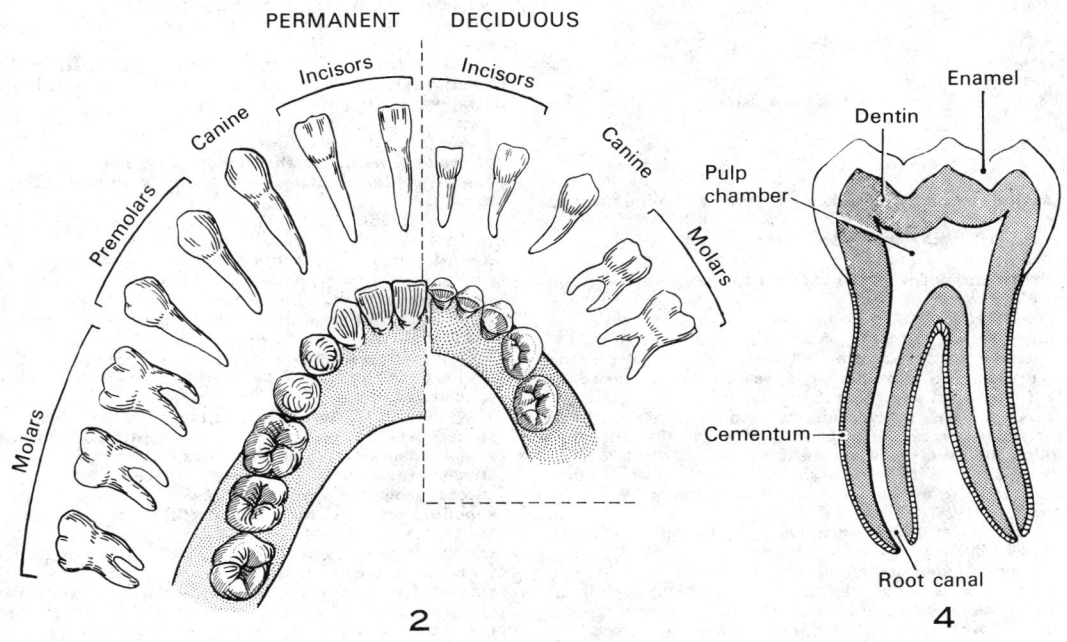

**Teeth**

*1,* Permanent and deciduous, upper jaw; *2;* permanent and deciduous, lower jaw; *3,* longitudinal section of the molar of a herbivore (horse); *4,* longitudinal section of the molar of a carnivore (human).

duplicate the anatomic forms of natural teeth.

**anterior teeth,** oral teeth; the central incisor, lateral incisor, and cuspid teeth, which comprise the organs for incision and are located in the front portion of the jaws.

**t. arrangement,** articulation (4); (1) the placement of teeth on a denture with definite objectives in mind; (2) the setting of teeth on temporary bases. See also subentries under articulation.

**au′ditory teeth** (of Huschke or Corti), *dentes* acustici.

**baby t.,** *dens* deciduus.

**back teeth,** all teeth posterior to the canines.

**bicuspid t.,** *dens* premolaris.

**buck t.,** an anterior t. in labioversion.

**canine t.,** *dens* caninus.

**cheek t.,** *dens* molaris.

**Corti's auditory teeth,** *dentes* acustici.

**cross-bite teeth,** posterior teeth designed to permit the modified cusps of the upper teeth to be positioned in the fossae of the lower teeth.

**cuspid t., cus′pidate t.,** *dens* caninus.

**cuspless t.,** (1) a t. devoid of cusp formation; (2) severe abrasion of an occlusal surface; (3) a type of artificial denture t.

**cutting teeth,** maxillary and mandibular anterior teeth.

**dead t.,** a misnomer, as what is being referred to is a pulpless t., *i.e.,* one from which the pulp has been removed, or one in which the pulp has died.

**deciduous t.,** *dens* deciduus.

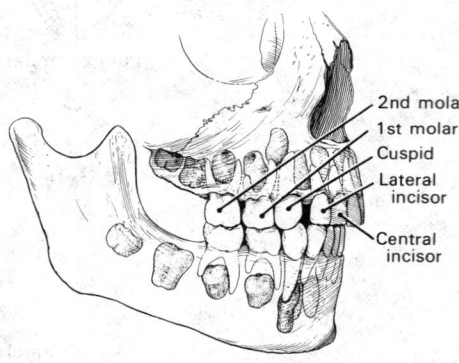

**Deciduous Teeth**

**devitalized t.,** a t. in which the pulp has been destroyed or removed.

**extruded teeth,** see under extrusion.

**eye t.,** *dens* caninus.

**fluoridated teeth,** teeth exposed to fluorine salts in the drinking water.

**fused teeth,** teeth joined by dentin as a result of embryological fusion or juxtaposition of two tooth germs.

**geminate teeth,** abnormally formed teeth, frequently the incisors, wherein the anomaly appears as though the result of a turning of anlage components.

**green t.,** one of the deciduous teeth of an infant, due to the deposition of altered blood pigment in the tooth bud following hemolysis when the mother's blood is Rh-negative and the child's is Rh-positive. The color of the t. varies from green to brown. The second dentition is not discolored.

**Horner's teeth,** incisor teeth having a hypoplastic groove running horizontally across them.

**Huschke's auditory teeth,** *dentes* acustici.

**Hutchinson's teeth,** the teeth of congenital syphilis in which the incisal edge is notched and narrower than the cervical area; see also Hutchinson's crescentic *notch*.

**impacted t.,** a t. whose normal eruption is prevented by adjacent teeth or bone.

**inci′sor t.,** *dens* incisivus.

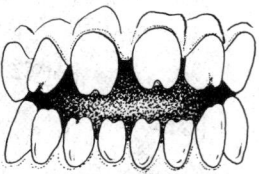

**Hutchinsons's Teeth**

**t. key,** an instrument formerly used for extracting a t. by grasping it and then twisting it by a movement similar to the turning of a key.

**malacot′ic teeth,** teeth comparatively soft in structure, white in color, and prone to decay.

**metal insert teeth,** prosthetic teeth containing metal cutting surfaces in the occlusal surfaces.

**migrating teeth,** teeth which are changing position under natural forces.

**milk t.,** *dens* deciduus.

**molar t., multicus′pid t.,** *dens* molaris; see also entries under molar.

**mottled t.,** see mottled *enamel.*

**nonanatomic teeth,** (1) teeth with occlusal surfaces not based on anatomic forms; (2) artificial teeth so designed that the occlusal surfaces are not copied from natural forms, but rather are given forms which in the opinion of the designer seem more nearly to fulfill the requirements of mastication, tissue tolerance, etc.

**nonvital t.,** a t. in which the pulp has died or has been removed.

**normally posed t.,** one in correct spatial relationship with its antagonist.

**notched teeth,** Hutchinson's teeth.

**oral teeth,** anterior teeth.

**pegged** or **pegtop teeth,** Hutchinson's teeth.

**permanent t.,** *dens* permanens.

**perpetually growing t.,** persistently growing t.; a physiologic phenomenon whereby the t. continually or constantly grows, calcifies, and erupts; rat incisor t. is an example.

**persistently growing t.,** perpetually growing t.

**plastic teeth,** artificial teeth constructed of synthetic resins.

**posterior teeth,** the bicuspid and molar teeth which comprise the organs of mastication and are located in the back part of the jaws.

**premo′lar t.,** *dens* premolaris.

**primary t.,** *dens* deciduus.

**protruding teeth,** teeth extending beyond the normal contour of the dental arches; usually in an anterior direction.

**sclerotic teeth,** teeth which are naturally hard, and usually yellowish in color.

**screwdriver t.,** malformed central or lateral incisor usually due to a congenital syphilitic condition.

**separation of teeth,** loss of proximal contact of teeth; in orthodontics, the creation of interproximal spaces for the fitting of an appliance.

**set of teeth,** usually refers to a full complement of maxillary and/or mandibular teeth, as they are carded by the manufacturer.

**snaggle-t.,** a t. which is out of line with the others.

**spaced teeth,** teeth which have separated and lost proximal contact with adjacent teeth.

**stomach t.,** one of the lower canine teeth.

**succedaneous t.,** *dens* permanens.

**syphilitic teeth,** Hutchinson's teeth.

**temporary t.,** *dens* deciduus.

**triangular′ity of the teeth,** a very well-marked indication of advancing age in the horse, shown by increasing depth from front to rear in the occlusal surfaces of the incisor teeth. At nine years, when the marks fail, this sign becomes of service in determining the age of the animal.

**tricuspid t.,** a t. having a crown with three cusps.

**tube teeth,** artificial teeth constructed with a vertical, cylindric aperture extending from the center of the base up into the body of the t. into which a pin may be placed or cast for the attachment of the t. to a denture base.

**unerupted t.,** (1) a t. prior to emergence; (2) a t. unable to break out or emerge from the dental alveolar tissues into the oral cavity.

**virgin t.,** 1. A tooth unmarked by wear or disease. 2. A horse's t. not yet worn down by attrition.

**vital t.,** a t. with a living pulp.

**wisdom t.,** *dens* serotinus.

**wolf t.,** a rudimentary first premolar t. of the horse, usually appearing in the upper jaw.

**zero degree teeth,** prosthetic teeth having no cusp angles in relation to the horizontal.

**toothache** (tooth' āk). Odontalgia; pain in a tooth due to involvement of the pulp or periodontal membrane as a result of caries, infection, or trauma.

**tooth-borne.** A term used to describe a prosthesis or part of a prosthesis which depends entirely upon the abutment teeth for support.

**top-.** See topo-.

**topagnosis** (top'ag-no'sis) [ top- + G. *a*- priv. + *gnosis,* recognition ]. Topoanesthesia; inability to localize tactile sensations.

**Topalanski's sign.** See under sign.

**topalgia** (to-pal'jī-ah) [ top- + G. *algos,* pain ]. Pain localized in one spot; a sympton occurring in neuroses whereby localized pain, without evident organic basis, is experienced.

**topectomy** (to-pek'to-mī) [ top- + G. *ektomē,* excision ]. Removal of a specific portion of the cerebral cortex.

**topesthesia** (top'es-the'zī-ah) [ top- + G. *aisthēsis,* sensation ]. The ability to localize a light touch applied to any part of the skin.

**Töpfer** (tĕp'fer), Alfred E., German physician, *1858. See T.'s *test.*

**tophaceous** (to-fa'shus) [ L. *tophaceus* ]. Sandy; gritty; pertaining to or manifesting the features of a tophus.

**tophi** (to'fi). Plural of tophus.

**tophus,** pl. **tophi** (to'fus, to'fi) [ L. a calcareous deposit from springs, tufa ]. 1. Gouty t. 2. A salivary calculus, or tartar.

**gouty t.,** chalkstone; arthritic calculus; a deposit of urates in periarticular fibrous tissue, cartilage of the external ear, or kidney, in gout.

**topica** (top'ī-kah) [ neut. pl. of Mod. L. *topicus,* local ]. Remedies for local external use.

**top'ical** [ G. *topikos,* fr. *topos,* place ]. Relating to a definite place or locality; local.

**Topinard** (top-e-nar'), Paul, French anthropologist, 1830–1912. See T.'s *angle, line.*

**topis'tic** [ G. *topos,* place ]. Denoting an anatomically defined region in the nervous system.

**topo-, top-** (top'o-, to'po-) [ G. *topos,* place ]. Combining forms denoting place, topical.

**topoanesthesia** (top'o-an-es-the'zī-ah, to-'po-) [ topo- + anesthesia ]. Topagnosis.

**topognosis, topognosia** (top'og-no'sis, -no'sī-ah) [ topo- + G. *gnōsis,* knowledge ]. The recognition of the location of a sensation; in the case of touch, topesthesia.

**topogometer** (top'o-gom'e-ter) [ topo- + G. *gonia,* angle, + *metron,* measure ]. A movable fixation target attached to the front of a keratometer, used in fitting contact lenses to measure the curvatures of the cornea in its peripheral zones.

**topography** (to-pog'rā-fī) [ topo- + G. *graphē,* a writing ]. In anatomy, the description of any part of the body, especially in relation to a definite and limited area of the surface.

**topology** (to-pol'o-jī) [ topo- + G. *logos,* study ]. 1. Regional anatomy. 2. The study of the dimensions of personality or the psyche.

**toponarcosis** (top'o-nar-ko'sis) [ topo- + narcosis ]. A localized cutaneous anesthesia.

**toponeurosis** (top'o-nu-ro'sis) [ topo- + neurosis ]. A localized neurosis.

**toponym** (to'po-nim) [ topo- + G. *onyma,* name ]. A regional term; one designating a region as distinguished from the name of a structure, system, or organ.

**toponymy** (to-pon'ī-mī) [ topo- + G. *onyma,* name ]. Topical or regional nomenclature, as distinguished from organonymy.

**topophobia** (to-po-fo'bī-ah) [ topo- + G. *phobos,* fear ]. A neurotic dread of or related to a particular place or locality.

**topophylaxis** (to-po-fi-lak'sis) [ topo- + G. *phylaxis,* protection ]. Prevention of arsphenamine shock by a tourniquet applied to the limb above the site of injection, and its slow release 5 or 6 minutes later.

**toposcope** (top'o-skōp) [ topo- + G. *skopeō,* to view ]. An apparatus to project the electrical activity of the cerebral cortex as a spatial coordinate visual system.

**topothermesthesiometer** (top-o-therm'es-the'zī-om'e-ter) [ topo- + G. *thermē,* heat, + *aisthēsis,* sensation, + *metron,* measure ]. A device for determining the temperature sense in different parts of the surface.

**topovaccinotherapy** (top'o-vak'sī-no-thĕr'ă-pī). Therapy with vaccine applied to the surface of the skin.

**torcular heroph'ili** [ L. wine-press of *Herophilus,* fr. *torqueo,* to twist ]. *Confluens* sinuum.

**Torek,** Franz J. A., American surgeon, 1861–1938. See T. *operation.*

**toric** (to'rik). Relating to, or having the curvature of, a torus.

**Torkildsen,** A., Norwegian neurosurgeon. See T. *shunt.*

**tor'men.** See tormina.

**tor'ment** [ L. *tormentum,* anguish, fr. *torqueo,* to twist. TORS- ]. Suffering; anguish; colic; ileus; tormina.

**tormina** (tor'mī-nah) [ L. pl. of *tormen,* the gripes, colic, fr. *torqueo,* to twist. TORS- ]. Severe colic or griping intestinal pain.

**tor'minal.** Relating to or marked by tormina.

**Tornwaldt** (torn'vahlt), Gustavus L., German physician, 1843–1910. See T.'s *disease.*

**to'rose, to'rous** [ L. *torosus,* fleshy, fr. *torus,* a knot, bulge ]. Bulging; tubercular; knobby.

**tor'pent** [ L. *torpeo,* pres. p. *-ens,* to be sluggish ]. 1. Torpid. 2. A benumbing agent.

**tor'pid** [ L. *torpidus,* fr. *torpeo,* to be sluggish ]. Inactive; sluggish.

**torpid'ity.** Torpor.

**tor'por** [ L. sluggishness, numbness ]. Inactivity, sluggishness, stupor, and insensibility.

**t. ret'inae,** a form of nyctalopia, the retina responding only to strong luminous stimuli.

**torque** (tork) [ L. *torqueo,* to twist ]. A rotatory force.

**torr** [ Evangelista *Torricelli* ]. A unit of pressure sufficient to support a 1-mm column of mercury at 0°C. against the standard acceleration of gravity at 45° north latitude (980.6 cm/sec$^2$); 1333.22 dynes/cm$^2$; 1.333 millibars; 1.36 cm H$_2$O; one standard atmosphere equals 760 t.

**Torre,** D. See T.'s *syndrome.*

**torrefaction** (tor'e-fak'shun) [ L. *torre-facio,* pp. *-factus,* to make dry by heat, fr. *torreo,* to parch ]. Parching or drying by heat; a pharmaceutical operation for rendering drugs friable.

**torrefy** (tor'e-fi). To parch.

**Torricelli,** Evangelista, Italian scientist, 1608–1647. See torr.

**torsiom'eter** (tor'sī-om'e-ter). An instrument for measuring ocular torsion, cycloductions, and cyclophorias.

**torsion** (tor'shun) [ L. *torsio,* fr. *torqueo,* to twist. TORS- ]. 1. A twisting or rotation of a part upon its axis. 2. Twisting of the cut end of an artery to arrest hemorrhage. 3. Rotation of the eye around its anteroposterior axis; see also intorsion, extorsion, dextrotorsion, levotorsion.

**t. of a tooth,** rotation of a tooth in its socket.

**torsionom'eter** (tor-shun-om+e-ter). A device for measuring the degree of rotation of the spinal column.

**tor'siver'sion.** A malposition of a tooth in which it is rotated on its long axis.

**tor'so** (tor'so) [ It. ]. The trunk; the body without relation to head or extremities.

**torsoclusion** (tor′so-klu′zhun) [ L. *torqueo*, to twist, + *claudo* or *cludo*, to close. CLAUS- ]. 1. Acupressure performed by entering the needle in the tissues parallel with the artery, then turning it so that it crosses the artery transversely, and passing it into the tissues on the opposite side of the vessel. 2. Torsiversion.

**torticollar** (tor′tĭ-kol′ar). Relating to or marked by torticollis.

**torticollis** (tor′tĭ-kol′is) [ L. *tortus*, twisted, + *collum*, neck ]. Wryneck; stiff-neck; a contraction, often spasmodic, of the muscles of the neck, chiefly those supplied by the spinal accessory nerve; the head is drawn to one side and usually rotated so that the chin points to the other side.

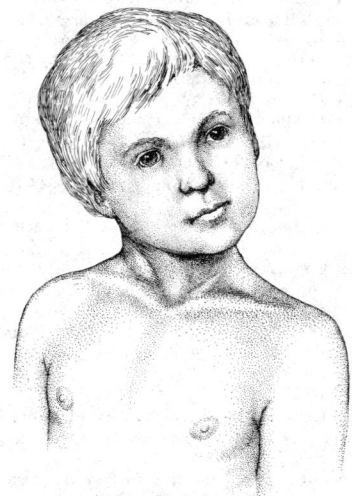

**Torticollis**

   **congenital t.,** t. due to unilateral fibrosis in the sternocleidomastoid muscle; a condition of unknown cause, present at the time of birth as a swelling that may subside or may lead to t. by shortening of the muscle.

   **dermatogenic t.,** painful stiff neck with limitation of motion due to extensive skin lesion in the area.

   **fixed t.,** persistent contracture of cervical muscles on one side.

   **intermit′tent t.,** t. spastica.

   **labyrinthine t.,** t. due to vestibular disorder.

   **mental t.,** spasmodic contractions of the muscles of the neck, of psychological origin or due to conditioning.

   **ocular t.,** t. incident to paralysis of an extraocular muscle, especially an oblique muscle; it is often accompanied by head rotation and tilt.

   **rheumat′ic t.,** symptomatic t.

   **spasmodic t.,** rotatory spasm or tic; t. due to intermittent contractions of the neck muscles.

   **t. spas′tica,** intermittent t.; stiff neck due to hypertonicity of the neck muscles.

   **spu′rious t.,** stiffness of the neck due to caries, malformation, or fracture of the cervical vertebrae.

   **symptomat′ic t.,** rheumatic t.; stiff neck due to rheumatism of the muscles of the neck, chiefly of the sternocleidomastoid, occurring especially in children.

**tor′tipel′vis.** Twisted pelvis.

**tortuous** (tor′chu-us) [ L. *tortuosus*, fr. *torqueo*, to twist ]. Having many curves, full of turns and twists.

**Torula** (tor′u-lah) [ L. *torulus*, *q.v.* ]. Old name for *Cryptococcus*.

   **T. capsula′tus, T. histolyt′ica,** old names for *Cryptococcus neoformans*.

**torulo′ma** [ fr. *Torula*, old name for *Cryptococcus*, + G. suffix *-oma*, tumor ]. Cryptococcoma.

**Torulop′sis.** A genus of yeasts morphologically similar to *Cryptococcus*, but characterized by the presence of small blastospores (2 to 4 mμ) and by the absence of mycelium.

   **T. glabra′ta,** a species that is the causative agent of torulopsosis.

   **T. neofor′mans,** see *Cryptococcus neoformans* or *Torula*.

**torulopsosis** (tor′u-lop′so-sis). A usually opportunistic infection in man caused by *Torulopsis glabrata*. The disease is usually seen in patients with severe underlying disease, *e.g.*, diabetes mellitus, or in patients treated with antibiotics, corticosteroids, or immunosuppressive agents; the pattern of disease may be bronchopulmonary, genitourinary, or septicemic.

**torulo′sis.** Cryptococcosis.

**torulus,** pl. **toruli** (tor′u-lus, -li) [ L. dim. of *torus*, a protuberance, swelling ]. A minute elevation; papilla.

   **toruli tactiles** [ NA ], tactile elevations; small areas in the skin of the palms and soles especailly rich in sensory nerve endings.

**torus,** pl. **tori** (to′rus, to′ri) [ L. swelling, knot, bulge ]. 1. A geometrical figure formed by the revolution of a circle round the base of any of its arcs, such as the convex molding at the base of a pillar. 2 [ NA ]. A rounded swelling, such as that caused by a contracting muscle. 3. *Tuber* cinereum.

   **t. bucca′lis,** a longitudinal mucosal fold stretching from the corner of the mouth to the level of the molar teeth; it is often irritated during mastication.

   **t. fronta′lis,** a slight prominence on the frontal bone at the root of the nose.

   **t. levator′ius** [ NA ], levator swelling; levator cushion; the bulge in the lateral wall of the nasopharynx, below the opening of the auditory tube, produced by the levator veli palatini muscle.

   **t. mandibula′ris,** a bony mass of variable shape and extent on the inner (lingual) surface of the mandibular corpus. It is not pathologic, and is most frequently found in the Eskimo.

   **t. ma′nus,** the carpal region.

   **t. occipita′lis,** an occasional ridge near the superior nuchal line of the occipital bone.

   **t. palati′nus** [ NA ], palatine t. or protuberance; a bony swelling sometimes present upon the median line (median palatine suture) of the roof of the oral cavity.

   **t. tuba′rius** [ NA ], Eustachian cushion; a ridge in the pharyngeal wall posterior to the opening of the auditory (Eustachian) tube, caused by the projection of the cartilaginous portion of this tube.

   **t. ureter′icus,** a smooth ridge in the bladder wall stretching between the ureteral orifices.

   **t. uteri′nus,** a transverse ridge on the back part of the cervix uteri, formed by the junction of the rectouterine folds.

**torutilin** (tor′u-til′in). Vitamin T.

**tosyl** (to′sil). Toluenesulfonyl radical.

**to′sylate.** USAN-approved contraction for *p*-toluenesulfonate.

**to′tem** [ Amer. Indian ]. An object (usually an animal or plant) serving as the emblem of a family or clan and often as a reminder of its ancestry; something that serves as a revered symbol.

**to′temism.** Belief in a kinship with, or a mystical relationship between, a group or individual and a totem.

**totemis′tic.** Relating to totemism.

**Toti** (to′te), Addeo, Italian ophthalmologist and laryngologist, *1861. See T.'s *operation*.

**totipotency, totipotence** (to′tĭ-po′ten-sĭ, to-tip′o-tens) [ L. *totus*, entire, + *potentia*, power ]. The ability of a cell to differentiate into any type of cell and thus form a new organism or regenerate any part of an organism. Examples are a fertilized ovum, also a small excised portion of a *Planaria*, which is capable of regenerating a complete new organism.

**totip′otent, to′tipoten′tial.** Relating to totipotency.

**touch** (tuch) [ Fr. *toucher*]. 1. The tactile sense; the sense by which slight contact with the skin or mucous membrane is appreciated. 2. Digital examination.

**Tourette.** See Gilles de la Tourette.

**Tournay's sign.** See under sign.

**tourniquet** (toor'nĭ-ket) [ Fr. fr. *tourner*, to turn ]. An instrument for arresting temporarily the flow of blood through a large artery in a limb; it consists of a broad band drawn tightly around the limb, with a pad over the artery, the pressure of which is increased by means of a screw.

**Dupuytren's t.,** an instrument for making compression on the abdominal aorta.

**Tourtual** (toor'tu-al), Caspar T., Prussian anatomist, 1802–1865. See T.'s *membrane, sinus.*

**Touton,** Karl, German dermatologist, *1858. See T. giant cell.

**tow** (to). The coarse and broken part of flax, unfit for spinning, used in surgical dressings.

**Towne projection roentgenogram.** See under roentgenogram.

**tox-.** See toxico-.

**toxanemia** (toks'ă-ne'mĭ-ah) [ G. *toxikon*, poison, + anemia ]. Anemia resulting from the effects of a hemolytic poison.

**tox'aphene.** A chlorinated hydrocarbon insecticide.

**Toxas'caris leonina** [ G. *toxon*, bow, + ascaris ]. An ascarid nematode of the dog, it differs from *Toxocara* in that the larvae do not migrate through the lungs; the entire developmental cycle occurs in the gut. This parasite has been found in man in a few instances and is a cause of visceral larva migrans in children, though less frequently implicated than is *Toxocara canis.*

**toxemia** (tok-se'mĭ-ah) [ G. *toxikon*, poison, + *haima*, blood ]. Toxicemia; toxicohemia; toxinemia. 1. Clinical manifestations observed during certain infectious diseases, assumed to be caused by toxins and other noxious substances elaborated by the infectious agent; in certain infections by Gram-negative bacteria, endotoxins probably play a role when the bacterial cell wall breaks down, releasing the complex lipopolysaccharide; however, the role of other bacterial substances in unclear, except in the case of the specific exotoxins such as those of diphtheria and tetanus. 2. The clinical syndrome caused by toxic substances in the blood. 3. An ill-defined term referring to metabolic disorders of pregnancy characterized by hypertension, edema, and albuminuria.

**toxe'mic.** Pertaining to, affected with, or manifesting the features of toxemia.

**toxi-.** See toxico-.

**toxic** (tok'sik) [ G. *toxikon*, an arrow-poison. TOX- ]. 1. Poisonous. 2. Pertaining to a toxin. 3. Caused by a poison.

**toxicant** (tok'sĭ-kant). 1. Toxic; poisonous. 2. Any poisonous agent, specifically an alcoholic or other poison, causing symptoms of what is popularly called intoxication.

**toxice'mia.** Toxemia.

**toxicity** (toks-is'ĭ-tĭ). A state of being poisonous; poisonousness.

**oxygen t.,** a body disturbance resulting from breathing high partial pressures of oxygen. Characterized by visual and hearing abnormalities, breathing difficulties, unusual fatigue, muscular twitching, anxiety, confusion, incoordination, action, and convulsions. Although the mechanism for the development of the condition is obscure, a disruption of enzymatic activity is commonly considered in the etiology.

**toxico-, tox-, toxi-, toxo-** [ G. *toxikon*, poison. TOX- ]. Combining form denoting poison, toxin.

**toxicoden'drol.** A fixed oil contained in the leaves of *Rhus toxicodendron.*

**Toxicodendron** (tok'sĭ-ko-den'dron) [ toxico- + G. *dendron*, tree ]. A genus of poisonous plants of the family Anacardiaceae; see also *Rhus.*

**T. diversiloba,** poison oak of the western United States.

**T. quercifolium,** poison oak in the eastern United States.

**T. radicans,** Nisfin vine or ivy; poison ivy.

**T. vernicifluum,** Asiatic lacquer tree; the source of Japan lacquer, obtained by incisions in the bark.

**T. vernix,** poison sumac; poison elder; poison ash, swamp dogwood, a shrub that grows in swamps, having leaves arranged in seven pairs on long stems; it is similar to *Rhus toxicodendron* in its toxication.

**toxicoderma** (tok'sĭ-ko-der'mah) [ toxico- + G. *derma*, skin ]. Toxicodermatosis; any skin disease caused by a poison or by a toxin-producing microorganism.

**toxicodermatitis** (tok'sĭ-ko-der'mă-ti'tis). Inflammation of the skin caused by the action of a poison.

**tox'icodermato'sis.** Toxicoderma.

**toxicogenic** (tok'sĭ-ko-jen'ik) [ toxico- + G. suffix *-gen*, producing ]. 1. Producing a poison. 2. Caused by a poison.

**toxicohe'mia.** Toxemia.

**toxicoid** (tok'sĭ-koyd) [ toxico- + G. *eidos*, resemblance ]. Having an action like that of a poison; temporarily poisonous.

**toxicologic** (tok'sĭ-ko-loj'ik). Relating to toxicology.

**toxicologist** (tok'sĭ-kol'o-jist). One who has a special knowledge of poisons and their antidotes.

**toxicology** (tok'sĭ-kol'o-jĭ) [ toxico- + G. *logos*, study ]. The science of poisons—their source, chemical composition, action, tests, and antidotes.

**toxicomania** (tok'sĭ-ko-ma'nĭ-ah) [ toxico- + G. *mania*, frenzy ]. An abnormal craving for a narcotic, intoxicant, or poison.

**toxicomu'cin.** A toxic mucin obtained from cultures of tubercle bacilli.

**toxicopath'ic.** Denoting any morbid state caused by the action of a poison.

**toxicopathy** (tok'sĭ-kop'ă-thĭ) [ toxico- + G. *pathos*, suffering ]. Any disease of toxic origin.

**tox'icopec'tic.** Relating to toxicopexis.

**toxicopexis** (tok'sĭ-ko-pek'sis) [ toxico- + G. *pēxis*, fixation ]. The neutralizing of a poison in the body, thus permitting its retention.

**toxicophobia** (tok'sĭ-ko-fo'bĭ-ah) [ toxico- + G. *phobos*, fear ]. Toxiphobia; a morbid fear of being poisoned.

**tox'icophylax'in.** An antitoxic phylaxin; an old and little used term for a protective protein that neutralizes a toxin or other noxious product from a microorganism.

**toxicosis** (tok'sĭ-ko'sis) [ toxico- + G. suffix *-osis*, condition ]. Toxicopathy; systemic poisoning; any disease of toxic origin.

**endogen'ic t.,** autointoxication.

**exogen'ic t.,** any disease caused by a poison introduced from without and not generated within the body.

**Frank's capillary t.,** a nonthrombocytopenic purpura of unknown cause.

**retention t.,** endogenic t.; nosotoxicosis; a disease due to the retention of waste products that are normally excreted as formed.

**T₃ t.,** triiodothyronine t.

**triiodothyronine t.,** T₃ t.; hyperthyroidism resulting from excessive circulating T₃ (3,5,3-triiodothyronine).

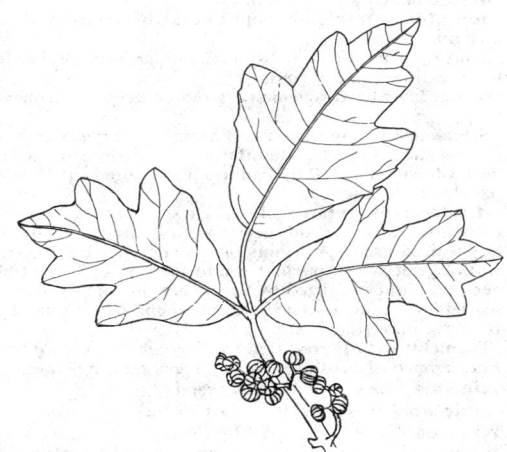

*Toxicodendron quercifolium* (Eastern Poison Oak)

(From Lampe, K. F., and Fagerström, R.: *Plant Toxicity and Dermatitis; A Manual for Physicians*, The Williams & Wilkins Co., Baltimore, 1968.)

**toxicosozin** (tok'sĭ-ko-so'zin). A sozin that destroys or neutralizes a toxin or other noxious substance from a microorganism.

**toxiferines** (tok-sif'er-ēnz). The most potent group of the curare alkaloids; the principle source is *Strychnos toxifera*.

**toxiferous** (tok-sif'er-us) [ toxi- + L. *fero*, to bear ]. Poisonous.

**tox'igenic.** Toxinogenic.

**toxigenicity** (tok'sĭ-jē-nis'ĭ-tĭ). Toxinogenicity.

**toximu'cin.** Toxicomucin.

**toxin** (tok'sin) [ G. *toxikon*, poison. TOX- ]. A noxious or poisonous substance that (1) is an integral part of the cell or tissue, or (2) is an extracellular product (exotoxin), or (3) represents a combination of the two situations, formed or elaborated during the metabolism and growth of certain microorganisms, as well as some of the higher plant and animal species; in general, t.'s are relatively complex antigenic molecules, and the chemical compositions are usually not precisely known.

    **animal t.,** zootoxin.

    **bacterial t.,** any intracellular or extracellular t. formed in or elaborated by bacterial cells.

    **botulinus t.,** botuline; botulismotoxin; potent neurotoxins from *Clostridium botulinum*, *q. v.*

    **cholera t.,** see *Vibrio cholerae*.

    **Dick test t.** streptococcus erythrogenic t.

    **dinoflagellate t.,** a potent neurotoxin that is thought to act similarly to botulinus t. by impairing the synthesis or the release of acetylcholine.

    **diphtheria t.,** see *Corynebacterium diphtheriae*.

    **diphtheria t., diagnostic,** Schick test t.

    **erythrogenic t.,** streptococcus erythrogenic t.

    **extracellular t.,** ectotoxin; exotoxin (or "true t."); a specific, soluble, antigenic, usually heat-labile, injurious substance elaborated by certain Gram-positive bacteria (rarely by Gram-negative species, *Shigella dysenteriae* and perhaps *Bordetella pertussis* being exceptions); it is formed within the cell, but is released into the environment, where it is rapidly active in extremely small amounts. Most t.'s of this type are protein in nature, with molecular weights ranging from 70,000 to 900,000, and the toxic portion of the molecule may be destroyed by means of heat (*e.g.*, 60°C. for 15 to 30 min.), prolonged storage, or treatment with certain chemicals (*e.g.*, formalin); the nontoxic, but antigenic form is termed *toxoid*.

    **fatigue t.,** ponogen; kinotoxin; a substance isolated by Weichardt from the body fluids, after excessive muscular exertion, believed to be the cause of the phenomena of fatigue; by methods analogous to those used in the case of bacterial t.'s Weichardt claims to have obtained a fatigue antitoxin possessing recuperative powers.

    **intracellular t.,** endotoxin.

    **normal t.,** a t. solution holding exactly 100 lethal doses in 1 ml.

    **plant t.,** phytotoxin; substance, similar in its properties to an extracellular bacterial t.

    **scarlet fever erythrogenic t.,** streptococcus erythrogenic t.

    **Schick test t.,** diphtheria t., diagnostic; *Corynebacterium diphtheriae* t. diluted so that the inoculated dose (0.1 or 0.2 ml.) will contain 1/50th of guinea pig minimal lethal dose; see also Schick *test*.

    **streptococcus erythrogenic t.,** Dick test t.; erythrogenic t.; scarlet fever erythrogenic t.; a culture filtrate of lysogenized group A strains of β-hemolytic streptococci, erythrogenic when inoculated into the skin of susceptible persons, and neutralized by antibodies that appear during scarlet fever convalescence; three immunological types (A, B, and C) are recognized.

    **Tunnicliff t.,** a t. produced by *Corynebacterium diphtheriae*, erroneously assumed pathogenic organism of measles.

**toxinemia** (tok'sĭ-ne'mĭ-ah). Toxemia.

**toxinic** (tok-sin'ik). Relating to a toxin.

**toxinogenic** (tok'sĭ-no-jen'ik) [ toxin + G. suffix *-gen*, producing ]. Toxigenic; producing a toxin (*e.g.*, a toxinogenic strain of *Corynebacterium diphtheriae*).

**toxinogenicity** (tok'sĭ-no-jē-nis'ĭ-tĭ). Toxigenicity; capacity to produce toxin.

**toxinology** (tok'sĭ-nol'o-jĭ) [ toxin + G. *logos*, study ]. The study of toxins, in a restricted sense, with reference to the relatively unstable proteinaceous substances of microbial, plant, or animal origins.

**toxinosis** (tok'sĭ-no'sis) [ toxin + G. suffix *-osis*, condition ]. Any disease or lesion caused by the action of a toxin.

**toxipath'ic.** Relating to any diseased state caused by a poison, *e.g.*, neuritis or hepatitis caused by arsenic.

**toxipathy** (tok-sip'ă-thĭ) [ toxi- + G. *pathos*, suffering ]. Any disease due to poisoning, especially chronic poisoning; toxicosis.

**toxiphobia** (tok-sĭ-fo'bĭ-ah). Toxicophobia.

**tox'is.** Poisoning.

**toxisterol** (tok-sis'ter-ol). Substance 248; a toxic substance formed by excessive irradiation of ergosterol or calciferol.

**toxitherapy** (tok'sĭ-thĕr'ă-pĭ). Treatment of an infectious disease by means of an antiserum.

**toxituberculid** (tok'sĭ-tu-ber'ku-lid). A cutaneous lesion believed to be due to the action of tuberculous toxin, the specific bacillus not being locally demonstrable.

**toxo-.** See toxico-.

**toxoalexin** (tok'so-ă-lek'sin). A defensive protein, protecting the cells from the action of a toxin.

**Toxocara** (tok'so-kār'ah) [ G. *toxon*, bow (TOX-), + *kara*, head ]. A genus of ascarid nematodes, chiefly found in carnivores, that cause toxocariasis.

    **T. ca'nis,** the common ascarid in the small intestine of the dog, where prenatal infection is a common mode of infection of pups; it is also reported from cats, wolves, foxes, coyotes, and badgers; the second-stage larva is the most frequent cause of visceral larva migrans in the liver of children.

    **T. mys'tax,** a common ascarid of cats, but not reported from dogs; prenatal infection of kittens does not occur, infection being by migration of second-stage larvae, as with *Ascaris lumbricoides* in man; mice and other vertebrates, and also some invertebrates (*e.g.*, earthworms, cockroaches) may serve as transport hosts.

**toxocariasis** (tok'so-kă-ri'ă-sis). Infection with nematodes of the genus *Toxocara*. Parenterally migrating larvae, chiefly of *Toxocara canis* may cause visceral larva migrans. Ocular involvement results in either a solitary granuloma in the retina, peripheral inflammatory masses, or chronic endophthalmitis.

**toxoid** (tok'soyd) [ toxin + G. *eidos*, resemblance ]. Anatoxin; a toxin that has been treated (commonly with formaldehyde) so as to destroy its toxic property but that still retains its antigenicity, *i.e.*, its capability of stimulating the production of antibodies and thus of producing an active immunity. For specific t.'s, see under vaccine.

**toxomu'cin.** Toxicomucin.

**tox'on, tox'one.** A hypothetical bacterial product, of feeble toxicity and weak affinity for antitoxin.

**toxoneme** (tok'so-nēm) [ G. *toxon*, bow, + *nema*, thread ]. Microneme.

**toxonoid** (tok'so-noyd). A hypothetical substance in cultures of the diphtheria bacillus, which has weak affinity for antitoxin; it is nontoxic to guinea pigs but causes paralysis in rabbits.

**toxonosis** (tok'so-no'sis) [ toxo- + G. *nosos*, disease ]. Toxicosis; toxicopathy; toxinosis.

**toxophil, toxophile** (tok'so-fil, -fĭl) [ toxo- + G. *philos*, fond ]. Susceptible to the action of a poison.

**toxophore** (tok'so-fōr) [ toxo- + G. *phoros*, bearing ]. Denoting the atomic group of the toxin molecule which carries the poisonous principle.

**toxophorous** (tok + sof'er-us). Relating to the toxophore group of the toxin molecule.

**toxophylaxin** (tok'so-fi-lak'sin). Toxicophylaxin.

**Toxoplasma gondii** (tok'so-plaz'mah) [ G. *toxon*, bow or arc, + *plasma*, anything formed ]. An abundant and widespread species of small, intracellular, non host-specific, protozoan parasites (family Toxoplasmatidae) causing toxoplasmosis. The vesicular nucleus is Feulgen-positive (DNA+) and the organism divides by means of longitudinal fission, forming ovoid or rounded cells that become crescentic (with one end rounded and the other slightly pointed); the mature forms range from 4 to 8 by 2 to 4 μ and manifest no distinction between ectoplasm and endoplasm. In tissues of the host, the parasites continue to multiply and result in bursting of the host cells, or the latter may be resistant and the cell wall remains tightly stretched as a covering for groups of parasites, thereby forming a pseudocyst.

**Toxoplasmatidae** (tok'so-plaz-mat'ĭ-de). A family of parasitic sporozoan protozoa in which host tissue reaction forms a pseudocyst around the parasite. It includes the genera *Toxoplasma* and *Encephalitozoon*.

**toxoplasmosis** (tok'so-plaz-mo'sis). Disease caused by presence of or reaction to *Toxoplasma gondii*, which may be found in the bloodstream (not in erythrocytes), in tissues, or within various cells, especially reticuloendothelial cells, leukocytes, and epithelial cells. Most infections acquired after birth are mild and little-noticed except for fever and swelling of lymph glands. Acute disease may develop, especially in immunologically compromised individuals, leading to generalized infection involving brain, lungs, liver and other organs. If death does not occur from gross damage to vital organs, especially the brain, a chronic latent phase develops with the formation of intracellular parasitic cysts. Infections occur sporadically in nearly all domestic and many wild animals as well as man; the manifestations vary widely, but chorioretinitis and uveitis are common. In prenatal infections, death or severe brain and eye damage usually occur, especially where the mother has not been previously exposed and acquires an infection during her pregnancy. Diagnosis is by finding parasites in smears, by animal inoculation, or by immunological test. Infection may be acquired from the feces of domestic cats, from raw or undercooked meat, especially mutton, and possibly by droplet aerosol or mucus contamination.

**acquired t. in adults,** may result in fever, encephalomyelitis, chorioretinopathy, maculopapular rash, arthralgia, myalgia, myocarditis, and pneumonitis; a lymphadenopathic form seems to be more prevalent in adults, and such persons may manifest (1) fever, lymphadenopathy, malaise, and headache, or (2) lymphadenopathy, malaise, and headache but no fever, or (3) only lymphadenopathy.

**congenital t.,** apparently resulting from parasites in an infected mother being transmitted *in utero* to the fetus; congenital t. may be observed as three syndromes: (1) acute, most of the organs containing foci of necrosis in association with fever, jaundice, encephalomyelitis, pneumonitis, cutaneous rash, ophthalmic lesions, hepatomegaly, and splenomegaly; (2) subacute, most of the lesions are partly healed or calcified, but those in the brain and eye seem to remain active, inasmuch as chorioretinitis is observed in more than 80 per cent of diseased infants; and (3) chronic, usually not recognized during the newborn period, but chorioretinitis and cerebral lesions may be detected weeks or months later.

**toxoso'zin.** Toxicosozin.

**Toynbee,** Joseph, English otologist, 1815–1866. See T.'s *corpuscles, experiment, law, muscle, otoscope.*

**TPC.** Abbreviation for thromboplastic plasma component; see *factor* VIII.

**TPI.** Abbreviation for *Treponema pallidum* immobilization *test.*

**TPN, TPNH.** Abbreviation for triphosphopyridine nucleotide and its reduced form (the oxidized form is TPN⁺); replaced by NADP, NADPH (NADPH⁺).

**TPP.** Abbreviation for thiamin pyrophosphate.

**TQ.** Abbreviation for tocopherolquinone (tocopherylquinone).

**tr.** Abbreviation for L. *tinctura,* or tincture.

**trabecula,** gen. and pl. **trabeculae** (tră-bek'u-lah, -le) [ L. dim. of *trabs,* a beam ] [ NA ]. One of the supporting bundles of fibers traversing the substance of a structure, usually derived from the capsule or one of the fibrous septa; a small piece of the spongy substance of bone usually interconnected with other similar pieces.

**trabec'ulae car'neae** [ NA ], columnae carneae; muscular bundles on the lining walls of the ventricles of the heart.

**trabeculae cor'poris spongio'si pe'nis** [ NA ], the fibrous bands interlacing between the vascular spaces of the corpus spongiosum and glans penis.

**trabec'ulae cor'porum cavernoso'rum** [ NA ], fibromuscular bands and cords given off from the fibrous envelopes and septum of the corpora cavernosa penis and which separate the cavernous veins.

**trabeculae cra'nii,** a pair of chondrification centers in the base of the embryonic cartilaginous neurocranium, lying in front of the developing hypophysis.

**trabec'ulae li'enis** [ NA ], small fibrous bands given off from the capsule of the spleen and constituting the framework of that organ.

**t. septomargina'lis** [ NA ], septomarginal t.; moderator band; Reil's band (1); one of the trabeculae carneae in the right ventricle of the heart; it carries the right branch of the A-V bundle from the septum to the opposite wall of the ventricle.

**t. tes'tis,** *septulum* testis.

**trabec'ular.** Relating to or containing trabeculae.

**trabec'ularism.** A state marked by the presence of trabeculae.

**trabec'ulate.** Trabecular.

**trabec'ula'tion.** The occurrence of trabeculae in the walls of an organ or part; the process of forming trabeculae, as in spongy bone.

**trace** (trās). 1. Evidence of the former existence, influence, or action of an object, phenomena, or event. 2. An extremely small amount or barely discernable indication of something.

**memory t.,** engram.

**tra'cer.** 1. An element or compound containing atoms that can be distinguished from their normal counterparts by physical means ( *e.g.,* radioactivity assay or mass spectrography or scintillation counter) and that can thus be used to follow (trace) the course of the normal substances in metabolism or similar chemical changes. A colored substance ( *e.g.,* a dye) can be used as a t. to follow the flow of water. However, most t.'s are radioactive or "heavy" nuclides ($^{32}$P, $^{14}$C, $^{2}$H, etc.). 2. An instrument used in dissecting out nerves and blood vessels. 3. A mechanical device with a marking point attached to one jaw and a graph plate or tracing plate attached to the other jaw; it is used to record the direction and extent of movements of the mandible; see also tracing.

**trache-.** See tracheo-.

**trachea,** pl. **tracheae** (tra'ke-ah, tra'ke-e) [ G. *tracheia artēria,* rough artery. TRACH-1 ] [ NA ]. Windpipe; the air tube extending from the larynx (sixth cervical vertebra) into the thorax (fifth or sixth thoracic vertebra) where it divides, the bifurcation of the t. The t. is composed of from 16 to 20 rings of hyaline cartilage connected by a membrane, the annular ligament; posteriorly the rings are deficient for one-fifth to one-third of their circumference, the interval forming the membranous wall being closed by a fibrous membrane containing smooth muscular fibers. Internally the mucosa is composed of a pseudostratified ciliated columnar epithelium with mucous goblet cells. Numerous small mixed mucous and serous glands occur, the ducts of which open to the surface of the epithelium.

**scabbard t.,** a deformity of the t. caused by flattening and approximation of the lateral walls, producing more or less pronounced stenosis.

**tracheal** (tra'ke-al). Relating to the trachea.

**trachealgia** (tra-ke-al'jĭ-ah) [ trachea + G. *algos,* pain ]. Pain in the trachea.

**trachealis** (tra-ke-a'lis). See under musculus.

**tracheitis** (tra-ke-i'tis) [ trachea + G. suffix *-itis,* inflammation ]. Tracheal catarrh; trachitis; inflammation of the lining membrane of the trachea.

**trachel-.** See trachelo-.

**trachelagra** (trak'ĕ-lag'rah) [ trachel- + G. *agra,* seizure ]. A gouty or rheumatic affection of the muscles of the neck, producing torticollis.

**trachelalis** (trak-ke-la'lis). *Musculus* longissimus capitis.

**trachelectomopexy** (trak'ĕ-lek'to-mo-pek'sĭ) [ trachel- + G. *ektomē,* excision, + *pēxis,* fixation ]. Partial excision, with fixation of the remaining portion of the cervix uteri.

**trachelectomy** (trak'ĕ-lek'to-mĭ) [ trachel- + G. *ektomē,* excision ]. Cervicectomy.

**trachelematoma** (trak'ĕ-le'mă-to'mah) [ trachel- + hematoma ]. A hematoma of the neck.

**trachelian** (tră-ke'lĭ-an) [ G. *trachēlos,* neck ]. Cervical.

**trachelism, trachelismus** (trak′ĕ-lizm, -liz′mus) [ G. *trachēlismos,* a seizing by the throat ]. A bending backward of the neck, such as sometimes ushers in an epileptic attack.

**trachelitis** (trak′ĕ-li′tis). Cervicitis.

**trachelo-, trachel-** (trak′ĕ-lo-) [ G. *trachēlos,* neck. TRACH-2 ]. Combining forms meaning neck.

**trachelocele** (trak′ĕ-lo-sēl) [ trachelo- + G. *kēlē,* tumor, hernia ]. Tracheocele.

**trachelocyrtosis** (trak′ĕ-lo-sur-to′sis) [ trachelo- + G. *kyrtos,* bent ]. Tuberculous *spondylitis.*

**trachelocystitis** (trak′ĕ-lo-sis-ti′tis) [ trachelo- + G. *kystis,* bladder, + suffix *-itis,* inflammation ]. Inflammation of the neck of the bladder.

**trachelodynia** (trak′ĕ-lo-din′ĭ-ah) [ trachelo- + G. *odynē,* pain ]. Cervicodynia; neck pain.

**trachelokyphosis** (trak′ĕ-lo-ki-fo′sis) [ trachelo- + G. *kyphōsis,* hump-back ]. Tuberculous *spondylitis.*

**trachelology** (trak-ĕ-lol′o-jī) [ trachelo- + G. *logos,* study ]. The study of the neck and its injuries and diseases.

**trachelomastoid** (trak′ĕ-lo-mas′toyd). *Musculus longissimus capitis.*

**trachelomyitis** (trak′ĕ-lo-mi-i′tis) [ trachelo- + G. *mys,* muscle, + suffix *-itis,* inflammation ]. Obsolete term for inflammation of the muscles of the neck.

**trachelooccipitalis** (trak′ĕ-lo-ok-sip′ĭ-ta′lis). *Musculus semispinalis capitis.*

**trachelopanus** (trak′ĕ-lo-pa′nus) [ trachelo- + L. *panus,* tumor, swelling ]. 1. Swelling of the lymphatic vessels of the neck. 2. Lymphatic engorgement of the cervix uteri.

**trachelopexia, trachelopexy** (trak′ĕ-lo-pek′sĭ-ah, -pek′-sĭ) [ trachelo- + G. *pēxis,* fixation ]. An operation for fixation of the cervix uteri.

**trachelophyma** (trak′ĕ-lo-fi′mah) [ trachelo- + G. *phyma,* tumor ]. A tumor or swelling of the neck.

**tracheloplasty** (trak′ĕ-lo-plas-tī) [ trachelo- + G. *plastos,* formed ]. Surgical repair of lacerations or other defects of the cervix uteri.

**trachelorrhaphy** (trak-ĕ-lor′ă-fī) [ trachelo- + G. + *rhaphē,* suture ]. Repair by suture of a laceration of the cervix uteri.

**trachelorrhectes** (trak-ĕ-lŏ-rek′tēz) [ trachelo- + G. *rhēktēs,* a breaker ]. An instrument used in embryotomy to crush the cervical vertebrae.

**trachelos** (trak′ĕ-los) [ G. *trachēlos* ]. The neck.

**tracheloschisis** (trak′ĕ-los′kĭ-sis) [ trachelo- + G. *schisis,* fissure ]. A congenital fissure in the neck.

**trachelotomy** (trak′ĕ-lot′o-mī) [ trachelo- + G. *tomē,* incision ]. Cervicotomy.

**tracheo-, trache-, trachi-** (tra′ke-o-) [ G. *tracheia,* windpipe, trachea (TRACH-1) ]. Combining form relating to the trachea.

**tracheoaerocele** (tra′ke-o-a′er-o-sēl) [ tracheo- + G. *aēr,* air, + *kēlē,* hernia ]. An air cyst in the neck caused by distention of a tracheocele.

**tra′cheobil′iary.** Relating to the trachea or bronchi and the biliary duct system.

**tracheobronchial** (tra′ke-o-brong′kĭ-al). Relating to both trachea and bronchi.

**tracheobronchitis** (tra′ke-o-brong-ki′tis). Inflammation of the mucous membrane of both trachea and bronchi. Bronchitis with extension of the inflammation to the trachea.

**tracheobronchoscopy** (tra′ke-o-brong-kos′ko-pī) [ tracheo- + bronchus, + G. *skopeō,* to view ]. Inspection of the interior of the trachea and bronchi.

**tracheocele** (tra′ke-o-sēl) [ tracheo- + G. *kēlē,* hernia ]. Trachelocele; a protrusion of the mucous membrane through a defect in the wall of the trachea.

**tracheoesophageal** (tra′ke-o-e-sof′ă-je′al). Relating to the trachea and the esophagus.

**tracheolaryngeal** (tra′ke-o-lă-rin′je-al). Relating to the trachea and the larynx.

**tracheomalacia** (tra′ke-o-mă-la′shī-ah) [ tracheo- + G. *malakia,* softness ]. Degeneration of elastic and connective tissue of trachea.

**tracheopath′ia osteoplas′tica.** A rare disease characterized by cartilaginous and bony growths in the trachea and bronchi which produce sessile polyps and plaques projecting into and partly obstructing the lumina. The symptoms are cough, hemoptysis, fever, and attacks of pneumonitis.

**tracheopharyngeal** (tra′ke-o-fă-rin′je-al). Relating to both trachea and pharynx; denoting an occasional band of muscular fibers passing from the inferior constrictor of the pharynx to the trachea.

**tracheophonesis** (tra′ke-o-fo-ne′sis) [ tracheo- + G. *phōnēsis,* a sounding ]. Auscultation of the heart sounds at the sternal notch.

**tracheophony** (tra-ke-of′o-nī) [ tracheo- + G. *phōnē,* voice ]. The hollow voice sound heard in auscultating over the trachea; see also bronchophony.

**tracheoplasty** (tra′ke-o-plas-tī) [ tracheo- + G. *plassō,* to form ]. Reparative or plastic surgery of the trachea.

**tracheopyosis** (tra-ke-o-pi-o′sis) [ tracheo- + G. + *pyōsis,* suppuration ]. Suppurative inflammation of the trachea.

**tracheorrhagia** (tra-ke-o-ra′jī-ah) [ tracheo- + G. *rhēgnymi,* to burst forth ]. Hemorrhage from the mucous membrane of the trachea.

**tracheoschisis** (tra-ke-os′kĭ-sis) [ tracheo- + G. *schisis,* fissure ]. A fissure into the trachea.

**tracheoscope** (tra′ke-o-skōp). An instrument used in tracheoscopy.

**tracheoscopic** (tra-ke-o-skop′ik). Relating to tracheoscopy.

**tracheoscopy** (tra-ke-os′ko-pī) [ tracheo- + G. *skopeō,* to examine ]. Inspection of the interior of the trachea.

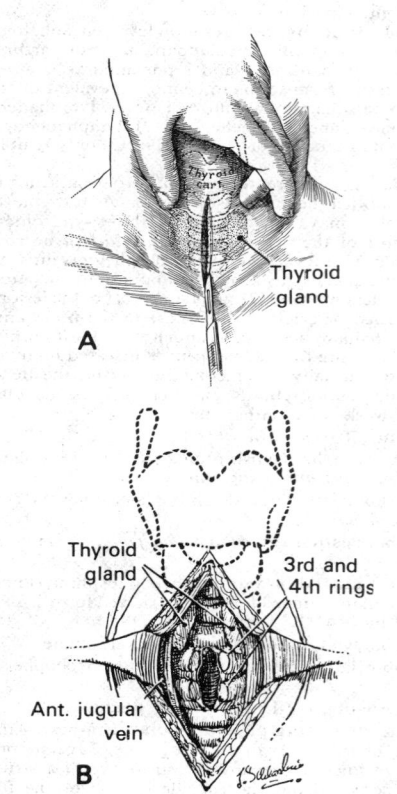

**Tracheotomy**

*A,* diagram showing the position of the fingers of the left hand grasping the larynx, and the index finger free for palpation of the midline; in emergencies the long incision illustrated is used for more complete exposure. *B,* the thyroid isthmus has been severed and window made. (From Proctor, D. F.: *Anesthesia and Otolaryngology,* The Williams & Wilkins Co., Baltimore, 1957.)

**tracheostenosis** (tra′ke-o-stĕ-no′sis) [ tracheo- + G. *stenōsis*, constrictior ]. Narrowing of the lumen of the trachea.

**tracheostoma** (tra′ke-os′to-mah) [ tracheo- + G. *stoma*, mouth ]. Opening into the trachea through the neck; generally applied to such an opening after tracheotomy or laryngectomy.

**tracheostomy** (tra′ke-os′to-mĭ) [ tracheo- + G. *stoma*, mouth ]. Formation of an opening into the trachea or that opening.

**tracheotome** (tra′ke-o-tōm). A knife used in the operation of tracheotomy.

**tracheotomize** (tra-ke-ot′o-mĭz). To perform tracheotomy upon.

**tracheotomy** (tra-ke-ot′o-mĭ) [ tracheo- + G. *tomē*, incision ]. The operation of opening into the trachea.

    **inferior t.,**  t. performed below the isthmus of the thyroid gland.

    **superior t.,**  t. performed above or through the isthmus of the thyroid gland.

**trachitis** (tra-ki′tis). Tracheitis.

**trachoma** (trã-ko′mah) [ G. *trachōma*, fr. *trachys*, rough, harsh ]. A chronic contagious viral inflammation, with hypertrophy, of the conjunctiva, marked by the formation of minute grayish or yellowish translucent granules caused by *Chlamydia trachomatis*. Also called contagious granular conjunctivitis; granular lids; granular ophthalmia; Egyptian ophthalmia.

    **Arlt's t.,**  granular *conjunctivitis.*

    **brawny t.,**  a condition in which there is a general granulation.

    **t. defor′mans,**  t. pudendorum characterized by shrinkage, infection, and fissuring of the mucous membrane with cicatricial contractions of the vulva.

    **diffuse t.,**  a form in which the granulations are of large size, approaching brawny t.

    **follic′ular t., granular t.,**  the ordinary form of t. marked by the presence of granulations on the conjunctiva.

    **pap′illary t.,**  a form in which the granulations are acuminate and red.

    **t. pudendo′rum, t. vulvae,**  *kraurosis* vulvae.

**trachomatous** (trã-ko′mã-tus). Relating to or suffering from trachoma.

**trachychromatic** (trak-ĭ-kro-mat′ik) [ G. *trachys*, rough, + *chrōmatikos*, chromatic ]. Denoting a nucleus with very deeply staining chromatin.

**trachypho′nia** (trak′ĭ-fo′nĭ-ah) [ G. *trachys*, rough, + *phōnē*, voice ]. Roughness of voice.

**tracing** (tra′sing). 1. Any graphic display of electrical or mechanical cardiovascular events, *e.g.*, electrocardiogram, phlebogram, etc.; curve. 2. In dentistry, a line or lines, scribed on a table or plate by a pointed instrument, representing a record of movements of the mandible; t.'s may be extraoral (made outside the oral cavity) or intraoral (made within the oral cavity).

    **arrow point t.,**  needle point t.

    **Gothic arch t.,**  needle point t.

    **needle point t.,**  stylus t.; Gothic arch t.; arrow point t.; a t. that resembles an arrowhead or a Gothic arch, made by means of a device attached to the opposing arches. The shape of the t. depends upon the relative location of the marking point and the t. table. The apex of a properly made t. is considered to indicate the most retruded unstrained relation of the mandible to the maxillare, *i.e.*, centric relation.

    **stylus t.,**  needle point t.

# TRACT

**tract** (trakt) [ L. *tractus, q.v.* ]. An elongated area, *e.g.*, path, track, way; see tractus and fasciculus.

    **alimen′tary t.,**  digestive t.

    **anterior corticospinal t.,**  *tractus* pyramidalis anterior.

    **anterior pyramidal t.,**  *tractus* pyramidalis anterior.

    **anterior spinocerebellar t.,**  *tractus* spinocerebellaris anterior.

    **anterior spinothalamic t.,**  *tractus* spinothalamicus anterior.

    **Arnold's t.,**  *tractus* temporopontinus.

    **association t.,**  see association *system.*

    **auditory t.,**  *lemniscus* lateralis.

    **Burdach's t.,**  *fasciculus* cuneatus.

    **central tegmental t.,**  *tractus* tegmentalis centralis.

    **cerebellorubral t.,**  *tractus* cerebellorubralis.

    **cerebellothalamic t.,**  *tractus* cerebellothalamicus.

    **Collier's t.,**  *fasciculus* longitudinalis medialis.

    **comma t. of Schultze,**  *fasciculus* semilunaris.

    **corticobulbar t.,**  *tractus* corticobulbaris.

    **corticopontine t.'s,**  *tractus* corticopontini.

    **corticospinal t.,**  *tractus* pyramidalis.

    **crossed pyramidal t.,**  *tractus* pyramidalis lateralis.

    **Deiterospinal t.,**  *tractus* vestibulospinalis.

    **dentatothalamic t.,**  *tractus* cerebellothalamicus.

    **descending t. of trigeminal nerve,**  *tractus* spinalis nervi trigemini.

    **digestive t.,**  alimentary t.; the passage leading from the mouth to the anus through the pharynx, esophagus, stomach, and intestine.

    **direct pyramidal t.,**  *tractus* pyramidalis anterior.

    **dorsal spinocerebellar t.,**  *tractus* spinocerebellaris posterior.

    **dorsolateral t.,**  *fasciculus* dorsolateralis.

    **fastigiobulbar t.,**  *tractus* fastigiobulbaris.

    **Flechsig's t.,**  *tractus* spinocerebellaris posterior.

    **frontopontine t.,**  *tractus* frontopontinus.

    **frontotemporal t.,**  *fasciculus* uncinatus.

    **geniculocalcarine t.,**  *radiatio* optica.

    **genital t.,**  genital duct; the genital passages of the urogenital apparatus.

    **t. of Goll,**  *fasciculus* gracilis.

    **Gowers' t.,**  *tractus* spinocerebellaris anterior.

    **habenulointerpeduncular t.,**  *fasciculus* retroflexus.

    **Hoche's t.,**  see *fasciculus* semilunaris.

    **hypothalamohypophysial t.,**  a fiber t. that connects the paraventricular and supraoptic nuclei of the hypothalamus with the neurohypophysis; the oxytocin synthetized by the paraventricular nucleus and the vassopressin synthetized by the supraoptic nucleus pass down the axons of the hypothalamohypophysial t. and are stored in the terminals of these fibers in the neurohypophysis, from which they can be released into the systemic circulation.

    **lateral corticospinal t.,**  *tractus* pyramidalis lateralis.

    **lateral pyramidal t.,**  *tractus* pyramidalis lateralis.

    **lateral spinothalamic t.,**  *tractus* spinothalamicus lateralis.

    **Lissauer's t.,**  *fasciculus* dorsolateralis.

    **Loewenthal's t.,**  *tractus* tectospinalis.

    **mamillothalamic t.,**  *fasciculus* mamillothalamicus.

    **Marchi's t.,**  *tractus* tectospinalis.

    **mesencephalic t. of trigeminal nerve,**  *tractus* mesencephalicus nervi trigemini.

    **Monakow's t.,**  *tractus* rubrospinalis.

    **t. of Münzer and Wiener,**  *tractus* tectopontinus.

    **nerve t.,**  a bundle or group of nerve fibers in the brain or spinal cord.

    **occipitopontine t.,**  *tractus* occipitopontinus.

    **olfactory t.,**  *tractus* olfactorius.

    **olivocerebellar t.,**  *tractus* olivocerebellaris.

    **olivospinal t.,**  Helweg's bundle; a slender bundle of nerve fibers in the peripheral zone of the lateral funiculus of the spinal cord, composed of spinoolivary fibers more likely than olivospinal fibers.

    **optic t.,**  *tractus* opticus.

    **parietopontine t.,**  *tractus* parietopontinus.

    **posterior spinocerebellar t.,**  *tractus* spinocerebellaris posterior.

    **prepyramidal t.,**  *tractus* rubrospinalis.

    **pyramidal t.,**  *tractus* pyramidalis.

    **respiratory t.,**  the air passages from the nose to the pulmonary alveoli, through the pharynx, larynx, trachea, and bronchi.

    **reticulospinal t.,**  *tractus* reticulospinalis.

    **rubrobulbar t.,**  that component of the rubrospinal t. which distributes its fibers to lateral parts of the rhombencephalic tegmentum rather than the spinal cord.

**rubroreticular t.,** fibers that pass from the red nucleus to the reticular formation of the pons and medulla.

**rubrospinal t.,** *tractus* rubrospinalis.

**t. of Schütz,** *fasciculus* longitudinalis dorsalis.

**sensory t.,** see lemniscus.

**septomarginal t.,** see *fasciculus* semilunaris.

**solitary t.,** *tractus* solitarius.

**sphincteroid t. of ileum,** basal *sphincter.*

**spinal t.,** any one of a multitude of fiber bundles ascending or descending in the spinal cord; see fig. under medulla spinalis.

**spinal t. of trigeminal nerve,** *tractus* spinalis nervi trigemini.

**spinocerebellar t.'s,** see entries under *tractus* spinocerebellaris.

**spinoolivary t.,** see olivospinal t.

**spinotectal t.,** *tractus* spinotectalis.

**spinothalamic t.,** *tractus* spinothalamicus.

**spiral foraminous t.,** *tractus* spiralis foraminosus.

**Spitzka's marginal t.,** *fasciculus* dorsolateralis.

**sulcomarginal t.,** collective term for those fiber t.'s which descend in the anterior funiculus of the spinal cord along the wall of the anterior median fissure: tectospinal t., medial longitudinal fasciculus, and anterior pyramidal t.

**supraopticohypophysial t.,** *tractus* supraopticohypophysialis.

**tectobulbar t.,** *tractus* tectobulbaris.

**tectopontine t.,** *tractus* tectopontinus.

**tectospinal t.,** *tractus* tectospinalis.

**temporofrontal t.,** *fasciculus* uncinatus.

**temporopontine t.,** *tractus* temporopontinus.

**thalamoolivary t.,** obsolete term for *tractus* tegmentalis centralis.

**tuberoinfundibular t.,** *tractus* tuberoinfundibularis.

**Türck's t.,** *tractus* frontopontinus.

**urinary t.,** the passage from the pelvis of the kidney to the urinary meatus through the ureters, bladder, and urethra.

**uveal t.,** *tunica* vasculosa bulbi.

**ventral spinocerebellar t.,** *tractus* spinocerebellaris anterior.

**ventral spinothalamic t.,** *tractus* spinothalamicus anterior.

**vestibulospinal t.,** *tractus* vestibulospinalis.

**Waldeyer's t.,** *fasciculus* dorsolateralis.

---

**tractellum,** pl. **tractella** (trak-tel'um, -ah) [ Mod. L. dim. of L. *tractus*]. An anterior locomotor flagellum of a protozoon.

**traction** (trak'shun) [ L. *tractio,* fr. *traho,* pp. *tractus,* to draw ]. 1. The act of drawing or pulling. 2. A pulling force. See also extension (2) and relevant subentries.

**axis t.,** t. upon the fetal head in the line of the birth canal by means of axis t. forceps; a rarely used procedure.

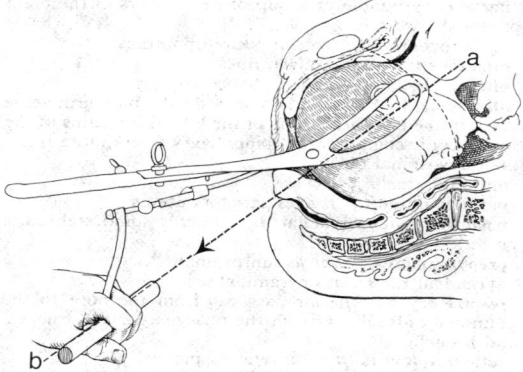

**Axis Traction**
*Dotted, curved line,* pelvic brim; *a-b,* line of traction.

**Bryant's t.,** t. upon the lower limb placed vertically, employed especially in fractures in children.

**external t.,** a pulling force created by using fixed anchorage (*e.g.,* a headcap or bed frame) outside the oral cavity; principally used in the management of midfacial fractures.

**intermaxillary t.,** maxillomandibular t.

**internal t.,** a pulling force created by using one of the cranial bones, above the point of fracture, for anchorage.

**maxillomandibular t.,** intermaxillary t.; a pulling force developed by using elastic or wire ligatures and interdental wiring or splints, or both.

**Russell t.,** an improvement of Buck's extension for fracture of femur.

**skeletal t.,** t. pull on a bone structure mediated through pin or wire inserted into the bone by means of metal pins or wires to reduce a fracture of long bones.

**tractor** [ Mod. L. a drawer, see traction ]. An instrument for making traction.

**Syms' t.,** a collapsible rubber bag attached to the extremity of a tube; the tube is introduced into the bladder through the perineal wound and the bag is inflated; traction now made brings the enlarged prostate into the wound where it is readily accessible.

**tractotomy** (trak-tot'o-mī) [ L. *tractus,* tract, + G. *tomē,* incision ]. Interruption of a nerve tract in the brain stem or spinal cord by laminectomy, craniotomy, or stereotaxy. Types include spinothalamic t., trigeminal t., and pyramidal t.

**anterolateral t.,** cordotomy.

**descending root t.,** trigeminal t.

**intramedullary t.,** sectioning of the descending trigeminal tract in the lateral aspect of the medulla.

**pyramidal t.,** division of a pyramidal nerve tract; may be mesencephalic (pedunculotomy or crusotomy), medullary (medullary pyramidotomy), or spinal (spinal pyramidotomy).

**Schwartz t.,** a medullary spinothalamic t.

**Sjöqvist t.,** trigeminal t.

**spinal t.,** cordotomy.

**spinothalamic t.,** division of a spinothalamic nerve tract; may be spinal (cordotomy), medullary (Schwartz t.), or mesencephalic (Walker t.).

**trigeminal t.,** Sjöqvist t., division of the descending root of the trigeminal nerve.

**Walker t.,** a mesencephalic spinothalamic t.

---

# TRACTUS

---

**tractus,** gen. and pl. **tractus** (trak'tus) [ L. a drawing, drawing out, extent, tract, fr. *traho,* pp. *tractus,* to draw ] [ NA ]. A tract; see tract and fasciculus.

**t. centra'lis tegmen'ti,** t. tegmentalis centralis.

**t. cerebellorubra'lis** [ NA ], cerebellorubral tract; that major component of the superior cerebellar peduncle (brachium conjunctivum) which distributes itself to the nucleus ruber of the opposite side.

**t. cerebellothalam'icus** [ NA ], cerebellothalamic tract; dentatothalamic tract; that component of the superior cerebellar peduncle (brachium conjunctivum) which, originating in the cerebellar nuclei and crossing over in the decussation of the brachia conjunctiva, bypasses the red nucleus and terminates in the thalamic nuclei ventralis anterior, ventralis lateralis, and centralis lateralis.

**t. corticobulba'ris,** corticobulbar tract; fibrae corticonucleares [ NA ]; corticonuclear fibers; collective term for those fibers which separate from the pyramidal tract in the course of the latter's descent through the pons and medulla oblongata, and innervate the motor nuclei of the trigeminal, facial, and hypoglossal nerves (perhaps also the nucleus ambiguus), either directly or by way of interneurons in the lateral part of the rhombencephalic tegmentum. No such supranuclear cortical innervation of the motor nuclei innervating the external eye muscles (oculomotor, trochlear, abducens) has been identified.

**t. corticoponti' ni** [ NA ], corticopontine tracts; collective term for the multitude of fibers which, originating in all of the major subdivisions of the cerebral cortex, descend in the internal capsule and cerebral peduncle to terminate in the nuclei pontis or pars ventralis pontis. Individual components of this massive fiber system are indicated, according to their origin in the cerebral cortex, as t. frontopontinus, t. parietopontinus, t. occipitopontinus, and t. temporopontinus.

**t. corticospina'lis** [ NA ], t. pyramidalis.

**t. corticospina'lis ante'rior** [ NA ], t. pyramidalis anterior.

**t. corticospina'lis latera'lis** [ NA ], t. pyramidalis lateralis.

**t. descen'dens ner'vi trigem'ini**, t. spinalis nervi trigemini.

**t. dorsolatera'lis** [ NA ], *fasciculus* dorsolateralis.

**t. fastigiobulba'ris**, fastigiobulbar tract; a fiber bundle originating in the nucleus fastigii (nucleus tecti) of both sides, passing out of the cerebellum in the inferior cerebellar peduncle (corpus restiforme) and distributing its fibers to the vestibular nuclei and other cell groups in the medulla oblongata. Part of its fibers loop over the dorsal surface of the superior cerebellar peduncle before turning ventrally into the restiform body, thus forming the uncinate bundle of Russell.

**t. frontoponti'nus** [ NA ], frontopontine tract; Türck's tract or bundle; a large group of fibers arising from the frontal lobe of the cerebral hemisphere, especially the precentral gyrus, descending in the capsula interna, farther caudalward composing the medial one-third of the cerebral peduncle in which they extend caudalward to end in the gray matter (pontine nuclei) of the pars ventralis pontis.

**t. haben'ulopeduncula'ris**, *fasciculus* retroflexus.

**t. iliotibia'lis** [ NA ], iliotibial band; Maissiat's band; a fibrous reinforcement of the fascia lata on the lateral surface of the thigh, extending from the crest of the ilium to the lateral condyle of the tibia.

**t. mesencephal'icus ner'vi trigem'ini** [ NA ], mesencephalic tract of the trigeminal nerve; located alongside the substantia grisea centralis and composed of primary sensory fibers, the cells of origin of which compose the mesencephalic nucleus of the trigeminus.

**t. occipitoponti'nus** [ NA ], occipitopontine tract; a group of fibers originating in the occipital lobe of the cerebral cortex and descending in the internal capsule and lateral one-third of the cerebral peduncle to the pontine nuclei or pars ventralis pontis.

**t. olfacto'rius** [ NA ], olfactory tract; olfactory peduncle (*q. v.*); olfactory nerve (obs.); a nervelike, white band composed primarily of nerve fibers originating from the mitral cells and tufted cells of the olfactory bulb but also containing the scattered cells of the anterior olfactory nucleus, possibly caudalward closely applied to the ventral surface of the frontal lobe, and attaching itself to the base of the cerebral hemisphere at the olfactory trigone, beyond which it extends in the form of the olfactory striae which distribute their fibers to the olfactory tubercle and, in largest number, to the olfactory cortex on and around the uncus of the parahippocampal gyrus.

**t. olivocerebella'ris** [ NA ], olivocerebellar tract; a large group of loosely arranged fiber fascicles emerging from the hilus of the olivary nucleus, crossing to the opposite side of the medulla oblongata through the stratum interolivare lemnisci and the contralateral olive, and joining the contralateral restiform body or inferior cerebellar peduncle; its fibers are distributed to all parts of the cerebellar cortex and are thought to terminate, in large part at least, as climbing fibers.

**t. op'ticus** [ NA ], optic tract; the continuation of the optic nerve beyond (behind) the latter's hemidecussation in the optic chiasm; each of the two symmetrical optic tracts is composed of fibers originating from the temporal half of the retina of the ipsilateral eye and a nearly equal number of fibers from the nasal half of the contralateral retina; it forms a compact, somewhat flattened fiber band passing caudolaterally alongside the base of the hypothalamus and over the basal surface of the cerebral peduncle; most of its fibers terminate in the lateral geniculate body, but a smaller number continue dorsomedially alongside the latter's medial side as the brachium of the superior

colliculus, to terminate in the superior colliculus and the pretectal region.

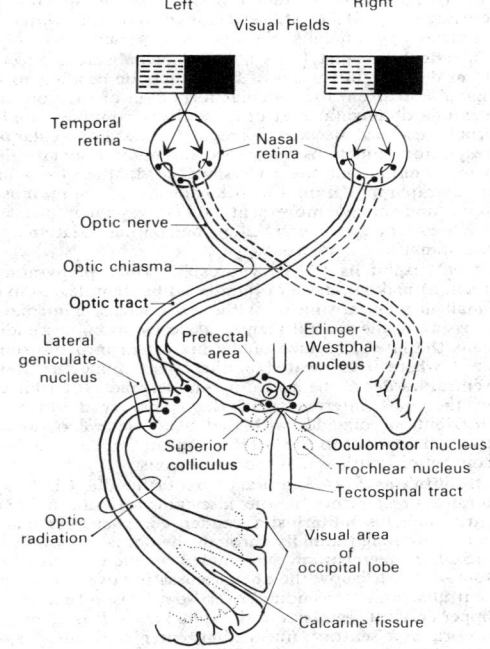

**Tractus Opticus (Optic Tract)**

**t. parietoponti'nus** [ NA ], parietopontine tract; a system of fibers originating in the parietal lobe of the cerebral cortex and descending in the internal capsule and lateral one-third of the cerebral peduncle to the nuclei pontis or pars ventralis pontis.

**t. pyramida'lis** [ NA ], t. corticospinalis [ NA ]; pyramidal or corticospinal tract; a massive bundle of fibers originating from large pyramidal cells (including Betz cells) in area 4 of the precentral motor cortex, to a lesser extent also in the postcentral gyrus, descending through the internal capsule, the middle third of the cerebral peduncle, and the pars ventralis pontis, to emerge on the ventral surface of the medulla oblongata as the pyramis. Continuing caudally, most (about 90 per cent) of the fibers cross to the opposite side in the pyramidal decussation to descend in the dorsal half of the lateral funiculus of the spinal cord as the t. pyramidalis lateralis (lateral pyramidal or lateral corticospinal tract), which distributes its fibers throughout the length of the spinal cord to interneurons of the zona intermedia of the spinal gray matter, in the (extremity-related) spinal cord enlargements, also directly to those (lateral) motoneuronal groups that innervate distal extremity muscles subserving in particular hand-and-finger or foot-and-toe movements. The uncrossed fibers form a small bundle, the t. pyramidalis anterior (anterior pyramidal or anterior or direct corticospinal tract, or Türck's column) which descends in the anterior funiculus of the spinal cord and terminates in synaptic contact with interneurons in the radial half of the anterior horn on both sides of the spinal cord. Interruption of the pyramidal tract at or below its cortical origin causes impairment of movement in the corresponding body-half, especially severe in the arm and leg: muscular weakness, spasticity and hyperreflexia, and a loss of the normal capacity to perform discrete finger and hand movements. Babinski's sign (dorsiflexion of the big toe) is associated with this condition of hemiplegia. See also t. corticobularis, and fig. under *medulla spinalis*.

**t. pyramida'lis ante'rior** [ NA ], t. corticospinalis anterior [ NA ]; anterior pyramidal or anterior corticospinal tract; direct pyramidal tract; Türck's column; fasciculus corticospinalis anterior; fasciculus pyramidalis anterior; see t. pyramidalis.

**t. pyramida'lis latera'lis** [ NA ], t. corticospinalis lateralis [ NA ]; lateral pyramidal or lateral corticospinal tract; crossed pyramidal tract; fasciculus corticospinalis lateralis; fasciculus pyramidalis lateralis; see t. pyramidalis.

**t. reticulospina'lis** [ NA ], reticulospinal tract; collective term denoting a variety of fiber tracts descending to the spinal cord from the reticular formation of the pons and medulla oblongata. Part of these fibers conduct impulses from the neural mechanisms regulating cardiovascular and respiratory functions to the corresponding somatic and visceral motor neurons of the spinal cord; others form links in extrapyramidal motor mechanisms affecting muscle tonus and somatic movement, and convey the influence of the premotor cortex, cerebellum, and corpus striatum upon the spinal motor neurons.

**t. rubrospina'lis** [ NA ], rubrospinal tract; prepyramidal tract; Monakow's tract or bundle; a fiber bundle, relatively small in man, arising from the red nucleus, immediately crossing in the ventral tegmental decussation, descending near the lateral surface of the brainstem into the spinal cord where it is located in the lateral funiculus at the ventral border of the lateral pyramidal tract. It terminates in the zona intermedia of the spinal cord where its distribution coincides with that of the lateral pyramidal tract; in contrast to the latter it appears not to have direct connections with spinal motor neurons.

**t. solita'rius** [ NA ], solitary tract or bundle; Gierke's or Krause's respiratory bundle; fasciculus rotundus or solitarius; funiculus solitarius; a slender, compact fiber bundle extending longitudinally through the dorsal region of the medullary tegmentum, surrounded by the nucleus of the solitary tract, below the obex decussating over the canalis centralis, and descending over some distance into the upper cervical segments of the spinal cord. It is composed of primary sensory fibers that enter with the vagus, glossopharyngeal, and facial nerves, and in part convey information from stretch receptors and chemoreceptors in the walls of the cardiovascular, respiratory, and intestinal tracts, in other part impulses generated by the receptor cells of the taste buds in the mucosa of the tongue. Its fibers are distributed to the nucleus of the solitary tract.

**t. spina'lis ner'vi trigem'ini** [ NA ], spinal tract of the trigeminal nerve; descending tract of the trigeminal nerve; t. descendens nervi trigemini; a compact fiber bundle, comma-shaped on transverse section, composed of primary sensory fibers of the portio major of the trigeminal nerve, descending from the level of the entrance of the trigeminus in the upper pons down through the dorsolateral region of the rhombencephalic tegmentum along the lateral side of the descending or spinal nucleus of the trigeminus, emerging on the dorsolateral surface of the lower medulla oblongata as the tuberculum cinereum, and continuing as far as the third or fourth cervical segment of the spinal cord. Its fibers are distributed to the descending or spinal nucleus of the trigeminus.

**t. spinocerebella'ris ante'rior** [ NA ], anterior spinocerebellar tract; ventral spinocerebellar tract; Gowers' tract or column; a bundle of fibers originating in the posterior horn and zona intermedia throughout the length of the spinal cord, crossing to the opposite side and ascending in a peripheral position in the ventral half of the lateral funiculus, accompanying the spinothalamic tract in its ascent through the rhombencephalon, then curving sharply dorsalward along the rostral border of the trigeminal motor necleus, entering the cerebellum in a caudal direction over the dorsal surface of the superior cerebellar peduncle, and terminating as mossy fibers in the granular layer of the cortex of the cerebellar vermis. The bundle conveys largely exteroceptive information from the opposite body half.

**t. spinocerebella'ris poste'rior** [ NA ], posterior or dorsal spinocerebellar tract; Flechsig's tract; a compact bundle of heavily myelinated fibers at the periphery of the dorsal half of the lateral funiculus of the spinal cord, consisting of thick fibers originating in the nucleus thoracicus (column of Clarke) on the same side of the cord and ascending by way of the inferior cerebellar peduncle to end as mossy fibers in the granular layer of the cortex of the cerebellar vermis. The bundle conveys largely proprioceptive infor-

mation originating, among others, in the annulospiral nerve endings surrounding muscle spindles.

**t. spinotecta'lis** [ NA ], spinotectal tract; the relatively small component of the t. spinothalamicus that terminates in the intermediate and deep layers of the superior colliculus.

**t. spinothalam'icus,** spinothalamic tract; lemniscus spinalis; a large ascending fiber bundle in the ventral half of the lateral funiculus of the spinal cord, composed of fibers that arise in the posterior horn at all levels of the cord, cross within their segments of origin in the commissura alba, and in their contralateral ascent are intermingled with numerous intersegmental fibers. The t. spinothalamicus continues from the spinal cord into the brainstem, occupying a ventrolateral position and issuing numerous fibers to the rhombencephalic and mesencephalic reticular formation, to the lateral part of the central gray substance of the mesencephalon, and to the deep and intermediate layers of the superior colliculus; the relatively few fibers (10 to 20 per cent) that remain form the true spinothalamic tract which enters the diencephalon and ends in the nucleus ventralis posterior and intralaminar nuclei of the thalamus. The tract in its ascent in the spinal cord is composed of a dorsal part, the t. spinothalamicus lateralis, which conveys impulses associated with pain and temperature sensation, and a more ventral part, the t. spinothalamicus anterior, involved in tactile sensation.

**t. spinothalam'icus ante'rior** [ NA ], anterior or ventral spinothalamic tract; see t. spinothalamicus.

**t. spinothalam'icus latera'lis** [ NA ], lateral spinothalamic tract; see t. spinothalamicus.

**t. spira'lis foramino'sus** [ NA ], spiral foraminous tract; openings in the cochlear area of the bottom of the internal acoustic meatus through which the fibers of the cochlear nerve leave the cochlea of the bony labyrinth to enter the cranial cavity.

**t. spira'lis foraminulo'sus,** *macula* cribrosa quarta.

**t. supraop'ticohypophysia'lis** [ NA ], supraopticohypophysial tract; a bundle of unmyelinated fibers originating from all cells of the supraoptic nucleus and an estimated 20 per cent of those of the paraventricular nucleus of the hypothalamus, and extending through the infundibulum and pituitary stalk to their endings in the posterior lobe of the hypophysis. The fibers convey a neurosecretory substance, the antidiuretic hormone, which is stored in (and can be released into the circulating blood from) their terminals. See also hypophysis; neurosecretion.

**t. tectobulba'ris,** tectobulbar tract; fibers originating in the deep layers of the superior colliculus and accompanying the t. tectospinalis but, unlike the latter, terminating in medial regions of the pontine and medullary tegmentum.

**t. tectoponti'nus,** tectopontine tract; tract of Münzer and Wiener; a fiber bundle arising in the superior colliculus, passing caudoventrally on the same side along the medial side of the lateral lemniscus, issuing fibers terminating in the lateral zone of the mesencephalic tegmentum, and ending in the lateral part of the gray matter of the pars ventralis pontis.

**t. tectospina'lis** [ NA ], tectospinal tract; predorsal bundle; Loewenthal's tract or bundle; Marchi's tract; a bundle of thick, heavily myelinated fibers originating in the deep layers of the superior colliculus, crossing to the opposite side in the dorsal tegmental decussation, descending along the median plane, between the medial longitudinal fasciculus dorsally, the medial lemniscus ventrally, into the anterior funiculus of the spinal cord. The tract ends in the medial region of the anterior horn of the cervical spinal cord, and appears to be involved in head movements during visual and auditory tracking. Throughout its course through the brainstem it is accompanied by fibers of the tectobulbar tract.

**t. tegmenta'lis centra'lis** [ NA ], t. centralis tegmenti; central tegmental tract or fasciculus; thalamoolivary tract (obs.); a large fiber bundle passing longitudinally through the mesencephalic and pontine tegmentum, distinct from adjacent longitudinal groups of fiber-fascicles of the reticular formation by a somewhat more compact composition. In transverse sections of the mesencephalon the bundle occupies a large triangular area lateral to the medial longitudinal fasciculus; farther caudally it expands ventralward and finally passes over the lateral side of the (inferior) olivary nucleus, becoming part of the latter's fiber capsule. The bundle is known to contain fibers descending from the subthalamic region and mesencephalic tegmentum to the olivary nucleus; it also includes numerous fibers ascending from the medullary, pontine, and mesencephalic reticular formation to the thalamus and subthalamus.

**t. temporoponti'nus** [ NA ], temporopontine tract; Arnold's tract or bundle; a fiber group originating in the cerebral cortex of the temporal lobe, particularly the superior and middle temporal gyri, following the sublenticular limb of the internal capsule into the lateral margin of the cerebral peduncle in which it descends to its termination in the pontine nuclei or pars ventralis pontis.

**t. tuberoinfundibula'ris**, tuberoinfundibular tract; a system of fine, unmyelinated fibers apparently originating from small-celled nuclei of the tuber cinereum, especially the nucleus arcuatus, and terminating in the median eminence of the infundibulum, in contact with modified ependymal cells and the capillary tufts from which the hypothalamohypophysial portal veins originate. See also hypophysis; neurosecretion.

**t. vestibulospina'lis** [ NA ], vestibulospinal tract; Deiterospinal tract; a fiber bundle originating from the lateral vestibular nucleus (nucleus of Deiters) of the medulla oblongata and descending, uncrossed, in the anterior part of the spinal cord's white matter, lateral to the anterior median fissure; the t. extends throughout the length of the cord, distributing fibers at all levels to the medial part of the anterior horn.

---

**tragacanth, tragacantha** (trag'ă-kanth, -santh, -kan'-thah) [ G. *tragakantha*, a gum-producing shrub, fr. *tragos*, goat, + *akanthos*, thorn ] (USP, BP). A gummy exudation from *Astragalus gummifer* and other species of *A.*, shrubs of the eastern end of the Mediterranean. It occurs as bands or strings of a tough gummy substance, forming a jelly-like mucilage with 50 parts of water. It is used as a demulcent and excipient, in emulsions and suspensions.

**tra'gal.** Relating to the tragus.

**tra'galism** [ G. *tragos*, a goat ]. Sensuality.

**tra'gi.** 1. Plural of tragus. 2 [ NA ]. The hairs growing at the entrance to the external acoustic meatus.

**tra'gicus.** See under musculus.

**tragomaschalia** (tră-go-mas-kal'ĭ-ah) [ G. *tragomaschalos*, with smelling armpits, fr. *tragos*, goat, + *maschalē*, the axilla ]. Bromidrosis of the axillae.

**tragophonia, tragophony** (trag'o-fo'nĭ-ah, tră-gof'o-nĭ) [ G. *tragos*, goat, + *phōnē*, voice ]. Egophony.

**tragopodia** (trag'o-po'dĭ-ah) [ G. *tragos*, goat, + *pous* (*pod*-), foot ]. Rarely used term for genu valgum.

**tra'gus**, pl. **tra'gi** [ G. *tragos*, goat, in allusion to the hairs growing on the park, like a goatee ] 1 [ NA ]. A tongue-like projection of the cartilage of the auricle in front of the opening of the external acoustic meatus and continuous with the cartilage of this canal. 2. See tragi (2).

**train** (trān) [ Fr. *trainer*, fr. L. *traho*, to draw ]. To increase the virulence of bacteria by successive inoculations in animals.

**train'ing.** An organized system of education, instruction, or discipline.

**toilet t.,** t. directed at teaching a child proper control of his bladder and bowel functions; in psychoanalytic personality theory, it is believed that the attitudes of both parent and child concerning this t. may have important psychological implications for the child's later development.

**trait** (trāt) [ Fr. from L. *tractus*, a drawing out, extension ]. A characteristic, especially one that distinguishes an individual from others.

**dominant t.,** (1) an outstanding mental or physical characteristic; (2) see dominance of genes, under gene.

**recessive t.,** see dominance of genes, under gene.

**sickle cell t.,** the heterozygous state of the gene for hemoglobin S; heterozygotes produce both hemoglobin S and hemoglobin A, a portion of their erythrocytes assume sickle shape on reduction of oxygen tension; heterozygotes have an increased risk for intravascular thrombosis in response to anoxia.

**trajector** (tră-jek'tor) [ L. fr. *tra-jicio*, pp. *-jectus*, to throw over or across. JAC- ]. An instrument for locating the course of a bullet in a wound.

**tralphium** (tral'fĭ-um). Helium-3.

**tram'adol hydrochloride** (USAN). (+)-*trans*-2-[ Dimethylamino)methyl ]-1-*m*-methoxyphenyl)cyclohexanol hydrochloride; analgesic.

**tramaz'oline hydrochloride** (USAN). RHINASPRAY; 2-[ (5,6,7,8-tetrahydro-1-naphthyl) amino ]-2-imidazoline hydrochloride; sympathomimetic, used for nasal decongestion.

**trance** (trans) [ L. *trans-eo*, to go across ]. An altered state of consciousness as in hypnosis, catalepsy, or ecstacy.

**death t.,** a condition of suspended animation, marked by unconsciousness and barely perceptible respiration and heart action.

**induced t.,** hypnotic or somnambulistic t.

**somnambulis'tic t.,** a state of somnambulism, paralysis, anesthesia, or catalepsy induced by suggestion in major hypnosis.

**trance-coma.** The deep sleep following major hypnosis.

**tranquilizer** (trang'kwĭ-li'zer). Ataractic; ataraxic; a drug that brings tranquility by calming, soothing, quieting, or pacifying without depressing patients.

**major t.,** antipsychotic *agent*.

**minor t.,** antianxiety *agent*.

**trans-** (trans-, tranz-) [ L. *trans*, through, across ]. 1. A prefix meaning across, through, beyond. 2. In genetics, denoting the location of two genes on opposite chromosomes of a homologous pair. 3. In organic chemistry, a form of isomerism in which the atoms attached to two carbon atoms, joined by double bonds, are located on opposite sides of the molecule; opposite of cis-. 4. In biochemistry, a prefix to group name in an enzyme name or a reaction denoting transfer of that group from one compound to another, *e.g.*, transformylase (transfers formyl group), transpeptidation.

$$\underset{cis\text{-}}{\overset{R-C-H}{\underset{R-C-H}{\vphantom{|}}}} \qquad \underset{trans\text{-}}{\overset{H-C-R}{\underset{R-C-H}{\vphantom{|}}}}$$

**transacet'ylase.** Acetyltransferase.

**transacet'yla'tion.** The transfer of an acetyl group ($CH_3CO—$), from one compound to another; such reactions, usually involving formation of acetyl-CoA, occur notably in the initiation of the tricarboxylic acid cycle by the transfer of an acetyl group to oxaloacetate to form citrate.

**transac'tion.** 1. Interaction arising from the encounter of two or more persons. 2. In transactional analysis, the unit of analysis involving a social stimulus and a response.

**transac'ylase.** Acyltransferase; see also *acetyl* t. and *malonyl* t.

**transal'dolase.** A transferase (EC 2.2.1.2), also known as dihydroxyacetonetransferase, interconverting sedoheptulose 7-phosphate plus glyceraldehyde 3-phosphate and erythrose 4-phosphate plus fructose 6-phosphate. See also transketolase.

**transal'dola'tion.** A reaction involving the transfer of an aldol group ($CH_2OHCOCHOH—$) from one compound to another; such reactions generally involve the sugar phosphates and occur in the phosphogluconate oxidation pathway of carbohydrate catabolism.

**transam'idinases.** Amidinotransferases.

**transam'idina'tion.** A reaction involving the transfer of an amidine group ($NH_2C=NH$) from one compound to another; the amidine donor is generally arginine and the reaction is of significance in the biosynthesis of creatine.

**transam'inases.** Aminotransferases.

**transam'ina'tion.** The reaction between an α- amino acid and an α-keto acid through which the amino group is transferred from the former to the latter.

**transanimation** (trans-an'ĭ-ma'shun) [ trans- + L. *anima*, breath, life ]. Resuscitation of a stillborn infant.

**transaudient** (trans-aw′dĭ-ent) [ trans- + L. *audio*, pres. p. *audiens*, to hear ]. Permeable to sound waves.

**transcalent** (trans-ka′lent) [ trans- + L. *caleo*, to be warm ]. Diathermanous.

**transcapsidation** (trans-kap′sĭ-da′shun). The phenomenon whereby the adenovirus capsid of the SV40 adenovirus "hybrid" is replaced by the capsid of another type of adenovirus; extended to include a similar phenomenon in other viruses.

**transcarbamoylase** (trans-kar-bam′o-il-ās). Carbamoyltransferase.

**transcarbox′ylase.** Carboxyltransferase.

**transcon′dylar.** Across or through the condyles; dentoing the line of bone incision in Carden's amputation.

**transcor′tical.** 1. Across or through the cortex of the brain, ovary, kidney, or other organ. 2. From one part of the cerebral cortex to another; denoting the various association tracts.

**transcor′tin.** Corticosteroid-binding globulin (CBG); corticosteroid-binding protein; an $\alpha_2$-globulin in blood that binds cortisol and corticosterone.

**trans′cuta′neous.** Percutaneous.

**transder′mic.** Percutaneous.

**transduce** (trans-dūs′). To effect transduction.

**transdu′cer** [ see transduction ]. A device designed to convert energy from one form to another; *e.g.*, a quartz crystal embedded in mercury can convert electrical energy to sound energy as is accomplished in sonic delay lines in computer storage systems.

    **pressure t.,** any of several devices designed to convert pressure differences into electrical current which can then be readily amplified and recorded.

**transdu′cing.** Pertaining to the mediation of transduction (*e.g.*, a transducing bacteriophage).

**transductant** (trans-duk′tant). A bacterium that has acquired a new character by means of transduction. T.'s may be *complete*, with integration of the transferred genetic fragment in its genome, or *abortive*, in which case the genetic fragment is not integrated and passes to only one of the two daughter cells on division.

**transduction** (trans-duk′shun) [ trans- + L. *duco*, pp. *ductus*, to lead across. DUC- ]. 1. The transfer of genetic material (and its phenotypic expression) from one bacterium to another by the mediation of bacteriophage. 2. The conversion of energy from one form to another.

    **abortive t.,** t. in which the genetic fragment from the donor bacterium is not integrated in the genome of the recipient bacterium, and, when the latter divides, is transmitted to only one of the daughter cells.

    **complete t.,** t. in which the transferred genetic fragment is fully integrated in the genome of the recipient bacterium.

    **general t.,** t. in which the transducing bacteriophage is able to transfer any gene of the donor bacterium.

    **high frequency t.,** specialized t. in which the donor bacterium contains not only the transducing, defective probacteriophage but also nondefective prophage that serves as "helper" virus, enabling most of the defective prophage particles to develop sufficiently to function as transducing agents.

    **low frequency t.,** specialized t. in which only a small portion of the prophage particles, because of their defectiveness, are able to develop sufficiently to serve as effective transducing agents.

    **specialized t.,** specific t.; t. in which the bacteriophage strain is able to transfer only some, or only one, of the donor bacterium genes.

    **specific t.,** specialized t.

**transection** (tran-sek′shun) [ trans- + L. *seco*, pp. *sectus*, to cut. SEC- ]. 1. A cross section. 2. Cutting across.

**trans′esterifica′tion.** Exchange of ester forms, as in conversion of glucose pentaacetate to glucose by sodium methylate with formation of methylacetate.

**transethmoidal** (trans′eth-moy′dal). Across or through the ethmoid bone.

**transfec′tion.** Infection of a bacterium or cell with nucleic acid (DNA or RNA) that has been isolated from bacteriophage or animal or plant virus, and that results in replication of complete virus.

**trans′fer** [ L. *trans-fero*, to bear across. FER- ]. A condition in which learning in one situation influences learning in another situation; a carry-over of learning; it may be positive in effect, as when learning one behavior facilitates the learning of something else, or it may be negative, as when one habit interferes with the acquisition of a later one.

**trans′ferases** Transferring enzymes; enzymes (EC class 2) transferring: one-carbon groups (2.1, including methyltransferases, 2.1.1; formyltransferases, 2.1.2; carboxyl- and carbamoyltransferases, 2.1.3, and amidinotransferases, 2.1.4); acyl residues (acyltransferases, 2.3); glycosyl residues (glycosyltransferases, 2.4, including hexosyltransferases, 2.4.1, and pentosyltransferases, 2.4.2); alkyl or aryl groups (2.5); nitrogenous groups (2.6); phosphorus-containing groups (2.7, phosphotransferases, *q.v.*); sulfur-containing groups (2.8, including sulfurtransferases, 2.8.1; sulfotransferases, 2.8.2; and CoA-transferases, 2.8.3).

**transfer′ence.** 1. The conveyance of an object from one place to another. 2. The shifting of symptoms from one side of the body to the other, as seen in certain cases of conversion hysteria. 3. The displacement of the affect from one person or one idea to another; in psychoanalysis, generally applied to the projection of feelings, thoughts and wishes onto the analyst, who has come to represent some person from the patient's past.

    **extrasensory thought t.,** telepathy; see also extrasensory *perception*.

    **t. love,** love expressed by the patient for the psychoanalyst as a manifestation of the t. situation.

    **negative t.,** t. characterized by predominantly hostile feelings on the part of the patient toward the analyst.

    **passive t.,** the passage of an immunity or allergic susceptibility by the injection of serum of an animal or individual who has acquired an active immunity to the disease.

    **positive t.,** t. characterized by predominantly friendly, respectful, and positive feelings on the part of the patient toward the analyst.

**transferrin** (trans-fĕr′in). Siderophilin; a $\beta_1$-globulin of the plasma, capable of associating reversibly with up to 1.25 μg. of iron per gm, and acting therefore as an iron transporting protein.

**transfer-RNA.** See under ribonucleic acid.

**trans′fix** [ L. *trans-figo*, pp. *-fixus*, to pierce through, fr. *figo*, to fasten ]. To pierce with a sharp instrument.

**transfixion** (trans-fik′shun) [ L. *transfixio* (see transfix) ]. A maneuver in amputation in which the knife is passed from side to side through the soft parts, close to the bone, and the muscles are then divided from within outward.

**transforate** (trans′fo-rāt) [ L. *trans-foro*, pp. *-atus*, to pierce through ]. To perforate; specifically, to bore through the base of the fetal skull as the first step in craniotomy.

**transforation** (trans′fo-ra′shun). Perforation of the base of the fetal skull in craniotomy.

**trans′forator.** An instrument for use in transforation.

**transform′ant.** A bacterium that has received genetic material (and its phenotypic expression) from another bacterium by means of transformation.

**transformation** (trans′for-ma′shun) [ L. *trans-formo*, pp. *-atus*, to transform ]. 1. Metamorphosis; change of form and shape. 2. A change of one tissue into another, as cartilage into bone. 3. Degeneration. 4. In metals, a change in phase and physical properties in the solid state caused by heat treatment. 5. In microbial genetics, transfer of genetic information between bacteria by means of "naked" intracellular DNA fragments derived from bacterial donor cells and incorporated into a competent recipient cell.

    **Haldane t.,** the multiplication of inspired oxygen concentration by the ratio of expired to inspired nitrogen concentrations in the calculation of oxygen consumption or respiratory quotient by the open circuit method.

    **Lobry de Bruyn-van Ekenstein t.,** the conversion of glucose to fructose and mannose in dilute alkali by enolization adjacent to the carbonyl group to form an enediol, a reaction analogous to certain biochemical transformations.

    **lymphocyte t.,** the t. into large, blastlike forms (immunoblasts) that occurs when lymphocytes are exposed to histoincompatible antigen either *in vitro* (mixed lymphocyte culture) or *in vivo* (organ transplant). See also mixed lymphocyte culture *test*.

**transfuse** (trans-fūz). To perform transfusion.

**transfusion** (trans-fu'zhun) [ L. *trans-fundo*, pp. -*fusus*, to pour from one vessel to another ]. 1. The transfer of blood from one person to another. 2. The injection into a vein of physiologic saline solution or, formerly, of other fluids such as milk.

  **arterial t.**, the passage of blood into an artery of the receptor or from an artery of the donor.

  **direct t.**, immediate t.; the transfer of blood from a vessel of one person (the donor) to one of another person (the receptor), either through a tube connecting the two vessles or by suturing the vessels together.

  **drip t.**, slow t. over a long time.

  **exchange t., exsanguina'tion t.**, substitution t.

  **immediate t.**, direct t.

  **indirect t.**, mediate t.; the donor is bled into a warmed vessel, the blood is defibrinated, and is then injected into a vein of the receptor.

  **intraarterial t.**, the injection of the transfusion fluid into an artery, radial, femoral, or the aorta, instead of into a vein, as is usual.

  **mediate t.**, indirect t.

  **peritoneal t.**, the injection of saline solution or other fluid into the peritoneal cavity whence it is absorbed into the circulation.

  **reciprocal t.**, an attempt to confer immunity by transfusing blood taken from a donor just recovered from an infectious disease into a receptor suffering from the same affection, the balance being maintained by transfusing an equal amount from the sick to the well person.

  **subcutaneous t.**, an infusion of absorbable solutions beneath the skin.

  **substitution t., total t.**, removal of most of the patient's blood followed by introduction of an equal amount, obtained from several donors, at least nine.

  **venous t.**, direct t. from a vein of the donor into a vein of the receptor.

**transglu'cosylase.** Glucosyltransferase.

**transgly'cosylase.** Glycosyltransferase.

**transient** (tran'shent, -zhent) [ L. *transiens*, pres. p. *transiens*, to cross over ]. A short-lived cardiac sound having little duration (less than 0.12 second) as distinct from a murmur; first, second, third, and fourth sounds, clicks, and opening snaps are t.'s.

**transient orange.** An orange intermediate compound formed in the bleaching of visual purple by light.

**transil'iac.** Extending from one ilium or iliac crest or spine to the other.

**transilient** (tran-sil'yent, -zil-) [ L. *trans-silio*, to leap across, fr. *salio*, to leap ]. Jumping across; passing over; pertaining to those cortical association fibers in the brain that pass from one convolution to another nonadjacent one.

**transillumination** (trans-ĭ-lu'mĭ-na'shun) [ trans- + L. *illumino*, pp. -*atus*, to light up ]. Method of examination by the passage of light through tissues or a body cavity.

**transin'sular.** Across the insula or island of Reil.

**transischiac** (trans-is'kĭ-ak). Extending from one ischium to the other.

**transisthmian** (trans-is'mĭ-an). Across any isthmus; specifically, across the isthmus of the gyrus fornicatus, denoting the gyrus transitivus.

**transition** (tran-sish'un, -zish'un) [ L. *transitio*, fr. *transeo*, pp. -*itus*, to go across ]. Change; passage from one condition or one part to another.

  **cervicothoracic t.**, the junction between the last cervical vertebra and first thoracic vertebra.

**transitional** (tran-sish'un-al, -zish-). Relating to or marked by a transition; transitory.

**transke'tolase.** Glycoaldehydetransferase; a transferase (EC 2.2.1.1) bringing about the interconversion of sedoheptulose 7-phosphate plus glyceraldehyde 3-phosphate and ribose 5-phosphate plus xylulose 5-phosphate; also other similar reactions, such as hydroxypyruvate and aldehyde into $CO_2$ and an extended hydroxypyruvate. See also transaldolase.

**transke'tola'tion.** A reaction involving the transfer of a ketol group ($CH_2OHCO$—) from one compound to another; see glycoaldehydetransferase.

**translation** (trans-la'shun) [ L. *translatio*, a transferring, fr. irreg. verb. *trans-fero*, pp. -*latus*, to carry across ]. Metastasis; transference.

**translocation** (trans'lo-ka'shun). The transposition of two segments between nonhomologous chromosomes as a result of abnormal breakage and refusion of reciprocal segments.

  **balanced t.**, the t. of the long arm of an acrocentric chromosome to another chromosome, accompanied by loss of the small fragment containing the centromere; an individual with a balanced t. is clinically normal but has a chromosome count of 45 and is capable of having children with an unbalanced t.

  **reciprocal t.**, t. without demonstrable loss of genetic material. See fig. under chromosome.

  **unbalanced t.**, condition resulting from fertilization of a gamete containing a t. chromosome by a normal gamete; if this abnormality is compatible with life, the individual would have 46 chromosomes but a segment of the t. chromosome would be represented three times in each cell and a partial or complete trisomic state would exist.

**translucent** (trans-lu'sent) [ L. *translucens*, fr. trans- + *luceo*, to shine through ]. Partially transparent; permitting light to pass through diffusely.

**transmem'brane.** Through or across a membrane.

**transmeth'ylase.** Methyltransferase.

**transmeth'yla'tion.** The transference of a methyl group from one compound to another; thus, homocysteine is converted to methionine by the transference to the latter of a methyl group derived from choline (*via* betaine and betaine-homocysteine methyltransferase, EC 2.1.1.5) or from *S*-adenosylmethionine (homocysteine methyltransferase, EC 2.1.1.10).

**transmigration** (trans-mi-gra'shun) [ L. *trans-migro*, pp. -*atus*, to remove from one place to another ]. Movement from one site to another; may entail the crossing of some usually limiting barrier, as in the passage of blood cells through the walls of the vessels (diapedesis).

  **o'vular t.**, the passage of an ovum from one ovary into the Fallopian tube of the other side; it is external, or direct, when it passes across the pelvic cavity, internal, or indirect, when it crosses the uterine cavity and so enters the tube of the opposite side.

**transmis'sible.** Capable of being transmitted (carried across) from one person to another, as a t. disease, an infectious or contagious disease.

**transmission** (trans-mish'un) [ L. *transmissio*, a sending across, fr. *trans-mitto*, pp. -*missus*, to send across ]. 1. Transfer. 2. The conveyance of disease from one person to another.

  **duplex t.**, the passage of impulses in both directions through a nerve trunk.

  **horizontal t.**, t. of infection by contact, in contradistinction to vertical t.

  **neurohumoral t.**, neurotransmission; a process by which a presynaptic cell, upon excitation, releases a specific chemical agent (a neurotransmitter) to cross a synapse to stimulate or inhibit the postsynaptic cell.

  **transovarial t.**, passage of a microorganism into the egg or embryo within the body of an infected female host, thus transferring an infection from mother to developing offspring; *e.g.*, *Rickettsia tsutsugamushi*, agent of tsutsugamushi disease, is transmitted by this manner to the developing eggs in the female vector, *Trombicula akamushi* or *Trombicula deliensis*.

  **vertical t.**, t. of a virus (*e.g.*, RNA tumor virus) by means of the genetic apparatus of a cell in which the viral genome is integrated.

**transmit'ter, transmit'tor.** See transmitter *substance*.

**transmu'ral** [ trans- + L. *murus*, wall ]. Through any wall, as of the body or of a cyst or any hollow structure.

**transmutation** (trans-mu-ta'shun) [ L. *trans-muto*, pp. -*atus*, to change, transmute ]. A change; transformation.

**transocular** (trans-ok'u-lar). Across the eye.

**transonance** (trans'o-nans) [ trans- + L. *sonans*, sounding ]. Transmission of a sound arising in one organ through another.

**transorbitome** (trans-or'bĭ-tōm) [ trans- + L. *orbita*, orbit, + G. *tomos*, cutting ]. A cutting instrument for piercing the roof of the orbit and performing transorbital lobotomy.

**transparietal** (trans-pă-ri'e-tal). Through or across a parietal region, area, or structure.

**transpep'tidase.** An enzyme catalyzing a transpeptidation reaction. Many proteolytic enzymes (*e.g.*, trypsin, papain) act as t.'s in the course of protolysis, forming an acylated enzyme as an intermediate in the process.

**transpep'tida'tion.** A reaction involving the transfer of one or more amino acids from one peptide chain to another as by "transpeptidase" action, or of a peptide chain itself, as in bacterial cell wall synthesis.

**transperitoneal** (trans-pĕr'ĭ-to-ne'al). Through the peritoneum; denoting, for example, a nephrectomy performed by abdominal section.

**transphos'phatase.** Phosphotransferase.

**transphosphorylase** (trans-fos-fōr'ĭ-lās). See phosphotransferase; phosphorylase; kinase.

**transphosphor'yla'tion.** A reaction involving the transfer of a phosphoric group from one compound to another, often with the involvement of adenosine triphosphate (ATP), as by the action of a phosphotransferase or kinase.

**transpinalis** (tran-spi-na'lis) [ L. ]. Any one of the muscular bands passing from one transverse process to another of the vertebrae.

**transpi'rable.** That can transpire or be transpired.

**transpiration** (tran-spī-ra'shun) [ trans- + L. *spiro*, pp. -*atus*, to breathe ]. The passage of watery vapor through the skin or any membrane; see also insensible *perspiration*.
  **pulmonary t.**, the passage of water vapor from the blood into the air via the respiratory tract.

**transpire** (tran-spīr) [ trans- + L. *spiro*, to breathe ]. To exhale vapor from the skin or respiratory mucous membrane.

**transplacen'tal.** Crossing the placenta.

**trans'plant** [ trans- + L. *planto*, to plant ]. 1. To transfer from one part to another, as in plastic operations or grafting. 2. The piece of tissue used in the operation of transplantation or grafting.
  **Gallie's t.**, narrow strips of the femoral fascia lata used for suture material.

**transplan'tar.** Across the sole of the foot; denoting certain muscular fibers or ligamentous structures.

**transplantation** (trans-plan-ta'shun) [ L. *trans-planto*, pp. -*atus*, to transplant ]. Grafting; implanting in one part a tissue or organ taken from another part or from another person. See also the subentries under graft.
  **heart t.**, replacement of severely damaged heart of a recipient with that of an otherwise healthy donor who died as a result of trauma, brain tumor, etc.
  **pancreaticoduodenal t.**, use of a homograft including both duodenum and pancreas as a method of treatment for diabetes mellitus, especially the severe juvenile type; pancreaticoduodenal transplants in man have shown that the procedure is technically feasible and that graft survival is possible within the limitations imposed by the rejection phenomenon.
  **renal t.**, use of a homograft obtained from an identical twin, a parent or sibling, a relative, or unrelated donors to restore kidney function in a recipient suffering from renal failure.
  **tendon t.**, tendon graft; the insertion of a slip from the tendon of a sound muscle into the tendon of a paralyzed muscle.
  **tooth t.**, the transfer of a tooth from one alveolus to another.

**transpleu'ral.** Through the pleura or across the pleural cavity; on the other side of the pleura.

**trans'port** [ L. *transporto*, to carry over, fr. trans- + *porto*, to carry ]. The movement or transference of biochemical substances.
  **active t.**, the passage of ions or molecules across a cell membrane, not by passive diffusion but by an energy-consuming process at the expense of catabolic processes

proceeding within the cell; in active t., movement takes place against an electrochemical gradient.

**transpose** (trans-pōz) [ L. *trans-pono*, pp. -*positus*, to place across, transfer ]. To transfer one tissue or organ to the place of another and *vice versa*.

**transposition** (trans-po-zish'un). 1. Removal from one place to another; transference; metathesis. 2. The state of being transposed or of being on the wrong side of the body, as in t. of the viscera, in which the viscera are on the side of the body opposite to that on which they are normally found, the liver being on the left, the apex of the heart on the right, etc.
  **t. of arterial stems**, t. of great vessels.
  **t. of the great vessels**, t. of arterial stems; a cyanotic form of congenital cardiovascular malformation in which the aorta arises from the right ventricle while the pulmonary artery arises from the left ventricle; for life to exist there must be an associated septal defect or patent ductus arteriosus to permit some crossflow between the two circulations.

**transsection** (trans-sek'shun). Transection.

**transsegmental** (trans-seg-men'tal). Across or through a segment.

**transseptal** (trans-sep'tal). Across or through a septum; on the other side of a septum.

**transsexual** (trans-sek'shu-al). 1. A person with the external genitalia and secondary sexual characteristics of one sex, but whose personal identification and psychosocial morphology is that of the opposite sex; a study of morphologic, genetic, and gonadal structure may be genitally congruent or incongruent. Such individuals often request surgery to relieve the conflict. 2. Denoting or relating to such a person. 3. Relating to medical and surgical procedures designed to alter a patient's external sexual characteristics so that they resemble those of the opposite sex.

**transsexualism** (trans-sek'shu-ă-lizm). 1. The state of being a transsexual. 2. Transsexual *surgery*.

**transsphenoidal** (trans'sfe-noy'dal). Through or across the sphenoid bone.

**transsulfurase** (trans-sul'fu-rās). Transulfurase; a descriptive term applied to the enzymes catalyzing, among others, the following reactions involving sulfur-containing compounds: (1) cystathionine → cysteine + α-ketobutyrate + NH₃ (cystathionine γ-lyase); (2) cystathionine → homocysteine + pyruvate + NH₃ (cystathionine β-lyase); (3) cystine → thiocysteine + pyruvate + NH₃ (cystathionine γ-lyase); (4) cystathionine → serine + homocysteine (cystathionine synthase).

**transsynaptic** (trans-sī-nap'tik). Indicating transmission of a nerve impulse across a synapse.

**transthalamic** (trans-thă-lam'ik). Passing across the thalamus.

**transther'mia** [ trans- + G. *thermē*, heat ]. Diathermy.

**transthoracic** (trans-tho-ras'ik). Passing through the thoracic cavity.

**transthoracotomy** (trans-tho'ră-kot'o-mĭ) [ trans- + thorax + G. *tomē*, incision ]. The operation of cutting through the chest.

**transubstantiation** (tran-sub-stan'shĭ-a'shun) [ trans- + L. *substantia*, substance ]. The substitution of one tissue for another, as in the experimental patching of an artery with peritoneal membrane.

**transudate** (tran'su-dāt) [ trans- + L. *sudo*, pp. -*atus*, to sweat ]. Term given to solvents and solutes that pass through membranes, such as the capillary wall, as a result of difference in hydrostatic pressure; the solvent filters through, and carries with it any solutes to which the membrane is permeable. Compare with exudate.

**transudation** (tran-su-da'shun) [ see transudate ]. The passage of a fluid or solute through a membrane by a hydrostatic or osmotic pressure gradient.

**transude** (tran-sūd'). To pass through a membrane; see transudation.

**transul'furase.** Transsulfurase.

**transurethral** (trans-u-re'thral). Through the urethra.

**transvaginal** (trans-vaj'ĭ-nal). Across or through the vagina.

**transvec′tor.** An animal that transmits a toxic substance that it does not produce, but that may be accumulated from animal (dinoflagellate) or plant (algae) sources; most commonly these are filter-feeding molluscs.

**transversa′lis** [ L. ] [ NA ]. Transverse.

**transverse** (trans-vers′) [ L. *transversus* ]. Crosswise; lying across the long axis of the body or of a part.

**transversectomy** (trans-ver-sek′to-mĭ) [ transverse + G. *ektomē*, excision ]. Exsection of the transverse process of a vertebra.

**transversion** (trans-ver′zhun). In dentistry, the eruption of a tooth in a position normally occupied by another; transposition of a tooth.

**transver′socos′tal.** Costotransverse.

**transversourethralis** (trans-ver-so-u-re-thra′lis). Denoting the transverse fibers of the sphincter urethrae muscle, arising from the arch of the pubes.

**transversus** [ L. fr. *trans*, across, + *verto*, pp. *versus*, to turn ] [ NA ]. Transverse.

**transvestism** (trans-ves′tizm) [ trans- + L. *vestio*, to dress ]. Transvestitism; the practice of dressing or masquerading in the clothes of the opposite sex.

    **male t.,** eonism; the adoption of feminine mannerisms and costume by a male.

**transvestite** (trans-ves tĭt). A person who practices transvestism.

**transvestitism** (trans-ves′tĭ-tizm). Transvestism.

**Trantas′ dots.** See under dot.

**Trantenroth,** Adolph A., German physician, *1867. See Bunge-T. *stain.*

**tranylcypromine sulfate** (tran′il-sip′ro-mēn). **(NF, BP).** PARNATE sulfate; (+)-*trans*-2-phenylcyclopropylamine sulfate; a monoamine oxidase inhibitor; an antidepressant used in the treatment of severe mental depression; hypertension, severe occipital headache, and intracranial bleeding may occur, particularly after eating tyramine-containing foods (*e.g.*, cheese).

**trape′zial.** Relating to any trapezium.

**trapeziform** (tră-pe′zĭ-form). Resembling a trapezium; trapezoid.

**trapeziometacarpal** (tră-pe′zĭ-o-met′ă-kar′pal). Relating to the trapezium and the metacarpus.

**trapezium,** pl. **trapezia, trapeziums** (tră-pe′zĭ-um, -ah) [ G. *trapezion*, a table or counter, a trapezium, dim. of *trapeza*, a table, fr. *tra-* (= *tetra-*), four, + *pous* (*pod-*), foot ]. 1. A four-sided geometrical figure having no two sides parallel. 2. *Os* trapezium.

**trape′zius.** *Musculus* trapezius.

**trapezoid** (trap′e-zoyd) [ G. *trapezōdēs*, fr. *trapezoin*, trapezium, + *eidos*, resemblance ]. 1. Trapeziform; resembling a trapezium. 2. A geometrical figure resembling a trapezium except that two of its opposite sides are parallel. 3. *Os* trapezoideum. 4. *Corpus* trapezoideum.

**Trapp,** Julius, Russian pharmaceutist, 1815–1908. See T.'s *formula*, T.-Häser *formula.*

**Traube** (trow′beh), Ludwig, German physician and pathologist, 1818–1876. See T.'s *bruit, corpuscles,* T.-Hering *curves,* T.'s *dyspnea, plugs, space,* double *tone,* T.-Hering *waves.*

**Traugott,** Carl, Frankfort internist, *1885. See Staub-T. *effect.*

**traum-, traumat-.** See traumato-.

**trauma,** pl. **traumata, traumas** (traw′mah, traw′mă-tah) [ G. wound ]. 1. Traumatism; an injury caused by rough contact with a physical object; accidental or inflicted wound. 2. In dentistry, an actual alteration of tissue produced by dental disharmony.

    **birth t.,** (1) physical injury to an infant during its delivery; (2) a psychological term that expresses the supposed emotional injury, inflicted by the events incident to birth, upon the psyche of the infant; sometimes appears in symbolic form in patients with mental disease.

    **occlusal t.,** abnormal occlusal stresses capable of producing or which have produced pathologic changes in the tooth and its surrounding structures.

    **psychic t.,** an upsetting experience precipitating or aggravating an emotional or mental disorder.

**traumasthenia** (traw-mas-the′nĭ-ah) [ traum- + G. *astheneia*, weakness ]. Nervous exhaustion following an injury.

**traumatic** (traw-mat′ik) [ G. *traumatikos* ]. Relating to or caused by a wound or injury.

**traumat′ic acid.** 2-Dodecenedioic acid; $HOOC(CH_2)_8CH = CHCOOH$; found in the tissues of certain plants after they have been cut or bruised; a plant hormone.

**traumatism** (traw′mă-tizm). Trauma.

**traumatize** (traw′mă-tize) [ G. *traumatizō*, to wound ]. To injure or wound.

**traumato-, traumat-, traum-** (traw′mă-to-) [ G. *trauma*, wound ]. Combining forms relating to a wound or injury.

**traumatology** (traw′mă-tol′o-jĭ) [ traumato- + G. *logos*, study ]. Accident surgery; the branch of surgery dealing with wounds.

**traumatonesis** (traw′mă-to-ne′sis, -ton′e-sis) [ traumato- + G. *neois*, a spinning ]. Surgical repair of an accidental wound.

**traumatopathy** (traw-mă-top′ă-thĭ) [ traumato- + G. *pathos*, suffering ]. Any pathologic condition resulting from violence or wounds.

**traumatophilia** (traw′mă-to-fil′ĭ-ah) [ traumato- + G. *phileō*, to love ]. The unconscious craving for, or tendency toward, sustaining injury; *cf.* masochism.

**traumatophobia** (traw′mă-to-fo′bĭ-ah) [ traumato- + G. *phobos*, fear ]. Morbid fear of injury.

**traumatopnea** (traw-mă-top-ne′ah) [ traumato- + G. *pnoē*, breath ]. The passage of air in and out through a wound of the chest wall.

**traumatopyra** (traw-mă-to-pi′rah) [ traumato- + G. *pyr*, fire, fever ]. Traumatic *fever.*

**traumatosepsis** (traw′mă-to-sep′sis) [ traumato- + sepsis, *q.v.* ]. Infection of a wound; septicemia following a wound.

**trau′matother′apy.** Treatment of trauma or the result of injury.

**Trautmann** (trowt′mahn), Moritz F., German surgeon, 1832–1902. See T.'s triangular *space.*

**tray.** A flat receptacle with raised edges.

    **acrylic resin t.,** a plastic impression t. used in dentistry; usually fashioned for the individual patient from an autopolymerizing acrylic resin.

    **annealing t.,** an electrically heated, thermostatically controlled device used to drive off the protective $NH_3$ gas coating from the surface of cohesive gold foil.

    **impression t.,** a receptacle.

**Treacher Collins.** See Collins, Edward Treacher.

**treacle** (tre′kl) [ G. *thēriakos*, theriaca, *q.v.* ]. 1. Molasses; a viscid syrup that drains from sugar refining molds. 2. A saccharine fluid. 3. Formerly, a remedy for poison, hence any effective remedy; see alo theriaca.

**treat** (trēt) [ Fr. *traiter*, fr. L. *tracto*, to drag, handle, perform ]. To attack a disease by medicinal, surgical, dietary, or other measures; to care for a patient medically or surgically.

**treatment** (trēt′ment) [ Fr. *traitement* (see treat) ]. Therapeutics; therapy; the medical or surgical care of a patient; the institution of measures or the giving of remedies designed to cure a disease. For types of treatment not listed here, see also subentries under therapy and under vaccine.

    **active t.,** energetic t. directly applied to the disease.

    **Allen's t.,** the so-called starvation t. of diabetes by means of certain days of absolute fasting followed by a spare diet with a minimum amount of carbohydrate.

    **Beauperthuy's t.,** t. of leprosy by mercury bichloride.

    **Carrel's t.,** t. of wounds by intermittent irrigation with Dakin's fluid by means of narrow tubes, the latter being made to flush every part of the surface, the wound having previously been freed from all foreign material and dead tissue. Also called Dakin-Carrel t.

    **causal t.,** t. directed to the removal of the cause of a disease.

    **conservative t.,** (1) abstention from the giving of remedies or from operative procedures until clear indications present themselves; (2) t. of an injured part by means directed to the preservation of the part, avoiding surgical mutilation.

**curative t.,** active t.; t. aiming at a cure of existing disease; distinguished from palliative and prophylactic t.

**Dakin-Carrel t.,** Carrel's t.

**drug t.,** pharmacotherapy; the use of drugs, as distinguished from water, air, heat, electricity, and other natural forces, exercise, diet, etc., in the t. of disease.

**empir'ical t.,** empiric medicine; empirical therapeutics; the use of remedies or measures which experience has shown to be of benefit in the disease in question, but for the success of which no scientific explanation can be given.

**expectant t.,** management of disease by t. of the symptoms as they arise, as distinguished from t. directed to the specific cause.

**Goeckerman t.,** a t. for psoriasis; the involved areas are painted with a solution of coal tar, or are covered with coal tar ointment and subsequently irradiated with ultraviolet.

**heat t.,** a method of controlled temperature handling of metals so as to change the microscopic structure and thus the physical properties; see also temper; anneal.

**heroic t.,** aggressive, daring t., which in itself may endanger the patient.

**hygien'ic t.,** t. by fresh air, cleanliness, and other nonmedicinal measures.

**insulin shock t.,** the t. of major mental illness by means of hypoglycemic convulsions induced by insulin; now rarely used.

**isoserum t.,** therapeutic use of serum taken from a person having or having had the same disease as the patient under treatment.

**Kenny's t.,** a method for the t. of anterior poliomyelitis. The affected parts are wrapped in woolen cloth wrung out of hot water. After the acute stage has passed, the limbs are passively exercised to reeducate the paralyzed muscles.

**light t.,** phototherapy.

**Mayo's t.,** of a bunion; a bunionectomy the principle feature of which is resection of the first metatarsal head.

**medical t.,** conservative t. of disease by hygienic and medicinal remedies, as distinguished from surgical t.

**medic'inal t.,** the use of drugs in therapy.

**milk t.,** t. by a diet containing nothing but milk.

**Mitchell's t.,** rest in bed, isolation, and a nourishing diet in the t. of neuroses.

**moral t.,** psychotherapy.

**Nauheim t.** (now'him) [ *Nauheim*, a city in Germany ], Nauheim bath; t. of certain cardiac affections by baths in water through which carbonic acid gas is bubbling, followed by resisting exercises and sometimes the terrain cure. Called also, after the originators, the Schott t.

**Oppenheimer t.,** a method of t. of alcoholism and drug addiction.

**pal'liative t.,** t. to alleviate symptoms without curing the disease.

**preventive t.,** prophylactic t.

**prophylac'tic t.,** preventive t.; the institution of measures designed to protect a person from an attack of a disease to which he has been, or is liable to be exposed.

**prolonged sleep t.,** Dauerschlaf; the treatment of certain mental disorders by means of prolonged sleep.

**rational t.,** t. based upon a knowledge of the nature of the disease and of the action of the remedies used to combat it; distinguished from empirical t.

**rest t.,** rest *cure*.

**root canal t.,** (1) the means by which painful or diseased teeth, in which the pulp is involved, are restored to a healthy state; (2) removal of a normal, diseased, or dead pulp by biochemical and mechanical means, enlargement and sterilization of the root canal, followed by filling the canal, to effect healing of diseased periapical tissues; (3) the diagnosis and t. of diseases of the pulp and their sequelae.

**sand t.,** psammotherapy.

**Schott t.,** Nauheim t.

**shock t.,** a form of psychiatric t., used in certain types of schizophrenia and mood disorders, in which a chemical substance or sufficient electric current is employed to produce a convulsive seizure and unconsciousness; the mechanism of action is still unknown.

**solar t.,** t. by sunlight.

**specific t.,** specific therapeutics; specific therapy; t. directed to the removal of the intrinsic cause of a disease; t. of a disease by a remedy acting especially against it or

its cause, as of malaria by quinine or of syphilis by mercury or arsphenamine.

**supporting t.,** t. directed toward maintaining the strength of the patient until the disease, self-limited in character, shall have spent its force.

**surgical t.,** t. by any manual or cutting operation.

**symptomat'ic t.,** expectant t.

**terrain t.,** see terrain *cure*.

**tonic t.,** t. of syphilis by the administration of small doses of mercury continued over a long period.

**Tweed edgewise t.,** see edgewise *appliance*.

**whey t.,** t. consisting of drinking large amounts of whey.

**trehala** (tre-hah'lah). A saccharine substance resembling manna, excreted by an insect, *Larinus maculatus*.

**trehalose** (tre'hah-lōs). Mycose; a nonreducing disaccharide, α-D-glucosido-α-D-glucoside, contained in trehala.

**Treitz** (tritz), Wenzel, Austrian physician, 1819–1872. See T.'s *arch, fascia, fossa, hernia, ligament, muscle.*

**Trélat** (tra-lah'), Ulysse, French surgeon, 1828–1890. See T.'s *sign, speculum, stools,* Leser-T. *sign.*

**trema** (tre'mah) [ G. *trēma*, a hole. TREM- ]. 1. Foramen. 2. The vulva.

**Trematoda** (trem'ă-to'dah) [ G. *trēmatōdēs*, full of holes, fr. *trēma*, a hole, + *eidos*, appearance ]. A class in the phylum Platyhelminthes (the flatworms), consisting of flukes with a leaf-shaped body and two muscular suckers, and an acoelomate parenchyma-filled body cavity. Circulatory system and sense organs are not present, but an incomplete alimentary canal is found (lacking an anus). Flukes of interest to human or veterinary medicine are members of the order Digenea, with complete life cycles involving embryonic multiplication in a mollusc first intermediate host. The other order, Monogenea, are chiefly parasites of fish and have a simpler pattern of direct development on a single host.

**trem'atode, trem'atoid.** 1. The common name for a parasitic worm of the class Trematoda, a fluke. 2. Relating to a fluke, or trematoid worm.

**trem'atol.** A toxic constituent of white snakeroot, *Eupatorium urticaefolium,* which causes trembles in domestic animals and milk sickness in man.

**trembles** (trem'blz) [ L. *tremulus,* trembling, fr. *tremo,* to tremble ]. An intoxication of cattle, caused by eating the white snakeroot or the rayless goldenrod; the active agent is supposed to be a higher alcohol, trematol. Intoxicated cows eliminate the poison in their milk, which causes milk sickness when ingested by man.

**tremb'ling.** Shaking; quaking; see also tremor.

**tremelloid, tremellose** (trem'ĕ-loyd, -lōs) [ L. *tremulus,* trembling ]. Jelly-like.

**tre'mens** [ L. pres. p. of *tremo,* to tremble ]. 1. Trembling; quaking. 2. *Delirium* tremens.

**trem'ogram.** The graphic representation of a tremor taken by means of the tremograph or kymograph.

**trem'ograph** [ L. *tremor,* a shaking, + G. *graphō,* to write ]. An apparatus for making a graphic record of a tremor.

**tremolabile** (tre'mo-la'bil, trem'o-) [ L. *tremor,* a shaking, + *labilis,* perishable ]. Inactivated or destroyed by shaking.

**tremophobia** (trem'o-fo'bĭ-ah) [ L. *tremor,* trembling, + G. *phobos,* fear ]. Morbid fear of trembling.

**trem'or** [ L. a shaking ]. Trembling; shaking.

**action t.,** intention t.

**alternating t.,** a form of hyperkinesia characterized by regular, symmetrical, to-and-fro movements (at about 4 per second) that are produced by patterned, alternating contraction of muscles and their antagonists.

**arsenical t.,** one caused by chronic poisoning by arsenic.

**t. ar'tuum,** trembling of the extremities, especially of the hands.

**benign essential t.,** heredofamilial t.

**coarse t.,** one in which the amplitude is large and the vibrations number not more than six or seven per second.

**continuous t.,** persistent t.

**epidemic t.,** avian infectious encephalomyelitis; a virus disease of very young chicks characterized by t., ataxia, somnolence, and finally death.

**fi'brillary t.,** isolated twitching of the fine strands or fasciculi of a muscle.

**fine t.,** one in which there are 10 or 12 vibrations per second.

**flapping t.,** asterixis.

**heredofamilial t.,** benign essential t.; status macrobioticus multiparus; t. inherited as a dominant character; it may be a rapid oscillation resembling that seen in thyrotoxicosis, a coarse t. during rest and inhibited by a voluntary effort, or one which appears only upon movement; it is benign in nature.

**intention t.,** action t.; volitional t. (2); a t. that occurs when a voluntary movement is made.

**kinetic t.,** t. occurring during active movement of the limb.

**mercu'rial t.,** one caused by chronic mercury poisoning.

**metal'lic t.,** t. caused by poisoning with metal.

**t. opiophago'rum,** a t. occurring in opium addicts.

**passive t.,** one that occurs when the subject is at rest, and diminishes or ceases during voluntary movement.

**persistent t.,** continuous t.; a t. that is constant, whether the subject is at rest or moving.

**postural t.,** static t.

**t. potato'rum,** a t. occurring in the subjects of chronic alcoholism.

**progressive cerebellar t.,** Hunt's *syndrome* (1).

**sat'urnine t.,** a t. caused by chronic lead poisoning.

**senile t.,** a t., usually an intention t., but sometimes a persistent t., occurring in the aged.

**static t.,** postural t.; a t. excited when the person makes an effort to hold a limb in a certain position.

**t. ten'dinum,** *subsultus* tendinum.

**volit'ional t.,** (1) one that can be arrested by a strong effort of the will; (2) intention t.

**trem'orgram.** Tremogram.

**trem'orine.** 1,4-Dipyrrolidino-2-butyne; an agent used experimentally to produce Parkinson-like tremors, salivation, diarrhea, and other parasympathomimetic effects. Can be counteracted by atropine and similar drugs.

**tremostable** (tre'mo'sta'bl, -trem'o-) [ L. *tremor*, a shaking, + *stabilis*, stable ]. Not subject to alteration or destruction by being shaken.

**trem'ulor.** An instrument for giving vibratory massage.

**trem'ulous.** Characterized by tremor.

**Trenaunay** (tren-o-ni'), Paul, French physician, *1875. See Klippel-T.-Weber *syndrome*.

**trend.** the general course or direction, or the prevailing tendency.

**psychiatric t.,** benign or malignant emotional interests and urges as revealed by postures, gestures, actions, or speech.

**t. of thought,** thinking with a tendency toward or centering on a particular idea with a particular affect.

**Trendel'enburg,** Freidrich, German surgeon, 1844–1924. See T.'s *operation, position, sign, symptom, test*.

**trepan** (tre-pan') [ G. *trepanon*, a borer. TRIB- ]. 1. A trephine. 2. To trephine.

**trepanation** (trep'ă-na'shun). Trephination.

**t. of the cornea,** the removal of a circular bit from the cornea in the treatment of anterior corneal staphyloma and corneal transplants.

**trepan'ner.** Trephiner.

**trephination** (tref'ĭ-na'shun). Trepanation; removal of a circular piece ("button") of cranium by a trephine.

**trephine** (tre-fīn', -fēn') [ contrived (Woodall, 1628) fr. L. *tres fines*, three ends; probably suggested by trepan, *q.v.* ]. 1. A cylindrical or crown saw used for the removal of a disc of bone, especially from the skull, or of other firm tissue as that of the cornea. 2. To remove a disc of bone or other tissue by means of a t.

**trephi'ner.** Trepanner; one who trephines.

**trephocyte** (tref'o-sīt) [ G. *trephō*, to nourish, + *kytos*, cell ]. Trophocyte.

**trep'idant** [ L. *trepidans*, pres. p. of *trepido*, to tremble, to be agitated ]. Trembling; marked by tremor.

**trepida'tio** [ L. ]. Trepidation.

**t. cordis,** palpitation.

**trepidation** (trep'ĭ-da'shun) [ L. *trepidatio*, fr. *trepido*, to tremble, to be agitated ]. 1. Trembling; tremor. 2. Anxious fear.

**Treponema** (trep'o-ne'mah) [ G. *trepō*, to turn, + *nēma*, thread ]. A genus of anaerobic bacteria (order Spirochaetales) consisting of cells, 3 to 8 μm in length, with acute, regular, or irregular spirals and no obvious protoplasmic structure. A terminal filament may be present. They stain with difficulty except with Giemsa's stain or silver impregnation. Some species are pathogenic and parasitic for man and other animals, generally producing local lesions in tissues. The type species is *T. pallidum*.

**T. callig'yrum,** a species found in lesions and membranes of the pudenda.

**T. carateum,** a species that causes pinta, or carate.

**T. cunic'uli,** a species which causes spirochaetosis in rabbits.

**T. genitalis,** a nonpathogenic species found on the genitalia of man.

**T. microden'tium,** a species found in the normal oral cavity.

**T. muco'sum,** a species found in pyorrhea alveolaris; it possesses pyogenic properties.

**T. pal'lidum,** a species which causes syphilis in man. This organism can be experimentally transmitted to anthrapoid apes and to rabbits. It is the type species of the genus *T.*

**T. perten'ue,** a species which causes yaws, tropica frambesia. Patients with this disease give a positive Wasserman test.

**trep'onemato'sis.** Treponemiasis.

**treponemiasis** (trep'o-ne-mi'ă-sis). Treponematosis; infection caused by *Treponema*.

**treponemicidal** (trep'o-ne'mĭ-si'dal) [ *Treponema* + L. *caedo*, to kill ]. Antitreponemal; destructive to any species of *Treponema*, but usually with reference to *T. pallidum*.

**trepopnea** (tre-pop'ne-ah) [ G. *trepō*, to turn, + *pnoē*, breathing ]. Selective orthopnea; the clinical situation in which breathing is comfortable in one position but not in another; *e.g.*, turning from the left to the right lateral recumbent position may relieve respiratory distress.

**treppe** (trep'eh) [ Ger. staircase ]. Staircase phenomenon; a phenomenon in cardiac muscle first observed by Bowditch; if a number of stimuli of the same intensity are sent into the muscle after a quiescent period, the first few contractions of the series show a successive increase in amplitude.

**Tresil'ian,** Frederick J., British physician, 1862–1926. See T.'s *sign*.

**tre'sis** [ G. *trēsis*, a boring. TREM- ]. Perforation.

**tret'inoin** (USP). *trans*-Retinoic acid; a ketolytic agent; see retinoic acid.

**Treves,** Frederick, English surgeon, 1853–1923. See T.'s *fold*.

**Treves,** Norman. See Stewart-T. *syndrome*.

**TRF.** Abbreviation for thyrotropin-releasing *factor*.

**tri-** [ L. and G. ]. A prefix denoting three.

**triace'tic acid.** 3,5-Dioxohexanoic acid; $CH_3COCH_2COCH_2COOH$; formed by condensation of acetyl and malonyl CoA's in the course of fatty acid synthesis.

**triacetin** (tri-as'ĕ-tin). Glyceryl triacetate.

**triacet'yloleandomy'cin.** Troleandomycin.

**triacylglycerol.** Triglyceride; glycerol esterified at each of its three hydroxyl groups by a fatty (aliphatic) acid; *e.g.*, tristearoylglycerol (formerly tristearin).

**triacylglycerol lipase** (EC 3.1.1.3). Pancreatic lipase; tributyrase; tributyrinase; steapsin; sometimes called simply lipase (*q.v.*); the fat-splitting enzyme in pancreatic juice.

**tri'ad** [ G. *trias (triad-)*, the number 3, fr. *tries*, three ]. 1. A collection of three things having something in common. 2. The transverse tubule and the terminal cisternae on each side of it in skeletal muscle fibers. 3. The father, mother, and child relationship projectively experienced in group psychotherapy.

**acute compression t.,** the rising venous pressure, falling arterial pressure, and small quiet heart of cardiac tamponade.

**Beck's t.,** acute compression t.

**Bezold's t.,** diminished perception of the deeper tones, retarded bone conduction, and negative Rinne's test, pointing, in the absence of objective signs, to otosclerosis.

**Charcot's t.,** in multiple (disseminated) sclerosis the three symptoms, nystagmus, tremor, and scanning speech.

**Fallot's t.,** *trilogy* of Fallot.

**Hull's t.,** the association of diastolic gallop, anasarca, and small pulse pressure.

**Hutchinson's t.,** parenchymatous keratitis, labyrinthine disease, and Hutchinson's teeth, significant of congenital syphilis.

**Saint's t.,** hiatal hernia, gallstones, and diverticulosis.

**triage** (tre′ahzh) [ Fr. sorting ]. The medical screening of patients to determine their priority for treatment; the separation of a large number of casualties, in military or civilian disaster medical care, into three groups: those who cannot be expected to survive even with treatment; those who will recover without treatment; and the priority group of those who need treatment in order to survive.

**triakaidekaphobia** (tri′ă-kai-dek-ă-fo′bĭ-ah). Triskaidekaphobia.

**trial and error.** The apparently random, haphazard, hit-or-miss exploratory activity which often precedes the acquisition of new information or adjustments; it may be overt, as in a rat running in a maze, or covert (vicarious), as when one thinks of various ways of coping with a situation.

**triamcinolone** (tri′am-sin′o-lōn). ARISTOCORT; KENACORT; 9α-fluoro-16α-hydroxyprednisolone. A glucocorticoid with actions and uses similar to those of prednisolone, but has greater anti-inflammatory potency and lacks the sodium-retaining and edema-producing properties characteristic of most glucocorticoids. May cause dizziness, weight loss, and muscular weakness.

**t. acetonide** (USP, BP), KENALOG; a potent glucocorticoid for topical treatment of dermatoses; USAN lists t. acetonide sodium phosphate (ARISTOSOL).

**t. diacetate** (NF). ARISTOCORT diacetate; an anti-inflammatory and antiallergic agent for parenteral use.

**triamelia** (tri′ă-me′lĭ-ah) [ tri- + G. *a-* priv. + *melos*, limb ]. Absence of three limbs.

**triamterene** (tri-am′ter-ēn) (USP, BP). DYRENIUM; 2,4,7-triamino-6-phenylpteridine; used in combination with thiazides to enhance their hypotensive and diuretic effects.

# TRIANGLE

**triangle** (tri′ang-gl) [ L. *triangulum*, fr. *tri-*, three, + *angulus*, angle ]. 1. A geometrical figure having three straight lines, joined two by two, forming three angles. 2. In anatomy and surgery, a more or less triangular area bounded by muscles, bony prominences, or other structures, within which are normally found certain important nerves or blood vessels; see also trigone and trigonum.

**Alsberg's t.,** an equilateral t. formed by lines passing through the long axis of the femoral diaphysis, the long axis of the femoral neck, and the base of the femoral head.

**anal t.,** *regio* analis.

**anterior t.,** a large area in the neck bounded by the mandible, the anterior border of the sternocleidomastoid muscle, and the anterior midline of the neck; it is subdivided into carotid, muscular, submandibular, and submental t.'s.

**Assézat's t.,** a t. formed by lines connecting the nasion with the alveolar and nasal points. Used to indicate prognathism in comparative craniology.

**auric′ular t.,** a t. formed by the base of the auricle and by lines drawn from the true tip of the auricle to the extremities of the base.

**t. of ausculta′tion,** space bounded by the lower border of the trapezius, the latissimus dorsi, and the rhomboideus major muscles.

**ax′illary t.,** a triangular area embracing the medial aspect of the arm, the axilla, and the pectoral region which is one of the seats of predilection for the petechial initial rash of smallpox.

**Béclard's t.,** area bounded by the posterior border of the hyoglossus muscle, the posterior belly of the digastric and the greater cornu of the hyoid bone.

**Bonwill t.,** an equilateral t. formed by lines from the contact points of the lower central incisors, or the medial line of the residual ridge of the mandible, to the condyle on either side and from one condyle to the other.

**Bryant's t.,** iliofemoral t.; a line (*a*) is drawn around the body at the level of the anterior superior iliac spines; from this line another (*b*) is drawn perpendicular to it to the great trochanter of the femur, and the t. is completed by a line (*c*) drawn from the trochanter to the iliac spine; upward displacement of the trochanter, in fracture of the neck of the femur, is measured along line *b.*

**car′diohepat′ic t.,** an area in the fifth intercostal space on the right side, marking the interval between the heart and the liver.

**carotid t.'s,** (1) inferior: muscular t.; (2) superior: *trigonum* caroticum.

**cephal′ic t.,** a t. on the cranium formed by lines connecting the metopion, the pogonion, and the occipital point.

**crural t.,** an area of predilection for the petechial initial rash of smallpox; it occupies the lower abdominal, inguinal, and genital regions and the inner aspects of the thighs, the base of the t. traversing the umbilicus.

**digas′tric t.,** *trigonum* submandibulare.

**Einthoven's t.,** an imaginary equilateral t. with the heart at its center, formed by lines representing the three standard limb leads of the electrocardiogram.

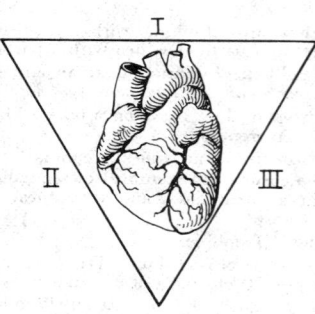

**Einthoven's Triangle**

**Elaut's t.,** t. formed by the iliac arteries and the promontory of the sacrum.

**t. of elbow,** a space between the pronator teres and the brachioradialis muscles on the flexor side of the elbow.

**facial t.,** a t. formed by lines connecting the basion, the prosthion, and the nasion.

**Farabeuf's t.,** the t. formed by the internal jugular and facial veins and the hypoglossal nerve.

**fem′oral t.,** *trigonum* femorale.

**t. of fillet,** *trigonum* lemnisci.

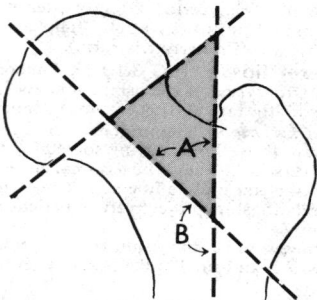

**Alsberg's Triangle (*shaded area*)**

*A,* Alsberg's angle (angle of elevation); *B,* angle of inclination (angle of depression).

**frontal t.,** a t. bounded above by the maximum frontal diameter and laterally by lines joining the extremities of this diameter with the glabella.

**Gombault's t.,** see *fasciculus* semilunaris.

**Grocco's t.,** paravertebral t.; a triangular patch of dullness at the base of the chest alongside the spinal column, on the side opposite a pleural effusion.

**Grynfeltt's t.,** Lesshaft's t.; a triangular space bounded above by the end of the last rib and the serratus posterior inferior muscle, anteriorly by the obliquus internus, and posteriorly by the quadratus lumborum; lumbar hernia occurs in this space.

**Hesselbach's t.,** *trigonum* inguinale.

**iliofem′oral t.,** Bryant's t.

**inferior carotid t.,** muscular t.

**inferior occip′ital t.,** has its apex at the external occipital protuberance; its base is formed by a line joining the two mastoid processes.

**infraclavic′ular t.,** trigonum deltoideopectorale; deltopectoral trigone; a t. bounded by the clavicle and the adjacent borders of the deltoid and pectoralis major muscles.

**in′guinal t.,** *trigonum* inguinale.

**Labbé's t.,** an area bounded below by a horizontal line touching the lower edge of the cartilage of the left ninth rib, laterally by the line of the false ribs, and to the right side by the liver; here the stomach is normally in contact with the abdominal wall.

**Langenbeck's t.,** a t. formed by lines drawn from the anterior superior iliac spine to the surface of the great trochanter and to the surgical neck of the femur; a penetrating wound in this area probably involves the joint.

**Lesser's t.,** the space between the bellies of the digastric muscle and the hypoglossal nerve.

**Lesshaft's t.,** Grynfeltt's t.

**Lieutaud's t.,** *trigonum* vesicae.

**lumbar t.,** *trigonum* lumbale.

**lum′bocos′toabdom′inal t.,** an irregular area bounded by the serratus posterior inferior, obliquus externus, obliquus internus, and erector spinae muscles.

**Macewen's t.,** suprameatal t.

**Malgaigne's t.,** *trigonum* caroticum.

**Marcille's t.,** an area bounded by the medial border of the psoas major, the lateral margin of the vertebral column, and the iliolumbar ligament below; it is crossed by the obturator nerve.

**muscular t.,** inferior carotid t.; bounded by the sternocleidomastoid muscle, the superior belly of the omohyoid muscle, and the anterior midline of the neck; the infrahyoid muscles occupy most of the t.

**occip′ital t.,** a t. of the neck bounded by the trapezius, the sternocleidomastoid, and the omohyoid muscles; see also inferior occipital t.

**omoclavicular t.,** *trigonum* omoclaviculare.

**pal′atal t.,** a triangular area bounded by the greatest transverse diameter of the palate and by lines converging from its extremities to the alveolar point.

**paraver′tebral t.,** Grocco's t.

**Petit's lumbar t.,** *trigonum* lumbale.

**Philippe's t.,** see *fasciculus* semilunaris.

**Pirogoff's t.,** formed by the intermediate tendon of the digastric muscle, the posterior border of the mylohyoid muscle, and the hypoglossal nerve.

**posterior t. of neck,** *regio* colli lateralis.

**pouboure′thral t.,** a t. in the perineum bounded by the transversus perinei, the ischiocavernosus, and the bulbocavernosus muscles.

**Reil's t.,** *trigonum* lemnisci.

**sacral t.,** the surface area over the sacrum.

**t. of safety,** the area at the lower left sternal border where the pericardium is not covered by lung.

**Scarpa's t.,** *trigonum* femorale.

**sternocostal t.,** *trigonum* sternocostale.

**subcla′vian t.,** *trigonum* omoclaviculare.

**subin′guinal t.,** *trigonum* femorale.

**submandib′ular t.,** *trigonum* submandibulare.

**submax′illary t.,** *trigonum* submandibulare.

**submen′tal t.,** a t. bounded on either side by the anterior belly of a digastric muscle, and below by the hyoid bone; the mylohyoid muscle forms its floor.

**suboccip′ital t.,** one bounded by the obliquus inferior, the obliquus superior, and the rectus capitis posterior major muscles.

**superior carot′id t.,** *trigonum* caroticum.

**suprame′atal t.,** Macewen's t.; a t. formed by the root of the zygomatic arch, the posterior wall of the bony external acoustic meatus, and an imaginary line connecting the extremities of the first two lines; used as a guide in mastoid operations.

**surgical t.,** see t. (2).

**tracheal t.,** inferior carotid t.

**umbil′icomam′millary t.,** a t. with apex at the umbilicus and base at the line joining the nipples.

**urogenital t.,** *regio* urogenitalis.

**ves′ical t.,** *trigonum* vesicae.

**Ward's t.,** an area seen within the trabecular of the neck of the femur evident by x-rays as well as by direct inspection.

**Weber's t.,** on the sole of the foot, an area indicated by the heads of the first and fifth metatarsal bone and the center of the plantar surface of the heel.

**Wilde's t.,** *cone* of light.

**Woelde's t.,** *cone* of light.

**triangula′ris** [ L. ]. See under musculus.

**triangulum** (tri-ang′u-lum) [ L. ]. Triangle; trigone.

**tri′azol′ogua′nine.** 8-Azaguanine.

**tribade** (trib′ād) [ G. *tribō*, to rub ]. A homosexual woman (lesbian), particularly designating one who obtains sexual pleasure by rubbing her external genitalia against those of another woman.

**trib′adism, trib′ady** [ G. *tribō*, to rub ]. Lesbianism, particularly as characterized by a tribade.

**triba′sic.** Having three titratable hydrogen atoms; denoting an acid with a basicity of 3.

**tribas′ilar.** Having three bases.

**tribe** [ L. *tribus* ]. In biological classification, an occasional division between the family and the genus; often the same as the subfamily.

**tribology** (trī-bol′o-jī) [ G. *tribō*, to rub, + *logos*, study ]. The study of friction and its effects in biological systems, notably in regard to articulated surfaces of the skeleton.

**triboluminescence** (trī′bo-lu′mī-nes′ens) [ G. *tribō*, to rub, + luminescence ]. Luminosity caused by friction.

**tribrachia** (tri-bra′kī-ah) [ tri- + G. *brachiōn*, arm ]. A condition seen in conjoined twins when the fusion has merged the adjacent arms to form a single one, so that there are only three arms for the two bodies.

**tribra′chius** (tri-bra′kī-us). Conjoined twins exhibiting tribrachia.

**tribro′moeth′anol.** $Br_3C$—$CH_2OH$; a crystalline hypnotic supplied as AVERTIN in a solution with amylene hydrate for rectal anesthesia.

**tribro′mohy′drin.** 1,2,3 Tribromopropane; allyl tribromide; $C_3H_5Br_3$. Used as a nematocide.

**tribro′mometh′ane.** Bromoform.

**tribulosis** (trib′u-lo′sis). Poisoning with the puncturevine, *Tribulus terrestris*, occurring particularly in sheep.

**tribu′tyrase.** Triacylglycerol lipase.

**tribu′tyrin.** Tributyrylglycerol.

**tributyrinase** (tri-bu′tī-rī-nās). Triacylglycerol lipase.

**TRIC.** Abbreviation for trachoma and inclusion conjunctivitis; see TRIC *agent*.

**tricalc′ium phosphate.** calcium phosphate, tribasic.

**tricarboxylic acid cycle** (tri-kar′bok-sil′ik). See under cycle.

**tricel′lular.** Three-celled.

**tricephalus** (tri-sef′ă-lus) [ tri- + G. *kephalē*, head ]. A fetus with three heads.

**tri′ceps** [ L. fr. *tri-*, three, + *capui*, head ]. Three-headed; denoting especially two muscles: **T. brachii** and **t. surae**, which see under musculus.

**trich-.** See tricho-.

**trichalgia** (trik-al′jī-ah) [ trich- + G. *algos*, pain ]. Trichodynia; pain produced by touching the hair.

**trichangiectasia, trichangiectasis** (trik′an-jī-ek-ta′zī-ah, -ek′tă-sis) [ trich- + G. *angeion*, vessel, + *ektasis*, extension ]. Telangiectasia.

**trichangion** (trik-an′jī-on) [ trich- + G. *angeion*, vessel ]. Telangion.

**trichatrophia** (trik′ă-tro′fī-ah) [ trich- + G. *atrophia*, atrophy ]. Atrophy of the hair bulbs, with brittleness, splitting, and falling of the hair.

**trichauxis** (trik-awk′sis) [ trich- + G. *auxis*, increase ]. Excessive growth of hair in length and quantity.

**trichi-.** See tricho-.

**-trichia** (-trik′ī-ah) [ G. *thrix* (*trich-*), hair, + suffix *-ia*, condition ]. Combining form denoting condition or type of hair, as in oligotrichia, schizotrichia.

**trichiasis** (trī-ki′ă-sis) [ trich- + G. suffix *-iasis*, condition ]. A condition in which the hair around a natural orifice turns in and causes irritation; *e.g.*, in inversion of an eyelid (entropion), eyelashes cause irritation of the conjunctiva.

**Trichina** (trī-ki′nah). Old name for a genus of nematode worms, correctly called *Trichinella*.

**trichina**, pl. **trichinae** (trī-ki′nah, -ne) [ Mod. L. fr. G. *thrix* (*trich-*), a hair ]. A larval worm of the genus *Trichinella*, infective form in pork.

**Trichinella** (trik′ī-nel′ah) [ Mod. L. fr. trichina + dim. suffix *-ella* ]. A nematode genus in the aphasmid group that causes trichinosis in man and a great many carnivores.

**T. spira′lis,** pork worm; trichina worm; causal parasite of trichinosis, found in most regions of the world but more frequently in the Northern Hemisphere; a white to gray-white, cylindroid worm with a gradually tapered anterior end; females vary from 2 to 4 by 0.06 mm., and males from 1 to 1.5 by 0.04 mm.; the female worm is viviparous, and bears approximately 1500 embryonic larvae that are from 80 to 100 $\mu$ in length and 5 or 6 $\mu$ in diameter; the larvae are laid deep in the mucosa so that they are picked up in the submucosal capillaries and are transported via the liver to the heart, lungs, and systemic circulation; eventually the larvae break out of the body capillaries, penetrate a muscle fiber, coil up, and encyst, thereby inducing the strong sensitization, pain, fever, edema, and eosinophilic reaction characteristic of trichinosis; transmission occurs as a result of ingesting raw or inadequately cooked meat (especially pork) that contains encysted larvae; the latter develop into adults that survive in the jejunum and ileum for approximately six weeks, during which time numerous larvae are born.

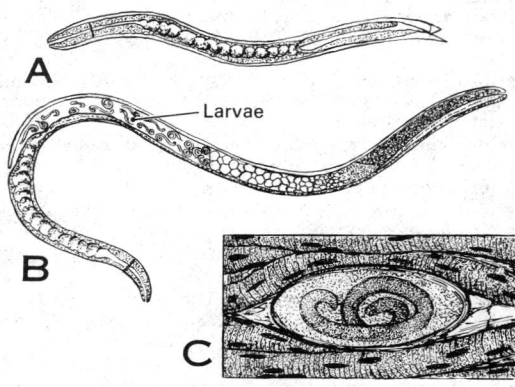

**Trichinella spiralis**

*A,* male (×30.5); *B,* female (×30.0); *C,* larvae encysted in muscle (×75).

**trichinelliasis** (trik′ī-nel-i′ă-sis). Trichinosis.

**Trichinelloidea** (trik′ī-nel-oy′de-ah). A superfamily of nematodes, including the following roundworms that are parasitic in man: *Trichinella spiralis,* the trichina worm; *Trichuris trichiura,* the human whipworm; *Capillaria hepatica,* the capillary liver worm.

**trichinellosis** (trik′ī-nel-o′sis). Trichinosis.

**trichiniasis** (trik′ī-ni′ă-sis). Trichinosis.

**trichiniferous** (trik′ī-nif′er-us). Containing trichina worms.

**trichiniza′tion** (trik′ī-nī-za′shun). Infection with trichina worms.

**trichinophobia** (trik′ī-no-fo′bī-ah) [ trichinosis + G. *phobos*, fear ]. Morbid fear of trichinosis.

**trichinoscope** (trik′ī-no-skōp) [ trichina + G. *skopeō*, to view ]. A magnifying glass used in the examination of meat suspected of being trichinous.

**trichinosis** (trik′ī-no′sis) [ *Trichinella* (trichina) + G. suffix *-osis*, condition ]. Trichinelliasis; trichiniasis; trichinellosis; the disease resulting from ingestion of raw or inadequately cooked meat (especially pork) that contains encysted viable larvae of *Trichinella spiralis.* Signs and symptoms may be related to the following conditions: (1) intestinal phase—poor appetite, abdominal discomfort, nausea (possibly vomiting), and loose stools, associated with inflammation caused by the adult worms in the jejunum and ileum; (2) phase of dissemination (second week)—superimposed on preceding, with fever, leukocytosis (and eosinophilia), and exaggeration of previous symptoms, associated with circulation of large numbers of larvae in the blood; (3) phase of widespread inflammation—a variety of signs and symptoms indicative of myositis, dermatitis, pneumonitis, meningitis, encephalitis, myocarditis, and so on, related to intense inflammatory reactions in sites where the larvae become degenerated and die; (4) phase of recession—increasingly less manifestation of the intestinal disorder, less conspicuous leukocytosis (although eosinophilia persists), less fever, and less pain in the muscles, but varying degrees of pain or discomfort may be noted for several weeks, and larvae coiled within oval cysts about 0.5 mm. long may be found in biopsies of skeletal muscle. Heavy infection will result in death in 5 to 6 weeks unless the patient has previously been exposed, in which case a strongly protective natural acquired immunity will usually develop.

**trichinous** (trik′ī-nus). Infected with trichina worms.

**trichite** (trik′īt). Trichocyst.

**trichitis** (trī-ki′tis) [ trich- + G. suffix *-itis,* inflammation ]. Inflammation of the hair bulbs.

**trichloral.** *m*-Chloral.

**tri′chlo′ride.** A chloride having three chlorine atoms in the molecule.

**tri′chlormethi′azide** (NF). NAQUA; 6-chloro-3-(dichloromethyl)-3,4-dihydro-2H-1,2,4-benzothiadiazine-7-sulfonamide; an orally effective benzothiazide diuretic and antihypertensive agent.

**tri′chloroace′tic acid** (USP, BP). CCl$_3$COOH; used as an astringent antiseptic in 1 to 5 per cent solution or as an escharotic for venereal and other warts; a widely used protein precipitant.

**tri′chloroeth′ane.** 1,1,1-Trichloroethane; methylchloroform; CH$_3$CCl$_3$; an industrial solvent with pronounced inhalation anesthetic activity.

**tri′chloroeth′anol.** 2,2,2-Trichloroethanol; trichloroethyl alcohol; C$_2$H$_3$Cl$_3$O; a hypnotic and sedative; as a metabolite of chloral hydrate, it contributes to the depressant activity of chloral hydrate.

**tri′chloroeth′ylene** (BP). TRILENE; trichloroethene; ethinyl trichloride; ClCH = CCl$_2$; an analgesic and inhalation anesthetic used in minor surgical operations, trigeminal neuralgia, and in obstetrical practice.

**tri′chloroflu′orometh′ane.** FREON 11; GENETRON 11; CCl$_3$F; trichloromonofluoromethane; widely used propellant for aerosol sprays; has anesthetic and arrhythmogenic activity if inhaled in high concentration.

**tri′chloromon′ofluorometh′ane** (NF). Trichlorofluoromethane.

**tri′chlorophe′nol.** Occurs as 2,4,5-t. and as 2,4,6-t.; used as an antiseptic, disinfectant, and fungicide.

**tricho-, trich-, trichi-** (trik′o-) [ G. *thrix* (*trich-*), hair. TRICH- ]. Combining form relating to the hair, or denoting a hairlike structure.

**trichobezoar** (trik′o-be′zōr) [ tricho- + bezoar, *q.v.* ]. A hairball or hair cast in the stomach or intestinal tract, common in cats.

**trichocardia** (trik′o-kar′dī-ah) [ tricho- + G. *kardia*, heart ]. Fibrinous *pericarditis.*

**Trichocephalus** (trik′o-sef′ă-lus) [ tricho- + G. *kephalē*, head ]. Incorrect name for *Trichuris.*

**trichocirsus** (tri-ko-ser′sus) [ tricho- + G. *kirsos*, varix ]. Telangiectasia.

**trichoclasia, trichoclasis** (trik′o-kla′zī-ah, trī-kok′lă-sis) [ tricho- + G. *klasis*, breaking off ]. *Trichorrhexis* nodosa.

**trichocryptomania** (trik′o-krip-to-ma′nī-ah) [ trichos- + G. *kryptos*, concealed, + *mania*, frenzy ]. Trichorrhexomania; an abnormal desire to break off hair of the scalp or face by nipping with the fingernail.

**trichocryptosis** (trik′o-krip-to′sis) [ tricho- + G. *kryptos*, concealed ]. Any disease of the hair follicles.

**trichocyst** (trik′o-sist) [ tricho- + G. *kystis*, bladder ]. One of a number of structures, in the form of minute elongated cysts, arranged radially around the periphery of a protozoan cell. The contained fluid, when discharged, serves for offense or defense. Found in the Ciliata, such as *Paramecium* species.

**Trichodectes** (trik′o-dek′tēz) [ tricho- + G. *dektēs*, a beggar ]. A genus of biting lice; see also *Bovicola* and *Damalinia.*

     **T. ca′nis,** *T. latus;* the biting louse of dogs that commonly serves as an intermediate host for the dog tapeworm, *Dipylidium caninum.*

     **T. cli′max,** *Bovicola caprae.*

     **T. la′tus,** *T. canis.*

     **T. parumpilo′sus,** *Bovicola equi.*

     **T. scala′ris,** *Bovicola bovis.*

     **T. sphaeroceph′alus,** *Bovicola ovis.*

**Trichoderma** (trik′o-der′mah) [ tricho- + G. *derma*, skin ]. A fungus in soil that furnishes the antibiotic gliotoxin.

**trichodophlebitis** (trik′o-do-flē-bi′tis) [ G. *trichōdes*, hair-like, + phlebitis ]. Inflammation of the venules.

**trichodyn′ia** [ tricho- + G. *odynē*, pain ]. Trichalgia.

**trichoepithelioma** (trik′o-ep-ĭ-the-lī′o′mah) [ tricho- + epithelioma ]. One of multiple small nodules, occurring mostly on the skin of the face, derived from basal cells of hair follicles enclosing keratin pearls; t.'s are benign and often familial. Also called acanthoma adenoides cysticum, benign cystic epithelioma; epithelioma adenoides cysticum; Brooke's tumor; Brooke's disease (1); hereditary multiple t.; t. papillosum multiplex.

**trichoesthesia** (trik′o-es-the′zī-ah) [ tricho- + G. *aisthēsis*, sensation ]. 1. The sensation felt when a hair is touched. 2. A form of paresthesia in which there is a sensation as of a hair on the skin, on the mucous membrane of the mouth, or on the conjunctiva.

**trichoesthesiometer** (trik′o-es-the-zī-om′e-ter) [ tricho- + G. *aisthēsis*, sensation, + G. *metron*, measure ]. A device for testing the sensibility of the scalp and other hairy parts.

**trichogen** (trik′o-jen) [ tricho- + suffix -*gen*, producing ]. An agent that promotes the growth of hair.

**trichogenous** (trī-koj′ĕ-nus). Promoting the growth of the hair.

**trichoglossia** (trik′o-glos′ī-ah) [ tricho- + G. *glōssa*, tongue ]. Hairy *tongue.*

**trichohyalin** (trik′o-hi′ă-lin). A substance of the nature of keratohyalin or eleidin, found in the hair.

**trichoid** (trik′oyd) [ tricho- + G. *eidos*, resemblance ]. Hairlike.

**tricholabis, tricholabium** (trī-kol′ă-bis, trik′o-la′bī-um) [ G. fr. trich- + *labis*, holder (pincers), or *labion*, dim. ]. Hair tweezers.

**tricholith** (trik′o-lith) [ tricho- + G. *lithos*, stone ]. A concretion on the hair; the lesion of piedra.

**trichologia** (trik′o-lo′jī-ah) [ G. *trichologeo*, to pluck hairs, fr. tricho- + *lego*, to pick out, gather ]. Trichology (2); a tic consisting of plucking at the hair.

**trichology** (trī-kol′o-jī). 1 [ tricho- + G. *logos*, study ]. The study of the hair—its anatomy, growth, and diseases.

2 [ G. *trichologeo*, fr. tricho- + *legō* to pick out ]. Trichologia.

**trichoma** (trī-ko′mah) [ tricho- + G. suffix -*oma*, tumor ]. 1. *Plica* polonica. 2. Trichiasis.

**trichomaphyte** (trī-ko′mă-fīt) [ trichoma + G. *phyton*, plant ]. A fungus found in plica polonica.

**trichomatose** (trī-ko′mă-tōs). Trichomatous.

**trichomatosis** (trī-ko′mă-to′sis). Trichoma.

**trichomatous** (trī-ko′mă-tus). Relating to or suffering from trichoma.

**trichomegaly** (trik′o-meg′ă-lī) [ tricho- + G. *megas*, large ]. A congenital condition characterized by abnormally long eyelashes.

**trichom′onad.** Common name for members of the family Trichomonadidae.

**Trich′omonad′idae.** A family of protozoan flagellates that includes the genera *Trichomonas, Pentatrichomonas, Tetratrichomonas,* and *Tritrichomonas.*

**Trichomonas** (trī-kom′o-nas) [ tricho- + G. *monas*, single (unit) ]. A genus of parasitic protozoan flagellates (subfamily Trichomonidinae, family Trichomonadidae, order Trichomonadorida) that have four anterior flagella and a posterior flagellum along the margin of an undulating membrane (which is not free posteriorly), a filamentous costa along the basal portion of the membrane, a typical pelta, a sausage-shaped parabasal body (Golgi body), a rodlike axostyle, and a large single anterior nucleus in a pyriform cell body with a pointed posterior end. Species cause trichomoniasis in man, other primates, and birds; specificity is more marked for precise microhabitat than for host species. This genus has been divided into several genera, *Trichomonas, Pentatrichomonas, Tetratrichomonas,* and *Tritrichomonas.*

     **T. bucca′lis,** *T. tenax.*

     **T. foe′tus,** see *Tritrichomonas foetus.*

     **T. gal′linae,** the cause of avian trichomoniasis; the pigeon is the natural host, but the organism also occurs in turkeys, chickens, doves, hawks, falcons, and other birds; infection is most serious in young domestic pigeons, who acquire it from pigeon milk produced in the pigeon crop; other birds are infected from contaminated water or by feeding on infected birds.

     **T. gallina′rum,** see *Tetratrichomonas gallinarium.*

     **T. hom′inis,** see *Pentatrichomonas hominis.*

     **T. o′vis,** see *Tetratrichomonas ovis.*

     **T. su′is,** see *Tritrichomonas suis.*

     **T. te′nax,** *T. buccalis;* lives as a commensal in the mouth of man and other primates, especially in the tartar around the teeth or in the defects of carious teeth; there is no evidence of direct pathogenesis, but it is frequently associated with pyogenic organisms in pus pockets or at the base of teeth.

     **T. vagina′lis,** frequently found in the vagina and urethra of women and in the urethra and prostate gland of men (the only known natural hosts), in whom it causes trichomoniasis vaginitis; considerable differences in pathogenicity exists among various strains of this species.

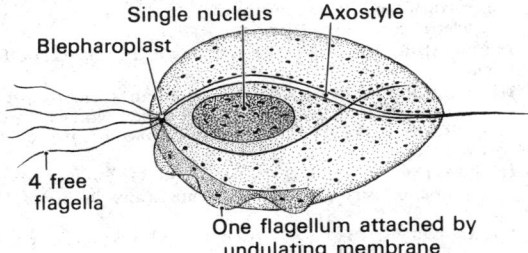

*Trichomonas vaginalis* (×1440)

**trichomoniasis** (trik′o-mo-ni′ă-sis). Trichomonosis; disease caused by infection with a species of *Trichomonas* or related genera; often used to designate t. vaginitis.

**avian t.,** occurs in the upper digestive tract in a variety of birds and is caused by *Trichomonas gallinae;* it causes caseous lesions in the mouth, esophagus, crop, and proventriculus, frequently with rapid weight loss and death.

**bovine t.** a venereal infection in cattle caused by *Trichomonas foetus;* in the bull, the infection is asymptomatic, the organisms being present in small or moderate numbers, chiefly on the glans penis; infection in the female may result in delayed conception, abortion early in pregnancy, or pyometra; transmission occurs during copulation or by artificial insemination from infected bulls.

**t. vaginitis,** acute or subacute vaginitis or urethritis caused by infection with *Trichomonas vaginalis,* which does not invade the mucosa or the tissue but provokes an inflammatory reaction, possibly as the result of physical irritation, production of toxic substances, or both; infection is venereal and is transmitted during coitus, but very rarely from contaminated toilet seats, towels, or bedding; widespread infection in human populations is usually asymptomatic but may produce vaginitis, with vaginal and vulvar pruritis, leukorrhea, and (rarely) purulent urethritis in males.

**trichomonosis** (trik'o-mo-no'sis). Trichomoniasis.

**trichomycetosis** (trik'o-mi'se-to'sis). Trichomycosis.

**trichomycosis** (trik'o-mi-ko'sis) [ tricho- + G. *mykēs,* fungus, + suffix -*osis,* condition ]. Formerly used to mean any disease of the hair caused by a fungus; presently used as synonymous with trichonocardiosis or t. axillaris. In present usage, t. is a misnomer because the causative agent of the disease is a *Nocardia* and not a fungus.

**t. axilla'ris,** Paxton's disease; lepothrix; t. nodosa; t. palmellina; t. chromatica; t. nodularis; trichonocardiasis axillaris; infection of axillary and pubic hairs with development of yellow (flava), black (nigra), or red (rubra) concretions around the hair shafts.

**t. chromat'ica,** t. axillaris.

**t. favo'sa,** favus.

**t. nodo'sa, t. nodula'ris,** t. axillaris.

**t. palmelli'na,** t. axillaris.

**t. pustulo'sa,** any parasitic disease of the hair marked by pustule formation at the orifices of the hair follicles.

**trichonocardiosis** (trik'o-no-kar'dĭ-o'sis) [ tricho- + *Nocardia* ]. An infection of hair shafts, especially of the axillary and pubic regions, with species of *Nocardia,* especially *N. tenuis.* Yellow, red, or black concretions develop around the infected hair shafts; the concretions contain the causative agent and frequently species of micrococci. The micrococci probably account for the variety of the colors of the concretions. probably accounts for the several varieties which have been described. See also trichomycosis, and trichomycosis axillaris.

**t. axillaris,** *trichomycosis* axillaris.

**trichonodosis** (trik'o-no-do'sis) [ tricho- L. *nodus,* node (swelling), + G. suffix -*osis,* condition ]. *Trichomycosis* axillaris.

**trichonosis** (trik'o-no'sis). Trichopathy.

**trichonosus** (trī-kon'o-sus) [ tricho- + G. *nosos,* disease ]. Trichopathy.

**t. furfura'cea,** *tinea* tonsurans.

**t. versic'olor,** ringed *hair.*

**trichopathic** (trik'o-path'ik). Relating to any disease of the hair.

**trichopathophobia** (trik'o-path-o-fo'bĭ-ah) [ tricho- + G. *pathos,* suffering, + *phobos,* fear ]. Excessive worry regarding disease of the hair, its color, or abnormalities of its growth.

**trichopathy** (trī-kop'ă-thī) [ tricho- + G. *pathos,* suffering ]. Trichonosus; trichonosis; trichosis; any disease of the hair.

**trichophagy** (trī-kof'ă-jī) [ tricho- + G. *phagein,* to eat ]. The tic of biting the hair.

**trichophobia** (trik'o-fo'bĭ-ah) [ tricho- + G. *phobos,* fear ]. A morbid disgust caused by the sight of loose hairs on the clothing or elsewhere.

**trichophytic** (trik'o-fit'ik). Relating to trichophytosis.

**trichophytid** (trī-kof'ĭ-tid, trik'o-fi'tid) [ tricho- + G. *phyton,* plant, + suffix -*id (1), q. v.* ]. An eruption which is the expression of allergic response to *Trichophyton* infection.

**trichophytin** (trī-kof'ĭ-tin). An extract of cultures of several species of *Trichophyton,* the ringworm fungus, formerly used in the diagnosis and treatment of the different varieties of ringworm.

**trichophytobezoar** (trik'o-fi'to-be'zōr) [ tricho- + G. *phyton,* plant, + *bezoar, q.v.* ]. A mixed hair- and food-ball, consisting of vegetable fibers, seeds and skins of fruits, and animal hair that are matted together to form a ball in the stomach of man or animals, especially ruminants.

**Trichophyton** (trik'o-fi'ton, trī-kof'ĭ-ton) [ tricho- + G. *phyton,* plant ]. A genus of pathogenic fungi causing dermatophytosis and trichophytosis.

**T. ajel'loi,** a geophilic species isolated worldwide from soil; there is some doubt as to its pathogenicity.

**T. arloin'gi,** T. quinckeanum.

**T. bennet'ti,** a species causing mouse favus, probably the same as *T. quinckeanum.*

**T. ceratoph'agus** [ G. *keras,* horn, + *phago,* to eat ], *T. schoenleinii.*

**T. concen'tricum,** an anthropophilic species closely resembling *T. schoenleinii,* but which is the causative agent of tinea imbricata.

**T. ec'tothrix, T. en'dothrix,** see *T. megalosporon.*

**T. equi'num,** a zoophilic species causing endothrix infections of hair in horses.

**T. galli'nae,** a zoophilic species that causes infection on the combs of fowl.

**T. gypseum,** a species of fungus that produces lesions on the nails and glabrous skin.

**T. in'terdigita'lis,** a cause of dermatophytosis of the feet or athlete's foot; a variant of *T. mentagrophytes.*

**T. megalos'poron** [ G. *megas (megal-),* large, + *sporos,* seed ], the large-spored ringworm fungus, common in France, but rare in England and the United States; it occurs in two forms: *T. m. ectothrix,* the spores of which are found usually outside the cuticle of the hair; and *T. m. endothrix,* which invades the substance of the hair.

**T. megnin'ii,** an anthropophilic species that has an absolute requirement for histidine.

**T. mentagrophy'tes,** a zoophilic species that causes infection of hair, skin, and nails.

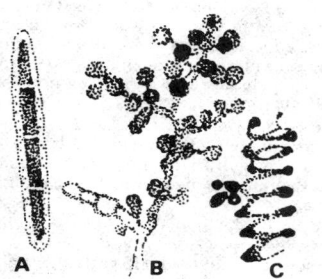 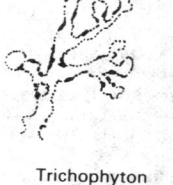

Trichophyton
mentagrophytes

Trichophyton
schoenleini

*Trichophyton*

*A,* clavate macroconidium; *B,* microconidium; *C,* coiled hypha.

**T. purpureum,** *T. rubrum.*

**T. quinckeanum,** *T. arloingi;* alpha fungus of Quincke, the pathogenic fungus of favus herpeticus.

**T. rosa'ceum,** members of the rosaceum group of fungi, such as *T. megnini* and *T. galli.*

**T. ru'brum,** *T. purpureum;* an anthropophilic species that causes recalcitrant lesions of the skin; infections of hair are rare.

**T. schoenleinii,** *T. ceratophagus;* an anthropophilic species that produces an endothrix infection of the hair, and is the common cause of favus.

**T. sim'ii,** a zoophilic species that causes infection in rhesus monkeys, dogs, and man; thus far, infections have had their origin in India.

**T. ton'surans,** an anthropophilic species that causes epidemic tinea tonsurans, as well as infections of the skin and nails.

**T. verrucos'um,** a zoophilic species that requires thiamin and inositol for growth; it causes tinea in cattle and other domestic animals, from which man becomes infected.

**T. viola'ceum,** an anthropophilic species that causes "black dot" ringworm or fungus infection of the scalp.

**trichophytosis** (trik'o-fi-to'sis) [ tricho- + G. *phyton*, plant, + suffix *-osis*, condition ]. Superficial fungus infection caused by species of *Trichophyton*.

    **t. bar'bae,** *tinea* sycosis.

    **t. cap'itis,** *tinea* tonsurans.

    **t. cor'poris,** *tinea* circinata.

    **t. cru'ris,** *tinea* cruris.

    **t. un'guium,** fungus infection of the nail plates; see also *tinea* unguium.

**Trichopleu'ris.** A genus of biting lice that infests ruminants, *e.g.*, *T. lipeuroides* and *T. parallelus* in American deer; considered by some to be a subgenus of *Damalinia*.

**trichopoliosis** (trik'o-po-li-o'sis) [ tricho- + G. *polios*, gray, + suffix *-osis*, condition ]. Canities.

**Trichoptera** (tri-kop'ter-ah) [ tricho- + G. *pteron*, wing ]. A group of flies (caddis flies) having hairy wings, that shed their hairs and epithelia, causing hay fever-like (allergic) symptoms in sensitive persons. The aquatic larvae construct a protective case (caddis) of bits of submerged material in a highly specific form; commonly found attached under stones in freshwater streams.

**trichoptilosis** (trik'o-ti-lo'sis, tri-kop'ti-lo'sis) [ tricho- + G. *ptilosis*, plumage, fr. *ptilon*, feathers, down ]. A condition of splitting of the shaft of the hair, giving it a feathery appearance.

**trichorrhexis** (trik'o-rek'sis) [ tricho- + G. *rhexis*, a breaking ]. Trichoschisis; a condition in which the hairs readily break or split.

    **t. invagina'ta,** bamboo *hair*.

    **t. nodo'sa,** trichoclasia; clastothrix; nodositas crinium; a condition in which minute nodes are formed in the hair shafts. Splitting and breaking, complete or incomplete, may occur at these points or nodes.

**trichorrhexomania** (trik'o-reks-o-ma'ni-ah) [ trichos- + G. *rhexis*, a breaking, + *mania*, frenzy ]. Trichocryptomania.

**trichoschisis** (tri-kos'ki-sis) [ tricho- + G. *schisis*, a cleaving ]. Trichorrhexis.

**trichoscopy** (tri-kos'ko-pi) [ tricho- + G. *skopeo*, to examine ]. Examination of the hair.

**trichosis** (tri-ko'sis) [ tricho- + G. suffix *-osis*, condition ]. Trichopathy.

    **t. carun'culae,** a growth of hair on the lacrimal caruncle.

    **t. sensiti'va,** hyperesthesia of the hairy parts.

    **t. seto'sa,** coarseness of the hair.

**trichosomatous** (trik'o-so'mă-tus) [ tricho- + G. *soma*, body ]. Having flagella with a small body; denoting certain protozoan organisms; see *Trichomonas*.

**Trichosporon** (tri-kos'po-ron, trik'o-spor'on) [ tricho- + G. *sporos*, seed (spore) ]. A genus of imperfect fungi that possess branching septate hyphae with arthrospores and blastopores; these organisms are part of the normal flora of the intestinal tract of man.

    **T. beigel'ii,** *T. cutaneum;* a species which is the causative agent of white piedra or trichosporosis.

    **T. capita'tum,** a species which may cause primary or secondary endogenous infections of man similar to those caused by *Geotrichum candidum*.

    **T. cuta'num,** *T. beigelii*.

**trichosporosis** (trik'o-spo-ro'sis) [ *Trichosporon* + G. suffix *-osis*, condition ]. A superficial mycotic infection of the hair in which nodular masses of causative fungi become attached to the hair shafts. This disease is commonly called piedra (*q. v.*). So-called black piedra is caused by *Piedraia hortai* and white piedra is caused by *Trichosporon beigelii*.

    **t. in'dica,** a mild form of piedra observed in India.

    **t. trop'ica,** piedra.

**trichostasis spinulosa** (tri-kos'tă-sis spi'nu-lo'sah) [ tricho- + G. *stasis*, a standing; L. *spinulosus*, thorny ]. A condition in which hair follicles are blocked with a keratin plug containing lanugo hairs.

**trichostrongyle** (trik'o-stron'jil). Common name for members of the family Trichostrongylidae.

**Trichostrongylidae** (trik'o-stron-jil'ĭ-de). A family of nematodes (suborder Strongylata, order Strongyloidea) that includes the genera *Trichostrongylus*, *Nematodira*, *Haemonchus*, *Teladosagia*, and *Ostertagia*.

**trichostrongylosis** (trik'o-stron-ji-lo'sis). Infection with *Trichostrongylus*.

**Trichostrongylus** (trik'o-stron'ji-lus) [ tricho- + G. *strongylos*, round ]. Hairworms; bankrupt worms; black scour worms; an economically important genus of small, slender nematodes (family Trichostrongylidae, suborder Strongylata) that inhabit the small intestine, in some cases the stomach, of a variety of herbivorous animals and gallinaceous birds; about 36 species have been described, of which two are from birds. They burrow into the mucosa and suck blood; in large numbers they do serious damage, especially to young hosts.

    **T. ax'ei,** occurs in the abomasum of sheep, horses; cattle, antelope, bison, llama, and deer, and in the stomach of pigs and horses, it is the most common species of *T.* in cattle.

    **T. capric'ola,** occurs in the small intestine and abomasum of sheep, goats, deer, and pronghorn.

    **T. colubrifor'mis,** occurs in anterior portions of the small intestine and sometimes in the abomasum of sheep, goats, cattle, camels, and some wild ruminants, and in the stomach of primates (including man), rabbits, and squirrels; it is distributed worldwide and is common in the United States, especially in sheep.

    **T. longispicula'ris,** found in the small intestine of cattle, sheep, and goats; it is distributed worldwide but uncommon in the United States.

    **T. ten'uis,** widespread pathogenic parasite of the ceca and small intestines of fowl, including ducks, geese, turkeys, pheasants, and partridges.

    **T. vitri'nus,** an important pathogen of lambs, it is found chiefly in the duodenum of sheep, camels, rabbits, and goats but has been reported from man and pigs.

**trichothecin** (trik'o-the'sin). $C_{19}H_{24}O_5$; an antifungal antibiotic obtained from cultures of the fungus *Trichothecium roseum*.

**Trichothe'cium.** A genus of imperfect fungi generally considered a common saprophyte; the species *T. roseum* is the source of trichothecin.

**trichotillomania** (trik'o-til'o-ma'ni-ah) [ tricho- + G. *tillo*, pull out, + *mania*, insanity ]. A compulsion to pull out one's own hair.

**trichotomy** (tri-kot'o-mi) [ G. *trichia*, threefold, + *tome*, a cutting ]. Division into three parts.

**trichotoxin** (trik'o-tok'sin). A cytotoxin having an injurious effect specifically for ciliated epithelium.

**trichotrophy** (tri-kot'ro-fi) [ tricho- + G. *trophe*, nourishment ]. Nutrition of the hair.

**trichroic** (tri-kro'ik). Relating to or marked by trichroism.

**trichroism** (tri'kro-izm) [ G. *trichroos*, three-colored, fr. tri- + *chroa*, color ]. The property of some crystals of presenting different colors in three different directions.

**trichromat** (tri-kro'mat) [ tri- + G. *chroma*, color ]. A person who sees three primary colors; hence, one with normal color vision.

**trichromatic** (tri-kro-mat'ik). Trichromic. 1. Having, or relating to, the three primary colors, red, blue, and green. 2. Capable of perceiving the three primary colors; having normal color vision.

**trichromatism** (tri-kro'mă-tizm) [ tri- + G. *chroma*, color ]. State of being trichromatic.

**trichromatopsia** (tri-kro'mă-top'si-ah) [ tri- + G. *chroma*, color, + *opsis*, vision ]. Normal color vision; the ability to perceive the three primary colors.

**trichromic** (tri-kro'mik). Trichromatic.

**trichterbrust** (tricht'er-broost) [ Ger. ]. *Pectus* excavatum.

**trichuriasis** (trik'u-ri'ă-sis). Infection with a species of Trichuris. In man, intestinal parasitization by *Tricuris trichuria* is usually asymptomatic and not associated with peripheral eosinophilia; it usually causes severe diarrhea or rectal prolapse.

**Trichuris** (tri-ku'ris) [ tricho- + G. *oura*, tail ]. Whipworm; a genus of aphasmid nematodes (sometimes, but improperly, termed *Trichocephalus*) related to the trichina worm, *Trichinella spiralis*, and having a body with a slender, elongated, anterior portion threaded into the mucosa of the colon or large intestine of the host and a thick posterior portion bearing reproductive organs and their products. *T.* contains about seventy species, all in mammals. Some systematists have divided the genus into two subfamilies, one with *T.* (as defined) and *Rudolphia*; the other with *Buckleyuris* and *Salamia*. However, most workers continue to use the single genus *T.*

**T. globulo'sa**, occurs in the cecum of cattle, sheep, goats, camels, and other ruminants; it is common in many regions but absent from North America, except for zoo records.

**T. o'vis**, occurs in the cecum and upper colon of sheep, goats, cattle, and other ruminants.

**T. su'is**, found in the cecum of swine and morphologically identical with *T. trichiura*, although probably distinct because of biological differences demonstrated in cross-infection studies.

**T. trichiu'ra**, the whipworm of man and the cause of trichuriasis in man; the body is filiform and slender in the anterior three-fifths, and more robust posteriorly; females are 4 or 5 cm. long, males are shorter (with coiled caudal extremity and a single eversible spicule); eggs are barrel-shaped, 50 to 56 by 20 to 22 $\mu$, with double shell and translucent knobs at each of the two poles; man is the only susceptible host and usually acquires infection by direct finger-to-mouth contact or by ingestion of soil, water, or food that contains larvated eggs (development takes 3 to 6 weeks under proper conditions of warmth and moisture, hence distribution is chiefly tropical); larvae escape from eggs in the ileum, mature in approximately a month, and then pass directly into the cecum without undergoing a parenteral migration as occurs with *Ascaris lumbricoides*; adults may persist for 2 to 7 years.

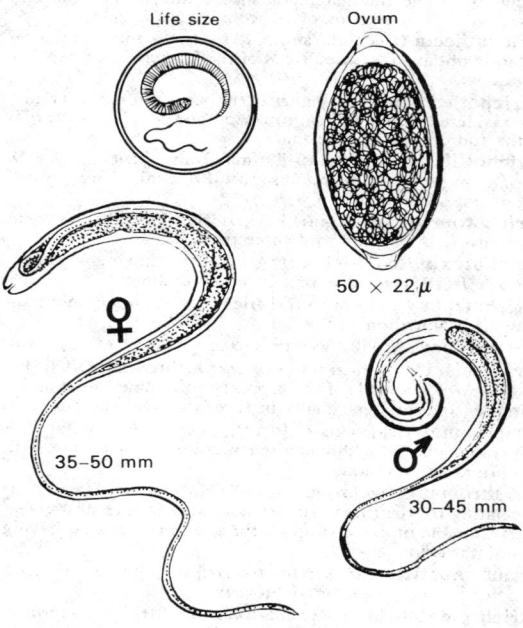

Life size      Ovum

♀

50 × 22 μ

35–50 mm

♂

30–45 mm

*Trichuris trichuria*

(From Jeffrey, H. C., and Leach, R. M.: *Atlas of Medical Helminthology and Protozoology*, Churchill Livingstone, Edinburgh, 1966.)

**T. vul'pis**, found in the cecum and large intestine of dogs, coyotes, and foxes throughout the world; most infections are light and asymptomatic, but heavy infections can cause severe symptoms, weight loss, and death.

**tricipital** (tri-sip'ĭ-tal). Having three heads; denoting a triceps muscle.

**triclobisonium chloride** (tri'klo-bĭ-so'nĭ-um). TRIB; TRIB-URON; hexamethylenebis[ dimethyl[ 1-methyl-3-(2,2,6-trimethylcyclohexyl)propyl ]ammonium chloride ]; a bis-quaternary ammonium compound used topically in the treatment of superficial infections of the skin and vagina (*e.g.*, impetigo contagiosa, folliculitis, furunculosis, infected burns, vulvitis, and vaginitis); a cationic antiseptic effective against both Gram-negative and Gram-positive organisms. It is inactivated by soap and pH changes.

**tri'clofen'ol piperazine** (USAN). RANESTOL; bis(2,4,5-trichlorophenol)piperazine; anthelmintic.

**triclofos sodium** (tri'klo-fōs) (BP, USAN). Monosodium salt of 2,2,2-trichloroethyl dihydrogen phosphate; a hypnotic.

**tricorn** (tri'korn) [ tri- + L. *cornu*, horn ]. 1. One of the lateral ventricles of the brain. 2. Tricornute.

**tricornute** (tri-kor'nūt) [ tri- + L. *cornutus*, horned, fr. *cornu*, a horn ]. Having three cornua or horns.

**tricre'sol**. A purified mixture of the three cresols; antiseptic.

**tri'cromyl**. CRODIMYL; 3-methylchromone; coronary vasodilator.

**tricrotic** (tri-krot'ik) [ tri- + G. *krotos*, a beat ]. Tricrotous; thrice-beating; marked by three waves in the arterial pulse tracing.

**tricrotism** (tri'kro-tizm). The condition of being tricrotic.

**tri'crotous**. Tricrotic.

**tricus'pid**. Having three points, prongs, or cusps.

**tricus'pidal, tricus'pidate**. Tricuspid.

**tricyclamol chloride** (tri-si'klă-mol) Procyclidine methochloride.

**tridactylous** (tri-dak'tĭ-lus). Tridigitate.

**tri'dent**. Tridendate.

**triden'tate** [ tri- + L. *dentatus*, toothed ]. Trident; three-toothed; three-pronged.

**trider'mic** [ tri- + G. *derma*, skin ]. Relating to or derived from the three primary germ layers of the embryo: ectoderm, endoderm, and mesoderm.

**tridermoma** (tri'der-mo'mah) [ tri- + G. *derma*, skin, + suffix *-oma*, tumor ]. A teratoid growth that includes tissue from all three germ layers.

    **adult** or **coeta'neous t.**, one in which the various elements resemble fully matured tissue.

    **embryonal t.**, one in which the various elements are of embryonal types.

**tridigitate** (tri-dij'ĭ-tāt) [ tri- + L. *digitus*, digit ]. Tridactylous; having three fingers.

**tridihexethyl chloride** (tri-di-heks-eth'il) (NF). PATHILON chloride; 3-diethylamino-1-phenyl-1-cyclohexyl 1-propanol ethylchloride; an anticholinergic drug that produces peripheral action of cholinergic block similar to that of atropine; used as an adjunct in the management of peptic ulcers, gastric hyperacidity, gastric and intestinal hypermotility.

**tridymite** (trid'ĭ-mīt) [ fr. G. *tridymos*, threefold ]. A form of silica used in dental casting investment.

**tridymus** (trid'ĭ-mus) [ G. *tridymos*, threefold, fr. tri- + suffix *-dymus*, fold (see *-dymus*) ]. Triplets.

**trielcon** (tri-el'kon) [ tri- + G. *helkō*, to draw ]. A long, three-jawed forceps for the extraction of foreign bodies from wounds or canals.

**triencephalus** (tri-en-sef'ă-lus). Triocephalus.

**triethanolamine** (tri-eth'ă-nol'a-mēn). (USP). A mixture of mono-, di-, and triethanolamine, used as an emulsifying agent in the preparation of medicated ointments and lotions and as an aid in the absorption of such medicaments through the skin.

**triethylamine** (tri-eth-il'ă-mēn). ($C_2H_5)_3N$; a colorless liquid with strong ammoniacal odor, formed in decaying fish; it is not violently poisonous. Used in the preparation of quaternary ammonium compounds.

**trieth'ylene gly'col**. 2,2'-Ethylenedioxybis(ethanol); $C_6H_{14}O_4$; used in the vapor state as an air-sterilizing agent; toxic to bacteria, fungi, and viruses in very low concentrations in air; variations in the humidity of the air limit the germicidal effectiveness.

**triethylenemelamine** (tri-eth'ĭ-lēn-mel'ă-mēn) (NF). TEM; 2,4,6-tris(ethyleneimino)-s-triazine; chemically related to the nitrogen mustards; used in the treatment of leukemia.

**trieth'ylenephos'phoramide.** TEPA; same actions and uses as triethylenemelamine in the treatment of leukemias.

**trieth'ylenethi'ophos'phoramide.** Thio-TEPA; tris(1-aziridinyl)phosphine sulfide; an alkylating agent used for the palliative treatment of malignant diseases such as leukemia, lymphoma, and carcinoma.

**trifa'cial** [ tri- + L. *facies*, face ]. Denoting the fifth pair of cranial nerves, nervus trigeminus.

**tri'fid** [ L. *trifidus*, three-cleft, fr. *tri-*, three, + *findo*, to split ]. Split into three.

**triflu'midate** (USAN). Ethyl *m*-benzoyl-N-[ (trifluoromethyl)sulfonyl ]carbanilate; an anti-inflammatory drug.

**trifluoperazine hydrochloride** (tri-flu'o-pĕr-ă-zēn) (NF, BP). STELAZINE; MODALINA; TRIFLURIN; 10-[ 3-(4-methyl-1-piperazinyl)propyl ]-2-(trifluoromethyl)- phenothiazine hydrochloride; an antipsychotic agent.

**trifluoroethyl vinyl ether.** Fluroxene.

**5-trifluoromethyldeoxyuridine** (tri-flu'or-o-meth'il-de-ok'sĭ-u'rĭ-dēn). A pyrimidine analogue used topically in the treatment of herpes simplex keratitis.

**trifluperidol hydrochloride** (tri'flu-pĕr'ĭ-dol) (USAN). TRIPERIDOL; PSICOPERIDOL hydrochloride; 4'-fluoro-4-[ 4-hydroxy-4-(α,α,α-trifluoro-*m*-tolyl)piperidino ]butyrophenone hydrochloride; a tranquilizer, possibly effective for highly agitated, manic patients.

**tri'flupro'mazine hydrochloride** (NF). VESPRIN; 10-[ 3-(dimethylamino) propyl ]-2-trifluoromethylphenothiazine hydrochloride; an antipsychotic agent, closely related chemically and pharmacologically to chlorpromazine.

**tri'fo'cal.** Having three foci; see t. *lens.*

**trifoliosis** (tri-fo'lĭ-o'sis) [ L. *trifolium*, trefoil, clover ]. Trefoil dermatitis; occurs in horses, cattle, sheep, and pigs from eating several types of clover as well as alfalfa. It is a form of photosensitization. It occurs only occasionally, in animals that are hypersensitive.

**trifolium** (tri-fo'lĭ-um) [ L. *trefoil*, clover ]. Red clover blossoms; the dried inflorescence of *Trifolium pratense* (family Leguminosae); has been used as expectorant and antispasmodic.

**trifurcation** (tri'fur-ka'shun) [ tri- + L. *furca*, fork ]. 1. A division into three branches. 2. The area where the tooth roots divide into three or more distinct portions.

**trigas'tric** [ tri- + G. *gastēr*, belly ]. Having three bellies; denoting a muscle with two tendinous interruptions.

**trigeminal** (tri-jem'ĭ-nal) [ L. *trigeminus*, threefold ]. Relating to the fifth cranial or trigeminus nerve.

**trigeminus** (tri-jem'ĭ-nus) [ L. threefold, fr. tri- + *geminus*, twin ]. Trigeminal.

**trigeminy** (tri-jem'ĭ-nĭ) [ L. *trigeminus*, threefold ]. Trigeminal *rhythm.*

**triglyceride.** Triacylglycerol.

**trigocephalus** (tri'go-sef'ă-lus). Trigonocephalus.

**trigona** (tri-go'nah) [ L. ]. Plural of trigonum.

**trig'onal.** Triangular; relating to a trigonum.

**trigone** (tri'gōn) [ L. *trigonum*, fr. G. *trigōnon*, triangle ]. 1. Triangle; trigonum. 2. The first three dominant cusps (protocone, paracone, and metacone), taken collectively, of an upper molar tooth.

   **t. of the auditory nerve,** trigonum acustici; acoustic tubercle; the slight prominence of the floor of the lateral recess of the fourth ventricle, corresponding to the underlying cochlear and vestibular nuclei.

   **t. of the bladder,** *trigonum* vesicae.

   **collateral t.,** *trigonum* collaterale.

   **t. of fillet,** *trigonum* lemnisci.

   **t. of the habenula,** *trigonum* habenulae.

   **t. of the hypoglossal nerve,** *trigonum* nervi hypoglossi.

   **inguinal t.,** *trigonum* inguinale.

   **Lieutaud's t.,** *trigonum* vesicae.

   **Müller's t.,** the floor of the supraoptic recess of the third ventricle.

   **olfactory t.,** *trigonum* olfactorium.

   **t. of the vagus nerve,** *trigonum* nervi vagi.

   **t. of the lateral ventricle,** *trigonum* collaterale.

**trigonel'line.** *N*-Methylnicotinic acid, the methyl betaine of nicotinic acid; a product of the metabolism of nicotinic acid; excreted in the urine.

**trigonid** (tri-gon'id) [ see *trigonum* ]. The first three dominant cusps, taken collectively, of a lower molar tooth. See also trigone.

**trigonitis** (tri'go-ni'tis) [ trigone + G. suffix *-itis*, inflammation ]. Inflammation of the urinary bladder, localized in the mucous membrane at the trigonum.

**trig'onocephal'ic.** Pertaining to trigonocephaly.

**trig'onoceph'alus.** Trigocephalus; an individual exhibiting trigonocephaly.

**trigonocephaly** (trig'o-no-sef'ă-lĭ, tri'go-no-) [ trigone + G. *kephalē*, head ]. A malformed condition characterized by a more or less triangular configuration of the skull. The distorted shape of the cranium is due in part to premature synostosis of the cranial bones and involves compression of the cerebral hemispheres.

**trigonum,** pl. **trigona** (tri-go'num, -nah) [ L. from G. *trigōnon*, a triangle ] [ NA ]. Trigone; any triangular area. See triangle (2).

   **t. acus'tici,** *trigone* of the auditory nerve.

   **t. carot'icum** [ NA ], carotid triangle; superior carotid triangle; a space bounded by the superior belly of the omohyoid muscle, anterior border of the sternocleidomastoid, posterior belly of the digastric; it contains the bifurcation of the common carotid artery.

   **t. cerebra'le,** fornix (2).

   **t. cervica'le,** t. colli.

   **t. collatera'le** [ NA ], collateral trigone; t. ventriculi; trigone of the lateral ventricle; a triangular prominence of the floor of the lateral ventricle at the transition between occipital and temporal horn, continuous rostrally with the collateral eminence and, like the latter, caused by the deep penetration of the collateral sulcus from the ventral surface of the temporal lobe.

   **t. col'li,** t. cervicale; any one of the triangles of the neck.

   **t. deltoid'eopectora'le,** infraclavicular *triangle.*

   **t. femora'le** [ NA ], femoral triangle; Scarpa's triangle; fossa scarpae major; a triangular space at the upper part of the thigh, bounded by the sartorius and adductor longus muscles and the inguinal (Poupart's) ligament.

   **trigona fibro'sa cor'dis** [ NA ], parts of the fibrous skeleton of the heart; the right trigone is located between the aortic fibrous ring and the rings surrounding the right and left atrioventricular ostia; the left trigone is in the interval between the left side of the left atrioventricular ring and the aortic ring.

   **t. haben'ulae** [ NA ], trigone of the habenula; a small triangular area on the dorsomedial surface of the thalamus at the posterior end of the stria medullaris, corresponding to the underlying habenula.

   **t. hypoglos'si,** t. nervi hypoglossi.

   **t. inguina'le** [ NA ], inguinal triangle; Hesselbach's triangle; the triangular area in the lower abdominal wall bounded by the inguinal ligament below, the border of the rectus abdominis medially and the inferior epigastric vessels laterally. It is the site of direct inguinal hernia.

   **t. lemnis'ci,** triangle of Reil; triangle or trigone of the fillet; a triangular area on the lateral surface of the caudal half of the mesencephalon, bordered caudally by the slight prominence of the lateral lemniscus, dorsally by the base of the inferior colliculus and brachium colliculi superioris, and ventrally by the cerebral peduncle.

   **t. lumba'le** [ NA ], lumbar triangle; Petit's lumbar triangle; an area in the posterior abdominal wall bounded by the edges of the latissimus dorsi and external oblique muscles and the iliac crest; herniations occasionally occur here.

   **t. ner'vi hypoglos'si** [ NA ], trigone of the hypoglossal nerve; t. hypoglossi; tuberculum hypoglossi; hypoglossal eminence; eminentia hypoglossi; a slight elevation in the floor of the inferior recess of the fourth ventricle, beneath which is the nucleus of origin of the 12th cranial nerve.

   **t. ner'vi va'gi** [ NA ], trigone of the vagus nerve; ala cinerea; ashen or gray wing; a prominence in the floor of the fovea inferior of the fourth ventricle that overlies the dorsal motor nucleus of the vagus.

   **t. olfacto'rium** [ NA ], olfactory trigone; a grayish triangular area corresponding to the attachment of the olfactory peduncle ("olfactory nerve" or tractus olfactorius) to the base of the brain, at the anterior border of the anterior perforated substance.

**t. omoclavicula're** [ NA ], omoclavicular triangle; subclavian triangle; fossa supraclavicularis major; the triangle bounded by the clavicle, the omohyoid muscle, and the sternocleidomastoid muscle; it contains the subclavian artery and vein.

**t. pala'ti,** palatal *triangle.*

**t. sternocosta'le,** sternocostal triangle; Larrey's cleft; a muscular defect in the diaphragm between the costal and the sternal portions.

**t. submandibula're** [ NA ], submandibular triangle; the triangle of the neck bounded by the mandible and the two bellies of the digastric muscle; it contains the submandibular gland.

**t. ventric'uli,** t. collaterale.

**t. vesi'cae** [ NA ], trigone of the bladder; Lieutaud's trigone or body; a triangular smooth area at the base of the bladder between the openings of the two ureters and that of the urethra.

**tri'hexyphen'idyl hydrochloride** (USP). ARTANE hydrochloride; PIPANOL; benzhexol hydrochloride; α-cyclohexyl-α-phenyl-1-piperidinepropanol hydrochloride; an anticholinergic, antispasmodic drug; used in the treatment of parkinsonism and drug-induced parkinsonism.

**trihybrid** (tri-hi'brid) [ tri- + L. *hybrida,* hybrid ]. The offspring of parents which differ in three Mendelian characters.

**trihy'dric.** Denoting a chemical compound containing three replaceable hydrogen atoms.

**trihydroxyes'trin.** Estriol.

**triiniodymus** (tri-in'i-od'i-mus) [ tri- + G. *inion,* nape of the neck, + *didymos,* twin ]. A grossly malformed fetus with three heads, joined at the occiput, and a single body.

**triiodide** (tri-i'o-did, -did). An iodide with three atoms of iodine in the molecule.

**triiodomethane** (tri-i'o-do-meth'ān). Iodoform.

**3,5,3'-triiodothyronine** (tri-i'o-do-thi'ro-nēn). Symbol T₃; liothyronine; triothyrone; a thyroid hormone normally synthesized in smaller quantities than thyroxin; it is present in blood and in thyroid gland and exerts the same biological effects as thyroxin but, on a molecular basis, is more potent and the onset of its effect is more rapid.

3,5,3'-Triiodothyronine

**triketohydrindene hydrate** (tri-ke'to-hi'drin-dēn). Ninhydrin.

**trike'topu'rine.** Uric acid.

**tri'labe** [ tri- + G. *labē,* a handle, hold. LAB- ]. A three-pronged forceps for removal of foreign bodies from the bladder.

**trilam'inar.** Having three laminae.

**trilat'eral.** Having three sides.

**trilo'bate, tri'lobed.** Having three lobes.

**triloc'ular.** Having three cavities or cells.

**trilogy** (tril'o-ji) [ G. *trilogia,* fr. tri- + *logos,* study, discourse ]. A triad.

**t. of Fallot,** Fallot's triad; atrial septal defect associated with pulmonic stenosis and right ventricular hypertrophy.

**triman'ual.** Performed by the aid of three hands; denoting certain obstetrical maneuvers.

**trimastigate** (tri-mas'ti-gāt) [ tri- + G. *mastix,* whip ]. Having three flagella. As observed in certain protozoan organisms.

**tri'mecaine hydrochloride.** MESOCAINE hydrochloride; 2-diethylamino-2',4',6'-trimethylacetanilide hydrochloride; local anesthetic.

**trimep'razine tartrate** (USP). TEMARIL; 10-[ 3-(dimethylamino)-2-methylpropyl ]phenothiazine tartrate; a phenothiazine compound related chemically and pharmacologically to promazine but with a more pronounced histamine-antagonizing action; used for the symptomatic relief of pruritus.

**trimester** (tri'mes-ter, tri-mes'ter) [ L. *trimestris,* of three-month duration ]. A period of 3 months; one-third of the length of a pregnancy.

**trimet'aphan camsylate** (BP). Trimethaphan camsylate.

**trimetaz'idine dihydrochloride.** VASTAREL; 1-(2,3,4-trimethoxybenzyl)piperazine dihydrochloride; coronary vasodilator.

**trimethadione** (tri'meth'ā-di'ōn) (USP). TRIDIONE; troxidone; 3,5,5-trimethyl-2,4-oxazolidinedione; an anticonvulsant used for the treatment of petit mal and psychomotor epilepsy.

**trimethaphan camsylate** (tri-meth'ā-fan) (USP). ARFONAD; trimetaphan camsylate; *d*-1,3-dibenzyldecahydro-2-oxoimidazo[ *c* ]thieno[ 1,2-α ]thiolium camphorsulfonate; a ganglionic blocking agent that produces vasodilation of brief duration; used in surgery, particularly neurosurgery, to produce a relatively bloodless operative field (controlled hypotension).

**tri'methid'ium methosulfate.** OSTENSIN; (+)-[ *N*-methyl-*N*-(γ-trimethylammoniumpropyl) ]-1,8,8-trimethyl-3-azabicyclo[ 3.2.1 ]octane dimethosulfate; a quaternary ammonium compound that blocks ganglionic transmission at sympathetic and parasympathetic ganglia; used in the treatment of severe hypertension.

**trimeth'oben'zamide hydrochloride** (NF). TIGAN hydrochloride; *N*-[ (2-dimethylaminoethoxy)benzyl ]-3,4,5-trimethoxybenzamide hydrochloride; an antiemetic agent.

**trimeth'oprim** (USP, BP). SYRAPRIM; 2,4-diamino-5-(3,4,5-trimethoxybenzyl)pyrimidine; antimicrobial agent that potentiates the effect of sulfonamides and sulfones.

**trimeth'ylamine.** N(CH₃)₃; a degradation product of nitrogenous plant and animal substances; originally obtained from herring brine by distillation with lime; used in the preparation of quaternary ammonium compounds.

**trimeth'ylcolchicin'ic acid.** An analogue of colchicine that appears to be less toxic than the parent compound; used in the treatment of gout.

**trimeth'ylene.** Cyclopropane.

**trimeth'ylomel'amine.** CEALYSIN; (*s*-triazine-2,4,6-triyltriimino)trimethanol; antineoplastic agent.

**5,7,8-trimeth'ylto'col.** α-Tocopherol.

**trimet'ozine** (USAN). TRIOXAZINE; 4-(3,4,5-trimethoxybenzoyl)morpholine; antianxiety agent.

**trimip'ramine maleate** (BP, USAN). STANGYL; SURMONTIL; 5-[ 3-(dimethylamino)-2-methylpropyl ]-10,11-dihydro-5*H*-dibenz[ *b,f* ]azepine maleate; antidepressant.

**trimor'phic.** Trimorphous.

**trimorphism** (tri-mor'fizm) [ tri- + G. *morphē,* form ]. Existence under three forms as in the case of certain insects that pass through the stages of larva, pupa, and imago.

**trimorphous** (tri-mor'fus). Existing under three forms; marked by trimorphism.

**trini'trocel'lulose.** Constituent of soluble guncotton. Used in the preparation of collodion and of pyroxylin.

**trini'troglyc'erin.** Nitroglycerin.

**trinitrotoluene** (tri-ni-tro-tol'u-ēn). TNT; trinitrotoluol; CH₃C₆H₂(NO₂)₃; an explosive made by the nitrification of toluene; it causes gastric and intestinal disturbances and dermatitis in workers in munition factories.

**trinu'cleotide.** A combination of three adjacent nucleotides in a polynucleotide or nucleic acid molecule; often used with specific reference to the unit (codon or anticodon) specifying a particular amino acid in expression of the genetic code.

**triocephalus** (tri'o-sef'ā-lus) [ tri- + G. *kephalē,* head ]. Triencephalus; a fetus having an imperfectly formed head without mouth, nose, or eyes. The head is small and rounded, and contains almost no brain.

**tri'oki'nase.** Triosekinase; a phosphotransferase (EC 2.7.1.28) catalyzing the phosphorylation of glyceraldehyde to glyceraldehyde 3-phosphate by ATP.

**triolein** (tri-o'le-in). Olein.

**triophthalmos** (tri'of-thal'moa) [ tri- + G. *ophthalmos*, eye ]. Conjoined twins with fusion in the facial region such that the eyes on the joined sides have merged to form a single one. A variety of opodidymus (see fig. under opodidymus).

**triopodymus** (tri'o-pod'ī-mus) [ tri- + G. *ōps*, face, + *didymos*, twin ]. A grossly malformed fetus exhibiting three more or less recognizable faces on a single head.

**triorchid, triorchis** (tri-or'kid, tri-or'kis) [ tri- + G. *orchis*, testis ]. One who has three testes.

**triorchism** (tri-or'kizm). Condition of having three testes.

**tri'ose.** A three-carbon monosaccharide.

**tri'oseki'nase.** Triokinase.

**tri'osephosphate isom'erase.** An isomerizing enzyme (EC 5.3.1.1) that catalyzes the interconversion of glyceraldehyde 3-phosphate and dihydroxyacetone phosphate, a reaction of importance in glycolysis.

**triothy'rone.** 3,5,3'-Triiodothyronine.

**triotus** (tri-o'tus) [ tri- + G. *ous*, ear ]. A diprosopic fetus with three ears.

**trioxsalen** (tri'-ok-sa'len) (USP). TRISORALEN; 4,5,8-trimethylpsoralen; 2,5,9-trimethyl- 7*H*-furo[ 3,2-g ] [ 1 ]benzopyran-7-one; an orally effective pigmenting, photosensitizing agent; used as a tanning agent and in the treatment of vitiligo.

**trioxymeth'ylene.** Paraformaldehyde.

**tripal'mitin.** Palmitin.

**tripara** (trip'ă-rah) [ tri- + L. *pario*, to bear ]. A woman who has borne three children in as many pregnancies.

**tripar'anol.** MER-29; 1-[ *p*-(2-diethylaminoethoxy)phenyl ]-1-(*p*-tolyl)-2-(*p*-chlorophenyl)ethanol; formerly used as inhibitor of cholesterol biosynthesis but withdrawn from market because of formation of cataract.

**tripe** [ O. Fr. ]. The muscular wall of the rumen and reticulum of cattle used as food.

   **honeycomb t.,** the muscular wall of the reticulum.

**tri'pelen'namine hydrochloride** (USP). PYRIBENZAMINE hydrochloride; 2-[ benzyl[ 2-(dimethylamino)ethyl ]amino ]pyridine monohydrochloride; histamine antagonizing agent used in allergic states. Also available (USP), with same actions; is t. citrate; it is less bitter than the hydrochloride salt, and is therefore used in elixir.

**triphalangia** (tri-fă-lan'jī-ah) [ tri- + phalanx, *q.v.* ]. A malformation consisting in the presence of three phalanges in the thumb or great toe.

**tripharmacon, tripharmacum** (tri-far'mă-kon, -kum) [ tri- + G. *pharmakon*, drug ]. A pharmaceutical compound containing three drugs.

**triphen'ylmeth'ane dyes.** Rosanilin dyes; a group of basic dyes effective against Gram-positive organisms and schistosomes.

**triphos'phopyr'idine nu'cleotide.** See nicotinamide adenine dinucleotide phosphate.

**Tripier** (tre-pe-a'), Léon, French surgeon, 1842–1891. See T.'s *amputation*.

**tri'plant.** See triplant *implant*.

**triplegia** (tri-ple'jī-ah) [ tri- + G. *plēgē*, stroke ]. Paralysis of an upper and a lower extremity and of the face, or of both extremities on one side and of one on the other.

**trip'let.** 1. One of three children delivered at the same birth. 2. A set of three similar objects, as a compound lens in a microscope, formed of three planoconvex lenses. 3. Codon.

   **nonsense t.,** a t. (codon) in which a base change results in premature termination of the growing polypeptide chain and, consequently, incomplete protein molecules.

**triploblastic** (trip'lo-blas'tik) [ G. *triploos*, threefold, + *blastos*, germ ]. Formed of three primary germ layers, or containing tissue derived from all three layers.

**triploid** (trip'loid) [ G. *triploos*, threefold, + *eidos*, form ]. See polyploidy.

**triplopia** (trip-lo'pī-ah) [ G. *triploos*, triple, + *opsis*, sight ]. A visual defect in which three images are seen of the same object.

**tri'pod** [ G. *tripous*, fr. tri- + *pous*, foot ]. 1. Three-legged. 2. A stand having three legs or supports.

   **Haller's t.,** *truncus* celiacus.

   **vital t.,** the brain, the heart, and the lungs, regarded as the three organs essential to life.

**tripodia** (tri-po'dī-ah) [ tri- + G. *pous*, foot ]. A condition seen in conjoined twins when fusion has merged the lower extremities on the joined sides to form a single foot so that there are only three feet for the two bodies.

**triprol'idine hydrochloride** (NF, BP). ACTIDIL; *trans*-2-[ 3-(1-pyrrolidinyl)-1-(*p*-tolyl) propenyl ]pyridine hydrochloride; an antihistaminic agent used in the management of allergic and pruritic conditions.

**triprosopus** (tri'pro-so'pus) [ tri- + G. *prosōpon*, face ]. A fetus with three heads fused, leaving only parts of three faces.

**trip'sis** [ G. a rubbing ]. 1. Trituration (1). 2. Massage.

**triquetrous** (tri-kwe'trus, -kwet-) [ L. *triquetrus*, three-cornered ]. Triangular.

**triquetrum** (tri-kwe'trum, -kwet-) [ L. *triquetrus*, three-cornered ]. *Os* triquetrum.

**tri'ra'dial, tri'ra'diate.** Radiating in three directions.

**triradius** (tri-ra'dī-us). Galton's delta (2); the figure at the base of each finger in the palm, produced by rows of papillae running in three directions so as to form a triangle.

**tris-.** Chemical prefix indicating three of the substituents that follow.

**Tris.** Abbreviation for tris(hydroxymethyl)aminomethane.

**tri'sac'charide.** A carbohydrate containing three monosaccharide residues (*e.g.*, raffinose).

**tris(2-chlo'roethyl)amine hydrochloride.** 2,2',2''-Trichlorotriethylamine hydrochloride; a nitrogen mustard used in the treatment of leukemia.

**tris(hydroxymethyl)aminomethane.** TRIS; THAM; TROMETHANE; tromethamine; 2-amino-2-(hydroxymethyl)-1,3-propanediol; $H_2N$—$C(CH_2OH)_3$; an alkalizing agent used intravenously in the treatment of metabolic acidosis, in $CO_2$ retention, and in salicylate and barbiturate intoxication. This weakly basic compound is also extensively used as a buffer in enzymic reactions.

**triskaidekaphobia** (tris'kai-dek-ă-fo'bī-ah) [ G. *triskaideka*, thirteen, + *phobos*, fear ]. Triakaidekaphobia; superstitious dread of the number thirteen.

**trismic** (triz'mik). Relating to or marked by trismus.

**trismoid** (triz'moyd) [ trismus + G. *eidos*, resemblance ]. 1. Resembling trismus. 2. Trismus nascentium, formerly regarded as a distinct variety due to pressure on the occiput during birth.

**trismus** (triz'mus) [ L. fr. G. *trismos*, a creaking, rasping ]. Lockjaw; ankylostoma; a firm closing of the jaw due to tonic spasm of the muscles of mastication from disease of the motor branch of the trigeminus; usually associated with and due to general tetanus.

   **t. capistra'tus** [ L. *capistrum*, a muzzle ], congenital adhesion of the cheeks to the gums.

   **t. dolorif'icus,** trigeminal *neuralgia*.

   **t. nascen'tium, t. neonato'rum,** tetanus neonatorum, which usually begins with stiffness of the jaw muscles.

   **t. sardon'icus,** *risus* sardonicus.

**trisomic** (tri-so'mik). Relating to an individual or cell containing an extra chromosome; in man a trisomic cell contains 47 chromosomes.

**trisomy** (tri'so-mī) [ tri- + (chromo)some ]. State of an individual or cell with an extra chromosome; instead of the normal pair of homologous chromosomes there are three of a particular chromosome; in man the state of a cell containing 47 normal chromosomes.

   **chromosome t. syndromes,** see trisomy *syndromes*.

**trisplanchnic** (tri-splangk'nik) [ tri- + G. *splanchnon*, viscus ]. Relating to the three visceral cavities: skull, thorax, and abdomen.

**tri'spo'ric acids.** Terpenoid $C_{18}$ carboxylic acids that serve as fungal ectohormones. Secreted by *Blakeslea trispora*, they stimulate carotene synthesis in members of this species and reproductive activity in *Mucor mucedo*. Two forms have been isolated to date and have been designated trisporic acid B and trisporic acid C.

**tristearin** (tri-ste'ă-rin). Stearin.

**tristichia** (tri-stik′ĭ-ah) [ G. *tristichos*, in three rows, fr. *tri-*, three, + *stichos*, row ]. The presence of three rows of eyelashes.

**tristimania** (tris-tĭ-ma′nĭ-ah) [ L. *tristis*, sad, + G. *mania*, frenzy ]. Melancholia (1).

**trisulcate** (tri-sul′kāt). Marked by three grooves.

**tritanope** (tri′tă-nōp). A person who exhibits tritanopia.

**tritanopia** (tri′tă-no′pĭ-ah) [ G. *tritos*, third, + *an*- priv. + *ōps*, eye ]. Blue blindness, blue being the third of the primary colors, red, green, and blue; see deuteranopia and protanopia.

**triter′penes.** Hydrocarbons or their derivatives formed by the condensation of six isoprene units (equivalent to three terpene units) and containing, therefore, 30 carbon atoms; *e.g.*, squalene.

**tritiated** (trit′ĭ-a-ted). Containing atoms of tritium ($^3$H) in the molecule.

**triticeoglossus** (tri-tish′e-o-glos′us) [ L. *triticeum*, *q.v.*, + G. *glōssa*, tongue ]. See under musculus.

**triticeous** (tri-tish′us) [ L. *triticeus*, fr. *triticum*, a grain of wheat ]. Resembling or shaped like a grain of wheat.

**triticeum** (tri-tish′e-um) [ L. *triticeus*, triticeous ]. *Cartilago* triticea.

**triticonucleic acid** (trit′ĭ-ko-nu-kle′ik). Nucleic acid in wheat.

**triticum** (trit′ĭ-kum) [ L. wheat ]. Agropyrum; dog-grass; quick-grass; couch-grass; the rhizome and roots of *Agropyron repens* (family Gramineae); the fluid extract was formerly used for cystitis.

 **t. sati′vum,** wheat.

**tritium** (trit′ĭ-um, trish′ĭ-um). Hydrogen-3.

**tritocal′ine.** Tritoqualine.

**tritopine** (trit′o-pēn, -pin, tri′to-). Laudanidine; $C_{20}H_{25}NO_4$; an alkaloid present in opium. Its action resembles that of strychnine.

**tritoqual′ine.** HYPOSTAMINE; tritocaline; 7-amino-4,5,6-triethoxy-3-(5,6,7,8-tetrahydro-4-methoxy-6-methyl-1,3-dioxolo[ 4,5-*g* ]isoquinolin-5-yl)-phthalide; antihistaminic.

**tri′tox′ide.** Trioxide.

**tri′totox′in.** A hypothetical form of toxin in certain bacterial cultures, which has less affinity for antitoxin than has deuterotoxin.

**Tri′trichom′onas** [ G. *tri-*, three, + *Trichomonas* ]. A genus of parasitic protozoan flagellates, formerly part of the genus *Trichomonas* but now separated as a distinct genus in a distinct subfamily (Tritrichomonadinae) by the absence of a pelta and the presence of three anterior flagella; see *Trichomonas*.

 **T. foe′tus,** formerly *Trichomonas foetus*; causes bovine trichomoniasis.

 **T. su′is,** formerly *Trichomonas suis*; occurs in the nasal passages, stomach, cecum, and colon of pigs.

**tri′tuber′cular.** Tricuspid; having three tubercles or cusps, as the second upper molar tooth occassionally, and the third upper molar usually.

**triturable** (trit′u-rā-bl). Capable of being triturated.

**triturate** (trit′u-rāt). 1. To accomplish trituration. 2. A triturated substance.

 **tablet t.,** a compressed tablet of a medicated powder rubbed up with milk sugar.

**trituration** (trit′u-ra′shun) [ L. *trituratio*, fr. *trituro*, to thresh, fr. *tero*, pp. *tritus*, to rub ]. 1. Tripsis (1); the act of reducing a drug to a fine powder and incorporating it thoroughly with sugar of milk by rubbing the two together in a mortar. 2. Mixing of dental amalgam in a mortar and pestle.

**triturium** (tri-tu′rĭ-um) [ see trituration ]. A vessel used to hold liquids of different densities, which rise to their respective levels and are then drawn off.

**tri′tyl.** The triphenylmethyl radical, $Ph_3C—$.

**trivalence** (tri-va′lens). The property of being trivalent.

**trivalent** (tri-va′lent) [ tri- + L. *valentia*, strength ]. Having a valence of 3.

**tri′valve.** Provided with three valves, as a speculum with three diverging blades.

**trivial name.** A name of a chemical, no part of which is used in a systematic sense. Such names are common for drugs, hormones, proteins and other biologicals (see also generic name, nonproprietary name). Trivial names, of themselves, give no clue as to chemical structure. Examples are water, aspirin, chlorophyll, heme, methotrexate, folic acid, caffeine, thyroxine, epinephrine, barbital, etc., also common abbreviations for chemically defined substances, such as ACTH, MSH, BAL, DDT, which are spoken as such and not in terms of the words they represent. The distinction between trivial and semitrivial names is seldom made; thus tetrahydrofolate, methylglycine, glucosamine, etc., are often termed trivial even though each contains a systematic part that is used in the correct systematic sense (tetrahydro for four hydrogen atoms, methyl for a —$CH_3$ group, amine for —$NH_2$ in the above). Trivial names are often assigned arbitrarily to chemical compounds, especially from natural sources, before the chemical structures, hence systematic names, can be assigned. Also, they afford useful shortenings of long systematic names even when these can be stated (although most such shortenings turn out to be semitrivial as they incorporate some portion of the systematic name).

**trizo′nal.** Having, or arranged in, three zones or layers.

**tRNA.** Abbreviation for transfer RNA; see under ribonucleic acid.

**trocar** [ Fr. *trocart*, fr. *trois*, three, + *carre*, side (of a sword blade) ]. An instrument for withdrawing fluid from a cavity, or for use in paracentesis; it consists of a metal tube (cannula), open at both ends, in which fits a rod with a sharp three-cornered tip, which is withdrawn after the instrument has been pushed into the cavity. The term t. is usually applied to the rod with sharpened tip alone, the entire instrument being designated t. and cannula.

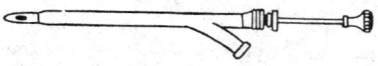

**Trocar and Cannula**

**troch.** Abbreviation of L. *trochiscus*, troche.

**trochanter** (tro-kan′ter) [ G. *trochantēr*, a rummer, fr. *trechō*, to run ]. One of the bony prominences developed from independent osseous centers near the upper extremity of the femur; there are two in man, three in the horse.

 **greater t.,** t. major.

 **lesser t.,** t. minor.

 **t. major,** [ NA ], greater t.; a strong process at the proximal and lateral part of the shaft of the femur, overhanging the root of the neck; it gives attachment to the gluteus medius and minimus, pyriformis, obturator internus and externus, and gemelli muscles.

 **t. minor** [ NA ], lesser t.; a pyramidal process projecting from the medial and proximal part of the shaft of the femur at the line of junction of the shaft and the neck; it receives the insertion of the psoas major and iliacus (iliopsoas) muscles.

 **small t.,** t. minor.

 **t. ter′tius** [ NA ], third t.; gluteal tuberosity (2); an occasional process at the proximal end of the lateral lip of the linea aspera of the femur, about on a level with the lesser t., giving insertion to the greater part of the gluteus maximus muscle.

 **third t.,** t. tertius.

**trochanterian, trochanteric** (tro-kan-tēr′ĭ-an, -tēr′ik). Relating to a trochanter; especially the trochanter major.

**trochanterplasty** (tro-kan′ter-plasty). Plastic surgery on trochanters and neck of femur.

**trochantin** (tro-kan′tin). *Trochanter* minor.

**trochantinian** (tro-kan-tin′ĭ-an). Relating to the trochanter minor.

**trochar** (tro′car). Trocar.

**troche** (trōk, tro′ke) [ L. *trochiscus*, *q.v.* ]. Lozenge; pastil; trochiscus; morsulus; a small, disk-shaped or rhombic body composed of solidifying paste containing an astringent, antiseptic, or demulcent drug, used for local treatment of the mouth or throat, the t. being held in the mouth until dissolved. The vehicle or base of the t. is usually sugar, made adhesive by admixture with acacia or tragacanth, fruit paste, made from black or red currants, confection of rose, or balsam of tolu.

**trochiscus,** pl. **trochisci** (tro-kis′kus) [ L. from G. *trochiskos*, a small wheel, a lozenge, fr. *trochos*, a wheel ]. Troche.

**trochlea,** pl. **trochleae** (trok′le-ah, -le-e) [ L. pulley, fr. G. *trochileia*, a pulley, fr. *trechō*, to run ]. [ NA ]. 1. A structure serving as a pulley. 2. A smooth articular surface of bone upon which another glides. 3. A fibrous loop in the orbit, near the nasal process of the frontal bone, through which passes the tendon of the superior oblique muscle of the eye.

    **t. fem′oris,** *facies* patellaris femoris.

    **t. fibula′ris calca′nei** [ NA ], official alternative term for t. peronealis.

    **t. hu′meri** [ NA ], t. or pulley of the humerus; the grooved surface at the lower end of the humerus articulating with the trochlear notch of the ulna.

    **t. muscula′ris** [ NA ], muscular pulley; a fibrous loop through which the tendon of a muscle passes; the intermediate tendon of the digastric and omohyoid pass through such a t.

    **t. mus′culi obli′qui superio′ris** [ NA ], t. of the superior oblique muscle; see trochlea (3).

    **t. peronea′lis** [ NA ], t. fibularis calcanei [ NA ]; peroneal pulley; trochlear process; processus trochlearis; a projection from the lateral side of the calcaneus between the tendons of the peroneus longus and brevis.

    **t. phalan′gis,** *caput* phalangis.

    **t. ta′li** [ NA ], pulley of the talus; the rounded articular surface of the talus articulating with the distal ends of the tibia and fibula.

**trochlear** (trok′le-ar). 1. Relating to a trochlea, especially the trochlea of the superior oblique muscle of the eye. 2. Trochleiform.

**trochleariform** (trok-le-ăr′if-orm). Trochleiform.

**trochlearis** (trok-le-a′ris) [ L. ]. Trochlear.

**trochleiform** (trok′le-ĭ-form). Trochleariform; trochlear (2); pulley-shaped.

**trochocardia** (trok-o-kar′dĭ-ah) [ G. *trochos*, wheel, + *kardia*, heart ]. A rotary displacement of the heart around its axis.

**trochoid** (tro′koyd) [ G. *trochōdēs*, fr. *trochos*, wheel, + *eidos*, resemblance ]. Revolving; rotating; denoting a revolving or wheel-like articulation.

**trochorizocardia** (trō-kor-i′zo-kar′dĭ-ah). Combined trochocardia and horizocardia.

**Troglotrema salmincola** (trog′lo-tre′mah sal-mingk′o-lah). *Nanophyetes salmincola.*

**Troisier** (trwah-ze-a′), Charles-Emile, French physician, 1844–1919. See T.'s *ganglion, node.*

**tro′lamine.** USAN-approved contraction for triethanolamine, N(CH₂CH₂OH)₃.

**tro′land** [ after L. T. *Troland* ]. Photon (1); a unit of visual stimulation at the retina equal to the illumination per square millimeter of pupil received from a surface of 1 lux brightness.

**Trolard** (trō-lar′), Paulin, French anatomist, 1842–1910. See T.'s *vein.*

**troleandomycin** (tro′le-an-do-mi′sin). CYCLAMYCIN; TAO; triacetyloleandomycin; the triacetyl ester of oleandomycin, with a potency of not less than 760 µg. per mg.; an orally effective antibiotic for infections produced by Gram-positive, penicillin-resistant bacteria.

**trolnitrate phosphate** (trol-ni′trāt). METAMINE; NITRE-TAMIN; triethanolamine trinitrate diphosphate; an organic nitrate with mild but persistent vasodilator action on smooth muscle of the smaller vessels of postarteriolar vascular beds; used in preventing attacks of angina pectoris.

**Tröltsch** (trëlch), Anton F. von, German otologist, 1829–1890. See T.'s *corpuscles, fold, pockets, recesses.*

**Trombicula** (trom-bik′u-lah). Chigger mite; a genus of mites (family Trombiculidae) whose larvae (chiggers, red bugs) include notorious pests of man and other animals and vectors of rickettsial and probably viral diseases.

    **T. akamu′shi** and **delien′sis** two species (subgenus *Leptotrombidium)* implicated in the transmission of *Rick-*

ettsia tsutsugamushi, agent of tsutsugamushi disease in Japan and elsewhere in the Orient; the larvae of these species are characteristic parasites of rodents, which therefore are reservoirs of human infections, although the mites themselves are also reservoirs, as their rickettsial parasites are transovarially transmitted from generation to generation (a requirement for transmission to man as the mites feed parasitically only once in their lifetimes).

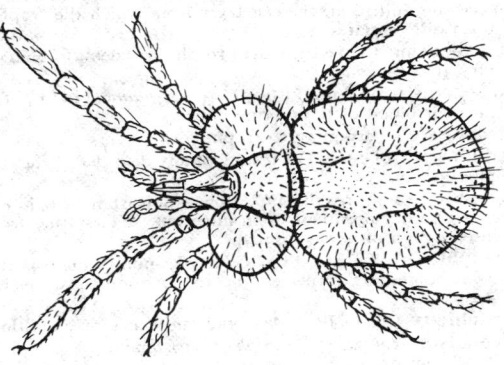

*Trombicula akamushi*
Adult (×30)

    **T. alfredduge′si,** common in North America, particularly in southeastern United States, in second growth and grassy brush areas; the larvae attack man (as well as reptiles, quail, rabbits, and domestic animals), causing an intensely itching dermatitis, especially in sensitized individuals.

**trombiculiasis** (trom-bik′u-li′ā-sis). Infestation by *Trombicula.*

**trombic′ulid.** Common name for members of the family Trombiculidae.

**Trombiculidae** (trom-bik-u-li′de). A family of mites whose larvae (redbugs, rougets, harvest mites, scrub mites, or chiggers) are parasitic on vertebrates and whose nymphs and adults are bright red, free-living mites that live on insect eggs or minute organisms in the soil. The six-legged larvae are barely visible red or orange parasites that attach to the skin for a few days to a month, producing an exceedingly irritating reaction. In the Orient, trombiculid chiggers transmit tsutsugamushi disease caused by *Rickettsia tsutsugamushi,* which is transovarially transmitted in these mites.

**Trombidiidae** (trom′bī-di′ī-de). A family of mites that formerly included the subfamily Trombiculinae, now raised to the family Trombiculidae (including the vectors of tsutsugamushi disease). T. larvae are characteristically parasitic on insects, not on invertebrates as with the larvae of Trombiculidae.

**tromethamine** (tro-meth′ā-mēn) (NF). Tris(hydroxymethyl)aminomethane.

**Trömmer,** Ernest L. O., German neurologist, *1868. See T.'s *reflex.*

**Trommer,** Karl A., German chemist, 1806–1879. See T.'s *test.*

**tromomania** (trom-o-ma′nĭ-ah) [ G. *tromos,* a trembling, + *mania,* frenzy ]. *Delirium* tremens.

**trona.** A native sodium carbonate.

**tropacocaine** (tro′pă-ko′kān). Benzoylpseudotropeine; an alkaloid obtained from Java coca leaves; a has been used as a local and spinal anesthetic.

**tro′pane.** A bicyclic hydrocarbon, the fundamental structure of tropine *(q.v.,* for structure), atropine, and other physiologically active substances.

**tro′pate.** A salt or ester of tropic acid.

**tropeine** (tro′pe-in). An ester of tropine; either a naturally occurring alkaloid or prepared synthetically.

**tropen′tane.** 1-Phenylcyclopentanecarboxylic acid 3α-tropanyl ester hydrochloride; antispasmodic with anticholinergic properties.

**tropeolins** (tro-pe'o-linz) [ G. *tropaios*, pertaining to a turning or change, fr. *tropē*, a turn ]. A group of azo-dyes used as indicators; *e.g.*, methyl orange and orange I.

**troph-.** See tropho-.

**trophectoderm** (trof-ek'to-derm) [ troph- + ectoderm ]. The outermost layer of cells in the mammalian blastodermic vesicle that will make contact with the endometrium and take part in establishing the embryo's means of receiving nutrition; the cell layer from which the trophoblast differentiates.

**trophedema** (trof'e-de'mah) [ troph- + edema ]. Hereditary *lymphedema*.

**trophema** (trof-e'mah) [ troph- + G. *haima*, blood ]. The nutrient blood of the uterine mucosa.

**trophe'sic.** Pertaining to trophesy.

**trophesy** (trof'e-sĭ). The results of any disorder of the trophic nerves.

**trophic** (trof'ik, tro'fik) [ G. *trophē*, nourishment ]. 1. Relating to or dependent upon nutrition. 2. Resulting from interruption of nerve supply.

**-trophic** (-trof'ik, -tro'fik) [ G. *trophē*, nourishment ]. Suffixed combining form relating to nutrition; also spelled -tropic.

**trophicity** (trŏ-fis'ĭ-tĭ). A trophic influence or condition.

**trophism** (trof'izm) [ G. *trophē*, nourishment ]. 1. Trophicity. 2. Nutrition.

**tropho-, troph-** (trof'o-, tro'fo-) [ G. *trophē*, nourishment ]. Combining forms relating to food or nutrition.

**trophoblast** (trof'o-blast, tro'fo-blast) [ tropho- + G. *blastos*, germ ]. The ectodermal cell layer covering the blastocyst which erodes the uterine mucosa and through which the embryo receives nourishment from the mother. The cells do not enter into the formation of the embryo itself but contribute to the formation of the placenta. The t. develops processes that later receive a core of vascular mesoderm and are then known as the chorionic villi. The t. soon becomes two-layered, the outer layer being a multinucleated protoplasmic mass or syncytium called the syncytiotrophoblast. In the deeper layer next to the mesoderm the cells retain their membranes and are therefore said to constitute the cytotrophoblast.
   **plasmodial t.,** syncytiotrophoblast.
   **syncytial t.,** syncytiotrophoblast.

**trophoblas'tic.** Relating to the trophoblast.

**trophoblasto'ma.** Choriocarcinoma.

**trophochromatin** (trof'o-kro'mă-tin). Trophochromidia.

**trophochromidia** (trof'o-kro-mid'ĭ-ah) [ tropho- + chromidia (see chromidium) ]. Trophochromatin; nongerminal or vegetative extranuclear masses of chromatin, found in certain protozoan forms; *e.g.*, the macronucleus of certain ciliates, such as *Paramecium*.

**trophocyte** (trof'o-sīt) [ tropho- + G. *kytos*, cell ]. A cell that supplies nourishment; *e.g.* Sertoli cells in the seminiferous tubules.

**trophoderm** (trof'o-derm) [ tropho- + G. *derma*, skin ]. The trophectoderm, or trophoblast, together with the vascular mesodermal layer underlying it. See also serosa (2).

**trophodermatoneurosis** (trof'o-der'mă-to-nu-ro'sis). Cutaneous trophic changes due to neural involvement.

**trophodynamics** (trof-o-di-nam'iks) [ tropho- + G. *dynamis*, power ]. Nutritional energy; the dynamics of nutrition or metabolism.

**trophoneurosis** (trof'o-nu-ro'sis) [ tropho- + G. *neuron*, nerve, + suffix -*osis*, condition ]. A trophic disorder, such as atrophy, hypertrophy, or a skin eruption, occurring as a consequence of disease or injury of the nerves of the part.
   **facial t.,** facial *hemiatrophy*.
   **lingual t.,** progressive lingual *hemiatrophy*.
   **muscular t.,** progressive muscular *atrophy*.
   **Romberg's t.,** facial *hemiatrophy*.

**trophoneurot'ic.** Relating to a trophoneurosis.

**trophono'sis, trophon'osus** [ tropho- + G. *nosos*, disease ]. Any disorder of nutrition or metabolism or disease resulting therefrom.

**trophonucleus** (trof-o-nu'kle-us). Macronucleus (2).

**trophopathia, trophopathy** (trof-o-path'ĭ-ah, trof'ă-thĭ) [ tropho- + G. *pathos*, suffering ]. 1. A disorder of nutrition. 2. A trophic disease, one due to excessive, deficient, or perverted nutrition, either local or general; trophonosis.

**trophoplasm** (trof'o-plazm) [ tropho- + G. *plasma*, a thing formed ]. An obsolete term referring to the achromatin or supposed formative substance of a cell.

**troph'oplast** [ tropho- + G. *plastos*, formed ]. A plastid.

**trophospongia** (trof'o-spon'jĭ-ah) [ tropho- + G. *spongia*, a sponge ]. 1. Canalicular structures described by Holmgren in the protoplasm of certain cells. 2. The highly vascular layer of the endometrium adjacent to the chorionic villi of the fetal portion of the placenta (obsolete).

**trophotaxis** (trof-o-tak'sis) [ tropho- + G. *taxis*, arrangement ]. Trophotropism.

**trophotonus** (tro-fot'o-nus) [ tropho- + G. *tonos*, tension ]. Rigidity of muscular or other contractile tissue due to disordered nutrition.

**trophotropic** (trof'o-trop'ik). Relating to trophotropism.

**trophotropism** (tro-fot'ro-pizm) [ tropho- + G. *tropē*, a turning ]. Trophotaxis; chemotaxis of living cells in relation to nutritive material; it may be positive (toward nutritive material) or negative (away from nutritive material.)

**trophozoite** (trof-o-zo'it) [ tropho- + G. *zōon*, animal ]. The ameboid, vegetative, asexual form of certain Sporozoa, such as the schizont of the plasmodia of malaria and related parasites.

**-trophy** [ G. *trophē*, nourishment ]. Suffix meaning food, nutrition.

**tro'pia** [ G. *tropē*, a turning ]. Abnormal deviation of the eye; see strabismus.

**-tropic** (-trop'ik, -tro'fik) [ G. *tropē*, a turning ]. 1. Suffixed combining form meaning a turning toward; having an affinity for. 2. An alternative spelling for the combining form -trophic, *q.v.*

**trop'ic acid.** Tropeic acid; tropaic acid; α-phenylhydracrylic acid; α-phenyl-β-hydroxypropionic acid; $C_6H_5$-$CH(CH_2OH)COOH$; a constituent of atropine and of scopolamine, in which it is esterified through its COOH to the 3-CHOH of tropine.

**tropicamide** (tro-pik'ă-mīd) (USP). MYDRIACYL; *N*-ethyl-2-phenyl-*N*-4-pyridylmethyl)hydracrylamide; an anticholinergic agent used to effect a rapid and brief mydriasis for eye examination.

**tro'pine.** 3α-Tropanol; 3α-hydroxytropane; the major constituent of atropine and scopolamine, from which it is obtained on hydrolysis.

**Tropine**

   **t. mandelate,** homatropine.

**tro'pism** [ G. *tropē*, a turning ]. The phenomenon observed in living organisms of moving toward (positive t.) or away from (negative t.) a focus of light, heat, or other stimulus; usually applied to the movement of a portion of the organism as opposed to taxis, the movement of an entire organism.

**tropocollagen** (tro'po-kol'ă-jen, trop'o-). The fundamental units of collagen fibrils consisting of three helically arranged polypeptide chains.

**tropom'eter** [ G. *tropē*, a turning, + *metron*, measure ]. Any instrument for measuring the degree of rotation or torsion, as of the eyeball, of the shaft of a long bone, etc.

**tropomy'osin B.** A fibrous protein extractable from dry powder of muscle.

**trot** [ M.E. ]. A gait of horses in which the diagonal legs act together.

**trough** (trof). A long, narrow, shallow channel or depression.

**gingival t.,** the formation of a crater as a result of destruction of interdental tissues so that, in effect, there exists a labial and lingual curtain of gingiva with no interproximal connection at all.

**Langmuir t.,** a t. with a movable surface barrier for studying the compression of surface films.

**synaptic t.,** the depression of the surface of the striated muscle fiber that accommodates the motor endplate.

**Trousseau** (troo-so'), Armand, French physician, 1801–1867. See T.-Lallemand *bodies,* T.'s *point, sign, spots, syndrome, test.*

**troxerutin.** PAROVEN; 7,3',4'-tris[ o-(2-hydroxyethyl) ]rutin; used for treatment of venous disorders.

**Trp.** Symbol for tryptophan and its radicals.

**truncal** (trung'kal). Relating to the trunk of the body or to any arterial or nerve trunk, etc.

**truncate** (trung'kāt) [ L. *trunco,* pp. *-atus,* to maim, cut off ]. Truncated; cut across at right angles to the long axis, or appearing to be so cut.

**truncus,** gen. and pl. **trunci** (trung'kus, -ki) [ L. stem, trunk ] [ NA ]. 1. The body (trunk or torso), excluding the head and extremities. 2. A primary nerve or vessel before its division. 3. A large collecting lymphatic vessel.

**t. arterio'sus commu'nis,** the common arterial trunk opening out of both ventricles in early fetal life, later destined to be divided into aorta and pulmonary artery by development of the bulbar septum.

**t. atrioventricula'ris** [ NA ], atrioventricular trunk; official alternate term for *fasciculus* atrioventricularis.

**t. brachiocepha'licus** [ NA ], brachiocephalic trunk; innominate artery; arteria anonyma; anonymous artery; *origin* arch of aorta; *branches,* right subclavian and right common carotid; occasionally it gives off the thyroidea ima.

**t. bronchiomediastina'lis** [ NA ], bronchomediastinal trunk; a lymphatic vessel arising from the union of the efferent lymphatics from the bronchial and mediastinal nodes on either side.

**t. celi'acus** [ NA ], celiac trunk; arteria celiaca; celiac artery; celiac axis; *origin,* abdominal aorta just below diaphragm; *branches,* left gastric, common hepatic, splenic.

**t. cor'poris callo'si** [ NA ], trunk of the corpus callosum; the main arched portion of the corpus callosum.

**t. costocervica'lis** [ NA ], costocervical trunk; costocervical artery; a short artery that arises from the subclavian artery on each side and divides into deep cervical and highest intercostal branches, the latter dividing usually to form the first and second posterior intercostal arteries.

**t. infe'rior** [ NA ], inferior trunk; the nerve bundle formed by the union of the ventral branches of the eighth cervical and first thoracic nerves; it provides fibers to the posterior and inferior cords (fasciculi) of the brachial plexus.

**trunci intestina'les** [ NA ], intestinal trunks; the vessels conveying lymph from the lower part of the liver, the stomach, spleen, pancreas, and small intestine; they discharge into the cisterna chyli and are sometimes duplicated.

**t. jugula'ris** [ NA ], jugular trunk or duct; lymphatic vessel on each side, conveying the lymph from the head and neck; that on the right side empties into the right lymphatic duct, that on the left into the thoracic duct.

**t. linguofacia'lis** [ NA ], the common trunk by which the lingual and facial arteries frequently arise from the external carotid artery.

**trunci lumba'les** [ NA ], lumbar trunks; two lymphatic ducts conveying lymph from the lower limbs, pelvic viscera and walls, large intestine, kidneys, and suprarenal capsules; they discharge into the cisterna chyli.

**t. lum'bosacra'lis** [ NA ], lumbosacral trunk; a large nerve, formed by the union of the fifth lumbar and first sacral, with a branch from the fourth lumbar nerve, which enters into the formation of the sacral plexus.

**t. me'dius** [ NA ], middle trunk; the continuation of the ventral branch of the seventh cervical nerve; it contributes fibers to the posterior and lateral cords (fasciculi) of the brachial plexus.

**persistent t. arterio'sus,** a congenital cardiovascular deformity resulting from failure of development of the bulbar septum and consisting of a common arterial trunk

opening out of both ventricles, the pulmonary arteries being given off from the ascending common trunk.

**trunci plex'us brachia'lis** [ NA ], trunks of the brachial plexus; the superior, middle, and inferior trunks; they divide distally to form the cords (fasciculi) of the plexus.

**t. pulmona'lis** [ NA ], pulmonary trunk; arteria pulmonalis; venous artery; pulmonary artery; *origin,* right ventricle of heart; *distribution,* it divides into the *arteria pulmonalis dextra* and the *arteria pulmonalis sinistra,* which enter the corresponding lungs and branch along with the segmental bronchi.

**t. subcla'vius** [ NA ], subclavian trunk or duct, formed by the union of the vessels draining the lymph nodes of either upper limb, emptying into the thoracic duct at the root of the neck on the left or into the right lymphatic duct.

**s. supe'rior** [ NA ], superior trunk; the nerve bundle formed by the union of the ventral branches of the fifth and sixth cervical nerves and some fibers from the fourth; it contributes fibers to the posterior and lateral cords (fasciculi) of the brachial plexus.

**t. sympath'icus** [ NA ], sympathetic trunk; gangliated cord; one of the two long ganglionated nerve strands alongside the vertebral column that extend from the base of the skull to the coccyx; they are connected to each spinal nerve by gray rami and receive fibers from the spinal cord through white rami connecting with the thoracic and upper lumbar spinal nerves.

**t. thyrocervica'lis** [ NA ], thyroid axis; a short arterial trunk arising from the subclavian and dividing generally into three branches: thyroidea inferior, transversa colli, and suprascapularis.

**t. vaga'lis** [ NA ], vagal trunk; one of the two nerve bundles, anterior and posterior, into which the esophageal plexus continues as it passes through the diaphragm.

**Trunecek** (troo'net-sek), Karel, Prague physician, *1865. See T.'s *symptom.*

**trunk** [ L. *truncus* ]. Truncus.

**atrioventricular t.,** *truncus* atrioventricularis.

**t.'s of brachial plexus,** *trunci* plexus brachialis.

**brachiocephalic t.,** *truncus* brachiocephalicus.

**celiac t.,** *truncus* celiacus.

**t. of corpus callosum,** *truncus* corporis callosi.

**costocervical t.,** *truncus* costocervicalis.

**inferior t.,** *truncus* inferior.

**intestinal t.'s,** *trunci* intestinales.

**jugular t.,** *truncus* jugularis.

**lumbar t.'s,** *trunci* lumbales.

**lumbosacral t.,** *truncus* lumbosacralis.

**middle t.,** *truncus* medius.

**nerve t.,** a collection of funiculi or bundles of nerve fibers enclosed in a connective tissue sheath, the epineurium.

**pulmonary t.,** *truncus* pulmonalis.

**subclavian t.,** *truncus* subclavius.

**superior t.,** *truncus* superior.

**sympathetic t.,** *truncus* sympathicus.

**vagal t.,** *truncus* vagalis.

**trusion** (tru'zhun) [ L. *trudo,* pp. *trusus,* to thrust ]. Displacement of a tooth forward.

**truss** [ Fr. *trousser,* to tie up, to pack ]. An instrument used to prevent the return of a reduced hernia or the increase in size of an irreducible hernia; it consists of a pad attached to a belt and kept in place by a spring or straps.

**Try.** Obsolete abbreviation for tryptophan; now Trp.

**try-in.** A preliminary insertion of a complete denture wax-up (trial denture), of a partial denture casting, or of a finished restoration to determine the fit, esthetics, maxillomandibular relation, etc.

**trypan** (trip'an, tri'pan). See t. blue, t. red.

**t. blue,** an acid azo dye, $C_{34}H_{34}N_6O_{14}S_4Na_4$, used for vital staining of the reticuloendothelial system, uriniferous tubules, and cells in tissue culture, and as an experimental teratogen; formerly used as a trypanocide.

**t. red,** an azo dye formerly used in the treatment of trypanosomiasis.

**trypanid** (trip'ă-nid). Trypanosomid.

**trypanocidal** (trī-pan'o-si'dal, trip'ă-no-). Destructive to trypanosomes.

**trypanocide** (trī-pan'o-sīd, trip'ă-no-) [ trypanosome L. *caedo,* to kill ]. Trypanosomicide; an agent that kills trypanosomes.

**Trypanoplasma** (trī-pan'o-plaz'mah, trip'ă-no-) [ G. *trypanon*, auger, + *plasma*, anything formed ]. A genus of flagellate Protozoa (family Cryptobiidae), the members of which have a body of varying shape with an undulating membrane and a flagellum projecting from either extremity. They are parasitic in the blood of fishes.

**Trypanosoma** (trī-pan'o-so'mah, trip'ă-no-) [ G. *trypanon*, an auger, + *sōma*, body ]. A genus of asexual, digenetic, protozoan flagellates (family Trypanosomidae) that have a spindle-shaped body with an undulating membrane on one side a single anterior flagellum, and a kinetoplast. These trypanosomes are parasitic in the blood plasma of many vertebrates (only a few being pathogenic) and as a rule have an intermediate host, a bloodsucking invertebrate, such as a leech, tick, or insect. The most important pathogenic forms cause trypanosomiasis in man and a number of other diseases in domestic animals.

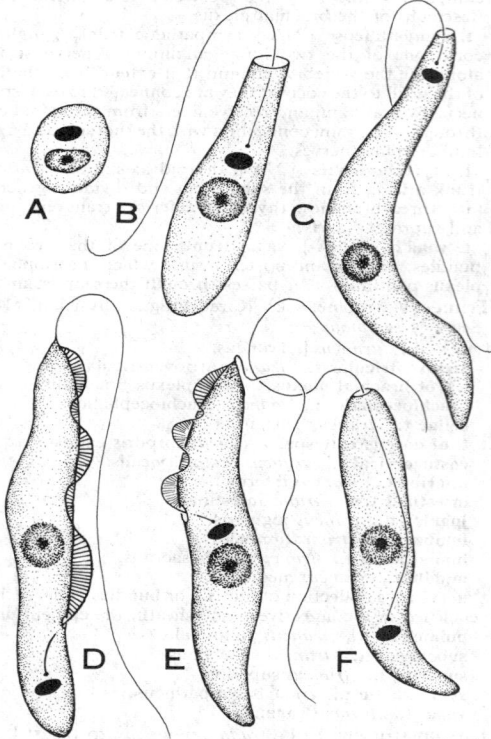

**Flagellate Body Forms in Family Trypanosomatidae**

*A*, amastigote (leishmanial form), genus *Leishmania; B*, choanomastigote (barleycorn form), genus *Crithidia; C*, promastigote (leptomonad form), genus *Leptomonas; D*, trypomastigote (trypanosomal or trypanosome form), genus *Trypanosoma; E*, epimastigote (crithidial or blastocrithidial form), genus *Blastocrithidia; F*, opisthomastigote (herpetomonad form), genus *Herpetomonas*. Parenthetical terms are old nomenclature.

**T. av'vium,** occurs in owls, crows, and other birds; various bloodsucking arthropods are the vectors, including mosquitoes, blackflies, and hippoboscids; this species was reported under a large number of names now considered to be physiologic strains of this species.

**T. bo'vis** *T. vivax.*

**T. bruce'i,** a common parasite of many types of domestic and wild mammals in tropical Africa, thought to be the source of the human strains *T. gambiense* and *T. rhodesiense;* it is nonpathogenic in African wild antelopes and other wild herbivores, but highly fatal in domestic cattle; it is one of the trypanosomes causing nagana and is generally transmitted by tsetse flies of the *Glossina morsi-*

*tans* group.

**T. congolen'se,** *T. pecorum;* the most common cause of nagana in Africa; it is highly pathogenic for cattle, but infection is also common and pathogenic in horses, pigs, sheep, goats and dogs; it is not pathogenic in native game; it is the most common *T.* species in Central Africa.

**T. cru'zi,** *T. escomelis; T. triatomae;* causes South American trypanosomiasis and is endemic in various countries of Central and South America, especially in Brazil, Chile, Argentina, and Venezuela; these organisms, but not the disease, are found also in reduviid bugs in parts of California, Texas, and Arizona; in man, trypomastigotes are found in the blood and amastigotes, indistinguishable from *Leishmania* that cause visceral and other leishmaniases, are found in the tissues; in South American trypanosomiasis, heart muscle fibers and cells of many other organs are attacked, the organisms not being restricted to marrow, spleen, liver, or lymph node macrophages as in visceral leishmaniasis; man, dogs, cats, house rats, armadillos, bats, certain monkeys, and opossums are the usual vertebrate hosts, and the organisms are transmitted by members of the family Triatomidae; also called *Schizotrypanum cruzi,* a distinct generic designation widely used in the endemic regions.

**T. dimor'phon,** an African species found in horses, cattle, sheep, goats, pigs and dogs, formerly thought to be the same as *T. congolense* but now recognized as a distinct and more pathogenic species in cattle, sheep, and dogs; it is spread by tsetse flies across Central Africa.

**T. equi'num,** the parasitic agent of mal de caderas of horses in South America; except for being akinetoplastic, it is identical to *T. evansi* and is transmitted in the same manner.

**T. equiper'dum,** *T. rougeti;* the parasitic agent of dourine.

**T. escome'lis.** *T. cruzi.*

**T. ev'ansi,** *T. hippicum; T. venezuelense;* a parasite chiefly of cattle, camels, horses and dogs, causing diseases, such as surra, murrina, and derrengadera; it is widely distributed outside of the tsetse belt, as it can be transmitted mechanically (without cyclical development) by tabanid flies.

**t. gambien'se,** *T. hominis; T. ugandense;* causes Gambian trypanosomiasis or African sleeping sickness; endemic in tropical regions of western and central Africa to its eastern limits of Lake Victoria and Tanzania; polymorphic forms are found in human blood that are related to the succession of antigenic forms found in man and to the development of the so-called "stumpy form" which infects the tsetse fly host; it is transmitted by several species of tsetse flies, particularly *Glossina palpalis,* whose habits determine the distribution of the human disease; natural reservoir hosts, other than man, are unknown.

**T. hip'picum,** *T. evansi.*

**T. hom'inis,** *T. gambiense.*

**T. igno'tum,** old name for *T. simiae.*

**T. lew'isi,** a worldwide nonpathogenic parasite in the blood of rats and widely used for laboratory study; it is transmitted by the rat flea, *Nosopsyllus fasciatus.*

**T. melopha'gium,** a nonpathogenic species (related to *T. theileri*) found in sheep throughout the world, and probably in goats as well; the vector is *Melophagus ovinus.*

**T. na'num,** old name for *T. congolense.*

**T. peco'rum,** *T. congolense.*

**T. por'ci,** *T. simiae.*

**T. range'li,** parasitizes a wide variety of mammals, including man, in South America and is transmitted by the triatomid bugs *Rhodnius prolixus* and *Tiratoma dimidiata,* and probably others; it is apparently nonpathogenic but may be pathogenic in the bug host.

**T. rhodesien'se,** causes Rhodesian trypanosomiasis, which is endemic in northeastern Zambia, Rhodesia, Malawi, Portuguese East Africa, and Tanzania—a distribution distinct from that of *T. gambiense* as a result of the habits of the vectors; it is morphologically identical to *T. gambiense* in man, but when *T. rhodesiense* is injected into rats, mice, and guinea pigs, the nuclei are frequently located in the posterior portion of the cell, a condition rarely observed in *T. gambiense* but characteristic of *T. brucei;* although *T. rhodesiense* and *T. gambiense* are considered to be subspecies of *T. brucei,* they are spearated as a matter of convenience because of their medical importance; the chief vector of *T. rhodesiense* is *Glossina morsitans*, also *Glossina swynnertoni* in some regions; the bushbuck, a small African antelope, is a reservoir host.

**T. rodhai'ni,** *T. simiae.*

**T. rouge'ti,** *T. equiperdum.*

**T. simi'ae,** *T. porci; T. rodhaini;* first described from monkeys, but normally found in warthogs; it is highly pathogenic in pigs and camels (causing death in a few days), slightly pathogenic in sheep and goats, and nonpathogenic in cattle, horses, and dogs.

**T. su'is,** a species of the *T. brucei* group occurring in swine in Africa; it causes acute and often fatal infection in young animals and less severe, chronic disease in older ones.

**T. thei'leri,** a large, relatively nonpathogenic trypanosome found in African antelopes and in cattle in many parts of the world; the parasites are spread by bloodsucking horseflies of the family Tabanidae.

**T. triatom'ae,** *T. cruzi.*

**T. uganden'se,** *T. gambiense.*

**T. venezuelen'se,** *T. evansi.*

**T. vi'vax,** *T. bovis;* a species characterized by very active motility; it occurs in cattle, horses, camels, sheep, goats, and antelope throughout the tsetse fly belt in Africa, and is most pathogenic in cattle, causing souma, a nagana-like disease; dogs, pigs, and monkeys are refractory to infection.

**Trypanosomatidae** (tri-pan-o-so-mat'ĭ-de). A protozoan family of hemoflagellates (order Kinetoplastida, class Zoomastiga, superclass Mastigophora) that are asexual blood and/or tissue parasites of leeches, insects, and vertebrates and are sap inhabitants of plants. They are characterized by a rounded or elongate form, single nucleus, elongate mitochondrion (its position in relation to the nucleus is a characteristic of each genus), and an anteriorly directed single flagellum (in some genera, it borders an undulating membrane). This family includes the genera *Crithidia, Herpetomanas, Leptomonas,* and *Blastocrithidia,* all of which are monogenetic and found in insects, and *Phytomonas, Endotrypanum, Leishmania,* and *Trypanosoma,* all of which are digenetic; *Leishmania* and *Trypanosoma* include important pathogens of man and animals. Many trypanosomes pass through developmental or life cycle stages similar to the body forms characteristic of the genera; these forms include amastigote, choanomastigote, opisthomastigote, promastigote, epimastigote, and trypomastigote.

**trypanosome** (trī-pan'o-sōm, trip'ă-no-). the common name for any member of the genus *Trypanosoma* or of its family Trypanosomatidae.

**trypanosomiasis** (trī-pan'o-so-mi'ă-sis, trip'ă-no-). Any disease caused by a trypanosome.

**African t.,** African sleeping *sickness.*

**Cruz t.,** South American t.

**Gambian t.,** sleeping sickness caused by *Trypanosoma gambiense* and transmitted from big game and domestic animals to man by tsetse flies; the chief features of the disease are skin affections, *e.g.,* erythematous patches and local edemas, neuralgic pains, cramps, and parasthesias, enlargement of the lymph glands, spleen, and liver; in the later stages (after invasion of trypanosomes into the central nervous system) there is lethargy, with somnolence deepening to coma in the terminal stage; see also trypanosomal *meningoencephalitis.*

**Rhodesian t.,** Rhodesian sleeping sickness, caused by *Trypanosoma rhodesiense* and transmitted by tsetse flies of the species *Glossina morsitans;* it occurs in northeastern Zambia, Rhodesia, Malawi, Portugese East Africa, and Tanzania and is similar to African sleeping sickness but runs a far more rapid, acute course; there may be maniacal symptoms, and death can result in a few weeks or months, whereas victims of gambian sleeping sickness may pass through a relatively benign chronic disease for months or years before reaching the terminal central nervous system stage.

**South American t.,** Chagas' or Chagas-Cruz disease; Cruz trypanosomiasis; caused by *Trypanosoma* (or *Schizotrypanum*) *cruzi* and transmitted by certain species of reduviid (triatomine) bugs which infest the huts of the residents. In its acute form, it is seen most frequently in young children; there is swelling of the skin at the site of

entry, most often the face, with regional lymph node enlargement. In its chronic form it assumes several aspects—cardiac, nervous, or myxedematous, according to the predominating symptoms; there may also be acute exacerbations.

**trypanosomic** (trī-pan'o-so'mik, trip'ă-no-). Relating to trypanosomes, especially denoting infection by such organisms.

**trypanosomicide** (trī-pan'o-so'mĭ-sīd). Trypanocide.

**trypanosomid** (trī-pan'o-so-mid) [ trypanosome + suffix -*id (1), q.v.* ]. Trypanid; a skin lesion resulting from immunologic changes from trypanosome disease.

**tryparsamide** (tri-par'să-mīd) (BP). Sodium *N*-carbamylmethyl-*p*-aminobenzenearsonate; used in the treatment of trypanosomic and spirochetal infections, especially neurosyphilis, and late stages of African sleeping sickness.

**trype'sis** [ G. a boring. TRYP- ]. Trephining.

**trypomastigote** (trip'o-mas'tĭ-gōt) [ G. *trypanon*, auger, + *mastix,* whip ]. Term to replace the older term, "trypanosome stage," which was often confused with the flagellate genus *Trypanosoma.* It denotes the stage (infective stage for South American trypanosomiasis and African trypanosomiasis, and the only stage found in man in the latter illness) in which the flagellum arises from a posteriorly located kinetoplast and emerges from the side of the body, with an undulating membrane running along the length of the body.

**trypsin** (trip'sin) (EC 3.4.21.4). A proteolytic enzyme formed in the small intestine from the inactive pancreatic precursor, trypsinogen, by the action of enterokinase, a peptidase from the duodenal mucosa. It is a serine proteinase (EC sub-subclass 3.4.21) that hydrolyzes peptides, amides, esters, etc., at bonds of the carboxyl groups of L-arginine or L-lysine. For medicinal uses, see crystallized t.

**crystallized t.** (NF), PARENZYME; TRYPTAR; a purified preparation of the pancreatic enzyme; used as an adjunct to surgery for débridement of necrotic wounds and ulcers.

**t. inhibitor,** (1) a peptide hydrolyzed off trypsinogen under the catalytic influence of enteropeptidase, with trypsin produced as a result; so called because the peptide masks or inhibits the active site of the trypsin molecule; (2) one of the polypeptides, from various sources (*e.g.,* human and bovine colostrum, soybeans, and egg white), that inhibit the action of trypsin.

**trypsinogen, trypsogen** (trip-sin'o-jen, trip'so-jen). Protrypsin; a substance secreted by the pancreas which is converted into trypsin by the action of enterokinase.

**tryptamine** (trip'tă-mēn, -min). 3-(2-Aminoethyl)indole; decarboxylation product of tryptophan; occurs in plants and certain foods (*e.g.,* cheese); if raises the blood pressure through vasoconstrictor action through the release of norepinephrine at postganglionic sympathetic nerve endings. Believed to be one of the agents responsible for hypertensive episodes following therapy with monoamine oxidase inhibitors (*e.g.,* pargyline hydrochloride, *q.v.*).

Tryptamine

**tryp'tamine-strophan'thidin.** A semisynthetic cardiac glycoside that is a condensation product of strophanthidin and tryptamine. Given orally, it has a rapid onset and short duration of cardiac action.

**tryp'tic.** Relating to trypsin, as t. digestion.

**tryp'tone'mia.** The presence of tryptone in the circulating blood.

**tryp'tophan.** 2-Amino-3-indolepropionic acid; a component of proteins.

**t. decarboxylase,** aromatic L-amino-acid decarboxylase.

**t. desmolase,** t. synthase.

**t. oxygenase,** tryptophan 2,3-dioxygenase.

**t. pyrrolase,** tryptophan 2,3-dioxygenase.

**t. synthase,** t. desmolase; t. synthetase; a hydro-lyase (EC 4.2.1.20) condensing L-serine (or glyceraldehyde phosphate) and indole (or indole-3-glycerol phosphate) to L-tryptophan. Pyridoxal phosphate is required.

**t. synthetase,** t. synthase.

**tryptophanase** (trip′to-fā-nās). 1. Tryptophan 2,3-dioxygenase. 2. An enzyme (EC 4.1.99.1), found in bacteria, that catalyzes the cleavage of tryptophan to indole, pyruvic acid, and ammonia; pyridoxal phosphate is a coenzyme.

**tryptophan 2,3-dioxygenase.** Tryptophan oxygenase; tryptophan pyrrolase; tryptophanase (1); an oxidoreductase (EC 1.13.11.11) catalyzing reductive closure of the side chain on the benzene ring in *N*-formylkynurenine to the pyrrole ring of tryptophan; an adaptive enzyme, the level (in liver) being controlled by adrenal hormones.

**tryptophanuria** (trip′to-fā-nu′rĭ-ah). Enhanced urinary excretion of tryptophan.

**t. with dwarfism,** a heritable condition believed to be caused by inadequate conversion of tryptophan to kynurenine; not associated with impaired tryptophan transport, for blood concentrations of tryptophan are high.

**tsetse** (tset′se, tse′tse) [ S. African native name ]. See *Glossina*.

**TSH.** Abbreviation for thyroid-stimulating *hormone.*

**TSH-RF.** Abbreviation for thyroid-stimulating hormone releasing factor (thyrotropin-releasing factor); see under factor.

**T. tet′anase** [ *t* = tetanizing ]. v. Behring's term for the constituent of tetanus toxin that stimulates the tetanic spasm.

**TTP.** Abbreviation for thymidine 5′-triphosphate.

**T.U.** Abbreviation for toxic *unit.*

**tu′aminohep′tane.** (NF). TUAMINE; 2-Aminoheptane; a sympathomimetic volatile amine, used by inhalation as a nasal decongestant; should be used cautiously in cardiovascular disease. Available also as t. sulfate (NF), with same actions, and more potent as a vasoconstrictor than ephedrine.

**tub.** To treat by means of a bath.

**tuba,** gen. and pl. **tubae** (tu′bah, tu′be) [ L. a straight trumpet ] [ NA ]. A tube, or a tubelike structure or canal.

**t. acus′tica,** t. auditiva.

**t. auditi′va** [ NA ], auditory tube; Eustachian tube; guttural duct; a tube leading from the tympanic cavity to the nasopharynx; it consists of an osseous (posterolateral) portion at the tympanic end, and a fibrocartilaginous (anteromedial) portion at the pharyngeal end; where the two portions join, in the region of the sphenopetrosal fissure, is the narrowest portion of the tube, the isthmus.

**t. eustachia′na, t. eusta′chii,** t. auditiva.

**t. fallopia′na, t. fallo′pii,** t. uterina.

**t. uteri′na** [ NA ], uterine tube; oviduct; Fallopian tube; salpinx; one of the tubes, leading on either side from the fundus of the uterus to the upper or outer extremity of the ovary; it consists of infundibulum, ampulla, isthmus, and uterine parts.

**tu′bage.** The introduction of a tube into a canal; intubation of the larynx.

**tu′bal.** Relating to a tube, especially the uterine tube.

**tubator′sion.** Tubotorsion.

**tubba, tubbae.** foot *yaws.*

**Tubbs′ dilator.** See under dilator.

# TUBE

**tube** [ L. *tubus* ]. 1. A hollow cylinder or pipe. 2. A canal or tubular organ; tuba; tubule.

**Abbott's t.,** Miller-Abbott t.

**air t.,** the trachea, or a bronchus or any of its branches conveying air to the lungs.

**auditory t.,** *tuba* auditiva.

**Babcock t.,** a t. in which milk, after treatment with sulfuric acid, is centrifuged and its fat content then determined in a graduated neck.

**Bouchut's t.,** a short cylindrical t. used in intubation of the larynx.

**bronchial t.'s,** bronchia; the smaller divisions of the bronchi.

**Cantor t.,** a long, single-lumen intestinal t. with a sealed rubber bag tip. Mercury is injected into the rubber bag with a needle and syringe.

**cardiac t.,** the primitive tubular heart in the embryo, before its division into chambers.

**Celestin t.,** a plastic tube introduced through a tumor in the esophagus; it permits maintenance of swallowing when the lesion is unresectable.

**Coolidge t.,** an x-ray t., in which the cathode consists of a tungsten wire spiral surrounded by a molybdenum t.; the tungsten spiral is heated by an electric current and the exact quality of the x-ray given off is regulated by varying the temperature of the cathode.

**corneal t.,** in stained corneal sections, a tubelike artifact between the lamellae of the cornea.

**digestive t.,** *canalis* alimentarius.

**Dominici t.,** a silver t. for the application of radium, allowing the passage of only the beta and gamma rays.

**drainage t.,** a t. of rubber or glass passed into a wound or cavity of the body to allow the escape of pus or blood.

**Durham's t.,** a jointed tracheotomy t.

**egg t.'s,** cords of potentially germinal cells growing into the ovarian stroma from the germinal epithelium; also called Pflüger's t.'s; ovarian t.'s.

**empyema t.,** a rubber drainage t. (see drain, 2) piercing a sheet rubber shield, passed through an opening in the chest wall in order to give exit to the pus as it is formed in a case of empyema.

**endobronchial t.,** a double-lumen t. that permits intubation of one bronchus or the other, thus effectively sealing off one lung from the other and allowing separate ventilation of each lung; used in bronchospirometry and in anesthesia for thoracic surgery.

**endotracheal t.,** a Portex or rubber catheter, inserted into the trachea as an airway in endotracheal intubation.

**Eustachian t.,** *tuba* auditiva.

**Fallopian t.,** *tuba* uterina.

**feeding t.,** a flexible t. passed through the esophagus into the stomach, through which liquid food is poured.

**Ferrein's t.,** *tubulus* renalis contortus.

**Geiger-Müller t.,** see Geiger-Müller counter.

**Haldane t.,** a t. for securing a sample of human alveolar air; it consists of a 3-foot length of hosepipe about 1 inch in diameter and a mouthpiece a short distance from which is a short narrow t. for the withdrawal of expired air at the end of a deep expiration.

**intuba′tion t.,** O'Dwyer's t.

**Levin t.,** a t. introduced through the nose into the upper alimentary canal, especially in conjunction with decompression following operations.

**Martin's t.,** a drainage t. with a cross piece near the extremity to keep it from slipping out of a cavity.

**medullary t.,** neural t.

**Miescher's t.'s,** elongate fusiform or cylindrical bodies forming the encapsulated cystic intramuscular stage of the protozoan *Sarcocystis.*

**Miller-Abbott t.,** Abbott's t.; a t. with two lumens, one ending in a small collapsible balloon, the other ending with numerous perforations and capped with metal; used in cases of intestinal distention.

**Moss t.,** (1) triple-lumen, nasogastric, feeding-decompression t.; the gastric balloon occludes cardioesophageal junction, with simultaneous esophageal aspiration and intragastric feeding; (2) double-lumen, gastric lavage t., providing continuous delivery of saline *via* small bore, with simultaneous aspiration of fluid and capsule-sized particles *via* large bore.

**Necheles' t.,** a double-lumen tube used in tests of bleeding in the alimentary canal.

**neural t.,** medullary t.; the epithelial t. formed from the neuroectoderm of the early embryo by the closure of the neural groove; by complex processes of cell proliferation and organization the neural t. develops into the spinal cord and brain.

**O'Dwyer's t.,** a metal t. used for intubation of the larynx after O'Dwyer's method.

**otopharyn′geal t.,** *tuba* auditiva.

ova'rian t.'s, egg t.'s.

Pflüger's t.'s, egg t.'s.

pharyng'otympan'ic t., *tuba* auditiva.

photomultiplier t., a detector which magnifies the signal (by as much as 106) received from the electromagnetic radiation by a system of electron acceleration from a photocathode through a series of dinodes.

Pitot t., a stationary L-shaped t. inserted in a fluid stream, with its opening upstream, and used for measuring the velocity of fluid movement at that point in terms of the pressure developed in the t. by the fluid impinging on it, compared to a second t. opening laterally or downstream.

pus t., pyosalpinx.

Rehfuss stomach t., a t. with a graduated syringe formerly used for aspiration of stomach contents in gastric analysis. Plastic disposable stomach t.'s are now used.

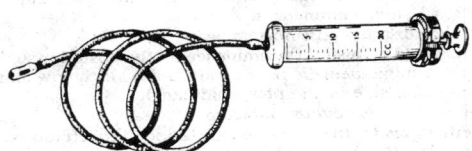

**Rehfuss Stomach Tube**

roll t., a modification of the plate culture; a seeded medium containing agar is placed in a test t. which is rolled or spun horizontally until the medium solidifies evenly on the interior of the t.

Ruysch's t., a minute tubular cavity opening in the lower and anterior portion of each surface of the nasal septum. It is best seen in the early fetal period when it is associated with the vomeronasal organ of Jacobson.

Ryle's t., a thin rubber t., with about the lumen of a no. 8 catheter, having an olive-pointed extremity, used in the giving of a test meal.

Schachowa's t., proximal convoluted tubule; see *tubulus* renalis contortus.

Sengstaken-Blakemore t., a t. with an attached inflatable balloon which is passed into and retained in the esophagus to arrest esophageal hemorrhage, as from a ruptured varix.

Southey's t.'s, cannulas of small, almost capillary, caliber, thrust by means of a trocar into the subcutaneous tissues to drain the same in case of anasarca.

stomach t., a flexible t. passed into the stomach for use in lavage or in forcible feeding.

T t., a t. with side extensions, shaped like a T.

test t., a t. of thin glass closed at one end, used in the examination of urine and other chemical operations, for bacterial cultures, etc.

tracheot'omy t., a curved t. used to keep the opening free after tracheotomy.

u'terine t., *tuba* uterina.

vacuum t., a glass t. from which the air has been nearly removed, used in the experimental passage of an electrical current or spark and in the production of x-rays.

Venturi t., a t. with a specially streamlined constriction to minimize energy losses in the fluid flowing through it while maximizing the fall in pressure in the constriction in accordance with Bernoulli's law; it is the basis of the Venturi meter.

Wangensteen t., see Wangensteen *suction.*

x-ray t., see x-ray, under ray.

tubectomy (tu-bek'to-mī) [ L. *tuba*, tube, + G. *ektomē*, excision ]. Salpingectomy.

tu'ber, pl. tu'bera [ L. protuberance, swelling ]. 1 [ NA ]. A localized swelling; a knob. 2. A short, fleshy, thick, underground stem of plants, such as the potato.

t. ante'rius, t. cinereum.

ashen t., t. cinereum.

calcaneal t., t. calcanei.

t. calca'nei [ NA ], calcaneal t. or tuberosity; t. calcis; the posterior extremity of the calcaneus, or os calcis, forming the projection of the heel.

t. calcis, t. calcanei.

t. cine'reum [ NA ], ashen or gray t.; t. anterius; a prominence of the base of the hypothalamus, bordered

caudally by the mamillary bodies, rostrally by the optic chiasm, and laterally by the optic tract, extending ventrally into the infundibulum and hypophysial stalk.

t. coch'leae, promontorium (3).

t. cor'poris callo'si, *splenium* corporis callosi.

t. dorsa'le, t. vermis.

Eustachian t., a slight projection from the labyrinthine wall of the middle ear below the fenestra vestibuli (ovalis).

frontal t., t. frontale.

t. fronta'le [ NA ], frontal t.; frontal eminence; eminentia frontalis; the most prominent portion of the frontal bone on either side.

gray t., t. cinereum.

t. ischiad'icum [ NA ], t. of the ischium; ischial tuberosity; the rough bony projection at the junction of the lower end of the body of the ischium and its ramus.

t. of ischium, t. ischiadicum.

t. maxil'lae [ NA ], maxillary tuberosity; the bulging lower extremity of the posterior surface of the body of the maxilla, behind the root of the wisdom tooth.

omental t., t. omentale.

t. omenta'le [ NA ], omental t.; (1) an eminence on the visceral surface of the left hepatic lobe to the left of the fossa for the ductus venosus; (2) a bulge on the anterior surface of the body of the pancreas to the left of the superior mesenteric vessels.

parietal t., t. parietale.

t. parieta'le [ NA ], parietal t.; parietal eminence; eminentia parietalis; a prominent portion of the parietal bone, a little above the center of its external surface, usually corresponding to the point of maximum width of the head.

t. ra'dii, *tuberositas* radii.

t. val'vulae, t. vermis.

t. ver'mis [ NA ], t. of the vermis; t. valvulae; t. dorsale; the posterior division of the inferior vermis of the cerebellum.

t. zygomat'icum, a slight prominence near the origin of the zygomatic process of the temporal bone.

tuberc-, tubercul-. See tuberculo-.

tubercle (tu'ber-kl) [ L. *tuberculum*, dim. of *tuber*, a swelling ]. 1. Tuberculum. 2. In dentistry, a small elevation arising on the surface of a tooth. 3. A granulomatous lesion due to infection by *Mycobacterium tuberculosis* or by certain noxious substances that are an integral part of the organism. Although somewhat variable in size (0.5 to 2 or 3 mm. in diameter) and in the proportions of various histologic components, t.'s tend to be fairly well circumscribed, spheroidal, firm lesions that usually consists of three, irregularly outlined but moderately distinct, zones: (a) an inner focus of necrosis—coagulative at first, and then becoming caseous; (b) a middle zone that consists of a fairly dense accumulation of large, mononuclear phagocytes (macrophages), frequently arranged somewhat radially (with reference to the necrotic material) in a sort of scalelike pattern that has a resemblance to epidermal cells—hence, are termed epithelioid cells; multinucleated giant cells of Langhans type may also be present; (c) an outer zone of numerous lymphocytes, and a few monocytes and plasma cells. In instances where healing has begun, a fourth zone may form at the periphery, *i.e.*, fibrous tissue. Morphologically indistinguishable lesions may occur in diseases caused by other agents, and many observers use the term nonspecifically, *i.e.*, with reference to any such

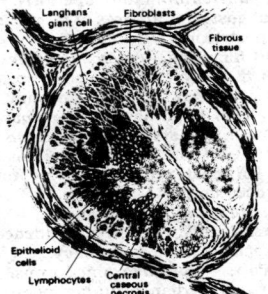

**Microscopic Structure of a Tubercle**

granuloma; others use the word t. only for tuberculous lesions, and then designate those of undetermined causes epithelioid-cell granulomas.

**acoustic t.,** *trigone* of the auditory nerve.

**adductor t.,** *tuberculum* adductorium.

**amygdaloid t.,** a projection from the roof of the anterior end-portion of the temporal horn of the lateral ventricle, marking the location of the amygdaloid nucleus.

**anatomical t.,** postmortem *wart.*

**anterior t. of atlas,** *tuberculum* anterius atlantis.

**anterior t. of cervical vertebrae,** *tuberculum* anterius vertebrarum cervicalium.

**t. of anterior scalene muscle,** *tuberculum* musculi scaleni anterioris.

**anterior t. of thalamus,** *tuberculum* anterius thalami.

**articular t.,** *tuberculum* articulare.

**ashen t.** *tuberculum* cinereum.

**auricular t.,** *tuberculum* auriculae.

**Carabelli t.,** a small t., resembling a supernumerary cuspid, found occasionally on the lingual surface of one or more of the molar teeth, near the mesial wall.

**carotid t.,** *tuberculum* caroticum.

**caseous t.,** soft t.

**Chassaignac's t.,** *tuberculum* caroticum.

**conoid t.,** *tuberculum* conoideum.

**corniculate t.,** *tuberculum* corniculatum.

**crown t.,** *tuberculum* dentis.

**t. of cuneate nucleus,** *tuberculum* nuclei cuneati.

**cuneiform t.,** *tuberculum* cuneiforme.

**Darwinian t.,** *tuberculum* auriculae.

**dental t.,** *tuberculum* dentis.

**dissection t.,** postmortem *wart.*

**dorsal t. of the radius,** Lister's t.; small prominence on the dorsal aspect of the distal end of the radius lateral to the groove for the extensor pollicis longus tendon.

**epiglottic t.,** *tuberculum* epiglotticum.

**Farre's t.'s,** nodules of cancerous tissue on the surface of the liver.

**fibrous t.,** one in which fibroblasts proliferate about the periphery (and into the cellular zones), eventually resulting in a rim or wall of cellular fibrous tissue or collagenous material around the t.

**genial t.,** *spina* mentalis.

**genital t.,** phallic t.; the median elevation just cephalic to the urogenital orifice of an embryo. It is the primordium of the penis of the male or the clitoris of the female.

**Gerdy's t.,** a t. on the lateral side of the upper end of the tibia giving attachment to the tractus iliotibialis and some fibers of the tibialis anterior muscle.

**Ghon's t.,** Ghon's focus; Ghon's primary lesion; the pulmonary lesion of primary tuberculosis.

**gracile t.,** *tuberculum* nuclei gracilis.

**gray t.,** *tuberculum* cinereum.

**greater t. of humerus,** *tuberculum* majus humeri.

**hard t.,** a t. lacking necrosis.

**hyaline t.,** a form of fibrous t. in which the cellular fibrous tissue and collagenous fibers become altered and merged into a fairly homogeneous, acellular, deeply acidophilic, firm mass.

**inferior thyroid t.,** *tuberculum* thyroideum inferius.

**infraglenoid t.,** *tuberculum* infraglenoidale.

**intercondylar t.,** *tuberculum* intercondylare.

**intervenous t.,** *tuberculum* intervenosum.

**jugular t.,** *tuberculum* jugulare.

**labial t.,** *tuberculum* labii superioris.

**lateral t. of posterior process of talus,** *tuberculum* laterale processus posterioris tali.

**lesser t. of humerus,** *tuberculum* minus humeri.

**Lisfranc's t.,** *tuberculum* musculi scaleni anterioris.

**Lower's t.,** *tuberculum* intervenosum.

**mamillary t. of hypothalamus,** *corpus* mamillare.

**mammillary t. of vertebrae,** *processus* mamillaris.

**marginal t.,** *tuberculum* marginale ossis zygomatici.

**medial t. of posterior process of talus,** *tuberculum* mediale processus posterioris tali.

**mental t.,** *tuberculum* mentale.

**Montgomery's t.'s,** elevated reddened areolar glands, usually associated with pregnancy.

**Morgagni's t.,** *cartilago* cuneiformis.

**Müller's t.,** a median protuberance projecting into the embryonic urogenital sinus from its dorsal wall; it is formed from the fused caudal ends of the paramesonephric ducts, and is the first evidence of the embryonic uterus and vagina.

**t. of nucleus gracilis,** *tuberculum* nuclei gracilis.

**nuchal t.,** *vertebra* prominens.

**obturator t.,** *tuberculum* obturatorium.

**olfactory t.,** *tuberculum* olfactorium.

**orbital t.,** *eminentia* orbitalis.

**pearly t.,** milium.

**phallic t.,** genital t.

**pharyngeal t.,** *tuberculum* pharyngeum.

**posterior t. of atlas,** *tuberculum* posterius atlantis.

**posterior t. of cervical vertebrae,** *tuberculum* posterius vertebrarum cervicalium.

**postmortem t.,** postmortem *wart.*

**Princeteau's t.,** a slight prominence on the temporal bone near the apex of the petrous part where the superior petrosal sinus commences.

**prosector's t.,** postmortem *wart.*

**pterygoid t.,** a slight prominence on the posterior surface of the lamina medialis of the sphenoid bone, below and to the medial side of the pterygoid canal.

**pubic t.,** *tuberculum* pubicum.

**reticulated t.,** the characteristic lesion of tuberculosis; see tubercle (3).

**t. of rib,** *tuberculum* costae.

**Rolando's t.,** *tuberculum* cinereum.

**t. of saddle,** *tuberculum* sellae.

**Santorini's t.,** *tuberculum* corniculatum.

**scalene t. of Lisfranc,** *tuberculum* musculi scaleni anterioris.

**t. of scaphoid bone,** *tuberculum* ossis scaphoidei.

**sebaceous t.,** milium.

**soft t.,** caseous t.; a t. showing caseous necrosis.

**superior thyroid t.,** *tuberculum* thyroideum superius.

**supraglenoid t.,** *tuberculum* supraglenoidale.

**supratragic t.,** *tuberculum* supratragicum.

**t. of tibia,** *tuberositas* tibiae.

**t. of upper lip,** *tuberculum* labii superioris.

**wedge-shaped t.,** *tuberculum* nuclei cuneati.

**Whitnall's t.,** *eminentia* orbitalis.

**Wrisberg's t.,** *tuberculum* cuneiforme.

**tuber'cula.** Plural of tuberculum.

**tubercular** (tu-ber'ku-lar). Tuberculate; nodular; pertaining to or characterized by tubercles or small nodules; *cf.* tuberculous.

**tuber'culate, tuber'culated.** Tubercular.

**tuberculation** (tu-ber'ku-la'shun). 1. The formation of tubercles or nodules. 2. The arrangement of tubercles or nodules in a part.

**tuberculid** (tu-ber'ku-lid) [ tubercul- + suffix -id (1), q.v. ]. Folliclis; a lesion of skin or mucous membrane seen in cases of tuberculosis and believed to be caused by an allergic response to tubercle bacilli or their products.

**papular t.,** papular scrofuloderma; lichen scrofulosorum; allergic manifestation to tuberculous infection in the body; small to medium-sized papules which have tuberculid architecture but do not contain the bacteria.

**papulonecrotic t.,** acne agminata; folliclis; tuberculosis papulonecrotica; tuberculosis cutis follicularis disseminata; acnitis; a papular eruption in which there is central necrosis of the lesions; this is a cutaneous allergic reaction in either active or dormant pulmonary tuberculosis.

**rosacea-like t.,** a facial t.; yellowish brown on diascopic pressure, with dermal tubercles not related to hair follicles.

**tuberculigenous** (tu-ber'ku-lij'ē-nus). Causing or predisposing to tuberculosis.

**tuberculin** (tu-ber'ku-lin). 1. A glycerin (5 per cent)-broth culture of *Mycobacterium tuberculosis* evaporated $1/_{10}$ volume at 100°C. and filtered; introduced by Robert Koch for the treatment of tuberculosis but now used chiefly for diagnostic tests; originally known as Koch's old t., OT, Koch's original t. 2. One or another of a relatively large number of extracts of *Mycobacterium tuberculosis* cultures, different from OT and now obsolete.

**Koch's old t.,** see t. (1).

**purified protein derivative of t.** abbreviated PPD; purified t. containing the active protein fraction; the t. from which it is prepared differs from OT (see t. (1)) chiefly in that the bacteria are grown in a synthetic rather than in a broth medium.

**tuberculitis** (tu-ber'ku-li'tis) [ tubercul- + G. suffix -itis, inflammation ]. Inflammation of any tubercle.

**tuber'culiza'tion.** The formation of tubercles.

**tuberculo-, tubercul-** (tu-ber'ku-lo-) [ L. tuberculum, tubercle ]. Combining forms relating to tubercle, tuberculosis.

**tuberculocele** (tu-ber'ku-lo-sēl) [ tuberculo- + G. kēlē, tumor, hernia ]. Tuberculosis of the testes.

**tuber'culochem'otherapeu'tic.** Relating to the treatment of tuberculosis by tuberculostatic or tuberculocidal drugs.

**tuber'culoci'dal.** Destructive to the tubercle bacillus.

**tuberculoderma** (tu-ber'ku-lo-der'mah). 1. Any tubercular process of the skin. 2. The cutaneous manifestation of tuberculosis.

**tuberculofibroid** (tu-ber'ku-lo-fi'broyd). A discrete, well circumscribed, usually spheroidal, moderately to extremely firm, encapsulated nodule that is formed during the process of healing in a focus of tuberculous granulomatous inflammation. As the active response of the reticuloendothelial tissue subsides, the proliferation of fibroblasts (and the formation of connective tissue elements) around and within the two outer zones of a tubercle (or a larger tuberculous nodule) results in a densely fibrous capsule, bands and small masses of collagen, and fairly homogeneous hyalin that enclose an inner zone of caseous and caseocalcified necrotic material.

**tuberculoid** (tu-ber'ku-loyd) [ tuberculo- + G. eidos, resemblance ]. Resembling tuberculosis, or a tubercle.

**tuberculoma** (tu-ber'ku-lo'mah) [ tuberculo- + G. suffix -oma, tumor ]. A rounded tumorlike but non-neoplastic mass, usually in the lungs or brain, due to localized tuberculous infection.

**tuberculophobia** (tu-ber'ku-lo-fo'bī-ah) [ tuberculo- + G. phobos, fear ]. Morbid fear of tuberculosis.

**tuber'culopro'tein.** Any one or a mixture of any or all of the proteins present in the body of the tubercle bacillus, all of which proteins have been found to possess certain properties of tuberculin.

**tuberculosis** (tu-ber'ku-lo'sis) [ tuberculo- + G. suffix -osis, condition ]. A specific disease caused by the presence of Mycobacterium tuberculosis; it may affect almost any tissue or organ of the body, the most common seat of the disease being the lungs; the anatomical lesion is the tubercle, which undergoes caseation. The local symptoms vary according to the part affected; the general symptoms are those of sepsis: hectic fever, sweats, and emaciation.

**acute t., acute miliary t.,** a rapidly fatal disease due to the general dissemination of tubercle bacilli in the blood, resulting in the formation of miliary tubercles in various organs and tissues, and producing symptoms of profound toxemia.

**adrenal t.,** Addison's disease.

**adult t.,** secondary t.

**anthracotic t.,** pneumoconiosis.

**arrested t.,** healed t.

**atten'uated t.,** a mild, chronic form, marked by caseous tubercles of the skin and the occurrence of cold abscesses.

**avian t.,** fowl t.; t. affecting birds.

**basal t.,** t. of the basilar portions of the lungs.

**bovine t.,** t. of cattle.

**cerebral t.,** (1) tuberculous meningitis; (2) cerebral tuberculoma.

**childhood type t.,** primary t.

**t. conclama'ta** [ L. conclamare, to cry aloud ], pronounced, fully developed, unmistakable t.

**cutaneous t.,** scrofuloderma; t. cutis; dermal t.; pathologic lesions of the skin caused by Mycobacterium tuberculosis.

**t. cutis,** cutaneous t.

**t. cutis follicularis disseminata,** papular necrotic tuberculid.

**t. cutis indurativa,** erythema induratum.

**t. cutis luposa,** lupus vulgaris.

**t. cutis orificia'lis,** t. ulcerosa; any tuberculous lesion in or about the mouth or anus.

**t. cu'tis verruco'sa,** lupus verrucosus; lupus papillomatosus; tuberculous wart; verrucous scrofuloderma; scrofulophyma; a tuberculous skin lesion having a warty surface with a chronic inflammatory base. See also postmortem wart.

**dermal t.,** cutaneous t.

**dissem'inated t.,** acute miliary t.

**fowl t.,** avian t.

**general t.,** miliary t.

**healed t.,** arrested or inactive t.; a scar or a calcified, fibrous, or caseous nodule in the pleura or lymph node resulting from previous t. that has regressed.

**inactive t.,** healed t.

**lymphat'ic t.,** scrofula.

**lym'phoid t.,** a form in which there is a diffuse embryonal cell infiltration instead of the ordinary tubercle.

**mil'iary t.,** general t.; a general dissemination of tubercle bacilli with the production of countless minute discrete tubercles in various organs and tissues.

**open t.,** pulmonary t., tuberculous ulceration, or other form in which the bacilli are cast out of the body in the excretions.

**t. papulonecrot'ica,** papular necrotic tuberculid.

**postprimary t.,** secondary t.

**primary t.,** childhood type t.; first infection by Mycobacterium tuberculosis; seen in children and, in recent decades, in adults; characterized in the lungs by the formation of a primary complex consisting of small peripheral pulmonary focus and hilar or paratracheal lymph node involvement; Primary t. may heal with calcification or progress, sometimes with miliary dissemination.

**pulmonary t.,** white plague; t. of the lungs.

**reinfection t.,** secondary t.

**secondary t.,** adult, postprimary, or reinfection t.; t. found in adults and characterized by lesions near the apex of an upper lobe, which may cavitate or heal with scarring; theoretically, secondary t. may be due to reinfection or to reactivation of a dormant endogenous infection.

**surgical t.,** t. of the bones or joints.

**t. ulcero'sa,** t. cutis orificialis.

**tuber'culostat.** A tuberculostatic agent.

**tuberculostatic** (tu-ber'ku-lo-stat'ik) [ tuberculo- + G. statikos, causing to stand ]. Relating to an agent that inhibits the growth of tubercle bacilli.

**tuber'culother'apist.** A physician who makes a special study of the treatment of tuberculosis.

**tuber'culother'apy.** 1. Treatment of tuberculosis. 2. An attempt at an immunizing treatment of tuberculosis by feeding with the raw flesh of tuberculous cattle.

**tuberculotoxin** (tu-ber'ku-lo-tok'sin). Any so-called toxin, intracellular or extracellular, of the tubercle bacillus.

**tuber'culotoxoid'in.** See under tuberculin.

**tuberculous** (tu-ber'ku-lus). Relating to or affected by tuberculosis; cf. tubercular.

---

# TUBERCULUM

**tuberculum,** pl. **tubercula** (tu-ber'ku-lum, -lah) [ L. dim. of tuber, a knob, swelling, tumor ] [ NA ]. 1. A tubercle or nodule, especially in an anatomical, not pathologic, sense. 2. A circumscribed, rounded, solid elevation on the skin, mucous membrane, or surface of an organ. 3. A slight elevation from the surface of a bone giving attachment to a muscle or ligament.

**t. adducto'rium** [ NA ], adductor tubercle; the prominence above the medial epicondyle of the femur to which the tendon of the adductor magnus attaches.

**t. ante'rius atlan'tis** [ NA ], anterior tubercle of the atlas; a conical protuberance on the anterior surface of the arm of the atlas.

**t. ante'rius thal'ami** [ NA ], anterior tubercle of the thalamus; a prominence at the anterior extremity of the thalamus which corresponds to the nuclei anteriores.

**t. ante′rius vertebra′rum cervica′lium** [ NA ], anterior tubercle of the cervical vertebrae; the anterior projection from the transverse processes.

**t. arthrit′icum,** (1) Heberden's *nodes.* (2) any gouty concretion in or around a joint.

**t. articula′re** [ NA ], articular tubercle or eminence; eminentia articularis; articular eminence of the temporal bone which bounds the mandibular fossa anteriorly; it forms the anterior root of the zygomatic process.

**t. auric′ulae** [ NA ], auricular tubercle; Darwinian tubercle; t. superius; a small projection from the upper end of the posterior portion of the incurved free margin of the helix.

**t. carot′icum** [ NA ], carotid tubercle; Chassaignac's tubercle; the anterior tubercle of the transverse process of the sixth cervical vertebra, against which the carotid artery may be compressed by the finger.

**t. cine′reum,** ashen or gray tubercle; Rolando's tubercle; a longitudinal prominence on the dorsolateral surface of the medulla oblongata along the lateral border of the tuberculum cuneatum; it is the surface profile of the tractus spinalis nervi trigemini, continuous caudally with the fasciculus dorsolateralis (Lissauer's tract).

**t. conoid′eum** [ NA ], conoid tubercle; the prominence near the lateral end of the inferior surface of the clavicle that gives attachment to the conoid ligament.

**t. cornicula′tum** [ NA ], corniculate tubercle; Santorini's tubercle; a rounded eminence on the posterior part of the aryepiglottic fold, formed by the underlying corniculate cartilages.

**t. coro′nae** [ NA ], crown tubercle; an alternate term for t. dentis.

**t. cos′tae** [ NA ], tubercle of a rib; the knob on a rib, near its head, which articulates with the transverse process of a vertebra.

**t. cuneifor′me** [ NA ], cuneiform tubercle; Wrisberg's tubercle; a rounded eminence on the posterior part of the aryepiglottic fold, formed by the underlying cuneiform cartilage.

**t. den′tis** [ NA ], tubercle of a tooth; t. coronae [ NA ]; crown or dental tubercle; a small elevation on some portions of a crown produced by an extra formation of enamel.

**tubercula doloro′sa,** multiple cutaneous myomas or neuromas, painful on pressure.

**t. epiglot′ticum** [ NA ], epiglottic tubercle; cushion of the epiglottis; a convexity at the lower part of the epiglottis over the upper part of the thyroepiglottic ligament.

**t. hypoglos′si,** *trigonum* nervi hypoglossi.

**t. im′par,** a small median protuberance on the floor of the oral cavity of the embryo, which plays a minor role in the development of the tongue.

**t. infraglenoida′le** [ NA ], infraglenoid tubercle; or tuberosity; a rough surface below the glenoid cavity of the scapula, giving attachment to the long tendon of the triceps.

**t. intercondyla′re** [ NA ], intercondylar tubercle; one of two projections, medial and lateral, springing from the central lip of each articular surface of the tibia on either side of the intercondylar eminence.

**t. interveno′sum** [ NA ], intervenous tubercle; tubercle of Lower; the slight projection on the wall of the right atrium between the orifices of the venae cavae.

**t. jugula′re** [ NA ], jugular tubercle; an oval elevation on the cerebral surface of the lateral part of the occipital bone, on either side of the foramen magnum.

**t. la′bii superio′ris** [ NA ], tubercle of the upper lip; labial tubercle; the slight projection on the free edge of the center of the upper lip.

**t. latera′le proces′sus posterio′ris ta′li** [ NA ], lateral tubercle of the posterior process of the talus; the prominence lateral to the groove for the flexor hallucis longus tendon.

**t. ma′jus hu′meri** [ NA ], greater tubercle or tuberosity of the humerus; the larger of the two tubercles next to the head of the humerus; it gives attachment to the supraspinatus, infraspinatus, and teres minor muscles.

**t. mal′lei,** *processus* lateralis mallei.

**t. margina′le os′sis zygomat′ici** [ NA ], marginal tubercle; a prominence on the temporal border of the zygomatic bone to which the temporal fascia is attached.

**t. media′le proces′sus posterio′ris ta′li** [ NA ], medial tubercle of the posterior process of the talus; the eminence medial to the sulcus for the flexor hallucis longus tendon.

**t. menta′le** [ NA ], mental tubercle; eminentia symphysis; a prominence on the lower border of the mandible on either side of the mental protuberance.

**t. mi′nus hu′meri** [ NA ], lesser tubercle or tuberosity of the humerus; the anterior of the two tubercles of the neck of the humerus on which the subscapularis is inserted.

**t. mus′culi scale′ni anterio′ris** [ NA ], tubercle of the anterior scalene muscle; Lisfranc's tubercle; scalene tubercle of Lisfranc; a small spine on the inner edge of the first rib, giving attachment to the scalenus anterior muscle.

**t. nu′clei cunea′ti** [ NA ], tubercle of the cuneate nucleus; wedge-shaped tubercle; the bulbous rostral extremity of the fasciculus cuneatus corresponding to the position of the nucleus cuneatus, lying lateral to the clava and separated from the t. cinereum on its lateral side by the posterior lateral sulcus.

**t. nu′clei gra′cilis** [ NA ], tubercle of the nucleus gracilis; gracile tubercle; clava; the somewhat expanded upper end of the fasciculus gracilis, corresponding to the position of the nucleus gracilis.

**t. obturato′rium** [ NA ], obturator tubercle; one of two processes, anterior and posterior, on the margin of the pubic portion of the obturator foramen, bounding the termination of the obturator groove.

**t. olfacto′rium,** olfactory tubercle; a small, oval area at the base of the cerebral hemisphere, between the diverging medial and lateral olfactory striae, in the anteromedial part of the anterior perforated substance; it is formed by a small area of allocortex characterized by the presence of the islands of Calleja. Corresponding to a much more prominent structure in nonprimate mammals (especially rodents and insectivores), the olfactory tubercle receives fibers from the olfactory bulb by way of the stria olfactoria intermedia; it has efferent connections with the hypothalamus and the mediodorsal nucleus of the thalamus.

**t. os′sis scaphoi′dei** [ NA ], tubercle of the scaphoid bone; a projection at the inferior lateral angle of the scaphoid (navicular) bone; it can be felt at the root of the thumb.

**t. os′sis trape′zii** [ NA ], oblique ridge of the trapezium; a prominent ridge on the trapezium (os multangulum majus) forming the lateral border of the groove in which runs the tendon of the flexor carpi radialis.

**t. pharyn′geum** [ NA ], pharyngeal tubercle; a projection from the under surface of the basilar portion of the occipital bone, giving attachment to the fibrous raphe of the pharynx.

**t. poste′rius atlan′tis** [ NA ], posterior tubercle of the atlas; a protuberance of the posterior extremity of the arch of the atlas, a rudiment of the spinous process giving attachment to the musculus rectus capitis posterior.

**t. poste′rius vertebra′rum cervica′lium** [ NA ], posterior tubercle of the cervical vertebrae; one of the posterior tips of the transverse processes of the cervical vertebrae.

**t. pu′bicum** [ NA ], pubic tubercle; pubic spine; a small projection at the anterior extremity of the crest of the pubis about 2 cm. from the symphysis.

**t. seba′ceum,** milium.

**t. sel′lae** [ NA ], tubercle of the saddle; the slight elevation in front of the pituitary fossa on the body of the sphenoid bone.

**t. sep′ti na′rium,** a flat elevation on the septum in each naris opposite the anterior end of the middle concha; it is due to an aggregation of glands.

**t. supe′rius,** t. auriculae.

**t. supraglenoida′le** [ NA ], supraglenoid tubercle; a rough surface above the glenoid cavity of the scapula, giving attachment to the tendon of the long head of the biceps.

**t. supratra′gicum** [ NA ], supratragic tubercle; a small nodule often present on the edge of the lamina just above the tragus.

**t. syphilit′icum,** gumma of the skin.

**t. thyroid′eum infe′rius** [ NA ], inferior thyroid tubercle; a slight lateral projection from the lower margin of the laminae of the thyroid cartilage on either side, at the inferior end of the oblique line.

**t. thyroid'eum supe'rius** [ NA ], superior thyroid tubercle; a blunt projection on the lamina of the thyroid cartilage on either side at the superior end of the oblique line.

---

**tuberiferous** (tu'ber-if'er-us) [ tuber + L. *ferro*, to bear ]. Tuberous.

**tu'berose.** Tuberous.

**tuberositas** (tu'ber-os'ĭ-tas) [ LL. fr. L., *tuberosus*, full of lumps, fr. *tuber* a knob ] [ NA ]. Tuberosity; a large tubercle or rounded elevation, especially from the surface of a bone.

    **t. coracoi'dea.** coracoid tuberosity; replaced by the NA terms *tuberculum* conoideum and *linea* trapezoidea, *q. v.*

    **t. costalis** [ NA ], *impressio* ligamenti costoclavicularis.

    **t. deltoi'dea** [ NA ], deltoid eminence; deltoid crest; a rough elevation about the middle of the lateral side of the shaft of the humerus, giving attachment to the deltoid muscle.

    **t. glu'tea** [ NA ], gluteal tuberosity (1); crista glutea; gluteal crest; the point of insertion in the upper portion of the shaft of the femur of the greater part of the gluteus maximus muscle; when markedly developed this tuberosity is called the third trochanter.

    **t. ili'aca** [ NA ], iliac tuberosity; a rough area above the auricular surface on the medial aspect of the ala of the ilium, giving attachment to the posterior sacroiliac ligament.

    **t. masseter'ica** [ NA ], masseteric tuberosity; a roughened surface on the external aspect of the angle of the mandible, giving attachment to fibers of the masseter muscle.

    **t. mus'culi scale'ni anterio'ris** [ NA ], tuberosity for the anterior scalene muscle; a roughened area on the superior margin of the second rib to which the anterior scalene muscle attaches.

    **t. mus'culi serra'ti anterio'ris** [ NA ], a rough oval area, about the middle of the outer surface and lower border of the second rib, for the attachment of the serratus anterior muscle.

    **t. os'sis cuboi'dei** [ NA ], tuberosity of the cuboid bone; a slight eminence on the lateral surface of the cuboid bone, capped with an articular facet for a sesamoid bone in the tendon of the peroneus longus muscle.

    **t. os'sis metatarsa'lis pri'mi** [ NA ], tuberosity of the first metatarsal; a tubercle at the base of the bone to which is attached the tendon of the peroneus longus muscle.

    **t. os'sis metatarsa'lis quin'ti** [ NA ], tuberosity of the fifth metatarsal; a tubercle at the base of this bone to the posterior part of which is attached the tendon of the peroneus brevis muscle.

    **t. os'sis navicula'ris** [ NA ], tuberosity of the navicular bone; scaphoid tuberosity; a rounded eminence on the medial surface of the navicular bone, giving attachment to a part of the tendon of the tibialis posterior muscle.

    **t. phalan'gis dista'lis** [ NA ], ungual tuberosity; t. unguicularis; a roughened raised surface of horseshoe shape on the palmar surface of the distal end of the terminal or ungual phalanx of each finger and toe, which serves to support the pulp of the digit.

    **t. pterygoi'dea** [ NA ], pterygoid tuberosity; a roughened area on the internal aspect of the mandible, giving attachment to fibers of the medial pterygoid muscle.

    **t. ra'dii** [ NA ], tuberosity of the radius; bicipital tuberosity; an oval projection from the medial surface of the radius just distal to the neck, giving attachment on its posterior half to the tendon of the biceps.

    **t. sacra'lis** [ NA ], sacral tuberosity; a prominence on the lateral surface of the sacrum posterior to the auricular surface.

    **t. tib'iae** [ NA ], tubercle of the tibia; an oval elevation on the anterior surface of the tibia about 3 cm. distal to the articular surface, giving attachment at its distal part to the ligamentum patellae.

    **t. ul'nae** [ NA ], tuberosity of the ulna; a prominence at the lower border of the anterior surface of the coronoid process, giving attachment to the brachialis muscle.

    **t. unguicula'ris**, t. phalangis distalis.

**tuberosity** (tu'ber-os'ĭ-tĭ). Tuberositas.

---

    **t. for anterior scalene muscle,** *tuberositas* musculi scaleni anterioris.

    **bicip'ital t.,** *tuberositas* radii.

    **calca'neal t.,** *tuber* calcanei.

    **cor'acoid t.,** see *linea* trapezoidea and *tuberculum* conoideum.

    **costal t.,** *impressio* ligamenti costoclavicularis.

    **t. of cuboid bone,** *tuberositas* ossis cuboidei.

    **t. of fifth metatarsal,** *tuberositas* ossis metatarsalis quinti.

    **t. of first metatarsal,** *tuberositas* ossis metatarsalis primi.

    **gluteal t.,** (1) *tuberositas* glutea; (2) *trochanter* tertius.

    **greater t. of humerus,** *tuberculum* majus humeri.

    **iliac t.,** *tuberositas* iliaca.

    **infraglenoid t.,** *tuberculum* infraglenoidale.

    **is'chial t.,** *tuber* ischiadicum.

    **lateral femoral t.,** *epicondylus* lateralis femoris.

    **lesser t. of humerus,** *tuberculum* minus humeri.

    **masseteric t.,** *tuberositas* masseterica.

    **max'illary t.,** *tuber* maxillae.

    **medial femoral t.,** *epicondylus* medialis femoris.

    **t. of navicular bone,** *tuberositas* ossis navicularis.

    **pterygoid t.,** *tuberositas* pterygoidea.

    **t. of radius,** *tuberositas* radii.

    **sacral t.,** *tuberositas* sacralis.

    **scaphoid t.,** *tuberositas* ossis navicularis.

    **t. of ulna,** *tuberositas* ulnae.

    **ungual t.,** *tuberositas* phalangis distalis.

**tu'berous** [ L. *tuberosus* ]. Knobby, lumpy; nodular; presenting many tubers or tuberosities.

**tu'bo-** [ L. *tubus, tuba*, tube ]. Combining form relating to a tube or tubes; see also salping-, salpingo-.

**tu'boabdom'inal.** Relating to a uterine (Fallopian) tube and the abdomen.

**tubocurarine chloride** (tu'bo-ku-rah'rēn, -rin). (USP, BP). *d*-Tubocurarine chloride; $C_{38}H_{44}Cl_2N_2O_6 \cdot 5H_2O$; an alkaloid (obtained from the stems of the genus *Chondodendron*, particularly *C. tomentosum*) that raises the threshold for acetylcholine at the myoneural junction by occupying the receptors competitively, and that also blocks ganglionic transmission and releases histamine. Used to produce muscular relaxation during surgical operations. Neostigmine is an effective antagonist.

**tu'boligamen'tous.** Relating to the uterine (Fallopian) tube and the broad ligament of the uterus.

**tu'bo-ova'rian.** Relating to the uterine (Fallopian) tube and the ovary.

**tubo-ovariectomy** (tu'bo-o-văr'ĭ-ek'to-mĭ). Salpingo-oophorectomy.

**tubo-ovaritis** (tu'bo-o'vă-ri'tis). Salpingo-oophoritis.

**tuboperitoneal** (tu'bo-pĕr-ĭ-to-ne'al). Relating to the uterine (Fallopian) tubes and the peritoneum.

**tu'boplasty.** Salpingoplasty.

**tubotorsion** (tu'bo-tor'shun) [ tubo- + L. *torsio*, torsion ]. Syringosystrophy; tubatorsion; twisting of a tubular structure, such as a uterine tube.

**tubotympanic, tubotympanal** (tu'bo-tim-pan'ik, -tim'-pă-nal). Relating to the auditory (Eustachian) tube and the tympanic cavity of the ear.

**tubouterine** (tu'bo-u'ter-in). Relating to a uterine (Fallopian) tube and the uterus.

**tubovaginal** (tu-bo-vaj'ĭ-nal). Relating to a uterine (Fallopian) tube and the vagina.

**tubular** (tu'bu-lar). Relating to or of the form of a tube or tubule.

**tubulature** (tu'bu-lă-chūr, -tūr). The short neck of a retort.

**tubule** tu'būl) [ L. *tubulus*, dim. of *tubus*, tube ]. A small tube. See also tubulus.

    **Albarran y Dominguez' t.'s,** Albarran's *glands.*

    **collecting t.,** *tubulus* renalis rectus.

    **connecting t.,** a narrow arching t. of the kidney joining the distal convoluted t. and the collecting t.

    **con'voluted t.,** (1) *tubulus* renalis contortus; (2) *tubulus* seminiferus contortus.

    **dental t.'s, dentinal t.'s,** *canaliculi* dentales.

    **discharging t.,** a urinary t. formed by the union of several collecting tubules and terminating as a papillary duct.

    **Henle's t.'s,** the straight portions of the uriniferous t.'s which form Henle's loop, distinguished as the descending and ascending tubules of Henle.

**Kobelt's t.'s,** Wolffian t.'s; remnants of the mesonephric t.'s in the female, contained within the epoophoron.

**Malpighian t.'s,** in insects, slender tubular or hairlike excretory structures that emerge from the alimentary canal between the mesenteron (midgut) and proctodeum (hindgut) in a region frequently termed the pylorus; the Malpighian t.'s vary in number from 1 to over 100, and may be assorted in equally sized bundles in some insects.

**mesonephric t.,** an excretory t. of the mesonephros.

**metanephric t.,** an excretory unit of the metanephros or permanent kidney; a nephron.

**paragenital t.'s,** remnants of embryonic mesonephric t.'s, some of which form the paradidymis.

**Pflüger's t.'s,** cordlike masses of cells in the secondary cortex of the embryonic ovary.

**pronephric t.,** an excretory unit of the pronephros, present only in vestigial form in human embryos.

**seminif'erous t.,** *tubulus* seminiferus.

**Skene's t.'s,** the embryonic urethral glands which are the female homologue of the prostate.

**spiral t.,** the segment of urinary t. coming next after the proximal convoluted t.

**straight t.,** (1) *tubulus* renalis rectus; (2) *tubulus* seminiferus rectus.

**T t.,** the transverse t. that passes from the sarcolemma across a myofibril of striated muscle; it is the intermediate t. of the triad.

**urinif'erous t.,** *tubulus* renalis.

**Wolffian t.'s,** Kobelt's t.'s.

**tu'buli.** Plural of tubulus.

**tubuliform** (tu'bu-lĭ-form). Tubular.

**tubulization** (tu'bu-lĭ-za'shun). Enclosing the joined ends of a divided nerve, after neurorrhaphy, in a cylinder of paraffin or of some slowly absorbable material to keep the surrounding tissues from pushing in and preventing union.

**tubulocyst** (tu'bu-lo-sist). Tubular cyst; a cyst formed by the dilation of any occluded canal or tube.

**tubulodermoid** (tu'bu-lo-der'moyd). A dermoid tumor arising from a persistent embryonal tubular structure.

**tubuloracemose** (tu'bu-lo-ras'e-mōs). Denoting a gland of combined tubular and racemose structure.

**tubulorrhexis** (tu'bu-lo-rek'sis) [ tubule + G. *rhēxis*, a breaking ]. A pathologic process characterized by necrosis of the epithelial lining in localized segments of renal tubules, with focal rupture or loss of the basement membrane.

**tu'bulose, tu'bulous.** Having many tubules.

**tubulus,** pl. **tubuli** (tu'bu-lus, -li) [ L. dim. of *tubus*, a pipe ] [ NA ]. Tubule; a small tube.

**t. bilif'erus,** *ductulus* biliferus.

**t. contor'tus,** (1) t. renalis contortus; (2) t. seminiferus contortus.

**tubuli denta'les,** *canaliculi* dentales.

**tubuli epooph'ori,** *ductuli* transversi epoophori.

**t. galactoph'orus, t. lactif'erus,** *ductus* lactiferus.

**tubuli parooph'ori,** *ductuli* paroophori.

**t. rec'tus,** (1) t. renalis rectus; (2) t. seminiferus rectus.

**t. rena'lis contor'tus** [ NA ], convoluted tubule of the kidney; the first, proximal, or primary leads from the capsule; the second or distal is formed from the ascending limb of Henle's loop which enters the labyrinth; it ends in a collecting tube.

**t. rena'lis rec'tus** [ NA ], one of the straight tubules of the kidney, present in the medulla and pars radiata of the cortex.

**t. seminif'erus contor'tus** [ NA ], convoluted seminiferous tubule; one of two or three twisted curved tubules in each lobule of the testis, in which spermatogenesis occurs.

**t. seminif'erus rec'tus** [ NA ], straight seminiferous tubule; the t. seminiferus contortus which becomes straight just before entering the mediastinum to form the rete testis.

**tu'bus,** pl. **tu'bi** [ L. ] [ NA ]. Tube; canal.

**t. digesto'rius,** *canalis* alimentarius.

**t. medulla'ris,** *canalis* centralis.

**t. vertebra'lis,** *canalis* vertebralis.

**Tucker-McLean forceps.** See under forceps.

**Tuffier** (tü-fe-a'), Marin T., French surgeon, 1857–1929. See T.'s *test.*

**Tuffnell,** Thomas J., English surgeon, 1818–1885. See T.'s *bandage.*

**tuft.** A cluster, clump, or bunch, as a tuft of hairs.

**Malpighian t.,** glomerulus (2).

**synovial t.'s,** *villi* synovialis.

**tug, tugging.** A pulling or dragging movement or sensation.

**tracheal t.,** (1) Cardarelli's sign; Oliver's sign; Oliver-Cardarelli sign; Porter's sign; a downward pull of the trachea, manifested by a downward movement of the thyroid cartilage, synchronous with the action of the heart; symptomatic of aneurysm of the aortic arch. The sign is elicited most easily by drawing the cricoid cartilage upward with the thumb and forefinger while the patient sits with head thrown back and mouth closed; (2) in anesthesiology, a jerky type of inspiration seen when the intercostal muscles and the sternocostal parts of the diaphragm are paralyzed by deep general anesthesia or muscle relaxant drugs; due to the unopposed action of the crura pulling on the dome of the diaphragm and thence on the pericardium, lung roots, and tracheobronchial tree during each inspiration.

**tularemia** (tu'lă-re'mĭ-ah) [ *Tulare*, Lake and County, Calif., + G. *haima*, blood ]. Deer fly fever; rabbit fever; Pahvant Valley plague or fever; a disease caused by *Francisella tularensis* and transmitted to man from rodents through the bite of a deer fly, *Chrysops discalis*, and other bloodsucking insects; it can also be acquired directly through the bite of a coyote or other infected animal or through handling of an infected animal's carcass. The symptoms are similar to those of undulant fever and the plague, consisting of a prolonged intermittent or remittent fever, and often swelling and suppuration of the lymph nodes in the neighborhood of the site of infection. The disease occurs in the United States, Canada, northern Europe, and Asia. Rabbits are an important reservoir host for the bacillus through bites of the deer fly or of other mechanical vectors, such as ticks.

**tulle gras** [ Fr. oily net ]. A dressing for wounds, used chiefly in France. It is a closed meshed curtain net, cut into squares and impregnated with soft paraffin (98 parts), balsam of Peru (1 part), and olive oil (1 part).

**Tulp (Tulpius),** Nicholas, Dutch physician, 1593–1674. See T.'s *valve.*

**tumefacient** (tu'me-fa'shent) [ L. *tume-facio*, to cause to swell, fr. *tumeo*, to swell ]. Swelling or swollen.

**tumefaction** (tu'me-fak'shun) [ see tumefacient ]. 1. A swelling. 2. The condition of becoming or of being swollen.

**tumefy** (tu'me-fi). 1. To swell. 2. To cause to swell.

**tumentia** (tu-men'shĭ-ah) [ L. fr. *tumeo*, to swell ]. Swelling.

**tumescence** (tu-mes'ens) [ L. *tumesco*, to begin to swell ]. Tumefaction.

**tumescent** (tu-mes'ent). Tumefying; swelling.

**tu'mid** [ L. *tumidus* ]. Swollen; tumefied.

# TUMOR

**tumor** [ L. *tumor*, a swelling ]. 1. Any swelling or tumefaction; one of the signs of inflammation enunciated by Celsus. 2. Neoplasm; an abnormal mass of tissue that grows more rapidly than normal and continues to grow after the stimuli which initiated the new growth cease.

**acute splenic t.,** acute splenitis, enlargement, and softening of the spleen, usually due to bacteremia or severe bacterial toxemia.

**adenoid t.,** adenoma, or neoplasm with glandlike spaces.

**adenomatoid t.,** adenofibromyoma; angiomatoid t.; benign mesothelioma of genital tract; a small, benign t. of the male and female genital tract, consisting of fibrous tissue or smooth muscle enclosing spaces lined by cells; the living cells may resemble endothelium, epithelium, or mesothelium.

**adenomatoid t. of the genital tract,** Recklinghausen's t.; adenoleiomyofibroma; a small benign t. of the wall of the Fallopian tube or myometrium, probably peritoneal (mesothelial) in origin.

**adipose t.,** lipoma.

**t. al'bus,** white *swelling.*

**ameloblastic adenomatoid t.,** adenoameloblastoma.

**amyloid t.,** see nodular *amyloidosis.*

**angiomatoid t.,** adenomatoid t.

**aortic body t.,** see chemodectoma.

**benign t.,** one that does not form metastases and does not invade and destroy adjacent normal tissue.

**blood t.,** (1) aneurysm; (2) hemorrhagic *cyst* or *hematoma.*

**Brenner t.,** a relatively infrequent, benign neoplasm of the ovary, consisting chiefly of fibrous tissue that contains nests of cells resembling transitional type epithelium, as well as glandlike structures that contain mucin; origin is controversial, but Brenner t.'s may arise from nests of Walthard's cells; ordinarily found incidentally in ovaries removed for other reasons, especially in postmenopausal women.

**Brooke's t.,** trichoepithelioma.

**brown t.,** a mass of fibrous tissue containing hemosiderin-pigmented macrophages and multinucleated giant cells, replacing and expanding part of a bone in primary hyperthyroidism.

**Buschke-Löwenstein t.,** giant *condyloma.*

**carcinoid t.,** carcinoid.

**Brown-Pearce t.,** an exceedingly malignant carcinoma of the skin, with irregular arrangement of the cells and almost total absence of stroma, and usually resulting in early and extensive metastases.

**t. car'neus,** sarcoma.

**carotid body t.,** see chemodectoma.

**cellular t.,** a t. composed mainly of cells embedded in a greater or lesser amount of homogeneous stroma, without distinct histoid structure, such as sarcoma.

**cerebellopontine angle t.,** acoustic *neurinoma.*

**chemoreceptor t.,** chemodectoma.

**chromaffin t.,** paraganglioma.

**Cock's peculiar t.,** a fungating mass of inflamed granulation tissue that may develop in adjacent tissue after the rupture of a suppurative sebaceous cyst.

**Codman's t.,** chondroblastoma.

**collision t.,** two originally separate t.'s, especially a carcinoma and a sarcoma, that appear to have developed by chance in close proximity, so that an area of mingling exists; ses also carcinosarcoma.

**connective t.,** histoid t.; any t. of the connective tissue group, such as osteoma, fibroma, etc., including also sarcoma.

**dermal duct t.,** eccrine *poroma.*

**dermoid t.,** dermoid (2).

**desmoid t.,** desmoid (2).

**eighth nerve t.,** acoustic *neurinoma.*

**em'bryonal t., embryon'ic t.,** embryoma; a neoplasm, usually malignant, that arises during intrauterine or early postnatal development from an organ rudiment or immature tissue. Embryonal t.'s include neuroblastoma and Wilms' t. They form immature structures characteristic of the part from which they arise, and may form other tissues as well. The term is also used to include certain neoplasms presenting in later life, this usage being based on the belief that such tumors arise from embryonic rests. See also teratoma.

**Erdheim t.,** craniopharyngioma.

**Ewing's t.,** Ewing's sarcoma; endothelioma of bone; endothelial myeloma; a malignant neoplasm in which the cell of origin is controvesial, but the most popular concept is that they are related to the multipotent parent reticulum cells. Histologically, there are conspicuous foci of necrosis in association with irregular masses of small, regular, rounded or ovoid cells (2 to 3 times the diameter of erythrocytes), with very scanty cytoplasm. The neoplasms occur usually before the age of 20 years, about twice as frequently in males; about 75 per cent involve bones of the extremities, including the shoulder girdle, and there is a predilection for the metaphysis.

**fecal t.,** coproma.

**fibroid t.,** old term for certain fibromas and leiomyomas.

**giant cell t. of bone,** giant cell myeloma; osteoclastoma; a soft, reddish brown, osteolytic t. composed of multinucleated giant cells and ovoid or spindle-shaped cells, occurring most frequently in an end of a long tubular bone of young adults; these t.'s are usually benign, but are sometimes malignant.

**giant cell t. of tendon sheath,** localized nodular tenosynovitis; a nodule, possibly inflammatory in nature, arising commonly from the flexor sheath of the fingers and thumb; composed of fibrous tissue, lipid- and hemosiderin-containing macrophages, and multinucleated giant cells.

**glomus t.,** angioneuromyoma; an unusual neoplasm composed of specialized pericytes (sometimes termed glomus cells) and neurites. The lesions are usually single, encapsulated, nodular masses that may be several millimeters in diameter, and they occur almost exclusively in the skin. Glomus t.'s are exquisitely tender, and may cause so much pain that patients voluntarily immobilize the extremity, sometimes leading to atrophy of muscles. Simple excision is curative.

**glomus jugulare t.,** see chemodectoma.

**granular cell t.,** granular cell myoblastoma; a microscopically specific, benign t. of uncertain histogenesis, often involving peripheral nerves in skin, mucosa, or connective tissue, which may be derived from Schwann cells; the abundant cytoplasm contains granules, the cells infiltrate between adjacent tissues although growth is slow, and adjacent surface epithelium may show hyperplasia.

**granulo'sa cell t.,** folliculoma; a t. of the ovary arising from the membrana granulosa of the Graafian follicle, frequently secreting estrogen. Granulosa cell t.'s are soft, solid, and white or yellow, consisting of small round cells sometimes enclosing small round spaces called Call-Exner bodies; larger lipid-containing cells may be present. The t.'s may be benign or malignant.

**Grawitz' t.,** renal *adenocarcinoma.*

**Gubler's t.,** a fusiform swelling on the wrist in lead palsy.

**heterol'ogous t.,** a t. composed of a tissue unlike that from which it springs.

**histoid t.,** a t. composed of a single tissue, such as a fibroma.

**homol'ogous t.,** a t. composed of tissue of the same sort as that from which it springs.

**Hürthle cell t.,** oxyphil adenoma or carcinoma of the thyroid; a neoplasm of the thyroid gland composed of polyhedral, acidophilic cells, thought by some to be oncocytes; the t.'s may be benign or malignant, the behavior of the latter depending on the general microscopic pattern, whether follicular, papillary, or undifferentiated.

**hylic t.,** hyloma.

**innocent t.,** benign t.

**Krompecher's t.,** rodent *ulcer.*

**Krukenberg t.,** a metastatic carcinoma of the ovary, usually bilateral and secondary to a mucous carcinoma of the stomach; they contain signet ring cells filled with mucus.

**Landschutz t.,** a transplantable, highly virulent neoplasm growing in any strain of mice; the host is killed in a few days by what is apparently an anaplastic carcinoma; the tumor may be isoantigenic.

**lepidic t.,** lepidoma.

**Lindau's t.,** hemangioblastoma.

**malignant t.,** cancer; a t. invading surrounding tissues and usually capable of producing metastases, likely to recur after attempted removal and to cause death of the host unless adequately treated.

**mar'garoid t.,** cholesteatoma.

**melanotic neuroectodermal t.,** melanoameloblastoma; retinal anlage t.; progonoma of the jaw; pigmented epulis; a benign t. of the jaw (especially the maxillae) of infants, containing melanin-pigmented cells.

**mixed t.,** a t. composed of two or more varieties of tissue.

**mixed mesodermal t.,** a sarcoma of the body of the uterus arising in older women, composed of more than one mesenchymal tissue, especially including striated muscle cells.

**mixed t. of salivary gland,** enclavoma; pleomorphic adenoma; a t. composed of salivary gland epithelium and fibrous tissue with mucoid or cartilaginous areas.

**mixed t. of the skin,** nodular *hidradenoma.*

**mucoepidermoid t.,** mucoepidermoid *carcinoma.*

**Nélaton's t.,** a fibrous t. or sarcoma lying between the peritoneum and the muscles of the abdominal wall.

**Nelson t.,** a pituitary t. causing symptoms (see Nelson *syndrome*) after an adrenalectomy for Cushing's syndrome.

**oil t.,** lipogranuloma.

**or'ganoid t.,** a t. of complex structure, glandular in origin, containing epithelium, connective tissue, etc.

**Pancoast t.,** superior pulmonary sulcus t.; an adenocarcinoma of a lung apex causing Pancoast syndrome.

**papillary t.,** papilloma.

**paraffin t.,** paraffinoma.

**pearl t.,** cholesteatoma.

**phantom t.,** accumulation of fluid in the interlobar spaces of the lung, secondary to congestive heart failure, radiologically simulating a neoplasm.

**pontine angle t.,** a t. growing in the proximal portion of the acoustic nerve, in the angle formed by the cerebellum and the lateral pons.

**potato t. of the neck,** a firm, nodular mass in the neck, usually a carotid body tumor (chemodectoma).

**Pott's puffy t.,** a circumscribed swelling of the scalp indicating an underlying osteitis of the skull or an extradural abscess.

**pregnancy t.,** *granuloma* gravidarum.

**ranine t.,** ranula.

**Rathke's pouch t.,** craniopharyngioma.

**Recklinghausen's t.,** adenomatoid t. of the genital tract.

**retinal anlage t.,** melanotic neuroectodermal t.

**rind t.,** lepidoma.

**Rokitansky's t.,** a multilocular ovarian cyst.

**Rous t.,** Rous *sarcoma.*

**sand t,** psammoma.

**Schmincke t.,** lymphoepithelioma.

**Schwann's t.,** (1) neurofibroma; (2) neurilemoma.

**scrotal t.,** elephantiasis of the scrotum.

**Sertoli cell t.,** androblastoma of the testis; see androblastoma (1).

**Steiner's t.,** Jeanselme's *nodules.*

**superior pulmonary sulcus t.,** Pancoast t.

**ter'atoid t.,** teratoma.

**theca cell t.,** thecoma; a rare ovarian t. of the theca folliculi closely related to granulosa cell t.'s.

**transmissible venereal t.,** canine venereal *granuloma.*

**turban t.,** cylindroma of the scalp which, when overgrown, may resemble a turban.

**villous t.,** papilloma.

**Warthin's t.,** papillary *cystadenoma* lymphomatosum.

**Wilms' t.,** adenomyosarcoma; embryoma of the kidney; mesoblastic nephroma; nephroblastoma; a malignant renal t. of young children; it is composed of small spindle cells and various other types of tissue, including tubules and, in some cases, structures resembling fetal glomeruli, and striated muscle and cartilage; Wilms' t. is radiosensitive, but may have already metastasized to the lungs or elsewhere when a renal mass or hematuria is noted.

**Yaba t.,** a virus-induced neoplasm; see Yaba monkey *virus.*

**Zollinger-Ellison t.,** a non-beta cell tumor of pancreatic islets causing the Zollinger-Ellison syndrome.

---

**tumoraffin** (tu'mor-af'in) [ tumor + L. *affinis,* related to ]. Oncotropic.

**tumoricidal** (tu'mor-ĭ-si'dal) [ tumor + L. *caedo,* to kill ]. Denoting an agent destructive to tumors.

**tumorigenic** (tu'mor-ĭ-jen'ik). Causing or producing tumors.

**tumorigenesis** (tu'mor-ĭ-jen'ĕ-sis) [ tumor + G. *genesis,* origin ]. The production of a new growth or growths.

**foreign body t.,** induction of malignant tumors in tissues by nonviable, nonabsorable solid material not known to contain a chemical carcinogen.

**tu'morlets.** Minute foci of atypical bronchiolar epithelial hyperplasia that are found multifocally; although now considered benign, they were once believed to be precursors of carcinoma.

**tumorous** (tu'mor-us). Swollen; tumor-like; protuberant.

**tumul'tus** [ L. tumult, fr. *tumeo,* to swell, be excited ]. A commotion; agitation; overaction; disturbed action.

**t. cordis,** palpitation and irregular action of the heart.

**t. sermo'nis,** extreme stuttering.

**Tunga penetrans** (tung'ah pen'e-tranz). Commonly known as chigger flea, sand flea, chigoe, jigger; a member of the flea family, Tungidae; the minute female penetrates the skin, frequently under the toenails, producing a painful local ulcer with inflammation as she becomes distended with eggs to about pea size.

**tungiasis** (tung-i'ă-sis). Infestation with sand fleas (*Tunga penetrans*).

**tung'sten** [ Swed. *tung,* heavy, + *sten,* stone ]. A metallic element, symbol W (*wolframium*), atomic no. 74, atomic weight 183.86, occurring as a gray powder of metallic luster.

**t. carbide,** one of the hardest known materials; used as an abrasive and in the manufacture of dental cutting instruments.

**tu'nic** [ L. *tunica* ]. Tunica.

**Bichat's t.,** the tunica intima of the blood vessels.

**Brücke's t.,** *tunica* nervea.

**fibrous t. of corpus spongiosum,** *tunica* albuginea corporis spongiosi.

**fibrous t. of eye,** *tunica* fibrosa bulbi.

**mucosal t.'s, mucous t.'s,** see entries under *tunica* mucosa.

**muscular t.'s,** see entries under *tunica* muscularis.

**serous t.'s,** see entries under *tunica* serosa.

**tunica,** pl. **tunicae** (tu'nĭ-kah, -ke) [ L. a coat ] [ NA ]. A coat or tunic; one of the enveloping layers of a part, especially one of the coats of a blood vessel or other tubular structure.

**t. abdomina'lis,** the aponeurosis of the abdominal muscles of quadrupeds.

**t. adventi'tia** [ NA ], membrana adventitia (1); the outermost fibrous coat of a vessel or an organ that is derived from the surrounding connective tissue.

**t. albugin'ea** [ NA ], a dense, white, collagenous tunic surrounding a structure.

**t. albugin'ea cor'porum cavernoso'rum** [ NA ], a strong, fibrous membrane enveloping each corpus cavernosum penis.

**t. albugin'ea cor'poris spongio'si** [ NA ], fibrous tunic of the corpus spongiosum; the thick layer of fibrous tissue surrounding the corpus spongiosum penis. It is thinner than the corresponding layer around each corpus cavernosum.

**t. albugin'ea oc'uli,** sclera.

**t. albugin'ea ova'rii,** the layer of dense connective tissue beneath the surface epithelium of the ovary.

**t. albugin'ea tes'tis** [ NA ], a thick white fibrous membrane forming the outer coat of the testis.

**t. car'nea,** t. dartos.

**t. conjuncti'va** [ NA ], the mucous membrane investing the anterior surface of the eyeball and the posterior surface of the lids.

**t. conjuncti'va bul'bi** [ NA ], conjunctival layer of the bulb; bulbar conjunctiva; it consists of the mucous membrane covering the anterior surface of the sclera and the surface epithelium of the cornea.

**t. conjuncti'va palpebra'rum** [ NA ], conjunctival layer of the eyelids; the mucous membrane that lines the posterior surface of the eyelids. It is continuous with the bulbar conjunctiva at the conjunctival fornices.

**t. dar'tos** [ NA ], t. carnea; a layer of smooth muscular tissue in the integument of the scrotum; see also *dartos* muliebris.

**t. elas'tica,** t. media of large arteries.

**t. exter'na** [ NA ], t. extima; (1) the outer of two or more enveloping layers of any structure; (2) specifically, the outer fibroelastic coat of a blood or lymph vessel.

**t. exter'na oc'uli,** t. fibrosa bulbi.

**t. exter'na the'cae follic'uli** [ NA ], theca externa; the external fibrous layer of the theca of a well developed vesicular ovarian follicle; the cells and fibers are arranged in a concentric fashion.

**t. ex'tima,** t. externa.

**t. fibro'sa** [ NA ], any fibrous envelope of a part.

**t. fibro'sa bul'bi** [ NA ], t. externa oculi; fibrous tunic of the eye; the outer layer of the eyeball composed of the sclera and cornea.

**t. fibro'sa hep'atis** [ NA ], the fibrous layer that surrounds the liver.

**t. fibro'sa li'enis** [ NA ], t. propria lienis; capsula lienis; the fibrous capsule of the spleen, containing collagen and elastic fibers and involuntary muscular tissue.

**t. fibro'sa re'nis,** *capsula* fibrosa renis.

**tunicae funic'uli spermat'ici et tes'tis** [ NA ], coverings of the spermatic cord and testis; these include external spermatic fascia, cremasteric muscle and fascia, internal spermatic fascia, and tunica vaginalis testis.

**Haller's t. vasculosa,** t. vasculosa bulbi.

**t. hyaloid'ea,** *membrana* vitrea.

**t. inter'na bulbi** [ NA ], retina.

**t. inter'na the'cae follic'uli** [ NA ], theca interna; the inner cellular and vascular layer of the vesicular ovarian follicle; there is evidence that the epithelioid cells produce estrogen and contribute to the formation of the corpus luteum after ovulation.

**t. in'tima** [ NA ], the innermost coat of a blood or lymphatic vessel; it consists of endothelium, usually a thin fibroelastic subendothelial layer, and an inner elastic membrane or longitudinal fibers.

**t. me'dia** [ NA ], the middle, usually muscular, coat of an artery or other tubular structure.

**t. muco'sa** [ NA ], mucous membrane; it consists of epithelium, lamina propria, and, in the digestive tract, a layer of smooth muscle.

**t. muco'sa bronchio'rum** [ NA ], the inner coat of the bronchi.

**t. muco'sa ca'vi tym'pani** [ NA ], the mucous layer of the tympanic cavity and the structures in it.

**t. muco'sa co'li** [ NA ], the inner mucous coat of the colon.

**t. muco'sa duc'tus deferen'tis** [ NA ], the inner layer of the ductus deferens.

**t. muco'sa esoph'agi** [ NA ], the inner coat of the esophagus.

**t. muco'sa intesti'ni ten'uis** [ NA ], the mucous coat of the small intestine.

**t. muco'sa laryn'gis** [ NA ], the mucous coat of the larynx.

**t. muco'sa lin'guae** [ NA ], mucous membrane of the tongue; the mucosa of the dorsum of the tongue appears velvety due to the presence of vast numbers of papillae; that of the inferior surface is smooth and thinner.

**t. muco'sa na'si** [ NA ], pituitary membrane; Schneiderian membrane; mucous membrane of the nose; it is continuous with the skin in the vertibule of the nose and with the mucosa of the nasopharynx, the paranasal sinuses and the nasolacrimal duct; and contains goblet cells. it is subdivided into the *regio* olfactoria and *regio* respiratoria, *q. v.*

**t. muco'sa o'ris** [ NA ], the mucous membrane of the oral cavity, including the gingiva.

**t. muco'sa pharyn'gis** [ NA ], the mucous coat of the pharynx.

**t. muco'sa tra'cheae** [ NA ], the inner mucous layer of the trachea.

**t. muco'sa tu'bae auditi'vae** [ NA ], the lining coat of the auditory tube.

**t. muco'sa tu'bae uteri'nae** [ NA ], the mucous layer of the uterine tube.

**t. muco'sa ure'teris** [ NA ], the inner layer of the ureter.

**t. muco'sa ure'thrae femini'nae** [ NA ], the inner mucosal layer of the female urethra.

**t. muco'sa u'teri** [ NA ], endometrium.

**t. muco'sa vagi'nae** [ NA ], the mucous membrane of the vagina.

**t. muco'sa ventric'uli** [ NA ], the mucous layer of the stomach.

**t. muco'sa ves'icae fel'leae** [ NA ], the inner coat of the gallbladder.

**t. muco'sa ves'icae urina'riae** [ NA ], the inner coat of the urinary bladder.

**t. muco'sa vesic'ulae semina'lis** [ NA ], the mucous membrane of the seminal vesicle.

**t. muscula'ris** [ NA ], the muscular, usually middle, layer of a tubular structure.

**t. muscula'ris bronchio'rum** [ NA ], muscular tunic of the bronchi.

**t. muscula'ris co'li** [ NA ], muscular tunic of the colon.

**t. muscula'ris duc'tus deferen'tis** [ NA ], muscular tunic of the ductus deferens.

**t. muscula'ris esoph'agi** [ NA ], muscular tunic of the esophagus.

**t. muscula'ris intesti'ni ten'uis** [ NA ], muscular tunic of the small intestine.

**t. muscula'ris pharyn'gis** [ NA ], muscular tunic of the pharynx.

**t. muscula'ris rec'ti** [ NA ], muscular tunic of the rectum.

**t. muscula'ris tra'cheae** [ NA ], muscular tunic of the trachea.

**t. muscula'ris tu'bae uteri'nae** [ NA ], muscular tunic of the uterine tube.

**t. muscula'ris ure'teris** [ NA ], muscular tunic of the ureter.

**t. muscula'ris ure'thrae femini'nae** [ NA ], muscular tunic of the female urethra.

**t. muscula'ris u'teri** [ NA ], muscular tunic of the uterus.

**t. muscula'ris vagi'nae** [ NA ], muscular tunic of the vagina.

**t. muscula'ris ventric'uli** [ NA ], muscular tunic of the stomach; it consists of smooth muscles arranged in three fairly well defined layers: an outer stratum longitudinale, comprising the musculus dilator pylori gastroduodenalis, a middle stratum circulare, continuous with the musculus sphincter pylori, and an inner incomplete layer consisting of fibrae obliquae arching over the cardiac notch.

**t. muscula'ris ves'icae fel'leae** [ NA ], muscular tunic of the gallbladder.

**t. muscula'ris ves'icae urina'riae** [ NA ], muscular tunic of the urinary bladder.

**t. ner'vea,** Brücke's tunic; an older term, formerly used to designate the retina exclusive of the layer of rods and cones.

**t. pro'pria,** the special envelope of a part as distinguished from the peritoneal or other investment common to several parts.

**t. pro'pria co'rii,** *stratum* reticulare corii.

**t. pro'pria li'enis,** t. fibrosa lienis.

**t. reflex'a,** the reflected layer of the t. vasculosa testis that lines the scrotum.

**t. sclerot'ica,** sclera.

**t. sero'sa** [ NA ], a serous tunic, coat, or membrane; serosa (1); the outermost coat of a visceral structure that lies in a body cavity; it consists of a surface layer of mesothelium reinforced by irregular fibroelastic connective tissue.

**t. sero'sa co'li** [ NA ], serous tunic of the colon.

**t. sero'sa hep'atis** [ NA ], serous tunic of the liver.

**t. sero'sa intesti'ni ten'uis** [ NA ], serous tunic of the small intestine.

**t. sero'sa peritone'i** [ NA ], serous tunic of the peritoneum.

**t. sero'sa tu'bae uteri'nae** [ NA ], serous tunic of the uterine tube.

**t. sero'sa u'teri** [ NA ], official alternate term for perimetrium.

**t. sero'sa ventric'uli** [ NA ], serous tunic of the stomach.

**t. sero'sa ves'icae fel'leae** [ NA ], serous tunic of the gallbladder.

**t. sero'sa ves'icae urina'riae** [ NA ], serous tunic of the urinary bladder.

**t. submuco'sa,** *tela* submucosa.

**t. vagina'lis commu'nis,** *fascia* spermatica interna.

**t. vagina'lis tes'tis** [ NA ], the serous sheath of the testis and epididymis, derived from the peritoneum; it consists of an outer and inner serous layer, lamina parietalis and lamina visceralis, respectively.

**t. vasculo'sa,** any vascular layer.

**t. vasculo'sa bul'bi** [ NA ], uvea; uveal tract; t. vasculosa oculi; Haller's t. vasculosa; the vascular, pigmentary, or middle coat of the eye, comprising the choroid, ciliary body, and iris.

**t. vasculo'sa len'tis,** a nutrient vascular layer enveloping the lens of the eye in the fetus.

**t. vasculo'sa oc'uli,** t. vasculosa bulbi.

**t. vasculo'sa tes'tis,** the vascular layer enveloping the testis beneath the t. albuginea.

**t. vit'rea,** *membrana* vitrea.

**tunicin** (tu'nĭ-sin) A substance resembling cellulose found in the outer envelope of the sea squirt and other tunicates; also called animal cellulose.

**tun'nel.** An elongated passageway, usually open at both ends.

**carpal t.,** the space bounded in front by the flexor retinaculum and behind by the anterior surfaces of the carpal bones; compression of the median nerve may occur at this site.

**Corti's t.,** Corti's canal; the spiral canal in the organ of Corti, formed by the outer and inner pillar cells or rods of Corti; it is filled with fluid and occasionally crossed by nonmedullated nerve fibers.

**Tunnicliff,** Ruth, Chicago physician, 1876–1946. See T. *toxin.*

**turanose** (tu'rȧ-nōs). 3-(α-D-Glucosido)-D-fructose; a reducing disaccharide.

**Turba'trix.** A genus of freeliving nematodes in the family Cephalobidae.

**T. ace'ti,** the vinegar eel, found in old vinegar or in rotting fruits and vegetables.

**tur'bid** [ L. *turbidus,* confused, disordered ]. Cloudy.

**turbidimeter** (tur'bĭ-dim'e-ter). An instrument for measuring turbidity.

**tur'bidimet'ric.** Pertaining to the measurement of turbidity.

**turbidimetry** (tur'bĭ-dim'e-trĭ) [ turbidity + G. *metron,* measure ]. A method for determining the concentration of a substance in a solution by the degree of cloudiness or turbidity it causes or by the degree of clarification it induces in a turbid solution.

**turbidity** (tur'bid'ĭ-tĭ) [ L. *turbiditas,* fr. *turbidus,* turbid ]. The quality of being turbid, of losing transparency because of sediment or insoluble matter.

**tur'binal.** Turbinated *body* (1).

**tur'binate.** 1. Turbinated. 2. *Concha* nasalis.

**tur'bina'ted** [ L. *turbinatus,* shaped like a top ]. Scroll-shaped.

**turbinectomy** (tur'bĭ-nek'to-mĭ) [ turbinate + G. *ektomē,* excision ]. Surgical removal of a turbinated bone.

**turbinotome** (tur'bĭ-no-tōm). An instrument for use in turbinotomy or turbinectomy.

**turbinotomy** (tur'bĭ-not'o-mĭ) [ turbinate + G. *tomē,* incision ]. Incision into or excision of a turbinated body.

**Türck,** Ludwig, Austrian neurologist, 1810–1868. See T.'s *bundle, column, degeneration, tract.*

**Turcot syndrome.** See under syndrome.

**turgescence** (tur-jes'ens) [ L. *turgesco,* to begin to swell, fr. *turgeo,* to swell ]. Swelling; inflation.

**turgescent** (tur-jes'ent). Swollen; turgid; tumid.

**turgid** (tur'jid) [ L. *turgidus,* swollen, fr. *turgeo,* to swell ]. Swollen; tumid; congested.

**turgometer** (tur-gom'e-ter) [ turgor + G. *metron,* measure ]. A device for measuring turgor, or turgescence, particularly of the skin.

**tur'gor** [ L. fr. *turgeo,* to swell ]. Fullness.

**t. vita'lis,** the normal fullness of the capillaries.

**Türk,** Wilhelm, Austrian hematologist, 1871–1916. See T.'s *cell, leukocyte, stain.*

**tur'key red.** Madder.

**turmeric** (tur'mĕ-rik). Curcuma.

**turn** [ A.S. *tyrnan* ]. 1. To revolve or cause to revolve; specifically, to change the position of the fetus in utero so as to convert a malpresentation into one permitting of normal delivery. 2. A change of position.

**Turner,** George Grey. See Grey Turner.

**Turner,** Henry H., American endocrinologist, *1892. See T.'s *syndrome,* pseudo-T.'s *syndrome.*

**Turner,** Sir William, English anatomist, 1832–1916. See T.'s *sulcus.*

**turn'ing.** In obstetrics, version.

**turn'over.** The quantity of a material metabolized or processed, usually within a given length of time.

**turpentine** (tur'pen-tĭn) [ G. *terebinthinos,* pertaining to *terebinthos,* the terebinth tree ]. An oleoresin from *Pinus palustris* and other species of *Pinus;* source of t. oil and a constituent of stimulating ointments.

**Canada t.,** Canada *balsam.*

**Chian t.,** an exudation from *Pistacia terebinthus,* a small tree of Chios and regions to the eastward. On exposure to air it thickens and forms translucent yellow masses similar to mastic.

**larch t.,** Venice t.; a transparent, yellowish, thick liquid, the oleoresin obtained from *Larix europaea* (family Pinaceae).

**t. oil** (BP), t. spirit; a volatile oil distilled from t.; has been used as a diuretic, carminative, vermifuge, expectorant, rubefacient, and counterirritant.

**t. oil, rectified,** obtained by treating t. oil with sodium hydroxide, and redistilling; used externally as a counterirritant.

**t. spirit,** t. oil.

**Venice t.,** larch t.

**white t.,** t. from *Pinus palustris.*

**turps.** A popular name for turpentine oil.

**turricephaly** (tur'ĭ-sef'ȧ-lĭ) [ L. *turris,* tower, + G. *kephalē,* head ]. Oxycephaly.

**turun'da,** pl. **turun'dae** [ L. ]. A surgical tent, gauze drain, or tampon.

**tush, tusk.** A canine tooth in the horse, pig, or musk-deer; an incisor in the elephant and walrus.

**tus'sal.** Tussive.

**tussicular** (tus-sik'u-lar) [ L. *tussicularis,* fr. *tussicula,* a slight cough, dim. of *tussis,* cough ]. Tussive.

**tussiculation** (tus-sik'u-la'shun). A hacking cough.

**tus'sis** [ L. ]. A cough.

**t. stomacha'lis,** stomach cough; a reflex cough due to irritation of the gastric mucous membrane.

**tussive** (tus'siv) [ L. *tussis,* a cough ]. Tussal; tussicular; relating to a cough.

**tuta'men,** pl. **tuta'mina** [ L. protection ]. Any defensive or protective structure.

**tuta'mina cer'ebri,** the scalp, cranium, and cerebral meninges.

**tuta'mina oc'uli,** the eyebrows, eyelids, and eyelashes.

**Tuttle,** Edward G., U. S. gynecologist, 1863–1920. See T.'s *mask.*

**Tuttle,** James P., American surgeon, 1857–1913. See T.'s *proctoscope.*

**TV** [ tuberculin + volutin ]. Behring's formula for the constituent of the tubercle bacillus soluble in pure water; it possesses the physical and chemical properties of volutin.

**Tweed,** C. H. See T. edgewise *treatment.*

**'tween-brain.** Obsolete term for diencephalon.

**tweezers** (twē'zers) [ A.S. *twisel,* fork ]. Vulsella *forceps.*

**twig** [ A.S. ]. One of the finer terminal branches of an artery; a small branch or small ramus.

**twilight** [ A.S. *twi-,* two ]. 1. The light existing when the sun is below the horizon. 2. A faint light; figuratively, faint or indistinct mental perception.

**twin** [ A.S. *getwin,* double ]. 1. One of two children born at one birth. 2. Double; growing in pairs; geminate.

**allan'toidoangiop'agous t.'s,** omphaloangiopagous t.'s; unequal monochorial t.'s with fusion of their allantoic vessels within the placenta. The lesser t. is essentially a parasite on the placental circulation of the larger.

**conjoined t.'s,** monozygotic t.'s with varying extent of union and different degrees of residual duplication. The various types of union are named by the use of a prefix designating the region that is united and adding the suffix -pagus, meaning fused (*e.g.,* craniopagus, thoracopagus). The various types of residual duplication are named by designating the parts duplicated and adding the suffix -didymus, or -dymus, meaning twin (*e.g.,* cephalodidymus, or cephalodymus).

**conjoined equal or symmetrical t.'s,** conjoined t.'s in which both members are approximately of the same size, and fairly normal except for the areas of fusion.

**conjoined unequal or asymmetrical t.'s,** conjoined t.'s with one member fairly normal (the host or autosite) and the other (the parasite) small, incomplete, and dependent for its nutrition upon the more nearly normal member.

**dichorial t.'s,** dizygotic t.'s.

**diovular t.'s,** dizygotic t.'s.

**dizygotic t.'s,** t.'s derived from two separate zygotes; also called dichorial, diovular, fraternal, or heterologous t.'s.

**enzygotic t.'s,** monozygotic t.'s.
**fraternal t.'s,** dizygotic t.'s.
**heterologous t.'s,** dizygotic t.'s.
**identical t.'s,** monozygotic t.'s.
**incomplete conjoined t.'s,** conjoined t.'s, the two components of which equal one another but are less than entire individuals.
**monoamniotic t.'s,** t.'s within a common amnion; such t.'s are monovular in origin and may be conjoined.
**monochorial t.'s,** monozygotic t.'s.
**monovular t.'s,** monozygotic t.'s.
**monozygotic t.'s,** type of t.'s resulting from a single fertilized ovum that at an early stage of development becomes separated into independently growing cell aggregations giving rise to two individuals of the same sex and identical genetic constitution; also called enzygotic, identical, monochorial, uniovular, or monovular t.'s.
**om'phaloangiop'agous t.'s,** allantoidoangiopagous t.'s.
**parasitic t.,** the smaller of unequal conjoined t.'s.
**placental parasitic t.,** omphalosite.
**polyzygotic t.'s,** type of t.'s resulting from fertilization of more than two ova which have been discharged in a single ovulating cycle.
**Siamese t.'s,** much publicized conjoined t.'s from Siam; these particular t.'s were xiphopagus. The term Siamese t.'s has since come into general lay usage for any type of conjoined t.'s.
**uniovular t.'s,** monozygotic t.'s.
**twinge** (twinj). A sudden momentary sharp pain.
**twin'ning.** The production of equivalent structures by division; the tendency of divided parts to assume symmetrical relations.
**twitch** [ A.S. *twiccian* ]. 1. To jerk spasmodically. 2. A momentary spasmodic contraction of a muscle fiber. 3. An instrument consisting of a stout wooden handle fitted at one end with a loop of strong rope. When the loop is placed around the upper lip of a horse and twisted by means of the handle, it pinches, causing pain. This distracts the animal's attention and makes it more amenable to examinations and even minor surgery.
**skin t.,** contraction of the skin muscle in certain animals in response to nocuous stimuli; the minimal response is used as a test in assaying the efficacy of anesthetic drugs.
**two-carbon fragment.** The acetyl group ($CH_3CO$—) taking part in transacetylation reactions with coenzyme A as carrier; also commonly referred to as acetate or as acetic acid.
**Twort,** Frederick W., British bacteriologist, 1877–1950. See T. *phenomenon,* T.-d'Herelle *phenomenon.*
**ty'bamate** (USAN). BENVIL; NOSPAN, SALACEN; SOLACIN; TYBATRAN; 2-(hydroxymethyl)-2-methylpentyl butylcarbamate carbamate; a tranquilizer related to meprobamate.
**ty'le** [ G. *tylē,* a swelling, a callus ]. Callosity.
**tylectomy** (ti-lek'to-mī) [ G. *tylē,* lump, + *ektomē,* excision ]. Lumpectomy; surgical removal of a tumor from the breast.
**tylion,** pl. **tylia** (til'ī-on, ti'lī-ah) [ G. a small pin, dim. of *tylē,* a lump ]. A craniometric point at the middle of the anterior edge of the sulcus chiasmatis.
**tyloma** (ti-lo'mah) [ G. a callus ]. Callosity.
**t. conjuncti'vae,** a localized cornification of the conjunctiva, occurring in xerosis of the conjunctiva.
**tylosis,** pl. **tyloses** (ti-lo'sis, -sēz) [ G. a becoming callous ]. The formation of a callosity (tyloma).
**t. cilia'ris,** pachyblepharon.
**t. ling'uae,** leukoplakia.
**t. palmaris et plantaris,** *keratosis* palmaris et plantaris.
**tylot'ic.** Callous; relating to or marked by tylosis (callosity).
**tyloxapol** (ti-lok'să-pol) (NF). SUPERINONE; oxyethylated *tert*-octylphenol formaldehyde polymer; a detergent and mucolytic agent used as an aerosol to liquify sputum.
**tymaz'oline.** 2-[ (Thymyloxy)methyl ]-2-imidazoline; nasal decongestant.
**tympan-, tympani-.** See tympano-.
**tympanal** (tim'pă-nal). Tympanic.
**tympanectomy** (tim'pă-nek'to-mī) [ tympan- + G. *ektomē,* excision ]. Excision of the tympanic membrane.
**tympania** (tim-pan'ī-ah). Tympanites.

**tympanic** (tim-pan'ik). Tympanal. 1. Relating to the tympanic cavity or membrane. 2. Resonant.
**tympanichord** (tim-pan'ī-kord). *Chorda* tympani.
**tympanichordal** (tim-pan-ī-kor'dal). Relating to the chorda tympani nerve.
**tympanicity** (tim'pă-nis'ī-tī). The quality of being tympanic or drumlike in tone.
**tympanism** (tim'pă-nizm). Tympanites.
**tympanites** (tim'pă-ni'tēz) [ L. fr. G. *tympanitēs,* a dropsy in which the belly is stretched like a drum, *tympanon* ]. Meteorism; tympanism; swelling of the abdomen from gas in the intestinal or peritoneal cavity.
**uterine t.,** physometra.
**tympanitic** (tim'pă-nit'ik). 1. Referring to tympanites. 2. Tympanic; denoting the quality of sound elicited by percussing over the inflated intestine or a large pulmonary cavity. See also resonance.
**tympanitis** (tim'pă-ni'tis). Myringitis.
**tympano-, tympan-, tympani-** (tim'pă-no-) [ G. *tympanon,* drum ]. Combining forms denoting tympanum or tympanites.
**tympanoeustachian** (tim'pă-no-u-sta'shun, -sta'kī-an). Relating to the tympanic cavity and the auditory (Eustachian) tube.
**tympanohyal** (tim'pă-no-hi'al). Relating to that part of the tympanic cavity developed from the second embryonic pharyngeal arch.
**tympanomalleal** (tim'pă-no-mal'e-al). Relating to the tympanic membrane and the malleus.
**tympanomandibular** (tim'pă-no-man-dib'u-lar). Relating to the tympanic cavity and the mandible.
**tympanomastoid** (tim'pă-no-mas'toyd). Relating to the tympanic cavity and the mastoid cells.
**tympanomastoiditis** (tim'pă-no-mas-toy-di'tis). Inflammation of the middle ear and the mastoid cells.
**tympanophonia, tympanophony** (tim'pă-no-fo'nī-ah, tim'pă-nof'o-nī) [ tympano- + G. *phōne,* sound ]. 1. *Tinnitus* aurium. 2. Autophony.
**tympanomeatomastoidectomy** (tim'pă-no-me'ă-to-mas-toy-dek'to-mī). Radical *mastoidectomy.*
**tympanoplasty** (tim'pă-no-plas'tī) [ tympano- + G. *plassō,* to form ]. Operative correction of a damaged middle ear.
**tympanosquamosal** (tim'pă-no-skwa-mo'sal). Relating to the tympanic and squamous parts of the temporal bone.
**tympanostapedial** (tim'pă-no-sta'pe'dī-al). Relating to the tympanic cavity and the stapes.
**tympanotemporal** (tim'pă-no-tem'po-ral). Relating to the tympanic cavity and the temporal region or bone.
**tympanotomy** (tim'pă-not'o-mī) [ tympano- + G. *tomē,* incision ]. Myringotomy.
**tympanous** (tim'pă-nus). Tympanitic.
**tympanum,** pl. **tympanums, tympana** (tim'pă-num, tim'pă-nah) [ L. fr. G. *tympanon,* a drum ]. Drum; frequently used to mean cavum tympani or middle ear, *q.v.*
**tympany** (tim'pă-nī). Low-pitched, resonant, drumlike note obtained by percussing the surface of a large air-containing space, such as the distended abdomen or the thorax with or without pneumothorax.
**Skoda's t.,** Skodaic *resonance.*
**Tyndall,** John, English physicist, 1820–1893. See T. *phenomenon.*
**tyn'dalliza'tion.** Fractional *sterilization.*
**type** [ G. *typos,* a mark, a model. TYP- ]. 1. The usual form, or a composite form, that all others of the class resemble more or less closely; a model; denoting especially a disease or a symptom complex giving the stamp or characteristic to a class. 2. In chemistry, a substance in which the arrangement of the atoms in a molecule may be taken as representative of other substances in that class. 3. See also personality and constitution.
**apoplectic t.,** see *habitus* apoplecticus.
**basic personality t.,** 1. An individual's unique, covert, or underlying personality propensities, whether or not they are behaviorally manifest or overt. 2. Personality characteristics of an individual which are also shared by a majority of the members of a social group.

**blood t.,** see under blood.

**nomenclatural t.,** the constituent element of a taxon to which the name of the taxon is permanently attached; the t. of a species is preferably a strain (in special cases it may be a description, a preserved specimen or preparation, or an illustration); the t. of a genus is a species; and the t. of an order, family, or tribe is the genus on whose name the name of the higher taxon is based.

**pyknic t.,** see pyknic.

**Tartar t.** [ Tartar, or Tatar, a Mongolian race in eastern and northern Asia ], mongolism.

**test t.,** see *test type*.

**vesanic t.,** a person with functional insanity without external cause.

**typhemia** (ti-fe′mĭ-ah). Typhoid bacillemia; the presence of typhoid bacilli (*Salmonella typhosa*) in the blood.

**typhia** (ti′fĭ-ah). Typhoid *fever*.

**typhinia** (ti-fin′ĭ-ah). Relapsing *fever*.

**typhization** (ti′fĭ-za′shun). 1. Infection with typhus or typhoid fever. 2. Preventive inoculation with typhoid vaccine.

**typhl-.** See typhlo-.

**typhlectasis** (tif-lek′tă-sis) [ G. *typhlon*, cecum, + *ektasis*, a stretching out ]. Dilation of the cecum.

**typhlectomy** (tif-lek′to-mĭ). Cecectomy.

**typhlenteritis** (tif′len-ter-i′tis). Cecitis.

**typhlitis** (tif′li′tis). Cecitis.

**typhlo-, typhl-** (tif′lo-). 1 [ G. *typhlon*, cecum ]. Combining form relating to the cecum; for words so beginning and not found here, see also those beginning with cec- and ceco-. 2 [ G. *typhlos*, blind ]. Combining form relating to blindness.

**typhlocele** (tif′lo-sēl). Cecocele.

**typhlodicliditis** (tif-lo-dik-lĭ-di′tis) [ G. *typhlon*, cecum, + *diklis* (*diklid*-), double-folding (of doors), + suffix *-itis*, inflammation ]. Inflammation of the ileocecal valve.

**typhloempyema** (tif′lo-em-pi-e′ma) [ G. *typhlon*, cecum, + *empyēma*, abscess ]. The presence of an abscess following typhlitis.

**typhloenteritis** (tif-lo-en-ter-i′tis). Cecitis.

**typhlolexia** (tif′lo-lek′sĭ-ah) [ G. *typhlos*, blind, + *lexis*, speech, a word ]. Alexia.

**typhlolithiasis** (tif′lo-lĭ-thi′ă-sis) [ G. *typhlon*, cecum, + *lithos*, stone ]. The presence of fecal concretions in the cecum.

**typhlology** (tif-lol′o-jĭ) [ G. *typhlos*, blind, + *logos*, study ]. The branch of science dealing with the causes and prevention of blindness, and the rehabilitation of those afflicted.

**typhlomegaly** (tif′lo-meg′ă-lĭ) [ G. *typhlon*, cecum, + *megas* (*megal*-), large ]. Enlargement of the cecum.

**typhlon** (tif′lon) [ G. TYPHL- ]. Cecum.

**typhlopexy, typhlopexia** (tif′lo-pek′sĭ, -pek′sĭ-ah). Cecopexy.

**typhloptosis** (tif′lop-to′sis). Cecoptosis.

**typhlorrhaphy** (tif-lor′ă-fĭ). Cecorrhaphy.

**typhlosis** (tif-lo′sis) [ G. TYPHL- ]. Blindness.

**typhlostomy** (tif-los′to-mĭ). Cecostomy.

**typhlotomy** (tif-lot′o-mĭ). Cecotomy.

**typhloureterostomy** (tif′lo-u-re′ter-os′to-mĭ) [ G. *typhlon*, cecum, + ureter, + *stoma*, mouth ]. Anastomosis of ureter into cecum.

**typho-** (ti′fo-) [ G. *typhos*. TYPH- ]. Combining form relating to typhus or typhoid.

**typhodes** (ti-fo′dēz) [ G. *typhōdēs*, like smoke, delirious, fr. *typhos*, smoke, + *eidos*, appearance ]. Typhoid.

**typhogenic** (ti′fo-jen′ik). Causing or predisposing to typhus.

**typhoid** (ti′foyd) [ typhus + G. *eidos*, resemblance ]. 1. Typhus-like; stuporous from fever. 2. Typhoid *fever*.

**ambulatory t.,** walking t.

**apyret′ic t.,** t. fever in which the temperature does not rise more than a degree or two.

**bilious t. of Griesinger,** relapsing *fever*.

**fowl t.,** an acute, septicemic disease of adult chickens and turkeys, caused by *Salmonella gallinarum;* some human infections with this organism have been reported.

**latent t.,** walking t.

**provocation t.,** an accelerated onset of t. fever, sometimes of unusual severity, resulting from T.A.B. vaccination late in the incubation period.

**walking t.,** ambulatory t.; latent t.; t. fever without much prostration, the patient being up and around and sometimes working.

**typhoid′al.** Typhoid; relating to or resembling typhoid fever.

**typholysin** (ti-fol′ĭ-sin). A hemolysin formed by *Salmonella typhosa*.

**typhomania** (ti-fo-ma′nĭ-ah) [ typho- + G. *mania*, frenzy ]. A muttering delerium characteristic of that in typhoid fever and typhus.

**typhopneumonia** (ti-fo-nu-mo′nĭ-ah). Pneumonia occurring during the course of typhoid fever.

**typhosepsis** (ti′fo-sep′sis). Typhoid *septicemia*.

**typhous** (ti′fus). Relating to typhus.

**typhus** (ti′fus) [ G. *typhos*, smoke, stupor. TYPH- ]. An acute infectious and contagious disease, caused by rickettsiae, and occurring in two chief forms, classical epidemic t. and endemic murine t. Also called sapropyra, saprotyphus, jail fever, typhus fever, war fever, camp fever, ship fever.

**endemic t.,** murine t.

**epidemic t.,** louse-borne t.; t. marked by high fever, mental and physical depression, and a macular and papular eruption; it lasts for about 2 weeks, is caused by *Rickettsia prowazekii*, is spread by body lice, and occurs when large crowds are brought together and personal hygiene is at a low ebb; recrudescences occur.

**flea-borne t.,** murine t.

**louse-borne t.,** epidemic t.

**mite t.,** tsutsugamushi *disease*.

**t. mit′ior,** a mild or abortive t.

**murine t.,** the form of t. that is transmitted to man by rat or mouse fleas; it is a milder disease than the louse-borne disease, but otherwise the two forms are similar. Also called endemic t., red fever, red fever of the Congo, Congolian red fever, bakandjia.

**North Queensland tick t.,** caused by *Rickettsia australis*.

**recrudescent t.,** Brill-Zinsser *disease*.

**scrub t.,** tsutsugamushi *disease*.

**tick t.,** eruptive fever; collective term for the tick-borne rickettsial diseases, found in many parts of the world, involving many strains (or species) placed in the subgenus *Dermacentroxenus;* identified by their immunological reactions and, in some cases, by their pathogenicity. The tick-borne rickettsiae invade the nuclei as well as cytoplasm of host cells (true typhus rickettsiae are found in cytoplasm only).

**tropical t.,** tsutsugamushi *disease*.

**typing** (ti′ping) [ see type ]. Classification according to type.

**bacteriophage t.,** a microbiological procedure, of epidemiological importance, for distinguishing types within a seemingly homogeneous bacterial species or strain by the use of type-specific bacteriophage.

**blood t.,** see blood grouping (under blood).

**typus** (ti′pus) [ L. impression, model. TYP- ]. Type.

**t. degenerativus amstelodamensis,** de Lange *syndrome*.

**Tyr.** Symbol for tyrosine and its radicals.

**tyraminase** (ti′ră-mĭ-nās, tīr-). Amine oxidase (flavin-containing).

**tyramine** (ti′ră-mēn, tīr-). 4-Hydroxyphenylmethylamine; decarboxylated tyrosine; a sympathomimetic amine having an action in some respects resembling that of epinephrine; present in ergot, mistletoe, ripe cheese, and putrefied animal matter.

**t. oxidase,** amine oxidase (flavin-containing).

**tyrannism** (tīr′ă-nizm) [ G. *tyrannos*, a tyrant ]. Sadism; a lust for domination and cruelty.

**tyremesis** (ti-rem′e-sis) [ G. *tyros*, cheese, + *emesis*, vomiting ]. The vomiting of curdy material by infants.

**tyrocidin, tyrocidine** (ti′ro-si′din). An antibacterial crystalline substance obtained from *Bacillus brevis*. It is a cyclopolypeptide; a mixture of t. with gramicidin is tyrothricin.

**Tyrode,** Maurice V., American pharmacologist, 1878–1930. See T.'s *solution.*

**tyrogenous** (ti-roj'ĕ-nus) [ G. *tyros,* cheese, + suffix -gen, producing ]. Produced by, or originating in, cheese.

**Tyroglyphus longior** (ti-rog'lĭ-fus, ti'ro-glif'us). *Tyrophagus putrescentiae.*

**ty'roid** [ G. *tyrōdēs,* fr. *tyros,* cheese, + *eidos,* resemblance ]. Cheesy; caseous.

**tyroketonuria** (ti'ro-ke-to-nu'rĭ-ah). The urinary excretion of ketonic metabolites of tyrosine, such as *p*-hydroxyphenylpyruvic acid.

**tyroma** (ti-ro'mah) [ G. *tyros,* cheese, + suffix -*oma,* tumor ]. A caseous tumor.

**tyromatosis** (ti-ro'mă-to'sis). Caseation.

**tyropanoate sodium** (ti'ro-pă-no'āt) (USAN). BILOPAQUE; 3-butyramido-α-ethyl-2,4,6-triiodohydrocinnamic acid sodium salt; radiographic medium for cholecystography.

**Tyrophagus putrescentiae** (ti-rof'ă-gus pu'tre-sen'tĭ-e). One of the grain mites, which cause ground itch, baker's itch, copra itch, miller's itch, barley itch, cottonseed itch, etc., forms of dermatitis resulting from infestation with grain mites among food and produce handlers.

**tyrosinase** (ti'ro-sĭ-nās, tīr-). Monophenol monooxygenase.

**β-tyrosinase.** Tyrosine phenol-lyase.

**tyrosine** (ti'ro-sēn, -sin). 2-Amino-3-(*p*-hydroxyphenyl)-propionic acid; β-(*p*-hydroxyphenyl)alanine; (HOC$_6$H$_4$)-CH$_2$CHNH$_2$COOH; an α-amino acid present in most proteins.

   **t. iodinase,** a postulated enzyme in thyroid catalyzing the iodination of t., a reaction important in the eventual biosynthesis of thyroxine. See also peroxidases and iodinase.

   **t. phenol-lyase,** β-tyrosinase; an enzyme (EC 4.1.99.2) cleaving L-tyrosine to phenol, pyruvate, and NH$_2$.

**tyrosinemia** (ti-ro-sĭ-ne'mĭ-ah) [ tyrosine + G. *haima,* blood ]. Hypertyrosinemia; a heritable disorder characterized by elevated blood concentrations of tyrosine, enhanced urinary excretion of tyrosine and tyrosyl compounds, hepatosplenomegaly, nodular cirrhosis of the liver, multiple renal tubular reabsorptive defects, and vitamin D-resistant rickets.

**tyrosinosis** (ti'ro-sĭ-no'sis) [ tyrosine + G. suffix -*osis,* condition ]. A very rare, possibly heritable disorder of tyrosine metabolism; may be caused by defective formation of *p*-hydroxyphenylpyruvic acid oxidase or of tyrosine transaminase; characterized by enhanced urinary excretion of *p*-hydroxyphenylpyruvic acid and of other tyrosyl metabolites upon ingestion of tyrosine.

**tyrosinuria** (ti'ro-sĭ-nu'rĭ-ah) [ tyrosine + G. *ouron,* urine ]. The excretion of tyrosine in the urine.

**tyrosis** (ti-ro'sis) [ G. *tyros,* cheese ]. 1. Tyremesis. 2. Tyromatosis.

**tyrosyluria** (ti'ro-sil-u'rĭ-ah). Enhanced urinary excretion of certain metabolites of tyrosine, such as *p*-hydroxyphenylpyruvic acid; present in tyrosinosis, scurvy, pernicious anemia, and other diseases.

**tyrothricin** (ti-ro-thri'sin). An antibacterial substance obtained from peptone cultures of *Bacillus brevis.* It yields the crystalline antibacterial agents gramicidin and tyrocidin; the gramicidin component is a polypeptide containing L-tryptophan, D-leucine, D-valine, L-valine, L-alanine, glycine, and an aminoethanol; the tyrocidin component is a cyclopolypeptide containing tyrosine, ornithine, and several other amino acids. T. is both bactericidal and bacteriostatic, and is active against Gram-positive bacteria.

**tyrotoxism** (ti'ro-tok'sizm) [ G. *tyros,* cheese, + *toxikon,* poison ]. Poisoning by cheese or any milk product.

**Tyrrell,** Frederick, English physician, 1797–1843. See T.'s *fascia, hook.*

**Tyson,** Edward, English anatomist, 1649–1708. See T.'s *glands.*

**Tyzze'ria.** A genus of coccidia (family Eimeriidae) in which the oocyst contains eight naked sporozoites.

   **T. anse'ris,** a relatively nonpathogenic species found in the small intestine of domestic and wild geese, whistling swans, and certain wild ducks.

   **T. pernicio'sa,** occurs in the small intestine of the domestic duck in North America and Europe, and is pathogenic in ducklings.

**Tzank,** Arnault, Russian dermatologist, 1886–1954. See T. *cells, test.*

# U

**U.** 1. Chemical symbol of the element uranium. 2. Abbreviation for unit. 3. Symbol for kilurane. 4. Symbol for uridine in polymers. 5. Symbol for urinary *concentration*, followed by subscripts indicating location and chemical species.

**u'berous** [ L. *uber*, fruitful ]. Fertile; prolific.

**u'berty** [ L. *ubertas*; fr. *uber*, fruitful ]. Fertility; fruitfulness.

**ubichromanol-9** **(-Q₉)** (u'bī-kro'mā-nol). Ubichromanol(50); the chroman form of ubiquinol-10 (ubihydroquinone-10), the reduced form of ubiquinone-10; abbreviated H₂Q-9-al.

**ubichromenol-9** **(-Q₉)** (u'bī-kro'me-nol). Ubichromenol(50); the chromene form of ubiquinone-10; abbreviated H₂Q-9-el.

**ubiquinol** (u'bĭ-ˌwi'nol, u-bik'wĭ-nol). Ubihydroquinone; the reduction product of ubiquinone; abbreviated Q-H₂ or H₂Q.

**ubiquinone** (u'bī-kwi'nōn, u-bik'wĭ-nōn). 2,3-Dimethoxy-5-methyl-1,4-benzoquinone with a multiprenyl side chain.

**ubiquinone-6 (-Q₆).** 2,3-Dimethoxy-5-methyl-6-hexaprenyl-1,4-benzoquinone; trivial name is coenzyme Q₆ or ubiquinone-30; abbreviated Q-6 or Q₆.

**ubiquinone-10** **(-Q₁₀).** 2,3-Dimethoxy-5-methyl-6-decaprenyl-1,4-benzoquinone; trivial name is coenzyme Q₁₀ or ubiquinone-50.

**ud'der** [ A.S., *üder* ]. The large complex of mammary glands of the cow and other ungulates.

**UDP.** Abbreviation for uridine diphosphate. See entries under uridine and under UDP.

**UDPG.** Abbreviation for uridine diphosphoglucose.

**UDPGal.** Abbreviation for uridine diphosphogalactose.

**UDPgalactose 4-epimerase.** UDPglucose epimerase.

**UDP-GlcUA.** Abbreviation for uridinediphosphoglucuronic acid.

**UDPglucose epimerase.** Galactowaldenase; UDPgalactose 4-epimerase; an enzyme (EC 5.1.3.2) that catalyzes the Walden inversion of UDPglucose to UDPgalactose.

**Uehlinger,** E. See U.'s *syndrome*, Meyenburg-Altherr-U. *syndrome*.

**Uffelmann** (oo'fel-mahn), Jules, German physician, 1837–1894. See U.'s *reagent.*

**Uhlenhuth** (oo'len-hoot), Paul, Berlin bacteriologist, 1870–1957. See U.'s *method.*

**ukambin** (oo-kam'bin). An African arrow poison from plants of the family Apocynaceae; a heart poison resembling digitalis or strophanthus in its action.

**ulcer** (ul'ser) [ L. *ulcus* (*ulcer-*), a sore, ulcer ]. A lesion on the surface of the skin or a mucous surface, caused by superficial loss of tissue, usually with inflammation. A wound with superficial loss of tissue from trauma is not primarily an u., but may become ulcerated if infection occurs.

**Aden u.,** (1) tropical u. of cutaneous leishmaniasis; (2) desert sore; an u. with a precipitous margin and a grayish base, caused by filth.

**amputating u.,** an u. encircling a limb.

**anastomotic u.,** u. of jejunum, after gastroenterostomy.

**aton'ic u.,** one that shows little or no tendency to heal.

**autoch'thonous u.,** chancre.

**buruli u.,** Searl's u.; an u. of the skin with widespread necrosis of subcutaneous fat, occurring in Uganda in persons living on the Nile river banks; due to mycobacterial infection.

**chiclero's u.,** a form of New World or American cutaneous leishmaniasis found among forest workers in parts of Mexico, Guatemala, and British Honduras. It is a zoonotic disease found in sylvatic rodents and transmitted by the night-biting sandfly, *Phlebotomus flaviscutellatus.* The agent is *Leishmania mexicana* (or *L. tropica* var. *mexicana*) and the disease is usually mild, commonly eroding the pinna of the ear over a long course of infection, which frequently is difficult to cure.

**chrome u.,** tanner's u.; one produced by exposure to chromium compounds.

**chronic u.,** a longstanding u. with fibrous scar tissue in the floor of the u.

**Clarke's u.,** (1) rodent u.; (2) u. of the cervix uteri.

**cockscomb u.,** one that may occur in association with condylomata acuminata.

**cold u.,** a small gangrenous u. on the extremities; due to imperfect circulation.

**constitutional u.,** symptomatic u.; one due to systemic disease, such as tuberculosis.

**corrosive u.,** noma.

**creeping u.,** serpiginous u.

**Curling's u.,** u. of the duodenum in a patient with extensive superficial burns or severe bodily injury.

**cystoscop'ic u.,** an u. of the bladder resulting from a burn of the mucous membrane by the lamp of a cystoscope.

**decu'bitus u.,** a chronic u. that appears in pressure areas in debilitated patients confined to bed; it is due to a circulatory defect in the area under pressure; also called bedsore; pressure sore; decubital, nosocomial, pressure, or hospital gangrene; sloughing phagedena; ulcus hypostaticum.

**decubitus u., acute,** a severe form of bedsore, occurring in hemiplegia, of neurotrophic origin.

**den'driform u.,** a linear u. of the cornea that sends out branches in various directions, occurring in herpetic keratitis.

**dental u.,** an irritable u. on the side of the tongue caused by rubbing against the projecting edge of a broken tooth or a rough coating of tartar.

**diphtheritic u.,** an u. covered with a gray, adherent membrane; caused by *Corynebacterium diphtheriae;* sometimes due to secondary invasion by diphtheria bacilli in yaws and in desert sores.

**distention u.,** an u. of the intestine in the dilated part above a stricture.

**duod'enal u.,** u. of the duodenum, usually a peptic u.

**dyspeptic u.,** recurrent ulcerative *stomatitis.*

**esophageal u.,** peptic u. of the lower end of the esophagus due to the regurgitation of acid gastric juice.

**Gaboon u.** [ *Gaboon*, a region in Africa ], a form of tropical u. affecting the residents of this region; it resembles a syphilitic u., especially in the appearance of its scar.

**gastric u.,** u. of the stomach, most commonly a peptic u. on or near the lesser curvature.

**gravitational u.,** a chronic u. of the leg that is prevented from healing because it is in a dependent position and the valves of the veins are incompetent due to varicosity; the venous return, in consequence, is defective; see also varicose u.

**groin u.,** *granuloma* inguinale tropicum.

**gummatous u.,** lesion of the skin occurring in late syphilis.

**hard u.,** chancre.

**healed u.,** an u. covered by epithelial regeneration, beneath which there may be scarring and absence of glands or appendages.

**Hunner's u.,** interstitial *cystitis* (*q. v.*); ulceration is not often present, and is superficial, but was described in the first reported cases.

**hypopyon u.,** (1) a creeping central suppurative u. of the cornea; see also hypopyon; (2) a corneal u. with pus in the anterior chamber; (3) serpiginous *keratitis.*

**indolent u.,** a chronic u., with hard elevated edges and few or no granulations, and showing no tendency to heal.

**inflamed u.,** one that has a purulent discharge and inflamed borders.

**Jacob's u.,** ulcerated basal cell carcinoma of the face.

**jejunal u.,** u. of the jejunum; see also stomal u.

**Kurunegala u.'s** (koo-roo-na-gah'lah) [ *Kurunegala*, a district in Ceylon ], *pyosis* tropica.

**Lipschütz' u.,** ulcus vulvae acutum; a simple acute ulceration of the vulvae or lower vagina of nonvenereal origin.

**lupoid u.,** an u. resembling that of cutaneous tuberculosis.

**Mann-Williamson u.,** see Mann-Williamson *operation.*

**marginal ring u.** **of the cornea,** a slowly creeping intermittent u. involving gradually the circumference of the corneal margin.

**Marjolin's u.,** warty u.; a malignant, verrucose, ulcerating growth occurring in cicatricial tissue or at the epithelial edge of a chronic benign u.

**Meleney's u.,** a rapidly burrowing u. in Meleney's synergistic *gangrene, q.v.*

**Mooren's u.,** basal cell carcinoma of the cornea.

**Parrott's u.,** u. occasionally seen in superficial moniliasis.

**penetrating u.,** an u. extending into deeper layers beneath the surface of an organ.

**peptic u.,** round u.; an u. of the alimentary mucosa, usually in the stomach or duodenum, exposed to acid gastric secretion.

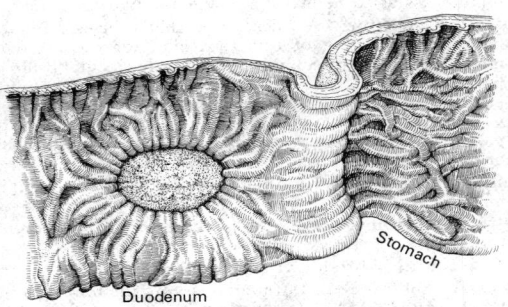

**Peptic Ulcer of the Duodenum**

**perambulating u.,** phagedenic u.

**perforated u.,** an u. extending through the wall of an organ.

**perforating u. of the foot,** malum perforans pedis; mal perforant; a round, deep, trophic u. of the sole of the foot, following disease or injury, in any part of its course from the center to the periphery of the nerve supplying the part.

**phageden'ic u.,** perambulating u.; ulcus ambulans; sloughing u.; a rapidly spreading u. attended by the formation of more or less extensive sloughing.

**phleg'monous u.,** one attended with inflammation of the neighboring tissues.

**Plaut's u.,** Vincent's *disease.*

**pneumococcus u.,** serpiginous *keratitis.*

**ring u.,** nonpyogenic marginal corneal u.

**rodent u.,** a slowly enlarging ulcerated basal cell carcinoma, usually on the face; also called rodent cancer, Krompecher's tumor; ulcus exedens; ulcus rodens; Clarke's u. (1); noli me tangere.

**round u.,** peptic u.

**Saemisch's u.,** a serpiginous u. of the cornea, frequently accompanied by hypopyon.

**Searl's u.,** buruli u.

**serpent u. of the cornea,** serpiginous *keratitis.*

**serpig'inous u.,** a creeping u.; an u. extending on one side while healing at the opposite edge.

**simple u.,** a local, not constitutional, u. attended with no marked pain or inflammation.

**sloughing u.,** phagedenic u.

**soft u.,** chancroid.

**stasis u.,** varicose u.

**ster'coral u.,** an u. of the colon due to pressure and irritation of retained fecal masses.

**stomal u.,** an intestinal u. occurring after gastrojejunostomy in the jejunal mucosa near the opening (stoma) between the stomach and the jejunum.

**stress u.'s,** acute peptic u.'s occurring in association with other conditions, including burns, cor pulmonale, intracranial lesions, and after surgery. The pathogenesis is unknown. Stress may be accompanied by increased secretion of corticosteroids; vasoactive substances affecting gastric mucosal vessels, or hypothalamic stimulation of gastric secretion.

**Sutton's u.,** a solitary, deep, painful u. of the buccal or genital mucous membrane.

**symptomat'ic u.,** a constitutional u.

**syphilitic u.,** chancre or other ulceration caused by syphilitic infection.

**Syr'iac u.,** diphtheria.

**tanner's u.,** chrome u.

**transparent u. of the cornea,** an u. of the cornea, occurring usually in children, that heals without opacity.

**trophic u.,** one due to impaired nutrition of the part.

**tropical u.,** (1) the tropical sore (dermal lesion) of Old World cutaneous leishmaniasis; (2) tropical phagedenic ulceration cuased by a variety of microorganisms, including mycobacteria; common in northern Nigeria.

**undermining u.,** a chronic cutaneous u. with overhanging margins; due to hemolytic streptococci or other bacteria.

**var'icose u.,** stasis u.; the loss of skin surface in the drainage area of a varicose vein, usually in the leg, resulting from stasis and infection.

**venereal u.,** chancroid.

**warty u.,** Marjolin's u.

**Zambesi u.,** an u., usually single, about the size of a half-dollar, seated on the foot or leg, occurring in laborers in the Zambesi Delta; it has a sloughing surface, but does not spread and produces no constitutional symptoms or glandular enlargement; it is associated with the presence of a spirillum and a large fusiform bacillus; one attack seems to confer a partial immunity.

**ul'cera.** Plural of ulcus.

**ulcerate** (ul'ser-āt). To form an ulcer.

**ulcerated** (ul'ser-a'ted). Having undergone ulceration.

**ulceration** (ul'ser-a'shun). 1. The formation of an ulcer. 2. An ulcer or aggregation of ulcers.

**lip and leg u.,** an infectious disease of sheep in which u. occurs between and around the base of the hooves and on the lips, the latter apparently being the result of biting the foot lesions; it is believed to be caused by *Actinomyces nodosus* working in association with *Spirochaeta penortha.*

**tracheal u.,** erosion of the tracheal mucous membrane with, in some cases, exposure of the rings, at the site at which a cuffed tracheostomy tube has been present for some time.

**ul'cera'tive.** Relating to, causing, or marked by an ulcer or ulcers.

**ulcerogenic** (ul'ser-o-jen'ik). Ulcer-producing.

**ul'ceroglan'dular.** Denoting a local ulceration at a site of infection followed by regional or generalized lymphadenopathy; the most common form of tularemia.

**ul'ceromem'branous.** Relating to or characterized by ulceration and the formation of a false membrane.

**ulcerous** (ul'ser-us) [ L. *ulcerosus,* fr. foll. ]. Relating to, affected with, or containing an ulcer.

**ulcus,** pl. **ulcera** (ul'kus, ul'ser-ah) [ L. ]. Ulcer.

**u. ambulans,** phagedenic *ulcer.*

**u. cancro'sum,** an obsolete term for (1) rodent *ulcer,* (2) chancre; (3) chancroid.

**u. cystoscop'icum,** cystoscopic *ulcer.*

**u. durum,** an obsolete term for chancre.

**u. ex'edens,** rodent *ulcer.*

**u. hypostat'icum,** decubitus *ulcer.*

**u. indura'tum,** an obsolete term for chancre.

**u. molle,** an obsolete term for chancroid.

**u. rodens,** rodent *ulcer.*

**u. serpens corneae,** serpiginous *keratitis.*

**u. terebrans,** a deeply invasive, ulcerating, basal cell carcinoma, usually around the eye, nose, or ear and extending to underlying bony tissue.

**u. vene'reum** (1) chancre; (2) chancroid.

**u. vulvae acu'tum,** Lipschütz' *ulcer.*

**ule-.** See ulo-.

**ulectomy** (u-lek'to-mī) [ G. *oulē,* scar, + *ektomē,* excision ]. Excision of cicatricial tissue.

**ulegyria** (u'le-ji'rī-ah) [ G. *oulē,* scar, + *gyros,* ring ]. A defect of the cerebral cortex characterized by narrow and distorted gyri. The condition may be congenital or the result of scars.

**ulerythema** (u'lĕr'ī-the'mah) [ G. *oulē,* scar, + *erythēma,* redness of the skin ]. Scarring with erythema.

**u. centrifugum,** *lupus* erythematosus.

**u. ophryog'enes,** folliculitis of the eyebrows resulting in scarring and alopecia.

**u. sycosifor'me,** lupoid *sycosis.*

**uletic** (u-let'ik) [ G. *oulē,* a scar ]. Relating to a scar; scarred; cicatricial.

**uletomy** (u-let'o-mĭ) [ G. *oulē,* scar, + *tomē,* incision ]. Cicatricotomy; incision of a cicatrix in order to relieve tension.

**U'lex europae'us.** Furze; gorse; a spiny shrub of the family Leguminosae; the seeds contain ulexine.

**ulexine** (u-lek'sēn). Cytisine; sophorine; baptitoxine; 1,2,3,4,5,6- hexahydro-1,5- methano-8*H*-pyrido [ 1,2-α ]-[ 1,5 ]diazocin-8-one; $C_{11}H_{14}N_2O$; an alkaloid present in the seeds of gorse (*Ulex europaeus*), laburnum, and other leguminous plants; formerly used as an antitussive and antiemetic.

**Ullmann's line.** See under line.

**Ullrich,** Otto, German physician, 1894–1957. See Morquio-U. *disease,* Bonnevie-U. *syndrome.*

**ulna,** gen. and pl. **ulnae** (ul'nah, ul'ne) [ L. elbow, arm, fr. G. *ōlenē* ] [ NA ]. Elbow bone; the medial and larger of the two bones of the forearm.

**ul'nad** [ ulna + L. *ad,* to ]. In a direction toward the ulna.

**ul'nar.** Relating to the ulna, or to any of the structures (artery, nerve, etc.) named from it.

**ulna'ris** [ Mod. L ] [ NA ]. Ulnar; relating to the ulna or to the ulnar or medial aspect of the upper limb.

**ul'nen** [ ulna + G. *en,* in ]. Relating to the ulna independent of other structures.

**ul'nocar'pal.** Relating to the ulna and the carpus, or to the ulnar side of the wrist.

**ul'nora'dial.** Relating to both ulna and radius; denoting the two articulations, ligaments, etc.

**ulo-, ule-** (u'lo-). 1 [ G. *oulē,* scar. UL-1 ]. Combining forms denoting scar or scarring. 2 [ G. *oulon,* gums. UL-2 ]. Combining forms (obsolete or rarely used) relating to the gums (gingivae).

**ulocarcinoma** (u'lo-kar'sĭ-no'mah) [ G. *oulon,* gum, + carcinoma ]. Carcinoma of the gums.

**ulodermatitis** (u-lo-der-mă-ti'tis) [ G. *oulē,* scar, + *derma,* skin, + suffix *-itis,* inflammation ]. Inflammation of the skin resulting in destruction of tissue and the formation of cicatrices.

**uloglossitis** (u'lo-glos-i'tis). Gingivoglossitis.

**u'loid** [ G. *oulē,* scar + *eidos,* resemblance ]. 1. Resembling a scar. 2. Uloid cicatrix; a scarlike lesion due to a degenerative process in deeper layers of skin.

**uloncus** (u-long'kus) [ G. *oulon,* gum, + *onkos,* mass (tumor) ]. Any tumor of the gums.

**ulosis** (u-lo'sis) [ G. *oulē,* scar, + suffix *-osis,* condition ]. Cicatrization.

**ulotic** (u-lot'ik) [ G. *oulē,* scar ]. Cicatricial.

**ulotomy** (u-lot'o-mĭ) [ G. *oulē,* scar, + *tomē,* incision ]. Section of contracting scar tissue to relieve deformity.

**ulotrichous** (u-lot'rĭ-kus) [ G. *oulotrichos,* curly haired, fr. *oulos,* wooly, + *thrix* (*trich-*), hair ]. Having short, curly hair, like the Negro; opposite of leiotrichous.

**ul'tex.** A one-piece bifocal or trifocal lens.

**ultimobranchial** (ul'tĭ-mo-brang'kĭ-al) [ L. *ultimus,* last, + G. *branchia,* gills ]. In embryology, relating to the caudal pharyngeal pouch.

**ultimogeniture** (ul'tĭ-mo-jen'ĭ-tūr, -chūr) [ L. *ultimus,* last, + *genitura,* birth, generation ]. Pertaining to the last born; also, reproductive exhaustion.

**ul'timum mo'riens** [ L. the last thing dying ]. 1. The upper portion of the trapezius, which often escapes involvement in progressive muscular atrophy. 2. The right atrium of the heart, said to contract after the rest of the heart is still.

**ultra-** (ul'trah-) [ L. beyond ]. A prefix denoting excess or exaggeration or beyond.

**ultrabrachycephalic** (ul-trah-brak-ĭ-sĕ-fal'ik). Denoting an extremely short skull, one with an index of at least 90.

**ultracen'trifuge.** A high speed centrifuge (up to ±100,000 rpm) by means of which large molecules, *e.g.,* of protein or nucleic acids are caused to sediment at practicable rates. Used for determinations of molecular weights, separation of large molecules, criteria of homogeneity of large molecules, etc.

**ultracy'tostome** [ ultra- + G. *kytos,* cell, + *stoma,* mouth ]. Former name for micropore.

**ultradolichocephalic** (ul-trah-dol-ĭ-ko-sĕ-fal'ik). Denoting a very long skull, one with a cephalic index of less than 65.

**ultrafil'ter.** A semipermeable membrane (collodion, fish bladder, or filter paper impregnated with gels) used as a filter to separate colloids and large molecules from water and small molecules, which pass through.

**ultrafiltration** (ul'trah-fil-tra'shun). Filtration through a semipermeable membrane or any filter that separates colloid solutions from crystalloids or separates particles of different size in a colloid mixture.

**ultraliga'tion.** Ligation of a blood vessel beyond the point where a branch is given off.

**ultrami'crobe.** A virus; a microorganism of such extreme minuteness as to be invisible under the light microscope.

**ultrami'croscope.** A microscope that utilizes refracted light for visualizing objects too small for the ordinary microscope when direct light is used. A horizontal beam of light passes through a slit in a shield to strike the minute particles of a solution contained in a small compartment with transparent side and top. The light thus striking the particles from the side is refracted and forms a bright point or ring.

**ultramicroscop'ic.** Too small to be visible under the light microscope.

**ultrami'crotome.** A microtome used in cutting sections 0.1 μ thick, or less, for electron microscopy.

**ultraquinine** (ul-trah-kwĭ-nēn'). Cupreine.

**ultrared** (ul'trah-red). Infrared; denoting the heat rays beyond the red end of the spectrum.

**ultrasonic** (ul'trah-son'ik) [ ultra- + L. *sonus,* sound ]. Relating to energy waves similar to those of sound but of higher frequencies (above 30,000 cycles per second). When they strike tissue with a different acoustical resistance, the waves are reflected and their energy is converted to heat; they may be used diagnostically, as in echoencephalography, or therapeutically, in treating joint disease, mainly for the purpose of producing local heat. In addition, by focusing them on particular areas of the brain by stereotactic instruments, these waves may selectively destroy these areas without injuring intervening tissue.

**ultrason'ogram.** The record obtained from ultrasonography.

**ultrasonography** (ul'trah-sŏ-nog'rā-fĭ) [ ultra- + L. *sonus,* sound, + G. *graphō,* to write ]. The location, measurement, or delineation of deep structures by measuring the reflection or transmission of ultrasonic waves.

**ultrasonosurgery** (ul'trah-son'o-sur'jer-ĭ). The use of ultrasound techniques to disrupt cells, tissues, or tracts, particularly in the central nervous system.

**ul'trasound.** Ultrasonic vibrations; see ultrasonic.

**ultrastruc'ture.** Fine structure; structures or particles seen with the ultramicroscope or the electron microscope.

**ultratherm** (ul'trah-therm) [ ultra- + G. *thermē,* heat ]. A short-wave diathermy machine.

**ultravi'olet.** Denoting the actinic or chemical rays beyond the violet end of the visible spectrum.

    **extravital u.** having wavelengths of 2900 to 1850 Å.

    **intravital u.,** having wavelengths of 3900 to 3200 Å.

    **vital u.,** rays necessary or helpful to normal growth, promoting calcium metabolism, and antirachitic in action, having wavelengths between 3200 and 2900 Å.

**ultravirus** (ul'trah-vi'rus). See under virus.

**ultromotiv'ity** [ L. *ultro,* beyond, on one's own part + L. *motio,* movement ]. Power of spontaneous movement.

**ululation** (u-lu-la'shun) [ L. *ululo,* pp. *-atus,* to howl ]. The inarticulate crying of emotionally disturbed persons.

**umbel'latine.** Berberine.

**umbel'lic acid.** Anisic acid.

**Umbelliferae** (um'bĕ-lif'er-e) [ L. *umbella,* a sunshade, dim. of *umbra,* shade, + *fero,* to bear ]. A family of plants to which the parsley, carrot, and parsnip belong; they bear white or yellow flowers in umbels.

**umbellif'erone.** 7-Hydroxycoumarin; skimmetin; hydrangin; $C_9H_6O_3$; the aglucon of skimmin, obtained from gum resins of many plants of the family Umbelliferae; used in sunscreen preparations.

**umbellif'erous** [ see *Umbelliferae* ]. Relating to umbel-bearing plants.

**umbilical** (um-bil'ĭ-kal). Relating to the umbilicus.

**umbil'icate, umbil'icated** [ L. *umbilicatus* ]. Of navel shape; pitlike; dimpled.

**umbil'ica'tion.** 1. A pit or navel-like depression. 2. The formation of a depression at the apex of a papule, vesicle, or pustule.

**umbilicus,** pl. **umbilici** (um-bil'ĭ-kus, um-bī-li'kus, -si, -ki) [ L. navel ] [ NA ]. Omphalos [ NA ]; omphalus; navel; belly-button; the pit in the center of the abdominal wall marking the point where the umbilical cord entered in the fetus.

**um'bo,** gen. **umbo'nis,** pl. **umbo'nes** [ L. boss of a shield, a knob ] [ NA ]. A projecting point of a surface.

  **u. membra'nae tym'pani** [ NA ], the projection on the inner surface of the tympanic membrane at the end of the manubrium of the malleus; this corresponds to the most depressed point of the membrane, viewed laterally, that is commonly called the umbo.

**UMP.** Abbreviation for uridine monophosphate (uridylic acid).

**uncal** (ung'kal). Denoting or relating to the uncus.

**uncia** (un'sĭ-ah) [ L. a twelfth part, an ounce ]. An ounce.

**unciform** (un'sĭ-form) [ L. *uncus*, hook, + *forma*, form ]. Uncinate.

**unciforme** (un-si-for'me) [ Mod. L. unciform ]. *Os* hamatum.

**Uncinaria** (un'sĭ-nār'ĭ-ah) [ LL. *uncinus*, a hook ]. A genus of Nematoda, formerly including the genera *Ancylostoma and Necator*, but now confined to worms (such as *U. stenocephala*) that infest various other mammals.

  **U. america'na,** *Necator americanus.*

  **U. duodena'lis,** *Ancylostoma duodenale.*

  **U. stenocephala,** the European hookworm of dogs, cats, and various wild carnivores; also found in North America, where it is much less common than *Ancylostoma caninum.*

**uncinariasis** (un-sĭ-nă-ri'ă-sis). Ancylostomiasis.

**uncinate** (un'sĭ-nāt) [ L. *uncinatus* ]. Unciform; hookline or hook-shaped.

**uncina'tum.** *Os* hamatum.

**un'cipressure** [ L. *uncus*, hook ]. Arrest of hemorrhage from a cut artery by pressure with a blunt hook.

**uncom'plemented.** Not united with complement and therefore inactive.

**unconscious** (un-kon'shus). 1. Not conscious; insensible. 2. In psychoanalysis, the psychic structure comprising the drives and feelings of which one is unaware.

  **collective u.,** in Jungian psychology, the combined engrams or memory potentials inherited from an individual's phylogenetic past.

**unconsciousness** (un-kon'shus-ness). An imprecise term used to describe impaired consciousness; see also consciousness.

**unco-ossified** (un-ko-os'ĭ-fīd). Not co-ossified; not united into one bone.

**uncouplers** (un-kup'lerz). Substances such as dinitrophenol that allow oxidation in mitochondria to proceed without the usual concomitant phosphorylation to produce ATP; these poisons thus "uncouple" oxidation and phosphorylation.

**unction** (ungk'shun) [ L. *unctio*, fr. *ungo*, pp. *unctus*, to anoint ]. The action of anointing or rubbing with an ointment or oil.

**unctuous** (ungk'shu-us, -chu-us) [ L. *unctuosus*, fr. *unctio*, unction ]. Greasy; oily.

**unc'ture.** Ointment; unguent.

**uncus,** pl. **unci** [ L. a hook. G. *onkos.* ONC-2 ]. 1 [ NA ]. Any hook-shaped process or structure. 2 [ NA ]. Uncinate gyrus; u. gyri parahippocampalis; the anterior, hooked extremity of the parahippocampal gyrus on the basomedial surface of the temporal lobe; the anterior face of the u. corresponds to the olfactory cortex, its ventral surface to the entorhinal area; in its depth lies the amygdala (corpus amygdaloideum).

  **u. gy'ri parahippocampa'lis,** u. (2).

**undecoylium chloride** (un-dĕ-ko-il'ĭ-um). Acyl-colaminoformylmethylpyridinium chloride; a topical antiseptic.

**undecoylium chloride-iodine.** VIRAC; a complex of iodine with undecoylium chloride; a cationic detergent used topically as a germicidal agent.

**undecylenate** (un-des'ĭ-lĭ-nāt). A salt of undecylenic acid.

**undecylenic acid** (un-des'ĭ-len'ik). (USP). Undecenoic acid (BP); $CH_2CH(CH_2)_8COOH$; an acid present in small amounts in sweat; used with its zinc salt in ointments, or as a powder in the treatment of fungus diseases of the skin, psoriasis, and certain other cutaneous affections.

**underachieve'ment.** The failure to achieve as well as one's abilities would seem to allow.

**underachiev'er.** A person who manifests underachievement.

**un'dercut.** 1. That portion of a tooth that lies between the survey line (height of contour) and the gingivae. 2. The contour of a cross-section of a residual ridge or dental arch which would prevent the insertion of a denture. 3. The contour of a flasking stone which interlocks in such a way as to prevent the separation of the parts.

**un'derhorn.** *Cornu* inferius.

**undernutri'tion.** A form of malnutrition resulting from a reduced supply of food or from inability to digest, assimilate, and utilize the necessary elements.

**un'dertoe.** A displacement of the great toe beneath the second toe.

**underventila'tion.** Hypoventilation.

**Underwood,** Michael, London pediatrician, 1737–1820. See U.'s *disease.*

**undescen'ded.** Not descended; denoting a testis that is retained within the abdomen.

**undifferentiated** (un-dif'er-en'shĭ-a-ted). Not differentiated; *e.g.*, primitive, embryonic, or immature.

**undine** (un'dēn, -dīn) [ Mod. L. *undina*, fr. L. *unda*, wave ]. A small glass flask used in irrigation of the conjunctiva.

**undinism** (un'dī-nizm) [ Mod. L. *undina*, fr. L. *unda*, wave ]. A condition in which sexual thoughts are aroused by water, urine, and urination.

**undo'ing.** In psychology and psychiatry, an unconscious defense mechanism by which one symbolically acts out in reverse some earlier unacceptable behavior.

**undulate** (un'du-lāt) [ Mod. L. *undula*, dim. of *unda*, wave ]. Having an irregular, wavy border; denoting the shape of a bacterial colony.

**ung.** Abbreviation of L. *unguentum,* ointment.

**ungual** (ung'gwal) [ L. *unguis*, nail ]. Unguinal; relating to a nail or the nails.

**unguent** (ung'gwent) [ L. *unguentum* ]. Ointment.

**Unguiculata** (ung-gwik'u-la'tah) [ L. *unguiculus*, nail or claw ]. A division of Mammalia including all mammals having nails or claws, as distinguished from the Ungulata.

**unguiculate** (ung-gwik'u-lāt). Having nails or claws, as distinguished from hooves.

**unguiculus** (un-gwik'u-lus) [ L. dim. of *unguis*, nail ]. A small nail or claw.

**unguinal** (ung'gwĭ-nal). Ungual.

**unguis,** pl. **ungues** (ung'gwis, -gwēz) [ L. ] [ NA ]. Onyx (1); nail (of finger or toe); one of the thin, horny, translucent plates covering the dorsal surface of the distal end of each terminal phalanx of fingers and toes. A nail consists of corpus or body, the visible part, and radix or root at the proximal end concealed under a fold of skin. The under part of the nail is formed from the stratum germinativum of the epidermis, the free surface from the stratum lucidum, the thin cuticular fold overlapping the lunula representing the stratum corneum. See fig. on p. 1510.

  **u. adun'cus,** ingrown *nail.*

  **u. a'vis,** *calcar* avis.

  **Haller's u.,** *calcar* avis.

  **u. incarna'tus,** ingrown *nail.*

**ungula,** pl. **ungulae** (ung'gu-lah, -le) [ L. a claw, hoof, fr. *unguis*, nail ]. 1. Hoof of the horse, ox, etc. 2. An instrument used for the extraction of a dead fetus from the uterus.

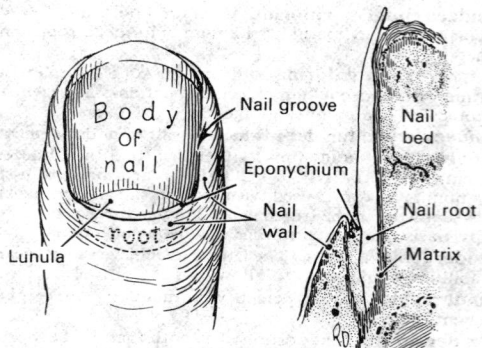

**Fingernail**

**Ungulata** (ung′gu-la′tah) A division of Mammalia containing the mammals with hooves, as distinguished from the Unguiculata.

**ungulate** (ung′gu-lāt) [ L. *ungulatus*, fr. *ungula*, hoof ]. Having hooves.

**unguligrade** (ung′gu-lĭ-grād) [ L. *ungula*, a hoof, + *gradus*, a step ]. Walking on hooves, as by horses, pigs, and ruminants.

**uni-** (u′nĭ-) [ L. *unus*, one ]. A prefix denoting one, single, not paired; equivalent to the Greek prefix *mono-*.

**uniartic′ular.** Monarticular.

**uniax′ial.** Having but one axis; growing chiefly in one direction.

**uniba′sal.** Having but one base.

**unicam′eral, unicam′erate.** Monolocular; consisting of a single cavity or chamber.

**unicel′lular.** Composed of but one cell, as the protozoons.

**unicen′tral.** Having a single center, as of growth or of ossification.

**unicep′tor** [ uni- + L. *capio*, to take ]. A supposed receptor that has only a haptophore group or a haptophore and a zymophore group, but no complementophil group.

**u′nicorn** (u′nĭ-korn). Unicornous.

**unicornous** (u′nĭ-kor′nus) [ L. *unicornis*, fr. uni- + *cornu*, horn ]. Having but one horn, or cornu.

**unicorn root.** Aletris.

**unicus′pid.** Provided with but one cusp, as a canine tooth.

**unicus′pidate.** Unicuspid.

**unifamil′ial.** Relating to or occurring in a single family; denoting especially a nervous disease attacking several of the children in the same family in which no hereditary taint is apparent.

**uniflagellate** (u-nĭ-flaj′ĕ-lāt). Monotrichous.

**unifo′rate.** Having but one foramen, pore, or opening of any kind.

**uniform** (u′nĭ-form) [ L. *uniformis*, fr. uni- + *forma*, form ]. 1. Having but one form; not variable in form. 2. Of the same form or shape as another structure or object.

**uniger′minal.** Relating to a single germ or ovum.

**uniglan′dular.** Involving, relating to, or containing but one gland.

**unigravida** (u′nĭ-grav′ĭ-dah). Primigravida.

**unilam′inar, unilam′inate.** Having but one layer or lamina.

**unilat′eral.** Confined to one side only.

**unilo′bar.** Having but one lobe.

**uniloc′ular** [ uni- + L. *loculus*, compartment ]. Having but one compartment.

**unimolec′ular.** Monomolecular.

**uninephrec′tomized.** Nephrectomized on one side. Incorrect neologism for mononephrectomized or seminephrectomized.

**uninephrec′tomy.** Removal of one kidney.

**uninu′clear, uninu′cleate.** Having but one nucleus.

**uniocular** (u-nĭ-ok′u-lar). 1. Relating to one eye only. 2. Having but one eye; one-eyed.

**union** (u′nyun) [ L. *unus*, one ]. 1. The joining or amalgamation of two or more bodies. 2. The structural adhesion or growing together of the edges of a wound.

**autogenous u.,** in dentistry, the u. of two pieces of metal without solder.

**faulty u.,** u. of fracture by fibrous tissue, without bone formation.

**fibrous u.,** a persisting fibrous callus forming between fractured bone.

**primary u.,** see healing or union of first intention, under intention.

**vicious u.,** u. of the ends of a broken bone in such a way as to cause a deformity, or a crooked limb; frequently used interchangeably with faulty u.

**unioval, uniovular** (u-nĭ-o′val, -ov′u-lar). Relating to or formed from a single ovum.

**unipara** (u-nip′ā-rah). Primipara.

**uniparous** (u-nip′ā-rus). Primiparous.

**unipen′nate** [ uni- + L. *penna*, feather ]. Having a feather arrangement on one side; resembling one-half of a feather.

**unipo′lar.** 1. Having but one pole; denoting a nerve cell from which the branches project from one side only. 2. Situated at one extremity only of a cell.

**unisep′tate.** Having but one septum or partition.

---

# UNIT

---

**u′nit** [ L. *unus*, one ]. 1. One; a single person or thing. 2. A standard of measure, weight, or any other quality, by multiplications or fractions of which a scale or system is formed. 3. A group of persons or things considered as a whole because of mutual activities or functions.

**absolute u.,** a u. whose value is constant regardless of place or time.

**absolute system of u.'s,** a system based on absolute u.'s accepted as being fundamental (length, mass, and time) and from which other u.'s (force, energy or work, and power) are derived; absolute systems of u.'s in common use are foot-pound-second (fps) system, the centimeter-gram-second (cgs) system, and the meter-kilogram-second (mks) system.

**alexin u.,** complement u.

**Allen-Doisy u.,** mouse u. (m.u.); the quantity of estrogen capable of producing in a spayed mouse a characteristic change in the vaginal epithelium, namely, disappearance of leukocytes and appearance of cornified cells, as determined by a vaginal smear. Equal approximately to one-half of an estrone u.

**alpha u.'s,** cytoplasmic glycogen granules arranged in rosettes.

**ambocep′tor u.,** hemolysin u.

**an′drogen u. (international),** the androgenic activity of 100 μg. (0.1 mg.) of crystalline androsterone as assayed by the comb growth response in capons.

**Ångström u.,** u. of wavelength; $10^{-10}$ meter; in the SI system, 0.1 nanometer (nm); abbreviated Å (sometimes A).

**an′tigen u.,** the smallest amount of antigen that, in the presence of specific antiserum, will fix 1 complement u.

**antitoxin u.,** antitoxin u.'s are defined with reference to a standard preparation of antitoxin preserved in the dried state, the former practice of definition in terms of standard toxin having been abandoned because of instability of toxin (*i.e.*, filtrate of a bacterial culture).

**antiven′ene u.,** the amount of antivenene which, injected in the ear vein, will protect 1 gram weight of rabbit against a fatal dose of snake venom.

**base u.'s,** the fundamental u.'s of length, mass, time, electric current, thermodynamic temperature, amount of substance, and luminous intensity in the International System of Units (SI). The names and symbols of the u.'s for these quantities are meter (m), kilogram (kg), second (s), ampere (A), kelvin (K), mole (mol), and candela (cd). See also International System of Units.

**bird u.,** a unit of prolactin activity, being the minimal quantity of the hormone which will cause a certain increase in weight of the crop gland of pigeons.

**Bodansky u.,** that amount of phosphatase that liberates 1 mg. of phosphorus as inorganic phosphate during the first hour of incubation with a buffered substrate containing sodium β-glycerophosphate.

**British thermal u.,** BTU; the quantity of heat required to raise one pound of water from 39°F. to 40°F; equal to 252 calories (*q. v.*).

**cat u.,** the dose of a drug (per kilogram of body weight of cat) which is just large enough to kill a cat when administered intravenously.

**CGS** or **cgs u.,** a system of absolute u.'s based on the centimeter, gram, and second; see also centimeter-gram-second *system.*

**chlorophyll u.,** the number of chlorophyll molecules required to reduce one molecule of carbon dioxide by photosynthesis.

**chorion′ic gonadotro′pin u. (international),** the specific gonadotropic activity of 0.1 mg. of the standard preparation of chorionic gonadotropin originating from the urine or placenta of pregnant women.

**Clauberg u.,** see Clauberg *test.*

**complement u.,** alexin u.; the smallest amount (highest dilution) of complement that will cause solution of the u. quantity of red blood cells in the presence of a hemolysin u.

**u. of convergence,** meter *angle.*

**Corner and Allen u.,** rabbit u. of progestational activity is the minimum dose which, divided into five equal daily portions, produces on the sixth day the uterine changes characteristic of the eighth day of normal pregnancy. The u. has about the same potency as the international u.

**coronary care u.,** a group of beds within a hospital set aside for the care of patients having or suspected of having myocardial infarction.

**corpus luteum hormone u.,** progesterone u.

**Dam u.,** a u. of activity of vitamin K; it is the smallest amount of vitamin K, per gm. of chick per day, capable of producing normal coagulability in the blood of K-avitaminotic chicks after 3 days of oral administration.

**digita′lis u. (international),** the activity of 0.1 gm. of the international standard powdered digitalis.

**diphtheria antitox′in u.,** Ehrlich's original diphtheria antitoxin u. was defined as the smallest amount of antitoxin that will neutralize 100 MLD of toxin, but was found to be unreliable because of the instability of toxin; see antitoxin u.

**dog u.,** the amount of adrenal cortical extract per kilogram of body weight which, given daily, will maintain an adrenalectomized dog in good condition for 7 to 10 days.

**electromagnetic u.'s,** emu; an absolute system (cgs) of u.'s dealing with the magnetic effects of current; see abampere, abfarad, abhenry, abohm, and abvolt.

**electrostatic u.** (esu), an absolute system (cgs) of u.'s dealing with static electricity; see statampere, statcoulomb, statfarad, stathenry, and statvolt.

**u.'s of energy or work,** (1) cgs u.'s: the erg and joule; (2) mks u.: the newton-meter; (3) fps u.: the foot-poundal; (4) gravitational u.'s: the gram-centimeter, gram-meter, kilogram-meter, and foot-pound.

**equine gonadotro′pin u. (international),** the specific gonadotropic activity of 0.25 mg. of standard preparation of the gonadotropic principle of pregnant mares' serum.

**estradi′ol ben′zoate u. (international),** the estrogenic activity of 0.1 μg. of a standard preparation of estradiol benzoate.

**estrone u. (international),** the estrogenic activity of 0.1 μg. (0.0001 mg.) of a standard preparation of crystalline estrone.

**Florey u.,** Oxford u.

**u. of force,** (1) cgs u.: the dyne; (2) fps u.: the poundal; (3) mks u.: the newton.

**fps u.'s,** a system of absolute u.'s based on the foot, pound, and second.

**G u. of streptomycin,** see streptomycin u.'s.

**gravitational u.,** abbreviated G.; gravitational units of energy are the gram-centimeter, gram-meter, kilogram-meter, and foot-pound.

**Hampson u.,** a u. of x-ray measurement, equal to ¼ erythema dose.

**u. of heat,** (1) calorie (gram calorie; kilocalorie); (2) British thermal u.; (3) joule.

**hemol′ysin u.,** hemolytic u.; amboceptor u.; the smallest quantity (highest dilution) of inactivated immune serum (hemolysin) that will sensitize the standard suspension of erythrocytes so that the standard complement will cause complete hemolysis.

**hemolyt′ic u.,** hemolysin u.

**heparin u.,** Howell u.; the quantity of heparin required to keep 1 ml. of cat's blood fluid for 24 hours at 0°C.; it is equivalent approximately to 0.002 mg. of pure heparin.

**Holzknecht u.,** a u. of x-ray dosage equal to one-fifth of the erythema dose

**Howell u.,** heparin u.

**insulin u. (international),** the activity contained in 1/22 mg. of the international standard of zinc-insulin crystals.

**intensive care u.,** a hospital facility with special equipment and personnel for the management of critically ill patients; abbreviated ICU.

**u. of interme′din,** based upon the action of the hormone in causing the expansion of the melanophores in a hypophysectomized frog; a u. equals 1 μg. of alkali-treated USP Posterior-pituitary Reference Standard.

**international u.,** abbreviated IU; a u. accepted by an international body such as a congress or unit of the United Nations.

**International System of Units (SI),** see under International.

**Jenner-Kay u.,** that amount of the enzyme, phosphatase, that liberates 1 mg. of phosphorus. One such u. equals approximately 2 Bodansky u.'s or 1 King u.

**Kienböck's u.,** a u. of x-ray dosage equivalent to 1/10 the erythema dose.

**King u.,** the quantity of phosphatase that, acting upon disodium phenylphosphate in excess, at pH 9 for 30 minutes, liberates 1 mg. of phenol.

**King-Armstrong u.,** see King u.

**L u. of streptomycin,** see streptomycin u.'s.

**u. of length,** in the metric system and SI, the meter; in the cgs system, centimeter; in the English system it is variable; the inch for short distances, the foot for moderate distances and for elevation, and the mile for long distances.

**light u.'s,** see candela (candle); footcandle; lumen; lux (meter-candle or candle-meter).

**u. of luminous intensity,** candela.

**lung u.,** (1) a respiratory bronchiole together with the alveolar ducts and sacs and pulmonary alveoli into which the respiratory bronchiole leads; (2) considered by some to include the terminal bronchiole and its subdivisions.

**u. of luteinizing activity (international),** progesterone u.

**Mache u.,** abbreviated M.u. (in German writings, M.E.); a u. of measure of radium emanation; one thousand Mache u.'s denote the amount of emanation in equilibrium with 1/2000 mg. of radium; 1 microcurie equals 2670 Mache u.'s.

**u.'s of magnetic field intensity,** see gauss; oersted.

**mks u.'s,** SI units (meter, kilogram, and second); see base u.'s.

**motor u.,** a single somatic motor neuron and the group of muscle fibers innervated by it.

**mouse u.,** Allen-Doisy u.

**nicotinic acid u.,** expressed in milligrams.

**nicotinic acid amide u.,** nicotinamide u., expressed in milligrams of the pure substance.

**Oxford u.,** Florey u.; the minimum amount of penicillin which will prevent the growth of *Staphylococcus aureus* over an area 26 mm. in diameter in a standard culture medium; 1 u. equals 0.6 μg. of crystalline sodium salt of penicillin.

**u. of oxyto′cin,** the oxytocic activity of 0.5 mg. of the USP Posterior-pituitary Reference Standard; 1 mg. of synthetic oxytocin corresponds to 500 International u.'s.

**pantothen′ic acid u.,** filtrate factor u., measured in milligrams of the synthetic substance.

**parathyroid u.,** each u. represents one one-hundredth of the amount required to raise the calcium content of 100 ml. of the blood serum of normal dogs 1 mg. within 16 to 18 hours after administration.

**u. of penicillin** (USP), the penicillin activity of 0.6 μg. of the Food and Drug Administration master standard; it is approximately equivalent to the original Oxford u.

**u. of penicillin (international),** the penicillin activity of 0.6 μg. of penicillin G.

**pepsin u.,** a measure of the pepsin content of the gastric juice; 100 u.'s in 1 ml. of a 1 per cent dilution of the gastric contents obtained after an Ewald test breakfast when added to 2 ml. of a 1 per cent solution of ricin will cause the latter to become clear.

**phosphatase u.,** see Bodansky u., Jenner-Kay u., King u.

**physiologic u.,** (1) the ultimate (hypothetical) vital u. of protoplasm, as conceived by Spencer; (2) the smallest division of an organ that will perform its function, e.g., the renal nephron.

**practical u.'s,** u.'s of magnitudes convenient for use in the practical applications of electricity; as originally defined they were absolute u.'s (multiples of cgs electromagnetic u.'s); they include the ampere, coulomb, farad, henry, joule, ohm, volt, and watt.

**u. of progestational activity (international),** progesterone u.

**proges'terone u. (international),** corpus luteum hormone u.; u. of luteinizing activity (international); the progestational activity of 1 mg. of u. of progestational activity (international); standard preparation of pure progesterone; see also Clauberg test and Corner and Allen u.

**prolac'tin u. (international),** the specific lactogenic activity contained in 0.1 mg. of the standard preparation of the lactogenic substance of the anterior pituitary gland.

**u. of radioactivity,** see Curie; roentgen; Mache u.; uranium u.

**riobofla'vin u.,** vitamin $B_2$ u.; potency usually expressed in terms of weight of pure riboflavin.

**roentgen u.,** roentgen.

**S u. of streptomycin,** see streptomycin u.'s.

**Sherman u.,** u. of vitamin C; minimum protective dose; the minimum amount of vitamin C which fed daily will protect a 300-gm. guinea pig from scurvy for 90 days; equivalent to 0.5 to 0.6 mg. of ascorbic acid.

**Sherman-Bourquin u. of vitamin $B_2$,** the amount of vitamin $B_2$ (G) required in the diet daily to sustain an average weekly gain of 3 gm. for 8 weeks in standard test rats; one such u. is equivalent to 1 to 7 μg. (0.001 to 0.007 mg.) of riboflavin depending on the deficiency diet used in the above assay.

**Sherman-Munsell u.,** a rat growth u.; the daily amount of vitamin A which sustains a rate of gain amounting to 3 gm. a week in standard test rats.

**SI u.'s,** see base u.'s; also International System of Units.

**Somogyi u.,** a term for expressing the level of activity of amylase in blood serum, as analyzed by means of the Somogyi method (the most frequently used procedure); one u. is equivalent to 1 mg. of reducing sugar liberated as glucose per 100 ml. of serum, when an aliquot of the latter is mixed with a standard starch substrate (plus sodium chloride for maximal activation) and incubated for a standard time. The normal range is 80 to 150 u.'s, but values are usually not regarded as clinically significant unless they are less than 200 u.'s.

**Steenbock u.,** a u. of vitamin D; the total amount of vitamin D which will produce within ten days a narrow line of calcium deposit in the rachitic metaphyses of the distal ends of the radii and ulnae of standard rachitic rats.

**streptomy'cin u.'s,** (1) G u.: equals 1 gm. of the crystalline material or about 1,000,000 of S u.'s; (2) L u.: equal to 1000 S u.'s; (3) S u.: the amount of s. which will inhibit the growth of a standard strain of Escherichia coli in 1 ml. of nutrient broth or other suitable medium.

**Svedberg u.,** a sedimentation constant of $1 \times 10^{-13}$ seconds; symbol, S.

**thi'amin hydrochloride u. (international),** vitamin $B_1$ hydrochloride u.; thiamin chloride u.; the antineuritic activity of 0.003 mg. of the standard crystalline vitamin $B_1$ hydrochloride.

**u. of thyrotroph'ic activity,** the activity of an amount of an extract of the anterior lobe of the hypophysis which, given daily for 5 days, will cause the thyroid of a guinea pig (weighing 200 gm.) to reach a weight of 600 mg.

**toxic u.,** see MLD, under dose.

**uranium u.,** a u. for the measurement of radioactivity, that of uranium being taken as 1.

**USP u.,** a u. as defined and adopted by the United States Pharmacopeia.

**u. of vasopres'sin,** the pressor activity of 0.5 mg. of the USP Posterior-pituitary Reference Standard; 1 mg. of synthetic vasopressin corresponds to 600 International u.'s.

**vitamin A u. (international) (USP),** the specific biologic activity of 0.3 μg. of vitamin A (alcohol form); see also Sherman-Munsell u.

**vitamin $B_1$ hydrochloride u.,** thiamin hydrochloride u.

**vitamin $B_2$ u.,** riboflavin u.; see also Sherman-Bourquin u.

**vitamin $B_6$ u.,** potency expressed in terms of weight of pure crystalline pyridoxine.

**vitamin C u. (international),** the vitamin C activity of 0.05 mg. of the standard crystalline levoascorbic acid; 1 mg. of crystalline vitamin C provides 20 USP units; see also Sherman u.

**vitamin D u. (international),** the antirachitic activity contained in 0.025 μg. of a preparation of crystalline vitamin $D_3$ (activated 7-dehydrocholesterol); see also Steenbock u.

**vitamin E u.,** potency usually expressed in terms of weight of pure α-tocopherol.

**vitamin K u.,** there is no international u. of vitamin K; see Dam u.

**u. of wavelength,** Ångström u.

**u. of weight,** in the English system, the pound; in the metric system, the gram; in the SI system, the kilogram.

**Wohlgemuth u.,** a set of terms for expressing the levels of activity of amylase in duodenal fluid, urine, and feces.

**u.'s of work,** see u.'s of energy.

---

**United States Adopted Names** (USAN). Designation for nonproprietary names (for drugs) adopted by the USAN Council (or its immediate predecessor, the American Medical Association-U. S. Pharmacopeia Nomenclature Committee) in cooperation with the manufacturers concerned; the designation USAN is applicable only to nonproprietary names coined since June 1961.

**United States Pharmacopeia.** See Pharmacopeia.

**univalence** (u-ni-va'lens). Monovalence.

**univalent** (u-ni-val'lent). Monovalent.

**unmed'ullated.** Unmyelinated.

**unmyelinated** (un-mi'ĕ-li-na'ted). Amyelinated; amyelinic; nonmyelinated; unmedullated; nonmedullated; refers to nerve fibers (axons) lacking a myelin sheath.

**Unna** (oo'nah), Paul G., German dermatologist, 1850-1929. See U.'s disease, mark, stain, U.-Pappenheim stain, U.-Taenzer stain.

**unofficial.** Denoting a drug that is not listed in the United States Pharmacopeia or the National Formulary.

**unospaston.** ALUTAN; triethyl(2-hydroxyethyl)ammonium bromide dicyclopentyl acetate; intestinal antispasmodic agent.

**unphysiolog'ic.** Pertaining to conditions in the organism which are abnormal; can be used to refer to subjecting the body to abnormal amounts of substances normally present.

**unsat'urated.** Not saturated; denoting a solution in which the solvent is capable of dissolving more of the solute; denoting also a chemical compound in which all the affinities are not satisfied, so that still other atoms or radicals may be added to it. In organic chemistry, denoting compounds containing double and triple bonds.

**unsex.** To castrate; to deprive of the gonads.

**unsound.** Unhealthy; morbid; defective.

**unsound'ness.** In a horse, any deviation in form or function from the normal that interferes with the animal's usefulness.

**unstri'ated.** Without striations; not striped; denoting the structure of the smooth or involuntary muscles.

**Unterberger's test.** See under test.

**unthrif'ty.** In animals, denoting a failure to grow or develop normally as a result of disease.

**ununited** (un'u-ni'ted). Not united or knit; denoting an unhealed fracture.

**Unverricht** (oon'fer-ikht), Heinrich, German physician, 1853–1912. See U.'s *disease*.

**upsiloid** (ŭp'sĭ-loyd). Hypsiloid.

**up'take.** A term used to indicate the absorption by a tissue of some substance, food material, mineral, etc. *e.g.*, iodine by the thyroid gland, and its permanent or temporary retention.

**urachal** (u'ră-kal). Relating to the urachus.

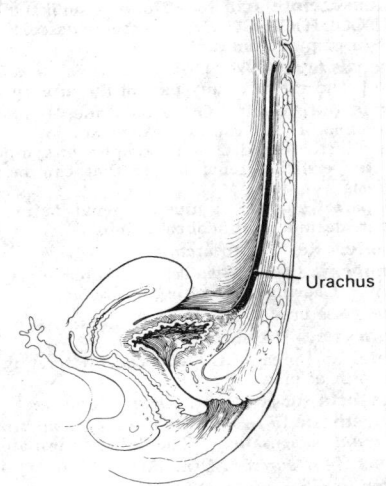

— Urachus

**Urachus**

**urachus** (u'ră-kus) [ G. *ourachos*, the urinary canal of a fetus. UR- ] [ NA ]. That portion of the reduced allantoic stalk between the apex of the bladder and the umbilicus. Postnatally it is normally merely a fibrous cord, but occasionally it is the old allantoic lumen may persist as a vesicoumbilical fistula.

**u'racil.** 2,4-Dioxopyrimidine; 2,4-(1*H*,3*H*)-pyrimidenedione; a pyrimidine (base) present in ribonucleic acid.

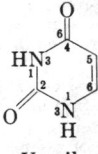

**Uracil**

*Inner numbering*, official international (IUPAC); *outer numbering*, original Fisher (abandoned).

   **u. dehydrogenase** (EC 1.2.99.1), u. oxidase; an oxidoreductase catalyzing oxidation of uracil to barbituric acid; also oxidizes thymine.

   **u. mustard** (NF), uramustine; 5-[ bis(2-chloroethyl-)amino ]uracil; alkylating antineoplastic agent.

   **u. oxidase,** u. dehydrogenase.

**uracrasia** (u'ră-kra'zĭ-ah) [ G. *ouron*, urine, + acrasia, *q.v.* ]. 1. A condition of foulness of the urine. 2. Enuresis; incontinence of urine.

**Uragoga.** *Cephaelis*; a genus of tropical plants (family Rubiaceae). *U. ipecacuanha* ( *Cephaelis ipecacuanha*) is the source of Rio or Brazilian ipecac; *U. acuminata* (*C. acuminata*) is the source of Cartagena, Nicaragua, or Panama ipecac.

**uragogue** (u'ră-gog) [ G. *ouron*, urine, + *agōgos*, drawing forth ]. Diuretic.

**uramus'tine.** Uracil mustard.

**uran'idine.** A yellow animal pigment found in coelenterates.

**u'ranine.** Fluorescein sodium.

**uraninite** (u-ran'ĭ-nit). Pitchblende.

**uranisco-.** See urano-.

**urisconitis** (u'ră-nis'ko-ni'tis). Palatitis.

**uraniscoplasty** (u'ră-nis'ko-plas'tĭ) [ uranisco- + G. *plassō*, to form ]. Palatoplasty.

**uraniscorrhaphy** (u'ră-nis-kor'ă-fĭ) [ uranisco- + G. *rhaphē*, suture ]. Palatorrhaphy.

**uraniscus** (u'ră-nis'kus) [ G. *ouraniskos*, roof of the mouth, dim. of *ouranos*, sky ]. Palatum.

**uranism** (u'ră-nizm) [ L. *Uranus*, G. *Ouranos*, god of the sky ]. Urningism; obsolete term for homosexuality.

**uranium** (u-ra'nĭ-um) [ after the planet Uranus ]. A metallic element, symbol U, atomic no. 92, atomic weight 238.03 occurring mainly in pitchblende from which it was first isolated by Klaproth in 1789; a hard, heavy metal of gray or black color, feebly radioactive; notable for its content of two isotopes: u.-238 and u.-235 (in 993-7 ratio), the latter of which was the first substance ever shown capable of supporting a self-sustaining chain reaction.

   **u. II,** a disintegration product of $^{238}$U; $^{239}$U, which gives off alpha particles to become ionium (thorium-230).

   **u. X$_1$,** a disintegration product of $^{238}$U; thorium-234, which gives off beta particles to become X$_2$, protactinium-239, which gives off beta particles to become u. II.

   **u. Y,** a disintegration product of $^{235}$U; thorium-231, which gives off beta particles to become protactinium-231.

**uranium-235** ($^{235}$U). Naturally occurring u. isotope, making 18 0.72 per cent of natural u.; alpha-emitter with half-life of 713 million years; notable for undergoing fission upon bombardment with thermal neutrons; hence acting as primary raw material for all fission power plants and fission bombs; also used as trigger for fusion bombs. Its fission in a reactor is used to create plutonium-239, also a fissionable material, from the nonfissionable major isotope of uranium, uranium-238.

**uranium-238** ($^{238}$U). Common, naturally occurring u. isotope, making up 99.27 per cent of natural u.; alpha-emitter with half life of 4.51 billion years; undergoes fission only after bombardment by fast neutrons, hence cannot form chain reaction; neutron bombardment, however, will convert it to plutonium-239 which can (basis of so called breeder reactions).

**urano-, uranisco-** (u'ră-no-) [ G. *ouranos*, sky vault, *ouraniskos*, roof of mouth (palate) ]. Combining forms relating to the palate (usually the hard palate); for words beginning thus and not found here, see palato-.

**uranolone.** 17a,β-Hydroxy-17α-methyl-5α-D-homoandrostane-3-one (a D-homoandrostane derivative; see sterods for structure). A steroid metabolite found in equine urine.

**uranoplasty** (u'ră-no-plas'tĭ). Palatoplasty.

**uranorrhaphy** (u'ră-nor'ă-fĭ) [ urano- + G. *raphē*, suture ]. Palatorrhaphy.

**uranoschisis** (u'ră-nos'kĭ-sis) [ urano- + G. *schisis*, fissure ]. Cleft of hard palate.

**uranostaphyloplasty** (u'ră-no-staf'ĭ-lo-plas'tĭ) [ urano- + G. *staphylē*, uvula, + *plassō*, to form ]. Uranostaphylorrhaphy; repair of a cleft of both hard and soft palate.

**uranostaphylorrhaphy** (u'ră-no-staf-ĭ-lor'ă-fĭ). Uranostaphyloplasty.

**uranostaphyloschisis** (u'ră-no-staf'ĭ-los'kĭ-sis) [ urano- + G. *staphylē*, uvula, + *schisis*, fissure ]. Uranoveloschisis; cleft of soft and hard palate.

**uranoveloschisis** (u'ră-no-vĕ-los'kĭ-sis). Uranostaphyloschisis.

**u'ranyl.** The ion, $UO_2^{2+}$, usually found in such salts as uranyl nitrate, $UO_2(NO_3)_2$.

**urari** (u-rah're). Curare.

**uraroma** (u'ră-ro'mah) [ G. *ouron*, urine, + *arōma*, spice ]. A spicy, aromatic odor of the urine.

**urarthritis** (u'rar-thri'tis) [ urate + arthritis ]. Gouty inflammation of a joint.

**u'rate.** A salt of uric acid.

   **u. oxidase** (EC 1.7.3.3), uricase; an oxygen oxidoreductase oxidizing uric acid.

**uratemia** (u′ra-te′mĭ-ah) [ urate + G. *haima*, blood ]. The presence of urates, especially sodium urate, in the blood.

**urateribonucleotide phosphorylase** (u′rāt-ri-bo-nu′kle-o-tĭd) (EC 2.4.2.16). A ribosyltransferase that phosphorylyzes urateribonucleotide to urate plus 1-phosphate.

**urat′ic.** Pertaining to a urate or to urates.

**uratolysis** (u′ra-tol′ĭ-sis) [ urate + G. *lysis*, solution ]. The decomposition or solution of urates.

**uratolytic** (u′ra-to-lit′ik). Causing the decomposition, or solution and removal of urates, from the tissues.

**uratoma** [ urate + G. suffix -*oma*, tumor ]. Tophus.

**urato′sis.** Any morbid condition due to the presence of urates in the blood or tissues.

**uraturia** (u′ra-tu′rĭ-ah) [ urate + G. *ouron*, urine ]. The passage of an increased amount of urates in the urine.

**Urbach,** Erich, U. S. dermatologist, 1893–1946. See U.-Wiethe disease.

**Urban,** Jerome A., U. S. surgeon, *1914. See U.'s *operation*.

**urce′iform** [ L. *urceus*, pitcher, + *forma*, form ]. Pitcher-shaped; urceolate.

**ur′ceolate** [ L. *urceolus*, dim. of *urceus*, pitcher ]. Urceiform.

**Urd.** Abbreviation for uridine.

**ur-defenses.** Fundamental beliefs essential for man's psychological integrity; for example, religion or science.

**ure-, urea-, ureo-** [ G. *ouron*, urine. UR- ]. Combining forms relating to urea and to urine; see also urin- and uro-

**urea** (u-re′ah) [ G. *ouron*, urine ]. (USP, BP). Carbamide; carbonyldiamide; NH₂—CO—NH₂; the chief end product of nitrogen metabolism in mammals, excreted in human urine in the amount of about 32 gm. (1 oz.) a day, about ⁶/₇ of the nitrogen excreted from the body. U. is formed in the liver, by means of the Krebs-Henseleit cycle in which arginine and arginase play the key role. It may be obtained artificially by heating a solution of ammonium cyanate. It occurs as colorless or white prismatic crystals, without odor but with a cooling saline taste, soluble in water; it forms salts with acids. It is used as a diuretic in kidney function tests, and topically for various skin disorders.

   **u. stib′amine,** a u. derivative of stibanilic acid. Used in the treatment of kala azar and certain other tropical diseases.

**urea frost.** Minute flakes of urea sometimes observed in the skin, particularly of the face, of patients with uremia.

**ure′al.** Ureic; relating to or containing urea.

**ureameter** (u′re-am′e-ter). A device for estimating the amount of urea in the urine.

**ureametry** (u′re-am′e-trĭ) [ urea + G. *metron*, measure ]. The determination of the amount of urea in the urine.

**Ureaplasma** (u-re′ah-plaz′mah). *T-mycoplasma;* a genus of microaerophilic to anaerobic, nonmotile bacteria (family Mycoplasmataceae) containing Gram-negative, predominantly coccoidal to coccobacillary elements, approximately 0.3 μm in diameter, which frequently grow in short filaments. They stain best by Giemsa or similar stains. The cells are bounded by a three-layered membrane. The colonies are generally small, 20 to 30 μm in diameter, and are normally without zones of surface growth; film and spots are absent. These organisms require urea and cholesterol for growth. Carbohydrates are not fermented. These organisms are found in the human genitourinary tract and occasionally in the pharynx and rectum. The pathogenicity of these organisms is questionable; in males they are associated with nongonococcal urethritis and prostatitis and, in females, with genitourinary tract infections and reproductive failure. The type species is *U. urealyticum.*

**ureapoiesis** (u-re′ah-poy-e′sis) [ urea + G. *poiēsis*, a making ]. Production of urea.

**urease** (u′re-ās) (EC 3.5.1.5). An amidohydrolase cleaving urea into CO₂ and NH₃.

**urecchysis** (u-rek′ĭ-sis) [ G. *ouron*, urine, + *ekchysis*, a pouring out. CHY- ]. Extravasation of urine into the tissues.

**uredema** (u-re-de′mah) [ G. *ouron*, urine, + *oidēma*, swelling ]. Infiltration of urine into the subcutaneous tissues.

**ure′do** [ L. a blight, a burning itch, fr. *uro*, pp. *ustus*, to burn ]. 1. Urticaria. 2. A burning sensation in the skin.

**ureide** (u′re-īd). Any compound of urea in which one or more of its hydrogen atoms have been substituted by acid radicals.

**3-ureidoisobutyric acid** (u-re′ĭ-do-i′so-bu-tīr′ik). H₂NCONH—CH₂CH(CH₃)COOH; an intermediate in thymine catabolism.

**3-ureidopropionic acid** (u-re′ĭ-do-pro-pĭ-on′ik). H₂NCONH—CH₂CH₂COOH; an intermediate in uracil catabolism.

**ureidosuccinic acid** (u-re′ĭ-do-suk-sin′ik). NH₂CONH—CH(COOH)CH₂COOH; *N*-carbamoylaspartic acid; a precursor of pyrimidines.

**urelcosis** (u′rel-ko′sis) [ G. *ouron*, urine, + *helkōsis*, ulceration ]. Ulceration of any part of the urinary tract.

**uremia** (u-re′mĭ-ah) [ G. *ouron*, urine, + *haima*, blood ]. Azotemia. 1. An excess of urea and other nitrogenous waste in the blood. 2. The complex of symptoms due to severe persisting renal failure that can be relieved by dialysis.

   **hy′percalce′mic u.,** due to renal failure caused by hypercalcemia with nephrocalcinosis.

**ure′mic.** Relating to uremia.

**uremigenic** (u-re-mĭ-jen′ik). 1. Of uremic origin or causation. 2. Causing or resulting in uremia.

**ureo-.** See ure-.

**ureom′eter.** Ureameter.

**ureotel′ic** [ urea + G. *telos*, end ]. Excreting nitrogen in the form of urea.

**urerythrin** (ūr-er′ĭ-thrin). Uroerythrin.

**uresiesthesia** (u-re′sĭ-es-the′zĭ-ah) [ G. *ourēsis*, a urinating, + *aisthēsis*, sensation ]. The desire to urinate.

**ure′sis** [ G. *ourēsis* ]. Urination.

**ureter** (u-re′ter, u′re-ter) [ G. *ourētēr*, urinary canal. UR- ] [ NA ]. The tube conducting the urine from the kidney to the bladder. It begins at the lower end of the renal pelvis and consists of a pars abdominalis and a pars pelvina. The thick wall of the u. is lined with transitional epithelium surrounded by smooth muscle, both circular and longitudinal, and covered externally by a tunica adventitia.

   **cur′licue u.,** term given to the twisted x-ray appearance of a u., herniated through the sciatic foramen; a very rare condition.

**ure′teral.** Ureteric; relating to the ureter.

**ureteralgia** (u-re′ter-al′jĭ-ah) [ ureter + G. *algos*, pain ]. Pain in the ureter.

**uretercystoscope** (u-re′ter-sis′to-skōp). A cystoscope with a ureteral catheter in a groove in its wall; the catheter is passed into the ureter when the orifice is brought into view with the cystoscope.

**ureterectasia** (u-re′ter-ek-ta′zĭ-ah) [ ureter + G. *ektasis*, a stretching out ]. Dilation of a ureter.

**ureterectomy** (u-re′ter-ek′to-mĭ) [ ureter + G. *ektomē*, excision ]. Exsection of a segment or all of a ureter.

**ureter′ic.** Ureteral.

**ureteritis** (u-re-ter-i′tis). Inflammation of a ureter.

**uretero-** (u-re′ter-o-) [ G. *ourētēr*, urinary canal ]. Combining form relating to the ureter.

**ureterocele** (u-re′ter-o-sēl) [ utero- + G. *kēlē*, hernia ]. The presence of a ureter amid the contents of a hernial sac.

**ure′terocer′vical.** Relating to a ureter and the cervix uteri; denoting a fistula between the two.

**ure′terocol′ic.** Relating to the ureter and the colon, especially to an anastomosis for lesions of the lower urinary tract.

**ureterocolostomy** (u′re′ter-o-ko-los′to-mĭ) [ uretero- + G. *kolon*, colon, + *stoma*, mouth ]. Implanting of ureter into colon.

**ure′terocyst′anastomo′sis.** Utererocystostomy.

**ureterocystoscope** (u-re′ter-o-sis′to-skōp). Uretercystoscope.

**ureterocystostomy** (u-re′ter-o-sis′tos′to-mĭ) [ uretero- + G. *kystis*, bladder, + *stoma*, mouth ]. Formation of an opening other than the natural one between a ureter and the bladder.

**ureterodialysis** (u-re′ter-o-di-al′ĭ-sis) [ uretero- + G. *dialysis*, separation ]. Rupture of a ureter.

**ureteroenteric** (u-re′ter-o-en-tĕr′ik). Relating to a ureter and the intestine; denoting a fistula uniting the two.

**ureteroenterostomy** (u-re′ter-o-en′ter-os′to-mĭ) [ uretero- + G. *enteron*, intestine, + *stoma*, mouth ]. The formation of an opening between a ureter and the intestine.

**ureterography** (u-re′ter-og′ră-fĭ) [ uretero- + G. *graphē*, a writing ]. Radiography of the ureter after the injection of collargol or argyrol or some similar substance.

**ure′terohy′dronephro′sis.** Hydronephrosis involving also the ureters.

**ureteroileostomy** (u-re′ter-o-il-e-os′to-mĭ) [ uretero- + ileum + G. *stoma*, mouth ]. Implantation of the ureter into the ileum.

**ureterolith** (u-re′ter-o-lith) [ uretero- + G. *lithos*, stone ]. A calculus in the ureter.

**ureterolithiasis** (u-re′ter-o-lĭ-thi′ă-sis) [ ureterolith + G. suffix *-iasis*, condition ]. The formation or presence of a calculus in a ureter.

**ureterolithotomy** (u-re′ter-o-lĭ-thot′o-mi) [ ureterolith + G. *tomē*, incision ]. Operation for the removal of a stone lodged in a ureter.

**ureterolysis** (u-re′ter-ol′ĭ-sis) [ uretero- + G. *lysis*, a loosening ]. Rupture of a ureter; ureterodialysis.

**ure′terone′ocystos′tomy** [ uretero- + G. *neos*, new, + *kystis*, bladder, + *stoma*, mouth ]. Ureterocystostomy.

**ure′terone′opyelos′tomy** [ uretero- + G. *neos*, new, + *pyelos*, pelvis, + *stoma*, mouth ]. The formation of an artificial opening between the ureter and the pelvis of the kidney.

**ureteronephrectomy** (u-re′ter-o-ne-frek′to-mĭ) [ uretero- + G. *nephros*, kidney, + *ektomē*, excision ]. Removal of a kidney with its ureter.

**ureteropathy** (u-re′ter-op′ă-thĭ) [ uretero- + G. *pathos*, suffering ]. Disease of the ureter.

**ureterophlegma** (u-re′ter-o-fleg′mah) [ uretero- + G. *phlegma*, phlegm ]. An accumulation of mucus in the ureter.

**ureteroplasty** (u-re′ter-o-plas′tĭ) [ uretero- + G. *plassō*, to form ]. Reparative or plastic surgery of the ureters.

**ureteroproctostomy** (u-re′ter-o-prok-tos′to-mĭ) [ uretero- + G. *prōktos*, rectum, + *stoma*, mouth ]. The establishment of an opening between a ureter and the rectum.

**ureteropyelitis** (u-re′ter-o-pi′ĕ-li′tis) [ uretero- + G. *pyelos*, pelvis, + suffix *-itis*, inflammation ]. Inflammation of the pelvis of a kidney with its ureter.

**ureteropyelography** (u-re′ter-o-pi′ĕ-log′ră-fĭ). Pyelography.

**ure′teropy′eloneos′tomy.** Ureteroneopyelostomy.

**ureteropyelonephritis** (u-re′ter-o-pi′ĕ-lo-ne-fri′tis). Ureteropyelitis.

**ureteropyelonephrostomy** (u′re′ter-o-pi′ĕ-lo-ne-fros′to-mĭ) [ uretero- + G. *pyelos*, pelvis, + *nephros*, kidney, + *stoma*, mouth ]. Formation of a junction of ureter and kidney.

**ureteropyeloplasty** (u-re′ter-o-pi′ĕ-lo-plas′tĭ) [ uretero- + G. *pyelos*, pelvis, + *plassō*, to form ]. Plastic surgery of the ureter and pelvis of the kidney.

**ureteropyelostomy** (u-re′ter-o-pi′ĕ-los′to-mĭ) [ uretero- + pelvis, + *stōma*, mouth ]. Formation of a junction of the ureter and the renal pelvis; a procedure for ureterovaginal ectopia.

**ureteropyosis** (u-re′ter-o-pi-o′sis) [ uretero- + G. *pyōsis*, suppuration ]. An accumulation of pus in the ureter.

**ure′terorec′toneos′tomy.** Ureteroproctostomy.

**ure′terorectos′tomy.** Ureteroproctostomy.

**ureterorrhagia** (u-re′ter-o-ra′jĭ-ah) [ uretero- + G. *rhēgnymi*, to burst forth ]. Hemorrhage from a ureter.

**ureterorrhaphy** (u-re′ter-or′ă-fĭ) [ uretero- + G. *rhaphē*, suture ]. Suture of a wounded ureter.

**ureterosigmoid** (u-re′ter-o-sig′moyd). Relating to the ureter and the sigmoid colon, especially to an anastomosis between the two.

**ure′terosigmoidos′tomy.** Implantation of the ureters into the sigmoid colon.

**ure′terostegno′sis** [ uretero- + G. *stegnōsis*, a making close ]. Ureterostenosis.

**ure′terosteno′ma** [ uretero- + G. *stenōma*, a narrow place, fr. *stenos*, narrow ]. The site of a stricture of a ureter.

**ure′terosteno′sis** [ uretero- + G. *stenōsis*, a narrowing ]. Stricture of a ureter.

**ureterostoma** (u-re′ter-os′to-mah) [ uretero- + G. *stoma*, mouth ]. A ureteral fistula.

**ureterostomy** (u-re′ter-os′to-mĭ) [ uretero- + G. *stoma*, mouth ]. The establishment of an external opening into the ureter.

**ureterotomy** (u-re′ter-ot′o-mĭ) [ uretero- + G. *tomē*, incision ]. Any cutting operation on a ureter.

**ureterotrigonoenterostomy** (u-re′ter-o-trī-go′no-en-ter-os′to-mĭ) [ uretero-, + trigone (of bladder), + enterostomy ]. Planting of ureter and its portion of trigone of bladder into the intestine.

**ure′tero-ure′teral.** Relating to two segments of the same ureter or to both ureters; denoting an artificial anastomosis between them.

**ure′tero-ure′teros′tomy.** The establishment of an anastomosis between the two ureters or between two segments of the same ureter.

**uretero-uterine** (u-re′ter-o-u′ter-in). Relating to a ureter and the uterus; denoting a fistula between the two.

**ureterovaginal** (u-re′ter-o-vaj′ĭ-nal). Relating to a ureter and the vagina; denoting a fistula, either surgical or pathologic, connecting the two.

**ure′teroves′ical.** Relating to the ureter and the bladder, specifically the junction of ureter with bladder.

**ureterovesicostomy** (u-re′ter-o-ves′ĭ-kos′to-mĭ) [ uretero- + L. *vesico*, bladder, + *stōma*, mouth ]. Surgical joining of ureter to bladder.

**u′rethan, urethane.** $NH_2COOC_2H_5$; ethyl carbamate; has antimitotic activity; formerly used medically as a hypnotic, but now more often used as an anesthetic for laboratory animals.

**urethr-.** See urethro-.

**urethra** (u-re′thrah) [ G. *ourēthra*. UR- ]. Urogenital canal; a canal leading from the bladder, discharging the urine externally.

  **female u.,** u. feminina.

  **u. femini′na** [ NA ], female u.; a canal about 4 cm. in length passing from the bladder, in close relation with the anterior wall of the vagina, opening in the vestibule behind the clitoris.

  **male u.,** u. masculina.

  **u. masculi′na** [ NA ], male u.; a canal about 20 cm. in length opening at the extremity of the glans penis; it gives passage to the spermatic fluid as well as the urine.

  **mem′branous u.,** *pars* membranacea urethrae masculinae.

  **u. muliebris,** u. feminina.

  **pe′nile u.,** *pars* spongiosa urethrae masculinae.

  **prostat′ic u.,** *pars* prostatica urethrae masculinae.

  **spongy u.,** *pars* spongiosa urethrae masculinae.

  **u. virilis,** u. masculina.

**ure′thral.** Relating to the urethra.

**urethralgia** (u-re-thral′jĭ-ah) [ urethr- + G. *algos*, pain ]. Pain in the urethra.

**urethram′eter.** Urethrometer.

**ure′thrascope.** Urethroscope.

**urethratresia** (u-re′thră-tre′zĭ-ah) [ urethr- + G. *a-* priv. + *trēsis*, a boring ]. Imperforation or occlusion of the urethra.

**urethrectomy** (u′re-threk′to-mĭ) [ urethr- + G. *ektomē*, excision ]. Excision of a segment or the whole of the urethea.

**urethremorrhagia** (u-re-threm′o-ra′jĭ-ah) [ urethr- + G. *haima*, blood, + *rhēgnymi*, to burst forth ]. Urethrorrhagia; bleeding from the urethra.

**urethremphraxis** (u-re-threm-frak′sis) [ urethr- + G. *emphraxis*, a stoppage ]. Obstruction, from any cause, to the free flow of urine through the urethra.

**urethreurynter** (u-re′thru-rin′ter) [ urethr- + G. *eurynō*, to dilate, fr. *eurys*, wide ]. An instrument for dilating the urethra.

**urethrism, urethrismus** (u're-thrizm, -thriz'mus). Urethrospasm; irritability or spasmodic stricutre of the urethra.

**urethritis** (u're-thri'tis) [ ureth- + G. suffix *-itis*, inflammation ]. Inflammation of the urethra.

**anterior u.,** inflammation of the portion of the urethra anterior to the triangular ligament.

**follicular u.,** granular u.; chronic u. with nodular lymphocytic infiltrations in the mucosa.

**gonococcal u.,** gonorrhea in males.

**granular u.,** follicular u.

**nonspecific u.,** simple u.; u. not resulting from gonococcal or other specific infectious agents.

**u. petrif'icans,** a form, sometimes of gouty origin, in which there is a deposit of calcareous matter in the wall of the urethra.

**posterior u.,** inflammation of the membranous and prostatic portions of the urethra.

**simple u.,** nonspecific u.

**specific u.,** gonorrhea.

**u. vene'rea,** gonorrhea.

**urethro-, urethr-** (u-re'thro-) [ G. *ourēthra*, urethra. UR- ]. Combining forms denoting urethra.

**ure'throbul'bar.** Bulbourethral.

**urethrocele** (u-re'thro-sēl) [ urethro- + G. *kēlē*, tumor, hernia ]. A prolapse of the female urethra.

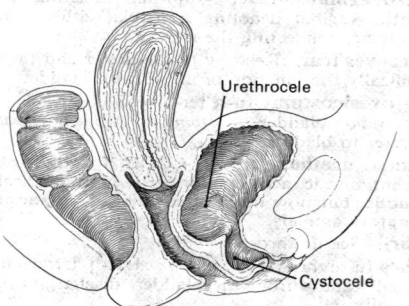

**Urethrocele Accompanied by Cystocele**

**urethrocystitis** (u-re'thro-sis-ti'tis) [ urethro- + G. *kystis*, bladder, + suffix *-itis*, inflammation ]. Inflammation of the urethra and bladder.

**ure'throcystom'etry** [ urethro- + G. *kystis*, bladder, + *metron*, measure ]. A procedure that simultaneously measures pressures in urinary bladder and urethra.

**ure'throcys'topexy** [ urethro- + G. *kystis*, bladder, + *pēxis*, fixation ]. Fixation of urethra and bladder for stress incontinence.

**urethrodynia** (u-re'thro-din'ī-ah) [ urethro- + G. *odynē*, pain ]. Pain in the urethra.

**ure'thrograph** [ urethro- + G. *graphō*, to write ]. A recording urethrometer, indicating graphically the location and extent of a stricture or strictures of the urethra.

**urethrometer** (u're-throm'e-ter) [ urethro- + G. *metron*, measure ]. An instrument for measuring the caliber of the urethra.

**urethropenile** (u-re'thro-pe'nil) Relating to the urethra and the penis.

**ure'throperine'al.** Relating to the urethra and the perineum.

**ure'throperine'oscro'tal.** Relating to the urethra, perineum, and scrotum.

**urethrophraxis** (u-re'thro-frak'sis). Urethremphraxis.

**urethrophyma** (u-re'thro-fi'mah) [ urethro- + G. *phyma*, a tumor ]. Any tumor or circumscribed swelling of the urethra.

**urethroplasty** (u-re'thro-plas'tī) [ urethro- + G. *plassō*, to form ]. Reparative or plastic surgery of the urethra.

**ure'throprostat'ic.** Relating to the urethra and the prostate.

**ure'throrec'tal.** Relating to the urethra and the rectum.

**urethrorrhagia** (u-re'thro-ra'jī-ah). Urethremorrhagia.

**urethrorrhaphy** (u-re-thror'ā-fī) [ urethro- + G. *rhaphē*, suture ]. Suture of a wound of the urethra.

**urethrorrhea** (u-re'thro-re'ah) [ urethro- + G. *rhoia*, a flow ]. An abnormal discharge from the urethra.

**urethroscope** (u-re'thro-skōp) [ urethro- + G. *skopeō*, to view ]. An instrument for affording a view, under electrical illumination, of the urethra.

**ure'throscop'ic.** Relating to the urethroscope or to urethroscopy.

**urethroscopy** (u-re-thros'ko-pī). The inspection of the urethra by means of the urethroscope.

**urethrospasm** (u-re'thro-spazm). Urethrism.

**urethrostaxis** (u-re'thro-stak'sis) [ urethro- + G. *staxis*, trickling ]. Oozing of blood from the mucous membrane of the urethra.

**urethrostenosis** (u-re'thro-stē-no'sis) [ urethro- + G. *stenōsis*, a narrowing ]. Stricture of the urethra.

**urethrostomy** (u-re-thros'to-mī) [ urethro- + G. *stoma*, mouth ]. Formation of a permanent opening into the membranous portion of the urethra through the perineum.

**urethrotome** (u-re'thro-tōm) [ urethro- + G. *tomos*, cutting ]. An instrument for dividing a stricture of the urethra.

**urethrotomy** (u're-throt'o-mī) [ urethro- + G. *tomē*, incision ]. Operation for division of a stricture of the urethra.

**anterior-posterior u.,** internal-external u.

**external u.,** Wheelhouse's operation; perineal u.; division of a stricture of the membranous urethra by an incision through the perineum.

**internal u.,** division of a stricture by means of an instrument passed through the urethra.

**internal-external u.,** anterior-posterior u.; an operation in which a stricture in the more anterior portion of the urethra is first divided by internal u., and one in the posterior urethra is subsequently divided by external u.

**perine'al u.,** external u.

**urethrovaginal** (u-re'thro-vaj'ī-nal). Relating to the urethra and the vagina.

**ure'throves'ical.** Relating to urethra and bladder.

**-uret'ic** [ G. *ourētikos*, relating to the urine ]. Combining form denoting relationship to urine.

**urgin'ea** [ L. *urgeo*, to press, referring to the shape of the seeds ]. The young bulbs of *Urginea indica* (Indian squill) and *Urginea maritima* (white or Mediterranean squill); the source of squill, *q. v.*

**urhidrosis** (u-ri-dro'sis). Uridrosis.

**uri-, uric-, urico-** [ G. *ouron*, urine ]. Combining forms relating to uric acid.

**u'rian.** Urochrome.

**uric** (u'rik). Relating to urine.

**u. acid,** lithic acid; 2,6,8-trioxypurine; white crystals, poorly soluble, contained in solution in the urine of mammals and in solid form in the urine of birds and reptiles. It is sometimes solidified in small masses as stones or crystals or in larger concretions as calculi. With sodium and other bases it forms urates.

**u. acid oxidase,** see urate oxidase.

**uricacidemia** (u'rik-as'ī-de'mī-ah) [ uric acid + G. *haima*, blood ]. Uricemia; lithemia; the presence of uric acid in excess in the blood.

**uricaciduria** (u'rik-as'ī-du'rī-ah) [ uric acid + G. *ouron*, urine ]. The presence of large amounts of uric acid in the urine.

**u'ricase.** Urate oxidase.

**uricemia** (u'rī-se'mī-ah). Uricacidemia.

**urico-.** See uri-.

**uricolysis** (u'rī-kol'ī-sis) [ urico- + G. *lysis*, a loosening ]. Decomposition of uric acid.

**uricolyt'ic.** Relating to or effecting the hydrolysis of uric acid.

**uricometer** (u'rī-kom'e-ter) [ urico- + G. *metron*, measure ]. An appliance for determining the amount of uric acid voided in the urine.

**u'rico-ox'idase.** Urate oxidase.

**uricosuria** (u'rī-ko-su'rī-ah) [ urico- + G. *ouron*, urine ]. Excessive amounts of uric acid in the urine.

**u'ricosu'ric.** Tending to increase the excretion of uric acid.

**u'ricotel'ic** [ urico- + G. *telos*, end ]. Producing uric acid as the chief excretory product of nitrogen metabolism.

**u'ridine.** 1-β-D-ribofuranosyluracil; uracil ribonucleoside.

**u. diphosphate,** UDP; uridine 5'-pyrophosphate. See also entries under UDP.

**u. diphosphogalactose,** UDPGal; a pyrophosphate group links the 5' position of uridine and the 1 position of galactose.

**u. diphosphoglucose,** UDPG or UDPGlc; a pyrophosphate group links the 5' position of uridine and the 1 position of glucose.

**u. nucleosidase** (EC 3.2.2.3), see nucleosidases.

**u. phosphorylase** (EC 2.4.2.3), a ribosyltransferase that catalyzes the phosphorolysis of uridine to uracil plus ribose 1-phosphate.

**uridinediphosphoglucuronic acid** (u'rī-dēn-di-fos'fo-glu-ku-ron'ik). UDP-GlcUA; uridine diphosphoglucose in which the 6 $CH_2OH$ of the glucose has been oxidized to —COOH (has become a glucuronyl residue).

**uridrosis** (u'rī-dro'sis) [ uri- + G. *hidrōs*, sweat ]. Urhidrosis; sudor urinosus; the excretion of urea or uric acid in the sweat.

**u. crystalli'na,** a deposit of a white powder of uric acid on the skin.

**uridyl'ic acid.** Uridine phosphate; uridine esterified by phosphoric acid on one or more sugar hydroxyl groups.

**u'ridyltrans'ferase.** Hexose-1-phosphate uridylyltransferase.

**uriesthesia** (u-rī-es-the'zī-ah). Uresiesthesia.

**urin-, urino-** (u'rin, u'rī-no-) [ G. *ouron*, urine. UR- ]. Combining forms relating to urine; see also ure- and uro-.

**urina** (oo-re'nah) [ L. fr. G. *ouron* ] [ NA ]. Urine.

**u. chy'li,** u. cibi.

**u. chylo'sa,** chylous *urine.*

**u. cibi** [ L. *cibus*, food ], the urine excreted after a meal.

**u. cruen'ta,** bloody urine.

**u. galacto'des** [ G. *gala*, milk ], chylous *urine.*

**u. hyster'ica,** hysterical urine; nervous u.; u. spastica; the pale urine secreted in large amount during a hysterical attack.

**u. jumento'sa** [ L. *jumentum*, a beast of burden ], cloudy urine like that of the horse.

**u. potus** [ L. *potus*, drink ], the urine excreted after the ingestion of a large amount of fluid.

**u. san'guinis** [ L. *sanguis*, blood ], the urine passed in the morning or after long abstinence from food and drink.

**u. spas'tica,** u. hysterica.

**urinaccelerator** (u'rin-ak-sel'er-a'tor). *Musculus bulbocavernosus.*

**u'rinal.** A vessel into which urine is passed.

**urinalysis** (u'rī-nal'ī-sis). Analysis of the urine.

**urinary** (u'rī-něr-ī). Relating to urine.

**urinaserum** (u'rī-nah-se'rum). Urinserum; urineserum; an antibody formed in response to the injection of albuminous urine; used in the precipitin test for albumin.

**urinate** (u'rī-nāt). To pass urine; to micturate.

**urination** (u'rī-na'shun). Micturition; the passing of urine.

**stuttering u.,** the passage of urine in jets caused by intermittent spasmodic contraction of the bladder.

**urine** (u'rin) [ L. *urina*; G. *ouron* ]. Urina; the fluid and dissolved substances excreted by the kidney.

**black u.,** black water; the u. of melanuria or hemoglobinuria.

**chylous u.,** urina chylosa; urina galactodes; u. of a milky appearance, containing chyle.

**cloudy u.,** nebulous u.; u. containing earthy phosphates in excess.

**crude u.,** pale u. of low specific gravity, with very little sediment.

**febrile u., feverish u.,** dark colored, concentrated u. of strong odor, passed by one suffering from fever.

**gouty u.,** u. of a high color containing uric acid in excess.

**honey u.,** old term for diabetes, not to be confused with the u. in maple syrup urine *disease.*

**milky u.,** chylous u.

**neb'ulous u.,** cloudy u.

**nervous u.,** *urina* hysterica.

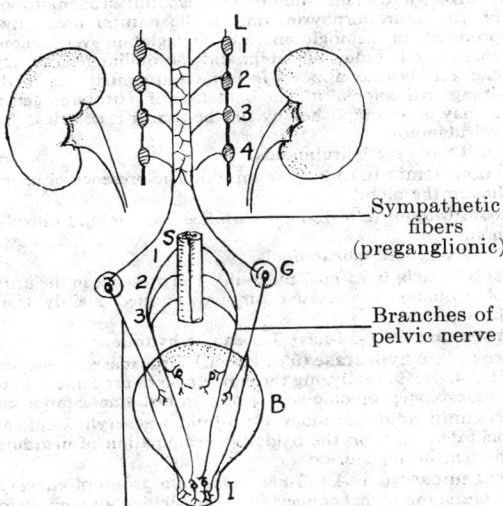

Sympathetic fibers (preganglionic)

Branches of pelvic nerve

Sympathetic (postganglionic)

**Innervation of the Act of Urination**

*B,* urinary bladder; *G,* hypogastric ganglion; *I,* internal sphincter; *L 1, 2, 3, 4* refer to the ganglia of the lumbar sympathetic chain; *S 1, 2, 3* indicate the sacral segments of the spinal cord from which the fibers of the pelvic nerve arise.

**resid'ual u.,** u. remaining in the bladder at the end of micturition in cases of enlarged prostate, paresis of the bladder, etc.

**urine'mia.** Obsolete term for uremia.

**urineserum** (u'rin-se'rum). Urinaserum.

**u'rinif'erous** [ urine + L. *fero*, to carry ]. Conveying urine; denoting the tubules of the kidney.

**u'rinif'ic** [ urine + L. *facio*, to make ]. Uriniparous.

**u'rinip'arous** [ urine + L. *pario*, to produce ]. Producing or excreting urine; denoting the Malpighian bodies and certain tubules in the renal cortex.

**u'rinogen'ital.** Genitourinary.

**urinogenous** (u'rī-noj'ě-nus). Urogenous. 1. Producing or excreting urine. 2. Of urinary origin.

**u'rinoglucosom'eter.** An apparatus for determining the amount of glucose in the urine.

**urinol'ogist.** Urologist.

**urinology** (u'rī-nol'o-jī). Urology.

**urinoma** (u'rī-no'mah). A cyst containing urine.

**urinometer** (u'rī-nom'e-ter) [ urine + G. *metron*, measure ]. Urometer; urogravimeter; a hydrometer for determining the specific gravity of the urine.

**urinom'etry.** The determination of the specific gravity of the urine.

**urinos'copy.** Uroscopy.

**urinosex'ual.** Genitourinary.

**u'rinous.** Relating to or of the nature of urine.

**urinserum** (u-rin-se'rum). Urinaserum.

**uriposia** (u'rī-po'sī-ah) [ urine + G. *posis*, drinking ]. Urine-drinking.

**uritis** (u-ri'tis) [ L. *uro*, pp. *ustus*, to singe, burn, + G. suffix *-itis*, inflammation ]. Dermatitis *ambustionis.*

**urningism** (oor'ning-izm) [ Ger. ]. Uranism.

**uro-** [ G. *ouron*, urine. UR- ]. Combining form relating to urine. See also ure- and urin-.

**uroacidimeter** (u-ro-as-ī-dim'e-tur). An apparatus for determining the degree of acidity of the urine.

**uroammoniac** (u-ro-am-o'nī-ak). Relating to uric acid and ammonia, denoting a variety of urinary calculus.

**uroanthelone** (u'ro-an'thě-lōn). Urogastrone.

**uroazotometer** (u-ro-az-o-tom'e-ter) [ uro- + Fr. *azote*, nitrogen, + G. *metron*, measure ]. Ureameter.

**urobilin** (u'ro-bi'lin, -bil'in). Urohematin; urohematoporphyrin; a uroporphyrin; one of the natural breakdown products of hemoglobin, *via* choleglobin, verdohemochrome, biliverdin, bilirubin, and *d*-urobilinogen; an acyclic tetrapyrrole; appears in urine and contributes to the orange-red color of it. The oxidation of *d*-urobilinogen to u. may be accomplished by air; the former is colorless. See bilirubinoids.

    **u. IX-α,** see bilirubinoids.

**urobilinemia** (u'ro-bi-li-ne'mi-ah). The presence of urobilins in the blood.

**urobilinogen** (u'ro-bi-lin'o-jen). See urobilin and bilirubinoids.

    **u. IX-α,** see bilirubinoids.

**urobilinuria** (u'ro-bi-li-nu'ri-ah). The presence in the urine of urobilins in excessive amount, formed mainly from hemoglobin.

**urocanase** (u'ro-kă-nās). Urocanate hydratase.

**urocanate hydratase** (u'ro-kă-nāt). Urocanase; an enzyme (EC 4.2.1.49) catalyzing the conversion of urocanic acid to imidazolonepropionic acid, a step in histidine catabolism.

**urocanic acid** (u'ro-kan'ik). 3-Imidazoleacrylic acid; an acid derived from the oxidative deamination of histidine; present in dog's urine.

**urocanicase** (u'ro-kan'i-kās). One of a group of enzymes (at least three) that converts urocanic acid to glutamic acid.

**urocanylcholine** (u'ro-kan'il-ko'lēn). Murexine.

**urocele** (u'ro-sēl) [ uro- + G. *kēlē,* hernia ]. Extravasation of urine into the scrotal sac.

**urocheras** (u-rok'er-as) [ uro- *cheras,* gravel (an incorrect form of *cherados,* gravel) ]. Uropsammus.

**urochesia** (u-ro-ke'zi-ah) [ uro- + G. *chezō,* to defecate ]. The passage of urine from the anus.

**urochrome** (u'ro-krōm). The principal pigment of urine, a compound of urobilin and a peptide of unknown structure.

**urochromogen** (u'ro-kro'mo-jen). Originally, a body in the urine that, on taking up oxygen, formed urochrome. Probably urobilinogen.

**urocrisia** (u'ro-kris'i-ah, -kriz'i-ah) [ uro- + G. *krinō,* to separate, judge. CRI- ]. 1. Urocrisis. 2. Diagnosis based upon the results of a urinary examination.

**urocrisis** (u'ro-kri'sis) [ uro- + G. *krisis,* crisis. CRI- ]. 1. The critical stage of a disease accompanied by a copious discharge of urine. 2. Severe pain in any of the urinary organs or passages occurring in tabes dorsalis.

**urocyanin** (u'ro-si'ă-nin) [ uro- + G. *kyanos,* a blue substance ]. Uroglaucin; an indigo blue pigment sometimes observed in the urine in certain diseases, especially scarlet fever.

**urocyanogen** (u-ro-si-an'o-jen). A blue pigment sometimes observed in the urine in cases of cholera.

**urocyanosis** (u'ro-si-ă-no'sis). A bluish discoloration of the urine in indicanuria.

**urocyst** (u'ro-sist) [ uro- + G. *kystis,* bladder ]. *Vesica urinaria.*

**urocystic** (u'ro-sis'tik). Relating to the urinary bladder.

**urocystis** (u'ro-sis'tis). *Vesica urinaria.*

**urocystitis** (u'ro-sis-ti'tis) [ uro- + G. *kystis,* bladder, + suffix *-itis,* inflammation ]. Inflammation of the urinary bladder.

**urodochium** (u-ro-dŏ-ki'um) [ uro- + G. *docheion,* a container ]. A urinal.

**urodynamics** (u'ro-di-nam'iks) [ uro- + G. *dynamis,* force ]. Hydrodynamics of the urinary tract.

**urodynia** (u'ro-din'i-ah) [ uro- + G. *odynē,* pain ]. Pain on urination; dysuria.

**u'rodysfunc'tion.** Urinary dysfunction.

**uroedema** (u'ro-e-de'mah) [ uro- + G. *oidēma,* swelling ]. Infiltration of urine.

**uroenterone** (u'ro-en'ter-ōn). Urogastrone.

**uroerythrin** (u'ro-ĕr'i-thrin). A urinary pigment that gives a pink color to deposits of urates; presumably derived from melanin; *cf.* bilirubin, uroflavin, urochrome, uromelanin, porphyrinuria.

**u'rofla'vin.** A fluorescent product of riboflavin catabolism, or perhaps riboflavin itself, found in mammalian urine and feces.

**urofuscohematin** (u'ro-fus'ko-hem'ă-tin). A brownish red pigment found in the urine in a case of leprosy.

**u'rogas'trone.** Anthelone; anthelone U; uroanthelone; uroenterone; a fluorescent pigment extracted from urine; an inhibitor of gastric secretion and motility; *cf.* enterogastrone.

**urogenital** (u'ro-jen'i-tal). Genitourinary.

**urogenous** (u-roj'ĕ-nus). Urinogenous.

**uroglaucin** (u-ro-glaw'sin) [ uro- + G. *glaukos,* bluish gray ]. Urocyanin.

**u'rogram.** The picture obtained by urography.

**urography** (u-rog'ră-fi) [ uro- + G. *graphō,* to write ]. Roentgenography of any part (kidneys, ureters, or bladder) of the urinary tract.

    **excretory u.,** x-ray examination of the urine passing through the ureters or in the bladder by means of a contrast fluid taken by the mouth; distinguished from **intravenous u.,** the fluid being injected into a vein, or **retrograde u., cystoscopic u.,** the fluid being injected into the bladder.

**urogravimeter** (u-ro-gră-vim'e-ter) [ uro- + L. *gravis,* heavy, + G. *metron,* measure ]. Urinometer.

**u'rohem'atin.** The urinary pigment that gives varying color to the urine according to its degree of oxidation. See urobilin; alkaptonuria.

**u'rohem'atopor'phyrin.** Urobilin.

**u'rohep'arin.** An inactive form of heparin excreted in the urine.

**urohypertensin** (u-ro-hi-per-ten'sin). A pressor substance derived from the urine.

**urohypophysis** (u-ro-hi-pof'i-sis). Caudal neurosecretory system; an enlargement at the caudal end of the spinal cord in teleost and elasmobranch fishes that contains neurosecretory cell bodies; its function has not been established.

**u'roki'nase.** 1. A proteinase (EC 3.4.99.26) found in mammalian urine, with the same action (cleaving plasminogen to plasmin) as streptokinase or staphylokinase. 2 (USAN). WIN-KINASE; used for treatment of pulmonary embolism.

**urolagnia** (u-ro-lag'ni-ah) [ uro- + G. *lagneia,* lust ]. A form of sexual stimulation in which the sight of a person urinating causes erethism.

**u'roleucin'ic** or **u'roleu'cic acid.** Name given to aromatic compounds excreted in the urine of persons with alkaptonuria; probably homogentisic acid and/or 5-hydroxyindoleacetic acid.

**u'rolith, u'rolite** [ uro- + G. *lithos,* stone ]. Urinary *calculus.*

**urolithiasis** (u-ro-li-thi'ă-sis). A state marked by or tending to the formation of urinary calculi.

**u'rolith'ic.** Relating to urinary calculi.

**urolithology** (u'ro-li-thol'o-ji) [ uro- + G. *lithos,* stone, + *logos,* study ]. The branch of science that has to do with the formation, composition, effects, and removal of urinary calculi.

**urological** (u'ro-loj'i-kal). Relating to urology.

**urol'ogist.** One versed in urology.

**urology** (u-rol'o-ji) [ uro- + G. *logos,* study ]. The branch of medical science that embraces the study, diagnosis, and treatment of diseases of the genitourinary tract.

**urolutein** (u-ro-lu'te-in). Name given to yellow pigment in the urine; see urochrome; uroporphyrin.

**uromel'anin.** A black pigment occasionally found in the urine, possibly a decomposition product of urochrome; see also homogentisic acid, uroerythrin.

**uromelus** (u-rom'e-lus) [ G. *oura,* tail, + *melos,* limb ]. Sirenomelus.

**urom'eter.** Urinometer.

**uroncus** (u-rong'kus) [ uro- + G. *onkos,* mass (tumor) ]. A urinary cyst; a circumscribed area of extravasation of urine.

**uronephrosis** (u'ro-ne-fro'sis). Hydronephrosis.

**uron'ic acids.** Acids derived from the monosaccharides by oxidation of the primary alcohol group (—CH$_2$OH) farthest removed from the carbonyl group to a carboxyl group (—COOH), *e.g.,* glucuronic acid.

**u'ronol'ogy.** Urology.

**uronophile** (u-ron'o-fīl) [ G. *ouron*, urine, + *philos*, fond ]. Denoting a microorganism growing best in urine or a medium in which urine is incorporated.

**u'ronos'copy.** Uroscopy.

**uropancreatone** (u'ro-pan'kre-ă-tōn). A principle in urogastrone preparations that inhibits pancreatic secretion. Whether it is separate and distinct from urogastrone itself is doubtful.

**u'ropar'otin.** A substance, isolated from human and animal urine, that exhibits weak parotin-line activity.

**uropathy** u'rop'ă-thī) [ uro- + G. *pathos*, suffering ]. Any affection involving the urinary tract.

**u'ropep'sin.** See urokinase.

**urophanic** (u'ro-fan'ik) [ uro- + G. *phainō*, to appear ]. Appearing in the urine; denoting any constituent, normal or pathologic, of the urine.

**urophein** (u'ro-fe'in) [ uro- + G. *phaios*, gray ]. A grayish pigment occasionally found in the urine, possibly identical with urobilin.

**uroplania** (u'ro-pla'nī-ah) [ uro- + G. *planē*, a wandering ]. Extravasation of urine.

**uropoiesis** (u'ro-poy-e'sis) [ uro- + G. *poiēsis*, a making ]. The production or secretion and excretion of urine.

**uropoietic** (u'ro-poy-et'ik). Relating or pertaining to uropoiesis.

**u'ropor'phyrin.** 1. Urochrome; porphyrin excreted in the urine in porphyrinuria; urobilin and its derivatives. 2. A class name for all porphyrins containing 4 acetic acid groups and 4 propionic acid groups in positions 1 through 8.

**uropsammus** (u-ro-sam'us) [ uro- + G. *psammos*, sand ]. Urocheras. 1. Gravel. 2. Any inorganic or uratic urinary sediment.

**uropterin** (u-rop'ter-in). Urothion.

**u'ropur'purin.** Purple pigment in the urine. See urochrome, uroerythrin, homogentisic acid.

**urorectal** (u'ro-rek'tal). Relating to the urinary tract and rectum.

**urorosein** (u-ro-ro'se-in). A chromogen in the urine that forms a red color on the addition of nitric acid; it normally exists in very minute quantity but is increased in tuberculosis and other wasting diseases. Related to ingestion of indole compounds (*cf.* alkaptonuria); see also uroporphyrin (1) and coproporphyrin.

**urorrhea** (u'ro-re'ah) [ uro- + G. *rhoia*, a flow ]. Enuresis.

**u'roru'bin.** A red pigment in urine made more visible by treatment with hydrochloric acid; *cf.* urorosein.

**urorubrohematin** (u'ro-ru'bro-hem'ă-tin). A reddish pigment occasionally present in the urine in various chronic diseases; see urorosein and uroporphyrin.

**uroscheocele** (u-ros'ke-o-sēl) [ uro- + G. *oscheon*, scrotum, + *kēlē*, tumor ]. Urocele.

**uroschesis** (u-ros'ke1sis) [ uro- + G. *schesis*, a checking ]. 1. Retention of urine. 2. Suppression of urine.

**u'roscop'ic.** Relating to uroscopy.

**uroscopy** (u-ros'ko-pī) [ uro- + G. *skopeō*, to view ]. Uronoscopy; urinoscopy; examination of the urine, usually by means of a microscope.

**urosemiology** (u'ro-sem-ī-ol'o-jī) [ uro- + G. *sēmeion*, a sign, + *logos*, study ]. The study of the urine as an aid to diagnosis.

**u'rosep'sin.** A substance formed by the decomposition of urine, supposed to be the cause of septic poisoning after urinary extravasation.

**urosepsis** (u'ro-sep'sis) [ uro- + G. *sēpsis*, decomposition ]. Sepsis resulting from the decomposition of extravasated urine.

**u'rosep'tic.** Relating to urosepsis.

**u'rospec'trin.** A pigment found in the urine, possibly the same as urohematoporphyrin.

**urostealith** (u-ros'te-ă-lith) [ uro- + G. *stear*, tallow, + *lithos*, stone ]. A renal calculus formed chiefly of a saponaceous material.

**urotheobromine** (u'ro-the-o-bro'mēn). 1,7-Dimethylxanthine; paraxanthine; isomer of theobromine sometimes present in the urine.

**urothion** (u'ro-thi'on). Uropterin; a sulfur-containing pteridine derivative isolated from urine.

**u'rotho'rax.** The presence of urine in the thoracic cavity, usually following complex multiple injuries.

**urotox'in.** An old term for a substance, or substances, thought to be responsible for the deleterious effects of urine when inoculated into normal animals.

**uroureter** (u-ro-u-re'ter). Hydroureter.

**uroxanthin** (u-ro-zan'thin). Indican.

**uroxin** (u-rok'sin). Alloxantin.

**ur'sin.** Arbutin.

**ursochol(an)ic acid.** See cholic acid.

**ursodeoxychol(an)ic acid.** See cholic acid.

**urtica** (ur-ti'kah, ur'tī-kah) [ L. a nettle, fr. *uro*, pp. *ustus*, to burn ]. The herb, *Urtica dioica* (family Urticaceae), nettle; a weed the leaves of which produce a stinging sensation when touching the skin. Has been used as a diuretic and hemostatic in metrorrhagia, epistaxis, and hematemesis.

**urticant** (ur'tī-kant) [ L. *urtica*, nettle; see urtica ]. Producing a wheal or other similar itching agent.

**urticaria** (ur'tī-kăr'ī-ah) [ L. *urtica*, *q.v.* ] Hives; nettle rash; cnidosis; an eruption of itching wheals usually of systemic origin. It may be due to a state of hypersensitivity to foods or drugs, foci of infection, physical agents (heat, cold, light, friction), or psychic stimuli.

**acute u., u. acu'ta,** febrile u.

**u. bullo'sa,** u. vesiculosa; an eruption of wheals capped with subepidermal vesicles.

**chronic u., u. chron'ica,** a form in which the wheals recur frequently, or persist.

**cold u.,** congelation u.; wheal formation that develops after exposure to lowered temperatures, with or without demonstrable passive-transfer antibodies.

**u. confer'ta,** a form of u. in which the wheals are aggregated in a group.

**congelation u.,** cold u.

**u., deafness, and amyloidosis,** Muckle-Wells *syndrome*.

**u. endem'ica, u. epidem'ica,** u. caused by the nettling hairs of certain caterpillars.

**u. evan'ida,** a form in which the eruption is of short duration.

**factitious u., u. facti'tia,** dermatographism.

**febrile u., u. febri'lis,** acute u.; u. accompanied by slight constitutional symptoms.

**giant u.,** angioneurotic *edema*.

**u. gi'gans, u. gigan'tea,** angioneurotic *edema*.

**u. hemorrhag'ica,** u. bullosa in which the serum contains blood.

**u. maculo'sa,** a chronic form of u. with lesions of a red color.

**u. mariti'ma,** u. occasionally produced in susceptible persons by salt water bathing.

**u. medicamento'sa,** an urticarial form of drug eruption.

**papular u.,** *lichen* urticatus.

**u. papulo'sa,** *lichen* urticatus.

**u. perstans** [ L. persisting ], a form of chronic u. in which the wheals persist unchanged for long periods.

**u. pigmento'sa,** Nettleship's disease; xanthelasmoidea; mastocytosis resulting from congenital excess of mast cells in the superficial dermis; a chronic eruption characterized by the eruption of brownish papules which urticate when stroked.

**solar u.,** a form of u. resulting from exposure to specific light spectra; some patients have passive-transfer antibodies and others do not.

**u. subcuta'nea,** u. in which itching is present without the wheals.

**u. tubero'sa,** angioneurotic *edema*.

**u. vesiculo'sa,** u. bullosa.

**urtica'rial, urtica'rious.** Relating to or marked by urticaria.

**urticate** (ur'tī-kāt) [ L. *urticatus* ]. 1. To perform urtication. 2. Marked by the presence of wheals.

**urtication** (ur'tī-ka'shun) [ L. *urticatio* ]. 1. Whipping with nettles to induce counterirritation, formerly used in the treatment of peripheral paralysis. 2. A burning sensation resembling that produced by urticaria or resulting from nettle poisoning. 3. Urticaria.

**urushiol** (oo′roo-shǐ-ōl) [ Jap. *urushi*, lac, + L. *oleum*, oil ]. A mixture of nonvolatile hydrocarbons, derivatives of catechol, constituting the active allergen of the irritant oil of poison ivy, *Rhus radicans*, and the Asiatic laquer tree, *Rhus vernicifera*.

   **u. oxidase,** monophenol monooxygenase.

**USAN.** Abbreviation for United States Adopted Names, *q. v.*

**U.S.D.** Abbreviation for United States Dispensatory.

**Usher,** C. H. See U.'s *syndrome.*

**Usher,** Barney, Canadian dermatologist, *1899. See Senear-U. *disease, syndrome.*

**Usnea** (us′ne-ah) [ A.S. *achneh*, lichen ]. A genus of lichens, tree-mosses (family Usneaceae).

**usnein** (us′ne-in). Usnic acid; usninic acid; antibacterial substance found in lichens, isolated from *Usnea barbata.*

**USP.** Abbreviation for *United States Pharmacopeia;* see Pharmacopeia.

**USPHS.** Abbreviation for United States Public Health Service.

**ustilaginism** (us′tǐ-laj′ǐ-nizm). Poisoning by *Ustilago maydis* (smut of maize) which produces burning, itching, hyperemia, acrocyanosis, and edema of the extremities. Resembles ergotism, pellagra, or infantile acrocynia.

**Ustilago** (us′tǐ-la′go) [ L. a kind of thistle, fr. *ustio*, a burning ]. A genus of smuts.

   **U. hypody′tes,** possible cause of friente.

   **U. may′dis,** corn-smut; corn ergot. Resembles ergot of rye in its ecbolic action.

   **U. zeae,** a corn smut parasite; its black spores on the ears of corn are dispersed by wind and can cause contamination of cultures.

**ustion** (us′chun) [ L. *ustio*, a burning ]. Cauterization by means of the actual cautery.

**ustulation** (us′tu-la′shun) [ L. *ustulo*, pp. *-atus*, to scorch ]. 1. The separation of compounds by heat, as in the process of freeing ores from sulfur by roasting. 2. The drying of a drug by heat to prepare it for pulverization.

**us′tus** [ L. pp. of *uro*, to burn ]. Calcined; roasted; burnt.

**usurpation** (u′sur-pa′shun) [ L. *usurpo*, pp. *-atus*, to seize ]. Assumption of pacemaker function of the heart by a subsidiary focus as a result of its own increased automaticity; *e.g.*, accelerated A-V nodal pacemaker takes command when it exceeds the sinus rate.

**uta** (oo′tah) [ Sp. ]. A form of New World or American cutaneous leishmaniasis caused by *Leishmania peruana*, occurring in the high Andean valleys of Peru and Bolivia. It is a mild disease with numerous small dermal lesions. The dog is an important reservoir. Unlike all other forms of American cutaneous leishmaniasis, this disease is found at high elevations (6000 to 8000 feet) in barren, open country, rather than in lowland tropical forests.

**uter-.** See utero-.

**uteralgia** (u′ter-al′jǐ-ah). Hysteralgia.

**uterectomy** (u′ter-ek′to-mǐ). Hysterectomy.

**uterine** (u′ter-in, u′ter-īn). Relating to the uterus.

**uterismus** (u′ter-iz′mus) [ uter- + L. suffix *-ismus*, action or condition, fr. G. *-ismos* ]. Painful spasmodic contraction of the uterus.

**uteritis** (u′ter-i′tis). Metritis.

**utero-, uter-** (u′ter-o-) [ L. *uterus* ]. Combining forms relating to the uterus.

**u′teroabdom′inal.** Relating to the uterus and the abdomen.

**u′terocer′vical.** Relating to the cervix uteri.

**uterocystostomy** (u′ter-o-sis-tos′to-mǐ) [ utero- + G. *kystis*, bladder, + *stoma*, mouth ]. The formation of a communication between the uterus (cervix) and the bladder.

**u′terofixa′tion.** Hysteropexy.

**uterogestation** (u′ter-o-jes-ta′shun) [ utero- + L. *gestatio*, fr. *gesto*, pp. *-atus*, to bear ]. Normal pregnancy; the development of the fetus within the uterus.

**uterolith** (u′ter-o-lith) [ utero- + G. *lithos*, stone ]. Uterine *calculus.*

**u′terom′eter.** Hysterometer.

**u′tero-ova′rian.** Relating to the uterus and an ovary.

**u′teropari′etal.** Relating to the uterus and the abdominal wall.

**u′teropel′vic.** Relating to the uterus and the pelvis.

**uteropexy** (u′ter-o-pek′sǐ). Hysteropexy.

**u′teroplacen′tal.** Relating to the uterus and the placenta.

**u′teroplas′ty** [ utero- + G. *plassō*, to form ]. Metroplasty; hysteroplasty; a plastic operation upon the uterus.

**u′terosa′cral.** Relating to the uterus and the sacrum.

**u′terosalpingog′raphy.** Hysterosalpingography.

**uteroscope** (u′ter-o-skōp). Hysteroscope.

**u′teros′copy.** Hysteroscopy.

**u′terotome.** Hysterotome.

**u′terot′omy.** Hysterotomy.

**uterotonic** (u′ter-o-ton′ik) [ utero- + G. *tonos*, tone, tension ]. 1. Giving tone to the uterine muscle. 2. An agent that overcomes relaxation of the muscular wall of the uterus.

**u′terotu′bal.** Pertaining to uterus and uterine tubes.

**u′terotubog′raphy.** Hysterosalpingography.

**uterovaginal** (u-ter-o-vaj′ǐ-nal). Relating to the uterus and the vagina.

**u′teroven′tral** [ utero- + L. *venter*, belly ]. Uteroabdominal.

**u′terover′dine.** Biliverdine.

**u′teroves′ical.** Relating to the uterus and the urinary bladder.

**uterus,** pl. **uteri** (u′ter-us, u′ter-i) [ L. ] [ NA ]. The womb; the hollow muscular organ in which the impregnated ovum is developed into the child; it is about 7.5 cm. in length in the nonpregnant woman, and consists of a main portion (corpus or body) with an elongated lower part (cervix or neck), at the extremity of which is the opening (os or mouth). The upper rounded portion of the u., opposite the os, is the fundus, at each extremity of which is the cornu or horn marking the part where the uterine (Fallopian) tube joins the u. and through which the ovum reaches the cavity of the womb after leaving the ovary. The organ is supported in the pelvic cavity by the broad ligaments, round ligaments, cardinal ligaments, and rectouterine and vesicouterine folds or ligaments.

   **u. acol′lis,** a u. with atresia or absence of the cervix.

   **anomalous u.,** a malformed u. caused by abnormal development or fusion of the paramesonephric ducts.

   **arcuate u., u. arcua′tus,** saddle-shaped u.; one with a depression at the fundus, an incomplete u. bicornis.

   **u. bicamera′tus vetula′rum** a condition in which fluid accumulates in and distends the cervix and body of the u., the two ora being sealed by adhesions.

   **bicornate u.,** u. bicornis.

   **u. bicor′nis,** bicornate or bifid u.; u. bifidus; one that is more or less completely divided into two lateral horns; it differs from u. septus, in which there is no external mark of separation; in u. bicornis the cervix may be single (u. bicornis unicollis) or double (u. bicornis bicollis).

   **bifid u., u. bi′fidus,** u. bicornis.

   **u. bifor′is** [ L. *bi-*, two, + *foris*, entrance ], double-mouthed u.; u. septus in which the cervix is divided into two by a septum.

   **u. bilocula′ris,** u. septus.

   **bipartite u., u. biparti′tus,** septate u.

   **capped u.,** a condition of tonic contraction of the fundus musculature of the u.

   **u. cordiform′is,** heart-shaped u.; an incomplete u. bicornis with a wedge-shaped depression at the fundus.

   **Couvelaire u.,** uteroplacental apoplexy; extravasation of blood into the uterine musculature and beneath the uterine peritoneum in association with severe forms of abruptio placentae.

   **u. didel′phys** [ G. *di-*, two, + *delphys*, womb ], dihysteria; double u. with double cervix and double vagina; due to failure of the ducts of Müller to unite.

   **u. duplex,** any u. with double lumen; it can be u. didelphys, u. bicornis bicollis, or u. septus.

   **gravid u.,** pregnant u.; *i.e.*, heavy with child.

**u. incudiform'is** [ L. of anvil form ], u. bicornis in which the fundus between the two cornua is broad and flat; also called u. planifundalis; u. triangularis.

**u. masculi'nus,** *utriculus prostaticus.*

**one-horned u.,** unicorn u.

**u. parvicol'lis,** a u. with an abnormal, disproportionately small cervix.

**Piskacek's u.,** asymmetrical enlargement of the corpus uteri by implantation of the blastocyst in one corner.

**u. planifunda'lis,** u. incudiformis.

**saddle-shaped u.,** arcate u.

**septate u., u. sep'tus,** one that is divided into two cavities by an anteroposterior septum; also called u. bilocularis, u. bipartitus.

**u. subsep'tus,** an incomplete u. septus.

**u. triangula'ris,** u. incudiformis.

**unicorn u., u. unicor'nis,** one-horned u.; one in which only one lateral half exists, the other half being undeveloped or absent.

**UTP.** Abbreviation for uridine triphosphate.

**utricle** (u'trĭ-kl) [ L. utriculus, *q.v.* ]. Utriculus.

**utricular** (u-trik'u-lar). Relating to or resembling a utricle.

**utriculitis** (u-trik-u-li'tis) [ utriculus + G. suffix *-itis*, inflammation ]. 1. Inflammation of the internal ear. 2. Inflammation of the utriculus prostaticus.

**utriculoplasty** (u-trik'u-lo-plas'tĭ) [ utriculus + G. *plassō*, to form ]. An operation for reducing the size of the uterus by excision of a wedge-shaped longitudinal strip the entire thickness of the wall of the organ.

**utriculosaccular** (u-trik'u-lo-sak'u-lar). Relating to the utricle and the saccule of the labyrinth.

**utriculus,** pl. **utriculi** (u'trik'u-lus, -li) [ L. dim. of *uter*, leather bag ] [ NA ]. Utricle; vestibular organ; the larger of the two membranous sacs in the vestibule of the labyrinth, lying in the elliptical recess; from it arise the semicircular ducts.

**u. prostaticus** [ NA ], prostatic utricle; alveus urogenitalis sinus pocularis; uterus masculinus; a minute pouch in the prostate opening on the summit of the seminal colliculus, the analogue of the uterus and vagina in the female, being the remains of the fused caudal ends of the paramesonephric (Müllerian) ducts.

**u'triform** [ L. *uter,* a skin bag, + *forma,* form ]. Shaped like a leather bottle.

**uva,** pl. **uvae** (u'vah, u've) [ L. grape. UV- ]. Grape; the fruit of *Vitus vinifera.*

**u. ur'si,** the dried leaves of *Arctostaphylos uva-ursi* (family Ericaceae), bearberry, mountain box, a common plant of the North Temperate zone; contains antiseptic glycosides, arbutin, methylarbutin, and tannins; used in chronic inflammations of the urinary tract.

**uvaefor'mis** [ L. *uva,* grape, + *forma,* form ]. *Lamina vasculosa* choroideae.

**uvea** (u've-ah) [ L. *uva,* grape ]. *Tunica vasculosa* bulbi.

**uveal** (u've-al). Relating to the uvea.

**uveitic** (u-ve-it'ik). Relating to or marked by uveitis.

**uveitides** (u-ve-it'ĭ-dēz). Plural of uveitis.

**uveitis,** pl. **uveitides** (u-ve-i'tis) [ uvea + G. suffix *-itis*, inflammation ]. Inflammation of the entire uveal tract: iris, ciliary body, and choroid.

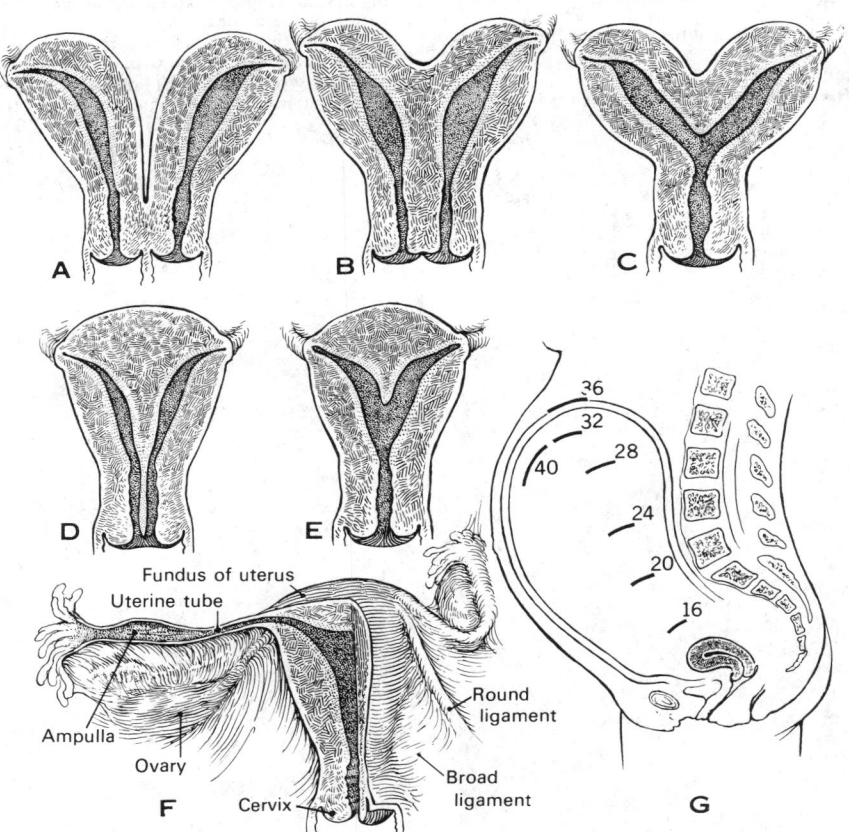

**The Uterus**

*A–E,* types of abnormal uteri: *A,* uterus didelphys; *B,* uterus bicornis bicollis; *C,* uterus bicornis unicollis; *D,* uterus septus; and *E,* uterus subseptus. *F,* normal uterus with adnexa. *G,* diagram showing changes in size and position of the uterus during pregnancy; the numbers indicate weeks on the basis of "menstrual age."

**anterior u.,** inflammation involving the ciliary body and iris.

**Förster's u.,** syphilitic changes in the entire uvea, with diffuse infiltration of nodules in the choroid and vascular changes in the retina.

**heterochromic u.,** pigmentary changes in the iris, with inflammation of the anterior uvea complicated by deposits on Descemet's membrane and by opacities in the vitreous.

**lens-induced u.,** phacoanaphylactic u.

**phacoanaphylactic u.,** lens-induced u.; intraocular inflammation occurring after extracapsular cataract extraction or needling operation; probably an autoallergic reaction to the patient's liberated lenticular proteins.

**posterior u.,** choroiditis.

**sympathetic u.,** a bilateral inflammation of the uveal tract due to a perforating wound of one eye in which damage to the uveal tract has occurred. Unless the exciting eye is enucleated within 10 days, the course is progressive until vision is lost.

**uveoencephalitis** (u've-o-en-sef-ă-li'tis). Harada's *syndrome.*

**uveoparotitis** (u've-o-păr-o-ti'tis). Uveitis associated with parotitis.

**uveoscleritis** (u've-o-skle-ri'tis). Inflammation of the sclera involved by extension from the uvea.

**u'viform** [ L. uva, grape, + *forma,* form ]. Resembling a grape or a bunch of grapes.

**uviofast** (u'vĭ-o-fast) [ uviol (ultraviolet), + fast ]. Not weakened or destroyed by subjection to ultraviolet radiation.

**uviol** (u'vĭ-ol) [ u(ltra)-viol(et) ]. A special kind of glass more than usually transparent to the ultraviolet or actinic rays.

**u'viom'eter.** An instrument for measuring ultraviolet radiation.

**uvioresis'tant.** Uviofast.

**u'viosen'sitive.** Sensitive to ultraviolet rays.

**uvul-.** See uvulo-.

**uvula,** pl. **uvuli** (u'vu-lah, -li) [ Mod. L. dim. of L. *uva,* a grape, the uvula. UV- ] [ NA ]. Appendant, fleshy mass; a structure bearing a fancied resemblance to the palatina u.

**bifid u.,** bifurcation of the u., constituting a partially cleft soft palate.

**u. cerebel'li,** u. vermis.

**Lieutaud's u.,** u. vesicae.

**u. palati'na** [ NA ], kion; cion; a conical projection from the posterior edge of the middle of the soft palate; it is composed of connective tissue containing a number of racemose glands, and some muscular fibers (musculus uvulae).

**u. ver'mis** [ NA ], u. cerebelli; a triangular elevation on the vermis of the cerebellum, lying between the two tonsils anterior to the pyramis.

**u. vesi'cae** [ NA ], Lieutaud's u.; a slight projection into the cavity of the bladder, usually more prominent in old men, just behind the urethral opening, marking the location of the middle lobe of the prostate.

**uvulaptosis** (u'vu-lap-to'sis). Uvuloptosis.

**uvular** (u'vu'lar). Relating to the uvula.

**uvularis** (u'vu-la'ris). *Musculus* uvulae.

**uvulatome** (u'vu-lă-tōm). Uvulotome.

**uvulectomy** (u'vu-lek'to-mĭ) [ uvula + G. *ektomē,* excision ]. Staphylectomy; excision of the uvula.

**uvulitis** (u'vu-li'tis). Staphylitis; inflammation of the uvula.

**uvulo-, uvul-** [ L. *uvula, q.v.* ]. Combining forms relating to the uvula (usually, the uvula palatina); see also staphylo-.

**uvuloptosis** (u'vu-lop'to'sis) [ uvulo- + G. *ptōsis,* a falling ]. Staphyloptosis; staphylodialysis; relaxation or elongation of the uvula.

**uvulotome** (u'vu-lo-tōm). Staphylotome; uvulatome; an instrument for cutting the uvula.

**uvulotomy** (u'vu-lot'o-mĭ) [ uvulo- + G. *tomē,* a cutting ]. Staphylotomy; any cutting operation on the uvula.

# V

**V.** 1. Abbreviation for vision or visual acuity. 2. Chemical symbol for the element vanadium. 3. With subscript 1, 2, 3, etc., the abbreviation for unipolar chest electrocardiogram leads. 4. Symbol for volume, frequently with subscripts denoting location, chemical species, and conditions.

**V$_{max}$.** Symbol for the maximum velocity in an enzymatic reaction, produced by increasing the substrate concentration to the point at which no further increase in velocity is obtained (see Michaelis-Menten *constant*). 2. Symbol for maximum velocity of contractile element shortening.

**V̇** [ volume + overdot denoting time derivative ]. 1. Symbol for gas *flow*, frequently with subscripts indicating location and chemical species. 2. Symbol for ventilation, frequently with a subscript; see subentries under ventilation.

**V̇CO$_2$.** Symbol for carbon dioxide *elimination*.

**V̇O$_2$.** Symbol for oxygen *consumption*.

**v.** 1. Abbreviation for volt. 2. As a subscript, refers to venous *blood*.

**v.** As a subscript, refers to mixed venous (pulmonary arterial) blood.

**vaccenic acid** (vak-sen'ik). 11-Octadecenoic acid, $CH_3(CH_2)_5CH = CH(CH_2)_9COOH$. An unsaturated fatty acid found in butter and other animal fats.

**vaccigenous** (vak-sij'en-us). Vaccinogenous.

**vaccina** (vak-si'nah). Vaccinia.

**vaccinable** (vak'si-nă-bl). Susceptible to the action of vaccine.

**vaccinal** (vak'si-nal). Relating to vaccine or vaccination.

**vaccinate** (vak'si-nāt). To administer a vaccine.

**vaccination** (vak'si-na'shun). 1. Inoculation with the virus of cowpox (vaccine, vaccinia) as a means of producing immunity against smallpox. 2. The injection of a killed culture of a specific microbe as a means of prophylaxis or cure of the disease caused by that microorganism.

**vaccinator** (vak'si-na-tor). 1. A person who vaccinates. 2. A scarifier or other instrument used in vaccination.

**vaccine** (vak'sēn) [ L. *vaccinus*, relating to a cow ]. Originally, the live vaccine (vaccinia, cowpox) virus inoculated in the skin as prophylaxis against smallpox, and obtained from the skin of calves inoculated with seed virus, but usage has extended the meaning to include essentially any preparation intended for active immunological prophylaxis—preparations of killed microbes of virulent strains or living microbes of attenuated (variant or mutant) strains; microbial, fungal, plant, protozoal, or metazoan derivatives or products. The method of administration varies according to the vaccine, inoculation being the most common, but ingestion is preferred in some instances and nasal spray is used occasionally.

**adjuvant v.,** a v. that contains an adjuvant; most often the antigen (immunogen) is included in a water-in-oil emulsion (Freund incomplete type adjuvant), or is adsorbed onto an inorganic gel (alum, aluminum hydroxide or phosphate).

**a'queous v.,** a v. having a liquid vehicle (*e.g.,* physiological salt solution), as distinguished from an emulsion.

**autog'enous v.,** a v. made from a culture of bacteria obtained from the patient himself.

**bacillus Calmette-Guérin v.,** BCG v.

**BCG v.,** bacillus Calmette-Guérin v.; a suspension of living, attenuated strain (bacillus Calmette-Guérin) of *Mycobacterium tuberculosis,* bovine type, which is inoculated into the skin for tuberculosis prophylaxis.

**brucella v.,** a living bacterial v. prepared from an attenuated variant strain of *Brucella abortus* (strain 19); used for vaccinating cattle.

**Calmette-Guérin v.,** BCG v.

**cholera v.,** an inactivated suspension of Inaba and Ogawa strains of *Vibrio cholerae* grown either on agar or in broth and preserved with phenol; the protective effect of the v., at best, is of short duration; **cholera toxoid** is the formalin-treated exotoxin (permeability factor) of *Vibrio cholerae.*

**crystal violet v.,** see hog cholera v.'s.

**Dakar v.,** yellow fever v. (2).

**diphtheria and tetanus toxoids and pertussis v.,** available in three forms: (1) diphtheria and tetanus toxoids plus pertussis vaccine (DTP); (2) tetanus and diphtheria toxoids, adult type (Td); (3) tetanus toxoid (T). Comparable amounts of tetanus toxoid are contained in all three preparations, but the adult type of diphtheria toxoid contains only about 15 to 20 per cent of that of the standard DTP material used in young children or in infants. They are prepared by treating the respective toxins with formaldehyde, and are usually adsorbed onto aluminum gel or other substances, but the fluid form (not adsorbed) is still sometimes used. Pertussis vaccine is prepared from a killed suspension of *Bordetella pertussis* or of a bacterial fraction, either fluid or adsorbed. It is recommended that vaccination begin at 2 to 3 months of age and include three intramuscular injections of DTP at 4- to 6-week intervals followed by a dose 1 year later, and again at the time of entrance to kindergarten or elementary school Afterward, Td should be given at intervals of approximately 10 years.

**duck embryo origin v.,** see rabies v., of duck embryo origin.

**Flury strain v.,** see rabies v., Flury strain egg-passage.

**foot and mouth disease virus v.'s,** v.'s either of inactivated virus from infected cattle tongue epithelium or, more recently, of live virus attenuated by embryonate egg or mouse passage and propagated in tissue culture.

**Haffkine's v.,** (1) a killed culture of *Vibrio cholerae* in two strengths, a weaker one for the initial inoculation and a stronger one for the second inoculation 7 to 10 days after the first; (2) a killed plague bacillus (*Yersinia pestis*) vaccine.

**heterog'enous v.,** v. that is not autogenous, but is prepared from the same species of bacterium.

**hog cholera v.'s,** v.'s either of virus from blood of infected swine, inactivated with crystal violet, or live virus attenuated in rabbits or tissue culture and frequently used in conjunction with hog cholera virus antiserum.

**influenza virus v.'s,** influenza virus grown in embryonate eggs and inactivated, usually by the addition of formalin. Because of the marked and progressive antigenic variation of the influenza viruses the strains included are regularly changed following various outbreaks of influenza in order to include most recently isolated epidemic strains of both type A influenza and type B influenza. Contraindicated in the case of persons sensitive (allergic) to eggs.

**live v.,** v. prepared from living, attenuated organisms.

**live oral poliovirus v.,** see poliovirus v.'s.

**measles virus v.,** (1) inactivated v., a suspension of the Edmondston strain of measles virus, propagated in monkey kidney or chick embryo tissue culture, inactivated by formaldehyde, precipitated with alum, and resuspended in buffered isotonic sodium chloride solution; now largely replaced by live v. (2) v. containing live, attenuated strains of measles virus prepared either with the attenuated strain, Edmondston B (chick embryo or canine renal cell culture), or with one of the further attenuated strains, Schwarz or Moraten (prepared only in chick embryo cell culture). The Edmondston B type is ordinarily used in combination with measles immune globulin, given in a different site with a separate syringe.

**multiv'alent v.,** polyvalent v.

**mumps v.,** (1) a suspension of mumps virus grown in chick embryo, inactivated by ultraviolet light or formaldehyde; (2) a live, attenuated virus v. prepared in chick embryo cell cultures, sprayed into the mouth.

**oil v.,** see adjuvant v.

**Pasteur v.,** see rabies v.

**pertussis v.,** see diphtheria and tetanus toxoids and pertussis v.

**plague v.,** the v. licensed for use in the United States is prepared from cultures of *Yersinia* (*Pasteurella*) *pestis,* inactivated with formaldehyde, and preserved with 0.5 per cent phenol; injections are made intramuscularly; booster inoculations are recommended every 6 to 12 months while individuals remain in an area of risk.

**poliomyelitis v.'s,** poliovirus v.'s.

**poliovirus v.'s,** inactivated poliovirus v.'s (IPV) have been largely replaced by v. of live, attenuated virus propagated in cultures of monkey kidney tissue (oral poliovirus v., OPV); and the trivalent OPV containing types I, II, and III has largely replaced use of the three types of monovalent OPV given at 6- to 8-week intervals. The primary series includes three adequately spaced doses of the trivalent OPV. It is recommended that the series start when the child is 6 to 12 weeks of age, and is commonly given with the first dose of diphtheria-tetanus-pertussis "vaccine," the second dose between 6 and 8 weeks later, and the third part, 8 to 12 months after the second. It is current practice to give a booster dose of the trivalent v. at the time the child enters school. Inactivated poliovirus v. is usually given in four parenteral doses, three at approximate intervals of 1 month, the fourth between 6 and 12 months after the third; a booster dose every several years is recommended.

**polyv'alent v.,** multivalent v.; a v. prepared from cultures of two or more strains of the same species or microorganism.

**rabies v.,** introduced by Pasteur in 1884-1885 as a method of treatment after exposure (bite of rabid animal). Daily (14 to 21) injections of virus that increased serially from noninfective to fully infective "fixed" virus were given to render the central nervous system refractory to infection by virulent virus. Pasteur's method, with but slight modification (*e.g.,* Semple v.), was used for about 75 years but had the serious defect that the large quantity of heterologous nervous tissue inoculated along with the virus occasionally gave rise to an allergic (immunological) demyelinization. It has been largely replaced, in the case of man, by rabies v. of duck embryo origin.

**rabies v., of duck embryo origin,** DEV; duck embryo origin v.; prepared from embryonate duck eggs infected with "fixed" virus inactivated with $\beta$-propiolactone; after its introduction in 1957 it largely replaced other types of v. in the United States for use in man.

**rabies v.'s, Flury strain egg passage,** (1) HEP (high egg passage) is a: living Flury strain rabies virus at the 180th to 190th level egg passage (embryonate eggs), used for vaccination of cattle and cats; (2) LEP (low egg passage) v.: at the 40th to 50th passage level, containing $10^3$ to $10^4$ mouse $LD_{50}$; nonpathogenic in dogs but retains some pathogenicity for cattle and cats.

**rabies v., Semple type,** a modification of the original Pasteur v., formerly widely used in the United States; prepared from rabbit "fixed" rabies virus and inactivated with phenol; administered in 14 to 21 daily injections.

**rickettsia v., attenuated,** see typhus v.

**Rocky Mountain spotted fever v.,** suspension of inactivated *Rickettsia rickettsii* prepared by growing the virus in the embryonate tissues of fowl eggs.

**rubella virus v., live,** a live virus v. prepared from tissue culture of avian or mammalian tissues infected with rubella virus; administered as a single subcutaneous injection. The live rubella virus v. is contraindicated in pregnancy.

**Sabin v.,** an orally administered v. containing live, attenuated strains of poliovirus; see poliovirus v.'s.

**Salk v.,** the original poliovirus v., of virus propagated in monkey kidney tissue culture and inactivated; see poliovirus v.'s.

**Semple v.,** see rabies v., Semple type.

**smallpox v.,** vaccine (vaccinia) virus suspensions prepared from cutaneous vaccinial lesions of calves (calf lymph) is the preferred v.; best inoculated into the skin by means of multiple pressure with the side of a needle or by jet injection. Contraindicated in case of skin disorders such as eczema, immunological dyscrasias, and pregnancy.

**staphylococcus v.,** a suspension of organisms from cultures of one or more strains of *Staphylococcus;* used for furunculosis, acne, and other suppurative conditions.

**stock v.,** a v. made from a stock microbial strain, in contradistinction to an autogenous v.

**T.A.B. v.,** typhoid-paratyphoid A and B v.

**tetanus v.,** see diphtheria and tetanus toxoids and pertussis v.

**tuberculosis v.,** BCG v.

**typhoid v.,** a suspension of *Salmonella typhi* inactivated either by heat or by chemical (acetone) with an added preservative; in the United States the combined typhoid and paratyphoid A and B v.'s have been largely replaced by the monovalent typhoid v. because of the lack of evidence of effectiveness of paratyphoid A and paratyphoid B ingredients.

**typhoid-paratyphoid A and B v.,** typhoid and paratyphoid v.; T.A.B. v.; a suspension of killed typhoid and paratyphoid A and B bacilli; see also typhoid v.

**typhus v.,** a formaldehyde-inactivated suspension of *Rickettsia prowazekii* grown in embryonate eggs; effective against louse-borne (epidemic) typhus; primary immunization consists of two subcutaneous injections 4 or more weeks apart; booster doses are required every 6 to 12 months, as long as the possibility of exposure exists. A v. containing living rickettsiae of an attenuated strain of *R. prowazekii* has also been used.

**whooping-cough v.,** pertussis v.

**yellow fever v.,** (1) a living, attenuated strain of yellow fever virus propagated in embryonate fowl eggs; (2) Dakar v.; Pasteur Institute Dakar; a suspension of dried mouse brain infected with French neurotropic strain of yellow fever virus, administered topically by the scratch method.

**vaccinia** (vak-sin'ĭ-ah) [ L. *vaccinus,* relating to a cow, fr. *vacca,* a cow ]. Variola vaccine; variola vaccina. 1. Cowpox; a contagious eruptive disease occurring in cattle caused by the vaccine (v.) virus; it is similar in its lesions to smallpox in man, but much milder, 2. Primary reaction; a disease, usually local and limited to the site of inoculation, induced in man by inoculation with the v. virus in order to confer resistance to smallpox. On about the third day after this vaccination, papules form at the site of inoculation which become transformed into umbilicated vesicles and later pustules; they then dry up, and the scab falls off on about the 21st day, leaving a pitted scar; in some cases there are more or less marked constitutional disturbances.

**v. gangrenosa,** progressive v.

**generalized v.,** secondary lesions of the skin following vaccination which may occur in subjects with previously healthy skin but are more common in the case of traumatized skin, especially in the case of eczema (eczema vaccinatum). In the latter instance, generalized v. may result from mere contact with a vaccinated person. Secondary vaccinial lesions may also occur following transfer of virus from the vaccination to another site by means of the fingers.

**progressive v.,** v. gangrenosa; a severe or even fatal form of v. occurring chiefly in subjects with an immunologic deficiency or dyscrasia and characterized by progressive enlargement of the initial and also of secondary lesions.

**vaccinial** (vak'sin'ĭ-al). Relating to vaccinia.

**vaccinid** (vak'sĭ-nid) [ vaccine + -id (1), q.v. ]. Allergic reaction to vaccination, with production of vesicles or papules about the area.

**vaccinifer** (vak'sin'ĭ-fer) [ vaccine + L. *fero,* to carry ]. The person from whom the vaccine was derived in the former practice of arm-to-arm vaccination.

**vacciniform** (vak'sin'ĭ-form). Resembling vaccinia (cowpox).

**vacciniola** (vak'sĭ-nĭ-o'lah) [ Mod. L. dim. of *vaccina* ]. An old term for generalized vaccinia.

**vaccinist** (vak'sĭ-nist). A vaccinator (1).

**vaccinization** (vak'sĭ-nĭ-za'shun). Vaccination repeated at short intervals until it will no longer take.

**vaccinogen** (vak-sin'o-jen). A source of vaccine, such as an inoculated heifer.

**vaccinogenous** (vak'sĭ-noj'ĕ-nus). Producing vaccine, or relating to the production of vaccine.

**vaccinoid** (vak'sĭ-noyd). Resembling vaccinia.

**vaccinophobia** (vak'sĭ-no-fo'bĭ-ah) [ vaccine + G. *phobos,* fear ]. Morbid fear of vaccination.

**vaccinostyle** (vak'sĭ-no-style). A pointed instrument used in vaccination.

**vaccinotherapy** (vak'sĭ-no-thĕr'ă-pĭ). Opsonic *therapy.*

**vaccinum** (vak'sĭ-num) [ L. ]. Vaccine.

**vacuolar** (vak'u-o'lar). Relating to or resembling a vacuole.

**vac'uolate, vac'uolated.** Having vacuoles.

**vacuolation** (vak'u-o-la'shun). Vacuolization; formation of vacuoles; the condition of having vacuoles.

**vacuole** (vak'u-ōl) [ Mod. L. *vacuolum,* dim. of L. *vacuum,* an empty space, ntr. of *vacuus,* empty, fr. *vaco,* to be empty ]. 1. A minute space in any tissue. 2. A clear space in the substance of a cell, sometimes degenerative in character, sometimes surrounding an englobed foreign body and serving as a temporary cell stomach for the digestion of the body.

  **autophagic v.,** cytolysome.

  **Barrier's v.'s,** peribronchitic abscesses.

  **contractile v.,** a cavity formed by the accumulation of fluid in the ectoplasm of a protozoan; after increasing for a time it empties itself externally by a sudden contraction; functions as a means of retaining water balance, especially in freshwater protozoans.

**vacuoliza'tion.** Vacuolation.

**vacuome** (vak'u-ōm) [ vacuole + L. noun suffix, *-oma* ]. A system of vacuoles which can be stained with neutral red in the living cell.

**vacuum** (vak'u-um) [ L. ntr. of *vacuus,* empty ]. An empty space, one practically exhausted of air or gas.

**va'dum** [ L. a ford ]. An occasional elevation from the bottom of a cerebral sulcus nearly obliterating it for a short distance.

**va'gal.** Relating to the vagus nerve.

**vagectomy** (va-jek'to-mǐ). Surgical removal of a segment of a vagus nerve.

**vagi** (va'gi, -ji). Plural of vagus.

**vagin-.** See vagino-.

**vagina,** gen. and pl. **vaginae** (vă-ji'nah, -ne) [ L. sheath, the vagina. VAGI- ] [ NA ]. 1. Any sheathlike structure. 2. The genital canal in the female, extending from the uterus to the vulva.

  **v. bul'bi** [ NA ], sheath of the eyeball; fascia bulbi; capsula bulbi; eye capsule; Tenon's capsule; a condensation of connective tissue on the outer aspect of the sclera from which it is separated by a narrow cleftlike space. The sheath is attached to the sclera near the sclerocorneal junction and blends with the fascia of the extraocular muscles.

  **v. carot'ica** [ NA ], carotid sheath; the dense fibrous investment of the carotid artery, internal jugular vein, and vagus nerve on each side; the layers of cervical fascia blend with it.

  **v. cellulo'sa,** the connective tissue sheath of a nerve or muscle (perineurium or perimysium, respectively).

  **v. exter'na ner'vi op'tici** [ NA ], the outer sheath around the optic nerve, continuous with the pachymeninx (dura mater).

  **vagi'nae fibro'sae digito'rum ma'nus** [ NA ], fibrous sheaths of the digits of the hand; the tubular fibrous layers that enclose the synovial sheaths and the superficial and deep flexor tendons and the tendon of the flexor pollicis longus in their passage along their respective digits; they are composed of annular and cruciform parts; see *pars* anularis vaginae fibrosae and *pars* cruciformis vaginae fibrosae.

  **vaginae fibro'sae digito'rum pe'dis** [ NA ], fibrous sheaths of the toes; the tubular fibrous layer enclosing the synovial sheath and the tendons of the long and short flexors of the toes and the flexor hallucis longus in the digits; they are composed of annular and cruciform parts; see *pars* anularis vaginae fibrosae and *pars* cruciformis vaginae fibrosae.

  **v. fibro'sa ten'dinis** [ NA ], fibrous sheath of a tendon.

  **v. fixu'ra,** fixation of the v.

  **v. inter'na ner'vi op'tici** [ NA ], the innermost sheath around the optic nerve, continuous with the leptomeninges (pia-arachnoid).

  **v. masculi'na,** *utriculus* prostaticus.

  **v. muco'sa ten'dinis,** v. synovialis tendinis.

  **v. mus'culi rec'ti abdo'minis** [ NA ], sheath of the rectus abdominis, formed by the aponeuroses of the three anterolateral muscles of the abdominal wall that split to enclose the rectus and fuse medially to form the linea alba. It consists of a lamina anterior and a lamina posterior, the latter being absent below the linea arcuata (semicircular line).

  **vagi'nae ner'vi op'tici,** sheaths of the optic nerve, formed by extensions of the central meninges; see v. interna nervi optici and v. externa nervi optici.

  **v. oc'uli,** v. bulbi.

  **v. proces'sus styloi'dei** [ NA ], sheath of the styloid process; vaginal process; a crest of bone (edge of the tympanic portion of the temporal bone) running from the front and medial side of the mastoid process to the spine of the sphenoid; it splits to ensheathe the base of the styloid process.

  **v. sep'ta,** a bipartite v. caused by the presence of a more or less complete longitudinal septum.

  **v. synovia'lis commu'nis musculo'rum flexo'rum** [ NA ], ulnar bursa; common synovial flexor sheath; the synovial sheath that surrounds the tendons of the superficial and deep flexors of the digits as they pass through the carpal canal; it is commonly continuous with the digital sheath of the little finger.

  **vagi'nae synovia'les digito'rum ma'nus** [ NA ], synovial sheaths of the digits of the hand; the synovial sheaths that enclose the flexor tendons of the fingers and line the inside of the fibrous tendon sheaths.

  **vagi'nae synovia'les digito'rum pe'dis** [ NA ], synovial sheaths of the digits of the foot; similar in structure to the corresponding sheaths of the hand.

  **v. synovia'lis intertubercula'ris** [ NA ], intertubercular synovial sheath; the extension of the synovial membrane of the shoulder joint downward in the intertubercular groove to surround the tendon of the long head of the biceps.

  **v. synovia'lis musculo'rum obli'qui superio'ris** [ NA ], synovial sheath of the superior oblique muscle; synovial trochlear bursa; v. synovialis trochleae; the synovial sheath enclosing the tendon of the superior oblique muscle as it passes through the trochlea.

  **v. synovia'lis musculo'rum perone'orum commu'nis** [ NA ], the synovial sheath that surrounds the tendons of the peroneus longus and brevis muscles in their passage across the ankle.

  **v. synovialis ten'dinis** [ NA ], synovial sheath of a tendon; vaginal synovial membrane; a sheath of synovial membrane enveloping certain of the tendons; it contains a small amount of synovial fluid.

  **v. synovia'lis ten'dinis mus'culi flexo'ris carpi radia'lis** [ NA ], the synovial sheath enclosing the tendon of the flexor carpi radialis as it crosses the wrist.

  **v. synovia'lis ten'dinis mus'culi flexo'ris hallu'cis longi** [ NA ], the synovial sheath that envelopes the tendon of the flexor hallucis longus as it passes into the foot deep to the flexor retinaculum.

  **v. synovia'lis ten'dinis mus'culi tibia'lis posterio'ris** [ NA ], the synovial sheath surrounding the tendon of the tibialis posterior as it passes into the foot deep to the flexor retinaculum.

  **v. synovia'lis troch'leae,** v. synovialis musculorum obliqui superioris.

  **v. ten'dinis mus'culi extenso'ris carpi ulna'ris** [ NA ], the synovial sheath surrounding the tendon of the extensor carpi ulnaris in its course deep to the extensor retinaculum.

  **v. ten'dinis mus'culi extenso'ris dig'iti min'imi** [ NA ], the synovial sheath surrounding the tendon of the extensor digiti minimi in its passage deep to the extensor retinaculum.

  **v. ten'dinis mus'culi extenso'ris hallu'cis lon'gi** [ NA ], the synovial sheath that surrounds the tendon of the extensor hallucis longus in its passage across the ankle.

  **v. ten'dinis mus'culi extenso'ris pol'licis lon'gi** [ NA ], the synovial sheath surrounding the extensor pollicis longus tendon in its passage deep to the extensor retinaculum.

  **v. ten'dinis mus'culi flexo'ris pol'licis lon'gi** [ NA ], radial bursa; the synovial sheath that envelopes the tendon of the flexor pollicis longus in its course through the carpal canal; it is continuous with the digital sheath of the thumb, the two generally being considered as one sheath.

  **v. ten'dinis mus'culi perone'i lon'gi planta'ris** [ NA ], the synovial sheath surrounding the tendon of the peroneus longus in its course across the sole of the foot.

  **v. ten'dinis mus'culi tibia'lis anterio'ris** [ NA ], the synovial sheath, deep to the extensor retinaculum, that surrounds the tendon of the tibialis anterior as it crosses the ankle.

  **v. ten'dinum mus'culi extenso'ris digito'rum pe'dis lon'gi** [ NA ], the synovial sheath that surrounds the tendons of the long extensor and the peroneus tertius in their passage across the ankle.

**v. ten′dinum mus′culi flexo′ris digito′rum pe′dis lon′gi** [ NA ], the synovial sheath that envelopes the flexor digitorum longus tendons as they pass into the foot deep to the flexor retinaculum.

**v. ten′dinum musculo′rum abducto′ris lon′gi et extenso′ris bre′vis pol′licis** [ NA ], the synovial sheath lining the compartment of the extensor retinaculum that contains the abductor pollicis longus and extensor pollicis brevis tendons.

**v. ten′dinum musculo′rum extenso′rum car′pi radia′lium** [ NA ], the synovial sheath lining the compartment of the extensor retinaculum containing the tendons of the extensor carpi radialis longus and brevis muscles.

**v. ten′dinum musculo′rum extenso′ris digitor′um et extenso′ris in′dicis** [ NA ], the synovial sheath that surrounds the four tendons of the extensor digitorum muscle and the tendon of the extensor indicis deep to the extensor retinaculum.

**vagi′nae vaso′rum,** sheaths of the vessels; fibrous envelopes ensheathing the arteries with their accompanying veins and sometimes nerves as well.

**vaginal** (vaj′ĭ-nal) [ Mod. L. *vaginalis* ]. Relating to the vagina or to any sheath.

**vaginalectomy** (vaj′ĭ-nă-lek′to-mĭ). Vaginectomy (2); excision of a portion of the tunica vaginalis testis.

**vaginalitis** (vaj′ĭ-nă-li′tis). Inflammation of the tunica vaginalis testis.

**vaginapexy** (vă-ji′nă-pek′sĭ). Vaginofixation.

**vaginate** (vaj′ĭ-nāt). 1. To ensheathe; to enclose in a sheath. 2. Ensheathed; provided with a sheath.

**vaginectomy** (vaj′ĭ-nek′to-mĭ) [ vagina + G. *ektomē*, excision ]. 1. Colpectomy; excision of the vagina, or a segment thereof. 2. Vaginalectomy.

**vaginicoline** (vaj′ĭ-nik′o-lĭn) [ vagina + L. *colo*, to inhabit ]. Inhabiting the vagina; denoting certain microorganisms normally there present.

**vaginism** (vaj′ĭ-nizm). Vaginismus.

**vaginismus** (vaj′ĭ-niz′mus) [ vagina + L. suffix *-ismus*, action, condition ]. Vaginism; vulvismus; painful involuntary spasm of the vagina preventing intromission or withdrawal of the penis; often associated with aversion to coitus.

    **mental v.,** v. caused by repugnance to the sexual act.

    **posterior v.,** spasmodic stenosis of the vagina caused by contraction of the levator ani muscle.

**vaginitis,** pl. **vaginitides** (vaj′ĭ-ni′tis, -ni′tĭ-dēz) [ vagina + G. suffix *-itis*, inflammation ]. Colpitis; elytritis; inflammation of the vagina.

    **v. adhesi′va,** inflammation of vaginal mucosa with adhesions of the vaginal walls to each other.

    **amebic v.,** v. caused by *Entamoeba histolytica.*

    **atrophic v.,** thinning and atrophy of the vaginal epithelium usually resulting from diminished endocrine stimulation; a common occurrence in postmenopausal women.

    **bovine granular v.,** a very common contagious disease of cattle transmitted by coitus and manifested by the appearance of small shotlike transparent nodules in the mucosa of the vagina of cows and of the penis of bulls; the mucosa is reddened and a mucopurulent exudate appears on the affected surfaces; the precise cause is not known.

    **v. cystica,** v. characterized by bullae in the vaginal wall.

    **desquamative inflammatory v.,** an acute inflammation of vagina of unknown cause, characterized by grayish psuedomembrane, free discharge, and easy bleeding on trauma. The discharge contains pus and immature epithelial cells, although estrogen levels are normal.

    **v. emphysemato′sa,** v. attended with an accumulation of gas in the connective tissue.

    **v. seni′lis,** v. occurring in old age, often assuming the form of v. adhesiva; atrophic v. resulting from withdrawal of estrogen stimulation of mucosa.

**vagino-, vagin-** (vaj′ĭ-no-) [ L. *vagina*, sheath. VAGI- ]. Combining forms relating to vagina. For some words beginning thus, and not found here, see colpo-, colp-.

**vaginoabdominal** (vaj′ĭ-no-ab-dom′ĭ-nal). Relating to the vagina and the abdomen.

**vaginocele** (vaj′ĭ-no-sēl). Colpocele.

**vaginodynia** (vaj′ĭ-no-din′ĭ-ah). Colpodynia; colpalgia; vaginal pain.

**vaginofixation** (vaj′ĭ-no-fik-sa′shun). Colpopexy; vaginopexy; vaginapexy; suture of a relaxed and prolapsed vagina to the abdominal wall.

**vaginogenic** (vaj′ĭ-no-jen′ik). Originating in the vagina.

**vaginohysterectomy** (vaj′ĭ-no-his-ter-ek′to-mĭ). Vaginal *hysterectomy.*

**vaginolabial** (vaj′ĭ-no-la′bĭ-al). Relating to the vagina and the pudendal labia.

**vaginomycosis** (vaj′ĭ-no-mi-ko′sis). Colpomycosis; colpitis mycotica; inflammation (infection) of the vagina due to a fungus.

**vaginopathy** (vaj′ĭ-nop′ă-thĭ) [ vagino- + G. *pathos*, suffering ]. Colpopathy; any diseased condition of the vagina.

**vaginoperineal** (vaj′ĭ-no-pĕr-ĭ-ne′al). Relating to or involving the vagina and perineum.

**vaginoperineoplasty** (vaj′ĭ-no-pĕr-ĭ-ne′o-plas′tĭ) [ vagino- + perineum, + G. *plassō*, to form ]. Colpoperineoplasty; plastic surgery for repair of a rupture of the perineum involving the vagina.

**vaginoperineorraphy** (vaj′ĭ-no-pĕr-ĭ-ne-or′ă-fĭ) [ vagino- + perineum, + G. *raphē*, suture ]. Colpoperineorrhaphy; sutural repair of the vagina and perineum in cases of laceration.

**vaginoperineotomy** (vaj′ĭ-no-pĕr-ĭ-ne-ot′′o-mĭ) [ vagino- + perineum + G. *tome*, incision ]. Division of the outlet of the vagina and adjacent portion of the perineum to facilitate childbirth.

**vaginoperitoneal** (vaj′ĭ-no-pĕr-ĭ-to-ne′al). Relating to the vagina and the peritoneum.

**vaginopexy** (vaj′ĭ-no-pek′sĭ). Vaginofixation.

**vaginoplasty** (vaj′ĭ-no-plas′tĭ). Colpoplasty; elytroplasty; plastic surgery involving the vagina.

**vaginoscope** (vaj′ĭ-no-skōp) [ vagino- + G. *skopeō*, to view ]. A vaginal speculum.

**vaginoscopy** (vaj′ĭ-nos′ko-pĭ). Inspection of the vagina, usually with an instrument.

**vaginotome** (vaj′ĭ-no-tōm). A device for cutting the tissues of the vaginal intractus or enlarging the vaginal entrance.

**vaginotomy** (vaj′ĭ-not′o-mĭ). Colpotomy; coleotomy (2); elytrotomy; a cutting operation in the vagina.

**vaginovesical** (vaj′ĭ-no-ves′ĭ-kal). Relating to the vagina and the urinary bladder.

**vaginovulvar** (vaj′ĭ-no-vul′var). Relating to the vagina and the vulva.

**vagitis** (va-gi′tis) [ vagus + G. suffix *-itis*, inflammation ]. Obsolete term for inflammation of the vagus nerve.

**vagitus** (vă-ji′tus) [ L. fr. *vagio*, to squall ]. The crying of an infant.

    **v. uteri′nus,** crying of the fetus while still within the womb, possible when the membranes have been ruptured and air has entered the uterine cavity.

**va′go-** [ L. *vagus, q.v.* ]. Combining form relating to the vagus nerve.

**vagoaccessorius** (va-go-ak-ses-so′rĭ-us). The vagus and the accessory portion of the spinal accessory nerve, regarded as one nerve.

**vagoglossopharyngeal** (va′go-glos′o-fă-rin′je-al). Relating to the vagus and glossopharyngeal nerves; denoting their adjacent nuclei of origin and termination, or regions innervated by both nerves such as the musculature of the pharynx.

**vagolysis** (va-gol′ĭ-sis) [ vago- + G. *lysis*, a loosening ]. Surgical destruction of the vagus nerve.

**va′golyt′ic.** 1. Pertaining to or causing vagolysis. 2. A therapeutic or chemical agent that has inhibitory effects on the vagus nerve.

**vagomimetic** (va′go-mĭ-met′ik). Mimicking the action of the efferent fibers of the vagus nerve.

**vagotomy** (va-got′o-mĭ) [ vago- + G. *tomē*, incision ]. Division of the vagus nerve.

**vagotonia** (va′go-to′nĭ-ah) [ vago- + G. *tonos*, strain ]. Irritability of the vagus nerve, often marked by excessive peristalsis and loss of the pharyngeal reflex; opposed to sympathicotonia.

**vagotonic** (va-go-ton′ik). Relating to or marked by vagotonia.

**vagotropic** (va-go-trop′ik) [ vago- + G. *tropos*, turning ]. Attracted by, hence acting upon, the vagus nerve.

**vagovagal** (va′go-va′gal). Pertaining to a process that utilizes both afferent and efferent vagal fibers.

**vagus**, gen. and pl. **vagi** (va′gus, va′gi, -ji) [ L. wandering, so-called because of the wide distribution of the nerve ]. *Nervus* vagus.

**vagusstoff** (va′gus-shtof, vah-goos-) [ vagus + Ger. *Stoff*, substance ]. A chemical substance liberated at the endings of the vagus when this nerve is stimulated; it has an action identical with that of acetylcholine and is generally believed to be the latter substance.

**Val.** Symbol for valine and its radicals.

**va′lence, va′lency** [ L. *valentia*, strength ]. Quantivalence; equivalence; the combining power of one atom of an element (or a radical), that of the hydrogen atom being the unit of comparison. Thus, in HCl, chlorine is monovalent; in $H_2O$, oxygen is bivalent (or divalent); in $NH_3$, nitrogen is trivalent, and so on. It is determined by the number of electrons in the outer shell of the atom, the v. electrons.

    **negative v.,** indicates the number of valence electrons an atom can take up.

    **positive v.,** indicates the number of valence electrons an atom can give up.

**va′lent.** Possessing valency.

**Valen′tin,** Gabriel G., German physiologist, 1810–1883. See V.'s *corpuscles, ganglion, nerve.*

**Valentine,** Ferdinand C., New York surgeon, 1851–1909. See V.'s *position, test.*

**val′eral, valeral′dehyde.** Valeric aldehyde; a colorless liquid, $CH_3(CH_2)_3CHO$, obtained by the oxidation of amyl alcohol. Used as a flavor and in the manufacture of synthetic resins.

**val′erate.** Valerianate, a salt of valeric or valerianic acid.

**valerian** (vă-lēr′ĭ-an). Vandal root; garden heliotrope; the rhizome and roots of *Valeriana officinalis* (family Valerianaceae), a herb native in Southern Europe and Northern Asia, cultivated also in England and America. Has been used as a sedative in hysteria and at the menopause.

**vale′rianate.** Valerate.

**valeric acid** (vă-lĕr′ik, vă-lēr′ik). Pentanoic acid; normal aliphatic acid; $C_4H_9COOH$; distilled from valerian root. Some of its salts are used in medicine.

**valeth′amate bromide.** MUREL; 2-diethylaminoethyl 3-methyl-2-phenylvalerate methylbromide; a quaternary ammonium compound predominantly anticholinergic in action; used as an antispasmodic.

**valetudinarian** (val′e-tu′dĭ-nĕr′ĭ-an) [ L. *valetudinarius*, sickly ]. An invalid or person in chronically poor health.

**valetudina′rianism.** A weak or infirm state due to invalidism.

**valgoid** (val′goyd) [ L. *valgus*, bowlegged, + G. *eidos*, resemblance ]. Relating to valgus; bowlegged (more commonly, knock-kneed); suffering from talipes valgus.

**val′gus** [ Mod. L. turned outward, fr. L. bowlegged ]. Bent or twisted outward.

**val′id** [ L. *valeo*, to be strong ]. Effective; producing the desired result.

**validation** (val-i-da′shun). The act or process of making valid.

    **consensual v.,** the confirmation of the experience or judgment of one person by another.

**val′ine.** 2-Aminoisovaleric acid; 2-amino-3-methylbutanoic acid; $(CH_3)_2CHCH(NH_2)COOH$; a constituent of most proteins.

**val′late** [ L. *vallo*, pp. *-atus*, to surround with, fr. *vallum*, a rampart ]. Cupped; surrounded with an elevation; circumvallate.

**vallecula**, pl. **valleculae** (vă-lek′u-lah, -le) [ L. dim. of *vallis*, valley ] [ NA ]. A crevice or depression on any surface.

    **v. cerebel′li** [ NA ], vallis; a deep hollow on the inferior surface of the cerebellum, between the hemispheres, in which the medulla oblongata rests.

    **v. epiglot′tica** [ NA ], a depression between the median and lateral glossoepiglottic folds on either side.

    **v. syl′vii,** *fossa* lateralis cerebri.

    **v. un′guis,** *sulcus* matricis unguis.

**Valleix** (val-a′e), François L. I., Paris physician, 1807–1855. See V.'s *points.*

**val′ley.** Vallecula.

**val′lis** [ L. valley ]. *Vallecula* cerebelli.

**vallum**, pl. **valla** (val′um, -ah) [ L. a rampart, fr. *vallus*, a stake ]. 1 [ NA ]. Any raised, more or less circular ridge. 2. The slightly raised outer wall of the circular depression, or fossa, surrounding a vallate papilla of the tongue.

    **v. un′guis** [ NA ], wall of the nail; the fold of skin overlapping the lateral and proximal margins of the nail.

**valnoc′tamide** (USAN). NIRVANIL; 2-ethyl-3-methylvaleramide; antianxiety agent.

**valoid** (val′oyd) [ L. *valeo*, to be strong ]. Equivalent *extract.*

**Valsal′va,** Antonio M., Italian anatomist, 1666–1723. See V.'s *experiment, ligaments, maneuver, muscle, sinus, teniae, test.*

**value** (val′u). A particular quantitative determination. Definitions of some chemical v.'s are given under specific names (*e.g.,* acetyl v., buffer v., caloric v., iodine v., saponification v.).

    **globular v.,** color *index.*

    **maturation v.,** an indicator of the level of maturation attained by the vaginal epithelium; derived from the maturation index (*q. v.*) by valuing the parabasal cells at 0.0, the intermediate cells at 0.5, and the superficial cells at 1.0; for special investigations, subtypes of a major cell type can be given different values. Used as one factor in cytohormonal evaluation.

**valva**, pl. **valvae** (val′vah, -ve) [ L. one leaf of a double door ] [ NA ]. Valve; valvula.

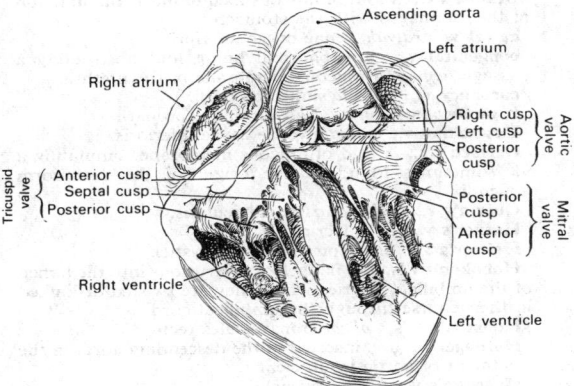

**Valves of the Heart**

    **v. aor′tae** [ NA ], aortic valve; the valve between the left ventricle and the ascending aorta, consisting of three fibrous semilunar cusps (valvulae semilunares), located in the adult as anterior, right posterior, and left posterior; they are named in the NA, however, in accordance with the embryonic arrangement in which the cusps are posterior, left, and right.

    **v. atrioventricula′ris dex′tra** [ NA ], valva tricuspidalis [ NA ]; right atrioventricular valve; tricuspid valve; the valve closing the orifice between the right atrium and right ventricle of the heart; its three cusps are called anterior, posterior, and septal.

    **v. atrioventricula′ris sinis′tra** [ NA ], valva mitralis [ NA ]; left atrioventricular valve; mitral valve; valvula bicuspidalis; the valve closing the orifice between the left atrium and left ventricle of the heart; its two cusps are called anterior and posterior.

    **v. ileoceca′lis,** [ NA ], ileocecal or ileocolic valve; valve of Bauhin, Tulp (Tulpius), or Varolius; ileocecal eminence; ileal papilla; the bilabial prominence of the terminal ileum into the large intestine at the cecocolic junction as seen in cadavers; in the living individual it appears as a truncated cone with a star-shaped orifice.

**v. mitra'lis** [ NA ], mitral valve; official alternate term for v. atrioventricularis sinistra.

**v. tricuspida'lis** [ NA ], tricuspid valve; official alternate term for v. atrioventricularis dextra.

**v. trun'ci pulmona'lis** [ NA ], valve of the pulmonary trunk; pulmonary valve; the valve at the entrance to the pulmonary trunk from the right ventricle; it consists of semilunar cusps (valvulae semilunares) which are usually arranged in the adult so that there is a right anterior, a left anterior, and a posterior cusp. The NA terminology names these cusps as right, left, and anterior, in conformity with their embryonic position.

**val'val, val'var.** Relating to a valve.

**val'vate.** Valvular; relating to or provided with a valve.

**valve** [ L. *valva, q.v.* ]. Valva; valvula. 1. A fold of the lining membrane of a canal or other hollow organ serving to retard or prevent a reflux of fluid. 2. Any reduplication of tissue or flaplike structure resembling a valve. See also valva, valvula, and plica.

**Amussat's v.,** *plica* spiralis ductus cystici.

**anal v.'s,** *valvulae* anales.

**anterior urethral v.,** a crescentic horizontal fold at the level of the penoscrotal junction.

**aor'tic v.,** *valva* aortae.

**atrioventricular v.'s,** *valva* atrioventricularis dextra and sinistra.

**Bauhin's v.,** *valva* ileocecalis.

**Béraud's v.,** Krause's v.; a small fold in the interior of the lacrimal sac at its junction with the lacrimal duct.

**Bianchi's v.,** a v. at the lower end of the nasolacrimal duct.

**bicuspid v.,** *valva* atrioventricularis sinistra.

**Bochdalek's v.,** Foltz' valvule; a fold of mucous membrane in the lacrimal canaliculus at the punctum lacrimale.

**Braune's v.,** a fold of mucous membrane at the junction of the esophagus with the stomach.

**ca'val v.,** *valvula* venae cavae inferioris.

**congenital v.,** an abnormal lining fold obstructing a passage, *e.g.,* of a mucous membrane in the urethra.

**coronary v.,** *valvula* sinus coronarii.

**v. of coronary sinus,** *valvula* sinus coronarii.

**Eustachian v.,** *valvula* venae cavae inferioris.

**Gerlach's v.,** a fold of mucous membrane, simulating a v., sometimes found at the origin of the vermiform appendix.

**Guérin's v.,** *valvula* fossae navicularis.

**Hasner's v.,** *plica* lacrimalis.

**Heister's v.,** *plica* spiralis ductus cystici.

**Hoboken's v.'s,** the flangelike protrusions into the lumen of the umbilical arteries where they are twisted or kinked in their course through the umbilical cord.

**Houston's v.'s,** *plicae* transversales recti.

**Hufnagel v.,** a v. inserted in the descending aorta in the treatment of aortic insufficiency.

**Huschke's v.,** *plica* lacrimalis.

**ileoce'cal v.,** *valva* ileocecalis.

**ileocolic v.,** *valva* ileocecalis.

**v. of the inferior vena cava,** *valvula* venae cavae inferioris.

**Kerckring's v.'s,** *plicae* circulares.

**Kohlrausch's v.'s,** *plicae* transversales recti.

**Krause's v.,** Béraud's v.

**left atrioventricular v.,** *valva* atrioventricularis sinistra.

**Mercier's v.,** an occasional fold of mucosa of the bladder partially occluding the ureteral orifice.

**mitral v.,** *valva* atrioventricularis sinistra.

**Morgagni's v.'s,** *valvulae* anales.

**nasal v.,** the variable aperture between the nasal septum and the moveable inferior margin of the lateral nasal cartilage.

**nonrebreathing v.,** a type of v. that prevents mixture of inhaled and exhaled gases; widely used in inhalation therapy and anesthesia.

**parachute mitral v.,** congenital deformity of the mitral v. in which there is only one papillary muscle present; the chordae of both v. leaflets converge to insert into this single muscle.

**posterior urethral v.'s,** anomalous folds occurring at the level of the verumontanum.

**pul'monary v.,** *valva* trunci pulmonalis.

**pylor'ic v.,** *valvula* pylori.

**rectal v.,** *plica* transversalis recti.

**reducing v.,** a v. designed to lower the pressure of a gas coming from a cylinder containing compressed gas under high pressure.

**right atrioventricular v.,** *valva* atrioventricularis dextra.

**Rosenmüller's v.,** *plica* lacrimalis.

**semilunar v.,** *valvula* semilunaris.

**spiral v.,** *plica* spiralis ductus cystici.

**Sylvian v.,** *valvula* venae cavae inferioris.

**Tarin's v.,** *velum* medullare inferius.

**Terrier's v.,** a valvelike fold between the gallbladder and the cystic duct.

**Thebesian v.,** *valvula* sinus coronarii.

**tricuspid v.,** *valva* atrioventricularis dextra.

**Tulp's** or **Tulpius' v.,** *valva* ileocecalis.

**urethral v.'s,** folds in the urethral mucous membrane; see also anterior urethral v. and posterior urethral v.'s.

**v. of Varolius,** *valva* ileocecalis.

**venous v.,** *valvula* venosa.

**vesicoureteral v.,** a lock mechanism in the wall of the intravesical portion of the ureter that normally prevents urinary reflux.

**Vieussens' v.,** *velum* medullare superius.

**valveless** (valv'les). Without valves; denoting certain veins, such as the portal, that are not provided with valves as are most of the veins.

**val'viform.** Valve-shaped.

**valvoplasty** (val'vo-plas'tǐ) [ valve + G. *plassō,* to form ]. Surgical reconstruction of a deformed cardiac valve, for the relief of stenosis or incompetence.

**valvotomy** (val-vot'o-mǐ) [ valve + G. *tomē,* incision ]. Valvulotomy. 1. Cutting through a valve; specifically, an incision of too large or rigid rectal folds. 2. Cutting through a stenosed cardiac valve to relieve the obstruction.

**rectal v.,** cutting through rectal folds that are too rigid or too large.

**valvula,** pl. **valvulae** (val'vu-lah, -le) [ Mod. L. dim of *valva* ] [ NA ]. Valvule; a valve, especially one of small size.

**Amussat's v.,** a fold of the urethral mucous membrane, generally conceded to be abnormal, seen below the prostatic sinuses on either side of the seminal colliculus.

**valvulae ana'les** [ NA ], anal valves; Morgagni's valves; delicate crescent-shaped mucosal folds that pass between the lower ends of neighboring anal columns; the small pocket thus formed is an anal sinus.

**v. bicuspida'lis,** *valva* atrioventricularis sinistra.

**v. conni'vens,** pl. **val'vulae conniven'tes,** *plicae* circulares.

**v. fora'minis ova'lis** [ NA ], falx septi; a fold projecting into the left atrium from the margin of the foramen ovale in the fetus; when, with beginning inspiration, the blood pressure within the left atrium increases, the valve closes and its edges become adherent to the margin of the foramen ovale, occluding it.

**v. fos'sae navicula'ris** [ NA ], Guérin's valve or fold; a fold of mucous membrane sometimes found in the root of the fossa navicularis urethrae.

**Gerlach's v.,** *ligamentum* pectinatum anguli iridocornea-lis.

**v. lymphat'ica** [ NA ], lymphatic valvule; one of the delicate semilunar valves found in lymphatic vessels; they are usually paired and similar in structure to venous valves and occur at close intervals along the vessel wall.

**v. proces'sus vermifor'mis,** a fold of mucous membrane at the opening of the vermiform appendix into the cecum.

**v. prostat'ica,** median *bar.*

**v. pylor'i,** pyloric valve; a prominent fold of mucous membrane at the gastroduodenal junction enclosing the gastroduodenal pylorus.

**v. semiluna'ris** [ NA ], semilunar valve; one of three semilunar segments serving as the three cusps of a valve preventing regurgitation at the beginning of the aorta; a similar valve guards the entrance of the pulmonary trunk the segments are named, respectively, anterior, right, and left in the right ventricle, and posterior, right, and left in the left ventricle.

**v. semiluna'ris tari'ni,** *velum* medullare inferius.

**v. si'nus corona'rii** [ NA ], valve of the coronary sinus; Thebesian valve; coronary valve; a delicate fold of endocardium at the opening of the coronary sinus into the right atrium.

**v. spiral'is,** *plica* spiralis ductus cystici.

**v. tricuspida'lis,** *valva* atrioventricularis dextra.

**v. ve'nae ca'vae inferio'ris** [ NA ], valve of the inferior vena cava; caval valve; Eustachian or Sylvian valve; an endocardial fold extending from the anterior inferior margin of the inferior vena cava to the anterior part of the limbus fossa ovalis.

**v. veno'sa,** (1) in the embryo, one of the pair of valves that guard the opening from the sinus venosus into the right atrium; (2) [ NA ] venous valve; a fold of the lining layer of a vein to prevent a reflux of blood.

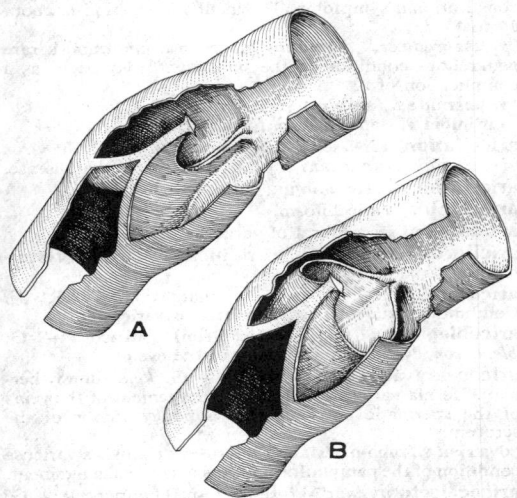

**Venous Valves in Femoral Vein**
*A*, closed; *B*, open.

**v. vestib'uli,** old term for valvulae venosae (1).

**val'vular.** Relating to a valve; valval; valvar.

**valvule** (val'vūl) [ L. *valvula, q.v.* ]. Valvula; a small valve.
   **Foltz' v.,** Bochdalek's *valve*.
   **lymphatic v.,** *valvula* lymphatica.

**valvulitis** (val'vu-li'tis) [ Mod. L. *valvula,* valve, + G. suffix *-itis,* inflammation ]. Inflammation of a valve, especially a heart valve.
   **rheumatic v.,** v. characterized in the acute stage by small fibrin vegetations along the lines of closure and by Aschoff bodies in the cusps; in the chronic stage, it is characterized by scarring, commissural adhesion, and stenosis or regurgitation.

**val'vuloplasty.** Valvoplasty.

**val'vulotome.** An instrument for sectioning a valve.

**valvulot'omy.** Valvotomy.

**val'yl.** The radical of valine.

**Van** or **van.** For some names with this prefix not found below, see the principal part of the name.

**van'adate.** A salt of vanadic acid.

**vanad'ic acid.** an acid, $H_3VO_4$, derived from vanadium, forming salts with various bases.

**vanadium** (vă-na′dĭ-um) [ *Vanadis,* a goddess of Scandinavian mythology ]. A metallic element, symbol V, atomic no. 23, atomic weight 50.95, of light gray color. The salts of v. have been used in various chronic diseases, but with doubtful beneficial effects.
   **v. group,** those elements resembling v. in chemical and metallurgical properties. Included with v. itself in this group are niobium (columbium) and tantalum.

**Van Allen,** James A., American physicist, *1914. See V. A. *phenomena.*

**van Bogaert,** Ludo, Belgian neuropathologist. See v. B.'s *encephalitis.*

**Van Buchem,** F. S. See V. B.'s *syndrome.*

**van Buren,** William H., New York surgeon, 1819–1883. See v. B.'s *disease.*

**vancomycin** (van'ko-mi'sin). Vancomycin hydrochloride (USP, BP); an antibiotic isolated from cultures of *Streptomyces orientalis* present in soil from India and Borneo. It is bactericidal and bacteriostatic against Gram-positive organisms.

**van Creveld,** S., Dutch physician, *1894. See Ellis-v. C. *syndrome.*

**van'dal root.** Valerian.

**van Deen** (dān), Izaak A., Dutch physiologist, 1804–1869. See v. D.'s *test.*

**van den Bergh,** A. A. H., Dutch physician, 1869–1943. See v. d. B.'s *test.*

**van der Kolk,** Jacobus L. C. S., Dutch physician, 1797–1862. See v. d. K.'s *law.*

**van der Spiegel.** See Spigelius.

**van der Velden,** Rienhardt, German physician, 1851–1903. See v. d. V.'s *test.*

**van der Waals,** Johannes D., Dutch physical chemist, *1837. See v. d. W.'s *forces.*

**van Ermengen,** Emile P., Belgian bacteriologist, 1851–1932. See v. E.'s *method.*

**van Gehuchten** (fahn ga-hoohk'ten), Arthur, Belgian anatomist, 1861–1915. See v. G.'s *fixative.*

**Vanghetti** (vahn-get'e), Giuliano, Italian surgeon, 1861–1940. See V.'s *prosthesis.*

**van Gieson** (ge'son), Ira, New York histologist and bacteriologist, 1865–1913. See v. G.'s *stain.*

**van Helmont,** Jean B., French physician and chemist, 1577–1644. See v. H.'s *mirror.*

**van Hoorne** (horn), Jan, Dutch anatomist, 1621–1670. See v. H.'s *canal.*

**vanilla** (vă-nil'ah) [ Sp. *vainilla,* little pod ] (NF). The cured, full-grown, unripe fruit of *Vanila planifolia* (Mexican or Bourbon v.) or of *V. tahitensis* (Tahiti v.), orchids (family Orchidaceae) native to Mexico and cultivated in other tropical countries; a flavoring agent.

**vanil'late.** A compound of vanillic acid; $C_8H_8O_4$.

**vanil'lic acid.** Methylprotocatechuic acid; 4-hydroxy-3-methoxybenzoic acid; $CH_3O—C_6H_3(OH)COOH$; a flavoring agent.

**vanil'lin** (USP). Methylprotocatechuic aldehyde; vanillic aldehyde; 4-hydroxy-3-methoxybenzaldehyde; obtained from vanilla and also prepared synthetically; a flavoring agent.

**vanil'lism.** 1. Symptoms of irritation of the skin, nasal mucous membrane, and conjunctiva from which workers with vanilla sometimes suffer. 2. Infestation of the skin by sarcoptiform mites found in vanilla pods.

**vanillylmandelic acid** (van'ĭ-lil-man-del'ik, vă-nil'il-). 4-Hydroxy-3-methoxymandelic acid; the major urinary metabolite of adrenal and sympathetic catecholamines. An abnormally elevated excretion in urine indicates the presence of a pheochromocytoma or other tumor with neurosecretory activity (some neuroblastomas and ganglioneuromas).

**Van Slyke,** Donald D., U. S. biochemist, 1883–1971, See V. S. *apparatus, formula.*

**van't Hoff,** Jacobus H., Dutch chemist, 1852–1911. See v. H.'s *laws,* Le Bel-v. H. *rule, theory.*

**Vanzetti** (vahn-tset'e), Tito, Italian surgeon, 1809–1888. See V.'s *sign.*

**vapocauterization** (va'po-kaw'ter-ĭ-za'shun). Cauterization by steam.

**va'por** [ L. steam ]. 1. The molecules in the gaseous phase of a solid or liquid substance exposed to a gas. 2. A visible emanation of fine particles of a liquid. 3. A medicinal preparation to be administered by inhalation.
   **anesthetic v.,** the gaseous phase of a liquid anesthetic with partial pressure great enough at room temperature to produce general anesthesia when inhaled.

**va'pora'rium.** Vaporium.

**va′porish.** Hypochondriacal; hysterical; melancholic; splenetic.

**vapo′rium** [ L. *vaporarium*, steam pipe ]. An apparatus for applying hot or cold or medicated vapors.

**va′poriza′tion.** 1. The change of a solid or liquid to a state of vapor. 2. The therapeutic application of a vapor.

**va′porize.** 1. To convert a solid or liquid into a vapor. 2. To apply a vapor therapeutically.

**va′porizer.** An apparatus for reducing medicated liquids to a state of vapor fit for inhalation or application to the accessible mucous membranes. See also nebulizer; atomizer.

**copper kettle v.,** a high thermal capacity v. for volatile anesthetic agents; it uses copper as a conductor and reservoir of heat and provides a large vaporizing interface by forcing the inflowing oxygen through a sintered bronze Porex disk.

**Fluotec v.,** a temperature-compensated drawover v. calibrated for halothane and permitting accurate concentrations down to 0.1 per cent to be delivered with the use of a wide range of carrier gas flows.

**Pentec v.,** a temperature-compensated drawover v. similar to the Fluotec v., but calibrated for methoxyflurane.

**Vernitrol v.,** a high thermal capacity v. for volatile anesthetic agents, similar to the copper kettle v., that makes possible accurate calculation of the percentage of vapor delivered to the patient if the vapor pressure of the volatile liquid, the oxygen flow into the v., and the diluent flow are known.

**va′pors.** Hypochondriasis; depression.

**vaporthorax** (va′por-tho′raks). The existence of large water vapor bubbles in the pleural space between the lungs and the chest wall in an unprotected person exposed to altitudes above 63,000 feet, where the barometric pressure is less than 47 mm. of Hg, where water at body temperature vaporizes from the liquid state.

**va′pother′apy.** Treatment of disease by means of vapor or spray.

**Vaquez** (vah-ka′), L. H., French physician, 1860–1936. See V.'s *disease*.

**var′iabil′ity.** The capability of being variable.

**variable** [ L. *vario*, to vary, change, differ ]. 1. That which is inconstant, which can or does change, as contrasted with a constant. 2. Deviating from the type in structure, form, physiology, or behavior.

**dependent v.,** in experiments, a v. that is influenced by or dependent upon changes in the independent v.

**independent v.,** in experiments, the v. controlled and manipulated by the experimenter.

**intervening v.,** an event, such as an attitude or emotion, inferred to occur within an organism between the stimulation and response in such a way as to influence or determine the response.

**var′iance.** The state of being variable, different, divergent, or deviate.

**ball v.,** swelling and changes in shape and consistency of the ball in a ball-valve prosthesis, especially in one replacing the aortic valve.

**var′iant.** 1. That which, or one who, is variable. 2. Having the tendency to alter or change, exhibit variety or diversity, not conform, or differ from the type.

**L-phase v.'s,** bacterial v.'s which do not have rigid cell walls but which may contain varying amounts of cell wall material. They are spherical to coccobacillary in shape and vary in size from small bodies that pass through filters which retain bacteria to bodies that are larger than the bacterial form. They are Gram-negative and resistant to penicillin. Some revert to the bacterial phase upon removal of the inducing substance, whereas others do not. The v.'s differ greatly from the parent bacterial cells in mode of reproduction, physiology, growth requirements, and individual and colonial morphology. L-phase v.'s are generally considered to be nonpathogenic, even if derived from a pathogenic bacterium. The term L-form was originally used by Klienberger-Nobel in honor of the Lister Institute, where she discovered and studied these v.'s.

**variation** (văr′ī-a′shun) [ L. *variatio*, fr. *vario*, to change, vary ]. Deviation from the type, especially the parent type, in structure, form, physiology, or behavior.

**continuous v.,** a series of very slight v.'s.

**inborn v.,** genetic v.

**meris′tic v.,** in heredity, v. in characters that can be counted.

**varication** (văr′ī-ka′shun). The formation or presence of varices.

**variceal** (văr′ī-se′al, vă-ris′e-al). Of or pertaining to a varix.

**varicella** (văr′ī-sel′ah) [ Mod. L. dim. of *variola*. VARI-2 ]. Chickenpox; an acute contagious disease; occurring usually in children only, marked by a sparse eruption of papules, becoming vesicles and then pustules, like that of smallpox although less severe; there are usually also mild constitutional symptoms. The incubation period is about 14 to 17 days.

**v. gangreno′sa,** *dermatitis* gangrenosa infantum; a rare gangrenous condition of the skin which may occur as a complication of v.

**v. pustulo′sa,** an old term for varioloid (2).

**var′ioloid v.,** an old term for alastrim.

**varicellation** (văr′ī-sĕ-la′shun). Inoculation with the virus of chickenpox as a means of protection against that disease.

**varicel′liform.** Resembling varicella.

**varicel′loid.** Varicelliform.

**varices** (văr′ī-sēz). Plural of varix.

**variciform** (văr′ī-sī-form, vă-ris′ī-form). Varicoid; resembling a varix.

**varico-** (văr′ī-ko-) [ L. *varix*, a dilated vein. VARI-1 ]. Combining form relating to a varix or varicosity.

**varicoblepharon** (văr′ī-ko-blef′ă-ron) [ varico- + G. *blepharon*, eyelid ]. A varicosity of the eyelid.

**varicocele** (văr′ī-ko-sēl) [ varico- + G. *kēlē*, tumor, hernia ]. Hernia varicosa; a varicose enlargement of the veins of the spermatic cord, causing a boggy tumor of the scrotum.

**ova′rian v., tubo-ova′rian v., u′tero-ova′rian v.,** a varicose condition of the pampiniform plexus in the broad ligament.

**varicocelectomy** (văr′ī-ko-se-lek′to-mī) [ varicocele + G. *ektomē*, excision ]. An operation for the relief of a varicocele by ligature and excision of the dilated veins.

**varicography** (văr′ī-kog′ră-fī) [ varico- + G. *graphō*, to write ]. Roentgenography of the veins after injection of a radiopaque medium into varicose veins.

**var′icoid.** Variciform.

**varicole** (văr′ī-kōl). Varicocele.

**varicomphalus** (văr′ī-kom′fā-lus) [ varico- + G. *omphalos*, navel ]. A swelling formed by varicose veins at the umbilicus.

**varicophlebitis** (văr′ī-ko-flĕ-bi′tis) [ varico- + G. *phleps*, vein, + suffix -*itis*, inflammation ]. Inflammation of varicose veins.

**varicose** (văr′ī-kōs). Relating to, affected with, or characterized by varices or varicosis.

**varicosis,** pl. **varicoses** (văr-ī-ko′sis, -sēz) [ varico- + G. suffix -*osis*, condition ]. A dilated or varicose state of a vein or veins.

**varicosity** (văr-ī-kos′ī-tī). 1. A varix. 2. A varicose condition.

**varicotomy** (văr-ī-kot′o-mī) [ varico- + G. *tomē*, a cutting ]. An operation for the cure of varicose veins by subcutaneous incision.

**varicula** (vă-rik′u-lah) [ L. dim. of *varix* ]. Conjunctival varix; a varicose condition of the veins of the conjunctiva.

**varicule** (văr′ī-kūl) [ L. *varicula*, dim. of *varix* ]. A small varicose vein ordinarily seen in the skin; it may be associated with venous stars, venous lakes, or larger varicose veins.

**variola** (vă-ri′o-lah) [ Mediev. L. dim. of L. *varius*, spotted. VARI-2 ]. Smallpox.

**v. benig′na,** varioloid (2).

**v. capri′na,** goat *pox*.

**v. crystalli′na,** an old term for varicella (chickenpox).

**v. hemorrha′gica,** hemorrhagic *smallpox*.

**v. major,** smallpox.

**v. malig′na,** malignant smallpox, usually of the hemorrhagic form.

**v. milia'ris,** a form of varioloid in which the eruption consists of miliary vesicles without the formation of pustules.

**v. minor,** alastrim; a mild form of smallpox, apparently caused by a less virulent strain of smallpox virus.

**v. pemphigo'sa,** a form of smallpox in which the eruption consists of pemphigus-like blebs.

**v. si'ne eruptio'ne,** an abortive form of smallpox in which the disease subsides without the appearance of any eruption, or at most a few papules that never go on to pustulation.

**v. vaccine,** vaccinia.

**v. vaccinia,** vaccinia.

**v. vera,** simple smallpox of ordinary severity in the unvaccinated.

**v. verruco'sa,** wartpox; a mild or abortive form of varioloid, the eruption of which consists mainly of papules, with occasionally minute vesicles at the apices, which persist for a time as wartlike lesions.

**variolar** (vă-ri'o-lar). Relating to smallpox.

**Variola'ria** [ Mediev. L. *variola,* smallpox (because the shields of the plant resemble smallpox spots) ]. A genus of lichens; some species are a source of litmus, and one, *V. amara,* has been used as an anthelmintic and febrifuge.

**variolate** (văr'ĭ-o-lāt). 1. To inoculate with smallpox. 2. Pitted or scarred, as if with smallpox.

**variolic** (văr'ĭ-ol'ik). Variolar; variolous.

**varioliform** (vă-ri'o-lĭ-form, văr'ĭ-o'lĭ-form) [ variola + L. *forma,* form ]. Resembling smallpox; varioloid (1).

**variolization** (văr'ĭ-o-lĭ-za'shun). Variolation.

**varioloid** (văr'ĭ-o-loyd) [ variola + G. *eidos,* resemblance ]. 1. Varioliform; resembling smallpox. 2. A mild form of smallpox occurring in persons who are relatively resistant, usually as a result of a previous vaccination; the course of the disease is materially shortened and the different stages of the eruption follow each other rapidly, or the lesions may abort at any stage. It is contagious and may cause virulent smallpox in a nonimmune contact.

**variolous** (vă-ri'o-lus). Variolar; variolic; relating to smallpox.

**variolovaccine** (vă-ri'o-lo-vak'sēn). A vaccine obtained from the eruption following inoculation of a heifer with smallpox from the human.

**varix,** pl. **varices** (văr'iks, văr'ĭ-sēz) [ L. *varix* (*varic-*), a dilated vein. VARI-1 ]. An enlarged and tortuous vein, artery, or lymphatic vessel.

   **v. anastomot'icus,** aneurysmal v.

   **aneurys'mal v.,** Pott's aneurysm; v. anastomoticus; dilation and tortuosity of a vein resulting from a direct communication with an adjacent artery.

   **cirsoid v.,** cirsoid *aneurysm.*

   **esophageal varices,** longitudinal venous varices at the lower end of the esophagus as a result of portal hypertension; they are superficial and liable to ulceration and massive bleeding.

   **gelat'inous v.,** a lumpy or nodular condition of the umbilical cord.

   **lymph v.,** the formation of varices or cysts in the lymph nodes in consequence of obstruction in the efferent lymphatics.

   **tur'binal v.,** a condition of permanent dilation of the veins of the turbinated bodies, especially of the inferior turbinate.

**varnish (dental).** Solutions of natural resins and gums in a suitable solvent, usually chloroform, acetone, or ether. A thin coating is applied over the surfaces of the cavity preparations before placement of restorations, to act as a protective agent for the tooth against constituents of restorative materials and thermal shock.

**Varo'lian.** Relating to Varolius.

**Varo'lius,** Constantius (Varolio, Costanzio), Italian anatomist, 1543–1575. See *pons* varolii, *valve* of V., V.'s *sphincter.*

**Varro,** Marcus Terentius, Roman writer, 234–149 B.C. Foreshadowed the theory of the bacterial origin of disease.

**va'rus** [ Mod. L. bent inward, fr. L. knock-kneed ]. Bent or twisted inward.

**vas-** [ L. *vas,* a vessel ]. Combining form relating to a vas, or blood vessel; see also vasculo- and vaso-.

**vas,** gen. **vasis,** pl. **vasa,** gen. pl. **vaso'rum** [ L. a vessel, dish ] [ NA ]. A vessel; a duct or canal conveying any liquid, such as blood, lymph, chyle, or semen.

   **v. aber'rans,** *ductulus* aberrans.

   **v. aber'rans hep'atis,** pl. **vasa aberran'tia hep'atis,** one of numerous irregularly coursing arterial twigs found along with blind bile ducts in the fibrous appendix and in the capsule of the liver.

   **v. af'ferens,** pl. **vasa afferentia** [ NA ], afferent vessel; (1) any artery conveying blood to a part; (2) the arteriole that enters a renal glomerulus; (3) a lymphatic vessel entering a lymph gland.

   **v. anastomot'icum** [ NA ], a vessel that establishes a connection between arteries, between veins, or between lymph vessels.

   **vasa aur'is inter'nae** [ NA ], vessels of the internal ear.

   **vasa bre'via,** *arteriae* gastricae breves.

   **v. capilla're** [ NA ], capillary vessel; see blood *capillary* and lymph *capillary.*

   **vasa chylif'era,** chyle vessels; see lacteal (2).

   **v. collatera'le** [ NA ], collateral vessel; a branch of an artery running parallel with the parent trunk.

   **v. def'erens,** pl. **vasa deferentia,** *ductus* deferens.

   **v. ef'ferens,** pl. **vasa efferentia,** [ NA ], efferent vessel; (1) a vein carrying blood away from a part; (2) the arteriole that carries blood out of a renal glomerulus; it passes to the capillary bed surrounding the renal tubules; (3) a lymphatic vessel leaving a lymph gland.

   **Ferrein's vasa aberrantia,** biliary canaliculi that are not connected with hepatic lobules.

   **Haller's v. aberrans,** *ductulus* aberrans.

   **vasa lymphat'ica** [ NA ], lymphatic vessels; the vessels that convey the lymph; they anastomose freely with each other.

   **vasa lymphat'ica profun'da** [ NA ], deep lymphatic vessels; the vessels that drain lymph from the deep structures of the body; they tend to follow the courses of blood vessels to reach regional lymph nodes.

   **vasa lymphat'ica superficia'lia** [ NA ], superficial lymphatic vessels; the lymphatic vessels that lie in the skin and subcutaneous tissues; they join the deep lymphatic vessels.

   **vasa nervor'um,** vessels supplying a nerve trunk.

   **vasa pre'via,** umbilical vessels presenting in advance of the fetal head, usually traversing the membranes and crossing the internal cervical os.

   **v. prom'inens** [ NA ], a blood vessel in the substance of the prominentia spiralis of the cochlea.

   **vasa rec'ta,** (1) *arteriolae* rectae; (2) *tubuli* seminiferi recti.

   **Roth's v. aberrans,** an occasional diverticulum of the rete testis.

   **v. sanguin'eum,** pl. **vasa sanguin'ea,** a blood vessel.

   **vasa sanguin'ea ret'inae** [ NA ], blood vessels of the retina.

   **v. spira'le** [ NA ], a blood vessel, larger than its fellows, in the basilar membrane just beneath the tunnel of Corti.

   **vasa vaso'rum** [ NA ], vessels of vessels; small arteries distributed to the outer and middle coats of the larger blood vessels, and their corresponding veins.

   **vasa vortico'sa,** *venae* vorticosae.

**vasa** (va'sah, vah'sah). Plural of vas.

**va'sal.** Relating to a vas or to vasa.

**vascular** (vas'ku-lar) [ L. *vasculum,* a small vessel, dim. of *vas* ]. Relating to or containing blood vessels.

**vascula'ris** [ L. ] [ NA ]. Vascular.

**vascular'ity.** The condition of being vascular.

**vascularization** (vas'ku-lar-ĭ-za'shun). Arterialization (2); the formation of new blood vessels in a part.

**vas'cularized.** Rendered vascular by the formation of new vessels.

**vasculature** (vas'ku-lă-chur). The vascular network of an organ.

**vasculitis** (vas'ku-li'tis). Angiitis.

   **nodular v.,** chronic or recurrent nodular nontuberculous lesions of subcutaneous tissue, especially of the legs of older women, with obliterative inflammation of the arteries and veins.

   **v. retinae syphilitica,** *retinitis* syphilitica.

**vasculo-** (vas'ku-lo-) [ L. *vasculum,* a small vessel, dim. of *vas* ]. Combining forms relating to the blood vessels; see also vas- and vaso-.

**vas'culocar'diac.** Relating to the heart and blood vessels.

**vas'culogen'esis** [ vasculo- + G. *genesis*, production ]. The formation of the vascular system.

**vas'culomo'tor.** Vasomotor.

**vasculum,** pl. **vascula** (vas'ku-lum, -lah) [ L. dim of *vas*, a vessel ]. A small vessel.

**vasec'tomized.** Having undergone vasectomy.

**vasectomy** (vă-sek'to-mĭ) [ vas- + G. *ektomē*, excision ]. Gonangiectomy; excision of a segment of the vas deferens.

**vas'icine.** Peganine; an alkaloid from *Adhotoda vasica* (family Acanthaceae), an East Indian shrub, and from *Peganum harmala;* destructive to low forms of animal and vegetable life; expectorant and anthelmintic.

**vasifac'tion.** Angiopoiesis.

**vasifac'tive.** Angiopoietic.

**vas'iform.** Having the shape of a vas or tubular structure.

**vasi'tis.** Deferentitis.

**vaso-** (vas'o-, va'so-, -zo-) [ L. *vas*, a vessel ]. Combining form relating to a vas, or blood vessel; see also vas- and vasculo-.

**vasoac'tive.** Influencing the tone and caliber of blood vessels.

**vasoconstric'tion.** Narrowing of the blood vessels.
**active v.,** reduced caliber of vessel caused by increased tonus in the smooth muscle in its walls.
**passive v.,** reduced caliber of vessel caused by decreased intraluminal pressure.

**vasoconstric'tive.** 1. Causing narrowing of the blood vessels. 2. Vasoconstrictor (1).

**vasoconstric'tor.** 1. Vasoconstrictive (2); an agent that causes narrowing of the blood vessels. 2. A nerve, stimulation of which causes vascular constriction.

**vasoden'tin.** Vascular dentin; dentin in which the primitive capillaries have remained uncalcified and so are wide enough to give passage to the formed elements of the blood.

**vasodila'tion.** Dilation of the blood vessels.
**active v.,** v. caused by decrease in tonus of smooth muscle in wall of vessel.
**passive v.,** v. related to increased pressure in lumen of vessel.

**vasodila'tive.** 1. Causing dilation of the blood vessels. 2. Vasodilator (1).

**vasodila'tor.** 1. Vasodilative (2); an agent that causes dilation of the blood vessels. 2. A nerve, stimulation of which results in dilation of the blood vessels.

**vasoepididymostomy** (vas'o-ep-ĭ-did-ĭ-mos'to-mĭ) [ vaso- + epididymis + G. *stoma*, mouth ]. Surgical anastomosis of the vasa deferentia to the epididymis.

**vasofac'tive.** Angiopoietic.

**vasoforma'tion.** Angiopoiesis.

**vasofor'mative.** Angiopoietic.

**vasoganglion** (vas'o-gang'glĭ-on). Glomus; a mass of blood vessels.

**vasography** (vă-sog'ră-fĭ). Roentgenography of blood vessels.

**vasohy'perton'ic** [ vaso- + G. *hyper*, over, + *tonos*, tone ]. Relating to increased arteriolar tension or vasoconstriction.

**vasohy'poton'ic** [ vaso- + G. *hypo*, under, + *tonos*, tone ]. Relating to reduced arteriolar tension or vasodilation.

**vasoinhibitor** (vas-o-in-hib'ĭ-tor). An agent that restricts or prevents the functioning of the vasomotor nerves.

**vasoinhib'itory.** Restraining vasomotor action.

**vasola'bile.** Characterizing the condition in which there is lability or active vasomotion of blood vessels.

**vasoliga'tion.** Ligation of the vas deferens.

**vasomo'tion.** Angiokinesis; change in caliber of a blood vessel.

**vasomo'tor.** Angiokinetic; vasculomotor. 1. Causing dilation or constriction of the blood vessels. 2. Denoting the nerves which have this action.

**vasomoto'rial, vasomotor'ic, vasomo'tory.** Vasomotor.

**vasoneuropathy** (vas'o-nu-rop'ă-thĭ) [ vaso- + G. *neuron*, nerve, + *pathos*, suffering ]. Any disease involving both the nerves and blood vessels.

**vasoneurosis** (vas'o-nu-ro'sis). Angioneurosis.

**vaso-orchidostomy** (vas'o-or'kĭ-dos'to-mĭ) [ vaso- + G. *orchis*, testis, + *stoma*, mouth ]. The reestablishment of the interrupted seminiferous channels by uniting the tubules of the epididymis or of the rete to the divided end of the vas deferens.

**vasoparal'ysis.** Angioparalysis; paralysis, atonia, or hypotonia of blood vessels.

**vasoparesis** (vas'o-pă-re'sis, -păr'e-sis) [ vaso- + G. *paresis*, weakness ]. Angioparesis; a mild degree of vasoparalysis.

**vasopressin** (va'so-pres'in, vas'o-) (USP, BP). PITRESSIN; β-hypophamine; the antidiuretic hormone of the neurohypophysis; a nonapeptide hormone related to oxytocin and vasotocin; synthetically prepared or obtained from the posterior lobe of the pituitary glands of healthy domestic animals used for food by man. In pharmacological doses it causes contraction of smooth muscle, notably that of all blood vessels; large doses may produce cerebral or coronary arterial spasm. Used parenterally in the treatment of diabetes insipidus and to stimulate intestinal motility. Many variants have been synthesized; see arginine vasopressin; lysine vasopressin, etc.

**vasopres'sor.** Producing vasoconstriction and a rise in blood pressure.

**vasopunc'ture.** The act of puncturing a vessel with a needle.

**vasore'flex.** A reflex that influences the caliber of blood vessels.

**vasorelaxation** (vas'o-re-lak-sa'shun). Reduction in tension of the walls of the blood vessels.

**vasosec'tion.** Vasotomy.

**vasosen'sory.** 1. Relating to sensation in the blood vessels. 2. Denoting sensory nerve fibers innervating blood vessels.

**vas'ospasm.** Angiospasm; angiohypertonia; contraction or hypertonia of the muscular coats of the blood vessels.

**vasospas'tic.** Angiospastic; relating to or characterized by vasospasm.

**vasostim'ulant.** 1. Exciting vasomotor action. 2. An agent that excites the vasomotor nerves to action. 3. Vasotonic (2).

**vasostomy** (vă-sos'to-mĭ) [ vaso- + G. *stoma*, mouth ]. Belfield's operation; an artificial opening into the deferent duct.

**vasothrom'bin.** Thrombin derived from the lining cells of the blood vessels.

**vasoto'cin.** A nonapeptide hormone, with vasopressin and oxytocin activities, of the neurohypophysis of subvertebrates; chemically identical with human vasopressin except for isoleucine at position 3; thus [ 3-isoleucine ]vasopressin or [ Ile³ ]vasopressin. See also arginine vasotocin.

**vasotomy** (vă-sot'o-mĭ) [ vaso- + G. *tomē*, incision ]. Vasosection; incision into or division of the vas deferens.

**vasotonia** (vas'o-to'nĭ-ah) [ vaso- + G. *tonos*, tone ]. Angiotonia; the tone of blood vessels, particularly the arterioles.

**vasoton'ic.** 1. Relating to vascular tone. 2. Vasostimulant (3); an agent that increases vascular tension.

**vasotribe** (vas'o-trĭb). Angiotribe.

**vasotripsy** (vas'o-trip'sĭ). Angiotripsy.

**vasotrophic** (vas'o-trof'ik) [ vaso- + G. *trophē*, nourishment ]. Angiotrophic.

**vasotropic** [ vaso- + G. *tropē*, a turning ]. Tending to act on the blood vessels.

**vasova'gal.** Relating to the action of the vagus nerve upon the blood vessels. See vasovagal *syndrome*.

**vasovasostomy** (vas'o-vă-sos'to-mĭ) [ vaso- + vaso- + G. *stoma*, mouth ]. Surgical anastomosis of vasa deferentia.

**vasovesic'ulec'tomy** [ vaso- + L. *vesicula*, vesicle, + G. *ektomē*, excision ]. Excision of the vas deferens and seminal vesicles.

**vastus** [ L. ] [ NA ]. Great; see under musculus.

**Vater** (fah'ter), Abraham, German anatomist and botanist, 1684–1751. See V.'s *ampulla*, V.-Pacini *corpuscle*, V.'s *fold*.

**vault** [ thr. O. Fr. fr. L. *volvo*, pp. *volutus*, to turn round ]. A part resembling an arched roof or dome, *e.g.*, the v. of the pharynx, the upper part or roof of the rhinopharynx; the palatine v., palatum; v. of the vagina, fornix.

**VC.** Abbreviation for (1) color *vision*, (2) vital *capacity*.

**VDRL.** 1. Abbreviation for Venereal Disease Research Laboratories. 2. See VDRL *test*.

**veal** (vēl) [ O.Fr. ]. Meat from milk-fed calves.

  **bob v.,** deacon; meat from calves under 3 weeks of age; such v. is pale, watery, and lower in nutriment than that from older animals.

**vection** (vek'shun) [ L. *vectio*, conveyance. VECT- ]. The transference of the agents of disease from the sick to the well by a vector.

**vectis** (vek'tis) [ L. a lever or bar ]. Lever; an instrument resembling one of the blades of an obstetrical forceps, used as an aid in delivery by making traction on the presenting part of the fetus.

**vector** (vek'tor) [ L. *vector*, a carrier. VECT- ]. 1. An insect or any living carrier that transports an infectious agent from an infected individual or its wastes to a susceptible individual or its food or immediate surroundings. The organism may or may not pass through any developmental cycle within the v. 2. Anything, *e.g.*, velocity, mechanical force, electromotive force, having magnitude, direction, and sense which can be represented by a straight line of appropriate length and direction. 3. Especially the electrical axis of the heart represented by an arrow whose length is proportional to the magnitude of the electrical force, whose direction gives the direction of the force, and whose tip represents the positive pole of the force.

  **biological v.,** a v., such as the mosquito for the malarial agents or the tsetse fly for the agents of African sleeping sickness, that is essential in the life cycle of the pathogenic organism.

  **instantaneous v.,** the resultant of the heart's action currents at any given moment, usually represented as an arrow of appropriate direction and magnitude.

  **manifest v.,** the projection of a spatial cardiac v. on a single plane.

  **mean v.,** a single cardiac v. representing the average of all v.'s present during a given time interval.

  **mechanical v.,** one that simply conveys pathogens to a susceptible individual without essential development by the pathogens in the v., as in the transfer of septic organisms on the feet or mouth parts of the housefly.

  **spatial v.,** a cardiac v. represented in more than one plane simultaneously; two- or three-dimensional orientation of a v.

**vectorcardiogram** (vek'tor-kar'dĭ-o-gram). A graphic representation of the magnitude and direction of the heart's action currents in the form of a vector loop.

**vectorcardiography** (vek'tor-kar-dĭ-og'ră-fĭ). 1. A variant of electrocardiography in which the heart's activation currents are represented by vector loops. 2. The study and interpretation of vectorcardiograms.

  **spatial v.,** three-dimensional v. in which vector loops are inscribed in frontal, sagittal, and horizontal planes.

**vecto'rial.** Relating in any way to a vector.

**vegan** (vej'an). A person who eats no animal food of any kind, not even milk, eggs, cheese, or seafood; see also vegetarian.

**veganism** (vej'an-izm). The dietary practices of a vegan; the state of being a vegan.

**vegetable** (vej'e-tă-bl) [ M.E. fr. L. *vegetabilis* (see vegetation) ]. 1. A plant, specifically one used for food. 2. Relating to plants, as distinguished from animals or minerals.

**vegetal** (vej'e-tal). 1. Vegetable; relating to plants. 2. Denoting the vital functions common to plants and animals, such as respiration, metabolism, growth, generation, etc., distinguished from those peculiar to animals, such as conscious sensation and the mental faculties.

**vegetality** (vej'e-tal'ĭ-tĭ). The aggregate of the vital functions common to both plants and animals.

**vegeta'rian.** One who lives wholly on vegetables, eschewing meat; a strict v. avoids tubers and everything except fruits and vegetables grown in the sunlight; a lactovegetarian eats tubers, milk, eggs, and anything except flesh food.

**vegeta'rianism.** The practice as to diet of a vegetarian.

**vegetation** (vej'e-ta'shun) [ Mod. L. *vegetatio*, growth, fr. *vegeto*, pp. *-atus*, to arouse, to animate, fr. *vegeo*, to rouse ]. 1. The process of growth in plants. 2. A condition of sluggishness, comparable to the inactivity of plant life. 3. A growth or excrescence of any sort. 4. Specifically, a clot, composed largely of fused blood platelets, fibrin, and bacteria, adherent to a diseased heart valve.

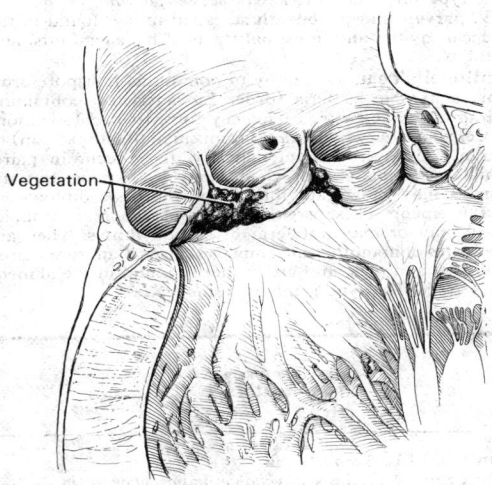

Vegetation—

**Vegetation on Aortic Valve**

**vegetative** (vej'e-ta'tiv) [ see vegetation ]. 1. Growing or functioning involuntarily or unconsciously after the assumed manner of vegetable life. 2. Resting; not active; denoting the stage of a cell or its nucleus in which the process of karyokinesis is quiescent.

**vegetoalkali** (vej-e-to-al'kă-li). An alkaloid.

**vegetoanimal** (vej-e-to-an'ĭ-mal). Relating to both plants and animals; denoting the vegetal functions.

  **v. matter,** gluten and albumin derived from plants.

**vehicle** (ve'hĭ-kl) [ L. *vehiculum*, a conveyance, fr. *veho*, to carry ]. An excipient; a menstruum; a substance, usually without therapeutic action, used as a medium, to give bulk, for the administration of medicines.

**veil** (vāl) [ L. *velum* ]. 1. Velum (1). 2. Caul (1).

  **Jackson's v.,** Jackson's *membrane*.

  **Sattler's v.,** a diffuse edema of the corneal epithelium that may develop with the use of contact lenses.

**Veillon** (va-yon'), Adrien, French bacteriologist, 1864–1931. Gave his name to *Veillonella*.

**Veillonel'la** (A. *Veillon*). A genus of nonmotile, nonsporeforming, anaerobic bacteria (family Veillonellaceae) containing small (0.3 to 0.5 μm in diameter), Gram-negative cocci which occur as diplococci and in masses. Carbon dioxide is required for growth, and carbohydrates are not fermented. These organisms are parasitic in the mouth and the intestinal and respiratory tracts of man and other animals. They produce serologically specific endotoxins (lipopolysaccharides) which induce pyrogenicity and the Schwarzman phenomenon in rabbits. The type species is *V. parvula.*

  **V. alcalescens,** a species found in the saliva of man and other animals.

  **V. alcalescens** subsp. **alcalescens,** a subspecies found primarily in the mouths of humans but occasionally in the buccal cavities of rabbits and rats. It is the type subspecies of the species *V. alcalescens.*

  **V. alcalescens** subsp. **criceti,** a subspecies found in the mouths of hamsters.

  **V. alcalescens** subsp. **dispar,** a subspecies found in the mouths and respiratory tracts of humans.

  **V. alcalescens** subsp. **ratti,** a subspecies found in the mouths and intestinal contents of rats.

**V. par'vula,** a species found normally as a harmless parasite in the natural cavities, especially the mouths and digestive tracts, of man and other animals. It is the types species of the genus *V.*

**V. parvula** subsp. **atypica,** a subspecies found in the buccal cavities of rats and humans.

**V. parvula** subsp. **parvula,** a subspecies found in the mouths or intestinal or respiratory tracts of humans. It is the type subspecies of the species *V. parvula.*

**V. parvula** subsp. **rodentium,** a subspecies found in the buccal cavities and intestinal tracts of hamsters, rats, and rabbits.

**Veillonella'ceae.** A family of nonmotile, nonsporeforming, anaerobic bacteria (order Eubacteriales) containing Gram-negative (with a tendency to resist decolorization) cocci which vary in diameter from small (0.3 to 0.5 μm) to large (2.5 μm). Characteristically, they occur in pairs; single cells, masses, or chains may also occur, but the chains may show gaps illustrating the basic diplococcal arrangement. These organisms are chemoorganotrophic; they may or may not ferment carbohydrates. They are parasites of homothermic animals such as man, ruminants, rodents, and pigs, and are primarily found in the alimentary tract. The type genus is *Veillonella.*

# VEIN

**vein** (vān) [ L. *vena* ]. Vena.

**accessory cephalic v.,** *vena* cephalica accessoria.
**accessory hemiazygos v.,** *vena* hemiazygos accessoria.
**accessory saphenous v.,** *vena* saphena accessoria.
**accessory vertebral v.,** *vena* vertebralis accessoria.
**accompanying v.,** vena comitans.
**anastomotic v.'s,** see entries under *vena* anastomotica.
**angular v.,** *vena* angularis.
**anonymous v.'s,** *venae* brachiocephalicae.
**anterior auricular v.,** *vena* auricularis anterior.
**anterior cardiac v.'s,** *venae* cordis anteriores.
**anterior cerebral v.,** *vena* cerebri anterior.
**anterior facial v.,** *vena* facialis.
**anterior intercostal v.'s,** *venae* intercostales anteriores.
**anterior jugular v.,** *vena* jugularis anterior.
**anterior labial v.'s,** *venae* labiales anteriores.
**anterior scrotal v.'s,** *venae* scrotales anteriores.
**anterior tibial v.'s,** *venae* tibiales anteriores.
**anterior vertebral v.,** *vena* vertebralis anterior.
**appendicular v.,** *vena* appendicularis.
**arciform v.'s of kidney,** *venae* arcuatae renis.
**arcuate v.'s of kidney,** *venae* arcuatae renis.
**arterial v.,** vena arteriosa; so called because it ramifies like an artery (portal vein) or because, while proceeding from the heart like an artery, it contains unaerated blood, like a vein (pulmonary artery).
**ascending lumbar v.,** *vena* lumbalis ascendens.
**auricular v.'s,** see entries under *vena* auricularis.
**axillary v.,** *vena* axillaris.
**azygos v.,** *vena* azygos.
**basal v.'s,** see entries under *vena* basalis.
**basal v. of Rosenthal,** *vena* basalis.
**basilic v.,** *vena* basilica.
**basivertebral v.,** *vena* basivertebralis.
**brachial v.'s,** *venae* brachiales.
**brachiocephalic v.'s,** *venae* brachiocephalicae.
**Breschet's v.,** *vena* diploica.
**bronchial v.'s,** *venae* bronchiales.
**Browning's v.,** *vena* anastomotica inferior.
**v. of bulb of penis,** *vena* bulbi penis.
**Burow's v.,** (1) an occasional v. passing from the inferior epigastric, sometimes receiving a tributary from the bladder, which empties into the portal v.; (2) one of the *venae* renis.
**capillary v.,** venula.
**cardiac v.'s,** see entries under *vena* cordis.
**cardinal v.'s,** the paired c. v.'s are the major systemic venous channels in adult primitive vertebrates and in the embryos of higher vertebrates; the **anterior** c. v.'s are the

major drainage channels from the cephalic part of the body, and the **posterior** c. v.'s, from the caudal part. The **common** c. v.'s, formed by the anastomosis of the anterior and posterior c. v.'s, are the main systemic return channels to the heart. In the older literature, sometimes called the ducts of Cuvier.
**central v.'s of liver,** *venae* centrales hepatis.
**central v. of retina,** *vena* centralis retinae.
**central v. of suprarenal gland,** *vena* centralis glandulae suprarenalis.
**cephalic v.,** *vena* cephalica.
**cerebellar v.'s,** see *venae* cerebelli inferiores and superiores.
**cerebral v.'s,** see entries under *vena* cerebri.
**cervical v.,** see *vena* cervicalis profunda.
**choroid v.,** *vena* choroidea.
**choroid v.'s of eye,** *venae* vorticosae.
**ciliary v.'s,** *venae* ciliares.
**circumflex v.'s,** see entries under *vena* circumflexa.
**v. of cochlear aqueduct,** *vena* aqueductus cochleae; see *vena* canaliculi cochleae.
**v. of cochlear canaliculus,** *vena* canaliculi cochleae.
**colic v.'s,** see entries under *vena* colica.
**common basal v.,** *vena* basalis communis.
**common facial v.,** vena facialis communis; a short vessel formed by the union of the facial v. and the retromandibular v., emptying into the jugular v.; considered to be a continuation of the facial v. in the NA.
**common iliac v.,** *vena* iliaca communis.
**companion v.** or **v.'s,** *vena* comitans, *venae* comitantes.
**condylar emissary v.,** *vena* emissaria condylaris.
**conjunctival v.'s,** *venae* conjunctivales.
**coronary v.,** *vena* gastrica sinistra.
**v. of corpus striatum,** *vena* thalamostriata.
**costoax'illary v.,** one of a number of anastomotic v.'s connecting the intercostal v.'s of the 1st to 7th intercostal spaces with the lateral thoracic or the thoracoepigastric v.
**cutaneous v.,** *vena* cutanea.
**Cuvier's v.'s,** the common cardinal v.'s of the embryo; see cardinal *veins.*
**cystic v.,** *vena* cystica.
**deep cervical v.,** *vena* cervicalis profunda.
**deep circumflex iliac v.,** *vena* circumflexa ilium profunda.
**deep v.'s of clitoris,** *venae* profundae clitoridis.
**deep dorsal v. of clitoris,** *vena* dorsalis clitoridis profunda.
**deep dorsal v. of penis,** *vena* dorsalis penis profunda.
**deep epigastric v.,** *vena* epigastrica inferior.
**deep facial v.,** *vena* faciei profunda.
**deep femoral v.,** *vena* profunda femoris.
**deep lingual v.,** *vena* profunda linguae.
**deep middle cerebral v.,** *vena* cerebri media profunda.
**deep v. of penis,** *vena* profunda penis.
**deep temporal v.'s,** *venae* temporales profundae.
**digital v.'s,** *venae* digitales.
**diploic v.,** *vena* diploica.
**dorsal v.'s of clitoris,** see *vena* dorsalis clitoridis profunda and *venae* dorsales clitoridis superficiales.
**dorsal digital v.'s of toes,** *venae* digitales dorsales pedis.
**dorsal lingual v.,** *vena* dorsalis linguae.
**dorsal metacarpal v.'s,** *venae* metacarpeae dorsales.
**dorsal metatarsal v.'s,** *venae* metatarseae dorsales.
**dorsal v.'s of penis,** see *vena* dorsalis penis profunda and *venae* dorsales penis superficiales.
**dorsispinal v.'s,** v.'s forming a plexus around the arches and processes of the vertebrae.
**em'issary v.'s,** see entries under *vena* emissaria.
**epigas'tric v.'s,** see entries under *vena* epigastrica.
**episcleral v.'s,** *venae* episclerales.
**esophageal v.'s,** *venae* esophageae.
**ethmoidal v.'s,** *venae* ethmoidales.
**external iliac v.,** *vena* iliaca externa.
**external jugular v.,** *vena* jugularis externa.
**external nasal v.'s,** *venae* nasales externae.
**external palatine v.,** *vena* palatina externa.
**external pudendal v.'s,** *venae* pudendae externae.
**v.'s of eyelids,** *venae* palpebrales.
**facial v.,** *vena* facialis.
**femoral v.,** *vena* femoralis.
**fibular v.'s,** *venae* peroneae.
**frontal v.'s,** *venae* supratrochleares.

**Galen's v.'s,** see *vena* cerebri magna and *venae* cerebri internae.

**gastric v.'s,** see entries under *vena* gastrica.

**gastroepiploic v.'s,** *vena* gastroepiploica dextra and sinistra.

**gluteal v.'s,** *venae* gluteae inferiores and superiores.

**great cardiac v.,** *vena* cordis magna.

**great cerebral v.,** *vena* cerebri magna.

**great v. of Galen,** *vena* cerebri magna.

**great saphenous v.,** *vena* saphena magna.

**hemiazygos v.,** *vena* hemiazygos.

**hemorrhoi'dal v.'s,** see entries under *venae* rectales.

**hepatic v.'s,** *venae* hepaticae.

**highest intercostal v.,** *vena* intercostalis suprema.

**hypogas'tric v.,** *vena* iliaca interna.

**ileal v.'s,** see *venae* jejunales et ilei.

**ileocolic v.,** *vena* ileocolica.

**iliac v.'s,** see entries under *vena* iliaca.

**iliolumbar v.,** *vena* iliolumbalis.

**inferior anastomotic v.,** *vena* anastomotica inferior.

**inferior basal v.,** *vena* basalis inferior.

**inferior cardiac v.,** *vena* cordis media.

**inferior cerebellar v.'s,** 12 *venae* cerebelli inferiores.

**inferior cerebral v.'s,** *venae* cerebri inferiores.

**inferior epigastric v.,** *vena* epigastrica inferior.

**v.'s of inferior eyelid,** *venae* palpebrales inferiores.

**inferior gluteal v.'s,** *venae* gluteae inferiores.

**inferior labial v.,** *vena* labialis inferior.

**inferior laryngeal v.,** *vena* laryngea inferior.

**inferior mesenteric v.,** *vena* mesenterica inferior.

**inferior ophthalmic v.,** *vena* ophthalmica inferior.

**inferior phrenic v.,** *vena* phrenica inferior.

**inferior rectal v.'s,** *venae* rectales inferiores.

**inferior thyroid v.,** *vena* thyroidea inferior.

**infrasegmental v.'s,** see *pars* infrasegmentalis.

**innominate v.'s,** *venae* brachiocephalicae.

**innominate cardiac v.'s,** Vieussens' v.'s; the small superficial v.'s of the heart.

**intercapitular v.'s,** *venae* intercapita'les.

**intercostal v.'s,** see entries under *venae* intercostales.

**interlobar v.'s of kidney,** *venae* interlobares renis.

**interlobular v.'s of kidney,** *venae* interlobulares renis.

**interlobular v.'s of liver,** *venae* interlobulares hepatis.

**internal auditory v.'s,** *venae* labyrinthi.

**internal cerebral v.'s,** *venae* cerebri internae.

**internal iliac v.,** *vena* iliaca interna.

**internal jugular v.,** *vena* jugularis interna.

**internal pudendal v.,** *vena* pudenda interna.

**internal thoracic v.,** *vena* thoracica interna.

**intersegmental v.'s,** see *pars* infrasegmentalis.

**intervertebral v.,** *vena* intervertebralis.

**intrasegmental v.'s,** *pars* infrasegmentalis.

**jejunal and ileal v.'s,** *venae* jejunales et ilei.

**jug'ular v.'s,** see entries under *vena* jugularis; see also posterior external jugular v.

**key v.,** a deep-seated, dilated v. causing a "spider burst" on the surface.

**v.'s of kidney,** *venae* renis.

**v.'s of knee,** *venae* genus.

**Krukenberg's v.'s,** *venae* centrales hepatis.

**Labbé's v.,** *vena* anastomotica inferior.

**labial v.'s,** *venae* labiales.

**labyrinthine v.'s,** *venae* labyrinthi.

**lacrimal v.,** *vena* lacrimalis.

**large v.,** a v., such as the inferior vena cava, characterized by having a reduced or absent tunica media and an adventitia with large bundles of longitudinally disposed smooth muscle.

**large saphenous v.,** *vena* saphena magna.

**laryngeal v.'s,** *vena* laryngea inferior and superior.

**Latarjet's v.,** *vena* prepylorica.

**lateral circumflex femoral v.'s,** *venae* circumflexae femoris laterales.

**lateral sacral v.'s,** *venae* sacrales laterales.

**lateral thoracic v.,** *vena* thoracica lateralis.

**left colic v.,** *vena* colica sinistra.

**left coronary v.,** *vena* cordis magna.

**left gastric v.,** *vena* gastrica sinistra.

**left gastroepiploic v.,** *vena* gastroepiploica sinistra.

**left hepatic v.'s,** *venae* hepaticae sinistrae.

**left inferior pulmonary v.,** *vena* pulmonalis inferior sinistra.

**left ovarian v.,** *vena* ovarica sinistra.

**left superior intercostal v.,** *vena* intercostalis superior sinistra.

**left superior pulmonary v.,** *vena* pulmonalis superior sinistra.

**left suprarenal v.,** *vena* suprarenalis sinistra.

**left testicular v.,** *vena* testicularis sinistra.

**left umbilical v.,** *vena* umbilicalis sinistra.

**levoatrio-cardinal v.,** the communication of a systemic v. with the left atrium, other than a left superior vena cava or coronary sinus; may be the right superior vena cava.

**lingual v.,** *vena* lingualis.

**long saphenous v.,** *vena* saphena magna.

**long thoracic v.,** *vena* thoracica lateralis.

**lumbar v.'s,** *venae* lumbales.

**Marshall's oblique v.,** *vena* obliqua atrii sinistri.

**masseter'ic v.'s,** plexiform v.'s, accompanying the masseteric artery that empty into the pterygoid venous plexus.

**mastoid emissary v.,** *vena* emissaria mastoidea.

**maxillary v.,** *vena* maxillaris.

**Mayo's v.,** *vena* prepylorica.

**medial circumflex femoral v.'s,** *venae* circumflexae femoris mediales.

**median antebrachial v.,** *vena* mediana antebrachii.

**median basilic v.,** *vena* mediana basilica.

**median cephalic v.,** *vena* mediana cephalica.

**median cubital v.,** *vena* mediana cubiti.

**median v. of forearm,** *vena* mediana antebrachii.

**median v. of neck,** occasionally present, owing to fusion of the two anterior jugular v.'s.

**median sacral v.,** *vena* sacralis mediana.

**mediastinal v.'s,** *venae* mediastinales.

**medium v.,** one characterized by having a thinner wall and larger lumen than its corresponding artery, and a media with small bundles of circular muscle separated by considerable connective tissue; also, valves occur.

**meningeal v.'s,** *venae* meningeae.

**mesenteric v.'s,** see *vena* mesenterica inferior and superior.

**metacarpal v.'s,** see subentries under *venae* metacarpeae.

**middle cardiac v.,** *vena* cordis media.

**middle colic v.,** *vena* colica media.

**middle hepatic v.'s,** *venae* hepaticae mediae.

**middle meningeal v.'s,** *venae* meningeae mediae.

**middle rectal v.'s,** *venae* rectales mediae.

**middle temporal v.,** *vena* temporalis media.

**middle thyroid v.,** *vena* thyroidea media.

**musculophrenic v.'s,** *venae* musculophrenicae.

**nasofrontal v.,** *vena* nasofrontalis.

**oblique v. of left atrium,** *vena* obliqua atrii sinistri.

**obturator v.,** *vena* obturatoria.

**occipital v.,** *vena* occipitalis.

**occipital emissary v.,** *vena* emissaria occipitalis.

**ophthalmic v.'s,** see *vena* ophthalmica inferior and superior.

**ovarian v.'s,** see *vena* ovarica dextra and sinistra.

**palatine v.,** *vena* palatina externa.

**palmar digital v.'s,** *venae* digitales palmares.

**palmar metacarpal v.'s,** *venae* metacarpeae palmares.

**pancreatic v.'s,** *venae* pancreaticae.

**pancreaticoduodenal v.'s,** *venae* pancreaticoduodenales.

**paraumbilical v.'s,** *venae* paraumbilicales.

**parietal emissary v.,** *vena* emissaria parietalis.

**parot'id v.'s,** *venae* parotideae.

**pectoral v.'s,** *venae* pectorales.

**perforating v.'s,** *venae* perforantes.

**pericardiacophrenic v.'s,** *venae* pericardiacophrenicae.

**pericardial v.'s,** *venae* pericardiacae.

**peroneal v.'s,** *venae* peroneae.

**petrosal v.,** see *sinus* petrosus superior and *sinus* petrosus inferior.

**pharyngeal v.'s,** *venae* pharyngeae.

**phrenic v.'s,** see entries under *vena* phrenica.

**plantar digital v.'s,** *venae* digitales plantares.

**plantar metatarsal v.'s,** *venae* metatarseae plantares.

**popliteal v.,** *vena* poplitea.

**portal v.,** *vena* portae.

**posterior anterior jugular v.,** a variable tributary of the external jugular v. arising in the upper posterior part of the neck.

**posterior auricular v.,** *vena* auricularis posterior.

**posterior facial v.,** *vena* retromandibularis.

**posterior intercostal v.'s,** *venae* intercostales posteriores.

**posterior labial v.'s,** *venae* labiales posteriores.

**posterior v. of left ventricle,** *vena* posterior ventriculi sinistri.

**posterior parotid v.'s,** *venae* parotideae.

**posterior scrotal v.'s,** *venae* scrotales posteriores.

**posterior tibial v.'s,** *venae* tibiales posteriores.

**prepyloric v.,** *vena* prepylorica.

**v. of pterygoid canal,** *vena* canalis pterygoidei.

**pudendal v.'s,** see *venae* pudendae externae and *vena* pudenda interna.

**pulmonary v.'s,** *venae* pulmonales.

**pyloric v.,** *vena* gastrica dextra.

**radial v.'s,** *venae* radiales.

**renal v.'s,** *venae* renales.

**retromandibular v.,** *vena* retromandibularis.

**Retzius' v.'s,** Ruysch's v.'s; v.'s arising in the walls of the intestine and passing to the branches of the vena cava instead of to those of the portal v.

**right colic v.,** *vena* colica dextra.

**right gastric v.,** *vena* gastrica dextra.

**right gastroepiploic v.,** *vena* gastroepiploica dextra.

**right hepatic v.'s,** *venae* hepaticae dextrae.

**right inferior pulmonary v.,** *vena* pulmonalis inferior dextra.

**right ovarian v.,** *vena* ovarica dextra.

**right superior intercostal v.,** *vena* intercostalis superior dextra.

**right superior pulmonary v.,** *vena* pulmonalis superior dextra.

**right suprarenal v.,** *vena* suprarenalis dextra.

**right testicular v.,** *vena* testicularis dextra.

**Rosenthal's v.,** *vena* basalis.

**Ruysch's v.'s,** Retzius' v.'s.

**sacral v.'s,** *venae* sacrales.

**Santorini's v.,** *vena* emissaria parietalis.

**saphenous v.'s,** see entries under *vena* saphena.

**Sappey's v.'s,** *venae* paraumbilicales.

**scrotal v.'s,** see entries under *venae* scrotales.

**v. of septum pellucidum,** *vena* septi pellucidi.

**short gastric v.'s,** *venae* gastricae breves.

**short saphenous v.,** *vena* saphena parva.

**sigmoid v.'s,** *venae* sigmoideae.

**small v.,** one in which the three tunics are poorly defined and thin; longitudinal elastic networks occur and the smooth muscle of the media, which is circularly arranged, may be incomplete or in one or two layers.

**small cardiac v.,** *vena* cordis parva.

**small saphenous v.,** *vena* saphena parva.

**smallest cardiac v.'s,** *venae* cordis minimae.

**spinal v.'s,** *venae* spinales.

**spiral v. of modiolus,** *vena* spiralis modioli.

**splenic v.,** *vena* lienalis.

**stellate v.'s,** *venulae* stellatae.

**Stensen's v.'s,** *venae* vorticosae.

**sternocleidomastoid v.,** *vena* sternocleidomastoidea.

**striate v.,** *vena* striata.

**stylomastoid v.,** *vena* stylomastoidea.

**subclavian v.,** *vena* subclavia.

**subcutaneous v.'s of abdomen,** *venae* subcutaneae abdominis.

**sublingual v.,** *vena* sublingualis.

**submental v.,** *vena* submentalis.

**superficial v.,** *vena* cutanea.

**superficial circumflex iliac v.,** *vena* circumflexa ilium superficialis.

**superficial dorsal v.'s of clitoris,** *venae* dorsales clitoridis superficiales.

**superficial dorsal v.'s of penis,** *venae* dorsales penis superficiales.

**superficial epigastric v.,** *vena* epigastrica superficialis.

**superficial middle cerebral v.,** *vena* cerebri media superficialis.

**superficial temporal v.'s,** *venae* temporales superficiales.

**superior anastomotic v.,** *vena* anastomotica superior.

**superior basal v.,** *vena* basalis superior.

**superior cerebellar v.'s,** *venae* cerebelli superiores.

**superior cerebral v.'s,** *venae* cerebri superiores.

**superior epigastric v.'s,** *venae* epigastricae superiores.

**v.'s of superior eyelid,** *venae* palpebrales superiores.

**superior gluteal v.'s,** *venae* gluteae superiores.

**superior labial v.,** *vena* labialis superior.

**superior laryngeal v.,** *vena* laryngea superior.

**superior mesenteric v.,** *vena* mesenterica superior.

**superior ophthalmic v.,** *vena* ophthalmica superior.

**superior phrenic v.'s,** *venae* phrenicae superiores.

**superior rectal v.,** *vena* rectalis superior.

**superior thyroid v.,** *vena* thyroidea superior.

**supraorbital v.,** *vena* supraorbitalis.

**suprarenal v.'s,** see *vena* suprarenalis dextra and sinistra.

**suprascapular v.,** *vena* suprascapularis.

**supratrochlear v.'s,** *venae* supratrochleares.

**temporal v.'s,** see entries under *vena* temporalis.

**v.'s of temporomandibular joint,** *venae* articulares temporomandibulares.

**temporomaxillary v.,** *vena* retromandibularis.

**terminal v.,** *vena* thalamostriata.

**testicular v.'s,** see *vena* testicularis dextra and sinistra.

**thalamostriate v.,** *vena* thalamostriata.

**Thebesian v.'s,** *venae* cordis minimae.

**thoracic v.'s,** see entries under *vena* thoracica.

**thoracoacro′mial v.,** *vena* thoracoacromialis.

**thoracoepigastric v.,** *vena* thoracoepigastrica.

**thymic v.'s,** *venae* thymicae.

**thyroid v.'s,** see entries under *vena* thyroidea.

**tracheal v.'s,** *venae* tracheales.

**transverse v. of face,** *vena* transversa faciei.

**transverse v.'s of neck,** *venae* transversae colli.

**transverse v. of scapula,** *vena* suprascapularis.

**Trolard's v.,** *vena* anastomotica superior.

**tympanic v.'s,** *venae* tympanicae.

**ulnar v.'s,** *venae* ulnares.

**umbil′ical v.,** see *vena* umbilicalis sinistra.

**uterine v.'s,** *venae* uterinae.

**varicose v.'s,** permanent dilation and tortuosity of v.'s, most commonly seen in the legs, probably as a result of congenitally incomplete valves; there is a predisposition to varicose v.'s among persons in occupations requiring long periods of standing, and in pregnant women.

**vertebral v.,** *vena* vertebralis.

**Vesalius' v.,** the emissary v. passing through Vesalius' foramen.

**vertical v.'s,** *venae* vesicales.

**vestibular v.'s,** *venae* vestibulares.

**v. of vestibular bulb,** *vena* bulbi vestibuli.

**Vidian v.,** *vena* canalis pterygoidei.

**Vieussens' v.'s,** innominate cardiac v.'s.

**vitelline v.'s,** v.'s returning blood from the yolk-sac to the embryo.

**vor′ticose v.'s,** *venae* vorticosae.

---

**veined** (vānd). Marked by veins or lines resembling veins on the surface.

**veinlet** (vān′let). Venula.

**Vejovis.** A genus of scorpions (the so-called devil scorpions of North America), including *V. spinigerus,* the stripe-tailed devil scorpion; *V. carolinianus,* the southern devil scorpion; and *V. flavus,* the slender devil scorpion.

**velamen,** pl. **velamina** (vĕ-la′men, vĕ-lam′ĭ-nah) [ L. a veil. VEL- ]. Velum.

 **v. vulvae,** hypertrophy of the labia minora; sometimes called Hottentot apron because of its frequency in this race.

**vel′amen′tous.** Expanded in the form of a sheet or veil.

**velamentum,** pl. **velamenta** (vel′ă-men′tum, -tah) [ L. a cover. VEL- ]. Velum.

**ve′lar.** Relating to any velum, especially the velum palati.

**vel′iform** [ L. *velum,* veil, + *forma,* form ]. Velamentous.

**Vella,** Luigi, Italian physiologist, 1825–1886. See V.'s *fistula,* Thiry-V. *fistula.*

**vellicate** (vel′ĭ-kāt) [ L. *vellico,* pp. *-atus,* to pluck, to twitch, fr. *vello,* to deprive of hair, pluck ]. To twitch; to contract spasmodically; said especially of fibrillary muscular spasms.

**vellication** (vel'ĭ-ka'shun) [ see vellicate ]. Twitching; fibrillary muscular spasm.

**vel'losine.** An alkaloid in the bark, fruit, and leaves of *Geissospermum vellozii* (family Apocynaceae), a plant of Brazil; antiperiodic.

**vel'lus** [ L. fleece ]. 1 [ NA ]. Fine body hair present before puberty. 2. A structure that is fleecy or soft and woolly in appearance.

 **v. oli'vae inferio'ris,** a stratum of nerve fibers surrounding the inferior olive.

**velocity** (vĕ-los'ĭ-tĭ) [ L. *velocitas,* fr. *velox (veloc-),* quick, swift ]. Rate of movement.

 **maximum v.,** see $V_{max}$.

 **nerve conduction v.,** the rate of impulse conductance in a peripheral nerve or its various component fibers, generally expressed in meters per second.

**velogen'ic** [ L. *velox,* rapid, + G. suffix *-gen,* producing ]. Denoting the virulence of a virus capable of inducing, after a brief incubation period, a fulminating and often lethal disease in embryonic, immature, and adult hosts; used in characterizing Newcastle disease virus.

**velonoskiascopy** (ve'lo-no-skī-as'ko-pĭ) [ L. *velum,* veil, + skiascopy ]. A subjective test for ametropia in which a thin rod is moved across the pupil while a distant light source is fixed; the shadow of the rod moves with the rod in myopia, and in the opposite direction in hyperopia.

**velopharyngeal** (ve'lo-fă-rin'je-al). Pertaining to the soft palate (velum palatinum) and the posterior nasopharyngeal wall.

**ve'losyn'thesis.** Staphylorrhaphy.

**Velpeau** (vel-po'), Alfred A. L. M., Paris surgeon, 1795–1867. See V.'s *bandage, canal, deformity, fossa, hernia.*

**velum,** pl. **vela** (ve'lum, -lah) [ L. veil, sail. VEL- ] 1 [ NA ]. Velamen; velamentum; veil (1); any structure resembling a veil or curtain. 2. Caul (1). 3. The *omentum majus.* 4. Any serous membrane or membranous envelope or covering.

 **anterior medullary v.,** v. medullaris superius.

 **inferior medullary v.,** v. medullare inferius.

 **v. interpos'itum,** *tela* choroidea ventriculi tertii.

 **v. medulla're infe'rius** [ NA ], inferior or posterior medullary v.; v. semilunare; v. tarini; Tarin's valve; valvula semilunaris tarini; a thin sheet of white matter, hidden by the tonsilla cerebelli, attached along the peduncle of the flocculus and, at and near the midline, to the nodulus of the vermis; it is continuous caudally with the lamina choroidea and plexus choroideus of the fourth ventricle.

 **v. medulla're supe'rius** [ NA ], superior or anterior medullary v.; valve of Vieussens; the thin layer of white matter stretching between the two superior cerebellar peduncles, forming the medial part of the roof of the superior recess of the fourth ventricle.

 **v. palati'num** [ NA ], official alternate name for *palatum molle.*

 **v. pendulum palati,** *palatum* molle.

 **posterior medullary v.,** v. medullare inferius.

 **v. semiluna're,** v. medullare inferius.

 **superior medullary v.,** v. medullaris superius.

 **v. tarini,** v. medullare inferius.

 **v. terminale,** *lamina* terminalis cerebri.

 **v. transver'sum,** a fold in the dorsal wall of the embryonic brain at the boundary between the telencephalon and diencephalon.

 **v. triangula're,** *tela* choroidea ventriculi tertii.

# VENA

**vena,** gen. and pl. **venae** (ve'nah, -ne) [ L. ] [ NA ]. Vein; a blood vessel carrying blood toward the heart; all the veins except the pulmonary carry dark or unaerated blood. See color plates 25 and 26.

 **v. ad'vehens,** pl. **venae advehentes,** veins carrying blood to capillaries as in the portal circulation of the liver.

 **v. anastomot'ica infe'rior** [ NA ], inferior anastomotic vein; vein of Browning or Labbé; an inconstant vein that passes from the superficial middle cerebral vein posteriorly over the lateral aspect of the temporal lobe to enter the transverse sinus.

 **v. anastomot'ica supe'rior** [ NA ], superior anastomotic vein; vein of Trolard; a large communicating vein between the superficial middle cerebral vein and the superior sagittal sinus; it passes upward from the lateral sulcus, often following the line of the sulcus centralis (Rolando's fissure).

 **v. angula'ris** [ NA ], angular vein; a short vein at the anterior angle of the orbit, formed by the supraorbital and supratrochlear veins and continuing as the facial.

 **v. appendicula'ris** [ NA ], appendicular vein; the branch of the ileocolic vein that accompanies the appendicular artery.

 **v. aqueduc'tus coch'leae** [ NA ], vein of the cochlear aqueduct; see v. canaliculi cochleae.

 **v. aqueduc'tus vestib'uli** [ NA ], vein of vestibular aqueduct; a small vein accompanying the endolymphatic duct; it terminates in the inferior petrosal sinus.

 **venae arcua'tae re'nis** [ NA ], arcuate or arciform veins of the kidney; they parallel the arcuate arteries, receive blood from interlobular veins and venulae rectae, and terminate in interlobar veins.

 **v. arterio'sa,** arterial *vein.*

 **venae articula'res temporomandibula'res** [ NA ], veins of the temporomandibular joint; several small tributaries to the retromandibular vein from the temporomandibular joint.

 **v. auricula'ris ante'rior** [ NA ], anterior auricular vein; v. preauricularis; one of several emptying into the retromandibular.

 **v. auricula'ris poste'rior** [ NA ], posterior auricular vein; a tributary to the external jugular vein, draining the region posterior to the ear.

 **v. axilla'ris** [ NA ], axillary vein; a continuation of the basilic and brachial veins running from the lower border of the teres major muscle to the outer border of the first rib where it becomes the subclavian.

 **v. az'ygos** [ NA ], azygos vein; v. azygos major; arises from the right ascending lumbar vein or the inferior v. cava, ascends through the aortic orifice of the diaphragm, lies in the posterior mediastinum, and terminates in the superior v. cava; receives blood from the right posterior intercostals, and the hemiazygos and accessory hemiazygos.

 **v. az'ygos major,** v. azygos.

 **v. az'ygos minor inferior,** v. hemiazygos.

 **v. azygos minor superior,** v. hemiazygos accessoria.

 **v. basa'lis** [ NA ], basal vein of Rosenthal; Rosenthal's vein; a large vein passing caudally and dorsally along the medial surface of the temporal lobe from which it receives tributaries; it empties into the vena cerebri magna of Galen from the lateral side.

 **v. basa'lis commu'nis** [ NA ], common basal vein; the tributary to the inferior pulmonary vein (right and left) that receives blood from the superior and inferior basal veins.

 **v. basa'lis infe'rior** [ NA ], inferior basal vein; tributary to the common basal vein draining the medial and posterior part of the inferior lobe in each lung.

 **v. basa'lis supe'rior** [ NA ], superior basal vein; tributary to the common basal vein draining the lateral and anterior part of the inferior lobe of each lung.

 **v. basilica** [ NA ], basilic vein; arises on the back of the hand from the ulnar side of the dorsal venous rete; it curves around the medial side of the forearm and passes up the medial side of the arm to join the axillary vein.

 **v. basivertebra'lis** [ NA ], basivertebral vein; one of a number of veins in the spongy substance of the bodies of the vertebrae, emptying into the anterior internal vertebral venous plexus.

 **Billroth's venae cavernosae,** *venae* cavernosae of spleen.

 **venae brachia'les** [ NA ], brachial veins; two veins in either arm accompanying the brachial artery and emptying into the axillary vein.

 **venae brachiocephal'icae** [ NA ], brachiocephalic veins; innominate veins anonymous veins; formed by the union of the internal jugular and subclavian; *tributaries:* the right brachiocephalic receives the right vertebral and internal thoracic, and the right lymphatic duct; the left receives the left vertebral, internal thoracic, superior intercostal, thyroidea ima, and various anterior pericardial, bronchial, and mediastinal veins.

**venae bronchia'les** [ NA ], many veins running in front of and behind the bronchi and uniting into two main trunks which empty on the right side into the azygos, on the left into the accessory hemiazygos or the left superior intercostal vein.

**v. bul'bi pe'nis** [ NA ], vein of the bulb of the penis; a tributary of the internal pudendal vein that drains the bulb of the penis.

**v. bul'bi vestib'uli** [ NA ], vein of the vestibular bulb; the vein draining the bulb of the vestibule; a tributary of the internal pudendal vein.

**v. canalic'uli coch'leae** [ NA ], v. aqueductus cochleae [ NA ], vein of the cochlear canaliculus or aqueduct; it drains the cochlea and the sacculus, and empties into the superior bulb of the jugular vein by accompanying the cochlear aqueduct through the cochlear canal.

**v. cana'lis pterygoid'ei** [ NA ], vein of the pterygoid canal; Vidian vein; a vein accompanying the nerve and artery through the pterygoid canal and emptying into the pharyngeal vein.

**v. cardi'aca mag'na,** v. cordis magna.

**v. ca'va infe'rior** [ NA ], inferior v. cava; receives the blood from the lower limbs and the greater part of the pelvic and abdominal organs; it begins at the level of the fifth lumbar vertebra on the right side, pierces the diaphragm at the level of the eighth thoracic vertebra, and empties into the back part of the right atrium of the heart.

**v. ca'va supe'rior** [ NA ], superior v. cava; returns blood from the head and neck, upper limbs, and thorax; formed by union of the two brachiocephalic veins; also the azygos vein.

**venae caverno'sae pe'nis** [ NA ], the cavernous venous spaces in the erectile tissue of the penis.

**venae cavernosae of the spleen,** Billroth's venae cavernosae; small tributaries of the splenic vein in the pulp of the spleen.

**v. centra'lis glan'dulae suprarena'lis** [ NA ], central vein of the suprarenal gland; the single draining vein of the gland; it receives a number of medullary veins; on the right side it empties directly into the inferior vena cava and on the left into the left renal vein.

**venae centra'les hep'atis** [ NA ], central veins of the liver; Krukenberg's veins; the terminal branches of the hepatic veins that lie centrally in the hepatic lobules and receive blood from the liver sinusoids.

**v. centra'lis ret'inae** [ NA ], central vein of the retina; formed by union of the retinal veins and accompanies the artery of the same name in the optic nerve.

**v. cephal'ica** [ NA ], cephalic vein; arises at the radial border of the dorsal venous rete of the hand, passes upward in front of the elbow and along the lateral side of the arm; it empties into the upper part of the axillary vein.

**v. cephal'ica accesso'ria** [ NA ], accessory cephalic vein; a variable vein that passes along the radial border of the forearm to join the cephalic vein near the elbow.

**venae cerebel'li inferio'res** [ NA ], inferior cerebellar veins; they drain the undersurface of the cerebellum and empty into the inferior petrosal and transverse sinuses.

**venae cerebel + li superio'res** [ NA ], superior cerebellar veins; they drain the upper surface of the cerebellum and empty into the straight and the transverse sinuses.

**v. cer'ebri ante'rior** [ NA ], anterior cerebral vein; a small vein that parallels the anterior cerebral artery and drains into the basal vein.

**venae cer'ebri inferio'res** [ NA ], inferior cerebral veins; numerous cerebral veins that drain the undersurface of the cerebral hemispheres and empty into the cavernous and transverse sinuses.

**venae cer'ebri inter'nae** [ NA ], internal cerebral veins; veins of Galen; two paired veins passing caudally near the midline in the tela choroidea of the third ventricle, formed by the union of the choroid vein, thalamostriate (terminal) vein, and vena septi pellucidi, and uniting caudally so as to form the v. cerebri magna.

**v. cer'ebri mag'na** [ NA ], great cerebral vein; great vein of Galen; a large, unpaired vein formed by the junction of the two internal cerebral veins in the caudal part of the tela choroidea of the third ventricle; it passes caudally between the splenium of the corpus callosum and the pineal gland, curving dorsally to continue into the sinus rectus.

**v. cer'ebri me'dia profun'da** [ NA ], deep middle cerebral vein; the vein that accompanies the middle cerebral artery in the depths of the Sylvian fissure and empties into the basal vein of Rosenthal.

**v. cer'ebri me'dia superficia'lis** [ NA ], superficial middle cerebral vein; a large vein passing along the line of the Sylvian fissure to join the cavernous sinus; it communicates with the superior sagittal sinus and transverse sinus via the superior and inferior anastomotic veins, respectively.

**venae cer'ebri superio'res** [ NA ], superior cerebral veins; numerous (8 to 10) veins that drain the dorsal convexity of the cortical hemisphere and empty into the superior sagittal sinus, curving rostralward in passing through the subdural space so as to enter the sinus at an acute forward angle.

**v. cervica'lis profun'da** [ NA ], deep cervical vein; it runs with the artery of the same name between the semispinalis capitis and semispinalis cervicis and empties into the brachiocephalic or the vertebral vein.

**v. choroi'dea** [ NA ], choroid vein; a tortuous vein that follows the choroid plexus of the lateral ventricle and unites with the thalamostriate vein and vena septi pellucidi to form the internal cerebral vein.

**venae choroi'deae oc'uli** [ NA ], choroid veins of the eye; official alternate term for venae vorticosae.

**venae cilia'res** [ NA ], ciliary veins; several small veins, anterior and posterior, coming from the ciliary body.

**venae circumflex'ae fem'oris latera'les** [ NA ], lateral circumflex femoral veins; the veins that accompany the lateral circumflex femoral artery.

**venae circumflex'ae fem'oris media'les** [ NA ], medial circumflex femoral veins; the venae comitantes that parallel the medial circumflex femoral artery.

**v. circumflex'a il'ium profun'da** [ NA ], deep circumflex iliac vein; corresponds to the artery of the same name, and empties, near or in a common trunk with the inferior epigastric, into the external iliac vein.

**v. circumflex'a il'ium superficia'lis** [ NA ], superficial circumflex iliac vein; corresponding to the artery of the same name, emptying usually into the greater saphenous, or sometimes into the femoral.

**v. col'ica dex'tra** [ NA ], right colic vein; the vein that parallels the right colic artery and drains blood from the ascending colon and right flexure.

**v. col'ica me'dia** [ NA ], middle colic vein; the tributary of the superior mesenteric vein that accompanies the middle colic artery.

**v. col'ica sinis'tra** [ NA ], left colic vein; a tributary of the inferior mesenteric vein that accompanies the left colic artery and drains the left flexure and descending colon.

**v. com'itans,** pl. **venae comitantes** [ L. accompanying vein ] [ NA ], companion vein or veins; (1) vena comitans; a vein accompanying another structure; (2) venae comitantes; a pair of veins, occasionally more, that closely accompany an artery in such a manner that the pulsations of the artery aid venous return.

**v. com'itans ner'vi hypoglos'si** [ NA ], runs with the hypoglossal nerve below and lateral to the hypoglossus muscle, emptying usually into the lingual vein.

**venae conjunctiva'les** [ NA ], conjunctival veins; the veins draining the conjunctiva.

**venae cor'dis anterio'res** [ NA ], anterior cardiac veins; two or three small veins in the anterior wall of the right ventricle opening into the right atrium independently of the coronary sinus.

**v. cor'dis mag'na** [ NA ], great cardiac vein; v. cardiaca magna; left coronary vein; a tributary of the coronary sinus, beginning at the apex and running in the anterior interventricular sulcus.

**v. cor'dis me'dia** [ NA ], middle cardiac vein; inferior cardiac or interventricular vein; begins at the apex of the heart and passes through the posterior interventricular sulcus to the coronary sinus.

**venae cor'dis min'imae** [ NA ], smallest cardiac veins; Thebesian veins; numerous small venous channels that open directly into the chambers of the heart from the capillary bed in the cardiac wall.

**v. cor'dis par'va** [ NA ], small cardiac vein; an inconstant vessel, accompanying the right coronary artery in the coronary sulcus, from the right margin of the right ventricle, and emptying into the coronary sinus or the middle cardiac vein.

**v. corona'ria ventric'uli,** v. gastrica sinistra.

**v. cuta'nea** [ NA ], cutaneous vein; superficial vein; one of a number of veins that course in the subcutaneous tissue and empty into deep veins; they form prominent systems of vessels in the limbs and are usually not accompanied by arteries.

**v. cys'tica** [ NA ], cystic vein; it drains the gallbladder, passing along the cystic duct to enter the right branch of the portal vein.

**venae digita'les dorsa'les pe'dis** [ NA ], dorsal digital veins of the toes; they receive intercapitular veins from the plantar venous arch, join to form four common dorsal digital veins, and terminate in the dorsal venous arch.

**venae digita'les palma'res** [ NA ], palmar digital veins; they form paired venae comitantes along the proper and common digital arteries and empty into the superficial palmar venous arch.

**venae digita'les planta'res** [ NA ], plantar digital veins; they arise in the toes and pass back to form four metatarsal veins that empty into the plantar venous arch.

**v. diplo'ica** [ NA ], diploic vein; Dupuytren's canal; one of the veins in the diploë of the cranial bones, connected with the cerebral sinuses by emissary veins; the main diploic veins are the frontal, anterior temporal, posterior temporal, and occipital.

**v. dorsa'lis clitor'idis profun'da** [ NA ], deep dorsal vein of the clitoris; a tributary of the vesical venous plexus; it runs a course deep to the fascia on the dorsum of the clitoris.

**venae dorsa'les clitor'idis superficia'les** [ NA ], superficial dorsal veins of the clitoris; a pair of veins on the dorsum of the clitoris, tributary to the external pudendal vein on either side.

**v. dorsa'lis lin'guae** [ NA ], dorsal lingual vein; a tributary of the lingual.

**v. dorsa'lis pe'nis profun'da** [ NA ], deep dorsal vein of the penis; a vein on the dorsum of the penis deep to the fascia penis; it is a tributary to the prostatic plexus.

**venae dorsa'les pe'nis superficia'les** [ NA ], superficial dorsal veins of the penis; a pair of veins on the dorsum of the penis superficial to the fascia penis; they are tributaries of the external pudendal veins on each side.

**v. emissa'ria,** pl. **venae emissa'riae** [ NA ], emissary vein; emissarium; one of the channels of communication between the venous sinuses of the dura mater and the veins of the diploë and the scalp.

**v. emissa'ria condyla'ris** [ NA ], condylar emissary vein; emissarium condyloideum; a vein that connects the sigmoid sinus and the external vertebral venous plexuses through the condylar canal of the occipital bone.

**v. emissa'ria mastoi'dea** [ NA ], mastoid emissary vein; emissarium mastoideum; the vein that connects the sigmoid sinus with the occipital vein or one of the tributaries of the external jugular by way of the mastoid foramen.

**v. emissa'ria occipita'lis** [ NA ], occipital emissary vein; emissarium occipitale; an inconstant vessel connecting the occipital veins with the confluens sinuum.

**v. emissa'ria parieta'lis** [ NA ], parietal emissary vein; emissarium parietale; Santorini's vein; the vein that connects the superior sagittal sinus with the tributaries of the superficial temporal vein and other veins of the scalp.

**v. epigas'trica infe'rior** [ NA ], inferior epigastric vein; deep epigastric vein; corresponds to the artery of the same name and empties into the external iliac vein.

**v. epigas'trica superficia'lis** [ NA ], superficial epigastric vein; drains the lower and medial part of the anterior abdominal wall and empties into the great saphenous vein.

**venae epigas'tricae superio'res** [ NA ], superior epigastric veins; the venae comitantes of the artery of the same name, tributaries of the internal thoracic.

**venae episcler'a'les** [ NA ], episcleral veins; a series of small venules in the sclera close to the corneal margin that empty into the anterior ciliary veins.

**venae esophage'ae** [ NA ], esophageal veins; several small venous trunks bringing blood from the esophagus and emptying into the brachiocephalic or the azygos.

**venae ethmoida'les** [ NA ], ethmoidal veins; veins that accompany the anterior and posterior ethmoidal arteries and pass into the superior ophthalmic vein; they drain the ethmoidal sinuses.

**v. facia'lis** [ NA ], facial vein; anterior facial vein; v. facialis anterior; a continuation of the angular vein at the medial angle of the orbit; passes diagonally downward and outward, uniting with the retromandibular below the border of the lower jaw before emptying into the internal jugular vein.

**v. facia'lis ante'rior,** v. facialis.

**v. facia'lis commu'nis,** common facial *vein*.

**v. facia'lis poste'rior,** v. retromandibularis.

**v. facie'i profun'da** [ NA ], deep facial vein; the communicating vein that passes from the facial vein to the pterygoid plexus in the infratemporal fossa; it is devoid of valves.

**v. femora'lis** [ NA ], femoral vein; it accompanies the femoral artery in the same sheath, being a continuation of the popliteal vein, and becomes the external iliac vein at the level of the inguinal (Poupart's) ligament.

**venae fibula'res** [ NA ], fibular veins; official alternate term for venae peroneae.

**venae fronta'les,** venae supratrochleares.

**venae gas'tricae bre'ves** [ NA ], short gastric veins; in the wall of the stomach emptying into the splenic vein.

**v. gas'trica dex'tra** [ NA ], right gastric vein; pyloric vein; it receives veins from both surfaces of the upper portion of the stomach, runs to the right along the lesser curvature of the stomach, and empties into the portal vein.

**v. gas'trica sinis'tra** [ NA ], left gastric vein; coronary vein; v. coronaria ventriculi; arises from a union of veins from both surfaces of the cardia of the stomach; it runs in the lesser omentum and empties into the portal vein.

**v. gastroepiplo'ica dex'tra** [ NA ], right gastroepiploic vein; a tributary of the superior mesenteric vein that parallels the right gastroepiploic artery along the greater curvature of the stomach.

**v. gastroepiplo'ica sinis'tra** [ NA ], left gastroepiploic vein; the vein that accompanies the left gastroepiploic artery along the greater curvature of the stomach; it empties into the splenic vein.

**venae ge'nus** [ NA ], veins of the knee; the veins that accompany the genicular arteries; they drain blood from the structures around the knee, terminating in the popliteal vein.

**venae glu'teae inferio'res** [ NA ], inferior gluteal veins; the venae comitantes of the inferior gluteal artery uniting at the sciatic foramen to form a common trunk which empties into the internal iliac vein.

**venae glu'teae superio'res** [ NA ], superior gluteal veins; the veins that accompany the gluteal artery, entering the pelvis as two veins which unite into one and empty into the internal iliac vein.

**v. hemiaz'ygos** [ NA ], hemiazygos vein; v. azygos minor inferior; the continuation of the left ascending lumbar vein; it pierces the left crus of the diaphragm, ascends along the left side of the bodies of the lower thoracic vertebrae, opposite the eighth vertebra, crosses the midline behind the aorta, thoracic duct, and esophagus, and empties into the azygos vein.

**v. hemiaz'ygos accesso'ria** [ NA ], accessory hemiazygos vein; v. azygos minor superior; formed by the union of the 4th to 7th left posterior intercostal veins, passes along the side of the bodies of the 5th, 6th, and 7th thoracic vertebrae, then crosses the midline behind the aorta, esophagus, and thoracic duct, and empties into the azygos vein.

**venae hemorrhoida'les inferio'res,** venae rectales inferiores.

**venae hemorrhoida'les me'diae,** venae rectales mediae.

**v. hemorrhoida'lis supe'rior,** v. rectalis superior.

**venae hepat'icae** [ NA ], hepatic veins; the veins that drain the liver; they collect blood from the central veins and terminate in three large veins opening into the inferior vena cava below the diaphragm and several small inconstant veins entering the vena cava lower down.

**venae hepat'icae dex'trae** [ NA ], right hepatic veins; veins draining the right lobe of the liver; they usually combine into one or two veins that empty into the inferior vena cava.

**venae hepat'icae me'diae** [ NA ], middle hepatic veins; the veins draining the caudate lobe of the liver; they usually form one trunk before emptying into the inferior vena cava.

**venae hepat'icae sinis'trae** [ NA ], left hepatic veins; the veins draining the left lobe of the liver; they usually form one or two veins that empty into the inferior vena cava.

**v. hypogas'trica,** v. iliaca interna.

**v. ileocol'ica** [ NA ], ileocolic vein; a large tributary of the superior mesenteric vein that runs parallel to the ileocolic artery and drains the terminal ileum, appendix, cecum, and the lower part of the ascending colon.

**v. ili'aca commu'nis** [ NA ], common iliac vein; formed by the union of the external and internal iliac veins at the brim of the pelvis and passes upward behind the internal iliac artery to the right side of the body of the fifth lumbar vertebra where it unites with its fellow of the opposite side to form the inferior v. cava; the left common iliac vein is submitted to a pulsating compression by the right common iliac artery against the vertebral column which may result in partial obstruction of the vein.

**v. ili'aca exter'na** [ NA ], external iliac vein; a direct continuation of the femoral above the inguinal ligament, uniting with the internal iliac to form the common iliac vein.

**v. ili'aca inter'na** [ NA ], internal iliac vein; hypogastric vein; v. hypogastrica; runs from the upper border of the greater sciatic notch to the brim of the pelvis where it joins the external iliac to form the common iliac; it drains most of the territory supplied by the internal iliac artery.

**v. iliolumba'lis** [ NA ], iliolumbar vein; accompanying the artery of the same name, anastomosing with the lumbar and deep circumflex iliac veins, and emptying into the internal iliac.

**inferior v. cava,** v. cava inferior.

**v. innomina'ta,** v. brachiocephalica.

**venae intercapita'les** [ NA ], intercapitular veins; the veins connecting the dorsal and palmar veins in the hand, or the dorsal and plantar veins in the foot.

**venae intercosta'les anterio'res** [ NA ], anterior intercostal veins; tributaries to the musculophrenic or internal thoracic veins from the intercostal spaces.

**v. intercosta'lis supe'rior dex'tra** [ NA ], right superior intercostal vein; a tributary of the azygos vein formed by the union of the right second, third and fourth posterior intercostal veins.

**v. intercosta'lis superior sinis'tra** [ NA ], left superior intercostal vein; the vein formed by the union of the left second, third and fourth intercostal veins; it passes forward across the arch of the aorta to empty into the left brachiocephalic vein and frequently communicates also with the accessory hemiazygos vein.

**v. intercosta'lis supre'ma** [ NA ], highest intercostal vein; the vein draining the first intercostal space into either the vertebral or the brachiocephalic vein.

**venae interloba'res re'nis** [ NA ], interlobar veins of the kidney; they parallel the interlobar arteries, receiving blood from arcuate veins, and terminate in the renal vein.

**venae interlobula'res hep'atis** [ NA ], interlobular veins of the liver; the terminal branches of the portal vein that course in the portal canals between liver lobules and empty into the liver sinusoids.

**venae interlobula'res re'nis** [ NA ], interlobular veins of the kidney; they parallel the interlobular arteries and drain the peritubular capillary plexus, emptying into arcuate veins.

**v. intervertebra'lis** [ NA ], one of numerous veins accompanying the spinal nerves, emptying in the neck into the vertebral, in the thorax into the intercostal, in the lumbar and sacral regions into the lumbar and sacral veins.

**venae jejuna'les et il'ei** [ NA ], jejunal and ileal veins; the veins that drain the jejunum and ileum; they terminate in the superior mesenteric vein.

**v. jugula'ris ante'rior** [ NA ], anterior jugular vein; it arises below the chin from veins draining the lower lip and mental region, descends the anterior portion of the neck superficially, and terminates in the external jugular at the lateral border of the scalenus anterior.

**v. jugula'ris exter'na** [ NA ], external jugular formed below the parotid gland by the junction of the posterior auricular and the retromandibular, it passes down the side of the neck superficial to the sternocleidomastoid muscle to empty into the subclavian vein.

**v. jugula'ris inter'na** [ NA ], internal jugular vein; a continuation of the sigmoid sinus of the dura mater, uniting, behind the cartilage of the first rib, with the subclavian to form the brachiocephalic; *tributaries:* superior thyroid, lingual, facial, retromandibular pharyngeal, meningeal, and the v. comitans nervi hypoglossi.

**venae labia'les anterio'res** [ NA ], anterior labial veins; they pass from the labia majora to the external pudendal veins.

**v. labia'lis infe'rior** [ NA ], inferior labial vein; a tributary of the facial vein draining the lower lip.

**venae labia'les posterio'res** [ NA ], posterior labial veins; they pass posteriorward from the labia majora to the internal pudendal veins.

**v. labia'lis supe'rior** [ NA ], superior labial vein; taking blood from the upper lip and discharging into the facial vein.

**venae labyrin'thi** [ NA ], labyrinthine veins; internal auditory veins; two veins accompanying each labyrinthine artery; they drain the internal ear, pass out through the internal acoustic meatus, and empty into the transverse sinus or the inferior petrosal sinus.

**v. lacrima'lis** [ NA ], lacrimal vein; it drains the lacrimal gland, passing posteriorly through the orbit with the lacrimal artery to empty into the superior ophthalmic vein.

**v. larynge'a infe'rior** [ NA ], inferior laryngeal vein; the vein passing from the lower part of the larynx to the plexus thyroideus impar.

**v. larynge'a supe'rior** [ NA ], superior laryngeal vein; it accompanies the superior laryngeal artery and empties into the superior thyroid vein.

**v. liena'lis** [ NA ], splenic vein; arises by the union of several small veins at the hilus on the anterior surface of the spleen, passes backward to the left kidney, then runs behind the upper border of the pancreas to the neck of the pancreas where it joins the superior mesenteric to form the portal.

**v. lingua'lis** [ NA ], lingual vein; receives blood from the tongue, sublingual and submandibular glands, and muscles of the floor of the mouth; empties into the internal jugular or the common facial.

**venae lumba'les** [ NA ], lumbar veins; five in number, these veins accompany the lumbar arteries, drain the posterior body wall and the lumbar vertebral venous plexuses, and terminate anteriorly as follows: the first and second in the ascending lumbar, the third and fourth in the inferior vena cava, and the fifth in the iliolumbar vein.

**v. lumba'lis ascen'dens** [ NA ], ascending lumbar vein; it arises from the sacral and lumbar veins and at the diaphragm becomes the azygos vein on the right side, the hemiazygos vein on the left.

**v. mamma'ria inter'na,** v. thoracica interna.

**v. maxilla'ris,** pl. **venae maxilla'res** [ NA ], maxillary vein; the posterior continuation of the pterygoid plexus; it joins the superficial temporal to form the retromandibular vein.

**v. media'na antebra'chii** [ NA ], median antebrachial vein; median vein of the forearm; it begins at the base of the dorsum of the thumb, curves around the radial side, ascends the middle of forearm, and just below the bend of the elbow divides into the median basilic and median cephalic veins; sometimes it divides lower down, one branch going to the basilic, the other to the median vein of the elbow.

**v. media'na basil'ica** [ NA ], median basilic vein; the medial branch of the median antebrachial vein which joins the basilic.

**v. media'na cephal'ica** [ NA ], median cephalic vein; the lateral branch of the median antebrachial vein that joins the cephalic near the elbow.

**v. media'na cu'biti** [ NA ], median cubital vein; a vein which passes across the bend of the elbow from the cephalic to the basilic; more commonly the vein in this location is called the median basilic.

**venae mediastina'les** [ NA ], several small veins from the mediastinum emptying into the brachiocephalic or the superior v. cava.

**venae menin'geae** [ NA ], meningeal veins; veins that accompany the meningeal arteries; they communicate with venous sinuses and diploic veins and drain into regional veins outside the cranial vault.

**v. menin'geae me'diae** [ NA ], middle meningeal veins; the venae comitantes of the middle meningeal artery that empty into the pterygoid plexus.

**v. mesenter'ica infe'rior** [ NA ], inferior mesenteric vein; is a continuation of the superior rectal at the brim of the pelvis, ascending to the left of the aorta behind the peritoneum and emptying into the splenic or into the superior mesenteric vein or rarely in the angle between these veins.

**v. mesenter'ica supe'rior** [ NA ], superior mesenteric vein; begins at the ileum in the right iliac fossa, ascends in the root of the mesentery, and unites behind the pancreas with the splenic vein to form the portal.

**venae metacar'peae dorsa'les** [ NA ], dorsal metacarpal veins; three veins on the dorsum of the hand draining blood from the four medial digits into the dorsal venous network of the hand.

**venae metacar'peae palma'res** [ NA ], palmar metacarpal veins; emptying into the deep venous arch from which the radial and ulnar veins arise.

**venae metatar'seae dorsa'les** [ NA ], dorsal metatarsal veins; arising from the dorsal digital veins forming the dorsal venous arch of the foot.

**venae metatar'seae planta'res** [ NA ], plantar metatarsal veins; formed from the plantar digital veins constituting the deep plantar venous arch, which empties into the medial and lateral plantar veins.

**venae mus'culophren'icae** [ NA ], musculophrenic veins; the veins that accompany the musculophrenic artery and drain blood from the upper abdominal wall, lower intercostal spaces, and the diaphragm.

**venae nasa'les exter'nae** [ NA ], external nasal veins; several vessels that drain the external nose, emptying into the angular or facial vein.

**venae intercosta'les posterio'res** [ NA ], posterior intercostal veins; veins draining the intercostal spaces posteriorly; from the 4th to the 11th spaces on the right they are tributaries of the azygos vein; on the left they empty into either the hemiazygos or accessory hemiazygos veins.

**v. nasofronta'lis** [ NA ], nasofrontal vein; the vein located in the anterior medial part of the orbit that connects the superior ophthalmic vein with the angular vein.

**v. obli'qua a'trii sinis'tri** [ NA ], oblique vein of the left atrium; oblique vein of Marshall; a small vein on the posterior wall of the left atrium, a tributary of the coronary sinus; it is developed from the left common cardinal vein.

**v. obturato'ria**, pl. **venae obturato'riae** [ NA ], obturator vein; formed by the union of tributaries draining the hip joint and the muscles of the upper and back part of the thigh; it enters the pelvis by the obturator canal and empties into the internal iliac vein.

**v. occipita'lis** [ NA ], occipital vein; drains the occipital region and empties into the internal jugular or the suboccipital plexus.

**v. ophthal'mica infe'rior** [ NA ], inferior ophthalmic vein; arises from the inferior palpebral and lacrimal and divides into two terminal branches, one of which runs to the pterygoid plexus while the other joins the superior ophthalmic or empties into the cavernous sinus.

**v. ophthal'mica supe'rior** [ NA ], superior ophthalmic vein; begins anteriorly from the nasofrontal vein, passes along the upper part of the medial wall of the orbit, passes through the superior orbital fissure, to empty into the cavernous sinus.

**v. ova'rica dex'tra,** [ NA ], right ovarian vein; begins at the pampiniform plexus at the hilus of the ovary and opens into the inferior v. cava.

**v. ova'rica sinis'tra** [ NA ], left ovarian vein; begins at the pampiniform plexus at the hilus of the ovary and empties into the left renal vein.

**v. palati'na exter'na** [ NA ], external palatine vein; drains the palatine regions and empties into the facial.

**venae palpebra'les** [ NA ], veins of the eyelids; veins draining the superior eyelid, tributaries of the superior ophthalmic vein.

**venae palpebra'les inferio'res** [ NA ], veins of the inferior or lower eyelid; veins originating in the inferior eyelid and emptying into the angular vein.

**venae palpebra'les superio'res** [ NA ], veins of the superior or upper eyelid; veins draining the superior eyelid into the angular vein.

**venae pancreat'icae** [ NA ], pancreatic veins; emptying into the superior mesenteric vein, one of the roots of the portal vein.

**venae pancreat'icoduodena'les** [ NA ], pancreaticoduodenal veins; veins that accompany the superior and inferior pancreaticoduodenal arteries, emptying into the superior mesenteric or portal vein.

**venae paraumbilica'les** [ NA ], paraumbilical veins; Sappey's vein; several small veins arising from cutaneous veins about the umbilicus running along the ligamentum teres of the liver, and terminating as accessory portal veins in the substance of this organ.

**venae parotide'ae** [ NA ], parotid veins; posterior parotid veins; parotid branches of the facial vein draining part of the parotid gland and emptying into the retromandibular vein.

**venae pectora'les** [ NA ], pectoral veins; veins draining the pectoral muscles and emptying directly into the subclavian vein.

**venae perforan'tes** [ NA ], perforating veins; the veins that accompany the perforating arteries; they drain blood from the vastus lateralis and the hamstring muscles and terminate in the v. profunda femoris.

**venae pericardi'acae** [ NA ], pericardial veins; several small veins from the pericardium emptying into the brachiocephalic or superior v. cava.

**venae pericardi'acophren'icae** [ NA ], pericardiacophrenic veins; the veins accompanying the pericardiacophrenic artery and emptying into the brachiocephalic or superior v. cava.

**venae perone'ae** [ NA ], venae fibulares [ NA ]; peroneal or fibular veins; the veins that accompany the peroneal artery; they join the posterior tibial veins to enter the popliteal vein.

**venae pharyn'geae** [ NA ], pharyngeal veins; several veins from the pharyngeal plexus emptying into the internal jugular.

**v. phren'ica infe'rior**, pl. **venae phren'icae inferio'res** [ NA ], inferior phrenic vein; drains the substance of the diaphragm and empties on the right side into the v. cava, on the left side into the left suprarenal vein. Often a second vein on the left side passes transversely across the diaphragm anterior to the esophageal hiatus to enter the inferior vena cava.

**venae phren'icae superio'res** [ NA ], superior phrenic veins; small veins that drain the upper surface of the diaphragm; they are tributaries of the azygos and hemiazygos veins.

**v. poplite'a** [ NA ], popliteal vein; arises at the lower border of the popliteus muscle by the union of the anterior and posterior tibial veins, ascends through the popliteal space, and pierces the adductor magnus muscle to become the femoral vein.

**v. por'tae** [ NA ], portal vein; a wide short vein formed by the superior mesenteric and splenic behind the pancreas, ascending in front of the inferior v. cava, and dividing at the right end of the transverse fissure of the liver into right and left branches, which ramify within the liver.

**v. poste'rior ventric'uli sinis'tri** [ NA ], posterior vein of the left ventricle; arises on the diaphragmatic surface of the heart near the apex, runs to the left and parallel to the posterior interventricular sulcus, and empties with the great cardiac vein.

**v. preauricula'ris**, v. auricularis anterior.

**v. prepylo'rica** [ NA ], prepyloric vein; vein of Latarjet; vein of Mayo; a tributary of the right gastric vein that passes anterior to the pylorus at its junction with the duodenum.

**venae profun'dae clitor'idis** [ NA ], deep veins of the clitoris; the veins that pass from the dorsum of the clitoris to join the vesical plexus.

**v. profun'da fem'oris** [ NA ], deep femoral vein; the vein that accompanies the deep femoral artery, receiving perforating veins from the posterior aspect of the thigh. It joins the femoral vein in the femoral triangle, usually in common with the medial and lateral circumflex femoral veins.

**v. profun'da lin'guae** [ NA ], deep lingual vein; the vein that accompanies the deep lingual artery and joins the lingual vein. It drains the body and apex of the tongue.

**v. profun'da pe'nis** [ NA ], deep vein of the penis; the vein deep to the deep fascia on the dorsum of the penis. It enters the prostatic plexus by passing through a gap between the arcuate pubic ligament and the transverse perineal ligament.

**venae puden'dae exter'nae** [ NA ], external pudendal veins; these correspond to the arteries of the same name; they empty into the great saphenous or directly into the femoral, and receive the superficial dorsal vein of the penis (clitoris) and the anterior scrotal (or labial) veins.

**v. puden'da inter'na** [ NA ], internal pudendal vein; a tributary of the internal iliac vein that accompanies the internal pudendal artery as a single or double vessel. It drains the perineum.

**venae pulmona'les** [ NA ], pulmonary veins; four veins, two on each side, conveying blood from the lungs to the left atrium of the heart. The former veins are known as intersegmental or infrasegmental veins, whereas the latter veins, which emerge from the segments, are named intrasegmental.

**v. pulmona'lis infe'rior dex'tra** right inferior pulmonary vein; the vein returning blood from the inferior lobe of the right lung to the left atrium.

**v. pulmona'lis infe'rior sinis'tra** [ NA ], left inferior pulmonary vein; the vein returning blood from the inferior lobe of the left lung to the left atrium.

**v. pulmona'lis supe'rior dex'tra** [ NA ], right superior pulmonary vein; the vein returning blood from the superior and middle lobes of the right lung to the left atrium.

**v. pulmona'lis supe'rior sinis'tra** [ NA ], left superior pulmonary vein; the vein returning blood from the left superior lobe of the lung to the left atrium.

**venae radia'les** [ NA ], radial veins; several veins continuing the deep palmar veins on the lateral side, and accompanying the radial artery.

**venae recta'les inferio'res** [ NA ], venae hemorrhoidales inferiores; inferior rectal or hemorrhoidal veins; veins that pass to the internal pudendal from the venous plexus around the anal canal.

**venae recta'les me'diae** [ NA ], venae hemorrhoidales mediae; middle rectal or hemorrhoidal veins; several veins that pass from the rectal venous plexus to the internal iliac vein.

**v. recta'lis supe'rior** [ NA ], v. hemorrhoidalis superior; superior rectal or hemorrhoidal vein; it drains the greater part of the rectal venous plexus, and ascends between the layers of the mesorectum to the brim of the pelvis, where it becomes the inferior mesenteric.

**venae rena'les** [ NA ], renal veins; they accompany the arteries of the same name, and open at right angles into the v. cava at the level of the second lumbar vertebra. The left renal vein receives the left suprarenal vein and the left gonadal vein.

**venae re'nis** [ NA ], veins of the kidney; the tributaries of the renal vein that drain the kidney; they parallel the arteries in the kidney and consist of interlobular, arcuate and interlobar veins.

**v. retromandibula'ris** [ NA ], retromandibular vein; posterior facial vein; temporomaxillary vein; v. facialis posterior; it is formed by the union of the temporal veins in front of the ear, runs behind the ramus of the lower jaw through the parotid gland, and unites with the facial vein.

**v. re'vehens**, pl. **venae revehen'tes**, veins in the embryo, passing from the sinusoidal vessels in the liver to the inferior v. cava. They develop into the hepatic veins.

**venae sacra'les latera'les** [ NA ], lateral sacral veins; several veins that accompany the corresponding artery and empty into the internal iliac vein on each side.

**v. sacra'lis media'na** [ NA ], median sacral vein; an unpaired vein accompanying the middle sacral artery emptying into the left common iliac vein.

**v. saphe'na accesso'ria** [ NA ], accessory saphenous vein; an occasional vein running in the thigh parallel to the great saphenous which it joins just before the latter empties into the femoral vein.

**v. saphe'na mag'na** [ NA ], great, large, or long saphenous vein; formed by the union of the dorsal vein of the great toe and the dorsal venous arch of the foot, ascends in front of the medial malleolus, behind the medial condyle of the femur, and empties into the femoral vein in the upper part of femoral (Scarpa's) triangle.

**v. saphe'na par'va** [ NA ], small or short saphenous vein; arises on the lateral side of the foot from a union of the dorsal vein of the little toe with the dorsal venous arch, ascends behind the lateral malleolus, along the lateral border of the calcanean tendon and then through the middle of the calf to the lower portion of the popliteal space where it empties into the popliteal vein.

**v. scapula'ris dorsa'lis** [ NA ], dorsal scapular vein; the vein accompanying the descending scapular artery; it is a tributary to the subclavian or the external jugular vein.

**venae scrota'les anterio'res** [ NA ], anterior scrotal veins; veins passing from the scrotum to the external pudendal veins.

**venae scrota'les posterio'res** [ NA ], posterior scrotal veins; veins passing posteriorward from the scrotum to the internal pudendal veins.

**v. sep'ti pellu'cidi** [ NA ], vein of the septum pellucidum; vein draining the septum pellucidum; it empties into the internal cerebral vein.

**venae sigmoi'deae** [ NA ], sigmoid veins; the several tributaries of the inferior mesenteric vein that drain the sigmoid colon.

**venae spina'les** [ NA ], spinal veins; the veins that drain the spinal cord; they form a plexus on the surface of the cord from which veins pass along the spinal roots to the internal vertebral venous plexus.

**v. spira'lis modi'oli** [ NA ], spiral vein of the modiolus; the vein running a spiral course in the modiolus of the cochlea; it is tributary to both the labyrinthine vein and the vein of the cochlear aqueduct.

**venae stella'tae,** *venulae* stellatae.

**v. sternocleidomastoi'dea** [ NA ], sternocleidomastoid vein; it arises in the sternocleidomastoid muscle and drains into the internal jugular vein.

**v. stria'ta** [ NA ], striate vein; any one of several veins embedded in the internal medullary lamina of the lentiform nucleus and in the capsula externa; in essence, anastomotic veins between the thalamostriate vein dorsally (superior striate veins), the v. cerebri media profunda and basal vein of Rosenthal below (inferior striate veins).

**v. stylomastoi'dea** [ NA ], stylomastoid vein; it drains the tympanic cavity and empties into the retromandibular vein.

**v. subcla'via** [ NA ], subclavian vein; the direct continuation of the axillary at the lateral border of the first rib; it passes medially to join the internal jugular and form the brachiocephalic vein on each side.

**venae subcuta'neae abdom'inis** [ NA ], subcutaneous veins of the abdomen; the network of superficial veins of the abdominal wall that empty into the thoracoepigastric, superficial epigastric, or superior epigastric veins.

**v. sublingua'lis** [ NA ], sublingual vein; a tributary of the lingualis.

**v. submenta'lis** [ NA ], submental vein; situated below the chin, anastomosing with the sublingual, connecting with the anterior jugular, and emptying into the facial.

**superior v. cava,** v. cava superior.

**v. supraorbita'lis** [ NA ], supraorbital vein; drains the front of the scalp and unites with the supratrochlear to form the angular.

**v. suprarena'lis dex'tra** [ NA ], right suprarenal vein; the short vein that passes from the hilus of the right suprarenal to the inferior vena cava.

**v. suprarena'lis sinis'tra** [ NA ], left suprarenal vein; the vein from the hilus of the left suprarenal gland that passes downward to open into the left renal vein. It usually is joined by the left inferior phrenic vein.

**v. suprascapula'ris** [ NA ], suprascapular vein; transverse scapular vein; v. transversa scapulae; a vein that accompanies the suprascapular artery; it empties into the external jugular vein.

**venae supratrochlea'res** [ NA ], supratrochlear veins; frontal veins; venae frontales; several veins that drain the front part of the scalp and unite with the supraorbital to form the angular.

**v. tempora'lis me'dia** [ NA ], middle temporal vein; it arises near the lateral angle of the orbit and joins the superficial temporal veins to form the retromandibular.

**venae tempora'les profun'dae** [ NA ], deep temporal veins, corresponding to the arteries of the same name; they empty into the pterygoid venous plexus.

**venae tempora'les superficia'les** [ NA ], superficial temporal veins; veins that pass from the temporal region to join the retromandibular vein.

**v. termina'lis,** v. thalamostriata.

**v. testicula'ris dex'tra** [ NA ], right testicular vein; it passes upward from the pampiniform plexus to join the inferior v. cava.

**v. testicula'ris sinis'tra** [ NA ], left testicular vein; originates from the pampiniform plexus and joins the left renal vein.

**v. thalamostria'ta** [ NA ], thalamostriate vein; terminal vein; v. terminalis; vein of the corpus striatum; a long vein passing forward in the groove between the thalamus and caudate nucleus, covered by the lamina affixa, receiving the transverse caudate veins along its lateral side, and joining at the caudal wall of Monro's foramen with the v. choroidea and v. septi pellucidi to form the v. cerebri interna.

**v. thora'cica inter'na,** pl. **venae thoracicae internae** [ NA ], internal thoracic vein; v. mammaria interna; usually two veins accompany each artery of the same name, fusing into one at the upper part of the thorax and emptying into the brachiocephalic of the same side.

**v. thora'cica latera'lis** [ NA ], lateral thoracic vein; long thoracic vein; a tributary of the axillary vein that drains the lateral thoracic wall and communicates with the thoraco-epigastric and intercostal veins.

**v. thoracoacromia'lis** [ NA ], thoracoacromial vein; thoracic axis; corresponding to the artery of the same name, empties into the axillary, sometimes by a common trunk with the cephalic vein.

**v. thoracoepigas'trica,** pl. **venae thoracoepigastricae** [ NA ], thoracoepigastric vein; one of two veins, sometimes a single vein, arising from the region of the superficial epigastric and opening into the axillary or the lateral thoracic vein.

**venae thy'micae** [ NA ], thymic veins; a number of small veins from the thymus emptying into the left brachiocephalic.

**v. thyroi'dea i'ma,** v. thyroidea inferior.

**v. thyroi'dea infe'rior** [ NA ], inferior thyroid vein; v. thyroidea ima; formed by veins from the isthmus and lateral lobe of the thyroid gland and from the plexus thyroideus impar; it terminates in the left brachiocephalic vein.

**v. thyroi'dea me'dia** [ NA ], middle thyroid vein; it passes from the thyroid gland across the common carotid artery to empty into the internal jugular vein.

**v. thyroi'dea supe'rior** [ NA ], superior thyroid vein; receives blood from the upper part of the thyroid gland and larynx, accompanies the artery of the same name, and empties into the internal jugular.

**venae tibia'les anterio'res** [ NA ], anterior tibial veins; the veins, usually two, that accompany the anterior tibial artery and empty into the popliteal vein.

**venae tibia'les posterio'res** [ NA ], posterior tibial veins; the veins, usually two, that accompany the posterior tibial artery and terminate in the popliteal vein.

**venae trachea'les** [ NA ], tracheal veins; several small venous trunks from the trachea, emptying into the brachiocephalic or the superior v. cava.

**venae transver'sae col'li** [ NA ], transverse veins of the neck; they accompany the corresponding arteries, emptying into the external jugular or sometimes into the subclavian.

**v. transver'sa facie'i** [ NA ], transverse vein of the face; a tributary of the retromandibular, anastomosing with the facial vein.

**v. transver'sa scap'ulae,** v. suprascapularis.

**venae tympan'icae** [ NA ], tympanic veins; veins exiting from the tympanic cavity through the petrotympanic fissure and emptying into the retromandibular vein.

**venae ulna'res** [ NA ], ulnar veins; veins that accompany the ulnar artery.

**v. umbilica'lis sinis'tra** [ NA ], left umbilical vein; the vein that returns the blood from the placenta to the fetus. Traversing the umbilical cord, it enters the fetal body at the umbilicus and passes thence into the liver, where it is joined by the portal vein. Its blood then goes by way of the ductus venosus and the inferior v. cava to the right atrium.

**venae uteri'nae** [ NA ], uterine veins; two veins on each side which arise from the uterine plexus, pass through a part of the broad ligament and then through a peritoneal fold, and empty into the internal iliac vein.

**v. vertebra'lis** [ NA ], vertebral vein, derived from tributaries which run through the foramina in the transverse processes of the first six cervical vertebrae and form a plexus around the vertebral artery; it empties as a single trunk into the brachiocephalic.

**v. vertebra'lis accesso'ria** [ NA ], accessory vertebral vein; a vein that accompanies the vertebral vein but passes through the foramen transversarium of the seventh cervical vertebra and opens independently into the brachiocephalic vein.

**v. vertebra'lis ante'rior** [ NA ], anterior vertebral vein; the small vein that accompanies the ascending cervical artery; it opens below into the vertebral vein.

**venae vesica'les** [ NA ], vesical veins; veins that drain the vesical plexus; they join the internal iliac veins.

**venae vestibula'res** [ NA ], vestibular veins; veins draining the saccule and utricle; they are tributaries of both the labyrinthine veins and the vein of the vestibular aqueduct.

**venae vortico'sae** [ NA ], vortex or vorticose veins; venae choroideae oculi [ NA ]; choroid veins of the eye; Stensen's veins; vasa vorticosae; several veins in the tunica vasculosa formed of branches from the posterior surface of the eye and the ciliary body emptying into the superior or inferior ophthalmic vein.

---

**vena'tion** [ L. *vena*, vein ]. The arrangement and distribution of veins.

**vene-.** 1 [ L. *vena*, vein ]. Combining form relating to the veins. 2 [ L. *venenum*, poison ]. Combining form relating to venom.

**ve'necta'sia.** Phlebectasia.

**venec'tomy.** Phlebectomy.

**venenation** (ven'e-na'shun, ve'ne-) [ L. *veneno*, pp. -*atus*, to poison, fr. *venenum*, poison ]. Poisoning.

**veneniferous** (ven'e-nif'er-us) [ L. *venenifer*, fr. *venenum*, poison, + *fero*, to carry ]. Conveying poison.

**Venenosa** (ven'e-no'sah, ve'nī-) [ L. *venenosus*, poisonous ]. Nocua; Thanatophidia; a former division or class of serpents including the distinctly venomous ones; the nonpoisonous serpents were classed as Innocua, and those the character of which was not known, as Suspecta.

**ven'enosal'ivary.** Venomosalivary; secreting a poisonous saliva, said of venomous reptiles.

**ven'enos'ity** [ L. *venenosus*, poisonous ]. The state of containing poison or being poisonous.

**ven'enous** [ L. *venenosus* ]. Poisonous.

**venereal** (vĕ-nēr'e-al) [ L. *Venus* (*vener-*), goddess of love ]. Relating to or resulting from sexual intercourse.

**venereology** (vĕ-nēr'e-ol'o-jī) [ venereal (disease) + G. *logos*, study ]. Cypridology; the study of venereal disease.

**venereophobia** (vĕ-nēr'e-o-fo'bī-ah) [ venereal (disease) + G. *phobos*, fear ]. Morbid fear of venereal disease.

**ven'ery** [ L. *veneria*, lust, fr. *Venus* (*vener-*), goddess of love ]. Excessive, especially illicit, sexual intercourse.

**venesec'tion** [ L. *vena*, vein, + *sectio*, a cutting ]. Phlebotomy.

**veni-.** See veno-, vene-.

**ven'in** [ see venom ]. Any poisonous substance found in snake venom.

**venipuncture** (ven'ī-punk'chur, ve'nī-) The puncture of a vein for any purpose.

**ven'isu'ture.** Phleborrhaphy; suture of a vein.

**veno-, vene-, veni-** [ L. *vena*, vein ]. Combining forms denoting vein.

**venoclysis** (ve-nok'lī-sis) [ veno- + G. *klysis*, a washing out ]. Drip *phleboclysis.*

**ve'nofibro'sis.** Phlebosclerosis.

**ve'nogram** [ veno- + G. *gramma*, a writing ]. 1. A radiogram of the veins. 2. Phlebogram.

**venography** (ve-nog'rǎ-fĭ) [ veno- + G. *grapho,* to write ]. Phlebography; visualization or skiagraphic recording of a vein, after the injection of a radiopaque substance.

   **splenic portal v.,** visualization of the splenic and portal veins after the injection of radiopaque material into the spleen through a large needle; intra- or extrahepatic portal obstruction may be thus revealed.

   **transosseous v.,** vertebral v.

   **vertebral v.,** transosseous v.; radiographic visualization of epidural venous plexus by injection of contrast media into the spinous process.

**ven'om** [ M. Eng. and O. Fr. *venim,* fr. L. *venenum,* poison ]. A poisonous fluid secreted by snakes, spiders, scorpions, etc.

   **kokoi v.,** a potent neurotoxin found in the frog *Phyllobates bicolor.* It is a nonprotein compound with a molecular weight of approximately 400. It is lethal in microgram quantities.

   **Russell's viper v.,** used as a coagulant in the arrest of hemorrhage from accessible sites in hemophilia.

**ven'omosal'ivary.** Venenosalivary.

**ve'nomo'tor** [ veno- + L. *motor,* a move ]. Causing change in the caliber of a vein.

**venoperitoneostomy** (ve'no-pĕr-ĭ-to-ne-os'to-mĭ) [ veno- + peritoneum + G. *stoma,* mouth ]. Ruotte's operation; the operation of inserting the cut end of the saphenous vein into the peritoneal cavity in cases of ascites; the vein is inverted so that the valves prevent regurgitation of blood into the cavity while the ascitic fluid readily flows away into the vein.

**ve'nopres'sor.** Relating to the venous blood pressure and consequently the volume of venous supply to the right side of the heart.

**ve'nosclero'sis.** Phlebosclerosis.

**venose** (ve'nos) [ L. *venosus* ]. Having veins; venous; veiny.

**ve'nosi'nal.** Pertaining to the vena cava and the atrial sinus of the heart.

**venosity** (ve-nos'ĭ-tĭ). 1. A venous state; a condition in which the bulk of the blood is in the veins at the expense of the arteries. 2. The unaerated condition of venous blood.

**venostasis** (ve'no-sta'sis, ve-nos'tă-sis) [ veno- + G. *stasis,* a standing ]. Phlebostasis.

**ve'nostat** [ veno- + G. *statos,* standing, stationary ]. Any instrument for arresting venous bleeding.

**venos'tomy.** Cutdown.

**venot'omy.** Phlebotomy.

**venous** (ve'nus) [ L. *venosus* ]. Relating to a vein or to the veins.

   **v. return,** the blood returning to the heart via the great veins.

**venovenostomy** (ve'no-ve-nos'to-mĭ) [ veno- + veno- + G. *stoma,* mouth ]. Phlebophlebostomy; the formation of an anastomosis between two veins.

**vent** [ O. Fr. *fente,* a chink, cleft ]. An opening into a cavity or canal, especially one through which the contents of such cavity are discharged, as the anus.

**ven'ter** [ L. *venter* (*ventr-*), belly. VENT- ]. 1 [ NA ]. The abdomen. 2 [ NA ]. The wide swelling part (belly) of a muscle. 3. One of the great cavities of the body. 4. The uterus.

   **v. ante'rior mus'culi digas'trici** [ NA ], the anterior belly of the digastric muscle, attached to the mandible.

   **v. fronta'lis** [ NA ], frontal belly; the anterior belly of the occipitofrontalis muscle.

   **v. infe'rior mus'culi omohyoi'dei** [ NA ], the inferior belly of the omohyoid muscle, attached to the superior border of the scapula.

   **v. occipita'lis** [ NA ], occipital belly; the posterior belly of the occipitofrontalis muscle.

   **v. poste'rior mus'culi digas'trici** [ NA ], the posterior belly of the digastric muscle, attached to the mastoid process.

   **v. propen'dens,** (1) anteversion of the uterus; (2) a pendulous abdomen.

   **v. supe'rior mus'culi omohyoi'dei** [ NA ], the superior belly of the omohyoid muscle, attached to the hyoid bone.

**ventilate** (ven'tĭ-lāt) [ L. *ventilo,* pp. *-atus,* to fan, fr. *ventus,* the wind ]. To aerate, or oxygenate, the blood in the pulmonary capillaries.

**ventilation** (ven'tĭ-la'shun) [ see ventilate ]. 1. Replacement of the air or other gas in a space by fresh air or gas. 2. Symbol V̇; in physiology, the tidal exchange of air between the lungs and the atmosphere that occurs in breathing. See also respiration.

   **alveolar v.,** symbol $V_A$; the volume of gas expired from the alveoli to the outside of the body per minute; calculated as the respiratory frequency (f) multiplied by the difference between tidal volume and the dead space ($V_T - V_D$); units: ml/min BTPS.

   **maximum voluntary v.,** maximum breathing *capacity.*

   **pulmonary v.,** respiratory minute volume, *i.e.,* the total volume of gas per minute inspired ($V_I$) or expired ($V_E$) expressed in liters per minute; it differs from alveolar v. in including the exchange of dead space gas.

**vent'plant.** An endo-osseous implant, usually made of titanium, utilized to provide support and fixation for a dental prosthesis by means of projections through the mucosa; a term used to designate a family of implants.

**ven'trad** [ L. *venter,* belly, + *ad,* to ]. Toward the ventral aspect; opposed to dorsad.

**ven'tral** [ L. *ventralis* ]. Relating to the belly or the abdomen; abdominal; as opposed to dorsal, posterior, or neural.

**ventra'lis** [ L. ] [ NA ]. Ventral.

**ventricle** (ven'trĭ-kl) [ L. *ventriculus,* dim. of *venter,* belly ]. Ventriculus.

   **Arantius' v.,** *calamus* scriptorius.

   **cerebral v.'s,** see *ventriculus* lateralis, *ventriculus* quartus, *ventriculus* tertius, and *cavum* septi pellucidi.

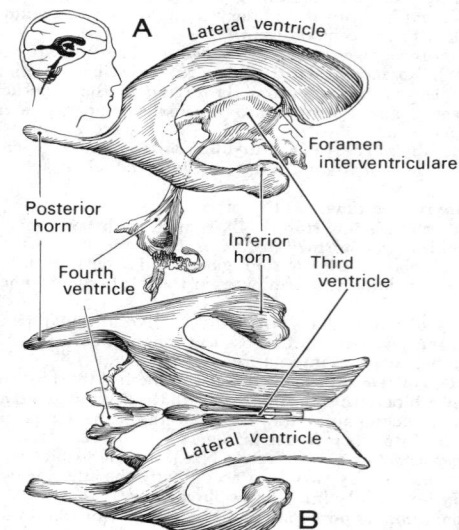

**Ventricles of the Brain**
*A,* lateral view; *B,* superior view

   **v. of cerebral hemisphere,** *ventriculus* lateralis.

   **v. of diencephalon,** *ventriculus* tertius.

   **Duncan's v.,** *cavum* septi pellucidi.

   **fifth v.,** *cavum* septi pellucidi.

   **fourth v.,** *ventriculus* quartus.

   **v.'s of heart,** see *ventriculus* cordis, dexter, and sinister.

   **laryngeal v.,** *ventriculus* laryngis.

   **lateral v.,** *ventriculus* lateralis.

   **left v.,** *ventriculus* sinister.

   **Morgagni's v.,** *ventriculus* laryngis.

   **v. of rhombencephalon,** *ventriculus* quartus.

   **right v.,** *ventriculus* dexter.

   **sixth v.,** Verga's v.

   **Sylvian v.,** *cavum* septi pellucidi.

   **terminal v.,** *ventriculus* terminalis.

   **third v.,** *ventriculus* tertius.

**Verga's v.,** cavum vergae; cavum psalterii; sixth ventricle; an inconstant, horizontal, slitlike space between the posterior one-third of the corpus callosum and the underlying commissura fornicis (commissura hippocampi; psalterium) resulting from failure of these two commissural plates to fuse completely during fetal development. Like the cavum septi pellucidi, the space is not a true v. in the sense that it did not develop from the central canal of the neural tube.

**Vieussens' v.,** cavum septi pellucidi.

**Wenzel's v.,** cavum septi pellucidi.

**ventricose** (ven'trĭ-kōs). Inflated; bellied; corpulent.

**ventricular** (ven-trik'u-lar). Relating to a ventricle, in any sense.

**ventricula'ris** [ Mod. L. fr. L. ventriculus. VENT- ]. 1. Ventricular. 2. Musculus thyroepiglotticus.

**ventric'ulariza'tion.** Transformation of an atrial phenomenon to simulate a ventricular, especially of the atrial (or venous) pulse tracing in tricuspid regurgitation.

**ventriculitis** (ven-trik'u-li'tis) [ ventricle + G. suffix -itis, inflammation ]. Inflammation of the ventricles of the brain.

**ventriculo-** (ven-trik'u-lo-) [ L. ventriculus, ventricle. VENT- ]. Combining form relating to a ventricle.

**ventric'ulocisternos'tomy** [ ventriculo- + L. cisterna, cistern, + G. stoma, mouth ]. An artificial opening between the ventricles of the brain and the cisterna magna; see also shunt (2).

**ventric'ulocordot'omy** [ ventriculo- + L. chorda, cord, + G. tomē, incision ]. The "debarking" operation on dogs, designed to lessen the noise by surgical removal of a portion of each vocal cord.

**ventriculography** (ven-trik-u-log'ră-fī) [ ventriculo- + G. graphē, a writing ]. Radiographic visualization of the ventricular system by direct injection of gaseous or radiopaque material.

**ventriculomastoidostomy** (ven-trik'u-lo-mas'toy-dos'to-mĭ) [ ventriculo- + mastoid, + G. stoma, mouth ]. The operation for the establishment of a communication between the lateral cerebral ventricle and the mastoid antrum by means of a polythene tube for the relief of hydrocephalus. See also shunt (2).

**ventriculonector** (ven-trik'u-lo-nek'tor) [ ventriculo- + L. necto, to join ]. Fasciculus atrioventricularis; see also conducting system of the heart.

**ventriculophasic** (ven-trik'u-lo-fa'zik). Influenced by ventricular contraction; applied to the atrial rhythm when this is modified by ventricular contraction; in v. sinus arrhythmia in complete A-V block the sinus impulse immediately following a ventricular contraction usually appears sooner than expected.

**ventric'uloplas'ty** [ ventriculo- + G. plassō, to form ]. Any surgical procedure to repair a defect of one of the ventricles of the heart, e.g., excision of a cardiac aneurysm.

**ventric'ulopunc'ture.** Insertion of a needle into a ventricle.

**ventriculoscopy** (ven-trik'u-los'ko-pī) [ ventriculo- + G. skopeō, to view ]. Direct inspection of a ventricle by means of an endoscope.

**ventric'ulos'tomy** [ ventriculo- + G. stoma, mouth ]. An operation to establish an opening usually from the third ventricle to the subarachnoid space to relieve hydrocephalus. See also third v.; shunt (2).

**third v.,** an operation to establish an opening from the third ventricle to the prechiasmal and interpeduncular cisterns (Stookey-Scarff operation) or from the third ventricle to the interpeduncular cistern (Dandy operation).

**ventriculosubarachnoid** (ven-trik'u-lo-sub-ă-rak'noyd) [ ventriculo- + subarachnoid ]. Relating to the space occupied by the cerebrospinal fluid.

**ventric'ulot'omy** [ ventriculo- + G. tomē, incision ]. Incision into a ventricle, e.g., into the third ventricle for the relief of hydrocephalus.

**ventriculus,** pl. **ventriculi** (ven-trik'u-lus, -lī) [ L. dim. of venter, belly. VENT- ]. Ventricle. 1 [ NA ]. The stomach. 2 [ NA ]. A normal cavity, as of the brain or heart. 3. The enlarged posterior portion of the mesenteron of the insect alimentary canal, in which digestion occurs.

**v. cor'dis** [ NA ], ventricle of the heart; one of the two lower chambers of the heart.

**v. dex'ter** [ NA ], right ventricle; the cavity on the right side of the heart which receives the venous blood from the right atrium and drives it by the contraction of its walls into the pulmonary artery.

**v. laryn'gis** [ NA ], laryngeal ventricle; sinus laryngeus; Morgagni's ventricle; the recess in each lateral wall of the larynx between the vestibular and vocal folds.

**v. latera'lis** [ NA ], lateral ventricle; the ventricle of the cerebral hemisphere, shaped somewhat like a horseshoe in conformity with the general shape of the hemisphere; it communicates with the third ventricle through the interventricular foramen of Monro, and expands from there forward into the frontal lobe as the cornu anterius (anterior or frontal horn) as well as caudalward over the thalamus as the pars centralis or cella media which, behind the thalamus, curves ventrally and laterally, then forward into the temporal lobe as the cornu inferius (inferior or temporal horn); from the apex of the curve a variably large cornu posterius (posterior or occipital horn) extends back into the white matter of the occipital lobe. The large choroid plexus of the lateral ventricle invades the cella media and the cornu inferius (but not the cornua anterius and posterius) from the medial side.

**v. quar'tus** [ NA ], fourth ventricle; the ventricle of the rhombencephalon; a cavity of irregular tentlike shape extending from the obex rostralward to its communication with the Sylvian aqueduct, enclosed between the cerebellum dorsally and the rhombencephalic tegmentum ventrally, having a rhomb-shaped floor, the fossa rhomboidea, and a tentlike roof which in its caudal part is formed by the tela choroidea and the velum medullare posterius, in its middle part by the white matter of the cerebellum, and in its narrowing rostral part (recessus superior) by the velum medullare anterius. The fourth ventricle reaches its greatest width at the pontomedullary transition where it expands laterally, behind the cerebellar peduncles, into the spoutlike recessus lateralis, its greatest height at the fastigial recess which reaches up into the cerebellar white matter. The only direct communication of the brain's ventricle system and the subarachnoid space is established at the level of the fourth ventricle by a median opening in the tela choroidea, the apertura mediana or foramen of Magendi, which opens into the cisterna magna, and on both sides by the apertura lateralis or foramen of Luschka, which connects the recessus lateralis with the cisterna basalis.

**v. quin'tus,** cavum septi pellucidi.

**v. sinis'ter** [ NA ], left ventricle; the cavity on the left side of the heart that receives the arterial blood from the left atrium and drives it by the contraction of its walls into the aorta.

**v. termina'lis** [ NA ], terminal ventricle; a dilation of the central canal of the spinal cord at the tip of the conus medullaris.

**v. ter'tius** [ NA ], third ventricle; diacele; the ventricle of the diencephalon; a narrow, vertically oriented, irregularly quadrilateral cavity, placed in the midplane and extending back from the lamina terminalis to the rostral opening of the Sylvian aqueduct, communicating at its rostrodorsal corner with each of the two lateral ventricles through the left and right interventricular foramen of Monro. Its narrow roof is formed by the tela choroidea which is attached on either side to the tenia thalami, its lateral wall by the medial surface of the thalamus and, below the sulcus hypothalamicus, by the hypothalamus which also forms its floor. In lateral profile, the third ventricle exhibits a number of recesses: in its floor, from before backward, (a) the preoptic recess in the acute angle between the base of the lamina terminalis and the dorsum of the optic chiasm, (b) the infundibular recess extending ventrally into the infundibulum but not (in man) into the hypophysial stalk, and (c) the mamillary or inframamillary recess caused by the protrusion of the mamillary bodies into the ventricle. From its dorsocaudal corner the pineal recess extends caudally into the pineal stalk.

**ven'triduct** [ L. venter, belly, + duco, pp. ductus, to lead ]. To draw toward the belly, as in flexion of the thigh.

**ventriduc'tion.** Drawing toward the belly.

**ventro-** [ L. venter, belly. VENT- ]. Combining form meaning ventral.

**ventrocystorrhaphy** (ven'tro-sis-tor'ă-fĭ) [ ventro- + G. kystis, cyst, + rhaphē, suture ]. Cystopexy.

**ventrodor'sad.** Dorsad; in a direction from the venter to the dorsum.

**ventroinguinal** (ven'tro-ing'gwĭ-nal). Relating to the abdomen and the groin.

**ventrolat'eral.** Both ventral and lateral.

**ventrome'dian.** Relating to the midline of the ventral surface.

**ventroptosis, ventroptosia** (ven'trop-to'sis, -to'sĭ-ah) [ ventro- + G. ptōsis, a falling ]. Gastroptosis.

**ventroscopy** (ven-tros'ko-pĭ) [ ventro- + G. skopeō, to view ]. Peritoneoscopy.

**ventrot'omy** [ ventro- + G. tomē, incision ]. Laparotomy (2).

**Venturi,** Giovanni B., Italian physicist, 1746–1822. See V. effect, meter, tube.

**venula,** pl. **venulae** (ven'u-lah, -le) [ L. dim. of vena, vein ] [ NA ]. Venule; veinlet; capillary vein; a minute vein; a venous radicle continuous with a capillary.

  **v. macula'ris infe'rior** [ NA ], inferior macular venule; a small tributary of the central vein of the retina that drains the lower part of the macula.

  **v. macula'ris supe'rior** [ NA ], superior macular venule; a small tributary of the central vein of the retina that drains the upper part of the macula.

  **v. media'lis ret'inae** [ NA ], medial venule of the retina; the small vein that passes from the medial part of the retina intermediate between the inferior nasal and superior nasal venules to join the central vein.

  **v. nasa'lis ret'inae infe'rior** [ NA ], inferior nasal venule of the retina; the small vein that passes from the inferior medial (nasal) part of the retina to join the central vein.

  **v. nasa'lis ret'inae supe'rior** [ NA ], superior nasal venule of the retina; the small vein that drains blood from the upper medial (nasal) part of the retina; it joins the central vein.

  **venulae rec'tae re'nis** [ NA ], straight venules of the kidney; venules that drain the medullary pyramids of the kidney; they open into arcuate veins.

  **venulae stella'tae** [ NA ], stellate venules or veins; venae stellatae; Verheyen's stars; the star-shaped groups of venules in the renal cortex.

  **v. tempora'lis ret'inae infe'rior** [ NA ], inferior temporal venule of the retina; the small vein that passes from the lower lateral (temporal) part of the retina to enter the central vein.

  **v. tempora'lis ret'inae supe'rior** [ NA ], superior temporal venule of the retina; the venule passes from the upper lateral (temporal) part of the retina to join the central vein.

**ven'ular.** Pertaining to venules.

**venule** (ven'ūl, ve'nūl). Venula.

  **macular v.'s,** see venula macularis inferior and superior.

  **medial v. of retina,** venula medialis retinae.

  **nasal v.'s of retina,** see venula nasalis retinae inferior and superior.

  **postcapillary v.'s,** v.'s in the lymph nodes and spleen with a high-walled endothelium, through which lymphocytes are believed to migrate; the postcapillary v.'s in lymph nodes are regarded as the site of reentry of blood lymphocytes into the lymphatic circulation.

  **stellate v.'s,** venulae stellatae.

  **straight v.'s of kidney,** venulae rectae renis.

  **temporal v.'s of retina,** see venula temporalis retinae inferior and superior.

**ven'ulous.** Venular.

**ve'nus** [ L. Venus, the goddess of love ]. Sexual intercourse.

**verap'amil** (USAN). ISOPTIN; iproveratril; 5-[ (3,4-dimethoxyphenethyl)methylamino ]-2-(3,4-dimethoxyphenyl)-2-isopropylvaleronitrile; coronary vasodilator.

**verat'ric acid.** 3,4-Dimethoxybenzoic acid; $C_9H_{10}O_4$; obtained by methylation and subsequent oxidation of protocatechuic acid; present in the seeds of Schoenocaulon officinale (Sabadilla officinarum).

**veratrine** (vĕr'ă-tren, -trin). A mixture of alkaloids from the seeds of Schoenocaulon officinale (Sabadilla officinarum) (family Liliaceae); a powder of acrid taste and intensely irritating to the nasal mucous membrane. It contains cevine, cevadine, cevadilline, sabadine, and verat-

ridine. Has been used as an anodyne counterirritant in neuralgias and arthritis.

**Veratrum** (vĕ-ra'trum) [ L. hellebore ]. A genus of toxic liliaceous plants.

  **V. album,** white or European hellebore; the rhizome has emetic and cathartic actions.

  **V. viride,** American or green hellebore; the dried rhizome and roots contains therapeutically important alkaloids (cevadine, veratridine, jervine, pseudojervine, rubijervine, and several ester alkaloids of the base germine) used in the treatment of hypertensive disorders.

**verbigeration** (ver-bij-er-a'shun) [ L. verbum, word, + gero, to carry about ]. Oral stereotypy; catalogia; the constant repetition of meaningless words or phrases.

**verbomania** (ver-bo-ma'nĭ-ah) [ L. verbum, word, + G. mania, frenzy ]. An abnormal talkativeness; a psychotic flow of speech.

**verdigris** (ver'dĭ-grēs, -gris, -grē) [ O. Fr. verd, green, de, of, Gris, Greeks ]. 1. Crystallized v.; normal cupric acetate. 2. Green v.; aerugo; copper subacetate.

**ver'dine** Biliverdine.

**verdohemochrome** (ver'do-he'mo-krōm). An intermediate stage in hemoglobin degradation to yield the bile pigments. Hemoglobin yields choleglobin (verdohemoglobin) and the loss of globin leaves verdohemochrome, the precursor of biliverdin.

**ver'dohemoglo'bin.** Choleglobin.

**ver'doperox'idase.** Myeloperoxidase; a peroxidase, occurring in leukocytes, that contains a greenish ferriheme (as does lactoperoxidase).

**Verga** (vair'gah), Andrea, Italian neurologist, 1811–1895. See cavum vergae, V.'s ventricle.

**verge.** Edge; margin.

  **anal v.,** the transitional zone between the moist, hairless, modified skin of the anal canal and the perianal skin.

**vergence** (ver'jens) [ L. vergo, to incline, to turn ]. Binocular disjugate movements, as of the eyes; see also convergence and divergence.

  **v. of lens,** the reciprocal of the principal focal distance used as a measure of the divergence or convergence of parallel rays.

**vergeture** (ver'jĕ-chūr) [ L. virga, a green twig, a stripe ]. Stria.

**Verheyen** (fer-hi'en), Philippe, Flemish anatomist, 1648–1710. See V.'s star, stellula verheyenii.

**Verhoeff,** Frederick H., American ophthalmologist, 1874–1968. See Agnew-V. incision, V.'s operation.

**Vermale** (ver-mal'), Raymond de, French surgeon, 18th century. See V.'s operation.

**Vermes** (ver'mēz) [ L. vermis, worm ]. Old term for the subkingdom of worms.

**vermi-** (ver'mĭ-) [ L. vermis, worm ]. Combining form for worm, wormlike.

**vermicidal** (ver'mĭ-si'dal) [ vermi- + L. caedo, to kill ]. Destructive to worms; specifically, destructive to the parasitic intestinal worms.

**vermicide** (ver'mĭ-sīd). An agent that kills intestinal parasitic worms.

**vermicular** (ver-mik'u-lar) [ L. vermiculus, dim. of vermis, worm ]. Relating to, resembling, or moving like a worm; vermiform.

**vermiculation** (ver-mik'u-la'shun). A wormlike movement, as in peristalsis.

**vermicule** (ver'mĭ-kūl) [ L. vermiculus, a small worm ]. 1. A small worm. 2. Ookinete.

**vermic'ulose, vermic'ulous.** 1. Wormy; infested with worms or larvae. 2. Wormlike; vermiform; vermicular.

**vermiculus** (ver-mik'u-lus) [ L. dim. of vermis, worm ]. Vermicule.

**ver'miform** [ vermi- + L. forma, form ]. Worm-shaped; resembling a worm in form.

**vermifugal** (ver-mif'u-gal). Anthelmintic (2).

**vermifuge** (ver'mĭ-fūj) [ vermi- + L. fugo, to chase away ]. Anthelmintic (1).

**vermilion** (ver-mil'yon). A red pigment made from cinnabar or red mercuric sulfide.

**vermilionectomy** (ver-mil'yon-ek'to-mĭ) [ vermilion border + G. *ektomē*, cutting out ]. Excision of vermilion border.

**ver'min** [ L. *vermis*, a worm ]. Parasitic insects, such as lice and bedbugs.

**ver'minal.** Verminous.

**vermination** (ver'mĭ-na'shun). 1. The production or breeding of worms or larvae. 2. Infestation with vermin.

**verminous** (ver'mĭ-nus) [ L. *verminosus*, wormy ]. Relating to, caused by, or infested with worms, larvae, or vermin.

**vermis,** pl. **vermes** (ver'mis, -mēz) [ L. worm ]. 1. A worm. 2. [ NA ]. V. cerebelli; the narrow middle zone between the two hemispheres of the cerebellum; the portion projecting above the level of the hemispheres on the upper surface is called the superior v.; the lower portion, sunken between the two hemispheres and forming the floor of the vallecula, is the inferior v.

**ver'mix.** *Appendix* vermiformis.

**Vernet,** Maurice, French neurologist, *1887. See V.'s *syndrome*.

**Verneuil** (ver-nĕ'e), Aristide A., Paris surgeon, 1823–1895. See Kümmell-V. *disease, hidradenitis* axillaris of V., V.'s *neuroma*.

**ver'nix** [ Mod. L. ]. Varnish.
   **v. caseo'sa,** the fatty substance, consisting of desquamated epithelial cells and sebaceous matter, which covers the skin of the fetus.

**Vernon,** William, English botanist, 17th century. Gave his name to *Vernonia*.

**Verno'nia** [ W. *Vernon* ]. A genus of plants of the family Compositae, the seeds of one species of which, *V. anthelmintica*, an East Indian plant, have vermifuge properties; the root of another species, *V. nigritiana* of West Africa, is a cardiac poison resembling digitalis, and contains a glycoside, vernonin.

**Verocay,** José, Prague pathologist, 1876–1927. See V. *bodies*.

**Veronica** (vĕ-ron'ĭ-kah) [ Mediev. L. fr. name of St. Veronica ]. A genus of plants of the family Scrophulariaceae.
   **V. virgin'ica,** leptandra.

**verruca,** pl. **verrucae** (vĕ-ru'kah, -ke) [ L. ]. Verruga; wart; a circumscribed hypertrophy of the papillae of the corium, with thickening of the Malpighian and granular layers of the epidermis, and a varying number and localization of vacuolated cells in these layers.
   **v. acumina'ta,** *condyloma* acuminatum.
   **v. digita'ta,** a wart in which the papillae project like fingers; these warts occur in groups, often on the scalp.
   **v. filifor'mis,** a wart composed of greatly elongated papillae; appears more commonly on the face and neck.
   **v. gla'bra,** a smooth wart.
   **v. molluscifor'mis,** condyloma.

   **v. necrogen'ica,** postmorten *wart.*
   **v. perua'na, v. peruvia'na,** *verruga* peruana.
   **v. pla'na juveni'lis,** a flat flesh-colored wart of small size, seen especially on the face of the young, and often associated with common warts of the hands.
   **v. plana seni'lis,** senile *keratosis.*
   **v. planta'ris,** plantar *wart.*
   **seborrheic v.,** seborrheic *keratosis.*
   **v. seni'lis,** senile *keratosis.*
   **v. sim'plex,** v. vulgaris; common wart; viral wart; a keratotic papilloma of the epidermis, occurring most frequently in young persons as a result of a localized viral infection and individual susceptibility or absence of immunity; the lesions are of variable duration, eventually undergoing spontaneous regression; epidermal cells in the lesion frequently contain inclusion bodies, and such warts have been called myrmecia; see also infectious warts *virus.*
   **v. vulga'ris,** v. simplex.

**verruciform** (vĕ-ru'sĭ-form) [ L. *verruca*, wart, + *forma*, form ]. Wart-shaped.

**verrucose, verrucous** (vĕr'u-kōs, -kus) [ L. *verrucosus* ]. Resembling a wart; denoting wartlike elevations.

**verrucosis** (vĕr'u-ko'sis) [ L. *verruca*, wart, + G. suffix *-osis*, condition ]. A condition marked by the appearance of multiple warts.
   **lymphostatic v.,** mossy *foot.*

**ver'rucous.** Verrucose.

**verruga** (vĕ-ru'gah) [ Sp. ]. Verruca.
   **v. perua'na, v. peruvia'na,** verruca peruana; Peruvian wart; hemorrhagic pian; a stage or cutaneous form of Oroya fever (Carrion's disease), characterized by an eruption of soft conical or pedunculated papules the size of a pea and larger, often following the systemic form of bartonellosis.

**versicolor** (ver'sĭ-kul'er) [ L. particolored, fr. *verso*, to turn, twist, + *color*, color ]. Variegated; marked by a variety of color.

**version** (ver'zhun, -shun) [ L. *verto*, pp. *versus*, to turn. VERT- ]. 1. A displacement of the uterus, consisting in a tilting of the entire organ without bending upon itself; the varieties of displacement are termed anteversion, forward, retroversion, backward, and lateroversion, to one or the other side. 2. Change of position of the fetus in the womb, occurring spontaneously or effected by the manipulations of the accoucheur. 3. Inclination. 4. Binocular conjugate movement; to the right, dextroversion; to left, levoversion; upward, supraversion; downward, infraversion.
   **biman'ual** or **bipo'lar v.,** turning of the baby *in utero,* performed by the hands acting upon both extremities of the fetus; it may be external or combined.
   **Braxton Hicks v.,** Hicks' v.
   **cephal'ic v.,** v. in which the fetus is turned so that the head presents.

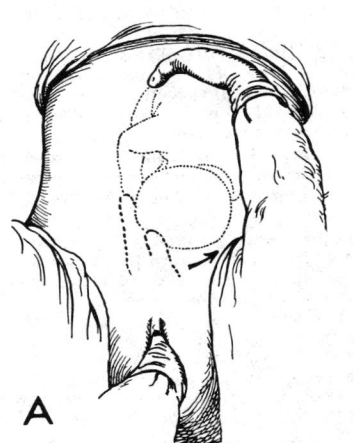 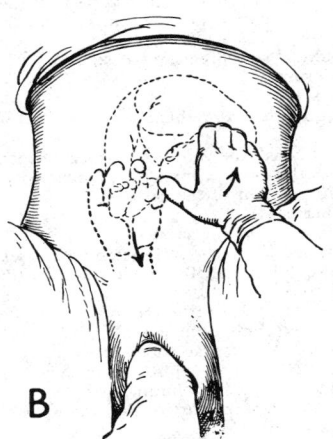

**Version and Podalic Extraction**
*A*, the head is forced upward; *B*, both feet are grasped and traction is made in the direction of the pelvic inlet. (From Taylor, E. S.: *Beck's Obstetrical Practice*, Ed. 9, The Williams & Wilkins Co., Baltimore, 1971.)

**combined v.,** bipolar v. by means of one hand in the vagina, the other on the abdominal wall.

**external v.,** v. performed entirely by external manipulation.

**Hicks' v.,** Braxton Hicks v.; a cephalic v. in which the head is guided into the pelvis by combined manipulation of a hand in the uterus and a hand on the abdomen.

**internal v.,** v. performed by means of one hand within the vagina.

**pelvic v.,** v. by means of which a transverse or oblique presentation is converted into a pelvic one by manipulating the buttocks of the fetus.

**podal'ic v.,** a manual procedure that results in a podalic extraction.

**postural v.,** nonmanual v. obtained by placing the mother in a certain position.

**Potter's v.,** a v. in which both feet are brought down until the buttocks are delivered, the back is then rotated to an anterior position, the arms and shoulders are delivered by twisting and downward movements.

**spontaneous v.,** turning of the fetus effected by the unaided contraction of the uterine muscle.

**Wright's v.,** a cephalic v. employed in cases of shoulder presentation when the shoulders are pushed upward while the breech is moved toward the center of the uterus by the other hand. The head is then guided into the pelvis.

**vertebra,** gen. and pl. **vertebrae** (ver'te-brah, -bre) [ L. joint, fr. *verto,* to turn. VERT- ] [ NA ]. One of the segments of the spinal column; in man there are usually 33 vertebrae, 7 cervical, 12 thoracic, 5 lumbar, 5 sacral (fused into one bone, the sacrum), and 4 coccygeal (fused into one bone, the coccyx).

**bas'ilar v.,** the lowest lumbar v.

**block vertebrae,** fused vertebrae which appear in radiographs as one bony mass.

**butterfly v.,** a hemivertebra or sagittally cleft v. that has a butterfly configuration in radiographs.

**caudal vertebrae,** see tail (1).

**cervical vertebrae,** vertebrae cervicales.

**vertebrae cervica'les** [ NA ], cervical vertebrae; the seven segments of the vertebral column located in the neck.

**vertebrae coccyg'eae** [ NA ], coccygeal vertebrae; tail vertebrae; the four terminal segments of the vertebral column, usually fused to form the coccyx.

**coccygeal vertebrae,** vertebrae coccygeae.

**codfish vertebrae,** the radiographic appearance of vertebrae in osteogenesis imperfecta tarda.

**cranial v.,** a segment of the skull regarded as homologous with a segment of the vertebral column.

**v. denta'ta,** axis (5).

**false vertebrae,** vertebrae spuriae; the fused vertebral segments of the sacrum and coccyx.

**hourglass vertebrae,** the radiographic appearance of some vertebrae in osteogenesis imperfecta tarda.

**vertebrae lumba'les** [ NA ], lumbar vertebrae; the vertebrae, usually five in number, located in the lumbar region of the back.

**lumbar vertebrae,** vertebrae lumbales.

**v. mag'na,** sacrum.

**odon'toid v.,** axis (5).

**v. pla'na,** spondylitis with reduction of vertebral body to a thin disk.

**v. prom'inens** [ NA ], the vertebra in the cervicothoracic region which has the most prominent spinous process (7th cervical v. in 70 per cent of the cases, 6th in 20 per cent, and 1st in 10 per cent).

**sacral vertebrae,** vertebrae sacrales.

**vertebrae sacra'les** [ NA ], sacral vertebrae; the segments of the vertebral column, usually five in number, that fuse to form the sacrum.

**ver'tebrae spu'riae,** false vertebrae.

**tail vertebrae,** vertebrae coccygeae.

**thoracic vertebrae,** vertebrae thoracicae.

**vertebrae thora'cicae** [ NA ], thoracic vertebrae; the segments of the vertebral column, usually 12, which articulate with ribs to form part of the thoracic skeleton.

**toothed v.,** axis (5).

**true v.,** v. vera; any one of the cervical, thoracic, or lumbar vertebrae.

**v. ve'ra,** true v.

**ver'tebral.** Relating to a vertebra or the vertebrae.

**vertebra'rium** [ Mod. L. ]. *Columna* vertebralis.

**Vertebrata** (ver'te-brah'tah, -bra'tah) [ L. *vertebratus,* jointed ]. Craniata; a major division of the phylum Chordata, the vertebrates, consisting of those animals with a dorsal hollow nerve cord enclosed in a cartilaginous or bony spinal column. It includes several classes of fishes, and the amphibians, reptiles, birds, and mammals.

**vertebrate** (ver'te-brāt). 1. Having a vertebral column. 2. An animal having vertebrae.

**notochordal v.,** a lower v. in which the notochord persists, unossified, in adult life.

**ver'tebra'ted.** Jointed; composed of segments arranged longitudinally, *e.g.,* v. catheter, v. probe.

**vertebrectomy** (ver'te-brek'to-mī) [ vertebra + G. *ektomē,* excision ]. Exsection of a vertebra.

**vertebro-, vertebr-** [ L. *vertebra, q.v.* ]. Combining forms for vertebra, vertebral.

**vertebroarterial** (ver'te-bro-ar-tēr'ĭ-al). Relating to a vertebra and an artery, or to the vertebral artery.

**vertebrochondral** (ver'te-bro-kon'dral) [ vertebro- + G. *chondros,* cartilage ]. Denoting the three false ribs (8th, 9th, and 10th), which are connected with the vertebrae at one extremity and the costal cartilages at the other, these cartilages not articulating directly with the sternum.

**ver'tebrocos'tal** [ vertebro- + L. *costa,* rib ]. 1. Costovertebral. 2. Vertebrochondral.

**vertebrofem'oral.** Relating to the vertebrae and the femur.

**vertebroiliac** (ver'te-bro-il'ĭ-ak). Relating to the vertebrae and the ilium.

**vertebrosa'cral.** Relating to the vertebrae and the sacrum.

**ver'tebroster'nal.** Sternovertebral.

**vertex,** pl. **vertices** (ver'teks, ver'tĭ-sēz) [ L. whirl, whorl. VERT- ]. 1 [ NA ]. The crown of the head; the topmost point of the vault of the skull, a landmark in craniometry. See fig. under craniometric *point.* 2. In obstetrics, the portion of the fetal head bounded by the planes of the trachelobregmatic and biparietal diameters, with the posterior fontanel at the apex.

**v. cordis,** *apex* cordis.

**v. cor'neae** [ NA ], vertex of the cornea; the central part of the cornea, slightly thinner than the peripheral part.

**ver'tical.** 1. Relating to the vertex, or crown of the head. 2. Perpendicular. 3. See verticalis.

**vertica'lis** [ L. ] [ NA ]. Vertical; denoting any plane or line that passes longitudinally through the body in the anatomical position.

**vertices** (ver'tĭ-sēz). Plural of vertex.

**ver'ticil** (ver'tĭ-sil) [ L. *verticillus,* the whirl of a spindle, dim. of *vertex,* a whirl. VERT- ]. A whorl; a collection of similar parts radiating from a common axis.

**verticillate** (ver'tĭ-sil'āt). Whorled; disposed in the form of a verticil.

**Verticillium** (ver'tĭ-sil'ĭ-um) [ L. *verticillus,* the whirl of a spindle. VERT- ]. A genus of hyphomycetous fungi often found in clinical specimens.

**V. graph'ii,** a mold occasionally found in the meatus in cases of otitis externa.

**verticomen'tal.** Relating to the crown of the head and the chin; denoting a diameter in craniometry.

**vertiginous** (ver-tij'ĭ-nus). Relating to or suffering from vertigo.

**vertigo** (ver'tĭ-go, ver-ti'go) [ L. *vertigo* (*vertigin-*), dizziness, fr. *verto,* to turn ]. A sensation of irregular or whirling motion, either of oneself (**subjective v.**) or of external objects (**objective v.**).

**v. ab aure laeso,** v. dependent upon chronic middle ear lesions.

**auditory v.,** Ménière's *disease.*

**aural v.,** v. caused by disease of the internal ear or pressure of cerumen on the drum membrane.

**Charcot's v.,** laryngeal *syncope.*

**chronic v.,** *status* vertiginosus.

**endem'ic paralyt'ic v.,** epidemic v.

**epidemic v.,** Gerlier's disease; kubisagari; paralyzing v.; endemic paralytic v.; v. of sudden onset with headache, vomiting, paralyses, diplopia, pupillary disturbances, nystagmus, and sometimes tinnitus, that attacks persons in the same locality.

**galvanic v.,** voltaic v.

**gastric v.,** Trousseau's syndrome (2); v. symptomatic of disease of the stomach.

**height v.,** dizziness experienced when looking down from a great height or in looking up a high building or cliff.

**horizontal v.,** dizziness experienced on lying down.

**labyrin'thine v.,** Ménière's *disease.*

**laryn'geal v.,** laryngeal *syncope.*

**lateral v.,** dizziness caused by watching the telegraph poles and fences from the window of a fast-moving vehicle.

**mechanical v.,** v. caused by continued rotation or vibration of the body.

**nocturnal v.,** a feeling of falling when dropping off to sleep.

**ocular v.,** dizziness attributed to refractive errors or imbalance of the extrinsic muscles.

**organic v.,** v. due to brain damage.

**paralyzing v.,** epidemic v.

**postural v.,** v. which occurs particularly in elderly people with change of position, usually from lying or sitting to standing position.

**rotary v.,** systematic v.; a form in which there is a sensation of rotation in a definite direction of the surrounding objects as well as oneself.

**sham-movement v.,** gyrosa; dizziness accompanied by an impression as if the body were rotating or as if objects were rotating about it.

**systematic v.,** rotary v.

**vertical v.,** that caused by looking down from a great height or looking up at a distant object.

**volta'ic v.,** galvanic v.; a lateral movement of the head upon galvanization of the vestibular nerve, the movement being in the direction opposed to the course of the current, *i.e.,* toward the positive pole.

**ertom'eter** [ vertex + G. *metron,* measure ]. Lensometer.

**erumontanitis** (vĕr'u-mon-tă-ni'tis). Colliculitis.

**erumonta'num** [ L. *veru,* a spit, + *montanus,* mountainous ]. *Colliculus* seminalis.

**e'rus** [ L. ] [ NA ]. True; genuine; as opposed to false.

**esalianum** (vĕ-sa'lī-a'num). *Os* vesaleanum.

**Vesa'lius,** Andreas [ *Vesalius,* Latinized form of Andre *Wesal* ], great Flemish anatomist of the Renaissance, born in Brussels, 1514–1564. Professor of anatomy at Padua and founder of modern anatomy; taught that anatomy could be learned only through the study of structures revealed by dissection. His great anatomical treatise, *De Humani Corporis Fabrica Libri Septem,* though bitterly attacked by the Galenists, revolutionized the teaching of anatomy and remained the authoritative text for two centuries. See V.'s *bones, foramen, ligament, vein.*

**esa'nia** [ L. fr. *vesanus,* insane, fr. *ve‑,* negative + *sanus,* sound ]. Insanity.

**esic-.** See vesico-.

**esica,** gen. and pl. **vesicae** (ves'ī-kah, -ke) [ L. ]. 1 [ NA ]. A bladder; a distensible musculomembranous organ serving as a receptacle for fluid, as the gallbladder. 2. Vesicle; blister; any hollow structure or sac, normal or pathologic, containing a serous fluid.

**v. fel'lea** [ NA ], gallbladder; vesicula fellis; cystis fellea; a pear-shaped receptacle on the inferior surface of the liver, in a hollow between the right lobe and the quadrate lobe; it serves as a storage reservoir for bile.

**v. prostat'ica,** *utriculus* prostaticus.

**v. urina'ria** [ NA ], urinary bladder; cystis urinaria; a musculomembranous elastic bag serving as a storage place for the urine.

**esical** (ves'ī-kal). Relating to any bladder, but usually the urinary bladder.

**esica'lis** [ L. ] [ NA ]. Vesical.

**es'icant.** Epispastic; vesicatory. 1. Blistering. 2. An agent that produces a blister.

**es'icate.** To blister.

**esication** (ves'ī-ka'shun). 1. The production of a blister. 2. A blister.

**es'icatory.** Vesicant.

**esicle** (ves'ī-kl) [ L. *vesicula,* a blister, dim. of *vesica,* bladder ]. 1. A small, circumscribed elevation on the skin,

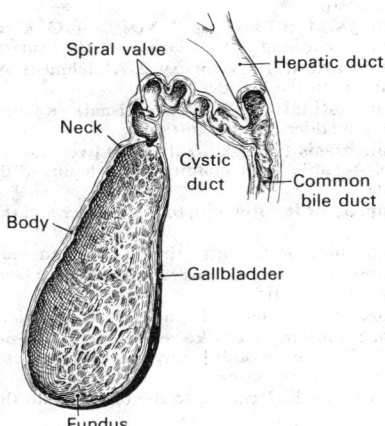

**Gallbladder (Vesica Fellea) and Bile Ducts**

containing serum. 2. A small sac containing liquid or gas.

**acous'tic v.,** auditory v.

**acrosomal v.,** *galea* capitis.

**air v.'s,** *alveoli* pulmonis.

**allanto'ic v.,** the hollow portion of the allantois.

**amniocardiac v.,** the rostral portion of the most primitive intraembryonic celom.

**auditory v.,** acoustic v.; otic v.; one of the paired sacs of invaginated ectoderm that develop into the membranous labyrinth of the internal ear.

**blastoder'mic v.,** blastocyst.

**cerebral v.,** encephalic v.; primary brain v.; each of the three divisions of the early embryonic brain; the anterior is the prosencephalon, the middle the mesencephalon, and the posterior the rhombencephalon.

**cervical v.,** an abnormally persisting vestige of the cervical sinus or its associated branchial grooves.

**encephalic v.,** cerebral v.

**forebrain v.,** prosencephalon.

**germinal v.,** archaic term for the nucleus of the ovum.

**hindbrain v.,** rhombencephalon.

**lens v.,** lenticular v.; in the embryo, the ectodermal invagination that forms opposite the optic cup. It is the primordium of the lens of the eye.

**lenticular v.,** lens v.

**Malpighian v.'s,** the minute air-filled v.'s on the surface of an expanded lung.

**midbrain v.,** mesencephalon.

**ocular v.,** *vesiculus* ophthalmica.

**optic v.,** *vesicula* ophthalmica.

**otic v.,** auditory v.

**pinocytotic v.,** a v. a fraction of a micron in diameter containing material being transported through a cell such as that of endothelium; see also pinocytosis.

**primary brain v.,** cerebral v.

**seminal v.,** *vesicula* seminalis.

**synaptic v.'s,** the small (average diameter 300 Å), intracellular, membrane-bound v.'s near the presynaptic membrane of a synaptic junction, containing the transmitter substance which, in chemical synapses, mediates the passage of nerve impulses across the junction; see also synapse.

**telencephalic v.,** a diverticulum arising from the prosencephalon, one on each side.

**umbilical v.,** yolk *sac.*

**vesico-, vesic-** (ves'ī-ko-) [ L. *vesica,* bladder ]. Combining forms for vesica, vesicle; see also vesiculo-.

**ves'icoabdom'inal.** Relating to the urinary bladder and the abdominal wall.

**ves'icobul'lous.** Denoting an eruption of lesions containing serum. The individual lesions range in size from 1 mm. to 2 cm. in diameter.

**vesicocele** (ves'ī-ko-sēl). Cystocele.

**vesicocer'vical.** Relating to the urinary bladder and the cervix uteri.

**vesicoclysis** (ves'i-kok'li-sis) [ vesico- + G. *klysis*, a washing out ]. Washing out, or lavage, of the urinary bladder.

**vesicofixa'tion.** 1. Cystopexy. 2. Attachment by suture of the uterus to the bladder wall.

**vesicointestinal** (ves'i-ko-in-tes'ti-nal). Relating to the urinary bladder and the intestine.

**vesicolithiasis** (ves'i -ko-li-thi'a-sis) [ vesico- + G. *lithos*, stone, + suffix -*iasis*, condition ]. Calculus in the urinary bladder.

**vesicoprostat'ic.** Relating to the bladder and the prostate gland.

**vesicopu'bic.** Relating to the bladder and the os pubis.

**vesicopustule** (ves'i-ko-pus'tul). A vesicle which is developing pus formation.

**vesicorec'tal.** Relating to the bladder and the rectum.

**vesicorectostomy** (ves'i-ko-rek-tos'to-mi) [ vesico- + rectum + G. *stoma*, mouth ]. Surgical urinary tract diversion, from bladder to rectum.

**vesicosig'moid.** Relating to the bladder and the sigmoid colon.

**vesicosigmoidostomy** (ves'i-ko-sig-moy-dos'to-mi) [ vesico- + sigmoid + G. *stoma*, mouth ]. The operative formation of a communication between the bladder and the sigmoid colon.

**vesicospi'nal.** Relating to the urinary bladder and the spinal cord; denoting the neural mechanisms that control retention and evacuation of urine by the bladder, located in the second lumbar and second sacral segment, respectively, of the spinal cord.

**vesicotomy** (ves'i-kot'o-mi). Cystotomy (1).

**vesicoumbilical** (ves'i-ko-um-bil'i-kal). Omphalovesical; relating to the urinary bladder and the umbilicus.

**vesicoureteral** (ves'i-ko-u-re'ter-al). Relating to the bladder and the ureters.

**vesicourethral** (ves'i-ko-u-re'thral). Relating to the bladder and the urethra.

**vesicouterine** (ves'i-ko-u'ter-in). Relating to the bladder and the uterus.

**vesicouterovaginal** (ves'i-ko-u'ter-o-vaj'i-nal). Relating to the bladder, uterus, and vagina.

**vesicovaginal** (ves-i-ko-vaj'in-al). Relating to the bladder and vagina.

**vesicovaginorectal** (ves'i-ko-vaj'i-no-rek'tal). Relating to the bladder, vagina and rectum.

**vesicovisceral** (ves'i-ko-vis'er-al). Relating to the urinary bladder and any other adjacent organ or viscus.

**vesicula,** gen. and pl. **vesiculae** (ve-sik'u-lah, -le) [ L. blister, vesicle, dim. of *vesica*, bladder ] [ NA ]. Vesicle; a small bladder or bladder-like structure.

    **v. fel'lis,** *vesica* fellea.

    **v. ophthal'mica** [ NA ], optic or ocular vesicle; in the embryo, one of the paired evaginations from the ventrolateral walls of the forebrain from which are developed the sensory and pigment layers of the retina.

    **v. semina'lis** [ NA ], seminal vesicle; seminal capsule; one of two folded, sacculated, glandular structures which is a diverticulum of the ductus deferens; its secretion is one of the components of the semen.

    **v. umbilica'lis,** yolk *sac.*

**vesic'ular.** 1. Relating to a vesicle. 2. Vesiculose; vesiculous; vesiculated; characterized by or containing vesicles.

**vesic'ulate.** 1. To become vesicular. 2. Vesiculated.

**vesic'ulated.** Vesicular (2); containing vesicles.

**vesiculation** (ve-sik'u-la'shun). 1. The formation of vesicles. 2. Inflation. 3. The presence of a number of vesicles.

**vesiculectomy** (ve-sik'u-lek'to-mi) [ L. *vesicula*, vesicle, + G. *ektome*, excision ]. Resection of a portion or all of each of the seminal vesicles; an operation for producing sterility.

**vesiculiform** (ve-sik'u-li-form). Resembling a vesicle.

**vesiculitis** (ve-sik'u-li'tis) [ L. *vesicula*, vesicle, + G. suffix -*itis*, inflammation ]. Inflammation of any vesicle; specifically, inflammation of a seminal vesicle.

**vesiculo-** (ve-sik'u-lo-) [ L. *vesicula*, vesicle ]. Combining form denoting vesicle.

**vesiculobronchial** (ve-sik'u-lo-brong'ki-al). Denoting an auscultatory sound partaking of both a vesicular and a bronchial character.

**vesiculocav'ernous.** Both vesicular and cavernous; denoting (1) an auscultatory sound partaking of both a vesicular and a cavernous quality, and (2) the structure of certain neoplasms.

**vesiculography** (ve-sik'u-log'ra-fi) [ vesiculo- + G. *grapho*, to write ]. X-ray of the seminal vesicles.

**vesiculopap'ular.** Pertaining to or consisting of a combination of vesicles and papules.

**vesiculoprostatitis** (ve-sik'u-lo-pros'ta-ti'tis) [ vesiculo- + prostate + G. suffix -*itis*, inflammation ]. Inflammation of the bladder and prostate.

**vesiculopus'tular.** Pertaining to a mixed eruption of vesicles and pustules.

**vesic'ulose.** Vesicular (2).

**vesiculotomy** (ve-sik'u-lot'o-mi) [ vesiculo- + G. *tome*, incision ]. Division of the seminal vesicles.

**vesic'ulotu'bular.** Denoting an auscultatory sound partaking of both a vesicular and a tubular quality.

**vesiculotympanic** (ve-sik'u-lo-tim-pan'ik). Denoting a percussion sound partaking of both a vesicular and a tympanic quality.

**vesic'ulous.** Vesicular (2).

**Veslingius,** Joannes, German anatomist, 1598–1649. See V.'s *line.*

**vespa'jus** [ L. *vespa*, wasp ]. Suppurative inflammation of the hair follicles of the scalp.

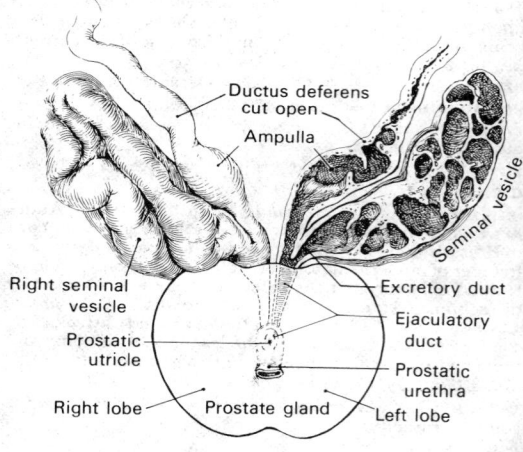

**Seminal Vesicles**

**ves'sel** [ O. Fr. fr. L. *vascellum*, dim. of *vas* ]. Vas; a duct or canal conveying any liquid, such as blood, lymph, chyle, or semen.

    **absorbent v.,** vas lymphaticum.

    **afferent v.,** *vas* afferens.

    **blood v.,** see *blood vessel.*

    **capillary v.,** vas capillare; see blood *capillary* and lymph *capillary.*

    **chyle v.,** lacteal (2).

    **collateral v.,** *vas* collaterale.

    **deep lymphatic v.'s,** *vasa* lymphatica profunda.

    **efferent v.,** *vas* efferens.

    **lac'teal v.,** lacteal (2).

    **lymph** or **lymphatic v.'s,** *vasa* lymphatica.

    **nutrient v.,** *arteria* nutricia.

    **superficial lymphatic v.'s,** *vasa* lymphatica superficialia.

**vestibular** (ves-tib'u-lar). Relating to a vestibule, especially the vestibule of the ear.

**vestibula'ris** [ L. ] [ NA ]. Vestibular.

**vestib'ulate.** Possessing a vestibule.

**vestibule** (ves'ti-bul) [ L. *vestibulum*, *q. v.* ]. Vestibulum.

    **aortic v.,** *vestibulum* aortae.

**buccal v.,** that part of the vestibulum oris related to the cheek.

**esophagogastric v.,** gastroesophageal v.

**gastroesophageal v.,** esophagogastric v.; the dilated aboral portion of the esophagus, just above the esophagogastric orifice; usually it corresponds to the lumen of pars abdominalis of the esophagus although its relation to the diaphragm is variable.

**labial v.,** that part of the vestibulum oris related to the lips.

**v. of larynx,** *vestibulum* laryngis.

**v. of mouth,** *vestibulum* oris.

**v. of nose,** *vestibulum* nasi.

**v. of omental bursa,** *vestibulum* bursae omentalis.

**Sibson's aortic v.,** *vestibulum* aortae.

**v. of vagina,** *vestibulum* vaginae.

**vestibulo-** (ves-tib'u-lo-) [ L. *vestibulum*, vestibule ]. Combining form denoting vestibule, vestibulum.

**vestibulocochlear** (ves-tib'u-lo-kok'le-ar). 1. Relating to the vestibulum and cochlea of the ear. 2. Statoacoustic.

**vestib'uloplas'ty** [ vestibulo- + G. *plassō*, to form ]. Any of a series of surgical procedures designed to restore alveolar ridge height by lowering muscles attaching to the buccal, labial, and lingual aspects of the jaws.

**vestib'ulospi'nal.** See *tractus vestibulospinalis.*

**vestibulotomy** (ves-tib'u-lot'o-mĭ) [ vestibulo- + G. *tomē*, incision ]. Operation for opening into the vestibule of the labyrinth; it is called *superior* or *inferior* according as the opening is made from above or from below.

**vestibulourethral** (ves-tib'u-lo-u-re'thral). Relating to vestibulum vaginae and urethra.

**vestibulum,** pl. **vestibula** (ves-tib'u-lum, -lah) [ L. antechamber, entrance court ] [ NA ]. Vestibule. 1. A small cavity or a space at the entrance of a canal. 2. Specifically, the central, somewhat ovoid, cavity of the osseous labyrinth communicating with the semicircular canals posteriorly and the cochlea anteriorly.

**v. aor'tae,** aortic vestibule; Sibson's aortic vestibule; the portion of the left ventricle of the heart immediately below the aortic orifice, having fibrous walls and affording room for the segments of the closed aortic valve.

**v. bur'sae omenta'lis** [ NA ], vestibule of the omental bursa; the upper part of the bursa omentalis, just within the epiploic foramen (of Winslow), behind the caudate lobe of the liver.

**v. laryn'gis** [ NA ], of the larynx; atrium glottidis; the upper part of the laryngeal cavity from the superior aperture to the vestibular folds.

**v. na'si** [ NA ], vestibule of the nose; the anterior part of the nasal cavity, practically that enclosed by cartilage.

**v. o'ris** [ NA ], vestibule of the mouth; buccal cavity (1); that part of the mouth bounded laterally by the lips and the cheeks, medially by the teeth and/or gums, and above and below by the reflections of the mucosa from the lips and cheeks to the gums.

**v. puden'di,** v. vaginae.

**v. vagi'nae** [ NA ], vestibule of the vagina; v. pudendi; the space behind the glans clitoridis between the labia minora, containing the openings of the vagina, urethra, and ducts of the greater vestibular glands.

**vestige** (ves'tij) [ L. *vestigium, q.v.* ]. Vestigium.

**v. of vaginal process,** *vestigium* processus vaginalis.

**vestigial** (ves-tij'ĭ-al). Relating to a vestige.

**vestigium,** pl. **vestigia** (ves-tij'ĭ-um, -ah) [ L. footprint (trace), fr. *vestigo*, to track, trace ] [ NA ]. Vestige; a trace; a rudimentary structure; the degenerated remains of any structure which occurs as an entity in the embryo or fetus.

**v. proces'sus vagina'lis** [ NA ], vestige of the vaginal process; incompletely obliterated remnants of the vaginal process of the peritoneum remaining in the spermatic cord.

**vesu'vine** [ *Vesuvius*, volcano in Italy ]. Bismarck brown Y.

**veterinarian** (vet'er-ĭ-nĕr'ĭ-an) [ see veterinary ]. One who is fitted by training and experience, and who is licensed by his government to minister to the ailments of animals both domestic and wild, and to advise livestock owners on the best methods of feeding, breeding, and caring for domesticated animals; a veterinary physician or surgeon.

**veterinarian's oath.** The official oath of the veterinary profession, adopted by the American Veterinary Medical Association in 1954: "Being admitted to the profession of veterinary medicine, I solemnly dedicate myself and the knowledge I possess to the benefit of society, to the conservation of our livestock resources and to the relief of suffering of animals. I will practice my profession conscientiously with dignity. The health of my patients, the best interest of their owners, and the welfare of my fellow man, will be my primary considerations. I will, at all times, be humane and temper pain with anesthesia where indicated. I will not use my knowledge contrary to the laws of humanity, nor in contravention to the ethical code of my profession. I will uphold and strive to advance the honor and noble traditions of the veterinary profession. These pledges I make freely in the eyes of God and upon my honor."

**veterinary** (vet'er-ĭ-nĕr-ĭ) [ L. *veterinarius*, fr. *veterina*, beast of burden ]. Relating to the diagnosis and therapeutics of the diseases of animals.

**via,** pl. **viae** (vi'ah, vē'ah, vi'e) [ L. way, road ]. Any passage in the body, as the intestine, the vagina, etc.

**per vi'as natura'les,** through natural channels; denoting the birth of a child through the vagina as distinguished from delivery by cesarean section.

**viability** (vi'ă-bil'ĭ-tĭ) [ Fr. *viabilité* fr. L. *vita*, life ]. Capability of living; the state of being viable; usually connotes a fetus that has reached 500 grams in weight and 20 gestational weeks.

**viable** (vi'ă-bl) [ Fr. fr. *vie*, life, fr. L. *vita* ]. Capable of living; denoting a fetus sufficiently developed to live outside of the uterus.

**vi'al** [ G. *phialē*, a drinking cup ]. Phial; a small bottle or receptacle for holding liquids, including medicines.

**vibesate** (vi'bes-āt). AEROPLAST; a mixture of polvinate and malrosinol in organic solvent and a propellant; a modified polyvinyl plastic used as a topical spray for wounds.

**vibration** (vi-bra'shun) [ L. *vibratio*, fr. *vibro*, pp. *-atus*, to quiver, shake ]. 1. A shaking. 2. A to-and-fro movement (oscillation).

**sonic v.,** a method for disrupting cell structures (*e.g.*, bacterial cell membranes) by producing waves of sound (ultrasonic) frequencies in an aqueous medium.

**ultrasonic v.,** see sonic v.

**vi'brative.** Vibratory.

**vi'brator.** An instrument used for imparting vibrations.

**vi'bratory.** Vibrative; marked by vibrations.

**Vibrio** (vib'rĭ-o) [ L. *vibro*, to vibrate ]. A genus of motile (occasionally nonmotile), nonsporeforming, aerobic to facultatively anaerobic bacteria (family Spirillaceae) containing short (0.5 to 3.0 μm), curved or straight rods which occur singly or which are occasionally united into S-shapes or spirals. Motile cells contain a single polar flagellum; in some species, two or more flagella occur in one polar tuft. These organisms are usually sensitive to 2,4-diamino-6,7-diisopropyl pteridine (0/129) and novobiocin. Some of these organisms are saprophytes in salt and fresh water and in soil; others are parasites or pathogens. The type species is *V. cholerae.*

**V. albensis,** a species of luminescent bacteria found in fresh water and in human feces and bile.

**V. cholerae,** cholera bacillus; comma bacillus; Koch's bacillus; *V. comma;* a species that produces a soluble exotoxin (permeability factor) that seems to be the cause of Asiatic cholera in human beings. It is the type species of the genus *V.*

**V. com'ma,** *V. cholerae.*

**V. fe'tus,** a species causing an infectious disease of sheep and cattle manifested principally by early abortions of pregnant females.

**V. fisheri,** a species of luminescent bacteria found in sea water.

**V. indicus,** a luminescent species of bacteria found in coastal sea water and in dead fish, crustacea, and other salt-water animals; also found in meat and on soldiers' wounds, where it produces no known harmful effects.

**V. jejuni,** a species causing diarrhea in cows and calves.

**V. leonard'ii,** a species highly pathogenic for the bee moth, *Galleria mellonela*, and the European corn borer, *Pyrausta nubialis.*

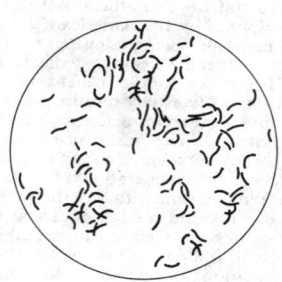

*Vibrio cholerae*
(Original magnification, ×2400)

**V. metsch'nikovii,** a species found in the intestinal contents of chickens, pigeons, and other animals with a cholera-like disease.

**V. pis'cium,** a species causing an epidemic infection in fish; also pathogenic for frogs.

**V. pro'teus,** a species found in the defecations of patients with cholera nostras and cholera infantum.

**V. sputorum,** a species found in the human oral cavity and in fusospirochetal diseases of the mouth.

**V. xenopus,** a species originally found in an abscess of the pectoral muscle of an African toad.

**vibrio** (vib'rĭ-o). A member of the genus *Vibrio.*

**El Tor v.,** a bacterium regarded as a biotype of *V. cholerae.* It was originally isolated from six pilgrims who died of dysentery or gangrene of the colon at the Tor quarantine station on the Sinai Peninsula.

**Nasik v.,** an organism differing from the cholera vibrio, being shorter and fatter and less comma-shaped; its cultures are very toxic to laboratory animals on intravenous injections.

**vibrion septique** (ve-bre-oṅ' sep-tēk) [ Fr. septic vibrio ]. *Clostridium septicum.*

**vibriosis** (vib'rĭ-o'sis). Infection caused by species of *Vibrio.*

**vibrissa,** gen. and pl. **vibrissae** (vi-bris'ah, vi-bris'e) [ L. found only in pl. *vibrissae,* fr. *vibro,* to quiver ] [ NA ]. One of the hairs growing at the anterior nares, or vestibulum nasi.

**vibris'sal.** Relating to the vibrissae.

**vibrocardiogram** (vi'bro-kar'dĭ-o-gram) [ L. *vibro,* to shake, + G. *kardia,* heart, + *gramma,* a drawing ]. A graphic record of chest vibrations produced by hemodynamic events of the cardiac cycle; the record provides an indirect, externally recorded measurement of isometric contraction and ejection times.

**vibromasseur** (vi'bro-mas-ër'). An instrument for giving vibratory massage; vibrator.

**vi'brotherapeu'tics.** Vibratory *massage.*

**Viburnum** (vi-bur'num) [ L. the way-faring tree ]. A genus of gamopetalous trees and shrubs of the family Caprifoliaceae.

**v. op'ulus,** the source of cramp bark, cranberry tree bark; has been used in functional uterine disorders.

**V. prunifo'lium,** black hawk; sheepberry; stag-bush; the bark of the root has been used in dysmenorrhea and as a general antispasmodic.

**vicarious** (vi-kăr'ĭ-us) [ L. *vicarius,* from *vicis,* supplying place of ]. Acting as a substitute; occurring in an abnormal situation.

**Vicat** (ve-kah'), L. J., French engineer, 1786–1861. See V. *needle.*

**vice** [ L. *vitium* ]. In pathology, a defect or imperfection, especially in physical conformation; an obsolete term.

**vic'ianose.** 6-β-L-Arabinosido)-D-glucose; a disaccharide of glucose and arabinose.

**vi'cine.** 2,5-Diamino-4,6-diketopyrimidine-3-β-D-glucoside; vicioside occurring in akta, a weed which contaminates *Lathyrus sativus* and is thought by some to be responsible for the symptoms of lathyrism.

**Vicq d'Azyr** (vik-daz-eer'), Félix, Paris anatomist, 1748–1794. See V. d'A.'s *bundle, centrum, foramen.*

**Victoria blue** [ Queen *Victoria* ]. Any of several blue di phenylnaphthylmethane derivatives; used as a stain in histology.

**Victoria orange.** An alkaline salt of dinitrocresol; aniline orange; English yellow; a reddish yellow stain; formerly used in histology.

**Vidal,** Jean Baptiste Emile, Paris dermatologist, 1825–1893. See V.'s *disease.*

**Vidal** (ve-dal') **de Cassis,** Auguste T., French surgeon, 1803–1856. See V.'s *operation.*

**Vid'ian.** Named after or described by Vidius.

**Vidius, Vidus** (vid'ĭ-us, vi'dus). Latinized form of Guido Guidi, Italian anatomist, 1500–1569. See Vidian *artery, canal, nerve, vein.*

**Vierordt** (feer'ort), Karl, German physiologist, 1818–1884. See V.'s *hemotachometer.*

**Vieussens** (vyĕ-saṅ'), Raymond, French anatomist, 1641–1715. See V.'s *ansa, anulus, centrum* ovale, *foramina, ganglion, isthmus, limbus, loop, ring, valve, veins, ventricle.*

**vigil** (vij'il) [ L. *vigilia,* wakefulness, alertness, fr. *vigeo,* to be active, to rouse ]. Wakefulness; sleeplessness; insomnia.

**coma v.,** a state of muttering delirium in which the person is lethargic and partly conscious, yet never actually sleeping or completely comatose.

**vigilambulism** (vij'ĭ-lam'bu-lizm) [ L. *vigil,* awake, alert, + *ambulo,* to walk about ]. A condition of unconsciousness regarding one's surroundings, with automatism, resembling somnambulism but occurring in the waking state.

**vigilance** (vij'ĭ-lans) [ L. *vigilantia,* wakefulness ]. Agrypnia; insomnia; pervigilium; an attentiveness, alertness, a watchfulness for whatever may occur.

**Villard** (ve-lar'), Eugène, French surgeon, *1868. See V.'s *button.*

**vil'li.** Plural of villus.

**villiki'nin** [ L. *villus,* shaggy hair (of beasts), + *kineō,* to move ]. A postulated hormone said to stimulate the movement of intestinal villi; preparations observed to exhibit such activity have been obtained from human plasma and from the intestinal mucosa of animals.

**villo'ma.** Papilloma.

**vil'lose.** Villous (2).

**villositis** (vil'o-si'tis) [ villous + G. suffix -*itis,* inflammation ]. Inflammation of the villous surface of the placenta.

**villosity** (vĭ-los'ĭ-tĭ). Shagginess; an aggregation of villi.

**vil'lous.** 1. Relating to villi. 2. Villose; shaggy; covered with villi.

**villus,** pl. **villi** (vil'us, vil'i) [ L. shaggy hair (of beasts) ]. 1 [ NA ]. A projection from the surface, especially of a mucous membrane. If the projection is minute, as from a cell surface, it is termed a microvillus. 2. An elongated dermal papilla projecting into an intraepidermal vesicle or cleft.

**anchoring v.,** a chorionic v. that is attached to the decidua basalis.

**arachnoid villi,** *granulationes* arachnoideales.

**chorion'ic villi,** vascular processes of the chorion of the embryo entering into the formation of the placenta.

**floating v.,** free v.

**free v.,** floating v.; a chorionic v. that is not attached to the decidua basalis, but is "free" in the maternal blood of the intervillous spaces.

**intestinal villi,** villi intestinales.

**villi intestina'les** [ NA ], intestinal villi; projections (0.5 to 1.5 mm. in length) of the mucous membrane of the intestine; they are leaf-shaped in the duodenum and become shorter, more finger-shaped, and sparser in the ileum.

**villi pericardi'aci,** pericardial villi; minute filiform projections from the surface of the serous pericardium.

**pericardial villi,** villi pericardiaci.

**peritoneal villi,** villi peritoneales.

**villi peritonea'les,** peritoneal villi; villi on the surface of the peritoneum.

**pleural villi,** villi pleurales.

**villi pleura'les,** pleural villi; shaggy appendages on the

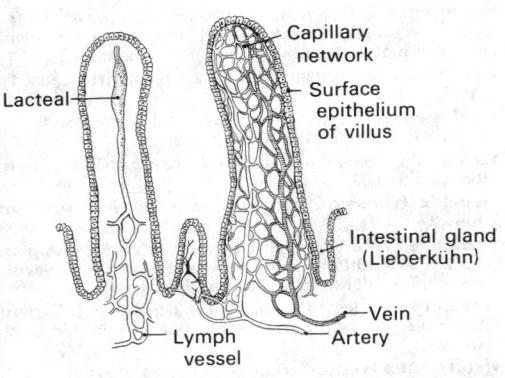

**Intestinal villus**
Vertical section through intestinal mucosa. (After Mall.)

pleura in the neighborhood of the costomediastinal sinus.
**primary v.,** the first stage of chorionic v. development, with columns of cytotrophoblastic cells covered by syncytiotrophoblast.
**secondary v.,** an intermediate stage of chorionic v. development following invasion by a connective tissue core.
**synovial villi,** villi synoviales.
**villi synovia'les** [ NA ], synovial villi; synovial tufts; synovial fringe; small vascular processes given off from a synovial membrane.
**tertiary v.,** the definitive chorionic v. with a vascular core separated from maternal blood by connective tissue, cytotrophoblast, and syncytiotrophoblast.
**villusectomy** (vil'us-ek'to-mĭ) [ villus + G. *ektomē,* excision ]. Synovectomy.
**Vim-Silverman needle.** See under needle.
**vinbar'bital.** DELVINAL; 5-ethyl-5-(1-methyl-1-butenyl)-barbituric acid; an intermediate-acting barbiturate used as a sedative and hypnotic. Also available as v. sodium (DELVINAL sodium), with same action and uses.
**vinblas'tine sulfate** (USP, BP). VELBAN; VLB; vincaleukoblastine; a dimeric alkaloid obtained from *Vinca rosea.* It arrests mitosis in metaphase (though vincristine is more active in this respect); it exhibits greater antimetabolic activity than vincristine. Used in the treatment of Hodgkin's disease, choriocarcinoma, acute and chronic leukemias, and other neoplastic diseases.
**vincaleukoblastine** (ving'kah-lu'ko-blas'tēn). Vinblastine sulfate.
**Vinca rosea** (ving'kah). Periwinkle; a species of myrtle (family Myrtaceae) used in various parts of the world as a home remedy. Four active dimeric alkaloids have been identified: vinblastine, vincristine, vinleurosine, and vinrosidine.
**Vincent,** Henri, Paris physician, 1862–1950. See V.'s *angina, bacillus, disease, infection, mycetoma, spirillum, stomatitis, tonsillitis.*
**vincristine sulfate** (vin-kris'tēn) (USP). ONCOVIN; VCR; a dimeric alkaloid obtained from *Vinca rosea.* Its antineoplastic activity is similar to that of vinblastine, but no cross-resistance develops between these two agents; it is more useful than vinblastine in lymphocytic lymphosarcoma and acute leukemia.
**vinculum,** pl. **vincula** (ving'ku-lum, -lah) [ L. a fetter, fr. *vincio,* to bind ] [ NA ]. A frenum, frenulum, or ligament.
**v. breve** [ NA ], short vinculum; a triangular band that extends from the dorsal surface of each of the flexor tendons of a digit to the capsule of the nearby interphalangeal joint and to the phalanx proximal to the insertion of the tendon; see also vincula tendinum.
**v. lin'guae,** *frenulum* linguae.
**vincula lin'gulae cerebell'i,** alae lingulae cerebelli; small lateral prolongations of the lingula of the vermis of the cerebellum resting on the dorsal surface of the superior cerebellar peduncle.

**long v.,** v. longum.
**v. lon'gum** [ NA ], long vinculum; a long, threadlike band that extends from the dorsal surface of each of the flexor tendons of a digit to the proximal phalanx; see also vincula tendinum.
**v. prepu'tii,** *frenulum* preputii.
**short v.,** v. breve.
**vincula ten'dinum** [ NA ], vincula of the tendons; synovial frenula or frena; tenacula tendinum; fibrous bands that extend from the flexor tendons of the fingers and toes to the capsules of the interphalangeal joints and to the phalanges; they convey small vessels to the tendons; see also v. breve and v. longum.
**vincula of tendons,** vincula tendinum.
**Vineberg procedure.** See under procedure.
**vinegar** (vin'e-gar) [ Fr. *vinaigre,* fr. *vin,* wine, + *aigre,* sour ]. Acetum; impure dilute acetic acid, made from wine, cider, malt, etc.
**mother of v.,** [ A.S. *modder,* mud ], a stringy sediment in v., the fungus of acetous fermentation.
**pyroligneous v.,** wood v.
**wood v.,** pyracetic acid; pyroligneous v.; crude pyroligneous acid; impure acetic acid produced by the destructive distillation of pine tar and wood.
**vin'etine.** Oxyacanthine.
**vi'nic** [ L. *vinum,* wine ]. Relating to or derived from wine.
**vinleurosine** (vin-lu'ro-sēn). VLR; a dimeric alkaloid obtained from *Vinca rosea.*
**vi'nous.** Relating to, containing, or of the nature of wine.
**vinrosidine** (vin-ro'zĭ-dēn). VRD; a dimeric alkaloid obtained from *Vinca rosea.*
**Vinson,** Porter P., American surgeon, *1890. See Plummer-V. *syndrome.*
**vi'num** [ L. ]. Wine.
**vi'nyl.** Ethenyl; the hydrocarbon radical, $CH_2 = CH—$.
**v. ether** (NF, BP), divinyl ether.
**vi'nylben'zene.** Styrene.
**vi'nylene.** The bivalent radical, $—CH = CH—$.
**vi'nyleth'yl ether.** Ethylvinyl ether.
**5-vinyl-2-thiooxazolidone.** Goitrin.
**Viola** (vi'o-lah) [ L. violet ]. A genus of flowering plants of the family Violaceae, including the pansies and violets.
**V. odora'ta,** the sweet or English violet, contains an alkaloid, violine, resembling emetine in action.
**V. tri'color,** pansy; hearts' ease; formerly used in cutaneous disorders and in tuberculosis.
**violaceous** (vi'o-la'shus) [ L. *viola,* violet ]. Denoting a purple discoloration, usually of the skin.
**violaxanthin** (vi'o-lah-zan'thēn). A widely distributed carotinoid plant pigment formed from zeaxanthin, a dihydroxy-$\beta$-carotene.
**violet** (vi'o-let) [ L. *viola* ]. 1. *Viola odorata.* 2. The color evoked by wavelengths of the visible spectrum shorter than 450 nm.
**crystal v.** (BP), methylrosaniline chloride.
**gentian v.** (USP), methylrosaniline chloride.
**Lauth's v.,** thionine.
**visual v.,** iodopsin.
**vi'omy'cin.** $C_{23}H_{36}N_{12}O_8$; an antibiotic agent obtained from *Streptomyces puniceus* var. *floridae;* active against acid-fast bacteria, including strains of tubercle bacilli resistant to streptomycin; may produce vestibular damage and deafness.
**viosterol** (vi-os'ter-ōl). Ergocalciferol.
**vi'per** [ L. *vipera,* serpent, snake ]. 1. A member of the family of venomous snakes, the true vipers and the adders, found in Europe, Africa, and Asia, such as *Vipera berus,* the common adder of Europe, or *Vipera russelli,* the highly poisonous Russell's viper. The family Crotalidae, or New World pit vipers, are differentiated by having a hollow, heat-sensitive pit between eye and nostril; includes the rattlesnake, copperhead, water moccasin, and fer-de-lance. The family Viperidae, or Old World vipers and adders, are distinguished from Crotalidae by not having a pit between eye and nostril; includes the genera *Vipera* (viper), *Cerastes* (horned viper), *Bitis* (puff-adder). 2. In a loose sense, any venomous or supposedly venomous snake.
**Russell's v.,** see v. (1).

**Viperidae** (vi-pĕr'ī-de) [ L. *vipera*, viper ]. An Old World family of poisonous snakes embracing the vipers and adders; see viper.

**Vipond** (ve-pawn'), French physician. See V.'s *sign.*

**vipryn'ium embonate** (BP). Pyrvinium pamoate.

**viraginity** (vĭr'ă-jin'ī-tĭ) [ L. *virago* (*viragin-*), a female warrior ]. The presence of pronounced masculine psychological qualities in a woman.

**vi'ral.** Virus (3).

**Virchow** (fēr'khō), Rudolf, great German pathologist, 1821–1902. He emphasized that the cell is the fundamental unit in pathology and as such should be studied intensively in order to gain an insight into diseased states. His views and a great collection of his observations were published in his *Cellular Pathologie.* See V.'s *angle*, V.-Holder *angle*, V.-Hassall *bodies*, V.'s *cells, corpuscles, crystals, granulations, law, node, psammoma*, V.-Robin *spaces.*

**viremia** (vi-re'mĭ-ah) [ virus + G. *haima*, blood ]. The presence, as in smallpox, of a virus in the blood stream.

**vi'res.** Plural of vis.

**virga** (vēr'gah) [ L. a rod ]. Penis.

**virgin** (ver'jin) [ L. *virgo* (*virgin-*), maiden ]. 1. A woman (or a man) who has never had sexual intercourse. 2. Fresh; unused; uncontaminated.

    **v. oil,** olive oil obtained by expression from the nearly ripe hand-picked fruit.

**virginal** (ver'jĭ-nal) [ L. *virginalis* ]. Relating to a virgin; innocent; virgin (2).

**virginity** (ver-jin'ī-tĭ) [ L. *virginitas* ]. The virgin state.

**virgophrenia** (ver'go-fre'nĭ-ah) [ L. *virgo*, maiden, + G. *phrēn*, mind ]. The receptive, capacious, and retentive mind of youth.

**viricidal** (vi'rĭ-si'dal). Virucidal.

**viricide** (vi'rĭ-sīd). Virucide.

**viridine** (vĭr'ĭ-dēn). Jervine.

**virile** (vĭr'il) [ L. *virilis*, masculine, fr. *vir*, a man ]. 1. Relating to the male sex. 2. Manly, strong, masculine. 3. Possessing masculine traits.

**virilescence** (vĭr'ĭ-les'ens). The assumption of male characteristics by the female, especially in the lower animals, and not infrequently in the human when past the reproductive age.

**virilia** (vĭ-ril'ĭ-ah) [ L. ntr. pl. of *virilis*, virile ]. The male sexual organs.

**virilism** (vĭr'ĭ-lizm) [ L. *virilis*, masculine ]. The possession of mature masculine somatic characteristics by a girl, woman, or prepubescent; may be present at birth or may appear first later in life, depending on its cause; it may be relatively mild (entailing, for example, just hirsutism) or may be severe. It is commonly the result of gonadal or adrenocortical dysfunction, or may be produced by androgenic therapy.

    **adrenal v.,** adrenal virilizing syndrome; v. produced by excessive or abnormal secretory patterns of adrenocortical steroids.

**virility** (vĭ-ril'ī-tĭ) [ L. *virilitas*, manhood, fr. *vir*, man ]. The reproductive age in the man; manhood.

**virilization** (vĭr'ĭ-lĭ-za'shun). The production, or the acquisition of virilism.

**virilizing** (vĭr'ĭ-li-zing). Causing virilism.

**virion** (vi'rĭ-on, vĭr'ĭ-on). An elementary virus particle; composed of a central, nucleic acid-containing core (nucleoid) surrounded by a protein covering (capsid); this nucleic acid-protein complex (nucleocapsid) may be the complete v. (as in the case of the adenoviruses and the picornaviruses) or may be surrounded by an "envelope" as in the herpesviruses and the myxoviruses. Capsids may be icosahedral or helical: the former are composed of capsomers, each of which consists either of five (pentamer, or pentagonal capsomer) or of six (hexamer, or hexagonal capsomer) protein units (monomers); helical capsids, not being in the form of icosahedrons, do not contain capsomers, the protein monomers forming simpler, cylindrical structures around the nucleic acid core. The envelope of an enveloped v. is a membrane-like structure containing lipids, proteins, and carbohydrates, and from the surface of which project structures resembling spikes.

**viripotent** (vĭr'ī-po'tent, vĭ-rip'o-tent) [ L. *viripotens*, fr. v man, + *potens*, having power ]. Obsolete term meanin sexually mature (denoting one of the male sex).

**virol'ogist.** A student of virology, or of virus-caused di eases.

**virology** (vi-rol'o-jĭ, vĭ-) [ virus + G. *logos*, study ]. Th study of viruses and of virus disease.

**virucidal** (vi'ru-si'dal) [ virus + L. *caedo*, to kill ]. Destru tive to a virus.

**virucide** (vi'ru-sīd). An agent active against virus infe tions.

**virulence** (vĭr'u-lens) [ L. *virutentia*, fr. *virulentus*, poiso ous ]. The quality of being poisonous; the disease-evokin power of a microorganism in a given host.

**virulent** (vĭr'u-lent) [ L. *virulentus*, poisonous ]. Extreme poisonous; denoting a markedly pathogenic microorgar ism.

**viruliferous** (vi'ru-lif'er-us). Conveying virus.

**viruria** (vi-ru'rĭ-ah) [ virus + G. *ouron*, urine ]. The pre ence of living viruses in the urine.

# VIRUS

**vi'rus**, pl. **viruses** [ L. poison ]. 1. Formerly, contagium the specific agent of an infectious disease. 2. Filtrable v ultravirus; specifically, a term for a group of microbe which with few exceptions are capable of passing throug fine filters that retain bacteria; they are incapable of growt or reproduction apart from living cells. V. particles vary i size from 15 to 300 mμ or more; are spherical, polyhedral occasionally rod-shaped or tadpole-shaped in form; an are composed of a coat of protein units arranged aroun a central nucleic acid core which consists of either ribonucleic acid (RNA) or deoxyribonucleic acid (DNA) this difference serving as the basis for division of v.'s int two major groups. Subgroups are classified according t their origin, mode of transmission, and manifestation produced in the host. Many are named for the geographi locations where they were first isolated. See also virion. 3 Viral; relating to or caused by a v.; *e.g.*, virus disease.

    **2060 v.,** JH v.; a strain of "common cold" v., seemingly identical to ECHO 28 v. and intermediate to ECHO v.' and rhinoviruses, but usually grouped with the latter.

    **adeno-associated v.,** AAV; v. particles that are antigeni cally unrelated to adenovirus and that require the presenc of replicating adenovirus in order to replicate in detectable quantities.

    **adenoidal-pharyngeal-conjunctival v.'s.,** adenoviruses.

    **ad'enovi'ruses** [ G. *adēn*, gland + virus ], adenoi dal-pharyngeal-conjunctival v.'s; a group of v.'s in which the particles are intranuclear, icosahedral in shape, and measure 70 to 90 mμ in diameter. Subunits or capsomeres are arranged around a DNA core. In man, there are many inapparent infections, certain types particularly being latent in adenoids and tonsils. Other types are associated with minor respiratory infections of children, pharyngitis conjunctivities, and pneumonia. Adenoviruses of simian bovine, porcine, canine, avian and murine origin are recognized.

    **African horse sickness v.,** an RNA v. apparently related to the reoviruses; the cause of a disease of horses, mules and donkeys, originally known only in Africa, but now occurring in several countries of southwestern and southern Asia. Infections may be mild, chronic or acute, with death resulting from pulmonary edema in the most severe cases. Nocturnal biting insects appear to be the vectors.

    **African swine fever v.,** a v. 175 to 215 mμ in size; may be a DNA v.; the etiologic agent of African swine fever, also called wart-hog disease, in domestic pigs in Africa, causing high fever, cough, diarrhea and high mortality; natural infections probably occur in wart-hogs and bush-pigs.

    **Aleutian disease (of mink) v.,** an unclassified filtrable agent, resistant to 0.3 per cent formalin; the cause of a fatal isease, especially of mink homozygous for the Aleutian gene which determines color.

**Allerton v.,** a herpesvirus that causes bovine ulcerative mammillitis.

**animal v.'s,** v.'s occurring in man and other animals, causing inapparent infection or producing disease.

**A-P-C v.'s,** adenoviruses.

**Apeu v.,** a group C arbovirus found in Brazil.

**arborviruses,** arboviruses.

**ar'bovi'ruses** [ *ar*, arthropod, + *bo*, borne, + virus ], arborviruses; a large group of RNA v.'s from 20 to 100 mμ, or more, in diameter, and divisible into antigenic groups on the basis of hemagglutination-inhibition tests; most are associated with arthropods which may serve as vectors; some cause infection in man or other animals, with or without disease, the manifestations of which are commonly encephalitic.

**atten'uated v.,** a variant strain of a pathogenic v., so modified as to excite the production of protective antibodies, yet not producing the specific disease.

**Aujeszky's disease v.,** pseudorabies v.

**Aura v.,** a group A arbovirus recovered from mosquitos in Brazil.

**Australian X disease v.,** Murray Valley encephalitis v.

**avian encephalomyelitis v.,** a picornavirus epidemic tremor in young chicks, characterized by ataxia, tremors of the head and neck, somnolence and death.

**avian erythroblastosis v.,** avian leukosis-sarcoma v.

**avian infectious laryngotracheitis v.,** a small v., probably of the herpes virus group, causing hemorrhagic tracheitis, associated with coughing and gasping, in fowl and pheasants. Not to be confused with the v. of infectious bronchitis.

**avian leukosis-sarcoma v.,** an RNA tumor v. currently thought to cause all of the expressions of infection referred to as the avian leukosis-sarcoma complex; also known as avian or fowl erythroblastosis v.; avian or fowl lymphomatosis v.; avian or fowl myeloblastosis v.; avian or Rous sarcoma v.

**avian lymphomatosis v.,** avian leukosis-sarcoma v.

**avian myeloblastosis v.,** avian leukosis-sarcoma v.

**avian neurolymphomatosis v.,** fowl neurolymphomatosis v.; the cause of neurolymphomatosis in chickens, and less frequently in turkeys, pheasants, and quails, with symptoms of progressive paralysis, usually of a wing or leg; the disease is also called fowl paralysis, range paralysis, and the nervous form of lymphoid leukosis, but the v. is believed to be distinct from those causing other forms of leukosis.

**avian pneumoencephalitis v.,** Newcastle disease v.

**avian sarcoma v.,** avian leukosis-sarcoma v.

**B v.,** a v.; the cause of a herpes-like infection of Asiatic monkeys; very similar morphologically to herpes simplex v.

**bacterial v.,** a v. which "infects" bacteria; a bacteriophage or a filamentous bacterial v.

**Batai v.,** an arbovirus of the Bunyamwera group.

**Bimiti v.,** one of the Guama group of miscellaneous arboviruses.

**blue comb v.,** an unclassified v. that causes diarrhea, hepatic lesions, and monocytosis in young turkeys and in pullets.

**bluetongue v.,** the agent of bluetongue of sheep, also called ovine catarrhal fever, originally known only in Africa but now occurring in many other countries including the United States. It is most pathogenic in young sheep, causing fever, inflammation and ulceration of buccal and lingual mucous membranes, and sometimes edema of the ears, lips, face, neck and lungs and lameness due to foot involvement. Cattle, pigs and goats are susceptible, but symptoms are much milder. The v. has been recovered from species of *Culicoides*. The v., like that of African horse sickness, resembles the reoviruses morphologically.

**Borna disease v.,** an unclassified v. that is the cause of Borna disease.

**Bornholm disease v.,** epidemic pleurodynia v.

**bovine papular stomatitis v.,** a poxvirus reported from North America, Africa and Europe causing oral lesions somewhat similar to those of foot and mouth disease, being first papular and later ulcerative.

**bovine virus diarrhea v.,** mucosal disease v.; a v., probably an RNA v., or possibly several v.'s, causing diarrhea, fever and oral ulcerations, and sometimes pneumonia in cattle, particularly calves; New York, Oregon and Indiana strains are recognized.

**Bukalasa v.,** a group B arbovirus from bats, with no known arthropod vector.

**Bunyamwera v.,** the type strain of the Bunyamwera group and of the Bunyamwera supergroup of arboviruses.

**Bussuguara v.,** a group B arbovirus.

**Bwamba v.,** a v. associated with cases of fever in Uganda, and one of about 40 miscellaneous arboviruses.

**CA v.,** croup-associated v.; parainfluenza 2 v.

**Cache Valley v.,** a strain of Bunyamwera group of arbovirus.

**California v.,** type strain of the California group of arboviruses, included in the Bunyamwera supergroup.

**canarypox v.,** a poxvirus closely related to fowlpox v., causing a fatal disease of canaries, and also infecting sparrows.

**canine distemper v.,** an RNA v. 115 to 160 mμ in diameter, resembling the v.'s of measles and rinderpest and antigenically related to them; causes canine distemper, a highly contagious disease of dogs, and also infecting foxes, wolves, ferrets, mink, and raccoons.

**Caraparu v.,** a group C arbovirus.

**cat distemper v.,** feline panleukopenia v.

**cattle plague v.,** rinderpest v.

**Catu v.,** an arbovirus of the Guama group.

**CCA,** chimpanzee coryza *agent*.

**CELO v.,** chicken embryo lethal orphan v.; a v. with characteristics of adenovirus, and similar to quail bronchitis v.

**Central European tick-borne encephalitis v.,** one of the tick-borne encephalitis v., one of the tick-borne encephalitis complex of group B arboviruses; the causative agent of central European tick-born encephalitis.

**Chenuda v.,** an arbovirus of the Kemerovo group.

**chicken embryo lethal orphan v.,** CELO v.

**chickenpox v.,** *Herpesvirus varicellae.*

**Chikungunya v.,** a group A, mosquito-transmitted arbovirus found in Tanganyika, Uganda, Congo, South Africa and Thailand causing an epidemic dengue-like disease of man. The name has to do with the "bent up" position of the subject.

**Clavelée v.,** sheep pox v.

**cocal v.,** a v. morphologically similar to vesicular stomatitis v., and related serologically to the Indiana strain; has been isolated from jungle rodents, mosquitos, and mites in Trinidad.

**Coe v.,** serologically identical with the A-21 strain of Coxsackie v.; cause of common-cold-like disease in recruits.

**coital exanthema of cattle v.,** infectious bovine rhinotracheitis v.

**cold v.,** common cold v.

**Colorado tick fever v.,** an arbovirus of the Rocky Mountain region of the United States causing a febrile disease of man which is transmitted by the tick, *Dermacentor andersoni.* The v. is antigenically unrelated to other v.'s.

**Columbia S. K. v.,** a strain of encephalomyocarditis v.

**common cold v.,** cold v.; any of the numerous strains of v. etiologically associated with the common cold; chiefly the rhinoviruses, but also strains of adenovirus, Coxsackie v., ECHO v., and parainfluenza v.

**contagious ecthyma (pustular dermatitis) v. of sheep,** orf v.; sore mouth v.; the poxvirus causing contagious ecthyma (pustular dermatitis) of sheep.

**contagious pustular dermatitis v.,** horsepox v.

**coro'navirus,** a type of common cold v., the surface of which appears in electron micrographs as a segmented ring, suggestive of a corona.

**coryzavirus,** rhinovirus.

**cowpox v.,** vaccinia (vaccine) v.

**Coxsack'ie v.'s,** a group of picornaviruses, spherical and about 28 mμ in diameter, first isolated at Coxsackie, N. Y., which cause myositis, paralysis, and death in young mice and are believed to be responsible for a variety of symptoms in man, but inapparent infections are common. They are divided antigenically into two groups (A and B), each of which includes a number of serological types.

**croup-associated v.,** CA v.; parainfluenza 2 v.

**cytomegalic inclusion disease v.,** a cytomegalovirus of man causing inapparent infection particularly of salivary glands, severe often fatal neonatal infections, or more chronic disease in older persons. Long-persisting inapparent infection is common.

**cytomegaloviruses,** visceral disease v.'s; a group of herpesviruses infecting man and other animals, many of them having special affinity for salivary glands and causing enlargement of cells of various organs and development of characteristic inclusions in the cytoplasm or nucleus. They are all species-specific and include cytomegalic inclusion disease v. of man, salivary gland v. of guinea pigs, salivary gland v. of mice, inclusion body rhinitis v. of pigs, and others.

**cytopathogenic v.,** a v. whose multiplication leads to degenerative changes in the host cell; see also cytopathic *effect.*

**Dakar bat v.,** a group B arbovirus, with no known arthropod vector.

**deer hemorrhagic fever v.,** a group-unassigned member of the Bunyamwera supergroup; the cause of fatal epizootics in Virginian white-tailed deer in middle and eastern United States, producing shock, multiple hemorrhages and coma preceding death.

**defective v.,** a v. particle that contains insufficient nucleic acid to provide for production of all essential viral components; consequently, infectious v. is not produced except under certain conditions (*e.g.,* when the host cell is infected with a "helper" v. also).

**dengue v.,** a group B arbovirus, about 20 m$\mu$ in diameter; the etiologic agent of dengue in man and also occurring in monkeys and chimpanzees, usually as inapparent infection. Four serotypes are recognized. Transmission is effected by mosquitoes of the genus *Aedes.*

**distemper v.,** see canine distemper v.; feline panleukopenia v.

**DNA v.'s,** deoxyviruses; v.'s; in which the core consists of deoxyribonucleic acid (DNA). A major group of animal v.'s which includes adenoviruses, papovaviruses, herpesviruses, poxviruses, and other unclassified DNA v.'s.

**dog distemper v.,** canine distemper v.

**duck hepatitis v.,** a picornavirus causing severe disease in young ducklings, involving especially the liver.

**duck influenza v.,** an influenza A v. distinct from human influenza A strains on bases of hemagglutination-inhibition.

**eastern equine encephalomyelitis v.,** EEE v.; a group A arbovirus occurring in eastern United States; normally present in certain wild birds as an inapparent infection, but capable of causing eastern equine encephalomyelitis in horses and man following transfer by the bites of culicine mosquitoes.

**EB v.,** Epstein-Barr v.; a herpes-like v. found by M. A. Epstein and Y. M. Barr in cell cultures of Burkitt lymphoma; also, antibodies reactive with EB v. have been reported in cases of infectious mononucleosis.

**ECBO v.,** enteric cytopathogenic bovine v.; a bovine picornavirus of the enterovirus group isolated from cattle; although capable of causing bloody diarrhea in colostrum-deprived calves, it is not known to be a natural pathogen for cattle.

**ECHO v.,** enteric cytopathogenic human orphan v.; an enterovirus, belonging to the picornavirus group, isolated from man; while there are many inapparent infections, certain of the several serotypes are associated with fever and aseptic meningitis, and some appear to cause mild respiratory disease.

**ECHO 28 v.,** see 2060 v.

**ECMO v.,** enteric cytopathogenic monkey orphan v.; simian picornavirus recovered from monkey kidney cells and stools.

**ECSO v.,** enteric cytopathogenic swine orphan v.; a picornavirus isolated from outbreaks of enteritis in swine, but not known to be a natural pathogen.

**ectromelia v.,** infectious ectromelia v.

**Edgehill v., Edge Hill v.,** a group B arbovirus isolated from mosquitos in Queensland.

**EEE v.,** eastern equine encephalomyelitis v.

**Egtved v.,** an RNA v., the cause of hemorrhagic septicemia in salmonids, especially rainbow trout.

**EMC v.,** encephalomyocarditis v.

**enceph'ali'tis v.,** any one of a variety of v.'s that cau encephalitis.

**enceph'alomyocardi'tis v.,** EMC v.; a picornavir probably of rodents; also isolated from blood and stools humans, other primates, pigs, and rabbits; occasiona causes febrile illness with central nervous system invol ment in man, and an often fatal myocarditis in chimpa zees, monkeys and pigs.

**enteric v.'s,** enteroviruses.

**enteric cytopathogenic bovine orphan v.,** ECBO v.

**enteric cytopathogenic human orphan v.,** ECHO v.

**enteric cytopathogenic monkey orphan v.,** ECMO v.

**enteric orphan v.'s,** enteroviruses isolated from man a other animals, the term orphan implying lack of kno association with disease when isolated. Many viruses of t group, however, are now known to be pathogenic. Th include ECBO v.'s of cattle, ECHO v.'s of man, ECSO v of swine, and enteric orphan v.'s of other animals.

**en'terovi'ruses,** v.'s infecting or propagating themselv in the alimentary canal and spread by fecal contaminatio *e.g.,* poliovirus or ECHO v.

**epidemic keratoconjunctivitis v.,** an adenovirus causi epidemic keratoconjunctivitis, especially among shipya workers, and also associated with outbreaks of swimmi pool conjunctivitis.

**epidemic myalgia v.,** epidemic pleurodynia v.

**epidemic parotitis v.,** mumps v.

**epidemic pleurodynia v.,** epidemic myalgia v.; Bornhol disease v.; Coxsackie B v., various types.

**Epstein-Barr v.,** EB v.

**equine abortion v.,** equine rhinopneumonitis v.

**equine arteritis v.,** infectious arteritis v. of horses; a unclassified RNA v. causing so-called equine influenz and probably the commonest cause, with symptoms fever, rhinitis, conjunctivitis, edema, gastrointestinal di turbances, and sometimes pneumonia; it is highly cont gious, affecting chiefly young animals, but is also frequent cause of abortion in mares. The essential lesior involve smaller arteries, with necrosis which may t followed by thrombosis, infarction, hemorrhages an edema.

**equine infectious anemia v.,** swamp fever v.; an unclass fied ether-sensitive v., the cause of a worldwide infectiou disease of horses and other Equidae (also called swam fever because of its prevalence in low-lying marshy areas infection is either acute or chronic, often with acute attack and remissions over months and even years, affecte animals developing fever, anemia, emaciation and areas subcutaneous edema. Horseflies and stable flies are be lieved to be mechanical vectors, but the v. can also b transmitted by contact, oral infection, or by the use unsterilized syringes and needles.

**equine influenza v.,** (1) influenza A v. of two serotype (A/Equi/1 and A/Equi/2) associated with one kind horse influenza; (2) equine rhinopneumonitis v.; (3) equin infectious arteritis v.

**equine rhinopneumonitis v.,** equine abortion v.; equin influenza v. (2); a herpesvirus reported in the United States Europe and South Africa causing mild upper respirator disease in horses, with fever, serous rhinitis and leukope nia, and also capable of causing abortion in mares Transmission is probably by the respiratory route.

**FA v.,** a strain of mouse encephalomyelitis v.

**feline infectious agranulocytosis v.,** feline panleukopeni v.

**feline panleukopenia v.,** feline infectious agranulocytosi v.; cat distemper v.; an unclassified DNA v., the cause o feline infectious agranulocytosis (also called feline infec tious enteritis, feline distemper, feline agranulocytosis, ca plague and cat fever). The v. infects all Felidae, raccoon and mink, but not dogs or other Canidae.

**fibromatosis v. of rabbits,** rabbit fibroma v.

**fibrous bacterial v.'s,** filamentous bacterial v.'s.

**filamentous bacterial v.'s,** fibrous bacterial v.'s; deox yribonucleoproteins that "infect" and replicate in Gram negative bacteria having sex pili and that, unlike bacterio phage, are released from infected bacteria without damag to the cell; they seem to be of two kinds, one of which ha a specificity for F pili and the other for I pili.

**fil'trable v.,** virus (2).

**...xed v.,** v. of rabies of the utmost possible virulence for ...bbits, obtained by numerous passages through this ...perimental host; see also street v.

**...landers v.,** a v. resembling the cocal v.

**...lury strain rabies v.,** see rabies v., Flury strain.

**...MD v.,** foot and mouth disease v.

**...oamy v.,** foamy *agent.*

**...oot and mouth disease v.,** FMD v.; a picornavirus ...using foot and mouth disease of cattle, swine, sheep, ...ats, and wild ruminants. It has wide distribution ...roughout Africa and Asia, causing serious economic ...sses. The v. is spread by contamination of the animal ...vironment with infected saliva and excreta.

**...owl erythroblastosis v.,** avian leukosis-sarcoma v.

**...owl lymphomatosis v.,** avian leukosis-sarcoma v.

**...owl myeloblastosis v.,** avian leukosis-sarcoma v.

**...owl neurolymphomatosis v.,** avian neurolymphomatosis

**...owlpox v.,** a poxvirus infecting chickens, turkeys, ...heasants and many other domestic and wild birds, ...ausing proliferative dermal lesions followed by scabbing ...hiefly on the head, but sometimes involving the feet and ...ent. The v. may also cause various eye lesions, lead to the ...rmation of caseous material in the infraorbital sinuses, or ...ffect the trachea causing so-called fowl diphtheria. Trans-...ission occurs by contact or mechanical transfer by ...iosquitoes.

**fox encephalitis v.,** infectious canine hepatitis v.

**Friend v., Friend leukemia v.,** Swiss mouse leukemia v.; ...strain of the splenic group of mouse leukemia v.'s, related ...o Moloney and Rauscher v.'s.

**Fujinami v.,** a strain of avian leukosis-sarcoma v. that is ...eadily infectious for ducks.

**GAL v.,** gallus adeno-like v.; a v. with characteristics of ...denovirus, not known to be associated with natural ...isease.

**gallus adeno-like v.,** GAL v.

**German measles v.,** rubella v.

**Germiston v.,** one of the Bunyamwera group of arbovi-...'uses.

**Getah v.,** Sagiyama v.; a group A arbovirus.

**goatpox v.,** the cause of pox in goats, chiefly in North ...Africa and the Middle East, producing generalized pocks ...n the skin and mucous membranes.

**Graffi's v.,** a mouse myeloleukemia v. from filtrates of ...transplantable tumors; possibly related to Gross' v.

**Gross' v., Gross' leukemia v.,** a strain of mouse leukemia ...v.

**Guama v.,** type strain of a subgroup of Bunyamwera ...supergroup of arboviruses.

**Guaroa v.** one of the Bunyamwera group of arboviruses.

**HA1 v.,** see parainfluenza 3 v.

**HA2 v.,** see parainfluenza 1 v.

**hand, foot, and mouth disease v.,** type A-16 or type A-5 ...Coxsackie v.

**hardpad v.,** probably canine distemper v., but v. ...sometimes is not recovered.

**Hart Park v.,** a v. resembling the cocal v.

**helper v.,** a v. whose replication renders it possible for a ...defective v. (also present in the host cell) to develop into ...fully infectious v.

**hemadsorption v. 1,** HA1 v.; see parainfluenza 3 virus.

**hemadsorption v. 2,** HA2 v.; see parainfluenza 1 virus.

**hepatitis v. A,** infectious hepatitis v.; the causative agent ...of viral hepatitis type A.

**hepatitis v. B,** serum hepatitis v.; the causative agent of ...viral hepatitis type B.

**herpes simplex v.,** *Herpesvirus hominis.*

**herpesvirus** (her'pēz-vi'rus), one of a group of v.'s causing ...herpes and also including several related v.'s. The v. ...particles have a DNA core, are icosahedral in form, range ...in size from 180 to 250 m$\mu$, and produce type A ...intranuclear inclusions. Many of them produce lesions ...which are first proliferative, later necrotic. The group ...includes the v.'s causing herpes in man and other primates; ...pseudorabies; varicella-zoster; infectious bovine rhinotra-...cheitis; and equine rhinopneumonitis. Other v.'s less ...certainly related to herpes but tentatively included in the ...group are those causing avian infectious laryngotracheitis, ...bovine malignant catarrh, and several cytomegaloviruses ...or salivary gland v.'s.

**Herpesvirus cunic'uli,** v. III of rabbits.

**Herpesvirus hominis,** herpes simplex v.; the pathogen of herpes simplex in man, causing acute stomatitis, especially in children, and so-called fever blisters, usually on the lips and external nares.

**Herpesvirus suis,** the causative agent of Aujeszky's disease; somewhat resembles *Herpesvirus hominis.*

**Herpesvirus varicel'lae,** varicella-zoster v.; chickenpox v.; herpes zoster v.; a herpesvirus causing varicella and herpes zoster in man. Varicella (chickenpox) is produced as a result of primary infection with the v.; herpes zoster, by secondary invasion by the same v. or by reactivation of latent infection.

**herpes zoster v.,** *Herpesvirus varicellae.*

**hog cholera v.,** swine fever v.; an unclassified RNA virus that may belong to the myxoviruses; the cause of hog cholera, a highly contagious and fatal disease of pigs of worldwide distribution; affected pigs show high fever, depression, diarrhea, cutaneous hemorrhages, and fre-quently encephalomyelitic symptoms. Pigs may die of the virus infection alone, or from complications of secondary bacterial infections. Transmission is by direct contact or ingestion of contaminated food, particularly garbage.

**horsepox v.,** contagious pustular dermatitis v.; the poxvirus causing contagious pustular dermatitis in the horse, in which papular, then vesicular, lesions form on the lips and buccal mucosa; the disease is now relatively rare.

**Hughes v.,** an unclassified arbovirus apparently carried by *Ornithodorus* ticks and associated with sea birds.

**IBR v.,** (1) infectious bovine rhinotracheitis v.; (2) inclusion body rhinitis v. of pigs.

**Icoaraci v.,** a *Phlebotomus*-borne arbovirus isolated from rodents in Brazil.

**Ilesha v.,** a Bunyamwera group arbovirus.

**Ilhéus v.,** a group B arbovirus first isolated in Brazil, later found in Colombia, Central America and the Caribbean, and the cause of occasional cases of encephalitis in man; related to St. Louis and Japanese B encephalitis v.'s, and to West Nile v.

**inclusion body rhinitis v. of pigs,** IBR v. (2); a v. morphologically resembling herpesvirus; infectious for young pigs.

**inclusion conjunctivitis v.'s,** see *Chlamydia trachomatis.*

**infectious arteritis v. of horses,** equine arteritis v.

**infectious bovine rhinotracheitis v.,** IBR v. (1); coital exanthema of cattle v.; a herpesvirus causing infectious bovine rhinotracheitis, also called necrotic rhinitis and red nose, the chief pathological lesions being acute inflamma-tion and necrosis of mucous membranes. The v. may also cause infectious pustular vulvovaginitis in older cattle and conjunctivitis in calves. Transmission is by contact.

**infectious bronchitis v.,** an unclassified RNA v., distinct from infectious laryngotracheitis v., causing infectious bronchitis or so-called gasping disease of chickens, being most pathogenic in chicks up to about 4 weeks of age; in laying hens there is severe drop in egg production. The infection causes profuse exudation and blocking in respira-tory passages, resulting in gasping and high mortality.

**infectious canine hepatitis v.,** fox encephalitis v.; Ru-barth's disease v.; an adenovirus causing infectious canine hepatitis (also known as Rubarth's disease) and fox encephalitis. The infection in dogs may be inapparent, but may cause symptoms of fever, vomiting, diarrhea, edema and frequently transient corneal opacities in weaned puppies; in foxes, the v. causes encephalitis, paralysis and death; coyotes, wolves and raccoons are also susceptible. The v. is spread via the respiratory tract or urine.

**infectious ectromelia v.,** mousepox v.; pseudo-lympho-cytic choriomeningitis v.; a poxvirus morphologically similar to vaccinia v. which occurs as a latent infection in laboratory mice, but which may be activated by stresses such as irradiation and transport to cause disease with various manifestations including conjunctivitis, hepatitis, meningitis or pneumonia. Inoculation into footpad results in edema and necrosis.

**infectious hepatitis v.,** hepatitis v. A.

**infectious porcine encephalomyelitis v.,** Teschen disease v.

**infectious warts v.,** verruca vulgaris v.; an icosahedral DNA v. (papovavirus), 45 m$\mu$ in diameter, causing certain kinds of warts in man; infection in the case of the deep type of wart with domed surface (myrmecia type) is associated with eosinophilic intranuclear and intracytoplasmic inclusion bodies which are lacking in the superficial, vegetating type (verruca vulgaris).

**influenza v.'s,** the myxoviruses causing influenza and influenza-like infections of man and other animals and transmitted chiefly by infected respiratory secretions; types A, B and C are recognized. **Influenza type A v.'s,** are the most important pathogens among the influenza v.'s, infecting man and many domestic animals and birds. Influenza A v. of man causes influenza and sometimes pneumonia and also naturally infects ferrets and pigs. Swine influenza v. causes influenza and pneumonia in domestic pigs, especially when associated with *Haemophilus influenzae suis.* Equine influenza v. is one of several v.'s, causing equine influenza, occurring especially in Central Europe, but recently identified in the United States. Fowl plague v. infects gallinaceous birds, passerine birds, pigeons, ducks and geese, causing dyspnea, edema of the head and neck, cyanosis, diarrhea, and sometimes disturbances of the central nervous system; it is most prevalent in North Africa, but occurs sporadically in Europe and certain other areas. Duck influenza v. has been described only in Czechoslavakia and Britain as a cause of sinusitis. **Influenza type B v.** causes influenza and sometimes pneumonia in man, the disease being more endemic than that caused by influenza A v. **Influenza type C v.** is thought to cause sporadic, mild influenza-like infections in man. The three types resemble each other in size and structure but are antigenically distinct, each type possessing a characterizing common nucleoprotein group ("soluble") antigen and a mosaic of surface antigens that varies from strain to strain.

**insect v.'s,** v.'s pathogenic for insects.

**Itaporanga v.,** a *Phlebotomus*-borne arbovirus isolated from rodents in Brazil.

**Itaqui v.,** a strain of group C arbovirus from Brazil.

**Japanese B encephalitis v.,** Russian autumn encephalitis v.; a group B arbovirus occurring particularly in Japan but probably widespread throughout southeast Asia. The v. is normally present in man, especially children, as inapparent infection, but may cause febrile response and sometimes encephalitis. It may cause encephalitis in horses and abortion in pigs. Wild birds are probably the natural hosts and culicine mosquitoes the vectors.

**JH v.,** 2060 v.

**Junin v.,** a Tacaribe group arbovirus; the cause of Argentinian hemorrhagic fever; also isolated from mites and rodents.

**K v.,** a DNA v. (papovavirus), spherical, approximately 50 mμ in diameter; causes pneumonia in young mice by various routes of inoculation.

**Kairi v.,** a Bunyamwera group arbovirus.

**Kelev strain rabies v.,** see rabies v., Kelev strain.

**Kisenyi sheep disease v.,** probably the same as Nairobi sheep disease v.

**Kokobera v.,** a group B arbovirus isolated from mosquitos in Queensland.

**Kyasanur Forest disease v.,** a group B arbovirus isolated from monkeys in India and capable of causing a severe febrile, nonencephalitic disease in man; the v. is spread by monkeys and birds having mild infections; the vectors are probably species of the tick *Haemaphysalis.*

**lactate dehydrogenase v.,** Riley v.; LDH agent; an RNA v. present, perhaps as a "passenger," in various transplantable mouse tumors.

**Lagos bat v.,** isolated from a pool of forest bats; possibly an arbovirus.

**Langat v.,** a group B arbovirus from ticks (*Ixodes granulatus*) in Malaya.

**Lassa v.,** an unclassified RNA v. that can cause severe or fatal infection in man, associated with prolonged viremia.

**latent rat v.,** an unclassified, small DNA v. causing inapparent infection in rats; also recoverable from rat tumors.

**LCM v.,** lymphocytic choriomeningitis v.

**louping-ill v.,** a group B arbovirus causing an encephalomyelitis called louping ill of sheep in the British Isles, transmitted by the tick *Ixodes ricinus.* Infection occurs

occasionally in cattle and in laboratory workers and pe in contact with sheep.

**Lucké's v.,** originally thought to cause adenocarcino of frogs' kidneys, but may be only a "passenger' probably a DNA virus of the herpesvirus group.

**Lukuni v.,** Anopheles A v., an unassigned arboviru

**Lumbo v.,** a California group arbovirus.

**lumpy skin disease v.'s,** several poxviruses isolated f cattle with lumpy skin disease in South and East Af causing fever and the formation of multiple nodules on skin; the Neethling v. has been most studied, an serologically closely related to the v. of African sheep

**Lunyo v.,** an atypical strain of Rift Valley fever v.

**lymphocytic choriomeningitis v.,** LCM v.; presemably RNA v. which probably occurs normally as inappa infection in house mice, but which also infects m monkeys, dogs and guinea pigs. It may cause an often f pneumonia in guinea pigs; in man, infection may inapparent, but sometimes causes influenza-like dise meningitis or rarely meningoencephalomyelitis. The les responsible for the name of the v. is lymphocytic infil tion around blood vessels and choroid plexuses.

**lymphogranuloma venereum v.,** see *Chlamydia tra matis.*

**Machupo v.,** a Tacaribe group arbovirus; the cause Bolivian hemorrhagic fever.

**Madrid v.,** a group C arbovirus.

**maedi v.,** medi v.; the cause of maedi, a disease of she it is very similar to the Visna v.

**Makonde v.,** Uganda S v.

**malignant catarrhal fever v.,** a herpesvirus of w distribution causing malignant catarrhal fever of cattle highly fatal, sporadic disease characterized by inflamm tion, ulceration and exudation of oral and upper respi tory mucous membranes, and sometimes eye lesions a nervous system disturbances; sheep and wildebeests h bor inapparent infections, and may transmit the v. cattle.

**mammary cancer v. of mice,** mammary tumor v.; mo mammary tumor v.; milk factor; Bittner agent; an RNA associated with adenocarcinomatous tumors of the ma mary gland, commonly latent in wild and laboratory m and causing cancer only in genetically susceptible strai under certain hormonal influences.

**mammary tumor v.,** mammary cancer v. of mice.

**Marcy v.,** a filtrable agent from stools in cases epidemic diarrhea; caused diarrhea without fever when to volunteers.

**Marituba v.,** a group C arbovirus.

**marmoset v.,** a herpes-like v. obtained repeatedly fro throat swabs and tissues of marmosets.

**masked v.,** a v. ordinarily occurring in the host in noninfective state, but which may be activated a demonstrated by special procedures such as blind passa in experimental animals.

**Mayaro v.,** a group A arbovirus causing an epidemic headache and fever among quarry and forest workers Brazil.

**measles v.,** rubeola v.; probably an RNA v. separate fro the myxovirus group; it causes measles, a widesprea disease, in man. The v. is transmitted via the respirato tract. It is related in several respects to canine distemp v., rinderpest v., and the parainfluenza v.'s.

**medi v.,** maedi v.

**Melao v.,** a California group arbovirus, isolated Trinidad.

**Mengo v.,** a strain of encephalomyocarditis v.

**Middelburg v.,** a group A arbovirus isolated fro mosquitos (*Aedes*) in South Africa; its relationship disease is uncertain.

**milker's nodes v.,** a poxvirus, antigenically distinct fro cowpox v. and vaccinia v.; the cause of lesions in cows an man similar to those of vaccinia; closely related to orf and papular stomatitis v.

**MM v.,** a strain of encephalomyocarditis v.

**Modoc v.,** a group B arbovirus with no known arthropo vector, isolated from a mouse in California.

**molluscum contagiosum v.,** the poxvirus causing mollus cum contagiosum of man, characterized by the formatio of pimples which become nodules containing white core transmission is by means of direct contact and fomites.

**Moloney's v.,** a lymphoid leukemia v. of mice, isolated originally during propagation of S 37 mouse sarcoma.

**monkey B v.,** B v.

**monkeypox v.,** a poxvirus causing an epidemic disease in captive monkeys, characterized by a generalized rash resembling that of variola; related to vaccinia v. but distinct from the Yaba v.

**mouse encephalomyelitis v.,** mouse poliomyelitis v., Theiler's v., T.O. (Theiler's Original); a picornavirus, normally associated with inapparent infections and found in the intestinal tracts of the infected mice, but causing a poliomyelitis-like disease in experimentally inoculated, susceptible mice.

**mouse hepatitis v.,** probably an RNA v., 80 to 120 m$\mu$, that in the presence of *Eperythrozoon coccoides* causes fatal hepatitis in newly weaned mice; otherwise causes inapparent infection.

**mouse leukemia v.'s,** several RNA rodent v.'s that produce leukemia and sometimes lymphosarcomas in mice, and include the Gross, Moloney, Friend, and Rauscher strains. They have been isolated from inbred mice having high incidence of spontaneous lymphoid leukemia. Friend's and Moloney's strains were isolated during propagation of tumors in mice and will induce lymphoid leukemia in certain strains of mice. Several other v.'s capable of causing mouse leukemia are recognized.

**mouse mammary tumor v.,** mammary cancer v. of mice.

**mouse parotid tumor v.,** polyoma v.

**mouse poliomyelitis v.,** mouse encephalomyelitis v.

**mousepox v.,** infectious ectromelia v.

**mouse thymic v.,** an unclassified ether-sensitive v., 75 to 100 m$\mu$ in diameter; causes necrosis of thymus in young mice.

**M-P v.,** an unclassified v. isolated from an Ehrlich mouse sarcoma; caused hepatitis and lymphocytopenia. Not to be confused with meningopneumonitis.

**mucosal disease v.,** bovine virus diarrhea v.

**mumps v.,** epidemic parotitis v.; a paramyxovirus causing parotitis in man, sometimes with complications of orchitis, oophoritis, pancreatitis, meningoencephalitis and others, and transmitted by infected salivary secretions.

**murine sarcoma v.,** a seemingly defective v. that produces sarcomas in mice when growing in the presence of a "helper" v.; *e.g.,* mouse leukemia v.

**Murray Valley encephalitis v.,** MVE v.; a group B arbovirus endemic in Australia and New Guinea that causes Australian X disease, an encephalitis of man resembling Japanese B encephalitis; transmitted by *Culex* mosquitos. The v. also infects birds and horses.

**Murutucu v.,** a group C arbovirus.

**MVE v.,** Murray Valley encephalitis v.

**myxomatosis v.,** rabbit myxoma v.

**myx'ovi'ruses** [ G. *myxa*, mucus, + virus ], a group of v.'s characterized by having special affinity for certain mucins and their ability to cause influenza or influenza-like infections in man, other primates, and domestic mammals and poultry. The v. particles in infected cells range in size from 80 to about 120 m$\mu$, with a nucleocapsid about 9 m$\mu$ in diameter, and are RNA-positive. They do not produce eosinophilic cytoplasmic inclusions. Transmission is by means of respiratory secretions of infected hosts. There are many inapparent infections. See also paramyxoviruses.

**Nairobi sheep disease v.,** An ungrouped arbovirus causing hemorrhagic gastroenteritis with high fever in sheep and goats in Kenya, Uganda and probably Congo and southeastern Africa; transmitted by the tick, *Rhipicephalus appendiculatus.*

**ND v.,** Newcastle disease v.

**Neethling v.,** see lumpy skin disease v.'s.

**Negishi v.,** one of the group B arboviruses of the tick-borne encephalitis complex, isolated from fatal infections in Japan.

**Nepuyo v.,** a group C arbovirus isolated in Trinidad.

**neurotrop'ic v.,** a v. that has an affinity for nervous tissue, *e.g.,* poliomyelitis v., neurotropic v. variant of yellow fever, and the "fixed" v. of rabies.

**Newcastle disease v.,** ND v.; avian pneumoencephalitis v.; a paramyxovirus causing disease in chickens, and to a lesser extent in turkeys and other birds, with either respiratory or nervous symptoms or both; it may occasionally infect laboratory and poultry workers, causing conjunctivitis and lymphadenitis.

**Ntaya v.,** a group B arbovirus from Uganda.

**Omsk hemorrhagic fever v.,** a group B arbovirus causing a diphasic disease of low mortality in man in central U.S.S.R., with fever, enlargement of lymph nodes, gastrointestinal disturbances, hemorrhages from the nose, stomach or uterus, and little or no central nervous disturbance; the vectors are species of *Dermacentor,* which may transmit the v. transovarially.

**oncornaviruses,** RNA tumor v.'s.

**O'nyong-nyong v.,** group A arbovirus found in Uganda, Kenya and Congo which causes a febrile, dengue-like disease of man. A severe epidemic affected thousands of people in Uganda in 1959. The vector appears to be *Anopheles.*

**orf v.,** contagious ecthyma v. of sheep.

**organized v.,** an old term for a pathogenic microorganism.

**Oriboca v.,** a group C arbovirus.

**ornithosis v.,** see *Chlamydia psittaci.*

**Oropouche v.,** a Simbu group arbovirus; cause of epidemic of fever in Trinidad and Brazil.

**orphan v.'s,** v.'s such as the enteric orphan v.'s which when originally found were not specifically associated with disease; a number of these, however, have since been shown to be pathogenic.

**Ossa v.,** a group C arbovirus isolated in Panama.

**Pacheco's parrot disease v.,** parrot v. (2); probably a herpesvirus, possibly related to the v. of infectious laryngotracheitis.

**panleukopenia v. of cats,** feline panleukopenia v.

**pantrop'ic v.,** the v. of yellow fever; the ordinary strain of yellow fever v., as distinguished from neurotropic strain.

**papilloma v.'s,** DNA v.'s (papovaviruses) causing infectious papillomatosis or warts; they include papilloma v. of man, rabbit papilloma v. (Shope papilloma v.), bovine papilloma v., and papilloma v.'s of pigs, dogs, horses, goats, chamois, and other animals.

**papo'vavi'ruses** [ *pa,* from *papilloma,* + *po,* from polyoma, + *va,* from vacuolating agent, + virus ], a group of v.'s related to rabbit papilloma and polyoma. They are mostly oncogenic v.'s. Particles are mainly intranuclear, measure 30 to 50 m$\mu$, and have basically icosahedral shape although some forms are filamentous. The group may prove not to be homogeneous.

**pappataci fever v.'s,** phlebotomus fever v.'s.

**papular stomatitis v. of cattle,** bovine papular stomatitis v.

**parainfluenza v.'s,** v.'s having myxovirus features but being larger and differing in other respects from typical influenza v.'s A and B. **Parainfluenza 1 v.** includes a Sendai strain known to cause pneumonia in pigs, and a hemadsorption v. 2 (HA2) which causes acute laryngotracheitis in children and occasionally adults; some strains may be latent in laboratory mice. **Parainfluenza 2 v.** is associated especially with acute laryngotracheitis or croup in young children and minor upper respiratory infections in adults. **Parainfluenza 3 v.** has been isolated from small children with pharyngitis, bronchiolitis and pneumonia, and causes occasional respiratory infection in adults; bovine strains have been isolated from cattle with shipping fever; originally described as hemadsorption v. 1 (HA1). **Parainfluenza 4 v.** has been isolated from a very few children with minor respiratory illness.

**paramyxoviruses,** RNA v.'s in some respects resembling myxoviruses, but they are about twice the diameter (150 to 220 m$\mu$) and have a nucleocapsid about 18 m$\mu$ in diameter; also, they produce eosinophilic cytoplasmic inclusions. Include the v.'s of mumps, the parainfluenza v.'s 1, 2, 3, and 4, the simian paramyxoviruses, and Newcastle disease v.

**paravaccinia v.,** pseudocowpox v.; the cause of a cowpox-like disease of the udders of cows capable of spreading to the hands of the milkers and producing pock lesions; the disease is called milkers' nodes in man. There is no cross-immunity with vaccinia v.

**parrot v.,** (1) an obsolete term for *Chlamydia psittaci;* (2) Pacheco's parrot disease v.

**Patois v.,** a group C arbovirus isolated in Panama.

**Peromyscus v.,** a hemadsorbing v., possibly a myxovirus from white-footed mice.

**pharyngoconjunctival fever v.,** one of several types of adenoviruses associated with outbreaks of fever and pharyngitis, sometimes with conjunctivitis, especially in service recruits and people in boarding schools.

**phlebotomus fever v.'s** pappataci fever v.'s; sandfly fever v.'s; a group of arboviruses transmitted by *Phlebotomus papataci* (sandfly) and causing fever, with pains in eyes and limbs. Naples and Sicilian serotypes are recognized.

**picor'navi'ruses** [ It. *piccolo,* very small, + RNA + virus ], a group of very small ether-resistant v.'s having RNA nucleic acid composition. The v. particles are arranged in closely packed spheres measuring 22 to 27 m$\mu$ in diameter in the cytoplasm of infected cells. The following v.'s are included in the group: poliomyelitis, Coxsackie and ECHO v.'s, rhinoviruses causing common colds, and v.'s causing foot and mouth disease, encephalomyocarditis, Teschen disease and vesicular exanthema of pigs, avian encephalomyelitis, mouse encephalomyelitis, and others.

**Pixuna v.,** a group A arbovirus isolated from mosquito and rodents.

**plant v.'s,** v.'s pathogenic to higher plants.

**pleurodynia v., epidemic,** epidemic pleurodynia v.

**pneumoencephalitis v. (avian),** Newcastle disease v.

**pneumonia v. of mice,** PVM v.; presumably an RNA v. occurring normally as latent infection in laboratory mice, but capable of activation by serial intranasal passage and causing pneumonia.

**poliomyelitis v.,** poliovirus hominis; the picornavirus causing poliomyelitis in man. The route of infection is the alimentary tract, but the v. may enter the blood stream and nervous system, sometimes causing paralysis of the limbs and rarely encephalitis. Many infections are inapparent. Serologic types 1,2 and 3 are recognized, type 1 being responsible for most paralytic poliomyelitis and most epidemics.

**poliovirus hominis,** poliomyelitis v.

**polyoma v.,** mouse parotid tumor v.; a papovavirus which normally occurs in inapparent infections in laboratory and wild mice, but after growth on tissue culture capable of producing parotid tumors in mice and sarcomas in hamsters as well as tumors in other laboratory animals.

**Pongola v.,** a Bwamba group arbovirus isolated in South Africa.

**porcine encephalomyelitis v., infectious,** Teschen disease v.

**Powassan v.,** a group B arbovirus, isolated from a fatal encephalitis in Ontario, and from *Ixodes* ticks.

**poxviruses,** a group of v.'s that characteristically propagate in epidermis, causing proliferative lesions which later become necrotic. They are rather large v.'s of rounded quadrangular form measuring approximately 200 to 300 m$\mu$, and have a DNA core. V. multiplication occurs within the cytoplasm of infected cells. Diseases caused by v.'s of this group include vaccinia, variola (smallpox), rabbitpox, monkeypox, cowpox, pseudocowpox (milkers' nodes), infectious ectromelia (mousepox), contagious pustular dermatitis of sheep (orf, sore mouth) goatpox, sheeppox, lumpy skin disease of cattle, horsepox, swinepox, camelpox, molluscum contagiosum of man, fowlpox, turkeypox, pigeonpox, canarypox, and myxomatosis and fibromatosis of rabbits.

**poxvirus officinalis,** vaccinia v.

**poxvirus variolae,** name suggested (International Congress of Microbiology) for the v. of smallpox.

**provirus,** precursor of an animal v.; analogous to the prophage in bacteria.

**pseudocowpox v.,** paravaccinia v.

**pseudo-lymphocytic choriomeningitis v.,** infectious ectromelia v.

**pseudorabies v.,** Aujesky's disease v.; a herpesvirus causing pseudorabies in swine (also called Aujeszky's disease, mad itch, and infectious bulbar paralysis). Infection in pigs is commonly inapparent, but in some cases causes fever, convulsions and paralysis; in sheep, cattle and carnivores, the v. causes intense pruritus and frequently encephalomyelitis with violent excitement and paralysis usually preceding death.

**psittacosis v.,** see *Chlamydia psittaci.*

**PVM v.,** pneumonia v. of mice.

**quail bronchitis v.,** an adeno-like v., closely relat antigenically to CELO v.

**Quaranfil v.,** an ungrouped arbovirus isolated fro human blood and from herons.

**v. III of rabbits** [ so named because the third stra isolated was used for study ], *Herpesvirus cuniculi;* herpesvirus causing latent infection of rabbits that can "activated" by "blind" passage; may be carried in tran planted tumors.

**rabbit fibroma v.,** fibromatosis v. of rabbits; Sho fibroma v.; a poxvirus causing subcutaneous, soft rubbe swellings, usually on the foot, in cotton rabbits (*Sylvilag* and European rabbits (*Oryctolagus*); the v. is closely relate to vaccinia and myxoma v.'s.

**rabbit myxoma v.,** myxomatosis v.; the poxvirus causi myxomatosis of rabbits, characterized by the formation subcutaneous gelatinous swellings (myxomata). The nat ral hosts are rabbits of the genus *Sylvilagus* in Californ (bush rabbit) and Brazil (local wild rabbit), in which t infection is not fatal and causes only local swelling; rabbits of the genus *Oryctolagus* in England and Australi the infection is nearly always fatal.

**rabbitpox v.,** causes epidemics of pox in laborato rabbits.

**rabies v.,** the causative agent of rabies; a rather lar bullet-shaped v., about 75 by 180 m$\mu$ in size, with regular spaced surface projections; probably an RNA-containin v., but sufficiently purified preparations have not bee studied to determine this with certainty.

**rabies v., Flury strain,** a v. isolated from human brai attenuated (fixed) by serial propagation in nonmammalia hosts, and subsequently established in chick embry culture.

**rabies v., Kelev strain,** an attenuated, embryonate fow egg-passaged strain.

**Rauscher's v.,** an RNA mouse leukemia v., similar t Friend's v.

**re'ovi'ruses** [ *respiratory enteric orphan virus*], a grou of RNA v.'s, 60 to 90 m$\mu$ in diameter, previously include with ECHO v.'s but now separated. They have bee isolated from children with mild fevers and sometime diarrhea, chimpanzees with coryza, dogs with respirator infection and enteritis, and from cattle feces. It is no known whether or not they cause these conditions. Ther are many inapparent natural infections.

**respiratory syncytial v.,** chimpanzee coryza agen (CCA); Rs v.; a v. 120 to 130 m$\mu$ in diameter, probabl RNA-containing, resembling in certain respects the para influenza v.'s; causes minor respiratory infection wit rhinitis and cough in adults, but is capable of causin bronchitis and bronchopneumonia in young children named for tendency to form syncytia in tissue culture. was first isolated from chimpanzees with respiratory disease.

**rhinovi'rus,** coryzavirus; a picornavirus, 20 to 30 m$\mu$ i diameter; one of a group of v.'s of worldwide distributio which cause common colds in man. Rhinoviruses wit similar properties have been isolated from calves and horses. R.'s usually are classified as M strains (culturable in rhesus monkey kidney cells) and H strains (growing onl in cultures of human cells).

**riboviruses,** RNA v.'s.

**Rida v.,** a v. from chronic encephalopathy of sheep resembling scrapie v.

**Rift Valley fever v.,** an ungrouped arbovirus occurring in Central and South Africa in sheep, goats and cattle and causing abortions and severe febrile disease, especially in young lambs. Man, especially herdsmen and veterinarians, may become infected through close contact with infected animals, developing a dengue-like disease. The v. also infects buffaloes, camels and antelopes. It is mosquito-borne, but also probably infects by contact and respiratory tract.

**Riley v.,** lactic dehydrogenase v.

**rinderpest v.,** cattle plague v.; an RNA v., 120 to 300 m$\mu$ in diameter, resembling the measles v.; causes so-called cattle plague in many parts of Africa and Asia. Virulent strains cause acute rinderpest, with high fever, constipation followed by severe diarrhea, nasal discharge, mucosal erosions, and frequently death, while milder strains may

:ause only subclinical infections. The v. also infects water ouffalo, sheep, goats, antelopes, swine and camels. It is :losely related to the measles and canine distemper v.'s.

**Rio Bravo v.,** a group B arbovirus from salivary glands of bats.

**RNA v.'s,** riboviruses; v.'s in which the core consists of ibonucleic acid (RNA); a major group of animal v.'s which includes picornaviruses, reoviruses, arboviruses, myxoviruses, paramyxoviruses, rabies v., avian leukosis-sarcoma v., and v.'s associated with mouse tumors.

**RNA tumor v.'s,** oncornaviruses; RNA v.'s resembling myxoviruses in structure and associated with various expressions of leukosis, sarcoma, or carcinoma in fowl and mammals; the various avian RNA tumor v.'s are commonly viewed as being strains of the avian leukosis-sarcoma v. that, according to circumstances, gives rise to the various expressions of infection included under avian leukosis-sarcoma complex; among the mammalian RNA tumor v.'s, there seems to be an antigenic relationship that closely links the leukemias and the sarcoma v.'s, and at the same time separates them as a group from the avian v.'s and the mammary cancer v. of mice; RNA tumor v. particles are morphologically of three types: type A, the significance of which if not clear; type B, associated with mouse mammary cancer; and type C, associated with the mouse leukoses.

**Rous-associated v.'s,** latent v.'s, normally present in chicken cells, that augment the development of the avian leukosis-sarcoma v.

**Rous sarcoma v.,** avian leukosis-sarcoma v.

**Rs v.,** respiratory syncytial v.

**Rubarth's disease v.,** infectious canine hepatitis v.

**rubella v.,** German measles v.; an RNA v. of fairly large size but still unclassified; the agent causing rubella (German measles) in man.

**rubeola v.,** measles v.

**Russian autumn encephalitis v.,** Japanese B encephalitis v.

**Russian spring-summer encephalitis v.,** a tick-borne group B arbovirus occurring in Central Europe and the U.S.S.R. in two subtypes causing two forms of Russian spring-summer encephalitis in man, a western form which is also called Central European tick-borne fever, and an eastern form, also called Far East Russian encephalitis; the vectors are ticks of the genus *Ixodes*.

**Sagiyama v.,** Getah v.

**Salisbury common cold v.'s,** strains of rhinovirus of historical interest because of early studies that established the viral etiology of common colds.

**salivary v., salivary gland v.,** a herpesvirus with particular affinity for the salivary gland tissue; highly species-specific.

**sandfly fever v.,** phlebotomus fever v.

**Sathuperi v.,** a Simbu group arbovirus isolated in India.

**scrapie v.,** a poorly characterized v., unusually resistant to physical agents; the cause of scrapie in sheep.

**Semliki forest v.,** a group A arbovirus, isolated from mosquitoes in Africa.

**Sen̄ii v.,** parainfluenza-1 v.

**serum hepatitis v.,** hepatitis v. B.

**sheep pox v.,** Clavelée v.; a poxvirus infecting sheep chiefly in parts of Asia, Africa, the Middle East and southern Europe, causing a generalized pock disease with mortality sometimes as high as 50 per cent.

**Shope fibroma v.,** rabbit fibroma v.

**Simbu v.,** type strain, Simbu group, Bunyamwera supergroup arbovirus.

**simian v.,** SV; any of a number of v.'s isolated from monkeys or from cultures of monkey cells; numbered serially (SV1, etc). They have been divided into groups on the basis of cytopathogenic effect (CPE), group I being adenoviruses; II, enteroviruses (mostly Coxsackie-like); III, mostly reoviruses; IV, unclassified; V, myxoviruses; VI, herpesvirus B; VII, vacuolating v. (SV40); VIII, unclassified.

**simian v. 40,** SV40; vacuolating v.; simian vacuolating v.; a small (40 to 45 mμ) DNA v. (papovavirus); the cause of seemingly inapparent infections in monkeys, especially rhesus, and a common contaminant of monkey cell cultures; may cause inapparent infection in man, and the v. may be excreted in stools of children for several weeks;

can produce fibrosarcoma in suckling hamsters, and transformation may occur in rhesus cell culture. May form "hybrid" v. in cells also infected with certain adenoviruses.

**simian vacuolating v.,** simian v. 40.

**Sindbis v.,** a group A arbovirus isolated from mosquito (*Culex*) and birds of several species.

**slow v.,** a v., or a virus-like agent, etiologically associated with a slow virus *disease, q.v.*

**smallpox v.,** variola v.

**sore mouth v.,** contagious ecthyma v. of sheep.

**Spondweni v.,** a group B arbovirus, isolated from mosquitoes in Africa; may cause disease in man.

**St. Louis encephalitis v.,** a group B arbovirus occurring in the United States except the eastern part, and in Trinidad and Panama; normally present as inapparent infection in man, but sometimes causes encephalitis. The v. has been isolated from birds in Panama and from several mosquito species, especially *Psorophora*.

**Stratford v.,** a group B arbovirus from mosquitos in Queensland.

**street v.,** the virulent rabies v. from a rabid domestic animal which has contracted the disease in the usual way, from a bite or scratch of another animal.

**SV,** simian v.

**SV40,** simian v. 40.

**swamp fever v.,** equine infectious anemia v.

**swine fever v.,** hog cholera v.

**swine fever v., African,** African swine fever v.

**swinepox v.,** a poxvirus, distinct from vaccinia v., the cause of a widespread, but low incidence, disease of pigs characterized by formation of generalized pocks, usually affecting younger animals. The pig louse plays an important role in transmission.

**Swiss mouse leukemia v.,** Friend v.

**Tacaribe v.,** the type v. of the Tacaribe group of arboviruses which includes the Junin v. and Machupo v. of Argentinian and Bolivian hemorrhagic fevers; isolated from bats and mosquitos in Trinidad.

**Tahyna v.,** a California group arbovirus from central Europe, known to infect man.

**Tensaw v.,** a Bunyamwera group arbovirus.

**Teschen disease v.,** infectious porcine encephalomyelitis v.; a picornavirus causing Teschen disease of pigs (also called infectious porcine encephalomyelitis). The v. is normally a harmless inhabitant of the intestinal tract, but virulent strains occur which cause epizootics in which affected pigs show stiffness, convulsions, paralysis and prostration. It is widespread in Europe, with most serious losses occurring in Poland and Czechoslovakia.

**TG v.,** transmissible gastroenteritis v. of pigs.

**Theiler's v., Theiler's original v.,** abbreviated T.O. or TO v.; see mouse encephalomyelitis v.

**TO v.,** Theiler's original strain of mouse encephalomyelitis v.

**trachoma v.,** see *Chlamydia trachomatis*.

**transmissible gastroenteritis v. of pigs,** TG v.; an unclassified v., possibly DNA, reported in the United States, Britain, Japan and U.S.S.R., causing a disease of young pigs characterized by diarrhea and vomiting and frequently death.

**Trivittatus v.,** a California group arbovirus.

**tumor v.'s,** particulates obtained from tumor tissue, notably from Rous chicken tumor, or from the milk of cancer-prone strains of mice, which resemble v.'s in molecular size and in nucleoprotein content; on injection into healthy tissue they are capable of inducing a cancerous change and therefore resemble v.'s in infective characteristics as well.

**turkey meningoencephalitis v.,** a group B arbovirus causing paralysis and enteritis in turkeys in Israel.

**Turlock v.,** an ungrouped arbovirus.

**Uganda S v.,** Makonde v.; a group B arbovirus from mosquitos.

**ultravirus,** virus (2).

**Umbre v.,** an arbovirus related serologically to the Turlock v.

**Una v.,** a group A arbovirus from mosquitoes in Trinidad and Brazil.

**Uruma v.,** a group A arbovirus from an epidemic of headache and fever in Bolivia.

**vaccine v.,** see vaccine.

vaccinia v., vaccinia variolae; poxvirus officinalis; the poxvirus used in the immunization of people against variola (smallpox), usually causing a local reaction but sometimes generalized vaccinia, especially in children. The v. is closely related serologically to the v.'s of variola and cowpox, but certain differences have been demonstrated which indicate that they are distinct v.'s.

vacuolating v., simian v. 40.

varicella-zoster v., *Herpesvirus varicellae.*

variola v., smallpox v.; a poxvirus, the pathogen of smallpox in man, causing a severe and often fatal disease (variola major), especially in Asia, Africa and Central America, and a mild, endemic pox (variola minor, alastrim) in other parts of the world.

VE v., vesicular exanthema v. of swine.

VEE v., Venezuelan equine encephalomyelitis v.

Venezuelan equine encephalomyelitis v., VEE v.; a group A arbovirus occurring in Venezuela and several other South American countries, and in Panama and Trinidad, causing Venezuelan equine encephalomyelitis in horses and man; this v. seems to be more viscerotropic than neurotropic; the natural vector is unknown, but the v. can be transmitted experimentally by mosquitoes; the reservoir host is also unknown.

verruca vulgaris v., infectious warts v.

vesicular exanthema v. of swine, VE v.; a single-stranded picornavirus which causes vesicular exanthema of swine, characterized by fever, loss of weight, and vesicles on the snout, tongue and feet.

vesicular stomatitis v., VS v.; apparently an RNA v., agent causing vesicular stomatitis in horses, cattle, sheep and pigs, with lesions similar to those of foot and mouth disease but milder clinical reaction. In countries, such as the United States, having no foot and mouth disease, differential diagnosis is of great importance. Raccoons and perhaps deer are reservoirs of infection. Laboratory infections occur in man.

visceral disease v., cytomegalovirus.

Visna v., possibly an RNA v., 85 mμ in diameter, and closely related antigenically to the similar maedi v.; causes a slow, demyelinating disease of sheep in Iceland; some authorities view the Visna v. and the maedi v. as strains of the same v., the former being neurotropic, the latter pneumotropic.

VS v., vesicular stomatitis v.

wart v., infectious, infectious warts v.

WEE v., western equine encephalomyelitis v.

Wesselsbron disease v., a group B arbovirus causing, in sheep, epizootic infection associated with abortion, hemorrhages, and jaundice; infection may be fatal to lambs and pregnant ewes.

West Nile v., a group B arbovirus reported in Egypt, Uganda, South Africa, Israel and India, usually occurring as silent infection in man, especially children, but capable of causing outbreaks of dengue-like disease with headache, adenopathy, rash, sore throat, and limb pains. Birds are probably the normal hosts, and culicine mosquitoes the vectors.

western equine encephalomyelitis v., WEE v.; a group A arbovirus occurring in the western United States and parts of South America; it occurs naturally, usually as symptomless infection in birds, but causes western equine encephalomyelitis in horses and man following transfer by the bites of mosquitoes, chiefly *Culex tarsalis.*

Wyeomyxia v., a Bunyamwera group arbovirus isolated from a man with fever.

Yaba monkey v., a poxvirus distinct from monkeypox v.; the agent causing so-called subcutaneous tumors in monkeys, the tumorlike growths occurring chiefly on the head and limbs; the natural disease has been reported only in Africa in monkeys kept out of doors.

yellow fever v., a group B arbovirus endemic in tropical Africa south of the Sahara and tropical South America, occasionally spreading to countries outside these areas, and the cause of yellow fever of man and other primates. The v. exists in wild primates, and probably also in edentates, marsupials and rodents, and is transmitted to man by *Aedes* mosquitoes. It is believed to be a v. of African origin brought to America with slave trade.

Zegle v., a group C arbovirus isolated in Panama.

Zika v., a group B arbovirus.

vis, pl. vi'res [ L. force ]. Force; energy; power.

v. a fron'te, a force acting from in front; an obstructiv restraining, or impeding force.

v. a tergo, a force acting from behind; a pushing accelerating force.

v. conserva'trix, the inherent power in the organis. resisting the effects of injury.

v. formati'va, the plastic or healing power in t organism.

v. medica'trix natu'rae, the healing force of nature; th which enables a condition to become corrected withou any special form of treatment.

v. vi'tae, v. vita'lis, vitalism.

viscance (vis'kans). A measure of the energy dissipatio due to a flow in a viscous system. In medicine an physiology, usually a measure of the energy dissipation the flow of liquids, sols, or gels within cells and tissues, of fluids (*e.g.,* blood, respiratory gases) in tubes. The v. the pressure gradient from one end to the other of the flo path when unit flow occurs. The relationship betwee viscosity and v. is of the same nature as that betwee specific resistance, or resistivity, of a conductor materia and the resistance of a particular conductor made fror that material.

viscera (vis'er-ah). Plural of viscus.

viscerad (vis'er-ad) [ viscera + L. *ad,* to ]. In a directio toward the viscera.

visceral (vis'er-al). Splanchnic; relating to the viscera.

visceralgia (vis-er-al'jī-ah) [ viscera + G. *algos,* pain ] Pain in any of the viscera.

viscerimo'tor. Visceromotor.

viscero- (vis'er-o-) [ L. *viscus,* pl. *viscera,* the internal or gans. VISC- ]. Combining form relating to the viscera. Se also splanchno-.

viscerocranium (vis'er-o-kra'nĭ-um) [ viscero- + cra nium ]. Splanchnocranium; jaw skeleton; that part of th skull derived from the embryonic pharyngeal arches; comprises the bones of the facial skeleton.

cartilaginous v., those elements of the fetal skull derived from the second and succeeding pharyngeal arch carti lages.

membranous v., membranous bones, developed in th fetal skull, that overlie maxillary and mandibular compo nents of the first pharyngeal arch cartilage.

viscerogenic (vis-er-o-jen'ik) [ viscero- + G. suffix *-gen* producing ]. Of visceral origin; denoting a number o sensory and other reflexes.

viscerograph (vis'er-o-graf) [ viscero- + G. *graphō,* to write ]. An instrument for recording the mechanica activity of the viscera.

visceroinhibitory (vis'er-o-in-hib'ĭ-to-rī). Restricting or arresting the functional activity of the viscera.

visceromegaly (vis'er-o-meg'ă-lī) [ viscero- + G. *megas,* large ]. Splanchnomegaly; organomegaly; abnormal en largement of the viscera, such as may be seen in acromeg aly.

visceromo'tor. Viscerimotor. 1. Relating to or controlling movement in the viscera; denoting the autonomic nerves innervating the viscera, especially the intestines. 2. Denot ing a movement having a relation to the viscera; referring to reflex muscular contractions of the abdominal wall in cases of visceral disease.

visceropari'etal [ viscero- + L. *paries,* wall ]. Relating to the viscera and the wall of the abdomen; denoting the operation of fixation of an unduly movable organ to the abdominal wall.

visceroperitoneal (vis'er-o-pĕr-ĭ-to-ne'al). Relating to the peritoneal and the abdominal viscera.

visceropleural (vis'er-o-plu'ral). Pleurovisceral; relating to the pleural and the thoracic viscera.

visceroptosis, visceroptosia (vis'er-op'to'sis, -to'sī-ah) [ viscero- + G. *ptōsis,* a falling ]. Splanchnoptosis; descent of the viscera from their normal positions.

viscerosen'sory. Relating to the sensory innervation of internal organs.

visceroskel'etal. Splanchnoskeletal; relating to the visceroskeleton.

**ceroskel'eton.** Splanchnoskeleton; visceral skeleton; 1. any bony formation in an organ, as in the heart, tongue, penis of certain animals; the term also includes according to some anatomists, the cartilaginous rings of the trachea and bronchi. 2. The bony framework protecting the viscera, such as the ribs and sternum, the pelvic bones, and the anterior portion of the skull.

**cerosomatic** (vis'er-o-so-mat'ik) [ viscero- + G. *sōma*, body ]. Splanchnosomatic; relating to the viscera and the body.

**cerotome** (vis'er-o-tōm) [ viscero- + G. *tomos*, cutting ]. An instrument by means of which a section of an organ, *e.g.*, liver, can be removed from a cadaver for examination without performing a general autopsy.

**ceroto'nia** [ viscero- + G. *tonos*, tone ]. Personality traits of love of food, sociability, general relaxation, friendliness, and affection.

**cerotrophic** (vis'er-o-trof'ik) [ viscero- + G. *trophē*, nourishment ]. Relating to any trophic change determined by visceral conditions.

**cerotropic** (vis'er-o-trop'ik) [ viscero- + G. *tropē*, a turning ]. Affecting the viscera.

**scid** (vis'id) [ L. *viscidus*, sticky, fr. *viscum*, birdlime. VISC- ]. Adhesive; sticky; glutinous.

**scidity** (vĭ-sid'ĭ-tĭ). Stickiness; adhesiveness.

**scidosis** (vis'ĭ-do'sis). Clarke-Hadfield syndrome; mucoviscidosis; a congenital metabolic disorder, inherited as a recessive trait, in which secretions of exocrine glands are abnormal; excessively viscid mucus causes obstruction of passageways, including pancreatic and bile ducts, intestines, and bronchi, and the sodium and chloride content of sweat are increased throughout the patient's life; symptoms usually appear in childhood; some of the manifestations are meconium ileus, poor growth despite good appetite, foul bulky stools, chronic cough, recurrent pneumonia, emphysema, clubbing of the fingers, and salt depletion in hot weather; the underlying metabolic defect is unknown and survival beyond childhood is uncommon; cystic fibrosis, or fibrocystic disease, of the pancreas are sometimes used as synonyms for v.

**scoelasticity** (vis'ko-e-las-tis'ĭ-tĭ). The property of a viscous material that also shows elasticity.

**scometer** (vis-kom'e-ter). Viscosimeter.

**scosimeter** (vis'ko-sim'e-ter). An apparatus for determining the viscosity of a fluid; in medicine, usually of the blood.

**scosimetry** (vis'ko-sim'e-trĭ) [ viscosity + G. *metron*, measure ]. The determination of the viscosity of a fluid, such as the blood.

**iscosity** (vis-kos'ĭ-tĭ) [ L. *viscositas*, fr. *viscosus*, viscous. VISC- ]. In general, the resistance to flow or alteration of shape, by any substance as a result of molecular cohesion; a term most frequently applied to liquids, *e.g.*, water, which flows freely, possesses a relatively low v., whereas glycerol, which flows with difficulty, possesses a relatively high v. It is the resistance of a fluid to flow due to a shearing force.

**absolute v.,** force per unit area applied tangentially to a fluid, causing unit rate of displacement of parallel planes separated by a unit distance; units in CGS system: poise.

**anomalous v.,** the viscous behavior of nonhomogenous fluids or suspensions, *e.g.*, blood, in which the apparent v. increases as flow or shear rate decreases toward zero.

**apparent v.,** the v. calculated from Poiseuille's law at any particular flow and tube diameter; it is used for suspensions, such as blood that exhibits anomalous v. and the Fähraeus-Lindqvist effect.

**coefficient of v.,** see under coefficient.

**dynamic v.,** symbol $\mu$; the internal or molecular frictional resistance of a fluid by Newton's law of v. as the ratio of the applied force per unit area to the relative velocity of adjacent fluid layers (produced by the force).

**kinematic v.,** symbol $\upsilon$; measure used in studies of fluid flow; the dynamic viscosity, $\mu$, in poises divided by the density of the material; units: stokes.

**Newtonian v.,** the v. characteristics of a Newtonian fluid.

**relative v.,** the ratio of the v. of a solution or dispersion to the v. of the solvent or continuous phase.

**iscous** (vis'kus) [ see viscid, viscosity ]. Viscid; sticky; adhesive; marked by high viscosity.

**viscum** (vis'kum). 1. Mistletoe; the berries of *Viscum album* (family Loranthaceae), a parasitic plant growing on apple, pear, and other trees; has been used as an oxytocic. 2. Herbage of *Phoradendron flavescens*, American mistletoe; has been used as an oxytocic and emmenagogue.

**viscus,** pl. **viscera** (vis'kus, vis'er-ah) [ L. the soft parts, internal organs. VISC- ] [ NA ]. An organ of the digestive, respiratory, urogenital, and endocrine systems as well as the spleen, the heart, and great vessels; hollow and multilayered walled organs studied in splanchnology.

**visile** (viz'il). 1. Denoting the type of mental imagery in which a person recalls most readily that which he has seen, as contrasted with audile and motile. 2. Visual.

**vision** (vizh'un) [ L. *visio*, fr. *video*, pp. *visus*, to see ]. Sight; the act of seeing.

**achromatic v.,** achromatopsia.

**binoc'ular v.,** v. with a single image, by both eyes simultaneously.

**blue v.,** cyanopsia.

**central v.,** direct v.; v. produced by the rays falling on the fovea centralis.

**chromatic v.,** chromatopsia.

**color v.,** chromatopsia.

**cone v.,** photopic v.

**direct v.,** central v.

**double v.,** diplopia.

**eccentric v.,** peripheral v.

**facial v.,** the presumed sensing of the proximity of objects by the nerves of the face in the case of the blind or when one is in the dark or blindfolded.

**field of v.,** see visual *field.*

**green v.,** chloropsia.

**halo v.,** a condition in which colored or luminous rings are seen around lights.

**haploscopic v.,** stereoscopic v. produced by the haploscope, or mirror-type stereoscope.

**indirect v.,** peripheral v.

**line of v.,** visual *axis.*

**linear v.,** the v. of a single row of graduated characters in contrast to groups of same.

**marginal v.,** perception of hand movements to 3/200.

**multiple v.,** polyopia.

**night v.,** v. that improves in dim light; see also scotopic v., and hemeralopia.

**v. null** [ Fr. *vision nulle* ], abnormal blind spots in the visual field in certain cases of lesion of the cortical center; the patient himself is unaware of them; see also v. obscure.

**v. obscure,** abnormal blind spots in the visual field in cases of lesion below the cortical center; the patient is himself aware of them; see also v. null.

**oscillating v.,** oscillopsia.

**peripheral v.,** indirect v.; eccentric v.; the v. resulting from retinal stimulation beyond the macula.

**photop'ic v.,** photopia; cone v.; v. when the eye is light-adapted; see light *adaptation,* light-adapted *eye.*

**pseudoscopic v.,** v. in reverse stereoscopic relief.

**red v.,** erythropsia.

**rod v.,** scotopic v.

**scotopic v.,** scotopia; rod v.; twilight v.; v. when the eye is dark-adapted; see also dark *adaptation,* dark-adapted *eye.*

**shaft v.,** tubular v.

**stereoscopic v.,** stereopsis; the perception of two images as one by means of fusing the impressions on both retinas; stereopsis is tested by spheroprism, mirror, or polaroid devices.

**subjective v.,** visual impressions due to conditions within the brain and sense organs and not due to external stimuli.

**triple v.,** triplopia.

**tubular v.,** shaft or tunnel v.; a narrowing of the visual field, as though one were looking through a hollow cylinder or tube; it may be a symptom of conversion hysteria or of malingering.

**tunnel v.,** tubular v.

**twilight v.,** scotopic v.

**yellow v.,** xanthopsia.

**visna** (vis'nah). A slow demyelinating leukoencephalitis caused by a virus, found in sheep in Iceland.

**visnadin.** CARDUBEN; 3,4,5-trihydroxy-2,2-dimethyl-6-chromanacrylic acid δ-lactone 4-acetate 3-(2-methylbutyrate); coronary vasodilator.

**vis'nagin.** VISNACORIN; 5-methoxy-2-methylfuranochromone; obtained from *Ammi visnaga* (family Umbelliferae); a coronary vasodilator.

**visual** (vizh'u-al) [ Late L. *visualis*, fr. *visus*, vision ]. Visile (2). 1. Relating to vision. 2. A person who learns and remembers more readily through sight than through hearing.

**visualize** (vizh'u-ă-līz). To make visible.

**visuoauditory** (vizh'u-o-aw'dĭ-to-rī). Relating to both vision and hearing; denoting nerves connecting the centers for these senses.

**visuognosis** (vizh'u-og-no'sis) [ L. *visus*, vision, + G. *gnōsis*, knowledge ]. The recognition and understanding of visual impressions.

**visuopsychic** (vizh'u-o-si'kik) [ L. *visus*, vision, + G. *psychē*, mind ]. Pertaining to the portion of the cerebral cortex concerned with the integration of visual impressions.

**visuosensory** (vizh'u-o-sen'so-rī). Pertaining to the perception of visual stimuli.

**vi'sus** [ L. ] [ NA ]. Vision.

    **v. amplifica'tus,** macropsia.
    **v. defigura'tus,** metamorphopsia.
    **v. dimidia'tus,** hemianopsia.
    **v. diminu'tus,** micropsia.
    **v. diur'nus,** nyctalopia.
    **v. duplica'tus,** diplopia.
    **v. lucidus,** photopsia.
    **v. musca'rum,** vision in which spots are seen before the eyes.
    **v. noctur'nus,** hemeralopia.
    **v. reticula'tus,** the occurrence of many scotomas, giving a sieve-like character to the field of vision.
    **v. triplex,** triplopia.

**visuscope** (viz'u-skōp). A modified ophthalmoscope which projects a black star on the patient's fundus (see euthyscope).

**vi'ta** [ L. ] [ NA ]. Life.

    **v. sexua'lis** sexual *life.*

**vi'tal** [ L. *vitalis*, fr. *vita*, life ]. Relating to life.

**vitalism** (vi'tal-izm) [ L. *vitalis*, pertaining to life ]. The theory that animal functions are dependent upon a special form of energy or force, the vital force, distinct from the physical forces.

**vi'talis'tic.** Pertaining to vitalism.

**vitality** (vi-tal'ĭ-tĭ). Vital force or energy.

**vi'talize.** To endow with vital force.

**vi'tals.** Viscera.

**vitamer** (vi'tă-mer). One of two or more similar compounds capable of fulfilling a specific vitamin function in the body; *e.g.,* niacin and niacinamide.

# VITAMIN

**vitamin** (vi'tă-min) [ L. *vita,* life, + amine ]. One of a group of organic substances, present in minute amount in natural foodstuffs, which are essential to normal metabolism and lack of which in the diet causes deficiency diseases.

    **antiberiberi v.,** thiamin.
    **antihemorrhagic v.,** v. K.
    **antineuritic v.,** thiamin.
    **antirachitic v.'s,** ergocalciferol (v. D$_2$), and cholecalciferol (v. D$_3$).
    **antiscorbutic v.,** ascorbic acid.
    **antisterility v.,** v. E.
    **fat-soluble v.'s,** those v.'s soluble in fat solvents (nonpolar solvents) and insoluble in water; marked in chemical structure by the presence of large hydrocarbon moieties in the molecule; *e.g.,* v.'s A, D, E, and K.
    **fertility v.,** v. E.

    **microbial v.,** a substance necessary for the growth certain microorganisms, *e.g.,* biotin, *p*-aminobenzoic ac
    **permeability v.,** v. P.
    **v. A,** (1) any β-ionone derivative, except provitamin carotenoids, possessing qualitatively the biological activ of retinol. Deficiency interferes with the production a resynthesis of rhodopsin (visual purple), thereby caus night blindness. Deficiency also produces pathologicall keratinizing metaplasia of epithelial cells and clinica xerophthalmia, keratosis, susceptibility to infections, a retarded growth. See also provitamin A; (2) original v. now known as retinol, *q.v.*
    **v. A$_1$,** retinol.
    **v. A$_1$ acid,** retinoic acid.
    **v. A$_1$ alcohol,** retinol.
    **v. A$_1$ aldehyde,** retinal(dehyde).
    **v. A$_2$,** dehydroretinol.
    **v. A$_2$ aldehyde,** dehydroretinal(dehyde).
    **v. B,** a group (see following subentries) of water-solu substances originally considered as one v.
    **v. B complex,** an old and erroneous term applied tc crude isolate similar to the v. B$_2$ complex, but includi thiamin (B$_1$).
    **v. B$_1$,** thiamin.
    **v. B$_2$,** an obsolete term for riboflavin.
    **v. B$_2$ complex,** An old and erroneous term applied crude isolates containing most or all of the v.'s B, includ thiamin (B$_1$); it is a simple mixture, not a complex in t chemical sense.
    **v. B$_3$,** obsolete term for nicotinamide.
    **v. B$_4$,** once believed to be a factor necessary for nutriti of the chick. Factor since identified simply as certa essential amino acids and/or adenine.
    **v. B$_5$,** obsolete; once used to describe biological activiti now ascribed to pantothenic acid or nicotinic acid.
    **v. B$_6$,** pyridoxine and related compounds (pyridox pyridoxamine); for uses, see pyridoxine.
    **v. B$_{10}$,** obsolete designation for a food factor later show to be folic acid or a related compound.
    **v. B$_{11}$,** obsolete designation for a food factor which, li v. B$_{10}$, was later identified as folic acid or a relate compound.
    **v. B$_{12}$,** cobinamide cyanide phosphate 3' ester wi 5,6-dimethyl-1-α-D-ribofuranosyl benzimidazole inn salt; generic descriptor for compounds exhibiting t biological activity of cyanocobalamin (cyanoco (III)alamin); the antianemia factor of liver extract; t most potent antipernicious anemia substance known. contains cobalt and a cyano group in a corrin (cobamid structure. Several substances with similar formulas an with the characteristic hematinic action have been isolate and designated: B$_{12a}$, hydroxocobalamin; B$_{12b}$, aquocoba lamin; B$_{12c}$, nitritocobalamin; B$_{12r}$, cob(II)alamin; B$_{12}$ cob(I)alamin; B$_{12III}$; also factors A and V$_{1a}$ (cobyric acid and pseudovitamin B$_{12}$. B$_{12b}$ has been obtained from cu tures of *Streptomyces aureofaciens;* B$_{12a}$ and B$_{12b}$ are know to be tautomeric compounds; B$_{12c}$ has been obtained fro cultures of *Streptomyces griseus* and is distinguishable fro B$_{12}$ by differences in its absorption spectrum. Vitami B$_{12III}$, factor A, and pseudovitamin B$_{12}$ are also coba mides, as are all the above except factor V$_{1a}$. Som synonyms for vitamin B$_{12}$ are: cyanocobalamin, cobami maturation factor, erythrocyte maturation factor, antiper nicious anemia factor, animal protein factor. See als cyanocobalamin.
    **v. B$_{12}$ with intrinsic factor concentrate** (USP), combina tion of v. B$_{12}$ with suitable preparations of the mucosa c the stomach or intestine of domestic animals used for foo by man. Administered in capsules or tablets in perniciou anemia.
    **v. B$_c$,** folic acid.
    **v. B$_c$ conjugase,** an enzyme catalyzing the hydrolysis o the pteroylpolyglutamic acids to pteroylmonoglutami acid, with consequent increase in vitamin activity; c$_c$ conjugase.
    **v. B$_T$,** carnitine.
    **v. B$_x$,** *p*-aminobenzoic acid.
    **v. C,** ascorbic acid.
    **v. D,** generic descriptor for all steroids exhibiting th biological activity of ergocalciferol (or cholecalciferol); th antirachitic v.'s; called popularly the sun-ray v.'s. They

romote the proper utilization of calcium and phosphorus, hereby producing growth in young children together with roper bone and tooth formation. Useful in tetany.

**v. D₁**, a lumisterol-ergocalciferol mixture originally mistaken for pure v. D.

**v. D₂**, ergocalciferol.

**v. D₃**, cholecalciferol.

**v. D₄**, activated 22,23-dihydroergosterol; 22,23-dihydrogocalciferol; less effective as an antirachitic than v. D₂ nd D₃.

**v. D₅**, irradiated 7-dehydrositosterol.

**v. E**, (1) α-tocopherol *q. v.;* (2) generic descriptor of tocol nd tocotrienol derivatives possessing biological activity of tocopherol; contained in various oils (wheat germ, otton-seed, palm, rice) and whole grain cereals where it onstitutes the nonsaponifiable fraction, also in animal issue (liver, pancreas, heart) and lettuce. Deficiency produces resorption or abortion in female rats and sterility n males, hence it is known as the antisterility or fertility actor or vitamin. Suggested in the treatment of habitual bortion and sterility in humans, also in certain cases of nuscular dystrophy.

**v. E₂(50)**, tocoquinone-10.

**v. F**, (1) a term sometimes applied to the essential nsaturated fatty acids, linoleic, linolenic, and arachidonic cids; (2) obsolete term for thiamin.

**v. G**, an obsolete term for riboflavin.

**v. H**, (1) biotin; (2) sometimes used incorrectly as a ynonym for v. B₆ or for *p*-aminobenzoic acid.

**v. K**, generic descriptor for compounds with the biological activity of phylloquinone (v. K₁); fat-soluble, thermostable compounds found in alfalfa, hog liver, fish meal, and vegetable oils. Essential for the formation of normal amounts of prothrombin. Its absorption in oily solution is facilitated by bile. It is used to diminish the clotting time in patients with obstructive jaundice and to decrease the incidence of hemorrhage in the newborn. Many quinone derivatives exhibit v. K activity. Also termed antihemorrhagic v.

**v. K₁**, or **K₁(20)**, phylloquinone.

**v. K₂**, or **K₂(30)**, menaquinone-6; v. K₂ is sometimes also used for other multiprenylmenaquinones.

**v. K₃**, menaquinone; menadione (see both).

**v. K₄**, 2-methyl-1,4-naphthohydroquinone; menadiol (diacetate or diphosphate); reduced menadione (v. K₃).

**v. K₅**, SYNKAMIN; 4-amino-2-methyl-1-naphthol hydrochloride.

**v. K₆**, 2-methyl-1,4-naphthalenediamine; a very potent antihemorrhagic compound but more toxic than the other v. K's.

**v. K₇**, 4-amino-3-methyl-1-naphthol. Turns violet on exposure to air and light.

**v. L**, factors of unknown chemical constitution, required for normal lactation; obtained from liver (v. L₁) and from yeast (v. L₂).

**v. M**, a factor, anticytopenic for monkeys; see folic acid.

**v. P**, citrin; permeability v.; capillary permeability factor; a mixture of bioflavonoids extracted from plants (especially citrus fruits). It reduces the permeability and fragility of capillaries and is useful in the treatment of certain cases of purpura that are resistant to v. C therapy. See also hesperidin; quercetin; rutin.

**v. T**, factor T; torutilin; name given to an extract from insects and from the fat of fungi and yeasts upon which they feed. When given to insects during their growing period giant types are produced; this substance, obtained from a type of yeast (*Torula*), is said to stimulate the growth and regeneration of diseased or injured human tissues. Probably a mixture of known factors.

**v. U**, anti-gizzard erosion factor; ulcer-preventive factor; term given to a factor in fresh cabbage juice that encourages the healing of peptic ulcer. Thought to be a methionine derivative.

**vi′taminol′ogy.** The study of vitamins.

**vitellarium** (vit′el-lăr′ĭ-um). Vitelline reservoir; in cestodes and trematodes, a common chamber receiving vitelline (yolk) material from the two vitelline ducts; the yolk material then passes into the ootype to surround the ovum and from the eggshell.

**vitel′liform.** Relating to or resembling the yolk of an egg.

**vitel′lin.** A protein combined with lecithin in the yolk of egg.

**vitelline** (vĭ-tel′in, -ēn). Relating to the yolk of an egg (vitellus).

**vitelliruptive** (vi-tel-ĭ-rup′tiv) [ L. *vitellus (vitelli-)*, yolk, + *ruptus*, broken ]. Relating to or resembling broken egg yolks, as in scrambled eggs.

**vitellogenesis** (vi-tel′lo-jen′ĕ-sis, vi′tĕ-lo-) [ L. *vitellus*, yolk, + G. *genesis*, production ]. Formation of the yolk and its accumulation in the yolk-sac.

**vitellolutein** (vi-tel′o-lu′te-in). Lutein from the yolk of egg.

**vitel′loru′bin.** A reddish pigment from the yolk of egg.

**vitellose** (vi-tel′ōs). A protein fragment from vitellin.

**vitellus** (vi-tel′us) [ L. ] [ NA ]. The yolk of an egg; see yolk (1).

**v. ovi**, yolk of egg; used in pharmacy for emulsifying oils and camphors.

**vitiation** (vish-ĭ-a′shun) [ L. *vitiatio* fr. *vitio*, pp. *vitiatus*, to corrupt, fr. *vitium*, vice ]. 1. Corruption. 2. Impairment; rendering useless or less efficacious.

**vitiliginous** (vit′ĭ-lij′ĭ-nus). Relating to or characterized by vitiligo.

**vitiligo**, pl. **vitiligines** (vit′ĭ-li′go, vit′ĭ-lij′ĭ-nēz) [ L. a skin eruption, fr. *vitium*, blemish, vice ]. Acquired leukoderma; acquired leukopathia; piebald skin; the appearance on the otherwise normal skin of loss of pigment with white patches of varied sizes, often symmetrically distributed; the skin bordering the affected sites is usually hyperpigmented, and hair in the affected areas is usually, but not always, white.

**v. cap′itis**, *alopecia* areata.

**Cazenave's v.**, *alopecia* areata.

**Celsus' v.**, *alopecia* areata.

**circumne′vic v.**, *leukoderma* acquisitum centrifugum.

**v. i′ridis**, small white patches of uniform size in brown irides.

**vitiligoidea** (vit′ĭ-li-goy′de-ah) [ vitiligo + G. *eidos*, appearance ]. Xanthoma.

**vitium**, pl. **vitia** (vish′ĭ-um, vish′ĭ-ah) [ L. vice ]. Defect; fault; vice.

**v. cordis**, an organic lesion of the heart.

**vitrectomy** (vĭ-trek′to-mī) [ vitreous + G. *ektomē*, excision ]. Removal of anterior vitreous and severance of vitreous strands; advocated in serious intraocular injuries with vitreous loss and intraocular hemorrhage to avoid the sequelae of fibrotic overgrowth.

**vitrein** (vit′re-in). Vitrosin; a collagen-like protein which, with the mucopolysaccharide hyaluronic acid, accounts for the gel state of the vitreous.

**vitreo-** (vit′re-o-) [ L. *vitreus*, glassy ]. Combining form for vitreous.

**vit′reoden′tin.** Dentin of a particular brittle hardness.

**vit′reoret′inal.** Relating to, pertaining to, or affecting the limit between the retina and the corpus vitreum, especially at the posterior pole of the fundus, at the macula.

**vit′reoretinop′athy.** Retinopathy with vitreous complications.

**exudative v.**, a familial, slowly progressive ocular disease occurring in otherwise healthy persons; characterized by posterior vitreous detachment, vitreous membranes, heterotopia of macula, retinal detachment, neovascularization, and recurrent hemorrhage.

**vitreous** (vit′re-us) [ L. *vitreus*, glassy, fr. *vitrum*, glass ]. 1. Glassy; resembling glass. 2. *Corpus* vitreum.

**persistent anterior hyperplastic primary v.**, a unilateral congenital abnormality occurring in full-term infants; characterized by a retrolental fibrovascular membrane formed by persistent primary v. plus remnants of the hyaloid artery and tunica vasculosa lentis, leukocoria, microphthalmos, shallow anterior chamber, and elongated ciliary processes.

**persistent posterior hyperplastic primary v.**, a unilateral congenital anomaly in full-term infants; associated with a congenital retinal fold and a v. membranous stalk containing remnants of hyaloid artery.

**primary v.,** the v. first formed in the embryo between the optic cup and the lens vesicle, and later vascularized by the hyaloid artery and its branches.

**secondary v.,** avascular v. formed around the primary v. which becomes restricted to the hyaloid canal.

**tertiary v.,** v. fibrils derived from the neuroepithelium of the ciliary body and forming the zonule of Zinn.

**vitreum** (vit're-um) [ L. ntr. of *vitreus,* glassy ]. *Corpus* vitreum.

**vit'reus** [ L. ] [ NA ]. Glassy; vitreous (1).

**vitricin.** An antibacterial substance extracted from vitrain, an ingredient of coal; it is active against *Bacillus subtilis.*

**vit'riol** [ L. *vitreolus,* glassy ]. Sulfuric acid.

**blue v.,** cupric sulfate.

**green v.,** ferrous sulfate.

**v. oil,** sulfuric acid.

**white v.,** zinc sulfate.

**vitrosin.** Vitrein.

**vit'ular, vit'ulary, vit'uline** [ L. *vitulus,* a calf ]. Relating to a calf.

**vivarium,** pl. **vivaria** (vi-vār'ī-um, -ah) [ L. *vivarius,* pertaining to living creatures ]. Quarters in which animals are housed, particularly animals used in medical research.

**vivi-** (viv'ī-) [ L. *vivus,* alive ]. Combining form meaning living, alive.

**vividialysis** (viv'ī-di-al'ī-sis). Removal by dialysis, as by lavage of peritoneal cavity.

**vividiffusion** (viv'ī-dī-fu'zhun) [ vivi- + diffusion ]. A term suggested by Abel, Rowntree, and Turner to denote a method by which the blood of a living animal may be submitted to dialysis outside the body and again returned to the natural circulation, without exposure to the air or to any noxious influences. The principle is used clinically today in the artificial kidney apparatus.

**vivification** (viv'ī-fī-ka'shun) [ L. *vivifico,* pp. *-atus,* fr. *vivus,* alive, + *facio,* to make ]. 1. The change of the protein of the food into living matter of the cells, in the final stage of assimilation. 2. Revivification (2).

**viviparity** (vīv'ī-pǎr'ī-tī). Zoogony; the quality or state of being viviparous, *i.e.,* producing offspring that are living at the time of birth.

**viviparous** (vi-vip'ǎ-rus) [ vivi- + L. *pario,* to bear ]. Zoogonous; giving birth to living young, in distinction to oviparous.

**viviperception** (viv-ī-per-sep'shun) [ vivi- + perception ]. Observation of the vital processes in the organism without the aid of vivisection.

**vivisect** (viv-ī-sekt'). To practice vivisection.

**vivisection** (viv-ī-sek'shun) [ vivi- + section ]. Biotomy; any cutting operation on a living animal for purposes of experimentation; extended to denote any form of animal experimentation.

**vivisec'tionist, vivisec'tor.** One who practices vivisection.

**vivisecto'rium.** A laboratory for animal experimentation.

**vivisepul'ture** [ L. *vivus,* living + *sepultura,* a burial ]. The burial of a person alive.

**Vladimiroff-Mikulicz amputation** or **operation.** See Mikulicz-Vladimiroff *amputation.*

**V.M.D.** See D.V.M.

**vocal** (vo'kal) [ L. *vocalis* ]. Pertaining to the voice or the organs of speech.

**voca'lis** [ L. ] [ NA ]. Vocal.

**Voges** (fo'ges), Otto, Berlin physician, *1867. See V.-Proskauer *reaction.*

**Vogt** (fōkht), Alfred, Swiss ophthalmologist, 1879–1943. See V.-Koyanagi *syndrome.*

**Vogt** (fōkht), Cécile, German neurologist, *1875. See V. *syndrome.*

**Vogt** (fōkht), Karl, German physiologist, 1817–1895. See V.'s *angle.*

**Vogt** (fōkht), Oskar, German neurologist, *1870. See Spielmeyer-V. *disease.*

**Vogt** (fōkht), Paul F. E., German surgeon, 1847–1885. See V.'s *point,* V.-Hueter *point.*

**voice** [ L. *vox* ]. The sound made by air passing out throu the larynx and upper respiratory tract, the vocal co being approximated and made tense.

**amphoric v.,** amphorophony; a sound having a holl blowing character heard over a pulmonary cavity when patient speaks or whispers.

**bronchial v.,** bronchophony.

**epigastric v.,** the delusion of a v. proceeding from epigastrium.

**eunuchoid v.,** high pitched v. in the adult male resembl the v. of an immature boy; usually functional in origi

**myxedema v.,** the forced, rough, raucous v. of subje of myxedema, probably due to myxedematous thickeni of the vocal cords.

**void.** To evacuate excrementitious matter.

**Voillemier** (vwal-me-a'), Léon C., French urologist, 1 century. See V.'s *point.*

**vola** (vo'lah) [ L. ] [ NA ]. Palm of the hand or sole of t foot.

**vo'lar.** Referring to the vola, the palm of the hand or s of the foot.

**volatilization** (vol'ǎ-til-ī-za'shun) [ fr. L. *volatilis,* volati fr. *volo,* pp. *volatus,* to fly ]. Evaporation; conversion o solid or liquid into a vapor.

**vol'atilize.** To cause or undergo volatilization or evapo tion.

**vole** (vōl). A heavy, mouselike rodent (a fieldmouse) of t genus *Microtus* (family Cricetidae). An acid-fast bacill isolated from the field v. of Great Britain has been used the preparation of a vaccine for use in tuberculosis of m and cattle.

**Volhard** (fōl'hart), Franz, German physician, 1872–195 See V.'s *test.*

**volition** (vo-lish'un) [ L. *volo* (irreg. verb), fut. p. *volitur* to wish ]. The conscious impulse to perform any act or abstain from its performance; voluntary action.

**volitional** (vo-lish'un-al). Voluntary; done by an act of wi relating to volition.

**Volkmann** (fōlk'mahn), Alfred W., German physiologis 1800–1877. See V.'s *canals.*

**Vol∤mann** (fōlk'mahn), Richard, German surgeon 1830–1889. See V.'s *cheilitis, contracture, deformity, spli spoon, subluxation.*

**vol'ley** [ Fr. *volée,* fr. L. *volo,* to fly ]. A synchronous grou of impulses induced simultaneously by artificial stimul tion of either nerve fibers or muscle fibers.

**antidromic v.,** a v. of impulses passing toward the centr nervous system in an efferent nerve fiber or toward th periphery of the body in an afferent nerve fiber; *i.e.,* passin in the reverse of the physiologic direction.

**Vollmer,** Herman, New York pediatrician, *1896. See \ *test.*

**volsella** (vol-sel'ah) [ see vulsella ]. Vulsella *forceps.*

**volt** [ A. *Volta* ]. The unit of electromotive force; the ele tromotive force that will produce a current of 1 ampere i a circuit which has a resistance of 1 ohm.

**Volta,** Allessandro, Italian physicist, 1745–1827. Gave hi name to volt and statvolt.

**voltage** (vōl'tej). The electromotive force; pressure or po tential expressed in volts.

**volta'ic.** Relating to Volta, who discovered the means o producing electricity by chemical action.

**voltaism** (vol'ta-izm). Galvanism.

**voltam'eter** [ volt + G. *metron,* measure ]. An apparatu for measuring the strength of a galvanic current by it electrolytic action.

**volt'ampere.** 1 watt; a unit of electrical power; the produc of 1 volt by 1 ampere; one-thousandth of a kilowatt.

**volt'meter.** An apparatus for measuring the electromotiv force or difference of potential.

**Voltolini** (vol-to-le'ne), Friedrich E. R., German laryngol ogist, 1819–1889. See V.'s *disease,* V.-Heryng *sign.*

**volume** (vol'yum) [ L. *volumen,* something rolled up, scroll fr. *volvo,* to roll ]. Symbol V; the space occupied by an form of matter, expressed usually in cubic millimeters cubic centimeters, liters, etc. See also fig. and subentrie under capacity.

**atomic v.,** the atomic weight of an element divided by its density in the solid state; the v. of the gram atomic weight of a solid element.

**closing v.,** the lung v. at which the flow from the lower parts of the lungs becomes severely reduced or stops during expiration, presumably because of airway closure; measured by the sharp rise in expiratory concentration of a tracer gas that had been inspired at the beginning of a breath that started from residual volume.

**distribution v.,** the v. throughout which an added tracer substance appears to have been evenly distributed, calculated by dividing the amount of tracer added by its concentration after equilibration.

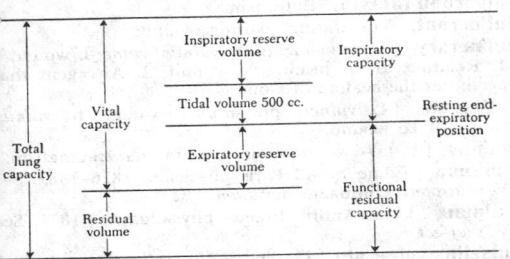

**Nomenclature of Lung Volumes**

(From Youmans, W. B.: *Fundamentals of Human Physiology*, Ed. 2, © Year Book Medical Publishers, Inc., 1962. Used by permission of Year Book Medical Publishers.)

**expiratory reserve v.,** abbreviated ERV; supplemental air; reserve air; the maximal v. of air (about 1000 cc.) that can be expelled from the lungs after a normal expiration.

**forced expiratory v.,** abbreviated FEV, with subscript indicating time interval in seconds; the maximal v. that can be expired in a specific time interval when starting from maximal inspiration.

**inspiratory reserve v.,** abbreviated IRV; complemental air; the maximal v. of air that can be inspired after a normal inspiration, less the tidal v.

**minute v.,** (1) the minute output of the heart equal to the stroke v. times the heart rate; (2) the minute v. of breathing, a product of tidal v. times the respiratory frequency.

**packed cell v.,** the v. of the blood cells in a sample of blood after it has been centrifuged in the hematocrit. Normally, it amounts to 45 per cent of the blood sample.

**partial v.,** the actual v. occupied by one species of molecule or particle in a solution; it is the reciprocal of the density of the molecule.

**resid'ual v.,** abbreviated RV; residual air; residual capacity; the v. of air remaining in the lungs after a maximal expiratory effort.

**standard v.,** the v. of a perfect gas at standard temperature and pressure, 22.414 liters.

**stroke v.,** the v. pumped out of one ventricle of the heart in a single beat.

**tidal v.,** symbol $V_T$; tidal air; the v. of air that is inspired or expired in a single breath during regular breathing.

**volumenometer** (vol'u-mē-nom'e-ter) [ volume + G. *metron*, measure ]. A device for determining the volume of a solid by measuring the amount of liquid which it displaces.

**volumetric** (vol'u-met'rik). Relating to measurement by volume; see v. analysis.

**volumometer** (vol'u-mom'e-ter). Volumenometer.

**voluntary** (vol'un-tĕr-ĭ) [ L. *voluntarius*, fr. *voluntas*, will, fr. *volo*, to wish ]. Relating or acting in obedience to the will; not obligatory.

**voluptuous** (vo-lup'tu-us) [ L. *voluptuosus*, fr. *voluptas*, pleasure ]. Causing or caused by sensual pleasure; given to gratification of the senses.

**volute** (vo-lūt) [ L. *voluta*, a scroll, fr. *volvo*, pp. *volutus*, to roll ]. Rolled up; convoluted.

**volutin** (vol'u-tin). A nucleoprotein complex found as cytoplasmic granules in certain bacteria, yeasts, and protozoa (such as trypanosome glagellates), and serving as food reserves; sometimes called metachromatic granules.

**Vol'vox** [ L. *volvo*, to roll ]. A genus of highly organized colonial green flagellates of the Phytomastigina.

**volvulosis** (vol'vu-lo'sis). Onchocerciasis.

**volvulus** (vol'vu-lus) [ L. *volvo*, to roll ]. A twisting of the intestine causing obstruction.

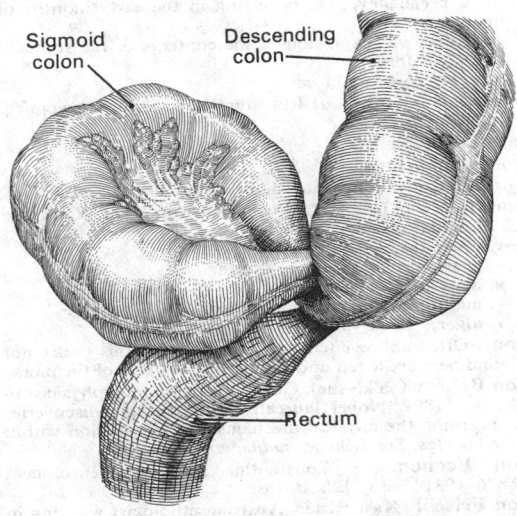

**Volvulus**

**gastric v.,** twisting of the stomach which results in obstruction and may impair blood supply to the organ; it occurs in paraesophageal hernia (upside-down stomach) and occasionally in eventration of the diaphragm.

**vo'mer,** gen. **vo'meris** [ L. ploughshare ] [ NA ]. A flat bone of trapezoidal shape forming the inferior and posterior portion of the nasal septum; it articulates with the sphenoid, ethmoid, two maxillae, and two palatine bones.

**v. cartilagin'eus,** *cartilago* vomeronasalis.

**vo'merine.** Relating to the vomer.

**vo'merobas'ilar.** Relating to the vomer and the base of the skull.

**vo'merona'sal.** Relating to the vomer and the nasal bone.

**vomica** (vom'ĭ-kah) [ L. an ulcer, boil, fr. *vomo*, to vomit ]. 1. A pulmonary cavity containing pus. 2. Profuse expectoration of purulent matter.

**vom'icine.** 12-Hydroxy-*N*-methylpseudostrychnine; an alkaloid found in nux vomica.

**vom'icose** [ L. *vomica*, an ulcer ]. Ulcerous; marked by many ulcers; profusely suppurating.

**vom'icus** [ L. ]. Vomica (2).

**vom'it** [ L. *vomo*, pp. *vomitus*, to vomit ]. 1. To eject matter forcibly from the stomach. 2. Matter thrown up from the stomach.

**Barcoo v.,** attacks of nausea and vomiting accompanied by bulimia affecting those living in the interior of the southern part of Australia.

**black v.,** coffee-ground v.; vomitus niger; the coffee-ground-colored material that is vomited, specifically, in severe yellow fever.

**coffee-ground v.,** black v.

**vomiting** (vom'ĭ-ting). The ejection of matter through the esophagus and mouth from the stomach.

**cyclic v.,** periodic v.

**dry v.,** retching; movements of v. without the ejection of matter from the stomach.

**epidemic v.,** nausea and v. that attacks a group of subjects (*e.g.*, in a school or small community). The onset of the v. is sudden, without prodromal illness or malaise; it is intense while it lasts, but ceases abruptly after a few hours or a day or so. There are headache, abdominal pain, giddiness, and diarrhea in most of the cases, and extreme prostration in about 75 per cent. The cause of the attack is unknown, but is probably a virus.

fecal v., stercoraceous v.; copremesis; the ejection of fecal matter, aspirated into the stomach from the intestine by the repeated spasmodic contractions of the gastric muscles.

**morning v.,** v. occurring on rising or immediately after breakfast in some women during early pregnancy.

**pernicious v.,** uncontrollable v.

**v. of pregnancy,** v. occurring in the early months of pregnancy.

**projectile v.,** expulsion of the contents of the stomach with great force.

**stercora'ceous v.,** fecal v.

**vomition** (vo-mish'un) [ L. *vomitio,* fr. *vomo,* to vomit ]. Vomiting.

**vom'itive.** Emetic.

**vom'itory.** Emetic.

**vomiturition** (vom-ĭ-tu-rish'un). Retching.

**vomitus** (vom'ĭ-tus) [ L. a vomiting, vomit ]. 1. Vomiting. 2. Vomited matter.

**v. cruen'tus,** hematemesis.

**v. gravida'rum,** *vomiting* of pregnancy.

**v. mari'nus,** seasickness.

**v. matuti'nus,** morning *vomiting.*

**v. niger,** black *vomit.*

**von.** Often abbreviated to v. Names with this prefix not found here are listed under the principal part of the name.

**von Békésy** (ba'ke-she), Georg, Hungarian biophysicist in U. S. *1899. Nobel laureate, 1961, for his discoveries concerning the physical mechanism of stimulation within the cochlea. See Békésy *audiometry.*

**von Economo,** Constantin, Austrian neurologist, 1876–1931. See v. E.'s *disease.*

**von Frisch,** Karl Ritter, Austrian ethologist working in Germany, *1886. Nobel laureate, 1973, with Konrad Lorenz and Nikolaas Tinbergen, for their discoveries concerning organization and elicitation of individual and social behavior patterns.

**von Hippel,** Eugen, German ophthalmologist, 1867–1939. See Hippel's *disease,* v. H.-Lindau *disease.*

**von Kossa stain.** See under stain.

**von Meyenburg,** H. See Meyenburg, H. von.

**von Spee** (spa), See Spee.

**von Willebrand,** E. A., Finnish physician, 1870–1949. See v. W.'s *disease.*

**Voorhees,** James D., U. S. obstetrician, 1869–1929. See V. *bag.*

**Voorhoeve,** N., Dutch radiologist. See V.'s *disease.*

**vortex,** pl. **vortices** (vor'teks, vor'tĭ-sēz) [ L. whirlpool, whorl, fr. *verto* or *vorto,* to turn around. VERT- ]. 1 [ NA ]. Whorl, *q.v.* 2. V. lentis; one of the stellar figures on the surface of the lens of the eye.

**v. coccyge'us,** coccygeal whorl; a spiral arrangement of coarse hairs sometimes present over the region of the coccyx.

**v. cordis** [ NA ], the whorl of muscular fibers at the apex of the heart.

**v. lentis,** v. (2).

**vortices pilo'rum** [ NA ], hair whorls; a spiral arrangement of the hairs, as at the crown of the head.

**Vorticella** (vor'tĭ-sel'ah) [ Mod. L. dim. of L. *vortex,* a whorl ]. A genus of Ciliata of the order Peritrichida, of bell shape and with a spiral of cilia around the adoral zone; various free-living species have been found at times in the feces, urine, and mucous discharges.

**vorticose** (vor'tĭ-kōs) [ L. *vorticosus,* fr. *vortex,* a whorl ]. Arranged in a whorl.

**vortico'sus** [ L. ] [ NA ]. Vorticose.

**Vossius' lenticular ring.** See under ring.

**voussure** (voo-sur') [ Fr. ]. Prominence of the precordium due to enlargement of the heart during childhood.

**vox** [ L. ]. Voice.

**v. cholera'ica,** a peculiar, hoarse, almost inaudible, voice of a sufferer in the last stage of Asiatic cholera.

**voyeur** (vwah-yer'). One who practices voyeurism.

**voyeurism** (vwah-yer'izm) [ Fr. *voir,* to see ]. Scopophilia; the practice of obtaining sexual pleasure by looking, especially at the naked body or genitals of another or at erotic acts between others.

**VR.** Abbreviation for vocal *resonance.*

**VS.** Abbreviation of volumetric *solution.*

**Vu.** A unit expressing the magnitude at a complex electric signal. The volume in Vu as measured by a volum indicator is equal to the number of decibels by which th wave differs from reference volume on the B scale.

**vulcanizing** (vul'kă-ni'zing) [ L. *Vulcanus,* Vulcan, god fire ]. The process of treating rubber to make it hard. I dentistry, used in connection with a denture base materi made of rubber impregnated with sulfur, so that when is heated under pressure a chemical reaction occurs and hard rigid mass is formed.

**vulga'ris** [ L. fr. *vulgus,* a crowd ]. Ordinary; of the usua type.

**vulgarobu'fotoxin.** Bufotoxin.

**vul'nerant.** Vulnerating; causing wounds.

**vul'nerary** [ L. *vulnerarius,* fr. *vulnus* (*vulner*-), wound 1. Relating to, or healing, a wound. 2. An agent tha promotes the healing of wounds.

**vul'nerate** [ L. *vulnero,* pp. -*atus,* to wound, fr. *vulnu.* wound ]. To wound.

**vul'nus** [ L. ]. A wound or injury; trauma; traumatism.

**Vul'pian,** Edme F. A., Paris physician, 1826–1887. Se V.'s *atrophy,* conjugate *deviation, test.*

**Vulpian,** Louis-André, French physiologist, *1871. Se V.'s *effect.*

**vulsella** (vul-sel'ah) [ L. pincers, fr. *vello,* pp. *vulsus,* t pluck ]. Vulsella *forceps.*

**vulsel'lum.** Vulsella *forceps.*

**vulva,** pl. **vul'vae** (vul'vah) [ L. a wrapper or covering seed covering, womb, fr. *volvo,* to roll ] [ NA ]. *Pudendun femininum* [ NA ]; pudendum muliebre; pudendum; cun nus; the external genitalia of the female, comprised of th mons pubis, the labia majora and minora, the clitoris, the vestibule of the vagina and its glands, and the opening o the urethra and of the vagina.

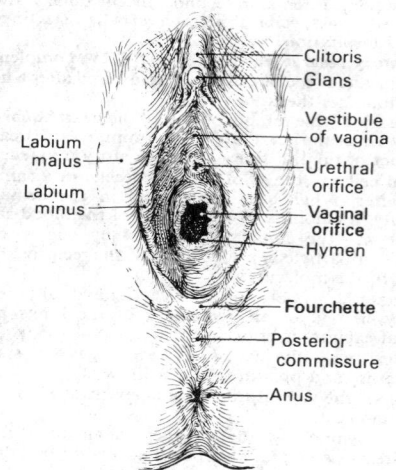

**The Vulva (Pudendum Femininum)**

**v. conni'vens,** a v. with very narrow opening.

**v. hi'ans,** a v. in which the labia are loosely approximated.

**vul'var, vul'val.** Relating to the vulva.

**vulvectomy** (vul-vek'to-mĭ) [ vulva + G. *ektomē,* exci sion ]. Excision (either partial, complete, or radical) of the vulva.

**vulvismus** (vul-viz'mus). Vaginismus.

**vulvitis** (vul'vi'tis) [ vulva + G. suffix -*itis,* inflammation ]. Aidoiitis; edeitis; inflammation of the vulva.

**chronic atrophic v.,** an inflammation of atrophic vulvar skin, usually with severe pruritus.

**chronic hypertrophic v.,** elephantiasis vulvae; swelling of the vulval tissues due to lymphatic obstruction; in some cases it may be caused by filariasis, with induration or ulceration of the skin.

**follic'ular v.,** inflammation of the vulvar follicles.

**leukoplakic v.,** *leukoplakia* vulvae.

**vulvo-, vulv-** [ L. *vulva, q.v.* ]. Combining forms relating to the vulva.

**vulvocrural** (vul'vo-kru'ral). Relating to the vulva and the clitoris.

**vulvouterine** (vul-vo-u'ter-in). Relating to the vulva and the uterus.

**vulvovaginal** (vul-vo-vaj'ĭ-nal). Relating to the vulva and the vagina.

**vulvovaginitis** (vul'vo-vaj'ĭ-ni'tis). Inflammation of both vulva and vagina, or of the vulvovaginal glands.

# W

**W.** Chemical symbol for the element tungsten (wolfram).

**Waardenburg,** Petrus Johannes, Dutch ophthalmologist, *1886. See W.'s *syndrome.*

**Wachendorf's membrane.** See under membrane.

**wadding** (wod'ing). Carded cotton or wool in sheets, used for surgical dressings.

**waddle** (wod'l). To walk with a side-to-side, swaying motion; occurring in pseudohypertrophic muscular dystrophy and certain other nervous conditions.

**Wadsworth,** Augustus B., American bacteriologist, *1872. See W.'s *method.*

**wa'fer.** A thin sheet of dried flour paste, used to enclose a powder, the wafer being moistened and folded over the drug, so that it can be swallowed without taste.

**Wagner,** H., Swiss ophthalmologist. See W.'s *disease.*

**Wagner** (vahg'ner), Wilhelm, German surgeon, 1848–1900. See W.'s *operation.*

**Wagner's line.** See under line.

**Wagner von Jauregg** (văg'ner von yow'reg), Julius, Austrian physician, 1857–1940. Nobel laureate, 1927, for treatment of paresis by fever therapy.

**Wagstaffe,** William W., English surgeon, 1843–1910. See W.'s *fracture.*

**wahoo** (wah'hoo) [ Am. Ind. name ]. Euonymus.

**waist** (wāst) [ A.S. *waext* ]. The portion of the trunk between the ribs and the pelvis.
**w. of the heart,** see under heart.

**wakam'ba.** A Zanzibar arrow poison that stimulates powerfully the vasomotor nerves, causing a marked rise of blood pressure.

**Waksman,** Selman A., U. S. microbiologist, *1888. Nobel laureate, 1952, for his discovery of streptomycin, the first antibiotic effective against tuberculosis.

**Walcher** (vahl'kher), Gustav A., German obstetrician, 1856–1935. See W. *position.*

**Wald,** George, U. S. biologist, *1906. Nobel laureate, 1967, with Ragnar Granit and Haldan K. Hartline, for their studies in visual physilogy.

**Waldenström,** J. H., Swedish physician, *1877. See W.'s *macroglobulinemia, purpura, syndrome, test.*

**Waldeyer** (vahl'di-er), Heinrich W. G., German anatomist, 1836–1921. See W.'s *fossae, glands,* zonal *layer,* throat *ring, tract.*

**wale** [ A.S. *walu* ]. A linear wheal, especially one produced by a blow with a stick or a whip.

**walk.** 1. To move on foot. 2. The characteristic manner in which one moves on foot; see also gait.

**Walker,** A. Earl, american neurologist, *1907. See Dandy-W. *syndrome,* W. *tractotomy.*

**Walker,** J. T. Ainslie, English chemist, 1868–1930. See Rideal-W. *coefficient, method.*

**Walker,** James, British gynecologist. See W.'s *chart.*

**Walker carcinoma** or **carcinosarcoma.** See under carcinosarcoma.

**wall** [ L. *vallum* ]. Paries; an investing part enclosing a cavity such as the chest or abdomen, or covering a cell or any anatomical unit.
**anterior w. of middle ear,** *paries* caroticus cavi tympani.
**anterior w. of stomach,** *paries* anterior ventriculi.
**anterior w. of vagina,** *paries* anterior vaginae.
**axial w.'s of the pulp chambers,** the w.'s parallel with the long axis of a tooth; these are the mesial, distal, buccal, and lingual.
**carotid w. of middle ear,** *paries* caroticus cavi tympani.
**cavity w.,** one of the surfaces bounding a cavity.
**cell w.,** the outer layer or membrane of some animal and plant cells; in the latter it is mainly cellulose.
**chest w.,** thoracic w.; in respiratory physiology, the total system of structures outside the lungs that move as a part of breathing; it includes the rib cage, diaphragm, abdominal w., and abdominal contents.
**enamel w.,** in dentistry, the part of the w. of a cavity consisting of enamel.

**external w. of cochlear duct,** *paries* externus ductus cochlearis.
**inferior w. of orbit,** *paries* inferior orbitae.
**inferior w. of tympanic cavity,** *paries* jugularis cavi tympani.
**jugular w. of middle ear,** *paries* jugularis cavi tympani.
**labyrinthic w. of middle ear,** *paries* labyrinthicus cavi tympani.
**lateral w. of middle ear,** *paries* membranaceus cavi tympani.
**lateral w. of orbit,** *paries* lateralis orbitae.
**mastoid w. of middle ear,** *paries* mastoideus cavi tympani.
**medial w. of middle ear,** *paries* labyrinthicus cavi tympani.
**medial w. of orbit,** *paries* medialis orbitae.
**membranous w. of middle ear,** *paries* membranaceus cavi tympani.
**membranous w. of trachea,** *paries* membranaceus tracheae.
**nail w.,** *vallum* unguis.
**parietal w.,** the body w. or the somatopleure from which it is formed.
**posterior w. of middle ear,** *paries* mastoideus cavi tympani.
**posterior w. of stomach,** *paries* posterior ventriculi.
**posterior w. of vagina,** *paries* posterior vaginae.
**pulpal w.,** one of the w.'s of the pulp cavity, *e.g.,* buccal pulpal w.
**splanchnic w.,** the w. of one of the viscera or the splanchnopleure from which it is formed.
**superior w. of orbit,** *paries* superior orbitae.
**tegmental w. of middle ear,** *paries* tegmentalis tympani.
**thoracic w.,** chest w.
**tympanic w. of cochlear duct,** *paries* tympanicus ductus cochlearis.
**vestibular w. of cochlear duct,** *paries* vestibularis ductus cochlearis.

**Wallenberg** (vah'len-bairg), Adolf, German physician, 1862–1949. See W.'s *syndrome.*

**Waller,** Augustus V., English physiologist, 1816–1870. See Wallerian *degeneration, law.*

**Walle'rian.** Relating to or described by A. V. Waller.

**wall'eye.** 1. Exotropia. 2. Absence of color in the iris, or leukoma of the cornea.

**Walsham forceps.** See under forceps.

**Walthard,** Max, Swiss gynecologist, 1867–1933. See W.'s cell *rest.*

**Walther** (vahl'ter), August F., German anatomist, 1688–1746. See W.'s *canals, ducts, ganglion, plexus.*

**Walton's law.** See under law.

**wan'dering** [ A.S. *wandrian,* to wander ]. Moving about; not fixed.

**Wang,** Chung T., Chinese pathologist, 1889–1931. See W.'s *test.*

**Wangensteen,** Owen H., American surgeon, *1898. See Braun-W. *graft,* W. *suction, tube.*

**warble** (war'bl) [ M. Sw. *varbulde,* boil ]. Small swelling in skin of back of cattle caused by the presence of the larvae of *Hypoderma bovis* or *H. lineata.*

**Warburg,** Otto, German biochemist, 1883–1970. Nobel laureate, 1931, for his discovery of the nature and mode of action of the respiratory enzyme. See W.'s *apparatus,* yellow *enzyme, theory,* W.-Lipmann-Dickens *shunt,* Barcroft-W. *apparatus,* Barcroft-W. *technique.*

**ward** [ A.S. *weard* ]. A room or hall in a hospital containing a number of beds.
**accident w., casualty w.,** a hospital w. for the reception of accident cases.
**isolation w.,** a w. in a hospital or institution, formerly in a separate pavilion, but now usually in the main hospital structure, where persons having or suspected of having a contagious disease are kept apart from others.
**psychopathic w.,** a w. in a general hospital for the reception and temporary treatment of mental patients.

**Ward's triangle.** See under triangle.

**Wardrop,** James, English surgeon, 1782–1869. See W.'s *disease, method.*

**warfarin sodium** (war'fă-rin) (USP, BP). COUMADIN sodium; PROTHROMADIN; PANWARFIN; [ [ 3-(α-acetonylbenzyl)-2-oxo-2 *H*-1-benzopyran-4-yl ]oxy ]sodium; an anticoagulant with the same actions as bishydroxycoumarin; also used as a rodenticide. The NF lists potassium warfarin, with same actions and uses as bishydroxycoumarin.

**warm-blooded.** Hemathermal.

**Warren's test.** See under test.

**wart** (wort). Verruca.

**anatomical w.,** postmortem w.

**asbestos w.,** asbestos *corn.*

**butcher's w.,** a nodular cutaneous growth of tuberculous nature.

**cattle w.'s,** infectious *papilloma* of cattle.

**common w.,** *verruca* simplex.

**fig w.,** *condyloma* acuminatum.

**flat w.,** *verruca* plana.

**fugitive w.,** a transitory w.; one that does not persist.

**Henle's w.'s,** Hassall-Henle *bodies.*

**infectious w.'s,** see infectious wart *virus.*

**moist w.,** *condyloma* acuminatum.

**mosaic w.,** plantar growth of numerous closely aggregated w.'s forming a mosaic appearance.

**necrogenic w.,** postmortem w.

**Peruvian w.,** *verruga* peruana.

**pitch w.,** a type of verruca common among workers in pitch and coal tar derivatives. It may progress to epithelioma.

**plantar w.,** verruca plantaris; a w. on the sole.

**pointed w.,** *condyloma* acuminatum.

**postmortem w.,** a tuberculous warty growth (tuberculosis cutis verrucosa) on the hand of one who performs postmorten examinations; also called verruca necrogenica; anatomical, dissection, postmortem, or prosector's tubercle; anatomical, necrogenic, or prosector's wart.

**prosector's w.,** postmortem w.

**seborrhe'ic w.,** seborrheic *keratosis.*

**senile w.,** senile *keratosis.*

**soft w.,** skin *tag.*

**soot w.,** chimney sweep's *cancer.*

**telangiectatic w.,** angiokeratoma.

**tuberculous w.,** *tuberculosis* cutis verrucosa.

**venereal w.,** *condyloma* acuminatum.

**viral w.,** *verruca* simplex.

**Wartenberg** (vahr'ten-bairg), Robert, German neurologist, *1887. See W.'s *symptom.*

**Warthin,** Aldred S., American pathologist, 1866–1931. See W.-Finkeldey *cells,* W.-Starry *stain,* W.'s *tumor.*

**wart'pox.** *Variola* verrucosa.

**wart'y.** Relating to or covered with warts.

**wash** (wosh). A lotion.

**black w.,** black *lotion.*

**eye w.,** collyrium; see ophthalmic *solution.*

**mouth w.,** collutorium.

**Wasmann,** Adolphus, German anatomist, 19th century. See W.'s *glands.*

**Wassén,** Erik, Danish physician, *1901. See W. *test.*

**Wassermann** (vah'ser-mahn), August P. von, Berlin bacteriologist, 1866–1925. See W. *antibody, reaction, test,* provocative W. *test.*

**Wassermann-fast.** A term used to designate a case in which the Wassermann reaction remains positive despite all treatment.

**waste** (wāst) [ thr. O.Fr fr. L. *vastus,* waste, desolate ]. 1. To emaciate; to grow thin. 2. Excrement.

**wasting** (wāst'ing). Emaciation.

**water** (waw'ter, wah'ter) [ A.S. *waeter* ]. 1. $H_2O$; a clear, odorless, tasteless liquid, solidifying at 32°F. (0°C. and R.), and boiling at 212°F. (100°C., 80°R.). It is present in all animal and vegetable tissues and in nearly all other substances; it is a solvent of more substances than any other liquid. 2. Euphemism for the urine. 3. A pharmacopeial preparation; w.'s or aromatic w.'s are clear, saturated aqueous solutions (unless otherwise specified) of volatile oils or other aromatic or volatile substances; aromatic w.'s

are prepared by processes involving distillation or solution (agitation followed by filtration).

**acid'ulous w.,** carbonic w.; carbonated w.; one that contains a considerable amount of carbonic acid in solution.

**w. of adhesion,** w. held by molecular attraction in contact with solid surfaces, but not forming an essential part of their constitution.

**alkaline w.,** one that contains appreciable amounts of the bicarbonates of calcium, lithium, potassium, or sodium.

**ammonia w.,** hartshorn.

**baryta w.,** a saturated aqueous solution of barium hydroxide. Used as an alkaline reagent.

**bitter w.,** a natural mineral w. containing Epsom salt.

**black w.,** *azoturia* of horses.

**bound w.,** w. held to colloids and other substances and not removed by filtration.

**bromine w.,** (1) one containing the bromides of magnesium, potassium, or sodium in therapeutic amounts; (2) bromine test solution; a saturated solution containing bromine in w.

**calcic w.,** one containing appreciable quantities of calcium salts in solution.

**car'bonated** or **carbon'ic w.,** acidulous w.

**carbon dioxide-free w.,** purified w. that has been boiled vigorously for 5 minutes or more.

**chalyb'eate w.,** one that contains salts of iron in appreciable quantities.

**chlorine w.,** (1) one that contains the chlorides of sodium, potassium, calcium, and magnesium in varying amounts; (2) chlorine test solution; a saturated solution of chlorine in w.

**combined w.,** w. that enters as an essential part in the constitution of a molecule; *e.g.,* the $H_2O$ of $C_6H_{12}O_6$, a hexose.

**w. of combustion,** w. of metabolism.

**w. of constitution,** w. held by a unit of structure as an essential part of its constitution, though not an ingredient of its molecules. See w. of crystallization.

**w. of crystallization,** w. of constitution that unites with certain salts and is essential to their arrangement in crystalline form; *e.g.,* $CuSO_4 \cdot 5H_2O$.

**distilled w.** (BP), w. purified by distillation.

**earthy w.,** one containing a large amount of mineral matter, chiefly sulfate, in solution.

**free w.,** w. in the body that can be removed by ultrafiltration and in which substances can be dissolved; see bound w.

**gentian aniline w.,** gentian violet with saturated aniline w., a more effective stain than simple gentian violet.

**hard w.,** w. containing ions, such as $Mg^{++}$ and $Ca^{++}$, that form insoluble salts with fatty acids so that ordinary soap will lather in it with difficulty or not at all.

**heavy w.,** deuterium oxide; HDO or $D_2O$; w. in which most of the hydrogen atoms are deuterium, or heavy hydrogen (2H); its properties differ noticeably from those of ordinary w. (it has higher boiling and freezing points).

**indifferent w.,** a mineral w. containing but a small quantity of saline matter.

**w. for injection** (USP, BP), w. purified by distillation for the preparation of products for parenteral use; it must meet USP requirements for purified w. (with the exception of bacteriological purity) and BP requirements for distilled w. The USP also lists sterile w. for injection and bacteriostatic w. for injection.

**w. of metabolism,** w. of combustion; the w. formed in the body by oxidation of the hydrogen of the food; the greatest amount is produced in the metabolism of fat, about 117 gm. per 100 gm. of fat.

**mineral w.,** one that contains appreciable amounts of certain salts which give to it therapeutic properties.

**potable w.,** a w. fit for drinking, being free from contamination and not containing a sufficient quantity of saline material to be regarded as a mineral w.

**purified w.** (USP, BP), w. obtained by distillation or deionization.

**Rhodesian red w.,** East Coast *fever.*

**saline w.,** one that contains neutral salts (chlorides, bromides, iodides, sulfates) in appreciable amounts.

**Selters** or **Seltzer w.** [ Nieder *Selters*, a mineral spring in Prussia ], a mineral w. containing carbonates of sodium, calcium, and magnesium, and chloride of sodium.

**soft w.,** w. lacking those ions that form insoluble salts with fatty acids, so that ordinary soap will lather in it easily. Opposite of hard w.

**sulfate w.,** one holding in solution appreciable quantities of the sulfates of calcium, magnesium, or sodium.

**sulfur w.,** one containing hydrogen sulfide or the metallic sulfides.

**waterborne.** Transported by drinking-water, as in diseases such as cholera and typhoid fever, spread largely by this means.

**Waterhouse,** Rupert, British physician, 1873–1958. See W.-Friderichsen *syndrome.*

**water-pang.** Pyrosis.

**waters.** Colloquialism for amniotic *fluid.*

   **bag of w.,** the amniotic sac and contained amniotic fluid.

   **false w.,** a leakage of fluid prior to or in beginning labor, before the rupture of the bag of w.

**Waters,** Charles Alexander, U. S. radiologist, 1888-1961. See W.'s view *roentgenogram.*

**Waters,** Edward G., U. S. obstetrician and gynecologist. See W.'s *operation.*

**Watson,** James D., U. S. geneticist, \*1928. Nobel laureate, 1962, with Francis H. C. Crick and Maurice H. F. Wilkins, for their discoveries concerning the molecular structure of nuclear acids and its significance for information transfer in living materials. See W.-Crick *helix.*

**Watson′ius watson′i.** An amphistome trematode fluke occasionally found in the intestine of Africans. Normal host is probably a monkey.

**Watt,** James, Scottish engineer, 1736–1819. Gave his name to the watt.

**watt** (wot) [J. *Watt*]. The unit of electrical power; the power available when the current is 1 ampere and the electromotive force is 1 volt. It is equal to 1 joule ($10^7$ ergs) per second.

**wattles** (wot′lz) [A.S.]. The fleshy appendages, generally bright red in color and featherless, that hang from the throat or chin of many birds. Some reptiles and goats have similar structures known by the same name.

**wave** [ A.S. *wafian*, to fluctuate ]. 1. A movement of particles in an elastic body, whether solid or fluid, whereby an advancing series of alternate elevations and depressions, or expansions and condensations, is produced. 2. The elevation of the pulse, felt by the finger, or represented graphically in the curved line of the sphygmogram. 3. The complete cycle of changes in the level of a source of energy that is repetitively varying with respect to time. In the electroencephalogram the w. is essentially a voltage-time graph. See also entries under rhythm.

   **acid w.,** acid *tide.*

   **alkaline w.,** alkaline *tide.*

   **alpha w.'s,** alpha *rhythm.*

   **arterial w.,** a w. in the jugular phlebogram due to transmission of carotid artery pulsation.

   **beta w.'s,** beta *rhythm.*

   **brain w.,** see electroencephalograph, and pertinent entries under rhythm.

   **cannon w.,** an exaggerated "a" w. in the jugular pulse caused by right atrial contraction occurring after ventricular contraction has closed the tricuspid valve, as in ventricular premature beats and in complete heart block.

   **delta w.,** (1) a slurring of the initial part of the upstroke of the R wave in the Wolff-Parkinson-White syndrome; (2) delta *rhythm.*

   **dicro′ic w.,** recoil w.; the second rise in the tracing of a dicrotic pulse.

   **electrocardiographic w.,** a deflection of special shape and extent in the electrocardiogram representing the activity of a portion of the heart muscle.

   **excitation w.,** a w. of altered electrical conditions that is propagated along a muscle fiber preparatory to its contraction.

   **f. or ff w.'s,** fibrillary w.'s; irregular undulations of the base line in the electrocardiogram, characterizing atrial fibrillation.

   **F or FF w.'s,** regular rapid atrial w.'s in the electrocardiogram characterizing atrial flutter.

**fibrillary w.'s,** ff w.'s.

**flat top w.'s,** activity in the electroencephalogram having a pattern suggesting a flat top. These w.'s are often found in temporal lobe discharges.

**fluid w.,** a sign of free fluid in the abdominal cavity; percussion on one side of the abdomen transmits a w. that is felt on the opposite side.

**microelectric w.'s,** microwaves.

**overflow w.,** the descending w. of the sphygmogram from the apex to the first anacrotic break.

**P w.,** the first complex of the electrocardiogram, representing depolarization of the atria. If the P w. is retrograde or ectopic in form it is labeled P′.

**percussion w.,** the main positive w. of an arterial pulse tracing.

**phrenic w.,** diaphragm *phenomenon.*

**postextrasystolic T w.,** the T w. of the sinus beat immediately following an extrasystole.

**pulse w.,** the progressive expansion of the arteries occurring with each contraction of the left ventricle of the heart.

**Q w.,** the initial deflection of the QRS complex when such deflection is negative (downward).

**R w.,** the first positive (upward) deflection of the QRS complex in the electrocardiogram. Successive upward deflections within the same QRS complex are labeled R′, R″, etc.

**radio w.'s,** Hertzian rays; electromagnetic radiation in the region beyond the infrared; the range of wavelengths is broad and the term can include radiation with wavelengths as low as 1 millimeter and as high as 30 kilometers; used commercially in radio, television, and radar.

**random w.'s,** w.'s in the electroencephalogram which occur paroxysmally and asynchronously.

**recoil w.,** dicrotic w.

**retrograde P w.,** the P w. pattern in the electrocardiogram representing retrograde depolarization of the atria, the impulse spreading from the A-V node upward.

**S w.,** a negative (downward) deflection of the QRS complex following an R w. Successive downward deflections within the same QRS complex are labeled S′, S″, etc.

**sonic w.'s,** audible sound w.'s, as distinguished from ultrasonic w.'s.

**Stephenson's w.,** congestion of the pelvic organs, gradually increasing prior to the menses, becoming stationary when the flow begins, and gradually subsiding at the termination of the menstrual period.

**supersonic w.'s,** see supersonic.

**T w.,** the next deflection in the electrocardiogram following the QRS complex; represents ventricular repolarization.

**theta w.'s,** theta *rhythm.*

**tidal w.,** the w. between the percussion w. and the dicrotic w. in the downward limb of the arterial pulse tracing.

**Traube-Herring w.'s,** Traube-Herring *curves.*

**U w.,** a positive w. following the T w. of the electrocardiogram.

**ultrasonic w.'s,** see ultrasonic.

**wavelength** (wāv-length). The distance from one point on a wave (shaped like a sine curve) to the next point in the same phase; *i.e.,* from peak to peak or from trough to trough.

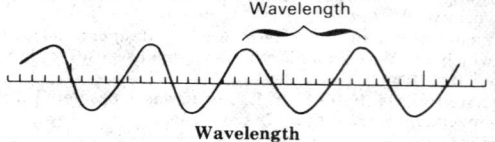

Wavelength

**wave′shape.** Wave *form.*

**wax** [ A.S. *weax* ]. 1. Cera; beeswax; a thick, tenacious substance, plastic at room temperature, secreted by bees for building their cells, or the honeycomb. 2. Any substance with physical properties similar to those of beeswax, of animal, vegetable, or mineral origin (oils, lipids, or fats that are solids at room temperature). 3. Chemical definition: esters of high molecular weight fatty acids with monohydric or dihydric alcohols (aliphatic or cyclic).

**animal w.,** beeswax, spermaceti, and any w. derived from the animal kingdom.

**bleached w.,** white w.

**bone w.,** Horsley's bone w.; a mixture of antiseptic agents, oil, and w. used to stop bleeding by plugging bone cavities or Haversian canals, especially of the skull.

**boxing w.,** w. used for boxing impressions; see also boxing.

**Brazil w.,** carnauba w.

**carnauba w.** (USP), Brazil w.; palm w.; a w. obtained from the Brazilian w. palm, *Copernica cerifera*.

**casting w.'s,** soft solids widely used in dentistry for patterns of all types and for many other purposes; most are basically paraffin but are modified by addition of gum dammar, carnauba w., or other ingredients, to meet various requirements.

**Chinese w.,** (1) a vegetable w.; (2) a w. secreted by a scale insect, *Coccus ceriferus* or *C. pela*, and deposited in the twigs of a species of ash trees. Used in China to make candles and also medicinally.

**ear w.,** cerumen.

**earth w.,** ceresin.

**emulsifying w.** (BP), a mixture of cetostearyl alcohol 9, and sodium lauryl sulfate 1, and water 0.4; a washable ointment base.

**grave w.,** adipocere.

**Horsley's bone w.,** bone w.

**Japan w.,** a vegetable w. derived from *Rhus succedanea* and *Toxicodendron verniciferum*.

**mineral w.,** (1) paraffin w.; (2) ozokerite.

**palm w.,** carnauba w.

**paraffin w.,** mineral w.; a w. derived from petroleum.

**vegetable w.,** palm w. or any w. derived from plants such as the bayberry.

**white w.** (USP), white beeswax (BP); bleached w.; yellow w. bleached by being rolled very thin and exposed to the light and air or bleached by chemical oxidants. Same uses as yellow w.

**yellow w.** (NF), a yellowish solid brittle substance prepared from the honeycomb of the bee, *Apis mellifera*. The chief constituent is myricin (myricyl palmitate); others are cerotic acid (cerin), melissic acid, heptacosane, and hentriacontane. Used in the preparation of ointments, cerates, plasters, and suppositories.

**wax'ing.** Waxing-up.

**waxing-up** Waxing; the contouring of a pattern in wax, generally applied to the shaping in wax of the contours of a trial denture.

**Way,** Stanley, British obstetrician-gynecologist. See Stanley Way *procedure*.

**wean** (wēn) [A.S. *wenian*]. To take from the breast; to deprive permanently of breast milk and nourish with other food.

**weaning** (we'ning). Ablactation; taking from the breast.

**weanling** (wēn'ling). A young animal that has become adjusted to food other than its mother's milk. Generally applied to foals.

**wear** (wăr). Wasting or deterioration caused by friction.

**occlusal w.,** attritional loss of substance on opposing occlusal units or surfaces; see also abrasion (3).

**web** [A.S.]. A tissue; a membrane; tela.

**esophageal w.,** a cribriform or w. formation in the esophagus caused by an irregular atrophy. See also Plummer-Vinson *syndrome*.

**terminal w.,** fibrillar cytoplasm, beneath the microvilli of intestinal absorbing cells, which is free of cytoplasmic organelles.

**web'bing.** A congenital condition apparent when adjacent structures are joined by a broad band of tissue that is not normally present to such a degree.

**Weber** (va'ber), Ernst H., German physiologist and anatomist, 1795–1878. See *W.'s experiment*, W.-Fechner *law*, W.'s *law*, *paradox*.

**Weber,** Frederick Parkes, English physician, 1863–1962. See W.-Christian *disease*, Rendu-Osler-W. *disease*, *syndrome*, Sturge-Kalischer-W. *syndrome*, Sturge-W. *disease*, *syndrome*, Klippel-Trenaunay-W. *syndrome*.

**Weber,** Sir Hermann, London physician, 1823–1918. See W.'s *sign*, *syndrome*.

**Weber** (va'ber), Moritz I., German anatomist, 1795–1875. See W.'s *gland*, *organ*.

**Weber** (va'ber), Wilhelm E., German physiologist, 1804–1891. See W.'s *point*, *triangle*.

**Webster,** John, English chemist, 1878–1927. See W.'s *test*.

**Webster,** John C., Chicago gynecologist, 1863–1950. See W.'s *operation*.

**Wechsler,** David, American psychologist, *1896. See W.-Bellevue and W. intelligence *scale*.

**Wedensky,** Nicolai I., Russian neurologist, *1844. See W. *inhibition*.

**wedge** (wej) [A.S. *weeg*]. A solid body having the shape of an acute-angled triangular prism.

**dental w.,** a double inclined plane used for separating the teeth, maintaining the separation once obtained, or holding a matrix in place.

**Weeks,** John E., New York ophthalmologist, 1853–1949. See Koch-W. *bacillus*, W.'s *bacillus*, Koch-W. *conjunctivitis*.

**Wegener,** F., German pathologist. See W.'s *granulomatosis*.

**Wegner** (veg'ner), Friedrich R. G., German pathologist, *1843. See W.'s *disease*, *sign*.

**Weichselbaum** (vīkh'zel-bowm), Anthony, Austrian pathologist, 1845–1920. See W.'s *coccus*, Fraenkel-W. *pneumococcus*.

**Weidel** (vi'del), Hugo, Austrian chemist, 1849–1899. See W.'s *reaction*.

**Weigert** (vi'gert), Karl, German pathologist, 1843–1904. See W.'s *law*, *solution*, *stains*.

**weight** (wāt) [A.S. *gewiht*]. The pull toward the center of the earth of a body at its surface; the product of the force of gravity, defined internationally as $980.665 \text{ cm/s}^1$, times the mass of the body. For comparative table of weights, see appendix 5.

**atomic w.,** the w. of an atom of a chemical element in relation to the w. of an atom of carbon-12 ($^{12}$C), which is set equal to 12.000; it is thus a ratio and therefore dimensionless (although the actual w., numerically the same, is sometimes expressed in daltons); not necessarily the w. of any individual atom of an element, since most elements are made up of several isotopes of different masses; *e.g.*, the atomic w. of chlorine is 35.457, because it is composed of $^{35}$Cl and $^{37}$Cl in proportions that give an average of 35.457. See also molecular w.

**birth w.,** in humans, the first w. of an infant obtained within less than the first 60 completed minutes after birth; a full-size infant is one weighing 2500 gm. or more; a low birth w. is considered to be less than 2500 gm.

**combining w.,** gram *equivalent*.

**equivalent w.,** gram *equivalent*.

**gram-atomic w.,** atomic w. expressed in grams (compare mole).

**gram-molecular w.,** molecular w. expressed in grams (compare mole).

**molecular w.,** the sum of the atomic w.'s of all the atoms constituting a molecule; the mass of a molecule relative to the mass of a standard atom, now $^{12}$C (taken as 12.0000 –). See also atomic w.

**weight'lessness.** The psychophysiologic experience of a person at zerogravity. An object's weight results from a gravitational force acting upon a supported mass. Anything deprived of support, falling freely in a vacuum, is weightless. A special case of the "free fall" is a satellite orbiting outside the earth's atmosphere. Within the earth's atmosphere a powered flight can traverse a parabolic curve similar to the curve for a "free fall" where gravitational pull and centrifugal force cancel each other out and one achieves a temporary state of simulated w.

**Weil** (vīl), Adolf, German physician, 1848–1916. See Larrey-W. *disease*, W.'s *disease*, *syndrome*.

**Weil** (vīl), Edmund, Austrian physician, 1880–1922. See W.-Felix *reaction*.

**Weil** (wīl), Richard, U. S. physician, 1876–1917. See W.'s *test*.

**Weill,** G. See W.-Marchesani *syndrome.*

**Weill,** Jean, French physician. See Leri-W. *syndrome.*

**Weinberg** (vīn'berg), Michel, French pathologist, 1868–1940. See W.'s *reaction.*

**Weingrow's reflex.** See under reflex.

**Weir** (weer), Robert F., U. S. surgeon, 1838–1927. See W.'s *operation, technique.*

**Weir Mitchell.** See Mitchell.

**Weisbach** (vīs'bahkh), Albin, Vienna anthropologist, 1837–1914. See W.'s *angle.*

**Weismann** (vīs'mahn), August F. L., German biologist, 1834–1914. See W.'s *theory.*

**Weismann's bundle,** see under bundle.

**weismannism.** The concepts of heredity introduced by August Weismann (1834–1914), particularly the noninheritance of acquired characters and the continuity of the germ plasm; see also Weismann's *theory.*

**Weiss** (vis), Leonhard, German physician, *1881. See Much-W. *stain,* W.'s *stain.*

**Weiss** (vīs), Leopold, Berlin oculist, 1849–1901. See W.'s *reflex.*

**Weiss** (vīs), Nathan, Austrian physician, 1851–1883. See W.'s *sign.*

**Weiss,** Soma, U. S. physician, 1898–1942. See Mallory-W. *syndrome.*

**Weitbrecht** (vīt'brekht), Josias, German anatomist in St. Petersburg, 1702–1747. See W.'s *cartilage, cord, fibers, foramen, ligament.*

**Welander,** L. See Kugelberg-W. *disease;* Wohlfart-Kugelberg-W. *disease.*

**Welch,** William H., American pathologist, 1850–1934. See W.'s *bacillus, stain.*

**Welcker's angle.** See under angle.

**Weller,** Thomas H., U. S. parasitologist, *1915. Nobel laureate, 1954, with John F. Enders and Frederick C. Robbins, for their discovery of the ability of poliomyelitis viruses to grow in cultures of various types of tissue.

**Wells,** M. See M.-Wells *syndrome.*

**Wells,** Sir Thomas Spencer, English surgeon, 1818–1897. See W.'s *facies, forceps.*

**welt** [ O.E. *waelt* ]. A wheal; particularly, a linear wheal resulting from a blow.

**Weltmann** (velt'mahn), Oskar, Austrian physician, 1885–1934. See W.'s coagulation *band.*

**wen** [ A.S. ]. Sebaceous *cyst.*

**explosive w.,** a sebaceous cyst that becomes secondarily infected.

**Wenckebach** (ven'kĕ-bahkh), Karel F., Dutch internist, 1864–1940. See W. *period, phenomenon.*

**Wenzel** (vent'sel), Joseph, German anatomist and physiologist, 1768–1808. See W.'s *ventricle.*

**Wepfer** (vep'fer), Johann J., 1620–1695. See W.'s *gland.*

**Werdnig** (verd'nig), Guido, Austrian neurologist, 19th century. See W.-Hoffmann *disease.*

**Werlhof** (verl'hof), Paul G., German physician, 1699–1767. See W.'s *disease.*

**Wermer,** Paul. See W.'s *syndrome.*

**Wernekinck** (ver'na-kink), Friedrich C. G., German anatomist, 1798–1835. See W.'s *commissure, decussation.*

**Werner** (ver'ner), Heinrich, German physician, *1874. See W.-His *disease.*

**Werner** (ver'ner), Otto, German physician, *1879. See W.'s *syndrome.*

**Wernicke** (ver'ne-keh), Karl, German neurologist, 1848–1905. See W.'s *aphasia, area, center, disease, encephalopathy,* W.-Korsakoff *encephalopathy,* W.'s *fibers, field, hypermetamorphosis, radiation, reaction, region, sign, syndrome, zone.*

**Wernicke,** Robert, Argentine pathologist, 19th century. See Posadas-W. *disease.*

**Wertheim** (vert'hīm), Ernst, Vienna gynecologist, 1864–1920. See W.'s *operation.*

**Westberg** (vest'berg), Friedrich, German physician, 19th century. See W.'s *space.*

**Westergren method.** See under method.

**Westphal,** Karl F. O., German neurologist, 1833–189 See W.'s *disease, phenomenon, pseudosclerosis,* pupilla *reflex, sign,* W.-Erb *sign,* W.-Piltz, W.-Strümpell *phenom non,* Edinger-W. *nucleus.*

**weth'er** [ A.S. ]. A male sheep (ram) castrated before se ual maturity.

**Wetzel,** Norman C., U. S. pediatrician, *1897. See W. *gri*

**Wever,** Ernest Glen, U. S. psychologist, *1902. Se W.-Bray *phenomenon.*

**Weyers,** Helmut, German pediatrician. See W.-Thier *sy drome,* Meyer-Schwickerath and W. *syndrome.*

**Wharton,** Thomas, English anatomist, 1614–1673. Se W.'s *duct, jelly.*

**whartonitis** (hwawr-ton-i'tis). Inflammation of the sub maxillary (Wharton's) duct.

**wheal** (hweel) [ A.S. *hwēle* ]. An acute, circumscribed, tran sitory area of edema of the skin; an urticarial lesio produced by intradermal injection or test.

**wheat germ oil.** An oil obtained by expression from th germ of the wheat seed, *Triticum aestivum* (family Gram neae); one of the richest sources of natural vitamin E; use as a nutritional supplement.

**Wheatstone,** Charles, English physicist, 1802–1875. Se W. *bridge, stereoscope.*

**Wheeler,** John M., U. S. ophthalmologist, 1879–1938. Se W. *method.*

**Wheeler-Johnson test.** See under test.

**Wheelhouse,** Claudius G., English surgeon, 1826–1909 See W.'s *operation.*

**wheeze** [ A.S. *hwēsan* ]. 1. To breathe with difficulty an noisily. 2. The sound made by air passing through th fauces, glottis, or narrowed tracheobronchial airways i difficult breathing; a puffing.

**asth'matoid w.,** a puffing sound heard in front of th patient's open mouth in a case of foreign body in th trachea or a bronchus.

**whelp** (hwelp) [ A.S. ]. The act of a female dog (bitch) o giving birth to puppies.

**whey** (hwā) [ A.S. *hwaeg* ]. Serum lactis; the watery par of milk remaining after the separation of the casein.

**alum w.,** w. produced by curdling milk by means o powdered alum.

**w. protein,** see under protein.

**whip'lash.** See whiplash *injury.*

**Whipple,** Allen O., U. S. surgeon, *1881. See W.'s *opera tion.*

**Whipple,** George H., U. S. pathologist, *1878. See Nobe laureate, 1934, with George R. Minot and William P. Murphy, for their discoveries concerning liver therapy in cases of anemia. See W's *disease.*

**whip'worm.** See *Trichuris.*

**whis'ky, whis'key** [ Gael, *usquebaugh,* water of life ]. Spiritus frumenti; an alcoholic liquid obtained by the distillation of the fermented mash of wholly or partly malted cereal grains, containing 47 to 53 per cent, by volume, of $C_2H_5OH$, at 15.56°C. It must have been stored in charred wood containers for not less than 2 years. The various grains used in the manufacture of w. are barley, maize, rye, and wheat.

**whis'per** [ A.S. *hwisprian* ]. 1. To speak without phonation. 2. The sound heard on auscultation of the chest when the subject whispers; called also whispering pectoriloquy and whispering resonance.

**whistle** (hwis'l) [ A.S. *hwistle* ]. 1. A sharp, shrill sound made by forcing air through a narrow opening. 2. An instrument for producing a w.

**Galton's w.,** a cylindrical w., attached to a compressible bulb, with a screw attachment that changes the note; used to test the hearing.

**White,** James C., U. S. dermatologist, 1833–1916. See W.'s *disease.*

**White,** Paul D., American physician, *1886. See Wolff-Parkinson-W. *syndrome.*

**white** [ A.S. *hwīt* ]. The color resulting from the perfect commingling of all the rays of the spectrum; the color of chalk or of snow.

**visual w.,** leukopsin.

**white'comb.** *Tinea* galli.

**Whitehead,** Walter, English surgeon, 1840–1913. See W.'s *operation.*

**whites.** Leukorrhea or blennorrhea.

**whi'ting.** Chalk ($CaCO_3$) used for polishing metals or plastic appliances.

**whitlow** (hwit'lo) [ M.E. *whitflawe* ]. Felon.

melanot'ic w., Hutchinson's disease (3); subungual melanoma; a pigmented sarcoma or melanoma beginning in the skin at the border of the nail.

thecal w., suppurative lesion of distal phalanx; may involve tendon sheath and bone.

**Whitman,** Royal, New York surgeon, 1857–1946. See W.'s *frame.*

**Whitmore,** Alfred, British surgeon, 1876–1946. See W. *bacillus.*

**Whitnall,** Samuel E., English anatomist, 1876–1952. See W.'s *tubercle.*

**whoop** (hōōp, hwōōp). The sonorous inspiration with which the paroxysm of coughing terminates in pertussis.

systolic w., systolic *honk.*

**whoop'ing cough.** Pertussis.

**whorl** (hwurl). 1. A turn of the spiral cochlea of the ear. 2. The *vortex* cordis. 3. A turn of a concha nasalis. 4. A verticil. 5. An area of hair growing in a radial manner suggesting whirling or twisting; see *vortices* pilorum. 6. Digital w.; one of the distinguishing patterns comprising Galton's system of classification of fingerprints (*q.v.*, under fingerprint).

coccygeal w., *vortex* coccygeus.

hair w.'s, *vortices* pilorum.

**whorled** (hwurld). Marked or arranged in by whorls; vorticose; turbinate; convoluted; verticillate.

**Whytt,** Robert, Scottish physician, 1714–1766. See W.'s *disease.*

**Wickham's striae.** See under stria.

**Widal** (ve-dal'), Fernand, Paris physician, 1862–1929. See Hayem-W. *anemia,* Hayem-W. *syndrome,* W.'s *reaction,* Gruber-W. *reaction,* W.'s *syndrome.*

**Widowitz' sign.** See under sign.

**widow's peak.** A sharp point of hair growth in the midline of the anterior scalp margin, usually resulting from recession of hair of the temple areas, or occurring as a congenital configuration of scalp hair.

**width.** Wideness; the distance from one side of an object or area to the other.

orbital w., the distance between the dacryon and the farthest point on the anterior edge of the outer border of the orbit (Broca), or between the latter point and the junction of the frontolacrimal suture and the posterior edge of the lacrimal groove.

**Wiedemann,** H. R. See Beckwith-W. *syndrome.*

**Wiener,** H. See *tract* of Münzer and W.

**Wigand,** J. Heinrich, German obstetrician and gynecologist, 1766–1817. See W.'s *maneuver.*

**Wij's method.** See under method.

**Wilde,** Sir William R. W., Dublin oculist and otologist, 1815–1876. See W.'s *cords, incision, triangle.*

**Wilder,** Burt G., American anatomist, 1841–1925. See W.'s *quadrant.*

**Wilder,** Joseph, U. S. neuropsychiatrist, *1895. See W.'s *law* (of initial value).

**Wilder,** Russell M., U. S. internist, 1885–1959. See Cutler-Power-W. *test.*

**Wilder,** William H., U. S. ophthalmologst, 1860–1935. See W.'s *sign.*

**Wildermuth** (vil'der-moot), Hermann A., German psychiatrist, 1852–1907. See W.'s *ear.*

**Wilhelmy,** Ludwig F., German scientist, 1812–1864. See W. *balance.*

**Wilkie,** David P. D., Scottish surgeon, 1882–1938. See W.'s *artery, disease.*

**Wilkins,** Maurice H. F., New Zealand biophysicist in England, *1916. Nobel laureate, 1962, with Francis H. C. Crick and James D. Watson, for their discoveries concerning the molecular structure of nuclear acids and its significance for information transfer in living materials.

**Wilkinson,** D. S. See Sneddon-W. *disease.*

**Willan,** Robert, English physician, 1757–1812. See W.'s *lepra, lupus.*

**Willebrand,** E. A. von. See von Willebrand.

**Willems** (vil'ems), Charles, Belgian surgeon, 19th century. See W.'s *method.*

**Willett,** J. Abernethy, London obstetrician, †1932. See W. *clamp, forceps.*

**Willi,** H. See Prader-W. *syndrome.*

**Williams,** Anna W., American bacteriologist, 1863–1955. See Park-W. *bacillus,* Park-W. *fixative,* W.'s *stain.*

**Williams,** George A., U. S. obstetrician and gynecologist. See W.'s *operation.*

**Williamson,** Carl S., American surgeon, 1896–1952. See Mann-W. *operation, ulcer.*

**Willis,** Thomas, English physician, 1621–1675. See W.'s *centrum* nervosum, *circle, cords, pancreas, paracusis, pouch.*

**Williston,** S. W. See W.'s *law.*

**willow** (wil'o) [ A.S. *welig* ]. A tree of the genus *Salix;* the bark of several species but especially *S. fragilis,* is a source of salicin.

**Wilms** (vilms), Max, German surgeon, 1867–1918. See W.'s *tumor.*

**Wilms' method, operation.** See the nouns.

**Wilson,** Clifford, English physician, *1906. See Kimmelstiel-W. *disease, syndrome.*

**Wilson,** James, English surgeon, 1765–1821. See W.'s *muscle.*

**Wilson,** M. G., U. S. pediatrician, *1922. See W.-Mikity *syndrome.*

**Wilson,** Samuel A. Kinnier, English neurologist, 1878–1937. See W.'s *disease, syndrome.*

**Wilson,** Sir William J. E., English dermatologist, 1809–1884. See W.'s *disease,* W.'s *lichen.*

**Wilson block.** See under block.

**Wilson's method.** See under method.

**Winckel** (ving'kel), Franz C. W. von, German obstetrician, 1837–1911. See W.'s *disease.*

**windage** (win'dej). Wind contusion; injury of an internal organ caused by a large missile, which produces no lesion of the skin; the injury is due to the compression of the air or to the fact that the missile does actually strike a glancing blow.

**wind-broken.** Heaving; asthmatic; said of a horse.

**wind'burn.** Erythema of face due to exposure to wind.

**windgall** (wind'gawl). A soft, pulpy swelling in the neighborhood of the fetlock joint of the horse, varying in size from a pinhead to a large hen's egg.

**window** (win'do). Fenestra.

aortic w., a radiolucent region below the aortic arch in the left anterior oblique view, formed by the bifurcation of the trachea and traversed by the left pulmonary artery.

cochlear w., *fenestra* cochleae.

oval w., *fenestra* vestibuli.

round w., *fenestra* cochleae.

**wind'pipe.** Trachea.

**wind'puffs.** An affection of horses marked by a collection of synovial fluid between the tendons of the legs, particularly just above the fetlock joint, the prominence appearing on both sides of the tendon. The condition is most common in hard-worked animals and may end in lameness.

**Windscheid** (vint'shit), Franz, German physician, 1802–1910. See W.'s *disease.*

**wind'sucker.** Cribber.

**wind'sucking.** Cribbing.

**wine** [ Fr. *vin;* L. *vinum* ]. 1. The fermented juice of the grape. 2. A group of preparations consisting of a solution of one or more medicinal substances in w., usually white w. because of its comparatave freedom from tannin. There are no official w.'s.

high w., the strong spirit obtained by rectification or redistillation of low w. in making whisky.

low w., the first weak distillate obtained from the mash in the process of making whisky.

red w., claret; an alcoholic liquor made by fermenting grapes, the fruit of *Vitis vinifera,* with their skins. Has been used as a tonic.

**sherry w.,** sherry; a w. of amber color obtained originally from Jerez, Spain; it contains about 20 per cent of alcohol. Used in preparation of medicinal w.'s.

**wing.** 1. The anterior appendage of a bird. 2. In anatomy, ala; a wing-shaped part.

**angel's w.,** a deformity in which both scapulae project conspicuously; see also winged *scapula.*

**ashen w.,** *trigonum* nervi vagi.

**w. of crista galli,** *ala* cristae galli.

**gray w.,** *trigonum* nervi vagi.

**great w. of sphenoid bone,** *ala* major ossis sphenoidalis.

**Ingrassia's w.,** *ala* minor ossis sphenoidalis.

**lesser w. of sphenoid bone,** *ala* minor ossis sphenoidalis.

**w. of nostril,** *ala* nasi.

**w. of vomer,** *ala* vomeris.

**Winiwarter** (ve′ne-var-ter), Alexander von, German surgeon, 1848–1916. See W.-Buerger's *disease.*

**wink** [ A.S. *wincian* ]. To close and open the eyes rapidly; an involuntary act by which the tears are spread over the conjunctiva, keeping it moist.

**Winkelman,** Nathaniel W., American neurologist, 1891–1956. See W.'s *disease.*

**wink′er.** Colloquialism for eyelash.

**Winkler's disease.** See under disease.

**Winslow,** Jacob B., Danish anatomist in Paris, 1669–1760. See W.'s *foramen, ligament, pancrease, stars, stellulae* Winslowii.

**Winterbottom's sign.** See under sign.

**win′tergreen.** Gaultheria.

**w. oil,** gaultheria oil.

**Winternitz** (vin′ter-nits), Wilhelm, Vienna physician, 1835–1917. See W.'s *sound.*

**Wintersteiner,** Hugo, Austrian ophthalmologist, 1865–1918. See W.'s *rosettes.*

**Wintersteiner's compounds.** See under compound.

**wire** (wir). Slender and pliable rod or thread of metal.

**Kirschner's w.,** an apparatus for skeletal traction in long bone fracture.

**wi′ring.** Fastening together the ends of a broken bone by wire sutures.

**circumferential w.,** fixation of mandibular fractures by passing wires around a section of bone with the ends exiting into the oral cavity; *i.e.,* circummandibular and circumzygomatic w.

**continuous loop w.,** Stout's w.; the formation of wire loops on both maxillary and mandibular teeth, for the placement of intermaxillary elastics; used in reduction and fixation of fractures.

**craniofacial suspension w.,** a method of w. using areas of bones not contiguous with the oral cavity for the support of fractured jaw segments (*e.g.,* pyriform aperture, zygomatic arch, zygomatic process of the frontal bone).

**Gilmer w.,** a method of intermaxillary fixation in which single opposing teeth are wired circumferentially, and the wires are twisted together.

**Ivy loop w.,** placement of a wire around two adjacent teeth to provide an attachment for intermaxillary elastics.

**perialveolar w.,** fixing a splint to the maxillary arch by passing a wire through the alveolar process from the buccal plate to the palate.

**pyriform aperture w.,** a method of wiring using the nasal bones at the area of the pyriform aperture for the stabilization of fractures of the jaws.

**Stout's w.,** continuous loop w.

**Wirsung** (veer′soong), Johann G., German anatomist in Padua, 1600–1643. See W.'s *canal, duct.*

**wi′ry.** Resembling or having the feel of a wire; filiform and hard; denoting a variety of pulse.

**Wiskott-Aldrich syndrome.** See Aldrich *syndrome.*

**Wistar,** Caspar, American biologist, 1760–1818. See W. *rat.*

**witch hazel.** Hamamelis.

**withdraw′al.** 1. The act of removal or retreating. 2. The discontinuance of an addicting agent or medication. 3. A pattern of behavior, observed in schizophrenia and depression, characterized by a pathological retreat from interpersonal contact and social involvement, and leading to self-preoccupation.

**With′ering.** William, English physician and medical botanist, 1741–1799. Learning of the popular use of foxglove (digitalis) as a remedy for dropsy, tested its action in the edema of heart disease with such success that he recommended it to the profession.

**with′ers** [ A.S. *wither,* against ]. The region of the back of an animal, particularly of the horse, which lies between the shoulder blades.

**fistulous w.,** a fistula, caused by bacterial infection, of the w.

**wit′kop.** White head; dikwakwadi; a favoid condition of the scalp seen in South Africans.

**witzelsucht** (vit′sel-zukht) [ Ger. *witzeln,* to affect wit, + *sucht,* mania ]. A morbid tendency to pun, make poor jokes, and tell pointless stories, while being oneself inordinately entertained thereby.

**wob′bler.** A disease of young horses showing progressive weakness and incoordination, most evident in the hind legs. It is associated with lesions in the cervical region of the spinal cord and is the result of compression of the spinal cord by malformed cervical vertebrae.

**Woelde's triangle.** See under triangle.

**Wohlfart,** G. See W.-Kugelberg-Welander *disease.*

**Wohlfartia** (vōl-far′tǐ-ah). A genus of dipterous flesh flies (family Sarcophagidae); the larvae of some species breed in ulcerated surfaces and flesh wounds of men and animals.

**W. opa′ca,** *W. vigil.*

**W. vig′il,** *W. opaca;* produces cutaneous myiasis in human infants in eastern North America; the larvae penetrate the skin and cause infected, boil-like or furuncular lesions; mink and fox pups in fur farms, and probably rabbits and rodents, are attacked.

**Wohlgemuth** (vōl′gem-oot), Julius, German physician, *1874. See W.'s *unit.*

**Wolf-Orton bodies.** See under body.

**Wolfe,** John R., Glasgow ophthalmologist, 1824–1904. See W.'s *graft, method.*

**Wolff** (volf), Julius, German anatomist, 1836–1902. See W.'s *law.*

**Wolff** (volf), Kaspar F., German embryologist in Russia, 1733–1794. See Wolffian *body, cyst, duct, rest, ridge, tubules.*

**Wolff,** Louis, American physician, *1898. See W.-Parkinson-White *syndrome.*

**Wolf′fian.** Relating to or described by one of the name Wolff, specifically Kaspar Wolff.

**Wölfler** (vĕl′fler), Anton, Austrian surgeon, 1850–1917. See W.'s *gland, operation, suture.*

**wolfram** (wŏŏlf′ram). Tungsten.

**Wolfring,** Emilij F. von, Polish ophthalmologist, 1832–1906. See W.'s *glands.*

**wolfs′bane.** See aconite.

**Wollaston,** William H., English physician and physicist, 1766–1828. See W.'s *doublet, theory.*

**Wolman,** M. See W.'s *disease.*

**womb** (wŏŏm) [ A.S. the belly ]. Uterus.

**falling of the w.,** prolapsus uteri; procidentia uteri; metroptosia; hysteroptosia.

**Wood,** I. J., Australian physician. See W.'s biopsy *instrument.*

**Wood,** Robert W., U. S. physicist, 1868–1955. See W.'s *glass, light.*

**wood alcohol** (wŏŏd). Methyl alcohol.

**wood oil.** Gurjun balsam (see under balsam).

**wood wool.** A specially prepared, not compressed, wood fiber used for surgical dressings.

**wool** (wŏŏl). Lana; the hair of the sheep; sometimes, when defatted, used as a surgical dressing.

**wool alcohols** (BP). Wool wax alcohols; may be prepared by saponification of the grease of the wool of sheep and separation of the fraction that contains cholesterol (not less than 30 per cent) and other alcohols. Used to prepare wool alcohols ointment.

**wool fat** (BP). Adeps lanae; anhydrous lanolin (USP); the purified, anhydrous, fatlike substance obtained from the wool of sheep. See also lanolin and subentries.

**hy′drous w. fat** (BP), lanolin.

**Woolner,** Thomas, English sculptor, 1826–1892. See W.'s *tip.*

**woo'rali, woo'rara, woo'rari.** Curare.

**word salad.** A jumble of meaningless and unrelated words emitted by persons with certain kinds of schizophrenia.

**working out.** In psychoanalysis, the state in the treatment process in which the patient's personal history and psychodynamics are uncovered.

**working through.** In psychoanalysis, the process of obtaining additional insight and personality changes in a patient through repeated and varied examination of a conflict or problem; the interactions between free association, resistance, interpretation, and working through constitute the fundamental facets of this process.

**Worm,** Ole, Danish anatomist, 1588–1654. See Wormian *bones.*

**worm** (wurm) [ A.S. *wyrm* ]. 1. Once used to designate any member of the invertebrate group or subkingdom Vermes, a collective term no longer used taxonomically, it is now commonly used to designate any member of the separate phyla Annelida (the segmented or true worms), the Nemathelminthes (roundworms), and the Platyhelminthes (flatworms). For some types of worms not listed as subentries here (because they are usually written as one word), see the full name. 2. In anatomy, any structure resembling a w., *e.g.,* the midline part of the cerebellum. 3. In veterinary anatomy, lyssa (1).

    **African eye w.,** *Loa loa.*
    **bankrupt w.,** see *Trichostrongylus.*
    **black scour w.,** see *Trichostrongylus.*
    **caddis w.,** aquatic larva in the insect order Trichoptera.
    **dragon w.,** *Dracunculus medinensis.*
    **eye w.,** see *Thelazia.*
    **fleece w.,** wool *maggot.*
    **forked w.,** *Syngamus trachea.*
    **guinea w.,** *Dracunculus medinensis.*
    **hair w.,** see *Trichostrongylus.*
    **kidney w. of swine,** *Stephanurus dentatus.*
    **lard w. of swine,** *Stephanurus dentatus.*
    **Manson's eye w.,** *Oxyspirura mansoni.*
    **meal w.,** the larva of beetles of the genus *Tenebrio;* both larvae and adults are important pests, destroying flour, meal and other cereal products; they are also intermediate hosts of the nematode parasite, *Gongylonema,* and of various tapeworms of the genus *Hymenolepis.*
    **Medi'na w.,** *Dracunculus medinensis.*
    **palisade w.,** see *Strongylus.*
    **pork w.,** *Trichinella spiralis.*
    **seat w.,** *Enterobius vermicularis.*
    **serpent w.,** *Dracunculus medinensis.*
    **stomach w.,** *Haemonchus contortus.*
    **thorny-headed w.'s,** see Acanthocephala; also *Moniliformis.*
    **tongue w.,** see *Pentastomida.*
    **trichina w.,** *Trichinella spiralis.*
    **twisted wire w.,** *Haemonchus contortus.*

**worm bark.** Andira.

**Wormley,** Theodore G., American chemist, 1826–1897. See W.'s *test.*

**Worm-Mueller** (vorm-mū'ler), Jacob, Norwegian physician, 1834–1889. See W.-M.'s *formula.*

**worm'seed.** 1. Santonica. 2. Chenopodium.

**worm'wood.** Absinthium.

**wort** [ A.S. *wyrt,* a plant ]. 1. A suffix in the popular names of many plants, such as liverwort, lungwort, woundwort, etc. 2. An infusion of malt.

**Worth,** Claud, British ophthalmologist, 1869–1936. See W.'s *amblyoscope.*

**Woulfe,** Peter, English chemist, 1727–1803. See W.'s *bottle.*

**wound** (wōōnd). 1. An injury or traumatism to any of the tissues of the body, caused by mechanical violence, with or without a solution of continuity. 2. A surgical incision.

    **abraded w.,** abrasion (1).
    **avulsed w.,** a w. caused by or resulting from avulsion.
    **blowing w.,** open *pneumothorax.*

    **contused w.,** an injury to the soft parts without a break in the skin. See also bruise and subentries under contusion.
    **crease w. of head,** tangential w. of head.
    **gunshot w.,** one made with a bullet or other missile projected by a firearm.
    **gutter w.,** a tangential glancing w. that merely makes a furrow on the side of the injured part, without perforating.
    **incised w.,** a clean cut made with a sharp instrument.
    **lacerated w.,** a tear of the tissues.
    **nonpenetrating w.,** injury within thorax or abdomen, without remarkable trauma to the surface of the body.
    **open w.,** one in which the affected tissues are freely exposed by an external opening.
    **penetrating w.,** one that extends into the abdomen or other cavity of the body.
    **penetrating w. of head,** an open w. in which the dura mater is pierced.
    **perforating w.,** a w. with hole of entrance and exit.
    **perforating w. of head,** a penetrating head w. that traverses the cranial cavity and the integument.
    **puncture w.,** one made by a narrow, pointed instrument.
    **puncture w. of head,** laceration in which the orifice is relatively small compared to the depth.
    **seton w.,** a tangential perforating w., the wounds of entrance and exit being on the same side of the body, head, or limb involved.
    **stab w.,** stab (2).
    **subcuta'neous w.,** one in which there is no opening or only a very small one in the skin.
    **sucking w.,** open *pneumothorax.*
    **tangen'tial w.,** a w., whether perforating (seton w.) or glancing (gutter w.), involving only one side of the injured part.
    **tangential w. of head,** a head w. made by a missile the trajectory of which is tangential to the curvature of the skull; also called gutter w., crease w.
    **traumatopneic w.,** open *pneumothorax.*

**W.r.** Abbreviation for Wassermann reaction.

**Wrᵃ.** Abbreviation for a very rare blood group antigen sometimes responsible for hemolytic disease of the newborn. See low frequency blood groups, in appendix 2.

**wreath** (rēth) [ A.S. *wraeth,* a bandage ]. 1. Spirem. 2. A structure resembling a wreath.
    **ciliary w.,** *corona* ciliaris.
    **daughter w.,** diaster, viewed from the surface.
    **mother w.,** aster, viewed from the surface.

**Wreden** (vra'den), Robert R., St. Petersburg otologist, 1837–1893. See W.'s *sign.*

**Wright,** James Homer, Boston pathologist, 1871–1928. See W.'s *stain.*

**Wright,** Marmaduke Burr, Cincinnati obstetrician, 1803–1879. See W.'s *version.*

**Wright respirometer.** See under respirometer.

**wrightine** (rīt'ēn). Conessine.

**wrinkle** (ring'kl). A furrow, fold, or crease in the skin.

**Wrisberg** (vriz'berg), Heinrich A., German anatomist, 1739–1808. See W.'s *cartilage, ganglia, ligament, nerve, tubercle.*

**wrist** (rist) [ A.S. wrist joint, ankle joint ]. Carpus (1).

**wrist-drop.** Carpoptosia; drop hand; paralysis of the extensors of the w. and fingers from lesion of the musculospiral nerve or from lead poisoning.

**wryneck** (ri'nek). Torticollis.

**Wuchereria** (vu-ker-ēr'ĭ-ah). A genus of filarial worms of man in the superfamily Filarioidea (class Nematoda, phylum Nemathelminthes); characterized by adult forms that live chiefly in lymphatic vessels and produce the widespread tropical infection, filariasis; the extreme form of this infection is elephantiasis. See also *Filaria,* the common name and also the former generic term for parasites now classified as *W,* and *Brugia,* a separate genus of filarial worms including *B. malayi,* formerly known as *W. malayi.*
    **W. bancrofti,** the Bancroftian filaria, formerly termed *Filaria bancrofti* or *F. nocturna;* endemic in South Pacific islands, coastal India and Burma, and throughout other tropical regions (including Caribbean islands); adults are white, cylindroid, threadlike worms (females, 70 to 100 by 0.2 to 0.4 mm.; males, 25 to 45 by 0.1 mm.), and the

microfilariae are ensheathed (150 to 300 by 7 to 10 μ), with rounded anterior end and tapered, non-nucleated tail. Transmitted to man (only definitive host) by mosquitoes, especially *Culex quinquefasciatus* and *Aedes pseudocutellaris*, but also several other species of *Culex, Aedes, Anopheles,* and *Mansonia.* The adult worms inhabit the larger lymphatic vessels (*e.g.,* in the extremities (especially lower), breasts, spermatic cord, and retroperitoneal tissues) and the sinuses of lymph nodes (*e.g.,* the popliteal, femoral, and inguinal groups, and also the epitrochlear and axillary nodes), where they sometimes cause (1) temporary obstruction to the flow of lymph, and (2) slight or moderate degrees of inflammation. The chief damage in filariasis results after death of the adult worms, inasmuch as this leads to granulomatous inflammation and permanent fibrosis causing obstruction of the lymphatic channels from dense, hyalinized scars in the subcutaneous tissues. The most serious consequence is elephantiasis or pachydermia, a form of chronic fibrosis of the affected tissues, controlled only by tight bandaging in early or moderate forms or by surgery in late cases. A characteristic of typical *W. bancrofti* microfilaremia is its sharp nocturnal periodicity, apparently tied to the nocturnal biting habits of the vector mosquitoes. In other areas, as in parts of Polynesia, mosquitoes are not strictly night-biters and the microfilarial periodicity is modified or absent.

**W. malayi,** *Brugia malayi.*

**wuchereriasis** (vu-ker'e-ri'ă-sis). Infestation with worms of the genus *Wuchereria;* also called filariasis.

**wu'rari.** Curare.

**Wurster** (voor'ster), Casimir, German chemist, 1856–1913. See W.'s *reagent, test.*

**Wyeth,** John A., U. S. surgeon, 1845–1922. See W.'s *operation.*

**Wyle's test.** See under test.

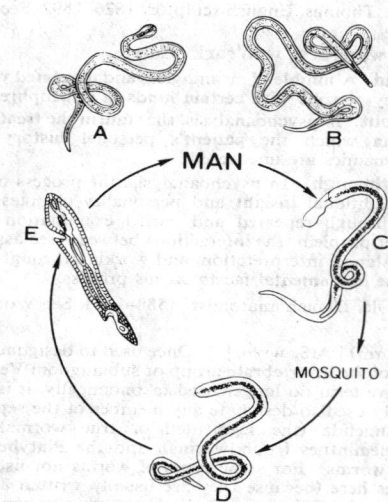

**Life Cycle of *Wuchereria bancrofti***

*A,* male, in man; *B,* female, in man; *C,* sheathed microfilaria; *D* and *E,* developmental cycle in mosquito.

**Wylie,** W. Gill, U. S. gynecologist, 1848–1923. See W.'s *drain, operation.*

**X.** Symbol for (1) Kienbock's *unit;* (2) reactance; (3) xanthosine.

**xanchromatic** (zan-kro-mat'ik). Xanthochromatic.

**xanth-.** See xantho-.

**xanthaline** (zan'thă-lēn). Papaveraldine; 6,7-dimethoxy-1-veratroylisoquinoline; an alkaloid, $C_{20}H_{19}NO_5$, derived from the mother liquor of morphine.

**xanthates** (zan'thāts). The *O* esters of xanthic acid.

**xanthelasma** (zan'the-laz'mah) [ xanth- + G. *elasma*, a beaten metal plate ]. Obsolete term for xanthoma.
  **x. palpebra'rum,** Obsolete term for *xanthoma* palpebrarum.

**xanthelas'mato'sis.** Obsolete term for xanthomatosis.

**xanthelasmoidea** (zan-the-laz-mo-id'e-ah) [ xanthelasma + G. *eidos*, resemblance ]. *Urticaria* pigmentosa.

**xanthematin** (zan'them'ă-tin). A yellow substance derived from hematin by treating with nitric acid.

**xanthemia** (zan-the'mī-ah) [ xanth- + G. *haima*, blood ]. Carotenemia.

**xanthene** (zan'thēn). The basic structure of many natural products, drugs, dyes (*e.g.,* fluorescein), indicators, pesticides, antibiotics, etc. Not to be confused with xanthine.

9*H*-Xanthene

**xanthic** (zan'thik). 1. Yellow; yellowish. 2. Relating to xanthine.
  **x. acid,** dithiocarbonic acid; HO—CS—SH.

**xanthine** (zan'thin). 2,6-Dioxopurine; 2,6(1*H*,3*H*)-purinedione; oxidation product of guanine and hypoxanthine, precursor of uric acid; occurs in many organs and in the urine, occasionally forming urinary calculi.
  **x. dehydrogenase,** an oxidoreductase (EC 1.2.1.37) oxidizing xanthine to uric acid with $NAD^+$ as the oxidant; see also x. oxidase.
  **x. nucleotide,** xanthosine phosphate.
  **x. oxidase,** hypoxanthine oxidase; Schardinger enzyme; a flavoprotein containing molybdenum; an oxidoreductase (EC 1.2.3.2) catalyzing oxidation by $O_2$ of xanthine to uric acid, producing $H_2O_2$; also oxidizes hypoxanthine, some other purines and pterins, and aldehydes. See also x. dehydrogenase.
  **x. ribonucleoside,** xanthosine.

**xanthinol niacinate** (zan'thī-nōl) (USAN). COMPLAMIN; 7-[ 2-hydroxy-3-[ (2-hydroxyethyl)-methylamino ]propyl ]-theophylline compound with nicotinic acid; peripheral vasodilator.

**xanthinuria** (zan'thī-nu'rī-ah) [ xanthine + G. *ouron*, urine ]. 1. The excretion of abnormally large amounts of xanthine in the urine. 2. A rare heritable disorder resulting from defective synthesis of xanthine oxidase; characterized by urinary excretion of xanthine in place of uric acid, hypouricemia, and, in some cases, the formation of xanthine stones.

**xanthism** (zan'thizm) [ G. *xanthos*, yellowish ]. Rufous albinism; a pigmentary anomaly of Negroes, characterized by red or yellow-red hair color, copper-red skin, and often dilution of iris pigment.

**xanthiu'ria.** Xanthinuria.

**xantho-, xanth-** (zan'tho-) [ G. *xanthos*, yellow ]. Combining forms meaning yellow or yellowish.

**xanthochroia** (zan-tho-kroy'ah). Xanthochromia.

**xanthochromatic** (zan-tho-kro-mat'ik). Xanthochromic; xanchromatic; yellow-colored.

**xanthochromia** (zan-tho-kro'mī-ah) [ xantho- + G. *chrōma*, color ]. The occurrence of patches of yellow color in the skin, resembling xanthoma, but without the nodules

or plates; also called xanthochroia; xanthopathy; xanthoderma (1); cholesteroderma; yellow disease (1).

**xanthochromic** (zan-tho-kro'mik). Xanthochromatic.

**xanthochroous** (zan-thok'ro-us) [ xantho- + G. *chroa*, complexion. CHROM- ]. Having a fair yellowish complexion; light-skinned; blond.

**xanthocyanopsia** (zan-tho-si-an-op'se-ah) [ xantho- + G. *kyanos*, blue substance, + *ops*, eye ]. Anomalous color vision in which yellow and blue are distinguished, but not red and green. See also red-green *blindness*.

**xanthoderma** (zan-tho-der'mah) [ xantho- + G. *derma*, skin ]. 1. Xanthochromia. 2. Any yellow coloration of the skin.

**xanthodont** (zan'tho-dont) [ xantho- + G. *odous*, tooth ]. One who has yellow teeth.

**xanthoerythrodermia perstans** (zan'tho-e-rith'ro-der'mī-ah per'stanz). Parapsoriasis.

**xanthogranuloma** (zan'tho-gran'u-lo'mah). A peculiar infiltration of retroperitoneal tissue by lipid macrophages; occurs most commonly in women, and etiology is uncertain.
  **juvenile x.,** nevoxanthoendothelioma.

**xanthogranulomatous** (zan'tho-gran'u-lo'mahtus). Relating to, of the nature of, or affected by xanthogranuloma.

**xanthoma** (zan'tho'mah) [ xantho- + G. suffix -*oma*, tumor ]. Fibroma lipomatodes; vitiligoidea; a yellow nodule or plaque, especially of the skin, composed of lipid-laden histiocytes.
  **x. diabetico'rum,** the eruption of cutaneous lesions of x. in some cases of diabetes.
  **x. dissemina'tum,** xanthomatosis.
  **fibrous x.,** dermatofibroma.
  **x. mul'tiplex,** xanthomatosis.
  **x. palpebra'rum,** soft, yellow-orange plaques found about the eyes; the most common type of x.
  **x. planum,** a form marked by the occurrence of yellow bands or rectangular plates in the corium.
  **x. tubero'sum,** x. tuberosum simplex; xanthomatosis associated with increased blood cholesterol and phospholipids.
  **x. tubero'sum sim'plex,** x. tuberosum.

**xanthomatosis** (zan-tho'mă-to'sis). Xanthoma disseminatum or multiplex; lipoid or lipid granulomatosis; cholesterosis cutis; widespread xanthomas, especially on the elbows and knees, that sometimes affect mucous membranes and are sometimes associated with metabolic disturbances.
  **x. bulbi,** ulcerative fatty degeneration of the cornea after injury.
  **cerebrotendinous x.,** cerebrotendinous cholesterinosis; a familial disorder associated with an accumulation of cholesterol in the brain and in tendon xanthomas, and with dementia and cataracts.
  **familial hypercholesteremic x.,** type II familial *hyperlipoproteinemia*.
  **normal cholestere'mic x.,** Hand-Schüller-Christian *disease*.

**xanthomatous** (zan-tho'mă-tus). Relating to xanthoma.

**xanthomycins** (zan'tho-mi'sinz). Antibiotics obtained from culture of unnamed strains of streptomyces; probably related to the actinomycins.

**xanthone** (zan'thōn). 9-Xanthenone; xanthen-9-one; benzophenone oxide; ovicide for moth eggs.

**xanthopathy** (zan-thop'ă-thī) [ xantho- + G. *pathos*, suffering ]. Xanthochromia.

**xanthophore** (zan'tho-fōr) [ xantho- + G. *phoros*, bearing ]. Lipophore; one of the cells of the skin of certain fish and other cold-blooded animals which contain mobile yellowish granules.

**xanthophose** (zan'tho-fōz) [ xantho- + G. *phōs*, light ]. A yellow phose.

**xanthophyll** (zan'tho-fil). 3,3'-Dioxy-α-carotene; lutein (2); luteol; a yellow plant pigment, occurring also in egg yolk.

**xanthopia** (zan-tho'pī-ah). Xanthopsia.

**xanthoplasty** (zan'tho-plas'tĭ) [ xantho- + G. *plassō*, to form ]. Xanthoderma.

**xanthoproteic** (zan-tho-pro'te-ik). Relating to xanthoprotein.

**x. acid,** a noncrystallizable yellow substance derived from proteins upon treating with nitric acid.

**xanthoprotein** (zan-tho-pro'te-in). The yellow product formed upon treating protein with hot nitric acid, probably from nitration of phenyl groups.

**xanthopsia** (zan-thop'sĭ-ah) [ xantho- + G. *opsis*, vision ]. Yellow vision; a state in which all objects appear of a yellow color. May occur in picric acid and santonin poisoning, in jaundice, and in digitalis intoxication.

**xanthopsin** (zan-thop'sin). Obsolete term for all-*trans*-retinal; see under retinal.

**xanthopsydracia** (zan-thop-sĭ-dra'sĭ-ah) [ G. *xanthos*, yellow, + *psydrax* (*psydrak-*), a blister on the tip of the tongue, a lie-blister, fr. *pseudō*, to lie, cheat ]. An eruption of small yellow pustules.

**xanthopterin** (zan-thop'ter-in). 2-Amino-4,6-pteridinediol; a pigment found in the wings of butterflies. Structurally similar to the pteridine component in folic acid; partially cures cytopenia in monkeys but is ineffective in pernicious anemia.

**xanthopuccine** (zan-tho-puk'sēn). Canadine.

**xanthosine** (zan'tho-sēn, -sin). 9-β-D-Ribosylxanthine; xanthine ribonucleoside; the deamination product of guanosine (O replacing —NH₂). Abbreviation, X or Xao.

**x. phosphate,** xanthine nucleotide; xanthylic acid; the phosphoric ester of xanthosine.

**xanthosis** (zan-tho'sis) [ xantho- + G. suffix -*osis*, condition ]. A yellowish discoloration of degenerating tissues, especially seen in malignant neoplasms.

**xanthous** (zan'thus) [ G. *xanthos*, yellow ]. Yellow.

**xanthoxylum** (zan-thoks'ĭ-lum) [ xantho- + G. *xylon*, wood ]. The dried bark or dried, fully grown berries of *Xanthoxylum americanum* or *X. clava-herculis* (family Rutaceae), northern and southern prickly ash, respectively; carminative and diaphoretic.

**xanthurenic acid** (zan'ther-re'nik). 4,8-Dihydroxyquinoline-2-carboxylic acid; 4,8-dihydroquinaldic acid; the sulfur-yellow crystals form a red compound with Millon reagent, or an intensely green one with ferrous sulfate; excreted in the urine of pyridoxine-deficient animals after the ingestion of tryptophan, and from rats fed almost exclusively with fibrin.

**xanthu'ria.** Xanthinuria.

**xanthyl** (zan'thil). A radical consisting of xanthine minus a hydrogen atom.

**xanthylic** (zan-thil'ik). Relating to xanthine.

**x. acid,** xanthosine phosphate.

**Xao.** Abbreviation for xanthosine (also denoted by the symbol or abbreviation, X).

**Xe.** Chemical symbol of the element xenon.

**xeno-** (zen'o-) [ G. *xenos*, guest, host, stranger, foreign. XEN- ]. Combining form meaning strange, or denoting relation to foreign material.

**xenodiagno'sis** (zen'o-di-ag-no'sis). 1. A method of diagnosing *Trypanosoma cruzi* infection (Chagas' disease) in man. Infection-free *Triatoma* bugs are fed on the suspected person and the trypanosome is identified by microscopic examination of the intestinal contents of the bug after a suitable incubation period. 2. A similar method of biological diagnosis based upon experimental exposure of a parasite-free normal host capable of allowing the organism in question to multiply, hence being more easily and reliably detected.

**xenogeneic** (zen'o-jen-e'ik). Xenogenic (2); heterologous, with respect to tissue grafts, especially when donor and recipient belong to widely separated species.

**xenogenic** (zen'o-jen'ik) [ xeno- + G. suffix -*gen*, producing ]. 1. Originating outside of the organism, or from a foreign substance that has been introduced into the organism. 2. Alternative spelling of xenogeneic, *q. v.*

**xenogenous** (zĕ-noj'ĕ-nus). Xenogenic.

**xenograft** (zen'o-graft). Heterograft, in the sense of a graft from an animal of a species of one order to that of another order.

**xenomenia** (zen-o-me'nĭ-ah) [ xeno- + G. *mēn*, month ]. Vicarious *menstruation.*

**xenon** (zen'on) [ G. *xenos*, a stranger ]. A gaseous element, symbol Xe, atomic no. 54, atomic weight 131.30; present in minute proportion in the atmosphere; produces general anesthesia in concentrations of 70 vol. per cent.

**xenon-133.** ¹³³Xe; a radioisotope of xenon with a gamma emission and a physical half-life of 5.27 days; used in the study of pulmonary function and organ blood flow.

**xenoparasite** (zen'o-păr'ă-sīt). An ecoparasite that becomes pathogenic in consequence of weakened resistance on the part of its host.

**xenophobia** (zen-o-fo'bĭ-ah) [ xeno- + G. *phobos*, fear ]. A morbid fear of meeting strangers.

**xenophonia** (zen-o-fo'nĭ-ah) [ xeno- + G. *phōnē*, voice ]. A speech defect marked by an alteration in accent and intonation.

**xenophthalmia** (zen'of-thal'mĭ-ah) [ xeno- + ophthalmia ]. Inflammation excited by the presence of a foreign body in the eye.

**Xenopsylla** (zen-op-sil'ah) [ xeno- + G. *psylla*, flea ]. A genus of fleas.

**X. cheo'pis,** the rat flea of tropical countries that transmits the plague bacillus; serves as a potent vector largely because its gut becomes "blocked" by a mass of the bacteria *Yersina pestis*, which prevents the flea from feeding normally, so that they are inclined to attack man and other hosts; an important source of infection in traditional epidemic areas such as India.

**Xenopus** (zen'o-pus) [ xeno- + G. *pous*, foot ]. A genus of clawed frogs or toads of the family *Pipidae.*

**xenyl** (zen'il). A radical consisting of biphenyl minus a hydrogen atom.

**xeransis** (ze-ran'sis) [ G. *xēransis*, fr. *xēros*, dry. XER- ]. Siccation; a gradual loss of moisture in the tissues.

**xerantic** (ze-ran'tik). Siccant; siccative; causing dryness.

**xerasia** (ze-ra'zĭ-ah) [ G. *xērasia*, fr. *xēros*, dry ]. A condition of the hair characterized by dryness and brittleness.

**xero-** [ G. *xeros*, dry. XER- ]. Combining form meaning dry.

**xerochilia** (zēr'o-ki'lĭ-ah) [ xero- + G. *cheilos*, lip ]. Dryness of lips.

**xeroderma** (zēr'o-der'mah) [ xero- + G. *derma*, skin ]. Dermatoxerasia; excessive dryness of the skin due to a slight increase of the horny layer and diminished cutaneous secretion; a mild form of ichthyosis.

**x. pigmento'sum,** Kaposi's dermatosis; atrophoderma pigmentosa; angioma pigmentosum et atrophicum; an eruption of exposed skin, occurring in childhood, characterized by numerous pigmented spots resembling freckles, larger atrophic lesions eventually resulting in glossy white thinning of the skin, surrounded by telangiectases, and multiple solar keratoses which undergo malignant change at an early age. The condition appears to result from an inherited hypersensitivity to the carcinogenic effect of ultraviolet light.

**xeroma** (ze-ro'mah). Xerophthalmia.

**xeromenia** (zēr'o-me'nĭ-ah) [ xero- + G. *mēniaia*, menses ]. The occurrence of the usual constitutional symptoms at the menstrual period without any show of blood.

**xeromycteria** (zēr'o-mik-tēr'ĭ-ah) [ xero- + G. *myktēr*, the nose ]. Extreme dryness of the nasal mucous membrane.

**xeronosus** (ze-ron'o-sus) [ xero- + G. *nosos*, disease ]. Xerosis.

**xerophagia** (zēr'o-fa'jĭ-ah) [ xero- + G. *phagein*, to eat ]. Xerophagy; the eating of dry food; subsisting on a dry diet.

**xerophagy** (ze-rof'ă-jĭ). Xerophagia.

**xerophthalmia** (zēr'of-thal'mĭ-ah) [ xero- + G. *ophthalmos*, eye ]. Xerophthalmus; conjunctivitis arida; xeroma; ophthalmoxerosis; extreme dryness of the conjunctiva, which loses its luster and becomes skinlike in appearance from a lack of intrinsic secretion; may be due to local disease or to a systemic deficiency of vitamin A.

**xerophthalmus** (zēr'of-thal'mus). Xerophthalmia.

**xeroradiography** (zēr'o-ra'dĭ-og'ră-fĭ). The making of a radiogram by means of a specially coated plate and developing without the use of liquid chemicals. The plate consists of a metal base that is coated with a layer of a semiconductor, such as selenium which holds an electric charge in the dark; the latter is dissipated by light. The plate is charged in a special chamber from a high voltage, direct current source. The plate is exposed in the usual way and then developed in the dark-room by dusting it with a powder that is taken up by the surface of the plate in proportion to the electric charge retained by the plate; thus an image is outlined.

**xerosis** (ze-ro'sis) [ xero- + G. suffix -osis, condition ]. 1. Pathologic dryness of the skin (xeroderma), the conjunctiva (xerophthalmia), or mucous membranes. 2. The normal evolutionary sclerosis of the tissues in old age.

  **x. parenchymatosus,** superficial drying of the conjunctiva due to diffuse scarring with closure of the openings of the lacrimal gland.

**xerostomia** (zēr'o-sto'mĭ-ah) [ xero- + G. *stoma*, mouth ]. A dryness of the mouth, having a varied etiology, resulting from diminished or arrested salivary secretion, or asialism.

**xerotes** (ze-ro'tēz) [ G. *xērotēs* ]. Dryness.

**xerotic** (ze-rot'ik). Dry; affected with xerosis.

**xerotocia** (zēr'o-to'sĭ-ah) [ xero- + G. *tokos*, labor ]. Dry *labor.*

**xerotripsis** (zēr'o-trip'sis) [ xero- + G. *tripsis*, a rubbing, fr. *tribō*, to rub ]. Dry friction.

**Xg blood group.** See appendix 2, Blood Groups.

**ximenynic acid.** Santalbic acid.

**xiphisternal** (zif-ĭ-ster'nal). Relating to the xiphisternum (xiphoid process).

**xiphisternum** (zif'ĭ-ster'num) [ xiphoid + G. *sternon,* chest ]. *Processus* xiphoideus.

**xipho-, xiph-, xiphi-** (zif'o-) [ G. *xiphos,* sword ]. Combining forms meaning xiphoid.

**xiphocostal** (zif'o-kos'tal) [ xipho- + L. *costa,* rib ]. Relating to the xiphoid process and the ribs.

**xiphodynia** (zif'o-din'ĭ-ah) [ xipho- + G. *odynē,* pain ]. Xyphoidalgia; pain of a neuralgic character, in the region of the xiphoid cartilage; see also hypersensitive xiphoid *syndrome.*

**xiphoid** (zif'oyd) [ xipho- + G. *eidos,* appearance ]. Sword-shaped; ensiform; applied to the processus xiphoideus.

**xiphoidalgia** (zif'oy-dal'jĭ-ah) [ xiphoid + G. *algos,* pain ]. Xiphodynia.

**xiphoi'deus** [ L. ] [ NA ]. Xiphoid.

**xiphoiditis** (zif'oy-di'tis) [ xiphoid + G. suffix -itis, inflammation ]. Inflammation of the ensiform cartilage of the sternum.

**xiphopagotomy** (zif'o-pă-got'o-mī) [ xiphopagus, + G. *tomē,* incision ]. Separation of twins joined at xiphoid.

**xiphopagus** (zĭ-fop'ă-gus) [ xipho- + G. *pagos,* something fixed ]. Conjoined twins united in the region of the xiphoid

process of the sternum.

**x-ray.** See under ray.

**xyl-, xylo-** [ G. *xylon,* wood ]. Combining forms relating to wood or to xylose.

**xylene** (zi'lēn). Xylol.

**xylenobacillin** (zi'le-no-bă-sil'in). A toxic substance extracted from cultures of the tubercle bacillus by treatment with xylol.

**xylenol** (zi'le-nol). $(CH_3)_2C_6H_3OH$; dimethylphenol; occurring in six isomeric forms. Used in the manufacture of coal tar disinfectants and synthetic resins.

**xylidine** (zi'lĭ-dēn). Aminoxylene, aminodimethylbenzene; $(CH_3)_2C_6H_3NH_2$. Used as a reagent and in the manufacture of dyes.

**xylobalsamum** (zi'lo-bawl'să-mum). The dried twigs of *Commiphora opobalsamum* (family Burseraceae).

**xyloidin** (zi-loy'din). Pyroxylin.

**xyloketose** (zi'lo-ke'tōs). Xylulose.

**xylol** (zi'lol). Xylene; dimethylbenzene; $C_6H_4(CH_3)_2$; a volatile liquid obtained from coal tar, having physical and chemical properties similar to those of benzene; it occurs as three isomers; *m-, o-,* and *p-*xylol; used as a solvent, in the manufacture of chemicals and synthetic fibers, and in histology and microscopy.

**xylometazoline hydrochloride** (zi'lo-mĕ-taz'o-lēn) (NF). OTRIVIN; 2-(4'-*tert*-butyl-2',6'-dimethylphenylmethyl)imidazoline hydrochloride; a sympathomimetic drug used as a nasal decongestant.

**xylopro'pamine.** ESANIN; α,3,4-trimethylphenethylamine; sympathomimetic drug.

**xylopyranose** (zi'lo-pi'ră-nōs). Xylose in pyranose form.

**xylose** (zi'lōs). Wood sugar; an aldopentose, isomeric with ribose (see structures under sugars); obtained by fermentation or hydrolysis of naturally occurring carbohydrate substances, *e.g.,* in wood fiber.

**xylulose** (zi'lu-lōs). *threo*-Pentulose; α-xyloketose; a 2-ketopentose. L-Xylulose appears in the urine in cases of essential pentosuria. D-Xylulose 5-phosphate is an intermediate in pentose metabolism.

**xylyl** (zi'lil). The radical consisting of xylene minus a hydrogen atom.

  **x. bromide,** $CH_3C_6H_4CH_2Br$; the *o-, m-,* and *p-* forms are powerful lacrimators.

**xylylene** (zi'lĭ-lēn). The radical consisting of xylene minus two hydrogen atoms.

**xyrospasm** (zi'ro-spazm) [ G. *xyron,* razor, fr. *xyō,* to scrape ]. Shaving *cramp.*

**xysma** (ziz'mah) [ G. filings, shavings, fr. *xyō,* to scrape ]. Membranous shreds in the feces.

**xyster** (zis'ter) [ G. scraper, fr. *xyō,* to scrape ]. A raspatory.

# Y

**Y.** Chemical symbol of the element yttrium.

**yanggona.** Yaqona.

**yaqona** (yang'go-nah) [ Fijian name ]. Kava (2); yanggona; a Fijian drink made from the powdered root of *Piper methysticum* (family Piperaceae); excessive drinking of it causes a state of hyperexcitability and a loss of power in the legs; chronic intoxication induces roughening of the skin and a state of debility. See also methysticum.

**yar'row.** *Achillea.*

**Yasuda's method.** See under method.

**yaw.** Frambesioma; an individual lesion of the eruption of yaws.

    **mother y.,** mamanpian; a large granulomatous lesion, usually considered to be the initial lesion in yaws, and usually occurring on the hand or foot.

**yawn** [ A.S. *gānian* ]. 1. To gape. 2. An involuntary opening of the mouth, usually accompanied by a movement of respiration; it may be a sign of drowsiness or of vital depression, as after hemorrhage, but is often caused by suggestion.

**yawn'ing.** The act of producing a yawn; pandiculation; chasma; gaping; oscitation.

**yaws** [ African, *yaw,* a raspberry ]. An infectious tropical disease caused by *Treponema pertenue;* characterized by the development of crusted, granulomatous ulcers on extremities; may involve bone, but, unlike syphilis, does not produce central nervous system or cardiovascular pathology. Also variously known as pian; rupia (2); boubas; bubas, Amboyna button; mycosis framboesiodes; frambesia; polypapilloma (2); granuloma tropicum; zymotic papilloma.

    **bosch y.,** *pian* bois.

    **bush y.,** *pian* bois.

    **crab y.,** foot y.

    **foot y.,** crab y.; tubba; tubbae; y. of the feet with keratoderma of the palms and soles and ulcer formation.

    **forest y.,** *pian* bois.

    **guinea corn y.,** a form in which the lesions resemble grains of Indian corn.

    **ringworm y.,** round, scaling, and crusted lesions that resemble ringworm.

**Yb.** Chemical symbol for the element ytterbium.

**yearling** (yēr'ling). An animal between one and two years of age. The term is generally applied to horses and cattle.

**yeast** (yēst) [ A.S. *gyst* ]. Y.'s are true fungi whose usual growth form is unicellular. Used properly the term y. refers to ascomycetes which possess a unicellular thallus, reproduce asexually by budding or transverse division and sexually by ascospore formation originating from a zygote or parthenogenetically from a somatic cell. The Saccharomycetaceae contain the y.'s *Saccharomyces cerevisiae* is a common species. As the name implies, the y.'s are active fermenters of carbohydrate. The term y.-like fungus is often applied to fungi which are not known to form ascospores, but otherwise possess the characteristics listed above; such forms include members of the genera *Candida, Geotrichum, Cryptococcus,* etc. Such asporogenous y.-like fungi are properly placed with the Fungi Imperfecti unless methods of sexual reproduction are known.

    **y. adenylic acid,** see adenylic acid.

    **brewers' y.,** y. produced by *Saccharomyces cerevisiae;* a by-product from brewing of beer.

    **compressed y.,** the moist living cells of *Saccharomyces cerevisiae* combined with a starchy or absorbent base.

    **cultivated y.,** a form propagated by culture and used in breadmaking, brewing, etc.

    **dried y.,** consists of the dry cells of a suitable strain of *Saccharomyces cerevisiae;* brewers' dried y., debittered brewers' dried y., or primary dried y. are the sources of dried y. It contains not less than 45 per cent of protein, and in each gram not less than 0.3 mg. of nicotinic acid, 0.04 mg. of riboflavin, and 0.12 mg. of thiamin hydrochloride; used as a dietary supplement.

    **y. nucleic acid,** ribonucleic acid.

    **primary dried y.,** source of dried y. obtained from suitable strains of *Saccharomyces cerevisiae* grown in media other than those required for the production of beer.

    **wild y.,** any of the uncultivated forms of y.'s, useless as ferments and sometimes pathogenic.

**yellow** (yel'o) [ A.S. *geolu* ]. 1. A color, that of gold or butter, occupying a position in the spectrum between green and orange. For individual yellow dyes see specific name. 2. Flavescent; xanthic; in combination, xantho-.

    **brilliant y.,** an indicator dye changing from y. to orange or red at pH 6.4 to 8.0.

    **indicator y.,** a compound formed from visual purple as a stage in the bleaching of this pigment by light; the name is derived from the fact that it changes color with a change in pH, being a deep chrome yellow between pH 3.3 and 4.0 and a pale lemon yellow between pH 9.0 and 10.0.

    **visual y.,** all-*trans*-retinal; see under retinal.

**yerba** (yer'bah) [ Sp. ]. Herb.

    **y. maté,** see maté.

    **y. santa,** eriodictyon.

**Yersinia** (yer-sin'ĭ-ah) [ A. J. E. *Yersin* ]. A genus of motile and nonmotile, nonsporeforming bacteria (family Enterobacteriaceae) containing Gram-negative, unencapsulated, ovoid to rod-shaped cells. These organisms are nonmotile at 37°C., but some species are motile at temperatures below 30°C.; motile cells are peritrichous. Citrate is not used as a sole source of carbon. These organisms are parasitic on man and other animals. The type species is *Y. pestis.*

    **Y. enterocolitica,** a species found in the feces and lymph nodes of sick and healthy animals, including man, and in material likely to be contaminated with feces; also found in the cadavers of cattle, rabbits, hares, dogs, guinea pigs, horses, monkeys, pigs, and sheep.

    **Y. pestis,** Kitasato's bacillus; *Pasteurella pestis;* a species causing plague in man, rats, ground squirrels, and other rodents. It is transmitted from rat to rat and from rat to man by the rat flea. It is the type species of the genus *Y.*

    **Y. pseudotuberculosis,** *Pasteurella pseudotuberculosis;* a species causing pseudotuberculosis in rodents, rarely in man, and some cases of acute mesenteric lymphadenitis in young people; also found in the intestines and lymph nodes of healthy carriers.

**-yl.** A chemical suffix signifying that the substance is a radical by loss of an H atom (*e.g.,* methyl, phenyl) or OH group (*e.g.,* acetyl, carbamoyl, ribosyl).

**-ylene.** A chemical suffix denoting a bivalent hydrocarbon radical (*e.g.,* methylene, —$CH_2$—) or possessing a double bond (*e.g.,* ethylene, $CH_2$=$CH_2$).

**yogurt, yoghurt** (yoh-ghoort) [ Bulg. ]. Fermented, partially evaporated, whole milk prepared by maintaining it at 50°C. for 12 hours after the addition of a mixed culture of *Lactobacillus bulgaricus, L. acidophilus,* and *Streptococcus lactis;* used as a food (a staple article of diet in Bulgaria). It has antibacterial properties.

**yohimbé, yohimbi** (yo-him'ba, yo-him'be) [ native African name ]. The bark of *Corynanthe yohimbi* (family Rubiaceae), an African tree supposed to possess aphrodisiac properties; it contains several alkaloids, the most important of which is yohimbine.

**yohimbine** (yo-him'bēn). An alkaloid, the active principle of yohimbé. It produces a competitive blockade, of limited duration, of adrenergic α-receptors; has been used as an aphrodisiac, but there is little convincing evidence for such an effect.

**yoke** (yōk) [ A.S. *geoc* ]. Jugum (1).

**yolk** (yōk, yōlk) [ A.S. *geolca; geolu,* yellow ]. 1. Vitellus; one of the types of nutritive material stored in the ovum for the nutrition of the embryo; it is particularly abundant and conspicuous in the eggs of birds. 2. The fatty material found in the wool of sheep; when extracted and purified it becomes lanolin.

    **y. sac,** see under sac.

    **y. stalk,** see under stalk.

    **white y.,** consisting of much finer particles than those of yellow y.; thin layers of it lie between the zones of yellow y. and form an outer layer with a flask-shaped central accumulation called the latebra.

yellow y., the chief constituent of the y. in a bird's egg; it is made up of relatively coarse particles of stored food materials and is laid down in concentric zones with interposed thin layers of white y.

**Yorke's autolytic reaction.** See under reaction.

**Young,** Thomas, English physician and physicist, 1773–1829. See Y.'s *rule*, Y.-Helmholtz *theory* of color vision.

**Young,** W. J. See Harden-Y. *ester.*

**yperite** (e'per-it) [ *Ypres*, a town in Belgium, where the Germans first used this gas ]. Dichlorodiethylsulfide; see mustard gas.

**ypsiliform** (ip'si-li-form) [ G. *ypsilon, upsilon*, the letter u

or y, + L. *forma*, form ]. Hypsiloid.

**ytterbium** (i-tur'bi-um) [ from *Ytterby*, a place in Sweden ]. A metal of the lanthanide ("rare earth") group; symbol Yb; atomic no. 70, atomic weight 173.04.

**yttrium** (it'ri-um) [ from *Ytterby*, a place in Sweden ]. A metallic element, symbol Y, atomic no. 39, atomic weight 88.92.

**yttrium-90.** A radioisotope which has been implanted in the pituitary fossa in the treatment of breast cancer by endocrine ablation.

**Yvon** (e-vawn'), Paul, French physician and chemist, 1848–1913. See Y.'s *test.*

# Z

**Z.** Abbreviation for benzyloxycarbonyl.

**Z0₂.** Symbol for microliters of oxygen taken up per hour by 10⁸ spermatozoa; can vary as a function of temperature.

**Zaglas' ligament.** See under ligament.

**Zahn,** Friedrich W., German pathologist, 1845–1904. See Z.'s *infarct, lines, striae.*

**Zambrini,** A. R., Argentinian physician. See Z. *ptyaloreaction.*

**Zappert** (tsah'pert), Julius, Vienna physician, 1867–1942. See Z.'s counting *chamber.*

**zea** (ze'ah) [ Mod. L. maize ]. Cornsilk; stigmata maydis; the styles and stigmas of *Zea mays* (family *Gramineae*), Indian corn. Formerly used as a diuretic and antispasmodic.

**zeatin** (ze'ă-tin). 6-(4-Hydroxy-3-methyl-*trans*-2-butenyl-amino)purine; a cytokinin first isolated from kernels of sweet corn.

**zeaxanthin** (ze-ă-zanth'in). β-Carotene-3,3'diol, a plant pigment isomeric with xanthophyll, derived from β-carotene by oxidation; ubiquitous in nature.

**Zeeman effect.** See under effect.

**ze'in.** A protein present in maize; it is lacking chiefly in the amino acids glycine and lysine and is low in cystine content.

**Zeis** (tsīs), Edward, Dresden ophthalmologist, 1807–1868. See Z.'s *gland,* Zeisian *sty.*

**ze'ism** [ Mod. L. *zea,* maize ]. Pellagra, on the assumption that it resulted from eating maize.

**Zeiss** (tsīs), Carl, German optician, 1816–1888. See Abbé-Z. *apparatus,* Thoma-Z. *hemocytometer.*

**ze'ist** [ Mod. L. *zea,* maize ]. An adherent of the theory that pellagra is due to the ingestion of Indian corn.

**Zellweger,** Hans U., U. S. pediatrician, *1909. See Z. *syndrome.*

**zelotypia** (ze-lo-tip'ĭ-ah) [ G. *zēlotypia;* rivalry, envy, fr. *zēlos,* zeal (ZE-), + *typtō,* to strike ]. Excessive zeal, carried to the verge of insanity, in the advocacy of any cause.

**Zenker** (tsenk'er), Friedrich A., German pathologist, 1825–1898). See Z.'s *degeneration, diverticulum, fluid,* formol-Z. *fluid, leiomyoma, myomalacia* cordis, *necrosis, paralysis.*

**ze'olite.** A naturally occurring hydrated sodium aluminum silicate, Na₂O·Al₂O₃·(SiO₂)ₓ·(H₂O)ₓ. Used as an ion-exchange medium for for softening of hard water, by exchanging its Na⁺ for the Ca⁺⁺ of the water; thus z. is an ion exchanger. Some synthetic ion exchangers are termed synthetic z.'s.

**zeoscope** (ze'o-skōp) [ G. *zeō,* to boil, + *skopeō,* to examine. ZE- ]. A device for determining the alcoholic content of a liquid by ascertaining its exact boiling point.

**ze'ro** [ Sp.; Ar. *sifr,* cipher ]. The figure 0, indicating nothingness. In thermometry, the point from which the figures on the scale start in one or the other direction; in the Centigrade and Réaumur scales z. indicates the freezing point for distilled water; in the Fahrenheit scale it indicates the degree of cold obtained by mixing ice and salt and is 32° below the freezing point.

**absolute z.,** the lowest possible temperature, that at which the form of motion constituting heat is assumed no longer to exist, reckoned as −273.2°C.

**zerogravity** (ze'ro-grav'ĭ-tī). A physical state existing in space or at a time in flight when the centrifugal thrust of a parabolic glide or turn exactly counteracts the force of gravity.

**zestocausis** (zes-to-kaw'sis) [ G. *zestos,* boiling hot, fr. *zeō,* to boil (ZE-), + *kausis,* a burning ]. Cauterization by means of hot steam.

**zestocautery** (zes-to-kaw'ter-ĭ). An appliance for zestocausis.

**Ziegler,** S. Louis, U. S. ophthalmologist, 1861–1925. See Z.'s *operation.*

**Ziehen** (tse'hen), Georg T., German psychiatrist, *1862. See Z.-Oppenheim *disease,* Z. *test.*

**Ziehl** (tseel), Franz, German bacteriologist, 1857–1926. See Z.-Neelsen *stain,* Z.'s *solution.*

**Ziemann** (tse'mahn), Hans R. P., German pathologist, *1865. See Z.'s *stippling.*

**Zieve,** Leslie, U. S. physician, *1915. See Z.'s *syndrome.*

**Zimmerlin** (tsim'er-lin), Franz, Swiss physician, 1858–1932. See Z.'s *atrophy.*

**Zimmermann** (tsim'er-mahn), Karl W., German histologist, 1861–1935. See Z.'s *corpuscle, granule,* elementary *particle, polkissen.*

**Zimmermann,** Wilhelm. See Z. *reaction, test.*

**zinc** (zingk) [ Ger. *zink* ]. A metallic element, symbol Zn, atomic no. 30, atomic weight 65.38, bluish white in color, malleable and ductile. A number of salts of z. are used in medicine. Crude commercial z. is called spelter.

**z. acetate** (USP), Zn(C₂H₃O₂)2H₂O; emetic, styptic, and astringent.

**z. cap'rylate,** a topical antifungal compound.

**z. carbonate,** calamine.

**z. chloride** (USP), butter of z.; ZnCl₂; formerly used as a caustic for the removal of cutaneous cancers, nevi, etc., and in weak solution in the treatment of gonorrhea and conjunctivitis.

**z. gelatin** (USP), contains z. oxide, gelatin, glycerin, and purified water; used topically as a protectant.

**globulin z. insulin,** see under insulin.

**z. iodide,** ZnI₂; has been used as an antiseptic and astringent.

**z. oxide** (USP, BP), ZnO; flowers of z.; z. white; used as a protective in ointment and as a dusting powder, and internally as an antispasmodic; also used in paint as a substitute for lead carbonate.

**z. oxide and eugenol,** used as a base material beneath metallic dental restorations and as a temporary filling material or impression material. Setting and hardening result from complex reactions between the powder and the eugenol.

**z. permanganate,** action is similar to that of potassium permanganate, but more astringent; used in urethritis, by injection or douche in a 1:4000 solution.

**z. peroxide,** ZPO; z. superoxide; ZnO₂; a yellowish white powder, insoluble in water; decomposed by acids; used in pharmaceutical preparations.

**z. peroxide, medicinal** (USP), a mixture of z. peroxide, z. carbonate, and z. hydroxide; topical disinfectant, astringent, and deodorant.

**z. phenolsulfonate,** z. sulfocarbolate; used as an intestinal antiseptic and locally as an astringent in chronic inflammation of the mucous membranes.

**z. phosphide,** Zn₃P₂; used as a bait poison for the extermination of rats and mice.

**z. silicate,** calamine.

**z. stearate** (USP), a z. compound with variable proportions of stearic and palmitic acids; a water-repellent, protective agent used in the treatment of eczema, acne, and other skin diseases.

**z. sulfate** (USP, BP), white vitriol; ZnSO₄·7H₂O; used as a local astringent in the treatment of gonorrhea, indolent ulcers, conjunctivitis, and various skin diseases; and internally as an emetic.

**z. sulfocarbolate,** z. phenolsulfonate.

**z. superoxide,** z. peroxide.

**z. undecylenate** (USP), z. undecenoate (BP); [ CH₂=CH(CH₂)₈COO ]₂Zn; the z. salt of undecylenic acid; used in the treatment of fungal and other affections of the skin, including psoriasis.

**z. white,** z. oxide.

**zinc-65.** ⁶⁵Z; radioactive z. isotope; decays mainly by K-capture with half-life of 245 days; used as tracer in studies of z. metabolism.

**zinciferous** (zing'kif'er-us). Containing zinc.

**zincoid** (zing'koyd) [ G. *eidos,* resemblance ]. Relating to or resembling zinc.

**zingiber** (zin'jĭ-ber). Ginger.

**Zinn** (tsin), Johann G., German anatomist, 1727–1759. See Z.'s *artery*, x-ray *cap*, vascular *circle, corona, ligament, membrane, ring, tendon, zonule.*

**zirconium** (zir-ko'nĭ-um) [ *zircon*, a mineral, fr. Ar. *zarkūn*, cinnabar ]. A metallic element, symbol Zr, atomic no. 40 atomic weight 91.22; it is widely distributed in nature, but never found in quantity in any one place.

**Zn.** Chemical symbol of the element zinc.

**zo-.** See zoo-.

**zoacanthosis** (zo'ă-kan-tho'sis) [ G. *zōon*, animal, + *acanthosis* ]. A cutaneous eruption due to introduction into the human skin of hair, bristles, stingers, etc., of lower animals.

**zoamylin** (zo-am'ĭ-lin) [ G. *zōē*, life, + *amylon*, starch ]. Glycogen.

**zo'anthrop'ic.** Relating to or marked by zoanthropy.

**zoanthropy** (zo-an'thro-pĭ) [ G. *zōon*, animal, + *anthrōpos*, man ]. A delusion that one is a horse or a dog or any other of the lower animals.

**zoescope** (zo'e-skōp) [ G. *zōē*, life, + *skopeō*, to examine ]. Stroboscope (2).

**zoetic** (zo-et'ik) [ G. *zōē*, life ]. Relating to life.

**zoetrope** (zo'e-trōp) [ G. *zōē*, life, + *tropē*, a turning ]. An optical toy in which figures on the inside of a revolving cylinder are viewed through slits in its circumference and appear like a single animated figure.

**zo'ic** [ G. *zōikos*, relating to an animal ]. Relating to living things; having life.

**zoite** (zo'īt) [ G. *zōon*, animal ]. Merozoite.

**Zollinger,** Robert M., American surgeon, *1903. See Z.-Ellison *syndrome, tumor.*

**Zöllner** (tsël'ner), Johann F., German physicist, 1834–1882. See Z.'s *lines.*

**zona,** pl. **zonae** (zo'nah, zo'ne) [ L. fr. G. *zōnē,* a girdle, one of the zones of the sphere ]. 1 [ NA ]. A zone; a segment; any encircling or beltlike structure, either external or internal, longitudinal or transverse. 2. *Herpes* zoster.

z. arcua'ta, arcuate zone; z. tecta; the inner third of the lamina basilaris ductus cochlearis extending from the tympanic lip of the osseous spiral lamina to the outer pillar cell of the spiral organ (of Corti).

z. cilia'ris, ciliary *zone.*

z. corona, costal *fringe.*

z. dermat'ica, a ridge of thickened skin surrounding the protrusion in spina bifida.

z. epithe'liosero'sa, the membranous ring, within the z. dermatica, surrounding the protrusion in spina bifida.

z. facia'lis, herpes zoster involving the face.

z. fascicula'ta, the layer of radially arranged cell cords in the cortical portion of the suprarenal gland, between the z. glomerulosa and z. reticularis.

z. glomerulo'sa, the outer layer of the cortex of the suprarenal gland just beneath the capsule.

z. hemorrhoida'lis [ NA ], anulus hemorrhoidalis; the part of the anal canal that contains the rectal venous plexus.

z. ig'nea, *herpes* zoster.

z. incer'ta [ NA ], a flat, horizontally disposed plate of gray matter in the subthalamus, interposed between the tegmental fields $H_1$ ventrally, $H_2$ dorsally, and H medially, continuous laterally with the nucleus reticularis thalami. It receives projections from the precentral motor cortex and cerebellum; its efferent connections are unknown.

z. medull'ovasculo'sa, the fissured segment of the spinal cord that closes dorsally the sac in meningomyelocele.

z. ophthal'mica, herpes zoster in the distribution of the ophthalmic nerve.

z. orbicula'ris [ NA ], orbicular zone; zonular band; ring ligament; fibers of the articular capsule of the hip joint encircling the neck of the femur.

z. pectina'ta, pectinate zone; the outer two-thirds of the lamina basilaris ductus cochlearis.

z. pellu'cida, a layer consisting of microvilli of the oocyte, cellular processes of follicular cells, and an intervening substance rich in glycoprotein; it appears homogeneous and translucent under the light microscope.

z. perfora'ta, *foramina* nervosa.

z. pupilla'ris, pupillary *zone.*

z. radia'ta, z. striata.

z. reticula'ris, the inner layer of the cortex of the adrenal gland, where the cell cords anastomose in a netlike fashion; see also fetal *cortex.*

z. serpigino'sa, *herpes* zoster.

z. stria'ta, z. radiata; striated membrane; the thickened cell membrane of the ovum in forms, such as certain amphibia, in which it appears radially striated under the light microscope. With the electron microscope the striations can be seen to be microvilli.

z. tec'ta, z. arcuata.

z. vasculo'sa, vascular zone; spongy spot; an area in the external acoustic meatus where a number of minute blood vessels enter from the mastoid bone.

z. volat'ica, *herpes* zoster.

**zo'nal.** Relating to a zone.

**zo'nary.** Relating to or having the form of a zone or belt.

**zo'nate.** zoned; ringed; having concentric layers of differing texture or pigmentation.

**Zondek,** Bernhardt, German obstetrician and gynecologist, 1891–1966. See Aschheim-Z. *test.*

---

# ZONE

---

**zone** (zōn) [ L. *zona, q.v.* ]. Zona (1). See also area, region, space, spot.

abdominal z.'s, *regiones* abdominis.

anacoustic z., the z. of silence in space; the region more than 100 miles above the earth's surface where the distance between the rarefied air molecules is greater than the wavelength of sound.

androgenic z., (1) X z. (1); (2) fetal *cortex (q.v.)*; named in the belief (as yet unsubstantiated) that the cells within this zone secrete androgens.

arcuate z., zona arcuata.

Barnes' z., cervical z.; the lower fourth of the pregnant uterus, attachment of the placenta to any part of which may cause dangerous hemorrhage.

cervical z., Barnes' z.

cervical z. of tooth, *collum* dentis.

Charcot's z.'s, hysterogenic z.'s.

ciliary z., zona ciliaris; the outer, wider z. of the anterior surface of the iris, separated from the pupillary z. by the collarette.

comfort z., the temperature range between 28 and 30°C. at which the naked body is able to maintain the heat balance without either shivering or sweating. In the clothed body the range is from 13 to 21°C.

z.'s of discontinuity, as seen in slitlamp biomicroscopy, concentric z.'s of varying optical density that reflect light, giving an onion-like appearance to the lens.

dolorogenic z., trigger z.; the area which, stimulated by touch, pressure, etc., sets up an attack of neuralgic pain.

entry z., the area of the dorsal funiculus of the spinal cord, medial to the tip of the posterior horn, in which the entering fibers of the posterior nerve root divide into an ascending and a descending branch.

ependymal z., ependymal *layer.*

epilep'togen'ic z., a cortical region that precipitates an epileptic seizure when stimulated.

erogenous z., erotogenic z.; a part of the body, stimulation of which excites the sexual feelings; *e.g.*, the oral, anal, and genital areas.

erotogen'ic z., erogenous z.

extravisual z., the portion of the optical mediums in which there is a dispersal of rays not properly focused.

fetal z., fetal *cortex.*

gingival z., that portion of the oral mucosa which surrounds the teeth and is firmly attached to the underlying alveolar bone.

Golgi z., part of the cytoplasm occupied by the Golgi apparatus (*q.v.*); in secretory cells of glands, a z. between the nucleus and the luminal surface.

Head's z.'s, Head's *lines.*

hypoacoustic z., the region in the upper atmosphere, between 60 and 100 miles above the earth's surface, where rarefied air molecules roughly equal the wave lengths of sound, transmitting it at a reduced volume.

**hysterogenic z.'s**, hysterogenic areas, spots, or points; Charcot's z.'s; various circumscribed areas on the body surface, pressure upon which excites a paroxysm of hysteria.

**interpalp'ebral z.**, the exposed area of the cornea and sclera between the lids of the open eye.

**isoelectric z.**, the range of H-ion concentration (pH) over which isoelectric precipitation occurs.

**language z.**, a large area of the cerebral cortex on the left side (in right-handed persons) embracing all the centers of memories and associations connected with language.

**latent z.**, that portion of the cerebral cortex a lesion of which produces no symptoms.

**Lissauer's marginal z.**, *fasciculus* dorsolateralis.

**Looser's z.'s**, a pseudofracture line usually seen in radiographs of persons with osteomalacia or ricketts.

**mantle z.**, mantle *layer*.

**Marchant's z.**, the area on the sphenoid and occipital bones at the base of the skull from which the dura mater is readily detached.

**marginal z.**, marginal *layer*.

**motor z.**, that portion of the cerebral cortex which when stimulated produces a movement and when injured produces spasticity or paralysis.

**neutral z.**, in dentistry, the potential space between the lips and cheeks on one side and the tongue on the other; natural or artificial teeth in this z. are subject to equal and opposite forces from the surrounding musculature.

**nucleolar z.**, nucleolar *organizer*.

**Obersteiner-Redlich z.**, Obersteiner-Redlich line; the narrow line along the course of a nerve (or nerve root) where the Schwann cells and connective tissue that support its axons are replaced by glia cells. The z. marks the true boundary between the central and the peripheral nervous system. Usually located at or near the surface of the spinal cord or brainstem, it can (*e.g.*, in the eighth nerve) lie several millimeters farther out along the nerve.

**orbicular z.**, *zona* orbicularis.

**pectinate z.**, *zona* pectinata.

**pellu'cid z.**, *zona* pellucida.

**polar z.**, the region in the vicinity of an electrode applied to the body; see also electrotonus.

**pupillary z.**, zona pupillaris; the central region of the anterior surface of the iris located between the collarette and the pupillary margin.

**reflexogenic z.**, the area or z. where stimulation will elicit a given reflex.

**secondary X z.**, an adrenocortical z., situated in the inner zona fasciculata, that appears upon postpubertal gonadectomy in some male rodents, most notably the mouse; the development of this z. is believed to be stimulated by pituitary gonadotropins.

**segmental z.**, in a young embryo, the thickened dorsal portion of the mesoderm; either side of the midline that becomes metamerically divided to form the mesodermic somites.

**Spitzka's marginal z.**, *fasciculus* dorsolateralis.

**sudanopho'bic z.**, a z. of cells, at the periphery of the zona fasciculata in the adrenal cortex of the rat, that is not stained by Sudan.

**tender z.'s**, Head's *lines.*

**thymus-dependent z.**, paracortex.

**trabecular z.**, trabecular *meshwork.*

**transitional z.**, (1) the region of the lens of the eye where the anterior epithelial capsule cells become transformed into the fibers composing the lens substance; (2) that portion of a scleral contact lens that joins the corneal and scleral sections.

**trigger z.**, dolorogenic z.

**trophotropic z. of Hess**, an area in the hypothalamus concerned with positive rewarding bodily sensations.

**vascular z.**, *zona* vasculosa.

**vermilion z., vermilion transitional z.**, vermilion *border.*

**Wernicke's z.**, Wernicke's *center.*

**X z.**, (1) a transient adrenocortical z. present in some rodents at birth, most notably in mice; situated between the zona reticularis and the adrenal medulla. It degenerates in males with the onset of androgen secretion at puberty and in females during their first pregnancy; slowly enlarges in unmated females after puberty and does not degenerate until middle age. The X z. appears to secrete no hormone; (2) misnomer for the fetal *cortex* (*q.v.*) of primates.

---

**zonesthesia** (zōn-es-the'zĭ-ah) [ G. *zōnē*, girdle, + *aisthēsis*, sensation ]. Girdle or cincture sensation; strangalesthesia; a sensation as if a cord were drawn around the body, constricting it.

**zonifugal** (zo-nif'u-gal) [ L. *zona*, zone, + *fugio*, to flee ]. Passing from any region outward; as in mapping out an area of disturbed sensation, when the stimulus is first applied to the affected region and is carried along into the part where sensation is normal.

**zo'ning.** A phenomenon observed sometimes in serologic tests employed in the diagnosis of syphilis; it is the occurrence of a stronger reaction in a less amount of suspected serum. The reaction is probably the result of high antibody titer.

**zonipetal** (zo-nip'ĕ-tal) [ L. *zona*, zone, + *peto*, to seek ]. Passing from without toward and into any region; as in mapping out an area of disturbed sensation, when the stimulus begins in the normal part and is carried into the affected region.

**zonoskeleton** (zo'no-skel'e-ton) [ L. *zona*, zone, skeleton ]. The proximal skeletal segments of the limbs, *i.e.*, scapula, clavicle, and hip bone.

**zonula**, pl. **zonulae** (zo'nu-lah, -le, zon'-) [ L. dim. of *zona*, zone ] [ NA ]. A small zone.

**z. adhe'rens**, the part of a terminal bar between epithelial cells where the plasmalemmas are separated by a space of 200 Å.

**z. cilia'ris** [ NA ], ciliary zonule; apparatus suspensorius lentis; zonule of Zinn; suspensory ligament of the lens; a series of delicate meridional fibers arising from the inner surface of the orbiculus ciliaris; these run in bundles between, and in a very thin layer over, the ciliary processes; at the inner border of the corona the fibers diverge into two groups that are attached to the capsule on the anterior and posterior surfaces of the lens close to the equator; the spaces between these two layers of fibers are filled with aqueous humor; they are known as spatia zonularia, or the canal of Petit.

**z. occlu'dens**, a tight junction between epithelial cells in which the plasmalemmas are often fused.

**zonular** (zon'u-lar, zo'nu-lar). Relating to a zonula.

**zonule** (zo'nūl, zon'ūl). Zonula.

**ciliary z.**, *zonula* ciliaris.

**Zinn's z.**, *zonula* ciliaris.

**zonuli'tis** [ zonule + G. suffix *-itis*, inflammation ]. Assumed inflammation of the zonule of Zinn, or suspensory ligament of the crystalline lens of the eye.

**zonulolysis** (zo'nu-lol'ĭ-sis) [ zonule + G. *lysis*, dissolution ]. Barraquer's method; disintegration of the zonula ciliaris by enzymes (α-chymotrypsin) instilled into the anterior chamber in selected cases of cataract extraction to facilitate surgical removal.

**zonuly'sin.** A highly purified, sterile, freeze-dried α-chymotrypsin, which is particularly indicated for dissolving the ciliary zonule.

**zonuly'sis.** Zonulolysis.

**zoo-** (zo'o-) [ G. *zōon*, animal. ZO- ]. Combining form denoting an animal or animal life.

**zooanthroponosis** (zo'o-an'thro-po-no'sis) [ zoo- + G. *anthrōpos*, man, + *nosos*, disease ]. A zoonosis maintained in nature by man (*e.g.*, amebiasis).

**zooblast** (zo'-o-blast) [ zoo- + G. *blastos*, germ ]. An animal cell.

**zoodermic** (zo-o-der'mik) [ zoo- + G. *derma*, skin ]. Relating to the skin of an animal; denoting the method of skin grafts in which the grafts are taken from the skin of an animal; see also dermatozooplasty.

**zooerastia** (zo'o-ĕ-ras'tĭ-ah) [ zoo- + G. *erastēs*, lover ]. Sexual practices with an animal.

**zo'oful'vin.** A yellow pigment obtained from the feathers of certain birds.

**zoogenesis** (zo-o-jen'ĕ-sis) [ zoo- + G. *genesis*, origin ]. Zoogeny; zoogony; the doctrine of animal production or generation.

**zo'ogen'ic, zo'ogenet'ic.** Zoogenous; relating to zoogenesis; produced or caused by animals.

**zoogenous** (zo-oj'ĕ-nus). Zoogenetic.

**zoogeny** (zo-oj'ĕ-nĭ). Zoogenesis.

**zoogeography** (zo-o-je-og'rä-fĭ). The geography of animals; the study of the distribution of animals on the earth's surface.

**zooglea** (zo-og'le-ah, zo'o-gle'ah) [ zoo- + G. *glia,* glue ]. In bacteriology, an old term for a mass of bacteria held together by a clear gelatinous substance.

**zoogonous** (zo-og'o-nus). Viviparous.

**zoogony** (zo-og'on-ĭ). Viviparity.

**zoograft** (zo'o-graft). A graft of tissue from one of the lower animals.

**zoografting** (zo-o-graf'ting). Zooplasty.

**zoography** (zo-og'rä-fĭ) [ zoo- + G. *graphō,* to write ]. A description of or treatise on animals.

**zoohormone** (zo'o-hor'mōn). An animal hormone, as distinguished from phytohormone.

**zooid** (zo'oyd) [ G. *zōodēs,* fr. *zōon,* animal, + *eidos,* resemblance ]. 1. Resembling an animal. 2. A unicellular organism of indefinite classification; a zoophyte. 3. An animal cell capable of independent existence or movement, as the ovum or a spermatozoon. 4. An individual of a colonial invertebrate, such as the z. of the freshwater bryozoan, *Plumatella.* 5. A term sometimes applied to hemoglobin because of its assumed vital properties.

**zoolagnia** (zo-o-lag'nĭ-ah) [ zoo- + G. *lagneia,* lust ]. Sexual attraction toward animals.

**zoolite, zoolith** (zo'o-lit, zo-o-lith) [ zoo- + G. *lithos,* stone ]. A petrified animal.

**zoologist** (zo-ol'o-jist). One who specializes in zoology.

**zoology** (zo-ol'o-jĭ) [ zoo- + G. *logos,* study ]. The science that deals with animals in all their relationships and categories.

**zoom.** The action of a varifocal lens system in a camera or microscope that maintains an object in focus while approaching it or receding from it; this effect may be obtained by moving two or more of the lens components at rates bearing a linear relation to one another. In the surgical microscope, the ratio of focal lengths (zoom ratio) is 5:1.

**zoomania** (zo'o-ma'nĭ-ah) [ zoo- + G. *mania,* frenzy ]. An excessive, abnormal love of animals.

**Zoomastigina** (zo'o-mas'tĭ-ji'nah) [ zoo- + G. *mastix,* whip ]. A class of Mastigophora, the flagellates; termed Zoomastigophorea in a recent classification.

**Zoomastigophorea** (zo'o-mas-tĭ-go-fo're-ah) [ zoo- + G. *mastix,* whip, + *phoros,* bearing ]. Zoomastigina.

**zoomylus** (zo-om'ĭ-lus) [ zoo- + G. *mylos,* stone ]. A dermoid *cyst.*

**zoonomy** (zo-on'o-mĭ) [ zoo- + G. *nōmos,* law ]. Animal physiology; the science dealing with the laws of the vital functions in animals.

**zoonosis** (zo-ŏ-no'sis) [ zoo- + G. *nosos,* disease ]. An infection or infestation shared in nature by man and lower vertebrate animals. See also anthroponosis, anthropozoonosis, cyclozoonosis, metazoonosis, saprozoonosis, zooanthroponosis.

   **direct z.,** a z. transmitted from an infected to a susceptible host by contact, by a mechanical vector, or by some vehicle of transmission. The agent requires a single vertebrate host for completion of its life cycle and does not develop or show significant change during transmission. May include anthropozoonoses (rabies), zooanthroponoses (diphtheria), and amphixinoses (certain streptococcoses).

**zoonotic** (zo'o-not'ik). Relating to a zoonosis.

**zooparasite** (zo-o-păr'ă-sīt). An animal parasite; an animal existing as a parasite.

**zoopathology** (zo-o-pă-thol'o-jĭ). The pathology of the lower animals; veterinary pathology.

**zoophagous** (zo-of'a-gus) [ G. *zōophagos,* fr. *zōon,* animal, + *phagein,* to eat ]. Subsisting on animal food; carnivorous.

**zoophile** (zo'o-fīl) [ zoo- + G. *philos,* fond ]. Zoophilist. 1. A lover of animals; especially one more fond of animals

than of people. 2. One opposed to any animal experimentation; an antivivisectionist.

**zoophilia** (zo-o-fil'ĭ-ah). Zoophilism.

**zoophilic** (zo'o-fil'ik). 1. Relating to or displaying zoophilism. 2. Animal-seeking or animal-preferring; denotes preference of a parasite for the animal host as a source of blood or tissues over the human host; *cf.* anthropophilic.

**zoophilism** (zo-of'ĭ-lizm). Zoophilia; fondness for animals, especially an extravagant fondness for them, as in antivivisectionism.

   **erot'ic z.,** the deriving of sexual pleasure by patting or stroking animals.

**zoophilist** (zo-of'ĭ-list). Zoophile.

**zoophobia** (zo-o-fo'bĭ-ah) [ zoo- + G. *phobos,* fear ]. A morbid fear of animals.

**zooplasty** (zo'o-plas-tĭ). Zoografting; the grafting of skin or other tissue from one of the lower animals.

**zooprecipitin** (zo-o-pre-sip'ĭ-tin). A precipitin obtained by repeated injection of an animal protein.

**zoopsia** (zo-op'sĭ-ah) [ zoo- + G. *opsis,* vision ]. Zooscopy; a delusion of seeing animals.

**zoopsychology** (zo-o-si-kol'o-jĭ). Animal psychology; the study of the mental processes or instincts and behavior of the lower animals.

**zoosadism** (zo-o-sa'dizm). Sexual pleasure from hurting animals.

**zooscopy** (zo-os'ko-pĭ) [ zoo- + G. *skopeō,* to view ]. Zoopsia.

**zoosmosis** (zo-oz-mo'sis) [ G. *zōos,* living, + osmosis, *q. v.* ]. The process of osmosis in living tissues.

**zoospore** (zo'o-spōr) [ zoo- + G. *sporos,* seed ]. A swarm-spore; among fungi a motile, asexually produced spore. Such spores are usually flagellated and produced as sporangiospores.

**zoosteroids** (zo'o-ster'oydz). Obsolete designation for steroids derived from animal sources.

**zoosterol** (zo-os'ter-ol). Obsolete designation for a sterol derived from animal life, *e.g.,* sex hormones, bile acids.

**zootechnics** (zo'o-tek'niks) [ zoo- + G. *technē,* art ]. The art of managing domestic or captive animals, including handling, breeding and keeping.

**zootherapy** (zo-o-thěr'ă-pĭ). Veterinary therapeutics.

**zootic** (zo-ot'ik). Pertaining to animals other than man.

**zootomist** (zo-ot'o-mist). A comparative anatomist.

**zootomy** (zo-ot'o-mĭ) [ zoo- + G. *tomē,* a cutting ]. Theriotomy. 1. Comparative *anatomy.* 2. Dissection of one of the lower animals.

**zootoxin** (zo'o-tok'sin). Animal toxin; a substance, resembling the bacterial toxins in its antigenic properties, found in the fluids of certain animals; snake venom, the secretions of poisonous insects, and eel-blood contain zootoxins.

**zootrophic** (zo-o-trof'ik) [ zoo- + Gr. *trophē,* nourishment ]. Relating to or serving for the nutrition of the lower animals.

**zoster** (G. *zōstēr,* a girdle ]. *Herpes* zoster.

**zoster'iform.** Zosteroid.

**zos'teroid** [ zoster + G. *eidos,* resemblance ]. Resembling herpes zoster; zosteriform.

**zoxazolamine** (zok'să-zo'lă-mēn). FLEXIN; 2-amino-5-chlorobenzoxazole; a skeletal muscle relaxant with actions similar to those of mephenesin; used in a variety of disorders associated with skeletal muscle spasticity, and as a uricosuric agent in the treatment of gout.

**Z-plasty.** A technique for lengthening contracted scar tissue.

**Zr.** Chemical symbol of the element zirconium.

**Zsigmondy** (sig'mon-de), Richard, German chemist, 1865–1929. See Z.'s *movements,* Brownian-Z. *movement,* Z.'s *test.*

**Zuckergussleber** [ Ger. ]. Frosted *liver.*

**Zuckerkandl** (tsoo'ker-kahn-del), Emil, Austrian anatomist, 1849–1910. See Z.'s *bodies, convolution, fascia, organs.*

**Zwenger's test.** See under test.

**Zwischenferment** (tsvēsh'en-fer-ment') [ Ger. ]. Glucose-6-phosphate dehydrogenase.

**zwitterions** (tsvit'er-i'onz) [ Ger. ]. See zwitter *hypothesis.*

**zyg-.** See zygo-.

**zy'gal.** Relating to or shaped like a zygon or yoke; H-shaped.

**zygapophysial, zygapophyseal** (zig'ă-po-fiz'ĭ-al, zig-ă-pof'ĭ-se'al). Relating to a zygapophysis or articular process of a vertebra.

**zygapophysis,** pl. **zygapophyses** (zig'ă-pof'ĭ-sis, -sēz) [ G. *zygon*, yoke, + *apophysis*, offshoot. PHYS ] [ NA ]. Official alternate term for *processus* articularis.

**zygion** (zig'ĭ-on) [ G. a later form of *zygon*, yoke ]. The point on the zygomatic arch on either side, at the extremity of the bizygomatic diameter.

**zygo-, zyg-** (zi'go-) [ G. *zygon*, yoke, *zygōsis*, a joining ]. Combining forms meaning yoke, a joining.

**zygocyte** (zi'go-sīt) [ zygo- + *kytos*, cell ]. Zygote.

**zygodactyly** (zi'go-dak'tĭ-lĭ). Syndactyly.

**zygoma** (zi-go'mah) [ G. a bar, bolt, the os jugale, fr. *zygon*, yoke ]. 1. *Os* zygomaticum. 2. *Arcus* zygomaticus.

**zygomatic** (zi'go-mat'ik). Relating to the os zygomaticum.

**zygomatico-** (zi'go-mat'ĭ-ko-) [ G. *zygoma*, *q. v.* ]. Combining form meaning zygomatic; relating usually to the zygomatic bone.

**zygomaticoauricular** (zi'go-mat'ĭ-ko-aw-rik'u-lar). Relating to the zygomatic bone and the auricle.

**zygomat'icoauricula'ris.** *Musculus* auricularis anterior.

**zygomaticofa'cial.** Relating to the zygomatic bone and the face.

**zygomaticofron'tal.** Relating to the zygomatic and frontal bones.

**zygomaticomax'illary.** Relating to the zygomatic bone and the maxilla.

**zygomatico-or'bital.** Relating to the zygomatic bone and the orbit.

**zygomaticosphenoid** (zi'go-mat'ĭ-ko-sfe'noyd). Relating to the zygomatic and sphenoid bones.

**zygomaticotem'poral.** Relating to the zygomatic and temporal bones.

**zygomat'icus** [ L. ] [ NA ]. Zygomatic.

**zygomax'illary.** Relating to the zygomatic bone and the maxilla.

**Zygomycetes** (zi'go-mi-se'tēz) [ zygo- + G. *mykēs* (*mykēt-*), fungus ]. A class of fungi characterized by sexual reproduction resulting in the formation of a zygospore, and asexual reproduction by means of nonmotile spores called sporangiospores or conidia.

**zy'gon** [ G. crossbar, yoke ]. The short crossbar connecting the branches of a zygal fissure.

**zygonema** (zi'go-ne'mah) [ zygo- + G. *nēma*, thread ]. Zygotene.

**zygopodium** (zi'go-po'di-um) [ zygo- + G. *podion*, small foot ]. The distal intermediate segment of the limb skeleton, *i.e.,* radius and ulna, tibia and fibula.

**zygosis** (zi-go'sis) [ G. a joining ]. True conjugation or sexual union of two unicellular organisms, consisting essentially in the fusion of the nuclei of the two cells.

**zygosity** (zi-gos'ĭ-tĭ). The nature of the zygotes from which individuals are derived; *e.g.,* whether, with respect to a particular gene, they are homozygous or heterozygous or whether, in the case of twins, they are monozygotic or dizygotic.

**zygosperm** (zi'go-sperm) [ zygo- + G. *sperma*, seed ]. Zygospore; a spore formed by the conjugation of two other spores.

**zygospore** (zi'go-spōr). Zygosperm.

**zygote** (zi'gōt) [ G. *zygōtos*, yoked ]. 1. The diploid cell resulting from union of a sperm and an ovum. 2. The individual that develops from a fertilized ovum.

**zygotene** (zi'go-tēn) [ zygo- + G. *tainia* (L. *taenia*), band ]. Zygonema; the stage of prophase in meiosis in which precise point for point pairing of homologous chromosomes begins; this pairing is often called synapsis or syndesis.

**zygot'ic.** Pertaining to a zygote, or to zygosis.

**zygo'toblast** [ G. *zygōtos*, yoked, + *blastos*, germ ]. Sporozoite.

**zygotomere** (zi-go'to-mēr) [ G. *zygōtos*, yoked, + *meros*, part ]. Sporoblast.

**zym-.** See zymo-.

**zy'mad.** The contagium vivum of a zymotic or infectious disease.

**zymase** (zi'mās). Obsolete term for enzyme; specifically, the intracellular enzyme of yeast that promotes alcoholic fermentation. This term was originally used by Buchner, who showed its presence in "yeast juice" obtained by grinding yeast and filtering free from cellular elements; it is actually a mixture of several enzymes.

**zyme** (zīm) [ G. *zymē*, leaven. ZE- ]. Obsolete term for (1) enzyme, (2) contagium vivum of an infectious disease.

**zymo-, zym-** (zi'mo-) [ G. *zymē*, leaven. ZE- ]. Combining forms relating to fermentation or to enzymes.

**zymochem'istry.** The study of chemical reactions catalyzed by yeast cells.

**zymogen** (zi'mo-jen). Proenzyme; see also z. *granules.*

**zymogenesis** (zi'mo-jen'ě-sis) [ zymo- + G. *genesis*, production ]. Transformation of a zymogen (or proenzyme) into an active enzyme.

**zymogen'ic.** Relating to a zymogen or to zymogenesis; causing fermentation.

**zymogenous** (zi-moj'ě-nus). Zymogenic.

**zymogram** (zi'mo-gram) [ zymo- + G. *gramma*, something written ]. A graphic demonstration of the enzyme content of tissues.

**zymohex'ase.** Fructose bisphosphate aldolase.

**zymohydrolysis** (zi'mo-hi-drol'ĭ-sis). Hydrolysis or cleavage of any compound under the influence of an enzyme.

**zymoid** (zi'moyd) [ G. *zymōdēs*, like leaven, fr. *zymē*, leaven, + *eidos*, resemblance ]. Resembling an enzyme.

**zy'molite.** Substrate.

**zymol'ogist.** Enzymologist.

**zymology** (zi-mol'o-jĭ). Enzymology.

**zymolysis** (zi-mol'ĭ-sis). Obsolete term for fermentation (enzymic digestion).

**zymometer** (zi-mom'e-ter) [ zymo- + G. *metron*, measure ]. An instrument for estimating the degree of fermentation.

**Zymonema** (zi-mo-ne'mah) [ zymo- + G. *nēma*, thread ]. An obsolete generic designation formerly applied to certain pathogenic fungi including members of the genera *Blastomyces* and *Cryptococcus.*

　　**Z. dermati'tidis,** a species of blastomycetes, the pathogen of North American blastomycosis.

　　**Z. farciminosum,** the cause of blastomycotic lymphangitis of horses.

**zymonematosis** (zi-mo-ne-mă-to'sis). Blastomycosis.

**zy'monucle'ic acid.** *Ribonucleic* acid.

**zymoplas'tic** [ zymo- + G. *plassō*, to form ]. Producing an enzyme.

**zymopro'tein.** Yeast protein.

**zy'mosan.** Anticomplementary factor; a carbohydrate (glucose polymer) obtained from the walls of yeast cells. Used in the assay of properdin.

**zymoscope** (zi'mo-skōp) [ zymo- + G. *skopeō*, to view ]. An instrument measuring $CO_2$ evolved and, therefore, the fermenting power of yeast.

**zy'mose.** Invertase.

**zymosim'eter, zymosiom'eter.** Zymometer.

**zymosis** (zi-mo'sis) [ G. ]. Obsolete term for fermentation (enzymic digestion).

**zymost'erol.** $5\alpha$-Cholesta-8,24-dien-3$\beta$-ol; a sterol isolated from yeast.

**zymosthen'ic** (zi'mo-sthen'ik) [ zymo- + G. *sthenos*, strength ]. Increasing the functional activity and power of an enzyme.

**zymotechny** (zi-mo-tek'nĭ) [ zymo- + G. *technē*, art ]. Any technique in which a process of fermentation is involved.

**zymurgy** (zi'mur-jĭ) [ zymo- + G. *ergon*, work ]. The branch of chemistry that deals with fermentation as applied to the manufacture of alcoholic beverages.

# Appendix 1: Alphabetical Index of Subentries

This index comprises a complete list of *Stedman* subentry titles, arranged alphabetically according to the first word or words of the titles. As such, it serves as a composite, "master" cross-referencing system for adjectival or descriptive terms in the vocabulary in lieu of such cross-referencing within the vocabulary. It not only provides a guide to the location of information that may be elusive (because of the *Stedman* format of alphabetically listed main entries with subordinately placed subentries), but also brings into focus the existence of related information.

The boldface words represent the adjectival or descriptive portions of the subentry titles; the lightface words following the colon are the nouns that complete the title and serve as vocabulary main entries under which the subentry definitions are located. For example, the index entry **cytologic** shows that in the *Stedman* vocabulary are definitions for **cytologic examination, cytologic screening, cytologic smear,** and **cytologic specimen,** each positioned as a subentry under the relevant noun main entry.

The boldface listings represent the exact wording of the subentry title in the vocabulary; that is, terms beginning with words such as acute, congenital, progressive, infectious, etc., are alphabetized in this index under those words. It is advisable (especially for disease names) to check the index under such descriptive words as well as under the specific name; for example, **bulbar paralysis** is listed under bulbar; **infectious bulbar paralysis,** under infectious. Similarly, anatomical terms beginning with words such as anterior, posterior, etc., are here alphabetized according to these words; however, where inclusion of every specific structure so designated would have greatly, and superfluously, increased the length of the index, guides to the relevant main entries, without the listing of specific structures, have been given (*e.g.,* see the entry, **anterior anatomical structures**).

Omitted from this index are subentry titles that are easily located in the vocabulary because the first word of the subentry is the same as its noun main entry. These include (1) all Latin nomenclature; (2) most chemical and pharmacological terms (see explanation on page xvi); and (3) "prepositional" terms such as **angle of declination** (found in the vocabulary under angle), **law of denervation** (under law), **base of the bladder** (under base). Also excluded are eponyms (*e.g.,* **Charcot's disease, Sylvian aqueduct**); for all eponymic terms the vocabulary itself provides cross-referencing from biographical main entries that identify the persons to whom the eponyms are attributed.

Significant adjectival terms in subentry titles are defined as main entries *per se* in the vocabulary, and these definitions may obviate the need for additional treatment in a subentry, or they may provide information that supplements that of the subentry; therefore, to locate the total amount of information provided in *Stedman's,* a check of both the vocabulary and this index will prove rewarding.

## A

α-: see alpha
A: band; bile; chain; cell; disk; esotropia; exotropia; fiber
A₂: thalassemia
aaa: disease
**abacterial thrombotic:** endocarditis
**abapical:** pole
**abarticular:** gout
**A.B.C.:** process
**abdominal:** angina; apoplexy; brain; canal; cavity; fissure; fistula; hernia; hysterectomy; hysteropexy; hysterotomy; migraine; myomyectomy; nephrectomy; pad; part; phthisis; pool; pregnancy; pulse; reflex; region; respiration; ring; sac; salpingectomy; salpingotomy; section; zone
**abdominal aortic:** plexus
**abdominal muscle deficiency:** syndrome
**abdominoanterior:** position
**abdominocardiac:** reflex
**abdominojugular:** reflux
**abdominoposterior:** position
**abdominothoracic:** arch
**abducens:** nucleus
**abducent:** nerve
**abductor:** muscle
**aberrant:** artery; bundle; complex; duct; ductule; ganglion; goiter

**aberrant bile:** duct
**aberrant ventricular:** conduction
**abnormal:** cleavage; occlusion
**ABO:** antigen; factor
**ABO hemolytic:** disease
**abomasal:** groove
**aborted:** systole
**aborted ectopic:** pregnancy
**abortion:** rate
**abortive:** epilepsy; neurofibromatosis; pneumonia; transduction
**abortus:** bacillus; fever
**abortus-Band-ring:** test
**ABR:** test
**abraded:** wound
**absolute:** accommodation; agraphia; alcohol; degree; dehydration; diet; glaucoma; hemianopsia; humidity; hydration; hyperopia; leukocytosis; scale; system; temperature; threshold; unit; viscosity; zero
**absolute increase of:** cells
**absolute refractory:** period
**absolute terminal innervation:** ratio
**absorbable:** gelatin
**absorbable gelatin:** sponge
**absorbable surgical:** suture
**absorbancy:** index
**absorbent:** cotton; point; system; vessel
**absorber:** head
**absorption:** band; cell; coefficient; fever; line; paper; spectrum

**absorptive:** cell
**abstinence:** symptom
**abstract:** intelligence; thinking
**a-c:** interval
**ac-:** globulin
**AC/A:** ratio
**acapnial:** alkalosis
**acarine:** dermatosis
**accelerated:** conduction; eruption; reaction
**accelerative:** epilepsy
**accelerator:** factor; fiber; globulin; nerve
**accessory:** adrenal; atrium; auricle; canal; cartilage; chromosome; cramp; flocculus; gland; ligament; nerve; organ; placenta; pocket; process; sign; spleen; symptom; thyroid
**accessory cephalic:** vein
**accessory cuneate:** nucleus
**accessory hemiazygos:** vein
**accessory lacrimal:** gland
**accessory nasal:** cartilage; sinus
**accessory obturator:** artery
**accessory olivary:** nucleus
**accessory pancreatic:** duct
**accessory parotid:** gland
**accessory phrenic:** nerve
**accessory plantar:** ligament
**accessory quadrate:** cartilage
**accessory saphenous:** vein
**accessory suprarenal:** gland

accessory thyroid: gland
accessory vertebral: vein
accessory volar: ligament
accident: neurosis; ward
accidental: abortion; albuminuria; hemorrhage; hypothermia; image; membrane; murmur; symptom
acclimating: fever
accolé: form
accommodation: iridoplegia; phosphene; reflex
accommodative: asthenopia; cyclophoria; strabismus
accompanying: vein
accordion: graft
accoucheur's: hand
accretion: line
accretionary: growth
A.C.E.: mixture
acentric: relation
acetabular: artery; fossa; notch
acetate replacement: factor
acetic: solution
acetone: body; chloroform; test
acetone-insoluble: antigen
acetous: fermentation
acetyl-activating: enzyme
achievement: age; motive; quotient; test
Achilles: bursa; reflex; tendon
achlorhydric: anemia
acholuric: jaundice
achondroplastic: dwarf
achrestic: anemia
achromatic: apparatus; lens; objective; threshold; vision
acid: agglutination; albumin; alcohol; cell; dyspepsia; fuchsin; gland; indigestion; intoxication; maltase; metaprotein; oxide; phosphatase; radical; reaction; ribonuclease; rigor; salt; stain; tartrate; tide; wave
acid-ash: diet
acid-base: balance; equilibrium
acid phosphatase: test
acidified serum: test
acidophil, acidophilic: adenoma; cell; granule; leukocyte; normoblast
acidophilus: milk
acidulous: element; water
acinar: carcinoma; cell
acinic cell: adenocarcinoma; carcinoma
acinose: carcinoma
acinotubular: gland
acinous: carcinoma; cell; gland
ackee: poisoning
acmastic: fever
acne: bacillus; keloid
acneform: syphilid
acoustic: agraphia; aphasia; area; cell; crest; lemniscus; nerve; neurilemoma; neurinoma; neuroma; papilla; radiation; schwannoma; spot; stria; tetanus; tolerance; tubercle; vesicle
acoustic trauma: deafness
acousticofacial: crest; ganglion
acousticopalpebral: reflex
acquired: agammaglobulinemia; character; drive; epilepsy; hyperlipoproteinemia; ichthyosis; immunity; leukoderma; leukopathia; methemoglobinemia; reflex; sensitivity; toxoplasmosis
acquired hemolytic: anemia; icterus
acrid: poison

acrocentric: chromosome
acrodynic: erythema
acrofacial: dysostosis; syndrome
acromegalic: gigantism
acromial: artery; network; process; reflex
acromial articular: facies; surface
acromioclavicular: disk; joint; ligament
acromion: presentation
acromiothoracic: artery
acroparesthesia: syndrome
acrosomal: cap, granule; vesicle
acrylic: resin
acrylic resin: base, tooth, tray
acting assistant: surgeon
actinic: cheilitis; conjunctivitis; dermatitis; elastosis; keratitis; keratosis; porokeratosis; ray
actinium: emanation
actinomycotic: appendicitis
action: current; pattern; potential; tremor
activated: atom; charcoal; epilepsy; hydrogen; resin
activated sludge: method
activation: analysis
active: acetate; algolagnia; anaphylaxis; caries; congestion; delirium; electrode; formyl; hyperemia; immunity; immunization; incontinence; methionine; methyl; movement; principle; prophylaxis; psychoanalysis; repressor; site; sulfate; transport; treatment; vasoconstriction; vasodilation
active chronic: hepatitis
active rosette: test
activity: coefficient
actual: cautery
acuminate papular: syphilid
acupuncture: anesthesia
acute: abdomen; abscess; alcoholism; anemia; angle; appendicitis; ataxia; cholecystitis; delirium; dementia; disease; glomerulonephritis; goiter; inflammation; malaria; melancholia; nephritis; nephrosis; pneumonia; porphyria; rhinitis; rickets; tuberculosis; urticaria
acute adrenocortical: insufficiency
acute anterior: poliomyelitis
acute articular: rheumatism
acute ascending: paralysis
acute atrophic: paralysis
acute bulbar: poliomyelitis
acute compression: triad
acute confusional: insanity
acute contagious: conjunctivitis
acute disseminated: encephalomyelitis; myositis
acute fulminating meningococcal: septicemia
acute hallucinatory: paranoia
acute hemolytic: anemia
acute hemorrhagic: encephalitis; glomerulonephritis; pancreatitis
acute infectious: paralysis
acute interstitial: nephritis; pneumonia
acute isolated: myocarditis
acute miliary: tuberculosis
acute necrotizing: encephalitis
acute necrotizing ulcerative: gingivitis
acute parenchymatous: hepatitis
acute promyelocytic: leukemia

acute pulmonary: alveolitis
acute radiation: syndrome
acute rheumatic: arthritis
acute scalp: cellulitis
acute serous: choroidopathy
acute splenic: tumor
acute transverse: myelitis
acute vascular: purpura
acute yellow: atrophy
acyclic: compound
acylmercaptan: bond
adaptation: disease
adaptive: behavior; enzyme; hypertrophy
addition: compound
additive: effect
adductor: canal; muscle; reflex; tubercle
Aden: fever; ulcer
adeno-associated: virus
adenoid: disease; facies; tissue; tumor
adenoid cystic: carcinoma
adenoidal-pharyngeal-conjunctival: virus
adenomatoid: tumor
adenomatous: goiter; polyp
adequal: cleavage
adequate: diet; stimulus
adherence: syndrome
adherent: leukoma; pericardium; placenta
adhesion: dyspepsia; phenomenon; test
adhesive: arachnoiditis; bandage; inflammation; pericarditis; peritonitis; phlebitis; pleurisy; pylephlebitis; tape
adient: behavior
adipokinetic: hormone
adipose: capsule; cell; degeneration; fossa; infiltration; tissue; tumor
adiposogenital: degeneration; dystrophy; syndrome
adjacent: angle
adjustable: articulator
adjustable axis: face-bow
adjustable occlusal: pivot
adjuvant: vaccine
admaxillary: gland
adnexal: adenoma; carcinoma
adobe: tick
adolescent: albuminuria; crisis; insanity; medicine; sterility
adrenal: androgen; apoplexy; body; capsule; cortex; crisis; gland; hermaphroditism; hypertension; rest; struma; tuberculosis; virilism
adrenal ascorbic acid depletion: test
adrenal cortical: adenoma; carcinoma; syndrome
adrenal virilizing: syndrome
adrenal weight: factor
adrenergic: amine; blockade; fiber; receptor
adrenergic blocking: agent
adrenergic neuronal blocking: agent
adrenocortical: hormone; insufficiency
adrenocorticotropic: hormone; peptide
adrenogenic: syndrome
adrenogenital: syndrome
adrenolytic: agent
adrenomimetic: agent; amine
adrenotropic: hormone
adsorption: analysis; theory
adult: rickets; tridermoma; tuberculosis
adventitial: cell; neuritis

amylic: fermentation
amylogenic: body
amyloid: body; corpuscle; degeneration; kidney; nephrosis; tumor
amyotrophic lateral: sclerosis
A-N: interval
anabiotic: cell
anacidotic: hyperglycemia
anaclitic: depression; psychotherapy
anacoustic: zone
anacrotic: limb; pulse
anadicrotic: pulse
anaerobic: dehydrogenase; respiration
anal: atresia; canal; cleft; column; erotism; fascia; fissure; fistula; gland; membrane; phase; pit; plate; reflex; region; sac; sinus; triangle; verge; valve
anal skin: tag
analeptic: enema
analgesic: abuse; nephritis; nephropathy
analytic: chemistry; psychiatry; psychology; therapy
analyzing: rod
anamnestic: reaction
anaphase: lag
anaphylactic: antibody; intoxication; shock
anaphylactoid: crisis; purpura; shock
anaplastic: cell
anarthritic rheumatoid: disease
anastomosed: graft
anastomosing: fiber
anastomotic: fiber; ulcer; vein
anatomic, anatomical: age; crown; element; neck; pathology; position; rigidity; root; sphincter; tooth; tubercle; wart
anatomical dead: space
anchor: band; splint
anchoring: villus
anchusin: paper
anconal: fosa
anconeus: muscle
ancylostome: anemia
ancylostomiasis: dermatitis
androgen: unit
androgenic: hormone; zone
android: pelvis
anechoic: chamber
anemic: anoxia; halo; infarct; murmur
anergastic: reaction
anergic: leishmaniasis
aneroid: manometer
anesthesia: machine
anesthetic: agent; circuit; depth; ether; gas; index; leprosy; shock; vapor
anestrous: ovulation
aneurysm: needle
aneurysmal: bruit; phthisis; sac; varix
aneurysmal bone: cyst
angel's: wing
angibromic: adenia
anginose: scarlatina
angioblastic: cell
angiodysgenetic: myelomalacia
angiofollicular mediastinal lymph node: hyperplasia
angiolithic: degeneration; sarcoma
angiomatoid: tumor
angioneurotic: edema; hematuria
angio-osteohypertrophy: syndrome

angiopathic: neurasthenia
angioplastic: infantilism
angiosclerotic: gangrene
angiospastic: anesthesia
angular: acceleration; aldehyde; aperture; artery; conjunctivitis; convolution; curvature; gyrus; methyl; notch; stomatitis; vein
anhematopoietic, anhemopoietic: anemia
anhidrotic ectodermal: dysplasia
anhydrocitrovorum: factor
anhydrous: alcohol; lanolin
anicteric virus: hepatitis
aniline: rash
aniline-water: solution
animal: charcoal; dextran; force; graft; gum; lymph; magnetism; pathology; pole; soap; starch; toxin; virus; wax
animal protein: factor
anion-exchange: resin
anionic: detergent
anisometropic: amblyopia
anisotropic: disk; lipoid
ankle: bone; clonus; jerk; joint; reflex
ankyloglossia superior: syndrome
ankylosing: spondylitis
annealing: lamp; tray
annectant: gyrus
annular: cartilage; ligament; pancreas; placenta; plexus; ring; scleritis; scotoma; sphincter; staphyloma; stricture; synechia; syphilid
annulate: lamella
annulospiral: ending; organ
anococcygeal: body; ligament; nerve
anocutaneous: line
anodal: current
anodal closure: contraction; tetanus
anodal duration: tetanus
anodal opening: contraction; tetanus
anode: ray
anogenital: band; raphe
anomalous: complex; correspondence; uterus; viscosity
anomalous mitral: arcade
anomeric: carbon
anomic: aphasia
anonymous: artery; vein
anorectal: abscess; junction; syndrome
anosognosic: seizure
anospinal: center
anovular: menstruation
anovular ovarian: follicle
anovulational: menstruation
anovulatory: cycle
anoxemia: test
anoxic: anoxia
ANS: angle
anserine: bursa
ansiform: lobule
antagonistic: muscle; reflex
antebrachial: fascia
antebrachiocarpal: joint
antecedent: sign
antecubital: space
antemortem: clot; thrombus
anterior: asynclitism; choroiditis; curvature; embryotoxon; guide; megalophthalmus; occlusion; rhinoscopy; rhizotomy; scleritis; sclerotomy; staphyloma; symblepharon; urethritis; uveitis

anterior anatomical structures (specific anterior anatomical and histological structures are listed under the following): arch; area; artery; border; bundle; canal; cell; chamber; column; commissure; convolution; crest; cusp; extremity; fissure; fontanel; foramen; fossa; funiculus; gland; groove; gyrus; horn; joint; layer; ligament; limb; lip; lobe; lobule; margin; membrane; muscle; naris; nerve; node; notch; nucleus; part; pillar; pituitary; plexus; pole; process; pyramid; recess; region; ring; root; segment; spine; substance; sulcus; surface; tract; triangle; tooth; tubercle; valve; vein; velum; wall
anterior chamber cleavage: syndrome
anterior component of: force
anterior facial: height
anterior myocardial: infarction
anterior pelvic: exenteration
anterior pituitary: gonadotropin; reaction
anterior pituitary-like: hormone; substance
anterior-posterior: urethrotomy
anterior spinal: paralysis
anterior tibial compartment: syndrome
anterograde: amnesia; block; conduction; memory
anteroinferior myocardial: infarction
anterolateral: column; fontanel; groove; sulcus; tractotomy
anterolateral myocardial: infarction
anteromedian: groove
anteroposterior: dysplasia
anteroseptal myocardial: infarction
antevesical: hernia
anthracotic: tuberculosis
anthrax: pneumonia
anthropoid: pelvis
antiacrodynia: factor
antialopecia: factor
antianemia: factor
antianemic: principle
antianthrax: serum
antianxiety: agent
anti-basement membrane: nephritis
antiberiberi: factor; vitamin
antibiotic: enterocolitis
anti-black-tongue: factor
antibody deficiency: disease; syndrome
anticoagulant: therapy
anticomplementary: factor; serum
antidiuretic: hormone
antidromic: conduction; volley
anti-egg-white-injury: factor
antiepithelial: serum
antifertility: factor
antifoaming: agent
anti-G: suit
antigen: unit
antigen-antibody: reaction
antigenic: competition; complex; determinant
antigen-responsive: cell
antigen-sensitive: cell
anti-gizzard erosion: factor
antiglobulin: test
antigonadotropic: hormone
antigravity: muscle
anti-gray-hair: factor
antihemophilic: factor; globulin; plasma

antihemorrhagic: factor; vitamin
anti-human globulin: test
anti-insulin: test
anti-intermediary: body
antiketogenic: diet
anti-kidney: antibody
antilymphocyte: serum
antimicrobial: spectrum
anti-Monson: curve
antineuritic: factor; vitamin
antinuclear: antibody; factor
antiophthalmic: factor
antipellagra: factor
antiperistaltic: anastomosis
antipernicious anemia: factor
antipodal: cone
antipsychotic: agent
antirabies: serum
antirachitic: vitamin
antireflection: coating
antireticular cytotoxic: serum
antiscorbutic: vitamin
antiseptic: dressing
antiserum: anaphylaxis
antisterility: factor; vitamin
anti-stiffness: factor
antitoxic: serum
antitoxin: rash; unit
antitragohelicine: fissure
antitrypsin: deficiency
antitryptic: index
antivenene: unit
antiviral: immunity
antixerophthalmic: factor
antral: pouch
anvil: sound
anxiety: dream; hysteria; neurosis; reaction; state; syndrome
anxious: delirium
aortic: arch; area; atresia; body; bulb; dwarfism; facies; foramen; incompetence; insufficiency; murmur; nerve; notch; plexus; reflex; regurgitation; sac; sinus; spindle; stenosis; sulcus; valve; vestibule; window
aortic arch: syndrome
aortic body: tumor
aortic septal: defect
aorticorenal: disease; ganglion
aortocoronary: bypass
aortoiliac: bypass
aortoiliac occlusive: disease
aortopulmonary: septum
apathetic: thyrotoxicosis
A-P-C: virus
ape: fissure; hand
aperiosteal: amputation
Apeu: virus
apex: beat; pneumonia
aphonic: pectoriloquy
aphthobullous: stomatitis
aphthous: fever
apical: abscess; area; complex; dendrite; foramen; gland; granuloma; infection; ligament; pericementitis; pneumonia; process; segment; space
apical ectodermal: ridge
apical lymph: node
apicoposterior: segment
aplanatic: lens
aplastic: anemia; lymph
apneic: oxygenation
apneustic: breathing

apochromatic: lens; objective
apocrine: adenoma; gland; metaplasia; miliaria
apolar: cell
aponeurotic: reflex
apophylactic: phase
apophysary: point
apophysial: fracture; point
apoplectic: cyst; retinitis; type
apoplectiform: myelitis; septicemia
apparent: viscosity
appendiceal: abscess
appendicular: abscess; artery; colic; muscle; skeleton; vein
apperceptive: mass
appetite: juice
applanation: tonometer
apple jelly: nodule
applied: anatomy; anthropology; chemistry
appliqué: form
apposition: suture
appositional: growth
approach-approach: conflict
approach-avoidance: conflict
approximate answers: syndrome (of)
approximation: suture
aptitude: test
APUD: cell
apyretic: tetanus; typhoid
aqueductal: intubation
aqueous: chamber; humor; phase; vaccine
aqueous influx: phenomenon
aquo-: ion
arachnoid, arachnoidal: cyst; foramen; granulation; membrane; villus
arborescent: cataract
arbo-, arbor-: virus
arborization: block
arc: light; perimeter
arc-flash: conjunctivitis
arc-welder's: disease
arch: bar; form
archaic-paralogical: thinking
arched: crest
archenteric: canal
arciform: artery; vein
arcuate: artery; crest; eminence; fasciculus; fiber; line; nucleus; vein; zone
arcuate popliteal: ligament
arcuate pubic: ligament
ardent: fever; spirit
areolar: choroidopathy; gland; tissue
argentaffin: cell; granule; syndrome
Argentinian hemorrhagic: fever
argyrophilic: cell; fiber
Arkansas: stone
arm: phenomenon
armed: tapeworm
armored: heart
aromatic: bitters; castor oil; compound; series; species
arousal: function; reaction
arrested: caries; tuberculosis
arrhenic: medication
arrow point: tracing
arsenic, arsenical: amblyopia; keratosis; pigmentation; tremor
arseniureted: hydrogen
arterial: arch; blood; bulb; canal; capillary; cone; circle; duct; groove; hyperemia; hypotension; ligament; murmur;

nephrosclerosis; sclerosis; spider; systole; tension; transfusion; vein; wave
arteriocapillary: fibrosis; sclerosis
arteriococcygeal: gland
arteriolar: nephrosclerosis; sclerosis
arteriolosclerotic: kidney
arteriolovenular: anastomosis; bridge
arteriosclerotic: aneurysm; kidney; psychosis; retinopathy
arteriovenous: anastomosis; aneurysm; communication; fistula; shunt
arteriovenous carbon dioxide: difference
arteriovenous oxygen: difference
artery: forceps; needle
arthritic: atrophy; calculus; cry
arthritic general: pseudoparalysis
arthrodial: cartilage; joint
articular: capsule; cartilage; chondrocalcinosis; corpuscle; crepitus; crescent; crest; disk; eminence; fossa; fracture; gout; lamella; leprosy; meniscus; muscle; nerve; network; process; sensibility; surface; tubercle
articular vascular: circle
articulated: skeleton
articulating: model; paper
artificial: anatomy; ankylosis; anus; crown; dentition; denture; eye; hibernation; insemination; kidney, melanin; pacemaker; pneumothorax; pupil; radioactivity; respiration; salt; selection; sphincter; stone
artificial active: immunity
artificial Carlsbad: salt
artificial Kissingen: salt
artificial passive: immunity
artistic: anatomy
aryepiglottic: fold
arytenoid: cartilage; gland; swelling
arytenoidal articular: surface
asbestos: acne; corn; liner; wart
ascending: artery; colon; current; degeneration; hemiplegia; myelitis; neuritis; paralysis; part; process
ascending cervical: artery
ascending frontal: convolution; gyrus
ascending lumbar: vein
ascending palatine: artery
ascending parietal: convolution; gyrus
ascending pharyngeal: artery; plexus
ascitic: agar
aseptic: fever; necrosis; surgery
asexual: dwarf; generation; reproduction
ashen: tuber; tubercle; wing
Asian: influenza
Asiatic: cholera; schistosomiasis
asiderotic: anemia
aspermatogenic: sterility
aspheric: lens
asphyxiating: gas
asphyxiating thoracic: dysplasia
aspirating: needle
aspiration: biopsy; pneumonia
Assam: fever
assident: sign; symptom
assimilation: pelvis; sacrum
assistant: surgeon
assisted: respiration
assistive: movement
associated: antagonist; movement
association: area; constant; fiber; mecha-

nism; neurosis; system; test; time; tract

**associative:** aphasia; reaction; strength

**associative automatic:** control

**assortative:** mating

**astacoid:** rash

**asteroid:** body; hyalosis

**asthenic:** orthophoria

**asthenic bulbar:** paralysis

**asthenic bulbospinal:** paralysis

**asthma:** crystal

**asthmatic:** bronchitis

**asthmatoid:** wheeze

**astigmatic:** dial

**astroglia:** cell

**Asturian:** leprosy

**asymmetric motor:** neuropathy

**asymmetrical:** chondrodystrophy; mitosis

**asynchronous pulse:** generator

**atactic, ataxic:** abasia; agraphia; aphasia; gait; nystagmus; paramyotonia; paraplegia

**atavistic:** epiphysis

**atelectatic:** rale

**ateliotic:** dwarf

**atheroma:** embolism

**atheromatous:** cyst; degeneration; plaque

**atherosclerotic:** aneurysm

**athlete's:** albuminuria; foot

**athletic:** heart

**atlantoaxial:** articulation

**atlantooccipital:** articulation; joint; membrane

**atmospheric:** pressure

**atom:** meter

**atomic:** core; heat; nucleus; number; pile; theory; volume; weight

**atomistic:** psychology

**atonic:** bladder; dyspepsia; epilepsy; impotence; ulcer

**atopic:** asthma; cataract; conjunctivitis; dermatitis; eczema; reagin

**atrabiliary:** capsule

**atrabilious:** temperament

**atraumatic:** needle; suture

**atresic:** teratosis

**atretic:** corpus; hormone

**atretic ovarian:** follicle

**atrial:** bigeminy; capture; complex; conduction; dissociation; extrasystole; fibrillation; flutter; gallop; kick; myxoma; sound; standstill; systole; tachycardia

**atrial septal:** defect

**atrial synchronous pulse:** generator

**atrial transport:** function

**atrial triggered pulse:** generator

**atrial-well:** technique

**atriocarotid:** interval

**atriodigital:** dysplasia

**atriosystolic:** murmur

**atrioventricular (or A-V):** band; block; bundle; canal; conduction; cushion; dissociation; extrasystole; gradient; groove; interval; nicking; node; rhythm; septum; sulcus; trunk; valve

**atrioventricular nodal:** bigeminy; extrasystole; rhythm; tachycardia

**atrophic:** arthritis; emphysema; excavation; fracture; gastritis; glossitis; inflammation; pharyngitis; rhinitis; thrombosis; vaginitis

**atrophic spinal:** paralysis

**atropine:** test

**attached:** craniotomy; gingiva

**attached cranial:** section

**attachment:** apparatus

**attention:** reflex

**attenuated:** tuberculosis; virus

**attitudinal:** reflex

**attraction:** sphere

**atypical:** insulin; mesolepidoma; pneumonia; pseudocholinesterase

**atypical verrucous:** endocarditis

**Au:** antigen

**auditory:** agnosia; alternans; amnesia; aphasia; area; canal; capsule; cartilage; cortex; fatigue; field; ganglion; hyperalgesia; hair; lemniscus; localization; nerve; nucleus; ossicle; pit; placode; process; reflex; stria; synesthesia; threshold; tooth; tract; tube; vertigo; vesicle

**auditory oculogyric:** reflex

**auditory receptor:** cell

**augmented histamine:** test

**augmenting:** factor

**augmentor:** fiber; nerve

**Aura:** virus

**aural:** aspergillosis; myiasis; nystagmus; vertigo

**auricular:** appendectomy; appendage; appendix; arc; canaliculus; cartilage; complex; extrasystole; fissure; ganglion; index; ligament; notch; point; reflex; standstill; systole; surface; tachycardia; triangle; tubercle; vein

**auriculocarotid:** interval

**auriculo-infraorbital:** plane

**auriculopalpebral:** reflex

**auriculopressor:** reflex

**auriculotemporal:** nerve

**auriculotemporal nerve:** syndrome

**auriculoventricular:** groove

**auropalpebral:** reflex

**auscultatory:** alternans; gap; percussion; sound

**aussage:** test

**Australia:** antigen

**Australian:** leech

**Australian X:** disease; encephalitis

**Australian X disease:** virus

**authoritarian:** personality

**authority:** figure

**autistic:** parasite

**autoallergic hemolytic:** anemia

**autochthonous:** idea; malaria; parasite; ulcer

**autodermic:** graft

**autoerythrocyte:** sensitization

**autogenous:** union; vaccine

**autogenous bone:** graft

**autoimmune:** disease

**autoimmune hemolytic:** anemia

**autokinetic:** effect

**autologous:** graft; protein

**autolytic:** enzyme

**automatic:** beat; chorea; contraction; epilepsy; plugger

**autonomic:** bladder; disorder; ganglion; imbalance; nerve; plexus

**autonomic diencephalic:** epilepsy

**autonomic motor:** neuron

**autonomic nervous:** system

**autonomous:** psychotherapy

**autoparenchymatous:** metaplasia

**autophagic:** vacuole

**autoplastic:** graft

**autopolymer:** resin

**autopolymerizing:** resin

**autoscopic:** phenomenon

**autoserum:** therapy

**autosomal:** gene

**autosomal recessive:** gargoylism

**autosynthetic:** cell

**autumn:** crocus; fever

**autumnal:** catarrh

**auxanographic:** method

**auxetic:** growth

**auxotrophic:** strain

**avalanche:** conduction

**average pulse:** magnitude

**aversive:** behavior

**avian:** diphtheria; erythroblastosis; leukosis; lymphomatosis; malaria; monocytosis; myeloblastosis; reticuloendotheliosis; spirochetosis; trichomoniasis; tuberculosis

**avian encephalomyelitis:** virus

**avian erythroblastosis:** virus

**avian infectious:** encephalomyelitis; laryngotracheitis

**avian infectious laryngotracheitis:** virus

**avian leukosis-sarcoma:** complex; virus

**avian lymphomatosis:** virus

**avian myeloblastosis:** virus

**avian neurolymphomatosis:** virus

**avian pneumoencephalitis:** virus

**avian sarcoma:** virus

**aviation:** medicine; otitis

**aviator's:** disease; ear

**avoidance:** conditioning

**avoidance-avoidance:** conflict

**avulsed:** wound

**avulsion:** fracture

**awareness of:** reality

**axial:** ametropia; aneurysm; angle; cataract; current; filament; hyperopia; illumination; muscle; myopia; neuritis; plate; skeleton; surface; wall

**axile:** corpuscle

**axillary:** anesthesia; arch; artery; cataract; cavity; fascia; fold; fossa; gland; line; nerve; plexus; region; space; triangle; vein

**axillary lymph:** node

**axillary sweat:** gland

**axioincisal:** angle

**axiolabiolingual:** plane

**axiomesiodistal:** plane

**axis:** cylinder; corpuscle; deviation; ligament; shift; traction

**axis-traction:** forceps

**axoaxonic:** synapse

**axodendritic:** synapse

**axon:** hillock; reflex; terminal

**axonal:** process

**axonal terminal:** bouton

**axosomatic:** synapse

**A.-Z.:** test

**azo:** itch

**azolitmin:** paper

**azotic:** diabetes

**azotobacter:** nuclease

**Aztec:** ear; idiocy

**azurophil:** granule

**azygos:** artery; vein

**azygos vein:** principle

## B

*β*-: see beta
**B**: bile; cell; chain; fiber; line; lymphocyte; virus
**B$_T$**: factor
**baby**: beef; tooth
**bacillary**: dysentery; layer; pyelonephritis
**bacillus Calmette-Guérin**: vaccine
**back**: knee; pressure; tooth
**back-action**: plugger
**back of foot**: reflex
**back vertex**: power
**backward**: caries; curvature; decay
**backward heart**: failure
**backwash**: ileitis
**bacon**: spleen
**bacterial**: allergy; aneurysm; antagonism; capsule endarteritis; endocarditis; hemolysin; persister; plaque; toxin; virus
**bacteriocin**: factor
**bacteriogenic**: agglutination
**bacteriolytic**: serum
**bacteriophage**: immunity; resistance; typing
**bacteriotropic**: substance
**bad**: breath
**badger**: leg
**Bagdad**: boil
**bait**: poison
**baked**: tongue
**baker's**: eczema; itch
**baking**: soda
**balance**: theory
**balanced**: anesthesia; articulation; bite; diet; occlusion; translocation
**balancing**: contact; side
**balancing occlusal**: surface
**balanic**: hypospadias
**balantidial**: dysentery
**BALB**: test
**bald**: tongue
**Balkan**: frame; splint
**ball**: thrombus; variance
**ball-and-socket**: joint
**ball-valve**: action; thrombus
**balloon**: atrioseptostomy; cell
**ballooning**: colliquation; degeneration
**bamboo**: hair
**bamie**: disease
**band**: cell; neutrophil
**band-shaped**: keratopathy
**bandage**: sign
**bandbox**: resonance
**bandy-**: leg
**banjo**: splint
**bankrupt**: worm
**bar**: clasp
**bar clasp**: arm
**bar joint**: denture
**Barbados**: aloe; leg
**barbed**: broach
**barber's**: itch
**barber's pilonidal**: sinus
**Barcoo**: rot; vomit
**bare**: area
**barium**: enema
**barometric**: pressure
**baroreceptor**: nerve
**barrel**: chest
**baryta**: water
**basal**: age; anesthesia; body; bone; cell;

corpuscle; diet; ganglion; granule; lamina; layer; metabolism; part; plate; ridge; rod; seat; sphincter; striation; surface; tuberculosis; vein
**basal cell**: carcinoma; epithelioma; hyperplasia; layer
**basal cell nevus**: syndrome
**basal joint**: reflex
**basal metabolic**: rate
**basal seat**: area
**basal skull**: fracture
**basal squamous cell**: carcinoma
**basaloid**: carcinoma; cell
**base**: hospital; line; material; metal; pair; plate; unit
**baseball**: finger
**basement**: lamina; membrane
**basibregmatic**: axis
**basic**: diet; fuchsin; metal; oxide; personality; salt; stain
**basic personality**: type
**basicranial**: axis
**basifacial**: axis
**basilar**: angle; apophysis; artery; bone; cartilage; cell; crest; impression; index; lamina; leptomeningitis; membrane; meningitis; part; plexus; process; prognathism; sinus; sulcus; vertebra
**basilic**: vein
**basinasal**: line
**basioccipital**: bone
**basipharyngeal**: canal
**basisquamous**: carcinoma
**basivertebral**: vein
**basket**: cell
**basophil**: adenoma; cell; granule; substance
**basophilic**: degeneration; leukemia; leukocyte; leukocytosis; leukopenia
**basosquamous**: carcinoma
**Bassora**: gum
**Batail**: virus
**basylous**: element
**bath**: itch; pruritus
**bathmic**: evolution
**battered child**: syndrome
**battle**: neurosis
**battledore**: placenta
**Bavarian**: splint
**BCG**: vaccine
**bayonet**: hair; leg
**Be$^a$ (Becker)**: antigen
**beaded**: hair
**beaked**: pelvis
**beaker**: cell
**beam**: therapy
**bearing-down**: pain
**bed**: sore
**beech-wood**: sugar
**beef**: tapeworm
**beer**: heart
**beer-drinker's**: cardiomyopathy
**beet**: sugar; tongue
**behavior**: chain; disorder; genetics; modification; reflex; therapist; therapy
**behavioral**: manifestation; psychology
**BEI**: test
**Belgian Congo**: anemia
**bell**: sound
**bell-shaped**: crown
**bellmetal**: resonance
**bellows**: murmur
**belly**: ache; band

**belt**: test
**benign**: albuminuria; glycosuria; hypertension; lymphadenosis; lymphoma; mesothelioma; nephrosclerosis; stupor; tumor
**benign bone**: aneurysm
**benign bovine**: theileriosis
**benign cystic**: epithelioma
**benign dry**: pleurisy
**benign essential**: tremor
**benign familial**: icterus
**benign inoculation**: lymphoreticulosis; reticulosis
**benign juvenile**: melanoma
**benign lymphoepithelial**: lesion
**benign mediastinal lymph node**: hyperplasia
**benign migratory**: glossitis
**benign mucosal**: pemphigoid
**benign myalgic**: encephalomyelitis
**benign ovine**: theileriosis
**benign paroxysmal**: peritonitis
**benign tertian**: malaria
**bent**: fracture
**benzidine**: test
**berlocque, berlock**: dermatitis
**berry**: aneurysm
**beryllium**: granuloma
**beta (*β*-)**: angle; cell; corynebacteriophage; factor; fungus; fiber; granule; hemolysin; hemolysis; leukocyte; oxidation; particle; phage; radiation; ray; receptor; rhythm; substance; thalassemia; wave
**beta-delta (*β-δ*)**: thalassemia
**beta-oxidation-condensation**: theory
**betel**: cancer
**B.-G.**: test
**BH**: interval
**Bi**: antigen
**biauricular**: axis
**biaxial**: joint
**bi-bi**: reaction
**bicameral**: abscess
**bicanalicular**: sphincter
**biceps**: muscle; reflex
**biceps femoris**: reflex
**bicipital**: bursitis; fascia; groove; rib; ridge; tuberosity
**bicipitoradial**: bursa
**biconcave**: lens
**biconvex**: lens
**bicornate**: uterus
**bicoudate**: catheter
**bicuspid**: tooth; valve
**bidirectional ventricular**: tachycardia
**bidiscoidal**: placenta
**bifid**: penis; rib; tongue; uvula
**bifidus**: factor
**bifocal**: lens; spectacles
**bifurcated**: ligament
**bifurcation**: operation
**big**: ACTH; head
**big liver**: disease
**bigeminal**: body; nerve; pregnancy; pulse; rhythm
**bilaminar**: blastoderm
**bilateral**: hemianopsia; hermaphroditism; lithotomy; synchrony
**bile**: capillary; cyst; duct; papilla; peritonitis; thrombus
**Bile's**: antigen
**bile pigment**: hemoglobin
**bilharzial**: appendicitis; dysentery

biliary: atresia; calculus; canaliculus; cirrhosis; colic; duct; ductule; fever; fistula; secretion; steatorrhea

bilious: colic; headache; temperament; typhoid

billious remittent: fever; malaria

bilirubin: encephalopathy

bill of: health

bilocular: joint; stomach

bimanual: percussion; version

bimaxillary: protrusion

Bimeter: gnathodynamometer

Bimiti: virus

binary: acid; alloy; combination; compound; fission; mixture; salt

binasal: hemianopsia

binaural: stethoscope

binding: energy

binocular: diplopia; fixation; hemianopsia; heterochromia; loupe; microscope; ophthalmoscope; parallax; rivalry; vision

binomial: distribution

biochemical: biopsy; block; genetics; metastasis; pharmacology

bioelectric: potential

biogenetic: law

biologic, biological: assay; chemistry; coefficient; evolution; half-life; hemolysis; time; vector

biomedical: engineering

biorbital: angle

biotic: community; factor; potential

biparietal: diameter

bipartite: uterus

bipennate: muscle

biphasic: insulin

bipolar: cautery; cell; lead; neuron; taxis; version

bird: arm; face; leg; tick; unit

bird-breeder's: disease; lung

bird-fancier's: lung

birth: control; palsy; rate; trauma; weight

biscuit: bite

Biskra: button

bite: analysis; block; fork; gauge; opening; plane; rim

bite-wing: film; radiograph

bitemporal: hemianopsia

biting: louse; pressure; strength

bitter: almond; apple; orange; tonic; water

bitterling: test

biundulant: meningoencephalitis

biuret: paper; reaction; reagent; test

bivalent: antibody; chromosome

bivalent gas gangrene: antitoxin

biventral: lobule

black: antimony; cataract; damp; death; disease; eye; fever; fly; hellebore; jaundice; lead; leg; leprosy; lung; measles; mustard; phthisis; piedra; plague; quarter; rat; scours; sickness; spore; tarantula; tongue; urine; vomit; wash; water

black currant: rash

black-dot: ringworm

black-legged: tick

black-pitted: tick

black-tongue: disease

blackwater: fever

bladder: reflex; schistosomiasis

blade: bone

blanching: phenomenon

bland: diet; embolism; embolus

blanket: suture

blast: cell; chest; injury

blastodermic: disk; layer; vesicle

blastomycetic: dermatitis; dermatomycosis

blastoporic: canal

BLB: mask

bleached: wax

bleaching: powder

blear-: eye

bleeding: polyp; time

blending: inheritance

blenorrheal: conjunctivitis

blighted: ovum

blind: boil; enema; fistula; foramen; gut; headache; spot; staggers; test

blind loop: syndrome

blind nasotracheal: intubation

blinding: disease

block: anesthesia; vertebra

block design: test

blocked: aerogastria

blocking: activity; agent; antibody

blood: agar; albumin; bath; blister; calculus; capillary; cast; cell; circulation; clot; corpuscle; count; crisis; crystal; cyst; disk; dyscrasia factor; fluke; island; line; lymph; mole; mote; plasma; plastid; plate; poisoning; pressure; quotient; serum; spavin; sugar; spot; tumor; type; typing; vessel

blood-air: barrier

blood-aqueous: barrier

blood-brain: barrier

blood-cerebrospinal fluid: barrier

blood group: agglutinin; agglutinogen; antibody; antigen; antiserum; system

blood group specific: substance

blood plasma: fraction

blood urea: nitrogen

blood-vascular: system

blood volume: nomogram

bloodless: amputation; decerebration; operation; phlebotomy

bloody: flux; sweat

blowing: wound

blow-out: fracture

blue: asphyxia; atrophy; baby; blindness; cataract; edema; fever; gum; line; nevus; pus; spot; stone; tongue; vision; vitriol

blue dome: cyst

blue pus: bacillus

blue rubber-bleb: nevus

blue-yellow: blindness

bluebottle: fly

bluecomb: disease; virus

bluetongue: virus

blunderbuss: prescription

blunt-: hook

boack scour: worm

board of: health

boat: form

bob: veal

body: cavity; image; language; mechanics; plethysmograph; schema; stalk

body righting: reflex

body-weight: ratio

bog: spavin

boiler-maker's: deafness

boiling: point

Bolivian hemorrhagic: fever

bolster: finger

bomb: calorimeter

bone: abscess; ache; age; architecture; ash; canaliculus; cell; chips; conduction; corpuscle; cyst; earth; flap; forceps; marrow; matrix; phosphate; plate; reflex; resorption; salt; sclerosis; sensibility; spavin; tissue; wax

bont: tick

bony: ankylosis; crepitus; heart; labyrinth; palate; part

bony semicircular: canal

boomerang: leg

booster: dose

Bordeaux: mixture

border: cell, molding; movement; rale; seal

border tissue: movement

borderline: ray

Borna: disease

Borna disease: virus

Borneo: camphor

Bornholm: disease

Bornholm disease: virus

bosch: yaws

Boston: exanthema; opium

bothropic, Bothrops: antitoxin

botulinum: antitoxin

botulinus: toxin

botulism: antitoxin

bound: water

boundary: membrane

bounding: mydriasis; pupil

bouquet: fever

boutonneuse: fever

bovine: antitoxin; babesiosis; brucellosis; colloid; epitheliosis; hemoglobinuria; hyperkeratosis; ketosis; mastitis; theileriosis; trichomoniasis; tuberculosis

bovine cancer: eye

bovine ephemeral: fever

bovine granular: vaginitis

bovine infectious: abortion

bovine milk: fever

bovine papular stomatitis: virus

bovine sporadic: encephalomyelitis

bovine virus: diarrhea

bovine virus diarrhea: virus

bow-: leg

Bowditch Island: ringworm

bowed: tendon

boxer's: ear; fracture

boxing: wax

brachial: anesthesia; artery; fascia; gland; muscle; plexus; vein

brachial birth: palsy

brachiocephalic: muscle; trunk; vein

brachioradial: muscle; reflex

brachypellic: pelvis

bracken: poisoning; staggers

bradykinetic: analysis

brain: abscess; cicatrix; concussion; congestion; contusion; edema; fever; hormone; laceration; lipoid; mantle; murmur; sand; sugar; swelling; syndrome; wave

brain wave: complex; cycle

brainstem: hemorrhage

branched chain: ketoaciduria

brancher: enzyme

brancher deficiency: amylopectinosis
branchial: apparatus; arch; cartilage; cell; cleft; cyst; duct; fissure; fistula; groove; mesoderm; pouch
branchial cleft: cyst
branchial cleft cyst: abscess
branchial efferent: column
branching: enzyme; factor
branchiomotor: nucleus
brandy: nose
branny: tetter
brass-worker's: ague
brassy: body; cough; eye
brawny: arm; scleritis; trachoma
Brazil: wax
Brazilian: blastomycosis
bread: pill
bread-and-butter: pericardium
break: shock
breakaway: phenomenon
breakbone: fever
breakoff: phenomenon
breast: bone; pang; pump
breath-holding: test
breathing: bag; reserve
breech: delivery; extraction; presentation
bregmatic: fontanel
bregmatolambdoid: arc
bregmocardiac: reflex
brephoplastic: graft
brewers': yeast
brick-dust: deposit
brickmaker's: anemia
bridge: corpuscle
bridle: stricture
brightness difference: threshold
brilliant: green; yellow
brilliant green bile salt: agar
brimstone: liver
brisket: disease
bristle: cell; probang
British: gum
British thermal: unit
brittle: bone; diabetes
broad: fascia; foot; ligament; spectrum; tapeworm
broad fish: tapeworm
broad spectrum: antibiotic
broadest: muscle
broken: dose; knee
bromide: acne
bromine: water
bromphenol: test
Bromsulphalein: test
bronchial: allergy; asthma; adenoma; artery; breathing; bud; fluke; fremitus; gland; hemorrhage; pneumonia; polyp; respiration; tube; voice; vein
bronchic: cell
bronchiolar: carcinoma
bronchitic: asthma
bronchoesophageal: fistula; muscle
bronchogenic: carcinoma
bronchopleural: fistula
bronchopulmonary: aspergillosis; segment; sequestration; spirochetosis
bronchopulmonary lymph: node
bronchoscopic: brush; smear; sponge
bronchovesicular: respiration
bronze: phlegmon
bronzed: diabetes; disease; skin
brood: capsule; cell

brow: ague
brown: atrophy; edema; fat; induration; stria; tumor
brown dog: tick
brucella: vaccine
brush: border; burn
brush burn: abrasion
brush heap: structure
bubble gum: dermatitis
bubbling: rale
bubonic: plague
buccal: angle; artery; cavity; curve; embrasure; flange; gingiva; gland; nerve; occlusion; pit; region; smear; surface; tablet; vestibule
buccal lymph: node
buccinator: artery; crest; nerve
buccocervical: ridge
buccogingival: ridge
buccolingual: diameter; dimension; relation
bucconasal: membrane
bucconeural: duct
bucco-occlusal: angle
buccopharyngeal: fascia; membrane; part
buck: tooth
bucked: shin
bucket-handle: fracture; tear
buckled: aorta
buckthorn: polyneuropathy
bud: fission
buddeized: milk
buffalo: gnat; neck
buffer: capacity; index
buffer salts: solution
buffy: coat
Bukalasa: virus
bulbar: apoplexy; myelitis; palsy; paralysis; pulse; ridge; septum
bulbocavernous: reflex
bulbosacral: system
bulbourethral: gland
bulboventricular: loop; ridge
bulboid: corpuscle
bulbomimic: reflex
bull: neck
bulldog: calf; forceps; head; scalp
bullet: bubo; forceps
bullous: edema; fever; impetigo; keratopathy; syphilid
bundle: bone
bundle-branch: block
Bunyamwera: virus
bur: drill
Burdwan: fever
Burgundy: pitch
buried: suture
Burmese: ringworm
burning drops: sign
burnt: alum
burr: cell
burrowing: hair
bursal: abscess; cyst; synovitis
buruli: ulcer
bush: sickness; yaws
buss: disease
Bussuguara: virus
butanol-extractable iodine: test
butcher's: wart
butter: cyst; stool
butterfly: adrenal; eruption; fracture; lung; patch; rash; vertebra

button: cautery; suture
buttonhole: fracture; iridectomy; stenosis
buttonmaker's: chorea
buttress: foot
buyo cheek: cancer
Bwamba: virus
By: antigen
Byzantine arch: palate

### C

C: bile; cell; factor; fiber
C1: esterase
C3: convertase; proactivator
c-a: interval
C-reactive: protein
CA: virus
cabbage: goiter
cable: graft; rash
cacao: butter
Cache Valley: virus
cachectic: edema; endocarditis; fever; infantilism; pallor
cadaveric: rigidity; spasm
caddis: fly; worm
café-au-lait: spot
Cagot: ear
Cain: complex
caisson: disease
cake: alum; kidney
caked: breast
Calabar: swelling
calcaneal: artery; bone; bursitis; region; sulcus; tuber; tuberosity
calcaneal articular: surface
calcanean: tendon
calcaneocuboid: joint; ligament
calcaneofibular: ligament
calcaneonavicular: ligament
calcaneotibial: ligament
calcareous: conjunctivitis; degeneration; infiltration; metastasis
calcarine: artery; fasciculus; fissure; sulcus
calcic: water
calcific nodular aortic: stenosis
calcification: inhibitor; line
calcified: cartilage
calcined: baryta; magnesia
calcinuric: diabetes
calcium: gout; rigor; time
calf: bone; diphtheria
caliciform, calyciform: cell; ending
California: disease; virus
California black-legged: tick
California psychological: test
caliper: micrometer
callosal: convolution; gyrus; sulcus
callosomarginal: fissure
calomel: electrode
caloric: nystagmus; quotient; test
calorigenic: action
calvarial: hook
cambium: layer
camel: pox
cameloid: anemia; cell
camp: fever; hospital
camphorated: menthol; phenol
camptomelic: dwarfism
Canada: balsam; snakeroot; turpentine
Canadian: hemp
canal: ray
canalicular: abscess; duct; sphincter

canarypox: virus
cancellous: bone; tissue
cancer: body; juice
cane: sugar
canefield: fever
canicola: fever
canine: babesiosis; eminence; fossa; leishmaniasis; prominence; spasm; tooth
canine distemper: virus
canine oral: papilloma
canine venereal: granuloma
canker: rash; sore
cannon: bone; sound; wave
cannonball: pulse
canon: bone
cantering: rhythm
canthal: hypertelorism
cantharidal: collodion
cantharis: camphor
cantilever: beam
caoutchouc: pelvis
cap: splint; stage
Cape: aloe; gum
capeline: bandage
capillary: angioma; apoplexy; arteriole; attraction; bed; bronchiectasis; bronchitis; circulation; drainage; embolus; fracture; hemangioma; lake; loop; nevus; pulse; pericyte; vein; vessel
capillary fragility: test
capillary resistance: test
capital: operation
capitate: bone
capitular: joint
capon-comb-growth: test
capped: elbow; hock; knee; uterus
capsular: advancement; antigen; cataract; cirrhosis; insufficiency; ligament; space
capsule: cell; forceps
capsulolenticular: cataract
capture: beat
car: sickness
Caraparu: virus
carbacrylamine: resin
carbocyclic: compound; ring
carbohydrate: metabolism
carbohydrate-induced: hyperlipemia
carbol-fuchsin: paint
carbolic: fuchsin
carbon: cycle
carbon dioxide: acidosis; alkalosis; cycle; electrode; elimination
carbon dioxide-free: water
carbon dioxide withdrawal seizure: test
carbon disulfide: poisoning
carbon monoxide: hemoglobin; poisoning
carbonated: water
carbonic: anhydrase
carbureted: hydrogen
carcinoembryonic: antigen
carcinogenic: hydrocarbon
carcinoid: syndrome; tumor
carcinomatous: implant; myopathy
cardiac: accident; albuminuria; aneurysm; arrest; asthma; calculus; catheter; cirrhosis; competence; cycle; decompression; diastole; diuretic; edema; failure; ganglion; gland; hemoptysis; heterotaxia; histiocyte; impression; impulse; incompetence; in-

dex; infarction; insufficiency; jelly; liver; lung; massage; monitor; murmur; muscle; neurosis; notch; opening; output; part; plexus; polyp; reflex; reserve; segment; skeleton; souffle; sound; symphysis; tamponade; telemetry; tube; vein
cardiac depressor: reflex
cardiac muscle: tissue
cardinal: ligament; point; symptom; vein
cardioarterial: interval
cardioesophageal: relaxation
cardiogenic: plate; shock
cardiohepatic: angle; triangle
cardioid: condenser
cardiomuscular: bradycardia
cardiopulmonary: bypass; murmur
cardiorespiratory: murmur
cardiothoracic: index; ratio
cardiotoxic: myolysis
cardiovascular: system
carinate: abdomen
cariniform: cartilage
carnauba: wax
carneous: degeneration; mole
β-carotene cleavage: enzyme
caroticoclinoid: ligament
caroticotympanic: artery; nerve
carotid: artery; body; bruit; bulb; canal; duct; foramen; ganglion; groove; shudder; sinus; sulcus; tubercle; triangle; wall
carotid body: tumor
carotid-cavernous: fistula
carotid sinus: reflex; syncope; syndrome
carpal: arch; artery; articulation; bone; canal; groove; joint; tunnel
carpal articular: surface
carpal tunnel: syndrome
carpometacarpal: joint; ligament
carpopedal: contraction; spasm
carrier: cell; state; strain
carrying: angle
cartilage: bone; capsule; cell; corpuscle; lacuna; matrix; space
cartilage-hair: hypoplasia
cartilaginous: joint; neurocranium; part; septum; tissue; viscerocranium
cascade: stomach
caseation: necrosis
caseous: abscess; degeneration; lymphadenitis; necrosis; osteitis; pneumonia; tubercle
cassia: cinnamon
cast gold: crown
cast iron: struma
Castile: soap
casting: flask; ring; wax
castor bean: tick
castrate: cell
castration: anxiety; cell; complex
cat: fever; flea; plague; unit
cat-bite: disease; fever
cat-cry: syndrome
cat distemper: virus
cat liver: fluke
cat-scratch: disease; fever
cat's-eye: pupil; syndrome
catacrotic: pulse
catadicrotic: pulse
catalactic: reaction
cataract: lens; needle; spoon

cataract-oligophrenia: syndrome
catarrhal: appendicitis; asthma; conjunctivitis; fever; gastritis; inflammation; jaundice; ophthalmia; pneumonia
catastrophic: reaction
catatonic: dementia; excitement; rigidity; schizophrenia; stupor
catatorulin: test
catchment: area
catecholamine: test
caterpillar: cell; dermatitis; rash
caterpillar-hair: ophthalmia
catgut: suture
catheter: embolus; fever; gauge
cathodal closure: contraction; tetanus
cathodal duration: tetanus
cathodal opening: clonus; contraction; tetanus
cathode: ray
cathode ray: oscillograph
cation-exchange: resin
cationic: detergent
cattle: grub; plague; tick; wart
cattle plague: virus
Catu: virus
cauda equina: syndrome
caudal: anesthesia; canal; flexure; ligament; retinaculum; sheath; vertebra
caudal neurosecretory: system
caudal pancreatic: artery
caudal pharyngeal: complex
caudal transtentorial: herniation
caudate: lobe; nucleus; process
caul: fat
cauliflower: ear; excrescence
causal: treatment
caustic: alkali; potash; soda
cautery: knife
caval: fold; pocket; valve
cavalry: bone
cavernous: angioma; artery; body; groove; hemangioma; lymphangiectasis; nerve; plexus; rale; resonance; respiration; rhonchus; sinus; syndrome; tissue
cavernous-carotid: aneurysm
cavernous voice: sound
caviar: lesion
cavity: margin; preparation; wall
cavity line: angle
cavosurface: angle
CB: lead
CCA: virus
CDE: antigen
ceasmic: teratosis
cecal: artery; foramen; fold; hernia; recess
cecocentral: scotoma
Celestin: tube
celiac: artery; axis; disease; ganglion; gland; plexus; rickets; syndrome; trunk
celiac lymph: node
celiac plexus: reflex
celiotomy: incision
cell: assembly; bridge; center; inclusion; line; membrane; nest; strain; wall
cell-color: index
cell-mediated: immunity; reaction
cellular: cartilage; embolus; immunity; infiltration; pathology; polyp; spill; tenacity; tumor
cellular immunity deficiency: syndrome

cellulitic: phlegmasia
cellulocutaneous: flap
CELO: virus
celomic: bay; pouch
celomic metaplasia: theory
cement: base; corpuscle; line; substance
cemental: ligament
cementifying: fibroma
cementodentinal: junction
cementum: hyperplasia
centigrade: scale
centimeter-gram-second: system
centinormal: solution
central: amputation; apparatus; artery;
    bearing; body; bone; bradycardia; cal-
    lus; canal; cataract; chromatolysis;
    deafness; ganglioneuroma; glare; gy-
    rus; illumination; implantation; inci-
    sor; inhibition; lacteal; lobule; necro-
    sis; neuritis; nystagmus; osteitis; pa-
    ralysis; pit; pneumonia; scotoma; spin-
    dle; sulcus; tendon; vein; vision
central angiospastic: retinitis; retinopa-
    thy
central areolar choroidal: sclerosis
central-bearing: device; point
central-bearing tracing: device
central core: disease
Central European tick-borne: fever
Central European tick-borne fever: vi-
    rus
central excitatory: state
central gray: substance
central lymph: node
central nervous: system
central pontine: myelinolysis
central serous: retinopathy
central tegmental: fasciculus; tract
central terminal: electrode
central transactional: core
centrencephalic: epilepsy
centric: checkbite; contact; occlusion; po-
    sition; relation
centric jaw: relation
centrifugal: casting; current; nerve
centrilobular: emphysema
centripetal: current; nerve
centroacinar: cell
centrodistal: joint
centrolecithal: egg; ovum
centromedian: nucleus
centronuclear: myopathy
cephalic: angle; delivery; flexure; index;
    pole; presentation; reflex; tetanus; tri-
    angle; vein; version
cephalometric: roentgenogram
cephalo-oculocutaneous: telangiectasia
cephalo-orbital: index
cephalopalpebral: reflex
cephalorrhachidian: index
cephalotrigeminal: angiomatosis
ceramide: saccharide
ceramo-metal: crown
ceratopharyngeal: part
cerebellar: ataxia; atrophy; artery; cor-
    tex; cyst; fissure; gait; hemisphere;
    notch; pyramid; rigidity; speech; syn-
    drome; sulcus; tonsil; vein
cerebellomedullary: cistern
cerebellomedullary malformation: syn-
    drome
cerebellopontine: angle; recess
cerebellopontine angle: syndrome; tu-
    mor

cerebellorubral: tract
cerebellothalamic: tract
cerebral: abscess; agraphia; anesthesia;
    aneurysmorrhaphy; angiography; an-
    thrax; arteriography; artery; claudica-
    tion; compression; cortex; crisis;
    death; decompression; decortication;
    diabetes; diataxia; edema; fissure; flex-
    ure; gigantism; hemisphere; hemor-
    rhage; hernia; hyperesthesia; index;
    layer; lipidosis; localization; palsy; pe-
    duncle; porosis; sinus; sphingolipi-
    dosis; sulcus; surface; tetanus; throm-
    bosis; tuberculosis; vein; ventricle; ve-
    sicle
cerebral vascular: accident
cerebrohepatorenal: syndrome
cerebropupillary: reflex
cerebroside: lipidosis
cerebrospinal: axis; fever; fluid; index;
    meningitis; pressure; system
cerebrospinal fluid: otorrhea; rhinor-
    rhea
cerebrotendinous: cholesterinosis; xan-
    thomatosis
cerebrovascular: disease
ceroid: lipofuscinosis
certified: milk
certified pasteurized: milk
ceruminous: gland
cervical: amputation; anesthesia; auri-
    cle; canal; carcinosis; diverticulum;
    duct; dysplasia; enlargement; fascia;
    fibrosis; fistula; flexure; fringe; gland;
    hydrocele; hyperesthesia; ligament;
    line; margin; myositis; myospasm;
    nerve; part; pleura; plexus; preg-
    nancy; rib; sinus; smear; spondylosis;
    vein; vertebra; vesicle; zone
cervical aortic: knuckle
cervical compression: syndrome
cervical disc: syndrome
cervical fusion: syndrome
cervical interspinal: muscle
cervical rib: syndrome
cervical rotator: muscle
cervical tension: syndrome
cervicolumbar: phenomenon
cervico-oculo-acoustic: syndrome
cervicothoracic: ganglion; transition
cervicovaginal: artery
cesarean: hysterectomy; operation; sec-
    tion
Ceylon: moss
CF: antibody; lead
CGS, cgs: unit
chain: reaction; reflex
chair: form
chalice: cell
chalybeate: water
chancriform: syndrome
chancroidal: bubo
character: analysis; disorder; neurosis
characterizing: group
charge: number; nurse
charge transfer: complex
check: ligament
cheek: bone; muscle; tooth
cheese: fly; maggot
cheesy: pneumonia; pus
chelating: agent
chemical: antidote; attraction; burn; car-
    tery; ceptor; conjunctivitis; dermatitis;
    energy; equation; equivalent; formula;

kinetics; mutagen; peritonitis; pneu-
    monia; prophylaxis; ray; solution; sym-
    pathectomy; thyroidectomy
chemoreceptor: apnea; tumor
chemotactic sexual: hormone
chemotherapeutic: index
Chenuda: virus
cherry: angioma
cherry-red: spot
cherubic: facies
chessboard: graft
chest: index; lead; wall
chewing: cycle; force
Chian: turpentine
chiasma: syndrome
chiasmatic: astrocytoma; sulcus
chick antidermatitis: factor
chick antipellagra: factor
chick nutritional: dermatosis
chicken: breast; cholera; pox
chicken embryo lethal orphan: virus
chicken fat: clot
chickenpox: virus
chiclero's: ulcer
chief: agglutinin; artery; cell
chigger: flea; mite
Chikungunya: virus
child: abuse
childbearing: age
childbed: fever
childhood muscular: dystrophy
childhood type: tuberculosis
Chilean: saltpeter
chimney sweep's: cancer
chimpanzee coryza: agent
chin: cap; jerk; reflex
chinchilla: giardiasis
Chinese: ginger; ringworm
Chinese liver: fluke
Chinese restaurant: syndrome
chip: syringe
chiral: crystal
chirognostic: feeling
chisel: fracture
chloride: depletion; shift
chlorinated: lime; paraffin
chlorine: water
chloropercha: method
chlorophyll: unit
chloroquine: retinopathy
chlorotic: anemia
choanal: atresia; polyp
chocolate: cyst
choke: damp
choked: disk
cholangiolitic: cirrhosis; hepatitis
cholecystoduodenal; fistula
choledoch: duct
choledochal: cyst; sphincter
choledochoduodenal: junction
cholemic: nephrosis
cholera: agar; bacillus; toxin; vaccine
choleraic: diarrhea
cholera-red: reaction
choleric: temperament
choleriform: syndrome
cholestatic: hepatitis; jaundice
cholesterinized: antigen
cholesterol: balance; cleft; embolism
cholestyramine: resin
cholinergic: blockade; fiber; receptor
chondrin: ball
chondrodystrophic: dwarfism
chondroectodermal: dysplasia

chondroid: tissue
chondromyxoid: fibroma
chondropharyngeal: part
chondroxiphoid: ligament
chop: amputation
chorda: saliva
chorda tympani: nerve
choreic: abasia; insanity; movement
chorioallantoic: graft; membrane; placenta
chorioamniotic: placenta
choriocapillary: layer
chorionic: gonadotropin; plate; sac; villus
chorionic gonadotropic: hormone
chorionic gonadotropin: unit
chorionic growth: hormone
chorioptic: mange
choriovitelline: placenta
choroid: fissure; glomus; plexus; skein; tela; vein
choroidal: cataract
Chr$^a$: antigen
Christchurch (Ch$^1$): chromosome
Christmas: disease; factor
chromaffin: body; cell; system; tissue; tumor
chromatic: aberration; apparatus; audition; fiber; granule; spectrum; vision
chromatin: body; network; nucleus; particle
chromatographic: adsorption; analysis
chromatophorotropic: hormone
chrome: alum; ulcer
chrome-cobalt: alloy
chromic: myopia
chromidial: apparatus; net; substance
chromophil: adenoma; granule; substance
chromophobe: adenoma; cell; granule
chromosome: aberration; satellite; trisomy
chronic: abscess; alcoholism; anaphylaxis; appendicitis; cholecystitis; dementia; disease; dysentery; gingivitis; glomerulonephritis; inflammation; malaria; melancholia; nephritis; periodontitis; pneumonia; rheumatism; rhinitis; shock; ulcer; urticaria; vertigo
chronic absorptive: arthritis
chronic acholuric: jaundice
chronic adrenocortical: insufficiency
chronic anterior: poliomyelitis
chronic atrophic: polychondritis; thyroiditis; vulvitis
chronic cicatrizing: enteritis
chronic coccogenic: sycosis
chronic constrictive: pericarditis
chronic cystic: mastitis
chronic desquamative: gingivitis; gingivosis
chronic discoid: lupus (erythematosus)
chronic endemic: fluorosis
chronic familial: icterus; jaundice; polyneuritis
chronic granulomatous: disease
chronic hemorrhagic villous: synovitis
chronic hypertensive: disease
chronic hypertrophic: vulvitis
chronic hyperventilation: syndrome
chronic hypocomplementemic: glomerulonephritis
chronic interstitial: hepatitis; salpingitis

chronic nonleukemic: myelosis
chronic progressive: chorea
chronic proliferative: arthritis
chronic respiratory: disease
chronic rheumatic: arthritis
chronic septic apical: pericementitis
chronologic: age
chyle: cistern; corpuscle; cyst; peritonitis; vessel
chyliform: ascites
chylous: arthritis; ascites; hydrothorax; urine
cicatricial: alopecia; conjunctivitis; horn; kidney; pemphigoid
cigarette: drain
cigarette-paper: scar
ciliary: blepharitis; body; canal; cartilage; crown; disk; fold; ganglion; gland; ligament; margin; movement; muscle; part; process; reflex; ·ing; staphyloma; vein; wreath; zone; zonule
ciliary ganglionic: plexus
ciliated: eipthelium
ciliospinal: center; reflex
cincture: sensation
cinema: eye
cinematic: amputation
cineplastic: amputation
cingulate: convolution; gyrus; herniation
circadian: rhythm
circinate: retinitis; retinopathy
circle absorption: anesthesia
circling: disease
circular: amputation; bandage; dichroism; fiber; fold; insanity; layer; psychosis; reaction; sinus; sulcus
circulation: time
circulatory: arrest; collapse; system
circumanal: gland
circumferential: cartilage; clasp; fibrocartilage; implantation; lamella; wiring
circumferential clasp: arm
circumflex: nerve; vein
circumflex fibular: artery
circumflex scapular: artery
circumnevic: vitiligo
circumscribed: edema; myxedema; peritonitis; pyocephalus; scleroderma
circumvallate: papilla
circus: movement; rhythm
cirrhotic: kidney
cirsoid: aneurysm; varix
cisternal: puncture
citrate: intoxication
citric acid: cycle
citrovorum: factor
CL: lead
clamp: band; forceps
clang: association
clasp: bar; guideline
clasping: reflex
clasp-knife: effect; rigidity; spasticity
classic, classical: conditioning; migraine
clastic: anatomy
clathrate: crystal
claustral: layer
clavate: papilla
Clavelée: virus
clavicular: notch; part; percussion
clavipectoral: fascia
claw: foot; hand

clay pigeon: poisoning
cleansing: cream
clear: cell; layer
clear cell: carcinoma; hidradenoma
clear liquid: diet
clearing: factor; medium
cleavage: cavity; cell; division; line; product; spindle
cleft: foot; hand; lip; nose; palate; spine; tongue
cleidocranial: dysostosis
clenched fist: sign
clergymen's sore: throat
clerical: spectacles
clicking: rale; tinnitus
clidocranial: dysostosis
client-centered: therapy
climacteric: melancholia; psychosis; syndrome
climatic: bubo; keratopathy
climbing: fiber
clinical: chemistry; crown; diagnosis; eruption; medicine; pathology; psychology; root; spectrometry; spectroscopy; thermometer
clinoid: process
clip: forceps
clipped: speech
cloacal: membrane; plate; theory
clonal: aging
clonal selection: theory
clonic: convulsion; spasm
close: bite
closed: bite; circle; drainage; fracture; hospital; reduction; surgery
closed chain: compound
closed chest: massage
closed circuit: method
closed loop: obstruction
closed plaster: method
closed skull: fracture
closing: contraction; snap; volume
closure: principle
clot retraction: time
clotting: enzyme; factor; time
clouding of: consciousness
cloudy: swelling; urine
clover: disease
club: foot; hair; hand; moss
clubbed: digit; finger; penis
cluster: analysis; headache
CM-: cellulose
CO$_2$: see carbon dioxide
coacervating: agent
coagulated: protein
coagulation: factor; necrosis; time
coal miner's: disease
coaptation: splint, suture
coarctate: retina
coarse: dispersion; tremor
coast: erysipelas
coastal: fever
coated: tongue
coat-sleeve: amputation
cobaltinitrate: method
cobbler's: chest; suture
cobra: hemotoxin
cobra venom: cofactor; factor
cocal: virus
cocarde: reaction
coccidioidal: granuloma
coccidioidin: test
coccygeal: body; bone; fistula; foveola; ganglion; gland; joint; nerve; plexus;

sinus; vertebra; whorl
**Cochin China:** diarrhea
**cochlear:** aqueduct; area; canal; canaliculus; duct; implant; joint; nerve; nucleus; recess; root; window
**cochlear hair:** cell
**cochleariform:** process
**cochleo-orbicular:** reflex
**cochleopalperbral:** reflex
**cochleopupillary:** reflex
**cochleostapedial:** reflex
**cockade:** reaction
**cockscomb:** ulcer
**coconut:** sound
**codfish:** vertebra
**Coe:** virus
**coenocytic:** mycelium
**coenzyme:** factor
**coetaneous:** tridermoma
**cofactor of:** thromboplastin
**coffee-ground:** vomit
**coffer:** dam
**coffin:** bone; joint
**cognitive:** psychology
**cognitive dissonance:** theory
**cogwheel:** phenomenon; respiration; rigidity
**cohesive:** gold
**coil:** gland
**coiled:** artery
**coin:** lesion; sign; test
**coital:** exanthema
**coital exanthema of cattle:** virus
**cold:** abscess; agglutination; agglutinin; allergy; autoantibody; bath; cautery; conization; cream; gangrene; hemolysin; infusion; light; nodule; pack; snare; sore; stage; test; ulcer; urticaria; virus
**cold bend:** test
**cold-blooded:** animal
**cold cure:** resin
**cold-curing:** resin
**cold hemagglutinin:** disease
**cold-rigor:** point
**coli:** granuloma; infection
**colic:** impression; intussusception; sphincter; surface; tenia; vein
**colitic:** arthritis
**collagen:** disease; fiber
**collagenous:** fiber
**collapse:** delirium; therapy
**collapsing:** pulse
**collar:** bone; crown
**collar-button:** abscess
**collar-stud:** chalazion
**collared:** flagellate
**collateral:** artery; circulation; eminence; fissure; hyperemia; inheritance; ligament; sulcus; trigone; vessel
**collateral digital:** artery
**collecting:** tubule
**collective:** unconscious
**collier's:** lung; phthisis
**colliquative:** albuminuria; degeneration; diarrhea; necrosis; sweat
**collision:** tumor
**collodion:** baby
**colloid:** adenoma; body; cancer; carcinoma; corpuscle; cyst; degeneration; goiter; milium; solution; system; theory
**colloidal:** dispersion; gel; gold; metal
**colloidoclastic:** shock

**colocutaneous:** fistula
**coloileal:** fistula
**colon:** bacillus
**colonic:** fistula; smear
**colony:** conception
**color:** amblyopia; blindness; hearing; hemianopsia; index; radical; scotoma; sense; spectrum; taste; vision
**color-contrast:** microscope
**Colorado tick:** fever
**Colorado tick fever:** virus
**colored:** sweat
**colorimetric:** analysis; titration
**colorimetric caries susceptibility:** test
**colostrum:** corpuscle
**colovaginal:** fistula
**colovesical:** fistula
**Columbia S. K.:** virus
**column:** cell
**columnar:** cell; epithelium; layer
**coma:** cast; vigil
**comb-growth:** test
**combination:** beat; filling
**"combination" oral:** contraceptive
**combined:** immunodeficiency; pregnancy; sclerosis; version; water
**combined fat- and carbohydrate-induced:** hyperlipemia
**combined system:** disease
**combining:** weight
**comblike:** septum
**combustion:** equivalent
**comedo:** nevus
**comfort:** zone
**comma:** bacillus; bundle; tract
**commemorative:** sign
**commensal:** parasite
**comminuted:** fracture
**commissural:** cell; cheilitis; fiber; myelotomy
**common:** limb; migraine; opsonin; wart
**common basal:** vein
**common carotid:** plexus
**common cold:** virus
**common facial:** vein
**common fibular:** nerve
**common hepatic:** artery; duct
**common iliac:** artery; vein
**common iliac lymph:** node
**common interosseous:** artery
**common palmar digital:** artery; nerve
**common peroneal:** nerve
**common plantar digital:** artery; nerve
**communicable:** disease
**communicated:** insanity
**communicating:** artery; hydrocephalus
**community:** dentistry; nurse; psychiatry; psychology
**community mental health:** center
**compact:** bone
**companion:** vein
**comparative:** anatomy; pathology; physiology; psychology
**comparator:** microscope
**compensated:** acidosis; alkalosis
**compensating:** curve; emphysema; ocular
**compensation:** neurosis
**compensatory:** atrophy; circulation; emphysema; hypertrophy; pause; polycythemia
**competitive:** antagonist; inhibition
**complement:** fixation; unit
**complement chemotactic:** factor

**complement-fixation:** reaction; test
**complement-fixing:** antibody
**complemental:** air
**complementary:** air; color; hypertrophy; role; strand
**complete:** abortion; amelia; antibody; antigen; ascertainment; cataract; cleavage; denture; disinfectant; fistula; hemianopsia; hernia; iridoplegia; metamorphosis; symblepharon; transduction
**complete A-V:** dissociation
**complete color:** blindness
**complete denture:** impression
**complete scalp:** avulsion
**complex:** cavity
**complex learning:** process
**complicated:** cataract; fracture
**complicating:** disease
**composite:** fracture
**compound:** anchorage; aneurysm; cavity; character; cyst; dislocation; eye; filling; fracture; gland; joint; lens; microsome; monster; nevus; pregnancy; protein
**compound granule:** cell
**compound hyperopic:** astigmatism
**compound myopic:** astigmatism
**compound skull:** fracture
**comprehensive medical:** care
**compressed:** sponge; tablet; yeast
**compressible cavernous:** body
**compression:** anesthesia; cough; cyanosis; molding; paralysis; syndrome; thrombosis
**compressive:** myelopathy; strength
**compulsive:** act; idea; insanity; neurosis; personality
**computer:** model; simulation
**concave:** lens
**concavoconcave:** lens
**concavoconvex:** lens
**concealed:** conduction; hemorrhage; hernia
**concentrated human red blood:** corpuscles
**concentration:** gradient
**concentric:** fibroma; hypertrophy; lamella
**concept:** formation
**conchal:** cartilage; crest
**concomitant:** strabismus; symptom
**concordant:** alternans; alternation
**concrete:** operation; seborrhea; thinking
**concussion:** edema; myelitis
**condensation:** compound
**condensed:** milk
**condensing:** enzyme; osteitis
**conditioned:** avitaminosis; hemolysis; reflex; response; stimulus
**conducting:** airway; system
**conduction:** analgesis; anesthesia; aphasia
**conductive:** deafness; heat
**conductive hearing:** impairment
**condylar:** articulation; axis; canal; fossa; guidance; joint; process
**condylar emissary:** vein
**condylar guidance:** inclination
**condyle:** cord; path; joint
**condyloid:** joint; process
**cone:** cell; fiber; granule; vision
**confluent:** articulation; smallpox
**confrontation:** method

confusion: color
confusional: insanity
congelation: urticaria
congenital: afibrinogenemia; agammaglobulinemia; amputation; anemia; baldness; cataract; conus; disease; dysphagocytosis; elephantiasis; glaucoma; hydrocele; hydrocephalus; hypophosphatasia; leukoderma; leukopathia; lymphedema; megacolon; methemoglobinemia; myxedema; nystagmus; pancytopenia; paramyotonia; pneumonia; stridor; syphilis; torticollis; toxoplasmosis; valve
congenital adrenal: hyperplasia
congenital aplastic: anemia
congenital aregenerative: anemia
congenital atonic: pseudoparalysis
congenital cerebral: aneurysm
congenital dyserythropoietic: anemia
congenital dysplastic: angiectasia; angiomatosis; angiopathy
congenital ectodermal: defect; dysplasia
congenital erythropoietic: porphyria
congenital hemolytic: anemia; icterus; jaundice
congenital hypoplastic: anemia
congenital ichthyosiform: erythroderma
congenital oral: leukokeratosis
congenital pyloric: stenosis
congenital sebaceous gland: hyperplasis
congenital spastic: paraplegia
congenital sutural: alopecia
congenital total: lipodystrophy
congestive: apoplexy; chill; failure; splenomegaly
Congo red: paper
Congolian red: fever
congruent: point
congruous: hemianopsia
conic: papilla
conical: cornea
conjoined: manipulation; tendon; twins
conjoint: therapy
conjugal: cancer; diabetes
conjugate: axis; deviation; diameter; disparity; foramen; focus; gaze; ligament; movement; paralysis
conjugated: compound; estrogen; protein
conjugated acid-base: pair
conjugated double: bond
conjunctival: artery; cul-de-sac; gland; layer; reaction; reflex; ring; sac; test; vein
connecting: cartilage; tubule
connective: tissue; tumor
connective tissue: cell; group
connector: bar
conoid: ligament; process; tubercle
consecutive: amputation; aneurysm; angiitis
consensual: reaction; validation
consensual light: reflex
conservation of: energy
conservative: surgery; treatment
consistency: principle
consonating: rale
constancy: phenomenon
constant: coupling; current

constant field: equation
constitutional: cause; disease; formula; hirsutism; psychology; reaction; symptom; thrombopathy; ulcer
constitutional hepatic: dysfunction
constriction: hyperemia; ring
constrictive: endocarditis
consulting: staff
consumption: coagulopathy
contact: allergy; cancer; catalysis; ceptor; dermatitis; illumination; lens; point; splint; surface
contact-type: dermatitis
contagious: abortion; agalactia; aphthae; disease; ecthyma
contagious ecthyma: virus
contagious pustular: dermatitis; stomatitis
contagious pustular dermatitis: virus
content: analysis
continued: fever
continuous: beam; capillary; clasp; eruption; murmur; phase; spectrum; suture; tremor; variation
continuous bar: retainer
continuous epidural: anesthesia
continuous gum: denture
continuous loop: wiring
continuous spinal: anesthesia
contour: height
contraceptive: factor
contracted: foot; heel; kidney; pelvis; tendon
contractile: stricture; vacuole
contractual: psychiatry; psychotherapy
contractural: diathesis
contralateral: hemiplegia; reflex; sign
contrary: sexual
contrast: bath; enema; medium; stain
contrecoup: injury
control: animal; experiment; gene; group
controlled: diet; hypertension; respiration
contused: wound
contusion: pneumonia
convalescent: carrier; diet; serum
convective: heat
convenience: form
conventional: sign
convergence: nucleus
convergent: evolution; strabismus
converging: meniscus
conversion: hysteria; reaction
conversion hysteria: neurosis
conversive: heat
convex: lens
convexoconcave: lens
convexoconvex: lens
convoluted: bone; gland; part; tubule
convulsant: threshold
convulsive: melancholia; reflex; state; tic
cool: bath
cooled-knife: method
coolie: itch
coordinate: convulsion
coordinated: reflex
copolymer: resin
copper: cataract; colic; nose
copper kettle: vaporizer
copper-sulfate: method
copra: itch

coracoacromial: ligament
coracobrachial: muscle
coracoclavicular: ligament
coracohumeral: ligament
coracoid: process; tuberosity
coral: calculus
coralliform: cararact
cord: bladder
cordate: pelvis
cordiform: pelvis
cordy: pulse
core: pneumonia
corneal: abscission; astigmatism; corpuscle; layer; lens; margin; microscope; pannus; reflex; space; spot; staphyloma; tube
corniculate: cartilage; tubercle
corniculopharyngeal: ligament
cornified: layer
corn-meal: disease
cornpicker's: pupil
cornual: pregnancy
corona-: virus
coronal: plane; pulp; section; suture
coronary: artery; band; bypass; cataract; endarterectomy; failure; insufficiency; ligament; node; occlusion; plexus; reflex; sinus; sulcus; tendon; thrombosis; valve; vein
coronary care: unit
coronary nodal: rhythm
coronary ostial: stenosis
coronary sinus: rhythm
coronoid: fossa; process
corpora lutea: cyst
corpuscular: lymph
corpus luteum: hormone
corpus luteum deficiency: syndrome
corpus luteum hormone: unit
corrected: dextrocardia
corrective emotional: experience
correlation: coefficient
correlational: method
correlative: differentiation
corridor: disease
corrosion: preparation
corrosive: sublimate; ulcer
corrugator: muscle
Corsican: moss
cortical: apraxia; arch; artery; blindness; bone; cataract; convexity; deafness; epilepsy; hormone; implantation; osteitis; sensibility; substance
cortical psychic: blindness
corticobulbar: fiber; tract
corticonuclear: fiber
corticopontine: fiber; tract
corticopupillary: reflex
corticoreticular: fiber
corticospinal: fiber; tract
corticosteroid-binding: globulin; protein
corticotropic: hormone
corticotropin-releasing: factor
corymbose: syphilid
coryza-: virus
cosmetic: dermatitis
cosmic: ray
costal: angle; arch; cartilage; chondritis; fringe; groove; notch; part; pit; pleurisy; process; respiration; surface; tuberosity
costal arch: reflex

costoaxillary: vein
costocervical: artery; trunk
costochondral: joint; syndrome
costoclavicular: ligament; line; syndrome
costocolic: ligament
costodiaphragmatic: recess
costomediastinal: recess; sinus
costopectoral: reflex
costophrenic septal: line
costotransverse: foramen; joint; ligament
costovertebral: joint
costoxiphoid: ligament
cottage: hospital
cotton-mill: fever
cotton-roll: gingivitis
cotton-wool: patch; spot
cotyledonary: placenta
cotyloid: cavity; joint; ligament; notch
couching: needle
cough: fracture; reflex
counseling: psychology
count: density
countercurrent: distribution
countercurrent multiplication: mechanism
counting: cell
coup: injury
coupled: beat; pulse; rhythm
coupling: defect; factor; interval
cover: glass
cow: face; hock; pox
cowl: muscle
cowpox: virus
cow's milk: anemia
coxal: bone
coxitic: scoliosis
Coxsackie: encephalitis; virus
CR: lead
crab: hand; yaws
cracked: heel
cracked-pot: resonance; sound
crackling: jaw
cradle: cap
craft: palsy
cranial: arteritis; bone; capacity; cavity; dysostosis; flexure; fontanel; fossa; index; nerve; root; sinus; suture; synchondrosis; vertebra
craniocardiac: reflex
craniocarpotarsal: dystrophy
craniofacial: angle; appliance; axis; dysostosis; notch
craniofacial dysjunction: fracture
craniofacial suspension: wiring
craniometaphysial: dysplasia
craniometric: point
craniopharyngeal: canal; duct
craniosinus: fistula
crater: arc
crazy chick: disease
crease: wound
creative: thinking
creeping: eruption; myiasis; palsy; thrombosis; ulcer
cremaster: muscle
cremasteric: artery; fascia; reflex
crepitant: rale
crescendo: murmur; sleep
crescent: cell
crescent cell: anemia
crescentic: lobule

cretinoid: dysplasia; idiocy
crevicular: epithelium
crib: death
cribbing: strap
cribriform: area; fascia; plate
cricoarytenoid: articulation; joint
cricoarytenoid articular: capsule
cricoid: cartilage
cricopharyngeal: ligament; part
cricosantorinian: ligament
cricothyroid: artery; articulation; joint; ligament; membrane; muscle
cricothyroid articular: capsule
cricotracheal: ligament; membrane
cricovocal: membrane
cri-du-chat: syndrome
Crimean hemorrhagic: fever
criminal: abortion; anthropology; hygiene; insanity; irresponsibility; psychology
crisis: intervention
criss-cross: inheritance
critical: angle; illumination; period; point; pressure; rate; temperature
critical flicker fusion: frequency
crocodile tears: syndrome
crooked: foot
crop: gland; milk
cross: agglutination; birth; bite; circulation; foot; infection; leg; reaction; tolerance
cross-bite: tooth
cross-linked: polymer; resin
cross-reacting: agglutinin; antibody
cross-sectional: method
crossed: anesthesia; cylinder; diplopia; embolism; embolus; eye; hemianesthesia; hemianopsia; hemiplegia; jerk; laterality; metastasis; paralysis; reflex
crossed adductor: reflex
crossed adductor knee: jerk
crossed extension: reflex
crossed knee: jerk
crossed phrenic: phenomenon
crossed pyramidal: tract
crossed spino-adductor: reflex
crossing over of: genes
crotalaria: poisoning
Crotalus: antitoxin
croup-associated: virus
croupous: bronchitis; conjunctivitis; inflammation; laryngitis; lymph; membrane; pharyngitis; pneumonia; rhinitis
crowing: inspiration
crown: bark; cavity; flask; glass; tubercle
crown-heel: length
crown-rump: length
CRST: syndrome
crucial: anastomosis; bandage; ligament
cruciate, cruciform: eminence; ligament; part
crude: drug; urine
crural: arch; artery; canal; fossa; hernia; ring; septum; sheath; triangle
crush: kidney; syndrome
crusted: ringworm; tetter
crutch: palsy; paralysis
cry: reflex
crypt: abscess
cryptogenic: cirrhosis; infection; pye-

mia; septicemia
cryptopthalamus: syndrome
crystal: cryoglobulinemia; rash; structure; violet
crystal violet: vaccine
crystalline: capsule; humor; lens
crystallized: trypsin
Cuban: itch
cubic: niter
cubital: bone; fossa; joint; nerve
cubital lymph: node
cuboid: bone
cuboidal: epithelium
cuboidal articular: surface
cuboideonavicular: joint; ligament
cuboidodigital: reflex
cuirass: respirator
cul-de-sac: smear
cultivated: yeast
cultural: anthropology; shock
culture: medium
cumulative: action; effect
cuneate: fasciculus; funiculus; nucleus
cuneiform: bone; cartilage; cataract; lobe; tubercle
cuneocuboid: joint; ligament
cuneometatarsal: joint
cuneonavicular: articulation; joint; ligament
cupping: glass
cupular: part
cupular blind: sac
Curaçao: aloe
curative: dose; treatment
curb: tenotomy
curby: hock
curd: soap
curdy: pus
curlicue: ureter
currant jelly: clot
curvature: hyperopia; myopia
cushingoid: sign
cusp: angle; height
cuspal: interference
cuspid: tooth
cuspidate: tooth
cuspless: tooth
cutaneomucous: muscle
cutaneomucouveal: syndrome
cutaneous: absorption; albinism; amputation; ancylostomiasis; anthrax; apoplexy; cyst; diphtheria; emphysema; fungus; gangrene; habronemiasis; hemorrhoids; horn; larva migrans; layer; leishmaniasis; leprosy; muscle; nerve; nodule; reaction; reflex; test; tuberculosis; vein
cutaneous cervical: nerve
cutaneous pupil: reflex
cutaneous tuberculin: test
cuticular: cyst
cutireaction: test
cutis: graft; plate
cutituberculin: reaction
cutting: edge; tooth
cuttlefish: disk
cyanide: poisoning
cyanotic: atrophy; induration; kidney
cyclic: albuminuria; compound; insanity; neutropenia; vomiting
cyclopean: eye
cyclothymic: personality
cylindric, cylindrical: bronchiectasis;

cell; epithelium; lens
**cylindroid:** aneurysm
**cylindromatous:** carcinoma
**cynic:** spasm
**Cyprus:** fever
**cystic:** acne; artery; cancer; carcinoma; diathesis; disease; duct; fibrosis; goiter; hyperplasia; kidney; maculopathy; mole; polyp; vein
**cystic duct:** cholangiography
**cystic gall:** duct
**cystic-glandular:** hyperplasia
**cystic heredomacular:** degeneration
**cystic medial:** necrosis
**cystic papillomatous:** craniopharyngioma
**cystine storage:** disease
**cystinotic:** leukocyte
**cystoduodenal:** ligament
**cystoscopic:** ulcer
**cythemolytic:** icterus
**cytogenic:** anemia; reproduction
**cytoid:** body
**cytologic:** examination; preparation; screening; smear; specimen
**cytomegalic:** cell
**cytomegalic inclusion:** disease
**cytomegalic inclusion disease:** virus
**cytomegalo-:** virus
**cytopathic:** effect
**cytopathogenic:** virus
**cytophil:** group
**cytophilic:** antibody
**cytophilic antibody:** test
**cytoplasmic:** bridge; inheritance; reticulum
**cytoplasmic inclusion:** body
**cytotrophoblastic:** shell

### D

**δ-:** see delta.
**D:** enzyme
**DA pregnancy:** test
**dactylographer's:** cramp
**daily:** dose
**Dakar:** vaccine
**Dakar bat:** virus
**dancing:** chorea; disease; mania; spasm
**dandy:** fever
**dark:** adaptation; reaction
**dark-adapted:** eye
**dark-field:** condenser; illumination; microscope
**dark-ground:** illumination
**dartoic:** tissue
**dartos:** muscle
**date:** boil; fever
**datum:** plane
**Datura:** poisoning
**daughter:** cell; colony; cyst; star; wreath
**day:** blindness; hospital; residue; sight
**dead:** finger; nerve; pulp; space; tooth
**dead fetus:** syndrome
**deadly:** nightshade
**DEAE-:** cellulose
**deamidizing:** enzyme
**deaminating:** enzyme
**death:** instinct; rate; trance
**debrancher, debranching:** enzyme; factor
**debrancher deficiency limit:** dextrinosis

**decanormal:** solution
**decapitation:** factor
**decay:** constant; theory
**decentered:** lens
**decerebrate:** rigidity
**decidual:** cast; cell; endometritis; fissure; reaction
**deciduate:** placenta
**deciduocellular:** sarcoma
**deciduoma:** test
**deciduous:** dentition; membrane; skin; tooth
**decinormal:** solution
**declamping:** phenomenon; shock
**decolorized:** sponge
**decomposition of:** movement
**decompression:** chamber; disease; operation; sickness
**decremental:** conduction
**decubital:** gangrene
**decubitus:** paralysis; ulcer
**deep:** bite; keratitis; percussion; reflex; sensibility
**deep abdominal:** reflex
**deep anatomical structures** (specific deep anatomical or histological structures are listed under the following): arch; artery; bursa; cell; cortex; fascia; gyrus; layer; ligament; muscle; nerve; node; nucleus; part; plexus; ring; space; vein; vessel
**deep punctate:** keratitis
**deer:** fly
**deer-fly:** disease; fever
**deer hemorrhagic:** fever
**deer hemorrhagic fever:** virus
**defective:** bacteriophage; phage; probacteriophage; prophage; virus
**defense:** mechanism; reflex
**defensive:** circle; protein
**deferent:** canal; duct
**deferential:** plexus
**deferred:** shock
**defervescent:** stage
**deficiency:** anemia; disease; symptom
**definitive:** callus; host; lysosome
**deflective occlusal:** contact
**degeneration:** cyst
**degenerative:** arthritis; chorea; index; inflammation; insanity; neuralgia
**degenerative joint:** disease
**deglutition:** apnea; pneumonia; reflex
**dehydrated:** alcohol
**dehydration:** fever
**dehydrocholate:** test
**Deiterospinal:** tract
**déjà entendu:** phenomenon
**déjà veçu:** phenomenon
**déjà vu:** phenomenon
**delayed:** allergy; conduction; dentition; epilepsy; eruption; graft; implantation; reaction; reflex; sensation; suture
**delayed reaction:** experiment
**deletion of:** chromosome
**Delhi:** boil
**delimiting:** keratotomy
**delirious:** shock
**delta:** cell; granule; rhythm; wave
**deltoid:** crest; eminence; impression; ligament; muscle; reflex; region
**delusional:** insanity
**demand:** pacemaker

**demand pulse:** generator
**demarcation:** current; potential
**demigauntlet:** bandage
**demilune:** body; cell
**demodectic:** acariasis; mange
**demyelinating:** disease; encephalopathy
**denarcotized:** opium
**denatured:** alcohol; protein
**dendriform:** keratitis; ulcer
**dendritic:** calculus; cell; depolarization; keratitis; process; spine; stone; thorn
**denervated eye:** test
**dengue:** fever; virus
**densimetric:** analysis
**density:** gradient
**density gradient:** centrifugation
**dental:** abscess; anatomy; anesthesia; ankylosis; apparatus; arch; articulation; biomechanics; biophysics; bulb; calculus; canal; cap; drill; dysfunction; engine; engineering; exostosis; fistula; floss; follicle; forceps; formula; furnace; geriatrics; granuloma; groove; hygienist; impaction; index; jurisprudence; lamina; ledge; lever; ligament; material; neck; nerve; orthopaedics; osteoma; pathology; periostitis; plaque; polyp; process; prophylaxis; prosthesis; prosthetics; pulp; pump; ridge; sac; senescence; shelf; star; surgeon; syringe; tubercle; tubule; ulcer; wedge
**dentate:** fascia; fissure; fracture; gyrus; line; nucleus; suture
**dentatothalamic:** tract
**denticulate:** ligament
**dentigerous:** cyst
**dentin:** globule
**dentinal:** canal; dysplasia; fiber; papilla; sheath
**dentinocemental:** junction
**dentinoenamel:** junction
**dentoalveolar:** abscess
**dentogingival:** lamina
**denture:** adhesive; base; border; brush; characterization; edge; esthetics; flange; flask; foundation; hyperplasia; packing; prognosis; retention; space; stability
**denture basal:** surface
**denture-bearing:** area
**denture foundation:** area; surface
**denture impression:** surface
**denture occlusal:** surface
**denture polished:** surface
**denture sore:** mouth
**denture-supporting:** area; structure
**Denver:** classification
**deodorized:** opium
**deoxy:** sugar
**department of:** health
**dependent:** beat; drainage; variable
**depletion:** response
**depot:** injection; reaction; therapy
**depressed:** fracture
**depressive:** delusion; stupor
**depressor:** fiber; muscle; nerve; reflex
**depth:** dose; perception; psychology; recording
**derby hat:** fracture
**derivative:** circulation
**derived:** albumin; protein
**dermal:** bone; leishmanoid; papilla; ridge; sinus; system; tuberculosis

dermatogenic: torticollis
dermatologic: paste
dermatomic: area
dermatopathic: lymphadenopathy
dermoepidermal: interface
dermoepidermic: graft
dermoid: cyst; system; tumor
dermolytic bullous: dermatosis
dermotuberculin: reaction
descending: artery; colon; current; degeneration; neuritis; nucleus; part; tract
descending palatine: artery
descending root: tractotomy
descending scapular: artery
descriptive: anatomy; myology; statistics
desensitizing: paste
desert: fever; rheumatism; sore
desiccated: liver
design: denture
desmoid: tumor
despeciated: antitoxin
desquamative: pneumonia
desquamative inflammatory: vaginitis
desquamative interstitial: pneumonia
destructive: distillation
detached: craniotomy
detached cranial: section
determinant: group
determinate: cleavage
developmental: age; anatomy; anomaly; line; physiology; psychology
deviation of: complement
devil: scorpion
devil's: grip
devital: pulp
devitalized: pulp; tooth
devitalizing: paste
Devonshire: colic
dew: claw; cure; point
dhobie: itch; mark
dhobie mark: dermatitis
Di: antigen
diabetic: amyotrophy; arthropathy; cataract; coma; dermopathy; diet; gangrene; gingivitis; glomerulosclerosis; lipemia; myelopathy; neuropathy; puncture; retinitis; retinopathy
diabetogenic: factor; hormone
diagnostic: anesthesia; cast
diagonal: conjugate
dial: manometer
dialysis: shunt; test
dialysis disequilibrium: syndrome
diamond: disk; fuchsin
diamond-cutting: instrument
diamond-shaped: murmur
diamond skin: disease
Diana: complex
diaper: dermatitis; rash
diaphragm: pessary; phenomenon
diaphragmatic: flutter; hernia; ligament; node; peritonitis; pleurisy; surface
diaphragmatic myocardial: infarction
diaphysial: aclasis; center; dysplasia
diaphysial juxtaepiphysial: exostosis
diarthrodial: cartilage; joint
diastatic skull: fracture
diastolic: murmur; pressure; shock; thrill
diastrophic: dwarfism

diathermic: therapy
diatomic: earth
diazo: reaction; reagent
dibasic: phosphate
dicarboxylic acid: cycle
dicentric: chromosome
dichorial: twins
dichorionic diamniotic: placenta
diclastic: amputation
dicrotic: notch; pulse; wave
didactic: analysis
diencephalic: syndrome
diestrous: cycle
diet: cure; therapy
dietetic: albuminuria
diethenoid: fatty acid
differential: adsorption; blood count; diagnosis; growth; stain; stethoscope; threshold
differential blood: pressure
differential spinal: anesthesia
diffuse: abscess; aneurysm; choroiditis; disease; ganglion; glomerulonephritis; goiter; peritonitis; phlegmon; sclerosis; trachoma
diffuse arterial: ectasia
diffuse infantile familial: sclerosis
diffuse waxy: spleen
diffused: reflex
diffusible: stimulant
diffusing: capacity
diffusion: anoxia; circle; method; respiration; shell; spot
digastric: fossa; muscle; notch; triangle
digenetic: fluke
digestive: fever; glycosuria; leukocytosis; system; tract; tube
digital: fossa; furrow; joint; pulp; reflex; vein
digital collateral: artery
digitalis: unit
digitate: impression
digitonin: reaction
dihydric: alcohol; phosphate
Dilantin hyperplastic: gingivitis
dilating: laryngotome
dilation: cyst; thrombosis
dilator: muscle
dilute, diluted: alcohol; hydrochloric acid; pentaerythritol; phosphoric acid
dilution: anemia
dimensional: stability
dimidiate: hermaphroditism
dimorphic: anemia
dineric: interspace
dinner: pad
dinoflagellate: toxin
Diogenes': cup
dioptric: aberration
diovular: twins
dip: phenomenon
diphasic: complex
diphasic milk: fever
diphtheria: antitoxin; toxin; vaccine
diphtheria antitoxin: unit
diphtheritic: conjunctivitis; endometritis; enteritis; membrane; neuropathy; paralysis; ulcer
diphyllobothrium: anemia
diplegic: idiocy
diplobacillary: conjunctivitis
diploic: canal; vein
diploid: nucleus

dipolar: ion
dipole: theory
direct: astigmatism; auscultation; calorimetry; current; diplopia; diuretic; embolism; fracture; illumination; image; immunofluorescence; injury; lead; metastasis; method; ophthalmoscopy; oxidase; percussion; ray; reflex; retainer; retention; technique; transfusion; vision; zoonosis
direct acrylic: filling
direct bone: impression
direct composite resin: filling
direct Coombs': test
direct filling: resin
direct method for: inlay
direct pulp: capping
direct pyramidal: tract
direct resin: filling
direct vision: spectroscope
directing: globule
directive: psychotherapy
disappearing bone: disease
disc (see also disk): electrophoresis; syndrome
discharging: tubule
disclosing: solution
discoid: lupus (erythematosus)
discoidal: cleavage
discontinuous: sterilization
discordant: alternans; alternation
discrete: smallpox
discrete colliquative: keratopathy
discriminant: stimulant
dish: face
dish-pan: fracture
disjugate: movement
disjunctive: absorption
disk: (see also disc)
disk sensitivity: method
dislocation: fracture
dispensing: tablet
disperse: placenta
dispersed: phase
dispersing: electrode
dispersion: colloid; medium; phase
displacement: threshold
disproportionating: enzyme
dissecting: aneurysm; cellulitis
dissection: tubercle
disseminated: choroiditis; lupus (erythematosus); sclerosis; tuberculosis
disseminated condensing: osteopathy
disseminated cutaneous: gangrene
dissociated: anesthesia; nystagmus
dissociation: constant; sensibility
dissociative: anesthesia; reaction
distal: cavity; centriole; end; extremity; ileitis; myopathy; occlusion; part; surface
distal bulbar: septum
distal radioulnar: articulation
distance: ceptor
distantial: aberration
distemper: virus
distention: cyst; ulcer
distilled: water
distobuccal: angle
distraction: conus
distributed: effort
distributing: artery
distribution: coefficient; curve; leukocytosis; volume

distributive: analysis
disulfide: bond
disuse: atrophy
diuretic: species
diurnal: rhythm
diver: goiter
diver's: palsy; paralysis
divergent: strabismus
diverging: meniscus
divided: dose
divisional: nursing
dizygotic: twins
DMF caries: index
D:N: quotient; ratio
DNA: helix; virus
doctrine of: signatures
dog: disease; flea; hookworm; nose; tick; unit
dog distemper: virus
dogmatic: school
dolichopellic: pelvis
doll's eye: sign
dolorogenic: zone
dome: cell
domestic: medicine; soap
dominance: hierarchy
dominance of: genes
dominant: character; eye; frequency; hemisphere; idea; inheritance; trait
dopa: reaction
dorsal: position; reflex
dorsal anatomical structures (specific dorsal structures are listed under the following): arch; artery; bone; column; decussation; fascia; fasciculus; flexure; ganglion; horn; ligament; mesocardium; muscle; nerve; network; nucleus; pancreas; part; root; spine; surface; tract; tubercle; vein
dorsalgic-gynecologic: syndrome
dorsispinal: vein
dorsoanterior: position
dorsolateral: fasciculus; placode; tract
dorsomedial: nucleus
dorsoposterior: position
dorsosacral: position
dorsum pedis: reflex
dotted: tongue
double: athetosis; bind; bond; chin; consciousness; fracture; helix; hemiplegia; insanity; knot; monster; parturition; penis; pneumonia; promontory; protrusion; quartan; refraction; salt; stain; tachycardia; tertian; vision
double antibody: immonoassay; method; precipitation
double aortic: stenosis
double-barreled: intussusception
double blind: experiment
double concave: lens
double congenital: athetosis
double contrast: enema
double convex: lens
double flap: amputation
double (gel) diffusion precipitin: test
double loop: hernia
double-point: threshold
double quotidian: fever
double-shock: sound
double tertian: malaria
doubly armed: suture
doubting: mania
douche: bath

dousing: bath
dragon: worm
drainage: tube
drain-trap: stomach
drawer: sign; test
dream: association; pain
dreamy: state
drepanocytic: anemia
dressing: forceps
dried: alum; gypsum; lemon (peel); yeast
dried human: albumin; plasma; serum
drip: phleboclysis; transfusion
driver's: thigh
dromedary: curve
drop: attack; finger; foot; hand; heart; jaw; phalangette; toe
droplet: infection; nucleus
dropped: beat
drug: abuse; addiction; allergy; disease; eruption; habit; insanity; pathogenesis; rash; tetanus; treatment
drug-induced: hepatitis
druggists': bark
drum: belly; membrane; shock
drumstick: appendage; finger
dry: abscess; amputation; beriberi; bronchiectasis; bronchitis; cup; distillation; gangrene; hernia; joint; labor; leprosy; nurse; pack; pleurisy; rale; socket; synovitis; tetter; vomiting
dual: personality
duck: sickness
duck embryo origin: vaccine
duck hepatitis: virus
duck influenza: virus
duckbill: speculum
duct: cancer; carcinoma; papilloma
ductal: carcinoma
ductless: gland
dumb: madness; rabies
dumbbell: ganglioneuroma
Dumdum: fever
dumping: syndrome
duodenal: ampulla; autacoid; bulb; cap; diverticulum; fistula; gland; impression; smear; sphincter; ulcer
duodenojejunal: angle; flexure; fold; fossa; hernia; recess; sphincter
duodenomesocolic: fold
duplex: transmission
duplication: cyst
duplication of: chromosomes
duplicity: theory
dural: sheath; sinus
duration: tetany
dust: ball; cell; corpuscle; disease
Dutch: cap
dwarf: pelvis; tapeworm
dwarf mouse: tapeworm
dyadic: psychotherapy; symbiosis
dye-dilution: curve
dynamic: aorta; compliance; demography; disease; ileus; murmur; psychiatry; psychology; psychotherapy; ray; refraction; relation; school; splint; viscosity
dynamite: head; headache
dyscrasic: fracture
dysenteric: arthritis; diarrhea
dysentery: antitoxin; bacillus
dysfunctional uterine: bleeding
dysgranular: cortex

dyshemopoietic: anemia
dysmenorrheal: membrane
dysmnesic: syndrome
dysmorphic: leprosy
dyspeptic: ulcer
dysspermatogenic: sterility
dysthyroidal: infantilism
dystocia-dystrophia: syndrome
dystrophic: calcification

E

ear: bone; cough; crystal; lobe; mange; sign; wax
early diastolic: murmur
earth: metal; wax
earthy: phosphate; water
East Coast: fever
eastern equine: encephalomyelitis
eastern equine encephalomyelitis: virus
eating: chancre
EB: virus
ECBO: virus
eccentric: amputation; checkbite; hypertrophy; occlusion; position; relation; vision
ecchymotic: mask
eccrine: gland; poroma; spiradenoma
ecdysial: gland
echinococcus: cyst
echo: beat; reaction; speech
ECHO: virus
eclamptic: idiocy; retinopathy
eclectic: medicine
eclipse: amblyopia; blindness; period; phase
ECMO: virus
ecological: ectocrine; system
ecphylactic: region
ECSO: virus
ectatic: aneurysm; emphysema
ECTEOLA: cellulose
ecthymatous: syphilid
ectocervical: smear
ectodermal: cloaca; dysplasia
ectogenic: teratosis
ectopic: beat; decidua; pacemaker; pinealoma; pregnancy; rhythm; tachycardia; teratosis; testis
ectopic ACTH: syndrome
ectoplacental: cavity
ectotrophoblastic: cavity
ectromelia: virus
eczematoid: seborrhea
eddy: sound
Edgehill, Edge Hill: virus
edge-strength of: amalgam
edge-to-edge: bite; occlusion
edgewise: appliance
educated: phagocyte
educational: psychology
EEE: virus
EEG: see electroencephalograph
effective: conjugate; dose; half-life; temperature
effective osmotic: pressure
effective refractory: period
effective renal blood: flow
effective renal plasma: flow
effective temperature: index
effector: cell
efferent: duct; fiber; lymphatic; nerve; vessel

efferent glomerular: arteriole
effervescent: salt; lithium
effort: syndrome
egg: albumin; cell; membrane; nest; tube
egg shell: nail
egg-white injury: syndrome
ego: analysis; ideal; identity; instinct
Egtved: virus
Egyptian: chlorosis; hematuria; ophthalmia; splenomegaly
Egyptian intestinal: fluke
eidetic: image
eighth cranial: nerve
eighth nerve: tumor
ejaculatory: duct
ejection: click; fraction; murmur; period; sound
elastic: artery; bandage; cartilage; dystrophy; fiber; lamella; lamina; layer; ligature; limit; membrane; skin; tissue
elastic band: fixation
elastoid: degeneration
elastotic: degeneration
elbow: bone; jerk; joint; reflex
elbowed: catheter
Electra: complex
electric: anesthesia; bath cataract; cautery; chorea; irritability; ophthalmia; probe; retinopathy; shock; sleep
electric cardiac: pacemaker
electric shock: therapy
electrical: alternans; alternation; axis; formula
electroacoustic: locator
electrocardiographic: complex; wave
electroconvulsive: therapy
electroencephalograph (EEG): activation
electroencephalographic: dysrhythmia
electrolyte: balance; metabolism
electrolytic: dissociation
electromagnetic: radiation; unit
electromagnetokinetic: phenomenon
electromechanical: dissociation; systole
electromotive: force
electromuscular: sensibility
electron: interferometer; interferometry; magneton; microscope; radiography
electronegative: element
electronic: charge; number; sterilization
electronic pacemaker: load
electron resonance: absorption
electron spin: resonance
electrophonic: effect
electrophrenic: respiration
electropositive: element
electroshock: therapy
electrostatic: unit
electrotherapeutic: bath; sleep
electrotherapeutic sleep: therapy
electrotonic: current; junction; synapse
elementary: body; granule; particle
elephant: leg
elephantoid: fever
elevator: disease; muscle
eleventh cranial: nerve
elfin: facies
elimination: diet
ellipsoidal: joint
elliptical: amputation; recess

elliptocytic: anemia
El Tor: vibrio
EMB: agar
embedding: agent
embolic: abscess; aneurysm; apoplexy; gangrene; nephritis; pneumonia
emboliform: nucleus
embolomycotic: aneurysm
embryonal: adenoma; area; carcinoma; cataract; leukemia; rhabdomyosarcoma; tridermoma
embryonic: anideus; axis; blastoderm; circulation; diapause; disk; membrane; shield
EMC: virus
emergency: theory
emergent: evolution
emery: disk
EMG: syndrome
emigration: theory
emissary: vein
emissary sphenoidal: foramen
emission: electron
emollient: species
emotional: age; amenorrhea; attitude; deprivation; disorder; disturbance; leukocytosis; overlay; tone
empathic: index
emphysematous: anthrax; cholecystitis; gangrene; phlegmon
empiric, empirical: formula; medicine; therapeutics; treatment
empty: sella
empyema: tube
empyemic: scoliosis
emulsifying: wax
emulsion: colloid
enamel: cap; cell; cleavage; cleaver; crypt; cuticle; dysplasia; eptihelium; fiber; fissure; fluorosis; germ; hypocalcification; hypoplasia; lamella; layer; ledge; membrane; niche; nodule; organ; pearl; pulp; prism; rod; wall
enamel rod: inclination; sheath
enarthrodial: joint
encephalic: angioma; vesicle
encephalitis: virus
encephaloclastic: microcephaly
encephalofacial: angiomatosis
encephaloid: cancer; sarcoma
encephalomyelonic: axis
encephalomyocarditis: virus
encephalotrigeminal: angiomatosis
encephalotrigeminal vascular: syndrome
encounter: group
encysted: pleurisy
end: artery; body; bud; bulb; gut; organ; plate; point; stage
end-on mattress: suture
end-position: nystagmus
end-to-end: bite; occlusion
endaural: incision
endemic: deafmutism; disease; funiculitis; goiter; hematuria; hemoptysis; hypertrophy; index; influenza; neuritis; osteoarthritis; typhus
endemic dental: fluorosis
endemic paralytic: vertigo
endergonic: reaction
endobronchial: tube
endocardial: cushion; fibroelastosis; murmur; sclerosis

endocardial cushion: defect
endocervical: smear
endochondral: bone; ossification
endocrine: adenomatosis; allergy; gland; ophthalmopathy; system
endocrine polyglandular: syndrome
endodermal: cell
endodontic: stabilizer
endogenic: toxicosis
endogenous: cycle; depression; fiber; infection
endoglobular: body
endolymphatic: duct; hydrops; sac
endometrial: cyst; implant; smear
endometrial stromal: sarcoma
endomyocardial: fibroelastosis; fibrosis
endo-osseous: implant
endopelvic: fascia
endoplasmic: reticulum
endoreduplication of: chromosome
endoscopic: biopsy
endoteric: bacterium
endothelial: cell; cyst; leukocyte; myeloma
endotheliochorial: placenta
endothelio-endothelial: placenta
endothermal: reaction
endothermic: compound; reaction
endothoracic: fascia
endotoxin: shock
endotracheal: anesthesia; intubation; stylet; tube
endovenous: septum
enema: rash
energy-rich: phosphate
engine: reamer
English: disease; position; rhinoplasty
English sweating: fever
ensheathing: callus
ensiform: cartilage; process
ensisternum: cartilage
enteric: fever; plexus; virus
enteric coated: pill
enteric cytopathogenic bovine orphan: virus
enteric cytopathogenic human orphan: virus
enteric cytopathogenic monkey orphan: virus
entericoid: fever
enterochromaffin: cell
enterocutaneous: fistula
enteroendocrine: cell
enterogastric: reflex
enterogenous: cyanosis; methemoglobinemia
enterohepatic: circulation
enterokinetic: agent
enteroptotic: habit
enterovaginal: fistula
enterovesical: fistula
entodermal: canal; cell; cloaca; pouch
entoptotic: pulse
entorhinal: area
entrance: block
entrapment: neuropathy
entry: zone
envelope: conformation; flap
enzootic: abortion; hepatitis
enzygotic: twins
enzymatic: synthesis
enzyme: antagonist
enzyme inhibition: theory

eosin-methylene blue: agar
eosinopenic: reaction
eosinophil, eosinophilic: adenoma; granule; granuloma; leukemia; leukocyte; leukocytosis; leukopenia; meningoencephalitis
epactal: bone; ossicle
epamniotic: cavity
eparterial: bronchus
ependymal: cell; cyst; layer; zone
ephemeral: fever; pneumonia
epibranchial: placode
epicondylar: ridge
epicranial: aponeurosis; muscle
epicritic: sensibility
epidemic: bronchitis; disease; dropsy; encephalitis; hemoglobinuria; hepatitis; hiccup; keratoconjunctivitis; myalgia; myositis; nausea; neuromyasthenia; paralysis; parotiditis; pleurodynia; rheum; roseola; stomatitis; tetany; tremor; typhus; vertigo; vomiting
epidemic benign dry: pleurisy
epidemic cerebrospinal: meningitis
epidemic diaphragmatic: pleurisy
epidemic gangrenous: proctitis
epidemic hemorrhagic: fever
epidemic keratoconjunctivitis: virus
epidemic myalgia: virus
epidemic myalgic: encephalomyelitis; encephalomyelopathy
epidemic parotitis: virus
epidemic pleurodynia: virus
epidemic transient diaphragmatic: spasm
epidermal: cyst
epidermal growth: factor
epidermic: cell; method
epidermic-dermic: nevus
epidermoid: cancer; carcinoma; cyst
epidermolytic: hyperkeratosis
epidural: abscess; anesthesia; cavity; hematoma; meningitis; space
epigastric: angle; fold; fossa; hernia; reflex; region; vein; voice
epigastric lymph: node
epiglottic: cartilage; tubercle
epihyal: bone; ligament
epilation: dose
epilemmal: ending
epileptic: cry; dementia; equivalent; idiocy; mania; temper
epileptiform: neuralgia
epileptogenic: zone
epimastical: fever
epinephrine: reversal
epinosic: gain
epiotic: center
epipapillary: membrane
epipericardial: ridge
epiphrenic: diverticulum
epiphysial: arrest; cartilage; eye; fracture; line; plate
epiphysial aseptic: necrosis
epiploic: abscess; appendage; foramen
epipteric: bone
episcleral: artery; lamina; space; vein
episternal: bone
epithelial: attachment; body; cancer; cast; cell; cyst; dysplasia; ectoderm; inlay; lamina; layer; migration; nest; outlay; pearl; plug; tissue
epithelial choroid: layer

epitheliochorial: placenta
epithelioid: cell
epithelioid cell: nevus
epithermal: chemistry; neutron
epitrichial: layer
epituberculous: infiltration
epitympanic: recess; space
epizoic: commensalism
epizootic: cellulitis
epizootic bovine: abortion
epoxy: resin
Epsom: salt
equal: cleavage
equation: division
equatorial: cleavage; plate; staphyloma
equilibrating: operation
equilibrium: constant; dialysis
equine: babesiosis; encephalitis; encephalomyelitis; gait: gonadotropin; influenza; rhinopneumonitis; syphilis
equine abortion: virus
equine arteritis: virus
equine biliary: fever
equine contagious pustular: stomatitis
equine gonadotropin: unit
equine infectious: anemia
equine infectious anemia: virus
equine influenza: virus
equine rhinopneumonitis: virus
equine serum: hepatitis
equine spinal: ataxia
equine swamp: fever
equine viral: arteritis
equine virus: abortion
equiphasic: complex
equisetum: poisoning
equivalent: extract; power; temperature; weight
equivalent form: reliability
equivocal: symptom
erect: illumination
erectile: tissue
erector: muscle
erector-spinal: reflex
erethistic: shock
erogenous: zone
erotic: zoophilism
erotogenic: zone
erroneous: projection
eruptive: fever; stage
erythema: dose; threshold
erythema nodosum: leprosy
erythematous: syphilid
erythredema: polyneuritis
erythremic: myelosis
erythroblastic: anemia
erythrocyte: mosaicism
erythrocyte adherence: phenomenon; test
erythrocyte maturation: factor
erythrocyte sedimentation: rate
erythrocytic: series
erythrogenic: toxin
erythroid: cell
erythronormoblastic: anemia
erythrophore: reaction
erythropoietic: hormone; porphyria; protoporphyria
escape: beat; conditioning; phenomenon
escape-capture: bigeminy
escaped: beat; contraction
escaped ventricular: contraction
Escherichia coli: enterotoxin; ribonu-

clease
esodic: nerve
esophageal: achalasia; artery; atresia; cardiogram; gland; groove; impression; lead; plexus; smear; speech; ulcer; varix; vein; web
esophagogastric: junction; orifice; vestibule
esophagosalivary: reflex; symptom
essential: albuminuria; amino acid; anemia; asthma; bradycardia; cyclophoria; dysmenorrhea; fever; fructosuria; hematuria; hypertension; oil; paralysis; pentosuria; phthisis; pruritus; tachycardia; telangiectasia; thrombocytopenia
essential food: factor
essential progressive: atrophy
established cell: line
esterified: estrogen
esthesiodic: system
estradiol benzoate: unit
estrogenic: hormone
estrone: unit
estrous: cycle
ether: apnea; cone; convulsion; epilepsy; fit; test
ethereal: oil; solution; tincture
ethmoid: angle; bone; infundibulum
ethmoidal: cell; crest; foramen; groove; labyrinth; notch; process; sinus; vein
ethmoidomaxillary: suture
ethmoverine: plate
eucalyptus: gum
eugnathic: anomaly
eunuchoid: gigantism; state; voice
euplastic: lymph
European: blastomycosis; hellebore; snakeroot; tarantula
eutectic: temperature
euthyroid: hypometabolism
evacuant: suppository
evacuation: hospital
evoked: response
examining: table
exanthematous: disease; fever
excentric: amputation
excess: lactate
excessive: appetite; hunger; sweat; thirst
exchange: transfusion
excitable: area
excitation: wave
excitatory: autacoid
excitatory postsynaptic: potential
exciting: cause; electrode; eye
excitor: nerve
excitoreflex: nerve
exclamation point: hair
exclusion of: pupil
excretory: duct; ductule; gland; urography
exercise: bone; test
exergonic: reaction
exertional: rhabdomyolysis
exfoliative: cytology; dermatitis; gastritis
exhaustion: atrophy; psychosis
existential: analysis; psychiatry; psychology; psychotherapy
exit: block; dose
exocardial: murmur
exoccipital: bone

exocelomic: membrane
exocrine: gland
exodic: nerve
exoerythrocytic: stage
exogenic: toxicosis
exogenous: cycle; fiber; hemochromatosis; hyperglyceridemia; ochronosis; pigmentation
exophthalmic: goiter; ophthalmoplegia
exophthalmos-producing: substance
exoteric: bacterium
exothermal, exothermic: compound; reaction
expansion: arch
expansive: delusion
expectant: treatment
expectation: neurosis
experimental: group; medicine; method; neurosis; psychology
experimental allergic: encephalomyelitis
experimenter: effect
expiratory: center; grunt; resistance; stridor
expiratory reserve: volume
expired: gas
exploratory: drive; incision; operation; puncture
exploring: electrode; needle
explosive: decompression; mixture; speech; wen
exposed: pulp
expressed skull: fracture
expressive: aphasia
expulsive: pain
exsanguination: transfusion
exsiccated: alum
exsiccation: fever
extemporaneous: mixture
extended family: therapy
extensor: aponeurosis; retinaculum; tetanus
external: absorption; defibrillator; fistula; hirudiniasis; hydrocephalus; medium; meningitis; nose; ophthalmopathy; pacemaker; phase; pyocephalus; respiration; strabismus; traction; urethrotomy; version
external anatomical structures (specific external structures are listed under the following): artery; axis; capsule; conjugate; crest; epithelium; fascia; fiber; fibrocartilage; foramen; genitalia; gland; ligament; lip; meatus; muscle; nerve; node; nose; nucleus; plexus; ridge; ring; sulcus; surface; vein; wall
external cardiac: massage
external carotid steal: syndrome
external enamel: epithelium
external oblique: reflex
external pin: fixation
exterofective: system
extinction: coefficient
extra-alveolar: crown
extra-amniotic: pregnancy
extracapsular: ankylosis; fracture; ligament
extracardiac: murmur
extracellular: enzyme; fluid; toxin
extrachorial: pregnancy
extrachromosomal: inheritance
extracoronal: retainer
extracorporeal: circulation

extracranial: pneumatocele; pneumocele
extracting: forceps
extraction: ratio
extradural: abscess; anesthesia; empyema; hemorrhage
extraembryonic: blastoderm: celom; mesoderm
extramembranous: pregnancy
extramural: practice
extranuclear: inheritance
extraperitoneal: fascia
extrapineal: pinealoma
extrapleural: pneumothorax
extrapyramidal: disease; dyskinesia; syndrome; system
extrasaccular: hernia
extrasensory: perception
extransensory thought: transference
extrauterine: pregnancy
extravasation: cyst
extravascular: fluid
extravisual: zone
extravital: ultraviolet
extreme: capsule
extrinsic: asthma; factor; sphincter
extrinsic allergic: alveolitis
extrusion: globule
exudation: cell; corpuscle; cyst
exudative: bronchiolitis; diathesis; glomerulonephritis; inflammation; retinitis; vitreoretinopathy
exudative discoid and lichenoid: dermatitis
exudative retinal: detachment
eye: capsule; cup; drops; gnat; lens; ointment; reflex; speculum; tooth; wash; worm
eye-closure: reflex
eye-ear: plane
eyelash: sign

**F**

F: agent; duction; factor; genote; thalassemia; wave
F': agent
f: wave
FA: virus
Fab: fragment
fabere: sign
face: ague; form
face-bow: fork; record
facial: angle; artery; axis; bone; canal; cleft; colliculus; diplegia; eczema; eminence; height; hemiatrophy; hemiplegia; hillock; index; nerve; neuralgia; palsy; paralysis; perception; plane; profile; reflex; root; spasm; surface; tic; triangle; trophoneurosis; vein; vision
facial motor: nucleus
facialis: phenomenon
facioscapulohumeral: atrophy
facioscapulohumeral muscular: dystrophy
factitious: purpura; urticaria
factor: analysis
factorial: experiment
facultative: anaerobe; hyperopia; parasite; saprophyte
fading: time
Fahrenheit: scale
faith: cure

falciform: cartilage; crest; ligament; lobe; margin; process
falciform retinal: fold
falciparum: fever; malaria
fallen: arch
falling: palate; sickness
falling of: womb
false: albuminuria; anemia; aneurysm; angina; ankylosis; branching; cast; conjugate; cyanosis; cyst; dextrocardia; diphtheria; diverticulum; glottis; hellebore; hematuria; hermaphroditism; hypertrophy; image; joint; knot; macula; masturbation; membrane; memory; mole; neuroma; nucleolus; pain; paracusis; pelvis; pregnancy; promontory; ptosis; rib; ringbone; suture; thirst; vertebra; waters
false-negative: reaction
false-positive: reaction
false vocal: cord
familial: amyloidosis; cystinuria; dysautonomia; encephalopathy; glycinuria; goiter; hyperbetalipoproteinemia; hypercholesterolemia; hyperchylomicronemia; hyperlipoproteinemia; hyperprebetalipoproteinemia; hypertriglyceridemia; hypoparathyroidism
familial benign chronic: pemphigus
familial erythroblastic: anemia
familial fat-induced: hyperlipemia
familial fibrous: dysplasia
familial high density lipoprotein: deficiency
familial hypercholesteremic: xanthomatosis
familial hypogonadotropic: hypogonadism
familial hypoplastic: anemia
familial intestinal: polyposis
familial juvenile: nephronophthisis
familial Mediterranean: fever
familial microcytic: anemia
familial nonhemolytic: jaundice
familial paroxysmal: polyserositis; rhabdomyolysis
familial periodic: paralysis
familial polyendocrine: adenomatosis
familial pseudoinflammatory: maculopathy
familial pseudoinflammatory macular: degeneration
familial recurring: polyserositis
familial spinal muscular: atrophy
familial splenic: anemia
familial vitamin D-resistant: rickets
familial white folded oral: dysplasia
family: therapy
famine: dropsy; edema; fever
fan: sign
fango: therapy
far: point; sight
far-and-near: suture
Far East Russian: encephalitis
far point of: convergence
farmer's: lung; skin
fascia: graft
fascial: hernia
fascicular: block; degeneration; keratitis; ophthalmoplegia; sarcoma
fasciculate: bladder
fasciolar: gyrus
fast: green; rhythm; smear

fastigiobulbar: tract

fat: body; cell; embolism; embolus; graft; indigestion; metabolism; necrosis; solvent; tide

fatality: rate

fatigue: antitoxin; fever; fracture; neurosis; reaction; test; toxin

fatty: acid; alcohol; ascites; atrophy; cast; change; cirrhosis; compound; degeneration; diarrhea; heart; hernia; infiltration; kidney; metamorphosis; oil; phanerosis; series; tissue

fatty acid oxidation: cycle

faucial: paralysis; reflex; tonsil

faulty: union

Fc: fragment

featural: surgery

febrile: albuminuria; crisis; psychosis; urine; urticaria

fecal: abscess; fistula; tumor; vomiting

federal: medicine

feedback: inhibition; mechanism; system

feeding: center; tube

feeling: tone

feline: agranulocytosis; pneumonitis

feline infectious: enteritis

feline infectious agranulocytosis: virus

feline panleukopenia: virus

female: catheter; gonad; hermaphroditism; homosexuality; hormone; prostate; pseudohermaphroditism; sterility; urethra

female prostatic obstructing: syndrome

femininity: complex

femoral: arch; artery; canal; fossa; hernia; muscle; nerve; plexus; reflex; ring; septum; sheath; triangle; vein

femoroabdominal: reflex

femoropatellar: joint

femoropopliteal: bypass

femoropopliteal occlusive: disease

femorotibial: joint

fenestrated: capillary; membrane

fenestration: operation

ferment: thrombus

fermentation *Lactobacillus casei*: factor

fermentative: dyspepsia

fern: test

ferric chloride: reaction; test

fertility: agent; factor; vitamin

fertilization: cone; membrane

fertilized: ovum

fescue: foot

festinating: gait

fetal: adenoma; age; bradycardia; circulation; cortex; death; distress; electrocardiography; habitus; hemoglobin; hydrops; inclusion; membrane; movement; ovoid; placenta; souffle; tachycardia; zone

fetal aspiration: syndrome

fetid: sweat

fetoplacental: anasarca

fever: blister; therapy

feverish: urine

FF, ff: wave

FGT cytologic: smear

fiber: optics

fibrillar: basket

fibrillary: chorea; contraction; myoclonia; neuroma; tremor; wave

fibrin: thrombus

fibrinogen-fibrin conversion: syndrome

fibrinoid: degeneration; necrosis

fibrinolytic: purpura

fibrinopurulent: inflammation

fibrinous: adhesion; bronchitis; cast; cataract; degeneration; inflammation; lymph; pericarditis; pleurisy; pneumonia; polyp; rhinitis

fibrin-stabilizing: factor

fibrocaseous: peritonitis

fibrocystic: disease

fibroepithelial: papilloma

fibrohyaline: tissue

fibroid: adenoma; cataract; degeneration; induration; inflammation; lung; phthisis; tumor

fibromatous: virus

fibromuscular: dysplasia; hyperplasia

fibrosing: adenomatosis; adenosis

fibrositic: headache

fibrous: adhesion; ankylosis; astrocyte; capsule; cavernitis; dysplasia; goiter; histiocytoma; joint; layer; membrane; pneumonia; polyp; protein; sheath; tissue; tubercle; tunic; union; xanthoma

fibrous articular: capsule

fibrous bacterial: virus

fibrous cortical: defect

fibular: artery; ligament; margin; notch; surface; vein

field: blocking; fever; hospital; lens

field block: anesthesia

field of: consciousness; fixation; vision

fifth: disease; finger; ventricle

fifth cranial: nerve

fifth venereal: disease

fig: wart

figure-of-8: abnormality, bandage; suture

filament-nonfilament: count

filament polymorphonuclear: leukocyte

filamentous: colony

filamentous bacterial: virus

filar: mass; micrometer; substance

filarial: arthritis; dermatosis; funiculitis; hydrocele; synovitis

filariform: larva

file-cutter's: phthisis

filial: generation

filiform: bougie; papilla; pulse

filigree: implantation

filler: graft

fillet: layer

filling: defect

filter: paper

filtering: cicatrix

filtrable: virus

filtrate: factor; nitrogen

filtration: angle; fraction; space

fimbriated: fold

fimbriodentate: sulcus

final: host; impression

fine: structure; tremor

finger: agnosia; percussion; phenomenon

finger-thumb: reflex

Finnish: bath

fire: damp

first: dentition; finger; messenger; molar

first arch: syndrome

first cranial: nerve

first cuneiform: bone

first duodenal: sphincter

first-order: reaction; receptor

first parallel pelvic: plane

first permanent: molar

first stage of: labor

first temporal: convolution

first visceral: cleft

fish: skin; test

fish tapeworm: anemia

fishmouth: meatus

fishmouth mitral: stenosis

fission: fungus; product

fissure: bur; cavity; sealant

fissured: fracture; tongue

fistula: knife; test

fistulous: withers

FIT: test

five-day: fever

five-year: survival

fixation: disparity; nystagmus; reaction

fixation of: complement

fixator: muscle

fixed: alkali; alkaloid; coupling; dressing; idea; oil; pupil; torticollis; virus

fixed drug: eruption

fixed rate: pacemaker

fixed rate pulse: generator

fixed virus: rabies

fixing: eye

flabby: tissue

flaccid: ectropion; membrane; part

flagellar: agglutinin; antigen

flail: chest; joint

flame: arc; spot

flammable: anesthetic

Flanders: virus

flange: contour

flank: bone

flannel: rash

flap: amputation; extraction; operation

flapless: amputation

flapping: tremor

flare of: nostril

flash: blindness; burn; dispersal; keratoconjunctivitis; method; point

flask: closure

flat: affect; bone; chest; condyloma; electroencephalogram; foot; hand; pelvis; wart

flat papular: syphilid

flat top: wave

flatulent: colic; dyspepsia

flatus: enema

flax-dresser's: phthisis

flea-bitten: kidney

flea-borne: typhus

fleck: dystrophy

fleece: worm

flesh: fly

fleshy: mole; polyp

flexible: collodion

flexor: reflex; retinaculum; tetanus

flexural: eczema

flicker: fusion; perimetry

flicker fusion frequency: technique

flight: blindness

flint: disease; glass

flittering: scotoma

floating: cartilage; kidney; organ; patella; rib; spleen; villus

floccular: degeneration; fossa

flocculation: reaction; test

flocculonodular: lobe

flood: fever
floor: cell; plate
floppy valve: syndrome
floriform: cataract
floss: silk
flotation: constant; method
flow of: amalgam
flower-spray: ending; organ
flowing: hyperostosis
fluid: balance; extract; lung; wave
fluorescein string: test
fluorescence: microscopy; quenching
fluorescent: microscope; screen; stain; test
fluorescent antibody: technique
fluorescent treponemal antibody-absorption: test
fluoridated: tooth
Fluotec: vaporizer
Flury strain: vaccine
Flury strain rabies: virus
flush: technique
fluted: tongue
flux: density; ratio
fluxionary: hyperemia
fly: agaric; blister
flying: blister
flying spot: microscope
FMD: virus
foam: cell
foamy: agent; virus
focal: amyloidosis; appendicitis; depth; distance; epilepsy; glomerulonephritis; infection; interval; myelitis; necrosis; nephritis; reaction; sclerosis
focal embolic: glomerulonephritis
focal lymphocytic: thyroiditis
focal sclerosing: glomerulopathy
folk: medicine
follicle-stimulating: hormone; principle
follicle-stimulating hormone-releasing: factor
follicular: abscess; adenoma; carcinoma; conjunctivitis; cyst; cystitis; gland; goiter; hormone; impetigo; iritis; lymphoma; mange; mucinosis; papule; pharyngitis; syphilid; trachoma; urethritis; vulvitis
follicular epithelial: cell
follicular ovarian: cell
food: ball; fever; impaction; poisoning
foot: mange; phenomenon; plate; plugger; process; rot; yaws
foot and mouth: disease
foot and mouth disease: virus
football: calf
footling: presentation
forage: poisoning
foraminal: herniation
forced: alimentation; beat; cycle; feeding; respiration
forced expiratory: volume
forced grasping: reflex
forceps: delivery
forebrain: vesicle
foreign: body; protein; serum
foreign body: salpingitis; tumorigenesis
foreign body giant: cell
foreign protein: therapy
forensic: dentistry; medicine; odontology; psychiatry; psychology
forequarter: amputation
forest: yaws

forked: worm
formal: operation
formaldehydogenic: corticoid
formative: cell; osteitis
formol: fluid; titration
Fort Bragg: fever
fortification: figure; spectrum
fortified: milk
forward: conduction
forward heart: failure
foudroyant: myelitis
fountain: decussation; syringe
fourth: disease; finger; nerve; ventricle
fourth parallel pelvic: plane
fourth stage of: labor
fourth venereal: disease
foveated: chest
foveolar: cell
fowl: cholera; erythroblastosis; leukemia; leukosis; lymphomatosis; myeloblastosis; paralysis; pest; plague; pox; tick; tuberculosis; typhoid
fowl erythroblastosis: virus
fowl lymphomatosis: virus
fowl myeloblastosis: virus
fowl neurolymphomatosis: virus
fowlpox: virus
fox: encephalitis
fox encephalitis: virus
fps: unit
fractional: anesthesia; distillation; dose; sterilization
fractional epidural: anesthesia
fractional gastric: analysis
fractional spinal: anesthesia
fracture: bed; box
fragility: test
fragmentation: myocarditis
fragmentation of: myocardium
frambesiform: syphilid
frame-shift: mutagen; mutation
franklinic: taste
fraternal: twins
free: association; energy; field; gingiva; graft; margin; radical; villus; water
free bone: flap
free-floating: anxiety
free inferior limb: joint
free nerve: ending
free superior limb: joint
free thyroxine: index
free-way: space
freezing: point
French: chalk; scale
frequency: curve; distribution
friction: knot; rub; sound
frictional: attachment
Friend: disease; virus
fright: reaction
fringed: tapeworm
frog: belly; face; tongue
frontal: angle; area; artery; axis; belly; bone; cortex; crest; eminence; fontanel; gyrectomy; horn; lobe; margin; nerve; notch; plane; plate; pole; process; region; sinus; sinusitis; suture; triangle; tuber; vein
frontoanterior: position
frontoethmoidal: suture
frontolacrimal: suture
frontomaxillary: suture
frontonasal: process; suture
fronto-occipital: fasciculus

fronto-orbital: area
frontopontine: tract
frontoposterior: position
frontosphenoidal: process
frontotemporal: tract
frontozygomatic: suture
front-tap: contraction; reflex
frost: itch
frosted: heart; liver
frozen: pelvis; section; shoulder
fruit: sugar
frustration: tolerance
frustration-aggression: hypothesis
FTA-ABS: test
fuchsin: agar; body
fuchsinophil: cell; granule; reaction
fugitive: swelling; wart
fugu: poison
Fujinami: virus
fulcrum: line
fulgurating: migraine
full: bath; denture
full liquid: diet
full thickness: graft
fuller's: earth
fulminant: anoxia; hyperpyrexia
fulminating: dysentery
functional: albuminura; aphasia; apoplexy; autonomy; blindness; castration; congestion; contracture; deafness; disease; disorder; dysmenorrhea; dyspepsia; group; hypertrophy; illness; murmur; occlusion; pathology; spasm; splint; stricture
functional chew-in: record
functional prepuberal castration: syndrome
functional residual: air; capacity
functional terminal innervation: ratio
fundamental: tone
fundiform: ligament
fundus: reflex
fungating: sore
fungiform: papilla
fungous: foot; synovitis
funicular: hydrocele; myelitis; myelosis; process
funnel: breast; chest
funnel-shaped: pelvis
furcal: nerve
furfurol: reaction
furious: rabies
furred: tongue
furrowed: tongue
fused: kidney; tooth
fusible: calculus; metal
fusiform: aneurysm; bacillus; cataract; cell; gyrus; layer; muscle
fusing: point
fusion: area; beat; point; temperature
fusion-inferred threshold: test
fusospirillary: gingivitis
fusospirochetal: disease
Fy: antigen

## G

γ-: see gamma
G: antigen; factor; force; unit
$G_{M1}$: gangliosidosis
$G_{M2}$: gangliosiodosis
g-: tolerance

G. vs. H.: disease
Gaboon: ulcer
gag: reflex
GAL: virus
galactagogue: factor
galactophorous: canal; duct
galactopoietic: factor; hormone
galactose: cataract; diabetes
galactose tolerance: test
gall: bladder; duct; sickness
gallbladder: fossa
gallop: rhythm; sound
gallstone: colic; ileus
gallus adeno-like: virus
galoche: chin
galvanic: cautery; threshold; vertigo
galvanic skin: reaction; reflex; response
galvanocaustic: snare
Gambian: fever; trypanosomiasis
gamekeeper's: thumb
gametic: nucleus
gametoid: theory
gametokinetic: hormone
gamma (γ-): angle; cell; efferent; fungus; fiber; hemolysis; loop; ray
gamma motor: neuron; system
gander: cough
gangliated: cord; nerve
ganglion: cell; ridge
ganglionic: blockade; crest; layer; saliva
ganglionic blocking: agent
ganglionic motor: neuron
ganglioside: lipidosis
gangrenous: appendicitis; pharyngitis; pneumonia; rhinitis; stomatitis
gap: arthroplasty; junction
garapata: disease
gargantuan: mastitis
gas: abscess; bacillus; cauterization; chromatography; constant; cyst; embolism; gangrene; peritonitis; phlegmon
gas gangrene: antitoxin
gas-liquid: chromatography
gaseous: acidosis; alkalosis; mediastinography; pulse
gasometric: analysis
gastral: mesoderm
gastrea: theory
gastric: analysis; calculus; canal; colic; crisis; diastole; digestion; dilation; dyspepsia; fever; fistula; fold; follicle; freezing; gland; groove; hemorrhage; impression; indigestion; juice; mucin; neurasthenia; pit; plexus; protease; secretin; smear; surface; tetany; ulcer; vein; vertigo; volvulus
gastric lymphatic: follicle
gastric remittent: fever
gastrocardiac: syndrome
gastrocolic: fistula; ligament; omentum; reflex
gastrocutaneous: fistula
gastrodiaphragmatic: ligament
gastroduodenal: artery; fistula; orifice
gastroduodenal lymph: node
gastroepiploic: vein
gastroesophageal: hernia; vestibule
gastrogenous: diarrhea
gastrohepatic: omentum
gastroileac: reflex
gastrointestinal: fistula; hormone
gastrojejunal loop obstruction: syndrome

gastrolienal: ligament
gastropancreatic: fold
gastrophrenic: ligament
gastrosplenic: ligament; omentum
gastrotoxic: serum
gate: theory
gauntlet: bandage
gauze: bandage
Ge: antigen
gel: diffusion; electrophoresis; filtration; structure
gel diffusion: reaction
gel diffusion precipitin: test
gelatin: sugar
gelatinous: ascites; infiltration; polyp; substance; tissue; varix
gemastete: cell
geminate: tooth
gemistocytic: astrocytoma; cell; reaction
genal: gland
gender: identity; role
general: anatomy; anemia; anesthesia; anesthetic; bloodletting; hospital; liposis; paralysis; peritonitis; physiology; sensation; stimulant; transduction; tuberculosis
general adaptation: reaction; syndrome
general duty: nurse; nursing
general somatic afferent: column
general somatic efferent: column
general visceral afferent: column
general visceral efferent: column
generalized: anaphylaxis; chondromalacia; epilepsy; gangliosidosis; glycogenosis; vaccinia
generalized cortical: hyperostosis
generalized Shwartzman: phenomenon
generated occlusal: path
generative: empathy
genesial: cycle
genetic: anemia; carrier; code; female; immunity; linkage; male; psychology; recombination
genetous: idiocy
genial: tubercle
genic: balance
geniculate: ganglion; neuralgia; otalgia
geniculocalcarine: radiation; tract
genioid: tubercle
genital: cord; corpuscle; duct; eminence; fold; furrow; gland; ligament; organ; phase; primacy; ridge; swelling; system; tract; tubercle
genitocrural: nerve
genitofemoral: nerve
genitoinguinal: ligament
genitourinary: fistula; system
genucubital: position
genupectoral: position
geographic, geographical: pathology; stippling; tongue
geometric: isomerism
geriatric: therapy
germ: cell; disease; layer; membrane; nucleus; theory
germ layer: theory
German: braxy; measles
German measles: virus
germinal: aplasia; area; cell; center; cord; disk; epithelium; localization; membrane; pole; rod; spot; vesicle
germinative: layer
Germiston: virus

gestalt: dissolution; phenomenon; psychology; theory; therapy
gestational: age; edema; proteinuria; psychosis
Getah: virus
ghatti: gum
Gheel: colony
ghost: cell; corpuscle
ghoul: hand
giant: cell; chromosome; colon; condyloma; fibroadenoma; urticaria
giant cell: aortitis; arteritis; carcinoma; hepatitis; myeloma; pneumonia; sarcoma; tumor
giant follicular: lymphoblastoma
giant hypertrophic: gastritis
giant osteoid: osteoma
gigantocellular: glioma
Gila: monster
gill: cleft
gill arch: skeleton
gin-drinker's: liver
ginger: paralysis
gingival: abrasion; abscess; architecture; atrophy; clamp; cleft; contour; crest; crevice; curvature; elephantiasis; enlargement; epithelium; festoon; fistula; flap; hyperplasia; hypertrophy; margin; massage; mucosa; pocket; proliferation; recession; resorption; retraction; septum; space; sulcus; tissue; trough; zone
gingivobuccal: groove; sulcus
gingivodental: ligament
gingivolabial: groove; sulcus
gingivolingual: groove; sulcus
ginglymoid: joint
girdle: anesthesia; pain; sensation
gitter: cell
glabrous: skin
glanders: bacillus
glandular: cancer; carcinoma; epithelium; fever; mastitis; pharyngitis; phthisis; plague; system; substance
glandulopreputial: lamella
glass: body; electrode; factor; pox; ray
glass bead: sterilizer
glass blower's: emphysema
glassworker's: cataract
glassy: degeneration; membrane; swelling
glaucomatocyclitic: crisis
glaucomatous: cup; excavation; halo; ring
glenohumeral: ligament
glenoid: cavity; fossa; ligament; surface
glia: cell
gliding: joint; occlusion
global: aphasia; paralysis
globe cell: anemia
globoid: body
globoid cell: leukodystrophy
globular: anemia; process; protein; sputum; thrombus; valve
glomangiomatous osseous malformation: syndrome
glomerular: crescent; cyst; layer; nephritis
glomerular filtration: rate
glomiform: gland
glomus: tumor
glomus jugulare: tumor
glossoepiglottic: ligament

glossolabiolaryngeal: paralysis
glossolabiopharyngeal: paralysis
glossopalatine: arch; fold
glossopharyngeal: nerve; part
glossy: skin
glove: anesthesia
glover's: suture
glucose oxidase paper strip: test
glucose 6-phosphatase hepatorenal: glycogenosis
glucose tolerance: test
glucose transport: maximum
gluteal: cleft; crest; fold; furrow; hernia; line; reflex; region; ridge; surface; tuberosity; vein
gluteofemoral: bursa
gluteus maximus: gait
gluteus medius: gait
glycerinated: gelatin; tincture
glycine succinate: cycle
glycogen: cardiomegaly
glycogen storage: disease
glycolipid: lipidosis
glycoprotein: hormone
glycotropic: factor; hormone
glycyl: chain
glyoxylic acid: cycle; reaction; test
G:N: ratio
gnathic: index
gnome's: calf
goat: pox
goatpox: virus
goat's milk: anemia
goblet: cell
gold: cure; equivalent; foil; inlay
gold sol: test
golf-hole ureteral: orifice
gompholic: joint
gonad: nucleus
gonadal: agenesis; aplasia; dysgenesis
gonadial: ridge
gonadotropic: hormone
gonococcal: conjunctivitis; urethritis
gonorrheal: ophthalmia; rheumatism; salpingitis
Good: antigen
good: object
goose: breathing; flesh; gait
Gothic: arch; palate
Gothic arch: tracing
gout: diet
gouty: arthritis; diathesis; pearl; tophus; urine
government: hospital
Gr: antigen
gracile: habitus; tubercle
gracilis: syndrome
graduate: nurse
graduated: bath; compress; tenotomy
graft versus host: disease; reaction
grain: itch
gram: calory; equivalent; ion
gram-atomic: weight
gram-molecular: weight
grand: climacteric; mal; multipara
grand mal: epilepsy
granddaughter: cyst
granny: knot
granular: cast; conjunctivitis; cortex; degeneration; induration; kidney; layer; leukoblast; leukocyte; lid; ophthalmia; pharyngitis; pit; urethritis
granular cell: myoblastoma; tumor

granular cytoplasmic: reticulum
granulation: tissue
granule: cell
granulocytic: leukemia; series
granulomatous: arteritis; colitis; encephalomyelitis; inflammation; nocardiosis
granulosa: cell
granulosa cell: tumor
granulosa lutein: cell
grape: cure; ending; mole; sugar
graphic: aphasia; formula
graphite: pneumoconiosis
graphomotor: aphasia
grasp: reflex
grasping: reflex
grass: bacillus; staggers; tetany
grave: delirium; wax
gravid: uterus
gravidic: retinitis; retinopathy
gravimetric: analysis
gravitation: abscess
gravitational: ulcer; unit
gray: atrophy; cataract; column; degeneration; eye; fiber; hepatization; induration; infiltration; matter; substance; tuber; tubercle; wing
grease: heel
greaseless: cream
greasy pig: disease
great: foramen; toe; vein; wing
great adductor: muscle
great alveolar: cell
great anastomotic: artery
great auricular: nerve
great cerebral: vein
great horizontal: fissure
great longitudinal: fissure
great pancreatic: artery
great saphenous: vein
great sciatic: nerve
great superior pancreatic: artery
great-toe: reflex
greater: circulation; cul-de-sac; horn; omentum; trochanter; tubercle; tuberosity
greater alar: cartilage
greater arterial: circle
greater multangular: bone
greater occipital: nerve
greater palatine: artery; canal; foramen; nerve
greater pectoral: muscle
greater peritoneal: sac
greater petrosal: nerve
greater posterior straight: muscle
greater psoas: muscle
greater rhomboid: muscle
greater sciatic: notch
greater splanchnic: nerve
greater superficial petrosal: nerve
greater supraclavicular: fossa
greater tympanic: spine
greater vestibular: gland
greater zygomatic: muscle
green: blindness; cancer; cataract; hellebore; hemoglobin; pus; sickness; soap; sputum; stain; tea; tooth; vision; vitriol
green-stick: fracture
grenz: ray
griffin-claw: hand
grinder's: asthma; disease; phthisis; rot

grinding: surface
grocer's: itch
groin: ulcer
grooved: tongue
gross: anatomy; lesion
Gross': virus
Gross' leukemia: virus
ground: bundle; itch; lamella; state; substance
ground itch: anemia
group: agglutination; agglutinin; antigen; dynamics; hospital; immunity; medicine; nursing; psychotherapy; reaction; test
growing: pain
growing ovarian: follicle
growth: factor; hormone; quotient; rate
growth hormone-releasing: factor; hormone
growth-onset: diabetes
guaiac: test
Guama: virus
guanidine: tetany
guanine: cell
guar: gum
Guaroa: virus
guide: plane
guillotine: amputation
guinea: worm
guinea corn: yaws
gum: contour; lancet; line; rash; resection; resin
gummatous: abscess; syphilid; ulcer
gun-barrel: enterostomy
gunshot: wound
gunstock: deformity
gurgling: rale
gurjun: balsam
gustatory: anesthesia; audition; bud; cell; hallucination; hyperesthesia; nucleus; organ; pore; rhinorrhea
gustatory-sudorific: reflex
gustatory sweating: syndrome
gut: glucagon
gutta percha: plugger; point
guttate: choroidopathy
gutter: dystrophy; fracture; wound
guttural: duct; pouch; pulse; rale
gymnocolon: bath
gynecoid: pelvis
gynecophoric: canal
gyrate: atrophy
gyrochrome: cell

## H

H: agglutinin; antigen; band; bone; colony; disease; disk; factor; field; ray; reflex; space; substance
H-shaped: ecchymosis
HA1: virus
HA2: virus
habenular: commissure; nucleus
habenulointerpeduncular: tract
habit: chorea; scoliosis; spasm; tic
habitual: abortion; aphthosis
Haff: disease
hafussi: bath
hair: ball; bulb; cast; cell; cross; cycle; follicle; papilla; root; shaft; stream; whorl; worm
hair-matrix: carcinoma
hairy: heart; mole; scorpion; tongue

**hairy cell:** leukemia
**half:** bath; time
**half-amplitude pulse:** duration
**half-chair:** form
**half-glass:** spectacles
**half-value:** layer
**hallucinatory:** neuralgia
**halo:** nevus; sign; vision
**halogen:** acne
**halothane:** hepatitis
**halothane-ether:** azeotrope
**hamate:** bone
**hammer:** finger; nose; toe
**hammock:** bandage; ligament
**hamstring:** muscle; tendon
**hamular:** notch; process
**hand:** eczema; ratio
**hand-and-foot:** syndrome
**hand-foot-and-mouth:** disease
**hand-foot-and-mouth disease:** virus
**hanging:** drop; heart; septum
**hanging block:** culture
**haploscopic:** vision
**Hapsburg:** jaw; lip
**hapten inhibition of:** precipitation
**hard:** cataract; chancre; corn; palate; papilloma; paraffin; pulse; ray; soap; solder; sore; tissue; tubercle; ulcer; water
**hardened:** pelvis
**hardness:** scale
**hard pad, hardpad:** disease; virus
**hare's:** eye
**harelip:** suture
**harlequin:** fetus; reaction
**harlequin color change:** syndrome
**harmonic:** suture
**harmonious:** correspondence
**Hartnup:** disease; syndrome
**Hart Park:** virus
**harvester:** ant
**hatchet:** excavator
**haunch:** bone
**haut:** mal
**Haverhill:** fever
**hay:** asthma; bacillus; fever
**He:** antigen
**head:** botfly; cavity; fold; gut; injury; kidney; mirror; nurse; process; stethoscope; tetanus; wound
**healed:** turberculosis; ulcer
**healing by 1st, 2nd, and 3rd:** intention
**health:** care; nurse
**heart:** antigen; beat; block; failure; hormone; position; rate; reflex; sac; sound; stroke; transplantation
**heart failure:** cell
**heart-lung:** preparation
**heat:** apoplexy; capacity; cramp; edema; exhaustion; hyperpyrexia; prostration; rash; rigor; stroke; treatment
**heat coagulation:** test
**heat-curing:** resin
**heat of:** combustion; crystallization; evaporation
**heat-rigor:** point
**heated globe:** thermometer
**heavy:** hydrogen; kaolin; nitrogen; oxygen; water
**heavy chain:** disease
**hebephrenic:** dementia; schizophrenia
**hebetic:** cough
**hectic:** fever; flush

**hederiform:** ending
**heel:** bone; fly; jar; tap; tendon
**heel-tap:** reaction; test
**height:** vertigo
**height-length:** index
**height of:** contour
**HeLa:** cell
**helicine:** artery
**helicoid:** ginglymus
**helicopod:** gait
**helium:** speech
**helminthic:** dysentery
**helper:** virus
**hemadsorption:** virus
**hemadsorption virus:** test
**hemagglutinating cold:** autoantibody
**hemagglutination:** inhibition
**hemal:** arch; gland; node; spine
**hemangiectatic:** hypertrophy
**hemangioma-thrombocytopenia:** syndrome
**hemapheic:** jaundice
**hematinic:** principle
**hematogenetic:** calculus
**hematogenous:** abscess; albuminuria; embolism; jaundice; osteitis; pigment; theory
**hematoid:** cancer
**hematopoietic, hemopoietic:** gland; system; tissue
**hematoxylin:** body
**hematoxylin and eosin:** stain
**hematoxyphil:** body
**hematuric bilious:** fever
**hemiazygos:** vein
**hemic:** calculus; distomiasis; murmur
**hemilateral:** chorea
**hemiopic:** reaction
**hemiopic pupillary:** reaction
**hemiplegic:** gait; idiocy; migraine
**hemisulfur:** mustard
**hemithoracic:** duct
**hemochorial:** placenta
**hemoclastic:** reaction
**hemoendothelial:** placenta
**hemoglobin C:** disease
**hemoglobin H:** disease
**hemoglobin Ringer:** solution
**hemoglobinuric:** fever; nephrosis
**hemohepatogenous:** jaundice
**hemolymph:** gland; node
**hemolysin:** unit
**hemolytic:** anemia; chain; disease; gas; jaundice; splenomegaly; streptococcus; unit
**hemolytic-uremic:** syndrome
**hemophilic:** arthritis; joint
**hemopleuropneumonia:** syndrome
**hemopoietic:** see hematopoietic
**hemorenal salt:** index
**hemorrhagic:** anemia; ascites; bronchitis; cyst; diathesis; disease; fever; gangrene; infarct; measles; nephritis; osteomyelitis; pachymeningitis; pian; plague; pleurisy; rickets; septicemia; shock; smallpox
**hemorrhoidal:** nerve; plexus; vein
**hemostatic:** collodion; forceps
**hemotoxic:** anemia
**hempseed:** calculus
**hen-cluck:** stertor
**heparin:** unit
**hepatic:** aloe; amebiasis; capsulitis;

colic; coma; cord; cyst; duct; encephalopathy; fistula; flexure; infantilism; insufficiency; lamina; lobule; plexus; segment; vein
**hepatic intermittent:** fever
**hepatic lymph:** node
**hepatic storage:** disease
**hepatitis:** antigen; virus
**hepatitis-associated:** antigen
**hepatitis B:** antigen
**hepatitis B core:** antigen
**hepatitis B surface:** antigen
**hepatocellular:** carcinoma; jaundice
**hepatocolic:** ligament
**hepatocystic:** duct
**hepatoduodenal:** ligament
**hepatoenteric:** recess
**hepatoesophageal:** ligament
**hepatogastric:** ligament
**hepatogenous:** jaundice; pigment
**hepatojugular:** reflex; reflux
**hepatolenticular:** degeneration; disease
**hepatolienal:** fibrosis
**hepatonephric:** syndrome
**hepatophosphorylase deficiency:** glycogenosis
**hepatopleural:** fistula
**hepatorenal:** ligament; pouch; recess; syndrome
**herald:** patch
**herd:** immunity; instinct
**hereditary:** arthrodysplasia; chorea; disease; hemiplegia; lymphedema; myokymia; nephritis; photomyoclonus; pseudohemophilia; spherocytosis
**hereditary cerebellar:** ataxia
**hereditary cutaneomandibular:** polyoncosis
**hereditary deforming:** chondrodysplasia; chondrodystrophy
**hereditary ectodermal:** dysplasia
**hereditary fructose:** intolerance
**hereditary hemorrhagic:** telangiectasis; thrombasthenia
**hereditary methemoglobinemic:** cyanosis
**hereditary multiple:** exostosis
**hereditary opalescent:** dentin
**hereditary progressive:** arthro-ophthalmopathy
**hereditary renal-retinal:** dysplasia
**hereditary sensory radicular:** neuropathy
**hereditary spinal:** ataxia
**heredofamilial:** tremor
**heredomacular:** degeneration
**hernia:** knife
**hernial:** aneurysm; sac
**herniated:** disk
**heroic:** treatment
**herpes:** encephalitis; virus
**herpetic:** fever; gingivostomatitis; keratitis; stomatitis
**herz:** hormone
**heterochromic:** cyclitis; uveitis
**heterocladic:** anastomosis
**heterocyclic:** compound; ring
**heterocytotropic:** antibody
**heterodermic:** graft
**heterogametic:** embryo
**heterogeneous:** system
**heterogenetic:** antibody; antigen
**heterogenous:** vaccine**

heterologous: antiserum; graft; insemination; protein; stimulus; tumor; twins
heteromeric: cell; peptide
heterometric: autoregulation
heteronomous: psychotherapy
heteronymous: diplopia; hemianopsia; image; parallax
heterophil: antibody; antigen; hemolysin; leukocyte
heteroplastic: graft
heterospecific: graft
heterotopic: bone; graft; pain; pregnancy
heterotropic: chromosome
heterotype: mitosis
heterotypic: cortex; division
heterotypical: chromosome
heterovaccine: therapy
hexacanth: embryo
hexaxial reference: system
hexone: base
HFR: strain
HG: factor
hiatal: hernia
hibernating: gland
hickory-stick: fracture
hidebound: disease
hidrotic ectodermal: dysplasia
high: convex; enema; lithotomy; wine
high altitude: chamber
high calorie: diet
high cell count: leukemia
high energy: compound; phosphate
high energy phosphate: bond
high fat: diet
high forceps: delivery
high frequency: current; deafness; transduction
high fusing: porcelain
high output: failure
high pressure: oxygen
high sodium: diet
high spinal: anesthesia
high steppage: gait
high tension: current
higher order: conditioning
highest intercostal: artery; vein
highest nuchal: line
highest thoracic: artery
hilar: dance
hill: diarrhea
hilus: cell
hind: gut; kidney
hindbrain: vesicle
hinge: axis; joint; movement; position
hip: bone; joint; phenomenon
hip-flexion: phenomenon
hippocampal: commissure; convolution; fissure; gyrus; sclerosis
Histalog: test
histamine: shock; test
histaminic: cephalalgia; headache
histiocytic: leukemia
histiocytic medullary: reticulosis
histocompatibility: gene
histoid: neoplasm; tumor
histo-latex: test
histologic: accommodation
histone: base
histotoxic: anoxia
histrionic: personality; spasm
HL-A: antigen

Ho: antigen
hobnail: liver; tongue
hoe: excavator; scaler
hog: cholera
hog-cholera: bacillus; vaccine; virus
holandric: gene; inheritance
holiday: syndrome
holistic: psychology
hollow: back; bone; foot
holoblastic: cleavage
holocrine: gland
hologynic: inheritance
holosystolic: murmur
homeometric: autoregulation
hemeostatic: equilibrium
homigrade: scale
hominal: physiology
homochronous: inheritance
homocladic: anastomosis
homocyclic: compound; ring
homocytotropic: antibody
homogametic: embryo
homogeneous: immersion; system
homolecithal: egg
homologous: antiserum; chromosome; graft; insemination; series; stimulus; tumor
homologous serum: jaundice
homonymous: diplopia; hemianopsia; image; parallax
homoplastic: graft
homosexual: panic
homotopic: pain
homotypic: cortex; division
homovanillic acid: test
homozygous: achondroplasia
honey: urine
honeycomb: lung; ringworm; scall; tetter; tripe
Hong Kong: foot; toe
hoof-and-mouth: disease
hook: bundle
hooked: bone; fasciculus
hookless: tapeworm
hookworm: anemia; disease
horizontal: atrophy; cell; fissure; fracture; heart; overlap; plane; sulcus; transmission; vertigo
hormonal: gingivitis
hormone pregnancy: test
horn: fly
horny: layer
horse: asthma; bots; leech; louse; pinworm; pox; tick
horsehair: probang
horsepox: virus
horseshoe: fistula; kidney; placenta
hospital: fever; gangrene; nurse; sister
hot: abscess; bath; flash; flush; gangrene; nodule; pack
hot atom: chemistry
hot house: lamb
hot salt: sterilizer
Hottentot: apron; tea
hound-dog: facies
hourglass: contraction; head; murmur; stomach; vertebra
house: physician; staff; surgeon
housemaid's: knee
housing: disease
Hu (He): antigen
huckle: bone
human: centrifuge; ecology; fibrinogen;

flea; pinworm; thrombin
human antihemophilic: factor; fraction
human chorionic: gonadotropin
human fibrin: foam
human gamma: globulin
human measles immune: serum
human menopausal: gonadotropin
human pertussis immune: serum
human placental: lactogen
human scarlet fever immune: serum
humanistic: psychology
humanized: lymph
humeral: artery; articulation
humeroradial: articulation; joint
humeroulnar: joint
humid: tetter
humoral: doctrine; immunity; pathology; theory
hunger: cure; contraction; pain; swelling; therapy
hunting: phenomenon; reaction
Hurloid: facies
H-V: interval
HVA: test
hyaline: body; cartilage; cast; degeneration; leukocyte; membrane; thrombus; tubercle
hyaline membrane: disease
hyaloid: body; canal; fossa; membrane
hyaloideoretinal: degeneration
hybrid: prosthesis
hydatid: cyst; fremitus; mole; polyp; pregnancy; rash; reasonance; sand; tapeworm; thrill
hydatidiform: mole
hydralazine: syndrome
hydrate: crystal
hydrate microcrystal: theory
hydremic: edema; plethora
hydroalcoholic: extract; tincture
hydrocephalic: idiocy
hydroelectric: bath
hydrogen: bond; electrode; number
hydrolytic: cleavage
hydrolyzing: enzyme
hydrophilic: colloid; petrolatum
hydrophobic: colloid; tetanus
hydropic: degeneration
hydrostatic: pressure; test
17-hydroxycorticosteroid: test
17-hydroxylase deficiency: syndrome
hygienic: treatment
hygienic laboratory: coefficient
hygroscopic: expansion
hylic: tumor
hyobranchial: cleft
hyoepiglottic: ligament
hyoglossal: membrane
hyoid: apparatus; arch; bone
hyomandibular: cleft
hyparterial: bronchus
hyperabduction: syndrome
hyperbaric: anesthesia; chamber; oxygen; oxygenation; pressure; solution
hyperbaric oxygen: therapy
hyperbaric spinal: anesthesia
hypercalcemic: sarcoidosis; uremia
hyperchromatic: anemia; macrocythemia
hyperchromic: anemia
hypercyanotic: angina
hyperemia: test
hyperergic: encephalitis

hyperextension-hyperflexion: injury
hyperfunctional: occlusion
hypergenic: teratosis
hyperglobulinemic: purpura
hyperglycemic-glycogenolytic: factor
hypergonadotropic: eunuchoidism
hyperkalemic periodic: paralysis
hyperkinetic: syndrome
hypermature: cataract
hypernatremic: encephalopathy
hyperosmolar hyperglycemic nonketonic: coma
hyperostotic: spondylosis
hyperplastic: arteriosclerosis; graft; inflammation; osteoarthritis; pulpitis; tissue
hyperquantivalent: idea
hypersegmented: neutrophil
hypersensitive: dentin
hypersensitive xiphoid: syndrome
hypersensitivity: angiitis
hypertensive: arteriopathy; arteriosclerosis; encephalopathy; retinopathy
hyperthyroid: asthma
hypertonic salt: solution
hypertrophic: arthritis; gastritis; pulpitis; rhinitis; ringworm
hypertrophic cervical: pachymeningitis
hypertrophic pulmonary: osteoarthropathy
hypertrophic pyloric: stenosis
hypertrophied frenula: syndrome
hyperventilation: syndrome; test; tetany
hyperviscosity: syndrome
hypnagogic: hallucination; image
hypnogenic: spot
hypnopompic: image
hypnotic: psychotherapy; relationship; sleep; state
hypoacoustic: zone
hypobaric: solution
hypobaric spinal: anesthesia
hypobranchial: eminence
hypochondriac: region
hypochondriacal: melancholia
hypochondrial: reflex
hypochromic: anemia
hypochromic microcytic: anemia
hypocytic: leukemia
hypodermic: implantation; injection; needle; syringe; tablet
hypoferric: anemia
hypogastric: artery; ganglion; nerve; reflex; vein
hypoglossal: canal; eminence; nerve; nucleus
hypogonadotropic: eunuchoidism; hypogonadism
hypokalemic: nephropathy
hypokalemic periodic: paralysis
hypomanic: reaction
hypometabolic: state; syndrome
hypoparathyroid: tetany
hypoparathyroidism: syndrome
hypopharyngeal: diverticulum
hypophysial: amenorrhea; cachexia; duct; fossa
hypophysiotropic: hormone
hypophysis: syndrome
hypoplastic: anemia; heart
hypoplastic left heart: syndrome
hypopyon: keratitis; keratoiritis; ulcer

hypostatic: abscess; congestion; ectasia; pneumonia
hypotensive: anesthesia
hypothalamic: infundibulum; obesity; sulcus
hypothalamohypophysial: tract
hypothalamohypophysial portal: system
hypothenar: eminence; prominence
hypothermic: anesthesia
hypothyroid: dwarf; infantilism
hypotonic salt: solution
hypovolemic: shock
hypoxemia: test
hypoxia warning: system
hypoxic: nephrosis
hypsiloid: angle; cartilage; ligament
hysterical: amblyopia; anesthesia; aphonia; chorea; convulsion; deafness; insanity; joint; personality; polydipsia; psychosis; syncope
hysterogenic: area; point; spot; zone
hysteroid: convulsion

# I

I: antigen; band; cell; disk; pilus
I cell: disease
$^{131}$I uptake: test
iatromathematical: school
IBR: virus
ice: bag; cap
Iceland: disease; moss
ichorous: pus
ichthyosiform: erythroderma
icing: heart; liver
Icoaraci: virus
iconic: sign
icteric: index
icterohemolytic: anemia
icterus: index
ideal alveolar: gas
ideational: agnosia; apraxia
identical: twins
identity: crisis
ideokinetic: apraxia
idiodynamic: control
idiographic: approach
idiohypophysial: diabetes
idiomuscular: contraction
idionodal: rhythm
idiopathic: anemia; bradycardia; cardiomyopathy; disease; dwarf; epilepsy; hirsutism; hypercalcemia; hyperlipemia; hypertension; infantilism; megacolon; neuralgia; proctitis; roseola; tetanus
idiopathic hypercalcemic: sclerosis
idiopathic hypertrophic: osteoarthropathy
idiopathic hypertrophic subaortic: stenosis
idiopathic hypochromic: anemia
idiopathic muscular: atrophy
idiopathic paroxysmal: myoglobulinemia
idiopathic retroperitoneal: fibrosis
idiopathic thrombocytopenic: purpura
idiophrenic: insanity
idioretinal: light
idiosyncratic: sensitivity
idioventricular: kick; rhythm
IKI: catgut

ileal: artery; bladder; conduit; intussusception; papilla; sphincter; vein
ileocecal: eminence; fold; intussusception; opening; valve
ileocecocolic: sphincter
ileocolic: artery; intussusception; valve; vein
ileocolic lymph: node
Ilesha: virus
Ilhéus: encephalitis; fever; virus
iliac: bone; bursa; colon; crest; fascia; fossa; horn; plexus; region; roll; spine; steal; tuberosity; vein
iliacosubfascial: fossa; hernia
iliococcygeal: muscle
iliofemoral: ligament; triangle
iliohypogastric: nerve
ilioinguinal: nerve
iliolumbar: artery; ligament; vein
iliopectineal: arch; bursa; eminence; fascia; fossa; ligament; line
iliopsoas: muscle
iliopubic: eminence
iliosciatic: notch
iliotibial: band
iliotrochanteric: ligament
ilosvay: reagent
imitative: tetanus
immature: cataract; granulocyte; neutrophil
immediate: agglutination; allergy; amputation; auscultation; contagion; denture; percussion; reaction; transfusion
immediate insertion: denture
immediate posttraumatic: automatism; convulsion
immersion: foot; lens; objective; system
immersion blast: injury
immobilizing: antibody
immovable: bandage; joint
immune: adsorption; agglutination; agglutinin; body; complex; deviation; hemolysin; hemolysis; inflammation; opsonin; precipitation; protein; reaction; response; serum; system
immune adherence: phenomenon
immune adhesion: test
immune complex: disease; nephritis
immune serum: globulin
immunochemical: assay
immunofluorescence: method; microscopy
immunofluorescent: stain
immunologic, immunological: competence; deficiency; enhancement; mechanism; paralysis; tolerance
immunological deficiency: syndrome
immunological pregnancy: test
immunologically activated: cell
immunologically competent: cell
immunoproliferative: disorder
immunoreactive: insulin
immunosuppressive: agent
impact: resistance
impacted: fracture; tooth
impedence: angle; method; plethysmography
imperative: conception
imperfect: stage
imperforate: anus
imperial: pint; quart
impetiginous: cheilitis; syphilid
implant: denture; technique

**implant denture:** substructure; superstructure
**implantation:** cone; cyst; dermoid; graft; metastasis; theory
**implanted:** suture
**implosive:** therapy
**imported:** malaria
**impression:** area; compound; material; tray
**impressive:** aphasia
**impulsive:** act; insanity; obsession
**impure:** flutter
**IMViC:** reaction
**in:** phase
**inactive:** repressor; tuberculosis
**inadequate:** diet; personality; stimulus
**inanition:** fever
**inappropriate:** affect
**inborn:** variation
**incarcerated:** hernia; placenta
**incarceration:** symptom
**incarial:** bone
**incasement:** theory
**incest:** barrier
**incident:** angle; ray
**incidental:** color; image; learning; parasite
**incipient:** abortion
**incisal:** angle; edge; guidance; guide; path; point; rest; surface
**incisal guide:** angle
**incised:** wound
**incisional:** hernia
**incisive:** bone, canal; duct; foramen; fossa; papilla; suture
**incisor:** canal; crest; foramen; tooth
**inclusion:** blenorrhea; body; compound; conjunctivitis; cyst; dermoid
**inclusion body:** disease; encephalitis
**inclusion body rhinitis:** virus
**inclusion cell:** disease
**inclusion conjunctivitis:** virus
**incompatible blood transfusion:** reaction
**incompetent cervical:** os
**incomplete:** abortion; antibody; antigen; ascertainment; cleavage; disinfectant; fistula; fracture; hemianopsia; metamorphosis; neurofibromatosis
**incomplete A-V:** dissociation
**incomplete conjoined:** twins
**incomplete scalp:** avulsion
**incongruent:** nystagmus
**incongruous:** hemianopsia
**incremental:** line
**incubative:** stage
**incudal:** fold; fossa
**incudomalleolar:** joint
**incudostapedial:** articulation; joint
**indentation:** hardness
**independent:** variable
**indeterminate:** cleavage
**index:** ametropia; finger; myopia
**indexical:** sign
**India:** ringworm
**India rubber:** jaw; pelvis
**Indian:** ginger; gum; hemp; method; operation; podophyllum; rhinoplasty; senna; sickness; squill
**Indian arrow:** poison
**Indian podophyllum:** resin
**indicator:** yellow
**indicator-dilution:** curve

**indifference to pain:** syndrome
**indifferent:** cell; electrode; gonad; oxide; tissue; water
**indirect:** calorimetry; diuretic; fracture; immunofluorescence; lead; method (for inlay); ophthalmoscopy; oxidase; placentography; ray; retainer; retention; technique; test; transfusion; vision
**indirect Coombs':** test
**indirect nuclear:** division
**indirect pulp:** capping
**indirect pupillary:** reaction
**individual:** difference; psychology; therapy; tolerance
**individuation:** field
**indolent:** bubo; ulcer
**indophenol:** method
**induced:** abortion; apnea; current; enzyme; glomerulonephritis; hypotension; insanity; lethargy; malaria; mutation; phagocytosis; radioactivity; symptom; trance
**inducible:** enzyme
**inducing:** current
**induction:** period
**inductive:** resistance
**indurative:** myocarditis; pneumonia
**industrial:** deafness; dermatitis; nursing; psychology
**industrial methylated:** spirit
**indwelling:** catheter
**inert:** gas
**inertia:** time
**inevitable:** abortion
**infant:** death
**infantile:** autism; cataract; convulsion; diplegia; dwarf; hemiplegia; hernia; hypothyroidism; leishmaniasis; liver; myxedema; osteomalacia; paralysis; pellagra; pseudoleukemia; scurvy; sexuality; tetany
**infantile cortical:** hyperostosis
**infantile muscular:** atrophy
**infantile progressive spinal muscular:** atrophy
**infantile purulent:** conjunctivitis
**infantile spastic:** paraplegia
**infantile spinal:** paralysis
**infection:** atrium; immunity
**infection-exhaustion:** psychosis
**infectious:** abortion; anemia; disease; endocarditis; enterohepatitis; granuloma; hepatitis; icterus; jaundice; mononucleosis; myoclonia; myositis; myxomatosis; nucleic acid; ophthalmoplegia; papilloma; polyneuritis; sinusitis; wart
**infectious arteritis:** virus
**infectious avian:** bronchitis
**infectious bovine:** keratitis; rhinotracheitis
**infectious bovine rhinotracheitis:** virus
**infectious bronchitis:** virus
**infectious bulbar:** paralysis
**infectious canine:** hepatitis
**infectious canine hepatitis:** virus
**infectious ectromelia:** virus
**infectious eczematoid:** dermatitis
**infectious hepatitis:** virus
**infectious necrotic:** hepatitis
**infectious porcine:** encephalomyelitis
**infectious porcine encephalomyelitis:** virus

**infectious warts:** virus
**infective:** disease; embolism; endocarditis; thrombus
**inferential:** statistics
**inferior:** laryngotomy; polioencephalitis; tracheotomy
**inferior anatomical structures** (specific inferior structures are listed under the following): angle; area; arteriole; artery; articulation; border; brachium; canal; colliculus; convolution; extremity; fascia; fasciculus; fissure; flexure; fold; foramen; fossa; ganglion; groove; gyrus; horn; joint; ligament; line; lobe; lobule; margin; muscle; nerve; node; notch; nucleus; olive; part; peduncle; pit; plexus; pole; recess; retinaculum; root; segment; sinus; strait; sulcus; surface; triangle; trunk; tubercle; vein; velum; vena; wall
**inferior myocardial:** infarction
**inferiority:** complex
**inferolateral:** margin
**inferolateral myocardial:** infarction
**inferomedial:** margin
**infiltrating:** lipoma
**infiltration:** anesthesia
**infinite:** distance
**inflamed:** ulcer
**inflammatory:** corpuscle; edema; exudate; lymph; rheumatism
**inflammatory fibrous:** hyperplasia
**inflammatory papillary:** hyperplasia
**influenza:** bacillus; virus
**influenza virus:** vaccine
**influenzal:** pneumonia
**information:** theory
**informational:** ribonucleic acid
**infrabony:** pocket
**infracardiac:** bursa
**infraclavicular:** fossa; infiltrate; part; region; triangle
**infraclinoid:** aneurysm
**infracostal:** line
**infraduodenal:** fossa
**infraglenoid:** tubercle; tuberosity
**infragranular:** layer
**infrahyoid:** bursa; muscle
**infralobar:** part
**infranatant:** fluid
**infranodal:** extrasystole
**infraorbital:** artery; canal; foramen; groove; nerve; region; suture
**infrapatellar:** fold
**infrapatellar fat:** body
**infrared:** light; microscope; ray; spectroscopy; thermography
**infrascapular:** artery; region
**infrasegmental:** part; vein
**infrasonic:** sound
**infraspinatus:** fascia
**infraspinous:** fossa
**infratemporal:** crest; fossa; region; surface
**infratrochlear:** nerve
**infundibular:** part; recess; stenosis
**infundibulo-ovarian:** ligament
**infundibulopelvic:** ligament
**infundibuloventricular:** crest
**infused:** graft
**ingravescent:** apoplexy
**ingrowing:** toenail
**ingrown:** hair; nail

inguinal: canal; crest; fold; fossa; gland; hernia; ligament; plexus; poradenitis; region; triangle; trigone
inguinal aponeurotic: fold
inguinocrural: hernia
inguinolabial: hernia
inguinoperitoneal: hernia
inguinoscrotal: hernia
inguinosuperficial: hernia
inhalation: anesthesia; anesthetic; therapy
inherent: immunity
inherited: character; disease
inherited variants of: albumin
inhibiting: antibody
inhibition: factor
inhibitory: autacoid; fiber; nerve; obsession
inhibitory postsynaptic: potential
initial: contact; dose; heat
injection: molding
injury: potential
innate: heat; immunity; reflex
inner skull: table
inner cell: mass
innermost intercostal: muscle
innervation: apraxia
innocent: murmur; tumor
innominate: artery; bone; cartilage; fossa; substance; vein
innominate cardiac: vein
inopectic: diathesis
inorganic: acid; chemistry; compound; murmur; orthophosphate; oxacid; pyrophosphatase
inquiline: parasite
insect: virus
insensible: perspiration
insoluble: soap
inspiratory: capacity; center; stridor
inspiratory reserve: volume
inspired: gas
instantaneous: vector
instantaneous electrical: axis
instrumental: conditioning
insufficiency: disease
insufflation: anesthesia
insular: area; cortex; hypothesis; sclerosis; scotoma
insulin: lipodystrophy; shock; unit
insulin-antogonizing: factor
insulin-like: acitivity
insulin shock: treatment
insulinopenic: diabetes
integumentary: system
intellectual: aura
intelligence: quotient; test
intensity of: sound
intensive: care; psychotherapy
intensive care: unit
intention: spasm; tremor
intentional: replantation
interaction process: analysis
interalveolar: pore; septum; space
interanular: segment
interarch: distance
interarticular: fibrocartilage; joint
interarytenoid: notch
interatrial: foramen; septum
intercalary: neuron; staphyloma
intercalated: disk; duct; nucleus
intercapillary: cell; glomerulosclerosis
intercapital: ligament

intercapitular: vein
intercarotid: body
intercartilaginous: part
intercavernous: sinus
intercellular: bridge; canaliculus; cement; digestion; junction; lymph
interceptive occlusal: contact
interchondral: articulation; joint; ligament
interclavicular: ligament; notch
interclinoid: ligament
intercolumnar: fascia; fiber
intercondylar: eminence; fossa; line; tubercle
intercondyloid: fossa; notch
intercornual: ligament
intercostal: anesthesia; ligament; membrane; nerve; neuralgia; node; space; vein
intercostobrachial: nerve
intercostohumeral: nerve
intercrural: fiber; ganglion
intercuneiform: joint; ligament
intercurrent: disease
intercuspal: position
interdental: canal; caries; papilla; septum; splint
interectopic: interval
interfacial: canal
interfacial surface: tension
interfascial: space
interfascicular: fasciculus
interference: beat; dissociation; microscope
interfoveolar: ligament
interglobular: space
interilioabdominal: amputation
interim: denture
interjudge: reliability
interlaminar: jelly
interlobar: duct; surface; vein
interlobular: artery; duct; ductule; emphysema; pleurisy; vein
interlocking: gyrus
intermaxillary: bone; fixation; relation; suture; traction
intermediary: body; movement; nerve; system
intermediate: abutment; amputation; body; disk; ganglion; heart; hemorrhage; host; lamella; line; mesoderm; nerve; part; ray
intermediate cuneiform: bone
intermediate dorsal cutaneous: nerve
intermediate great: muscle
intermediate sacral: crest
intermediate supraclavicular: nerve
intermediolateral: nucleus
intermediolateral cell: column
intermediomedial: nucleus
intermembranous: part
intermenstrual: fever; pain
intermesenteric: plexus
intermetacarpal: joint; ligament
intermetatarsal: articulation; joint; ligament
intermittent: albuminuria; arthralgia; claudication; cramp; hydrarthrosis; insanity; malaria; pulse; sterilization; tetanus; torticollis
intermittent acute: porphyria
intermittent malarial: fever
intermittent positive pressure: breath-

ing
intermuscular: septum
internal: antigen; attachment; decompression; fistula; fixation; hemorrhage; hirudiniasis; hydrocephalus; medicine; meningitis; ophthalmopathy; phase; pyocephalus; resorption; respiration; strabismus; secretion; traction; urethrotomy; version
internal anatomical structures (specific internal structures are listed under the following): artery; axis; capsule; conjugate; crest; fascia; fiber; fibrocartilage; foramen; gland; ligament; lip; meatus; muscle; nerve; node; plexus; sulcus; surface; vein
internal adhesive: pericarditis
internal capsule: syndrome
internal-external: urethrotomy
internal vaginal testicular: hernia
internasal: suture
international: system; unit
interneuromeric: cleft
internodal: segment
internuncial: neuron
interocclusal: clearance; distance; gap; record
interocclusal rest: space
interofective: system
interosseous: bursa; cartilage; crest; fascia; groove; ligament; margin; membrane; nerve
interpalpebral: zone
interpapillary: ridge
interparietal: bone; sulcus; suture
interpeduncular: cistern; fossa; ganglion; nucleus
interpelviabdominal: amputation
interphalangeal: articulation; joint
interpleural: space
interpolated: extrasystole
interposition: arthroplasty
interproximal: papilla; space
interpubic: disk
interradicular: alveoloplasty; septum; space
interrenal: body; gland
interridge: distance
interrupted: respiration; suture
interscapular: gland; hibernoma
interscapulothoracic: amputation
intersegmental: fasciculus; vein
interseptovalvular: space
intersheath: space
intersigmoid: hernia; recess
interspecific: graft
interspinal: line; muscle
interspinous: ligament
interspongioplastic: substance
intersternebral: joint
interstitial: absorption; atrophy; cystitis; cell; disease; emphysema; fluid; gastritis; gland; growth; hernia; implantation; inflammation; keratitis; lamella; mastitis; myositis; nephritis; neuritis; nucleus; pneumonia; pregnancy; tissue
interstitial cell-stimulating: hormone
interstitial plasma cell: pneumonia
intersystolic: peroid
intertarsal: articulation; joint
interthalamic: adhesion
intertragic: notch

**intertransverse:** ligament; muscle
**intertrochanteric:** crest; line
**intertropical:** anemia; hyphemia
**intertubercular:** bursitis; groove; line; sulcus
**interureteric:** fold
**interval:** gout; operation; scale
**intervening:** variable
**intervenous:** tubercle
**interventricular:** foramen; groove; septum
**intervertebral:** disk; foramen; ganglion; notch; vein
**intervertebral disk:** injury
**intervillous:** lacuna; space
**interzonal:** mesenchyme
**intestinal:** anastomosis; angina; anthrax; artery; atresia; calculus; capillariasis; digestion; dysepepsia; emphysema; fistula; fluke; follicle; gland; hemorrhage; infantilism; intoxication; juice; lipodystrophy; metaplasia; myiasis; portal; rotation; sand; schistosomiasis; sepsis; steatorrhea; surface; trunk; villus
**intra-arterial:** transfusion
**intra-articular:** cartilage; fracture; ligament
**intra-atrial:** block; conduction
**intrabony (infrabony):** pocket
**intrabronchial:** electrocardiography
**intrabulbar:** fossa
**intracanalicular:** fibroadenoma
**intracapsular:** ankylosis; fracture; ligament
**intracapsular temperomandibular joint:** arthroplasty
**intracardiac:** catheter; lead
**intracardiac pressure:** curve
**intracellular:** canaliculus; digestion; enzyme; fluid; hormone; toxin
**intracerebral:** abscess; hemorrhage
**intrachondral:** joint
**intracoronal:** retainer
**intracranial:** abscess; aneurysm; ganglion; hematoma; hemorrhage; hypotension; pneumatocele; pressure
**intracutaneous:** reaction
**intracystic:** papilloma
**intradermal:** nevus
**intraductal:** carcinoma; papilloma
**intradural:** abscess
**intraembryonic:** mesoderm
**intraepidermal:** carcinoma
**intraepiploic:** hernia
**intraepithelial:** carcinoma; gland
**intrafusal:** fiber
**intrailiac:** hernia
**intrajugular:** process
**intralaminar:** nucleus
**intralobar:** part
**intramedullary:** anesthesia; tractotomy
**intramembranous:** ossification
**intramural:** hematoma; practice; pregnancy
**intranasal:** anesthesia
**intraocular:** fluid; neuritis; pressure; tension
**intraoral:** anesthesia
**intraosseous:** anesthesia; fixation
**intraparietal:** sulcus
**intrapartum:** hemorrhage; period
**intrapelvic:** hernia

**intraperiosteal:** fracture
**intraperitoneal:** pregnancy
**intrapyretic:** amputation
**intraretinal:** space
**intrasegmental:** part; vein
**intraspinal:** anesthesia
**intrathecal:** injection
**intrathyroid:** cartilage
**intratracheal:** anesthesia; intubation
**intrauterine:** amputation; device; fracture; pneumonia
**intrauterine contraceptive:** device
**intravascular:** lymph
**intravenous:** anesthesia; anesthetic; drip
**intravenous regional:** anesthesia
**intraventricular:** block; conduction; hemorrhage
**intravital:** stain; ultraviolet
**intrinsic:** albuminuria; asthma; deflection; dysmenorrhea; factor; fiber; light; reflex; sphincter
**intrinsicoid:** deflection
**introduced:** malaria
**intromittent:** organ
**introspective:** method
**intubation:** tube
**intuitive:** stage
**intumescent:** cataract
**intussusceptive:** growth
**inulin:** clearance
**inundation:** fever
**invaginate:** planula
**invasive:** carcinoma
**inverse:** anaphylaxis; symmetry; syntropy
**inversed jaw-winking:** syndrome
**inversion of:** chromosomes
**invert:** sugar
**inverted:** image; pelvis; reflex; testis
**inverted cone:** bur
**inverted radial:** reflex
**investigatory:** reflex
**investing:** cartilage; tissue
**investment:** cast
**invisible:** differentiation; spectrum
**involuntary:** muscle
**involuntary nervous:** system
**involution:** cyst; form
**involutional:** melancholia; psychosis
**iodate:** reaction; test
**iodide transport:** defect
**iodinated:** albumin; glycerol
**iodine:** cyst; eruption; number; reaction; test
**iodized:** collodion
**iodophil:** granule
**iodotyrosine deiodinase:** defect
**ion-exchange:** resin
**ionic:** medication; ray; strength
**ionization:** chamber
**ionized:** atom
**ipomea:** resin
**ipsilateral:** reflex
**iridial:** part
**iridocorneal:** angle
**iridocorneal mesodermal:** dysgenesis
**Irish:** moss
**Irish moss:** gelatin
**iron:** index; lung
**iron deficiency:** anemia
**iron storage:** disease
**irradiated:** milk

**irreducible:** hernia
**irregular:** astigmatism; gout
**irresistible:** impulse
**irreversible:** colloid; hydrocolloid; reaction; shock
**irritable:** breast; colon; heart; testis
**irritation:** cell
**irruption:** canal
**ischemic:** lumbago; necrosis
**ischemic muscular:** atrophy
**ischiadic:** plexus; spine
**ischial:** bone; bursa; tuberosity
**ischiatic:** hernia; notch
**ischiocapsular:** ligament
**ischiofemoral:** ligament
**ischiopubic:** ramus
**ischiorectal:** abscess; fossa
**island:** disease; fever; flap
**islet:** cell; tissue
**islet cell:** adenoma
**isobaric:** solution
**isobaric spinal:** anesthesia
**isochromic:** anemia
**isocyclic:** compound; ring
**isodiphasic:** complex
**isodynamic:** law
**isoelectric:** line; period; point; zone
**isogeneic:** graft; homograft
**isogenic:** strain
**isogenous:** chondrocyte
**isoionic:** point
**isolated:** dextrocardia
**isolated parietal:** endocarditis
**isolation:** hospital; ward
**isolecithal:** egg; ovum
**isologous:** graft
**isomeric:** function
**isometric:** contraction; interval; period; relaxtion; ruler; scale
**isomorphic:** response
**isomorphous:** gliosis
**isoniazid:** neuropathy
**isoperistaltic:** anastomosis
**isoplastic:** graft
**isoprene:** rule
**isorhythmic:** dissociation
**isoserum:** treatment
**isotonic:** coefficient; contraction
**isotonic sodium chloride:** solution
**isotropic:** disk; lipoid
**isovolume pressure-flow:** curve
**isovolumetric:** relaxation
**isovolumic:** relaxation
**Italian:** leprosy; method; operation
**Itaporanga:** virus
**Itaqui:** virus
**ivory:** exostosis; membrane

## J

**J:** point
**J-sella:** deformity
**jacket:** crown
**jail:** fever
**jake:** paralysis
**jalap:** resin
**Japan:** wax
**Japanese:** disease; schistosomiasis
**Japanese B:** encephalitis
**Japanese B encephalitis:** virus
**Japanese river:** fever
**jargon:** aphasia
**jaw:** bone; jerk; joint; movement; reflex;

repositioning; separation; skeleton
jaw-winking: phenomenon; syndrome
jaw-working: reflex
jejunal: artery; ulcer; vein
jejunogastric: intussusception
jejunoileal: bypass; shunt
jenghol: poisoning
Jericho: boil
jerk: finger; nystagmus
jerky: respiration
jet: injection; injector; nebulizer
jet ejector: pump
JH: virus
jimmy: legs
jitter: legs
Jk: antigen
Job: syndrome
Jobbins: antigen
Jocasta: complex
jock: itch
joint: capsule; cry; evil; ill; mice; sense
Js: antigen
jugal: bone; ligament; point
jugular: arch; bulb; embryocardia; foramen; fossa; ganglion; gland; nerve; notch; plexus; process; pulse; sinus; trunk; tubercle; vein; wall
jugular foramen: syndrome
jugulodigastric: node
jugulo-omohyoid lymph: node
jump: flap; graft
jumped process: complex
jumper: disease
jumping: thrombosis
jumping the: bite
junction: nevus
junctional: complex; cyst; extrasystole
jungle: fever
jungle yellow: fever
Junin: virus
justifiable: abortion
juvenile: angiofibroma: arrhythmia; cataract; cell; chorea; cirrhosis; diabetes; hemangiofibroma; hormone; neutrophil; pattern; pelvis; polyp; retinoschisis; xanthogranuloma
juvenile muscular: atrophy
juvenile rheumatoid: arthritis
juxta-articular: nodule
juxtacortical osteogenic: sarcoma
juxtaglomerular: apparatus; body; cell; complex
juxtarestiform: body

### K

κ-: see kappa
K: antigen; complex; radiation; region; virus
k: antigen
K:A: ratio
kabure: itch
Kaffir: pox
kang: cancer
kangaroo: tendon
kangri: cancer
kangri burn: carcinoma
kappa (κ-): angle; factor; granule; particle
karaya: gum
karyochrome: cell
Katayama: disease; syndrome
edani: disease; fever

keeled: chest
Kelev strain rabies: virus
keloidean: blastomycosis
Kelvin: scale
kennel: cough
kerasin: histiocytosis
keratic: precipitate
keratin: pearl
keratogenous: membrane
keratoid: exanthema
keratose: cuticle
keratosic: cone
kern-plasma relation: theory
ketogenic: diet; hormone; threshold
ketogenic-antiketogenic: ratio
ketogenic corticoids: test
17-ketogenic steroid assay: test
ketone: body
ketosis: threshold
17-ketosteroid assay: test
Kew garden: fever
key: attachment; vein
key-in-lock: maneuver
keyhole: pupil
keyway: attachment
kidney: worm
kilogram: calorie
kinematic: face-bow; viscosity
kineplastic: amputation
kinesiodic: system
kinesthetic: aura; sense
kinetic: ataxia; drive; energy; perimetry; strabismus; system; tremor
king's: evil
kinked: aorta
Kinkiang: fever
kinky: hair
kinky-hair: disease
kinoplasmic: droplet
Kisenya sheep disease: virus
Klieg: conjunctivitis: eye
knee: jerk; joint; phenomenon; reflex
knee-chest: position
knee-elbow: position
knee-jerk: reflex
knife: needle
knife-rest: crystal
knock-: knee
knock-out: drops
knuckle: pad
Kobobera: virus
kokoi: venom
Korean hemorrhagic: fever
kukuruku: disease
Kurungala: ulcer
Kuskokwim: syndrome
Kyasanur forest: disease
Kyasanur forest disease: virus
kyphoscoliotic: pelvis
kyphotic: pelvis

### L

L: dose; form; radiation; unit
L⁺ or L₀: dose
L-phase: variant
lab-: enzyme
labial: arch; bar; embrasure; flange; gingiva; gland; hernia; occlusion; paralysis; part; splint; sulcus; surface; swelling; tubercle; vestibule; vein
labile: current; element; factor
labiogingival: angle; lamina

labiolingual: plane
labioscrotal: fold; swelling
labor: pain; stages (of)
laboratory: diagnosis
labyrinthic: wall
labyrinthine: angiospasm; nystagmus; placenta; reflex; torticollis; vein; vertigo
labrinthine righting: reflex
lacerated: foramen; wound
lacinate: ligament
lacis: cell
lacrimal: artery; bay; bone; calculus; duct; fascia; fistula; fold; fossa; gland; groove; lake; margin; nerve; notch; papilla; process; reflex; sac; vein
lacrimoconchal: suture
lacrimogustatory: reflex
lacrimomaxillary: suture
lactacid oxygen: debt
lactate dehydrogenase: virus
lactated Ringer's: injection; solution
lactation-amenorrhea: syndrome
lacteal: cyst; fistula; vessel
lactic acid: bacillus; fermentation
lactiferous: duct; gland; sinus
lactobacillary: milk
Lactobacillus: factor
lactogenic: factor; hormone
lactose: intolerance
lactose-litmus: agar
lacunar: abscess; amnesia; ligament; tonsilitis
lady: fern
lag: phase
lagophthalmic: keratitis
Lagos bat: virus
laky: blood
lamb: dysentery
lambda: angle
lambdoid: margin; suture
lambing: sickness
lamellar: bone; cataract; exfoliation; ichthyosis; keratoplasty
lamellated: corpuscle
laminar: flow
laminar cortical: necrosis; sclerosis
laminate: induration
laminated: clot; cortex; epithelium; thrombus
lampbrush: chromosome
Lan: antigen
lancet: fluke
land: quarantine; scurvy
Langat: virus
language: game; zone
lanugo: hair
larch: turpentine
lard: worm
lardaceous: degeneration; kidney; liver; spleen
large: artery; muscle; pelvis; vein
large pudendal: lip
large red: kidney
large saphenous: vein
large white: kidney
larval: conjunctivitis; epilepsy; plague; pneumonia; therapy
laryngeal: atresia; chorea; crisis; epilepsy; gland; granuloma; part; pharynx; phthisis; polyp; pouch; reflex; sinus; stridor; syncope; tonsil; vein; ventricle; vertigo

laryngospastic: reflex
laryngotracheal: groove
laser: microscope; photocoagulator
Lassa: virus
late: chlorosis; reaction; rickets; systole
late apical systolic: murmur
late diastolic: murmur
latency: period; phase
latent: allergy; carcinoma; coccidioidomycosis; content; diabetes; empyema;
energy; epilepsy; gout; heat; homosexuality; hyperopia; hyperthyroidism;
jaundice; learning; microbism; nystagmus; period; reflex; schizophrenia;
stage; tetany; typhoid; zone
latent adrenocortical: insufficiency
latent rat: virus
lateral: aberration; abscess; aneurysm;
chain; checkbite; curvature; column;
excursion; hemianopsia; hermaphroditism; illumination; line; lithotomy;
movement; nystagmus; occlusion; vertigo
lateral anatomical structures (specific
lateral structures are listed under the
following): angle; aperture; arch; artery; body; bone; bundle; column; commissure; condyle; cord; fillet; fissure;
fold; fossa; funiculus; ginglymus;
groove; gyrus; horn; incisor; joint;
lake; lamina; layer; ligament; limb;
margin; meniscus; mesoderm; muscle;
nerve; node; nucleus; part; peduncle;
plate; pole; process; recess; region; retinaculum; root; segment; sinus; stria;
sulcus; surface; swelling; tract; tubercle; tuberosity; vein; ventricle; wall
lateral alveolar: abscess
lateral condylar: inclination
lateral ground: bundle
lateral line: system
lateral line sense: organ
lateral lingual: swelling
lateral myocardial: infarction
lateral oblique: roentgenogram
lateral ramus: roentgenogram
lateral recumbent: position
lateral skull: roentgenogram
lateral spinal: sclerosis
lateral sympathetic: line
lateral vaginal wall: smear
lateral ventral: hernia
latex: test
latrine: fly
lattice corneal: dystrophy
latticed: layer
laudable: pus
laughing: disease; gas; sickness
laughter: reflex
laurel: fever
laxative: species
LCAT: deficiency
LCL: body
LCM: virus
L-D: body
LDH: agent
L.E.: body; cell; factor; phenomenon
Le: antigen
lead: anemia; colic; encephalitis; encephalopathy; gout; line; neuropathy;
palsy; paralysis; poisoning; stomatitis
lead-pipe: colon; fracture; rigidity
leapfrog: position

leaping: ill
Lear: complex
learned: drive
learning: set; theory
leather-bottle: stomach
lechuguilla: fever; poisoning
left anatomical structures (specific left
structures are listed under the following): appendage; artery; auricle; crus;
duct; flexure; heart; ligament; lobe;
node; plate; valve; vein; ventricle
left axis: deviation
left dorsoanterior: position
left dorsoposterior: position
left frontoanterior: position
left frontoposterior: position
left occipitoanterior: position
left occipitoposterior: position
left-to-right: shunt
left ventricular: failure
left ventricular ejection: time
leg: phenomenon
legal: dentistry; medicine; psychiatry
length-breadth: index
length-height: index
lengthening: reaction
lens: pit; placode; star; suture; vesicle
lens-induced: uveitis
lenticular: ansa; apophysis; astigmatism; bone; capsule; cataract; colony;
fossa; ganglion; knife; loop; nucleus;
papilla; process; sling; syphilid; vesicle
lenticular progressive: degeneration
lenticulostriate: artery
lentiform: nucleus
Lentulo: plugger
leonine: facies
leopard: fundus; retina
leper: juice
lepidic: tumor
Lepore: thalassemia
lepra: cell
lepromatous: leprosy
lepromin: reaction
leprosy: bacillus
leprous: neuropathy
leptomeningeal: fibrosis
leptospiral: jaundice
lesser: circulation
lesser anatomical structures (specific
lesser structures are listed under the
following): artery; bone; cartilage; circle; cul-de-sac; foramen; fossa; gland;
horn; muscle; nerve; notch; omentum;
pancreas; sac; spine; trochanter; tubercle; tuberosity; wing
lethal: coefficient; dose; dwarfism; factor; gene
lethal midline: granuloma
lethality: rate
lethargic: hypnosis
letter: blindness
leucine: hypoglycemia
leukemic: leukemia; myelosis; reticuloendotheliosis; reticulosis; retinitis;
retinopathy
leukemic hyperplastic: gingivitis
leukemoid: reaction
leukocyte: cream; inclusion
leukocytic: sarcoma
leukocytosis-promoting: factor
leukoerythroblastic: anemia

leukopenic: factor; index; leukemia;
myelosis
leukoplakic: vulvitis
levator: cushion; hernia; swelling
Levay: antigen
levoatrio-cardinal: vein
Lf, L$_f$: dose
libido: theory
lichenoid: dermatosis; eczema
lid: reflex
lienomyelogenous: leukemia
lienophrenic: ligament
lienteric: diarrhea
life: cycle; instinct
ligature: sign
light: adaptation; bath; cell; diet; difference; green; kaolin; metal; reflex;
sense; threshold; treatment; unit
light-adapted: eye
light liquid: petrolatum
light-touch: palpation
light wire: appliance
ligneous: conjunctivitis; struma; thyroiditis
ligneous pelvic: cellulitis
Lilliputian: hallucination
lily: rash
limb: bud; lead
limb-girdle muscular: dystrophy
limb-kinetic: apraxia
limber: neck
limbic: lobe; system
liminal: stimulus
limit: dextrin; dextrinase, dextrinosis
limiting: angle; layer; membrane; sulcus
line: angle, test
linear: acceleration; accelerator; amputation; atrophy; craniectomy; fracture;
phonocardiograph; vision
linear skull: fracture
lingual: aponeurosis; arch; artery; bar;
bone; crypt; flange; follicle; gingiva;
goiter; gyrus; lobe; nerve; occlusion;
papilla; plate; plexus; quinsy; rest;
splint; surface; titubation; tonsil; trophoneurosis; vein
lingual lymph: node
lingual tongue: flap
linguocervical: ridge
linguogingival: angle; fissure; groove;
ridge
linguo-occlusal: angle
linin: network
lining: cell
lion-jaw bone-holding: forceps
lip: line; reflex; sulcus
lip and leg: ulceration
lipid: granulomatosis; hystiocytosis;
pneumonia; proteinosis
lipoatrophic: diabetes
lipoblastic: lipoma
lipogenous: diabetes
lipoid: dermatoarthritis; granuloma;
granulomatosis; nephrosis; pneumonia; theory
lipomatous: polyp
lipomelanic: reticulosis
lipophagic: granuloma
lipophagic intestinal: granulomatosis
lipoprotein: polymorphism
lipotropic: factor
liquefaction: degeneration
liquefactive: necrosis

liquefied: phenol
liquid: air; extract; glucose; paraffin; petrolatum; pitch
liquid human: serum
lissive: agent
Listeria: meningitis
literal: agraphia
lithiasis: conjunctivitis
lithotomy: position
litigious: paranoia
litmus: paper
little: ACTH; finger
littoral: cell
live: vaccine
liveborn: infant
livedoid: dermatitis
liver: acinus; bud; flap; fluke; palm; rot; spot; starch
liver cell: carcinoma
liver filtrate: factor
liver Lactobacillus casei: factor
liver residue: factor
living: anatomy
L-L: factor
Lo, L₀: dose
lobar: pneumonia; sclerosis
lobster-claw: deformity; hand
lobular: carcinoma; glomerulonephritis; pneumonia
local: anaphylaxis; anemia; anesthesia; anesthetic; asphyxia; bloodletting; chorea; death; disease; glomerulonephritis; immunity; pyrexia; reaction; sign; stimulant; symptom; syncope; tetanus; tic
local anesthetic: reaction
local excitatory: state
localization: agnosia
localized: amnesia; osteitis; peritonitis
localized nodular: tenosynovitis
localizing: electrode; symptom
lock-: finger; jaw
locked: bite; facet; knee
locomotor: ataxia
loco weed: disease
loculated: empyema
loculation: syndrome
logarithmic: phase; phonocardiograph
logistic: curve
loin: disease
Lombardy: leprosy
London: force
Lone Star: tick
long: axis; bone; chain; pulse; process; root; sight; vinculum
long abductor: muscle
long-acting thyroid: stimulator
long adductor: muscle
long buccal: nerve
long ciliary: nerve
long cone: technique
long extensor: muscle
long incubation: hepatitis
long palmar: muscle
long peroneal: muscle
long plantar: ligament
long posterior ciliary: artery
long saphenous: nerve; vein
long subscapular: nerve
long thoracic: artery; nerve; vein
longitudinal: aberration; arch; arc; canal; dissociation; duct; fissure; fold; fracture; layer; lie; ligament; method;

sinus; study; sulcus
loose: body; cartilage; fracture; skin
lop: ear
lordosis: reflex
lordotic: albuminuria; pelvis
louping: ill
louping-ill: virus
louse: fly
louse-borne: typhus
low: convex; delirium; fever; wine
low calorie: diet
low fat: diet
low flow: principle
low forceps: delivery
low frequency: transduction
low output: failure
low potassium: diet
low salt: syndrome
low sodium: diet; syndrome
low spinal: anesthesia
low tone: deafness
low tone loss of: hearing
lower: extremity; eyelid; jaw; lip; lobe
lower abdominal periosteal: reflex
lower lateral cutaneous: nerve
lower motor: neuron
lower nephron: nephrosis
lower nodal: extrasystole
lower respiratory tract: smear
lower slope of: ridge
lower uterine: segment
lowest lumbar: artery
lowest splanchnic: nerve
lowest thyroid: artery
Lr, L_r: dose
Lu: antigen
lubricating: cream
lucid: interval
luetic: mask
lug: rest
Lukuni: virus
lumbar: appendicitis; artery; enlargement; flexure; ganglion; hernia; nerve; part; plexus; puncture; region; rheumatism; rib; triangle; trunk; vein; vertebra
lumbar interspinal: muscle
lumbar lymph: node
lumbar puncture: needle
lumbar quadrate: muscle
lumbar rotator: muscle
lumbar splanchnic: nerve
lumberman's: itch
Lumbo: virus
lumbocostal: ligament
lumbocostoabdominal: triangle
lumbodorsal: fascia
lumboinguinal: nerve
lumbosacral: angle; joint; plexus; trunk
luminous: flux; intensity; ophthalmoscope
lumpy: jaw
lumpy skin: disease
lumpy skin disease: virus
lunar: caustic
lunate: bone; fissure; sulcus; surface
lung: abscess; bud; fluke; reflex; unit
lunger: disease
Lunyo: virus
lupoid: hepatitis; sycosis; ulcer
lupus: nephritis
lupus erythematosus: see L.E.
luteal: cell; phase

luteal phase: defect; deficiency
lutein: cell
luteinizing: hormone; principle
luteinizing hormone-releasing: factor
luteotropic: hormone
luting: agent
luxus: breathing; heart
lying-down: dysentery
lymph: capillary; cell; circulation; corpuscle; embolism; follicle; gland; node; nodule; sac; scrotum; sinus; space; varix; vessel
lymph node permeability: factor
lymphadenoid: goiter
lymphatic: angina; cachexia; corpuscle; duct; dyscrasia; edema; fistula; follicle; infantilism; leukemia; plexus; pseudoleukemia; reaction; sarcoma; sinus; stroma; system; tissue; tuberculosis; valvule; vessel
lymphatic dissemination: theory
lymphedematous: keratoderma
lymphoblastic: leukemia
lymphocyte: transformation
lymphocytic: choriomeningitis; leukemia; leukemoid reaction; leukocytosis; leukopenia; series
lymphocytic choriomeningitis: virus
lymphocytotoxic: antibody
lymphogenous: embolism
lymphogranuloma venereum: antigen; virus
lymphoid: cell; corpuscle; hemoblast; leukemia; leukosis; polyp; ring; series; tissue; tuberculosis
lymphosarcoma cell: leukemia
lymphosarcomatous: leukemia
lymphostatic: verrucosis
lyophilic: colloid
lyophobic: colloid
lyotropic: series
lysogenic: bacterium; conversion; induction
lytic: cocktail

## M

M: antigen; band; line; protein
machinery: murmur
Machupo: virus
macrocytic: anemia; hyperchromia
macrocytic achylic: anemia
macrofollicular: adenoma
macroglia: cell
macro-Kjeldahl: method
macromolecular: chemistry
macrophage migration inhibition: test
macroscopic: anatomy; sphincter
macular: area; artery; atrophy; degeneration; erythema; leprosy; retinopathy; syphilid; venule
maculofibrinous: stomatitis
maculopapular: erythroderma
mad: itch; staggers
Madrid: virus
Madura: boil; foot
maedi: virus
magenta: tongue
maggot: therapy
magical: thinking
magnet: operation; reaction; reflex
magnetic: attraction; field; implant
main sensory: nucleus

median retruded: relation
mediastinal: emphysema; part; space; vein
mediate: agglutination; auscultation; contagion; percussion; therapeutics; transfusion
medical: anatomy; aneurysm; care; chemistry; diathermy; ethics; examiner; jurisprudence; ophthalmoscopy; pathology; selection; tetanus; treatment
medical record: linkage
medicinal: chemistry; eruption; rash; soap; treatment
Medina: worm
mediocolic: sphincter
mediodorsal: nucleus
mediopubic: reflex
mediotarsal: amputation
Mediterranean: anemia; fever; squill
Mediterranean exanthematous: fever
Mediterranean-hemoglobin E: disease
medium: artery; vein
medullary: artery; bone; cancer; carcinoma; cavity; center; chemoreceptor; cone; cord; groove; layer; leukemia; membrane; plate; pyramidotomy; ray; sarcoma; sheath; space; substance; tenia; tube
medullary sponge: kidney
medullated nerve: fiber
Medusa: head
meerschaum: probe
megacystic: syndrome
megakaryocytic: leukemia
megaloblastic: ahemia
megalocytic: anemia
meiotic: division; phase
melamine: resin
melancholic: temperament
melanocyte-stimulating: hormone
melanoflocculation: test
melanophore-expanding: principle
melanotic: cancer; carcinoma; freckle; pigment; progonoma; sarcoma; whitlow
melanotic neuroectodermal: tumor
Melao: virus
melon-seed: body
melting: point; temperature
membrane: bone; potential
membranoproliferative: glomerulonephritis
membranous: ampulla; cataract; cochlea; conjunctivitis; dysmenorrhea; labyrinth; laryngitis; layer; neurocranium; ossification; part; pharyngitis; rhinitis; septum; stomatitis; urethra; viscerocranium; wall
memory: loop; span; trace
Mengo: encephalitis; virus
meningeal: hernia; plexus; vein
meningitic: respiration; streak
meningocerebral: cicatrix
meningococcal: meningitis
meningotyphoid: fever
meningovascular: syphilis
meniscofemoral: ligament
meniscus: lens; sign
menopausal: syndrome
menstrual: colic; cycle; edema; intoxication; leukorrhea; molimen; sclerosis
ntal: aberration; age; agraphia; al-

lergy; apparatus; artery; assimilation; canal; chronometry; deficiency; diplopia; disease; fog; foramen; health; hospital; hygiene; illness; image; impairment; impression; nerve; point; process; region; retardation; scotoma; spine; torticollis; tubercle; vaginismus
mentoanterior: position
mentolabial: furrow
mentoposterior: position
mephitic: gas
mercurial: cachexia; line; manometer; stomatitis; tremor
mercury: arc; poisoning
meridional: aberration; cleavage; fiber
meristic: variation
mermaid: deformity
meroblastic: cleavage
merocrine: gland
mesameboid: cell
mesangial: cell
mesatipellic: pelvis
mesencephalic: flexure; nucleus; tegmentum; tract
mesenchymal: cell; epithelium; hyloma; tissue
mesenteric: gland; hernia; vein
mesenteric artery: occlusion
mesentericoparietal: fossa; recess
mesh: graft
mesial: angle; displacement; drifting; occlusion; surface
mesiobuccal: angle
meso: compound
mesoblastic: nephroma; segment; sensibility
mesocaval: shunt
mesoglia: cell
mesomelic: dwarfism
mesometanephric: carcinoma
mesometric: pregnancy
mesonephric: duct; fold; rest; ridge; tissue; tubule
mesothelial: cell; hyloma
mesovarian: margin
messenger: ribonucleic acid
metabolic: acidosis; alkalosis; craniopathy; pool
metabolized vitamin D: milk
metacarpal: index; ligament; vein
metacarpohypothenar: reflex
metacarpophalangeal: articulation; joint
metacarpothenar: reflex
metacentric: chromosome
metachromatic: body; granule; leukodystrophy; stain
metafacial: angle
metahypophysial: diabetes
metal: base
metal fume: fever
metal insert: tooth
metallic: rale; tremor
metameric nervous: system
metanephric: bud; cap; diverticulum; duct; tubule
metanephrogenic: tissue
metaphysial: dysplasia; dysostosis
metaplastic: anemia; malacia; ossification
metapneumonic: pleurisy
metastatic: abscess; calcification; carcinoma; mumps; ophthalmia; pneu-

monia; retinitis
metastatic carcinoid: syndrome
metatarsal: artery; ligament; reflex
metatarsophalangeal: articulation; joint
metatropic: dwarfism
meter: angle
methacrylate: resin
methionine-activating: enzyme
methodical: chorea
3-methoxy-4-hydroxymandelic acid: test
methylated: spirit
methylene blue: test
metopic: point; suture
metrial: gland
metric: ophthalmoscopy; system
metroperitoneal: fistula
metrotrophic: test
Mexican: scammony; tea
Mexican hat: cell; corpuscle
Mi²: antigen
mianeh: disease; fever
micro-Astrup: method
microbial: genetics; persistence; vitamin
microbiallergic: reaction
microbiotic: diet
microcephalic: idiocy
micrococcal: nuclease
microcrystalline: cellulose
microcystic: disease
microcytic: anemia
microdrepanocytic: anemia
microelectric: wave
microfilarial: sheath
microfollicular: adenoma; goiter
microglia: cell
micrognathia with peromelia: syndrome
microinvasive: carcinoma
micro-Kjeldahl: method
microlecithal: egg
micromelic: dwarf
micromyeloblastic: leukemia
microprecipitation: test
microscopic: anatomy; field; hematuria; section; sphincter
microwave: therapy
micturition: reflex; syncope
midaxillary: line
midbrain: tegmentum; vesicle
midclavicular: line
Middleburg: virus
mid-diastolic: murmur
middle: pain
middle anatomical structures (specific middle structures are listed under the following): artery; bone; cell; convolution; fascia; finger; fold; fossa; ganglion; gyrus; joint; ligament; lobe; nerve; node; peduncle; plexus; sulcus; trunk; vein
middle lobe: syndrome
midforceps: delivery
midgastric transverse: sphincter
midget bipolar: cell
midland: disease
midline: myelotomy
midnodal: extrasystole
midsagittal: plane
midsigmoid: sphincter
midtarsal: joint

mignon: lamp
migraine: headache
migrating: abscess; tooth
migration: theory
migration inhibition: test
migration-inhibitory: factor
migratory: ophthalmia; pneumonia
mika: operation
mild: gallsickness
miliary: abscess; aneurysm; embolism; fever; gland; tuberculosis
miliary papular: syphilid
milieu: therapy
military: medicine; neurosis
milk: abscess; anemia; colic; corpuscle; crust; cyst; duct; factor; fever; gland; leg; line; pox; ridge; scall; sickness; spot; sugar; tetter; tooth; treatment
milk-alkali: syndrome
milk-ejection: reflex
milk-ring: test
milker's: node; nodule; spasm
milker's nodes: virus
milky: ascites; urine
mill: fever
mill wheel: murmur
milled-in: curve; path
miller's: asthma
millet: seed
millinormal: solution
mimetic: chorea; paralysis
mimic: convulsion; gene; spasm; tic
Minamata: disease
mind: blindness; pain
miner's: anemia; asthma; cramp; disease; elbow; lung; nystagmus; phthisis
mineral: water; wax
Minerva: jacket
miniature: stomach
miniature scarlet: fever
minimal: air; dose
minimal alveolar: concentration
minimal infecting: dose
minimum: temperature
Minnesota multiphasic personality inventory: test
minor: agglutinin; amputation; connector; hypnosis; hysteria; operation; surgery; tranquilizer
minor duodenal: papilla
minor sublingual: duct
minus: lens; strand
minute: output; volume
miostagmin: reaction
mirror: haploscope; image; speech
mirror-image: cell
missed: abortion; labor; period
missense: mutation
mist: bacillus
mite: typhus
mitochondrial: matrix; myopathy; sheath
mitogenetic: radiation
mitotic: cycle; division; figure; period
mitral: area; atresia; cell; click; commissurotomy; facies; gradient; incompetence; insufficiency; murmur; orifice; regurgitation; stenosis; tap; valve
mixed: agglutination; aphasia; astigmatism; beat; chancre; gland; glioma; glyceride; hyperlipemia; infection; leukemia; nerve; paralysis; thrombus; tumor

mixed agglutination: reaction; test
mixed cell: leukemia
mixed expired: gas
mixed lymphocyte: culture
mixed lymphocyte culture: reaction; test
mixed mesodermal: tumor
Miyagawa: body
mks: unit
MLD, mld: dose
$MLD_{50}$, $mld_{50}$: dose
MM: virus
M'Naghten: rule
mnemic: hypothesis; theory
MNSs: antigen
mobile: spasm
modal: alteration
model: game
modeling: composition; compound; plastic
moderate: hypothermia
moderator: band
modified: milk; smallpox; tetanus
modified radical: hysterectomy
Modoc: virus
modulation transfer: function
mogen: clamp
moist: gangrene; papule; rale; tetter; wart
molal: solution
molar: absorptivity; behavior; concentration; gland; pregnancy; solution; tooth
molar absorbancy: index
molar absorption: coefficient
molar extinction: coefficient
mold: guide
mole: fraction
molecular: anemia; behavior; biology; disease; dispersion; distillation; formula; heat; layer; movement; pathology; rotation; sieve; weight
molecular dispersed: solution
molecular dissociation: theory
molluscum: body; conjunctivitis; corpuscle
molluscum contagiosum: virus
molting: hormone
Monday morning: sickness
mongolian: idiocy; idiot; macula; spot
moniliasis: pneumonia
moniliform: hair
monkey antianemia: factor
monkey B: virus
monkeypox: virus
monoamniotic: twins
monobasic: phosphate
monobromated: camphor
monochorial: twins
monochorionic diamniotic: placenta
monochorionic monoamniotic: placenta
monochromatic: ray
monocrotic: pulse
monocular: diplopia; heterochromia; strabismus
monocytic: angina; leukemia; leukemoid reaction; leukocytosis; leukopenia
monocytoid: cell
monohydric: alcohol; phosphate
monoleptic: fever
monomolecular: layer; reaction
monophasic: complex
monophyletic: theory

monopolar: cautery
monorecidive: chancre
monostotic fibrous: dysplasia
monovalent: antiserum
monovular: twins
monozygotic: twins
Montana chronic progressive: pneumonia
monthly: flux; nurse; period
moon: blindness; face
moor: bath
moral: ataxia; imbecile; insanity; treatment
morbid: anatomy; fear; impulse; obesity; thirst
morbidity: rate
morning: diarrhea; paralysis; ptosis; sickness; vomiting
morning glory: anomaly
morphogenetic: movement
morphogenic: hormone
morphologic: element
Morse: finger
mortality: rate
mortise: joint
mosaic: achondroplasia; fungus; inheritance; wart
mosaicism of: chromosome; gene
mosquito: forceps
mossed: bark
mossy: cell; fiber; foot
moth: patch
moth-eaten: alopecia
mother: cell; colony; cyst; fixation; liquor; star; surrogate; wreath; yaw
mother of: vinegar
mother superior: complex
motile: leukocyte
motion: sickness
motor: abreaction; agraphia; aphasia; apraxia; area; ataxia; cell; cortex; decussation; endplate; fiber; image; impersistence; nerve; neuron; nucleus; paralysis; plate; point; root; unit; zone
motor neuron: disease
motor speech: center
mottled: enamel; tooth
mountain: anemia; balm; fever; sickness
mounting: medium
mouse: cancer; encephalomyelitis; leprosy; pinworm; poliomyelitis; pox; septicemia; unit
mouse antialopecia: factor
mouse encephalomyelitis: virus
mouse hepatitis: virus
mouse leukemia: virus
mouse mammary tumor: virus
mouse parotid tumor: virus
mouse poliomyelitis: virus
mouse thymic: virus
mouse-tooth: forceps
mousepox: virus
mousetail: pulse
mouth: breathing; mirror; rehabilitation; speculum; wash
mouth-to-mouth: respiration
movable: heart; joint; kidney; pulse; spleen
Mozart: ear
M-P: virus
MR: test
MRD, mrd: dose
MS-1: agent

MS-2: agent
Mu (Mi²): antigen
mucilaginous: gland
mucinogen: granule
mucinoid: degeneration
mucinous: carcinoma; plaque
muciparous: gland
mucoalbuminous: cell
mucobuccal: fold
mucocutaneous: junction; leishmaniasis; muscle
mucoepidermoid: carcinoma; tumor
mucoid: adenoma; colony; degeneration
mucoid medial: degeneration
mucoperiosteal: flap
mucosal: disease; fold; graft; layer; tunic
mucosal disease: virus
mucosal relief: roentgenography
mucoserous: cell
mucous: cast; cell; colic; colitis; cyst;
diarrhea; enteritis; gland; membrane;
ophthalmia; patch; plug; polyp;
plaque; rale; sheath
mucous connective: tissue
mucous neck: cell
mud: fever
muffle: furnace
mulberry: calculus; molar; ovary; rash;
spot
mule-spinner's: cancer
multiangular: bone
multiaxial: joint
multicuspid (molar): tooth
multifocal: osteitis
multiform: layer
multilamellar: body
multilocular: cyst; fat
multilocular adipose: tissue
multilocular hydatid: cyst
multinodular: goiter
multipartial: serum; vaccine
multiple: amputation; embolism; endocrinopathy; exostosis; fibroma; fission;
fracture; gangrene; myeloma; myelomatosis; myositis; neuritis; neurofibroma; parasitism; personality; pregnancy; sclerosis; serositis; stain; vision
multiple ego: state
multiple epiphysial: dysplasia
multiple idiopathic hemorrhagic: sarcoma
multiple intestinal: polyposis
multiple mucosal neuroma: syndrome
multiple puncture tuberculin: test
multiplicative: division; growth
multipolar: cell; mitosis; neuron
multivalent: vaccine
multivariate: study
multivesicular: body
mummification: necrosis
mummified: pulp
mumps: meningoencephalitis; vaccine;
virus
mumps sensitivity: test
mumps skin test: antigen
mumu: fever
Munchausen: syndrome
mung bean: nuclease
municipal: hospital
mural: aneurysm; cell; endocarditis;
pregnancy; thrombosis; thrombus
murine: leprosy; typhus
murine sarcoma: virus

Murrary Valley: encephalitis
Murray Valley encephalitis: virus
Murutucu: virus
muscle: bundle, column; curve; epithelium; fascicle; hemoglobin; plasma;
plate; relaxant; repositioning; serum;
sound; spasm; spindle
muscle-tendon: attachment; junction
muscular: anesthesia; artery; asthenopia; atrophy; dystrophy; fibril; hyperesthesia; incompetence; insufficiency;
movement; murmur; process; rheumatism; sense; substance; system; tissue;
triangle; trophoneurosis; tunic
muscular subaortic: stenosis
musculocutaneous: amputation; nerve
musculophrenic: artery; vein
musculospiral: groove; nerve; paralysis
musculotubal: canal
mushroom: poisoning
mushroom-worker's: lung
music: blindness
musical: agraphia; murmur
musician's: cramp
muskeag: moss
mustard: gas
mutagenic: agent
mutase: effect
mutton-fat keratic: precipitate
MVE: virus
myasthenic: facies; reaction
mycoplasma: pneumonia
mycotic: abscess; aneurysm; endophthalmitis; keratitis; stomatitis
mydriatic: rigidity
myelin: body; figure; sheath
myelinated nerve: fiber
myelinic: degeneration
myeloblastic: leukemia; leukosis
myelocytic: crisis; leukemia; leukemoid
reaction; leukosis
myelogenic, myelogenous: leukemia;
pseudoleukemia; sarcoma
myeloid: cell; leukemia; metaplasia; reticulosis; sarcoma; series; tissue
myelomonocytic: leukemia
myelopathic: anemia
myelophthisic: anemia
myeloplastic: malacia
myeloproliferative: syndrome
myenteric: plexus; reflex
mylohyoid: fossa; groove; line; nerve;
ridge
mylopharyngeal: part
myocardial: infarction; ischemia; insufficiency
myoclonus: epilepsy
myoelastic: theory
myoepicardial: mantle
myoepithelial: cell
myofacial pain-dysfunction: syndrome
myogenic: paralysis; theory
myoid: cell
myomatous: polyp
myometrial arcuate: artery
myometrial radial: artery
myoneural: blockade; junction
myopathic: atrophy; facies; scoliosis
myophosphorylase deficiency: glycogenosis
myopic: astigmatism; choroidopathy;
conus; crescent
myotatic: contraction; irritability; reflex

myotonic: dystrophy
myotubular: myopathy
myovascular: sphincter
myovenous: sphincter
myxedema: heart; voice
myxedematous: infantilism
myxoid: cystoma; degeneration
myxomatosis: virus
myxomatous: degeneration
myxomembranous: colitis

### N

nacreous: ichthyosis
nail: extension; fold; horn; matrix; plate;
pulse; skin; wall
nail-patella: syndrome
Nairobi: disease
Nairobi sheep disease: virus
nanoid: enamel
nape: nevus
napkin: rash
narcoleptic: tetrad
narcotic: blockade; hunger
narrow angle: glaucoma
nasal: bone; calculus; capsule; catarrh;
cavity; crest; duct; feeding; foramen;
ganglion; gland; glioma; height; hemorrhage; index; margin; muscle; myiasis; nerve; notch; part; pharynx; pit;
point; placode; polyp; process; reflex;
region; sac; septum; spine; surface;
valve; venule
nasal venous: arch
Nasik: vibrio
nasion-postcondylar: plane
nasobasilar: line
nasobregmatic: arc
nasociliary: nerve
nasofrontal: vein
nasolabial: groove
nasolacrimal: canal; duct
nasomandibular: fixation
nasomental: reflex
nasooccipital: arc
nasopalatine: groove; nerve
nasopharyngeal: groove; leishmaniasis
nasotracheal: intubation
Natal: aloe
natal: cleft
natiform: skull
native: albumin; protein
natriuretic: hormone
natural: antibody; dentition; hemolysin;
immunity; mutation; selection
nature-nurture: issue
Nauheim: bath; treatment
navel: ill
navicular: abdomen; bone; disease; fossa
navicular articular: surface
ND: virus
near: point; reflex; sight
near point of: convergence
nebulous: urine
neck: reflex; sign; syndrome
necrogenic: wart
necrogranulomatous: keratitis
necrosis: bacillus
necrotic: angina; cirrhosis; cyst; inflammation; rhinitis
necrotic infectious: conjunctivitis
necrotizing: angiitis; arteriolitis; encephalitis; papillitis

**necrotizing ulcerative:** gingivitis
**needle:** bath; biopsy; culture
**needle point:** tracing
**negation:** delusion (of)
**negative:** accommodation; anemia; catalyst; chronotropism; convergence; electrode; electrotaxis; feedback; meniscus; phase; pole; politzerization; pressure; reinforcer; scotoma; stain; taxis; thermotaxis; transference; valence
**negatively:** bathmotropic; dromotropic; inotropic
**Negishi:** virus
**negligible:** glycosuria
**nemaline:** myopathy
**neokinetic:** system
**neonatal:** anemia; apoplexy; hepatitis; isoerythrolysis; tetany
**neoplastic:** arachnoiditis; meningitis
**neotype:** culture; strain
**nephric:** duct
**nephritic:** colic; diet; syndrome
**nephrogenic:** cord; diabetes; tissue
**nephronic:** loop
**nephrotic:** syndrome
**nephrotomic:** cavity
**Neptune's:** girdle
**Nepuyo:** virus
**nerve:** blocking; cell; ceptor; conduction; deafness; decompression; ending; energy; fascicle; fiber; force; ganglion; graft; implantation; pain; papilla; plexus; root; suture; tract; trunk
**nerve block:** anesthesia
**nerve cell:** body
**nerve conduction:** velocity
**nerve growth:** factor
**nerve growth factor:** antiserum
**nerve-point:** massage
**nervous:** asthenopia; asthma; bladder; breakdown; dyspepsia; exhaustion; force; glycosuria; indigestion; prostration; system; temperament; tissue; urine
**net:** flux; knot
**nettle:** rash
**nettling:** hair
**neural:** arch; axis; canal; crest; cyst; deafness; fold; ganglion; groove; layer; plate; segment; spine; tube
**neuralgic:** amyotrophy
**neurasthenic:** asthenopia
**neurenteric:** canal
**neurilemma:** cell
**neuritic:** atrophy
**neurobiotactic:** movement
**neurocentral:** joint; suture; synchondrosis
**neurochronaxic:** theory
**neurocirculatory:** asthenia
**neurocutaneous:** melanosis; syndrome
**neuroectodermal:** junction
**neuroendocrine:** cell
**neuroepithelial:** cell; layer
**neurofibrillary:** degeneration
**neurogenic:** bladder; fracture; theory
**neuroglia:** cell
**neurohumoral:** secretion; transmition
**neurolemma:** cell
**neuroleptic:** agent
**neuromast:** organ
**neuromuscular:** cell; hypertension; junction; spindle; system

**neuroparalytic:** keratitis; ophthalmia
**neuropathic:** albuminuria; arthropathy; diathesis
**neuropsychologic:** disorder
**neurosecretory:** cell; substance
**neurosomatic:** junction
**neurotendinous:** organ; spindle
**neurotic:** gangrene; manifestation
**neurotonic:** reaction
**neurotrophic:** atrophy
**neurotropic:** attraction; virus
**neutral:** element; fat; occlusion; oxide; point; reaction; stain; zone
**neutral axis of straight:** beam
**neutralization:** test
**neutralizing:** antibody
**neutropenic:** angina
**neutrophil:** granule
**neutrophilic:** leukemia; leukocyte; leukocytosis; leukopenia
**nevocytic malignant:** melanoma
**nevoid:** amentia; cyst; elephantiasis; hypertrichosis
**new:** growth; tuberculin
**New Hampshire:** rule
**New World:** hookworm; leishmaniasis
**new yellow:** enzyme
**Newcastle:** disease
**Newcastle disease:** virus
**nickel:** dermatitis
**nicotinic acid:** maculopathy; unit
**nicotinic acid amide:** unit
**nictitating:** membrane; spasm
**nictitating membrane:** test
**night:** blindness; cry; hospital; palsy; sight; sweat; vision
**nihilistic:** delusion
**nine mile:** fever
**ninhydrin:** reaction
**ninth cranial:** nerve
**ninth-day:** erythema
**nipple:** line; shield
**nirvana:** principle
**nitritoid:** reaction
**nitrogen:** balance; cycle; equivalent; mustard; narcosis
**nitrogenous:** equilibrium
**nitroid:** shock
**nitroprusside:** test
**noble:** cell; element; gas; metal
**nociceptive:** reflex
**nocifensor:** reflex
**nocturnal:** amblyopia; diarrhea; epilepsy; myoclonus; vertigo
**nodal:** bigeminy; bradycardia; escape; extrasystole; fever; point; rhythm; tachycardia; tissue
**nodding:** spasm
**nodose:** ganglion; rheumatism
**nodular:** amyloidosis; arteriosclerosis; disease; fasciitis; glomerulosclerosis; headache; hidradenoma; leprosy; mesoneuritis; panencephalitis; sclerosis; syphilid; vasculitis
**nodular nonsuppurative:** panniculitis
**nodular subepidermal:** fibrosis
**noduloulcerative:** syphilis
**noetic:** anxiety
**nomenclatural:** type
**nominal:** aphasia
**nomothetic:** approach
**nonabsorbable surgical:** suture
**nonan:** malaria

**nonanatomic:** tooth
**nonbacterial regional:** lymphadenitis
**nonbacterial thrombotic:** endocarditis
**nonbacterial verrucous:** endocarditis
**nonchromaffin:** paraganglioma
**noncohesive:** gold
**noncommunicating:** hydrocephalus
**noncompetitive:** inhibition
**noncomplementary:** role
**nondeciduous:** placenta
**nondepolarizing neuromuscular:** agent
**nondirective:** psychotherapy
**nonessential:** amino acid
**nonfenestrated:** forceps
**nonfilament polymorphonuclear:** leukocyte
**nongranular:** leukocyte
**nonhomologous:** chromosome
**nonimmune:** agglutination
**noninfiltrating lobular:** carcinoma
**noninflammatory:** edema
**nonketotic:** hyperglycemia
**nonlamellar:** bone
**nonlipid:** histiocytosis
**nonmedullated:** fiber
**nonmotile:** leukocyte
**non-Newtonian:** fluid
**nonobstructive:** jaundice
**nonossifying:** fibroma
**nonovulational:** menstruation
**nonparasitic:** sycosis
**nonparticipant:** observer
**nonpedunculated:** hydatid
**nonpenetrating:** wound
**nonphasic sinus:** arrhythmia
**nonpolar:** compound; solvent
**nonprecipitable:** antibody
**nonprecipitating:** antibody
**nonprotein:** nitrogen
**nonrebreathing:** anesthesia; mask; valve
**nonrenal:** azotemia
**nonsense:** mutation; syndrome; triplet
**nonseptate:** mycelium
**nonsexual:** generation
**nonspecific:** anergy; cholinesterase; immunity; protein; system; therapy; urethritis
**nonthrombocytopenic:** purpura
**nontoxic:** goiter
**nontropical:** sprue
**nonverbal:** communication
**nonvital:** pulp; tooth
**noogenic:** neurosis
**Nordhausen:** sulfuric acid
**normal:** animal; antibody; antithrombin; antitoxin; axis; bite; concentration; distribution; dwarf; hearing; occlusion; opsonin; ovariotomy; phosphate; serum; solution; tartrate; temperature; toxin
**normal cholesteremic:** xanthomatosis
**normal horse:** serum
**normal human:** plasma; serum
**normal human serum:** albumin
**normally posed:** tooth
**normochromic:** anemia
**normocytic:** anemia
**normoglycemic:** glycosuria
**normokalemic periodic:** paralysis
**normospermatogenic:** sterility
**North American:** blastomycosis
**North Queensland tick:** fever; typhus

Norway: itch
Norwegian: scabies
nose: fly
nose-bridge-lid: reflex
nose-eye: reflex
nosocomial: gangrene
notched: tooth
note: blindness
no-threshold: concept
notochordal: canal; plate; process; sheath; vertebrate
notoedric: mange
NPH: insulin
Ntaya: virus
nuchal: fascia; ligament; plane; tubercle
nuclear: atom; bag; cataract; chemistry; combustion; energy; envelope; fusion; hyaloplasm; jaundice; layer; magneton; medicine; membrane; ophthalmoplegia; pore; reaction; ribonucleic acid; sap; spindle; stain
nuclear-cytoplasmic: ratio
nuclear inclusion: body
nuclear magnetic: resonance
nucleate: endonuclease
nucleinic: base
nucleolar: chromosome; organizer; satellite; zone
nucleoplasmic: index
nucleoside diphosphate: sugar
nucleotide: pair
numerical: aperture; hypertrophy
nummular: sputum; syphilid
nun's: murmur
nurse: cell
nutmeg: liver
nutrient: agar; artery; canal; enema; foramen; vessel
nutrition: nucleus
nutritional: amblyopia; anemia; cirrhosis; edema; encephalomalacia; hemosiderosis; polyneuropathy
nutritive: equilibrium; ratio
nymphocaruncular: sulcus
nymphohymeneal: sulcus
nystagmus: test
NZB: mouse

## O

O: agglutinin; antigen; colony
oat: cell
oat cell: carcinoma
obeliar: area
obesity: index
object: blindness; choice; constancy; glass; libido; relationship
objective: optometer; psychology; sensation; sign; symptom
obligate: aerobe; anaerobe; parasite
oblique: amputation; bandage; bundle; cord; diameter; fiber; fissure; fracture; illumination; lie; line; muscle; part; ridge; sinus; vein
oblique arytenoid: muscle
oblique facial: cleft
oblique lateral jaw: roentgenogram
oblique popliteal: ligament
obliterative: arachnoiditis; bronchitis
obsessive: behavior
obsessive-compulsive: neurosis
obstacle: sense
obstetric, obstetrical: binder; conju-

gate; forceps; hand; paralysis; position
obstructive: appendicitis; dysmenorrhea; jaundice; murmur; thrombus
obturating: embolus
obturator: artery; canal; crest; fascia; foramen; groove; hernia; membrane; nerve; tubercle; vein
occipital: angle; artery; belly; bone; fissure; fontanel; groove; gyrus; horn; lobe; margin; neuralgia; neuritis; operculum; plane; plexus; point; pole; region; sinus; somite; triangle; vein
occipital emissary: vein
occipital lymph: node
occipitoanterior: position
occipitoaxial: ligament
occipitofrontal: fasciculus; muscle
occipitoiliac: position
occipitolevoanterior: position
occipitolevoposterior: position
occipitomastoid: suture
occipitopontine: tract
occipitoposterior: position
occipitotemporal: sulcus
occipitothalamic: radiation
occluding: frame; ligature; paper; relation
occluding centric relation: record
occlusal: adjustment; analysis; balance; cavity; clearance; correction; curvature; disharmony; embrasure; equilibration; force; form; harmony; path; pattern; pivot; plane; position; pressure; radiograph; rim; scheme; surface; system; trauma; wear
occlusal rest: bar
occlusal vertical: dimension
occlusion: rim
occlusion of: pupil
occlusive: dressing; ileus; meningitis
occult: bleeding; blood; carcinoma; fracture; jaundice
occupation: neurosis; spasm
occupational: deafness; dermatitis; disease; therapy
ochre: mutant
ochronotic: arthritis
ocular: albinism; ataxia; bobbing; cone; crisis; cup; flutter; humor; hypertelorism; lens; lymphomatosis; micrometer; muscle; myiasis; myopathy; nystagmus; ochronosis; onchocerciasis; paralysis; pemphigus; prosthesis; sparganosis; scoliosis; torticollis; vertigo; vesicle
ocular-mucous membrane: syndrome
oculoauriculovertebral: dysplasia
oculobuccogenital: syndrome
oculocardiac: reflex
oculocephalic: reflex
oculocephalogyric: reflex
oculocerebrorenal: syndrome
oculocutaneous: syndrome
oculodentodigital: dysplasia; syndrome
oculodermal: melanosis
oculoencephalic: angiomatosis
oculogyric: crisis
oculomotor: nerve; nucleus; response; system
oculopharyngeal: reflex; syndrome
oculovertebral: dysplasia; syndrome
oculovestibulo-auditory: syndrome
odd: chromosome

odontoblastic: layer
odontogenic: cyst
odontoid: ligament; process; vertebra
odoriferous: gland
Oedipal: neurosis; period; phase
Oedipus: complex
OFD: syndrome
official: formula
17-OH-corticoids: test
oil: cyst; embolism; embolus; gland; immersion; pneumonia; red; tumor; vaccine
oily: granuloma
old: sight
Old World: hookworm; leishmaniasis
old yellow: enzyme
olecranon: fossa; process; reflex
olefiant: gas
olfactory: anesthesia; angle; area; brain; bulb; bundle; cortex; epithelium; esthesioneurocytoma; foramen; gland; glomerulus; groove; hallucination; membrane; mucosa; nerve; neuroblastoma; neuroepithelioma; organ; peduncle; pit; placode; pyramid; region; root; stria; sulcus; tract; trigone; tubercle
olfactory receptor: cell
oligemic: shock
oligodendroglia: cell
olivary: body; eminence
olivocerebellar: tract
olivocochlear: bundle
olivopontocerebellar: atrophy; degeneration
olivospinal: tract
Olympian: forehead
omasal: groove
omega: oxidation
omega-oxidation: theory
omental: abscess; bursa; enterocleisis; sac; tuber
omoclavicular: triangle
omphaloangiopagus: twins
omphalomesenteric: artery; duct
Omsk hemorrhagic: fever
Omsk hemorrhagic fever: virus
oncofetal: antigen
oncorna-: virus
oncotic: pressure
one-child: sterility
one-horned: uterus
onion: body
onium: compound
O'nyong-nyong: virus
oophoritic: cyst
opacifying: gallstone
opaline: patch
opaque: microscope
open: biopsy; bite; drainage; fracture; hospital; joint; pneumothorax; reduction; tubercusis; wound
open angle: glaucoma
open chain: compound
open chest: massage
open circuit: method
open drop: anesthesia
open heart: surgery
open skull: fracture
opening: axis; contraction; movement; snap
opera-glass: hand
operant: behavior; conditioning

operating: microscope; table
operational: definition
operative: dentistry; myxedema
operator: gene
opercular: fold
ophryospinal: angle
ophthalmic: artery; hyperthyroidism; migraine; nerve; ointment; plexus; reaction; solution; test; vein
ophthalmoplegic: migraine
ophthalmovascular: choke
opium: addiction; habit
opossum: encephalitis
opportunistic: pathogen
opposer: muscle
opsonic: index; technique; therapy
optic: agnosia; agraphia; anesthesia; angle; aphasia; axis; canal; capsule; center; chiasm; cup; decussation; disk; foramen; gland; groove; keratoplasty; layer; nerve; neuritis; papilla; part; placode; radiation; recess; stalk; tract; vesicle
optic nerve: hypoplasia
optical: aberration; activity; allachesthesia; antipode; density; illusion; image; iridectomy; isomerism; maser; pachymeter; rotation; test
optical-corneal pressure: ophthalmodynamometer
optical righting: reflex
optical rotatory: dispersion
opticofacial: reflex
opticokinetic: nystagmus
optimum: dose; pH; temperature
optokinetic: nystagmus
oral: cavity; coitus; contraceptive; fissure; hygiene; membrane; part; pathology; pharynx; phase; physiotherapy; plate; primacy; pyoderma; region; smear; stereotypy; surgeon; surgery; tooth
oral-facial-digital: syndrome
orbicular: bone; ligament; muscle; process; zone
orbicularis: phenomenon
orbicularis oculi: reflex
orbicularis pupillary: reflex
orbital: abscess; apex; axis; decompression; eminence; fascia; gyrus; height; index; lamina; layer; muscle; nerve; ophthalmoplegia; part; periostitis; plane; plate; process; region; sulcus; surface; tubercle; width
orbital space: laboratory
orbitofrontal: cortex
orbitosphenoid: cartilage
orcin: test
orcinol: reaction; test
orf: virus
organ-specific: antigen
organic: acid; catalyst; chemistry; compound; contracture; delirium; disease; evolution; headache; murmur; oxacid; pain; phosphate; principle; stricture; vertigo
organification: defect
organized: pneumonia; virus
organoid: tumor
orgastic: impotence
Oriboca: virus
Oriental: boil; button; fluke; ringworm; schistosomiasis; sore

orienting: reflex; response
orificial: surgery
ornithine: cycle
ornithosis: virus
oroantral: fistula
orodigitofacial: dysostosis; syndrome
orofacial: fistula
oronasal: fistula; membrane
oropharyngeal: membrane
Oropouche: virus
orotracheal: intubation
orphan: virus
orthodontic: therapy
orthodromic: conduction
orthogenic: evolution
orthograde: degeneration
orthomolecular: therapy
orthopaedic: surgery
orthostatic: albuminuria; hypopiesis; hypotension; proteinuria
orthotopic: graft
oscillating: vision
osmotic: diuresis; nephrosis; pressure; shock
Ossa: virus
osseous: ampulla; cell; labyrinth; lacuna; polyp; rheumatism; tissue
osseous hydatid: cyst
osseous spiral: lamina
ossicular: chain
ossific: center
ossification: center
osteochondrogenic: cell
osteocollagenous: fiber
osteogenetic: fiber; layer
osteogenic: cell; sarcoma; tissue
osteoid: osteoma; sarcoma; tissue
osteomalacic: pelvis
osteomyelofibrotic: syndrome
osteopathic: physician; scoliosis
osteoplastic: amputation; craniotomy; necrotomy
osteosclerotic: anemia
ostial: sphincter
Ot: antigen
Othello: syndrome
otic: abscess; barotrauma; capsule; ganglion; placode; vesicle
otitic: hydrocephalus; meningitis
otodectic: mange
otolithic: membrane
otomandibular: dysostosis; syndrome
otopalatodigital: syndrome
otopharyngeal: tube
out of: breath; phase
oval: amputation; area; corpuscle; fasciculus; fossa; window
ovale: malaria
ovale tertian: malaria
ovalocytic: anemia
ovarian: amenorrhea; artery; colic; cycle; cyst; dysmenorrhea; follicle; fossa; hormone; ligament; plexus; pregnancy; tube; varicocele; vein
ovarian ascorbic acid depletion: test
ovarian hyperemia: test
ovarioabdominal: pregnancy
overeating: disease
overflow: wave
overhanging: filling
overlay: denture
overproduction: theory

overriding: aorta
overt: homosexuality
ovigerous: cord
ovine: mastitis
ovine virus: abortion
ovular: membrane; transmigration
ovulational: sclerosis
ovulocyclic: porphyria
own: control
ox: bots
oxalic acid: diathesis
Oxford: unit
oxidase: reaction
oxidation-reduction: indicator; potential; reaction; system
oxidative: phosphorylation
oxidized: cellulose
oxygen: capacity; consumption; debt; deficit; electrode; poisoning; tent; therapy; toxicity
oxygen deprivation: therapy
oxygen utilization: coefficient
oxygenated: hemoglobin
oxyntic: cell; gland
oxyphil: adenoma; cell; granule
oxyphilic: leukocyte

### P

P: antigen; cell; enzyme; factor; wave
P-A: interval
P and P: test
pacemaker: failure; output; sensitivity
Pacheco's parrot disease: virus
pachydermoperiostosis: syndrome
Pacific: tick
pacing: catheter
packed cell: volume
packing: process
Pahvant Valley: fever; plague
pain: principle; reaction
pain-pleasure: principle
painful: heel; point
painful-bruising: syndrome
painless: jaundice
painter's: colic
paired: allosome; associate; beat
pajaroella: tick
palatal: abscess; bar; index; myoclonus; nystagmus; process; reflex; seal; shelf; triangle
palate: hook; myograph
palatine: aponeurosis; bone; groove; gland; papilla; process; ridge; surface; tonsil; vein
palatoethmoidal: suture
palatoglossal: arch
palatoglossus: muscle
palatomaxillary: index; suture
palatopharyngeal: arch; muscle
palatouvularis: muscle
palatovaginal: canal; groove
pale: bark; hypertension; infarct; thrombus
paleokinetic: system
paleostriatal: syndrome
palindromic: encephalopathy
palisade: layer; worm
pallesthetic: sensibility
palliative: treatment
pallidal: syndrome
palm: grasp; wax
palm-chin: reflex

palmar: fascia; fibromatosis; ligament; reflex; space; surface; syphilid
palmar carpometacarpal: ligament
palmar digital: artery; vein
palmar interosseous: artery
palmar metacarpal: artery; vein
palmar radiocarpal: ligament
palmar ulnocarpal: ligament
palmate: fold
palmin, palmitin: test
palomental: reflex
palpable: kidney; rale
palpatory: albuminuria; percussion
palpebral: artery; fissure; gland; part
paludal: fever
pampiniform: body; plexus
Panama: fever
pancervical: smear
pancreatic: abscess; amylase; calculus; colic; deoxyribonuclease; diabetes; digestion; diverticulum; dornase; duct; encephalopathy; hormone; infantilism; island; islet; juice; lipase; lithiasis; notch; plexus; ribonuclease; sphincter; steatorrhea; vein
pancreatic hyperglycemic: hormone
pancreaticuduodenal: transplantation; vein
pancreaticoenteric: recess
pancreaticosplenic lymph: node
pancreatogenous: diarrhea
pancreozymin-secretin: test
pandemic: disease
panleukopenia: virus
pannicular: hernia
panniculus carnosus: muscle
panoptic: stain
panoramic: roentgenogram
panoramic rotating: machine
panphobic: melancholia
pansystolic: murmur
pantaloon: embolus
pantoscopic: spectacles
pantothenic acid: unit
pantropic: virus
paper: chromatography; plate
papillary: adenocarcinoma; adenoma; carcinoma; cystadenoma; duct; ectasia; foramen; hidradenoma; layer; muscle; process; stasis; trachoma; tumor
papillary cystic: adenoma
papillary muscle: dysfunction; syndrome
papilloma: virus
papillotonic: pseudotabes
papova-: virus
pappataci: fever
pappataci fever: virus
papular: fever; mucinosis; scrofuloderma; syphilid; tuberculid; urticaria
papular stomatitis: virus
papulonecrotic: tuberculid
papulosquamous: tuberculid
papyraceous: plate; scar
paraaortic: body
parabasal: body; filament
parabiotic: phenomenon
paraboloid: condenser
paracaseous: lymphadenitis
paracentral: fissure; lobule; nucleus; scotoma
paracervical block: anesthesia
parachordal: cartilage; plate

parachute mitral: valve
paracinar: emphysema
paracoccidioidal: granuloma
paracolic: recess
paracolon: bacillus
paracyclic: ovulation
paracystic: pouch
paradental: cyst
paradoxical: contraction; embolism; embolus; incontinence; metastasis; pulse; pupil; reflex; respiration; sleep
paradoxical diaphragm: phenomenon
paradoxical extensor: reflex
paradoxical flexor: reflex
paradoxical patellar: reflex
paradoxical pupillary: phenomenon; reaction; reflex
paradoxical triceps: reflex
paraduodenal: fold; fossa; recess
paradysentery: bacillus
paraesophageal: hernia
paraffin: cancer; prosthetic; tumor; wax
parafollicular: cell
parafrenal: abscess
paraganglionic: cell
paragenital: tubule
paraglenoid: groove; sulcus
Paraguay: tea
parahippocampal: gyrus
parainfluenza: virus
parajejunal: fossa
parallax: method; test
parallel: attachment; ray
paralobular: emphysema
paraluteal: cell
paralysis: tick
paralytic: abasia; chorea; ectropion; idiocy; ileus; miosis; mydriasis; myoglobinuria; rabies; scoliosis
paralyzing: vertigo
paramastoid: process
paramedian: incision
paramesonephric: duct
parametric: abscess
parametritic: abscess
paramyxo-: virus
paranasal: sinus
paranephric: abscess; body
paraneural: infiltration
paranoid: personality; schizophrenia
paranosic: gain
paranuclear: body
paraperitoneal: hernia; nephrectomy
parapharyngeal: space
paraphysial: cyst
paraplegic: idiocy
pararectal: fossa; pouch
parasaccular: hernia
paraseptal: cartilage; emphysema
parasinoidal: sinus
parasite-host: ecosystem
parasitic: cyst; disease; granuloma; hemoptysis; leiomyoma; melanoderma; monster; otitis; sycosis; thyroiditis; twin
parasol: insertion
parasternal: hernia; line
parasternal lymph: node
parastriate: area; cortex
parasympathetic: ganglion; nerve; part
parasympathetic nervous: system
parataxic: distortion
paratenic: host

paraterminal: body; gyrus
parathyroid: gland; hormone; insufficiency; osteosis; struma; tetany; unit
parathyroprival: tetany
parathyrotropic: hormone
paratracheal: node
paratuberculous: lymphadenitis
paratyphoid: bacillus; fever
paraumbilical: vein
paraurethral: duct; gland
paravaccinia: virus
paravaginal: hysterectomy
paraventricular: nucleus
paravertebral: anesthesia; ganglion; triangle
paravesical: fossa; pouch
paraxial: mesoderm
parchment: heart; induration; skin
parenchymatous: cell; degeneration; goiter; hemorrhage; inflammation; keratitis; mastitis; nephritis; neuritis; pneumonia; tonsillitis
parent: cell; cyst
parental: generation; rejection
parenteral: absorption; hyperalimentation; therapy
parenteric: fever
paretic: impotence; melancholia
parietal: abscess; angle; bone; cell; eminence; eye; fistula; foramen; hernia; layer; lobe; margin; notch; plate; region; thrombus; tuber; wall
parietal emissary: vein
parietomastoid: suture
parietooccipital: fissure; sulcus
parietopontine: tract
Paris: line
paroccipital: process
parolfactory: area
paroophoritic: cyst
parotid: abscess; bubo; duct; fascia; gland; notch; papilla; plexus; recess; vein
parotid lymph: node
parotideomasseteric: region
paroxysmal: albuminuria; disease; sleep; tachycardia
paroxysmal cerebral: dysrhythmia
paroxysmal nocturnal: dyspnea; hemoglobinuria
paroxysmal trepidant: abasia
parrot: disease; fever; jaw; mouth; virus
parrot-beak: nail
parry: fracture
partial: agglutinin; aneuploidy; anodontia; antigen; denture; enterocele; epilepsy; group; infantilism; insanity; pressure; symblepharon; volume
partial adrenocortical: insufficiency
partial color: blindness
partial denture: impression; retention
participant: observer
particulate: inheritance
partition: chromatography; coefficient
parturient: canal; paralysis; paresis
parvilocular: cyst
passed assistant: surgeon
passional: attitute
passive: agglutination; algolagnia; anaphylaxis; clot; congestion; duction; hemagglutination; hyperemia; immunity; immunization; incontinence; interval; learning; medium; movement;

prophylaxis; transference; tremor; vasoconstriction; vasodilation
**passive-aggressive:** behavior; personality
**passive cutaneous:** anaphylaxis
**pastern:** bone
**pastil:** radiometer
**pastoral:** counseling
**patch:** test
**patchy:** amnesia
**patellar:** ligament; network; reflex; surface
**patellar-tendon:** reflex
**patello-adductor:** reflex
**patent:** ductus; medicine
**path of:** insertion
**pathematic:** aphasia
**pathetic:** nerve
**pathogenic:** occlusion
**pathognomonic:** symptom
**pathologic:** absorption; amenorrhea; amputation; anatomy; diagnosis; glycosuria; myopia; physiology; rigidity; sphincter
**pathologic retraction:** ring
**Patois:** virus
**pavement:** epithelium
**paving-stone:** nevus
**PBI:** test
**peak:** magnitude
**pear-shaped:** area
**pearl:** cyst; disease; moss; tumor
**pearl-worker's:** disease
**pearly:** tubercle
**peccant:** humor
**pecking:** order
**pecten:** band
**pectinate:** fiber; ligament; line; muscle; zone
**pectineal:** ligament; line; muscle
**pectiniform:** septum
**pectoral:** fascia; gland; nerve; reflex; ridge; species; vein
**pedal:** bone; system
**pedicle:** flap; graft
**peduncular:** ansa; loop
**pedunculated:** hydatid; polyp
**peg-and-socket:** joint
**pegged:** tooth
**pegtop:** tooth
**peliosis:** hepatitis
**pellagra-preventing:** factor
**pellet:** implantation
**pellucid:** zone
**pelvic:** abscess; brim; canal; cavity; cellulitis; diaphragm; exenteration; ganglion; girdle; hematocele; index; inlet; kidney; limb; outlet; part; peritonitis; plane; plexus; pole; presentation; promontory; spot; surface; version
**pelvic inflammatory:** disease
**pelvic splanchnic:** nerve
**pelvirectal:** achalasia; sphincter
**pelvivertebral:** angle
**pelvofemoral muscular:** dystrophy
**pemphigoid:** syphilid
**pen:** grasp
**pencil:** tenderness
**pendular:** movement; nystagmus
**pendulous:** abdomen; heart; palate
**pendulum:** rhythm
**penetrating:** ulcer; wound
**penile:** reflex; urethra

**penis:** bone; envy; spine; thorn
**pennate:** muscle
**penoscrotal:** hypospadias
**pension:** neurosis
**Pentec:** vaporizer
**pep:** pill
**pepsin:** unit
**peptic:** cell; digestion; esophagitis; gland; ulcer
**peptide:** bond
**peptonized:** iron
**peracute:** mania
**perambulating:** ulcer
**percept:** analysis
**perceptive:** deafness
**perceptual:** expansion
**percussion:** sound; wave
**percutaneous:** cholangiography
**perfect:** stage
**perforated:** space; ulcer
**perforating:** artery; fiber; ulcer; vein; wound
**performance:** test
**perfusion:** cannula
**perhydrase:** milk
**perialveolar:** wiring
**parianal odoriferous:** gland
**periapical:** abscess; curettage; roentgenogram; tissue
**periappendiceal:** abscess
**periarterial:** pad; plexus; sympathectomy
**periarticular:** abscess
**pericanalicular:** fibroadenoma
**pericapillary:** cell
**pericardiacophrenic:** artery; vein
**pericardial:** cavity; decompression; fremitus; knock; murmur; poudrage; reflex; rub; vein; villus
**pericardial friction:** sound
**pericardioperitoneal:** canal
**pericardiopleural:** fold; membrane
**pericemental:** abscess; attachment
**perichondral:** bone
**perichoroid:** space
**periclaustral:** lamina
**pericolic membrane:** syndrome
**periconchal:** sulcus
**pericoronal:** abscess; flap
**pericorpuscular:** synapse
**peridental:** membrane
**peridontal:** atrophy
**peridural:** anesthesia
**peri-infarction:** block
**perilimbal suction:** cup
**perilymphatic:** duct; space
**perimuscular:** fibrosis
**perineal:** artery; body; flexure; hernia; lithotomy; membrane; muscle; nerve; region; section; space; urethrotomy
**perineovaginal:** fistula
**perinephric:** abscess
**perineuronal:** satellite
**perinuclear:** cataract; space
**periodic:** abdominalgia; arthralgia; disease; edema; insanity; law; neutropenia; ophthalmia; paralysis; peritonitis; system
**periodic acid-Schiff:** stain
**periodic migrainous:** neuralgia
**periodontal:** abscess; anesthesia; ligament; membrane; pocket; probe
**periodontal membrane:** fiber

**perioplic:** band
**periorbital:** membrane
**periosteal:** bone; elevator; ganglion; graft; implantation; reflex
**periosteoplastic:** amputation
**periotic:** bone; cartilage
**peripheral:** aneurysm; cataract; chemoreceptor; glare; iridectomy; resistance; scotoma; seal; tabes; vision
**peripheral nervous:** system
**periportal:** space
**perirectal:** abscess
**perirenal:** fascia; insufflation
**periscopic:** lens; meniscus
**perisinusoidal:** space
**peristatic:** hyperemia
**peristriate:** area; cortex
**peritarsal:** network
**perithelial:** cell
**peritoneal:** button; cavity; fossa; transfusion; villus
**peritonsillar:** abscess
**peritracheal:** gland
**periureteral:** abscess
**periurethral:** abscess
**periventricular:** fiber
**perivisceral:** cavity
**perivitelline:** space
**permanent:** cartilage; filling; stricture; tooth
**permeability:** theory; vitamin
**perna:** disease
**pernicious:** anemia; malaria; vomiting
**pernicious anemia type:** metarubricyte; prorubricyte; rubriblast
**Peromyscus:** virus
**peroneal:** artery; phenomenon; vein
**peroneal communicating:** nerve
**peroneal muscular:** atrophy
**peroxidase:** reaction
**perpendicular:** fasciculus; plate
**perpetually growing:** tooth
**persecution:** complex
**Persian:** tick
**Persian relapsing:** fever
**persistent:** cloaca; tremor; truncus (arteriosus)
**persistent atrioventricular:** canal
**persistent hyperplastic primary:** vitreous
**persistent penile:** erection
**persistently growing:** tooth
**personal:** equation; motivation
**personal growth:** laboratory
**personality:** disorder; formation; integration; inventory; profile; test
**perspiratory:** gland
**pertrochanteric:** fracture
**pertussis:** vaccine
**pertussis immune:** globulin
**Peruvian:** wart
**perverted:** appetite
**pessary:** cell; corpuscle
**petechial:** angioma; fever; hemorrhage
**petit:** mal
**petit mal:** epilepsy
**petrolatum:** gauze
**petrooccipital:** joint
**petrosal:** bone; fossa; ganglion; sinus; vein
**petrosquamous:** fissure; suture
**petrotympanic:** fissure
**petrous:** bone; pyramid

PGSR: audiometry
pH: scale
phacoanaphylactic: uveitis
phacolytic: glaucoma
phagedenic: ulcer
phagocytic: index
phalangeal: cell; joint
phallic: phase; tubercle
phantom: aneurysm; corpuscle; limb; pregnancy; tumor
phantom limb: pain
pharaonic: circumcision
pharmaceutical: chemistry
pharyngeal: anesthesia; arch; bursa; canal; fistula; gland; groove; hypophysis; isthmus; membrane; opening; pituitary; plexus; pouch; reflex; space; tonsil; tubercle; vein
pharyngobasilar: fascia
pharyngobranchial: duct
pharyngoconjunctival: fever
pharyngoconjunctival fever: virus
pharyngoepiglottic: fold
pharyngoesophageal: cushion; diverticulum
pharyngomaxillary: space
pharyngonasal: cavity
pharyngopalatine: arch
pharyngotympanic: groove; tube
phase: microscope; rule
phasic: reflex
phasic sinus: arrhythmia
PHC: syndrome
pheasant-hunter's: toe
phenol: coefficient
phenolphthalein: agar
phenolsulfonphthalein: test
phenoltetrachlorphthalein: test
phenotypic: mixing
phentolamine: test
phenylalanyl: chain
phenylpyruvic: amentia
phenylthiocarbamoyl: peptide; protein
pheochrome: cell
phi: phenomenon
Philadelphia: chromosome; cocktail
philanthropic: hospital
philosopher's: stone
phlebotomus: fever
phlebotomus fever: virus
phlegmatic: temperament
phlegmonous: abscess; cellulitis; enteritis; erysipelas; gastritis; mastitis; ulcer
phlogiston: theory
phlorizin, phloridzin: diabetes; glycosuria
phloroglucin-HCl: test
phlyctenular: conjunctivitis; keratitis; ophthalmia; pannus
phocomelic: dwarf
phonemic: regression
phonic: spasm
phosphatase: unit
phosphate: tetany
phosphatic: diabetes
phosphorescent: sweat
phosphoroclastic: cleavage; reaction
phosphorylase: phosphatase
phosphorylated: hesperidin
phosphureted: hydrogen
phossy: jaw
photechic: effect

photic: driving; stimulation
photoallergic: sensitivity
photochromic: lens
photodynamic: sensitization
photoelectric: effect; nystagmography
photogenic: epilepsy
photomultiplier: tube
photon: density
photopic: adaptation; eye; vision
photoreactivating: enzyme
photosensor: oculography
photostress: test
phototoxic: sensitivity
phrenic: avulsion; ganglion; nerve; node; phenomenon; plexus; vein; wave
phrenic pressure: test
phrenicocolic: ligament
phrenicocostal: sinus
phrenicosplenic: ligament
phrenogastric: ligament
phrenopericardial: angle
phrenosplenic: ligament
phrygian: cap
phthalein: test
phthinoid: chest
physaliphorous: cell
physical: age; allergy; anthropology; diagnosis; elasticity; fitness; half-life; medicine; sign; therapist; therapy
physiologic, physiological: age; albuminuria; amenorrhea; anatomy; anemia; antidote; chemistry; congestion; cup; drive; dwarf; elasticity; equilibrium; excavation; hypertrophy; icterus; incompatibility; jaundice; leukocytosis; occlusion; respiration; saline; sclerosis; scotoma; sphincter; unit
physiologic dead: space
physiologic rest: position
physiologic retraction: ring
physiologic salt: solution
physiologically balanced: occlusion
pial: funnel
pial-glial: membrane
pianist's: cramp
Pickwickian: syndrome
picorna-: virus
piebald: skin
pig: skin
pigeon: breast; tick; toe
pigeon's: milk
pigeon-breeder's: disease
pigment: cell; epitheliopathy; epithelium; induration
pigmentary: cirrhosis; glaucoma; retinopathy; syphilid
pigmented: epithelium; epulis; layer
pigmented keratic: precipitate
pigmented purpuric lichenoid: dermatosis
pigmented villonodular: synovitis
pilar: cyst
piliferous: cyst
pillar: cell
piloid: astrocytoma; gliosis
pilomotor: fiber; reflex
pilonidal: cyst; fistula; sinus
pilonidal cyst: abscess
pilous: gland
pilular: mass
pin: amalgam; bone; implant
pincer nail: syndrome
pinch: graft

pineal: body; cell; cyst; eye; gland; habenula; recess; stalk
pineapple: test
ping-pong: bone; fracture; mechanism
pinhole: pupil
pink: disease; eye
pinocytotic: vesicle
pipe: bone
pipe-smoker's: cancer
pipe-stem: artery
piqûre: diabetes
piriform, pyriform: area; cortex; fossa; muscle; opening; recess; sinus
pisiform: bone
pisohamate: ligament
pisometacarpal: ligament
pisotriquetral: joint
pisouunciform: ligament
pisouncinate: ligament
pistol-shot femoral: sound
piston: pulse
pit: cavity
pitch: poisoning; wart
pitch-worker's: cancer
pithecoid: idiot; theory
pitting: edema
pituitary: adamantinoma; adiposity; basophilia; basophilism; cachexia; diverticulum; dwarfism; eunuch; fossa; gigantism; gland; infantilism; membrane; myxedema; nanism; struma
pituitary gonadotropic: hormone
pituitary growth: hormone
pituitary stalk: section
pivot: joint
Pixuna: virus
P-J: interval
place: theory
placenta: protein
placental: barrier; circulation; dystocia; hormone; membrane; plasmodium; polyp; presentation; septum; sign; souffle; thrombosis
placental dysfunction: syndrome
placental growth: hormone
placental parasitic: twin
placental stage of: labor
plague: bacillus; pneumonia; vaccine
plane: joint; suture
planoconcave: lens
planoconvex: lens
plant: agglutinin; antitoxin; dermatitis; hormone; pathology; ribonuclease; sterol; toxin; virus
plantar: arch; cushion; fascia; fibromatosis; flexion; ligament; muscle; reflex; space; surface; syphilid; wart
plantar calcaneocuboid: ligament
plantar calcaneonavicular: ligament
plantar digital: vein
plantar metastarsal: artery; vein
plantar muscle: reflex
plantar quadrate: muscle
plasma: cell; layer; membrane; protein; stain; therapy
plasma accelerator: globulin
plasma cell: hepatitis; leukemia; mastitis; myeloma
plasma iodoprotein: disorder
plasma labile: factor
plasma protein: fraction
plasma thromboplastin: factor
plasmacrit: test

plasmatic: stain
plasmic: stain
plasmin prothrombins conversion: factor
plasmocytic: leukemoid reaction
plasmodial: trophoblast
plaster: bandage; splint
plaster of Paris: disease
plastic: anatomy; base; bronchitis; corpuscle; cyclitis; filling; induration; iritis; lymph; motor; operation; pleurisy; surgery; tooth
plate: thrombosis
plateau: pulse
platelet: cofactor; factor; thrombosis
platelet tissue: factor
platinum: foil
platypellic: pelvis
platypelloid: pelvis
play: therapy
pleasure: curve; principle
pleomorphic: adenoma
plethysmographic: goggle
pleural: cavity; epilepsy; fluid; fremitus; pneumonia; poudrage; pressure; recess; ring; shock; sinus; space; villus
pleuritic: pneumonia; rub
pleurodynia: virus
pleuroesophageal: line; muscle
pleuropericardial: canal; hiatus; membrane; murmur
pleuroperitoneal: canal; cavity; fold; hiatus; membrane
pleuropneumonia-like: organism
plexiform: layer; neurofibroma; neuroma
plugging: instrument
plural: pregnancy
pluriglandular: adenomatosis
pluripotent: cell
plus: lens; strand
PMA: index
pneocardiac: reflex
pneopneic: reflex
pneumatic: bone; cabinet; space; tonometer
pneumatoenteric: recess
pneumococcal: pneumonia
pneumococcus: polysaccharide; ulcer
pneumoencephalitis: virus
pneumoenteric: recess
pneumogastric: nerve
pneumogenic: osteoarthropathy
pneumonia: virus
pneumonic: plague
pneumotaxic: localization
PNP: syndrome
P/O: ratio
podalic: extraction; version
podophyllum: resin
point: angle; mutation
point system: test types
pointed: condyloma; wart
poker: back; spine
polar: anemia; body; cataract; cell; compound; coordinate; globule; hypogenesis; plate; presentation; ring; solvent; star; zone
polarized: light
polarizing: microscope
pole: ligation
polio-: virus
poliomyelitis: vaccine; virus

poliomyelitis immune: globulin
poliovirus: vaccine
polishing: brush
polka: fever
poll: evil
pollen: antigen; coryza; extract
polyamine-methylene: resin
polyaxial: joint
polycarboxylate: cement
polychromatic: cell
polychromatophil: cell
polycystic: disease; kidney; ovary
polycystic ovary: syndrome
polydystrophic: dwarfism
polyleptic: fever
polymer fume: fever
polymorphic light: eruption
polymorphocytic: leukemia
polymorphonuclear: leukocyte
polymorphous: layer; perversion
polyneuritic: psychosis
polyoma: virus
polyostotic fibrous: dysplasia
polyovular ovarian: follicle
polyphyletic: theory
polypoid: adenoma; degeneration
polypous: endocarditis; gastritis
polytropous: enteronitis
polytene: chromosome
polyuria: test
polyvalent: allergy; antiserum; serum; vaccine
polyzygotic: twin
Pomona: fever
pond: fracture
ponderal: index
Pongola: virus
pontile: apoplexy
pontine: angle; cistern; flexure; hemorrhage; nucleus
pontine angle: tumor
pontine gray: matter
pontocerebellar: cisternography; recess
pooled: serum
poor man's: gout
popliteal: artery; fascia; fossa; groove; line; muscle; notch; plane; plexus; space; surface; vein
popliteal communicating: nerve
popliteal lymph: node
porcelain: inlay
porcine: parakeratosis
porcine encephalomyelitis: virus
porcupine: skin
pork: tapeworm; worm
portacaval: shunt
portal: canal; circulation; cirrhosis; hypertension; lobule; pyemia; system; vein
portal-systemic: encephalopathy
portasystemic vascular: shunt
port-wine: mark; stain
position: agnosia; effect
positional: hypotension
positive: accommodation; anergy; catalyst; chronotropism; column; convergence; electrode; electrotaxis; feedback; feeling; meniscus; phase; pole; ray; reinforcer; scotoma; taxis; thermotaxis; transference; valence
positive end-expiratory: pressure
positive-negative pressure: breathing
positive-pressure: breathing; respira-

tion
positively: bathmotropic; dromotropic; inotropic
post: dam; implant
post-: crown
postadrenalectomy: syndrome
postage stamp: graft
postanal: gut
postbasic: stare
postcapillary: venule
postcardiotomy: syndrome
postcentral: area; fissure; gyrus; sulcus
postcholecystectomy: syndrome
postcloacal: gut
postcommissurotomy: syndrome
postconcussion: neurosis; syndrome
postcostal: anastomosis
post-dam: area
postdiphtheritic: paralysis
posterior: asynclitism; discission; embryotoxon; occlusion; rhinoscopy; rhizotomy; rachischisis; scleritis; sclerosis; sclerotomy; staphyloma; urethritis; uveitis; vaginismus
posterior anatomical structures (specific posterior structures are listed under the following): arch; area; artery; border; bundle; canal; cell; chamber; column; commissure; convolution; cord; crest; cusp; extremity; fauces; fissure; fontanel; foramen; fossa; funiculus; groove; gyrus; horn; layer; ligament; limb; lip; lobe; lobule; margin; membrane; muscle; naris; nerve; node; notch; nucleus; part; pillar; pituitary; plexus; pole; pyramid; recess; region; ring; root; segment; spine; substance; sulcus; surface; tooth; tract; triangle; tubercle; valve; vein; velum; wall
posterior inferior cerebellar artery: syndrome
posterior myocardial: infarction
posterior palatal: seal
posterior palatal seal: area
posterior spinal: sclerosis
posterior tooth: form
posterolateral: fissure; fontanel; groove; sulcus
postextrasystolic: pause; wave
postganglionic motor: neuron
postgastrectomy: syndrome
postglenoid: foramen
posthemiplegic: athetosis; chorea
posthemorrhagic: anemia
posthepatitic: cirrhosis
posthippocampal: fissure
posthypnotic: amnesia; psychosis; suggestion
posticus: palsy; paralysis
postinfectious: bradycardia; psychosis
post-kala azar dermal: leishmanoid
postlingual: fissure
postlunate: fissure
postmeiotic: phase
postmeningitic: hydrocephalus
postmenopausal: atrophy
postmortem: clot; delivery; examination; pustule; rigidity; thrombus; tubercle; wart
postmyocardial infarction: syndrome
postnasal: drip
postnatal: circulation; life

postnecrotic: cirrhosis
postnormal: occlusion
postoperative: parotiditis; pneumonia; tetany
postoperative cerebral: anemia
postoperative pressure: alopecia
postoral: arch
postpalatal: seal
postpalatal seal: area
postpartum: amenorrhea; cardiomyopathy; estrus; hemorrhage; hypertension; psychosis; tetanus
postpartum pituitary necrosis: syndrome
postparturient: hemoglobinuria
postperfusion: lung
postpericardiotomy: syndrome
postpharyngeal: space
postphlebitic: syndrome
postprandial: lipemia
postprimary: tuberculosis
postpyloric: sphinter
postpyramidal: fissure
postreduction: phase
postrenal: albuminuria
postrhinal: fissure
postrubella: syndrome
postsphenoid: bone
postsphygmic: interval; period
postsynaptic: membrane
post-term: infant
posttraumatic: delirium; dementia; epilepsy; hydrocephalus; neurosis; psychosis; syndrome
posttraumatic arterial or venous: thrombosis
posttraumatic leptomeningeal: cyst
posttraumatic neck: syndrome
posttussis suction: sound
posttussive: suction
postural: albuminuria; contraction; hypotension; ischemia; myoneuralgia; position; proteinuria; reflex; set; syncope; version; vertigo
posture: sense
postvaccinal: encephalitis
potable: water
potassium: inhibition
potato: nose; tumor
potential: cautery; energy
potentiometric: titration
potter's: asthma; phthisis
poultryman's: itch
Powassan: virus
powder: head
powdered: belladona; caraway; coriander; gold; ipecac; opium; stomach
power: failure; point
pox-: virus
P-P: interval
P-Q: interval
P-R: interval; segment
PR: enzyme
practical: anatomy; nurse; unit
practice of: medicine
Prague: maneuver; pelvis
prairie: conjunctivitis; itch
preagonal: ascites
preanesthetic: medication
preauricular: point; sulcus
preautomatic: pause
precancerous: lesion; melanosis
precapillary: anastomosis

precentral: area; gyrus; line; sulcus
precervical: sinus
prechordal: plate
precipitate: labor
precipitated: sulfur
precipitating: antibody
precipitin: reaction; test
precision: attachment; rest
precocious: pseudopuberty; puberty
precollagenous: fiber
precommissural: bundle; septum
precommissural septal: area
preconceptual: stage
preconscious: system
precordial: lead
precordial catch: syndrome
precorneal: film
precostal: anastomosis
precursory: cartilage
predisposing: cause
predorsal: bundle
preejection: period
preen: gland
preexcitation: syndrome
preextraction: cast; record
preformation: theory
prefrontal: area; cortex; leukotomy; lobotomy
preganglionic motor: neuron
pregenital: organization; phase
pregnancy: cell; diabetes; disease; gingivitis; luteoma; tumor; test
pregnant mare's serum: gonadotropin
pregranulosa: cell
prehyoid: gland
preinfarction: syndrome
preinterparietal: bone
preliminary: impression
prelogical: thinking
premammary: abscess
premature: alopecia; beat; birth; contact; contraction; delivery; ejaculation; labor; systole
premature senility: syndrome
premaxillary: bone; suture
premeiotic: phase
premenstrual: edema; intoxication
premenstrual salivary: syndrome
premenstrual tension: syndrome
premixed: gas
premolar: tooth
premotor: area; cortex; syndrome
prenatal: life
preoccipital: notch
pre-Oedipal: phase
preoperative: cast; record
preoptic: area; region
preoral: gut
prepapillary: sphincter
preparatory: iridectomy
prepared: chalk; coal tar; ipecacuanha; suet
prepatellar: bursa; bursitis
preputial: calculus; gland; sac
prepyloric: sphincter; vein
prepyramidal: tract
prepyriform: gyrus
prerectal: lithotomy
prereduction: phase
prerenal: albuminuria
prerubral: field; nucleus
presacral: anesthesia; nerve; neurectomy; sympathectomy

prescribed: occupation
presenile spontaneous: gangrene
presomite: embryo
presphenoid: bone
presphygmic: interval; period
presplenic: fold
pressor: amine; base; fiber; nerve; substance
pressoreceptive: area; mechanism
pressoreceptor: nerve; reflex; system
pressure: anesthesia; area; atrophy; epiphysis; fracture; gangrene; palsy; plethysmograph; point; sense; sore; stasis; transducer
pressure-controlled: respirator
presternal: notch
prestriate: area
presumptive: region
presynaptic: membrane
presystolic: gallop; murmur; thrill
pretectal: area; region
preterm: infant
preternatural: anus
pretibial: fever; myxedema
pretracheal: fascia; layer; node
preventive: dentistry; dose; medicine; treatment
prevertebral: fascia; ganglion; layer
previllous: embryo
prickle: cell
prickle cell: layer
prickly: heat
primal: repression; scene
primaquine: sensitivity
primary: abutment; adhesion; aerodontalgia; agammaglobulinemia; alcohol; amenorrhea; amputation; amyloidosis; anemia; anesthetic; assimilation; atelectasis; bronchus; bubo; carcinoma; cardiomyopathy; caries; cataract; cementum; choana; coccidioidomycosis; color; complex; current; dementia; dentin; dentition; deviation; digestion; drive; dysmenorrhea; fissure; gain; hemorrhage; hydrocephalus; hyperoxaluria; hyperparathyroidism; hypertension; hyperthyroidism; hypogammaglobulinemia; hypogonadism; impression; irritant; lymphedema; lysosome; mesoderm; methemoglobinemia; myocardiopathy; narcissism; oocyte; organizer; palate; pentosuria; process; proteose; pyoderma; ray; reaction; reinforcement; screwworm; sensation; sequestrum; shock; spermatocyte; syphilis; tooth; tuberculosis; union; villus; vitreous
primary biliary: cirrhosis
primary brain: vesicle
primary dental: lamina
primary dried: yeast
primary embryonic: cell
primary erythroblastic: anemia
primary irritant: dermatitis
primary macular: atrophy
primary medical: care
primary mental: ability
primary ovarian: follicle
primary progressive cerebellar: degeneration
primary refractory: anemia
primary renal tubular: acidosis
primary sex: character

primary visual: area; cortex
primitive: aorta; chorion; circulation; furrow; groove; knot; node; ovum; palate; pit; ridge; streak
primitive costal: arch
primitive reticular: cell
primordial: cartilage; cell; dwarf; dwarfism; gigantism
primordial germ: cell
primordial ovarian: follicle
primo-secondary: suture
princeps cervicis: artery
principal: artery; cell; focus; islet; point
principal optic: axis
printer's: asthma
prism: diopter
prism vergence: test
prismatic: spectacles
prison: psychosis
private: antigen; hospital
private duty: nurse
privet: cough
pro-: virus
proacrosomal: granule
proactive: inhibition
probability: curve
probationer: nurse
probe: gorget; patency
procaryotic: cell
procerus: muscle
process: schizophrenia
prochordal: plate
procursive: chorea; epilepsy
prodromal: myopia; stage
prodromic: sign
product-moment: correlation
productive: inflammation
profile: line; record
profound: hypothermia
profuse: sweat
progeria: syndrome
progestational: hormone
progesterone: unit
prognathian, prognathic: dilation
progressive: cataract; cleavage; hypocythemia; lipodystrophy; process; vaccinia
progressive bacterial synergistic: gangrene
progressive bulbar: paralysis
progressive cerebellar: tremor
progressive cerebral: poliodystrophy
progressive choroidal: atrophy
progressive emphysematous: necrosis
progressive lingual: hemiatrophy
progressive multifocal: leukoencephalopathy
progressive muscular: atrophy; dystrophy
progressive pernicious: anemia
progressive pigmentary: dermatosis
progressive spinal: amyotrophy
progressive subcortical: encephalopathy
progressive supranuclear: palsy
progressive systemic: sclerosis
progressive tapetochoroidal: dystrophy
progressive torsion: spasm
projectile: vomiting
projection: fiber; perimeter; system
projective: test
prokaryotic: cell
prolactin: unit

prolactin-inhibiting: factor
proliferating: pleurisy
proliferation: cyst
proliferative: arthritis; cyst; dermatitis; fasciitis; gingivitis; glomerulonephritis; inflammation; intimitis
proliferous: cyst
proligerous: cyst; disk; membrane
prolonged nasotracheal: intubation
prolonged sleep: treatment
prominent: heel
pronator: reflex; ridge
prone: position
pronephric: duct; tubule
proof: spirit
propagated: thrombus
proper: fasciculus; ligament
proper hepatic: artery
proper palmer digital: nerve
proper planter digital: artery; nerve
properdin: factor; system
properitoneal inguinal: hernia
prophylactic: membrane; odontotomy; treatment
proportional: counter; limit
proportionate: infantilism
proprietary: hospital; medicine
proprioceptive: mechanism; reflex; sensibility
prosecretion: granule
prosector's: tubercle; wart
proserum prothrombin conversion: accelerator
prostate: gland
prostatic: calculus; catheter; concretion; duct; ductule; fluid; plexus; sinus; urethra
prostatic venous: plexus
prostaticovesical: plexus
prosthetic: dentistry; group
prosthetic speech: aid
prostomial: mesoderm
protamine zinc: insulin
protection: test
protective: block; colloid; ferment; protein
protective laryngeal: reflex
protein: factor; fever; metabolism; quotient; shock; synthesis
protein-bound: iodine
protein-bound iodine: test
protein-losing: enteropathy
protein shock: therapy
proteomorphic: theory
prothoracic: gland
prothoracic gland: hormone
prothoracotropic: hormone
prothrombin: test; time
prothrombin and proconvertin: test
prothrombin conversion: factor
protochordal: knot
protodiastolic: gallop
protopathic: sensibility
protoplasmic: astrocyte; astrocytoma; movement
prototrophic: strain
protozoan: cyst
protruded: disk
protruding: tooth
protrusive: checkbite; excursion; occlusion; position; record; relation
protrusive jaw: relation
proud: flesh

provisional: callus; cortex; denture; ligature
provocation: typhoid
provocative: test
proximal: cavity; centriole; contact
proximal bulbar: septum
proximal radioulnar: articulation
proximate: cause; contact; principle
proximobuccal: angle
proximolabial: angle
proximolingual: angle
prozone: reaction
"prune-belly": syndrome
prune-juice: expectoration; sputum
psalterial: cord
psammoma: body
pseudoachondroplastic spondyloepiphysial: dysplasia
pseudobulbar: paralysis
pseudocholinesterase: deficiency
pseudochylous: ascites
pseudocowpox: virus
pseudoepitheliomatous: hyperplasia
pseudoexfoliative capsular: glaucoma
pseudo-Graefe: sign
pseudohypertrophic muscular: atrophy; dystrophy; paralysis
pseudolepromatous: leishmaniasis
pseudolobster-claw: deformity
pseudolymphocytic choriomeningitis: virus
pseudolysogenic: strain
pseudomembranous: bronchitis; colic; colitis; conjunctivitis; enteritis; enterocolitis; gastritis; inflammation; rhinitis
pseudometatropic: dwarfism
pseudomucinous: cyst
pseudomuscular: hypertrophy
pseudoneurotic: schizophrenia
pseudo-osteomalacic: pelvis
pseudoplastic: fluid
pseudorabies: virus
pseudosarcomatous: fasciitis
pseudoscopic: vision
pseudostratified: epithelium
pseudotuberculous: ophthalmia
pseudotubular: degeneration
pseudo-Turner's: syndrome
pseudounipolar: cell; neuron
pseudoxanthoma: cell
psi: phenomenon
psittacosis: virus
psittacosis inclusion: body
psoas: abscess
psoriatic: arthritis
psoroptic: acariasis; itch; mange
psychedelic: therapy
psychiatric: deviance; medicine; nosology; trend
psychic: blindness; contagion; deafness; determinism; energy; epilepsy; equivalent; force; impotence; inertia; overtone; seizure; tic; trauma
psychoanalytic: psychiatry; psychotherapy; situation; therapy
psychocardiac: reflex
psychogalvanic: reaction; reflex; response
psychogalvanic skin: reaction; reflex; response
psychogenic: deafness; pain; polydipsia; purpura

psychographic: disturbance
psychological: test
psychomotor: epilepsy; retardation; test
psychopathic: personality; ward
psychophysiologic: disorder; manifestation
psychosensory: aphasia
psychosexual: development
psychosomatic: disorder; medicine
psychotic: manifestation
PTA: factor
PTC: factor; peptide; protein
pterygoid: canal; chest; depression; fissure; fossa; lamina; nerve; notch; pit; plate; plexus; process; ridge; tubercle; tuberosity
pterygomandibular: ligament; space
pterygomaxillary: fissure; fossa; notch
pterygopalatine: canal; fossa; ganglion; groove; nerve
pterygospinal: ligament
pterygospinous: ligament; process
ptotic: organ
puberty: melancholia
pubic: angle; arch; artery; body; bone; crest; ramus; region; spine; tubercle
public: antigen; hospital
public health: nurse
pubocapsular: ligament
pubococcygeal: muscle
pubofemoral: ligament
puboprostatic: ligament; muscle
puborectal: muscle
pubourethral: triangle
pubovaginal: muscle
pubovesical: ligament; muscle
pudding: opium
puddle: sign
pudendal: anesthesia; canal; cleavage; hematocele; nerve; sac; vein
pudic: nerve
puerile: respiration
puerperal: convulsion; eclampsia; fever; hemoglobinemia; hemoglobinuria; mania; mastitis; period; phlebitis; psychosis; sepsis; septicemia; tetanus
pullet: disease
pullorum: disease
pulmonary: acariasis; acinus; adenomatosis; anthrax; apoplexy; arc; area; artery; aspergillosis; atresia; bulla; circulation; collapse; cone; conus; distomiasis; edema; embolism; emphysema; fistula; glomangiosis; heart; hemorrhage; hemosiderosis; hypertension; incompetence; insufficiency; ligament; lobule; murmur; opening; osteoarthropathy; pleurisy; plexus; pressure; pulse; ridge; salient, stenosis; sulcus; surface; transpiration; trunk; tuberculosis; valve; vein; ventilation
pulmonary alveolar: microlithiasis; proteinosis
pulmonary dysmaturity: syndrome
pulmonary lymph: node
pulmonic: incompetence; murmur
pulmonocoronary: reflex
pulp: abscess; amputation; calcification; calculus; canal; capping; cavity; chamber; horn; nodule; polyp; stone; test
pulpal: wall
pulpar: cell
pulpit: spectacles

pulpy: kidney; testis
pulpy kidney: disease
pulsating: empyema; metastasis; neurasthenia
pulse: curve; deficit; duration; generator; period; pressure; rate; wave
pulseless: disease
pulsion: diverticulum
pumiced: foot
pump: failure; substance
punch: biopsy
punchdrunk: syndrome
punctata albescens: retinopathy
punctate: basophilia; cataract; hemorrhage; hyalosis; keratitis; retinitis
puncture: diabetes; wound
pupillary: athetosis; axis; distance; membrane; reflex; zone
pupillary-skin: reflex
pure: color; culture; cyclitis; line
pure red cell: anemia
pure tone: audiogram
purified: cotton; ether; ozokerite; water
purified placental: protein
purified protein derivative of: tuberculin
purine: base; body
purine-free: diet
purse-string: suture
purulent: cyclitis; encephalitis; inflammation; ophthalmia; pleurisy; synovitis
pus: basin; cell; corpuscle; tube
push-back: procedure
pustular: miliaria; psoriasis; syphilid
putrescent: pulp
putrid: bronchitis
putrid sore: throat
PVM: virus
pyemic: abscess; embolism
pyknic: type
pyloric: artery; canal; cap; gland; incompetence; insufficiency; orifice; part; sphincter; stenosis; valve; vein
pyloric lymph: node
pyogenic: fever; infection; membrane; pachymeningitis; salpingitis
pyramid: sign
pyramidal: bone; cataract; cell; decussation; eminence; fiber; fracture; lobe; muscle; process; radiation; tract; tractotomy
pyramidal cell: layer
pyridinoprotein: enzyme
pyriform: (see also piriform)
pyriform aperture: wiring
pyrimidine: base
pyrogen: test
pyroligneous: spirit; vinegar
pyroxylic: spirit
pyrrol, pyrrhol: cell
pyruvate kinase: deficiency
pyruvate oxidation: factor

## Q

Q: band; disk; enzyme; fever; wave
Q-R: interval
Q-RB: interval
QRS: complex; interval
Q-S₂: interval
Q-T: interval
quack: medicine

quadrangular: cartilage; lobule; membrane; therapy
quadrantic: hemianopsia
quadrate: ligament; lobe; lobule; muscle; part
quadriceps: artery; muscle; reflex
quadrigeminal: body; plate; pulse; rhythm
quandripedal extensor: reflex
quadruple: amputation; rhythm
quail bronchitis: virus
qualitative: alteration; analysis
quantitative: alteration; analysis; hypertrophy; perimetry
quantum: limit; theory
Quaranfil: virus
quartan: ague; fever; malaria; parasite
quarter: evil; ill
quartz: glass
quaternary: carbon; compound; syphilis
quaternary ammonium: base
quellung: phenomenon; reaction
quick cure: resin
quiet: iritis; lung
quiet hip: disease
quilled: suture
quilted: suture
quinhydrone: electrode
quinine: amblyopia
quinine carbacrylic: resin
quinine carbacrylic resin: test
quotidian: ague; fever; malaria

## R

R: enzyme; factor; wave
R-on-T: phenomenon
rabbit: fever; papilloma; pinworm; septicemia; snuffles; tick
rabbit fibroma: virus
rabbit myxoma: virus
rabbit oral: papilloma
rabbitpox: virus
rabies: vaccine; virus
racemose: aneurysm; gland; hemangioma
rachitic: pelvis; rosary; scoliosis
racial: melanoderma
racket: amputation; nail
radial: acceleration; artery; border; bursa; eminence; fossa; nerve; notch; phenomenon; reflex; surface; vein
radial collateral: artery; ligament
radial compression: test
radial flexor: muscle
radial index: artery
radial recurrent: artery
radial styloid: tendovaginitis
radiant: energy; heat
radiate: crown; layer; ligament
radiation: anemia; biology; burn; cataract; chemistry; chimera; myelopathy; sickness
radical: cure; hysterectomy; mastoidectomy; operation
radicular: artery; cyst; odontoma; pulp; syndrome
radio: wave
radioactive: atom; constant; cyanocobalamin; equilibrium; iodine; isotope; thyroxine
radioactive colloidal gold: test
radioactive iodide uptake: test

**radiobicipital:** reflex
**radiocarpal:** articulation; joint
**radiochemical:** purity
**radioisotopic:** purity
**radiological:** anatomy; sphincter
**radionuclide:** angiography; generator
**radionuclidic:** purity
**radioperiosteal:** reflex
**radiopharmaceutical:** purity
**radiotelemetering:** capsule
**radioulnar:** disk; joint
**radium:** emanation
**radium beam:** therapy
**rag-sorter's:** disease
**RAI:** test
**railroad:** nystagmus
**railway:** medicine; spine
**rain:** bath
**rainbow:** symptom
**random:** mating; sample; wave
**range:** paralysis
**range of:** convergence
**Ranikhet:** disease
**ranine:** artery; tumor
**rank-difference:** correlation
**raphe:** nucleus
**rapid:** decompression
**rapid biplane:** angiocardiography
**rapid eye:** movement
**rapid eye movement:** sleep; state
**rapid plasma reagin:** test
**rapidly progressive:** glomerulonephritis
**rare:** earth
**rare earth:** element; metal
**raspberry:** polyp; tongue
**rat:** flea; leprosy; pinworm
**rat bite:** fever
**rat mite:** dermatitis
**rate:** constant; meter
**ratio:** scale
**rational:** formula; medicine; therapeutics; therapy; treatment
**ray:** fungus; therapeutics
**reaction:** center; formation; time
**reaction of:** degeneration
**reactive:** astrocyte; cell; depression; hyperemia; schizophrenia
**reading frame-shift:** mutation
**reaginic:** antibody
**real:** focus; image
**reality:** adaptation; awareness; principle
**reaper's:** keratitis
**rebound:** phenomenon; tenderness
**rebreathing:** anesthesia; technique
**recapitulation:** theory
**receptive:** aphasia
**receptor:** amblyopia; protein; site
**recessive:** character; gene; inheritance; trait
**reciprocal:** arm; beat; bigeminy; inhibition; innervation; rhythm; transfusion; translocation
**reciprocating:** rhythm
**reclotting:** phenomenon
**recognition:** time
**recoil:** atom; wave
**recombinant:** strain
**reconstructive:** psychotherapy
**record:** base; rim
**recovery:** room; score
**recrudescent:** typhus
**recruiting:** response

**rectal:** alimentation; anesthesia; fold; plexus; reflex; shelf; suppository; sinus; valvotomy
**rectal venous:** plexus
**rectangular:** amputation
**rectified:** birch; spirit; tar
**rectocardiac:** reflex
**rectococcygeal:** muscle
**rectolabial:** fistula
**rectolaryngeal:** reflex
**rectosigmoid:** sphincter
**rectourethral:** fistula; muscle
**rectouterine:** fold; pouch
**rectovaginal:** fistula; pouch; septum
**rectovesical:** fascia; fistula; fold; muscle; pouch; septum
**rectovestibular:** fistula
**rectovulvar:** fistula
**recurrent:** albuminuria; bandage; encephalopathy; fever; melancholia; nerve; stricture
**recurrent aphthous:** stomatitis
**recurrent canker:** sore
**recurrent interosseous:** artery
**recurrent laryngeal:** nerve
**recurrent meningeal:** nerve
**recurrent ulcerative:** stomatitis
**recurrent ulnar:** artery
**red:** atrophy; bark; blindness; corallin; corpuscle; degeneration; fever; gum; half-moon; hepatization; hypertension; induration; infarct; lead; mange; marrow; neuralgia; nucleus; precipitate; pulp; quebracho; sweat; test; thrombus; vision; wine
**red blood:** cell
**red cell adherence:** phenomenon; test
**red-green:** blindness
**red pulp:** cord
**redox:** see oxidation-reduction
**reduced:** eye; hemoglobin
**reduced enamel:** epithelium
**reducible:** hernia
**reducing:** agent; diet; enzyme; sugar; valve
**reduction:** deformity; division; nucleus; phase
**reduction of:** chromosome
**reduplicated:** cataract
**redwater:** fever
**reed instrument:** theory
**reedy:** nail
**reef:** knot
**reel:** foot
**reentry:** phenomenon; theory
**reference:** electrode
**referred:** pain; sensation
**reflected:** light; ray
**reflecting:** ophthalmoscope; stereoscope
**reflection:** coefficient
**reflex:** action; akinesia; angina; arc; asthma; control; cough; dyspepsia; epilepsy; headache; inhibition; iridoplegia; ligament; movement; otalgia; sensation; symptom; therapy
**reflexogenic:** pressosensitivity; zone
**refracted:** light
**refractive:** dose; index
**refractory:** cast; flask; investment; period; state
**refrigeration:** anesthesia
**regional:** anatomy; anesthesia; enteritis; enterocolitis; hypothermia; ileitis;

perfusion
**registered:** nurse
**regressive-inspirational:** psychotherapy
**regressive-reconstructive:** approach
**regular:** astigmatism; insulin; practitioner
**regulator:** gene
**regulatory:** albuminuria
**regurgitant:** murmur
**regurgitation:** jaundice
**reinfection:** tuberculosis
**relapsing:** fever; malaria; perichondritis
**relational:** threshold
**relative:** accommodation; dehydration; hemianopsia; humidity; immunity; incompetence; leukocytosis; polycythemia; scotoma; sterility; viscosity
**relaxation:** factor; suture
**release:** phenomenon
**released:** substance
**releasing:** factor; hormone
**reliability:** coefficient
**relief:** area; chamber
**religious:** insanity; mania
**reminiscent:** neuralgia
**remittent:** malaria
**remittent malarial:** fever
**remitting spinal:** atrophy
**remote:** memory
**removable:** bridge
**renal:** adenocarcinoma; agenesis; amyloidosis; anacidogenesis; artery; asthma; ballottement; calculus; carbuncle; carcinosarcoma; cast; colic; collar; corpuscle; cortex; column; diabetes; epistaxis; fascia; ganglion; glycosuria; hematuria; hemophilia; hemorrhage; hypertension; impression; infantilism; insufficiency; labyrinth; lobe; osteodystrophy; osteitis; papilla; pelvis; plexus; pyramid; reflex; retinopathy; rickets; segment; sinus; surface; threshold; transplantation; vein
**renal cell:** carcinoma
**renal cortical:** adenoma; lobule
**renal fibrocystic:** osteosis
**renal papillary:** necrosis
**renal-splanchnic:** steal
**renal-splenic venous:** shunt
**renal tubular:** acidosis
**renewed:** bark
**reniform:** pelvis
**renin-angiotensin:** system
**renovascular:** hypertension
**reo-:** virus
**reparative giant cell:** granuloma
**repetition:** rate
**repetition-compulsion:** principle
**replacement:** bone; fibrosis; therapy
**replicative:** form
**repressible:** enzyme
**reproductive:** assimilation; cycle; mycelium; nucleus; system
**reserve:** air; force
**reserve tooth:** germ
**reservoir:** bag; host
**residual:** abscess; affinity; air; body; capacity; cleft; lumen; ridge; urine; volume
**residual ovary:** syndrome
**resistance:** factor; form; pyrometer; thermometer

resistance-inducing: factor
resistance-transfer: episome; factor
resistive: movement
resolving: power
resonance: theory
resorcinol-HCl: test
resorption: lacuna
respirable: aerosol
respiration: rate
respiratory: acidosis; airway; alkalosis; arrhythmia; bronchiole; capacity; center; coefficient; enzyme; epithelium; frequency; hippus; insufficiency; lobule; metabolism; metal; mucosa; murmur; pulse; pigment; quotient; region; scleroma; sound; system; tract
respiratory exchange: ratio
respiratory syncytial: virus
respondent: behavior; conditioning
response: hierarchy
response-produced: cue
rest: area; bacillus; bite; body; cure; nitrogen; pain; position; relation; seat; treatment
rest jaw: relation
rest vertical: dimension
restiform: body; eminence
resting: cell; saliva; stage
resting wandering: cell
restless: legs
restless legs: syndrome
restorative: dentistry
restorative dental: material
restored: cycle
restrained: beam
retained: menstruation; placenta; testis
retarded: dentition
rete: cord; cyst; peg; ridge
rete ovarian: cyst
retention: area; arm; cyst; form; groove; jaundice; point; polyp; toxicosis
retentive: arm
reticular: cartilage; cell; degeneration; formation; fiber; groove; lamina; layer; membrane; nucleus; substance; tissue
reticular activating: system
reticulated: bone, corpuscle; tubercle
reticulating: colliquation
reticuloendothelial: cell; system
reticulospinal: tract
reticulum cell: sarcoma
retiform: cartilage; tissue
retinal: abiotrophy; adaptation; asthenopia; camera; cone; detachment; dysplasia; embolism; epilepsy; image
retinal anlage: tumor
retinocerebral: angiomatosis
retraction: syndrome
retroactive: inhibition
retroauricular lymph: node
retrobulbar: abscess; neuritis
retrocecal: abscess; recess
retrocedent: gout
retrocochlear: deafness
retrocolic: spasm
retroduodenal: artery; fossa; recess
retroflex: fasciculus
retrogasserian: neurectomy; neurotomy
retrograde: amnesia; aortography; block; chromatolysis; conduction; degeneration; embolism; embolus; hernia; intussusception; memory; men-

struation; metamorphosis; metastasis
retrograde P: wave
retrohyoid: bursa
retroinguinal: space
retrolental: fibroplasia
retrolenticular: limb
retromammary: mastitis
retromandibular: fossa; vein
retromolar: fossa; pad
retromylohyoid: space
retroperitoneal: fibrosis; hernia; space
retropharyngeal: abscess; space
retropharyngeal lymph: node
retropubic: hernia; space
retrospective: falsification
retrosternal: hernia; struma
retrotarsal: fold
retrusive: occlusion
return: extrasystole
return of the: repressed
returning: cycle
reverberating: circuit
reverse: bandage; curve
reverse Eck: fistula
reverse Kingsley: splint
reversed: anaphylaxis; astigmatism; coarctation; current; peristalsis; shunt
reversed paradoxical: pulse
reversed passive: anaphylaxis
reversed reciprocal: rhythm
reversible: calcinosis; colloid; decortication; disease; hydrocolloid; reaction; shock
Rh: antigen; hapten
Rh blocking: test
Rh₀ (D) immune: globulin
rhagiocrine: cell
rhegmatogenous retinal: detachment
rheumatic: arteritis; carditis; chorea; disease; endocarditis; fever; pericarditis; pneumonia; tetanus; tetany; torticollis; valvulitis
rheumatic heart: disease
rheumatismal: edema
rheumatoid: arteritis; arthritis; disease; factor; nodule; spondylitis
rhinal: fissure; sulcus
rhino-: virus
rhizomelic: spondylosis
Rhodesian: trypanosomiasis
Rhodesian red: water
Rhodesian tick: fever
rhombencephalic: isthmus
rhombic: groove; lip
rhomboid: fossa; impression; ligament
rhomboidal: sinus
rhonchal: fremitus
rhus: dermatitis
Rhus toxicodendron: antigen
Rhus venenata: antigen
rhythmic: chorea
rib: spreader
ribbed: tongue
ribbon: arch
ribo-: virus
riboflavin: deficiency; unit
ribosomal: ribonucleic acid
rice: body; diet
rice-water: stool
ricefield: fever
rickettsia: vaccine
rickettsial: pox
Rida: virus

rider's: bone; bursa; leg; muscle; tendon
ridge: extension; relation; resorption
riding: embolus
Rift Valley: fever
Rift Valley fever: virus
right anatomical structures (specific right structures are listed under the following): appendage; artery; auricle; crus; duct; flexure; heart; ligament; lobe; node; part; plate; valve; vein; ventricle
right axis: deviation
right dorsoanterior: position
right dorsoposterior: position
right frontoanterior: position
right frontoposterior: postion
right occipitoanterior: position
right occipitoposterior: position
right ovarian vein: syndrome
right-to-left: shunt
right ventricular: failure; hypoplasia
righting: reflex
Riley: virus
rind: tumor
rinderpest: virus
ring: abscess; bone; chromosome; compound; finger; ligament; pessary; scotoma; test; ulcer
ring precipitin: test
ring-wall: lesion
ringed: hair
ringworm: yaws
Rio Bravo: virus
Rio Grande: fever
ripe: cataract
rise: time
risorius: muscle
ritualistic: behavior
RNA: virus
RNA tumor: virus
Rochelle: salt
rock: fever
Rocky Mountain: tick
Rocky Mountain spotted: fever
Rocky Mountain spotted fever: vaccine
rod: cell; granule; myopathy; vision
rod nuclear: cell
rodent: cancer; ulcer
roentgen: ray; unit
role: conflict; deviance
roll: sulfur; tube
roll-tube: culture
roller: bandage; forceps
Roman: fever
roof: nucleus; plate
room: temperature
root: abscess; amputation; apex; canal; dehiscence; end; foramen; filament; resection; resorption; sheath; tip
root canal: file; filling; orifice; plugger; spreader; therapy; treatment
rope: graft
rosacea-like: tuberculid
rose: cold; rash; spot
rose bengal radioactive (¹³¹I): test
rosette-forming: cell
rostral: lamina; layer
rostral transtentorial: herniation
rostrate: pelvis
rotary: joint; vertigo
rotation: center
rotational: axis
rotator: cuff; muscle

rotatory: joint; nystagmus; spasm; tic
rote: learning
rotten: stone
rough: colony
rough-surfaced cytoplasmic: reticulum
rouleaux: formation
round: bur; eminence; foramen; ligament; muscle; ulcer; window
round cell: sarcoma
Rous-associated: virus
Rous sarcoma: virus
rowing: method
R-R: interval
Rs: virus
RS-T: segment
rubber: dam; pelvis; tissue
rubber-bulb: syringe
rubber dam: clamp
rubber dam clamp: forceps
rubbing: alcohol
rubella: retinopathy; virus
rubella HI: test
rubella virus: vaccine
rubeola: virus
rubrobulbar: tract
rubroreticular: tract
rubrospinal: decussation; tract
ruby: spot
rufous: albinism
rum: nose
rumen: fluke
runt: disease
rupial: syphilid
ruptured: disk
Russian: bath; fly
Russian autumn: encephalitis
Russian autumn encephalitis: virus
Russian spring-summer: encephalitis
Russian spring-summer encephalitis: virus
Russian tick-borne: encephalitis
rusty: sputum

S

S: antigen; factor; parotin; peptide; potential; protein; wave
S-A: node
saber, sabre: leg; shin; tibia
sabot: heart
sabural: amaurosis
saccadic: movement
sacciform: recess
saccular: aneurysm; gland; nerve; spot
sacculated: aneurysm; bronchiectasis; pleurisy
sacral: anesthesia; canal; crest; flexure; foramen; ganglion; horn; index; nerve; plexus; region; triangle; tuberosity; vein; vertebra
sacral lymph: node
sacral splanchnic: nerve
sacral venous: plexus
sacred: bone; disease
sacroanterior: position
sacrococcygeal: disk; joint
sacrogenital: fold
sacroiliac: articulation; joint
sacropelvic: surface
sacroposterior: position
sacrosciatic: notch
sacrospinous: ligament
sacrotuberous: ligament

saddle: back; embolus; head; joint; nose
saddle block: anesthesia
saddle-shaped: uterus
sadomasochistic: relationship
safe: period
safety: lens
sagittal: axis; border; crest; fontanel; groove; line; plane; section; sulcus; suture
Sagiyama: virus
sago: spleen
Saigon: cassia
sail: sound
sailor's: skin
Saint (see also St.)
Saint Agatha's: disease
Saint Aignan's: disease
Saint Anthony's: dance
Saint Avertin's: disease
Saint Blaize's: disease
Saint Claire's: disease
Saint Dymphna's: disease
Saint Erasmus': disease
Saint Fiacre's: disease
Saint Francis': fire
Saint Gervasius': disease
Saint Gete's: disease
Saint Gile's: disease
Saint Guy's: disease
Saint Hubert's: disease
Saint Ignatius': itch
Saint John's: dance; evil
Saint Main's: evil
Saint Martin's: evil
Saint Mathurin's: disease
Saint Modestus': disease
Saint Roch's: disease
Saint Rose's: disease
Saint Valentine's: disease
Saint Vitus': dance
Saint With's: dance
Saint Zachary's: disease
sakushu: fever
salaam: convulsion; spasm
salicylic acid: collodion
saline: agglutinin; purgative; solution; water
Salisbury common cold: virus
saliva: ejector; parotin; pump
salivary: amylase; calculus; colic; corpuscle; digestion; duct; fistula; gland; virus
salivary gland: hormone
salivary taste: hormone
salmon: patch; poisoning
Salmonella food: poisoning
salol: test
Salonica, Saloniki: fever
salpingopalatine: fold
salpingopharyngeal: fold; muscle
salt: action; depletion; dye; edema; fever; loading; poisoning; sensitivity; solution
salt depletion: syndrome
salt-free: diet
salt-losing: nephritis
salt water: boil; soap
saltatory: chorea; conduction; evolution; spasm
salted: plasma
Samoan eye: disease
San Joaquin: fever
sand: bath; body; flea; fly; treatment;

tumor
sandal strap: dermatitis
sandfly: fever
sandfly fever: virus
sandpaper: disk; gallbladder
sandworm: disease
sanguine: temperament
sanguineous: cyst
sanious: pus
saphenous: nerve; opening; vein
saponification: number
sarcogenic: cell
sarcomatoid: carcinoma
sarcomatous: osteitis
sarcoplasmic: reticulum
sarcoptic: acariasis; itch; mange
Sassoon hospital: syndrome
satellite: abscess; cell
Sathuperi: virus
satiety: center
saturated: color; compound; fat; fatty acid; hydrocarbon; solution
saturation: index
saturnine: cachexia; colic; encephalopathy; gout; tremor
sausage: finger; poisoning
sausage-shaped: roll
scabbard: trachea
scalded skin: syndrome
scalene: tubercle
scalenus-anticus: syndrome
scalp: contusion; emphysema; laceration; muscle
scalpriform: incisor
scaly: leg; ringworm; tetter
scamping: speech
scanning: speech
scanning electron: microscope
scanty: sweat
scaphoid: abdomen; bone; fossa; scapula; tuberosity
scapular: notch; reflex; region
scapulocostal: syndrome
scapulohumeral: atrophy; periarthritis; reflex
scapuloperiosteal: reflex
scar: pterygium
scarf: bandage; skin
scarification: test
scarlatinal: nephritis
scarlatiniform: erythema
scarlet: fever; rash
scarlet fever: antitoxin
scarlet fever erythrogenic: toxin
scavenger: cell; enzyme
scent: gland
schematic: eye
schindyletic: joint
schistosome: dermatitis
schizencephalic: microcephaly
schizo-affective: psychosis
schizoid: personality
schizophrenic: decompensation
school: nurse; phobia
sciatic: foramen; hernia; nerve; neuralgia; neuritis; plexus; scoliosis
scimitar: syndrome
scintillating: scotoma
scintillation: counter; scanning
scirrhous: cancer; carcinoma
scissor: gait; leg
scleral: roll; spur; staphyloma
scleral buckling: operation

sclerocorneal: junction
sclerocystic: disease
sclerosing: adenosis; agent; hemangioma; inflammation; keratitis; mastoiditis; osteitis; therapy
sclerotic: coat; degeneration; gastritis; kidney; stomach; tooth
scoliotic: pelvis
scotopic: adaptation; eye; vision
scrapie: virus
scratch: reflex; test
screen: defense; memory
screening: test
screw: artery; elevator; joint
screwdriver: tooth
screwworm: fly
scrivener's: palsy
scrofulous: abscess; keratitis; ophthalmia; rhinitis
scroll: bone; ear
scrotal: artery; hernia; septum; swelling; tongue; tumor; vein
scrub: nurse; typhus
scurf (scarf): skin
scurvy: rickets
Scythian: disease
sea: scurvy; sickness
sea gull: murmur
sea urchin: granuloma; sting
Seabright bantam: syndrome
seal-fin: deformity
sealed jar: technique
seamstress's: cramp
seat: worm
sebaceous: adenoma; crypt; cyst; flux; follicle; gland; horn; tubercle
seborrheic: dermatitis; dermatosis; eczema; keratosis; verruca; wart
seclusion of: pupil
second: finger; incisor; law; messenger; molar; sight
second cranial: nerve
second cuneiform: bone
second gas: effect
second-order: conditioning; receptor
second signaling: system
second stage of: labor
second temporal: convolution
second tibial: muscle
secondary: adhesion; aerodontalgia; agammaglobulinemia; alcohol; amenorrhea; amputation; amyloidosis; anemia; atelectasis; axis; buffer; carcinoma; cardiomyopathy; caries; cartilage; cataract; cementum; choana; coccidioidomycosis; current; cyst; degeneration; dementia; dentin; dentition; deviation; dextrocardia; digestion; disease; drive; dysmenorrhea; elaboration; encephalitis; failure; fissure; follicle; fracture; gain; glaucoma; gout; hemorrhage; host; hydrocephalus; hyperparathyroidism; hyperthyroidism; hypogammaglobulinemia; hypogonadism; hypothyroidism; infection; lysosome; mark; mesoderm; methemoglobinemia; narcissism; nodule; oocyte; palate; pellagra; pneumonia; process; proteose; pyoderma; ray; reinforcement; saturation; screwworm; shock; spermatocyte; suture; syphilid; syphilis; thrombus; tuberculosis; villus; vitreous

secondary abdominal: pregnancy
secondary adrenal: insufficiency
secondary antibody: deficiency
secondary generalized: epilepsy
secondary medical: care
secondary refractory: anemia
secondary renal tubular: acidosis
secondary sensory: cortex; nucleus
secondary sex: character
secondary visual: area; cortex
secondary spiral: plate
secondary tympanic: membrane
secondary X: zone
secretin: test
secretor: factor
secretory: canaliculus; cyst; nerve
sectional: impression; roentgenography
sedimentary: cataract
sedimentation: constant; rate; reaction; test
seed: corn
seedy: toe
seesaw: murmur; nystagmus
segmental: anesthesia; glomerulonephritis; neuritis; neuropathy; plate; sphincter; zone
segmentation: cavity; nucleus; sphere
segmented: cell; leukocyte; neutrophil
segmenting: body
segregation of: gene
Seidlitz powder: test
selection: coefficient; pressure
selective: angiocardiography; arteriography; grinding; inattention; inhibition; stain
selenium: poisoning
self-curing: resin
self-registering: thermometer
self-retaining: catheter
semantic: aphasia
semicircular: canal; duct
semiclosed: anesthesia; circle
semidirect: lead
semihorizontal: heart
semilunar: bone; cartilage; fascia; fasciculus; fibrocartilage; fold; ganglion; line; notch; valve
semilunar conjunctival: fold
semimembranosus: muscle
semimembranosus and semitendinosus: reflex
seminal: capsule; colliculus; cyst; duct; fluid; granule; hillock; lake; vesicle
seminiferous: epithelium; tubercle
seminiferous tubule: dysgenesis
seminormal: solution
semi-open: anesthesia
semioval: center
semipermeable: membrane
semipolar: bond
semiprone: position
semispinal: muscle
semitendinous: muscle
semivertical: heart
Semliki forest: virus
Sendai: virus
Seneca: snakeroot
senegal: gum
senile: amyloidosis; arteriosclerosis; atrophy; cataract; chorea; degeneration; delirium; dementia; deterioration; dwarf; ectasia; elastosis; emphysema; fibroma; gangrene; heman-

gioma; insanity; involution; keratoma; keratosis; lentigo; memory; nephrosclerosis; osteomalacia; paraplegia; psychosis; reflex; retinoschisis; tremor; wart
senile dental: caries
senile guttate: choroidopathy
senile lenticular: myopia
sensation: time
sense: organ
sensible: heat; perspiration; temperature
sensitive: dentin
sensitivity training: group
sensitized: antigen; cell; culture
sensitizing: dose; injection; substance
sensorial: area; idiocy
sensorimotor: area; theory
sensorineural: deafness
sensorineural loss of: hearing
sensory: amusia; aphasia; area; cortex; crossway; deafness; decussation; deprivation; epilepsy; ganglion; image; nerve; paralysis; receptor; root; tract
sensory speech: center
sentinal: gland; pile; tag
separating: medium
separation: anxiety
separation of: tooth
septal: area; artery; bone; cartilage; cell; cusp; dermatoplasty; gingiva
septate: mycelium; uterus
septic: abortion; endocarditis; fever; intoxication; pneumonia; shock
septic sore: throat
septicemic: abscess; plague
septomarginal: fasciculus; tract
sequence: hypothesis
"sequential" oral: contraceptive
sequestration: cyst; dermoid
serial: roentgenography; section
serofibrinous: inflammation; pleurisy
seromucous: cell; gland
serous: abscess; albuminuria; apoplexy; atrophy; cell; cyclitis; cyst; diarrhea; demilune; gland; hemorrhage; inflammation; iritis; membrane; meningitis; otitis; pleurisy; pulpitis; retinitis; synovitis; tunic
serpent: ulcer; worm
serpentine: aneurysm
serpiginous: keratitis; syphilid; ulcer
serrate: suture
Sertoli cell: tumor
"Sertoli cell only": syndrome
serum: accelerator; accident; agar; agglutinin; albumin; disease; eruption; hepatitis; nephritis; rash; reaction; shock; sickness; test; therapy
serum accelerator: globulin
serum hepatitis: virus
serum prothrombin conversion: accelerator
serumal: calculus
sesamoid: bone; cartilage
sessile: hydatid; polyp; receptor
set of: teeth (see tooth)
seton: operation; wound
setting: expansion
seven-day: fever
seven-year: itch
seventh: sense
seventh cranial: nerve

**sewing:** spasm
**sex:** cell; chromatin; chromosome; cord; factor; hormone; linkage; object; reversal; skin
**sex chromosome:** imbalance
**sex-linked:** character; gene; inheritance
**sexual:** anesthesia; deviance; dimorphism; dwarf; generation; gland; infantilism; instinct; intercourse; life; melancholia; neurasthenia; neurosis; perversion; potency; reproduction; selection
**sexual receptivity:** test
**shadow:** cell; corpuscle; nucleus; test
**shaft:** vision
**shaggy:** chorion; pericardium
**shagreen:** skin
**shake:** culture
**shaking:** palsy
**shallow:** breathing
**sham:** feeding; rage
**sham-movement:** vertigo
**shank:** bone; fever
**sharp:** spoon
**shaving:** cramp
**shawl:** muscle
**shear:** flow; rate; thinning
**shearing:** edge
**sheath:** ligament; process
**sheathed:** artery
**sheep:** bots; fever; pox
**sheep liver:** fluke
**sheep pox:** virus
**shelf:** procedure
**shell:** shock
**shellac:** base
**shelving:** operation
**sherry:** wine
**shifting:** dullness; pacemaker
**shilling:** scar
**shimamushi:** disease
**shin:** bone; splint
**ship:** fever
**shipping:** fever
**shipyard:** eye
**shirt-stud:** abscess
**shock:** antigen; therapy; treatment
**shocking:** dose
**shoe:** boil
**shoe dye:** dermatitis
**Shope:** fibroma; papilloma
**Shope fibroma:** virus
**short:** bone; chain; gyrus; process; sight; vinculum
**short abductor:** muscle
**short adductor:** muscle
**short ciliary:** nerve
**short extensor:** muscle
**short flexor:** muscle
**short gastric:** artery; vein
**short incubation:** hepatitis
**short luteal:** phase
**short palmar:** muscle
**short peroneal:** muscle
**short posterior ciliary:** artery
**short saphenous:** nerve; vein
**short term:** memory
**short wave:** diathermy
**shortening:** reaction
**shotgun:** prescription; quarantine
**shot-silk:** phenomenon; reflex; retina
**shotted:** suture
**shoulder:** bursitis; girdle; joint; presentation; tick

**shoulder-hand:** syndrome
**show:** fever
**shuffle:** foot
**shut-in:** personality
**SI:** unit
**Siamese:** twins
**sibilant:** rale
**sibling:** rivalry
**sicca:** syndrome
**sick:** headache; nurse; role
**sick sinus:** syndrome
**sickle:** cell; form
**sickle cell:** anemia; crisis; dactylitis; disease; hemoglobin; retinopathy; syndrome; test; trait
**sickle cell-thalassemia:** disease
**side:** chain; effect
**side chain:** theory
**sideropenic:** dysphagia
**siderotic:** nodule
**sieve:** bone; graft; plate
**sight:** meter
**sigma:** effect; peptide
**sigmoid:** artery; colon; flexure; fossa; groove; notch; sinus; sulcus; vein
**sigmoidovesical:** fistula
**sign:** blindness
**signal:** node
**signet:** ring
**signet ring:** cell
**signet ring cell:** carcinoma
**silent:** area; electrode; gap; gallstone; period
**silent myocardial:** infarction
**silicate:** cement; filling
**silicon:** granuloma
**siliculose, siliquose:** cataract
**silk:** peptone
**silkworm:** gut
**silo-filler's:** disease
**silver:** cell; point; poisoning; protein
**silver fork:** deformity; fracture
**silver-tin:** alloy
**silverized:** catgut
**Simbu:** virus
**simian:** fissure; malaria; virus
**simple:** beam; color; diplopia; dislocation; epithelium; fission; fracture; goiter; hypertrophy; joint; microscope; necrosis; obesity; protein; schizophrenia; ulcer; urethritis
**simple continued:** fever
**simple hyperopic:** astigmatism
**simple membranous:** limb
**simple myopic:** astigmatism
**simple skull:** fracture
**simple squamous:** epithelium
**simulated:** hypertrophy
**simultaneous:** contrast; insanity
**Sindbis:** virus
**singer's:** node; nodule
**single:** ascertainment; bond; microscope
**single (gel) diffusion precipitin:** test
**singlet:** oxygen; state
**sinoatrial:** block; node
**sinuatrial:** chamber
**sinus:** arrest; arrhythmia; balloon; barotrauma; block; bradycardia; nerve; node; pause; phlebitis; reflex; rhythm; septum; standstill; tachycardia
**sinusoidal:** capillary
**sinuvertebral:** nerve
**siren:** limb

**SISI:** test
**situation:** anxiety
**situational:** psychosis; test
**sitz:** bath
**sixth:** disease; sense; ventricle
**sixth cranial:** nerve
**sixth venereal:** disease
**sixth-year:** molar
**skein:** cell
**skeletal:** extension; muscle; traction
**skeletal muscle:** fiber; tissue
**skeleton:** hand
**skew:** deviation; form; pupil
**skim, skimmed:** milk
**skin:** botfly; diabetes; dose; factor; graft; groove; heart; reaction; reflex; ridge; stone; tag; test; twitch
**skin-muscle:** reflex
**skin-puncture:** test
**skin-pupillary:** reflex
**skinbound:** disease
**skip:** area
**skull:** cap; fracture
**slab-off:** lens
**slant:** culture
**slaty:** anemia
**sleep:** disorder; dissociation; drunkeness; epilepsy; paralysis; spindle
**sleeping (African):** sickness
**sleeve:** graft
**slender:** fasciculus; lobule; process
**slide:** micrometer
**sliding:** flap; hernia
**sliding esophageal hiatal:** hernia
**sliding filament:** hypothesis
**sliding hiatal:** hernia
**slime:** fungus
**sling:** psychrometer
**slipped:** tendon
**slipped (sliding):** hernia
**slipped tendon:** disease
**slipping:** patella; rib
**slipping rib:** cartilage
**slit-:** lamp
**slitlamp:** microscope
**slope:** culture
**slotted:** attachment
**sloughing:** phagedena; ulcer
**slow:** combustion; fever; virus
**slow-reacting:** substance
**slow virus:** disease
**sludged:** blood
**sluggish:** layer
**slurring:** speech
**Sm:** antigen
**small:** artery; canal; pancreas; pelvis; trochanter; vein
**small cardiac:** vein
**small deep petrosal:** nerve
**small increment sensitivity:** index
**small pudendal:** lip
**small red:** kidney
**small saphenous:** vein
**small sciatic:** nerve
**smaller:** muscle
**smaller white:** snakeroot
**smallest cardiac:** vein
**smallest scalene:** muscle
**smallest splanchnic:** nerve
**smallpox:** vaccine; virus
**smear:** culture; test
**smell:** brain
**smelling:** salt

smoker's: patch; tongue
smoker's respiratory: syndrome
smooth: broach; chorion; colony; diet; leprosy; muscle
smooth muscle: relaxant; tissue
smooth muscular: sphincter
smooth-surfaced cytoplasmic: reticulum
smudge: cell
SNA: angle
snaggle-: tooth
snail: fever
snap: attachment; finger
snapping: hip; reflex
sneezing: gas
snout: reflex
snow: blindness; conjunctivitis
snowball: opacity
soap: cyst
soapsuds: enema
social: adaptation; control; deviance; disease; instinct; intelligence; maladjustment; psychiatry; therapy
social network: therapy
socialized: medicine
socio-experiential: method
sociometric: distance
socket: joint
socotrine: aloe
sodium: pump
sodium-responsive periodic: paralysis
soft: cataract; chancre; corn; diet; gold; palate; papilloma; part; pulse; ray; soap; sore; sulfur; tubercle; ulcer; wart; water
soil: disease
solar: blindness; cauterization; dermatitis; energy; fever; ganglion; keratosis; plexus; retinopathy; therapy; treatment; urticaria
soldier's: heart; patch
sole: nucleus; plate; reflex
sole-plate: ending
sole tap: reflex
solid: angle; edema; hidradenoma
solitary: bundle; follicle; foramen; gland; nodule; tapeworm; tract
solitary bone: cyst
solitary osteocartilaginous: exostosis
soluble: glass, ligature; ribonucleic acid; soap, starch; tartar
soluble gum: cotton
soluble specific: substance
solution: pressure
solvent: drag; ether; inhalation
somatic: agglutinin; antigen; artery; cell; death; delusion; layer; mesoderm; mitosis; mutation; nerve; nucleus; reproduction; teniasis
somatic motor: neuron; nucleus
somatic mutation: theory
somatic sensory: cortex
somatotropic: hormone
somatotropin release-inhibiting: factor
somatotropin-releasing: factor
somesthetic: area; system
somite: cavity
somnambulic: epilepsy
somnambulistic: trance
sonic: vibration; wave
sonomotor: response
sonorous: rale

soot: wart
sore: head; mouth; shin; throat
sore mouth: virus
soul: pain
sour-milk: diet
South African genetic: porphyria
South African tick-bite: fever
South American: blastomycosis; trypanosomiasis
space: capsule; maintainer; medicine; nerve; retainer; sense; simulator; suit
spaced: teeth (see tooth)
spade: finger; hand
spagiric: medicine
spallation: product
Spanish: fly
sparing: action
spasmodic: apoplexy; asthma; diathesis; dysmenorrhea; mydriasis; rabies; stricture; tic; torticollis
spasmophilic: diathesis
spastic: abasia; anemia; aphonia; diplegia; gait; hemiplegia; ileus; miosis; mydriasis; paraplegia; speech; syndrome
spastic flat: foot
spastic spinal: paralysis
spatial: formula; localization; vector; vectorcardiography
spatula: needle
special: anatomy; hospital; nurse; nursing; sensation; sense
special somatic afferent: column
special visceral efferent: column; nucleus
specialized: transduction
species: tolerance
species-specific: antigen
specific: absorbance; action; activity; anergy; antiserum; antigen; bactericide; cause; cholinesterase; compliance; disease; epithet; extinction; gravity; heat; hemolysin; immunity; opsonin; parasite; protein; reaction; rotation; serum; therapeutics; therapy; transduction; treatment; urethritis
specific absorption: coefficient
specific active: immunity
specific capsular: substance
specific dynamic: action
specific innate: immunity
specific soluble: polysaccharide; sugar
spectacle: eye
spectral: phonocardiograph
spectrophotometric: analysis
spectroscopic: analysis
specular: image
speculum: forceps
speech: audiogram; center
speeding: electron
sperm: aster; cell; crystal; nucleus
spermatic: cord; duct; filament; fistula; plexus
sphagnum: moss
sphenoethmoidal: recess; suture
sphenofrontal: suture
sphenoid: angle; bone; crest; process
sphenoidal: border; fissure; fontanel; herniation; sinus
sphenoidal turbinated: bone
sphenomandibular: ligament
sphenomaxillary: fissure; fossa; suture
sphenooccipital: suture

sphenoorbital: suture
sphenopalatine: artery; foramen; ganglion: notch
sphenoparietal: sinus; suture
sphenopetrosal: fissure
sphenosquamous: suture
sphenotic: center; foramen
sphenozygomatic: suture
spherical: aberration; amalgam; lens; nucleus; recess
spherical form of: occlusion
spherocylindrical: lens
spherocytic: anemia; jaundice
spheroid: articulation; colony; joint
spherophakia-brachymorphia: syndrome
sphincter: muscle
sphincteral: achalasia
sphincteroid: tract
sphingomyelin: lipidosis
sphygmic: interval; period
spica: bandage
spider: angioma; cancer; cell; finger; mole; nevus; pelvis; telangiectasia
spike: potential
spike and wave: complex
spinach: stool
spinal: acuology; analgesia; anesthesia; anesthetic; angiography; apoplexy; arteriography; ataxia; atrophy; canal; caries; column; concussion; cord; curvature; decompression; fusion; ganglion; headache; hypotension; induction; marrow; muscle; nerve; nucleus; paralysis; point; puncture; pyramidotomy; quotient; reflex; root; sign; tap; tract; tractotomy; vein
spindle: cataract; cell; fiber
spindle cell: carcinoma; nevus; sarcoma
spindle-celled: layer
spindle-shaped: muscle
spine: cell; sign
spinning: disk
spinning disk: nebulizer
spino-adductor: reflex
spinocerebellar: tract
spinoglenoid: ligament
spinoolivary: tract
spinotectal: tract
spinothalamic: tract; tractotomy
spinous: layer; process
spiral: artery; bandage; crest; canal; fold; fracture; ganglion; groove; hypha; joint; ligament; line; membrane; organ; plate; suture; tubule; valve; vein
spiral foraminous: tract
spiral reverse: bandage
spirillar: dysentery
spirillum: fever
spirit: lamp
spirituous: liquor
spiro-: index
spirochetal: icterus
spironolactone: test
spiruroid: larva migrans
splanchnesthetic: sensibility
splanchnic: anesthesia; cavity; ganglion; layer; mesoderm; nerve; wall
splay-: foot
spleen: deoxyribonuclease; endonuclease; phosphodiesterase

splenial: gyrus
splenic: anemia; apoplexy; artery; cell; cord; corpuscle; fever; flexure; index; leukemia; plexus; pulp; recess; sinus; vein
splenic flexure: syndrome
splenic lymph: follicle
splenic portal: venography
splenius: muscle
splenomedullary: leukemia
splenomyelogenous: leukemia
splenorenal: shunt
splint: bone
splinter: hemorrhage
splintered: fracture
split: foot; hand; parturition; pelvis; personality; papule; tolerance
split cast: method; mounting
split-thickness: graft
splitting: enzyme
spodogenous: splenomegaly
Spondweni: virus
spondyloepiphysial: dysplasia
spondylolisthetic: pelvis
spong: biopsy; graft; tent
spongiform: pustule
spongiose: part
spongy: body; bone; degeneration; iritis; polyp; spot; urethra
spontaneous: abortion; agglutination; amputation; combustion; evolution; fracture; gangrene; generation; phagocytosis; pneumothorax; recovery; remission; version
spoon: nail
sporadic: disease
sporotrichositic: chancre
spot-film: roentgenography
spotted: fever; sickness
spotted-fever: tick
sprain: fracture
spread: foot
spreading: depression; factor
spring: conjunctivitis; finger; lancet; ligament; ophthalmia
spurious: ankylosis; cast; meningocele; pregnancy; torticollis
sputum: smear
squamocolumnar: junction
squamomastoid: suture
squamoparietal: suture
squamotympanic: fissure
squamous: cell; margin; metaplasia; pearl; suture
squamous cell: carcinoma
square: knot
square wave: stimulus
squatting: facet
squint: angle; hook
squinting: eye
squirrel plague: conjunctivitis
S-T: junction; segment
St.: see also Saint
St. Louis encephalitis: virus
stab: cell; culture; drain; neutrophil; wound
stabilized: baseplate
stable: colloid; factor; fly; isotope
staccato: speech
staff: cell
staff of: Aesculapius
Staffordshire: knot

stag-horn: calculus
stagnant: anoxia
stagnation: mastitis
stainless: steel
staircase: phenomenon
stalked: hydatid
stammering of: bladder
standard: cell; deviation; lead; pressure; score; solution; temperature; volume
standard error of: difference; mean
standard urea: clearance
standby pulse: generator
standing: test
stapedial: artery; fold
stapedius: muscle
stapes: mobilization
stapes mobilization: operation
staphylococcal: enterotoxin; pneumonia
staphylococcus: antitoxin; vaccine
staphylococcus food: poisoning
staphylo-opsonic: index
starch: endophthalmitis; equivalent; glycerite; gum; sugar
startle: reaction; reflex
starvation: diabetes
stasis: cirrhosis; dermatitis; eczema; ulcer
state: hospital; medicine
static: arthropathy; ataxia; compliance; convulsion; gangrene; hysteresis; infantilism; medicine; perimetry; reflex; refraction; relation; scoliosis; sense; system; tremor
station: hospital; test
stationary: cataract; phase
statistical: genetics
statoconial: membrane
statokinetic: reflex
statotonic: reflex
stave of: thumb
stay: knot
steady: state
steal: phenomenon
steam: cauterization; cautery
steam-fitter's: asthma
steel-grinder's: disease
steeple: skull
stellate: abscess; block; cataract; cell; fracture; ganglion; hair; ligament; reticulum; retinopathy; vein; venule
stellate skull: fracture
stem: bronchus; cell
stem cell: leukemia
stenopeic, stenopaic: disk; iridectomy; spectacles
stenosal: murmur
steppage: gait
stepping: reflex
stercoraceous: vomiting
stercoral: abscess; appendicitis; fistula; ulcer
sterculia: gum
stereochemical: formula; isomerism
stereoscopic: microscope; parallax; pelvimetry; vision
stereotactic, stereotaxic: instrument; surgery
sterile: abscess; cyst
sterilized surgical: catgut
sternal: angle; artery; bar; cartilage; joint; line; membrane; muscle; notch; part; plane; puncture; synchondrosis

sternal articular: surface
sternobrachial: reflex
sternochondroscapular: muscle
sternoclavicular: angle; disk; joint; ligament; muscle
sternocleidomastoid: muscle; region; vein
sternocostal: articulation; joint; ligament; part; surface; triangle
sternohyoid: muscle
sternomastoid: artery
sternopericardial: ligament
sternothyroid: muscle
steroid: diabetes; fever; hormone
steroid metabolic clearance: rate
steroid production: rate
steroid secretory: rate
steroid withdrawal: syndrome
stethoscopic: phonocardiograph
stichochrome: cell
sticktight: flea
stiff: neck; pupil; sickness; toe
stiff lamb: disease
stiff-man: syndrome
stiffneck: fever
stifle: bone; joint
still: layer
stillborn: infant
stimulus: control; generalization; substitution; threshold
stippled: epiphysis; tongue
stitch: abscess
Stobo: antigen
stock: culture; strain; vaccine
stocking: anesthesia
stoker's: cramp
stomach: ache; cough; drops; pump; reefing; tooth; tube; worm
stomal: ulcer
stomatognathic: system
stone: asthma; mole
stone-cutter's: phthisis
stone-mason's: disease
stop-: needle; speculum
storage: disease
strabismic: amblyopia
straboscopic: disk
straddling (riding): embolus
straight: gyrus; muscle; part; sinus; tubule; venule
straight back: syndrome
strain: fracture; gauge
strait: jacket
strangulated: hernia
strap: cell; muscle
Stratford: virus
stratified: epithelium; thrombus
stratified ciliated columnar: epithelium
straitified squamous: epithelium
stratiform: fibrocartilage
stratographic: adsorption; analysis
straw: itch
straw-bed: itch
strawberry: birthmark; gallbladder; mark; nevus; tongue
strawberry-cream: blood
streak: culture; hyperostosis
streaming: movement
street: virus
street virus: rabies
strength-duration: curve
streptococcal: pneumonia

streptococcus erythrogenic: toxin
Streptococcus M: antigen
streptomycin: unit
stress: fracture; immunity; pseudodiabetes; reaction; ulcer
stress-bearing: area
stress-strain: curve
stretch: receptor; reflex
striate: area; atrophy; body; keratopathy; vein
striated: border; membrane; muscle
striated muscular: sphincter
string: galvanometer; test
stringed instrument: theory
strip: area
stripped: atom
stripper's: asthma
stroboscopic: disk; microscope
stroke: output; volume
stroma: plexus
stromal: endometriosis
structural: formula; gene; isomerism
strumous: abscess
stuck: finger
student: nurse
student's: aneurysm
study: cast; model
stump: foot; hallucination; neuralgia
stuttering: urination
Stuttgart: disease
styloglossus: muscle
stylohyoid: ligament; muscle
styloid: cornu; process
stylomandibular: ligament
stylomastoid: artery; foramen; vein
stylomaxillary: ligament
stylopharyngeal: muscle
styloradial: reflex
stylus: tracing
stypic: collodion; colloid; cotton
subacromial: bursa; bursitis
subacute: abscess; disease; glomerulonephritis; hepatitis; inflammation; nephritis; rheumatism
subacute combined: degeneration
subacute granulomatous: thyroiditis
subacute inclusion body: encephalitis
subacute necrotizing: myelitis
subacute sclerosing: leukoencephalitis; panencephalitis
subadventitial: fibrosis
subanconeus: muscle
subaortic: stenosis
subapical: segment
subarachnoid: anesthesia; cistern; cavity; hemorrhage; space
subarcuate: fossa
subastragalar: amputation
subcallosal: area; fasciculus; gyrus
subcapital: fracture
subcapsular: cataract
subcecal: fossa
subchorial: lake; space
subchronic: disease
subclavian: artery; groove; loop; muscle; nerve; plexus; steal; triangle; trunk; vein
subclavian steal: syndrome
subclinical: diabetes
subcommissural: organ
subconscious: memory
subcorneal pustular: dermatitis; dermatosis

subcostal: artery; groove; line; muscle; nerve; plane
subcranial: abscess
subcrepitant: rale
subcrestal: pocket
subcrural: muscle
subcutaneous: emphysema; myiasis; operation; part; ring; saw; tissue; transfusion; vein; wound
subcutaneous fat: necrosis
subcutaneous infrapatellar: bursa
subcuticular: suture
subdeltoid: bursa; bursitis
subdiaphragmatic: abscess; pyopneumothorax
subdigastric: node
subdural: abscess; cavity; empyema; hematoma; hemorrhage; hygroma; space
subendocardial myocardial: infarction
subendothelial: layer
subenergetic: phonation
subepidermal: abscess
subgaleal: abscess; emphysema; hemorrhage
subgerminal: cavity
subgingival: calculus; curettage; space
subhepatic: abscess; recess
subhyoid: bursa
subinguinal: fossa; triangle
subjective: fremitus; psychology; sensation; sign; symptom; vision
sublenticular: limb
subleukemic: leukemia; myelosis
sublimed: sulfur
subliminal: self; stimulus
sublingual: artery; crescent; cyst; fold; fossa; ganglion; gland; nerve; pit; tablet; vein
submammary: mastitis
submandibular: duct; fossa; ganglion; gland; triangle
submandibular lymph: node
submaxillary: duct; fossa; ganglion; gland; triangle
submental: artery; triangle; vein
submental lymph: node
submental vertex: roentgenogram
submerged: tonsil
submetacentric: chromosome
submucosal: implant; plexus
subnasal: point
subneural: apparatus
suboccipital: decompression; nerve; neuralgia; neuritis; triangle
suboccipital venous: plexus
suboccluding: ligature
subocclusal: surface
subpapillary: layer; network
subparietal: sulcus
subpellicular: fibril; microtubule
subpelvic: tendon
subperiosteal: amputation; fracture; implant
subperitoneal: appendicitis; fascia
subphrenic: abscess; recess
subpopliteal: recess
subpubic: angle
subquadricipital: muscle
subsartorial: canal
subscapular: artery; bursa; fossa; muscle; nerve
subscapular lymph: node
subserous: plexus

substantive: emphysema
substernal: goiter; struma
substitution: compound; product; therapy; transfusion
substitutive: therapy
substrate: mycelium
subsuperior: segment
subsurface: cisterna
subsynovial: cyst
subtaler: joint
subtemporal: decompression
subthalamic: nucleus
subthreshold: stimulus
subtotal: hysterectomy
subungual: abscess; melanoma
subvalvular: stenosis
subvocal: speech
succedaneous: dentition; tooth
succenturiate: placenta
successive: contrast
succinic acid: cycle
sucking: cushion; pad; wound
suckling: reflex
suction: cup; ophthalmodynamometer; plate
suctorial: pad
sudanophobic: zone
sudden death: syndrome
sudomotor: fiber
sudoriferous: duct; gland
sudoriparous: abscess
suffocating: gas
suffocative: goiter
sugar: acid; alcohol
sugar of: lead
sugar-coated: spleen
sugar-icing: liver
sugar loaf: shoulder
suggestive: psychotherapy; therapeutics
suicidal: melancholia
suicide: gesture
suicide prevention: center
sulcal: artery
sulcomarginal: tract
sulcular: epithelium
sulcus: chancre
sulfate: water
sulfatide: lipidosis
sulfation: factor
sulfosalicylic acid turbidity: test
sulfur: water
sulfurated: lime; potash
sulfureted: hydrogen
sullen: rabies
summation: beat; gallop
summation of: stimulus
summer: asthma; bronchitis; cell; complaint; diarrhea; disease; itch; prurigo; rash; sore
sump: drain
sun: bath; cauterization; stroke
superciliary: arch; ridge
superenergetic: phonation
superfatted: soap
superficial: angioma; cleavage; ectoderm; fascia; implantation; layer; reflex; tonsillitis; vein
superficial anatomical structures (specific superficial structures are listed under the following): arch; artery; ligament; muscle; nerve; node; plexus; ring; vein; vessel
superficial punctate: keratitis

**superficial pustular:** perifolliculitis
**superficial scalp:** infection
**superimposed:** preeclampsia
**superior:** intelligence; laryngotomy; paraplegia; polioencephalitis; tracheotomy
**superior anatomical structures:** (specific superior structures are listed under the following): angle; area; arteriole; artery; articulation; border; brachium; colliculus; convolution; extremity; fascia; fasciculus; fissure; fold; flexure; fossa; ganglion; gyrus; horn; joint; ligament; limb; line lobe; lobule; margin; muscle; nerve; node; notch; nucleus; olive; part; pedunculus; pit; plexus; pole; process; recess; retinaculum; root; segment; sinus; strait; sulcus; surface; triangle trunk; tubercle; vein; velum; vena; wall
**superior cerebellar artery:** syndrome
**superior hemorrhagic:** polioencephalitis
**superior limbic:** keratoconjunctivitis
**superior mesenteric artery:** syndrome
**superior pulmonary sulcus:** tumor
**superior vena caval:** syndrome
**superiority:** complex
**supernatant:** fluid
**supernormal recovery:** phase
**supernumerary:** organ; placenta
**superolateral:** surface
**supermedial:** margin
**supersaturated:** solution
**supersonic:** ray; syndrome; wave
**supersonic vibration:** technique
**supertemporal:** fissure
**supertraction:** conus
**supination:** reflex
**supinator:** crest; jerk; muscle; reflex
**supinator longus:** reflex
**supine:** position
**supine hypotensive:** syndrome
**supplemental:** air; lobe; ridge
**supplementary:** menstruation
**supplementary motor:** cortex
**supporting:** area; cell; reaction; reflex; treatment
**supportive:** psychotherapy
**suppressed:** menstruation
**suppressor:** mutation
**suppurating:** gingivitis
**suppurative:** appendicitis; arthritis; cerebritis; encephalitis; hepatitis; hyalitis; inflammation; mastitis; necrosis; nephritis; periodontitis; pleurisy; pneumonia; pulpitis; synovitis
**supra-arytenoid:** cartilage
**supra-auricular:** point
**supracallosal:** gyrus
**supracervical:** hysterectomy
**suprachoroid:** layer
**supraclavicular:** fossa; muscle; node; part
**supraclinoid:** aneurysm
**supracondylar:** aneurysm; fracture; process; ridge
**supraduodenal:** artery
**supragingival:** calculus
**supraglenoid:** tubercle
**suprahepatic:** space
**suprahyoid:** gland; muscle

**suprainterparietal:** bone
**supramarginal:** convolution; gyrus
**supramastoid:** crest; fossa
**supramaximal:** stimulus
**suprameatal:** spine; triangle
**supranasal:** point
**supranuclear:** lesion; paralysis
**supraoptic:** commissure; nucleus
**supraopticohypophysial:** tract
**supraorbital:** arch; artery; foramen; nerve; neuralgia; notch; point; reflex; ridge; vein
**suprapatellar:** bursa; reflex
**suprapineal:** recess
**suprapleural:** membrane
**suprapubic:** cystotomy; lithotomy
**suprarenal:** body; capsule; cortex; gland; impression; plexus; vein
**suprarenogenic:** syndrome
**suprascapular:** artery; ligament; nerve; notch; vein
**suprasellar:** cyst
**supraspinatus:** syndrome
**supraspinous:** fossa; ligament; muscle
**suprasternal:** bone; notch; plane; space
**supratonsillar:** tubercle
**supratragic:** tubercle
**supratrochlear:** artery; nerve; vein
**supraumbilical:** reflex
**supravalvular aortic stenosis:** syndrome
**supraventricular:** crest; extrasystole
**supravesical:** fossa
**supravital:** stain
**sural:** artery; nerve
**surface:** analgesia; anatomy; catalysis; cell; demarcation; tension; thermometer
**surface-active:** agent; material
**surface tension:** theory
**surgeon-:** apothecary
**surgeon's:** knot
**surgical:** abdomen; anatomy; anesthesia; aneurysm; diathermy; diphtheria; emphysema; eruption; erysipelas; gut; hospital; kidney; ligation; mask; microscope; neck; orthodontics; pathology; prosthesis; shock; silk; splint; template; treatment; triangle; tuberculosis
**surging:** faradism
**surplus:** field
**survey:** line
**survival:** time
**suspended:** animation; heart
**suspension:** colloid; laryngoscopy; stability
**suspensory:** bandage; ligament; muscle
**sustentacular:** cell; fiber
**sutural:** bone; cataract; ligament
**suture:** joint
**SV, SV40:** virus
**Sw$^a$:** antigen
**swallowing:** reflex; threshold
**swamp:** fever; itch
**swamp fever:** virus
**Swann:** antigen
**sweat:** duct; gland; pore; test
**sweat duct:** adenoma
**sweating:** sickness; stage; test
**Swedish:** gymnastics; movement
**sweet:** balm; birch; fern; orange; precipitate

**sweet clover:** disease; poisoning
**swell-:** foot; head
**swelled:** head
**swim:** bladder
**swimmer's:** itch
**swimming:** test
**swimming pool:** conjunctivitis; granuloma
**swine:** cholera; dysentery; erysipelas; fat; fever; icteroanemia; influenza; pest; plague; pox
**swine edema:** disease
**swine fever:** virus
**swineherd's:** disease
**swinepox:** virus
**Swiss cheese:** endometrium
**Swiss mouse leukemia:** virus
**Swiss type:** agammaglobulinemia
**swordfish:** test
**syllabic:** speech
**sylvatic:** plague
**symbiotic fermentation:** phenomenon
**symmetric, symmetrical:** asphyxia; gangrene
**symmetric distal:** neuropathy
**sympathetic:** agent; amine; blockade; ganglion; hormone; hypertonia; imbalance; iridoplegia; iritis; nerve; ophthalmia; part; plexus; saliva; segment; symptom; trunk; uveitis
**sympathetic formative:** cell
**sympathetic nervous:** system
**sympathetic reflex:** dystrophy
**sympathicotropic:** cell
**sympathizing:** eye
**sympathochromaffin:** cell
**sympatholytic:** agent
**sympathomimetic:** agent; amine
**symphysial:** surface
**symphysic:** teratosis
**symptom:** complex; formation; group; substitution
**symptomatic:** anemia; anthrax; asthma; epilepsy; erythema; fever; headache; impotence; leukemia; nanism; neuralgia; paramyotonia; porphyria; pruritus; reaction; roseola; torticollis; treatment; ulcer
**synaptic:** cleft; conduction; ending; phase; resistance; terminal; trough; vesicle
**synarthrodial:** joint
**synchondrodial:** joint
**synchronous:** reflex
**synclonic:** spasm
**syncytial:** bud; knot; sprout; trophoblast
**syndesmochorial:** placenta
**syndesmodial:** joint
**synergic:** control
**synergistic:** muscle
**syngeneic:** graft; homograft
**synovial:** bursa; cell; chondromatosis; crypt; cyst; fluid; fold; frenulum; frenum; fringe; gland; hernia; joint; ligament; membrane; mesenchyme; sarcoma; sheath; tuft; villus
**synovial trochlear:** bursa
**syntactial:** aphasia
**synthetic:** chemistry
**syntonic:** personality
**syphilitic:** abscess; aneurysm; aortitis; chancre; fever; leukoderma; meningoencephalitis; nephritis; roseola;

tooth; ulcer
**Syriac:** ulcer
**syringomyelic:** dissociation
**system:** disease
**systematic:** anatomy; bacteriology; vertigo
**systematized:** delusion; nevus
**systemic:** anaphylaxis; anatomy; circulation; death; desensitization; heart; lupus (erythematosus); myelitis
**systolic:** click; gallop; gradient; honk; murmur; pressure; shock; thrill; whoop
**systolic time:** interval

### T

**T:** agglutinogen; antigen; bandage; cell; coliphage; enzyme; group; lymphocyte; Mycoplasma; phage; splint; system; tube; tubule; wave
**t:** test
**T₃:** toxicosis
**T₃ uptake:** test
**T-even:** phage
**T.A.B.:** vaccine
**tabby-cat:** striation
**tabetic:** arthropathy; crisis; cuirass; dissociation; osteoarthropathy
**tablet:** triturate
**Tacaribe:** virus
**tactile:** agnosia; amnesia; anesthesia; cell; corpuscle; disk; elevation; fremitus; hair; hyperesthesia; image; meniscus; papilla; sense
**tagged:** atom
**Tahyna:** virus
**tail:** bone; bud; fold; gut; sheath; vertebra
**tailor's:** bunion; cramp; muscle; spasm
**talar:** sulcus; surface
**talc:** operation; pneumoconiosis
**tallow:** soap
**talocalcaneal, talocalcanean:** joint; ligament
**talocalcaneocentral:** joint
**talocalcaneonavicular:** joint
**talocrural:** articulation
**talonavicular:** ligament
**tambour:** sound
**tampan:** tick
**tangent:** plane
**tangential:** wound
**Tangier:** disease
**tanned red:** cell
**tanner's:** ulcer
**tapetal light:** reflex
**tapetoretinal:** degeneration
**tapeworm:** anemia
**tapir:** mouth
**tar:** acne; camphor
**tarbagan:** plague
**tardive:** cyanosis
**tardive oral:** dyskinesia
**tardy:** epilepsy
**target:** behavior; cell; gland; organ; patient; response
**target cell:** anemia
**tarry:** cyst
**tarsal:** arch; asthenopia; bone; canal; cartilage; cyst; gland; joint; ligament; plate; sinus

**tarsal tunnel:** syndrome
**tarsocrural:** joint
**tarsometatarsal:** joint; ligament
**tarsophalangeal:** reflex
**tarsotibial:** amputation
**tart:** cell
**Tartar:** type
**tartrated:** antimony
**task-oriented:** group
**taste:** blindness; bud; bulb; cell; corpuscle; deficiency; hair; organ; pore; ridge
**tautomeric:** fiber
**teacher's:** node
**TEAE-:** cellulose
**tear:** gas; sac; stone
**teardrop:** fracture; heart
**tectobulbar:** tract
**tectonic:** keratoplasty
**tectopontine:** tract
**tectorial:** membrane
**tectospinal:** decussation; tract
**tegmental:** decussation; field; syndrome; wall
**telangiectatic:** angioma; cancer; cystosarcoma; fibroma; fibromyoma; lipoma; wart
**telegrapher's:** cramp
**telencephalic:** flexure; vesicle
**telephone:** theory
**telephonic:** probe
**teleradium:** therapy
**telescopic:** denture
**television:** microscope
**telocentric:** chromosome
**telolecithal:** egg; ovum
**temperate:** bacteriophage; bath
**temperature:** coefficient; sense; spot
**template:** ribonucleic acid
**temporal:** aponeurosis; apophysis; arteritis; bone; canal; dispersion; fascia; fissure; fossa; fovea; horn; line; lobe; muscle; plane; pole; process; region; ridge; surface; vein; venule
**temporal lobe:** epilepsy
**temporary:** base; callus; cartilage; denture; filling; leukemia; parasite; stricture; tooth
**temporofrontal:** tract
**temporomandibular:** arthrosis; articulation; joint; ligament; nerve; syndrome
**temporomandibular joint pain-dysfunction:** syndrome
**temporomaxillary:** vein
**temporoparietal:** muscle
**temporopontine:** tract
**temporozygomatic:** suture
**tenaculum:** forceps
**tender:** line; point; zone
**tendinous:** arch; cord; inscription; spot; synovitis
**tendo achillis:** reflex
**tendon:** advancement; bundle; cell; graft; recession; reflex; suture; transplantation
**tendon sheath:** syndrome
**tennis:** elbow; leg; thumb
**tense:** part; pulse
**tensile:** strength; stress
**tension:** cavity; curve; headache; pneumothorax; suture
**tensor:** muscle
**tenth cranial:** nerve

**tentorial:** angle; nerve; sinus
**tepid:** bath
**teratoid:** tumor
**teratomatous:** cyst
**teres major:** muscle
**teres minor:** muscle
**term:** infant
**terminal:** artery; bar; bouton; bronchiole; cisterna; crest; dementia; endocarditis; filum; ganglion; hair; ileitis; ileus; infection; leukocytosis; notch; nerve; nucleus; plate; pneumonia; sinus; stria; sulcus; thread; vein; ventricle; web
**terminal jaw relation:** record
**terminal nerve:** corpuscle
**termino-terminal:** anastomosis
**ternary:** acid; alloy; complex; compound
**terrain:** cure; treatment
**tertian:** fever; malaria; parasite
**tertiary:** alcohol; amputation; cortex; syphilid; syphilis; villus; vitreous
**tertiary medical:** care
**Teschen:** disease
**Teschen disease:** virus
**tesselated:** epithelium; fundus
**test:** meal; object; paper; solution; skein; tube; type
**test handle:** instrument
**test-retest:** reliability
**testicular:** artery; cord; duct; fluid; hormone; plexus; vein
**testicular feminization:** syndrome
**testicular tubular:** adenoma
**testis:** cord
**testoid:** hyperthecosis
**tetanic:** contraction; convulsion
**tetanoid:** chorea; paraplegia
**tetanus:** antitoxin; vaccine
**tetanus and gas gangrene:** antitoxin
**tetanus immune:** globulin
**tentanus-perfringens:** antitoxin
**tetany:** cataract
**tetracyclic:** steroid
**tetraethyl:** lead; poisoning
**Texas:** snakeroot
**Texas cattle:** fever
**Texas fever cattle:** tick
**text:** blindness
**TG:** virus
**thalamic:** animal; brain; epilepsy; syndrome; tenia
**thalamoolivary:** tract
**thalamostriate:** vein
**thallium:** poisoning
**thanatophoric:** dwarfism
**theater:** nurse; sister
**theca:** cell
**theca cell:** tumor
**theca interna:** cone
**theca-lutein:** cell
**thecal:** abscess; cyst; whitlow
**thematic:** paralogia; paraphasia
**thematic apperception:** test
**thenar:** eminence; prominence; space
**therapeutic:** abortion; agent; alliance; anesthesia; community; carbon; crisis; electrode; fever; group; incompatibility; index; iridectomy; nihilism; optimism; pessimism; pneumothorax; ratio
**therapeutic ratio of:** dose

thermal: analysis; anesthesia; burn; capacity; sense; spectrum
thermic: anesthesia; fever; sense
thermodynamic: potential; theory
thermoelectric: pile
thermogenic: action
thermolabile: opsonin
thermoluminescence: dosimetry
thermometer: scale
thermoprecipitin: reaction
thermostable opsonin: test
theta: rhythm; wave
thiamin hydrochloride: unit
thiazide: diabetes
thick-split: graft
thigh: bone; joint
thin-layer: chromatography; electrophoresis
thinking: compulsion
thiochrome: method
thioclastic: cleavage
thiocyanogen: number
thioridazine: retinopathy
third: corpuscle; disease; eyelid; finger; molar; ovary; tonsil; trochanter; ventricle; ventriculostomy
third and fourth pharyngeal pouch: syndrome
third cranial: nerve
third cuneiform: bone
third occipital: nerve
third order: receptor
third parallel pelvic: plane
third party: medicine
third peroneal: muscle
third sacral: nerve
third stage of: labor
third temporal: convolution
thirst: cure; enema; fever
thoracic: axis; cage; cavity; choke; duct; fistula; ganglion; girdle; gland; goiter; index; limb; nerve; nucleus; part; respiration; spine; stomach; vertebra; vein; wall
thoracic aortic: plexus
thoracic cardiac: nerve
thoracic interspinal: muscle
thoracic intertransverse: muscle
thoracic outlet: syndrome
thoracic rotator: muscle
thoracoacromial: artery; vein
thoracodorsal: artery; nerve
thoracoepigastric: vein
thoracolumbar: aponeurosis; system
thoracolumbar venous: line
thorium: emanation
thorn: apple
thorn apple: crystal
thorny-headed: worm
thought process: disorder
thread: fungus; galvanometer
thready: pulse
threatened: abortion
three-cornered: bone
three-day: fever; measles; sickness
three-dimensional: record
three-glass: test
thresher's: lung
threshold: body; differential; percussion; shift; stimulus; substance
thrombocytic: series
thrombocytopenic: purpura

thrombopathic: syndrome
thrombopenic: purpura
thromboplastic component of: plasma
thrombotic: apoplexy; gangrene; hydrocephalus; microangiopathy; phlegmasia
thrombotic thrombocytopenic: purpura
through: drainage; illumination
through-and-through myocardial: infarction
thrush: fungus
thumb: forceps; lancet; reflex
thunder: disease; humor
thyme: camphor
thymergastic: reaction
thymic: abscess; alymphoplasia; factor; stridor; vein
thymol turbidity: test
thymotrophic: hormone
thymus: corpuscle; gland
thymus-dependent: zone
thyroarytenoid: muscle
thyrocardiac: disease
thyroepiglottic: ligament; muscle
thyroglossal: diverticulum; duct
thyroglossal duct: cyst
thyrohyoid: ligament; membrane; muscle
thyrohypophysial: syndrome
thyroid: axis; body; bruit; cartilage; colloid; crisis; diverticulum; eminence; follicle; foramen; gland; hormone; insufficiency; storm; therapy; vein
thyroid-stimulating hormone: test
thyroidal articular: surface
thyrolingual: cyst; duct
thyropharyngeal: part
thyrotoxic: coma; crisis; encephalopathy; myopathy; serum
thyrotoxic complement-fixation: factor
thyrotropic: hormone
thyrotropin-releasing: factor
thyroxine-binding: globulin; prealbumin; protein
tibial: border; crest; nerve; phenomenon; surface
tibial collateral: ligament
tibial communicating: nerve
tibial intertendinous: bursa
tibiocalcaneal: part
tibiofemoral: index
tibiofibular: articulation; joint; ligament
tibionavicular: ligament; part
tic-tac: rhythm; sound
tick: fever; paralysis; typhus
tick-borne: encephalitis
tidal: air; drainage; respiration; volume; wave
tiger: heart
tigroid: body; fundus; mass; retina; striation; substance
tilt: table
time: characteristic; constant; marker; sense
time-zone: syndrome
tin-: foil
tine: test
tinted denture: base
tip: foot
tissue: adhesive; basophil; culture; displaceability; displacement; fluid;

lymph; molding; registration; respiration; tension; thromboplastin
tissue-bearing: area
tissue-specific: antigen
Tj: antigen
TO: virus
to-and-fro: anesthesia; murmur
toasted: shin
tobacco: heart
Tobruk: splint
toe: clonus; itch; phenomenon; reflex
toilet: training
tolerance: dose
Tolu: balsam
tone: color
tone decay: test
tongue: bone; depressor; phenomenon; traction; worm
tonic: contraction; control; convulsion; epilepsy; pupil; reflex; spasm; treatment
tonoclonic: spasm
tonsil: position
tonsillar: calculus; crypt; fossa; herniation; ring
tonsillolingual: sulcus
tooth: abrasion; avulsion; band; bud; cement; cough; form; germ; ligation; migration; plane; polyp; pulp; rash; sac; socket; spasm; transplantation
tooth-and-nail: syndrome
tooth-borne: base
toothed: vertebra
toper's: nose
tophaceous: gout
topical: anesthesia
topographic: anatomy; diagnosis
toric: lens
tornado: epilepsy
torsion: forceps; fracture; neurosis; spasm
torsional: deformity
torsive: occlusion
torus: fracture
total: acidity; albinism; aphasia; biopsy; cataract; elasticity; energy; excision; hyperopia; necrosis; symblepharon; synechia
total body: hypothermia
total catecholamine: test
total lung: capacity
total pelvic: exenteration
total peripheral: resistance
total push: therapy
total refractory: period
total spinal: anesthesia
totipotent: cell
totipotential: protoplasm
touch: cell; corpuscle
tourniquet: poditis; test
tow-glass: test
tower: skull
toxemic: jaundice; retinopathy
toxic: amaurosis; amblyopia; anemia; cataract; cirrhosis; cyanosis; delirium; dementia; equivalent; goiter; hemoglobinuria; hydrocephalus; insanity; megacolon; nephrosis; neuritis; psychosis; tetanus; unit
toxic epidermal: necrolysis
toxicogenic: conjunctivitis
toxin: spectrum

**TPI:** test
**Tr<sup>a</sup>:** antigen
**trabecular:** bone; meshwork; network; zone
**trace:** conditioning; element
**trace conditioned:** reflex
**tracheal:** cartilage; fenestration; fistula; gland; node; pain; ring; triangle; tugging; ulceration; vein
**trachelobregmatic:** diameter
**tracheloclavicular:** muscle
**tracheobiliary:** fistula
**tracheobronchial:** dyskinesia; groove
**tracheobronchial lymph:** node
**tracheoesophageal:** fistula
**tracheotomy:** hook; tube
**trachoma:** body; forceps; gland; virus
**trachomatous:** conjunctivitis; keratitis
**traction:** aneurysm; atrophy; diverticulum; epiphysis; fiber
**trained:** nurse; reflex
**training:** analysis; group
**trainwheel:** rhythm
**transactional:** analysis; psychotherapy
**Transcaucasian:** fever
**transcellular:** fluid
**transcendental:** anatomy
**transcervical:** fracture
**transcondylar:** fracture
**transcortical:** aphasia; apraxia
**transcranial:** roentgenogram
**transcutan:** bath
**transduodenal:** sphincterotomy
**transfer:** coping; factor; ribonucleic acid
**transference:** neurosis
**transferred:** ophthalmia; sensation
**transferring:** enzyme
**transfixion:** suture
**transformed:** lymphocyte
**transforming:** agent; factor
**transfusion:** hepatitis; nephritis
**transient:** agammaglobulinemia; albuminuria; hypertension
**transient ischemic:** attack
**transition:** mutation; ray
**transitional:** cell; convolution; denture; epithelium; gyrus; leukocyte; zone
**transitional cell:** carcinoma; papilloma
**transitory:** mania
**translatory:** movement
**translocation:** carrier; mongol
**translocation of:** chromosome
**translumbar:** aortography
**transmembrane:** potential
**transmethylation:** factor
**transmissible:** enteritis; gastroenteritis
**transmissible gastroenteritis:** virus
**transmissible venereal:** tumor
**transmitted:** light
**transmitter:** substance
**transmural:** pressure
**transmural myocardial:** infarction
**transneuronal:** atrophy
**transorbital:** leukotomy; lobotomy
**transosseous:** venography
**transovarial:** transmission
**transparent:** septum
**transparent corneal:** ulcer
**transplant lung:** syndrome
**transplantation:** metastasis
**transporionic:** axis
**transport:** host; maximum; number; tetany

**transpulmonary:** pressure
**transpyloric:** plane
**transsexual:** surgery
**transsynaptic:** chromatolysis; degeneration
**transthoracic:** pressure
**transureteroureteral:** anastomosis
**transurethral:** resection
**transverse:** amputation; fracture; hermaphroditism; lie; myelitis; plane; presentation; test
**transverse anatomical structures** (specific transverse structure are listed under the following): arch; artery; articulation; colon; convolution; crest; diameter; disk; ductule; fasciculus; fiber; fissure; fold; foramen; fornix; gyrus; joint; ligament; muscle; nerve; part; plane; process; ridge; septum; sinus; sulcus; suture; vein
**transverse facial:** fracture
**transversion:** mutation
**transversovertical:** index
**trapezium:** bone
**trapezius:** muscle
**trapezoid:** body; bone; ligament; line; ridge
**trapped:** placenta
**traumatic:** amnesia; amputation; anemia; anesthesia; aneurysm; asphyxia; cataract; dermatitis; encephalopathy; fever; gastritis; hysteria; idiocy; meningocele; neurasthenia; neuritis; neuroma; neurosis; occlusion; orchitis; pneumonia; psychosis; spondylopathy; tetanus
**traumatic cervical:** discopathy
**traumatic progressive:** encephalopathy
**traumatogenic:** occlusion
**traumatopneic:** wound
**traveler's:** diarrhea
**treatment:** denture
**trefoil:** dermatitis; tendon
**trembling:** disease
**tremulous:** iris
**trench:** fever; foot; hand; leg; lung; mouth; nephritis; shin
**trephine:** biopsy
**treponema-immobilizing:** antibody
**Treponema pallidum immobilization:** reaction; test
**treponemal:** antibody
**triadic:** symbiosis
**trial:** base; case; denture; frame; lens; plate
**triangular:** bandage; bone; cartilage; crest; disk; fold; fossa; lamella; ligament; recess; ridge
**triangularity of:** tooth
**triaxial reference:** system
**tribasilar:** synostosis
**TRIC:** agent
**tricarboxylic acid:** cycle
**triceps:** muscle; reflex
**triceps surae:** reflex
**trichilemmal:** cyst
**trichina:** worm
**trichorhinophalangeal:** syndrome
**trichrome:** stain
**tricuspid:** area; atresia; incompetence; insufficiency; murmur; orifice; stenosis; tooth; valve
**trident:** hands

**trifacial:** nerve; neuralgia
**trifid:** stomach
**trifocal:** lens
**trigeminal:** cavity; cough; crest; decompression; ganglion; impression; lemniscus; nerve; neuralgia; pulse; rhizotomy; rhythm; tractotomy
**trigeminofacial:** reflex
**trigger:** action; area; finger; point; zone
**trihydric:** alcohol
**triiodothyronine:** toxicosis
**triiodothyronine uptake:** test
**triketohydrindene:** reaction
**trilaminar:** blastoderm
**trimalleolar:** fracture
**Trinidad:** disease
**triphammer:** pulse
**triphyllomatous:** teratoma
**triplant:** implant
**triple:** bond; phosphate; quartan; response; rhythm; vision
**triple symptom:** complex
**triplet:** monster; state
**triquetral:** bone
**triquetrous:** cartilage
**trisomy 13:** syndrome
**trisomy 13–15:** syndrome
**trisomy17:** syndrome
**trisomy 17–18:** syndrome
**trisomy 18:** syndrome
**trisomy 21:** syndrome
**trisomy D:** syndrome
**trisomy D$_1$:** syndrome
**trisomy E:** syndrome
**trisomy E$_1$:** syndrome
**tritiated:** thymidine
**Trivittatus:** virus
**trochanter:** reflex
**trochanteric:** bursa; bursitis; crest; fossa; syndrome
**trochlear:** fossa; nerve; notch; nucleus; pit; process; spine
**trochlear synovial:** bursa
**trochoid:** articulation; joint
**trophic:** change; fracture; gangrene; hormone; nucleus; ulcer
**trophoblastic:** lacuna; operculum
**trophoneurotic:** anemia; atrophy; leprosy
**trophotropic:** zone
**tropic:** hormone
**tropical:** abscess; anemia; boil; chlorosis; diarrhea; eczema; eosinophilia; lichen; liver; mask; measles; medicine; myositis; neurasthenia; pyomyositis; sore; splenomegaly; sprue; typhus; ulcer
**tropical horse:** tick
**true:** albuminuria; aneurysm; ankylosis; chancre; cholinesterase; conjugate; diverticulum; dwarf; glottis; hermaphroditism; hypertrophy; knot; mole; pelvis; reversion; rib; thirst; vertebra
**truncate:** ascertainment
**truth:** serum
**trypanosomal:** meningoencephalitis
**trypanosome:** fever; stage
**tsetse:** fly
**TSH:** test
**tsutsugamushi:** disease; fever
**tubal:** abortion; cartilage; colic; dysmenorrhea; extremity; infantilism; insuf-

flation; pregancy; tonsil
**tubal air:** cell
**tube:** cast; tooth
**tubed pedicle:** flap
**tuberal:** nucleus
**tubercle:** bacillus
**tubercular:** syphilid
**tuberculin:** test
**tuberculoid:** leprosy
**tuberculo-opsonic:** index
**tuberculosis:** vaccine
**tuberculous:** abscess; bronchopneumonia; meningitis; nephritis; peritonitis; polyarthritis; rheumatism; scrofuloderma; spondylitis; wart
**tuberoinfundibular:** tract
**tuberosity:** reduction
**tuberous:** root; sclerosis
**tuboabdominal:** pregnancy
**tubo-ovarian:** abscess; pregnancy
**tubotympanic:** canal; recess
**tubouterine:** pregnancy
**tubular:** adenoma; aneurysm; cyst; degeneration; forceps; gland; hyposthenuria; maximum; respiration; vision
**tubular excretory:** mass
**tubuloacinar:** gland
**tubuloalveolar:** gland
**tufted:** phalanx
**tularemic:** chancre; conjunctivitis; pneumonia
**tumor:** embolus; virus
**tuning:** fork
**tunnel:** anemia; cell; disease; vision
**turban:** tumor
**turbinal:** varix
**turbinated:** body; bone; crest
**turkey-meningoencephalitis:** virus
**Turkish:** bath; manna; saddle
**turpentine:** enema
**tussive:** fremitus
**twelfth cranial:** nerve
**twelfth-year:** molar
**twilight:** blindness; sleep; state; thirst; vision
**twin:** cone; crystal; helix; monster; placenta; pregnancy
**twist:** form
**twisted:** hair
**twisted wire:** worm
**two-dimensional:** chromatography
**two-step exercise:** test
**two-sympathin:** theory
**two-way:** catheter
**tympanic:** antrum; body; bone; canal; cell; cavity; crest; ganglion; gland; groove; incisure; intumescence; lip; membrane; nerve; notch; opening; plate; plexus; promontory; ring; scute; sinus; vein; wall
**tympanitic:** resonance
**tympanohyal:** bone
**tympanomastoid:** fissure; suture
**tympanosquamous:** fissure
**tympanostapedial:** junction
**type:** culture; species; strain
**type 1-4:** dextrocardia
**type 1-6:** glycogenosis
**type I-V familial:** hyperlipoproteinemia
**type I-VII:** mucopolysaccharidosis
**type IS:** mucopolysaccharidosis
**typh:** fever

**typhoid:** bacillus; bacteriophage; cholera; fever; pleurisy; pneumonia; septicemia; spine; vaccine
**typhoid-paratyphoid:** vaccine
**typhus:** fever; vaccine
**typical:** formula; mesolepidoma
**Tzaneen:** disease

## U

**U:** wave
**Uganda S:** virus
**ulcer-preventive:** factor
**ulcerated sore:** throat
**ulcerating pudendal:** granuloma
**ulcerative:** colitis; pulpitis; scrofuloderma; stomatitis
**ulceromembranous:** angina; gingivitis
**ulnar:** artery; bursa; eminence; margin; nerve; notch; reflex; surface; vein
**ulnar collateral:** ligament
**ulnar flexor:** muscle
**uloid:** cicatrix
**ultimate:** principle
**ultimobranchial:** body; pouch
**ultra-:** microscope; virus
**ultrafiltration:** hemodialyzer
**ultrasonic:** cephalometry; cleaning; cutting; lithotresis; microscope; nebulizer; ray; therapy; vibration; wave
**ultrasound:** cardiography
**ultrastructural:** anatomy
**ultraviolet:** lamp; microscope; ray
**ultropaque:** method
**Ulysses:** syndrome
**umbilical:** artery; cord; cyst; duct; fissure; fistula; fossa; fungus; hernia; notch; part; region; ring; souffle; vein; vesicle
**umbilical prevesical:** fascia
**umbilicomammilary:** triangle
**umbilicovesical:** fascia
**Umbre:** virus
**Una:** virus
**unarmed:** tapeworm
**unavoidable:** hemorrhage
**unbalanced:** translocation
**uncal:** herniation
**unciform:** bone; fasciculus; process
**uncinate:** attack; bundle; epilepsy; fasciculus; gyrus; pancreas; process
**uncompensated:** acidosis; alkalosis
**unconditioned:** reflex; response; stimulus
**unconscious:** homosexuality
**uncoupling:** factor
**uncus:** band
**undercut:** gauge
**undermining:** ulcer
**undescended:** testis
**undetermined:** nitrogen
**undifferentiated:** cell
**undulant:** fever
**undulating:** membrane; purse
**unequal:** cleavage
**unerupted:** tooth
**ungual:** phalanx; tuberosity
**uniaxial:** joint
**unicameral:** cyst
**unicameral bone:** cyst
**unicanalicular:** sphincter
**unicellular:** gland; sclerosis

**unicorn:** uterus
**unidirectional:** block; flux
**unilateral:** anesthesia; hemianopsia; hermaphroditism
**unilocular:** cyst; fat; joint
**unilocular hydatid:** cyst
**unimolecular:** reaction
**uninterrupted:** suture
**uniocular:** hemianopsia; strabismus
**uniovular:** twins
**unipennate:** muscle
**unipolar:** cell; electrocardiogram; lead; neuron
**unit:** character; fibril; membrane
**uniting:** canal; cartilage; duct
**univalent:** antibody
**universal:** donor; infantilism; solvent
**universal incomplete:** albinism
**unmyelinated:** fiber
**unpaired:** allosome
**unproductive:** mania
**unresolved:** pneumonia
**unsaturated:** alcohol; compound; fat; fatty acid
**unstable:** colloid; hemoglobin
**unstrained jaw:** relation
**unstriated:** muscle
**unsystematized:** delusion
**ununited:** fracture
**upper:** extremity; eyelid; jaw; lip; lobe
**upper abdominal periosteal:** reflex
**upper lateral cutaneous:** nerve
**upper motor:** neuron
**upper nodal:** extrasystole
**upper uterine:** segment
**ur-:** defense
**urachal:** cyst; fistula; fold; ligament
**uracil:** mustard
**uranium:** nephritis; unit
**urea:** clearance; concentration; cycle; index; nitrogen
**urea clearance:** test
**uremic:** amblyopia; colitis; lung; pericarditis; pneumonia; pneumonitis; polyneuropathy
**ureteral:** meatoscopy; neocystostomy; opening
**ureteric:** bud; dysmenorrhea; fold; plexus
**ureteroileal:** neocystotomy
**ureterorenal:** reflux
**ureterotubal:** anastomosis
**ureteroureteral:** anastomosis
**urethral:** apoplexy; artery; caruncle; crest; fever; gland; groove; hematuria; opening; papilla; plate; suppository; surface; valve
**uric acid:** diathesis; infarct
**uricolytic:** index
**urinary:** apparatus; bladder; calculus; cast; cyst; fever; fistula; nitrogen; reflex; schistosomiasis; smear; stuttering; system; tract
**urinary exertional:** incontinence
**urinary stress:** incontinence
**uriniferous:** tubule
**urinous:** abscess
**urobilin:** jaundice
**urogenital:** canal; diaphragm; fistula; membrane; region; ridge; septum; sinus; system; triangle
**uropoietic:** organ; system

uropygial: gland
urorectal: fold; membrane; septum
urticarial: fever
Uruma: virus
USP: unit
"usual": pseudocholinesterases
uterine: apoplexy; appendage; artery; calculus; colic; dysmenorrhea; extremity; fluid; gland; inertia; insufficiency; mask; milk; part; pregnancy; sinus; sinusoid; souffle; tetanus; tube; tympanites; vein
uterine venous: plexus
uteroabdominal: pregnancy
uteroepichorial: membrane
uteropelvic: obstruction
uterperitoneal: fistula
uteroplacental: sinus
uterosacral: ligament
uterovaginal: canal; plexus
uterovesical: fold; pouch
utilization: time
utricular: nerve; reflex; spot
utriculoampullar: nerve
utriculosaccular: duct
uveal: staphyloma; tract
uveocutaneous: syndrome
uveo-encephalitic: syndrome
uveomeningitis: syndrome
uveoparotid: fever
uviol: lamp
Uzbekistan hemorrhagic: fever

## V

V: antigen; esotropia; exotropia; lead
V-2: carcinoma
vaccine: body; lymph; therapy; virus
vaccinia: lymph; virus
vaccinoid: reaction
vacuolar: degeneration; nephrosis
vacuolating: virus
vacuum: cast; desiccator; extractor; flask; headache; investing; tube
vagabond's: disease
vagal: apnea; attack; trunk
vaginal: artery; atresia; celiotomy; column; dysmenorrhea; hernia; gland; hysterectomy; hysteropexy; hysterotomy; lithotomy; myomectomy; nerve; opening; plug; pool; process; smear; suppository; synovitis
vaginal cornification: test
vaginal mucification: test
vaginal venous: plexus
vagolytic: agent
vagovagal: reflex
vagrant's: disease
vagus: area; nerve; pulse
valence: electron
vallate: papilla
vallecular: dysphagia
valley: fever
valvotomy: knife
valvular: endocarditis; incompetence; insufficiency; pneumothorax; thrombus
vampire: bat
vanillylmandelic acid: test
vanishing: cream
vapor: density; pressure
variable: coupling
varicella: encephalitis

varicella-zoster: virus
varicelloid: smallpox
varicose: aneurysm; eczema; ulcer; vein
variegate: porphyria
variola: virus
varioliform: syphilid
varioloid: varicella
vascular: arch; bud; circle; cone; dentin; fold; headache; hemophilia; keratitis; layer; leiomyoma; murmur; nerve; papilla; plexus; polyp; sclerosis; spider; spur; system; zone
vasculocardiac: syndrome
vasculonebulous: keratitis
vasoformative: cell
vasogenic: shock
vasomotor: ataxia; epilepsy; imbalance; nerve; paralysis; rhinitis; spasm
vasopressin-resistant: diabetes
vasopressor: reflex
vasovagal: attack; epilepsy; syncope; syndrome
VCE: smear
VDRL: test
VE: virus
veal: skin
vector: cardiography; loop
VEE: virus
vegetable: acid; albumin; alkali; base; calomel; charcoal; gelatin; mercury; pathology; sulfur; wax
vegetal: pole
vegetarian: diet
vegetative: bacteriophage; endocarditis; life; mycelium; pole; stage
vegetative nervous: system
veiled: puff
veiling: glare
vein: stone
Vel: antigen
velamentous: insertion
veldt: sore
vellus: hair
velocity: coefficient; constant
velopharyngeal: closure; insufficiency
velvet: ant
Ven: antigen
venereal: bubo; disease; lymphogranuloma; sore; ulcer; wart
Venezuelan equine: encephalitis
Venezuelan equine encephalitis: virus
Venice: turpentine
venom: hemolysis
veno-occlusive: disease
venorespiratory: reflex
venous: angle; artery; blood; calculus; canal; capillary; circle; congestion; duct; embolism; gangrene; groove; heart; hum; hyperemia; insufficiency; lake; ligament; murmur; plexus; pulse; segment; sinus; star; transfusion; valve
venous occlusion: plethysmography
venous-stasis: retinopathy
ventilation: meter
ventral: aorta; column; gland; hernia; horn; mesocardium; nucleus; pancreas; part; plate; root
ventral sacrococcygeal: ligament; muscle
ventral sacroiliac: ligament
ventral spinocerebellar: tract

ventral spinothalamic: tract
ventral splanchnic: artery
ventral thalamic: peduncle
ventricular: aberration; afterload; aneurysm; band; bigeminy; bradycardia; capture; complex; conduction; diverticulum; escape; extrasystole; fibrillation; fluid; flutter; fold; gradient; ligament; loop; plateau; rhythm; septum; standstill; systole; tachycardia
ventricular inhibited pulse: generator
ventricular septal: defect
ventrcular synchronous pulse: generator
ventricular triggered pulse: generator
ventriculoatrial: conduction
ventriculoradial: dysplasia
ventrobasal: nucleus
ventromedial: nucleus
verbal: agraphia; amnesia
vermian: fossa
vermicular: colic; movement; pulse
vermiform: appendage; process
vermilion: border; zone
vermilion transitional: zone
verminous: abscess; aneurysm; appendicitis; bronchitis; ileus
vernal: conjunctivitis; encephalitis; fever
Vernitrol: vaporizer
verruca vulgaris: virus
verrucous: carcinoma; endocarditis; scrofuloderma
vertebra prominens: reflex
vertebral: arch; artery; canal; column; foramen; formula; fusion; ganglion; groove; nerve; notch; part; plexus; polyarthritis; pulp; region; rib; vein; venography
vertebral-basilar: system
vertebral cervical: dislocation; instability; sprain; strain; subluxation
vertebral venous: plexus; system
vertebrated: catheter; probe
vertebroarterial: foramen
vertebrochondral: rib
vertebropelvic: ligament
vertebrosternal: rib
vertex: presentation
vertical: axis; dimension; heart; hymen; illumination; index; muscle; nystagmus; opening; parallax; plate; strabismus; transmission; vein; vertigo
vertical retraction: syndrome
vesanic: type
vesical: calculus; diverticulum; fistula; gland; hematuria; plexus; reflex; surface; triangle
vesicating: gas
vesicocelomic: drainage
vesicocolic: fistula
vesicointestinal: fistula
vesicoumbilical: ligament
vesicoureteral: reflux; valve
vesicourethral: canal
vesicouterine: ligament; pouch
vesicovaginal: fistula
vesicovaginorectal: fistula
vesicular: bronchiolitis; bronchitis; emphysema; exanthema; keratitis; mole; murmur; rale; resonance; respiration;

stomatitis
vesicular exanthema: virus
vesicular ovarian: follicle
vesicular stomatitis: virus
vesiculocavernous: respiration
vesiculotympanitic: resonance
vestibular: anus; area; crest; fissure; fold; fossa; ganglion; gland; ligament; lip; membrane; nerve; nucleus; nystagmus; organ; root; surface; vein; wall
vestibular blind: sac
vestibular hair: cell
vestibulocochlear: nerve
vestibulo-equilibratory: control
vestibulospinal: reflex; tract
vestigial: fold; muscle; organ
Veterans Administration: hospital
veterinary: anatomy; medicine; surgery
Vi: antibody; antigen
vibrating: line; reed
vibration: tolerance
vibratory: massage; sensibility
vicarious: diarrhea; hypertrophy; menstruation; respiration
vicious: cicatrix; circle; union
villonodular pigmented: tenosynovitis
villous: adenoma; carcinoma; papilloma; placenta; tenosynovitis; tumor
vinous: liquor
violinist's: cramp
viral (see also virus): dysentery; hemagglutination; hepatitis; strand; wart
virgin: generation; silk; tooth
virginal: membrane
Virginia: snakeroot
viridans: hemolysis
virile: member; reflex
virtual: cautery; focus; image
virulent: bacteriophage; bubo
virus (see also viral): abortion; blockade; encephalomyelitis; hepatitis; keratoconjunctivitis; pneumonia
virus A: hepatitis
virus B: hepatitis
virus X: disease
visceral: anatomy; anesthesia; arch; brain; cavity; cleft; disorder; epilepsy; inversion; larva migrans; layer; leishmaniasis; lymphomatosis; mesoderm; plate; pleurisy; ptosis; sense; skeleton; surface
visceral disease: virus
visceral motor: neuron
visceral nervous: system
visceral traction: reflex
viscerogenic: reflex
visceromotor: reflex
visceropannicular: reflex
viscerosensory: reflex
viscerotrophic: reflex
visible: spectrum
visiting: nurse
Visna: virus
visual: acuity; allesthesia; alternans; amnesia; angle; aphasia; area; axis; blackout; cortex; cycle; efficiency; field; image; pigment; purple; threshold; violet; white; yellow
visual evoked: potential
visual orbicularis: reflex
visual receptor: cell
visual-spatial: agnosia

vita: glass
vital: capacity; center; force; index; knot; node; pulp; red; stain; sign; spirit; statistics; tooth; tripod; ultraviolet
vitality: test
vitamin: unit
vitamin $B_c$: conjugase
vitamin $B_{12}$: neuropathy
vitamin C: test
vitamin D: milk
vitamin D-resistant: rickets
vitelliform: degeneration
vitelline: duct; fistula; membrane; pole; reservoir; sac; vein
vitelliruptive macular: degeneration
vitellointestinal: cyst; duct
vitiated: air
vitreo-: retinopathy
vitreoretinal traction: syndrome
vitreous: body; camera; chamber; degeneration; humor; lamella; membrane; table
vivax: fever; malaria
VMA: test
vocal: amusia; cord; fold; fremitus; ligament; muscle; resonance; shelf
volar carpal: ligament
volar interosseous: artery; nerve
volatile: alkali; anesthetic; oil
vole: bacillus
Volhynia: fever
volitional: tremor
voltaic: taste; vertigo
volume: index
volume-controlled: respirator
volume-displacement: plethysmograph
volumetric: analysis; flask
voluntary: dehydration; hospital; muscle; nystagmus
volutin: granule
vomerine: canal; cartilage
vomerobasilar: canal
vomeronasal: organ
vomerovaginal: canal; groove
vomiting: gas; reflex
vorticose: vein
VS: virus
vulnerable: period
vulnerable child: syndrome
vulsella: forceps
vulvovaginal: cystectomy; gland
Vw: antigen

## W

W: chromosome; factor; ray
"w": hernia
waiter's: cramp
waking: numbness
waking (morning): ptosis
walking: typhoid
wallet: stomach
wandering: abscess; cell; goiter; kidney; liver; organ; pacemaker; pneumonia; rash
war: edema; fever; medicine; nephritis; neurosis
warble: botfly; fly
ward: sister
warehouseman's: itch
warm: agglutinin; autoantibody; bath

warm-blooded: animal
warm-cold: hemolysin
wart: virus
wart-hog: disease
warty: dyskeratoma; horn; ulcer
wash-: bottle
washed: sulfur
washed field: technique
washerman's: mark
washerwoman's: itch
washing: soda
washout: cannula
wasserhelle: cell
wasting: disease; palsy; paralysis
watchmaker's: cramp
water: aspirator; balance; bath; bed; brash; cancer; canker; cure; depletion; diuresis; dressing; flea; gas; glass; intoxication; itch; pox; sore; stroke
water-clear: cell
water-gurgle: test
water-hammer: pulse
water-trap: stomach
water wheel: murmur
water-whistle: sound
watering-can: scrotum
watering-pot: perineum
watershed: infarction
watery: diarrhea; eye
wattle: gum
wave: analyzer; form; number
wax: bougie; expansion; form; inlay; pattern
wax model: denture
waxed: sponge
waxy: cast; degeneration; finger; kidney; liver; spleen
weak: foot
weaning: brash
wear-and-tear: pigment
weaver's: cough
web: eye
Webb: antigen
webbed: finger; neck; penis; toe
wedge: biopsy; bone; pressure; resection
wedge-and-groove: joint
wedge-shaped: fasciculus; tubercle
WEE: virus
weekend: hospital
weeping: eczema
welder's: conjunctivitis; lung
Wesselsbron disease: virus
West African: fever
West Indian: smallpox
West Nile: fever; virus
western equine: encephalomyelitis
western equine encephalomyelitis: virus
wet: beriberi; compress; cup; dream; gangrene; lung; nurse; pack; pleurisy; shock; tetter
wet-bulb: thermometer
wettable: sulfur
wharf: rat
wheat: poisoning
whetstone: crystal
whey: alum; protein; treatment
whip: bougie
whiplash: injury
whispered: bronchophony; pectoriloquy
whistle-tip: catheter
whistling: rale

whistling face: syndrome
white: arsenic; beeswax; bile; birch; bole; commissure; corpuscle; diarrhea; eye; fat; fiber; finger; flux; gangrene; head; hellebore; infarct; lead; leg; leprosy; line; matter; mustard; petrolatum; piedra; pine; plague; pneumonia; pox; precipitate; pulp; quebracho; scours; snakeroot; spot; squill; substance; swelling; thrombus; turpentine; vitriol; wax; yolk
white blood: cell
white folded: gingivostomatosis
white muscle: disease
white of: egg; eye
white-out: syndrome
white soft: paraffin
white spot: disease
whole: blood
whooping: cough
whooping-cough: vaccine
whorled: enamel
wide: plane; spectrum
wide field: ocular
wild: ginger; ipecac; jalap; yeast
wild-type: strain
wildfire: rash
willow: fracture
wind: contusion
Windigo, Wittigo: psychosis
window: resection
wine: spirit
wing: cell; plate
winged: catheter; scapula
wink: reflex
winking: spasm
winter: cough; dysentery; eczema; itch; sleep; tick
winter-vomiting: disease
wire: arch; splint
wire-loop: lesion
wiry: pulse
wisdom: tooth
Wistar: rat
witch's: milk
withdrawal: reflex; symptom
wolf: tooth
womb: stone
wood: charcoal; naphtha; spirit; sugar; tick; vinegar
woodcutter's: encephalitis
wooden: resonance; tongue
wooden-shoe: heart
wool: ball; maggot
wool-sorter's: disease; pneumonia

woolly: hair
woolly-hair: nevus
word: blindness; deafness
working: bite; contact; occlusion; side
working occlusal: surface
worm: abscess; aneurysm
worsted: test
wound: dehiscence; fever; hormone; myiasis
woven: bone
Wr$^a$: antigen
Wright: antigen
wrinkled: tongue
wrinkler: muscle
wrist: clonus; ganglion; joint; sign
wrist clonus: reflex
writer's: cramp
writing: hand
wry: neck
Wyeomyxia: virus

## X

X: chromosome; disease; zone
x-: body; esotropia; exotropia; leg; radiation; ray
x-linked: gene; ichthyosis
x-linked recessive: gargoylism
x-ray: cap; dermatitis; microscope; tube
xanthine: base
xanthogranulomatous: cholecystitis; pyelonephritis
xanthoproteic: reaction; test
xenogeneic: graft
xenon-arc: photocoagulator
Xenopus: test
xerotic: keratitis
Xg: antigen
xiphisternal: joint
xiphisternal crunching: sound
xiphoid: cartilage; process
Xiphophorus: test
XO: syndrome
XXY: syndrome
xylose: test

## Y

Y: cartilage; chromosome; factor
y-: angle
y-linked: gene
y-shaped: ligament
Yaba: tumor
Yaba monkey: virus
Yangtze: edema
Yangtze Valley: fever

yeast: fungus
yeast eluate: factor
yellow: atrophy; bark; blindness; body cartilage; cinchona; disease; fever; fiber; hepatization; ligament; marrow precipitate; skin; spot; vision; wax yolk
yellow fever: vaccine; virus
yellow nail: syndrome
yellow soft: paraffin
yield: stress
yogurt: diet
yoke: bone
yolk: cell; cleavage; membrane; plug sac; stalk
yolk-sac: chorion
Yt$^a$: antigen

## Z

Z: band; chromosome; disk; line
Zambesi: ulcer
zero: gravity
zero degree: tooth
zero-order: reaction
Zika: fever; virus
zinc: colic; gelatin
zinc-eugenol: cement
zinc-phosphate: cement
zirconium: granuloma
zonal: necrosis
zonary: placenta
zonular: band; cataract; fiber; layer; space
zoogeneic: infection
zooplastic: graft
zoster: encephalomyelitis
zwitter: hypothesis
zygal: fissure
zygapophysial: joint
zygomatic: arch; bone; diameter; fossa; margin; nerve; process; region
zygomaticoauricular: index
zygomaticofacial: foramen
zygomaticomaxillary: suture
zygomatico-orbital: artery; foramen
zygomaticotemporal: foramen
zygomaxillary: point
zymatic: disease
zymogen: granule
zymogenic: cell
zymoplastic: substance
zymotic: doctrine; papilloma; principle; theory
zymotoxic: group

# Appendix 2: Blood Groups

In this appendix, and in related terms defined in the dictionary proper, the term "blood group" is used to refer to an entire blood group system consisting of erythrocyte antigens whose specificity is controlled by a series of allelic genes, or by a series of genes so closely linked on a single chromosome that they cannot be distinguished from alleles by available genetic methods. The terms "blood type" and "phenotype" are used to refer to a specific reaction pattern to testing antisera within a system. This usage is not universal. It should be noted that in current literature a single system may be referred to in the plural (*i.e.*, ABO blood groups) and the term "blood group" may be assigned to a single phenotype (*i.e.*, blood group A).

Each blood group is defined in terms of reaction to the original antiserum with which the system was discovered, with modification or extension as required by the discovery of additional antisera proved to be related to the same system. A "new" blood group antigen can be defined by showing that it is detected by an antiserum with reactions different from those of previously known antisera. If it can be shown that the "new" antigen is genetically independent of known blood group systems, it may qualify as the prototype antigen of a new blood group. If it can be shown that the "new" antigen is controlled by a gene allelic to one or more known blood group genes, it is assigned to the blood group of its alleles. Many known antigens have not been shown to be either genetically independent or related to certain other known antigens, and their status remains in doubt.

In the blood group definitions emphasis has been placed on identification of symbols for genes, antigens, antisera and phenotypes. These often appear in the literature without specification that they refer to a blood group. Attention is called to the general convention, followed here, that symbols for genes and genotypes are set in italics, whereas symbols for gene products or antigens, antisera and phenotypes are set in Roman type. In the Rh-Hr terminology for the Rh blood group, Roman type is used to designate antigenic substances, and bold face type is used to designate serologic factors and their corresponding antibodies. These conventions are in wide usage, but are not consistently followed by all authors.

## ABO blood group

The classical blood group system defined by the agglutination reactions of erythrocytes to the natural isoantibodies anti-A and anti-B and related antisera (Landsteiner, 1900). In normal human blood there is a reciprocal relationship between the ABO antigens or agglutinogens on the surface of the erythrocyte and the natural antibodies or isoagglutins found in serum. Individuals of type O do not have either the A or B antigens on the erythrocytes, but their serum contains both anti-A and anti-B agglutinins. Individuals of type A have antigen A on the erythrocytes and anti-B in the serum. Individuals of type B have antigen B on the erythrocytes and anti-A in the serum. Individuals of type AB have both A and B antigens on the erythrocytes, but no isoagglutinins in the serum. Types A and AB may be subdivided by anti-$A_1$ serum into types $A_1$ and $A_2$, and $A_1B$ and $A_2B$. The $A_2$ antigen is weaker in reaction than $A_1$, but their difference is also qualitative. Production of ABO antigens is controlled by a series of allelic genes $A_1$, $A_2$, $B$ and $O$ (sometimes designated $I^{A_1}$, $I^{A_2}$, $I^B$ and $i$; $i^{A_1}$, $i^{A_2}$, $i^B$ and $i$ or $A_1$, $A_2$, $a^B$ and $a$). $A_1$ is dominant to $A_2$ and both are dominant to $O$; there is no dominance between $A_1$ and $B$ or $A_2$ and $B$.

In the usual typing method a strong anti-A serum is used that agglutinates cells containing $A_1$ or $A_2$ antigen; cells agglutinated by this serum but not by anti-B are of type A, but may be of genotype $A_1A_1$, $A_1A_2$, $A_1O$, $A_2A_2$ or $A_2O$. Cells of persons of type A that are agglutinated by anti-$A_1$ are of type $A_1$ and may be of genotype $A_1A_1$, $A_1A_2$ or $A_1O$; type A cells not agglutinated by anti-$A_1$ are of type $A_2$ and may be of genotype $A_2A_2$ or $A_2O$. Cells agglutinated by anti-B but not anti-A are type B, and may be genotype $BB$ or $BO$. Cells agglutinated by both anti-A and anti-B are type AB and can be divided into types $A_1B$ (genotype $A_1B$) and $A_2B$ (genotype $A_2B$) by anti-$A_1$. Cells not agglutinated by either anti-A or anti-B are of type O and genotype $OO$. Cells of type O do not simply lack antigenic substance; the vast majority possess an antigen called H that is chemically similar to antigens A and B and is probably the precursor antigen that is modified under influence of genes $A_1$, $A_2$ and $B$ into their corresponding antigens.

Rare individuals fail to form H antigen and, regardless of ABO genotype, do not produce A, B or H antigens; such persons seem to be homozygous for a recessive gene called $h$ or $x$. The postulated allele $H$ or $X$ is apparently necessary to convert a mucopolysaccharide precursor into H antigen. The term "Bombay" phenotype was assigned to such persons whose cells lack A, B and H antigen, and whose serum contains anti-A, anti-B and anti-H; they are also referred to as the "Oh" phenotype. In addition, weak variants of antigen A have been described with phenotypes designated $A_3$, $A_4$, $A_5$, $A_x$ and $A_z$ ; more rarely weak variants of B have been found. The ABO types are of prime importance with respect to blood transfusion, and maternal-fetal incompatibility is a frequent cause of fetal death and erythroblastosis fetalis.

### Auberger blood group

The erythrocyte antigen defined by reaction to an antibody designated anti-Au$^a$ found in the serum of a Madame Auberger who had received many transfusions (Salmon, Salmon, Liberge, Andre, Tippett and Sanger, 1961). The Au$^a$ antigen is inherited as a dominant trait and occurs in about 80 per cent of Caucasians and Negroes.

### Diego blood group

The erythrocyte antigen defined by anti-Di$^a$ antibody first found in Venezuela where it had been the cause of erythroblastosis fetalis (Layrisse, Arends and Dominguez, 1955). An antibody with antithetical reactions, anti-Di$^b$, was discovered in 1967. The antigen system is controlled by two alleles, $Di^a$ and $Di^b$. The Di$^a$ antigen is common in American Indians and in Asiatics, but is apparently absent in Caucasians. This distribution is considered strong anthropological evidence to support the thesis that American Indians are derived from Mongolian or Asiatic ancestors.

### Dombrock blood group

The erythrocyte antigen defined by reaction to anti-Do$^a$ antibody (Swanson, Polesky, Tippett and Sanger, 1965). The Do$^a$ antigen exhibits autosomal dominant inheritance and is found in about 65 to 66 per cent of Northern Europeans, U. S. Caucasians, and Israelis, in about 45 to 55 per cent of U. S. Negroes and American Indians, and in about 13 per cent of Thais.

### Duffy blood group

The erythrocyte antigens defined by reactions to an immune serum called anti-Fy$^a$, first found in a hemophilic patient named Duffy who had received many .transfusions (Cutbush, Mollison and Parkin, 1950), and a serum with antithetical reactions, anti-Fy$^b$ (Ikin, Mourant, Peffenkofer and Blumenthal, 1951). The bloods of practically all Caucasians are agglutinated by one, the other, or both of these antisera, but bloods of the majority of Negroes and some Yemenite Jews give negative reactions to both antisera. It is therefore assumed that production of Duffy antigens is controlled by a series of at least three allelic genes, $Fy^a$, $Fy^b$ and $Fy$, with antibodies specific for only the first two of the series being now known. Persons with blood reacting positively to anti-Fy$^a$ and negatively to anti-Fy$^b$ are of phenotype Fy(a+b−) and their genotype may be either $Fy^aFy^a$, or $Fy^aFy$. Persons of phenotype Fy(a+b+) are of genotype $Fy^aFy^b$. Those of phenotype Fy(a−b+) may be of genotype $Fy^bFy^b$ or $Fy^bFy$. Those of phenotype Fy(a−b−) are of genotype $FyFy$. Duffy antibodies occasionally cause transfusion reactions or erythroblastosis fetalis.

### High frequency blood groups

A group of antigens that are found in almost all individuals, but are absent in members of a very few families. Because of very high frequency they are often called "public" antigens. The antibodies usually have been found in the serum of a patient lacking the antigen who has become immunized by transfusion or pregnancy. Names or symbols applied to public antigens include: Vel, Yt$^a$, Ge, Lan and Sm. See also low frequency blood groups.

### I blood group

The erythrocyte antigens defined by reactions to antibodies designated anti-I (Wiener, Unger, Cohen and Feldman, 1956) and anti-i. Antigen I differs from other blood group antigens in the slowness of its development and in its wide range of strength in different individuals; the range approximates a normal distribution curve. Anti-I occurs in a wide range of strength and in two forms: autoanti-I is the antibody usually found in the serum of patients with acquired hemolytic anemia of the "cold agglutinin" type and in sera described as containing "nonspecific complete cold autoagglutinin"; natural anti-I or isoanti-I occurs regularly in the serum of persons of phenotype i. Phenotype i may be divided into types $i_1$ and $i_2$ , both rare in adults.

### Kell blood group

The erythrocyte antigens defined by an immune antibody, anti-K, first found in the serum of a Mrs. Kell (Coombs, Mourant and Race, 1946), and by anti-k (Levine, Backer, Wigod and Ponder, 1949). Anti-k was known as anti-Cellano until its antithetical reactions to anti-K were established. An antiserum originally designated anti-Si was found to be identical to anti-K. The antigens K and k are controlled by a pair of allelic genes without dominance, hence three genotypes ($KK$, $Kk$, $kk$) may be recognized by agglutination of erythrocytes by anti-K alone, both anti-K and anti-k, or anti-k alone. Variant antigens of this system detected by human sera have been designated Kp$^a$ and Kp$^b$. Very rare families have been found in which erythrocytes of certain persons give negative reactions with all antisera of the Kell group; this phenotype is designated K-k-Kp(a−b−). As a cause of transfusion reactions and erythroblastosis fetalis, the Kell blood group is next in clinical importance after the ABO and Rh blood groups.

### Kidd blood group

The erythrocyte antigens defined by reactions to an antibody designated anti-Jk$^a$ discovered in the serum of a Mrs. Kidd who had delivered an infant with erythroblastosis (Allen, Diamond and Niedziela, 1951), and by reactions to its anthetical serum, anti-Jk$^b$ (Plaut, Ikin, Mourant, Sanger and Race, 1953). The antigens are controlled by a pair of genes without dominance, $Jk^a$ and $Jk^b$, that are genetically independent of other blood group genes. Persons with erythrocytes that are agglutinated by anti-Jk$^a$ but not by anti-Jk$^b$ are of phenotype Jk(a+b−) and genotype $Jk^aJk^a$; agglutination by both antisera indicates phenotype Jk(a+b+) and genotype $Jk^aJk^b$; agglutina-

TABLE 1. *Secretor-Lewis Interactions**

| Genotypes | Antigens | | | | |
|---|---|---|---|---|---|
| | Of saliva | | | | Of erythrocytes |
| | ABH | Le$^a$ | Le$^{bL}$ | Le$^{bH}$ | |
| SeSe LeLe<br>SeSe Lele<br>Sese LeLe<br>Sese Lele | + | + | + | + | Le(a−b+) |
| sese LeLe<br>sese Lele | − | + | − | − | Le(a+b−) |
| SeSe lele<br>Sese lele | + | − | − | + | Le(a−b−) |
| sese lele | − | − | − | − | Le(a−b−) |

* From Race, R. R., and Sanger, R.: *Blood Groups in Man*, Ed. 4, Blackwell Scientific Publications, Ltd., Oxford, England, 1962.

tion by only anti-Jk$^b$ indicates phenotype Jk(a−b+) and genotype $Jk^bJk^b$. The possibility that there may be a third allele at this locus, or a modifier capable of suppressing the action of genes at this locus, has been raised by the discovery of rare individuals (usually of Asiatic or South American Indian ancestry) whose erythrocytes give negative reactions to both antisera. Kidd antibodies occasionally cause transfusion reactions or erythroblastosis fetalis.

### Lewis blood group

The antigens of erythrocytes, saliva and certain other body fluids defined by reactions to anti-Le$^a$ antibody, first found in the serum of a Mrs. Lewis (Mourant, 1946), by reactions to related sera particularly anti-Le$^b$, and by interactions with the secretor factor. The Lewis antigens are formed in tissue under control of genes designated Le and le (Le dominant to le) and released into body fluids where they may be absorbed onto the surface of erythrocytes and determine the reactions of erythrocytes to antisera. The Lewis erythrocyte types of children may not develop fully until about age six years. The Lewis genes are genetically independent of those controlling the secretor factor (Se and se), but their products interact in certain phenotypic effects. Several theories have been proposed to account for the complex immunologic and genetic observations. The theory of Grubb and Ceppellini was summarized by Race and Sanger (1962) as shown in table 1.

Variant antibodies of this system include anti-Le$^X$ (originally called anti-X), which seems to be anti-Le$^a$ plus anti-Le$^b$; anti-Le$^c$, an immune rabbit serum that agglutinates Le(a−b−) cells; the Magard antiserum, obtained from a patient with carcinoma of the stomach, that agglutinates strongly the cells of A$_1$ Le(a−b−) secretors and less strongly those of A$_2$ Le(a−b−) secretors. Lewis antibodies have occasionally been implicated as a cause of transfusion reactions.

### Low frequency blood groups

A group of erythrocyte antigens, each defined by a specific antiserum, and each found only in members of a very few families. Because of their rarity they are often referred to as "private" antigens. The antibodies usually have been found in the sera of patients who have received transfusions or in mothers of erythroblastotic infants. They are often named for the family in which they were first discovered. The names or symbols assigned to some private antigens are: Levay, Jobbins, Becker, Ven, Chr$^a$, Wright or Wr$^a$, Be$^a$, By, Swann or Sw$^a$, Good, Biles or Bi, Tr$^a$, Stobo, Ot, Ho, and Webb. See also high frequency blood groups.

### Lutheran blood group

The blood group antigens defined by reactions to an antibody designated anti-Lu$^a$ first found in serum of a patient who had received many transfusions (Callender, Race and Paykoc, 1945) and its reciprocal, anti-Lu$^b$ (Cutbush and Chanarin, 1956). Production of the antigens is controlled by a pair of allelic genes, Lu$^a$ and Lu$^b$, without dominance. The erythrocytes of persons with genotype $Lu^aLu^a$ are agglutinated by anti-Lu$^a$ but not by anti-Lu$^b$, those of genotype $Lu^aLu^b$ are agglutinated by both antisera, and those of genotype $Lu^bLu^b$ are agglutinated by anti-Lu$^b$ but not by anti-Lu$^a$. These antibodies are an uncommon cause of transfusion reactions.

### MNSs blood group

The system of erythrocyte antigens originally defined by reactions to immune rabbit sera designated anti-M and anti-N (Landsteiner and Levine, 1927) and since extended by reactions to sera anti-S, anti-s and certain others. When tested with the readily available anti-M and anti-N sera only, the erythrocytes of all individuals may be assigned to one of three classes, M, N or MN, depending on whether they are agglutinated by one, the other or both antisera. Production of M and N antigens is controlled by two allelic genes, M and N; persons of genotype MM are type M, those of genotype NN are type N, and those of the heterozygous genotype MN are type MN. As anti-M and anti-N sera are commercially available and the reactions are simple and reliable, they are widely used for medicolegal

TABLE 2. *MNSs Phenotypes and Genotypes*

| Antisera | | | | Genotypes |
|---|---|---|---|---|
| M | N | S | s | |
| + | − | + | − | MS/MS |
| + | − | + | + | MS/Ms |
| + | − | − | + | Ms/Ms |
| + | + | + | − | MS/Ns |
| + | + | + | + | MS/Ns or Ms/NS |
| + | + | − | + | Ms/Ns |
| − | + | + | − | NS/NS |
| − | + | + | + | NS/Ns |
| − | + | − | + | Ns/Ns |

TABLE 3. *P Blood Group**

| Phenotypes | | Phenotype symbol | Genotypes |
|---|---|---|---|
| anti-P + $P_1$ ($Tj^a$) | anti-$P_1$ (P) | | |
| + | + | $P_1$ | $P_1P_1$ ; $P_1P_2$ ; $P_1p$ |
| + | − | $P_2$ | $P_2P_2$ ; $P_2p$ |
| − | − | p | $pp$ |

* From Race, R. R., and Sanger, R.: *Blood Groups in Man*, Ed. 4, Blackwell Scientific Publications, Ltd., Oxford, England, 1962.

TABLE 4. *Rh Gene Designations in Three Nomenclature Systems**

| Rh-Hr (Wiener) | CDE (Fisher-Race) | Numerical (Rosenfield *et al.*) |
|---|---|---|
| $r$ | *cde* | $R^{-1, -2, -3, 4, 5}$ |
| $R^1$ | *CDe* | $R^{1, 2 -3, -4, 5}$ |
| $R^2$ | *cDE* | $R^{1, -2, 3, 4, -5}$ |
| $R^o$ | *cDe* | $R^{1, -2, -3, 4, 5}$ |
| $r'$ | *Cde* | $R^{-1, 2, -3, -4, 5}$ |
| $r''$ | *cdE* | $R^{-1, -2, 3, 4, -5}$ |
| $R^z$ | *CDE* | $R^{1, 2, 3, -4, -5}$ |
| $r^y$ | *CdE* | $R^{-1, 2, 3, -4, -5}$ |
| (Paired combinations of the above give rise to 36 genotypes) | | |

* Tables 4 and 5 are modified from Rosenfield, R. E., Allen, F. H., Jr., Swisher, S. N., and Kochwa, S.: A review of Rh serology and presentation of a new terminology. *Transfusion*, **2:** 287, 1962 (official journal of the American Association of Blood Banks, J. B. Lippincott Co., publisher).

blood testing in disputed paternity actions and for genetic linkage and population studies. The *MN* locus is not genetically linked to loci of other major blood group systems. The MNSs antigens are only rarely the cause of hemolytic reactions to transfusion.

With the discovery of anti-S serum (1947) and its reciprocal anti-s (1951) it was shown that the MNSs group is complex and that nine phenotypes representing ten genotypes may be defined by the four antisera (table 2). In addition, nearly 1 per cent of blood samples of Negroes lack both S and s. An antibody designated as anti-U has been found that reacts with both S and s antigens. Weak variants of the M and N antigens that react with some anti-M or anti-N sera but not with others have been designated $M_2$ and $N_2$. A qualitative variant of M has been designated $M_1$. An antigen that gives intermediate reactions has been designated $M^c$. An extremely rare variant of M detected with a special serum has been designated $M^g$. Antigens designated Hu and He are detected by sera obtained from rabbits immunized with blood of certain Negroes and are found almost entirely in persons of African ancestry; anti-Hu gives distinct reactions only with cells that also contain N, and most positives to anti-He possess both N and S. Other rare antigens that are associated with or are variants of the MNSs group have been designated $Mi^2$, Vw (identical with Gr) and Mu.

### P blood group

The system of erythrocyte antigens originally defined by reaction to immune rabbit serum designated anti-P (Landsteiner and Levine, 1927), but since extended to include related antigens. An antibody previously known as anti-$Tj^a$ was shown to be related to anti-P in 1955, and the terminology presented in table 3 was proposed by Sanger. In this terminology, $P_1$ is the phenotype previously called P+, $P_2$ is the phenotype previously called P−, and p the phenotype previously called Tj(a−). A rare variant designated $P^k$ has also been found.

### Rh blood group

The complex system of erythrocyte antigens defined originally by reactions to serum from rabbits or guinea pigs immunized with blood of the rhesus monkey (Landsteiner and Wiener, 1940) but now defined by reactions to a series of human antisera usually obtained from persons immunized by transfusion or pregnancy. The nomenclature of genes, antigens and antisera of this system has undergone an evolution reflecting the aquisition of new knowledge since 1940, and conflicting systems of nomenclature have been in use. The most widely used nomenclatures are those proposed by Wiener (Rh-Hr system) and by Fisher and Race (CDE system), both of which have been frequently modified and extended, and that proposed in 1962 by Rosenfield, Allen, Swisher and Kochwa (numerical system). Certain differences of theoretic interpretations of both immunology

TABLE 5. *Rh Antiserum Designations in Three Nomenclature Systems*

| Rh-Hr (Wiener) | CDE (Fisher-Race) | Numerical (Rosenfield *et al.*) |
|---|---|---|
| Standard antisera | | |
| $\mathbf{Rh_0}$ | D | Rh1 |
| **rh′** | C | Rh2 |
| **rh″** | E | Rh3 |
| **hr′** | c | Rh4 |
| **hr″** | e | Rh5 |
| Other antisera | | |
| **hr** | f, ce | Rh6 |
| **rh** | Ce | Rh7 |
| $\mathbf{rh^{w1}}$ | $C^w$ | Rh8 |
| $\mathbf{rh^x}$ | $C^x$ | Rh9 |
| $\mathbf{hr^v}$ | V, $ce^s$ | Rh10 |
| $\mathbf{rh^{w2}}$ | $E^w$ | Rh11 |
| $\mathbf{rh^G}$ | G | Rh12 |
| $\mathbf{Rh^A}$ | No term | Rh13 |
| $\mathbf{Rh^B}$ | No term | Rh14 |
| $\mathbf{Rh^C}$ | No term | Rh15 |
| $\mathbf{Rh^D}$ | No term | Rh16 |
| $\mathbf{Hr_0}$ | No term | Rh17 |
| **Hr** | No term | Rh18 |
| $\mathbf{hr^s}$ | No term | Rh19 |
| $\mathbf{Hr^H}$ plus $\mathbf{hr^v}$ | VS, $e^s$ | Rh20 |
| No term | $C^G$ | Rh21 |

and genetics are associated with the different nomenclatures. It is agreed that production of Rh antigens is controlled by a complex series of genes located on a single chromosome, that there are eight major genes or gene complexes that control production of qualitatively different antigens, that the paired arrangements of these eight genes give rise to 18 qualitative phenotypes or erythrocyte patterns that can be recognized by reactions with five standard antisera which are commercially available, that many more antigens or antigen combinations exist, with both qualitative and quantitative differences which can be recognized by a series of other antisera not generally available with reaction specificities that reflect wide immunologic and genetic variation. The Rh-Hr nomenclature implies that all Rh genes constitute a single set of multiple alleles located at a single chromosome locus and that a single gene may control production of an erythrocyte antigen or agglutinogen possessing many factors each of different antibody specificity. The CDE nomenclature implies that there are three contiguous chromosome loci, or areas of genetic information, each with a series of two major and probably several minor alleles, each controlling production of a specific erythrocyte antigen. The numerical system assigns an arbitrary number to each known antiserum, using numbers 1 through 5 for the five standard antisera and higher numbers for others, and classifies individuals by positive or negative reactions to the antisera used. The correspondence of the three nomenclatures with respect to designations for genes, phenotypes and antisera are given in tables 4, 5, and 6.

The symbol $D^u$ is used in the CDE nomenclature to designate antigens that are agglutinated by some anti-D sera and not by others, and these apparently represent weak or incomplete forms of the D antigen. Many varieties of $D^u$ exist. Individuals possessing $D^u$ may be mistyped as D-negative (d), but $D^u$ blood may stimulate the formation of anti-D if transfused to a D-negative recipient. Some $D^u$ persons have made anti-D when transfused with D-positive blood. In the Rh-Hr nomenclature, weak variants are indicated by using Germanic type (for example, $\mathfrak{Rh_o}$). The Rh-Hr nomenclature also designates the extremely rare phenotypes that lack the factor pairs rh'-hr' and rh"-hr" by placing a double bar above the appropriate symbol ($\overline{\overline{Rh}}_o$ ; $\overline{\overline{Rh}}^w$); the corresponding phenotype in the CDE nomenclature is designated —D—.

## Sutter blood group

The erythrocyte antigen defined by reaction to an antibody designated anti-$Js^a$ found in the serum of a Mr. Sutter who had been previously transfused (Giblett, 1958). The $Js^a$ antigen is inherited as a dominant trait. It occurs in about 20 per cent of American Negroes but is rare in other ethnic groups.

## Xg blood group

The erythrocyte antigen defined by reaction to an antibody designated anti-$Xg^a$ (Mann, Cahan, Gelb, Fisher, Hamper, Tippett, Sanger, and Race, 1962) which was found in the serum of a patient who had received many transfusions. In contrast to all other known blood group antigens, $Xg^a$ proved to be controlled by a gene located on the X chromosome and is thus the only known sex-linked blood group. Anti-$Xg^a$ has been used for genetic linkage studies of diseases caused by sex-linked genes.

TABLE 6. *Rh Phenotypes Defined by Five Standard Antisera*

| Antiserum reactions | | | | | Phenotypes | | |
|---|---|---|---|---|---|---|---|
| $Rh_o$ D Rh1 | $rh'$ C Rh2 | $rh''$ E Rh3 | $hr'$ c Rh4 | $hr''$ e Rh5 | Rh-Hr | CDE | Numerical |
|   |   |   | + | + | rh | cde/cde | Rh: −1, −2, −3, 4, 5 |
| + | + | − | + | + | $Rh_1rh$ | CDe/cde* | Rh: 1, 2, −3, 4, 5 |
| + | + | − | − | + | $Rh_1Rh_1$ | CDe/CDe* | Rh: 1, 2, −3, −4, 5 |
| + | + | + | + | + | $Rh_2Rh_0$ | CDe/cDE* | Rh: 1, 2, 3, 4, 5 |
| + | − | + | + | + | $Rh_2rh$ | cDE/cde* | Rh: 1, −2, 3, 4, 5 |
| + | − | − | + | + | $Rh_0$ | cDe/cde* | Rh: 1, −2, −3, 4, 5 |
| + | − | + | + | − | $Rh_2Rh_2$ | cDE/cDE* | Rh: 1, −2, 3, 4, −5 |
| − | + | − | + | + | rh'rh | Cde/cde | Rh: −1, 2, −3, 4, 5 |
| − | − | + | + | + | rh"rh | cdE/cde | Rh: −1, −2, 3, 4, 5 |
| + | + | + | − | + | $Rh_zRh_1$ | CDE/CDe* | Rh: 1, 2, 3, −4, 5 |
| + | + | + | + | − | $Rh_zRh_2$ | CDE/cDE* | Rh: 1, 2, 3, 4, −5 |
| − | + | + | + | + | $rh_yrh$ | Cde/cdE* | Rh: −1, 2, 3, 4, 5 |
| − | + | − | − | + | rh'rh' | Cde/Cde | Rh: −1, 2, −3, −4, 5 |
| − | − | + | + | − | rh"rh" | cdE/cdE | Rh: −1, −2, 3, 4, −5 |
| − | + | + | − | + | $rh_yrh'$ | CdE/Cde | Rh: −1, 2, 3, −4, 5 |
| − | + | + | + | − | $rh_yrh''$ | CdE/cdE | Rh: −1, 2, 3, 4, −5 |
| + | + | + | − | − | $Rh_zRh_z$ | CDE/CDE* | Rh: 1, 2, 3, −4, −5 |
| − | + | + | − | − | $rh_yrh_y$ | CdE/CdE | Rh: −1, 2, 3, −4, −5 |

* Expressed as most common of two or more genotypes of this phenotype.

# Appendix 3: Common Latin Terms Used in Prescription Writing

(From *Drug Topics Red Book, 1964;* reprinted by permission of the Topics Publishing Company, Inc., New York.)

| Latin word or phrase | Latin abbreviation | English meaning |
|---|---|---|
| A, ab | | From |
| Ad | | To, up to |
| Adde | add | Add |
| Ad libitum | ad lib | Freely |
| Admove | admov | Apply |
| Ad saturandum | ad. sat | To saturation |
| Ad tertiam vicem | ad tert. vic | Three times |
| Ad usum externum | ad us. exter | For external use |
| Adversum | adv | Against |
| Agita ante usum | agit. a. us. | Shake before using |
| Agita bene | agit. bene. | Shake well |
| Alternis horis | | Every other hour |
| Ana | aa | Of each |
| Ante cibum | a. c | Before meals |
| Ante jentaculum | ant. jentac | Before breakfast |
| Ante prandium | ant. prand | Before dinner |
| Aqua bulliens | aq. bull | Boiling water |
| Aqua fervens | aq. ferv | Warm water |
| Auris, aures | aur | The ear, ears |
| Balneum vaporis | b. v. | A vapor bath |
| Bibe | bib | Drink |
| Bihorium | bihor | During two hours |
| Bis in die | b. i. d | Twice a day |
| Bulliat | bull | Let it boil |
| Capiat | cap | Let him take |
| Capsula mollis | cap. moll | Soft capsule |
| Caute | | Cautiously |
| Cibus | cib | Food, meal |
| Cito | | Quickly |
| Cito dispensetur | cito disp | Dispense quickly |
| Cochleare | coch | Spoonful |
| Cochleare amplum | coch. amp | Tablespoonful |
| Cochleare magnum | coch. mag. | Tablespoonful |
| Cochleare medium | coch. med. | Dessertspoonful |
| Cochleare parvum | coch. parv | Teaspoonful |
| Cola, colatus | col | Strain |
| Collunarium | collun | Nose wash |
| Collutorium | collut | Mouth wash |
| Compositus | co., comp. | Compound |
| Congius | cong | Gallon |
| Conserva | cons | Conserve, to keep |
| Conspergere | consperg | Dust or sprinkle |
| Contere | conter | Rub together |
| Continuentur remedia | cont. rem. | Continue the medicines |
| Coque | coq | Boil |

| Latin word or phrase | Latin abbreviation | English meaning |
|---|---|---|
| Cras | cr | Tomorrow |
| Crastinus | crast | Of tomorrow |
| Cras vespere | cr. vesp | Tomorrow evening |
| Cujus libet | cuj. lib | Of any you please |
| Curatio | curat | A dressing |
| Cyathus | cyath | Cup, wineglass |
| Da, detur | d., det | Give |
| Debita spissitudo | deb. spiss. | Proper consistence |
| Decem, decimus | | Ten, the tenth |
| De die in diem | de d. in d. | From day to day |
| Deglutiatur | deglut | Swallow |
| Dentur tales doses | d. t. d | Give of such doses |
| Detur in duplo | d. in dup | Give twice as much |
| Dexter, dextra | | The right |
| Diebus alternis | dieb. alt. | Every other day |
| Diebus secundis | dieb. secund | Every second day |
| Diebus tertiis | dieb. tert. | Every third day |
| Dies | d | A day |
| Dimidius | dim | One-half |
| Directione propria | dir. prop | With proper direction |
| Divide in partes aequales | d. in p. aeq. | Divide into equal parts |
| Durante dolare | dur. dol | While pain lasts |
| Eadem | ead | The same |
| Ejusdem | ejusd | Of the same |
| Emplastrum | emp | Plaster |
| Epistomium | epistom | A stopper |
| Etiam | | Also, besides |
| Ex or E | e | Out of, with |
| Ex modo praescripto | e. m. p. | In the manner prescribed |
| Extende | ext | Spread |
| Fac, fiat, fiant | ft | Make |
| Febris | feb | Fever |
| Fervens | ferv | Hot |
| Fiat gargarisma | ft. garg | Make a gargle |
| Fiat infusum | ft. infus | Make an infusion |
| Fiat mistura | ft. mist | Make a mixture |
| Fiat pulvis | ft. pulv | Make a powder |
| Fiat trochisci | ft. troch | Make lozenges |
| Fiat unguentum | ft. ung | Make an ointment |
| Gargarisma | garg | A gargle |
| Gradatim | grad | Gradually |
| Granum, grana | gr | Grain, grains |
| Gutta, guttae | gtt | Drop, drops |
| Guttatim | guttat | Drop by drop |
| Haustus | haust | A drink |
| Hic, haec, hoc | | This |

| Latin word or phrase | Latin abbreviation | English meaning | Latin word or phrase | Latin abbreviation | English meaning |
|---|---|---|---|---|---|
| Hoc vespere.... | hoc vesp.. | Tonight (evening) | Pondere........ | pond.... | By weight |
| Hora decubitus. | h. d...... | At bedtime | Post aurem..... | post aur... | Behind the ear |
| Hora somni.... | h. s. or h. som.... | Just before sleep | Post cibum, cibos......... | p. c...... | After meals |
| Horae unius spatio.......... | hor. un. spat.... | At the end of an hour | Potus......... | pot...... | A drink |
| | | | Prandium...... | prand.... | Dinner |
| | | | Primus......... | ........ | The first |
| | | | Prius.......... | ........ | Before, former |
| Horis intermediis.......... | hor. interm.. | In the intermediate hours | Pro dose...... | pro dos... | For a dose |
| | | | Pro ratione aetatis.......... | pro rat. aet.... | According to age |
| Ibidem......... | ibid..... | In the same place | Pro re nata..... | p. r. n.... | As occasion arises |
| Idem.......... | ........ | The same | Pro usu externo. | pro. us. ext.... | For external use |
| Identidem...... | ........ | Repeatedly | | | |
| Illico legena obturatur....... | illic. leg. obturat. | Stopper the bottle at once | Quantum libet, Quantum placet.......... | q. l., q. p. | As much as you please |
| Incide.......... | incid.... | Cut | Quantum sufficiat.......... | q. s....... | A sufficient quantity |
| In die.......... | in d..... | In a day | | | |
| Infunde........ | infund... | Pour in | Quaque........ | qq...... | Each or every |
| Injectio........ | inj...... | An injection | Quaque hora... | q. h....... | Every hour |
| Inter cibos.... | int. cib.. | Between meals | Quartus........ | quart..... | Fourth |
| Inter noctem... | int. noct.. | During the night | Quater........ | quat..... | Four times |
| Involve........ | involv.... | Coat | Quater in die.. | q. i. d.... | Four times a day |
| Ita........... | ........ | In such manner | Quoque........ | q.q...... | Also |
| Jam........... | ........ | Now | Quorum........ | quor..... | Of which |
| Jentaculum..... | jentac... | Breakfast | Quotidie....... | quotid.... | Daily |
| Lateri dolente.. | lat. dol... | To the painful side | Quoties........ | quot..... | As often as needed |
| Leniter........ | lenit..... | Gently | Recens........ | rec....... | Fresh, recent |
| Leviter........ | levit..... | Lightly | Redactus in pulverem........ | red. in pulv.... | Reduce to a powder |
| Luce primo..... | luc. prim.. | At daybreak | | | |
| Mane......... | man..... | In the morning | | | |
| Massa........ | mass.... | A mass | Renovetur semel | ren. sem.. | Renew once |
| Misce......... | M....... | Mix | Saepe.......... | ........ | Often, frequently |
| Mistura........ | mist..... | Mixture | Satis.......... | ........ | Enough |
| Mitte tales.... | mitt. tal.. | Send such | Secundum artem | s. a...... | According to art |
| Mollis........ | moll..... | Soft | Semel......... | ........ | Once |
| Moro dicto.... | mor. dict.. | As directed | Semel in die.... | semel in d. | Once a day |
| Moro solito..... | mor. sol... | In the usual way | Semi, semis.... | sem..... | One-half |
| Ne tradas sine nummo....... | ne tr. s. num.... | Cash on delivery | Semidrachma... | semidr.... | Half a drachm |
| | | | Semihora...... | semih..... | Half an hour |
| Nisi.......... | ........ | Unless | Semissem....... | ss........ | One-half |
| Nocte......... | noct...... | At night | Semper........ | ........ | Always |
| Nocte maneque. | noct. maneq..... | Night and morning | Septimana...... | ........ | A week |
| Nunc.......... | ........ | Now | Sescuncia..... | ........ | An ounce and a half |
| Octarius........ | oct...... | A pint | | | |
| Oculo dextro.. | O.D..... | In the right eye | Sesquihora.... | sesquihor. | An hour and a half |
| Oculo sinistro.. | O.S...... | In the left eye | Sex, sextus..... | ........ | Six, sixth |
| Oculo utro...... | O.U..... | In each eye | Sic........... | ........ | So |
| Omni die ...... | o. d...... | Every day | Siccus......... | ........ | Dry, dried |
| Omni hora.... | omn. hor.. | Every hour | Signa......... | Sig..... | Write, label |
| Omni mane..... | omn. man. | Every morning | Simul.......... | ........ | Together |
| Omni nocte.... | omn. noct. | Every night | Sine.......... | ........ | Without |
| Pars, partis.... | part..... | A part | Si opus sit..... | s. o. s.... | If needed |
| Partes aequales. | part. aeq.. | Equal parts | Sit........... | ........ | Let it be |
| Partes dolentes. | part. dolent.... | Painful parts | Solve......... | solv..... | Dissolve |
| Partitis vicibus. | part. vic.. | In divided parts | Spiritus vini rectificatus...... | S.V.R.... | Alcohol |
| Per os......... | ........ | By mouth | Statim........ | stat...... | Immediately |
| Perstetur....... | pt....... | Let it be continued | Stillatim...... | stillat.... | By drops, or in small quantities |
| Phiala prius agitata....... | p. p. a.... | Having first shaken the bottle | | | |

| Latin word or phrase | Latin abbreviation | English meaning | Latin word or phrase | Latin abbreviation | English meaning |
|---|---|---|---|---|---|
| Stratum super stratum | s. s. s. | Layer on layer | Ter in die | t. i. d. | Three times a day |
| Sumat talem | sum. tal. | Take one like this | Ut dictum | ut dict. | As directed |
| Sume | sum | Take | Ut supra | ut supr. | As above |
| Talis, tales | | Such, like this | Utendus | utend. | To be used |
| Tandem | | At last, finally | Uto, uti | | To make use of |
| Tantum | | Only | Vas vitreum | vas vitr. | A glass vessel |
| Ter | t. | Three times | Vel | | Or |
| Tere | ter. | Rub | Vices | vic. | Times |

# Appendix 4: Proofreaders' Marks

| | |
|---|---|
| ✗ Change bad letter | ⌐ Raise |
| ↧ Push down space | ⌐ Lower |
| ↻ Turn over | ≡ Straighten lines |
| ℛ Take out (*dele*) | ⊙ Period |
| ⋀ Left out; insert | ⋀ Comma |
| # Insert space | :/ Colon |
| ✔ Equalize spacing | ;/ Semicolon |
| ⌣ Less space | ⋎ Apostrophe |
| ⊂ Close up | ❧ Quotation |
| | = Hyphen |

| | |
|---|---|
| ⋎ Superior figure | *w.f.* Wrong font |
| ⋀ Inferior figure | .... Let it stand |
| ⌐ Move to left | *stet* Let it stand |
| ⌐ Move to right | *tr.* Transpose |
| *out,s.c.* Out, see copy | *cap* Capital letters |
| ▢ Em quad space | *Sm.cap* Small caps |
| ⊥/m One-em dash | *lc.* Lower case |
| # Paragraph | *ital.* Italics |
| *no#* No paragraph | *rom.* Roman |
| | *b.f.* Bold Face |

# Appendix 5: Weights and Measures

There are, unfortunately, several systems of weights and measures in use among the English speaking peoples—the metric, the avoirdupois, the troy, and the apothecaries' weights, and the Imperial and the United States measures of quantity, in addition to the common British and American linear, square, and cubic measures. The metric system is universally employed by laboratory workers throughout the world and its use commercially and in pharmacy is legal in the United States and permissible in Great Britain; the U.S.P. and B.P. employ it together with their national weights and measures, and it will probably eventually supersede the latter in prescription writing as it has in the laboratory.

## THE METRIC SYSTEM

### Linear Measures

The unit of the metric system is the meter, which is the one ten-millionth part of the meridian quadrant of the earth, the circumference of the earth at the equator being therefore 40,000,-000 meters, or 40,000 kilometers, or roughly 25,000 miles. In the nomenclature of the system multiples of the meter are indicated by prefixes derived from the Greek, as follows:

Meter; decameter, 10 meters; hectometer, 100 meters; kilometer, 1000 meters; myriameter, 10,000 meters.

Fractions of the meter are indicated by prefixes derived from the Latin, as follow:

Meter; decimeter, $\frac{1}{10}$ meter; centimeter, $\frac{1}{100}$ meter; millimeter, $\frac{1}{1000}$ meter.

In microscopy, the unit of the measure is $\frac{1}{1000}$ of a millimeter, called micron (symbol $\mu$), or, incorrectly, micromillimeter; the prefix micro- properly notes the one-millionth of the measure to which it is attached, the micron being therefore correctly called micrometer.

### Square Measures

A square meter, in land measure, is called a centiare; 100 sq. meters = 1 are; 100 ares (10,000 sq. meters) = 1 hectare.

### Cubic Measures or Volumes

The unit of volume is the cubic decimeter, called a liter; one liter of water weighs practically 1 kilogram. It is divided into the deciliter, $\frac{1}{10}$ liter (weight 100 grams); centiliter, $\frac{1}{100}$ liter (weight 10 grams); and milliliter, formerly abbreviated in U.S.P. and N.F. to mil cubic centimeter), $\frac{1}{1000}$ liter (weight 1 gram).

Theoretically there are also multiples of the liter: decaliter, 10 liters; hectaliter, 100 liters; kiloliter, 1000 liters; practically, however, the hectaliter (weight of water 100 kilograms) is the only multiple in use.

### Weights

The unit of weight is the gram, or gramme, abbreviation gr. (in English speaking countries usually g. or gm. to distinguish it from grain). It is practically the weight of one cubic centimeter of distilled water at its maximum density (4°C.); exactly, it is one-thousandth the weight of a mass of platinum, called *kilogramme des archives*, preserved as the standard in Paris. Multiples of this unit are designated by prefixes derived from the Greek numerals, as follows:

Gram; decagram, 10 grams; hectogram, 100 grams; kilogram (abbr. kilo), 1000 grams. In France, multiples of the kilo are sometimes called: 100 kilos, quintal; 1000 kilos, tonne or millier. One-half a kilo is popularly called a livre (pound).

Fractions of the gram are designated by prefixes, derived from the Latin numerals, as follows:

Gram; decigram, $\frac{1}{10}$ gram; centigram, $\frac{1}{100}$ gram; milligram, $\frac{1}{1000}$ gram.

In pharmacy and laboratory work the unit of volume is the cubic centimeter, abbr. cc. (called mil in the U.S.P.IX), that of weight is the gram. In the countries where the metric system is in use, liquid medicinal preparations are dispensed by weight and not by volume, by grams and not by cubic centimeters. In prescription writing, fractions of the cubic centimeter or of the gram are expressed by decimals, or by figures written to the right of a vertical line; thus:

| 2 | cubic centimeters | or | 2 | gm., | 2 | or | 2 | |
| $\frac{1}{10}$ | cubic centimeter | or | $\frac{1}{10}$ | gm., | 0.1 | or | | 1 |
| $\frac{3}{100}$ | cubic centimeter | or | $\frac{3}{100}$ | gm., | 0.03 | or | | 03 |
| $\frac{2}{1000}$ | cubic centimeter | or | $\frac{2}{1000}$ | gm., | 0.002 | or | | 002 |
| $1\frac{35}{100}$ | cubic centimeters | or | $1\frac{35}{100}$ | gm., | 1.35 | or | 1 | 35 |

## BRITISH AND AMERICAN MEASURES

### Linear Measures

| mile | furlongs | rods | yards | feet | inches |
|------|----------|------|-------|------|--------|
| 1 = | 8 = | 320 = | 1760 = | 5280 = | 63360 |
| | 1 = | 40 = | 220 = | 660 = | 7920 |
| | | 1 = | 5½ = | 16½ = | 198 |
| | | | 1 = | 3 = | 36 |
| | | | | 1 = | 12 |

Other measures are: league, 3 miles; cable, 10 fathoms = 60 feet; fathom, 6 feet; chain, 22 yards = 66 feet = 100 links; link, 7.92 inches; cubit, 2 quarters = 18 inches; quarter, 9 inches; hand, 4 inches; palm, 3 inches; ell, 1.25 yards = 45 inches; line, 12 inch.

### Square Measure

| acre | perches | sq. yards | sq. feet | sq. inches |
|------|---------|-----------|----------|------------|
| 1 = | 160 = | 4840 = | 43,560 = | 6,560,640 |
| | 1 = | 30.25 = | 272.25 = | 39,204 |
| | | 1 = | 9 = | 1296 |
| | | | 1 = | 144 |

A square mile = 640 acres = 5400 square chains, 10 square chains (each 4356 square feet) = 1 acre.

## TROY OR APOTHECARIES' AND AVOIRDUPOIS WEIGHTS

In the United States the weights used in prescription writing and the compounding of drugs are those of the apothecaries' system; the weights of the British Pharmacopoeia are those of the avoirdupois system. In both, the weight of the grain is the same, but the drachm, ounce, and pound differ.

### Troy Weights

| pound | ounces | pennyweights | grains |
|-------|--------|--------------|--------|
| 1 = | 12 = | 240 = | 5760 |
| | 1 = | 20 = | 480 |
| | | 1 = | 24 |

### Apothecaries' Weights (U.S.P.)

| pound | ounces | drachms | scruples | grains |
|-------|--------|---------|----------|--------|
| 1 = | 12 = | 96 = | 288 = | 5760 |
| | 1 = | 8 = | 24 = | 480 |
| | | 1 = | 3 = | 60 |
| | | | 1 = | 20 |

### Avoirdupois Weights (B.P.)

| pound | ounces | drachms | grains |
|-------|--------|---------|--------|
| 1 = | 16 = | 256 = | 7000 |
| | 1 = | 16 = | 437.5 |
| | | 1 = | 27.34375 |

To convert troy ounces to avoirdupois, add 10 per cent; to convert avoirdupois ounces to troy, subtract $\frac{1}{11}$. These are approximate equivalents.

Other weights are: quarter, 28 pounds; hundredweight, 112 pounds; ton, 20 hundredweight = 2240 pounds; in America there is also the "short ton" of 2000 pounds, with the corresponding hundred weight of 100 pounds, and quarter of 25 pounds. The stone is 14 pounds for the weight of man, but varies in value for different commodities.

## LIQUID MEASURES

### United States Apothecaries' Measures

| gallon | | quarts | | pints | | fluid ounces | | fluid drachms | | minims |
|---|---|---|---|---|---|---|---|---|---|---|
| 1 | = | 4 | = | 8 | = | 128 | = | 1024 | = | 61440 |
| | | 1 | = | 2 | = | 32 | = | 256 | = | 15360 |
| | | | | 1 | = | 16 | = | 128 | = | 7680 |
| | | | | | | 1 | = | 8 | = | 480 |
| | | | | | | | | 1 | = | 60 |

### Imperial Apothecaries' Measures

| gallon | | quarts | | pints | | fluid ounces | | fluid drachms | | minims |
|---|---|---|---|---|---|---|---|---|---|---|
| 1 | = | 4 | = | 8 | = | 160 | = | 1280 | = | 76800 |
| | | 1 | = | 2 | = | 40 | = | 320 | = | 19200 |
| | | | | 1 | = | 20 | = | 160 | = | 9600 |
| | | | | | | 1 | = | 8 | = | 480 |
| | | | | | | | | 1 | = | 60 |

The minim, fluidrachm, and fluidounce of the U.S. apothecaries' measure are slightly larger than the corresponding denominations in the Imperial (British) measure; the pint, quart, and gallon, on the other hand, are materially smaller.

| | U.S. | Imp. | | Imp. | U.S. |
|---|---|---|---|---|---|
| minim, fluidrachm, fluidounce | 1 = | 1.0406 | | 1 = | 0.9609 |
| pint, quart, gallon | 1 = | 0.8325 | | 1 = | 1.2011 |

### EQUIVALENTS

Tables of exact equivalents of metric and apothecaries' and avoirdupois weights, and metric and English and American measures are given below, but for rough calculations the following will suffice:

#### Linear Measures

One kilometer = $\frac{5}{8}$ mile or 3281 feet; 8 kilometers = 5 miles; 1 meter = 39 inches; 1 centimeter = $\frac{2}{5}$ inch; 1 millimeter = $\frac{1}{25}$ inch or $\frac{1}{2}$ line; 1 micron = $\frac{1}{25000}$ inch.

One mile = $1\frac{3}{5}$ kilometers; 1 yard = 92 centimeters; 1 foot = 30.5 centimeters; 1 inch = 25 millimeters; 1 line = 2 millimeters.

To convert kilometers to miles, multiply by 5 and divide by 8; to convert miles to kilometers multiply by 8 and divide by 5.

To convert meters to yards, multiply by 70 and divide by 64; to convert yards to meters multiply by 64 and divide by 70.

To convert centimeters to feet, multiply by 10 and divide by 307; to convert feet to centimeters multiply by 307 and divide by 10.

To convert millimeters to inches, multiply by 10 and divide by 254; to convert inches to millimeters multiply by 254 and divide by 10.

#### Weights

One kilogram = $2\frac{1}{5}$ pounds, or $35\frac{1}{3}$ ounces, avoirdupois; or $2\frac{7}{10}$ pounds, or $32\frac{1}{5}$ ounces, troy; 1 gram = $15\frac{1}{2}$ grains.

One pound avoirdupois = 453.6 grams; 1 pound troy = 373.2 grams; 1 ounce avoirdupois = 28.4 grams; 1 ounce troy = 31.1 grams; 1 drachm = 3.89 grams; 1 grain = 0.065 gram.

To convert kilograms to pounds avoirdupois multiply by 1000 and divide by 454; to convert pounds avoirdupois to kilograms,

multiply by 454 and divide by 1000; to convert kilograms to pounds troy, multiply by 1000 and divide by 371; to convert pounds troy to kilograms multiply by 371 and divide by 100.

To convert grams to ounces avoirdupois, multiply by 20 and divide by 567; to convert grams to ounces troy, multiply by 20 and divide by 622; or in both cases simply divide by 30; to convert ounces avoirdupois to grams, multiply by 567 and divide by 20; to convert ounces troy to grams, multiply by 622 and divide by 20; or in both cases simply multiply by 30.

To convert grams to drachms, divide by 4; to convert drachms to grams multiply by 4.

To convert grams or fractions of a gram to grains, multiply by 155 and divide by 10, or simply multiply by 15; to convert grains to grams, multiply by 10 and divide by 155; or divide by 15.

To convert centigrams to grains, divide by 6; to convert grains to centigrams, multiply by 6.

To convert milligrams to grains, divided by 60; to convert grains to milligrams, multiply by 60.

#### Fluid Measures

One liter = 1.76 imperial pints or 2.1 U.S. pints; 1 cubic centimeter = 17 minims (B.P.) or $16\frac{1}{4}$ minims (U.S.P.).

One imperial gallon = 4.55 liters; 1 U.S. gallon = 3.79 liters; 1 imperial pint = 568 cubic centimeters; 1 U.S. pint = 473 cubic centimeters; 1 fluid ounce (B.P.) = 28.4 cubic centimeters; 1 fluidounce (U.S.P.) = 29.5 cubic centimeters; 1 fluid drachm (B.P.) = 3.5 cubic centimeters; 1 fluidrachm (U.S.P.) = 3.7 cubic centimeters; 1 minim = 0.065 cubic centimeter.

To convert liters to imperial gallons, multiply by 22 and divide by 100; to convert liters to U.S. gallons, multiply by 265 and divide by 1000 (by moving the decimal point three places to the left): to convert imperial gallons to liters, divide by 22 and multiply by 100; to convert U.S. gallons to liters divide by 265 and multiply by 1000.

To convert liters to imperial pints, multiply by 88 and divide by 50; to convert liters to U.S. pints, multiply by 21 and divide by 10; to convert imperial pints to liters, multiply by 50 and divide by 88; to convert U.S. pints to liters, multiply by 100 and divide by 21.

To convert cubic centimeters to fluid drachms (B.P.), multiply by 2 and divide by 7; to convert cubic centimeters to fluidrachms (U.S.P.), multiply by 20 and divide by 74; or in both cases simply divide by 4; to convert fluid drachms (B.P.) to cubic centimeters, multiply by 7 and divide by 2; to convert fluidrachms (U.S.P.) to cubic centimeters, multiply by 74 and divide by 20; or in both cases simply multiply by 4.

To convert cubic centimeters, or fractions thereof, to minims, multiply by 100 and divide by 6; to convert minims to cubic centimeters, multiply by 6 and divide by 100 (by moving the decimal point two places to the left).

#### METRIC EQUIVALENTS OF APOTHECARIES' WEIGHTS

| grains | grams | grains | grams |
|---|---|---|---|
| $\frac{1}{120}$ | 0.000539 | 7 | 0.453586 |
| $\frac{1}{100}$ | 0.000648 | 8 | 0.518384 |
| $\frac{1}{60}$ | 0.001079 | 9 | 0.583182 |
| $\frac{1}{50}$ | 0.001296 | 10 | 0.647980 |
| $\frac{1}{30}$ | 0.002159 | 15 | 0.971970 |
| $\frac{1}{25}$ | 0.002592 | 20 | 1.295960 |
| $\frac{1}{20}$ | 0.003237 | 30 | 1.943940 |
| $\frac{1}{12}$ | 0.005399 | drachms | grams |
| $\frac{1}{10}$ | 0.006479 | 1 | 3.88788 |
| $\frac{1}{8}$ | 0.008098 | 2 | 7.77576 |
| $\frac{1}{6}$ | 0.010798 | 3 | 11.66364 |
| $\frac{1}{4}$ | 0.016197 | 4 | 15.55152 |
| $\frac{1}{3}$ | 0.021597 | ounces | grams |
| $\frac{1}{2}$ | 0.032395 | 1 | 31.10394 |
| 1 | 0.064798 | 2 | 62.20788 |
| 2 | 0.129596 | 3 | 93.31182 |
| 3 | 0.194394 | 4 | 124.41576 |
| 4 | 0.259192 | 6 | 186.62364 |
| 5 | 0.323990 | 12 | 373.24728 |
| 9 | 0.388788 | | |

## METRIC EQUIVALENTS OF AVOIRDUPOIS WEIGHTS

The equivalents for grams and fractions of a grain are the same as those of apothecaries' weights.

| drachms | grams | ounces | grams |
|---|---|---|---|
| 1 | 1.77182 | 1 | 28.34912 |
| 2 | 3.54364 | 2 | 56.69824 |
| 3 | 5.31546 | 8 | 226.79296 |
| 4 | 7.08728 | 16 | 453.58592 |
| 8 | 14.17456 | | |

## EQUIVALENTS OF METRIC IN APOTHECARIES' OR AVOIRDUPOIS WEIGHTS

| grams | grains | grams | grains |
|---|---|---|---|
| 0.001 | 0.01543 | 0.2 | 3.08678 |
| 0.002 | 0.03086 | 0.3 | 4.63017 |
| 0.003 | 0.04629 | 0.4 | 6.17359 |
| 0.004 | 0.06173 | 0.5 | 7.71699 |
| 0.005 | 0.07716 | 0.6 | 9.26039 |
| 0.006 | 0.09261 | 0.7 | 10.80379 |
| 0.007 | 0.10803 | 0.8 | 12.34719 |
| 0.008 | 0.12347 | 0.9 | 13.89059 |
| 0.009 | 0.13891 | 1.0 | 15.43399 |
| 0.01 | 0.15433 | 2.0 | 30.86798 |
| 0.02 | 0.30866 | 3.0 | 46.30197 |
| 0.03 | 0.46301 | 4.0 | 61.73598 |
| 0.04 | 0.61735 | 5.0 | 77.16995 |
| 0.05 | 0.77169 | 6.0 | 92.60394 |
| 0.06 | 0.92603 | 7.0 | 108.03793 |
| 0.07 | 1.08037 | 8.0 | 123.47196 |
| 0.08 | 1.23471 | 9.0 | 138.90591 |
| 0.09 | 1.38905 | 10.0 | 154.33991 |
| 0.1 | 1.54339 | | |

| kilograms | ounces (avoirdupois) | ounces (troy) |
|---|---|---|
| 1 | 35.27 | 32.15 |
| 2 | 70.55 | 64.31 |
| 5 | 176.37 | 160.77 |
| 10 | 352.74 | 321.54 |

| kilograms | pounds (avoirdupois) | pounds (troy) |
|---|---|---|
| 1 | 2.2048 | 2.6792 |
| 2 | 4.4096 | 5.3584 |
| 5 | 11.0240 | 13.3960 |
| 10 | 22.0480 | 26.7920 |

## METRIC EQUIVALENTS OF U. S. APOTHECARIES' MEASURES

| minims | cubic centimeter | minims | cubic centimeters |
|---|---|---|---|
| 1/120 | 0.000513 | 1 | 0.061618 |
| 1/100 | 0.000616 | 2 | 0.123236 |
| 1/60 | 0.001027 | 3 | 0.184854 |
| 1/50 | 0.001232 | 4 | 0.246472 |
| 1/30 | 0.002054 | 5 | 0.308091 |
| 1/25 | 0.002464 | 6 | 0.369708 |
| 1/20 | 0.003081 | 7 | 0.431326 |
| 1/12 | 0.005135 | 8 | 0.492944 |
| 1/10 | 0.006161 | 9 | 0.554562 |
| 1/8 | 0.007703 | 10 | 0.616181 |
| 1/6 | 0.010271 | 15 | 0.924272 |
| 1/4 | 0.015405 | 20 | 1.232362 |
| 1/3 | 0.020542 | 30 | 1.848543 |
| 1/2 | 0.030809 | | |

| fluid drachms | cubic centimeters | fluid ounces | cubic centimeters |
|---|---|---|---|
| 1 | 3.697086 | 1 | 29.576686 |
| 2 | 7.394172 | 2 | 59.153372 |
| 3 | 11.091258 | 3 | 88.730058 |
| 4 | 14.788344 | 4 | 118.306744 |
| 5 | 18.485431 | 6 | 177.460116 |
| 6 | 22.182516 | 12 | 354.920232 |
| 7 | 25.876602 | 16(pt.) | 473.226976 |

## METRIC EQUIVALENTS OF IMPERIAL APOTHECARIES' MEASURES

| minims | cubic centimeters | minims | cubic centimeters |
|---|---|---|---|
| 1/120 | 0.000493 | 1 | 0.059205 |
| 1/100 | 0.000592 | 2 | 0.118410 |
| 1/60 | 0.000985 | 3 | 0.177615 |
| 1/50 | 0.001184 | 4 | 0.236820 |
| 1/30 | 0.001971 | 5 | 0.296025 |
| 1/25 | 0.002368 | 6 | 0.355230 |
| 1/20 | 0.002961 | 7 | 0.414435 |
| 1/12 | 0.004934 | 8 | 0.473640 |
| 1/10 | 0.005920 | 9 | 0.532845 |
| 1/8 | 0.007395 | 10 | 0.592050 |
| 1/6 | 0.009849 | 15 | 0.888075 |
| 1/4 | 0.014790 | 20 | 1.184100 |
| 1/3 | 0.019718 | 30 | 1.776150 |
| 1/2 | 0.029601 | 45 | 2.664225 |

| fluid drachms | cubic centimeters | fluid ounces | cubic centimeters |
|---|---|---|---|
| 1 | 3.5523 | 1 | 28.4184 |
| 2 | 7.1046 | 2 | 56.8368 |
| 3 | 10.6569 | 3 | 85.2552 |
| 4 | 14.2092 | 4 | 113.6736 |
| 5 | 17.7615 | 5 | 142.0920 |
| 6 | 21.3138 | 6 | 170.5104 |
| 7 | 24.8661 | 10 | 284.1840 |
| | | 20(pt.) | 568.3680 |

## EQUIVALENTS OF METRIC IN U. S. APOTHECARIES' MEASURES

| cubic centimeters | minims | cubic centimeters | minims |
|---|---|---|---|
| 0.001 | 0.01623 | 0.2 | 3.24682 |
| 0.002 | 0.03246 | 0.3 | 4.87023 |
| 0.003 | 0.04871 | 0.4 | 6.49364 |
| 0.004 | 0.06493 | 0.5 | 8.11706 |
| 0.005 | 0.08117 | 0.6 | 9.74047 |
| 0.006 | 0.09741 | 0.7 | 11.36388 |
| 0.007 | 0.11363 | 0.8 | 12.98729 |
| 0.008 | 0.12987 | 0.9 | 14.61071 |
| 0.009 | 0.14611 | 1.0 | 16.23412 |
| 0.01 | 0.16234 | 2.0 | 32.46824 |
| 0.02 | 0.32468 | 3.0 | 48.70236 |
| 0.03 | 0.48702 | 4.0 | 64.93648 |
| 0.04 | 0.64936 | 5.0 | 81.17061 |
| 0.05 | 0.81171 | 6.0 | 97.40473 |
| 0.06 | 0.97404 | 7.0 | 113.63885 |
| 0.07 | 1.13638 | 8.0 | 129.87297 |
| 0.08 | 1.29872 | 9.0 | 146.10709 |
| 0.09 | 1.46107 | 10.0 | 162.34122 |
| 0.1 | 1.62341 | | |

| liter | fluidounces | pints |
|---|---|---|
| 1 | 33.82108 | 2.11381 |

## EQUIVALENTS OF METRIC IN IMPERIAL APOTHECARIES' MEASURES

| cubic centimeters | minims | cubic centimeters | minims |
|---|---|---|---|
| 0.001 | 0.01689 | 0.2 | 3.37822 |
| 0.002 | 0.03378 | 0.3 | 5.06733 |
| 0.003 | 0.05067 | 0.4 | 6.75644 |
| 0.004 | 0.06756 | 0.5 | 8.44556 |
| 0.005 | 0.08445 | 0.6 | 10.13467 |
| 0.006 | 0.10134 | 0.7 | 11.82378 |
| 0.007 | 0.11823 | 0.8 | 13.51289 |
| 0.008 | 0.13512 | 0.9 | 15.20200 |
| 0.009 | 0.15202 | 1.0 | 16.89112 |
| 0.01 | 0.16891 | 2.0 | 33.78224 |
| 0.02 | 0.33782 | 3.0 | 50.67336 |

| cubic centimeters | minims | cubic centimeters | minims |
|---|---|---|---|
| 0.03 | 0.50673 | 4.0 | 67.56448 |
| 0.04 | 0.67564 | 5.0 | 84.45560 |
| 0.05 | 0.84455 | 6.0 | 101.34672 |
| 0.06 | 1.01346 | 7.0 | 118.23784 |
| 0.07 | 1.18237 | 8.0 | 135.12896 |
| 0.08 | 1.35128 | 9.0 | 152.02008 |
| 0.09 | 1.52020 | 10.0 | 168.91123 |
| 0.1 | 1.68911 | | |

| liters | fluid ounces | pints |
|---|---|---|
| 1 | 35.19691 | 1.75984 |

### Approximate Liquid Measures

In America a teaspoonful is reckoned as 1 fluidrachm, or 4 cc.; a dessertspoonful as 2 fluidrachms, or 8 cc.; a tablespoonful as half an ounce, or 16 cc. Elsewhere a teaspoonful is regarded as approximately the equivalent of 5 cc. (85 minims B.P.); a tablespoonful as three teaspoonfuls or 15 cc. (255 minims B.P.).

A wineglassful is 2 fluidounces, or 64 cc.; a teacupful = 2 wineglassfuls, 4 fluidounces, 125 cc.; a tumblerful = 4 wineglassfuls, 8 fluidounces, half a pint, 250 cc.

A drop is a measure of very uncertain quantity, varying in size not only according to the nature of the liquid but also according to the shape of the container, and its aperture, from which it falls.

### Energy Measures

One kilogrammeter is the energy or force expended in raising a weight of 1 kilogram to a height of 1 meter. One foot-pound is the energy or force expended in raising a weight of 1 pound avoirdupois to a height of 1 foot.

One kilogrammeter = 7.24 foot-pounds.

One foot-pound = 0.1381 kilogrammeter.

# Appendix 6: Symbols

(See also appendix 10, Glossary of Abbreviations.)

♏ minim.
℈ scruple.
ʒ drachm.
℥ ounce.
O pint.
℔ pound.
℞ recipe, take.
m̄ misce, mix.
′ foot; minute; primary accent; univalent.
″ inch; second; bivalent.
‴ line (1/12 inch); trivalent.
μ micron.
μμ micromicron.
+ plus; excess; acid reaction; positive. In noting the result of the Wassermann test for syphilis, complete inhibition of hemolysis is usually indicated by ++++ (or 4+); 75 per cent by +++ (or 3+); 50 per cent by ++ (or 2+), and less than 50 per cent by +.
— minus; deficiency; alkaline reaction; negative.
± plus or minus; either positive or negative; indefinite.
÷ divided by.
× multiplied by; in microscopy, magnification.
= equal to.
> greater than; whence, from which is derived.
< less than; from, derived from.
√ root; square root; radical.
$\sqrt[2]{}$ square root.
$\sqrt[3]{}$ cube root.
∞ infinity.
: ratio; "is to."
:: equality between ratios; "as."
* birth.
† death.
♀ Venus; female; copper.
○ female.
♂ Mars; male; iron.
□ male.
◯ undetermined sex.
⊙ the sun; gold.
☿ mercury.
♃ Jupiter; tin.
♄ Saturn, lead.
☾ the moon, silver.
° degree
% per cent.

# Appendix 7: Laboratory Analyses and Observations; Normal or Usual Results When No Disease Is Recognized

| Qualitative or quantitative analysis, test, or observation performed | Body fluid, tissue, or other material used | "Normal" or usual amount, or "normal" observation |
|---|---|---|
| Acetone | Serum | |
|   Qualitative | | Negative |
|   Quantitative | | 0.3–2.0 mg/100 ml |
| Addis count | 12-hr urine | White cells (white blood cells and renal epithelial cells): 1,800,000; children, slightly lower |
| | | Red blood cells: 500,000; children slightly lower |
| | | Casts (hyaline): 0–5000; children slightly higher |
| Agglutination | Serum | |
|   Widal | | Fourfold rise in titer between acute and convalescent sera |
|   Weil-Felix | | Fourfold rise in titer between acute and convalescent sera |
|   Brucella | | Less than 1:80 |
|   Strep. Mg | | Less than 1:20 |
|   Tularemia | | Less than 1:80 |
|   Trichinosis | | Negative |
| Albumin | | |
|   Qualitative | Random urine | Negative |
|   Quantitative | 24-hr urine | 10–100 mg/24 hr |
| Alcohol (ethyl) | Serum or whole blood | Negative |
| Aldolase | Serum | 3–8 Sibley-Lehninger units/ml; children and newborn, higher levels |
| Aldosterone | 24-hr urine | 2–23 µg/24 hr |
| | Serum | 1–21 ng/100 ml |
| Alkapton bodies | Random urine | Negative |
| α-Amino acid nitrogen | Serum | 4–6 mg/100 ml |
| | 24-hr urine | 0.1–0.29 g/24 hr |
| δ-Aminolevulinic acid | 24-hr urine | 1.3–7.0 mg/24 hr |
| Ammonia | Plasma | 20–150 µg/100 ml (diffusion) |
| | | 40–80 µg/100 ml (enzymatic) |
| | | 12–48 µg/100 ml (resin) |
| Ammonia nitrogen | 24-hr urine | 0.14–1.47 g/24 hr |
| Amylase | Serum | 60–150 Somogyi units/100 ml |
| | Random urine | 35–260 Somogyi units/hr |
| Anti-DNA antibodies | Serum | Less than 1:8 |
| Antimitochondrial antibody | Serum | Negative |
| Antinuclear antibody (ANA) | Serum | Negative |
| Anti-smooth muscle antibody | Serum | Negative |
| Antistreptohyaluronidase | Serum | Less than 1:256 |
| Antistreptolysin O | Serum | Less than 166 Todd units |
| Antithyroid antibodies | Serum | |
|   Antithyroglobulin | | Less than 1:32 |
|   Antithyroid microsomal | | Less than 1:56 |
|   Bentonite particle test | | Less than 1:5 |
|   Sensitized red cell method | | Less than 1:40 |
| α-1-Antitrypsin | Serum | 200–400 mg/100 ml |
| Ascorbic acid (vitamin C) | Plasma | 0.6–1.6 mg/100 ml |
| Australian antigen (hepatitis-associated antigen) | Serum | Negative |
| Barbiturates | Serum or urine | Negative |

| Qualitative or quantitative analysis, test, or observation performed | Body fluid, tissue, or other material used | "Normal" or usual amount, or "normal" observation |
|---|---|---|
| Basal acid output (1 hr) | Gastric fluid | 0–6 mEq/hr |
| Basal acid output to maximal acid output (ratio) | Gastric fluid | Less than 0.40 |
| Base, total | Serum | 145–160 mEq/liter |
| Bence Jones protein (see Protein) | | |
| Bile, qualitative | Random stool | Negative in adults, positive in children |
| Bilirubin | Serum | |
| Direct | | Up to 0.3 mg/100 ml |
| Indirect | | 0.1–1.0 mg/100 ml |
| Total | | Up to 1.2 mg/100 ml |
| Bilirubin (bile), qualitative | Random urine | Negative |
| Blood count, complete | Whole blood | |
| Hematocrit | | Male, 40–54 vol %; female, 37–47 vol % |
| Hemoglobin | | Male, 14–18 g/100 ml; female, 12–16 g/100 ml |
| Red blood cell | | Male, 4.6–6.2 million/cu mm; female, 4.2–5.4 million/cu mm |
| White blood cell | | 5,000–10,000/cu mm |
| Platelet count | | 150,000–450,000/cu mm |
| Blood indices | Whole blood | |
| Mean corpuscular hemoglobin | | 27–31 $\mu\mu$g |
| Mean corpuscular volume | | 82–92 cu $\mu$ |
| Mean corpuscular hemoglobin concentration | | 32–36% |
| Blood, occult, qualitative | Random urine | Negative |
| Blood-synovial glucose difference | Synovial fluid | Less than 10 mg/100 ml |
| Bromide | Serum | 0.8–1.5 mg/100 ml |
| BSP (see Sulfobromophthalein) | | |
| Calcium | | |
| Ionized | Serum | 2.1–2.6 mEq/liter; 4.2–5.2 mg/100 ml |
| Quantitative | 24-hr urine | Average diet, 100–250 mg/24 hr; low-calcium diet, less than 150 mg/24 hr; high-calcium diet, 250–300 mg/24 hr |
| Sulkowitch | Random urine | 1+, moderate turbidity |
| Total | Serum | 4.5–5.3 mEq/liter; 9.0–10.6 mg/100 ml; infants, 11–13 mg/100 ml |
| Carbon dioxide content | Serum | Adults, 24–30 mmoles/liter; infants, 20–28 mmoles/liter |
| Carbon dioxide partial pressure ($pCO_2$) | Whole blood (arterial) | 35–40 mm Hg |
| | Whole blood (venous) | 40–45 mm Hg |
| Carboxyhemoglobin | Whole blood | Less than 5% |
| $\beta$-Carotene | Serum | 40–200 $\mu$g/100 ml |
| Catecholamines | Random urine | 0–14 $\mu$g/100 ml |
| | 24-hr urine | 100 $\mu$g/24 hr (varies with muscular activity) |
| Cell count | Cerebrospinal fluid | 0–10 cells/$\mu$l |
| Ceruloplasmin | Serum | 23–50 mg/100 ml |
| Chloride | Cerebrospinal fluid | 118–132 mEq/liter |
| | Serum | 95–103 mEq/liter |
| | Sweat | 4–60 mEq/liter |
| | 24-hr urine | 110–250 mEq/24 hr |
| Cholesterol | Serum | |
| Esters | | 65%–75% of total |
| Total | | 150–250 mg/100 ml |
| Coagulation tests | Whole blood | |
| Bleeding time | | Ivy, 1–6 min; Duke, 1–3 min |

| Qualitative or quantitative analysis, test, or observation performed | Body fluid, tissue, or other material used | "Normal" or usual amount, or "normal" observation |
|---|---|---|
| Clot retraction | | One-half the original mass in 2 hr |
| Dilute blood clot lysis time | | Clot lysis in over 6 and under 10 hr |
| Euglobulin clot lysis time | | Clot lysis in over 2 and under 6 hr |
| Factor XIII (fibrin-stabilizing factor) | | Clot insoluble in 5 M urea or 2% monochloroacetic acid in 16–24 hr |
| Partial thromboplastin time | | 60–70 sec; kaolin-activated, 35–45 sec |
| Prothrombin time | | 12–14 sec |
| Prothrombin utilization | | Over 20 sec at 60 min |
| Venous clotting time | | 3 tubes, 5–15 min; 2 tubes, 5–8 min |
| Whole blood clot lysis | | None in 24 hr |
| Colloidal gold curve | Cerebrospinal fluid | All zero, or 0001111000 |
| Congo red test | Serum | More than 60% at 1 hr |
| Cold agglutinins | Serum | Less than 1:32 |
| Copper | Serum | 70–140 μg/100 ml |
| Coproporphyrin | Random urine | Adults, 20 μg/100 ml |
| | 24-hr specimen | 50–160 μg/24 hr; children, 0–80 μg/24 hr |
| Cortisol | Plasma | 8 a.m., 6–18 μg/100 ml; 4 p.m., one-half to one-third the a.m. volume |
| C-reactive protein (*see* Protein, C-reactive) | | |
| Creatine | Serum | Male, 0.2–0.6 mg/100 ml; female, 0.6–1.0 mg/100 ml |
| | 24-hr urine | Male, 0–40 mg/24 hr; female, 0–100 mg/24 hr; higher in children and during pregnancy |
| Creatine phosphokinase (CPK) | Serum | Male, 5–50 IU; female, 5–30 IU |
| Creatinine | Serum | 0.5–1.2 mg/100 ml |
| | 24-hr urine | Male, 1000–1900 mg/24 hr; female, 800–1700 mg/24 hr, or 5–15 mg/kg of body wt/24 hr |
| Creatinine clearance Endogenous | Serum and urine | Male. 97–137 ml/min: female. 88–128 ml/min 150–180 liters/24 hr |
| Cryoglobulins | Serum | Negative |
| Cystine, qualitative | Random urine | Negative or trace |
| Diacetic acid, qualitative | Random urine | Negative |
| Diagnex test (tubeless gastric) | Urine | Free HCl present |
| Differential cell count | Synovial fluid | Granulocytes less than 25% of nucleated cells |
| Dilution and concentration | Urine | Concentrated specimen, 1.025 or higher; first diluted specimen, 1.001–1.003 |
| Double refractile bodies | Random urine | Negative |
| Duodenal drainage | Duodenal contents | Variable—consult reference books |
| Electrophoresis (*see* Hemoglobin; Protein) | | |
| Eosinophil count | Whole blood | 100–300/cu mm |
| Estrogens | 24-hr urine specimen | Male, 4–25 μg/24 hr; female, 4–60 μg/24 hr; pregnancy, up to 45,000 μg/24 hr |
| Fasting residual volume | Gastric fluid | Up to 50 ml |
| Fat | Stool | Total fat, 10–25% of dry matter and less than 5.0 g/24 hr |
| Neutral fat | | 1–5% of dry matter |
| Free fatty acids | | 5–13% of dry matter |
| Combined fatty acids | | 5–15% of dry matter |
| Fat, qualitative | Random urine | Negative |
| Fatty acids, total | Serum | 9–15 mmoles/liter |
| α-Fetoprotein | Serum | Negative |

| Qualitative or quantitative analysis, test, or observation performed | Body fluid, tissue, or other material used | "Normal" or usual amount, or "normal" observation |
| --- | --- | --- |
| Fibrin clot | Synovial fluid | Absent |
| Fibrinogen | Plasma | 0.2–0.4 g/100 ml |
| Fluorescent treponemal antibody (FTA) | Serum | Negative |
| Folic acid (folate) | Serum | 7–16 ng/ml |
| Follicle-stimulating hormone (see Gonadotropic hormone) | | |
| Fragility test, osmotic | Whole blood | Begins 0.45–0.39%; complete 0.33–0.30% |
| Globulin | | |
|   Qualitative (Pandy) | Cerebrospinal fluid | Negative |
|   Quantitative | Cerebrospinal fluid | 6–16 mg/100 ml |
|   Total | Serum | 2.3–3.5 g/100 ml |
| γ-Globulin | Serum | 0.5–1.6 g/100 ml |
| Glucose | Cerebrospinal fluid | 45–75 mg/100 ml |
| Glucose, fasting | Serum or plasma | 70–110 mg/100 ml |
| | Whole blood | 60–100 mg/100 ml |
| Glucose, qualitative | Random urine | Negative |
| Glucose, quantitative | | |
|   Copper-reducing substances | 24-hr specimen | 0.5–1.5 g/24 hr |
|   Total sugars | 24-hr specimen | Average, 250 mg/24 hr |
|   Glucose | 24-hr specimen | Average, 130 mg/24 hr |
| Glucose tolerance | | |
|   Oral | Serum | Fasting, 70–110 mg/100 ml; 30 min, 30–60 mg above fasting; 60 min, 20–50 mg above fasting; 120 min, 5–15 mg above fasting; 180 min, fasting level or below |
|   Intravenous | Serum | Fasting, 70–110 mg/100 ml; 5 min, max of 250 mg/100 ml; 60 min, significant decrease; 120 min, below 120 mg/100 ml; 180 min, fasting level |
| Glucose-6-PO$_4$-dehydrogenase | Serum | 5–10 IU/g Hgb |
| Gonadotropic hormone, pituitary | 24-hr urine | 10–50 mouse uterine units/24 hr |
| Haptoglobin | Serum | 60–200 mg Hgb binding capacity/100 ml |
| Hemoglobin | Random urine | Negative |
|   Free | Serum or plasma | Negative |
| Hemoglobin, electrophoresis | Whole blood | Hemoglobin A |
| Hemoglobin, fetal (Singer) | Whole blood | Less than 2% |
| Hepatitis-associated antigen (see Australia antigen) | | |
| 17-Hydroxycorticosteroids | Plasma | Male, 7–19 µg/100 ml; female, 9–21 µg/100 ml; 35–55 µg/100 ml after i.m. ACTH (25 USP units). |
| | 24-hr urine | Male, 5.5–14.5 mg/24 hr; female, 4.9–12.9 mg/24 hr; lower in children; 200–400% increase after i.m. ACTH (25 USP units). |
| 5-Hydroxyindoleacetic acid | | |
|   Qualitative | Random urine | Negative |
|   Quantitative | 24-hr urine | Less than 9 mg/24 hr |
| Immunoglobulins | Serum | |
|   IgA | | 50–250 mg/100 ml |
|   IgD | | 0.5–3.0 mg/100 ml |
|   IgE | | 0.01–0.04 mg/100 ml |
|   IgG | | 800–1500 mg/100 ml |
|   IgM | | 40–120 mg/100 ml |

| Qualitative or quantitative analysis, test, or observation performed | Body fluid, tissue, or other material used | "Normal" or usual amount, or "normal" observation |
|---|---|---|
| Insulin tolerance | Serum | Fasting, 70–110 mg glucose/100 ml; 30 min, 50% of fasting; 90 min, fasting level |
| Iodine | | |
|   Butanol-extractable | Serum | 3.5–6.5 µg/100 ml |
|   Protein-bound | Serum | 4.0–8.0 µg/100 ml |
| Iron | Serum | 60–280 µg/100 ml |
| Iron-binding capacity | Serum | 250–425 µg/100 ml |
| Ketone bodies | Random urine | Negative |
| 17-Ketosteroids | Plasma | 25–125 µg/100 ml |
| | 24-hr urine | Male, 8–15 mg/24 hr; female, 6–11.5 mg/24 hr; children, 12–15 yr, 5–12 mg/24 hr; children less than 12 yr, less than 5 mg/24 hr; 50–100% increase after i.m. ACTH (25 USP units). |
| Lactic acid | Whole blood (venous) | 5–20 mg/100 ml |
| Lactic dehydrogenase (LDH) | Serum | Varies with test method, less than 300 IU/liter |
| L. E. preparation | Whole blood | Negative |
| Lead | Whole blood | 0–50 µg/100 ml |
| | 24-hr urine | Less than 100 µg/24 hr |
| Leucine aminopeptidase | Serum | 75–200 Goldbarg-Rutenburg units/ml |
| Lipase | Serum | 0–1.5 Cherry-Crandall units |
| Lipids, total | Serum | 400–800 mg/100 ml |
|   Cholesterol | | 115–290 mg/100 ml |
|   Fatty acids | | 9–15 mmoles/liter |
|   Neutral fat | | 0–200 mg/100 ml |
|   Phospholipid-P | | 8–11 mg/100 ml |
|   Phospholipids | | 150–380 mg/100 ml |
|   Triglycerides | | 50–175 mg/100 ml |
| Liquefaction | Seminal fluid | Within 20 min |
| Lithium | Serum | Negative |
| | | Therapeutic level, 0.5–1.5 mEq/liter |
| Magnesium | Serum | 1.5–2.5 mEq/liter; 1.8–3.0 mg/100 ml |
| Maximal histamine stimulation: acid output (1 hr) | Gastric fluid | Male, 10–40 mEq/hr; female, 5–30 mEq/hr |
| Melanin, qualitative | Random urine | Negative |
| Metanephrines | 24-hr urine | Less than 1.3 mg/24 hr |
| Methemoglobin, quantitative | Whole blood | 0–0.24 g/100 ml (average, 0.06 g/100 ml) |
| Microscopic examination | Random urine | Acid urine: may show small amounts of uric acid, calcium oxalate, or urate |
| | | Alkaline urine: may show small amounts of ammonium biurate, phosphate crystals, or amorphous phosphate |
| Morphology | Seminal fluid | More than 70% normal, mature spermatozoa |
| Motility | Seminal fluid | More than 60% |
| Mucin clot | Synovial fluid | Abundant |
| Nitrogen, total | 24-hr stool | 10% of intake (1–2 g/24 hr) |
| Nonprotein nitrogen | Serum | 20–35 mg/100 ml |
| Nucleated cell count | Synovial fluid | Less than 200 cells/cu mm |
| Osmolality | Serum | 280–290 mOsmoles/kg |
| | Random urine | 38–1400 mOsmoles/kg water; 500–800 mOsmoles/kg water (normal fluid intake) |
| Oxygen pressure | Whole blood (arterial) | 95–100 mm Hg |

| Qualitative or quantitative analysis, test, or observation performed | Body fluid, tissue, or other material used | "Normal" or usual amount, or "normal" observation |
| --- | --- | --- |
| Oxygen saturation | Whole blood (arterial) | 94–100% |
| Pandy's test | Cerebrospinal fluid | Negative |
| pH | Whole blood | 7.35–7.45 |
| | Gastric fluid | Less than 2.0 |
| | Seminal fluid | More than 7.0 (average, 7.7) |
| | Random urine | 4.6–8.0 (mean, 6.3) |
| Phenolsulfonphthalein excretion (6 mg dye) | | |
| Dye administered i.v. | 15-min urine | 20–50% dye excreted |
| | 30-min urine | 16–24% dye excreted |
| | 60-min urine | 9–17% dye excreted |
| | 120-min urine | 3–10% dye excreted |
| Dye administered i.m. | 60-min urine | 40–60% dye excreted |
| | 130-min urine | 20–25% dye excreted |
| Phenylalanine | Serum | 3.0–5.0 mg/100 ml |
| Phenylpyruvic acid, qualitative | Random urine | Negative |
| Phosphatase | Serum | |
| Acid | | 0–1.1 Bodansky units; 1–4 King-Armstrong units; 0.13–0.63 Bessey-Lowry units |
| Alkaline | | Adults: 1.5–4.5 Bodansky units; 0.8–2.3 Bessey-Lowry units; 4.0–13.0 King-Armstrong units |
| | | Children: 5.0–14.0 Bodansky units; 2.8–6.7 Bessey-Lowry units; 15.0–30.0 King-Armstrong units |
| Phosphorus | Serum | Adults: 1.8–2.6 mEq/liter; 3.0–4.5 mg/100 ml |
| | | Children: 2.3–4.1 mEq/liter; 4.0–7.0 mg/100 ml |
| | 24-hr urine | 0.9–1.3 g/24 hr (varies with intake) |
| Phospholipids (see lipids) | | |
| Porphobilinogen, qualitative | Random urine | Negative |
| Potassium | Plasma | 3.8–5.0 mEq/liter |
| | 24-hr urine | 25–100 mEq/24 hr |
| Pregnancy tests | | |
| Frog test | Concentrated morning urine or serum | Positive in a normal pregnancy or tumors producing chorionic gonadotropin |
| Latex pregnancy test | Concentrated morning urine | Same as above |
| Rabbit (Friedman) test | Concentrated morning urine | Same as above |
| Mouse (Ascheim-Zondek) test | Concentrated morning urine | In pregnancy, positive in dilutions up to 1 to 10 (10,000 mouse units) |
| Pregnanediol | Urine | Male, 0–1 mg/24 hr; female, 1–8 mg/24 hr (peak, 1 week after ovulation; peak during pregnancy, 60–100 mg/24 hr); children, negative |
| Pregnanetriol | 24-hr urine | Male, 1.0–2.0 mg/24 hr; female, 0.5–2.0 mg/24 hr; children, less than 0.5 mg/24 hr |
| Protein | | |
| Qualitative | Random urine | Negative |
| Quantitative | 24-hr urine | 10–150 mg/24 hr |
| Protein, total | Serum | 6.0–7.8 g/100 ml |
| Albumin | | 3.2–4.5 g/100 ml |
| Globulin | | 2.3–3.5 g/100 ml |

| Qualitative or quantitative analysis, test, or observation performed | Body fluid, tissue, or other material used | "Normal" or usual amount, or "normal" observation |
| --- | --- | --- |
| Protein, total | Cerebrospinal fluid | 15–45 mg/100 ml |
|   Albumin | | 52% |
|   $\alpha_1$-Globulin | | 5% |
|   $\alpha_2$-Globulin | | 14% |
|   $\beta$-Globulin | | 10% |
|   $\gamma$-Globulin | | 19% |
| Protein, Bence Jones | First morning urine | Negative |
| Protein, C-reactive | Serum | Negative |
| Protein, fractionation (electrophoresis) | Serum | |
|   Albumin | | 3.2–5.6 g/100 ml |
|   $\alpha_1$-Globulin | | 0.1–0.4 g/100 ml |
|   $\alpha_2$-Globulin | | 0.4–1.2 g/100 ml |
|   $\beta$-Globulin | | 0.5–1.1 g/100 ml |
|   $\gamma$-Globulin | | 0.5–1.6 g/100 ml |
| Reticulocyte count | Whole blood | 0.5–1.5% |
| Rheumatoid arthritis factor | Serum | |
|   Latex | | Less than 1:80 |
|   Sensitized sheep cell | | Less than 1:160 |
|   Bentonite | | Less than 1:32 |
| Salicylates | Serum | Negative; therapeutic level, 20–25 mg/100 ml; toxic level, more than 30 mg/100 ml |
| Sedimentation rate (Westergren) | Whole blood | Men under age 50, less than 15 mm/hr; men over age 50, less than 20 mm/hr; women under age 50, less than 20 mm/hr; women over age 50, less than 30 mm/hr |
| Serotonin (*see* 5-Hydroxyindoleacetic acid) | | |
| Sickle cell preparation | Whole blood | Negative (no sickling) |
| Sodium | Plasma | 136–142 mEq/liter |
| | Sweat | 10–80 mEq/liter |
| | 24-hr urine | 130–260 mEq/24 hr (diet-dependent) |
| Solids, total | 24-hr urine | 55–70 g/24 hr; decrease with age to 30 g/24 hr |
| Specific gravity | Random urine | 1.001–1.035 (1.016–1.022, normal fluid intake) |
| Sperm count | Seminal fluid | 60–150 million/ml |
| Sugars (excluding glucose) | Random urine | Negative |
| Sulfate | Serum | 0.2–1.3 mEq/liter |
| Sulfobromophthalein (BSP) | Serum | 0–5% (45 min) |
| Sulfonamides | Serum or whole blood | Negative |
| $T_3$ test (see Thyroid hormone test) | | |
| $T_4$ tests (see under Thyroxine) | | |
| Testosterone | Serum | Male, 200–1000 ng/100 ml; female, 20–80 ng/100 ml |
| Thiocyanate | Serum | Negative |
| Thymol flocculation | Serum | 0–5 units |
| Thyroid hormone test ($T_3$ test) | Serum | 24–35 relative % uptake |
| Thyroid $^{131}$I uptake | Thyroid gland | 7.5–25% in 6 hr |
| Thyroid-stimulating hormone (TSH) | Serum | 0–15 microunits/ml |
| Thyroxine | Serum | Expressed as thyroxine |
|   $T_4$ (Murphy-Pattee) | | 6.0–11.8 $\mu$g/100 ml |
|   $T_4$ by column | | 5.0–11.0 $\mu$g/100 ml |
|   Free $T_4$ | | 0.9–2.3 ng/100 ml |
| Thyroxine-binding globulin | Serum | 10–26 $\mu$g/100 ml |
| Titratable acidity | Random or 24-hr urine | 200–500 ml 0.1 N NaOH/24-hr urine |

| Qualitative or quantitative analysis, test, or observation performed | Body fluid, tissue, or other material used | "Normal" or usual amount, or "normal" observation |
|---|---|---|
| Transaminase | Serum | |
|   Glutamic oxaloacetic | | Less than 40 IU |
|   Glutamic pyruvic | | Less than 20 IU |
| Trypsin, semiquantitative | Random stool | Positive (2+ to 4+) |
| Urea clearance | Serum and urine | Maximal clearance, 64–99 ml/min; standard clearance, 41–65 ml/min, or more than 75% of normal clearance |
| Urea nitrogen | Serum | 9–20 mg/100 ml |
| | 24-hr urine | 6–17 g/24 hr |
| Uric acid | Serum | Male, 2.1–7.8 mg/100 ml; female, 2.0–6.4 mg/100 ml |
| | 24-hr urine | 250–750 mg/24 hr |
| Urobilinogen | | |
|   Qualitative | Random stool | Positive |
|   Quantitative | 24-hr stool | 40–200 mg/24 hr, or 30–280 Ehrlich units/24 hr |
| | 24-hr urine | 0.05–2.5 mg/24 hr, or 0.5–4.0 Ehrlich units/24 hr |
|   Semiquantitative | 2-hr urine | 0.05–2.5 mg/24 hr |
| Uroporphyrin | 24-hr urine | 10–30 µg/24 hr |
| Vanillylmandelic acid (VMA) | 24-hr urine | 2–9 mg/24 hr |
| Viscosity | Synovial fluid | High |
| Vitamin A | Serum | 15–60 µg/100 ml |
| Vitamin A tolerance | Serum | Fasting, 15–60 µg/100 ml; 3 hr or 6 hr, increase to 200–600 µg/100 ml; 24 hr, fasting values or slightly above |
| Vitamin $B_{12}$ | Serum | 200–900 pg/ml |
| Vitamin C (*see* Ascorbic acid) | | |
| Volume | Seminal fluid | 1.5–5.0 ml |
| Volume | Synovial fluid | Less than 3.5 ml |
| Volume, total | 24-hr urine | 600–1600 ml/24 hr |
| Xanthochromia | Cerebrospinal fluid | Negative |
| Xylose absorption | Serum | 25–40 mg/100 ml between 1 and 2 hr (maximum is approximately 10 mg/100 ml in malabsorption) |
| Zinc | 24-hr urine | 0.15–1.2 mg/24 hr |
| Zinc sulfate turbidity | Serum | Less than 12 units |

# Appendix 8: Comparative Temperature Scales

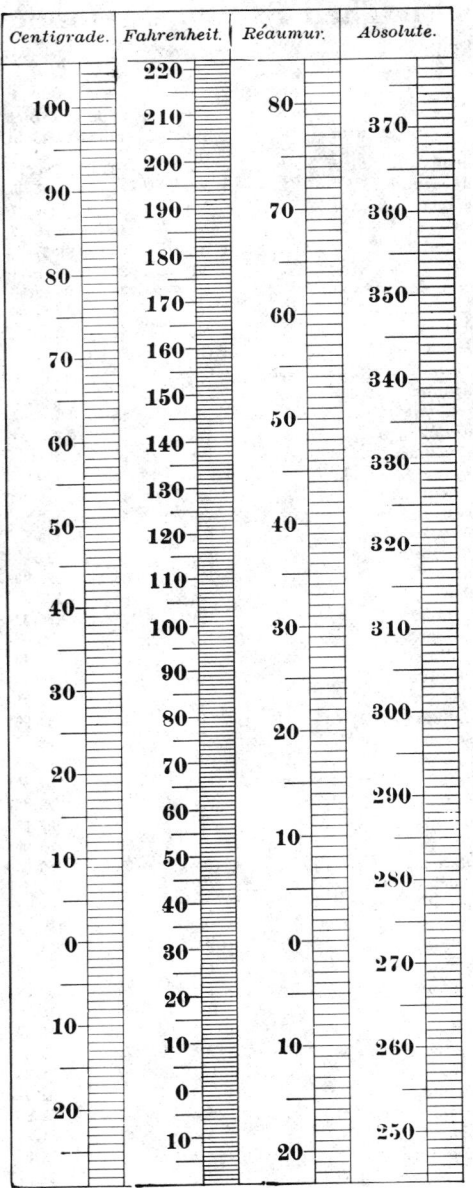

| Centigrade. | Fahrenheit. | Réaumur. | Absolute. |
|---|---|---|---|

solute zero, which is the point at which the form of motion which constitutes heat ceases, or the point of absence of all heat; it is calculated to be 273.16° below zero of the centigrade scale; −459.69°F., or −218.53°R. The centigrade scale is now often called the Celsius scale after its inventor, after the precedent set by the Fahrenheit and Réaumur scales. Similarly, the absolute scale is often referred to as the Kelvin scale and a temperature on such a scale may be abbreviated °A or °K. An absolute scale beginning at absolute zero, but using Fahrenheit degrees rather than centigrade, is named the Rankine scale.

The zero of the centigrade and Réaumur scales marks the temperature of melting ice (32°F.); the zero of the Fahrenheit scale is an arbitrary point, that of the lowest temperature observed by the deviser of the scale during the winter of 1709, practically the temperature of a mixture of ice and salt; it corresponds to −17.77°C., −14.22°R. The temperature of boiling water, at sea-level, is marked 100° on the centigrade scale (hence the name), 80° on the Réaumur scale, and 212° on the Fahrenheit scale. A degree F. is therefore ⁵⁄₉ degree C. and ⁴⁄₉ degree R.; a degree R. is ⁵⁄₄ degree C.

The following are rules for the conversion of the temperature of one scale into that of one of the others:

### I. Above 0°C. and R., or 32°F.

F. to C.: subtract 32, multiply by 5, divide by 9.
F. to R.: subtract 32, multiply by 4, divide by 9.
C. to F.: multiply by 9, divide by 5, add 32.
C. to R.: multiply by 4, divide by 5.
R. to F.: multiply by 9, divide by 4, add 32.
R. to C.: multiply by 5, divide by 4.

### II. Between 0° and 32°F.; −17.77° and 0°C., −14.22° and 0°R.

F. to C.: subtract from 32, multiply by 5, divide by 9.
F. to R.: subtract from 32, multiply by 4, divide by 9.
C. to F.: multiply by 9, divide by 5, subtract from 32.
C. to R.: multiply by 4, divide by 5.
R. to F.: multiply by 9, divide by 4, subtract from 32.
R. to C.: multiply by 5, divide by 4.

### III. Below 0°F., −17.77°C., −14.22°R.

F. to C.: add 32, multiply by 5, divide by 9.
F. to R.: add 32, multiply by 4, divide by 9.
C. to F. multiply by 9, divide by 5, subtract 32.
C. to R.: multiply by 4, divide by 5.
R. to F.: multiply by 9, divide by 4, subtract 32.
R. to C.: multiply by 5, divide by 4.

#### EXAMPLES:

I. 63°F. to C.: 63 − 32 = 31 × 5 = 155 ÷ 9 = 17.2°C.
   63°F. to R.: 63 − 32 = 31 × 4 = 124 ÷ 9 = 13.8°R.
   37°C. to F.: 37 × 9 = 333 ÷ 5 = 66.6 + 32 = 98.6°F.
   37°C. to R.: 37 × 4 = 148 ÷ 5 = 29.6°R.
   34°R to F.: 34 × 9 = 306 ÷ 4 = 76.5 + 32 = 108.5°F.
   34°R. to C.: 34 × 5 = 170 ÷ 4 = 42.5°C.
II. 10°F. to C.: 32 − 10 = 22 × 5 = 110 ÷ 9 = −12.2°C.
   10°F. to R.: 32 − 10 = 22 × 4 = 88 ÷ 9 = −9.8°R.
   −12°C. to F.: 12 × 9 = 108 ÷ 5 = 21.6; 32 − 21.6 = 10.4°F.
   −12°R. to F.: 12 × 9 = 108 ÷ 4 = 27; 32 − 27 = 5°F.
III. −10°F. to C.: 10 + 32 = 42 × 5 = 210 ÷ 9 = −23.3°C.
   −10°F. to R.: 10 + 32 = 42 × 4 = 168 ÷ 9 = −18.7°R.
   −18°C. to F.: 18 × 9 = 162 ÷ 5 = 32.4 − 32 = 0.4°F.
   −18°R. to F.: 18 × 9 = 162 ÷ 4 = 40.5 − 32 = −8.5°F.

*Special note:*

To convert C. to A.: add 273.16. To convert F. or R. to A., convert to C. first, then add 273.16. Examples:—72°C. to A.: 72 + 273.16 = 345.16°A. 63°F. to A.: 63°F. = 17.2°C. as above, 17.2 + 273.16 = 290.36°A. (round off to the proper number of significant figures).

There are three temperature scales in more or less general use, *viz.*, the centigrade; the Fahrenheit, and the Réaumur. The Réaumur is in popular use in Russia and some parts of Germany, but is giving way to the centigrade; the Fahrenheit is in popular use in Holland and in English speaking countries; the centigrade is in popular use on the Continent of Europe and in Latin America, and is generally employed everywhere in laboratories and in scientific work. A fourth scale, the absolute, is used in physics and physical chemistry, and is particularly used to indicate very low temperatures; it is based on the ab-

# Appendix 9: Chemical Elements (with Their Symbols, Atomic Numbers, and Atomic Weights)

| Element | Symbol | Atomic Number | Atomic Weight* | Element | Symbol | Atomic Number | Atomic Weight* |
|---|---|---|---|---|---|---|---|
| Actinium | Ac | 89 | 227 | Mercury | Hg | 80 | 200.61 |
| Aluminum (Aluminium) | Al | 13 | 26.98 | Molybdenum | Mo | 42 | 95.95 |
| Americium | Am | 95 | [243] | Neodymium | Nd | 60 | 144.27 |
| Antimony | Sb | 51 | 121.76 | Neon | Ne | 10 | 20.179 |
| Argon | Ar (A) | 18 | 39.944 | Neptunium | Np | 93 | [237] |
| Arsenic | As | 33 | 74.92 | Nickel | Ni | 28 | 58.71 |
| Astatine | At | 85 | [210] | Niobium (Columbium) | Nb | 41 | 92.90 |
| Barium | Ba | 56 | 137.36 | Nitrogen | N | 7 | 14.006 |
| Berkelium | Bk | 97 | [247] | Nobelium | No | 102 | [253] |
| Beryllium | Be | 4 | 9.012 | Osmium | Os | 76 | 190.2 |
| Bismuth | Bi | 83 | 208.98 | Oxygen | O | 8 | 16.0000 |
| Boron | B | 5 | 10.82 | Palladium | Pd | 46 | 106.4 |
| Bromine | Br | 35 | 79.904 | Phosphorus | P | 15 | 30.973 |
| Cadmium | Cd | 48 | 112.40 | Platinum | Pt | 78 | 195.09 |
| Calcium | Ca | 20 | 40.08 | Plutonium | Pu | 94 | [247] |
| Californium | Cf | 98 | [249] | Polonium | Po | 84 | 210 |
| Carbon | C | 6 | 12.011 | Potassium | K | 19 | 39.100 |
| Cerium | Ce | 58 | 140.13 | Praseodymium | Pr | 59 | 140.91 |
| Cesium | Cs | 55 | 132.91 | Promethium | Pm | 61 | [145!] |
| Chlorine | Cl | 17 | 35.457 | Protactinium | Pa | 91 | 231 |
| Chromium | Cr | 24 | 51.996 | Radium | Ra | 88 | 226.03 |
| Cobalt | Co | 27 | 58.93 | Radon | Rn | 86 | 222 |
| Columbium (Niobium) | Cb | 41 | 92.90 | Rhenium | Re | 75 | 186.22 |
| Copper | Cu | 29 | 63.54 | Rhodium | Rh | 45 | 102.91 |
| Curium | Cm | 96 | [245] | Rubidium | Rb | 37 | 85.46 |
| Dysprosium | Dy | 66 | 162.51 | Ruthenium | Ru | 44 | ·101.1 |
| Einsteinium | Es | 99 | [254] | Samarium | Sm | 62 | 150.35 |
| Erbium | Er | 68 | 167.27 | Scandium | Sc | 21 | 44.96 |
| Europium | Eu | 63 | 151.96 | Selenium | Se | 34 | 78.96 |
| Fermium | Fm | 100 | [252] | Silicon | Si | 14 | 28.08 |
| Fluorine | F | 9 | 18.99 | Silver | Ag | 47 | 107.868 |
| Francium | Fr | 87 | [223] | Sodium | Na | 11 | 22.991 |
| Gadolinium | Gd | 64 | 157.26 | Strontium | Sr | 38 | 87.63 |
| Gallium | Ga | 31 | 69.72 | Sulfur | S | 16 | 32.066† |
| Germanium | Ge | 32 | 72.60 | Tantalum | Ta | 73 | 180.95 |
| Gold | Au | 79 | 196.96 | Technetium | Tc | 43 | [98.91] |
| Hafnium | Hf | 72 | 178.49 | Tellurium | Te | 52 | 127.61 |
| Helium | He | 2 | 4.002 | Terbium | Tb | 65 | 158.93 |
| Holmium | Ho | 67 | 164.93 | Thallium | Tl | 81 | 204.39 |
| Hydrogen | H | 1 | 1.0080 | Thorium | Th | 90 | 232.03 |
| Indium | In | 49 | 114.82 | Thulium | Tm | 69 | 168.93 |
| Iodine | I | 53 | 126.90 | Tin | Sn | 50 | 118.70 |
| Iridium | Ir | 77 | 192.2 | Titanium | Ti | 22 | 47.90 |
| Iron | Fe | 26 | 55.85 | Tungsten (Wolfram) | W | 74 | 183.86 |
| Krypton | Kr | 36 | 83.80 | Uranium | U | 92 | 238.03 |
| Lanthanum | La | 57 | 133.905 | Vanadium | V | 23 | 50.941 |
| Lawrencium | Lr | 103 | | Wolfram (Tungsten) | W | 74 | 183.86 |
| Lead | Pb | 82 | 207.21 | Xenon | Xe | 54 | 131.30 |
| Lithium | Li | 3 | 6.940 | Ytterbium | Yb | 70 | 173.04 |
| Lutetium | Lu | 71 | 174.97 | Yttrium | Y | 39 | 88.91 |
| Magnesium | Mg | 12 | 24.35 | Zinc | Zn | 30 | 65.38 |
| Manganese | Mn | 25 | 54.93 | Zirconium | Zr | 40 | 91.22 |
| Mendelevium | Md | 101 | [256] | | | | |

* An atomic weight is given in brackets for those elements that do not occur in nature in appreciable quantities, and represents the mass number of the most stable isotope.

† Due to variations in the large number of isotopes of sulfur, the atomic weight of sulfur has a range of ±0.003.

# Appendix 10: Glossary of Abbreviations

The following list is a compilation of the usages preferred by a selected group of medical and scientific journals. Unless otherwise indicated, the same abbreviation is used for the plural form as for the singular. The use of periods varies, depending on editorial preference. Most journal editors request that terms of measurement be abbreviated only when used with numerals.

International System of Units (SI) proposals for some basic, supplementary, and derived units for general international scientific and technological use are included in the following list; these are also discussed in the vocabulary section, in the definition of International System of Units, and some are defined as individual vocabulary entries. Some symbols commonly used in scientific writing, in general, are presented in Appendix 6. Abbreviations or contractions of the names of many chemical or biochemical substances, respiratory physiology terms, and clinical and laboratory terms not found here are listed in the vocabulary, where they are alphabetized as written, letter-for-letter.

| | |
|---|---|
| about (*circa*) | *ca.* |
| absolute | abs. |
| absorbance, absorbancy | *A* |
| afternoon (*post meridiem*) | p.m. |
| against (*versus*) | *vs.* |
| alternating current | a.c. |
| altitude | alt. |
| amount | amt. |
| ampere | A |
| analysis, analytical(ly) | anal. |
| and others (*et alii*) | *et al.* |
| Ångstrom unit | Å |
| *ante meridiem* (before noon) | a.m. |
| antilogarithm | antilog |
| approximate, approximately | approx. |
| aqueous | aq. |
| atmosphere | atm |
| atomic mass unit | amu |
| atomic weight | at. wt. |
| atto- ($10^{-18}$) | a- |
| audiofrequency | af |
| average | av. |
| avoirdupois | avdp. |
| Baumé | Bé. |
| biological oxygen demand | BOD |
| body weight | body wt. |
| boiling point | b.p. |
| British thermal unit | Btu |
| calculate | calc. |
| calorie, small | gm cal; cal |
| calorie, large | kg cal, kcal; Cal |
| candela | cd |
| Celsius | C |

| | |
|---|---|
| centi- ($10^{-2}$) | c- |
| centigrade | C |
| centigram | cg |
| centimeter | cm |
| centimeter, square | sq cm; cm² |
| centimeter, cubic | cc; cu cm; cm³ |
| centimeter-gram-second | cgs |
| chemical(ly) | chem. |
| chemically pure | CP |
| *circa* (about) | *ca.* |
| coefficient | coeff. |
| composition | compn. |
| compound | compd. |
| concentrate, concentrated, concentration | conc. |
| configuration | D-, L-, DL- (see these entries in the dictionary) |
| constant | const. |
| corrected | cor. |
| cosine | cos |
| coulomb | coul. |
| counts per minute | cpm; counts/min |
| counts per second | cps; counts/sec |
| crystalline | cryst. |
| cubic | cu (cu centimeter, foot, meter, etc., see the nouns) |
| curie | Ci |
| cycles per minute | cpm; cycles/min |
| cycles per second | cps; cycles/sec |
| deca- ($10^1$) | da |
| deci- ($10^{-1}$) | d |
| decibel | db |
| decigram | dg |

| | | | |
|---|---|---|---|
| deciliter | dl | for example (*exempli gra-* | |
| decimeter | dm | *tia*) | *e.g.* |
| decompose | decomp. | forenoon (*ante meridiem*) | a.m. |
| decomposition | dec.; decompn. | freezing point | f.p. |
| degree (temperature) | Examples:9°C;30°F, | fusion point | fn. p.; fu. p. |
| | 287°K; or 9 C, | gallon | gal |
| | 30 F, 287 K | gamma | see microgram |
| degree (angular) | Use symbol: 30° an- | generations | see filial generations |
| | gle | giga- (10⁹) | G- |
| density | *D;* or *d* | grain | gr; or spell out |
| derivative | deriv. | gram | gm; g |
| determine | det. | gram calorie | see calorie, small |
| dextrorotatory | *d-; dextro-;* (+) (see | gram molecule | see mole |
| | *d-* in the diction- | gravity, centrifugal | *g* |
| | ary) | gravity, specific | sp. gr. |
| diameter | diam. | half-value layer | HVL |
| diffusion coefficient | *D* | half-value thickness | HVT |
| dilute | dil. | hecto- (10²) | h- |
| direct current | d.c. | hectometer | hm |
| disintegration per minute | dpm | horsepower | hp |
| disintegration per second | dps | hour | hr |
| dissociate | dissoc. | hundredweight | cwt |
| dissociation constant, neg- | | hydrogen ion concentra- | |
| ative log of, | *pK'* | tion | pH |
| distilled | distd. | inch | spell out |
| dozen | doz | infective dose, median | $ID_{50}$ |
| dram | dr | infrared | ir |
| dry weight | dry wt. | inorganic | inorg. |
| effective dose, median | $ED_{50}$ | insoluble | insol. |
| electric, electrical(ly) | elec. | international unit | IU |
| electrode potential | *E* | intracutaneous(ly) | i.c. |
| electromagnetic unit | emu | intramuscular(ly) | i.m. |
| electromotive force | emf | intraperitoneal(ly) | i.p. |
| electron paramagnetic res- | | intravenous(ly) | i.v. |
| onance | EPR | irradiation | irradn. |
| electron spin resonance | ESR | joule | J |
| electron volt | eV | Kelvin | K |
| electrostatic unit | esu | kilo- (10³) | k- |
| equilibrium(s) | equil. | kilocalorie | see calorie, large |
| equivalent | Eq; eq; equiv. | kilocycle | kc |
| erg | spell out | kilocycles per second | kc/sec |
| estimate | est. | kiloelectron volt | keV |
| *et alii* (and others) | *et al.* | kilogram | kg |
| *et cetera* (and so forth) | etc. | kiloliter | kl |
| evaporate | evap. | kilometer | km |
| examined | examd. | kiloroentgen | kr |
| experiment | expt. | kilovolt | kV |
| extinction coefficient | *E* | kilowatt | kW |
| extract | ext. | lambda | see microliter, and |
| Fahrenheit | F | | wavelength |
| faraday, farad | F | Lambert | L |
| female | F; ♀; ○ | latitude | lat. |
| femto (10⁻¹⁵) | f | lethal dose, median | $LD_{50}$ |
| filial generations | $F_1$, $F_2$, $F_3$, etc. | levorotatory | *l-, levo;* see *l-*, in the |
| foot (feet) | ft | | dictionary |
| foot, square | sq ft; ft² | liquid | liq. |
| foot, cubic | cu ft; ft³ | liter | l |
| foot-candle | ft-c | logarithm | log; ln |

longitude................. long.
magnified by............. ×
male..................... M; ♂; □
mathematical(ly)........ math.
maximum................. max.
mega- (10⁶)............ M-
melting point............. m.p.
melts at, melting at..... m.
meter.................... m
meter, cubic............. cu m; m³
meter, square........... sq m; m²
mho (reciprocal ohm)..... mho
micro- (10⁻⁶)........... μ
microcurie............... μCi
microfarad.............. μf
microgram............... μg (use of gamma is not preferred)
microliter............... μl (use of lambda is not preferred)
micrometer.............. μm
micromicrogram (picogram)................. μμg (pg)
micromicron............. μμ
micromolar (unit of concentration)............. mм
micromole (unit of mass).. μmole, pl. μmoles
micron.................. μ
microunit ............... μU
microvolt............... μV
microwatt............... μW
mile.................... spell out
miles per hour........... mph
milli- (10⁻³)............. m-
milliampere............. mA
millicurie............... mCi
milliequivalent.......... mEq; meq
milligram.............. mg
milliliter............... ml
millimeter.............. mm
millimeter, square....... sq mm; mm²
millimeter, cubic........ cu mm; mm³
millimicron............. mμ
millimolar (unit of concentration................ mм
millimole (unit of mass)... mmole
million electron volts..... meV
milliosmole............. mOsmole; or (preferred) spell out
milliosmolar............. mOsм; or (preferred) spell out
millivolt................ mV
millivolt-second......... mV-sec
minimum................. min
minimum lethal dose...... MLD
minute.................. min
minute (angular measure). ′
miscellaneous........... misc.
mixture................. mixt.

molal.................... $m$
molar (unit of concentration)................... м; $M$; M
mole (unit of mass)....... mole, pl. moles
molecular or molar extinction coefficient.......... ε (lower case Greek epsilon)
molecular weight........ mol wt
molecule, molecular...... mol.
month.................... mo
morning (*ante meridiem*).. a.m.
nano- (10⁻⁹)............. n-
nanogram ................ ng
nanometer............... nm
negative(ly)............. neg.
newton.................. N
normal (concentration)... N; $N$; N
nuclear magnetic resonance................. NMR
number.................. no.
observed................. obsd.
optical density.......... O.D.
optical rotatory dispersion................... ORD
optimal................. opt.
organic................. org.
osmole.................. spell out
ounce................... oz
oxidation............... oxidn.
paralysis, median....... PD₅₀
parts per million........ ppm
peak electron volts...... peV
per cent................ %
physical(ly)............. phys.
pico- (prefix, 10⁻¹²)...... p-
picogram (micromicrogram)................. pg
positive(ly)............. pos.
*post meridiem*........... p.m.
pound................... lb
pounds per square inch... psi
pounds per square inch absolute.................. psia
pounds per square inch gauge................. psig
precipitate.............. ppt.
precipitated............. pptd.
precipitation............ pptn.
prepare................. prep.
probability............. $p$, or $P$
proton magnetic resonance PMR
qualitative(ly).......... qual.
quantitative(ly)......... quant.
radian.................. rad
radiation, ionizing....... rad
radiofrequency.......... rf
reduction............... redn.
reference............... ref.

| | | | |
|---|---|---|---|
| refractive index | $n$ | steradian | sr |
| respective(ly) | resp. | subcutaneous(ly) | s.c. |
| respiratory quotient | RQ | Svedberg unit | S |
| revolutions per minute | rpm; rev/min | symmetrically | sym. |
| roentgen | R | tangent | tan |
| roentgen equivalent man | rem | technical | tech. |
| roentgen equivalent phys- | | temperature | temp. |
| ical | rep | tera- ($10^{12}$) | T- |
| saponification | sapon. | tertiary (with alkyl groups | |
| saturate | sat. | only) | *tert* |
| second (time) | sec or s | tissue culture dose, 50% in- | |
| second (angular measure) | ″ | fectivity | $TCD_{50}$ |
| secondary (with alkyl | | ultraviolet | uv |
| groups only) | *sec* | viscosity | $\eta$ (lower case Greek |
| sedimentation coefficient | *s* | | eta) |
| separate(ly) | sep. | volt | V |
| sine | sin | volume | vol |
| soluble | sol. | volume for volume | v/v |
| solution | soln. | watt | W |
| specific | sp. | wavelength | $\lambda$ (lower case Greek |
| specific gravity | sp. gr. | | lambda) |
| square | sq (sq centimeter, foot, meter, etc., see the nouns) | week | wk |
| | | weight | wt |
| | | weight for weight | w/w |
| standard | std. | weight per volume | w/v |
| standard deviation | S.D. | year | yr |
| standard error | S.E. | | |